Holland-Frei Cancer Medicine

Ninth Edition

Dedication

From the preparation for the first edition throughout the next eight editions, Emil Frei III, Tom to us and to his legion of friends, was an Editor extraordinaire. His deep knowledge of cancer, his extensive professional and personal contacts, and his vision gave strength to the book and its production. He was a towering figure in world oncology, and through his participation in it and in this treatise promoted its creation as a medical discipline. He was a consummate clinician who trained many of the major oncologists of the United States during his leadership at the National Cancer Institute, MD Anderson Cancer Center and the Dana Farber Cancer Institute of Harvard University. He was a pioneer of translational research. His writings, lectures, and open friendship made him a valued, virtual companion to every working oncologist. His influence will outlive him.

We editors who treasured his fraternity miss him sorely, and dedicate this ninth edition of Cancer Medicine to this great man.

James F. Holland
Robert C. Bast Jr.
Donald W. Kufe
Ralph R. Weichselbaum
Raphael E. Pollock
William N. Hait
Waun Ki Hong

Holland-Frei Cancer Medicine

Ninth Edition

EDITORS

Robert C. Bast Jr., MD

Vice President for Translational Research, MD Anderson Cancer Center, Houston, Texas

Carlo M. Croce, MD

Distinguished University Professor, The John W. Wolfe Chair in Human Cancer Genetics, Professor and Chair, Department of Molecular Virology, Immunology and Medical Genetics, The Wexner Medical Center, The Ohio State University, Columbus, Ohio

William N. Hait, MD, PhD

Global Head, Research and Development, Janssen Pharmaceutical Companies of Johnson and Johnson, Raritan, New Jersey

Waun Ki Hong, MD, DMSc (Hon)

Professor of Thoracic/Head and Neck Medical Oncology, American Cancer Society Professor, Samsung Distinguished University Chair in Cancer Medicine Emeritus, The University of Texas MD Anderson Cancer Center, Houston, Texas

Donald W. Kufe, MD

Distinguished Physician, Dana-Farber Cancer Institute, Professor of Medicine, Harvard Medical School, Leader, Translational Pharmacology and Early Therapeutic Trials Program, Dana-Farber/Harvard Cancer Center, Boston, Massachusetts

Martine Piccart-Gebhart, MD, PhD

Professor of Oncology, Université Libre de Bruxelles (ULB), Head of the Medicine Department, Jules Bordet Institute, Brussels, Belgium

Raphael E. Pollock, MD, PhD, FACS

Professor and Director, Division of Surgical Oncology, Surgeon in Chief, James Comprehensive Cancer Center, Surgeon in Chief, The Ohio State University Health System, The Ohio State University Wexner Medical Center, Columbus, Ohio

Ralph R. Weichselbaum, MD

Daniel K. Ludwig Distinguished Service Professor of Radiation and Cellular Oncology, Chair, Department of Radiation and Cellular Oncology, University of Chicago, Hospital Director, Chicago Tumor Institute, Chicago, Illinois

Hongyang Wang, MD

Professor and Director, National Center for Liver Cancer, China; Eastern Hepatobiliary Surgery Hospital, Shanghai, China

James F. Holland, MD, ScD (hc)

Distinguished Professor of Neoplastic Diseases, Director Emeritus of Derald H. Rutttenberg Cancer Center, Icahn School of Medicine at Mount Sinai, New York, New York

ASSOCIATE EDITOR

Fadlo R. Khuri, MD

Executive Associate Dean for Research, Emory University School of Medicine, Atlanta, Georgia; President, the American University of Beirut, Beirut, Lebanon

Published in collaboration with 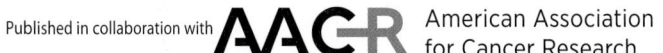 American Association for Cancer Research

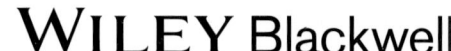

Published by John Wiley & Sons, Inc., Hoboken, New Jersey

Published simultaneously in Canada

The contents of this work are intended to further general scientific research, understanding, and discussion only and are not intended and should not be relied upon as recommending or promoting a specific method, diagnosis, or treatment by health science practitioners for any particular patient. The publisher and the author make no representations or warranties with respect to the accuracy or completeness of the contents of this work and specifically disclaim all warranties, including without limitation any implied warranties of fitness for a particular purpose. In view of ongoing research, equipment modifications, changes in governmental regulations, and the constant flow of information relating to the use of medicines, equipment, and devices, the reader is urged to review and evaluate the information provided in the package insert or instructions for each medicine, equipment, or device for, among other things, any changes in the instructions or indication of usage and for added warnings and precautions. Readers should consult with a specialist where appropriate. The fact that an organization or Website is referred to in this work as a citation and/or a potential source of further information does not mean that the author or the publisher endorses the information the organization or Website may provide or recommendations it may make. Further, readers should be aware that Internet Websites listed in this work may have changed or disappeared between when this work was written and when it is read. No warranty may be created or extended by any promotional statements for this work. Neither the publisher nor the author shall be liable for any damages arising herefrom.

For general information on our other products and services or for technical support, please contact our Customer Care Department within the United States at (800) 762-2974, outside the United States at (317) 572-3993 or fax (317) 572-4002.

Wiley also publishes its books in a variety of electronic formats. Some content that appears in print may not be available in electronic formats. For more information about Wiley products, visit our web site at www.wiley.com.

Library of Congress Cataloging-in-Publication Data

Names: Bast, Robert C., Jr. (Robert Clinton), 1943- editor.

Title: Holland-Frei Cancer Medicine / editors, Robert C. Bast, Jr, Carlo M. Croce, William Hait, Waun Ki Hong, Donald W. Kufe, Martine Piccart-Gebhart, Raphael E. Pollock, Ralph R. Weichselbaum, Hongyang Wang, James F. Holland.

Other titles: Cancer Medicine

Description: 9th edition. | Hoboken, New Jersey : John Wiley & Sons, Inc., 2016. | Preceded by Holland-Frei Cancer Medicine 8, 2010. | Includes bibliographical references and index.

Identifiers: LCCN 2016017204 (print) | LCCN 2016018267 (ebook) | ISBN 9781118934692 (hardback) | ISBN 9781119000846 (pdf) | ISBN 9781119000839 (epub)

Subjects: | MESH: Neoplasms

Classification: LCC RC261 (print) | LCC RC261 (ebook) | NLM QZ 200 | DDC 616.99/4–dc23

LC record available at https://lccn.loc.gov/2016017204

Cover images:

gettyimages.com/photos/85757113 by Science Photo Library – SteveGS

gettyimages.com/photos/91560125 by Science Photo Library – SteveGS

gettyimages.com/photos/179706497 by Photostock israel

gettyimages.com/photos/186600576 by 2p2play

gettyimages.com/photos/511794063 by Everythingpossible

10 9 8 7 6 5 4 3 2 1

Printed and bound in Malaysia by Vivar Printing Sdn Bhd

Contents

Part 12: MANAGEMENT OF CANCER COMPLICATIONS

List of contributors

Stuart A. Aaronson, MD
Aron Professor
Department of Oncological Sciences
Icahn School of Medicine at Mount Sinai
New York, NY
USA

Amy Abernethy, MD, PhD
Professor of Medicine, Division of Medical Oncology
Director, Center for Learning Health Care
Duke University Medical Center & Duke Clinical
Research Institute
Durham, NC
USA

David H. Abramson, MD
Chief
Ophthalmic Oncology Service, Department of Surgery
Memorial Sloan Kettering Cancer Center
New York, NY
USA

Jeremy S. Abramson, MD, MMSc
Assistant Professor, Medicine, Harvard Medical School
Dana-Farber Cancer Institute
Boston, MA
USA

Ala Abudayyeh, MD
Assistant Professor, Division of Internal Medicine
Section of Nephrology
The University of Texas MD Anderson Cancer Center
Houston, TX
USA

Mario Acunzo, PhD
Research Scientist
James Comprehensive Cancer Center
The Ohio State University
Columbus, OH
USA

Roberto Adachi, MD
Associate Professor
Department of Pulmonary Medicine
The University of Texas MD Anderson Cancer Center
Houston, TX
USA

Ranjana H. Advani, MD
The Saul A. Rosenberg, MD, Professor of Lymphoma
Department of Medicine/Medical Oncology
Stanford University
Stanford, CA
USA

Judy U. Ahrar, MD
Associate Professor
Department of Interventional Radiology, Division of
Diagnostic Imaging
The University of Texas MD Anderson Cancer Center
Houston, TX
USA

Jaffer A. Ajani, MD
Professor
Department of Gastrointestinal (GI) Medical Oncology
Division of Cancer Medicine
The University of Texas MD Anderson Cancer Center
Houston, TX
USA

James P. Allison, PhD
Professor and Chair
Department of Immunology
The University of Texas MD Anderson Cancer Center
Houston, TX
USA

Edward P. Ambinder, MD
Tisch Cancer Institute
Clinical Professor of Medicine
Icahn School of Medicine at Mount Sinai
New York, NY
USA

Kenneth C. Anderson, MD
Professor of Medicine
Medical Oncology
Dana-Farber Cancer Institute/Harvard Medical School
Boston, MA
USA

Ana Aparicio, MD
Associate Professor
Genitourinary Medical Oncology
The University of Texas MD Anderson Cancer Center
Houston, TX
USA

James Armitage, MD
Professor, Internal Medicine
Division of Hematology & Oncology
UNMC Oncology-Hematology Division
Omaha, NE
USA

Sarah T. Arron, MD, PhD
Associate Professor
Department of Dermatology
University of California
San Francisco, CA
USA

Rony Avritscher, MD
Associate Professor
Department of Interventional Radiology
The University of Texas MD Anderson Cancer Center
Houston, TX
USA

Diwakar D. Balachandran, MD
Associate Professor
Department of Pulmonary Medicine
The University of Texas MD Anderson Cancer Center
Houston, TX
USA

Jacqueline C. Barrientos, MD
Assistant Professor
Medicine
Hofstra Northwell School of Medicine
New Hyde Park, NY
USA

Lara Bashoura, MD
Associate Professor
Department of Pulmonary Medicine
The University of Texas MD Anderson Cancer Center
Houston, TX
USA

Robert C. Bast Jr., MD
Vice President for Translational Research
The University of Texas MD Anderson Cancer Center
Houston, TX
USA

Susan Bates, MD
Professor of Medicine
Division of Hematology/Oncology
Columbia University Medical Center
New York, NY
USA

Stephen B. Baylin, MD
Deputy Director
The Sidney Kimmel Comprehensive Cancer Center
Johns Hopkins University
Baltimore, MD
USA

Georgia M. Beasley, MD
Duke University Medical Center
Durham, NC
USA

Jonathan S. Berek, MD, MMS, FASCO
Laurie Kraus Lacob Professor
Fellow, Stanford Distinguished Careers Institute
Director, Special Programs, Stanford Cancer Institute
Director, Stanford Women's Cancer Center
Director, Stanford Health Care Communication Program
Stanford University School of Medicine
Stanford, CA
USA

Ross S. Berkowitz, MD
William H. Baker Professor of Gynecology
Director of Division of Gynecologic Oncology at Brigham and Women's Hospital and Dana Farber Cancer Institute
Director of New England Trophoblastic Disease Center
Harvard Medical School
Boston, MA
USA

Leslie Bernstein, PhD
Professor and Director
Division of Cancer Etiology, Department of Population Sciences
Beckman Research Institute and the City of Hope Comprehensive Cancer Center
Duarte, CA
USA

Donald A. Berry, PhD
Professor
Department of Biostatistics
The University of Texas MD Anderson Cancer Center
Houston, TX
USA

Joseph R. Bertino, MD
Professor
Medicine and Pharmacology
Robert Wood Johnson Medical School
Rutgers, The State University of New Jersey
New Brunswick, NJ
USA

Teena Bhatla, MD
Assistant Professor of Pediatrics
Division of Pediatric Hematology-Oncology
New York University Medical Center
The Stephen D. Hassenfeld Children's Center for Cancer and Blood Disorders
New York, NY
USA

Boris Blechacz, MD, PhD
Assistant Professor
Department of Gastroenterology, Hepat, & Nutr
Division of Internal Medicine
The University of Texas MD Anderson Cancer Center
Houston, TX
USA

Mark Bloomston, MD, FACS
Professor
Division of Surgical Oncology
Department of Surgery
The Ohio State University
Wexner Medical Center
Columbus, OH
USA

Otis W. Brawley, MD, MACP
Chief Medical Officer
American Cancer Society, Inc.
Atlanta, GA
USA

Freddie Bray, PhD
Head
Section of Cancer Surveillance
International Agency for Research on Cancer
Lyon
France

Malcolm Brenner, MB, PhD
Professor
Center for Gene Therapy
Baylor College of Medicine
Houston, TX
USA

Robert S. Bresalier, MD
Professor, Gastroenterology, Hepatology & Nutrition
Division of Internal Medicine
The University of Texas MD Anderson Cancer Center
Houston, TX
USA

Kristin Brogaard, PhD
Project Manager
Institute for Systems Biology
Seattle, WA
USA

Lionel Brookes, 3rd, PhD
Postdoctoral student
Department of Dermatology
University of California
San Francisco, CA
USA

Kristoffer W. Brudvik, MD, PhD
Postdoctoral Fellow
Department of Surgical Oncology
The University of Texas MD Anderson Cancer Center
Houston, TX
USA

Alan H. Bryce, MD
Assistant Professor of Medicine
Department of Hematology/Oncology
Mayo Clinic Arizona
Scottsdale, AZ
USA

Earle F. Burgess, MD
Attending Physician, Medical Oncology
Levine Cancer Institute, Carolinas HealthCare System
Charlotte, NC
USA

Meredith Buxton, PhD
Assistant Professor
Department of Surgery
UCSF School of Medicine
San Francisco, CA
USA

Aman U. Buzdar, MD, FACP
Professor of Medicine and Internist
Department of Breast Medical Oncology, Division of Cancer Medicine
The University of Texas MD Anderson Cancer Center
Houston, TX
USA

Maria E. Cabanillas, MD
Associate Professor
Department of Endocrine Neoplasia and Hormonal Disorders
The University of Texas MD Anderson Cancer Center
Houston, TX
USA

Guangwen Cao, MD, PhD
Professor
Department of Epidemiology
Second Military Medical University
Shanghai
China

William L. Carroll, MD
Julie and Edward J. Minskoff Professor of Pediatrics and Pathology
Chief, Division of Pediatric Hematology-Oncology at NYU Langone Medical Center
Stephen D. Hassenfeld Children's Center for Cancer and Blood Disorders
New York, NY
USA

Tina Cascone, MD, PhD
Fellow, Cancer Medicine
The University of Texas MD Anderson Cancer Center
Houston, TX
USA

A. P. Chahinian, MD
Professor
Department of Medicine
Mount Sinai School of Medicine
New York, NY
USA

Richard Champlin, MD
Chair, Professor of Medicine
Department of Stem Cell Transplantation and Cellular Therapy
The University of Texas MD Anderson Cancer Center
Houston, TX
USA

Martin C. Chang, MD, PhD, FCAP, FRCPC
Assistant Professor
Lab Med and Pathobiology
Mount Sinai Hospital
Toronto, ON
Canada

Joe Y. Chang, MD, PhD
Director, Stereotactic Radiotherapy Program
Department of Radiation Oncology
The University of Texas MD Anderson Cancer Center
Houston, TX
USA

Alejandro Chaoul, PhD
Assistant Professor
Department of Palliative, Rehabilitation & Integrative Medicine
The University of Texas MD Anderson Cancer Center
Houston, TX
USA

Brian F. Chapin, MD
Assistant Professor
Department of Urology, Division of Surgery
The University of Texas MD Anderson Cancer Center
Houston, TX
USA

Sai-Juan Chen, MD, PhD
Professor of Hematology
State Key Laboratory of Medical Genomics
Shanghai Institute of Hematology
Rui-Jin Hospital affiliated to Shanghai Jiao Tong University School of Medicine
Shanghai
China

Zhu Chen, PhD
Vice-Chairman, 12th Standing Committee of the National People's Congress
President, Chinese Medical Association
Beijing
China

Anne Chiang, MD, PhD
Assistant Professor
Department of Medicine, Section of Medical Oncology
Yale School of Medicine, Yale Cancer Center, and Smilow Cancer Hospital
New Haven, CT
USA

Steven J. Chmura, MD, PhD
Associate Professor of Radiation and Cellular Oncology
The University of Chicago Pritzker School of Medicine
Chicago, IL
USA

James E. Cleaver, PhD
Professor Emeritus
Department of Dermatology
University of California
San Francisco, CA
USA

Steven K. Clinton, MD, PhD
Professor
Department of Internal Medicine
College of Medicine
The Ohio State University Comprehensive Cancer Center
Arthur G. James Cancer Hospital and Richard J. Solove Research Institute (OSUCCC – James)
Columbus, OH
USA

Jeffrey I. Cohen, MD
Chief, Laboratory of Infectious Diseases
National Institute of Allergy and Infectious Diseases
National Institutes of Health
Bethesda, MD
USA

Carmel J. Cohen, MD
Professor, Division of GYN Oncology
Department of Obstetrics and Gynecology
Ruttenberg Cancer Center, Icahn School of Medicine at Mount Sinai Medical Center
New York, NY
USA

Harvey J. Cohen, MD
Division Chief of Geriatrics, Director of the Center for the Study of Aging and Human Development
Duke University Medical Center
Durham, NC
USA

Lorenzo Cohen, PhD
Professor and Director
Integrative Medicine Program
Department of Palliative, Rehabilitation and Integrative Medicine
The University of Texas MD Anderson Cancer Center
Houston, TX
USA

Peter D. Cole, MD
Associate Professor
Pediatrics
Albert Einstein College of Medicine
The Children's Hospital at Montefiore
Bronx, NY
USA

Elizabeth Comen, MD
Medical Oncologist
Breast Medicine Service
Memorial Sloan Kettering Cancer Center
New York, NY
USA

Philip P. Connell, MD
Associate Professor
Department of Radiation and Cellular Oncology
University of Chicago Hospital
Chicago, IL
USA

Laurence J. Cooper, MD, PhD
Visiting Scientist
Pediatrics Research
The University of Texas MD Anderson Cancer Center
Houston, TX
USA

Carlos Cordon-Cardo, MD, PhD
Professor and Chair
Department of Pathology
Icahn School of Medicine at Mount Sinai
New York, NY
USA

Christopher L. Corless, MD, PhD
Medical Director of the Cancer Pathology Share Resource
Oregon Health & Science University
Portland, OR
USA

Jorge Cortes, MD
Professor of Medicine
Chair CML and AML Section
Department of Leukemia
The University of Texas MD Anderson Cancer Center
Houston, TX
USA

David Cosgrove, MB, BCh
Assistant Professor, Department of Oncology
Johns Hopkins University
Baltimore, MD
USA

Richard Cote, MD, FRCPath
Professor & Joseph R. Coulter Jr. Chair, Department of Pathology
Professor, Department of Biochemistry and Molecular Biology
Chief of Pathology
Jackson Memorial Hospital
University of Miami Miller School of Medicine
Miami, FL
USA

Kenneth H. Cowan, MD, PhD
Director, Fred and Pamela Buffett Cancer Center
University of Nebraska Medical Center
Omaha, NE
USA

Christopher H. Crane, MD
Professor with Tenure
Department of Radiation Oncology
The University of Texas MD Anderson Cancer Center
Houston, TX
USA

Carlo M. Croce, MD
Distinguished University Professor
The John W. Wolfe Chair in Human Cancer Genetics
Professor and Chair
Department of Molecular Virology, Immunology and Medical Genetics
The Wexner Medical Center
The Ohio State University
Columbus, OH
USA

Christopher P. Crum, MD, FRCP
Professor of Pathology, Harvard Medical School
Department of Pathology
Brigham and Women's Hospital
Boston, MA
USA

William Cruz-Munoz, PhD
Postdoctoral Fellow
Biological Sciences Platform
Sunnybrook Research Institute
Toronto, ON
Canada

Steven A. Curley, MD, FACS
Professor of Surgery and Chief
Division of Surgical Oncology
Baylor College of Medicine
Houston, TX
USA

Timothy A. Damron, MD, FACS
Professor of Orthopedic Surgery
Upstate University Hospital
Syracuse, NY
USA

Siamak Daneshmand, MD
Associate Professor of Urology (Clinical Scholar)
Director of Urologic Oncology, USC Institute of
Urology
Los Angeles, CA
USA

John W. Davis, MD, FACS
Associate Professor, Department of Urology
Division of Surgery
The University of Texas MD Anderson Cancer Center
Houston, TX
USA

**Shaheenah Dawood, MD, MBBch,
FACP, FRCP, MPH, CPH**
Head of Medical Oncology
Dubai Hospital
Dubai
United Arab Emirates

Lisa M. DeAngelis, MD, FAAN
Neuro-Oncologist
Chair, Department of Neurology
Lillian Rojtman Berkman Chair in Honor of Jerome B.
Posner
Memorial Sloan Kettering Cancer Center
New York, NY
USA

Yadwinder S. Deol, PhD
Postdoctoral Research Fellow
University of Michigan Comprehensive Cancer Center
Ann Arbor, MI
USA

Maria T. De Sancho, MD, MSc
Associate Professor of Clinical Medicine
Non-Malignant Hematology Program at Weill Cornell
Medicine's Center for Blood Disorders
New York, NY
USA

Summer B. Dewdney, MD
Assistant Professor
Division of Gynecologic Oncology
Rush University Medical Center
Chicago, IL
USA

Radwa G. Diab, MD, MBBCH, PhD
Lecturer of Medical Parasitology
Faculty of Medicine, Alexandria University
Alexandria
Egypt

Robert B. Diasio, MD
Director, Mayo Clinic Cancer Center
William J. and Charles H. Mayo Professor
Departments of Molecular Pharmacology &
Experimental Therapeutics and Oncology
Rochester, MN
USA

Burton F. Dickey, MD
Professor
Department of Pulmonary Medicine
The University of Texas MD Anderson Cancer Center
Houston, TX
USA

Zeliha Gunnur Dikmen, MD, PhD
Faculty of Medicine
Department of Biochemistry
Hacettepe University
Ankara
Turkey

Michaela A. Dinan, PhD
Medical Instructor, Division of Medical Oncology
Duke University Medical Center
Durham, NC
USA

Nicholas C. Dracopoli, PhD
Vice President and Head of Oncology Biomarkers
Janssen Research & Development, LLC.
Raritan, NJ
USA

Anthony Dragun, MD
Assistant Professor
Department of Radiation Oncology
James Graham Brown Cancer Center
Louisville, KY
USA

Madeleine M. Duvic, MD
Professor, Dermatology
The University of Texas MD Anderson Cancer Center
Houston, TX
USA

George A. Eapen, MD
Professor
Department of Pulmonary Medicine
The University of Texas MD Anderson Cancer Center
Houston, TX
USA

John M. L. Ebos, PhD
Assistant Professor of Oncology
Department of Cancer Genetics
Department of Medicine
Department of Pharmacology and Therapeutics
(Graduate Program)
Roswell Park Cancer Institute
Buffalo, NY
USA

Joseph P. Eder, MD
Professor of Medicine (Medical Oncology)
Yale-New Haven Hospital
New Haven, CT
USA

Eleni Efstathiou, MD, PhD
Associate Professor, Department of Genitourinary
Medical Oncology, Division of Cancer Medicine
The University of Texas MD Anderson Cancer Center
Houston, TX
USA

Suhendan Ekmekcioglu, PhD
Professor
Melanoma Medical Oncology – Research
The University of Texas MD Anderson Cancer Center
Houston, TX
USA

Mervat Z. El Azzouni, MD, PhD
Professor of Medical Parasitology
Faculty of Medicine
Alexandria University
Alexandria
Egypt

Lawrence Einhorn, MD
Professor of Medicine, Division of
Hematology-Oncology/Department of Urology
Indiana University School of Medicine
Melvin and Bren Simon, Cancer Center, IN
USA

Carmen P. Escalante, MD
Professor and Chairman
Department of General Internal Medicine, Ambulatory
Treatment and Emergency Care
The University of Texas MD Anderson Cancer Center
Houston, TX
USA

Laura Esserman, MD, MBA
Professor, Departments of Surgery and Radiology, and
Affiliate Faculty, Institute for Health Policy Studies
University of California
San Francisco, CA
USA

David S. Ettinger, MD, FACP, FCCP
Alex Grass Professor of Oncology
The Sidney Kimmel Comprehensive
Cancer Center at Johns Hopkins
Baltimore, MD
USA

Douglas B. Evans, MD
Ausman Family Foundation Professor of Surgery
Chairman, Department of Surgery
Medical College of Wisconsin
Milwaukee, WI
USA

Scott E. Evans, MD
Associate Professor
Department of Pulmonary Medicine
The University of Texas MD Anderson Cancer Center
Houston, TX
USA

Steven M. Ewer, MD
Division Cardiovascular Medicine
University of Wisconsin School of Medicine of Public
Health
Madison
WI, USA

Michael S. Ewer, MD, MPH, JD, LLM, MBA
Special Assistant to the Vice President of Medical
Affairs
The University of Texas MD Anderson Cancer Center
Houston, TX
USA

Stefan Faderl, MD
Chief
John Theurer Cancer Center's Leukemia Division
Hackensack, NJ
USA

Saadia A. Faiz, MD
Associate Professor
Department of Pulmonary Medicine
The University of Texas MD Anderson Cancer Center
Houston, TX
USA

Mark K. Ferguson, MD
Professor of Surgery
Department of Surgical Oncology
University of Chicago Medical Center
Chicago, IL
USA

Jacques Ferlay, MSc, ME
Informatics Officer
Section of Cancer Surveillance
International Agency for Research on Cancer
Lyon
France

Renata Ferrarotto, MD
Assistant Professor of Medicine
Department of Thoracic-Head and Neck Medical
Oncology
The University of Texas MD Anderson Cancer Center
Houston, TX
USA

William D. Figg Sr, Pharm D
Deputy Chief
Genitourinary Malignancies Branch Center for Cancer
Research, National Cancer Institute, National Institutes
of Health
Bethesda, MD
USA

Lisa Figueiredo, MD
Assistant Professor
Pediatrics
Albert Einstein College of Medicine
The Children's Hospital at Montefiore
Bronx, NY
USA

Tito Fojo, MD, PhD
Professor of Medicine
Division of Hematology/Oncology
Columbia University Medical Center
New York, NY
USA

Patrick M. Forde, MD, MBBCh
Assistant Professor of Oncology
Sidney Kimmel Comprehensive Cancer Center
Johns Hopkins
Baltimore, MD
USA

Adolfo Firpo-Betancourt, MD, MPA
Professor of Pathology
The Mount Sinai Hospital
New York, NY
USA

Jasmine H. Francis, MD
Assistant Attending
Ophthalmic Oncology Service, Department of Surgery
Memorial Sloan-Kettering Cancer Center
New York, NY
USA

Arthur E. Frankel, MD
Professor in the Department of Internal Medicine
UT Southwestern Medical Center
Dallas, TX
USA

Milo Frattini, MD, PhD
Head
Laboratory of Molecular Pathology
Institute of Pathology
Locarno
Switzerland

Arnold S. Freedman, MD
Professor of Medicine
Harvard Medical School
Dana Farber Cancer Institute
Boston, MA
USA

Michael L. Friedlander, MD, MBChB, PhD
Conjoint Professor of Medicine
Director of Medical Oncology
The Prince of Wales Hospital
Consultant Medical Oncologist
Royal Hospital for Women
Sydney, NSW
Australia

Emil Frei III, MD (deceased)
Director and Physician-in-Chief
Dana-Farber Cancer Institute
Boston, MA
USA

Jing Fu, MD, PhD
Research Assistant
International Lab on Signaling Transduction
Eastern Hepatobiliary Surgery Hospital
Shanghai
China

Valentin Fuster, MD, PhD
Professor, Icahn School of Medicine
Physician-in-Chief
Mount Sinai Hospital
New York, NY
USA

Robert F. Gagel, MD
Head, Division of Internal Medicine
The University of Texas MD Anderson Cancer Center
Houston, TX
USA

Robert C. Gallo, MD
Homer & Martha Gudelsky Distinguished Professor in
Medicine & Director, Institute of Human Virology
University of Maryland School of Medicine
Baltimore, MD
USA

Jianjun Gao, MD, PhD
Assistant Professor, Department of Genitourinary
Medical Oncology, Division of Cancer Medicine
The University of Texas MD Anderson Cancer Center
Houston, TX
USA

M. Kay Garcia, DrPH, MSN, LAc
Associate Professor
Department of Palliative, Rehabilitation and Integrative
Medicine
The University of Texas MD Anderson Cancer Center
Houston, TX
USA

Adam S. Garden, MD
Professor, Department of Radiation Oncology
The University of Texas MD Anderson Cancer Center
Houston, TX
USA

Chirag D. Gandhi, MD, FACS, FAANS
Associate Professor of Neurosurgery, Neurology, and
Radiology
Program Director, Neurointerventional Fellowship
Associate Program Director, Neurosurgical Residency
Rutgers University – New Jersey Medical School
Chief and Division Director, Neurological Surgery
Newark Beth Israel Medical Center
Newark, NJ
USA

Teresa A. Gilewski, MD
Professor of Clinical Medicine
Weill Cornell Medical College
Memorial Sloan-Kettering Cancer Center
New York, NY
USA

Edward L. Giovannucci, MD, ScD
Professor of Nutrition and Epidemiology
Department of Nutrition & Department of
Epidemiology
Harvard T.H. Chan School of Public Health
Boston, MA
USA

Donald P. Goldstein, MD
Founder and Director Emeritus
Brigham and Women's Hospital
Boston, MA
USA

Daniel R. Gomez, MD
Assistant Professor
Radiation Oncology Department
The University of Texas MD Anderson Cancer Center
Houston, TX
USA

Sangeeta Goswami, MD, PhD
Internal Medicine Resident
University of Pittsburg Medical Center
Pittsburg, PA
USA

Elizabeth M. Grainger, PhD, RD
Professor, Department of Emergency Medicine
Division of Internal Medicine
The University of Texas MD Anderson Cancer Center
Houston, TX
USA

Jill Granger, BSc, MSc
Research Supervisor
Cancer Stem Cell Laboratory
Department of Internal Medicine-
Hematology/Oncology
University of Michigan
Ann Arbor, MI
USA

Joe W. Gray, PhD
Professor and Gordon Moore Endowed Chair,
Department of Biomedical Engineering
Director, OHSU Center for Spatial Systems Biomedicine
Associate Director for Biophysical Oncology, Knight
Cancer Institute
Oregon Health & Science University
Portland, OR
USA

David J. Grdina, PhD
Professor of Radiation and Cellular Oncology
Department of Radiation and Cellular Oncology
The University of Chicago
Chicago, IL
USA

F. Anthony Greco, MD
Director, Sarah Cannon Cancer Center
Senior Investigator
Department of Oncology
Sarah Cannon Research Institute and Tennessee
Oncology, PLLC
Nashville, TN
USA

Iqbal Grewal, PhD, DSc, FRCPath
Vice President, Head of Immuno-Oncology in the
Oncology Therapeutic Area
Janssen Research & Development, LLC
Raritan, NJ
USA

Elizabeth A. Grimm, PhD
Professor, Department of Melanoma Medical Oncology
Waun Ki Hong Distinguished Chair in Translational
Oncology
The University of Texas MD Anderson Cancer Center
Houston, TX
USA

Horiana B. Grosu, MD
Assistant Professor
Department of Pulmonary Medicine
The University of Texas MD Anderson Cancer Center
Houston, TX
USA

Luca Grumolato, PhD
Associate Professor
INSERM U982-Department of Biology
University of Rouen Normandie
Mont Saint Aignan
France

Jian Gu, PhD
Associate Professor
Department of Epidemiology, Division of OVP, Cancer
Prevention and Population Sciences
The University of Texas MD Anderson Cancer Center
Houston, TX
USA

Eric Guerin, MD
Scientist
Laboratoire de Biochimie et Biologie Moléculaire
Hôpital de Hautepierre - Hôpitaux Universitaires de
Strasbourg
Strasbourg
France

Jose G. Guillem, MD
Colorectal Service, Department of Surgery
Memorial Sloan Kettering Cancer Center
New York, NY
USA

Radhika Gulhar, BA
Medical student
Department of Dermatology
University of California
San Francisco, CA
USA

James L. Gulley, MD, PhD, FACP
Chief
Genitourinary Malignancies Branch
Center for Cancer Research
National Cancer Institute
National Institutes of Health
Bethesda, MD
USA

Michael Haake, MD
Medical Director
Department of Radiation Oncology
Levine Cancer Institute at Carolinas Medical Center
and Senior Physician
Southeast Radiation Oncology
Charlotte, NC
USA

John D. Hainsworth, MD
Senior Investigator
Department of Oncology
Sarah Cannon Research Institute and Tennessee
Oncology, PLLC
Nashville, TN
USA

William N. Hait, MD, PhD
Global Head, Research and Development
Janssen Pharmaceutical Companies of Johnson and
Johnson
Raritan, NJ
USA

Douglas Hanahan, PhD
Director, Swiss Institute for Experimental Cancer
Research
Professor, Department of Molecular Oncology
Swiss Federal Institute of Technology
Lausanne
Switzerland

Axel-R. Hanauske, MD, PhD, MBA
Senior Medical Fellow, Medical Oncology, Global Early
Drug Development
Eli Lilly and Company
Indianapolis, IN
USA

Eric K. Hansen, MD
Radiation Oncologist
The Oregon Clinic
Portland, OR
USA

Curtis C. Harris, MD
Chief
Laboratory of Human Carcinogenesis
National Cancer Institute, National Institutes of Health
Bethesda, MD
USA

Harold A. Harvey, MD
Director, Hematology/Oncology Fellowship Program
Penn State Hershey Cancer Institute
Hershey, PA
USA

Saima Hassan, MD, PhD, FRCSC
Postdoctoral Research Fellow
Department of Biomedical Engineering
Oregon Health & Science University
Portland, OR
USA

Laura M. Heiser, PhD
Assistant Professor
Department of Biomedical Engineering
Affiliated Faculty
OHSU Center for Spatial Systems Biomedicine
Oregon Health & Science University
Portland, OR
USA

William P. D. Hendricks, PhD
Assistant Professor
Integrated Cancer Genomics Division
Translational Genomics Research Institute
Phoenix, AZ
USA

Bryan T. Hennessy, MD
Senior Lecturer
RCSI and Consultant Medical Oncologist
Beaumont Hospital
Our Lady of Lourdes Hospital
Dublin
Ireland

Roy S. Herbst, MD, PhD
Professor (Ensign Professor of Medicine)
Department of Medicine, Section of Medical Oncology
Yale School of Medicine, Yale Cancer Center, and
Smilow Cancer Hospital
New Haven, CT
USA

Michael F. Herfs, PhD
Principal Investigator
GIGA-Cancer
Laboratory of Experimental Pathology
Department of Pathology
University of Liege
Liege
Belgium

H. Franklin Herlong, MD
Professor of Medicine
Department of Gastroenterology, Hepatology and
Nutrition
The University of Texas MD Anderson Cancer Center
Houston, TX
USA

James G. Herman, MD
Professor of Medicine
Co-Leader, UPCI Lung Cancer Program
University of Pittsburgh Cancer Institute
Pittsburgh, PA
USA

John V. Heymach, MD, PhD
Chair, Department of Thoracic Head and Neck
The University of Texas MD Anderson Cancer Center
Houston, TX
USA

Teru Hideshima, MD, PhD
Institute Scientist
Department of Medical Oncology
Dana-Farber Cancer Institute
Principal Associate in Medicine
Harvard Medical School
Boston, MA
USA

Bradford R. Hirsch, MD, MBA
Department of Medicine
Adjunct Assistant Professor
Duke University Medical Center
Durham, NC
USA

James W. Hodge, PhD, MBA
Senior Investigator
Laboratory of Tumor Immunology and Biology
Center for Cancer Research
National Cancer Institute
National Institutes of Health
Bethesda, MD
USA

Lorne J. Hofseth, PhD
Professor and Graduate Director, College of Pharmacy
University of South Carolina
Professor, Drug Discovery & Biomedical Sciences
South Carolina College of Pharmacy
Columbia, SC
USA

James F. Holland, MD, ScD (hc)
Distinguished Professor of Neoplastic Diseases
Director Emeritus of Derald H. Ruttenberg Cancer
Center
Icahn School of Medicine at Mount Sinai
New York, NY
USA

Jimmie C. Holland, MD
Wayne E. Chapman Chair in Psychiatric Oncology
Memorial Sloan-Kettering Cancer Center
New York, NY
USA

Waun Ki Hong, MD, DMSc (Hon)
Professor of Thoracic/Head and Neck Medical
Oncology
American Cancer Society
Professor, Samsung Distinguished University Chair in
Cancer Medicine Emeritus
The University of Texas MD Anderson Cancer Center
Houston, TX
USA

Leroy Hood, MD, PhD
Providence Health & Services
Institute for Systems Biology
Seattle, WA
USA

Richard T. Hoppe, MD
The Henry S. Kaplan-Harry Lebeson Professor in
Cancer Biology
Department of Radiation Oncology
Stanford University
Stanford, CA
USA

Neil S. Horowitz, MD
Assistant Professor
Obstetrics and Gynecology
Brigham and Women's Hospital
Boston, MA
USA

Arti Hurria, MD
Professor, Department of Medical Oncology and
Therapeutics Research
City of Hope
Altadena, CA
USA

Ilya Iofin, MD
Assistant Professor of Orthopedics
Mount Sinai Hospital
New York, NY
USA

Nitin Jain, MD, MSPH
Associate Professor, Physical Medicine and
Rehabilitation and Orthopaedics, Director of PM&R
Research and Co-Director of Orthopaedic Sports
Medicine Research
Vanderbilt Stallworth Rehabilitation Hospital
Nashville, TN
USA

Anuja Jhingran, MD
Professor
Department of Radiation Oncology
Section of Gynecology
The University of Texas MD Anderson Cancer Center
Houston, TX
USA

Carlos A. Jimenez, MD
Professor
Department of Pulmonary Medicine
The University of Texas MD Anderson Cancer Center
Houston, TX
USA

Roy Jones, MD, PhD
Professor, Cancer Medicine, Department of Stem Cell
Transplantation & Cellular Therapy
The University of Texas MD Anderson Cancer Center
Houston, TX
USA

**Virgil Craig Jordan, OBE, PhD,
DSc, FMedSci**
Professor of Breast Medical Oncology and Professor of
Molecular and Cellular Oncology
The University of Texas MD Anderson Cancer Center
Houston, TX
USA

Roshni D. Kalachand, MBBCh, MD
Specialist Registrar in Medical Oncology
Beaumont Hospital and Royal College of Surgeons
Dublin
Ireland

Hagop M. Kantarjian, MD
Professor and Chairman, Department of Leukemia
The University of Texas MD Anderson Cancer Center
Houston, TX
USA

Michael Karin, PhD
Distinguished Professor of Pharmacology
Pharmacology
University of California, San Diego
La Jolla, CA
USA

Ahmed O. Kaseb, MD
Associate Professor, Department of Gastrointestinal
(GI) Medical Oncology, Division of Cancer Medicine
The University of Texas MD Anderson Cancer Center
Houston, TX
USA

Richard M. Kaufman, MD
Assistant Professor of Pathology
Harvard Medical School
Medical Director, Adult Transfusion Service
Brigham and Women's Hospital
Boston, MA
USA

Ronan J. Kelly, MD
Director of the Gastroesophageal Cancer Therapeutics
Program
Johns Hopkins University School of Medicine
Baltimore, MD
USA

Robert S. Kerbel, PhD
Senior Scientist, Biological Sciences Platform
Sunnybrook Research Institute
Professor, Department of Medical Biophysics
University of Toronto
Toronto, ON
Canada

Merrill S. Kies, MD
Professor of Medicine
Department of Thoracic–Head and Neck Medical
Oncology
The University of Texas MD Anderson Cancer Center
Houston, TX
USA

Youn H. Kim, MD
The Joanne and Peter Haas, Jr., Professor for Cutaneous
Lymphoma Research
Department of Dermatology
Stanford University
Stanford, CA
USA

Jeri Kim, MD
Associate Professor, Department of Genitourinary
Medical Oncology, Division of Cancer Medicine
The University of Texas MD Anderson Cancer Center
Houston, TX
USA

Catherine E. Klein, MD
Professor of Medicine
Division of Medical Oncology
University of Colorado
Aurora, CO

Chief, Hematology/Oncology
Eastern Colorado Health Care
Denver Veterans Affairs
Denver, CO
USA

Justin M. Ko, MD, MBA, FAAD
Clinical Associate Professor, Dermatology
Stanford Medical
Redwood City, CA
USA

**Christian Kollmannsberger, MD,
FRCPC**
Clinical Associate Professor of Medicine
Division of Medical Oncology
University of British Columbia
BCCA Vancouver Cancer Centre
Vancouver, BC
Canada

Ritsuko K. Komaki, MD
Professor
Department of Radiation Oncology
The University of Texas MD Anderson Cancer Center
Houston, TX
USA

Scott Kopetz, MD, PhD
Associate Professor, GI Medical Oncology
The University of Texas MD Anderson Cancer Center
Houston, TX
USA

Michael Kroll, MD
Professor
Department of Pulmonary Medicine
The University of Texas MD Anderson Cancer Center
Houston, TX
USA

**Deborah Kuban, MD, FACR,
FASTRO**
Professor, Department of Radiation Oncology
The University of Texas MD Anderson Cancer Center
Houston, TX
USA

Donald W. Kufe, MD
Distinguished Physician, Dana-Farber Cancer Institute
Professor of Medicine, Harvard Medical School
Leader, Translational Pharmacology and Early
Therapeutic Trials Program
Dana-Farber/Harvard Cancer Center
Boston, MA
USA

Anita Kumar, MD
Assistant Attending, Lymphoma Service
Department of Medicine
Memorial Sloan-Kettering Cancer Center and
Instructor of Clinical Medicine
Weill Cornell Medical College
New York, NY
USA

Michael E. Kupferman, MD
Associate Professor
Department of Head and Neck Surgery
The University of Texas MD Anderson Cancer Center
Houston, TX
USA

Ann S. LaCasce, MD
Assistant Professor of Medicine
Harvard Medical School
Boston, MA
USA

Stephen Y. Lai, MD, PhD
Associate Professor
Department of Head and Neck Surgery
The University of Texas MD Anderson Cancer Center
Houston, TX
USA

Raymond S. Lance, MD
Urologist
Deaconess Medical Center-Spokane
Spokane, WA
USA

Robert S. Langer, ScD
David H. Koch Institute Professor
Department of Chemical Engineering
Massachusetts Institute of Technology
Cambridge, MA
USA

Peter F. Lebowitz, MD, PhD
Global Therapeutic Area Head, Oncology
Janssen Research & Development, LLC.
Raritan, NJ
USA

Michelle M. Le Beau, PhD
Arthur and Marian Edelstein Professor of Medicine
Director, University of Chicago Comprehensive Cancer
Center
Chicago, IL
USA

J. Jack Lee, PhD, MS, DDS
Associate Vice Provost, Quantitative Research
The University of Texas MD Anderson Cancer Center
Houston, TX
USA

Richard T. Lee, MD
Assistant Professor
Department of Medicine
University Hospitals and Case Western Reserve
University
Cleveland, OH
USA

Donghui Li, PhD
Professor of Medicine
Department of Gastrointestinal Medical Oncology
The University of Texas MD Anderson Cancer Center
Houston, TX
USA

Scott M. Lippman, MD
Professor
Moores Cancer Center
University of California San Diego
La Jolla, CA
USA

Virginia R. Litle, MD
Associate Professor of Surgery
Boston University School of Medicine
Boston, MA
USA

Jennifer K. Litton, MD
Associate Professor
Breast Medical Oncology
The University of Texas MD Anderson Cancer Center
Houston, TX
USA

Danny Liu
Research Assistant
Brigham and Women's Hospital
Harvard Medical School
Boston, MA
USA

Yanlan Liu, PhD
Post-doctoral Researcher
Brigham and Women's Hospital
Harvard Medical School
Boston, MA
USA

Christopher J. Logothetis, MD
Chairman & Professor
Genitourinary Medical Oncology
The University of Texas MD Anderson Cancer Center
Houston, TX
USA

Gabriel Lopez, MD
Assistant Professor
Department of Palliative, Rehabilitation and Integrative
Medicine
The University of Texas MD Anderson Cancer Center
Houston, TX
USA

Charles Lu, MD, SM
Professor, Department of Thoracic/Head and Neck
Medical Oncology, Division of Cancer Medicine
The University of Texas MD Anderson Cancer Center
Houston, TX
USA

Karen Lu, MD
Chair, Department of Gynecologic Oncology and
Reproductive Medicine, Division of Surgery
The University of Texas MD Anderson Cancer Center
Houston, TX
USA

Guishuai Lv, MD
Research Assistant
International Lab on Signaling Transduction
Eastern Hepatobiliary Surgery Hospital
Shanghai
China

Donald F. Lynch, Jr., MD
Urologist
Eastern Virginia Medical School
Norfolk, VA
USA

Anirban Maitra, MD
Professor of Pathology
Department of Pathology
The University of Texas MD Anderson Cancer Center
Houston, TX
USA

Melanie Majure, MD
HS Clinical Instructor
UCSF School of Medicine
San Francisco, CA
USA

Robert G. Maki, MD, PhD, FACP
Professor of Medicine, Pediatrics, and Orthopaedics
Mount Sinai Medical School
New York, NY
USA

Shan Man, BSc
Senior Technician/Lab Manager
Biological Sciences Platform
Sunnybrook Research Institute
Toronto, ON
Canada

Alberto M. Marchevsky, MD
Director, Pulmonary and Mediastinal Pathology
Cedars-Sinai Medical Center
West Hollywood, CA
USA

Kim A. Margolin, MD
Director, Multi-disciplinary Melanoma Program
City of Hope Department of Medical Oncology and
Comprehensive Cancer Center
Duarte, California
USA

Megan E. McNerney, MD, PhD
Assistant Professor of Pathology
Department of Pathology
University of Chicago
Chicago, IL
USA

Jeffrey I. Mechanick, MD
Clinical Professor of Medicine
Division of Endocrinology, Diabetes, and Bone Disease
Icahn School of Medicine at Mount Sinai
New York, NY
USA

Stephanie C. Melkonian, PhD
Postdoctoral Research Fellow
Department of Epidemiology
The University of Texas MD Anderson Cancer Center
Houston, TX
USA

Ilgen Mender, PhD
Postdoctoral Researcher
Department of Cell Biology
The University of Texas Southwestern Medical Center
Dallas, TX
USA

Department of Biochemistry
Faculty of Medicine, Hacettepe University
Ankara
Turkey

Matthew Meyerson, MD, PhD
Professor
Department of Pathology
Dana-Farber Cancer Institute
Boston, MA
USA

Eric A. Millican, MD
Fellow, Procedural Dermatology
Vanderbilt University
Nashville, TN
USA

Gordon B. Mills, MD, PhD
Professor
Department of Systems Biology
The University of Texas MD Anderson Cancer Center
Houston, TX
USA

Bruce D. Minsky, MD
Professor of Radiation Oncology
Frank T. McGraw Memorial Chair
Department of Radiation Oncology
The University of Texas MD Anderson Cancer Center
Houston, TX
USA

David L. Mitchell, PhD
Professor
Department of Carcinogenesis
Science Park-Research Division
Department of Carcinogenesis
The University of Texas MD Anderson Cancer Center
Smithville, TX
USA

Francesca Molinari, PhD
Scientific collaborator
Laboratory of Molecular Pathology
Institute of Pathology
Locarno
Switzerland

Daniel Morgensztern, MD
Associate Professor
Department of Medicine, Division of Medical Oncology
Washington University School of Medicine St. Louis
Missouri, MO
USA

Rodolfo C. Morice, MD
Professor
Department of Pulmonary Medicine
The University of Texas MD Anderson Cancer Center
Houston, TX
USA

Donald L. Morton, MD, FACS (deceased)
Chief of the Melanoma Program and Co-Director of the Surgical Oncology Fellowship Program
John Wayne Cancer Institute (JWCI)
Santa Monica, CA
USA

Jeffrey A. Moscow, MD
Pediatric Hematologist-Oncologist
Senior Investigator, National Cancer Institute
Bethesda, MD
USA

Judy S. Moyes, MA (Cantab), MB, BChir, FRCPC, FRCPCH
Technical Writer
Pediatrics Research
The University of Texas MD Anderson Cancer Center
Houston, TX
USA

Mariela Blum Murphy, MD
Assistant Professor
Department of Gastrointestinal Medical Oncology
The University of Texas MD Anderson Cancer Center
Houston, TX
USA

Muhammed Murtaza, MBBS, PhD
Assistant Professor
Co-Director, Center for Noninvasive Diagnostics
Translational Genomics Research Institute
Phoenix, AZ
USA

Hyman B. Muss, MD
Mary Jones Hudson Distinguished Professorship in Geriatric Oncology
School of Medicine
UNC-Chapel Hill
Chapel Hill, NC
USA

Serge Patrick Nana-Sinkam, MD
Associate Professor
Division of Pulmonary, Allergy, Critical Care and Sleep Medicine
Department of Molecular Virology, Immunology & Medical Genetics
James Comprehensive Cancer Center
The Ohio State University
Columbus, OH
USA

Vignesh Narayanan, MD
Fellow, Hematology-Oncology
University of Colorado
Aurora, CO
USA

Victor A. Neel, MD, PhD
Assistant Professor, Department of Dermatology
Harvard Medical School
Boston, MA
USA

Lior Nesher, MD
Infectious Disease Institute
Soroka University Medical Center
Senior lecturer, Faculty of Health Sciences
Ben-Gurion University of the Negev
Beersheba
Israel

Craig R. Nichols, MD
Director-Testicular Cancer Commons
Co-Director Testicular Cancer Multidisciplinary Clinic
Virginia Mason Medical Center
Seattle, WA
USA

Monique Nilsson, PhD
Senior Research Scientist, Department of Thoracic Head and Neck
The University of Texas MD Anderson Cancer Center
Houston, TX
USA

Larry Norton, MD
Deputy Physician-in-Chief for Breast Cancer Programs
Memorial Sloan Kettering Cancer Center
New York, NY
USA

Daniel P. Nussbaum, MD
Resident, General Surgery
Department of Pharmacology and Cancer Biology
Duke University Medical Center
Durham, NC
USA

Susan O'Brien, MD
Professor
Department of Leukemia
Division of Cancer Medicine
The University of Texas MD Anderson Cancer Center
Houston, TX
USA

Takao Ohnuma, MD, PhD
Professor of Medicine
Division of Hematology and Oncology
Tisch Cancer Institute
Icahn School of Medicine at Mount Sinai
New York, NY
USA

Amir Onn, MD
Head, Institute of Pulmonary Medicine
Sheba Medical Center
Ramat Gan
Israel

Susana Ortiz-Urda, MD, PhD, MBA
Assistant Professor
Department of Dermatology
University of California
San Francisco, CA
USA

Brian O'Sullivan, MD, FRCPI, FRCPC
Professor, Department of Radiation Oncology
University of Toronto
Head, Radiation Oncology Sarcoma Site Group
Princess Margaret Cancer Centre
Toronto, ON
Canada

Jamie S. Ostroff, PhD
Chief, Behavioral Sciences Service
Director, Tobacco Treatment Program
Memorial Sloan Kettering Cancer Center
New York, NY
USA

Marta Paez-Ribes, PhD
Research Associate
Department of Pathology
University of Cambridge
Cambridge
UK

Margaret Pain, MD
Neurosurgical Resident
Icahn School of Medicine at Mount Sinai
New York, NY
USA

Ben Ho Park, MD, PhD
Professor, Department of Oncology, Johns Hopkins University
Professor of Oncology, Breast and Ovarian Cancer Program
Associate Director, Hematology/Oncology Fellowship Training Program
Associate Director for Research Training and Education
The Sidney Kimmel Comprehensive Cancer Center at Johns Hopkins
Baltimore, MD
USA

Harvey I. Pass, MD
Stephen E. Banner Professor of Thoracic Oncology
Professor of Surgery and Cardiothoracic Surgery
Director, General Thoracic Division
Chief, Thoracic Oncology
NYU Langone Medical Center
New York, NY
USA

Anisha B. Patel, MD
Assistant Professor of Dermatology
The University of Texas MD Anderson Cancer Center
Houston, TX
USA

Krina K. Patel, MD
Assistant Professor
Stem Cell Transplantation and Cellular Therapy
The University of Texas MD Anderson Cancer Center
Houston, TX
USA

Natalya N. Pavlova, PhD
Postdoctoral Research Fellow
Cancer Biology and Genetics Program
Memorial Sloan Kettering Cancer Center
New York, NY
USA

Karl Peggs, MD, MA, MRCP, FRCPath
Senior Lecturer in Stem Cell Transplantation and Immunotherapy
University College Hospital London
London
UK

Errol J. Philip, PhD
Chief Clinical Research Fellow in the Department of
Psychiatry and Behavioral Sciences
Memorial Sloan Kettering Cancer Center
New York, NY
USA

**Martine Piccart-Gebhart, MD,
PhD**
Professor of Oncology
Université Libre de Bruxelles (ULB)
Head of the Medicine Department
Jules Bordet Institute
Brussels
Belgium

Marco A. Pierotti, PhD
Scientific Directorate
Fondazione Istituto Ricerche Pediatriche Città della
Speranza
Padova
Italy

Head
Molecular Genetics of Cancer Unit
Fondazione Istituto FIRC di Oncologia Molecolare
Milan
Italy

**Raphael E. Pollock, MD, PhD,
FACS**
Professor and Director, Division of Surgical Oncology
Surgeon in Chief, James Comprehensive Cancer Center
Surgeon in Chief, The Ohio State University Health
System
The Ohio State University Wexner Medical Center
Columbus, OH
USA

Yves Pommier, MD, PhD
Chief
Developmental Therapeutics Branch, National Cancer
Institute, National Institutes of Health
Bethesda, MD
USA

Carol S. Portlock, MD
Attending Physician
Lymphoma Service, Department of Medicine
Memorial Sloan-Kettering Cancer Center and
Professor of Clinical Medicine
Weill Cornell Medical College
New York, NY
USA

**Kalmon D. Post, MD, FACS,
FAANS**
Chairman Emeritus Department Neurosurgery
Professor Neurosurgery & Medicine
Icahn School of Medicine at Mount Sinai
Program Director Department Neurosurgery
Mount Sinai Health System
New York, NY
USA

**Selvaraj E. Pravinkumar, MD,
FRCP**
Associate Professor
Department of Critical Care
The University of Texas MD Anderson Cancer Center
Houston, TX
USA

Nathan D. Price, PhD
Professor and Associate Director
Institute for Systems Biology
Seattle, WA
USA

Xia Pu, PhD
Instructor
Department of Epidemiology
The University of Texas MD Anderson Cancer Center
Houston, TX
USA

Sergio Quezada, PhD
Professorial Research Fellow
UCL Cancer Institute
London
UK

**Derek Raghavan, MD, PhD, FACP,
FRACP, FASCO**
President, Levine Cancer Institute &
Professor-Medicine, UNC School of Medicine,
Charlotte Campus, Carolinas HealthCare System
Charlotte, NC
USA

Kristjan T. Ragnarsson, MD
Professor and Chairman
Department of Rehabilitation Medicine
Icahn School of Medicine at Mount Sinai
New York, NY
USA

Jamal Rahaman, MD
Associate Clinical Professor
The Mount Sinai Hospital
New York, NY
USA

Kanti R. Rai, MD
Professor of Medicine and Professor of Molecular
Medicine
Joel Finkelstein Cancer Foundation
Hofstra Northwell School of Medicine
New Hyde Park, NY
USA

Noopur Raje, MD
Director, Center for Multiple Myeloma
Rita Kelley Chair in Oncology
Massachusetts General Hospital Cancer Center
Associate Professor of Medicine
Harvard Medical School
Boston, MA
USA

Pilar Ramos, PhD
Postdoctoral Fellow
Integrated Cancer Genomics Division
Translational Genomics Research Institute
Phoenix, AZ
USA

Jacob H. Rand, MD
Hematologist
Montefiore Medical Center
Bronx, NY
USA

Mark J. Ratain, MD
Leon O. Jacobson Professor of Medicine
Department of Medicine and Committee on Clinical
Pharmacology and Pharmacogenomics
University of Chicago
Chicago, IL
USA

**Chandrajit P. Raut, MD, MSc,
FACS**
Associate Surgeon, General and Gastrointestinal
Surgery
Brigham and Women's Hospital
Harvard Medical School
Boston, MA
USA

John C. Reed, MD, PhD
Pharmaceutical Research & Early Development
Roche Innovation Center
Basel
Switzerland

Marvin S. Reitz, PhD
Adjunct Professor
School of Medicine
Institute of Human Virology
Baltimore, MD
USA

**David C. Rice, MB, BCh, BAO,
FRCSI**
Professor
Department of Thoracic and Cardiovascular Surgery
Division of Surgery
The University of Texas MD Anderson Cancer Center
Houston, TX
USA

Stephen B. Riggs, MD
Attending Surgeon, Department of Urology and Levine
Cancer Institute
Carolinas HealthCare System
Charlotte, NC
USA

Brian I. Rini, MD, FACP
Professor of Medicine
Department of Solid Tumor Oncology
Cleveland Clinic Taussig Cancer Institute
Cleveland, OH
USA

Ana M. Rodriguez, MD, MPH, FACOG
Assistant Professor
Department of Obstetrics & Gynecology
University of Texas Medical Branch
Galveston, TX
USA

Kenneth V. I. Rolston, MD, FACP
Adjunct Professor, Department of Medicine/Infectious Diseases Section
The University of Texas MD Anderson Cancer Center
Houston, TX
USA

Bruce J. Roth, MD
Professor of Medicine
Division of Oncology, Section of Medical Oncology
Washington University School of Medicine
Missouri, MO
USA

Jacob Rotmensch, MD
Oncologist
Department of Gynecologic Oncology
Rush University Medical Center
Chicago, IL
USA

Eric K. Rowinsky, MD
Adjunct Professor, Department of Medicine
NYU School of Medicine
New York, NY
USA

Julia H. Rowland, PhD
Director, Office of Cancer Survivorship
Division of Cancer Control and Population Sciences, National Cancer Institute, NIH-DHHS
Bethesda, MD
USA

Hope S. Rugo, MD
Clinical Professor, Department of Medicine (Hematology/Oncology)
University of California San Francisco School of Medicine
San Francisco, CA
USA

Rachel A. Sanford, MD
Fellow, Division of Cancer Medicine Fellowship Program
The University of Texas MD Anderson Cancer Center
Houston, TX
USA

David T. Scadden, MD
Massachusetts General Hospital
Director, MGH Center for Regenerative Medicine
Boston, MA
USA

Amy C. Schefler, MD, FACS
Attending
Retina Consultants of Houston
Houston, TX
USA

Charles A. Schiffer, MD
Professor of Medicine and Oncology
Joseph Dresner Chair for Hematologic Malignancies
Department of Oncology
Karmanos Cancer Center
Wayne State University School of Medicine
Detroit, MI
USA

Jeffery Schlom, PhD
Chief
Laboratory of Tumor Immunology and Biology
National Cancer Institute
National Institutes of Health
Bethesda, MD
USA

Carl Schmidt, MD
Associate Professor
Department of Surgery
The Ohio State University Wexner Medical Center
Columbus, OH
USA

Leslie R. Schover, PhD
Professor of Behavioral Science
The University of Texas MD Anderson Cancer Center
Houston, TX
USA

Lawrence H. Schwartz, MD
James Picker Professor of Radiology
Department of Radiology
University of Columbia
Columbia, OH
USA

Aleksandar Sekulic, MD, PhD
Associate Professor of Dermatology
Vice Chair, Department of Dermatology
Chair, Cutaneous Oncology Disease Group
Mayo Clinic Arizona
Scottsdale, AZ
USA

Boris Sepesi, MD
Assistant Professor
Thoracic and Cardiovascular Surgery
The University of Texas MD Anderson Cancer Center
Houston, TX
USA

Vickie R. Shannon, MD
Professor
Department of Pulmonary Medicine
The University of Texas MD Anderson Cancer Center
Houston, TX
USA

Padmanee Sharma, MD, PhD
Professor, Department of Genitourinary Medical Oncology, Division of Cancer Medicine
The University of Texas MD Anderson Cancer Center
Houston, TX
USA

Manish R. Sharma, MD
Assistant Professor of Medicine
Department of Medicine and Committee on Clinical Pharmacology and Pharmacogenomics
University of Chicago
Chicago, IL
USA

Jerry W. Shay, PhD
Professor, Department of Cell Biology
UT Southwestern Medical Center
Dallas, TX
USA

Professor
Center for Excellence in Genomics Medicine Research
King Abdulaziz University
Jeddah
Saudi Arabia

Steven I. Sherman, MD
Associate Vice Provost, Clinical Research
Chair and Naguib Samaan Distinguished Professor in Endocrinology
Department of Endocrine Neoplasia and Hormonal Disorders
The University of Texas MD Anderson Cancer Center
Houston, TX
USA

Jinjun Shi, PhD
Assistant Professor of Anaesthesia
Department of Anaesthesia
Brigham and Women's Hospital
Harvard Medical School
Boston, MA
USA

Junichi Shindoh, MD, PhD
Associate Professor
Department of Hepatobiliary and Pancreatic Surgery
The University of Tokyo
Tokyo
Japan

Elizabeth Shpall, MD
Professor, Department of Stem Cell Transplantation and Cellular Therapy
The University of Texas MD Anderson Cancer Center
Houston, TX
USA

Zahid H. Siddik, PhD
Professor of Medicine (Pharmacology)
The University of Texas MD Anderson Cancer Center
Houston, TX
USA

Branimir I. Sikic, MD
Professor of Medicine (Oncology)
Stanford Medicine
Stanford, CA
USA

Richard T. Silver, MD
Professor of Medicine, Division of Hematology-Oncology
Department of Medicine
Weill Cornell Medical College
New York, NY
USA

Lewis R. Silverman, MD
Associate Professor
Department of Medicine, Hematology and Medical
Oncology
Mount Sinai Hospital
New York, NY
USA

Richard Simon, DSc
Associate Director
Division of Cancer Treatment and Diagnosis
National Cancer Institute
Bethesda, MD
USA

Cardinale B. Smith, MD, MSCR
Assistant Professor of Medicine
Associate Program Director of Research, Internal
Medicine Residency
Division of Hematology/Medical Oncology and
Brookdale Department of Geriatrics and Palliative
Medicine
Icahn School of Medicine at Mount Sinai
New York, NY
USA

Vernon K. Sondak, MD
Chief of the Division of Cutaneous Oncology and
Director of Surgical Education
H. Lee Moffitt Cancer Center and Research Institute
Tampa, FL
USA

Stephen T. Sonis, DMD, DMSc
Clinical Professor of Oral Medicine and Diagnostic
Sciences
Harvard School of Dental Medicine
Brigham and Women's Hospital
Boston, MA
USA

Gabriella Sozzi, PhD
Head
Tumor Genomics Unit
Department of Experimental Oncology and Molecular
Medicine
Fondazione IRCCS Istituto Nazionale dei Tumori
Milan
Italy

Margaret R. Spitz, MD, MPH
Professor
Dan L. Duncan Cancer Center
Baylor College of Medicine
Houston, TX
USA

William G. Stebbins, MD
Assistant Professor of Dermatology
Vanderbilt University
Nashville, TN
USA

Richard M. Stone, MD
Chief of Staff
Program Director, Adult Leukemia
Professor of Medicine
Harvard Medical School Center/Program
Boston, MA
USA

Michael D. Stubblefield, MD
National Medical Director for Cancer Rehabilitation
Select Medical
Medical Director for Cancer Rehabilitation
Kessler Institute for Rehabilitation
West Orange, NJ
USA

Sumit K. Subudhi, MD, PhD
Assistant Professor
Department of Genitourinary Medical Oncology
Division of Cancer Medicine
The University of Texas MD Anderson Cancer Center
Houston, TX
USA

Zhifei Sun, MD
Research Assistant
Department of Leukemia
University of Texas Medical Center
Dallas, TX
USA

Max W. Sung, MD
Associate Professor of Medicine, Hematology and
Medical Oncology
The Mount Sinai Hospital
New York, NY
USA

Thomas Suter, MD
Professor of Medicine
Department of Cardiology
University Hospital Bern
Basel
Switzerland

Susan M. Swetter, MD
Professor of Dermatology
Palo Alto Veterans Affairs Health Care System and the
Stanford University Medical Center
Stanford, CA
USA

Stephen G. Swisher, MD, FACS
Division Head, Division of Surgery
The University of Texas MD Anderson Cancer Center
Houston, TX
USA

Chris H. Takimoto, MD, PhD, FACP
Vice President, Translational Medicine Early
Development
Janssen Research & Development, LLC.
Raritan, NJ
USA

Kenneth K. Tanabe, MD, FACS
Associate Professor
Director, Mesothelioma Program
Director, Thoracic Chemo-Radiation Program
The University of Texas MD Anderson Cancer Center
Department of Thoracic-Head & Neck Medical
Oncology
Houston, TX
USA

Koji Taniguchi, MD, PhD
Assistant Project Scientist
Pharmacology
University of California, San Diego
La Jolla, CA
USA

Nizar M. Tannir, MD, FACP
Professor and Deputy Chairman
Department of Genitourinary Medical Oncology
The University of Texas MD Anderson Cancer Center
Houston, TX
USA

Haruko Tashiro, MD, PhD
Post-doctoral fellow
Baylor College of Medicine
Houston, TX
USA

Ayalew Tefferi, MD
Professor of Medicine and Hematology
Department of Internal Medicine Mayo Clinic
Rochester, MN
USA

Anish Thomas, MBBS, MD
Staff Clinician
Thoracic and Gastrointestinal Oncology Branch, Center
for Cancer Research
National Cancer Institute
National Institutes of Health
Bethesda, MD
USA

Melanie B. Thomas, MD, MS
Associate Center Director for Experimental
Therapeutics
Gibbs Cancer Center & Research
Institute –Spartanburg
Spartanburg, SC
USA

David C. Thomas, MD, MHPE
Professor of Medicine, Medical Education and
Rehabilitation Medicine
Vice Chair for Education
Samuel Bronfman Department of Medicine

Associate Dean for CME
Icahn School of Medicine at Mount Sinai
New York, NY
USA

Craig B. Thompson, MD
President and CEO-Member
Cancer Biology and Genetics Program
Memorial Sloan Kettering Cancer Center
New York, NY
USA

Jelena Todoric, MD, PhD
Postdoctoral Researcher
Pharmacology
University of California, San Diego
La Jolla, CA
USA

Jeffrey M. Trent, PhD
Professor
Integrated Cancer Genomics Division
Translational Genomics Research Institute
Phoenix, AZ
USA

Susan Tsai, MD
Assistant Professor of Surgery
Department of Surgery
Medical College of Wisconsin
Milwaukee, WI
USA

Anne S. Tsao, MD
Associate Professor
Department of Thoracic-Head & Neck Medical
Oncology
The University of Texas MD Anderson Cancer Center
Houston, TX
USA

David A. Tuveson, MD, PhD
Professor
Cold Spring Harbor Laboratory
Cold Spring Harbor, NY
USA

Douglas S. Tyler, MD
John Woods Harris Distinguished Chair in Surgery
University of Texas Medical Branch
Galveston, TX
USA

Marc Uemura, MD
Fellow in Hematology and Medical Oncology
Anderson Cancer Center
Houston, TX
USA

Atsushi Umemura, MD, PhD
Assistant Professor
Department of Molecular Gastroenterology and
Hepatology, Graduate School of Medical Science
Kyoto Prefectural University of Medicine
Kyoto
Japan

David J. Vander Weele, MD, PhD
Section of Hematology-Oncology, Department of
Medicine
Comprehensive Cancer Center
University of Chicago
Chicago, IL
USA

Ara A. Vaporciyan, MD
Professor and Chairman
Director of Clinical Education and Training
Department of Thoracic and Cardiovascular Surgery
M.G. & Lillie A. Johnson Chair for Cancer Treatment &
Research
The University of Texas MD Anderson Cancer Center
Houston, TX
USA

Jean-Nicolas Vauthey, MD
Professor, Department Surgical Oncology
Chief, Hepato-Pancreato-Biliary Section
The University of Texas MD Anderson Cancer Center
Houston, TX
USA

Michael A. Via, MD
Assistant Professor of Medicine
Associate Fellowship Director
Director of Metabolic Support
Division of Endocrinology, Diabetes, and Bone Disease
Mount Sinai Beth Israel Medical Center
Icahn School of Medicine at Mount Sinai
New York, NY
USA

**Srinivas R. Viswanathan, MD,
PhD**
Director
Department of Gynecologic Radiation Oncology
Dana-Farber Cancer Institute
Boston, MA
USA

Bert Vogelstein, MD
Professor, Department of Oncology
Johns Hopkins University
Baltimore, MD
USA

Daniel D. Von Hoff, MD, FACP
Director, AHSC Cancer Therapeutics Program
Department of Medicine
University of Arizona College of Medicine
Physician in Chief and Distinguished Professor
Translational Genomics Research Institute
Phoenix, AZ
USA

Evan Vosburgh, MD
Clinical Associate Professor of Medicine
Department of Medicine
Yale University School of Medicine
New Haven, CT
USA

Michael J. Wallace, MD
Professor
Department of Interventional Radiology
The University of Texas MD Anderson Cancer Center
Houston, TX
USA

Hongyang Wang, MD
Professor and Director
National Center for Liver Cancer
China

Eastern Hepatobiliary Surgery Hospital
Shanghai
China

Ralph R. Weichselbaum, MD
Daniel K. Ludwig Distinguished Service Professor of
Radiation and Cellular Oncology
Chair, Department of Radiation and Cellular Oncology
University of Chicago
Hospital Director, Chicago Tumor Institute
Chicago, IL
USA

Robert A. Weinberg, PhD
Professor of Biology
Whitehead Institute
Massachusetts Institute of Technology
Cambridge, MA
USA

John N. Weinstein, MD, PhD
Professor and Chair, Department of Bioinformatics and
Computational Biology, Division of Quantitative
Sciences
The University of Texas MD Anderson Cancer Center
Houston, TX
USA

Ainsley Weston, PhD
Associate Director for Science
Division of Respiratory Disease Studies
Centers for Disease Control and Prevention (CDC)
Morgantown, WV
USA

Max S. Wicha, MD
Madeline and Sidney Forbes Professor of Oncology
University of Michigan Comprehensive Cancer Center
Ann Arbor, MI
USA

Talia W. Wiesel, PhD
Assistant Professor
Psychiatry
Icahn School of Medicine at Mount Sinai
New York, NY
USA

Christopher P. Wild, PhD
Director, International Agency for Research on Cancer
Lyon
France

William N. William, Jr., MD
Associate Professor
Department of Thoracic / Head and Neck Medical
Oncology
The University of Texas MD Anderson Cancer Center
Houston, TX
USA

Ignacio I. Wistuba, MD
Professor and Chair
Department of Translational Molecular Pathology
Anderson Clinical Faculty Chair for Cancer Treatment
and Research
The University of Texas MD Anderson Cancer Center
Houston, TX
USA

Robert A. Wolff, MD
Professor of Medicine
Department of Gastrointestinal Medical Oncology
The University of Texas MD Anderson Cancer Center
Houston, TX
USA

Scott E. Woodman, MD, PhD
Assistant Professor
Department of Melanoma Medical Oncology, Division
of Cancer Medicine
The University of Texas MD Anderson Cancer Center
Houston, TX
USA

Woodring E. Wright, MD, PhD
Department of Cell Biology
University of Texas Southwestern Medical Center
Dallas, TX
USA

Xifeng Wu, MD, PhD
Professor and Department Chair
Department of Epidemiology
The University of Texas MD Anderson Cancer Center
Houston, TX
USA

Ping Xu, PhD
Research Associate
Biological Sciences Platform
Sunnybrook Research Institute
Toronto, ON
Canada

Xiao-Jing Yan, MD
Physician and Research Fellow
Shanghai Institute of Hematology
Rui Jin Hospital
Shanghai Jiao Tong University School of Medicine
Shanghai
China

Haining Yang, PhD
Associate Professor
Cancer Biology Program
University of Hawaii Cancer Center
Honolulu, HI
USA

James C. Yao, MD
Professor with Tenure
Department of Gastrointestinal Medical Oncology
The University of Texas MD Anderson Cancer Center
Houston, TX
USA

Andrew J. Yee, MD
Instructor in Medicine
Massachusetts General Hospital Cancer Center
Harvard Medical School
Boston, MA
USA

Sai-Ching Jim Yeung, MD, PhD, FACP
Professor, Department of Emergency Medicine,
Division of Internal Medicine
The University of Texas MD Anderson Cancer Center
Professor, Department of Emergency Medicine and
Department of Endocrine Neoplasia and Hormonal
Disorders
The University of Texas MD Anderson Cancer Center
Houston, TX
USA

Anthony F. Yu, MD
Cardiologist
Memorial Sloan Kettering Cancer Center
Department of Medicine, Cardiology Service
New York, NY
USA

Anna Yuan, DMD
Oral Medicine Fellow
Brigham and Women's Hospital
Boston, MA
USA

Jonathan S. Zager, MD
Professor
Moffitt Cancer Center
Tampa, FL
USA

Michael R. Zalutsky, PhD, MA
Professor of Radiology
Department of Research
Duke University School of Medicine
Durham, NC
USA

Sarina van der Zee, MD
Fellow, The Zena and Michael A. Wiener
Cardiovascular Institute
The Mount Sinai Medical Center
New York, NY
USA

Guang-Biao Zhou, MD
Professor of Institute of Zoology
State Key Laboratory of Biomembrane and Membrane
Biotechnology
Institute of Zoology
Chinese Academy of Sciences
Beijing
China

Amado Zurita-Saavedra, MD
Assistant Professor, Genitourinary Medical Oncology
The University of Texas MD Anderson Cancer Center
Houston, TX
USA

Preface

Our understanding of cancer at the molecular, cellular, and clinical levels continues to expand. Translation of molecular diagnostics and therapeutics to the clinic has begun to realize the promise of precision medicine with the development and approval of dozens of new targeted drugs, antibodies, and predictive biomarkers. Assimilating this knowledge poses an acute challenge for students, residents, fellows, and established practitioners of oncology. Laboratory-based investigators seeking to translate their discoveries to human application require an accurate overview of clinical oncology, informed by cancer biology. As new therapies and diagnostics may now be applicable across multiple disease sites, it is essential that Pharma and Biotech understand the new advances and the unmet needs across the entire field of oncology.

This 9th Edition of *Cancer Medicine* provides a comprehensive synthesis of clinical oncology and the principles underlying approaches to detection, diagnosis, and cancer management. Biological hallmarks of cancer and the clinical manifestations of neoplastic diseases are described. Oncologists must now be familiar with pathways and processes that explain the origin and pathogenesis of neoplasms. Transformational technologies are discussed in depth to provide oncologists with an understanding of technical procedures such as deep sequencing, methods for measuring epigenetic modification of DNA and histones, transcriptional profiling, ncRNAs, specific functions of RNAs, proteomics, and metabolomics. The heterogeneity within and between cancers and their metastases are described and implications for clinical management are discussed. Quantitative oncology is explained in understandable terms providing an introduction not only to biostatistics and novel trial design, but also to bioinformatics and systems biology.

This work includes concise guidelines for the use of both conventional and novel drugs. As in the past editions, there is an emphasis on multidisciplinary patient care including surgical and radiation oncology, psycho-oncology, and population science. This volume should be of value to oncologists of every discipline. *Cancer Medicine*, 9th Edition, includes electronic web-based access with links to relevant references that will be regularly updated.

The editors have chosen experts who have written authoritatively about the disciplines and diseases covered in their respective chapters. Given the global importance of oncology, editors have now been included from Europe and Asia. As the world of science and medicine chip away the unknowns of the cancer process and its prevention and therapy, we believe the contents of this work will provide a platform for understanding the current state of accomplishment and preparing the reader for a critical evaluation of discoveries still to come.

The Editors
2016

Acknowledgments

The editors gratefully acknowledge the exceptional contributions of Jene' Reinartz whose tireless efforts have been critical to the organization of CM9. We greatly appreciate our assistants Cheryl Ashorn, Michelle Denney, Guishuai Lv, Kate Charlesworth-Miller, Sharon Palko, Kathy Profrock, Ruby Robinson, Catherine Rotsaert, Mary Werowinski, and Elizabeth Wilkins who have helped to make this volume possible. We thank Nancy Hubener for her efforts in completing this edition. We thank Dr. Michael Ewer for his effort and expertise in reviewing multiple chapters.

Working with John Wiley, Inc., has been a particular pleasure. Our initial editor, Thom Moore, was instrumental in establishing the project and in acquiring the rights to CM9. His vision and persistence were essential. Claire Bonnet has been truly outstanding in bringing the book to completion. The Wiley staff has been most helpful.

Our authors have utilized their extraordinary knowledge, experience, and judgment to capture the critical points regarding each topic and disease site. The editors are grateful for their efforts and are proud of each chapter.

Finally, we must acknowledge the contribution of our patients from whom we have learned. It is their courage, equanimity, and strength in coping with illness that inspires us every day. For patients still to come, we hope that *Cancer Medicine*, 9th Edition, will benefit them by helping their doctors.

PART 1

Introduction

1 Cardinal manifestations of cancer

James F. Holland, MD, ScD (hc) ▪ Waun Ki Hong, MD, DMSc (Hon) ▪ Donald W. Kufe, MD ▪
Robert C. Bast Jr., MD ▪ William N. Hait, MD, PhD ▪ Raphael E. Pollock, MD, PhD, FACS ▪
Ralph R. Weichselbaum, MD

Overview

Cancer is asymptomatic at its initiation. Symptoms arise when a conduit is impaired, when cancer cells impinge on nerve fibers causing pain or dysfunction, when secretory products of the tumor cause systemic symptoms such as fever, weight loss, or fatigue, when ulceration and bleeding occur, or upon recognition of a mass. Indeed any symptom that lasts two weeks, even intermittently, could be a symptom of cancer, the great imitator. Cancer always belongs in the differential diagnosis.

Cancer is a singular word that embraces a vast diversity of diseases that can occur in any organ system throughout the animal kingdom. The unique characteristic of cancer is the proliferation of cells of a type different from, if ever so slightly, the normal complement of the organism. The proliferation of cancer cells may be rapid or slow, and the accumulation of cells may be massive or miniscule. The essence of the matter, however, is that aberrant cells, distinct from the ordinary evolution of cell types, appear and accumulate. Thus, a cancer differs from hypertrophy and hyperplasia, which involve normal cells.

A cancer cell does not obey the complex rules of architecture and function that govern the usual placement and behavior of cells within a tissue. The wondrous coexistence of cells and tissues of multiple types that make up the eye, the finger, or the kidney, for example, each with appropriate anatomic location with all connections intact to fulfill their appointed tasks, is part of the miracle we call life. The explanation for this marvelous organization is the field of continuing exploration seeking the messages and the exquisite controls that exist in multicellular organisms.

Cancer is distinguished from other abnormal cellular growths that lead to benign tumors in its characteristic independence from the restrictions present in normal tissues. Benign tumors expand and compress, but do not attack or invade adjacent tissues. Accumulated cancer cells make a tissue that ignores the anatomic barriers of adjacent cell membranes and basement membranes. Through chemical and mechanical means, the cancer cell insinuates itself between and into the space of the normal cells, killing them by chemical and physical means, the grand usurper. Even though the placenta in mammals shows this behavior, there is self-limitation in location and in survival of the placental invasion. Although leukocytes normally extravasate and permeate tissues, they do not share the other characteristics of cancer. The cancer cell is partially or absolutely insensitive to such normal constraints and may continue its invasiveness indefinitely.

Upon reaching a circulatory conduit, either lymphatic or capillary vessel, a process that may not be entirely haphazard, cancer cells often penetrate the wall as part of their invasive behavior. They then may be carried by the lymphatic or the venous circulation to remote sites where the possibility of adherence, extravasation, and colonization can occur, establishing metastases. In the absence of an intervening event, and given enough time, with few exceptions, the cancer process, as described, can lead to such anatomic or functional distortions that death ensues.

The cancer process does not start with a fully invasive cancer cell. A disorder in molecular instructions for protein synthesis is the common precursor lesion, nearly always because of qualitatively or quantitatively aberrant ribonucleic acid (RNA) messages transcribed from nuclear deoxyribonucleic acid (DNA). This occurs because of a mutation of the DNA, or because of overexpression of particular genes that encode proteins important as catalysts in pathways for stimulating growth, or because of under expression of genes whose coded proteins control and inhibit growth. Portions of genes may be lost, translocated, or amplified. Indeed, entire chromosomes may be deleted, replicated, or fused in abnormal ways. All such distortions of DNA can give rise to abnormal or unbalanced RNA messages, leading to qualitative or quantitative differences in proteins that result in disordered cellular function. Sometimes the functional abnormality is so extreme as to be lethal to the cell, initiating the suicidal mechanism of apoptosis. In other instances, the functional abnormality results in disease. Some of these diseases display the characteristics of cancer. Mutation, overexpression, and underexpression of genes can result from a wide spectrum of intrinsic and extrinsic causes, with various pathways that lead not to one final common pathway, but by several converging routes to cells with the phenotypic characteristics of cancer. When these cells are limited to an epithelial layer above the basement membrane, they are called carcinoma-in-situ or intraepithelial neoplasia. Similar changes probably occur, but are more difficult to recognize, in the mesenchymal tissues. Even cancer cells that do not penetrate the basement membrane, and thus lack one of the cardinal features of true cancer, represent a long series of antecedent molecular abnormalities that eventually lead to this optically recognizable cellular change. Furthermore, these evolving cancer cells are the common, if not the exclusive, precursor of invasive cancer.

In their initial stages, as proliferating cells accumulate, cancers are almost always asymptomatic. Cancers cause symptoms as they advance as a consequence of their mass, because they ulcerate on an epithelial surface, or because of change in function of the affected structure or organ. Nearly all the symptoms that can be caused by cancer can also be caused more commonly by noncancerous diseases. The astute clinician must include cancer in the differential diagnosis of virtually every symptom, albeit a benign disease may usually explain it. Doctors never diagnose diseases they do not think of. Cancers occur at any age. A longer life span provides greater opportunity for intrinsic organic events or an encounter

Holland-Frei Cancer Medicine, Ninth Edition. Edited by Robert C. Bast Jr., Carlo M. Croce, William N. Hait, Waun Ki Hong, Donald W. Kufe, Martine Piccart-Gebhart, Raphael E. Pollock, Ralph R. Weichselbaum, Hongyang Wang, and James F. Holland.
© 2017 John Wiley & Sons, Inc. ISBN: 978-1-118-93469-2

with environmental carcinogens, however, and greater opportunity for initial DNA mutations to be fully realized as invasive cancers. Thus, age is the principal risk factor for most, but not all, cancers.

Common symptoms such as sore throat, runny nose, or a chest cold can sometimes be a result of cancers of pharynx, sinuses, or bronchi, respectively. Indeed, patients with these cancer diagnoses usually have been treated, often repeatedly and for extended periods, for the benign disease because cancer was not considered in the differential diagnosis and appropriate observations were not made. Cancer symptoms such as diarrhea, constipation, or mild pain often seem commonplace. Cancer symptoms may be intermittent, with spontaneous temporary improvement, a phenomenon that is usually misinterpreted by patients and often by physicians as evidence against the diagnosis of cancer. In fact, recurrent appearance or chronicity of a symptom which in short duration is characteristic of a common benign disease markedly heightens the possibility of an underlying dysfunction caused by cancer.

Cancers cause their symptoms by a few readily understandable mechanisms.

Occlusion of an essential conduit, partial or complete, can be caused by tumor. A tumor mass grows to such size that it partially or completely occludes an essential conduit. Classic presentations are cancer of the bronchus where partial bronchial occlusion causes cough, diminishes ciliary clearance of secretion, and sometimes leads to bronchopneumonia. Complete bronchial occlusion leads to atelectasis and chronic pneumonia. Compromise of the esophageal lumen by tumor mass or muscular dysfunction resulting from infiltration causes dysphagia, which, in its early presentation, is far too often attributed to benign cause. Gastric tumors rarely cause complete obstruction, but often impair normal gastric motility. This defect may lead to easy satiety, anorexia, indigestion, and nausea. Decrease in caliber of the transverse and descending colon, sigmoid, or rectum by tumor mass can lead to change in bowel habit, including diminished caliber of stools, constipation, and bouts of cramps and/or diarrhea from peristaltic efforts of the proximal gut. Compromise of the lumen of the common bile duct by carcinoma of the head of the pancreas or of the bile duct itself produces obstructive jaundice, not infrequently after minor antecedent digestive complaints or unexplained pruritus ascribed to accumulated bile salts.

Ureteral obstruction by compression from retroperitoneal masses or bladder tumor leads to hydroureter and hydronephrosis, often asymptomatic or revealed by vague discomfort in flank or loin, or by urinary tract infection. Bilateral obstruction leads to uremia with its protean symptomatology. Compromise of the urethra as it courses through the prostate causes diminished urinary stream, inadequate bladder emptying, frequency, urgency, nocturia, and when severe, obstructive uropathy and uremia.

Tumors in the cecum and ascending colon and in the urinary bladder, because their content is not solid and because of greater luminal diameter, uncommonly cause obstruction, but may distort normal function enough to alter bowel or urinary habits.

A *mass* discovered by palpation or X-ray may be a presenting finding, as in breast carcinoma. Dysfunction from replacement of the substance of a parenchymatous organ by tumor is a subset of mass presentation. The classic example is primary or, more commonly, metastatic brain tumor, which becomes identified by abnormal brain function. Seizure or paralysis, sensory or coordination abnormality, memory defect, and personality change may all be consequences of space occupation. These changes may occur not only because a specific area of the brain is affected but also because of increased intracranial pressure as the calvarium is not distensible. Similar dysfunction of the spinal cord with distal motor and sensory phenomena can reflect space occupation by a mass within or impinging on the cord or cauda equina. Hepatic dysfunction from space occupation by primary or metastatic tumor, often with related intrahepatic bile duct compression, can present as jaundice. Sometimes the liver enlarges to enormous size, causing digestive disorders, pain, and a visible and palpable mass in the upper abdomen. Thyroid cancer usually presents as a mass, and uncommonly this results in hypothyroid laboratory values, but rarely in clinical hypothyroidism.

A sarcoma of the soft tissues usually presents as a palpable mass. Testicular cancer ordinarily presents as a mass: the testicle may only be slightly larger than its fellow, but harder and heavier in the examiner's hand. Ovarian cancer may be detected as an adnexal mass.

A new lump or mass, or a changing one, requires exclusion of cancer based on clinical examination, imaging studies, or a biopsy. Most lipomas, and self-discovery of the xiphoid, are two types of lumps that can usually be dismissed on clinical grounds. A dominant breast mass, or even a questionable one, requires assessment by appropriate imaging—often by cytologic or histologic means. A thyroid nodule, an enlarged lymph node that is hard, a node that remains enlarged without infectious explanation for 2 weeks, a skin mass with the characteristics of melanoma or carcinoma, especially if ulcerated, and a new subcutaneous or abdominal or scrotal mass all require consideration of cancer and appropriate diagnostic study.

Ulceration on the skin or on an epithelial surface can lead to blood loss and occasionally can serve as a portal of infection. Skin ulcerations are commonly ignored for weeks or months and are often interpreted as a common injury of unremembered origin that did not heal. Bronchial ulceration results in hemoptysis, usually blood-tinged sputum, and only rarely massive bleeding. Any of the upper alimentary canal cancers can ulcerate and bleed. Usually the bleeding is slow, intermittent, and silent, leading to iron-deficiency anemia. Hematemesis or massive melena is uncommon. Carcinomas of the cecum and ascending colon often present with the symptoms of anemia because of ulceration and bleeding.

Carcinoma of the bladder and carcinoma of the kidney commonly manifest hematuria. Sometimes this is fortuitously discovered as a microscopic or chemical abnormality on routine urinalysis. Clots from renal bleeding can lead to ureteral colic. Hematuria less often heralds prostate cancer, but hematospermia implies prostate disease, benign or malignant, because carcinoma of the seminal vesicle is exceedingly rare.

Endometrial carcinoma most often presents as postmenopausal vaginal bleeding, although any vaginal bleeding outside the normal menstrual cycle is worthy of suspicion. Contact bleeding during intercourse is suggestive of cervical ulceration, most commonly a result of cancer.

Pain is commonly thought of as a surrogate for early cancer, although this is mistaken. Most cancers are initially painless. Pain occurs when a tumor invades, presses on, or stretches a nerve, or when proximal smooth muscle contracts in an attempt to bypass an obstructed or dysfunctional distal segment of a conduit. Most pains of short duration that disappear are not caused by cancer. Cancer must enter the differential diagnosis, however, when pain is recurrent or persistent without ready explanation, or atypical, or present when there is no other recognizable cause. New pain, not necessarily severe, must be carefully interpreted. Abdominal pain and skeletal pain distinct from joint symptomatology deserve particular attention and early rather than late studies to establish a cause. Pain in a breast mass does not exclude its being cancer.

Weight loss may first indicate an unsuspected cancer, and when combined with grumbling low-grade discomforts, malaise, and fatigue is a cause for particular scrutiny. A wide variety of other diseases can also cause these common symptoms, but cancer should not be at the bottom of the list. If a diagnosis is not established after initial studies, a second complete history and physical examination after a short interval is imperative.

Effusion caused by cancer in the pleural, pericardial, or peritoneal cavities can lead to dyspnea and discomfort. Increasing abdominal girth, often with malaise, oliguria, constipation, and weight gain, is a cardinal symptom of ascites. In the thorax, bronchogenic carcinoma, mesothelioma, metastatic breast or ovarian cancer, and primary carcinoma of serous membranes are the frequent causes of malignant effusion. Ascites as a presenting symptom is characteristic of ovarian cancer and cancer of the serous membranes. Pancreatic cancer, mesothelioma, metastatic carcinoma on the peritoneum and in the liver and several non-neoplastic diseases also enter the differential diagnosis.

Perforation caused by invasion of the wall of a hollow viscus causes pain, usually sudden. Cancer is not suspected in most cases when this rare event occurs. Pneumothorax from perforation of the pleura by a primary or metastatic pulmonary tumor is an uncommon emergency. Fistulization of gastric cancer into the transverse colon leads to vague abdominal discomfort, which is misinterpreted or neglected, and then sudden onset of diarrhea with prominent gastrocolic reflex. Appendiceal cancer, albeit a rare tumor, frequently presents as acute appendicitis with peritonitis because of rupture. Perforation of the colon is more frequently caused by diverticulitis than by colon cancer. Ruptured ectopic pregnancy due to choriocarcinoma has been reported. Tracheoesophageal fistulization in the course of esophageal or bronchogenic cancers is almost always late in the course.

Fever of unknown origin that persists for more than 1 week must include cancer among its possible causes. Hodgkin disease, other lymphomas, acute leukemia, cancer of the kidney, and cancers of the liver are high on the list of neoplasms that can cause fever. Certain cancers predispose to infections because of ulceration, obstruction, or disordered leukopoiesis.

Endocrine hyperactivity syndromes may occasionally turn out to be caused by cancer. Hyperadrenalism, sometimes first manifest as hirsutism, can indicate adrenal cancer. Cushing syndrome can also result from small cell carcinoma of the lung. Hyperparathyroidism rarely comes from parathyroid cancer but can be mimicked by ovarian cancer and squamous carcinomas. Tumors that secrete thyroid hormone, estrogens, insulin, glucagon, aldosterone, epinephrine, or norepinephrine are often benign tumors of the parent endocrine organ, but cancer must always be considered. Functional neuroendocrine tumors may secrete serotonin and other vasoactive principles that cause the carcinoid syndrome.

Paraneoplastic syndromes may be early symptoms of cancer. Myasthenia gravis, Raynaud syndrome, hypertrophic osteoarthropathy and clubbing, and refractory anemia may herald thymoma, myeloma, lung cancer, and hematologic dyscrasia (and thymoma), respectively. A diligent search must be made for these and other causes.

Absence of cardinal manifestations is usual for cancers detected by screening by Papanicolaou smears, human papillomavirus (HPV) identification, mammography, prostate-specific antigen determinations, colonoscopy, computed tomography, lung scanning, and total skin examination. Asymptomatic cancers discovered by these methods are generally far less advanced than those that cause symptoms. Occasionally, routine chemical or hematologic laboratory data in asymptomatic patients suggest cancer or leukemia. Such incidental discovery reinforces the proposition that early in their pathogenesis most cancers are asymptomatic.

Predisposition to cancer characterizes a broad spectrum of diseases, exposures, and lifestyle behaviors. Patients who have had inflammatory bowel disease, HPV infection of the cervix, hepatitis B or C infection; those with prior radiation exposure, earlier treatment with alkylating agents, anthracyclines, or podophyllotoxin derivatives, or specific environmental exposures such as asbestos; those who have smoked, heavily imbibed alcohol, or sun worshipped, and those with a strong family history of cancer, particularly those neoplasms known in part to be heredofamilial all are in groups that deserve special consideration for the particular cancers that occur in them at a higher frequency than normal.

Cancerophobia does not predispose to cancer. Depression occurs more frequently with carcinoma of the pancreas than with gastric carcinoma, however, and may be an early symptom of pancreatic neoplasia.

The present

By the time cancer is diagnosed, it is often past the stage of easy curability. Frequently, the earliest symptoms were ignored or rationalized. Technical improvements in imaging, early surgery, and hormonal, chemotherapeutic, and immunologic treatment have decreased mortality from breast cancer; viral discovery, cytology, and early treatment have diminished cervical cancer mortality; and colonoscopy and polypectomy have decreased colon cancer mortality. Other screening programs portend similar promise by diagnosing cancers before they become symptomatic. Cancer has replaced syphilis as the great imitator. Many symptomatic patients with cancer are still curable with today's therapies. Delay cannot possibly help, however, once an early symptom occurs that eventually proves to be caused by cancer. Inclusion of cancer as a possibility in every differential diagnosis can save lives.

The future

The expansion of diagnostic techniques based on genomics and proteomics augurs well for earlier identification of cancers. Not only is it reasonable to believe that clinical diagnosis will be accelerated by laboratory methods, but genomic and proteomic discoveries are likely to alter our understanding of the cancer process as it occurs in humans. It is hoped that the consequent impact of this knowledge on cancer prevention and on cancer therapy will be revolutionary. The cardinal manifestations of cancer may then become principally of historical interest, while laboratory abnormalities are instrumentally detectable well before clinical presentation. Indeed, departure from a population norm may be less significant than departure from an individual's prior proteomic profile taken as a baseline during health. If such a blue-sky future ever unfolds, public understanding and compliance will still be critical determinants of cancer prevention and early diagnosis.

2 Biological hallmarks of cancer

Douglas Hanahan, PhD ▪ *Robert A. Weinberg, PhD*

Overview

An enigma for cancer medicine lies in its complexity and variability, at all levels of consideration. The hallmarks of cancer constitute an organizing principle that provides a conceptual basis for distilling the complexity of this disease in order to better understand it in its diverse presentations. This conceptualization involves eight biological capabilities—the hallmarks of cancer—acquired by cancer cells during the long process of tumor development and malignant progression. Two characteristic traits of cancer cells facilitate the acquisition of these functional capabilities. The eight distinct hallmarks consist of sustaining proliferative signaling, evading growth suppressors, resisting cell death, enabling replicative immortality, inducing angiogenesis, activating invasion and metastasis, deregulating cellular energetics and metabolism, and avoiding immune destruction. The principal facilitators of their acquisition are genome instability with consequent gene mutation and tumor-promoting inflammation. The integration of these hallmark capabilities involves heterotypic interactions among multiple cell types populating the "tumor microenvironment" (TME), which is composed of cancer cells and a tumor-associated stroma, including three prominent classes of recruited support cells—angiogenic vascular cells (AVC), various subtypes of fibroblasts, and infiltrating immune cells (IIC). In addition, the neoplastic cells populating individual tumors are themselves typically heterogeneous, in that cancer cells can assume a variety of distinctive phenotypic states and undergo genetic diversification during tumor progression. Accordingly, the hallmarks of cancer—this set of necessarily acquired capabilities and their facilitators—constitute a useful heuristic tool for elucidating mechanistic bases and commonalties underlying the pathogenesis of diverse forms of human cancer, with potential applications to cancer therapy.

Distilling the dauntingly complex manifestations of cancer

As outlined in the preceding chapter, and comprehensively described elsewhere in this encyclopedic textbook, the manifestations of cancer are disconcertingly complex and diverse. Cancers affecting different organs vary dramatically, in regard to genetics, histopathology, effects on systemic physiology, prognosis, and response to therapeutic intervention, explaining why the discipline of oncology is largely balkanized into organ-specific specialties, and why the chapters of this textbook are largely aligned as individualistic descriptions of organ-specific cancers.

In the face of this disconcerting diversity and complexity of disease manifestations, one might ask whether there are underlying principles—mechanistic commonalities—masked by the genetic and phenotypic complexities that span the multitude of cancer types and forms. In 2000, and again in 2011, we put forward a hypothesis that the vast complexity of human cancers reflects different solutions to the same set of challenges, namely that the lesions we observe in the forms of symptomatic neoplastic disease

have all necessarily acquired, by various strategies, a common set of distinct functional capabilities that enable inappropriately chronic cell proliferation, and the focal or disseminated growth of populations of neoplastic cancer cells. We proposed to call this set of acquired capabilities "hallmarks of cancer."[1,2] We further suggested that two characteristic traits of neoplastic growths—elevated mutability of cancer-cell genomes and inflammation by complex arrays of immune cells—are the key facilitators used by incipient neoplasias to acquire essential hallmark capabilities. Our current conceptualization of the biological hallmarks of cancer incorporates the eight distinct functional capabilities and the two enabling facilitators, these being schematized in Figure 1.

The following sections describe these 10 key aspects of cancer pathophysiology. Then we introduce the observation that cancer cells recruit a variety of normal cell types that contribute in various ways the acquisition of hallmark functionalities. We conclude with a brief discussion on potential clinical implications of the hallmarks concept. For further detail and background, the reader is referred to our initial publications laying out the concept of the hallmarks of cancer,[1,2] as well as to another perspective that expands on the roles of stromal cells in enabling the hallmarks of cancer.[3] Notably, only a few recent publications not cited in these three perspective articles are referenced herein. A textbook on the biology of cancer[4] may provide additional details on many of the mechanisms of cancer pathogenesis described in outline in this chapter.

Acquired functional capabilities embody biological hallmarks of cancer

In our current conceptualization, there are eight hallmark capabilities that are common to many, if not most forms of human cancer (Figure 1). Each capability serves a distinct functional role in supporting the development, progression, and persistence of tumors and their constituent cells, as summarized briefly in the following sections.

Hallmark 1: sustaining proliferative signaling

The defining criterion of cancer as a disease is chronic, inappropriate cell proliferation, which results from corruption of cellular regulatory networks that normally orchestrate (transitory) proliferation of cells during embryonic development, physiological growth, and homeostatic maintenance of tissues throughout the body. Both positive (inductive) and negative (repressive) signals govern cell division and proliferation. Thus, this first hallmark capability embodies a complex set of inductive signals that instruct entry into and progression through the cell growth-and-division cycle to produce daughter

Holland-Frei Cancer Medicine, Ninth Edition. Edited by Robert C. Bast Jr., Carlo M. Croce, William N. Hait, Waun Ki Hong, Donald W. Kufe, Martine Piccart-Gebhart, Raphael E. Pollock, Ralph R. Weichselbaum, Hongyang Wang, and James F. Holland.
© 2017 John Wiley & Sons, Inc. ISBN: 978-1-118-93469-2

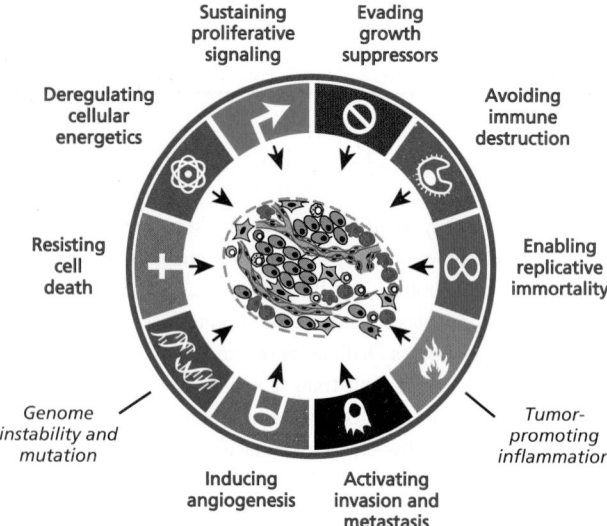

Figure 1 **The biological hallmarks of cancer.** The schematic illustrates what are arguably necessary conditions to manifest malignant disease—the hallmarks of cancer—comprising eight distinct and complementary functional capabilities and two facilitators (in black italics) of their acquisition.[1,2] These halllmark traits may be acquired at different stages in the multistep development of cancer, via markedly distinctive mechanisms in different forms of human cancer. Two aberrant characteristics of cancerous lesions are demonstrably involved in facilitating the acquisition during tumorigenesis of these functional capabilities: genome instability and the resultant mutation of regulatory genes, and the infiltration of immune inflammatory cells endowed by their biology—for example involvement in wound healing—to contribute to one or another hallmark capability. Different forms of cancer may be more or less dependent on a particular hallmark. Thus, adenomatous tumors typically lack the capability for invasion and metastasis. Leukemias may not require angiogenesis or invasive ability, although progression to lymphoma almost certainly requires both. The necessity of evading tumor immunity may be less important for certain cancers but is increasingly appreciated to be widespread.

cells. In the context of cancer, such stimulatory signals are activated and, in contrast to normal situations in which proliferative signaling is transitory, the signals are sustained chronically.

The most well-established and widespread mechanism of sustaining proliferative signaling involves mutational alteration of genes within cancer cells that convert such genes into active drivers of cell proliferation. These activated genes—defined as oncogenes—render otherwise transitory proliferation-promoting signals chronic. Such oncogenes typically encode proteins altered in structure and function or abundance compared to their normal cellular counterparts, which are responsible for receiving proliferative signals from extracellular sources and transmitting the signals through complex regulatory circuits operating within the cell.

Prominent examples of mutated driver oncogenes that sustain proliferative signaling in human cancers include the epidermal growth factor (EGF) receptor and signal transducers in the downstream KRAS–RAF–MEK–MAPK pathway that process and transmit growth-stimulatory signals via a succession of protein phosphorylations to the cell-division machinery operating in the nucleus. Mutations that render one or another of these proteins chronically active are found in many forms of human cancer, including the aforementioned *EGFR* and related receptor tyrosine kinases such as *HER2* and *ALK*; similarly acting mutations result in chronic activation of the downstream signal transducers *KRAS*, *BRAF*, and *MEK*. We note, however, that activation in cancer

of this central mitogenic pathway does not invariably depend on genetic changes acquired during the course of tumor progression. In certain instances, epigenetic deregulation of autocrine (autostimulatory) and paracrine (cell-to-cell) signaling circuits can also provide cancer cells with chronic growth-promoting signals, doing so in the apparent absence of underlying somatic mutations.

Hallmark 2: evading growth suppressors

The essential counterbalance to proliferative signals in normal cells are braking mechanisms that either overrule the initiation of, or subsequently block, the cell-division process instigated by such signals. The genes encoding these proteins are often termed tumor suppressor genes (TSGs). The most prominent brakes are the direct regulators of progression through the cell growth-and-division cycle, embodied in the retinoblastoma protein (pRb) and several "cyclin-dependent" kinase-inhibitor proteins. The activity of this molecular-braking system is itself normally regulated by the integration of extracellular pro- and antigrowth signals transduced by receptors on the cell surface, along with monitors of the intracellular physiologic state of the cell, in order to regulate tissue homeostasis and orchestrate transitory physiological proliferation.

An intracellular monitoring system, which is centered upon the p53 protein, serves to ensure that cells only advance through their growth-and-division cycles when the physiologic state of the cell is appropriate. Thus, p53 detects unrepaired damage to a cell's genome as well as stressful physiologic imbalances that could impair accurate genome duplication, chromosomal segregation, and cell division. In response to cellular stress alarms, p53 then proceeds to activate inhibitors of the cell-cycle machinery. In cases of severe genomic damage or stressful physiological abnormalities, p53 and its associates can instead induce programmed cell death (see below), an extreme form of putting on the brakes to cell proliferation.

A number of component genes in both of these generic braking mechanisms—the Rb and p53 pathways—are classified as TSGs by virtue of their frequent loss-of-function via deletion or intragenic mutations; alternatively, other mechanisms may achieve the same end by shutting down expression of these genes through epigenetic mechanisms, notably those involving DNA and histone methylation. Thus the p53 gene is mutated in ~40% of all human cancers, and many of the remaining tumors with wild-type p53 instead carry genetic lesions or epigenetic alterations that compromise p53 signaling in other ways.

Genetic profiling of genomes and transcriptomes indicates that a majority of human tumors contain defects—genetic or epigenetic—in the functions of the Rb and p53 tumor-suppressor pathways. Moreover, a large body of functional studies involving manipulation of these pathways in cultured cancer cells and mouse models of tumor initiation, growth, and malignant progression have clearly established the critical importance of TSGs in these pathways as significant barriers to the development of cancer. As such, evasion of growth suppressors is clearly a hallmark capability, necessary to ensure that continuing cancer cell proliferation and consequent tumor growth is not halted by braking mechanisms that, under normal circumstances, limit the extent of cell proliferation in order to maintain tissue homeostasis.

Hallmark 3: resisting cell death

There exists a second, fundamentally distinct barrier to aberrant cell proliferation, which involves intrinsic cellular mechanisms that can orchestrate the programmed death of cells deemed to be either aberrant or, in the case of normal development and homeostasis, superfluous. The most prominent form of programmed cell death is apoptosis, the genetically programmed fragmentation of a cell destined to die. Included among the situations where normal cells activate their apoptotic program to die are ones where the cell is damaged in various ways, mislocalized, or inappropriately migrating or proliferating. The apoptotic program can be triggered by cell intrinsic and non-cell-autonomous signals that detect different forms of cellular abnormality.

The apoptotic cell-death program involves the directed degradation of the chromosomes and other critical cellular organelles by specialized enzymes (e.g., caspases), the shriveling and fragmentation of the cell, and its engulfment, either by its neighboring cells or by tissue-surveying phagocytes, notably macrophages. The apoptotic cascade is completed in less than an hour in mammalian tissues, explaining why apoptotic cells are often surprisingly rare when visualized in tissue sections, even in a population of cells experiencing apoptosis-inducing environmental conditions, such as cancer cells in tumors subjected to cytotoxic chemotherapy or to acute hypoxia consequent to vascular insufficiency.

The rapid engulfment of apoptotic cell bodies ensures that their death does not release subcellular components that would otherwise provoke an immune response; this "immune silence" contrasts with a second form of programmed cell death: necroptosis. Long known as necrosis and envisioned as the passive dissolution of a dying cell, necrosis can also be an active, programmed process that is governed by cellular regulators and effectors distinct from those regulating apoptosis. Necroptosis can be activated by various conditions, including oxygen and energy deprivation, viral infection, and inflammation.[5] Cells dying by necroptosis (or passive necrosis) rupture, releasing their contents and leaving their carcasses as immunogenic debris that can attract (or exacerbate) an immune inflammatory response, which, as discussed below, can have both tumor-promoting and tumor-antagonizing effects.

A third program capable of inducing cell death, termed autophagy, serves as a recycling system for cellular organelles that can help cells respond to conditions of nutrient deprivation, by degrading nonessential cellular organelles and recycling their component parts. Thus, autophagy generates metabolites and nutrients necessary for survival and growth that cells may be unable to acquire from their surroundings. In addition, while generally a survival system, extreme nutrient deprivation or other acute cellular stresses can lead to a hyperactivation of autophagic recycling that drives a cell to a point-of-no return, in which its complement of organelles falls below the minimum level required for viability; as a consequence, the cell dies via "autophagy-associated" cell death, distinct in its characteristics from both apoptosis and necroptosis. Stated differently, depending on the physiologic state of a neoplastic cell, autophagy may either sustain its survival and facilitate further proliferation or eliminate it via autophagy-associated cell death.[6]

These three distinct mechanisms for triggering cell death must be variably circumvented or attenuated by cancer cells if they and their descendants are to continue their proliferative expansion and phenotypic evolution to states of heightened malignancy.

Hallmark 4: enabling replicative immortality

A third intrinsic barrier to chronic proliferation is integral to the linear structure of mammalian chromosomes: the telomeres at the ends of chromosomes record—by progressive reduction of their length during each cell-division cycle—the number of successive cell generations through which a cell lineage has passed. The telomeres are composed of thousands of tandem copies of a specific hexanucleotide DNA sequence located at the ends of every chromosome that are associated with a specialized set of DNA-binding proteins. Operating together, these nucleoprotein complexes protect the ends of chromosomes both from degradation by the DNA-repair machinery, which is designed to detect DNA damage, and from end-to-end fusions with other chromosomes catalyzed by naked DNA ends.

Notably, when the number of telomere repeats erodes below a certain threshold, a tripwire is triggered, causing cell-cycle arrest or apoptosis mediated by the p53 tumor-suppressor protein, operating in its role to sense DNA damage. Circumventing these p53-induced antiproliferative responses (e.g., by mutational inactivation of the p53 gene) allows cancer cells with eroding telomeres to ignore the short-telomere checkpoint and continue proliferating, but only transiently. Sooner or later, the continuing erosion of telomeric DNA leads to loss of the protective nucleoprotein caps protecting the chromosomal DNA ends, which allows end-to-end fusions of chromosomes, breakage–fusion–bridge cycles during mitosis, and resultant karyotypic chaos that leads to cell death instead of cell division.

The cancer cells in many fully developed tumors circumvent the proliferative barrier presented by telomere erosion and the imminent mitotic catastrophe of telomere dysfunction by activating a system for telomere maintenance and extension that is normally used to preserve the replicative capacity of normal embryonic and tissue stem cells. This system involves expression of the telomere-extending enzyme named telomerase. Less frequently, they engage an alternative interchromosomal recombination-based mechanism for preserving telomere length. Thus, through one strategy or another, cancer cells acquire the capability to maintain their telomeres, avoiding the barrier of intolerably shortened telomeres, thereby enabling the unlimited replicative potential—termed cellular immortality—that is required for continuing expansion of populations of cancer cells.

Hallmark 5: inducing angiogenesis

Like normal organs, tumors require a steady supply of oxygen, glucose, and other nutrients, as well as a means to evacuate metabolic wastes, in order to sustain cell viability and proliferation. The tumor-associated vasculature serves these purposes. The deleterious effect that ischemia has in normal tissue is well established clinically and experimentally: cells die, via one form of programmed cell death or another, causing tissue and organ degradation and dysfunction. Similarly, the growth of developing nests of cancer cells halts when their ability to acquire blood-borne nutrients becomes inadequate, typically when the nearest capillary is more than $200\,\mu$ away. Angiogenesis—the formation of new blood vessels—is commonly activated and demonstrably beneficial for many tumor types.

Cells at the diffusion limit from the nearest capillary activate various stress-response systems, of which the most prominent involves the hypoxia-inducible transcription factors (HIF), which regulate hundreds of genes, including ones that directly or indirectly induce angiogenesis and other stress-adaptive capabilities. Much like cells in ischemic tissues, cancer cells lacking sufficient oxygen and glucose will typically die by necrosis/necroptosis, apoptosis, or rampant autophagy. This explains why most vigorously growing tumors are well vascularized with evidence of ongoing angiogenesis.

Of note, the tumor-associated neovasculature is usually aberrant both morphologically and functionally. Tumor blood vessels are tortuous, dilated, and leaky, with erratic flow patterns and "dead zones" in which no blood flow is detectable, in marked contrast to the seamless blood flow operating in the normal vasculature. Moreover, the degree of vascularity varies widely from one tumor type to another, ranging from intensely vascularized renal carcinomas to poorly vascularized pancreatic ductal adenocarcinomas.

Finally, we note that while chronic angiogenesis is a hallmark of most solid tumors, some may devise an alternative means to acquire access to the vasculature: in certain cases, cancers coopt normal tissue vasculature, by employing the hallmark capability for invasion and metastasis. Thus, particular types of cancer cells can proliferate and grow along normal tissue capillaries, creating sleeves whose outer diameters are dictated by the 200-μ diffusion limit. While vascular cooption is evident in certain cases (e.g., glioblastoma) and in some tumors treated with potent angiogenesis inhibitors, most tumors rely to a considerable extent on chronic angiogenesis to support their expansive growth. Still others may adapt to living in quasi-hypoxic environments where most cancer cells would perish.

Hallmark 6: activating invasion and metastasis

The five hallmarks detailed above stand as logical necessities for the chronic proliferative programs of cancer cells. The sixth is less intuitive: high-grade cancer cells become invasive and migratory. Invasive growth programs enable cancer cells to invade into adjacent tissue as well as into blood and lymphatic vessels (intravasation); these vessels serve thereafter as pipelines for dissemination to nearby and distant anatomical sites. The tissue-draining lymphatic vasculature can transport cancer cells to lymph nodes, where metastatic growths—lymph node metastases—can form; such cell colonies may serve, in turn, as staging areas for further dissemination by entering the bloodstream. Cells entering the bloodstream by direct intravasation within a tumor or indirectly via lymph nodes may soon become lodged in the microvessels of distant organs and extravasate across the vessel walls into the nearby tissue parenchyma. The resulting seeded micrometastases may die or lay dormant in such ectopic tissue locations or, with extremely low efficiency, generate macroscopic metastases—the process of "colonization."

The regulation of the intertwined capabilities for invasion and metastasis is extraordinarily complex, involving both cell-intrinsic programs and assistance from accessory cells in the tissue microenvironment. Prominent among the cancer cell-intrinsic regulatory mechanisms is the activation in epithelial cancer cells (carcinomas) of a developmental program termed the epithelial–mesenchymal transition (EMT),[2,4] which is associated with cell migrations and tissue invasions during normal organogenesis. An interconnected regulatory program induced by the microenvironment in some tumors is the aforementioned hypoxia response system, which triggers the activation of the HIFs, HIF1α and HIF2α, consequently altering expression of hundreds of genes,[7,8] including components of the EMT program. Both transcriptional regulatory systems control genes that can facilitate invasive migration as well as survival in the blood and lymphatic systems, and in ectopic tissue locations.

Notably, the acquisition of this hallmark capability can occur at various points along the pathways of multistep tumor development and progression that lead incrementally from normal cells of origin to those found in aggressive high-grade malignancies. In some cases, the capability for invasion and metastasis arises late, reflecting mutational or epigenetic evolution of the cancer cell, whereby rare subsets of cells populating such primary tumors are enabled to become invasive/metastatic. In other cases, this capability is acquired early, such that many cancer cells within a tumor may already be capable of invasion and metastasis. Moreover, there are indications that the EMT program may in some cases be transiently

active and functionally important for dissemination and seeding, but then switched off in macrometastatic colonies.[9,10] It remains unclear whether the acquired traits of invasion and metastasis are beneficial and hence actively selected during the evolution of primary tumors; alternatively, these malignancy-defining capabilities may represent incidental byproducts of activating global regulatory networks (e.g., proliferative signaling, EMT, and HIF) that are initially selected because they facilitate primary tumor formation by contributing to the acquisition of other hallmark functions.

Hallmark 7: deregulating cellular energetics and metabolism

The concept that cancer cells alter their utilization of energy sources—notably glucose—to support their proliferation was introduced almost 90 years ago by Otto Warburg, who observed that certain cultured-cancer cells have enhanced uptake of glucose, which is metabolized via glycolysis, even in the presence of oxygen levels that normally should favor oxidative phosphorylation. The result was counterintuitive, as glycolysis is far less efficient at producing ATP, the primary currency of intracellular energy. However, we now appreciate that the "aerobic glycolysis" described by Warburg produces, in addition to ATP, many of the building blocks for the cellular macromolecules that are required for cell growth and division. Indeed, the metabolism of cancer cells resembles that of actively dividing normal cells rather than being a novel invention of neoplasia. Moreover, it is important to appreciate that there is not a binary switch from oxidative phosphorylation to aerobic glycolysis in cancer cells; rather, cancer cells continue to utilize oxidative phosphorylation in addition to incorporating differing rates of glycolysis, the proportions of which may well prove to be dynamic in time, variable among the cancer cells in different subregions within a tumor and in different tissue microenvironments.

Aerobic glycolysis can be indirectly monitored by positron-emission tomography (PET) using radiolabeled analogs as tracers. PET involving [^{18}F]-fluorodeoxyglucose is commonly used to visualize glycolytic tumors via their elevated expression of glucose transporters and a resulting increase in the uptake of glucose. Although glucose is the primary fuel source used by most cancer cells, glutamine is also emerging as another key blood-borne source of energy and a precursor of lipids and amino acids. In most cases, glutamine likely supplements and enhances glucose in supplying energy and biomaterials for growth and proliferation of cancer cells, although in some cases of glucose insufficiency, glutamine uptake and metabolism may be able to compensate.[11]

A third player in metabolic fueling is lactate. While long considered to be toxic waste that is secreted by cells undergoing aerobic and anaerobic glycolysis, lactate is now appreciated to have diverse tumor-promoting capabilities.[12] In certain cancer cells, particularly those suffering glucose deprivation, extracellular lactate can be imported via specific transporters and used as fuel for generation of ATP and biomaterials. Similarly, some cancer-associated fibroblasts (CAF) can utilize lactate. Hence, metabolic symbioses may be operative in some tumors, involving partnerships between glucose-importing/lactate-exporting cells and lactate-importing cells.[12]

Finally, we note a still unresolved question, about whether this hallmark is significantly independent of the six cited above in terms of its regulatory mechanisms, or conversely is concordantly regulated under the auspices of these other hallmark traits. Thus, oncogenes such as KRAS and cMYC, as well as the loss of function of TSGs such as p53, can serve to reprogram the energy metabolism of cancer cells. For this reason, the reprogramming of cellular energetics and metabolism was initially defined as an "emerging hallmark."[2] Irrespective of this qualification, it is clearly a crucial property of the neoplastic cell phenotype.[13]

Hallmark 8: avoiding immune destruction

The eighth hallmark has been on the horizon for decades, originally conceived as the proposition that incipient neoplasias must find ways to circumvent active surveillance by the immune system that would otherwise eliminate aberrantly proliferating premalignant cells. While clearly demonstrable in highly antigenic tumors in mouse models, and implicated in virus-induced human cancers, the generality of immune surveillance of incipient cancer as a barrier to neoplastic progression is unresolved. One factor is immune self-tolerance: the vast majority of antigens expressed by spontaneously arising cancer cells are likely shared with those expressed by their cells-of-origin in normal tissues and thus are ignored, reflecting the tolerance of the immune system for self-antigens. Nonetheless, some cancer cells demonstrably express antigens for which the immune system has failed to develop tolerance, including embryonic antigens, and novel antigens produced by rampant mutation of the genome; such antigens can indeed elicit antitumor immune responses and are an increasing focus for strategies aimed to elicit efficacious tumor immunity.

By contrast, the immune response to the ~20% of virus-induced human tumors is clear: oncogenic viruses express foreign antigens (including oncoproteins responsible for driving cell transformation) to which the immune system is not tolerant, resulting in humoral and cellular immune responses that can kill virus-infected precancer cells and thereby eradicate incipient neoplasias. The fact that virus-transformed cells can nevertheless succeed in evading immune elimination to produce overt cancer testifies to immune-evasive capabilities evolved by such tumor viruses or selected for in virus-transformed cancer cells. Nevertheless, the immune system likely serves as a significant barrier to virus-induced tumors, as indicated by the increased rates of cancer in individuals who are immune-compromised for various reasons, including organ-graft recipients and AIDS patients.

Although the incidence of nonvirus-induced human cancers is not markedly increased in the context of immunodeficiency—suggesting a lack of immune surveillance of incipient neoplasias in the other 80% of human cancers—various lines of evidence suggest that some tumor types must indeed deal with immune recognition and attack during later stages of tumor progression and, in response, acquire immune-evasive strategies. Here, histopathological analyses of human tumor biopsies have shed light on the potential role of immune attack and immune evasion. For example, among patients with surgically resected colorectal carcinomas, those whose tumors contained dense infiltrates of cytotoxic T lymphocytes (CTLs) have a better prognosis than patients with tumors of similar grade and size that have comparatively few infiltrating CTLs.[14] Such data implicate the actions of the immune system as a significant obstacle to the progressive growth and dissemination of cancer cells, one that is necessarily blunted or circumvented in some aggressive tumor types.[14] Indeed, immune phenotyping of tumors, including their associated stroma, is being evaluated as a new metric in the diagnosis of tumors that may enable, when combined with traditional criteria, more accurate assessments of prognosis and more effective treatment decisions.[15,16] Accordingly, it is reasonable to view antitumor immune responses as a significant barrier to be circumvented during the lengthy multistage development of many forms of human cancer.

Nevertheless, the rules of immune engagement remain ambiguous when viewing the spectrum of human cancers. Thus, it is generally unclear when during different organ-specific tumor development pathways the attention of the immune system is attracted, or what the precise characteristics and efficacy of resultant immune responses are, or how the genetic constitutions of patients and the tumors that they harbor affect the development of antitumor immunity. Nevertheless, evading immune destruction seems increasingly to be an important mandate for developing tumors and thus an evident hallmark of cancer.

Taken together, we envision that these eight distinct capabilities define a necessary condition for malignancy (Figure 1), along with the two associated facilitators of their acquisition described below. Importantly, however, one cannot ignore the complex mechanisms underlying this conceptual simplicity: different tumors acquire these hallmarks by diverse mechanisms, doing so by coopting and subverting a diverse array of mechanisms normally responsible for cell, tissue, and organismic homeostasis.

Aberrations that enable acquisition of the necessary functional capabilities

The lengthy process of tumor development and malignant progression, long appreciated to involve a succession of rate-limiting steps, reflects the need of evolving neoplastic cells to acquire the eight hallmark capabilities discussed earlier. How then are these functional capabilities acquired? Currently, there are two clearly established means by which the hallmarks are acquired: (1) genome instability and the resulting mutation of hallmark-enabling genes in the overt cancer cells and (2) inflammation by cells of the immune system that help provide these capabilities cooperatively.

Genome instability and the consequent mutation of hallmark-enabling genes

Genome instability and the consequent mutation of hallmark-enabling genes is the primary modality of acquiring hallmark capabilities. The cell genome is subject to routine DNA damage, from a variety of chemically reactive products of normal metabolism, from environmental insults, and from its replication during every cell division. The resulting defects, if left unrepaired, become cell-heritable mutations, explaining the need of an elaborate consortium of proteins that continuously monitor DNA integrity and, in response to damage, undertake repair. Irreparable damage provokes the elimination of cells, a task orchestrated by the p53 TSG, which has for this reason been dubbed the "guardian of the genome."

This highly efficient genome-integrity machine normally keeps the rates of gene mutation and genome rearrangement at low levels, which is likely incompatible with the efficient acquisition of hallmark functions by genetic evolution and phenotypic selection for these necessary capabilities. This dichotomy provides a compelling explanation for the frequent observation of genome instability in cancer cells. Indeed, many tumor types contain neoplastic cells that carry readily identifiable defects in the complex machinery designed to monitor and repair genomic damage. Most apparent are the frequently documented mutant alleles of p53 that have been found in perhaps 40% of all cancers; without p53 on duty, damaged DNA can persist unrepaired, and mutant cells can survive and pass their damaged genomes on to their progeny. Numerous other specialized DNA repair and genome-maintenance enzymes are also found to be defective in many tumors, and inherited familial defects in DNA repair often lead to elevated risk of cancer development, again by enabling the acquisition of tumor-promoting mutations.

The elevated rates and persistence of proliferation in neoplastic lesions create cell lineages that have undergone far more successive growth-and-division cycles than is typical of cells in normal tissues, further increasing the potential for mutagenic errors occurring during DNA replication. Among these consequences is one that we described earlier: critically shortened and thus dysfunctional, telomeres can trigger chromosomal rearrangements and fusions that can affect gene function in various ways. Mutant cancer cells that survive this karyotypic chaos may have acquired advantageous phenotypes and thus the capability to undergo clonal expansion.

The foundation of cancer in genetic mutation is being further substantiated by the development of high-throughput DNA-sequencing technologies and the consequent ability to systematically analyze large numbers of independently arising cancer-cell genomes. Complemented by other methods for genome scanning, such as comparative genomic hybridization to identify copy number variations and "chromosome painting" to detect translocations, the derangements of the cancer-cell genome are being revealed in unprecedented detail.[17–20] The results substantiate the fact that almost every form of human cancer involves cancer cells whose genomes have been mutated either through chromosomal rearrangements or more localized intragenic mutations or both. The density of genetic alterations varies over many orders of magnitude, from very low numbers detected in certain pediatric cancers to the blizzards of mutations present in the genomes of UV-induced melanomas and tobacco-induced lung cancers. Thus, the aberrations can range from dozens of point mutations to hundreds of thousands, and from quasi-diploid chromosomal karyotypes to widespread aneuploidy, translocations, and multiple large-scale amplifications and deletions.

The data generated by these increasingly high-throughput genomic technologies is presenting a major challenge to clarify which of the plethora of mutational alterations in the cancer-cell genome actually contribute causally to the acquisition of hallmark capabilities. The numbers of mutations that are being cataloged in many cancer cells greatly exceed those that are likely to be important in reshaping cell phenotype. The recurrence of specific mutations in cohorts of patients with the same cancer type or subtype provides one indication of functional involvement. Many other mutations, however, may reflect alternative solutions utilized in one individual's tumor but not another's, and thus are less frequently recurrent. And yet other mutations—often the great majority in a cancer cell's genome—may simply be ancillary consequences of genomic instability, having been carried along for the ride with other function-enabling mutations that do indeed afford selective advantage and thus clonal expansion during tumor growth and progression. Thus, the concept is emerging that cancer cells contain two classes of mutations: drivers and passengers. One future imperative will be to leverage such genome-profiling data to identify the driver mutations and their mechanistic contributions to the acquisition of hallmark capabilities, not only mutations that are frequent in a particular cancer type, but also others that are infrequent but nonetheless functionally important for an individual patient's tumor growth and progression. A second imperative will be to clarify the potential of both recurrent and rare driver mutations as therapeutic targets in different tumor types. An added complexity is that advantageous hallmark traits conferred by driver mutations in some tumors may be acquired in other tumors by changes in the epigenome—the spectrum of cell-heritable changes in chromatin that are not reflected by changes in nucleotide sequence.[21,22] Indeed, it has been argued that all eight of the hallmark capabilities can

be conveyed by epigenetic changes in gene regulation, occurring both in the overt cancer cells and in the supporting cells of the tumor-associated stroma.[23] While the prevalence of epigenetic mechanisms as primary orchestrators of tumorigenesis is currently unresolved, genomic instability may prove to play less prominent roles in some tumors, where mutational alterations in DNA may be consequences of hallmark functions rather than causal of them.

The field of cancer genetics is poised for an extraordinary decade during which tens of thousands of cancer-cell genomes will be comprehensively analyzed for multiple parameters, including alterations in DNA sequence and copy number, changes in gene transcription, splicing, and translation, as well as repatterning of histone and DNA methylation (and other modifications) that mediate regional alterations in chromatin structure, thereby governing gene accessibility for transcription. The challenge and the opportunity will be to distill the identity and contributions of specific alterations—genetic and epigenetic—to hallmark-enabling functions from increasingly massive datasets, and to exploit such knowledge for improved detection, evaluation, and informed treatment of human cancers.

Tumor-promoting immune cell infiltration (inflammation)

Tumor-promoting immune cell infiltration (inflammation) is the second important modality through which developing cancers acquire hallmark capabilities. Strikingly, most tumors are infiltrated by a variety of cell types of the immune system (the so-called infiltrating immune cells, or IIC[3]). While the inflammation caused by IIC might reasonably be considered a failed attempt to eradicate a tumor, recent evidence now clearly makes a far more insidious point: IIC help convey in paracrine fashion multiple functional capabilities, encompassing seven of the eight hallmarks.[3] Thus, IIC can variously supply proliferative and survival signals, proangiogenic factors, and facilitate local invasion and blood-borne metastasis. In addition, some of these IIC (T-regulatory cells and myeloid-derived suppressor cells) can actively suppress the cytotoxic T lymphocytes that have been dispatched by the immune system to eradicate cancer cells.

Tumor-promoting IIC are recruited by a variety of means in different tumor types and at various stages of multistep tumorigenesis. The roster of the recruiting signals—including an ensemble of chemokine and cytokine signaling factors—is still incompletely understood. In some cases, the nature of the neoplastic lesion may trigger tissue abnormality or damage signals that attract IIC, represent the adaptive and innate immune systems. In other cases, oncogenic signaling, by activating transcriptional networks, induces expression of cytokines and chemokines that recruit IIC. In early-stage lesions, the recruited IIC can help incipient cancer cells to proliferate, survive, evade antigrowth controls, or activate angiogenesis. At later stages of progression, IIC at the margins of tumors can facilitate invasiveness. Some experiments reveal that IIC can pair with cancer cells as they migrate through the circulation and become established in distant locations.[24] Additionally, certain IIC, such as macrophages, can subject cancer cells to DNA-damaging reactive oxygen species, thereby contributing to the mutational alteration and evolution of the cancer-cell genome.

Most types of solid tumor are associated with tumor-promoting immune infiltrations that range from histologically subtle to the obvious inflammatory responses recognized by pathologists. In addition, the long-appreciated epidemiologic association between chronic inflammation and carcinogenesis supports the proposition that pre-existing inflammatory conditions can be fertile breeding grounds for the inception and progression of certain forms of cancer. Chronically inflamed tissues share features with wound healing; both involve induction of angiogenesis and stimulation of cell survival, proliferation, and migration/invasion, involving the inflammatory IIC and other cell types (e.g., fibroblasts) that they activate in the affected tissue. These acquired traits represent hallmark capabilities, reinforcing the notion that IIC can inadvertently foster neoplastic initiation and/or progression of incipient cancer cells present in inflammatory tissue microenvironments.

The histopathological complexity of cancer, manifested in tumor microenvironments (TMEs)

Pathologists have long recognized that solid tumors are complex histological structures, incorporating not only cancer cells but also a variety of morphologically distinct cells, recognizable because they are similar to constituents of noncancerous tissues, both normal and affected by conditions such as infections or wound healing. In analogy to the stroma that supports epithelia in many normal tissues, the apparently noncancerous component of tumors has been labeled as the tumor stroma. As in normal tissue stroma, the tumor-associated stroma can be seen to contain blood vessels, assemblages of fibroblastic cells, and in many cases IIC. Historically, a simplistic view of the tumor stroma posited that endothelial cells, through the process of angiogenesis that produced a tumor neovasculature, provided oxygen and nutrients, while cancer-associated fibroblasts (CAFs) were either passengers or provided structural support, and the IIC, discussed earlier, represented ineffectual antitumoral immune responses. As described above, we now appreciate the fact that the diverse stromal cells inside tumors can contribute functionally to the acquisition of seven of the eight hallmarks.[3]

In analogy to normal tissues, tumors are often conceptually compartmentalized into the parenchyma (formed by the cancer cells) and the stroma (formed by the ostensibly normal supporting cells); the assemblage of these two compartments, incorporating as well extracellular material (including extracellular matrix, ECM, and basement membrane, BM) is increasingly referred to as the "tumor microenvironment" (TME), as illustrated in Figure 2; some also refer to the TME exclusively as the noncancerous stromal compartment, although conceptually the microenvironment incorporates the entirety of the tumor, that is, both its neoplastic and stromal compartments.

The three classes of stromal cell—angiogenic vascular cells (AVC), consisting of endothelial cells and supporting pericytes; CAF; and IIC—constitute the bulk of the stromal component of the TME.[3] These simple classifications, however, mask important diversity in cellular phenotypes. Thus, there are a number of CAF subtypes, of which the two most prevalent are derived either from myofibroblasts, mesenchymal stem cells, and tissue stellate cells that all characteristically express alpha-smooth muscle actin, or from connective tissue-derived fibroblasts that do not. Both subtypes of CAF arise via epigenetic reprogramming of their respective normal cells of origin by paracrine signals emanating from the TME; these inductive signals reflect similar signaling circuits used to engage fibroblasts in wound healing or inflammatory responses. A growing number of IIC subtypes are being recognized, each with distinctive functions and characteristics; some may be lineage derived (e.g., expressed by definition in immune-cell progenitors recruited from the bone marrow) and others the result of "local education" by particular inductive signals in the TME. The list of tumor-promoting IIC includes forms (subtypes) of macrophages, neutrophils, partially differentiated myeloid progenitors, and in some cases specialized subtypes of B and T lymphocyte. The endothelial cells and pericytes of the

tumor vasculature are comparatively less diverse, although both epitope and gene-expression profiling have revealed tissue and tumor type-specific features of both endothelial cells and pericytes, likely with subtle functional implications in regard to tumor biology. A second distinct class of endothelial cells forms the lymphatic vascular network, which becomes enlarged via lymphangiogenesis proximal to many tumors and is implicated in lymphatic metastasis.

This recent and more nuanced view of stromal cells elevates their importance in understanding disease pathogenesis by virtue of their hallmark-enabling functional contributions.[2,3] CAFs, as an example not discussed earlier, can in different neoplastic contexts secrete proteases, proliferative signaling ligands, and/or other bioactive molecules that contribute to different tumor phenotypes. CAFs have been variously documented to liberate epithelial cells from the growth-suppressive effects imposed by normal tissue architecture, to induce tumor-promoting inflammation, to facilitate both local invasion and metastatic seeding, and to provide cancer cells with metabolic fuel. CAFs can also induce angiogenesis and, remarkably, act in an immune-suppressive manner to blunt the attacks of tumoricidal CTLs.

Looking to the future, an important goal will be to continue mapping the multidimensional landscape of stromal cell types and subtypes operative within different forms of cancer, and at different stages of progression.

Another dimension of the TME involves genetic and functional heterogeneity within populations of cancer cells. Indeed, the cancer cells within individual neoplastic lesions have long been recognized to be morphologically and genetically heterogeneous. Genome-profiling technologies (karyotyping, comparative genomic hybridization, allelic loss analysis, exome (gene) sequencing, and more recently whole-genome sequencing, now at the single-cell level) have documented the mutational evolution of the genome as nascent cancer cells in incipient neoplasias progress to spawn the genetically diverse subpopulations that coexist within high-grade tumors.

A second dimension of intratumoral heterogeneity is evident at the epigenetic level. Thus, in many carcinomas, cancer cells at the margins of invasive tumors are phenotypically distinct, having undergone an EMT that renders them more fibroblastic, with attendant capability for invasion. Others retain various degrees of differentiation characteristic of the cell type from which they originated, for example, squamous epithelia. In addition, the regional variation in histological characteristics seen in various tumor types is now realized to reflect (at least in some cases) genetically distinct clones of cancer cells, the result of mutational alteration of unstable genomes and clonal outgrowth, presumably reflecting different genetic solutions within the same neoplasia to the challenge of acquiring hallmark-enabling capabilities that enable malignant progression.

In addition, most tumors are now appreciated to contain distinct subpopulations—comparatively rare—of cancer cells exhibiting phenotypic similarity, at least superficially, to normal tissue stem cells. These cancer stem-like cells (CSC) typically proliferate comparatively slowly, express cell-surface markers diagnostic of tissue stem cells, and have enhanced capability to form new cancers upon ectopic transplantation of small numbers of cells into appropriate animal hosts, as compared to their more abundant counterparts, who proliferate more rapidly but are inefficient at or incapable of seeding transplant tumors.[9,25] (This latter assay operationally defines such cells as tumor-initiating cells, TIC.) One hypothesis was that the cell of origin of a cancer was a normal tissue stem or progenitor cell, which underwent neoplastic transformation into a CSC that in turn spawned cancer cells much like normal tissue

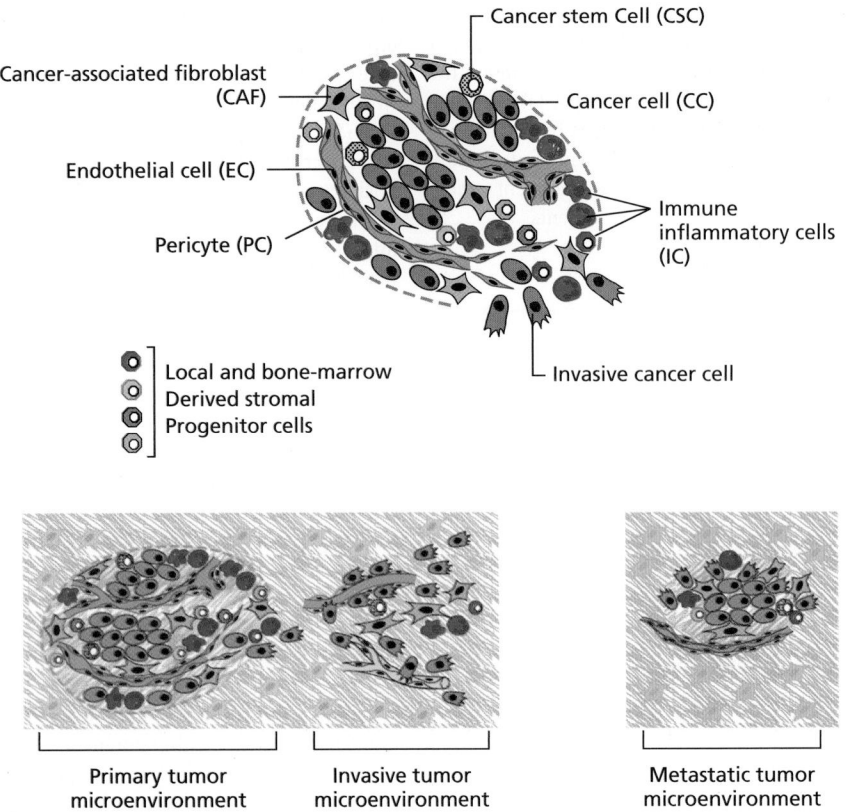

Figure 2 The constitution of the hallmark-enabling tumor microenvironment. An assemblage of distinct cell types constitutes the TME of most solid tumors, involving two distinct compartments—the parenchyma of cancer cells and the stroma of supporting cells. Both compartments contain distinct cell and subcell types that collectively enable tumor growth and progression.[2,3] Notably, the immune inflammatory cells present in tumors can include both tumor-promoting and/or immuno-suppressive as well as tumor-killing subclasses. The lower panels illustrate an important characteristic: the TME is dynamic, varying both in composition and abundance of constituent cell types (and sub-cell types) and in their effects on the histologically distinct stages in multistep tumorigenesis, namely premalignant stages (not shown) and malignant stages, including the cores of primary tumors, invasive margins and frankly invasive lesions, and metastases.

stem cells spawn differentiated cell types, and indeed there are indications of such cases. For example, the CSCs in squamous cell carcinomas of the skin produce partially differentiated cancer cells with features of squamous cells much as normal skin stem cells produce the squamous epithelium. A number of hematopoeitic malignancies evidently also arise from transformation of normal stem/progenitor cells into CSCs. In certain other cases, however, it appears that a dynamic interconversion operates between CSCs and their non-CSC counterparts, whereby CSCs can be converted into non-CSCs and vice versa, such that cancer cells can be converted into CSCs, and vice versa; in some such cases, the EMT appears to switch on the CSC phenotype in cancer cells, while its converse (the mesenchymal-to-epithelial transition, MET) reduces the abundance of CSCs in tumors.[9,25] There are indications that the comparatively less proliferative CSC may be more resistant to some genotoxic anticancer drugs, providing an avenue for drug resistance and clinical relapse. As such, therapeutic targeting of CSCs may be crucial to achieving enduring cancer therapies.

Therapeutic targeting (and cotargeting) of cancer hallmarks

An important question for cancer medicine is whether there are clinical applications of the hallmarks conceptualization? One possible benefit of this concept may come from helping cancer researchers appreciate common principles and thereby rationalize the diverse molecular and cellular mechanisms by which particular forms of human cancer develop and progress to malignancy. A wealth of data is being generated by multiplatform analysis—whole genome sequencing, and genome-wide profiling of RNA transcripts, proteins and phospho-proteins, and DNA and histone methylations—of cancer cells and neoplastic lesions in different tumor types (see, e.g., Ref. 26 and chapters throughout this textbook). Moreover, there will be other extrapolations of these increasingly powerful analytic technologies, including the profiling of lesional stages in tumorigenesis and tumor progression, in particular metastases; additionally, these technologies will likely provide insights into the adaptations that occur in tumors and metastases during the response and relapse phases to mechanism-targeted therapies. The challenge will be to integrate all of this information in order to understand the key determinants of particular carcinogenesis pathways; to identify new therapeutic targets; to identify modes of adaptive resistance to therapy; and then to use the data for diagnosis, prognosis, and treatment decisions. It is possible, although as yet unproven, that the hallmarks of cancer will prove useful in this integration and distillation: perhaps by filtering such cancer "omics" data—of the genome, the transcriptome, the proteome and phosphoproteome, and the methylome—through the growing knowledge base of regulatory pathways, it will be possible to identify the genetic and epigenetic signatures that underlie the acquisition of various hallmarks, potentially informing more precise management of disease.

We also envision that the hallmarks concept will prove useful in the design of future clinical treatment protocols. Notably, there are either approved drugs or drugs in late-stage clinical trials that target each of the eight hallmark capabilities and both of the enabling facilitators of those hallmarks (Figure 3); moreover, for most of the 10, there are multiple distinctive drugs targeting the same mechanistic effectors of these hallmarks. Although this is a provocative development in cancer therapeutics, these mechanism-based therapies targeting individual hallmarks have not in general been transformative for the treatment of late stage, aggressive forms of human cancer. An exception to this rule may be in the exciting ascendance of therapeutic immunomodulation to activate and sustain antitumoral immunity, involving most notably inhibitors of immune checkpoint receptors expressed on T lymphocytes (CTLA4 and PD1). Signaling from these checkpoint receptors can disable cytotoxic T cells, evidently rendering antitumoral immune responses ineffectual, thereby contributing to the hallmark capability for evading immune destruction. Notably, exciting clinical responses are being observed in melanoma and other selected tumors[27,28] treated with therapeutic antibodies that inhibit checkpoint activation, particularly when both checkpoints are cotargeted with therapeutic antibody cocktails.[29] Nevertheless, not all patients respond to such immunotherapies, and the duration of response remains to be ascertained, as does the prevalence of adaptive resistance to such immunotherapies.

For other hallmark-targeting therapies, it is typical, after a period of response, to see adaptive resistance mechanisms kick in, enabling the surviving cancer cells (and cancer stem cells) to circumvent the mechanistic blockade imposed by the treatment and resume progressive growth. Various solutions can be proposed to overcome the failures of currently employed, targeted therapies. We suggest that a fruitful therapeutic strategy might involve applying the concept of functionally distinct hallmarks traits, more specifically by targeting multiple hallmarks concomitantly. This multi-targeting may reduce the likelihood of acquired resistance to treatment, thereby yielding significant improvements in initial responses and in long-term survival.[30] Certainly, an important issue will be effectively managing the toxicities of such combinations. Thus, in addition to simple cocktails, it may be necessary to use hallmark-targeting drugs sequentially, episodically, or in layers, fine-tuned to maximize efficacy while managing toxicity and limiting adaptive resistance. It is further envisioned that refined preclinical mouse models—both genetically engineered *de novo* and patient-derived xenograft (PDX) transplants—will have utility in testing alternative therapeutic trials designs aimed to reduce the matrix of possibilities to clinically feasible numbers, taking the best-performing trial arms from preclinical trials into clinical trials and personalized treatments.[31–33]

In conclusion, the hallmarks of cancer may provide the student of modern oncology with a foundation and a framework for absorbing the subsequent topical chapters of this textbook, and more generally for investigating and interpreting pathogenic mechanisms and applying such knowledge toward the development of more effective diagnosis and treatment of human cancers.

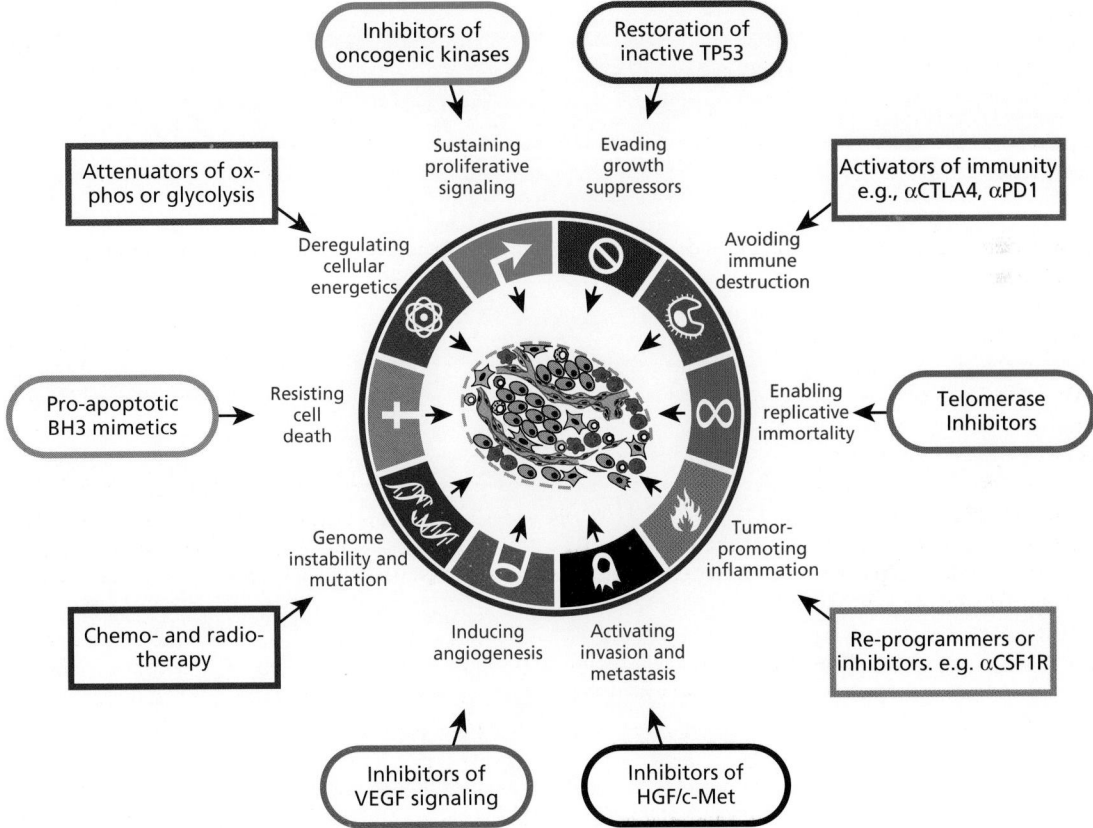

Figure 3 Therapeutic targeting of the hallmarks of cancer. Drugs have been developed that disrupt or interfere with all eight of the hallmark capabilities, and with the two enabling facilitators (genome instability and tumor-promoting inflammation). Some of these hallmark-targeting drugs are approved for clinical use, while others are being tested in late-stage clinical trials; moreover, there is a pipeline full of new hallmark-targeting drugs in development and preclinical evaluation. Recognizing that eventual adaptive resistance during therapeutic treatment is apparent for virtually all of these hallmark-targeting drugs, a hypothesis has emerged: perhaps, by cotargeting multiple independent hallmarks, it will be possible to limit or even prevent the emergence of simultaneous adaptive resistance to independent hallmark-targeting drugs;[30] clinical and preclinical trials are beginning to assess the possibilities.

References

1 Hanahan D, Weinberg RA. The hallmarks of cancer. *Cell*. 2000;**100**:57–70.

2 Hanahan D, Weinberg RA. Hallmarks of cancer: the next generation. *Cell*. 2011;**144**:346–674.

3 Hanahan D, Coussens LM. Accessories to the crime: functions of cells recruited to the tumor microenvironment. *Cancer Cell*. 2012;**21**:309–322.

4 Weinberg RA. *The Biology of Cancer*. New York: Garland Press; 2013.

5 Vanden Berghe T, Linkermann A, Jouan-Lanhouet S, et al. Regulated necrosis: the expanding network of non-apoptotic cell death pathways. *Nat Rev Mol Cell Biol*. 2014;**15**:135–147.

6 Rebecca VW, Amaravadi RK. Emerging strategies to effectively target autophagy in cancer. *Oncogene*. 2015. doi: 10.1038/onc.2015.99 (Epub ahead of print).

7 Keith B, Johnson RS, Simon MC. HIF1α and HIF2α: sibling rivalry in hypoxic tumour growth and progression. *Nat Rev Cancer*. 2011;**12**:9–22.

8 Semenza GL. Hypoxia-inducible factors: mediators of cancer progression and targets for cancer therapy. *Trends Pharmacol Sci*. 2012;**33**:207–214.

9 Baccelli I, Trumpp A. The evolving concept of cancer and metastasis stem cells. *J Cell Biol*. 2012;**198**:281–293.

10 Savagner P. Epithelial-mesenchymal transitions: from cell plasticity to concept elasticity. *Curr Top Dev Biol*. 2015;**112**:273–300.

11 Daye D, Wellen KE. Metabolic reprogramming in cancer: unraveling the role of glutamine in tumorigenesis. *Semin Cell Dev Biol*. 2012;**23**:362–369.

12 Dhup S, Dadhich RK, Porporato PE, Sonveaux P. Multiple biological activities of lactic acid in cancer: influences on tumor growth, angiogenesis and metastasis. *Curr Pharm Des*. 2012;**18**:1319–1330.

13 Ward PS, Thompson CB. Metabolic reprogramming: a cancer hallmark even Warburg did not anticipate. *Cancer Cell*. 2012;**21**:297–308.

14 Fridman WH, Pagès F, Sautès-Fridman C, Galon J. The immune contexture in human tumours: impact on clinical outcome. *Nat Rev Cancer*. 2012;**12**:298–306.

15 Galon J, Mlecnik B, Bindea G, et al. Towards the introduction of the 'Immunoscore' in the classification of malignant tumours. *J Pathol*. 2014;**232**:199–209.

16 Galon J, Angell HK, Bedognetti D, Marincola FM. The continuum of cancer immunosurveillance: prognostic, predictive, and mechanistic signatures. *Immunity*. 2013;**39**:11–26.

17 https://tcga-data.nci.nih.gov/tcga/tcgaHome2.jsp

18 http://www.sanger.ac.uk/research/projects/cancergenome/

19 http://icgc.org/

20 http://www.ncbi.nlm.nih.gov/sky/

21 You JS, Jones PA. Cancer genetics and epigenetics: two sides of the same coin? *Cancer Cell*. 2012;**22**:9–20.

22 Easwaran H, Tsai HC, Baylin SB. Cancer epigenetics: tumor heterogeneity, plasticity of stem-like states, and drug resistance. *Mol Cell*. 2014;**54**:716–727.

23 Azad N, Zahnow CA, Rudin CM, Baylin SB. The future of epigenetic therapy in solid tumours – lessons from the past. *Nat Rev Clin Oncol*. 2013;**10**:256–266.

24 Labelle M, Hynes RO. The initial hours of metastasis: the importance of cooperative host-tumor cell interactions during hematogenous dissemination. *Cancer Discov*. 2012;**2**:1091–1099.

25 Visvader JE, Lindeman GJ. Cancer stem cells: current status and evolving complexities. *Cell Stem Cell*. 2012;**10**:717–728.

26 The Cancer Genome Atlas Network. Comprehensive molecular portraits of human breast tumours. *Nature*. 2012;**490**:61–70.

27 Sharma P, Allison JP. The future of immune checkpoint therapy. *Science*. 2015;**348**:56–61.

28 Topalian SL, Drake CG, Pardoll DM. Immune checkpoint blockade: a common denominator approach to cancer therapy. *Cancer Cell*. 2015;**27**:450–461.

29 Sharma P, Allison JP. Immune checkpoint targeting in cancer therapy: toward combination strategies with curative potential. *Cell*. 2015;**161**:205–214.

30 Hanahan D. Rethinking the war on cancer. *Lancet*. 2013;**383**:558–563.

31 De Palma M, Hanahan D. The biology of personalized cancer medicine: facing individual complexities underlying hallmark capabilities. *Mol Oncol*. 2012;**6**:111–127.

32 Das Thakur M, Pryer NK, Singh M. Mouse tumour models to guide drug development and identify resistance mechanisms. *J Pathol*. 2014;**232**:103–111.

33 Siolas D, Hannon GJ. Patient-derived tumor xenografts: transforming clinical samples into mouse models. *Cancer Res*. 2013;**73**:5315–5319.

PART 2

Tumor Biology

3 Molecular biology, genomics, proteomics, and mouse models of human cancer

Srinivas R. Viswanathan, MD, PhD ▪ *David A. Tuveson, MD, PhD* ▪ *Matthew Meyerson, MD, PhD*

Overview

Cancer is a genetic disease. It is typified by abnormalities in genes that control cellular proliferation and lead to the unrestrained growth that characterizes a malignant cell. Thus, to gain the initiative in cancer detection and treatment, oncologists must begin to understand the molecular roots of the disease: genes, their messenger ribonucleic acids (mRNAs), and the proteins they produce. In short, oncologists should be conversant with the tools of molecular biology.

This chapter is a basic survey of molecular biology and is directed toward the clinician or trainee who wants a fundamental understanding of this discipline. It is "methods oriented" and will serve as a frame of reference for other chapters in this book. It describes the principles that underlie the procedures used most commonly by molecular biologists and provides examples of clinically relevant situations that draw on particular techniques. Molecular biology already plays an important role in clinical cancer medicine, both in terms of diagnosis (e.g., in the analysis of tumors for prognostic or pathogenetic information) and in treatment (e.g., in the production of pharmacologic and biologic agents, such as recombinant growth factors and monoclonal antibodies).

We begin with an overview of genes, gene expression, and gene cloning. Our discussion of techniques follow the flow of genetic information as we explain the procedures used to analyze gene expression at the levels of DNA, RNA, and protein. Good general overviews of these topics can be found in several books.[1-3]

Overview: gene structure

Genes and gene expression

The gene is the fundamental unit of inheritance and the ultimate determinant of all phenotypes. The DNA of a normal human cell contains an estimated 20,000–25,000 protein-coding genes, but only a fraction of these are expressed in any particular cell at any given time. For example, genes specific for erythroid cells, such as the hemoglobin genes, are not expressed in brain cells. The identity of each gene expressed in a particular cell at a given time and its level of expression are defined as the "transcriptome."

According to the central dogma of molecular biology, a gene exerts its effects by having its DNA transcribed into an mRNA, which, in turn, is translated into a protein, the final effector of the gene's action. Thus, molecular biologists often investigate gene expression or activation, by which is meant the process of transcribing DNA into RNA or translating RNA into protein. The process of transcription involves creating an RNA copy (a "transcript") of the gene using the DNA of the gene as a template. The mRNA transcript is then translated into a protein by the ribosome, which decodes the sequence information contained within the transcript to build a corresponding protein composed of amino acids.

Functional components of the gene

Every gene consists of several functional components, each involved in a different facet of the process of gene expression (Figure 1). Broadly speaking, however, there are two main functional units: the promoter region and the coding region.

The promoter region controls when and in what tissue a gene is expressed. For example, the promoter of the hemoglobin gene is responsible for its expression in erythroid cells and not in brain cells. How is this tissue-specific expression achieved? In the DNA of the gene's promoter region, there are specific structural and sequence elements (see section titled "Structural Considerations") that permit the gene to be expressed only in an appropriate cell. These are the elements in the hemoglobin gene that instruct an erythroid cell to transcribe hemoglobin mRNA from that gene. These structures are referred to as "cis-acting elements" because they reside on the same molecule of DNA as the gene. In some cases, other tissue-type-specific cis-acting elements, called enhancers, reside on the same DNA molecule but at a great distance from the coding region of the gene.[4,5] In the appropriate cell, the cis-acting elements bind protein factors that are physically responsible for transcribing the gene. These proteins are called trans-acting factors because they reside in the cell's nucleus, separate from the DNA molecule bearing the gene. For example, brain cells would not have the right trans-acting factors that bind to the hemoglobin promoter and activate gene expression; therefore, brain cells would not express hemoglobin. They would, however, have trans-acting factors that bind to neuron-specific gene promoters.

The structure of a gene's protein is specified by the gene's coding region. The coding region contains the information that directs an erythroid cell to assemble amino acids in the proper order to make the hemoglobin protein. How is this order of amino acids specified? As described in detail later, DNA is a linear polymer consisting of four distinguishable subunits called nucleotides. In the coding region of a gene, the linear sequence of nucleotides encodes the amino acid sequence of the protein. This genetic code is in triplet form so that every group of three nucleotides encodes a single amino acid. The 64 triplets that can be formed by four nucleotides exceed the 20 distinct amino acids used to make proteins. This makes the code degenerate and allows some amino acids to be encoded by several different triplets.[6] As discussed in the section titled "Nucleotide Sequencing", the nucleotide sequence of any gene can be determined using a variety of methods (see below). By translating the code, one can therefore derive a predicted amino acid sequence for the protein encoded by a gene.

Structural considerations

Fine structure

The basic repeating units of the DNA polymer are nucleotides (Figure 2). Nucleotides consist of an invariant portion, a five-carbon

Holland-Frei Cancer Medicine, Ninth Edition. Edited by Robert C. Bast Jr., Carlo M. Croce, William N. Hait, Waun Ki Hong, Donald W. Kufe, Martine Piccart-Gebhart, Raphael E. Pollock, Ralph R. Weichselbaum, Hongyang Wang, and James F. Holland.

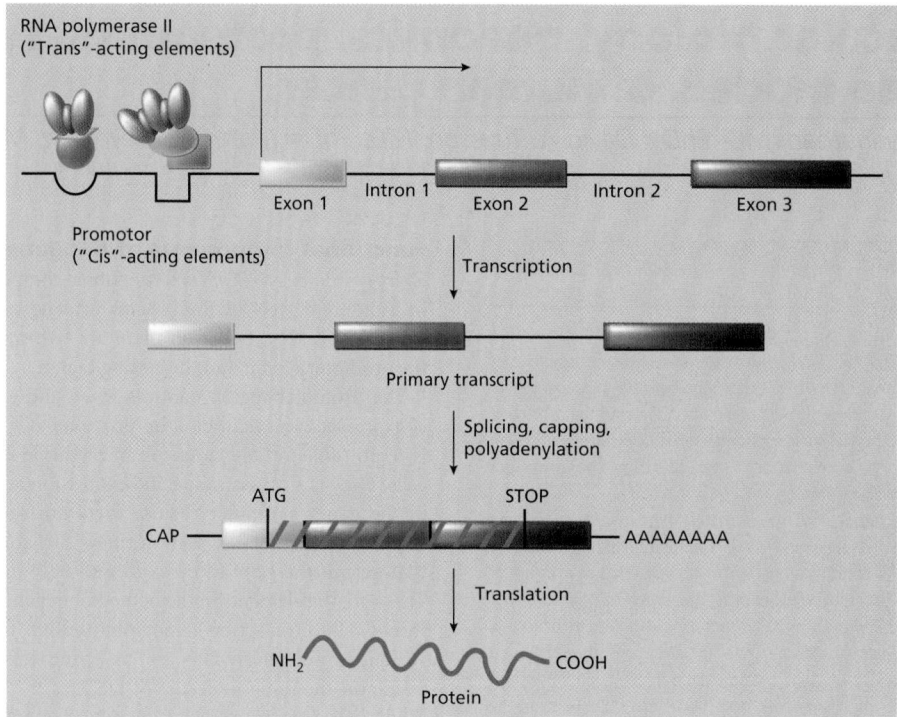

Figure 1 Gene expression. A gene's DNA is transcribed into messenger ribonucleic acid (mRNA), which, in turn, is translated into protein. The functional components of a gene are schematically diagrammed here. Areas of the gene destined to be represented in mature mRNA are called exons, and intervening areas of DNA between exons are called introns. The portion of the gene that controls transcription, and therefore expression, is the promoter. This control is exerted by specific nucleotide sequences in the promoter region (so-called cis-acting factors) and by proteins (so-called trans-acting factors) that must interact with promoter DNA and/or ribonucleic acid (RNA) polymerase II for transcription to occur. The primary transcript is the RNA molecule made by RNA polymerase II that is complementary to the entire stretch of DNA containing the gene. Before leaving the nucleus, the primary transcript is modified by splicing together exons (thus removing intronic sequences), adding a cap to the 5′ end and adding a poly-A tail to the 3′ end. Once in the cytoplasm, mature mRNA undergoes translation to yield a protein.

deoxyribose sugar with a phosphate group, and a variable portion, the base. Of the four bases that appear in the nucleotides of DNA, two are purines, adenine (A) and guanine (G), and two are pyrimidines, cytosine (C) and thymine (T). Nucleotides are connected to each other in the DNA polymer through their phosphate groups, leaving the bases free to interact with each other through hydrogen bonding. This base pairing is specific, so that A interacts with T and C interacts with G. DNA is ordinarily double stranded; that is, two linear polymers of DNA are aligned so that the bases of the two strands face each other. Base pairing makes this alignment specific, so that one DNA strand is a perfectly complementary to the other. This complementarity means that each DNA strand carries the information needed to make an exact replica of itself.

In every strand of a DNA polymer, the phosphate substitutions alternate between the 5 and 3 carbons of the deoxyribose molecules. Thus, there is directionality to DNA: the genetic code reads in the 5–3 direction. In double-stranded DNA, the strand that carries the translatable code in the 5–3 direction is called the sense strand, whereas its complementary partner is termed the antisense strand.[7]

Gross structure

In eukaryotes, the coding regions of most genes are not continuous. Rather, they consist of areas that are transcribed into mature mRNA (exons) interrupted by stretches of DNA that do not appear in mature mRNA (introns) (Figure 1). The exact functions of introns are not known with certainty. Some may contain regulatory sequences, and certainly an important purpose is implied by their conservation across evolution. There is reason to believe that the overall physical structure of introns might be more important than their specific nucleotide sequences, because the nucleotide sequences of introns diverge more rapidly in evolution than do the sequences of exons. Overall, the DNA that ultimately encodes for protein comprises only a tiny minority of total DNA. Between genes, there are vast stretches of untranscribed DNA that are assumed to play an important structural role. There are also many regions that give rise to transcribed "noncoding" RNA species—these regulatory RNAs are transcribed and functionally active without being translated into proteins.[8–10]

In the nucleus, DNA is not present as naked nucleic acid. Rather, it is found in close association with a number of accessory proteins, such as the histones, and in this form is called chromatin.[11] A multitude of accessory DNA proteins allow for the correct packaging of DNA. For example, DNA's double helix is ordinarily twisted on itself to form a supercoiled structure.[12] This structure must partially unwind during DNA replication and transcription.[13] Accessory proteins such as topoisomerases, histone acetylases, and histone deacetylases, are involved in regulating this process.

Summary

Genes specify the sequence and structure of proteins that are responsible for their phenotype. Although the nucleus of every human cell contains 20,000–25,000 genes, only a tiny fraction of them are expressed in any given cell at any given time. The promoter (with or without an enhancer) is the part of the gene that determines when and where it will be expressed. The coding region is the part of the gene that dictates the amino acid sequence of the protein encoded by the gene. In addition to the proportion of the DNA

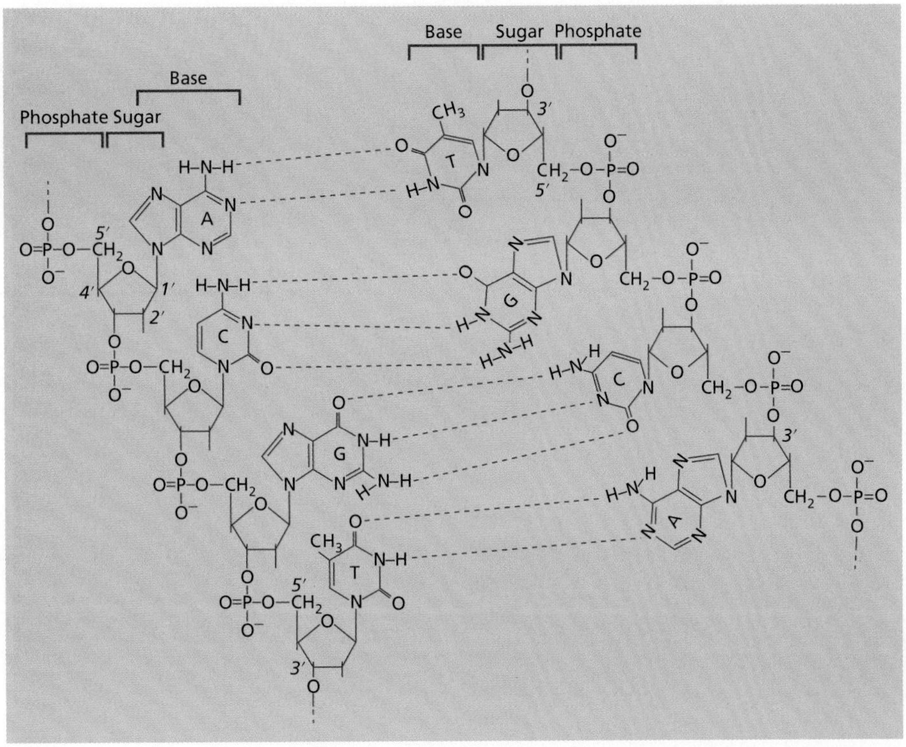

Figure 2 Structure of base-paired double-stranded DNA. Each strand of DNA consists of a backbone of five-carbon deoxyribose sugars connected to each other through phosphate bonds. Note that as one follows the sequence down the left-hand strand (A to C to G to T), one is also following the carbons of the deoxyribose ring, going from the 5′ carbon to the 3′ carbon. This is the basis for the 5′ to 3′ directionality of DNA. The 1 carbon of each deoxyribose is substituted with a purine or pyrimidine base. In double-stranded DNA, bases face each other in the center of the molecule and base pair via hydrogen bonds (dotted lines). Base pairing is specific so that adenine pairs with thymine and guanine pairs with cytosine.

that contains genes encoding for proteins, the genome contains vast stretches of regulatory sequences and noncoding RNA sequences. DNA is a linear polymer of nucleotides. Ordinarily, the nucleotide bases of one strand of DNA pair with those of the complementary strand (A with T, C with G) to make double-stranded DNA. In the cell's nucleus, DNA is associated with accessory proteins and packaged into the higher order form known as chromatin

General techniques

Restriction endonucleases and recombinant DNA

In eukaryotic chromosomes, individual molecules of DNA are several million base pairs long. Because these molecules are far too large to analyze directly, scientists are usually interested in cutting DNA into fragments of more manageable size. Fortunately, for molecular biologists, bacteria have evolved a highly diverse set of enzymes, the restriction endonucleases, which cleave DNA internally within the polymer[14]

In nature, these enzymes have evolved to protect bacteria from invasion by foreign species, such as bacteriophages. To discriminate between "domestic" and "foreign" DNA, these enzymes recognize specific nucleotide sequences. DNA without such specific sequences is left undisturbed by the enzymes. However, when a restriction endonuclease spots a recognition site, it binds to the site and cleaves both strands of the DNA to which it has bound. Individual restriction endonucleases recognize specific sequences, usually in the order of four to six bases in length, and these sequences are often palindromes (i.e., the 5–3 sequence in the upper strand is identical to the 5–3 sequence in the lower strand) (Figure 3).[15]

Although restriction endonucleases cut DNA into smaller fragments, there is a lower limit to the size of useful fragments. One would not want to cut DNA into such small pieces that the informational content of each piece is negligible. Statistically, the longer a restriction endonuclease's recognition sequence, the less frequently this sequence will occur in a stretch of DNA. Therefore, the enzymes most commonly used to cut DNA into usefully large fragments are those that recognize a 6-nt recognition site (so-called six-base cutters). For example, an endonuclease isolated from *Escherichia coli*, called EcoRI, recognizes the sequence GAATTC, and wherever this occurs in double-stranded DNA, it will cleave between the G and A (Figure 3). (Note that the antisense strand, which reads CTTAAG in the 3′–5′ direction, will also read GAATTC in the 5′–3′ direction. This is what is meant by a palindromic sequence.)

Gene cloning

Mechanics

The most powerful technique available for gene analysis, and the one technique that is the cornerstone for all others, is gene cloning (Figure 3). In the gene cloning process, a discrete piece of DNA is faithfully replicated in the laboratory. Cloning provides quantities of specific DNA sufficient for biochemical analysis or for any other manipulation, including joining to a foreign piece of DNA. In the early 1970s, Cohen et al.[16] drew on two fundamental properties of bacteria and their viruses (phages) that made this innovation possible: plasmids and DNA ligases.

Plasmids are circular molecules of DNA that replicate in the cytoplasm of bacterial cells, separate from the bacteria's own DNA. In

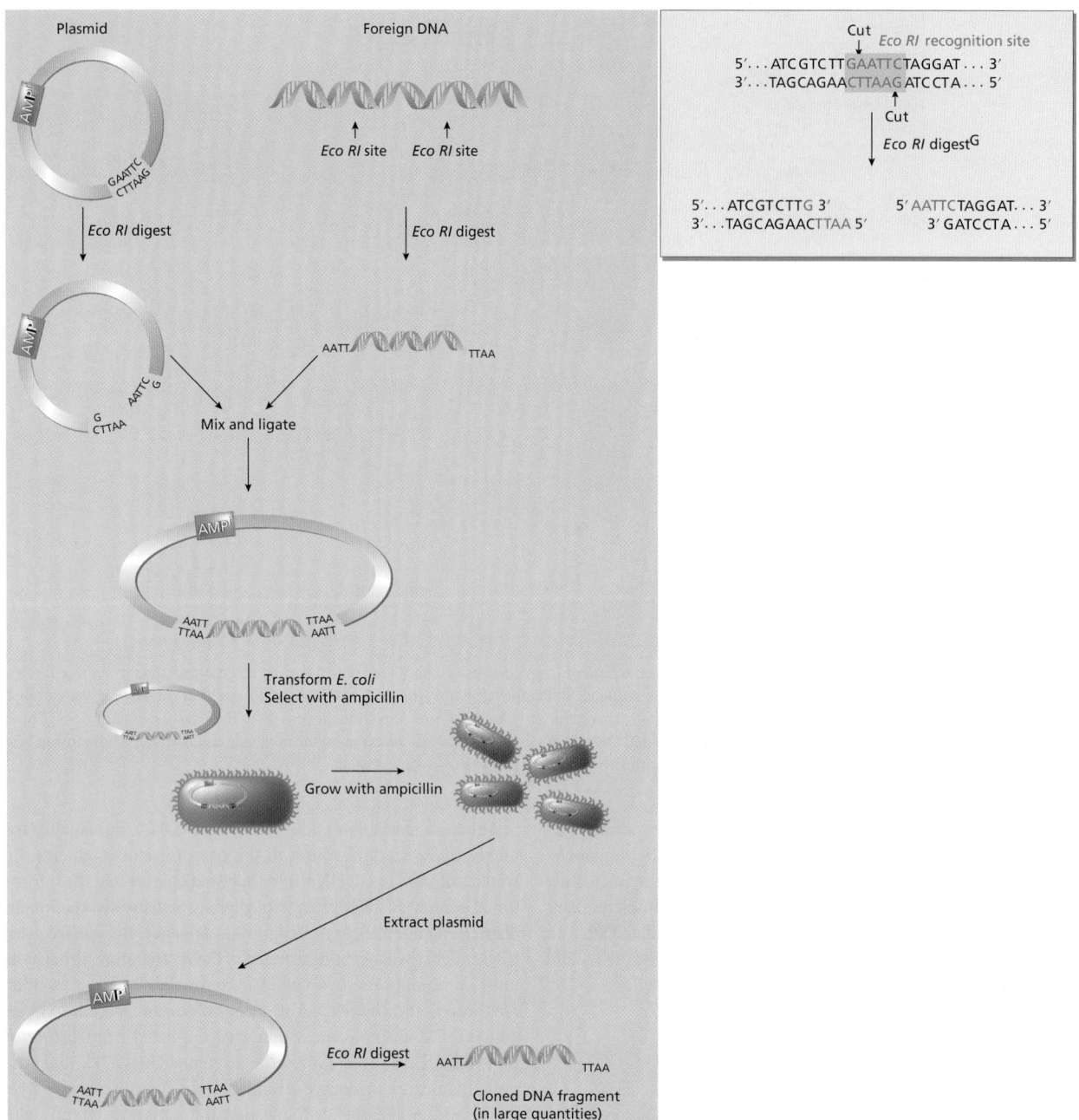

Figure 3 Digestion of DNA with the restriction endonuclease EcoRI and gene cloning. In this example, a small amount of foreign DNA (a few nanograms) is digested with EcoRI. The nucleotide sequence of this stretch of DNA contains the recognition sequence for EcoRI, GAATTC (boxed). EcoRI cuts the DNA in both strands between the indicated nucleotides, resulting in fragments with five single-stranded tails. This foreign DNA can come from any source, the only requirement being that it contains the same restriction endonuclease recognition sites as the vector. Plasmid vector is also digested with EcoRI to create a linear DNA molecule. The "sticky" single-stranded ends of the foreign DNA can align and base pair with the complementary "sticky ends" of the plasmid, after which DNA ligase covalently bonds foreign DNA to plasmid DNA. This recombinant DNA is introduced into *E. coli* by a process called transformation. Because the bacteria themselves are not resistant to ampicillin, growth in ampicillin will select only those bacteria that have taken up the plasmid DNA (which carries an ampicillin resistance gene). The plasmid contains a bacterial origin of replication so that as the bacterial culture grows, plasmids replicate, resulting in several copies in each bacterium. When the culture has grown to sufficient size, plasmid DNA can be isolated biochemically, foreign DNA can be cut from the plasmid using EcoRI, and the resulting yield will often be milligrams of DNA, that is, greater than a 10^6-fold amplification.

nature, plasmids often carry genetic information useful to the host bacterium, such as genes that confer resistance to antibiotics. For the purposes of gene cloning, plasmids are important because they contain all of the information necessary for directing bacterial enzymes to replicate the plasmid DNA, in some cases, to many thousands of copies per bacterium.

DNA ligases are enzymes produced by bacteria (and some phages when they infect bacteria) that can link or ligate together separate pieces of DNA. The nucleotide sequence in a piece of DNA does not influence the activity of a DNA ligase so that a DNA ligase can join any two pieces of DNA together, even ones that are not ordinarily connected to each other in nature. Indeed, the power of cloning comes in the ability to "mix and match" segments of DNA in a fashion tailored to the desired use.

Cloning with restriction endonucleases

In the traditional form of gene cloning, one uses a restriction endonuclease to cut open the circular plasmid DNA in a region of the plasmid not necessary for replication (Figure 3). Suppose, for example, that the enzyme EcoRI cuts open the plasmid in such a nonessential area. EcoRI recognizes the sequence GAATTC and cuts both DNA strands between the G and the A nucleotides. Protruding from the cut ends will be single-stranded DNA "tails" with the sequence AATT. (Note that the tail's sequence in the sense strand is the same as the sequence in the antisense strand when the nucleotides are read in the 5′–3′ direction.) Any other piece of DNA that has been cut with EcoRI will also have single-stranded AATT tails, and the AATT tails on this foreign piece of DNA can base pair with the complementary TTAA tails (reading 3′–5′) on the cut plasmid. When this happens, the foreign DNA piece physically closes the gap in the plasmid, forming a closed circular plasmid again (which is necessary for plasmid propagation).

Although the nucleotides at the ends of the plasmid and foreign DNA now abut each other, they are not covalently connected. This is an unstable situation that the DNA ligase rectifies. The DNA ligase covalently joins the plasmid and foreign DNA to create a recombinant plasmid, which still has all of the information needed to be replicated in a bacterium but which also contains a foreign DNA insert. Obviously, the EcoRI-cut ends of the plasmid can also base pair with themselves again to reform the native plasmid, but molecular biologists have developed a number of tricks to suppress this phenomenon. It should be pointed out that single-stranded tails are not always necessary for making recombinant DNA. Under certain conditions, the DNA ligase can join together two fragments of blunt-ended DNA without these tails.

When a recombinant plasmid is reintroduced into a host bacterium (by a process called transformation), the plasmid will replicate normally. Now, however, its foreign DNA insert is replicated along with the plasmid into which it was inserted. The transformed bacteria can then be grown to large numbers in liquid culture. With each bacterial cell division, the progeny bacteria contain plasmid molecules that continue to replicate. When the bacterial culture contains the desired quantity of this plasmid (this may be milligrams of plasmid DNA in a 1 L culture), it can be reisolated as pure DNA. The cloned foreign piece of DNA can then be cut out (with EcoRI, in our example) for further analysis or manipulation. One can also use bacterial viruses (or phages) in the same manner by infecting host bacteria with recombinant phage-bearing foreign DNA sequences. In all of these experiments, the plasmid or phage that houses the foreign DNA is called a vector because it is the vehicle that directs the foreign DNA into the host bacterium.

These extraordinarily powerful tools, which are now part of the standard armamentarium of all molecular biology laboratories, have been responsible for the development of nearly all of the analytic techniques described later. Several excellent manuals that describe these techniques in detail have been published.[17,18]

Gateway cloning

Gateway cloning is a proprietary commercial system that has gained widespread popularity for the ease with which it allows researchers to transfer DNA fragments between plasmids. In Gateway cloning, a DNA fragment of interest is first appended with specific Gateway sequences on the 5′ and 3′ ends (termed "attB1" and "attB2", respectively). A proprietary recombinase named BP Clonase that recognizes these Gateway sequences is then used to recombine the fragment into a so-called Gateway Donor vector, to generate a clone in which sequences termed "attL1" and "attL2" flank the fragment of interest. Once in the Gateway Donor vector, the fragment (now termed an "entry clone") can be transferred to any one of thousands of available Gateway Destination vectors using another recombinase mix termed "LR Clonase".[19] This recombinase-based technology therefore allows gene fragments to be easily shuttled between plasmids without the need for restriction digestion and purification steps (Figure 4a).

Gibson cloning

A recent development in cloning has been termed the Gibson Assembly method. This allows for the facile assembly of multiple overlapping DNA fragments. In this method, two or more fragments to be assembled are mixed together with a combination of three DNA enzymes—an exonuclease, a polymerase, and a ligase. The exonuclease removes the 5′ ends of the fragments to be joined, thereby exposing a 3′ single-stranded DNA overhang. Overlapping fragments then anneal via their 3′ overhangs, and the gaps and nicks are filled in by the DNA polymerase and DNA ligase, respectively. These fragments can be joined together in a one-step isothermal reaction. This powerful synthetic biology method can be routinely used to enzymatically assemble multiple DNA fragments of up to several hundred kilobases.[20] For example, it was recently applied to synthesize the complete mouse mitochondrial genome, a size of 16.3 kilobases, using 600 overlapping fragments (Figure 4b).[21]

Gene probes and hybridization

We shall see in the following sections that what lies at the heart of gene analysis is the ability to identify a specific gene (or mRNA) in a complex mixture of all of the DNA (or RNA) in a cell or tissue. This can be done only when one already has a cloned fragment of DNA from the gene of interest. Such fragments are usually obtained from gene libraries constructed from genomic DNA or complementary deoxyribonucleic acid (cDNA) or generated using polymerase chain reaction (PCR, to be described below). These DNA fragments can be almost any size, from a fraction of the size of the gene (a few hundred or even fewer nucleotides) to the size of an entire gene (several thousand nucleotides). These cloned gene fragments are called probes because they are used to probe native DNA or RNA for the gene of interest.

To be useful, a gene probe must contain a sufficient number of nucleotides so that it will recognize the sequences of its corresponding gene. Recognition occurs by a process called nucleic acid hybridization, in which two pieces of DNA can align themselves (or "anneal") by base pairing. Hybridization occurs by the specific pairing of A to T bases and of G to C bases (Figure 2). Perfectly matched sequences pair more tightly than sequences containing mismatches, and long-matched sequences pair more tightly than shorter matched sequences. Hybridization is the concept that underlies many molecular biology methods, such as Southern blotting, Northern blotting, microarray analysis, PCR, and others (see below).

Summary

Total genomic DNA can be cut into smaller pieces using restriction endonucleases that recognize specific nucleotide sequences. Individual genes can be captured from total genomic DNA and replicated in bulk for detailed analysis. This process is called cloning and employs bacterial plasmids and viruses (phage) as carriers for the cloned genes. Enzymes called DNA ligases join foreign DNA to plasmid or phage vectors, which can then replicate within bacterial

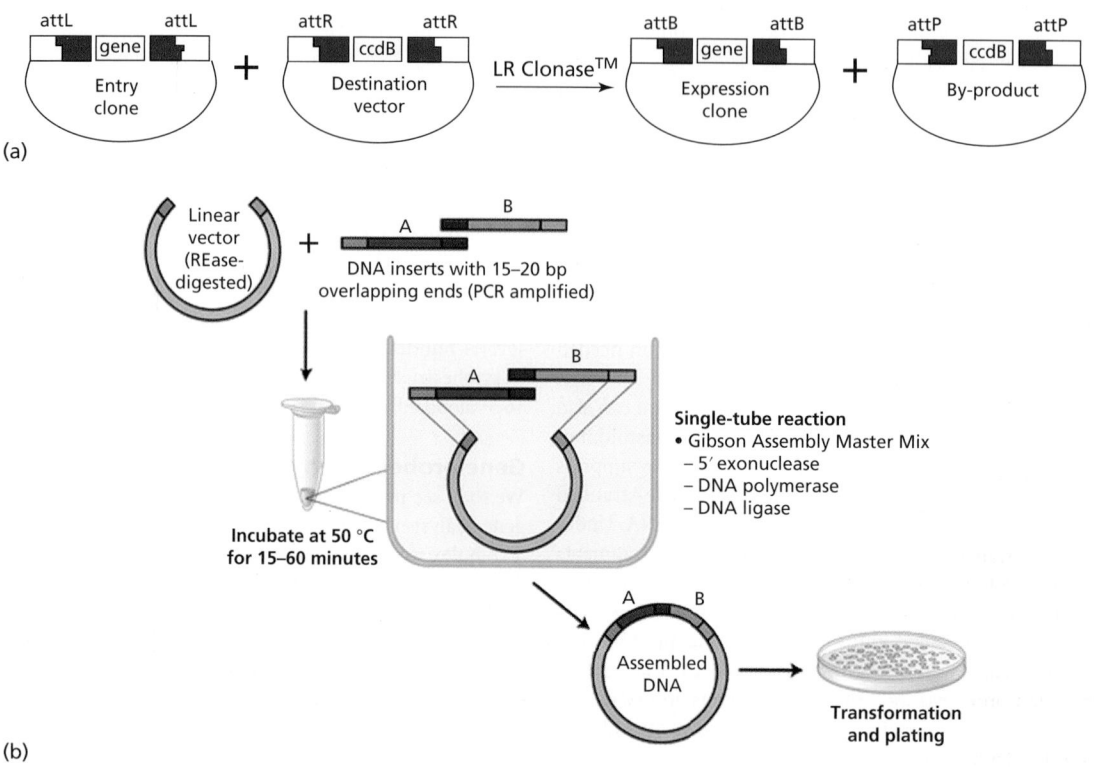

BP Reaction: Facilitates recombination of an *att*B substrate (*att*B-PCR product or a linearized *att*B expression clone) with an *att*P substrate (donor vector) to create an *att*L-containing entry clone (see diagram below). This reaction is catalyzed by BP Clonase™ enzyme mix.

LR Reaction: Facilitates recombination of an *att*L substrate (entry clone) with an *att*R substrate (destination vector) to create an *att*B-containing expression clone (see diagram below). This reaction is catalyzed by LR Clonase™ enzyme mix.

Figure 4 (a) Gateway cloning. Source: Gateway Technology Manual from: http://www.thermofisher.com/us/en/home/life-science/cloning/gateway-cloning/gateway-technology.html, page 16. ccdB, negative selection cassette included in donor and destination vectors. (b) Gibson cloning. Source: Gibson (NEB). https://www.neb.com/applications/cloning-and-synthetic-biology/dna-assembly-and-cloning/gibson-assembly.

cells to create gene libraries. Using nucleic acid hybridization, cloned genes can be used as probes to detect the presence of their native counterparts in complex mixtures of DNA or RNA.

Gene analysis: DNA

Southern blotting

One of the most useful techniques for analyzing a gene at the level of genomic DNA is Southern blotting, named for its inventor, E. M. Southern.[22] In general, it allows one to determine whether specific nucleotide sequences in a cloned probe are present in a sample of genomic DNA. The presence of these sequences usually means that the gene itself is present in the genomic DNA. Figure 5 diagrams the technique. Purified genomic DNA is digested with a specific restriction endonuclease, which, as described earlier, will produce an array of differently sized DNA fragments. Electrophoresis through an agarose gel then separates these fragments according to size. (Because the phosphate groups in DNA make the molecules negatively charged, they will migrate toward the anode in an electric field. The semiporous agarose will allow molecules of DNA to pass with varying degrees of ease, at a rate inversely proportional to their size. At any time after electrophoresis begins, smaller molecules will be closer to the anode than larger molecules.)

The final goal of Southern blotting is to identify specific fragments of cut DNA using nucleic acid hybridization. Because the agarose gel used in electrophoresis is thick and the DNA fragments can move within it, DNA in the gel is not in a suitable form for further analysis. The DNA fragments must therefore be transferred to a solid support to which they are irreversibly bound to carry out nucleic acid hybridization studies. Thus, after electrophoresis, a paper-thin membrane microfilter (made of nitrocellulose or nylon) is placed over the flat portion of the gel. Liquid is then forced through the agarose gel in a direction perpendicular to the direction in which the DNA moved during electrophoresis. As the liquid perfuses the gel, it carries DNA fragments with it, depositing them on the membrane filter, to which the DNA sticks. After transfer, the DNA fragments are arrayed by size on the solid support.

At this point, a fragment of cloned DNA (the probe) is radiolabeled by using any of a variety of techniques. The membrane

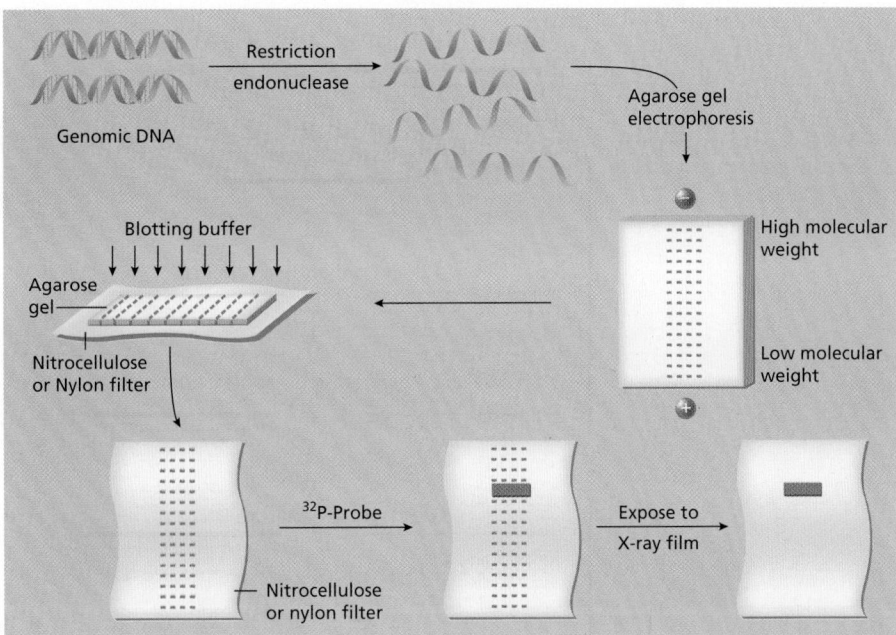

Figure 5 Genomic Southern blotting. Genomic DNA is digested with a single-restriction endonuclease, resulting in a complex mixture of DNA fragments of different sizes, that is, molecular weights. Digested DNA is arrayed by size using electrophoresis through a semisolid agarose gel. Because DNA is negatively charged, fragments will migrate toward the anode, but their progress is variably impeded by interactions with the agarose gel. Small fragments interact less and migrate farther; large fragments interact more and migrate less. The arrayed fragments are then transferred to a sheet of nitrocellulose- or nylon-based filter paper by forcing buffer through the gel as shown. The DNA fragments are carried by capillary action and can be made to bind irreversibly to the filter. Now the DNA fragments, still arrayed by size on the filter, can be probed for specific nucleotide sequences using a ³²P-radiolabeled nucleic acid probe. The probe will hybridize to complementary sequences in the DNA, and the position of the fragment that contains these sequences can be revealed by exposing the filter to X-ray film.

containing the transferred DNA is then soaked in a solution containing the radiolabeled probe. If there are any sequences in the genomic DNA that are complementary to those in the probe, the probe will hybridize to those sequences on the filter. The unbound probe can be washed away, and the remaining specifically hybridized probe can be visualized by exposing the filter to X-ray film.

What results from these studies is a pattern of one or more bands on an X-ray film. Each band corresponds to a restriction endonuclease-generated DNA fragment containing nucleotide sequences complementary to those in the radioactive probe. For any particular gene probe, the size (i.e., length) of the band it identifies will be the same from individual to individual (see below for a discussion of restriction fragment length polymorphisms [RFLPs], an important exception). Therefore, if a gene has undergone a structural rearrangement, the pattern may change.

As an example, suppose that the c-abl probe ordinarily recognizes a 2000-base EcoRI fragment in normal genomic DNA. If the translocation break point in a chronic myelogenous leukemia (CML) patient occurs within that fragment, part of the c-abl gene and one of its EcoRI sites will move to chromosome 22 from chromosome 9. Southern blot analysis of the patient's DNA may now detect either (1) a larger fragment than normal if the recipient chromosome has an EcoRI site farther away than the old EcoRI site or (2) a smaller fragment if it has an EcoRI site closer than the old one. Southern blotting is thus a sensitive technique for detecting large structural rearrangements in the genome, such as those that are occasionally associated with malignancy.

Because the amount of the radiolabeled probe that hybridizes to a Southern blot is proportional to the number of copies of the specific gene present in the target DNA, this technique can also be used quantitatively. For example, in an analysis of primary breast

cancer tissue, Southern blotting was used to determine that 30% of these samples contained multiple copies of HER-2/neu oncogene DNA—that is to say, the gene was amplified.[23]

Polymerase chain reaction (PCR)

To detect gene sequences by Southern blotting, at least 1–2 mg of genomic DNA are required. This translates into several milligrams of tissue that must be used fresh or freshly frozen. PCR is a powerful technique that can be used to amplify specific fragments of DNA, thus lowering the theoretic limit of detectable DNA sequences in a sample to a single molecule of DNA. With some advance knowledge of the nucleotide sequences in the DNA to be detected, microscopically small amounts of tissue, even a single cell, contain enough DNA to be amplified, and the amplified DNA can be easily used for downstream analysis. Even fixed tissue in paraffin blocks or on slides can yield sufficient DNA for analysis using PCR.[24] The concepts underlying PCR are diagrammed in Figure 6. Two short single-stranded DNA fragments, called primers, are designed with sequences complementary to those that flank the stretch of DNA to be amplified. Primers and target DNA are mixed, the mixture is heated to dissociate the paired double strands of target DNA, and the temperature is then lowered to permit hybridization, or annealing, of the primers to their complementary sequences on the target DNA. A DNA polymerase enzyme is added to the mixture, which will add nucleotides to the 3′ end of the primers using the target DNA as a sequence template. This step generates one copy of each strand of one target DNA molecule. The mixture is heated again to dissociate the strands and then cooled to allow more primers to anneal to the target sequences on both the original and new pieces of DNA. DNA polymerase is added again and now generates four copies of the target sequences. These steps are

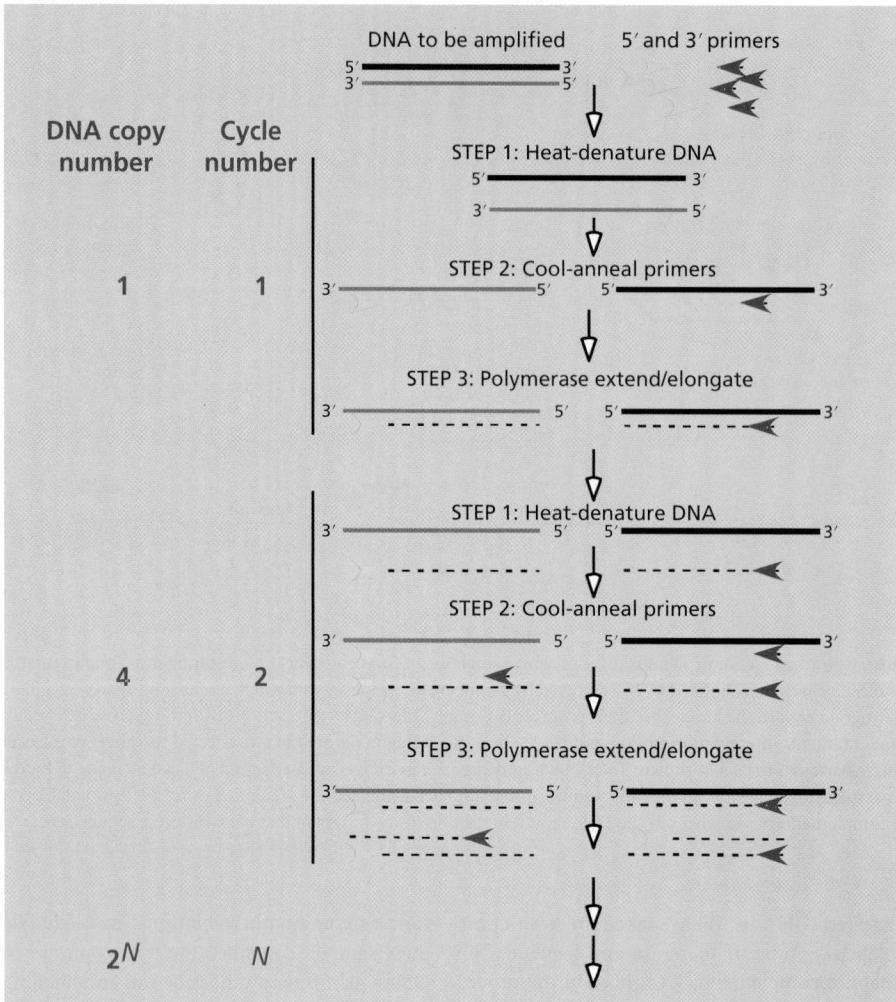

DNA copy number / Cycle number

1 / 1

4 / 2

2^N / N

Figure 6 Polymerase chain reaction. DNA is mixed with short (10–20 base) single-stranded oligonucleotide primers that are complementary to the 5′ and 3′ ends of the sequence to be amplified. The mixture is heated to denature or "melt" all double-stranded DNA and then cooled to permit the primers to anneal to their complementary sequences on the DNA to be amplified. Note that the 5′ primer will anneal to the lower strand and the 3′ primer will anneal to the upper strand. A heat-resistant (thermostable) DNA polymerase (Taq polymerase; see text) was present in the original mixture, and it now synthesizes DNA by starting at the primers and using the strands to which the primers are annealed as a template. This results in the formation of two double-stranded DNA copies for every molecule of double-stranded DNA in the original mixture. The reaction is then heated to melt double-stranded DNA and cooled to allow reannealing, and the polymerase makes new double-stranded DNA again. There are now four double-stranded DNA copies for each original DNA molecule. This process can be repeated times (usually 20–50) to result in 2n copies of double-stranded DNA.

repeated, resulting in a geometrically increasing amount of target DNA, that is, a chain reaction. With the discovery and cloning of the DNA polymerase from the thermophilic bacterium *Thermus aquati* (the "Taq polymerase"), which retains activity after being heated to 95°C, heating and cooling steps could be carried out on the same mixture without adding a new enzyme for each cycle.[25,26] This allowed the PCR procedure to be automated. There are now automated thermal cyclers in every molecular biology laboratory and in many clinical laboratories; these thermocyclers can take PCR mixtures through 20 to 50 cycles, producing large amounts of synthetic DNA from a tiny quantity of starting sample, to be used for subsequent analysis.

DNA polymorphisms

A genetic polymorphism (which literally means "many forms") is defined as the occurrence of two or more relatively common normal alleles for a single locus. The difference between a polymorphism and a mutation is that a polymorphism occurs more commonly and is associated with a normal variant phenotype. The usual distinction is that a gene is polymorphic when its least frequent manifestation appears in at least 1% of the population. Examples include blood types and major histocompatibility complex molecules.

Polymorphisms need not necessarily be associated with an obvious phenotype. For example, changes in nucleotide sequence within introns or in regions between genes would not necessarily result in altered proteins and could therefore be "silent." However, if these changes are polymorphic and frequent enough, then there is a high probability that an individual might be heterozygous for the polymorphism. In other words, it would be possible for the two chromosomes of a diploid pair to each carry a different version of the polymorphism. Then, if the chromosomal position of the polymorphic change were known, it could be used as a marker for mapping other genes. There are several varieties of DNA polymorphisms, and they provide the basis for gene mapping techniques that have identified the genomic locations of several important cancer genes.

RFLPs appear as differences among individuals in the pattern of bands on a Southern blot probed with a single cloned DNA.

There are two mechanisms whereby DNA polymorphisms are detectable by Southern blotting. First, a single nucleotide change might either create or destroy the recognition site for a restriction endonuclease. This would cause an alteration in the Southern blot pattern of that gene when the DNA is digested with a particular restriction endonuclease. For example, if a stretch of DNA with the sequence … AGGATTTCGA … in one individual contained a single nucleotide change in a second individual so that the sequence was … AGGAATTCGA … , the recognition site for EcoRI (GAATTC) would be created in the second individual. Digesting the second individual's DNA with EcoRI would generate two new restriction fragments and remove one old one when compared with the first individual's DNA (Figure 3).

The second mechanism of RFLP involves one of the more mysterious features of genomic DNA in eukaryotes, namely, that it is replete with repeated sequences of unknown function. The sequences often stretch themselves along the DNA polymer, one set of sequences after the other, in so-called tandem repeats. In humans, the best known repetitive sequence is called Alu (because it contains recognition sites for the restriction endonuclease AluI); its nucleotide sequence is so specific to humans that it can be used to identify human DNA in a mixture of DNAs from many species. In many cases, the number of tandem Alu repeats varies among individuals.[27] Therefore, if one does a Southern blot with a DNA probe that recognizes a restriction fragment containing tandem repeats, the size of that fragment may vary from one individual to the next. This type of RFLP is also called variable number of tandem repeats (VNTRs).

Both of these types of RFLPs are stably inherited in a Mendelian fashion, which permits them to be used in gene mapping. RFLPs occur at specific positions (loci) in genomic DNA. If all of the affected individuals in a family with a particular genetic disease inherit the same RFLP, there is presumptive evidence that the gene for the disease is close (or "linked") to the RFLP locus. Linking a disease locus to an RFLP maps the location of the gene for that disease and is the first step toward cloning the gene responsible for the disease. These are the tools of reverse genetics, which have also led to the identification of many of the genes associated with malignant transformation. A prime example is the BRCA1 gene on chromosome 17, whose mutations are responsible for a relatively significant fraction of heritable breast cancer.[28]

RFLPs have also been used to demonstrate gene loss in cancer (Figure 7a). This approach relies on an individual being heterozygous for an RFLP, that is, having one polymorphism on one chromosome and another polymorphism on the other. If an individual with cancer is heterozygous for a particular RFLP (termed an informative individual), his or her tumor can be analyzed by Southern blotting, using the probe that recognizes the polymorphism, and compared with normal tissue analyzed the same way. If one of the RFLPs present in the heterozygous individual's normal DNA is missing from the tumor cell DNA, the tumor is said to have undergone a reduction to homozygosity, or a loss of heterozygosity (LOH). This implies a loss of genetic material from the tumor, specifically the DNA that includes the missing RFLP. This is the hallmark of tumor suppressor genes, such as Retinoblastoma (Rb) or TP53.[29,30]

Another type of interesting type of polymorphism is known as a microsatellite. For unknown reasons, about 50,000 copies of the repetitive sequence dC-dA (tandemly repeated 10–60 times) are dispersed throughout the human genome.[31] Because the longer tandem repeats (VNTRs, as mentioned earlier) have been called minisatellite DNA, the shorter dC-dA repeats are called microsatellite DNA. (The term satellite refers to the fact that the buoyant density

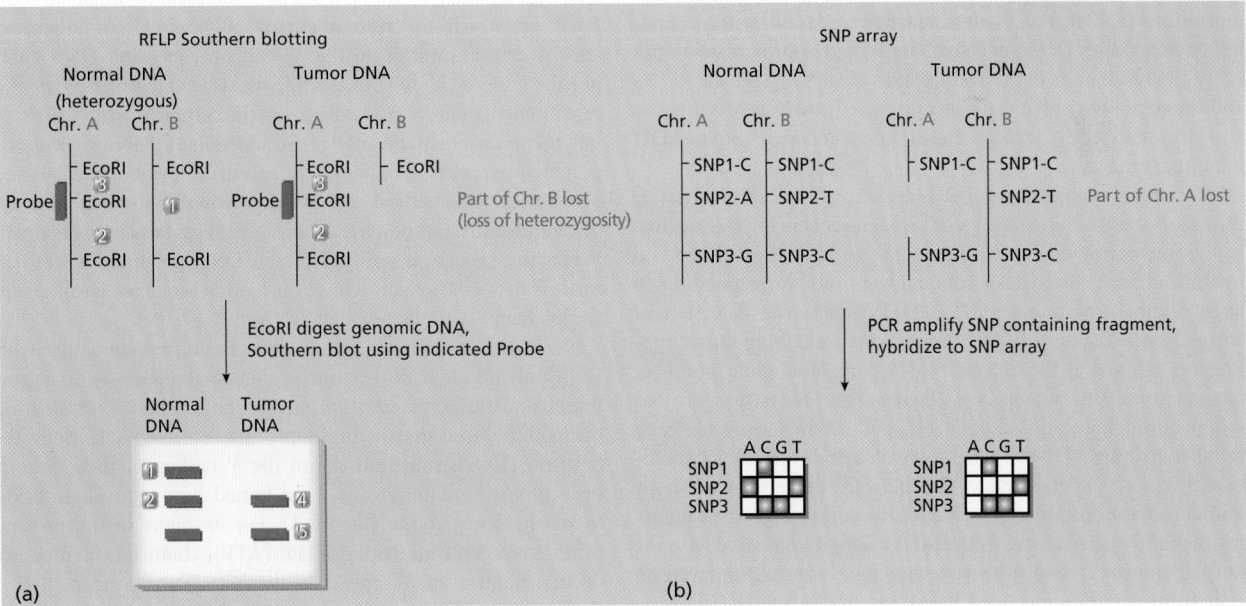

Figure 7 Methods to detect loss of heterozygosity in tumor tissue. (a) Restriction fragment length polymorphism (RFLP) and Southern blotting. In this example, an individual is heterozygous for an EcoRI recognition site: the second EcoRI site on chromosome A is absent on its diploid partner, chromosome B. The individual's tumor is assumed to be clonal and to have arisen from a cell that lost the region of chromosome B displayed in the figure. Southern blotting can then be performed using genomic DNA from the individual's normal DNA and tumor DNA in separate lanes of the agarose gel. Probing the DNA with the probe (indicated on the figure) reveals a heterozygous banding pattern in normal DNA (reflecting the presence of both polymorphisms, one on each chromosome pair) and a loss of that pattern in the tumor DNA. This is one of the hallmarks of a tumor suppressor gene. (b) Single nucleotide polymorphism (SNP) array. In this example, an individual is heterozygous for SNPs 2 and 3 and homozygous for SNP 1. Following the polymerase chain reaction (PCR) amplification of genomic fragments containing each SNP individually, these fragments are hybridized to an array composed of oligonucleotides complementary to the ones amplified. The loss of a heterozygous SNP signal on the array indicates loss of the chromosomal region containing this SNP.

of repetitive DNA is different from the majority of genomic DNA. This leads to the appearance of small satellite bands distinct from the main DNA band when genomic DNA is purified by density gradient centrifugation.) The number of repeats at a particular locus varies in a polymorphic way among individuals, and because these sequences are stably inherited, they can serve as polymorphic markers. The difference in the number of repeat units between two polymorphic microsatellites can be as small as a few nucleotides. These differences cannot be detected by Southern blotting, which has a resolution of 100 nt. However, these differences can easily be resolved using PCR. Primers that flank the repeat region are used in a PCR in the presence of radiolabeled deoxynucleotides, and the products are separated on a DNA-sequencing-style polyacrylamide gel. Mini- and microsatellite polymorphic markers are much more useful in gene mapping than RFLPs because, unlike RFLPs, which usually have only two alleles, the variable number of repeats creates multiple alleles for each locus, significantly raising the likelihood that an individual will be heterozygous for the marker.

Although the number of repeats in a microsatellite marker is usually stable, in some cancers, most notably colorectal cancer, the number of microsatellite repeats in the tumors differs from that in normal colorectal tissue from the same patient. Because the variability in repeat number occurs at all positions throughout the genome of the tumor, this suggests that the tumors experience overall genetic instability.[32,33] The basis of this instability is believed to be a mutation in the human homologs of DNA "proofreading" genes that, when mutated in yeast, lead to the appearance of unstable numbers of dCdA repeats. One of these human genes, MSH2, which maps to chromosome 2, is responsible for hereditary nonpolyposis colorectal cancer.[34,35]

Of course, a polymorphism need not create a restriction site, tandem repeat, or other obvious marker. Indeed, most common polymorphisms within the genome are so-called single nucleotide polymorphisms (SNPs).[36] SNPs are single base variations within a coding or noncoding DNA sequence; they occur approximately once every 1350 base pairs in the average individual.[37–39] Like the RFLPs and microsatellite polymorphisms discussed, analysis of SNPs can also be used to localize cancer-causing genes and to determine LOH in human cancers.

The major approach for LOH detection by SNP analysis is through the use of microarrays, or through sequencing (see below). In the microarray approach, genomic DNA is PCR amplified and hybridized to a microarray containing probes corresponding to large numbers of human SNPs. This permits the detection of chromosomal regions of LOH (i.e., regions containing tumor suppressors) as well as the detection of regions of amplification (i.e., regions containing oncogenes) (Figure 7b). SNP arrays provide a high-throughput and automatable method for large-scale copy number analysis.[40,41] Next-generation nucleotide sequencing methods (discussed in detail below) also allow for the inference of copy number alterations, which are characterized by changes in sequencing depth for a given locus in the cancer sample compared with the normal control.[42] Both of these technologies can be employed on cells from paraffin-embedded tissue specimens, thereby allowing genomic studies on standard pathologic specimens.[43]

Nucleotide sequencing

Sanger sequencing

The nucleotide sequence within a gene's coding region encodes the amino acid sequence of its corresponding protein. Thus, the nucleotide sequence of a gene can be used to predict the structure and function of its protein product. Historically, the major

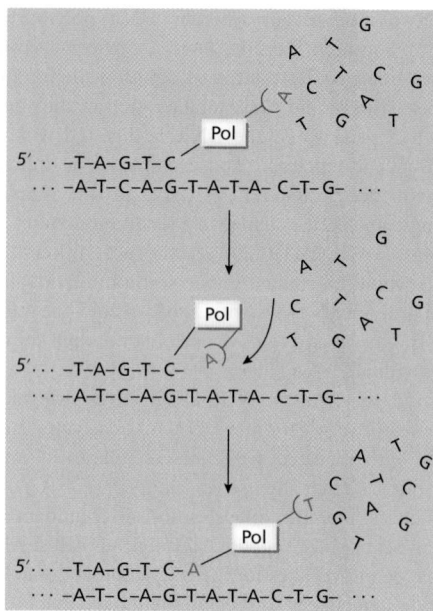

Figure 8 DNA polymerase. In this schematic, the enzyme DNA polymerase is creating a new DNA chain (upper strand) using a template (lower strand). Specific nucleotides are added from the 5′ to the 3′ direction as determined by the next nucleotide in the template.

method used for sequencing DNA has been the "enzymatic chain termination" method devised by Sanger and colleagues.[44] The chain termination method relies on properties of enzymes called *DNA polymerases* (Figure 8). These are enzymes that create new DNA polymers starting from individual nucleotides. However, for a DNA polymerase to work, it needs a template of single-stranded DNA on which to create the new polymer. DNA polymerase adds a new nucleotide to the 3′ end of a growing DNA chain, but the base of the new nucleotide must be able to base pair (i.e., be complementary) to the base on the template over which the polymerase is positioned. After the addition of that nucleotide, the polymerase moves to the next nucleotide on the template and adds a new nucleotide to the 3′ end of the growing chain. Again, the new nucleotide must be complementary to the next base in the template. When the process is completed, the DNA polymerase will have made a new DNA chain whose nucleotide sequence is completely complementary to the template DNA.

Nucleotide sequencing is based on the observation that when DNA polymerase adds a synthetic abnormal nucleotide to a growing chain, the polymerization stops. The synthetic "terminating" nucleotides used most commonly are dideoxynucleotides that have no alcohol substitutions on the 3′ carbon of their deoxyribose groups and thus cannot be joined by a phosphate bridge to the next nucleotide (Figure 2). For example, in the presence of dideoxyadenosine triphosphate (ATP), chain termination will occur wherever an A appears in the new DNA sequence (a T in the template) (Figure 9). These reactions are performed *in vitro* in a test tube, where millions of new DNA molecules are being made at once. If normal deoxy-ATP is mixed with dideoxy-ATP in the proper proportion, only a few of these molecules will terminate at each T in the template. This will generate a series of new DNA polymers, each one stretching from the beginning of the chain to the position of an A (i.e., a T in the template). If the newly formed DNA is fluorescently labeled, the products can be separated electrophoretically in a polyacrylamide gel or capillary gel (see below). Each step of the ladder is a fragment of DNA that stretches from

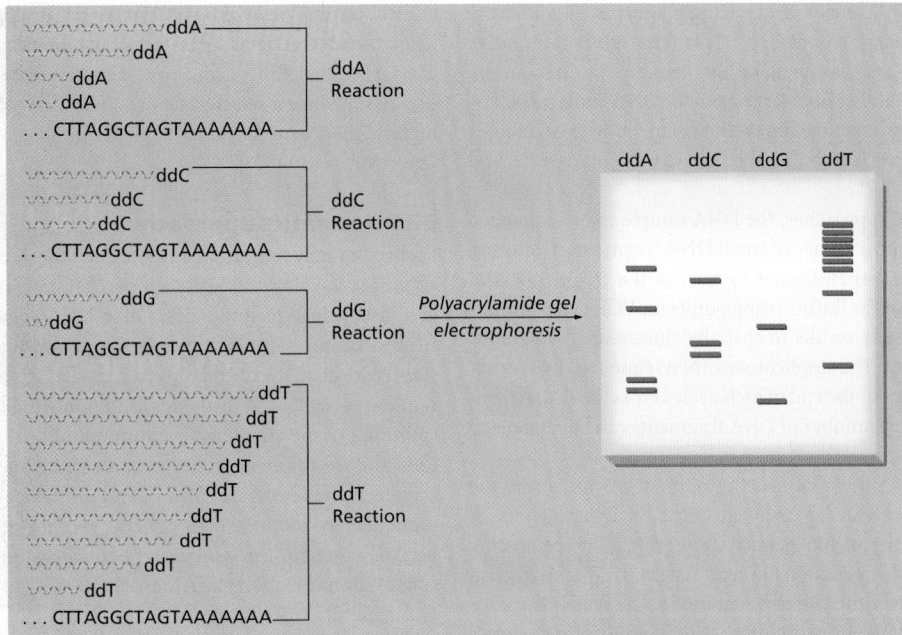

Figure 9 DNA sequencing using the chain termination method. In this example, DNA ending with the sequence CTTAGGCTAGTAAAAAAA is being analyzed. Four reactions are performed, each using this DNA as a template for a DNA polymerase reaction and each containing one of the four dideoxynucleotides (dideoxyadenosine triphosphate [ddA], dideoxycytidine triphosphate [ddC], dideoxyguanosine triphosphate [ddG], and dideoxythymidine triphosphate [ddT]). In each reaction, chain elongation will terminate when the dideoxynucleotide is incorporated at the position of its complementary nucleotide in the template. This will result in a family of chains of differing lengths that correspond to the position at which polymerization terminated. In this example, these chains can be resolved by electrophoresis through a urea-containing polyacrylamide gel, in which longer chains run near the top of the gel and shorter chains near the bottom. Each new chain is radioactively labeled, and after autoradiography, the pattern of bands can be read from X-ray film. By noting the order in which bands appear, starting at the bottom of the gel, one can read the sequence of the template by substituting the complement of each dideoxynucleotide at every position. Reading from the bottom yields GAATCCGATCATTTTTTT, and substituting the complementary base at each position yields CTTAGGCTAGTAAAAAAA, the sequence of the template. The use of fluorescent labels in capillary gel electrophoresis is conceptually similar.

the start of the new polymer to the position of an A. Four separate reactions are performed using each of the four dideoxynucleotides, each coded with a distinct fluorescent color. The four reactions are run together in a capillary gel, and the order of nucleotides is read by the order of the different colors.

Sanger sequencing has served as the backbone for a generation of biological discovery, and was instrumental to the Human Genome Project, which launched in 1990 and was completed in 2003. Following the successful assembly of the human genome sequence, genome researchers shifted their efforts from *de novo* to comparative sequencing. These studies have aimed to sequence the genome in both its normal and diseased states, with the aim of understanding the genomic changes associated with disease.

Perhaps the most active area of comparative sequencing has been in cancer genomics. Early sequencing studies targeted to particular genes or gene families identified key differences between the cancer and normal genomes; in many cases, these discoveries provided the rationale for targeted therapeutics. For example, the discovery of mutations in the c-kit protein tyrosine kinase gene by DNA sequencing of gastrointestinal stromal tumors (GISTs)[45] led to the successful treatment of GIST with the c-kit inhibitor STI-571 or Gleevec.[46] In lung adenocarcinoma, activating mutations in the epidermal growth factor receptor (*EGFR*) tyrosine kinase gene are common, especially in East Asian populations.[47–49] These activating mutations have been shown to predict response to the kinase inhibitors gefitinib and erlotinib.[47–49] Activating mutations in the *BRAF* serine-threonine kinase gene have been found in over half of all melanomas[50] and subsequently in other cancer

types, including colorectal, lung, and thyroid carcinomas. The *BRAF* inhibitor Vemurafenib leads to improved overall survival in patients with metastatic melanoma harboring an activating BRAF *V600E* mutation.[51] Mutations in the phosphatidylinositol 3-kinase catalytic subunit gene *PIK3CA* mutations have been discovered in colorectal carcinoma, glioblastoma,[52] and breast carcinomas. And in myeloproliferative diseases such as polycythemia vera, the *JAK2* V617F activating mutation is a pathognomonic finding.[53–55]

Next-generation sequencing

More recent cancer genomics studies have employed "next-generation" sequencing technologies, which far surpass traditional Sanger sequencing in throughput, scale, and resolution. Next-generation sequencing methods allow for millions of short-fragment sequencing reactions to proceed in parallel.[56–59] One of the biggest advantages of next-generation sequencing with respect to cancer genomics is the ability to effectively detect the numerous mutations present in a heterogeneous cancer sample,[60] without the need for purification of a clonal DNA template. Indeed, next-generation sequencing assays have become the technology of choice for cancer mutation detection in the research arena and are beginning to be incorporated in clinical diagnostic testing as well.

Next-generation sequencing was employed to sequence the first cancer genome, acute myeloid leukemia, in 2008.[61] Since then, the coding regions (exomes) or whole genomes of a number of other tumor types have been sequenced. Many of these efforts have been coordinated through the Cancer Genome Atlas (TCGA) and the International Cancer Genome Consortium (ICGC) initiatives.[64]

Most commercially available sequencing platforms fall under the category of "cyclic array sequencing." This term refers to iterative cycles of enzymatic-based sequencing and imaging-based sequence detection, done in parallel on a large array of DNA molecules.[58] A number of cyclic array sequencing methods currently exist, including those by Illumina (Solexa), Pacific Bio, 454/Roche, SOLiD, and Ion Torrent.

In all of the above approaches, the DNA sample to be sequenced is initially sheared into a library of small DNA fragments. Common adapter sequences are then ligated to each of the fragments, and these adapters are used as the initiating points for PCR-based amplification. This ultimately results in spatially clustered clonal amplicons of each fragment. The amplicons are then sequenced by synthesis, with imaging done at the end of each cycle across the entire array. In this manner, a large number of DNA fragments can be sequenced in parallel in a high-throughput fashion.[58]

Each of the cyclic array sequencing approaches differs in the method used to generate spatially-clustered PCR amplicons of DNA fragments and in the biochemistry underlying the sequencing process. There are also variations in read length, throughput, cost, and accuracy between the different methods. Currently, the Illumina sequencing platform is the most widely used for a majority of applications.[62] Illumina sequencing generates clonal amplicons through a method known as "bridge PCR." In this method, forward and reverse primers complementary to the adapter sequences are immobilized to a glass slide. PCR-based amplification results in a spatial cluster of approximately 1000 copies of each DNA fragment. Cyclic sequencing then occurs. In each cycle of sequencing, a DNA polymerase incorporates fluorescently labeled dNTPs with a reversible 3′ termination moiety. Similar to the Sanger sequencing concept, the 3′ termination moiety allows only a single base to be added to each fragment. All fragments (or "features") are then imaged in four colors, with each color corresponding to one of the dNTP species. The reversible 3′ termination moiety is then cleaved, and then next cycle of sequencing begins anew. At the end of this process, one is able to obtain the DNA sequence for each of the many fragments, all sequenced in parallel (Figure 10).[58]

Target enrichment and clinical panel testing
While the methodology described above can be used to sequence an entire genome, this is not always technically or computationally feasible, cost-effective, or necessary. "Target enrichment" refers to the process whereby a nucleotide library is enriched for particular genomic regions of interest prior to sequencing. Target enrichment can be performed through a variety of methods, including PCR, molecular inversion, and hybrid capture; hybrid capture has emerged as the most popular method in most situations. An excellent review is available on this topic.[63]

In hybrid-capture target enrichment, oligonucleotide probes for genomic regions of interest are hybridized to a fragmented DNA library, and nonbinding fragments are washed away. The hybridization reaction may occur either on a surface (i.e., a slide) or in solution. In cancer genomics, hybrid capture technology is commonly used to reduce a full genome library to only those fragments that correspond to "exomes," or the protein-coding genomic regions. So-called whole-exome sequencing reduces the total amount of DNA to be sequenced from 3 Gb to 30 Mb. This reduces computational demands, cost, and sequencing time while still elucidating the majority of somatic mutations likely to occur in human cancers.[63,64]

As next-generation sequencing has decreased in cost and increased in reliability, it is being increasingly incorporated into clinical testing. Several institution-specific and commercially marketed targeted gene panel tests are currently available. These panels use target enrichment and next-generation sequencing technologies to sequence a selected set of cancer-driving genes with the aim of providing genomic data likely to influence prognostication or choice of therapy.

Bioinformatics approaches
Perhaps equally important as the sequencing technologies described above are the bioinformatics approaches for analyzing the data generated by those technologies. Once DNA sequences are obtained from a tumor sample and a matched germline control, the first step is to quality control the raw reads by removing low-quality sequences (usually at read ends) and removing the sequences corresponding to the adapters. The tumor and normal sample reads are then aligned to the reference genome using one of several available sequence alignment algorithms, and differences from the reference sequence are identified. In general, bioinformatics tools are then used to assess for three major types of alterations: single nucleotide substitutions or small insertion-deletions, copy number alterations, and structural rearrangements (Figure 11).[42,64]

Single-nucleotide substitutions and small insertion-deletions
A single-nucleotide substitution or small insertion-deletion ("indel") is detected as a change in the tumor sequence that varies in frequency from the germline control and from the reference genome. For example, germline mutations are generally found in a frequency of either 50% (if heterozygous) or 100% (if homozygous), but single-base substitutions within a tumor sample may be found at a range of frequencies, depending on the mutant allele fraction within the tumor tissue, the purity of the tumor sample, and the ploidy of the tumor. Ultimately, mutation calling is a statistical task and is based in the statistical significance of the number of mutation counts in the cancer sequence compared with the matched normal.[42,64] A number of somatic mutation calling tools exist, including MuTect,[65] Varscan2,[66] JointSNVMix,[67] and MutSigCV.[68] These and other mutation callers differ in their precise methodologies, but the general goal of all of them is to apply statistical methods to detect somatic mutations with low allele fractions with a high degree of specificity. The major causes of missed mutation calls include tumor admixture with normal tissue, intratumoral heterogeneity, and differences in ploidy. A fundamental advantage of next-generation sequencing over Sanger sequencing is that it is digital, rather than analog. This means that the same stretch of DNA can be read multiple times, allowing for "oversampling" or sufficient depth of coverage necessary to confidently call somatic alterations at a statistically significant level.[42,64]

Copy-number variations
Next-generation sequencing affords the ability to interrogate copy-number changes at single-nucleotide levels, a significant increase in resolution over array-based technologies. In simplistic terms, copy number can be inferred from next-generation sequencing data by comparing the number of reads at a locus in the tumor sample to that in the normal control. Several bioinformatics tools for inferring copy number from next-generation sequencing data exist. These tools take into account the fact that copy-number reads within a given window must be normalized for sequence coverage in that region. This is critical, since coverage can vary across the genome based on GC content, ambiguously mapped reads, and other factors.[64,69]

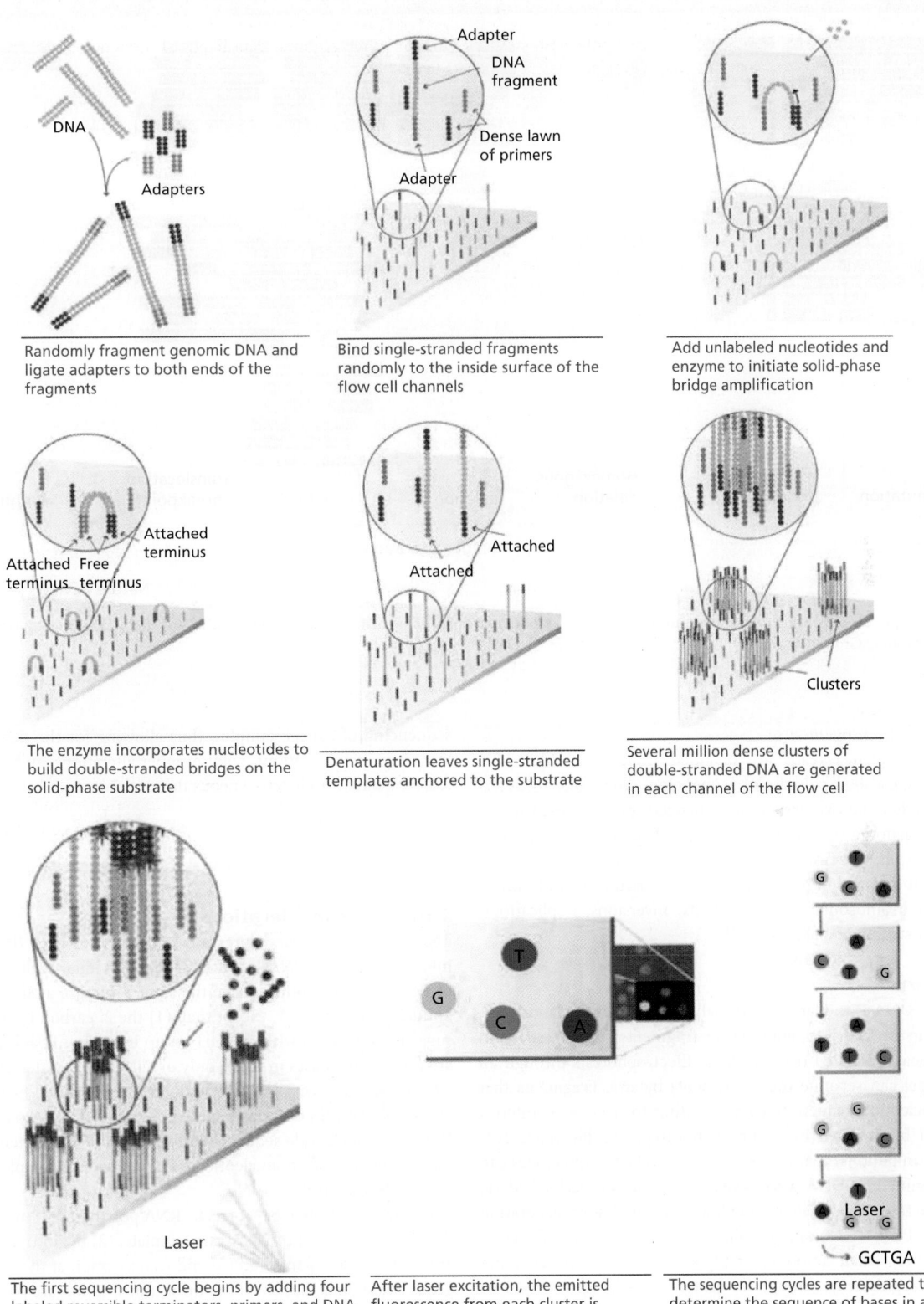

Randomly fragment genomic DNA and ligate adapters to both ends of the fragments

Bind single-stranded fragments randomly to the inside surface of the flow cell channels

Add unlabeled nucleotides and enzyme to initiate solid-phase bridge amplification

The enzyme incorporates nucleotides to build double-stranded bridges on the solid-phase substrate

Denaturation leaves single-stranded templates anchored to the substrate

Several million dense clusters of double-stranded DNA are generated in each channel of the flow cell

The first sequencing cycle begins by adding four labeled reversible terminators, primers, and DNA polymerase

After laser excitation, the emitted fluorescence from each cluster is captured and the first base is identified

The sequencing cycles are repeated to determine the sequence of bases in a fragment, one base at a time

Figure 10 Next generation sequencing using Illumina platform. Source: http://openwetware.org/images/d/de/Illumina_sequencing.pdf. Used under CC BY-SA 3.0 http://creativecommons.org/licenses/by-sa/3.0/.

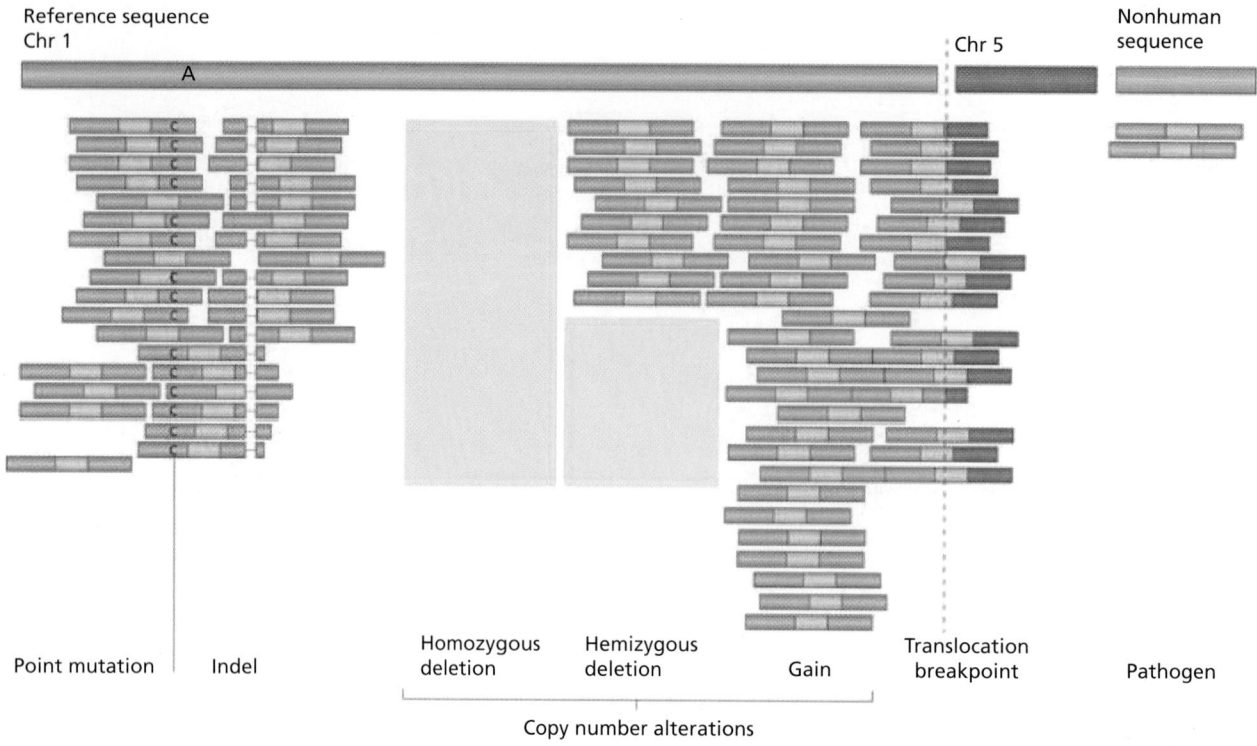

Reference sequence
Chr 1

Chr 5

Nonhuman
sequence

| Point mutation | Indel | Homozygous deletion | Hemizygous deletion | Gain | Translocation breakpoint | Pathogen |

Copy number alterations

Nature Reviews | Genetics

Figure 11 Types of genome alterations that can be detected by second-generation sequencing. Source: Meyerson 2010.[42] Reproduced with permission of Nature Publishing Group.

Structural rearrangements

Typically, sequence reads are obtained from both sides of a sequence. So-called paired-end sequencing allows one to determine whether the two ends of a sequenced fragment map to the reference genome at an expected distance from each other. When reads are "split," the two ends of the read map to distinct parts of the genome. Interrogation of split reads can be used to identify intra- and interchromosomal rearrangements, inversions, duplications, and other structural changes.[42,70,71]

Summary

Genomic DNA is too large to be analyzed easily in the laboratory, but it can be cut into manageable fragments using restriction endonucleases isolated from bacteria. Electrophoresis through an agarose gel can separate these fragments by size. Fragments that carry nucleotide sequences corresponding to a gene of interest can then be detected by Southern blotting. Specific nucleotide changes (mutations) that give rise to stable genetic differences can be determined by DNA sequencing, which can be performed via either the traditional "Sanger" method or through next-generation methods. PCR technology permits the detection of specific genes in extremely small amounts of tissue. There are various types of polymorphic sites throughout genomic DNA; some create or destroy restriction endonuclease sites leading to RFLPs; others contain a variable number of tandemly repeated sequences and are called microsatellites; a third group, SNPs, represents single base variations. Nucleotide polymorphisms can be interrogated by microarray technology or next-generation sequencing methods to allow for gene mapping and cancer diagnostics. Next-generation sequencing can be used for high-throughput and high-resolution sequencing of cancer samples, thus allowing for the detection of low-frequency mutations, copy-number alterations, and structural rearrangements in heterogeneous tumor tissue.

Gene expression: mRNA transcript analysis

Structural considerations

The first step in gene expression is transcription of the genetic information from DNA into RNA. The individual building blocks of RNA, ribonucleotides, have the same structure as the deoxyribonucleotides in DNA, except that: (1) the 2′ carbon of the ribose sugar is substituted with an -OH group instead of H and (2) there are no thymine bases in RNA, only uracil (demethylated thymine), which also pairs with adenine by hydrogen bonding. Just like the DNA polymerases described earlier, the enzyme RNA polymerase II uses the nucleotide sequence of the gene's DNA as a template to form a polymer of ribonucleotides with a sequence complementary to the DNA template.

For transcription to be "correct," RNA polymerase II must (1) use the antisense strand of DNA as a template, (2) begin transcription at the start of the gene, and (3) end transcription at the end of the gene. The signals that ensure faithful transcription are provided to the RNA polymerase II by DNA in the form of specific nucleotide sequences in the promoter of the gene. After reading and interpreting these signals, the RNA polymerase generates a primary RNA transcript that extends from the initiation site to the termination site in a perfect complementary match to the DNA sequence used as a template. However, not all transcribed RNA is destined to arrive in the cytoplasm as mRNA. Rather, sequences complementary to introns are excised from the primary transcript, and the ends of exon sequences are joined together in a process termed splicing.[72] In addition to splicing, the primary transcript is further modified by the addition of a methylated guanosine triphosphate "cap" at the 5′ end[73] and by the addition of a stretch of anywhere from 20 to 40 adenosine bases at the 3′ end (poly-A tail).[74] These modifications appear to promote the translatability[75,76] and relative stability of mRNAs and help direct the subcellular localization of mRNAs destined for translation.

Northern blotting

The fundamental question in the analysis of gene expression at the RNA level is whether RNA sequences derived from a gene of interest are present in a cell type of interest under conditions of interest. Detecting specific RNA sequences can be accomplished by Northern blotting, the whimsically named RNA analog of Southern blotting. RNA can be isolated from cells in its intact form, free from significant amounts of DNA.[77] mRNA is much smaller than genomic DNA, so it can be analyzed by agarose gel electrophoresis without the enzymatic digestion steps that are necessary for the analysis of high-molecular-weight DNA.

RNA is single stranded and has a tendency to fold back on itself. This allows complementary bases on the same stretch of RNA to base pair with each other and to form what is termed secondary structure. Because secondary structure can lead to aberrant electrophoretic behavior, RNA is electrophoretically separated by size in the presence of a denaturing agent, such as formaldehyde or glyoxal/dimethyl sulfoxide. After electrophoresis through a denaturing agarose gel, the RNA is transferred to a nitrocellulose or nylon-based membrane in the same manner as DNA for Southern blotting (Figure 5). Hybridization schemes and blot washing are essentially the same for Northern blotting as for Southern blotting. In this manner, specific RNA sequences corresponding to those in cloned DNA probes can easily be identified.

There is a lower limit to the sensitivity of Northern blotting so that only moderately abundant mRNAs can be detected using this technique. One way to increase the sensitivity of Northern blotting is to enrich the RNA preparation for mRNA. Ordinarily, mRNA makes up <10% of the total RNA content of a cell or tissue; the remainder is made up primarily of ribosomal RNA and transfer RNA. An RNA preparation can be enriched for mRNA species by removing all RNA molecules that lack the 3 poly(A) tail.[78] This can be done by exposing the RNA preparation to a tract of poly(U) or poly(T) bound to an immobilized support, such as a plastic bead. The poly(A) portion of mRNA will bind to the poly(U) or poly(T) material, and non-poly(A)-containing RNA can be washed away. After washing, the poly(A)-containing mRNA can be recovered from the solid support and used in Northern blot analysis. This procedure improves the sensitivity of Northern blotting by nearly two orders of magnitude.

A dramatic use of Northern blotting in cancer research has been the demonstration of oncogene expression in some human tumors. RNA was isolated from human tumor samples and analyzed by Northern blotting using cloned DNA probes derived from various oncogenes. The earliest observations included expression of c-abl and c-myc in human tumor cell lines and leukemic blasts.[79,80] Since these early discoveries, a large number of proto-oncogenes have been shown to be transcribed in primary human tumor tissue.

Complementary deoxyribonucleic acid

The flow of genetic information usually runs from DNA to RNA to protein, according to the so-called central dogma of molecular biology. There are, however, exceptions to this rule, the most prominent

of which involves the life cycle of retroviruses. These viruses encode their genetic information in RNA rather than in DNA. When they invade a susceptible host cell, they direct the synthesis of a DNA intermediate that is a complementary copy of their genomic RNA. The enzyme that accomplishes this task, reverse transcriptase, is a DNA polymerase (see above) that uses RNA, rather than DNA, as a template to form a cDNA copy of the RNA.[81,82] This enzyme can be used *in vitro* to make cDNA copies of any available RNA.

One important application of cDNA synthesis has been the construction of cDNA libraries, which are basically gene libraries consisting only of the genes that are expressed in a cell or tissue of interest.[83,84] Most of the time, one is not really concerned with all of the DNA in the genome, as a large proportion of the cell's DNA is composed of intronic sequences, promoters, and vast regions of "noncoding" DNA that lies between genes. Therefore, one way to construct a library comprising only tissue-specific expressed genes is to clone all of the mRNA in a specific cell or tissue of interest. Practically speaking, this is done by using all of the mRNA in a cell as a template for making double-stranded cDNA, which can then be inserted into a cloning vector.

To make a cDNA library, one isolates all of the mRNA from a cell or tissue. Then, using this mRNA as a template, reverse transcriptase is used to make cDNA copies of each mRNA molecule in the mixture. The cDNA is ligated into a plasmid or phage vector as described earlier (Figure 3), and the recombinant vectors are introduced into bacteria. After growth on agar plates, each bacterial colony or phage plaque of a cDNA library houses a unique recombinant vector containing the cDNA copy of a single mRNA transcript. Desired clones can be detected by nucleic acid hybridization to the plaques or colonies using a radiolabeled gene probe.[85,86] Alternatively, if the vector containing the cDNA molecules can direct transcription of mRNA by host bacterial cells, mRNA will be synthesized, and that mRNA will be translated. In this case, each bacterial colony or plaque will produce a different protein, and each protein will have been encoded by an mRNA from the original cell or tissue being investigated. If an antibody directed against a protein of interest is available, the cDNA clone corresponding to the mRNA that encodes that protein can be identified by binding the antibody to the colonies or plaques of the cDNA library. This technique, called expression cloning, often employs the bacteriophage λgt11 as the cloning vector.[87]

cDNA libraries can be used to clone cDNA for a known gene to discover the sequence of the mRNA it encodes. One application of this is the generation of expressed sequence tag databases by sequencing clones of various cDNA libraries. Alternatively, cDNA libraries can also be used to identify previously unknown genes. In a process called differential screening, cDNAs that owe their existence to a particular differentiation or activation state in the cell of origin can be discovered. For example, this technique has been used to identify genes whose expression is turned on by hormones or by growth factors.[88]

Sequence-based gene expression profiling

The most comprehensive way to display a unique pattern of gene expression that determines the identity of a cell or tissue would be to construct a cDNA library from it and sequence every clone. This was originally thought to be an impossible task and, historically, a technique called serial analysis of gene expression (SAGE) was developed to approximate this goal. In SAGE, the investigator sequences a small and unique fragment (10–17 nucleotides in length) of each expressed gene (called a SAGE tag) and quantifies the number of

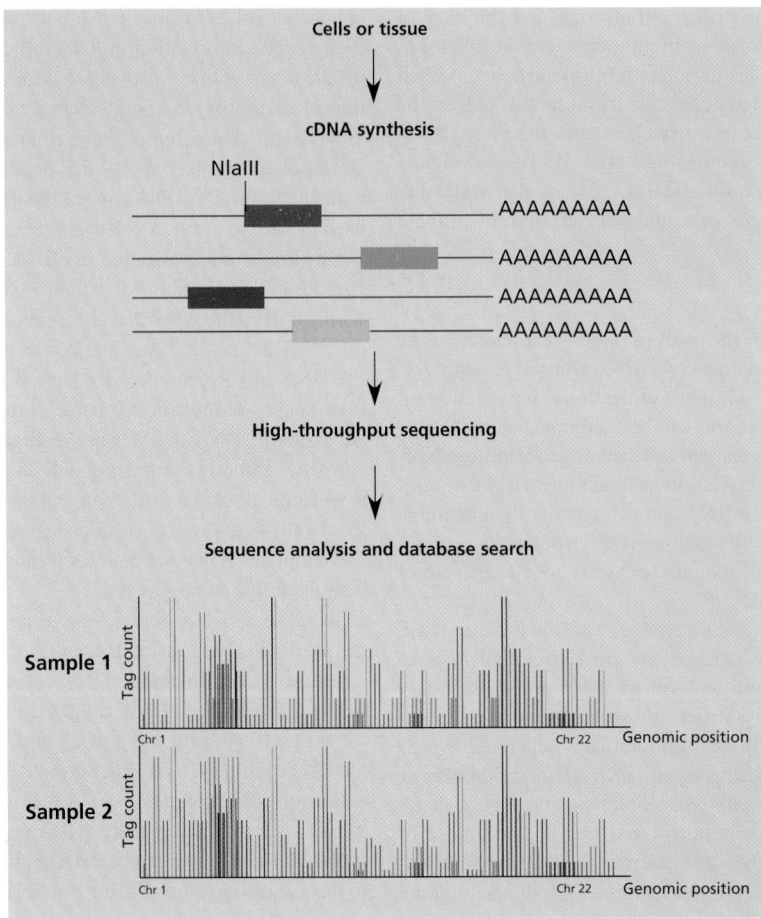

Figure 12 Construction and analysis of serial analysis of gene expression (SAGE) libraries. In step 1, a complementary deoxyribonucleic acid (cDNA) library is constructed from the cells or tissue of interest, and the cDNAs are immobilized on magnetic beads at their three ends. In step 2, the cDNAs are subjected to restriction enzyme digestion with a so-called anchoring enzyme. This anchoring enzyme is a frequent cutter restriction endonuclease (usually NlaIII) that ensures that all of the cDNAs are cut at least once. Subsequently another linker that contains a recognition site for a tagging enzyme is ligated to the cDNA ends. This tagging enzyme is a type two restriction endonuclease (usually MmeI) that cuts at some distance to the three sides of the actual recognition site. These tags are then directly processed for single-molecule DNA sequencing platform. Data are analyzed by using software that reads the sequence obtained, derives the tags, matches them to their cognate cDNA, and gives the gene expression profile in a numeric format.

times it appears (called the SAGE tag number). The SAGE tag numbers, therefore, directly reflect the abundance of the corresponding transcript.

The sensitivity and the quantitative accuracy of SAGE are theoretically unlimited. The generation of a SAGE library does not require any prior knowledge of what genes are expressed in the cell of interest. Therefore, SAGE is able to detect and quantify the expression of previously uncharacterized genes.

The generation of a SAGE library used to be a technically challenging multistep procedure that has been described in detail elsewhere.[89] However, it has become much more feasible with (and, in many cases, has been replaced by) the emergence of single-molecule sequencing platforms.[56] Figure 12 outlines the essence of the method.

SAGE has been used for the comparison of gene expression profiles of different cell types from normal and tumor tissue[90] and is one of the techniques that was used by the National Cancer Institute–funded Cancer Gene Anatomy Project (CGAP),[91] an international database aimed at cataloging the genes expressed in various normal and cancerous tissue types. SAGE libraries generated as part of the CGAP project are deposited on the National Center for Biotechnology Education/CGAP SAGE map Web site (http://cgap.nci.nih.gov/SAGE).[91,92]

DNA microarray analysis

Another approach to comparative gene expression profiling employs the use of DNA microarrays, often referred to as DNA chips. Two basic types of DNA microarrays are currently available: oligonucleotide arrays[93,94] and cDNA arrays.[95,96] Both approaches involve the immobilization of DNA sequences in a gridded array on the surface of a solid support, such as a glass microscope slide or a silicon wafer. In the case of oligonucleotide arrays, 25-nt-long fragments of known DNA sequence are synthesized *in situ* on the surface of the chip using a series of light-directed coupling reactions similar to photolithography. Using this method, as many as 400,000 distinct sequences representing over 18,000 genes can be synthesized on a single 1.3 × 1.3 cm microarray. In the case of cDNA microarrays, cDNA fragments are deposited onto the surface of a glass slide using a robotic spotting device. For both microarray approaches, the next step involves the purification of RNA from the source of interest (e.g., from a tumor), enzymatic fluorescent labeling of the RNA, and hybridization of the fluorescently labeled material to the microarray. Hybridization events are then captured by scanning the surface of the microarray with a laser-scanning device and measuring the fluorescence intensity at each position in the microarray. The fluorescence intensity of each spot on the array

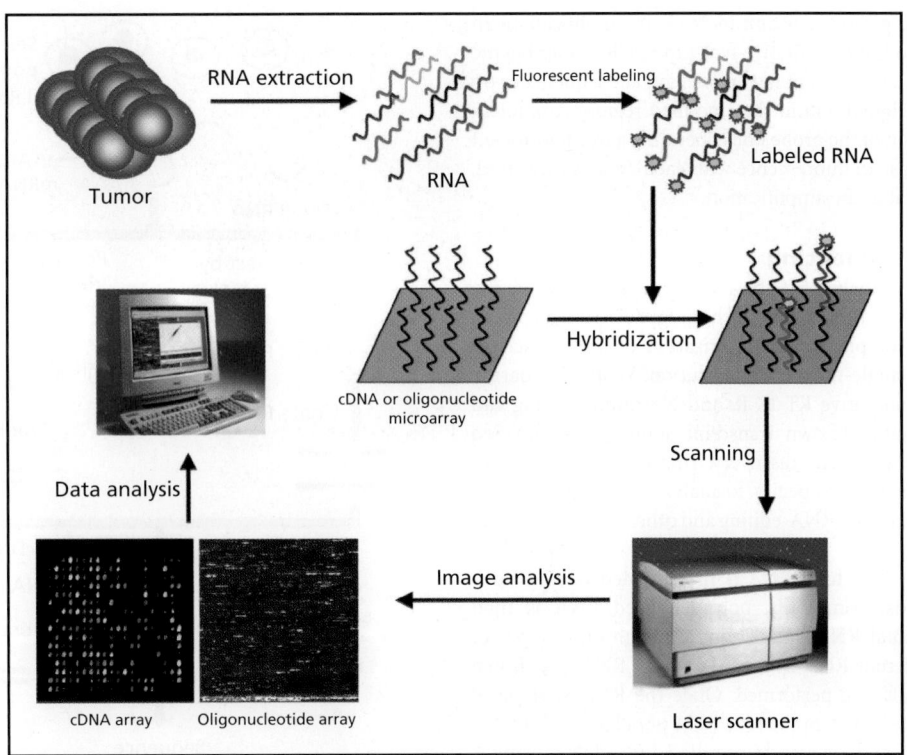

Figure 13 DNA microarray analysis. In this example, RNA extracted from a tumor is end labeled with a fluorescent marker and then allowed to hybridize to a chip derivatized with complementary DNA (cDNAs) or oligonucleotides, as described in the text. The precise location of RNA hybridization to the chip can be determined using a laser scanner. Because the position of each unique cDNA or oligonucleotide is known, the presence of a cognate RNA for any given unique sequence can be determined.

is proportional to the level of expression of the gene represented by that spot. This process is illustrated in Figure 13.

Microarray analysis has proved to be a powerful method for the analysis of gene expression patterns in human cancer and for cancer classification. Gene expression profiles have been used for class prediction, for determining which samples belong to which tumor class, and for class discovery of new tumor types. The first proof of principle for gene expression analysis in cancer was the demonstration that acute myeloid leukemias and acute lymphoid leukemias could be accurately distinguished on the basis of their gene expression profile[97] Since then, new cancer classes have been discovered in leukemias,[98] lymphomas,[99,100] brain cancer,[101] breast cancer,[102,103] prostate cancer,[104,105] lung cancer,[106,107] and others.

The challenge in interpreting microarray data is in recognizing meaningful gene expression patterns and in distinguishing those patterns from noise. Such noise (random gene expression levels) can be generated by (1) variability among microarrays, (2) variability in RNA labeling and hybridization methods, and, perhaps most importantly (3) biologic variability among samples. It is likely that all of the above sources of variability are significant. Many of the problems associated with array-based technologies are eliminated with the use of sequence-based methods described below in the section titled "Transcriptomic Sequencing". Thus, as sequencing technologies have improved and become more affordable and widely available, microarray technology has become less used.

Reverse-transcriptase polymerase chain reaction (RT-PCR)

Another important use of cDNA technology has allowed PCR to be applied to RNA. Because the Taq polymerase is a DNA polymerase (see above), it cannot use RNA as a template. Therefore, simply

adding primers and Taq polymerase to an RNA preparation will not result in amplification. However, if an RNA of interest is made into cDNA, then PCR can proceed as usual.

The first step in this analysis is generating a cDNA copy of the mRNA of interest using reverse transcriptase. This can be done using a primer consisting of Ts (complementary to the poly(A) tail) or of another sequence complementary to some portion of the 3′ region of the mRNA. Once the single-stranded cDNA is produced, it can be amplified in a standard PCR reaction using Taq polymerase as described earlier (Figure 6). In one of the first applications of this technique, Philadelphia-chromosome-positive leukemias were diagnosed by identifying chimeric bcr-abl mRNA species in clinical material using PCR. Since then, so-called reverse transcriptase polymerase chain reaction (RT-PCR) has come into widespread clinical and laboratory use.[108]

One inherent problem in using standard PCR to monitor mRNA expression is quantitation of the amplified PCR products. In Northern blotting analysis, the intensity of the hybridization signal is directly proportional to the amount of target RNA in the sample. Thus, one can compare the number of RNA molecules in one sample with another. With PCR, however, a slight change in the efficiency of polymerization in an early cycle in one sample will lead to a geometrically increasing discrepancy between the amount of amplified product in that sample compared with another sample, and the amounts of PCR product when the reaction reaches saturation can also differ significantly. Fortunately, a number of techniques have been described for normalizing the products of PCRs to allow quantitative comparisons.

Most notably, quantitative real-time PCR[109] is a method for continuous monitoring of amplification. This method makes quantitative comparisons of amplifications during the unbiased linear range in which each cycle gives a constant increase in amplification. In one common method of quantitative real-time PCR, a fluorogenic probe that contains a fluorescent tag on one end and a quencher on the other end is designed within the amplified region. Amplification leads to digestion of the probe, thus liberating a free fluorescent molecule; the increase in fluorescence with each cycle is measured, and it is proportional to the amplification.

Transcriptomic sequencing

A major advance in analysis of the transcriptome has been the development of RNA-sequencing technology. RNA-sequencing (RNA-Seq) allows for precise characterization of the transcripts present in a cell at single-nucleotide resolution. While microarray analysis, SAGE, quantitative RT-PCR, and Northern blotting can all be used to quantify known transcript abundance, RNA-Seq also allows for *novel* transcript discovery. This affords the ability to discover new classes of RNA species, to analyze alternative-splicing patterns, and to interrogate RNA-editing and other RNA-processing events.

To perform RNA-Seq, total RNA is first isolated from a sample of interest. Most commonly, polyadenylated RNA is then selected from the total RNA population, although other types of enrichment for different RNA species (i.e. small RNAs, as shown in Figure 14) can also be performed. Once the RNA subtype of interest has been selected from the total RNA population, this RNA is then fragmented and reverse transcribed into cDNA using a reverse transcriptase. Once cDNA is produced, it can be amplified and sequenced using the next-generation platforms described above. Typically, 50–200 million short reads are produced from an RNA-Seq run, with most read lengths in the 50–250 bp range (Figure 14).[110]

After these short RNA sequences have been obtained, they must be "assembled" to reconstruct the transcripts that comprise the transcriptome. This is usually done by aligning the reads to a reference genome. The use of paired-end reads—or fragments that are sequenced from both ends—allows for higher quality sequencing data, and is more likely to produce faithful alignments to the reference genome. Read alignments are then assembled into transcript models using computational methods, and expression levels of individual transcripts are then quantified. A common unit used to quantify transcript expression level is "RPKM," or reads per kilobase per million mapped reads.[111–113]

RNA-Seq offers the ability to quantify transcript abundance, as well as the opportunity to identify unannotated transcripts, splice variants, gene fusions, nonhuman transcripts, and somatic mutations, among other events. This is a significant advantage over microarray analysis, which is limited by a defined set of predesigned probes.[110] Therefore, RNA-Seq has begun to supplant microarray technology as a method for studying transcriptomes.

Clinical application of gene expression profiling

A number of gene-expression-profiling-based diagnostic tests have been approved by the Federal Drug Administration (FDA), and these are increasingly being incorporated into the clinical management of patients diagnosed with early-stage breast cancer.[114,115] Examples include the Oncotype DX,[116] Mammaprint,[117] PAM50,[118] and the H : I ratio Breast Cancer Index.[119] Each of these tests uses the expression level of a set of genes (ranging in number from two genes in the Breast Cancer Index to 70 genes in the Mammaprint assay) to provide prognostic information about a patient's breast cancer recurrence risk. These and other expression-based tests vary in their clinical utility, indications, and diagnostic validity. Of these tests, the Oncotype DX, or 21-gene recurrence score, is

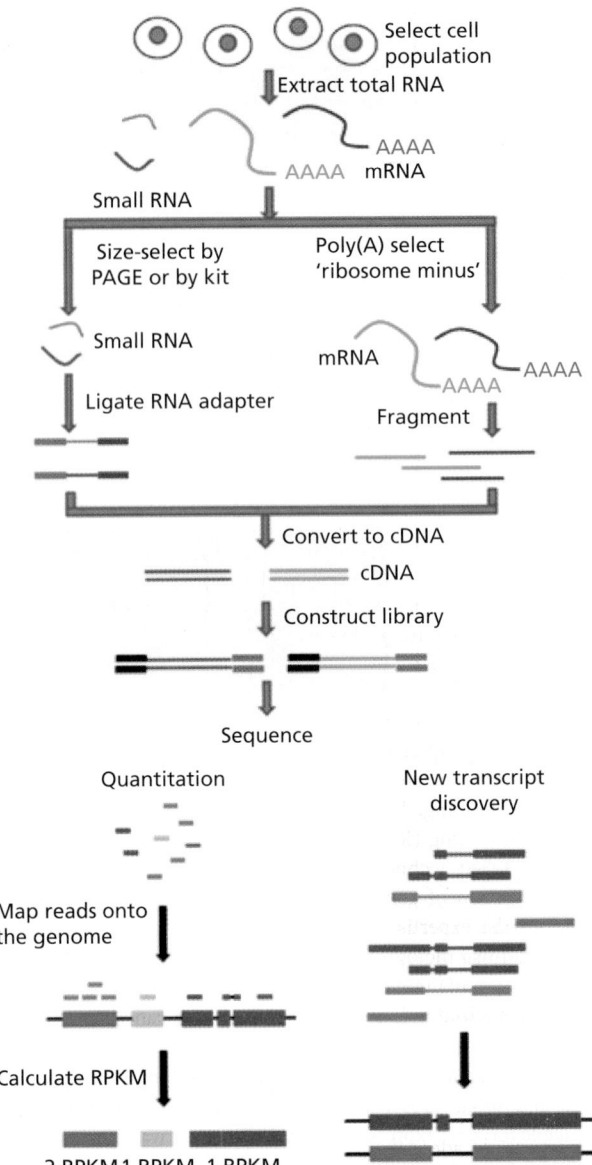

Figure 14 RNA-seq work flow. Source: Zeng 2012.[110] Reproduced with permission of Nature Publishing Group. RPKM, reads per kilobase per million mapped reads.

the most widely used and has been incorporated into management guidelines from the American Society of Clinical Oncology (ASCO).

The Oncotype DX score was developed on the basis of testing of the expression of a candidate gene set (250 cancer-related genes) by quantitative real-time PCR in fixed tissue from a large number of patients collected from three different datasets. The score was then validated in an independent dataset derived from samples banked on the NSABP B-14 trial, a large prospective randomized trial designed to test the benefit of adjuvant tamoxifen in hormone-receptor-positive, node-negative breast cancer.[116] It was found that a gene signature composed of 21 genes predicted 10-year breast cancer recurrence. The expression levels of these 21 genes measured by quantitative RT-PCR are fed into an algorithm and used to produce a number between 0 and 100, which is termed the recurrence score. The recurrence score is categorized into low (score <18), intermediate (score >18 but <30), and high (score

≥30). Several follow-up studies in various cohorts have confirmed that the Oncotype DX recurrence score is among the best-validated prognostic assays available. It is currently used to guide prognosis in women with node-negative, estrogen receptor (ER)-positive breast cancer, and to inform the decision about whether these women are likely to glean benefit from adjuvant chemotherapy. In practice, those women with a low recurrence score have a favorable prognosis and are unlikely to derive a significant absolute benefit from adjuvant chemotherapy.

As more and more genomic and transcriptomic data is generated and curated, there has been increasing effort placed on developing molecular prognostic tests for a variety of tumor types. It is important to carefully consider the clinical utility, exact indications, and precisely defined patient population for application of these tests. At present, the molecular prognostic profiles available can supplement, but not replace, clinical prognostic factors.

Summary

The genetic information in DNA is copied, or transcribed, into mRNA by the enzyme RNA polymerase II. Before being transported to the cytoplasm, primary transcripts in the nucleus are modified by splicing out introns, adding a 5′ cap and adding a 3′ poly(A) tail. A retroviral enzyme called reverse transcriptase can be used to make cDNA copies of mRNA transcripts. These cDNAs can be cloned into cDNA libraries, which are useful for isolating and analyzing expressed genes. The expression level of cytoplasmic mRNA can be interrogated using a variety of techniques, including Northern blotting, RT-PCR, microarray analysis, and transcriptomic sequencing (RNA-Seq). Rapid developments in microarray and RNA-Seq technologies have made clear that the successful elucidation of genetic networks through expression profiling requires the expertise of a new generation of scientists, namely, computational biologists. Gene expression profiles of tumors may be used to guide treatment planning of individual cancer patients in a personalized fashion.

Epigenetic regulation

In recent decades, the search for genes implicated in tumorigenesis focused on genes that are genetically altered in tumors. However, recent progress in understanding the role of epigenetic regulation of tumor suppressor genes and oncogenes suggests that epigenetic modifications are also likely to play a role in tumorigenesis. Epigenetic modifications affect the expression of genes without causing any alterations in DNA sequence. Epigenetic regulatory programs depend on DNA methylation, chromatin (histone) modification, and noncoding RNAs. Each of these mechanisms has been shown to play a role in regulating cellular differentiation and tumorigenesis. For example, DNA methylation has been demonstrated to play an important role in silencing gene expression, imprinting, and X-chromosome inactivation.[120–122] Inherited defects in DNA methylation and imprinting result in developmental defects and increase the risk of tumorigenesis. Recent data also implicate DNA methylation and chromatin changes as initiating events in neoplasia preceding the occurrence of genetic alterations.[123–125] This was experimentally proved in mice by introducing into the germline a hypomorphic allele of the DNA methyltransferase gene DNMT1, which led to 90% decrease in DNA methylation and subsequently to cancer development.[126]

The increased interest in analyzing epigenetic modifications led to the development of novel technologies that allow the analysis of these changes in a comprehensive manner and at a genome-wide scale. Methylation-sensitive arbitrarily primed polymerase chain reaction (MS-AP-PCR),[127] methylated CpG island amplification followed by restriction difference analysis (MCARDA),[128] CpG island arrays coupled with differential methylation hybridization (DMH),[129] restriction length genome scanning (RLGS) using methylation-sensitive enzymes,[130] methyl-CpG-binding domain affinity chromatography,[131] and gene expression profiling following demethylation/deacetylation treatment,[132] all have been successfully used for the identification of novel methylated loci in different cancer types.[133] Methylation-specific digital karyotyping (MSDK) is a sequence-based technology that enables comprehensive and unbiased genome-wide DNA methylation analysis.[134] Using a combination of a methylation-sensitive mapping enzyme (e.g., EagI) and a fragmenting enzyme (e.g., NlaIII), short sequence tags can be obtained and uniquely mapped to genome location. The number of MSDK tags obtained from a sample reflects the methylation status of the mapping enzyme sites.

DNA methylation and chromatin modification are interrelated processes and noncoding RNAs may link the two processes together.[133,135] In the past several years, the number and type of known histone modifications increased dramatically, and a large set of enzymes that play a role in mediating these processes has been identified. The four core histones (H2A, H2B, H3, and H4) have been found to subject to various posttranslational modifications, including acetylation, methylation, phosphorylation, ubiquitination, sumoylation, ADP ribosylation, deimination, and proline isomerization. Most of these modifications regulate transcription by influencing the recruitment of other proteins, and a few of them are also involved in DNA repair and chromatin condensation. Using antibodies specifically recognizing methylated histone H3-lys9 and the recently developed ChIP-on-chip,[136] GMAT (genome-wide mapping technique),[137] and ChIP-Seq[138] technologies, it is now possible to analyze heterochromatin changes at a genome-wide scale.

Several recent studies suggest that cancers display a profound genome-wide epigenetic dysregulation.[139] Interestingly, several large-scale cancer genome sequencing projects have also revealed somatic mutations in epigenetic modifier proteins. Examples include mutation of the DNA methyltransferase DNMT3A in acute myeloid leukemia,[140,141] mutation of enzymes involved in DNA demethylation (e.g., TET2, IDH1, IDH2) in myeloid leukemias and gliomas,[142–144] mutation of the histone methylatransferase SETD2 in renal cell carcinoma,[145] mutation of the histone demethylase KDM6A in bladder cancer,[146] and many others. This highlights the fact that tumorigenesis is likely promoted through cooperation between aberrant epigenetic modifications and genetic mutations, with the genetic mutations at times occurring in the epigenetic modifiers themselves.

Summary

The role of epigenetic programs in tumor initiation and progression is becoming increasingly clear. It is likely that epigenetic alterations may precede genetic events and promote the acquisition of genetic changes. Rapidly evolving technology now allows for analysis of epigenetic marks on a genome-wide scale. Cancer genome sequencing initiatives have identified recurrent mutations in a number of epigenetic modifier proteins. Because epigenetic programs are reversible and targetable with inhibitors of DNA and histone modifier enzymes, the efficacy of epigenetic therapy is currently being tested in several different cancer types.

Gene expression: protein analysis

Structural considerations

Proteins are polymeric molecules consisting of amino acids linked by peptide bonds. The sequence of amino acids in a protein is dictated by the sequence of nucleic acids in the mRNA that encodes the protein. Because amino acids are joined to each other in a linear polymer, there is directionality to proteins, just as there is to DNA and RNA. The 5′ end of the mRNA corresponds to the amino end of its cognate protein and the 3′ end corresponds to the carboxy end (Figure 1).

For many proteins, the linear polymer of amino acids must undergo a number of alterations to be functional. These alterations are referred to as posttranslational modifications. For example, proteins destined to be secreted from a cell initially exist as propeptides with a 20- to 30-amino acid sequence at their amino ends. This highly hydrophobic tail, called a leader sequence, remains embedded in the membranes of the endoplasmic reticulum and secretory granule until the protein is to be secreted, at which point, the leader sequence is cleaved. There are many examples of propeptides that undergo cleavage of specific amino acids before they become mature, functional proteins.

Other posttranslational modifications include the addition of various nonpeptide substituents to the side chains of amino acids. These include simple and complex carbohydrate chains, sulfate groups, and phosphate groups. Phosphorylation of intracellular proteins, usually on serine, threonine, or tyrosine residues, plays an important regulatory role in protein function. For example, many of the cell surface receptors for growth factors, such as the platelet-derived growth factor (PDGF) receptor[147] and the receptor for macrophage colony-stimulating factor (M-CSF)[148,149] are themselves protein tyrosine kinases. When this type of receptor binds its ligand, the receptor undergoes a conformational change that activates its kinase activity. The activated receptor then adds phosphate groups to some of its own tyrosine residues and to tyrosines in other proteins. These phosphorylations are part of the signal transduction process, whereby a message is sent from the cell surface receptor to the nucleus. The importance of tyrosine phosphorylation in cell growth may be reflected in the fact that tyrosine kinases form the largest functional subset of oncogenes. Tyrosine kinase inhibitors, such as imatinib mesylate or Gleevec, which blocks the action of the c-abl and c-kit tyrosine kinases, have been proved as effective anticancer chemotherapeutic treatments.[46,150]

Sodium dodecyl sulfate-polyacrylamide gel electrophoresis

As with nucleic acids, the most common analytic technique applied to proteins is separation by size using electrophoresis. However, unlike nucleic acids, not all proteins are anionic, and they do not have a uniform charge-to-mass ratio. In the presence of an electric field, a mixture of unmodified and uncharacterized proteins would migrate in an unpredictable way, providing little or no information about their structures. This problem has been overcome by performing protein electrophoresis in the presence of the anionic detergent sodium dodecyl sulfate (SDS). SDS binds to proteins in a uniform way, at approximately one molecule of SDS for every two amino acids. Thus, all proteins become polyanions in the presence of SDS, and the number of negative charges (supplied by the sulfate group in SDS) is directly proportional to the size, or molecular weight, of the protein.

Because proteins are generally smaller than the most commonly analyzed nucleic acids, electrophoresis is performed through a solid support made of polyacrylamide, which resolves low-molecular-weight molecules better than agarose. In the presence of an electric field, proteins in SDS will migrate toward the anode at a rate inversely proportional to the log of their molecular weights.[151] Proteins can be analyzed by sodium dodecyl sulfate-polyacrylamide gel electrophoresis (SDS-PAGE) in the presence or absence of β-mercaptoethanol (β-ME), which reduces sulfhydryl groups on the side chains of cysteines that can bind two separate protein chains together. Electrophoresis in the presence of β-ME permits the analysis of protein subunits, whereas electrophoresis in the absence of β-ME can reveal multimeric protein associations. SDS-PAGE is routinely employed to test the purity of a protein preparation. It is also an integral component of the techniques of immune precipitation and Western blotting, discussed below.

Immunoblotting

One of the most valuable immunologic identification techniques is immunoblotting (Figure 15a).[152] A mixture of proteins can be electrophoretically separated by SDS-PAGE, and the separated proteins can be transferred to a nitrocellulose or nylon-based filter by electrophoresis in a direction perpendicular to that of the first electrophoresis. The proteins will remain bound to the membrane support. By analogy to Southern blotting for DNA and Northern blotting for RNA, this technique for protein transfer has been called Western blotting. The protein blot can be soaked in a solution that contains a specific antibody that binds to the protein of interest. The presence of the bound antibody on the blot can then be detected if the antibody is labeled. The label can be an enzyme that reveals its presence by catalyzing a color or light-emitting reaction, or it can be a radionuclide, such as ^{125}I, that can be detected by autoradiography. Alternatively, an unlabeled antibody can be detected by washing the blot in a solution that contains a labeled anti-immunoglobulin antibody. This technique has been used to demonstrate overexpression of the HER2/protein in some breast cancers in which Southern blotting revealed no gene amplification.[23] Because the protein is the effector of gene function and the determinant of phenotype, overexpression of the protein can be highly significant and a Western blot is often considered to be the "gold standard" technique for detecting overexpression.

Immune precipitation

A primary goal of molecular biology is to use gene probes to detect the presence of a particular gene in a complex mixture of DNAs or RNAs. In a similar way, a specific antibody can be used as a probe to detect the presence of a particular protein in a complex mixture of proteins. An antibody directed against a protein of interest can be added to a mixture of proteins under conditions that allow the antibody to bind to its target protein (Figure 15b). One can then collect all of the immunoglobulins in that mixture by adding a protein that binds to immunoglobulins, such as anti-immunoglobulin antibodies or staphylococcal protein A. These proteins are often bound to a solid support, such as polystyrene beads, which can be removed from the solution by gentle centrifugation. As the beads collect at the bottom of the centrifuge tube, their attached immunoglobulin and target proteins collect there as well. When boiled in SDS and β-ME, the protein complexes dissociate, and they can be electrophoretically separated by SDS-PAGE. This process is called immune precipitation. To document the specificity of the antibody, a second immune precipitation is usually performed with a control antibody that does not bind the protein of interest. The two precipitations can be run side by side on SDS-PAGE, and the protein of interest can be identified by its presence in the experimental lane and its absence from the control lane. The proteins can be identified by staining

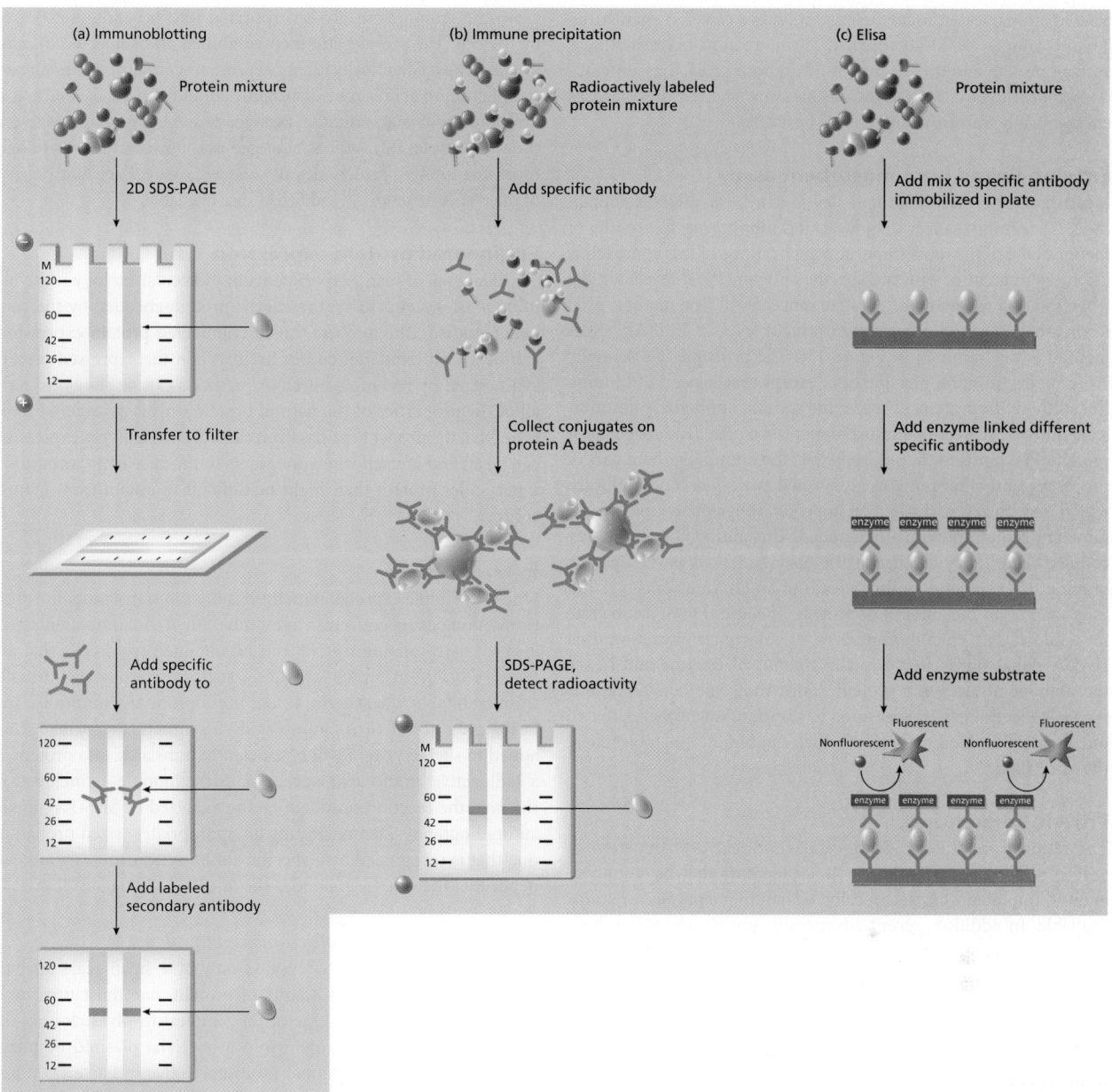

Figure 15 Methods of protein identification and detection. (a) Immune (Western) blotting. A complex mixture of proteins can be separated by size using electrophoresis (SDS-PAGE). The separated proteins are then transferred to a nitrocellulose or nylon filter in an electric field, maintaining their size-specific spatial orientation on the filter. Antibodies directed against one specific protein (in this case, the gray ellipsoid) in the original mixture are added to the filter and bind to the specific protein. Bound antibodies can be radiolabeled or enzymatically labeled themselves, or they can be visualized by incubating the filter with labeled anti-immunoglobulin antibodies. (b) Immunoprecipitation. A complex mixture of radiolabeled proteins (indicated by different geometric shapes) is incubated with antibodies specific for one of those proteins (in this case, the gray ellipsoid). After the antibodies have bound to their protein, small polystyrene or agarose beads containing staphylococcal protein A are added to the mixture. Protein A binds to the antibodies, and when centrifuged, the beads to which the protein A is bound will sediment to the bottom of the centrifuge tube, taking along the antibodies and the specific protein to which they have bound. The unbound proteins remain in the supernatant and can be removed. After boiling to dissociate the protein A/antibody/protein complex, specifically precipitated radiolabeled protein can be visualized by electrophoresis (SDS-PAGE) and autoradiography. (c) Enzyme-linked immunosorbent assay (ELISA). To perform ELISA, one needs to develop two independent antibodies that bind to the protein to be detected (gray ellipsoid in this example) with high specificity and affinity. One of these antibodies is then coupled to a plate, which is then incubated with the protein mix to be analyzed (this can be tissue, blood, or another body fluid). The specifically bound protein is retained on the plate and is detected with the second antibody generated against it, which is coupled to an enzyme or isotope, allowing quantitation of the bound protein. ELISAs are usually very sensitive and can detect picomolar amounts of proteins.

reactions or, if the protein preparation is radiolabeled, by autoradiography.

An important application of this technique was the demonstration that the protein product of the retinoblastoma susceptibility gene (Rb) binds to proteins encoded by DNA tumor viruses.

Antibodies directed against adenovirus proteins were used in an immune precipitation of proteins from cells transformed or infected by adenovirus. In addition to the adenovirus proteins, the precipitated proteins contained another protein that was proved to be the protein encoded by the retinoblastoma susceptibility gene.[153] Similar experiments using antibodies directed against the large T antigen of SV40 revealed an interaction between the T antigen protein and the RB protein.[154] In both cases, these interactions appear to be central to the mechanisms whereby these viruses oncogenically transform susceptible host cells.

Enzyme-linked immunosorbent assay

Measurement of serum protein levels can be a valuable tool in cancer screening, cancer diagnosis, and monitoring the results of therapy. One of the most important applications of this approach is the measurement of prostate-specific antigen (PSA) levels for the detection and follow-up of prostate cancer.[155,156] The method used to measure PSA and other serum protein levels is ELISA.[157] This method is diagrammed in Figure 15c. The principle is essentially the same as immune precipitation, except that instead of binding the antibody to protein A beads, the specific antibody is immobilized onto the surface of a transparent plastic plate. The specific test protein then binds to the antibody (i.e., the immunosorbent part of the assay), and other proteins are washed away. A second antibody, which recognizes a distinct epitope or antigenic region of the same antigenic protein, is then added. This antibody is covalently coupled to an enzyme (hence the enzyme-linked part). Specific binding of the second antibody leads to an enzyme concentration proportional to the amount of protein. The addition of a substrate for a fluorescent, chemiluminescent, or colorimetric reaction then gives a signal proportional to the amount of enzyme and hence the amount of antigenic protein. Small molecule concentrations (i.e., drug levels) can be measured in the same way if there are two independent antibodies, both of which can bind to the molecule at the same time.

Protein sequencing

The ultimate in protein identification is direct determination of amino acid sequence. Automated sequenators that have considerably simplified this technically demanding analysis are now available. In addition, recent advances in protein chemistry have permitted sequencing to be performed on mere picomoles of protein. In fact, Western blotting can be used to purify small amounts of protein, and the fragment of the blot containing the stained protein of interest can be used directly in an automated sequenator.[158]

Direct protein sequencing was responsible for ushering in the modern era of molecular oncology. The protein encoded by the oncogene v-sis, the transforming gene of the simian sarcoma virus, was found to be nearly identical to the empirically determined amino acid sequence of the B chain of human PDGF.[159,160] This was the first demonstration of a connection between oncogenes and the components involved in normal cellular proliferation.

Mass spectrometry

Dramatic advances in mass spectrometric methods in recent years have made mass spectrometry a preferred method for protein analysis and offer promise for use in diagnostic analysis as well. Mass spectrometry is a technique to convert molecules into ions and then to measure their mass. The distinct mass of a given protein is a method to identify that protein in a mixture. Furthermore, proteins can be identified unambiguously by tandem mass spectrometry, in which the proteins are first fragmented into peptides and separated, and then the peptides are fragmented further for sequencing.[161,162] Mass spectrometry is summarized briefly in Figure 16. A recent application of mass spectroscopy has been a technique known as SILAC,[163] or stable isotope labeling by amino acids in cell culture. In SILAC, cells are cultured in the presence of medium containing either a normal or a heavy (nonradioactive) amino acid. As the cells grow, the amino acids are incorporated into proteins synthesized by the cell. The samples are then combined and subjected to mass spectroscopy. Chemically identical proteins containing either heavy or light amino acid can be distinguished on the basis of their mass. This allows for a quantitative assay of protein abundance between the two samples. SILAC has emerged as a powerful means to perform quantitative proteomics in cancer biology. Excellent reviews of mass spectroscopy[164] and SILAC are available.[165]

Engineered protein expression

The final goal of many experiments in molecular biology is the use of biologic systems to synthesize the protein encoded by the gene being studied. This process, called engineered protein expression, can be an experimental end in itself. When the expressed protein synthesized by recombinant DNA methods can be shown to have all of the properties of the natural protein, this is considered to be proof that the proper gene has been cloned. Alternatively, expression can be an end in itself when one wants to produce large amounts of a particular protein that might be difficult to obtain from natural sources.

In vitro *translation*

One very simple expression method is *in vitro* translation, in which translation occurs entirely in a test tube. All of the components necessary for translating mRNA can be obtained from cells that are highly efficient in protein synthesis, such as reticulocytes (usually from rabbits) or wheat germ. Under the appropriate conditions, and in the presence of all 20 amino acids, a synthetic or purified RNA added to such a system will be efficiently translated into protein. If a radioactive amino acid, such as [^{35}S]methionine, is included in the mix, the reaction products can be analyzed by SDS-PAGE and autoradiography. Demonstrating an appropriately sized protein or one that is recognized by a specific antibody constitutes good evidence that the mRNA in hand is the one the investigator desires.

Large-scale production of recombinant proteins

In vitro translation can be applied only at a small-scale analytic level. To produce large amounts of protein, one must turn to *in vivo* expression systems. One of the simplest involves cloning the cDNA for the desired protein into a bacterial plasmid or phage that contains a transcriptional promoter active in bacteria. When introduced into the appropriate bacterial host, large amounts of mRNA will be transcribed, which, in turn, will be translated into protein. The recombinant protein can then be purified away from all of the bacterial proteins. This is the way in which some clinically available interferons[166–168] have been produced.

As noted earlier, many eukaryotic proteins require posttranslational modifications for maximal activity. Bacteria do not have the machinery required to accomplish complex modifications, such as the addition of specific carbohydrate groups. Moreover, the interior milieu of a bacterial cell is a reducing environment so that disulfide bonds essential to the structure and function of many eukaryotic proteins cannot form. When these modifications are required, mammalian cells can be used for expression. The basic concept is the same as in bacterial systems: a cDNA is cloned into a vector with a eukaryotic transcriptional promoter, and the resulting recombinant DNA is introduced into mammalian cells.[169] However, there are still significant disadvantages in the use of mammalian cells for large-scale recombinant protein production. Mammalian cells are expensive to grow *in vitro* because they require a medium rich in nutrients and growth factors. Yeast cells, insect cells, and even plant cells are being exploited as an attractive compromise between

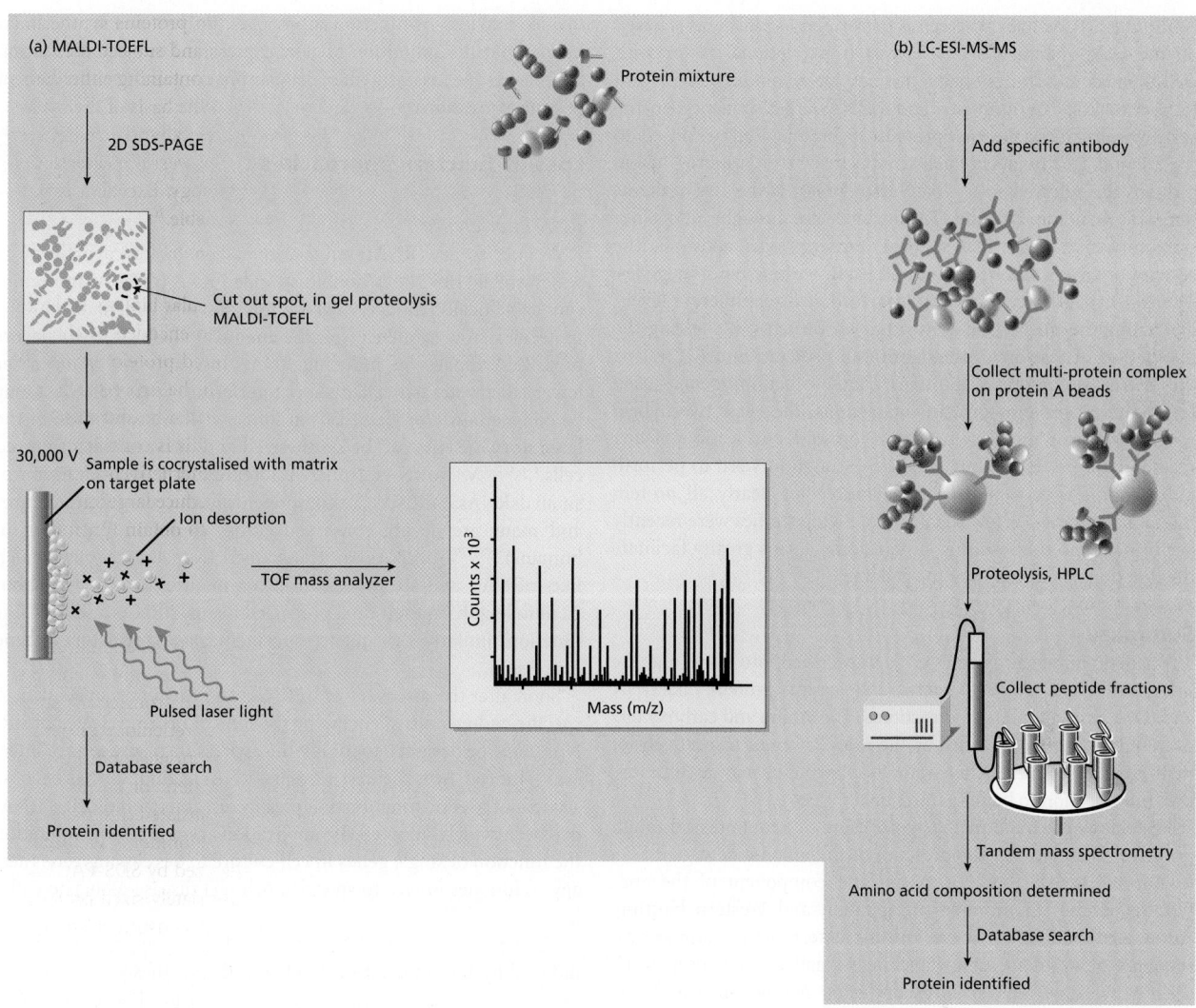

Figure 16 Mass spectrometry. (a) Matrix-assisted laser desorption ionization time-of-flight mass spectrometry (MALDI-TOF). For organisms whose genome sequence is known, the identification of "interesting" protein spots from a two-dimensional gel is routinely performed using MALDI-TOF. A complex mixture of proteins is separated by size and charge using two-dimensional electrophoresis. Protein spots are excited from the gel, digested with a protease, mixed with a matrix solution, and allowed to cocrystallize on a target plate. When a laser is fired at the target plate, the matrix absorbs the laser light's energy and vaporizes, carrying some of the sample with it into a vacuum space. At the time the laser is fired, a high voltage is applied to the target plate to accelerate the ionized sample's movement toward the time-of-flight (TOF) mass analyzer. The resulting peptide fingerprint can then be used to search databases to determine the identity of the protein. (b) The liquid chromatography electrospray ionization tandem mass spectrometry (LC-ESIMS-MS) can be used to obtain amino acid sequence information, allowing highly refined database searches. The approach employs capillary high-performance liquid chromatography (HPLC), which allows very slow (submicroliter/min) flow rates that are essential for obtaining high-sensitivity ESI-MS-MS of peptides. Following the liquid chromatography and electrospray ionization, the ions are analyzed by linearly linked tandem mass spectrometers that yield amino acid composition information.

mammalian cell culture and bacterial culture for protein expression. These eukaryotic cells can execute most of the posttranslational modifications required by mammalian proteins, including disulfide bonding. At the same time, these cells are easier and more economical to grow *in vitro*. A number of expression vectors analogous to those described here for bacteria and animal cells have been developed for these alternative eukaryotic hosts. Interested readers are referred to other sources for in-depth descriptions.[170,171]

Methods for analyzing protein–protein interactions

An important and challenging task in post-genomic biology is to understand the function of proteins encoded by the genome and to determine their involvement in signaling pathways and cellular networks. One approach to understanding protein function is to investigate its interaction with other proteins of known function. By performing such analysis at a genome-wide level, one can create protein–protein physical interaction networks.[172] These networks can be combined with gene expression or other genomic data to generate regulatory and signaling networks at the cellular level. Several methods allow the characterization of protein–protein interactions at a genome-wide scale. These include comprehensive protein pull-down assays, protein chips, and two-hybrid screens. Comprehensive protein pull-down assays use the combination of immunoprecipitation and mass spectrometric methods discussed earlier, whereas protein chips are the application of the microarray technology originally used for DNA or RNA profiling (see above) for protein interaction analysis.

The classic two-hybrid screen is performed in yeast and is based on the Gal4 system. Gal4 is a yeast transcriptional factor with well-defined and functionally distinct DNA binding (DB) and trans-activator (TA) domains and a DNA target sequence. In the two-hybrid screen, the two proteins to be analyzed are fused to the DB and TA domains of Gal4, respectively. The resulting fusion proteins are referred to as "bait" and "prey." If the two proteins interact, then the DB and TA domains are brought into close proximity and create a functional transcriptional activator, the activity of which can be monitored using various reporter genes. The two-hybrid screen can be performed at three different levels: (1) testing the interaction of two known proteins, (2) testing the interaction of a known protein with all proteins, and (3) testing the interaction among all proteins. Unlike other approaches used for analyzing protein–protein interactions, the yeast two-hybrid screen does not require the expression and purification of any recombinant proteins. Thus, it is fairly straightforward to perform at a genome-wide scale and is applicable for nearly all protein interaction studies. A few such genome-wide studies were recently performed, and the resulting "interactome" maps greatly facilitate the functional annotation of the genome.[173–175]

Summary

The genetic information in DNA is transcribed into RNA, and the information in RNA is ultimately translated into protein. Like DNA and RNA, proteins are also directional. The amino and carboxy termini of proteins are specified by the 5′ and 3′ ends, respectively, of their cognate mRNAs. After translation, proteins may require further modification to be fully functional.

Proteins can be fractionated by size using electrophoresis through polyacrylamide gels in the presence of the anionic detergent SDS (SDS-PAGE). SDS-PAGE is an integral component of the analytic techniques of immune precipitation and Western blotting. Automated analyzers that can directly determine the amino acid sequence of a protein using vanishingly small amounts of material are now available. Mass spectroscopy using methods such as SILAC allows for large-scale quantitative proteomics.

The mRNA that encodes a protein can be translated *in vitro* using cellular extracts of rabbit reticulocytes or wheat germ. For expressing larger quantities of protein, bacterial cells are a simple and economical option, but they cannot perform many of the posttranslational modifications required by mammalian proteins. Vectors that permit mammalian cells to express foreign proteins with great efficiency and fidelity have been designed. Eukaryotic expression systems using yeast cells, insect cells, or plant cells also provide excellent alternatives.

Global analysis of protein interactions is used for the generation of interactome maps that reveal regulatory and functional networks, greatly facilitating our understanding of cellular function at the systemic level.

Functional screens for the identification of therapeutic targets in cancer

One consequence of the sequencing of the human genome is that we now have a comprehensive catalog of all of the genes that can be expressed. Cancer genome sequencing efforts have also given us a catalog of the genes most commonly mutated in cancer. The challenge going forward is to integrate this data with functional studies, and to systematically compile a list of genes whose mutation or aberrant expression drives cancer initiation or maintenance. Recent technical advances provide the means to search systematically for genes involved in cancer development. Broadly, these efforts can be divided into loss-of-function approaches (i.e., assessment of cellular phenotype after inhibition of gene expression) or gain-of-function approaches (i.e., assessment of cellular phenotype after enforcement of gene expression).

Loss-of-function approaches

RNA interference

RNA interference (RNAi) refers to an ancient biological pathway by which small (18–21 nt), double-stranded RNA (dsRNA) molecules can catalytically induce degradation of complementary mRNA molecules in a sequence-specific manner. There are two flavors of dsRNA capable of inducing RNAi. In plants and some other lower eukaryotes, so-called short interfering RNAs (siRNAs) may be endogenously processed from longer dsRNA substrates; in the laboratory, siRNAs can be synthesized and delivered into cultured cells.[176,177] MicroRNAs (miRNAs) represent a second flavor of small dsRNAs; miRNAs are components of the eukaryotic genome, and many are deeply conserved across evolution (including in humans).[178,179] miRNAs are transcribed from the genome, much like mRNAs, and are processed into a mature form that is about 22 nt in length. In their final processed forms, siRNAs and miRNAs function similarly, as sequence-specific negative regulators of gene expression.

Soon after the discovery of miRNAs and the report of sequence-specific endogenous silencing by dsRNAs, it became clear that siRNAs could be designed to inhibit the expression of any gene of interest.[180] Indeed, over the past 15 years, RNAi technology has become a staple of loss-of-function analyses in research laboratories. RNAi has been widely adopted for applications ranging from inhibiting the function of single genes in cell culture to developing gene therapy techniques *in vivo* to specifically target disease-associated alleles.

In mammalian cells, RNAi-mediated gene suppression can be induced by the transfection of chemically synthesized siRNAs, or by the use of plasmids expressing short hairpin RNAs (shRNAs), which get processed to siRNAs endogenously by the Drosha and Dicer ribonucleases.[181,182] The shRNAs can be either expressed from a plasmid containing an RNA polymerase III promoter, or can be expressed from within a miRNA-like context as part of a longer transcript, under the control of an RNA polymerase II promoter.[183] In either case, the siRNA becomes incorporated into the RNA-induced silencing complex (RISC) and directs sequence-specific degradation or translational suppression of the target mRNA, resulting in decreased protein expression.[184] Athough siRNAs are easily synthesized and highly effective in inducing gene knockdown, such oligonucleotide reagents are relatively expensive and can only be used for transient loss-of-function experiments. Vector-based systems offer the possibility of adding selectable markers, such as drug resistance, stable expression of the RNAi construct, as well as being a renewable resource through propagation in bacteria. More recently, inducible RNAi vectors have also been developed, allowing fine temporal and spatial regulation of RNAi-induced gene knockdown.[185]

Both siRNA and shRNA libraries have been used successfully in transfection-based arrayed screens looking at phenotypes that develop shortly after gene suppression, such as apoptosis, cell signaling events, or cell cycle distribution.[186–188] For many other cancer-related phenotypic assays, such as anchorage-independent colony formation, bypass of senescence, or tumor xenografts, long-term gene suppression is essential, requiring stable integration and expression of the RNAi vector. An additional significant advantage of the retroviral-based libraries is the ability to work with cells that are refractory to transfection. This is particularly true for the lentiviral-based systems, which can even be used to infect post-mitotic and other difficult-to-transduce cells, including primary cells or differentiated cells.[189,190]

CRISPR/CAS9

A major discovery in the past 5 years has been the observation that aspects of the microbial adaptive immune system can be exploited to engineer changes into the genomes of mammalian cells. It had been observed for many years that microbial genomes contain clusters of repeat elements with intervening spacer sequences.[191,192] These clusters were termed CRISPR, or *c*lustered *r*egularly *i*nterspaced *s*hort *p*alindromic *r*epeats. Adjacent to these repeat elements, were CRISPR-associated (Cas) genes. It had also been observed that many of the spacer sequences that intervene CRISPR repeats are of phage origin, suggesting that the CRISPR-Cas system represents a form of bacterial adaptive immunity against phage infection. Indeed, mechanistic studies have now shown that the CRISPR array is transcribed as a noncoding RNA transcript known as a crRNA, which is then processed and associated with a Cas protein complex. In the most widely studied type of CRISPR/Cas system, known as the Type II CRISPR, the crRNA associates with another trans-activating RNA (known as a tracrRNA) as well as the Cas9 DNA nuclease. The crRNA and tracrRNA form an RNA hybrid that recognizes DNA containing a protospacer-adjacent motif (PAM) sequence, and mediates cleavage near the recognition site. The CRISPR/Cas system has now been established as the basis for an adaptive immune system in many archaea and bacteria that protects against foreign genetic elements (i.e., bacteriophages or plasmids). Readers are directed to an excellent reviews for further detail on this rapidly evolving field.[193,194]

A watershed moment in this field was the realization that the Type II CRISPR/Cas9 system could be modified and transferred to other cell types for use as an exceptionally powerful genome editing tool. The tracrRNA:crRNA hybrid can be engineered as a single RNA chimera,[195] or sgRNA, and the spacer (or guide) sequence can be modified to target a desired sequence of DNA for cleavage. This allows for an RNA-programmable molecular machine that can be directed to cleave near almost any desired site in the genome. Indeed, it has been shown that CRISPR/Cas9 cleavage can be engineered in mammalian cells in a highly generalizable fashion.[196,197] The double-strand breaks induced by Cas9 are most often repaired by the error-prone process of nonhomologous end joining (NHEJ), which frequently introduces small indels (which may induce frameshifts) at the site of cleavage. Thus, CRISPR/Cas9 technology offers a powerful means of inducing loss of function of a gene of interest. In addition, when Cas9 is used in conjunction with a homology-directed repair template, the cuts induced by Cas9 can be repaired via homologous recombination, allowing for precise genome-editing.

Recent studies have reported genome-scale lentiviral libraries of sgRNAs, analogous to the genome-wide RNAi libraries discussed above.[198] These CRISPR libraries allow one to target each gene in the genome and assess the effect on a phenotype of interest. As compared with shRNAs, CRISPR-mediated inhibition of gene expression is often more robust, and possibly accompanied by fewer "off-target" effects. Thus, it is likely that genome-scale screening with CRISPR/Cas9 libraries will become a cornerstone of functional genomics that builds upon and refines previous advances made by shRNA screening efforts (Figure 17).

Gain-of-function approaches

Most gain-of-function screens involve introduction of a cDNA library into cells either transiently or stably, ideally resulting in the hyperactivation of pathways positively regulated by the gene corresponding to the introduced cDNA. Several large collections of cloned cDNAs have been used successfully to this end.[200,201] Several of these are compatible with recombination-mediated transfer systems, allowing shuttling of the open reading frames (ORFs) of interest into different vectors, facilitating adaptation of the system to individual needs.

Gain-of-function approaches have been used for a variety of purposes, including to identify modulators of signal transduction pathways as assessed by transcriptional reporters,[202] to identify genes whose expression can bypass senescence,[201] and to identify genetic programs conferring drug resistance phenotypes.[203] Depending on the goal of the screen, the cDNA can either be transiently expressed by transfection (an approach that works well with transcriptional reporter-driven systems focused on short-term events) or stably integrated by using a viral cDNA expression vector (an approach that is often needed for many screens relevant to oncogenic transformation that require long-term expression and selection.)

Another type of gain-of-function approach utilizes miRNA expression libraries to screen using phenotypic assays. As discussed above, miRNAs are endogenous small RNAs that function by downregulating expression of their target genes, either through induction of transcript degradation or translational inhibition. miRNAs implicated in cancer include let-7, a negative regulator of RAS, c-Myc and other oncogenes[204]; the miR-17-92 cluster, which is upregulated in lymphomas and can promote lymphomagenesis[205]; and miR-15 and miR-16, negative regulators of BCL2, that are downregulated in chronic lymphocytic leukemia.[206] These examples suggest that full extent of the contribution of miRNAs to tumorigenesis is not yet known. Thus, further functional studies are necessary. For example, work using a retroviral expression library of miRNAs identified miR-372 and miR-373 in a Ras-induced senescence bypass screen, suggesting possible oncogenic function for these miRNAs.[207] Future applications of this approach will likely yield many more cancer-relevant miRNAs and the identification of their respective targets are also likely to provide further insight into the oncogenic process.

Summary

Increasingly, unbiased genome-wide functional screens have been used for the identification and validation of novel therapeutic targets in cancer. Most of these screens are performed in cell culture models, with the hits then validated by analysis of primary human tumor samples. RNA interference and CRISPR/Cas9 screens represent the main loss-of-function approaches while ORF screens represent the predominant gain-of-function approach. Several of these screens have resulted in the discovery of genes with key roles in tumorigenesis. Improvements in culture models and the application of these technologies in animal models increase the likelihood that the findings are validated in human cancer patients.

Mouse models of human cancer

Despite advances in our understanding of the biology of cancer at the molecular level, the application of this knowledge to the clinical management of cancer patients has been lagging. One of the factors limiting the translation of discoveries made in the laboratory to the clinic has been the availability of *in vivo* animal models of cancer that faithfully reproduce the human disease. Animals, particularly rodents, have been used in cancer research for decades to explore fundamental biological properties of tumors and to evaluate anti-neoplastic therapies.[208] Initially, such rodent models were largely limited to spontaneous or carcinogen-induced neoplasms, or, more commonly, the ectopic or orthotopic transplantation of murine or human tumor cells into syngeneic or immunodeficient mice. Although none of these approaches accurately represents the complexity of human cancer, preclinical studies with these models are nonetheless traditionally required during the regulatory approval of investigational antineoplastic agents.

Improved animal cancer models became available with the advent of genetically engineered mouse models (GEMMs) of cancer following advances in molecular biology and embryology in the early 1980s. GEMMs enabled the direct investigation of potential tumorigenic genes *in vivo*, and, today, models that accurately represent nearly every major human cancer exist.[209] The first generation of GEMMs was transgenic tumor-prone mice produced through the ectopic introduction of activated oncogenes. Indeed, such "oncomice" confirmed the tumorigenic properties of c-Myc, Ras, and several viral oncoproteins; mice transgenic for these oncogenes developed lymphoma, breast cancer, and pancreatic cancer.[210] Although many early oncomouse models were informative, most human cancers could not be accurately modeled using this approach, likely due to the nonphysiological properties

inherent in ectopic expression cassettes and tissue mosaicism. An alternative early approach to model human cancer was through the disruption or "knockout" (KO) of endogenous putative tumor suppressor alleles that were identified in cancer-prone kindreds. Indeed, KO mice confirmed Knudsen's hypothesis of tumor suppressor gene function, although the tumor spectrum in such KO mice oftentimes was quite distinct from the cognate human condition. A detailed description of the basic methodologies required for the generation of transgenic and KO mice can be found in an excellent manual on the manipulation of the mouse embryo.[211] These early mouse models were very powerful in validating the cancer-relevant role of particular genes or their combination in tumorigenesis and allowed the identification of cooperating genetic alterations by insertional mutagenesis. However, a major drawback of these early mouse models is that genetically engineered mutations are present in every cell of the mouse. This is problematic for multiple reasons. First, it can lead to embryonic lethality or abnormalities if the affected oncogene or tumor suppressor gene is required for normal development. Second, with the exception of hereditary cancer predisposition syndromes, the modus operandi of these mutational events does not reproduce the human disease because the majority of human tumors evolve owing to acquired somatic genetic changes. Third, it does not allow the interrogation of the role of cancer-relevant genes in

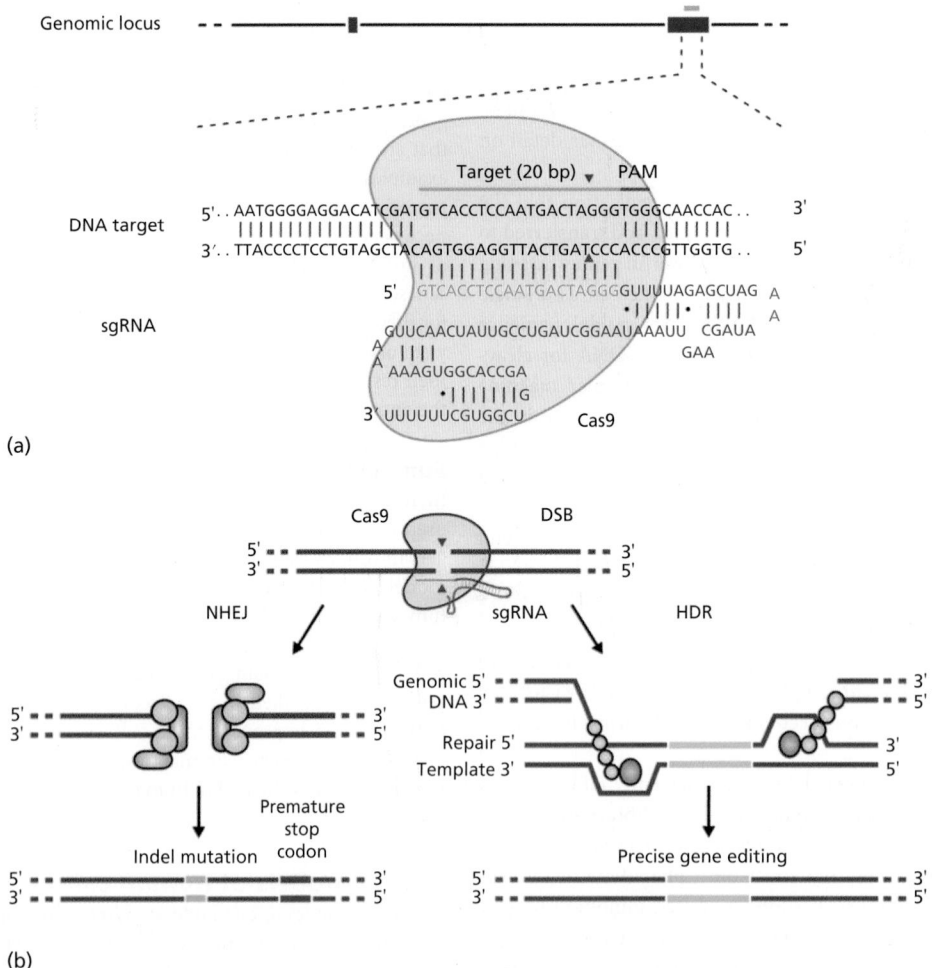

(a)

(b)

Figure 17 (a) Schematic of the RNA-guided Cas9 nuclease, which is directed to its DNA target by a 20-nt guide sequence (blue). The red triangle represents the approximate nucleotide position where Cas9 would be expected to initiate a DSB. (b) DSBs created by Cas9 can be repaired either via error-prone NHEJ or homologous recombination. Source: Ran 2013.[199] Reproduced with permission of Nature Publishing Group.

a particular organ type or stage of tumorigenesis. Recognizing these deficiencies, investigators have been developing ever more sophisticated mouse models that more faithfully reflect the human disease.

Current state-of-the-art mouse models employ new genetic tools to address the shortcomings of classic oncomice and KO mice.[212] Indeed, the advent of inducible and conditional mutant alleles enables the sophisticated spatial and temporal control of cancer gene expression. A common type of inducible cancer allele is transcriptionally regulated by variants of the *E. coli* Tetracycline operon, usually with the chemical analog doxycycline. It has two different variations, TET-OFF and TET-ON, depending on whether the expression of the targeted gene (regulated by a TET-responsive TA) is expressed in the presence (TET-ON) or absence (TET-OFF) of doxycycline.[213] Doxycycline-sensitive alleles can include putative oncogenes, and such alleles were used to demonstrate a causal role for oncogenes in the development and maintenance of many tumor types in mouse models.[209,214] In addition, doxycycline-dependent alleles can reversibly suppress gene expression through the expression of dominant-negative tumor suppressor genes and short hairpin interfering RNA constructs.[215] To control the cell lineage in which the doxycycline-dependent genetic element is expressed, cell-type-specific promoters are used to encode the tetracycline TA.[213] Another inducible gene expression system utilizes chimeric proteins containing the gene of interest fused to the ligand binding portion of the estrogen receptor (ER). Such fusion proteins are held in a latent state in the cytoplasm in complex with heat shock proteins and are released following the addition of estrogenic analogs such as Tamoxifen. ER fusions with Myc and P53 have been used to generate a variety of clever mouse models of various cancer types.[216,217] Conditional mutant alleles are employed to directly modulate gene expression through either deleting putative tumor suppressor genes or expressing a single allele of an activated oncogene from its endogenous promoter. Conditional mutant alleles are controlled by the Bacteriophage P1 Cre/loxP system, whereby the Cre recombinase will direct the looping and excision of DNA elements that are flanked by 34 bp LoxP sites. Conditional tumor suppressor alleles thus consist of genes that contain exons surrounded by intronic LoxP sites, and these alleles are expressed at diploid levels until Cre recombinase is introduced and mediates the deletion of the gene with loss of mRNA and protein. Conditional oncogenes are latent alleles that are not expressed until Cre recombinase causes the removal of transcriptional silencing or "Stop" elements; and in this scenario, the gene dosage changes from haploid to diploid with half of the gene dosage consisting of the oncogenic alleles. There are additional recombinases now available for mouse modeling, and there are a variety of related strategies to control conditional gene expression. Inducible cancer alleles can be used alone, or in tandem with conditional mutant alleles such that added ligands can control the expression of Cre recombinase, enabling exquisite spatial and temporal control of cancer gene expression.[218,219] Using these state-of-the-art strategies, GEMMs that faithfully model the development of preinvasive and invasive carcinomas of the lung, pancreas, prostate, ovary, and breast have now been developed.[209] Such models oftentimes demonstrate additional pathophysiological sequelae, including cachexia and metastasis, and somatic biochemical and genomic alterations that are common in the cognate human malignancy. A major advance using these GEMMs is the identification of new pathways in human cancers by cross-species comparisons.[220] Investigations are now under way to determine the role of GEMMs of cancer in diagnostic and therapeutic development. Unanswered questions about GEMMs

include the absence of evidence demonstrating a superior predictive therapeutic utility of GEMMs to xenografted tumor models, and whether species-specific differences in drug metabolism, the tumor microenvironment, and cell intrinsic pathways will preclude the translation of information in GEMMs to the clinical setting. Nonetheless, several publications suggest that these models will be informative in the preclinical assessment of antineoplastic agents.

Recently, developments in CRISPR/Cas9-based genome editing (see above) have also been extended to animal models. For example, a recent report used hydrodynamic injection to directly deliver CRISPR plasmids and sgRNAs to the mouse liver in order to target the tumor suppressor genes Pten and p53. The result was a loss of Pten and p53 function comparable to that achieved by genetic KO, with the mice developing liver tumors.[221] In another study, CRISPR/Cas9-mediated genome editing of tumor suppressor genes was overlaid on a Kras-driven lung cancer model to functionally characterize a panel of potential tumor suppressor genes.[222] In the coming years, it is likely that CRISPR/Cas9 technology will become more widely used as a complement to traditional genetic manipulation methods in an effort to create mouse models of cancer that faithfully recapitulate the human disease.

Summary

Rodent models are required components in anticancer drug development. Several GEMMs faithfully recapitulate the human disease and are useful for studying disease biology and for preclinical testing of potential therapeutics. CRISPR/Cas9 technology can complement traditional genetic manipulation methods, and will likely help further refine the degree to which current GEMMs recapitulate the human disease.

Key references

The complete reference list can be found on the Wiley Companion Digital Edition of this title (see inside front cover for login instructions).

2 Alberts B (ed). *Molecular Biology of the Cell*, 5th ed. New York: Garland Science; 2008.

6 Nirenberg M, Leder P. RNA codewords and protein synthesis. The effect of trinucleotides upon the binding of sRNA to ribosomes. *Science*. 1964;**145**(**3639**):1399–1407.

7 Watson JD, Crick FH. Molecular structure of nucleic acids; a structure for deoxyribose nucleic acid. *Nature*. 1953;**171**(**4356**):737–738.

16 Cohen SN, Chang AC, Boyer HW, Helling RB. Construction of biologically functional bacterial plasmids in vitro. *Proc Natl Acad Sci U S A*. 1973;**70**(**4594039**):3240–3244.

18 Green MR. *Molecular Cloning: A Laboratory Manual*, 4th ed. Cold Spring Harbor, NY: Cold Spring Harbor Laboratory Press; 2012. 3 p.

20 Gibson DG, Young L, Chuang R-Y, Venter JC, Hutchison CA, Smith HO. Enzymatic assembly of DNA molecules up to several hundred kilobases. *Nat Methods*. 2009;**6**(**5**):343–345.

22 Southern EM. Detection of specific sequences among DNA fragments separated by gel electrophoresis. *J Mol Biol*. 1975;**98**(**1195397**):503–517.

23 Slamon DJ, Godolphin W, Jones LA, et al. Studies of the HER-2/neu proto-oncogene in human breast and ovarian cancer. *Science*. 1989;**244**(**2470152**):707–712.

26 Mullis KB, Faloona FA. Specific synthesis of DNA in vitro via a polymerase-catalyzed chain reaction. *Methods Enzymol*. 1987;**155**:335–350.

27 Nakamura Y, Leppert M, O'Connell P, et al. Variable number of tandem repeat (VNTR) markers for human gene mapping. *Science*. 1987;**235**(**3029872**):1616–1622.

28 Miki Y, Swensen J, Shattuck-Eidens D, et al. A strong candidate for the breast and ovarian cancer susceptibility gene BRCA1. *Science*. 1994;**266**(**5182**):66–71.

36 Wang DG, Fan JB, Siao CJ, et al. Large-scale identification, mapping, and genotyping of single-nucleotide polymorphisms in the human genome. *Science*. 1998;**280**(**9582121**):1077–1082.

37 Sachidanandam R, Weissman D, Schmidt SC, et al. A map of human genome sequence variation containing 1.42 million single nucleotide polymorphisms. *Nature*. 2001;**409(6822)**:928–933.

38 Altshuler D, Pollara VJ, Cowles CR, et al. An SNP map of the human genome generated by reduced representation shotgun sequencing. *Nature*. 2000;**407(6803)**:513–516.

44 Sanger F, Nicklen S, Coulson AR. DNA sequencing with chain-terminating inhibitors. *Proc Natl Acad Sci U S A*. 1977;**74(12)**:5463–5467.

46 Joensuu H, Roberts PJ, Sarlomo-Rikala M, et al. Effect of the tyrosine kinase inhibitor STI571 in a patient with a metastatic gastrointestinal stromal tumor. *N Engl J Med*. 2001;**344(11287975)**:1052–1056.

47 Lynch TJ, Bell DW, Sordella R, et al. Activating mutations in the epidermal growth factor receptor underlying responsiveness of non-small-cell lung cancer to gefitinib. *N Engl J Med*. 2004;**350(21)**:2129–2139.

48 Pao W, Miller V, Zakowski M, et al. EGF receptor gene mutations are common in lung cancers from "never smokers" and are associated with sensitivity of tumors to gefitinib and erlotinib. *Proc Natl Acad Sci U S A*. 2004;**101(36)**:13306–13311.

49 Paez JG, Jänne PA, Lee JC, et al. EGFR mutations in lung cancer: correlation with clinical response to gefitinib therapy. *Science*. 2004;**304(5676)**:1497–1500.

51 Chapman PB, Hauschild A, Robert C, et al. Improved survival with vemurafenib in melanoma with BRAF V600E mutation. *N Engl J Med*. 2011;**364(26)**:2507–2516.

56 Hodges E, Xuan Z, Balija V, et al. Genome-wide in situ exon capture for selective resequencing. *Nat Genet*. 2007;**39(17982454)**:1522–1527.

61 Ley TJ, Mardis ER, Ding L, et al. DNA sequencing of a cytogenetically normal acute myeloid leukaemia genome. *Nature*. 2008;**456(7218)**:66–72.

65 Cibulskis K, Lawrence MS, Carter SL, et al. Sensitive detection of somatic point mutations in impure and heterogeneous cancer samples. *Nat Biotechnol*. 2013;**31(3)**:213–219.

66 Koboldt DC, Zhang Q, Larson DE, et al. VarScan 2: somatic mutation and copy number alteration discovery in cancer by exome sequencing. *Genome Res*. 2012;**22(3)**:568–576.

68 Lawrence MS, Stojanov P, Polak P, et al. Mutational heterogeneity in cancer and the search for new cancer-associated genes. *Nature*. 2013;**499(7457)**:214–218.

72 Sharp PA. Split genes and RNA splicing. *Cell*. 1994;**77(7516265)**:805–815.

81 Baltimore D. RNA-dependent DNA polymerase in virions of RNA tumour viruses. *Nature*. 1970;**226(5252)**:1209–1211.

82 Temin HM, Mizutani S. RNA-dependent DNA polymerase in virions of Rous sarcoma virus. *Nature*. 1970;**226(5252)**:1211–1213.

89 Velculescu VE, Zhang L, Vogelstein B, Kinzler KW. Serial analysis of gene expression. *Science*. 1995;**270(7570003)**:484–487.

95 Schena M, Shalon D, Davis RW, Brown PO. Quantitative monitoring of gene expression patterns with a complementary DNA microarray. *Science*. 1995;**270(5235)**:467–470.

97 Golub TR, Slonim DK, Tamayo P, et al. Molecular classification of cancer: class discovery and class prediction by gene expression monitoring. *Science*. 1999;**286(10521349)**:531–537.

113 Trapnell C, Williams BA, Pertea G, et al. Transcript assembly and quantification by RNA-Seq reveals unannotated transcripts and isoform switching during cell differentiation. *Nat Biotechnol*. 2010;**28(5)**:511–515.

122 Herman JG, Baylin SB. Gene silencing in cancer in association with promoter hypermethylation. *N Engl J Med*. 2003;**349(21)**:2042–2054.

126 Gaudet F, Hodgson JG, Eden A, et al. Induction of tumors in mice by genomic hypomethylation. *Science*. 2003;**300(12702876)**:489–492.

138 Mikkelsen TS, Ku M, Jaffe DB, et al. Genome-wide maps of chromatin state in pluripotent and lineage-committed cells. *Nature*. 2007;**448(17603471)**:553–560.

150 Druker BJ, Sawyers CL, Kantarjian H, et al. Activity of a specific inhibitor of the BCR-ABL tyrosine kinase in the blast crisis of chronic myeloid leukemia and acute lymphoblastic leukemia with the Philadelphia chromosome. *N Engl J Med*. 2001;**344(11287973)**:1038–1042.

176 Fire A, Xu S, Montgomery MK, Kostas SA, Driver SE, Mello CC. Potent and specific genetic interference by double-stranded RNA in Caenorhabditis elegans. *Nature*. 1998;**391(9486653)**:806–811.

178 Lee RC, Feinbaum RL, Ambros V. The C. elegans heterochronic gene lin-4 encodes small RNAs with antisense complementarity to lin-14. *Cell*. 1993;**75(5)**:843–854.

179 Wightman B, Ha I, Ruvkun G. Posttranscriptional regulation of the heterochronic gene lin-14 by lin-4 mediates temporal pattern formation in C. elegans. *Cell*. 1993;**75(5)**:855–862.

195 Jinek M, Chylinski K, Fonfara I, Hauer M, Doudna JA, Charpentier E. A programmable dual-RNA-guided DNA endonuclease in adaptive bacterial immunity. *Science*. 2012;**337(6096)**:816–821.

197 Cong L, Ran FA, Cox D, et al. Multiplex genome engineering using CRISPR/Cas systems. *Science*. 2013;**339(6121)**:819–823.

198 Shalem O, Sanjana NE, Hartenian E, et al. Genome-scale CRISPR-Cas9 knockout screening in human cells. *Science*. 2014;**343(6166)**:84–87.

214 Chin L, Tam A, Pomerantz J, et al. Essential role for oncogenic Ras in tumour maintenance. *Nature*. 1999;**400(6743)**:468–472.

4 Oncogenes

Marco A. Pierotti, PhD ▪ Milo Frattini, MD, PhD ▪ Francesca Molinari, PhD ▪ Gabriella Sozzi, PhD ▪ Carlo M. Croce, MD

Overview

The initiation and progression of human neoplastic diseases is a multistep process involving the accumulation of genetic changes in somatic cells. These genetic changes typically consist of the activation of cooperating oncogenes and the inactivation of tumor suppressor genes, which both appear necessary for a complete neoplastic phenotype. Oncogenes are altered versions of normal cellular genes called proto-oncogenes, usually involved in the regulation of cell growth and activated by mutation, chromosomal rearrangement, or gene amplification. In this chapter, at first we will describe the methods that have been applied by the researchers for the discovery and the identification of oncogenes. Then we will present the genetic mechanisms of proto-oncogenes activation (point mutations, gene amplifications, chromosomal rearrangements) with several examples, and we will describe the role played by oncogenes in the initiation and progression of various cancers.

The identification of oncogene abnormalities has provided tools for the molecular diagnosis and monitoring of cancer. Most important, oncogenes represent potential targets for new types of cancer therapies, which are continuously discovered and tested in clinical trials. The goal of these new drugs is to kill cancer cells selectively while sparing normal cells. These new therapies display an evident benefit for the treatment of several neoplastic diseases that were, before targeted therapies development, very hard to be treated and cured. However, they are not able to kill 100% of neoplastic cells, essentially due to the occurrence of mechanisms of secondary resistance. In the last part of the chapter, we will review all the genes for which a targeted therapy has been developed.

Since the early proposal of Boveri more than a century ago, multiple experimental evidence have confirmed that, at the molecular level, cancer is due to lesions in the cellular DNA. First, it has been observed that a cancer cell transmits to its daughter cells the phenotypic features characterizing the "cancerous" state. Second, most of the recognized mutagenic compounds are also carcinogenic. Finally, the karyotyping of several types of human tumors, particularly those belonging to the hematopoietic system, led to the identification of recurrent chromosomal aberrations, reflecting pathologic rearrangements of the cellular genome. Taken together, these observations suggest that the molecular pathogenesis of human cancer is due to structural and/or functional alterations of specific genes whose normal function is to control cellular growth and differentiation or, in different terms, cell birth and cell death.[1,2]

The identification and characterization of the genetic elements playing a role in the scenario of human cancer pathogenesis have been made possible by the development of DNA recombinant techniques during the past decades, enhanced by the possibility to sequence even the whole genome. One milestone was the identification of the cellular origin of the "viral oncogenes" followed by the possibility to transfer the tumorigenic properties to the RNA tumor viruses also known as retroviruses.[3,4] Lastly, it was discovered that most cellular transforming genes do not have a viral counterpart. Besides the source of their original identification, viral or cellular genome, these transforming genetic elements have been designated as proto-oncogene in their normal physiologic version and oncogene when altered in cancer.[5] A second relevant experimental approach has regarded the identification and characterization of clonal and recurrent cytogenetic abnormalities (including translocations and inversions) in cancer cells, especially those derived from the hematopoietic system. Additional oncogenes have been identified through the analysis of anomalously stained chromosomal regions (homogeneously staining regions (HSRs), representing gene amplification.[6] Furthermore, the detection of chromosome deletions has been instrumental in the process of identification and cloning of a second class of cancer-associated genes, the tumor suppressors (which act in the normal cell as negative controllers of cell growth and are inactive in tumor cells).[5,6] Lastly, using automated sequencing instruments, it has been demonstrated that also point mutations are a frequent mechanism of oncogene activation.[7] In the last subgroup, we can also number those obtained by the analysis of the protein kinases (kinome)[8] or phosphatases (phosphatome)[9] of the human genome or of several isoforms of a relevant protein involved in cancer development (such as PI3K).[10]

In this chapter, the methods by which oncogenes were discovered will be first briefly described. The various functions of cellular proto-oncogenes will then be presented, and the genetic mechanisms of proto-oncogene activation will be summarized. Then, the role of specific oncogenes in the initiation and progression of human tumors will be discussed. Lastly, the discovery that oncogenes may represent relevant target for new drugs will be described.

Discovery and identification of oncogenes

The first oncogenes were discovered through the study of *retroviruses*, RNA tumor viruses whose genomes are reverse transcribed into DNA in infected animal cells.[11] During the course of infection, retroviral DNA is inserted into the chromosomes of host cells. The integrated retroviral DNA, called the provirus, replicates along with the cellular DNA of the host, leading to the production of viral progeny that bud through the host cell membrane to infect other cells.[11] Acutely transforming retroviruses can rapidly cause tumors within days after injection. Chronic or weakly oncogenic retroviruses can cause tissue-specific tumors in susceptible strains of experimental animals after a latency period of many months.

Retroviral oncogenes are altered versions of host cellular proto-oncogenes that have been incorporated into the retroviral genome by recombination with host DNA, a process known as retroviral *transduction*.[5] This surprising discovery was made through study of the Rous sarcoma virus (RSV) (Figure 1), revealing that the transforming gene of RSV was not required for viral

Holland-Frei Cancer Medicine, Ninth Edition. Edited by Robert C. Bast Jr., Carlo M. Croce, William N. Hait, Waun Ki Hong, Donald W. Kufe, Martine Piccart-Gebhart, Raphael E. Pollock, Ralph R. Weichselbaum, Hongyang Wang, and James F. Holland.
© 2017 John Wiley & Sons, Inc. ISBN: 978-1-118-93469-2

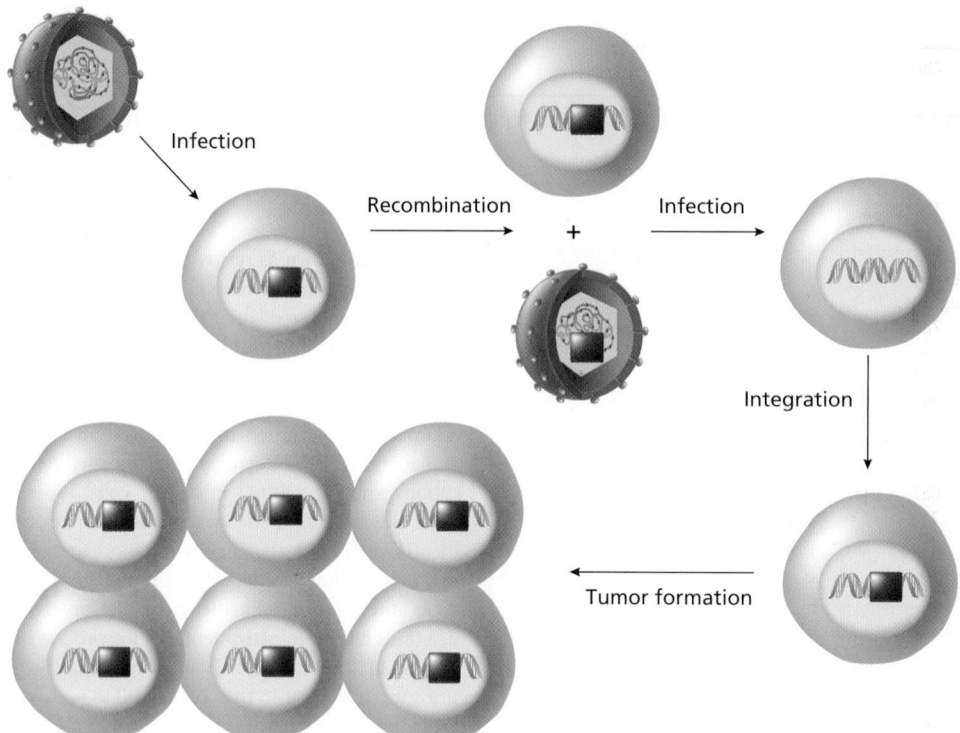

Figure 1 Retroviral transduction. An RNA tumor virus infects a human cell carrying an activated *src* gene (red box). After the process of recombination between retroviral genome and host DNA, the oncogene *c-src** is incorporated into the retroviral genome and is renamed *v-src*. When the retrovirus carrying *v-src* infects a human cell, the viral oncogeneis rapidly transcribes and is responsible for the rapid tumor formation.

replication.[12] Molecular hybridization studies then showed that the RSV transforming gene (designated *v-src*) was homologous to a host cellular gene (*c-src*) that was widely conserved in eukaryotic species.[13] Studies of many other acutely transforming retroviruses from fowl, rodent, feline, and nonhuman primate species have led to the discovery of dozens of different retroviral oncogenes (Table 1). In every case, these retroviral oncogenes are responsible for the rapid tumor formation and efficient *in vitro* transformation activity, characteristic of acutely transforming retroviruses.

In contrast, weakly oncogenic retroviruses do not carry viral oncogenes. These retroviruses, which include mouse mammary tumor virus (MMTV) and various animal leukemia viruses, induce tumors by a process called *insertional mutagenesis* (Figure 2).[6] This process results from the integration of the provirus DNA into the host genome in infected cells and acquires relevance when (rarely) the provirus is inserted near a proto-oncogene, whose expression is then abnormally driven by the transcriptional regulatory elements contained within the long terminal repeats of the provirus.[6] Therefore, proviral integration represents a mutagenic event that activates a proto-oncogene. The long latent period of tumor formation of weakly oncogenic retroviruses is therefore due to the rarity of the provirus insertional event that leads to tumor development from a single transformed cell. Insertional mutagenesis by weakly oncogenic retroviruses, first demonstrated in bursal lymphomas of chickens, frequently involves the same oncogenes (such as *myc*, *myb*, and *erb B*) that are carried by acutely transforming retroviruses.[6,14] In many cases, however, insertional mutagenesis has been used as a tool to identify new oncogenes, including *int-1, int-2, pim-1,* and *lck*.[6]

The demonstration of activated proto-oncogenes in human tumors was first shown by the DNA-mediated transformation technique.[15,16] This method, also called *gene-transfer* or *transfection*

assay, verifies the ability of donor DNA from a tumor to transform a recipient strain of rodent cells called NIH 3T3, an immortalized mouse cell line (Figure 3).[17] This sensitive assay, which can detect the presence of single-copy oncogenes in a tumor sample, also enables the isolation of the transforming oncogene by molecular cloning techniques.[18] Overall, approximately 20% of individual human tumors have been shown to induce transformation of NIH 3T3 cells in gene-transfer assays. The value of transfection assay was reinforced by Weinberg's laboratory, which showed that the ectopic expression of the telomerase catalytic subunit (hTERT), in combination with the simian virus 40 large T product and a mutated oncogenic H-ras protein, resulted in the direct tumorigenic conversion of normal human epithelial and fibroblast cells.[19] Many of the oncogenes identified by gene-transfer studies are identical or closely related to oncogenes transduced by retroviruses.[20] A number of new oncogenes (such as *neu, met,* and *trk*) have also been identified by the gene-transfer technique.[21] In many cases, however, oncogenes identified by gene transfer were shown to be activated by rearrangement during the experimental procedure and are not activated in the human tumors that served as the source of the donor DNA, as in the case of *ret* that was subsequently found genuinely rearranged and activated in papillary thyroid carcinomas.[22]

Chromosomal translocations have served as guideposts for the discovery of new oncogenes, especially in many hematological and solid tumors.[23,24] These abnormalities include chromosomal rearrangements as well as the gain or loss of whole chromosomes or chromosome segments. The first consistent karyotypic abnormality identified in a human neoplasm was a characteristic small chromosome in the cells of patients with chronic myelogenous leukemia (CML).[23] Later identified as a derivative of

Table 1 Oncogenes.

Oncogene	Chromosome	Identification	Method neoplasm mechanism of activation	Protein function	
Growth factors					
V-SIS	22q12.3–13.1	Sequence homology	Glioma/fibrosarcoma	Constitutive production	B-chain PDGF
INT2	11q13	Proviral insertion	Mammary carcinoma	Constitutive production	Member of FGF family
KS3	11q13.3	DNA transfection	Kaposi sarcoma	Constitutive production	Member of FGF family
HST	11q13.3	DNA transfection	Stomach carcinoma	Constitutive production	Member of FGF family
Growth factor receptors					
Tyrosine kinases: integral membrane proteins					
EGFR	7p1.1–1.3	DNA amplification/DNA sequencing	Squamous cell carcinoma	Gene amplification/protein/point	EGF receptor
v-FMS	5q33–34 (FMS)	Viral homolog	Sarcoma	Constitutive activation	CSF1 receptor
v-KIT	4q11–21 (KIT)	Viral homolog/DNA sequencing	Sarcoma/GIST	Constitutive activation/point mutation	Stem cell factor receptor
v-ROS	6q22(ROS)	Viral homolog	Sarcoma	Constitutive activation	Chimeric protein
MET	7p31	DNA transfection	MNNG-treated human osteocarcinoma cell line	DNA rearrangement/ligand-independent constitutive activation (fusion proteins)	HGF/SF receptor
TRK	1q32–41	DNA transfection	Colon/thyroid carcinomas	DNA rearrangement/ligand-independent constitutive activation (fusion proteins)	NGF receptor
NEU	17q11.2–12	Point mutation/DNA amplification	Neuroblastoma/breast carcinoma/NSCLC	Gene amplification/point mutation	Unknown ligand
RET	10q11.2	DNA transfection	Carcinomas of thyroid Men 2A/Men 2B	DNA rearrangement/point mutation (ligand-independent constitutive activation/fusion proteins)	GDNF/NTT/ART/PSP receptor
Receptors lacking protein kinase activity					
MAS	6q24–27	DNA transfection	Epidermoid carcinoma	Rearrangement of 5' noncoding region	Angiotensin receptor
Signal transducers					
Cytoplasmic tyrosine kinases					
SRC	20p12–13	Viral homolog	Colon carcinoma	Constitutive activation	Protein tyrosine kinase
v-YES	18q21–23 (YES)	Viral homolog	Sarcoma	Constitutive activation	Protein tyrosine kinase
v-FGR	1p36.1–36.2 (FGR)	Viral homolog	Sarcoma	Constitutive activation	Protein tyrosine kinase
v-FES	15q25–26 (FES)	Viral homolog	Sarcoma	Constitutive activation	Protein tyrosine kinase
ABL	9q34.1	Chromosome translocation	CML	DNA rearrangement (constitutive activation/fusion proteins)	Protein tyrosine kinase
Membrane-associated G proteins					
HRAS	11p15.5	Viral homolog/DNA transfection	Colon, lung, pancreas carcinomas	Point mutation	GTPase
KRAS	12p11.1–12.1	Viral homolog/DNA transfection	AML, thyroid carcinoma, melanoma/colon/lung	Point mutation	GTPase
NRAS	1p11–13	DNA transfection	Carcinoma, melanoma	Point mutation	GTPase
BRAF	6	DNA sequencing	Melanoma, thyroid, colon, ovary	Point mutation	Ser/Thr kinase
GSP	20	DNA sequencing	Adenomas of thyroid	Point mutation	Gs alpha
GIP	3	DNA sequencing	Ovary, adrenal carcinoma	Point mutation	Gi alpha
GTPase exchange factor (GEF)					
DBL	Xq27	DNA transfection	Diffuse B-cell lymphoma	DNA rearrangement	GEF for Rho and Cdc42Hs
VAV	19p13.2	DNA transfection	Hematopoietic cells	DNA rearrangement	GEF for Ras?
Serine/threonine kinases: cytoplasmic					
v-MOS	8q11 (MOS)	Viral homolog	Sarcoma	Constitutive activation	Protein kinase (ser/thr)
v-RAF	3p25 (RAF-1)	Viral homolog	Sarcoma	Constitutive activation	Protein kinase (ser/thr)
PIM-1	6p21 (PIM-)	Insertional mutagenesis	T-cell lymphoma	Constitutive activation	Protein kinase (ser/thr)
Cytoplasmic regulators					
v-CRK	17p13 (CRK)	Viral homolog	—	Constitutive tyrosine phosphorylation of cellular substrates (e.g., paxillin)	SH-2/SH-3 adaptor

(continued overleaf)

Table 1 (Continued)

Oncogene	Chromosome	Identification	Method neoplasm mechanism of activation		Protein function
Transcription factors					
v-MYC	8q24.1 (MYC)	Viral homolog	Carcinoma myelocytomatosis	Deregulated activity	Transcription factor
N-MYC	2p24	DNA amplification	Neuroblastoma: lung	Deregulated activity	Transcription factor
L-MYC	1p32	DNA amplification	Carcinoma of lung	Deregulated activity	Transcription factor
v-MYB	6q22−24	Viral homolog	Myeloblastosis	Deregulated activity	Transcription factor
v-FOS	14q21−22	Viral homolog	Osteosarcoma	Deregulated activity	Transcription factor API
v-JUN	p31−32	Viral homolog	Sarcoma	Deregulated activity	Transcription factor API
v-SKI	1q22−24	Viral homolog	Carcinoma	Deregulated activity	Transcription factor
v-REL	2p12−14	Viral homolog	Lymphatic leukemia	Deregulated activity	Mutant NF-kappa B
v-ETS-1	11p23−q24	Viral homolog	Erythroblastosis	Deregulated activity	Transcription factor
v-ETS-2	21q24.3	Viral homolog	Erythroblastosis	Deregulated activity	Transcription factor
v-ERB A1	17p11−21	Viral homolog	Erythroblastosis	Deregulated activity	T3 Transcription factor
v-ERB A2	3p22−24.1	Viral homolog	Erythroblastosis	Deregulated activity	T3 Transcription factor
Others					
BCL2	18q21.3	Chromosomal translocation	B-cell lymphomas	Constitutive activity	Antiapoptotic protein
MDM2	12q14	DNA amplification	Sarcomas	Gene amplification/increased protein	Complexes with p53

Abbreviations: AML, acute myeloid leukemia; CML, chronic myelogenous leukemia; GTPase, guanosine triphosphatase; PDGF, platelet-derived growth factor.

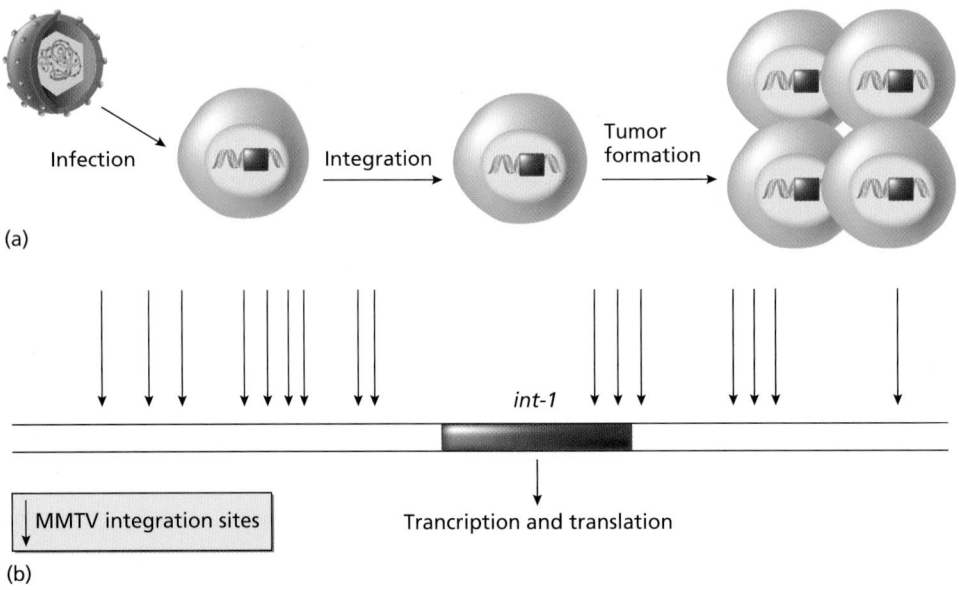

Figure 2 Insertional mutagenesis. (a) The process is independent from genes carried by the retrovirus. Retrovirus, for example, MMTV, infects a human cell. The proviral DNA is integrated into the host genome in infected cells. Rarely, the provirus inserts near a proto-oncogene (e.g., *int-1*) and activates the proto-oncogene. Activated proto-oncogene results in cell transformation and in tumor formation. (b) Sites of integration of MMTV retrovirus near the proto-oncogene *int-1*. All sites determine *int-1* activation.

chromosome 22, this abnormality was designated the Philadelphia chromosome, after its city of discovery. The application of chromosome banding techniques in the early 1970s enabled the precise cytogenetic characterization of many chromosomal translocations in human leukemia, lymphoma, and solid tumors.[25] The subsequent development of molecular cloning techniques then enabled the identification of proto-oncogenes at or near chromosomal breakpoints in various neoplasms. Some of these proto-oncogenes, such as *myc* and *abl*, had been previously identified as retroviral oncogenes. In general, however, the cloning of chromosomal breakpoints has served as a rich source of discovery of new oncogenes involved in human cancer. More recently, the use of high-throughput sequencing technologies and bioinformatics

from the Human Genome Project led to the discovery of new genes involved in cancer development, such as *BRAF* and *PIK3CA*.[7,10]

Oncogenes, proto-oncogenes, and their functions

Proto-oncogenes encode proteins that are involved in the control of cell growth. Alteration of the structure and/or expression of proto-oncogenes can activate them to become oncogenes capable of inducing in susceptible cells the neoplastic phenotype. Oncogenes can be classified into five groups based on the functional and biochemical properties of protein products of their normal counterparts (proto-oncogenes). These groups are (1) growth factors, (2) growth factor receptors, (3) signal transducers, (4) transcription factors, and (5) others, including programmed cell death regulators.

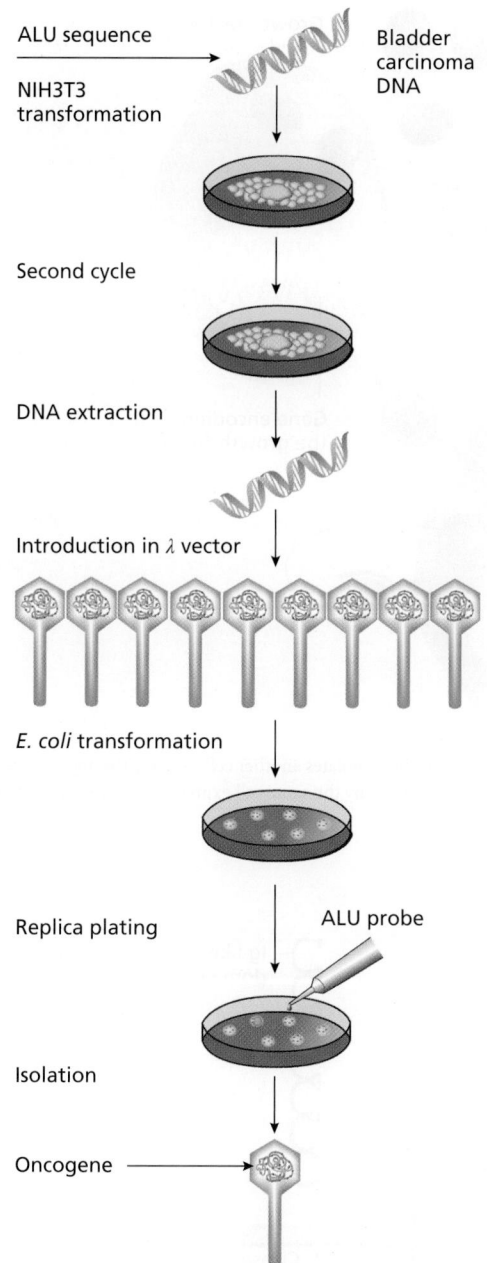

Figure 3 Transfection assay. DNA from a tumor (e.g., bladder carcinoma) is used to transform a rodent immortalized cell line (NIH3T3). After serial cycles, DNA from transformed cells was extracted and then inserted into p vector that was subsequently used to transform an appropriate *Escherichia coli* strain. Using a specific probe (Alu in the figure), it was possible to isolate and then characterize the involved human oncogene.

Table 1 lists examples of oncogenes according to their functional categories.

Growth factors

Growth factors are secreted polypeptides that function as extracellular signals to stimulate the proliferation of target cells that possess a specific receptor in order to respond to a specific type of growth factor.[2] A well-characterized example is platelet-derived growth factor (PDGF), an approximately 30-kDa protein consisting of two polypeptide chains.[26] PDGF, released from platelets during the process of blood coagulation, stimulates the proliferation of fibroblasts, a cell growth process that plays an important role in

wound healing. Other well-characterized examples of growth factors include nerve growth factor (NGF), epidermal growth factor, and fibroblast growth factor.

The link between growth factors and retroviral oncogenes was revealed by study of the *sis* oncogene of simian sarcoma virus, a retrovirus first isolated from a monkey fibrosarcoma. Sequence analysis showed that *sis* encodes the beta chain of PDGF.[26] This discovery established the principle that inappropriately expressed growth factors may constitutively activate their receptor, resulting in self-sustained aberrant cell proliferation and therefore functioning as oncogenes. The mechanism behind is called *autocrine stimulation* (Figure 4).[26] This model, derived from experimental animal systems, has been demonstrated in a human tumor, dermatofibrosarcoma protuberans (DP), an infiltrative skin tumor that was demonstrated to present specific cytogenetic features: reciprocal translocation and supernumerary ring chromosomes, involving chromosomes 17 and 22.[26] Molecular cloning of the breakpoints revealed a fusion between the *collagen type Ia1 (COL1A1)* gene and PDGF-B gene. The fusion gene resulted in a deletion of PDGF-B exon 1 and a constitutive release of this growth factor. Subsequent experiments of gene transfer of DP's genomic DNA into NIH 3T3 cells directly demonstrated the occurrence of an autocrine mechanism by the human rearranged PDGF-B gene involving the activation of the endogenous PDGF receptor.[26] Another example of a growth factor that can function as an oncogene is *int-2*, a member of the fibroblast growth factor family. *Int-2* is sometimes activated in mouse mammary carcinomas by MMTV insertional mutagenesis.[27]

Growth factor receptors

Some viral oncogenes are altered versions of normal growth factor receptors that possess intrinsic tyrosine kinase (TK) activity.[28] Receptor tyrosine kinases (RTKs), as these growth factor receptors are collectively known, have a characteristic protein structure consisting of three principal domains: (1) the extracellular ligand-binding domain, (2) the transmembrane domain, and (3) the intracellular TK catalytic domain (Figure 5). RTKs are molecular machines that transmit information in a unidirectional manner across the cell membrane. The binding of a growth factor to the extracellular ligand-binding domain of the receptor results in the activation of the intracellular TK catalytic domain, usually after dimerization, leading to the activation of downstream proteins that physically interact with RTK, mainly represented by the mitogen-activated protein kinases (MAPKs) pathway, by the PI3K/AKT axis and by STAT proteins. These pathways are activated differently, depending on the specific RTK, overall resulting in abnormal cell duplication and in escaping from programmed cell death (apoptosis).[28]

The list of RTK includes *ERB B1*, *ERB B2*, *FMS*, *KIT*, *MET*, *RET*, *ROS*, *ALK*, and *TRK*, which can be converted into oncogenes through different mechanisms, often depending on tumor type.[28] *ERB B1* (the epidermal growth factor receptor—EGFR) can be oncogenically activated by deletion of the ligand-binding domain, by point mutations in the TK domain in a subgroup of patients affected by non-small-cell lung cancer (NSCLC) (more commonly in Japan than in other western countries, suggesting that ethnic differences may have a significant impact on *ERB B1* activation),[29] or at germ-line level in patients showing multiple lung adenocarcinomas,[30] by overexpression of ligands or by gene amplification in colorectal cancer (CRC) patients.[31,32]

Another example is represented by *ERB B2*, whose growth factor is still unknown, which is altered by gene amplification in breast and gastric cancers and by point mutations in gastric, colorectal,

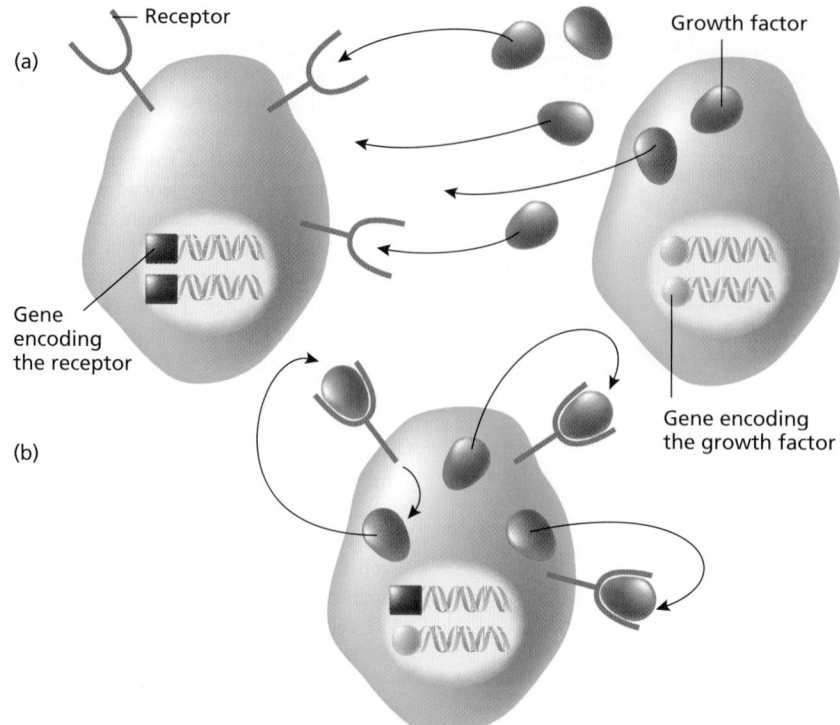

Figure 4 Paracrine and autocrine stimulation. (a) A growth factor produced by the cell on the right stimulates another cell carrying the appropriate receptor (left) on cell membrane. This process is named paracrine stimulation. (b) A growth factor is produced by the same cell expressing the cognate receptor. This process is designated autocrine stimulation.

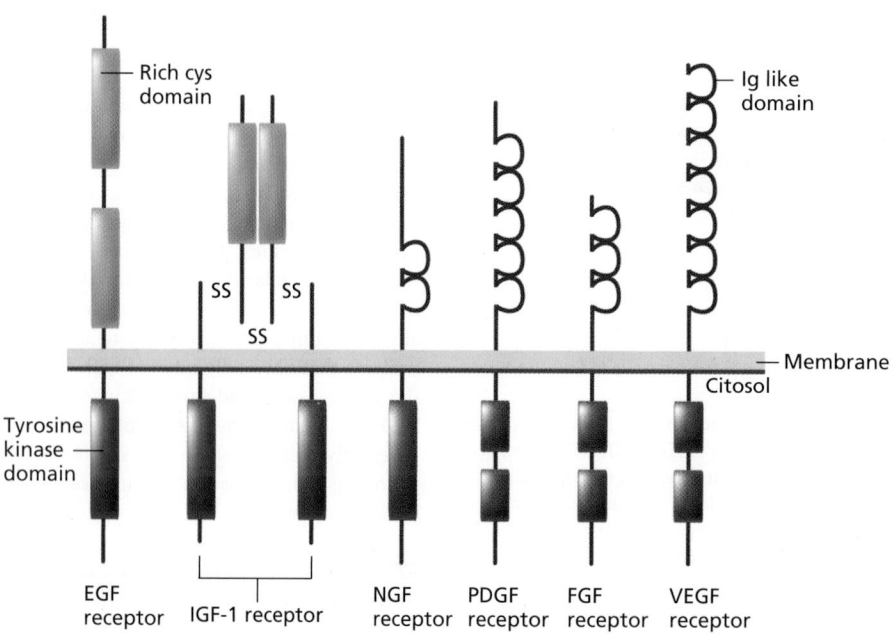

Figure 5 Representative examples of tyrosine kinase receptor families.

and breast cancers. Interestingly, immunohistochemical staining for *ERB B2* revealed no differences between tumors with or without *ERB B2* mutations, indicating that overexpression probably does not accompany the mutation.[33]

Last example is *KIT*, whose activation in tumor cells can be due to three different mechanisms: (1) autocrine and/or paracrine stimulation of the receptor by its ligand, stem cell factor (SCF); (2) cross-activation by other kinases and/or loss of

regulatory phosphatase activity; and (3) acquisition of activating mutations of several different exons of the *KIT* gene.[34] *KIT* mutations (typically in exon 17) are most commonly found in mastocytosis/mast cell leukemia, acute myelogenous leukemia (AML), seminoma/dysgerminoma, and sinosal natural killer/T-cell lymphoma. In gastrointestinal stromal tumors (GISTs), more heterogeneous mutations are described: mutations most commonly occur in exon 11 (encoding the juxtamembrane region) (in about

65% of all GISTs), whereas about 10% of GISTs have kit exon 9 mutations and 2% exon 13 or exon 17 mutations. In GIST showing any alterations in the *KIT* gene, point mutations may occur in *PDGFRA*, a gene belonging to the same family as *KIT*. Approximately 5% of GIST have a constitutively activating mutations in *PDGFRA*, mostly (80%) found in exon 18 and the rest either in exon 12 (10–15%) or 14 (1–5%).[34] *KIT* and *PDGFRA* mutations are mutually exclusive. Gastric GISTs with exon 11 deletions are more aggressive than those with substitutions. The less common *KIT* exon 9 codons 502–503 duplication occurs predominantly in small intestinal GISTs. *PDGFRA* mutations are associated with gastric GISTs, epithelioid morphology and a less malignant course of disease.[34] Germ-line mutations in *KIT* gene have been found in patients manifesting multiple GIST arising at earlier age, urticaria pigmentosa, melanocytic nevi, melanomas, achalasia, or neuronal hyperplasia of the mesentheric plexus.

Signal transducers

Mitogenic signals are transmitted from RTK on the cell surface to the cell nucleus through a series of complex interlocking pathways collectively referred to as the signal transduction cascade.[28] This relay of information is accomplished in part by the stepwise phosphorylation of interacting proteins in the cytosol. Signal transduction also involves guanine nucleotide-binding proteins and second messengers such as the adenylate cyclase system. The first retroviral oncogene discovered, *SRC*, was subsequently shown to be involved in signal transduction.[13,28]

Many proto-oncogenes are members of signal transduction pathways.[35] These consist of two main groups: nonreceptor protein kinases and guanosine triphosphate (GTP)-binding proteins. The nonreceptor protein kinases are subclassified into TKs (e.g., *ABL*, *LCK*, and *SRC*) and serine/threonine kinases (e.g., *RAF-1*, *MOS*, and *PIM-1*). GTP-binding proteins with intrinsic guanosine triphosphatase (GTPase) activity are subdivided into monomeric and heterotrimeric groups. Monomeric GTP-binding proteins are members of the important *RAS* family of proto-oncogenes that includes *HRAS*, *KRAS*, and *NRAS*.[36] Heterotrimeric GTP-binding proteins (G proteins) implicated as proto-oncogenes currently include *GSP* and *GIP*. Signal transducers are often converted to oncogenes by mutations that lead to their unregulated activity, which in turn leads to uncontrolled cellular proliferation.[36]

Transcription factors

Transcription factors are nuclear proteins that regulate the expression of target genes or gene families.[37] Transcriptional regulation is mediated by protein binding to specific DNA sequences or DNA structural motifs (such as zinc fingers), usually located upstream of the target gene. The mechanism of action of transcription factors also involves binding to other proteins, sometimes in heterodimeric complexes with specific partners. Transcription factors are the final link in the signal transduction pathway that converts extracellular signals into modulated changes in gene expression.

Many proto-oncogenes are transcription factors that were discovered through their retroviral homologs.[37] Examples include *ERB A*, *ETS*, *FOS*, *JUN*, *MYB*, and *C-MYC*. Together, fos and jun form the AP-1 transcription factor, which positively regulates a number of target genes whose expression leads to cell division.[38] *ERB A* is the receptor for the T3 thyroid hormone, triiodothyronine.[39] Proto-oncogenes that function as transcription factors are often activated by chromosomal translocations in hematologic and solid neoplasms. In certain types of sarcomas, chromosomal translocations cause the formation of fusion proteins involving the association of *EWS* gene with various partners and resulting in an

aberrant tumor-associated transcriptional activity. Interestingly, a role of the adenovirus *E1A* gene in promoting the formation of fusion transcript fli1/ews in normal human fibroblasts was recently reported.[40] An important example of a proto-oncogene with a transcriptional activity in human hematologic tumors is the *C-MYC* gene, which helps to control the expression of genes leading to cell proliferation.[41] As will be discussed later in this chapter, the *C-MYC* gene (which is encoded for a nuclear DNA-binding protein belonging to the helix-loop-helix/leucine zipper superfamily, involved in transcriptional regulation) is frequently activated by chromosomal translocations in human leukemia and lymphoma.

Programed cell death regulation

Normal tissues exhibit a regulated balance between cell proliferation and cell death. Programmed cell death is an important component in the processes of normal embryogenesis and organ development. A distinctive type of programmed cell death, called apoptosis, has been described for mature tissues.[42] Studies of cancer cells have shown that both uncontrolled cell proliferation and failure to undergo programmed cell death can contribute to neoplasia and insensitivity to anticancer treatments.

The first proto-oncogene shown to regulate programmed cell death is *BCL-2*, discovered in human lymphomas. Experimental studies show that *BCL-2* activation inhibits (in a dominant mode) programmed cell death in lymphoid cell populations. The *BCL-2* gene encodes a protein localized to the inner mitochondrial membrane, endoplasmic reticulum, and nuclear membrane. The mechanism of action of the bcl-2 protein has not been fully elucidated, but studies indicate that it functions in part as an antioxidant that inhibits lipid peroxidation of cell membranes,[43] and in part through protein–protein interaction with homolog proteins. Site-directed mutagenesis of BH1 and BH2 domains showed that these two regions are important for binding of bcl-2 to bax, a member of the bcl-2-family that promotes cell death and whose interaction with bcl-2 is necessary to regulate the apoptotic pathway (Figure 6). Although translocation is the main mechanism of *BCL-2* gene activation, *BCL-2* point mutations (in high-grade B-cell lymphomas) and amplification (in about 30% of high-grade diffuse large cell lymphomas (DLCL) lacking bcl-2 translocation) have been reported.[44] Clinical relevance of BCL-2 expression has

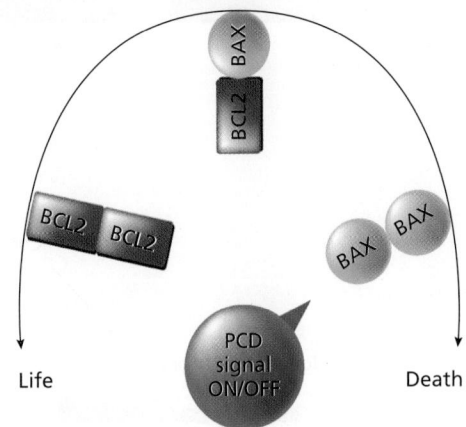

Figure 6 Effect of bcl-2 activity on the control of the cell life. In the presence of BAX only, the cell goes to apoptosis. bcl-2 regulates the cycle of the cell by the interaction with BAX. When bcl-2 is overexpressed, the cell cycle is deregulated and the apoptosis is prevented, eventually leading to tumor formation. This is an important cause for tumor formation. *Abbreviations*: PCD, program cell death or apoptosis.

been shown in solid tumors, such as breast, prostate, thyroid, and lung.[45,46]

The second oncogene involved in apoptosis is caspase-9, which is activated by the following intrinsic pathway. Release of cytochrome c into the cytosol results in activation of the caspase adaptor Apaf-1 and procaspase-9, which form a holoenzyme complex named apoptosome.[47] Caspase-9, in turn, activates downstream caspases, especially caspase-3 and also caspase-6, 7, and 8, leading to DNA fragmentation and apoptosis. It has been demonstrated that Akt may regulate apoptosome function by phosphorylation of caspase-9 at the Ser-196 level.[48] This phosphorylation event has relevant functional consequences, leading to the suppression of apoptosis caspase-9-mediated. The Akt suppression is specific for caspase-9 and probably is due to the inactivation of the intrinsic catalytic activity. More recently, it has been demonstrated that bax is also involved, leading to caspase-9 stimulation (through Apaf-1) in response to mitochondrial membrane damage.[49]

Mechanisms of oncogene activation

The activation of oncogenes involves genetic changes to cellular proto-oncogenes. The consequence of these genetic alterations is to confer a growth advantage to the cell. Four genetic mechanisms activate oncogenes in human neoplasms: (1) mutation, (2) gene amplification, (3) chromosome rearrangements, and (4) overexpression. The first three mechanisms result in either an alteration of proto-oncogene structure or an increase in proto-oncogene expression (Figure 7). Because neoplasia is a multistep process, more than one of these mechanisms may occur, leading to a combination of proto-oncogene activation and tumor-suppressor gene loss or inactivation.

Mutation

Mutations activate proto-oncogenes through structural alterations in their encoded proteins. These alterations, which usually involve critical protein regulatory regions or directly the catalytic domain,

often lead to the uncontrolled, continuous activity of the mutated protein. Various types of mutations, such as base substitutions, deletions, and insertions, are capable of activating proto-oncogenes.[50] Retroviral oncogenes, for example, often have deletions that contribute to their activation. Examples include deletions in the amino-terminal ligand-binding domains of the *ERB B*, *KIT*, *ROS*, *MET*, and *TRK* oncogenes. In human tumors, however, most characterized oncogene mutations are base substitutions (point mutations) that change a single amino acid within the protein.

Point mutations are frequently detected in the ras family of protooncogenes (*KRAS*, *HRAS*, and *NRAS*). The human *ras* genes encode for membrane-bound 21 kd proteins (189 amino acids) involved in signal transduction, with a guanine nucleotide-binding activity as well as an intrinsic GTPase activity. When activated, ras proteins transduce the signal by linking TKs to downstream serine/threonine kinases, such as raf, and MAP kinases (Figure 8).[51] Stabilization of ras proteins in their active state causes a continuous flow of signal transduction, which results in malignant transformation. This status can be achieved after point mutation, mainly at codon 12 (in *KRAS* gene), 13 and 61 (mainly in *NRAS* gene) level. Rare mutations can be detected in codons 59, 117, and 146.[52] Mutations of *ras* in human tumors have been linked to carcinogen exposure: for example, the occurrence of *KRAS* mutations in NSCLC seems to be due to smoking exposure, in particular to benzoapyrene.[53] It has been estimated that as many as 15–20% of unselected human tumors may contain a *RAS* mutation. Mutations in *KRAS* predominate in tumors derived from endodermal tumors, including carcinomas of pancreas (90%), colorectal (40%) and lung.[36,51] This finding is due to the fact that *KRAS*, but not *HRAS* or *NRAS*, promotes the expansion of an endodermal stem/progenitor cell and blocks its differentiation.[54] *NRAS* mutations are preferentially found in hematologic malignancies, with up to a 25% incidence in AMLs and myelodysplastic syndromes, or in melanoma and in a subgroup of CRC.[55] The majority of thyroid carcinomas have been found to have *RAS* mutations distributed among *KRAS*, *HRAS*, and *NRAS*, without preference for a single

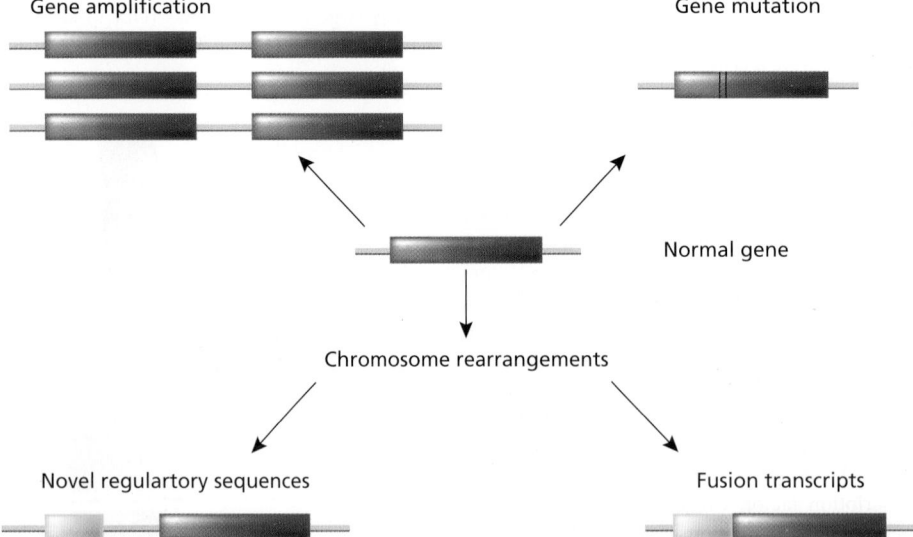

Figure 7 Schematic representation of the main mechanisms of oncogene activation (from proto-oncogenes to oncogenes). The normal gene (proto-oncogene) is depicted with its transcribed portion (rectangle). In the case of gene amplification, the latter can be duplicated 100-fold, resulting in an excess of normal protein. A similar situation can occur when following chromosome rearrangements such as translocation, the transcription of the gene is now regulated by novel regulatory sequences belonging to another gene. In the case of point mutation, single amino acid substitutions can alter the biochemical properties of the gene product, causing, in the example, its constitutive enzymatic activation. Chromosome rearrangements, such as translocation and inversion, can then generate fusion transcripts resulting in chimericoncogenic proteins.

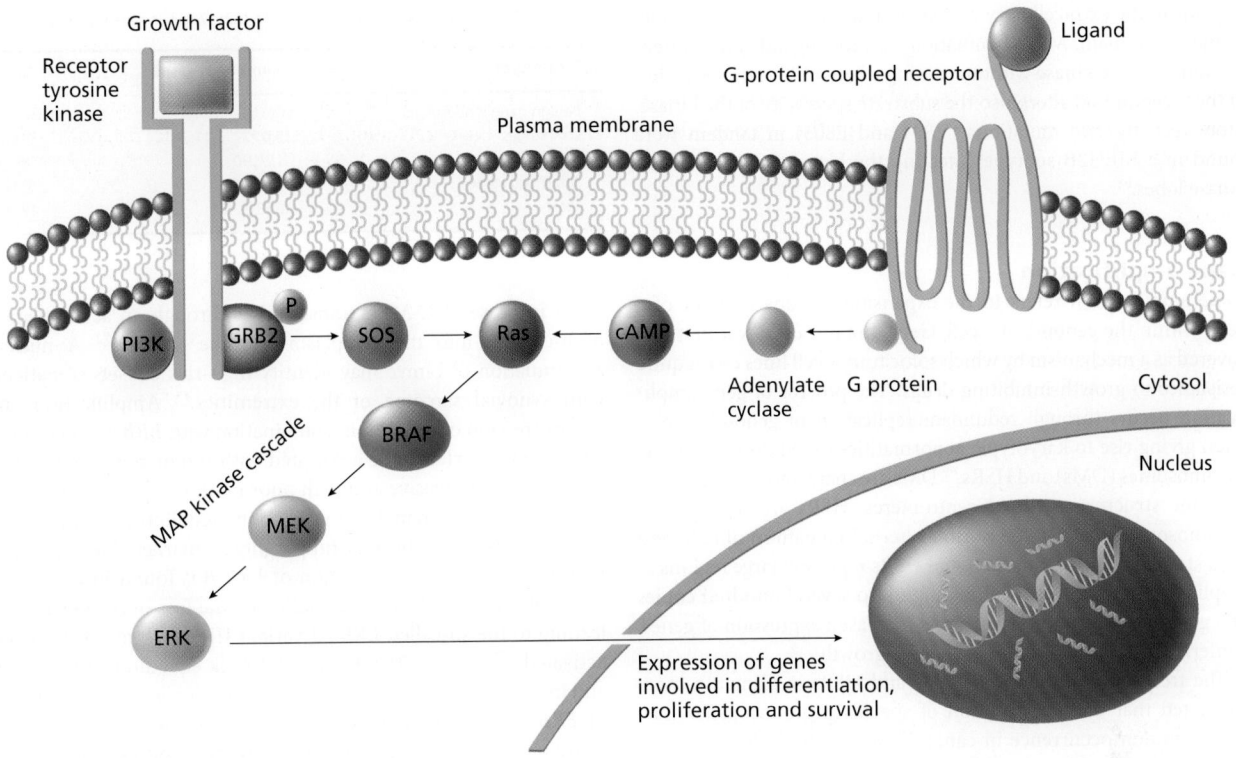

Figure 8 The ras–raf–MAPK signaling pathway.

RAS family member, but showing an association with the follicular type of differentiated thyroid carcinomas. Moreover, again in CRC, the identification of *KRAS* mutations in stool samples may be used in early diagnosis,[56] and in plasma samples for monitoring patients' follow-up.[57]

In addition to cancer, *RAS* mutations are involved in other diseases. Specifically, *NRAS* mutations cause a human autoimmune lymphoproliferative syndrome,[58] while *HRAS* and *KRAS* germ-line mutations underlie disorders of the Noonan syndrome spectrum.[51] The last data, coupled with the evidence that cancers rarely occur in these individuals, is leading to a re-evaluation of the effective role played by *RAS* genes in carcinogenesis.

Another example of activating point mutations is represented by those occurring in *BRAF* gene, the first result of the human genome project in the screening of cancer genes using high-throughput genomic technologies.[7] The *BRAF* gene product is recruited to the plasma membrane upon binding to ras-GTP and represents a key point in the signal transduction through the MAP kinase pathway (Figure 8). The most common oncogenic mutation of *BRAF*, occurring in more than 90% of cases, is the valine to glutamic acid change at codon 600, which mimics the phosphorylation of threonine 599 and serine 602, required for BRAF activation.[7] In tissue specimens, *BRAF* mutations occur in melanomas (75%), thyroid (45%), colorectal (12%), and ovarian cancer (14%)[59] and in acute lymphoblastic leukemia (ALL).[60] Furthermore, it has been shown that *BRAF* mutations occur in CRC only when tumors do not carry mutations in the *KRAS* gene, and in papillary thyroid carcinoma when *RET* or *TRK* rearrangements are absent. These mutual exclusions have led to the assumption that *BRAF* and *K-ras* alterations, or *BRAF*, *RET,* and *TRK* alterations, could have the same functional effect in colorectal or in thyroid carcinogenesis, respectively.[59,61] As regards CRC, *BRAF* mutations are frequently present in sporadic cases with methylated h*MLH1* promoter but not in HNPCC-related cancers, thus representing a possible strategy

for exclusion criteria for HNPCC.[62] Moreover, *BRAF* mutations are frequently found in hyperplastic polyps and serrated adenomas,[63] suggesting that they represent an early and critical event in these types of lesions. *BRAF* mutations may have an influence on patients' prognosis depending on the tumor type where they occur: in ovarian cancer, *BRAF* mutations are associated with type I tumors that are slow growing and generally confined to the ovary at diagnosis[64] and with the aggressive papillary thyroid and colorectal carcinomas.[59] *BRAF* mutations, especially the V600E change that is very easy to investigate, are now acquiring a role in early diagnosis or disease monitoring in patients' follow-up: indeed, they are investigated to improve the diagnosis in fine-needle aspiration biopsy with cytological findings suspicious for papillary thyroid carcinomas.[65] On the contrary, in melanoma, *BRAF* mutations could be only used to monitor in serum the follow-up of patients receiving biochemotherapy[66] and not for early diagnosis because they even precede the neoplastic transformation, as all types of nevi besides Spitz and Blue nevi show *BRAF* alterations at a high frequency.[67]

Another significant example of activating point mutations is represented by those affecting the *RET* proto-oncogene in multiple endocrine neoplasia (MEN) type 2 (2A and 2B) syndrome and familial medullary thyroid carcinomas (FMTC). MEN 2A is associated most frequently with mutations of codon 634 (85%), particularly C634R. This germ-line point mutation affecting one of the cysteine residues located in the juxtamembrane domain of the ret receptor has been found to confer an oncogenic potential through the abnormal formation of intermolecular disulfide bonding, resulting in a ligand-independent activation of the TK activity of the receptor. Most MEN2B patients carry the M918T mutation in the kinase domain, which confers an aggressive phenotype to MEN2B subtype. Sporadic mutations of V804, M918, and E768 occur in about 50% of sporadic medullary thyroid carcinomas, whereas FMTC mutations are evenly distributed among the various cysteins in the extracellulary cysteinerich domain and occasionally in the TK domain. M918T mutation lead to a ligand-independent activation of the kinase without causing a constitutive dimerization of the receptor and alters also the substrate specificity of the kinase. More recently, two mutations (V804 and E805) in tandem were found in a MEN2B subtype, affecting the hinging motion of the kinase lobes.[68]

Gene amplification

Gene amplification refers to the expansion in copy number of a gene within the genome of a cell. Gene amplification was first discovered as a mechanism by which some tumor cell lines can acquire resistance to growth-inhibiting drugs. The process of gene amplification occurs through redundant replication of genomic DNA, often giving rise to karyotypic abnormalities called double-minute chromosomes (DMs) and HSRs.[69] DMs are characteristic minichromosome structures without centromeres. HSRs are segments of chromosomes that lack the normal alternating pattern of light and dark staining bands. Both DMs and HSRs represent large regions of amplified genomic DNA, containing up to several hundred copies of a gene. Amplification leads to the increased expression of genes, conferring a selective advantage for cell growth.

The frequent observation of DMs and HSRs in human tumors suggested that the amplification of specific protooncogenes may be a common occurrence in cancer.[69] Studies then demonstrated that three proto-oncogene families—MYC, ERB B, and RAS—are amplified in a significant number of human tumors (Table 2). About 20–30% of breast and ovarian cancers show C-MYC amplification.[69] N-MYC was discovered as a new member of the MYC proto-oncogene family through its amplification in neuroblastomas.[70] Amplification of N-MYC correlates strongly with advanced tumor stage in neuroblastoma (Table 3), suggesting a role for this gene in tumor progression.[70] L-MYC was discovered through its amplification in small-cell lung carcinoma and bladder neoplasia.[71] Furthermore, C-MYC activation may be mediated by APC and/or b-catenin alterations in several tumors, leading

to an increase of C-MYC transcription through an accumulation of b-catenin into the cytoplasm and the nucleus.[72] A nuclear accumulation of c-myc may identify high-risk subsets of patients with synovial sarcoma of the extremities.[73] Amplification and overexpression of C-MYC, in combination with ERB B2 alterations, have been reported to be associated with tumor progression from noninvasive to invasive and with poor prognosis[74] in patients with breast carcinoma. In melanoma[75] and in medulloblastoma,[76] c-myc expression seems to be a useful prognostic marker able to identify high-risk patients. Amplification of ERB B is found in up to 50% of glioblastomas (often accompanied by the loss of the exons 2–7, leading to the so-called ERB B1 variant III, which is constitutively activated),[77] in 10–20% of head and neck squamous carcinomas, and in about 50% of CRC.[78] Gene amplification and overexpression of ERB B2 have been reported in approximately 25% of breast, ovarian, endometrial, gastric, and salivary gland carcinomas.[33] It was detected also in 16% of non-small-cell lung carcinoma and in a subset of malignant pancreatic endocrine tumor (gastrinoma). Overexpression of the ERB B2, performed at immunohistochemical level, was detected in thick melanoma, pancreatic carcinoma, and prostatic tumors.[33]

In breast cancer, ERB B2 amplification correlates with advanced stage and poor prognosis. Members of the RAS gene family, including KRAS and NRAS, are sporadically amplified in various carcinomas.[33]

Chromosomal rearrangements

Recurring chromosomal rearrangements are often detected in hematological malignancies and some solid tumors.[79] These rearrangements consist mainly of chromosomal translocations and, less frequently, chromosomal inversions. Chromosomal rearrangements can lead to hematological malignancy by two different mechanisms: (1) the transcriptional activation of proto-oncogenes or (2) the creation of fusion genes. Transcriptional activation results from chromosomal rearrangements that move a proto-oncogene close to an immunoglobulin or T-cell receptor (TCR) gene (Figure 7). Therefore, the proto-oncogene is constitutively activated in blood cells, leading to cancer development.

Fusion genes can be created by chromosomal rearrangements when the chromosomal breakpoints fall within the loci of two different genes, leading to a composite structure consisting of the head of one gene and the tail of another gene. Fusion genes encode chimeric proteins with transforming activity. In general, both genes involved in the fusion contribute to the transforming potential of the chimeric oncoprotein. Mistakes in the physiologic rearrangement of immunoglobulin or TCR genes are thought to give rise to many of the recurring chromosomal rearrangements found in hematologic malignancy.[80] Examples of molecularly characterized chromosomal rearrangements in hematologic and solid malignancies are given in Table 4. In some cases, the same proto-oncogene is involved in several different translocations (i.e., C-MYC, EWS, and RET).

Table 3 Correlation of N-myc copy number with stage and survival in neuroblastoma.

Tumor type	Number of cases	%
Benign ganglioneuromas	0/64	(0)
Low stages	31/772	(4)
Stage 4-S	15/190	(8)
Advanced stages	612/1.974	(31)
Total	658/3000	(22)

Table 2 Oncogene amplification in human cancers.

Tumor type	Gene amplified	%
Neuroblastoma	MYCN	20–25
Small-cell lung cancer	MYC	15–20
Glioblastoma	ERB B1 (EGFR)	33–50
Breast cancer	MYC	20
	ERB B2 (EGFR2)	~20
	FGFR1	12
	FGFR2	12
	CCND1 (cyclin d1)	15–20
Esophageal cancer	MYC	38
	CCND1 (cyclin d1)	25
Gastric cancer	KRAS	10
	CCNE (cyclin e)	15
Hepatocellular cancer	CCND1 (cyclin d1)	13
Sarcoma	MDM2	10–30
	CDK4	11
Cervical cancer	MYC	25–50
Ovarian cancer	MYC	20–30
	ERB B2 (EGFR2)	15–30
	AKT2	12
Head and neck cancer	MYC	7–10
	ERB B1 (EGFR)	10
	CCND1 (cyclin d1)	~50
Colorectal cancer	MYB	15–20
	HRAS	29
	KRAS	22

Table 4 Molecularly characterized chromosome rearrangements in tumors.

Affected gene	Rearrangements	Disease	Protein type
Hematopoietic tumor			
Gene fusion			
C-ABL (9q34)	t(9:22)(q34:q11)	Chronic myelogenous leukemia and acute leukemia	Tyrosine kinase activated by BCR
BCR (22q11)			
ALK (2p23)	t(2;5)(p23;q35)	Anaplastic large cell lymphomas	Tyrosine kinase activated by NPM
NPM (5q35)			
PDGFR-B (5q33)	t(5;12)(q33;p13)	Chronic myelomonocytic leukemia	Tyrosine kinase activated by tel
TEL (12p13)			
PBX1(1q23)	t(1:19)(q23:p13.3)	Acute pre-B-cell leukemia	Homeodomain (HLH)
E2A (19p13.3)			
PML(15q21)	t(15:17)(q21:q11−22)	Acute myeloid leukemia	Zn finger
RAR (17q21)			
CAN (6p23)	t(6:9)(p23:q34)	Acute myeloid leukemia	No homology
DEK (9q34)			
REL	ins(2:12)(p13:p11.2−14)	Non-Hodgkin's lymphoma	NF-κB family
NRG		No homology	
Oncogenes juxtaposed with IG loci			
C-MYC	t(8:14)(q24:q32)	Burkitt's lymphoma. BL-ALL	HLH domain
	t(2:8)(p12:q24)		
	t(8:22)(q24:q11)		
BCL-1 (PRADI?)	t(11:14)(q13:q3	B-cell chronic lymphocyte leukemia	PRADI-GI cyclin
BCL-2	t(14:18)(q32:21)	Follicular lymphoma	Inner mitochondrial membrane
BCL-3	t(14:19)(q32:q13.1)	Chronic B-cell leukemia	CDC10 motif
IL-3	t(5:14)(q31:q32)	Acute pre-B-cell leukemia	Growth factor
Oncogenes juxtaposed with TCR loci			
C-MYC	t(8:14)(q24:q11)	Acute T-cell leukemia	HLH domain
LYLA	t(7:19)(q35:p13)	Acute T-cell leukemia	HLH domain
TALA/SCL/TCL-5	t(1:14)(q32:q11)	Acute T-cell leukemia	HLH domain
TAL-2	t(7:9)(q35:q34)	Acute T-cell leukemia	HLH domain
Rhombotin 1/TTG-1	t(11:14)(p15:q11)	Acute T-cell leukemia	LIM domain
Rhombotin 2/TTG-2	t(11:14)(p13:q11)	Acute T-cell leukemia	LIM domain
	t(7:11)(q35:p13)		
HOX 11	t(10:14)(q24:q11)	Acute T-cell leukemia	Homeodomain
	t(7:10)(q35:q24)		
TAN-1	t(7:9)(q34:q34.3)	Acute T-cell leukemia	Notch homolog
TCL-1	t(7q35-14q32.1) or inv t(14q11-14q32.1) or inv	B-cell chronic lymphocyte leukemia	
Solid tumors			
Gene fusions in sarcomas			
FLI1,EWS	t(11:22)(q24:q12)	Ewing's sarcoma	Ets transcription factor family
ERG,EWS	t(21:22)(q22:q12)	Ewing's sarcoma	Ets transcription factor family
ATV1,EWS	t(7:21)(q22:q12)	Ewing's sarcoma	Ets transcription factor family
ATF1,EWS	t(12:22)(q13:q12)	Soft-tissue clear cell sarcoma	Transcription factor
CHN,EWS	t(9:22)(q22 31:q12)	Myxoid chondrosarcoma	Steroid receptor family
WT1,EWS	t(11:22)(p13:q12)	Desmoplastic small round cell tumor	Wilms' tumor gene
SSX1,SSX2,SYT	t(X:18)(p11.2:q11.2)	Synovial sarcoma	HLH domain
PAX3,FKHR	t(2:13)(q37:q14)	Alveolar	Homeobox homolog
PAX7,FKHR	t(1:13)(q36:q14)	Rhabdomyosarcoma	Homeobox homolog
CHOP,TLS	t(12:16)(q13:p11)	Myxoid liposarcoma	Transcription factor
VAR,HMG1-C	t(var:12)(var:q13-15)	Lipomas	HMG DNA-binding protein
HMG1-C?	t(12:14)(q13-15)	Leiomyomas	HMG DNA-binding protein
Gene fusions in thyroid carcinomas			
RET/PTC1	inv(10)(q11.2:q2.1)	Papillary thyroid carcinomas	Tyrosine kinase activated by H4
RET/PTC2	t(10:17)(q11.2:q23)	Papillary thyroid carcinomas	Tyrosine kinase activated by RIa(PKA)
RET/PTC3	inv(10)(q11.2)	Papillary thyroid carcinomas	Tyrosine kinase activated by ELE1
TRK	inv(1)(q31:q22-23)	Papillary thyroid carcinomas	Tyrosine kinase activated by TPM3
TRK—T1(T2)	inv(1)(q31:q25)	Papillary thyroid carcinomas	Tyrosine kinase activated by TPR
TRK—T3	t(1q31:3)	Papillary thyroid carcinomas	Tyrosine kinase activated by TFG
Hematopoietic and solid tumors			
Oncogenes juxtaposed with other loci			
PTH deregulates PRAD1	inv(11)(p15:q13)	Parathyroid adenoma	PRADI-GI cyclin
BTG1 deregulates MYC	t(8:12)(q24:q22)	B-cell chronic lymphocytic	MYC-HLH domain

Abbreviations: IG, immunoglobulin; TCR, T-cell receptor; HLH, helix−loop−helix structural domain; zn, zinc; HMG, high mobility group; H4; ELE1; TPR and 1TFG, partially uncharacterized genes with a dimerizing coiled-coil domain; RIa, regulatory subunit of PKA enzyme; TPM3, isoform of nonmuscle tropomyosin.

Gene activation

The t(8;14)(q24;q32) translocation, found in about 85% of cases of Burkitt's lymphoma, is a well-characterized example of the transcriptional activation of a proto-oncogene. This chromosomal rearrangement places the *C-MYC* gene, located at chromosome band 8q24, under the control of regulatory elements from the immunoglobulin heavy-chain locus located at 14q32. The *C-MYC* gene is also activated in some cases of Burkitt's lymphoma by translocations involving immunoglobulin light-chain genes. These are t(2;8)(p12;q24), involving the *k* locus located at 2p12, and t(8;22)(q24;q11), involving the λ locus at 22q11 (Figure 9). The position of the chromosomal breakpoints relative to the *C-MYC* gene may vary considerably in individual cases of Burkitt's lymphoma, but with the same effect. An alternative mechanism of *C-MYC* alteration is represented by gene mutations, which can occur in the gene transactivation domain and in the coding region after translocation into the *Ig* gene[81] or in the noncoding gene exon 1 and at the exon 1/intron 1 boundary with or without *C-MYC* gene translocation.[82] In T-cell ALL (T-ALL), the *C-MYC* gene is activated by the t(8;14)(q24;q11) translocation, when it is placed under the control of regulatory elements within the TCR.[83] In this tumor, several other proto-oncogenes encoding nuclear proteins are activated by various chromosomal translocations involving α or β loci of the TCR. These include *HOX11, TAL1, TAL2,* and *RBTN1/TGT1*.[84] The proteins encoded by these genes are thought to function as transcription factors through DNA-binding and protein–protein interactions, whose inappropriate expression leads to uncontrolled cellular proliferation.

A number of other proto-oncogenes are also activated by chromosomal translocations in leukemia and lymphoma.

Gene fusion

The first example of gene fusion was discovered through the cloning of the breakpoint of the Philadelphia chromosome in CML.[25] The t(9;22)(q34;q11) translocation in CML fuses the *C-ABL* gene, normally located at 9q34, with the *BCR* gene at 22q11 (Figure 10). The *BCR/ABL* fusion, created on the der(22) chromosome, encodes a chimeric protein of 210 kD with increased TK activity and abnormal cellular localization.[25] The precise mechanism by which the *BCR/ABL* fusion protein contributes to the expansion of the neoplastic myeloid clone is not yet known. The t(9;22) translocation is also found in up to 20% of cases of ALL. In these cases, the breakpoint in the *BCR* gene differs somewhat from that found in CML, resulting in a 185-kD bcr/abl fusion protein.[85] It is unclear at this time why the slightly smaller bcr/abl fusion protein leads to such a large difference in neoplastic phenotype. Inhibition of bcr/abl TK activity has been introduced as a chemotherapeutic approach in patients with CML. Administration of imatinib resulted in an antileukemic effect in CML patients in whom treatment with standard chemotherapy had failed.[86] However, cases of imatinib-resistance have also been recently documented.[87] Cause of such a failure is due to either *BCR/ABL* gene amplification or single amino acid substitutions affecting residues that are in direct contact with ATP or are within the ATP pocket of the kinase domain of abl, resulting in structural changes that could influence inhibition sensitivity. Strategies for overcoming resistance have

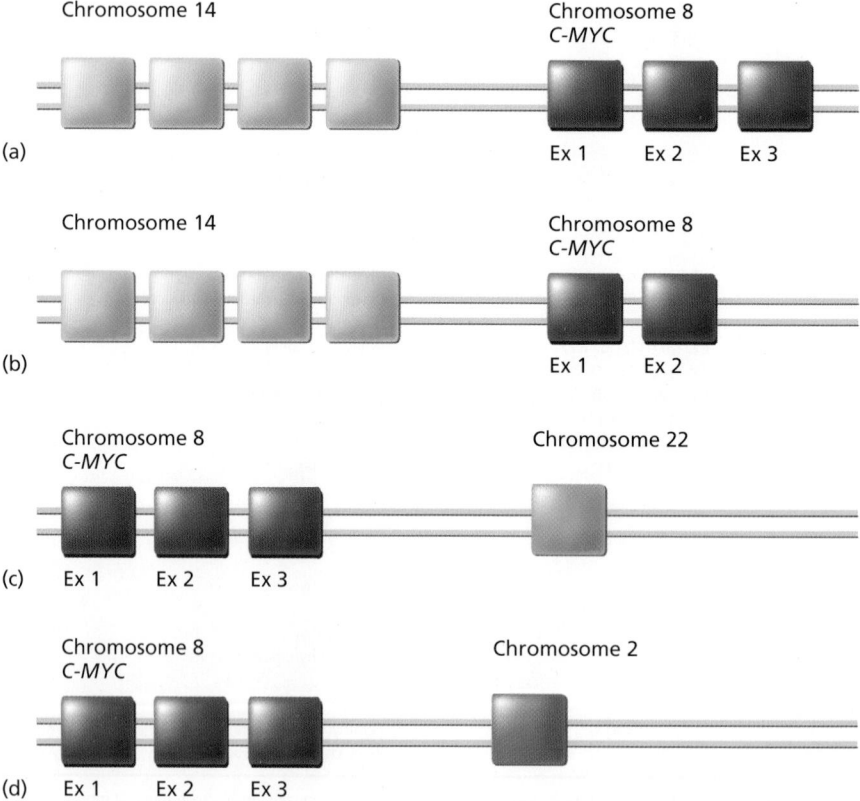

Figure 9 *C-MYC* translocations found in Burkitt lymphoma. (a) t(8;14)(q24;q32) translocation involving the locus of immunoglobulin heavy chain gene located at 14q32. (b) t(8;14)(q24;q32) translocation where only two exons of *C-MYC* are translocated under regulatory elements from the immunoglobulin heavy chain locus located at 14q32. (c) t(8;22)(q24;q11) translocation involving the *l* locus of immunoglobulin light chain gene at 22q11. (d) t(2;8)(p12;q24) translocation involving the *k* locus of immunoglobulin light chain gene located at 2p12.

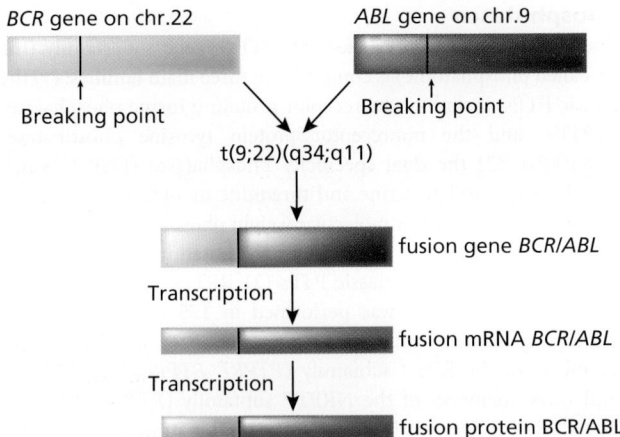

Figure 10 Gene fusion. The t(9;22)(q34;q11) translocation in CML determines the fusion of the *ABL* gene with the *BCR* gene. Such a gene fusion encodes an oncogenic chimeric protein of 210 KD.

been suggested, exploiting dependence of bcr/abl protein on the molecular chaperone heat shock protein 90.[87]

Additional genes encoding TKs involved in gene fusion events in hematologic malignancy are represented by the t(2;5)(p23;q35) translocation in anaplastic large cell lymphomas fusing the *NPM* gene (5q35) with the *ALK* gene (2p23)[88] and the t(5;12)(q33;p13) translocation fusing the *tel* gene (12p13) with the TK domain of the *platelet-derived growth factor receptor* b gene (*PDGFR-B* at 5q33) in chronic myelomonocytic leukemia (CMML) (Table 4).[89]

Gene fusions sometimes lead to the formation of chimeric transcription factors.[90] The t(1;19)(q23;p13) translocation, found in childhood pre-B-cell ALL, fuses the *E2A* transcription factor gene (19p13) with the *PBX1* homeodomain gene (1q23).[91] The E2A/PBX1 fusion protein consists of the amino-terminal transactivation domain of the E2A protein and the DNA-binding homeodomain of the PBX1 protein. Another gene fusion leading to a chimeric transcription factor is represented by the t(15;17)(q22;q21) translocation in acute promyelocytic leukemia, fusing the *PML* gene (15q22) with the *RARA* gene at 17q21.[92] Leukemia patients with the *PML/RARA* gene fusion respond well to retinoid treatment. In these cases, treatment with all-trans retinoic acid induces differentiation of promyelocytic leukemia cells.

The *ALL1* gene, located at chromosome band 11q23, is involved in approximately 5–10% of acute leukemia cases overall in children and adults.[93] *ALL1* is unique because it participates in fusions with a large number of different partner genes on the various chromosomes. Over 20 different reciprocal translocations involving the *ALL1* gene at 11q23 have been reported, the most common of which are those involving chromosomes 4, 6, 9, and 19. In approximately 5% of cases of acute leukemia in adults, the *ALL1* gene is fused with a portion of itself. This special type of gene fusion is called self-fusion.[94] Self-fusion of the *ALL1* gene, which is thought to occur through a somatic recombination mechanism, is found in high incidence in acute leukemias with trisomy 11 as a sole cytogenetic abnormality. The *ALL1* gene encodes a large protein with DNA-binding motifs, a transactivation domain, and a region with homology to the *Drosophila trithorax* protein (a regulator of homeotic gene expression). The various partners in *ALL1* fusions encode a diverse group of proteins, some of which appear to be nuclear proteins with DNA-binding motifs.[94] The ALL1 fusion protein consists of the amino terminus of ALL1 and the carboxyl terminus of one of a variety of fusion partners. It appears that the critical feature in all *ALL1* fusions, including self-fusion, is

the uncoupling of the ALL1 amino-terminal domains from the remainder of the ALL1 protein.

Solid tumors, especially sarcomas, sometimes have consistent chromosomal translocations that correlate with specific histological types of tumors.[95] In general, translocations in solid tumors result in gene fusions that encode chimeric oncoproteins. Studies thus far indicate that in sarcomas, the majority of genes fused by translocations encode transcription factors.[96] Table 4 summarizes translocations in solid tumors, with the most relevant represented by the t(12;16)(q13;p11) translocation fusing the *FUS (TLS)* gene at 16p11 with the *CHOP* gene at 12q13 in myxoid liposarcomas,[97] and the t(11;22)(q24;q12) translocation, fusing the *EWS* gene at 22q12 with the *FLI1* gene at 11q24 in Ewing's sarcoma.[98]

In DP, both a reciprocal translocation t(17;22)(q22;q13) and supernumerary ring chromosomes derived from the t(17;22) have been described.[99]

Although early successful studies in this field have been performed with lymphomas and leukemia, as we have discussed before, the first chromosomal abnormality in solid tumors to be characterized at the molecular level as a fusion protein was an inversion of chromosome 10 found in papillary thyroid carcinomas.[100] In this tumor, two main recurrent structural changes have been described, including inv(10)(q112.2; q21.2), as the more frequent alteration, and a t(10;17)(q11.2; q23). These two abnormalities represent the cytogenetic mechanisms that activate the proto-oncogene *RET* on chromosome 10, forming the oncogenes *RET/PTC1* and *RET/PTC2*, respectively. Moreover, other chromosomal rearrangements leading to ret activation were recently described, especially in children of the Chernobyl-contaminated areas.[101,102] Virtually, all breakpoints in the *RET* gene occur within intron 11, leading intact the TK domain of the receptor and enabling the *RET/PTC* oncoprotein to bind to SHC via Y1062 and activate the downstream cascade.[103] Somatic chromosomal rearrangements involving the *RET* gene represent the most frequent genetic alteration in *PTC*, although wide variations in frequency ranging from 5% to 70% have been observed in different geographic areas.[104] Recent results suggest that a broad variability in the reported prevalence of *RET/PTC* rearrangements is at least in part a result of the use of different detection methods and tumor genetic heterogeneity.[105] Alterations of chromosome 1 in the same tumor type have then been associated to the activation of NTRK1 (chromosome 1), an NGF receptor, which, like *RET,* forms chimeric fusion oncogenic proteins in PTC.[106] A comparative analysis of the oncogenes originated from the activation of these two TK receptors has allowed the identification and characterization of common cytogenetic and molecular mechanisms of their activation. In all cases, chromosomal rearrangements fuse the TK portion of the two receptors to the 5′-end of different genes that, because of their general effect, have been designated as "activating genes." In the majority of cases, the latter belong to the same chromosome where the related receptor is located, 10 for RET and 1 for NTRK1.

Furthermore, although functionally different, the various activating genes share the following three properties:
1. They are ubiquitously expressed.
2. They display domains demonstrated or predicted to be able to form dimers or multimers.
3. They translocate the signal from the membrane to the cytoplasm.

These characteristics can explain the mechanism(s) of oncogenic activation of *RET* and *NTRK1* proto-oncogenes. In fact, following the fusion of their TK domain to the activating gene (1) *RET* and *NTRK1,* whose tissue-specific expression is restricted to subsets of neural cells, become expressed in the epithelial thyroid cells; (2) their dimerization triggers a constitutive, ligand-independent trans-autophosphorylation of the cytoplasmic domains and, as a consequence, the latter can recruit SH2- and SH3-containing cytoplasmic effector proteins, such as Shc and Grb2 or phospholipase C gamma (PLC), thus inducing a constitutive mitogenic pathway; and (3) the relocalization in the cytoplasm of *RET* and *NTRK1* enzymatic activity could allow their interaction with unusual substrates, perhaps modifying their functional properties. *RET* rearrangements are mutually exclusive with *NTRK1* rearrangements and *BRAF* mutations and show similar but distinct gene expression patterns in PTC.[59] Overall, papillary carcinomas with *RET/PTC* rearrangements typically present at younger age and have a high rate if lymph-node metastases, clinical papillary histology, and possibly more favorable prognosis.[103]

Protein overexpression and constitutive phosphorylation

Protein overexpression refers to a general deregulation driven by a mechanism not understood or not investigated. An example is Akt, three serine-threonine kinases that represent major effectors mediating survival signal. Generally, Akt proteins possess six sites of phosphorylation: Ser124 and Thr450 are basally phosphorylated, Tyr315 and Tyr316 depend on Src, Thr308 represents the major site of regulation and is phosphorylated by 3-phosphoinositides-dependent protein kinase 1, Ser473 is only required for maximal Akt activity but the mechanism by which it is phosphorylated remains controversial. Akt is phosphorylated and therefore activated after cell stimulation from different growth factors and a series of interleukins, while its action is inhibited by PTEN. Once activated, Akt dissociates from the plasma membrane and translocates to both the cytoplasm and the nucleus. Akt inhibits directly, through phosphorylation of Bad and caspase-9, and indirectly, by inducing *de novo* gene expression of IKK protein kinase and transcription factors. Akt determines cell survival also by virtue of its involvement in cell-cycle progression.[107] Analyses of tissue specimens pointed out that the protein encoded by *AKT3* is overexpressed in poorly differentiated breast and prostate cancers and may contribute to the progression of sporadic melanoma.[108] Akt1 is especially involved in the pathogenesis of sporadic thyroid cancer, whereas Akt2 seems to be the isoform that plays a pivotal role in ovarian, pancreatic, thyroid, and CRC. Mutations in *AKT* genes are rare.[109]

New markers from large-scale genomic analysis

Kinases

A recent analysis organized the protein kinase complement of the human genome (the so-called kinome) into a dendrogram containing nine broad groups of genes.[110] Using high-throughput sequencing technologies and bioinformatics from the human genome project, one major branch of the histogram, containing three of the nine major groups, was selected for mutational analysis. The selected groups included the 90 tyrosine kinase genes (TK group), the 43 tyrosine kinase-like genes (TKL group), and the 5 receptor guanylate cyclase genes (RGC group). The analysis took into consideration all exons encoding their predicted kinase domains in 35 CRC cell lines and in 147 colorectal specimens.[8] Thirty-five different types of somatic mutations were identified in seven genes (*NTRK3, FES, KDR, EPHA3, NTRK2* belonging to the TK group, *MLK4* to *TKL*, and *GUCY2F* to *RGC*), representing an attractive target for chemotherapeutic intervention.[8]

Phosphatases

The protein tyrosine phosphatases (PTPs), gene superfamily (the so-called phosphatome) is composed of three main families: (1) the classic PTPs, including the receptor protein tyrosine phosphatases (RPTPs) and the nonreceptor protein tyrosine phosphatases (NRPTPs); (2) the dual specificity phosphatases (DSPs), which can dephosphorylate serine and threonine in addition to tyrosine residues; and (3) the low molecular weight phosphatases (LMPs).[111] Using high-throughput technologies, a mutational analysis of all the coding exons of 53 classic PTPs (21 RPTPs and 32 NRPTPs), 32 DSPs, and 1 LMP was performed in 175 CRCs.[9] Six genes containing somatic mutations were identified, including three members of the RPTP subfamily (*PTPRF, PTPRG,* and *PTPRT*), and three members of the NRPTP subfamily (*PTPN3, PTPN13,* and *PTPN14*). Overall, 77 mutations were identified, in aggregate, affecting 26% of colorectal tumors analyzed. The great majority of the mutations would result in proteins devoid of phosphatase catalytic activity.[9] The identification of protein phosphatases mutated could lead to reactivation of their activity through new targeted pharmacologic treatments or, better, inactivate the corresponding kinases that phosphorylate substrates normally regulated by the mutant phosphatases.

PI3K isoforms

Phosphatidylinositol 3-kinases (PI3K) belong to the lipid kinase family that regulate signal transduction.[112] Hidden-Markov models identified eight *PI3K* and *PI3K*-like genes, including two uncharacterized genes, in the human genome. By the analysis of the predicted kinase domains, it has been found that *PIK3CA* was the only gene with somatic mutations.[10] Hyperactivating *PIK3CA* mutations were also identified in several cancers from the colon, the lung, the ovaries, the liver, the brain, the stomach, and the breast.[113-115] The analysis of *PIK3CA* mutations in patients affected by hereditary CRCs revealed alteration in 21% of FAP invasive carcinomas, 21% of HNPCC invasive carcinomas, and 15% of sporadic invasive carcinomas, thus demonstrating that *PIK3CA* mutations are involved in both types of familial colorectal carcinogenesis (FAP and HNPCC) without an evident segregation (at odds with *BRAF*) and with a similar extent that seen in sporadic patients.[116] In addition to point mutations, *PIK3CA* may be altered through gene amplification, especially in ovarian cancer.[117]

Oncogenes in the initiation and progression of neoplasia

Human neoplasia is a complex multistep process involving sequential alterations in proto-oncogenes (activation) and in tumor-suppressor genes (inactivation). Statistical analysis of the age incidence of human solid tumors indicates that five or six independent mutational events may contribute to tumor formation. In human leukemias, only three or four mutational events may be necessary, presumably involving different genes.

The study of chemical carcinogenesis in animals provides a foundation for our understanding of the multistep nature of cancer.[118] In the mouse model of skin carcinogenesis, tumor formation involves three phases, termed *initiation, promotion,* and *progression.* Initiation of skin tumors can be induced by chemical mutagens such as 7,12-dimethyl-benzanthracene (DMBA) (Figure 11). After application of DMBA, the mouse skin appears normal. If the skin is then continuously treated with a promoter, such as the phorbol ester TPA, precancerous papillomas will form. Chemical promoters such as TPA stimulate growth but are not mutagenic substances. Over a

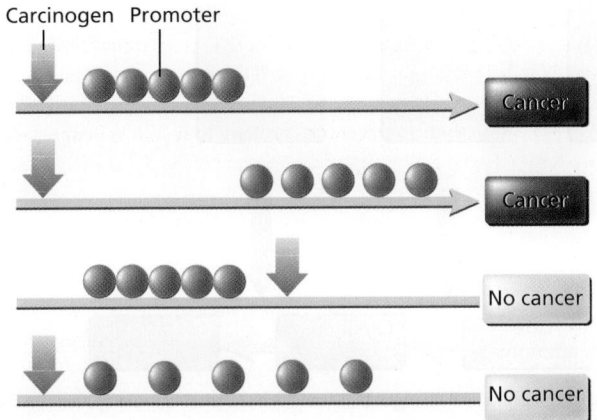

Figure 11 Some possible ways of exposure to a mutagen and a tumor promoter and their effects. Cancer develops exclusively when the exposure to promoter follows the exposure to carcinogen (mutagen, e.g., DMBA) and only when the intensity of the exposure to promoter is higher than a threshold.

period of months of continuous application of the promoting agent, some of the papillomas will progress to skin carcinomas. Treatment with DMBA or TPA alone does not cause skin cancer. Mouse papillomas initiated with DMBA usually have *HRAS* oncogenes with a specific mutation in codon 61 of the *HRAS* gene. The mouse skin tumor model indicates that initiation of papillomas is the result of mutation of the *HRAS* gene in individual skin cells by the chemical mutagen DMBA. For papillomas to appear on the skin, however, growth of mutated cells must be continuously stimulated by a promoting agent. Additional unidentified genetic changes must then occur for papillomas to progress to carcinoma.

Although a single oncogene is sufficient to cause tumor formation, transformation by a single oncogene is not usually seen in experimental models of cancer. On the contrary, different oncogenes frequently cooperate in producing the neoplastic phenotype.[119] Cooperation between oncogenes can also be demonstrated by *in vitro* transformation studies using nonimmortalized cell lines. For example, studies have shown cooperation between the nuclear myc protein and the cytoplasmic-membrane-associated ras protein in the transformation of rat embryo fibroblasts.[120]

Collaboration between two different categories of oncogenes (e.g., nuclear and cytoplasmic) can often be demonstrated but is not strictly required for transformation.[121] These transgenic mice strains, in fact, generally show an increased incidence of neoplasia and the tumors that result frequently are clonal, implying that other events are necessary.[122]

Cytogenetic studies of the clonal evolution of human hematologic malignancies have provided much insight into the multiple steps involved in the initiation and progression of human tumors.[123] The evolution of CML from chronic phase to acute leukemia is characterized by an accumulation of genetic changes seen in the karyotypes of the evolving malignant clones. The early chronic phase of CML is defined by the presence of a single Philadelphia chromosome. The formation of the *BCR/ABL* gene fusion as a consequence of the t(9;22) translocation is thought to be the initiating event in CML.[25] The biologic progression of CML to a more malignant phenotype corresponds with the appearance of additional cytogenetic abnormalities such as a second Philadelphia chromosome, isochromosome 17, or trisomy 8.[124] Although the karyotypic changes in evolving CML are somewhat variable from patient to patient, the accumulation of genetic changes always correlates with progression

from differentiated cells of low malignancy to undifferentiated cells of high malignancy.

The initiation and progression of human neoplasia involve the activation of oncogenes and the inactivation or loss of tumor-suppressor genes. The mechanisms of oncogene activation and the time course of events, however, vary among different types of tumors. In hematologic malignancies, soft-tissue sarcomas, and the papillary type of thyroid carcinomas, initiation of the malignant process predominantly involves chromosomal rearrangements that activate various oncogenes.[90] Many of the chromosomal rearrangements in leukemia and lymphoma are thought to result from errors in the physiologic process of immunoglobulin or TCR gene rearrangement during normal B-cell and T-cell development. Late events in the progression of hematologic malignancies involve oncogene mutation, mainly of the *RAS* family, inactivation of tumor-suppressor genes such as *TP53*, and sometimes additional chromosomal translocations.[125]

In lung cancers, the initiation of neoplasia has been shown to involve oncogene and tumor-suppressor gene mutations. These mutations are generally thought to result from chemical carcinogenesis, especially in the case of tobaccorelated lung cancers, where a novel tumor-suppressor gene (designated *FHIT*) has been found to be inactivated in the majority of cancers, particularly in those from smokers.[126] Later, *KRAS* (especially in the adenocarcinoma subtype) and *TP53* alterations drive the malignant transformation of lung cancer.[127]

As far as CRC is concerned, intensive screening for genetic alteration led to the identification of two major types of CRC that are distinct by their carcinogenic process. One is characterized by normal karyotype, normal DNA index, and genetic instability at microsatellite loci (MSI) and was called RER-positive tumor for replicative error-positive phenotype and now is called MSI-positive cancer.[128] The second one is represented by alterations of *APC*, *KRAS*, and *TP53* genes and genetic losses at MSI.[129] The second type led to the association between the stepwise progression from normal to dysplastic epithelium to carcinoma and the accumulation of multiple clonally selected genetic alterations. This model, first proposed by Vogelstein in 1990,[130] suggests that APC (or, better, the APC-b-catenin pathway) represents the initial mutational event that determines hyperplastic proliferation and then early adenoma formation. The stage of late adenoma is achieved with K-ras protein stabilization. Loss of tumor-suppressor genes at chromosome 18q (such as *DCC*) and mutations in the *TP53* gene lead to carcinoma *in situ* formation (Figure 12).[128–130]

In melanoma, *BRAF* mutations occur in the vast majority of cases and represent a very early event, as they were also detected in preneoplastic lesions such as Spitz and Blue nevi.[7,67]

Although there is variability in the pathways of human tumor initiation and progression, studies of various types of malignancy have clearly confirmed the multistep nature of human cancer.

Oncogenes as target of new drugs

Several oncogenes act in key points of cell life. Most of them, in fact, codify for growth factor receptors or are involved in the signal transduction. Therefore, they represent a natural target for the development of new drugs that are able to block selectively the cells carrying a deregulation in the drug target. The new insights in targeted therapies are summarized here.

ERB B2

ERB B2 gene amplification occurs in a consistent fraction of breast cancers. A monoclonal antibody (MoAb) against erb B2 receptor,

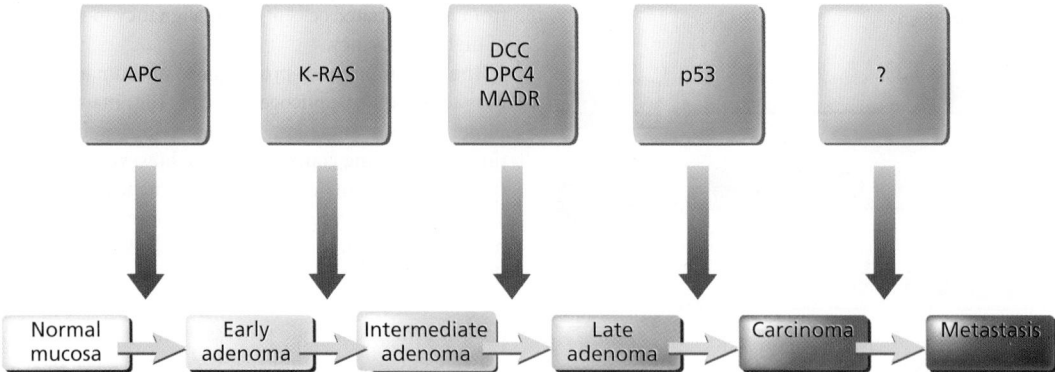

Figure 12 Colorectal cancer development. Colorectal cancer results from a series of pathological changes that transform normal colonic epithelium into invasive carcinoma. Specific genetic events, shown by vertical arrows, accompany this multistep process.

trastuzumab, was the first anti-erb B2 drug that entered clinical practice, with evident benefit for patients harboring *ERB B2* gene amplification/overxpression. Trastuzumab is indicated for patients affected by a metastatic breast cancer and, more recently, also for the adjuvant and neo-adjuvant setting. Currently, additional targeted therapies, both MoAbs (pertuzumab and a second-generation trastuzumab named T-DM1, with trastuzumab conjugated with emtansine) and small-molecule tyrosine kinase inhibitors (TKIs) (lapatinib) have been developed and are routinely used for the treatment of metastatic patients and in the neo-adjuvant setting. Unfortunately, not all patients showing *ERB B2* gene amplification may benefit from trastuzumab administration. This is probably due to the deregulation of *ERB B2* downstream members. Indeed, at preclinical level, it has been demonstrated that activating point mutations in the *PIK3CA* gene as well as the loss of expression of PTEN protein lead to trastuzumab resistance.[33]

More recently, it has been demonstrated that *ERB B2* can be deregulated in other solid tumors, with a putative relevant clinical role. *ERB B2* gene amplification or protein overexpression occur in up to 34% of patients affected by an advanced gastric or gastroesophageal junction cancers, and trastuzumab is approved for erb B2 positive patients (as evaluated by fluorescent *in situ* hybridization or immunohistochemistry).[33] In CRC, *ERB B2* gene amplification is a rare phenomenon (observed in <5% of cases), linked to resistance to EGFR-targeted therapies.[131] However, the efficacy of trastuzumab in CRC, proposed in *in vivo* models (xenografts), deserves additional confirmatory studies. In lung adenocarcinoma, a recent retrospective study showed that patients with *ERB B2* gene mutations (occurring in about 1% of cases) may benefit from the administration of trastuzumab. Furthermore, the occurrence of *ERB B2* gene mutations or amplification seems to be represented by a mechanism of secondary resistance to anti-EGFR therapies.[33]

ERB B1

ERB B1 codify for a receptor TK playing an important role in cancer cell proliferation, angiogenesis, and metastasis. Therefore, targeting erb B1 is a valuable molecular approach in cancer therapy. Two classes of erb B1 antagonists have been successfully tested in phase III trials and are now in clinical use: MoAbs and TKIs. MoAbs, represented by cetuximab and panitumumab, are able to bind to the extracellular domain of the receptor when it is in the inactive configuration, compete for receptor binding by occluding the ligand-binding region, and thereby block ligand-induced TK of the receptor. TKIs, represented by gefitinib and erlotinib, compete reversibly with ATP to bind to the intracellular catalytic domain of

the receptor and, therefore, inhibit receptor autophosphorylation and downstream signaling.[77]

In NSCLC, only 10–20% of patients have a partial response to gefitinib/erlotinib. Several retrospective and prospective studies confirmed that patients carrying an *EGFR* mutation were particularly sensitive to gefitinib/erlotinib, with a response rate up to 80% of mutated patients. Many types of mutations in the *ERB B1* have been reported, but so far, only four drug-sensitive mutations have been ascertained, including exon 19 deletions, and exon 18 (G719A/C), exon 21 L858R and exon 21 L861Q substitutions. In addition, *ERB B1* gene copy number gain (chromosome 7 high polysomy or gene amplification) is emerging as another relevant method for patients' selection.[132] Patients characteristics associated with increased responsiveness to gefitinib/erlotinib are never smoking history, Asian ethnicity, female gender, and adenocarcinoma histology. Acquisition of drug resistance in patients initially responsive to gefitinib/erlotinib has been linked to a specific secondary somatic mutation (*T790M*) occurring in exon 20 of the *ERB B1* gene. In addition, *MET* and *ERB B2* gene amplification represents alternative mechanisms of TKIs resistance (Takezawa et al., 2012). Novel inhibitors are currently under evaluation to specifically act against the T790M mutation: these drugs are named "irreversible inhibitors."[134,135]

In CRC, the class of erb B1 inhibitors showing clinical efficacy is represented by MoAbs. Cetuximab or panitumumab monotherapy is associated with response rates of 9–12%, that increase to 20–30% when the drugs are used in combination with irinotecan in patients who did not benefit from a previous therapy with irinotecan. Recent data indicate that erb B1 protein expression as evaluated by immunohistochemistry as well as *ERB B1* gene status by fluorescent *in situ* hybridization cannot be used to predict the efficacy of EGFR-targeted therapies (in contrast with earlier studies), essentially due to the fact that these two methodologies are not reproducible. On the contrary, *KRAS* and *NRAS* gene mutations are negative predictors of EGFR-targeted therapies efficacy and are mandatory to be tested before MoAbs administration.[136] In addition, the detection of gene or protein alterations of other *ERB B1* downstream members, such as *BRAF* and *PIK3CA* point mutations, and the loss of expression of PTEN protein, has been proposed to be additional mechanisms of the resistance to cetuximab/panitumumab, but the data reported so far are controversial and therefore their test is not required before drug administration.[137]

Cetuximab and panitumumab are effective also in 10–13% of patients affected by head and neck squamous cell carcinoma, and EGFR-targeted therapy is the first and only molecularly targeted therapy to demonstrate a survival benefit for patients with recurrent or metastatic disease.[138]

KIT and PDGFRA

It has been clearly demonstrated that imatinib, an inhibitor of TK activity in bcr-abl-positive leukemia, was effective in treating GIST (Figure 13). In this pathology, *KIT* and *PDGFRA* mutational status predicts for the likelihood of achieving response to such a targeted drug. Patients with a *KIT* exon 11 mutation have a partial response rate up to 85–90%, while those with a *KIT* exon 9 mutation have a partial response rate of around 50%. Recent data points out that for patients with *KIT* exon 9 mutation the better treatment is represented by a double dose of imatinib. Patients who have GIST with *KIT* exon 11 mutation also have longer median time to treatment failure as compared to those with GIST harboring other types of mutations. Patients who have no detectable mutation of *KIT* or *PDGFRA* respond less frequently to imatinib than those with exon 11 mutants, but still up to 39% do respond. The rare patients who have GIST with *KIT* exon 13 or 17 mutation of *PDGFRA* mutation may also respond to imatinib. The rare patients who have GIST with a mutation known to be resistant to imatinib, such as D842V *PDGFRA* exon 18 mutation, may be the only exception to this rule. Interestingly, the D842V *PDGFRA* exon 18 mutation is functionally equivalent to the D816V *KIT* exon 17 mutation, never found in GIST, but which confers resistance to imatinib treatment in leukemia.[139] A majority of patients with a GIST metastatic disease ultimately cease to respond to imatinib. The reasons for failure usually include secondary mutations at the ATP/imatinib binding pocket (exon 13 or exon 14) or in the activation loop (exon 17) of the kit protein kinase that prohibit imatinib binding. Patients who progress despite imatinib dose escalation are candidates for a trial with other TK inhibitors. Sunitinib (SU11248) is an inhibitor of kit, pdgfra, fms-like TK-3 and vascular EGFR-2, and has been approved by the Food and Drug Administration for the treatment of GIST patients whose disease has progressed on imatinib or are unable to tolerate treatment with imatinib.

More recently, the clinical role of *KIT* mutations has expanded to melanoma. It has been showed that *KIT* mutations occurs in specific subtypes of melanoma patients, in the majority of uveal, in up to in 39% of mucosal, 36% of acral, and 28% of melanomas arising from chronically sun-damaged skin, but not in any (0%) cutaneous melanomas without chronic sun damage.[140] The typical alteration is represented by the L576P point mutation. Results from case reports and from human uveal melanoma cell lines demonstrated that imatinib inhibits cell proliferation and invasion rates.[141] These results justify the need for clinical trials (which are now under evaluation) to investigate in vivo the response of uveal melanoma to imatinib.

RET

Recently, various kinds of therapeutic approaches, including TKIs, gene therapy with dominant negative *RET* mutants, MoAbs, and nuclease-resistant aptamers that recognize and inhibit RET, have been developed. The use of these strategies in preclinical models has provided evidence that RET is indeed a potential target for selective cancer therapy. In clinical cases, in addition to papillary thyroid cancers where they play a relevant role, *RET* rearrangements have been found in a small subgroup of lung cancers (1–2%). Two specific gene fusions (*CCDC6-RET* and *KIF5B-RET*) have been described. *RET* rearrangements appear limited to adenocarcinoma histology and are not seen concurrently with *ERB B1* or *KRAS* mutations, or *ALK* rearrangements. There are currently at least six marketed TKIs against RET (vandetanib, sorafenib, sunitinib, cabozantinib, regorafenib, and ponatinib), but the efficacy of these agents in RET rearranged lung cancers has not been completely established.[81,142]

RAS

A number of different approaches aimed at abrogating *KRAS* activity have been explored in clinical trials. Usually, the inhibitors directly addressed to K-RAS are too toxic for human cells. Currently, the most promising agents are represented by aminobiphosphonates that have entered clinical practice in the treatment of bone

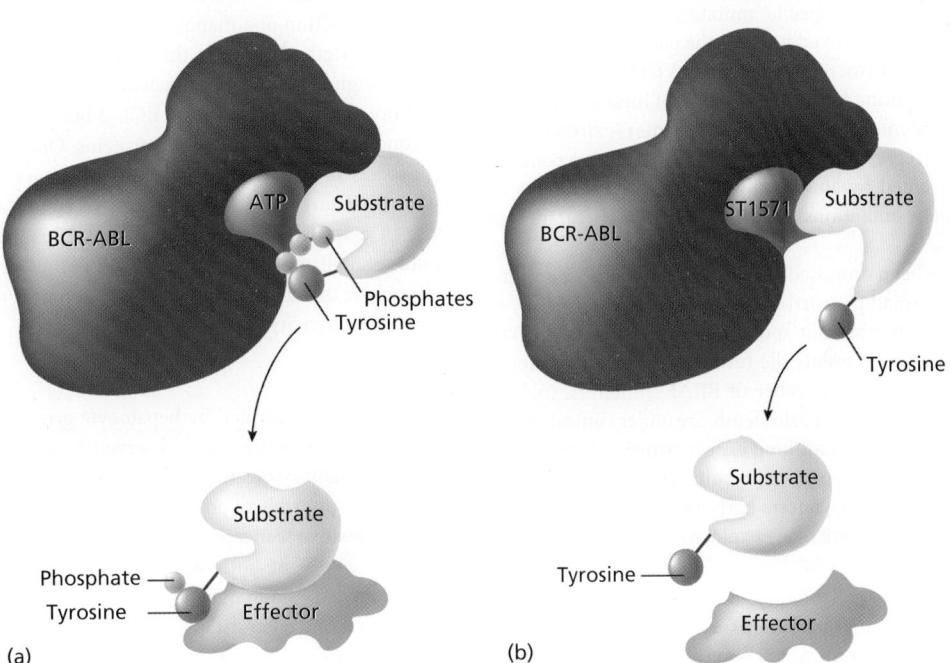

Figure 13 Mode of action of imatinib. In (a), the effect of ATP binding on the oncoprotein BCR-ABL isdepicted. The fusion protein binds the molecule of ATP in the kinase pocket. Afterward, it can phosphorylate a substrate that can interact with the downstream effector molecules. When imatinib is present (b), the oncoprotein binds imatinib in the kinase pocket (competing with ATP) and then the substrate cannot be phosphorylated.

metastases from several neoplasms, including breast and prostate adenocarcinomas.

KRAS mutations play also a role in the prediction of efficacy of treatment targeted to upstream activated RTK, such as EGFR. Indeed, *KRAS* mutations represent an independent predictive factor in cetuximab- or panitumumab-treated advanced CRC patients.[137] Until 2013, only the characterization of *KRAS* codons 12 and 13, located in exon 2, was mandatory before the administration of EGFR-targeted therapies. However, starting from the evidence that also different *KRAS* mutations (at codons 59, 61, 117, and 146, located in exons 3 and 4, which can be cumulatively found in up to 5% of cases) can be detected in CRC and that also these regions are important for K-ras activity, the analysis of large cohorts demonstrated that also *KRAS* exons 3-4 mutations are negative predictors of efficacy of MoAbs against EGFR.[136,143,144] Furthermore, *NRAS* mutations may occur in CRC patients (in up to 5% of cases, in the same codons altered in *KRAS* gene), and recently, it has been demonstrated that also patients carrying mutations in this gene are resistant to anti-EGFR therapies.[55,136,145] Overall, therefore, the combined analysis of *KRAS* and *NRAS* gene mutations is now mandatory before the administration of EGFR-targeted therapies in CRC patients with a metastatic disease. As far as the clinical role of *KRAS* mutations in the prediction of efficacy of TKIs against EGFR in lung adenocarcinoma patients is concerned, at odds with preliminary data, essentially obtained in preclinical models and in few selected cohorts, the current hypothesis is that *KRAS* mutations cannot predict the efficacy of these drugs.

BRAF

BRAF now provides a critical new target for drugs treating malignant melanoma, including antisense oligonucleotides and small molecules. These inhibitors block the expression of BRAF protein, block the BRAF/ras interaction, block its kinase activity, or the kinase activity of the BRAF target protein MAP kinase. Besides these approaches, vemurafenib is a selective BRAF TKI inhibitor approved for the treatment of melanoma patients. The Food and Drug Administration approved this drug for the administration to patients carrying the V600E specific mutation, whereas the European Medicine Agency approved it for all the patients carrying any mutation at codon 600 (therefore including V600K, V600D, and V600G, overall accounting for more than 10% of melanoma cases). The effect of vemurafenib on *BRAF* mutant patients is extremely fast in terms of tumor regression, but after 10–12 months, secondary alterations (represented by abnormally spliced BRAF proteins or other *BRAF* somatic mutations) lead to a rapid reappearance of metastatic lesions.[146]

A recent role has been proposed also in NSCLC. *BRAF* mutations occur not only in a small proportion of cases (up to 2%), mainly at codon 600, but also in other hot-spot codons (466, 469, and 594); therefore, lung cancer represents the tumor with the widest spectrum of *BRAF* mutations. A number of BRAF inhibitors, including sorafenib, vemurafenib, and dabrafenib, are under clinical development in V600E *BRAF* mutant lung cancer patients, with vemurafenib showing the most promising results, at least on the basis of few case reports. For lung cancers harboring non-V600E *BRAF* mutations, MEK inhibitors are being explored.[81,147]

AKT

Deregulation of AKT expression seems to be involved into AKT drug response and radioresistance in several tumors,[148] especially in metaplastic cancer, where it confers resistance to hormone therapy,[149] and in ovarian cancer, where it confers resistance to cisplatin by modulating the direct action of p53 on the caspase-dependent mitochondrial death pathway.[150] Moreover, recent efforts have been made in the development of small-molecule inhibitors that directly bind to AKT, such as triciribine and pyridine derivatives. However, several drawbacks have been found because of toxicity issues owing to the involvement of AKT in insulin signaling.[108]

PIK3CA

Owing to the relevance in carcinogenesis, PIK3CA represents a natural target with specific drugs. Most of these have been developed, but many of these showed high toxicity for human cells. Some PIK3CA inhibitors entered clinical trials and the evaluation is awaited. *PIK3CA* mutations are linked, at least at preclinical level, to resistance against trastuzumab in metastatic breast cancers,[151] whereas it has been proposed that only specific mutations (i.e., those occurring at exon 20) represent a mechanism of primary resistance to cetuximab or panitumumab in metastatic CRC patients, but this data deserves additional confirmation.[137] Furthermore, the clinical efficacy of selective inhibitors in *PIK3CA* mutant ovarian cancers is under investigation in on-going clinical trials. However, the major clinical application of *PIK3CA* mutations in clinical diagnosis is in CRC patients before the administration of aspirin in an adjuvant setting. Aspirin, in fact, is a drug efficiently preventing colorectal adenomas and carcinomas, and the effect is thought to be driven by the inhibition of cyclooxygenase enzymes. This anticancer effect has reported to be restricted to patients with cyclooxygenases overexpression. Two large prospective studies demonstrated that a stronger effect is observed in patients additionally carrying a *PIK3CA* mutation, probably because it seems that *PIK3CA* gene product further induces cyclooxygenases expression. A more recent study based on retrospective analysis has confirmed the predictive value of *PIK3CA* mutations for patients treated with aspirin in an adjuvant setting. Interestingly, this effect could not be observed in patients taken the specific cyclooxygenase inhibitor rofecoxib.[152,153]

BCL-2

Many groups have been working to develop anticancer drugs that block the function of antiapoptotic BCL-2 members, thus favoring cell death. Methods include the downregulation of BCL-2 expression through antisense oligonucleotides, or the use of peptides or small organic molecules to the BCL-2 binding pocket, preventing its sequestration of proapoptotic proteins. One of the most promising aspects of these small-molecule inhibitors in treating cancer is that their targets and mechanisms of action are different from those of cytotoxic drugs and radiation. This makes it feasible to combine small-molecule inhibitors with other treatments, creating a synergistic therapy, without likely development of cross-resistance or increased toxicity.[154]

MET

MET is an RTK activated by hepatocyte growth factor. MET protein overexpression has been observed in a number of neoplastic diseases, usually associated with poor prognosis. *MET* gene amplification is responsible of protein overexpression in only a subgroup of MET-positive cancers. In NSCLC, *MET* gene amplification occurs in 2–4% of both squamous and nonsquamous cancers. Interestingly, *MET* amplification represents one of the major mechanisms of secondary resistance to TKI against EGFR. Several MET inhibitors have been developed, both TKI (such as crizotinib and tivantinib) and MoAbs (such as onartuzumab), but the efficacy of these compounds has to be still proven in lung as well as in other cancers.[81,155]

FGFR

FGFR family includes four members, with FGFR1 showing the most promising clinical role in cancers. In particular, in NSCLC, *FGFR1* gene amplification occurs in approximately 20% of cases with a squamous histology but in <2% of adenocarcinoma. These amplifications appear to confer an FGFR1-addiction to tumoral cells. FGFR1 inhibitors (such as AZD4547, JNJ-42756493, BGJ398, and ponatinib) are under evaluation.[81,156]

DDR2

Discoidin death receptor 2 (DDR2) is an RTK mutated in approximately 4% of squamous NSCLCs and in about 1% of lung adenocarcinoma. The multitarget kinase inhibitor dasatinib, the sole DDR2 promising inhibitor, has demonstrated good efficacy in both preclinical models and few patients.[81,157]

ALK

Rearrangements of ALK primarily occur as fusion to *EML4* gene. These fusion proteins can be found in approximately 3–7% of lung adenocarcinoma. Among EML4-ALK fusion proteins, several *EML4* breakpoints have been described. In rare cases, other fusion partners have been observed, including *TFG* and *KIF5B* genes.[81] The first ALK-selective inhibitor was represented by the multitargeted inhibitor crizotinib. The first clinical trial including ALK-positive patients showed very attractive results: 61% of overall survival, 71% of disease control rate, and increased progression-free survival, leading a rapid approval of crizotinib by the Food and Drug Administration for the treatment of lung adenocarcinomas characterized by *ALK* translocation, as evaluated by fluorescent *in situ* hybridyzation.[158] Unfortunately, the duration of clinical benefit of crizotinib is limited, owing to the occurrence of variable systemic resistance mechanisms: occurrence of secondary mutations in ALK active site, erb B family pathway activation, *ALK* copy number gain, *KIT* gene amplification, and *KRAS* mutations. Currently, a major effort is on the development of second-generation ALK inhibitors, capable of blocking lung adenocarcinoma that developed crizotinib resistance.[81] ALK rearrangements are also considered one (but not the most frequent) of the mechanisms of acquired resistance to TKI against EGFR in *ERB B1*-mutant lung adenocarcinoma.[81]

ROS1

Rearrangements of *ROS1* oncogene appear to occur in approximately 1–2% of lung adenocarcinoma. *ROS1* has a high degree of homology with *ALK* (49% within the TK domain and 77% with the ATP-binding site) and patients with *ROS1* rearrangements display superimposable clinicopathological features with whom carrying *ALK* translocations.[81] The multitargeted inhibitor crizotinib have demonstrated efficacy in *ROS1* rearranged patients, with preliminary response rate of 57% and disease control rate of 79%. Consequently, *ROS1* rearrangements have entered clinical diagnosis for lung adenocarcinoma patients.[159]

Summary and conclusions

The initiation and progression of human neoplasia is a multistep process involving the accumulation of genetic changes in somatic cells. These genetic changes then consist of the activation of cooperating oncogenes and the inactivation of tumor-suppressor genes, both of which appear necessary for a complete neoplastic phenotype. Oncogenes are altered versions of normal cellular genes called proto-oncogenes. Proto-oncogenes are a diverse group of genes involved in the regulation of cell growth. The functions of proto-oncogenes include growth factors, growth factor receptors, signal transducers, transcription factors, and regulators of programmed cell death. Proto-oncogenes may be activated by mutation, chromosomal rearrangement, or gene amplification. Chromosomal rearrangements that include translocations and inversions can activate proto-oncogenes by deregulation of their transcription (e.g., transcriptional activation) or by gene fusion. Tumor-suppressor genes, which also participate in the regulation of normal cell growth, are usually inactivated by point mutations or truncation of their protein sequence coupled with the loss of the normal allele.

The discovery of oncogenes represented a breakthrough for our understanding of the molecular and genetic basis of cancer. Oncogenes have also provided important knowledge concerning the regulation of normal cell proliferation, differentiation, and programmed cell death. The identification of oncogene abnormalities has provided tools for the molecular diagnosis and monitoring of cancer. Most important, oncogenes represent potential targets for new types of cancer therapies. The goal of these new drugs will be to kill cancer cells selectively while sparing normal cells. One promising approach entails using specific oncogene targets to trigger programmed cell death. The first example of the accomplishment of such a goal is represented by the inhibition of the tumor-specific TK bcr/abl in CML, by imatinib. The same compound has been proven active also in a different tumor type, GIST where it inhibits the TK receptor *c-KIT* and in chordomas, where it switches off the PDGFR. Another example is represented by gefitinib and cetuximab, which inhibit the intracellular TK and the extracellular domain, respectively, of ERB B1. Thereafter, a plethora of new targeted drugs has entered clinical trials, with evident benefit for the treatment of several neoplastic disease that were, before targeted therapies development, very hard to be treated and cured. The use of high-throughput technologies for the identification of new oncogenes and the rapidly expanding knowledge of the molecular mechanisms of cancer hold great promise for the development of better combined methods of cancer therapy in the near future.

Key references

The complete reference list can be found on the Wiley Companion Digital Edition of this title (see inside front cover for login instructions).

1 Bernards R, Weinberg RA. A progression puzzle. *Nature.* 2002;**418**:823.
2 Hanahan D, Weinberg RA. Hallmarks of cancer: the next generation. *Cell.* 2011;**144**:646–674.
3 Bishop JM. Retroviruses and oncogenes II. In: *Les Prix Nobel.* Stockholm: Almqvist and Wiksell; 1989:220–238.
4 Varmus HE. Retroviruses and oncogenes I. In: *Les Prix Nobel.* Stockholm: Almqvist and Wiksell; 1989:194–212.
5 Todd R, Wong DT. Oncogenes. *Anticancer Res.* 1999;**19**:4729–4746.
8 Bardelli A, Parsons DW, Silliman N, et al. Mutational analysis of the tyrosine kinome in colorectal cancers. *Science.* 2003;**300**:949.
9 Wang Z, Shen D, Parsons DW, et al. Mutational analysis of the tyrosine phosphatome in colorectal cancers. *Science.* 2004;**304**:1164–1166.
11 Mahalingam S, Meanger J, Foster PS, Lidbury BA. The viral manipulation of the host cellular and immune environments to enhance propagation and survival: a focus on RNA viruses. *J Leukoc Biol.* 2002;**72**:429–439.
12 Rubin H. The early history of tumor virology: Rous, RIF, and RAV. *Proc Natl Acad Sci U S A.* 2011;**108**:14389–14396.
14 Sanchez-Beato M, Sanchez-Aguilera A, Piris MA. Cell cycle deregulation in B-cell lymphomas. *Blood.* 2002;**101**:1220–1235.
15 Krontiris TG, Cooper GM. Transforming activity of human tumor DNAs. *Proc Natl Acad Sci U S A.* 1981;**78**:1181–1184.
16 Dayaram T, Marriott SJ. Effect of transforming viruses on molecular mechanisms associated with cancer. *J Cell Physiol.* 2008;**216**:309–314.
20 Macaluso M, Russo G, Cinti C, et al. Ras family genes: an interesting link between cell cycle and cancer. *J Cell Physiol.* 2002;**192**:125–130.

23 Falini B, Mason DY. Proteins encoded by genes involved in chromosomal alterations in lymphoma and leukemia: clinical value of their detection by immunocytochemistry. *Blood*. 2002;**99**:409–426.

27 Grimm SL, Nordeen SK. Mouse mammary tumor virus sequences responsible for activating cellular oncogenes. *J Virol*. 1998;**72**:9428–9435.

29 Paez JG, Janne PA, Lee JC, et al. EGFR mutations in lung cancer: correlation with clinical response to gefitinib therapy. *Science*. 2004;**304**:1497–1500.

35 Cantley LC, Auger KR, Carpenter C, et al. Oncogenes and signal transduction. *Cell*. 1991;**64**:281–302.

36 Malumbres M, Barbacid M. RAS oncogenes: the first 30 years. *Nat Rev Cancer*. 2003;**3**:459–465.

37 Darnell JE Jr. Transcription factors as targets for cancer therapy. *Nat Rev Cancer*. 2002;**2**:740–749.

41 Boxer LM, Dang CV. Translocations involving c-myc and cmyc function. *Oncogene*. 2001;**20**:5595–5610.

42 Konopleva M, Zhao S, Xie Z, et al. Apoptosis. Molecules and mechanisms. *Adv Exp Med Biol*. 1999;**457**:217–236.

43 Danial NN. BCL-2 family proteins: critical checkpoints of apoptotic cell death. *Clin Cancer Res*. 2007;**13**:7254–7263.

46 Mazaris E, Tsiotras A. Molecular pathways in prostate cancer. *Nephrourol Mon*. 2013;**5**:792–800.

57 Frattini M, Gallino G, Signoroni S, et al. Quantitative and qualitative characterization of plasma DNA identifies primary and recurrent colorectal cancer. *Cancer Lett*. 2008;**263**:170–181.

69 Storlazzi CT, Lonoce A, Guastadisegni MC, et al. Gene amplification as double minutes or homogeneously staining regions in solid tumors: origin and structure. *Genome Res*. 2010;**20**:1198–1206.

77 Ciardiello F, Tortora G. EGFR antagonists in cancer treatment. *N Engl J Med*. 2008;**358**:1160–1174.

81 Gerber DE, Gandhi L, Costa DB. Management and future directions in non-small cell lung cancer with known activating mutations. *Am Soc Clin Oncol Educ Book*. 2014:e354–e365. doi: 0.14694/EdBook_AM.2014.34.e353.

95 Skapek SX, Chui CH. Cytogenetics and the biologic basis of sarcomas. *Curr Opin Oncol*. 2000;**12**:315–322.

97 Xia SJ, Barr FG. Chromosome translocations in sarcomas and the emergence of oncogenic transcription factors. *Eur J Cancer*. 2005;**41**:2513–2527.

103 Ciampi R, Nikiforov YE. RET/PTC rearrangements and BRAF mutations in thyroid tumorigenesis. *Endocrinology*. 2007;**148**:936–941.

104 Arighi E, Borrello MG, Sariola H. RET tyrosine kinase signaling in development and cancer. *Cytokine Growth Factor Rev*. 2005;**16**:441–467.

118 Weinberg RA. Oncogenes and multistep carcinogenesis. In: Weinberg RA, ed. *Oncogenes and the Molecular Origins of Cancer*. New York, NY: Cold Spring Harbor; 1989:307–326.

120 Land H, Parada LF, Weinberg RA. Tumorigenic conversion of primary embryo fibroblasts requires at least two cooperating oncogenes. *Nature*. 1983;**304**:596–602.

122 Pelengaris S, Khan M, Evan G. c-MYC: more than just a matter of life and death. *Nat Rev Cancer*. 2002;**2**:764–776.

123 Nowell PC. The clonal evolution of tumor cell populations. *Science*. 1976;**194**:23–28.

130 Fearon ER, Vogelstein B. A genetic model for colorectal tumorigenesis. *Cell*. 1990;**61**:759–767.

136 Douillard JY, Oliner KS, Siena S, et al. Panitumumab-FOLFOX4 treatment and RAS mutations in colorectal cancer. *N Engl J Med*. 2013;**369**:1023–1034.

137 Custodio A, Feliu J. Prognostic and predictive biomarkers for epidermal growth factor receptor-targeted therapy in colorectal cancer: beyond KRAS mutations. *Crit Rev Oncol Hematol*. 2013;**85**:45–81.

146 Tronnier M, Mitteldorf C. Treating advanced melanoma: current insights and opportunities. *Cancer Manag Res*. 2014;**6**:349–356.

153 Domingo E, Church DN, Sieber O, et al. Evaluation of PIK3CA mutation as a predictor of benefit from nonsteroidal anti-inflammatory drug therapy in colorectal cancer. *J Clin Oncol*. 2013;**31**:4297–4305.

5 Tumor suppressor genes

David Cosgrove, MB, BCh ▪ Ben Ho Park, MD, PhD ▪ Bert Vogelstein, MD

Overview

Cancer is a genetic disease. Mutations and other alterations in growth promoting genes (oncogenes) and tumor suppressor genes can accumulate during the lifetime of a normal cell resulting in cancer. Unlike oncogenes, tumor suppressor genes generally require biallelic inactivation in order to demonstrate a cancerous phenotype. Importantly, the discovery of heritable tumor suppressor gene mutations that lead to familial forms of cancer has revealed great insight into tumor suppressor function. This has clinical screening implications for individuals with a family history of cancer and has led to newer therapies to target cancer cells with loss of specific tumor suppressors.

A genetic basis for the development of cancer has been hypothesized for over a century, supported by familial, epidemiologic, and cytogenetic studies. However, only in the past 40 years has definitive evidence emerged that cancer is a genetic disease. It is now known that cancers arise through a multistage process in which inherited and somatic mutations of cellular genes lead to repeated waves of clonal selection in which cells with the most robust and aggressive growth properties prevail. Two classes of genes, oncogenes and tumor suppressor genes, are primary targets for the mutations as these genes control the ratio of cell birth and cell death. In all normal tissues of the adult, this ratio is exactly 1.0; mutations increase the ratio. A third class of genes, called genomic stability genes, do not alter the ratio when mutated, but it can indirectly contribute to tumorigenesis through an acceleration of mutations in oncogenes and tumor suppressor genes.

The vast majority of the mutations that contribute to the development and behavior of cancer cells are somatic (i.e., arising during tumor development) and are present only in the neoplastic cells of the individual. A small fraction of mutations in cancer cells are constitutional, present in all somatic cells and can be passed on to progeny, increasing cancer risk in subsequent generations.

The identification and function of oncogenes are reviewed in other chapters of this book. We provide a brief summary of their general properties as a comparison to tumor suppressor genes. In general, oncogenes have critical roles in a variety of growth regulatory pathways, and their protein products are distributed throughout many subcellular compartments. The mutant alleles present in cancers have sustained gain-of-function alterations resulting from point mutations, chromosomal rearrangements, gene amplifications, or other changes to the oncogene sequence. In the overwhelming majority of cancers, mutations in oncogenes arise somatically in the tumor cells, although germline mutations have been described, notably in *RET* (rearranged during transfection) and *MET* (metastasis), leading to familial medullary thyroid cancer and hereditary papillary renal cell carcinoma, respectively.

Although oncogenic alleles harbor activating mutations, tumor suppressor genes are defined by their inactivation in human cancer, and, as with oncogenes, the cellular functions of tumor suppressor genes appear to be diverse.

Defects in genomic stability genes have also been implicated in a broad spectrum of human cancers. Like tumor suppressor genes, the genomic stability genes are inactivated in human cancers. However, unlike the mutations in tumor suppressor genes, mutations in genomic stability genes are more often inherited in mutant form. For example, inherited mutations in the breast cancer 1 (*BRCA1*) early-onset or breast cancer 2 (*BRCA2*) early-onset genes play a key role in hereditary breast and ovarian cancers, but these genes are rarely mutated somatically in nonfamilial forms of breast cancers.

Enormous progress has been made in the identification of inherited and somatic mutations in oncogenes, tumor suppressor genes, and genomic stability genes in human cancers. The function of these genes has been elucidated, in part, through the analysis of a variety of model systems employing mice, flies, worms, and other organisms, and through the investigation of human cancer cell lines and sequencing of human cancer cells. The principal aims of this chapter are to review the somatic cell genetic and epidemiologic studies that established the existence of tumor suppressor genes; to describe the identification and cloning of representative tumor suppressor genes; to highlight selected studies of the function of tumor suppressor genes in the regulation of cell birth and cell death; and to illustrate an example of a genomic stability gene that plays a causal role in common human cancers.

Genetic basis for tumor development

The inherited basis of human cancer has been appreciated for almost 150 years. In 1866, Broca described a family in which many members developed breast or liver cancer, and he proposed that an inherited abnormality within the affected tissue allowed for tumor development.[1] Following the rediscovery of Mendel's work, studies of the rates of spontaneous mammary tumor formation in various inbred strains of mice led Haaland to argue that tumorigenesis could behave in a formal sense as a Mendelian genetic trait.[2] Similarly, Warthin's analysis of the pedigrees of cancer patients at the University of Michigan Hospital between 1895 and 1913 identified four multigenerational families with susceptibilities to specific cancer types that appeared to be transmitted as autosomal dominant Mendelian traits (Figure 1).[3] Although these and other studies suggested the existence of an inherited genetic basis for some cancers, other explanations for familial clustering were certainly possible (e.g., shared exposure to a carcinogenic agent in the environment or diet). Furthermore, it was highlighted that most cancers in humans appeared to arise as sporadic, isolated cases.

Holland-Frei Cancer Medicine, Ninth Edition. Edited by Robert C. Bast Jr., Carlo M. Croce, William N. Hait, Waun Ki Hong, Donald W. Kufe, Martine Piccart-Gebhart, Raphael E. Pollock, Ralph R. Weichselbaum, Hongyang Wang, and James F. Holland.
© 2017 John Wiley & Sons, Inc. ISBN: 978-1-118-93469-2

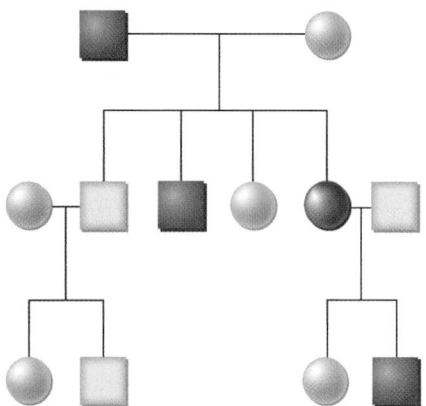

Figure 1 The inheritance of cancer in a family. The affected members with cancer are indicated by shaded squares (males) or circles (females). This family demonstrates a dominant pattern of inheritance, meaning that each offspring has a 50% chance of inheriting a germline mutation that predisposes to a high probability of developing cancer.

A role for somatic mutations in the development of cancer was first proposed by Boveri,[4] who noted that, in sea urchin eggs fertilized by two sperms, abnormal mitotic divisions leading to the loss of chromosomes occurred in daughter cells, and atypical tissue masses could be seen in the resulting gastrula. He believed that these abnormal tissues appeared physically similar to the poorly differentiated tissue masses seen in tumors and hypothesized that cancer arose from a cellular aberration producing abnormal mitotic figures. Boveri's hypothesis apparently did not gain favor at the time, initially because of the lack of direct experimental support from studies of the karyotypes of animal and human tumors. Such karyotypes were impossible to obtain with the available technology. Once the karyotypic studies were performed decades later, and appeared to support his hypothesis, Boveri was still doubted because of uncertainty about whether the changes in chromosome number in tumors were a cause or an effect of the neoplastic process.

A landmark observation in the search to identify a genetic basis for cancer was reported by Rous in 1911, when he showed that sarcomas could be reproducibly induced in chickens by cell-free filtrates of a sarcoma that had previously arisen in another chicken.[5] Although this observation provided strong evidence that neoplasms could be virally induced, the observation also provided support for the view that cancer could be attributed to discrete genetic elements. Sixty years after Rous's initial report, the oncogenic region of the Rous sarcoma virus was identified. Further characterization and cloning of the transforming sequences demonstrated that the oncogenicity of the virus depended on *vsrc*, a transduced and mutated copy of the *csrc* cellular oncogene. Subsequently, all oncogenes of acutely transforming ribonucleic acid (RNA) tumor viruses have been found to be transduced cellular genes. (In fact, they were defined as oncogenes.) The viral oncogenes cause transformation because they are mutated versions of cellular oncogenes or are expressed at abnormally high levels. In human cancers, somatic mutations generate oncogenic alleles from oncogenes.

Oncogenes play a role in most forms of human cancer, but are particularly prominent in "liquid" tumors, such as leukemias and lymphomas, as well as in sarcomas. Such cancers often have characteristic chromosomal translocations that alter oncogenes at the breakpoints, fusing them with unrelated genes and endowing the fusion product with new properties that increase cell birth or decrease cell death.

Somatic cell genetic studies of tumorigenesis

The studies of Ephrussi et al.[6] and Harris[7] provided compelling evidence that the ability of cells to form a tumor behaves as a recessive trait at the cellular level. They observed that the growth of murine tumor cells in syngeneic animals could be suppressed when the malignant cells were fused to nonmalignant cells, although reversion to tumorigenicity often occurred when the hybrids were propagated for extended periods in culture. The reappearance of malignancy was found to be associated with specific chromosome losses. The interpretation of those authors, that malignancy can be suppressed in somatic cell hybrids, was subsequently supported by additional studies on mouse, rat, and hamster intraspecies somatic cell hybrids, as well as by interspecies hybrids between rodent tumor cells and normal human cells.[8,9] The karyotypic instability of the rodent human hybrids, however, complicated the analysis of the human chromosomes involved in the suppression process. Stanbridge and his colleagues overcame this problem by studying hybrids made by fusing human tumor cell lines to normal, diploid human fibroblasts.[10,11] Their analysis confirmed that hybrids retaining both sets of parental chromosomes were suppressed, with tumorigenic variants arising only rarely after chromosome losses in the hybrids. Moreover, it was demonstrated that the loss of specific chromosomes, and not simply chromosome loss in general, correlated with the reversion to tumorigenicity. Tumorigenicity could be suppressed even if activated oncogenes, such as mutant *ras* genes, were expressed in the hybrids.[11,12]

The observation that the loss of specific chromosomes was associated with the reversion to malignancy suggested that a single chromosome (and perhaps even a single gene) might be sufficient to suppress tumorigenicity. To directly test that hypothesis, the technique of microcell-mediated chromosome transfer was used to transfer single chromosomes from normal cells to tumor cells. It was found that the transfer of a single chromosome 11 into the HeLa cervical carcinoma cell line suppressed the tumorigenic phenotype of the cells.[13] Similarly, transfer of chromosome 11 into a Wilms tumor cell line was found to suppress tumorigenicity, whereas the transfer of several other chromosomes had no effect.[14] Many studies have demonstrated that transfer of even very small chromosome fragments will specifically suppress the tumorigenic properties of certain cancer cell lines.

Although tumorigenic growth in immunocompromised animals can often be suppressed in hybrids resulting from fusion between malignant and normal cells or by transfer of unique chromosome fragments, other traits characteristic of the parental tumor cells, such as immortality and anchorage-independent growth *in vitro*, may be retained. This observation is consistent with the notion that most malignant tumors arise as a result of multiple genetic alterations. Suppression of tumorigenicity following cell fusion or microcell chromosome transfer might thus represent correction of only one of many alterations.

In summary, somatic cell genetic approaches provided early and persuasive evidence for the existence of critical growth-regulating genes in normal cells that can suppress phenotypic traits of immortal or even fully cancerous cells.

Retinoblastoma: a paradigm for tumor suppressor gene function

Essentially concurrent with the initial cell fusion experiments of Harris and colleagues, Knudson's analysis of the age-specific incidence of retinoblastoma led him to propose that two "hits" or mutagenic events were necessary for retinoblastoma development.[15] Retinoblastoma occurs sporadically in most cases, but, in some families, it displays an autosomal dominant inheritance. In an individual with the inherited form of the disease, Knudson proposed that the first hit is present in the germline, and thus in all cells of the body. However, the presence of a mutation at the susceptibility locus was argued to be insufficient for tumor formation, and a second somatic mutation was hypothesized to be necessary for promoting tumor formation. Given the high likelihood of a somatic mutation occurring in at least one retinal cell during development, the dominant inheritance pattern of retinoblastoma in some families could be explained. In the non-hereditary form of retinoblastoma, both mutations were proposed to arise somatically within the same cell. Although each of the two hits could theoretically have been in different genes, subsequent studies (see later) led to the conclusion that both hits were at the same genetic locus, ultimately inactivating both alleles of the retinoblastoma 1 (*RB1*) susceptibility gene. Knudson's hypothesis served not only to illustrate mechanisms through which inherited and somatic genetic changes might collaborate in tumorigenesis but also to link the notion of recessive genetic determinants for human cancer to somatic cell genetic findings on the recessive nature of tumorigenesis.

The first clue to the location of a putative gene responsible for inherited retinoblastoma was obtained from karyotypic analyses of patients with retinoblastoma. Constitutional deletions of chromosome 13 were observed in some cases.[16] Subsequent cytogenetic studies of patients with retinoblastoma identified detectable germline deletions of chromosome 13 in only about 5% of all patients. However, in cases where deletions were observed, the common region of deletion was centered around chromosome band 13q14.[17] When compared with karyotypically normal family members, patients with deletions of 13q14 were found to have reduced levels of esterase D, an enzyme of unknown physiologic function.[18] This finding implied that the esterase D gene might be contained within chromosome band 13q14. Indeed, analysis of the segregation patterns of esterase D isozymes and retinoblastoma development in families with inherited retinoblastoma established that the esterase D and *RB1* loci were genetically linked.[19]

Subsequently, a child with inherited retinoblastoma was found to have esterase D levels approximately one-half of normal, although no deletion of chromosome 13 was seen in karyotype studies of his blood cells and skin fibroblasts.[20] Interestingly, tumor cells from this patient had a complete absence of esterase D activity, despite harboring one apparently intact copy of chromosome 13. Based on these findings, it was proposed that the copy of chromosome 13 retained in the tumor cells had a submicroscopic deletion of both the esterase D and *RB1* loci. Moreover, it was concluded that the initial *RB1* mutation in the child was recessive at the cellular level (i.e., cells with inactivation of one *RB1* allele had a normal phenotype). However, the effect of the predisposing mutation could be unmasked in the tumor cells by a second event, such as the loss of the chromosome 13 carrying the wild-type *RB1* allele. This proposal was entirely consistent with Knudson's two-hit hypothesis.[15,21]

To establish the generality of these observations, Cavenee and colleagues undertook studies of retinoblastomas, both inherited and sporadic, by using deoxyribonucleic acid (DNA) probes from chromosome 13. Probes detecting DNA polymorphisms were used, so that the two parental copies of chromosome 13 in the cells of the patient's normal and tumor tissues could be distinguished from one another. By using such markers to compare paired normal and tumor samples from each patient, the Cavenee group was able to demonstrate that loss of heterozygosity (LOH—i.e., the loss of one parental set of markers) for chromosome 13 alleles had occurred during tumorigenesis in more than 60% of the cases studied.[22] LOH

for chromosome 13, and specifically for the region of chromosome 13 containing the *RB1* gene, occurred via a number of different mechanisms (Figure 2). In addition, through study of inherited cases, it was shown that the copy of chromosome 13 retained in the tumor cells was derived from the affected parent and that the chromosome carrying the wild-type *RB1* allele had been lost.[22,23] These data established that the unmasking of a predisposing mutation at the *RB1* gene, whether the initial mutation had been inherited or had arisen somatically in a single developing retinoblast, occurred by the same chromosomal mechanisms.

Patients with the inherited form of retinoblastoma were known to be at an increased risk for the development of a few other cancer types, particularly osteosarcomas. LOH for the chromosome 13q region containing the *RB1* locus was seen in osteosarcomas arising in patients with the inherited form of retinoblastoma, suggesting that inactivation of both *RB1* alleles was critical to the development of osteosarcomas in those with inherited retinoblastoma.[24,25] Chromosome 13q LOH was also frequently observed in sporadic osteosarcomas. These molecular studies of retinoblastomas and osteosarcomas provided strong support for Knudson's two-hit hypothesis and suggested that a variety of tumors might arise through the inactivation of various tumor suppressor loci.[11,21,23] In addition, the studies demonstrated that the inherited and sporadic forms of a specific tumor type both appeared to arise as a result of genetic alterations in the same gene.

Cloning and analysis of the *RB1* gene

The molecular cloning of the *RB1* gene was facilitated by the identification in the chromosome 13q14 region of an anonymous DNA marker that detected DNA rearrangements in retinoblastomas.[26] Analysis of the DNA sequences flanking this DNA marker revealed a gene with the properties expected of RB1.[27-29] The *RB1* gene has a complex organization, with 27 exons spanning more than 200 kb of DNA, and an RNA transcript of about 4.7 kb. The *RB1* gene appears to be expressed ubiquitously rather than to be restricted to retinoblasts and osteoblasts.

Cloning of *RB1* allowed study of mutations that inactivate the gene. Although gross deletions of *RB1* sequences are observed in a small subset of retinoblastoma and osteosarcoma cases, most tumors appear to express full-length *RB1* transcripts and lack detectable gene rearrangements when analyzed by Southern blotting.[30-33] Hence, the detection of inherited and somatic mutations in the *RB1* gene in most cases requires detailed characterization of its sequence. Extensive analysis of mutant *RB1* alleles has provided definitive molecular evidence supporting Knudson's two-hit model. As predicted, patients with inherited retinoblastoma have been found to have one mutated and one normal allele in their constitutional (blood) cells. In retinoblastomas of such individuals, the remaining *RB1* allele has been found to be inactivated by somatic mutation, usually by loss of the normal allele through a gross chromosomal event (Figure 2), but in some cases by point mutation. Multiple tumors arising in an individual patient with inherited retinoblastoma were all found to contain the same germline mutation, but different somatic mutations affected the remaining *RB1* allele. The vast majority of patients with a single retinoblastoma and no family history of the disease have two somatic mutations in their tumors and two normal alleles in their constitutional cells.

The observation that *RB1* is ubiquitously expressed is rather puzzling, given the restricted spectrum of tumors that develop in patients with germline *RB1* mutations. Patients with germline mutations of *RB1* are at elevated risk only for the development of a rather limited number of tumor types, including retinoblastoma in childhood, osteosarcoma, soft-tissue sarcoma, and melanoma

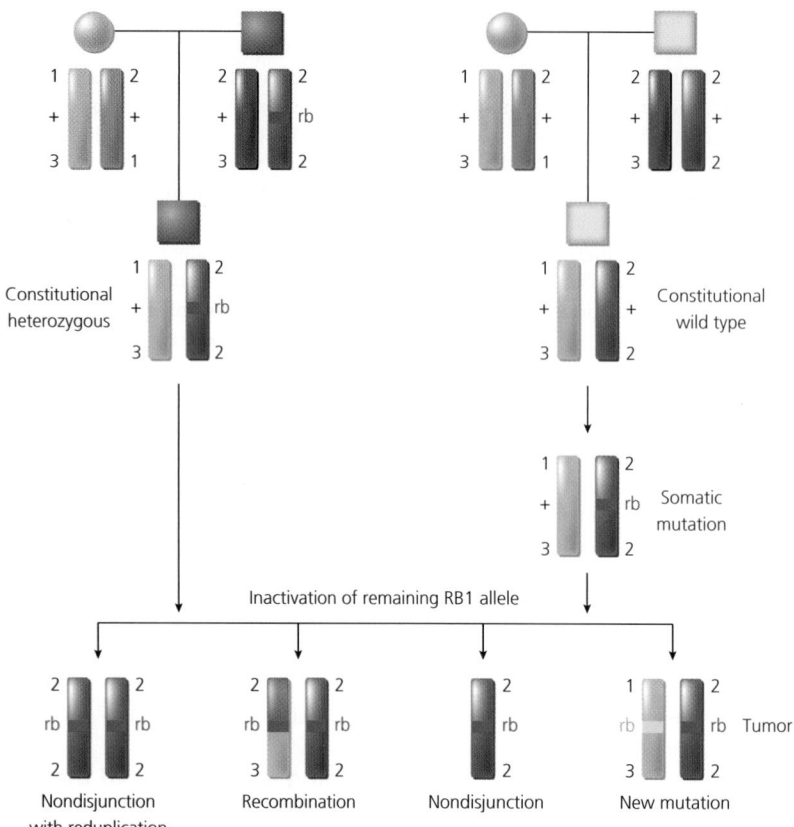

Figure 2 Chromosomal mechanisms that result in loss of heterozygosity for alleles at the retinoblastoma predisposition (RB1) locus at chromosomal band 13q14. In the inherited form of the disease (*top left*), the affected son inherits a mutant *RB1* allele *(rb)* from his affected father and a normal RB1 allele (+) from his mother. Thus, he has one wild-type and one mutant *RB1* allele in all his cells (i.e., constitutional genotype for *RB1* is *rb/+*). The two copies of chromosome 13 in his normal cells (one from each parent) can be distinguished using polymorphic DNA markers flanking the *RB1* locus (the polymorphic alleles are designated by number). A retinoblastoma can arise after inactivation of the remaining wild-type *RB1* allele. Among the genetic mechanisms found to inactivate the remaining wild-type *RB1* allele during tumor development are chromosome nondisjunction and reduplication of the remaining copy of chromosome 13, mitotic recombination, nondisjunction, and new RB mutations that inactivate the remaining *RB1* allele. Shown at the *top right* is the situation in the noninherited (sporadic) form of the disease. A somatic mutation arises in a developing retinal cell and inactivates one of the *RB1* alleles. A retinoblastoma will develop if the remaining *RB1* allele is inactivated by one of the mechanisms shown.

later in life. *RB1* germline mutations fail to predispose to most common cancers, despite the fact that somatic *RB1* mutations have been observed in a wide variety of cancer types, including breast, small cell lung, bladder, pancreas, and prostate cancers.[34] It is possible that retinoblastoma protein functions differently in retinal epithelial cells than in other cell types, so that the *RB1* gene acts as a "gatekeeper" in retinal cells but not in other cell types.

Function of retinoblastoma protein P105-RB

The protein product of the *RB1* gene is a nuclear phosphoprotein known as p105-Rb or, more commonly, pRB. Its molecular weight is about 105,000 Da. Studies by Whyte and colleagues provided critical insights into pRB function, connecting human tumorigenesis with experimental tumors caused by DNA tumor viruses. They demonstrated that pRB formed a complex with the E1A oncoprotein encoded by the murine DNA tumor virus adenovirus type 5.[35] Prior studies of E1A had established that it had many effects on cell growth, including cell immortalization and cooperation with other oncogenes (e.g., mutated ras oncogene alleles) in neoplastic transformation. It was thus hypothesized that functional inactivation of pRB through its interaction with E1A might contribute to some of E1A's transforming functions. Additional support for that proposal was provided by data establishing that mutations inactivating the ability of E1A to bind to pRB also inactivated E1A's transforming

function.[36,37] The significance of physical interaction between pRB and a DNA tumor virus oncoprotein was further supported by the subsequent demonstration that other DNA tumor virus oncoproteins also formed complexes with pRB, including SV40 T antigen and the E7 proteins of human papillomavirus (HPV) types 16 and 18 (Figure 3).[38,39] Many of the mutations that inactivated the transforming activities of these oncoproteins also inactivated their ability to interact with pRB. Furthermore, E7 proteins from "high-risk" HPVs (i.e., those linked to cancer development), such as HPV 16 and 18, formed complexes more tightly with pRB than did E7 proteins of "low-risk" viruses (e.g., HPV types 6 and 11). These studies of pRB provided compelling evidence that DNA tumor viruses might transform cells at least in part by inactivating tumor suppressor gene products. In addition, given the critical dependence of DNA tumor viruses on harnessing the cell's machinery for replication of the viral genome, the studies also provided support for the hypothesis that pRB might control normal cell growth by interacting with cellular proteins that regulate the cell's decision to enter into the DNA synthesis (S) phase of the cell cycle.

The functional activity of pRB is regulated by phosphorylation during normal progression through the cell cycle. Accordingly, pRB appears to be predominantly unphosphorylated or hypophosphorylated in the G1 phase of the cell cycle and maximally phosphorylated in G2 (Figure 4). The critical phosphorylation events regulating the

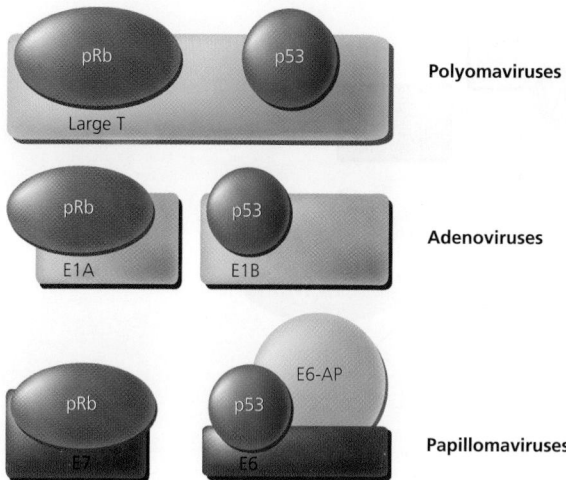

Polyomaviruses

Adenoviruses

Papillomaviruses

Figure 3 Schematic representation of interactions between tumor suppressor gene products and proteins encoded by DNA tumor viruses. Large T antigen from polyomaviruses [such as simian virus 40 (SV40)] bind both the retinoblastoma (pRB) and p53 proteins. For the adenoviruses and the high-risk human papillomaviruses (HPV types 16 and 18), various viral protein products complex with pRB and TP53. A cellular protein known as E6-associated protein (E6-AP) cooperates with the HPV E6 protein to complex and degrade TP53.

function of pRB are likely to be mediated at the boundary between the G1 and S phases of the cell cycle by cyclin and cyclin-dependent kinase (Cdk) protein complexes.[34,40] When it is not phosphorylated, pRB forms complexes with proteins in the E2F family and inhibits transcription by recruiting proteins involved in transcriptional repression.[40] When phosphorylated, pRB can no longer efficiently form complexes with E2Fs (Figure 4). The E2F proteins, when dimerized with their differentiation-regulated transcription factor partner (DP) proteins, are then capable of activating the expression of a number of genes that are likely to regulate or promote entry into S-phase, including DNA polymerase a, thymidylate synthase, ribonucleotide reductase, cyclin E, and dihydrofolate reductase.[40] The E2F family members that directly affect cellular proliferation were shown in conditional mouse knockout models.[41] Several other cellular proteins that bind to pRB have been identified, but their functions and the significance of their interactions with pRB remain less-well characterized than the interactions of pRB with E2Fs. Future studies will undoubtedly shed further light on the means by which loss of pRB function and that of pRB homologs p107 and p130[42] contribute to cancer development.

TP53 gene

Studies in the late 1970s revealed that a cellular phosphoprotein with a relative molecular mass of about 53,000 Da formed a tight complex with SV40 T antigen; hence, the name of the p53 protein.[43-45] Further work established that TP53 also formed a complex with other viral oncogene products, including the adenovirus E1B protein, and that TP53 was present at low levels in normal cells and high levels in many tumors and tumor cell lines.[43,46-48] These initial findings suggested that increased levels of TP53 might contribute to cancer. Consistent with that notion, gene transfer studies provided data demonstrating that TP53 functioned as an oncogene in *in vitro* experiments.[47,49-51] However, subsequent studies in human tumors showed that TP53 was in reality a tumor suppressor gene.[52]

The rationale for the human cancer studies was the observation that chromosome 17p LOH was common in a number of tumor types, including colorectal, bladder, breast, and lung cancer.[53,54]

Detailed mapping showed that region 17p, which was lost in colorectal cancers, included the *TP53* gene.[52] Analysis of the sequence of the *TP53* alleles retained in those cancers with 17p LOH demonstrated that the remaining *TP53* allele was mutated,[52] in perfect accord with Knudson's hypothesis for the alterations expected in tumor suppressor genes. These observations were soon extended to other cancer types, and they explained many previous observations concerning TP53 that had been confusing when *TP53* was believed to be an oncogene.[55-59] Additional evidence that *TP53* functions as a tumor suppressor gene in human cancer is provided by gene transfer studies, but such overexpression studies cannot be easily interpreted, as many genes with no role in neoplasia can inhibit the growth of transfected cells.[60-63] Based on genome-wide sequencing of multiple tumor types, it is now clear that *TP53* is believed to be the most frequently mutated gene in human cancers in general.[64]

Germline mutations in the *TP53* gene have been seen in those affected by Li–Fraumeni syndrome (LFS) and in a small subset of pediatric patients with sarcomas or osteosarcomas that do not meet the more strict criteria for diagnosis of LFS.[65-67] Those with LFS are at risk for developing a number of tumors, including soft-tissue sarcoma, osteosarcoma, brain tumors, breast cancer, and leukemia. Between one-half and two-thirds of patients with LFS have germline mutations in the central core domain of the *TP53* coding sequences that resemble the somatic mutations frequently seen in sporadic cancers.[68] Some LFS patients and families with phenotypic features of LFS have germline mutations in a gene termed *hCHK2* that phosphorylates *TP53* and controls the cell's response to DNA-damaging events.[69]

In addition to somatic and inherited mutations in the gene, *TP53* function can be inactivated by other mechanisms. As noted earlier, most cervical cancers contain high-risk or cancer-associated HPV genomes (i.e., HPV type 16 or 18). The *E6* gene product of high-risk, but not low-risk, HPV types binds to a cellular protein known as E6-AP (for E6-associated protein) and stimulates TP53 degradation.[70-74] A cellular TP53-binding protein known as mouse double minute 2 (MDM2) is overexpressed in a subset of soft-tissue sarcomas as a result of gene amplification involving chromosome 12q sequences.[75] More recent studies have identified another TP53-binding protein, MDM4, which is overexpressed in a variety of cancers as a result of gene amplification of chromosome 1q sequences.[76] DNA transfection studies have shown that both the *MDM2* and *MDM4* genes can function as oncogenes when overexpressed. The oncogenic function is presumably mediated through their binding to and inactivation of TP53. Both proteins mask TP53's transcriptional activation domain and promote TP53's ubiquitination and subsequent degradation by the proteasome.[77-79] Consistent with the notion that MDM2 is a critical inhibitor of TP53 function, sarcomas with *MDM2* amplification and overexpression rarely harbor somatic mutations in *TP53*.[80] Disruption of the *MDM2* and *MDM4* genes in the germline of mice is lethal, probably because such disruption allows unregulated activity of *TP53*. Accordingly, disruption of the murine *TP53* gene rescues MDM2-deficient and MDM4-deficient mice from embryonic lethality.[81,82] Other mechanisms of regulating TP53 function have also been described, including mutation of a nuclear-cytoplasmic shuttle protein called nucleophosmin in almost 100% of adult acute myelogenous leukemias that demonstrate cytoplasmic localization of this protein, with the notable exception of acute promyelocytic leukemia.[83]

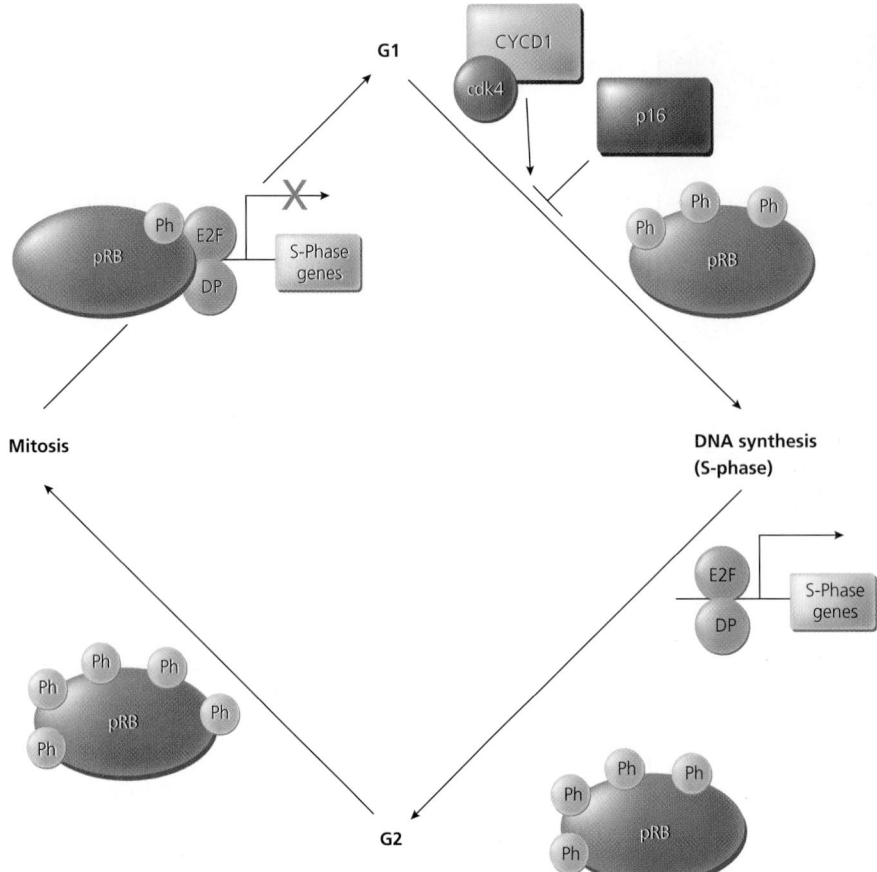

Figure 4 The function of the retinoblastoma protein (pRB) is regulated during the cell cycle by phosphorylation. The pRB protein is hypophosphorylated in the G1 phase of the cell cycle, and phosphorylation (Ph) of specific sites appears to increase during progression through the cell cycle. A protein complex that appears to phosphorylate pRB before DNA synthesis (S-phase) includes a cyclin (Cyc) and a cyclin-dependent kinase (Cdk)—for example, cyclin D1 and Cdk4. The CycD1/Cdk4 complex is regulated by the p16 inhibitor protein, which is itself the product of a tumor suppressor gene on chromosome 9p, known as *CDKN2* (see text). In its hypophosphorylated state, pRB binds to E2F transcriptional regulatory proteins. When pRB is brought to the promoter regions of genes via its interaction with E2F proteins, pRB represses the expression of the E2F/DP target genes. Phosphorylation of pRB releases it from the E2F/DP protein complex and results in gene activation, including those genes involved in DNA synthesis. The figure also indicates that pRB phosphorylation increases in G2 with pRB dephosphorylated at or near anaphase.

TP53 function

The p53 protein has been shown to function as a transcriptional regulatory protein[84,85] though other, nontranscriptional functions for p53 have been described (ref. to recent review). In its wild-type state, the p53 protein is capable of binding to specific DNA sequences with its central core domain (Figure 5). The amino terminal sequences of p53 function as a transcriptional activation domain, and the carboxyl terminal sequences appear to be required for TP53 to form dimers and tetramers with itself. TP53 activates transcription of a number of genes with roles in the control of the cell cycle, including *WAF1/CIP1/p21* (which encodes a regulator of Cdk activity),[86] *MDM2* (as noted earlier, encoding a protein that is a known negative regulator of *TP53*), and 14-3-3 (a regulator of G2/M progression),[87] and various genes that likely function in apoptosis, including *PUMA* and *NOXA*. Experimental disruption of these genes by targeted homologous recombination can re-create some of the phenotypes associated with *TP53* inactivation.[88,89]

The vast majority of the somatic mutations in TP53 are missense mutations leading to amino acid substitutions in the central portion of the protein (exons 5–9).[90] Consistent with the structure of the p53 protein, these missense mutations have marked effects on the p53 protein's ability to bind to its cognate DNA recognition sequence through either of two mechanisms.[91] Some mutations

(e.g., mutations at codons 248 or 273) alter *TP53* sequences that are directly responsible for sequence-specific DNA binding. Other mutations (e.g., codon 175) appear to affect the folding of *TP53* and thus indirectly affect its ability to bind to DNA. Evidence that these missense mutations can confer "gain of function" rather than a dominant negative effect was demonstrated via "knock in" mouse models, whereby precise missense mutations were introduced into the endogenous *TP53* gene.[92–96]

Under some circumstances, TP53 acts at the G1/S checkpoint to regulate the cell's decision to synthesize DNA, although TP53 also appears to have a critical function at G2/M.[97,98] In other settings, TP53 appears to exert control over the cell's decision to undergo apoptosis or programmed cell death.[85] Of particular interest with regard to cancer treatment are data suggesting that some tumor cells lacking TP53 function are less sensitive to irradiation and chemotherapeutic agents such as cisplatin.[92,99,100] However, studies of other tumor cells suggest that *TP53* status shows a very different relationship to chemotherapeutic response, with cells that lack functional TP53 being markedly sensitive to DNA-damaging agents but resistant to 5-fluorouracil.[101] Thus far, studies of primary human cancers have emphasized that a rather complex relationship is likely to exist between *TP53* mutational status and the responsiveness of cancer cells to chemotherapy or radiation therapy, or

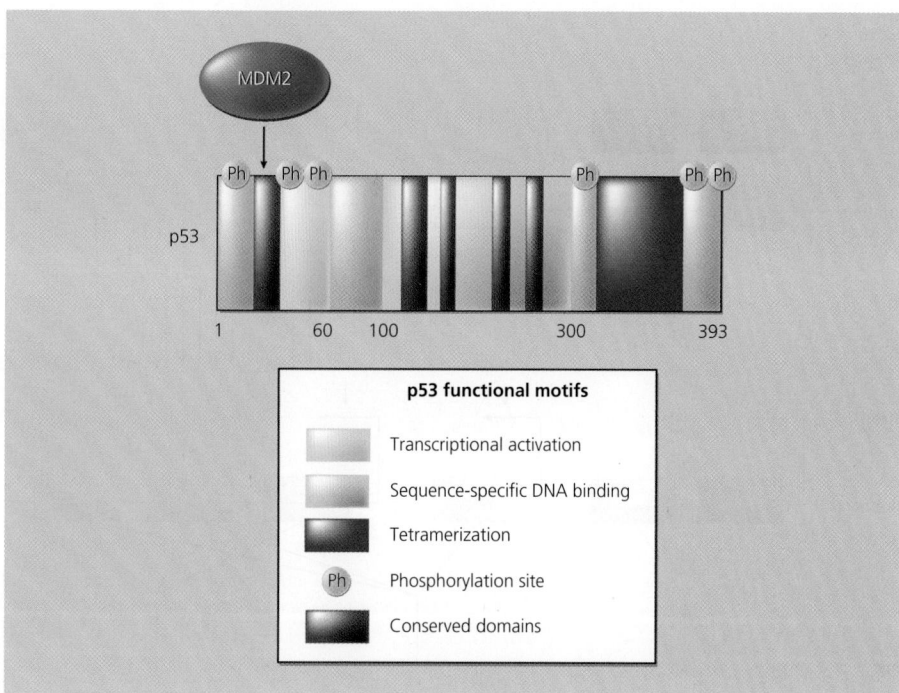

Figure 5 TP53 functional motifs. Sequences of TP53 involved in transcriptional activation, sequence-specific DNA binding, tetramerization, and binding by the MDM2 protein are indicated. The five distinct regions of TP53 sequence that are highly conserved between p53 proteins of diverse species are indicated. In addition, the locations of several sites in the protein that are phosphorylated (Ph) and that regulate TP53 function are indicated.

both. In particular, it is difficult to distinguish the effects of *TP53* mutation on the natural progression of disease from its effects on responses to treatment and other cellular stresses.[102,103] Hopefully, further research on *TP53* will clarify our understanding of its normal functions, the basis for its frequent inactivation in many different cancers, and the consequences of its inactivation on tumor growth and response to therapy.

Cyclin-dependent kinase inhibitor 2A locus

Studies of the cyclin-dependent kinase inhibitor 2A (CDKN2A) locus on chromosome 9p illustrate well how observations from initially disparate lines of investigation often converge to implicate a particular locus as a critical factor in cancer development. The LOH of chromosome 9p was frequently found in many different tumor types, including melanoma, glioma, nonsmall cell lung, bladder, head and neck cancers, and leukemia.[104–107] Of considerable interest were observations establishing that a subset of such tumors had homozygous (complete) deletions affecting the 9p21 region,[108–110] strongly supporting the existence of a tumor suppressor gene in the region. In addition to the frequent somatic alterations of chromosome 9p sequences in cancers, linkage studies of some families with inherited melanoma indicated a melanoma predisposition gene mapped to essentially the same region of 9p.[111] These observations stimulated great interest in the chromosome 9p region presumed to contain the tumor suppressor gene or genes. One of the genes identified in the region as a result of positional cloning efforts was initially termed multiple tumor suppressor 1 (MTS1).[112] Sequence analysis of *MTS1* showed that it was identical to a previously described gene that encoded the Cdk inhibitor protein known as p16.[113] Because the p16 protein functioned by inhibiting Cdk4 and Cdk6, it was termed an inhibitor of cyclin-dependent kinase 4 (INK4) protein. Another highly related gene, mapping immediately next to the *p16/MTS1* gene on chromosome 9p, was found to encode a second INK4 protein, known as p15 (Figure 6). The gene

encoding the p16 protein is most often termed *INK4A*, and the gene for p15 is *INK4B*.[114,115] The approved symbols are *CDKN2A* and *CDKN2B*, respectively.

Subsequent studies show that heterozygous mutations in *CDKN2A* are present in some families with inherited predispositions to melanoma or pancreatic cancer.[116–119] Somatic mutations in *CDKN2A* are present in many different cancer types, including but not limited to melanoma, glioma, pancreatic and bladder cancers, and leukemia. In some tumors, deletions affecting the *CDKN2A* gene also involve the *CDKN2B* gene. In rare tumors, deletions inactivate *CDKN2B* but not *CDKN2A*.[120] The prevalence and specific nature of *CDKN2A* mutations vary markedly from one tumor type to another. In contrast to other tumor suppressor genes, such as *RB1* and *TP53*, homozygous deletion is a fairly common mechanism of *CDKN2A* inactivation in cancer.[121]

Detailed studies of the *CDKN2A* locus led to the identification of a novel alternative transcript containing nucleotide sequences identical to those in transcripts for the p16[INK4A] protein, but with unique 5′ sequences (Figure 6).[114,115,122] The alternative CDKN2A locus transcript encodes a protein known as p14 alternative reading frame (p14[ARF]). Of note, human p14[ARF] is the same product as the originally identified mouse protein p19[ARF], which was designated as p19 due to its apparent weight.

The p14[ARF] protein contains sequences from a distinct first exon (exon 1β). Exon 1β is located upstream of exon 1α, the first exon present in transcripts for p16 (Figure 6). Exon 1β is spliced to exon 2, which, along with exon 3, is present in the transcripts for both the p14[ARF] and p16[INK4A] proteins. However, the p14[ARF] protein shares no sequence similarity with the p16[INK4A] protein because p14[ARF] synthesis initiates at a unique methionine codon in exon 1β and continues through exon 2, using an alternative open reading frame with no similarity to the p16[INK4A] open reading frame. Careful studies of somatic and inherited mutations at the *CDKN2A* locus indicate that localized mutations inactivating the p16[INK4A]

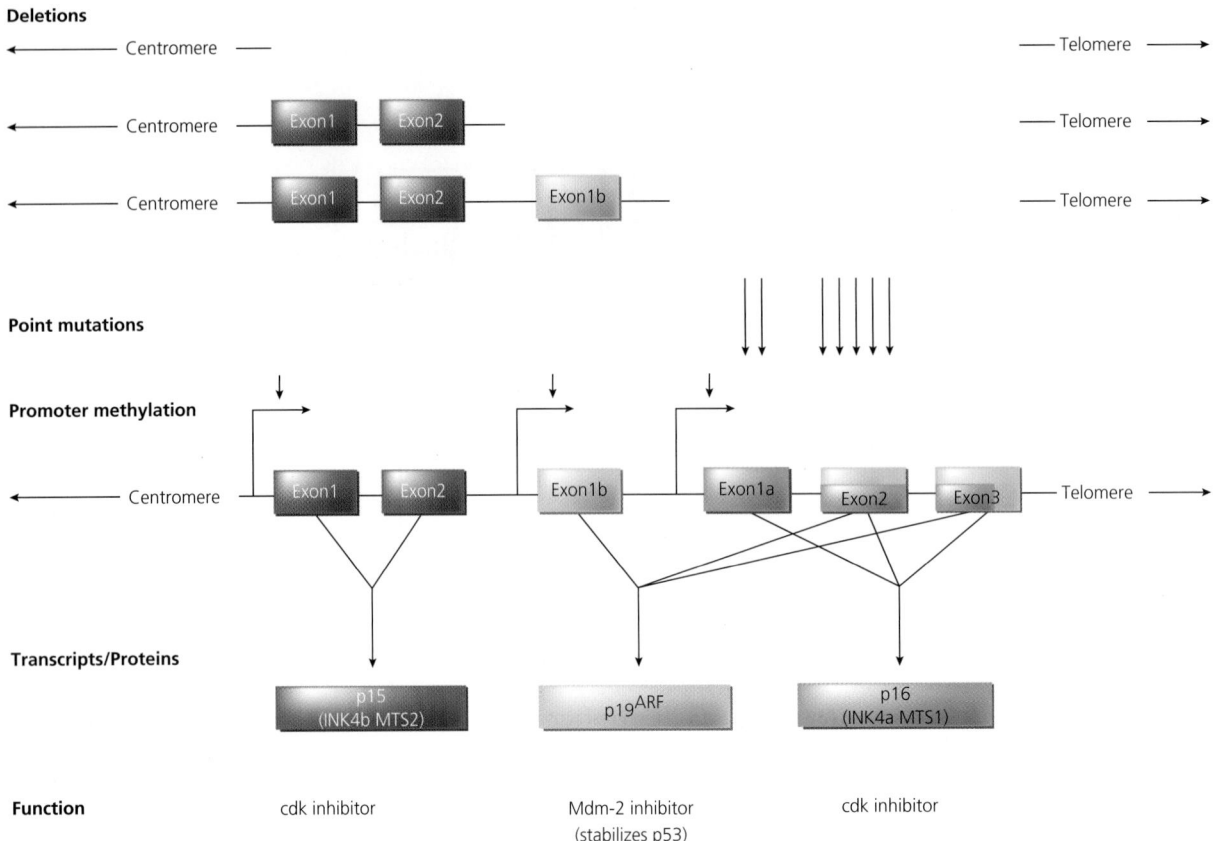

Figure 6 Genomic structure, mutations, and transcripts of the *CDKN2B* (p15) and *CDKN2A* (p16/p19ARF) locus. The origins of the p15, p16, and p19ARF transcripts are shown schematically, along with a representative depiction of genomic deletions, point mutations *(arrows)*, and promoter methylation *(arrowheads)* noted in human cancers. The exons of the *CDKN2B* and *CDKN2A* loci are shown as *rectangles*. The transcripts/proteins and presumed functions of the transcripts/proteins are indicated. The *red rectangles* indicate the open reading frame in transcripts encoding p15; the *yellow rectangles* indicate the open reading frame present in transcripts encoding p19ARF; and the *lavender rectangles* indicate the open reading frame present in transcripts encoding p16. The size of the locus, exons, and transcripts are not shown to scale.

protein are common in human cancer, with more than 60 germline mutations identified, but that localized mutations inactivating p14[ARF] are uncommon.[114,115] However, the frequent occurrence of homozygous deletions at the *CDKN2A* locus implies that mutational inactivation of both proteins—and of p15[INK4B]—may be strongly selected for during tumor development (Figure 6). Other findings suggest that p16[INK4A] and p14[ARF] expression may be lost in some tumor types as a result of methylation of DNA regulatory sequences at the *CDKN2A* locus (Figure 6).[123–125] Recent studies have demonstrated the importance of DNA methyltransferases in initiating and maintaining epigenetic silencing of the p16 tumor suppressor.[126,127] Furthermore, studies of mice with germline inactivation of p14[ARF] and p16[INK4A] indicate that these proteins function as tumor suppressor genes *in vivo*.[128–130]

The mechanism through which the p16[INK4A] protein controls tumorigenic growth is apparently through its inhibition of Cdk4 activity. As indicated earlier, phosphorylation of pRB impedes its ability to transcriptionally regulate E2F-target genes (Figure 4). The cyclin D1/Cdk4 complex has a critical role in regulating pRB phosphorylation and function.[124] Hence, the p16[INK4A] protein, by virtue of its regulation of Cdk4 activity, is, in turn, a critical factor in regulating pRB phosphorylation. Presumably, inactivation of p16[INK4A] results in inappropriate phosphorylation of pRB and a subsequent inability of hyperphosphorylated pRB to bind E2Fs and appropriately regulate gene expression at the G1–S transition. p14[ARF] functions as a tumor suppressor by direct binding to the

MDM2 protein, inhibiting the MDM2-induced degradation of TP53, thus maintaining appropriate function of TP53 in cells,[115] much like p16INK4A maintains normal pRB function.

Contrary to this interpretation, however, is the fact that alterations of p14[ARF] and TP53 often coexist in cancer cells, suggesting that they do not alter the same pathway, whereas Rb and p16INK4A alterations are mutually exclusive, supportive of the fact that they affect the same pathway.[131] Nevertheless, these findings emphasize the concept that oncogenes and tumor suppressor genes do not function in isolation. Rather, they function in intricately linked cascades or networks that have important consequences for both tumorigenesis and therapy (Figure 7).[85,132]

Adenomatous polyposis coli gene

Identification and germline mutations
Colon cancers arising in a minority of hereditary syndromes do so from a state of polyposis. One of the polyposis syndromes is known as familial adenomatous polyposis (FAP) or adenomatous polyposis coli (APC). FAP is an autosomal dominant disorder affecting about 1 in 8000 individuals in the United States. The syndrome is characterized by the development of hundreds of adenomatous polyps in the colon and rectum of affected individuals by early adulthood. The lifetime risk of colorectal cancer in those with the classic form of FAP is extremely high, approaching 100% by age 60 years.

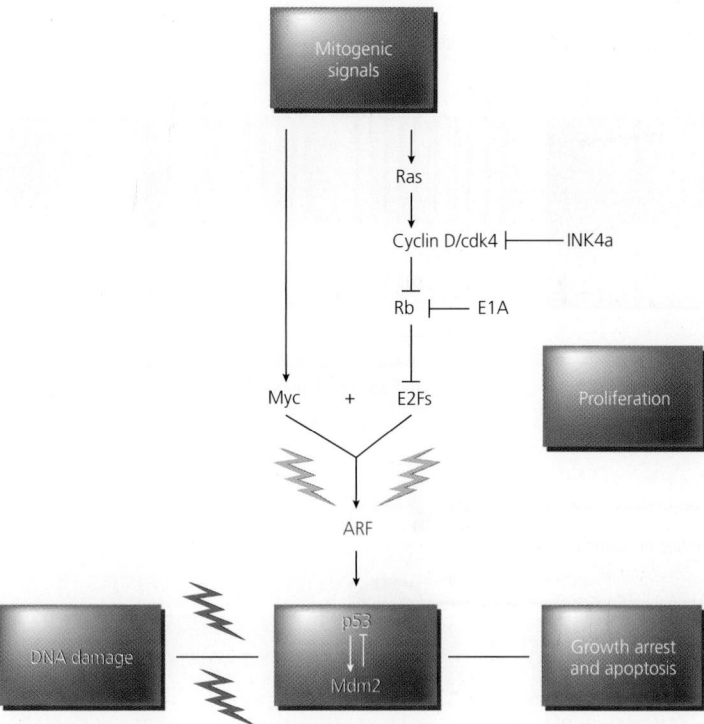

Figure 7 Role of the p19*^{RF} protein in checkpoint control. The p19^{ARF} protein (ARF) responds to proliferative signals normally required for cell proliferation. When these signals exceed a critical threshold, the ARF-dependent checkpoint *(yellow lightning bolts)* is activated, and ARF triggers a TP53-dependent response that induces growth arrest or apoptosis, or both. Signals now known to induce signaling via the ARF-TP53 pathway include Myc, E1A, and E2F-1. In principle, "upstream" oncoproteins, such as products of mutated *ras* alleles, constitutively activated receptors, or cytoplasmic signal transducing oncoproteins, might also trigger ARF activity via the cyclin D-Cdk4-RBE2F or Myc-dependent pathways, both of which are normally necessary for S-phase entry. In inhibiting cyclin D-dependent kinases, p16^{INK4A} can dampen the activity of mitogenic signals. In the figure, E1A is shown to work, at least in part, by opposing RB function. For simplicity, Myc and E2F-1 are shown to activate only TP53 via the effects on ARF, though highly overexpressed levels of these proteins can activate TP53 in ARF-negative cells, albeit with an attenuated efficiency. ARF activation of TP53 likely depends on inactivation of Mdm2-specific function(s). DNA damage signals (e.g., ionizing and ultraviolet radiation, hypoxic stress) activate *(blue lightning bolts)* TP53 through multiple signaling pathways.

An interstitial deletion of chromosome 5q in a patient with features of FAP, but without any family history of the syndrome, greatly aided localization of the *APC* gene.[133] Subsequent DNA linkage studies confirmed that, in multiple kindreds with FAP, or the related condition known as Gardner syndrome, the polyposis phenotype segregated with DNA markers near 5q21.[134,135] In 1991, positional cloning efforts identified the *APC* gene as the specific gene responsible for FAP.[136–139] The *APC* gene is large, with more than 15 exons, and alternative splicing affects the 5′ untranslated portion of transcripts. The predominant *APC* transcript encodes a 2843-amino acid protein expressed in many adult tissues.

In the great majority of individuals with FAP, heterozygous germline mutations can be identified in the *APC* gene.[140–142] All of the germline *APC* mutations in those with FAP appear to inactivate APC protein function. The overwhelming majority of these germline mutations are localized nonsense or frameshift mutations in the 5′ half of the coding region of *APC* (Figure 8). Consistent with Knudson's two-hit hypothesis, inactivation of the remaining wild-type APC allele by somatic mutation in those carrying a germline *APC* mutation is observed in the cancers that arise.[143,144] Correlations between the location of a particular germline *APC* mutation and clinical features have been found,[145] although clear insights into the molecular basis for the predisposition to extracolonic tumors (e.g., jaw osteomas and desmoid tumors) in FAP patients with variant phenotypes are lacking. However, some light has been shed on the variability in polyp number seen in families with polyposis.[143,146] Mutations in the 5′ region of the *APC* gene

appear to be correlated with an attenuated phenotype attributable to reentry of the ribosome on the APC transcript downstream of the premature stop codon, resulting in an APC protein that retains some of its normal activity.[146] Mutations in 3′ third of the *APC* gene are also associated with a milder polyposis phenotype than mutations in the central third of the gene, perhaps because the mutated APC proteins similarly retain some tumor suppressor activity. Unexpectedly, extracolonic features such as desmoid tumors appear to be more common in patients with 3′ mutations.[143] Finally, a missense mutation in the middle of the *APC* gene has been found to predispose to colorectal cancers in Ashkenazi Jewish families.[147] This mutation does not alter the function of the gene product, but creates a "hot spot" that appears to be highly mutable, resulting in somatic deletions or insertions of surrounding nucleotides that produce truncations.

Somatic mutations in sporadic colon tumors

Although germline *APC* mutations are an uncommon cause of colorectal cancer in the general population and are present in only about 0.5% of all colon cancers, somatic *APC* mutations are present in the vast majority of sporadic colorectal adenomas and carcinomas.[148] The initial observation suggesting that *APC* inactivation might be common in colon tumors was the observation that the chromosome 5q region containing the *APC* gene was affected by LOH in many sporadic colorectal adenomas and carcinomas.[54,149] Since the identification of the *APC* gene, detailed analyses of the

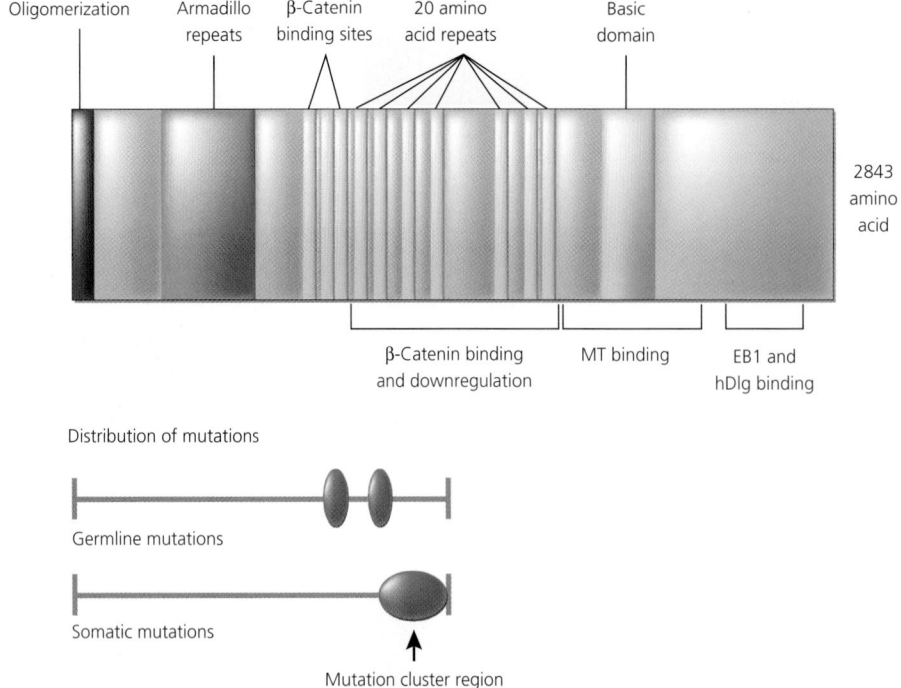

Figure 8 Schematic representation of Apc protein domains with respect to mutational analysis results. The relative positions of various Apc domains. A putative domain involved in homo-oligomerization of Apc is located at the amino-terminus. Also noted are a series of repeats of unknown function with similarity to the *Drosophila* armadillo protein, sequences known to mediate binding to p-catenin and its downregulation, a basic domain in the carboxy-terminal third of the protein that appears to facilitate complexing with microtubules (MT), and sequences near the carboxy terminus of Apc that are known to interact with the EB1 and human homolog of the *Drosophila* disc large (hDlg) protein. Germline mutations in the *APC* gene (predominantly chain terminating) are dispersed throughout the 5′ half of the sequence, with two apparent "hot spots" at codons 1061 and 1309. Somatic mutations in the *APC* gene in colorectal cancer appear to cluster in a region termed the "mutation cluster region," and mutations at codons 1309 and 1450 are most common.

somatic mutations inactivating the *APC* gene in colorectal tumors have been carried out. The somatic *APC* mutations in sporadic tumors are similar in nature and location to the germline *APC* mutations found in those with FAP (Figure 8). Present findings suggest that up to 90% of colorectal tumors, regardless of their size or particular histopathologic features, harbor somatic mutations that inactivate APC. [143–150]

Function
The *APC* gene encodes a large protein of roughly 300 kDa that is hypothesized to regulate cell adhesion, cell migration, or apoptosis in the colonic crypt. The localization of the APC protein in the basolateral membrane of colonic epithelial cells, with an apparent increase in APC expression in cells near the top of the crypt, implies that APC may regulate shedding or apoptosis of cells as they reach the crypt apex.[151] Perhaps consistent with this view, restoration of APC protein expression in colorectal cancer cells lacking endogenous APC expression has been reported to promote apoptosis.[152,153]

The APC protein binds to a number of proteins, including β-catenin, Y-catenin (also known as plakoglobin), glycogen synthase kinase 3β (GSK3β), end-binding protein 1 (EB1), human Drosophila large discs (hDLG), microtubules, and the related proteins axin and conductin.[154] With the exception of β-catenin, GSK3β, and the conductin and axin proteins, the significance and role of APC's interactions with its various binding partners are not well understood. Several lines of evidence imply that APC has a critical function in regulating β-catenin.[154,155] β-Catenin is an abundant cellular protein, first identified because of its role

in linking the cytoplasmic domain of the E-cadherin cell–cell adhesion molecule to the cortical actin cytoskeleton, via β-catenin's binding to α-catenin. The truncated (mutant) APC proteins present in many colorectal cancers lack some or all of the repeat motifs crucial for binding to β-catenin. APC not only binds to β-catenin, but, in collaboration with the GSK3β enzyme and other proteins, such as axin and conductin, it appears to regulate the abundance of β-catenin in the cytosol via phosphorylation. In colorectal cancers in which *APC* is mutated and unable to bind or effectively coordinate the regulation of β-catenin, β-catenin accumulates in the cell, complexes with the transcription factor T-cell factor-4 (Tcf-4), and translocates to the nucleus (Figure 9). Once there, β-catenin functions as a transcriptional coactivator, activating expression of Tcf-4-regulated genes, typically bypassing regulatory proteins, such as Wnt. Consistent with the notion that β-catenin is a critical target of *APC* regulation, somatic mutations in β-catenin have been found in the small fraction of colorectal cancers lacking *APC* mutations.[156–158] These mutations consistently alter GSK3β phosphorylation consensus sites near the amino terminus of the β-catenin protein, and the mutations presumably render the defective β-catenin proteins oncogenic as a result of their resistance to degradation by APC and GSK3β. Although somatic mutations in *APC* appear to be rare in cancers arising outside the colon and rectum, oncogenic mutations in β-catenin's *N*-terminus have been observed in many different cancer types.[159,160]

Wilms tumor gene
Wilms tumors are the most common renal neoplasm in children, accounting for approximately 6% of all pediatric cancers.[161] Wilms tumors are similar to retinoblastomas in a number of ways: both can

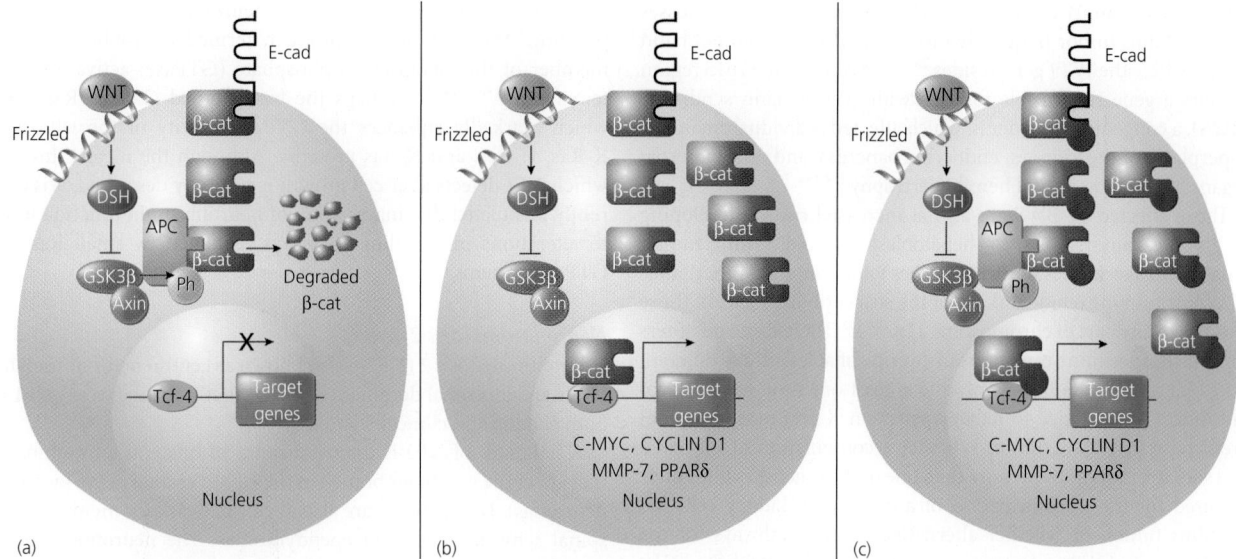

Figure 9 A model indicating the function of the Apc, axin, and Gsk3p proteins in the regulation of p-catenin (p-cat) in normal cells, and the consequence of Apc or p-cat defects in cancer cells. p-Cat is an abundant cellular protein, and much of it is often bound to the cytoplasmic domain of the E-cadherin (E-cad) cell–cell adhesion protein. (a) In normal cells, the proteins glycogen synthase kinase 3p (Gsk3p), Apc, and axin function to promote degradation of free cytosolic p-cat, probably as a result of phosphorylation of the *N*-terminal sequences of p-cat by Gsk3p. Gsk3p activity and p-cat degradation are inhibited by activation of the wingless (Wnt) pathway, as a result of the action of the Frizzled receptor and disheveled (Dsh) signaling protein. (b) Mutation of Apc in colorectal and other cancer cells results in accumulation of p-cat, binding to Tcf-4, and transcriptional activation of Tcf-4 target genes, such as *c-myc*, cyclin D1, *MMP-7*, and PPARS (see text). (c) Point mutations and small deletions in p-cat in cancer cells inhibit phosphorylation and degradation of p-cat by Gsk3p and Apc, with resultant activation of *c-myc* and other Tcf-4 target genes.

occur bilaterally or unilaterally, with single or multiple foci, and in a sporadic or inherited fashion. The two mutation model originally proposed for retinoblastoma was also proposed to explain Wilms tumor.[162] However, hereditary cases are not as common among Wilms tumor patients as they are in retinoblastoma patients. Almost all patients inheriting a mutation at the *RB1* locus develop a retinoblastoma, but only approximately 50% of individuals carrying a germline mutation predisposing to Wilms tumor develop the disease (i.e., lower penetrance).[161]

Perhaps the first finding to offer insight into an inherited genetic basis for Wilms tumor was a report describing six patients with Wilms tumor and sporadic aniridia (i.e., congenital absence of the iris).[163] It was proposed that the simultaneous occurrence of these two very rare conditions might result from chromosomal aberrations affecting two or more loci, a situation now often called a contiguous gene syndrome—mutation of one locus presumably leading to aniridia and mutation of another leading to Wilms tumor. This hypothesis was subsequently supported by the discovery of interstitial deletions of chromosome 11p13 in peripheral blood samples from children with the WAGR syndrome (Wilms tumor with aniridia, genitourinary abnormalities, and mental retardation) of Wilms tumor.[164] Cytogenetic studies of tumor tissues in a few cases of sporadic-type Wilms tumors revealed deletions or translocations of chromosome band 11p13.[165,166] Subsequent studies of paired samples of Wilms tumor and normal cells from patients, using probes that detect restriction fragment length polymorphisms (RFLPs) on chromosome 11p, revealed that LOH of 11p occurred frequently in Wilms tumors of both the inherited and sporadic types.[167–170]

The Wilms tumor 1 (*WT1*) gene was identified in 1990 by virtue of mutations inactivating the gene in patients with the WAGR syndrome and by analysis of somatic mutations in the gene in tumors from a minority of patients with unilateral Wilms tumor

and no associated congenital malformation.[171] *WT1* is encoded by 10 exons and its transcripts are subject to alternative splicing.[172,173] In contrast to the rather ubiquitous expression of the *RB1*, *TP53*, and *APC* genes, expression of the *WT1* gene appears to be restricted to embryonic kidney and a small subset of other tissues.[174,175] *WT1* messenger ribonucleic acids (mRNAs) encode proteins with molecular masses of 45,000–49,000 Da and 4 zinc-finger motifs. Based on their predicted amino acid sequences, the WT1 proteins were suspected from the outset to function in transcriptional regulation.[174] Several studies provide evidence to support that notion, although some WT1 isoforms may have a role in RNA processing, rather than in transcription regulation.[173,174] WT1 proteins suppress the transcriptional activity of promoter elements from a number of growth-inducing genes, including the genes for early growth response (EGR1), insulin-like growth factor-2 (IGF-2), and platelet-derived growth factor A (PDGFA) chain, suggesting that WT1 may function in gene repression.[176] Other studies suggest that WT1 can activate or repress gene expression, depending on the cell type and promoter context.[177] Consistent with the notion that WT1 may have a physiologic function in transcriptional activation, recent work indicates that WT1 activates expression of amphiregulin, a member of the epidermal growth factor family.[178] Loss of amphiregulin expression may contribute to loss of appropriate differentiation during Wilms tumor development. Adding to the complex nature of WT1's role as a transcriptional regulator, recent studies suggest that certain *WT1* splice variants have dramatically different effects in their ability to regulate gene expression,[179,180] including acting as an oncogene in a variety of adult cancers.

WT1 inactivation clearly contributes to Wilms tumor development in those with the WAGR syndrome. Moreover, approximately 10% of apparently sporadic Wilms tumors harbor detectable somatic mutations in the *WT1* gene.[181] Nevertheless, much evidence indicates that Wilms tumors arise through mutations in genes other than *WT1*. First, the chromosome 11p allelic losses seen in Wilms tumor frequently involve band 11p15, but not band 11p13, where the *WT1* gene resides.[181-183] Second, the 11p15 region harbors a gene responsible for Beckwith–Wiedemann syndrome (BWS), a congenital disorder in which affected individuals manifest hyperplasia of the kidneys, endocrine pancreas, and other internal organs; macroglossia; and hemihypertrophy.[184,185]

Those affected by BWS are also at increased risk of developing embryonic tumors, such as hepatoblastoma and Wilms tumor. Finally, linkage studies of three families with dominant inheritance of Wilms tumor exclude linkage of the susceptibility locus in those families to any part of chromosome 11p.[186,187] These data and others suggest that germline mutations in any one of at least three different genes (i.e., *WT1*, the *BWS* gene, and at least one gene not on chromosome 11p reference to haber's paper on X-chromosome gene) predispose to Wilms tumor. Whether a combination of inherited and somatic mutations in more than one of those genes is ultimately required for the transformation of a developing kidney cell into a Wilms tumor, or whether alternative genetic pathways for the development of Wilms tumors exist, remains to be established. The genetic heterogeneity observed among Wilms tumors provides an important contrast to the apparently less complex genetic pathway of retinoblastoma.

Neurofibromatosis 1 and 2 genes

Neurofibromatosis 1 gene
Von Recklinghausen's disease, also called neurofibromatosis 1 (NF1), is a dominantly inherited syndrome with variable disease manifestations. The consistent feature is that tissues derived from the neural crest are commonly affected. In addition to the nearly uniform development of neurofibromas, NF1 patients are at elevated risk for developing pheochromocytomas, schwannomas, neurofibrosarcomas, and primary brain tumors.[188-190] The *NF1* gene was initially localized to the pericentromeric region of chromosome 17q by linkage analyses.[191,192] Subsequently, karyotype studies of two NF1 patients identified germline chromosomal rearrangements involving band 17q11.[193,194] In further work, both patients were found to have genetic alterations of a localized region of band 17q11. Intensive positional cloning efforts in this chromosome region led to the identification of the *NF1* gene in 1991.[195-197] The *NF1* gene is large, spanning roughly 350 kb of DNA, and it encodes a protein product with a molecular mass of about 300 kDa.[188,190,198] Although germline mutations in the *NF1* gene are believed to underlie the development of the associated disease features in all or nearly all NF1 patients, specific germline *NF1* mutations have been identified in approximately one-half to two-thirds of NF1 patients. [188,190,198,199] Difficulties in identifying germline mutations in the *NF1* gene in the remaining NF1 patients may be a result of the inherent inefficiencies and insensitivity associated with mutation detection strategies in such a large gene, and over 1500 distinct mutations have thus far been described.

In addition to germline *NF1* mutations in those patients with NF1, the *NF1* gene is affected by somatic mutations in a fraction of colon cancers, melanomas, neuroblastomas, and bone marrow cells from patients with the myelodysplastic syndrome.[188,198,200-202] Consistent with its presumed tumor suppressor role, the mutations inactivate *NF1*. Studies of leukemias arising in pediatric neurofibromatosis patients provide the clearest evidence that both copies of the *NF1* gene are inactivated during tumorigenesis,[203] as predicted by the Knudson model. Like the *RB1*, *TP53*, and *APC* genes, the *NF1* gene is expressed ubiquitously. Thus, as for other inherited cancer syndromes, the basis for the tissue specificity of

the malignant tumors observed in neurofibromatosis patients is puzzling. The NF1 protein product, termed neurofibromin, is a member of the guanosine triphosphate (GTPase)-activating protein family.[188,204-206] Perhaps the best studied GAP is Ras-GAP, which markedly enhances the GTPase activity of the wild-type K-Ras, H-Ras, and N-Ras proteins. Although the means through which *NF1* defects alter cell growth is not fully described, it is currently postulated that inactivation of neurofibromin function leads to alterations in signaling pathways regulated by small Ras-like GTPase proteins.[207]

Neurofibromatosis 2 gene
Neurofibromatosis 2 (NF2—also known as central neurofibromatosis) is an autosomal dominant disorder that is distinct from NF1 in both genetic and clinical features.[188,208,209]

A hallmark of NF2 is the occurrence of bilateral schwannomas that affect the vestibular branch of the eighth cranial nerve (acoustic neuromas). NF2 patients are also at elevated risk for meningiomas, spinal schwannomas, and ependymomas. The neurofibromatosis 2 (*NF2*) gene was mapped to chromosome 22q by a combination of linkage analyses and LOH studies[210-212] and was cloned in 1993 using positional cloning approaches.[213,214] Germline mutations inactivating the *NF2* gene were observed in those patients with NF2, and somatic *NF2* mutations were also observed in a subset of sporadic schwannomas and meningiomas. Somatic *NF2* mutations in most other tumor types appear to be infrequent. However, preliminary studies indicate that the *NF2* gene may be frequently affected by somatic mutations in malignant mesotheliomas[215,216] despite this tumor type not being seen at increased frequency in patients with NF2.[209] The *NF2* gene encodes a protein, Merlin, with a high sequence homology to a cytoskeletal protein family [ERM (Ezrin/Radixin/Moesin)], which acts as linker proteins between integral membrane proteins and scaffolding proteins of the filamentous submembrane lattice.[214] Consequently, *NF2* gene alterations might contribute to tumor development, at least in part, by effects on cell shape, cell–cell interactions, or cell movement (or a combination).

von Hippel–Lindau gene
von Hippel–Lindau (VHL) syndrome is a rare dominant disorder predisposing affected individuals to the development of hemangioblastomas of the central nervous system and retina, renal carcinomas of clear cell type, and pheochromocytomas.[217-219] The *VHL* gene was mapped to chromosome 3p by linkage analysis. As with many other inherited cancer genes, LOH studies established that the *VHL* gene behaves as a typical tumor suppressor gene, with both alleles inactivated during tumorigenesis.[218,220] Positional cloning efforts identified the *VHL* gene in 1993.[221] Germline mutations inactivating one *VHL* allele are seen in the majority of individuals in families displaying features of the VHL syndrome.[217-219] As with some other inherited cancer syndromes, preliminary genotype–phenotype relationships have been observed. Specifically, a certain class of *VHL* germline mutations is associated with the development of renal cancer only, a second class is linked to predisposition to both renal cancer and pheochromocytoma, and yet a third mutation class is associated only with pheochromocytoma.[218] Somatic mutations in the *VHL* gene are also seen in more than 80% of sporadic renal cell carcinomas of the clear cell type, but not in renal cell carcinomas of other histopathologic types (e.g., papillary type).[218,219] Approximately, 20% of sporadic clear cell renal cancers do not carry a detectable mutation in the *VHL* gene. However, in many of these cases, the *VHL* gene may be inactivated by epigenetic silencing,[222] a mechanism noted earlier in

this chapter in connection with inactivation of the *CDKN2A* locus. In tumor types other than clear cell renal cancer, inactivation of the *VHL* gene appears to be uncommon.[218]

The *VHL* gene encodes a 213-amino acid protein whose major function appears to be in the regulation of angiogenesis through protein degradation. The protein encoded by *VHL* is part of a ubiquitin ligase complex that degrades hypoxia-inducing factor 1a (HIF-1a) in the presence of oxygen. In the absence of oxygen in normal cells, or when *VHL* is mutated in tumor cells, the HIF-1a transcription factor is stabilized, leading to the expression of cytokines such as vascular endothelial growth factor and the stimulation of angiogenesis. Further biochemical and cell biology studies on *VHL* and renal cell carcinomas are likely to offer definitive insights into angiogenesis, one of the most important stromal processes associated with neoplasia.[223,224]

Genomic stability genes

Several recessive cancer predisposition syndromes resulting from inactivation of genes that function in DNA damage recognition and repair have been described, including ataxia telangiectasia (AT), Bloom syndrome, xeroderma pigmentosum, and Fanconi anemia. In each case, the specific cancer type and the DNA-damaging agents that increase cancer risk are distinct. Although AT heterozygotes may subtly increase the risk of breast cancer,[225] in other recessive cancer syndromes, only homozygotes appear to clearly increase cancer risk. This observation contrasts sharply with the picture in the dominant cancer predisposition syndromes discussed earlier (e.g., inherited retinoblastoma, FAP, NF1, and NF2), where heterozygotes have a clearly elevated cancer risk. Homozygous mutations in tumor suppressor genes rarely if ever exist, probably because the condition is lethal during embryogenesis. It is important to remember that the tumor suppressor genes do not only function as guardians against cancer; their main function is the control of normal cell balance, and their inactivation is expected to be incompatible with normal embryonic development.

Because recessive cancer syndromes are quite rare, this discussion of the role of genomic stability genes in cancer will focus on syndromes that are inherited in an autosomal dominant fashion. These syndromes include the most common types of familial cancers, predisposing to tumors of the colon, breast, and other organs.

DNA mismatch repair gene defects and hereditary nonpolyposis colorectal cancer

Familial clustering of colon cancer has long been recognized, with approximately 5% of all colon cancers attributable to inheritance of a gene defect with a strong effect on cancer risk and another 10–15% with a moderate effect on risk. Germline *APC* mutations are responsible for 0.5–1% of colorectal cancer cases in the Western world, and hereditary nonpolyposis colorectal cancer (HNPCC) is responsible for 2–4%.[226–228]

Diagnostic criteria for identifying those individuals and families most likely to be affected by HNPCC have been determined,[226–229] despite the absence of overt clinical findings before cancer diagnosis, and the potential for chance clustering of colon cancer within a family. Representative diagnostic criteria include (1) exclusion of familial polyposis; (2) colorectal cancer in at least three relatives, one of them being a first-degree relative of the others; (3) two or more successive generations affected; and (4) at least one of the affected individuals being younger than 50 years of age at the time of diagnosis. Although not all individuals affected by HNPCC meet these criteria, familial aggregations of colorectal cancer that are likely to have a genetic basis distinct from that underlying the majority of HNPCC cases can be excluded.[226,228]

Several genes responsible for HNPCC have been identified, including two on chromosome 2p [mutS homologs 2 and 6 (MSH2, MSH6)], another on chromosome 3p [mutS homolog 1 (MLH1)], and another on chromosome 7p [postmeiotic segregation 2 (PMS2)]. Together, germline mutations in these four genes account for virtually all classic HNPCC cases.[226,228–231] The protein products of the *MSH2* and *MLH1* genes appear to have critical roles in the recognition and repair of DNA mismatches (Figure 10). In cells with one normal and one mutant allele of a DNA mismatch repair (MMR) gene, DNA repair is minimally impaired, if at all. However, inactivation of the remaining allele can occur as a result of somatic mutation in a normal epithelial cell. This "second hit" abrogates MMR function, and hundreds to thousands of mutations may thereby occur during each subsequent cell-division cycle. Because these mutations preferentially arise in mononucleotide, dinucleotide, and trinucleotide repeat tracts (i.e., microsatellite sequence tracts), the phenotype is often called the microsatellite instability (MSI) phenotype.[226]

Germline mutations in the known MMR genes have been detected in only 2–4% of colorectal cancer patients, although approximately 15–20% of all colon cancers display the MSI phenotype.[226,229–234] Clearly, only a small fraction of the sporadic colorectal cancers with the MSI phenotype develop as the result of a germline mutation in a known MMR gene. Somatic mutations in MMR genes have been found in some sporadic colorectal cancers with the MSI phenotype.[235] In most sporadic cases, however, inactivation of the *MLH1* gene occurs as a result of epigenetic inactivation.[236,237]

Many of the mutations arising in cells with MMR deficiency are likely to be detrimental to cell growth. A small fraction of the total mutations that arise presumably activate oncogenes or inactivate tumor suppressor genes. Some genes are preferentially mutated in MMR-deficient cancers, presumably because the mutations confer a selective growth advantage. For instance, genes that contain repetitive DNA sequences, such as microsatellite tracts, might be expected to be targets of mutation in these cancers, and data support this prediction.

BRCA1 and BRCA2 genes

As in the case of colorectal cancers, family history has long been hypothesized to be a major risk factor in breast cancer. The greatest risk is seen in those who have a history of breast cancer in multiple first-degree relatives. However, only in the late 1980s was evidence obtained that predisposition to breast cancer in some families could be attributed to a highly penetrant autosomal dominant allele. In 1990, Hall and colleagues reported the localization of one such breast cancer predisposition gene, *BRCA1*, on chromosome 17q21.[238] Others found that germline *BRCA1* mutations substantially increase the risk not only of breast cancer but also of ovarian cancer.[239,240] Intensive research efforts were focused on the region of chromosome 17q harboring *BRCA1*, and the gene was ultimately identified by positional cloning approaches in 1994.[241,242]

Studies of germline *BRCA1* mutations in breast cancer patients have yielded important results. In studies of families with four or more cases of breast or ovarian cancer (or both) diagnosed before age 60 years, germline *BRCA1* mutations were identified in nearly 50% of families studied.[243–245] In fact, germline *BRCA1* mutations may account for cancer predisposition in roughly 75% of families who manifest both breast and ovarian cancer.[243,244] Many distinct germline *BRCA1* mutations have been identified, although most of the mutations result in the synthesis of a truncated BRCA1 protein.[243,244] Although most germline *BRCA1* mutations have been identified in only one or a few families, some mutations have

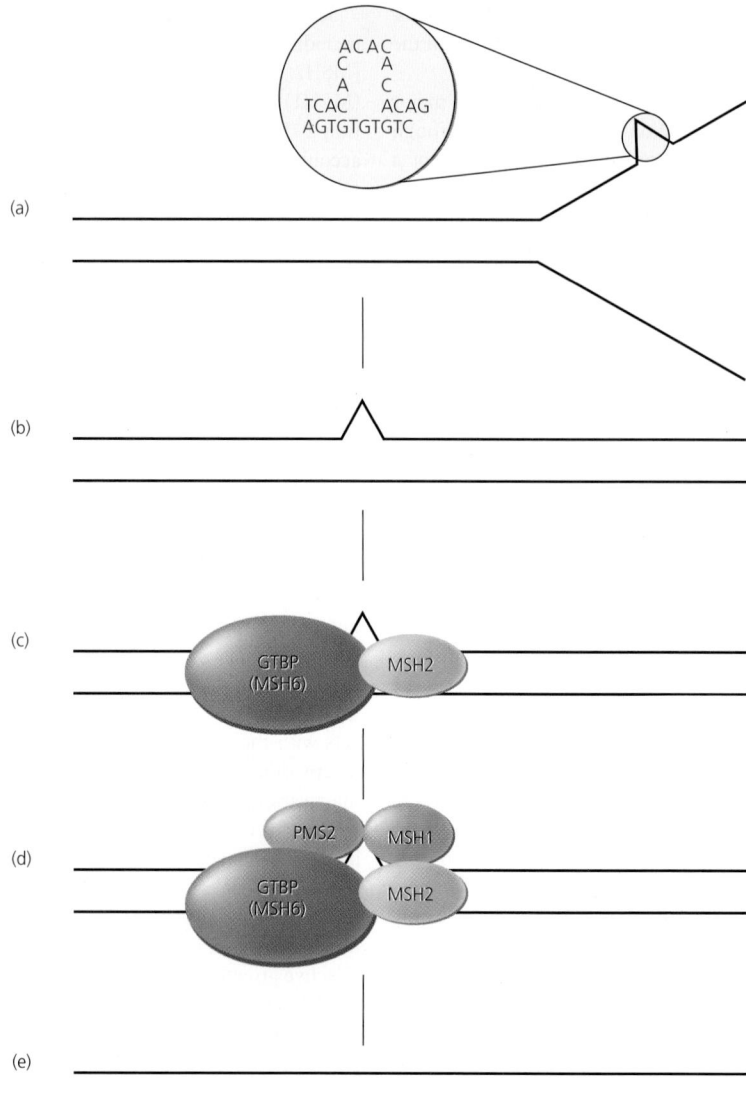

Figure 10 Mismatch repair pathway in human cells. (a,b) During DNA replication, DNA mismatches may arise, such as from strand slippage (shown) or misincorporation of bases (not shown). (c) The mismatch is recognized by MutS homologs, perhaps most often Msh2 and GTBP/Msh6, although another MutS homolog, Msh3, may substitute for GTBP/Msh6 in some cases. (d,e) MutL homologs, such as Mlh1 and Pms2, are recruited to the complex, and the mismatch is repaired through the action of a number of proteins, including an exonuclease, helicase, DNA polymerase, and ligase.

been found recurrently. The 11 most common mutations account for about 45% of the total BRCA1 mutations observed.[244,245] In fact, the two most common mutations in *BRCA1* (185delAG and 5382insC) account for approximately 10% of the total. Of note, the 185delAG frameshift mutation at codon 185 of *BRCA1*, involving a deletion of two bases (adenine and guanine), has been identified in more than 20 Jewish families with familial breast or ovarian cancer. Moreover, population surveys of Ashkenazi Jews, chosen without regard to a family history of cancer, indicate that approximately 1% carry the 185delAG mutation.[244–246] Based on studies of families with germline *BRCA1* mutations, the lifetime risks of breast cancer and ovarian cancer in those carrying an inactivating mutation are estimated to be 85% and 50%, respectively.[243,244,247] Whether specific germline *BRCA1* mutations confer a greater risk of breast and ovarian cancer than do other mutations remains uncertain.

As with most tumor suppressor genes and their associated familial cancer syndromes, germline mutations of *BRCA1* lead to the presence of a mutant allele in every cell of the body. Cancers then arise through inactivation of the second wild-type allele by the mechanisms outlined in Figure 2. In the case of *BRCA1* (and *BRCA2*), LOH of the remaining wild-type allele is usually responsible for the second "hit" leading to inactivation of the *BRCA1* gene. In addition, LOH of the *BRCA1* locus was found in approximately 50% of unselected breast cancers and 65–80% of unselected ovarian cancers.[244,248] Because most breast and ovarian cancers are not associated with a hereditary predisposition (i.e., they are sporadic), these studies of unselected cancers led investigators to hypothesize that BRCA1 would play an important role in the development of sporadic breast and ovarian cancers. However, despite these LOH data, sporadic breast and ovarian cancers rarely harbor mutations in the *BRCA1* gene, demonstrating that at least one wild-type allele is still present in most of these sporadic cancers.[244,248] Somewhat surprisingly, this finding would suggest that BRCA1 does not have a role in the genesis of the more common, nonfamilial forms of breast and ovarian cancers. However, it is still possible that downstream

Table 1 Select tumor suppressor and stability genes associated with inherited cancer predisposition syndromes.

Gene[a]	Syndrome	Hereditary pattern	Pathway[b]	Major hereditary tumor types[c]
APC	FAP	Dominant	APC	Colon, thyroid, stomach, intestine
AXIN2	Attenuated polyposis	Dominant	APC	Colon
CDH1 (E-cadherin)	Familial gastric carcinoma	Dominant	APC	Stomach
GPC3	Simpson–Golabi–Behmel syndrome	X-linked	APC	Embryonal
CYLD	Familial cylindromatosis	Dominant	APOP	Pilotrichomas
EXT1, EXT2	Hereditary multiple exostoses	Dominant	GLI	Bone
PTCH	Gorlin	Dominant	GLI	Skin, medulloblastoma
SUFU	Medulloblastoma predisposition	Dominant	GLI	Skin, medulloblastoma
FH	Hereditary leiomyomatosis	Dominant	HIF1	Leiomyomas
SDHB, SDHC, SDHD	Familial paraganglioma	Dominant	HIF1	Paragangliomas, pheochromocytomas
VHL	von Hippel–Lindau	Dominant	HIF1	Kidney
TP53 (p53)	Li–Fraumeni	Dominant	TP53	Breast, sarcoma, adrenal, brain, and so on
WT1	Familial Wilms tumor	Dominant	TP53	Wilms
STK11 (LKB1)	Peutz–Jeghers	Dominant	PI3K	Intestinal, ovarian, pancreatic
PTEN	Cowden	Dominant	PI3K	Hamartoma, glioma, uterus
TSC1, TSC2	Tuberous sclerosis	Dominant	PI3K	Hamartoma, kidney
CDKN2A (p16INK4A, p14ARF)	Familial malignant melanoma	Dominant	RB	Melanoma, pancreas
CDK4	Familial malignant melanoma	Dominant	RB	Melanoma
RB1	Hereditary retinoblastoma	Dominant	RB	Eye
NF1	Neurofibromatosis	Dominant	RTK	Neurofibroma
BMPR1A	Juvenile polyposis	Dominant	SMAD	Gastrointestinal
MEN1	Multiple endocrine neoplasia type I	Dominant	SMAD	Parathyroid, pituitary, islet cell, carcinoid
SMAD4 (DPC4)	Juvenile polyposis	Dominant	SMAD	Gastrointestinal
BHD	Birt–Hogg–Dube	Dominant	?	Renal, hair follicle
HRPT2	Hyperparathyroidism jaw-tumor	Dominant	?	Parathyroid, jaw fibroma
NF2	Neurofibromatosis	Dominant	?	Meningioma, acoustic neuromas
MUTYH	Attenuated polyposis	Recessive	BER	Colon
ATM	Ataxia telangiectasia	Recessive	CIN	Leukemias, lymphomas, brain
BLM	Bloom	Recessive	CIN	Leukemias, lymphomas, skin
BRCA1, BRCA2	Hereditary breast cancer	Dominant	CIN	Breast, ovary
FANCA, FANCC, FANCD2, FANCE, FANCF, FANCG	Fanconi anemia A, C, D2, E, F, and G	Recessive	CIN	Leukemias
NBS1	Nijmegen breakage	Recessive	CIN	Lymphomas, brain
RECQL4	Rothmund–Thomson	Recessive	CIN	Bone and skin
WRN	Werner	Recessive	CIN	Bone and brain
MSH2, MLH1, MSH6, PMS2	HNPCC	Dominant	MMR	Colon, uterus
XPA, XPC; ERCC2, ERCC3, ERCC4, ERCC5; DDB2	Xeroderma pigmentosum	Recessive	NER	Skin

[a]Representative genes of all major pathways and hereditary cancer predisposition types are listed. Approved gene symbols are provided for each entry; alternative names are in parentheses.

[b]In many cases, the gene has been implicated in several pathways. The single pathway that is listed for each gene represents a "best guess" (when one can be made) and should not be regarded as conclusive.

[c]In most cases, the nonfamilial tumor spectrum caused by somatic mutations of the gene includes those occurring in familial cases but also additional tumor types. For example, mutations of TP53 and CDKN2A are found in many more tumor types than those to which Li–Fraumeni and familial malignant melanoma patients, respectively, are predisposed.

Abbreviations: APC, adenomatous polyposis coli; APOP, apoptotic pathway; BER, base excision repair; CIN, chromosomal instability; FAP, familial adenomatous polyposis; GLI, glioma-associated oncogene; HIF1, hypoxia-inducing factor 1; MMR, mismatch repair; NER, nucleotide excision repair; PI3K, phosphatidylinositol 3-kinase; RB, retinoblastoma; RTK, receptor tyrosine kinase pathway; SMAD, SMA- and MAD-related protein 4; wt, wild type.

Source: Adapted from Vogelstein and Kinzler 2004.[131] Reprinted by permission from Macmillan Publishers Ltd.

effectors of the BRCA1 protein are altered in sporadic breast and ovarian cancers, suggesting that the pathway, rather than the gene, is an important contributor to the carcinogenic process of these cancers.[249]

Although germline mutations in the BRCA1 gene underlie cancer predisposition in roughly 40–50% of families with multiple breast cancer cases, another highly penetrant autosomal dominant susceptibility gene termed BRCA2 plays a critical role in a significant fraction of the families with multiple breast cancer cases lacking BRCA1 mutations. The BRCA2 gene was mapped to chromosome 13q12-13 in 1994[250] and identified by positional cloning strategies in 1995.[251] Although germline mutations in BRCA1 and BRCA2 appear to confer essentially similar lifetime risks of female breast cancer (i.e., ~80%), the risk of ovarian cancer is reduced to approximately 10% in those with BRCA2 mutations compared with approximately 40–50% in those with BRCA1 mutations. The risk of male breast cancer is markedly elevated in BRCA2 mutation carriers, with a lifetime risk of approximately 7%, as opposed to a 1% lifetime risk of in BRCA1 mutation carriers.[252] There also appears to be an elevated risk of pancreatic and several other cancers in both male and female BRCA2 mutation carriers.[244] As is the case for BRCA1, LOH of the BRCA2 locus at 13q12, but not at the RB1 locus at 13q14, has been observed in some sporadic breast, pancreatic, head and neck, and other cancers, suggesting that BRCA2 may be a target for somatic mutations in cancer. However, as with BRCA1, detections of somatic BRCA2 mutations in sporadic cancers have been few,[244] once again suggesting that perhaps the pathway, rather than the gene, is the target of genetic alteration in sporadic forms of these cancers.

The *BRCA1* and *BRCA2* genes each encode a large nuclear protein. The amino acid sequences of the two proteins have only short regions of similarity with one another or other well-characterized proteins. Although their lack of obvious functional motifs stymied initial attempts to define the cellular functions of BRCA1 and BRCA2, several lines of evidence indicate that both proteins interact directly or indirectly with homologs of yeast Rad51, a protein that functions in the repair of double-stranded DNA breaks.[253–260] Moreover, the BRCA1, BRCA2, and Rad51 proteins all appear to be present in a stable multiprotein complex in the cell's nucleus. Consequently, it has been suggested that BRCA1 and BRCA2 may function in the response to or repair of DNA damage, particularly double-strand DNA breaks.[261] Other findings imply that BRCA1 and perhaps BRCA2 may have a role in regulating transcription.[262] Although the DNA repair and transcription regulation functions may be distinct, it is entirely possible that the two functions are linked in a process sometimes called transcription-coupled DNA repair.[255] There is precedent for this idea, in that some nucleotide excision repair genes causing xeroderma pigmentosum can also function in transcription,[263] and repair of certain types of DNA damage is known to be coupled to transcription.[264]

Candidate tumor suppressor genes

The tumor suppressor genes discussed earlier and others summarized in Table 1 are distinguished by the fact that germline-inactivating mutations in the genes are associated with inherited cancer predisposition. The link between germline mutation and elevated cancer risk provides incontrovertible evidence of the gene's role in tumorigenesis. Other findings, such as the demonstration in sporadic cancers of LOH of one tumor suppressor gene allele accompanied by somatic mutation of the remaining allele, offer evidence for a more widespread role for many of the inherited cancer genes. Although the tumor suppressor genes in Table 1 are definitively linked to inherited cancer syndromes, it is possible that germline mutations in other bona fide tumor suppressor genes may be associated with a more modest cancer risk, as has already been demonstrated for the I1307K mutation in *APC*. A complete listing of all documented tumor suppressor genes is beyond the scope of this chapter and is ever-evolving as new data come to light from detailed sequencing studies of human cancers. Based on the prevalence of inactivating mutations identified in such studies, it is estimated that there are approximately 100 tumor suppressor genes that play a role in human cancers of various types.[64] The majority of these genes are only inactivated somatically and do not give rise to inherited cancer predisposition syndromes.

Studies of RNA have revealed a large number of genes whose transcription is reduced in cancers. Some of these genes were initially termed tumor suppressors solely on the basis of this reduced expression. A small subset of these genes may, indeed, have critical roles in growth regulation, but expression data provide insufficient evidence to invoke causality. The altered expression of genes in cancers more often reflects the effect rather than the cause of the neoplastic process (i.e., the altered growth and differentiation properties of cancer cells and their abnormal microenvironment compared with normal cells in the tissue or organ from which the cancer arose). Moreover, many genes that play no role in cancer can dramatically alter cell growth when expressed exogenously at high, unphysiologic levels, rendering functional analyses of such candidates problematic. In the end, the functional evidence should be carefully weighed before a conclusion can be drawn that a gene has a causal role in tumorigenesis and that it should appropriately be designated a tumor suppressor gene. The only definitive way to identify a tumor suppressor gene at present is to document a highly statistically significant number of inactivating mutations in it in specific cancer types.[64]

Summary

There is now overwhelming evidence that mutations in tumor suppressor genes are major molecular determinants for most common human cancers. Thus far, dozens of confirmed tumor suppressor genes have been identified by molecular cloning techniques. In some cases, these genes are inactivated in the germline, and their inactivation predisposes to cancer. Far more frequently, these same tumor suppressor genes are inactivated by somatic mutations during tumor development.

Although much has been learned about tumor suppressor genes, a great deal of work remains. Advancements in our understanding of tumorigenesis will continue with the detailed characterization of their normal cellular functions and the mechanisms through which mutations of these genes subvert these normal functions. It is essential to point out that tumor suppressor genes, unlike oncogenes, are in general not directly targetable by drugs: all drugs inactivate their target proteins and tumor suppressor genes are already inactivated in cancers. Therefore, the best hope for exploiting tumor suppressor gene mutations in cancers is through targeting downstream pathways that are consequently upregulated. Understanding the pathways through which these genes act is therefore of paramount importance.

Key references

The complete reference list can be found on the Wiley Companion Digital Edition of this title (see inside front cover for login instructions).

1 Broca P. Etiologie des productions accidentelles. *Traite des Tumerus.* 1866: 147–157.

4 Boveri T. *The Origin of Malignant Tumors.* Baltimore, MD: Williams and Wilkins; 1929.

10 Stanbridge EJ, Der CJ, Doersen CJ, et al. Human cell hybrids: analysis of transformation and tumorigenicity. *Science.* 1982;**215**(**4530**):252–259.

15 Knudson AGJ. Mutation and cancer: statistical study of retinoblastoma. *Proc Natl Acad Sci U S A.* 1971;**68**(**4**):820–823.

19 Sparkes RS, Murphree AL, Lingua RW, et al. Gene for hereditary retinoblastoma assigned to human chromosome 13 by linkage to esterase D. *Science.* 1983;**219**(**4587**):971–973.

21 Knudson AG Jr. Hereditary cancer, oncogenes, and antioncogenes. *Cancer Res.* 1985;**45**(**4**):1437–1443.

22 Cavenee WK, Dryja TP, Phillips RA, et al. Expression of recessive alleles by chromosomal mechanisms in retinoblastoma. *Nature.* 1983;**305**(**5937**):779–784.

26 Dryja TP, Rapaport JM, Joyce JM, Petersen RA. Molecular detection of deletions involving band q14 of chromosome 13 in retinoblastomas. *Proc Natl Acad Sci U S A.* 1986;**83**(**19**):7391–7394.

35 Whyte P, Buchkovich KJ, Horowitz JM, et al. Association between an oncogene and an anti-oncogene: the adenovirus E1A proteins bind to the retinoblastoma gene product. *Nature.* 1988;**334**(**6178**):124–129.

43 DeLeo AB, Jay G, Appella E, Dubois GC, Law LW, Old LJ. Detection of a transformation-related antigen in chemically induced sarcomas and other transformed cells of the mouse. *Proc Natl Acad Sci U S A.* 1979;**76**(**5**):2420–2424.

52 Baker SJ, Fearon ER, Nigro JM, et al. Chromosome 17 deletions and p53 gene mutations in colorectal carcinomas. *Science.* 1989;**244**(**4901**):217–221.

54 Vogelstein B, Fearon ER, Hamilton SR, et al. Genetic alterations during colorectal-tumor development. *N Engl J Med.* 1988;**319**(**9**):525–532.

69 Bartek J, Falck J, Lukas J. CHK2 kinase—a busy messenger. *Nat Rev Mol Cell Biol.* 2001;**2**(**12**):877–886.

75 Oliner JD, Kinzler KW, Meltzer PS, George DL, Vogelstein B. Amplification of a gene encoding a p53-associated protein in human sarcomas. *Nature.* 1992;**358**(**6381**):80–83.

76 Marine JC, Jochemsen AG. Mdmx and Mdm2: brothers in arms? *Cell Cycle.* 2004;**3**(**7**):900–904.

85 Vogelstein B, Lane D, Levine AJ. Surfing the p53 network. *Nature.* 2000;**408**(**6810**): 307–310.

86 el-Deiry WS, Tokino T, Velculescu VE, et al. WAF1, a potential mediator of p53 tumor suppression. *Cell.* 1993;**75**(**4**):817–825.

88 Waldman T, Kinzler KW, Vogelstein B. p21 is necessary for the p53-mediated G1 arrest in human cancer cells. *Cancer Res.* 1995;**55**(**22**):5187–5190.

89 Yu J, Wang Z, Kinzler KW, Vogelstein B, Zhang L. PUMA mediates the apoptotic response to p53 in colorectal cancer cells. *Proc Natl Acad Sci U S A.* 2003;**100**(**4**):1931–1936.

90 Hollstein M, Hergenhahn M, Yang Q, Bartsch H, Wang ZQ, Hainaut P. New approaches to understanding p53 gene tumor mutation spectra. *Mutat Res.* 1999;**431**(**2**):199–209.

92 Jeffers JR, Parganas E, Lee Y, et al. Puma is an essential mediator of p53-dependent and -independent apoptotic pathways. *Cancer Cell.* 2003;**4**(**4**):321–328.

101 Bunz F, Hwang PM, Torrance C, et al. Disruption of p53 in human cancer cells alters the responses to therapeutic agents. *J Clin Invest.* 1999;**104**(**3**):263–269.

112 Kamb A, Gruis NA, Weaver-Feldhaus J, et al. A cell cycle regulator potentially involved in genesis of many tumor types. *Science.* 1994;**264**(**5157**):436–440.

121 Cairns P, Polascik TJ, Eby Y, et al. Frequency of homozygous deletion at p16/CDKN2 in primary human tumours. *Nat Genet.* 1995;**11**(**2**):210–212.

124 Jacobs JJ, Kieboom K, Marino S, DePinho RA, van Lohuizen M. The oncogene and Polycomb-group gene bmi-1 regulates cell proliferation and senescence through the ink4a locus. *Nature.* 1999;**397**(**6715**):164–168.

126 Bachman KE, Park BH, Rhee I, et al. Histone modifications and silencing prior to DNA methylation of a tumor suppressor gene. *Cancer Cell.* 2003;**3**(**1**):89–95.

131 Vogelstein B, Kinzler KW. Cancer genes and the pathways they control. *Nat Med.* 2004;**10**(**8**):789–799.

132 Schmitt CA, Fridman JS, Yang M, et al. A senescence program controlled by p53 and p16INK4a contributes to the outcome of cancer therapy. *Cell.* 2002;**109**(**3**):335–346.

136 Groden J, Thliveris A, Samowitz W, et al. Identification and characterization of the familial adenomatous polyposis coli gene. *Cell.* 1991;**66**(**3**):589–600.

143 Kinzler KW, Vogelstein B. Lessons from hereditary colorectal cancer. *Cell.* 1996;**87**(**2**):159–170.

145 Nieuwenhuis MH, Vasen HF. Correlations between mutation site in APC and phenotype of familial adenomatous polyposis (FAP): a review of the literature. *Crit Rev Oncol Hematol.* 2007;**61**(**2**):153–161.

152 Morin PJ, Vogelstein B, Kinzler KW. Apoptosis and APC in colorectal tumorigenesis. *Proc Natl Acad Sci U S A.* 1996;**93**(**15**):7950–7954.

162 Knudson AG Jr, Strong LC. Mutation and cancer: a model for Wilms' tumor of the kidney. *J Natl Cancer Inst.* 1972;**48**(**2**):313–324.

167 Fearon ER, Vogelstein B, Feinberg AP. Somatic deletion and duplication of genes on chromosome 11 in Wilms' tumours. *Nature.* 1984;**309**(**5964**):176–178.

171 Call KM, Glaser T, Ito CY, et al. Isolation and characterization of a zinc finger polypeptide gene at the human chromosome 11 Wilms' tumor locus. *Cell.* 1990;**60**(**3**):509–520.

181 Haber DA, Housman DE. The genetics of Wilms' tumor. *Adv Cancer Res.* 1992;**59**:41–68.

188 Gutman D. Neurofibromatosis type 1. In: Kinzler KW, ed. *The Genetic Basis of Human Cancer.* New York, NY: McGraw-Hill; 1998:423–442.

203 Shannon KM, O'Connell P, Martin GA, et al. Loss of the normal NF1 allele from the bone marrow of children with type 1 neurofibromatosis and malignant myeloid disorders. *N Engl J Med.* 1994;**330**(**9**):597–601.

207 Patrakitkomjorn S, Kobayashi D, Morikawa T, et al. NF1 tumor suppressor, neurofibromin, regulates the neuronal differentiation of PC12 cells via its associating protein, collapsin response mediator protein-2. *J Biol Chem.* 2008;**283**(**14**):9399–9413.

218 Linehan WM. Renal carcinoma. In: Kinzler KW, ed. *The Genetic Basis of Human Cancer.* New York, NY: McGraw-Hill; 1998:455–474.

226 Boland CR. Hereditary nonpolyposis colorectal cancer. In: Kinzler KW, ed. *The Genetic Basis of Human Cancer.* New York, NY: McGraw-Hill; 1998:333–346.

229 Lynch HT, de la Chapelle A. Genetic susceptibility to non-polyposis colorectal cancer. *J Med Genet.* 1999;**36**(**11**):801–818.

236 Herman JG, Umar A, Polyak K, et al. Incidence and functional consequences of hMLH1 promoter hypermethylation in colorectal carcinoma. *Proc Natl Acad Sci U S A.* 1998;**95**(**12**):6870–6875.

238 Hall JM, Gryfe R, Kim H, et al. Linkage of early-onset familial breast cancer to chromosome 17q21. *Science.* 1990;**250**(**4988**):1684–1689.

243 Collins FS. BRCA1—lots of mutations, lots of dilemmas. *N Engl J Med.* 1996;**334**(**3**):186–188.

6 Epigenetic contributions to human cancer

James G. Herman, MD ▪ Stephen B. Baylin, MD

Overview

Over the past 20 years, an exciting advance in our understanding of the mechanisms underlying cancer development has been our growing appreciation that these diseases are not driven solely by genetic changes, but also by epigenetic changes.[1–4] Strictly speaking, the term epigenetic refers to heritable changes in gene expression, in dividing somatic cells, which are mediated by alterations other than changes in the primary base sequence of DNA.[5–7] This definition encompasses two critical translational characteristics concerning epigenetic alterations in cancer and their clinical importance. First, the coding and noncoding genes affected by epigenetic changes in cancer remain wild type for DNA sequence rather than harboring irreversible mutations. Second, and closely related, the changes are, then, potentially reversible if normal gene expression can be restored such that the wild-type gene function can emerge.[1,2,4,7–10]

This recognition of epigenetic changes, which are fundamental to cancer initiation and progression, is occurring in the midst of a dynamic explosion of knowledge as to how the human genome is normally controlled, via chromatin packaging of DNA, to regulate gene expression in different tissues and during development.[5–7,11] For example, epigenetic processes play a fundamental role during normal embryonic development and adult-cell renewal. As such, these processes control the emergence of different cellular phenotypes, all with the exact underlying DNA sequence, which occur during development and differentiation. While this knowledge of gene regulation continues to grow rapidly, our understanding of the complete spectrum of epigenetic changes that are key to cancer development is expanding rapidly but could even still, relatively, be in its early stages. However, there is much that has already been learned, and this knowledge in the understanding of basic cancer biology and carcinogenesis already has palpable translational implications, which are discussed in this chapter.

Mechanisms involved in epigenetic regulation of gene expression

Formation of chromatin

While all of the fundamental information for gene expression lies in the primary base sequence of DNA, which can be viewed as a "hard drive" for storage of this essential coding, the patterns of gene expression in cells are determined by how this DNA is modified following synthesis and replication and how it is packaged into the nucleus by the proteins, or chromatin, by which it is arranged.[5–7,11] The latter processes of packaging might, then, be viewed as the "software," which provides the readout of the hard-drive information contained in the DNA sequence. The primary role of the DNA modification and chromatin packaging is required to balance the genome such that the majority of DNA is encompassed in a silent or low-transcription state to guard against unwanted expression of repeat sequences, potential transposable elements, and viral

insertions accrued over evolution.[5,6,12] The first element of DNA packaging is its interactions with proteins forming chromatin. The fundamental scaffolding proteins for chromatin are the histone proteins, and their assembly with DNA, in turn, forms the key element, or nucleosomes (Figure 1), which are essential for arranging DNA in the nucleus.[13,14]

Nucleosomes consist of ~146 bp of DNA wrapped twice around an octamer of the core histone proteins, H2A, H2B, H3, and H4.[13,14] For functional mediation of gene expression profiles from DNA, nucleosomes must not only be properly distributed linearly along DNA, but must also be arranged into higher-order, multinucleosome structures[13,14] (Figure 2). These dynamics are mediated by chromatin-remodeling proteins, and the more widely and irregularly spaced the nucleosomes are in their linear placement along DNA, and the less compacted the higher-order structures, the more "open" the chromatin is and the more available the DNA is for active-gene transcription (Figure 2). This is often the case in areas in and around active-gene promoters. Conversely, the more regular and evenly the nucleosomes are spaced, and the more compacted their higher-order structures (Figure 2), the more "closed" is the chromatin and the more repressive for gene transcription. This latter configuration dominates most of the human genome, as noted earlier, to prevent unwanted gene expression and to facilitate chromosome structure.

Integrally involved with this dynamic chromatin structure is a dependency of nucleosome function on states of chromatin, which are determined by differing ratios of active and repressive histone "modifications."[6,7,11,14,15]

These consist of additions or modifications to key amino acids, primarily located in the tails of the histones that stick out from the nucelosome assembly, in the form of lysine acetylation, lysine and arginine methylation, serine and threonine phosphorylation, glutamic acid ADP-ribosylation, and lysine ubiquitination and sumoylation.[6,7,11,14,15]

The balance of these marks form what was initially termed a "histone code," now realized to be more complex than envisioned, that participates, along with nucleosome positioning, in packaging the genome such that both constitutive and cell type-dependent chromatin patterns of open and/or closed configurations are maintained from cell division to cell division and ensuring that these patterns remain stable in nondividing cells.[6,7,11] It is in this way that cells maintain a "memory" for patterns of gene expression and chromosome structure that facilitate normal patterns of development and the maintenance of mature-cell renewal and differentiation states.[14,15]

The best characterized of the histone modifications, mentioned earlier, are lysine methylation and acetylation, which are most closely associated with either high or low states of gene transcription. These marks in turn are established by families of enzymes consisting of histone methyltransferases (HMTs) that catalyze the methylation, histone demethylases that remove these

Holland-Frei Cancer Medicine, Ninth Edition. Edited by Robert C. Bast Jr., Carlo M. Croce, William N. Hait, Waun Ki Hong, Donald W. Kufe, Martine Piccart-Gebhart, Raphael E. Pollock, Ralph R. Weichselbaum, Hongyang Wang, and James F. Holland.
© 2017 John Wiley & Sons, Inc. ISBN: 978-1-118-93469-2

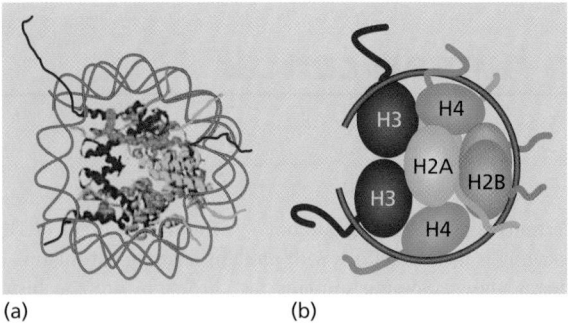

(a)   (b)

Figure 1 Nucleosome structure. (a) Model of the double helix wound around the protein structure of the constituent histones as outlined in the text. (b) The schematic representation shows the organization of the H3/H4 tetramer on the DNA, followed by two sets of H2A/H2B dimers forming the histone core with the DNA (*black line*) wrapped around. The amino-terminal histone tails are shown extruding from the nucleosome core of the eight histone proteins.

methyl additions, and histone acetylases or (HATs) and histone deacetylases (HDACs), which place and remove the acetyl groups, respectively.[7,11,15–17] For these dynamic events, examples of key methylation marks associated with gene states are methylation of lysine 4 of histone 3 (H3K4me3), which is associated with open chromatin typical of active transcription, and methylation of lysine 9 or lysine 27 (H3K9me3, H3K27me3), which is characteristic of repressed-gene expression.[6,15] Adding to the information contained in this histone code is the fact that lysine methylation may be present in either monomeric, dimeric, or trimeric, states.[6,7,11,15] There is also a regulated balance for histone acetylation in which enzymatic activities of the HATs and HDACs determine the states of histone–lysine acetylation that are typical of open, transcriptionally active chromatin, and deacetylation, more associated with closed chromatin and repressed transcription.[7,11,15] Key examples of such active marks at gene promoters are H3K9acetyl and H4K16acetyl.[7,11,15]

DNA methylation

While not present in all multicellular organisms, humans, other mammals, and other higher organisms add an additional layer of epigenetic regulation. Working in close concert with chromatin states to package the human genome is a key modification consisting of methylation added directly to postreplicated DNA.[7,10,17,18] This step consists of attachment of a methyl moiety to the C5 position of the base, cytosine, only when it is located preceding a guanine or in a "CpG" dinucleotides context. The methyl group is transferred from S-adenosyl methionine to DNA through catalysis by a family of DNA methyltransferase (DNMT) enzymes.[17–19]

The role of this DNA methylation[19] is closely tied to the distribution of the CpG dinucleotide in human and other genomes. This is a nonrandom and uneven distribution in which there has been a global and progressive depletion of CpGs over evolution because the deamination of methylated CpGs results in changing the cytosines (Cs) to thymidines (Ts).[7,17,18] Failure to repair these thymidines then results in transition of the Cs to Ts. However, there remains interspersed conservation of nondepleted, CpG-rich stretches (∼0.4 to several thousand kb) or the so-called "CpG islands," which are particularly important to the DNA-methylation patterns.[17,18] These islands, especially when found in the 5′ end of about 50–60% of human genes,[17,18] remain non-DNA methylated, while the majority of the CpG′ sites in the remainder of DNA are methylated[4,7,17,18] (Figure 2).

This pattern of DNA methylation, depicted in Figure 2, works in tight concert with the nucleosome positioning and histone modifications previously discussed to determine the epigenetic regulation of the genome. Thus, methylated DNA associates with, and helps maintain in a tight heritable state, the relatively transcriptionally inert status of the majority of the genome, which is most apparent in the closed chromatin or "heterochromatic regions" concentrated in pericentromeric parts of chromosomes. In contrast, the non-DNA-methylated CpG islands associated with gene-start sites appear to reflect and facilitate a transcriptional ready and/or active transcription state.[4,7,17] This tight interaction between histone modifications and DNA methylation is reflected in the fact that transcriptional repression is associated with DNA methylation, which serves to help maintain the repression of many closed chromatin states. Thus, deacetylated histone lysines, such as for H3K9, and repressive methylation marks, such as H3K9me3, associate with methylated DNA.[17–19] In turn, such marks, and particularly H3K9me, appear important for targeting of DNA methylation.[17–19]

It is important to note that an important exception to the above role of DNA methylation in repression of gene transcription has been recently noted. Thus, one common site of 5mC is in the body of active and not repressed genes. This methylation appears to work with the mark of H3K36 me3 to allow transcriptional elongation and enhanced gene expression.[7,10,20,21]

There have been recent and most important advances in our understanding of how DNA-methylation patterns are established and maintained for inserting and maintaining DNA methylation in the epigenome. It has long been recognized that three biologically active enzymes, DNA methyltransferases (DNMTs), are responsible for establishing and maintaining sites of DNA methylation.[19] In this regard, DNMT 1 is predominantly a maintenance DNMT, which is responsible for preserving patterns of established DNA methylation during DNA replication. DNMT3A and DNMT3B are predominantly de novo DNMTs, which can establish new sites of DNA methylation. However, much data suggests a more complex scenario in which there can be cooperativity between the three DNMTs and interacting proteins such that they can, in some instances, replace one another in function when stress situations require this.[22] For example, DNMT3A and DNMT3B may function to repair errors made by DNMT1 during DNA synthesis.[14]

While the above scenarios for establishing DNA-methylation patterns have been appreciated, it was long thought that removal of this modification is a passive event accomplished only by failure to replace methylation sites during DNA replication. However, an exciting new era has emerged in which we appreciate that, as for histone modifications, there are distinct active steps for erasing DNA methylation. A family of enzymes, termed TET (ten-eleven translocations) family proteins, can, through oxidative steps, convert 5-methyl cytosine (5MT) to 5-hydroxylmethyl cytosine (5hMT), which, through subsequent DNA repair steps, convert 5MT back to cytosine.[19,23,24] These conversions are important during normal development and adult-cell functions, and later we outline their importance for cancer.[25–27]

Altered DNA methylation and chromatin in cancer or the "cancer epigenome"

Loss of DNA methylation

Virtually all cancer types harbor what appears to be a marked shift away from the normal epigenetic patterns, described in the previous sections, for normal cells[4,7,8] (Figure 2). This has been best studied to date for DNA methylation, where there are at least

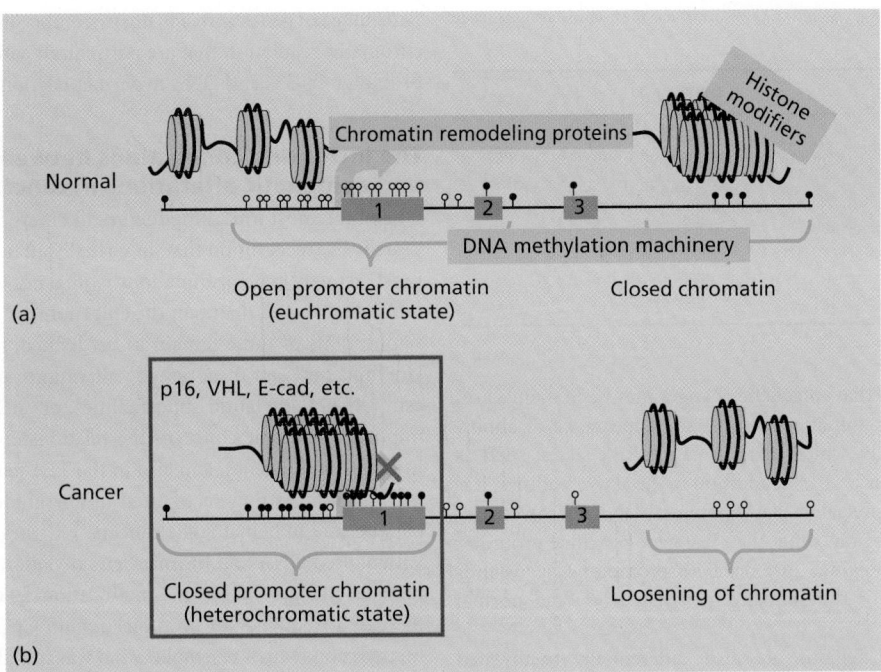

Figure 2 Depiction of the packaging arrangement of human DNA (straight black line). Panel (a) shows, for normal cells, a more linear arrangement of nucleosomes (yellow circles with DNA wrapped around as outlined in Figure 1) depicting the "open" arrangement of chromatin around most gene promoters containing CpG islands (unmethylated CpG sites shown as white lollipops), which are being actively transcribed or can be induced to transcribe (large light-blue arrow). Exons 1–3 of the model gene are depicted by the numbered light-blue boxes. Regions of DNA within the body of the gene and extending beyond the third exon are depicted as being in the closed, transcriptionally repressed, conformation typical of the majority of the normal human genome. This closed structure is represented by the more packed, three-dimensional organization of the nucleosomes, and the CpG sites in the closed regions are depicted as being methylated (black lollipops). The text in yellow squares depicts the chromatin remodeling protein complexes, histone-modifying enzymes, and enzymes performing DNA methylation (DNA-methylation machinery), which are responsible for DNA packaging as discussed in the text. Panel (b) depicts the altered chromatin patterns present in a typical cancer cell with a switch in positions of the normal closed and open chromatin regions in the genome. Many closed regions now have an open chromatin with loss of DNA methylation, while a large group of gene promoters have assumed a closed chromatin with abnormal, CpG island DNA methylation and repressed transcription (large red X over the transcription start site depicted by the light-blue arrow.

two major changes that are now well appreciated. First, there are global losses of this modification from the widespread regions of the genome, which harbor DNA methylation in normal cells[1,2,7,8,10] (Figure 2). Indeed, this was the first chromatin abnormality well cataloged for cancer[28] although much remains to be learned about the ramifications of this change. As these are generally areas of closed chromatin where the DNA methylation helps to maintain transcriptionally repressed DNA, such losses could associate with abnormal transcription.[1–4] Indeed, a number of genes with oncogenic potential, and which normally have low expression in normal cells, have now been reported to be upregulated in association with cancer-specific decreases in promoter DNA methylation.[1] Moreover, pericentromeric regions are a target for DNA-methylation losses in multiple cancer types and this may play a role in the genesis of chromosomal instability in neoplasia.[1–4,29] Most recently, losses of DNA methylation from gene body regions have also been observed in tumors. This can have an opposite effect on gene expression to those above as methylation in these regions, as discussed earlier, actually facilitates gene expression through enhancing transcriptional elongation.[7,20,21]

Gene promoter DNA hypermethylation

The best-studied chromatin change associated with epigenetic abnormalities in cancer, and the one with the most-recognized ramifications, to date, entails localized increases in DNA methylation in gene promoter CpG islands, which are protected from this change, as discussed earlier, in normal cells (Figure 2).[1–4,7,8]

This change is associated with tight transcriptional repression of genes and can, thus, serve in a process that provides an alternative to gene mutations for loss of function of a number of well-characterized tumor-suppressor genes.[1–4,7,8] In addition to these classic-suppressor genes, data derived from random screens of cancer-cell DNA for DNA-hypermethylated genes, such as in the Cancer Genome Atlas Project (TCGA), indicate that hundreds of such genes appear to exist, for multiple cancer types analyzed, in a given patient's tumor.[1–4,7,8,30–33] While all of these gene changes may not be pivotal for driving the initiation or progression of the particular cancers that harbor them, many, including the classic-suppressor genes, do encode for genes for which loss of function would be important for tumor development.[3,4,7,8] Many genes, which are seldom or never mutated in cancers, may still have important roles in tumorigenesis, as they undergo promoter DNA hypermethylation and silencing during tumor progression.[4,7,8] In this regard, virtually every critical pathway known to play a role in tumorigenesis is now known to be involved with genes bearing cancer-specific DNA hypermethylation in one or more tumor types[3,4,7,8] (Table 1). Finally, many of the genes involved exhibit the DNA-methylation change in preinvasive lesions, which have the potential for malignant progression, as demonstrated by "benign" colon polyps.[1,2,4,7,8,34] In these preinvasive colon lesions, multiple hypermethylated genes are already present and encode for key genes that, when inactivated, would deregulate key pathways, such as the Wnt pathway, which are well known to drive the initiation and progression of all colon cancers.[1,2,4,7,8,34] These findings have

Table 1 Examples of pathways altered by gene-promoter hypermethylation and gene silencing in cancer.

Pathway	Genes 3–5
Wnt pathway	APC, SFRP family, SOX17
Altered cell-cycle control	Rb, p16, p15, p14, p73
Repair of DNA damage	MLH1, O6-MGMT, GST-Pi, BRCA1
Apoptosis	DAP kinase, caspase 8, TMS-1
Tumor-cell invasion, angiogenesis	THBS1, E-cadherin, VHL, APC, LKB1, TIMP3,
Tumor architecture	Growth-factor response ER, RAR-beta, SOCS-1*

led to the hypothesis that epigenetic changes may be in many cases important for tumor initiation and for the appearance of abnormally expanding cells, which arise in cancer-risk states, such as chronic inflammation.[4,7,34–36] In addition to the above findings, it is now increasingly appreciated that differential DNA increases may affect key genomic regions other than just gene proximal promoter regions.[3,4,7,14,19,37,38] Regions just distal to promoter CpG islands called "shores" can be differentially methylated between normal and cancer tissues.[37,38]

The above shore regions are also differentially methylated between normal tissues, so the meaning for cancer per se, and especially as reflective of associated gene expression changes, is less clear than for proximal promoter, CpG island regions. Similarly, there is a building body of data for increased methylation in gene-enhancer regions, or DNA-regulatory sequences, which through binding of key proteins and histone modifications are master regulators of gene expression. These sequences can lie at variable, and often large, distances away from gene proximal promoters.[39–41] De novo DNA-methylation changes at enhancers may also contribute key gene expression abnormalities in cancer and especially for increasing cancer-risk states.[42,43] While the theme of differential enhancer DNA methylation in cancer is under more and more investigation, the role of these changes, and their balance with gene promoter CpG island hypermethylation, is still being clarified.

Long-range changes in DNA methylation and chromatin in cancer

A recent exciting advance in studying both normal and cancer epigenomes, stemming from in-depth analyses of CpG methylation and chromatin throughout the genome, is that there are nonrandom regional configurations that can be altered between cancer and normal cells. These occupy megabase regions in many chromosomes (100 kb to 10 Mb).[3,4,7,8,44–46] These are largely CpG poor regions, and the constituent CpGs are heavily methylated but to degrees that vary significantly throughout different normal tissues leading to the term partially methylated domains.[3,4,7,8,44–46] Cancers characteristically have losses of normal DNA methylation throughout these areas, creating the so-called megabase islands or canyons of hypomethylated domains as particularly defined to date in colon and other cancers.[3,4,7,8,44–46] Within these blocks of sequence, cancers can establish long-range appearance of repressive histone modifications, such as for H3K9 methylation as well.[3,4,7,8,44–46] In some regions, there may be long-range areas of nonrepressive or more open chromatin.[45,47–50] Intriguingly, much smaller-embedded genes within these large domains, which harbor promoter CpG islands, can have the de novo gains in DNA methylation discussed in detail earlier.[3,4,7,8,45] Thus, in essence, hypomethylated canyons in cancer often exhibit many of the cancer-associated losses and more focal CpG island gains of DNA methylation in cancer.[3,4,45] Moreover, these large domains may harbor a much higher than expected

percentage of genes with a history of embryonic and adult stem cell chromatin regulation that are particularly vulnerable to abnormal, promoter CpG island DNA hypermethylation.[3,4,7,8,35,45,51,52]

The increasing connections between genetic and epigenetic alterations in cancer

One of the most intriguing themes to emerge over the past several years is the recognition that, in virtually all tumor types, one of the most frequent type of mutations is in genes encoding for proteins that establish and maintain the epigenome.[3,4,7,53,54] While the exact implications of these remain to be defined, there are now several key links between these genetic alterations and either tumorigenesis, DNA-methylation abnormalities, or chromatin changes. One important example concerns the relationships between mutations in IDH 1 and 2 genes, and also in the TET genes, and DNA hypermethylation. As now recognized in low-grade gliomas in younger patients and in hematologic cancers,[55–57] these mutations associate with altered DNA and histone-demethylation pathways. These can include changes in histone-methylation levels and a pattern of increased frequency of promoter region CpG island DNA hypermethylation, which resembles what was initially characterized, in a subset of colon cancers, as the CpG island methylator phenotype or CIMP.[56–59] Much is coming to be understood about why the IDH mutations, especially, produce chromatin and DNA-methylation changes. The mutated genes lead to the massive accumulation of 2-hydroxy-glutarate formed from, and leading to depletion of, ketoglutarate.[60–62] The latter is a key cofactor for multiple enzymes that help regulate and maintain key chromatin marks and the previously mentioned TET proteins that can protect against abnormal DNA methylation.[63,64] These changes are thought to incite, over time, a molecular progression from increases in repressive-histone marks and subsequently the above DNA hypermethylation.[60–62] Recent mouse studies indicate that IDH mutations are drivers for early tumor-progression events[65] by blocking normal differentiation of normal stem/progenitor cells and thus facilitating abnormal self-renewal and diminished lineage commitment and differentiation.[57,60,66] Importantly, drugs directly targeting the IDH mutations have been developed and are now undergoing trials in AML and brain tumors.

Another fascinating set of mutations has been delineated in a pediatric subtype of brain tumor in a key repressive, histone mark itself. Thus, mutations in H3K27, present in only one allele of the multiple copies of histone H3, block the activity of the enzyme, EZH2, which catalyzes H3K27 methylation. Accordingly, the tumors have a marked loss of H3K27me3,[3,67,68] and this is postulated to induce abnormal activation of genes to drive initiation and/or progression of the tumors.

Clinical implications of altered DNA methylation in cancer

Although the full impact of understanding chromatin alterations in cancer is still to emerge, important progress is being made in at least two broad categories of translational application. First is the use of DNA-hypermethylated gene promoter sequences as tumor biomarkers, and second is the use of epigenetic therapies, which may be efficacious because they target reversal of abnormal gene silencing.[1,2,9,69–71]

Cancer DNA methylation biomarkers

There are some simple advantages that the detection of DNA-methylation changes in cancer allows over other molecular approaches. First, the overall frequencies of methylation changes appear to be greater in many instances than mutational changes.[3,7,30,69] This appears to be true for all major solid and liquid cancer types examined thus far, although the specific genes altered are different among tumor types. A second advantage of the detection of DNA-methylation changes associated with gene silencing is that this change is confined to the promoter region for many genes, making this alteration easily targeted for assays that can potentially serve as molecular markers for cancer. The large numbers of these genes allow for construction of gene panels for which DNA-hypermethylation markers essentially cover cancer genomes providing for high chance of marker detection in any given patient.[72] The fact that the abnormality arises for many genes in early, preinvasive stages of cancer and for others later in progression allows for potential uses of such markers in cancer-risk assessment, early diagnosis, molecular restaging of tumors, and prediction of tumor behavior. Thus, the high frequency, early occurrence of such changes, and the ability to assay methylation of each gene with a single assay, facilitate the use of such approaches for the early detection of cancer. Examples of each of the marker possibilities mentioned earlier include those listed in Table 2. Thus, for cancer-risk assessment, detection of DNA-hypermethylated gene sequences in sputum DNA now holds considerable promise for predicting which individuals at high risk for developing lung cancer will actually manifest this disease within a defined period after initiation of marker monitoring.[2,73] Detection of colon cancer has been explored by detection of altered DNA methylation in either the blood or stool and these are emerging as especially useful when added to mutation detection.[74–79] Detection of such genes in urine can potentially stratify the risk for, or provide for early diagnosis of, bladder cancer[80] and in prostate biopsies for improvement in the diagnosis of prostate cancer.[81,82] Several of the tests, for stool, and prostate biopsies are now available to clinicians via CLIA-approved tests.

A second area in which the changes of DNA methylation may be used in the management of cancer follows the observation that these genes are part of key pathways in the development of cancer. This allows the use of DNA methylation in these genes to potentially be used as prognostic or predictive biomarkers (Table 2). In general, the presence of DNA methylation for most genes has been associated with adverse outcome, thus providing a prognostic biomarker. This is consistent with the role that silencing of key tumor-suppressor genes can play in altering key signaling pathways. Thus, tumors with alterations of single genes, or multiple genes, are more aggressive or molecularly advanced, and thus lead to worse outcomes.[83,84] Recently, detection of a small panel of DNA-hypermethylated genes simultaneously in tumor and mediastinal lymph node DNA provides an extremely promising approach to restaging of stage 1 lung cancer patients to stage 3, thus predicting which of these individuals has a high risk of rapid recurrence.[85]

Another useful tool for the management of patients by medical oncologists is the possibility that DNA methylation in specific genes may affect the cancer-cell sensitivity to different therapies. For example, silencing of a DNA repair gene may increase likelihood of tumor response to DNA-damaging agents that would be repaired by this protein. The most clear example of this has been demonstrated for patients with the virulent brain tumor, glioblastoma, where detection of tumor DNA hypermethylation for the DNA damage-repair gene, *O6MGMT*, predicts for higher likelihood of response and post-treatment period of freedom from disease recurrence, for patients treated with the DNA-alkylating agent, Temazolamide.[86–88] Other studies have suggested that sensitivity to cisplatin may be mediated by silencing of *FANCF* in ovarian cancer[89,90] and sensitivity of colon cancer to topoisomerase inhibitors may be mediated by silencing of the Werner syndrome gene (*WRN*).[91] Recently, the promoter methylation of SMAD1 has been reported to predict resistance to doxorubicin, for patients with diffuse large B-cell lymphoma (DBCL).[92] Low doses of DNMT inhibitors reverse the repression of this gene, and this was found to relieve the chemoresistance.[92] These preclinical findings are being tested in a phase I clinical trial with early findings suggesting that the DNMT inhibitor used can prime for better chemotherapy responses.[92] Before clinical use, all of these studies need to be confirmed in additional populations and ideally in prospectively evaluated patients. However, such developments might greatly aid in optimizing the therapeutic choices offered to patients, who only have one opportunity for first-line therapy. An ever-increasing number of larger and larger clinical trials seek to validate the marker approaches and push their incorporation into standard oncology practice. Finally, other DNA-methylation changes, such as losses of normal DNA methylation in tumor DNA, and changes in chromatin marks for active or repressed-gene function, will almost certainly appear as promising molecular cancer markers.

Table 2 Examples of using gene-promoter DNA-hypermethylated sequences as cancer biomarkers: nearing clinical use.

Early diagnosis and/or detection of high-risk states:
  Detection of CpG-island DNA hypermethylation of gene panels in sputum from individuals at high risk for lung cancer[5,22]
  Detection of **GSTP1** DNA hypermethylation in prostate biopsies and urine specimens for prostate cancer[27,28]

Prognosis:
  Detection of DNA hypermethylation in gene panels in tumor, and lymph node DNA, to restage stage 1 non-small-cell lung carcinoma and predict early recurrences[31]
  Detection of DNA hypermethylation to predict sensitivity of glioblastomas to Temazolamide[32–34]
  Hypermethylation of specific genes Whole DNA-methylome profiles
  Histone-modification maps

Prediction:
  CpG-island hypermethylation as a marker of response to chemotherapy, hormone therapy, and targeted therapy, for example, MGMT in patients with glioma and temozolomide treatment

"Epigenetic" cancer therapy

This type of therapy refers to cancer treatments based on the concept of reverting abnormal gene expression patterns toward normal as a means of cancer treatment. To date, two classes of drugs, which may achieve this goal, those which can experimentally induce DNA demethylation (5-aza-cytidine, azacytidine and 5-aza-2′-deoxycytidine, or decitabine) and those which inhibit histone deacetylases (SAHA), have been approved by the FDA for treatment of the preleukemic state, myelodysplasia (MDS), and cutaneous T-cell lymphoma, respectively. Both azacitidine[93] and decitabine[7,94–96] have shown clinical benefit, and most recently, in a randomized phase III trial, azacitidine has shown a survival benefit.[97] Although, in both instances, these drugs achieve impressive response rates, and durable responses, in previously refractory diseases, it must be cautioned that their exact mode of efficacy remains to be proven—that is, they may not work clinically, solely, or partially—through the epigenetic effects, they mediate experimentally.[70,95,98,99] Thus, use of these drugs in other hematologic malignancies is the focus of many ongoing trials, and potentially promising results are being seen especially for the DNA-demethylating agents in acute myelogenous leukemias (AML) and chronic myelogenous leukemias (CML).[94,100] In addition, there is experimental evidence for synergy of DNA demethylating, and histone deacetylase inhibition, for re-expression of DNA hyper-methylated cancer genes.[101] Thus, multiple trials are exploring the clinical potential of using combination therapies with these agents. Most of these trials are joined with studies trying to examine whether DNA demethylation and re-expression of abnormally silenced genes corresponds with, or predicts, therapeutic response. Probably, over the next few years, all of these clinical studies will establish the true position of these drugs and their mechanism of clinical efficacy, in the clinical arena.

The use of epigenetic therapy in solid tumors, while less well explored, has been introduced in the past[102,103] and is now becoming a major focus with some promising and important results.[70,71] The universal presence of the therapeutic targets, as discussed in multiple sections of this chapter, makes the potential for such approaches as compelling in these cancers as in the hematologic malignancies. Recent preclinical studies have investigated how low doses of DNMT inhibitors can affect solid tumor cells and suggest that nanomolar doses of both Vidaza and Dacogen can yield antitumor responses, which may reflect the ability of these drugs to "reprogram" cancer cells with little off-target effects.[104] Using such low-dose approaches, plus the availability of new DNA-demethylating agents, such as SGI-110, which acts as a prodrug for DAC,[105,106] clinical trials are increasing. These include combining these drugs with other epigenetic therapy agents such as histone deacetylase inhibitors (HDACis). For example, such a combination, in recent trials in 65 patients with advanced, pretreated, non-small-cell lung cancer resulted in robust, durable responses in a small subset of patients.[107] In addition, results in these same trials suggest that the epigenetic therapy could prime a larger group of patients for better responses to subsequent therapies,[107] including standard chemotherapies and exciting new forms of immunotherapy.[108,109] With respect to the immunotherapy, preclinical work suggests that the DNA-methylation inhibitors can, in lung cancer cells and other solid tumor types, induce complex immune cell attraction pathways involving hundreds of genes.[110] The potential for the above sensitization of NSCLC patients to chemotherapy and immunotherapy is now undergoing testing in larger in larger trials. In addition to these studies in NSCLC, others are finding that DNA-methylation inhibitors can prime patients with advanced serous ovarian cancer to subsequent chemotherapy.[111]

It is certain that, over the next few years, many trials will appear for epigenetic-therapy approaches in solid tumors and, as in the leukemias, these will include studies to elucidate the precise mechanisms underlying clinical efficacy. All of these investigations, plus those in the hematologic malignancies, will not only guide the use of currently existing agents, but foster the development of newer and possibly more potent and specific drugs, as well. As we learn more about what precisely mediates abnormal DNA methylation and the components of chromatin that collaborate to initiate and maintain such changes, new molecular targets will almost surely emerge. Combination therapies exploiting these targets will likely follow. In this regard, small molecule inhibitors for several key steps in chromatin assembly have been developed and several of these are already in clinical trials.[4,70,71,112–116]

Summary

Work over the past decade, especially for DNA-methylation changes, has amply established that, from initiation through progression to advanced stages, cancer is a disease of epigenetic as well as genetic alterations. These studies, closely entwined with an explosion of basic knowledge about how chromatin constituents package the human genome to regulate gene-expression patterns, are providing a rich substrate for new cancer biomarker and therapy strategies. There is enormous potential for these strategies to enter usage in the cancer clinical arena over the next decade.

Key references

The complete reference list can be found on the Wiley Companion Digital Edition of this title (see inside front cover for login instructions).

1 Esteller M. Epigenetics in cancer. *N Engl J Med.* 2008;**358**(**11**):1148–1159.

3 Shen H, Laird PW. Interplay between the cancer genome and epigenome. *Cell.* 2013;**153**(**1**):38–55.

4 Baylin SB, Jones PA. A decade of exploring the cancer epigenome - biological and translational implications. *Nat Rev Cancer.* 2011;**11**(**10**):726–734.

5 Allis C, Jenuwein T, Reinberg D (eds) Caparros M (associate editor). *Epigenetics.* Cold Spring Harbor, NY: Cold Spring Harbor Laboratory Press; 2007.

8 Jones PA, Baylin SB. The epigenomics of cancer. *Cell.* 2007;**128**(**4**):683–692.

9 Egger G, Liang G, Aparicio A, Jones PA. Epigenetics in human disease and prospects for epigenetic therapy. *Nature.* 2004;**429**(**6990**):457–463.

13 Kornberg RD, Lorch Y. Twenty-five years of the nucleosome, fundamental particle of the eukaryote chromosome. *Cell.* 1999;**98**(**3**):285–294.

14 Jones PA. Functions of DNA methylation: islands, start sites, gene bodies and beyond. *Nat Rev Genet.* 2012;**13**(**7**):484–492.

15 Allis CD, Jenuwein T, Reinberg D. Overview and concepts. In: Allis CD, Jenuwein T, Reinberg D, eds. *Epigenetics.* Cold Spring Harbor, NY: Cold Spring Harbor Laboratory Press; 2007.

18 Li E, Bird A. DNA methylation in mammals. In: Allis CD, Jenuwein T, Reinberg D, eds. *Epigenetics.* Cold Spring Harbor, NY: Cold Spring Harbor Laboratory Press; 2007.

22 Rhee I, Bachman KE, Park BH, et al. DNMT1 and DNMT3b cooperate to silence genes in human cancer cells. *Nature.* 2002;**416**(**6880**):552–556.

23 Tahiliani M, Koh KP, Shen Y, et al. Conversion of 5-methylcytosine to 5-hydroxymethylcytosine in mammalian DNA by MLL partner TET1. *Science.* 2009;**324**(**5929**):930–935.

31 Hammerman PS, Hayes DN, Wilkerson MD, et al. Comprehensive genomic characterization of squamous cell lung cancers. *Nature.* 2012;**489**(**7417**):519–525.

35 Ohm JE, McGarvey KM, Yu X, et al. A stem cell-like chromatin pattern may predispose tumor suppressor genes to DNA hypermethylation and heritable silencing. *Nat Genet.* 2007;**39**(**2**):237–242.

36 Feinberg AP, Ohlsson R, Henikoff S. The epigenetic progenitor origin of human cancer. *Nat Rev Genet.* 2006;**7**(**1**):21–33.

45 Berman BP, Weisenberger DJ, Aman JF, et al. Regions of focal DNA hypermethylation and long-range hypomethylation in colorectal cancer coincide with nuclear lamina-associated domains. *Nat Genet.* 2012;**44**(**1**):40–46.

50 Timp W, Feinberg AP. Cancer as a dysregulated epigenome allowing cellular growth advantage at the expense of the host. *Nat Rev Cancer.* 2013;**13**(**7**):497–510.

51 Schlesinger Y, Straussman R, Keshet I, et al. Polycomb-mediated methylation on Lys27 of histone H3 pre-marks genes for de novo methylation in cancer. *Nat Genet.* 2007;**39**(**2**):232–236.

52 Widschwendter M, Fiegl H, Egle D, et al. Epigenetic stem cell signature in cancer. *Nat Genet.* 2007;**39**(**2**):157–158.

53 You JS, Jones PA. Cancer genetics and epigenetics: two sides of the same coin? *Cancer Cell.* 2012;**22**(**1**):9–20.

54 Garraway LA, Lander ES. Lessons from the cancer genome. *Cell.* 2013;**153**(**1**):17–37.

56 Noushmehr H, Weisenberger DJ, Diefes K, et al. Identification of a CpG island methylator phenotype that defines a distinct subgroup of glioma. *Cancer Cell.* 2010;**17**(**5**):510–522.

58 Issa JP. Aging and epigenetic drift: a vicious cycle. *J Clin Invest.* 2014;**124**(**1**):24–29.

60 Lu C, Ward PS, Kapoor GS, et al. IDH mutation impairs histone demethylation and results in a block to cell differentiation. *Nature.* 2012;**483**(**7390**):474–478.

67 Chan K-M, Fang D, Gan H, et al. The histone H3.3K27M mutation in pediatric glioma reprograms H3K27 methylation and gene expression. *Genes Dev.* 2013;**27**(**9**):985–990.

68 Lewis PW, Muller MM, Koletsky MS, et al. Inhibition of PRC2 activity by a gain-of-function H3 mutation found in pediatric glioblastoma. *Science.* 2013;**340**(**6134**):857–861.

69 Laird PW. The power and the promise of DNA methylation markers. *Nat Rev Cancer.* 2003;**3**(**4**):253–266.

70 Ahuja N, Easwaran H, Baylin SB. Harnessing the potential of epigenetic therapy to target solid tumors. *J Clin Invest.* 2014;**124**(**1**):56–63.

71 Azad N, Zahnow CA, Rudin CM, Baylin SB. The future of epigenetic therapy in solid tumours-lessons from the past. *Nat Rev Clin Oncol.* 2013;**10**(**5**): 256–266.

79 Imperiale TF, Ransohoff DF, Itzkowitz SH, et al. Multitarget stool DNA testing for colorectal-cancer screening. *N Engl J Med.* 2014;**370**(**14**):1287–1297.

85 Brock MV, Hooker CM, Ota-Machida E, et al. DNA methylation markers and early recurrence in stage I lung cancer. *N Engl J Med.* 2008;**358**(**11**):1118–1128.

86 Esteller M, Garcia-Foncillas J, Andion E, et al. Inactivation of the DNA-repair gene MGMT and the clinical response of gliomas to alkylating agents. *N Engl J Med.* 2000;**343**(**19**):1350–1354.

87 Hegi ME, Diserens AC, Gorlia T, et al. MGMT gene silencing and benefit from temozolomide in glioblastoma. *N Engl J Med.* 2005;**352**(**10**):997–1003.

93 Silverman LR, Demakos EP, Peterson BL, et al. Randomized controlled trial of azacitidine in patients with the myelodysplastic syndrome: a study of the cancer and leukemia group B. *J Clin Oncol.* 2002;**20**(**10**):2429–2440.

96 Issa JP. Optimizing therapy with methylation inhibitors in myelodysplastic syndromes: dose, duration, and patient selection. *Nat Clin Pract Oncol.* 2005; **2**(**Suppl 1**):S24–S29.

101 Cameron EE, Bachman KE, Myohanen S, Herman JG, Baylin SB. Synergy of demethylation and histone deacetylase inhibition in the re-expression of genes silenced in cancer. *Nat Genet.* 1999;**21**(**1**):103–107.

104 Tsai HC, Li H, Van Neste L, et al. Transient low doses of DNA-demethylating agents exert durable antitumor effects on hematological and epithelial tumor cells. *Cancer Cell.* 2012;**21**(**3**):430–446.

107 Juergens RA, Wrangle J, Vendetti FP, et al. Combination epigenetic therapy has efficacy in patients with refractory advanced non-small cell lung cancer. *Cancer Discov.* 2011;**1**(**7**):598–607.

108 Brahmer JR, Tykodi SS, Chow LQ, et al. Safety and activity of anti-PD-L1 antibody in patients with advanced cancer. *N Engl J Med.* 2012;**366**(**26**):2455–2465.

109 Topalian SL, Hodi FS, Brahmer JR, et al. Safety, activity, and immune correlates of anti-PD-1 antibody in cancer. *N Engl J Med.* 2012;**366**(**26**):2443–2454.

7 Cancer genomics and evolution

William P. D. Hendricks, PhD ▪ Aleksandar Sekulic, MD, PhD ▪ Alan H. Bryce, MD ▪ Muhammed Murtaza, MBBS, PhD ▪ Pilar Ramos, PhD ▪ Jeffrey M. Trent, PhD

Overview

Over 100 years ago, the Nobel Prize in Physiology or Medicine was given to Paul Ehrlich for postulating that "magic bullets" could specifically target and kill cells such as cancer cells based on their unique molecular features. The completed Human Genome Project and the cancer genomics revolution have now mapped the specific genetic changes underlying unique features of many common malignancies. However, although cancer has long been recognized to be heterogeneous in its clinical presentation, course, and pathology, we now recognize that it is far more molecularly heterogeneous than anticipated and that such variability will require an individualized approach to patient care. Rather than a single magic bullet, we will need an arsenal and this arsenal will require precise delivery. While inter- and intratumoral genomic heterogeneity present significant challenges to cancer management and drug discovery, a number of developments foster hope for accelerated progress in the war on cancer. First, our catalog of genomic targets underlying diverse cancers is rapidly growing. Second, we are beginning to understand how diverse mutations converge on a small number of druggable pathways. Third, we continue to develop drugs and biologic agents (e.g., immune checkpoint inhibitors) that target an increasingly wide array of genomic subtypes of cancer. Finally, advances in next-generation sequencing technologies now enable far earlier detection of disease recurrence than ever before. This chapter will focus on these developments and how their integration is aiding in the precise delivery of "magic bullets."

Precis

Cancer is a genetic disease in which the stepwise accumulation of oncogene and tumor suppressor gene (TSG) mutations in clonally expanding cell populations drives malignant transformation. Throughout the twentieth century, overwhelming evidence steadily accumulated in support of this model while a growing understanding of the mutations underlying cancer subtypes helped to guide innovation in clinical cancer management. The genomics revolution begun in the twenty-first century has now transformed our understanding of cancer by generating exhaustive catalogs of cancer-driving mutations and identifying the great genomic diversity existing between and within individual tumors. These data are enabling targeted drug development, genomics-guided clinical management, and new approaches to early disease detection. Yet, gaps nonetheless remain in our knowledge of the causative mutations underlying some cancers, in our understanding of the biology of the mutations we have identified, in developing drugs capable of targeting many of these diverse mutations, and in fending off the inevitable emergence of drug resistance. In this chapter, we review the history and methods of cancer genetics and genomics, summarize current knowledge of the spectrum of mutations in cancers, discuss emerging concepts in cancer evolution and genomic heterogeneity, and present a case study on the clinical impact of melanoma genomics.

Introduction

As detailed in the previous chapters, cancer is a genetic disease resulting from the stepwise accumulation of mutations that confer upon cells a selective growth advantage.[1] Such mutations alter the birth and death rate as well as the genomic stability of cells as they undergo waves of clonal expansion. With the accumulation of mutations in cancer genes, cell populations acquire increasingly malignant phenotypes in successive generations. These hallmark cancer phenotypes include sustained proliferation, evasion of growth suppression, evasion of the immune system, promotion of inflammation, activation of invasion and metastasis, induction of genomic instability, immortal replication, induction of angiogenesis, deregulation of cellular energetics, and resistance to cell death.[2] Cancer genes in which mutation confers a growth advantage are classified as oncogenes or TSGs. Oncogenes, when activated through mutation in recurrent hotspots, drive constitutive activation of cell signaling pathways accelerating the cell birth rate. TSGs, when mutationally inactivated, are no longer able to promote cell death and thereby decrease the cell death rate. This model has been well characterized in colorectal cancer in which mutations in the *APC* tumor suppressor have been shown in most cases to drive adenoma formation. Additional mutations in cancer genes comprising proliferative, cell cycle, and apoptosis pathways then result in the formation of malignant tumors capable of invasion and metastasis.[3,4] Multiple other cancers have also been shown to follow this model, although we now know that there are many disparate evolutionary paths to malignancy even within the same cancer type (Figure 1).

While some mutations in cancer genes occur in the germ line and are heritable, the majority (90%) arise sporadically in somatic tissues over an individual's lifetime (i.e., they are tumor specific) owing to replication error, genotoxic stress, and/or environmental damage.[5] These mutations may result from subtle sequence alterations (single-base substitutions and insertions or deletions of one or a few bases), changes in chromosome copy number (amplification, deletion, chromosome loss, or duplication), or changes in chromosome structure (inter- and intrachromosomal translocation, inversion, or other types of rearrangement). For the remainder of this chapter, we will refer to these alterations as somatic single nucleotide variants (SNVs), copy number variants (CNVs), or structural variants (SVs). Classic examples of SNVs, CNVs, and SVs are shown in Figure 2 and include an activating missense SNV in NRAS (one of the most commonly mutated oncogenes), an inactivating homozygous deletion CNV in one of the most commonly inactivated tumor suppressors *TP53*, and an activating translocation SV involving *BCR* and *ABL*. Epigenomic

Holland-Frei Cancer Medicine, Ninth Edition. Edited by Robert C. Bast Jr., Carlo M. Croce, William N. Hait, Waun Ki Hong, Donald W. Kufe, Martine Piccart-Gebhart, Raphael E. Pollock, Ralph R. Weichselbaum, Hongyang Wang, and James F. Holland.
© 2017 John Wiley & Sons, Inc. ISBN: 978-1-118-93469-2

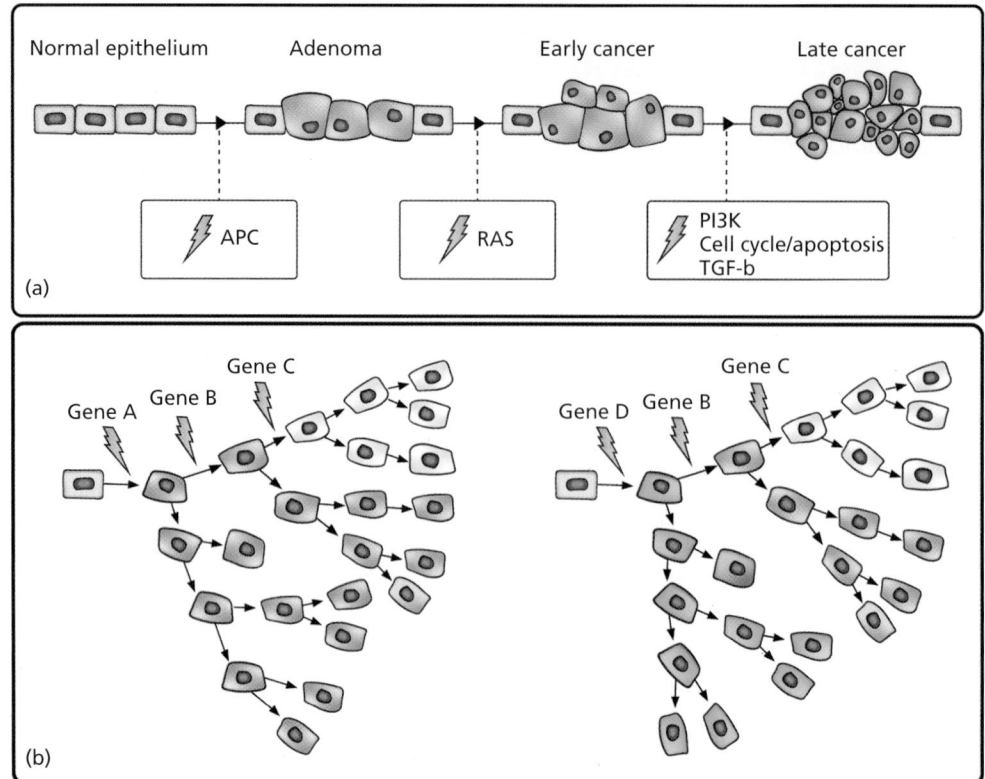

Figure 1 Cancer results from the stepwise accumulation of diverse, branching mutations. (a) "Vogelgram" model of progressive development of colorectal cancer.[3] Inactivation of the tumor suppressor *APC* is commonly observed in colorectal cancer precursor lesions. Subsequent mutational activation of the *RAS* oncogene is associated with transition from early adenoma to early cancer. Progressive accumulation of molecular alterations eventually leads to a malignant tumor that can invade the basement membrane and metastasize to lymph nodes and distant organs. (b) Expanded model depicting disparate cancer-initiating mutations as well as stepwise branching evolution in which cells accumulate secondary mutations followed by clonal expansion leading to both inter- and intratumoral heterogeneity.

modifications of cancer genes can also significantly alter gene function. These modifications of DNA, while not altering the DNA sequence itself, can include DNA methylation changes, chromatin modifications, or noncoding RNA-dependent gene regulation that may be heritable and play a role in tumorigenesis. This increasingly important area of study will be discussed in other chapters. We will focus here on DNA sequence-altering mutations.[6–9] In this chapter, we use specific examples to highlight the state of cancer genomics knowledge by describing current methods in genomic analysis, compiling results from landmark cancer genomic studies, and assessing the role of cancer evolution in determining its clinical management. We then conclude with a detailed case study of melanoma genomics, evolution, and genomics-guided medicine.

The history and methods of cancer genomics

The early history of cancer genetics

The elucidation of cancer's genetic etiology and breadth of its diversity has paralleled seminal advances in genetics and genetic technology (Figure 3a). Many landmark studies in the late nineteenth and early twentieth century laid the groundwork for cancer genomics—development of the theory of evolution by natural selection,[10] discovery of heritable biological units,[11] identification of chromosomes,[12] chromosomal heredity[13,14] and chromosomal genes,[15] and modern evolutionary synthesis linking biology,

genetics, and evolutionary theory.[16] The subsequent discovery of DNA's structure then provided a framework for understanding the genetic code and the mechanism for molecular transmission of genetic information.[17] Meanwhile, reports of heritable breast and colorectal cancers had arisen[18] and cancer was increasingly understood to be able to be caused by chemical agents such as coal tar[19] and cigarette smoke,[20] physical agents such as radiation,[21] and biological agents such as viruses.[22] Discovery that these carcinogenic agents were also mutagenic drove speculation that cancer was a disease of mutation. Ultimately, although cancer had been suggested by some to be a chromosomal disease or a disease of mutation, the concept of cancer as a genetic disease did not gain traction until later in the twentieth century when cytogenetic and sequencing technology alongside experimental transformation of normal cell lines with oncogenes enabled assessment of cancer gene mutations at the molecular level and establishment of their causal role in tumorigenesis. Some of these landmark studies are shown in Figure 3a.

Molecular cytogenetics: Identification of recurrent chromosomal alterations in cancer

Mid-twentieth century developments in the field of cytogenetics such as chromosome staining in fixed leukocytes from peripheral blood finally enabled empirical observation of the chromosomal complement of a cell.[23,24] Using this approach, Nowell was the first to discover a specific recurrent genetic change associated with a

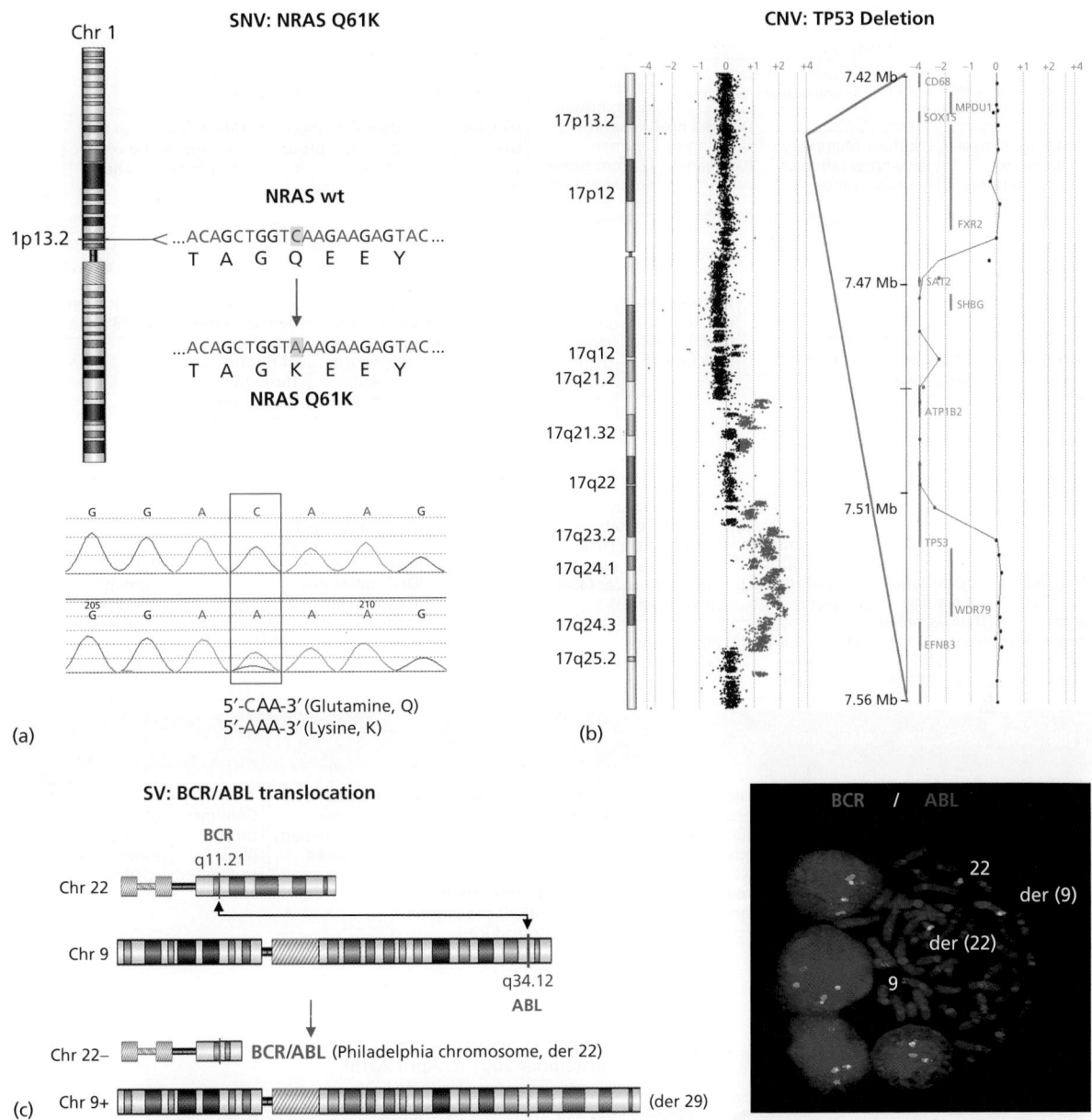

Figure 2 Examples of cancer mutation types. (a) The *NRAS* oncogene, located on chromosome 1, is commonly mutationally activated in diverse cancers. A single nucleotide variant (SNV) results in a codon alteration and substitution of lysine (K) for glutamine (Q) at amino acid 61—Q61K (top figure). Shown below is the chromatogram from Sanger sequencing analysis of a tumor sample harboring the *NRAS* Q61K mutation. (b) CGH log2 ratio data are plotted for chromosome 17 (left), as well as a focal region of homozygous deletion with a breakpoint within the TP53 tumor suppressor (right). Regions of DNA copy loss are plotted to the left of the axis and regions of gain are plotted to the right. Individual log2 ratio data (dots) and log2 ratio moving average (line) are shown. (c) Schematic of the DNA translocation that occurs between the genes *BCR* and *ABL*, leading to the formation of the *BCR-ABL* gene fusion known as the Philadelphia chromosome (left). Shown on the right is interphase and metaphase FISH detection of the t(9;22) BCR-ABL gene fusion using fluorescently labeled genomic probes for *BCR* (green) and *ABL* (red). Note that the fusion of *BCR* and *ABL* probes results in a yellow signal indicating colocalization of the red and green probes as a result of the t(9;22). Source: The *BCR-ABL* micrograph is courtesy of Dr. Susana Raimondi of St. Jude Children's Research Hospital.

cancer type—the "Philadelphia chromosome" fragment occurring in nearly all evaluated cases of chronic myelogenous leukemia (CML).[25] Over a decade later, Rowley then used chromosome banding to map the components of this fragment, determining the Philadelphia chromosome to be a balanced reciprocal translocation between chromosomes 9 and 22.[26,27] These discoveries drove a search for recurrent structural aberrations both within and across cancer types. They led to identification of characteristic translocations in sarcomas, leukemias, and lymphomas. However, most carcinomas were found to possess few recurrent alterations, instead displaying great variety in the number and type of chromosome aberrations.[28]

After Nowell and Rowley's discoveries, rapid innovation in chromosomal banding and spectral karyotyping (SKY) allowed progressively detailed views of chromosome aberrations in cancer cells using techniques based on fluorescence *in situ* hybridization (FISH), which relies on fluorescent DNA probes that hybridize to specific chromosomal regions.[29–38] Approaches for genome-wide cytogenetic analysis have also been developed including SKY,[29] multiplex-fluorescence *in situ* hybridization

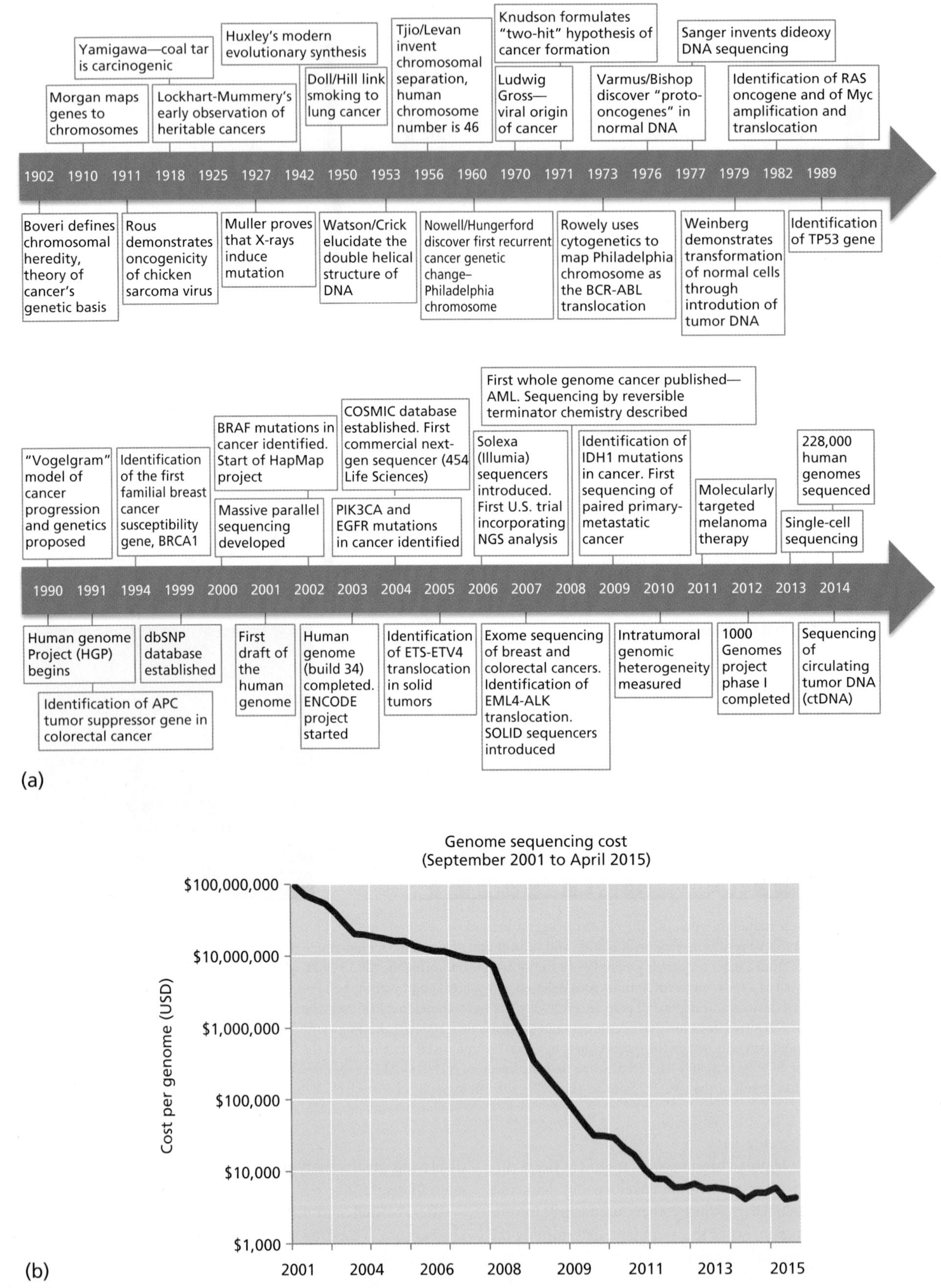

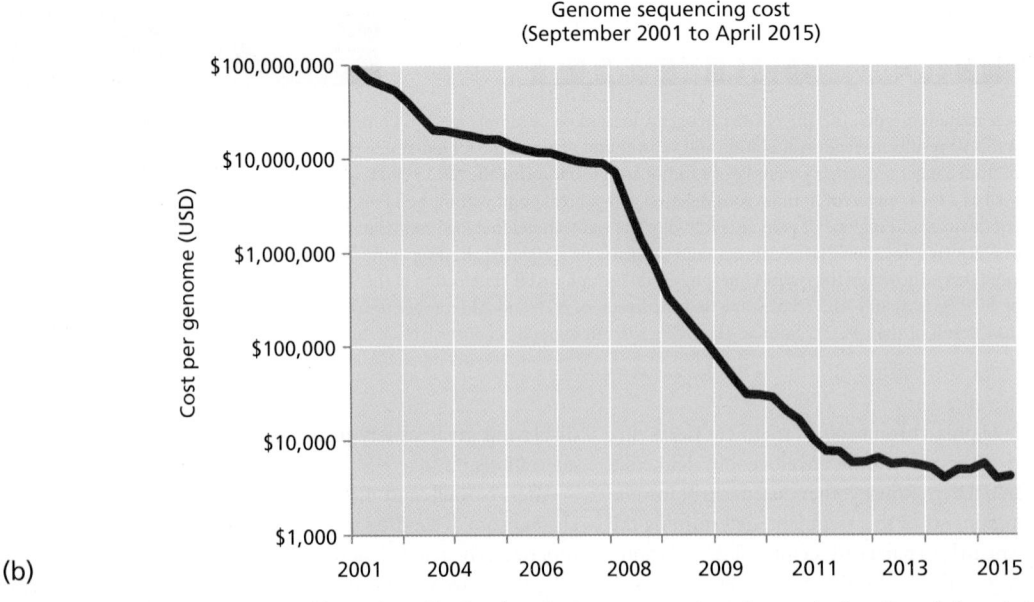

Figure 3 The history of cancer genomics. (a) Timeline of landmark studies in cancer genetics and genomics from Boveri's formulation of the chromosomally aberrant nature of cancer in 1902 to the advent of 228,000 human genomes sequenced in 2014. (b) Cost of sequencing a 3000 Mb genome (i.e., the size of the human genome) over time. Source: Data from the NHGRI Genome Sequencing Program (Wetterstrand KA; see http://www.genome.gov/sequencingcosts/).

(M-FISH),[39] chromosome microdissection,[38] and comparative genomic hybridization (CGH).[40] CGH is a particularly powerful fluorescent molecular cytogenetic technique for screening genome-wide chromosomal copy number changes in tumor genomes.

Novel approaches to printing nucleic acids on slides (microarrays) soon revolutionized molecular cytogenetics by reducing cost and increasing throughput. Array comparative genomic hybridization (aCGH) originally involved spotting large probes (large-insert clones or artificial chromosomes)[41,42] onto slides in intervals (1–3 Mb resolution) across chromosomal regions. Now, high-resolution genome-wide platforms consisting of small, customizable oligonucleotide probes[43,44] have demonstrated increased throughput and sensitivity in characterizing cancers such as breast,[45–47] melanoma,[48–50] B-cell lymphoma,[51,52] and many others. Similarly, oligonucleotide arrays designed to genotype thousands of single nucleotide polymorphisms (SNPs) are useful for characterizing tumor genome complexity with rapid genotyping of over millions of SNPs now possible (Affymetrix, Illumina). Similar to CGH arrays, SNP arrays quantitate locus-specific hybridization signal and can be used to estimate copy number or loss of heterozygosity (LOH).[53–55] Notable cancer studies incorporating SNP arrays include genotyping of the NCI-60 cell line panel[56] as well as lung cancer,[57] AML,[55,58] neuroblastoma,[59] melanoma,[56,60,61] basal cell carcinoma,[54] breast cancer,[62] colorectal cancer,[62–64] glioblastoma,[65,66] and pancreatic cancer.[67]

Both SVs and CNVs can be characterized using the tools of molecular cytogenetics and cytogenomics. Translocations are some of the most common SVs observed in cancer and, as in the case of the Philadelphia Chromosome in CML, are signature aberrations for many liquid cancers and sarcomas. They involve the movement of a chromosomal segment from one position to another, either within the same chromosome (intrachromosomal) or a different chromosome (interchromosomal). Other types of SV include chromosomal deletions, duplications, inversions, insertions, rings, and isochromosomes. These SVs may result from errors in double-stranded break (DSB) repair or other means of intra- or interchromosomal recombination.[68] Translocations and other SVs can either activate oncogenes (such as when the *ABL* tyrosine kinase is constitutively activated by fusion with the *BCR* gene) or inactivate TSGs (such as when translocations involving the *TP53* tumor suppressor interrupt the gene and lead to loss of function). CNVs involving a gain or loss of an entire chromosome are some of the simplest and most common chromosomal aberrations. They result from defective chromosomal segregation. The functional consequence of CNVs can be difficult to establish because the aberrations may extend over tens of thousands of megabases and may affect hundreds to thousands of genes. It has been easier to establish the cancer relevance of more limited regions of chromosomal gain and loss, created by amplification or deletion, as these smaller aberrations have been shown to alter the dosage of known oncogenes or TSGs. Classic examples of oncogene amplification in solid tumors discovered through molecular cytogenetics include *ERBB2* in breast cancers and *MYC* in a variety of tumor types, while loss of specific regions of the genome is often associated with loss of TSGs such as *TP53*, *RB1*, *PTEN*, and *CDKN2A*. Such deletions of TSGs are critical for promotion of tumorigenesis both in cases of heritable cancers in which germline mutation of a single TSG allele must be coupled with loss of the wild-type allele as well as in sporadic cancers in which both alleles must be inactivated.

Molecular genetics: Identification of recurrent sequence alterations in cancer

While some molecular cytogenetic techniques are capable of detecting chromosomal breakpoints at base pair resolution, advances in molecular genetics were required to allow detection of subtle sequence changes in DNA itself. These advances were enabled by developments in molecular cloning and invention of the polymerase chain reaction (PCR) capable of generating the millions of DNA copies necessary for detection of these mutations.[69] Coupled with the Sanger sequencing method based on dideoxynucleotide chain termination and agarose gel electrophoresis,[70] progressive advances in this methodology, including fluorescently labeled nucleotides, capillary electrophoresis, paired-end sequencing, shotgun sequencing, and improved laboratory automation have allowed scaling to sequence entire genomes. This technology enabled the Human Genome Project (HGP), launched in 1990 as a $3 billion dollar publicly funded international collaboration. The rough draft of the human genome, covering 94% of the genome, was published in 2001[71,72] with the complete draft finished ahead of schedule in 2003.[73] In addition to establishing genome-wide ground truth for the locations, organization, and sequences of all human genes, the technical and informatic lessons learned in the course of this project made possible the first ambitious cancer mutation screens on the level of entire gene families[74–77] and the majority of the protein-coding genome.[62,65–67] Nonetheless, genome sequencing projects using Sanger-based sequencing continued to be expensive and logistically challenging and thereby limited the application of this approach toward large-scale characterization of cancer genomes until the advent of massively parallel sequencing.

Gene expression microarrays: Cancer signatures and pathways

Microarrays such as those employed in aCGH studies were originally developed for high-throughput gene expression studies. Complementary DNA (cDNA formed from reverse transcription of RNA) and later oligonucleotide microarrays were implemented in high-throughput quantitation of mRNA transcripts. Advances in this technology paralleled improvements in automated Sanger sequencing in the 1990s and the turn of the millennium. They provided some of the first insights into gene signatures and pathways correlating to specific cancer subtypes. A parallel method, serial analysis of gene expression (SAGE) was developed to enable high-throughput digital quantitation of transcripts.[78] While originally designed to assay the expression of individual genes, gene expression profiling methods were later adapted to profile and map global transcription on the exon and genome levels,[79] as well as to profile the expression of mature human micro-RNAs (miRNAs).[80] Gene expression patterns have been widely used to subclassify cancers into homogeneous entities not easily discernible using traditional histopathologic or cytogenetic techniques, for instance, in diffuse large B-cell lymphoma (DLBCL),[81,82] lung cancer,[83] melanoma,[84] and breast cancer.[85,86] In some instances, subgroups have been shown to represent distinct disease states responding differently to standard therapies. Gene expression profiles have also been widely mined to specifically identify sets of genes predictive of disease progression, response to therapy, or metastasis,[87–89] as well as the presence of specific recurrent cytogenetic abnormalities,[90–92] or gene mutations.[93–96] Although advances in massively parallel sequencing have largely supplanted microarrays in sensitivity and robustness, if not cost and clinical readiness, gene expression profiling continues to play a significant role in cancer biology and medicine. In fact, commercially available clinical tests based on microarray signatures (OncoType DX and MammaPrint) are available for breast cancer profiling.

Massively parallel sequencing: Charting cancer genome landscapes

Explosive growth in our understanding of cancer genomics has been built on the backbone of the advances that emerged from the completion of the human genome at the turn of the twenty-first century. However, although these advances had driven the cost of one genome down from an estimated $1 billion to the $1 million mark at the time of the HGP's completion, this extraordinary cost nonetheless held back large-scale genomic studies.[97] Thus, the National Human Genome Research Institute initiated a $70 million sequencing technology program intended to drive the price down to the $1000 mark. The cost of a human genome sequence now lies slightly below $2000 and is steadily approaching $1000 (Figure 3b).

The quest for the $1000 genome required fundamental rethinking of the approach to DNA sequencing. Sanger sequencing, even in its most expert execution, faced insurmountable bottlenecks including (1) the need for molecular cloning steps and/or individual PCR reactions to generate sequencing templates and (2) every sequencing reaction can only accommodate a relatively small genomic region. Therefore, cloning/amplifying and sequencing many regions, even when run in parallel in multiwell plates, requires large amounts of materials, equipment, and analysis time. The paradigm shift in sequencing cost and throughput was brought about by the invention of approaches that allowed generation of sequencing templates without cloning or individual PCR reactions, immobilization of entire sequencing libraries in a single reaction chamber, and massively parallel sequencing of millions of templates in that chamber. The ability of this approach to collect data on clonal populations derived from single DNA molecules additionally provides great power for detection of rare variants from heterogeneous tumor samples. These rapid, accurate, and inexpensive approaches are also referred to as next-generation sequencing (NGS).

Key inventions in the 1990s and early 2000s such as sequencing-by-synthesis, pyrosequencing, colony sequencing, and emulsion PCR enabled development of the first NGS platforms.[98–101] The first such platform was developed by Lynx Therapeutics (later acquired by Solexa) in 2000, although it did not achieve widespread adoption.[102] 454 Life Sciences offered the first commercially available system—the 454 FLX Pyrosequencer—in 2004,[103] followed by the Solexa (now Illumina) Genome Analyzer in 2006, and the Supported Oligonucleotide Ligation and Detection (SOLiD) System from Applied Biosystems in 2007 that also incorporated polony sequencing.[104,105] The Solexa system was used in 2008 to sequence James Watson's genome within a single laboratory in only 2 months.[106] These platforms at last made the possibility of sequencing and assembling multiple cancer genomes a reality as evidenced by the characterization of genome-wide SVs in two lung cancer genomes.[107] This study utilized a paired-end approach, demonstrating strikingly complex genomic rearrangements including those resulting in previously unreported fusion transcripts. Importantly, this study also demonstrated that DNA copy number can be estimated by the relative local abundance of genomic fragments sequenced, providing sensitivity comparable to aCGH platforms while at the same time providing DNA sequence information. Massively parallel sequencing methods have now dramatically decreased the cost of sequencing while greatly increasing throughput. Presently, sequencing of 500 billion bases (e.g., sequencing the equivalent of 156 human genomes or 156X average genome coverage) within a single 6-day commercial instrument run is standard, with throughput still steadily increasing.

Many massively parallel sequencing platforms exist today and are reviewed in more detail elsewhere.[108] Table 1 provides an overview of some of the most common platforms in use today. They have been adapted to a variety of purposes ranging from diverse DNA sequence, copy number, and structural analyses to transcriptomics and epigenomics. DNA sequencing applications include *de novo* sequencing, such as the first such application in determining the previously unknown genomic sequence of *Acinetobacter baumannii*.[109] In addition, resequencing of human genomes is performed in order to characterize normal variation or variation in specific disease states such as cancer. Resequencing is undertaken by mapping NGS sequencing reads to the reference genome and identifying differences between the sample and reference.[65] Of course, it is not always necessary or informative to assess whole genomes, and thus, a number of target-enrichment strategies have been conceived that enable more cost-effective and focused analyses. The first of these—direct genomic selection—was based on hybridizing defined genomic regions to biotinylated BACs and capturing these sequences on streptavidin beads before sequencing.[110] New enrichment methods such as hybridization-based capture (using oligonucleotides either in solution or on microarrays), highly multiplexed PCR, and microdroplet PCR are common.[111–114] A relatively small fraction of the human genome has been functionally characterized, and therefore, it is often most expedient to assess the 1% of the genome containing coding regions (all exons—the exome). Thus, a number of commercially available human exome and other targeted capture kits (such as panels of common cancer genes) are available. This ability to target specific genes to enable rapid, accurate, affordable sequencing is aiding not only in biological discovery but also in clinical laboratory testing by enabling practical complex testing.

Cancer genome landscapes

Landmark cancer genomic studies

Despite commonalities observed within and between individual types of cancer in historic genetic studies, the high-throughput genomic studies of the past decade have provided a much more complex view of cancer. The first large-scale cancer mutation screens implemented high-throughput Sanger sequencing of individual genes such as *BRAF* in large cohorts[115,116] or focused on gene families such as protein kinases in diverse cancer types.[74–77,117,118] Notably, such screens have led to the identification of activating *BRAF* mutations in a large percentage of human melanomas[115] and nevi,[119] as well as *ERBB2* mutations in human breast cancer.[118] The first cancer gene panels (110 exons from 12 target genes) were completed in 140 acute myeloid leukemia (AML) samples in 2003.[120] This study identified six previously described and, strikingly, seven previously unknown coding mutations in AML genomes. Soon after, results of Sanger-based exome sequencing of 13,023 genes in 11 breast and 11 colorectal cancers were published in 2006.[121] This study revealed a surprising total of 189 frequently mutated genes with an average of 90 mutant genes per tumor, although only a subset was thought to be causally related to tumorigenesis or progression (an average of 11 per tumor). In a follow-up analysis of an additional 7000 genes in the same tumors, it was confirmed that a handful of commonly mutated genes (the "mountains" in the genomic landscape) existed among a large number of less frequently mutated "hills". In 2008, four Sanger-based exome projects additionally characterized over 20,000 genes in glioblastoma multiforme[62,65,66] and pancreatic cancer.[67] Amidst an average of 63 and 47

Table 1 Massively parallel sequencing platforms.

Company	System platform[a]	Latest release	Template preparation	Sequencing chemistry	Maximum read length	Bases per run (Gb)	Accuracy	Run time	Application
Illumina	Illumina HiSeq 4000	2015	Emulsion PCR	Reversible terminator	150	1500	>99%	<1–3.5 days	WGS, E-S, RNA-S, T-S, C-S, MG
	Illumina HiSeq 3000	2015	Emulsion PCR	Reversible terminator	150	750	>99%	<1–3.5 days	WGS, E-S, RNA-S, T-S, C-S, MG
	Illumina HiSeq 2500	2014	Solid-phase	Reversible terminator	125	500	> 99%	6 days	WGS, E-S, RNA-S, T-S, C-S, MG, DN-S
	Illumina HiSeq X (Ten/Five)	2014	Solid-phase	Reversible terminator	150	1800	>99%	<3 days	WGS
	Illumina MiSeq	2014	Solid-phase	Reversible terminator	300	15	>99%	4 h	E-S, RNA-S, T-S, C-S, DN-S
	Illumina NextSeq 500	2014	Solid-phase	Reversible terminator	150	120	>99%	30 h	WGS, E-S, RNA-S, T-S, C-S, MG
Life Technologies	IonTorrent Personal Genome Machine	2014	Emulsion PCR	Proton detection	400	2	>99%	2 h	Microbial WGS, E-S, RNA-S, T-S, C-S, MG
	IonTorrent Proton	2014	Emulsion PCR	Proton detection	200	10	>99%	2–4 h	Microbial WGS, E-S, RNA-S, T-S, C-S, MG
	SOLiD	2014	Emulsion PCR	Sequencing by ligation	75	120	99.99%	8 days	WGS, DN-S, E-S, RNA-S, T-S, C-S, MG
Pacific Biosciences	PacBio RS II	2014	Single molecule	Real-time sequencing	15,000	3	85%	20 min	DN-S, T-S
Roche	454 GS Junior	2014	Emulsion PCR	Pyro-sequencing	400	0.07	>99%	10 h	Microbial DN-S, E-S
	454 GS FLX	2014	Emulsion PCR	Pyro-sequencing	700	0.7	100%	24 h	Microbial DN-S, E-S

WGS, whole genome sequencing; E-S, exome sequencing; RNA-S, RNA sequencing; T-S, targeted sequencing; C-S, ChIP-sequencing; MG, MetaGenomics; and DN-S, *de novo* sequencing.
[a]Additional versions are available for some models.

mutations per pancreatic tumor or glioblastoma, these studies identified novel genes bearing low-frequency mutations such as *IDH1* and *PIK3R1* mutations in glioblastoma. Strikingly, they uncovered few unknown genes recurrently mutated at high rates. In these and future studies, it was found that the high-frequency mountains had already largely been identified using the low-throughput genetic technologies of the past decades. The growing challenge has since been interpretation and characterization of the many hills. However, these studies all show that multiple genes within core signaling pathways, rather than single genes, tend to be mutated in these cancers, suggesting an avenue for treating tumors based on aberrant pathways instead of individual aberrant genes.

Following these landmark studies, the number, breadth, and size of cancer genome projects rapidly accelerated in keeping with the advent of massively parallel sequencing. The first cancer whole genome sequences generated by massively parallel sequencing were those of two lung cancers published in 2008[107] followed shortly by those of individual AML cases published in 2008 and 2009.[122,123] These studies focused on assessment of genome-wide SVs and missense mutations, respectively. The first analysis of paired primary and metastatic tumors enabling genome-wide assessment of evolution was conducted in breast cancer in 2009, identifying both shared and exclusive mutations in each sample.[124] The first studies to systematically assess genome-wide mutations of all classes, published in 2010, were conducted in the melanoma cell line COLO-829[125] and a small cell lung cancer cell line.[126] These studies uncovered an extraordinary mutation burden (over 33,000 mutations in melanoma and 23,000 in lung) and mutational signatures supporting ultraviolet (UV) radiation etiology and tobacco smoke etiology in melanoma and lung, respectively. Discovery has since continued at a rapid pace and, as discussed later, large genomic analyses having been completed in all common cancers, many rare cancers, primary/recurrent/metastatic matched cohorts, and even cancers undergoing treatment.

Large-scale cancer genomic studies have also been powered by national and international consortia. The US National Cancer Institute (NCI) and National Human Genome Research Institute (NHGRI) launched a large collaborative project in 2005, the Cancer Genome Atlas (TCGA; see http://cancergenome.nih.gov/). Using

multiple state-of-the-art genomic technologies to comprehensively identify all genomic alterations associated with multiple cancer types, the TCGA effort began with large pilot studies of glioblastoma multiforme[65] ovarian cancer,[127] and squamous cell lung cancer.[128] TCGA studies have since included colorectal,[129] breast,[130] endometrial,[131] AML,[132] clear cell renal cell,[133] expanded glioblastoma,[134] urothelial bladder,[135] lung adenocarcinoma,[136] gastric,[137] chromophobe renal cell,[138] papillary thyroid,[139] head and neck squamous cell,[140] low-grade glioma,[141] cutaneous melanoma,[142] and a suite of 18 pan-cancer studies.[143] Across 34 cancer types, data have been collected from more than 11,000 cases. Similarly ambitious studies have been undertaken by members of the International Cancer Genome Consortium (ICGC; see http://icgc.org)[144] launched in 2010 to comprehensively catalog all genomic aberrations associated with at least 50 different cancers. This consortium currently encompasses 55 projects covering 33 cancer types with over 13,000 donors and has produced publications on bisulfite sequencing techniques,[145,146] DLBCL,[147] Burkitt lymphoma,[148] X chromosome hypermutation,[149] signatures of mutational processes,[150] and primary CNS lymphoma.[151] The ultimate success of these comprehensive, large-scale projects will continue to rapidly advance our understanding of cancer genetics and genomics and will potentially revolutionize our approach to the diagnosis and treatment of cancer.

Cancer genomic data repositories and analysis tools

Data generated by the TCGA, ICGC, and other curated genomic repositories are publicly available. Systematic analysis of these data remains challenging, but improved web-based tools for both novices and experienced bioinformaticians are greatly democratizing cancer genomics research (Table 2). One of the oldest and most comprehensive resources for mining such data is the Catalogue of Somatic Mutations in Cancer (COSMIC; see http://www.sanger.ac.uk/genetics/CGP/cosmic) maintained by the Wellcome Trust Sanger Institute Cancer Genome Project.[152] COSMIC is manually curated from publications and therefore entails a broad reach across targeted studies and genome projects (currently more than 20,000). The current build (August 2014) describes over

Table 2 Cancer genomics databases.

Name	Detail	Link
canEvolve	Analysis of mRNA, miRNA, protein expression, and CNV data in 10,000 patient samples from TCGA, GEO, and Array Express	www.canevolve.org
canSAR	Integrated analysis of biological, chemical, and pharmacological data from COSMIC, chEMBl, UniProt, BindingDB, Array Express, and STRING	https://cansar.icr.ac.uk
cBioPortal	TCGA data portal; graphical visualization and analysis	http://www.cbioportal.org
CGAP	Graphical summary and analysis of gene expression; integration of cytogenetic data	http://cgap.nci.nih.gov
CGHub	Secure, comprehensive data repository; TCGA, CCLE, and TARGET projects	https://cghub.ucsc.edu
CPRG	Integrative analysis tools for cancer research	http://www.broadinstitute.org/software/cprg
COSMIC	Largest genomics data repository; manually curated publications and output from large sequencing studies	http://www.sanger.ac.uk/genetics/CGP/cosmic
EBI Array Express	Annotated functional genomics data; data generated via microarray and high-throughput sequencing projects	http://www.ebi.ac.uk/microarray-as/ae
EGA	Comprehensive data repository; restricted access; ICGC output; SNV and CNV data	https://www.ebi.ac.uk/ega
GDAC	Pipelines for genomic analysis; user-friendly interface	http://gdac.broadinstitute.org
GEO	Gene expression microarray and functional genomics data repository	http://www.ncbi.nlm.nih.gov/geo
ICGC	Visualization tool; genomic, transcriptomic, and epigenomic characterization of 50 tumor types	http://dcc.icgc.org
MethylCancer	Methylation database; interprets the correlation of methylation, gene expression, and cancer biology	http://methycancer.psych.ac.cn
SomamiR	Archive of experimentally validated somatic mutations in noncoding RNA	http://compbio.uthsc.edu/SomamiR
UCSC Cancer Genome Browser	Multipurpose data viewer incorporating multiple data types including clinical information	https://genome-cancer.soe.ucsc.edu

2 million mutations in more than 1 million samples encompassing 12,000 cancer genomes. In addition to SNVs, it details over 6 million noncoding mutations, 10,000 fusions, 61,000 SVs, 700,000 CNVs, and 60 million expression variants. These data are easily queried using key words or by gene or cancer type. COSMIC also includes more advanced tools that are in some cases linked to other databases. These include a detailed census of all human genes that have been causally linked to tumorigenesis (Cancer Gene Census; see http://www.sanger.ac.uk/genetics/CGP/Census)[5,153] as well as tools to assess mutation signatures and drug sensitivity. Another highly versatile data portal is the cBioPortal for Cancer Genomics maintained by Memorial Sloan-Kettering Cancer Institute.[154] This portal primarily contains highly processed Cancer Cell Line Encyclopedia (CCLE) and TCGA data sets but also provides a powerful, intuitive web interface enabling queries by gene or cancer type as well as more advanced analysis through an application programming interface and also integration with R and MATLAB. A similar portal is available for ICGC data (see http://dcc.icgc.org).

While the above-mentioned portals enable advanced analysis with only modest bioinformatics training, additional repositories exist for advanced users to access various levels of raw data. The Cancer Genomics Hub (CGHub), hosted by the University of California Santa Cruz (UCSC), is a secure central repository for data generated through the NCI including TCGA, CCLE, and Therapeutically Applicable Research to Generate Effective Treatments (TARGET).[155] The European Genome-phenome Archive (see http://ega.crg.eu) similarly collects and distributes sequencing and genotyping data, primarily cancer data emerging from the ICGC. Data repositories and analysis tools are also available for other data types. Cytogenetic aberrations and fusions observed in over 65,000 human tumors have been compiled and are maintained online (The Mitelman Database of Chromosome Aberrations in Cancer at the US National Cancer Institute [NCI] Cancer Genome Anatomy Project [CGAP] Web site: http://cgap.nci.nih.gov).[28] Data from numerous gene expression microarray studies are warehoused by multiple entities, including the US National Center for Biotechnology Information (NCBI Gene Expression Omnibus; see http://www.ncbi.nlm.nih.gov/geo/) and the European Bioinformatics Institute (EBI Array Express; see http://www.ebi.ac.uk/microarray-as/ae/). Additional data repositories and web resources are outlined in Table 2.

The vast and varied landscapes of human cancers

Although few new mutational "mountains" have been discovered in the past 10 years, systematic study of cancer genomes has revealed many new "hills" as well as mutational processes and dysregulated pathways. The total mutation burden itself can reflect cancer etiology and have bearing on clinical course. This burden is much more variable than originally anticipated. In some pediatric cancers such as rhabdoid tumors[156] and small cell carcinoma of the ovary,[157] cases with only a single coding SNV have been discovered, while leukemias such as AML bear a median of nine coding SNVs (Figure 4). Conversely, cancers with mutagenic etiology such as bladder, lung, and melanoma bear high mutation rates with medians of 148, 217, and 254 coding SNVS, respectively, while tumors with mismatch repair defects can contain thousands of coding SNVs. Distinct mutational signatures can also reflect these external and internal mutagenic factors such as enrichment for C > T transition in dipyrimidines as seen in cancers from UV-damaged sites.[150] Overall, coding SNVs are generally more common in cancers than coding CNVs and SVs, although broad variability in CNV and SV profiles also exists across cancer types. Thirty-seven percent of cancers experience whole-genome doublings with a quarter of most

solid tumor genomes containing large-scale chromosomal variations and 10% containing focal CNVs. Over 140 genomic regions have been found to contain recurrent CNVs, only 38 of which contain known cancer genes.[158-160] Most solid tumors also contain dozens of SVs although many of these occur in regions that do not contain genes and are likely passengers. Whole genome sequencing has also recently uncovered "chromothripsis" events, occurring in 2–3% of cancers when errors in chromosome segregation during mitosis lead to shattering of a single or a few chromosomes and massive rearrangement in a single cell generation.[161-163]

In addition to mutagenic etiology, variability in mutation burden is the likely result of mutation timing, patient age, and the number of divisions that have occurred in precursor cells with mutations accumulating in dividing cells over time, although a "punctuated evolution" model has also been proposed.[164-166] Ultimately, only a few such mutations can "drive" cancer (driver mutations) insofar as they confer a selective growth advantage on the cells that carry them. Other mutations are "passengers" with no phenotypic effect on cell growth.[167] Several methods have been developed to classify mutations as drivers or passengers based on the pattern and frequency with which they arise across cancers,[4,168,169] but experimental validation is required to confirm the role of these mutations in cancer.

It has been estimated that more than 138 cancer driver genes exist[4] with 571 genes causally implicated in cancer catalogued in the Cancer Gene Census (see http://cancer.sanger.ac.uk/census).[5] The top 10 most commonly mutated cancer genes are given in Table 3, while cancer genes associated with the most lethal cancers in the United States are given in Table 4. While this vast array of mutations may seem overwhelmingly complex, particularly from the therapeutic perspective, there is nonetheless some hope. For example, dramatic clinical responses are seen with agents targeting mutant proteins in highly complex cancers such as mutant BRAF and ALK in melanoma and lung cancer.[194,195] Further, multiple cancer genes often converge on an individual pathway and may be functionally equivalent. Thus, specific pathways may collectively be subject to genomic aberrations at a frequency far higher than any of their individual gene components. Indeed, most driver genes converge on the hallmark pathways and can ultimately be reduced to those impacting cell differentiation, cell proliferation, cell death, and genomic maintenance.[2] Thus, the integration of multiple types of genomic data will clearly be necessary to unravel the complexity of somatic cancer genetics.

While it seems possible that the majority of cancer genes have now been discovered, new genes are occasionally implicated in cancer, although at low frequency across many cancer types or at high frequency in a rare and previously uncharacterized cancer. However, most cancers require 5–8 driver mutations based on epidemiological studies[196] and only 3–6 drivers have been found in most cancers with notable exceptions (such as pediatric cases) in which three or fewer drivers have been discovered.[4] Remaining knowledge gaps are likely due to both technical limitations of sequencing technology and study design as well as limitations in our growing understanding of mutations occurring in noncoding regions of DNA or through epigenomic mechanisms. Clearly, the catalogue of cancer-driving mutations is still incomplete and although the maps of cancer genome landscapes have been broadly charted, much work remains to characterize these vast landscapes in detail in order to guide clinical cancer management.

Clinical implications of cancer genome landscapes

Exhaustive information now available from cancer genomics projects has greatly improved our comprehension of the development, progression, and clinical behavior of human neoplasms. These

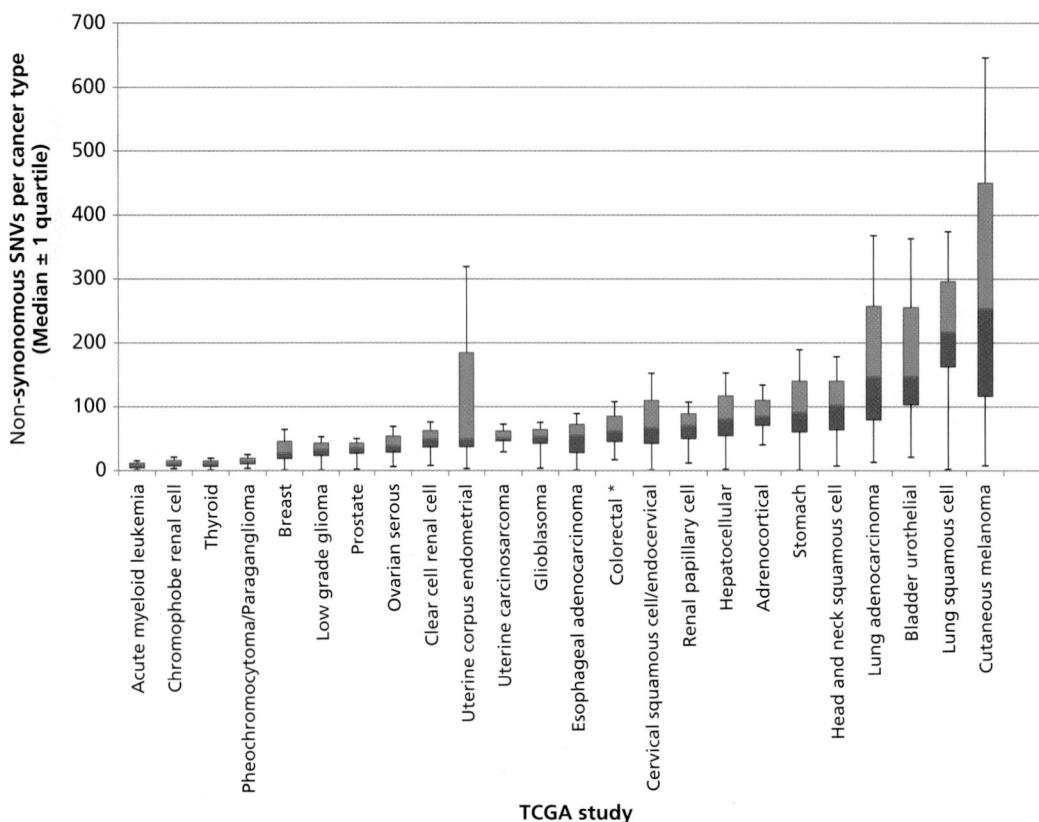

Figure 4 Number of coding single nucleotide variants (SNVs) per tumor type across a selection of human cancers. DNA sequencing data obtained from published TCGA studies were used to calculate the distribution and median number of coding SNVs mutations in each cancer type. Colored bars indicate the 25% and 75% quartiles. Outlier values (values below Q1 − 1.5 × IQR or above Q3 + 1.5 × IQR) are not shown and asterisks represent studies with more than 10% outliers.

Table 3 Ten most commonly mutated oncogenes and tumor suppressor genes (TSG) in the COSMIC database.

Gene	Classification[a]	SNVs in COSMIC	Homozygous deletions (TSGs) or amplifications (oncogenes) in COSMIC[b]	Fusions in COSMIC
TP53	TSG	28,253	17	1
NPM1	TSG	5224	1	319
CDKN2A	TSG	4836	1046	0
APC	TSG	4351	10	0
PTEN	TSG	3296	275	0
VHL	TSG	2443	2	0
TET2	TSG	2085	3	0
NOTCH1	TSG	2009	12	0
NF2	TSG	1076	12	0
CEBPA	TSG	706	3	0
JAK2	Oncogene	42,963	109	35
BRAF	Oncogene	41,637	105	625
KRAS	Oncogene	32,021	231	1
EGFR	Oncogene	24,189	646	0
FLT3	Oncogene	15,789	102	0
IDH1	Oncogene	8508	11	0
PIK3CA	Oncogene	7983	425	0
KIT	Oncogene	7413	106	0
CTNNB1	Oncogene	5372	12	22
NRAS	Oncogene	4278	31	0

[a]Oncogene and TSG status were determined by the 20/20 rule[4] using sample data in the COSMIC database (see http://www.sanger.ac.uk/genetics/CGP/cosmic/).
[b]Amplifications shown for samples in which average genome ploidy ≤ 2.7 and total gene copy number ≥ 5 or average genome ploidy > 2.7 and total gene copy number ≥ 9. Homozygous deletions shown for samples in which the average genome ploidy ≤ 2.7 and total gene copy number = 0 or average genome ploidy > 2.7 and total copy number < (average genome ploidy − 2.7).

Table 4 Commonly mutated cancer genes in the deadliest cancers.

Cancer[a]	Familial cancer genes	Common somatically mutated genes	References
Breast	BRCA1, BRCA2, PTEN, TP53	PIK3CA, TP53, MAP3K1, GATA3, MLL3, CDH1, PTEN, ERBB2, MAP2K4, CDKN2A, PTEN, RB1	62,121,130,170–172
Colorectal	APC, MSH2, MLH1, MSH6, PMS2, MUTYH, LKB1, SMAD4, BMPR1A, PTEN, KLLN	APC, TP53, KRAS, PIK3CA, FBXW7, SMAD4, TCF7L2, NRAS, ARID1A, SOX9, FAM123B, ERBB2, IGF2, NAV2, TCF7L1	62,121,129,173,174
Liver	HFE, SLC25A13, ABCB11, FAH, HMBS, UROD	TP53, CTNNB1, AXIN1, RPS6KA3, RB1, FAM123A, CDKN2A, MYC, RSPO2, CCND1, FGF19, ARID1A, ARID1B, ARID2, MLL, MLL3	175–178
Lung	EGFR, BRAF, KRAS, TP53	TP53, KRAS, STK11, EGFR, ALK, BRAF, AKT1, DDR2, HER2, MEK1, NRAS, PIK3CA, PTEN, RET, ROS1, EML4, NTRK1, FHIT, FRA3B, FGFR1, HER2	57,75,116,118,126,128,136,179
Pancreatic	BRCA2, PALB2	KRAS, TP53, CDKN2A, SMAD4, MLL3, TGFRB2, ARID1A, SF3B1, ROBO2, KDM6A, PREX2	67,180–183
Prostate	BRCA2, BRCA1, HOXB13	EPHB2, ERG, TMPRSS2, PTEN, TP53, SPOP, FOXA1, MED12, NKX3-1	166,184–188
Ovarian	STK11, BRCA1, BRCA2	FBXW7, AKT2, ERBB2, TGFBR1, TGFBR2, BRAF, KRAS, PIK3CA, PTEN, ARID1A, BRCA1, MMP-1, BRCA1, BRCA2, MLPA, MAPH	127,189–192

[a]The seven cancers estimated to cause the greatest number of deaths in the United States in 2015.[193]

data and the technology used to generate them are also impacting cancer screening, diagnostics, and treatment. As sequencing costs continue to decline, exome- and genome-wide population screening becomes increasingly viable and it is likely that each patient's personal genome sequence will comprise a key component of their medical record. Such screening may reveal *de novo* mutations that would otherwise go undiagnosed until disease presentation and the power of this approach will grow exponentially as we continue to connect genetic variants to disease phenotypes. The NIH has acknowledged the importance of this new healthcare approach through the establishment of the Precision Medicine Initiative.[197] Targeted Sanger sequencing of small gene panels is already commonly used in familial cancer screening. In cases such as germline *BRCA1/2* or *MLH1/MSH2* mutations, which dramatically increase lifetime risk for breast/ovarian or colorectal cancer, genomic testing can guide clinical decisions about surveillance and prophylactic surgery. Now, NGS-based sequencing of hundreds of genes can be completed at a similar cost and thereby enable detection of lower penetrance rare variants not detectable with smaller panels. For example, in a study of 141 *BRCA1/2*-negative patients with a family or personal history of breast cancer, a panel of 40 additional genes identified 16 patients with pathogenic variants in nine genes other than *BRCA1/2* such as *TP53* and *PTEN*.[198] These findings have shaped new guidelines from the National Comprehensive Cancer Network recommending targeted panels for patients' breast or ovarian cancer family history who are negative for common hereditary mutations.[199] Targeted NGS panels have also shown greater sensitivity and specificity than traditional diagnostic tools in genetic testing of familial cancer genes such as *BRCA1/2*, *TP53*, and *APC* in additional studies.[170,200–202] NGS panels may also facilitate differential diagnosis and patient stratification given that the diagnostic yield of NGS panels, exomes, or even whole genomes has been shown in multiple studies to outperform small Sanger-based panels.[203,204]

Cancer genetics discoveries have driven targeted drug development since the first report of a recurrent chromosomal abnormality—the BCR-ABL translocation in CML. The selective tyrosine kinase inhibitor imatinib, designed to target the BCR-ABL chimeric fusion gene and its constitutively active tyrosine kinase protein product in CML, was the first successful targeted therapy.[205–207] The paradigm of targeting cancer-specific mutations to vastly improve the therapeutic index of chemotherapy has now been repeated with dramatic success. Examples include expansion of imatinib to *PDGFR*- and *KIT*-mutated gastrointestinal stromal tumors (GIST) and hypereosinophilic syndromes[208–210]; dasatinib and nilotinib in primary and imatinib-resistant CML[211–213]; trastuzumab, a neutralizing antibody targeted to the Her2/ErbB2 tyrosine kinase receptor whose encoding gene *ERBB2* is amplified and overexpressed in 25–30% of breast carcinomas[214,215]; sunitinib in renal cell carcinoma, GIST, and pancreatic neuroendocrine tumors[216–218]; gefitinib and erlotinib with striking efficacy in the 5–10% of lung adenocarcinoma patients with European ancestry and 25–30% of Japanese patients who harbor activating mutations in *EGFR*[219,220]; crizotinib in *ALK*-rearranged lung cancer[221,222]; vismodegib in basal-cell carcinoma bearing hedgehog pathway mutations[223]; and vemurafenib in *BRAF*-mutant melanoma.[224] Cancer gene mutations have also been associated with innate or acquired resistance to these targeted therapies. For example, amplification of the *BCR-ABL* gene is common in CML patients resistant to imatinib.[205,225] Preclinical studies and clinical trials are ongoing for numerous novel therapeutic agents directed against genomic targets in cancer in addition to agents capable of circumventing or treating drug-resistant disease.

The fundamental goal of oncology practice is recommendation of the most effective treatment supported by scientific evidence for an individual patient. Genomic data would be expected to provide just such data. However, although the HGP was completed in 2003, genomic medicine's entrance into the care stream has been painstakingly slow. In 2010, results from one of the first pilot studies using personalized molecular profiling to guide treatment selection in refractory metastatic cancer were published. Despite considerable challenges including the absence of a precedent for the novel trial design, overall patient attrition, and a diverse pharmacopeia, it was found that in 27% of 68 patients, treatment selection guided by molecular profiling (gene expression microarray analysis) resulted in a longer progression-free survival than that during the most recent regimen on which the patient had progressed.[226] The next major step in bringing genomic tools to the patient was a novel study combining whole genome sequencing and comprehensive RNA sequencing to individualize treatment of metastatic triple-negative breast cancer (TNBC) patients.[227] TNBC is characterized by the absence of expression of estrogen receptor (ER), progesterone receptor (PR), and HER-2. This study identified somatic mutations in the RAS/RAF/MEK and PI3K/AKT/mTOR signaling pathways that have led to clinical trials combining agents targeting MEK and mTOR genes with encouraging results.

New trial designs, such as those above and including adaptive, basket, and umbrella trials, are aimed at extending individualized therapy to all cancer patients. Multiple large academic observational and interventional trials have now appeared in publication[228–233] or are ongoing (see http://clinicaltrials.gov). These include adaptive trials such as I-SPY 2 (Investigation of Serial Studies to Predict your therapeutic response with imaging and molecular analysis) in which treatment arms are modified in the course of the study based on patient response.[234] Basket trials such as the NCI MATCH trial assign patients with various advanced cancers to treatment baskets based on mutational profiles, then treat with agents matched to their tumor's mutations.[231] Umbrella trials are also ongoing in which multiple drugs are studied in a single disease. For example, the ongoing Stand Up To Cancer and the Melanoma Research Alliance Dream Team Clinical trial is assessing molecularly guided therapy in a single-histology patient population that lacks a universal therapeutic target—non-V600 *BRAF* metastatic melanoma. In a nontreatment pilot study (now a randomized treatment study), a combination of whole genome and whole transcriptome sequencing was used to identify molecular aberrations matched to an appropriate clinical treatment from a pharmacopeia comprised standard of care, FDA-approved and investigational agents.[230] The challenge of returning actionable information during a clinically relevant time period is considerable. This includes patient consent, tumor biopsy, quality DNA/RNA extraction, DNA- and RNA sequencing, data integration, report generation, and tumor board review to formulate a treatment plan (Figure 5). Streamlining this process will be critical to expansion of these tools beyond major academic research centers.

Large-scale genomic characterization of tumors in the context of clinical trials has allowed identification of predictive biomarkers—recurrent genomic alterations that identify patients most likely to benefit from a particular drug. These provide tremendous clinical value by allowing patient stratification to the most relevant treatment option and have been rapidly commercialized. A broadening array of sequencing tests that may aid in diagnosis and treatment decisions is available to oncologists and their patients. Over 100 academic centers and 50 commercial laboratories have made such tests available. Examples of such commercial tests are provided in Table 5. Although cost is still prohibitive for widespread use, expanded panel-, exome-, or whole genome-based sequencing will continue to transform screening and diagnostics in coming years. However, routine clinical use will not only require further cost reduction but also more comprehensive data supporting genomics-correlated clinical outcomes to illustrate the benefit of such testing and off-label drug use. Accordingly, commercial sequencing laboratories will need to acquire FDA and Medicare approval. These data will ensure that insurance companies will cover these tests. Promising signs already include the addition of procedural terminology codes and a preliminary list of 21 sequencing tests included in the fee schedule of the Centers for Medicare and Medicaid Services. Finally, germline genomic analysis (whether part of hereditary cancer testing or conducted in tumor-matched normal tissue) entails the high likelihood of incidental secondary findings of putatively pathogenic genomic variants with unclear disease association and therefore presents a challenge. Widespread controversy exists over the balance between patient autonomy and the perception that patients knowledge of this information would result in physical or mental harm.[235]

Unlike relative differences in mRNA or protein expression between tumor and normal tissue, somatic mutations in cancer genes are exclusive and specific markers of cancer cells. This fact has been recently leveraged to use cell-free tumor-specific DNA in plasma (ctDNA) as an accurate circulating biomarker of tumor burden. The value of ctDNA for monitoring tumor burden, treatment response, and recurrence was first recognized in colorectal cancer.[236] This study identified somatic mutations in patient tumors in recurrently mutated colorectal cancer genes (*TP53*, *PIK3CA*, *APC*, and *KRAS*) and retrospectively analyzed plasma samples using highly sensitive assays specifically design for each patient. The results showed ctDNA levels reflect changes in tumor burden during treatment when compared with imaging and carcinoembryonic antigen. The challenges in implementation of ctDNA as a routine biomarker for tumor monitoring include the need to identify somatic alterations in each patient, design of patient-specific molecular assays, and low abundance of mutations in circulation, particularly in early stages of disease. Another recent study used NGS of tumors and digital PCR and found ctDNA levels during treatment reflected disease progression in metastatic breast cancer.[237] In these results, ctDNA was found to be more responsive and applicable to the largest fraction of patients when compared with enumeration of circulating tumor cells or CA-125, a glycoprotein biomarker of breast cancer. Similar results supporting the role of serial analysis of ctDNA for monitoring tumor burden have been published for lung cancer,[238,239] melanoma,[240] and osteosarcoma.[241]

Advances in molecular methods including the use of high-depth noise-corrected targeted NGS assays are enabling the study of patients with localized, potentially resectable cancers.[242,243] Recent work in localized breast cancer shows ctDNA can predict post-operative recurrence of cancer a median of 8 months before tumors become detectable on imaging.[244] This study and additional papers describing ctDNA in localized cancers demonstrate novel opportunities for optimizing treatment of cancer with curative intent by individualizing therapeutic strategies.[245]

Prospective trials are needed to establish benefit of guiding clinical cancer management using ctDNA as a biomarker. Nevertheless, observational studies reported so far show superior performance of ctDNA to monitor tumor burden compared to a number of circulating tumor cell or glycoprotein biomarkers.[246] With some variations between cancer types, ctDNA has wide applicability across patients as shown in a recent comprehensive survey of 640 patients.[246] The same study found ctDNA was detectable in 55% of patients with potentially curable disease. These results suggest that improved molecular assays may enable detection of ctDNA in presymptomatic individuals with cancer, potentially leading to a screening test with higher specificity than traditional methods.[247–250]

Cancer evolution

The ability to sequence cancer genomes has shed light on the process of molecular evolution and its importance for understanding cancer biology and treatment. Although not new, historical consideration of this concept has largely been confined to a process of linear clonal evolution driving the development of an increasingly malignant cancer phenotype.[1] However, it is increasingly clear that cancer evolution generates tremendous heterogeneity by continuously generating clonal diversity. As a result, multiple related, but distinct clonal lineages may coexist within a single patient.[251] These lineages differ in their ability to progress and metastasize[252] as well as to respond to or resist therapy.[253] The implications of this complex, branched evolution model will be critically important for understanding cancer biology and developing better treatment approaches.

The cornerstone of cancer evolution lies in the accumulation of genomic mutations, ultimately impacting cellular phenotype.

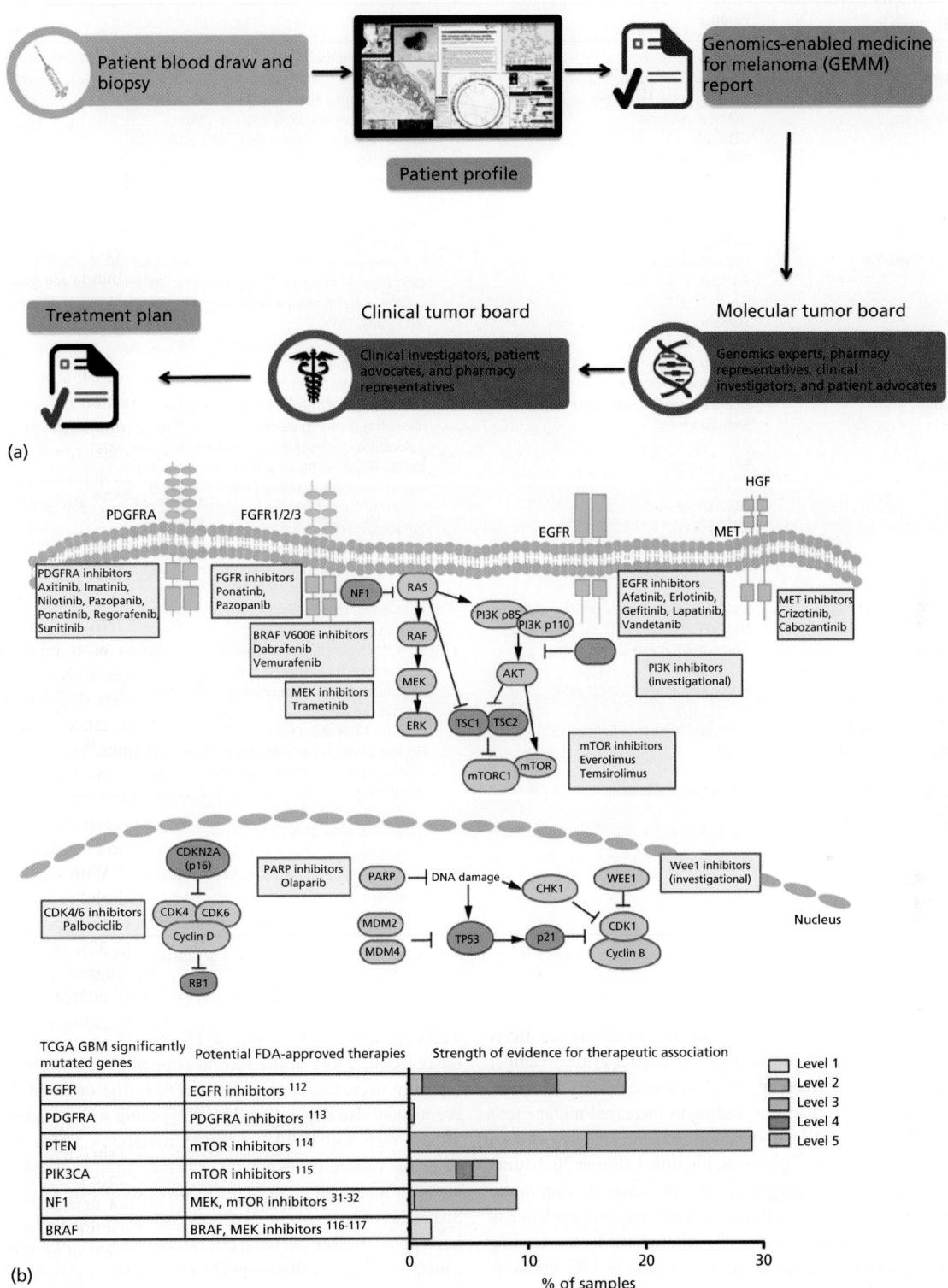

(a)

(b)

Figure 5 Precision Medicine clinical trials. (a) Process diagram depicting key steps from patient consent through molecular profiling and treatment plan generation. The entire process from biopsy to treatment plan is designed to be performed in less than 5 weeks. Source: From LoRusso, P et al. Pilot Trial of Selecting Molecularly Guided Therapy for Patients with Non-V600 BRAF-Mutant Metastatic Melanoma: Experience of the SU2C/MRA Melanoma Dream Team. Molecular Cancer Therapeutics. 2015 Aug 14(8): 1962–1971. Reprinted with permission. (b) Potential therapeutic implications of significantly mutated genes identified in the primary glioblastoma TCGA data set. (Top) Pathway representation of frequently altered pathways and selected potential therapeutic agents. (Bottom) Table of frequently mutated genes from TCGA mapped to potential FDA-approved therapeutic agents. (Right) Bar chart of level of evidence for the association between an alteration and therapeutic implication. Source: Prados 2015.[228] Reproduced with permission of Oxford University Press.

Table 5 Commercial cancer genome tests.

Provider	Product	Description[a]
Ambry Genetics	Exome Next	Full exome + mitochondrial genome, SNVs, CNVs
Ambry Genetics	*BRCA1* and *BRCA2* gene sequencing	SNVs, CNVs, *BRCA1/2* SVs
Arup Laboratories	Gastrointestinal hereditary cancer panel	15 genes + intron/exon junctions, SNVs, CNVs
Ashion Analytics	GEM Cancer Panel	562 genes, tumor/germline, SNVs, CNVs
	GEM GW	Whole exome, tumor/germline, SNVs, CNVs, SVs
	RNA sequencing	RNA, tumor/germline. Gene expression, fusions, alternative splicing, SNVs
Cancer Genetics Incorporated (CGI)	FOCUS:CLL	Seven actionable CLL targets
	FOCUS:Myeloid	54 genes, prognostic and therapeutic assessment
Caris	MI Profile	47 genes, SNVs
Foundation Medicine	Foundation One	236 genes, 47 introns from 19 genes associated with SV. SNVs, CNVs, SVs
	Foundation One Heme	405 genes, 31 introns associated with SV, and RNA-seq of 265 genes. SNVs, CNVs, SVs, fusions, and gene expression in hematologic tumors
GeneDx	XomeDx	Full exome, SNVs
	XomeDx Plus	Full exome + mitochondrial genome, SNVs
	XomeDx Slice	Targeted exome, SNVs
	Comprehensive cancer panel	29 genes, SNVs, CNVs
GPS@WUSTL	Comprehensive Cancer Gene Set Analysis	Sequencing of 42 genes. Mutation analysis
Agendia	Mammaprint	Microarray gene expression analysis of 70 genes. Predicts chemotherapy benefit and risk of recurrence of breast cancer
Myriad Genetics	BRACAnalysis	Sanger, *BRCA1/2*, breast and ovarian cancer risk
	COLARIS	Sanger, six genes, hereditary colorectal cancer
	COLARIS AP	Sanger, *APC* and *MYH* genes, adenomatous polyposis colon cancer risk
	MELARIS	Sanger, *CDKN2A*, hereditary melanoma
	PANEXIA	Sanger, *PALB2* + *BRCA2* genes, pancreatic cancer risk
	Myriad myRisk Hereditary Cancer	Sanger, 25 genes, breast, ovarian, gastric, colorectal, pancreatic, melanoma, prostate, and endometrial cancer risk
NeoGenomics Laboratories	NeoTYPE Cancer Exome Profile	4813 genes, identify SNVs
	NeoTYPE Profiles	Custom gene panels, SNVs
OncotypeDX	OncotypeDX Breast Cancer Assay	RT-PCR, 21 genes, gene expression, chemotherapy benefit, and likelihood of recurrence for invasive breast cancer
	OncotypeDX Colon Cancer Assay	RT-PCR, 18 genes, gene expression, recurrence risk in stage II and stage III colon cancer
	OncotypeDX Prostate Cancer Assay	RT-PCR <17 genes, gene expression, treatment selection for prostate cancer
Paradigm	PCDx	Number of genes not specified, DNA and RNA analysis, SNVs, CNVs, SVs, gene expression, fusions, alternative splicing
Personal Genome Diagnostics (PGDX)	Whole Genome Analysis	Whole genome, tumor or ctDNA and germline, SNVs, CNVs, SVs
	CancerXome	Full exome, SNVs, CNVs, SVs
	Cancer Select (R88, R203)	88 or 203 genes, SNVs, CNVs, SVs
	ImmunoSelect-R	Exome, ineoantigen prediction to asses utility of immunotherapy
	PlasmaSelect-R	58 genes in ctDNA, SNVs
Quest Diagnostics	OncoVantage	34 genes, SNVs

[a]These descriptions are derived from company web sites and may not be complete. They also do not constitute endorsement of any particular product.

Although the majority of acquired cancer mutations are likely to be passengers, a small proportion will impact critical cellular pathways and processes, thereby acting as disease drivers. However, the exact molecular mechanisms leading to increased mutagenesis in cancer are incompletely understood. Recent analysis, carried out on thousands of cancer genomes, identified at least 20 distinct mutational signatures pointing to diverse processes driving mutagenesis in various cancers, with most cancers showing evidence of more than one such process at play.[150] Although the factors leading to several identified mutational signatures such as UV, smoking, or exposure to chemotherapy agents are well known, many are not associated with a known causative processes. Elucidating such novel mechanisms of mutagenesis will be important for facilitating development of better prevention and treatment strategies.

The accumulation of mutations clearly provides the raw material (population diversity) for cancer evolution. However, this accumulation often contributes to the process of clonal evolution within temporal and spatial constrains. The order in which mutations are acquired can dramatically impact cell fate. For example, a loss of *BRCA1* or *BRCA2* leads to cell cycle arrest in the context of normal

TP53 but not in the setting of *TP53* loss.[254] Consistent with this observation, a loss of the second copy of *BRCA1* in breast cancer typically occurs after the loss of *TP53*. The order of mutational events may also depend on the cell type and state of differentiation. This is seen with *KRAS* or *NRAS* mutations, which occur early in colon cancer development, whereas similar *NRAS* mutations are seen mainly at a late stage in myelodysplastic syndrome.[255,256] Spatial constraints of clonal diversification, on the other hand, have been noted in clear cell renal cell carcinoma and non-small-cell lung cancer,[257,258] where divergent clones develop in specific geographic locations of the tumor. In fact, such spatial separation could lead to "parallel evolution" characterized by distinct mutations arising independently in individual clones, but targeting the same gene or the same pathway, as observed in a variety of cancers.[259] An important practical implication of such parallel evolution is that an effective targeted therapy would have to be capable of simultaneously inhibiting independent and molecularly distinct clones within a single patient.

Although clonal diversification is crucial, recent data indicates that simple outgrowth of the most aggressive clones does not fully account for the extent of clonal evolution in cancer. Indeed, similar to the principles of evolutionary biology in general, where no species evolves in isolation, cancers seem to evolve within an ecosystem of interactions not only with the host but also with other coexisting tumor clones. For example, in an experimental model of glioblastoma, a minor clone harboring an *EGFR* mutation appears to support the major *EGFR*-wt clone through paracrine mechanisms.[260] Similarly, within heterogeneous tumors in zebrafish melanoma xenograft models, a phenomenon of "cooperative invasion" is seen. Here, the presence of an invasive clone enables invasion by another, otherwise poorly invasive clone.[261] Such clonal cooperation does not only apply to tumor survival and progression but also extends into the realm of therapeutic resistance. In a model of colon cancer, for instance, the presence of an EGFR inhibitor-resistant, *KRAS*-mutated minor clone appears to support the survival of a drug-sensitive, *KRAS*-wt clone through paracrine mechanisms involving transforming growth factor α and amphiregulin.[253]

On the basis of the above-mentioned temporal and spatial constraints as well as clonal interactions, several models of clonal evolution have been proposed.[259] These range from (1) a simple model of linear evolution, where successive accumulation of mutations leads to increasingly aggressive clones that outcompete their predecessors, to (2) models of allopatric speciation, where subpopulations evolve in geographically distinct areas of the tumor, to the models incorporating clonal interactions including (3) a model of clonal competition with distinct clones competing for growth advantages in the form of antagonistic evolution and (4) a model of clonal cooperation with a symbiotic relationship between individual clones (Figure 6).

Understanding of the molecular spectrum and mechanisms of cancer evolution impacts our ability to treat cancer. Molecular heterogeneity and clonal evolution limit the benefits derived from targeted treatments. The repertoire of clones with distinct molecular signatures within each patient's tumor(s) allows for treatment-driven selection, manifesting as acquired therapeutic resistance even in patients who initially respond to treatment. Pre-existing somatic mutations (even passenger events) or new mutations acquired during therapy can drive therapeutic resistance. While improvements in experimental models have enhanced our ability to understand and perturb complex patterns of clonal evolution in the laboratory, development of methods such as ctDNA analysis in plasma can allow monitoring of clonal evolution in the clinic.[262] In patients who progress on targeted therapies, multiple studies have shown that somatic mutations driving resistance are detectable in plasma. For instance, lung cancer patients treated with erlotinib or gefitinib (an EGFR inhibitor) most often develop acquired treatment resistance owing to a second mutation in *EGFR* p.T790M that affects drug binding. This resistance-driving mutation is detectable in ctDNA up to 16 weeks before disease progression is evident on routine imaging.[239] Similar data has been reported for patients with colorectal cancer who progress on cetuximab (an anti-EGFR antibody) where *KRAS* mutations are evident weeks before disease progression.[263] A recent study of colorectal

(a) Linear evolution

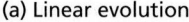

(b) Clonal separation (allopartic speciation)

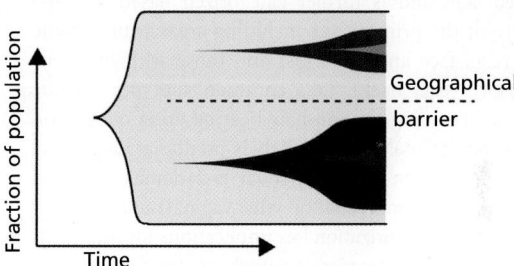

(c) Clonal competion (antaganonist evolution) (d) Clonal cooperation (symbiotic evolution)

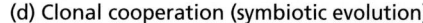

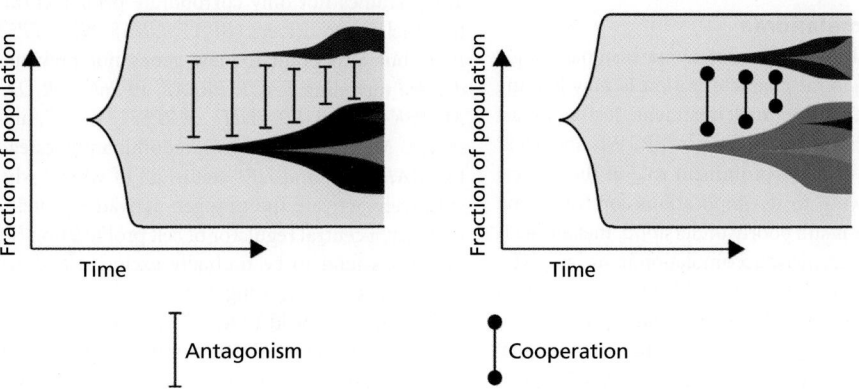

Figure 6 (a) Linear evolution involves sequential accumulation of mutations over time. As can be seen, linear evolution can result in heterogeneity if a subclone has failed to outcompete its predecessors. (b) Tumor subclones may evolve through a process equivalent to allopatric speciation when subclonal populations are geographically distinct within a tumor. (c) Clonal competition can occur between subclonal populations, where distinct subclones compete for growth advantages (equivalent to an antagonistic relationship). (d) Subclonal populations may cooperate, resulting in a symbiotic relationship. Source: McGranahan 2015.[259] Reproduced with permission of Elsevier.

cancer patients confirmed that if targeted therapy is discontinued upon disease progression (a drug holiday) and replaced with chemotherapy, circulating levels of the KRAS mutation in ctDNA recede (suggesting recession of KRAS-mutation bearing tumor subclone).[264] While these studies used deep targeted sequencing strategies to investigate hypothetical genes driving treatment resistance, hypothesis-free genome-wide analysis to discover novel drivers of treatment resistance has also been described.[265] These proof of principle results describing ctDNA analyses to track clonal evolution warrant investigation of ctDNA-based, personalized adaptive, sequential, or combination treatment strategies.

Cancer genomics and evolution in clinical practice: A case study in melanoma

Background

Malignant melanoma is the sixth most common cancer in the United States and is one of few that is increasing in incidence.[266] Although detection and surgical resection of early-stage disease can be curative, a tumor thickness of merely 4 mm portends metastatic disease and an abysmal prognosis. Dramatic recent progress in melanoma precision medicine powerfully illustrates the potential for genomics to impact clinical cancer management. In this section, we will focus on this progress and its impact on melanoma treatment while clinical features will be discussed in detail in Chapter 111. Melanoma is a disease of transformed melanocytes and is clinically subdivided by anatomic location, histopathology, sun exposure, and progression (using tumor-node-metastasis staging).[267] By site, cutaneous melanoma most commonly originates on sun-exposed skin and is further categorized based on type of sun exposure of the primary site including areas with chronic sun exposure (e.g., face and forearms) and those with intermittent sun exposure (e.g., back). Less common subtypes include acral melanoma, occurring on non-hair-bearing areas of skin on hands and feet; ocular melanoma, which is predominantly uveal with a smaller proportion of conjunctival melanomas; mucosal (nasopharyngeal, bowel, anorectal, or vulvovaginal) and primary CNS melanoma. This categorization has implications for prognosis and treatment, although it is sometimes unable to predict outcome or treatment response. Further, until the discoveries of the past decade, metastatic melanoma was uniformly treated with cytotoxic chemotherapy to limited effect.[268]

The genetic basis of melanoma

Where variation in clinical course by melanoma histopathologic subtype is confounding, genomic characterization is now helping to clarify etiology, biology, and optimal treatment. Just as breast cancer can best be characterized according to ER, PR, and Her2 status, genotype should now take a prominent role in the clinical approach to melanoma owing to its implications for treatment. Although melanomagenesis is still poorly understood, melanoma is known to occur through the stepwise accumulation in melanocytes of mutations in cancer genes (Figure 7).[269] Most melanomas are sporadic with 5–10% of cases due to familial predisposition predominantly driven by germline variants in the first familial melanoma gene identified—the tumor suppressor CDKN2A (40% of familial cases).[270-272] Additional rare variants in other cancer genes have since been found in familial cases (CDK4, BRCA2, BAP1, TERT promoter, MITF, and POT1).[273-278] Beyond heredity, UV radiation is recognized as the greatest risk factor for cutaneous melanomas, although not for sun-shielded mucosal, acral, or ocular

disease.[279] In keeping with UV etiology, additional melanoma risk factors include fair skin, increased freckling and benign nevi, MC1R germline variants, and tanning.[280-283]

Early genetic and functional characterization of melanoma determined that it is driven both by mutations that inactivate cell cycle gatekeepers and by those that activate cell proliferation pathways. Building on discovery of familial mutations in CDKN2A, a locus that regulates the p53 and RB proteins, these tumor suppressors were found to be frequently disrupted by disparate mutations that enable unconstrained cell growth such as CDKN2A, CDK4, RB1, TP53, and MDM2 mutations.[284-288] Meanwhile frequent mutations in the proliferation pathway genes BRAF, KIT, NRAS, and PTEN were identified and found to cooperate with inactivation of cell cycle tumor suppressors to promote malignancy.[115,119,289-302] Cytogenetic and molecular studies further pointed to as-yet unidentified genes in recurrently altered regions of chromosomes 1p, 6q, 7p, and 11q.[288,303-311] As with many early genetic analyses of human cancers, these studies were typically performed in disparate small cohorts or model systems, focused on only one or several genes in a single clinical subtype, and often produced inconclusive results.

Melanoma genomic landscapes

The striking genetic complexity between subtypes and within individual tumor genomes revealed by the above analyses was soon confirmed at high resolution through a succession of genomic studies. Genome-wide aCGH profiling and targeted sequencing of BRAF and NRAS in 126 tumors first revealed distinct patterns of somatic mutation based on subtype. BRAF and NRAS mutations were found to be enriched in intermittently sun-exposed and cutaneous melanoma but rare in chronically sun-exposed, mucosal, and acral melanoma. Patterns of mutation also varied by subtype with CNVs enriched in mucosal melanoma. Subsequent analyses identified patterns of CNV correlating with poor prognosis[49,289] as well as subtype-specific KIT mutations occurring in 10–20% of mucosal and acral as well as at low frequency in cutaneous melanoma in sun-damaged sites.[48,312] The existence of molecular subsets of disease was also borne out by gene expression microarray studies[84,313,314] and such molecular subsetting of clinical melanoma categories seeded hope that these types could be tied to clinical outcome or exploited for therapeutic targeting.[315]

A spate of massively parallel sequencing studies beginning in 2011 spurred explosive growth in the genomic understanding of cutaneous melanoma, recently culminating in two large multiplatform studies that jointly span over 500 cases.[142,275,315-325] These studies not only corroborate prior identification of important melanoma drivers (BRAF, NRAS, NF1, TP53, CDKN2A, and RB1) but also point to new genes not previously linked to the disease including RAC1, PREX2, PPP6C, ARID2, TACC1, GRM3, MAP3K4, MAP3K9, IDH1, MRPS31, RPS27, and the TERT promoter. Melanoma is now predominantly categorized according to BRAF, RAS, and NF1 status, all of which, when mutated, constitutively activate the mitogen-activated protein kinase (MAPK) pathway, a central regulator of cell proliferation (Figure 8).[142] These mutations tend to be mutually exclusive and account for all but 10% of cases, suggesting four genomic subtypes: BRAF, NRAS, NF1, and triple wild type (TWT). Genome-wide sequencing has also enabled characterization of mutation signatures in melanoma, shedding further light on the role of UV radiation in various subtypes. Melanomas on sun-exposed skin are characterized by UV signature mutations—cytosine to thymine (C > T) substitutions occurring in dipyrimidines as more than 60% of the total mutation burden.[142,318,326] Curiously, most common mutations in BRAF and NRAS are not C > T substitutions despite their driver roles in the

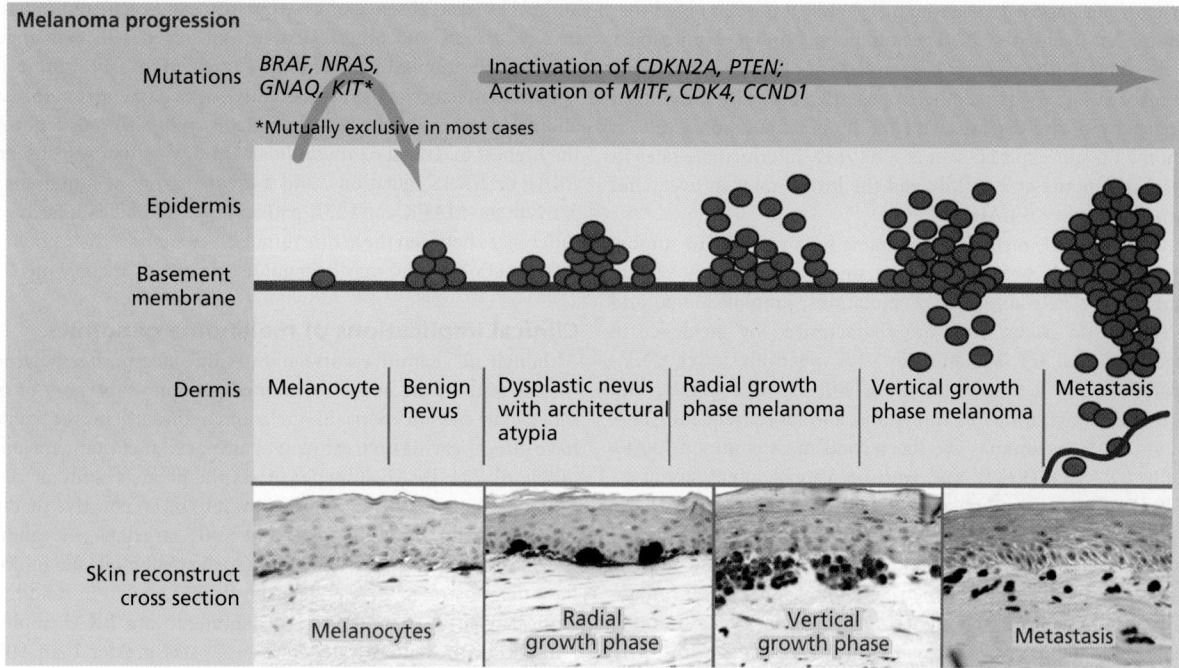

Figure 7 The genetic basis of cutaneous melanoma. Melanoma, the deadliest of skin cancers, is caused by the transformation of melanocytes (pigment-producing cells) that accumulate genetic alterations, leading to abnormal proliferation and dissemination. Clinically, melanoma lesions can be classified based on location and progression, ranging from benign nevi to metastatic melanoma. Important driver genes in melanomas are shown in the figure. MAPK signaling is often constitutively activated through alterations in membrane receptors or through mutations of RAS or BRAF. Source: Vultur 2013.[269] Reproduced with permission of Elsevier.

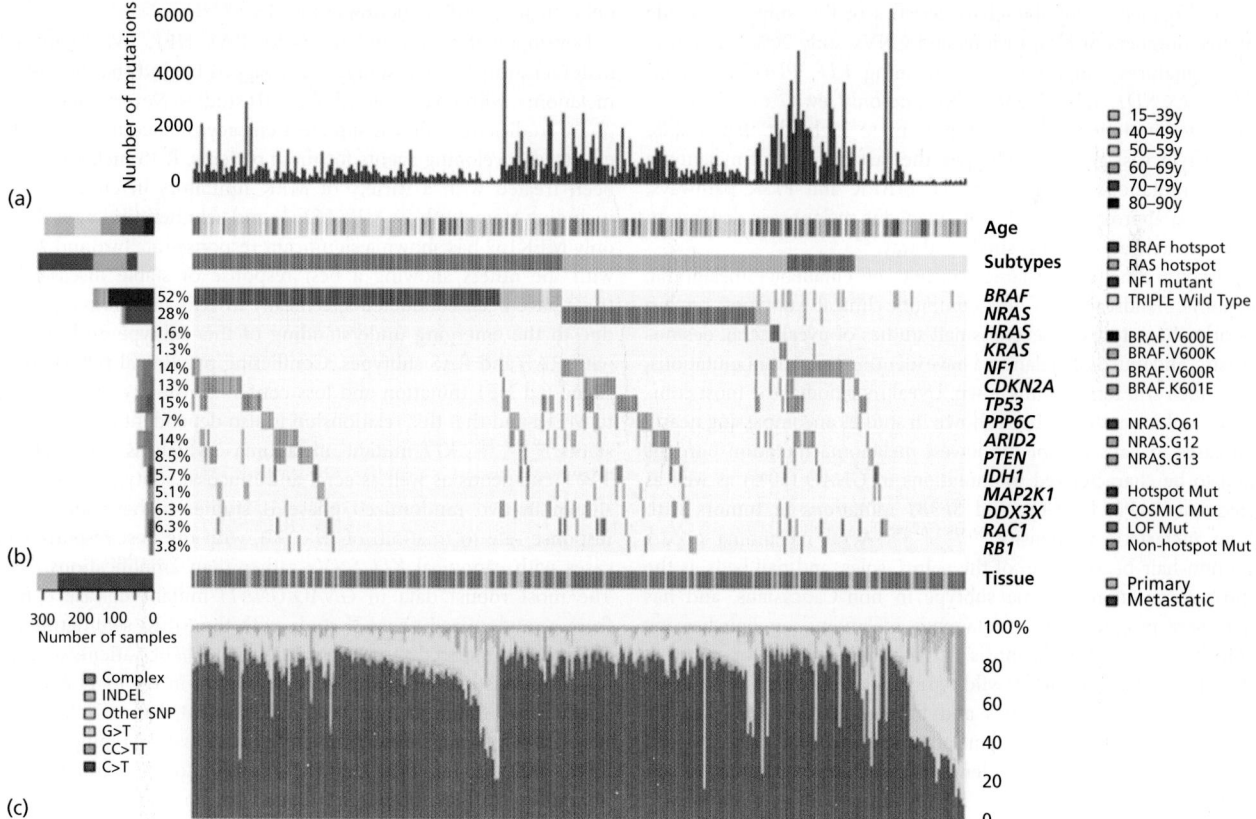

Figure 8 The genomic landscape of cutaneous melanoma. Total number of mutations, age at melanoma accession, and mutation subtype (BRAF, RAS [N/H/K], NF1, and Triple-WT) are indicated for each sample (a). (Not shown are one hypermutated and one co-occurring NRAS BRAF hot-spot mutant). Color-coded matrix of individual mutations (specific BRAF and NRAS mutations indicated) (b), type of melanoma specimen (primary or metastasis), and mutation spectra for all samples (c) are indicated. For the two samples with both a matched primary and metastatic sample, only the mutation information from the metastasis was included. Source: The Cancer Genome Atlas Network. 2015.[142] Reproduced with permission of Elsevier.

majority of sun-exposed melanomas.[317] While it is often noted that melanoma has the highest average mutational burden of any cancer type, the mutation frequency can range from 0.1–100 mutations per megabase.[169] This marked heterogeneity tracks with the clinical heterogeneity of the disease, with the highest mutational rate in melanoma on sun-exposed skin at >100/Mb, intermediate rates in mucosal melanoma at 2–5/Mb, and the lowest rates in uveal and CNS melanoma at <0.1/Mb.[316,327,328]

Cutaneous BRAF melanomas account for over 50% of tumors and predominantly bear the hotspot missense mutation V600E, although other activating *BRAF* mutations, amplifications, and even fusions do occur. They are characterized by incidence in younger patients, UV signature in 91%, relatively fewer CNVs compared to TWT, amplifications of *BRAF*, *MITF*, PD-1, and PD-L1, enrichment for *TP53* mutations, and more frequent *PTEN* deletions. RAS melanomas are the second most common (30%), typically *NRAS* Q61R/K/L and with occasional mutations in *K-* or *H-RAS*. These mutations are nearly always mutually exclusive with *BRAF* mutations although molecular features of this category otherwise resemble the BRAF subtype. NF1 melanomas comprise 15% of cases, the majority of which contain inactivating *NF1* mutation. This subtype bears the highest SNV burden, occurs in older patients, and contains a UV signature. It can co-occur with *BRAF* and *NRAS* mutations and tends to show a pattern of co-occurrence with other mutated "RASopathy" genes such as *RASA2*.[319] Similar to *BRAF* and *RAS* mutations, most NF1 mutations drive RAS and MAPK pathway activation. Finally, TWT melanoma is a heterogeneous subtype that lacks recurrent driver mutations although *KIT*, *CTNNB1*, *GNAQ*, *GNA11*, and *EZH2* mutations have been found at low frequency. Notable characteristics of this subtype include higher numbers of SVs, fusions and CNVs, only 30% containing UV signatures, amplifications containing *KIT*, *PDGFRA*, *KDR*, *CDK4*, *CCND1*, *MDM2*, and *TERT*, and only few (7%) with *TERT* promoter mutations.[142] It is important to highlight that despite diversity across genomic subtypes, the vast majority of melanoma driver mutations converge on the MAPK and PI3K pathways, such that approximately 91% of cutaneous melanomas depend on aberrant activation of this single pathway.[329]

Despite exhaustive characterization of cutaneous melanoma, genomic landscapes of less-common clinical subtypes remain poorly characterized. Several small studies of uveal, acral, desmoplastic, and mucosal melanoma have identified recurrent mutations, but much still remains unknown. Uveal melanoma, the most common ocular tumor, has been shown in studies encompassing nearly 80 cases to have one of the lowest melanoma mutation burdens and to be characterized by mutations in *GNAQ* (50%) as well as frequent *BAP1*, *EIF1AX*, and *SF3B1* mutations in tumors with high metastatic propensity.[324,325,330–332] Acral melanoma occurs on non-hair-bearing skin of the palms, soles, and nail beds, is the most common melanoma subtype in non-Caucasians, and has a poorer prognosis than cutaneous melanoma on hair-bearing skin owing to later diagnosis.[333] Although known for nearly a decade to be largely *BRAF* wild type, it is rarely included in larger cutaneous genomics studies and limited focused data sets are available. In total, 38 acral melanomas have been characterized across six studies that have identified the following characteristics: about 30% *KIT*-mutant, 20% *BRAF*-mutant, 10% *NRAS*-mutant, low SNV burden, high CNV and SV burden, and absence of UV signature.[49,316–318,332,334,335] Data on mucosal melanoma, another rare and aggressive subtype that is predominantly *BRAF* wild type, is more sparse with only 10 cases comprehensively assessed in a single study.[327] This study largely confirmed prior targeted and cytogenomic analyses, showing a low SNV frequency, high CNV

and SV burden, absence of UV signature, and recurrent mutations in *KIT*, *PTEN*, and other putative cancer genes in two or fewer samples. Desmoplastic melanoma, a rare and invasive fibrous form of dermal melanoma has also recently been characterized (62 cases) and preliminary results reveal a notably high SNV burden (one of the highest to date at 62 mutations/Mb), UV signatures, absence of *BRAF* or *NRAS* mutations, and a diverse array of mutations that activate the MAPK and PI3K pathways.[336] Notable similarities and differences between these rare tumor types support their potentially distinct etiology and may help guide therapeutic management.

Clinical implications of melanoma genomics

Although no definitive correlation with outcome has been identified based on the above-mentioned genomic subtyping or other molecular classifications in melanoma, these genomic subtypes have direct bearing on treatment of advanced metastatic melanoma (Table 6). The BRAF subtype carries the greatest array of clinical options. Mutant *BRAF* has now proven to be an effective therapeutic target, with *BRAF*V600E/K and K601 targetable by inhibitors of BRAF or MEK. As of 2015, three such small molecule inhibitors have demonstrated an overall survival (OS) benefit in randomized clinical trials. Vemurafenib and dabrafenib are BRAF inhibitors (BRAFi) with demonstrated response rates greater than 90% in BRAF melanoma.[224,337] Trametinib is a MEK inhibitor (MEKi) which, while less dramatically effective than BRAFi, nevertheless triples progression-free survival (PFS) versus chemotherapy.[338] The best results to date from trials of targeted agents in BRAF melanoma have come from combined BRAFi and MEKi with dabrafenib and trametinib, a combination with marked improvement in PFS and OS with an overall reduction in toxicity.[339,340]

Development of targeted agents for RAS, NF1, TWT, and rare histological melanoma subtypes has lagged behind that for BRAF melanoma, with no completed phase III studies. Nevertheless, early phase studies have shown sufficient efficacy to encourage ongoing efforts at developing agents for these patients. RAS melanoma has been treated with a variety of MEK inhibitors in clinical trials including trametinib,[341] MEK162,[342] and selumetinib.[343] Of these, only MEK162 has shown a significant response rate (around 20%), with the others showing a best response of stable disease. No trials have been conducted specifically in NF1 melanoma, in part due to the emerging understanding of this subtype and overlap with RAF and RAS subtypes. Conflicting preclinical reports have suggested NF1 mutation and loss confers sensitivity or resistance to MEKi and that this relationship is also dependent on RAF/RAS status.[319,344–346] *KIT*-mutant melanoma (which is common in TWT cutaneous as well as acral and mucosal subtypes) has been shown in two randomized phase II studies to have an overall response rate to imatinib of 19–29%, with the best responses in cases with canonical *KIT* SNVs rather than amplifications.[286,347] The most robust data in *GNAQ*/*GNA11*-mutant disease comes from a randomized phase II study with the MEKi selumetinib.[348] Selumetinib induced tumor regression in 49% of patients and led to a nonstatistically significant improvement in OS to 11.8 versus 9.1 months. Additional agents in development that are relevant to many subtypes and/or may motivate additional subtyping include CDK, MDM2, and PI3K/Akt/mTOR inhibitors in clinical trials in addition to ERK, IDH1, EZH2, and aurora kinase inhibitors in preclinical development.[142]

Little is known about the impact of genomics on immunotherapy. Immunotherapy with the CTLA-4 inhibitor ipilimumab and the PD1 inhibitors pembrolizumab and nivolumab have revolutionized melanoma care with long-term survival even in advanced disease, but the role of genomics as predictive or prognostic for

Table 6 Therapeutic options in melanoma by genomic subtype.

Genotype	Approved treatments	Selected phase I or II data
BRAF mutant	Targeted—vemurafenib, dabrafenib, and trametinib	Cobimetinib
	Immunotherapy[a]—ipilimumab, nivolumab, and pembrolizumab	
RAS mutant	Targeted therapy—none	Trametinib, MEK162
	Immunotherapy[a]—ipilimumab, nivolumab, and pembrolizumab	
NF1 mutant	Targeted therapy—none	None
	Immunotherapy[a]—ipilimumab, nivolumab, and pembrolizumab	
Triple wild type (TWT)[b]	Targeted therapy—none	None
	Immunotherapy[a]—ipilimumab, nivolumab, and pembrolizumab	
TWT — KIT mutant or overexpressed	Targeted therapy—none	Imatinib, nilotinib
	Immunotherapy[a]—ipilimumab, nivolumab, and pembrolizumab	
TWT — GNAQ/GNA11 mutant	Targeted therapy—none	Selumetinib, trametinib, MEK 162
	Immunotherapy[a]—ipilimumab, nivolumab, and pembrolizumab	

[a]Phase III studies for immunotherapy have not included genotyping beyond BRAF. FDA approval for these does not specify genotype and thus is inclusive of all genotypes.
[b]No trials to date have specifically identified TWT patients, although KIT and GNAQ/GNA11 cases do occur in this category.

immunotherapy remains to be fully elucidated.[349–351] While there is interest in mutational burden as a predictor of response to immunotherapy based on the hypothesis that immunogenicity is a probabilistic aggregate that increases in proportion to total mutation burden, to date no prospective data bears this out. While the hypothesis is supported by the fact that PD1 inhibitors were first approved in melanoma and then lung cancer (the two cancers with the highest mutational burdens), renal cell carcinoma has a very low mutational burden but has demonstrated responsiveness to PD1 inhibitors in phase II studies. Only a minority of patients on the registration studies for pembrolizumab and nivolumab had noncutaneous melanoma and ocular melanomas were excluded. While 20–35% of patients had *BRAF* V600 mutations, genotyping was not routinely done so that the rate of *NRAS* mutant and TWT patients is unknown.

Drug resistance and evolution in melanoma

Despite the activity of targeted agents in BRAF melanoma, drug resistance (both innate and acquired) remains a key challenge. Only about 50% of patients respond to BRAFi and in those who do respond, acquired resistance to BRAFi invariably develops.[224] BRAFi resistance is driven by a diverse range of mechanisms, most of which reactivate MAPK activity or redirect proliferative signaling through the PI3K pathway. Resistance can occur through further mutation in *NRAS*,[352] *MEK1*,[353,354] *MEK2*,[354] *NF1*,[344] or *BRAF* (via amplification).[355] *BRAF* splice variants,[356] *EGFR* activation,[357,358] and *COT* activation[359] have also been implicated. Activation of other receptor tyrosine kinases such as *PDGFR-β* and *IGF-1R* or loss of *PTEN* has also been demonstrated in laboratory models.[354,360–364] Clinical trials are ongoing to test whether identification of these resistance mechanisms in the clinical setting will allow for targeted therapeutic approaches that may circumvent resistance to BRAFi. Hypothetical approaches to circumvent specific resistance mechanism after progression on dual inhibition with BRAFi and MEKi are given in Table 7.

With the recent approval of new targeted and immunologic therapies for metastatic disease, it is now critically important that the clinician clearly identify the genetic signature of the patient's disease in order to optimize outcomes. Similarly, genomic testing can accelerate new drug development and target identification for the less common subtypes of melanoma and potentially lead to identification of resistance pathways to guide drug selection in individual patients. Thus, the genomic landscape of melanoma conforms to the clinical heterogeneity of the disease, with melanomas of different locations having markedly different genotypic signatures that speak

Table 7 Hypothetical treatment approaches to acquired BRAFi/MEKi resistance.

Mechanism of resistance	Therapeutic strategy
EGFR activation	EGFR inhibitor—erlotinib, gefitinib, afatinib, and dasatinib PIK3 inhibitor—in trials
IGF-1R activation *PTEN* loss *PTEN* mutation PIK3CA activation	PIK3Ca inhibitor—in trials
cMET activation	cMET inhibitor—crizotinib
PDGFR-β activation	RTK inhibitor—dasatinib, sunitinib
FGFR activation	FGFR inhibitors—ponatinib, dasatinib
COT activation	ERK inhibitor—in trials

to distinct etiologies. The challenge, then, is to use available genomic technologies in a real time clinical setting. In theory, one could identify the evolutionary mechanisms active in the individual patient to guide treatment selection.

In addition to molecular diversity across melanoma subtypes and even between individual patients with the same disease subtype, a higher order of complexity is becoming apparent. As outlined in the previous section on cancer evolution, recent data indicates that development of melanoma cannot be fully explained by a linear model of accumulating mutations leading to an increasingly aggressive phenotype. Instead, an emerging picture points to cancer as a complex ecosystem driven by the process of branched clonal evolution. As a result, multiple related, but distinct clonal lineages may exist within a single patient,[251] with some lineages being more likely to progress and metastasize.[252] Furthermore, this diversity may provide an escape mechanism leading to therapeutic resistance. This is well illustrated by almost universal development of resistance to BRAF inhibition in melanoma, where rapidly relapsing disease can harbor multiple resistance mechanisms differing between individual subclones even within a single patient.[365] This challenge is potentiated by the fact that, while some mechanisms of resistance are driven by mutations, others appear to be mediated through epigenetic or posttranslational processes.[366] The obvious and critical question raised by these observations is whether a single tumor biopsy in a metastatic setting can capture the full spectrum of disease heterogeneity, its drivers, and potential therapeutic targets. The solution to this conundrum may lie in approaches with the potential to monitor the clonal complexity on a larger scale, such as "liquid biopsies" that attempt to molecularly characterize circulating tumor DNA in the patient's bloodstream. Emerging data describing detection of ctDNA and concordance of BRAF mutation status between tumor and plasma samples is encouraging.[246,367,368] In addition, anecdotal evidence suggests that serial ctDNA analysis may be a useful marker of treatment response to immunotherapy.[240]

Summary

Detailed characterization of the genomic lesions underlying cancer has led to identification of biological pathways driving tumorigenesis, improved cancer diagnosis through molecular classification, enhanced selection of therapeutic targets for drug development, promoted the development of faster and more efficient clinical trials using targeted agents and sophisticated biomarkers, and created markers for early detection and recurrence surveillance. Yet, gaps nonetheless remain in our knowledge of the causative mutations underlying some cancers, in our understanding of the biology of the mutations we have identified, in developing drugs capable of targeting many of these diverse mutations, and in fending off the inevitable emergence of drug resistance. As summarized in this chapter, genomics has already made extraordinary contributions to our understanding of cancer biology and cancer medicine. Nevertheless, the enormous potential of cancer genomics has only just begun to be realized.

Acknowledgments

The authors thank the patients who have supported these studies. We also thank Matthew Taila and Victoria Zismann for assistance in preparation and proofreading of this chapter as well as Jeffrey Watkins for assistance in creation of figures. WPDH, AS, AHB, and JMT received research support from a Stand Up To Cancer—Melanoma Research Alliance/Melanoma Dream Team Translational Cancer Research Grant (SU2C-AACR-DT0612). Stand Up To Cancer is a program of the Entertainment Industry Foundation administered by the American Association for Cancer Research (AACR). WPDH, AS, PR, and JMT are supported by NIH R01CA195670. AS is additionally supported by the Pardee Foundation, NIH R01CA179157, and NIHR01CA185072. MM is additionally supported by a grant from the Science Foundation Arizona. JMT is additionally supported by the Komen Breast Cancer Foundation KG111063 and the Melanoma Research Alliance VUMC42693-R with additional generous support from The Entertainment Industry Foundation, Dell, Inc. through the Dell Powering the Possible Program, and Yale Cancer Center's UM1 CA186689.

Glossary

Array comparative genomic hybridization (CGH)	Microarray platform optimized to identify genome-wide DNA copy number changes.
Chromothripsis	Phenomenon by which extensive chromosomal rearrangements occur in a single event in one or a few chromosomes.
Copy number variant (CNV)	Change in DNA copy number such as amplification or deletion relative to a reference sequence.
Driver mutation	A mutation that confers a selective growth advantage on the cell in which it occurs.
Epigenomics	Global study of epigenetic changes throughout the genome.
Exome sequencing	Application of NGS for the parallel sequencing of many exons (coding areas of the genome).
Fluorescence *in situ* hybridization (FISH)	Cytogenetic technique for detecting specific DNA sequences on chromosomes using fluorescent probes.
Gene expression array	Oligonucleotide microarray platform designed to probe for the transcriptome-wide abundance of RNA messages.
Genomics	Study of the structure, function, evolution, and sequence of genomes.
Germline mutation	Mutation in the germ cell lineage present in all cells of the body and transmitted to offspring.
Loss of heterozygosity	Loss of the normal, functional allele at a heterozygous locus via deletion or other mutational event.
Massively parallel sequencing (also known as next generation sequencing or NGS)	High-throughput sequencing methodologies based on simultaneous sequencing of large numbers of genes or entire genomes.
Mutational hills	Mutations that occur at low frequency.
Mutational mountains	Mutations such as BRAF V600E that are frequent in a single cancer type or across multiple cancer types.
Single nucleotide polymorphism (SNP) array	Microarray platform that probes for genome-wide SNPs used to characterize allelic variation, LOH, or CNVs in cancers.
Oncogene	Gene that, when activated by mutations, promotes cancerous phenotype.
Passenger mutation	A mutation that does not confer a selective growth advantage to the cell in which it occurs.
Sanger sequencing	An approach for targeted DNA sequencing of individual genes or sets of genes using dideoxy chain termination and agarose gel electrophoresis.
Single nucleotide polymorphism (SNP)	Single nucleotide sequence difference occurring in germ lines of individuals across populations.
Single nucleotide variant (SNV)	Change in the DNA sequence relative to a reference sequence including point mutation and small insertions and deletions.
Somatic mutation	Mutation acquired somatically in a subset of cells (e.g., in a cancer).
Structural variant (SV)	Structural DNA changes such as rearrangements, translocations, inversions, etc.

| Transcriptomics | Study of all RNA transcripts in a cell or population of cells. |
| Tumor suppressor | A gene safeguarding cellular processes that, when inactivated, facilitates oncogenesis. |

Key references

The complete reference list can be found on the Wiley Companion Digital Edition of this title (see inside front cover for login instructions).

2 Hanahan D, Weinberg RA. Hallmarks of cancer: the next generation. *Cell.* 2011;**144**(**5**):646–674.

3 Fearon ER, Vogelstein B. A genetic model for colorectal tumorigenesis. *Cell.* 1990;**61**(**5**):759–767.

4 Vogelstein B, Papadopoulos N, Velculescu VE, Zhou S, Diaz LA, Kinzler KW. Cancer genome landscapes. *Science.* 2013;**339**(**6127**):1546–1558.

8 Jones PA, Baylin SB. The fundamental role of epigenetic events in cancer. *Nat Rev Genet.* 2002;**3**(**6**):415–428.

9 Calin GA, Croce CM. MicroRNA signatures in human cancers. *Nat Rev Cancer.* 2006;**6**(**11**):857–866.

25 Nowell P. A minute chromosome in human granulocytic leukemia. *Science.* 1960;**132**:1497.

27 Rowley JD. Letter: a new consistent chromosomal abnormality in chronic myelogenous leukaemia identified by quinacrine fluorescence and Giemsa staining. *Nature.* 1973;**243**(**5405**):290–293.

42 Pinkel D, Segraves R, Sudar D, et al. High resolution analysis of DNA copy number variation using comparative genomic hybridization to microarrays. *Nat Genet.* 1998;**20**(**2**):207–211.

71 Lander ES, Linton LM, Birren B, et al. Initial sequencing and analysis of the human genome. *Nature.* 2001;**409**(**6822**):860–921.

84 Bittner M, Meltzer P, Chen Y, et al. Molecular classification of cutaneous malignant melanoma by gene expression profiling. *Nature.* 2000;**406**(**6795**):536–540.

87 van't Veer LJ, Dai H, van de Vijver MJ, et al. Gene expression profiling predicts clinical outcome of breast cancer. *Nature.* 2002;**415**(**6871**):530–536.

107 Campbell PJ, Stephens PJ, Pleasance ED, et al. Identification of somatically acquired rearrangements in cancer using genome-wide massively parallel paired-end sequencing. *Nat Genet.* 2008;**40**(**6**):722–729.

115 Davies H, Bignell GR, Cox C, et al. Mutations of the BRAF gene in human cancer. *Nature.* 2002;**417**(**6892**):949–954.

119 Pollock PM, Harper UL, Hansen KS, et al. High frequency of BRAF mutations in nevi. *Nat Genet.* 2003;**33**(**1**):19–20.

142 The Cancer Genome Network. Genomic classification of cutaneous melanoma. *Cell.* 2015;**161**(**7**):1681–1696.

157 Ramos P, Karnezis AN, Hendricks WP, et al. Loss of the tumor suppressor SMARCA4 in small cell carcinoma of the ovary, hypercalcemic type (SCCOHT). *Rare Dis.* 2014;**2**(**1**):e967148.

165 Tomasetti C, Vogelstein B. Variation in cancer risk among tissues can be explained by the number of stem cell divisions. *Science.* 2015;**347**(**6217**):78–81.

174 Lipson D, Capelletti M, Yelensky R, et al. Identification of new ALK and RET gene fusions from colorectal and lung cancer biopsies. *Nat Med.* 2012;**18**(**3**):382–384.

197 Collins FS, Varmus H. A new initiative on precision medicine. *N Engl J Med.* 2015;**372**(**9**):793–795.

206 Druker BJ, Talpaz M, Resta DJ, et al. Efficacy and safety of a specific inhibitor of the BCR-ABL tyrosine kinase in chronic myeloid leukemia. *N Engl J Med.* 2001;**344**(**14**):1031–1037.

219 Paez JG, Janne PA, Lee JC, et al. EGFR mutations in lung cancer: correlation with clinical response to gefitinib therapy. *Science.* 2004;**304**(**5676**):1497–1500.

223 Sekulic A, Migden MR, Oro AE, et al. Efficacy and safety of vismodegib in advanced basal-cell carcinoma. *N Engl J Med.* 2012;**366**(**23**):2171–2179.

226 Von Hoff DD, Stephenson JJ, Rosen P, et al. Pilot study using molecular profiling of patients' tumors to find potential targets and select treatments for their refractory cancers. *J Clin Oncol.* 2010;**28**(**33**):4877–4883.

230 LoRusso PM, Boerner SA, Pilat MJ, et al. Pilot trial of selecting molecularly guided therapy for patients with non–V600 BRAF-mutant metastatic melanoma: experience of the SU2C/MRA melanoma dream team. *Mol Cancer Ther.* 2015;**14**(**8**):1962–1971.

231 Conley BA, Doroshow JH. Molecular analysis for therapy choice: NCI MATCH. Seminars in oncology; 2014: Elsevier.

246 Bettegowda C, Sausen M, Leary RJ, et al. Detection of circulating tumor DNA in early- and late-stage human malignancies. *Sci Transl Med.* 2014;**6**(**224**):224ra24.

263 Diaz LA Jr, Williams RT, Wu J, et al. The molecular evolution of acquired resistance to targeted EGFR blockade in colorectal cancers. *Nature.* 2012;**486**(**7404**):537–540.

265 Murtaza M, Dawson SJ, Tsui DW, et al. Non-invasive analysis of acquired resistance to cancer therapy by sequencing of plasma DNA. *Nature.* 2013;**497**(**7447**):108–112.

272 Kamb A, Gruis NA, Weaver-Feldhaus J, et al. A cell cycle regulator potentially involved in genesis of many tumor types. *Science.* 1994;**264**(**5157**):436–440.

278 Zuo L, Weger J, Yang Q, et al. Germline mutations in the p16INK4a binding domain of CDK4 in familial melanoma. *Nat Genet.* 1996;**12**(**1**):97–99.

287 Albino A, Vidal M, McNutt N, et al. Mutation and expression of the p53 gene in human malignant melanoma. *Melanoma Res.* 1994;**4**(**1**):35–45.

323 Huang FW, Hodis E, Xu MJ, Kryukov GV, Chin L, Garraway LA. Highly recurrent TERT promoter mutations in human melanoma. *Science.* 2013;**339**(**6122**):957–959.

339 Flaherty KT, Infante JR, Daud A, et al. Combined BRAF and MEK inhibition in melanoma with BRAF V600 mutations. *N Engl J Med.* 2012;**367**(**18**):1694–1703.

349 Hodi FS, O'Day SJ, McDermott DF, et al. Improved survival with ipilimumab in patients with metastatic melanoma. *N Engl J Med.* 2010;**363**(**8**):711–723.

351 Weber JS, D'Angelo SP, Minor D, et al. Nivolumab versus chemotherapy in patients with advanced melanoma who progressed after anti-CTLA-4 treatment (CheckMate 037): a randomised, controlled, open-label, phase 3 trial. *Lancet Oncol.* 2015;**16**(**4**):375–384.

8 Chromosomal aberrations in cancer

David J. Vander Weele, MD, PhD ▪ Megan E. McNerney, MD, PhD ▪ Michelle M. Le Beau, PhD

Overview

The malignant cells of most patients who have leukemia, lymphoma, or a solid tumor have acquired clonal chromosomal abnormalities, the identification of which can aid in establishing the correct diagnosis and prognosis and in the selection of therapy. Today, our arsenal of approaches to characterize an individual's malignant disease combines pathologic evaluation, cytogenetic analysis, and molecular studies, typically focused on a few key genes. The advent of high-throughput methods, such as next-generation sequencing, capable of surveying the entire genome or large panels of cancer-related genes, presents new options for a revolutionary change in the way we diagnose, characterize, and treat cancer. The vision for the future entails an integrated molecular profile, that is, chromosomal pattern, gene/miRNA expression, DNA methylation/epigenomic pattern, gene mutation status, and chemosensitivity of each patient's tumor, as well as predisposition to disease, facilitating the development of an individualized treatment plan with decreased toxicities and prolonged survival.

Introduction

Cancer is a heterogeneous group of diseases caused by the stepwise accumulation of numerous genetic and epigenetic aberrations altering the function of genes that regulate genome stability, cell proliferation and differentiation, cell death, adhesion, angiogenesis, invasion, and metastasis in complex cell and tissue microenvironments. The analysis of metaphase chromosomes provided our first broad glimpse into the genetic anatomy of a malignant cell and identified many of the basic abnormalities that characterize cancer, such as deletions, translocations, and gene amplifications. Specific cytogenetic abnormalities have been identified that are very closely, and sometimes uniquely, associated with morphologically distinct subsets of leukemia, lymphoma, or solid tumors.[1,2] The detection of one of these recurring abnormalities is helpful in establishing the diagnosis and adds information of prognostic importance. In the hematologic malignancies, patients with favorable prognostic features benefit from standard therapies with a well-known spectra of toxicities, whereas those with less favorable clinical and cytogenetic characteristics may be better treated with more intensive or investigational therapies. The disappearance of an abnormal clone is an important indicator of complete remission following treatment, whereas the appearance of new abnormalities signals clonal evolution and, often, more aggressive behavior. Similarly, in solid tumors, the detection of a recurring cytogenetic abnormality or genetic change may inform the selection of targeted therapy or an investigational clinical trial. Given the rapid progress in genomic analysis, one can envision a new approach to patients with cancer based on molecular profiling of the malignant cells as well as host factors that influence the development and treatment of the disease.[3] This chapter focuses on the key role of cytogenetic analysis in the context of diagnosis, prognosis, and molecular pathobiology of human tumors.

Genetic consequences of genomic rearrangements

Recurring chromosomal translocations result in alterations of the genes located at the breakpoints and play an integral role in the process of malignant transformation.[2] The altered genes fall into several functional classes, including tyrosine or serine protein kinases, cell surface receptors, growth factors and, the largest class, transcription regulators, which regulate growth and differentiation via the induction, or repression of gene transcription. There are two general mechanisms by which chromosomal translocations result in altered gene function in a dominant manner. The first is deregulation of gene expression, characteristic of the translocations in lymphoid neoplasms that involve the immunoglobulin genes in B lineage tumors and the T cell receptor genes in T lineage tumors, that results in the inappropriate or constitutive expression of an oncogene. The second mechanism is the expression of a novel, fusion protein, resulting from the juxtaposition of coding sequences from two genes, typically located on different chromosomes. Thus, these tumor-specific fusion proteins are therapeutic targets. Examples are the chimeric BCR-ABL1 protein resulting from the t(9;22) in chronic myelogenous leukemia (CML) or the anaplastic lymphoma kinase (ALK) fusion proteins in lung cancer.

A number of human tumors, particularly solid tumors, result from homozygous, recessive mutations. The hallmark of these genes, known as "tumor suppressor genes" (TSGs), whose normal role(s) is to limit cellular proliferation, promote differentiation, or repair DNA, is the loss of genetic material, resulting from chromosomal loss or deletion, as well as by other genetic mechanisms.[2] A growing number of TSGs act by haploinsufficiency, whereby loss of one allele results in a reduction in the level of the protein product by half, perturbing normal cellular processes.[4] This mechanism is common in the recurring deletions in myeloid neoplasms. Conversely, alterations in copy number resulting from gain of a whole, or part of a chromosome, or from gene amplification, for example, *ERBB2/HER2* in breast cancer, result in increased expression of one or more critical genes.

More than one mutation is required for the pathogenesis of human tumors; thus, an important aspect of cancer biology is the elucidation of the spectrum of chromosomal and molecular mutations that cooperate in the pathways leading to disease. Where known, we describe the cooperating mutations associated with specific cytogenetic subsets of leukemia, lymphoma, or solid tumors.

Holland-Frei Cancer Medicine, Ninth Edition. Edited by Robert C. Bast Jr., Carlo M. Croce, William N. Hait, Waun Ki Hong, Donald W. Kufe, Martine Piccart-Gebhart, Raphael E. Pollock, Ralph R. Weichselbaum, Hongyang Wang, and James F. Holland.
© 2017 John Wiley & Sons, Inc. ISBN: 978-1-118-93469-2

Chromosome nomenclature

Chromosomal abnormalities are described according to the International System for Human Cytogenetic Nomenclature (Table 1).[5] The total chromosome number is listed first, followed by the sex chromosomes, and numerical and structural abnormalities in ascending order. The observation of at least two cells with the same structural rearrangement, for example, translocations, deletions, or inversions, or gain of the same chromosome, or three cells each showing loss of the same chromosome, is considered evidence for the presence of an abnormal clone. An exception to this is a single cell characterized by a recurring structural abnormality, which likely represents the karyotype of the malignant cells. One cell with a normal karyotype is considered evidence for a normal cell line.

Methods that complement karyotype analysis

Fluorescence *in situ* hybridization (FISH)

Fluorescence *in situ* hybridization (FISH) is widely used in cancer diagnostics and is based on the ability of a labeled DNA probe to anneal to complementary DNA from interphase cells or metaphase chromosomes that are affixed to a glass microscope slide.[6] FISH can be performed on marrow or blood smears, or fixed and sectioned tissue, for example, formalin fixed paraffin-embedded (FFPE) tissue, as it does not require dividing cells. Probes are now commercially available for most clinically relevant abnormalities, such as centromere-specific probes to detect numerical abnormalities as well as the sex chromosome complement in the stem cell transplant setting, and locus-specific probes to detect translocations, deletions, and amplifications (Figure 1a–e). Advantages of FISH include (1) the rapid nature of the method; (2) its high sensitivity and specificity—cytogenetic abnormalities have been identified by FISH in samples that appeared to be normal by conventional cytogenetic analyses; and (3) the ability to obtain cytogenetic data from samples with a low mitotic index or terminally differentiated cells. The major disadvantage is the inability to interrogate more than a few abnormalities. FISH is often used to assess therapeutic efficacy by evaluating abnormalities identified by karyotyping at diagnosis, for example, detection of the *BCR-ABL1* fusion in CML patients following therapy with an oral tyrosine kinase inhibitor (TKI). Applications in solid tumors include the detection of gene amplificaton, for example, *ERBB2* in breast cancer and *EGFR* or *ALK* in lung cancer, or the UroVysion™ test in bladder cancer.

Table 1 Glossary of cytogenetic and genetic terminology[a].

Amplification	An increase in the number of copies of a DNA segment
Aneuploidy	An abnormal chromosome number, owing to either gain or loss
Banded chromosomes	Each chromosome pair has a unique pattern of alternating dark and light segments due to special stains or pretreatment with enzymes before staining
Breakpoint	A specific site on a chromosome that is involved in a structural rearrangement, such as a translocation or deletion
Centromere	The chromosome constriction that is the site of the spindle fiber attachment, enabling chromatid separation by shortening of the spindle fibers attached to opposite poles during mitosis
Clone	Defined as two cells with the same additional or structurally rearranged chromosome, or three cells with loss of the same chromosome
Deletion	A segment of a chromosome is missing, typically as the result of two breaks and loss of the intervening piece (interstitial deletion)
Diploid	Normal chromosome number and composition of chromosomes
Epigenetics	The study of the heritable changes in gene function that result from modifications to the genome, such as DNA or histone methylation, rather than changes in the primary DNA sequence
Fluorescence *in situ* hybridization	A molecular-cytogenetic technique based on the visualization of fluorescently labeled DNA probes hybridized to complementary DNA sequences from metaphase or interphase cells, used to detect numerical and structural abnormalities
Haploid	Only one-half the normal complement, that is, 23 chromosomes
Hyperdiploid	Additional chromosomes; therefore, the modal number is 47 or greater
Hypodiploid	Loss of chromosomes with a modal number of 45 or less
Inversion	Two breaks occur in the same chromosome with rotation of the intervening segment
Isochromosome	A chromosome that consists of identical copies of one chromosome arm (separated by the centromere) with loss of the other arm
Karyotype	Arrangement of chromosomes from a cell according to a internationally established system, such that the largest chromosomes are first and the smallest ones are last. A normal female or male karyotype is described as 46,XX or 46,XY, respectively
Loss of heterozygosity (LOH)	Typically results from a gross chromosomal abnormlity, such as a deletion, that results in loss of one parental copy of a locus or segment (also called hemizygosity). Copy-neutral LOH is the presence of two copies of a chromosome (or segment) originating from one parent, with loss of the copy contributed by the other (also called uniparental disomy)
Single nucleotide polymorphisms (SNPs)	These are common, heritable DNA sequence variations that occur when a single nucleotide (A, T, C, or G) is changed, occurring every 100–300 base pairs
Pseudodiploid	A diploid number of chromosomes accompanied by structural abnormalities
Recurring abnormality	A numerical or structural abnormality noted in multiple patients who have a similar neoplasm
Translocation	A break in at least two chromosomes with exchange of material
Nomenclature symbols	
p	Short arm
q	Long arm
+	Indicates a gain of a whole chromosome (e.g., +8)
−	Indicates a loss of a whole chromosome (e.g., −7)
t	Translocation
del	Deletion
inv	Inversion
i	Isochromosome
mar	Marker chromosome
r	Ring chromosome

[a]Modified from Ref. 2.

Other low-throughput methods

In addition to FISH, other low-throughput tests, such as ISH, RT-PCR (reverse transcription polymerase chain reaction), and immunohistochemistry (IHC), comprise the bulk of clinical molecular tests to detect translocations or copy number aberrations (CNAs). For example, they provide rapid diagnosis of acute promyelocytic leukemia (APL), diagnosis of ER/PR and *ERBB2* status in breast cancer. The main disadvantage of these assays is that the number of clinically relevant gene alterations per tumor has grown to the extent that high-throughput assays are becoming more efficient and cost-effective.

Single nucleotide polymorphism (SNP) arrays

Single nucleotide polymorphism (SNP) arrays probe for the presence of common SNPs genome wide. They provide sensitive detection of CNAs, on the order of kilobases, providing higher resolution than karyotyping (3–5 Mb resolution) (Figure 1f). Unlike karyotyping, they do not require dividing cells, an advantage for solid tumors. SNP arrays also detect copy-number neutral loss-of-heterozygosity (CN-LOH) but not balanced translocations. SNP arrays are available as an adjunct test to karyotyping and FISH analysis of leukemias and lymphomas, and they facilitate detection of genomic abnormalities in a substantial proportion of cases with a normal karyotype.

Next-generation sequencing (NGS)

Next-generation sequencing (NGS) is sequencing in a massively parallel manner, analyzing over one billion DNA fragments simultaneously, and has revolutionized clinical cancer diagnosis. NGS enables the most comprehensive testing, providing data on the spectrum of genetic alterations, including CNAs, LOH, translocations, single nucleotide mutations, small insertions and deletions (indels), germ-line predisposition variants, pharmacogenomic information, and oncogenic virus identification. Assays are evolving rapidly, driven by advances in instrumentation, design, software, and decreasing cost. NGS is routine at some centers and is expected to become widely used in oncology.

DNA or RNA can be obtained from fresh tissue, FFPE tissue, slide scrapings, or biopsies. Generally, small amounts of material are required, and some tests are available even for fine needle aspirates. High tumor cellularity is preferred, although lower cellularity can be compensated for by greater sequencing depth.[7] Extracted nucleic acids are converted into sequencing libraries and 75–250 bp paired-end reads are generated, which are then aligned to the reference genome.

CNAs are detected by counting the number of reads that align to a region, and comparing that number to data collected from a panel of normal diploid samples (Figure 2a). Regions of LOH are determined by examining SNP allele frequencies within the region. Homozygous deletions and amplifications greater than seven have been detected with 99% sensitivity and 100% specificity by NGS, comparing favorably to IHC and FISH.[7] Of note, NGS provides average DNA content, similar to arrays. In contrast, ISH is performed on a cell-by-cell basis; thus, ISH may have higher sensitivity for samples with low tumor cellularity. Translocations can be characterized by (1) read pairs that map to discordant portions of the genome or (2) reads that map directly to a breakpoint (Figure 2b). Although NGS can achieve comparable sensitivity and specificity as FISH and provides finer-scale information,[8] FISH is currently the gold standard for translocation identification.

Targeted gene panels

Targeted gene panels cover <0.05% of the genome and are composed of tens to hundreds of clinically significant genes. Some panels are comprehensive, whereas others are tailored for the tumor type. Compared to whole genome sequencing, they are cost-effective, provide greater sequencing depth, high sensitivity, the shortest turn-around-time, and decreased bioinformatics burden, as well as circumventing issues of incidental findings.

For identification of CNAs, target genes are typically enriched from DNA by probe hybridization. Targeting translocations is less straightforward because most translocations have breakpoints in introns, which can be significantly longer than NGS reads. Thus, capture probes for DNA must target introns, which increases the territory of DNA surveyed (Figure 2a). RNA-based sequencing avoids the problem of intervening introns, but is limited to detecting expressed chimeric fusion transcripts, and will fail to detect common translocations such as *IGH/MYC*. In addition, RNA suffers degradation in FFPE specimens.

Exome sequencing

Exome capture is enrichment by hybridization capture of all protein coding DNA, ~1% of the genome. Some clinical laboratories offer this as an unbiased assay of mutations and CNAs in all potentially pathogenic genes. The cost is lower than whole genome sequencing, but there is limited utility in detecting translocations.

Whole genome sequencing (WGS)

Whole genome sequencing (WGS) is sequencing of the entire tumor genome without a prior enrichment step and identifies all structural changes in coding and noncoding regions. Although used for research purposes and some clinical trials,[9] WGS is encumbered by cost, data size, and computational requirements. As sequencing costs decrease and laboratories gain more experience with NGS data, WGS may become more widely used.

Specific clonal disorders

Chronic myelogenous leukemia (CML)

The first consistent chromosomal abnormality in any malignant disease was identified in CML.[10] The Philadelphia (Ph) chromosome results from a reciprocal t(9;22)(q34.1;q11.2) (Figures 1a,b, 4a) and arises in a pluripotent stem cell that gives rise to both lymphoid and myeloid lineage cells. The standard t(9;22) is identified in about 92% of CML patients, whereas 7% have variant translocations that also involve a third chromosome. The genetic consequences are to move the 3′ portion of the *ABL1* oncogene on chromosome 9 next to the 5′ portion of the *BCR* gene on 22. Rare patients with CML who lack the t(9;22) have a rearrangement involving *ABL1* and *BCR* that is detectable only at the molecular level (~0.5% of cases).[11]

The t(9;22) and resultant *BCR-ABL1* fusion is the *sine qua non* of CML.[11] The BCR-ABL1 fusion protein acquires a novel function in transmitting growth-regulatory signals to the nucleus via the RAS/MAPK, PI3K/AKT, and JAK/STAT pathways. The tyrosine kinase activity of BCR-ABL1 can be inhibited by several commercially available oral TKIs: imatinib mesylate (Gleevec/STI571, Novartis Pharmaceuticals), dasatinib (Sprycel, BMS-354825, Bristol-Myers Squibb), and nilotinib (Tasigna, AMN107, Novartis Pharmaceuticals).[12,13] Additional oral agents are being tested in clinical trials.[14] Imatinib has shown remarkable activity in all phases of CML and is the preferred therapy for most patients with newly diagnosed CML, who can be monitored by FISH analysis or qRT-PCR.[15,16] Several types of genetic changes are associated with imatinib resistance, including point mutations leading to amino acid substitutions in the ABL1 kinase domain that interfere with

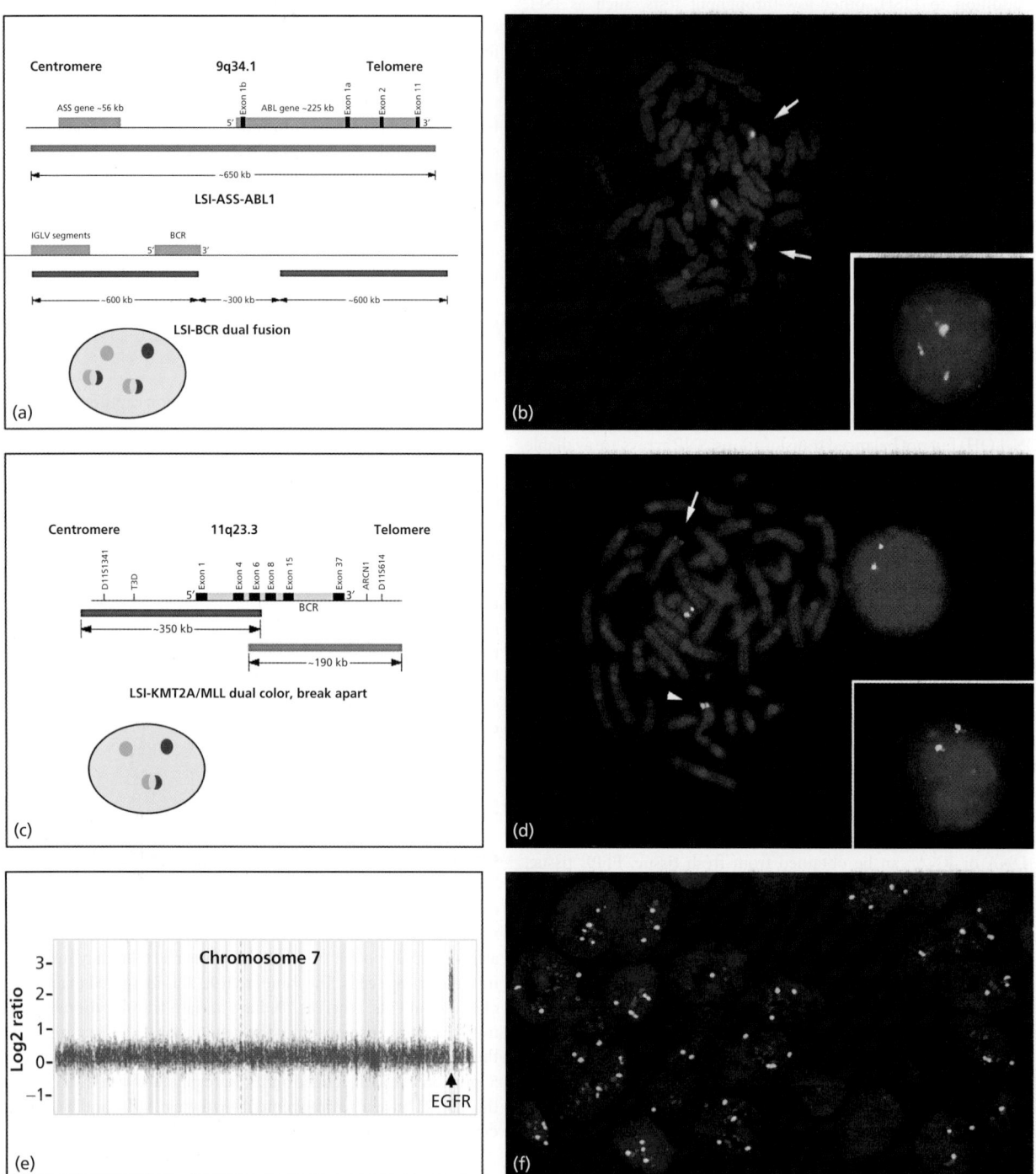

Figure 1 Fluorescence *in situ* hybridization and SNP array analysis. Panels (b), (d), and (e) illustrate images of metaphase or interphase cells following FISH; the cells are counterstained with 4,6-diamidino-2-phenylindole-dihydrochloride (DAPI). (a) Schematic diagram of the genomic origin of the *BCR* and *ABL1* dual fusion probe (Abbott Molecular), and configuration of signals in interphase cells. (b) In cells with the t(9;22), one green and one red signal is observed on the normal 9 and 22 homologs, and two yellow fusion signals (arrows) are observed on the der(9) and the der(22) (Ph) chromosomes as a result of the juxtaposition of the *ABL1* and *BCR* sequences. (c) Schematic diagram of the *KMT2A/MLL* break-apart probe (Abbott Molecular), and configuration of signals in interphase cells. (d) In cells with a translocation of 11q23.3, a yellow fusion signal is observed for the germ-line configuration on the normal chromosome 11 homolog, a green signal is observed on the der(11) chromosome, and a red signal is observed on the partner chromosome. (e,f) Detection of gene amplification. (e) SNP array analysis for DNA copy number aberrations in a glioblastoma reveals amplification of the *EGFR* locus. (f) FISH analysis for *ERBB2/HER2* amplification in breast carcinoma. The probe labeled with Spectrum Green (green signal) is a centromere-specific probe for chromosome 17 (CEP17). Most cells have two copies of the centromere of chromosome 17; however, polyploid cells have more copies. The probe labeled with spectrum orange (red signal) is a locus-specific probe for the *ERBB2/HER2* gene, with an estimated average of 10–20 copies per cell (Abbott Molecular). The *ERBB2/HER2*:CEP17 ratio was reported as ≥2.0. Source: Dr. Carrie Fitzpatrick, Department of Pathology, University of Chicago.

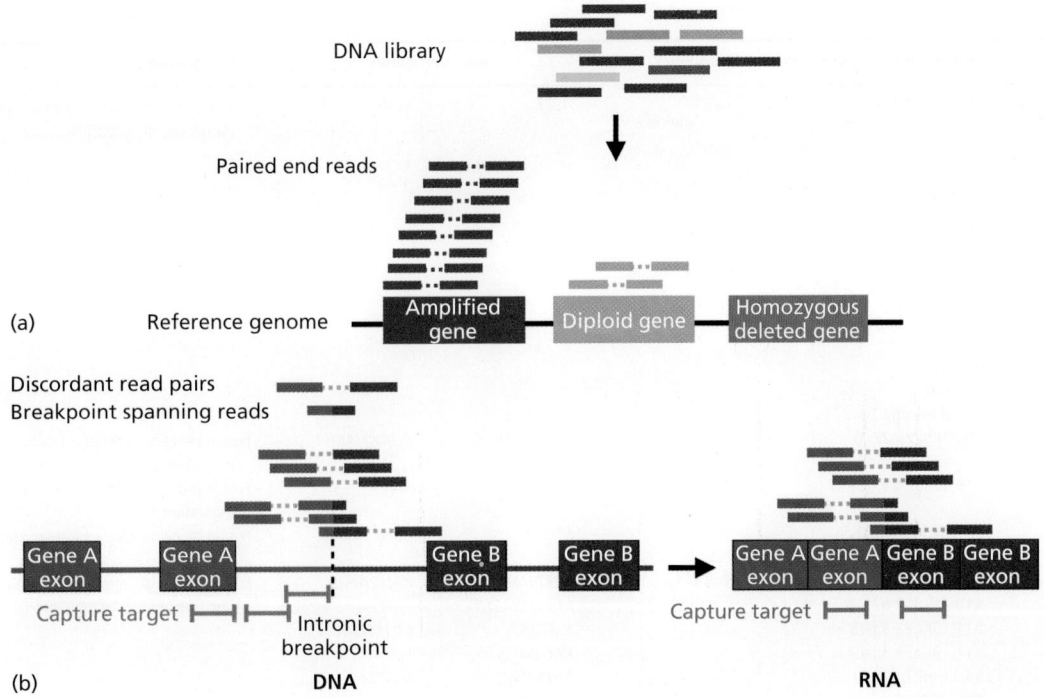

DNA library

Paired end reads

(a) Reference genome

Discordant read pairs
Breakpoint spanning reads

(b) DNA RNA

Figure 2 Detection of chromosomal aberrations by next-generation sequencing (NGS). (a) Copy number alterations are determined from a DNA library, that can be derived from whole genome DNA, or enriched by exome capture or a smaller, targeted gene panel. Paired-end or single-end (not shown) NGS is performed on the tumor sample, and reads are aligned to a reference human genome. The number of reads that align to a region are compared to either normal tissue from the same patient, or a database of normal, diploid patient samples. Regions of amplification will have a higher number of reads as compared to normal. Regions with heterozygous or homozygous deletions will have relatively fewer reads than expected. (b) Translocations can be identified by discordant read pairs that map to two different regions of the genome, or from reads that span breakpoints. Structural changes can be detected from DNA (left panel) or RNA (right panel). In the case of DNA, translocations can be identified by whole genome sequencing or by an initial capture step. As translocations involving two genes often have heterogenous breakpoints occurring in large regions of intronic sequence, capture probes have to be designed to span this intervening sequence. The advantage of using RNA is that the introns are spliced out; thus, capture probes are only required for exons, which are shorter than introns.

imatinib binding, as well as the acquisition of additional copies of the Ph chromosome or *BCR-ABL1* gene amplification, both of which can be detected by FISH.[15]

Historically, most CML patients in the accelerated or acute phases (80%) showed karyotypic evolution, commonly a gain of chromosomes 8 or 19, or a second Ph (by gain of the first), or an i(17q), as well as mutations in the *TP53, RB1, MYC, CDKN2A (p16), KRAS/NRAS,* or *RUNX1/AML1* genes.[11] With the advent of TKI therapy, the natural history of CML has been altered, and the karyotype in blast phase differs, but is not yet well described.

Interestingly, because each of the oral TKIs blocks kinase activities in addition to ABL1, they have proven to be effective in other hematologic malignancies, including myeloproliferative neoplasms (MPNs) with rearrangements of *PDGFRB*, a myeloproliferative variant of hypereosinophilic syndrome that expresses the FIP1L1-PDGFRA fusion protein, and in patients with mast cell malignancies that demonstrate *KIT* activation, as well as in some solid tumors, for example, *KIT*-mutated melanoma and GIST.[17]

Other myeloproliferative neoplasms (MPNs)

A cytogenetically abnormal clone is present in 15% of untreated and 40% of treated polycythemia vera (PV) patients, compared with 100% when the disease progresses to acute myeloid leukemia (AML) (Table 2).[18,19] Common changes are +8 or +9, del(13q), or del(20q), noted in 30% of patients.[18] A del(5q) (40%) or −7 (20%) is often observed in the leukemic phase. Cytogenetic analysis has revealed clonal abnormalities in 60% of primary myelofibrosis (MF), commonly +8, −7, or a del(7q), del(11q), del(13q), and del(20q).[18] A

change in the karyotype may signal evolution to AML. *JAK2*[V617F] mutations leading to activation of the STAT, PI3K, and MAPK signaling pathways occur in PV (90–95%), essential thrombocythemia (ET, 50–70%), and MF (40–50%).[20,21] More recently, the majority of ET and MF cases with nonmutated *JAK2* have been shown to carry somatic mutations in the calreticulin gene (*CALR*).[22,23]

Primary myelodysplastic syndromes (MDS)

The myelodysplastic syndromes (MDSs) are a heterogeneous group of diseases.[24,25] Clonal chromosome abnormalities can be detected in marrow cells of 40–60% of patients with primary MDS at diagnosis, including refractory cytopenia with unilineage dysplasia (25%), refractory anemia with ring sideroblasts (RARS, 10%), refractory cytopenia with multilineage dysplasia (RCMD, 50%), refractory anemia with excess blasts (RAEB–1,2, 50–70%), MDS with isolated del(5q) (100%), MDS unclassifiable, and childhood MDS (Table 2).[26–28] The common changes, +8, del(5q), −7/del(7q), and del(20q), are similar to those seen in AML *de novo* (Figure 3a). The recurring translocations that are closely associated with the distinct morphologic subsets of AML *de novo* are almost never seen in MDS.

MDS with isolated del(5q) occurs in a subset of older patients, frequently women, with RA, generally low blast counts, and normal or elevated platelet counts.[30] These patients have an interstitial deletion of 5q as the sole abnormality or with one additional abnormality and typically have a relatively benign course that extends over several years.[29] Haploinsufficiency of *RPS14*, encoding an essential component of the 40S ribosomal subunit, appears to be

Table 2 Recurring chromosomal abnormalities in malignant myeloid diseases.

Disease[a]	Chromosome abnormality	Frequency	Involved genes[b]		Consequence
CML	t(9;22)(q34.1;q11.2)	~99% [c]	ABL1	BCR	Fusion protein—altered cytokine signaling pathways, genomic instability
PV	+8	20% (combined)	—	—	—
	+9				
	del(20q)				
	del(13q)				
	Partial trisomy 1q				
MF	+8	30% (combined)	—	—	—
	+9				
	−7/del(7q)				
	del(5q)/t(5q)				
	del(20q)				
	del(13q)				
	Partial trisomy 1q				
AML	t(8;21)(q22;q22.1)	10%	RUNX1T1/ETO	RUNX1/AML1	Fusion protein—altered transcriptional regulation
	t(15;17)(q24.1;q21.2)	9%	PML	RARA	Fusion protein—altered transcriptional regulation
	inv(16)(p13.1q22) or t(16;16)(p13.1;q22)	5%	MYH11	CBFB	Fusion protein—altered transcriptional regulation
	t(9;11)(p21.3;q23.3)	5–8% for all	MLLT3/AF9	KMT2A/MLL	Fusion proteins—altered chromatin structure and transcriptional regulation
	t(10;11)(p12;q23.3)	t(11q23.3)	MLLT10/AF10	KMT2A	
	t(11;19)(q23.3;p13.3)		KMT2A	MLLT1/ENL	
	t(11;19)(q23.3;p13.1)		KMT2A	ELL	
	t(6;11)(q27;q23.3)		MLLT4/AF6	KMT2A	
	Other t(11q23.3)		KMT2A		
	del(11)(q23)				
	+8	8%			
	−7 or del(7q)	14%			
	del(5q)/t(5q)	12%			
	t(6;9)(p23;q34.1)	1%	DEK	NUP214/CAN	Fusion nuclear pore protein
	inv(3)(q21.3q26.2) or t(3;3)	2%	MECOM/EVI1		Overexpression of MECOM
	del(20q)	5%			
Therapy-related MN	−7 or del(7q)	45%			
	del(5q)/t(5q)	40%			
	der(1;7)(q10;p10)	2%			
	dic(5;17)(q11.1-13;p11.1-13)	5%		TP53	Loss of function—DNA damage response
	t(9;11)(p21.3;q23.3)/t(11q23)	3%	MLLT3	KMT2A	Fusion proteins—altered transcriptional regulation
	t(11;16)(q23.3;p13.3)	2% (t-MDS)	KMT2A	CREBBP	
	t(21q22.1)	2%	RUNX1/AML1		
	t(3;21)(q26.2;q22.3)	3%	MECOM	RUNX1	Overexpression of MECOM
MDS (unbalanced)	+8	10%			
	−7/del(7q)[d]	12%			
	del(5q)/t(5q)[d]	15%			
	del(20q)	5–8%			
	−Y	5%			
	i(17q)/t(17p)[d]	3–5%	TP53	—	Loss of function, DNA damage response
	−13/del(13q)[d]	3%			
	del(11q)[d]	3%			
	del(12p)/t(12p)[d]	3%			
(balanced)	t(1;3)(p36.3;q21.2)[d]	1%	MMEL1	RPN1	Deregulation of MMEL1—transcriptional activation?
	t(2;11)(p21;q23.3)/t(11q23.3)[d]	1%		KMT2A	KMT2A fusion—altered transcriptional regulation
	inv(3)(q21.3q26.2)/t(3;3)[d]	1%	RPN1	MECOM/EVI1	Altered transcriptional regulation by MECOM
CMML	t(5;12)(q32;p13.2)	~2%	PDGFRB	ETV6/TEL	Fusion protein—altered signaling pathways

[a]AML, acute myeloid leukemia; CML, chronic myelogenous leukemia; CMML, chronic myelomonocytic leukemia; MDS, myelodysplastic syndrome.

[b]Genes are listed in order of citation in the karyotype, for example, for CML, ABL1 is at 9q34.1 and BCR at 22q11.2.

[c]Rare patients with CML have an insertion of ABL1 adjacent to BCR in a normal appearing chromosome 22.

[d]Considered in the WHO 2008 Classification as presumptive evidence of MDS in patients with persistent cytopenias(s), but with no dysplasia or increased blasts.

responsible for the defect in erythropoiesis,[31] whereas two adjacent micro-RNAs, miR-145 and miR-146a, cooperate with loss of RPS14 and mediate the megakaryocytic dysplasia seen in this disease.[32,33]

SNP microarrays can detect abnormalities in 10–15% of cases with a normal karyotype. Of these, LOH of 7q, 11q, and 17p are associated with a poor outcome.[34,35] As defined by the International Prognostic Scoring System Revised, patients with a "very good outcome" have −Y or del(11q) as the sole abnormality; those with a "good outcome" have normal karyotypes, del(5q) alone or with one additional abnormality, del(12p) alone, or del(20q) alone; those with an "intermediate outcome" have del(7q), +8, +19, i(17q) or any other single or double abnormality; those with a "poor outcome" have −7, inv(3q)/t(3;3) double abnormalities, including −7/del(7q), and complex karyotypes with 3 abnormalities; and those with a "very poor outcome" have complex karyotypes with >3 abnormalities, typically with abnormalities of chromosome 5.[26,36,37]

Acute myeloid leukemia (AML) *de novo*

Clonal chromosomal abnormalities are detected in ~75% of patients with AML and have prognostic and therapeutic implications.[38–41] The most frequent abnormalities are +8 and −7 (Figure 3a).[2] The recurring translocations occur in younger patients with a median age in the 30s, whereas other abnormalities, such as del(5q) or −7/del(7q), occur in patients with a median age over 50. The WHO classification now recognizes specific recurring abnormalities together with their molecular counterparts as

separate disease entitites within AML (Table 2).[2] These entities include the core-binding factor (CBF) leukemias characterized by the t(8;21)(q22;q22.1) (Figure 4b) occurring in 5% of AML, and the inv(16)(p13.1q22) (Figure 4c) in 5% of AML (25% of AMMoL), the t(15;17)(q24.1;q21.2) (Figure 4d) in APL, and the t(9;11)(p21.3;q23.3) (Figure 4e).[2] At the molecular level, CBF rearrangements disrupt the two genes encoding the subunits of the CBF transcription factor (*RUNX1* at 21q22.1 and *CBFB* at 16q22) essential for hematopoiesis.[42] CBF-AML has a favorable prognosis in adults (overall 5-year survival of 70% for t(8;21); 60% for inv(16)), but the outcome in children with a t(8;21) is poor.[42] Secondary mutations of *KIT, KRAS,* and *NRAS* are common in CBF-AML, although only *KIT* mutations confer a poor prognosis.[42]

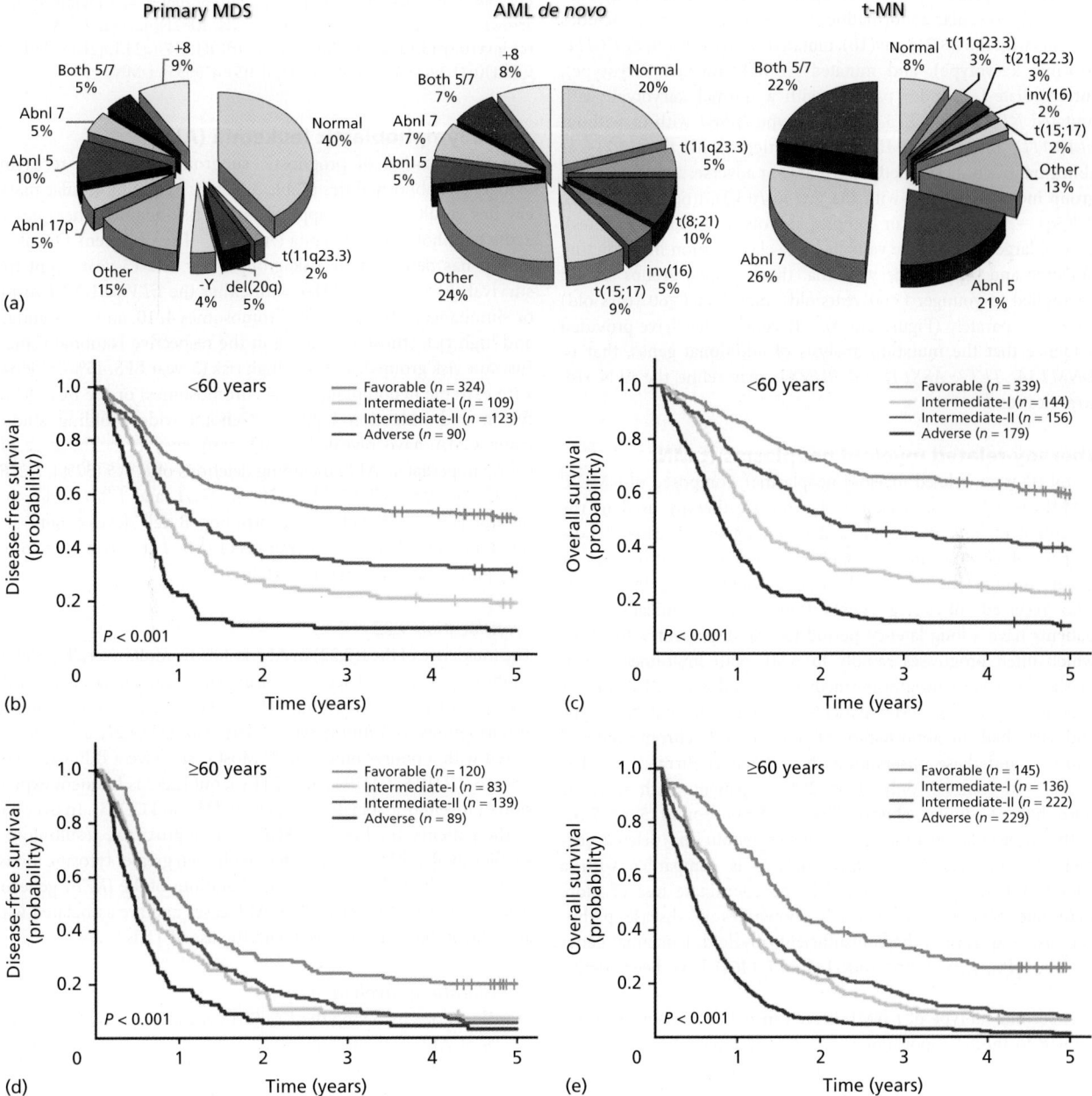

Figure 3 (a) Frequency of recurring chromosomal abnormalities in MDS, AML *de novo*, and t-MN. (b–e) Outcome of patients with AML classified according to the four European LeukemiaNet groups. (b) Disease-free survival and (c) overall survival of AML patients younger than 60 years of age. (d) Disease-free survival and (e) overall survival of patients aged 60 years or older. Source: Mrozek et al.[29] Reproduced with permission of American Society of Clinical Oncology.

The t(15;17) results in a fusion retinoic acid receptor-alpha protein (PML-RARA), the oncogenic potential of which results from the aberrant repression of RARA-mediated gene transcription through histone deacetylase (HDAC)-dependent chromatin remodeling.[43] *FLT3* internal tandem duplications (ITDs) are observed in 35% of patients. Establishing the diagnosis of APL with the typical t(15;17) is important because this disease is sensitive to therapy with all-trans retinoic acid (ATRA). Translocations of 11q23.3 are associated with acute monoblastic leukemia and are 4-times more common in children less than 1 year of age than in adults.[41,44] They result in fusion proteins of *KMT2A/MLL*, which encodes a histone methyltransferase that regulates transcription of target genes, for example, *HOX* genes, via chromatin remodeling.[45]

In an international effort, the European LeukemiaNet (ELN) has recently proposed a standardized system integrating cytogenetic and molecular abnormalities.[38] The favorable group includes patients with the t(8;21), inv(16), mutated *NPM1* without *FLT3-ITD* (normal karyotype), and mutated *CEBPA* (normal karyotype); Intermediate-I includes patients with a normal karyotype with mutated *NPM1* and *FLT3-ITD*, wild-type *NPM1* with or without *FLT3-ITD*; Intermediate-II includes patients with the t(9;11) or abnormalities not classified as favorable or adverse; and the adverse group includes patients with the inv(3q)/t(3;3), t(6;9), t(11q23.3), del(5q), −7, loss of 17p, or complex karyotype (≥3 abnormalities). Several large studies have validated this classification in predicting outcome and support the view that these genetic groups should be applied to younger (<60 years old) and older (≥60 years old) patients separately (Figure 3b–e).[29] Recent studies have provided evidence that the mutation analysis of additional genes, that is, *DNMT3A, TET2, ASXL1,* and *RUNX1,* may refine the ELN risk stratification.[46–49]

Therapy-related myeloid neoplasms (t-MN)

t-MN (therapy-related myeloid neoplasms), composed of t-MDS/t-AML, is a late complication of cytotoxic therapy used in the treatment of both malignant and nonmalignant diseases.[50] Loss of part of chromosome 5, del(5q) (Figure 4f), and/or part or all of chromosome 7 [−7/del(7q)] are characteristic in patients who received alkylating agents (Figure 3a). Clinically, these patients have a long latency period (5 years), present with MDS, which often progresses rapidly to AML with multilineage dysplasia and a poor prognosis (median survival 8 months). In our experience, 92% of t-MN patients had an abnormal karyotype and 70% had an abnormality of one or both chromosomes 5 and 7,[51] and these observations have been confirmed in other series.[52] In contrast, only about 20% of patients with AML *de novo* have a similar abnormality of chromosomes 5 or 7 or both.[2] Molecular analysis of the genes within the deleted segment of chromosome 5 (band 5q31.2) is compatible with a haploinsufficiency model in which the coordinate loss of more than one gene on 5q in HSCs cooperates in disease pathogenesis, and several haploinsufficient myeloid leukemia genes (*EGR1, APC, RPS14,* and *miR-145/miR-146a*) have been identified.[53,54]

A second subtype of t-AML is seen in patients receiving drugs known to inhibit topoisomerase II, for example, etoposide, teniposide, and doxorubicin. Clinically, these patients have a shorter latency period (1–2 years), present with overt leukemia, often with monocytic features, without an antecedent MDS, and have a more favorable response to intensive induction therapy. Translocations involving *KMT2A* at 11q23.3 or *RUNX1* at 21q22.1 are common in this subgroup.[50]

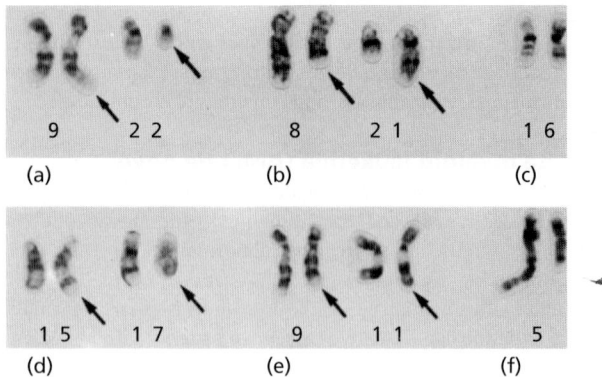

Figure 4 Partial karyotypes from trypsin-Giemsa-banded metaphase cells depicting select recurring chromosomal rearrangements observed in myeloid leukemias. The rearranged chromosomes are identified with arrows. (a) t(9;22)(q34.1;q11.2), CML. (b) t(8;21)(q22;q22.1), AML-M2. (c) inv(16)(p13.1q22), AMMoL-M4Eo. (d) t(15;17)(q24.1;q21.1), APL. (e) t(9;11)(p21.3;q23.3), AMoL-M5. (f) del(5)(q15q35), t-MN.

Acute lymphoblastic leukemia (ALL)

The identification of prognostic subgroups based on recurring cytogenetic abnormalities (Table 3, Figure 5) and molecular markers has resulted in the application of risk-adapted therapies in acute lymphoblastic leukemia (ALL).[55,56] The Children's Oncology Group has defined four risk groups: low risk (5-year event-free survival (EFS), at least 85%), with either the *ETV6-RUNX1* fusion or simultaneous trisomies of chromosomes 4, 10, and 17; standard and high risk (those remaining in the respective National Cancer Institute risk groups); and very high risk (5-year EFS, 45% or below) with extreme hypodiploidy (<44 chromosomes) or the *BCR-ABL1* fusion and induction failure.[57] Genome-wide profiling studies using CMA have revealed a high frequency of submicroscopic CNAs in pediatric ALL, including deletions of *PAX5* (32%), *IKZF1* (*IKAROS,* 29%), *CDKN2A/B* (50%), *BTG1,* and *EBF1* (8%), that disrupt genes and pathways controlling B cell development and differentiation.[58] Genetic alterations of *IKZF1* are associated with a very poor outcome in B cell progenitor ALL.[59]

Translocation 9;22

The incidence of the t(9;22) in ALL is 30% in adults overall, ~50% in adults over 60 years of age, and 5% in children and is associated with a very poor prognosis. About 70% of the patients show additional abnormalities, commonly with +der(22)t(9;22),+21, or −7 (associated with a poorer outcome).[60] Most cases have a B lineage phenotype (CD10+, CD19+, and TdT+), but there is frequent expression of myeloid-associated antigens (CD13 and CD33). In over half of the patients, the break in *BCR* is more proximal, resulting in a smaller BCR-ABL1 fusion protein with even greater tyrosine kinase activity (BCR-ABL1^{p190}). Genetic alterations of the *IKZF1* gene are detectable in up to 80% of Ph+ ALL cases and are associated with an unfavorable outcome even with the use of TKIs.[61]

Translocations involving 11q

Translocations involving the *KMT2A* gene at 11q23.3 are observed in 5% of ALL patients but in 80% of ALL in infants.[62] Of these, the most common is the t(4;11)(q21.3;q23.3) (Figure 6a), followed by the t(11;19)(q23;p13.3). Patients with the t(4;11) have a pro B phenotype (CD10−, CD19+), with co-expression of monocytic (CD15+) or, less commonly, T cell markers, and a poor response to conventional chemotherapy (adults: remission rate of 75% with EFS of only 7 months).[62]

Table 3 Cytogenetic-immunophenotypic correlations in malignant lymphoid diseases.

Disease[a]	Chromosome abnormality	Frequency[b]	Involved genes[c]		Consequence[d]
Acute lymphoblastic leukemia					
Precursor B	t(12;21)(p13.2;q22.1)	25%	ETV6/TEL	RUNX1/AML1	Fusion protein—TF
	t(9;22)(q34.1;q11.2)	10%[e]	ABL1	BCR	Fusion protein—altered cytokine signaling pathways
	t(4;11)(q21.3;q23.3)	5%	AFF4	KMT2A	Fusion protein—TF
Pre-B	t(1;19)(q23;p13.3)	6% (30%)	PBX1	TCF3 (E2A)	Fusion protein—TF
B (SIg+)	t(8;14)(q24.2;q32.3) or variant	7% (100%)	MYC	IGH	Deregulated expression—TF
Other	Hyperdiploidy (50–60)	10%	—	—	—
	del(12p),t(12p)	10%			
T	t(11;14)(p15.4;q11.2)	1%	LMO1	TRA	Deregulated expression-TF
	t(11;14)(p13;q11.2)	3%	LMO2	TRA	Deregulated expression-TF
	t(10;14)(q24.3;q11.2)	3%	TLX1	TRA	Deregulated expression-TF
	del(9p),t(9p)	<1% (10%)	CDKN2A, CDKN2B		Tumor suppressor gene—cell cycle regulation
Non-Hodgkin's lymphoma					
B cell NHL					
Burkitt	t(8;14)(q24.2;q32.3)	95%	MYC	IGH	Deregulated expression—TF
	t(2;8)(p12;q24.2)	1%	IGK	MYC	Deregulated expression—TF
	t(8;22)(q24.2;q11.2)	4%	MYC	IGL	Deregulated expression—TF
Follicular SNCL DLBCL	t(14;18)(q32.3;q21.3)	80% 20%	IGH	BCL2	Deregulated expression—anti-apoptosis protein
DLBCL	t(3;22)(q27;q11.2)	45% for all	BCL6	IGL	Deregulated expression—TF
	t(3;14)(q27;q32.3)	t(3q27)	BCL6	IGH	Deregulated expression—TF
MCL	t(11;14)(q13.3;q32.3)	~100%	CCND1	IGH	Deregulated expression—TF
LPL	t(9;14)(p13.2;q32.3)	—	PAX5	IGH	Deregulated expression—TF
MALT	t(11;18)(q22.2;q21.3)	40–50%	BIRC3/API2	MALT1	Fusion protein—NFkB activation
	t(1;14)(p22.3;q32.3)	10%	BCL10	IGH	Deregulated expression—increased NFkB activation
	t(14;18)(q32.3;q21.3)	10–20%	IGH	MALT1	Deregulated expression—increased NFkB activation
	t(3;14)(p13;q32.3)	10%	FOXP1	IGH	Deregulated expression—TF
PCFCL	t(14;18)(q32.3;q21.3)	40%	IGH	BCL2	Deregulated expression—anti-apoptosis protein
T cell NHL					
ALK+ ALCL	t(2;5)(p23.2;q35.1)	75%	ALK	NPM1	Deregulated expression Tyrosine kinase
ALK− ALCL	t(6;7)(p25.3;q32.3)	10–15%	IRF4, DUSP22	—	Deregulated expression of TF (IRF4) and phosphatase (DUSP22)
Nasal/NK cell	i(1q), i(7q), i(17q)	—	—	—	—
Hepatosplenic	i(7q)	>95%	—	—	—
Peripheral	t(5;9)(q33.3;q22.2)	15%	ITK	SYK	Constitutively active tyrosine kinase (SYK)
Chronic lymphocytic leukemia					
B	t(11;14)(q13.3;q32.3)	10%	CCND1	IGH	Deregulated expression—cell cycle regulation
	t(14;19)(q32.3;q13.2)	5%	IGH	BCL3	Deregulated expression—increased NFkB activation
	t(2;14)(p13;q32.3)	5%		IGH	
	t(14q32.3)	15%	IGH		
	del(13q)	30%			
	+12	25%			
T	t(8;14)(q24.2;q11.2)	5%	MYC	TRA	Deregulated expression—TF
	inv(14)(q11.2q32.3)	5%	TRA/TRD	IGH	Deregulated expression
	inv(14)(q11.2q32.1)	5%	TRA/TRD	TCL1A	Deregulated expression—TF
Multiple myeloma					
B	−13/del(13q)	40%			
	t(4;14)(p16.3;q32.3)	15%	FGFR3 WHSC1 /MMSET	IGH IGH	Deregulated expression—growth factor receptor and histone methyltransferase
	t(14;16)(q32.3;q23)	5%	IGH	MAF	Deregulated expression—TF
	t(6;14)(p21.3;q32.3)	4%	CCND3	IGH	Deregulated expression—cell cycle regulation
	t(11;14)(q13.3;q32.3)	15%	CCND1	IGH	Deregulated expression—cell cycle regulation
	t(14q32.3)	50%	IGH		
	del(17p)/t(17p)	30%	TP53		Loss of DNA damage response
	gain of 1q	20%			
	hyperdiploidy: +3, +5, +7, +9, +11				
Adult T-cell leukemia/lymphoma					
—	t(14;14)(q11.2;q32.3)	—	TRA	IGH	Deregulated expression
	inv(14)(q11.2q32.3)		TRA/TRD	IGH	Deregulated expression
	+3				

[a]DLBCL, diffuse large B cell lymphoma; MCL, mantle cell lymphoma; LPL, lymphoplasmacytoid lymphoma; MALT, mucosa-associated lymphoid tumor; PCFCL, primary cutaneous follicular center lymphoma; ALCL, anaplastic large cell lymphoma.
[b]The percentage refers to the frequency within the disease overall. The number in the parentheses refers to the frequency within the morphological or immunological subtype of the disease.
[c]Genes are listed in order of citation in the karyotype, for example, for precursor B ALL, ETV6 is at 12p13.2 and RUNX1 is at 21q22.3.
[d]TF, transcription factor.
[e]By cytogenetic analysis, the frequency in children is about 5% and in adults is about 25%; using molecular probes, this frequency is 30% in adults overall and 50% in adults over 60 years of age.

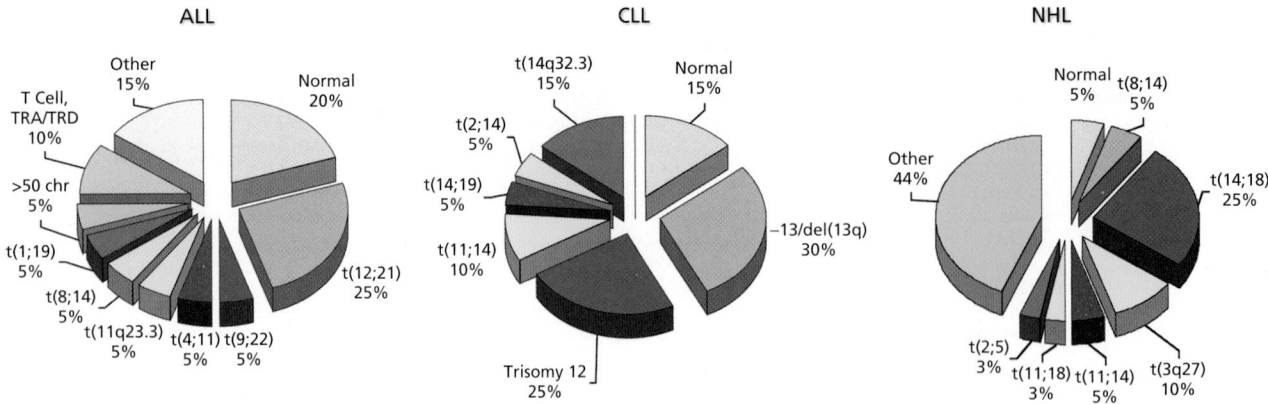

Figure 5 Frequency of recurring chromosomal abnormalities in ALL, CLL, and NHL.

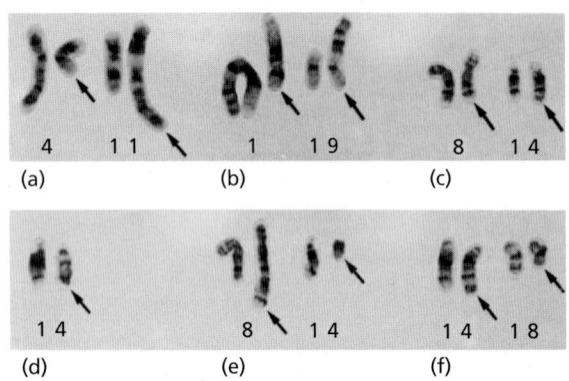

Figure 6 Partial karyotypes of trypsin-Giemsa-banded metaphase cells depicting select recurring chromosomal rearrangements observed in lymphoid neoplasms. The rearranged chromosomes are identified with arrows. (a) t(4;11)(q21.3;q23.3) in ALL. (b) t(1;19)(q23;p13.3) in pre-B cell ALL. (c) t(8;14)(q24.2;q32.3) in B cell ALL and Burkitt lymphoma. (d) inv(14)(q11.2q32.3) in T cell leukemia/lymphoma. (e) t(8;14)(q24.2;q11.2) in T cell leukemia/lymphoma. (f) t(14;18)(q32.3;q21.3) in B cell lymphoma.

Translocation 12;21

The t(12;21)(p13.2;q22.3) has been identified in a high proportion (~25%) of childhood precursor B leukemia but is uncommon in adults (~4% of ALL cases).[63] This cryptic translocation is not detectable by cytogenetic analysis but can be detected reliably using RT-PCR or FISH analysis. The t(12;21) defines a distinct subgroup of patients aged 1–10 years, with a B lineage immunophenotype (CD10+, CD19+, HLA-DR+), and a favorable outcome (5-year EFS of 91% vs 65% for other ALL). The t(12;21) results in a fusion protein containing the N-terminus of ETV6/TEL, a transcriptional repressor of the ETS family, and most of the RUNX1 transcription factor.

Hyperdiploidy

The leukemia cells of some patients with ALL are characterized by a gain of many chromosomes. Two distinct subgroups are recognized: a group with 1–4 extra chromosomes,[47–50] and the more common group with >50 chromosomes (typically 51–60 chromosomes). The latter subgroup is common in children (~30%) but is rarely observed in adults (<5%). Certain additional chromosomes are common (X chromosome, and chromosomes 4, 6, 10, 14, 17, 18, and 21). Patients with >50 chromosomes with +4, +10, and +17 have favorable clinical features, including age between 1 and 9

years, low white blood cell count (median 6700/L), and favorable immunophenotype (early pre-B or pre-B).[64]

Translocation 1;19 and translocation 8;14

The t(1;19)(q23;p13.3) is associated with a good prognosis and has been identified in about 6% of children with a B lineage leukemia (Figure 6b). The leukemia cells have cytoplasmic immunoglobulin and are CD10+, CD19+, CD34−, and CD9+. The t(8;14)(q24.2;q32.3) is observed in mature B cell ALL (Figure 6c). These patients have a high incidence of central nervous system involvement and/or abdominal nodal involvement at diagnosis. Historically, the outcome has been poor, but the use of high-intensity chemotherapy has markedly improved the outcome (EFS of 80% in children).

Ph-like ALL

Ph-like ALL is a novel subgroup of high-risk ALL (15% of pediatric and 30% of adult ALL), characterized by increased expression of HSC genes, a similar gene expression profile to Ph-positive ALL, and by a high frequency of *IKZF1* deletions and mutations, which confer a poor prognosis. Genetic alterations responsible for the activated kinase and cytokine receptor signaling signature in Ph-like ALL include point mutations and gene fusions affecting *CRLF2, JAK2, ABL1, PDGFRB, EPOR, EBF1, FLT3, IL7R, SH2B3*, and other genes.[65,66]

T-cell acute lymphoblastic leukemia

T lymphoblastic leukemia/lymphoma has a distinct pattern of recurring abnormalities, involving the T cell receptor loci at 14q11.2 (Figure 6d,e) and two regions of chromosome 7 (7q34) and 7p14) (Table 3).[67,68] The most common are the t(10;11)(q24.3;q11.2) (7% of childhood and 30% of adult patients, *TLX1* gene) and the cryptic t(5;14)(q35.1;q32.1) (*TLX3*, 20% of childhood, and 10–15% of adult cases). About 30% of patients have activating mutations of the *NOTCH1* gene. Patients with T-cell ALL are most often young males and often have a mediastinal tumor mass, high white blood cell count, and leukemia cells in the cerebrospinal fluid.

Chronic lymphocytic leukemia (CLL)

Only 50% of chronic lymphocytic leukemia (CLL) patients have detectable abnormalities by cytogenetic analysis, which increases to 80% when FISH analysis is used (Table 3, Figure 5).[69] The most frequent changes seen by FISH are: −13/del(13q) (55%), deletion of *ATM* on 11q (18%), +12 (16%), deletion of *TP53* on 17p, and deletion of 6q (6%).[70] The median survival is shorter in patients with 17p (32 months) or 11q (79 months) loss, than in those with no detectable abnormality (111 months), +12 (114 months), or −13/del(13q) (133 months). ZAP-70, an enzyme critical for T cell activation, is upregulated in CLL cells that contain unmutated *IGH* genes, conferring a poor prognosis.[71] Patients whose CLL cells have mutated *IGH* and lack expression of ZAP-70 and CD38 have the longest treatment-free period after diagnosis.[72]

T-cell CLL and large granular lymphocytic leukemia are uncommon disorders. Rearrangements involving 14q11.2, with or without an accompanying break in 14q32.3, have been reported in T-CLL as well as in T-cell lymphomas (Table 3).[67] The most common is inv(14)(q11.2q32.3) (Figure 6d).

Non-Hodgkin lymphoma (NHL)

More than 90% of non-Hodgkin lymphoma (NHL) cases are characterized by clonal chromosomal abnormalities, which correlate with histology and immunophenotype (Table 3, Figure 5).[73,74] For example, the t(14;18) is observed in a high proportion of follicular small cleaved cell lymphomas (70–90%). Most patients with a t(3;22)(q27;q11.2) or t(3;14)(q27;q32.3) have diffuse large B cell lymphomas (DLBCLs), and patients with a t(8;14)(q24.2;q32.3) have either small noncleaved cell or DLBCL. *IGH* at 14q32.3 is frequently involved in translocations in B-cell neoplasms (~70%). Similarly, a large proportion of T cell neoplasms are characterized by rearrangements of the TCR genes at 14q11.2, 7q34, or 7p14. Gene expression profiling has proven useful in distinguishing unique genetic subtypes of lymphoma.[75] For example, gene expression profiling has shown that DLBCL comprises at least three different subtypes (Germinal Center B-cell like, activated B-cell like, and primary mediastinal B-cell lymphoma), each with a distinct oncogenic mechanism, prognosis, and response to therapies.[76]

The t(8;14) or variant t(2;8) or t(8;22) is characteristic of both endemic and nonendemic Burkitt tumors, as well as Epstein–Barr virus-negative and -positive tumors (Figure 6c). Moreover, the t(8;14) has been observed in other lymphomas, particularly small noncleaved cell (non-Burkitt) and large cell immunoblastic lymphomas, HIV-associated BL (100%) and HIV-related DLBCL (30%).[77] The t(8;14) results in constitutive expression of *MYC* (8q24.2) via juxtaposition of the coding exons with *IGH* sequences (14q32.3). MYC is a transcription factor that plays a critical role in a number of cellular processes, including DNA replication, proliferation, and apoptosis.

Between 70% and 90% of follicular lymphomas and 20% of DLBCL have the t(14;18) (Figure 6f), in which the *BCL2* gene at 18q21.3 is juxtaposed to the *IGH* J segment, leading to the deregulated expression of BCL2, an anti-apoptotic mitochondrial membrane protein.[78] Common secondary abnormalities include −7, +18, and del(6q). Double-hit lymphomas arising from the progression of a follicular lymphoma to a DLBCL have both a *BCL2* and *MYC* translocation.[79]

The t(11;14) (q13.3;q32.3) is observed in virtually all cases of mantle cell lymphoma (MCL), a poor prognostic group with a median survival of 3 years, in 3% of myeloma, and in up to 20% of prolymphocytic leukemias.[80] This translocation results in the activation of the cyclin D1 (*CCND1*) gene, located 100–130 kb away from the breakpoint, by the *IGH* gene. The D-type cyclins act as growth factor sensors, regulating cell division via phosphorylation and inactivation of RB1.

Rearrangements leading to overexpression of *BCL6* at 3q27 occur in 40% of DLBCL and in up to 10% of follicular lymphomas and result most commonly from a t(3;22)(q27;q11.2) or t(3;14)(q27;q32.3).[73] BCL6 is a 96 kD POZ/Zn finger transcriptional repressor and may suppress genes involved in lymphocyte activation, differentiation, cell cycle arrest, and apoptosis. Somatic mutations have been identified in the 5′ regulatory regions of *BCL6* in ~20% of DLBDL without translocations, suggesting that overexpression of *BCL6* is more broadly involved than initially recognized.[81]

Extranodal marginal zone B-cell lymphomas of mucosa-associated lymphoid tissue (MALT lymphoma) are composed of several genetic subgroups, one characterized by +3 plus other abnormalities (60%), and another by the t(11;18)(q21.2;q21.3) (25–50%) and its variants.[82] The t(11;18) results in the fusion of the apoptosis-inhibitor gene *BIRC3 (API2)* to a novel gene at 18q21.3, *MALT1*, whose product activates the NFkB pathway.

Anaplastic large cell lymphoma (ALCL) is characterized by a young age at presentation and skin and/or lymph node infiltration by large, often bizarre lymphoma cells, which preferentially involve the paracortical areas and lymph node sinuses. The majority of such tumors express one or more T-cell antigens, a minority express B-cell antigens, and some express both T- and B-cell antigens (the null phenotype). The t(2;5)(p23.2;q35.1), t(1;2)(q25;p23), or variant rearrangement involving the *ALK* tyrosine kinase gene at 2p23 occurs at a high frequency in ALCL of either T-cell or null phenotype.[83] The tumor cells are positive for CD30 on the cell membrane and in the Golgi region, and ALK expression is detectable in 60–85% of cases, where it confers a more favorable outcome (5 year survival, 80% in ALK+ vs 40% in ALK−tumors).

Multiple myeloma

The application of FISH in combination with plasma cell enrichment techniques has led to the discovery of abnormalities in a high proportion of myeloma, a monoclonal malignancy of post-follicular B cells, preceded by a premalignant monoclonal gammopathy of undetermined significance (MGUS) (Table 3).[84,85] MGUS is characterized by chromosomal aneuploidy, *IGH* translocations (45%), hyperdiploidy, and deletions of 13q (15–50%), leading to dysregulation of the cyclin D/RB1 pathway, also seen as the earliest changes in plasma cell myeloma.[84,86–88]

A molecular cytogenetic classification for myeloma recognizes three major groups: (1) nonhyperdiploid with *IGH* translocations (40% of myeloma patients and 10% of MGUS patients); (2) hyperdiploid; and (3) other abnormalities.[84,86] The t(11;14)(q13.3;q32.2) is found in 15% of cases and results in *CCND1* overexpression. The t(4;14)(p16.3;q32.3) is noted in about 15% of patients and deregulates the expression of the fibroblast growth factor receptor 3 gene *(FGFR3)* translocated to the der(14), and the *WHSC1/MMSET* domain remaining on the der(4) chromosome. The t(14;16)(q32.3;q23), noted in 5% of cases, results in the overexpression of the *MAF* transcription factor gene. The t(4;14) and t(14;16) are both associated with a poor clinical outcome, whereas the t(11;14) confers a favorable prognosis. Nearly half of myeloma cases are hyperdiploid (45%), most commonly with 49–56 chromosomes, including trisomy for three or more odd-numbered chromosomes (chromosomes 3, 5, 7, 9, 11, 15, 19, or 21), a genetic subgroup that is associated with older patients and a more favorable outcome.

Deletions of *TP53* on 17p are noted by FISH in 10% of myeloma and are associated with a poor prognosis (37% of these patients also have mutations of *TP53*). Chromosome 1 abnormalities frequently resulting in both gain of 1q and loss of 1p (*CDKN2C*) are associated with a shorter survival.[89] Thus, a comprehensive FISH testing panel for myeloma should include probes for 1p and, particularly, 1q.

Additional events occur with disease progression in myeloma, including mutations of *NRAS* and *KRAS* (30–40%), *MYC* deregulation, and epigenetic alterations. Several genes are silenced through aberrant promoter hypermethylation in both MGUS and multiple myeloma, including *DAPK1 (67%), SOCS1, CDKN2B (p15),* and *CDKN2A (p16).*[86]

Solid tumors

In contrast to the hematologic malignancies, our understanding of the contribution of chromosomal alterations to solid tumors has lagged behind, largely due to technical constraints. With recent advances in genetic analysis, however, chromosomal changes clearly play a significant role in solid tumors (Table 4). Although simple karyotypes with disease-specific gene fusions are the norm in hematologic malignancies and sarcomas, chromosomal aberrations in other solid tumors often involve a larger fraction of the genome. Indeed, the median number of somatic CNAs in solid tumors is 39, a much higher number than in hematologic malignancies.[90] Extreme cases of CNAs have been described as "chromothripsis" and "chromoplexy," involving highly complex rearrangements,[91,92] that are frequently associated with *TP53* mutations and a poor prognosis.[93] As with hematologic malignancies, many recurring alterations in solid tumors involve genes encoding transcriptional regulators or tyrosine kinases, the latter creating potentially druggable proteins. In addition to providing potential therapeutic targets, chromosomal alterations can give insight into the biology of solid tumors, improve disease classification, predict response to therapy, and inform our understanding of prognosis. Representative diseases and associated recurring chromosomal aberrations are discussed in the following sections.

Sarcomas

Sarcomas are a heterogeneous group of diseases that over time have come to be recognized as comprising an increasing number of distinct entities. Histologic similarity does not always translate to similar clinical behavior, and knowledge of the genetic basis of these diseases has assisted in improving disease classifications and contributed to our understanding of how these separate diseases are related.

In 1983, the t(11;22)(q24.3;q12.2) was identified in Ewing sarcomas.[94,95] This translocation results in an in-frame fusion of Ewing Sarcoma Breakpoint Region 1 (*EWSR1*), a member of the FET family, and Friend Leukemia Virus Integration Site 1 (*FLI1*), a member of the ETS transcription factor family. The resultant EWS-FLI1 fusion protein consists of the *N*-terminal transactivation domain of EWS fused with the DNA-binding domain of FLI1, forming an oncogenic transcription factor that upregulates or downregulates thousands of genes and is required for tumorigenesis.[96–98] The fusion breakpoint is variable and the functional significance of the different fusion products is not entirely characterized.[99]

A decade later, the *EWSR1* and ETS-related gene (*ERG*) fusion was identified in ~10% of Ewing sarcomas. *ERG* encodes another ETS family member that has 98% identity with *FLI1* in the DNA-binding ETS domain.[100] Together with EWS-FLI1, these account for 95% of Ewing sarcomas. The remaining 5% contain other fusions of FET family members, particularly *EWSR1* or *FUS*, with ETS family members, including *FLI1, ERG, ETV1, ETV4,* or *FEV*.[101] These fusions are mutually exclusive, suggesting that the resulting proteins function in a similar manner.

Ewing-like sarcomas are histologically similar to Ewing sarcomas but do not contain a detectable FET/ETS chromosomal rearrangement. They are characterized by other rearrangements, involving *EWSR1* and non-ETS family members.[102] It is likely that diagnostic definitions of these diseases will change as we improve our understanding of the fusion genes and the associated disease. Complicating the diagnostic challenge is the association of *EWSR1*

rearrangements with other sarcomas, including *EWSR1-ATF1* and clear cell sarcoma, *EWSR1-WT1* and desmoplastic round cell tumor, *EWSR1-NR4A3* and extraskeletal myxoid chondrosarcoma, *EWSR1-DDIT3* and myxoid liposarcoma, and *EWSR1-ZNF278* and small round cell sarcoma. As with Ewing Sarcoma, a single rearrangement is most common for each diagnosis, but one or both of the genes involved can also form fusion partners with other genes.

A translocation involving *SS18* at 18q11.2 and *SSX1* at Xp11.23 was identified in synovial sarcoma in 1986.[103] A large family of genes and pseudogenes is homologous with *SSX1* and many of them can form fusion oncogenes with *SS18*. The resulting fusion proteins regulate transcription through interactions with the SWI-SNF chromatin remodeling complex and the polycomb group protein complex.[104–106] The various fusion gene products appear to have subtle functional differences and result in morphologically distinct tumor variants.

Renal cell carcinoma

Conventional renal cell carcinoma (RCC) refers to clear cell carcinoma, which comprises ~85% of cases. Almost all clear cell RCCs are associated with disruption of *VHL*, through deletion, mutation, and/or epigenetic silencing. It is typically altered in every cell within the tumor, indicating that these genetic changes occur in the parental clone and are likely to be essential for tumor initiation.[107] In addition to loss of *VHL*, 90% or more of clear cell RCCs harbor a deletion of other genes located on 3p, including *PBRM1, SETD2,* and *BAP1*.[108]

Oncocytomas and chromophobe RCCs are thought to originate from the intercalated cells of the collecting ducts and they can be difficult to distinguish histologically. Oncocytomas rarely metastasize, however, suggesting that prior reports of metastatic oncocytomas may have been diagnosed incorrectly.[109] Both can harbor a variety of chromosomal abnormalities; oncocytomomas, but not chromophobe RCC, frequently have rearrangements leading to overexpression of *CCND1* (11q13). Identifying these alterations can have a major impact on predicting risk of metastatic potential and, therefore, clinical management.[110]

Gliomas

Oligodendrogliomas are well-differentiated tumors that are associated with an unbalanced translocation involving 1q and 19p, with subsequent loss of 1p and 19q. Anaplastic oligodendrogliomas and oligoastrocytomas are somewhat less differentiated, and their prognosis appears to be related to the presence of the codeletion. Among oligodendrogliomas, those that harbor this codeletion are sensitive to chemotherapy and patients have a median survival that exceeds 10 years. In contrast, tumors without these changes are more likely to have astrocytic features and shorter survival (2–3 years).[111] Thus, assessment for the codeletion is recommended for all oligodendrogliomas at the time of diagnosis.

Non-small-cell lung cancer (NSCLC)

In addition to predicting response to cytotoxic therapy, the protein products resulting from many chromosomal alterations have emerged as drug targets. A decade ago, small molecule inhibitors of EGFR were found to be effective for ~10% of patients with non-small-cell lung cancer (NSCLC), a subset that appeared to be composed of never-smokers with adenocarcinoma, especially in Asian patients.[112,113] Subsequently, most responders were found to have *EGFR* mutations with frequent amplification of the mutated allele.[114] Before this discovery, *KRAS* mutations were the sole driver

Table 4 Recurring chromosomal abnormalities in solid tumors.

Tumor type	Chromosome abnormality	Frequency	Fusion product or candidate gene affected[a]		Consequence
Bladder	t(4;4)(p16.3;p16.3)	3%	FGFR3	TACC3	Kinase activation
	t(12;17)(q13.1;q12)	3%	DIP2B	ERBB2	Kinase activation
	add(6p22.3)	20%	E2F3/SOX4		
	add(7p12)	10–15%	EGFR		Kinase activation
	add(3q26.3)	20%	PIK3CA		
	add(12q13.2)	10–15%	ERBB3		Kinase activation
	del(9p21.3)	50%	CDKN2A		
	del(17p11.2)	25%	NCOR1		
	del(10q23.3)	10–15%	PTEN		Kinase activation
	del(13q14.2)	15%	RB1		
	del(9q34.1)	5–10%	TSC1		Kinase activation
Breast	t(1;1)(p12;q44)	2%	MAGI3	AKT3	Kinase activation
	add(11q13.3)	15%	CCND1		Luminal subtype
	add(8p11.23)	15%	ZNF703		Luminal subtype
	add(8q24.2)	20%	MYC		Basal-like subtype
	add(17q12)	15%	ERBB2		Kinase activation
	add(7p12)	3%	EGFR		Kinase activation
	del(8q23.2)	10%	CSMD1		
	del(13q14.2)	5%	RB1		
	del(10q23.3)	5%	PTEN		Kinase activation
Cervical	add(8q24.2)	8%	MYC	—	
	add(11q13.3)	3%	CCND1		
	add(7p12)	3%	EGFR		Kinase activation
	add(17q12)	3%	ERBB2		Kinase activation
Colon	t(2;11)(p11.2;p15.1)	3%	TCF7L1	NAV2	
	t(10;10)(q25.2;25.3)	3%	VTI1A		
	add(17q12)	5%	ERBB2	TCF7L2	Kinase activation
	add(8q24.2)	6%	MYC		
	add(11p15.5)	4%	IGF2, miR-483		
	add(1q)	17%			
	del(3p14.2)	10%	FHIT		
	del(16p13.3)	25%	RBFOX1		
	del(6q26)	10%	PARK2		
	del(5q22.2)	2%	APC		
	del(14q)	30%			
	del(15q)	30%			
Endometrial	i(1)(q10)			—	
	add(15q26.3)	2%	IGF1R		Poor prognosis
	add(8q24.2)	5%	MYC		Serous-like
	add(17q12)	4%	ERBB2		Serous-like
	add(19q12)	4%	CCNE1		Serous-like
Esophagus	add(11q13.3)	—	CCND1	—	—
Head and neck	t(4;4)(p16.3;p16.3)	<5%	FGFR3	TACC3	
	add(3q26.3)	20%	SOX2		
	add(7p12)	15%	EGFR		Kinase activation
	add(11q13.3)	35%	CCND1		
	del(9p21.3)	25%	CDKN2A		
Lung cancer, small cell	inv(1)(p32p34.3)	10%	RLF	MYCL1	—
	add(3q26.2)	25–30%	SOX2		
	add(1p34.3)		MYCL		
	add(8q24.2)		MYC		
	add(6p22.3)		SOX4		
	add(19q12)		URI1		
	del(13q14.2)		RB1		
	del(8p21.1)		ESCO2		
	del(5q31.3)		ANKHD1		
	del(5q12.1)		KIF2A		
Lung cancer, non-small-cell	inv(2)(p21p23.2)	5%	EML4	ALK	Kinase activation
	t(4;6)(p15.2;q22.1)	all ROS1 2%	SLC34A2	ROS1	Kinase activation
	t(6;20)(q22.1;q12)		ROS1	SDC4	Kinase activation
	t(5;6)(q32;q22.1)		CD74	ROS1	Kinase activation
	inv(10)(p11.2q11.2)	all RET 1%	KIF5B	RET	Kinase activation
	inv(6)(q22.1q25)		ROS1	EZR	Kinase activation
	inv(10)(q11.2q21.2)		RET	CCDC6	Kinase activation
	add(12q15)	5–10%	MDM2		
	add(7p12)	8%	EGFR		Kinase activation
	del(9p21.3)	25%	CDKN2A		

(continued overleaf)

Table 4 (*Continued*)

Tumor type	Chromosome abnormality	Frequency	Fusion product or candidate gene affected[a]		Consequence
Prostate	t(1;7)(q32.1;p21)	1%	*SLC45A3*	*ETV1*	
	t(7;7)(q32;q34)	1%	*NRF1*	*BRAF*	Kinase activation
	t(1;17)(q32.1;q21.3)	1%	*SLC45A3*	*ETV4*	
	t(21;21)(q22.3;q22.3)	all TMPRSS2-ERG	*TMPRSS2*	*ERG*	ETS family member
	del(21)(q22.3q22.3)	45%	*TMPRSS2*	*ERG*	fusions—altered
	t(1;21)(q32.1;q22.3)	1%	*SLC45A3*	*ERG*	transcription
	t(3;21)(q27.2;q22.3)	1%	*ETV5*	*TMPRSS2*	
	t(7;21)(p21;q22.3)	1%	*ETV1*	*TMPRSS2*	
	t(17;21)(q21;q22)	1%	*ETV4*	*TMPRSS2*	
	t(1;7)(q32.1;q34)	1%	*SLC45A3*	*BRAF*	Kinase activation
	trisomy 7				
	monosomy 8				
Renal cell	t(X;17)(p11.2;q23.1)	all TFE	*TFE3*	*CLTC*	
	t(X;1)(p11.2;p34.3)	translocations	*TFE3*	*SFPQ*	
	inv(X)(p11.2q13.1)	~2%	*TFE3*	*NONO*	
	t(X;17)(p11.2;q25)		*TFE3*	*ASPSCR1*	
	add(5q)	69%			
	add(7q)	20%			
	del(3p25.3)	95%	*VHL*		
	del(14q)	42%			
	del(8p)	32%			
	del(9p)	29%			
Thyroid carcinoma	inv(10)(q11.2q21)	25%	*RET*	*CCD6*	Kinase activation
	Inv(10)(q11.2q11.2)	10%	*RET*	*NCOA4*	Kinase activation
	t(10;17)(q11.2;q24.2)	2%	*RET*	*PRKAR1A*	Kinase activation
	inv(1)(q21.3q23.1)		*TPM3*	*NTRK1*	
	t(1;3)		*NTRK1*	*TPR/TFG*	
	inv(7q21.2q34)		*AKAP9*	*BRAF*	Kinase activation
Salivary gland mucoid carcinoma	t(11;19)(q21;p13.2)	35–70%	*MAML2*	*MECT1/CRTC1*	Good prognosis
Lipoma	add(12q)	80–90%	*HMGA2, MDM2*		—
Synovial sarcoma	t(X;18)(p11.2;q11.2)	—	*SSX1*	*SS18/SYT*	Altered chromatin remodeling
Rhabdomyosarcoma, alveolar type	t(2;13)(q36.1;q14.1)	—	*PAX3*	*FOXO1*	—
	t(1;13)(p36.1;q14.1)		*PAX7*	*FOXO1*	
Extraskeletal myxoid chondrosarcoma	t(9;22)(q22;q12.2)	50–60%	*NR4A3*	*EWSR1*	—
	t(9;17)(q22;q12)	15–20%	*NR4A3*	*TAF15*	
Myxoinflammatory fibroblastic scarcoma	t(1;10)(p22.1;q24.3)	~95%	*TGFBR3*	*MGEA5*	—
	add(3p12.1)		*VGLL3*		
Congential fibrosarcoma	t(12;15)(p13.2;q25.3)	~95%	*ETV6*	*NTRK3*	Altered transcription
Fibromyxoid sarcoma	t(7;16)(q34;p11.2)	~95%	*CREB3L2*	*FUS*	—
Anaplastic astrocytoma	trisomy 7	30%	—	—	—
	del(9p)	30%			
	del(10q)	30–40%			
Glioblastoma	trisomy 7	50–60%	—	—	—
	del(9p)	30–40%			
	monosomy 10	50–60%			
	monosomy 13	30–40%			
Schwannoma	del(22q12.2)	45%	*NF2*	—	—
	add(9q34)	10%			
	add(17q)	5%			
Ewing tumor	t(11;22)(q24.3;q12.2)	85%	*FLI1*	*EWSR1*	Altered transcription
	t(21;22)(q22.3;q12.2)	10%	*ERG*	*EWSR1*	Altered transcription
Medulloblastoma	monosomy 6	—			Good prognosis
	add(8q24)				Poor prognosis
	i(17q)				
Neuroblastoma	add(2p24.3)	60%	*MYCN*	—	—
	add(2p23.2)	10%	*ALK*		
Wilms tumor	add(1q)	25–30%		—	Poor prognosis
	del(11p13)	10–30%	*WT1*		
	del(Xq11.1)	13%	*AMER1*		
	del(16q)	10–15%			
Mesoblastic nephroma	t(12;15)(p13.2;q25.3)	—	*ETV6*	*NTRK3*	Cellular subtype
Retinoblastoma	del(13q14.2)	~3%	*RB1*	—	
Clear cell sarcoma of soft parts	t(12;22)(q13.1;q12.2)	—	*ATF1*	*EWSR1*	Altered transcription
	t(2;22)(q33.3;q12.2)		*CREB1*	*EWSR1*	Altered transcription
Testicular tumors	i(12p)	together nearly	—	—	—
	add(12p)	100%			
Dermatofibrosarcoma protuberans	t(17;22)(q21.3;q13.1)	—	*COL1A1*	*PDGFB*	Kinase activation
	ring chromosome				

[a]Genes are listed in order of citation in the karyotype, for example, for bladder cancer, *DIP2B* is at 12q13.1 and *ERBB2* at 17q12.

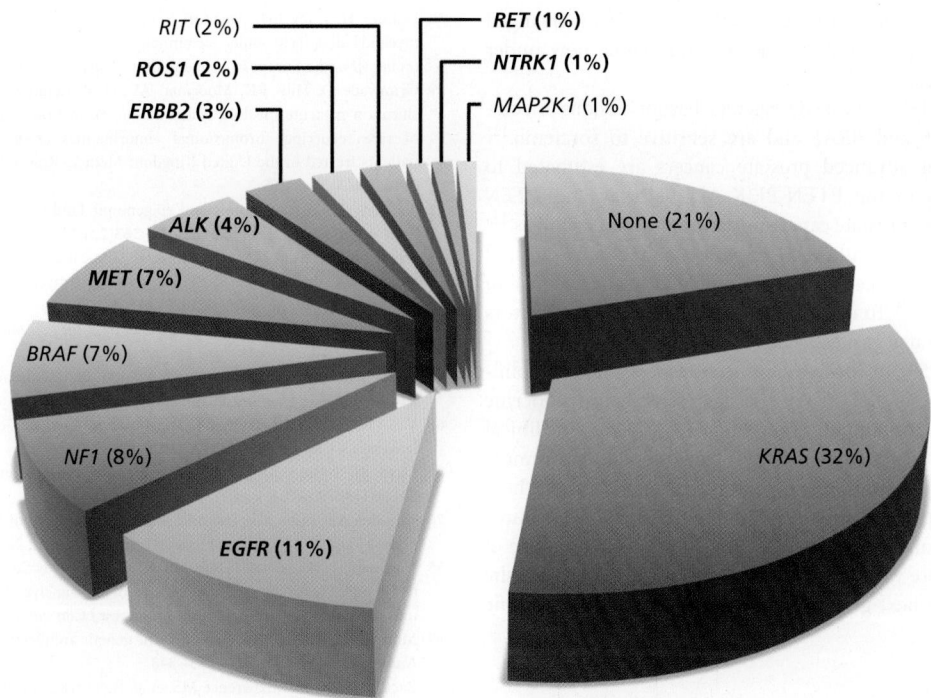

Figure 7 Frequency of driver gene alterations in lung adenocarcinoma. Genes that are involved in chromosomal abnormalities are identified with bold text.

mutation identified in NSCLCs, presenting a challenging drug target. In 2007, the *EML4-ALK* fusion oncogene was identified in ~5% of patients, typically in young, never or light smokers.[115] Just 4 years later, crizotinib was approved by the FDA for patients with *EML4-ALK* translocations. In patients with genetic alterations predicting response, targeted inhibitors of EGFR and ALK are preferred over cytotoxic therapy.

Although the percent of patients with each driver oncogene is low, there is a growing number of driver oncogenes in adenocarcinomas (Figure 7). These include fusions of *ALK* with other fusion partners; *CD74-ROS1, SLC34A2-ROS1,* and other fusions involving *ROS1*; *KIF5B-RET* and other *RET* fusions; fusions involving *NTRK1*; and others. Recent sequencing efforts have identified amplifications of *MET* and *ERBB2*.[116] *FGFR3-TACC3* mutations were first identified in glioblastoma but have been found also in squamous cell carcinoma of the lung and urothelial cancers.[117] Patients with fusions involving *ALK, ROS1,* and, possibly, *NTRK1* respond to crizotinib. Various RET inhibitors are being tested in patients with *RET* fusions and tumors with *FGFR* family fusions are likely to be sensitive to FGFR inhibitors. Testing for alterations of driver genes is recommended for patients with newly diagnosed NSCLC, especially those with adenocarcinoma or young age at diagnosis. As the number of identified driver mutations has grown, multiplex evaluation or more comprehensive sequencing techniques have replaced PCR-based assays of individual genes.

Prostate cancer

Given the high prevalence of prostate cancer, the *TMPRSS2-ERG* fusion found in ~40–50% of patients with prostate cancer is the most common gene fusion in human neoplasms.[118,119] It leads to high expression of *ERG*, driven by the androgen receptor-regulated *TMPRSS2* promoter, which is otherwise expressed at very low levels. Similar to the *EWSR1* fusion genes in sarcoma, multiple other *ETS* family members also form fusion genes in prostate cancer, including *ETV1, ETV4, ETV5,* and *ELK4*, and these fusions are mutually exclusive. Each of these *ETS* family members can form fusions with

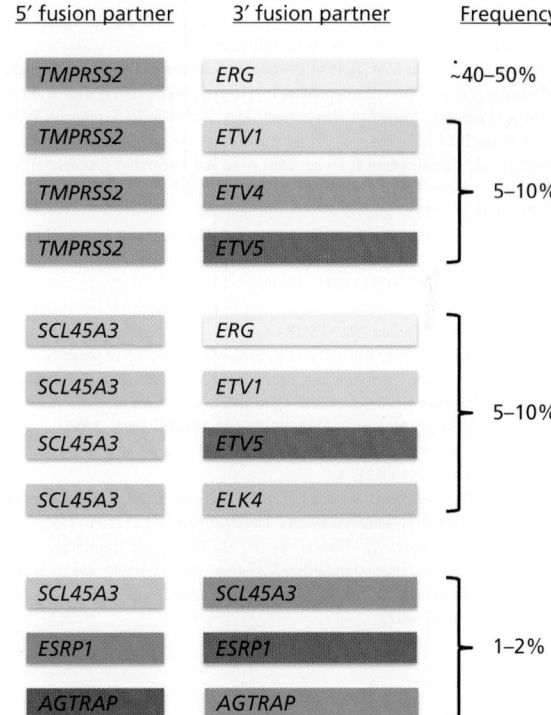

Figure 8 Fusion genes identified in prostate cancer.

5′ fusion partners, including *TMPRSS2* or *SCL45A3* or other fusion partners. In total, 60% of prostate cancers harbor *ETS*-family fusions (Figure 8).

ETS-family rearrangements appear to be an early event in tumor initiation and have been demonstrated in preneoplastic prostatic intraepithelial neoplasm (PIN) lesions.[120] Initially, ETS-family rearrangements were associated with a poor prognosis; subsequent reports refuted this finding and it remains a topic of debate. Recent preclinical data have demonstrated sensitivity of *ETS*-rearranged cell lines and xenograft models to PARP1 inhibitors, now under evaluation in clinical trials.[121]

Approximately 1% of prostate cancers harbor fusions involving each of *CRAF* and *BRAF* and are sensitive to sorafenib.[122] Virtually, 100% of advanced prostate cancers are estimated to harbor alterations in the PTEN-PI3K-Akt pathway and *PTEN* deletion in localized prostate cancer portends a worse prognosis.[123] *PTEN* deletion together with *MYC* amplification predicts a 50-fold increase in prostate cancer mortality compared to the absence of both abnormalities.[124] To date, however, PI3K and AKT inhibitors have not demonstrated clinical benefit.

Approximately 5% of localized prostate cancers have amplifications of *AURKA* or *MYCN*. In the aggressive neuroendocrine variant, however, the amplification rate is ~40%.[125] Preclinical models have demonstrated sensitivity of neuroendocrine tumors to AURKA inhibitors and ongoing clinical trials are testing these agents for this aggressive subtype. Although evaluation for chromosomal aberrations in prostate cancer seldom occurs outside of a clinical trial, more widespread analysis will likely occur with the implementation of next-generation sequencing and fusion-specific panels.

Key references

The complete reference list can be found on the Wiley Companion Digital Edition of this title (see inside front cover for login instructions).

1 Heim S, Mitelman F. *Cancer Cytogenetics: Chromosomal and Molecular Genetic Aberrations of Tumor Cells*. New York: Wiley; 2011.

2 Ouyang KJ, Le Beau MM. Role of cytogenetic analysis in the diagnosis and classification of hematopoietic neoplasms. In: Orazi A, Weiss LM, Foucar K, Knowles DM, eds. *Knowles' Neoplastic Hematopathology*. Philadelphia: Lippincott Williams & Wilkins; 2014:232–264.

3 Godley LA, Cunningham J, Dolan ME, et al. An integrated genomic approach to the assessment and treatment of acute myeloid leukemia. *Semin Oncol.* 2011;**38**(2):215–224.

7 Frampton GM, Fichtenholtz A, Otto GA, et al. Development and validation of a clinical cancer genomic profiling test based on massively parallel DNA sequencing. *Nat Biotechnol.* 2013;**31**(11):1023–1031.

9 Shyr D, Liu Q. Next generation sequencing in cancer research and clinical application. *BiolProced Online.* 2013;**15**(1):4.

12 Druker BJ, Guilhot F, O'Brien SG, et al. Five-year follow-up of patients receiving imatinib for chronic myeloid leukemia. *N Engl J Med.* 2006;**355**(23):2408–2417.

24 Bejar R, Stevenson K, Abdel-Wahab O, et al. Clinical effect of point mutations in myelodysplastic syndromes. *N Engl J Med.* 2011;**364**(26):2496–2506.

25 Lindsley RC, Ebert BL. Molecular pathophysiology of myelodysplastic syndromes. *Annu Rev Pathol.* 2013;**8**:21–47.

26 Greenberg PL, Tuechler H, Schanz J, et al. Revised international prognostic scoring system for myelodysplastic syndromes. *Blood.* 2012;**120**(12):2454–2465.

29 Mrozek K, Marcucci G, Nicolet D, et al. Prognostic significance of the European LeukemiaNet standardized system for reporting cytogenetic and molecular alterations in adults with acute myeloid leukemia. *J Clin Oncol.* 2012;**30**(36):4515–4523.

38 Dohner H, Estey EH, Amadori S, et al. Diagnosis and management of acute myeloid leukemia in adults: recommendations from an international expert panel, on behalf of the European LeukemiaNet. *Blood.* 2010;**115**(3):453–474.

39 Grimwade D, Hills RK, Moorman AV, et al. Refinement of cytogenetic classification in acute myeloid leukemia: determination of prognostic significance of rare recurring chromosomal abnormalities among 5876 younger adult patients treated in the United Kingdom Medical Research Council trials. *Blood.* 2010;**116**(3):354–365.

48 Network TCGAR. Genomic and epigenomic landscapes of adult de novo acute myeloid leukemia. *N Engl J Med.* 2013;**368**(22):2059–2074.

51 Smith SM, Le Beau MM, Huo D, et al. Clinical-cytogenetic associations in 306 patients with therapy-related myelodysplasia and myeloid leukemia: the University of Chicago series. *Blood.* 2003;**102**(1):43–52.

55 Harrison CJ. Acute lymphoblastic leukemia. *Clin Lab Med.* 2011;**31**(4):631–647, ix.

58 Mulligan CG. Genomic characterization of childhood acute lymphoblastic leukemia. *Semin Hematol.* 2013;**50**(4):314–324.

68 Van Vlierberghe P, Ferrando A. The molecular basis of T cell acute lymphoblastic leukemia. *J Clin Invest.* 2012;**122**(10):3398–3406.

74 Dave BJ, Nelson M, Sanger WG. Lymphoma cytogenetics. *Clin Lab Med.* 2011;**31**(4):725–761, x–xi.

76 Alizadeh AA, Eisen MB, Davis RE, et al. Distinct types of diffuse large B-cell lymphoma identified by gene expression profiling. *Nature.* 2000;**403**(6769):503–511.

85 Hartmann L, Biggerstaff JS, Chapman DB, et al. Detection of genomic abnormalities in multiple myeloma: the application of FISH analysis in combination with various plasma cell enrichment techniques. *Am J Clin Pathol.* 2011;**136**(5):712–720.

87 Morgan GJ, Walker BA, Davies FE. The genetic architecture of multiple myeloma. *Nat Rev Cancer.* 2012;**12**(5):335–348.

91 Baca SC, Prandi D, Lawrence MS, et al. Punctuated evolution of prostate cancer genomes. *Cell.* 2013;**153**(3):666–677.

92 Stephens PJ, Greenman CD, Fu B, et al. Massive genomic rearrangement acquired in a single catastrophic event during cancer development. *Cell.* 2011;**144**(1):27–40.

96 Delattre O, Zucman J, Plougastel B, et al. Gene fusion with an ETS DNA-binding domain caused by chromosome translocation in human tumours. *Nature.* 1992;**359**(6391):162–165.

97 Ouchida M, Ohno T, Fujimura Y, et al. Loss of tumorigenicity of Ewing's sarcoma cells expressing antisense RNA to EWS-fusion transcripts. *Oncogene.* 1995;**11**(6):1049–1054.

102 Ordonez JL, Osuna D, Herrero D, et al. Advances in Ewing's sarcoma research: where are we now and what lies ahead? *Cancer Res.* 2009;**69**(18):7140–7150.

108 Cancer Genome Atlas Research Network. Comprehensive molecular characterization of clear cell renal cell carcinoma. *Nature.* 2013;**499**(7456):43–49.

111 Cairncross G, Wang M, Shaw E, et al. Phase III trial of chemoradiotherapy for anaplastic oligodendroglioma: long-term results of RTOG 9402. *J Clin Oncol.* 2013;**31**(3):337–343.

115 Soda M, Choi YL, Enomoto M, et al. Identification of the transforming EML4-ALK fusion gene in non-small-cell lung cancer. *Nature.* 2007;**448**(7153):561–566.

116 Cancer Genome Atlas Research Network. Comprehensive molecular profiling of lung adenocarcinoma. *Nature.* 2014;**511**(7511):543–550.

121 Brenner JC, Ateeq B, Li Y, et al. Mechanistic rationale for inhibition of poly(ADP-ribose) polymerase in ETS gene fusion-positive prostate cancer. *Cancer Cell.* 2011;**19**(5):664–678.

123 Taylor BS, Schultz N, Hieronymus H, et al. Integrative genomic profiling of human prostate cancer. *Cancer Cell.* 2010;**18**(1):11–22.

125 Beltran H, Rickman DS, Park K, et al. Molecular characterization of neuroendocrine prostate cancer and identification of new drug targets. *Cancer Discov.* 2011;**1**(6):487–495.

9 MicroRNA expression in cancer

Serge Patrick Nana-Sinkam, MD ▪ Mario Acunzo, PhD ▪ Carlo M. Croce, MD

Overview

In the last two decades, researchers have identified a novel group of non-coding RNAs (ncRNAs) classified according to their function and size. The best studied of these ncRNAs termed microRNAs (miRNAs) are short non-coding RNAs that are approximately 22 nucleotides in length and play a key role in the regulation of a large number of biological processes and diseases, including cancer. Since the initial description of an association between miRNA and cancer in 2002, miRNAs have emerged as central regulators of processes fundamental to the initiation and progression of cancer. More recently, miRNAs have been detected in bodily fluids including blood, sputum, and urine, thus making them potential noninvasive diagnostic and prognostic biomarkers of disease. The application of miR-NAs in human cancer therapy has become a fascinating field of study, representing one of the newest frontiers for cancer treatment. However, our knowledge for these small molecules and their application to human cancers is still growing. In this chapter, we provide an overview of the connection between miRNAs and cancer with a focus on translation to human application.

Background

As investigators increasingly recognize the inherent complexities of cancer, they continue to search for novel molecular pathways in cancer that may be leveraged for the development of novel biomarkers and therapeutics, with the ultimate goal of saving lives. For decades, investigators have held the belief that a large percentage of the human genome was composed of "junk-DNA" or "dark matter" due to its inability to code for proteins. In the last two decades, researchers have now identified functions for regions of the human genome previously considered to be nonfunctional. Some genes located within these regions indeed encode for noncoding RNAs (ncRNAs), with microRNAs (miRNAs) representing the most researched member of this group. Since their initial discovery two decades ago in *Caenorhabditis elegans*, miRNAs have emerged as key regulators of biological processes fundamental to the initiation and progression of cancers.[1,2] Approximately, 22 nucleotides (nt) in length, miRNAs tend to be highly conserved across species and often demonstrate global deregulation in solid and hematological malignancies.[3,4] By directly binding to either the 3′ or 5′ untranslated region (UTR) of target mRNAs, miRNAs can either degrade target mRNA or inhibit translation. In addition, based on their relatively short size, miRNAs have the capacity for the simultaneous regulation of tens to hundreds of genes, thus interdicting in numerous biological pathways. In fact, the estimate that miRNAs may regulate up to 60% of the human genome is probably wrong and miRNA may regulate over the 90% of the protein-coding genes[4,5]). miRNAs are often located in fragile regions of the chromosome and thus susceptible to regulation through chromosomal amplifications,

deletions, or rearrangements.[6] The mechanisms for the regulation of miRNAs in the setting of cancer are complex and remain only partially understood. However, increasing lines of investigation indicate that miRNA regulation may occur by several mechanisms including alterations in key components of processing, epigenetic silencing, and polymorphisms in either miRNAs or target mRNAs interfering with binding and regulation.[7] The mechanisms for miRNA regulation and function are further complicated by their tumor and cell specificity. We are now approaching the identification of nearly 3000 miRNAs. miRNAs may function either as tumor suppressors or oncogenes depending on tumor and cell type and regulate processes fundamental to tumorigenesis (hallmarks of cancer) including differentiation, proliferation, and angiogenesis.[8] The mechanisms that regulate miRNAs in cancer, as well as their roles in cancer initiation and progression, are only beginning to be uncovered. While the use of high-throughput profiling strategies for the identification of clinically relevant miRNA-based biomarkers has been useful, this approach to miRNA investigation remains limited by issues of reproducibility and the need for improved algorithms for miRNA-target prediction and validation. Thus, there is still considerable work required to translate miRNAs into markers for clinical decision-making. One must also consider the inherent difficulties in achieving tumor-specific miRNA delivery. As miRNA biology transitions to the clinic, there is encouraging evidence suggesting that human applications for miRNAs, particularly as therapeutics, are in the not-too-distant future. For instance, nanotechnology-based carriers for miRNA delivery represent a new promising tool for the effective shuttling of miRNAs in the human body. Santaris/miRNA Therapeutics Inc. has tested human delivery of an antagomir against miR-122 for the treatment of hepatitis C. More recently, investigators have initiated trials testing human delivery of miR-34 in hepatocellular carcinoma as well as a phase I trial testing miR-16 replacement in recurrent malignant mesothelioma. Such studies represent the first of hopefully a series of future applications for the treatment of human cancer.

Biogenesis and production of microRNAs

miRNAs are short ncRNAs with a length of approximately 22 nucleotides encoded by evolutionarily conserved genes. miR-NAs are more frequently located within the introns or exons of protein-coding genes (about the 70%), or in intergenic regions (30%). The expression of intergenic miRNAs is related to their host gene expression, all intragenic miRNAs having independent transcription units.[9] miRNAs are processed and generated through a well-orchestrated series of interrelated steps, each of which is currently being investigated (Figure 1). In the first step, a long primary transcript termed the (pri)-miRNA undergoes transcription by RNA polymerase II. The pri-miRNAs are then bound to the double-stranded RNA-binding domain (dsRBD)

Holland-Frei Cancer Medicine, Ninth Edition. Edited by Robert C. Bast Jr., Carlo M. Croce, William N. Hait, Waun Ki Hong, Donald W. Kufe, Martine Piccart-Gebhart, Raphael E. Pollock, Ralph R. Weichselbaum, Hongyang Wang, and James F. Holland.

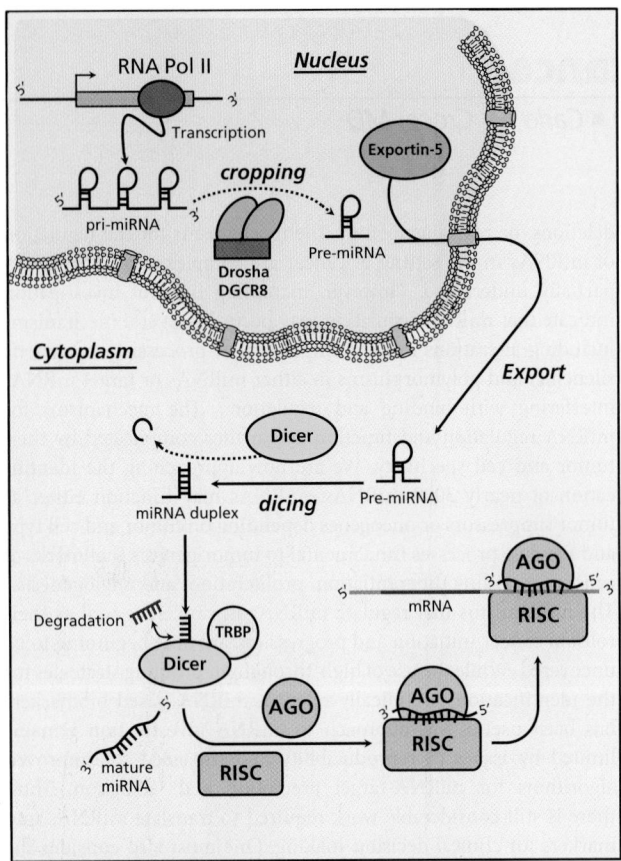

Figure 1 MicroRNA biogenesis.

protein known as DiGeorge syndrome critical region gene 8 (DGCR8) for vertebrates.[10] (An RNase III endonuclease termed The Drosha/DGCR8 complex cleaves the pri-miRNA into a smaller stem-loop ~70-nucleotide (nt) precursor miRNA (pre-miRNA). Pre-miRNAs are then exported from the nucleus to the cytoplasm using the double-stranded RNA-binding protein, Exportin 5 (XPO5).[11] Once in the cytoplasm, the pre-miRNA is cleaved into a mature 18–25 nucleotide miRNA by a complex that includes RNAase Dicer, Argonaute 2 (Ago 2), and transactivation-responsive RNA-binding protein (TRBP). The Ago2 protein belongs to the Argonaute family of proteins that bind fragments to guide RNA (including miRNAs). The resultant miRNA sequence, which consists of two strands, is then loaded into the RNA-induced silencing complex (RISC), with the mature strand being maintained while the complementary strand is degraded. The remaining strand possesses complementarity either to the 3' or 5' UTR of a target gene leading to degradation through endonuclease activity or to translational inhibition. Recently, investigators have shown that an miRNA can also bind to the coding sequence of a transcript, leading to translational repression.[12] The degree of complementarity between the "seed" sequence of the mature miRNA and the target is the primary determinant of the biological effect. It is important to recognize that investigators have now identified additional mechanisms for miRNA biogenesis, suggesting that we are just beginning to understand the complexities of this process.

MicroRNA deregulation in cancer

Calin et al.[13] made the first observations linking miRNA deregulation to cancer in a study. While investigating the mechanisms

for chronic lymphocytic leukemia (CLL), this team of investigators made the startling observation that a pair of miRNAs, miR-15a/16-1 which, along with the deleted in leukemia (DLEU) gene, are located at the chromosomal region 13q14.3, was either deleted or downregulated in 68% of patients with CLL.[13] In addition, both of these miRNAs were highly expressed in normal CD5+ B cells. Both findings suggested that these miRNAs were in fact important to the pathogenesis of the disease. This initial observation was corroborated by independent investigators who identified a functional link between miR-15a/16-1 and the prosurvival molecule Bcl2. They validated *in vitro* that miR-15a/16-1 targeted Bcl2 to induce apoptosis. Since this initial discovery of miRNAs in CLL, investigators have observed patterns of global dysregulation of miRNAs across both solid and hematological malignancies. In the last few years, researchers have determined that the causes for such dysregulation are multifactorial. For instance, the altered expression and/or function of the proteins involved in the biogenesis of miRNAs, such as Drosha and Dicer, can lead to an aberrant expression of miRNAs and thus to cancer.[14] A decreased expression level of Drosha and Dicer has been found in a high percentage of ovarian cancer patients.[15] Moreover, epigenetic changes within miRNA promoters such as changes in their methylation can also induce changes in miRNA expression levels.[16] Like other deregulated genes that cover an important role as oncogenes or tumor suppressors, the epigenetic deregulated expression of a single miRNA can be the triggering event for carcinogenesis. One such example involves the intensely studied miR-155 whose dysregulation can induce leukemia in miR-155 transgenic mice.[17] The tumor-suppressor miR-127 in primary prostate cancer and bladder tumors causes the upregulation of the proto-oncogene BCL6, which is a direct target of miR-127.[18] On the other hand, miRNAs can also act as protagonists in the control of the global cellular methylation status by acting on the enzymes responsible for epigenetic control. For example, the miR-29 family is able to modulate methylation levels by affecting the *ex-novo* expression of DNA methyltransferases DNMT3a and DNMT3B in lung cancer.[16] Another important and complex regulative mechanism of miRNAs is related to the transcriptional control of gene expression.[19] The activation of the miR-17/92 cluster induced by the MYC oncogene modulates the anti-apoptotic action of E2F1, thus mediating the MYC proliferative effect.[20] Recently, the effect of the membrane tyrosine-kinase receptors on miRNA expression has been studied. For instance, the hepatocyte growth factor receptor c-MET is able, through the transcriptional factor AP1, to induce the expression of the onco-miRNA miR-221/222 cluster, suggesting that the important effect of deregulated c-MET in cancer is at least in part linked to a deregulated miRNA expression pathway.[21] Finally, considering that the loss of p53 is one of the most represented genetic abnormalities in cancer, the link between the miR-34a family and p53 is another important example of miRNA transcriptional regulation.[22] p53 stimulates the transcription of the miR-34 family, inducing apoptosis and senescence. The loss of p53 function induces the downregulation of the miR-34 family in a very high percentage of ovarian cancer patients with a p53 mutation.[23] Hence, the primary theme is that patterns of miRNA expression are globally deregulated in cancer, this event being potentially a cause as well as a consequence of cancer itself. The global deregulation of miRNA in cancer has a dramatic effect on downstream targets of several cellular pathways.

Recently, investigators have also determined that miRNA function may be altered through mutations in target gene seed sequences. Such mutations can render an miRNA incapable of regulating a given mRNA and have been identified as biomarkers of clinical outcome. Mutations in the 3' UTR have been identified in several solid malignancies including ovarian, lung, breast, and colon cancers. Conversely, SNPs in miRNA gene sequences can change miRNA functions. We know that mRNA functional regulation by miRNAs is highly sensitive to base pair mismatches within nucleotides 2–8 of the miRNA, which have been defined as the seed region.[24] Therefore a single point mutation on an miRNA gene or a post-transcriptional modification such as RNA editing, can change the function or modify the targetome of an miRNA.[25,26] For example, it was determined that a single nucleotide polymorphism (SNP) in a let-7 (lethal-7) miRNA complementary site in the KRAS 3′ UTR increases nonsmall-cell lung cancer risk.[27] A mutation of let-7 binding site in the Kras 3′ UTR has been detected also in juvenile myelomonocytic leukemia (JMML).[28]

MicroRNA as biomarkers in cancer

Over the last several years, miRNAs have been implicated in virtually every type of cancer. Early studies have focused on applying high-throughput platforms as a means for linking patterns of miRNA deregulation to clinical parameters. One of the first such approaches was made in 2005 by Volinia and colleagues who profiled the miRNA signatures of six human solid tumors, detecting miR-21, miR-17-5p, and miR-191 overexpressed in some tumors.[29] Since that initial study, investigators have conducted similar multiple studies with the primary goals of identifying a prognostic miRNA signature. Yanaihara and colleagues conducted high-throughput profiling of cases of stage 1 adenocarcinoma of the lung. They identified over 40 miRNAs that distinguished lung tumors from adjacent uninvolved lung.[30] A broader study conducted on 22 different tumor types showed how an miRNA expression profile is able to classify tumors according to tissue of origin with high accuracy.[31] Studies have also focused on preselected miRNAs as potential prognostic markers. For example, Nadal et al.[32] examined the tumor-suppressive miR-34 as a prognostic biomarker in early-stage adenocarcinoma of the lung. They identified methylation and reduced expression of miR-34b/c in nearly half (46%) of early-stage lung adenocarcinomas and determined that reduced expression and methylation of miR-34b/c correlated with shorter disease-free survival and overall survival. For example, in a separate study, investigators showed that miRNA expression levels may correlate with BCR-ABL kinase activity in chronic myeloid leukemia (CML),[33] suggesting, therefore, a potential application in the adjustment of the therapy during treatment to improve the outcome. Another very intriguing application of miRNAs as biomarkers consists of the integration of both protein-coding and noncoding gene expressions in order to develop a prognostic signature in early stages of cancer. Akagi et al.[34] examined 148 cases of stage 1 lung adenocarcinoma for 42 preselected genes as predictive biomarkers. Through testing and subsequent validation in independent cohorts, the authors developed a four-gene classifier (DLC1, XPO1, HIF1A, and BRCA1) that correlates to survival in stage 1 lung adenocarcinoma. In addition, they determined that miR-21 expression was independently associated with survival in the same cohorts. Lastly, the combination of the four-gene classifier and miR-21 expression was superior to either biomarker alone. Despite the multitude of very encouraging miRNA profiling studies, investigators have yet to reach consensus on which miRNAs confer the most accurate prognostic information. A primary reason for the lack of reproducibility is that, similarly to other high-throughput analyses, miRNA profiling studies are susceptible to certain biases, including small cohort sizes, varying platforms (array, sequencing, RT-PCR), and variability in data interpretation.

MicroRNAs as noninvasive biomarkers in cancer

The development of noninvasive biomarkers in cancer that may inform clinical decision-making remains elusive and the subject of continued study. Several studies have demonstrated that miRNAs exist in body fluids (serum, plasma, urine, sputum, cerebrospinal fluid, and bronchoalveolar lavage) in a relatively stable form at different conditions of pH and temperature.[35–37] miRNAs are also present in blood, where they were detected in plasma, platelets, erythrocytes, and nucleated blood cells. One of the earliest studies revealed that miRNAs were detectable in circulation in prostate cancer.[38] Shen et al.[39] demonstrated that plasma-based miRNAs could be used as biomarkers to distinguish solitary lung nodules. A subsequent larger study further validated the concept that circulating miRNAs could be used in the setting of lung cancer early detection.[40]

The compartment specific location of miRNAs in circulation remains the subject of debate. However, circulating miRNAs have been found packaged in extracellular vesicles (EVs) as well as associated with RNA-binding proteins like Argonaute 2 or lipoprotein complexes, which prevent their degradation (Figure 2).[41–44] EVs are small membrane-encapsulated fluid particles comprised of a family shedding vesicles and exosomes that are released from a wide variety of cell types by entirely independent cellular mechanisms.[45] Investigators to date have focused primarily on exosomes, which are ~40 to 100 nm vesicles. These particles consist of a lipid bilayer, generated from secretory multivesicular bodies (MVB) that fuse with the plasma membrane for release into the extracellular environment. Exosomes contain various molecular constituents of their cell of origin including lipids, proteins, messenger RNA (mRNA), and miRNA, which may be transferred from donor to target cells to facilitate direct cell-to-cell contact and subsequent reprogramming of the tumor microenvironment.[42] In pathological states, such as cancer, exosomes cross-talk, and/or influence major tumor-related pathways such as epithelial-mesenchymal transition (EMT), cancer stemness, angiogenesis, and metastasis involving many cell types within the tumor microenvironment.[46–49] Exosomes have also been detected in a number of human body fluids including plasma, urine,

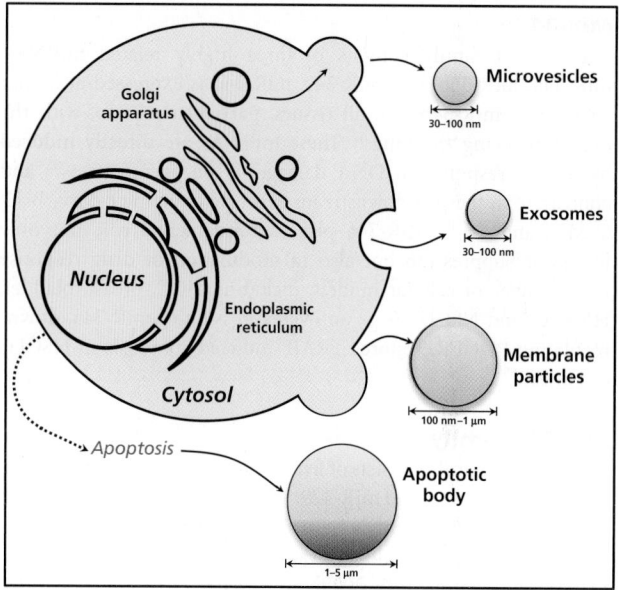

Figure 2 Process of extracellular vesicles release from cells. Apoptotic cells release apoptotic bodies.

breast milk, amniotic fluid, malignant ascites, and bronchoalveolar lavage fluid, suggesting their potential importance as biomarkers of disease.[50]

Selected miRNAs implicated in cancer

Following a multitude of miRNA in cancer studies, several miRNAs, including miR-155, let-7, miR-21, and miR-34, for example, have emerged as fundamental contributors to tumor development. These miRNAs are now being integrated into clinical trials as biomarkers for clinical diagnosis and therapy.

LET-7

The let-7 gene was first discovered in *C. elegans* as a key regulator of development.[51] The mature form of let-7 family members is highly conserved across species. let-7 miRs family plays an essential role in regulating cell proliferation and differentiation during development in different species. In addition, let-7 is a marker of fully differentiated cells while undetectable in stem cells.[52] The human let-7 family contains 12 members located on nine different chromosomes, they map to fragile sites associated with different types of solid cancers.[53] Indeed, the deregulation of these miRs has been shown as a feature of many types of cancer.[54–56] One of the most studied let-7 targets and regulators is the c-Myc oncogene, given, moreover, the well-known double-negative feedback between them.

MiR-21

MiR-21 is one of most studied oncomiRs, as most of its validated targets are tumor suppressors (i.e., PTEN, Bcl2, and Sprouty1 and 2). This miR is probably one of the most dynamic miRNAs, being responsive to various stimuli given its involvement in positive and negative feedback loops. miR-21 is one of the most altered miRNAs in solid tumors including breast, ovaries, cervix, colon, lung, liver, brain, esophagus, prostate, pancreas, and thyroid.[29,57–59] miR-21 is also upregulated in leukemic cancers,[60] indicating an important key role for this miRNA in cancer development and progression. Moreover, a recent study established circulating miR-21 as a biomarker of various carcinomas, unveiling its potential as a tool for cancer diagnosis.[61]

MiR-34

The miR-34 family consists of three highly related miRNAs: miR-34a, miR-34b, and miR-34c. miR-34a is expressed at higher levels than miR-34b/c in all tissues, particularly brain, with the exception being the lung.[62] These miRNAs are directly induced by p53 in response to DNA damage or oncogenic stress[63] and contribute to the p53 downstream effect by targeting c-Myc, Bcl2, C-Met, and Src.[64] MiR-34a plays a fundamental role not only in tumor suppression but also in modulation of drug response in a number of cellular models, including HCC, breast, bladder, HNSCC, and NSCLC (e.g., an overexpression of miR-34a, down-regulating PDGFR, restores TRAIL-induced apoptosis in NSCLC cell lines).[65]

MiR-200 family

The miR-200 family consists of five members: miR-200a, miR-200b, miR-200c, miR-141, and miR-429. These miRs are highly expressed in epithelial tissues and are involved in tumor suppression by inhibiting EMT, migration, invasion, tumor cell adhesion, and metastasis.[66] Among miR-200 family targets, ZEB1 and ZEB2, two central mediators of EMT, are two of the most studied. Moreover, there is a double-negative ZEB/miR-200 feedback loop, given the ability of ZEB1 to suppress the expression of miR-200 family members.[67] Furthermore, there is evidence that breast cancer metastases may be under the control of the Akt-miR200-E-cadherin axis. Specifically, the balance of the three Akt isoforms can control the expression of miR-200 and that of the E-cadherin mRNA in primary and metastatic human breast cancers.[68]

Therapeutic targeting and miRNA

Given that deregulation of a single or group of miRNAs can drive malignancy, it is hypothesized that through directed targeting of their deregulation, at least *in vitro*, one can attenuate carcinogenesis. Alternatively, patterns of miRNA deregulation may drive chemoresistance to traditional agents. For example, strategies aimed at using global miRNA expression profiling of selectively created drug-resistant cell lines have been utilized to identify which specific miRNAs are responsible for the acquired resistance. These findings have translated to miRNAs serving both as directed targets and predictors of response to chemotherapeutic agents. Importantly, the contribution of specific miRNAs to chemoresistance can be highly cell tumor specific. As mentioned, miRNAs have the capacity to simultaneously target and regulate multiple biological pathways. In the case of CLL, selected patterns of miRNA expression could clinically predict which patients would respond to the selected agent fludarabine.[69] In solid tumors such as lung cancer, miRNAs including miR-21, miR-30, miR-221, and miR-222 have been associated with response to chemotherapeutic agents. Recently, Vecchione et al.[70] profiled an miRNA signature that is able to define chemoresistance in ovarian cancer. It has been reported that an miRNA profiling is useful to identify a subtype of temozolomide-resistant glioblastoma.[71]

In the last few years, the majority of applications of miRNAs as directed therapies in human disease have taken place in *in vitro* and murine models of disease settings. The primary goal of directed therapeutics is to manipulate miRNAs that are known to be deregulated in tumors and thus alter their downstream targets and biological pathways. This approach may occur through the selected targeting of an miRNA or as a strategy for augmenting the effects of an established therapeutic agent. The manipulation of miRNAs via either selective gain of function (e.g., mimics) for the purposes of repletion or silencing (e.g., antagonists) has been applied with variable results. miRNAs may be delivered by several modalities including viral vectors and nanoparticles (NPs). Viral-based carriers have been effectively used to deliver miRNAs in solid tumors including let-7 in lung cancer.[72] However, viral carriers for small molecule delivery are not without limitations including the potential immunogenic and toxic effects of the carrier to the host. More recently, investigators have employed lipid-based NPs as carriers for small molecules including miRNA. NPs represent smaller engineered particles that are particularly suitable for drug delivery based on their modifiable composition allowing for optimal binding and absorption. Several recent studies have demonstrated the efficacy of NPs as vehicles for miRNA delivery *in vivo*. For example, Wu et al. recently showed that lipid-based NPs could be utilized to effectively deliver miR-29 in lung cancer both *in vitro* and *in vivo*.[73] In an independent study, Trang et al. showed that delivery of let-7 could reduce tumor growth and many oncogenes.[74] Issues of off-target effects, stability of carriers, and toxicity all remain germane to miRNA-based therapeutics. The use of miRNA sponges represents an alternative strategy to antagomirs. RNA sponges are able to simultaneously repress a large number of miRNA molecules. The existence of circular RNA (circRNA) has been already established in nature and can represent an example of miRNA sponge. circRNA is a type of RNA, which forms a covalently closed continuous loop, forming a circRNA whereby the 3′ and 5′ ends are attached together forming a round RNA molecule. This structural characteristic confers stability to circRNAs in the cytosol, while also ensuring the ability to bind simultaneously a variable number of miRNA molecules thus inhibiting their action. circRNAs are derived from protein-coding genes but do not encode for any protein and are thus classified as ncRNA.[75] Recently, investigators determined that a circRNA called R1as/CiRS-7 could serve as sponge for miR-7. This circRNA was able to downregulate miR-7 by acting as a specific sponge for it through 63 miR-7 binding sites.[76] The design of synthetic sponges able to mimic natural circRNA action represents a novel approach for the modulation of aberrant miRNA expression in cancer. This technology is very useful in satisfying the need to simultaneously downregulate several miRNAs or miRNA families.[77]

Recently, investigators have developed novel computational tools for the design of synthetic miRNAs capable of effectively and simultaneously targeting multiple specific mRNAs of choice (multitarget, multisite targeting). Lagana et al.[78] in 2014 developed and validated a bioinformatic tool termed "miR-Synth," which represents a single synthetic miRNA able to simultaneously target MET and EGFR. Interestingly, this tool can be applied to create synthetic miRNAs for a wide variety of different target combination choices. The concept of modulating miRNA in cancer through the reintroduction or the repression of deregulated miRNAs combined with the use of synthetic technology for the modulation of miRNA expression (miRNA sponges) and, finally, the employment of synthetic miRNA that can modulate simultaneously the expression of different genes of choice does not represent a strategy void of issues. The off-target problem and difficulties in delivery make miRNA-centered cancer therapy a promising technology not yet applicable.

Human applications for miRNAs

While the majority of miRNA-focused lines of investigation have been laboratory based, an increasing number of human clinical trials have begun to incorporate miRNAs as with predictive/therapeutic biomarkers or as directed therapeutics. Currently, there are over 100 clinical trials incorporating miRNAs that are either actively recruiting or completed recruiting. The majority of such studies are utilizing miRNAs as potential clinical biomarkers. However, in the last few years, we have witnessed the emergence if clinical studies directed at utilizing miRNAs as therapeutics in humans. The most recognized such study involves the application of an antagomir for miR-122 to treat hepatitis C.[79] Both phase I and phase II trials have been completed using the agent SPC3649 (Miravirsen) in both healthy volunteers and those with chronic Hepatitis C.[80] Currently, studies are ongoing to examine the utility of Miravirsen in chronic Hepatitis C nonresponders. In the area of cancers, there are two exciting studies on the horizon that have potential for clinical application. The first such study is an ongoing phase I trial, which is a multicenter phase I trial using a liposomal formulation of miR-34 (MRX34) for primary unresectable liver cancer or advanced metastatic solid malignancies with or without metastases. The second study identified as MesomiR-1 is a phase I trial involving the use of an EGFR-targeting delivery vehicle harboring miR-16 in individuals with malignant pleural mesothelioma or advanced nonsmall-cell lung cancer who have failed previous therapies.

References

1 Lee RC, Feinbaum RL, Ambros V. The *C. elegans* heterochronic gene lin-4 encodes small RNAs with antisense complementarity to lin-14. *Cell.* 1993;75:843–854.

2 Ambros V. The functions of animal microRNAs. *Nature.* 2004;431:350–355.

3 Croce CM. Causes and consequences of microRNA dysregulation in cancer. *Nat Rev Genet.* 2009;10:704–714.

4 Lagos-Quintana M, Rauhut R, Lendeckel W, Tuschl T. Identification of novel genes coding for small expressed RNAs. *Science.* 2001;294:853–858.

5 Miranda KC, Huynh T, Tay Y, et al. A pattern-based method for the identification of MicroRNA binding sites and their corresponding heteroduplexes. *Cell.* 2006;126:1203–1217.

6 Calin GA, Croce CM. MicroRNA signatures in human cancers. *Nat Rev Cancer.* 2006;6:857–866.

7 Nana-Sinkam SP, Hunter MG, Nuovo GJ, et al. Integrating the MicroRNome into the study of lung disease. *Am J Respir Crit Care Med.* 2009;179:4–10.

8 Nana-Sinkam SP, Croce CM. Non-coding RNAs in cancer initiation and progression and as novel biomarkers. *Mol Oncol.* 2011;5:483–491.

9 Rodriguez A, Griffiths-Jones S, Ashurst JL, Bradley A. Identification of mammalian microRNA host genes and transcription units. *Genome Res.* 2004;14:1902–1910.

10 Gregory RI, Yan KP, Amuthan G, et al. The Microprocessor complex mediates the genesis of microRNAs. *Nature.* 2004;432:235–240.

11 Bohnsack MT, Czaplinski K, Gorlich D. Exportin 5 is a RanGTP-dependent dsRNA-binding protein that mediates nuclear export of pre-miRNAs. *RNA.* 2004;10:185–191.

12 Helwak A, Kudla G, Dudnakova T, Tollervey D. Mapping the human miRNA interactome by CLASH reveals frequent noncanonical binding. *Cell.* 2013;153:654–665.

13 Calin GA, Dumitru CD, Shimizu M, et al. Frequent deletions and down-regulation of micro- RNA genes miR15 and miR16 at 13q14 in chronic lymphocytic leukemia. *Proc Natl Acad Sci U S A.* 2002;99:15524–15529.

14 Karube Y, Tanaka H, Osada H, et al. Reduced expression of Dicer associated with poor prognosis in lung cancer patients. *Cancer Sci.* 2005;96:111–115.

15 Merritt WM, Lin YG, Han LY, et al. Dicer, Drosha, and outcomes in patients with ovarian cancer. *N Engl J Med.* 2008;359:2641–2650.

16 Fabbri M, Garzon R, Cimmino A, et al. MicroRNA-29 family reverts aberrant methylation in lung cancer by targeting DNA methyltransferases 3A and 3B. *Proc Natl Acad Sci U S A.* 2007;104:15805–15810.

17 Costinean S, Sandhu SK, Pedersen IM, et al. Src homology 2 domain-containing inositol-5-phosphatase and CCAAT enhancer-binding protein beta are targeted by miR-155 in B cells of Emicro-MiR-155 transgenic mice. *Blood.* 2009;114:1374–1382.

18 Saito Y, Liang G, Egger G, et al. Specific activation of microRNA-127 with downregulation of the proto-oncogene BCL6 by chromatin-modifying drugs in human cancer cells. *Cancer Cell.* 2006;9:435–443.

19 Lee Y, Kim M, Han J, et al. MicroRNA genes are transcribed by RNA polymerase II. *EMBO J.* 2004;23:4051–4060.

20 O'Donnell KA, Wentzel EA, Zeller KI, Dang CV, Mendell JT. c-Myc-regulated microRNAs modulate E2F1 expression. *Nature.* 2005;435:839–843.

21 Garofalo M, Romano G, Di Leva G, et al. EGFR and MET receptor tyrosine kinase-altered microRNA expression induces tumorigenesis and gefitinib resistance in lung cancers. *Nat Med.* 2012;18:74–82.

22 He L, He X, Lowe SW, Hannon GJ. microRNAs join the p53 network—another piece in the tumour-suppression puzzle. *Nat Rev Cancer.* 2007;7:819–822.

23 Corney DC, Flesken-Nikitin A, Godwin AK, Wang W, Nikitin AY. MicroRNA-34b and microRNA-34c are targets of p53 and cooperate in control of cell proliferation and adhesion-independent growth. *Cancer Res.* 2007;67:8433–8438.

24 Brennecke J, Stark A, Russell RB, Cohen SM. Principles of microRNA-target recognition. *PLoS Biol.* 2005;3:e85.

25 Nigita G, Alaimo S, Ferro A, Giugno R, Pulvirenti A. Knowledge in the investigation of A-to-I RNA editing signals. *Front Bioeng Biotechnol.* 2015;3:18.

26 Kawahara Y, Zinshteyn B, Sethupathy P, Iizasa H, Hatzigeorgiou AG, Nishikura K. Redirection of silencing targets by adenosine-to-inosine editing of miRNAs. *Science.* 2007;315:1137–1140.

27 Chin LJ, Ratner E, Leng S, et al. A SNP in a let-7 microRNA complementary site in the KRAS 3′ untranslated region increases non-small cell lung cancer risk. *Cancer Res.* 2008;68:8535–8540.

28 Steinemann D, Tauscher M, Praulich I, Niemeyer CM, Flotho C, Schlegelberger B. Mutations in the let-7 binding site - a mechanism of RAS activation in juvenile myelomonocytic leukemia? *Haematologica.* 2010;95:1616.

29 Volinia S, Calin GA, Liu CG, et al. A microRNA expression signature of human solid tumors defines cancer gene targets. *Proc Natl Acad Sci U S A.* 2006;103:2257–2261.

30 Yanaihara N, Caplen N, Bowman E, et al. Unique microRNA molecular profiles in lung cancer diagnosis and prognosis. *Cancer Cell.* 2006;9:189–198.

31 Rosenfeld N, Aharonov R, Meiri E, et al. MicroRNAs accurately identify cancer tissue origin. *Nat Biotechnol.* 2008;26:462–469.

32 Nadal E, Chen G, Gallegos M, et al. Epigenetic inactivation of microRNA-34b/c predicts poor disease-free survival in early-stage lung adenocarcinoma. *Clin Cancer Res.* 2013;19:6842–6852.

33 Ferreira AF, Moura LG, Tojal I, et al. ApoptomiRs expression modulated by BCR-ABL is linked to CML progression and imatinib resistance. *Blood Cells Mol Dis.* 2014;53:47–55.

34 Akagi I, Okayama H, Schetter AJ, et al. Combination of protein coding and noncoding gene expression as a robust prognostic classifier in stage I lung adenocarcinoma. *Cancer Res.* 2013;**73**:3821–3832.

35 Creemers EE, Tijsen AJ, Pinto YM. Circulating microRNAs: novel biomarkers and extracellular communicators in cardiovascular disease? *Circ Res.* 2012;**110**:483–495.

36 Shen J, Liao J, Guarnera MA, et al. Analysis of microRNAs in sputum to improve computed tomography for lung cancer diagnosis. *J Thorac Oncol.* 2014;**9**:33–40.

37 Xing L, Todd NW, Yu L, Fang H, Jiang F. Early detection of squamous cell lung cancer in sputum by a panel of microRNA markers. *Mod Pathol.* 2010;**23**:1157–1164.

38 Mitchell PS, Parkin RK, Kroh EM, et al. Circulating microRNAs as stable blood-based markers for cancer detection. *Proc Natl Acad Sci U S A.* 2008;**105**:10513–10518.

39 Shen J, Liu Z, Todd NW, et al. Diagnosis of lung cancer in individuals with solitary pulmonary nodules by plasma microRNA biomarkers. *BMC Cancer.* 2011;**11**:374.

40 Boeri M, Verri C, Conte D, et al. MicroRNA signatures in tissues and plasma predict development and prognosis of computed tomography detected lung cancer. *Proc Natl Acad Sci U S A.* 2011;**108**:3713–3718.

10 Aberrant signaling pathways in cancer

Luca Grumolato, PhD ▪ Stuart A. Aaronson, MD

Overview

Most, if not all, human cancers harbor aberrant activation of one or several signaling pathways, contributing to tumor initiation and/or progression. In this chapter, we describe how growth factors signal to receptors with intrinsic tyrosine kinase activity to promote cell proliferation and survival, largely through activation of the phosphatidylinositol-3′-kinase(PI-3-K)/Akt and Ras/MAP kinase pathways. Using different paradigmatic examples of oncogenic alterations in growth factor signaling, we discuss functional implications and relevance of these pathways for human cancer. General cell signaling principles in both normal and tumor cells will be addressed, and we briefly discuss how the initiation and progression of specific cancer types can be affected by the deregulation of certain other pathways, including those mediated by cytokines, the transforming growth factor-β (TGFβ) family, Wnt, Hedgehog, Notch, and nuclear receptors.

Finally, we discuss the concepts of oncogene addiction and targeted therapy and provide a few representative examples to illustrate how increased understanding of the mechanisms underlying signaling pathway aberrations in cancer can been translated to the clinic.

Intercellular communication in multicellular organisms is required for processes such as embryonic development, tissue differentiation, and systemic responses to wounds and infections. These complex signaling networks are in large part mediated by growth factors, cytokines, and hormones. Such factors can influence cell proliferation in positive or negative ways, as well as induce a series of differentiated responses in appropriate target cells. Cytoplasmic molecules that mediate these responses have been termed second messengers. The eventual transmission of biochemical signals to the nucleus leads to effects on the expression of genes involved in mitogenic and differentiation responses.

The pathogenic expression of critical genes in growth factor signaling pathways can also contribute to altered cell growth associated with malignancy. The v-*sis* oncogene of simian sarcoma virus, which encodes a growth factor homologous to the B chain of human platelet-derived growth factor (PDGF-B), is the paradigm for such genes.[1] The normal counterparts of other retroviral oncogenes were subsequently shown to encode membrane-spanning growth factor receptors.[2,3] Other genes that act early in intracellular pathways of growth factor signal transduction have been implicated as oncogenes as well. Present knowledge indicates that the constitutive activation of growth factor signaling pathways through genetic alterations affecting these genes contributes to the development and progression of most, if not all, human cancers.

Because of space limitations, this chapter primarily focuses on growth factor signaling mediated by receptors with intrinsic tyrosine (Tyr) kinase activity. However, we briefly highlight other ligand-triggered pathways relevant to cancer biology.

Growth factor receptors with Tyr kinase activity

Hormones that act at great distances from the cells producing them have been known for many years. Hormones as signaling molecules were isolated from tissue fluids and readily characterized by their *in vivo* effects. The initial discoveries of growth factors indicated more subtle activities capable of stimulating the growth of chicken embryonic nerve cells in the case of nerve growth factor (NGF)[4] or promotion of eyelid opening and incisor eruption in the case of epidermal growth factor (EGF).[5] An important discovery concerning growth factors came from the demonstration of a unique enzymologic activity associated with binding of EGF to its receptor.[5] Studies of the product of the viral oncogene, v-*src*, had led to the demonstration of its ability to act as a protein kinase.[6,7] Many protein kinases had been previously identified, but these had the capacity to phosphorylate serine (Ser) and/or threonine (Thr) residues. Moreover, it was well established that phosphorylations and dephosphorylations affected the activities of a variety of proteins. However, the *src* product was subsequently shown to have a unique specificity as a protein kinase in that it was capable of phosphorylating Tyr residues.[8] Cohen then showed that addition of EGF led to phosphorylation of its purified receptor on Tyr residues.[5] Subsequent studies have demonstrated that Tyr kinase activity is central to the functions of a large number of mitogenic signaling molecules.

More than 50 receptor Tyr kinases (RTKs) belonging to at least 18 different receptor families have been identified[9,10] (Figure 1). All RTKs contain a large, glycosylated, extracellular ligand-binding domain, a single transmembrane region, and a cytoplasmic portion with a conserved protein Tyr kinase domain. In addition to the catalytic domain, a juxtamembrane region and a carboxyl-terminal tail can be identified in the cytoplasmic portion. Because of their structure, RTKs can be visualized as membrane-associated allosteric enzymes with the ligand-binding and protein Tyr kinase domains separated by the plasma membrane. Their role is to catalyze the transfer of the γ-phosphate of adenosine triphosphate (ATP) to Tyr residues of exogenous substrates, as well as within their own polypeptide chain. Tyr phosphorylation represents the language that these receptors use to transduce the information carried by the growth factor.

RTKs are activated by their ligands through receptor oligomerization, which stabilizes interactions between adjacent cytoplasmic domains and controls the activation of kinase activity.[10] Dimerization can take place between two identical receptors (homodimerization), between different members of the same receptor family, or, in some cases, between a receptor and an accessory protein (heterodimerization),[10] thus expanding both the repertoire of ligands recognized by each receptor and the diversity of effector pathways stimulated by a given receptor.

How ligands bind to induce receptor oligomerization varies for each class of RTKs.[10,11] PDGF, for example, induces receptor dimerization by virtue of its dimeric nature.[12] EGF induces instead

Holland-Frei Cancer Medicine, Ninth Edition. Edited by Robert C. Bast Jr., Carlo M. Croce, William N. Hait, Waun Ki Hong, Donald W. Kufe, Martine Piccart-Gebhart, Raphael E. Pollock, Ralph R. Weichselbaum, Hongyang Wang, and James F. Holland.
© 2017 John Wiley & Sons, Inc. ISBN: 978-1-118-93469-2

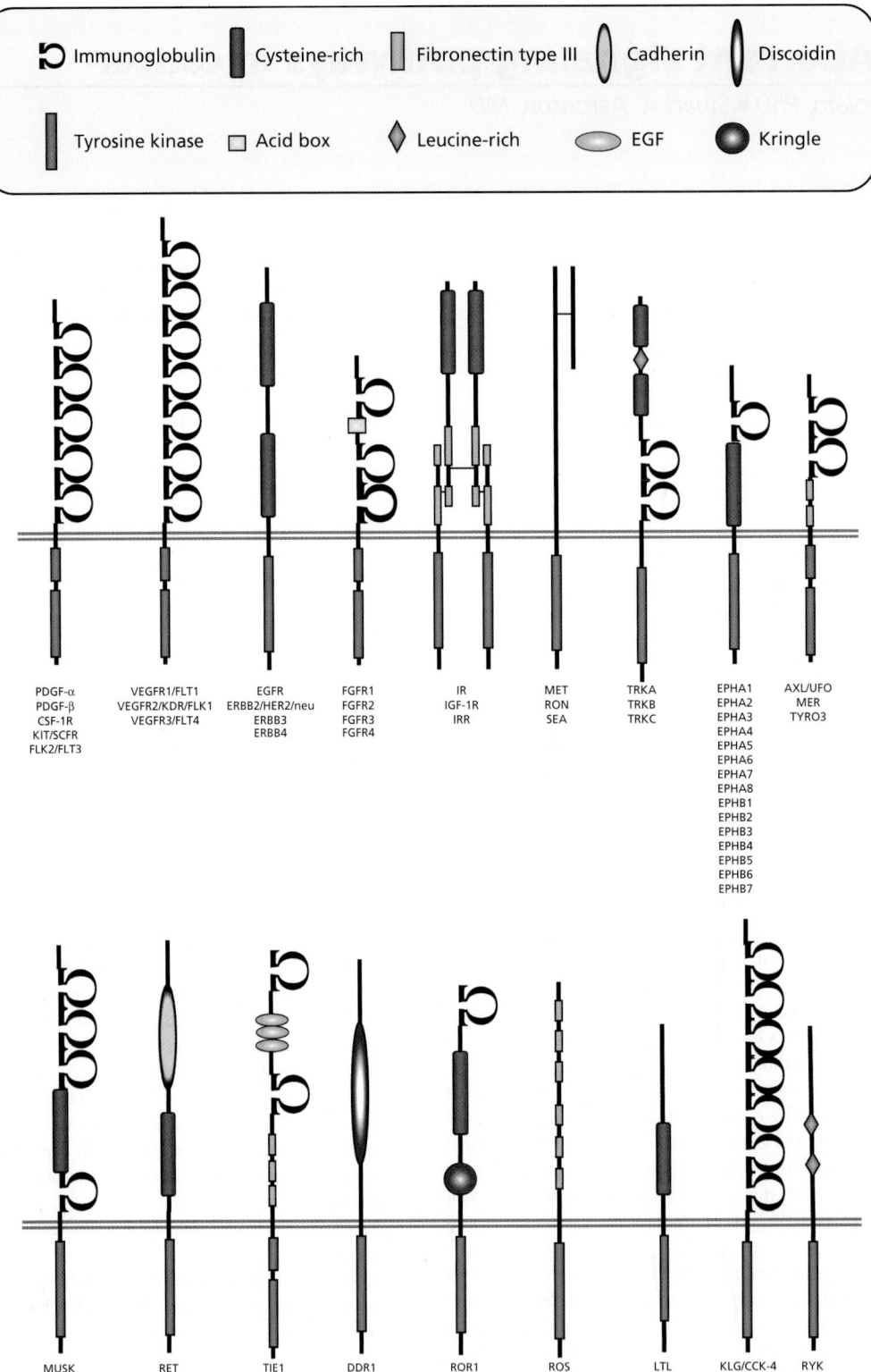

Figure 1 Families of receptor tyrosine kinases.

a conformational change in the extracellular domain of the epidermal growth factor receptor (EGFR), resulting in the exposure of a dimerization domain that is masked in the absence of the ligand.[10] Fibroblast growth factor, which is a monomeric ligand like EGF, needs an accessory molecule, heparan sulfate proteoglycan, to induce receptor dimerization.[13,14] In contrast, the insulin receptor family exists as disulfide-bonded homo- or heterodimers

of receptor subunits, and ligand binding causes a conformational change in the preformed dimeric receptor, which leads to receptor activation.[15,16]

The activation of intrinsic protein kinase activity results in autophosphorylation of specific Tyr residues in the cytoplasmic portion of the RTK. Moreover, Tyr phosphorylation in the kinase domain stimulates the intrinsic catalytic activity of the receptor.

Biochemical and structural studies have revealed some of the molecular mechanisms that mediate such activation. There is substantial evidence that autophosphorylation occurs in *trans* by a second RTK after dimerization induced by ligand binding. In the unphosphorylated state, the receptor possesses a low catalytic activity due to the particular conformation of a specific domain in the kinase region, which interferes with the phosphotransfer event. Phosphorylation of the kinase domain removes this inhibition, and the catalytic activity is enhanced and persists for some time independently of the presence of the ligand. Although kinase activity is at a low basal level in the monomeric state, this activity is sufficient to induce *trans*-autophosphorylation once the dimer forms. In addition to this mechanism, different RTKs contain *cis*-inhibitory elements outside the kinase domain, such as in the juxtamembrane domain (e.g., in KIT and MuSK) or the C-terminal tail (e.g., in Tie2), that can be disrupted by trans-phosphorylation following receptor dimerization. Besides the regulation of receptor catalytic activity, the other major function of RTK autophosphorylation is to create specific docking sites for downstream molecules that participate in the transduction of the signal (see the following section).

Aberrations affecting growth factor receptors in tumor cells

Although growth factor receptors can be constitutively activated by autocrine/paracrine loops, a number of other mechanisms have been identified by which growth factor receptors can become transforming. The paradigm for such alterations is the avian erythroblastosis viral oncogene *v-erbB*, which corresponds to a truncated form of EGFR, in which deletion of the ligand-binding domain results in the constitutive activation of the receptor.[2] Alterations affecting a large number of RTKs have been implicated in different human malignancies. One mechanism involves the amplification or overexpression of a normal receptor, such as in the case of EGFR, ErbB-2, and MET.[17-20] *ErbB-2* was initially identified as an amplified gene in a primary human breast carcinoma and a salivary gland tumor.[21,22] Clinical studies have indicated that the normal *ErbB-2* gene is frequently amplified and/or overexpressed in human breast carcinomas and in ovarian carcinomas,[23] and detection in breast carcinomas of high ErbB-2 levels was initially a prognostic indicator of poor survival.[17,18] While ErbB-2 overexpression has been observed primarily in adenocarcinomas, the overexpression of a normal EGFR has been reported frequently in squamous cell carcinomas and glioblastomas.[17,24] In many cases, the EGFR appears to be activated by autocrine stimulation by one of its ligands, most commonly transforming growth factor-α.

Genomic alterations, such as mutation or rearrangement, have also been shown to activate the transforming capacity of RTKs in different human malignancies.[25] For example, deletions within the external domain of the EGFR receptor or mutations in its Tyr kinase domain[26,27] are associated with its constitutive activation in some glioblastomas, lung and breast cancers.[17,24] The *ret* gene is activated by rearrangement, as a somatic event, in about one-third of papillary thyroid carcinomas, whereas germline mutations of cysteine residues in the extracellular region, which affect receptor dimerization, are responsible for multiple endocrine neoplasia (MEN) 2A and for the familial medullary thyroid carcinoma syndrome. Of note, point mutations in the RET kinase domain are associated with MEN 2B,[28] indicating that the catalytic function of an RTK can be upregulated by oncogenic alterations affecting distinct domains of the receptor. Another example of an RTK activated by genetic alterations in the germline is the receptor for hepatocyte growth factor, MET, which is responsible for hereditary papillary renal carcinomas. Aberrant activation of MET

through amplification/overexpression or mutations is also found in a variety of sporadic tumors including renal, liver, and gastric cancer.[20] Finally, several other receptors, including the anaplastic lymphoma kinase (ALK), ROS1 and TrkA, have been shown to be oncogenically activated in human malignancies by chromosomal rearrangements that lead to fusion products containing the activated TK domain.[25]

> **KEY POINTS**
> - RTKs are activated by growth factors through receptor dimerization and subsequent trans-phosphorylation.
> - Tyr phosphorylation represents the language used by these receptors to transduce their signals, allowing specific recruitment of different effector or adaptor proteins.
> - Different mechanisms are responsible for constitutive RTK activation in tumor cells. These include receptor/ligand overexpression, RTK amplification/mutation, and chromosomal translocation, which results in the formation of constitutively active fusion protein.

Signaling pathways of Tyr kinase receptors

Molecules, known as adaptor and scaffolding proteins,[29] play an integral role in intracellular signaling by both recruiting various proteins to specific locations and assembling networks of proteins particular to RTK cascades. These adaptor proteins often contain a variety of motifs that mediate protein–protein interactions, including Src homology 2 (SH2) and phosphoTyr-binding domains, which bind to specific phosphorylated Tyr containing sequences, or SH3 domains, which recognize and bind to proline-rich sequences in target proteins.[29,30] One such adaptor, Grb2, is important in the activation of the small G-protein Ras (Figure 2).

The PDGF system has served as the prototype for identification of the components of signaling cascades. Certain molecules become physically associated and/or phosphorylated by the activated PDGF receptor (PDGFR) kinase. These include phospholipase C-γ,[31] PI-3-K regulatory subunit (p85),[32] NCK,[33] the phosphatase SHP-2,[34] Grb2,[35] CRK,[36] RAS p21 GTPase-activating protein (GAP),[37] SRC, and SRC-like Tyr kinases.[38] Many of these molecules contain SH2 or SH3 domains.

PI-3-K and survival signaling

The regulation of cell survival and cell death is essential for both normal development and tissue homeostasis in adult organisms, where damaged cells must be removed and terminally differentiated cells must be sustained. A failure for this to occur may result either in the accumulation of mutations leading to cancer or to degenerative diseases.

PI-3-K is a lipid kinase that catalyzes the transfer of the γ-phosphate from ATP to the D3 position of the phosphoinositide (PtdIns), generating PtdIns(3,4,5)P3. These lipids can act in a variety of cascades, promoting the activation of several proteins (Figure 2). PI-3-K activation has been demonstrated to play an important role in survival signaling in a number of cell types.[39,40] The prototypical class 1 PI-3-K consists of two tightly associated subunits encoded by two distinct loci: a regulatory and a catalytic subunit. The classic mode of PI-3-K activation involves binding of the regulatory subunit to the phosphorylated Tyr residues of RTKs through SH2 domains, resulting in a conformational change that facilitates activation of the catalytic subunit. There are several known downstream effectors of PI-3-K. These include Rac, certain isoforms of protein kinase C, and, most relevant to cell survival,

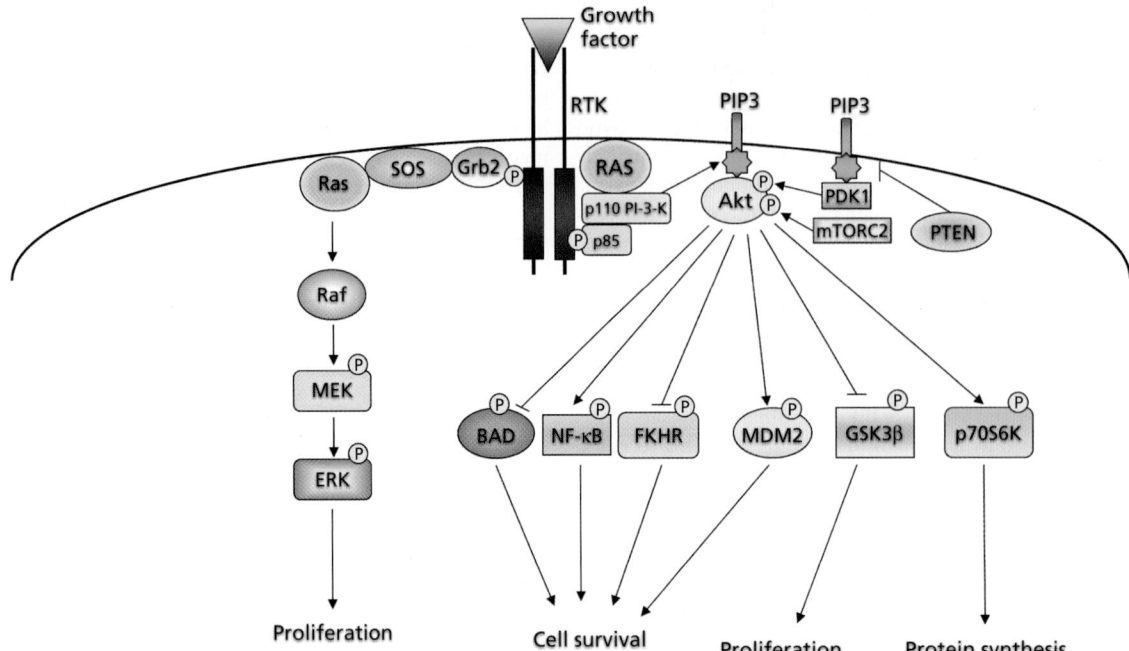

Figure 2 Intracellular effectors of receptor tyrosine kinases.

Akt, the cellular homolog of the viral oncogene *v-Akt*.[39,40] Three human homologs encode 57 kDa Ser/Thr kinases that contain an *N*-terminal pleckstrin homology (PH) domain, which binds to the activated PtdIns products of PI-3-K. These lipids are believed to mediate the localization of Akt to the plasma membrane. In addition, phosphorylation of two residues, Thr 308 and Ser 473, is required for its full activation.[39,40]

Akt promotes survival and prevents apoptosis in various cell types through the regulation of different downstream pathways and effectors[41] (Figure 2). Akt phosphorylates the pro-apoptotic protein BAD (BCL2-associated agonist of cell death), thus creating a docking site for the cytosolic protein 14-3-3, which sequesters BAD and inhibits its activity. Akt also phosphorylates FOXO transcription factors creating a binding site for 14-3-3, which retains them in the cytoplasm and inhibits their transcriptional targets, including pro-apoptotic proteins such as BIM and FAS ligand. Moreover, Akt can increase p53 degradation through phosphorylation of MDM2, and there is evidence that Akt can increase the pro-survival functions of the nuclear factor-κB (NF-κB) transcription factor complex and inhibit the pro-apoptotic c-Jun *N*-terminal kinase (JNK) and p38 pathways.[41] Besides promoting cell survival, Akt can also exert positive effects on cell growth through inhibitory phosphorylations of the tuberous sclerosis complex 2, resulting in the activation of the mTOR pathway, or GSK3, which normally targets cyclin D1 for degradation[41,42] (Figure 2).

PI-3-K signaling in cancer

PIK3CA, which encodes the p110α catalytic subunit, was originally found to be amplified in a high percentage of ovarian tumors and ovarian tumor cell lines.[43] Later studies revealed that PIK3CA is one of the most frequently mutated oncogenes in human cancer, particularly in colon, breast, endometrial, brain, and gastric tumors.[44,45] While far less frequently mutated in cancer, Akt can also play a role in human malignancies. Akt1 was found to be amplified 20-fold in a primary gastric adenocarcinoma.[46] Additional studies have shown genomic amplification and overexpression of Akt2 in pancreatic and ovarian carcinoma cell lines, as well as in some ovarian and breast

carcinomas.[47] Overexpression of Akt2 occurs more frequently in undifferentiated and, thus, more aggressive tumors. Missense mutations in the Akt1 PH domain were identified in breast, colon, and ovarian cancers, resulting in prolonged Akt activation owing to its pathological localization to the plasma membrane.[48]

Further evidence of the involvement of the PI-3-K/Akt pathway in cancer stems from the discovery of the phosphatase and tensin homolog (PTEN) tumor suprressor, a gene inactivated by mutation in a high fraction of glial and endometrial tumors, as well as in melanoma, prostate, renal, and small-cell lung carcinomas.[42,45,49] By dephosphorylating the three position of phosphatidylinositol, PTEN directly opposes PI-3-K activity, thus inhibiting Akt activation.

Ras

Ras proteins are a major point of convergence in RTK signaling and are important components of the cellular machinery necessary to transduce extracellular signals (Figure 2). These small GTP-binding proteins are membrane-bound intracellular signaling molecules that mediate a wide variety of cellular functions, including proliferation, differentiation, and survival. Ras acts as a molecular switch alternating from an inactive GDP-bound state to an active GTP-bound state. The paradigm for Ras activation involves the recruitment of a guanine nucleotide exchange factor (GEF) to the membrane in response to growth factor binding and subsequent activation of an RTK.[50] GEFs promote the release of GDP from the catalytic pocket of Ras, and the relative abundance of intracellular GTP as compared to GDP ensures preferential binding of GTP. The best example of a Ras GEF is son of sevenless, which is brought to the membrane by its stable association with the adaptor protein Grb2.[51] Although Ras is a GTPase, its intrinsic GTPase activity is actually quite low and requires additional proteins known as GAPs to promote GTP hydrolysis. GAPs can accelerate GTP hydrolysis by several orders of magnitude and are, thus, negative regulators of Ras functions.[50,52] An example of a Ras GAP is neurofibromin, encoded by the *NF1* gene, which is frequently inactivated by mutation in different types of cancer, including glioblastoma and lung cancer, as well as in patients with the familial tumor syndrome, neurofibromatosis type I.[50,53]

Ras mediates its multitude of biologic effects via a number of downstream effectors. Several proteins have been shown to directly bind to Ras in a GTP-dependent manner, including Raf, Ral, and PI-3-K.[52] In fact, Ras can activate PI-3-K independently of RTKs, providing a direct connection between Ras and PI-3-K prosurvival signaling.[50]

Ras and cancer

Ras has been shown to be oncogenically activated by mutations in over 15% of all human tumors, and in some cancers, such as pancreatic carcinoma, the frequency is as high as 60%.[52,54] The initial evidence for Ras involvement in cancer came from the discovery of transforming retroviruses, Harvey and Kirsten sarcoma viruses, which contained *H-* and *K-ras* cellular-derived oncogenes. The first human oncogenes were identified by transfecting genomic DNA from human tumor cell lines into NIH3T3 mouse fibroblasts and isolating the DNA fragments from the transformed foci. These were shown to be the human homologs of the viral *ras* genes.[55]

The major hotspots for activating Ras mutations decrease the intrinsic rate of GTP hydrolysis by Ras and make the molecule significantly less sensitive to GAP-stimulated GTP hydrolysis. Thus, the outcome is a predominantly GTP-bound form that is constitutively active and essentially independent of growth factor stimulation.[52,54]

Signaling downstream of Ras: Ras>Raf>MAPKinase cascade

The most well-studied effector of Ras is the Ser/Thr kinase Raf. Raf has been shown to bind to Ras and, in many cases, has been demonstrated to be indispensable for Ras functions, such as cellular transformation.[56,57] There are three known mammalian Raf isoforms, designated A-, B-, and C-Raf (also known as Raf-1), displaying distinct expression patterns.[57] Ras-GTP binds to the amino terminus of Raf and promotes its activation, resulting in Raf homo- or heterodimerization and the phosphorylation of different Ser/Thr and Tyr residues participating in the regulation of Raf activity.[57,58] Once activated, Raf can phosphorylate the mitogen/extracellular-signal regulated kinase (MEK), also known as MAP kinase kinase (MKK), a dual specificity kinase, leading to its activation[56,58] (Figure 2). MEK can, in turn, activate MAP kinase or extracellular signal-regulated kinase (ERK) through tandem phosphorylations on both Thr 183 and Tyr 185. ERK then translocates to the nucleus, where it can activate a variety of proteins through phosphorylation on Ser or Thr, including the ETS family of transcription factors and the kinase p90 RSK, involved in protein translation.[58,59] Activation of the Ras-Raf-MAPK pathway results in an increase of DNA synthesis and cell proliferation, exemplified by the induction of cyclin D1,[60] a major regulator of early cell cycle progression. In fact, cyclin D1 is also one of the most frequently amplified genes in cancer.[61]

Raf and cancer

The direct implication of Raf in human cancer came relatively recently with the identification of B-Raf mutations in more than half of melanoma cell lines and primary tumors.[62] B-Raf mutations, which generally affect few specific residues, such as valine 600, were subsequently found in other malignancies, including thyroid (60%), colorectal (10%), and lung (6%) cancer.[56] While B-Raf is one of the most commonly activated oncogenes, mutated in about 8% of all cancers, the frequency of A-Raf and C-Raf mutations is far lower, probably because of their weaker basal kinase activity compared to B-Raf.[56] Of note, oncogenic activation of B-Raf can also occur following chromosome translocations, which result in

the expression of fusion proteins containing the catalytic carboxy terminus of B-Raf. Such translocations have been found in pediatric astrocytoma, glioma, and thyroid cancers.[56]

Other MAP kinases

In addition to the ERKs, there are other MAP kinases belonging to distinct MAPK cascades with both different upstream activators and downstream effectors. JNK and p38 are stress-activated kinases involved in the cellular responses to a wide variety of extracellular stimuli, including mitogens, inflammatory cytokines, and UV irradiation.[63] In contrast to its ability to activate the MAPK/ERK cascade, Ras only minimally perturbs JNK and p38, whose activity is mainly induced by the Rho family of small G-proteins, including Rac1, Cdc42, and RhoA. The pathways leading to JNK or p38 activation mirror those seen for ERK, with a variety of MKKs that can phosphorylate the various JNK isoforms.[63]

As with the ERKs, the end result of JNK and p38 activation is the phosphorylation of different transcription factors, resulting in increased expression of their target genes. Examples of transcription factors directly phosphorylated by either JNK or p38, or both, include ATF2, ELK1, JUN, MYC, and MEF2.[63,64] Of note, some of these factors were initially discovered as retroviral oncogenes.

KEY POINTS

- Activated RTKs promote PI-3-K-mediated synthesis of PtdIns3P, resulting in the recruitment and activation of the kinase Akt. Through the regulation of different downstream effectors, Akt promotes survival in various cell types.

- RTKs stimulate cell proliferation largely through activation of the Ras/Raf/MAPK pathway.

- In human cancer, these downstream pathways can be frequently activated independently of RTKs, generally through mutations in the genes encoding various key effectors, including PI-3-K, Ras, and Raf.

Other signaling pathways aberrantly deregulated in cancer

While activation of the RTK pathway is common in most, if not all, types of cancer, other signaling pathways can also play instrumental roles in tumor initiation and progression. During embryonic development and in adulthood, these pathways exert diverse physiological functions, but, as with RTK signaling, they can be aberrantly activated (or inactivated) in cancer, as a result of mutations, chromosomal rearrangements or other mechanisms.

Although RTKs represent the largest family of cell surface receptors possessing an enzymatic activity, there are other classes of receptors with such activities. For example, transforming growth factor-β (TGFβ) induces the formation of a tetrameric complex containing two type I and two type II TGFβ receptors, both Ser/Thr kinases. Type II receptors then phosphorylate type I receptors, which propagate the signal through binding and phosphorylation of the SMAD transcription factors, resulting in SMAD activation.[65] Depending on cellular context, the TGFβ pathway can play a role in either tumor suppression or progression. In pre-malignant cells, TGFβ signaling can promote apoptosis, thus explaining the frequent inactivating mutations of TGFβ receptors or SMADs found in certain tumors, including colorectal and pancreatic carcinomas. Other tumors, including glioma, melanoma, and breast carcinoma, can use other mechanisms to circumvent this tumor-suppressive activity of TGFβ, while maintaining a functional pathway, which, in more advanced tumors, can favor progression and metastasis through crosstalk between tumor cells and their microenvironment.[65]

Other surface receptors lack an intrinsic catalytic activity but instead directly interact with enzymatic adaptor proteins that mediate propagation of the signal. This is the case, for example, with cytokine receptors, which bind to the Janus kinase (JAK) family of Tyr kinases.[66] Upon cytokine-induced dimerization of their receptors, JAKs transphosphorylate each other, as well as the *C*-terminus of the receptors, thus creating docking sites for a family of transcription factors, the signal transducers and activators of transcriptions (STATs). Following JAK-mediated phosphorylation, STATs form homo- or heterodimers through their SH2 domains and translocate to the nucleus to transcriptionally activate their target genes.[66,67] Activating mutations of JAK2 are common in patients with different types of myeloproliferative neoplasms, including polycythemia vera and essential thrombocythemia, resulting in cytokine hypersensitivity and cytokine-independent proliferation.[68] While STAT mutations are far less common, different mechanisms have been shown to promote STAT3 and STAT5 activation in various cancers, affecting tumor growth and invasion, as well as tumor interactions with the immune system.[67] Another example of receptors directly interacting with proteins possessing enzymatic activity are the G-protein-coupled receptors (GPCRs), a large family of seven membrane-spanning domain proteins, which are activated by very different types of ligands, including hormones, neurotransmitters, and chemokines.[69] While certain tumors contain mutations in GPCRs or their G proteins, the most common mechanism of aberrant activation of this signaling pathway in cancer is through receptor overexpression and autocrine stimulation.[69] The GPCR pathway is particularly relevant in tumors of the endocrine system, and ligands signaling through these receptors, such as certain chemokines, are major modulators of the tumor microenvironment.[70]

Activation of other signaling pathways with well-established roles in cancer occurs through more complex mechanisms involving different co-receptors, adaptor proteins and cytoplasmic complexes with or without enzymatic activity. This is the case with Wnt, Hedgehog, Hippo, Notch, and tumor necrosis factor (TNF)/NF-κB signaling. A common feature of these diverse signaling pathways is that ligand activation of the receptor results in stabilization or activation at or near the cell membrane of a transcription or co-transcription factor, for example, NF-κB (TNF),[71] GLI (Hedgehog),[72] YAP/TAZ (Hippo)[73] and β-catenin (Wnt).[74] A variation on this theme is represented by the Notch pathway, where binding by Delta/Jagged ligands induces cleavage of the Notch receptor and release of its cytoplasmic domain, which translocates to the nucleus and activates the CBF1, Suppressor of Hairless, Lag-1 transcription factors.[75] These highly conserved signaling pathways regulate fundamental physiological processes required for normal embryonic development and stem/progenitor cell maintenance in the adult. Their capacity to regulate cell proliferation, survival, and differentiation helps to explain why these pathways are frequently targeted in tumorigenesis. For example, mutations of different genes resulting in aberrant activation of Wnt/β-catenin signaling can be found in almost all colorectal carcinomas.[74,76,77] Of note, aberrant activation of Wnt signaling through different mechanisms has also been identified at significant frequency in diverse tumor types including breast, adrenocortical, and hepatocellular carcinoma.[74,78–80]

A different class of signaling molecules can cross the cell membrane and binds in the cytoplasm or in the nucleus to a large family of transcription factors, which serve as receptors for such ligands. Once bound to their ligands, these nuclear receptors can activate, as homo- or hetero-dimers, the expression of specific target genes through interaction with different co-activators.[81] The nuclear receptor family includes around 50 members and regulates diverse physiological processes, which can play a crucial

role in some types of cancer. For example, the proliferation and growth of a large fraction of breast and prostate tumors depends on sex hormone receptors, that is, estrogen/progesterone and androgen receptors, respectively. These findings have important implications for the treatment of such tumors, which respond to sex hormone antagonists or inhibitors of sex hormone synthesis.[82–84] Another example of the involvement of nuclear receptors in cancer is the chromosomal translocation of the *promyelocytic leukemia* (*PML*) and the *retinoid acid receptor* α (*RARα*) genes resulting in a PML-RAR fusion protein. This fusion protein enhances the recruitment of co-repressors to the regulatory regions of RARα target genes, inhibiting normal differentiation of the myeloid lineage. This results in accumulation of immature granulocytes precursors and to a deadly form of blood malignancy, acute promyelocytic leukemia (APL). The discovery of this tumorigenic mechanism translated into the design of a new therapy based on treatment with all-trans RA, which can result in cure of 70–80% of APL patients.[85] The example of APL illustrates how signaling pathways aberrantly activated in cancer can be specifically targeted in the clinic to block or restrain the growth and/or the spread of tumors, a concept discussed further in the following text.

KEY POINTS

- Other ligand families signal through their receptors to activate diverse effector pathways.

- In most cases, such receptors directly or indirectly activate specific transcription factors at or near the cell surface, and these factors regulate the expression of specific target genes.

- Certain ligands penetrate the cell to bind their cognate receptors, which function as bona fide transcription factors.

- These pathways control a wide range of physiological processes, and their aberrant deregulation through different mechanisms plays an instrumental role in the initiation and/or progression of various tumors.

Growth factor signaling and cancer therapy

As many of the signaling pathways involved in cellular transformation by oncogenes have been elucidated, efforts have been made to develop therapeutic strategies that target such oncogenically activated signaling molecules or their downstream effectors. One of the important advantages of rationally based targets is that approaches are generally available to monitor *in vivo* inhibition of the target molecule. This makes correlation of clinical response with pharmacodynamic analysis of target suppression feasible to speed the process of clinical testing. Another advantage is that some of these agents appear to have less inherent toxicities than standard chemotherapeutic regimens. Such approaches rely on the concept of "oncogene addiction," which implies that tumor cells, despite their complex pattern of mutational events, can become particularly dependent on one or a few signaling pathways for their growth and/or survival.[86] These pathways are thought to counterbalance other pro-apoptotic signals also triggered by oncogenic alterations in the tumor: once the pro-survival signal is blocked, the tumor cell undergoes what has been defined as "oncogenic shock" and dies.[87] This idea is supported by studies with tumor cell lines,[88] as well as in genetically modified mice, in which complete regression of tumors induced by oncogenes, such as K-Ras, was achieved by switching off expression of the oncogene.[89] Treatments targeting aberrantly activated signaling pathways, either alone or in combination with traditional chemo- or radiation therapy, have yielded extraordinary clinical benefit for certain types of malignancies.

However, additional genetic lesions, often activating the same signaling pathway, have been shown in many cases to eventually by-pass the targeted oncogene with associated disease progression (see the following sections).

Monoclonal antibodies

One possible target for therapeutic intervention is the initial triggering of growth factor signaling at the surface of tumor cells. Monoclonal antibodies have been generated to specifically neutralize the activities of growth factors or interfere with ligand receptor interactions. Monoclonal antibodies have also been applied to interfere with receptors overexpressed in certain types of cancer[90] (Table 1). Trastuzumab (herceptin, Genentech), a humanized monoclonal antibody against ErbB2, became the first clinically approved drug targeting an oncogene product. Experimental evidence further indicated that trastuzumab enhances the responsiveness of ErbB2 overexpressing breast cancer cells to taxanes, anthracyclines, and platinum compounds.[91] Cetuximab (erbitux, ImClone Systems), a chimeric monoclonal antibody against the EGFR has been approved for the treatment of colorectal and head and neck cancers in combination with chemotherapy and radiotherapy, respectively.[91–93] Of note, it was shown that cetuximab

Table 1 Cancer therapeutics targeting aberrant signaling pathways.

Cancer drug	Target	Disease
Monoclonal antibodies		
Bevacizumab (Avastin)	VEGF	Colorectal cancer, NSCLC, RCC, glioblastoma, and cervical cancer
Cetuximab (Erbitux)	EGFR	Colorectal cancer, head, and neck cancer
Denosumab (Xgeva)	RANKL	Giant cell tumor of the bone
Panitumumab (Vectibix)	EGFR	Colorectal cancer
Pertuzumab (Perjeta)	ErbB2	Breast cancer
Ramucirumab (Cyramza)	VEGFR2	Stomach adenocarcinoma
Siltuximab (Sylvant)	IL-6	Lymphoma
Trastuzumab (Herceptin)	ErbB2	Breast cancer and gastric cancer
Fusion protein		
Aflibercept (Zaltrap)	VEGFA, VEGFB, and PGF	Colorectal cancer
Small molecule inhibitors		
Abiraterone (Zytiga)	Testosterone synthesis	Prostate cancer
Afatinib (Gilotrif)	EGFR, ERBB2, and ERBB4	NSCLC
Anastrozole (Arimidex)	Estrogen synthesis	Breast cancer
Axitinib (Inlyta)	VEGFR, PDGFR, and c-KIT	RCC
Bosutinib (Bosulif)	Abl, Src	CML
Cabozantinib (Cometriq)	c-Met, RET, VEGFR, c-KIT, FLT-3, TIE-2, TRKB, and AXL	Thyroid cancer
Ceritinib (Zykadia)	ALK	NSCLC
Crizotinib (Xalkori)	ALK and c-Met	NSCLC
Dabrafenib (Tafinlar)	B-Raf	Melanoma
Dasatinib (Sprycel)	Abl and Src	CML, ALL
Enzalutamide (Xtandi)	AR	Prostate cancer
Erlotinib (Tarceva)	EGFR	NSCLC, pancreatic carcinoma
Everolimus (Afinitor)	mTOR	RCC, astrocytoma, PNET, breast cancer
Exemestane (Aromasin)	Estrogen synthesis	Breast cancer
Fulvestrant (Faslodex)	ER	Breast cancer
Gefitinib (Iressa)	EGFR	NSCLC
Ibrutinib (Imbruvica)	BTK	CLL, mantle cell lymphoma
Idelalisib (Zydelig)	PI-3-K	CLL
Lapatinib (Tykerb)	EGFR and ERBB2	Breast cancer
Letrozole (Femara)	Estrogen synthesis	Breast cancer
Imatinib (Gleevec)	Abl, PDGFR, and c-Kit	CML, GIST, ALL, and dermatofibrosarcoma protuberans
Nilotinib (Tasigna)	Abl, PDGFR, and c-Kit	CML
Pazopanib (Votrient)	VEGFR, PDGFR, and c-KIT	RCC, soft tissue sarcoma
Regorafenib (Stivarga)	VEGFR, Ret, Kit, PDGFR, and Raf	Colorectal cancer, GIST
Sorafenib (Nexavar)	VEGFR, PDGFR, FLT3, c-Kit, Raf, and Ret	RCC, hepatocellular carcinoma, and thyroid cancer
Sunitinib (Sutent)	VEGFR, PDGFR, FLT3, c-Kit, and Ret	GIST, RCC, and PNET
Tamoxifen	ER	Breast cancer
Temsirolimus (Torisel)	mTOR	RCC
Toremifene (Fareston)	ER	Breast cancer
Trametinib (Mekinist)	MEK	Melanoma
Vandetanib (Caprelsa)	VEGFR, EGFR, and Ret	Thyroid cancer
Vemurafenib (Zelboraf)	B-Raf	Melanoma
Vismodegib (Erivedge)	Smoothened	BCC
Ligand analogs		
Alitretinoin (Panretin)	RAR and RXR	Kaposi sarcoma
Bexarotene (Targretin)	RXR	Cutaneous T-cell lymphoma
Tretinoin (Vesanoid)	RAR	APL

ALK, anaplastic lymphoma kinase; ALL, acute lymphoblastic leukemia; APL, acute promyelocytic leukemia; AR, androgen receptor; BCC, basal cell carcinoma; BTK, Bruton's tyrosine kinase; CLL, chronic lymphocytic leukemia; CML, chronic myeloid leukemia; ER, estrogen receptor; GIST, gastrointestinal stromal tumor; IL6, interleukin 6; MEK, mitogen/extracellular signal-regulated kinase; NSCLC, non-small-cell lung carcinoma; PGF, placental growth factor; PI-3-K; phosphatidylinositol-3′-kinase; PNET, pancreatic neuroendocrine tumor; RAR, retinoic acid receptor; RANKL, receptor activator of NF-κB ligand; RCC, renal cell carcinoma; and RXR, retinoid X receptor.
Drugs included in this table have been approved by the Food and Drug Administration (FDA).

significantly increased the survival of colorectal cancer patients with wild-type *K-Ras*. However, it had no benefit in the presence of *K-Ras* mutations, accounting for 40% of the tumors,[94] thus emphasizing the need to identify the particular genetic context required for successful therapeutic intervention.

Another example is bevacizumab (avastin, Genentech), a monoclonal antibody targeting vascular endothelial growth factor (VEGF), a ligand that promotes angiogenesis. The FDA has approved bevacizumab for treatment of glioblastoma, colorectal, renal, and lung cancer. Contrary to trastuzumab and cetuximab, bevacizumab acts on vascular endothelial cells in the tumor microenvironment. Advantages include that drug resistance in such normal cells is less likely to develop than in genetically unstable tumor cells and that such therapy may be applicable to a wider range of tumors.[95] Of note, recent findings suggest that targeting VEGF may also directly affect some tumor cells, which express VEGF receptors.[96]

Tyr kinase inhibitors

Increased understanding of the important role of growth factor signal transduction in cancer has also led to intensive efforts focused on the development of small molecule inhibitors of constitutively activated Tyr kinases (Table 1). The most striking example is imatinib (gleevec, Novartis), a small molecule inhibitor of the non-RTK Abl. *Abl* is translocated in chronic myelogenous leukemia (CML) as part of the Philadelphia chromosome to create the *Bcr-Abl* oncogene.[97] Imatinib interacts with the ATP-binding pocket of the Abl kinase domain and stabilizes a catalytically inactive conformation of this oncogene product.[98] Clinical trials rapidly confirmed the efficacy of this agent in CML and Bcr-Abl as a therapeutic target in this disease. Remarkable responses were observed in the chronic phase of the disease with complete clearing of Ph+ cells from the circulation in 95% of patients, who had failed standard therapy. Only 9% of patients relapsed over a median follow-up of 18 months,[99] leading to regulatory approval. Imatinib is most effective in the chronic phase, with fewer responses and more relapses with patients in myeloid blast crisis. Unfortunately, during the progression of the disease, tumor cells often develop resistance, either through mutations that interfere with the binding of imatinib to Abl or by *Bcr-Abl* gene amplification.[98] Imatinib was subsequently shown to inhibit related RTKs, in particular Kit and PDGFR, for which activating mutations have been identified in gastrointestinal stromal tumor (GIST), leading to FDA approval for its use in therapy of this tumor type as well.

Examples of other small molecules targeting RTKs include gefitinib (iressa, AstraZeneca) and erlotinib (tarceva, OSI/Genentech), which were approved for the treatment of lung cancers displaying EGFR mutations.[100] Crizotinib (xalkori, Pfizer) inhibits ALK, a receptor activated by chromosome translocations or mutations in tumors including lung cancer and neuroblastoma.[101] Other more promiscuous small molecule inhibitors that target different Tyr kinases involved in both tumorigenesis and angiogenesis, such as sorafenib (nexavar, Bayer) and sunitinib (sutent, Pfizer), have been approved for the treatment of certain cancers, including advanced renal cell carcinoma, hepatocellular carcinoma, and imatinib-refractory GIST (Table 1).

Inhibition of growth factor downstream signaling

Downstream components of growth factor signaling pathways activated in cancer cells are also potential therapeutic targets. While extensive efforts to generate efficient and specific Ras inhibitors for the clinic have not been successful, this approach has paid off with the recent approval of new small molecules targeting downstream effectors of RTK signaling (Table 1). One striking example

is vemurafenib (zelboraf, Plexxikon/Roche), approved in 2011 for the treatment of melanomas harboring B-Raf V600E mutations. Vemurafenib is paradigmatic in that it was specifically developed to selectively block the mutant, but not wild-type B-Raf. Similar to other targeted therapeutic agents, after an initial response, these tumors often become unresponsive to the inhibitor. Several mechanisms have been described for the acquired resistance to vemurafenib, including mutation of Ras, expression of particular B-Raf splice-variants or the overexpression of RTKs, such as the PDGFR.[56] Recent evidence indicates that melanoma cells resistant to vemurafenib may show a decreased fitness in the absence of the B-raf inhibitor. Thus, intermittent vemurafenib dosing may forestall the clonal expansion of resistant cells, preventing or delaying the onset of drug-resistant disease.[102]

The recent advances in targeting specific growth factor signaling aberrations in human cancer cells argue strongly that knowledge gained on the important role of growth factor signaling in cancer is leading to a promising new era in cancer therapeutics. Increasing understanding of the molecular basis for the selectivity of the successful targeted drugs, as well as the mechanisms of acquired resistance to these therapies, strongly suggests that therapies will be individually tailored based on the genetic profile of the tumor. The astonishing advances in genome sequencing,[103] combined with the ability to isolate and DNA sequence primary tumors and circulating cancer cells,[104,105] offer powerful new approaches in this regard that would be deemed to belong in the realm of fantasy only a decade ago.

KEY POINTS

- Tumor cells can become dependent or addicted to a particular signaling pathway for their growth and survival.

- The pathways aberrantly deregulated in tumor cells may be specifically targeted in the clinic through different therapeutic strategies, including monoclonal antibodies, Tyr kinase inhibitors, and inhibitors of downstream effectors.

Summary

In multicellular organisms, physiological processes are regulated through a complex and interconnected network of signaling pathways, generally mediated by hormones, cytokines, and growth factors. These molecules normally act in a timely and precise manner to specifically control the phenotype of a well-defined population of cells, including their proliferation, differentiation, survival, and motility. When a signaling pathway goes awry, this tight regulation is lost, resulting in an aberrant cell behavior that can lead to cell transformation. Most, if not all, human cancers contain aberrant activation (or, less commonly, inhibition) of more than one such pathway, contributing to increased proliferation, survival, invasiveness, and metastatic spread. Such aberrations occur through different mechanisms, including autocrine/paracrine deregulation or genetic alterations affecting a particular component of the pathway. In this chapter, we discuss growth factor signaling through receptors exhibiting intrinsic tyrosine kinase activity and focus on two major downstream pathways activated by these receptors to promote cell proliferation and survival, that is, the PI-3-K/Akt and Ras/MAP kinase pathways. We will provide different paradigmatic examples, with special emphasis on the functional implications of such aberrations for tumorigenesis. General principles in cell signaling in both normal and tumor cells are addressed, and we briefly discuss how the initiation and progression of particular types of cancer can be affected by the deregulation of several other signaling pathways, including those mediated by cytokines, the TGFβ family of ligands, Wnt, Hedgehog, Notch, and nuclear receptors.

Finally, we discuss the concepts of oncogene addiction and targeted therapy, providing representative examples to illustrate how increased understanding of the mechanisms responsible for aberrant deregulation of particular signaling pathways in cancer can be translated to the clinic.

Acknowledgments

L.G. is supported by a Chair of Excellence program from INSERM and the University of Rouen and by a grant from "La Ligue contre le Cancer." SAA is supported by grants from the NCI, NICHD, and Breast Cancer Research Foundation.

Key references

The complete reference list can be found on the Wiley Companion Digital Edition of this title (see inside front cover for login instructions).

9 Aaronson SA. Growth factors and cancer. *Science.* 1991;**254**(**5035**):1146–1153.

10 Lemmon MA, Schlessinger J. Cell signaling by receptor tyrosine kinases. *Cell.* 2010;**141**(7):1117–1134.

16 Pollak M. The insulin and insulin-like growth factor receptor family in neoplasia: an update. *Nat Rev Cancer.* 2012;**12**(3):159–169.

17 Citri A, Yarden Y. EGF-ERBB signalling: towards the systems level. *Nat Rev Mol Cell Biol.* 2006;**7**(7):505–516.

18 Arteaga CL, Engelman JA. ERBB receptors: from oncogene discovery to basic science to mechanism-based cancer therapeutics. *Cancer Cell.* 2014;**25**(3):282–303.

19 Trusolino L, Bertotti A, Comoglio PM. MET signalling: principles and functions in development, organ regeneration and cancer. *Nat Rev Mol Cell Biol.* 2010;**11**(12):834–848.

20 Gherardi E, Birchmeier W, Birchmeier C, Vande WG. Targeting MET in cancer: rationale and progress. *Nat Rev Cancer.* 2012;**12**(2):89–103.

24 Tebbutt N, Pedersen MW, Johns TG. Targeting the ERBB family in cancer: couples therapy. *Nat Rev Cancer.* 2013;**13**(9):663–673.

25 Shaw AT, Hsu PP, Awad MM, Engelman JA. Tyrosine kinase gene rearrangements in epithelial malignancies. *Nat Rev Cancer.* 2013;**13**(11):772–787.

26 Lynch TJ, Bell DW, Sordella R, et al. Activating mutations in the epidermal growth factor receptor underlying responsiveness of non-small-cell lung cancer to gefitinib. *N Engl J Med.* 2004;**350**(21):2129–2139.

27 Paez JG, Janne PA, Lee JC, et al. EGFR mutations in lung cancer: correlation with clinical response to gefitinib therapy. *Science.* 2004;**304**(**5676**):1497–1500.

29 Wagner MJ, Stacey MM, Liu BA, Pawson T. Molecular mechanisms of SH2- and PTB-domain-containing proteins in receptor tyrosine kinase signaling. *Cold Spring Harb Perspect Biol.* 2013;**5**(12):a008987.

39 Engelman JA, Luo J, Cantley LC. The evolution of phosphatidylinositol 3-kinases as regulators of growth and metabolism. *Nat Rev Genet.* 2006;**7**(8):606–619.

40 Vanhaesebroeck B, Stephens L, Hawkins P. PI3K signalling: the path to discovery and understanding. *Nat Rev Mol Cell Biol.* 2012;**13**(3):195–203.

41 Manning BD, Cantley LC. AKT/PKB signaling: navigating downstream. *Cell.* 2007;**129**(7):1261–1274.

42 Fruman DA, Rommel C. PI3K and cancer: lessons, challenges and opportunities. *Nat Rev Drug Discov.* 2014;**13**(2):140–156.

44 Samuels Y, Wang Z, Bardelli A, et al. High frequency of mutations of the PIK3CA gene in human cancers. *Science.* 2004;**304**(**5670**):554.

45 Kandoth C, McLellan MD, Vandin F, et al. Mutational landscape and significance across 12 major cancer types. *Nature.* 2013;**502**(**7471**):333–339.

50 Karnoub AE, Weinberg RA. Ras oncogenes: split personalities. *Nat Rev Mol Cell Biol.* 2008;**9**(7):517–531.

52 Pylayeva-Gupta Y, Grabocka E, Bar-Sagi D. RAS oncogenes: weaving a tumorigenic web. *Nat Rev Cancer.* 2011;**11**(11):761–774.

56 Holderfield M, Deuker MM, McCormick F, McMahon M. Targeting RAF kinases for cancer therapy: BRAF-mutated melanoma and beyond. *Nat Rev Cancer.* 2014;**14**(7):455–467.

62 Davies H, Bignell GR, Cox C, et al. Mutations of the BRAF gene in human cancer. *Nature.* 2002;**417**(**6892**):949–954.

63 Wagner EF, Nebreda AR. Signal integration by JNK and p38 MAPK pathways in cancer development. *Nat Rev Cancer.* 2009;**9**(8):537–549.

65 Massague J. TGFbeta signalling in context. *Nat Rev Mol Cell Biol.* 2012;**13**(10):616–630.

66 Stark GR, Darnell JE Jr. The JAK-STAT pathway at twenty. *Immunity.* 2012;**36**(4):503–514.

70 Lappano R, Maggiolini M. G protein-coupled receptors: novel targets for drug discovery in cancer. *Nat Rev Drug Discov.* 2011;**10**(1):47–60.

71 Perkins ND. The diverse and complex roles of NF-kappaB subunits in cancer. *Nat Rev Cancer.* 2012;**12**(2):121–132.

72 Briscoe J, Therond PP. The mechanisms of Hedgehog signalling and its roles in development and disease. *Nat Rev Mol Cell Biol.* 2013;**14**(7):416–429.

73 Harvey KF, Zhang X, Thomas DM. The Hippo pathway and human cancer. *Nat Rev Cancer.* 2013;**13**(4):246–257.

74 Clevers H, Nusse R. Wnt/beta-catenin signaling and disease. *Cell.* 2012;**149**(6):1192–1205.

75 Guruharsha KG, Kankel MW, Artavanis-Tsakonas S. The Notch signalling system: recent insights into the complexity of a conserved pathway. *Nat Rev Genet.* 2012;**13**(9):654–666.

81 Evans RM, Mangelsdorf DJ. Nuclear receptors, RXR, and the big bang. *Cell.* 2014;**157**(1):255–266.

82 Jordan VC. Chemoprevention of breast cancer with selective oestrogen-receptor modulators. *Nat Rev Cancer.* 2007;**7**(1):46–53.

84 Mills IG. Maintaining and reprogramming genomic androgen receptor activity in prostate cancer. *Nat Rev Cancer.* 2014;**14**(3):187–198.

87 Sharma SV, Settleman J. Oncogene addiction: setting the stage for molecularly targeted cancer therapy. *Genes Dev.* 2007;**21**(24):3214–3231.

96 Goel HL, Mercurio AM. VEGF targets the tumour cell. *Nat Rev Cancer.* 2013;**13**(12):871–882.

98 Druker BJ. Translation of the Philadelphia chromosome into therapy for CML. *Blood.* 2008;**112**(13):4808–4817.

100 Sharma SV, Bell DW, Settleman J, Haber DA. Epidermal growth factor receptor mutations in lung cancer. *Nat Rev Cancer.* 2007;**7**(3):169–181.

101 Hallberg B, Palmer RH. Mechanistic insight into ALK receptor tyrosine kinase in human cancer biology. *Nat Rev Cancer.* 2013;**13**(10):685–700.

103 Vogelstein B, Papadopoulos N, Velculescu VE, Zhou S, Diaz LA Jr, Kinzler KW. Cancer genome landscapes. *Science.* 2013;**339**(**6127**):1546–1558.

11 Differentiation therapy

Sai-Juan Chen, MD, PhD ▪ Xiao-Jing Yan, MD ▪ Guang-Biao Zhou, MD ▪ Zhu Chen, PhD

Overview

Abnormal differentiation is one of the main features of human cancers, especially in hematological malignancies. Many aberrant genetic and epigenetic factors have been shown to disrupt the regulation of cell differentiation in a variety of cancers and play an important role in oncogenesis. Differentiation therapy refers to the application of therapeutic agents selectively targeting the key molecules involved in the process of cell differentiation, leading to the restoration of normal cellular homeostasis and the eventual clearance of cancer cells. Over the past four decades, investigations of the molecular mechanisms underlying cancer cell differentiation arrest or blockage have allowed the identification of an array of drug targets. On the other hand, many physiological or pharmacological agents have been tested using in vitro and in vivo systems as the inducers of differentiation and maturation of cancer cells. The translational research in this field has gradually turned the differentiation therapy from a concept to clinical practices. The most successful model of cancer differentiation therapy is the development of synergistic targeted treatment of acute promyelocytic leukemia (APL) with all-trans-retinoic acid (ATRA) and arsenic trioxide (ATO). This chapter discusses the basic theories of differentiation therapy and the clinical achievements of this therapeutic approach.

Molecular mechanisms underlying differentiation blockage in cancer

It has long been recognized that in human cancers, there exist some relationship between the clinical aggressiveness and their differentiation status, with poorly differentiated tumors being usually more aggressive. To understand the biology of differentiation arrest or blockage in cancer, it is necessary to elucidate how the related functions are regulated in normal cells and how they become disrupted in cancer cells. These studies are of importance for identifying meaningful therapeutic targets.

It is well established that pluripotent embryonic stem cells are capable of self-renewal and differentiating into various cells with specific functions in an organism. These cells can then develop into distinct cell types, tissues, and organs, which are under accurate regulation in a finely organized manner. A large body of evidence has been obtained that the underlying mechanisms entail the sequential action of cell-/tissue-specific or time-specific transcription factors (TFs) that activate or repress the differentiation-associated genes under appropriate conditions.[1–3] The transcriptional expression of genes is also orchestrated by complex mechanisms designated as epigenetic regulation. Notably, many pathways and networks that regulate cell differentiation during normal development are affected by genetic and epigenetic abnormalities during tumorigenesis. As a result, cancer cell population generally bears an aberrant expression of regulators for embryonic morphogenesis and maintains a subset with properties of stem cells. Meanwhile, cancer cells often show defects in programs that keep cells in differentiated state (Figure 1).

Transcriptional factors (TFs)

Cellular differentiation can be defined by a sequential process of acquisition of different functions, and cell fate is largely determined by control of gene expression through the combination of TFs and epigenetic modifiers.[3,4] TFs are nuclear proteins capable of DNA binding and trans-activating or trans-repressing the transcription of target genes. They are often assembled into multiprotein complex with cofactors (activators or repressors) and play decisive roles in regulating the gene expression profiles of stem/progenitor cells and determining their ability to differentiate into mature cell lineages.[5] TFs are also essential for control of cell proliferation and programmed cell death (apoptosis). Recently, cellular reprogramming and induction of pluripotency across differentiated lineages have been achieved using combinations of TFs, which provide strong evidence for the key role that TFs play in the decisions of cell fate.[6–11] In addition, that cell differentiation can be directed by lineage-specific TFs has also been supported by a large amount of experimental data.[3,5,12] In contrast, abnormalities of differentiation-associated TFs due to dysregulated expression or aberrant functions imposed by gene point mutations or fusions may disturb the differentiation program of normal stem/progenitor cells.[5] As a result, immature descendants with growth and survival advantages may be produced, eventually leading to the development of cancer.

The cancer-associated TFs can be divided into distinct classes according to structural and/or functional features,[12] such as leucine zipper factors (bZIP, e.g., c-JUN), helix-loop-helix factors (bHLH, e.g., MYC), Cys4 zinc fingers [e.g., nuclear receptors (NRs), GATA factors], helix-turn-helix factors (HTH, e.g., HOX family, OCT-1/2), and Rel homology region (e.g., NF-κB). These TFs are considered as key regulators of cell proliferation, differentiation, and apoptosis, and their mutations and/or aberrant expression have been shown to play an essential role in malignant transformation. A special class of ligand-activated zinc finger proteins known as superfamily of NRs is worth particular attention, as they are major regulators in the initiation and/or maintenance of differentiated status of many cell/tissue types.[13] This family contains the receptors for different ligands including steroid/thyroid hormones, retinoids, vitamin D3, and certain fatty acids. Notably, many of these receptors are subject to dysregulated expression or structural abnormalities in various cancers. These abnormalities subsequently lead to undesired activation of the normally hormone-regulated genes in a hormone-independent way, or even activation of some genes unrelated to hormone regulation, which will be discussed in detail in the section entitled "Agents targeting aberrant TFs."

For long time, hematopoiesis has been at the frontline of research in the biology of normal and abnormal cell differentiation[5,14,15] owing to the discoveries of hematopoietic hormones and related signaling pathways and the specific TFs that regulate the fate of

Holland-Frei Cancer Medicine, Ninth Edition. Edited by Robert C. Bast Jr., Carlo M. Croce, William N. Hait, Waun Ki Hong, Donald W. Kufe, Martine Piccart-Gebhart, Raphael E. Pollock, Ralph R. Weichselbaum, Hongyang Wang, and James F. Holland.
© 2017 John Wiley & Sons, Inc. ISBN: 978-1-118-93469-2

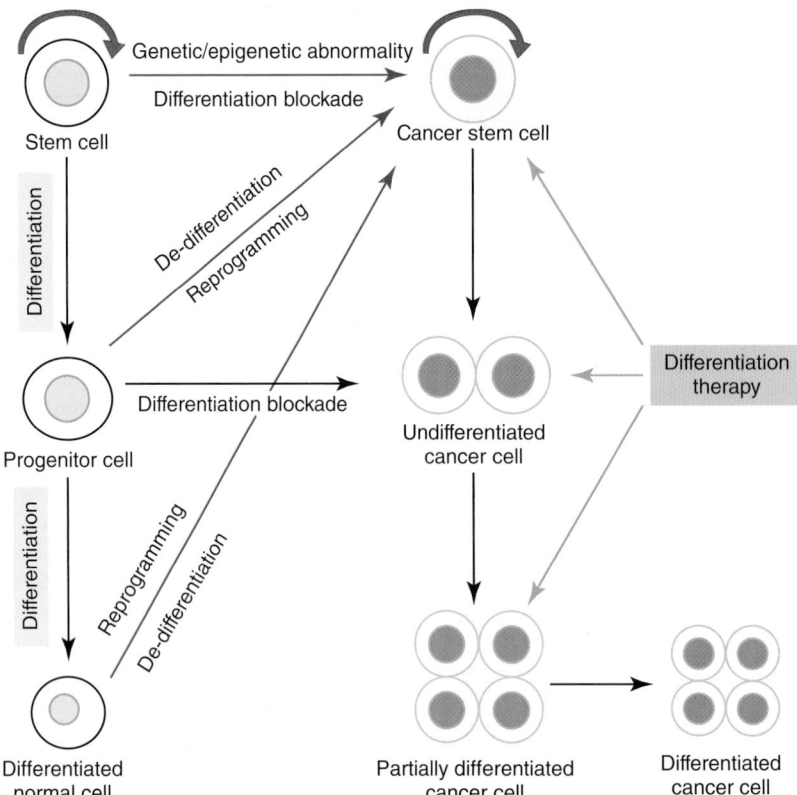

Figure 1 Differentiation blockade and differentiation therapy in cancer. In addition to self-renewal, normal stem cells are capable of differentiating into specific mature cells, while differentiation blockade may lead to the development of cancer. Cancer stem cells may originate from normal stem cells acquiring genetic and/or epigenetic abnormalities, or from normal progenitor or differentiated cells undergoing de-differentiation and reprogramming also due to genetic and/or epigenetic abnormalities. Differentiation therapy exerts therapeutic efficacy by inducing differentiation of cancer stem cells and undifferentiated cancer cells.

hematopoietic stem/progenitor cells (HSPC) (Figure 2). Each stage of myeloid and lymphoid differentiation shows particular TFs signatures that function in networks. For example, RUNX1, GATA1, C/EBPα, C/EBPβ, MYB, E2A, PAX5, TAL1/SCL, or PU.1 are turned on or turned off in an orchestrated manner to ensure blood cell lineage specification.[3,15] Some of these TFs were originally identified following the molecular characterization of gene point mutations or fusion in leukemia, such as C/EBPα in *CEBPA* mutation of acute myeloid leukemia (AML), RUNX1 in the *RUNX1(AML1)–ETO* fusion gene of t(8;21) AML, and SCL(TAL1) in t(1;14) T-cell acute lymphoblastic leukemia (ALL).[16–18] Disruption of these hematopoietic TFs in leukemia blocks hematopoietic cells in their early stages of differentiation.

The fact that abnormal TFs disturbing cell differentiation are "drivers" in oncogenesis has aroused interest for these proteins to be potential targets for therapeutic intervention. However, most current anticancer research activities are concentrated on cell-surface receptors because they offer a relatively straightforward way for drugs to affect cellular behavior, whereas agents acting at the level of transcription need to penetrate the cell membrane and enter into the nucleus. Efforts should be supported to design drugs affecting cancer-associated transcriptional patterns for re-establishing differentiation. Small molecule drugs directed against well-defined interacting sites between TFs and DNA or between TFs and other proteins in transcription machinery can be developed, so as to modulate the key TF target genes. On the other hand, the re-introduction of differentiation-related wild-type TFs with gene therapy might also serve as a strategy for cancer differentiation therapy.

Epigenetic modifiers

Epigenetic regulation constitutes crucial mechanisms governing the variability in gene expression, which is heritable through mitosis and potentially also meiosis, without changes of genomic sequence.[19,20] All cells of an organism share the same genome information but exhibit different phenotypes with diverse functions. This phenotypic diversity is due to distinct gene expression patterns among different cell types. It is well established that chromatin states are primary determinants for the turn-on or turn-off of genes. The assembly and compaction of chromatin require multiple regulatory mechanisms, including DNA methylation (cytosine methylation and hydroxymethylation) or demethylation, post-translational modifications of histones (phosphorylation, acetylation, methylation, and ubiquitylation), and noncoding RNA-mediated pathways.[20–22] A large number of enzymes have been identified to be regulatory factors in the mechanisms, such as DNA methyltransferases (DNMTs) and DNA demethylases (DNDMs), histone deacetylases (HDACs) and histone acetyltransferases (HATs), and histone methyltransferases (HMTs) and histone demethylases (HDMs) (Figure 3a and b). The different modifications of DNA or histones are closely interrelated and can both reinforce each other and inhibit each other. Many histone-modifying enzymes are components of cofactor complexes and function cooperatively with TFs to modulate gene expression (Figure 3c).

Recently, new technological platforms have allowed comprehensive epigenomic map to be made in pluripotent and differentiated cells, which provide further support to the concept that cell differentiation is accompanied by dynamic features of chromatin

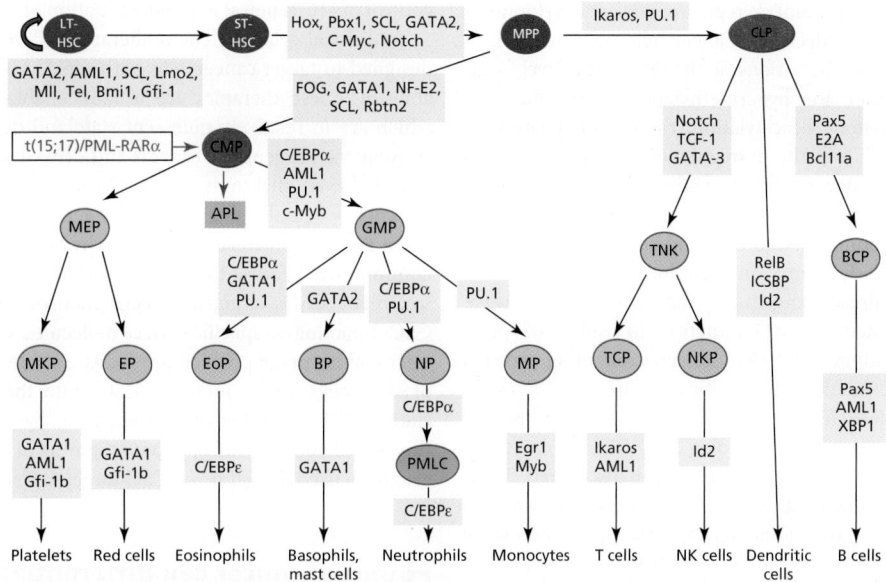

Figure 2 Signaling pathways and transcriptional factors (TFs) regulating the differentiation of hematopoietic stem/progenitor cells (HSPC). Differentiation block may result in leukemia, exemplified by development of acute promyelocytic leukemia (APL), a subtype of acute myeloid leukemia (AML) characterized by accumulation of abnormal promyelocytes in bone marrow/peripheral blood, the presence of t(15;17)/PML-RARα fusion gene, and severe bleeding syndrome. In fact, almost all the listed signaling molecules and TFs are subject to mutations (gene fusions, point mutations, gene amplifications/deletions) and/or dysregulation of expression in hematological malignancies.

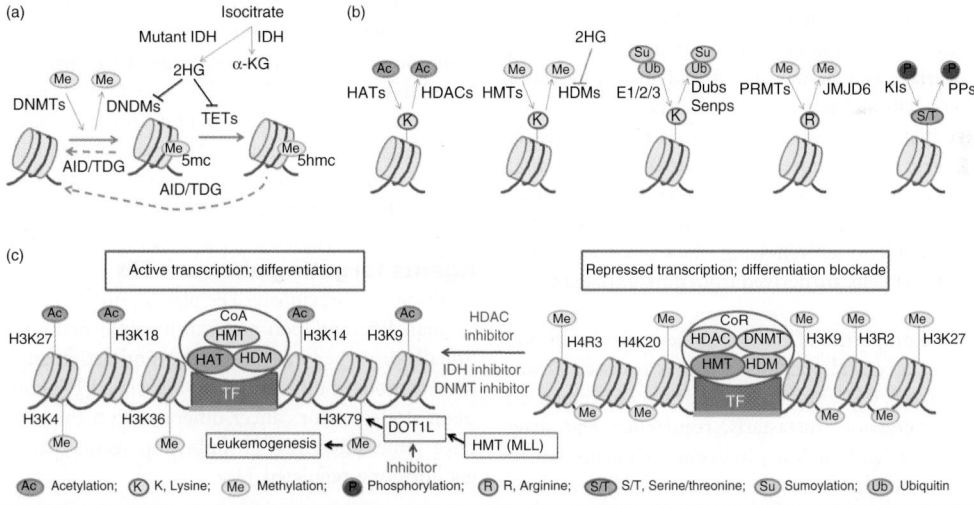

2HG, 2-hydroxyglutarate; 5mc, 5-cytosine methylation; 5hmc, hydroxylmethylcytosine; α-KG, a-ketoglutarate; AID, activation-induced deamination; CoA, co-activator; CoR, co-repressor; DNDMs, DNA demethylases; DNMT, DNA methyltransferase; Dubs, deubiquitinating enzymes; E1/2/3, ubiquitin-activating enzyme E1, ubiquitin-conjugating enzyme E2, ubiquitin ligase E3; H, histone; HAT, histone acetyltransferase; HDAC, histone deacetylase; HDM, histone demethylase; HMT, histone methyltransferase; IDH, isocitrate dehydrogenase; KIs, kinases; PPs, phosphatases; PRMTs, protein arginine methyltransferases; JMJD6, Fe(II) and 2-oxoglutarate-dependent dioxygenase Jumonji domain-6 protein; Senps, sumo-specific proteases; TDG, thymine-DNA glycosylase; TET, ten-eleven translocation; TF, transcription factor

Figure 3 Epigenetic regulation involved in the cell differentiation and tumorigenesis. (a) DNA methylation (cytosine methylation and hydroxymethylation) are regulated by different enzymes DNMTs, TETs, and IDH. (b) Post-translational modifications of histones include phosphorylation, acetylation, methylation, and ubiquitylation or sumoylation, which are regulated by a variety of factors HATs, HDACs, HMTs, HDMs, and so on. Notably, most of these epigenetic modifier genes have been found to be mutated in human cancers including solid tumors and hematological malignancies. (c) Gene expression is controlled in the promoter regions by a combination of chromatin modification and transcriptional factor (TF). In tumor cells, gene expression is silenced by condensing chromatin, methylating DNA, and deacetylating histones, which results the differentiation blockade. Inhibition of HDACs, DNMTs, and IDH may result in active transcription and differentiation of cancer cells. Some HMTs (e.g., MLL and related fusion proteins) may enhance H3K79 methylation by promoting DOT1L to activate transcription of some leukemogenic genes, and inhibitor of DOT1L may suppress the leukemogenic genes to treat leukemia.

states.[22–25] Genetic studies in different model organisms have shown the importance of chromatin regulators in key developmental transitions and cell fate decision. Cancer cells are characterized by typical genome-wide aberrations at the epigenetic level, such as the hypomethylation, the hypermethylation of specific promoter regions, the histone deacetylation, the downregulation of microRNAs (miRNAs), and the dysregulation of certain components of epigenetic machinery.[20,21,26] Recently, somatic alterations of many epigenetic modifiers have been identified as common genetic events in cancers including solid tumors and hematopoietic malignancies.[27–30] In acute leukemia and myelodysplastic syndrome (MDS), besides the already known aberrations of mixed lineage leukemia (*MLL1*) located on 11q23, mutations in a subset of epigenetic modifiers, including other SET domain-containing proteins (*MLL2*, *SETD2*),[31] tet methylcytosine dioxygenase 2 (*TET2*),[32–34] isocitrate dehydrogenase (*IDH1*/*IDH2*),[35] additional sex combs-like 1 (*ASXL1*),[36,37] enhancer of zeste homolog 2 (*EZH2*),[38,39] and DNA methyltransferase 3A (*DNMT3A*),[40,41] have been discovered. These mutations have been shown not only to contribute to the leukemogenesis but also serve as the biomarker of clinical prognosis since they often predict a poor overall survival (OS) of patients.[28–30] The aberrations of epigenetic modification together with those of genetic regulation result in permanent changes in the gene expression patterns that confer a selective advantage to differentiation block, apoptotic deficiency, and uncontrolled cell growth. Because the epigenetic modifications are usually reversible, therapies targeting epigenetic modifiers hold the promise of being clinically effective.

Cancer stem cells (CSCs)

Most cancers are heterogeneous in terms of cell proliferation and differentiation status. In recent years, evidence has been accumulated to suggest the existence of less-differentiated, stem cell–like cells within the cancer cell population in solid tumors (lung, colon, prostate, ovarian, and brain cancers and melanoma) and leukemia.[42–45] These cells are now referred to as cancer stem cells (CSCs) or tumor-initiating cells capable of self-renewal and giving rise to the entire cancer bulk.[46] Indeed, a single leukemia-initiating cell (LIC) from human being can cause a full-blown AML in animal model.[47] As a result, malignant cells in a given cancer are highly hierarchical, with the unique self-renewing CSCs at the top of the hierarchy, while all other cells are derived from differentiated CSCs (Figure 1).

Investigation of the properties of CSCs and their roles in disease mechanisms occupies a central position in cancer research nowadays. Generally speaking, CSCs represent the driving force behind cancer initiation, progression, metastasis, recurrence, and drug resistance.[43,48] It is nevertheless not easy to define the phenotypes of CSCs in that they are variable from one cancer to another and are affected by the initial transformation as well as different stages of neoplastic development. Currently, fluorescence-activated cell sorting using cell surface markers or intracellular molecules represents the common method to identify CSCs.[42,43] There are still problems to be tackled: CSC biomarkers are lacking in some cancers; not all CSCs express the markers or marker sets; some differentiated cancer cells also express the same marker sets as CSCs do; some currently used marker sets are not specific to CSC since they are also expressed by stem/progenitor cells in normal tissues. On the other hand, gene expression patterns may be of value because dysregulation of certain pathways or networks can be seen in CSCs but not in differentiated cancer cell compartments, which can eventually be used as new CSC markers. So far, PI3K/Akt, PTEN, JAK/STAT, TGF-β, Wnt/β-catenin, hedgehog, Notch, NF-κB, and

Bcl-2 have been included into the pathways that are involved in the control of self-renewal and differentiation of CSCs.[42,43]

Traditional cytotoxic chemotherapy (CT) or radiation therapy is designed to target cancer cells with rapid proliferative or dividing abilities. These therapies are usually unable to eliminate CSCs, which are in relatively quiescent state and divide slowly, and can consequently regenerate cancers and drive disease recurrence.[48–50] It is believed that only when CSCs are eradicated can cancer patients be actually cured. In recent years, great attention has been given to the characteristics of CSCs by both scientific and medical communities because these cells provide a unique target for cancer treatment. CSCs-targeted strategy focuses on the elimination of CSCs by acting on specific surface molecules, signaling pathways, or microenvironments, which are indispensable for the maintenance of stem cells, or by inducing CSCs into the more differentiated state.[4,45,48,49] A number of existing agents have been investigated in this regard and high-throughput screening of chemical libraries has also been used to find novel CSC-targeted chemicals.[51,52]

Potential cancer cell differentiation-inducing agents

Cancer differentiation therapy aims at using appropriate therapeutic agents to induce cell cycle arrest and a commitment to the cell differentiation program toward terminal cell division, specific function gaining, and ultimately apoptosis.[53] This concept applies relatively clearly to hematologic malignancies, whereas "authentic" differentiation therapy for solid tumors is sometimes difficult to define and often refers to the processes that convert malignant cells to a more benign phenotype, accompanied by diminished proliferative and metastatic abilities and the expression of mature cell markers.[4] Interestingly, some initially defined differentiation inducers have turned out to be compounds targeting oncoproteins, while some newly developed targeting therapeutics have been found to trigger significant differentiation of cancer cells. Thus far, about 80 agents of differentiation induction have been identified and biosynthesized, and most of them are under investigations *in vitro* or on animal models, among which only a fraction have been used in clinical practice.

Agents targeting aberrant TFs

As discussed previously, TFs play a powerful role in physiological cellular differentiation and can be abnormally regulated or functionally disturbed in cancers. The modulation and/or restoration of the functions of differentiation-associated TFs constitute one of the main strategies for cancer differentiation therapy. Here, we introduce some differentiation-induction agents, which specifically target hormone-regulated TFs.

Retinoids

Retinoids are a group of vitamin A derivatives. Retinoic acids (RAs) are the physiologically existing active metabolite of retinol, which regulate a wide range of biological processes including development, differentiation, proliferation, and apoptosis in normal or cancer cells.[13,54–56] The most important isomers of RAs are all-trans-retinoic acid (ATRA), 13-cis-retinoic acid (13-cRA), and 9-cis-retinoic acid (9-cRA), which have different spectrums of biological activity and ligand affinity.[57,58] Synthetic retinoids include bexarotene and fenretinide. The effects of RAs on cell differentiation are exerted mostly via their NRs. Two types of receptors, the retinoic acid receptors (RARs, with three major isoforms RAR-α/-β/-γ) and the retinoid X receptors (RXRs, with three main isoforms RXR-α/-β/-γ), mediate RA signaling as heterodimer RAR/RXR.[13,56] These receptor heterodimers are able to bind, at genomic level, to the specific motifs defined as retinoic acid response elements (RAREs) on the promoters of target genes. RAR/RXR differentially activates or represses gene transcription while recruiting co-activators (CoA) or co-repressors (CoR) complexes. These different modes of action depend on the presence or absence of the ligands, RAs. Physiological concentrations of RA (1 pmol/L) are able to release CoR (such as N-CoR/SMRT complex and the chromatin remodeling complexes, e.g., HDACs, DNMTs) from the RAR/RXR and recruit CoA (such as p300/CBP complex with HAT activity), leading to the transcriptional activation of genes involved in cell differentiation (e.g., C/EBPα and PU.1), growth, and apoptosis.[56,59-65]

Retinoid signaling is often disrupted during carcinogenesis, suggesting that restoration of this pathway may be a viable option for cancer treatment.[54,55,58,66] The effects of RA-induced differentiation are particularly observed on promyelocytic leukemia cell-like cell lines such as HL60 and NB4, or fresh primary APL (acute promyelocytic leukemia) cells.[67,68] These cells can undergo terminal differentiation to morphologically and functionally mature granulocytes after incubation with pharmacological concentrations (0.1–1 μmol/L) of RAs, especially ATRA.[67] Myeloblasts from other AML subtypes are generally not affected by RAs, whereas only limited differentiating effects of retinoids are seen on cell lines such as THP-1 (monoblastic leukemia), K562 (blastic phase of CML), HEL (erythroleukemia), and U937 (monocytic leukemia).[59,68] Until now, the most successful clinical practice of differentiation therapy is the use of ATRA in APL, which will be discussed in details in the following section.

Retinoids have been reported to induce the differentiation of many solid tumor cell lines *in vitro* and suppress carcinogenesis in tumorigenic animal models, including human teratoma, melanoma, neuroblastoma, osteosarcoma, and rhabdomyosarcoma.[57,69,70] In thyroid carcinoma cell lines, retinoids were shown to induce the expression of type I iodothyronine-5′-deiodinase and sodium/iodide symporter, which are the thyroid differentiation markers.[71-73] In early clinical studies, patients with poorly differentiated, inoperable thyroid carcinoma with lacking or insufficient iodine uptake were treated with 13-cRA at oral doses of 0.3–1.5 mg/kg/day over 5 weeks and up to 9 months. The results showed an increased radio iodide uptake in 20–40% of patients.[73-75] In some of these trials, afluorine-18 fluorodeoxyglucose positron emission tomography (18 F-FDG PET) was used for the evaluation of therapy with 13-cRA in thyroid cancer. These data indicate retinoids as promising differentiation therapy agents for the treatment of thyroid cancer.

In addition to induction of differentiation, retinoids exert antitumor effects through other modes of action: repressing cell proliferation, promoting cell apoptosis, and inhibiting angiogenesis and metastasis.[56,57] Notably, retinoids are used effectively in the treatment of certain cutaneous premalignancies and malignancies with good results.[76] Bexarotene, the first synthetic highly selective RXR agonist, has been shown to induce apoptosis of cutaneous T-cell lymphoma (CTCL) cells with downregulation of its receptors and of survivin, an inhibitor of apoptosis.[77]

In clinical practice, systemic retinoids are approved by the US Food and Drug Administration (FDA) for the treatment of APL and CTCL.

Vitamin D compounds

Vitamin D is known to have a variety of actions at cell proliferation and differentiation.[78] These actions are mainly mediated by vitamin D receptor (VDR), a member of NR superfamily. While performing physiological functions, VDR forms heterodimer with RXR. The VDR/RXR heterodimer binds to vitamin D response elements (VDREs) in the promoter regions of target genes.[79] In the absence of physiologically active form of vitamin D, 1,25 dihydroxy vitamin D3 $[1,25(OH)_2D_3](1,25D)$, the VDR/RXR heterodimer recruits co-repressors including HDACs and results in transcriptional repression.[66] However, once the ligand binds to VDR/RXR, the resultant conformational change of the receptor heterodimer triggers the transcriptional activation of the target genes. It has been demonstrated that the recruitment of several coactivators to VDR/RXR is indispensable for this trans-activation. The VDR also directly interacts with a number of other proteins (e.g., β-catenin) and regulate their activities.[80] Besides, 1,25D can trigger "rapid responses" via activating membrane initiated signaling pathways, such as MAPK pathways, the lipid signaling pathways, or PI3K/AKT pathway.[79,81,82]

Similar to the differentiation-inducing effects of retinoids, 1,25D has been shown to dispose differentiating actions on various types of human AML cells,[78] including HL-60, U937, NB4, THP-1, and KG-1. Animal model studies have shown that 1,25D strongly promotes cell differentiation and thereby significantly prolongs the survival of mice transplanted with leukemic cells. However, the results of clinical trials are unsatisfactory. Neither 1,25D nor vitamin D analogs (VDAs) show clear beneficial effects on patients with AML or MDS.[83,84] An important issue for these failures could be the heterogeneous nature of the diseases. The clinical utility of 1,25D has also been limited by the severe toxicity of its therapeutic doses, primarily due to fatal drug-induced hypercalcemia.[85]

Some types of solid tumors, such as colon, breast, and prostate cancers and osteosarcoma, were also reportedly to respond to *in vitro* applied VDAs.[86,87] Nevertheless, little is known about how VDAs mediate their antiproliferation or pro-differentiation activity.[86] Moreover, the results of clinical trials of VDAs across a variety of cancers have been disappointing with regard to efficacy.[88] Thus, the routine recommendation of vitamin D for cancer treatment is premature.

PPARγ agonists

Peroxisome proliferator-activated receptor gamma (PPARγ) is also a member of the NR superfamily.[89] PPARγ forms heterodimer with RXR, which then binds to PPARγ response elements in the promoter regions of target genes. It is well established that PPARγ is important in the regulation of proliferation, differentiation, and apoptosis in many cell types.[89] Synthetic PPARγ agonists have been developed, including drugs used in the treatment of type 2 diabetes [e.g., troglitazone, rosiglitazone (TGZ)] and nonsteroidal anti-inflammatory agents (e.g., indomethacin).[59,69]

Activation of PPARγ with agonists can suppress the growth and induce the differentiation of several types of tumors *in vitro* and in animal models for colon, breast, prostate, and thyroid cancers, liposarcoma (LPS), pituitary adenomas, and acute leukemia.[90-92] Antitumor effects of PPARγ agonists may also be associated with regulation of cell cycle, apoptosis, and expression of tumor suppressor genes (TSGs, e.g., *PTEN* and *BRCA1*).[59,93,94] Besides, there has been evidence for "off-target" effects of PPARγ agonists, which is independent on the PPARγ receptor activity.[59]

Clinical trials of PPARγ agonists have been carried out in several human malignancies. A few studies have reported that TGZ could induce the differentiation of cancer cells in patients with LPS.[95] It was initially found that terminal adipocytic differentiation was induced in a few patients with intermediate to high-grade LPS.

However, such responses and clinical benefit could not be confirmed in a subsequent trial.[96] Clinical investigations in breast, prostate, colon, lung, and thyroid cancers and LPS did not reveal a meaningful benefit of TGZ therapy.[59,73,96–98] Although the clinical effects of PPARγ agonists have not been convincing, their low toxicity profile and potential additive or synergistic effects combined with other anticancer agents such as retinoids make them reasonable candidates in combination therapy trials.

Agents targeting epigenetic modifiers

It has been shown that the aberration of epigenetic regulation and TFs governing differentiation occurs in many cancers. Recurrent somatic alterations in epigenetic modifiers are also observed in solid tumors and hematological malignancies. Hence, there has been substantial interest in preclinical and clinical studies for epigenetic regulating agents to be considered as differentiation inducers.[99] A large amount of epigenetic agents are currently under investigation and a few have received FDA approval. Promising results have been already yielded in certain cancer types.

DNMTs inhibitors

DNA methylation is the most characterized epigenetic modification and is described as a stable epigenetic marker.[100] The enzymes catalyzing DNA methylation are known as DNMTs. As hypermethylation of TSGs and over-expression of DNMTs have been established as the key factors in carcinogenesis, demethylating agents seem to be especially promising as anticancer drugs.[101,102] To date, 5-azacytidine (5-Aza) and 5-aza-2′-deoxycytidine (decitabine) are the most successful DNMTs inhibitors, already approved by FDA for the treatment of patients with MDS or AML, and 5-Aza has also been approved by the FDA and the European Medicines Agency (EMA) for the treatment of chronic myelomonocytic leukemia (CMML).[101] The mode of action seems dose-dependent and a "dual mechanism" has been identified: the cytotoxicity and/or the inhibition of cell proliferation at high doses, and the DNA hypomethylation effect on the induction of gene expression at low doses.[101,102] Numerous studies have described terminal differentiation of AML cells treated with 5-Aza or decitabine.[102–104] Moreover, it has been demonstrated that decitabine-induced killing of myeloid leukemia cells is independent on DNA damage and apoptosis.[102] In some solid tumor cells, 5-Aza or decitabine induces cancer cell apoptosis and senescence through multiple mechanisms.[105]

Recent clinical studies indicated that repeated exposure at low doses (decitabine: $20\,mg/m^2$ for 5 days every 28 days; 5-Aza: $75\,mg/m^2$ for 7 days every 28 days) to these agents can induce DNA demethylation with a better antineoplastic effect than when used at higher doses (decitabine: $45\,mg/m^2$ for 3 days every 42 days).[102,106–109] In MDS patients, 5-Aza induces an overall response rate of 20–30% and significantly improves survival compared with standard care, while decitabine induces cytogenetic remission (Cyto-CR) rates of 35–50% at optimal doses and prolongs survival when compared with historical controls.[102,106–108,110,111] Clinical trials of DNMTs inhibitors in combination with other agents have also obtained promising results in solid tumors such as nonsmall-cell lung cancer and refractory ovarian cancer.[105,112,113] Therefore, rational use of the existing DNMTs inhibitors are to be encouraged and efforts to develop new compounds targeting more selectively DNMTs and with less toxicities should be continued.

HDAC inhibitors

As enzymes catalyzing the deacetylation of histones, HDACs are involved in the control and regulation of cell growth and differentiation. Abnormal expression or mutations of HDACs, together with aberrant histone acetylation patterns, have been found in a broad range of cancer types.[114] HDACs have thus become a novel class of targets in cancer therapy (Figure 3c). Histone deacetylase inhibitors (HDACIs) comprise diverse compounds such as suberoylanilide hydroxamic acid (SAHA, vorinostat) or valproic acid (VPA). It has been reported that HDACIs promote growth arrest, differentiation, and apoptosis of many solid tumor cells (e.g., lung, prostate, thyroid, and breast cancers, chondrosarcoma, and glioblastoma) and cell lines of hematopoietic malignancy, and exhibit only minimal effects on normal tissues.[69,115–121] For instances, SAHA and VPA are able to induce in vitro myeloid differentiation and early apoptosis of Kasumi-1 AML cells, which express AML1-ETO. Similar effects were also reported in a murine xenograft tumor model.

Inspired by preclinical data, many researchers have investigated the effects of HDACIs in clinical trials. Early study of SAHA showed efficacy in a panel of hematologic diseases.[122] The compound has been successfully applied to the treatment for refractory CTCL and becomes the first HDACI approved by FDA for this disease. A pilot study combining VPA and ATRA in eight refractory or high-risk AML patients demonstrated clinical benefits in seven cases, with myelomonocytic differentiation of circulating blasts. Although promising results have been obtained in hematological malignancies, clinical data for HDACIs in patients with solid tumors are inadequate.[123] In future, the effects of the combination of HDACI with conventional cancer treatment should be explored in solid tumor.

DOT1L inhibitor

MLL gene is one of the epigenetic modifier genes identified through molecular cloning of chromosomal translations involving 11q23. This gene encodes a SET domain histone methyltransferase, which catalyzes the methylation of lysine 4 of histone H3 (H3K4) at specific gene loci.[124] MLL is essential for fetal and adult hematopoiesis in that it regulates the expression of HOX genes and some cofactors key to the expansion and differentiation of HSPCs.[125–127] Abnormalities of MLL gene account for over 70% of infant leukemia and approximately 10% of adult AML, and are correlated to a particularly worse clinical outcome.[128] In addition to MLL translations, MLL partial tandem duplication (PTD) is also reported as a recurrent genetic defect. In the chimerical genes, the catalytic SET domain of MLL is lost and the fusion partners are capable of interacting with a histone H3K79 methyltransferase DOT1L.[129,130] As a result, fusion products not only retain gene-specific recognition elements within the MLL moiety, but also gain the ability to recruit DOT1L to these locations. The ectopic H3K79 methylation due to recruitment of DOT1L leads to enhanced expression of leukemogenic genes, such as HOXA9 and MEIS1.[131] Of particular interest is that DOT1L contributes to the transforming activity of MLL fusion and thus functions as a catalytic driver of leukemogenesis.

It has been proposed that inhibition of DOT1L may provide a pharmacologic basis for therapeutic intervention in MLL-related leukemia (Figure 3c). In vitro and in vivo experiments have demonstrated that EPZ-5676, a specific inhibitor of DOT1L, can selectively kill cells carrying on the MLL gene translocation by causing cell cycle arrest and promoting cell differentiation.[132] Data of phase 1 clinical trial of EPZ-5676 for the treatment of refractory or relapsed MLL rearranged acute leukemia patient reported that the compound was generally safe and well tolerated (NCT01684150). Eight of the 34 MLL-related patients showed biological or clinical responses,[133] including two complete responses (CRs) and one partial response (PR). Other DOT1L inhibitors such as EPZ4777 and SYC-522 also have been documented to promote differentiation and apoptosis.[134–136] Interestingly, bioinformatics analysis suggested that DOT1L may play a role in the pathogenesis of breast cancer. *In vitro* study has shown that DOT1L inhibition selectively inhibited proliferation, self-renewal, and metastatic potential of breast cancer cells and induced cell differentiation.[137]

Inhibitors of isocitrate dehydrogenase (IDH)

Somatic mutations of the metabolic enzyme IDH have recently been reported in human glioma, melanoma, thyroid cancer, chondrosarcoma, and AML.[35,138–140] All mutations are located at arginine residues in the catalytic pockets of IDH1 (R132) or IDH2 (R140 and R172) and thus confer on the enzymes a new activity: catalysis of α-ketoglutarate (α-KG) to 2-hydroxyglutarate (2-HG).[140,141] High concentrations of 2-HG, known as an "oncometabolite," have been shown to inhibit α-KG-dependent dioxygenases, including histone and DNA demethylases, which are main modifiers of the epigenetic state of cells (Figure 3a).[140–143] It has been suggested that cancer-associated IDH mutations may induce a block of cellular differentiation to promote tumorigenesis and therefore may be potential targets of differentiation therapy.[143,144] Indeed, it has been shown that a selective IDH1/R132H inhibitor (AGI-5198) induces the expression of genes associated with gliogenic differentiation and triggers astroglial differentiation of IDH1/R132H mutant (mIDH1) cells.[145] Moreover, blockade of mIDH1 suppresses the growth of glioma cells with IDH1/R132H, but not those with wild-type IDH1 *in vitro* or in IDH1/R132H glioma xenograft mice. It is worth noting that AGI-6780, a small molecule that potently and selectively inhibits the tumor-associated mutant IDH2/R140Q, has also been developed. AGI-6780 is capable of inducing differentiation of TF-1 erythroleukemia and primary human AML cells *in vitro*.[146] These findings provide proof-of-concept that inhibitors targeting mutant IDH1 or IDH2 may have potential applications as cancer differentiation inducers.

Recently, promising results of early phase clinical studies on AG-120 (the first inhibitor of mutated IDH1) and AG-221 (the inhibitor of the mutated IDH2 protein) were reported (https://www.clinicaltrials.gov/).[144] AG-120 was well tolerated and showed encouraging clinical efficacy in patients with advanced *IDH1*-mutation positive AML. The compound seemed able to reduce 2-HG levels in diseased cells to normal levels and allow leukemia cells to mature into granulocytes. Among 14 evaluable cases out of 17 patients, 7 patients responded to the drug, with 4 CR (Daniel Pollyea, the 26th European Organization for Research and Treatment of Cancer Symposium). Consistent with the clinical observation, AG-120 reduces intracellular 2-HG and induces cellular differentiation in TF-1 R132 cells and primary human *IDH1* mutant AML patient samples treated *ex vivo* (56th ASH meeting, abstract 70455). The ongoing phase 1 study of AG-221 as a single agent in patients with *IDH2*-mutant positive advanced hematologic malignancies also showed a favorable safety profile as well as durable clinical benefits (56th ASH meeting, abstract 70721). Out of 48 patients enrolled, 20 patients achieved objective responses, including 12 CRs and 8 PRs. Responses were durable, with durations up to 8 months. Interestingly, AG-221 induces differentiation and impairs self-renewal of IDH2-mutant leukemia cells in murine models of IDH2-mutant leukemia and primary human AML xenograft models (56th ASH meeting, abstract 70656 and 76334).

Actually, the studies on cancer differentiation inducers gradually take momentum. Of particular interest is the model disease APL, where differentiation-inducing agents have been demonstrated to exert a curative effect in the great majority of patients. Besides, some other differentiation-induction agents have shown promising effects in preclinical experiments and clinical trials. Differentiation therapy for cancers, although still in its relative infancy, has given hope to millions of cancer patients.

APL as a successful model of cancer differentiation therapy

APL is the M3 subtype of AML, characterized not only by distinct clinical manifestations but also by unique molecular pathogenesis and effective target-based differentiation therapy.

Clinical treatment strategies in APL

APL was first described in 1957 as the most malignant form of acute leukemia.[147] Patients with APL show specific features: a very rapid fatal natural course of only a few weeks' duration, an accumulation of abnormal promyelocytes in bone marrow, and a severe bleeding syndrome due to disseminated intravascular coagulation (DIC) or hyperfibrinolysis. In the era before ATRA-based therapy, only 23–35% of the APL patients could have a 5-year survival by CT.[148] Inspired by the Chinese philosophy of educational approach in health maintenance and the Western medical science of induction of cancer cell differentiation, scientists from Shanghai Institute of Hematology (SIH) carried out the research on leukemia differentiation therapy since the late 1970s.[148]

In 1980, a group from United States published the results of *in vitro* terminal differentiation of HL-60 cells upon the effect of 13-cRA.[67] Clinical improvement or CR after treatment with 13-cRA in a few isolated cases of APL were then reported, accompanied by maturation of promyelocytes with disappearance of signs of coagulopathy.[149–151] The SIH group, on the other hand, was focused on the potential therapeutic effects of ATRA. The first clinical trial of ATRA was reported in 24 APL cases (16 newly diagnosed and 8 anthracycline refractory cases) who were treated with ATRA alone.[152] CR was achieved in all patients and the evidence of *in vivo* blast differentiation with Auer's rods in polynucleated granulocytes was documented. The results have been quickly confirmed by a large amount of clinical practices around the world.[59,148] ATRA therapy became the standard for induction of newly diagnosed APL patients, which was then further improved stepwise through the effective combination regimen of ATRA with CT. Moreover, the roles of ATRA and CT in consolidation or maintenance therapy have been verified to reduce the incidence of relapse. By using this protocol, 5-year OS was up to about 70%.[69,148,153–155] The routine prescription of ATRA is 45 mg/m^2/day, while the recommendation dosage of ATRA in the SIH is 25 mg/m^2/day. The reason to reduce the initial dose of ATRA is to avoid ATRA toxicity but to achieve the same therapeutic effects as the conventional dosage.[156]

Even though the ATRA/CT combination was considered very efficient anti-APL therapy, up to about 30% of APL patients still ended with relapse.[157–159] The introduction of arsenic trioxide (ATO) since the early 1990s has further changed the clinical landscape of APL. *In vitro* studies showed that ATO exerts dose-dependent effects on APL cells including differentiation and apoptosis, although the differentiation is only a partial one compared with that induced by ATRA.[160] Clinically, refractory or relapsed APL after ATRA/CT therapy as well as newly diagnosed APL could achieve CR, suggesting an absence of cross-resistance between ATRA and ATO.[161] Therefore, new therapeutic strategies have focused on minimizing CT and administering ATRA plus ATO as primary therapy. Indeed, the ATRA-/ATO-based protocol yielded a much longer survival in newly diagnosed APL compared with therapy with ATRA or ATO alone.[148,162,163] These outcomes

Table 1 Sanz score for APL risk stratification.

Characteristic	Low risk	Intermediate risk	High risk
WBC ($\times 10^9$/L)	≤10	≤10	>10
Platelets ($\times 10^9$/L)	>40	≤40	≤40

Source: Data from Ref. 165.

were even not influenced by FLT3 mutation status, which was a poor prognostic factor in APL patients treated with ATRA and CT.[164] Combination of ATRA and ATO have obtained about 95% of CR rate and 5-year DFS and OS were near 90%.[162] Of note, the combination therapy without CT was associated with very high 2-year EFS and OS rates (97% and 99%, respectively) in nonhigh-risk APL by Sanz Score (Table 1).[158,165] Thus, in some newly updated authoritative guidelines, the ATRA-/ATO-based therapy has been the first-line strategy for APL patients. Although consensus has not yet been reached on the details of specific consolidation or maintenance therapy, it has been widely accepted that ATRA, ATO, and anthracycline-based CT should be given sequentially. The recommendation of APL treatment is listed in Tables 2 and 3.

The conventional administration of ATO is the intravenous route. An oral formulation of ATO was also found to be active in relapsed APL and has subsequently been evaluated in upfront management. Another formulation of arsenic in advanced clinical investigation is tetra-arsenic tetra-sulfide (AS_4S_4) and an oral AS_4S_4-containing formula named the Realgar–Indigo naturalis formula (RIF) in traditional Chinese Medicine was used in APL patients.[167,168] No significant differences were noted between the RIF and intravenously administered ATO groups with regard to the CR rate, the 3 year of OS or the 2 years of DFS at 2 years.[169,170] These two trials have established the feasibility and safety of prolonged oral arsenic administration, but long-term safety data are still required. Oral arsenic formulations are not currently available in the United States or Europe.

As the prognosis of APL patients is getting much better, the issues of early mortality [related to bleeding, differentiation syndrome (DS), or infection] and relapse [including central nerve system (CNS) relapse] becomes increasingly important. In patients with clinical and pathologic features of APL, ATRA should be started upon first suspicion of APL without waiting for genetic confirmation of the diagnosis.[166] Early initiation of ATRA may prevent the lethal complication of bleeding. DS is a common complication in the ATRA or ATO treatment, with a frequency being around

Table 2 The recommendation of APL treatment (in China).

	Nonhigh-risk APL	High-risk APL
Induction therapy	ATRA 25 mg/m²/d × 28–42 or until clinical remission	ATRA 25 mg/m²/d × 28–42 or until clinical remission
	ATO 0.16 mg/kg/d × 28–35 or until BM remission	ATO 0.16 mg/kg/d × 28–35 or until BM remission
	HU 20–40 mg/kg/d (when WBC > 10 × 10⁹/L)	IDA 6–8 mg/m²/d × 3 or DNR 45 m/m²/d × 3
Consolidation therapy	DA: DNR 45 mg/m²/d × 3 + Ara-C 100–200 mg/m²/d × 7	DA or (DNR + Ara-C 1.5–2.5 g/m²/d × 3)
	MA: MTZ 6–8 mg/m²/d × 3 + Ara-C 100–200 mg/m²/d × 7	MA or (MTZ + Ara-C 1.5–2.5 g/m²/d × 3)
	HA: HHT 2–3 mg/m²/d × 3 + Ara-C 100–200 mg/m²/d × 7	HA or (HHT + Ara-C 1.5–2.5 g/m²/d × 3)
Maintenance therapy	ATRA 25 mg/m² × 28	ATRA 25 mg/m² × 28
	ATO 0.16 mg/kg × 28	ATO 0.16 mg/kg × 28
	6-MP + MTX: 6-MP 100 mg/d on days 1–7, 15–21	6-MP + MTX: 6-MP 100 mg/d on days 1–7, 15–21
	MTX 20 mg/d on days 1, 8, 15, 21	MTX 20 mg/d on days 1, 8, 15, 21
	5 cycles of sequential use of ATRA, ATO, and CT	5 cycles of sequential use of ATRA, ATO, and CT

Abbreviations: Ara-C, cytarabine; ATO, arsenic trioxide; ATRA, all-trans-retinoic acid; BM, bone marrow; HU, hydroxyurea; IDA, idarubicin; DNR, daunorubicin; MTZ, mitozantrone; HHT, homoharringtonine; 6-MP, 6-mercaptopurine; MTX, methotrexate.
Source: Data from Ref. 166.

Table 3 The recommendation of APL treatment (NCCN guideline 2015).

	Induction therapy	Consolidation therapy
High-risk APL	ATRA 45 mg/m²/d until clinical remission + DNR 50 m/m²/d × 4 + Ara-C 200 mg/m²/d × 7	ATO 0.15 mg/kg/d × 5 days/week × 5 weeks × 2 cycles, then (ATRA 45 mg/m²/d × 7 + DNR 50 mg/m²/d × 3) × 2 cycles
	ATRA 45 mg/m²/d until clinical remission + DNR 60 m/m²/d × 3 + Ara-C 200 mg/m²/d × 7	(DNR 60 mg/m²/d × 3 + Ara-C 200 mg/m²/d × 7), then (DNR 45 mg/m²/d × 3 + Ara-C 1.5–2 g/m² Q12h × 3)
	ATRA 45 mg/m²/d until clinical remission + Idarubicin 12 mg/m²/d on days 2, 4, 6, 8	(ATRA 45 mg/m²/d × 15 + IDA 5 mg/m²/d × 3 + Ara-C 1 g/m²/d × 4), then (ATRA 45 mg/m²/d × 15 + MTZ 10 mg/m²/d × 5), then (ATRA 45 mg/m²/d × 15 + IDA 12 mg/m²/d × 1 + Ara-C 150 mg/m² Q8h × 4)
Nonhigh-risk APL	ATRA 45 mg/m²/d × 1–36 + Idarubicin 6–12 mg/m²/d on days 2, 4, 6, 8 + ATO 0.15 mg/kg/d × 9–26	(ATRA 45 mg/m²/d × 28 + ATO 0.15 mg/kg/d × 28), then (ATRA 45 mg/m²/d × 7 d/2 wk × 3 + ATO 0.15 mg/kg/d × 5 d/wk × 5 wk)
	ATRA 45 mg/m²/d until clinical remission + ATO 0.15 mg/kg/d until BM remission	ATO 0.15 mg/kg/d × 5 d/wk × 4 wk/8 wk × 4 cycles + ATRA 45 mg/m²/d × 2 wk/4 wk × 7 cycles
	ATRA 45 mg/m²/d until clinical remission + DNR 50 m/m²/d × 4 + Ara-C 200 mg/m²/d × 7	ATO 0.15 mg/kg/d × 5 d/wk × 5 wk × 2 cycles, then (ATRA 50 mg/m²/d × 7 + DNR 50 mg/m²/d × 3) × 2 cycles
	ATRA 45 mg/m²/d until clinical remission + DNR 60 m/m²/d × 3 + Ara-C 200 mg/m²/d × 7	(DNR 60 mg/m²/d × 3 + Ara-C 200 mg/m²/d × 7) × 1 cycle, then (DNR 45 mg/m²/d × 3 + Ara-C 1 g/m² Q12h × 4) × 1 cycle
	ATRA 45 mg/m²/d until clinical remission + Idarubicin 12 mg/m²/d on days 2, 4, 6, and 8	(ATRA 45 mg/m²/d × 15 + IDA 5 mg/m²/d × 3), then (ATRA 45 mg/m²/d × 15 + MTZ 10 mg/m²/d × 5), then (ATRA 45 mg/m²/d × 15 + IDA 12 mg/m²/d × 1)

Abbreviations: Ara-C, cytarabine; ATO, arsenic trioxide; ATRA, all-trans-retinoic acid; BM, bone marrow; DNR, daunorubicin; HHT, homoharringtonine; IDA, idarubicin; 6-MP, 6-mercaptopurine; MTZ, mitozantrone; MTX, methotrexate; NCCN, US National Comprehensive Cancer Network.
Source: Data from http://www.nccn.org/professionals/physician_gls/f_guidelines.asp.

25% both in United States and in Europe,[171,172] but relatively rare in East Asian populations (5–10%).[154,162] Signs and symptoms of this syndrome include hyperleukocytosis, dyspnea with interstitial pulmonary infiltrates, peripheral edema, unexplained fever, weight gain, hypotension, and acute renal failure. The mortality could be down to 3% or lower if DS is recognized early and treated promptly with CT and high dose of dexamethasone (10 mg twice daily).[172,173] In addition, patients with a high white blood cell count (WBC > 30×10^9/L) at diagnosis may benefit from prophylactic steroids. A common practice to avoid CNS prophylaxis (methotrexate 5–10 mg, cytarabine 40–50 mg, and dexamethasone 5 mg) for APL patients are recommended, 4–6 times for nonhigh-risk APL and 6–8 times for the patients with high WBC counts.[166] Another issue is side effects of ATO because the compound has long been considered as a very strong poison. In fact, the protocol incorporating ATO proves to be quite safe. The common adverse effects such as minor bone marrow myelosuppression, hepatotoxicity, gastrointestinal reactions, and neurotoxicity can be controlled and are generally reversible without need of the discontinuation of the drug.[162,166] In very rare situation, clinically significant arrhythmias due to prolongation of the QT interval on the ECG are observed, which can be avoided with appropriate precautions and withdrawal of the medicine.[174] At the same time, arsenic concentrations in the urine of patients who had ceased maintenance treatment for 2 years were below the safety limits recommended by government agencies in several countries or regions, whereas arsenic levels in plasma, nails, and hair were only slightly higher than those found in healthy controls.[162]

Leukemogenesis and therapeutic mechanisms of APL

It has been well known that PML-RARα resulting from t(15;17)(q22;q21) translocation is the key driver of APL leukemogenesis, which exerts dominant negative effects on RARα- and PML-related pathways.[175] The fusion protein represses the transcriptional expression of target genes essential for hematopoietic differentiation and yields an increasing proliferation and self-renewal of LICs.[175–177] The PML-RARα fusion protein binding to RXR co-receptor functions as a constitutive transcriptional repressor at RAREs of target genes through recruitment of CoR, which leads to the characteristic differentiation block.[148,176,178] In normal cells, PML proteins multimerize to form multiprotein subnuclear structures called PML-nuclear bodies (PML-NBs).[179] PML-NBs have been shown to play an important role in DNA damage repair, apoptosis, growth, senescence, and angiogenesis, and more recently, in the maintenance of HSPCs. In APL cells, PML-NBs are disrupted owing to the formation of PML/PML-RARα heterocomplex, interfering with the normal biological functions of PML.[180] This mechanism probably cooperates with the disruption of RAR/RXR pathway to enforce the APL-specific differentiation block and acquisition of self-renewal, thus transforming the committed HSPCs into immortal, fully transformed LICs (Figure 4).

Combining the discovery of PML-RARα in APL pathogenesis with special effective treatment of ATRA and ATO has pointed to a possible molecular mechanism underlying PML-RARα-specific therapy. Indeed, a large number of studies have revealed that ATRA and ATO act through distinct but complementary mechanisms, providing a biologic rationale for the two agents to be used in combination to achieve synergistic efficacy with low toxicity.

At pharmacological level (10^{-7}–10^{-6} mol/L), ATRA binds to the ligand-binding domain (LBD) of RARα portion in the fusion protein and induces a conformational change of the chimerical receptor.[181,182] This leads to displacement of CoR complexes and recruitment of CoA complexes and clearance of PML-RARα from promoters of target genes, thereby restoring wild-type RARα function and subverting the differentiation block.[63,148,178,183] ATRA also leads to the degradation of PML-RARα oncoprotein,[184–186] which may contribute to the response, and generate a restoration of nuclear architecture with reformation of PML-NBs. Re-establishment of RARα signaling allows differentiation of APL blasts and yields short-term disease management. Even though ATRA and anthracyclines are very efficient anti-APL therapies, APL patients can relapse, perhaps due to ATRA failing to affect LICs.

ATO exerts dose-dependent effects on APL cells in initial cellular and molecular mechanistic studies.[160,187] At low concentrations, ATO induces partial morphologic differentiation in APL cells, whereas at high concentrations, apoptosis induction occurs predominantly. Both effects are associated with a degradation of PML-RARα. ATO efficiently triggers the degradation of PML-RARα and PML through direct binding to the RBCC domain of PML moiety, which induces the conformational changes of PML proteins, leading to protein–protein aggregation and sumoylation of these proteins.[188] In addition, ATO-induced oxidative stress promotes PML homodimerization by cross-linking PML via disulfide bonds.[189] Sumoylated PML and PML-RARα recruit the ubiquitin ligase RNF4 and subject to proteasome-mediated proteolysis.[190,191] Besides, arsenic can act through other mechanisms independent of PML-RARα status, such as pro-apoptotic effects mediated by the mitochondria-mediated pathway, DNA damage, telomerase activity, autophagy, and so on.[148,192] Notably, ATO could induce LIC eradication in APL through several pathways, which may be a key factor in the success of ATO for APL patients.[148,177,183,192,193] Sufficient and rapid degradation of PML and PML-RARα is required for LIC clearance and long-term disease eradication,[194,195] which can be obtained by ATO treatment. Arsenic can also facilitate elimination of LICs through inhibiting Notch pathway, antagonizing the Hedgehog–Gli pathway, and repressing NF-κB and β-catenin. The pleiotropic behaviors may be the reason why arsenic is very active in APL, as a single agent as well as in combination.

Because ATRA and ATO target respectively the *C*- and *N*-terminals of PML-RARα, enhanced degradation of PML-RARα oncoprotein might provide a plausible explanation for the superior efficacy of combination therapy in patients. Intriguingly, consistent with the mechanistic researches, genetic mutations in the LBD of the RARα moiety that interfere with ATRA binding or nuclear coregulators binding are observed in about 40% of relapsed APL patients treated with ATRA/CT,[196–198] while genetic mutations in the PML moiety of the PML-RARα oncogene that probably impair the direct binding of ATO to PML-RARα in patients with clinical ATO resistance have been described after treatment with ATRA/ATO/CT.[199,200] A small number of APL patients harbor PLZF-RARα fusion gene resulting from t(11;17)(q23;q21), which are resistant to ATRA and ATO therapy.[201,202] These data further support that PML-RARα is the direct target of both ATRA and ATO. Several groups have shown that ATRA and ATO display a synergy in many pathways including TFs and cofactors, activation of calcium signaling, stimulation of the IFN pathway, activation of the proteasome system, cell cycle arrest, gain of apoptotic potential, downregulation of telomerase and telomere length, upregulation of cAMP/PKA activity, and enhanced arsenic uptake by APL cells through induced expression of cell membrane arsenic transporter (AQP9).[148,176,203,204] Recent studies have shown that the ATRA/ATO

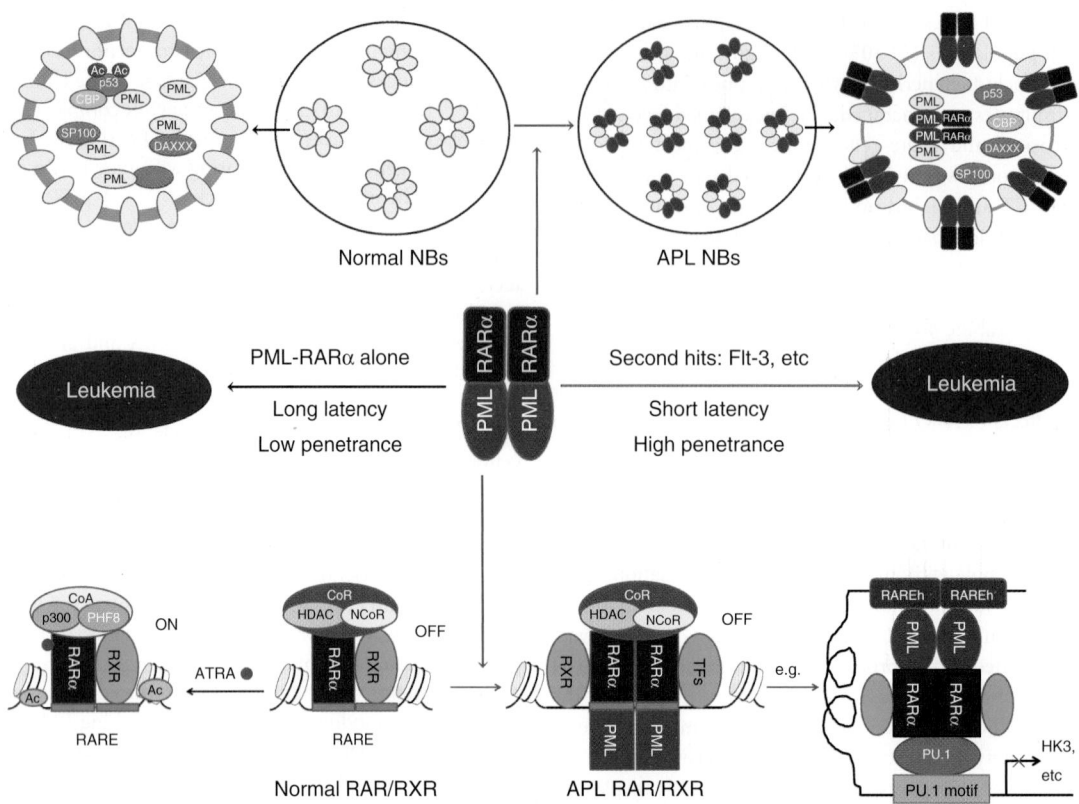

Figure 4 Molecular pathogenesis of APL. PML-RARα plays a key role in leukemogenesis of APL, which exerts dominant negative effects on RARα- and PML-related pathways. Under physiological condition, RAR/RXR heterodimers bind to the specific motifs defined as retinoic acid response elements (RAREs) on the promoters of target genes and differentially activates or represses gene transcription while recruiting co-activators (CoA) or co-repressors (CoR) complex depend on the presence or absence of the ligands, such as ATRA. The fusion protein binding to RXR co-receptor functions as a constitutive transcriptional repressor at RAREs of target genes through recruitment of CoR. In other hand, PML proteins multimerize to form multiprotein subnuclear structures called PML-nuclear bodies (PML-NBs) in normal cells. In APL cells, PML-NBs are disrupted owing to the formation of PML/PML-RARα heterocomplex.

combination rapidly clears PML-RARα + LICs, resulting in APL eradication and dramatically prolong survival in murine models.[177,194] All these findings may contribute to the dramatically improved response from APL patients under the treatment of ATRA and ATO combination.

In conclusion, ATRA and ATO exert different but cross-linked actions on APL cells. ATRA mainly works through transcriptional modulation, and the main effects of ATO occur at the protein level, while both agents target PML-RARα. These data may further explain the lack of cross-resistance between the two agents (Figure 5). Therapy of APL with ATRA and ATO is to date the most successful example of cancer differentiation therapy, and key factor can be the synergistic targeting of the oncoprotein by the two agents. This scientific history may hence serve as a template for subsequent development of similar treatments in other leukemias and solid tumors. More importantly, the story of APL provides new way for thinking that differentiation therapy is essentially target therapy on the molecules affecting differentiation pathway and combination or synergistic targeting strategy is highly effective to eliminate CSCs.

Perspectives

Taken together, differentiation therapy against cancer has the potential to make tumor cells convert from a malignant path to a benign course, which has given hope to scientists and clinicians on a much better cancer treatment outcome. However, interest and application of differentiation-based therapy for solid tumors and

hematological malignancies other than APL are just at the beginning. One major challenge is the complexity of histopathological subtypes and clinical stages of cancers, resulting in the absence of developmental models of cancer progression. The re-establishment of the genotype that characterizes the original tissue types and the morphological transformation of tumor cells to the normal cells may help to determine more successful differentiation induction. In addition, there have not yet been definite markers for evaluating the effects of differentiation inducers. Assessment of the precise therapeutic role of agents is often hampered by the difficulties in distinguishing *in vivo* cytotoxicity from differentiation. The classic evaluation of therapeutic responses mainly focuses on the shrinkage of the tumor mass, but this is not suitable for the response evaluation of differentiation therapy that just restores the differentiation program of tumor cells. Consequently, identifying accurate novel biomarker sets of response to differentiation therapy becomes urgent for clinical application. Recent evidence suggests that targeting of leukemia driver proteins other than PML-RARα can induce cell differentiation in some other types of AML and can eventually yield high-quality CR, paving the way of enlarging this approach in hematological malignancies. Nevertheless, solid tumors are still viewed as much more heterogeneous aberrant tissues than most leukemia, and much more complex molecular mechanisms are involved in their pathogenesis. Hence, the development of differentiation therapy in solid tumors may need more comprehensive approach to combine CT, immunotherapy, and differentiation agents in order to produce multiplied synergistic targeting effects.

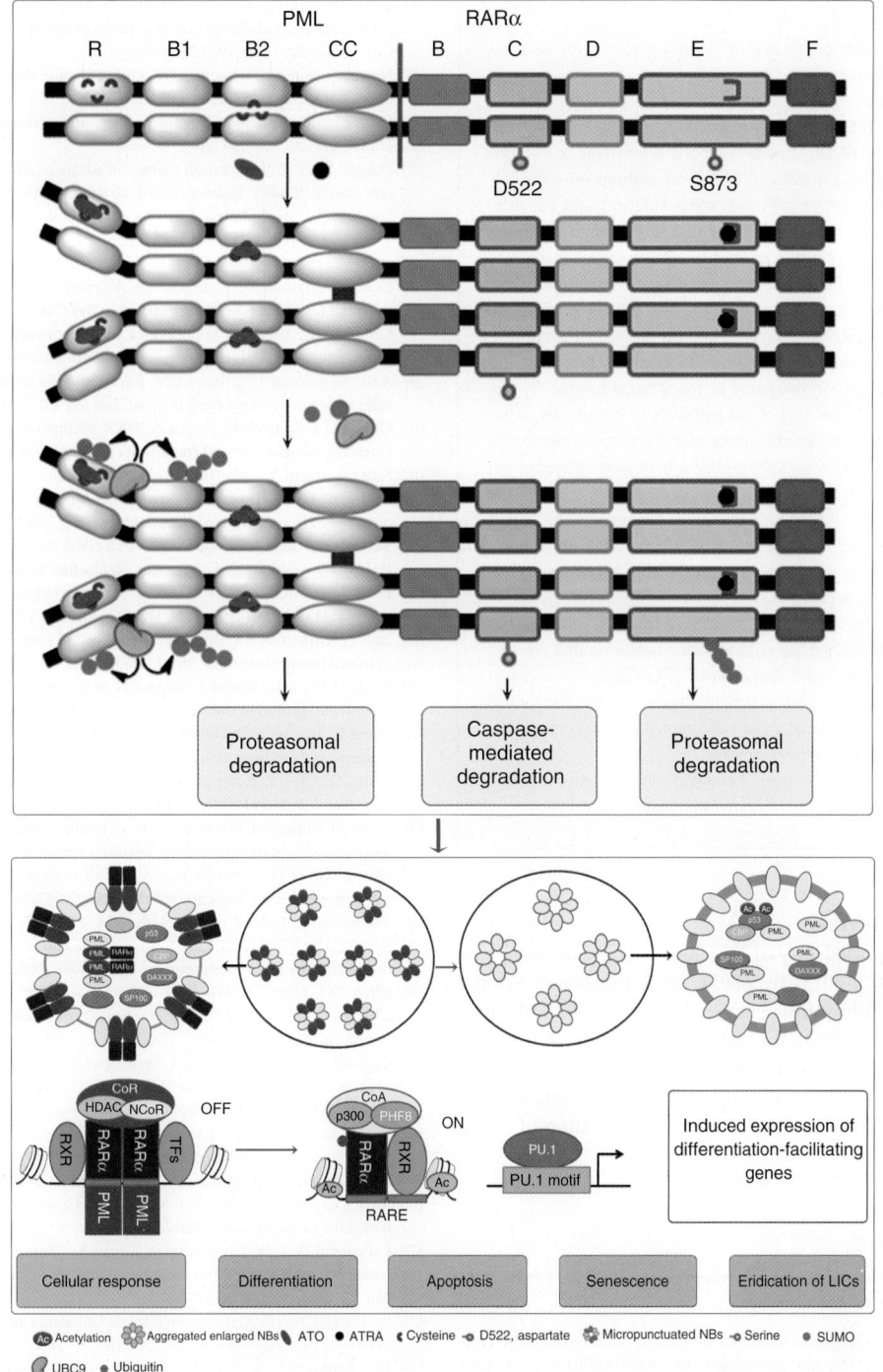

Figure 5 Therapeutic mechanism of APL. ATRA and ATO target respectively the *C*- and *N*-terminals of PML-RARα, enhancing degradation of PML-RARα oncoprotein. ATRA binds to the ligand-binding domain (LBD) of RARα portion in the fusion protein and ATO binds to the RBCC domain of PML moiety, which induces the conformational change and the consequential degradation of the fusion protein. The degradation of PML-RARα generates a restoration of nuclear architecture with reformation of PML-NBs. ATRA binding also leads to displacement of CoR complexes and recruitment of CoA complexes and clear PML-RARα from promoters of target genes, thereby restoring wild-type RARα function. The synergistic effects of ATRA and ATO result in a variety of cellular response including differentiation, apoptosis, and senescence of leukemic cells, and importantly, the eradication of leukemia-initiating cell (LIC).

Summary

Most human cancers show characteristics of abnormal cell differentiation, often coupled with dysregulation of proliferation and/or apoptosis. Cancer cells may be blocked at a particular stage of differentiation along

with the involved cellular lineage, or they may differentiate into an inappropriate cell type. Hence, cancer differentiation therapy represents the approach aimed at the re-activation of endogenous differentiation programs or subverting differentiation/maturation blockage within cancer cells, often accompanied by the loss of malignant phenotype and the restoration, at least in part, of the normal phenotype.

The concept of differentiation therapy was pioneered by the work of Pierce and Verneyin 1961 when they observed differentiation of teratocarcinoma cells.[205] In 1970s, important reports were made to demonstrate the differentiating capability of DMSO on erythropoiesis, the differentiation of neuroblastoma cells with some inducers, and the morphologic and functional maturation of leukemia cells induced by certain agents.[59,67,206–208] Many substances have thus been shown to possess the potential of cancer differentiation inducer with *in vitro* cell line experiments. To trigger malignant cells to overcome their differentiation block and to enter the apoptotic pathways has become an elegant alternative to the therapies simply killing malignant cells. However, differentiation therapy had historically been hampered by many factors, especially due to the insufficient understanding of the pathways of normal cell differentiation and the much higher complexity of the process of cancer cell reversion to "normal" cells/tissues induced by differentiation therapy than the cytotoxic approaches.[69]

The advancement of differentiation therapy to a real successful clinical practice was not realized until the use of ATRA and ATO in the treatment of APL.[53] This breakthrough has transformed APL from once a fatal disease to one of the most curable human cancers, with 5-year OS rates of 85–90%.[148] In addition, over the past several years, progress has been made in understanding the differentiation pathways that are also cross-talking with those of the regulation of cell proliferation and survival, and the development of some targeted therapies on other types of leukemia has already yielded promising differentiation-inducing effects, which need to be further explored clinically.

This chapter focuses on the basic theories of differentiation therapy, and the clinical achievements of this novel therapeutic approach.

Acknowledgments

This work was supported in part by Chinese National Key Basic Research Project (973: 2013CB966803), Mega-projects of Science Research for the 12th Five-Year Plan (2013ZX09303302), Ministry of Health Grant (201202003), the State Key Laboratories Project of Excellence Grant (81123005), the National Natural Science Foundation of China (81170519), and Program for New Century Excellent Talents in Universities of the Ministry of Education of China (NCET-13-1037).

Key references

The complete reference list can be found on the Wiley Companion Digital Edition of this title (see inside front cover for login instructions).

3 Regalo G, Leutz A. Hacking cell differentiation: transcriptional rerouting in reprogramming, lineage infidelity and metaplasia. *EMBO Mol Med.* 2013;5:1154–1164.

4 Xu WP, Zhang X, Xie WF. Differentiation therapy for solid tumors. *J Dig Dis.* 2014;15:159–165.

5 Sive JI, Gottgens B. Transcriptional network control of normal and leukaemic haematopoiesis. *Exp Cell Res.* 2014;329:255–264.

20 Taby R, Issa JP. Cancer epigenetics. *CA Cancer J Clin.* 2010;60:376–392.

22 Chen T, Dent SY. Chromatin modifiers and remodellers: regulators of cellular differentiation. *Nat Rev Genet.* 2014;15:93–106.

28 Shih AH, Abdel-Wahab O, Patel JP, Levine RL. The role of mutations in epigenetic regulators in myeloid malignancies. *Nat Rev Cancer.* 2012;12:599–612.

42 Pattabiraman DR, Weinberg RA. Tackling the cancer stem cells – what challenges do they pose? *Nat Rev Drug Discov.* 2014;13:497–512.

43 Chen K, Huang YH, Chen JL. Understanding and targeting cancer stem cells: therapeutic implications and challenges. *Acta Pharmacol Sin.* 2013;34:732–740.

53 Pettersson F, Miller WH Jr, Nervi C, et al. The 12th international conference on differentiation therapy: targeting the aberrant growth, differentiation and cell death programs of cancer cells. *Cell Death Differ.* 2011;18:1231–1233.

56 Ablain J, de The H. Retinoic acid signaling in cancer: the parable of acute promyelocytic leukemia. *Int J Cancer.* 2014;135:2262–2272.

57 Connolly RM, Nguyen NK, Sukumar S. Molecular pathways: current role and future directions of the retinoic acid pathway in cancer prevention and treatment. *Clin Cancer Res.* 2013;19:1651–1659.

59 Nowak D, Stewart D, Koeffler HP. Differentiation therapy of leukemia: 3 decades of development. *Blood.* 2009;113:3655–3665.

69 Cruz FD, Matushansky I. Solid tumor differentiation therapy – is it possible? *Oncotarget.* 2012;3:559–567.

73 Haugen BR. Redifferentiation therapy in advanced thyroid cancer. *Curr Drug Targets Immune Endocr Metabol Disord.* 2004;4:175–180.

79 Hughes PJ, Marcinkowska E, Gocek E, Studzinski GP, Brown G. Vitamin D3-driven signals for myeloid cell differentiation – implications for differentiation therapy. *Leuk Res.* 2010;34:553–565.

86 Deeb KK, Trump DL, Johnson CS. Vitamin D signalling pathways in cancer: potential for anticancer therapeutics. *Nat Rev Cancer.* 2007;7:684–700.

90 Grommes C, Landreth GE, Heneka MT. Antineoplastic effects of peroxisome proliferator-activated receptor gamma agonists. *Lancet Oncol.* 2004;5:419–429.

99 Azad N, Zahnow CA, Rudin CM, Baylin SB. The future of epigenetic therapy in solid tumours—lessons from the past. *Nat Rev Clin Oncol.* 2013;10:256–266.

101 Gnyszka A, Jastrzebski Z, Flis S. DNA methyltransferase inhibitors and their emerging role in epigenetic therapy of cancer. *Anticancer Res.* 2013;33:2989–2996.

102 Saunthararajah Y. Key clinical observations after 5-azacytidine and decitabine treatment of myelodysplastic syndromes suggest practical solutions for better outcomes. *Hematol Am Soc Hematol Educ Prog.* 2013;2013:511–521.

123 Ververis K, Hiong A, Karagiannis TC, Licciardi PV. Histone deacetylase inhibitors (HDACIs): multitargeted anticancer agents. *Biologics.* 2013;7:47–60.

129 Bernt KM, Zhu N, Sinha AU, et al. MLL-rearranged leukemia is dependent on aberrant H3K79 methylation by DOT1L. *Cancer Cell.* 2011;20:66–78.

130 Neff T, Armstrong SA. Recent progress toward epigenetic therapies: the example of mixed lineage leukemia. *Blood.* 2013;121:4847–4853.

145 Rohle D, Popovici-Muller J, Palaskas N, et al. An inhibitor of mutant IDH1 delays growth and promotes differentiation of glioma cells. *Science.* 2013;340:626–630.

146 Wang F, Travins J, DeLaBarre B, et al. Targeted inhibition of mutant IDH2 in leukemia cells induces cellular differentiation. *Science.* 2013;340:622–626.

148 Wang ZY, Chen Z. Acute promyelocytic leukemia: from highly fatal to highly curable. *Blood.* 2008;111:2505–2515.

151 Flynn PJ, Miller WJ, Weisdorf DJ, et al. Retinoic acid treatment of acute promyelocytic leukemia: in vitro and in vivo observations. *Blood.* 1983;62:1211–1217.

152 Huang ME, Ye YC, Chen SR, et al. Use of all-trans retinoic acid in the treatment of acute promyelocytic leukemia. *Blood.* 1988;72:567–572.

155 Tallman MS, Andersen JW, Schiffer CA, et al. All-trans retinoic acid in acute promyelocytic leukemia: long-term outcome and prognostic factor analysis from the North American Intergroup protocol. *Blood.* 2002;100:4298–4302.

156 Chen GQ, Shen ZX, Wu F, et al. Pharmacokinetics and efficacy of low-dose all-trans retinoic acid in the treatment of acute promyelocytic leukemia. *Leukemia.* 1996;10:825–828.

160 Chen GQ, Shi XG, Tang W, et al. Use of arsenic trioxide (As_2O_3) in the treatment of acute promyelocytic leukemia (APL): I. As_2O_3 exerts dose-dependent dual effects on APL cells. *Blood.* 1997;89:3345–3353.

162 Hu J, Liu YF, Wu CF, et al. Long-term efficacy and safety of all-trans retinoic acid/arsenic trioxide-based therapy in newly diagnosed acute promyelocytic leukemia. *Proc Natl Acad Sci U S A.* 2009;106:3342–3347.

166 Mi JQ, Li JM, Shen ZX, Chen SJ, Chen Z. How to manage acute promyelocytic leukemia. *Leukemia.* 2012;26:1743–1751.

175 Lallemand-Breitenbach V, Zhu J, Kogan S, Chen Z, de The H. Opinion: how patients have benefited from mouse models of acute promyelocytic leukaemia. *Nat Rev Cancer.* 2005;5:821–827.

176 de The H, Chen Z. Acute promyelocytic leukaemia: novel insights into the mechanisms of cure. *Nat Rev Cancer.* 2010;10:775–783.

177 Dos Santos GA, Kats L, Pandolfi PP. Synergy against PML-RARa: targeting transcription, proteolysis, differentiation, and self-renewal in acute promyelocytic leukemia. *J Exp Med.* 2013;210:2793–2802.

180 de The H, Le Bras M, Lallemand-Breitenbach V. The cell biology of disease: acute promyelocytic leukemia, arsenic, and PML bodies. *J Cell Biol.* 2012;198:11–21.

183 Nichol JN, Garnier N, Miller WH Jr. Triple A therapy: the molecular underpinnings of the unique sensitivity of leukemic promyelocytes to anthracyclines, all-trans-retinoic acid and arsenic trioxide. *Best Prac Res Clin haematol.* 2014;27:19–31.

188 Zhang XW, Yan XJ, Zhou ZR, et al. Arsenic trioxide controls the fate of the PML-RARalpha oncoprotein by directly binding PML. *Science.* 2010;328:240–243.

192 Chen SJ, Zhou GB, Zhang XW, et al. From an old remedy to a magic bullet: molecular mechanisms underlying the therapeutic effects of arsenic in fighting leukemia. *Blood.* 2011;117:6425–6437.

12 Cancer stem cells

Yadwinder S. Deol, PhD ▪ Jill Granger, BSc, MSc ▪ Max S. Wicha, MD

Overview

There is substantial evidence that many if not most tumors contain a sub-population of cells that display stem cell properties. These "cancer stem cells" (CSCs) play an important role in tumor initiation and propagation. Furthermore, these cells may mediate resistance to cancer therapeutic agents and therefore play a fundamental role in cancer relapse. This highlights the importance of developing therapeutic approaches to target this cell population. In this chapter, we will review current thoughts on the role of tissue stem cells in carcinogenesis, the pathways that regulate these cells, and current progress in development of CSC targeting therapeutic agents. We will then review clinical implications of CSC models.

Cancer stem cell hypothesis

The idea that cancer originated from "primitive embryonic-like cells" dates back over a hundred years.[1] However, it is only within the past several decades that cellular and molecular technologies have permitted the direct testing of these concepts. The "cancer stem cell (CSCs) hypothesis" consists of two separate but inter-related concepts. The first concerns the cellular origins of cancer and the second the cellular organization of established cancers.

Models of carcinogenesis and cellular origin of cancer

Currently, two main models of carcinogenesis have been proposed, which are summarized in Figure 1. The classical "stochastic" model proposes that cancer may arise from any cell and that carcinogenesis evolves through random "stochastic" processes of mutation followed by clonal selection. As illustrated in the sequential accumulation of mutations during carcinogenesis (Figure 1b), disease development is driven by Darwinian selection of the fittest clones of cancer cells. In contrast to stochastic models, the CSC model posits that this process originates in those cells that possess or acquire the stem cell property of self-renewal. It is important to emphasize that the CSC model does not hold that tissue stem cells are the sole cellular source of cancer initiation. Although cancers may arise in normal tissue stem cells,[2,3] there is evidence that some cancers arise in tissue progenitor cells through mutations that endow these cells with self-renewal capabilities.[4] This process generates tumors that display a degree of hierarchical organization. At the apex of this hierarchy are CSCs, which are operationally defined as cancer cells that maintain the ability to self-renew (Figure 1a). These CSCs are capable of generating tumors that recapitulate the phenotypic heterogeneity of the original tumor when transplanted into mouse models.

Although the "stochastic" and "CSC model" were initially described as mutually exclusive, more resent research suggests that elements drawn from both models might better describe tumor development. Recent reports by the Vogelstein suggest that the incidence of cancers in many organs is directly proportional to their number of tissue stem cell divisions.[5] The latter is reflective of their stem cell frequency and division rate. As tissue stem cell mutations are themselves stochastic, this work provides a unifying model of carcinogenesis, whereby stem cells may be a functional unit of mutation and subsequent clonal selection. Furthermore, CSCs may undergo mutation during tumor evolution, generating tumors that contain multiple CSCs and their clonal progeny. The combination of these concepts, derived from both models of carcinogenesis, may provide a molecular explanation for the generation of intra-tumor heterogeneity; a phenomenon with considerable therapeutic implications.

Cancer stem cells as a unifying concept in multiple cancers

CSCs were first identified in human leukemia in 1997.[6] In seminal studies, John Dick et al. demonstrated that only a small fraction of primary human leukemia cells were capable of regenerating the leukemia when transplanted into immune-suppressed NOD/SCID (nonobese diabetic/severely compromised immunodeficient) mice.[6] Further, these tumor-initiating leukemia cells were prospectively identified by virtue of their phenotypic characterization as CD34+/CD38−, a phenotype resembling that found on normal hematopoietic stem cells. Although the frequency of these leukemia initiating cells was found to be approximately 1 in 250,000, the leukemias generated in transplanted mice recapitulated the phenotypic heterogeneity of the initial tumor. Utilizing similar tumor transplantation technologies, investigators have subsequently identified CSC in a wide variety of solid tumors. These include cancers of the breast,[7] brain,[8] prostate,[9,10] colon,[11,12] pancreas,[13] liver,[14,15] lung,[16] melanoma,[17] and head and neck.[18] In fact, evidence suggests that the majority of tumors are hieratically organized and contain cell populations that display stem cell properties.

Isolation, identification, and characterization of CSCs

In order to study the basic attributes of CSCs, it is necessary to first identify, isolate, purify, and characterize these cells by employing techniques that enable one to distinguish them from the bulk tumor cell population. The functional characteristics of CSCs, including self-renewal capability and differentiation potential, can be exploited by various *in vitro* and *in vivo* assays to identify and characterize this important cell population. Several methods or techniques exist to identify and isolate stem cell-like cancer cells; flow cytometry detecting expression of CSC-related markers, dye exclusion, ALDH (aldehyde dehydrogenase) assay, label retention (PKH staining), and a recent novel method of using autofluorescence in presence of riboflavin. CSCs, enriched by these techniques,

Holland-Frei Cancer Medicine, Ninth Edition. Edited by Robert C. Bast Jr., Carlo M. Croce, William N. Hait, Waun Ki Hong, Donald W. Kufe, Martine Piccart-Gebhart, Raphael E. Pollock, Ralph R. Weichselbaum, Hongyang Wang, and James F. Holland.
© 2017 John Wiley & Sons, Inc. ISBN: 978-1-118-93469-2

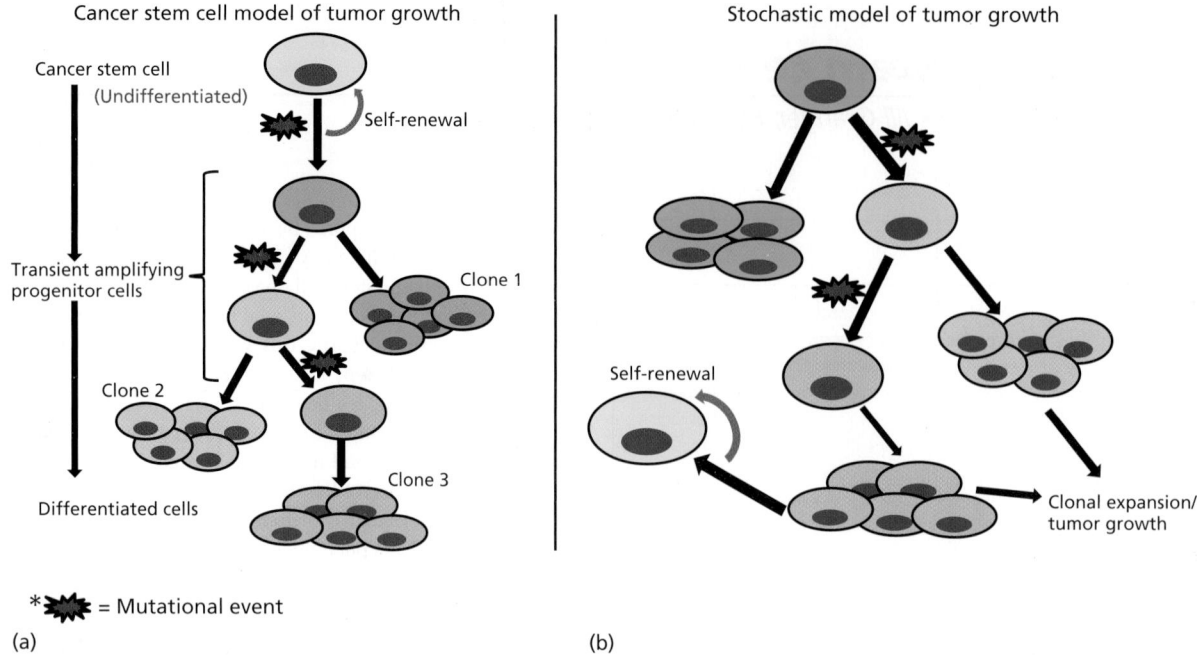

Figure 1 Schematic representation of two models of tumorogenesis. (a) Depicts "cancer stem cell" model where tumors arise in cells with stem cell properties generating hierarchically organized tumors driven by "cancer stem cells" at the top of hierarchy. These cells then generate differentiated clonal progeny that form the tumor bulk. (b) Depicts stochastic or classical model of tumorogenesis where random mutations in any cell generates cancerous clonal populations, which evolve through further mutation.

may be functionally validated by sphere formation assays or serial transplantation assays *in vivo* for evaluation of tumorigenic and self-renewal potential. The details of the methods are listed in the following sections.

CSC marker expression

The first CSCs in solid tumors were described in human breast cancer based on cellular expression of CD44 and lack of expression of CD24 (i.e., CD44+/CD24−).[7] Interestingly, these markers have proven useful for the isolation of CSC from a variety of other solid tumors. In parallel, CD133 has been shown to be useful in enriching for CSC in brain and lung cancers.[8,16] Another stem cell marker, ALDH, is also used along with CD44/CD24 or CD133 to identify the CSC population in several tumors. ALDHs are a family of enzymes that are involved in the oxidation of retinol to retinoic acid.[19] ALDH activity can be readily determined using the commercially available Aldefluor assay and was shown to be a useful CSC marker in cancers of the breast,[20] ovary,[21] colon,[22] head and neck,[23] and recently melanoma.[24]

Dye exclusion assays

Dye exclusion is based on the ability of stem cells to efflux lipophilic dyes, such as Rhodamine or Hoechst, owing to the high expression of the ATP-binding cassette transporter proteins such as ABCG2/BCRP1.[25] Utilizing flow cytometry analysis, cells that do not retain dye are observed as a side population.[26] Several studies have demonstrated that such side populations are enriched in cells with tumor-initiating capacity and are capable of regenerating heterogeneous cell populations.[27] This stem cell-like side population has been observed in several cancer types, as well as bone marrow and normal solid tissues.[28,29] The cellular toxicity of Hoechst dye limits their ability to be combined with functional studies.

Label retention

Another dye-based method used to characterize CSCs *in vitro* is the cell membrane, label-retaining assay using fluorescent PKH dye. This dye consists of a fluorophore that binds to the cell membrane lipid bilayer.[30] Upon cell division, the dye becomes distributed equally among daughter cells. Subsequent continuous cell divisions lead to decreased intensity.[31] Stem cells, including CSCs, normally undergo an asymmetric self-renewal process generating a stem cell and a daughter cell. The generated stem cells are quiescent and thus retain PKH dye for a longer time period, whereas the daughter cells proliferate and differentiate leading to decreased intensity of PKH dye. These daughter cells are then identified and sorted by flow cytometry. This method has been used successfully to isolate murine hematopoietic and mammary stem cells.[32]

Recently, it was reported that CSCs demonstrate autofluorescence in the presence of riboflavin.[33] The authors isolated this population using flow cytometry, distinguished these cells from the side population, and demonstrated that these putative CSCs had a greater tumor sphere-forming ability, increased chemo-resistance, were highly metastatic, and possessed long-term *in vivo* tumorogenecity. Further, in support of the cancer stem model, this autofluorescent CSC-like population was detected in several cancers.[33]

Sphere formation assays

The sphere formation assay is another *in vitro* assay that has proven useful for the identification of CSC populations. This is based on a property shared by both normal and malignant stem cells: survival when cultured in suspension and generation of spheroids at clonal density.[34] These spheres can be serially passaged and display stem cell properties with each passage. It has also been possible to combine a number of *in vitro* CSC assays. For instance, the addition of PHK dye during sphere formation results in the formation of spheres that often contain a single label-retaining sphere-initiating cell.[35]

In vivo serial dilution CSC assays

Although the use of CSC markers and *in vitro* assays has proven useful in the isolation and characterization of CSC, all of these techniques have limitations. The expression of CSC markers is variable and may be influenced by culture conditions or the tumor microenvironment.[36] Further, sphere formation assays may not correlate with tumor initiation capacity.[37] In light of these limitations, the "gold standard" for CSC identification is demonstration of tumor initiation upon implantation into immunosuppressed mice.[37] The tumor-initiating frequency in any cell population may be assessed by the ability of cells to initiate tumor development in mice using limiting dilution of cell suspensions. Thus, the definition of "CSCs" is ultimately an operational one.

It is important to note that immunosuppressed mouse models also have limitations. In human melanoma, the frequency of tumor-initiating cells was strongly influenced by the degree of immune competence of the mouse model utilized.[38] Recent studies have indicated that the immune system may actually play an important role in CSC regulation.[39,40] Studies elucidating these roles have been carried out in mouse tumors transplanted into syngeneic immune-competent mice. Such studies have confirmed the existence of CSC as determined by serial transplantation.[41]

Lineage tracing studies

One criticism of all transplantation studies is that they perturb the normal microenvironment where tumors develop. To circumvent this limitation, a series of studies using cell markers and lineage tracing have been performed. Such studies have confirmed the existence of CSC in tumors of the skin,[42] brain,[43] and colon.[44]

EMT/MET and cancer stem cells

Epithelial–mesenchymal transition (EMT) is a physiological process of particular importance during embryonic development whereby epithelial cells acquire mesenchymal properties, are characterized by a loss of cell adhesion and the acquisition of invasive properties. The EMT process was initially described during development, where it induced the migration of mesodermal cells during gastrulation or the delamination of the neural crest cells from the dorsal neural tube.[45] Similarly in cancer, EMT has been associated with the process of metastasis where epithelial cells from the primary tumor acquire mesenchymal phenotype and invade to other tissues.[46]

EMT is regulated by signals from the microenvironment that mediate epigenetic alterations driven by core transcription factors. Microenvironmental factors include tissue hypoxia, TGF-β (transforming growth factor-β), and other inflammatory molecules with subsequent induction of EMT-related transcription factor expression such as TWIST1, TWIST2, SNAI1, SNAI2, ZEB1, and ZEB2, among others.[47,48] Overexpression of these transcription factors induce a mesenchymal and invasive phenotype through repression of cell adhesion molecules, such as E-cadherin.[49] Twist1, which is involved in mesenchymal development during embryogenesis, has been shown to induce metastasis in breast cancer.[50] Several studies suggest that the EMT process generates CSC-like cells.[51,52] In this regard, overexpression of SNAI1 or TWIST1 alone was shown to induce EMT in MCF10A and immortalized human mammary epithelial cells.[53] In addition, there was increased expression of the stem cell marker CD44 and a decrease in CD24 expression, which suggests induction of CSC-like phenotype. Moreover, TWIST1 has been associated with an increased ability of breast cancer cells to form mammospheres and secondary tumors in an oncogenic

HRAS-g12V model.[54] Based on the molecular classification of breast cancer, a basal subtype, particularly claudin-low are known to possess an EMT-like gene expression signature. Such cancers have a high proportion of CD44+/24− cells that are locked within the mesenchymal state. These tumors display a highly aggressive behavior accompanied by a greater propensity to develop metastasis. Further, TWIST1 upregulated BMI expression, when suppressed by the miR-200 microRNA cluster, decreased CSC self-renewal, and cellular differentiation. Similarly, BMP signaling induced MET via induction of miR-205 and the miR-200 family of microRNAs that are key regulators of MET.[55]

The aforementioned studies strongly suggest the role of EMT in the acquisition of a stem cell phenotype. It is plausible that the CSC possesses alternative phenotypes; one involved in tumor invasion and metastasis while another state maintains the bulk of the tumors. This is evident from the recent study that used gene expression analysis to compare ALDH+ and CD44+/24− BCSCs isolated from different subtypes of breast cancer. This comparative gene expression analysis suggested that, although each population was independently capable of tumor initiation in NOD/SCID mice, yet they were quite distinct both functionally and anatomically in the original primary tumors. ALDH+ CSCs usually populated the interior of the tumors where they self-renewed and proliferated at a higher rate, whereas CD44+/24− CSCs were more mesenchymal, displayed an EMT phenotype located on the tumor margins or invasive front, and were more quiescent.[56] Further characterization of these two populations showed that CD44+/24− cells were highly vimentin positive and E-cadherin negative, whereas an ALDH+ population was highly positive for E-cadherin and negative for vimentin. Therefore, these CD44+/24− cells were more EMT-like, and may be poised to invade the blood vessels when triggered by stromal factors such as hypoxia, TGF-β, and other inflammatory agents.

These studies also demonstrated that BCSCs maintain the plasticity to transition between EMT and MET states in a process regulated by the tumor microenvironment. The interconversion of BCSCs from the EMT-like to MET-like state has also been shown to be regulated by microRNA networks. Such networks included EMT-inducing mir-9, mir-100, mir-221, and mir-155 as well as MET-inducing mir-200, mir-205, and mir-93.[57] The plasticity of BCSCs from a quiescent mesenchymal state to a proliferative epithelial-like state is critical for formation of tumor metastases at distant sites. The knockdown of TWIST1 in a spontaneous squamous-cell carcinoma model reversed EMT and allowed cells to proliferate and form metastasis.[58] Similarly, the loss of the EMT inducer Prrx1 was required for cancer cells to form lung macrometastasis.[59] In addition, MET-promoting factors, such as miR-200 family members, were found to promote metastatic colonization of breast cancer cells and induce epithelial differentiation.[60] Furthermore, expression of Id1 gene in breast cancer cells reconverted EMT cells into MET by downregulating TWIST1, which is required for establishing macrometastasis.[61] The above studies provide evidence that two alternative states of CSCs display plasticity and are regulated by microenvironmental factors that modulate the genetic regulators and several transcription factors. The existence of multiple CSC states has important therapeutic implications as elimination of CSC may require successful targeting of multiple CSC populations.

Signal transduction pathways in cancer stem cells and their therapeutic targeting

Like their normal counterparts, a number of evolutionarily conserved developmental pathways play a significant role in the regulation of CSCs in several cancer types. The conservation of these pathways in CSCs of different tumor types further strengthens the cancer stem model. Moreover, these pathways could provide common potential therapeutic targets irrespective of the tumor type.

Hedgehog signaling

The Hedgehog (Hh) family of proteins controls cell growth, survival, pattern of the vertebrate body, and stem/progenitor cell maintenance. Dysregulation of Hh signaling, including that arising from somatic mutation, has been linked to several cancer types. The binding of Hh proteins to the receptor Patched (Ptc) activates a signaling cascade that leads to the upregulation of a zinc-finger transcription factor GLI1–3 and its downstream gene targets.[62–64] Of the three mammalian Hh ligands, sonic hedgehog (SHH), Indian hedgehog (IHH), and desert hedgehog (DHH), SHH is the most highly expressed Hh signaling molecule and is involved in the regulation of many epithelial tissues. Aberrant activation of Hh signaling has been linked to basal cell carcinoma,[65,66] medulloblastoma,[67,68] rhabdomyosarcoma,[69] and other cancers, such as glioma, breast, esophageal, gastric, pancreatic, prostate, and small-cell lung carcinoma.[70] GLI1 amplifications are also known to occur in gliomas.[71]

The Hh signaling pathway plays a major role in mammary gland development both in humans and in mice. In mice, constitutive activation of Gli1 or inactivation of Gli3 resulted in mammary bud formation defects.[72] Ectopic expression of Gli1 has been shown to induce the nuclear Snail expression resulting in loss of E-cadherin expression in mouse mammary glands tissue during pregnancy.[73] In addition, the transcription factor FOXC2 also promoted mesenchymal differentiation via the Hh pathway and Snail upregulation.[74] Similarly, SHH overexpression in mouse mammary glands leads to mammary bud defects.[75] Perturbation of other Hh pathway molecules, such as activation of SMO or loss of PTCH1, has resulted in terminal end bud abnormalities.[76] Normal human mammary stem cells expressed PTCH1, Gli1, and Gli2 during mammosphere formation, a pathway that is downregulated during the process of differentiation. Hh signaling played an important role in stem cell regulation as activation of Hh signaling through Hh ligand, or Gli1/Gli2 overexpression, increased mammosphere formation and size through activation of BMI-1, a member of the polycomb gene family.[77] The similar activation of SMO, driven by an MMTV (mouse mammary tumour virus) promoter, increased mammosphere formation of primary mammary epithelial cells in transgenic mice.[76] Hh ligands are also known to exert mitogenic effects on mammary stem cells through paracrine interactions. This process may be involved in the regulation of mammary differentiation during pregnancy, in a process regulated by TP63.[78] Apart from TP63, the transcription factor Runx2 has been shown to regulate the expression of Hh ligands.[79]

Hh signaling pathway members SHH, PTCH1, and GLI1 were highly expressed in invasive breast carcinomas suggesting a role for this pathway in human breast cancers.[80] Further, Hh ligand expression was associated with basal-like breast cancer; an aggressive phenotype with relatively poor outcome. These findings were corroborated in mouse models where ectopic expression of Hh ligand in BLBC mice induced high-grade invasive tumors.[81] Similarly, SHH upregulation due to hypomethylation of the SHH promotor has been observed in breast carcinomas that were associated with expression of NF-κB in breast cancer clinical samples.[82] Hh signaling has also been linked to bone metastasis in this disease. In bone metastases, secretion of Hh ligand by tumor cells activates the transcription of osteopontin (OPN) by bone osteoclasts. This

further promotes osteoclast maturation and resorptive activity, facilitating metastasis.[83]

The most commonly used antagonist of the Hh pathway is the plant alkaloid cyclopamine that binds to SMO and downregulates Gli1.[84] Other antagonists that bind to SMO include SANTs 1–4;[85] KAAD-cyclopamine,[84] compound-5 and compound-Z,[86] and Cur-61414.[87] Further, 5E1 monoclonal antibody targeting SHH treated tumors in small-cell lung carcinoma.[88] GDC-0449 (Vismodegib, trade name: Erivedge®), the first Hh pathway inhibitor approved by FDA, was used in clinical trials in combination with the Notch signaling inhibitor RO4929097 (a γ-secretase inhibitor, GSI).[89]

Notch signaling

Notch is another evolutionarily conserved signaling pathway that is involved in the regulation of cell fate determination, proliferation, and differentiation in many tissues. The core components of the Notch signaling cascade include the ligands-Delta-like-1, -3, and -4 (DLL1, DLL3, and DLL4), Jagged-1 and -2 (JAG1 and JAG2), and four transmembrane receptors (Notch 1 to Notch 4). After ligand binding, the receptor undergoes two proteolytic events. First, cleavage occurs in close proximity to the extracellular side of the plasma membrane. This is followed by a second cleavage within the transmembrane domain, mediated by a γ-secretase complex, which leads to the release of the intracellular domain of the receptor from the membrane. Upon cleavage, the intracellular Notch domain translocates to the nucleus where it forms a complex with the ubiquitously expressed transcription factor CSL and recruits co-activators such as mastermind-like (MAML-1, -2, and -3).[90] The transcriptional targets of Notch signaling include not only differentiation-related factors, such as Hairy/enhancer of split (Hes) and Hes-related (HRT/HRP/Hey) families, but also cell cycle regulators (p21 and cyclin D1) and regulators of apoptosis.[90,91]

The oncogenic role of Notch 1 was first discovered in T-ALL where the translocation of t(7;9)(q34;q34.3) led to juxtaposition of Notch 1 with TCR-β (T cell receptor-beta). This translocation led to the ligand-independent activity and deregulated expression of intracellular Notch 1 regulated by TCR-β that impacted T-cell differentiation.[92] Overexpression of Notch 4 in mouse mammary glands utilizing an MMTV promotor blocked cellular differentiation with aberrant lactation and poorly differentiated mammary and salivary adenocarcinomas occurred between two and seven months of age.[93] This evidence again underscores the role that Notch signaling plays in the differentiation and tumorigenesis of several tissues. A correlation between Ras overexpression and elevated Notch 1 levels has been reported.[94] Furthermore, expression of Numb, a negative regulator of Notch signaling, was lost in approximately 50% of primary human mammary carcinomas and these tumors showed increased Notch 1 activity.[95] Overexpression of several Notch signaling molecules was reported in several tumors such as pancreatic cancer, renal cell carcinoma, prostate cancer, multiple myeloma, and Hodgkin's and anaplastic lymphoma.[96–100] In lung cancer, Notch signaling had a differential effect based on the cell type: in small lung cancer, Notch signaling is inactive but Hes1 and Hash1 are active[101] and introduction of constitutively active intracellular Notch induces Notch signaling resulting in growth arrest.[102] In contrast, Notch signaling is active in nonsmall lung cancer with high expression of Hes1 and Hey1.[101]

CD24+/24– breast CSCs has been reported to display Notch pathway activation.[103] Notch 3 was found to be upregulated in CD44+ populations of normal and breast cancer cells via SAGE analysis.[104] Other studies have suggested that Notch 4 is the most important regulator of breast stem cells.[105] Moreover, aberrant activation of Notch signaling is an early event in breast cancer, as this has been observed in ductal carcinoma *in situ* (DCIS). Treatment of primary DCIS tissue with a γ-secretase inhibitor significantly reduced the mammosphere formation.[103] Similarly, in an *in vitro* mammosphere culture system, activation of Notch signaling via a DSL peptide promoted self-renewal and branching morphogenesis in three-dimensional Matrigel cultures,[106] a process that was inhibited by a Notch 4 blocking antibody or a γ-secretase inhibitor. Therefore, activated Notch signaling may maintain the epithelial cells in a proliferative state instead of differentiation leading to carcinoma.

Regulation of Notch pathways has also been attributed to epigenetic regulation through hypermethylation and hypomethylation. Notch ligand DLL1 gene is hypermethylated resulting in decreased NOTCH1 expression.[107] Similarly, reduced methylation of NOTCH4 gene promoter in tumors compared to surrounding tissue was observed.[108] Overexpression of JAG2 in multiple myeloma cells was correlated with hypomethylation in malignant cells from multiple myeloma patients and cell lines.[109] Knockdown of the canonical Notch effector Cbf-1 in mammary stem cells increased stem cell activity, whereas constitutive Notch signaling increased luminal progenitor cells, leading to hyperplasia and tumorigenesis.[110] In addition, co-expression of JAG1 and NOTCH1 was associated with poor overall survival.[111] In ESA+ CD24-CD44+ BCSCs, activity of Notch 4 and Notch 1 were eightfold and fourfold higher, respectively, compared to the differentiated bulk tumor cells and inhibition of this activity resulted in reduce tumor growth.[105]

The complexity of the Notch pathway increases through interaction with other oncogenic pathways such as ErbB2, Jak/Stat, TGF-β, NF-κB, Wnt, and Hh.[112] As ErbB2 induces Notch 1 activity through Cyclin D1,[113] combined treatment of DAPT and Lapatinib targeted stem/progenitor cells both *in vitro* and *in vivo* in DCIS.[114] The Wnt pathway also interacts with Notch through Jagged-1 (target of WNT/TCF pathway) and Mel-18, a negative regulator of Bmi-1. Knockdown of Mel-18 has been shown to enhance the self-renewal of BCSCs through upregulation of Jagged-1, consequently activating the Notch pathway.[115] The activation of Notch activity further activates the Hh pathway and increases expression of Ptch and Gli.[77] Taken together, these studies suggest that treatments aimed at targets affecting multiple stem cell pathways could present a novel strategy for targeted therapies. A variety of agents that inhibit Notch signaling are in early phase clinical trials. These include γ-secretase inhibitors that block Notch processing,[116] antibodies against specific Notch receptors,[117,118] and antibodies against the Notch ligand DLL4.[119,120]

Wnt signaling

The Wnt/β-catenin/TCF pathway is another complex evolutionarily conserved pathway involved not only in development and maintenance of adult tissue homeostasis but also cell proliferation, differentiation, migration, and apoptosis.[121] It also regulates the self-renewal and maintenance of embryonic and tissue-specific stem cells.[122-124] Dysregulation of Wnt signaling is a hallmark of several cancers where molecules involved in pathway could act as either tumor suppressors or enhancers depending on their activation status.[125-127] Wnt signaling involves both canonical and noncanonical pathways. The canonical Wnt pathway involves activation of β-catenin/TCF complex, resulting in its dissociation from APC (adenomatous polyposis coli) with subsequent translocation into the nucleus leading to activation of transcriptions including TCF/LEF.[128] This in turn leads to upregulation of oncogenic targets such as c-myc and cyclin D1. This canonical pathway has been extensively studied and found to be deregulated in many cancers.

Noncanonical Wnt signaling involves a planer-cell polarity pathway that regulates the cytoskeleton and a Wnt-calcium-dependent pathway that regulates intracellular calcium levels.[129,130] Mutation of APC (Wnt pathway molecule regulating β-catenin stability) is associated with the majority of sporadic colorectal cancers.[131,132] Germline mutations in APC have been shown to be involved in familial polyposis syndromes, a condition associated with development of numerous intestinal polyps with a high propensity for further neoplastic transformation. In addition to colon cancer, oncogenic mutations in β-catenin have been described in cancers of the liver and colon, as well as in melanoma, thyroid, and ovarian cancers.[133] Epigenetic silencing through methylation of Wnt antagonist genes such as the secreted frizzled-related proteins (SFRPs) has been reported in colon, breast, prostate, lung and other cancers.[121]

Wnt signaling has been shown to be involved in maintenance of CSCs in several cancers. In a transgenic mouse model, LRP5 (a key component of the Wnt co-receptor group) knockdown significantly reduced stem/progenitor cells.[134] In addition, transgenic mice overexpressing Wnt-1 developed mammary glands that were enriched for epithelial cells expressing keratin 6 and Sca1 markers of mammary stem cells. This suggests that mammary carcinogenesis may involve stem cell expansion secondary to Wnt activation. Wnt/β-catenin signaling is also involved in EMT regulation through downregulation of E-cadherin and upregulation of Snail and Twist.[135] EMT has been shown to induce stem cell-like phenotype in breast cancer cells.[52] Wnt signaling has also been demonstrated to maintain pluripotency and neural differentiation of embryonic stem cells.[136] Wnt signaling may also contribute to stem cell expansion induced by tumor hypoxia, a process mediated by Hif 1-α.[137]

A number of drugs that inhibit Wnt signaling are in development. In preclinical models, two nonsteroidal anti-inflammatory drugs (NSAIDs), sulindac[138] and celecoxib,[139,140] have been found to inhibit Wnt signaling by targeting Dvl and cyclo-oxygenase, respectively. Sulindac is currently being investigated in phase II trials.[141] In addition, several non-NSAID inhibitors such as NSC668036 and PCN-N3, among others, have been shown to degrade β-catenin by inhibiting DVL and hence, stabilizing the destruction complex.[142,143] Further, antibodies targeting Wnt pathway members are also under development. A Wnt3A neutralizing antibody was shown to reduce proliferation and enhance apoptosis in prostate cancer mouse models.[144] Another monoclonal antibody-OMP-54F28 has been shown to inhibit patient-derived xenograft tumor growth by specifically targeting CSCs. A Wnt decoy receptor[145] and an antibody to the Wnt co-regulator R spondin[122] are also in development. These aforementioned Wnt inhibiting drugs are currently being tested in several early phase clinical trials.

Clinical significance of cancer stem cells and future perspectives

There is now substantial evidence that CSC plays an important role in treatment resistance; in addition to their role in tumor propagation and tumor metastasis, resistance of CSC to cytotoxic chemotherapy was first demonstrated in preclinical models[146,147] and later confirmed in clinical trials.[148] The relative resistance of CSC to radiation therapy has been demonstrated in a number of tumor types. In patients, it has been shown that the relative proportion of cells expressing CSC markers increases following chemotherapy or radiation therapy.[148] A number of mechanisms have been described that contribute to this resistance. These include alterations in cell cycle kinetics, increased expression of anti-apoptotic proteins, increased in cellular transporters, and increased efficiency of DNA repair, as reviewed in Ref. 149. In addition to the relative therapeutic resistance of CSC, these cells may actually be stimulated by chemotherapy via stimulation of cytokine loops activated by these treatments. These inflammatory cytokines include IL-8 and IL-6. Inhibitors to these cytokines and their receptors have been developed, and several are entering clinical trials.

The CSC model has significant clinical implications. In addition to emphasizing the importance of successfully targeting these cells, acknowledgement of their existence implies a critical role in the tumor microenvironment, which merits thoughtful consideration for the future design of therapeutic trials and development of appropriate clinical endpoints. Currently, tumor shrinkage as accessed by RECIST (response evaluation criteria in solid tumors) is considered an important endpoint for accessing treatment efficacy. However, tumor shrinkage is only poorly correlated with ultimate patient survival across a wide spectrum of tumor types.[150] Tumor shrinkage is a measure of effects of treatments on bulk tumor populations. As CSC constitute only a minority of the tumor bulk, successful targeting of these cells will not necessarily lead to tumor shrinkage. For that reason, the current approach for CSC drug development involves accessing toxicity in Phase I trials followed by combining CSC-targeting drugs with more traditional agents that target bulk populations. As many of the pathways utilized by CSC are shared with normal tissue stem cells, caution is required when introducing such therapeutics in the clinic to access their safety profile. With this cautionary note, a number of CSC-targeting drugs summarized in Figure 2 are now in early phase clinical testing. Interestingly, preliminary data suggests that these agents are well tolerated at doses that reduce CSC number in serial biopsies.[151] This suggests that CSC may be more dependent on these pathways than their normal tissue stem cells counterparts, providing an advantageous therapeutic window. Novel methods are under development to

achieve more direct measurement of CSC targeting agents' effects. These include accessing CSC by marker expression in circulating tumor cells (CTC) assays. Studies have demonstrated that CTCs are highly enriched for CSCs supporting the important role these cells play in mediating tumor metastasis.[152–154]

Another important prediction of the CSC model is that CSC-targeted therapies should have their greatest effect when they are deployed in the adjuvant setting. This is the case because the CSCs are unique in that they possess a sufficient self-renewal capacity to generate clinically significant disease from micrometastases. The efficacy of adjuvant therapies is directly related to their ability to eliminate micrometastasis. This concept is supported by studies demonstrating the remarkable ability of Her 2-targeting drugs, such as trastuzumab, to prevent recurrence when utilized in the adjuvant setting in Her2+ breast cancer.[148] The clinical importance of Her2 in breast cancer may be due to its role as an important regulator of CSC in these tumors.[155]

One of the most exciting areas in cancer therapy is the development of cancer immunotherapies including immune checkpoint blockers. Interestingly, there is evidence that CSC may be particularly competent at evading immune surveillance. Several mechanisms have been proposed, including the high expression of PDL-1 or secretion of immunosuppressive TGF-β. A number of approaches utilizing the immune system to target CSCs are being developed to circumvent these processes. These include CSC-based vaccines and peptides. In the future, such approaches may be combined with immune checkpoint blockers to more effectively target CSCs.

Worldwide, there are currently over 70 clinical trials utilizing novel CSC targeting agents. Most of these studies are in their early stages but the next several years should yield exciting and potentially significant results. Ultimately, carefully controlled randomized clinical trials will be required to conclusively determine if the successful targeting of CSCs improves patient outcome.

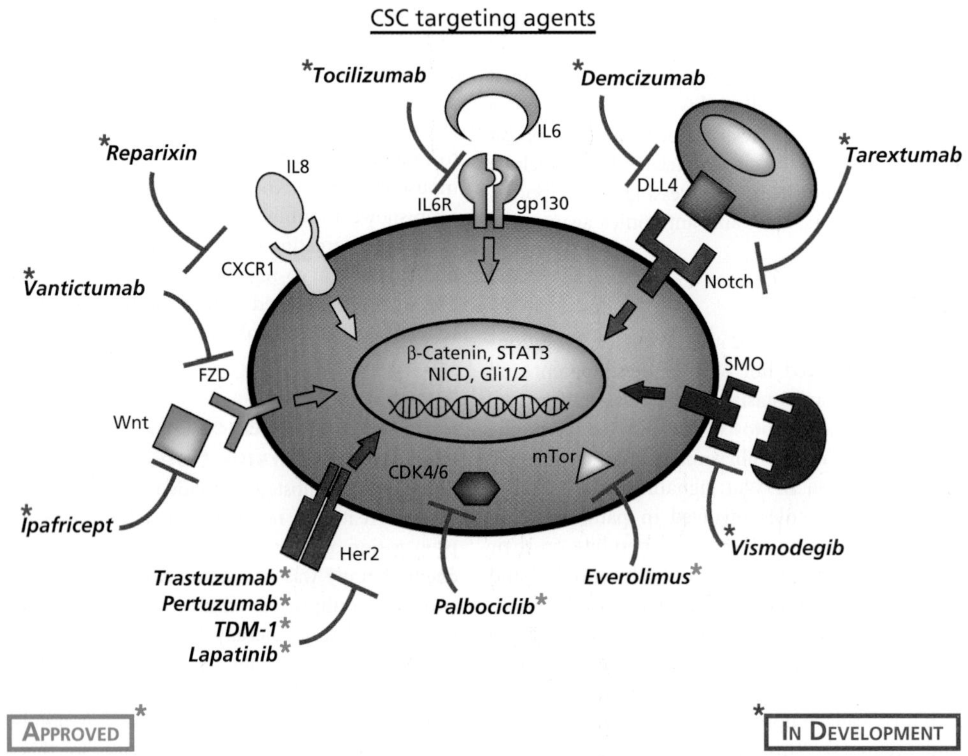

Figure 2 Cancer stem cell-targeted drugs and their cellular targets currently being evaluated in early phase clinical trials or FDA approved for other purposes.

Summary

Despite considerable progress in delineating the molecular underpinnings of cancer, this increased understanding has yet to translate into significant improvements in survival for patients with advanced disease. For most common cancers, the development of metastasis renders them incurable. There is now substantial evidence that many cancers are hierarchically organized and driven by a population of cells that display stem cell properties. These properties include the ability to self-renew and differentiate, forming the cells that constitute the tumor bulk. These cells, termed "tumor-initiating cells" or "cancer stem cells," may mediate tumor metastasis and contribute to treatment resistance. The existence of as well as understanding of molecular mechanisms regulating cancer stem cells is of clinical significance in that additional therapies targeting stem cell populations may be required to limit metastasis and significantly improve patient survival.

Key references

The complete reference list can be found on the Wiley Companion Digital Edition of this title (see inside front cover for login instructions).

1 Huntly BJ, Gilliland DG. Cancer biology: summing up cancer stem cells. *Nature.* 2005;**435**(**7046**):1169–1170. PubMed PMID: 15988505.

2 Sell S. On the stem cell origin of cancer. *Am J Pathol.* 2010;**176**(**6**):2584–2594. PubMed PMID: 20431026. Pubmed Central PMCID: 2877820.

3 Reya T, Morrison SJ, Clarke MF, Weissman IL. Stem cells, cancer, and cancer stem cells. *Nature.* 2001;**414**(**6859**):105–111. PubMed PMID: 11689955.

4 Pattabiraman DR, Weinberg RA. Tackling the cancer stem cell - what challenges do they pose? *Nat Rev Drug Discov.* 2014;**13**(**7**):497–512. PubMed PMID: 24981363. Pubmed Central PMCID: 4234172.

5 Tomasetti C, Vogelstein B. Cancer etiology. Variation in cancer risk among tissues can be explained by the number of stem cell divisions. *Science.* 2015;**347**(**6217**):78–81. PubMed PMID: 25554788. Pubmed Central PMCID: 4446723.

6 Bonnet D, Dick JE. Human acute myeloid leukemia is organized as a hierarchy that originates from a primitive hematopoietic cell. *Nat Med.* 1997;**3**(**7**):730–737. PubMed PMID: 9212098.

7 Al-Hajj M, Wicha MS, Benito-Hernandez A, Morrison SJ, Clarke MF. Prospective identification of tumorigenic breast cancer cells. *Proc Natl Acad Sci U S A.* 2003;**100**(**7**):3983–3988. PubMed PMID: 12629218. Pubmed Central PMCID: 153034.

8 Singh SK, Hawkins C, Clarke ID, Squire JA, Bayani J, Hide T, et al. Identification of human brain tumour initiating cells. *Nature.* 2004;**432**(**7015**):396–401. PubMed PMID: 15549107.

9 Collins AT, Berry PA, Hyde C, Stower MJ, Maitland NJ. Prospective identification of tumorigenic prostate cancer stem cells. *Cancer Res.* 2005;**65**(**23**):10946–10951. PubMed PMID: 16322242.

10 Patrawala L, Calhoun T, Schneider-Broussard R, Li H, Bhatia B, Tang S, et al. Highly purified CD44+ prostate cancer cells from xenograft human tumors are enriched in tumorigenic and metastatic progenitor cells. *Oncogene.* 2006;**25**(**12**):1696–1708. PubMed PMID: 16449977.

11 O'Brien CA, Pollett A, Gallinger S, Dick JE. A human colon cancer cell capable of initiating tumour growth in immunodeficient mice. *Nature.* 2007;**445**(**7123**):106–110. PubMed PMID: 17122772.

12 Ricci-Vitiani L, Lombardi DG, Pilozzi E, Biffoni M, Todaro M, Peschle C, et al. Identification and expansion of human colon-cancer-initiating cells. *Nature.* 2007;**445**(**7123**):111–115. PubMed PMID: 17122771.

13 Li C, Heidt DG, Dalerba P, Burant CF, Zhang L, Adsay V, et al. Identification of pancreatic cancer stem cells. *Cancer Res.* 2007;**67**(**3**):1030–1037. PubMed PMID: 17283135.

14 Ma S, Chan KW, Hu L, Lee TK, Wo JY, Ng IO, et al. Identification and characterization of tumorigenic liver cancer stem/progenitor cells. *Gastroenterology.* 2007;**132**(**7**):2542–2556. PubMed PMID: 17570225.

16 Kim CF, Jackson EL, Woolfenden AE, Lawrence S, Babar I, Vogel S, et al. Identification of bronchioalveolar stem cells in normal lung and lung cancer. *Cell.* 2005;**121**(**6**):823–835. PubMed PMID: 15960971.

17 Schatton T, Murphy GF, Frank NY, Yamaura K, Waaga-Gasser AM, Gasser M, et al. Identification of cells initiating human melanomas. *Nature.* 2008;**451**(**7176**):345–349. PubMed PMID: 18202660. Pubmed Central PMCID: 3660705.

18 Prince ME, Sivanandan R, Kaczorowski A, Wolf GT, Kaplan MJ, Dalerba P, et al. Identification of a subpopulation of cells with cancer stem cell properties in head and neck squamous cell carcinoma. *Proc Natl Acad Sci U S A.* 2007;**104**(**3**):973–978. PubMed PMID: 17210912. Pubmed Central PMCID: 1783424.

20 Ginestier C, Hur MH, Charafe-Jauffret E, Monville F, Dutcher J, Brown M, et al. ALDH1 is a marker of normal and malignant human mammary stem cells and a predictor of poor clinical outcome. *Cell Stem Cell.* 2007;**1**(**5**):555–567. PubMed PMID: 18371393. Pubmed Central PMCID: 2423808.

21 Silva IA, Bai S, McLean K, Yang K, Griffith K, Thomas D, et al. Aldehyde dehydrogenase in combination with CD133 defines angiogenic ovarian cancer stem cells that portend poor patient survival. *Cancer Res.* 2011;**71**(**11**):3991–4001. PubMed PMID: 21498635. Pubmed Central PMCID: 3107359.

22 Huang EH, Hynes MJ, Zhang T, Ginestier C, Dontu G, Appelman H, et al. Aldehyde dehydrogenase 1 is a marker for normal and malignant human colonic stem cells (SC) and tracks SC overpopulation during colon tumorigenesis. *Cancer Res.* 2009;**69**(**8**):3382–3389. PubMed PMID: 19336570. Pubmed Central PMCID: 2789401.

23 Clay MR, Tabor M, Owen JH, Carey TE, Bradford CR, Wolf GT, et al. Single-marker identification of head and neck squamous cell carcinoma cancer stem cells with aldehyde dehydrogenase. *Head Neck.* 2010;**32**(**9**):1195–1201. PubMed PMID: 20073073. Pubmed Central PMCID: 2991066.

24 Luo Y, Dallaglio K, Chen Y, Robinson WA, Robinson SE, McCarter MD, et al. ALDH1A isozymes are markers of human melanoma stem cells and potential therapeutic targets. *Stem Cells.* 2012;**30**(**10**):2100–2113. PubMed PMID: 22887839. Pubmed Central PMCID: 3448863.

34 Dontu G, Abdallah WM, Foley JM, Jackson KW, Clarke MF, Kawamura MJ, et al. In vitro propagation and transcriptional profiling of human mammary stem/progenitor cells. *Genes Dev.* 2003;**17**(**10**):1253–1270. PubMed PMID: 12756227. Pubmed Central PMCID: 196056.

35 Pece S, Tosoni D, Confalonieri S, Mazzarol G, Vecchi M, Ronzoni S, et al. Biological and molecular heterogeneity of breast cancers correlates with their cancer stem cell content. *Cell.* 2010;**140**(**1**):62–73. PubMed PMID: 20074520.

38 Quintana E, Shackleton M, Sabel MS, Fullen DR, Johnson TM, Morrison SJ. Efficient tumour formation by single human melanoma cells. *Nature.* 2008;**456**(**7222**):593–598. PubMed PMID: 19052619. Pubmed Central PMCID: 2597380.

46 Kang YB, Massague J. Epithelial-mesenchymal transitions: twist in development and metastasis. *Cell.* 2004;**118**(**3**):277–279. PubMed PMID: WOS: 000223353100004. English.

56 Liu S, Cong Y, Wang D, Sun Y, Deng L, Liu Y, et al. Breast cancer stem cells transition between epithelial and mesenchymal states reflective of their normal counterparts. *Stem Cell Rep.* 2014;**2**(**1**):78–91. PubMed PMID: 24511467. Pubmed Central PMCID: 3916760.

71 Kinzler KW, Bigner SH, Bigner DD, Trent JM, Law ML, O'Brien SJ, et al. Identification of an amplified, highly expressed gene in a human glioma. *Science.* 1987;**236**(**4797**):70–73. PubMed PMID: 3563490.

77 Liu S, Dontu G, Mantle ID, Patel S, Ahn NS, Jackson KW, et al. Hedgehog signaling and Bmi-1 regulate self-renewal of normal and malignant human mammary stem cells. *Cancer Res.* 2006;**66**(**12**):6063–6071. PubMed PMID: 16778178. Pubmed Central PMCID: 4386278.

83 Kang Y, Siegel PM, Shu W, Drobnjak M, Kakonen SM, Cordon-Cardo C, et al. A multigenic program mediating breast cancer metastasis to bone. *Cancer Cell.* 2003;**3**(**6**):537–549. PubMed PMID: 12842083.

103 Farnie G, Clarke RB, Spence K, Pinnock N, Brennan K, Anderson NG, et al. Novel cell culture technique for primary ductal carcinoma in situ: role of Notch and epidermal growth factor receptor signaling pathways. *J Natl Cancer Inst.* 2007;**99**(**8**):616–627. PubMed PMID: 17440163.

105 Harrison H, Farnie G, Howell SJ, Rock RE, Stylianou S, Brennan KR, et al. Regulation of breast cancer stem cell activity by signaling through the Notch4 receptor. *Cancer Res.* 2010;**70**(**2**):709–718. PubMed PMID: 20068161. Pubmed Central PMCID: 3442245.

106 Dontu G, Jackson KW, McNicholas E, Kawamura MJ, Abdallah WM, Wicha MS. Role of Notch signaling in cell-fate determination of human mammary stem/progenitor cells. *BCR.* 2004;**6**(**6**):R605-R615. PubMed PMID: 15535842. Pubmed Central PMCID: 1064073.

137 Conley SJ, Gheordunescu E, Kakarala P, Newman B, Korkaya H, Heath AN, et al. Antiangiogenic agents increase breast cancer stem cells via the generation of tumor hypoxia. *Proc Natl Acad Sci U S A.* 2012;**109**(**8**):2784–2789. PubMed PMID: 22308314. Pubmed Central PMCID: 3286974.

150 Reddy RM, Kakarala M, Wicha MS. Clinical trial design for testing the stem cell model for the prevention and treatment of cancer. *Cancer.* 2011;**3**(**2**):2696–2708. PubMed PMID: 24212828. Pubmed Central PMCID: 3757438.

151 Schott AF, Landis MD, Dontu G, Griffith KA, Layman RM, Krop I, et al. Preclinical and clinical studies of gamma secretase inhibitors with docetaxel on human breast tumors. *Clin Cancer Res.* 2013;**19**(**6**):1512–1524. PubMed PMID: 23340294. Pubmed Central PMCID: 3602220.

155 Korkaya H, Paulson A, Iovino F, Wicha MS. HER2 regulates the mammary stem/progenitor cell population driving tumorigenesis and invasion. *Oncogene.* 2008;**27**(**47**):6120–6130. PubMed PMID: 18591932. Pubmed Central PMCID: 2602947.

13 Cancer and cell death

John C. Reed, MD, PhD

Overview

Cell death is a normal facet of human physiology, ensuring tissue homeostasis by offsetting cell production with cell demise. Neoplasms arise in part because of defects in physiological cell death mechanisms, contributing to pathological cell expansion when genetic or epigenetic alternations impart a selective survival advantage to premalignant or malignant cells. Defects in normal cell death pathways also contribute to cancer progression by permitting progressively aberrant cell behaviors, while also desensitizing tumor cells to immune-mediated attack, radiation, and chemotherapy. Multiple mechanisms that account for dysregulation of cell death mechanisms in human malignancies have been identified, providing insights into cancer pathogenesis and suggesting targets for therapeutic intervention based on the concept of restoring sensitivity to natural pathways for triggering cell suicide.

Introduction

Evasion of endogenous cell death processes represents one of the cardinal characteristics of cancer.[1] Enormous amounts of cell death occur on a daily basis within the human body, estimated at 50–70 billion cells per day for the average adult. In bulk terms, this amounts to a mass of cells equal to an entire body weight annually. This "programmed" cell death offsets daily cell production resulting from cell division, achieving tissue homeostasis. Cell death can proceed by several distinct mechanisms. Apoptosis and necrosis are the two broadest categories of cell death mechanisms, but specialized forms of cell death have also been described, including necroptosis, pyroptosis, ferrotopsis, and autophagic cell death. Apoptosis is the most common nonpathological route of cell demise in the context of normal tissue homeostasis and mammalian development.[2-4]

During recent years, numerous examples have been delineated whereby cancer cells place roadblocks in the way of endogenous cell death mechanisms, thus endowing neoplastic cells with a selective survival advantage. Several molecules that create barriers to cell death within tumors have been identified, providing insights into pathogenic mechanisms of human neoplasia and cancer—in addition to suggesting targets for drug discovery, with the aim of restoring the integrity of natural pathways for cell suicide and thereby stimulating auto-destruction of cancer cells.[5,6] Alternatively, malignant cells can escape demise by silencing or neutralizing endogenous activators of cell death, with several examples of such mechanisms already elucidated. Replacing or reawakening these endogenous stimulators of programmed cell death (PCD) defines another emerging strategy for potentially eradicating tumors.[7,8]

Defects in the natural mechanisms regulating cell death aid cancers in many ways.[2,5,6] First, activation of oncogenes such as *C-MYC* drives proliferation of transformed cells and also promotes apoptosis, unless counteracted by cell survival proteins—thus constituting a type of oncogene "complementation."[9] A second, closely related, benefit to tumors of defective cell death is that various cell cycle "checkpoints" trigger apoptosis of cells undergoing aberrant cell replication or division. Thus, defects in apoptosis and other cell death mechanisms can permit aberrant cell division. Third, genomic instability is also aided by defects in cell death mechanisms because mutations introduced by DNA replication errors and chromosome segregation errors would normally trigger cell suicide. Fourth, defects in cell death mechanisms allow growth factor (or hormone)-independent cell survival, thus helping transformed cells to escape normal paracrine and endocrine growth control mechanisms. Fifth, cell death induced by hypoxia and metabolic stress, conditions that occur in the microenvironments of most rapidly growing solid tumors, are neutralized by defects in cell death machinery that occur in cancers. Sixth, invasion and metastasis of solid tumors may also be enabled by defects in cell death mechanisms, given that epithelial cells normally undergo apoptosis when they lose their attachment to extracellular matrix through integrins.[10] Seventh, defects in cell death mechanisms contribute to avoidance of immune surveillance mechanisms by making it more difficult for cytolytic T-cells (CTLs) and natural killer (NK) cells to kill tumor cells.

In this chapter, the major pathways for cell death are reviewed and examples of their defects in cancers are described, including hypoexpression (hypoactivity) of pro-death genes and overexpression (hyperactivity) of cytoprotective genes. Insights into the mechanisms that lead to cell death dysregulation in cancers have also sparked a variety of oncology drug discovery and development efforts, which are also described briefly. With apology to the many contributors to the field of cell death biology, only representative references are cited for purposes of brevity.

Pathways for cell death

Several endogenous pathways for triggering cell suicide have been delineated and a variety of ways for cataloging these cell death mechanisms have been utilized by the research community.[11,12] A general construct for categorizing cell death mechanisms can be attributed to the essential involvement of a family of intracellular proteases called "Caspases" (cysteine-dependent aspartate-specific proteases).[13] Broadly, cell death mechanisms can thus be divided into Caspase-dependent versus Caspase-independent, though mixtures of these two basic mechanisms are commonly observed in various settings.

Caspase-dependent cell death

Caspase-dependent cell death culminates in the constellation of morphological changes meeting criteria for "apoptosis," where cells detach from extracellular matrix, become rounded and

Holland-Frei Cancer Medicine, Ninth Edition. Edited by Robert C. Bast Jr., Carlo M. Croce, William N. Hait, Waun Ki Hong, Donald W. Kufe, Martine Piccart-Gebhart, Raphael E. Pollock, Ralph R. Weichselbaum, Hongyang Wang, and James F. Holland.
© 2017 John Wiley & Sons, Inc. ISBN: 978-1-118-93469-2

Table 1 Domains associated with cell death proteins.

Domain	Proteins (examples)
Caspase catalytic domain	Caspase family cysteine proteases
Caspase-associated recruitment domain (CARD)	Caspases-1, -4, -5, -9; Apaf1; ASC; NLRP1, 4
Death domain (DD)	TNFR1, FAS, DR4, DR5, TRADD, RAIDD, RIP1
Death effector domain (DED)	Caspases-8, -10; FADD; c-FLIP
Baculovirus IAP repeat (BIR)	XIAP, c-IAP1, c-IAP2, Livin, Apollon, ML-IAP, NAIP
Bcl-2 homology (BH)	Bd-2, Bcl-XL, Mcl-1, Bax, Bak, Bim, Bid

shrunken in volume, with nuclear chromatin condensation, nuclear fragmentation, and the membrane "bubbling" with membrane protrusions (blebs) that can bud off to create apoptotic bodies. These morphological changes can be attributed directly or indirectly to the multitude of proteolytic cleavage events mediated by Caspases, a full accounting of which is still under investigation using comprehensive proteomics methods.[14]

Caspases operate in hierarchical networks of upstream initiators and downstream effectors, where they cleave and activate each other to create amplifiable cascades of proteolysis.[15,16] These proteases are present as inactive zymogens within the cytosol of essentially all animal cells. Activation of the most proximal Caspases typically occurs through protein interactions that encourage clustering of the inactive zymogens.[16] Once activated, these upstream initiators then cleave and activate downstream effector Caspases. The upstream initiator Caspases contain N-terminal prodomains that mediate protein interactions with other proteins involved in Caspase regulation—namely, CARDs (Caspase-associated recruitment domains) and DEDs (death effector domains) (Table 1). Genomic mutations that inactivate Caspases have been described in a variety of cancers, though overall they are relatively rare.

Multiple pathways that lead to Caspase activation and that thereby cause apoptosis or variations of apoptosis have been delineated (Figure 1). For example, CTLs and NK cells introduce apoptosis-inducing proteases, particularly Granzyme B (a serine protease), into target cells via perforin-mediated pores.[17] Enzymologically, Granzyme B is a serine rather than a cysteine protease. However, similar to the Caspases, Granzyme B cleaves its substrates at Asp residues.[18] Granzyme B is capable of cleaving and activating multiple Caspases. Tumors overcome this pathway for cell death by expressing various immune ligands for checkpoint receptors expressed on T cells (PD1, Tim3, LAG3, etc.) that suppress T-cell activation or by expressing ligands for inhibitory NK receptors (killer immunoglobulin-like receptors (KIRs)).

Another Caspase-activation pathway is stimulated by tumor necrosis factor (TNF)-family receptors. Eight of the ~30 known members of the TNF family in humans contain a so-called death domain (DD) in their cytosolic tails.[19,20] Several of these DD-containing TNF-family receptors use Caspase activation as a signaling mechanism, including TNF receptor-1 (TNFR1)/CD120a; Fas/APO1/CD95; death receptor-3 (DR3)/Apo2/Weasle; DR4/TrailR1; DR5/TrailR2; and DR6. Ligation of these receptors at the cell surface results in receptor clustering and recruitment of several intracellular proteins, including certain pro-Caspases, to the cytosolic domains of these receptors, forming a "death-inducing signaling complex" (DISC) that triggers Caspase activation and leads to apoptosis.[21] The specific Caspases recruited to the DISC are Caspase-8 and, in some cases, Caspase-10. These Caspases contain DEDs in their N-terminal prodomains that bind to a corresponding

DED in FADD, a bipartite adapter protein containing a DD and a DED. FADD functions as a molecular bridge between the DD and DED domain families, and is in fact the only protein in the human genome with this dual domain structure. Consequently, cells from mice in which the *fadd* gene has been knocked out are resistant to apoptosis induction by TNF-family cytokines and their receptors. Cells derived from *Caspase-8* knockout mice also fail to undergo apoptosis in response to ligands or antibodies that activate TNF-family death receptors, demonstrating an essential role for this Caspase in this pathway.[22,23] However, mice lack the highly homologous protease, Caspase-10, which is found in humans, having arisen from an apparent gene duplication on chromosome 2.[15] Thus, Caspases-8 and -10 may play redundant roles in human cells. Genomic mutations in genes encoding TNF-family ligands or receptors have been documented in some types of cancer. For example, somatic mutations in the *FAS (CD95)* gene have been found in lymphoid malignancies.[24,25] Missense mutations within the DD of Fas (CD95) are associated with retention of the wild-type allele, suggesting a dominant-negative mechanism, whereas missense mutations outside the DD are associated with allelic loss.

Mitochondria also play important roles in apoptosis, releasing Cytochrome-c (Cyt-c) into the cytosol, which then causes assembly of a multiprotein Caspase-activating complex, referred to as the *apoptosome*.[26-29] The central component of the apoptosome is Apaf1, a Caspase-activating protein that oligomerizes upon binding Cyt-c and which specifically binds pro-Caspase-9. Apaf1 and pro-Caspase-9 interact with each other via their CARDs. Such CARD–CARD interactions play important roles in many steps in apoptosis pathways. The central importance of the Cyt-c-dependent pathway for apoptosis is underscored by the observation that cells derived from mice in which either the *apaf1* or *pro-Caspase-9* genes have been ablated are incapable of undergoing apoptosis in response to agents that trigger Cyt-c release from mitochondria.[30,31] Nevertheless, such cells can die by non-apoptotic routes,[32] demonstrating that mitochondria control both Caspase-dependent and Caspase-independent cell death pathways (see below). Mitochondria can also participate in cell death pathways induced via TNF-family death receptors, through cross-talk mechanisms involving proteins such as Bid, which become activated upon proteolytic cleavage by Caspase-8 and then stimulate Cyt-c release from mitochondria.[33] However, mitochondrial *("intrinsic")* and death receptor *("extrinsic")* pathways for Caspase activation are fully capable of independent operation in most types of cells.[34] Tumor cells can evolve a variety of mechanisms for averting mitochondria-dependent apoptosis, as outlined below.

Activation of Caspase-1 in the context of infection and inflammation has been shown to stimulate a Caspase-dependent form of cell death called *pyroptosis*.[35] Caspase-1 has a CARD-containing prodomain that can bind directly to the CARDs of NLR (nucleotide-binding domain and leucine-rich repeat domain) proteins, such as NLRP1 (NALP1). Alternatively, the CARD of Caspase-1 can bind the CARD of a bipartite adapter protein ASC (Pycard), which also contains a PRYIN domain (PYD) that binds PYDs of NLR family proteins such as NLRP3 (NALP3) or proteins such as AIM2. NLRs oligomerize in response to binding components of pathogens or molecules elaborated during tissue injury, forming *"inflammasomes"* that recruit and activate Caspase-1.[36-38] The relevance of pyrotopsis to cancer biology is largely unknown.

Caspase-2 is another CARD-carrying member of the Caspase family. Its CARD interacts specifically with the CARD of the bipartite adapter protein RAIDD, which additionally carries a DD.[39] Caspase-2 activation has been linked to genotoxic stress

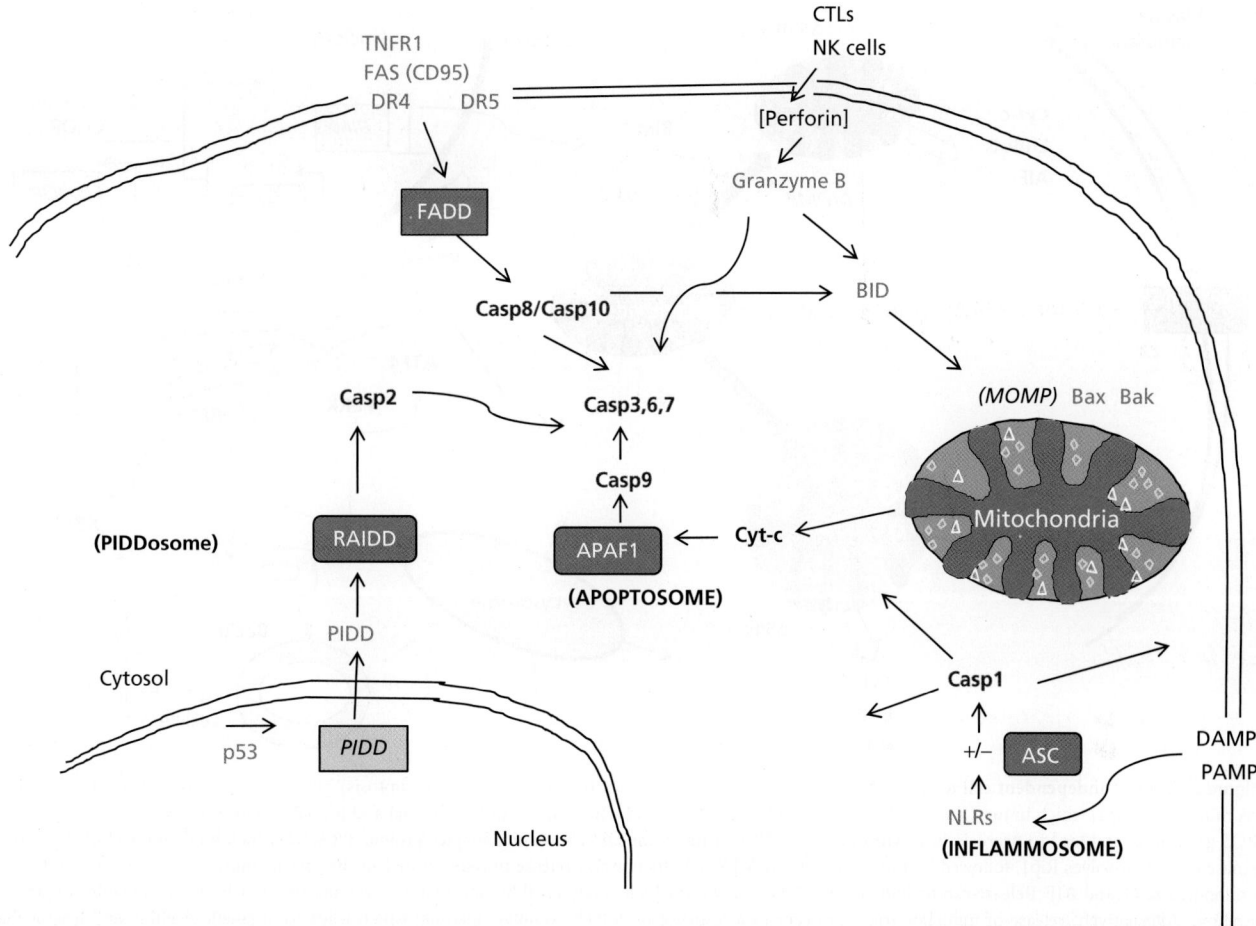

Figure 1 Caspase activation pathways. The major pathways for Caspase activation in mammalian cells are presented. The schematic represents an over-simplification of the events that occur *in vivo*. The extrinsic (left, upper) is induced by members of the TNF- family of cytokine receptors such as TNFR1, Fas, and the TRAIL Receptors, DR4 and DR5. These proteins recruit adapter proteins to their cytosolic DDs, including FADD, to assemble "death-inducing signaling complexes" (DISCs), which bind DED-containing pro-Caspases, particularly pro-Caspase-8, inducing their activation. Caspase-8 (and Caspase-10 in humans) cleaves downstream effector proteases, such as Caspases-3, -6, and -7, as well as pro-apoptotic Bcl-2 family member Bid, which is an agonist of MOMP-inducing Bax and Bak. CTLs and NK cells introduce the protease Granzyme B into target cells (right, upper). This protease cleaves and activates multiple members of the Caspase-family, as well as Bid. The intrinsic pathway (left, lower) is initiated by release of Cyt-c from mitochondria, induced by various stimuli, including elevations in the levels of pore-forming pro-apoptotic Bcl-2 family proteins such as Bax and Bak. In the cytosol, Cyt-c binds and activates Apaf-1, allowing it to associated with and activate pro-Caspase-9, forming "apoptosomes." Active Caspase-9 directly cleaves and activates the effector proteases, Caspase-3 and -7. Exogenous pathogen-associated molecular patterns (PAMPs) and endogenous danger-associated molecular patterns (DAMPs) activate NLR family proteins to cause their oligomerization and assembly of "inflammasomes" that may contain PYD-containing adapter protein ASC in many cases, which binds pro-Caspase-1. Activated Caspase-1 cleaves a variety of cellular proteins, including cytokines as well as plasma membrane proteins that promote osmotic stress and cell death.

via a pathway whereby tumor suppressor p53 induces expression of PIDD, a DD-containing protein that binds the DD of RAIDD, oligomerizes, and assembles into a multiprotein complex termed the "PIDDosome".[40]

Additional Caspase activation mechanisms have been elaborated, though it is less clear how prominently they figure in the pathophysiology of cell death.[41–44]

Caspase-independent cell death

Multiple Caspase-independent cell death mechanisms have been identified, with a few prominent examples mentioned here (Figure 2). *Necrosis* can be initiated by many stimuli. It occurs when cells are incapable of maintaining osmotic equilibrium such that plasma membrane integrity is compromised, resulting in cell swelling and rupture. Organelles within cells during necrosis also typically swell and rupture, including mitochondria and lysosomes,

releasing molecules that promote cell death. Initiators of necrosis include circumstances that compromise bioenergetics such as hypoxia and hypoglycemia, resulting in inadequate adenosine triphosphate (ATP) concentrations for powering plasma membrane ionic pumps, as well as insults to the plasma membrane such as serum complement factors that create pores. Necrosis is relevant to cancer biology in the context of rapidly growing tumors that outstrip their vascular supply (insufficient angiogenesis), creating regions of hypoxia and nutrient insufficiency.

Mitochondria-initiated cell death pathways can also lead to Caspase-independent cell death, in addition to the aforementioned Caspase-dependent pathway downstream of Cyt-c.[45] In addition to Cyt-c, mitochondria also release several other proteins of relevance to apoptosis, including Endonuclease G, AIF (an activator of nuclear endonucleases), and Smac (Diablo) and Omi (HtrA2), antagonists of a family of Caspase-inhibitory proteins known as the inhibitor of apoptosis proteins (IAP)s (see below).[46,47] Moreover, distinguishing

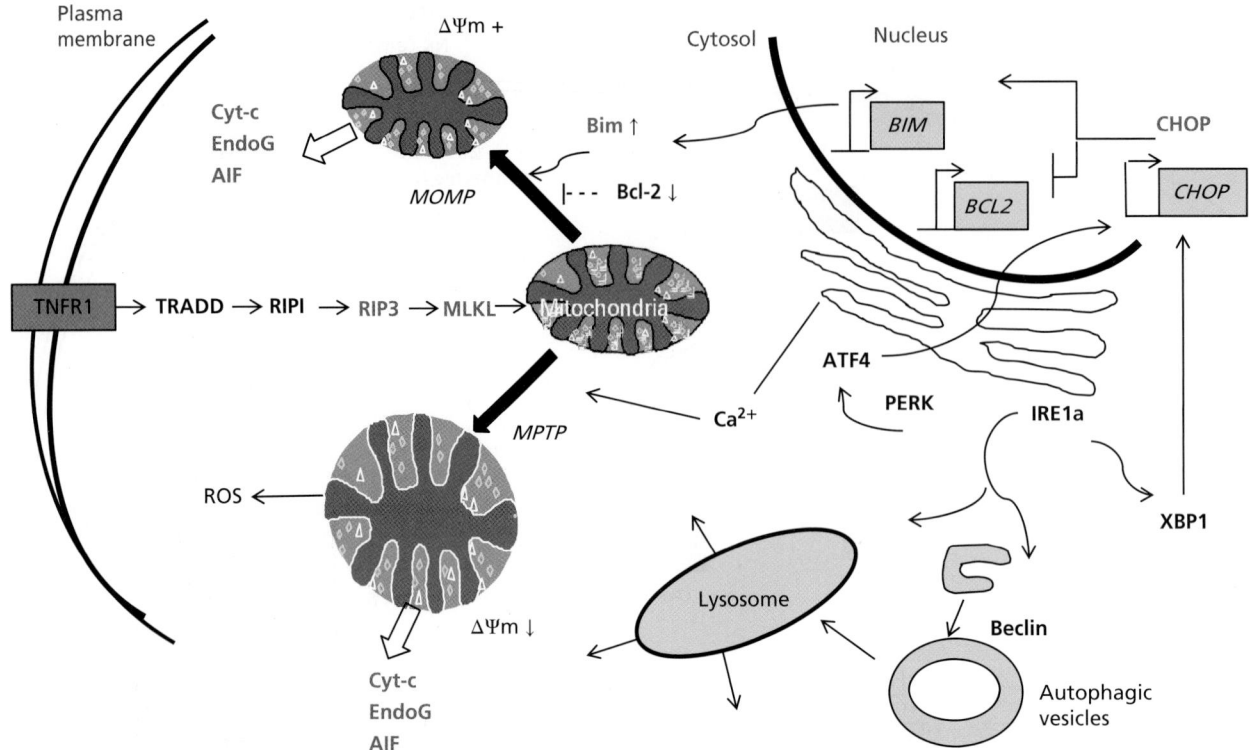

Figure 2 Caspase-independent cell death pathways. The TNFR1-mediated pathway for necrosis (necroptosis) involves a cascade of events that include recruitment of Rip1, which in turn activates Rip3, which activates MLKL and which causes mitochondrial and probably lysosomal changes that stimulate ROS generation and lead to necrosis. The cytosolic DD of TNFR1 binds the DD-containing adapter protein TRADD, which binds the DD of Rip1. The kinase cascade involves Rip1, followed by Rip3, followed by MLKL. Mitochondria release proteins stored in the intermembrane space, including Cyt-c, Endonuclease G, and AIF. Release can be induced by MOMP (*upper*), which is regulated by Bcl-2 family proteins and which does not involve organelle swelling. Alternatively, release of mitochondrial can occur as a result of by MPTP complex opening, which leads to organelle swelling and loss of the electrochemical gradient ($\Delta\Psi_m$). MPTP opening is induced by Ca^{2+} influx and oxidative stress, among other stimuli. Accumulation of unfolded proteins in the ER results in UPR signaling, including activation of IRE1α, which splices XBP1 mRNA to generate XBP1 protein (transcription factor) and activation of the kinase PERK, which stimulates phosphorylation events that promote ATF4 mRNA translation and production of transcription factor ATF4. The UPR transcription factors (XBP1, ATF4, and (not shown) ATF6) converge on the promoter of the *CHOP* gene, which encodes a transcription factor that upregulates pro-apoptotic gene *BIM* and downregulates anti-apoptotic gene *BCL-2*. Autophagic vesicles emerge from the ER, form double membrane vesicles, which fuse with lysosomes (*bottom, right*).

mitochondria-driven apoptotic from non-apoptotic cell death can be challenging in many contexts due to the similar morphological features caused probably by some of the proteins released from these organelle such as EndoG and AIF, which promote chromatin condensation and DNA fragmentation. The mitochondrial mechanisms for apoptotic and non-apoptotic cell death are activated by myriad stimuli, including growth factor deprivation, oxidants, Ca^{2+} overload, DNA-damaging agents, microtubule-modifying drugs, and much more. In this sense, mitochondria are sometimes viewed as central integrators of cell stress signals that ultimately dictate cell life and death decisions.[48-50]

Uniformly, these mitochondrial cell death mechanisms involve compromises of mitochondrial membrane integrity, but the membrane permeability change can occur via different mechanisms.[51] In the context of insults such as ischemia-reperfusion injury (where oxidative stress occurs due to reactive oxygen species (ROS) and nitrosyl free radicals) and Ca^{2+} dysregulation where cytosolic free Ca^{2+} levels rise (due to loss of plasma membrane integrity or escape from the endoplasmic reticulum [ER]), osmotic homeostasis of mitochondria is perturbed due to opening of the *mitochondrial permeability transition pore* (MPTP) complex that spans inner and outer membranes at contact sites where they come into close apposition.[52-54] The change in permeability in the inner membrane of mitochondria allows water and electrolytes to enter the

protein-rich matrix of mitochondria, resulting in swelling of the organelle and eventually popping of the outer membrane, whose surface area is smaller than the extensively folded inner membrane with its cristae. During pathological opening of the MPTP complex, the electrochemical gradient (proton gradient) that is essential for ATP production is lost, and thus bioenergetics is severely compromised. An essential component of the MPTP complex is the adenine nucleotide translocator (ANT), which is thought to be chiefly responsible for the permeability transition that leads to mitochondrial swelling.

Alternatively, cell death mechanisms can involve the phenomenon of *mitochondrial outer membrane permeabilization* (MOMP), where the outer membrane becomes selectively permeabilized, allowing release of Cyt-c and other proteins that reside in the intermembrane space.[51,55,56] With MOMP, the electrochemical gradient is preserved and mitochondrial osmotic homeostasis is maintained. MOMP is caused by pro-apoptotic members of the Bcl-2 family (see below), namely Bax and Bak (possibly also Bok).[57-60] Though others may exist, an established mechanism for triggering MOMP entails interaction of pro-apoptotic proteins such as Bid, Bim, and Puma with Bax and/or Bak, causing oligomerization of Bax and Bak in the mitochondrial outer membrane and the formation of ill-defined pores that permit escape of Cyt-c and other proteins. MOMP induced by Bax and/or Bak thus initiates the mitochondrial pathway for Caspase-dependent cell death and apoptosis by releasing Cyt-c, but it also secondarily causes Caspase-independent necrotic cell death by uncoupling of oxidative phosphorylation (when Cyt-c becomes limiting) and causing diversion of electrons from the respiratory chain into production of toxic free radicals.[61]

Given the diversity of cell death mechanisms initiated by mitochondria, it is not surprising that tumors evolve a variety of alternations in these organelles and their regulation. The metabolic changes that convert the bioenergetic signature of tumor cells from dependence on aerobic respiration to non-aerobic glycolysis are well known (Warburg effect), and could be argued to make tumor cells less dependent on mitochondria. Indeed, some tumors seem to have a diminution in the numbers of mitochondria compared to normal cells of the same cell lineage.[62]

Cell death induced by CTCs and NK cells can also occur via Caspase-independent mechanism. In this regard, Granzyme B directly cleaves some of the same substrates as Caspases,[63,64] thereby potentially bypassing the need for Caspases to cause proteolytic events associated with apoptosis. Also, the cytotoxic granules of CTLs and NK cells contain several other death-promoting molecules besides Granzyme B.[17] Moreover, the perforin-mediated pores created in the plasma membrane of target cells by CTLs and NK cells can also lead to osmotic disequilibrium and thus Caspase-independent cell death. The diversity of cytolytic mechanisms invoked by CTLs and NK cells bodes well for attempts to harness the immune system as a weapon for attacking cancers, since specific blocks to cell death in tumors (see below) might be overwhelmed by the multiple parallel cytotoxic mechanisms initiated by these immune cells.

Necroptosis is the term that has been applied to a Caspase-independent cell death mechanism initiated by TNFR1. When Caspase-8 is incapacitated, TNFR1 can stimulate a non-apoptotic cell death signaling pathway that involves the serine/threonine protein kinases Rip1, Rip3, and MLKL (mixed lineage kinase domain-like).[65-67] Rip3-dependent necroptosis occurs through a process involving ROS generated by mitochondria. Necroptosis was initially identified by studies of tumor cells where TNFα was shown to kill via a Caspase-independent mechanism, suggesting that this cell death pathway could provide a conduit for attacking cancers.

Both Caspase-dependent and Caspase-independent cell death signaling mechanisms have been implicated in endoplasmic reticulum stress (*ER stress*). A wide variety of microenvironmental conditions (including those relevant to the tumor microenvironment) can cause the accumulation of unfolded proteins in the ER, triggering an adaptive signal transduction response called the *unfolded protein response* (UPR).[68-70] Among these UPR events is increased transcription of a gene encoding the pro-apoptotic transcription factor CHOP, which in turn stimulates expression of the gene encoding DR5 (death receptor 5; TRAIL Receptor-2), causing Caspase-8-dependent apoptosis. In addition, CHOP has been reported to directly stimulate transcription of the gene encoding Bim, a pro-apoptotic member of the Bcl-2 family (see below) that stimulates Bax/Bak oligomerization in mitochondrial membranes to induce MOMP and release Cyt-c and other proteins from mitochondria. Thus, ER stress has multiple potential routes of stimulating both Caspase-dependent and Caspase-independent cell death, with the predominant pathway probably varying among cell types and pathophysiological contexts.

Furthermore, the important role that the ER plays in regulating intracellular Ca^{2+} homeostasis provides another potential link to cell death mechanism where changes in cytosolic free Ca^{2+} contribute (reviewed in[70-72]). When extreme, liberation of Ca^{2+} from the lumen of the ER can trigger a variety of downstream signaling events that promote cell death. Also, the ER collaborates with mitochondria in many ways that can either promote cell life or cause death. ER membranes from close contacts with mitochondria to create structures where Ca^{2+} effluxes from ER into mitochondria, aiding bioenergetics. However, too much Ca^{2+} entry into mitochondria triggers opening of the MPTP complex, such that mitochondria swell and eventually rupture.

Autophagy ("self-eating") is a catabolic mechanism where senescent proteins and organelles become entrapped in double membrane vesicles that bud off from the ER and that are transported to lysosomes for degradation of their contents. The physiological roles of autophagy include protein homeostasis, supplementing the ubiquitin-proteasome system for removal of unfolded, defective, and aged proteins, as well as providing a source of substrates for maintaining metabolism during times of nutrient deprivation.[73,74] In the context of nutrient deprivation, autophagy can contribute to cell survival and is thought to aid tumors at some points in their evolution. However, when taken to an extreme, mechanisms that rely on components of the autophagy machinery have been reported to cause cell death via a process called autophagic cell death, which is Caspase independent.[75] Under some conditions, exposure of tumor cells to cytotoxic chemotherapeutic drugs can trigger autophagic cell death.[76]

Additional Caspase-independent cell death mechanisms have been described, including lysosome-dependent cell death,[77] iron-dependent cell death (ferroptosis),[78] and others,[11] which are not reviewed here. All of them may be relevant to cancer biology at some level in some contexts.

Cell death resistance mechanisms used by cancers

Cancer cells have been shown to put the brakes on Caspases and thereby suppress apoptosis by at least three fundamental mechanisms—(1) preventing activation of Caspase zymogens (pro-enzymes); (2) neutralizing active Caspases (active enzymes); and (3) suppressing expression of genes encoding Caspases or Caspase-activating proteins (see below). Malignant cells also develop a variety of ways of counteracting Caspase-independent cell death mechanisms. Some of the more prominent examples understood to date are outlined here.

IAPs

Endogenous suppressors of Caspases include IAPs ($n = 8$ in humans),[15,79,80] an evolutionarily conserved family of proteins that directly bind active Caspases and that either suppress their protease activity or that target active Caspases for destruction.[79,81,82] Overexpression of IAPs occurs in cancers and leukemias, making it more difficult to propagate the Caspase-dependent proteolytic events necessary for apoptotic cell death.

IAPs are characterized by the presence of protein interaction domains called BIRs (baculovirus internal repeats), numbering between 1 and 3 per protein[83] (Table 1). Most IAPs also carry RING domains that endow them with E3 ligase activity through interactions with ubiquitin-conjugating enzymes (UBCs). Some of the apoptogenic proteins released from mitochondria, notably SMAC and HtrA2,[84,85] bind certain BIRs and thereby compete for protein interactions on the surface of IAPs. In many cases, Smac binding to IAPs induces their polyubiquitination and proteasomal degradation. Thus, factors that cause MOMP take the brakes off the Caspases by eliminating various IAP family proteins.

The most established Caspase inhibitor among the IAP family members is XIAP (so called because its encoding gene resides on the X-chromosome). The XIAP protein contains 3 BIR domains. BIR2 of XIAP (and an adjacent segment) binds downstream effector proteases, Caspases-3 and -7, to potently suppress apoptosis at a distal point. BIR3 of XIAP binds upstream initiator protease, Caspase-9, to suppress an apical step in the mitochondrial pathway for apoptosis. Overexpression of XIAP mRNA and protein has been reported in cancers and leukemias, apparently caused by epigenetic mechanisms rather than genomic lesions to the *XIAP* gene. XIAP protein stability may also be increased in tumors with Akt hyperactivity.[86]

The c-IAP-1 (BIRC2) and c-IAP2 (BIRC3) proteins are also capable of binding to Caspases-3, -7, and -9, though they are far less potent as direct enzymatic inhibitors and may rely on their E3 ligase activity for controlling Caspase degradation. However, these IAP family members also participate in other cell-death-relevant mechanisms by impacting signal transduction by TNF-family receptors.[65,66,87] Binding of cytokine TNFα to TNFR1 can trigger at least three different signaling pathways, each involving overlapping but distinct protein complexes that are assembled at the receptor.[88] In addition to the pathways for Caspase-dependent and Caspase-independent cell death outlined above, TNFR1 also stimulates a cell survival pathway in which c-IAP1 and c-IAP2 participate. In this regard, the BIR3 domains of c-IAP1 and c-IAP2 directly bind the kinase Rip1. In the TNFR1-mediated survival pathway, Rip1 forms protein complexes that contain the E3 ligases c-IAP1, c-IAP2, and TRAF2, stimulating noncanonical (lysine 63, rather than lysine 48) ubiquitination of Rip1 to initiate a signal transduction pathway that causes activation of transcription factor NF-κB.[89,90] NF-κB influences the expression of many target genes involved in host defenses and immune regulation, among which are several genes that suppress apoptosis[91] (see below). As a result, this NF-κB pathway nullifies the Caspase pathway, negating apoptosis, in addition to accounting for the untoward inflammatory actions of this cytokine. In addition, the Rip3-dependent pathway for necrotoposis is suppressed by c-IAP1 and c-IAP2, probably via their roles as E3 ligases and possibly involving ubiquitin-/proteasome-mediated reductions in Rip3 protein levels. In human cancers, chromosomal translocations that deregulate c-IAP2 by creating a chimeric protein mucosa-associated lymphoid tissue (MALT-c-IAP2) have been described in lymphomas.[92,93] In addition, the genomes of some cancers have amplification of the gene encoding TRAF2, the c-IAP1/c-IAP2-binding protein implicated in TNF-family receptor signaling. Overexpression of c-IAP1 and c-IAP2 mRNAs and proteins, presumably via epigenetic mechanisms, is also reported. In this regard, *c-IAP2* is among the direct transcriptional targets of NF-κB, and hyperactivity of the canonical (RelA) and alternative (RelB) pathways is well established in human malignancies of various types.

Additional members of the IAP family, not described here (Survivin, Apollon/Bruce, ML-IAP, etc.), also have interesting mechanisms of interacting with components of cell death pathways; and they can have other roles beyond cell death regulation. For example, the Survivin protein plays a fundamental role in chromosome segregation and cytokinesis.[94]

c-FLIP

The c-FLIP protein provides another example of an endogenous modulator of Caspases whose overexpression is a common occurrence in tumors.[95,96] FLIP is structurally similar to certain Caspases, containing a pair of DEDs analogous to Caspases-8 and -10. It directly binds and suppresses activation of Caspases-8 and -10 in the context of TNF-family death receptor signaling. However, the role of c-FLIP is more complex than merely suppressing Caspase-8 or -10 activation, as it also collaborates with these Caspases in poorly understood ways (probably involving Caspase-8, MALT, and Bcl-10) to promote NF-κB activation.[97] Testimony to this complex interaction is also found in the observation that knockout of the genes encoding either c-Flip or Caspase-8 in mice results in similar embryonic lethal phenotypes. In addition to promoting NF-κB activation, the *c-FLIP* gene is itself also a direct transcriptional target of NF-κB, whose expression is strikingly upregulated (positive feedback).[98]

Bcl-2

Among the central regulators of MOMP are members of the Bcl-2 family, evolutionarily conserved proteins that either promote (e.g., Bax; Bak) or suppress (e.g., Bcl-2, Bcl-XL) MOMP.[99–101] The Bcl-2-family proteins ($n = 26$ in humans)[15] physically interact with each other, forming complex networks of homo- and heterodimers that steer the cell toward either life or death.[102,103] Numerous examples of altered expression and function of Bcl-2-family proteins have been identified in cancers, accounting for intrinsic resistance to cell death induced by myriad stimuli, including most cytotoxic anticancer drugs and x-irradiation, growth factor deprivation and therapeutic inhibitors of growth factor receptor signal transduction pathways.

Many members of the Bcl-2-family have a hydrophobic stretch of amino acids near their carboxyl-terminus that anchors them in the outer mitochondrial membrane. In contrast, other Bcl-2-family members such as Bid, Bim, and Bad lack these membrane-anchoring domains, but dynamically target to mitochondria in response to specific stimuli. Still others have the membrane-anchoring domain but keep it latched against the body of the protein, until stimulated to expose it (e.g., Bax).

Based on their predicted (or experimentally determined) three-dimensional structures, Bcl-2 family proteins can be broadly divided into two groups. One subset of these proteins is probably similar in structure to the pore-forming domains of bacterial toxins, such as the colicins and diphtheria toxin.[104–106] These α-helical pore-like proteins include both anti-apoptotic proteins (Bcl-2, Bcl-X$_L$, Mcl-1, Bfl-1, Bcl-W, Bcl-B), as well as pro-apoptotic proteins (Bax, Bak, Bok, and Bid). Most of the proteins in this subcategory can be recognized by conserved stretches of amino acid sequence homology, including the presence of Bcl-2 homology (BH) domains, BH1, BH2, BH3, and sometimes BH4 (Table 1). However, this is not uniformly the case, as the Bid protein contains only a BH3 domain but has been determined to share the same overall protein-fold with Bcl-X$_L$, Bcl-2, and Bax. Where tested to date, these proteins have all been shown to form ion-conducting channels in synthetic membranes in vitro, including Bcl-2, Bcl-X$_L$, Bax, and Bid,[107] but the significance of this pore activity remains largely unclear. The other subset of Bcl-2 family proteins appears to have in common only the presence of the BH3 domain, including Bad, Bik, Bim, Hrk, Bcl-G$_S$, p193, APR (Noxa), and PUMA. These "BH3-only" proteins are uniformly pro-apoptotic. Their cell-death-inducing activity depends, in most cases, on their ability to dimerize with anti-apoptotic Bcl-2 family members, functioning as trans-dominant inhibitors of proteins such as Bcl-2 and Bcl-X$_L$.[101,102] However, a select group of them (Bim, Bid, Puma) interact with pro-apoptotic proteins Bax and Bak, functioning as agonists that induce their oligomerization in mitochondrial membranes to stimulate MOMP.

The BH3 domains mediate dimerization among Bcl-2 family proteins (Figure 3). This domain consists of an amphipathic α-helix of

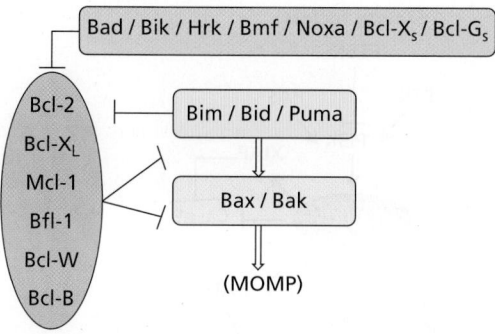

Figure 3 Network of interactions among Bcl-2-family proteins. The functional and physical interactions among pro-apoptotic and anti-apoptotic Bcl-2-family proteins are depicted as pertains to their regulation of MOMP.

~16 amino acids length that inserts into a hydrophobic crevice on the surface of anti-apoptotic proteins such as Bcl-2 and Bcl-X$_L$.[104,105] The BH3-only proteins link a wide variety of environmental and iatrognic stimuli to the mitochondrial pathway for apoptosis (see below).

While Bcl-2 family members clearly regulate MOMP, it has been proposed that they also regulate other aspects of mitochondrial biology. For example, components of the MPTP complex, including ANT and the voltage-dependent anion channel (VDAC), reportedly interact with Bcl-2 family members, with anti-apoptotic proteins suppressing and pro-apoptotic facilitating MPTP complex opening.[108] In addition, VDAC has been proposed as a facilitator of Cyt-c release from mitochondria, via a Bcl-2 suppressible mechanism[109] while Bcl-XL has been reported to enhance delivery of ATP to the cytosol via effects on ANT and thereby support cell survival in the context of growth factor deprivation.[110] Anti-apoptotic Bcl-XL also may regulate mitochondrial metabolism through poorly understood mechanisms to reduce production of acetyl-CoA.[111] The significance of this reduction in acetyl-CoA has been attributed to reduce N-acetylation of apoptosis-relevant proteins, including certain Caspases, which may make it more difficult to activate these proteases. Bcl-2 has also been proposed to regulate mitochondrial redox metabolism, though mechanistic details remain largely unclear.[112]

In addition to mitochondria, mechanistic links for Bcl-2 family proteins to ER stress have also been delineated.[113] For example, Bax and Bak can bind the ER stress signaling protein, IRE-1α, a central component of UPR signaling.[114] IRE-1α spans the ER membranes and possesses a protein kinase domain and a ribonuclease domain that reside on the cytosolic face of the ER membrane. Bax and Bak stimulate the intrinsic autokinase activity and the endoribonuclease activity of IRE1α, thus stimulating production of CHOP-inducing transcription factor XBP-1 (by RNA splicing mechanisms) and also stimulating stress kinase activation (Ask1, p38MAPK, JNK1, etc.). Pro-apoptotic (Bak/Bax) and anti-apoptotic (Bcl-2/Bcl-XL) family members also have opposing effects on basal ER Ca^{2+} levels, probably via effects on Ca^{2+} channel proteins in ER membranes (e.g., IP$_3$Rs, BI-1 and TmBim3).[72]

In addition to mitochondria- and ER-initiated cell death pathways, Bcl-2-family proteins have also been implicated in control of autophagic cell death. Anti-apoptotic protein Bcl-2 binds the autophagy protein Beclin, preventing it from forming complexes with downstream autophagy proteins (e.g., ATG5) and apparently sequestering Beclin to preclude its participation in autophagy.[115] During nutrient deprivation, Bcl-2 can suppress cell death mechanisms that depend on components of the autophagy pathway.[116] Beclin has recently been recognized as a haplo-insufficient tumor

suppressor gene,[117] suggesting that suppression of autophagy contributes to tumorigenesis. These recent findings concerning links between autophagy, tumorigenesis, and anti-apoptotic Bcl-2-family proteins indicate a master-switch role for Bcl-2-family proteins in controlling cell life and death decisions.

Genomic lesions involving members of the Bcl-2 family are well documented in human cancers.[6,118–120] These mechanisms include hyperactivation of anti-apoptotic Bcl-2 family members by chromosomal translocations that cause overproduction of transcripts and proteins (Bcl-2), gene amplification (Bcl-2, Bcl-X, Mcl-1), and deletion/mutational inactivation of microRNAs (miRs) that suppress expression of anti-apoptotic Bcl-2 family genes (miR15-16 targeting Bcl-2 mRNA). Conversely, mutations inactivating pro-apoptotic members of the Bcl-2 family also occur in some human cancers (Bax). In addition, a wide and diverse array of epigenetic mechanisms contribute to dysregulation of Bcl-2 family gene expression in cancers and leukemias, some of which are outlined below.

Signal transduction pathway alterations in cancers—impact on cell death machinery

Various receptor-mediated signal transduction pathways converge on the core components of the cell death machinery outlined above, including tyrosine kinase growth factor receptors and their downstream signaling pathways that become deregulated in many cancers. Some examples of the intimate links between growth factor receptor–mediated signal transduction and cell death pathways are described here (Figure 4).

Protein kinases

By catalyzing phosphorylation of tyrosines on themselves and on various substrates, protein tyrosine kinase (PTK) growth factor receptors uniformly transduce signals that lead to activation of the (1) phosphatidyl inositol 3′ kinase (PI3K) and Akt pathway and (2) Raf/MEK/Erk pathway (*reviewed elsewhere in this book*). One or both of these pathways is also activated by most non-receptor PTKs (Src-family, Jak-family, c-Abl, etc.) and Ras-family GTPases.

The murine gene encoding Akt was first discovered by virtue of its similarity to the *v-akt* oncogene found in some murine leukemia viruses, where it becomes activated in thymomas caused by retrovirus insertions near the *c-akt* gene.[122] Humans contain three *AKT* genes. Akt can phosphorylate multiple proteins within the core apoptosis machinery.[123] For example, the pro-apoptotic Bcl-2 family member Bad is a target of Akt, where phosphorylation of Bad causes its sequestration by 14-3-3 family proteins, thus inhibiting Bad from heterodimerizing with Bcl-X$_L$.[124] Akt also phosphorylates Bax on serine 184, inhibiting its translocation from cytosol to mitochondrial membranes,[125] as well as Bim, suppressing its pro-apoptotic activity.[126] Akt also can phosphorylate human Caspase-9, blocking apoptosis downstream of mitochondria.[127] Forkhead transcription factors (FKHDs) are another class of substrates of Akt relevant to apoptosis. Some FKHD family members such as Foxo-3 appear to control apoptosis, perhaps by affecting transcription of genes encoding Fas-ligand (FasL) and Bim.[128] Phosphorylation of FKHD by Akt prevents its entry into the nucleus. Akt also reportedly causes phosphorylation of XIAP, promoting stability of the XIAP protein probably by reducing ubiquitin-dependent proteasomal degradation.[86]

Several growth factor receptors and lymphokine receptors signal via Jak/STAT pathways. STAT family transcription factors are known to stimulate transcription of the *BCL-X* gene as at least one of their mechanisms of suppressing apoptosis.[129] In addition, Jak

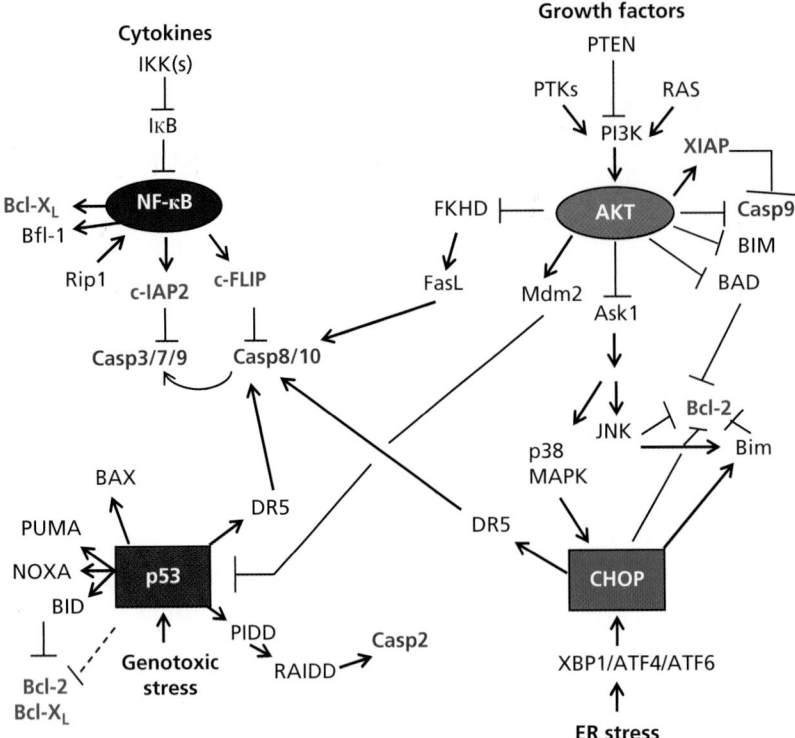

Figure 4 Signal transduction and cell death regulation. Some of the transcription factors and kinases that play prominent roles in apoptosis regulation are depicted, including kinases Akt (PKB) and the transcription factors p53, NF-κB, and CHOP. Illustrative examples of the connections to apoptosis-regulating proteins and genes are shown, without attempting to be comprehensive. The protein kinase Akt (PKB) is activated in response to second messengers produced by PI3K, a lipid kinase that is activated by many growth factor receptors and oncoproteins. PTEN is a lipid phosphatase that prevents accumulation of these second messengers, the expression of which is lost in many tumors through gene deletions, gene mutations, and other mechanisms.[89] Akt can phosphorylate and either activate (arrows) or inactivate (⊣) multiple proteins directly or indirectly relevant to apoptosis.[121] Expression of the transcription factor CHOP is stimulated by transcription factors that are elaborated during ER stress, including XBP1, ATF4, and ATF6. See text for additional details.

family non-receptor PTKs are capable of stimulating PI3K activity, which in turn causes activation of Akt family kinases. These signaling mechanisms are also relevant various oncogenes such as BCR-ABL, the oncogenic driver of certain types of leukemia.[130]

The Raf/MEK/Erk signaling pathway has important links to the cell death machinery. For example, phosphorylation by Erk of pro-apoptotic protein Bim on serine 69 promotes Bim protein degradation via proteasomal-dependent mechanisms.[131] Inhibitors of the Raf/MEK/Erk pathway therefore help promote apoptosis by enabling accumulation of Bim protein levels. MEK-dependent phosphorylation of anti-apoptotic protein Bcl-2 has also been described, purportedly enhancing its survival-promoting function through unclear mechanisms.[132]

Protein acetylation

Acetylation of lysines in histones is a well-established mechanism for controlling chromatin structure and thus transcription of genes. However, acetylation of non-histone proteins is increasingly recognized as a mechanism for impacting biological processes through diverse mechanisms. In terms of cell death regulations, examples of dysregulated protein acetylation impacting the core components of the cell death machinery are only just emerging. For example, acetylation of transcription factor FoxO1 was reported to be required for induction of Bim expression in the context of treatment of cancer cells with histone deacetylase (HDAC) inhibitors.[133] Acetylation also indirectly impacts the expression of multiple apoptosis and cell-death-relevant genes through modification of lysines on a variety of other transcription factors, including STATs, NF-κB,

and p53.[134] In addition, acetylation of tumor suppressor p53 has also been reported to be required for a transcription-independent mechanism of Bax activation.[135] Acetylation of DNA damage repair protein Ku70 neutralizes its anti-apoptotic functions by interfering with interactions with proteins constituting core components of the cell death machinery (see below). As mentioned above, via effects on mitochondrial acetyl-CoA production, Bcl-XL may also broadly impact N-alpha-acetylation of proteins, including certain Caspases that require this post-translational modification for interactions with upstream activators.[111]

Transcription factors

As expected, epigenetic dysregulation of expression of cell death genes is a common occurrence in human cancers, with mechanisms too abundant to catalog here. Among the cancer-relevant connections are steroid hormone receptors including estrogen, androgen, and vitamin D receptors, which regulate the expression of various cell death and cell survival genes. For example, estrogen receptor (ER) is a prominent transcriptional regulator of the *BCL-2* gene expression in mammary epithelial cells and in ER-positive breast adenocarcinomas.[136] Retinoid receptors and other nuclear receptors also regulate the expression of various cell death and cell survival genes through transcriptional mechanisms.[137] The roles of transcription factors such as FKHD family members (Foxo-3, FoxO1), CHOP, NF-κB family members, and p53 have been cited above. Precedence also exists for nontranscriptional mechanisms of regulating cell death proteins, where transcription factors leave the nucleus and physically interact with Bcl-2 family members on the surface of mitochondria.[138] Chromatin-modifying enzymes responsible for histone acetylation and deacetylation have also been implicated in controlling core components of the cell death machinery. Therefore, cancer-associated aberrations in the regulation of transcription factors and chromatin-modifying enzymes are connected ultimately to perturbations in the core cell death machinery.

Cytotoxic chemotherapeutic oncology drugs

Chemotherapeutic cytotoxic drugs remain a foundational component of cancer therapy today, though giving way to more targeted agents. These chemical agents were designed to interfere with replication of rapidly dividing cells by inhibiting DNA synthesis, inducing DNA damage, or crippling microtubules. The cellular injuries induced by classical chemotherapeutic anticancer drugs, and x-irradiation, trigger molecular events with connections to the core cell death machinery. Some examples are described here. Cytoprotective proteins that blunt cell death pathways thus play important roles in chemoresistance.

Radiotherapy and DNA-damaging anticancer drugs potently stimulate activation of the tumor suppressor p53, one of the principal mediators of apoptosis induced by genotoxic stress. The p53 protein is a tetrameric transcription factor, whose levels are controlled by the E3 ligase Mdm2. This transcription factor directly induces expression of BH3-only proteins Bim, Bid, and PUMA, and the MOMP-inducing protein Bax, thus linking p53 to the death machinery.[139-142] Active p53 also stimulates transcription of DR5, a TNF-family death receptor, thus rendering tumor cells more sensitive to its ligand TRAIL.[143] Loss of p53 activity occurs in many human malignancies by a variety of mechanisms, including gene deletion, gene mutations that result in mutant p53 proteins lacking transcriptional activity, and *MDM2* gene amplification. Small-molecule drugs that block Mdm2 protein interaction with p53 have shown promising preclinical activity against hematological malignancies[144] and are synergistic with Bcl-2 inhibitors.[145]

Interestingly, in addition to its role as a nuclear transcription factor, evidence has emerged suggesting that p53 may promote apoptosis also via nontranscriptional mechanisms under some circumstances. Specifically, a cytoplasmic pool of p53 reportedly associates with mitochondria, directly inducing activation of the Bax and inhibiting Bcl-2 and Bcl-XL.[146,147] Importantly, even mutant p53 is capable of activating this cell death pathway, raising hopes of finding pharmacological interventions that agonize this mechanism for promoting cell death.

DNA damage is also linked to regulation of the core cell death machinery via p53-independent mechanisms. For example, Ku70 plays an important role in repairing double-strand DNA breaks. Ku70 binds Bax and suppresses its translocation to mitochondria; but after DNA damage, Ku70 becomes acetylated and dissociates from Bax.[148,149] Ku70 also interacts with c-FLIP and suppresses its ubiquitation and proteasomal degradation, where Ku70 acetylation releases c-FLIP and allows its degradation to promote apoptosis.[150] Another DNA repair protein RAD9 has been reported to translocate from nucleus to mitochondria following DNA damage, where it reportedly binds and neutralizes anti-apoptotic proteins Bcl-2 and Bcl-XL to promote cell death.[151]

Anti-microtubule drugs impact the cell death machinery via a variety of mechanisms. For example, the pro-apoptotic Bcl-2 family member Bmf-1 is sequestered on microtubules. When microtubules are disrupted by anticancer drugs, Bmf is released from microtubule-binding proteins (dynein light chains), allowing it to engage and neutralize anti-apoptotic members of the Bcl-2 family.[152] A role for Bim in cell death induced by microtubule-targeting drugs has also been identified, facilitated perhaps by other BH3-only proteins Bmf and Puma.[153] Microtubule-targeting drugs also stimulate a stress kinase cascade that results in multisite phosphorylation of Bcl-2, which is proposed to impair its anti-apoptotic function.[154,155]

Cancer drug discovery by targeting the cell death machinery

Multiple efforts have been made to devise therapeutics that neutralize anti-apoptotic or activate pro-apoptotic components of the core cell death machinery. All drug targets can be approached by at least three means, involving attack at the level of the gene, mRNA, or protein. The relative attractiveness of these alternative strategies depends on the nuances of the target and its biology. Discussion here is limited to therapeutic strategies that modulate protein targets, though nucleic acid–based therapeutics (RNA therapeutics, gene therapy) have been explored preclinically and some even taken into advanced clinical trials. Also, while a wide variety of signal transducing proteins (e.g., protein kinases, transcription factors) provide inputs into cell death pathways described above and thus are attractive targets for indirectly promoting tumor cell death, the focus here is limited to direct modulators of components of the core cell death machinery.

Bcl-2-family inhibitors

In humans, six anti-apoptotic members of the Bcl-2-family have been identified (Bcl-2, Bcl-XL, Mcl-1, Bcl-W, Bfl-1, Bcl-B), with overexpression of various individuals occurring in a variety of cancers. Simultaneous overexpression of two or more anti-apoptotic members of the Bcl-2 family in tumors has also been documented in some cases, raising the issue of redundancy. Overexpression of Bcl-2 or other anti-apoptotic members of the Bcl-2 family has been associated with chemoresistant states, due to the ability of these proteins to block cell death induced by DNA-damaging agents, microtubule-modifying drugs, and antimetabolites. Thus, restoring chemosensitivity by nullifying Bcl-2 and related proteins has emerged as an attractive strategy for improving cancer therapy.

Chemicals that bind regulatory sites on anti-apoptotic Bcl-2-family proteins and that directly neutralize the cytoprotective actions of these proteins have been identified and brought into clinical development. Some have progressed into advanced human clinical trials, and at least one molecule (venetoclax) has produced sufficiently compelling data that the U.S. Food & Drug Administration (FDA) has granted approval for treatment of some forms of leukemia. The compounds described to date target a crevice on the surface of anti-apoptotic Bcl-2-family proteins that serves as a receptor for the BH3 peptidyl motif present in endogenous antagonists of the anti-apoptotic Bcl-2 family proteins.[6,104,120] Compounds that mimic the BH3 peptidyl structure suppress anti-apoptotic Bcl-2-family proteins, tapping into a natural pathway for defending against excessive Bcl-2. Several natural products and synthetic chemicals have been reported to occupy the BH3-binding site on Bcl-2 or Bcl-XL, and some of them have been shown to promote apoptosis of tumor cells in culture and to suppress tumor growth in mouse models.[156-162] The strategies for generating chemical antagonists of anti-apoptotic Bcl-2 family proteins have ranged from highly selective inhibitors, which neutralize only 1 of the 6 human anti-apoptotic Bcl-2 family proteins, to broad-spectrum that cross-react with multiple family members. The trade-offs with these opposing strategies are efficacy versus drug safety. For example, development of a chemical inhibitor with activity against Bcl-2, Bcl-XL, and Bcl-W (navitoclax) was stalled because of thrombocytopenia—which has been attributed to the requirement of Bcl-XL for longevity of platelets.[163–165] In contrast, a selective Bcl-2 inhibitor (venetoclax) is free of the thrombocytopenia side effect; but with a narrower spectrum of activity, its efficacy is likely to be more limited to tumors where Bcl-2 is the major driver of cell survival.

Other approaches to tackling Bcl-2 family proteins for cancer therapy have been proposed, though most of those concepts are less validated. For example, direct agonists of Bax and Bak that mimic the actions of Bid, Bim, and Puma could be envisioned,[166] though this has not been reduced to practice to date. Alternatively, indirect mechanisms for upregulating pro-apoptotic Bcl-2 family members are actively being explored. Small-molecule antagonists of Mdm2, such as idasanutlin, cause an accumulation of p53 protein, which in turn stimulates transcription of several pro-apoptotic Bcl-2 family genes including *BAX, NOXA, BID,* and *PUMA.* Mdm2 antagonists have progressed to advanced clinical trials, following displays of promising activity for some types of malignancy such as acute leukemia. It remains to be seen whether the Mdm2 inhibitor strategy is applicable only to tumors that retain wild-type p53 versus whether it may also benefit some patients whose malignancies harbor mutants of p53 that still retain the ability to exit the nucleus and directly modulate Bcl-2 family protein activity at the surface of the mitochondria (see above). In addition, chemical inhibitors of MEK (Trametinib, Cobimetinib, etc.) can produce elevations in the levels of Bim protein by reducing its ubiquitination and proteasomal degradation. In an analogous fashion, small-molecule inhibitors of Akt that are currently in advanced clinical development also would be expected to help restore the activity of pro-apoptotic Bcl-2 family proteins that are phosphorylated by this protein kinase (e.g., Bad, Bax, etc.). Finally, compounds that stimulate an orphan member of the nuclear receptor family, Nur77 (NR4A1), have been described; and they cause this transcription factor to exit the nucleus and translocate to mitochondria, where it interacts with Bcl-2, Bfl-1, and Bcl-B to promote cell death.[138,167–169]

TRAIL

Cytokines of the TNF family have been extensively evaluated in preclinical studies for anticancer activity. Two general strategies for exploiting this endogenous mechanism for triggering apoptosis have been tested clinically, involving parenteral administration of either recombinant proteins constituting functional fragments of the cytokine ligands or agonistic monoclonal antibodies that bind the TNF-family death receptors and trigger their activation.

Attempts to apply TNFα, the founding member of the TNF family, as a cancer therapy provided highly toxic, due to the proinflammatory activity of this cytokine. At present, TNFα is employed only in rare circumstances for treatment of melanomas and soft tissue sarcomas confined to specific limbs using turnicate-based methods to prevent systemic exposure.[170] TRAIL (TNF-related apoptosis-inducing ligand) emerged as a possible alternative, owing to its ability to induce tumor cell apoptosis without inducing signals that cause inflammation. Preclinical studies, including data from primates, indicated that a soluble fragment of TRAIL (produced as a recombinant protein) was nontoxic, apparently sparing normal tissues, while showing potent preclinical activity against tumor xenografts in mice.[171] Moreover, TRAIL is sometimes synergistic when used in combination with cytotoxic anticancer drugs, at least in preclinical mouse models. Based on these promising data, a recombinant version of TRAIL was taken into clinical trials but lack of efficacy resulted in its eventual termination. Postulated reasons

for the poor efficacy of TRAIL in the clinic are myriad, including intrinsic blocks in cancers to the downstream apoptotic signaling pathways, expression of "decoy" receptors that compete for TRAIL binding to function death receptors on tumor cells, insufficient expression levels of DR4 (TRAIL-R1) and DR5 (TRAIL-R2), and other explanations.[171]

Agonistic antibodies that bind DR4, DR5, or both have been reported, and several were taken into clinical development.[172,173] Clinical responses when tested as monotherapy were rare, and some of these antibodies showed hepatotoxicity,[174,175] which was theorized to be due to FcR binding to Kupfer cells in the liver. In this regard, the agonists antibodies were uniformly dependent on FcR-binding to achieve crosslinking of receptors tumor cells, and thus reliant on macrophages, NK cells, or other types of FcR-expressing immune cells to achieve the desired apoptotic signaling. More recently, highly engineered antibodies that utilize FcR-independent mechanisms to achieve death receptor crosslinking have been advanced into clinical studies, awaiting results at the time of this writing.

TRAIL and TRAIL Receptors can induce apoptosis via either mitochondria-dependent or mitochondria-independent pathways, depending on the specifics of how apoptosis pathways are regulated in a given tumor.[176] The mitochondrial-dependent route of signaling entails cleavage by Caspase-8 of and Bid, which activates the protein such that it can interact with Bax and Bak to induce MOMP. The possible advantage of mitochondria-independent apoptosis is that roadblocks to apoptosis created by survival proteins such as Bcl-2 are bypassed, an attractive feature for chemorefractory cancers that often have defects in the mitochondrial pathway. Unfortunately, predicting whether TRAIL operates via a mitochondria-dependent versus mitochondria-independent mechanism in a given tumor is still an empirical process, as no single predictive biomarker has emerged.

Among the roadblocks to TRAIL-induced apoptosis is c-FLIP, a protein that is produced as either longer and shorter isoforms (due to mRNA splicing) that associate with the Caspases normally recruited into the TRAIL receptor complex. The longer c-FLIP proteins is overexpressed in many cancers, and is capable of squelching signaling by TNF-family death receptors by modulating Caspase activation.[95] Chemical compounds that reduce c-FLIP protein levels have been identified, including HDAC inhibitors such as suberoylanilide hydroxamic acid (SAHA)[177] and synthetic triterpenoids such as Bardoxolone (1[2-Cyano-3,12-dioxooleana-1,9(11)-dien-28-oyl]imidazole [CDDO]) and its analogs.[178–183] Preclinical studies have shown that Bardoxolone analogs used in combination with recombinant TRAIL can synergistically suppress growth of human tumor xenografts in mice, where the human tumor cells were resistant to treatment with TRAIL alone.[184] Thus, compounds such as CDDO can restore sensitivity of cancer cells to TRAIL (and agonistic anti-TRAIL Receptor antibodies), and therefore might serve as adjuncts to TRAIL therapy. At least in mice, the combination of TRAIL and CDDO analogs is a nontoxic therapy,[184] suggesting that combining these two targeted therapies provides a promising direction for future research. Bardoxolone (CDDO analog) was brought into the clinic for a non-oncology indication but development terminated.

IAP inhibitors

The most common strategy employed for generating small-molecule inhibitors of IAPs is to mimic the effects of endogenous antagonists of IAPs, particularly the proteins SMAC and HtrA2. SMAC- and HtrA2-mimicking agents bind the BIRs of multiple IAP family members, thus disrupting their interactions with Caspases

(Caspase-3, -7, -9) and kinases (Rip1, Rip2).[185] The active region of SMAC and HtrA2 has been reduced to a 4 amino acid peptide that is necessary and sufficient to bind IAPs, displace Caspases or kinases, and promote apoptosis or inhibit signal transduction.[186] Several peptidyl compounds that occupy the same tetramer-binding site on IAPs have been described,[187–189] as well as at least one natural product. Several of the synthetic compounds were taken into clinical development, and some of them remain actively under investigation at the time of this writing. These SMAC-mimicking compounds show only occasional single-agent activity as apoptosis inducers when applied against cultured tumor cell lines, which has been the reason for termination of several of these drug development programs. However, SMAC mimics often sensitize transformed cells very potently to apoptosis induced by cytotoxic anticancer drugs and TNF-family death receptors such as TRAIL and agonistic antibodies targeting TRAIL Receptors. In this sense, IAP antagonists take the breaks the cell death pathways induced by TNF-family death receptor, providing a solid rationale for combination therapy.

An alternative approach to deriving chemical inhibitors of IAPs involves screening compound libraries using an enzyme derepression assay, where recombinant IAPs are mixed with active Caspases, forming an inhibited enzyme complex, and where chemicals displacing the Caspase are then revealed by cleavage of fluorogenic substrates.[190,191] Compounds derived by the latter approach, however, have failed to yield molecules with sufficient affinity (potency) to progress into clinical development.

Finally, an additional strategy for attacking IAPs has been suggested by interrogation of the actions of another apoptogenic protein released from mitochondria called ARTS.[192] The ARTS protein binds certain IAPs, including XIAP, c-IAP1, and c-IAP2. It has been shown to recruit an E3 ligase (Siah-1) to IAPs and promote their degradation.[193] Short peptides from ARTS purportedly can induce apoptosis,[194] though the translation of these observations into drug-like molecules remains an ambition to date. The structural nature of the ARTS binding site on IAPs also remains to be determined, which would presumably provide important insights into the "druggability" of this protein–protein interface.

Some tumors overexpress simultaneously two or more members of the IAP family, suggesting that broad-spectrum inhibitors that address multiple IAPs may be preferable to selective agents. More extensive comparisons of the therapeutic indices of selective versus broad-spectrum inhibitors are needed to reveal the best path forward.

Conclusions

Dysregulation of PCD mechanisms plays critical roles in cancer pathogenesis and progression. Elaboration of the complex cell death pathways and the networks of proteins that modulate these pathways has provided insights into the underlying mechanisms of cell life–death decisions—though many mechanistic details remain still to be revealed. In several cases, the available information has already sparked efforts to translate the base of information into therapeutic strategies, with new agents for cancer treatment nearing or already reality.

List of abbreviations

BH	Bcl-2 homology domain
CARDs	Caspase recruitment domains
Caspases	Cysteine aspartyl proteases
Cyt-c	Cytochrome-c
CTL	Cytolytic T cells
DD	Death domain
DEDs	Death effector domains
DISC	Death-inducing signaling complex
DR	Death receptor
ER	Endoplasmic reticulum
FasL	Fas-ligand
FKHD	Forkhead transcription factors
IAP	Inhibitor of apoptosis
miRs	microRNAs
MOMP	Mitochondrial outer membrane permeabilization
MPTP	Mitochondrial permeability transition pore
MLKL	Mixed lineage kinase domain-like
MALT	Mucosa-associated lymphoid tissue
MMs	Multiple myelomas
NK	Natural killer
NHLs	non-Hodgkin lymphomas
PI3K	Phosphatidylinositol-3′kinase
PCD	Programmed cell death
ROS	Reactive oxygen species
TNFR1	TNF receptor-1
TNF	Tumor necrosis factor
UBCs	Ubiquitin conjugating enzymes

Key references

The complete reference list can be found on the Wiley Companion Digital Edition of this title (see inside front cover for login instructions).

2 Green DR, Evan G. A matter of life and death. *Cancer Cell.* 2002;**1**:19–30.

3 Danial NN, Korsmeyer SJ. Cell death: critical control points. *Cell.* 2004; **116(2)**:205–219.

5 Reed JC. Apoptosis-targeted therapies for cancer. *Cancer Cell.* 2003;**3**:17–22.

11 Kroemer G, El-Deiry WS, Golstein P, et al. Classification of cell death: recommendations of the nomenclature committee on cell death. *Cell Death Differ.* 2005;**12(Suppl 2)**:1463–1467.

12 Galluzzi L, Maiuri MC, Vitale I, et al. Cell death modalities: classification and pathophysiological implications. *Cell Death Differ.* 2007;**14(7)**:1237–1243.

15 Reed JC, Doctor KS, Godzik A. The domains of apoptosis: a genomics perspective. *Sci STKE.* 2004;**2004(239)**:re9.

20 Kersse K, Verspurten J, Vanden Berghe T, Vandenabeele P. The death-fold superfamily of homotypic interaction motifs. *Trends Biochem Sci.* 2011;**36(10)**:541–552.

21 Peter ME, Krammer PH. The CD95(APO-1/Fas) DISC and beyond. *Cell Death Differ.* 2003;**10(1)**:26–35.

28 Adams JM, Cory S. Apoptosomes: engines for caspase activation. *Curr Opin Cell Biol.* 2002;**14**:715–720.

33 Korsmeyer SJ, Wei MC, Saito M, Weiler S, Oh KJ, Schlesinger PH. Pro-apoptotic cascade activates BID, which oligomerizes BAK or BAX into pores that result in the release of cytochrome c. *Cell Death Differ.* 2000;**7**:1166–1173.

35 Bergsbaken T, Fink SL, Cookson BT. Pyroptosis: host cell death and inflammation. *Nat Rev Microbiol.* 2009;**7(2)**:99–109.

46 Green DR, Galluzzi L, Kroemer G. Mitochondria and the autophagy-inflammation-cell death axis in organismal aging. *Science.* 2011;**333(6046)**:1109–1112.

48 Kroemer G, Reed JC. Mitochondrial control of cell death. *Nat Med.* 2000;**6**: 513–519.

53 Marzo I, Brenner C, Zamzami N, et al. The permeability transition pore complex: a target for apoptosis regulation by caspases and Bcl-2-related proteins. *J Exp Med.* 1998;**187**:1261–1271.

55 Green DR, Kroemer G. The pathophysiology of mitochondrial cell death. *Science.* 2004;**305**:626–629.

58 Vaux D, Korsmeyer S. Cell death in development. *Cell.* 1999;**96**:245–254.

69 Kaufman RJ. Orchestrating the unfolded protein response in health and disease. *J Clin Invest.* 2002;**110**:1389–1398.

70 Kim I, Xu W, Reed JC. Cell death and endoplasmic reticulum stress: disease relevance and therapeutic opportunities. *Nat Rev Drug Discov.* 2008;**7(12)**:1013–1030.

71 Giorgi C, Romagnoli A, Pinton P, Rizzuto R. Ca2+ signaling, mitochondria and cell death. *Curr Mol Med.* 2008;**8(2)**:119–130.

72 Sano R, Reed J. ER stress-induced cell death mechanisms. *Biochim Biophys Acta.* 2013;**1833(12)**:3460–3470.

73 Mizushima N, Levine B, Cuervo AM, Klionsky DJ. Autophagy fights disease through cellular self-digestion. *Nature*. 2008;**451**(**7182**):1069–1075.

75 Kroemer G, Marino G, Levine B. Autophagy and the integrated stress response. *Mol Cell*. 2010;**40**(**2**):280–293.

79 Deveraux QL, Reed JC. IAP family proteins: suppressors of apoptosis. *Genes Dev*. 1999;**13**:239–252.

80 LaCasse EC, Mahoney DJ, Cheung HH, Plenchette S, Baird S, Korneluk RG. IAP-targeted therapies for cancer. *Oncogene*. 2008;**27**(**48**):6252–6275.

91 Baud V, Karin M. Is NF-kappaB a good target for cancer therapy? Hopes and pitfalls. *Nat Rev Drug Discov*. 2009;**8**(**1**):33–40.

96 Yu JW, Shi Y. FLIP and the death effector domain family. *Oncogene*. 2008;**27**(**48**):6216–6227.

101 Chipuk JE, Moldoveanu T, Llambi F, Parsons MJ, Green DR. The BCL-2 family reunion. *Mol Cell*. 2010;**37**(**3**):299–310.

102 Strasser A. The role of BH3-only proteins in the immune system. *Nat Rev Immunol*. 2005;**5**:189–200.

104 Fesik SW. Insights into programmed cell death through structural biology. *Cell*. 2000;**103**:273–282.

116 Shimizu S, Kanaseki T, Mizushima N, et al. Role of Bcl-2 family proteins in a non-apoptotic programmed cell death dependent on autophagy genes. *Nat Cell Biol*. 2004;**6**(**12**):1221–1228.

119 Calin GA, Croce CM. Chromosomal rearrangements and microRNAs: a new cancer link with clinical implications. *J Clin Invest*. 2007;**117**(**8**):2059–2066.

120 Huang J, Fairbrother W, Reed J. Therapeutic targeting of Bcl-2 family for treatment of B-cell malignancies. *Expert Rev Hematol*. 2015;**8**(**3**):283–297.

121 Testa JR, Bellacosa A. AKT plays a central role in tumorigenesis. *Proc Natl Acad Sci U S A*. 2001;**98**(**20**):10983–10985.

132 Konopleva M, Contractor R, Tsao T, et al. Mechanisms of apoptosis sensitivity and resistance to the BH3 mimetic ABT-737 in acute myeloid leukemia. *Cancer Cell*. 2006;**10**(**5**):375–388.

166 Czabotar P, Westphal D, Dewson G, et al. Bax crystal structures reveal how BH3 domains activate Bax and nucleate its oligomerization to induce apoptosis. *Cell*. 2013;**152**(**3**):519–531.

171 Ashkenazi A. Targeting death and decoy receptors of the tumour-necrosis factor superfamily. *Nat Rev Cancer*. 2002;**2**:420–430.

173 Lemke J, von Karstedt S, Zinngrebe J, Walczak H. Getting TRAIL back on track for cancer therapy. *Cell Death Differ*. 2014;**21**(**9**):1350–1364.

185 Fesik SW, Shi Y. Structural biology. Controlling the caspases. *Science*. 2001;**294**:1477–1478.

186 Shi Y. A conserved tetrapeptide motif: potentiating apoptosis through IAP-binding. *Cell Death Differ*. 2002;**9**:93–95.

191 Wu TY, Wagner KW, Bursulaya B, Schultz PG, Deveraux QL. Development and characterization of nonpeptidic small molecule inhibitors of the XIAP/caspase-3 interaction. *Chem Biol*. 2003;**10**:759–767.

14 Cancer cell immortality: targeting telomerase

Ilgen Mender, PhD ▪ Zeliha Gunnur Dikmen, MD, PhD ▪ Woodring E. Wright, MD, PhD ▪ Jerry W. Shay, PhD

Overview

Finding specific targeted agents for cancer therapy remains a challenge. One of the hallmarks of cancer is the limitless proliferation (immortalization) of cancer cells, which correlates with the activation of the ribonucleoprotein enzyme complex called telomerase. As 85–90% of primary human cancers express telomerase activity, while most normal cells do not, telomerase is a unique and almost universal therapeutic target for cancer. Although there have been several approaches developed for telomerase-targeted therapies, there is still no agent that has been approved. This chapter focuses on the pros and cons of the different approaches to target telomerase and summarizes preclinical and clinical results. We will also review novel telomerase-mediated telomere uncapping approaches that target telomerase-expressing cancer cells, but not normal cells.

Telomerase: a universal target for cancer therapy

Telomeres (TTAGGG)$_n$ are repetitive hexameric nucleotide repeats that are found at the ends of linear chromosomes. Telomere length varies in different organisms such as humans (2–15 kb) and mice (up to 100 kb).[1] Telomeres are protected from being recognized as damaged or broken chromosomes by a special protein complex. This is termed the shelterin complex that stabilizes the chromosomal ends with 6 protein components (TRF1, TRF2, Rap1, TIN2, TPP1, and POT1) to protect the telomeric ends from exonuclease activity and DNA damage recognition.[1-3] Shelterin proteins also have a role in the generation of a special lariat-like loop structure at each telomere end called the telomere loop (T-loop). The single-stranded telomeric DNA overhang at the ends of each chromosome bends backward and is believed to strand invade into the telomere DNA duplex structure disrupting the double-stranded TTAGGG repeats and forming a triple-stranded structure called the displacement loop (D-loop). The D-loop is bound by a single-stranded TTAGGG-binding protein called POT1 and this entire T-loop and D-loop structure functions in part by hiding or masking the single- and double-stranded telomeric DNA from being recognized as broken DNA and thus is important in telomere maintenance.[4]

G-quadruplex formation is a secondary structure that is generated between guanine bases in telomeric DNA and is also proposed to protect the ends of chromosomes from degradation.[5] As normal somatic cells have a limited capacity to divide in culture, they stop proliferating after a finite number of cell doublings (the so-called Hayflick limit), which is related to DNA replication turnover.[6] Because DNA polymerase is unable to replicate the 3′ end of the DNA lagging strand (often referred to as the end replication problem), in the absence of a maintenance mechanism, telomeres shorten with each cell division until they become "uncapped."[7] In addition to the end replication problem, oxidative stress and/or other unknown processes may accelerate telomeric shortening *in vitro* and *in vivo*. It is believed that only a few short telomeres with uncapped ends are sufficient to trigger a p53-dependent G1/S cell cycle arrest, which is known as replicative senescence. When cells enter senescence, the fate of normal cells is to remain in a quiescent phase. If other alterations occur in important cell cycle checkpoint genes such as TP53 or pRB, then senescence can be bypassed and cells continue to proliferate (extended lifespan phase) until many telomere ends become critically shortened leading to end fusions and chromosome bridge fusion breakage cycles (also referred to as crisis). Senescence and crisis are two fundamental mechanisms that protect cells against the early development of cancer. The cells that escape from crisis almost universally express the enzyme telomerase; a ribonucleoprotein cellular reverse transcriptase (Figure 1a), which has two essential components for the elongation of telomeres: the catalytic component hTERT (telomerase reverse transcriptase) and the telomerase RNA component (hTR or hTERC) (Figure 1b).[8,9] Telomerase is active during early human fetal development, then becomes silent in most tissues (Figure 2a) except embryonic stem cells and some but not all proliferating progenitors (e.g., male germline spermatocytes, activated lymphocytes, and a few other transient amplifying cell types).[10] Telomerase is not absolutely required for cells to become malignant; however, 85–90% of primary human tumors have telomerase activity (Figure 2a), while the vast majority of normal tissues do not have detectable enzyme activity.[9] A rarer (3–10%) mechanism to maintain telomere length is called ALT (alternative lengthening of telomeres) and involves intratelomeric recombination and perhaps T-loop resolution.

There have been several studies on changes in telomerase expression/activation in normal and cancer cells. DNA rearrangement breakpoints within the TERT promoter region correlate with increased TERT expression in some cancers.[11] In addition, mutations in the TERT promoter can lead to activated telomerase in immortalized, nontumorigenic fibroblasts.[12] Different studies show that the mutations in the TERT promoter[13] and gene amplifications in TERT[14,15] correlate with increased TERT transcriptional activation and expression of telomerase activity. While it is difficult to regulate very low abundant transcripts such as TERT, it has been reported that another mechanism for telomerase regulation is by alternative splicing. Precursor mRNA (pre-mRNA) that is transcribed from DNA is processed to exclude introns (noncoding sequences) and join exons (coding sequences) in order to produce mRNA for mature protein translation. However, during RNA splicing, exons may be included or excluded from the pre-mRNA to create diverse proteins with multifunctional roles. This process is known alternative splicing[16] and may be important in the regulation of telomerase.

Holland-Frei Cancer Medicine, Ninth Edition. Edited by Robert C. Bast Jr., Carlo M. Croce, William N. Hait, Waun Ki Hong, Donald W. Kufe, Martine Piccart-Gebhart, Raphael E. Pollock, Ralph R. Weichselbaum, Hongyang Wang, and James F. Holland.

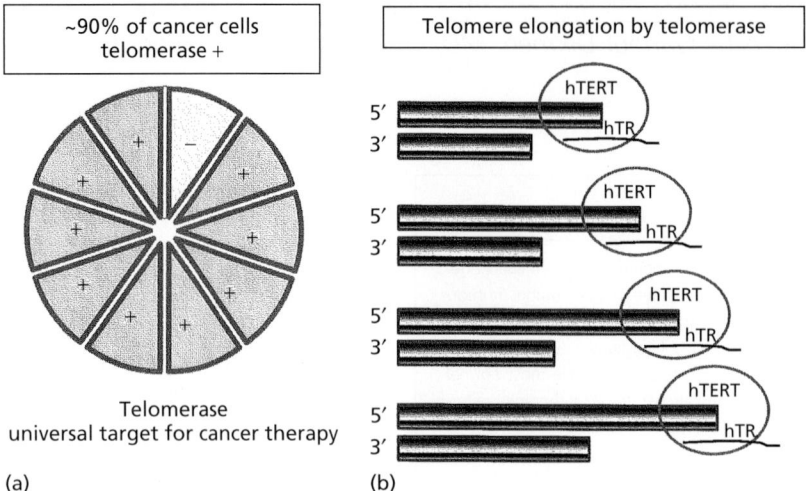

Figure 1 Normal cells that do not express telomerase activity cannot elongate their telomeres, hence their life span is limited whereas telomerase-expressing cancer cells (~90% of cancer cells, a) can elongate their telomeres by telomerase (with hTERT and hTR subunits, b) resulting in unlimited proliferative lifespan (a hallmark of cancer). This important difference between normal and cancer cells make telomerase an almost universal therapeutic target.

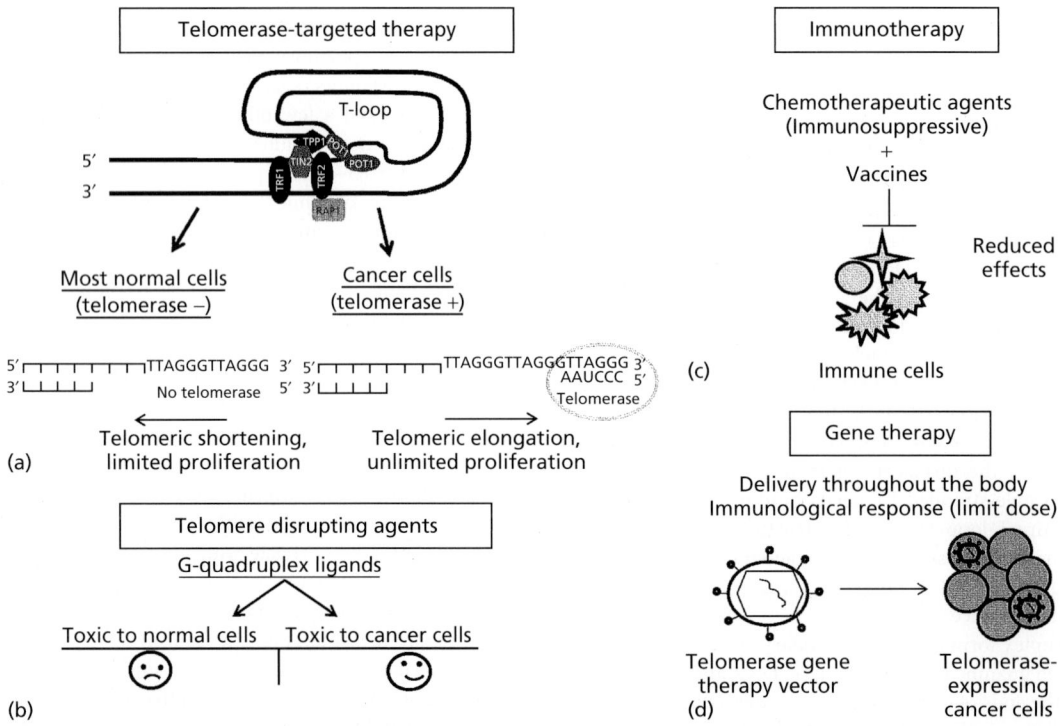

Figure 2 Diagram of hypothetical telomere demonstrating the t-loop structure. This structure is similar in normal and cancer cells but as normal cells generally do not express telomerase, telomeres shorten progressively while cancer cells expressing telomerase can maintain their telomeres (a). There are disadvantages of G-quadruplex stabilizers (b), immunotherapy (c), and gene therapy approaches (d). G-quadruplex stabilizers show their toxic effects by binding and stabilizing T-loop structures and they are also found at the other regions of chromosomes beside telomeres. Thus, these agents are likely to be toxic for both normal and cancer cells (b). One of the most important disadvantages for immunotherapy is that when combination chemotherapy is used with vaccines for cancer patients, some agents can block the effect of immunization as most chemotherapeutic agents are immunosuppressive (c). The main challenge for gene therapy is the delivery of the gene vector to the cancer cells (d) throughout the body. In addition, immunologic responses to therapy can also limit dosing. Gene therapies generally require more invasive approaches to delivery and are generally not orally available for systemic delivery.

Induction of hTERT cDNA into most normal cells causes reactivation of telomerase and unlimited cell proliferation,[17,18] indicating that repression of telomerase activity is primarily regulated by transcriptional mechanisms and generation of full-length hTERT is likely responsible for activation of telomerase.[19,20] However, it is also known that posttranscriptional and epigenetic alterations may play an important role in this dynamic process.[19] There remains no known consensus mechanism to repress telomerase during human developmental and to reactivate telomerase during cancer progression. Alternative splicing is one of the potential mechanisms for repression or reactivation of telomerase.[21,22] Several groups have found that there are different hTERT splice forms such as minus alpha, minus beta, or minus alpha beta,[16,21,23,24] which may have a role on regulation of telomerase activity.[16,20] hTERTα is one of the known splice variants that inhibits telomerase activity by acting as a dominant-negative inhibitor. Thus, the balance between hTERTα form and full-length hTERT and other splice variants may be important in the regulation of active telomerase.[19,25] Recent papers showed that a 1.1-kb region of a 38-bp variable number tandem repeats (conserved among Old World primates) is essential for exclusion of exon 7 and 8 to produce the minus beta splicing form and that RNA:RNA pairing between these repetitive sequences may be used to regulate decisions on hTERT splicing.[26,27] Importantly, misregulation of alternative splicing is a hallmark of nearly all cancers. In addition, a recent shift in our understanding of telomerase regulation has occurred. The common paradigm in the field was that hTERT was transcriptionally silenced in normal differentiated human tissues. However, there is increased evidence that hTERT is transcribed in normal cells but spliced to variants that do not have telomerase activity (Andrew Ludlow, unpublished observations). Although hTR (hTERC) is expressed in almost all cells, hTERT is only detected at extremely low levels even in cancer cells. How TERT is regulated to produce an optimal level for telomerase function in stem cells and cancer cells is still largely unknown. However, one could speculate that targeting hTERT at the splicing level may be a novel approach to reduce telomerase activity in cancer cells perhaps with minimal toxicity to normal cells.[16]

Compared to normal cells with long telomeres, the vast majority of cancer cells have relatively short telomeres. As normal stem cells generally have longer telomeres compared to cancer cells, this may facilitate cancer cells undergoing apoptosis with telomerase-targeted drug administration without a significant effect on normal cells.[28] As an example, the transfection of an hTERT dominant-negative mutant into tumor cell lines resulted in apoptosis and reduced tumorigenic capacity.[29,30] The death by apoptosis in tumor cells correlates with initial telomere length, the tumor cells with short telomeres die before those with longer telomeres.[31] In addition, it has been proposed that tumors are less likely to develop resistance against telomerase-based therapies compared to other cancer targets.[32] However, this has not been experimentally observed in ALT or other telomere maintenance mechanisms. All of these factors suggest that targeting telomerase is not only a unique and almost universal cancer target, but it is likely to be a relatively safe anticancer treatment approach with fewer side effects compared to standard chemotherapy. Thus, a more complete understanding of the relationships between telomeres, telomerase, aging, and cancer may increase our knowledge and contribute to new approaches to cancer therapy and basic tumor biology research (Figure 1).

Table 1 Telomere/telomerase-targeted strategies.

Therapeutic approach	Inhibitors
G-quadruplex stabilizers	BRACO19, RHPS4, Telomestatin, porphyrin, TMPyP4, CX-3543/quarfloxin, AS1411/ Cytarabine/Ara-C
Immunotherapy	GV1001, VX-001, GRNVAC1/2
Gene therapy	Telomelysin, Ad-hTERT-NTR/CB1954, hTERTp-HRP/IAA
Telomere and telomerase-associated proteins	Geldanamycin (GA), Curcumin
T-oligo approach	PARP inhibitors
Small-molecule inhibitors	BIBR1532
Oligonucleotides	GRN163L
Telomerase-mediated telomere uncapping approaches	Lentiviral mutant hTERC, 6-thio-2′ deoxyguanosine

There are no telomere/telomerase-targeted drugs approved by the Food and Drug Administration (FDA)

Although proof of concept of different approaches against telomerase-based therapies has repeatedly been achieved in the preclinical setting, there are no telomerase inhibitors in clinical trials that have been approved by FDA. The most promising telomere/telomerase-targeted strategies are reviewed in Table 1.

G-quadruplex stabilizers

G-quadruplexes are formed by the ability of guanosine self-assembly together with monovalent cations (e.g., potassium) in the presence of guanine tandem repeats. G-quadruplexes may form in telomeres, oncogene promoter sequences, and other biologically relevant regions of the genome.[33] It has been demonstrated that small molecules that target G-quadruplex structure in human telomeres cause telomerase inhibition (perhaps indirectly) and telomeric end disruption.[34] Thus, this secondary structure is a popular target to design small-molecule ligands.

Telomestatin is isolated from *Streptomyces anulatus* 3533-SV4 and reported to be a telomerase inhibitor that interacts with G-quadruplex structures.[35,36] Nakajima and co-workers[37] showed that telomestatin causes telomerase inhibition and induces apoptosis in primary leukemic blasts that were isolated from bone marrow of acute myeloid leukemia (AML-M2) patients. The other reported G-quadruplex ligand is termed TMPyP4. Hurley and colleagues showed that telomestatin caused telomerase inhibition by stabilizing of intramolecular G-quadruplex structures and eventually telomere shortening, whereas TMPyP4 suppressed the proliferation of ALT-positive cells as well as telomerase-positive cells by facilitating the formation of intermolecular G-quadruplexes leading to the induction of anaphase bridges. They also reported that telomestatin more tightly and specifically binds to the intramolecular G-quadruplexes compared to other G-quadruplex interactive compounds such as TMPyP4.[38] Another investigated telomeric G4 ligand is termed RHPS4 (pentacyclic acridine). RHPS4 reduces telomerase activity at submicromolar levels through stabilization of G-quadruplex structures formed by single-stranded telomeric DNA.[39] Others reported that RHSP4 causes telomere capping alterations in a telomere length-independent manner.[40] *In vivo* experiments demonstrate that RHSP4 is even more effective when compared with other antineoplastic drugs in terms of antitumoral and antimetastatic effects.[41] Although BRACO19 (trisubstituted acridine) is classified in the class of G-quadruplex stabilizers due to *in vitro* and *in vivo* anticancer effects,[31] the utility of this compound is limited because of its low permeability for biological barriers in the airways or intestinal epithelial cell cultures *in vitro*.[42] Several ligands induce growth inhibition of various cancer cells *in vitro* by causing cellular senescence and/or apoptosis. These ligands also exert short-term effects with telomere uncapping.[43] Over the past decade, many G-quadruplex ligands have been described including fluorenons, bisubstituted acridines, cationic porphyrins, a perylenetetracarboxylic diimide derivative, indolo-quinolines. However, the evidence for specificity of these compounds for telomerase is very limited and they poorly bind to the quadruplex structures compared to double DNA.[31] Thus, many of these compounds may affect quadruplex structures in normal cells as well as cancer cells (Figure 2b). Any compound that inhibits cell growth will decrease telomerase activity, so it is not sufficient to show telomerase inhibition to suggest specificity without also testing these compounds on normal cells without telomerase.

Some of the proteins that interact with G-quadruplex stabilizers also have the ability to induce senescence and/or apoptosis. Although G-quadruplex structures appear to be good targets for anticancer therapy, they are also observed during replication in chromosome regions besides telomeres. Because G-quadruplexes also have a large planar surface formed by terminal G-tetrad, most of the small molecules designed so far target this common structure instead of a specific target for a particular G-quadruplex. Thus, a general concern about these compounds is safety: while small-molecule ligands toward G-quadruplex structures affect cancer cells, they may also affect the telomere structure of normal cells[44,45] (Figure 2b).

Although there are two quadruplex-related small molecules that have already entered into clinical trials, there remains lack of direct evidence that these small molecules are specific for telomerase-targeted therapy. The first agent CX-3543 (quarfloxin/quarfloxacin, Cylene Pharmaceuticals, San Diego, CA, USA) is a fluoroquinolone derivative, that selectively disrupts nucleolin/rDNA G-quadruplex complexes in the nucleolus by inhibiting Pol1 transcription, resulting in decreased cancer cell proliferation and induction of apoptosis.[46,47] However, CX-3543 also interacts with MYC G-quadruplexes,[46] so the *in vitro* antiproliferative and *in vivo* antitumoral activity in xenograft models may not be related to G quadruplexes at telomeres. In addition, CX-3543 selectively targets Pol1, rather than telomere function, which further suggests that CX-3543 may have indirect or even no effect on telomere function.[47] The other quadruplex forming agent in clinical trials is AS1411 (Cytarabine/Ara-C, Antisoma Research, London, UK), which specifically targets nucleolin.[48]

Immunotherapy

Tumor-associated antigens (TAAs)-specific immunotherapy has been investigated for several decades. However, as most TAAs immunotherapies have been restricted to only a few tumor types, telomerase-based immunotherapy would theoretically be a good approach owing to the ubiquitous expression of telomerase in most tumor cells.[49] Degradation of hTERT in proteasomes by E3 ubiquitin ligase generates protein fragments/peptides that may be presented on the tumor cell surface as antigens by the major histocompatibility complex (MHC) class I pathway. Thus, targeting these antigens by a patient's own immune system (CD8+ T lymphocytes) is a direct way to kill the telomerase-expressing tumor cells[50,51] (reviewed in Ref. 52). Several hTERT vaccines have already been developed, but GV1001 and GRNVAC1 are the most promising vaccines that are in clinical trials (Table 2). GV1001 is a 16-mer TERT peptide (aa 611–626) that binds multiple HLA class II molecules. Recent studies showed that vaccination with hTERT-transfected dendritic cells helped to induce telomerase-specific CD4+ and CD8+ T-cell responses[53] and also vaccination with GV1001-induced hTERT-specific T-cell responses in nonresectable pancreatic cancer patients and nonsmall lung cancer patients.[54,55] The combination treatment of GV1001 and cyclophosphamide in hepatocellular carcinoma failed to show partial or complete responses to treatment in a phase 2 clinical trial.[56] GV1001 vaccination with chemotherapy together did not improve overall survival in advanced or metastatic pancreatic cancer in a phase 3 clinical trial.[57] GRNVAC1 was also designed to induce CD4 and CD8 responses. GRNVAC1 was prepared from autologous dendritic cells transduced with mRNAs encoding a near full-length hTERT protein *ex vivo*. The dendritic cells are reintroduced into the patient and can potentially recognize any hTERT peptide in a patient's tumor.[32] Currently, GRNVAC1 is in phase 2 clinical trials for acute myelogenous leukemia patients. As monotherapy is likely to have limited efficacy, combination therapy might be a more effective approach to kill the heterogeneous nature of tumor cells. However, most chemotherapeutic agents are immunosuppressive and they might preclude the immunization effect. For this reason, vaccines should probably not be used in combination with chemotherapeutic agents[58] (Figure 2c). Hence, new strategies are required to improve clinical efficacy with enhanced immune response effects of telomerase vaccination during chemotherapy.

Gene therapy

Gene therapy is a technique that treats diseases such as cancer by delivering therapeutic DNA into the patient's cells. DNA that encodes a therapeutic effect can be delivered to the target cells. DNA becomes expressed by the cell machinery that ultimately makes a protein that can result in apoptosis. Genes can be delivered via oncolytic viral vectors and can include enzymes metabolizing prodrugs or suicide genes.[59] Although gene therapy can be highly tumor specific, there are challenges including manufacture/formulation, which is often complex and clinical trials

Table 2 Telomerase-targeted vaccines in clinical trials.

Vaccines	ClinicalTrials.gov Identifier/phase	Condition	Drug intervention	Status
GV1001	NCT01223209/phase 1	Carcinoma	GV1001, LTX-315	Completed
	NCT01247623/phase1/2	Advanced malignant melanoma	GV1001	Completed
	NCT01342224/phase 1	Locally advanced pancreatic adenocarcinoma	Tadalafil and vaccination	Active, not recruiting
	NCT00425360/phase 3	Locally advanced or metastatic pancreatic cancer	Gemcitabine, capecitabine, GV1001	Completed
	NCT01579188/phase 3	Inoperable stage 3 nonsmall-cell lung cancer	GV1001	Not yet recruiting
	NCT00509457/not provided	Nonsmall-cell lung cancer	GV1001	Completed
	NCT00444782/phase 2	Hepatocellular carcinoma	GV1001	Completed
	NCT00358566/phase 3	Advanced unresectable pancreatic cancer	GV1001, gemcitabine	Terminated
GRNVAC1	NCT00510133/phase 2	Acute myelogenous leukemia	GRNVAC1	Active, not recruiting
VX001	NCT01935154/phase 2	Nonsmall-cell lung cancer metastatic	VX001	Recruiting

requiring special expertise[60] (Figure 2d). Some studies showed the proof of concept in treating cancer, but there are some concerns about off-target effects. Targeting tumor cells in order to have a reduction of tumor burden and durable responses is the main purpose for successful therapy.[61,62] There are adenoviral vectors that have been engineered to kill cancer cells by only entering cells that have telomerase activity. These adenoviral vectors have a TERT promoter driving replication of the adenovirus. In this instance, the virus uniquely replicates in telomerase-positive cells, thus sparing most normal cells.[63] After replication and amplification of the virus, the tumor cell will lyse and viral particles will spread to adjacent cells.[63–66] This approach is known as a tumor-specific replication-competent adenoviral (hTERTp-TRAD) gene therapy approach.[61,67] One example for telomerase-mediated virus therapy is Telomelysin (OBP-301), which is an hTERT promoter driven modified oncolytic adenovirus. Preclinical studies demonstrated antitumor activity of telomelysin (and similarly engineered adenoviruses) in various cancer cells.[64,66,68,69] Phase 1 clinical trials did not show significant related toxic events but there were multiple manageable adverse events such as fever, chills, fatigue, and injection site pain. Some patients with solid tumors developed a decreased asymptomatic transient lymphocyte.[70] Systemic treatment also has the potential effects on telomerase-positive proliferating normal stem cells. Therefore, systemic hTERTp-TRAD may affect transient amplifying stem cells such as proliferating cells in the crypts of the intestine, hematological cells, and a subset of cells in the basal and suprabasal layer of the epidermis.[8,60] The other concern is that intratumoral injections may not be sufficient to reduce the tumor burden.[71]

Suicide gene therapy (Ad-hTR-NTR), also called "gene directed enzyme prodrug therapy," targets only tumor cells without affecting normal cells, similar to oncolytic gene therapy.[32,72] Three general steps are required for this approach: first is targeting the vector, second is transfecting the vector carrying an enzyme-encoding gene driven by hTERT into the cells, third is a prodrug that is activated by an enzyme, resulting in a release of toxins into the cytoplasm causing death of telomerase-positive cells.[72] Although gene therapy (suicide gene or oncolytic vector) show some promising results, they do not appear to be as effective as vaccines or oligonucleotides.[73] Future directions would be to make multifunctional viral vectors such as those replicating only in p53 mutant cells with telomerase expression. This would potentially reduce the effects on normal proliferating stem cells.

Small-molecule inhibitors and antisense oligonucleotides

Although millions of compounds have been screened during the past decade to identify small-molecule inhibitors of telomerase, there are currently no potent/specific small-molecule inhibitors except one candidate compound, BIBR1532. While BIBR1532 showed promising results in some preclinical models,[74,75] it was not effective enough to enter clinical trials perhaps owing to its short binding on/off rate with telomerase.[76,77] After many years of screening new drugs, GRN163L (Imetelstat, Geron Corporation) was found as a parallel approach to small-molecule inhibitors. This telomerase-targeted oligonucleotide approach uses a lipid-modified N3′ → P5′ thio-phosphoramidate oligonucleotide and has shown highly potent telomerase inhibition as a competitive enzyme inhibitor by being designed to complement the hTR template of telomerase that recognizes telomeres.[78] GRN163L, 13-mer oligonucleotide (not antisense) was generated as a second improved generation of GRN163 to increase cellular uptake with a conjugating lipophilic palmitoyl (C16) group attached to the 5′ terminal.[28]

The effects of GRN163L have been investigated in different cancer cell lines and xenograft models. GRN163L demonstrates both *in vivo* and *in vitro* effects by inhibiting telomerase activity and resulting in progressive telomere shortening in a variety of cancer cell lines such as hepatocellular carcinoma,[79] lung cancer,[80] breast cancer,[81,82] bladder cancer,[71] multiple myeloma,[83] pancreatic cancer,[84] colorectal cancer,[85] glioblastoma,[86] and esophageal adeno-carcinoma.[87] *In vivo* antimetastatic effects of GRN163L were tested in tumor xenograft models. When A549 lung cancer cells were injected into the nude mice via the tail vein, lung tumor formation was not observed in the animals treated with 15 mg/kg GRN163L (intraperitoneal, three times per week for 3 weeks).[80] In mice having implanted hepatoma cancer cells, GRN163L inhibited tumor growth and also sensitized tumor cells to conventional chemotherapy.[79] In a xenograft model of breast cancer and lung metastasis, administration of 30 mg/kg GRN163L for 12 treatments (three times per week, 4 weeks total) effectively reduced the proliferation of breast cancer cells and metastasis to the lungs.[82] Different studies showed that GRN163L reduced tumor size as well as improved survival in a human myeloma cell-derived xenograft model.[83] Although there are many studies showing promising effects of GRN163L *in vitro* and *in vivo*, GRN163L has not succeeded in most clinical trials owing to hematological side effects and liver function abnormalities as well as other adverse events. When patients had dose-limiting toxicities such as thrombocytopenia, owing to GRN163L, interruption of dosing until their platelet numbers returned to the normal range resulted in telomere re-elongating during the drug holiday period.

GRN163L (Imetelstat), is the first telomerase inhibitor in clinical trials, and 17 studies have been completed, including 10 phase 1 and 6 phase 2 trials. These are summarized in Table 3. The preliminary data in 50- to 74-year-old patients with advanced solid tumors (6 colorectal, 3 lung, 2 mesothelioma, 2 pancreas, 7 others) showed aPTT prolongation (active prolonged thromboplastin), gastrointestinal side effects, fatigue, anemia, GGT elevation, and peripheral neuropathy. Although thrombocytopenia is a dose-limiting toxicity at 4.8 mg/kg, one death from unknown reasons was observed at 3.2 mg/kg dose.[88] Locally recurrent or metastatic breast cancer (MBC) patients were treated with GRN163L in combination with paclitaxel and bevacizumab (3 of 14 patients with *de novo* MBC and 6 of 14 patients with prior (neo) adjuvant taxane). Phase 1 clinical trials showed that the most common toxicities were cytopenia. The majority of patients had dose reduction or delays in treatments with GRN163L and/or paclitaxel owing to neutropenia and/or thrombocytopenia or other adverse effects.[73] Main outcome from pediatric patients with solid tumors in phase 1 clinical trials was that the reduction of telomerase activity in PBMCs (peripheral blood mononuclear cells) and telomerase-positive tumors with the recommended phase 2 dose, which is 285 mg/m^2 (MTD, maximum tolerated dose). In this study intravenous injection was conducted for 2 h on days 1 and 8 of a 21-day cycle. As a result, dose-limiting toxicity levels (DLT; 360 mg/m^2) caused myelosuppression leading to a delay in the therapy of more than 14 days. Some patients had anemia, lymphopenia, neutropenia, thrombocytopenia, and catheter related infections depending on their grade level and cycle number of treatment.[89] The advanced breast cancer phase 2 trial (NCT01256762) was stopped owing to poorer overall survival in patients treated with GRN163L.[49] As GRN163L is administered on days 1 and 8 of a 21-day cycle, it is possible that telomerase cannot be inhibited sufficiently during this schedule, so that a new telomere equilibrium length for cancer cells emerges.

Table 3 GRN163L in clinical trials.

ClinicalTrials.gov Identifier/phase	Condition	Drug intervention	Status
NCT01568632/phase 1	Refractory or recurrent solid tumors/lymphoma	GRN163L	Withdrawn
NCT01273090/phase 1	Refractory or recurrent solid tumors/lymphoma	GRN163L	Completed
NCT01243073/phase 2	Essential thrombocythemia/polycythemia vera (ET/PV)	GRN163L, standard of care	Suspended
NCT00594126/phase 1	Refractory or relapsed multiple myeloma	GRN163L	Completed
NCT01916187/phase 1	Neuroblastoma	GRN163L, 13-cis retinoic acid	Withdrawn
NCT00732056/phase 1	Recurrent or metastatic breast cancer	GRN163L, paclitaxel, bevacizumab	Completed
NCT00310895/phase 1	Refractory or relapsed solid tumor malignancies	GRN163L	Completed
NCT00718601/phase 1	Multiple myeloma	GRN163L, bortezomib, dexamethasone	Completed
NCT01242930/phase 2	Multiple myeloma	GRN163L, standard of care	Active, not recruiting
NCT00510445/phase 1	Advanced or metastatic nonsmall-cell lung cancer	GRN163L, paclitaxel, carboplatin	Completed
NCT01265927/phase 1	Her2+ breast cancer	GRN163L, trastuzumab	Active, not recruiting
NCT00124189/phase 1	Chronic lymphoproliferative disease (CLD)	GRN163L	Completed
NCT02011126/phase 2	Relapsed or refractory solid tumors	GRN163L	Withdrawn
NCT01137968/phase 2	Nonsmall-cell lung cancer	GRN163L, bevacizumab	Completed
NCT01731951/Not provided	Primary or secondary myelofibrosis	GRN163L	Active, not recruiting
NCT01256762/phase 2	Recurrent or metastatic breast cancer	GRN163L, paclitaxel, w/wo bevacizumab	Completed
NCT01836549/phase 2	Recurrent or refractory brain tumors	GRN163L	Recruiting

Challenges for developing telomerase inhibitors

The other potential challenge for telomerase inhibitors, such as GRN163L, is that the response time that is needed to induce senescence or crisis is long as telomere attrition occurs following each cell replication cycle. Therefore, this delayed response limits its utility as a first-line treatment for advanced cancer. It has been suggested that telomerase inhibitors following conventional therapy might be a good option to block the growth of residual cancer cells.[65] A phase 2 study used GRN163L in a maintenance therapy setting after initial standard of care doublet chemotherapy for advanced nonsmall-cell lung cancer (NSCLC) has been completed (clinicaltrials.gov: NCT01137968). This study was designed to evaluate whether or not GRN163L, given as maintenance therapy, prolonged progression-free survival (PFS) in NSCLC. Eligible stage IV or recurrent locally advanced NSCLC patients were randomized to GRN163L (9.4 mg/kg over a 2-h IV infusion on day 1 and day 8 of each 21-day cycle) with or without bevacizumab on day 1 of each 21-day cycle, vs. standard of care alone (patients who had received bevacizumab before randomization were continued with bevacizumab maintenance or had no follow-up maintenance treatment). This study, while not achieving statistical significance showed a trend in PFS in the GRN163L arm, most apparent in the cohort of patients with the shortest telomeres at the initiation of the trial.[90] Experience with these types of trials is important to more fully understand how to provide antitelomerase therapies going forward.

Overexpression of mutant hTERC and wild-type hTERC-targeted siRNA by lentiviral vectors are different types of gene therapy strategies for telomerase-targeted therapies

The other strategy to disrupt telomere maintenance in cancer cells is to express mutant hTR (hTERC) in the template region (mutant-template human telomerase RNA; MT-hTERC). Wild-type telomere repeats contain DNA binding sites for direct telomeric binding proteins such as POT1, TRF1, and TRF2 in humans.[91,92] It is predicted that mutated DNA that is directly synthesized by MT-hTERC disrupts the binding of telomeric proteins,[93–95] which might lead to telomere uncapping. Studies showed that

the uncapping of human telomeres by mutating TRF2 can induce growth arrest (p53 dependent) and apoptosis in cells.[96,97] Introduction of MT-hTERC via lentiviral vectors into telomerase-positive human cancer cells causes an alteration in the cancer cellular phenotype and reduced tumor growth in xenografts.[94,95] In another approach using siRNA (a hairpin short-interfering RNA) expressed from a lentiviral vector-targeted wild-type human telomerase RNA (WT-hTERC) also caused cell growth inhibition and apoptosis (these effects are telomere length independent). Coexpression of MT-hTERC and anti-WT-hTERC-siRNA showed additive or perhaps synergistic effects on cancer cells. Therefore, mutant hTERC and siRNA present promising anticancer therapy strategies owing to the lack of dependency on p53, initial telomere length, or progressive telomere shortening.[98] However, these are still gene therapy approaches and require high efficiency in targeting to the cancer cells to be effective in the clinical setting.

6-Thio-dG is a small molecule that is a telomerase-based telomere uncapping target that may overcome some of the problems with gene therapy

Ideal cancer targets are those that are expressed in cancer cells, but not in normal cells. Compared to other targets, telomerase is one of the most universal targets expressed in almost all tumor cells, but not in normal cells except some proliferative progenitor stem cells. Therefore, telomerase is an important target to focus on for new therapeutic strategies.

So far, there have been two different therapeutic strategies in telomere biology: telomere or telomerase-targeted strategies. The strategy that targets telomerase inhibition is correlated with telomere length, whereas telomere-targeted approach is independent from initial telomere length (Figure 3). This makes an important difference between these two approaches. With only telomerase inhibition, a long lag period is expected (the time between enzyme inhibition and biological effect). Thus treatments will generally be long and depend on significant reduction of telomere length before reduction of tumor growth, senescence, or apoptosis is observed.[29,30]

Some approaches that target telomeres (not directly telomerase) lead to telomere uncapping (e.g., G-quadruplex), which is independent of p53 status and initial telomere length. However, normal

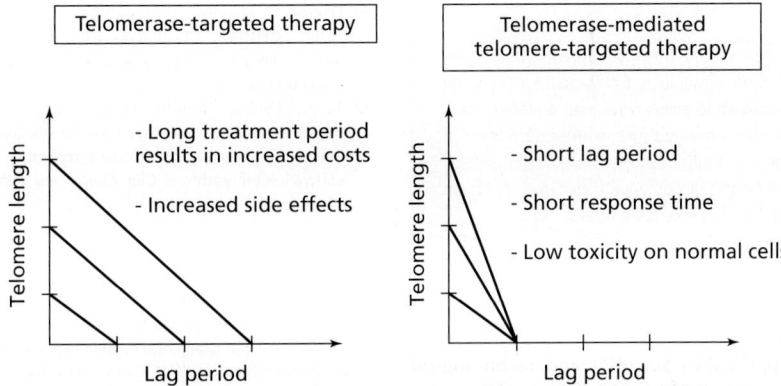

Figure 3 Telomerase-targeted therapeutic responses (such as Imetelstat/GRN163L) are dependent on the initial tumor cell telomere length. Cancer cells have variable telomere lengths. Therefore, cells with long telomeres are predicted to take a longer treatment period to be sensitive to telomerase inhibitors compared to cells with shorter telomeres (left side). As a result, any long-term treatment for telomerase may lead to unwanted side effects, high costs, and potentially re-establishing feedback loops establishing a stable new telomere length. In contrast to telomerase-targeted therapies, telomerase-mediated telomere targeting therapies (such as 6-thio-dG or MT-hTERC gene therapy) do not need long treatment periods as they are independent of the initial telomere length, therefore short response time to tumor burden reduction is a key advantage of these approaches (right side). The other most important advantage is that they may be less toxic to normal cells as most do not express telomerase. However, the MT-hTERC approach has the same obvious limitations of all gene therapy approaches of needing to reach almost all cells and delivery concerns. However, new approaches such as 6-thio-dG nucleoside may be orally available with minimal side effect and have the obvious advantage that all small molecules have.

tissue toxicity remains a major concern owing to quadruplex formation in other regions of the genome and in normal cells.[99] Thus, approaches that do not target through telomerase may not have a therapeutic window of efficacy. In addition, using direct telomerase inhibitors or telomere-targeted therapies may need to be combined with other cytotoxic drugs to reduce the potential resistance capacity of heterogeneous tumor cells.[99] For example, the cells from mTR knock-out mice showed telomere dysfunction by sensitizing cells to some anticancer drugs (e.g., doxorubicin).[100] This result shows that telomerase-targeted therapy in combination with other chemotherapeutic agents may sensitize cells to other chemotherapeutics by resulting in reduced resistant capacity.

In recent work, we focused on a novel approach to identify a small molecule that would uncap telomeres but only in telomerase-positive cells. This theoretical approach using a small molecule obviates some of the problem with gene therapy and also could reduce the lag phase from initiation of treatment to tumor burden reduction. To test this concept, we decided to focus on nucleoside analogs that are good substrates for telomerase (not inhibitors of telomerase) and also more specific for telomerase than for other polymerases. 6-Thio-2′deoxyguanosine (6-thio-dG) is a new telomere-targeted nucleoside analog that is recognized by telomerase and is used by telomerase as a substrate.[101] In our recent studies, we showed that 6-thio-dG causes telomere dysfunction by causing altered telomere structures called telomere dysfunction-induced foci (TIFs) in telomerase-expressing cancer cells of varying telomere lengths and comparing these to normal and ALT cells. Interestingly, beside short-term cell killing effects, 6-thio-dG caused rapid and progressive telomere shortening in surviving cancer cells but not in normal cells. These studies demonstrated that 6-thio-dG targets telomeres by being preferentially used by telomerase as a substrate. In human xenograft models in immunodeficient mice, 6-thio-dG reduced lung cancer growth (no observed side effects, e.g., no death, no weight loss) and caused telomere dysfunction. There were no long-term side effects on normal tissues and hematological, liver, and kidney functions were in the acceptable range. Thus, 6-thio-dG is a promising "telomeric poison" targeting telomeres by using telomerase as a catalyst to

change telomeres so they are recognized as DNA damage. Additional, perhaps more potent nucleoside analogs will be the new direction for targeting the cell immortality cancer hallmark.

Summary

Telomeres are protective structures that are found at the ends of linear chromosomes. Telomeres shorten with each cell division owing to the end replication problem. However, telomerase maintenance mechanisms can counteract this progressive shortening process. While most normal cells do not express telomerase activity, it is detected in almost all primary human tumors. Therefore, telomerase is a unique and almost universal target for cancer.

Although there have been promising approaches targeting telomerase for cancer therapies, there are no drugs that have been approved. G-quadruplex stabilizers that target the G-rich DNA sequences in human telomeres cause telomerase inhibition and telomeric end disruption. However, the specificity of these compounds is very limited and may affect quadruplex structures in normal cells as well as cancer cells.

Immunotherapy approaches in clinical trials utilize hTERT GV1001 (peptide vaccine) and GRNVAC1 (dendritic cell priming *ex vivo*). The utility of these vaccines in combination with conventional therapy may be limited owing to immunosuppressive effect of chemotherapeutic drugs.

GRN163L (Imetelstat) is a telomerase-targeted oligonucleotide approach. GRN163L shows highly potent telomerase inhibition, resulting in progressive telomere shortening in cancer cells. Owing to adverse hematological events, clinical trials in solid tumors have not progressed. One of the potential challenges for GRN163L is the response (long lag) time that is needed to induce senescence/apoptosis.

Gene therapy is a well-established technique that targets cancer by delivering therapeutic DNA. Mutant hTERT (dominant-negative approach) or siRNA directed at hTERT are some of the different gene therapy approaches in preclinical studies. In addition, introduction of a mutant hTERC via lentiviral transfer is a telomerase-dependent telomere "upcapping" approach. Gene therapy is a promising anticancer therapy approach but requires high efficiency to target the vast majority of cancer cells.

Typical telomerase inhibitors (GRN163L) require a long lag period between enzyme inhibition and biological effect. In contrast, telomerase-mediated telomere-targeted therapy is predicted to have a much shorter lag period. One example is 6-thio-dG, a nucleoside analog. 6-thio-dG is a new approach to target telomeres, is preferentially recognized by telomerase and incorporated into telomeres resulting in TIFs. This small-molecule approach results in short-term cell killing effects on telomerase-expressing cells (short lag time) with minimal effects on telomerase silent normal cells (e.g., quiescent stem cells).

Acknowledgments

I. Mender was partially supported by Scientific and Technological Research Council of Turkey (TUBITAK). These studies were also supported in part by NCI SPORE P50CA70907, the Simmons Cancer Center Support Grant 5P30 CA142543 and support from the Southland Financial Corporation Distinguished Chair in Geriatric Research. This work was performed in space constructed with support from National Institute of Health grant C06 RR30414.

Key references

The complete reference list can be found on the Wiley Companion Digital Edition of this title (see inside front cover for login instructions).

1 de Lange T. How shelterin solves the telomere end-protection problem. *Cold Spring Harb Symp Quant Biol*. 2010;**75**:167–77.

2 Shay JW. Are short telomeres predictive of advanced cancer? *Cancer Discov*. 2013;**3**:1096–8.

4 Palm W, de Lange T. How shelterin protects mammalian telomeres. *Annu Rev Genet*. 2008;**42**:301–34.

5 Gilson E, Geli V. How telomeres are replicated. *Nat Rev Mol Cell Biol*. 2007;**8**:825–38.

9 Shay JW, Wright WE. Role of telomeres and telomerase in cancer. *Semin Cancer Biol*. 2011;**21**:349–53.

11 Davis CF, Ricketts CJ, Wang M, et al. The somatic genomic landscape of chromophobe renal cell carcinoma. *Cancer Cell*. 2014;**26**:319–30.

12 Zhao Y, Wang S, Popova EY, et al. Rearrangement of upstream sequences of the hTERT gene during cellular immortalization. *Genes Chromosomes Cancer*. 2009;**48**:963–74.

13 Huang FW, Hodis E, Xu MJ, et al. Highly recurrent TERT promoter mutations in human melanoma. *Science*. 2013;**339**:957–9.

16 Wong MS, Wright WE, Shay JW. Alternative splicing regulation of telomerase: a new paradigm? *Trends Genet*. 2014;**30**:430–8.

18 Bodnar AG, Ouellette M, Frolkis M, et al. Extension of life-span by introduction of telomerase into normal human cells. *Science*. 1998;**279**:349–52.

28 Herbert BS, Gellert GC, Hochreiter A, et al. Lipid modification of GRN163, an N3′—>P5′ thio-phosphoramidate oligonucleotide, enhances the potency of telomerase inhibition. *Oncogene*. 2005;**24**:5262–8.

31 Gowan SM, Harrison JR, Patterson L, et al. A G-quadruplex-interactive potent small-molecule inhibitor of telomerase exhibiting in vitro and in vivo antitumor activity. *Mol Pharmacol*. 2002;**61**:1154–62.

32 Harley CB. Telomerase and cancer therapeutics. *Nat Rev Cancer*. 2008;**8**:167–79.

35 Kim MY, Vankayalapati H, Shin-Ya K, et al. Telomestatin, a potent telomerase inhibitor that interacts quite specifically with the human telomeric intramolecular G-quadruplex. *J Am Chem Soc*. 2002;**124**:2098–9.

38 Kim MY, Gleason-Guzman M, Izbicka E, et al. The different biological effects of telomestatin and TMPyP4 can be attributed to their selectivity for interaction with intramolecular or intermolecular G-quadruplex structures. *Cancer Res*. 2003;**63**:3247–56.

39 Gowan SM, Heald R, Stevens MF, et al. Potent inhibition of telomerase by small-molecule pentacyclic acridines capable of interacting with G-quadruplexes. *Mol Pharmacol*. 2001;**60**:981–8.

40 Leonetti C, Amodei S, D'Angelo C, et al. Biological activity of the G-quadruplex ligand RHPS4 (3,11-difluoro-6,8,13-trimethyl-8H-quino[4,3,2-kl]acridinium methosulfate) is associated with telomere capping alteration. *Mol Pharmacol*. 2004;**66**:1138–46.

42 Taetz S, Baldes C, Murdter TE, et al. Biopharmaceutical characterization of the telomerase inhibitor BRACO19. *Pharm Res*. 2006;**23**:1031–7.

43 Kelland L. Targeting the limitless replicative potential of cancer: the telomerase/telomere pathway. *Clin Cancer Res Off J Am Assoc Cancer Res*. 2007;**13**:4960–3.

49 Mocellin S, Pooley KA, Nitti D. Telomerase and the search for the end of cancer. *Trends Mol Med*. 2013;**19**:125–33.

52 Liu JP, Chen W, Schwarer AP, et al. Telomerase in cancer immunotherapy. *Biochim Biophys Acta*. 1805;**2010**:35–42.

56 Greten TF, Forner A, Korangy F, et al. A phase II open label trial evaluating safety and efficacy of a telomerase peptide vaccination in patients with advanced hepatocellular carcinoma. *BMC Cancer*. 2010;**10**:209.

57 Middleton G, Silcocks P, Cox T, et al. Gemcitabine and capecitabine with or without telomerase peptide vaccine GV1001 in patients with locally advanced or metastatic pancreatic cancer (TeloVac): an open-label, randomised, phase 3 trial. *Lancet Oncol*. 2014;**15**:829–40.

58 Kyte JA, Gaudernack G, Dueland S, et al. Telomerase peptide vaccination combined with temozolomide: a clinical trial in stage IV melanoma patients. *Clin Cancer Res Off J Am Assoc Cancer Res*. 2011;**17**:4568–80.

60 Shay JW, Keith WN. Targeting telomerase for cancer therapeutics. *Br J Cancer*. 2008;**98**:677–83.

61 Keith WN, Bilsland A, Hardie M, et al. Drug insight: cancer cell immortality-telomerase as a target for novel cancer gene therapies. *Nat Clin Pract Oncol*. 2004;**1**:88–96.

63 Fujiwara T, Urata Y, Tanaka N. Therapeutic targets and drugs IV: telomerase-specific gene and vector-based therapies for human cancer. In: Hiyama K, ed. *Telomeres and Telomerase in Cancer*. Menlo Park, CA: Geron Corporation; 2009:293–312.

65 Ouellette MM, Wright WE, Shay JW. Targeting telomerase-expressing cancer cells. *J Cell Mol Med*. 2011;**15**:1433–42.

67 Keith WN, Thomson CM, Howcroft J, et al. Seeding drug discovery: integrating telomerase cancer biology and cellular senescence to uncover new therapeutic opportunities in targeting cancer stem cells. *Drug Discov Today*. 2007;**12**:611–21.

70 Nemunaitis J, Tong AW, Nemunaitis M, et al. A phase I study of telomerase-specific replication competent oncolytic adenovirus (telomelysin) for various solid tumors. *Mol Ther*. 2010;**18**:429–34.

73 Ruden M, Puri N. Novel anticancer therapeutics targeting telomerase. *Cancer Treat Rev*. 2013;**39**:444–56.

84 Burchett KM, Yan Y, Ouellette MM. Telomerase inhibitor Imetelstat (GRN163L) limits the lifespan of human pancreatic cancer cells. *PLoS One*. 2014;**9**:e85155.

86 Marian CO, Cho SK, McEllin BM, et al. The telomerase antagonist, imetelstat, efficiently targets glioblastoma tumor-initiating cells leading to decreased proliferation and tumor growth. *Clin Cancer Res*. 2010;**16**:154–63.

88 Molckovsky A, Siu LL. First-in-class, first-in-human phase I results of targeted agents: highlights of the 2008 American society of clinical oncology meeting. *J Hematol Oncol*. 2008;**1**:20.

89 Thompson PA, Drissi R, Muscal JA, et al. A phase I trial of imetelstat in children with refractory or recurrent solid tumors: a Children's Oncology Group Phase I Consortium Study (ADVL1112). *Clin Cancer Res*. 2013;**19**:6578–84.

98 Li S, Rosenberg JE, Donjacour AA, et al. Rapid inhibition of cancer cell growth induced by lentiviral delivery and expression of mutant-template telomerase RNA and anti-telomerase short-interfering RNA. *Cancer Res*. 2004;**64**:4833–40.

99 Kelland LR. Overcoming the immortality of tumour cells by telomere and telomerase based cancer therapeutics—current status and future prospects. *Eur J Cancer*. 2005;**41**:971–9.

100 Lee KH, Rudolph KL, Ju YJ, et al. Telomere dysfunction alters the chemotherapeutic profile of transformed cells. *Proc Natl Acad Sci U S A*. 2001;**98**:3381–6.

101 Mender I, Gryaznov S, Dikmen ZG, et al. Induction of telomere dysfunction by the telomerase substrate precursor, 6-thio-2′ deoxyguanosine. *Cancer Discov*. 2015;**5**:82–95.

15 Cancer metabolism

Natalya N. Pavlova, PhD ▪ Craig B. Thompson, MD

Overview

Successful cell proliferation is dependent on a profound remodeling of cellular metabolism, required to support the biosynthetic needs of a growing cell. Constitutive signaling through aberrantly activated oncogenes activates pro-growth metabolic circuits that can lock cancer cells into net macromolecular synthesis and resistance to cell death. Oncogenic signaling can induce cellular uptake of metabolic substrates, such as glucose and glutamine, as well as utilization of unconventional nutrient sources. In contrast to nonproliferating tissues, which preferentially oxidize acquired metabolic substrates in mitochondria to fuel the oxidative phosphorylation and energy production, cancer cells prioritize the use of acquired metabolic substrates in anabolic processes, including fatty acid, cholesterol, nonessential amino acid, and nucleotide biosynthesis. The accumulation of these precursors supports the synthesis of the macromolecules necessary to sustain cell growth. Oncogene-directed increases in levels of select metabolites can also influence cellular processes beyond metabolic circuits, resulting in changes to the cellular epigenetic state as well as long-ranging effects on cells within the tumor microenvironment. Recent studies suggest these alterations in tumor cell metabolism can be exploited to improve the diagnosis and treatment of a wide variety of cancers.

Malicious builders

A unifying characteristic of cancer is loss of extrinsic controls over cell proliferation. In normal tissues, the quantities of cells, as well as their relative positions, are maintained by extracellular signaling, which include tissue-specific soluble growth factors as well as signals from the extracellular matrix to which cells adhere. Together, these mechanisms control the timing and the extent of cell survival and proliferation. Basal level of signaling enables day-to-day tissue maintenance, while the upregulation of growth signaling in response to tissue perturbations leads to enhanced production of terminally differentiated cells—for instance, epidermal keratinocytes and dermal fibroblasts in a setting of a cutaneous injury, or T cells in response to infection. In this manner, cell proliferation only takes place in response to a cell-type-specific signal of a sufficient strength and duration, which ensures that the overall structural and biochemical integrity of a metazoan organism is maintained.

In contrast to normal cells, genetic and epigenetic alterations acquired by cancer cells allow them to accumulate within tissues in a manner that is independent of extrinsic growth stimuli, at the same time becoming resistant to antigrowth signals.[1] Together, these adaptations enable survival and proliferation of cancer cells in settings where normal cell proliferation is strictly regimented. Mutations, copy number amplifications, and translocations targeting growth factor receptors are among the most frequently seen growth-promoting genetic alterations in tumors and are thus termed "driver alterations." For example, activating mutations in EGFR (epidermal growth factor receptor) are found in 10% of nonsmall cell lung carcinoma in United States and up to 35% in Japan,[2] and amplifications of HER2 are found in 25–30% of breast carcinomas.[3] In addition to growth factor receptors, downstream integrators of growth factor and matrix attachment signals are often aberrantly activated in cancer as well: for instance, up to 70% of breast cancers have mutations in the PI-3 kinase pathway,[4] up to 90% of pancreatic tumors are driven by activating mutations in KRAS,[5] and amplification of c-Myc is seen in up to 50% of human cancers regardless of tissue of origin.[6]

A cell that had received a proper growth signal commits to creating two daughter cells. To accomplish this, it must synthesize a complete set of biomolecules sufficient to build a new, functional cell. This set of biomolecules is extremely diverse and includes not only a vast array of proteins, but also lipids and their derivatives for building plasma and organelle membranes, hexose sugars for glycosylation of proteins, as well as pentose sugars and nucleotide bases for genome replication. To ensure that a cell does not attempt to replicate itself without having ample supply of biomolecules, the same signals that control proliferation are in control of nutrient uptake and the biosynthesis of macromolecular precursors. Thus, a growth-factor-stimulated cell undergoes remodeling of its metabolism in order to support the required biosynthesis. First, this remodeling involves acquiring a sufficient amount of building materials from the surrounding environment. Second, a proliferating cell must prioritize the use of these materials for biosynthesis, as opposed to catabolizing them for energy.

> **KEY POINTS**
>
> Constitutive signaling via aberrantly activated oncogenes allows cancer cells to perpetually receive pro-growth stimuli, which for normal tissues are only transient in nature. As a consequence, cancer metabolism is constitutively geared toward supporting proliferation.

This chapter will describe the mechanisms of how oncogenic transformation reshapes cellular metabolism toward nutrient acquisition and biosynthesis. Furthermore, this chapter will demonstrate how altered metabolic state of cancer cells, in turn, exerts profound effects on cellular epigenetic state and on tumor microenvironment, driving tumor expansion and dissemination. To this end, we will explore how alterations in tumor metabolism can be exploited in cancer detection and therapy.

From yeast to mammals—same means to different ends

Metabolic pathways and enzymes that drive their progression are remarkably conserved throughout evolution, yet the way the

Holland-Frei Cancer Medicine, Ninth Edition. Edited by Robert C. Bast Jr., Carlo M. Croce, William N. Hait, Waun Ki Hong, Donald W. Kufe, Martine Piccart-Gebhart, Raphael E. Pollock, Ralph R. Weichselbaum, Hongyang Wang, and James F. Holland.
© 2017 John Wiley & Sons, Inc. ISBN: 978-1-118-93469-2

metabolism of metazoan cells is regulated is fundamentally distinct from unicellular organisms. Unicellular organisms, such as bacteria or yeast, use external nutrient abundance as a signal to begin proliferating.[7] By attuning their proliferation to the environmental conditions, this strategy allows them to maximize their evolutionary success. For a metazoan organism, on the other hand, an evolutionary goal is not to multiply its cells to no end—which would lead to a physiologic chaos—but to maintain the functionality and structural integrity of its organs and tissues, repair injuries, and fight infections. To serve this goal, metazoans have developed complex and tissue-specific control mechanisms, which regulate cell survival and proliferation, yet allow for rapid induction of proliferation of specific cell populations when needed. Accordingly, the pro-proliferative metabolic state of cancer cells, driven by the loss of tissue-specific control mechanisms, can be best understood by first examining the differences in metabolic regulation in metazoans and in unicellular eukaryotes.

Metabolism of living cells is centered on the acquisition and stepwise biochemical transformation of molecules, which consist of reduced carbon and nitrogen. Glucose is a major metabolic substrate that can be utilized by all living cells as a source of (1) bioenergetic equivalents in a form of high-energy phosphate bonds of adenosine triphosphate (ATP) and (2) carbon building blocks, which can be used to produce a variety of biomolecules. One key chemical constituent that a glucose molecule does not provide is nitrogen. Nitrogen is required for the biosynthesis of amino acids and nucleotide bases, thus, an access to a source of reduced nitrogen is critical for both unicellular eukaryotes and metazoans. Although some bacteria can reduce atmospheric nitrogen to ammonia, most species must acquire a reduced form of nitrogen from the environment. Unicellular organisms can use free ammonia (NH_4^+) as a source of reduced nitrogen. For example, a wild-type, or prototrophic, yeast culture can proliferate in a so-called synthetic complete medium, which consists purely of glucose as a sole carbon source and ammonia as a sole nitrogen source. A yeast cell has all metabolic enzymes to synthesize a complete spectrum of biomolecules from the materials provided.

Metazoan organisms rely on glucose as a preferred carbon source and amino acids as the primary source of reduced nitrogen. In contrast to unicellular organisms, metazoans have lost the ability to synthesize 9 out of 20 amino acids required for protein synthesis (these nine amino acids are termed "essential," while the rest are termed "nonessential"). The amino acid glutamine, a carrier of two nitrogen atoms, is the predominant "nitrogen currency" for metazoan organisms. Because of its special importance as a reduced nitrogen source, glutamine is a "conditionally essential" amino acid for most proliferating metazoan cells.[8]

The significance of glucose and glutamine as key metabolic substrates for metazoan cells can be illustrated by the fact that in a mammalian organism, nearly constant levels of these two nutrients are maintained in plasma at all times: glucose levels are within the range of 4–6 mM and glutamine, the most abundant amino acid in plasma, ranges within 0.6–0.9 mM.[9] These steady levels of glucose and glutamine are maintained by a combination of hormone-mediated utilization of glycogen stores in muscle and liver, *de novo* synthesis of glutamine and glucose, as well as the stimulation of feeding behavior.

Unicellular organisms do not have steady levels of carbon and nitrogen sources around them at all times. Instead, they rely on nutrient sensing mechanisms to assess the availability of nutrients in their environment. In yeast, for instance, glucose limitation leads to Snf1 kinase [a homolog of adenosine monophosphate (AMP)-activated protein kinase (AMPK) in mammalian cells]

activation, which promotes energy production and suppresses biosynthetic processes.[10] Addition of glucose to a yeast culture triggers a shift toward biosynthetic metabolism and proliferation.[11,12] When glucose is abundant, Ras1 and Ras2 GTPases, homologs of the mammalian RAS protein family, become active and promote cell cycle progression. Another signaling mediator downstream of glucose is Sch9 kinase, which is related to Akt and S6 kinases in mammals and plays a role in promoting the use of glucose for biosynthetic processes.[13] Concurrently, the amino acid status of a yeast cell is measured through Gcn2 serine/threonine kinase, which is homologous to mammalian GCN2. Gcn2 is activated by uncharged tRNA, which accumulates in cells when amino acid levels are insufficient. Activated Gcn2, in turn, inhibits protein translation rates and induces Gcn4 (ATF4 in mammals), a transcription factor that controls expression of a number of enzymes involved in *de novo* synthesis of amino acids.[14] In the absence of glucose, however, active Snf1 represses Gcn4 expression, thus coordinating the metabolism of nitrogen and carbon.[15] As intracellular amino acid levels rise, they, in turn, activate TOR1/2 (mTOR in mammalian cells), which acts as a coordinator of a number of anabolic processes, including protein translation and biosynthesis of fatty acids. If nutrient sources remain plentiful, cell growth is converted into cell division and the process is repeated until the extracellular nutrient supply falls below the necessary threshold.

Cells within a metazoan organism are surrounded by ample glucose and glutamine in plasma and interstitial fluid, yet in contrast to yeast, they do not proliferate unless a proper extrinsic growth signal is present. First of all, the very access of cells to the extracellular pools of glucose and glutamine is controlled by receptor tyrosine kinases, proteins that are absent in unicellular eukaryotes. We now appreciate that stimulation by a cytokine or a growth factor, for example, directs a cell to take up nutrients, providing it with a supply chain of metabolic substrates. To this end, signals from receptor tyrosine kinases converge on PI-3 kinase/Akt, activation of which triggers rapid translocation of glucose transporters (GLUTs) from the cytosol-localized endosomal vesicles to the plasma membrane,[16,17] as well as stimulates GLUT gene expression,[18] driving the entry of glucose into cells. In illustration of this paradigm, PI-3 kinase/Akt signaling facilitates glucose uptake by populations of cells that are induced to undergo proliferative expansion, for example, activated T cells mounting an immune response,[19] or those induced to synthesize massive amounts of macromolecules, such as milk-producing cells of the mammary gland during lactation.[20]

In addition to effects on glucose transport, growth-factor-stimulated mammalian cells rapidly induce transcription of a set of immediate-early genes, one of which is the transcription factor c-Myc. C-Myc drives expression of a large set of metabolic genes and plays a role as a gatekeeper of cellular access to glutamine—the major metazoan source of nitrogen.[21] To this end, c-Myc facilitates the expression of glutamine transporters, ASCT2 and SN2,[22] as well as a glutaminase enzyme, GLS1, which catalyzes the breakdown of glutamine to glutamate and free ammonia.[23] Through facilitation of glutamine acquisition, c-Myc also indirectly influences the uptake of essential amino acids by the cell. Essential amino acid transport into cells is coupled to the efflux of glutamine into the extracellular space.[24] This mechanism allows cells to coordinate the import of essential amino acids to intracellular glutamine status.

Besides signals from receptor tyrosine kinases, cellular anchorage to the extracellular matrix is also needed to facilitate glucose uptake. Glucose consumption is suppressed in cells that are deprived of the matrix attachment even in the presence of soluble growth factors.[25]

This ensures that not only proliferation, but also positions of cells within the tissue are controlled on a metabolic level.

Taken together, pro-growth signaling through receptor tyrosine kinases has emerged as a control point for nutrient acquisition. Although conserved from yeast to mammals, mammalian RAS is no longer governed by glucose abundance, but by tissue-specific receptors. Similarly, mammalian TOR, while retaining its sensitivity to amino acid levels, have been harnessed by growth signaling control via Akt-dependent phosphorylation and inactivation of TSC2, a negative regulator of mTOR. Next, we will next examine how genetic alterations in growth signaling pathways influence the nutrient uptake in cancer cells.

KEY POINTS

Nutrient abundance is sufficient to stimulate proliferation of unicellular organisms, but not of metazoan cells, which has relegated the control over the ability to access nutrients around them to extrinsic growth stimuli.

Bad table manners of cancer cells

Discovery of the fundamental differences in rates of nutrient uptake between tumors and nontransformed tissues was among the earliest in modern cancer research, predating the discovery of the oncogenes and the role of carcinogens in tumorigenesis. In the 1920s, biochemical characterization of cancer cells from peritoneal ascites and slices of normal, nonproliferating tissues by German physiologist Otto Warburg revealed that the rate of consumption of glucose by tumors far exceeds that of normal tissues.[26] Some 30 years later, American pathologist Harry Eagle showed that glutamine requirements of HeLa cells in culture exceed the needs for other amino acids by 10- to a 100-fold, far surpassing the quantity needed for protein synthesis.[27]

On a signaling level, cellular glucose uptake is controlled through PI-3 kinase/Akt, which targets GLUTs to plasma membrane, as well as promotes their expression on a transcriptional level.[17] Thus, cancer-specific alterations in PI-3 kinase/Akt signaling allow cancer cells to consume glucose constitutively. Activated RAS and c-Src can promote GLUT1 expression as well.[28] To match the supply of carbon with a supply of nitrogen, tumor cells concurrently increase their uptake of glutamine. As described previously, the key driver of glutamine uptake and utilization in mammalian cells is c-Myc.[22,29] With c-Myc levels aberrantly elevated, cancer cells continuously import and utilize available glutamine for bioenergetic support, nucleotide biosynthesis, and to coordinate essential amino acid uptake and nonessential amino acid biosynthesis in support of protein production.

Tumors originate within the confines of a normal tissue, which is not suited to sustain uncontrolled cellular proliferation. Thus, tumors often lack adequate vasculature, as *de novo* angiogenesis within tissues is negatively regulated by tissue-specific factors.[30] Capillaries that do form in response to tumor-secreted pro-angiogenic molecules tend to be underdeveloped and inefficient in delivering oxygen and nutrients to a growing tumor. As proliferation of cancer cells depletes the microenvironment around them of amino acids and glucose, growing tumors face increasingly unfavorable conditions for proliferation. One adaptation that cancer cells use to withstand nutrient limitations is *autophagy*—a regulated process of self-catabolism of proteins, lipids, and even whole organelles as a temporary means of sustaining viability during starvation.[31] A major cellular bioenergetic sensor, AMPK, initiates the process of autophagy in response to falling ATP/AMP levels,

whereas mTOR, on the other hand, acts as an autophagy inhibitor.[32] The significance of autophagy for tumor growth *in vivo* has been demonstrated in mutant Kras[G12D] and Braf[V600E]-driven lung tumors, in which the genetic knockout of the autophagy machinery component Atg7 dramatically limits tumor cell accumulation and aggressiveness.[33,34]

Although autophagy can serve as a temporary means to survive nutrient shortages and maintain cellular bioenergetics, it cannot be used as a source of new biomass. In addition to intracellular proteins, KRAS- and c-Src-transformed cells have been recently shown to recover amino acids from proteins dissolved in extracellular fluid, which are consumed via large (up to $1–2$ μm in diameter) vesicles at sites of plasma membrane ruffling.[35] These vesicles are called macropinosomes (from latin *pino*—"to drink"). Under conditions of nutrient depletion, macropinosomes are targeted to lysosomes, where engulfed cargo is degraded. This alternative, "scavenging" form of nutrient uptake allows cells to survive amino acid limitations by unlocking otherwise inaccessible amino acid stores. RAS-driven macropinocytosis is an evolutionarily ancient mechanism of acquiring nutrients. In fact, it can be a primary pathway of nutrient acquisition in slime molds, such as *Dictyostelium*.[36] Thus, reactivation of macropinocytosis in oncogene-transformed cells can be viewed as yet another example of how cancer cells utilize evolutionarily ancient mechanisms of nutrient uptake.

Another problem that stems from the inadequacies of tumor vasculature is reduced supply of oxygen, or hypoxia. Lack of sufficient oxygen has a profound effect on cellular metabolism as it inhibits those biochemical reactions in which oxygen is consumed. One reaction that becomes inhibited in hypoxic conditions is stearoyl-CoA desaturase 1 (SCD1)-catalyzed desaturation of fatty acid carbon bonds to create unsaturated fatty acids, which are essential for proper fluidity of plasma and organelle membranes. To circumvent this problem, Ras-transformed cells were shown to be able to bypass the need for SCD1-catalyzed desaturation reaction by scavenging unsaturated lipids from the extracellular environment.[37]

KEY POINTS

Oncogene signaling allows cancer cells to use conventional metabolic sources, glucose and glutamine, in an unrestricted manner, as well as enables cells to access unconventional sources of biomolecules.

The traveling electrons

Most biochemical reactions within living cells are energetically unfavorable and require catalysis by specific metabolic enzymes. Metabolic reactions can be divided into two types: (1) *catabolic*—in which complex biochemical substrates are degraded to simpler constituents and (2) *anabolic*—in which complex biomolecules, such as amino acids, fatty acids, and nucleotides, are produced from simpler constituents. Catabolic processes involve reactions in which substrates undergo oxidation. Electrons derived from these oxidative steps are captured in a form of hydride anions ($:H^-$), which are carried by specialized enzyme cofactors NAD+ and FAD (NADH and FADH2 in their reduced forms), or NADP+ (NADPH in its reduced form). The chemical energy of electrons from NADH and FADH2 is then utilized by a series of enzyme complexes of *the electron transport chain*, which is located at the inner membrane of mitochondria. NADH/FADH2-derived electrons travel down the electron transport chain until they react with oxygen to produce water. The chemical energy of electrons that are being passed along the electron transport chain is used to create a proton gradient between the mitochondrial matrix and the mitochondrial intermembrane space. The resulting build-up of electrochemical potential across the inner mitochondrial membrane, in turn, fuels the activity of ATP synthase, a supramolecular complex that regenerates high-energy phosphate bonds of ATP from ADP. The coupling of electron transport to ADP conversion to ATP is termed *oxidative phosphorylation*.

In living cells, the ratio of ATP to ADP provides the thermodynamic driving force for a myriad of energetically unfavorable cellular processes, as well as for protein and lipid phosphorylation by kinases—a versatile mode of regulating functions of a variety of proteins and transmitting signals within a cell.

The maintenance of an electrochemical proton gradient through the electron transport chain is dependent on the availability of oxygen—the terminal acceptor of electrons, and ADP—a substrate for the ATP synthase. An excessive influx of electrons from NADH/FADH2 can deplete the supply of either of these, stopping the oxidative phosphorylation. Consequently, electrons that become stalled in the electron transport chain can be lost over time from their intramembrane carriers, reacting with the aqueous environment of the cell to produce reactive oxygen species (ROS). ROS are avid oxidants, which readily react with a wide spectrum of biomolecules—including lipids, proteins, and nucleotides. To control their redox state, cells produce a variety of ROS-neutralizing molecules, or antioxidants. However, when ROS become elevated beyond the cellular antioxidant capacity, they can cause widespread damage to cellular organelles and DNA.

As noted previously, most catabolic reactions couple the oxidation of their substrates to the reduction of NAD+ and FAD to NADH and FADH2. In contrast, a few metabolic reactions result in a transfer of electrons to a structurally related cofactor, NADP+, reducing it to NADPH. Whereas NADH and FADH2 are mainly used for energy production, NADPH replenishes the cellular antioxidant pool by sustaining the reduced state of glutathione and related sulfhydryl-containing molecules. In addition, the reducing power of NADPH is used in biosynthesis of complex biomolecules, such as fatty acids and nucleotides, which require sequences of reductive reactions. How does a cell choose to prioritize one class of such reactions over others? As it turns out, the allocation of substrates into processes that support bioenergetics versus those with biosynthetic outcomes is coordinated by many of the same pro-growth signals that promote the uptake of biochemical substrates by cells in the first place.

> **KEY POINTS**
>
> A living cell maintains its viability by oxidizing biochemical substrates acquired from the environment. Catabolic reactions produce simple building blocks, which can be consecutively utilized in biosynthetic reactions. In addition, catabolic reactions serve as sources of reducing power to fuel cellular energy production, enable biosynthetic reactions, and bolster the antioxidant defense.

Warburg effect—how to play safe while looking sloppy

Glucose catabolism takes place in two cellular compartments: its first stage, glycolysis, occurs in the cytosol, while the second stage is localized to mitochondria and involves a series of reactions of the tricarboxylic acid cycle (TCA cycle, which is also called citric acid or Krebs cycle). Phosphorylation of glucose by a hexokinase (HK) to produce glucose 6-phosphate is the first committed step

of glycolysis (Figure 1a). The HK reaction prevents the exit of glucose back into the extracellular space. A second committed step of glycolysis is an irreversible phosphorylation catalyzed by phosphofructokinase enzyme (PFK1). Along with targeting the GLUT1 transporter to the plasma membrane, Akt potentiates the action of both HK[38] and PFK1,[39] thus acting as a coordinator of glucose progression through glycolysis. In fact, the ability of Akt to suppress apoptosis in response to growth factor withdrawal is dependent on glucose;[40] moreover, overexpression of GLUT1 and HK alone is sufficient to suppress growth factor withdrawal-induced cell death.[39] PFK1 activity in cancer cells is further enhanced by frequent overexpression of PFKFB3,[41] an enzyme that produces fructose 2,6-bisphospate, an allosteric activator of PFK1.

Downstream of glucose capture and degradation, the various intermediates of glycolysis and the TCA cycle provide the backbones of essentially all the amino acids, acyl groups, and nucleotides a cell can synthesize *de novo* to support macromolecular synthesis. When it was discovered that oncogenic mutations resulted in flooding the cell with glucose that can maintain a supply of these precursors, it became clear why the Warburg effect was selected for during tumorigenesis. A cell engaged in excessive glucose uptake becomes resistant to apoptosis, has virtually unlimited supply of macromolecular precursors, and simply secretes any carbon in excess of its needs by converting the end product of glycolysis, pyruvate, into lactate, which is expelled from the cell. This form of gluttony exhibited by tumors harboring mutations that increase glucose uptake became known as *aerobic glycolysis*—to distinguish it from the well-established increase in glucose uptake exhibited by normal cells when depleted of oxygen, or *anaerobic glycolysis*.

Recently, it has been shown that aerobic glycolysis is not restricted to tumor cells. When stimulated with growth factors, normal cells too, begin to display Warburg-like metabolism.[42] The discovery that the Warburg effect is a growth-factor-driven phenomenon and not a peculiar "abnormality" of cancer cells warranted exploring whether it may be in fact, a part of a metabolic reprogramming aimed at increasing the cellular capacity for biosynthesis. Thus, it is now becoming appreciated that maximization of the bioenergetic yield from glucose catabolism would run contrary to the biosynthetic priorities of a growth-factor-stimulated cell.[43]

How can glycolysis help biosynthesis? There are several ways through which glycolytic intermediates can act as substrates for producing both biosynthetic precursors and NADPH (Figure 1a). One such pathway is the *pentose phosphate pathway* (PPP), which begins with glucose 6-phosphate. Glucose 6-phosphate is oxidized to produce two NADPH molecules, and after a series of interconversions, it produces ribose 5-phosphate—a structural component of nucleotides. Significantly, the PPP enzyme transketolase-like 1 (TKTL1) is required for growth of a number of cancer cell lines and is predictive of poor prognosis in patients.[44]

Another key branch point of glycolysis is at the level of 3-phosphoglycerate. In a series of three consecutive reactions, 3-phosphoglycerate is converted to the amino acid serine. As metabolic studies demonstrate, serine biosynthesis is massively upregulated in tumors beyond the amount necessary for protein biosynthesis.[45] Moreover, PHGDH gene, encoding the enzyme that catalyzes the limiting step in serine biosynthesis, is frequently amplified in breast cancer and in melanoma, predicts tumor aggressiveness and is required for tumor growth *in vivo*.[46,47] Why do tumors produce so much serine? Serine is not only used as a building block in protein translation, but is also a key substrate in a so-called *one-carbon*, or *folate cycle*, where a serine-donated carbon is passed on to a tetrahydrofolate (THF) molecule. The folate cycle involves a complex series of oxidative–reductive transformations,

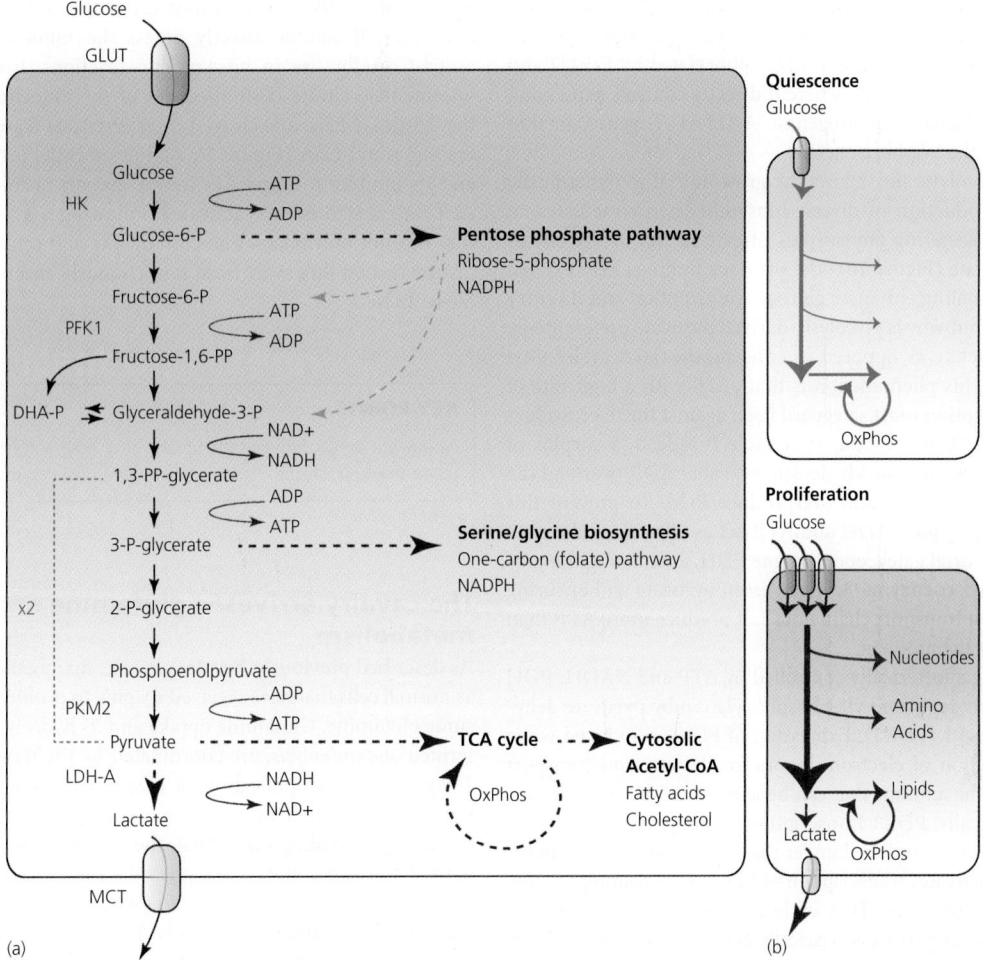

Figure 1 Glycolysis. (a) Catabolism of one glucose molecule via glycolysis yields two molecules of pyruvate, which can then be transported to the mitochondria and used as a source of acetyl-CoA for the TCA cycle. Alternatively, pyruvate can be reduced to lactate and excreted out of the cell. Besides its bioenergetic uses, glycolysis also provides biosynthetic power to cells. Glucose-6-phosphate can be utilized in the PPP to generate NADPH and ribose 5-phosphate for nucleotide biosynthesis; or, its intermediates can be shunted back into glycolysis (shown by gray dashed arrows). In addition, 3-phosphoglycerate can be converted to serine, a carbon donor for the folate (one-carbon) cycle. Folate cycle generates NADPH, as well as provides one-carbon units for the biosynthesis of nucleotide bases and for methylation reactions. GLUT, glucose transporter, HK, hexokinase, PFK1, phosphofructokinase 1, PKM2, pyruvate kinase M2, LDH-A, lactate dehydrogenase A, MCT, monocarboxylate transporter, OxPhos, oxidative phosphorylation. (b) Quiescent cells consume moderate amount of glucose and preferentially catabolize it to pyruvate to fuel oxidative phosphorylation in mitochondria. In proliferating cells, growth factor signaling or constitutively active oncogenes facilitate the increase in glucose uptake. In contrast to a quiescent cell, the majority of glucose consumed by a growth-stimulated cell goes into biosynthetic pathways to produce nucleotides, amino acids, and lipids—or is expelled as lactate.

which involve serine-donated methyl group, and is indispensable for a number of processes that affect cellular growth and proliferation.[48] In particular, serine-derived carbon is used as (1) a carbon donor for purine synthesis; (2) a donor of methyl groups onto S-adenosylmethionine (SAM), a substrate for histone and DNA methyltransferase enzymes, and (3) a donor of reducing power for the production of NADPH. As a recent study has demonstrated, up to 50% of all cellular NADPH may be generated via one-carbon pathway.[49] Taken together, diversion of glycolytic intermediates into the pentose phosphate shunt and into the serine biosynthesis pathway both provide building blocks for nucleotide generation as well as produce NADPH.

How does a cell regulate the rate at which glycolytic intermediates are diverted into biosynthetic pathways? Exploration of the interplay between growth factor signaling pathways and metabolism have led to a seminal discovery that has shed light on this question. Specifically, tumor cells express an M2 splice variant of pyruvate kinase M (called PKM2), while their normal counterparts preferentially express the M1 variant.[50] Pyruvate kinase is a rate-limiting enzyme that catalyzes the conversion of phosphoenolpyruvate (PEP) to pyruvate (Figure 1a). Intriguingly, the PKM2 isoform is a less active form of pyruvate kinase than PKM1. Moreover, PKM2, but not PKM1, is susceptible to further inhibition via binding to phosphorylated tyrosine residues through its unique C-terminal sequence.[51] Thus, the activity of PKM2 becomes dampened even further in response to increased tyrosine kinase signaling. Replacement of PKM2 with a PKM1 isoform reduces the tumorigenic potential of cancer cells, promotes oxygen consumption, and inhibits production of lactate.[50] The lower rate of catalysis by PKM2 creates a "traffic jam" at the level of PEP, facilitating the entry of accumulated glycolytic intermediates into the two pathways described previously.[52] Reciprocally, products downstream of both PPP (succinylaminoimidazolecarboxamide ribose 5′-phosphate or SAICAR)[53] and serine biosynthetic pathway (serine itself)[54] act as allosteric activators of PKM2, which allows a cell to balance the biosynthetic and bioenergetic uses of glycolysis.

Besides its function as a gatekeeper of glycolysis, PKM2 also promotes glucose utilization at the level of gene expression. Thus, in EGF-treated cells, PKM2 becomes phosphorylated by Erk1/2 and is translocated to the nucleus, where it directly controls expression of GLUT1 and lactate dehydrogenase A (LDH-A) genes, further contributing to the Warburg effect.[55]

Increased glycolytic flux allows the growing cell to dynamically regulate the production of diverse biosynthetic intermediates, at the same time secreting any surplus of carbon out of the cell in the form of lactate (Figure 1b). The previous findings help explain why growth signaling enhances glucose consumption and its entry into glycolysis, but why is glycolysis-derived pyruvate preferentially converted to lactate as opposed to entering the TCA cycle? One explanation of this phenomenon is that a cell with a high rate of glucose consumption must safeguard itself against the overproduction of $NADH/FADH2$ in the TCA cycle.[56] Indeed, a surplus of electron donors would quickly deplete available ADP, overload the electron transport chain, and overproduce ROS. To prevent this from happening, both NADH and ATP act as allosteric inhibitors of the mitochondrial gatekeeper enzyme PDH, attenuating the production of acetyl-coenzyme A (CoA) from pyruvate and ensuring that the electron transport chain does not produce more ATP than a cell can use at the moment.

Besides being allosterically controlled by ATP and NADH, PDH is also negatively regulated via phosphorylation by pyruvate dehydrogenase kinase 1 (PDK1). Expression of PDK1 is induced when cellular production of electron donors for the electron transport chain exceeds the amount that can be assimilated by the available oxygen. Specifically, PDK1 transcription is upregulated by HIF1α, a transcription factor induced under these conditions.[57,58] Concurrently, HIF1α activates transcription of LDH-A, re-routing the flux of carbon away from the TCA cycle and toward lactate production.[59] Even though HIF1α is classically activated by oxygen deficit, transformed cells exhibiting excess glycolysis induce HIF1α even in normoxic conditions.[60] Nor is HIF1α the only transcriptional activator of PDK1. Indeed, another commonly activated pathway in cancer, the Wnt/β-catenin pathway, has been shown to promote the Warburg effect by upregulating the expression of PDK1, as well as the lactate transporter MCT1.[61]

A damaging effect of an unrestricted pyruvate catabolism has been recently proposed as a metabolic mechanism of oncogene-induced senescence (OIS). OIS is a phenomenon in which overexpression of mutant oncogenes, such as RAS or BRAF, triggers growth arrest, overproduction of ROS, and DNA damage response.[62] Interestingly, the onset of OIS is dependent on PDH activity. To this end, the modulation of the PDH activity by expressing PDK1 or inhibiting PDH phosphatase PDP2 was found to facilitate cellular escape from OIS.[63]

A decade ago, it was discovered that the role of mitochondria in the successful evolution of the eukaryotic cells depended more on their contributions to macromolecular biosynthesis than to ATP production. In an evolutionary sense, mitochondria became essential organelles because they supplied a variety of precursors for biosynthetic reactions. In what is referred to as cataplerosis, TCA cycle intermediates exit the mitochondria to be used as precursors for a variety of anabolic reactions—including biosynthesis of sugars, nonessential amino acids, and fatty acids. In addition, mitochondria support the synthesis of iron–sulfur (Fe–S) clusters, which are central for the function of a variety of mitochondrial as well as cytosolic enzymes.

Cytosol-localized biosynthesis of fatty acids and cholesterol is particularly essential for proliferating cells. A universal precursor for fatty acid and cholesterol biosynthesis is acetyl-CoA, but because the bulky CoA cannot cross the mitochondrial membrane, a cell cannot directly access the mitochondrial pool of acetyl-CoA for use in biosynthetic reactions. Instead, the TCA intermediate citrate is shuttled out of the mitochondria and into the cytosol, where it is cleaved by ATP-citrate lyase (ACL), regenerating acetyl-CoA (Figure 2). ACL is essential for tumorigenesis, and its inhibition suppresses tumor growth in mice.[64,65] Notably, ACL enzyme becomes activated following Akt induction,[66] so that Akt not only enables glucose uptake and catabolism, but also diverts carbon flux away from mitochondria and toward fatty acid biosynthesis.

KEY POINTS

Pro-growth signals facilitate the uptake of glucose and remodel the glycolytic flux to satisfy the increased biosynthetic demands of a growing cell.

The cavalry arrives!—glutamine and anabolic metabolism

As described previously, besides glucose, many cancer cells (as well as normal cells that have received a signal to proliferate) avidly consume glutamine. Glutamine uptake and its hydrolysis to glutamate, termed *glutaminolysis*, are coordinated by the transcription factor c-Myc; in fact, amplification of c-Myc was shown to make cells critically dependent on glutamine supply. Why is glutamine so essential for dividing cells? First, the carbon skeleton of glutamine is used to restock the TCA cycle when its intermediates exit the mitochondria to participate in anabolic synthesis. Because proliferating cells continuously borrow TCA cycle intermediates, such as citrate, to support biosynthesis, cataplerotic processes must be balanced by the influx of carbons elsewhere in the cycle in a process termed *anaplerosis*. Two major anaplerotic inputs have been described: one is via glutamine-derived α-ketoglutarate and another is via pyruvate carboxylase (PC)-catalyzed carboxylation of pyruvate into oxaloacetate (Figure 2). Though glutamine is a preferential anaplerotic substrate in cancer cells, cells with high PC activity can use a PC-derived oxaloacetate to survive glutamine deprivation or glutaminase suppression.[67] In addition, besides replenishing the TCA cycle, glutamine-derived α-ketoglutarate can exit the TCA cycle halfway in the form of malate and become oxidized by malic enzyme (ME) in the cytosol to produce NADPH.[68] Together, ME, PPP, and folate cycle produce virtually all of the cellular NADPH.

As discussed previously, the entry of glycolysis-derived pyruvate into the TCA cycle may be restricted by negative regulatory inputs into PDH—for example, as a result of upregulated HIF1α or activation of Wnt signaling. This, however, creates a quandary—if pyruvate is diverted away from the TCA cycle by the coordinate inhibition of pyruvate dehydrogenase and activation of LDH-A and MCT, how can the TCA cycle produce enough citrate for biosynthesis? In fact, some cancer cells have found an unexpected solution to this problem by using glutamine-derived α-ketoglutarate to run a section of the TCA cycle in reverse, producing citrate for fatty acid biosynthesis in conditions where pyruvate-derived acetyl-CoA levels are limiting (Figure 2).[69,70]

Besides contributing its carbon skeleton to the TCA cycle, glutamine is a major donor of reduced nitrogen for cellular needs. Although its amine nitrogen is used primarily in nonessential

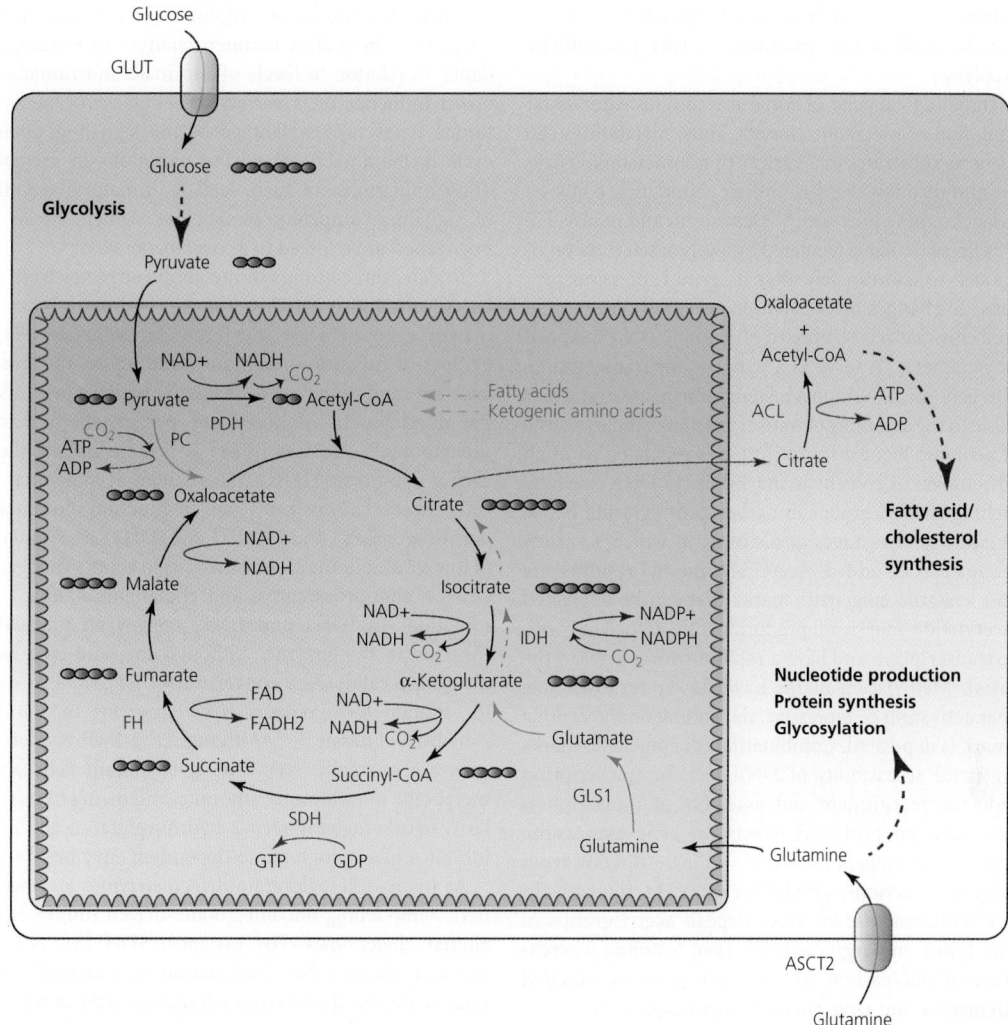

Figure 2 Carbon metabolism in mitochondria. Glycolysis-derived pyruvate serves as a donor of acetyl-CoA for the tricarboxylic acid (TCA) cycle. Cataplerotic efflux of citrate into the cytosol (shown by a maroon arrow) allows maintaining the extramitochondrial pool of acetyl-CoA for fatty acid and cholesterol biosynthesis. Glutamine and pyruvate function as anaplerotic substrates to restock the TCA cycle intermediates (shown by solid green arrows). In conditions when acetyl-CoA is limiting, citrate can be produced from the reductive carboxylation of glutamine-derived α-ketoglutarate (shown by dashed green arrows). Pink circles represent a number of carbon atoms in a molecule. GLUT, glucose transporter, PDH, pyruvate dehydrogenase, PC, pyruvate carboxylase, IDH, isocitrate dehydrogenase, SDH, succinate dehydrogenase, FH, fumarate hydratase, ACL, ATP-citrate lyase, GLS1, glutaminase, ASCT2, glutamine transporter.

amino acid biosynthesis, amide nitrogen of glutamine contributes to the biosynthesis of purine and pyrimidine bases. Thus, one molecule of glutamine is needed to build a thymine or a uracil, adenine and cytosine use two, and guanine synthesis requires three glutamine molecules. Notably, together with promoting glutamine uptake for synthesis of nucleotide bases, c-Myc also controls the expression of a number of nucleotide biosynthetic enzymes—namely, thymidylate synthase (TS), inosine monophosphate dehydrogenase 2 (IMPDH2), and phosphoribosyl pyrophosphate synthetase 2 (PRPS2), a rate-limiting enzyme in the biosynthesis of nucleotides.[71,72]

In conclusion, the notion that pro-growth signaling is a central facilitator of the acquisition and use of extracellular nutrients by metazoan cells has overturned a long-held view that cellular metabolic networks are self-regulating and exist independently from signaling inputs. However, metabolic circuits themselves are not merely passive recipients of cellular signals. In fact, a cell continuously monitors rising and falling levels of select metabolites

and integrates this information so as to coordinate global decisions including growth and differentiation.

> **KEY POINTS**
>
> Glutamine fuels anabolic metabolism by serving as both a source of carbon to replenish the TCA cycle intermediates and maintain its biosynthetic capacity, as well as providing reduced nitrogen for the biosynthesis of nucleotides and nonessential amino acids.

The nucleus smells what's cooking

Metabolites are known to act as allosteric modulators of specific metabolic enzymes, providing regulatory feedback that allows a cell to adjust the output of its catabolic and anabolic reactions in response to fluctuations in metabolite levels. An example of such regulation is allosteric activation of glycolysis gatekeeper enzyme PKM2 by SAICAR and serine, products of two biosynthetic branches of glycolysis.

Notably, the signaling capacity of some metabolites extends far beyond the regulation of metabolic circuits. Thus, metabolites can act as cofactors or as substrates in a variety of nonmetabolic enzymatic reactions, and through changes in their abundance, convey a regulatory message to these processes.[73] Deposition and removal of epigenetic marks in particular is regulated by levels of select metabolites, allowing a cell to coordinately alter its gene expression programs in response to changes in its nutritional status.[74]

Eukaryotic cell chromatin is composed of genomic DNA wrapped around histone octamers. To serve as a template for transcription, select loci within genomic DNA must be temporarily unwound and become accessible to the assembly of transcriptional complexes. The accessibility of genomic loci for transcription is regulated through deposition and removal of epigenetic marks on (1) DNA itself, by covalently attaching methyl groups to carbon 5 of cytosine bases, and (2) select amino acid residues of histones, to which a variety of chemical groups can be added. Acetyl and methyl residues are among the most versatile epigenetic marks that can be deposited on histones. Acetylation marks are predominantly associated with enhanced gene transcription and have a rapid turnover rate (in the order of minutes). Methylation marks have slower turnover rate and can be either activating or repressive, depending on the residue on which the mark is deposited. Combinations of epigenetic marks influence the general accessibility of DNA loci for transcription as well as guide the recruitment and assembly of transcription complexes, thus exerting profound effects on gene expression. Both acetyl and methyl epigenetic marks originate directly from products of metabolic reactions, acetyl-CoA and SAM, respectively. Thus, histone acetyltransferase enzymes deposit acetyl groups of acetyl-CoA onto lysine and arginine residues of histones, whereas SAM, a product of one-carbon (folate) cycle, provides methyl groups for both histone and DNA methyltransferases.

Using metabolic intermediates as precursors for epigenetic marks allows a cell to respond to its "fed" status with targeted upregulation of metabolic genes. As an example, targeted depletion of extramitochondrial acetyl-CoA through genetic repression of ACL profoundly affects histone acetylation patterns, resulting in attenuated expression of GLUTs, HK, PFK1, and LDH-A.[75] In this manner, by affecting histone acetylation, high levels of acetyl-CoA can promote the utilization of glucose and reinforce the Warburg effect.

Not only the deposition, but the removal of acetyl and methyl marks from histones is guided by the cellular metabolic status as well. Thus, sirtuin deacetylases, which catalyze the removal of acetyl groups from histones, as well as a variety of nonhistone proteins, use an oxidized form of NAD+ as a cofactor;[76] similarly, oxidized FAD serves as a cofactor for a histone demethylase LSD1.[77] By sensing a shift in NAD+/NADH ratio, sirtuins coordinate multiple genetic and post-translational changes aimed at maximizing energy conservation and extraction from metabolic substrates.

A whole host of enzymes—some of which are epigenetic regulators, while others are involved in post-translational modifications of nonhistone proteins—are regulated by the abundance of TCA cycle metabolites: α-ketoglutarate, succinate, and fumarate. Specifically, α-ketoglutarate acts as a cofactor for Jumonji C domain-containing family of histone demethylases, a TET family of methylcytosine hydroxylases, as well as prolyl hydroxylases, a class of enzymes that regulate HIF1α levels, among other processes. In the course of reactions catalyzed by these enzymes, α-ketoglutarate itself is converted to succinate. Importantly, both succinate and its downstream product fumarate act as inhibitors of α-ketoglutarate-dependent enzymes.[78] In such a manner, changes in α-ketoglutarate abundance in relation to levels of succinate and fumarate may exert a broad influence on a variety of cellular processes. In fact, select tumor types take advantage of the signaling potential of TCA cycle metabolites by acquiring mutations in metabolic enzymes. These mutations, in turn, lead to unnatural elevations in levels of signaling-competent metabolites, which, in an analogy with oncogenes, are referred to as *oncometabolites*.[79]

To date, three groups of metabolic enzymes have been found to be recurrently mutated in cancer. TCA cycle enzymes succinate dehydrogenase (SDH) and fumarate hydratase (FH) are targeted by loss-of-function mutations, leading to the accumulation of succinate and fumarate, respectively. Biallelic loss of SDH underlies the development of hereditary paragangliomas and pheochromocytomas,[80] and loss of FH is responsible for the rare familial cancer syndrome HLRCC (hereditary leiomyomatosis and renal cell cancer).[81] Conversely, gain-of-function mutations in isocitrate dehydrogenases 1 and 2 (IDH1 and IDH2) are found in the majority of low-grade glioma cases, as well as in acute myelogenous leukemia (AML), chondrosarcoma, and cholangiosarcoma.[82-85] Oncogenic mutations in IDH1 and IDH2 convey an unusual neomorphic function to the enzyme. Although the wild-type isocitrate dehydrogenase catalyzes a conversion of isocitrate to α-ketoglutarate, the mutant form reduces α-ketoglutarate to a D-enantiomer of 2-hydroxyglutarate.[86,87] Although D-2-hydroxyglutarate levels in cells are normally very low, IDH-mutant cells accumulate this metabolite to millimolar amounts, and owing to its structural similarity to α-ketoglutarate, D-2-hydroxyglutarate acts as a competitive inhibitor of α-ketoglutarate-dependent enzymes.[88]

As many α-ketoglutarate-driven enzymes are involved in epigenetic remodeling, oncometabolite-driven tumors have profoundly altered epigenomes. For instance, SDH loss is associated with the increase in DNA methylation (a so-called hypermethylator phenotype) in SDH-driven paragangliomas as well as in sporadic gastrointestinal stromal tumors, a fraction of which harbors SDH mutations as well.[89,90] Similarly, mutant alleles of IDH1 and IDH2 are strongly associated with the hypermethylator phenotype in glioma and AML.[91,92] In AML in particular, IDH mutations are mutually exclusive with the loss-of-function mutations in methylcytosine hydroxylase TET2, further strengthening the mechanistic link between the two enzymes.[92] In various cellular settings, introduction of mutant IDH, or treatment with D-2-hydroxyglutarate, was sufficient to trigger alterations in DNA and histone methylation and suppress cell differentiation.[93,94] Conversely, targeted inhibition of mutant IDH enzymes promoted differentiation in glioma and AML cell models.[95,96] Taken together, through global remodeling of DNA and histone methylome, oncometabolites may contribute to tumorigenesis through locking cells in an undifferentiated state.

KEY POINTS

Metabolic adaptations of cancer cells do not only facilitate macromolecular biosynthesis, but can also exert profound nonmetabolic effects on cellular fate.

From petty thieves to ringleaders—how cancer cells corrupt their neighbors

Even though composed of genetically stable cells, the tissue microenvironment in the vicinity of a tumor becomes profoundly altered during tumorigenesis. Most strikingly, its constituents—fibroblasts, endothelial cells, and components of innate and adaptive immunity—convert from being pro-homeostatic into active enablers of tumor growth.[97] Tumors use a variety of signals to corrupt normal cells, including secreted factors, cell–cell interactions, as well as changes in metabolite levels. Two prominent examples illustrating how altered tumor metabolism affects its microenvironment are discussed as follows.

Increased nutrient consumption by tumors is coupled to the secretion of large amounts of lactate into the extracellular fluid, which has wide-ranging effects on tumor microenvironment. Thus, lactate contributes to the induction of angiogenesis by stabilizing HIF1α in endothelial cells[98] and potentiating pro-angiogenic NF-κB and PI3-kinase signaling,[99–101] as well as by promoting VEGF (vascular endothelial growth factor) secretion from macrophages.[102] At the same time, lactate attenuates local antitumor immune responses by suppressing migration of monocytes[103] and activation of T cells and dendritic cells,[104,105] as well as affecting the polarization state and localization patterns of tumor-associated macrophages.[106,107] Tumor-associated macrophages can assume two functional subtypes: M1, which is associated with secretion of pro-inflammatory cytokines, and M2 subtype, which is involved in immunosuppression and wound repair. Tumor-associated macrophages are predominantly M2-polarized, and M2 subtype has been shown to be directly induced by lactate.[106] Finally, accumulation of lactate contributes to a decreased pH of the tumor extracellular fluid, which, in turn, promotes the activity of numerous matrix-degrading enzymes and promotes invasion.[108,109]

Another strategy used by cancer cells to attenuate antitumor immune responses is through the selective depletion of the amino acid tryptophan from their microenvironment.[110] To this end, tumors upregulate the expression of tryptophan-degrading enzymes, indoleamine 2,3-dioxygenase (IDO) and tryptophan 2,3-dioxygenase (TDO), which both degrade tryptophan to its derivative kynurenine. Insufficient levels of tryptophan trigger apoptosis of effector T cells;[111] in addition, accumulation of kynurenine promotes the emergence of immune-suppressive regulatory T cells.[112] Finally, kynurenine-mediated signaling enhances invasiveness and extracellular-matrix-degrading capacity of tumor cells themselves.[113]

KEY POINTS

Cancer cells use the signaling capacity of select metabolites to influence the state of cells in their microenvironment and promote tumorigenesis.

Cancer metabolism comes into the clinic

For over three decades, increased uptake of glucose by cancer cells has been successfully exploited in tumor imaging, where the uptake of 2-deoxyglucose conjugated to ^{18}F, a radioactive isotope of fluorine, is detected by positron emission tomography (PET).[114] ^{18}F-Fluorodeoxyglucose (^{18}F-FDG) is transported into cells and is phosphorylated by HK in the same manner as glucose, yet cannot be further catabolized, which leads to its intracellular accumulation. A noninvasive tumor detection approach, ^{18}F-FDG-PET is widely used in the clinic for tumor detection and staging as well as for monitoring tumor response to therapy. However, ^{18}F-FDG-PET has a number of limitations, which include false-positive signals from tissue infiltration by immune cells (for instance, in autoimmune thyroiditis), or inability to detect those tumors that are

not markedly glycolytic (as is often the case in prostate cancer). In addition, some tissues, especially brain, exhibit high constitutive levels of glucose uptake, which precludes the detection of tumors localized to brain. Following the success of ^{18}F-FDG, other metabolite-based tracers, such as ^{18}F-fluoroglutamine,[115] ^{11}C-acetate,[116] and α-^{11}C-methyl-L-tryptophan,[117,118] are currently being developed. Other metabolic imaging approaches, such as ^{1}H magnetic resonance spectroscopy (MRS) are being developed for the use in the clinic. MRS can detect endogenously abundant metabolites in select tissues. For instance, MRS has been adapted to the detection of gliomas with IDH1 mutation, by using accumulation of D-2-hydroxyglutarate as a marker.[119]

In addition to tumor imaging, at least two metabolic cancer therapies have been successfully used in the clinic for decades. L-Asparaginase, a recombinant form of a bacterial enzyme that degrades the amino acid asparagine, was approved by the Food and Drug Administration in 1978 as an effective therapy for childhood acute lymphoblastic leukemia.[120] Leukemic cells lack the capacity to synthesize sufficient asparagine, so that the depletion of plasma asparagine (as well as, potentially, glutamine) sensitizes them to cell death. A class of drugs, which inhibit nucleotide biosynthesis, is another example of a successful metabolic therapy. These agents include 5-fluorouracil, an inhibitor of thymidine synthesis, gemcitabine and hydroxyurea, deoxyribonucleotide synthesis blockers, and an antifolate drug methotrexate, which interferes with dihydrofolate reductase-mediated synthesis of THF, disrupting the folate-cycle-driven synthesis of nucleotides. The therapeutic efficacy of antifolate drugs was first demonstrated by Sidney Farber in Boston in 1940s,[121] followed by the discovery of their mechanism of action in 1958.[122]

Dependence of cancer cells on glucose metabolism had prompted extensive testing of therapies that target the uptake of glucose or various steps in the glycolysis pathway. However, antiglycolytic interventions, such as, for example, inhibition of HK by a nonmetabolizable glucose analog 2-deoxyglucose or a drug lonidamine, had shown mixed results in trials, and lonidamide had undesirable systemic effects.[123] Furthermore, 2-deoxyglucose was shown to trigger compensatory activation of IGF-I receptor-mediated signaling.[124] A snapshot of therapeutic agents targeting metabolic pathways that are currently being developed are shown in Table 1.

Metformin, a standard-of-care antidiabetes drug, had shown clinical promise as both a therapeutic and a chemopreventive anticancer agent. A number of retrospective studies indicate that

Table 1 Cancer metabolic therapies currently undergoing clinical development.

Enzyme target	Targeting compound	Metabolic pathway
GLUT family of glucose transporters	Phloretin and silybin	Glucose uptake
MCT (lactate transporter)	AZD3965	Glycolysis
PDK1	Dichloroacetate	Pyruvate catabolism
Mitochondrial complex I	Metformin	Oxidative phosphorylation
Glutaminase (GLS1)	CB-839	Glutaminolysis
Fatty acid synthase	TVB-2640	Fatty acid biosynthesis
HMGCR	Statins	Sterol biosynthesis
IDH1	AG-120	Oncometabolite production
IDH2	AG-221	Oncometabolite production
IDO/TDO	INCB024360 and indoximod	Tryptophan degradation

patients, who were taking metformin as a part of their antidiabetes regimen, had both reduced cancer risk and better treatment outcomes. Effects of metformin were further confirmed in nondiabetic patients.[125] The mechanism of anticancer activity of metformin is likely to be complex. Metformin impairs mitochondrial oxidative phosphorylation via inhibition of electron transport chain complex I, which leads to an increase in AMP/ATP ratio and activation of AMPK.[126] In addition, metformin attenuates the production of ROS and reduce DNA damage, which may contribute to its cancer-preventive effects.[127] Finally, systemic effects of metformin, such as reduction of circulating IGF-I levels and liver gluconeogenesis, may play a role in its anticancer properties as well.

KEY POINTS

The dependence of tumor cells on various aspects of its altered metabolism has formed a basis for a number of imaging and therapeutic strategies.

Conclusions

Discoveries of modern cancer metabolism has elucidated how tumor cells reprogram their metabolism to sustain growth, circumvent nutrient and oxygen limitations, and alter their own fate as well as the fate of neighboring cells. There is, conceivably, a lot more left to learn about how a cell gauges the levels of its many metabolites and the complex ways in which it converts this information into decisions about nutrient acquisition, execution of cell death and differentiation programs, and a cross-talk with the microenvironment as well as the organism as a whole. In addition to macronutrients, the contribution of micronutrients, such as vitamins and metal ions, to metabolism and signaling of cancer cells is only beginning to be unraveled. Our growing understanding of cancer metabolism has already been translated into innovative imaging and therapeutic tools, and the arsenal of these applications will continue to grow in the foreseeable future.

Summary

Proliferation of cells within a metazoan organism is governed by external stimuli, including signals from soluble growth factors as well as from cellular attachments to the extracellular matrix. Pro-growth signals induce a profound shift in the metabolic state of a responding cell, increasing its capacity for de novo synthesis of macromolecules—namely, proteins, lipids, and nucleic acids, required for growth. Pro-growth signals directly facilitate the uptake of metabolic substrates from the surrounding environment, ensuring that a proliferating cell has an adequate supply of macromolecular precursors to grow. Pro-growth signals also dictate the downstream metabolic fate of acquired substrates, directing them toward the generation of precursors for a variety of biosynthetic reactions, which include fatty acid, cholesterol, nonessential amino acid, and nucleotide biosynthesis. In contrast to normal tissues, in which pro-growth signals are transient in nature, aberrantly activated oncogenes accumulated by cancer cells lock their metabolism in a constitutive state of nutrient acquisition and macromolecule biosynthesis.

Although pro-growth signals influence the uptake of metabolic substrates and their progression through cellular metabolic pathways, changes in levels of select metabolites, in turn, affect a diverse range of nonmetabolic processes in the cell. For example, intracellular metabolites act either as substrates or as cofactors for several classes of epigenetic

enzymes. As a consequence, changes in levels of select metabolites exert changes upon the cellular epigenetic state. Some tumor types take advantage of this form of regulation by acquiring mutations in metabolic enzymes, leading to a newly discovered class of cancer-inducing intermediates, termed oncometabolites. In addition, metabolic alterations of cancer cells influence other cells within the tumor microenvironment, resulting in increased tumor expansion and dissemination.

A number of imaging and therapeutic agents that exploit cancer-specific metabolic alterations have been used in the clinic, and our developing understanding of the complexity of tumor-specific metabolic adaptations holds a promise for expanding the arsenal of such applications in the future.

Key references

The complete reference list can be found on the Wiley Companion Digital Edition of this title (see inside front cover for login instructions).

1 Hanahan D, Weinberg RA. Hallmarks of cancer: the next generation. *Cell.* 2011;**144**(5):646–674.
7 Broach JR. Nutritional control of growth and development in yeast. *Genetics.* 2012;**192**(1):73–105.
9 Hensley CT, Wasti AT, DeBerardinis RJ. Glutamine and cancer: cell biology, physiology, and clinical opportunities. *J Clin Invest.* 2013;**123**(9):3678–3684.
12 Zaman S, Lippman SI, Schneper L, Slonim N, Broach JR. Glucose regulates transcription in yeast through a network of signaling pathways. *Mol Syst Biol.* 2009;**5**:245.
17 Wieman HL, Wofford JA, Rathmell JC. Cytokine stimulation promotes glucose uptake via phosphatidylinositol-3 kinase/Akt regulation of Glut1 activity and trafficking. *Mol Biol Cell.* 2007;**18**(4):1437–1446.
19 Jacobs SR, Herman CE, Maciver NJ, et al. Glucose uptake is limiting in T cell activation and requires CD28-mediated Akt-dependent and independent pathways. *J Immunol.* 2008;**180**(7):4476–4486.
20 Boxer RB, Stairs DB, Dugan KD, et al. Isoform-specific requirement for Akt1 in the developmental regulation of cellular metabolism during lactation. *Cell Metab.* 2006;**4**(6):475–490.
22 Wise DR, DeBerardinis RJ, Mancuso A, et al. Myc regulates a transcriptional program that stimulates mitochondrial glutaminolysis and leads to glutamine addiction. *Proc Natl Acad Sci U S A.* 2008;**105**(48):18782–18787.
25 Schafer ZT, Grassian AR, Song L, et al. Antioxidant and oncogene rescue of metabolic defects caused by loss of matrix attachment. *Nature.* 2009;**461**(7260):109–113.
26 Warburg O. On the origin of cancer cells. *Science.* 1956;**123**(3191):309–314.
27 Eagle H. The minimum vitamin requirements of the L and HeLa cells in tissue culture, the production of specific vitamin deficiencies, and their cure. *J Exp Med.* 1955;**102**(5):595–600.
29 Yuneva M, Zamboni N, Oefner P, Sachidanandam R, Lazebnik Y. Deficiency in glutamine but not glucose induces MYC-dependent apoptosis in human cells. *J Cell Biol.* 2007;**178**(1):93–105.
32 Kim J, Kundu M, Viollet B, Guan KL. AMPK and mTOR regulate autophagy through direct phosphorylation of Ulk1. *Nat Cell Biol.* 2011;**13**(2):132–141.
35 Commisso C, Davidson SM, Soydaner-Azeloglu RG, et al. Macropinocytosis of protein is an amino acid supply route in Ras-transformed cells. *Nature.* 2013;**497**(7451):633–637.
39 Rathmell JC, Fox CJ, Plas DR, Hammerman PS, Cinalli RM, Thompson CB. Akt-directed glucose metabolism can prevent Bax conformation change and promote growth factor-independent survival. *Mol Cell Biol.* 2003;**23**(20):7315–7328.
40 Elstrom RL, Bauer DE, Buzzai M, et al. Akt stimulates aerobic glycolysis in cancer cells. *Cancer Res.* 2004;**64**(11):3892–3899.
43 Vander Heiden MG, Cantley LC, Thompson CB. Understanding the Warburg effect: the metabolic requirements of cell proliferation. *Science.* 2009;**324**(5930):1029–1033.
45 Locasale JW, Grassian AR, Melman T, et al. Phosphoglycerate dehydrogenase diverts glycolytic flux and contributes to oncogenesis. *Nat Genet.* 2011;**43**(9):869–874.
46 Possemato R, Marks KM, Shaul YD, et al. Functional genomics reveal that the serine synthesis pathway is essential in breast cancer. *Nature.* 2011;**476**(7360):346–350.
50 Christofk HR, Vander Heiden MG, Harris MH, et al. The M2 splice isoform of pyruvate kinase is important for cancer metabolism and tumour growth. *Nature.* 2008;**452**(7184):230–233.

51 Christofk HR, Vander Heiden MG, Wu N, Asara JM, Cantley LC. Pyruvate kinase M2 is a phosphotyrosine-binding protein. *Nature*. 2008;**452**(**7184**):181–186.

57 Kim JW, Tchernyshyov I, Semenza GL, Dang CV. HIF-1-mediated expression of pyruvate dehydrogenase kinase: a metabolic switch required for cellular adaptation to hypoxia. *Cell Metab*. 2006;**3**(**3**):177–185.

60 Lum JJ, Bui T, Gruber M, et al. The transcription factor HIF-1alpha plays a critical role in the growth factor-dependent regulation of both aerobic and anaerobic glycolysis. *Genes Dev*. 2007;**21**(**9**):1037–1049.

63 Kaplon J, Zheng L, Meissl K, et al. A key role for mitochondrial gatekeeper pyruvate dehydrogenase in oncogene-induced senescence. *Nature*. 2013;**498**(**7452**):109–112.

64 Bauer DE, Hatzivassiliou G, Zhao F, Andreadis C, Thompson CB. ATP citrate lyase is an important component of cell growth and transformation. *Oncogene*. 2005;**24**(**41**):6314–6322.

65 Hatzivassiliou G, Zhao F, Bauer DE, et al. ATP citrate lyase inhibition can suppress tumor cell growth. *Cancer Cell*. 2005;**8**(**4**):311–321.

69 Wise DR, Ward PS, Shay JE, et al. Hypoxia promotes isocitrate dehydrogenase-dependent carboxylation of alpha-ketoglutarate to citrate to support cell growth and viability. *Proc Natl Acad Sci U S A*. 2011;**108**(**49**):19611–19616.

70 Metallo CM, Gameiro PA, Bell EL, et al. Reductive glutamine metabolism by IDH1 mediates lipogenesis under hypoxia. *Nature*. 2012;**481**(**7381**):380–384.

73 Wellen KE, Thompson CB. A two-way street: reciprocal regulation of metabolism and signalling. *Nat Rev Mol Cell Biol*. 2012;**13**(**4**):270–276.

74 Lu C, Thompson CB. Metabolic regulation of epigenetics. *Cell Metab*. 2012;**16**(**1**):9–17.

75 Wellen KE, Hatzivassiliou G, Sachdeva UM, Bui TV, Cross JR, Thompson CB. ATP-citrate lyase links cellular metabolism to histone acetylation. *Science*. 2009;**324**(**5930**):1076–1080.

76 Imai S, Armstrong CM, Kaeberlein M, Guarente L. Transcriptional silencing and longevity protein Sir2 is an NAD-dependent histone deacetylase. *Nature*. 2000;**403**(**6771**):795–800.

86 Ward PS, Patel J, Wise DR, et al. The common feature of leukemia-associated IDH1 and IDH2 mutations is a neomorphic enzyme activity converting alpha-ketoglutarate to 2-hydroxyglutarate. *Cancer Cell*. 2010;**17**(**3**):225–234.

87 Dang L, White DW, Gross S, et al. Cancer-associated IDH1 mutations produce 2-hydroxyglutarate. *Nature*. 2010;**465**(**7300**):966.

92 Figueroa ME, Abdel-Wahab O, Lu C, et al. Leukemic IDH1 and IDH2 mutations result in a hypermethylation phenotype, disrupt TET2 function, and impair hematopoietic differentiation. *Cancer Cell*. 2010;**18**(**6**):553–567.

93 Lu C, Ward PS, Kapoor GS, et al. IDH mutation impairs histone demethylation and results in a block to cell differentiation. *Nature*. 2012;**483**(**7390**):474–478.

95 Rohle D, Popovici-Muller J, Palaskas N, et al. An inhibitor of mutant IDH1 delays growth and promotes differentiation of glioma cells. *Science*. 2013;**340**(**6132**):626–630.

106 Colegio OR, Chu NQ, Szabo AL, et al. Functional polarization of tumour-associated macrophages by tumour-derived lactic acid. *Nature*. 2014;**513**(**7519**):559–563.

113 Opitz CA, Litzenburger UM, Sahm F, et al. An endogenous tumour-promoting ligand of the human aryl hydrocarbon receptor. *Nature*. 2011;**478**(**7368**):197–203.

119 Choi C, Ganji SK, DeBerardinis RJ, et al. 2-hydroxyglutarate detection by magnetic resonance spectroscopy in IDH-mutated patients with gliomas. *Nat Med*. 2012;**18**(**4**):624–629.

125 Rizos CV, Elisaf MS. Metformin and cancer. *Eur J Pharmacol*. 2013;**705**(**1-3**):96–108.

16 Modeling therapy of late or early-stage metastatic disease in mice

Robert S. Kerbel,PhD ▪ Marta Paez-Ribes, PhD ▪ Shan Man, BSc ▪ Ping Xu, PhD ▪ Eric Guerin, MD ▪ William Cruz-Munoz, PhD ▪ John M. L. Ebos, PhD

Overview

An ongoing problem in oncology drug development is the frequent failure of preclinical therapy models involving treatment of tumor-bearing mice, which show positive results, to predict similar success in patients enrolled in clinical trials. There are numerous possible reasons for causing such high rates of false positives. One is the failure to reproduce the clinical circumstances of treating systemic metastatic disease, whether microscopic or macroscopic in nature—but especially the latter. Thus, it is still common practice to treat mice with established primary tumors, whether they are transplanted or spontaneous, of mouse or human origin, or derived from cell lines or tumor tissue grafts—including human patient-derived xenografts (PDXs). In this chapter, we summarize recent progress in developing mouse models of spontaneous metastases, especially of late-stage disease, after surgical resection of primary tumors, including the use of human tumor cell lines, PDXs, and genetically engineered mouse models (GEMMs). Some limited therapy results using such models, and how they retrospectively or prospectively correlated with relevant phase III clinical trial outcomes, are discussed. A limited database indicates the possible benefits of using such models for predictive investigational therapeutic studies relevant to the treatment of patients with metastatic disease. Some limitations of such models are also discussed.

Introduction

The development of new cancer drugs is a painstakingly complex, laborious, and expensive undertaking, associated with an ultimate failure rate much higher than any other therapeutic area; indeed, it has been reported that greater than 60% of all phase III trials in oncology fail to meet their primary endpoint and are thus considered failures.[1] Such long-term and hugely expensive trials almost invariably follow what were highly encouraging preclinical results—usually undertaken in mice—as well as subsequent small phase I and II clinical trials that also suggested encouraging results, thus bolstering the decision to proceed with further development at the pivotal double-blind placebo-controlled randomized phase III clinical trial level. The subsequent high failure rate at the phase III trial level has therefore resulted in a number of critical questions, and among them include the following: (1) what are the reasons for the tendency of preclinical models involving therapy of tumors in mice to overpredict encouraging outcomes, and how might such models be improved for predicting future clinical trial outcomes? (2) what are the reasons for the failure to reproduce positive results detected in phase II clinical trials in subsequent phase III trials—and how might the design of such smaller phase II trials be improved to better predict what will happen at the phase III level?

This chapter will focus with the first question beginning with a discussion of the numerous possible factors that lead to highly exaggerated "false positives" of therapeutic outcomes obtained in mouse therapy studies, followed by an analysis of some strategies designed to overcome current mouse tumor therapy model limitations. Special emphasis will be placed on one particular approach to improve clinical relevance of mouse tumor models, namely, recapitulating clinical treatment of systemic metastatic disease, early (microscopic) or (overt) late stage, especially the latter.

Some factors that reduce the clinical relevance and hence translatability of most mouse tumor therapy models

Many reviews or commentaries have been published on the limitations of preclinical mouse tumor therapy models for assessing cancer drug activity, at least with respect to clinical relevance and predictive potential.[2-4] Some factors are well known, but others less so, and hence less appreciated. Among them include the following: (1) it is virtually unknown for therapy studies in mice to be initiated in older animals that would be equivalent to the age of the majority of cancer patients, that is, middle age or elderly.[5] Instead, it is typical for therapy to be initiated in mice (at least when using transplanted tumor models) at 6–10 weeks of age. As such, this would be the roughly equivalent of undertaking a pediatric oncology clinical trial. However, it is well known that the impact of cancer drugs in children can be vastly different when compared to adults because of critical parameters that impact cancer drug activity such as drug metabolism and pharmacokinetics; (2) in contrast to a typical clinical trial where every patient enrolled is genetically distinct, mouse studies using inbred mouse strains obviously involve a high degree of homogeneity with respect to the population under study. This essentially eliminates or severely reduces the impact in humans of pharmacogenomic heterogeneity on such vital parameters as drug half life and metabolism, which can strongly impact therapeutic outcomes[6]; (3) either the optimal, or maximum tolerated doses (MTDs) of drugs can be very different between mice and humans; for example, the MTD of many different chemotherapy drugs may be much higher in a mouse compared to humans.[6] This can cause potent tumor response artifacts, especially when using human tumor xenografts for the therapeutic studies; (4) many commonly used transplanted mouse tumor models are highly immunogenic and as a result, this can facilitate the immune system (provided an immunocompetent mouse is used as a host for the therapeutic investigations) to have an influence on therapeutic outcome—but in a way that could distort or exaggerate the degree of efficacy obtained[7]; (5) the endpoints used in preclinical studies are often clinically irrelevant or inappropriate.[8] For example, a common clinical endpoint, such as progression free survival (PFS) based on imaging, is rarely used to assess efficacy in mice and yet PFS is increasingly used as a primary or secondary endpoint in most phase III clinical trials. Instead, it is typical, especially

Holland-Frei Cancer Medicine, Ninth Edition. Edited by Robert C. Bast Jr., Carlo M. Croce, William N. Hait, Waun Ki Hong, Donald W. Kufe, Martine Piccart-Gebhart, Raphael E. Pollock, Ralph R. Weichselbaum, Hongyang Wang, and James F. Holland.
© 2017 John Wiley & Sons, Inc. ISBN: 978-1-118-93469-2

when using tumor transplants, to simply detect an effect on tumor growth per se, usually involving established primary tumors. A growth delay is often noted in such studies in the absence of any overt tumor regression. From a clinical perspective, growth delays would be viewed as "treatment failure"/progressive disease, and yet such results are often viewed as encouraging by cancer researchers because there is a nontreated control group allowing the benefit between the treated and untreated groups to be observed; (6) as any quick glance through current cancer research journals will indicate, the main way cancer drugs are tested in mice remains very much the same as what was half a century or more ago: tumor cells are transplanted into mice, often subcutaneously, to establish a "primary" ectopic tumor, which is then "staged" to a certain size, and treatment of the tumor-bearing mice subsequently initiated. These transplanted tumors can be of either mouse or human origin. In both cases, especially when using mouse tumors, doubling times can be extremely short owing to a very high tumor cell proliferative rate. This can render the tumor hypersensitive to various cancer drugs, especially cytotoxic chemotherapeutic agents that preferentially target cells in cycle replicating DNA or activating intracellular machinery such as microtubules or various enzymes involved in DNA replication. Moreover, tumor cells in cycle might also have an impact on their sensitivity to other types of drug such as signal transduction inhibitors. However, such high cell proliferative rates are not typical of most spontaneous human cancers; (7) the clinical circumstance of treating advanced systemic disease in multiple organ sites such as the lungs, liver, brain, and bones is rarely undertaken in preclinical mouse model studies.[4] Compared to therapy of primary tumors in mice—be they transplanted or spontaneously arising—treating mice with overt metastatic disease is more cumbersome, expensive, and time consuming. However, it is well known that late-stage systemic disease in humans in common solid malignancies is difficult to successfully treat—indeed, it is essentially incurable and associated with very modest gains in PFS or overall survival in "positive" phase III clinical trials. Such gains may be statistically significant and associated with a respectable hazard ratio—but the clinical meaningfulness of such results and their associated cost effectiveness are often marginal.[9]

What follows is a discussion of some of the current attempts to model therapy of metastatic disease in mice; with the emphasis on advanced-stage disease, and also some comment is provided on early-stage (micrometastatic) disease, utilizing transplanted tumors established from either human tumor cell lines or patient-derived xenografts (PDXs) as well as spontaneously arising tumors in genetically engineered mouse models (GEMMs) of cancer.

On the development of postsurgical human tumor xenograft models of advanced visceral metastatic disease using established cell lines

Beginning about a decade ago, attempts were made to develop models of advanced "spontaneous" metastatic disease from resected established primary tumors, virtually the first of their kind.[10] The basic methodology employed involved a variation of the pioneering studies of Fidler[11] who first reported the derivation of variant sublines from the B16 mouse melanoma capable of more aggressive metastatic spread, especially to the lungs, after serial selection *in vivo* involving successive intravenous tumor cell inoculations and recovery of resultant "artificial" or "experimental" lung metastases. In these studies, 10 successive intravenous-mediated cell selections were undertaken, thus generating successive sublines of increasing metastatic properties after intravenous inoculation, for example, the B16F1 and B16F10 sublines.[11] In our case, we made an attempt to select similar variants capable of spontaneous metastatic spread

from an established, but resected orthotopic primary tumor[10] so that the metastatic cells would need to accomplish all of the early and late steps necessary for establishment of a distant metastasis. To achieve this, an established human breast cancer cell line, for example, the "triple-negative" MBA-MD-231 cell line, was implanted into the mammary fat pads of female immune deficient (SCID) mice, a procedure known to promote the rate and extent of distant metastatic spread to sites such as the lungs, compared to ectopic injection of cells into the subcutaneous space.[12,13] Once the primary tumors attained a predesignated volume/size, for example, 500 mm³, resection was undertaken. This was considered necessary to allow the mice to survive for a longer period of time, thus increasing the probability that tumor cells seeded from the primary tumor would have sufficient time to establish macroscopic metastases in distant organs, for example, the lungs. Such metastases could be detected by gross inspection beginning after a period of about 4 months, or longer, post surgical resection of the primary tumors.[10] Several such lung metastases were harvested and a cell line established from the pooled population of metastases. These cells were then reinjected once more into the mammary fat pads and the subsequent primary tumors resected approximately 4 weeks later. This resulted in an accelerated rate and degree of pulmonary metastases (and sometimes, variably, extrapulmonary metastases). An individual lung metastasis was harvested and a subline established from it, for example, a more aggressive metastatic variant called LM2.4.[10] It would then be used for experimental therapeutic studies by once again injecting the cells orthotopically, resecting the resultant primary tumors, allowing the mice to develop overt metastatic disease, which now occurred within about 1 month—mostly confined to the lungs but sometimes involving other sites such as the lymph nodes or liver.[10] It would be at such a late stage of tumor progression that an experimental therapy would be initiated, with survival used as a primary endpoint for assessing therapeutic efficacy.[10] In addition, such variant pro-metastatic sublines can be tagged with markers to monitor disease burden and response to therapy over time. Such markers include luciferase that permits whole body optical/bioilluminscent imaging[14] as well as undertaking transduction of the gene for the β subunit of human choriogonadotropic protein (β-hCG), levels of which can be detected in urine as a molecular surrogate of tumor burden.[15] These same procedures have been successfully employed to develop models of advanced metastatic disease not only for human breast cancer but also for human malignant melanoma,[16] renal cell carcinoma,[17] and colorectal carcinoma.[18] In addition, models of advanced intraperitoneal metastatic ovarian cancer had been developed, which did not involve prior serial selection *in vivo*[19] as well as locally advanced orthotopic hepatocellular carcinoma.[20]

The rationale underlying development of these models was that most experimental therapies would likely have reduced (if any) efficacy when used to treat advanced metastatic disease, when compared to treating the same tumor line in control mice as an established (nonresected) primary tumor. However, we speculated that there might be occasional exceptions to this trend, that is, where a particular drug or therapy could cause meaningful efficacy in the advanced metastatic setting but not, counterintuitively, in the primary tumor treatment setting, or which caused good efficacy in both treatment settings. Such a therapy, it was reasoned, might have a greater probability of showing efficacy (although not necessarily to the same degree) when subsequently tested in patients with advanced metastatic disease. We also adopted a similar strategy for studying adjuvant therapy of earlier-stage microscopic disease.[14] Thus, once the primary tumor was resected, therapy could be initiated very soon after resection at a time when whole body imaging indicated the absence of overt systemic metastases, but where a proportion of the mice would be at risk for developing subsequent metastatic disease.[14,17,18]

A limited body of evidence has suggested the tentative validity of this experimental approach as an improved strategy to assess drug activity for predicting future activity of a given drug or therapy in patients. There are, however, limitations that must also be considered. With respect to the former, that is, supportive evidence for the concept, two observations are particularly noteworthy.

The first observation, or series of results, concerns an attempt to reproduce prior phase III clinical trial outcomes, in particular negative/failed outcomes that were preceded by highly encouraging positive results using conventional mouse tumor therapy models involving treatment of established primary tumors.[21] Thus, a highly compelling example of phase III clinical trial failures is the combination of an oral antiangiogenic tyrosine kinase inhibitor (TKI) plus conventional chemotherapy.[21] There are by now over 15 such phase III trials that failed to meet their primary or secondary endpoints and thus considered failures in breast, colorectal, and lung cancers, among others.[22–24] Perhaps the most discouraging examples are four separate phase III trials evaluating sunitinib in combination with different chemotherapy backbone partners, or when used alone, as reviewed by Guerin et al.[24] These trials represent either first or second line therapies. The first line trials were preceded by positive preclinical results involving mostly treatment of established primary tumors in multiple and different models.[25] As shown in

Figure 1, three different antiangiogenic drugs, namely, sunitinib, another oral TKI (pazopanib), or an antibody that targets vascular endothelial growth factor (VEGF) receptor-2 called DC101 all showed the typical growth delay[25] when treating established orthotopic primary tumor xenografts of the LM2.4 metastatic variant obtained from the MDA-MB-231 breast cancer cell line.[24,25] In contrast, in another group of mice where the primary tumors were resected and treatment initiated at the stage of advanced metastatic disease, the efficacy results were assessed to be negative based on a lack of statistically significant benefit in median overall survival.[24] Moreover, the results remain negative when an antiangiogenic drug, for example, sunitinib, was combined with standard of care paclitaxel chemotherapy.[24] If instead of an oral TKI, the anti-VEGFR-2 antibody was used in conjunction with the same chemotherapy, a benefit in median overall survival was observed, compared to control untreated mice. Although the benefit compared to the paclitaxel treatment group was not statistically significant in terms of an overall survival benefit,[24] there was a trend that likely would have translated into a PFS, had this been measured. As such, this particular result seemed to recapitulate a number of positive phase III clinical trials of the VEGF antibody, bevacizumab, combined with chemotherapy, especially with paclitaxel where small but statistically significant benefit in PFS was observed.[24]

The second observation concerns the development of spontaneous brain metastases in mice with systemic metastatic disease—either of malignant melanoma or breast cancer—and

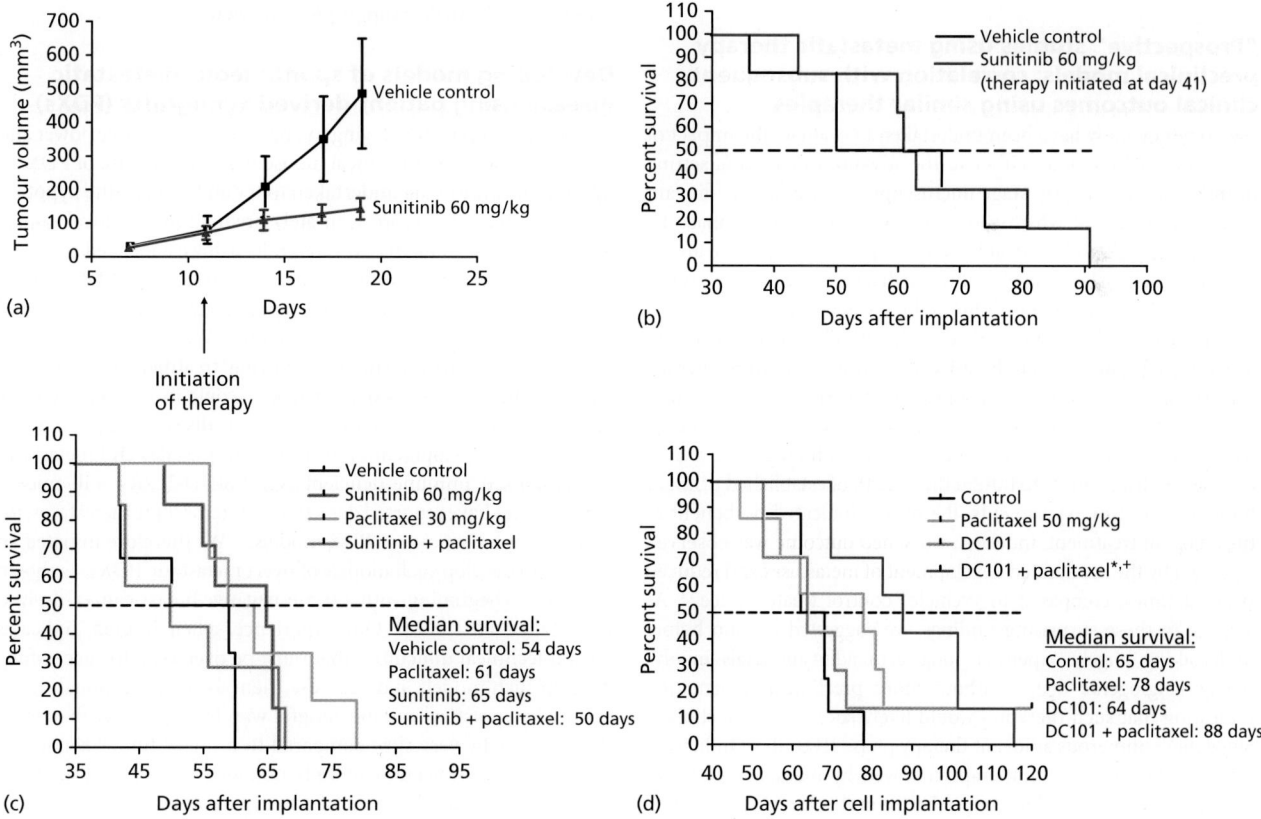

Figure 1 Contrasting outcomes of sunitinib versus DC101 (a VEGF receptor-2 targeting antibody, with or without chemotherapy when treating primary tumors vs overt metastases). A spontaneous metastatic variant of MDA-MB-231 called LM2.4[10] was injected into the mammary fat pads of mice to establish primary tumors (a), or the tumors were resected and the mice allowed to develop extensive metastases, at which point therapy was initiated usually ~20 days after tumor resection (b–d). (a) Sunitinib is active against primary tumors once therapy is initiated (arrow), whereas (b) no impact based on survival using the same dose and schedule of sunitinib in postsurgical mice with advanced metastatic disease. Combination of sunitinib with standard paclitaxel does not improve efficacy of paclitaxel, and in fact worsens outcome (c). In contrast, the DC101 VEGFR-2 antibody improves paclitaxel efficacy (d). Similar results to sunitinib were obtained using pazopanib, which are not shown here. Statistical results and experimental details provided in Guerin et al.[24]

whose survival was prolonged by a particular treatment strategy. This recapitulates a clinical treatment circumstance that is increasingly being observed, namely, the emergence of CNS metastases in patients with systemic metastatic disease whose survival is prolonged by a particular therapy, for example, trastuzumab plus chemotherapy in women with metastatic breast cancer.[26] The basis for the emergence of a higher rate of relapse of brain metastases in such circumstances is that patients with microscopic metastatic disease in the brain developed overt symptomatic lesions as a result of their prolonged survival, this allowed sufficient time for the microscopic metastases to develop into macroscopic lesions. The emergence of spontaneous brain metastases in these therapeutic models resulted in the establishment of models of spontaneous brain metastasis in which cell lines developed from melanoma brain metastases could maintain the spontaneous brain metastatic phenotype upon retransplantation, and moreover, do so without any therapeutic intervention to prolong survival.[16] This indicated the selection of a subpopulation of metastatic tumor cells capable of spontaneous brain metastasis.[16] Additional studies uncovered some possible molecular drivers of spontaneous brain metastasis, one of which involves increased expression of endothelin receptor B.[27] Interestingly, endothelin receptors and endothelins have been implicated as a survival mechanism fostering the growth of brain tumors and metastases as well as their resistance to therapy by Fidler's group.[28] As a result, endothelin receptor antagonists are now being evaluated as a potentially promising strategy to treat brain tumors, for example, glioblastomas, and possibly in the future CNS metastatic disease.

"Prospective" studies using metastatic therapy preclinical models: correlation with subsequent clinical outcomes using similar therapies

Two types of study have been undertaken to evaluate the impact of investigational therapies either in the advanced metastatic setting or in the setting of early-stage microscopic disease (as an adjuvant therapy) versions of which were then later evaluated in phase III clinical trials. This allowed, at least to a degree, a prospective analysis of the possible benefits of evaluating drug activity in postsurgical models of metastatic disease. One of these studies involved adjuvant therapy using an antiangiogenic drug (sunitinib) for the treatment of early-stage microscopic breast cancer where sunitinib therapy was initiated on resected LM2.4 primary breast tumors soon after surgical resection, when no overt metastases could be detected by whole body imaging.[14] Using a short course of therapy, and a high dose of the drug known to inhibit the growth of established primary tumors in control experiments, the results indicated no benefit of the adjuvant treatment; indeed, a worsened outcome was observed as shown by the accelerated development of metastases and reduced survival times, compared to "vehicle" control treated mice.[14] As a result of these surprising findings, we suggested caution before undertaking hugely expensive long-term adjuvant trials involving antiangiogenic drugs without more preclinical information indicating that such therapies would likely succeed in the clinic.[14] Since then, numerous adjuvant therapy phase III trials of induction bevacizumab plus chemotherapy followed by maintenance bevacizumab have been undertaken in breast and colorectal cancer[29,30] as well as with sorafenib in hepatocellular carcinoma and sorafenib or sunitinib in renal cell carcinoma without any chemotherapy. All of these trials failed to show a benefit in disease free survival and in one case, the outcome was actually worse in the bevacizumab containing arm compared to chemotherapy only.[30] Thus, while there is admittedly little evidence for consistent worsened outcomes in these trials, the clinical findings nevertheless support our original

contention, based on the preclinical adjuvant therapy model results that it was premature to undertake such adjuvant trials, especially in the absence of preclinical experimental results supporting the concept of adjuvant antiangiogenic therapy.

A second example of (tentative) prospective validation studies stems from the results evaluating low-dose "metronomic" chemotherapy either alone or in combination with an antiangiogenic drug for the treatment of advanced metastatic disease. A number of such preclinical studies have shown the surprisingly potent efficacy of metronomic chemotherapy-based regimens when treating advanced metastatic disease in mice despite the fact that the same therapy showed less-impressive effects when treating primary established tumors,[4,10] or similar effects on both primary tumor-bearing mice and mice with advanced metastatic disease.[4] Such results have helped contribute to the decision to initiate phase II and even randomized phase III clinical trials evaluating metronomic chemotherapy-based regimens. The first such reported phase III trial, called CAIRO3, evaluated metronomic daily lower dose capecitabine plus bevacizumab as a maintenance therapy in first line metastatic colorectal cancer patients.[31] A marked benefit was noted in PFS, the primary endpoint using the maintenance regimen compared to observation only.[31] While it is true that this particular regimen was not evaluated in prior preclinical studies, the results nevertheless would appear to make a case for the preclinical results evaluating metronomic chemotherapy in the advanced metastatic setting as being a harbinger of possible future phase III clinical trial success when treating metastatic patients.[32] Additional ongoing phase III trials evaluating metronomic chemotherapy should provide further support for this view—or not.

Developing models of spontaneous metastatic disease using patient-derived xenografts (PDXs)

A major development in trying to improve the predictive power and clinical relevance of preclinical mouse models is the use of PDXs.[33] Many studies are being undertaken to try and validate the hypothesis that such models more accurately predict future clinical impact of cancer drugs, compared to xenografts using established cell lines, as described earlier or other models.[33] Virtually, all PDX studies, however, involve growth and therapeutic response of established primary tumors in immune-deficient mice. We are unaware of PDX investigational therapy studies involving treatment of metastatic disease, whether microscopic or macroscopic in nature. There are only a few reports documenting metastatic disease in PDX models, for example, development of ovarian cancer ascites and metastases in humanized immune-deficient NOD-SCID-IL2Rγ null mice.[34] Some studies have reported detection of microscopic metastases, for example, in breast cancer PDX models.[35] We therefore initiated an attempt to develop such models of overt metastatic PDXs, as shown in Figure 1, beginning with a triple-negative breast-cancer-derived PDX called HCI-002.[35] Our experience, albeit limited, indicates several technical difficulties that must be overcome to successfully develop such models and then use them for investigational therapeutics in a practical and meaningful way. First, the growth of most PDXs is usually very slow compared to primary tumor xenografts generated from injection of cells obtained from established cell lines. Thus, the development of overt metastases—if they occur at all in mice whose primary tumors have been resected—can take exceedingly long to emerge. In the case shown in Figure 1, this took 9 months and only occurred in one of 55 mice evaluated. Second, detection of distant metastases, which is easily done using techniques such as whole body bioluminescent imaging of luciferase tagged tumor cell lines, cannot be done using PDX tissues. Thus, other sophisticated imaging methods, for example, MRI using

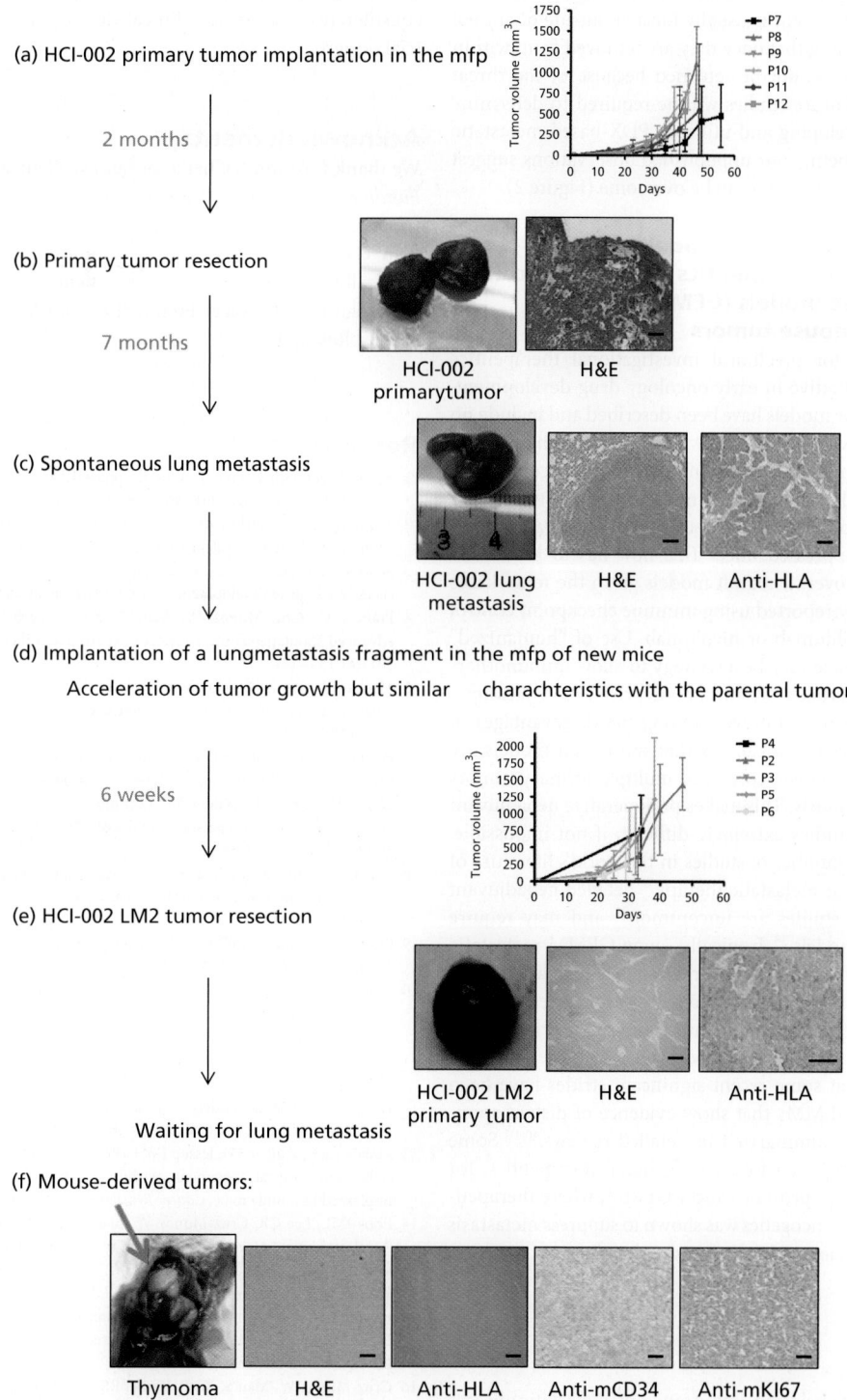

(a) HCI-002 primary tumor implantation in the mfp

2 months

(b) Primary tumor resection

7 months

HCI-002 primarytumor

H&E

(c) Spontaneous lung metastasis

HCI-002 lung metastasis

H&E

Anti-HLA

(d) Implantation of a lungmetastasis fragment in the mfp of new mice

Acceleration of tumor growth but similar charachteristics with the parental tumor

6 weeks

(e) HCI-002 LM2 tumor resection

HCI-002 LM2 primary tumor

H&E

Anti-HLA

Waiting for lung metastasis

(f) Mouse-derived tumors:

Thymoma

H&E

Anti-HLA

Anti-mCD34

Anti-mKI67

Figure 2 Developing a spontaneous metastatic variant from a breast cancer PDX. (a) Tumor fragments of the triple-negative PDX breast cancer tumor called HCI-002[35] were implanted in the mammary fat pads (mfp) of SCID mice. The tumor growth rate remained similar after successive passages. (b) After 2 months, primary tumors were resected and the mice maintained for observation of development of distant overt metastases. (c) After 7 months, one mouse (among 55 examined) developed a lung metastasis that was positive for the human leukocyte antigen (HLA) big enough to be implanted into the mfp of new mice. (d) Fragments of this lung metastasis were implanted in the mfp of new SCID mice. These new tumors grew with an accelerated rate when compared to the parental HCI-002 (tumor volumes of 1000 mm^3 were reached after 6 weeks). (e) The tissue architecture of this new variant remained similar to that of the parental tumor. The growth rate of this new variant was also consistently maintained after successive passages. (f) Mouse-derived thymic lymphomas also appeared in the 15.9% of the mice implanted with PDX tumors. These tumors (which were negative for HLA, with no human component) showed high rates of proliferation and were positive for the hematopoietic progenitor cell antigen CD34. The arrow shows a mouse thymoma. Scale bars, 150 μm. Thus, the results indicate the rarity of development of overt distant metastases using PDXs, the protracted time frame for an overt spontaneous metastasis to develop and the complication of the appearance of the novo mouse thymomas in older SCID mice. Source: Adapted from R.S. Kerbel, Accepted. Used under CC-BY http://creativecommons.org/licenses/by/4.0/.[36]

specialized equipment capable of small animal imaging, would be required, and such equipment is usually located outside of animal holding facilities, meaning that once they are removed from within a holding facility they cannot be returned because of the threat of causing infection. Future studies will be required to determine the practicality of developing and utilizing PDX-based metastatic models. For the time being, our unpublished observations suggest serious practical hurdles may have to be overcome (Figure 2).

Development of metastatic models for investigational therapeutics using genetically engineered mouse models (GEMMs) of spontaneous mouse tumors

The use of GEMMs for preclinical investigational therapeutics represents a major initiative in early oncology drug development. The advantages of these models have been described and include no species difference between the tumors which arise in such mice and the host stroma, and the fact that such mice are immune competent, thus making it possible to undertake immunotherapy studies in a more practical way compared to human tumor xenograft models involving immune suppressed mice. This now has to be viewed as a major advantage over xenograft models given the remarkable clinical results recently reported using immune checkpoint control antibodies such as ipililumab or nivolumab. Use of "humanized" immune suppressed mice may be a strategy to allow immunotherapy studies to be undertaken in immune-deprived mice lacking a murine immune system.[34] However, among the disadvantages of using GEMMs, at least historically, is that most such models are nonmetastatic, and moreover, consist of multiple primary tumors that emerge asynchronously. This makes perioperative neoadjuvant or adjuvant therapy studies extremely difficult, if not impossible. Similar to the limited number of studies in the world's literature of postsurgical adjuvant or metastatic therapy[37] detailed neoadjuvant (presurgical therapy) studies are uncommon[38] and may require transplanted tumor models.[38] Ironically, some GEMM metastatic models involve transplantation of the fragments of primary tumors into secondary syngeneic hosts followed by surgical resection of the resultant primary tumors in a manner similar for transplanted human tumor xenografts,[39] as described earlier.

It is noteworthy that some recent significant strides have been made in developing GEMMs that show evidence of distant spontaneous metastasis, as summarized in detailed reviews.[40,41] Some of these are now being used for investigational therapeutics, for example, the "RapidCap" prostate cancer GEMM, where therapeutic targeting of the myc oncogenes was shown to suppress metastasis in a lethal PTEN-deficient model, after development of castration resistance.[42]

Conclusions

Considering the overwhelming importance of metastatic disease in the morbidity and mortality of cancer, it is somewhat disappointing and surprising that efforts to model the clinical treatment of metastasis—especially of late-stage overt systemic (visceral) metastatic disease—have been so limited over the past half century using various mouse tumor therapy models. As summarized here, this is now beginning to change, and the small data sets currently available would appear to indicate that the therapy results obtained from studies utilizing these more clinically relevant models of metastasis—including those involving surgical resection of primary tumors—may be a promising strategy to reduce "false-positive" results with respect to subsequent clinical translation. Such models may not be practical for routine drug screening, but could be

helpful in making more informed "go–no go" decisions before consideration of further clinical development, as well as clinical trial design.

Acknowledgments

We thank Cassandra Cheng for her excellent secretarial assistance. *Funding Information*: The work summarized in this review was supported by multiple grant sources to RSK including the Canadian Cancer Society Research Institute, the Canadian Institutes of Health Research, the National Institutes of Health, USA, the Canadian Breast Cancer Foundation, and the Ontario Institute for Cancer Research.

References

1 Amiri-Kordestani L, Fojo T. Why do phase III clinical trials in oncology fail so often? *J Natl Cancer Inst*. 2012;**104**:568–569.

2 Talmadge JE, Singh RK, Fidler IJ, Raz A. Murine models to evaluate novel and conventional therapeutic strategies for cancer. *Am J Pathol*. 2007;**170**:793–804.

3 Sharpless NE, DePinho RA. The mighty mouse: genetically engineered mouse models in cancer drug development. *Nat Rev Drug Discov*. 2006;**5**:741–754.

4 Francia G, Cruz-Munoz W, Man S, Xu P, Kerbel RS. Mouse models of advanced spontaneous metastasis for experimental therapeutics. *Nat Rev Cancer*. 2011;**11**:135–141.

5 Meehan B, Garnier D, Dombrovsky A, et al. Ageing-related responses to antiangiogenic effects of sunitinib in atherosclerosis-prone mice. *Mech Ageing Dev*. 2014;**140**:13–22.

6 Peterson JK, Houghton PJ. Integrating pharmacology and in vivo cancer models in preclinical and clinical drug development. *Eur J Cancer*. 2004;**40**:837–844.

7 Hewitt HB, Blake ER, Walder AS. A critique of the evidence for active host defence against cancer, based on personal studies of 27 murine tumours of spontaneous origin. *Br J Cancer*. 1976;**33**:241–259.

8 Singh M, Lima A, Molina R, et al. Assessing therapeutic responses in Kras mutant cancers using genetically engineered mouse models. *Nat Biotechnol*. 2010;**28**:585–593.

9 Ocana A, Tannock IF. When are "positive" clinical trials in oncology truly positive? *J Natl Cancer Inst*. 2011;**103**:16–20.

10 Munoz R, Man S, Shaked Y, et al. Highly efficacious non-toxic treatment for advanced metastatic breast cancer using combination UFT-cyclophosphamide metronomic chemotherapy. *Cancer Res*. 2006;**66**:3386–3391.

11 Fidler IJ. Selection of successive cell lines for metastasis. *Nat New Biol*. 1973;**242**:148–149.

12 Kubota T. Metastatic models of human cancer xenografted in the nude mouse: the importance of orthotopic transplantation. *J Cell Biochem*. 1994;**56**:4–8.

13 Morikawa K, Walker SM, Jessup JM, Fidler IJ. In vivo selection of highly metastatic cells from surgical specimens of different primary human colon carcinomas implanted into nude mice. *Cancer Res*. 1988;**48**:1943–1948.

14 Ebos JML, Lee CR, Cruz-Munoz W, Bjarnason GA, Christensen JG, Kerbel RS. Accelerated metastasis after short-term treatment with a potent inhibitor of tumor angiogenesis. *Cancer Cell*. 2009;**15**:232–239.

15 Francia G, Emmenegger U, Lee CR, et al. Long term progression and therapeutic response of visceral metastatic disease non-invasively monitored in mouse urine using beta-hCG choriogonadotropin secreting tumor cell lines. *Mol Cancer Ther*. 2008;**7**:3452–3459.

16 Cruz-Munoz W, Man S, Xu P, Kerbel RS. Development of a preclinical model of spontaneous human melanoma CNS metastasis. *Cancer Res*. 2008;**68**:4500–4505.

17 Jedeszko C, Paez-Ribes M, Di Desidero T, et al. Orthotopic primary and postsurgical adjuvant or metastatic renal cell carcinoma therapy models reveal potent anti-tumor activity of minimally toxic metronomic oral topotecan with pazopanib. *Sci Transl Med*. 2015;**7**:282ra50.

18 Hackl C, Man S, Francia G, Milsom C, Xu P, Kerbel RS. Metronomic oral topotecan prolongs survival and reduces liver metastasis in improved preclinical orthotopic and adjuvant therapy colon cancer models. *Gut*. 2013;**62**:259–271.

19 Hashimoto K, Man S, Xu P, et al. Potent preclinical impact of metronomic low-dose oral topotecan combined with the antiangiogenic drug pazopanib for the treatment of ovarian cancer. *Mol Cancer Ther*. 2010;**9**:996–1006.

20 Tang TC, Man S, Lee CR, Xu P, Kerbel RS. Impact of UFT/cyclophosphamide metronomic chemotherapy and antiangiogenic drug assessed in a new preclinical model of locally advanced orthotopic hepatocellular carcinoma. *Neoplasia*. 2010;**12**:264–274.

21 Kerbel RS. A decade of experience in developing preclinical models of advanced or early stage spontaneous metastasis to study antiangiogenic drugs, metronomic chemotherapy and the tumor microenvironment. *Cancer Journal.* 2015;**21**:274–283.

22 Gori B, Ricciardi S, Fulvi A, Del Signore E, de Marinis F. New oral multitargeted antiangiogenics in non-small-cell lung cancer treatment. *Future Oncol.* 2012;**8**:559–573.

23 Mackey JR, Kerbel RS, Gelmon KA, et al. Controlling angiogenesis in breast cancer: a systematic review of anti-angiogenic trials. *Cancer Treat Rev.* 2012;**38**:673–688.

24 Guerin E, Man S, Xu P, Kerbel RS. A model of postsurgical advanced metastatic breast cancer more accurately replicates the clinical efficacy of antiangiogenic drugs. *Cancer Res.* 2013;**73**:2743–2748.

25 Abrams TJ, Murray LJ, Pesenti E, et al. Preclinical evaluation of the tyrosine kinase inhibitor SU11248 as a single agent and in combination with "standard of care" therapeutic agents for the treatment of breast cancer. *Mol Cancer Ther.* 2003;**2**:1011–1021.

26 Lin NU, Winer EP. Brain metastases: the HER2 paradigm. *Clin Cancer Res.* 2007;**13**:1648–1655.

27 Cruz-Munoz W, Jaramillo ML, Man S, et al. Roles for endothelin receptor B and BCL2A1 in spontaneous CNS metastasis of melanoma. *Cancer Res.* 2012;**72**:4909–4919.

28 Kim SW, Choi HJ, Lee HJ, et al. Role of the endothelin axis in astrocyte- and endothelial cell-mediated chemoprotection of cancer cells. *Neuro Oncol.* 2014;**16**:1585–1598.

29 Cameron D, Brown J, Dent R, et al. Adjuvant bevacizumab-containing therapy in triple-negative breast cancer (BEATRICE): primary results of a randomised, phase 3 trial. *Lancet Oncol.* 2013;**14**:933–942.

30 de Gramont A, Van Cutsem E, Schmoll HJ, et al. Bevacizumab plus oxaliplatin-based chemotherapy as adjuvant treatment for colon cancer (AVANT): a phase 3 randomised controlled trial. *Lancet Oncol.* 2012;**13**:1225–1233.

31 Simkens LHJ, van Tinteren H, May A, et al. Maintenance treatment with capecitabine and bevacizumab in metastatic colorectal cancer, the phase 3 CAIRO3 study of the Dutch Colorectal Cancer Group (DCCG). *Lancet.* 2015 [Epub head of print].

32 Kerbel RS, Grothey A. Gastrointestinal cancer: Rationale for metronomic chemotherapy in phase III trials. *Nat Rev Clin Oncol.* 2015;**12**:313–314.

33 Tentler JJ, Tan AC, Weekes CD, et al. Patient-derived tumour xenografts as models for oncology drug development. *Nat Rev Clin Oncol.* 2012;**9**:338–350.

34 Bankert RB, Balu-Iyer SV, Odunsi K, et al. Humanized mouse model of ovarian cancer recapitulates patient solid tumor progression, ascites formation, and metastasis. *PLoS ONE.* 2011;**6**:e24420.

35 DeRose YS, Wang G, Lin YC, et al. Tumor grafts derived from women with breast cancer authentically reflect tumor pathology, growth, metastasis and disease outcomes. *Nat Med.* 2011;**17**:1514–1520.

36 Paez-Ribes M, Man S, Xu P, et al. Development of patient derived Xenograft models of overt spontaneous breast cancer metastasis: a cautionary note. *PLoS One.* 2016;**11**:e0158034.

37 Ebos JML, Kerbel RS. Impact of antiangiogenic therapy on invasion, disease progression, and metastasis. *Nat Rev Clin Oncol.* 2011;**8**:210–221.

38 Ebos JM, Mastri M, Lee CR, et al. Neoadjuvant antiangiogenic therapy reveals contrasts in primary and metastatic tumor efficacy. *EMBO Mol Med.* 2014;**6**:1561–1576.

39 Doornebal CW, Klarenbeek S, Braumuller TM, et al. A preclinical mouse model of invasive lobular breast cancer metastasis. *Cancer Res.* 2013;**73**:353–363.

40 Rampetsreiter P, Casanova E, Eferi R. Genetically modified mouse models of cancer invasion and metastasis. *Drug Discov Today Dis Models.* 2011;**9**:67–74.

41 Saxena M, Christofori G. Rebuilding cancer metastasis in the mouse. *Mol Oncol.* 2013;**7**:283–296.

42 Cho H, Herzka T, Zheng W, et al. RapidCaP, a novel GEM model for metastatic prostate cancer analysis and therapy, reveals myc as a driver of Pten-mutant metastasis. *Cancer Discov.* 2014;**4**:318–333.

17 Tumor angiogenesis

John V. Heymach, MD, PhD ▪ Amado Zurita-Saavedra, MD ▪ Scott Kopetz, MD, PhD ▪ Tina Cascone, MD, PhD ▪ Monique Nilsson, PhD

Overview

Angiogenesis, the growth of new capillary blood vessels, is central to cancer growth and metastasis and is recognized to be a potential therapeutic target for the treatment of cancer. Antiangiogenic agents have become part of the standard treatment armamentarium for many solid tumors, providing significant clinical benefits for some cancers (e.g., renal cell, colorectal) and modest or no benefit for others. This chapter is focused on principles of tumor angiogenesis that are intrinsic to the behavior of human cancer, and lessons that can be gleaned from the clinical testing and use of angiogenesis inhibitors to date.

Tumor angiogenesis

Angiogenesis, the growth of new capillary blood vessels, is central to the growth and metastatic spread of cancer. More than four decades ago, it was recognized to be a potential therapeutic target for the treatment of cancer.[1] Since that seminal observation, the field has undergone explosive growth that has taken it from theory to clinical validation of angiogenesis as a therapeutic target, and antiangiogenic therapy is now in routine clinical use. Bevacizumab, a monoclonal antibody targeting vascular endothelial growth factor (VEGF), has undergone the most extensive clinical evaluation to date and is now a standard agent for the treatment of colorectal, lung, renal cell, and other malignancies. Several other antiangiogenic agents are also in routine use for other cancers including ramucirumab, an antibody targeting VEGF receptor-2; the VEGF- and placental-growth factor (PlGF) targeting protein aflibercept; and a number of tyrosine kinase inhibitors targeting angiogenic pathways including sunitinib, pazopanib, sorafenib, vandetanib, and axitinib.

While the progress of the field is encouraging, the clinical benefits of antiangiogenic agents have been relatively modest thus far, and key questions remain unanswered: How should antiangiogenic therapy be combined with other therapeutic regimens and treatment modalities? In what tumor types, and at what stage(s), should these agents be used? Can markers be developed to identify patients most likely to benefit, or experience toxicities, from treatment? The ultimate impact of antiangiogenic therapy in the treatment of cancer will be determined at least in part by the ability of basic researchers and clinicians to address these questions.

An understanding of the cellular and molecular basis of tumor angiogenesis is therefore important for clinicians who diagnose and treat cancer by whatever modalities. This chapter is focused on certain general principles of tumor angiogenesis that are intrinsic to the behavior of human cancer, and lessons that can be gleaned from the clinical testing and use of angiogenesis inhibitors to date.

Rationale for targeting tumor vasculature

The enormous progress that has been made in understanding molecular and genetic events that underlie the transformation of a normal cell to a cancer cell is reflected in many chapters in this book. Not surprisingly, most therapeutic approaches that have arisen from this research are targeted at the cancer cell, with a number of notable successes, such as therapies targeting BCR-ABL oncogene in CML or mutated c-KIT in gastrointestinal stromal tumors. In these cases it appears that cell survival and other key processes are highly dependent on a single activated pathway. For the vast majority of solid tumors, targeting a single molecular pathway in the cancer cell has produced much more modest benefits. Experimental and clinical evidence reviewed in this chapter indicates that it is prudent to develop cancer therapies against another target, the microvascular endothelial cell, with the understanding that the two targets are not mutually exclusive.

Consider a cancer cell that has progressed through a series of mutations so that by activation of certain oncogenes and by loss of specific suppressor genes, it has become self-sufficient in growth signals, insensitive to antigrowth signals, unresponsive to apoptotic signals, capable of limitless replicative potential, and tumorigenic.[2] Current evidence argues that these neoplastic properties may be necessary but not sufficient for a cancer cell to expand into a population that is symptomatic, clinically detectable, metastatic, and lethal. For a tumor to develop a metastatic and/or a lethal phenotype, it must first recruit and sustain its own private blood supply, a process called tumor angiogenesis.[2]

A tumor can recruit vessels through at least four mechanisms: (1) co-option of existing vessels; (2) sprouting from existing vessels (angiogenesis); (3) formation of new vessels de novo, typically from bone marrow-derived cells in the adult (vasculogenesis); (4) intussusception, the insertion of interstitial tissue columns into the lumen of preexisting vessels (reviewed in Ref. 3).

Nonangiogenic tumors are harmless

There is an early stage of neoplastic development when tumors are not yet able to recruit new microvascular endothelial cells and cannot induce angiogenesis. As a result, most human tumors remain *in situ* and dormant at a microscopic size and are harmless to the host.[4]

Cancer without disease: prolonged survival with nonangiogenic, dormant tumors

Nonangiogenic tumors in humans stop expanding at a microscopic size of ~1 mm or less. For over 100 years, pathologists performing autopsies on individuals who died of accidental causes have found that for a given age group, a large number of individuals harbor *in situ* carcinomas, while a very small percentage in that age group are diagnosed with cancer during life.[5] For example, carcinoma *in situ* is found in the breasts of 39% of women aged 40–50 years

Holland-Frei Cancer Medicine, Ninth Edition. Edited by Robert C. Bast Jr., Carlo M. Croce, William N. Hait, Waun Ki Hong, Donald W. Kufe, Martine Piccart-Gebhart, Raphael E. Pollock, Ralph R. Weichselbaum, Hongyang Wang, and James F. Holland.
© 2017 John Wiley & Sons, Inc. ISBN: 978-1-118-93469-2

who died of trauma, but only 1% are ever diagnosed with cancer in this age range. Carcinoma *in situ* of the prostate is diagnosed in 46% of men aged 60–70 years who died of trauma, but only 15% are diagnosed during life. One mechanism that keeps these *in situ* carcinomas in check may be host-derived factors that prevent switching to the angiogenic phenotype. Physiologic levels of endogenous angiogenesis inhibitors (see later sections) may serve this function.[6]

Disease of cancer requires expansion of tumor mass
Expansion of the tumor mass beyond the initial microscopic size of a nonangiogenic tumor, resulting in the disease of cancer, is usually dependent on recruitment of endothelial cells. Such endothelial cell recruitment begins when tumor cells undergo a switch to the angiogenic phenotype.[7–9] The angiogenic phenotype is driven by a number of changes which may include (1) increased expression by tumor cells of angiogenic proteins such as VEGF and basic fibroblast growth factor (bFGF); (2) increased expression of angiogenic proteins from stromal cells (i.e., stromal fibroblasts), a process induced by the tumor itself; (3) decreased expression of endogenous angiogenesis inhibitors (i.e., thrombospondin [TSP]-1) by the tumor and by stromal fibroblasts; and (4) recruitment of bone marrow-derived endothelial cell precursors (see below for a detailed discussion of the switch to the angiogenic phenotype). Other mechanisms will unquestionably be uncovered. Absence of tumor angiogenesis prevents expansion of the tumor mass beyond a microscopic size, thereby avoiding metastatic spread and tumor-related symptoms, and hence, "cancer without disease".[6] The therapeutic implications of this concept are profound. Therapeutic blockade of angiogenesis may not only slow the growth of clinically evident tumors, but also may help prevent the emergence of microscopic lesions into clinically evident tumors.

Recruitment of microvascular endothelial cells is also necessary for expansion of a normal tissue mass and for expansion of an organ mass, for example, after partial hepatectomy.[10] In fact, angiogenesis is fundamental to reproduction, development, and repair, but such physiologic angiogenesis occurs mainly as short-lived capillary blood vessel growth that usually lasts only days (ovulation angiogenesis), weeks (wound healing angiogenesis), or months (fetal and placental angiogenesis) but then it is always downregulated spontaneously and on a predictable timetable.[11,12] These physiological roles for angiogenesis help explain below some of the toxicities observed from use of angiogenesis inhibitors in the clinic.

Historic background
More than 100 years ago, it was observed that tumors were often more vascular during surgery than corresponding normal tissues.[13] This was explained by simple dilation of existing host blood vessels.[14] Vasodilation was thought to be a side effect of metabolites or of necrotic tumor products escaping from the tumor. Three reports, although largely overlooked, suggested that tumor hyperemia could be related to neovascularization and not solely to vasodilation.[15, 16] Nonetheless, debate continued in the literature for two more decades about whether a tumor could expand to a large size (centimeters) by simply living on preexisting vasculature (vessel co-option).[17] Even the few investigators who accepted the concept of tumor-induced neovascularization generally assumed that this was an inflammatory reaction, a side effect of tumor growth, not a requirement for tumor growth.[18] It is now recognized that the two processes are often linked and that the recruitment of inflammatory cells plays a key role in initiating and promoting tumor angiogenesis.

Beginning of angiogenesis research

Hypothesis: tumor growth depends on angiogenesis
In 1971, Folkman proposed a new hypothesis that tumor growth is angiogenesis dependent.[1] This hypothesis suggested that tumor cells and vascular endothelial cells within a neoplasm may constitute a highly integrated ecosystem and that endothelial cells may be switched from a resting state to a rapid growth phase by a "diffusible" chemical signal from tumor cells. An additional speculation was that angiogenesis could be a relevant target for tumor therapy (i.e., antiangiogenic therapy). These ideas were based on experiments Folkman and Frederick Becker performed in the early 1960s, which revealed that tumor growth in isolated perfused organs was severely restricted in the absence of tumor vascularization (Figure 1).[19–23]

These concepts were not widely accepted at the time. Another obstacle to research on tumor angiogenesis was the conventional wisdom at that time that any new vessels induced by a tumor, 'such as new vessels in a wound, would become established and thus could not be made to involute. From this assumption, scientists concluded that antiangiogenic therapy could never regress a tumor; therefore, it would be fruitless to try to discover angiogenesis inhibitors. Eventual acceptance of Folkman's 1971 hypothesis, and the development of angiogenesis research as a field, was subsequently facilitated by a number of advances including the ability to reproducibly culture vascular endothelial cells, the discovery of endogenous angiogenesis proteins, and the identification of drugs able to block angiogenesis *in vitro* and *in vivo*.[24–28]

Throughout the 1970s, laboratory studies were devoted to demonstrating that tumor vessels were new proliferating capillaries; the sequential steps of the angiogenic process could be identified; qualitative and quantitative bioassays for angiogenesis could be developed; viable tumor cells released diffusible angiogenic factors that stimulated new capillary growth and endothelial mitosis *in vivo*, despite the arrest of tumor cell proliferation by irradiation; necrotic tumor products were not angiogenic per se; and angiogenesis itself could be inhibited.[29–32] Today the field has broadened to include a wide spectrum of basic science disciplines, from developmental biology to molecular genetics, as well as a variety of clinical specialties, including oncology, cardiology, dermatology, gynecology, ophthalmology, and rheumatology.

Experimental evidence
By the mid-1980s, considerable experimental evidence had been assembled to support the hypothesis that tumor growth is angiogenesis dependent. The idea could now be stated in its simplest terms: "Once tumor take has occurred, every further increase in tumor cell population must be preceded by an increase in new

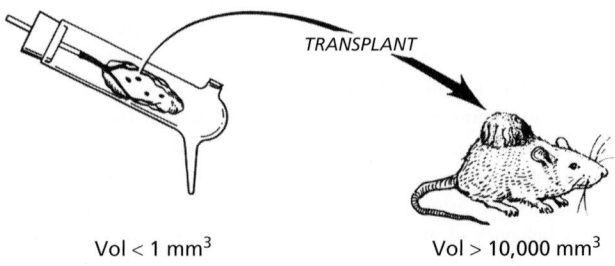

TRANSPLANT

Vol < 1 mm³   Vol > 10,000 mm³

Figure 1 Tumors remain avascular in isolated perfused organs.[20] Whole organs, supported by perfusion, allow growth of tumors in isolation from a host. The tumor remains very small, less than 1 mm³, in an avascular environment compared to growth in mice which can exceed 10,000 mm³.

capillaries that converge upon the tumor".[33] The hypothesis predicted that if angiogenesis could be completely inhibited, tumors would become dormant at a small, possibly microscopic, size.[22] It forecasted that while the presence of neovascularization would be necessary but not sufficient for expansion of a tumor, the absence of neovascularization would prevent expansion of a primary tumor mass beyond $1-2\,mm^3$ and restrict a metastasis to a microscopic dormant lesion (Figure 1).

The hypothesis that tumors are angiogenesis dependent has been supported by a large body of preclinical evidence,[34] including pharmacological and genetic studies, as well as clinical studies discussed in a later section. Some of the observations supporting the angiogenic hypothesis included:

1. Tumors implanted into subcutaneous transparent chambers grow slowly before vascularization, and tumor volume increases linearly. After vascularization, tumor growth is rapid and tumor volume may increase exponentially.[35,36]

2. Tumors grown in the vitreous of the rabbit eye remain viable but are restricted to diameters of less than 0.50 mm for as long as 100 days. Once such a tumor reaches the retinal surface, it becomes neovascularized and within 2 weeks can undergo a 19,000-fold increase in volume over the avascular tumor.[37]

3. The limit of oxygen diffusion is approximately $100-200\,\mu m$. Tumor cells that exceed these distances from a capillary vessel become necrotic, as determined by intravital microscopy of tumors in transparent skin chambers in mice (Figure 2).[38]

4. In transgenic mice that develop carcinomas of the β cells in the pancreatic islets, large tumors arise from a subset of preneoplastic hyperplastic islets but only after they have become vascularized.[8]

5. In colon carcinomas arising in rats after carcinogen exposure, there is an early phase (tumor diameter < 3.5 mm) during which the tumor is temporarily supplied by preexisting host microvessels that are dilated and widened.[39] This stage is similar to "co-option" of blood vessels.[40] Subsequently, new capillary vessels sprout and proliferate (angiogenesis), which leads to increasing microvessel density and is accompanied by rapid tumor growth.

6. A neutralizing antibody to VEGF was administered to mice bearing tumors that induced angiogenesis solely by VEGF.[41] Tumor growth was inhibited by more than 90%. The antibody had no effect on the tumor cells *in vitro*.[42] This observation

has been replicated using a variety of different means to block VEGF, including a fusion protein engineered from VEGF receptors (VEGF trap).[43] Similar results were seen with an antibody directed against another angiogenic factor, bFGF.[44]

Biology of tumor angiogenesis

The role of angiogenesis in preneoplasia and early tumorigenesis

In the experiments with isolated perfused organs by Folkman and colleagues more than four decades ago, the growth of tumors was severely restricted in diameter in the absence of angiogenesis.[20,45] This and other studies led to the proposal that the growth of solid tumors is dependent on new capillary sprouts (termed angiogenesis), and that without angiogenesis solid tumors might become completely dormant.[1] This raised the possibility that angiogenesis might be a therapeutic target not only for the treatment of advanced cancers, but potentially for chemoprevention as well. In recent years, angiogenesis has been validated as a therapeutic target for advanced cancers through a growing body of preclinical and clinical studies. The study of angiogenesis inhibitors for blocking the earliest steps in the development of cancer (chemoprevention) has lagged behind, despite the strong support for the concept provided by preclinical studies (reviewed in Refs 46 and 47).

Preclinical studies demonstrating a role for angiogenesis in early tumorigenesis

In the 1970s it was shown by Gullino[48] that precancerous tissues demonstrate signs of early angiogenesis, and it was suggested that blocking this process may be used to prevent cancer. Later, using transgenic mouse models of tumorigenesis, Hanahan and colleagues demonstrated that some premalignant lesions undergo "angiogenic switch" early in carcinogenesis, reflecting a change in the net balance between angiogenic stimulators and inhibitors.[8,9] VEGF and matrix metalloproteinase-9 (MMP-9) were shown to play important roles in the angiogenic switch in these models.[49-51] In a murine model of pancreatic islet carcinoma, four different antiangiogenic agents were tested (TNP-470, endostatin, angiostatin, or the MMP inhibitor BB-94) and had distinct activity profiles in terms of their ability to prevent tumor formation

Human melanoma

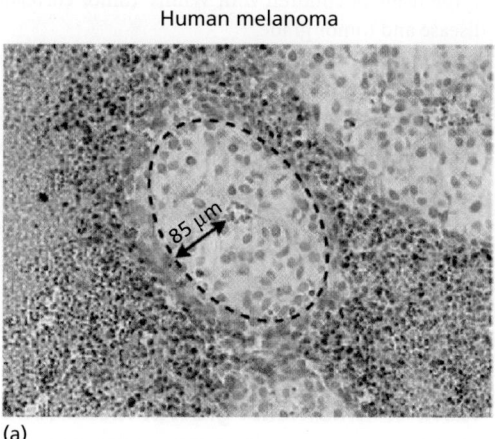

Rat prostate cancer

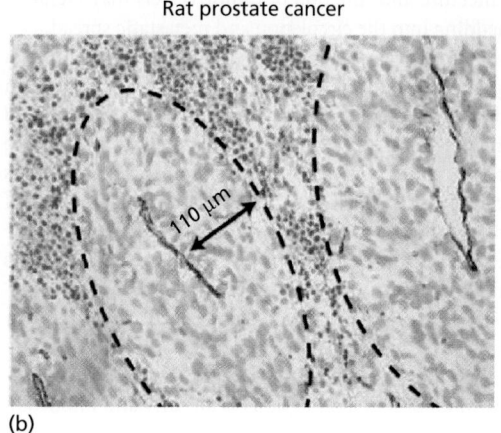

(a)   (b)

Figure 2 (a) A cuff of viable tumor cells surrounding a microvessel in a human melanoma growing in a SCID mouse has an average radius of 85 μm. The appearance of an ellipsoid is a result of the way the section is cut. (b) A cuff of rat prostate cancer cells surrounding a microvessel has an average radius of 110 μm.

(chemoprevention), slow the growth of small tumors (early intervention), and regress established tumors.[8,52,53] In another study, established mammary cancer cells (i.e., previously transformed cells but not primary tumors) were implanted in a dorsal skinfold window chamber in rats, and were found to induce angiogenesis long before the tumor population would have reached the limiting size of a nonneovascularized tumor, that is, 0.2–2 mm. These and other preclinical studies suggest that angiogenesis is an early and critical step in tumorigenesis, and that antiangiogenic agents may inhibit tumor progression and growth.

Preneoplasia is associated with increased angiogenesis in human tumors

Studies from human clinical specimens provide further support for the hypothesis that angiogenesis occurs early in tumor progression, typically during the preneoplastic stage. In cervix cancer, an initial mild increase in vessel density has been detected in the early dysplastic [cervical intraepithelial neoplasia (CIN) I] stage. Mid–late dysplasias (CIN II–III) exhibited a readily apparent angiogenic switch, wherein new vessels became densely apposed along the basement membrane underlying the dysplastic epithelium.[54,55] Biopsies from lung cancer patients and high risk individuals have shown that preneoplastic lesions ranging from hyperplasia and metaplasia to carcinoma in situ are associated with increased microvessel density in the surrounding mucosa.[56–58] A distinctive pattern known as angiogenic squamous dysplasia[57] has also been identified. The specific angiogenic stimulators in bronchial preneoplastic lesions have not been established but elevated levels of VEGF,[56] EGFR (epidermal growth factor receptor),[59] and COX-2[60] have been observed.

Role of angiogenesis in the metastatic spread of cancer

In addition to its role in enabling the growth of small premalignant or malignant lesions, angiogenesis contributes to the hematogenous metastatic spread of tumors. This spread may be facilitated by the presence of "mosaic" blood vessels in tumors, in which both endothelial and tumor cells form the luminal blood surface, facilitating the shedding of tumor cells into the circulation. In one study, approximately 15% of vessels in a colon cancer xenograft model were mosaic vessels in which tumor cells appeared to directly contact the luminal vessel surface without endothelial cells acting as a barrier.[61] Similar numbers of mosaic tumor vessels were detected in human tumor biopsies. These observations suggest that the irregular architecture and function of tumor vessels may facilitate tumor cell shedding into the circulation and metastatic spread.

Micrometastases also appear to be dependent on angiogenesis in order to progress into clinically evident tumors. They may remain dormant in distant sites for an extended period of time but a small fraction of these acquire an adequate blood supply to permit the development of tumors; angiogenesis inhibitors can inhibit this process in a variety of murine models.[62–67] The continued growth of both the primary tumor and metastases thereafter depends on the maintenance of an adequate blood supply. In theory, angiogenesis inhibitors may therefore offer benefit when used for chemoprevention as well as in treatment of early stage, occult metastatic, or advanced disease.[46,68,69]

Taken together, these preclinical and clinical studies provide evidence that the induction of angiogenesis is an early and important step in tumor progression, likely occurring in precancerous lesions, and is involved in metastatic spread. For these reasons, angiogenesis is a rational target for chemoprevention. Additional studies will be needed to elucidate the key regulators of early angiogenesis,

and to identify the different types of antiangiogenic agents that may be optimal for chemoprevention, advanced disease, and other applications.

Regulators of angiogenesis

The discovery of diffusible factors stimulating tumor angiogenesis

The observation in the 1970s that tumors implanted into the avascular cornea or onto the vascularized chick chorioallantoic membrane induced an ingrowth of new capillaries indicated that tumors released diffusible angiogenic factors.[9] This result motivated the development of in vitro and in vivo bioassays to guide the search for tumor-derived angiogenic factors.[70]

Fibroblast growth factors

bFGF (or FGF-2) was the first angiogenic protein to be isolated and purified from a tumor (1982), followed shortly by acidic FGF (aFGF or FGF-1).[28,71,72] Acidic and bFGFs stimulate endothelial cell mitosis and migration in vitro and are among the most potent angiogenic proteins in vivo. They have high affinity for heparin and heparan sulfate.[73] The expression of bFGF receptors is very low. A wide variety of cancer types secrete bFGF, including those of the central nervous system, sarcomas, genitourinary tumors, and even endothelial cells in the tumor vasculature. Identification of an FGF-binding protein secreted by tumors into the extracellular matrix may illuminate a mechanism of tumor mobilization of stored FGFs.[74–76] Furthermore, some tumors recruit macrophages[77] and activate them to secrete bFGF,[78] whereas others attract mast cells, which, because of their high content of heparin, could sequester bFGF. In spontaneous tumors that arise in transgenic mice, aFGF and bFGF are exported into conditioned medium by angiogenic tumor cells but not by preangiogenic cells in earlier stages of tumor progression.[38,79] bFGF also interferes with adhesion of leukocytes to endothelium, and it has been suggested that tumors that elaborate bFGF may produce a form of local immunologic tolerance.[80–82] In mouse models of cancer, inhibition of the FGFR signaling pathways results in inhibited tumor angiogenesis and reduced tumor growth.[83]

Abnormally elevated levels of bFGF are found in the serum and urine of cancer patients and in the cerebrospinal fluid of patients with different types of brain tumors.[84,85] High bFGF levels in renal carcinoma correlated with a poor outcome.[86] Moreover, bFGF levels in the urine of children with Wilms' tumor correlate with stage of disease and tumor grade.[87]

In addition to contributing to tumor angiogenesis, multiple FGFR fusion proteins have been identified on diverse cancers including lung squamous cell, bladder, glioblastoma, and thyroid cancer, and appear to be oncogenic drivers as pharmacologic inhibition of FGFR suppresses the growth of FGFR fusion-positive tumor models.[88] Additional reports have shown FGFR1 to be amplified in a subset of small cell lung cancers among other malignancies, and tumor cells harboring FGFR amplification are sensitive to target inhibition.[89] In these settings, inhibition of FGFRs will therefore have both direct antitumor cell effects and indirect tumor cell effects through targeting of the tumor vasculature.

Vascular endothelial growth factor (VEGF) family

Dvorak first proposed that tumor angiogenesis is associated with increased microvascular permeability.[90] This led to the identification of vascular permeability factor (VPF).[91–93] VPF was subsequently sequenced by Ferrara and colleagues and in 1989 was

Table 1 Examples of regulators of angiogenesis.

Proangiogenic molecules	Antiangiogenic molecules	Transcription factors, oncogenes, and other regulators
Vascular endothelial growth factor (VEGF)	Interferon–α,β,γ	Hypoxia-inducible factor (HIF)-1α, 2α
Basic fibroblast growth factor (bFGF)	Thrombospondin-1,2	Nuclear factor-κB (NFκB)
Transforming growth factor-α (TGF-α)	Angiopoietin 2	Epidermal growth factor receptor (EGFR)
Platelet-derived growth factor (PDGF)	Tissue inhibitors of MMPs (TIMPs)	Ras
Epidermal growth factor (EGF)	Endostatin	p53
Angiopoietins	Angiostatin	von Hippel-Lindau
Interleukin-6	Interleukin-12	Cadherin
Interleukin-8	Endostatin	Integrin
Matrix metalloproteinases (MMPs)	Thrombospondin-1	Semaphorin
Hepatocyte growth factor (HGF)		Id1, Id2
Stromal cell-derived factor-1α (SDF-1α)		Prolyl hydroxylases
Delta-like ligand 4 (DLL4)		myc
Ephrins		
Monocyte chemoattractant protein-1 and other chemokines		

reported to be a specific inducer of angiogenesis called VEGF.[92–94] At the same time, a novel angiogenic protein was first isolated and purified from a tumor (sarcoma 180) in the Folkman lab, and in a collaboration with Ferrara was shown to be VEGF.[94] Since then, more than 40 angiogenic inducers have been identified, most as tumor products (Table 1).[3,95] VEGF is an endothelial cell mitogen and motogen that is angiogenic *in vivo*.[96–98] Its expression correlates with blood vessel growth during embryogenesis and is essential for development of the embryonic vascular system.[99,100] VEGF expression also correlates with angiogenesis in the female reproductive tract, and in tumors.[49,101–103] VEGF is a 40–45 kDa homodimeric protein with a signal sequence secreted by a wide variety of cells and the majority of tumor cells. VEGF exists as five different isoforms of 121, 145, 165, 189, and 206 amino acids, of which VEGF$_{165}$ is the predominant molecular species produced by a variety of normal and neoplastic cells. Two receptors for VEGF are found mainly on vascular endothelial cells, the 180 kDa fms-like tyrosine kinase (Flt-1)[104] and the 200 kDa human kinase insert domain-containing receptor (KDR) and its mouse homolog, Flk-1.[105] VEGF binds to both receptors, but KDR/Flk-1 transduces the signals for endothelial proliferation and chemotaxis.[106–109] Other structural homologs of the VEGF family include VEGF-B, VEGF-C, VEGF-D, and VEGF-E.[110,111] VEGF-C and VEGF-D bind to Flt-4, which is preferentially expressed on lymphatic endothelium.[112,113]

Klagsbrun et al. discovered that neuropilin-1, a neuronal guidance molecule, is a coreceptor for VEGF$_{165}$, but not for VEGF.[114,115] This finding provides a molecular mediator that coordinates growth in the vascular system with the nervous system. Other neuronal guidance proteins and/or their receptors are also angiogenesis regulators. For example, neuropilin is a receptor for VEGF and for semaphorin. Semaphorin repels neurite outgrowth and is also an angiogenesis inhibitor. Ephrins are neural guidance molecules, but also genetically determine arteries and veins during embryogenesis. EphrinB2 is expressed by tumor vascular endothelium. Perhaps in part because of the overlap between regulators of the nervous and vascular systems, angiogenesis in brain tumors has distinctive characteristics such as high interstitial fluid pressure (IFP) and low oxygen tension that contribute to the malignant behavior of these tumors.[116]

Neuropilin is not a tyrosine kinase receptor and is expressed on nonendothelial cells, including tumor cells. This allows VEGF that is synthesized by tumor cells to bind to their surface. Surface-bound VEGF could make endothelial cells chemotactic to tumor cells, or it could act in a juxtacrine manner to mediate co-option of microvessels by tumor cells. Neuropilin also binds placenta growth factor-2

(PlGF-2), and heparin is essential for the binding of VEGF$_{165}$ and PlGF-2 to neuropilin-1.[40,117] The natural cell surface polysaccharide *in vivo* is heparan sulfate, not heparin. Heparan sulfate may act as a template to accelerate the interaction of VEGF or PlGF-2 with VEGF. VEGF expression by tumors is upregulated by hypoxia and is often elevated near areas of tumor necrosis.[118–121] Hypoxia activates hypoxia-inducible factor-1 (HIF-1), which binds to the hypoxia response element (HRE sequence) in the VEGF promoter, which leads to VEGF mRNA transcription.[106,120] Independent of this, hypoxia stabilizes the VEGF mRNA.

VEGF signal transduction

While VEGF-A binds VEGFR1 with a higher affinity than VEGFR-2, the majority of biological effects of VEGF-A on tumor endothelium are thought to be mediated through VEGFR-2. Upon ligand binding, VEGFR-2 dimerizes, resulting in activation of the tyrosine kinase and autophosphorylation of residues including Tyr^{951}, Tyr^{996}, Tyr^{1054}, Tyr^{1175}, and Tyr^{1214}.[122] Phosphorylation of these residues induces the activation of signal transduction molecules including PI3K, phospholipase C-γ (PLC-γ), Akt, Src, Ras, and MAPK (Figure 3). Phosphorylation of Tyr^{1175} results in the binding and phosphorylation of PLC-γ, which subsequently promotes the release of Ca^{2+} from internal stores and activation of protein kinase C (PKC). PKC activation and Ca^{2+} mobilization are considered to be critical for VEGF-A-induced cell proliferation and nitric oxide production, respectively.[123]

The PI3K pathway is paramount in the regulation of cell proliferation, survival, and migration. VEGF-A has been shown to promote phosphorylation of the p85 subunit of PI3K and enhance PI3K enzymatic activity. The mechanism by which VEGF-A results in activation of PI3K remains unclear, although studies have implicated a role for Src kinases, β-catenin, and VE-cadherin.[124,125] VEGFR-2-induced activation of PI3K results in accumulation of phosphatidylinositol-3,4,5-trisphosphate (PIP$_3$), which induces phosphorylation of Akt/PKB. Once activated, Akt/PKB phosphorylates and thus inhibits proapoptotic proteins BAD and caspase-9.

Members of the Src family kinases, Src, Fyn, and Yes, are expressed in endothelial cells. Following VEGFR-2 autophosphorylation, T cell-specific adapter (TSAd) binds Tyr^{951} and then associates with Src. Src kinases control actin stress fiber organization and may mediate VEGF-A-induced PI3K activation. Ligand binding to VEGFR-2 also initiates activation of the Ras pathway, triggering signaling through the Raf-1–MEK–ERK signal cascade[122] known to be important in growth factor-induced

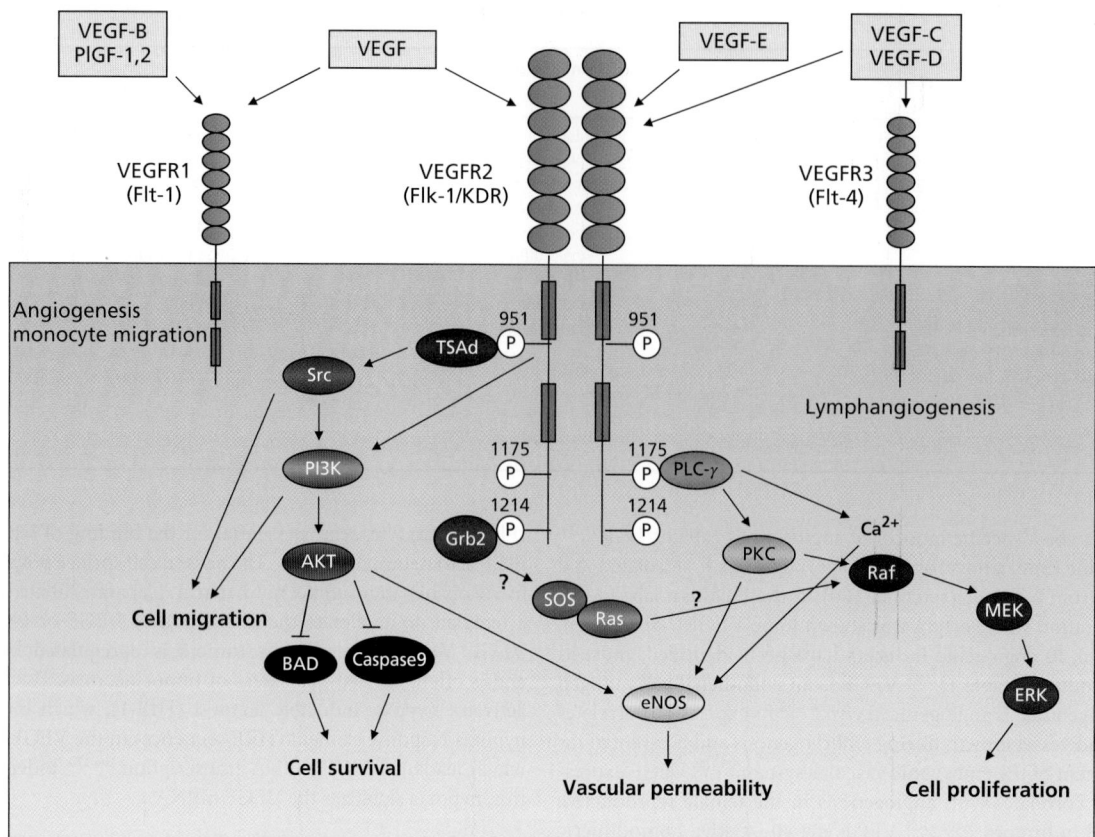

Figure 3 VEGFR signal transduction. VEGF family members, VEGF, VEGF-B, VEGF-C, VEGF-D, VEGF-E, and PlGF bind three VEGFR tyrosine kinases, resulting in dimerization, receptor autophosphorylation, and activation of downstream pathways. Signal transduction via VEGFR2 is shown. Ligand binding to VEGFR2 activates signal-transduction molecules phospholipase C-[γ] (PLC-[γ]), PI3K, Akt, Ras, Src, and MAPK and regulates cell proliferation, migration, survival, and vascular permeability.

cell proliferation. This activation may occur through multiple routes.[122,126]

Biological function of VEGF

In its initial discovery, VEGF was identified as a mediator of vessel permeability.[110,127] This capacity to render small veins and venules hyperpermeable is a critical function of VEGF. VEGF is indeed one of the most potent regulators of vascular permeability, and the observation that tumor-associated blood vessels are hyperpermeable is attributed to tumor-secreted VEGF. While the mechanisms by which VEGF increases microvascular permeability are incompletely understood, it may be at least in part due to VEGF-induced endothelial fenestrations,[100] opening of junctions between adjacent endothelial cells,[128] and through a calcium-dependent pathway involving nitric oxide (NO) production.[129–131]

In addition to its effect on vascular permeability, VEGF is a survival factor for endothelial cells, inhibiting endothelial cell apoptosis through activation of the PI3K–Akt pathway[132] and increases in the antiapoptotic protein bcl-2.[133] *In vivo*, VEGF blockade has been demonstrated to cause increases in apoptosis of immature, nonpericyte-covered vessels.[134] VEGF is an endothelial cell mitogen though VEGFR-2 mediates signal transduction through Erk1/2, JNK/SAPK, and possibly PKC.[133,135] While VEGF is not as potent an endothelial cell mitogen as other factors such as bFGF, it has a broader range of activity for processes critical for angiogenesis. VEGF induces expression of MMPs and serine proteinases involved in degradation of the basement membrane, which is necessary for endothelial cell sprouting and invasion.[133] In addition, VEGF facilitates endothelial cell migration through FAK and p38 MAPK-induced actin reorganization.[3,128,133,136]

Circulating VEGF may be one of the angiogenic signals by which tumors recruit bone marrow-derived cells, including endothelial progenitors and myeloid cells whose recruitment is thought to be mediated by VEGFR-2 and VEGFR-1, respectively.[137–141] A growing body of evidence suggests that VEGFR-bearing bone marrow-derived cells contribute to initiating tumor formation, by creating a "metastatic niche", and/or help promote tumor angiogenesis[142–146] although there appear to be VEGFR-1-independent mechanisms as well.[147] Circulating endothelial and myeloid cells are further being studied as potential biomarkers, as noted later in the chapter, and may contribute to resistance to VEGF pathway inhibitors.[148,149] It is worth noting that not all VEGF in the circulation may be tumor derived. VEGF serum concentrations closely correlate with platelet counts in cancer patients. VEGF is stored in platelets, and is transported by and released from them.[150] Furthermore, Pinedo and colleagues report that higher platelet counts correlate with a worse prognosis for cancer patients.[151,152] Therefore, it is possible that for those types of tumors that recruit bone marrow-derived endothelial cells, communication from tumor to bone marrow may be mediated in part by the VEGF in circulating platelets.

Angiopoietins

Angiopoietin-1 (Ang1) is a 70 kDa ligand that binds to a specific tyrosine kinase expressed only on endothelial cells, called Tie2 (also called Tek). Ang1 ligand binds Tie2 expressed on ECs, and

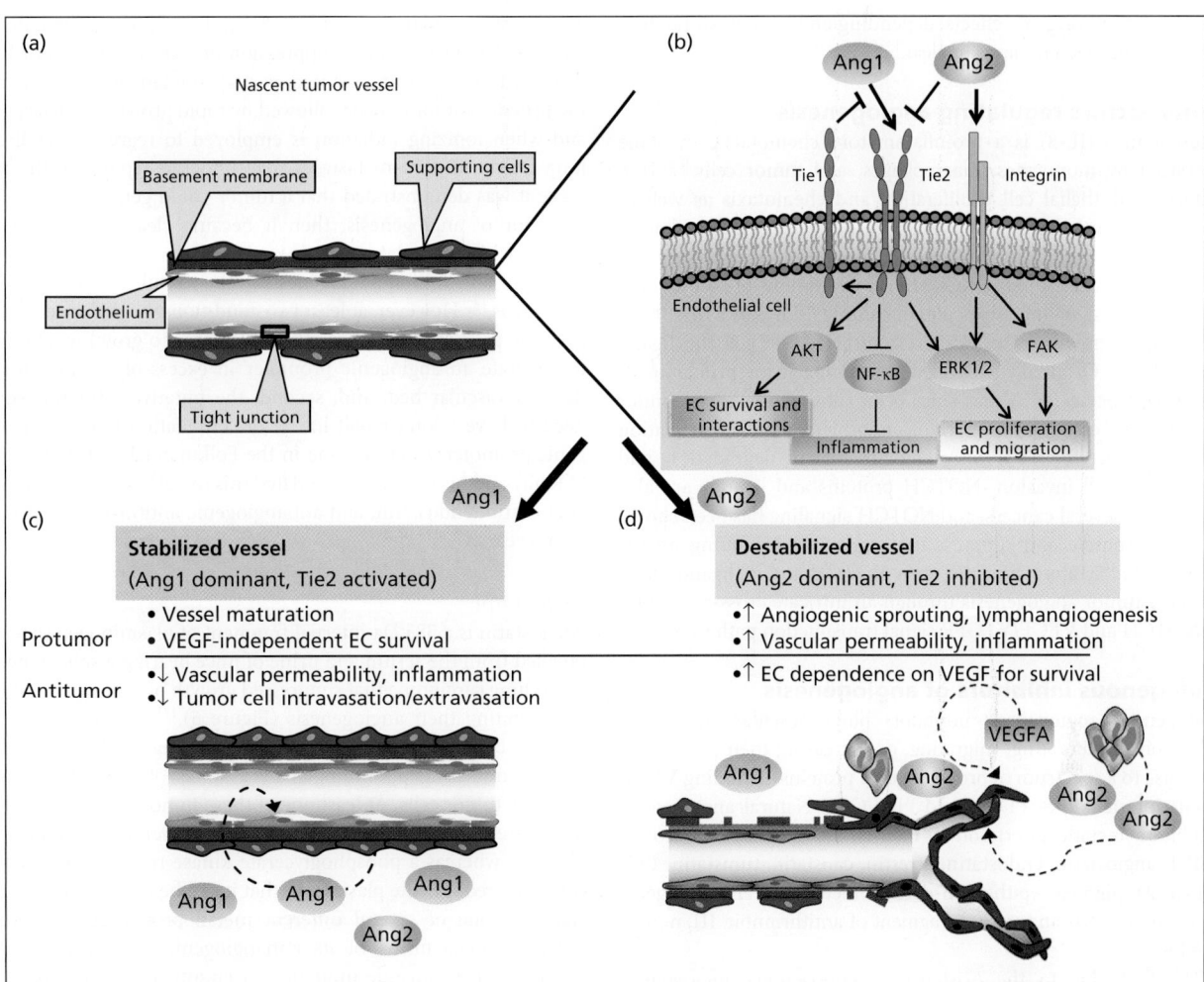

Figure 4 Ang/Tie2 signaling pathway. (a) Representation of nascent tumor blood vessel structure in quiescent state. Endothelial cells (ECs; green) are organized to form vessel lumen and tightly interact with perivascular cells (blue), separated by basement membrane. (b) Ang1 ligand binds Tie2 localized on ECs; Tie2 subsequently dimerizes and is phosphorylated. Activated Tie2 activates phosphatidylinositol 3-kinase and Ras/Raf/MEK, promoting EC survival and proliferation/migration. Generally, Ang2 functions as an Ang1 antagonist by inducing increased vascular permeability, sprouting vascularization. Autophosphorylated Tie2 activates Tie1, the extracellular domain of which in turn interferes with Ang1/Tie2 binding, therefore antagonizing Ang1 signaling. Ang1 has anti-inflammatory properties, whereas Ang2 plays a proinflammatory role. Ang1-activated Tie2 inhibits nuclear factor-κB–mediated inflammatory gene expression, whereas Ang2 promotes expression through blockade of Ang1 function. (c) Perivascular cells secrete Ang1, which binds Tie2 expressed on ECs. In this interaction, Ang1 contributes to vessel integrity, reduces vessel permeability, and maintains vasculature quiescence. (d) Ang2 plays a major role in angiogenesis by mediating dissociation of pericytes and destabilizing cellular junctions. In the presence of other proangiogenic factors (e.g., VEGF), ECs proliferate and/or migrate to form new sprouting, disorganized blood vessels. In the absence of proangiogenic factors, Ang2 signaling results in EC apoptosis and regression. Source: Cascone and Heymach 2012.[153] Reprinted with permission. © 2012 American Society of Clinical Oncology. All rights reserved.

Tie2 subsequently dimerizes and is phosphorylated. Activated Tie2 triggers activation of PI3K and Ras/Raf/MEK, promoting EC survival and proliferation/migration (Figure 4).[153] A ligand for Tie1 has not been elucidated.[114,154–157] Like VEGF, Ang1 is an endothelial cell-specific growth factor. Ang1, however, is not a direct endothelial mitogen *in vitro*. Rather, it induces endothelial cells to recruit pericytes and smooth muscle cells to become incorporated in the vessel wall. Pericyte and smooth muscle recruitment is mediated by endothelial production of PDGF-BB (and probably other factors) when Tie2 is activated by Ang1.[158] There is increased vascularization in mice that overexpress Ang1 in the skin.[157] The vessels are significantly larger than normal and the skin is reddened. The vessels are not leaky and there is no skin edema, in contrast to dermal vessels of mice overexpressing VEGF. In double transgenic mice expressing both Ang1 and VEGF in the skin, dermal angiogenesis is increased in an additive manner, but the vessels do not leak.[159] This model closely approximates angiogenesis in healing

wounds (i.e., relatively nonleaky vessels with pericytes and some perivascular smooth-muscle cells contained in the vascular wall). In contrast, tumor vessels are leaky and thin walled with a paucity of pericytes. Angiopoietin-2, produced by vascular endothelium in a tumor bed, blocks the Tie-2 receptor and acts to repel pericytes and smooth muscle.[154] Nevertheless, tumor vessels remain thin "endothelium-lined tubes" even though some of these microvessels reach the diameter of venules. High levels of Ang2 are associated with metastases in melanoma patients, and in preclinical models, Ang2 promotes metastatic formation.[160,161] A key point is that angiopoietins and VEGF together play a role in angiogenesis, and the activity of both is context dependent with different activities observed in angiogenic versus mature vessels. Because VEGF plays a key role in the proangiogenic activity of Ang2, using combination inhibitors targeting both the Ang/Tie2 and VEGF receptor pathways may provide clinical benefit, a concept that has begun to be explored. However, given that angiopoietins can apply either pro- or antitumorigenic effects, depending on the context, the best targeting approach remains unclear.[153]

Other factors regulating angiogenesis

Interleukin-8 (IL-8) is a proinflammatory chemotactic cytokine produced by monocytes, macrophages, and tumor cells.[162] IL-8 induces endothelial cell proliferation and chemotaxis as well as promotes endothelial cell survival.[162,163] The effects of IL-8 are mediated through interactions with two cell-surface G protein-coupled receptors, CXCR1 and CXCR2, and activation of subsequent downstream signaling molecules including PI3K and MAPK.[164] Hepatocyte growth factor/scatter factor (HGF/SF) is the ligand for c-Met.[165] Originally identified as a mitogen for primary cultured hepatocytes, HGF has since been shown to facilitate tumor angiogenesis. c-Met is expressed on endothelial cells, and activation by tumor-secreted HGF/SF augments matrix degradation and endothelial cell invasion. NOTCH proteins and ligands are also elevated in several cancers, and NOTCH signaling has been shown to both promote and suppress tumor growth depending on the tumor type.[166] Interactions between NOTCH and its ligand DLL4 promote tumor angiogenesis through an intricate cross-regulation of NOTCH and VEGF/VEGFR signal transduction pathways.[167,168]

Endogenous inhibitors of angiogenesis

Endogenous angiogenesis inhibitors block vascular endothelial cells from proliferating, migrating, or increasing their survival in response to a spectrum of proangiogenic proteins, including VEGF, bFGF, interleukin-8, PDGF, and PD-ECGF. Natural angiogenesis inhibitors include interferon-α, interleukin-12, platelet factor 4, TSP-1, angiostatin, endostatin, arrestin, canstatin, tumstatin, PEX (MMP-2), pigment epithelium-derived factor, and antiangiogenic antithrombin III (an internal fragment of antithrombin III, named aaAT).[27,169–175]

The first clue to the existence of endogenous angiogenesis inhibitors came from the discovery that interferon-α inhibited endothelial cell migration and that platelet factor 4 inhibited endothelial proliferation.[176–178] Both were subsequently shown to inhibit angiogenesis.[176–180] However, Bouck and her colleagues were the first to show that a tumor could generate an angiogenesis inhibitor; they subsequently proposed that the angiogenic phenotype was the result of a net balance of endogenous inhibitors and stimulators of angiogenesis.[181] A nontumorigenic hamster cell line became tumorigenic in association with the loss of a suppressor gene and concomitant with the onset of angiogenic activity. The nontumorigenic line secreted high levels of an angiogenesis inhibitor, a truncated form of TSP-1, that decreased by about 96% in the tumorigenic cells.[182] TSP-1 was shown to be regulated by the wild-type tumor suppressor p53 in fibroblasts and in mammary epithelial cells.[183,184] Loss of p53 function in the transformed derivatives of these cells dramatically decreased the level of the angiogenesis inhibitor. Restoration of p53 upregulated TSP-1 and raised the antiangiogenic activity of the tumor cells. Deletion of TSP-1 led to accelerated growth of breast cancers that arise spontaneously in neu-transgenic mice.[185] The demonstration that the switch to an angiogenic phenotype involved a negative regulator of angiogenesis generated by the tumor per se suggested to Folkman a unifying angiogenic mechanism to explain a well-recognized but previously unsolved clinical and experimental phenomenon: the inhibition of tumor growth by the tumor mass. In this phenomenon, "the removal of certain tumors, for example, breast carcinomas, colon carcinomas, and osteogenic sarcomas can be followed by rapid growth of distant metastases".[186,187] Postoperative chemotherapy was introduced mainly to prevent or delay the growth of secondary metastases. Several studies in terminally ill patients demonstrated the suppression of a secondary tumor by a primary tumor.[188] In melanoma, partial spontaneous regression of the primary tumor may be followed by rapid growth of metastases, and when ionizing radiation is employed to regress a small cell lung cancer, distant metastases may undergo rapid growth.[173,189] Once it was demonstrated that a tumor could generate a negative regulator of angiogenesis, then it became clear that a primary tumor, while stimulating angiogenesis in its own vascular bed, could possibly inhibit angiogenesis in the vascular bed of a distant metastasis.[182] However, at least two conditions would be necessary: first, the primary tumor (i.e., the first tumor to grow) would need to generate an angiogenic promoter in excess of an inhibitor in its own vascular bed, and, second, the putative inhibitor would need to have a longer half-life in the circulation than the angiogenic promoter. After arriving in the Folkman laboratory in 1991, O'Reilly and his colleagues validated this hypothesis by discovering angiostatin, endostatin, and antiangiogenic antithrombin over the next 8 years.[171–173,190,191]

Angiostatin

Angiostatin is a 38 kDa internal fragment of plasminogen that was purified from the serum and urine of mice bearing a subcutaneous Lewis lung carcinoma that suppressed growth of its lung metastases by inhibiting their angiogenesis (Figure 5).[171] Angiostatin is not secreted by tumor cells but is generated through proteolytic cleavage of circulating plasminogen by a series of enzymes released from the tumor cells. At least one of these tumor-derived enzymes, urokinase plasminogen activator (uPA), converts plasminogen to plasmin, whereas a phosphoglycerate kinase from hypoxic tumor cells then reduces the plasmin so that it can be converted to angiostatin by one of several different metalloproteinases.[192] Several potential mechanisms of its antiangiogenic activity have been reported. These include induction of endothelial apoptosis[193–195]; suppression of endothelial cell migration induced by plasmin binding to $\alpha_v\beta_3$-integrin[196,197]; inhibition of HGF-induced signaling via c-MET, Akt, and ERK-1/2[198]; and downregulation of VEGF expression in tumor cells.[199] This implies that angiostatin may act as a direct and an indirect inhibitor of angiogenesis. In support of this, when angiostatin was delivered to mice bearing a variety of tumors, it showed significant efficacy either alone or in combination with endostatin, as a fusion protein of angiostatin and endostatin, or in combination with interleukin-12.[199–202]

Endostatin

A strategy similar to the one that uncovered angiostatin (e.g., suppression of tumor growth by tumor mass) was employed with murine hemangioendothelioma and human small cell lung cancer to discover endostatin and the antiangiogenic conformation of antithrombin-IIIAT.[172,173,191] Both endostatin and aaAT are generated from larger parent proteins by enzymes released by tumor cells. Endostatin is a 20–22 kDa internal fragment of collagen XVIII.[172,191,203,204] It is the first of a group of endogenous angiogenesis inhibitors that are predominantly extracellular proteins, which generally require proteolytic processing to become active.[3,205] Like angiostatin, endostatin appears to have both direct and indirect effects on tumor endothelium, and a number of different mechanisms have been proposed. It is a specific inhibitor of endothelial cell proliferation and migration,[206,207] and blocks the binding of $VEGF_{121}$ and $VEGF_{165}$ to the KDR/ Flk-1 receptor and subsequent downstream signaling events.[208] Although endostatin does not bind to VEGF,[208] it does downregulate VEGF expression in tumor cells.[199] In bFGF-treated endothelial cells,

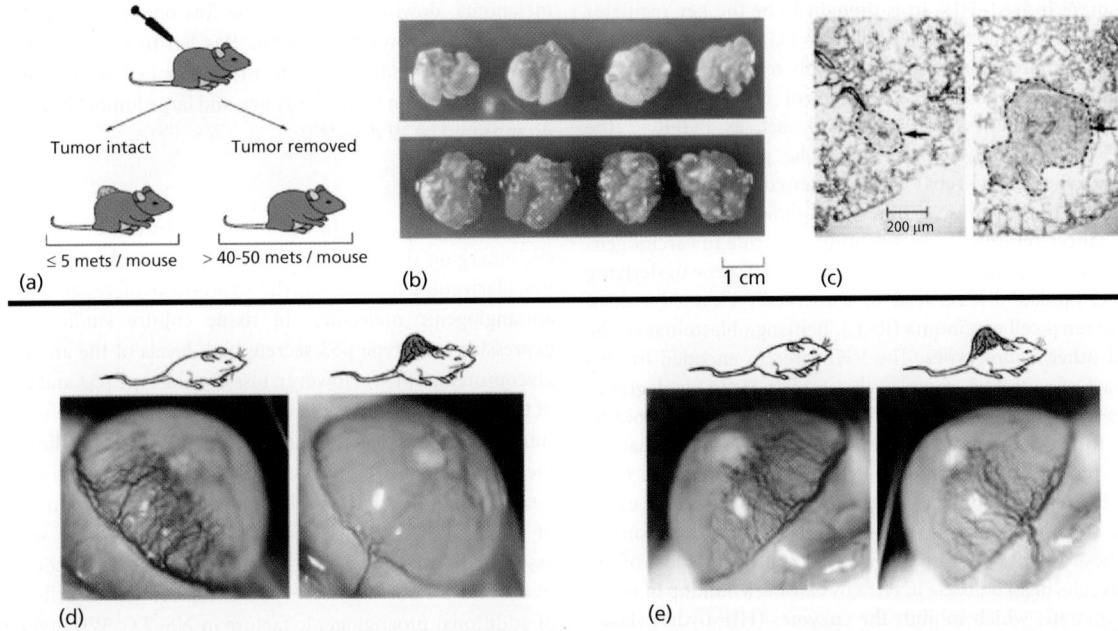

Figure 5 (a) Mice bearing Lewis Lung carcinoma.[499] Tumors were resected when tumor size reached 1.5–2 cm² and the animals were killed after 5 or 15 days. (b) Upper panel: lungs from animals still bearing the primary tumor. Lower panel: lungs removed at the same time from animals in which the tumor had been resected and the animals killed 15 days later. (c) Left panel: microscopic pulmonary metastasis in an animal in which a primary tumor is in place at the same time as the right panel. There is no evidence of angiogenesis as only a single central microvessel stained with antibody to von Willebrand factor. This dormant metastasis is 200 μm in its longest diameter. Right panel: lung metastasis from an animal euthanized 5 days after the primary tumor was removed, showing eight or nine new vessels in an enlarging metastasis. (d) A human prostate carcinoma (LNCaP) growing on the dorsum of an SCID mouse inhibits cornea neovascularization induced by an implanted sustained release pellet of bFGF (80 ng) (right panel). Left panel depicts bFGF-induced corneal neovascularization at 5 days in the absence of a primary tumor. LNCaP prostate cancer generates angiostatin. (e) A human colon cancer that does not produce an angiogenesis inhibitor, growing in an SCID mouse as a control for (d).

endostatin induces endothelial cell apoptosis, in part by activating tyrosine kinase signaling of the Shb adaptor protein.[209] Endostatin decreases formation of VEGF-induced microvessels sprouting from aortic rings *in vitro*[210] and inhibits the catalytic activity of MMP-2.[211,212] As a result, endothelial cell invasion is inhibited and tumor cell invasion may also be decreased. Endostatin also inhibits integrin-dependent endothelial cell migration because it binds to α_5- and α_v-integrins on the endothelial cell surface, in particular $\alpha_5\beta_1$.[213] It has been proposed that $\alpha_5\beta_1$-integrin may be a functional receptor for endostatin.[34]

A wide variety of tumors in many different laboratories have been inhibited by endostatin in mice and rats.[214] These include lung adenocarcinoma, thyroid carcinoma, colon carcinoma, leukemia, human non-small cell lung cancer (NSCLC), human pancreatic cancer, human neuroblastoma, breast cancer, and spontaneous pancreatic islet carcinomas.[215–222]

Tumstatin

Tumstatin (28 kDa) is the NC1 domain fragment of the α_3 collagen molecule and exhibits antiangiogenic activity in both *in vitro* and *in vivo* assays.[223–227] Tumstatin (α_3(IV)NC1) binds to endothelial cells via $\alpha_v\beta_3$-integrin and $\alpha_6\beta_1$-integrin[223,224,226,227] and induces apoptosis of proliferating endothelial cells.[225] Cell biologic experiments demonstrated that the antiangiogenic activity of tumstatin is dependent on $\alpha_v\beta_3$-integrin binding to proliferating endothelial cells.[223,227] These experiments support the notion that through the action of endogenous inhibitors such as tumstatin, $\alpha_v\beta_3$-integrin could also function as a negative regulator of angiogenesis.[223,228–230]

Antiangiogenic conformation of antithrombin III

A human small cell lung carcinoma suppressed angiogenesis and tumor growth at remote sites in immunodeficient mice. These cells generated an enzyme *in vitro* that converted the 58 kDa conformation of circulating antithrombin III to a 53 kDa form of the protein in which the externally configured stressed loop of antithrombin was retracted into the body of the molecule. The 53 kDa "cleaved" form is a specific endothelial inhibitor and a potent angiogenesis inhibitor and has no thrombin-binding activity. Antithrombin III has no antiendothelial or antiangiogenic activity. The enzymes that induce this conformational change have not yet been elucidated. Human pancreatic cancer also generates the 53 kDa cleaved antiangiogenic antithrombin.[215]

Other pathways regulating angiogenesis

Hypoxia-inducible factor-1

Expression of angiogenic factors including VEGF is positively regulated by hypoxia through the stabilization of the transcription factor hypoxia-inducible factor 1 (HIF-1).[231,232] HIF-1 is a transcription factor comprised of two subunits, HIF-1α and HIF-1β. While HIF-1β is expressed constitutively, expression of HIF-1α is tightly regulated. The stability of HIF-1α is primarily controlled by hypoxia. When oxygen is abundantly present, prolyl hydroxylases modify proline residues 402 and 564 on HIF-1α allowing it to bind the VHL tumor suppressor gene which targets it for degradation.[232] Following binding of the HIF-1α and -β subunits, HIF-1 transverses to the nucleus and modulates the expression of numerous genes involved in angiogenesis, cell survival, invasion, and glucose metabolism.[232] Indeed, HIF-1α is thought to be the key regulator of potent proangiogenic factors including VEGF.

Although initially thought to be primarily regulated by hypoxia, recent studies have revealed a number of nonhypoxic regulators including receptor tyrosine kinases such as EGFR,[233] the PI3K/AKT/mTOR pathway, and metabolic pathways including the tricarboxylic acid (Krebs) cycle (reviewed in Ref. 234, 235). Alterations in these pathways have been shown to contribute to inherited cancer syndromes, highlighting their role in carcinogenesis. For example, germline mutations in the VHL gene underlying von Hippel–Lindau disease lead to a markedly elevated risk of developing renal cell carcinoma (RCC), hemangioblastomas of the CNS, and other tumor types. The VHL protein encoded by this gene is part of a protein complex that targets HIFs for degradation.[234] Sporadic mutations in the VHL gene also occur in sporadic clear-cell RCC. A second syndrome, hereditary leiomyomatosis and RCC, results from mutations in the fumarate hydratase (FH) gene.[236] FH is a mitochondrial protein involved in the TCA cycle. Although the mechanism(s) by which FH mutations promote tumorigenesis is still under investigation, it appears that loss of FH function results in an increase in HIFs by causing a buildup of intracellular fumarate, which inhibits the enzymes (HIF hydroxylases, also known as EGLNs) that hydroxylate HIFs and target them for VHL-mediated degradation. A third hereditary syndrome, tuberous sclerosis complex, is caused by mutations in the tuberous sclerosis complex, resulting in elevated HIFs via the mTOR pathway.[237,238] Several other syndromes have also been identified that resulted in elevated levels of HIFs and downstream HIF-regulated gene products, causing a "pseudohypoxic" state.[235,237] The observations that multiple inherited cancer syndromes involve pathways that converge on HIFs support the hypothesis that dysregulation of the pathways regulating angiogenesis is likely to play a role in driving early tumorigenesis. Several drugs targeting HIFs are currently in clinical development.

Oncogenes as regulators of angiogenesis

It is widely established that activation of proto-oncogenes can induce tumorigenesis. In tissue culture, expression of activated oncogenes increases cell proliferation and decreases apoptosis.[239] While these changes contribute to tumorigenesis by altering the equilibrium between cell proliferation and apoptosis, there is considerable evidence that this alone is not sufficient to produce expansive tumor growth.[240,241] Rather, tumors must also acquire an adequate vascular supply to grow beyond 1–2 mm in diameter. In support of this concept, published reports have demonstrated that transfection of tumor cells with oncogenes results in enhanced production of proangiogenic molecules,[242] and the *in vivo* growth of oncogene-driven tumors can be restricted with angiogenesis inhibitors.[243] In lung cancer patients, for example, mutations in K-Ras, p53, and EGFR are among the oncogenes that have been linked to angiogenesis. Oncogenes shown to play a role in regulating angiogenic factors include:

Ras

Ras is one of the most commonly activated oncogenes, occurring in 17–25% of all human tumors.[244] In tissue culture studies, transfection of transformed murine endothelial cells with the Ras oncogene results in elevated production of VEGF, and treatment of these cells with the PI3K inhibitor, wortmannin, abrogates VEGF expression, indicating that mutated Ras regulates VEGF expression in a PI3K-dependent manner.[245] K-Ras gene mutations were positively associated with high VEGF expression in human NSCLC specimens[246] and other disease types. In a transgenic model of

melanoma, downregulation of the Ras oncogene in a melanoma driven by doxycycline-inducible Ras led to massive apoptosis of microvascular endothelium in the tumor bed starting within 6 h. Tumor cells began to die days later, and large tumors had completely disappeared by 12 days.[247]

p53

In addition to its role in the regulation of cell cycle and apoptosis, emerging data indicates that p53 indirectly promotes tumor vascularization by altering the expression of proangiogenic and antiangiogenic molecules. In tissue culture studies, fibroblasts expressing wild-type p53 secrete high levels of the antiangiogenic glycoprotein, TSP-1. However, loss of wild-type p53 and expression of the mutant form result in diminished TSP-1 mRNA and protein. Immunohistochemical evaluation of 73 NSCLC clinical specimens revealed a strong statistical association between p53 nuclear localization and microvessel count.[248] Additionally, in an analysis of 107 NSCLC patients, p53 was determined to be significantly associated with VEGF expression and microvessel count.[249] It is likely that loss of wild-type p53 enhances tumor cell expression of additional proangiogenic factors in NSCLC. Wild-type p53 has been demonstrated to promote Mdm2-mediated ubiquitination and degradation of HIF-1α.[250] The loss of wild-type p53 is associated with elevated levels of HIF-1α in tissue culture and augments hypoxia-induced VEGF expression.[250]

Myc

Myc is a pleiotropic transcription factor overexpressed in many cancer types, which plays a role in regulating angiogenesis, inflammation, and many other processes. Myc activity has been shown to be regulated by RAS pathway activation,[242] which in turn regulates angiogenesis at least in part through effects on TSP-1. Myc has also been shown to interact with the HIF-1α pathway to induce angiogenesis by an hypoxia-independent mechanism[251] and regulate the recruitment of mast cells required for myc-driven tumorigenesis in a transgenic mouse model.[252]

EGFR family

EGFR is a member of the erbB family of receptor tyrosine kinases, which also includes HER2/Neu, HER3 (ErbB3), and HER4 (ErbB4). An expanding body of evidence indicates that activation of EGFR leads to enhanced production of proangiogenic molecules. Initial experiments using prostate cancer cell lines demonstrated that stimulation of tumor cells with EGF elevated HIF-1α expression.[253] EGF has been shown to increase VEGF production in some tumor cell lines[254,255] and, conversely, treatment of tumor cells with EGFR inhibitors can decrease VEGF expression in various tumor types.[233,255–257] In NSCLC cell lines, EGF activates HIF-1α and induces expression of the chemokine receptor CXCR4 in tissue culture.[258] Moreover, in an immunohistochemical study of 172 NSCLC patients, expression of EGFR was associated with HIF-1α positivity,[259] and EGFR mutations causing constitutive receptor activation led to upregulated HIF-1α protein and increased VEGF levels.[260]

Like EGFR, HER2/Neu has also been shown to play a role in regulating angiogenesis. Blockade of HER2 using the monoclonal antibody trastuzumab (Herceptin) has been shown to block the production of multiple angiogenic factors and induce vessel normalization and regression in a murine model of human breast cancer, and enhance the effects of VEGF pathway blockade.[261,262]

Therapeutic approaches to targeting tumor vasculature

Angiogenesis inhibitors versus vascular targeting agents

Angiogenesis is the formation of new vessels from preexisting vasculature. Angiogenesis inhibitors are therefore typically targeted at the early stages in this process, including endothelial sprouting and survival mechanisms, which are often VEGF dependent. Vascular targeting agents (VTAs), also known as vascular disrupting agents (VDAs), differ from angiogenesis inhibitors in that they target established abnormal tumor vasculature.[263] VTAs can induce rapid collapse of tumor vasculature, and their effects on normal vasculature can cause a host of side effects including acute coronary syndromes, thrombophlebitis, and tumor pain. None of these agents are currently in routine clinical use for cancer but several have undergone clinical testing. Vadimezan (ASA404) initially demonstrated positive results in combination with chemotherapy as treatment for patients with lung cancer in a phase II trial.[264] Unfortunately, these findings were not validated in a subsequent phase III study evaluating vadimezan in combination with carboplatin/paclitaxel as first-line treatment in NSCLC, as no significant differences were demonstrated in overall survival (OS) between vadimezan and placebo arms [median OS 13.4 vs 12.7 months, respectively (hazard ratio; HR = 1.01; $p = 0.535$)]. Given the lack of clinical benefit, the development of vadimezan in lung cancer has been discontinued by Novartis.[265] ABT-751 is another VDA with preclinical anticancer activity, which has failed to demonstrate an improvement in progression-free survival (PFS) in a phase I/II study in combination with docetaxel as second-line treatment for NSCLC.[266]

Antiangiogenic effects of chemotherapy and other therapeutic agents

Multiple preclinical studies have suggested that several "classical" chemotherapeutic agents may also have potent antiangiogenic or vascular-targeting effects, which may be enhanced by low dose, frequent dosing schedules (metronomic dosing).[267–269] Several of these regimens are undergoing clinical evaluation. It also appears that certain chemotherapy agents, particularly taxanes and vinca alkaloids, may have relatively more potent antiangiogenic effects than other drugs,[269] which may help explain why there are differences in the degree of enhancement observed when antiangiogenic agents such as bevacizumab are added to chemotherapy. This prompted further examination of a wide variety of drugs which were initially thought to target primarily tumor cells. Many of these were subsequently found to also have antiangiogenic effects, prompting the term "accidental antiangiogenics".[270]

Targeting VEGF pathway

VEGF is the prototypic member of a family of structurally related, homodimeric growth factors that includes PlGF, VEGF-B, VEGF-C, VEGF-D, and VEGF-E. As described earlier, VEGF family members bind to a family of transmembrane receptor tyrosine kinases that include VEGFR-1 (Flt-1), VEGFR-2 (KDR, Flk-1), and VEGFR-3 (Flt-4) (Figure 3). The effects of VEGF or VEGFR on vascular permeability and endothelial proliferation, migration, and survival are thought to be primarily mediated by VEGFR-2, while VEGFR-3 is primarily expressed on lymphatic endothelium (reviewed in Ref. 122, 129). Agents targeting the VEGF pathway include monoclonal antibodies that bind the ligand (i.e., bevacizumab) or block

the receptor (ramucirumab). In addition, many small molecule receptor tyrosine kinase inhibitors (RTKIs) have been developed to target critical signaling pathways involved in angiogenesis. These RTKs, which include vatalanib (PTK787), vandetanib (ZD6474), sunitinib (SU11248), axitinib (AG-013736), and nintedanib (BIBF 1120), have been the focus of many preclinical and clinical studies. Because of the structural similarity of the different receptor tyrosine kinase domains, RTKIs typically inhibit multiple receptors such as PDGFR, c-KIT, FGFR, and Axl in addition to VEGFR. These multitargeting agents have demonstrated higher anticancer activity compared to agents with single targets. Furthermore, they are orally available, and thus more convenient for patients. Conversely, the off-target effects may have additive toxicities. These profiles of receptor specificity for each inhibitor, as well as their pharmacokinetics and potency for receptor inhibition, are likely to be the key determinants of their clinical activity. Representative agents targeting the VEGF pathway that are currently FDA approved are listed in Table 2.

Combinations of antiangiogenics with chemotherapy: mechanisms for enhanced antitumor activity

Preclinical and clinical studies have demonstrated that antiangiogenic therapy improves the outcome of cytotoxic therapies.[271,272] This finding is paradoxical. It was initially expected that targeting the tumor vasculature would drastically diminish the delivery of oxygen and therapeutics to the solid tumor, producing hypoxia that would cause many chemotherapeutics, as well as radiation, to be less effective.[271,272] Tumor vasculature is known to be structurally and functionally abnormal, with tortuous, highly permeable vessels. Blood flow within these intratumoral vessels is nonuniform. Proliferating tumor cells compress blood and lymphatic vessels resulting in a microenvironment typified by interstitial hypertension (elevated hydrostatic pressure outside the blood vessels), acidosis, and hypoxia.[273,274] This deficient vascular network and interstitial hypertension impair drug delivery to tumor cells. Moreover, hypoxia renders tumor cells resistant to radiation and several cytotoxic agents, and increases genetic instability selecting for tumor cells that have a greater metastatic potential. In addition to the direct effects on tumor cells, hypoxia leads to vascular abnormalization by signaling via PHD2 in tumor endothelial cells[275] and, along with the low pH within the tumor microenvironment, weakens the cytotoxic functions of tumor infiltrating immune cells. Collectively, the abnormal vasculature within solid tumors creates a significant barrier to delivery and efficacy of cancer therapeutics.

One proposed mechanism to explain the enhancement in efficacy of chemotherapy by antiangiogenic therapy is that these agents have the potential to "normalize" tumor vessels. In animal models of cancer, inhibition of VEGF signaling results in a vasculature network that more closely resembles vessels within normal tissue. This "normalized" vasculature is less leaky, is less dilated, and has less tortuous vessels with a more normal basement membrane and increased pericyte coverage. Concurrent with these changes in vascular morphology, within the tumor there is a decrease in IFP, increased oxygenation, and improved delivery of concurrently administered chemotherapeutics (Figure 6).[276–284] Evidence from a Phase I/II clinical trial in locally advanced rectal carcinoma patients receiving bevacizumab and chemotherapy (with radiation) corroborates preclinical findings. Bevacizumab treatment was associated with a decrease in tumor IFP and an increase in mature, pericyte-covered vessels.[285,286]

Table 2 Approved VEGF pathway inhibitors.

Type	Agent	Target	Approval
Monoclonal antibody	Bevacizumab (Avastin)	VEGF-A	FDA approved for CRC, breast cancer, NSCLC, platinum-resistant ovarian carcinoma, and late-stage cervical cancer
	IMC-1121B Ramucirumab	VEGFR-2 extracellular domain	FDA approved for advanced gastric or gastro-esophageal junction adenocarcinoma; metastatic NSCLC
Soluble decoy receptor	VEGF Trap (Aflibercept)	VEGF-A, VEGF-B, and PlGF	FDA approved for metastatic colorectal cancer
RTKIs	Vandetanib	VEGFR-2, EGFR, and RET	FDA approved for progressive medullary thyroid carcinoma
	Sorafenib	VEGFR-2 and 3, PDGFR-β, Flt-3, c-Kit, and B-Raf	FDA approved for renal cell, hepatocellular cancers, and metastatic differentiated thyroid carcinoma
	Sunitinib	VEGFR-1,2, PDGFR, c-Kit, RET, and Flt-3	FDA approved for renal cell carcinoma, gastrointestinal stromal tumors, and neuroendocrine tumors of the pancreas
	AG-013736 (axitinib)	VEGFR-1,2,3 and PDGFR	FDA approved for RCC
	Lenvatinib	VEGFR-2,3	FDA approved for thyroid cancer
	BIBF 1120 (Nintedanib)	VEGFR-1,2,3, PDGFR, and FGFR-1/3	Approved by FDA and EU for idiopathic pulmonary fibrosis, Approved by EU for NSCLC
	GW786034 (pazopanib)	VEGFR2	FDA approved for RCC, and soft tissue sarcoma

AML, acute myelogenous leukemia; CRC, colorectal cancer; EGFR, epidermal growth factor receptor; FDA, Food and Drug Administration; EU, European Union; GBM, glioblastoma multiforme; NSCLC, non-small cell lung cancer; PlGF, placental growth factor; PDGFR, platelet-derived growth factor receptor; RCC, renal cell carcinoma; RTKI, small molecule receptor tyrosine kinase inhibitor; VEGF, vascular endothelial growth factor; VEGFR, vascular endothelial growth factor receptor.

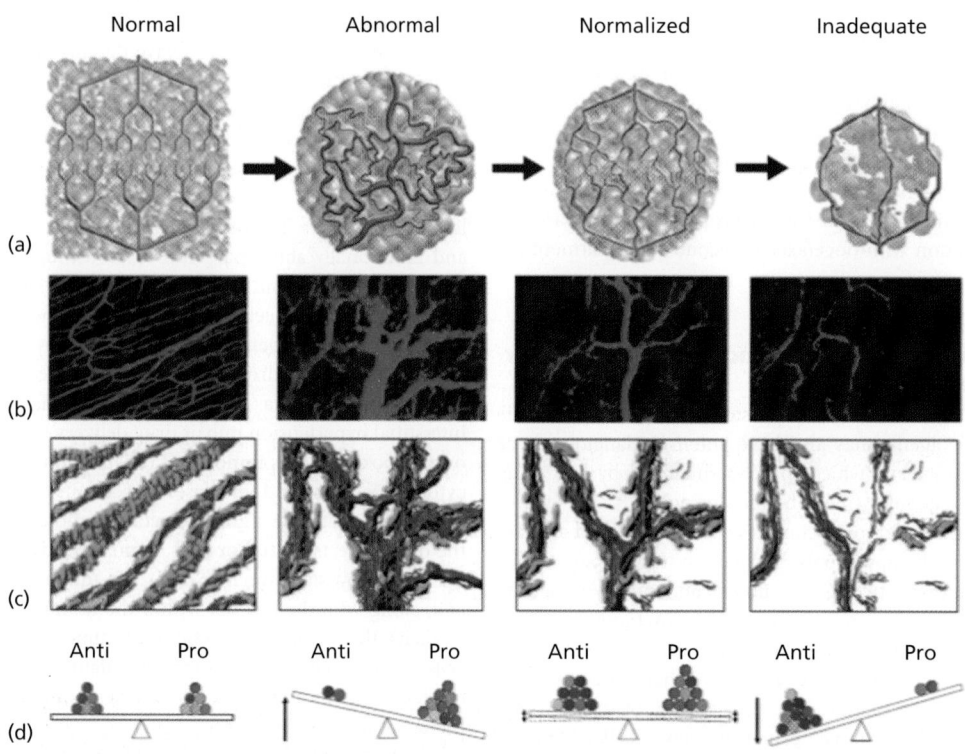

Figure 6 Changes in tumor vasculature during treatment with antiangiogenic agents.[271] (a) The tumor vascular network is structurally and functionally abnormal. Antiangiogenic therapies might initially improve both the structure and the function of tumor vessels. Continued or aggressive antiangiogenic regimens may eventually result in a vascular supply that is inadequate to support tumor growth. (b) Vascular normalization due to inhibition of VEGFR2. On the left is a two-photon image depicting normal blood vessels in skeletal muscle; subsequent representative images show human colon carcinoma vasculature in mice at day 0, day 3, and day 5 after treatment with a VEGR2-specific antibody. (c) Diagram illustrating the concomitant changes in basement membrane (blue) and pericyte (red) coverage during vessel normalization. (d) These changes in the vasculature may reflect changes in the balance of pro- and antiangiogenic factors in the microenvironment.

Antiangiogenic agents in combination with radiotherapy

A growing body of evidence suggests that antiangiogenic therapy may enhance the efficacy of radiotherapy for solid tumors. There are several proposed mechanisms through which this enhancement may occur. First, radiotherapy may act by "normalizing" the disorganized and hyperpermeable vasculature in tumors.[271,287] Vessel

normalization would permit a more effective delivery of oxygen to tumor tissue, resulting in a reduction in tumor hypoxia and augmenting radiation-induced cytotoxicity in part by increasing the formation of oxygen-free radicals. This reduction in hypoxia may be transient, however, as prolonged use of antiangiogenic agents may eventually also reduce the "normalized" vessels within tumors resulting in an inadequate intratumoral vascular supply, such that the tumor would again be hypoxic with reduced radiosensitivity. This concept is supported by mouse xenografts showing the existence of a period of time ("normalization window") during which radiation therapy used in conjunction with an antiangiogenic agent is most effective.[283,288]

Antiangiogenic therapy may act to enhance the antiendothelial effects of radiotherapy. While it was initially assumed that the antitumor effect of radiotherapy was due to direct action on tumor cells, more recent evidence has demonstrated that radiotherapy also induces endothelial cell apoptosis.[288-290] Other studies have confirmed these results.[291] Thus, the exact mechanism(s) of interaction between antiangiogenic agents and radiation remains unclear.

Nevertheless, several preclinical studies demonstrate that antiangiogenic agents can synergize with or potentiate the effects of radiotherapy.[292-296] Blockade of VEGF signaling on endothelial cells may render the tumor-associated vasculature more sensitive to radiotherapy. In addition, radiation induces VEGF expression, which contributes to radioresistance by blocking radiation-induced endothelial cell apoptosis.[297,298]

One possible cause for concern in testing combinations of antiangiogenic therapy and radiotherapy is the observation from preclinical studies that at least some of the toxicities of radiotherapy such as intestinal radiation damage may also be due to endothelial apoptosis.[299] In lung cancer patients treated with the combination of bevacizumab, chemotherapy, and radiotherapy, tracheoesophageal fistulas have been observed.[300] Clearly additional studies will be needed to assess the feasibility and efficacy of these combinations.

Clinical advances in the use of antiangiogenic therapy

The hypothesis that tumor angiogenesis could serve as a target for cancer therapy is now strongly supported by results of a number of randomized phase III clinical trials across multiple different tumor types. Bevacizumab, a monoclonal antibody targeting VEGF, is now a standard therapy for metastatic colorectal, non-small cell lung, and other tumor types[301,302]; VEGFR TKIs such as sunitinib, pazopanib, axitinib, and sorafenib are now approved for RCC and other diseases.[303,304] These advances, coupled with our increased understanding of the biological pathways underlying tumor angiogenesis and the development of improved agents for targeting these pathways, have led to a dramatic increase in the number of clinical trials employing antiangiogenic therapy either alone or in combination with other therapeutic modalities. Currently, the majority of these agents target the VEGF pathway because of its role as a key regulator of tumor angiogenesis.

VEGF pathway inhibitors as anticancer therapy: clinical experience. Clinical trials of one of the earliest VEGF pathway inhibitors, bevacizumab, began in 1997. When used as monotherapy for the treatment of advanced solid tumors, the clinical activity of these agents, as judged by objective tumor responses, has generally been low with the exception of RCC. For example, no partial or complete remissions were observed in 25 patients treated in a phase I trial of bevacizumab.[305] Furthermore, in 243 previously treated patients with colorectal cancer, objective response rates (ORR) were 3% for bevacizumab monotherapy, 9.2% for FOLFOX4 chemotherapy (fluorouracil, oxaliplatin, leucovorin), and 21.8% for the combination. Low response rates have also been reported for VEGFR TKIs when used as single agents as discussed below. For this reason, VEGF pathway inhibitors have often been developed as part of combination regimen with chemotherapy or other targeted therapeutics. Major findings in the clinical development of VEGF

pathway inhibitors for several common tumor types are reviewed below.

Renal cell cancer

One tumor type for which VEGF pathway inhibitors are particularly useful, even when used as monotherapy, is metastatic RCC. These tumors are often marked by inactivation of the von Hippel-Lindau gene leading to overexpression of VEGF and other angiogenesis mediators (reviewed in Ref. 306). In randomized studies, bevacizumab, sorafenib, and pazopanib have been shown to significantly prolong time to progression compared to placebo controls.[307-309] Sunitinib and axitinib also demonstrated substantial antitumor activity in metastatic RCC, with 25-45% ORR in phase III testing.[304,310,311]

Cytokine therapies (interferon-α- and interleukin-2-based therapies) had long been the mainstay of therapy for RCC, so it was rational to evaluate anti-VEGF therapy in the context of such agents. Phase III trials examining four small molecule RTKIs of VEGF receptors (sorafenib, sunitinib, pazopanib, and axitinib) and monoclonal anti-VEGF therapy (bevacizumab) have been reported, and consistently favor the use of anti-VEGF therapy compared to interferon.

Trials of anti-VEGF therapy versus cytokine therapy
Motzer and colleagues compared the use of sunitinib (at a dose of 50 mg orally daily for 4 weeks, followed by 2 weeks without treatment) or interferon α (9 MU subcutaneously three times weekly) in patients with previously untreated, metastatic RCC.[304] The primary endpoint of PFS was significantly improved in patients receiving sunitinib (11 vs 5 months, $p < 0.001$). Patients receiving sunitinib also experienced higher response rates, longer OS, and improved quality of life.[310]

Trials of cytokine therapy with or without anti-VEGF therapy
Escudier et al.[312] and the Cancer and Leukemia Group B performed placebo-controlled Phase III trials comparing the use of interferon α-2a to interferon-α-2a plus bevacizumab in patients with previously untreated metastatic RCC.[313] PFS was significantly longer in patients receiving the combined biologic approach. There was a trend to improved OS favoring the bevacizumab-containing treatments.[314,315] More than 50% of the patients received second-line therapy including VEGF-targeted agents, potentially affecting the survival difference.[315,316]

Trials of anti-VEGF therapy following cytokine therapy
Escudier et al.[303] performed a Phase III trial of sorafenib (400 mg twice daily) versus placebo in patients who had progressed following first-line cytokine therapy for advanced RCC. Median PFS was 5.5 months in the sorafenib group and 2.8 months in the placebo group ($p < 0.01$). Analysis of OS showed that sorafenib reduced the risk of death (HR, 0.88; 95% CI, 0.74-1.04; $p = 0.146$).[317] Although this benefit was not statistically significant, censoring of placebo-assigned patients who crossed over to sorafenib uncovered a significant result (17.8 vs 14.3 months, respectively; HR = 0.78; 95% CI, 0.62-0.97; $p = 0.0287$).

Therapy following initial anti-VEGF treatment
The demonstration of a beneficial effect for anti-VEGF therapy in RCC has fundamentally altered the treatment landscape for this disease. Nevertheless, anti-VEGF therapy is not curative and only modestly prolongs survival, leaving room for substantial therapeutic improvement. Patients progressing on one VEGF-targeting agent may still respond to another.[318-320] Whether

this cross-sensitivity is a function of the promiscuity of RTKIs, of differential pharmacokinetics, or of varying affinities for VEGF receptors is unknown.

mTOR inhibition in RCC

Two trials[321,322] examined the role of mTOR inhibition in patients with advanced RCC. While mTOR has several biologic roles, one is as a downstream effector of VEGF signaling. In a trial comparing the mTOR inhibitor temsirolimus versus interferon α versus the combination of temsirolimus plus interferon α as front-line therapy, Hudes et al.[321] demonstrated the superiority of temsirolimus to interferon α, with a significant improvement in OS (10.9 months vs 7.3 months, $p = 0.008$); the combination arm was not superior to interferon monotherapy. In addition, the temsirolimus group had fewer serious adverse events than the interferon α group. In a placebo-controlled randomized Phase III trial in the post-VEGF TKI setting, the mTOR inhibitor everolimus significantly prolonged PFS when compared to placebo (4 vs 1.9 months, $p < 0.001$).[322] OS was not significantly different, perhaps due to the fact that crossover was allowed for patients progressing on placebo. Though toxicities were generally mild, significant increases in severe (grade 3 or 4) toxicities were seen for stomatitis, $p = 0.03$; infections, $p = 0.03$; hypercholesterolemia, $p = 0.03$; hyperglycemia, $p < 00001$; lymphopenia, $p = 0.002$; and hypophosphatemia, $p = 0.01$. No prospective data is available that directly compares everolimus with a VEGF RTKI in patients whose disease has progressed on prior treatment with a VEGF inhibitor, but, OS was shown inferior for temsirolimus as compared with sorafenib (12.3 vs 16.6 months, respectively; stratified HR, 1.31; 95% CI, 1.05–1.63; two-sided $p = 0.01$) after disease progression on sunitinib.[323] Moreover, one randomized phase II clinical trial suggested that everolimus is inferior to sunitinib regarding PFS, particularly when used in first line.[324] There is no evidence to support the use of combinations of agents with different mechanisms of action as compared to sequential use, and toxicity may be increased, as shown for the combination of bevacizumab with temsirolimus (compared to bevacizumab and interferon).[325]

Antiangiogenic therapy as adjuvant therapy in RCC

The advent of multiple active antiangiogenic agents led to the development of several adjuvant trials in RCC. Early results of one, E2805, in which patients were randomly assigned to 1 year of treatment with sorafenib (400 mg twice daily), sunitinib (50 mg/day for 4 of every 6 weeks), or placebo, indicated that neither sorafenib nor sunitinib prolonged time to disease recurrence after surgery (5.6 years with either sorafenib or sunitinib vs 5.7 years with placebo).[326]

Prediction of therapeutic benefit in RCC

It has been established that relatively high VEGF levels are associated with worse tumor stage and grade, performance status, and overall prognosis.[317,327,328] Moreover, in a phase III trial of sorafenib versus placebo, patients with VEGF in the highest concentration quartile obtained greater relative benefit from sorafenib than those with lower concentrations.[327] However, studies addressing whether VEGF is a predictive marker for identifying RCC patients who are likely to benefit from VEGF-targeted therapies have yielded inconsistent results.[329] A recent study in samples from two subsequent phase II and III studies identified interleukin (IL)-6 as predictive of PFS benefit from pazopanib versus placebo.[330] Unfortunately, no biomarkers that are predictive of differential benefit between available and active drugs in RCC have yet been validated.

Future directions in RCC

While FGF and VEGF receptor inhibition with dovitinib failed to improve PFS relative to sorafenib in third line after progression to VEGF and mTOR inhibition,[331] coinhibition of other pathways of potential escape to VEGF signaling blockade such as cMET remains promising. Given very promising results of novel immunotherapeutic agents such as checkpoint inhibitors in RCC, multiple clinical trials are now evaluating their combination with angiogenesis inhibitors.

Colorectal cancer

Advanced colorectal cancer represented the first human cancer in which a Phase III trial demonstrated clinical benefit, and to this day represents among the best studied of human solid tumors with regard to antiangiogenic therapy. In 2004, results of a phase III, randomized, placebo-controlled study were reported comparing standard IFL chemotherapy (irinotecan, fluorouracil, and leucovorin) with or without bevacizumab in patients with previously untreated metastatic colorectal cancer.[301] Patients treated with IFL plus bevacizumab had a significantly longer OS and PFS as well as a higher ORR. This trial provided definitive evidence that the addition of an angiogenesis inhibitor to chemotherapy could prolong survival and, based on the results of this trial, bevacizumab received approval from the US Food and Drug Administration (FDA) for use in combination with fluorouracil-containing chemotherapy as first-line treatment for metastatic colorectal cancer.

Subsequent studies have built upon this original finding. In a trial of previously treated patients with colorectal cancer, patients treated with bevacizumab combined with FOLFOX4 chemotherapy had a prolonged survival compared to those treated with FOLFOX4 alone,[332] although the magnitude of this benefit (2.1 months) appeared to be smaller than that observed in the first-line trial (4.7 months), presumably related to the more advanced nature of the disease.

First-line studies of bevacizumab or placebo in combination with either FOLFOX or XELOX failed to demonstrate an improvement in OS (21.3 vs 19.9 months) despite improvements in PFS (9.4 vs 8.0 months).[333] The mechanism for the discrepancy between this study and the pivotal IFL study has been attributed to the different cytotoxic backbone or practice patterns of treatment until progression of disease versus regimen interruptions for cumulative oxaliplatin toxicities. Several studies have evaluated the role of bevacizumab after an initial course of oxaliplatin- and fluoropyrimidine-based first-line chemotherapy. These "maintenance" regimens have demonstrated the benefit of bevacizumab when combined with fluoropyrimidines. The CAIRO-3 randomized study demonstrated that continued bevacizumab either alone or in combination with capecitabine provided a survival benefit compared to observation alone.

Cohort studies had suggested a benefit from continued VEGF inhibition after progression on first-line therapy with bevacizumab. The TML study evaluated second-line therapy with FOLFIRI or FOLFOX (as determined by the treating physician) with or without bevacizumab for patients who had previously progressed on first-line bevacizumab-containing regimen. The study demonstrated a modest but statistically significant survival advantage of 1.4 months, resulting in the addition of bevacizumab continuation to treatment guidelines.

A similar study was conducted with ziv-aflibercept, a fusion protein utilizing the extracellular domains of VEGFR1 and VEGFR2, thereby providing inhibition of both VEGF-A and PlGF. Patients who had been previously treated with an oxaliplatin regimen (which may have included bevacizumab) were randomized to

FOLFIRI with bevacizumab or placebo.[334] The primary endpoint of OS was met with a 1.4 month improvement (13.5 months vs 12.1 months), with an improvement in PFS and response rate. Grade 3 and 4 diarrhea and stomatitis were substantially higher in the ziv-aflibercept arm, consistent with the established role for PlGF in mucosal lining repair.[335] The result of these two studies is the addition of new treatment options for second-line antiangiogenic therapy in combination with chemotherapy for patients who have previously progressed on bevacizumab-based first-line regimens.

Biomarker analyses of colorectal cancer trials have been largely unavailing. Expression levels of VEGF-A, thrombospondin, and microvessel density performed in a subset analysis of the original Hurwitz trial were not associated with clinical outcome.[336] Similarly, analysis of oncogenes known to play a role in colorectal cancer (e.g., K-Ras, b-raf, and p53) failed to demonstrate an association with clinical outcome.[337] As in metastatic breast cancer, the presence of clinically significant hypertension has been associated with clinical outcome in a Phase II trial analysis.[338]

Though monoclonal antibodies are the best-studied antiangiogenic agents in advanced colorectal cancer, TKIs with various selectivity for VEGFRs have also been examined in randomized Phase III trials. A notable initial randomized phase III trial compared FOLFOX4 chemotherapy alone or in combination with the oral small molecule RTKI vatalanib (PTK787) as first-line therapy for metastatic colorectal cancer. This study failed to demonstrate improvements in PFS or OS.[339] Similar studies with sunitinib and cediranib, among others, have failed to demonstrate a benefit. The outlier is the approval of regorafenib, a multikinase inhibitor that inhibits VEGFR, which has been shown to improve OS by 1.4 months when compared to placebo in the CORRECT study.[340] While toxicities are generally higher with TKIs, the reason for the general success of large molecule inhibitors and limited success of TKIs in combination with chemotherapy is not known.

Gastric and gastroesophageal junction cancer

Antiangiogenic therapy for advanced gastric cancer was initially evaluated in the AVAGAST study, which evaluated bevacizumab in first-line therapy in combination with cisplatin-capecitabine.[341] Despite improvements in PFS and response rate, there was no difference in OS, and further development of bevacizumab in gastric or gastroesophageal junction (GEJ) cancer has not been pursued.

In contrast, a second-line study of 355 patients with gastric or GEJ adenocarcinoma demonstrated benefit of ramucirumab compared to placebo, leading to US FDA approval. Ramucirumab, a monoclonal antibody that binds VEGFR2 at the N-terminus and prevents ligand binding and receptor conformational changes,[342] was identified from phage display library and is notable for its picomolar binding affinity to VEGFR2.[343,344] This pivotal trial (the REGARD study) demonstrated a survival benefit of second-line ramucirumab when compared to placebo, with median OS of 5.2 months compared to 3.8 months.[345] The agent was well tolerated with modestly higher risk of grade 3 hypertension (8% vs 3%) but no increased risk for thromboembolic events.

Two additional studies were subsequently conducted to further evaluate the role of antiangiogenic therapy in advanced gastroesophageal cancer. As the clinical practice for many oncologists is to provide cytotoxic chemotherapy in second line, the RAINBOW trial was designed to evaluate the addition of ramucirumab or placebo to paclitaxel in patients who had previously progressed on first-line platinum and fluoropyrimidine-based chemotherapy.[346] This 655-patient international study met its primary endpoint with improved OS (9.6 vs 7.3 months). A subgroup analysis found that the survival benefit was notably higher in Caucasian patients

than in Asian sites. The same regional differences were seen in the AVAGAST study, suggesting differences in disease biology or treatment patterns between Asian and Caucasian patients. The potential biological mechanism, if any, for this discrepancy is currently awaited.

A phase 2 study was conducted to evaluate the activity of ramucirumab or placebo in combination with FOLFOX chemotherapy in previously untreated advanced gastroesophageal cancer patients. In this setting there was no difference in OS or PFS despite improved rates of disease control. As a result, ramucirumab use is currently limited to patients with advanced gastric or GEJ adenocarcinomas with disease progression on or after prior therapy with fluoropyrimidine- or platinum-containing chemotherapy.

VEGFR TKIs have likewise been evaluated in gastric cancer. Sunitinib was evaluated in second line in a randomized study of docetaxel with placebo or sunitinib. This smaller phase II study failed to demonstrate an improvement in time to progression or OS, despite a meaningful increase in response rate (41% vs 14%).[347] In contrast, the VEGFR TKI apatinib, at two different doses, was evaluated in a randomized phase III study in patients progressing on two or more lines of prior therapy. Both doses of afatinib demonstrated benefit compared to placebo in PFS (1.4 vs 3.7/3.2 months) and OS (2.5 vs 4.8/4.3 months).[348] Toxicities included hypertension and hand–foot syndrome, consistent with the mechanism of action for the agent. Confirmatory studies are awaited.

Non-small cell lung cancer (NSCLC)

Angiogenesis inhibitors as single agents for advanced NSCLC
When tested as monotherapy for advanced NSCLC, inhibitors directed at VEGF have generally led to low rates of objective tumor responses. In a phase II trial of chemotherapy with or without bevacizumab, 19 patients in the control arm received high-dose, single-agent bevacizumab on progression, and although five had disease stabilization, there were no objective responses.[349] VEGFR TKIs have demonstrated clear evidence of antitumor activity as single agents in NSCLC, although to date there are no studies demonstrating that they prolong OS compared to chemotherapy or other targeted agents.

Vandetanib (ZD6474), a dual VEGFR/EGFR inhibitor, has been one of the most extensively tested thus far. In a randomized phase II trial involving 168 patients with locally advanced or metastatic, platinum-refractory NSCLC, a statistically significant but modest improvement in median PFS was observed in patients receiving vandetanib compared to gefitinib (11.0 vs 8.1 weeks, $p = 0.011$).[350] Vandetanib was also directly compared to chemotherapy (carboplatin and paclitaxel), or the combination of vandetanib with chemotherapy, in a phase II study in 181 previously untreated NSCLC patients.[351] A trend toward inferior PFS was observed in the vandetanib arm compared to chemotherapy alone (11.5 vs 23.1 weeks, $p = $ NS). Phase III trials of vandetanib in NSCLC patients have been completed.[352] In a phase III study testing the efficacy of vandetanib compared to standard second-line erlotinib (ZEST), no significant improvement in PFS was detected for patients treated with vandetanib versus erlotinib (median PFS of 2.6 vs 2.0 months). No significant differences were detected for the secondary endpoints of OS (HR = 1.01; $p = 0.83$), ORR (both 12%), and time to deterioration of symptoms for pain (HR = 0.92; $p = 0.28$). In a noninferiority analysis, both agents showed similar PFS and OS.[353]

Sorafenib has also shown evidence of single-agent activity in advanced, recurrent NSCLC. In a randomized discontinuation phase II clinical trial (ECOG2501), NSCLC patients with stable disease during treatment with sorafenib ($N = 97$) were randomized to either continue sorafenib or receive placebo.[354] Patients on the sorafenib arm had a significantly longer PFS compared to those receiving placebo (3.6 vs 1.9 months, $p = 0.01$). Interestingly, only a single patient had an objective response, illustrating that for NSCLC, as in RCC,[303] objective tumor response rates may not be the most appropriate metric for benefit in early testing.

Sunitinib has also demonstrated encouraging single-agent activity in patients with recurrent NSCLC.[355] Objective tumor responses were observed in 7 of 63 patients (ORR 11.1%), and 70% of patients demonstrated at least some degree of tumor shrinkage. The safety profile was considered acceptable overall, but two patients, both with squamous cell histology, died of treatment-related pulmonary hemorrhage. This toxicity has been seen with other angiogenesis inhibitors, as described below, and has led to the exclusion of patients with squamous histology from treatment with bevacizumab and several other agents.

Pazopanib (GW786034, GlaxoSmithKline), a TKI targeting VEGFRs, PDGFRs, FGFR-1, and FGFR-3, has produced encouraging responses as neoadjuvant therapy in patients with stage I/II NSCLC,[356] with tolerable toxicity profile including hypertension, diarrhea, and fatigue. The activity and efficacy of this agent are currently under investigation in the adjuvant and advanced setting.[357] Other VEGFR TKIs that have demonstrated single-agent activity in advanced NSCLC include vatalanib (PTK787), axitinib (AG-013736),[358] and XL647.[359]

Bevacizumab with chemotherapy for advanced NSCLC

Given their modest single-agent activity, angiogenesis inhibitors have most commonly been tested in combination with chemotherapy for NSCLC. Initial phase II testing in chemo-naïve, advanced NSCLC patients suggested that bevacizumab improved ORR and time to progression when added to the standard doublet chemotherapy regimen of carboplatin and paclitaxel.[349] This study also revealed an unanticipated and concerning side effect: severe pulmonary hemorrhage, which occurred in six out of 67 patients who received bevacizumab, and was fatal in four cases. Tumor characteristics associated with significant hemoptysis were central location, proximity to major blood vessels, necrosis and cavitation before or during therapy, and squamous histology. As squamous cell tumors are more commonly located centrally and have a greater tendency to cavitate than adenocarcinomas, it is unclear whether histology alone is the primary risk factor for hemoptysis, or simply a surrogate for other risk factors.

On the basis of the promising outcomes with bevacizumab in this phase II trial, a randomized phase II/III trial was conducted by the Eastern Cooperative Oncology Group (ECOG), E4599, comparing standard carboplatin and paclitaxel for six cycles with or without bevacizumab in 878 patients with previously untreated, advanced (stage IIIB or IV) nonsquamous NSCLC.[302] Patients receiving carboplatin–paclitaxel with bevacizumab had a significantly improved median OS (12.3 vs 10.3 months, HR 0.77, $p = 0.003$), PFS (6.2 vs 4.5 months, $p < 0.0001$), and response rate (35% vs 15%, $p < 0.001$) compared to carboplatin–paclitaxel alone. The main grade 3 or higher toxicities associated with bevacizumab were clinically significant bleeding (4.4% vs 0.7% in the standard chemotherapy arm), febrile neutropenia, and hypertension. The overall rate of fatal hemoptysis with bevacizumab when squamous histology was excluded was approximately 1%. This may be considered an acceptable risk in light of the absolute improvements in survival of 7% and 8% at 1 and 2 years, respectively.

Interestingly, unplanned subset analyses of E4599 found that the survival benefit was confined primarily to male participants,

although females did benefit in terms of response and PFS.[360] The reason for this apparent gender-based difference in benefit is unclear. In elderly patients, defined as >70 years old, there also appeared to be an increase in toxicity but no obvious improvements in OS.[361]

This was the first randomized phase III study in advanced NSCLC that demonstrated superior OS when targeted therapy is combined with standard chemotherapy. A similar randomized III trial testing bevacizumab in combination with another standard doublet of cisplatin and gemcitabine has been reported (AVAIL).[362] In this study, a total of 1043 patients were randomized to either low (7.5 mg/kg) or high (15 mg/kg) dose bevacizumab one every 3 weeks with cisplatin–gemcitabine, compared to cisplatin–gemcitabine alone. In this study PFS and ORR were significantly improved in the bevacizumab-containing arms compared to cisplatin–gemcitabine but OS was not improved. There were no significant differences in efficacy or toxicity between the low and high doses of bevacizumab. This clinical result is consistent with the vascular normalization hypothesis.[363]

At present, the use of bevacizumab in combination with chemotherapy is being tested in the neoadjuvant or adjuvant settings. The BEACON phase II study is being conducted to determine whether the addition of bevacizumab to a cisplatin-based chemotherapy in the neoadjuvant setting improves response rates. ECOG trial E1505, a phase III randomized study of adjuvant chemotherapy with or without bevacizumab for patients with resected stage IB–IIIA NSCLC has completed accrual and the results are awaited.

On the basis of these results, some oncologists regard bevacizumab in combination with carboplatin–paclitaxel as a new standard of care for patients with nonsquamous NSCLC. Given the results of the AVAIL trial, however, it remains an open question as to whether a similar degree of benefit can be expected when bevacizumab is combined with any platinum-containing doublet for untreated NSCLC patients, and whether additional clinical criteria such as sex or age should be used in selecting patients for treatment.

Ramucirumab with chemotherapy for refractory NSCLC

Ramucirumab has recently received FDA approval for the treatment of relapsed NSCLC patients in combination with second-line docetaxel. The approval was based on the results of the phase III REVEL trial, an international study that involved 1253 patients with nonsquamous and squamous cell NSCLC who had experienced disease progression after treatment with platinum-based chemotherapy for locally advanced or metastatic disease.[364] Patients were randomized to treatment with ramucirumab plus docetaxel or placebo plus docetaxel. Median OS was significantly improved in the ramucirumab group compared with the placebo group (10.5 vs 9.1 months; HR 0.857; $p = .0235$), as was median PFS (4.5 vs 3.0 months; HR, 0.762; $p < .0001$). The ORR was also improved in the ramucirumab group (23% vs 14%; $p < .0001$). The most common grade ≤ 3 toxicities that were more frequent in patients in the ramucirumab than in the placebo group were neutropenia (48.8% vs 39.8%), febrile neutropenia (15.9% vs 10.0%), fatigue (14.0% vs 10.5%), leukopenia (13.7% vs 12.5%), and hypertension (5.6% vs 2.1%). Patients in the ramucirumab group experienced more bleeding/hemorrhage events of any grade compared with patients in the placebo group, but the rate of grade 3 or higher bleeding events was similar among the two groups.

VEGFR TKIs with chemotherapy as first-line NSCLC therapy

VEGFR TKI/chemotherapy combinations are also being evaluated in randomized trials for first-line treatment of advanced NSCLC treatment. The phase III trial ESCAPE (Evaluation of Sorafenib, Carboplatin and Paclitaxel Efficacy in NSCLC) comparing the efficacy of carboplatin–paclitaxel, with and without sorafenib, in 926 patients failed to demonstrate a significant advantage in terms of OS with the addition of sorafenib in nonsquamous histotype, and, in a planned subgroup analysis, showed a detrimental effect in patients with squamous cell carcinoma.[365] The NExUS phase III trial (NCT00449033) evaluated cisplatin–gemcitabine with and without sorafenib and was stopped early owing to failure in meeting its primary endpoint of OS.

Cediranib (AZD2171), an oral VEGFR, PDGFRs, and KIT TKI, was tested with carboplatin–paclitaxel in a planned phase II/III trial by the National Cancer Institute of Canada (NCIC trial BR24)[366] in 296 patients. Although evidence of improved PFS and ORR was observed in the cediranib arm, the trial was discontinued at a preplanned analysis at the end of the phase II component because of an excess of dose-related adverse effects including dehydration, diarrhea, and fatigue. A similar phase II N0528 study evaluated the safety and efficacy of gemcitabine–carboplatin with or without cediranib (45 mg orally daily). The trial failed to show significant differences in terms of response rate (RR; 20% vs 18%; $p = 1.0$), median PFS (6.3 vs 4.5 months; HR, 0.69; $p = 0.15$), and median OS (11.8 vs 9.9 months; HR, 0.66; $p = 0.16$), Grade 3 and higher toxicities were increased in the arm containing cediranib (71% vs 45%; $p = 0.01$).[367]

Given the concern of intolerable toxicity, the NCIC BR29 phase III trial was similarly designed to further evaluate cediranib 20 mg in combination with carboplatin–paclitaxel. An interim analysis demonstrated insufficient efficacy, thus the study was closed.[368]

As noted previously, vandetanib with carboplatin–paclitaxel (VCP) was compared to carboplatin–paclitaxel or vandetanib alone in 181 patients.[351] VPC could be safely administered, even in patients with squamous cell histology and treated brain metastases. Patients receiving VPC had trend toward improved ORR (32% vs 25%) and longer PFS (24 vs 23 weeks; HR = 0.76, one-sided $p = .098$) compared to carboplatin–paclitaxel.

Nintedanib (BIBF 1120), which has activity against PDGFR and FGFR in addition to VEGFR, has shown single agent activity in a phase II study of pretreated NSCLC with 48% of patients achieving disease stabilization.[369] Phase II trials testing the efficacy of nintedanib in combination with chemotherapy are underway. Taken together, trials of VEGFR TKIs with chemotherapy for first-line NSCLC treatment have been somewhat disappointing thus far, with modest gains, at most, in efficacy and significant toxicities in some cases.

VEGFR TKIs with chemotherapy for recurrent NSCLC

Vandetanib has also been evaluated in combination with docetaxel for patients previously treated with platinum-containing chemotherapy.[370] One hundred and twenty seven patients were randomized to receive docetaxel with either low dose (100 mg once daily) or high dose (300 mg once daily) vandetanib. This study met its primary endpoint of prolonged median PFS in the vandetanib arm, although, interestingly, a trend toward greater benefit was observed in the low dose arm (19, 17, and 12 weeks in low dose, high dose, and control arms, respectively). On the basis of these results, a randomized, phase III trial of vandetanib 100 mg daily with docetaxel versus docetaxel was conducted (ZODIAC). The primary endpoint of this study was achieved, with a prolongation in PFS in the vandetanib arm (PFS HR = 0.79, $p < 0.001$), but this did

not translate into significantly improved OS.[352] A biomarker analysis from this study suggested that patients with EGFR copy number gains had greater benefit from the addition of vandetanib.[371]

Nintedanib (BIBF1120) has also recently completed clinical testing in patients with platinum-refractory NSCLC. In the LUME-Lung 1 randomized phase III trial comparing docetaxel combined with either nintedanib or placebo, PFS was prolonged in the nintedanib arm compared with the placebo arm, regardless of histology (HR 0.79; $p = 0.0019$; squamous HR 0.77, $p = 0.02$; adeno HR 0.77, $p = 0.0019$).[372] Furthermore, significantly prolonged OS was observed in patients with adenocarcinoma (HR 0.83; $p = 0.0359$; median 12.6 vs 10.3 months), but not in the squamous subgroup. Preliminary reports of the LUME-Lung 2A study testing nintedanib in combination with pemetrexed indicate that a significant PFS, but not OS, advantage was observed for patients with platinum-refractory nonsquamous disease.[373] On the basis of these results, nintedanib has recently received approval in the European Union (EU) for NSCLC. Furthermore, it is approved by the FDA and in the EU for the treatment of idiopathic pulmonary fibrosis on the basis of two randomized phase III trials.[374,375]

Antiangiogenic agents in combination with other targeted therapies for NSCLC

The molecular pathways regulating tumor angiogenesis and tumor cell survival are complex and somewhat redundant.[241,376] It is not surprising, therefore, that therapeutic approaches targeting a single pathway do not typically provide long-term disease control and tumor resistance inevitably develops. Combinations of targeted agents may therefore improve clinical outcomes while avoiding the toxicities associated with chemotherapy. In NSCLC and several other diseases, dual blockade of the EGFR and VEGF pathways is being studied clinically because both are validated therapeutic targets that are known to be interrelated. VEGF is downregulated by EGFR inhibition, likely through both HIF-α-dependent and -independent mechanisms,[233,257,259,260,377–379] and EGFR, like VEGFR-2, may be expressed on tumor-associated endothelium.[380–382] Acquired resistance to the EGFR inhibitor was found to be associated with increased VEGF levels and increased tumor angiogenesis in preclinical studies.[383]

Clinically, inhibition of both VEGF and EGFR has been investigated using combinations of individual drugs, or a single multitargeted TKIs such as vandetanib as discussed above. In a randomized phase II trial, bevacizumab and erlotinib were compared to chemotherapy alone (docetaxel or pemetrexed) or chemotherapy with bevacizumab in patients with refractory or recurrent NSCLC.[384] A trend toward improved PFS, and improved tolerability, was observed in the bevacizumab–erlotinib arm compared to chemotherapy. A randomized phase III study of bevacizumab–erlotinib compared to erlotinib (BETA trial, for BEvacizumab/TArceva) was subsequently conducted in 636 second-line patients. Patients in the bevacizumab–erlotinib arm had improved PFS (3.4 vs 1.7 months) and ORR compared to the erlotinib arm, but OS was not prolonged (9.3 vs 9.2 months). There did, however, appear to be greater benefit for the combination in patients bearing EGFR mutations. This observation was confirmed in a phase III study of erlotinib with or without bevacizumab in EGFR-mutant NSCLC.[385] The molecular basis underlying the greater sensitivity of the EGFR-mutant subgroup to bevacizumab is not completely understood, but may be related to the constitutive activation of HIF-1α and hence greater VEGFR dependence of these tumors.[260] Furthermore, in preclinical models, EGFR TKI resistance is associated with a rise in VEGF.[386] Finally, the ATLAS phase III trial of bevacizumab–erlotinib versus bevacizumab and placebo as maintenance therapy after first-line treatment was stopped early as an interim analysis revealed that the combination led to a significant improvement in PFS.[387] Together these data support the use of combined VEGF and EGFR inhibition in patients bearing EGFR mutations.

Antiangiogenic therapy for operable NSCLC

The use of angiogenesis inhibitors in the neoadjuvant or adjuvant setting is also being investigated in NSCLC patients with operable disease. In one preoperative trial, the VEGFR TKI pazopanib was found to have significant antitumor activity, with 87% of patients demonstrating a reduction in tumor volume.[388] A phase III randomized trial testing is also underway testing whether the addition of bevacizumab to four cycles of standard chemotherapy improves outcomes compared to chemotherapy alone for fully resected stage IB–IIIA NSCLC (ECOG1505).

Breast cancer

Antiangiogenic agents in breast cancer have failed to reproducibly demonstrate improvements in OS in metastatic disease, and no agents are currently FDA approved. Bevacizumab received accelerated approval in 2008 on the basis of a randomized study of paclitaxel with or without bevacizumab in 715 previously untreated women with metastatic HER2-negative breast cancer.[389] This study demonstrated statistically significant improvements in response rate from 37% to 21%, and PFS from 5.9 to 11.8 months, but no difference in OS. The accelerated approval was conditional on further evidence of improved survival from additional studies. The AVADO study of docetaxel with or without bevacizumab saw similarly improved response rates and PFS, but no improvements in OS in HER2-negative patients.[390] Similarly, the RIBBON-1 study of chemotherapy with or without bevacizumab produced similar incremental benefits in response rates and PFS without improved OS.[391] A study in the HER2-positive population of docetaxel, trastuzumab, with or without bevacizumab improved response rates (66% vs 77%) but failed to improve PFS or OS.[392] On the basis of the available data, the FDA revoked the agency's approval of bevacizumab for breast cancer in 2011. Similarly disappointing results were seen in the ROSE study, which evaluated ramucirumab in combination with docetaxel, and failed to demonstrate an improvement in PFS.[393]

Subsequent analyses of the AVADO study demonstrated the potential for high VEGF-A plasma levels to be a predictive biomarker for benefit from bevacizuamb.[394] This hypothesis is being prospectively evaluated in the MERiDiAN study with a coprimary endpoint of PFS in the high VEGF-A population.

Hepatoma

Hepatoma (hepatocellular carcinoma) is an important cancer on a global basis, and has been characterized by remarkably poor prognosis and few active agents for decades. The advent of antiangiogenic therapy has reinvigorated therapeutic attacks on hepatoma.

In a randomized placebo-controlled Phase III trial, sorafenib prolonged OS compared with control (5.5 vs 2.5 months).[395] Multiple antiangiogenic agents are currently under investigation.

Other malignancies

Antiangiogenic therapies (particularly anti-VEGF therapies) have been examined in numerous other human malignancies, with initial positive results (and a few signal failures) in several cancers. Many of these approaches are discussed elsewhere in this book, and will be summarized only briefly here.

Pancreatic cancer: A large Phase III trial comparing gemcitabine plus bevacizumab versus gemcitabine plus placebo was reported as a negative trial. Pancreatic cancer continues to elude our best therapeutic efforts.

Soft-tissue sarcoma: In 2012, the FDA approved pazopanib for the treatment of metastatic nonadipocytic soft tissue sarcoma following positive results from the phase III PALETTE clinical study (NCT00753688).[396]

Ovarian cancer: In the phase III AURELIA clinical study, the addition of bevacizumab to chemotherapy significantly improved PFS and ORR in platinum-resistant ovarian cancer patients, prompting FDA approval in 2014.[397]

Cervical cancer: Results from a phase III trial (GOG 240) testing the efficacy of bevacizumab and nonplatinum combination chemotherapy in patients with advanced cervical cancer led to the FDA approval of bevacizumab to treat patients with persistent, recurrent or late-stage cervical cancer.[398]

Glioblastoma: While early clinical studies testing the efficacy of bevacizumab in patients with glioblastoma appeared promising,[399,400] in further phase III testing, bevacizumab did not improve OS in patients with newly diagnosed glioblastoma.[401] The phase III study (REGAL) testing the efficacy of cediranib as monotherapy or in combination with lomustine versus lomustine alone in patients with recurrent glioblastoma was also negative.[402]

Glioma: Several Phase II trials of anti-VEGF therapy as monotherapy have suggested that bevacizumab has therapeutic activity in advanced gliomas. These promising results have led to a submission to the FDA for accelerated approval, and to the development of a proof-of-concept Phase III trial.

Non-Hodgkin Lymphoma: Positive early results for anti-VEGF therapy have been reported from several Phase II trials, and have led to the development of Phase III trials, which are ongoing.

Toxicities of antiangiogenic therapy

Angiogenesis inhibitors have been developed with the hope that they would provide a relatively nontoxic means to slow or prevent tumor growth that could be used over long periods of time, toward the goal of converting cancer into a manageable, chronic condition. On the basis of the clinical experience to date, it appears that they do in fact have a generally favorable side effect profile that is nonoverlapping with chemotherapy. Certain toxicities have emerged, however, that appear to be specific to entire classes of agents and, in some cases, potentially life threatening.

Pure VEGF antagonists (e.g., bevacizumab) offer an important window into the physiologic and pathophysiologic effects of VEGF blockade; agents that combine VEGF blockade with blockade of other kinases (e.g., sorafenib and sunitinib) add side effects specific to the kinases blocked. Additional drug-specific idiosyncratic side effects may also occur. In addition, as antiangiogenic agents are regularly combined with chemotherapeutic agents across a broad array of diseases, and frequently prolong PFS, chemotherapy-related side effects may be increased related to increased duration of their use. For instance, in the E2100 Phase III breast cancer trial, patients receiving bevacizumab and paclitaxel-based chemotherapy suffered statistically significant increases in VEGF-related side effects such as hypertension, cerebrovascular ischemia, headache, and proteinuria, and in Grade 3 and 4, infection, fatigue, and sensory neuropathy.[389] It seems likely that the latter were a function of prolonged exposure to chemotherapy, as patients receiving bevacizumab not only had prolonged PFS, but also received increased duration of taxane-based chemotherapy.

The availability of multiple Phase III trials allows us to gauge these toxicities across large populations, while smaller studies have focused on individual toxic effects. In this section we will focus on toxicities that are VEGF related and mechanistic in nature (i.e., a function of a ligand–receptor interaction in a normal tissue organ). These side effects include toxicities that are seen across most diseases treated with anti-VEGF therapy, as well as side effects that—while mechanistic—are seen more commonly with specific diseases (e.g., bowel perforation and pulmonary hemorrhage). Side effects unrelated to VEGF inhibition observed with nonspecific RTKIs will not be discussed here.

Hypertension
The most commonly reported toxicity in patients receiving anti-VEGF therapies is hypertension. It is generally mild-to-moderate in nature, though very rarely severe (malignant) hypertension has been reported. Hypertension is thought to be related to alterations in endothelial function related to blockade of the nitric oxide pathway downstream from the VEGF receptor.[403] In contrast to anti-VEGF therapy, VEGF infusions are associated with decreases in blood pressure. Management of anti-VEGF-related hypertension has not been carefully studied in the clinic, though it appears responsive to standard antihypertensive agents, and is reversible upon discontinuation of anti-VEGF therapy. For patients experiencing mild-to-moderate degrees of hypertension, anti-VEGF therapy may be continued in the presence of appropriate antihypertensive therapy. Recent data suggests that the presence of hypertension may be associated with improved outcome, and as such hypertension may represent a type of pharmacokinetic or pharmacodynamic surrogate biomarker of response.[404] Analysis of the E2100 Phase III breast cancer trial demonstrated a relationship between hypertension and particular single-nucleotide polymorphisms for VEGF, though this finding awaits and requires confirmation.[405] The results of a recently reported subgroup analysis of the phase III ECOG 4599 trial of bevacizumab and chemotherapy in NSCLC revealed a positive correlation between the onset of hypertension and improved clinical outcomes in bevacizumab-treated patients.[406] Similarly, the analysis of data derived from six phase II trials evaluating axitinib in patients with various solid tumor types indicated the potential role of diastolic blood pressure > 90 mmHg as biomarker of prolonged survival.[325] Prospective studies to validate hypertension as a reliable biomarker of response in clinical practice are warranted.

Arterial thromboembolic events
An increased incidence of thromboembolic and cardiovascular events has been observed in some but not all clinical trials of VEGF inhibitors. These events, while uncommon, may be serious and life threatening. Data pooled from five Phase III trials with bevacizumab (all of which excluded patients with recent history of stroke or heart attack) demonstrated a HR of 2.0 for such events, with an increase in absolute risk from 1.7% in control patients to 3.8% in bevacizumab-treated patients. There was no associated increase in venous thromboembolic events. Cerebrovascular ischemia reported with bevacizumab may involve either transient ischemic attacks or stroke; myocardial infarction and angina have also been reported to occur with increased frequency.[407] These toxicities are more common in the elderly (age >65) and in patients with a prior history of arterial thromboembolic events. Management of these complications is similar to those in patients not receiving anti-VEGF therapy. In contrast to hypertension, which is generally readily managed with antihypertensive therapy, discontinuation of VEGF-targeted therapy in the presence of arterial thromboembolic events seems appropriate.

Patients receiving VEGF-targeted therapy frequently experience headaches, with severe headaches occurring ~3% of the time in Phase III trials. These headaches are typically migraine-like in nature, and anecdotally respond to antimigraine agents such as serotonin receptor-active agents. Headaches may recur, and patients may require chronic antimigraine medications such as β-blockers therapy if their cancer continues to respond to anti-VEGF therapy. The relationship of such headaches to more severe central nervous system ischemic events is unknown.

Reversible posterior leukoencephalopathy syndrome (RPLS)
RPLS is a rare central nervous system complication of anti-VEGF therapy. RPLS is a subacute neurologic syndrome typically consisting of headache, cortical blindness, and seizures, and has been reported anecdotally in patients receiving VEGF-targeting therapy. The etiology of RPLS is not well understood at present, nor is its relationship to VEGF inhibition; though it has been suggested that vasospasm of the posterior cerebral arteries may be important. Immediate cessation of anti-VEGF therapy and appropriate antihypertensive management (a potential predisposing factor) are indicated.[408,409]

Nephrotoxicity
Nephrotoxicity, in the form of proteinuria, is common in patients receiving prolonged anti-VEGF therapy with as many as 40% of patients having at least some degree of proteinuria. More severe protein loss (e.g., nephrotic syndrome) is rare, occurring in approximately 1–2% of patients. While not well studied, proteinuria is reversible when anti-VEGF therapy is held, and patients may be rechallenged. A standard approach has been to discontinue bevacizumab temporarily if urine protein excretion is ≥2 g/24 h and resume when protein excretion is <2 g/24 h. Bevacizumab treatment should be discontinued if nephrotic-range proteinuria develops. From a mechanistic standpoint, VEGF is important in renal glomerular homeostasis, so the renal effects of anti-VEGF therapy are perhaps unsurprising.[410] A recent investigation has associated bevacizumab-induced proteinuria with renal thrombotic microangiopathy, suggesting that VEGF plays a critical role in protection against this condition.[411]

Pulmonary hemorrhage
Pulmonary hemorrhage was reported in the initial Phase II trial of lung cancer patients, where fatal hemorrhagic events were observed.[349] This trial suggested that patients with squamous cell cancer histology were at increased risk for this complication, and along with patients with gross hemoptysis (1/2 tsp or more per event) and those being treated with anticoagulant therapy or nonsteroidal anti-inflammatory agents were excluded from the proof-of-concept Phase III NSCLC trial E4599. Despite these exclusions, the rate of life-threatening pulmonary hemorrhage was 1.9% (with 1.2% fatal events), suggesting that we remain imperfect at predicting which patients will experience this complication.[302] The discussion of pulmonary hemorrhagic events should be part of the informed consent discussion for all lung cancer patients receiving bevacizumab or other VEGF-targeting agents. The mechanism of this side effect is unknown as is its dose–response relationship. The relationship with squamous cell lung carcinoma may be related to the tendency of these cancers to undergo central necrosis; central cavitation is common in lung cancers treated with anti-VEGF therapy.

Bowel perforation

Bowel perforation has been seen predominantly in patients with advanced colorectal cancer and ovarian cancer, though it has been reported to occur in virtually every cancer treated with bevacizumab, albeit less commonly in cancers not involving the abdomen or pelvis. One recent analysis has suggested a 30-day mortality of 12.5% for patients undergoing this complication, suggesting its seriousness.[412] A recent review has suggested that the incidence of bowel perforation seems to be higher in patients with an intact primary tumor, recent history of sigmoidoscopy or colonoscopy, or previous abdominal or pelvic radiotherapy. Interestingly, a prior history of peptic ulcer disease, diverticulosis, or use of nonsteroidal anti-inflammatory drugs was not obviously associated with an increased risk of bowel perforation.[413] At present we lack any useful exclusion factors that might prevent patients from developing this complication. The etiology of this side effect is uncertain, though preclinical evidence suggests that anti-VEGF therapy may greatly reduce the vascular density of normal intestinal villi.[414] This may be exacerbated when anti-VEGF therapy is combined with radiation.[294]

The management of bowel perforation involves awareness and recognition of symptoms and emergent surgical intervention. Surgical intervention in the face of anti-VEGF therapy may itself be associated with an increased risk of postsurgical complications such as further bowel perforation and abdominal fistulae. These, however, should not prevent a lifesaving surgical intervention.[191,415]

Lessons from clinical studies of antiangiogenic therapy and future directions

Reconciling differences in preclinical and clinical efficacy of antiangiogenic therapy

While antiangiogenic agents have had dramatic effects on tumor growth as single agents in preclinical animal models, in patient trials the majority of antiangiogenic agents must be given in combination with other treatment regimens to be effective. This difference in antitumor activity is linked to key differences between mouse tumor models and cancer patients. Human patients have extensive variability in tumor heterogeneity and genetic background compared to experimental models. Furthermore, in mouse models of cancer, the tumor growth rate is frequently extremely high, potentially heightening the sensitivity to antiangiogenic agents. In preclinical models, therapy is frequently initiated early in tumor development, whereas in the clinical setting, tumors may have been present for years before treatment begins, and clinical trials often include patient populations with advanced, metastatic disease.[416]

Mechanisms of resistance to VEGF pathway inhibitors

The therapeutic efficacy of conventional chemotherapy for most solid tumors is limited in part by the emergence of drug resistance in rapidly mutating tumor cells. Because antiangiogenic agents are directed against tumor endothelium, which was presumed to be diploid and genetically stable, it was initially thought that tumors will not develop resistance to antiangiogenic therapy[191,415] as they do to cytotoxic chemotherapy. Clinical experience thus far, however, suggests that virtually all tumors do eventually progress despite treatment with a VEGF inhibitor. Studies have suggested several potential mechanisms by which tumors may initially have

or acquire resistance, or at least decreased sensitivity, to VEGF pathway inhibitors.[149,417]

Incomplete target inhibition

Drugs may not be present at sufficiently high concentrations at their targets for a sufficiently long time to cause a sustained inhibition of VEGF receptor signaling and tumor angiogenesis. In trials of VEGFR inhibitors SU5416 and SU6668, tumor biopsies taken before and during treatment revealed that VEGFR phosphorylation was inhibited by <50% in all cases, providing a potential explanation for the lack of significant clinical activity observed in these trials.[418,419] For other TKIs such as gefitinib and imatinib, incomplete target inhibition has been shown to result from genetic changes, for example, secondary mutations in EGFR or BCR-ABL, or epigenetic changes reducing the intracellular concentrations of the inhibitor.[420–422] It is not yet known whether mutations may be present within VEGFR in tumor endothelium.

Bypass of the VEGF pathway through expression of additional angiogenic factors

Genetic mutations or the activation of pathways such as HIF-1 may lead to the expression of additional angiogenic factors (or the loss of angiogenic inhibitors) by malignant cells in the tumor.[232,423] In turn, these changes may promote the proliferation and survival of tumor endothelial cells even in the presence of VEGF blockade. It has been observed, for example, that advanced-stage breast cancers express a greater number of proangiogenic factors than early-stage cancers do,[424] which may help explain why previously untreated patients with metastatic breast cancer appeared to have a greater benefit from the addition of bevacizumab to standard chemotherapy than previously treated patients.[425,426]

Recently, Cascone et al.[427] have shown that gene expression changes associated with acquired resistance to bevacizumab occurred predominantly in stromal and not tumor cells in mouse xenograft models of human lung adenocarcinoma. Specifically, the EGFR and FGFR signaling pathways were upregulated in the stroma, and increased expression of activated EGFR was detected on pericytes of xenografts that acquired resistance to VEGF inhibition and on endothelium of tumors with relative primary resistance. Furthermore, changes in the vasculature pattern characterize the phenotype of resistance. Murine models of human NSCLC that acquired resistance to bevacizumab were characterized by a pattern of pericyte-covered, normalized revascularization, whereas tortuous, uncovered vessels were observed in models of relative primary resistance. Dual VEGF and EGFR pathway blockade reduced pericyte coverage and increased PFS of tumor-bearing animals, suggesting that alterations in tumor stromal pathways may contribute to VEGF-inhibitor resistance in NSCLC and that targeting these pathways may improve therapeutic efficacy. In a phase II trial evaluating the regimen FOLFIRI in combination with bevacizumab for the treatment of patients with colorectal cancer, increased baseline levels of IL-8 correlated with poorer PFS. In the same study, before the radiographic development of disease progression, circulating levels of several proangiogenic cytokines known to be associated with angiogenesis and myeloid recruitment increased compared to baseline, such as FGF, HGF, PlGF, SDF, and MCP.[428]

Numerous studies have provided additional evidence that tumors can escape VEGFR pathway inhibition by increasing other angiogenic factors. In preclinical models, inhibition of FGFR signaling can restore sensitivity to VEGF-targeting agents.[83] Galectin-1 (Gal1) has also been shown to play a role in resistance to antiangiogenic therapies. Gal1 is upregulated in hypoxic conditions, modulates trafficking of EGFR and VEGF, and promotes tumor angiogenesis. In cultured endothelial cells, GAL1 binds to neutral branched N-glycans on VEGFR2, resulting in VEGFR2 signaling and enhanced cell surface retention. In animal studies, anti-VEGF refractory tumors exhibit increased hypoxia and increased Gal1 expression compared to anti-VEGF sensitive tumors. Targeting of Gal1 along with anti-VEGF therapy improved antitumor activity.[429]

Increased infiltration of myeloid cells has also been linked to antiangiogenic therapy resistance.[430] Elevated numbers of CD11b + Gr1+ myeloid-derived suppressor cells (MDSCs) have been observed in refractory tumors compared to tumors sensitive to antiangiogenic agents.[148] In a recent report, IL-17, produced by T helper type 17 cells, was shown to facilitate IL-17-dependent but VEGF-independent angiogenesis through upregulation of G-CSF, which in turn leads to the mobilization and recruitment of MDSCs from the bone marrow and spleen to the tumor.[431] In mice, the efficacy of anti-VEGF therapy in refractory tumors was improved when IL-17 was targeted.

Altered threshold for hypoxia-induced apoptosis
Certain changes within a tumor cell may make it less sensitive to the diminished vascular supply and resulting hypoxia induced by antiangiogenic therapy. For instance, it has been demonstrated in murine xenograft models that tumor cells bearing mutated p53 are less sensitive to hypoxic conditions *in vitro* and respond somewhat less well to a VEGFR2 inhibitor.[432] Studies performed in tissue biopsies obtained from patients with recurrent high-grade glioma treated with bevacizumab and irinotecan revealed that high expression levels of carbonic anhydrase 9 (CAIX), a marker of hypoxia, were significantly associated with poor 1-year survival.[433] Similarly, findings of another tumor tissue study of patients with malignant glioma revealed that low CAIX expression and increased VEGF expression were associated with improved PFS in those patients who received metronomic etoposide and bevacizumab.[434]

Genetic alterations within tumor endothelium
The assumption that tumor endothelium are normal diploid cells and therefore presumably genetically stable has been challenged by observations from murine studies.[435] Furthermore, in biopsies from patients with B-cell non-Hodgkin lymphoma with specific genetic aberrations, the endothelial cells of the cancer microvasculature acquired the same specific chromosomal translocations.[436] Genetically unstable tumor endothelial cells might derive from a common progenitor cell,[437] or may be the product of an endothelial phenotype differentiation, under the pressure of angiogenic factors within the tumor microenvironment. Fusion between neoplastic and endothelial cells has also been hypothesized. Overall, the functional significance and relevance of this finding to other tumor types are not yet known, but it supports the mounting evidence that tumor endothelial cells, like tumor cells, are likely to be a complex therapeutic target.

Genetic variability in host
Recent studies have suggested that polymorphisms in the VEGF gene are associated with the risk of developing cancer[438–440] and may also influence the response to bevacizumab when given with chemotherapy in breast cancer[405] and glioblastoma patients.[441] Polymorphisms in other genes regulating angiogenesis, such as IL-8 and the HIF family, have also been described. The availability of high throughput methods for analyzing polymorphisms on a genome-wide basis should facilitate the analysis of genetic differences in the host and their impact on response to angiogenesis inhibitors.

Potential biomarkers for VEGF pathway inhibitors

The critical need for biomarkers for VEGF pathway inhibitors
Despite significant progress, the benefits of antiangiogenic therapy to date have been modest, are seen only in subsets of patients, and inevitably yield to therapeutic resistance. The mechanisms by which tumors develop resistance to VEGF inhibition are not fully understood, and understanding them is critical for identifying patients with resistance and building combination regimens to overcome it. Furthermore, the biological activity of these agents remains difficult to assess because they do not typically lead to objective responses as judged by tumor shrinkage when used as monotherapy. As an illustration of this point, in a phase I trial of bevacizumab, no objective responses were observed among 25 patients.[442] Thus, there is an urgent need for biomarkers to identify which patients are most likely to respond to treatment or develop therapeutic resistance, select the optimal drug dosage, and determine whether the intended molecular target has been effectively inhibited.[443–445] Ideally such methods should be noninvasive and practical for routine clinical care. There are currently no validated biomarkers for routine clinical use, but a number of markers are under investigation in clinical and preclinical studies (Table 3). These can be divided into invasive markers that assess changes in tissue or vasculature directly, circulating markers detectable in blood or urine, and radiographic markers. Several of these are discussed below.

Invasive markers
Serial biopsies taken before and during treatment have the potential to directly demonstrate drug effects on tumors and other tissues at the cellular and molecular level but are typically not practical to obtain outside the setting of a clinical trial. This approach has been used to demonstrate that bevacizumab induces changes in microvessel density, tumor-cell apoptosis, and proliferation in rectal cancer patients.[285,286,446] Changes in tumor IFP, a key parameter impacting vascular function, have also been demonstrated.[286,287] This approach may also provide insights into the lack of significant clinical activity seen for some agents. For example, in clinical trials of the VEGFR TKIs SU5416 and SU6668, it was observed that VEGFR and other key targets were incompletely inhibited in post-treatment tumor biopsies,[418,419] suggesting that higher drug concentrations, or more potent inhibitors, may be required. In addition, studies of changes in gene expression in cancer cells and tumor-associated macrophages (TAMs) after VEGF blockade with bevacizumab have shown upregulation of the SDF1α–CXCR4 pathway and of the VEGF receptor NRP1 in rectal cancer patients.[447]

The expression of TAMs within the tumor microenvironment of cancer treated with anti-VEGF therapies has been shown to correlate with outcomes following treatment with antiangiogenic therapies. A retrospective autopsy study of patients with recurrent glioblastoma treated with various VEGF inhibitors, including bevacizumab, showed that increased expression of CD68+ and CD11+ TAMs is associated with poor survival, suggesting a potential role as biomarker of escape.[448]

Circulating markers in blood and urine
Tumor angiogenesis is regulated by a balance between pro- and antiangiogenic factors and cytokines released by tumor cells,

Table 3 Surrogate markers under investigation for the evaluation of efficacy of antiangiogenic agents.

Marker	Parameter evaluated	Comments/limitations	References
Tumor-based			
Tissue biopsy	Immunohistochemistry: • Protein expression as a marker • Microvascular density • Perivascular cell coverage of tumor vessels • Cell proliferation/apoptosis Genomic analyses	Not easily available in some tumors	285,286,358,418,486,487
Interstitial fluid pressure measurement	Tumor interstitial fluid pressure	Limited accessibility in some tumors	285,286,488,489
Measurements of tissue oxygenation	Tumor oxygen tension	Difficult accessibility in some tumors	490
Skin wound healing	Wound healing time	Investigated as biomarker of efficacy and indicator of side effects	491
Circulating markers in blood or urine			
Blood CECs, CPCs, or CEPs	Concentration of viable CEC/CPCs/CEPs	Unclear origin, viability, and surface phenotype of the circulating cells	285–288,458,463,470,471,475,492
Circulating proteins (cytokines, angiogenic factors, etc.)	Concentration of levels of cytokines, angiogenic factors, markers of hypoxia, endothelial damage, and other factors in the blood	Can be done using commercially available multiplexed assays, ELISAs	288,453,458–460,462,493,494
Protein level in urine	Urine MMPs, VEGF, and so on	Limited to excreted proteins and depends on factors that might be altered by treatment such as renal function (e.g., proteinuria)	495
Radiographic			
CT imaging	Blood flow and volume, permeability-surface area product mean transit time	Resolution, measurement of composite parameters	285,286,496
PET imaging	Tracer uptake	Resolution, measurement of composite parameters	285–287,496
MRI	Blood flow, permeability	Resolution, measurement of composite parameters	288,481,497,498

CAF, circulating angiogenic factor; CECs, circulating endothelial cells; CEPs circulating endothelial progenitors; CT, computer tomography; MMPs, matrix metalloproteinases; MRI, magnetic resonance imaging; PET, positron emission tomography; VEGF, vascular endothelial growth factor.

stroma, and by inflammatory cells. Many of these factors can be detected in circulation and other biologic fluids and serve as biomarkers for monitoring anti-VEGF therapies.[417,443–445]

Plasma and serum levels of VEGF and soluble VEGFR-2 have been investigated as pharmacodynamic biomarkers of activity of VEGF inhibitors, prognostic markers, and predictive markers of clinical benefit. In preclinical models, rapid increases of plasma VEGF, and decreases in soluble VEGFR-2, have been observed in both nontumor- and tumor-bearing mice.[449–451] These increases were induced in a dose-dependent manner, and correlated with the treatment efficacy, suggesting that they may be useful for selecting the appropriate drug dosage.

These markers have also been evaluated in clinical trials. Bevacizumab (alone and with cytotoxics) has been shown to increase both serum and plasma total VEGF levels.[285,287,305,307] Interestingly, free serum VEGF concentrations decreased to undetectable levels even with low doses of bevacizumab in one of the studies.[305] Most VEGFR TKIs have been shown to induce similar changes. The most widely studied is sunitinib maleate (SU11248, Sutent®, and Pfizer), which along with other TKIs has been shown to consistently induce on-therapy increases in VEGF plasma levels, and decreases in soluble (s)VEGFR-2, that are rapidly reversible when the therapy is stopped.[288,452–457] In one study, changes in sVEGFR-2 correlated with plasma levels of the drug.[458] Collectively, these findings suggest that VEGF and sVEGFR-2 may be useful pharmacodynamic markers.

Baseline levels of VEGF may also be predictive of benefit for some drugs although this has not been consistently observed in all studies. NSCLC patients with high VEGF were more likely to respond to the combination of bevacizumab with chemotherapy compared to chemotherapy alone.[459] Interestingly, a trend in the opposite direction was observed for the TKI vandetanib, as patients with low VEGF appeared to derive a greater clinical benefit from

the vandetanib containing arm compared to the control arm in three randomized phase II studies.[460] It appears that the predictive value of markers such as VEGF will depend on the specific drug and disease setting.

Recent technological advances such as multiplex bead assays have permitted investigators to assess a much wider variety of factors. A signature derived from a profile of 35 cytokines and angiogenic factors was shown to be predictive of vandetanib benefit in a randomized phase II study.[461] Among these circulating biomarkers, PlGF has been shown to be consistently increased by anti-VEGF therapy in cancer patients regardless of the tumor type or agent used, suggesting that it might be an additional pharmacodynamic biomarker for antiangiogenic therapy.[285,287,288,453,462,463] Future studies will establish if PlGF levels have any predictive value for this therapy. Finally, this approach may also prove to be useful for identifying potential mechanisms of therapeutic resistance. Several candidates are SDF1α–CXCR4 pathways, bFGF, Il-6, HGF, and IL-8.[287,288,461,463,464]

VEGF single-nucleotide polymorphisms (SNPs)

VEGF genotype and VEGF SNPs are also being investigated as potential markers of response to VEGF-targeting agents. It is believed that SNPs may affect the responses to drugs through alterations in gene expression or post-transcriptional modifications. An analysis of 133 patients with advanced NSCLC in the ECOG 4599 trial revealed that an SNP signature of VEGFA—634GG, ICAM1 469T/C, and IL8-251T/A—was the best predictor of OS and PFS.[465] In the E2501 randomized phase II study of sorafenib versus placebo in patients with metastatic NSCLC, analysis of DNA collected from 88 plasma samples showed that VEGFA-1498CC and -634CC genotypes correlated with improved PFS.[466] In patients with advanced breast cancer, benefit from bevacizumab correlated with certain genetic polymorphisms in *VEGF* and *VEGFR-2/KDR*.[405]

More recently, in a phase II study of bevacizumab and sorafenib for the treatment of patients with relapsed glioblastoma, SNPs in the *VEGF* and *VEGFR2* promoters correlated with prolonged 6-month PFS. Furthermore, SNPs in the *VEGF* promoter were shown to correlate with higher grade of toxicities.[441]

Circulating endothelial cells (CECs) and progenitors (CEPs)

Mature CECs (derived from existing vessels) and bone marrow-derived circulating precursor cells (CPCs) or circulating endothelial precursors (CEPs), which can differentiate into mature endothelial cells and contribute to neovascularization, have been investigated as biomarkers for antiangiogenic therapy.[139,140,143,288,458,467–470] Consistent with preclinical models,[471,472] increases during treatment in mature CECs, which have a large percentage of apoptotic cells and are thought to represent cells shed from tumor endothelium, may be associated with benefit in patients treated with antiangiogenic or VTAs.[458,473–475] In one study evaluating patients with metastatic breast cancer who were treated with low-dose metronomic chemotherapy using cyclophosphamide and methotrexate, the CEC count after 2 months of continuous therapy correlated with DFS and OS at more than 2-year follow up.[475] CPCs, by contrast, appear to decrease with bevacizumab[285–287] or sunitinib treatment.[463] Despite these encouraging results, the clinical application of circulating cells as biomarkers will require standardization and further phenotypic definition of cell populations.[476–478]

Imaging

A number of different techniques are under investigation for assessing parameters related to tumor vasculature such as perfusion, permeability, hypoxia, and metabolic activity. These include dynamic contrast-enhanced MRI (DCE-MRI), CT, and positron emission tomography (reviewed in Ref. 444, 445, 479–485). These methods have the important advantage of permitting longitudinal assessments noninvasively. There are a number of limitations for each of these methods, however. There is significant heterogeneity in blood flow and permeability within tumors, and the currently available methods generally lack the spatial resolution to assess this. Furthermore, most assess composite parameters, which depend on both tumor blood flow and permeability.[417] The cost of these studies may also limit their use, particularly for large randomized clinical trials needed to validate their utility.

Concluding remarks

Nearly four decades ago, tumor angiogenesis was recognized as a potential therapeutic target for the treatment of cancer.[1] Since that seminal observation, the field has moved from conception to the clinical testing of dozens of new agents. Angiogenesis inhibitors are now part of the standard treatment regimens for lung, colorectal, renal, breast, and several other types of cancers. While these recent advances have validated antiangiogenic therapy as a treatment modality and provided benefit to countless patients, it is also true that the clinical gains thus far have been modest. As the field moves from infancy into adolescence, a number of key issues will need to be addressed in order for antiangiogenic therapy to realize its therapeutic potential for cancer patients. Among these issues are understanding the mechanism(s) by which antiangiogenic therapy enhances the efficacy of chemotherapy and radiotherapy, and designing combinations appropriately; identifying critical pathways driving angiogenesis other than VEGF, and developing drugs to inhibit them; creating biomarkers to identify which patients will benefit (or experience toxicity) from a given agent; and exploring the application of angiogenesis inhibitors to earlier stages of cancer, with the goal of rendering microscopic tumors dormant.

Acknowledgments

This chapter is dedicated to Judah Folkman, MD, for his pioneering work in tumor angiogenesis and for his generous mentorship. We would also like to acknowledge Rakesh Jain, PhD and George Sledge, MD for their contributions to earlier versions of this chapter.

Key references

The complete reference list can be found on the Wiley Companion Digital Edition of this title (see inside front cover for login instructions).

1 Folkman J. Tumor angiogenesis: therapeutic implications. *N Engl J Med.* 1971;**285**:1182–1186.

2 Hanahan D, Weinberg RA. The hallmarks of cancer. *Cell.* 2000;**100**:57–70.

3 Carmeliet P, Jain RK. Angiogenesis in cancer and other diseases. *Nature.* 2000;**407**:249–257.

4 Achilles EG, Fernandez A, Allred EN, et al. Heterogeneity of angiogenic activity in a human liposarcoma: a proposed mechanism for "no take" of human tumors in mice. *J Natl Cancer Inst.* 2001;**93**:1075–1081.

8 Folkman J, Watson K, Ingber D, Hanahan D. Induction of angiogenesis during the transition from hyperplasia to neoplasia. *Nature.* 1989;**339**:58–61.

9 Hanahan D, Folkman J. Patterns and emerging mechanisms of the angiogenic switch during tumorigenesis. *Cell.* 1996;**86**:353–364.

18 Folkman J. Toward an understanding of angiogenesis: search and discovery. *Perspect Biol Med.* 1985;**29**:10–36.

19 Folkman J, Long DM Jr, Becker FF. Growth and metastasis of tumor in organ culture. *Cancer.* 1963;**16**:453–467.

20 Folkman J, Cole P, Zimmerman S. Tumor behavior in isolated perfused organs: in vitro growth and metastases of biopsy material in rabbit thyroid and canine intestinal segment. *Ann Surg.* 1966;**164**:491–502.

21 Folkman J. Anti-angiogenesis: new concept for therapy of solid tumors. *Ann Surg.* 1972;**175**:409–416.

40 Holash J, Maisonpierre PC, Compton D, et al. Vessel cooption, regression, and growth in tumors mediated by angiopoietins and VEGF. *Science.* 1999;**284**:1994–1998.

47 Williams WN, Kim ES, Heymach JV, Lippman SL. Molecular Targets for Cancer Chemoprevention. *Nat Rev Drug Discov.* 2009;**8(3)**:213–225.

53 Parangi S, O'Reilly M, Christofori G, et al. Antiangiogenic therapy of transgenic mice impairs de novo tumor growth. *Proc Natl Acad Sci U S A.* 1996;**93**:2002–2007.

67 Naumov GN, Bender E, Zurakowski D, et al. A model of human tumor dormancy: an angiogenic switch from the nonangiogenic phenotype. *J Natl Cancer Inst.* 2006;**98**:316–325.

68 Herbst RS, Hidalgo M, Pierson AS, Holden SN, Bergen M, Eckhardt SG. Angiogenesis inhibitors in clinical development for lung cancer. *Semin Oncol.* 2002;**29**:66–77.

123 Nilsson M, Heymach JV. Vascular endothelial growth factor (VEGF) pathway. *J Thorac Oncol.* 2006;**1**:768–770.

139 Asahara T, Murohara T, Sullivan A, et al. Isolation of putative progenitor endothelial cells for angiogenesis. *Science.* 1997;**275**:964–967.

144 Lyden D, Young AZ, Zagzag D, et al. Id1 and Id3 are required for neurogenesis, angiogenesis and vascularization of tumour xenografts. *Nature.* 1999;**401**:670–677.

153 Cascone T, Heymach JV. Targeting the angiopoietin/Tie2 pathway: cutting tumor vessels with a double-edged sword? *J Clin Oncol.* 2012;**30**:441–444.

154 Maisonpierre PC, Suri C, Jones PF, et al. Angiopoietin-2, a natural antagonist for Tie2 that disrupts in vivo angiogenesis. *Science.* 1997;**277**:55–60.

173 O'Reilly MS, Pirie-Shepherd S, Lane WS, Folkman J. Antiangiogenic activity of the cleaved conformation of the serpin antithrombin. *Science.* 1999;**285**:1926–1928.

174 Moses MA, Sudhalter J, Langer R. Identification of an inhibitor of neovascularization from cartilage. *Science.* 1990;**248**:1408–1410.

241 Nilsson M, Hanrahan E, Heymach J. Angiogenesis inhibitors for the Treatment of Lung Cancer. In: Teicher BA, Ellis LM, eds. *Antiangiogenic Agents in Cancer Therapy,* 2nd ed. Totowa, NJ: Humana Press; 2008.

260 Xu L, Nilsson MB, Saintigny P, et al. Epidermal growth factor receptor regulates MET levels and invasiveness through hypoxia-inducible factor-1α in non-small cell lung cancer cells. *Oncogene.* 2010;**29(18)**:2616–2627.

265 Lara PN Jr, Douillard JY, Nakagawa K, et al. Randomized phase III placebo-controlled trial of carboplatin and paclitaxel with or without the vascular disrupting agent vadimezan (ASA404) in advanced non-small-cell lung cancer. *J Clin Oncol.* 2011;**29**:2965–2971.

266 Rudin CM, Mauer A, Smakal M, et al. Phase I/II study of pemetrexed with or without ABT-751 in advanced or metastatic non-small-cell lung cancer. *J Clin Oncol.* 2011;**29**:1075–1082.

271 Jain RK. Normalization of tumor vasculature: an emerging concept in antiangiogenic therapy. *Science.* 2005;**307**:58–62.

273 Jain RK. Normalizing tumor vasculature with anti-angiogenic therapy: a new paradigm for combination therapy. *Nat Med.* 2001;**7**:987–989.

301 Hurwitz H, Fehrenbacher L, Novotny W, et al. Bevacizumab plus irinotecan, fluorouracil, and leucovorin for metastatic colorectal cancer. *N Engl J Med.* 2004;**350**:2335–2342.

304 Motzer RJ, Hutson TE, Tomczak P, et al. Sunitinib versus interferon α in metastatic renal-cell carcinoma. *N Engl J Med.* 2007;**356**:115–124.

310 Motzer RJ, Hutson TE, Tomczak P, et al. Overall survival and updated results for sunitinib compared with interferon α in patients with metastatic renal cell carcinoma. *J Clin Oncol.* 2009;**27**:3584–3590.

312 Escudier B, Pluzanska A, Koralewski P, et al. Bevacizumab plus interferon α-2a for treatment of metastatic renal cell carcinoma: a randomised, double-blind phase III trial. *Lancet.* 2007;**370**:2103–2111.

330 Tran HT, Liu Y, Zurita AJ, et al. Prognostic or predictive plasma cytokines and angiogenic factors for patients treated with pazopanib for metastatic renal-cell cancer: a retrospective analysis of phase 2 and phase 3 trials. *Lancet Oncol.* 2012;**13**:827–837.

351 Heymach JV, Paz-Ares L, De Braud F, et al. Randomized phase II study of vandetanib alone or with paclitaxel and carboplatin as first-line treatment for advanced non-small-cell lung cancer. *J Clin Oncol.* 2008;**26**:5407–5415.

352 Herbst RS, Sun Y, Eberhardt WE, et al. Vandetanib plus docetaxel versus docetaxel as second-line treatment for patients with advanced non-small-cell lung cancer (ZODIAC): a double-blind, randomised, phase 3 trial. *Lancet Oncol.* 2010;**11**:619–626.

370 Heymach JV, Johnson BE, Prager D, et al. Randomized, placebo-controlled phase II study of vandetanib plus docetaxel in previously treated nonsmall-cell lung cancer. *J Clin Oncol.* 2007;**25**:4270–4277.

371 Heymach JV, Lockwood SJ, Herbst RS, Johnson BE, Ryan AJ. EGFR biomarkers predict benefit from vandetanib in combination with docetaxel in a randomized phase III study of second-line treatment of patients with advanced non-small cell lung cancer. *Ann Oncol.* 2014;**25**:1941–1948.

376 Byers LA, Heymach JV. Dual targeting of the vascular endothelial growth factor and epidermal growth factor receptor pathways: rationale and clinical applications for non-small-cell lung cancer. *Clin Lung Cancer.* 2007;**8**(**Suppl 2**): S79–S85.

384 Herbst RS, O'Neill VJ, Fehrenbacher L, et al. Phase II study of efficacy and safety of bevacizumab in combination with chemotherapy or erlotinib compared with chemotherapy alone for treatment of recurrent or refractory non small-cell lung cancer. *J Clin Oncol.* 2007;**25**:4743–4750.

386 Naumov GN, Nilsson MB, Cascone T, et al. Combined vascular endothelial growth factor receptor and epidermal growth factor receptor (EGFR) blockade inhibits tumor growth in xenograft models of EGFR inhibitor resistance. *Clin Cancer Res.* 2009;**15**:3484–3494.

418 Heymach JV, Desai J, Manola J, et al. Phase II Study of the Antiangiogenic Agent SU5416 in Patients with Advanced Soft Tissue Sarcomas. *Clin Cancer Res.* 2004;**10**:5732–5740.

427 Cascone T, Herynk MH, Xu L, et al. Upregulated stromal EGFR and vascular remodeling in mouse xenograft models of angiogenesis inhibitor-resistant human lung adenocarcinoma. *J Clin Invest.* 2011;**121**:1313–1328.

428 Kopetz S, Hoff PM, Morris JS, et al. Phase II trial of infusional fluorouracil, irinotecan, and bevacizumab for metastatic colorectal cancer: efficacy and circulating angiogenic biomarkers associated with therapeutic resistance. *J Clin Oncol.* 2010;**28**:453–459.

443 Zurita A, Wu H, Heymach J. Blood-based biomarkers for VEGF inhibitors. In: Davis D, Herbst R, Abbruzzese J, eds. *Antiangiogenic Cancer Therapy*. Boca Raton, FL: CRC Press; 2007:517–531.

444 Jain RK, Duda DG, Clark JW, Loeffler JS. Lessons from phase III clinical trials on anti-VEGF therapy for cancer. *Nat Clin Pract Oncol.* 2006;**3**:24–40.

474 Heymach J, Kulke M, Fuchs C, et al. Circulating endothelial cells as a surrogate marker of antiangiogenic activity in patients treated with endostatin. *Proc Am Soc Clin Oncol.* 2003;**22**:979.

PART 3

Quantitative Oncology

18 Cancer bioinformatics

John N. Weinstein, MD, PhD

Overview

Bioinformatics is a rapidly developing scientific field in which computational methods are applied to the analysis and interpretation of biological data, usually at the cell or molecular level and usually in the form of large, multivariate datasets. In the context of cancer, the most frequent scenario is molecular profiling at the DNA, RNA, protein, and/or metabolite level for basic understanding of the biology, for identification of potential therapeutic targets, and/or for clinical prediction. The new massively-parallel sequencing technologies are generating a data deluge—literally quadrillions of numbers in all—that strain the capacity of our hardware, software, and personnel infrastructures for bioinformatics; hence, the computational aspect of a sequencing project is now generally more expensive and time-consuming than the laboratory work.

Bioinformatic analysis can be hypothesis-generating or hypothesis-testing. When it is hypothesis-generating, the assumption is that one can afford a large number of false-positive findings in order to identify one or a few evocative or useful ones; when it is hypothesis-testing, the full rigor of statistical inference should be applied. A large number of statistical and machine-learning algorithms, scripts, and software packages are now available for the analysis, and options are multiplying rapidly. Because the datasets are often so large, however, an important aspect of bioinformatics is data visualization, for example display of data arrayed along the length of the genome or, most commonly, in the form of a clustered heat map.

Cancer biologists and clinical researchers should preferably take the lead in biological interpretation of the massive datasets, but statistical analysis should be done by (or under the vigilant aegis of) a professional in informatics; when there are more variables (e.g., genes) than cases (e.g., patients), there is a tendency for the untrained to obtain overly optimistic p-values or see false patterns in even randomized datasets. In addition, subtle errors that arise in the unglamorous tasks of data management and pre-processing often lead to misleading or frankly wrong conclusions from the data.

As high-throughput molecular profiling projects have become cheaper and easier, they have been incorporated progressively into the work of individual institutions, both academic and commercial. However, there are also growing numbers of large-scale public projects in the domain. At the level of cell lines, the first was the NCI-60, a panel of 60 human cancer lines used since 1990 by the U.S. National Cancer Institute to screen more than 100,000 chemical compounds plus natural products for anticancer activity. That panel was followed more recently by the Cancer Cell Line Encyclopedia, the Genomics of Drug Sensitivity in Cancer project, and others. At the clinical level, The Cancer Genome Atlas project has been center-stage, profiling more than 10,000 human cancers of 33 different types, and there is an alphabet-soup of acronyms for other such projects that are in progress or on the drawing board. Those projects, which require massive bioinformatics support, have spawned robust communities of bioinformatics expertise and served as testbeds for the development of new algorithms, software, and visualizations.

I can assure you that data processing is a fad that won't last out the year.
– Editor for a major publishing house, 1957

A generation ago, the results of most laboratory studies on cancer could be processed in a simple spreadsheet and the results written into a laboratory notebook. The data were generally analyzed by experimentalists themselves, using very basic statistical algorithms. That landscape shifted progressively with the advent of microarrays in the mid-1990s and then massively parallel "second-generation" (or "next-generation") sequencing a decade later. At the turn of the millennium, there was a prediction—only half in jest—that most biomedical researchers would soon abandon the wet laboratory and be hunched over their computers, mining the data produced by "biology factories." That has not happened, of course; small wet laboratories are thriving. But we do see increasing numbers of biology factories, prominent among them the high-throughput sequencing centers. And, overall, the trend toward computation is unmistakable. That trend is largely a result of new, robotically-enhanced technologies that make it faster, cheaper, and more reliable to perform the *laboratory portions* of large-scale molecular profiling projects and screening assays. As a result, large centers and also small laboratories can churn out increasingly robust streams of data. Those trends have conspired to produce massive datasets that often contain many billions or trillions of entries, requiring more complex, larger-scale, often subtler statistical analyses and "biointerpretive" resources.

Just as the 'Light-Year' was introduced for astronomical distances too large to be comprehended in miles or kilometers, the 'Huge' (Human Genome Equivalent; about 3.3 billion base-pairs) can be defined for genomics. All of Shakespeare's writings (plays, sonnets, and poems) contain a little over 5 million letters, less than 0.002 Huge. Storage, management, transmission, analysis, and interpretation of data are now most often the bottlenecks, not wet-laboratory data generation itself. The data deluge has variously been likened to an avalanche, a flood, a torrent, or a tsunami. Hence the rise and kaleidoscopic advance of bioinformatics, a multidisciplinary field based on statistics, computer science, biology, and medicine—a field crucial to current biomedical research and clinical progress but still in what might be characterized as an awkward adolescent phase.

The aim of this chapter is not to provide a comprehensive treatment of the sprawling, rapidly evolving arena of cancer bioinformatics. That would, in any case be impossible to do at any depth in the space available. Some sub-fields, for example analysis of the metabolome and the structural analysis of proteins and nucleic acids, will, unfortunately, be short-changed.

The aim is also not (with apologies) to give due credit to pioneers in the field or to cite all of the tools and resources that deserve mention. Rather, the aims are (1) to illuminate some generic aspects of cancer bioinformatics in its current and likely future states; (2) to highlight a sample of the statistical algorithms, computational tools, and data resources available; and (3) to showcase some issues that should be borne in mind by the nonspecialist who is trying to navigate the bioinformatics literature, to comprehend what bioinformatician collaborators are doing, or to use bioinformatics

Holland-Frei Cancer Medicine, Ninth Edition. Edited by Robert C. Bast Jr., Carlo M. Croce, William N. Hait, Waun Ki Hong, Donald W. Kufe, Martine Piccart-Gebhart, Raphael E. Pollock, Ralph R. Weichselbaum, Hongyang Wang, and James F. Holland.
© 2017 John Wiley & Sons, Inc. ISBN: 978-1-118-93469-2

in a project for a better understanding of cancer or for the direct benefit of cancer patients and their families.

The definition and scope of bioinformatics

Definition of "bioinformatics"

The term "bioinformatics" is not new. It first appeared in print in 1970 with a very broad meaning,[1] but its definition, as applied currently, is a matter of almost Talmudic debate. Multiple committees, academic surveys, and publications have struggled with the subject, even attempting to distinguish between "bioinformaticians" and "bioinformaticists".[2] For present purposes, an extended definition of bioinformatics attributed to the U.S. National Center for Biotechnology Information (NCBI) will suffice: "*Bioinformatics is the field of science in which biology, computer science, and information technology merge into a single discipline. There are three important sub-disciplines within bioinformatics: the development of new algorithms and statistics with which to assess relationships among members of large data sets; the analysis and interpretation of various types of data including nucleotide and amino acid sequences, protein domains, and protein structures; and the development and implementation of tools that enable efficient access and management of different types of information.*"

There can be no definitive line of demarcation between bioinformatics and related or overlapping disciplines such as computational biology and medical informatics. Computational biology "*involves the development and application of data-analytical and theoretical methods, mathematical modeling and computational simulation techniques to the study of biological, behavioral, and social systems.*"[3] It includes, but extends far beyond, the focus on biological molecules characteristic of bioinformatics. Medical informatics has been defined as "*the field of information science concerned with the analysis and dissemination of medical data through the application of computers to various aspects of health care and medicine.*"[4] Medical informatics is closely tied to the practical needs of clinical research and clinical practice, whereas bioinformatics is more closely allied with pre-clinical research. However, the two meet—and should synergize—in such projects as biomarker-driven clinical trials.

In the end, a word means what we collectively choose it to mean, and the best way to get a feel for the extent of the field is to list some key words associated with it. As per the famous dictum of U.S. Supreme Court Justice Potter Stewart, "I know it when I see it." The ingredients of most bioinformatics projects include biological molecules, large databases, multivariate statistical analysis, high-performance computing, graphical visualization of the molecular data, and biological or biomedical interpretation. Typical sources of data for bioinformatic analysis include microarrays, DNA sequencing, RNA sequencing, mass spectrometry of proteins and metabolites, histopathological descriptors, and clinical records. Some of the salient datasets originate within studies being conducted in particular laboratories, but large, publicly available databases and search resources are playing ever-larger roles.

Questions typically addressed by bioinformatic analysis and interpretation

Questions addressed by bioinformatic analysis relate to biological mechanisms, pathways, networks, biomarkers and biosignatures, macromolecular structures, subsetting of cancer types, early detection, and prediction of clinical outcome variables such as risk, survival, metastasis, response to therapy, and recurrence. The paradigmatic bioinformatics project—the type that will be cited throughout this chapter—involves the design, statistical analysis,

and biological interpretation of molecular profiles. Figure 1 shows a schematic view of the specimen and information flows in a generic sequencing project whose aim is to identify mutational and/or DNA copy number aberrations as possible biomarkers. The data from such studies can also be used to subset cancers or to make direct comparisons such as tumor versus paired normal tissue, tumor type versus tumor type, responder versus nonresponder, metastatic versus nonmetastatic, or primary versus recurrent cancer.

One frequent aim has been the identification of "prognostic" biomarkers for survival, time to recurrence, or metastasis. However, the interest in such biomarkers has been declining, in part because they do not specify a therapy and in part because the landscape of cancer therapy is changing so rapidly that natural history of the disease has lost much of its meaning. Instead, the focus has turned to "predictive" biomarkers. The term is curiously non-specific, and its etymology is unclear, but it has gained currency for molecular markers that predict which subpopulations of patients will respond to a particular therapy. An allied concept is that of the "actionable" biomarker. An actionable, predictive biomarker may be a target for therapy or it may simply be correlated with response. Historically, bioinformatic analysis has identified associations and correlations more often than it has identified causal relationships, but "bioperturbing" technologies such as siRNA, shRNA, CRISPR, and consequent synthetic lethal pharmacological screens are producing large datasets with immediate causal implications.

The analog (microarray) to digital (sequencing) transition

We are witnessing a transition from the primacy of microarrays (fundamentally analog technologies) to the primacy of DNA and RNA sequencing (fundamentally digital technologies). The digital revolution took hold in computing, then in television, in watches, in cameras and cars, and now in biomedical research. DNA and RNA sequencing provide more precise, incisive, and extensive information about the molecular profiles of cancers than could be obtained from microarrays. For example, sequencing the mixture of mRNAs in a tumor (RNA-seq) can yield information on mRNA splicing, mRNA editing, clonal heterogeneity and evolution, viral insertion, fusion gene expression, and allelic components of the overall expression level. In contrast, expression microarrays generally indicate only the relative amounts of the mRNA species present in a sample. However, the transition is not without its growing pains. As of 2015, sequencing is still generally more expensive than gene expression microarrays. And massively-parallel second-generation sequencing currently challenges the bioinformatics community at the levels of hardware, software, and "wetware" (i.e., personnel).

Hardware challenges

Moore's law[5] is familiar. It relates to the number of transistors that can be crammed into unit surface area on a very large integrated circuit. That number has increased in a remarkably consistent way, two-fold every other year since the 1960s. As a consequence, and because the speed of transistors has increased, the cost of computing power has been cut in half every 18 months. However, the Moore's law decrease has not kept up with the decline in sequencing cost, which was cut 1,000-fold (from about $10 million per human genome to about $10 thousand) in the 4 years from late 2007 to late 2011 as second-generation sequencing became available (Figure 2). The decline in price has slowed dramatically since that time as we await cost-effectiveness of "third-generation" sequencing technologies such as those based on single-molecule

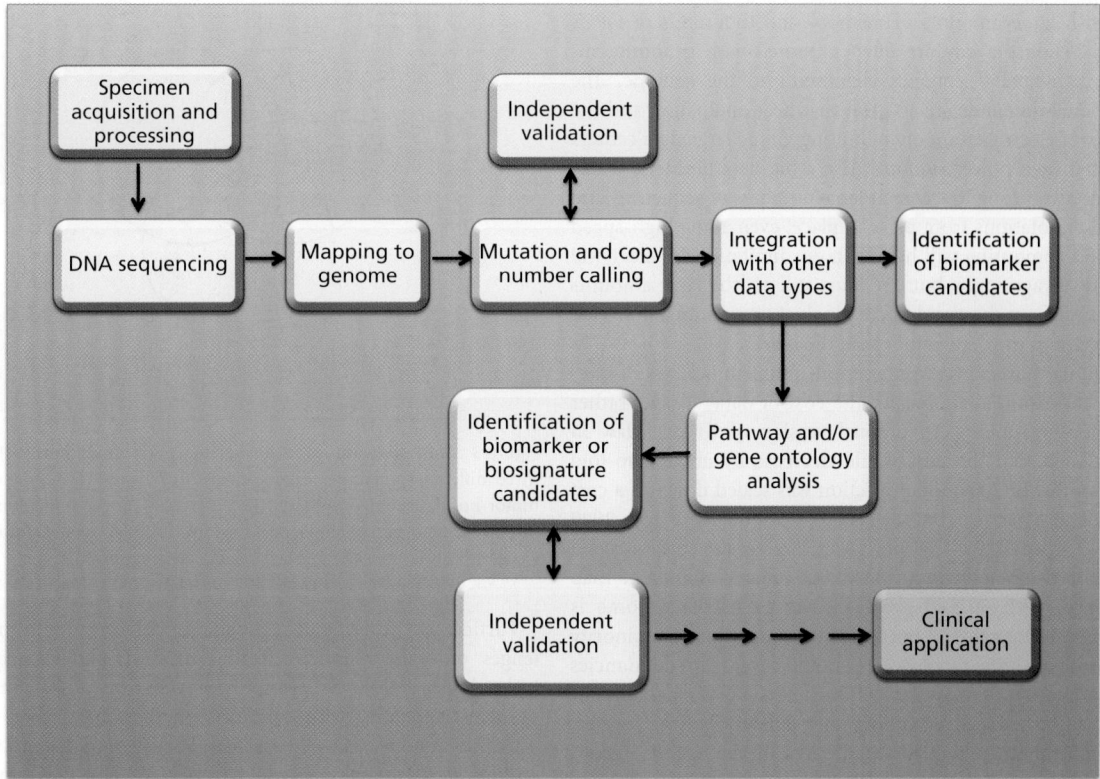

Figure 1 Schematic view of specimen and information flows for sequencing of cancers to identify mutations and/or copy number aberrations as possible biomarkers for clinical application. Amber boxes indicate downstream "biointerpretive" aspects of the pipeline. As indicated by the multiple arrows, many hurdles (scientific, technical, logistical, ethical, and regulatory) must be overcome before possible clinical application. Analogous schematics can be drawn for other data types at the DNA, RNA, protein, and metabolomic levels (including studies based on microarrays, rather than sequencing).

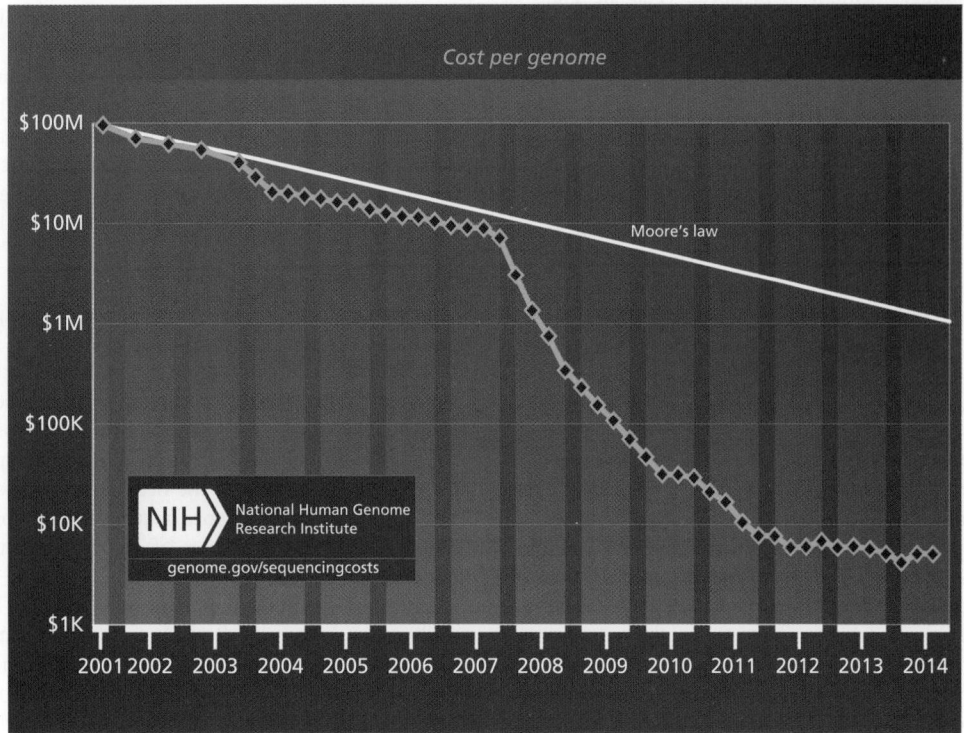

Figure 2 Cost per genome for human whole-genome sequencing. The figure shows an inflection point in late 2007 as massively-parallel sequencing came into practice. We are awaiting the maturation and cost-effectiveness of "third-generation" technologies, principally based on sequencing of single molecules. Source: genome.gov/sequencingcosts (The National Human Genome Research Institute).

sequencing. Nonetheless, even our high-performance computer clusters with large amounts of memory and thousands of CPUs operating 24 hours a day are often saturated with genomic calculations, principally sequence alignments to the genome. The computational demands are so great that heat dissipation and the availability of electricity are often limiting. Some large data centers require their own power stations. Also a big-data problem, it can take prohibitively long to transmit large numbers of sequences and associated annotations from place to place, even along high-speed lines. Cloud computing will help with our limitations of electrical power and storage space, but one must still get the large amounts of data to and from the cloud. Increasingly, computational tools are being brought to the data, rather than the reverse.

Less familiar but an even more serious problem is Kryder's law,[6] analogous to Moore's law but for the cost of data storage, rather than computing power. An original version of Kryder's law in 2004 predicted that the cost would decrease by about two-fold every 6 months. In 2009, the projection was scaled down to a cost decrease of 40% per year, but the actual rate of decrease from 2009 through 2014 was only 15% per year. The storage space needed for a standard whole-genome BAM file (binary alignment map file/sequence) with 30-fold average coverage of the genome is "only" about 100 gigabytes, but to identify mutations in minority clones within a tumor can require genome coverage redundancies in the hundreds (if they can be identified at all). The storage space required can be reduced by coding only differences from a reference standard, but the reduction is limited by the need to record quality-control information and other types of annotations. Even large institutions are running out of storage space. It may be less expensive to re-sequence samples than to store sequencing data from them over time.

However, there are new possibilities for mass storage on the horizon, paradoxically including DNA itself. DNA may be the most compact storage medium in prospect. A single gram of DNA could encode about 700,000 gigabytes of data (roughly 7,000 whole-genome BAM files). One team has encoded all of Shakespeare's sonnets in DNA and another has encoded an entire book—with an intrinsic error rate of only two per million bits, far better than magnetic hard drives or human proof-readers can achieve.[7] They then replicated the DNA to produce 70 billion copies of the book—enough for each person in the world to own 10 copies (without taking up space on their bookshelves). Under the right storage conditions, DNA can remain stable, potentially for hundreds of thousands of years, even at room temperature. If you were faced with the challenge of passing knowledge down to future civilizations, DNA storage would be your best bet. The technology for getting information into and out of DNA is far too expensive for large-scale use at this time, but the price is decreasing rapidly.

Software challenges
Creative ideas are flowing through the field of bioinformatics software development. Many hundreds of capable software packages are being developed and deployed, some of them commercial but most of them academically developed, open-source, and publicly available. The range of choices for any given computational function is almost paralyzing. One result is fragmentation of the community of users, who, for the most part, have not yet coalesced around particular algorithms, software, or websites. Among bioinformaticians, the "not-invented-here" syndrome often applies. As a consequence, Bioinformatics is a classic Tower of Babel in which software packages usually fail to communicate nicely with each other. Various annotation schemes and data formats remain mutually incompatible, despite major international efforts at standardization.

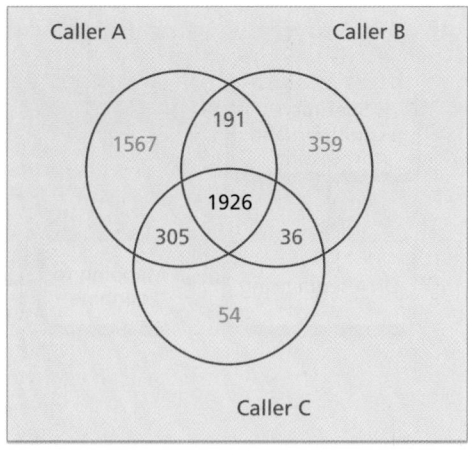

Figure 3 Venn diagram of the somatic point mutations detected by three different mutations callers circa 2013 on 20 TCGA endometrial tumor-normal exome-seq pairs. The differences for point mutations would be smaller now, but an analogous diagram for indels or structural variants would still show considerable lack of concordance. From[9]

Particularly in terms of sequencing, there are algorithmic challenges of major import.[8] If the massively-parallel sequencing technologies and the data from them were truly digital, one should be able to identify with certainty whether there is or is not a mutation at a given DNA base-pair. However, that is not the case, as indicated in Figure 3, which shows a Venn diagram for the consistency of somatic mutation calls on the same sequencing data by three major sequencing centers. The differences are considerable, perhaps in part because of clonal heterogeneity, low percentage of tumor cells, poor coverage in some regions of the genome, and/or degradation of the DNA. An additional reason is probabilistic. If each of two callers were 99.999% accurate in identifying mutation at a given base-pair in a genome of three billion bases, then they would still disagree on tens of thousands of calls. Important calls, for example calls of driver mutations and other cancer biomarkers, must be validated by an independent technology. Three such strategies are (1) validation of DNA and RNA calls against each other for the same samples, (2) use of a consensus of calls by different sequencing centers,[9] and (3) follow up with a different technology such as polymerase chain reaction focused on particular bases.

Wetware challenges
At the present time, personnel (wetware) and expertise are even more seriously limiting than the hardware or software issues. Bioinformatics is highly multidisciplinary, at the interface of computer science, statistics, biology, and medicine. There are not many individuals with expertise in all of those disciplines to operate across the interfaces among them. Despite stereotyped pipelines for some parts of the necessary analyses—generally the steps from raw data to mapped sequence—bioinformatics projects usually require customization of analyses and the efforts of a multidisciplinary team.

The bioinformatics components of a typical large molecular profiling project can be divided roughly into data management, statistical analysis, and biointerpretation. Data management sounds mundane, but for a project that includes data from multiple molecular technologies and clinical data sources, it can be challenging in the extreme. When the Hubble telescope was launched in 1990, it was initially crippled by a 1.3-mm error in its mirror because a custom "null corrector" was substituted for the conventional one during final testing. In 1999, the Mars Climate Orbiter was lost because computer software produced output in pound-seconds instead of newton-seconds (metric units); the orbiter's incorrect trajectory brought it too close to Mars, and it disintegrated in the atmosphere. Analogous data mismatch problems are endemic to bioinformatics. Missing or carelessly composed annotations often result in puzzlement or wrong conclusions about the exact meaning of a data field.

Roles in the multidisciplinary bioinformatics team: an opinion
Statistical analysis of highly multivariate data, unlike that of the simple laboratory experiment, generally calls for specialist expertise in computational analysis. The biomedical researcher should be *involved in* the statistical analysis, equipped with a basic understanding of the methods employed and the potential pitfalls. He or she should be prepared to provide the analyst with (1) questions to be asked of the data, (2) biomedical domain information, and (3) information on idiosyncrasies of the technologies and experimental design that may affect analysis. If a data analyst is not given those types of information, he or she will often generate the right answer to the wrong question or an answer based on incorrect premises. It is dangerous, however, for those untrained in statistics to perform the data management tasks and statistical analyses alone or without very close supervision. Experience has shown a remarkable tendency for the untrained to make mistakes, generally mistakes of over-optimism.[10] They often achieve apparently positive, even ground-breaking, results that later prove to be meaningless. "Unnatural selection" plays a role in that phenomenon; there is a human tendency, reinforced by wishful thinking, to do analyses different ways until one of them gives the desired result. There is also a remarkable, highly tuned tendency for the human mind to find patterns in data where none exist. The analogy of allowing a statistician to perform brain surgery (or a brain surgeon to perform statistical analyses) overstates the case, but not dramatically so.

In biointerpretation and medical interpretation, to the contrary, the biomedical researcher should preferably take the lead on the basis of specific domain expertise and general knowledge of cancer biology. Every basic, translational, or clinical cancer researcher should be able to use a selection of the available tools of biointerpretation to explore the genes, pathways, networks, cell biological entities, and clinical correlates that come into focus on the basis of large-scale molecular datasets. Training researchers in the use of such tools can be considered a primary responsibility of the bioinformatician. The bioinformatician should be prepared to explain the essence of statistical or machine-learning algorithms that he or she is using and to do so in visual, nonmathematical terms. That is *always* possible to do. However, the bioinformatician is likely to have the broader knowledge necessary for selection of the optimal tools and data resources for a project and can do the programming that is often necessary to customize an algorithm or a graphical visualization of the data.

Bioinformatic analysis, visualization, and interpretation

Table 1 lists some molecular data types and phenomena that can be significant in the analysis of cancers, often for early detection or for prediction of cancer risk, diagnosis, prognosis, response to treatment, recurrence, or metastasis. The "omic" terminology sometimes seems strained, but it is compact, convenient, and etymologically justified. The suffix "-ome" is from the Greek for an "abstract entity, group, or mass," so omics is the study of entities in aggregate.[11] (A curiosity: we have genetics for the single-gene counterpart of genomics but not protetics for the single-gene counterpart

of proteomics or metaboletics for the single-compound counterpart of metabolomics.)

Many of the statistical principles, algorithms, and software used in the field are agnostic to the type of data, but each type has its own peculiarities that require customized attention. Issues like background level, normalization, filtering for variation, distributional properties, thresholds, and representation as continuous or dichotomized values all require careful attention. Poor choices of procedure in those matters can lead to fundamentally wrong results in the analysis. In fact, the most important and most challenging, often unresolvable problems in bioinformatics arise from the most mundane, least glamorous tasks: pre-processing of the data to

Table 1 A potpourri of bioinformatic data types, phenomena, and data sources

Data types	Immunomic
Genomic—germline, somatic (DNA level)	Epitope-mapping
	Immune cell profiling
Single-nucleotide variation (SNV)	Immune regulatory network modeling
Insertion/Deletion (Indel)	Connectomic
Copy number variation	
Loss of heterozygosity (LOH)	Co-occurring and mutually exclusive elements
Translocation	Hub nodes
Repeat element	Random vs. scale-free properties
Functional motif	Disassortivity
Domain structure	
Fusion gene	Pathological
Viral insertion	
Pseudogene	Classification, subclassification
	Grade
Epigenomic	Percent tumor cells
	Clonal heterogeneity (microscopic, macroscopic)
DNA methylation (CpG island)	Marker studies (by immunohistochemistry, in situ hybridization, etc.)
DNA methylation (non-CpG island)	
DNA modification (other)	
Histone modification (acetylation, methylation, etc.)	Clinical
Transcriptomic (RNA level)	Survival
	Disease-free survival
mRNA expression	Time to Relapse
microRNA expression	Response to therapy
long non-coding RNA expression	
Transcript splice variation	**Data sources**
RNA editing	Bulk measurement
Allele-specific indices	
	Whole exome sequencing (WES)
Proteomic	Whole genome sequencing (WGS)
	Bisulfite sequencing
Protein expression	Low-coverage copy number sequencing
Post-translational modification	Reverse-phase protein arrays
Protein complexes and interactions	Mass spectrometry
Metabolomic	Antibody arrays
	Nucleic acid microarrays
Metabolite flux	
Metabolite expression level	Single-cell measurement
Targeted identification (MRM)	Single-cell sequencing (DNA, RNA)
Chromosomic	Flow cytometry (fluorescence, mass-tagging)
Transcription factor target	
Histone modifier target	Clinical
Replication start site and kinetics	
Transcription start site and kinetics	Medical records
Accessibility of chromosome location	Clinical trials
Microsatellite instability (MSI)	Other
Chromosomal instability (CIN)	
3D chromosomal arrangement	siRNA, shRNA
Long-range genomic regulation	CRISPR
Choreography of mitosis and meiosis	Mass spectrometry
	Microdissection, tumor disaggregation
Pharmacomic	Microscopy
	Imaging
Response to treatment	Circulating exosomes, tumor cells (CTC)
Natural and acquired resistance	
Pharmacokinetics	

minimize noise without eliminating signal. Also important, there is a tremendous loss of opportunity and a real danger of uncorrected or uncorrectable error if the datasets and analytical procedures used on them cannot be reproduced months or years later for cross-checking and independent analysis.

"Data integration" is a term that rolls easily off the tongue, but it hides an entire field of intensive study. There are many methods for making disparate data types commensurate with each other and therefore able to be integrated, but none of them are totally satisfactory. Table 2 lists a small sample of the many web-based tools that are available and widely used for analysis, visualization, integration, and interpretation of bioinformatic data.

Visual pattern recognition is a strength of humans, and even the mathematically talented can generally interpret patterns in data better if they are visual. Accordingly, a large number of graphical representations are central tools in bioinformatics. Hierarchical cluster analysis is the data-mining method most frequently used. It builds trees of similarity and difference analogous to those in phylogenetics. For example, a typical gene expression profiling study across a set of patients' samples produces a rectangular matrix of values in which each column represents a patient, each row represents a gene, and each entry in the matrix is the expression level of a gene in a particular patient's tumor. The patients can be clustered to show patterns of similarity and difference in their profiles, and the genes can be clustered to show the similarities and differences in their patterns across the patient samples.

Clustered heat maps (CHMs)

Clustered Heat Maps (CHMs) are the most frequently used graphics for summarizing patterns in bioinformatic data. Hierarchical clustering in *both* horizontal and vertical directions serves to illuminate patterns in the data. CHMs were introduced into bioinformatics in the early 1990s (see[19]), and they have since become the ubiquitous graphic for visualizing patterns in omic data. They have appeared in many thousands of publications. The first CHM known to have influenced medical practice (in 1993) is shown in Figure 4. It reflects drug activity correlations in a study of platinum-containing compounds in the NCI-60 anti-cancer cell line screen. It tipped the balance in favor of clinical development of oxaliplatin, now a standard agent for treatment of colorectal cancer.

Hypothesis-generating and hypothesis-driven research

Through most of its history, biology was predominantly an observational science. Darwin formulated his hypothesis about

Table 2 A sample of web-based bioinformatics tools and data resources useful in bioinformatics

The UCSC Genome Browser[12]—Offers interactive online access to a database of genomic sequences and rich annotation data for a wide variety of organisms. Genome sequence is displayed horizontally, accompanied by a set of annotation tracks (which can be user-selected). For example, there are tracks that give the locations of predicted genes, transcription factor targets, DNA repeat elements, microRNAs, and cross-species comparative genomic information. There is an associated Cancer Genomics Browser for displaying and analyzing cancer genomic data along with associated clinical data[13] (http://genome.ucsc.edu/).

The cBioportal[14]—A resource for intuitive, interactive exploration of multiple cancer genomic datasets and correlative information from many different public molecular profiling projects, including TCGA (http://www.cbioportal.org/).

Cytoscape—A flexible open source software platform for analyzing, visualizing, and annotating complex interaction networks. (http://www.cytoscape.org/)

Bioconductor—An extensive open-source, open-development collection of programs (934 of them as of March 2015), mostly written in R, for analysis, graphical visualization, and annotation of bioinformatic data[15] (http://www.bioconductor.org).

Ingenuity pathway analysis—Integrated analysis of pathway, regulatory, and disease data (available in public and commercial versions) (http://www.ingenuity.com).

Pathway studio—A resource of molecular interactions and associated tools, based in part on natural language processing of biological and medical literature (commercial product) (http://www.elsevier.com/solutions/pathway-studio).

Oncomine—An integrated collection of hundreds of public microarray gene expression studies on cancers, with associated tools for meta-analysis of the data, for example to identify tumor subtypes, biomarkers, and therapeutic targets (available in public and commercial versions)[16] (http://www.lifetechnologies.com/us/en/home/life-science/cancer-research/cancer-genomics/cancer-genomics-data-analysis-compendia-bioscience/oncomine-cancer-genomics-data-analysis-tools/oncomine-gene-browser.html)).

The Gene Ontology (GO)[17]—Product of an international initiative to unify the annotations of genes and gene products by imposing a controlled vocabulary and hierarchical structure of categories (or terms). Formally, the structure is an "acyclic graph" in which each category in the hierarchy can have more than one parent category. There are three independent ontologies: biological process, molecular function, and cellular component. GO is frequently used to identify categories that are relatively enriched with overexpressed or under-expressed genes in a comparison of two gene expression profiles. The many tools for statistical assessment of the enrichment include AmiGo, David, GoMiner, and OBO-Edit (http://geneontology.org/).

Compendium of TCGA Next-Generation Clustered Heat Maps (NG-CHMs)—CHMs are the graphical visualizations ubiquitous in bioinformatics for identifying patterns in molecular profile databases. However, they are generally static images. NG-CHMs are highly interactive versions in which one can zoom and navigate using a Google-Maps-like technology; link out to pertinent public data resources including pathway programs, the UCSC Genome Browser, and the cBio Portal; re-color the map on the fly; access a statistical toolbox for detailed analysis of the data; produce high-resolution graphics; and store all metadata necessary to reproduce the map months or years later (http://bioinformatics.mdanderson.org/main/TCGA/NGCHM).

The Cancer Genome Atlas (TCGA) Data Portal—A primary source for access to non-restricted TCGA data (http://cancergenome.nih.gov).

The Cancer Proteome Atlas (TCPA) Portal—A collection of proteomic databases and tools for analysis and visualization of proteomic data, principally but not exclusively from TCGA (http://cancergenome.nih.gov).

Firehose—An analysis infrastructure that coordinates the flow of gigabyte- or terabyte-scale datasets through dozens of analysis algorithms for cancer genome projects including TCGA. An add-on, Nozzle, provides user-friendly formats for the results (http://gdac.broadinstitute.org).

Regulome Explorer—A suite of tools for exploration and visualization of large complex datasets, featuring a machine-learning algorithm (random forest) plus a circular ideogram layout, a linear multi-track browser, and 2D plots (http://explorer.cancerregulome.org).

Paradigm—A program that infers patient-specific genetic activities on the basis of curated pathway interactions among genes. It incorporates multiple types of omic data on tumor samples and predicts a pathway's activity level based on probabilistic inference (http://sbenz.github.com/Paradigm).[18] A related program, Paradigm-Shift (http://github.org/paradigmshift) uses a belief-propagation algorithm to infer gene activity from gene expression and copy number data in the context of a set of pathway interactions.

NCI Genomic Data Commons—Comprehensive computational infrastructure under development to store and harmonize genomic data on cancer generated through NCI-funded research programs.

GenBank—The NIH/NLM genetic sequence database, an annotated collection of all publicly available DNA sequences (http://www.ncbi.nlm.nhi.gov/genbank).

GEO (Gene Expression Omnibus)—A functional genomics data repository of curated microarray- and sequence-based gene expression datasets (http://www.ncbi.nlm.nih.gov/geo).

Cancer Genomics Hub (CGHub)—A secure repository for storing, cataloging, and accessing cancer genome sequences, alignments, and mutation information (including restricted-access personally identifiable data) from The Cancer Genome Atlas consortium and related projects. (https://cghub.ucsc.edu/).

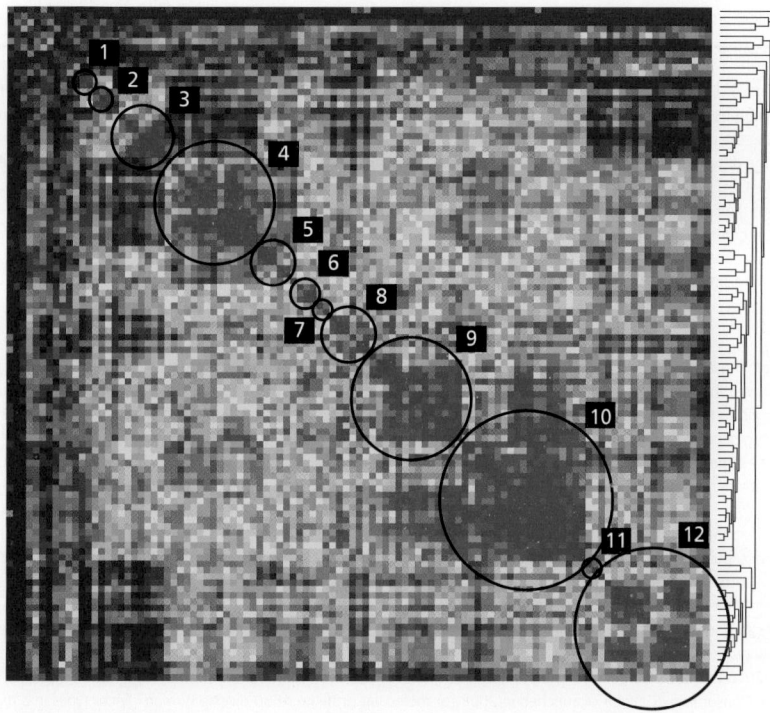

Figure 4 Drug versus drug clustered heat map for the activity of platinum-containing compounds against the NCI-60 panel of human cancer cell lines. Drugs are listed on both axes in the same clustered order, hence the heat map is symmetrical around the diagonal. Red indicates high correlation of activity profiles, blue indicates low correlation. The data define 12 families (which are highly correlated with the chemical structures of the compounds). Cluster #4 drugs, which consisted entirely of diaminocyclohexyl derivatives, including oxaliplatin, were selectively active against colorectal cell lines. That information tipped the balance for clinical development of oxaliplatin, now a standard agent for treatment of colorectal cancers (due to T Fojo, T Myers, JN Weinstein).

natural selection by unbiased observation of the Galapagos finches and other archipelago species, not by experimenting on them. By the middle of the 20th century, however, the dominant research paradigm in biology had shifted to tightly-focused, hypothesis-driven experiments. Taking a lesson from the concept in physics of a critical experiment, *patterns* of experimental result in biology were relegated to the background. In the 1990s, with the maturation of microarrays and other high-throughput molecular technologies, the balance shifted again—toward a synergistic relationship between hypothesis-driven experiments and hypothesis-generating omic research. Announcement in 2000 of the draft human genome sequence solidified that trend, serving as motivation and justification for additional large-scale molecular profiling programs such at The Cancer Genome Atlas (TCGA) and International Cancer Genome Consortium (ICGC) projects. As noted in the introduction, the trend toward high-throughput omic research was responsible for the emergence of bioinformatics as a prominent player in biomedical science.

The multiple-hypothesis testing trap

This is the most common error in bioinformatic analysis made by those without training in statistics. When mining large molecular or clinical databases for biomarkers, p-values <0.05 are not hard to find. Consider, for example, a database of 20,000 gene expression values generated by microarray or by RNA sequencing for tumors from 50 patients who responded to a particular drug and 50 who did not respond. If the aim is to discover a gene whose expression in the tumor is positively correlated with response to the drug (therefore a potential predictive biomarker), then ~20,000 different hypotheses are being tested in parallel, one for each gene. As the p-value (for rejection of the null hypothesis that there is *no* difference) will be less

than 0.05 about one in 20 times, even if the data are simply random, there will appear to be about 1,000 potential biomarkers just by chance. More subtle versions of the multiple-hypothesis problem occur, for example, any time multiple statistical algorithms, subsets of genes, or subsets of sample are analyzed. If one tries five different algorithms before finding one that yields a p-value less than 0.05, then the p-value is misleading because it was chosen among the five possibilities. Conceptually the simplest, but overly conservative, remedy is the Bonferroni correction in which the critical p-value (e.g., 0.05) is divided by the number of independent hypotheses to get a corrected critical value. For 20,000 genes, viewed as independent, that would be $p = 0.05/20,000 = 2.5 \times 10^{-6}$ before one would accept the p-value as statistically significant. Most popular for the corrections are algorithms based on false discovery rate (FDR), the fraction of apparently positive results (i.e., apparent rejections of the null hypothesis) that are expected actually to be *false* positives. The statistical nuances are complex, and dozens of different algorithms for the correction have been proposed.[20] A popular approach in bioinformatics is the Statistical Analysis of Microarrays (SAM) algorithm, which takes correlation structures in the data into account.[21]

The multiple-hypothesis problem brings into sharp focus the important difference between *hypothesis generation* and *hypothesis testing* in bioinformatics. For the latter, the strict rules of statistical inference must be observed or the results will be incorrect. For example, about 1,000 genes in the above case would spuriously be identified as biomarkers if the investigator were simply mining for genes with uncorrected p < 0.05. However, if the investigator started, before looking at the data, with a single-minded focus on one single gene out of the 20,000, then the critical level for that gene would be p = 0.05, regardless of how many other genes were present in the dataset.

Table 3 Some major molecular profiling projects on human cancers, normal tissues, and cell lines

---

Cultured cancer cells

The NCI-60—A panel of 60 human cell lines used since 1990 by the NCI to screen >100,000 chemical compounds plus large numbers of natural products for anticancer activity.[22] This was the first large public project to link pharmacology to multi-faceted molecular profiling of diverse cancer cells. One byproduct was development of new tools for bioinformatics including the clustered heat map[19] and other statistical and machine-learning innovations.[23] The NCI-60 provided a template for the design of CCLE, GDSC, and it informed the design of TCGA (see below). The project is continuing (data at http://discover.nci.nih.gov/cellminer/home.do).

The Cancer Cell Line Encyclopedia (CCLE)—Gene expression, DNA copy number, and sequencing data on 947 diverse human cancer cell lines, with metabolic inhibition assays of 24 anticancer drugs in 479 of the lines. Naïve Bayes and elastic net algorithms were used to predict response profiles on the basis of cell lineage, genetic defects, and gene expression.[24] The project is continuing (http://www.broadinstitute.org/ccle).

The Genomics of Drug Sensitivity in Cancer (GDSC)—Point mutations, indels, microsatellite instability, DNA rearrangements, and gene expression for 639 diverse human cancer cell lines, with metabolic inhibition assays of 130 anticancer gents on 275–507 cell lines per agent. Elastic net regression was used to predict drug sensitivity from the molecular profiles.[25] The project is continuing (http://www.cancerrxgene.org/).

Clinical tumors and tissues

The Human Genome Project—Planning began in 1986,[26] and articles announcing the draft sequence were published in 2001.[27,28] Surprisingly to many investigators at the time, bioinformatic analysis showed that there are only about 23,000 human genes, not the >50,000 expected. The sequence was pronounced 99% complete in 2004,[29] but a major pain for bioinformatics is the necessity of updates in software and databases to keep in sync with continuing refinements of the reference sequence, now in its 38th version (http://www.cancerrxgene.org/).

The International HapMap Project—Initiated in 2002 to define common DNA sequence variations among subsets of the human population. Unrelated individuals are ~99.9% identical in sequence, but the remaining sequence and copy number polymorphisms are both useful and a nuisance for bioinformatic analysis[30] (http://hapmap.ncbi.nlm.nih.gov/).

The Cancer Genome Atlas (TCGA)—Initiated in 2005 for molecular profiling of 10,000 human cancers of 25 types at the genomic, epigenomic, transcriptomic, pathologic, and clinical levels. The first project, published in 2008, was on glioblastoma.[31] More than 10,000 tumors in all from 33 cancer types have been profiled, more than meeting the initial goals. A "Pan-Cancer" project[32,33] summarized similarities and differences among the first 12 tumor types studied. It addressed (1) the commonality of particular functional themes (e.g., driver mutations, aberrant pathways, and drug resistance genes) across multiple tumor types, and (2) the extent to which tumor types can be subdivided into finer and finer categories in ways that may lead to more precise, targeted clinical management. TCGA originally focused on DNA and RNA profiles, but protein studies by reverse-phase protein array (RPPA) and mass spectrometry were later added.[34,35] A comprehensive Pan-Cancer analysis covering all 33 TCGA tumor types is scheduled for completion in 2016 (http://cancergenome.nih.gov/).

The International Cancer Genome Consortium (ICGC)[36]—Launched in 2008 for molecular profiling of 50 diverse human cancer types in a manner similar to the profiling in TCGA. The TCGA Research Network and ICGC are collaborating on whole-genome sequencing and analysis of diverse cancers from 2,000 patients (https://icgc.org/).

The Adjuvant Lung Cancer Enrichment Marker Identification and Sequencing Trials (ALCHEMIST)—Launched in 2014 by the NCI's National Clinical Trials Network to identify early-stage lung cancer patients with tumors that have genetic changes (EGFR mutations or ALK rearrangements) to evaluate drug treatments targeted against those changes (http://www.cancer.gov/types/lung/research/alchemist).

The Exceptional Responders Initiative—Launched by the NCI in 2014 to explore the molecular underpinnings of exceptional responses to treatment. The primary technologies to be used are whole exome- and mRNA sequencing (http://www.nih.gov/news/health/sep2014/nci-24.htm).

Genotype-Tissue Expression Project (GTEx)—Initiated in 2006 by the National Human Genome Research Institute to assess the correlation between genotype and expression levels in multiple normal tissues from up to 900 volunteer cadaver-donors—to serve as an aid to genome-wide association studies and as a base of normal background data for studies of cancer and other diseases (http://www.gtexportal.org/home/).

1000 Genomes Project—Launched in 2008 as an international effort to establish the most detailed catalogue available on human germline genomic variation[37] (http://www.gtexportal.org/home).

The Encyclopedia of DNA Elements (ENCODE)—An international consortium launched by the NHGRI as a follow-up to the Human Genome Project. Its ultimate aim was to identify all functional elements in the human genome, particularly those not located in RNA-coding regions.[38] (https://www.encodeproject.org).

The Therapeutically Applicable Research to Generate Effective Treatments (TARGET)—Multi-institutional molecular profiling of genetic changes (gene expression, DNA copy number, DNA methylation, and microRNA expression) that affect the initiation, progression, and response of pediatric cancers to therapy (https://ocg.cancer.gov/programs/target).

Hypothesis generation would consist of asking for each gene whether it is a plausible enough candidate biomarker to warrant further study. The FDR provides a metric of that plausibility. One can list the genes in order of their FDR values, from lowest to highest, and keep as candidates all of the genes at the top of the list, extending as far down the list as desired. There is a tendency to select an FDR cutoff of 0.05 by analogy with the usual p-value criterion, but that may be too conservative. How often in biology or medical science do we expect to be correct 19 out of 20 times? As a practical matter, the number of candidates accepted as positive should depend on a balance between the "cost" of independently validating a candidate and the "cost" of missing a *true* positive. If the validation step is a simple assay, one can afford many false positives; if the next step is major surgery, then few if any false positives can be tolerated. The issue of false positives, true positive, and "positive predictive values" is familiar from many areas of public health and clinical practice, for example in the controversies over PSA screening. The issues arise repeatedly throughout bioinformatic analysis. It is, therefore, important that anyone doing a statistical analysis know the question being asked, the reason why it is being asked, and the cost/benefit ratio of follow-up.

Analysis and biointerpretation in major molecular profiling projects

Large-scale molecular profiling projects have provided important arenas for application of bioinformatics and also rich testbeds for innovation in the field. Table 3 lists some of the more prominent large, publicly sponsored molecular profiling projects. The first waves of large-scale projects have focused on cancer cell lines and bulk samples of primary tumors paired with blood or normal tissue controls. However, additional projects are asking, or will be asking, incisive questions based on microdissection, single-cell sequencing,[39] archived formalin-fixed paraffin-embedded samples, pre-treatment/post-treatment pairs, primary tumor/metastasis pairs, comparison of samples from different parts of the same primary tumor, comparison of different metastases from the same patient, primary/recurrent pairs, and samples from responders and non-responders. Those next waves of projects make use of many of the current algorithms and programs for data analysis and interpretation, but they are also motivating the development of novel bioinformatics tools. For example, single-cell sequencing, particularly at the DNA level, imposes a new set of requirements as well as providing a new set of opportunities for incisive analysis. Because recurrent tumors can reflect clones that were

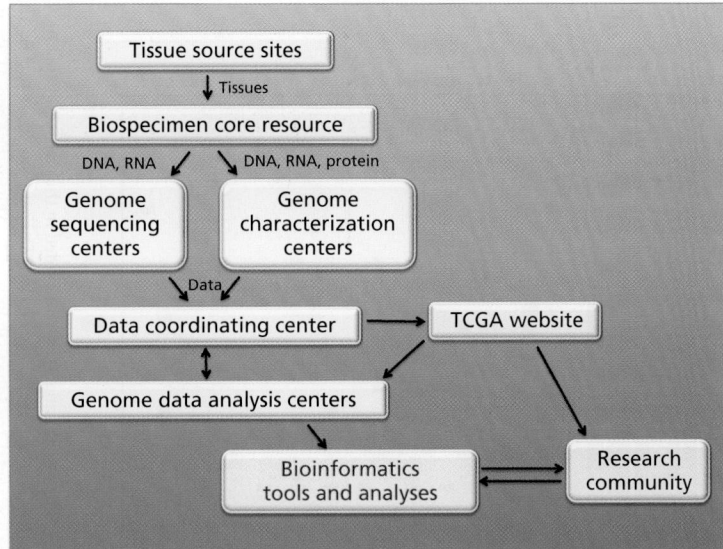

Figure 5 Simplified generic view of the flow of samples and information in The Cancer Genome Atlas program. Tumor plus normal blood and/or "normal tumor-adjacent tissue" specimens were collected with consent by tissue source sites and handled according to defined protocols for submission to the project. The Biospecimen Core Resource vetted the specimens and accompanying clinical data, generated DNA, RNA, and protein samples, quality-controlled the samples, and sent them to the Genome Sequencing and Genome Characterization Centers. Those Centers profiled the samples by sequencing, microarray analysis, or other technologies and sent the data to the Data Coordinating Center. As soon as feasible, non-restricted forms of the data were made public on TCGA's website for use by the research community, including TCGA's Genome Data Analysis Centers. Omitted here for simplicity are many additional components of the information flow such as the Broad Institute's Firehose, which performs and presents large numbers of analyses on the data; Sage Bionetics' Synapse, which provides an environment and tools that facilitate wide collaborative use of the data; Memorial Sloan-Kettering's cBio, which presents the data in a form accessible to nonspecialists; and MD Anderson's compendia of clustered heat maps for pattern recognition in the DNA, RNA, and protein datasets. Also not shown are the expert reviews of clinical data and pathology.

minor in the primary but important for choice of therapy, the logistical, fiscal, and ethical barriers to re-biopsy will probably continue to decrease for more and more tumor types and clinical contexts.

Figure 5 shows schematically the flows of tissue and information in the most prominent molecular profiling project to date, TCGA. Over 50 Tissue Source Sites provided paired tumor and normal samples (blood and/or tumor-adjacent "normal" tissue) plus information on the pathology and clinical history for 33 tumor types. Analysis of the samples by a panel of pathologists with specialist expertise in the particular tumor type has proved critical. The samples were processed in the Biospecimen Core Resource to produce DNA, RNA, and protein preparations, which were then profiled (principally by microarray or sequencing) in the Genome Sequencing and Genome Characterization Centers. Data generation was completed in 2015, but data analysis and interpretation will be the work of many years. The Data Coordinating Center organized and further quality-controlled the data, then made "non-restricted" datasets publicly available as soon as feasible on the TCGA Data Portal. "Restricted" data—those types that might be sufficient to identify an individual patient—are accessible only to researchers who have gone through a registration and vetting process to ensure confidentiality and appropriate use. Raw DNA and RNA sequences, for example, are restricted because they are considered personally identifiable. Central to analysis and interpretation are the seven designated Genome Data Analysis Centers (GDACs), which have matured as a TCGA community of shared, progressively more sophisticated bioinformatic expertise.

A major spin-off of TCGA has been the coalescence of a large bioinformatics community around the disease-specific and Pan-Cancer Analysis Working Groups (PCAWGs). Each Analysis

Working Group (AWG) represents a self-assembled aggregate of the multidisciplinary expertise required for data analysis and biological/medical interpretation. At the center are the GDACs, but many other individuals and institutions join in. Because everyone in an AWG is drilling down into the same datasets and data types, the result is a powerfully creative environment for development of new, innovative tools for analysis, visualization, and interpretation. Figure 6 is based on TCGA's multifaceted Urothelial Bladder Cancer profiling. Figure 6a shows a compact graphical visualization of the DNA-sequencing data, Figure 6b shows an interactive "next-generation" CHM for the RNA expression levels, and Figure 6c shows a particular representation of key pathways.

TCGA was originally designed as a series of disease-focused projects, but similarities and differences in profile across tumor types, as identified by the PCAWGs, have proved extraordinarily valuable. Figure 7 represents the Pan-Cancer project schematically as a 3D matrix of results.

Statistical methods and associated pitfalls

Table 4 is a list, by no means comprehensive, of statistical and machine-learning algorithms commonly used in bioinformatics. The descriptions in the table are intended to give the reader a general sense of how the algorithm can be used in bioinformatics, rather than to be rigorous or complete for the statistically trained. In this section, two of the most common will be considered in somewhat more detail with the principal aim of pointing out limitations and frequent errors in their use or interpretation in bioinformatics. Even the simplest univariate statistics can frequently be misused or misleading. The descriptions here, as in Table 4, will focus on issues that should be considered by biologists and clinical researchers,

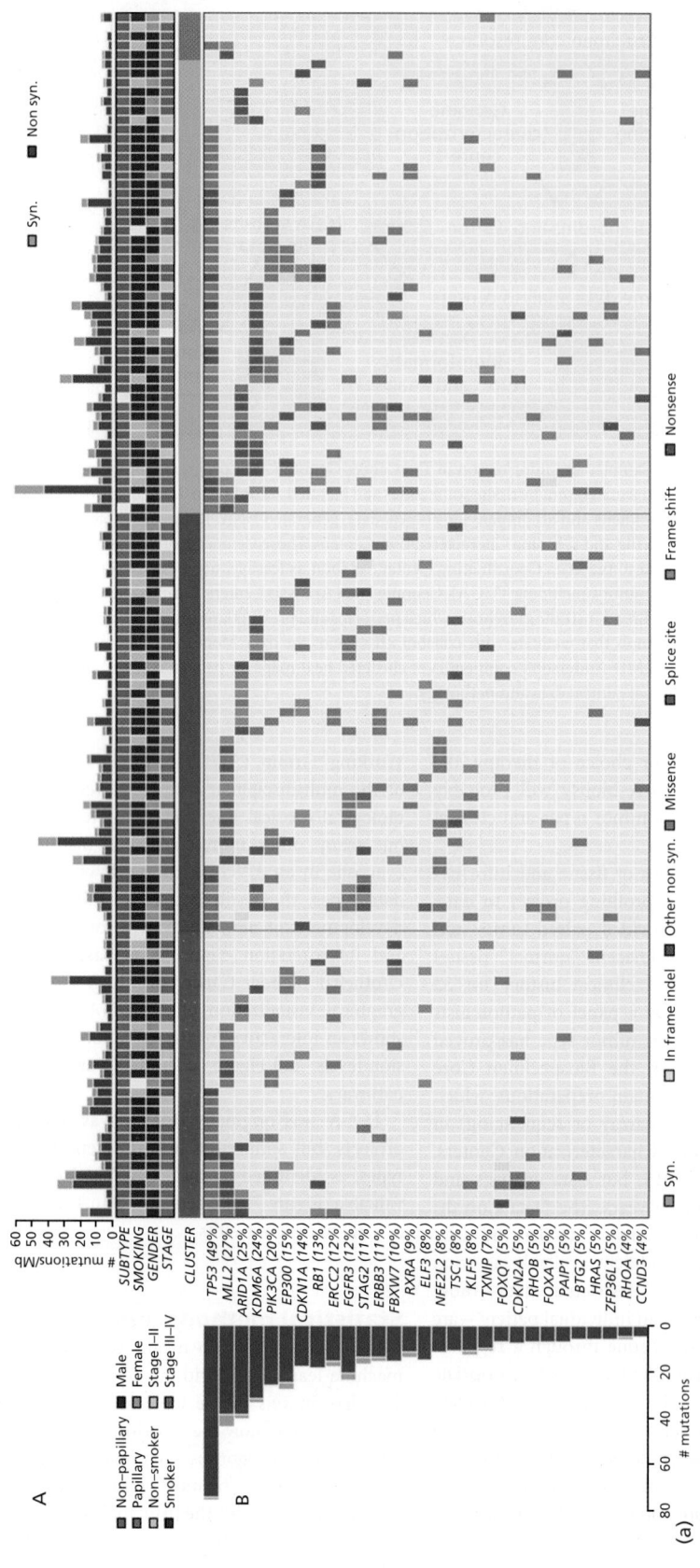

Figure 6 Data visualizations in TCGA's Urothelial Bladder Cancer Project. Source: The Cancer Genome Atlas Research Network 2014.[40] Tumor specimens from 131 patients were included in the analyses. Panel A: A compact visualization of mutation profiles across the bladder cancer specimens for genes scored by the MutSig 1.5 algorithm as significantly mutated (due to J. Kim, A. Cherniack, G. Getz, D. Kwiatkowski). **Panel B**: An interactive Next-Generation Clustered Heat Map representation of the mRNA expression data. Genes are on the vertical axis; patient specimens are on the horizontal axis (due to B. Broom, R. Akbani, D. Kane, M. Ryan, C. Wakefield, J. Weinstein). **Panel C**: Representation of four pathways found to be altered at the DNA level in urothelial bladder cancer. Somatic mutations and copy number alterations (CNAs) were found in the p53/Rb pathway, RTK/RAS/PI(3)K pathway, histone modification system, and SWI/SNF complex. Red, activating genetic alterations; blue, inactivating genetic alterations. Percentages shown denote activation or inactivation of at least one allele (due to C. Creighton, D. Kwiatkowski, L Donehower, P Laird).

(a)

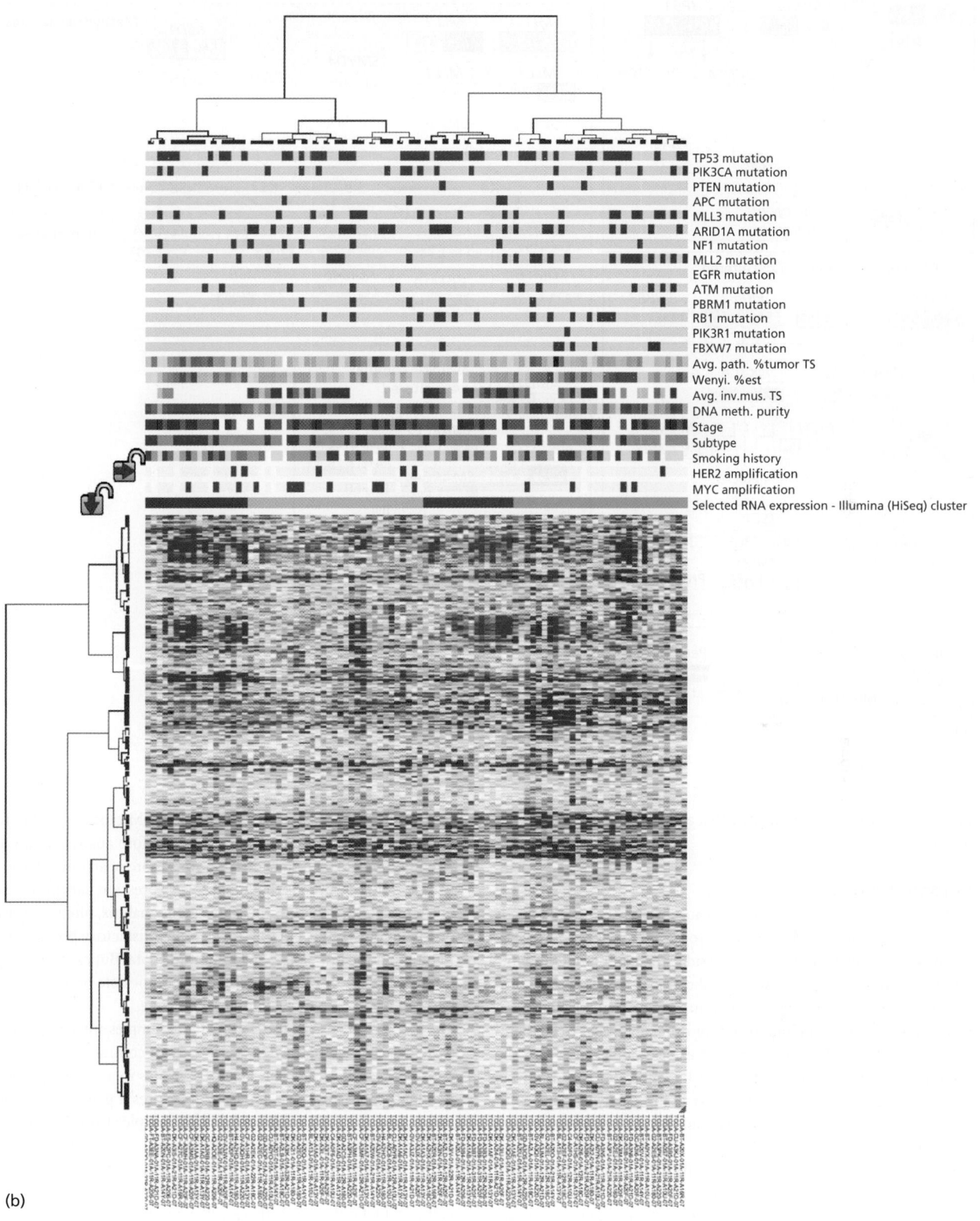

(b)

Figure 6 (*Continued*)

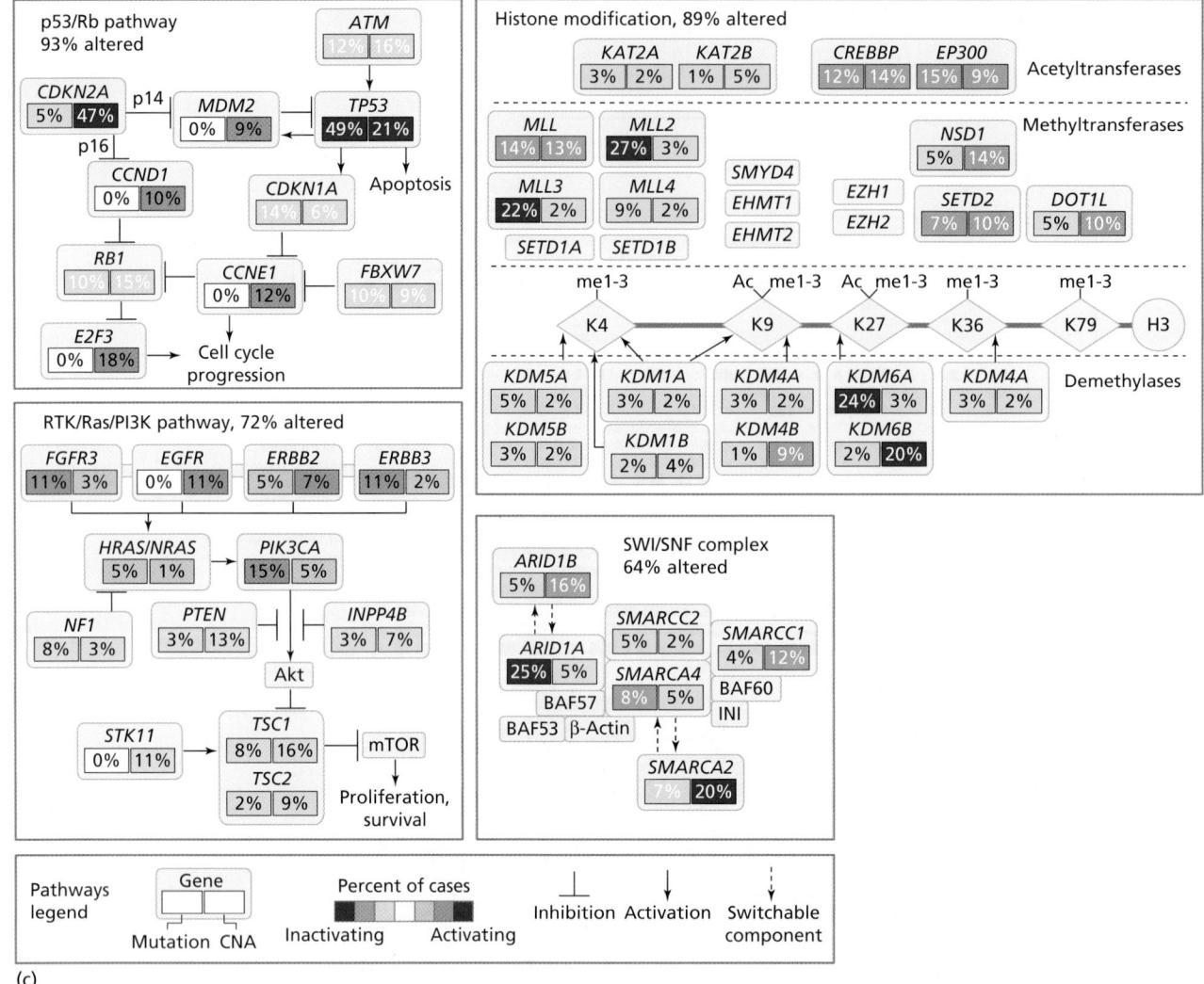

(c)

Figure 6 (*Continued*)

ignoring many of the complexities that a biostatistician would want to consider.

Student's t-test

Student's t-test was not so named because it is geared to the needs of neophyte trainees. Rather, it was introduced in 1908 by a brewery chemist/academic who published it under the pen name "Student" because company policy forbade publication. The t-test is used in cancer bioinformatics, for example, to assess whether the mean expression of a gene in blood or tumor differs between treated and untreated patients. If treated and untreated samples are from the same patient, the paired t-test (which has more statistical power) can be invoked. Every bench biologist is intimately familiar with the t-test, but two limitations deserve note because they are ignored with regularity:

- The t-test statistic (paired or unpaired) can always be calculated for sets of specimens, but, if the sample size is not large, a correct p-value can be calculated only if both sets of sample values are approximately normally distributed. An extension of the original Student's t-test permits the standard deviations of the two groups to be different, but the distributions must still be normal for calculation of a correct p-value. The problem is that data encountered in bioinformatics are rarely normally distributed,

so t-test p-values are often misleading. Microarray data, for example, are generally log-transformed before analysis in a vain attempt to make their data distributions more nearly normal. The usual result, however, is that noisy low-expression data points are given *too much* weight in the subsequent analysis, often seriously distorting the results obtained. The only satisfactory procedure is to filter out the low-noisy, low-amplitude data. But exactly how to do that without throwing out too much of the data or introducing bias can be an extremely complex challenge.

- The p-value can also be misleading if the samples are not independent of each other in the necessary sense. A common mistake is to consider technical replicates (say, triplicates in an assay) as independent. If, for example, an assay measures a gene's expression before and after treatment in triplicate samples from 10 patients, the number of actual samples in each group will be 30. However, if the variation in expression among *patients* is much greater than the variation among *replicates* from the same patient (and that will usually be the case), there will actually be only 10 independent values for treated patients and 10 for untreated. The statistical power of the t-test is dependent on N, the number of samples. Hence, if N = 30 is inserted into the standard formula, the p-value calculated will be too optimistic; the null hypothesis that the treatment had no effect may be rejected spuriously.

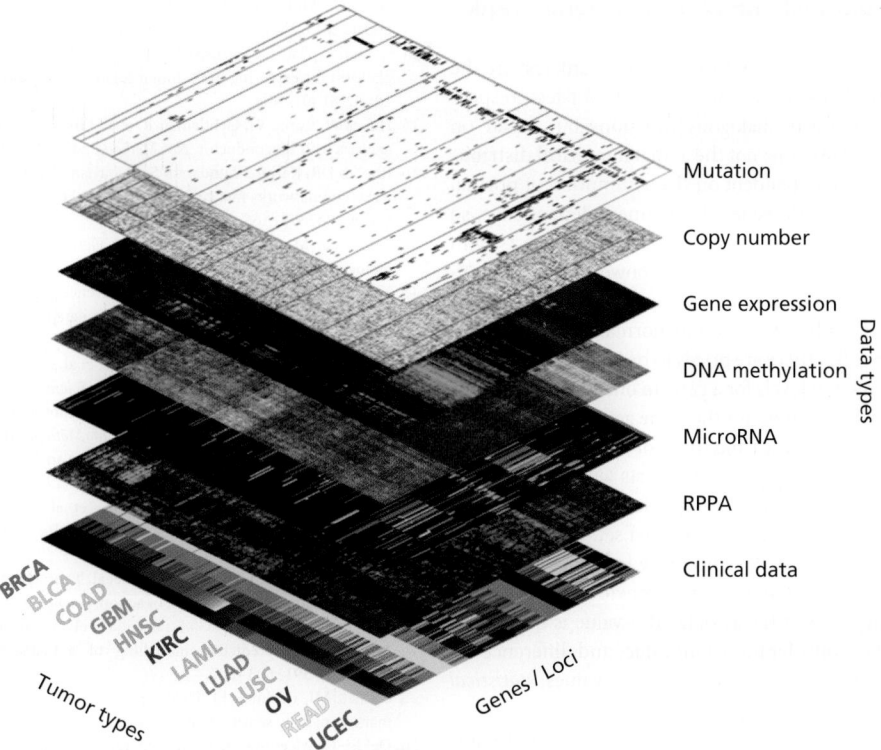

Figure 7 Representation of the Pan-Cancer TCGA project as a 3-dimensional matrix in which the axes are tumor type, data type, and gene or locus. Source: The Cancer Genome Atlas Research Network 2013.[32]

Table 4 A sample of statistical algorithms commonly used in bioinformatics.

Univariate analysis

t-test (unpaired): A statistical examination of two sample means. A two-sample t-test examines whether two samples are different and is commonly used when the variances of two normal distributions are unknown and when an experiment uses a small sample size.

t-test (paired): A version of the t-test in which samples are paired (e.g., with tumor specimens before and after treatment)

Permutation t-test: A version of the t-test applicable without assuming normal distribution (but assuming that the distributions of the two samples are the same). Almost all "parametric" statistical tests (i.e., ones in which the reference distributions are obtained from a theoretical probability distribution, e.g. normal distribution) have non-parametric equivalents in which the p-value is obtained by permuting the samples in an appropriate way.

Wilcoxon signed-rank test: Non-parametric equivalent of the paired t-test (based on ranks so normality not necessary)

Wilcoxon rank-sum (Mann–Whitney test): Non-parametric equivalent of the unpaired t-test (based on ranks so normality not necessary.

Multivariate analysis

Analysis of variance (ANOVA): Various forms of ANOVA extend the t-test to situations in which multiple variables are involved and normal distribution is assumed (e.g., multiple characteristics of more than two types of tumor specimens are being compared).

Multivariate analysis of variance (MANOVA): Like ANOVA but taking into account the interactions (dependencies) among variables.

Cross-validation: Useful in predicting an outcome (e.g., survival) on the basis of expression of one or more genes in a set of samples. A predictive model is trained on, say, 90%, of the patients and then tested on the other 10%. Different sets of 10% are then left out iteratively in order to pile up statistics on the model's success on patient samples it has not "seen" during the particular round of training and testing. However, if the model is "tweaked" in any way to optimize it on the basis of the cross-validation, it must then be validated against a separate set of samples to avoid overly optimistic conclusions about the algorithm. For most purposes, the model must be validated using an independent dataset anyway.

Bootstrap: Finds statistical confidence limits for a calculated statistic (e.g., a Pearson or Spearman correlation coefficient between two patients' tumors based on similarities and differences in their expression patterns across N genes). To proceed, we select *with replacement* a random sample of size N from the set of genes to produce a "pseudo-sample" of N values, then calculate the Pearson correlation coefficient for that sample. We do that many times, say 10,000 times, to build a histogram of estimates of the Pearson correlation coefficient and pick 95% confidence limits on the basis of that histogram. Because the sampling is done with replacement, any given gene may appear in a given sample 0, 1, 2, 3, or more times (according to the Poisson distribution with a mean of 1).

ROC (Receiver-Operator Characteristic): A plot of sensitivity versus 1-specificity that indicates the performance of a binary classifier (for example expression of a particular gene as a predictor of recurrence) as the discrimination threshold of expression is varied from low to high. The area under the ROC curve is directly related to the (non-parametric) Wilcoxon rank sum test.

Hierarchical cluster analysis: The clustering brings similar profiles (e.g., across tumor specimens or across genes) together in a tree-like structure to illuminate patterns of similarity and difference among them. Clustering (supervised or unsupervised) is often used to define subcategories of tumor types.

Fisher's exact test: A permutation test for the independence of variables in a contingency table. For example, if each patient in a clinical trial is labeled as a responder or non-responder to a treatment and labeled as wild-type or mutant with respect to a particular gene, the results of the study can be expressed in a 2×2 contingency table. Fisher's exact test (one- or two-tailed) gives a p-value for the null hypothesis that the gene's status has no effect on response. The word "exact" indicates that the p-value is accurate for even very small sample sizes. The test can be extended to larger (i.e., $m \times n$) contingency tables.

Bayesian methods: Statistical methods that assign probabilities or distributions to (a posteriori) outcomes or parameters based on a priori experience or best guesses specified before the data are analyzed. Bayes' theorem is then applied to revise the a posteriori probabilities. Bayesian methods differ in concept from the more common "frequentist" ones. An example is a multi-arm, biomarker-driven clinical trial in which accumulating experience is used to reassess the likelihood that a particular biomarker predicts response—and then using that information to put more patients on the arm with the most promising biomarker-predicted therapy.

Wilcoxon rank-sum test and Wilcoxon signed-rank test

The Wilcoxon rank-sum test and Wilcoxon signed-rank test are the non-parametric equivalents of the t-test and paired t-test, respectively. That is, they perform analogous functions but based on rank-ordering of the data points, not the actual numerical distributions. Hence, they are not dependent on the assumption of normal distribution. However, they do generally assume independence, so they are subject to the same issue as noted above for t-tests with replicates. They have somewhat less statistical power than the equivalent t-test when the samples are indeed normal, but they are less sensitive to outliers and other types of non-normality. They are less likely to be misleading. But there are prices to be paid for the choice. Imagine that the expression levels for a gene in one set of specimens range from 1 to 2 units, and those for the same gene in the other set of specimens differs dramatically from those of the first set, ranging from 101 to 102 units. The non-parametric tests will give the same answers as if the second set's values ranged from 2.1 to 2.2 units, i.e., differing only slightly from those of the first set. Only the ranks count, so very large differences have no more influence than relatively small ones. Hence, the t-statistic may provide a metric more reflective of the reality, even if the associated p-value is unreliable. It is always advisable to consider the *actual* values and differences in addition to p-values or quantities related to the p-values; *statistical* significance does not imply *biological* significance.

The *t*-test and its nonparametric and permutation-based equivalents are among the simplest statistical tests one can encounter in bioinformatics. They are much simpler in principle and in practice than the multivariate and machine-learning analyses. Nonetheless, the foregoing examples indicate the gross mistakes that can be made in using them and the advisability of professional expertise for the statistical analysis of most data in bioinformatics.

References

1 Hesper B, Hogeweg P. Bioinformatica: een werkconcept. *Kameleon*. 1970;**1**:28–29.

2 Luscombe NM, Greenbaum D, Gerstein M. What is bioinformatics? A proposed definition and overview of the field. *Methods Inf Med*. 2001;**40(4)**:346–358.

3 http://bioinformaticsweb.tk. Bioinformatics definition - a review 2015

4 Mosby. *Mosby's Dental Dictionary*, 2nd ed. Maryland Heights: Elsevier B.V.; 2008.

5 Moore GE. Cramming more components onto integrated circuits. *Electronics*. 1965;**38(8)**:114–117.

6 Kryder MH, Kim CS. After hard drives - What comes next? *IEEE T MAGN*. 2009;**45(10)**:3406–3413.

7 Church GM, Gao Y, Kosuri S. Next-generation digital information storage in DNA. *Science*. 2012;**337(6102)**:1628.

8 Lawrence MS, Stojanov P, Polak P, et al. Mutational heterogeneity in cancer and the search for new cancer-associated genes. *Nature*. 2013;**499(7457)**:214–218.

9 Kim SY, Speed TP. Comparing somatic mutation-callers: beyond Venn diagrams. *BMC Bioinformatics*. 2013;**14**:189.

10 Baggerly KA, Coombes KR. Deriving chemosensitivity from cell lines: forensic bioinformatics and reproducible research in high-throughput biology. *Ann Appl Stat*. 2009;**3**:1309–1334.

11 Weinstein JN. Fishing expeditions. *Science*. 1998;**282(5389)**:628–629.

12 Kent WJ, Sugnet CW, Furey TS, et al. The human genome browser at UCSC. *Genome Res*. 2002;**12(6)**:996–1006.

13 Goldman M, Craft B, Swatloski T, et al. The UCSC Cancer Genomics Browser: update 2013. *Nucleic Acids Res*. 2013;**41(Database issue)**:D949–D954.

14 Cerami E, Gao J, Dogrusoz U, et al. The cBio cancer genomics portal: an open platform for exploring multidimensional cancer genomics data. *Cancer discovery*. 2012;**2(5)**:401–404.

15 Huber W, Carey VJ, Gentleman R, et al. Orchestrating high-throughput genomic analysis with Bioconductor. *Nat Methods*. 2015;**12(2)**:115–121.

16 Rhodes DR, Kalyana-Sundaram S, Mahavisno V, et al. Oncomine 3.0: genes, pathways, and networks in a collection of 18,000 cancer gene expression profiles. *Neoplasia*. 2007;**9(2)**:166–180.

17 Ashburner M, Ball CA, Blake JA, et al. Gene ontology: tool for the unification of biology. The Gene Ontology Consortium. *Nat Genet*. 2000;**25(1)**:25–29.

18 Vaske CJ, Benz SC, Sanborn JZ, et al. Inference of patient-specific pathway activities from multi-dimensional cancer genomics data using PARADIGM. *Bioinformatics*. 2010;**26(12)**:i237–i245.

19 Weinstein JN, Myers TG, O'Connor PM, et al. An information-intensive approach to the molecular pharmacology of cancer. *Science*. 1997;**275(5298)**:343–349.

20 Farcomeni A. A review of modern multiple hypothesis testing, with particular attention to the false discovery proportion. *Stat Methods Med Res*. 2008;**17(4)**:347–388.

21 Tusher VG, Tibshirani R, Chu G. Significance analysis of microarrays applied to the ionizing radiation response. *Proc Natl Acad Sci U S A*. 2001;**98(9)**:5116–5121.

22 Shoemaker RH, Monks A, Alley MC, et al. Development of human tumor cell line panels for use in disease-oriented drug screening. *Prog Clin Biol Res*. 1988;**276**:265–286.

23 Weinstein JN, Kohn KW, Grever MR, et al. Neural computing in cancer drug development: predicting mechanism of action. *Science*. 1992;**258(5081)**:447–451.

24 Barretina J, Caponigro G, Stransky N, et al. The Cancer Cell Line Encyclopedia enables predictive modelling of anticancer drug sensitivity. *Nature*. 2012;**483(7391)**:603–607.

25 Garnett MJ, Edelman EJ, Heidorn SJ, et al. Systematic identification of genomic markers of drug sensitivity in cancer cells. *Nature*. 2012;**483(7391)**:570–575.

26 DeLisi C. Meetings that changed the world: Santa Fe 1986: Human genome baby-steps. *Nature*. 2008;**455(7215)**:876–877.

27 McPherson JD, Marra M, Hillier L, et al. A physical map of the human genome. *Nature*. 2001;**409(6822)**:934–941.

28 Venter JC, Adams MD, Myers EW, et al. The sequence of the human genome. *Science*. 2001;**291(5507)**:1304–1351.

29 International Human Genome Sequencing C. Finishing the euchromatic sequence of the human genome. *Nature*. 2004;**431(7011)**:931–945.

30 International HapMap C, Altshuler DM, Gibbs RA, et al. Integrating common and rare genetic variation in diverse human populations. *Nature*. 2010;**467(7311)**:52–58.

31 Cancer Genome Atlas Research N. Comprehensive genomic characterization defines human glioblastoma genes and core pathways. *Nature*. 2008;**455(7216)**:1061–1068.

32 Cancer Genome Atlas Research N, Weinstein JN, Collisson EA, et al. The Cancer Genome Atlas Pan-Cancer analysis project. *Nat Genet*. 2013;**45(10)**:1113–1120.

33 Hoadley KA, Yau C, Wolf DM, et al. Multiplatform analysis of 12 cancer types reveals molecular classification within and across tissues of origin. *Cell*. 2014;**158(4)**:929–944.

34 Li J, Lu Y, Akbani R, et al. TCPA: a resource for cancer functional proteomics data. *Nat Methods*. 2013;**10(11)**:1046–1047.

35 Akbani R, Ng PKS, Werner HMJ, et al. *Nat Commun*. 2014;**5(3887)**. doi: 10.1038/ncomms4887 PMID: 24871328.

36 International Cancer Genome C, Hudson TJ, Anderson W, et al. International network of cancer genome projects. *Nature*. 2010;**464(7291)**:993–998.

37 Genomes Project C, Abecasis GR, Altshuler D, et al. A map of human genome variation from population-scale sequencing. *Nature*. 2010;**467(7319)**:1061–1073.

38 Consortium EP. The ENCODE (ENCyclopedia Of DNA Elements) Project. *Science*. 2004;**306(5696)**:636–640.

39 Navin N, Kendall J, Troge J, et al. Tumour evolution inferred by single-cell sequencing. *Nature*. 2011;**472**:90–94.

40 Cancer Genome Atlas Research Network. Comprehensive molecular characterization of urothelial bladder carcinoma. *Nature*. 2014;**507(7492)**:315–322.

19 Systems biology and genomics

Saima Hassan, MD, PhD, FRCSC ■ *Laura M. Heiser, PhD* ■ *Joe W. Gray, Ph.D.*

Overview

Cancers are complex, adaptive systems comprised of cancer cells, the proximal and distal cells, and soluble and insoluble proteins that influence the behavior of the cancer cells. Features pertaining to the cancer are referred to as intrinsic to the cancer and those comprising the proximal and distal microenvironments are referred to as extrinsic to the cancer. Genomics studies seek to develop comprehensive cellular and molecular profiles of cancers and cancer systems biology studies seek to develop the experimental and theoretical methods needed to understand how the components work together to determine cancer function. The overall goal of these efforts is to develop the ability to predict the behavior of cancers—including progression and response to therapy—from measurements of the intrinsic and extrinsic molecular and cellular components of the cancers. Here, we review recent progress in international efforts to measure the genomic, epigenomic, and proteomic features (aka omic features) of major tumor types. We summarize work on establishing associations between omic features and cancer behavior. Finally, we summarize the computational and experimental models that are currently being used to understand and manipulate the behavior of complex cancer systems.

Introduction

Studies of the behavior of biological systems have traditionally been reductionist, focusing on specific genes or pathways. Today, efforts to generate molecular profiles of cancers are well established, momentum is building to establish associations between features and biomedical behavior, and efforts to establish mechanistic theoretical models are beginning. Systems biology approaches to cancer include studies of the intrinsic molecular features of cancer cells, as well as studies of how signals from the extrinsic microenvironment influence cancer cell signaling and phenotypic response (Figure 1).

Intrinsic cancer systems biology, the study of malignant cells that comprise the tumor mass, has evolved with advancements in genomic and epigenomic profiling technologies. These technologies produce comprehensive measurements of the genomic aberrations, and transcriptional and proteomic levels that comprise individual tumors. Several recent studies have identified recurrent events that define cancer subsets, have led to a better understanding of cancer heterogeneity, have identified prognostic subgroups and predictors of response to therapy, and have facilitated discovery of novel therapeutic targets.[1,2]

Extrinsic systems biology focuses on understanding external signals that alter the behavior of tumor cells. Extrinsic signals may come from microenvironments in close proximity to the tumor cells (e.g., invading immune cells, cancer-associated fibroblasts (CAFs), and vascular endothelial cells)[3] as well as from distal organs, especially the brain.[4,5] Several recent observations point to the clinical importance of the tumor microenvironment (TME):

stromal components can predict outcome,[6] the TME can mediate therapeutic response and resistance,[7] and the immune microenvironment has been shown to mediate tumorigenesis, disease progression,[8] and therapeutic response.[9–11]

Together, intrinsic and extrinsic systems biology approaches strive to enable an all-encompassing understanding of the cancer cell and its interactions with its environments. This chapter will discuss both intrinsic and extrinsic systems biology. The intrinsic systems biology section will focus on the clinical impact of high-throughput genomics and the use of cancer cell lines as predictive models of therapeutic response in patients. The extrinsic systems biology section will discuss its different constituents, the clinical significance, and how the microenvironment can be incorporated into preclinical models.

KEY POINTS

Potential of omics

- TCGA studies have used patient samples to identify new tumor classifications that have prognostic significance and novel therapeutic targets
- Panels of cancer cell lines have been used to identify gene signatures that are predictive of therapeutic response and present in patient samples
- Data analytical tools are being developed and validated in order to integrate different "omic" data types

Intrinsic systems biology and genomics in cancer

Since the mapping of the human genome, numerous technological advancements have enabled the "omics" era in which high-throughput profiling efforts provide comprehensive assessment of changes in DNA, RNA, and protein level in tumors and associated stroma that occur during cancer genesis, progression and response to therapy.[12] Much work today is aimed at developing strategies to use these data to improve the clinical management of cancer. The bottleneck now lies in data processing and interpretation.[13] Removing the bottleneck will require novel bioinformatic approaches that can effectively identify actionable molecular events and druggable therapeutic targets. Although the robustness of platforms and validation of gene signatures are some of the major concerns regarding their clinical utility,[14,15] there are multiple pragmatic issues that must be addressed to better integrate genomic platforms into the clinic. For example, next-generation tumor banks now require greater infrastructure with a larger team of health-care providers that acquire and manage relevant tissue and associated clinical metadata.[16] Tissues for study include surgical specimens, tissue biopsies, and blood samples, each requiring different standard operating protocols and sample preparation

Holland-Frei Cancer Medicine, Ninth Edition. Edited by Robert C. Bast Jr., Carlo M. Croce, William N. Hait, Waun Ki Hong, Donald W. Kufe, Martine Piccart-Gebhart, Raphael E. Pollock, Ralph R. Weichselbaum, Hongyang Wang, and James F. Holland.
© 2017 John Wiley & Sons, Inc. ISBN: 978-1-118-93469-2

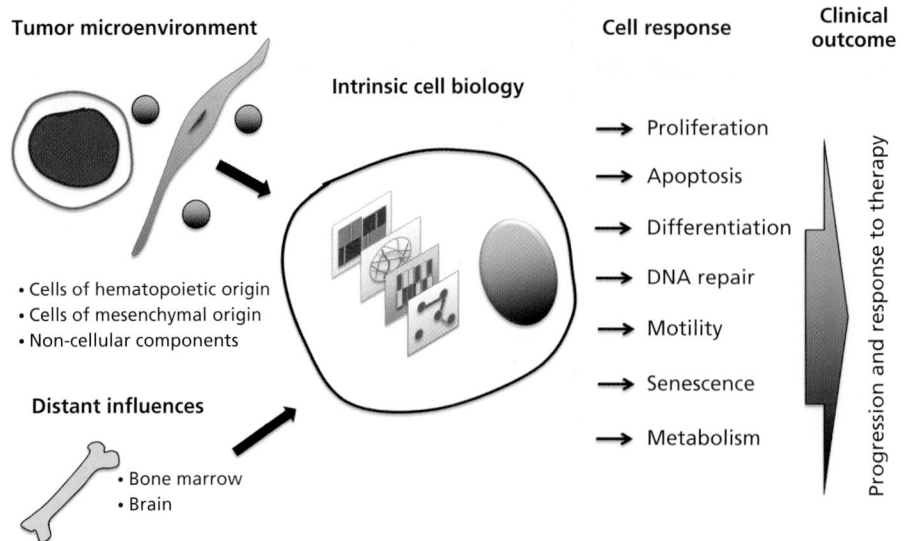

Figure 1 A schematic illustration of the influence of extrinsic and intrinsic systems biology upon cellular function with the potential to identify progression and response to therapy in patients. The extrinsic systems biology component consists of the tumor microenvironment including cells of hematopoetic origin, mesenchymal origin, and noncellular components, in addition to distant influences, from the bone marrow and other multiple organs. Together, with a systems biology approach, cellular function can be studied using various endpoints, including cellular proliferation, apoptosis, differentiation, DNA repair, motility, senescence, and metabolism. Our laboratory is striving to combine these endpoints to better understand tumor progression and response to therapy in the laboratory, and how this may correlate to patients in the clinic.

techniques.[16] Nonetheless, several institutions have been using genomic platforms to guide clinical trials or in clinical contexts, particularly for diseases where there is little evidence supporting current management practices such as tumors of unknown origin.[12,17,18]

This section is divided into three parts: (1) Genomic analyses of patient samples to provide a better understanding of cancer biology and help fuel future clinical trials. (2) Preclinical models to select cancer subtypes that will better respond to therapy. (3) Bioinformatics approaches to integrate the different genomic platforms.

High-throughput genomics

High-resolution genome analysis techniques are being used in international cancer genome analysis efforts to catalog aberrations driving the pathophysiology of nearly all major cancer types. Together, The Cancer Genome Atlas[19] (TCGA, http://cancergenome.nih.gov/) project and the International Cancer Genome Consortium[20,21] (ICGC, http://www.icgc.org/) have assessed aberrations in over 12,000 samples in 55 separate tumor lineages.[22] The broad goal of these efforts is to improve the prevention, diagnosis, and treatment of cancer patients.[19] In these projects, patient samples have been profiled on multiple platforms that examined whole-genomes and whole-exomes,[23–26] mRNA, DNA methylation,[27] miRNA,[28,29] and protein and phosphoprotein levels.[30] Results for several cancers are already publically available[25,31–33] and several recent papers have described integrative analyses of the characteristics of a dozen human cancer types.[34–36] Genome aberrations[37] found to be important in human cancers include (1) somatic changes in DNA copy number that increase or decrease the levels of important coding and noncoding RNA transcripts; (2) somatic mutations that alter gene expression, protein structure, and protein stability and/or change the way transcripts are spliced, (3) structural changes that change transcript levels by altering gene-promoter associations or create new fusion genes,[38,39] and (4) epigenomic modifications that alter gene expression.[40,41]

Analysis of these rich datasets has yielded clinically relevant insights into how we may better treat different cancers. For example, urothelial bladder cancers were found to be enriched in mutations in chromatin-regulatory genes, suggesting the potential use of therapeutic agents that target chromatin modifications.[23] Half of the high-grade serous ovarian cancers analyzed were found to be defective in homologous recombination, increasing their likelihood to be more susceptible to poly (ADP-ribose) polymerase (PARP) inhibitors.[25] Classification systems are now emerging that stratify tumors into biologically distinct subtypes and are demonstrating greater prognostic and predictive significance in comparison to the commonly used histologic classifications. Illustrative classification systems are now emerging for cancers of the breast,[42,43] colon,[44] pancreas,[45] ovary,[25] lung,[46] and gastric cancer.[24] The METABRIC cohort is a particularly well-developed cohort comprised of nearly 2000 breast tumors that were profiled to assess changes in copy number and gene expression.[49] Analysis of the copy number profiles identified 10 breast cancer subpopulations, each with a unique spectrum of alterations and disease-specific survival rate.

Our understanding of the molecular landscape of breast cancer is particularly advanced. A key observation from the TCGA breast cancer study[33] is that there are a few common mutations that occur in >5% of tumors (e.g., TP53, PIK3CA, CDH1, MLL3, GATA3, and MED12) and hundreds more that occur in <1% of breast cancers. The genomic aberrations in an individual tumor are comprised of a mix of "driver" and "passenger" aberrations. Driver aberrations are selected during tumor progression because they enable one or more aspects of the cancer pathophysiology that allow initiation, progression, and determination of cancer behavior, including response to therapy.[48] Passenger aberrations do not contribute to cancer pathophysiology but arise by chance during progression in a genomically unstable tumor.

Recent analyses of glioblastoma have illustrated the strong interplay between the genome and treatment. The initial TCGA studies[31,50] demonstrated a link between MGMT promoter methylation and a hypermutator phenotype consequent to mismatch repair deficiency in temozolomide-treated glioblastomas. Johnson et al.[51] performed exome sequencing for initial and recurrent low-grade gliomas. Of 10 tumors treated with adjuvant temozolomide, 6 were hypermutated when they recurred and carried driver mutations involving the AKT-mTOR pathways. This suggests a role for therapeutic agents that target the AKT-mTOR pathways in patients with recurrent low-grade gliomas previously treated with temozolomide. In many cases, the genome landscapes of the recurrent tumors were dramatically different than those of the primary tumor, illustrating the need for longitudinal following of patients during treatment.

A pan-cancer approach was launched in 2012 to analyze genomic aberrations among the panel of TCGA cancers[36] with the goal of identifying genomic features common to multiple cancer types. Initial studies have focused on 13 cancers.[52,53] Integrative analysis of genomic and proteomic platforms identified novel cancer subtypes that were associated with survival.[34] Interestingly, the pan-cancer approach to proteomic profiling revealed an elevated expression of HER2 in several cancers, including endometrial cancer, bladder cancer, and lung adenocarcinoma.[30] Because endometrial cancer has a higher expression of HER2 in comparison to breast cancer, this suggests that anti-HER2 agents, such as T-DM1, may be effective in treating endometrial cancer.[30] The pan-cancer approach lends itself to basket-style clinical trials, which are guided by specific molecular aberrations across different tumor types, as opposed to the traditional clinical trial designs that use large populations based on histologic classifications.[54]

Organization of these large-scale data for convenient visual and computational analysis is critical to enable community-wide. Useful tools for this are now emerging, and several of the most popular are listed in Table 1.

Gene signatures—prognostic and predictive biomarkers of response

Tissue histology and locally invasive properties are still commonly used as surrogate markers for distant metastatic spread and indicators of outcome. However, in the last decade, conventional classification strategies have been supplemented by omic-based strategies. These efforts began in 1999 with the demonstration that gene expression analysis could be used to distinguish between acute myeloid leukemia and acute lymphoblastic leukemia.[55] This was quickly followed by an analysis of gene expression in breast cancer that identified intrinsic breast cancer subtypes, designated as hormone receptor-positive luminal A and luminal B, HER2-enriched, basal-like, and normal-like.[56] The classification of these subtypes was validated in several independent cohorts and was found to have strong prognostic significance.[56]

Several efforts are now underway to use this information to develop clinically validated prognostic signatures. In breast cancer, for example, van't Veer et al.[57] identified a 70-gene signature that

could predict recurrence in a select group of younger patients with early breast cancers. This signature, now marketed by Agendia BV as MammaPrint, was validated in independent cohorts and outperformed Adjuvant! Online software in clinicopathologic risk assessment.[58,59] Although smaller retrospective studies have demonstrated the use of MammaPrint as a prognostic marker,[59,60] no prospective data is yet available that demonstrates its benefit in the adjuvant setting. Another test, marketed by Genomic Health as OncotypeDx, was developed in 2004 using an RT-PCR assay on RNA extracted from formalin-fixed paraffin-embedded tumor blocks. This 21-gene assay was tested retrospectively in two clinical trials, and was found to have prognostic significance. It is now widely used in the clinic to inform patients with estrogenreceptor-positive and early breast cancer of their risk of distant recurrence and potential benefit from chemotherapy.[61,62] Several competing prognostic and predictive gene expression signatures have been published[63,64] including a 17-gene signature for estrogen receptor-positive, node-negative breast cancer,[65] a 50-gene PAM50 risk of recurrence signature,[66] and a 44-gene Rotterdam signature.[67]

Not surprisingly, cancer subtype signatures are being developed for a growing number of other cancers. In colon cancer, for example, three unique gene signatures have been identified: Oncotype Dx colon cancer assay (Genomic Health, Inc.), ColoPrint (Agendia), and ColDx (Almac).[71] Although these tests have been shown to be independent prognostic biomarkers, their predictive value is still unknown.[72] In a positive move, academic efforts are now underway to reconcile diverse colorectal cancer classification schemes-based gene expression signatures.[44] For example, gene expression analysis identified basal-like and luminal subtypes associated with overall and disease-specific survival.[73] A pancreatic cancer classifier has been reported that identified three subtypes of pancreatic ductal adenocarcinoma that demonstrated a differential prognosis response to therapy.[45] Importantly, an ongoing community-wide classification effort is now underway that is attempting to integrate genomic and proteomic profiles to identify subtypes that transcend tumor origin. A recent report from this group defined a unified classification of tumors into 11 major subtypes.[34] This approach will become more powerful as additional tumor types are added to the analysis.

Experimental models of patient tumors for pharmacogenomics studies

Identification of molecular features that are causally related to clinical outcomes such as cancer progression or response to therapy requires experimental models in which cells carrying aberrant genes and networks can be manipulated. Collections of cell lines derived from patient tumors are widely used as laboratory models of cancer.[74] Cell lines are an attractive model system for studying cell-intrinsic biology for several reasons, including that they are: (1) a renewable resource; (2) can be manipulated in the laboratory setting; (3) are amenable to genomic profiling; and (4) can be used to assess therapeutic responses can be quickly assessed.[74,75] Although the first tumor-derived cell lines were established in the 1950s, their use as an experimental tool gained traction with the development of the National Cancer Institute 60 (NCI60) platform.[76,77] The NCI60 consists of 60 human tumor cell lines, representing nine cancer types, and has been used to screen over 100,000 compounds for therapeutic efficacy.[78] Analysis of these data with the COMPARE algorithm has provided a quantitative method for identifying associations between molecular features of cells and sensitivity to particular compounds.[78]

Table 1 Computational and visual analytical tools available for community wide use.

Tool	Uniform resource locator (url)
UCSC Cancer Genome Browser	https://genome-cancer.ucsc.edu/
cBioPortal for Cancer Genomics	http://www.cbioportal.org
Sage Synapse	https://www.synapse.org
Catalog of Somatic Mutations in Cancer	http://cancer.sanger.ac.uk/cosmic
The Cancer Proteome Atlas	http://app1.bioinformatics.mdanderson.org/tcpa/_design/basic/index.html

Since the demonstration of the utility of the NCI60, several other groups have developed panels of cancer cell lines, including pan-cancer[79–81] and tissue-specific collections (e.g., breast,[82] lung,[83,84] and melanoma[85]). One of the most well-developed panels, comprised of ~70 breast cancer cell lines, has been used to assess gene function and to identify mechanisms of therapeutic response and resistance.[82,86,87] Recently, very large cell line collections representing multiple tumor types have been used to identify associations between molecular features and response to molecular perturbants across tumor types.[80,81,88] Comparison of the genomic and epigenomic features of cell lines with those measured from primary tumors showed that the cell lines mirror many aspects of "omic" diversity in primary tumors that are likely to influence therapeutic response. Cell line and tumor similarities include: (1) recurrent copy number changes and mutations,[82,86,89] (2) transcriptional subtypes,[86,89] and (3) pathway activity.[86] However, there are significant exceptions. For example, cell lines grown on plastic have been reported to change epigenomic status[90] and some cell lines fail to retain genomic aberrations that were present in the tumors from which they were derived. Glioblastoma is a notable example of the latter, as cells grown on plastic usually fail to retain a region of amplification involving the EGFR oncogene that is frequently present in primary tumors.[91]

In breast cancer, analysis of correlations between drug sensitivity and molecular features revealed that approximately 30% of the compounds tested are associated with subtype or genome copy number aberration,[86] and robust integrated predictive signatures of sensitivity can be identified for ~50% of compounds.[86,87] Importantly, many of the *in vitro* signatures can be observed in primary patient samples[80,81,87] suggesting that cell line studies may be used to guide the development of signatures that can be used to stratify patients in the clinic. Evidence from other tissue types also supports the notion that cell lines are a powerful system for studying the molecular underpinnings of therapeutic response. For example, *in vitro* model systems accurately recapitulated several clinical observations, including that (1) lung cancers with EGFR mutations respond to gefitinib,[92] (2) breast cancers with HER2/ERBB2 amplification respond to trastuzumab and/or lapatinib,[82,93] and (3) tumors with mutated or amplified BCR-ABL respond to imatinib mesylate.[94] Of course, cell lines grown on plastic do not model many aspects of human cancers. A particular weakness is that they do not model the impact of the microenvironment on cancer cell behavior. Models the include signals from the microenvironment as covered later in this chapter.

Principles of integrative analysis

Several computational tools have been developed to identify molecular signatures associated with biological behavior. One of the first of these is gene set enrichment analysis (GSEA).[95] The rationale behind GSEA is to analyze the expression of predefined groups of genes that share a common biological function, chromosomal location, or regulation, to determine whether they show wholesale differences in gene expression between comparator populations. For example, GSEA analysis identified the RAS, NGF, and IGF1 pathways as differentially expressed in TP53 mutant versus TP53 wild-type cancers.[95]

The network analysis tool PARADIGM[96] was designed to identify pathways whose activities differ between comparator populations. PARADIGM integrates multiple omic data types, including DNA copy number and gene expression, to calculate integrated pathway levels (IPLs) for over 1300 curated signal transduction, transcriptional, and metabolic pathways from publicly available databases (e.g., the NCI Pathway Interaction Database KEGG, Reactome, and BioCarta). These IPLs can then be used to identify subnetworks that differ between comparator populations (e.g., responsive versus resistant tumors). The subnetworks are composed of interlinked *pathway features* (genes, proteins, complexes, families, processes, etc.) that take on activities distinctive in one class of tumors compared to another. For example, PARADIGM analysis of TCGA breast cancer samples identified HIF1-α/ARNT pathway activity as high in basal-like breast cancers, suggesting that these malignancies might be susceptible to angiogenesis inhibitors and/or bioreductive drugs that become activated under hypoxic conditions.[33]

One problem with tools that incorporate pathway information is that some genes and networks have been more extensively studied than others, and so there is inherent bias in the resultant pathways. HotNet2 is an algorithm to find aberrant networks using a strategy that tries to avoid curation bias. HotNet2 uses a modified diffusion process and considers the source, or directionality, of heat flow in the identification of subnetworks that reduces the impact of curation bias. This tool was applied in recent pan-cancer network analyses to identify 16 frequently mutated networks that affect well-known cancer phenotypes.[97]

Crowd sourcing to rapidly advance systems biology

Advances in profiling technologies and subsequent generation of large, complex datasets require robust analytical methods to facilitate the conversion of "big data to knowledge" (http://bd2k.nih.gov/). This effort is still in its infancy; many competing methods are being developed so it is difficult to determine which perform best. One novel approach to identify effective algorithms is using crowd-sourced community-wide challenges. The DREAM project (http://dreamchallenges.org) is one example of the power of this approach. DREAM brings communities of researchers together to address complex problems in systems biology, while also developing methods for identifying the most effective novel algorithms. A key aspect of these challenges is to eliminate the "self-assessment trap" in which data generation, data analysis, and model validation are combined within the same study.[98] Moreover, the advancements that arise through these collaborative efforts come at a much more rapid pace than can be achieved through traditional single-team research approaches.

Two recent DREAM challenges demonstrate the power of this crowd-sourcing approach. In the NCI-DREAM7 challenge, unpublished drug sensitivity measurements along with transcriptional and proteomic profiles for a panel of breast cancer cell lines were made freely available to the scientific community.[99] Over 40 international groups developed predictors of drug response using a broad range of machine learning and statistical algorithms. A meta-analysis of all methods demonstrated that modeling nonlinear relationships and incorporating existing knowledge are essential features for generating robust predictive biomarkers. Another DREAM challenge sought to assess the ability of computational strategies to predict breast cancer survival from clinical features, gene expression, and copy number profiles in breast cancer.[100] This challenge used data from the METABRIC breast cancer cohort,[49] and in multiple rounds of blinded evaluations, assessed the performance of more than 1400 models. It showed that the best-performing modeling strategy significantly outperformed a benchmark first-generation 70-gene risk predictor.[58] Interestingly, this study also demonstrated the "wisdom of the crowd" as the aggregation of the predictions from all the models performed as well or better than the best model. These results demonstrate the power of crowd sourcing to advance algorithm development and identify clinically relevant biomarkers.

Tumor microenvironment

Constituents of the tumor microenvironment

There are different ways of categorizing the TME,[7] and one approach divides the TME into three main groups: cells of hematopoetic origin, cells of mesenchymal origin, and noncellular components.[101] Cells of hematopoietic origin populate two cell lymphoid and myeloid lineages. The lymphoid cell lineage consists of T cells, B cells, and natural killer cells, whereas the myeloid cell lineage consists of macrophages, neutrophils, and myeloid-derived suppressor cells. Cells of mesenchymal origin include fibroblasts, myofibroblasts, mesenchymal stem cells, adipocytes, and endothelial cells. The two major components of this group are CAFs and endothelial cells. CAFs are fibroblasts that have been co-opted by the tumor to promote tumor growth, angiogenesis, and distant metastasis.[102,103] Endothelial cells and pericytes have also been shown to play an important role in vessel growth formation needed for tumor progression.[104] The most important player of the noncellular group is the extracellular matrix (ECM). The ECM can be further subdivided in two parts: the basement membrane, which consists of type IV collagen, laminin, and fibronectin, and the interstitial matrix, which is made up of fibrillar collagens, proteoglycans, and glycoproteins. The ECM has been shown to play roles in maintaining tissue architecture, cell invasion, tumor progression, and angiogenesis.[105]

Tumor microenvironment and the hallmarks of cancer

Hanahan and Weinberg[106] defined six essential capabilities, termed the hallmarks of cancer, that are essential for tumor growth. These include (1) evading apoptosis, (2) self-sufficiency in growth signals, (3) insensitivity to anti-growth signals, (4) tissue invasion and metastasis, (5) limitless replicative potential, and (6) sustained angiogenesis. Eleven years later, an update of these six hallmarks was published, with recognition of the TME as an important player in tumor growth, and the addition of two hallmarks: reprogramming of energy metabolism and evading immune destruction. However, categorizing the cancer hallmarks into two distinct categories of origin—tumor cell and TME—is an artificial classification, as the majority of the cancer hallmarks (7/8) are in fact a product of the cross-talk between stromal and cancer cells.[107]

Role of tumor microenvironment in modulating therapeutic response and predicting recurrence and survival

The TME can serve as a mediator of either response or resistance to therapeutic agents. One classic example is that of vessel normalization, wherein tumor vasculature can be manipulated to improve delivery of chemotherapy.[7,108] Vasculature associated with tumors is abnormal and consists of immature vessels with increased permeability as well as compromised ability to deliver nutrients and therapeutics. The administration of anti-angiogenic therapy leads to pruning of immature vessels, resulting in a "normalized vasculature" that allows for more effective delivery of chemotherapy agents.[108] Furthermore, the TME may serve as a predictive biomarker of localized and long-term response to therapy. For example, melanoma has a distinct type of metastasis called in-transit disease, wherein patients develop locoregional metastases in the skin and subcutaneous tissues more than 2 cm from the primary lesion but not beyond the regional nodal basin. One of the treatments for this type of disease is intralesional injection of interleukin (IL)-2, which can be administered in the office. One of our co-authors (SH) studied the immune response at the site of disease, from tissue biopsies 6–8 weeks post-treatment and found that patients who developed a pathologic complete response to treatment demonstrated an increased peritumoral infiltrate of CD8+ T cells and an improved overall survival. This is suggestive, along with other studies, that a localized response in the TME can be an important factor in mediating a systemic response, which in turn can impact overall survival.[109,110]

Resistance to therapy can either be an innate process, mediated by intrinsic properties of the TME, or an acquired process, which is an adaptive host response to therapeutic intervention.[7,111] Several mechanisms have been proposed to explain intrinsic resistance to therapy, including survival signals from protective niches in the TME, impaired drug delivery from vascular impairments and leakage, paracrine signaling with secretion of chemokines from stromal cells, and immunosuppression.[7,112] Immune responses are important factors in mediating acquired therapeutic resistance. Resistance to paclitaxel has been shown to result in part by enhanced expression of IL-34, colony-stimulating factor (CSF)-1, and macrophage infiltration.[113] Indeed, a monoclonal antibody has been identified, RG7155 (Roche), which targets macrophages and CSF-1 receptor activation, and has demonstrated response in patients with diffuse-type giant-cell tumors.[114] Other mechanisms that have been implicated in acquired resistance include the induction of senescence-associated secretory phenotype and changes in cell differentiation.[7]

Studies of the TME have yielded predictive markers of local recurrence in mouse models and prognostic markers in patients. An inflammatory signature has been identified, which was associated with recurrence of clinically detectable disease but not advanced recurrent disease. This inflammatory signature was characterized by an increase in serum concentrations of IL-6 and vascular endothelial growth factor (VEGF). The progression of minimal residual disease to a recurrence occurred through an evasion of the immune response by the cancer cells.[115,116] Park et al. established the importance of the TME as a prognostic marker in breast cancer.[6] They used laser capture microdissection to isolate stromal cells from the primary tumor of patients. A gene signature derived from the stroma was found to be a strong prognostic marker of overall survival and relapse-free survival. Immune cells were an important component of this gene signature, with the good-outcome patients demonstrating an enrichment of T-cell and NK-cell markers, suggesting a T_H1-type immune response. The prognostic significance of the amount of stroma within the primary tumor, termed tumor-stroma ratio has also been demonstrated in colon cancer and breast cancer.[117] Furthermore, the prognostic value of immune cells has since been demonstrated in breast cancer and colon cancer.[118–121] A stromal lymphocytic infiltrate was found to be an independent prognostic marker associated for overall survival in two randomized controlled trials with triple negative breast cancer patients.[120] In colon cancer, a score that measures the presence of certain lymphocyte populations, termed Immunoscore, was shown to be a stronger prognostic marker than current AJCC (American Joint Committee on Cancer) prognostic markers, including T stage (tumor depth) and N stage (nodal involvement).[122] Interestingly, the Immunoscore may have great potential in patients with localized colorectal cancer with no detectable spread or lymph node involvement on pathology of imaging, of which 25% of such patients go on to develop recurrence.[123] In two independent cohorts, Immunoscore was able to identify a group of patients that were at higher risk of developing recurrence and may have otherwise benefited from adjuvant therapy.[123,124] Given the prognostic significance of stromal gene signatures, it is important to consider the composition and extent of the stroma in tumor samples when tumor-derived gene signatures are being generated.[125]

Modeling the tumor microenvironment

The majority of pharmacologic agents targeting aspects of the microenvironment suggested by laboratory studies have not been successful in clinical trials.[126,127] This may be due to intrinsic tumor factors or limitations associated with preclinical models. A common criticism about preclinical models is that cancer cell lines alone do not encompass the complexity inherent to heterotypic signaling associated with cancer cells and their microenvironment. Table 2 summarizes a few of the chemosensitivity models that have been proposed to better model the complex interactions between the tumor and its microenvironment.

Two-dimensional (2D) models in which cancer cells are grown as monolayers on plastic are commonly used to assess therapeutic response.[128] These 2D models have been instrumental in driving the development of many therapeutic agents that are currently used in the clinic. Several approaches have been developed to add microenvironmental signaling. One approach employs 2D

co-cultures in which cancer cell lines are grown together with stromal cells. Co-culture models have identified changes in tumor genotype, phenotype, and response to therapy that result from interaction with microenvironmental signals.[136,137] Alternately, cells can be grown on substrates comprised of soluble and insoluble proteins from the diverse microenvironments to which cancer cells are known to spread. This can be accomplished efficiently by arranging microarrays comprised of thousands of individual array elements carrying one or more microenvironment proteins. These are referred to hereafter as microenvironmental microarrays (MEArrays). MEArrays are produced by printing combinations of ECM, growth factors, and other proteins onto substrata as ~200 μm diameter spots that support cell adhesion and growth. Live cells are then added and grown to assess the impact on growth of the proteins.[130,138] Cells grown on MEArray can also be treated with therapeutic compounds to assess the impact of the microenvironmental proteins on therapeutic response. Typically, cells that are grown are immunofluorescently stained using an affinity reagent that report on cancer-related phenotypes (e.g., proliferation, apoptosis, differentiation status, and senescence) of interest and then quantified using high-content imaging[130,139] (Figure 2).

Three-dimensional (3D) culture methods establish cells in 3D environments comprised of extracellular proteins and sometimes other cell types.[7,128,140] Matrix components such as matrices (e.g., matrigel) or scaffolds (e.g., collagen, laminin, and alginate) can be added to 3D models in order to better model tissue architecture. Isolated from mouse sarcoma cells, matrigel is a basement membrane-derived hydrogel that has been commonly used in cancer models and shown to support tumor growth and angiogenesis.[141,142] However, one of the challenges in the use of matrigel is its relatively undefined molecular composition and high lot-to-lot

Table 2 Summary of advantages and disadvantages of several pre-clinical chemosensitivity models

Model	Advantages	Disadvantages
Cell lines	• Unlimited source of self-replicating material • Easy to use • Amenable to high-throughput screening	• Generated from more aggressive tumors • Do not model the complex paracrine and endocrine influences upon tumor growth
2-Dimensional	• Easy to use • Amenable to high-throughput screening	• Differences in cell morphology, polarity, receptor expression, oncogene expression, between 2D monolayers and *in vivo*[128]
3-Dimensional	• 3D spheroids may better model the hypoxic core and drug diffusion found in solid tumors • Differential response to therapy in comparison to 2D models	• May be variability in cell size and shape • May require more specialized equipment and cost • More labor-intensive • If using matrigel, need to take into account lot-to-lot variability[129]
Microenvironment microarray	• Amenable to high-throughput screening • Influence of different microenvironment proteins upon therapeutic response and resistance	• Difficult to model tumor heterogeneity • Statistical analytical approaches are being developed[130] • Validation still required[130]
Mouse models	• Can be used to test therapeutic response upon primary tumor growth and distant metastasis • Both transgenic mice and xenografts can be used to observe response alongside clinical trials[131,132]	• Difficult to use on a larger scale to test multiple therapeutic compounds
Xenografts	• Easier to use, as cancer cell lines can either be easily injected or transplanted	• Use immunodeficient mice and cancer cell lines that often represent more aggressive tumors
Transgenic	• Can better model human tumor progression[133]	• Difficult to use in the preclinical setting as the age of mice need to be synchronized in order to administer treatment to similar sized-tumors
Patient-derived xenografts	• Renewable tissue resource[134,135] • Similar genomic properties as in patient tumors[131] • Therapeutic response in PDX models is similar to clinical outcome achieved in patients[131]	• Requires set-up to acquire patient samples and to grow tumors in mice • Requires immunodeficient mice[131] • Engraftment failure can be high and time to treatment long in some tumor types[131]

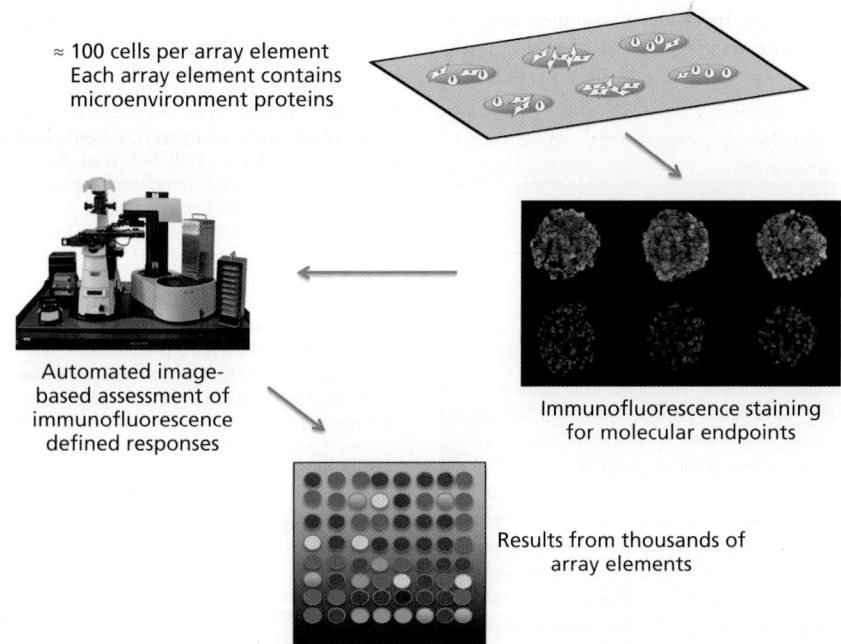

≈ 100 cells per array element
Each array element contains
microenvironment proteins

Automated image-
based assessment of
immunofluorescence
defined responses

Immunofluorescence staining
for molecular endpoints

Results from thousands of
array elements

Figure 2 Schematic illustration of the use of microenvironment microarrays to assess the impact of diverse microenvironments on cancer cell growth. Several thousand microenvironmental proteins printed as ~250 micrometer diameter spots host the growth of cancer cells. Changes in immunofluorescence staining pattern induced by the microenvironmental proteins are recorded using fluorescence image analysis.

variability therein.[129] Microfluidic systems, consisting of 3 connected wells, an inlet reservoir, a cell culture chamber, and an outlet reservoir, have been developed for 2D and 3D models, in addition to high-throughput platforms.[128] 3D co-culture models have also been developed. One such promising model has demonstrated the formation of larger sized breast tumors within 24 h.[143] The fidelity with which co-culture models mirror *in vivo* microenvironments is increasing as 3D cell-printing techniques[144,145] are used to arrange multiple cell types into laboratory cancer "tissues".

The importance of the TME has also been well established from mouse models. In xenograft mouse models, cancer cell lines are injected into immunocompromised mice. Metastasis develops infrequently when cell lines are injected subcutaneously ectopic sites. With a favorable microenvironment, tumors grown in orthotopic models tend to grow faster than their ectopic counterparts and have a greater propensity to metastasize.[146] Although xenograft models are useful tools to study tumor growth and metastasis inhibition, they are limited by the immunocompromised status of the host mice and the use of cell lines that are derived from more aggressive tumors.[131] Efficacy of therapeutic agents in xenograft models has not been shown to correlate well with efficacy in clinical trials.[147] As a result, there has been an effort to develop genetically engineered or transgenic mice as more realistic models. The advantage of this model is that the mice are immunocompetent and tumors progress from preinvasive, invasive, and distant metastasis, in a manner akin to human tumor progression.[133] Some transgenic mouse models develop tumors with short latency and have been used as chemosensitivity models.[127,132,148] However, these models are difficult to use on a large scale, owing to the need to synchronize the generation of pups, onset of tumors, and subsequent administration of therapy.[148]

More recently, patient-derived xenograft (PDX) models are being used to study therapeutic efficacy. PDXs are established from patient biopsies engrafted into immunocompromised mice.[131] The rate of engraftment is variable ranging from as low as 13%[149] to as high as 71%.[150] PDX models enable transplantability of human tissue

from mouse to mouse and are thus a renewable tissue resource.[134] Whole-genome sequencing has revealed high similarity between PDX tumors and human tumors in terms of copy number and structural variations. PDXs have been used as a model to better understand clonal evolution in the growth of breast cancers.[151] PDXs are currently being used to assess chemosensitivity for breast cancer, lung cancer, melanoma, and pancreatic cancer.[131,152] Preliminary studies, albeit with a small number of patients, have identified a good correlation with therapeutic response in PDX models and clinical outcome.[150,152] Therefore, PDX models are gradually being integrated into the later stages of preclinical development for therapeutic agents. The PDX models are also being considered in co-clinical trials, in which therapeutic agents are tested patients in a clinical trial alongside in mice in order to better understand how best to strategize against therapeutic resistance.[131]

Conclusion

The long-term goal of cancer systems biology is to develop the experimental and theoretical methods needed to understand and manipulate the behavior of the complex and adaptive cancers with which we are confronted. This will require that we be able to measure the molecular composition, cellular organization, and anatomic locations of these cancers and that we develop the theoretical framework needed to predict the behavior of cancer cells including the effect of the proximal and distal environmental signals that influence their behavior. International cancer genome efforts are now providing increasingly detailed information about the molecular components of cancers, imaging strategies are emerging that allow assessment of the multiscale organization of cancerous tissues, and increasingly accurate biological models are being developed that enable identification of molecular features that are causally related to cancer cell behavior. It now remains to develop cancer analytics that can be used to predict the behavior of complex adaptive systems so that this information can be used to more accurately predict cancer behavior and to devise more durable treatment strategies.

Summary

Cancer genomics and systems biology studies seek to describe molecular and cellular features that are intrinsic and extrinsic to cancer cells and to interpret the resulting data in ways that allow prediction of the behavior of individual cancers. These studies guide several aspects of precision medicine including prediction of cancer behavior, identification of optimal therapeutic targets, and development of strategies for durable control of individual cancers. International omic analysis efforts are now yielding comprehensive omic profiles of hundreds to thousands of tumors of most major cancer types and the data are generally available to the scientific community. Computational scientists are making good progress in establishing associations between cancer omic profiles and cancer behavior—especially aspects of cancer progression and response to therapy. Systems biologists are now developing experimental and theoretical strategies to understand and predict the behavior of the complex systems. These studies focus both on the behavior of the cancer cells themselves and the influence of distal and proximal environments on the behavior of the cancer cells. This chapter highlights work in all of these areas and provides illustrative examples of recent progress in each.

Acknowledgments

We would like to thank our funding organizations: for SH, the Canadian Breast Cancer Foundation, the Young Investigator Award of the Conquer Cancer Foundation of ASCO, endowed by the Breast Cancer Research Foundation and Evelyn H. Lauder family, Banting Postdoctoral Fellowship from CIHR, and support from the Ontario Institute for Cancer Research through funding by the Government of Ontario. JG and LH received support from the Susan G. Komen Breast Cancer Foundation, NIH/NCI U54 CA112970 and the Knight Cancer Institute.

Key references

The complete reference list can be found on the Wiley Companion Digital Edition of this title (see inside front cover for login instructions).

1 Werner HM, Mills GB, Ram PT. Cancer systems biology: a peek into the future of patient care? *Nat Rev Clin Oncol.* 2014;**11**(3):167–176.
2 Zou J, Zheng MW, Li G, Su ZG. Advanced systems biology methods in drug discovery and translational biomedicine. *Biomed Res Int.* 2013;**2013**:742835.
3 Hanahan D, Coussens LM. Accessories to the crime: functions of cells recruited to the tumor microenvironment. *Cancer Cell.* 2012;**21**(3):309–322.
5 Antoni MH, Lutgendorf SK, Cole SW, et al. The influence of bio-behavioural factors on tumour biology: pathways and mechanisms. *Nat Rev Cancer.* 2006;**6**(3):240–248.
6 Finak G, Bertos N, Pepin F, et al. Stromal gene expression predicts clinical outcome in breast cancer. *Nat Med.* 2008;**14**(5):518–527.
7 Klemm F, Joyce JA. Microenvironmental regulation of therapeutic response in cancer. *Trends Cell Biol.* 2015;**25**(4):198–213.
12 Tran B, Dancey JE, Kamel-Reid S, et al. Cancer genomics: technology, discovery, and translation. *J Clin Oncol.* 2012;**30**(6):647–660.
13 Good B, Ainscough B, McMichael J, Su A, Griffith O. Organizing knowledge to enable personalization of medicine in cancer. *Genome Biol.* 2014;**15**(8):438.
14 Chibon F. Cancer gene expression signatures – the rise and fall? *Eur J Cancer.* 2013;**49**(8):2000–2009.
15 Hatzis C, Bedard PL, Birkbak NJ, et al. Enhancing reproducibility in cancer drug screening: how do we move forward? *Cancer Res.* 2014;**74**(15):4016–4023.

16 Basik M, Aguilar-Mahecha A, Rousseau C, et al. Biopsies: next-generation biospecimens for tailoring therapy. *Nat Rev Clin Oncol.* 2013;**10**(8):437–450.
17 Manolio TA, Chisholm RL, Ozenberger B, et al. Implementing genomic medicine in the clinic: the future is here. *Genet Med.* 2013;**15**(4):258–267.
18 Sameek R, Chinnaiyan AM. Translating genomics for precision cancer medicine. *Annu Rev Genomics Hum Genet.* 2014;**15**(1):395–415.
34 Hoadley KA, Yau C, Wolf DM, et al. Multiplatform analysis of 12 cancer types reveals molecular classification within and across tissues of origin. *Cell.* 2014;**158**(4):929–944.
35 Omberg L, Ellrott K, Yuan Y, et al. Enabling transparent and collaborative computational analysis of 12 tumor types within The Cancer Genome Atlas. *Nat Genet.* 2013;**45**(10):1121–1126.
36 Cancer Genome Atlas Research Network, Weinstein JN, Collisson EA, et al. The Cancer Genome Atlas Pan-Cancer analysis project. *Nat Genet.* 2013;**45**(10):1113–1120.
37 Collisson EA, Cho RJ, Gray JW. What are we learning from the cancer genome? *Nat Rev Clin Oncol.* 2012;**9**(11):621–630.
48 Vogelstein B, Papadopoulos N, Velculescu VE, Zhou S, Diaz LA Jr, Kinzler KW. Cancer genome landscapes. *Science.* 2013;**339**(6127):1546–1558.
54 Sleijfer S, Bogaerts J, Siu LL. Designing transformative clinical trials in the cancer genome era. *J Clin Oncol.* 2013;**31**(15):1834–1841.
56 Perou CM, Børresen-Dale A-L. Systems biology and genomics of breast cancer. *Cold Spring Harb Perspect Biol.* 2011;**3**(2):a003293. doi:10.1101/cshperspect.a003293.
74 Sharma SV, Haber DA, Settleman J. Cell line-based platforms to evaluate the therapeutic efficacy of candidate anticancer agents. *Nat Rev Cancer.* 2010;**10**(4):241–253.
78 Holbeck SL, Collins JM, Doroshow JH. Analysis of FDA-approved anti-cancer agents in the NCI60 Panel of human tumor cell lines. *Mol Cancer Ther.* 2010;**9**(5):1451–1460.
80 Barretina J, Caponigro G, Stransky N, et al. The cancer cell line encyclopedia enables predictive modelling of anticancer drug sensitivity. *Nature.* 2012;**483**(7391):603–607.
81 Garnett MJ, Edelman EJ, Heidorn SJ, et al. Systematic identification of genomic markers of drug sensitivity in cancer cells. *Nature.* 2012;**483**(7391):570–575.
82 Neve RM, Chin K, Fridlyand J, et al. A collection of breast cancer cell lines for the study of functionally distinct cancer subtypes. *Cancer Cell.* 2006;**10**(6):515–527.
86 Heiser LM, Sadanandam A, Kuo WL, et al. Subtype and pathway specific responses to anticancer compounds in breast cancer. *Proc Natl Acad Sci U S A.* 2012;**109**(8):2724–2729.
87 Daemen A, Griffith O, Heiser L, et al. Modeling precision treatment of breast cancer. *Genome Biol.* 2013;**14**(10):R110.
88 CTD2 Data Portal: National Cancer Institute, Office of Cancer Genomics, 6 April 2015. Available from: https://ctd2.nci.nih.gov/dataPortal/CTD2_DataPortal.html.
100 Margolin AA, Bilal E, Huang E, et al. Systematic analysis of challenge-driven improvements in molecular prognostic models for breast cancer. *Sci Transl Med.* 2013;**5**(181):181re1.
107 Hanahan D, Weinberg RA. Hallmarks of cancer: the next generation. *Cell.* 2011;**144**(5):646–674.
120 Adams S, Gray RJ, Demaria S, et al. Prognostic value of tumor-infiltrating lymphocytes in triple-negative breast cancers from two phase III randomized adjuvant breast cancer trials: ECOG 2197 and ECOG 1199. *J Clin Oncol.* 2014;**32**(27):2959–2966.
121 Pages F, Berger A, Camus M, et al. Effector memory T cells, early metastasis, and survival in colorectal cancer. *N Engl J Med.* 2005;**353**(25):2654–2666.
126 Kelland LR. Of mice and men: values and liabilities of the athymic nude mouse model in anticancer drug development. *Eur J Cancer.* 2004;**40**(6):827–836.
127 Sharpless NE, Depinho RA. The mighty mouse: genetically engineered mouse models in cancer drug development. *Nat Rev Drug Discov.* 2006;**5**(9):741–754.
128 Breslin S, O'Driscoll L. Three-dimensional cell culture: the missing link in drug discovery. *Drug Discov Today.* 2013;**18**(5–6):240–249.
130 Labarge MA, Parvin B, Lorens JB. Molecular deconstruction, detection, and computational prediction of microenvironment-modulated cellular responses to cancer therapeutics. *Adv Drug Deliv Rev.* 2014;**69–70**:123–131.
131 Hidalgo M, Amant F, Biankin AV, et al. Patient-derived xenograft models: an emerging platform for translational cancer research. *Cancer Discov.* 2014;**4**(9):998–1013.
132 Lunardi A, Pandolfi PP. A co-clinical platform to accelerate cancer treatment optimization. *Trends Mol Med.* 2015;**21**(1):1–5.
138 Rantala J, Kwon S, Korkola J, Gray J. Expanding the diversity of imaging-based RNAi screen applications using cell spot microarrays. *Microarrays.* 2013;**2**(2):97–114.
140 Bissell MJ, Rizki A, Mian IS. Tissue architecture: the ultimate regulator of breast epithelial function. *Curr Opin Cell Biol.* 2003;**15**(6):753–762.

20 Statistical innovations in cancer research

J. Jack Lee, PhD, MS, DDS ▪ *Donald A. Berry, PhD*

Overview

Cancer research is rapidly changing, with fast-growing numbers of possible cancer targets and cancer drugs to investigate and no end in sight. Advances in genomics, proteomics, and epigenetics provide remarkably detailed profiles of each patient's tumor and, as a result, allow science to consider each patient as unique, with the goal of delivering precision medicine to each patient. The low success rates of late-phase clinical oncology trials and high costs of bringing new drugs to market, however, have necessitated changes in the drug-development process. Statistical innovations can help in the design and conduct of clinical trials to facilitate the discovery and validation of biomarkers and streamline the clinical trial process. The application of Bayesian statistics provides a sound theoretical foundation that can encourage the development of adaptive designs to improve trial flexibility and efficiency while maintaining desirable statistical-operating characteristics.

The principal goals of the innovations presented in this chapter are to (1) use information from clinical trials more efficiently in drawing conclusions about treatment effects, (2) use patient resources more efficiently while treating patients who participate in clinical trials as effectively as possible, and (3) identify better drugs and therapeutic strategies more rapidly, moving them more quickly through the development process. The underlying premise is to exploit all available evidence, placing information gleaned from an ongoing clinical trial into the context of what is already known. The innovations considered are intuitively appealing. However, some are controversial. Some are being used in actual clinical trials while others are still being developed and evaluated for such use.

This chapter addresses two types of innovations. One is a natural extension of the traditional practice of frequentist statistics. The other type is based on a Bayesian statistical philosophy. The Bayesian approach is tailored to real-time learning (as data accrue), and the frequentist approach is tied to particular experiments and to the experiment's design. However, there is substantial overlap between these complementary approaches.

The main topics covered in this chapter include the following. The introduction of basic probability theory and Bayesian approach is explained through examples. Differences between frequentist and Bayesian methods are compared and contrasted. The development of adaptive designs by applying outcome adaptive randomization, predictive probability, interim and extraim analyses, and factorial design is discussed. In addition, hierarchical modeling can be utilized to synthesize information available from the trial as well as external to the trial. Seamless phase I/II and II/III designs can be applied to shorten the drug-development period. Platform designs can be constructed to evaluate many drugs simultaneously. The application of these statistical innovations is illustrated in the BATTLE trials and I-SPY 2 trial. Finally, information on computing resources for the design and implementation of innovative trials is given.

Cancer research (and medical research, in general) is rapidly changing; the number of possible cancer targets and cancer drugs to investigate is growing, with no end in sight. Advances in genomics, proteomics, and epigenetics provide remarkably detailed profiles for each patient's tumor and, as a result, allow science to consider each patient as unique. Modern computing has supported these advances, allowing statisticians to simulate trials with complicated designs and to evaluate design properties such as statistical power and false-positive rate. The basic requirement is that the design be specified prospectively.

The low success rates of late-phase clinical oncology trials[1-3] and high costs of bringing new drugs to market[4] have necessitated changes in the drug-development process. Recognizing the need to modernize, the FDA issued its *Critical Path Opportunities Report* in March 2006, identifying biomarker development and streamlining clinical trials as essential changes to be made in this process.[5] Further guidance was then issued by centers within the FDA: The Center for Devices and Radiological Health (CDRH) published initial guidelines for using Bayesian statistics in medical device clinical trials in 2006 and final guidelines in 2010.[6] The Center for Biologics Evaluation and Research (CBER) and the Center for Drug Evaluation and Research (CDER) issued a joint guidance document for planning and implementing adaptive designs in clinical trials.[7] In addition, CDRH released a draft guidance on adaptive designs for medical device clinical studies in 2015.[8]

The principal goals of the innovations presented in this chapter are to (1) use information from clinical trials more efficiently in drawing conclusions about treatment effects, (2) use patient resources more efficiently while treating patients who participate in clinical trials as effectively as possible, and (3) identify better drugs and therapeutic strategies more rapidly, moving them more quickly through the development process. The underlying premise is to exploit all available evidence, placing information gleaned from an ongoing clinical trial into the context of what is already known. The innovations considered are intuitively appealing. However, some are controversial. Some are being used in actual clinical trials while others are still being developed and evaluated for such use.

This chapter addresses two types of innovations. One is a natural extension of the traditional practice of frequentist statistics. The other type is based on a Bayesian statistical philosophy. Readers who are familiar with Bayesian ideas may wish to skip some Bayesian sections. The Bayesian approach is tailored to real-time learning (as data accrue), and the frequentist approach is tied to particular experiments and to the experiment's design. However, there is substantial overlap between these complementary approaches. Much of this chapter's development of clinical trial design employs the Bayesian approach as a tool for finding designs that tend to treat patients in the clinical trial more effectively and that identify better drugs more rapidly. However, the frequentist

Holland-Frei Cancer Medicine, Ninth Edition. Edited by Robert C. Bast Jr., Carlo M. Croce, William N. Hait, Waun Ki Hong, Donald W. Kufe, Martine Piccart-Gebhart, Raphael E. Pollock, Ralph R. Weichselbaum, Hongyang Wang, and James F. Holland.
© 2017 John Wiley & Sons, Inc. ISBN: 978-1-118-93469-2

properties (such as false-positive rate and power) of the design thus derived can always be found, often requiring simulation. Ensuring that a design has prespecified frequentist properties means that the Bayesian approach can be used to design trials with good frequentist properties.

Preliminaries

The basis of all experimentation is comparison. Evaluating an experimental therapy in a clinical trial requires information about the outcomes of the patients had they received some other therapy. The best way to address this issue is to randomize patients to the experimental therapy and to some comparison therapy. Although there are ways to learn without randomizing, there are limitations to approaches that do not employ randomization. Moreover, randomization does not require equal assignment probabilities to the therapeutic strategies, or "arms," being compared. Unbalanced randomization is possible, either with fixed ratios or adaptive ratios, that is, such that assignment probabilities depend on data accumulating in the trial. (The latter possibility is the principal focus of this chapter.)

Most clinical trials are conducted in accord with a protocol, which aims to evaluate the treatment effect as a whole.[9] Protocols may refer to retrospective or sporadic collection of data, but they are usually prospective. Clinical trials are always prospective. A prospective protocol describes how the trial is to be conducted, including how patients will be assigned to a therapy and when the trial will end. Deviations from a protocol may make scientific inferences from the trial difficult or impossible (although they may be necessary at times to avoid exposing participants to unnecessary risks). Valid inference can only be made based on sound statistical theory in properly conducted trials.

Bayesian approach

This section shows how Bayesian learning takes place and how the Bayesian approach relates to the more traditional frequentist approach. It is necessarily superficial. Further reading includes a comprehensive but elementary introduction to Bayesian ideas and methods,[10] discussions of their role in medical research,[11] and of clinical trials in particular,[12–15] and books describing more advanced Bayesian methods.[16,17]

Bayesian updating

The defining characteristic of any statistical approach is how it deals with uncertainty. In the Bayesian approach, uncertainty is measured by probability. Any event whose occurrence is unknown has a probability. The frequentist approach uses probabilities as well, but in a more restricted manner, as described hereafter. Examples of probabilities in the Bayesian approach that do not have frequentist counterparts include the following: The probability that the drug is effective, the probability that patient Smith will respond to a particular chemotherapy, and the probability that the future results in the trial will show a statistically significant benefit for a particular therapy.

The Bayesian paradigm is one of learning. As information becomes available, one updates one's knowledge about the unknown aspects of the process that is producing the information. The fundamental tool for learning under uncertainty is Bayes' rule. Bayes' rule relates inverse probabilities. An example that will be familiar to many readers is finding the positive predictive value (PPV) of a diagnostic test: In view of a positive test result, what is the probability that the individual being tested has the disease in question? It can be considered as the "inverse probability" of a positive test given the presence of the disease, which is called the test's sensitivity. PPV also depends on the test's specificity, which is the probability of a negative test, given that the individual does not have the disease. Moreover, PPV depends on the prevalence of the disease in the population. In applying Bayes' rule to statistical inference, the analog of PPV is the "posterior probability" that a hypothesis is true, given the experimental results. The analog of disease prevalence is the "prior probability" that the hypothesis is true.

Consider an overly simplified numerical example, one with only two possible response rates (r): $r = 0.75$ and $r = 0.50$. If you are accustomed to thinking about PPV for diagnostic tests, consider one of these to be that the "patient has the disease" and the other to be that the "patient does not have the disease." The question is this: Is r equal to 0.75 or 0.50? Before any experimentation, these two possibilities are regarded to be equally likely: $P(r = 0.75) = P(r = 0.50) = 1/2$.

The focus of the Bayesian approach is learning. Probabilities are calculated as new information becomes available, and is taken to be "given." Statisticians have a notation that facilitates thinking about and calculating probabilities as new information accrues. They use vertical bars to separate the unknown event of interest from known quantities (or taken to be given): $P(A|B)$ is read "probability of A given B." Assign R for tumor response and N for nonresponse. Using this notation, for example, $P(R|r = 0.75) = 0.75$. More interesting is the probability of $r = 0.75$, given a tumor response: $P(r = 0.75|R)$. These two expressions are reciprocally inverse, with the roles of the event of interest and the event being assumed. Bayes' rule connects the relationship between these two expressions, namely that the updated (posterior) probability of $r = 0.75$ is as follows:

$$P(r = 0.75|R) = P(R|r = 0.75)P(r = 0.75)/P(R)$$

The denominator on the right-hand side of the equation follows from the law of total probability:

$$P(R) = P(R|r = 0.75)P(r = 0.75) + P(R|r = 0.50)P(r = 0.50)$$
$$= (0.75)(1/2) + (0.5)(1/2) = 5/8$$

That is, $P(R)$ is the average of the two response rates under consideration, 0.75 and 0.50, where the average is with respect to the corresponding prior probabilities—half each in this example. Substituting the numerical values into Bayes' rule, the posterior probability of $r = 0.75$ is as follows:

$$P(r = 0.75|R) = (0.75)(1/2)/(5/8) = 3/5$$

Therefore, the new evidence boosts the probability of $r = 0.75$ from 1/2 (or 50%) to 60%. As the total probability is 100%, the evidence in a single response lowers the probability of $r = 0.50$ from 50% to 40%.

Consider a second independent observation. The probability of r before this second observation is the posterior probability of the first observation. If the second observation is also a response, then a second application of Bayes' rule applies to give $P(r = 0.75|R, R) = 9/13 = 69\%$, which is a further increase from the previous values of 50% and 60%. On one hand, if the second observation is a nonresponse, then $P(r = 0.75|R, N) = 3/7 = 43\%$, a decrease from 60%. This process can go on indefinitely, updating either after each observation or all at once on the basis of whatever evidence is available. The current probabilities of the various possible values of response rate r can be found at any time. These probabilities depend on the original prior probability and on the intervening observed data. This process of updating and real-time learning is an important advantage of the Bayesian approach to designing and conducting clinical trials.

The example mentioned previously considered only two possible values of r. More realistically, the response rate r may be any number between 0 and 1. The left-hand panel in Figure 1a shows a constant or flat curve that is a candidate for prior distribution. The flat curve indicates that the probability is spread equally over this range of values of r. This might be termed an "open-minded prior distribution" because the posterior distribution depends almost entirely on the evidence from the experiment at hand. After a single-tumor response, Bayesian updating serves to change the probability distribution to the one shown in the right-hand panel of Figure 1a—that is, the right-hand panel is the posterior distribution after observing R when the prior distribution is the one shown in the left-hand panel. The shift in the distribution to larger values of r corresponds to the intuitive notion that larger response rates become more likely after observing R. Bayes' rule quantifies this intuition.

There are many candidate prior distributions other than the first one shown in Figure 1a. Three other prior/posterior pairs are shown in Figure 1b–d. The right-hand panel within each pair is the posterior distribution after observing R when the prior distribution is the one shown in the left-hand panel. Moreover, the left-hand curves in Figure 1b–d are themselves posterior distributions for the right-hand curves in Figure 1a–c, respectively, but in the situation when the observation is an N. Intuitively, after a nonresponse, the concentration of probabilities shifts to smaller values of r. Mathematically, observing R means to multiply the current distribution by r (the response rate) and renormalize it so that the area under the curve is 1. Similarly, observing an N means to multiply by $(1-r)$, the rate of nonresponse.

An implication is that moving left to right and top to bottom in Figure 1 corresponds to starting with the prior distribution in the left-hand panel of Figure 1a and observing RNRNRNR. The eight curves shown in Figure 1 are proportional to the following respective functional forms: 1, r, $r(1-r)$, $r^2(1-r)$, $r^2(1-r)^2$, $r^3(1-r)^2$, $r^3(1-r)^3$, and $r^4(1-r)^3$. Each observation of response increases the exponent of r by 1, and each observed N increases the exponent of $(1-r)$ by 1. As is evident in the figure, additional observations lead to narrower distributions. As the number of observations increases, the distribution tends to concentrate about a single point, which is the "true" value of r, the response rate that produces the observations. Free software that provides a visual demonstration of the Bayesian update in the context of the so-called beta-binomial distribution can be downloaded at https://biostatistics.mdanderson.org/SoftwareDownload/SingleSoftware.aspx?Software_Id=96.

The principal message of this section is not the numerical calculation defining the updated distribution, but the fact that updated distributions can be found using the Bayesian approach at any time during a clinical trial.

Prior probabilities

Bayesian updating requires a starting point: a prior distribution of the various parameters. In the example, one must have a probability distribution for response rate r in advance of or separate from the experiment in question. This prior distribution may be subjectively assessed or based explicitly on the results of previous experiments. In some settings, such as some regulatory scenarios, an appropriate default distribution is noninformative or open-minded[10,13] in the sense that all possible values of the parameters are assigned the same prior probabilities. The left-hand panel of Figure 1a is an example.

Noninformative or flat prior distributions limit the benefits of taking a Bayesian approach when they ignore information that is available from outside the experiment. However, the benefit of employing Bayesian updating may be substantial even if one starts with a flat distribution that does not reflect anyone's assessment of the prior information. Flat prior distributions serve some important roles. One is that it may be helpful to distinguish the evidence in the data in the experiment under consideration from that present before the experiment. Another is that the Bayesian conclusions that arise from using flat prior distributions are often the same as the corresponding frequentist conclusions.

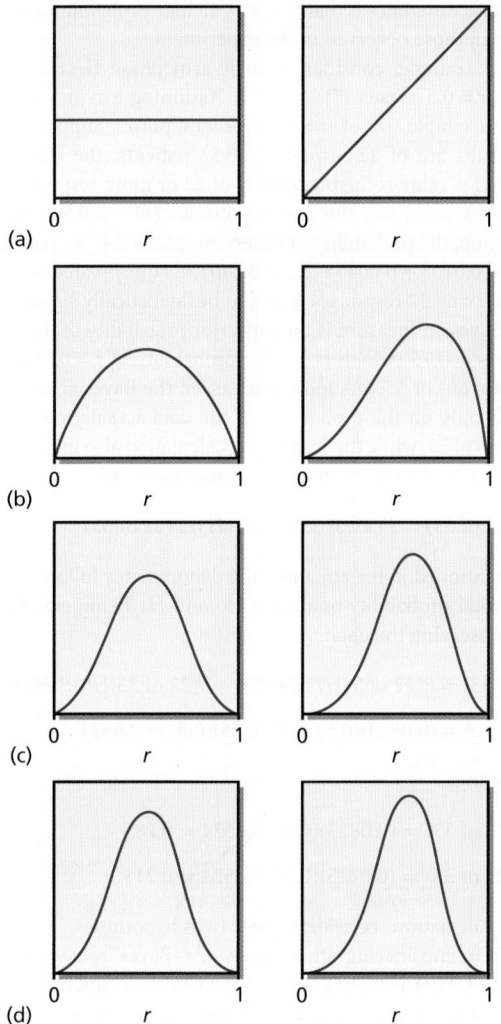

Figure 1 Prior distributions of response rate r. The left-hand panel in each pair is the prior distribution of response rate r. The right-hand panel is the posterior distribution of r after having observed a response in a single patient. The (predictive) probability of a response for each left-hand panel is 0.500, increasing in the right-hand panels to 0.667, 0.600, 0.571, and 0.556 in cases (a), (b), (c), and (d), respectively. Changes are greater and learning is more rapid when the prior distribution reflects greater uncertainty.

Prior distributions are usually based on historical data. Suppose that a similar drug (or the same drug in a possibly different patient population) gave a response rate of 50% in 20 patients: 10 responders and 10 nonresponders. The corresponding likelihood of response rate r (see the section titled "Frequentist/Bayesian Comparison") is $r^{10}(1-r)^{10}$. Given that there may be differences between the historical setting and that of the current trial, it would not be reasonable to use this information directly without any modification as a prior distribution for r, but it would be appropriate to somehow exploit this relevant information. One possibility (another is described in the section titled "Hazards over Time") is to discount the historical evidence as it applies to the context of the current trial. For example, weighing an historical observation as having the information equivalent of 30% of that of a current observation would mean using a prior distribution proportional to $r^3(1-r)^3$. This is the distribution shown in Figure 1d, left-hand panel.

Robustness

In the presence of enough data, essentially all observers will have similar posterior distributions; this is robustness. An implication is that the particular prior distribution assumed does not matter much when the sample size is moderate or large. As an example, consider the eight distributions shown in Figure 1 and think of each of them in turn as being the prior distribution of a different person. Parameter r is the response rate to a particular drug. Suppose that 40 patients are treated in a trial and 20 of them respond. Applying the principle of robustness, the eight people in question will come to very nearly the same conclusion about the drug's response rate. The eight posterior distributions are shown in Figure 2. The curves are nearly superposed. The eight 95% probability intervals will also be very similar. The data outweigh any of the prior distributions shown in Figure 1.

If two prior distributions are markedly different and the corresponding information contained in the prior distribution is strong,

then robustness still applies, but it could take a good deal of data to bring two disparate distributions close together.

Frequentist/Bayesian comparison

In the frequentist approach, hypotheses and parameters do not have probabilities. Rather, probability assignments apply only to data, with particular values assumed for given unknown parameters in calculating these probabilities. For example, the ubiquitous p-value is the probability of data as or more extreme than the observed data assuming that the null hypothesis is true. In symbols:

- Frequentist p-value: $P(\text{observed or more extreme data} \mid H0)$
- Bayesian posterior probability: $P(H0 \mid \text{observed data})$

It is easy to confuse these two concepts. A p-value is commonly interpreted as the probability of no effect, and 1 minus the p-value as the probability of an effect. This interpretation is wrong. This is trying to have a Bayesian posterior probability without a prior probability, which is impossible.

There are two important differences between a frequentist p-value and a Bayesian posterior probability. One is the inversion of the conditions: what is assumed in the former has a probability in the latter. The second difference is that p-values include probabilities of results other than those observed in the experiment.

As an example, consider a single-arm phase II trial for testing $H0$: $r = 0.5$ versus $H1$: $r = 0.75$. Assuming a type I error rate $\alpha = 5\%$, a sample size of $n = 33$ gives 90% power. Suppose that the final results are of 22 responses of 33 patients, the (frequentist) one-sided p-value is the probability of 22 or more responses of the 33 patients, assuming the null hypothesis, $H0$: $r = 0.5$. Under this assumption, the probability of observing 22, 23, 24, … responses is $0.0225 + 0.0108 + 0.0045 + \ldots = 0.0401$. As this p-value is less than 5%, observing 22 responses is said to be "statistically significant."

The Bayesian measure is the posterior probability of the hypothesis that $r = 0.75$ (which is $1 -$ the probability of $r = 0.5$) given 22 responses out of 33. (As indicated earlier, the Bayesian calculation depends only on the probability of the data actually observed, 22 responses of 33, while the frequentist calculation also includes probabilities of 23, 24, etc., responses.) Using Bayes' rule:

$$P(H1 \mid 22 \text{ of } 33) = P(22 \text{ of } 33 \mid H1)P(H1)/P(22 \text{ of } 33)$$

As mentioned in the equation, the denominator follows from the law of total probability assuming $H0$ and $H1$ being equally likely before observing the data:

$$P(22 \text{ of } 33) = P(22 \text{ of } 33 \mid H1)P(H1) + P(22 \text{ of } 33 \mid H0)P(H0)$$

$$= (0.0823)(0.5) + (0.0225)(0.5) = 0.0524$$

Therefore,

$$P(H1 \mid 22 \text{ of } 33) = (0.0823)(0.5)/0.0524 = 0.785$$

$$P(H0 \mid 22 \text{ of } 33) = (0.0225)(0.5)/0.0524 = 0.215$$

The calculation considers just two hypotheses, $r = 0.5$ and $r = 0.75$. In considering other values of r, Bayes' rule weighs them by $P(22 \text{ of } 33 \mid r)$, which is called the likelihood function of r. The likelihood function is pictured in Figure 3. It indicates the degree of support for response rate r provided by the observed data. Values of r having the same likelihood are equally supported by the data. Only relative likelihoods matter. For example, conclusions about $r = 0.5$ versus 0.75 depend only on the ratio of their likelihoods, 0.0823 and 0.0225, values that are highlighted in Figure 3. Because $0.0823/0.0225 = 3.66$, the data lend 3.66 times as much support to $r = 0.75$ as they do to $r = 0.5$.

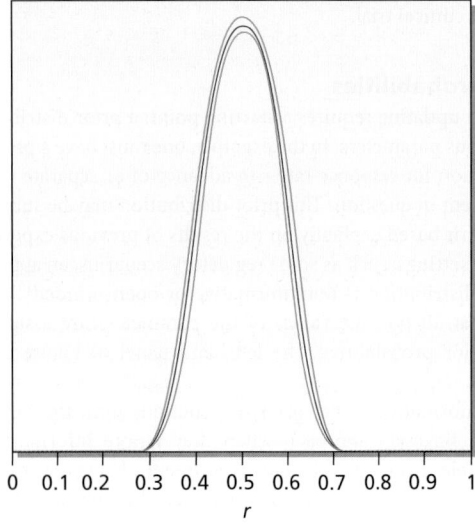

Figure 2 Posterior distributions for response rate r based on an experiment with 20 responses and 20 failures. The eight prior distributions considered are the eight distributions shown in Figure 1. Except for proportionality constants, these are 1, r, $r(1-r)$, $r^2(1-r)$, $r^2(1-r)^2$, $r^3(1-r)^2$, $r^3(1-r)^3$, and $r^4(1-r)^3$. The corresponding posterior distributions are proportional to $r^{20}(1-r)^{20}$, $r^{21}(1-r)^{20}$, $r^{21}(1-r)^{21}$, $r^{22}(1-r)^{21}$, $r^{22}(1-r)^{22}$, $r^{23}(1-r)^{22}$, $r^{23}(1-r)^{23}$, and $r^{24}(1-r)^{23}$. These eight posterior distributions are very similar, demonstrating the robustness principle.

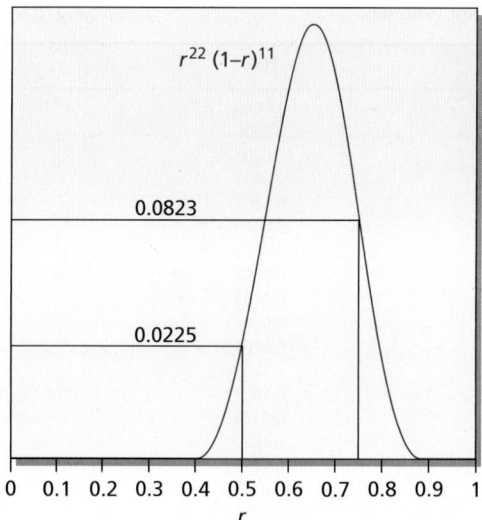

Figure 3 Likelihood of r for 22 responses out of 33 observations. The likelihood is $P(22 \text{ of } 33|r)$, which is proportional to $r^{22}(1-r)^{11}$. The likelihoods at $r = 0.5$ and 0.75 are highlighted. These values are used in the calculational example in the text.

The conclusions of the two approaches are different conceptually and numerically. In the frequentist approach, the results are statistically significant, with p-value $= 0.0401$. Some researchers interpret statistical significance to mean that $H0$ is unlikely to be true. That is not what it means. It means that the observed data are unlikely when $H0$ is true. The Bayesian posterior probability of $H0$ directly addresses the question of the probability that $H0$ is true. This probability is 0.215. Although smaller than the prior probability of 0.50 (because the data point somewhat more strongly to $H1$ than to $H0$), it is five times as large as the p-value!

Interval estimates also have different interpretations in the two approaches. In the Bayesian approach, one can find the probability that a parameter lies in any given interval. In the frequentist approach, confidence intervals have a long-run frequency interpretation for fixed and given parameters. So it is not correct to say that a 95% confidence interval has a probability of 95% containing the parameter of interest. Despite the different interpretations, there is a point of agreement between the two approaches. In other words, if the prior distribution is flat (e.g., the left-hand panel of Figure 1a), then the Bayesian posterior probability of a confidence interval is essentially the same as the frequentist level of confidence. For example, if the prior distribution is flat, then the Bayesian posterior probability, indicating that a parameter lies in its 95% confidence interval, is in fact 95%. For prior distributions that are not flat, the posterior probability of a 95% confidence interval may be greater than or less than 95%. If the historical data upon which the prior distribution is based are consistent with those from the current experiment, then the posterior probability indicating that the parameter is in the 95% confidence interval will be >95%. If the historical data are different from those in the current experiment, then the probability that the 95% confidence interval contains the true parameter will typically be <95%.

Predictive probabilities

The ability to predict the future—with the requisite uncertainty—is important for designing and monitoring trials. The Bayesian approach allows for calculating probabilities of future results without having to assume that any particular hypothesis is true. The process is straightforward, at least logically if not mathematically.

For a specified experimental design, one finds the conditional probabilities of the future data for each parameter value and averages them with respect to the current probabilities of the various parameter values. Predictive probabilities are exploited extensively in this chapter.

Consider the 33-patient trial described earlier. Suppose that the first 16 patients have been treated, with 13 responses and 3 nonresponses. What will be the results after the full complement of 33 patients is available? The number of responses will be between 13 and 30, but not all events are equally likely. In particular, it seems most unlikely that there will be no responses in the next 17 patients after having seen 13 of the first 16 patients, and it is.

It might seem reasonable to use an estimate of r (e.g., the current rate, $13/16 = 0.81$) and calculate the probabilities of the results of the next 17 patients, assuming this value of r, but this could be wrong. Such a calculation incorporates the uncertainty in the future data for the given r, but fails to incorporate uncertainty in r. Bayesian predictive probabilities incorporate both types of uncertainty. Table 1 shows the results, assuming just two values of r, 0.5 and 0.75. The first column (the leftmost column) lists the possible numbers (S) of responses after 33 patients. The second and third columns show the probabilities of the possible values of S for these two values of r. The corresponding probabilities without conditioning on r are shown in the fourth column. This is a weighted average of the second and third columns. The weights are the respective probabilities of the two values of r conditional on having observed 13 responses in the first 16 patients: 0.039 for $r = 0.5$ and 0.961 for $r = 0.75$. The fourth column evinces greater variability (greater standard deviation) than either of the previous two columns. Typically, when all values of r between 0 and 1 are considered (i.e., all values have positive probability), predictive probabilities reflect greater uncertainty about future results than when conditioning on a particular value of r. (The rightmost column of Table 1 is discussed in the next section.)

For convenience in this example, equal prior probabilities are assumed: $P(H1) = P(H0) = 0.5$. Although there is no vertical bar "|" in these expressions, these probabilities can depend on other available evidence, such as results of earlier clinical and preclinical trials. There may be additional information from biological assessments, such as when considering targeted therapies. These overall conditions are taken to be understood in setting down $P(H0)$ and $P(H1)$.

Bayesian versus frequentist interim analyses

There are numerous commonalties and a few differences between the Bayesian and frequentist approaches. This section addresses a principal difference. In the Bayesian approach, one makes an observation and updates the probabilities of the various hypotheses. This simple process implies a degree of flexibility that is difficult to mimic in the frequentist approach.

Consider the trial design described previously, with $n = 33$ patients and testing $H0$: $r = 0.5$ versus $H1$: $r = 0.75$. Observing 22 or more responses will be sufficient to reject $H0$ in favor of $H1$ (with a one-sided 5% type I error rate). However, assigning 33 patients to an experimental therapy without assessing interim results is ethically problematic and would likely be questioned by institutional review boards. If the results are conclusive (either positive, strongly suggesting $r > 0.5$, or negative, suggesting $r \leq 0.5$) part of the way through the trial, then the trial should be stopped. Suppose that after 16 patients, one finds that 13 respond and 3 do not, from a Bayesian perspective, the updated probability of $H1$ is 96.1% (assuming prior probability $P(H0) = 0.5$).

Whether this probability is "conclusive" is not clear. The decision as to whether to continue a trial is complicated. It depends on the

Table 1 Predictive probabilities of number *S* of responses after 33 patients, given 13 responses in the first 16 patients.

S(of 33)	P(S|r = 0.5)	P(S|r = 0.75)	P(S)	P(HI)
13	0.0000	0.0000	0.0000	0.0002
14	0.0001	0.0000	0.0000	0.0006
15	0.0010	0.0000	0.0000	0.0017
16	0.0052	0.0000	0.0002	0.0050
17	0.0182	0.0000	0.0007	0.0148
18	0.0472	0.0001	0.0019	0.0432
19	0.0944	0.0005	0.0042	0.1192
20	0.1484	0.0025	0.0082	0.2887
21	0.1855	0.0093	0.0162	0.5491
22	0.1855	0.0279	0.0341	0.7851
23	0.1484	0.0668	0.0701	0.9164
24	0.0944	0.1276	0.1263	0.9705
25	0.0472	0.1914	0.1857	0.9900
26	0.0181	0.2209	0.2129	0.9966
27	0.0052	0.1893	0.1820	0.9989
28	0.0010	0.1136	0.1091	0.9996
29	0.0001	0.0426	0.0409	0.9999
30	0.0000	0.0075	0.0072	1.0000

Note: Columns $P(S\|r = 0.5)$ and $P(S\|r = 0.75)$ assume the indicated value of *r* in calculating the probability. Column *P(S)* is the weighted average of the two previous columns, where the respective weights are 0.039 and 0.961. The last column gives *P(HI)*, the probability of *HI* (*r* = 0.75), given *S* responses after 33 patients.

consequences of the trial, given the current results and also given the future results. In the Bayesian approach, the consequences of future results can be weighed by their predictive probabilities; for example, suppose that the impact of the trial depends on whether the posterior probability of *H*1 is > 95% when the data from the full complement of 33 patients become available, then one can calculate the predictive probability of this event. The rightmost column in Table 1 shows the posterior probability of *H*1 assuming *S* responses of 33 patients. To achieve >95% posterior probability requires at least 24 responses in the 33 patients. The probability of this event is the sum of the probabilities for $S \geq 24$ (the fourth column in Table 1), which is 0.8642. Although the current probability of *H*1 is > 95%, owing to the uncertainty in *S* and in *r*, this characteristic will be lost with probability $1 - 0.8642 = 0.1358$. That this has moderate probability indicates the tentative nature of the current conclusion. The possibility that the current conclusion is moderately likely to change can be factored into the decision to continue the trial.

If the predictive probability that the current conclusion will be maintained is sufficiently high, then one may reasonably decide to stop a trial. This is true for both claims of futility and superiority. The possibility of stopping a trial early on the basis of predictive probability should be stated explicitly in the trial's protocol.

The focus of the frequentist perspective is the type I error rate, α. This is the probability of rejecting *H*0 when *H*0 is true, which depends on the trial design. For a fixed sample size of 33 patients, the calculation is straightforward. Rejecting *H*0 for ≥ 22 responses means $\alpha = 0.0401$ (see the previous section). The calculation becomes more complicated when there is a possibility of stopping the trial early. In the example, if the trial is stopped and *H*0 is rejected, when there are 12 or more responses in the first 16 patients, then α is increased because there is additional opportunity for rejecting *H*0. Assuming $r = 0.5$, the probability of rejecting *H*0 is now 0.0640. Because this is greater than 0.05, the convention is to modify the stopping and rejection criteria to reduce α to about 0.05. For example, rejecting only if there are 13 responses or more out of 16 patients treated, or if there are 22 or more responses after 33 patients are treated, gives an overall type I error rate of 0.0450.

It follows that it is more difficult to draw a conclusion of statistical significance when there are interim analyses. The reason is that the type I error rates are calculated assuming that a particular hypothesis (the null hypothesis of no effect) is true. In a sense, an investigator is penalized for interim analyses in the frequentist approach. There are no such penalties for interim analyses in a Bayesian perspective. The reason is that Bayesian probabilities are not conditional on the basis of any particular hypothesis.

Although it is not a Bayesian quantity, the type I error rate of any Bayesian design, however complicated, can be evaluated. If the design has interim analyses, then such a calculation incorporates appropriate penalties. This calculation is straightforward in a simple example such as that given earlier. In more complicated settings, it can require Monte Carlo simulations.

A breast cancer trial illustrates some advantages of a Bayesian design.[18] Women with breast cancer who were at least 65 years of age were randomized to receive either standard chemotherapy or capecitabine. The sample size was expected to be 600–1800. After the 600th patient had enrolled in the trial, and following the protocol, predictive probabilities were calculated. Calculations were made of the predictive probability of statistical significance given the present sample size and with additional patient follow-up at the present sample size. If that achieved a predetermined level, patient accrual would stop, but observations of the existing patients would continue. The predictive probability cutoff point was achieved at the first interim analysis and so accrual stopped (the final sample size was 633). Indeed, the study later showed that the women in this study population who were treated with standard chemotherapy had a lower risk of breast cancer recurrence and death than women treated with capecitabine.[19]

Analysis issues

The purpose of this section is to consider two types of analytical issues. The first is an extension of the previous section. The second is unrelated to the first and deals with a particular aspect of survival analysis.

Hierarchical modeling: synthesizing information

When analyzing data from a clinical trial, other information is usually available about the treatment under consideration. This section deals with a method called hierarchical modeling. One of its uses is synthesizing information from different sources. The method applies in many settings, including meta-analysis and incorporating historical information. A hierarchical model is a random-effects model. In a meta-analysis, one level of the experimental unit is the patient (within a trial) and the second level is the trial itself. Hierarchical models also apply for design issues such as combining results across diseases or disease subtypes and for such seemingly disparate issues such as cluster randomization. Design issues for hierarchical modeling are considered in the next section.

Consider a phase II trial in which 21 of 33 patients responded. The one-sided p-value is 0.08 for the null hypothesis $H0$: $r = 0.50$, and so the results are not statistically significant at the 5% level. Now consider an earlier phase I trial using the same treatment in which 15 of 20 patients responded. This information seems relevant, even if the population being treated might have been somewhat different and the trial might have been conducted at a different institution. However, it is not obvious how to incorporate the information into an analysis. The frequentist approach is experiment specific, which requires imagining that the two trials are part of some larger experiment. If one assumes that the entire set of data resulted from a single trial involving 53 patients with 36 responses, then from a frequentist perspective this would lead to a p-value of 0.0063, which is highly statistically significant. However, this conclusion is wrong because the assumption is wrong. Moreover, it is not clear how to make it right.

Any Bayesian analysis that assumes the same response rate applies in both trials would be similarly flawed. Response rate r may be reasonably expected to vary from one trial to another. Two response rates for the same therapy may be different even if the eligibility criteria in the two trials are the same. For one thing, the eligibility criteria may be applied differently in the two settings. However, even if the patients accrued are apparently similar, their accruals differ in time and place. Our understanding of cancer and its detection changes over time. Moreover, there are differences in the use of concomitant therapy and variations in the ability to assess clinical and laboratory variables. A way to repair the analysis is to explicitly consider two values of r, say $r1$ for the first trial and $r2$ for the second.

Recapitulating, there are two extreme assumptions that lead to analyses that are easier to carry out, but both are wrong. One is to assume that $r1$ and $r2$ are unrelated and to base any inferences about $r2$ on the results of the second trial alone. The other is to assume that $r1 = r2$ and combine the results in the two trials.

The two r-values may be the same or different. In a Bayesian hierarchical model, both possibilities are allowed, but neither is assumed. In other words, $r1$ and $r2$ are regarded as having come from a population of r-values. The population may have little variability (homogeneity) or substantial variability (heterogeneity). The observed response rates give information concerning the extent of heterogeneity, with disparate rates suggesting greater heterogeneity. When the observed rates are similar, the precision of estimates of $r1$ and $r2$ will be greater than when the observed rates are disparate. In the former case, there will be greater "borrowing of strength" across the trials. If it happens that the results of the trials are very different, then there will be little borrowing and the information from any one trial will not apply much beyond that trial.

More generally, there may be any number of related studies or databases that provide supportive information regarding a particular therapeutic effect. The studies may be heterogeneous and may consider different patient populations. The next example is generic but it is more complicated than the previous example because it includes nine studies.[20] The only commonalty in the studies is that all addressed the efficacy of the same therapy.

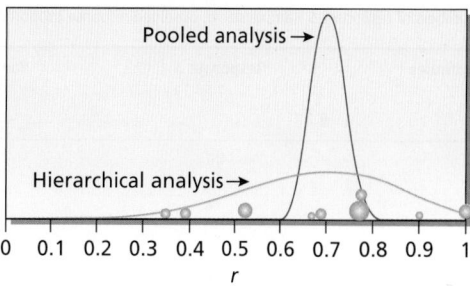

Figure 4 Response comparisons. The dot plot on the r-axis shows the observed response proportions given in Table 2. The areas of the dots are approximately proportional to sample sizes n. The pooled-analysis curve shows the distribution of response rate r assuming no study effect. The hierarchical analysis curve shows the Bayesian estimate of the distribution of response rates allowing for heterogeneity across the various studies.

The response rates can take any value between 0 and 1. The number S of responses and sample size n are shown for each study in Table 2 and Figure 4. There are nine response rates, $r1$, $r2$, up to $r9$, one for each study. Each of the nine sample response proportions S/n is an estimate of the corresponding r. There were 106 responses among 150 patients. If all nine of the response rates are assumed to be equal, then the posterior distribution of the common response rate r (assuming a flat prior distribution) is that shown in Figure 4, labeled "pooled analysis."

Even though this pooled analysis is wrong, the overall estimate of 106/150 may be quite reasonable. However, the precision associated with this estimate is too great (equivalently, its standard error is too small). In contrast, the "hierarchical analysis" curve in Figure 4 is a Bayesian estimate of the distribution of the response rates in the population of studies. (This curve is the mean posterior distribution assuming a noninformative prior for the parameters in a particular class of distributions for r-values, called *beta distributions*.) As is typical of hierarchical analyses, this curve shows greater variability than does the analogous curve under the assumption of homogeneity.

In a hierarchical analysis, an individual study's r has a distribution that depends on the data from that study, but it also depends on the data from the other studies. The rightmost column in Table 2 shows the mean of the distribution of each study's response rate. This is also the predictive probability of the response for a future patient in that study. The individual study probabilities are shrunk toward the overall mean. This shrinkage is greater for smaller studies, and for studies with observed proportions further from the overall mean. Hierarchical borrowing is defensible because it does not make the assumption that all studies had the same true response rate, and because the extent of borrowing is determined by the data.

Figure 5 provides a pictorial comparison of the rightmost two columns in Table 2, demonstrating shrinkage. The Bayesian estimates are intermediate between simple pooling (complete shrinkage) and each trial standing alone. The amount of shrinkage—including the two extremes mentioned previously—depends on the prior distribution of the population of trials. This aspect of the prior distribution should be set in advance, or varied to allow for assessing the sensitivity of the overall conclusion.

Shrinkage is a consequence of hierarchical modeling. The motivation for such modeling is to use the available information appropriately in improving precision or in decreasing the required sample size. Consider study number 1 in Table 2. Simply pooling the data from the other eight studies would greatly increase the precision of its estimated response rate. For example, the standard error would be reduced from 0.116 to 0.037. However, in view of the possibility of heterogeneity in the studies, such pooling would

Table 2 Numbers of responses S, sample size n, observed response proportions (including its standard error), and adjusted estimates of response rates by study.

Study number	Responses S	Sample size n	Observed response proportions (standard error)	Bayes estimate (standard deviation)
1	11	16	0.69 (0.116)	0.69 (0.094)
2	20	20	1.00 (0.000)	0.90 (0.064)
3	4	10	0.40 (0.155)	0.53 (0.121)
4	10	19	0.53 (0.115)	0.57 (0.094)
5	5	14	0.36 (0.128)	0.48 (0.109)
6	36	46	0.78 (0.061)	0.77 (0.058)
7	9	10	0.90 (0.095)	0.80 (0.097)
8	7	9	0.78 (0.139)	0.73 (0.110)
9	4	6	0.67 (0.192)	0.68 (0.125)
Total	106	150	0.71 (0.037)	0.68 (0.064)

Note: The Bayes estimate column is described in the text.

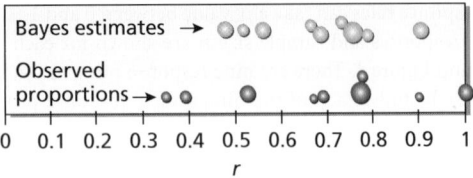

Figure 5 Observed response proportions compared to the adjusted response rate estimates. Values are given in the two rightmost columns in Table 2. The dot plot on the r-axis shows the observed response proportions, just as in Figure 4. The Bayes estimates assume a hierarchical model and show shrinkage toward the overall mean.

not be justified. Borrowing hierarchically also strengthens the conclusion, but not as much. The standard deviation of the Bayes estimate is only about 20% smaller, from 0.116 to 0.094. Although smaller than the reduction with unabashed pooling, this reduction implies that >50% savings in sample size is necessary to carry out a clinical trial (in the setting of study number 1 in Table 2) with the same precision: $(0.116/0.094)^2 - 1 = 52\%$. For example, to achieve the same standard error in a stand-alone study would require 25 as opposed to 16 patients in study number 1 of Table 2.

Patient covariates can be incorporated into a hierarchical analysis, thus adjusting for known differences in the studies but still accounting for unknown effects. In this example and in more complicated hierarchical settings as well,[21] modeling allows for borrowing from other studies and databases. If the results are consistent across studies, then the amount of borrowing will be greater. If the results are sufficiently different (after accounting for covariates), then this suggests heterogeneity among the studies and there is little borrowing.

Hierarchical modeling in trial design

There are many settings in which trials can be set up to borrow strength from related, but not necessarily identical, experimental units.

Consider designing a trial for a therapy for a disease that has several subtypes, such as several different histologies that exist for one type of tumor. The response rates will likely differ for the different subtypes. The setting is essentially the same as that of the previous section. The focus is then the tumor response rate within the individual subtype. These have a distribution, just as in the previous section. Recognizing the possibility of borrowing across subtypes means greater precision for estimating each individual response rate and therefore that the sample size within each subtype can be smaller.

The extent of borrowing depends on the results, just as in the previous section. In other words, the savings in terms of sample size cannot be predicted with certainty. However, this is not a problem if the interim results can be monitored. The interim results can be used to determine the precision associated with the estimates of the various response rates. If the interim results will not be available when the decision to stop the trial must be made, then the uncertainties regarding heterogeneity across subtypes can be assessed at the trial design stage and the sample size chosen accordingly, recognizing that the eventual precisions cannot be predicted perfectly.

Hazards over time

Time-to-event (TITE) analyses/survival analyses are ubiquitous in cancer research. In this section, we focus on a narrow aspect of survival analysis that enables greater understanding of cancer and its treatment. For illustration, we use data from a clinical trial, protocol 8541 of the Cancer and Leukemia Group B (CALGB).[22]

This trial considered three different dose schedules of cyclophosphamide, doxorubicin, and 5-fluorouracil (CAF) in the treatment of node-positive breast cancer: high, moderate, and low. These are, respectively, four cycles of CAF at 600, 60, and 600 mg/m², six cycles at 400, 40, and 400 mg/m², and four cycles at 300, 30, and 300 mg/m². The primary endpoint was disease-free survival, which is shown in Figure 6 for the three dose groups using Kaplan–Meier plots. We provide no p-values for the comparisons (high vs moderate; high vs low) because the statistical significance is not relevant to our purpose.

Although TITE curves such as those in Figure 6 are standard, they do not tell the whole story regarding any benefit of increasing dose and dose intensity. A clearer picture is contained in hazard plots over time. Hazards are the proportions of events within a particular time period as a fraction of those patients who are at risk at the beginning of the period. For example, suppose that the event is a recurrence and there are 100 patients in a group that are at risk in the first year. If 10 of these patients experience a recurrence of the disease in the first year, then the first-year hazard is 10%. Going into the second year there are 90 patients at risk. If another 18 experience recurrences in the second year, then the second-year hazard is $18/90 = 20\%$. When calculating the hazards from survival plots such as those in Figure 6, one subtracts the current year's survival proportion from the previous year's survival proportion and divides by the previous year's survival proportion. The resulting yearly hazards are shown in Figure 7.

A striking observation from Figure 7 is that the hazards decrease over time (after the second year) for all three treatment arms. This is a reflection of the heterogeneity of this disease. The most aggressive

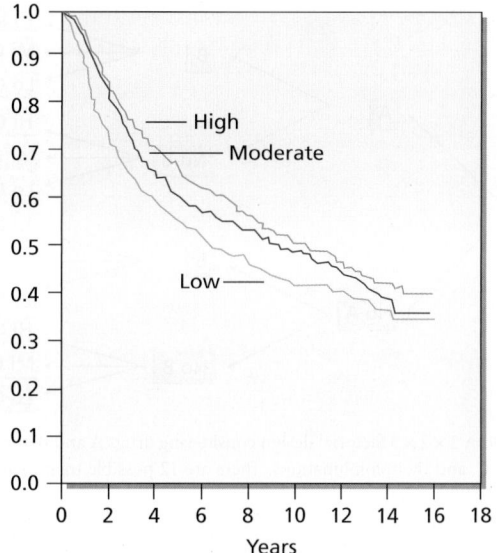

Figure 6 Disease-free survival proportions for the three CAF dose groups of CALGB 8541.

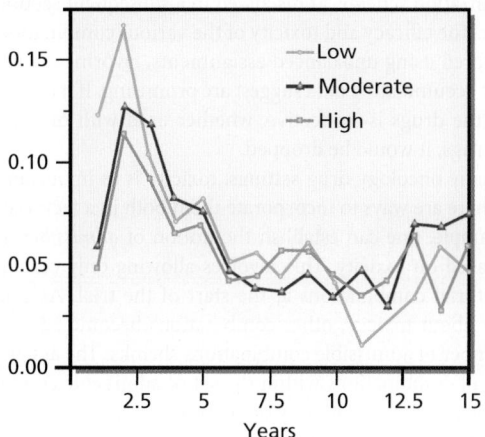

Figure 7 Hazards for the three CAF dose groups of CALGB 8541, derived from Figure 6.

tumors recur early, giving the high hazards evident in the first few years. Once their tumors have recurred, patients are removed from the at-risk population. The remaining tumors are less aggressive and so they recur at a lower rate.

Regarding a treatment arm effect, the apparent benefit of the high-dose schedule is restricted to the first 5 years or so. Actually, the hazard for patients on the high-dose schedule is lower than those of the other two arms in each of the first 6 years. (Although it is not much lower in the last few of these 6 years, and it is not much lower than that of the moderate-dose schedule at any time.) This observation is impressive because each year is like a new study, with previous recurrences not counted when starting a new year.

A final comment regarding hazards relates to the common problem of predicting survival results into the future for patients already accrued to a trial. This differs from the general problem of prediction discussed in "Predictive Probabilities." Consider Figure 6. Some of the patients have as little as 10 years of follow-up information. As more follow-up information becomes available, there will be no change in these curves before the 10-year time point. However, the curves are subject to change beyond 10 years. Because the focus is on patients for whom the tumor has not yet recurred, the way the curves will change depends on the hazards

beyond 10 years. The information available about these hazards is shown in Figure 7. For predicting when and whether a patient's disease will recur, consider hazards 1 year at a time, always building on the patient's current year of follow-up. Each incremental hazard prediction depends on the data for the corresponding year.

Principles of statistical design: decision analysis and factorial experiments

Decision analysis

Clinical practice and clinical research involve making decisions. A list of the possible results, probabilities, and consequences of each decision, pros and cons expressed as utilities, allows for choosing one decision over another. Predictive probabilities play a central role in the decision-making process, which makes the Bayesian approach ideal. Choosing the trial design and selecting the optimal sample size are decisions that benefit from the use of decision analysis, which is described in greater detail in other references.[23–32]

Factorial experiments

Most comparative drug trials in oncology test one experimental agent against a control. The patients in both treatment arms may receive additional therapy based on the current standard of care for the type and stage of their cancer, and on their prior treatment. They may have surgery and receive concomitant radiation and other chemotherapy, which may include several drugs. If the experimental drug is shown to be sufficiently effective, then it will be incorporated into the standard therapy. This approach is simple and clean, but it has a number of drawbacks. One is that it is not possible to assess the individual contributions of the various components of polychemotherapy or combination therapy that are developed in this way. Another is that the approach provides a mechanism for adding drugs to standard regimens but not for subtracting them. An experimental agent's effectiveness may or may not require all other components of the standard regimen. Adding an experimental drug to a standard regimen, however, may make other components of the regimen unnecessary. In the latter case, there is no way of identifying these components.

To some extent this conundrum is inevitable. Studying the possible removal of a component of standard chemotherapy is difficult, and for ethical reasons this is so, even if the component has never been proven to contribute to the overall effectiveness of the combination. However, better approaches for developing drugs would alleviate the problem and could lead to more rapid development of better therapies. A fundamental principle of optimal experimental design in statistics is to change the various contributing factors in such a way as to learn efficiently about their impact on outcome. This impact may involve interactions between the factors and it is important to learn about such interactions. What is required is to model relationships and exploit the available data to inform the model.

An alternative to varying one factor at a time in separate studies is using factorial designs.[33] In the simplest example, patients would be assigned to one of four regimens: A alone, B alone, A and B in combination, and neither. (The last of these does not mean "no therapy" because all patients receive standard therapy.) These four possibilities are shown schematically in Figure 8, where "A" means that the patient receives A and "No A" means the patient does not receive A. The factors may be drugs, or other interventions ("A" could be radiation therapy, or surgery before rather than after chemotherapy, or a high dose as opposed to a low dose of a drug). Reading

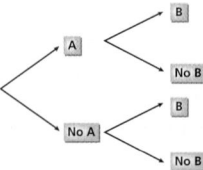

Figure 8 A 2 × 2 factorial design considering drugs A and B and their combination. There are four possible treatment combinations.

from left to right in Figure 8 may not indicate time. The two drugs may be given concurrently or sequentially, A before B or B before A. Indeed, sequential versus concurrent administration of drugs could be another factor in a factorial design.[34,35]

An advantage of factorial designs is that they enable estimating the "main effects" of the individual drugs and therefore a single trial answers two (or more) questions, while using the same sample size as a two-arm trial. Another advantage is that factorial designs allow for assessing interactions between the factors. For example, comparing the difference between the top two cases in Figure 8 with the difference between the bottom two cases addresses whether the effect of B is the same when it is given with drug A as when it is given without drug A. Table 3 shows the types of interactions that are possible for the four combinations of drugs A and B considered in Figure 8, assuming that the endpoint is the response rate. For negative interactions, the effect of the combination is less than the sum of the individual drug effects. For positive interactions, the effect of the combination is greater than the sum of the individual drug effects.

A limitation of factorial designs is that some treatment combinations may not be ethically or practically possible. For example, one of the combinations in Figure 8 is neither of the two drugs. In some oncology settings it may not be possible to have such a treatment arm. Including only three arms in the trial is better than having only two, but then individual drug effects cannot be assessed and the sample size advantages of the factorial design are lost.

When a two-arm trial is designed to have a particular power, a second factor can be added without increasing the sample size. The power for assessing the interaction between the factors is not as great as for assessing a main effect, but there will be some information about interactions. The sample size can be increased if high power for assessing an interaction is required, but a reasonable and usually a more realistic alternative is to keep the sample size the same and accept modest power for assessing interactions. Learning about interactions is essential, both clinically and scientifically, and interactions cannot be identified from a single two-arm trial. Factorial designs can consider more than two factors and more than two levels per factor. Figure 9 shows a more complicated example, a 2 × 2 × 3 factorial design. Now there are three doses of drug C. Data from every patient contribute in estimating the main effects of A, B, and C separately and so there is no increase in sample size. Estimating three-way interactions has less power than estimating two-way interactions, but the results from the factorial design in Figure 9 will

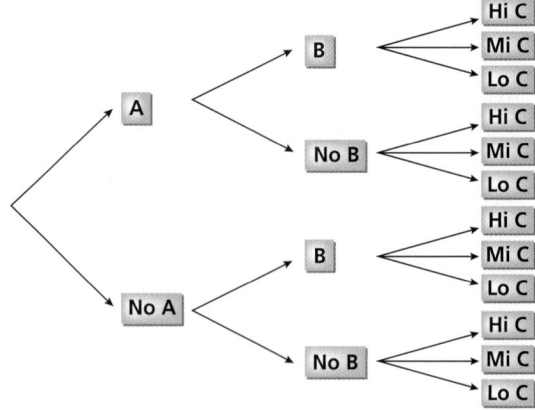

Figure 9 A 2 × 2 × 3 factorial design considering drugs A and B, three levels of drug C, and their combinations. There are 12 possible treatment combinations.

contain some information about the three-way interaction of drugs A, B, and C.

A modification for a large factorial design is to use an adaptive randomization scheme, as discussed in a subsequent section of this chapter. The efficacy and toxicity of the various combinations could be explored using unbalanced assignments, favoring combinations that the accumulating data suggest are promising. If it turns out that one of the drugs is ineffective, whether used with or without the other drugs, it would be dropped.

In many oncology drug settings, toxicity is as important as efficacy. There are ways to incorporate them both in a factorial design. For example, one can establish the notion of *admissible combinations* based on toxicity. This involves allowing only certain of the full factorial combinations at the start of the trial. As experience accrues about toxicity, other combinations become admissible, or the number of admissible combinations shrinks. The assignment to treatment combinations within the set of admissible combinations can be made either randomly or adaptively based on accumulating information about efficacy.

Adaptive designs of clinical trials

The focus of this section is a family of designs that are adaptive or dynamic in the sense that observations made during the trial can affect the subsequent course of the trial. The focus is clinical trials, but the ideas also apply to the preclinical setting.

Designs of clinical trials are usually static in that the sample size and any prescription for assigning treatment, including randomization protocols, are fixed in advance. Results observed during the trial are not used to guide its course. There are exceptions. Some phase II cancer trials have two stages, with stopping after the first stage possible if the results are not sufficiently promising. Moreover, most phase III protocols specify interim analyses that determine whether the trial should be stopped early for sufficiently strong evidence of a

Table 3 Response rates (%) for the four treatment combinations in a factorial design in which drugs A and B are added to standard therapy (hypothetical effects).

Treatment combination	Neither effective	A effective B not	B effective A not	Additive effects	Negative interaction	Positive interaction (Example I)	Positive interaction (Example II)
A and B	20	30	30	40	30	50	40
A, no B	20	30	20	30	30	30	20
B, no A	20	20	30	30	30	30	20
Neither	20	20	20	20	20	20	20

difference between competing treatment arms. However, traditional early stopping criteria are very conservative and so few trials stop early.

The simplicity of trials with static designs makes them solid inferential tools. Their sample sizes tend to be large, at least in comparison with the alternatives to be discussed in this section. In addition, they usually consider two therapeutic strategies, or arms, thus enabling straightforward treatment comparisons. That is not to say that static trials always give clear answers as to whether one arm is better than the other, but only that they usually allow for an unambiguous quantification of the uncertainty regarding whether one arm is better.

Despite their virtues, static trials result in slow and unnecessarily costly drug development. The number of cancer drugs available for development is increasing exponentially. It is inefficient to focus on a single drug when myriad others are sitting on the sidelines waiting to be evaluated. Pharmaceutical companies and medical researchers generally must be able to consider hundreds or thousands of drugs for development at the same time. Static trials inhibit the simultaneous processing of many drugs. Moreover, they cannot efficiently address dose–response questions when many drugs are under consideration. Dynamic designs that are integrated with the drug-development process are necessary for reasonable progress in medical research.

Using an adaptive design means examining the accumulating data periodically, or even continually, with the goal of modifying the trial's design. These modifications depend on what the data show about the unknown hypotheses. Among the modifications possible are stopping early, restricting eligibility criteria, expanding accrual to additional sites or inclusion of certain subgroups of patients, extending accrual beyond the trial's original sample size if its conclusion is still not clear, dropping arms or doses, and adding arms or doses. All of these possibilities are considered in the light of the accumulating information. Adaptive designs also include unbalanced randomization where the degree of imbalance depends on the accumulating data. For example, arms that give more information about the hypothesis in question or that are performing better than other arms can be weighted more heavily.[36]

Adaptation is not limited to the data accumulating in the trial. Information that is reported from other ongoing trials can also be used. This is easier to implement if one takes a Bayesian approach, possibly using hierarchical modeling as described in the previous section.

Adaptive designs are increasingly being used in cancer trials. This is true for trials sponsored by pharmaceutical companies, and more generally. For example, a variety of trials conducted at The University of Texas MD Anderson Cancer Center are prospectively adaptive.[37] Examples of commonly used adaptive designs are given below.

Continual reassessment method (CRM) in phase I trials

The purpose of phase I cancer trials is to identify the maximum-tolerated dose (MTD). Phase I trial designs generally use either a rigid, algorithm-based up-and-down design or an adaptive design that is based on a statistical model. Variants of the so-called 3 + 3 design[38] and the accelerated titration design[39] are forms of the up-and-down design that are commonly used in phase I trials. Variants of the continual reassessment method (CRM) are forms of model-based dose-finding design.

The 3 + 3 design enrolls patients in groups of three. If none of the three patients experiences toxicity, the dose is increased one level for the next group of three. If two or three of the three patients

experience toxicity, then the next lower dose is the MTD, providing that at least six patients have been treated at that dose. If one of the three experiences toxicity, then three more patients are added at the same dose level. If two or more of the six patients at that dose experience toxicity, then again the next lower dose with at least six patients treated is the MTD.[40] This algorithm-based design is crudely adaptive and is likely to assign low doses and to select an ineffective MTD. Moreover, the decision of the next dose depends on only the result of the current dose and ignores the information accumulating from all other doses administered in the trial. In other words, dose assignments are myopic and not based on sufficient statistics.[41]

The CRM and its extensions[42–44] use Bayesian updating, which assumes a particular model of the relationship between dose and toxicity (such as the logistic function). The CRM assigns each patient to the dose that has the probability of toxicity closest to some predetermined target value. This is the Bayesian posterior probability calculated from the data available up to that point (and so is based on sufficient statistics). Variations of the CRM include the escalation with overdose control (EWOC) design[45] and the Bayesian model averaging continual reassessment method (BMA-CRM).[46]

The CRM more effectively finds the MTD than does the 3 + 3 design. Although the CRM-type of design has been the preferred design for phase I trials at MD Anderson Cancer Center, it is being improved in a number of ways. One of these uses the fundamental principle that ignoring information is wrong. (A catch, of course, is that taking information into account is work, and it can require modeling.) There is some information that accrues about efficacy in a phase I trial. This information is limited, especially regarding the dose–efficacy relationship. However, at a minimum, in proceeding to phase II with a particular dose (usually the MTD), one should use the efficacy information from those patients in phase I who were assigned to that dose. This notion leads to using a phase I/II design that addresses safety and efficacy simultaneously, or one that focuses on efficacy after an initial focus on toxicity. Such an approach is efficient from the perspective of both time and patient resources.

In terms of trial conduct in which both 3 + 3 and CRM designs are suboptimal is the need to pause the accrual while waiting for toxicity information. Such pauses are inefficient and cause logistical problems. Trials should be paused or stopped if there are safety concerns, not because the design cannot get out of its own way. When obtaining information about toxicity (or efficacy), there is seldom a magical dose that the next patient must receive. All doses are potentially informative. Rather than stopping, one should use a design that models dose response (toxicity and efficacy) by the look-ahead principle or the TITE-CRM, which is able to assign a next dose even though patients previously treated are not yet fully evaluable.[47,48] Other designs for when the toxic effects of a new drug are not expected to be observable soon after the dose is administered, but only after a delay, include the expectation-maximization CRM[49] and the data augmentation CRM.[50] Model-based dose-finding designs have also been developed for trials that evaluate drugs in combination.[51–55]

Additional limitations of a phase I design, in which both 3 + 3 and CRM designs are constrained, are the assumption that toxicity is dichotomous and the exclusion of efficacy from consideration. A better approach—again because of using all available information—would be to account for both the severity of toxicity and the efficacy in a phase I/II design.[56–62]

As more biologics are evaluated in clinical trials, dose-finding trials shift from determining the MTD (based on the use of highly toxic chemotherapies) to determining the optimal biological dose (OBD). Biologics are expected to have low toxicity within the range of therapeutic doses, and the optimal dose is generally defined as the lowest safe dose of the targeted agent that has the highest rate of efficacy. Several approaches have been proposed for determining the OBD in phase I dose-finding trials.[52,62–64] Readers may refer to Braun[65] for a comprehensive review of adaptive designs for phase I dose-finding trials.

Adaptive phase II trials

In many diseases, the standard phase II dose-finding design allocates a fixed number of patients to each of a number of doses in a grid. Such questions are of less interest in cancer chemotherapy trials because of the goal of administering as much of the drug as the patient can tolerate. However, with increased use of biological agents, dose finding for efficacy is becoming more important in cancer research.

After seeing the results of a dose-finding trial, investigators usually wish they had assigned patients in some other manner. Perhaps the dose–response curve was shifted more to the left or right than anticipated. If so, then the assignment of a bulk of the patients on one end or the other was wasted. Or perhaps the slope of the dose–response curve is greater than anticipated and the response of patients assigned to the flat regions of the curve would have been more informative if the doses assigned had been in the region where the slope is apparently greatest. Or perhaps, the results for the early patients made it clear that the dose–response curve was flat over the entire range and therefore the trial could have stopped earlier. Or perhaps, the results of the trial show that the standard deviation of the outcome of interest is greater or less than anticipated and so the trial should have been larger or could have been smaller.

Sequential designs for phase II studies have been developed to evaluate the efficacy of new treatments within a prespecified range of doses. This dose-ranging stage continues until a decision is made that the drug is not sufficiently effective to pursue future development or that the optimal dose for the confirmatory phase III trial is sufficiently well known. Early single-arm designs used two stages to reach a predetermined efficacy rate while controlling the type I and type II error rates.[66,67] Bayesian adaptive trial design for a binary outcome measure have been proposed with efficacy and/or futility-stopping rules.[68] The design of Berry et al.[69] also proceeds sequentially, analyzing the data as they accumulate (see also additional approaches[70,71]) as well as applying predictive probability for utility early stopping in phase II design.[72] Further discussion of group sequential designs can be found in the work of Jennison and Turnbull.[73]

The example trial of Berry et al.[69] involves a biological neuroprotective agent for stroke. However, the same principles of trial design apply in cancer research. Each patient entering the trial is assigned the dose (1 of 16, including a placebo) that maximizes the information about the dose–response relationship, given the results observed so far. This dose could be in the region of the greatest apparent slope, or it could be the placebo or a high dose. However, future patients are not assigned to doses in any region where accumulating evidence suggests that the dose–response curve is flat.

In the dose-ranging stage, neither the number of patients assigned to any particular dose nor the total number of patients assigned in this stage are fixed in advance. The dose-ranging sample size will be large when the data suggest that the drug has moderate benefit, when the dose–response curve is gently sloping, or when the standard deviation of the responses is moderately large. It will tend to be small if the drug has substantial benefit, if the drug has no benefit, if the dose–response curve rises over a narrow range of doses, or if the standard deviation of the responses turns out to be small. (In addition, and somewhat nonintuitively, the dose-ranging stage

will be small if the standard deviation of the responses is very large. The reason is that a sufficiently large standard deviation means that a very large sample size would be required to demonstrate a beneficial drug effect. The required sample size may be so large that it would be impossible to study the drug and so the trial stops in the dose-ranging phase before it consumes substantial resources.)

In the stroke trial considered by Berry et al.,[69] the ultimate endpoint is an improvement in the stroke scale from baseline to 13 weeks. If the accrual rate is large, then the benefit of adaptive assignment can be limited by delays in obtaining the endpoint information. (Note: a "sweet spot" optimizing the accrual rate and the time of endpoint evaluation can be found.[74]) To minimize the effects of delayed information, each patient's stroke scale is assessed weekly between baseline and week 13. Within-patient measurements are correlated, with correlations greater if they are closer together in time. We incorporate a longitudinal model into the analysis of the trial and carry out Bayesian predictions of the ultimate endpoint based on the current patient-specific information, and we update the probability distributions of the treatment effect accordingly.

A design with adaptive dosing is more effective than the standard design at identifying the right dose. In addition, it usually identifies the right dose with a smaller sample size than when using fixed-dose assignments. Another advantage is that many more doses can be considered in an adaptive design. (Even though some doses will be little used and some may never be used, these cannot be predicted in advance.) An adaptive design therefore has some ability to distinguish responses at adjacent doses and to estimate the nuances of the dose–response curve.

The circumstances of the stroke trial are similar to those in many other types of trials. Finding the right dose is a ubiquitous problem in pharmaceutical development, and it is seldom done well or efficiently. The adaptive nature of the stroke trial would be less advantageous if we had not exploited early endpoints. Cancer, too, is characterized by the availability of information about a patient's performance (local control of the disease, biomarkers, etc.) before reaching the primary endpoint. Furthermore, Bayesian adaptive design can be applied to screen efficacious combination therapies in phase II trials by formulating the selection procedure as a Bayesian hypothesis testing problem and using the current values of the posterior probabilities to adaptively allocate patients to treatment combinations.[75] Finally, the possibility of moving seamlessly from phase I to phase II or from phase II to phase III, contingent upon promising results, exists for many types of drugs. That issue leads naturally to the subject of the next section.

Seamless phase I/II and phase II/III designs

The convention of discretizing drug development into phases is unfortunate. We proceed from one phase to the next when we think we know something: the MTD from phase I, or that a drug's impact on a phase II endpoint will translate into a benefit in phase III, and at the phase II dose. In the Bayesian approach, one never takes a quantity to be perfectly known. Instead, the Bayesian perspective is to carry along uncertainty with whatever knowledge is available. Phases of drug development are arbitrary labels that describe a process that is, or should be, continuous.

One of the consequences of partitioning drug development into phases is that there are delays between phases. For example, there is a pause between phases II and III to set up one or more pivotal studies. As mentioned in the context of the stroke trial, its design allows for avoiding such a hiatus. At each time point, say weekly, the algorithm that guides the conduct of the trial carries out a decision analysis and recommends either (1) continue the dose-ranging stage of the trial, (2) stop the trial for lack of efficacy (inadequate slope of the dose–response curve or, more accurately, evidence of a positive dose–response that is insufficient to justify continuing the trial), or (3) shift into a confirmatory trial. This shift can be made seamlessly, with no break in the accrual. Indeed, it is even theoretically possible to implement such a shift in a double-blind trial without informing the investigators: they simply continue to randomize doses, but unbeknownst to them, the only two being assigned are the phase III dose and the placebo.

Many trial designs have encompassed both phases I and II.[37,57–61,64,76–80] Such designs allow for addressing toxicity and efficacy throughout the trial. Only "admissible" doses or combinations of doses are used, and doses are escalated as others become admissible. All the while, the designs allow for learning about the relationship between dose and efficacy as well as about dose and toxicity.

Trials designed to encompass both phases II and III use a seamless switch to phase III.[81–85] The seamless aspect is as follows. Patients are accrued to a trial, which we can think of as phase II. If the accumulating data are sufficiently strong in suggesting that the drug/treatment has no effect on local control or survival, then the trial stops. If the data suggest that the drug may have an impact on local control and that this impact translates into a survival benefit, then the trial will be expanded and the accrual rate will increase accordingly. During such an expansion, patients continue to accrue at the initial site so that there is no downtime in the local accrual while other centers prepare to join the trial. This is an efficient use of patient resources because data from the patients who enrolled early contribute to the eventual inferences about survival. These patients are the most informative of all those enrolled because their follow-up times are the longest.

The trial continues until stopping occurs because (1) continuing would be futile, judged by predictive probabilities, (2) the maximum sample size is reached, or (3) the predictive probability of eventually achieving statistical significance becomes sufficiently large. If the third event occurs, the accrual ceases and the pharmaceutical company prepares a marketing application.

For example, the sample size of a conventional phase III trial with the desired operating characteristics is 900. This is taken to be the maximum sample size in the seamless design as well. Actual accrual is very likely to be much less than this maximum sample size, particularly, when the experimental treatment is either very promising or not promising at all. On the other hand, incorporating the same number of interim analyses in a conventional design using a conventional type of stopping boundary allows for only a slight decrease in the average sample size. A Bayesian design occasionally leads to a relatively large trial (close to 900 patients). However, a pleasant aspect of the design is that the sample size is large precisely when a large trial is necessary. Conventional trials may well (and sometimes do!) come to their predetermined end with an ambiguous conclusion. In a Bayesian approach, one may choose to continue such a trial to resolve the ambiguity, and this option has substantial utility. (Carrying this argument to the maximum sample size, there may be times for which stopping at 900 is ill advised, but for logistical reasons we specified a maximum size.) Within a seamless adaptive design, one can use the data accumulating in the trial to re-estimate the sample size, which can result in reduced sample sizes.[86–90]

A conventional drug-development strategy involves running a phase I trial to identify the MTD, then, following that by a phase II trial to address local control; digesting the results, and if the results are positive, starting to develop a phase III trial with survival as the primary endpoint. In comparison with such a strategy, a seamless

approach can greatly reduce the sample size. In addition, a seamless design minimizes the pauses between phases, which greatly shorten the total drug-development time.

Adaptive randomization

The adaptive designs discussed so far are motivated by the desire to learn efficiently and as rapidly as possible. Another kind of adaptive design aims to assign patients to treatments as effectively as possible. Adaptive randomization encompasses two primary approaches: covariate-adjusted adaptive randomization and outcome-adaptive randomization. A covariate-adjusted adaptive randomization scheme may assign patients to a treatment arm on the basis of baseline measurements of particular characteristics that are associated with prognosis (prognostic markers). This balances the determinant factors among the treatment arms.[91,92] In contrast, an outcome-adaptive randomization scheme assigns patients to a treatment arm on the basis of the responses to treatment that are accumulating from patients already enrolled in the trial, which tends to assign more participants to treatments that are achieving better patient responses.[93,94] Outcome-adaptive randomization increases the likelihood that more patients will receive the more efficacious treatment. This strategy benefits the individuals participating in the trial, which strengthens the "individual ethics" of the trial.[95] Equal randomization, on the other hand, maximizes the statistical power, which emphasizes the "group" or "collective ethics" of the trial, with the goal of identifying effective treatments from the trial and then applying that information to benefit future patients. In addition to making clinical trials more attractive to patients and thereby increasing participation in clinical trials, outcome-adaptive randomization strategies have the important side benefit of being efficient, and so they result in rapid learning.

The purpose of adaptive randomization is to shift the probability weight toward better performing arms as the trial proceeds and the results accumulate. Other allocation algorithms can be considered, for example, assigning doses in proportion to the powers of these probabilities. Many of these trials have more than two treatment arms. The arms may be distinct or closely related therapies. An example of the latter is a trial to determine the dose of an additional prophylactic agent that would inhibit acute graft-versus-host-disease (GVHD) in leukemia patients who received bone marrow transplants.[96] The trial evaluated five doses (including 0) of a drug (pentostatin) added to the standard prophylaxis regimen. The problem was that the drug might inhibit the successful engraftment of the transplant, which was necessary for survival. Such inhibition might be related to dose. A combination endpoint was used in the trial: survival at 100 days free of GVHD. The conflict between engraftment and freedom from GVHD meant that the dose–response curve might not be monotone. In particular, it might increase for small doses and then decrease. Doses were initially assigned in a graduated manner, slowly climbing the dose ladder. However, as doses became admissible, more patients were assigned to the doses that were performing well.

Consider a patient who qualifies for the trial. To decide which pentostatin dose to assign, one calculates the current (Bayesian) probabilities that each admissible dose is better than the placebo. This calculation uses all the information from the patients treated to date. Doses are allocated randomly, with weights proportional to these probabilities. Doses that are doing sufficiently poorly become inadmissible in the sense that their assignment weight becomes 0. When and if it is learned that the drug is effective, the trial is stopped. When and if it is learned that the drug is ineffective, then again the trial is stopped. Patients in the trial benefit from data collected in the trial. The explicit goal is to treat patients more effectively as well as to learn more efficiently. Each design's frequentist operating characteristics are evaluated using Monte Carlo simulation, with possible modification of the parameters of the assignment algorithm to achieve desired characteristics.

Outcome-adaptive randomization can be constructed under either a frequentist or a Bayesian framework. A frequentist approach has been used to derive the optimal randomization probability under various criteria,[97,98] and interim data available at the time of patient allocation have been used to estimate the response rates.[99] The "doubly adaptive biased coin" design[100,101] extends this approach by considering the proportion of patients assigned to each treatment and the current estimate of the desired allocation proportion to compute the randomization probability to achieve optimal design properties with less variability.

The most intuitive approach is standard Bayesian adaptive randomization, which assigns patients to treatment arm 1 with $\phi_1 = \mathrm{Prob}(\theta_1 > \theta_2)$, where θ_i is the posterior probability of p_i for $i = 1,2$ at the time of randomization. This approach has been extended by applying a power transformation, $\phi_1 = \mathrm{Prob}(\theta_1 > \theta_2)^c / (\mathrm{Prob}(\theta_1 > \theta_2)^c + \mathrm{Prob}(\theta_1 < \theta_2)^c)$, and using $c = n/(2N)$, where n is the number of currently enrolled patients and N the maximum number of patients in the trial, to decrease the variability of the randomization probability.[102] Thus, the randomization probability is approximately 0.5 at the start of the trial, and varies as more data accumulate, particularly if the data show a large difference in the response rates between the treatment arms. The randomization probability can be restricted to a range around 0.5 to decrease its variability. Other schemes use the posterior mean (or median) of the treatment effect to determine the randomization probability: $\phi_1 = \hat{\theta}_1 / (\hat{\theta}_1 + \hat{\theta}_2)$, where $\hat{\theta}_i$ is the posterior mean (or median) of θ_i for $i = 1,2$.[103,104]

One can design a clinical trial to begin with an equal randomization scheme and then transition to an adaptive randomization scheme after observing patient responses to the treatment. The adaptive randomization strategy can be combined with early stopping rules for futility and/or efficacy based on predictive probability. This format can result in a sensible drug-development process. (1) When the trial starts, equal randomization is applied as there is not much information on treatment efficacy. (2) After a reasonable amount of data are accumulated, one can switch to adaptive randomization so more patients can be assigned to the better-performing arms based on the available data. (3) The trial continues to accrue patients toward the maximum sample size, but allows for interim monitoring such that the trial can be stopped early when sufficient evidence has accrued that will allow for the inference of treatment efficacy. The flexible format of the trial illustrates the advantages of the Bayesian adaptive clinical trial design.[105]

Using adaptive randomization to evaluate multiple treatments requires the trial statistician to carefully check for population drift to prevent biased comparisons of the various treatments. This is of concern when using an adaptive randomization scheme that tends to assign more patients to the better-performing treatments because the scheme may cause imbalance in the patient characteristics across the treatment arms.[106] The trial can be designed to partially correct for population drift by including a control arm and placing limits on the randomization probability to achieve a nonnegligible randomization probability for each treatment arm. A marked population drift can invalidate proper inference. This issue can be resolved using regression analysis, for example, to account for the imbalance in prognostic covariates among the treatment arms. Recommendations for monitoring adaptive trials are provided by Marchenko et al.[107]

The advantages and disadvantages of incorporating outcome-adaptive randomization strategies in a clinical trial have prompted numerous discussions and may depend on the specific scenario under which the strategy is applied. Equal randomization has been preferred in a two-arm trial with a binary endpoint because it is easier to implement, and results in smaller sample sizes and fewer nonresponders.[106] A recent analysis of outcome-adaptive randomization questioned the ethics of using this strategy for two-arm trials.[108] Adaptive randomization strategies can increase the favorable response rate and achieve better statistical power when a large difference exists between the effects of the different treatments tested in a trial.[109] Adding an early stopping rule to the trial design will somewhat decrease this advantage. Compared to equal randomization strategies, adaptive randomization strategies may be advantageous in trials that evaluate a rare disease. Adaptive randomization is advantageous in trials that evaluate multiple treatments and which combine multiple stages of study, and particularly when one treatment is much more beneficial than the others.[69,104,109]

Extraim analyses

A common circumstance is that a clinical trial ends without a clear conclusion. For example, a statistical significance level of 5% in the primary endpoint may be required for drug registration, and the p-value may turn out to be 6%. The regulatory agency then suggests that the trial was "underpowered" and that the company should carry out another trial. It would be much more efficient to simply increase the sample size in the present trial. The problem is that the possibility of such an extension increases the type I error rate. The principle is identical to that for interim analyses.

The solution is to build into the design the possibility of continuing the trial depending on the results, and suitably adjusting the significance levels. In contrast to the adjustments for interim analyses, the adjustments for "extra-im" (extraim) analyses are reversed, with much of the overall significance level "spent" at the originally planned sample size. For example, taking equal significance levels at each possible termination point is preferable to O'Brien-Fleming stopping boundaries because the latter are too conservative for extraim analyses. Allowing for extending the trial increases the maximal sample size and also the average sample size. However, a modest increase in the average sample size (such as 20%) comes with a substantial increase in statistical power (such as 80% increasing to 95%). The reason for this beneficial tradeoff is that the trial is extended only when such an extension is worthwhile.

The "penalty" in the significance level can be either partially or fully offset by including futility analyses as part of the design, Namely the trial would be stopped for sufficiently negative results at preset interim time points. The reason such analyses offset the penalty for extraim analyses is that the null hypothesis is never rejected when the trial stops for futility. The increment in sample size depends on the available data at the time the decision is made to continue the accrual. It also depends on the number of possible extensions. In trials we have designed, we have based each extension on the predictive power. The usual definition of power assumes a particular value of the parameter of interest, say r. Predictive power considers all possible values of r. The data available at the time of the extraim analysis plays two roles. First, they count in the final results of the trial. Second, they are used to update the (Bayesian) probability distribution of r. Fix the total sample size n and calculate the power for detecting each possible value of r. Average this power with respect to the probability distribution of r to give the predictive power for sample size n. Extend the accrual by the minimum sample size that will achieve a total sample size having a prespecified predictive power. If there is no such value of *n*, then continuing the accrual may be unwise.

There is no need to stop a trial just because some of the endpoint information is unavailable. Early information (biomarkers and performance status) that is correlated with the endpoint of interest can be used to inform the prediction. Processes that can be completely and precisely described can be simulated. An advantage of simulations is that each iteration provides data from a fully accrued trial. Therefore, it is possible to check any characteristic of interest regarding the trial's design by calculating the proportion of the trials that have that characteristic. Characteristics of interest include the power, the actual sample size, and the probability of extending the accrual.

The Bayesian framework is ideally suited for incorporating information from outside the trial to make inference. For example, hierarchically commensurate priors and power priors can be applied to adaptively incorporate historical information into clinical trials.[110,111] Historical data on similar therapies or devices can be readily available in many settings. The efficient and appropriate use of such historical information to strengthen the inference for a new trial has been demonstrated in the development of medical devices.[112]

Process or trial? Evaluating many drugs simultaneously in platform trials with or without adaptive allocation

The greatest need for innovation in drug development is the process of effectively dealing with the enormous numbers of potential drugs that are available for development. The notion of developing drugs one at a time is changing. Companies that are able to screen many drugs simultaneously and effectively will survive and others will not.

The platform-based clinical trial design is an example of innovation in the process of developing new agents and therapies.[113,114] A platform is an operational and statistical framework that is specific to a particular disease or condition rather than being specific to a particular clinical protocol. Each new agent or therapy can be considered as a "module" that can be plugged in and out of the "platform" that targets a particular disease or condition. These new treatments can be simultaneously screened as they are developed as an alternative to conducting several separate phase II trials to evaluate multiple treatment arms. Bayesian modeling and randomization can be easily incorporated into the platform-based design. It can be shown that the platform design is much more efficient than running multiple, separate trials. Once the appropriate dose of a new agent has been determined in a phase I trial, that new agent may be added to the platform. An agent may also be dropped from the platform if the data accumulating in the screening process demonstrate that the agent is not producing the desired results. An agent that is dropped from the platform can be returned to a phase I study to re-examine the optimal treatment dose or schedule of doses. If that phase I trial determines that an alternative dose or schedule of doses may be beneficial, then the agent previously dropped from the platform may re-enter the screening process.

The platform-based design brings important statistical challenges to the conduct of such screening trials. The Bayesian posterior distributions and predictive probabilities are computationally intensive to calculate; however, after the predictive probabilities are calculated, boundaries can be specified for the continuous monitoring of the platform-based designs. Sequential adaptive strategies must be properly implemented to monitor the futility of the many experimental agents while maintaining the predetermined type I error rate. The platform-based design bases its futility stopping rule on the posterior predictive probability of achieving a successful trial. The design uses a Bayesian model to account for the uncertainty emanating from interim estimations of the model parameters, and uses simulations to calibrate the design parameters. A Bayesian model is also used to account for the variability resulting from the treatment responses of future patients in the trial.

Much of the research on multiarm and/or multistage trial designs includes similar strategies for improving the efficiency of drug development.[115-119] The platform-based design and the related master protocol, umbrella trials, and basket trials, with particular application to biomarker studies, are discussed by Berry.[120] The platform-based design has potential advantages that include decreasing the overall duration of the treatment screening process; substantially decreasing the number of patients allocated to the control arm; increasing the number of treatments that can be screened, thereby expanding the treatment options available to patients in the trial; decreasing the bias arising from the heterogeneity of separate trials; improving the control of inherent multiplicities; and better informing decisions about subsequent confirmatory trials.

Application of statistical innovation in clinical oncology trials

This section briefly describes two clinical oncology trials that employ statistical innovations: the "Biomarker-integrated approaches of targeted therapy of lung cancer elimination" (BATTLE) trial and the "Investigation of serial studies to predict your therapeutic response with imaging and molecular analysis" (I-SPY 2) trial.

The BATTLE trial[121,122] evaluated four targeted therapies in patients with stage IV recurrent non-small-cell lung cancer, matching each therapy with one of the four biomarker profiles evaluated (defined by expressions of genes, gene mutations, copy numbers, and proteins measured by immunohistochemistry). The outcome was the 8-week disease control rate. The trial incorporates outcome-adaptive randomization and a futility stopping rule under the probit hierarchical model. The stopping rule may exclude specific agents from randomization possibilities for a given patient when that patient's biomarker profile indicates that he/she will not benefit from that agent. The BATTLE-2 trial uses the results from the first trial to screen patients for 10–15 candidate biomarkers. It incorporates adaptive randomization in a two-stage design to evaluate four treatments for non-small-cell lung cancer. The trial is a process, involving training, test, and validation procedures to select the most appropriate biomarkers to use in the trial. The design uses group lasso and adaptive lasso methods to identify prognostic and predictive markers.[123,124]

The multicenter I-SPY 2 trial[125] employs adaptive randomization within each biomarker-based patient group and uses a futility or efficacy stopping rule. The I-SPY 2 trial evaluates neoadjuvant treatments in breast cancer in addition to the administration of up to 12 experimental drugs.[126] This trial has randomized more than 700 patients, transferred two experimental agents to confirmatory studies, and successfully demonstrated that this adaptive trial design can reduce drug-development costs and improve the efficiency of screening new drugs.[125-127]

Clinical trial software

Numerous software programs to use in planning and implementing clinical trials are available online as propriety products or as free offerings.[128] Many useful computer programs for the design, conduct, and analysis of innovative trials can be found at the MD Anderson software download site. (https://biostatistics.mdanderson.org/SoftwareDownload/). Software developed for the CRM[129] in a phase I dose-finding trial includes the CRM simulator, the BMA-CRM, and the TITE-CRM. The CRM simulator uses the prior means of toxicity to select the optimal dose level and permits the user to vary the parameters until achieving the desired output. The BMA-CRM[46] uses multiple sets of probabilities of the prior means for toxicity to select the optimal dose. Software developed for the TITE-CRM[48] has comparable application for determining the optimal dose of an agent when delayed toxicity is expected.

For a dose-finding cancer trial, software developed to determine dose EWOC[45,130] employs adaptive learning. This method has been shown to allocate fewer patients to subtherapeutic or severely toxic doses, treat more patients at doses near the MTD, and estimate that dose with lower average bias and mean squared error when compared to the CRM. Another method uses modified toxicity posterior intervals (mTPI) and Bayesian decision theory to determine the optimal dose of an oncology drug.[131]

Another method that minimizes the likelihood of assigning patients to subtherapeutic or overly toxic doses is the Bayesian optimal interval (BOIN) design.[132] Used in phase I clinical trials, the R function (BOIN.r) computes the optimal probability interval to determine the MTD, optimizing the dose assignment for each patient who enrolls in the trial. After specifying the design parameters, the BOIN design uses an algorithm and can be implemented similarly to the traditional 3 + 3 design. The BOIN design is comparable to the CRM in selecting the MTD, but the BOIN has a much lower risk of assigning patients to subtherapeutic or overly toxic doses.

The predictive probability design[72] can determine the cutoff values of the predictive probability and calculate the stopping boundary needed for continuous trial monitoring on the basis of the input of the type I and type II error rates. The BFDesigner[133] is useful for creating efficient stopping rules. Other computational tools that are helpful when using adaptive designs are the *parameter solver*, which calculates the distribution parameters of a random variable given either two quantiles or the mean and variance, and *predictive probabilities* for a two-arm trial with a binary endpoint, which calculates the posterior predictive probabilities of finding one treatment arm to be superior to the other or of stopping for futility.[16] With more software available for the design and conduct of novel clinical trials, more rapid translation of statistical innovation from theory to practice can be achieved.

Acknowledgments

The authors thank the Cancer and Leukemia Group B for permission to use data from CALGB 8541 and LeeAnn Chastain for editorial assistance. This work was supported in part by Grant CA016672 from the National Cancer Institute.

Key references

The complete reference list can be found on the Wiley Companion Digital Edition of this title (see inside front cover for login instructions).

12 Berry DA. Introduction to Bayesian methods III: use and interpretation of Bayesian tools in design and analysis. *Clin Trials*. 2005;2:295–300.

13 Berry DA. Bayesian clinical trials. *Nat Rev Drug Discov*. 2006;5:27–36.

14 Lee JJ, Chu CT. Bayesian clinical trials in action. *Stat Med*. 2012;31:2955–2972.

15 Speigelhalter DJ, Abrams KR, Myles JP. *Bayesian Approaches to Clinical Trials and Healthcare Evaluation*. Chichester, UK: John Wiley & Sons, Ltd; 2004.

16 Berry SM, Carlin BP, Lee JJ, Muller P. *Bayesian Adaptive Methods for Clinical Trials*. Boca Raton: Chapman and Hall/CRC Press; 2010.

31 Ventz S, Trippa L. Bayesian designs and the control of frequentist characteristics: a practical solution. *Biometrics*. 2015;71:218–226.

33 Simon R, Freedman LS. Bayesian design and analysis of two x two factorial clinical trials. *Biometrics*. 1997;53:456–464.

37 Biswas S, Liu DD, Lee JJ, Berry DA. Bayesian clinical trials at the University of Texas MD Anderson Cancer Center. *Clin Trial*. 2009;6:205–216.

46 Yin G, Yuan Y. Bayesian model averaging continual reassessment method in phase I clinical trials. *J Am Stat Assoc*. 2009;104:954–968.

48 Cheung YK, Chappell R. Sequential designs for phase I clinical trials with late-on-set toxicities. *Biometrics*. 2000;56:1177–1182.

52 Mandrekar SJ, Cui Y, Sargent DJ. An adaptive phase I design for identifying a biologically optimal dose for dual agent drug combinations. *Stat Med*. 2007;26:2317–2330.

59 Zhang W, Sargent DJ, Mandrekar SJ. An adaptive dose-finding design incorporating both toxicity and efficacy. *Stat Med*. 2006;25:2365–2383.

62 Zang Y, Lee JJ, Yuan Y. Adaptive designs for identifying optimal biological dose for molecularly targeted agents. *Clin Trials*. 2014;11:319–327.

64 Hoering A, LeBlanc M, Crowley J. Seamless phase I-II trial design for assessing toxicity and efficacy for targeted agents. *Clin Cancer Res*. 2011;17:640–646.

65 Braun TM. The current design of oncology phase I clinical trials: progressing from algorithms to statistical models. *Chin Clin Oncol*. 2014;3:1.

69 Berry DA, Mueller P, Grieve AP, et al. Adaptive Bayesian designs for dose-ranging drug trials. In: Gatsonis C, Carlin B, Carriquiry A, eds. *Case Studies in Bayesian Statistics V*. New York, NY: Springer-Verlag; 2001:99–181.

72 Lee JJ, Liu DD. A predictive probability design for phase II cancer clinical trials. *Clin Trials*. 2008;5:93–106.

74 Gajewski BJ, Berry SM, Quintana M, et al. Building efficient comparative effectiveness trials through adaptive designs, utility functions, and accrual rate optimization: finding the sweet spot. *Stat Med*. 2015;34:1134–1149.

75 Cai C, Yuan V, Johnson VE. Bayesian adaptive phase II screening design for combination trials. *Clin Trials*. 2013;10:353–362.

78 Yin G, Li Y, Ji Y. Bayesian dose-finding in phase I/II trials using toxicity and efficacy odds ratio. *Biometrics*. 2006;62:777–784.

79 Huang X, Biswas S, Oki Y, et al. A parallel phase I/II clinical trial design for combination therapies. *Biometrics*. 2007;63:429–436.

80 Yuan Y, Yin G. Bayesian phase I/II drug-combination trial design in oncology. *Ann Appl Stat*. 2011;5:924–942.

81 Inoue LYT, Thall P, Berry DA. Seamlessly expanding a randomized phase II trial to phase III. *Biometrics*. 2002;58:264–272.

97 Hu F, Rosenberger W. Optimality, variability, power: evaluating response-adaptive randomization procedures for treatment comparisons. *J Am Stat Assoc*. 2003;98:671–678.

102 Thall PF, Wathen KJ. Practical Bayesian adaptive randomisation in clinical trials. *Eur J Cancer*. 2007;43:859–866.

103 Lee JJ, Gu X, Liu S. Bayesian adaptive randomization designs for targeted agent development. *Clin Trials*. 2010;7:584–597.

105 Yin G, Chen N, Lee JJ. Phase II trial design with Bayesian adaptive randomization and predictive probability. *J R Stat Soc: Ser C: Appl Stat*. 2012;61:219–235.

107 Marchenko O, Fedorov V, Lee JJ, Nolan C, Pinheiro J. Adaptive clinical trials: overview of early-phase designs and challenges. *Ther Innov Regul Sci*. 2014;48:20–30.

108 Hey SP, Kimmelman J. Are outcome-adaptive allocation trials ethical? *Clin Trials*. 2015;12:102–106.

109 Lee JJ, Chen N, Yin G. Worth adapting? Revisiting the usefulness of outcome-adaptive randomization. *Clin Cancer Res*. 2012;18:4498–4507.

110 Hobbs BP, Carlin BP, Mandrekar SJ, Sargent DJ. Hierarchical commensurate and power prior models for adaptive incorporation of historical information in clinical trials. *Biometrics*. 2011;67:1047–1056.

112 Campbell G. Bayesian statistics in medical devices: innovation sparked by the FDA. *J Biopharm Stat*. 2011;21:871–887.

117 Wason JMS, Jaki T. Optimal design of multi-arm multi-stage trials. *Stat Med*. 2012;31:4269–4279.

118 Wason JM, Trippa L. A comparison of Bayesian adaptive randomization and multi-stage designs for multi-arm clinical trials. *Stat Med*. 2014;33(13):2206–2221.

119 Parmar MKB, Carpenter J, Sydes MR. More multiarm randomised trials of superiority are needed. *Lancet*. 2014;384:283–284.

120 Berry DA. The brave new world of clinical cancer research: adaptive biomarker-driven trials integrating clinical practice with clinical research. *Mol Oncol*. 2015;9:951–959.

121 Zhou X, Liu S, Kim ES, et al. Bayesian adaptive design for targeted therapy development in lung cancer—a step toward personalized medicine. *Clin Trial*. 2008;5:181–193.

122 Kim ES, Herbst RS, Wistuba II, et al. The BATTLE trial: personalizing therapy for lung cancer. *Cancer Discov*. 2011;1:44–53.

124 Gu X, Chen N, Wei C, et al. Bayesian two-stage biomarker-based adaptive design for targeted therapy development. *Stat Biosci* 2015. http://link.springer.com/article/10.1007/s12561-014-9124-2

127 Quantum Leap. *I-SPY 2 Breast Cancer Clinical Trial Graduates Two Promising Drugs*. 2013. Available at: http://www.quantumleaphealth.org/spy-2-trial-graduates-2-new-drugs-press-release/ (accessed 17 July 2015).

128 Lee JJ, Chen N. Software for design and analysis of clinical trials. In: Crowley J, Hoering A, eds. *Handbook of Statistics in Clinical Oncology*, 3rd ed. Boca Raton, FL: Chapman & Hall/CRC Press; 2012:305–324.

132 Liu S, Yuan Y. Bayesian optimal interval designs for phase I clinical trials. *J R Stat Soc: Ser C: Appl Stat*. 2015;64:507–523.

21 Biomarker-based clinical trial design in the era of genomic medicine

Richard Simon, DSc ▪ Martine Piccart-Gebhart, MD, PhD

Overview

The increasingly recognized molecular heterogeneity of human cancers together with the growing availability of powerful tools providing "molecular portraits" of this heterogeneity require the development of new paradigms for the development of a reliable basis for "personalized" medicine. We review new approaches to the design and analysis of clinical trials for the development of "targeted" therapeutics and diagnostics to inform their use.

Introduction: why we need new designs and analysis paradigms for biomarker-driven clinical trials

Randomized clinical trials have enabled the development of a reliable evidence-based medicine. They have generally evaluated a treatment relative to a control regimen for a broadly defined population of patients defined by primary site, histology, stage, and number of prior treatments. In recent years, sequencing of human tumor DNA has established that cancers of a primary site often represent a heterogeneous collection of diseases that differ with regard to the genomic aberrations that cause them and drive their invasion.[1] The tumors are often heterogeneous with regard to the genes and pathways that can be inhibited by molecularly targeted therapy. Broad eligibility clinical trials are severely underpowered for detecting benefit for the subset of patients whose tumors are most susceptible to the action of the new drug. In the broad eligibility clinical trials that are "positive" because the sample size has been increased to such an extent that even small average treatment effects are statistically significant, only a small proportion of the intent to treat population actually benefits from treatment resulting in toxicity for patients who do not benefit and a large societal economic cost for overtreatment of the population.

Today, we have powerful tools for characterizing the tumors biologically and using this characterization to prospectively structure the design and analysis of more informative clinical trials that result in larger treatment effects for a larger portion of the treated patients. In this chapter, we discuss these modern designs and analyses that should better respond to the needs of "personalized" oncology.

Phase II trials of molecularly targeted agents with companion diagnostics

Nowadays, most of the cancer drugs are being developed for defined molecular targets. In some cases, the targets are well understood, and there is a compelling biological basis and evidence from phase I clinical trials for restricting development to the subset of patients whose tumors are characterized by deregulation of the drug target. For other drugs, there are multiple targets and more uncertainty about how to measure whether a drug target is driving tumor biology in an individual patient.[2]

The ideal approach in the former situation is the codevelopment of the drug and a companion diagnostic that measures the deregulation of the drug target in a robust way.

In the era of molecular oncology, not only must the phase II trial determine whether there is activity of the drug overall in a histologic type, but it also must determine whether the subsequent phase III trial should be restricted based on a candidate companion diagnostic. Freidlin et al.[3] have described a design for use with a single binary candidate biomarker in a randomized phase II design. Their design enables one to determine whether the drug should be (1) developed in a phase III enrichment trial, (2) developed in an analysis stratified all comers' trial, (3) developed in an all comers' trial without measurement of the biomarker, or (4) dropped from further development. This design is shown in Figure 1. The sample size is determined so that the treatment effect on progression-free survival (PFS) in the marker-positive subset has power 0.9 for detecting a doubling of median PFS at a one-sided significance level of 0.10. This will generally provide at least as many events for evaluating treatment effect in the marker-negative subset. If the treatment effect in the marker-positive subset is not significant, then the overall treatment effect is tested at a one-sided 0.05 significance level. If that treatment effect is not statistically significant, then the drug is not recommended for phase III development. If the overall treatment effect is significant, then a traditional phase III trial without measurement of the candidate biomarker is recommended. If the treatment effect in the marker-positive subset is significant, then one examines an 80% confidence interval for the hazard ratio of treatment effect in the marker-negative subset. If the upper confidence interval is below 1.3, then one concludes that the treatment is not active in the marker-negative patients and an enrichment phase III trial is recommended. If the lower confidence limit is above 1.5, then one concludes that the treatment works well in the marker-negative patients and a traditional phase III trial in which the biomarker is not even measured is recommended. Otherwise, a biomarker-stratified phase III trial is recommended.

Other phase II designs for evaluation of a treatment within marker subsets in single-arm phase II studies have been described by Pusztai and Hess[4] and Jones and Holmgren.[5] These designs are focused primarily on ensuring that promising activity of the drug is not missed in cases where its activity is restricted to test-positive patients, and yet excessive numbers of patients are not required in cases where its activity is sufficiently broad that the marker is not needed.

There are more complicated phase II settings, where no natural cut-point of the biomarker is known in advance, or where there are multiple candidate biomarkers. The BATTLE I trial in NSCLC

Holland-Frei Cancer Medicine, Ninth Edition. Edited by Robert C. Bast Jr., Carlo M. Croce, William N. Hait, Waun Ki Hong, Donald W. Kufe, Martine Piccart-Gebhart, Raphael E. Pollock, Ralph R. Weichselbaum, Hongyang Wang, and James F. Holland.
© 2017 John Wiley & Sons, Inc. ISBN: 978-1-118-93469-2

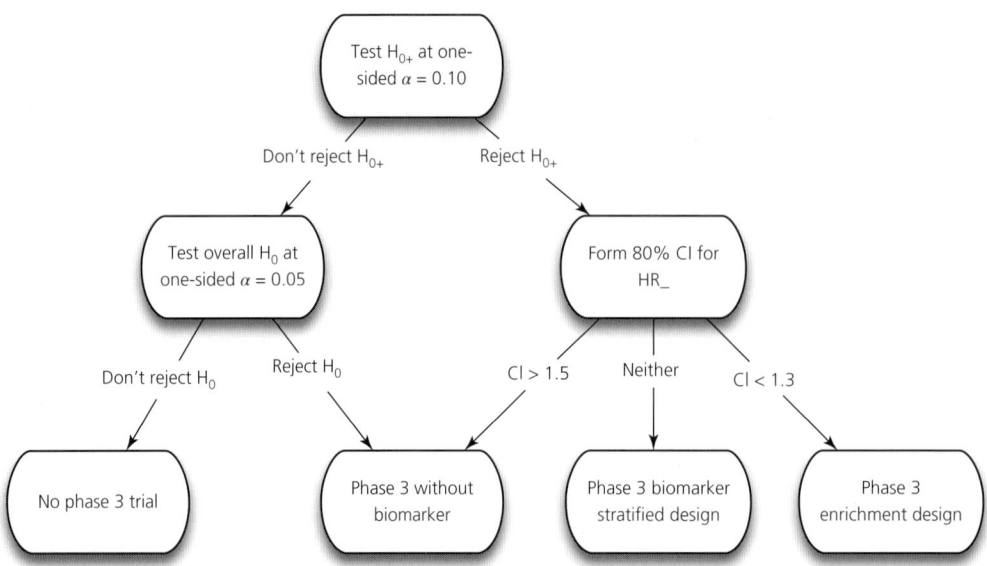

Figure 1 Analysis strategy for randomized phase II design to decide whether phase III trial should be restricted to biomarker-positive population, should include positives and negatives, whether biomarker should not even be measured or whether the conduct of a phase III trial is not supported by phase II results. Data from [3]. HR_+ is hazard ratio in biomarker-positive group. HR_- is hazard ratio for treatment in biomarker-negative group. H_{0+} is null hypothesis that $HR_+ = 1$. H_0 is null hypothesis that overall $HR = 1$.

(nonsmall cell lung cancer) is an example of a phase II clinical trial using a response-adaptive randomization,[6] which is discussed in another chapter of this book. Of note, some statisticians have raised doubts about the effectiveness of such adaptive randomization designs.[7]

Phase IIa basket and umbrella discovery trials

Large tumor sequencing studies such as the Cancer Genome Project in the United Kingdom and the Cancer Genome Atlas (TCGA) in the United States have identified recurrent genomic aberrations in a variety of primary tumor sites.[1] These data provide a scientific basis for treatment of individual patients based on the biological characterization of their tumors. There are, however, many challenges in moving tumor genomics to clinical oncology and the first one is the tremendous heterogeneity of the genomic landscapes of the tumors, implying the existence of multiple, rare genomic segments within a given tumor type.

Developing a single targeted drug in a single small genomic segment of one disease is a lengthy, inefficient, and costly exercise. Let us take the example of HER2 mutations that, contrary to HER2 gene amplification, occur at a low frequency of 1–2% in advanced breast cancer. There is preliminary evidence that these mutations are "actionable" using a potent irreversible tyrosine kinase inhibitor such as neratinib.[8] Conducting a "confirmatory" phase II trial of around 40 patients would require the screening of 2000–4000 women with advanced breast cancer. Moreover, at the end of this exercise, the potential value of the new drug versus standard of care or in other tumor types harboring similar mutations would remain unknown. Figure 2 highlights the challenges of a registration path of such a drug in a "small" genomic segment of the breast cancer (BC) population. This genomic aberration, therefore, would be best matched with its candidate drug in the context of an "umbrella" discovery trial, where a panel of genomic aberrations would be screened and investigated in the context of several breast cancer phase II arms. Alternatively, a basket trial could examine HER2 mutations across several tumor types and investigate the activity of

the TKI (tyrosine kinase inhibitor) in each of them with "early stopping rules" in case of lack of antitumor activity. These increasingly popular forms of clinical trials are described later.

"Basket" discovery trials include patients with advanced cancer of multiple primary sites that are resistant to standard treatment.[9] A sequencing assay is used to evaluate the tumor DNA of a patient and it is determined whether an actionable aberration is present. "Actionable" means that a drug is available whose range of molecular targets overlap with the genomic alterations of the tumor in a way that suggest treatment may result in benefit for that patient. Various kinds of evidence may be used to determine whether a drug is a reasonable candidate for a given mutation. It will include biological understanding of the targets of the drug and the role of those targets in the disease. It may involve using the COSMIC (Catalog of Somatic Mutations in Cancer) database to determine whether the gene is mutated frequently enough in that histologic type to be considered a "driver" mutation. It may involve using algorithms to determine whether mutations found in a gene are predicted to alter protein function. It may also involve using preclinical data about drug activity in cell lines, tumor grafts bearing that mutation in mice, or clinical data in a different tumor type. The rules of actionability should be prospectively defined. Defining levels of evidence for actionability of a drug and a genomic aberration may help trial organizers resolve difficult binary decisions of whether there is sufficient evidence to warrant considering a drug actionable.

The term "basket trial" is often reserved for clinical trials of a single drug with multiple histologic types of patients and multiple types of mutations of either a single gene or several genes. The trials with multiple drugs involved are often called "umbrella trials." Both types of trials are early discovery trials and attempt to identify the genomic characterization of tumors for which there is evidence of substantial anticancer activity of a drug. These positive signals should be confirmed in later expanded phase II or II/III trials.

Some umbrella trials are randomized; outcome for patients who receive drugs based on actionability rules are compared to outcomes on a control drug or on drugs selected based on physicians' choice without genomic characterization. Both the MPACT

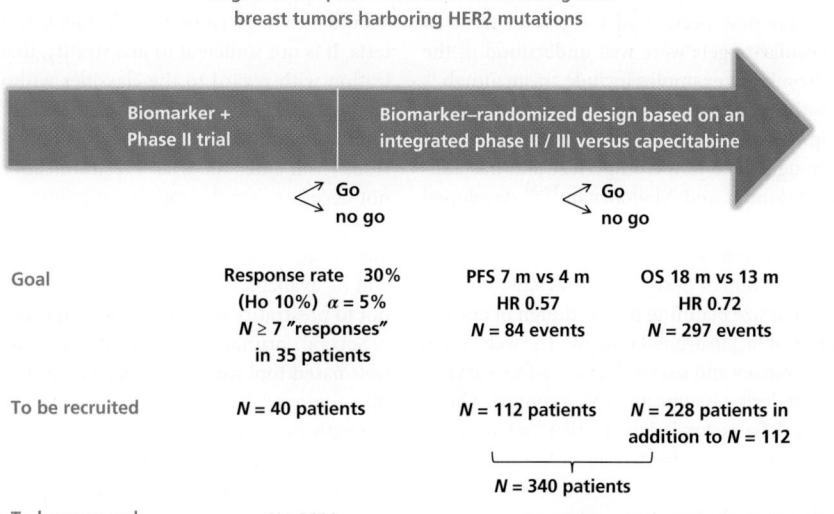

Registration "path" for a HER2-TKI used against
breast tumors harboring HER2 mutations

Statistical assumptions by J. Bogaerts (EORTC)

Figure 2 Schema for phase II and III clinical trials for developing a drug that inhibits a target, which is mutated in only 1–2% of cases. Although the number of patients required for the clinical trials are reasonable, the number screened is very large. It is more efficient to incorporate development of such a drug in an infrastructure of common national and international screening with regard to multiple targets and then triaging patients to clinical trials for which they are eligible.

(molecular profiling based assignment of cancer therapeutics) clinical trial being conducted by the National Cancer Institute and the Stand-Up-To-Cancer sponsored clinical trial in BRAF^WT melanoma use 2 : 1 randomization plans.[10] The randomized umbrella designs address two distinct questions.[10] One is testing the null hypothesis that the policy of trying to match the drug to the genomics of the tumor is no more effective than a treatment strategy that does not use any tumor characterization beyond that used for standard of care. Although most traditional randomized clinical trials evaluate a single drug or regimen, the null hypothesis here relates to a matching policy for a given set of drugs and biomarkers available for the study. This makes it particularly important to obtain a broad enough menu of potent inhibitors of the selected targets. The matching policy is also determined by the type of genomic characterization performed and by the "rules" for matching drug to tumor. If matching is done by a tumor board and is not rule based or if the rules change frequently, the pragmatic value of the clinical trial will be limited. It may also be difficult for regulatory bodies to approve investigational drugs for use as decided by a tumor board rather than in a more rule-based manner. The use of a randomized control group facilitates the use of PFS as endpoint. The proof-of-principle embodied by the null hypothesis may be more meaningful, however, in a trial of a single histologic category than in cases where a wide range of primary sites of disease are included.

A second objective of randomized umbrella studies is the screening of individual drugs used in specific genomic and histologic contexts. For some primary sites, a gene such as "NRAS" may be mutated sufficiently frequently for the study to provide an adequate phase II evaluation of the drug for that new indication. In many cases, however, the numbers will not be adequate for a proper phase II evaluation. Nevertheless, the trial may serve to screen for drug-mutation matches for which there is a substantial degree of activity, larger than is usually tested for in traditional phase II trials. These leads should be confirmed in an expanded cohort of a follow-up trial.[8] In this discovery mode, assessment of activity of a drug against tumors with a given gene mutated must take into account the possibility that the cell type in which the mutation

occurs or the histology of the tumor may modulate activity of the drug against the alteration. This was the case for BRAF inhibitors in colorectal cancer.[11]

New statistical designs specifically for basket or umbrella trials have not yet been introduced. Many such trials incorporate a traditional two-stage design for drug-mutation strata that will have sufficient patients to be separately analyzed. A traditional two-stage design for distinguishing a response rate of 10% from one of 35% with 85% power and 10% type I error requires only five first stage patients and has a 60% chance of terminating at the first stage if the true response probability is only 10%.[12] Such designs can be computed online at http://brb.nci.nih.gov.

LeBlanc et al.[13] previously introduced a design for multiple histology phase II trials that can be used in some basket or umbrella clinical trials. It combines statistical significance tests of drug activity within histology strata with a combined analysis that borrows information from all the patients in the study. Sequential futility analyses are conducted once each strata or the overall group reaches a specified minimum amount. Thall et al.[14] developed a hierarchical Bayesian method for evaluating treatment effects in discrete strata of a phase II trial while accounting for the relatedness of the strata. This approach has been critiqued by Freidlin and Korn[15] who concluded that "there appears to be insufficient information in the outcome data to determine whether borrowing across subgroups is appropriate."

Phase III designs with a single binary biomarker

Targeted (enrichment) designs

Designs in which eligibility is restricted to those patients considered most likely to benefit from the experimental drug are called "targeted designs" or "enrichment designs" and are illustrated in Figure 3a. With an enrichment design, the analytically validated diagnostic test is used to restrict eligibility for a randomized clinical trial comparing a regimen containing a new drug to a control regimen. This approach has now been used for pivotal trials of many drugs whose molecular targets were well understood in the context of the disease. Prominent examples include trastuzumab,[16] vemurafenib,[17] and crizotinib.[18]

The enrichment design was very effective for the development of trastuzumab, even though the test was imperfect and has subsequently been improved. Simon and Maitournam[19,20] developed general formulas for comparing the enrichment design to the standard design with regard to the number of randomized and screened patients. They found the enrichment design very efficient and have made the methods of sample size planning for the design of enrichment trials available online at http://brb.nci.nih.gov. The web-based programs are available for binary and survival/disease-free survival endpoints. The enrichment design is appropriate for contexts where there is a strong biological basis for believing that test-negative patients will not benefit from the new drug.

All comers' (stratification) designs

When a predictive biomarker has been developed but there is not compelling biological or phase II data that test-negative patients do not benefit from the new treatment, it is often best to include both classifier positive and classifier negative in the phase III clinical trials comparing the new treatment to the control regimen. This is shown in Figure 3b. The biomarker is measured in all patients at entry to the trial, and then all patients are randomized to the test treatment or the control regimen. In this case, it is essential that an analysis plan be predefined in the protocol for how the predictive classifier will be used in the analysis. The analysis plan will generally define the testing strategy for evaluating the new treatment in the test-positive patients, the test-negative patients, and overall.[21] The testing strategy must preserve the overall type I error of the trial. The overall type I error is the probability that a claim for a statistically significant difference is made from any of the comparisons when in fact the treatments are equivalent both overall and within the biomarker-specific subsets. Controlling the overall type I error often requires that a threshold of significance <0.05 is used

for interpreting the individual significance tests. The clinical trial should also be sized to provide adequate statistical power for these tests. It is not sufficient to just stratify, that is, balance, the randomization with regard to the classifier without specifying a complete analysis plan. The main value of "stratifying" (i.e., balancing) the randomization is that it assures that only patients with adequate test results will enter the trial. Prestratification of the randomization is not necessary for the validity of inferences to be made about treatment effects within the test-positive or test-negative subsets.[22] If an analytically validated test is not available at the start of the trial but will be available by the time of analysis, then it may be preferable not to prestratify the randomization process.

Several primary analysis plans have been described and a web-based tool for sample size planning for some of these analysis plans is available at http://brb.nci.nih.gov. If one has moderate strength evidence that the treatment, if effective at all, is likely to be more effective in the test-positive cases, one might first compare treatment versus control in test-positive patients using a threshold of significance of 5%. Only if the treatment versus control comparison is significant at the 5% level in test-positive patients, the new treatment will be compared to the control among test-negative patients, again using a threshold of statistical significance of 5%. This sequential approach controls the overall type I error at 5%.[23] In the situation where one has limited confidence in the predictive marker, it can be effectively used for a "fallback" analysis. Outcomes for the new treatment group is first compared to those for the control group overall. If that difference is not significant at a reduced significance level such as 0.03, then the new treatment is compared to the control group just for test-positive patients. The latter comparison uses a threshold of significance of 0.02, or whatever portion of the traditional 0.05 not used by the initial test.[23] In situations where one has an intermediate level of confidence in the candidate biomarker, one can use the MAST analysis plan.[24] At the final analysis, one first tests the null hypothesis of no treatment effect for the marker-positive patients. The threshold of significance for this test is prespecified as some value α_+ less than the total type I error 0.05 of the design. For example, α_+ may be 0.04. If

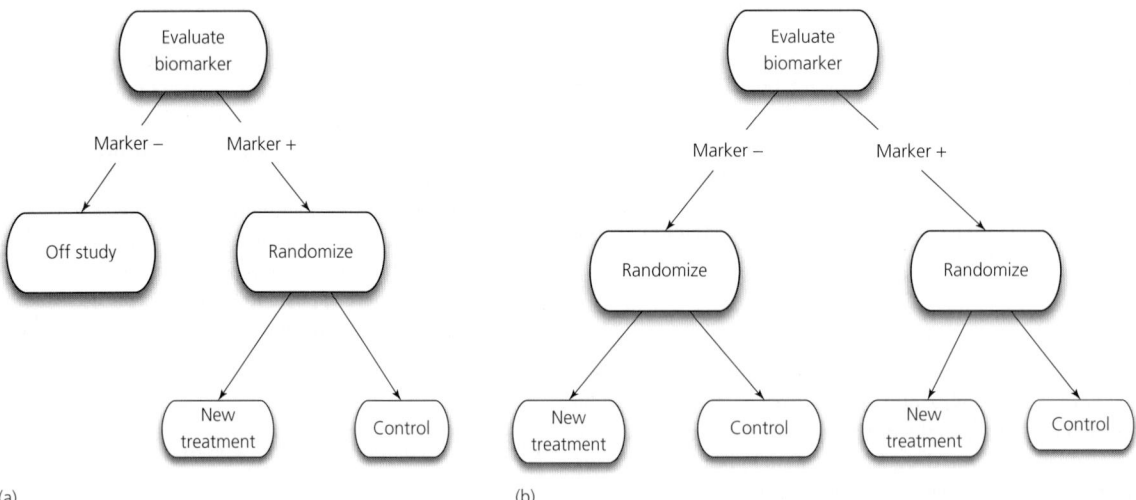

(a)   (b)

Figure 3 (a) The targeted enrichment design is used for evaluating a new treatment in the population of patients who are identified using a predictive biomarker as best candidates for benefit from the new treatment. It is primarily for settings where there is a compelling basis for believing that "marker-negative" patients will not benefit from the new treatment and an analytically validated test is available. (b) The "all comers' design" or "marker stratification design" is used for evaluating the effectiveness of a new treatment versus a control in a population prospectively characterized by a binary predictive marker. A detailed prospective analysis plan should describe the primary comparison of treatment to control, in the marker-positive, marker-negative, and overall populations. With a focused analysis plan that limits the study-wide type I error to the traditional 5% level, claims of treatment effectiveness in marker-positive patients need not be restricted to cases where the treatment is effective overall or there is a significant interaction.

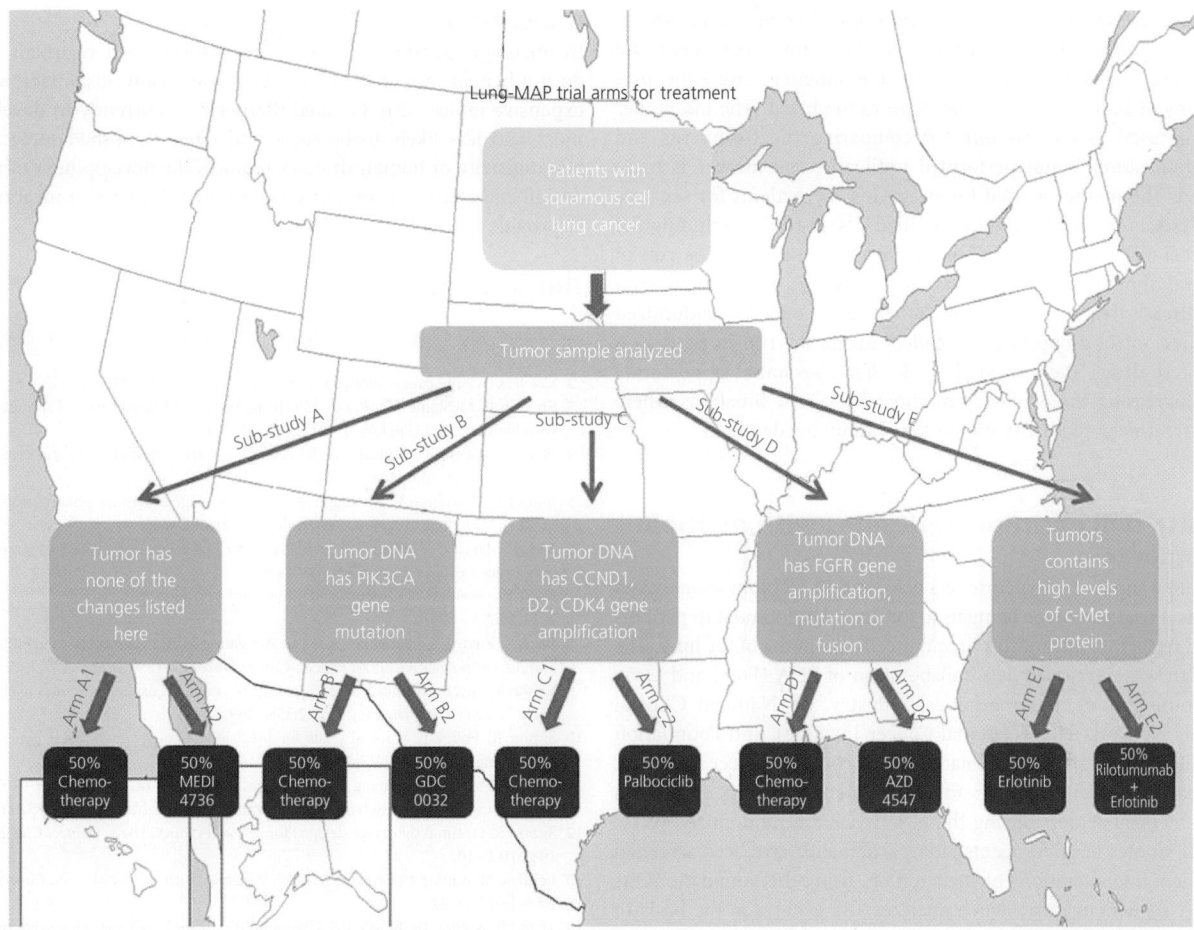

Figure 4 Lung-MAP clinical trial master design. Patients with squamous cell carcinoma of the lung are screened for genomic mutations in their tumors. Depending on the genomic alterations found, patients are enrolled on one of six randomized clinical trials. Each component trial compares the same control treatment to a treatment specially designed for patients with a class of genomic alterations. Each component clinical trial is a randomized phase II/III clinical trial, which may serve as a pivotal trial for approval of the test drug for the selected patient population. Source: National Cancer Institute, http://www.lung-map.org.

that null hypothesis is rejected, then the null hypothesis for the marker-negative patients is tested using a significance threshold of 0.05. If the null hypothesis for the marker-positive patients is not rejected, then the null hypothesis for the pooled overall population is tested using a significance threshold of $0.05 - \alpha_+$, 0.01 in this example.

Other "real-world" experience with stratification and enrichment designs are described by Freidlin et al.[25] and Mandrekar and Sargent.[26] Adaptive forms of the enrichment design in which one starts with "all comers" and adaptively restricts the eligibility are described by Wang et al.,[27] Rosenblum and VanDerLaan,[28] and Simon and Simon.[29]

Prospective–retrospective designs

In some cases, a completed randomized clinical trial with archived tumor specimens can be used to evaluate treatment effect in a subset determined by a new candidate biomarker. For example, the hypothesis that the effectiveness of anti-EGFR antibodies in colorectal cancer would be limited to patients whose tumors did not contain K-RAS mutations was evaluated in randomized clinical trials that had been planned before this hypothesis was suggested by other investigators. Simon et al.[30] described a prospective–retrospective approach to using archived tumor specimens for a focused re-analysis of a randomized phase III

trial with regard to a predictive biomarker. The approach requires that archived specimens be available on most patients, and that an analysis plan focused on a single marker be developed before performing the blinded assays. The finding must also be evaluated in two such prospective–retrospective trials in order to be considered type I evidence. It is not necessary that the randomization should have used the marker as a stratification variable. This is not relevant to the validity of the analysis of treatment effect in marker-positive patients.[22] Simon[22] has also pointed out that there is no critical minimum proportion of the tumors archived necessary for the retrospective–prospective approach. The key factor is that there should be no bias between treatment groups with regard to availability of archived specimens. Lack of such bias can be assured if patient and physician agreement for tissue archival is established before randomization.

Run-in designs

Predictive biomarkers are usually thought of as biological measurements that are obtained from the tumor or the patient before the start of treatment. Hong and Simon[31] developed a run-in design that permits a pharmacodynamic, immunologic, or intermediate response endpoint measured after a short run-in period on the new treatment or the control to be used as the predictive biomarker. After measuring the biomarker during the run-in period, either all patients are randomized between continuing the new treatment or switching to control or just the "marker-positive" patients, those showing substantial change in the measurement from the pre-treatment baseline measurement are randomized. The biomarker is not used as an endpoint for comparing the treatments and randomization is not performed until after the marker is measured. The marker is used for stratifying the patients for separate analysis as in the all comers' stratified design or for excluding the marker-negative patients as in the enrichment design. The run-in period should be short because one does not want the survival or disease-free survival of the patients subsequently randomized to the control group to be extended during the run-in period on the test drug. The run-in designs offer substantial opportunity for increasing the efficiency of clinical trials in situations where pre-treatment-predictive biomarkers cannot be identified.

Phase II/III enrichment designs with multiple biomarkers

Figure 4 shows the structure of a new lung-MAP biomarker-driven clinical trial prototype being used for drug development in patients with refractory advanced squamous cell carcinoma of the lung. The design was developed as a collaboration of FDA (Food and Drug Administration), pharmaceutical industry, US National Clinical Trials Network, NCI (National Cancer Institute), and Foundation Medicine under the coordination of Friends of Cancer Research. Plans call for enrolling up to 5000 patients through more than 200 medical centers during the next 5 years in randomized phase II/III studies of novel agents after participants have been screened for genomic alterations of their tumors using the FoundationOne DNA sequencing test, which analyzes 182 genes. On the basis of the results of the screening, patients will be channeled to one of five randomized phase II/III trials. Each of the five randomized trials will have a phase II stage and will progress to the phase III stage if results are promising. The primary endpoint is PFS. These trials are all potentially pivotal phase III enrichment clinical trials with companion diagnostics for different patient subsets. As the evaluations of these drugs are completed, an additional five to seven agents will be tested.

The new models of collaboration required by clinical trials of the "genomic era" and the challenges ahead

We are still at the start of a "learning curve" in classifying cancers molecularly in a therapeutically relevant manner. It is likely that we will soon be moving from simple classifications relying on aberrations at the DNA level toward more complex classifications also incorporating critical information generated by RNA sequencing and (phospho)protein platforms. It can also be foreseen that "pathway-directed" treatment strategies will replace single-target-directed strategies, as aiming at the latter is likely to fail in view of the plasticity of the cancer cell. Moving "genomics" to "therapeutics" implies dealing with uncertainty and statisticians will continue to play a critical role in this regard.

At the same time, it is clear that achieving the benefits of "personalized" oncology requires paradigm changes in academic clinical investigation, with the setup of large collaborative teams, in industry drug development, with less walls between drug development paths when it comes to combination strategies, and in regulatory evaluation, with more adaptive licensing routes for new compounds or innovative drug combinations.

Conclusion

In oncology, treatment of broad populations with regimens that do not benefit most patients is less economically sustainable with expensive molecularly targeted therapeutics currently in development and less likely to be successful. The established molecular heterogeneity of human diseases requires the development of new design and analysis paradigms for using randomized clinical trials to provide a reliable basis predictive medicine.

References

1 Stratton MR, Campbell PJ, Futreal PA. The cancer genome. *Nature.* 2009;**458**: 719–724.

2 Sawyers CL. The cancer biomarker problem. *Nature.* 2008;**452**:548–552.

3 Freidlin B, McShane LM, Polley MY, Korn EL. Randomized phase II trial designs with biomarkers. *J Clin Oncol.* 2012;**30**:3304–3309.

4 Pusztai L, Hess KR. Clinical trial design for microarray predictive marker discovery and assessment. *Ann Oncol.* 2004;**15**:1731–1737.

5 Jones CL, Holmgren E. An adaptive Simon two-stage design for phase 2 studies of targeted therapies. *Contemp Clin Trials.* 2007;**28**:654–661.

6 Kim ES, Herbst JJ, Wistuba II, et al. The BATTLE trial: personalizing therapy for lung cancer. *Cancer Discov.* 2011;**1**:44–53.

7 Korn EL, Freidlin B. Outcome-adaptive randomization: is it useful? *J Clin Oncol.* 2011;**29**:771–776.

8 Bose R, Kavuri S, Searleman A, et al. Activating HER2 mutations in HER2 gene amplification negative breast cancer. *Cancer Discov.* 2013;**3**(2):224–237.

9 Simon R, Roychowdhury S. Implementing personalized cancer genomics in clinical trials. *Nat Rev Drug Discov.* 2013;**12**:358–369.

10 Simon R, Polley E. Clinical trials for precision oncology using next generation sequencing. *Pers Med.* 2013;**10**:485–495.

11 Prahallad A, Sun C, Huang S, et al. Unresponsiveness of colon cancer to BRAF (V600E) inhibition through feedback activation of EGFR. *Nature.* 2012;**483**:100–103.

12 Simon R. Optimal two-stage designs for phase II clinical trials. *Control Clin Trials.* 1989;**10**:1–10.

13 LeBlanc M, Rankin C, Crowley J. Multiple histology phase II trials. *Clin Cancer Res.* 2009;**15**:4256–62.

14 Thall PF, Wathen JK, Bekele BN, Champlin RE, Baker LO, Benjamin RS. Hierarchical Bayesian approaches to phase II trials in diseases with multiple subtypes. *Stat Med.* 2003;**22**:763–80.

15 Freidlin B, Korn EL. Borrowing information across subgroups in phase II trials: Is it useful? *Clin Cancer Res.* 2013;**19**:1326–34.

16 Shak S. Overview of the trastuzumab (Herceptin) anti-HER2 monoclonal antibody clinical program in HER2-overexpressing metastatic breast cancer. *Semin Oncol.* 1999;**26**:71–77.

17 Chapman PB, Hauschild A, Robert C, et al. Improved survival with vemurafenib in melanoma with BRAF V600E mutation. *N Engl J Med.* 2011;**364**:2507–2516.

18 Shaw AT, Yeap BY, Solomon BJ, et al. Effect of crizotinib on overall survival in patients with advanced non-small-cell lung cancer harbouring ALK gene rearrangement: a retrospective analysis. *Lancet Oncol.* 2011;**12**:1004–1012.

19 Simon R, Maitournam A. Evaluating the efficiency of targeted designs for randomized clinical trials. *Clin Cancer Res.* 2005;**10**:6759–6763.

20 Maitournam A, Simon R. On the efficiency of targeted clinical trials. *Stat Med.* 2005;**24**:329–339.

21 Simon RM. *Genomic Clinical Trials and Predictive Medicine.* Cambridge, MA: Cambridge University Press; 2013.

22 Simon R. Stratification and partial ascertainment of biomarker value in biomarker driven clinical trials. *J Biopharm Stat.* 2014;**2**(5):1011–1021.

23 Simon R. Using genomics in clinical trial design. *Clin Cancer Res.* 2008;**14**: 5984–5993.

24 Freidlin B, Korn EL. Biomarker enrichment strategies: matching trial design to biomarker credentials. *Nat Rev Clin Oncol.* 2014;**11**:81–90.

25 Freidlin B, McShane LM, Korn EL. Randomized clinical trials with biomarkers: design issues. *J Natl Cancer Inst.* 2010;**102**:152–160.

26 Mandrekar SJ, Sargent DJ. Predictive biomarker validation in practice: lessons from real trials. *Clin Trials.* 2010;**7**:567–573.

27 Wang SJ, Hung HMJ, O'Neill RT. Adaptive patient enrichment designs in therapeutic trials. *Biom J.* 2009;**51**:358–374.

28 Rosenblum M, VanDerLaan MJ. Optimizing randomized trial designs to distinguish which subpopulations benefit from treatment. *Biometrika.* 2011;**98**:845–860.

29 Simon N, Simon R. Adaptive enrichment designs in clinical trials. *Biostatistics.* 2013;**14**:613–625.

30 Simon RM, Paik S, Hayes DF. Use of archived specimens in evaluation of prognostic and predictive biomarkers. *J Natl Cancer Inst.* 2009;**101**:1–7.

31 Hong F, Simon R. Run-in phase III trial designs with pharmacodynamic predictive biomarkers. *J Natl Cancer Inst.* 2013;**105**:1628–1633.

22 Clinical informatics

Edward P. Ambinder, MD

Overview

Informatics is the integration of information technology into health care. For oncology, the need to understand informatics is critical because of the need to keep up with the rapidly changing basic, translational and clinical cancer research findings, therapeutic interventions using panomic data required for precision medicine, latest practice guidelines, shifting reimbursement practices, and the dominating and at times frustrating electronic health record (EHR) that is the repository of our health data and window into the health care system. All of this must take place in a value-enhanced practice environment that constantly measures our quality of care in a well-coordinated system for our engaged patients who are digitally connected to multiple practices, their hospital, their smartphones and medical devices, their personal health record and multiple EHRs. Oncologists will soon have a well-defined "Oncology Digital Health Information Technology System" that will redefine cancer research by capturing meaningful and actionable patient data in every cancer patient. They will continue to participate in the mobile computing revolution that is just beginning to have a transformative effect on all of medicine where computers will do our work, apps work with other apps and EHRs to educate us and our patients and use real electronically shareable and reusable medical data. Today, the majority of patients have their cancer care documented in EHRs. As rapid learning systems (RLSs) such as ASCO's CancerLinQ capture all this data and use Big Data analytic tools for capturing and comparing similar cancer patients as to the best treatments and outcomes, we will have real precision medicine. The evolving "Internet of Things" where medical devices and health care platforms will give us the unprecedented ability to measure in real time the health and wellness of our cancer patients undergoing chemotherapy treatments on a 24-h basis will provide huge monetary savings for the health system, improved quality of care, and innovative medical research as cancer care develops into a RLS.

Introduction

Oncologists and their patients are facing disruptive changes in health care practice, research, governmental oversight, business practices, communication, and reimbursement—changes brought on by the individual growth and merging of the fields of information technology with medical technology, medical practice, biology, and physics. We now practice in large hospital systems or accountable care organizations rather than in small group practice silos; deal with changing reimbursement methods as we transition from fee-for-service to bundling payments and defined encounters of care; document our patient care using electronic media rather than paper; and see the doctor–patient relationship become more patient-centric. We are increasingly communicating electronically with all health care stakeholders, including our patients.

This dramatic increase in the quantity, quality, and ease of finding information—brought about by the use of computers and the effortlessness of connecting everyone and everything—all of which has been brought about by the Internet, has changed our lives forever. However, we remain frustrated with our electronic devices needed to communicate with our health care system because they still require typing or dictation for data entry, and the data entered are not easily understood by the computer or able to be shared, reused, or reported easily because of the absence of seamless data interoperability where data entered into one device could be understood, used, and reused effectively in another device.

Clayton Christensen presciently warned us about the disruptive effects of this transformation in 1997,[1] and he warned us specifically about its effects on health care in 2008.[2] Indeed, for the first time, this new, disruptive digital world of medicine is increasingly defined by information becoming electronically mobile, cheap, available to all, and consumer-oriented to such an extent that almost all recent information technology advances in hardware and software begin with the consumer rather than business. Oncologists and their patients must begin to understand this transformative event that will directly address our current frustrations.

An oncology digital health information technology system

Common data elements and value sets

Common data elements define the data to be collected in the medical record by specifically identifying the label of each data field and the appropriate value set to choose for data entry. When possible, the value set choice should reference a standard code system such as a clinical vocabulary used to describe the clinical encounter (e.g., SNOMED-CT), the laboratory data (e.g., LOINC), the terms describing basic and clinical research activities [e.g., cancer Biomedical Informatics Grid (caBIG)], and the elements and codes that define specific disease classifications used for billing and registry reporting purposes (e.g., ICD-9 and ICD-10 codes).

Data types

Computers capture electronic *structured* and *unstructured* data. Data can be structured using data elements and value sets that are machine readable, reusable, shareable, actionable, multiuser-able, and multipurposeful. Unstructured or narrative data are entered by typing or dictation and adds context making it is understood by humans but not by computers unless sophisticated natural language processing tools are used or the data can be tagged by metadata that renders them searchable. Searchable or machine-readable data would permit the EHR (electronic health record) to provide clinical decision support (CDS), user education, and secondary reporting purposes. In reality, both types of data are important in capturing the complete patient's health record.

Holland-Frei Cancer Medicine, Ninth Edition. Edited by Robert C. Bast Jr., Carlo M. Croce, William N. Hait, Waun Ki Hong, Donald W. Kufe, Martine Piccart-Gebhart, Raphael E. Pollock, Ralph R. Weichselbaum, Hongyang Wang, and James F. Holland.
© 2017 John Wiley & Sons, Inc. ISBN: 978-1-118-93469-2

Table 1 EHR functional elements defined by ASCO's Electronic Health Record Workgroup.

EHR functional element	How it is used in the practice
View patient information	Review patient's symptoms or chief complaints, medication list, test results, and other clinical documentation
Gather data	Build electronic patient charts that are searchable. Build patient charts from customizable templates
Compile data	Pull together patient or practice population, histories, and graph it or map it for analysis. Report generation
Query patient or practice data to generate standard and/or custom reports	Assist in evaluating, diagnosing, and reviewing acute or chronic diseases and treatment regimens and provide appropriate clinical alerts and warnings based on established guidelines. Interoperability with other systems
Clinical decision support	Interact with internal practice management and other internal information systems (e.g., laboratory information system—LIS); interface with external hospital, lab, imaging, pharmacies, and payers
Search capabilities	Query the database for reports on clinical issues and costs
Patient management	Manage the individual patient's acute and chronic diseases and conditions
Practice marketing	Provide information regarding types of services you perform most often. Provide analysis on your patients' clinical conditions, referral base, and patient population
Standardization	Standardize disease management goals and treatment regimens for patient groups within your practice
Billing and coding	Provide internal checks and balances with ICD and CPT codes to details of the patient encounter; integrate E&M coding and HCPCS codes. Order entry, order labs, imaging, referrals, and other nonmedications
Chemotherapy ordering	Initiate chemotherapy orders, associated ancillary therapies, and dose modifications with proper authorization and confirmation
e-Prescribing	Authorize and manage prescription refills. Access formulary information. Route new prescriptions online to pharmacy
Communication	Communicate online with patients, colleagues, payers, hospitals, and pharmacies
Provide built-in compliance and regulatory guidance	Compliance
Clinical trials	Conduct research, registry, and clinical trial activities
Patient interaction	Incorporate information originating from the patient, including data from a personal health record (PHR) and medical and patient devices
Quality measurement	Use data to participate in quality measurement programs

Table 2 Oncology-specific documentation required in an oncology EHR.

Provide menu-driven site/histology/pathology findings
Manage patient response to treatment on flow sheets
Document intent and goals of adjuvant/curative versus palliative therapy
Document patient performance status per standardized guidelines
Maintain list of co-morbid conditions and major toxicities expected to complicate chemotherapy
Plan and manage chemotherapy/biotherapy regimens
Manage and automate body surface area (BSA), starting doses, and dose adjustments
Manage chemotherapy delivery—IV and oral, number of cycles, duration
Document drug administration process
Track duration of treatment and number of planned cycles
Schedule and document radiation therapy and/or maintain results
Assess pain and supportive care needs
Manage patients on clinical trials
Clinical Oncology Treatment Plan and Summary and Survivorship Report

Software functionalities and documentation

Software functionalities refer to the capabilities that a software program should provide. For all EHRs, ePrescription software is necessary, whereas for medical oncology, EHRs chemotherapy administration is required. Table 1 lists EHR functional elements defined by ASCO's EHR workgroup and Table 2 lists oncology-specific documentation required in an oncology EHR.

Internet

The Internet serves as the communication and messaging component of the digital health care system. The development of the Internet can be separated into four stages. At its inception, the Internet was used for "searching" for information and "communicating" with text, files and pictures, and any media. Users were mostly academicians and business people. E-mail and bulletin boards were popular. Next, we were able to "do" things using web sites. Consumers discovered the Internet and commerce exploded. Then, we were able to "socialize" and "collaborate" using social media sites like Facebook. Apps exploded as mobile computing dominated the Internet. Now, we are entering the Internet of "Things," where any medical device can inexpensively communicate over the Internet with other devices and computers.

Computer interoperability and data exchange

Computer interoperability and data exchange or the sharing of data requires that the data created in one EHR be sent to another EHR with full understanding and context so that it will be placed in the appropriate data field of the receiving program. ASCO and the National Cancer Institute's caBIG and Community Cancer Center Program created the Clinical Oncology Requirements for the EHR (CORE) that delineated the core common data elements, functionalities, and interoperability standards for oncology that helped to define the original oncology EHR certification criteria used by the Certification Commission for Healthcare Information Technology (CCHIT).[3] Seamless interoperability standards have foundational importance by defining and transmitting medical information in a way that will make our data entry, computerized workflows, and result reporting dramatically simplified and efficient.

Most of the data elements that we use in medicine have been defined, standardized, and harmonized into code sets and SNOMED-CT, a clinical vocabulary. Meaningful Use Stage 1 brought some interoperability to public health reporting. Meaningful use stage 2 brought additional interoperability to well-defined content, vocabulary, and transport standards for transitions of care. Our leading Standards Developing Organization (SDO), Health

Level Seven International (HL7®) has defined and standardized the use of clinically useful summary documents known as consolidated clinical document architecture (C-CDA) documents.[4,5]

ASCO's Data Standards and Interoperability Task Force, which I chair, has developed two oncology-specific interoperable technology standards. We have taken two ASCO Treatment Plan and Summary paper templates developed for adjuvant breast cancer and adjuvant colorectal cancer[6–8] and transformed them into implementation guides (IGs). The IGs can be used to create an interoperable document that can be electronically exchanged between any computer system that adheres to the HL7 C-CDA standard.[9] CDAs define content and transport of a document that can be large. This document standard [entitled Clinical Oncology Treatment Plan and Summary (COTPS)] summarizes cancer data from almost all medical reports that are created by physicians, hospitals, laboratories, imaging centers, pharmacies, and patients during the cancer journey and gives review and guidance to the patient and their providers involved with their care. We plan on creating similar C-CDA documents for other common cancers, patient-reported outcomes, and cancer survivorship plans.

At the HIMSS Interoperability Showcase for 2014, ASCO's COTPS was used to demonstrate how the use of common data elements, standardized reports, adherence to interoperability standards, and use of innovative data entry tools can make provider workflows more efficient and our notes and reports sharable, actionable, and multipurposeful. There, 10 vendors used these standards for exchanging data in real time. Novel data entry tools including voice-recognition transcription to text to data to structured data, a care plan manager, medical devices in the patient's home demonstrating data capture and alerting capabilities, patient education, patient-reported outcomes and questionnaires, and actionable reports for quality, research, population health, and big data analytic registries were shown. A health information exchange captured and displayed the compilation of clinical reports in real time and made them available to all vendor systems while recording the cancer journey of a woman given adjuvant treatment for her breast cancer. The care plan manager was able to electronically create the ASCO COTPS for the patient, caregivers, and all providers.

HL7 is closer to approving a new, nimble, and simpler interoperability and data exchange standard called Fast Healthcare Interoperability Resources (FHIR).[10] FHIR can represent granular or discrete data elements and documents. Part of the enthusiasm surrounding FHIR is due to the elegant simplicity of the technology. It combines the best features of HL7 V2, HL7 V3, and CDA, while leveraging the latest web service technologies. The major technology change embodied in FHIR is a fundamental move away from a document-centric approach to a data-level access approach using application programming interfaces (APIs). The ability of this interface to exchange data with any software including the EHR using a public API can foster an ecosystem of interoperability among health IT systems. Specifically, FHIR features a modular concept called *Resources* that can be extended and adapted as a step forward from today's document-based exchange architecture using a very basic set of structured data like a medication list or lab result. FHIR provides for a plug-and-play platform working within and between systems that is conceptually similar to the Apple app system. FHIR would also allow developers to create new and innovative apps by using the public APIs and following a well-defined set of rules. Most vendors would likely embrace a public API offering a unified approach to share data with any application. Systems can easily read the extensions using the same framework as other resources, and when FHIR and the SMART

platform are combined, we have a nimble interoperable standard that can capture the functionalities of Apple's App model. Recently, many EHR vendors and health care organizations have formed the Argonaut Project to accelerate query/response interoperability under the auspices of ANSI-certified HL7 standards development organization processes for sharing electronic health care information, a most promising change from groups that have in the past encouraged being proprietary.[11]

For the oncologist, we will have true interoperability and data exchange whereby small nimble apps will be able to accept data from another app or an enterprise-wide EHR, use that data effectively, send it to another app and eventually return it to the originating application source with updated data that can be understood and incorporated into the originating program's database. Efficient data entry tools, educational links for the oncologist or for their patients (think CDS), wellness data incorporation and useful personal health records (PHRs) creation, important current and meaningful alerts, and automated secondary uses of data can be reported such as quality measures, state registry data, and rapid learning systems (RLSs). Enterprise-wide EHRs that takes years for updates and do very little in educating the user can rely on these nimble apps from trusted sources to enhance their products. Centers for Medicare and Medicaid Services (CMS) has made interoperability a major goal for the country in its recent report "Connecting Health and Care for the Nation."[12]

Electronic health record database and repository

The EHR is a systematic database that collects longitudinal, attributable, secure, nonmodifiable digital health information and data about an individual patient or population. It should be capable of being shared across all health care settings, providers, and with the patient. It should represent data that accurately captures and presents the latest health status of the patient and their clinical encounters. It does a superb job in documenting EHR-defined clinical activities and administrative requirements, but today it is unacceptable in providing efficient data entry, educational and safety features, effective provider workflows, helpful CDS, seamless interoperability across all EHRs, plug-and-play modular designs and automated registry, and other secondary reporting needs. This is because the initial EHR creators modeled it after a paper chart that was passive and a nonparticipant in health care. It lacked an understanding of the clinical workflow or a provider's or the health care system's needs. Today, government financial incentives for purchasing EHRs and meeting meaningful use that require some interoperability, quality improvement, CDS, and registry reporting have persuaded the majority of oncologists to adopt them. Unfortunately, they are frustrated because these meaningful use functionalities are poorly designed into today's EHRs. EHR data must not only document our clinical activities with relevance, succinctness, and context that paper systems may have more easily captured in the past, but it also must be used for secondary purposes such as clinical and population research, quality measurements, registry reporting, reimbursement documentation, and RLS analytics to name a few that current EHRs do not effectively address. We spend less face-to-face interaction time with our cancer patients, more time with the computer screen using menus, interfaces, and alerts,[13] and our workdays are averaging 48 min longer due to EHR use.[14]

EHRs must become more adept in data entry providing voice to text to data functionality (dictate and have the computer use natural language and machine reading skills to place the dictated material into corresponding data fields). Also, by opening up their software, EHR vendors could unleash a creative army of developers that could help their users and improve the product.

Table 3 American College of Physicians proposed basic documentation for electronic health records.

Primary purpose of clinical documentation should be to support patient care and improve clinical outcomes through enhanced communication
Physicians should define standards for documentation, and information exchange should be facilitated by standards set by individual specialties
EHRs should facilitate seamless patient care that improves outcomes and support data analysis that enables value-based care
Collecting structured data should only be done when useful for care or important for quality improvement
Prior authorizations should not require unique data and format requirements
Patient engagement and care quality will be enhanced when patients are able to access their progress notes as well as the rest of their record
Research is needed to improve the processes involved in documenting care and facilitating technological advancements that allow better, more accurate record of observations
EHR development should be optimized for longitudinal team-based care
Cognitive processes during documentation should be supported in EHR design
When reusing data, embedded tags should be included to identify the original source
Checkboxes to indicate something that has already been documented should be eliminated
Patient-generated data should be incorporated into their medical record and the source identity maintained

Source: Data from Ref. 15.

The Medical Informatics Committee of the American College of Physicians has recently explored EHR documentation issues and written an excellent position paper with cogent recommendations for changes that are listed in Table 3. Yet, computers will remain our individual link to our health care system for the foreseeable future. We must find more efficient ways to capture and reuse data and have computers do more of our work.

Personal health records

Patients will continue to take a more responsive role in health care as they pay a larger share of its cost, make known their values and wishes, and help make key decisions. With the unlimited educational resources of the Internet, our patients have access to the same medical literature and textbooks that we have. With meaningful use requirements for providing electronic patient reports to the patient, with the CMS proposing that patients have access to their laboratory test results, with e-mailing between patients and oncologists becoming commonplace (and reimbursable with some payers), and with most medical reports becoming available in digitized form, patients will be in control of their medical record. A pilot project that makes almost the entire medical record electronically available to patients has been successfully implemented at the MD Anderson Cancer Center; the majority of patients are more than satisfied, and most doctors, many of whom were skeptical initially, have become converted proponents of "open access" care.[16] The highly successful OpenNotes project is an example of how eager patients are receiving more of their medical information.[17]

Knowledge and education

Oncology knowledge bases
After aggregating a cancer patient's actionable health data into our EHR using our data gathering and entry tools, we need to have our EHR assist us with CDS tools to search our available knowledge bases today and prepare for contributing to a RLS for oncology with our EHRs to hopefully provide us with a "technology to aggregate individual patient data across populations that share common characteristics defining a health state in order to generate knowledge and learning" into improving patient outcomes, quality, and health care value utilizing practice guidelines or algorithms as so eloquently discussed by Yu.[18] Our knowledge bases in oncology consist of clinical trials data, systems biology data, patient-sourced data (health and wellness), and health systems data on operational processes and patient outcomes.

Clinical trials data come from being published in peer-reviewed journals or systematic reviews of the medical literature and being vetted and weighed for quality and knowledge gaps by experts gathered by a professional society and published as a clinical practice guideline.

Systems biology data in oncology help us characterize the molecular, cell growth regulatory and immunologic changes found in different cancers as they progress, permitting us to understand their causation, classification, and therapies. As computational biology and their analytical tools begin to deal with the terabytes of panomic data from an individual patient whose genome, transcriptome, proteome, and metabolome could be routinely assessed in the near future, nimble resources such as The Cancer Genome Atlas[19] and the Global Alliance for Genomics and Health[20] will support providers and researchers in their quest for providing personalized medicine and improved patient outcomes. These knowledge bases working together will permit a more rapid drug evaluation and approval process for targeted drugs by identifying exceptional cancer responses associated with specific panomic aberrations.

Finally, the Digital Health Information Technology System will use our EHR clinical data, patient-reported data, laboratory information systems and data repositories, administrative claim data, cancer registries, wellness, activity and nutritional data, and postmarketing surveillance data to capture health care systems data that reflect the real-world patient population experience with our therapies.

Clinical decision support systems (CDSS)
CDSS (clinical decision support systems) are user-chosen or situational awareness invoking application tools that have access to knowledge bases or practice guidelines that are used by EHRs to educate and/or alert their users about patient-specific clinical decision making and health management at the point of service. Musen et al. have described the following three types of CDSS[21]:

• Information management (direct link to a textbook section or Internet site or a tool such as an Infobutton that is a context-sensitive link embedded within an EHR, which allows easy retrieval and subsequent electronic reuse of the relevant information residing in the EHR or at an Internet link)[22]
• Situational awareness (alerts or patient dashboards)
• Patient specific logic-based guidance on diagnostic and therapeutic choices such as could be derived from Knowledge bases or a RLS like CancerLinQ.[18]

Rapid learning systems
As cancer patients increasingly have their medical records digitized, it becomes obvious that there is a treasure trove of clinical data in these records that have the potential to benefit society by opening up what happens to the 97% of cancer patients who do not go

on clinical trials. By learning about the comparative benefits or harm of our new treatments and procedures in nonclinical trial patients after these therapies have been granted regulatory approval, we can apply findings and improve treatments on a continuous, ongoing basis. The National Cancer Policy Forum of the Institute of Medicine workshop entitled "A Foundation for Evidence-Driven Practice: A Rapid Learning System for Cancer Care" examined the elements of a RLS for cancer.[23] It recommended that the elements of such a system include registries and databases, emerging information technology, tools for patient-centered and patient-driven CDS and patient engagement, ways of accommodating culture change, clinical practice guidelines, point-of-care needs in clinical oncology, and federal policy issues and implications. ASCO and others have begun to define a RLS for cancer called CancerLinQ.[24,25] It will use these tools to develop a more thorough understanding of cancer biology, defining a cancer based on a molecularly driven diagnosis; it will also incorporate a therapeutic development system that uses oncology EHR registries to produce smarter and faster clinical trials. Because of its more seamless integration of clinical and translational research, it has the potential to ensure that every cancer patient's experience can inform research and improve care.

RLS will require computational tools for data compilation and analysis from pooled massive databases combining machine learning, data visualization, statistics, and programming. For our cancer patients, this *Big Data* operation could incorporate all clinical data, genomic data, wellness and health data derived from medical devices and medical payment data obtained from Medicare and the private payers. ASCO's CancerLinQ hopes to obtain all EHR and clinical knowledge base data for all cancer patients residing in the United States from our offices, cancer centers, and hospitals. An oncologist could enter all the clinical information on his patient and ask CancerLinQ to electronically match the patient to the closest group of patients with similar clinical characteristics and reveal the treatments that produced the best outcomes for these similar patients. In addition, it could generate knowledge for improving quality and cost effectiveness of care by creating an informatics infrastructure for practice-based research networks to collect practice-based evidence using CDSS functionality built into our EHRs to link machine-readable oncology knowledge bases and guidelines repositories as originally described by Sim et al.[26]

The mobile computing revolution

Today, general-purpose Windows and Mac OS X computers are the devices most commonly used for EHRs, but they carry the burden of 30 years of rapid, unplanned change. Many physicians and patients are frustrated with a lot of the existing EHR software choices that rely on the existing PC and Mac paradigm that uses windows, icons, menus, and pointers for human–computer interaction.

With the introduction of the iPhone by Apple in 2007, Apple introduced a natural human-like interface that could sense touch, touch force, voice, vision, hearing, location, body position, height, and direction. It could communicate over Wi-Fi, Bluetooth, cellular, and NFC (near field communication). It has become the most easily learned and most efficient mobile operating system available. Most EHR vendors today are providing access to their programs via iPhones, iPads, and Android devices, and others are calling for an Apple-like app platform for EHRs.[27]

Government and medical leadership consensus on a mobile HIT evolution

For the first time, our thought leaders in health information technology (HIT), governmental groups overseeing health information

and EHR technology, Congress, our President and his expert panels, our medical leaders and specialty organizations, medical standards organizations, informatic experts, the health care industry and even many, vendors/developers agree that the technologic infrastructure, and recent advances in hardware, software, and services can provide a new relationship between physicians and their computers where computers serve us as an efficient, up to date, personalized, customizable, secure, shareable, and knowledgeable assistant. Halamka popularized the term "electronic medicine"[28] to urge EHRs to adopt these mobile computing advances in 2011, and I have taken the liberty to include additional items that have been developed over the past 4 years that will help oncologists participate in a true Oncology Digital Health Information Technology System.

Cloud computing

Cloud computing refers to storing patient data in centralized servers connected to the Internet rather than in our offices and provides the ability to scale up complex software that can be updated frequently and simultaneously with all software users at different sites thus removing the need of our offices to deal with database administration, server hosting, and data security at great financial savings. By being Internet connected, EHRs can more easily share data with patients and other physicians, send reports to external registries and have sophisticated tools to assist with learning the software initially and later on with updates.

Apps

Apps are versatile, small programs that use web-based APIs, that have extensions which can work with data passed on from another app or an EHR program. Apps could provide new functionalities for the EHR or could collect data from the EHR and send it to registries or RLSs that could analyze this new data and provide CDS for the EHR program. APIs are simply a collection of functions that a programmer can call to use another programs services and data. APIs contain tiny, atomistic chunks of data that must use consistent units and terminology that are handled much more efficiently. Natural language processing is being used to extract these tiny chunks of data from our narrative dictations and create structured machine-readable content that can be used more effectively by the computer for any purpose. It is an ideal method for permitting a medical specialty society to provide specialty-specific updated tools for EHRs that find it hard to keep their software up to date with the needs of the medical specialist.

Modular software and application programming interfaces (APIs)

The SMART (substitutable medical apps and reusable technology) platform designed by Mandl and Kohane[27] is an ideal platform to bring Apple's App model system into the EHR ecosystem. Mandl recently pointed out how this platform could work in an emergency situation to permit the Center for Disease Control and Prevention (CDC) to create an App that could work with any cooperating EHR and reshape ER triage workflows to emphasize travel history and recommend rapidly updated assessment and isolation guidelines for handling patients who present to an ER with fever and recent travel to an Ebola-affected region.[29] The App could be immediately used by all EHRs, updated easily, and specific data about all patients quarantined by a hospital could be sent back to the CDC for monitoring and reporting purposes on a national level. He points out that this hypothetical app could be rapidly written once and run nearly everywhere.

Engaged, digitally connected digitized patients, medical devices, and the Internet of Things

Over this time period, our health system has been transformed so that patients instead of being passive participants in the health care system are now very engaged as they have access to the same medical literature that we have on the Internet and their complete medical record permitting joint decision making with their providers leading to better outcomes and fewer malpractice suits. Using digital educational tools now available on web sites or in Apps, patient have a better understanding of their diseases, treatments, upcoming procedures, suitable clinical trials, informed consent, and can provide their values, wishes, and misconceptions directly to shared EHRs in some institutions.

As we enter the Internet of Things stage with inexpensive, accurate, intelligent medical devices, disease prevention and early medical interventions along with the increasing interest in the wellness of the patient will lead to the rapid uptake of these medical devices and wearable computing garments that connect wirelessly with our smartphones, facilitating reimbursable telemedicine consults with our patients with chronic illnesses at home and early detection of adverse events from our therapies or their diseases. Using digital devices to measure vital signs and digital EKGs, stethoscopes, cameras, ophthalmoscopes, otoscopes, and ultrasound devices attached to our smartphone, the physical exam can be completed remotely.[30] Monitoring and analyzing this digital data will require Big Data tools that are rapidly being developed to transform medicine as it is currently practiced. Also, certain regulatory and compliance issues arise when using medical devices such as security, auditability, and the need for provenance that are currently being addressed.

Precision medicine

Precision medicine is the prevention and treatment strategies that take individual variability into account using large-scale biologic databases (such as the human genome sequence), powerful methods for characterizing patients (such as proteomics, metabolomics, genomics, diverse cellular assays, and even mobile health technology), and computational tools for analyzing large sets of data. Whole genome sequencing is reaching the $1000 threshold and we are fast approaching the ability to sequence the "digital" patient's germ line DNA, RNA, microbiome, epigenome along with their environment, anatomical, and clinical features.[31] The breadth of this digital human data will permit President Obama to launch his Precision Medicine Initiative that supports a common medical data set, true interoperability of medical data that remains private and secure and a value- and quality-based payment system.[32,33]

Apple-ization of medicine

Apple, through its unique ability to create, market, and integrate the best hardware, software, and computer services and its ability to work with other leading companies in many diverse fields, has caused a revolutionary transformation of many industries. Now with its latest mobile operating system, platform kits, mobile computing architecture and app models of software and their recent alliances with many of the largest health care industrial stakeholders, it has the ability to do the same for health care. Apple's HealthKit that synchronizes health and wellness data, PHRs and medical device data, is a platform that resides on the iPhone that interfaces with cooperating medical devices. The iPhone gathers information on vital signs, body position, activity, behavior, nutrition, pulmonary function, and sleep using its accelerometer, microphone, gyroscope, and GPS (global positioning system) sensors and links to other medical devices to gain insight into a patient's gait, motor impairment, fitness, speech, nutrition, memory, asthma inhaler use, and biomedical analytics such as glucose and oxygen. Data are safe, secure, and HIPPA compliant and is presented to the patient in a pleasant, graphic manner. It is a two-way medical communication platform that patients control. Data can be electronically sent to any cooperating EHR, analytics warehouse repository, or provider group and cannot be sold, misused, or seen by Apple.

Apple's medical ResearchKit platform is an open-source software tool that will empower consumers and patients to decide if they want to participate in a medical study and how their data are to be shared with researchers. It is designed to give medical researchers a new way to gather information on patients residing anywhere in the world by using their iPhones and Apple Watch. The ResearchKit platform is designed to work hand in hand with Apple's HealthKit software. Patients can digitally sign up for a trial, sign consent forms, communicate directly with the research center, have up to date information on the study, and have their results and pooled results. Innovative research apps are able to monitor the physical, mental, and behavioral effects of disease along with monitoring adverse events to treatments. A Stanford cardiac study signed up over 10,000 patients in 3 days compared with their expectation of getting 50 patients per institution over 1 year!

For oncologists, these innovative developments will permit our patients to wear devices that can be used to measure and send data over the Internet to their smartphones that will have health platform software for HIPAA compliant storage, analytic and graphical representation of the captured data that can then be sent to an individual's providers, hospitals or medical alert capture stations all chosen by the patient.

Mobile computing, actionable, and shareable data provided by seamless interoperability standards and an oncologic RLS will continue to provide us with the tools to efficiently and effectively produce a health care system that "just works" for all stakeholders.

References

1 Christensen CM. *The Innovator's Dilemma: When New Technologies Cause Great Firms to Fail.* Boston, MA: Harvard Business School Press; 1997.
2 Christensen CM, Grossman JH, Hwang J. *The Innovator's Prescription: A Disruptive Solution for Health Care.* New York, NY: McGraw-Hill; 2008.
3 American Society of Clinical Oncology. Clinical oncology requirements for the EHR (CORE). October 6, 2009. Available from: http://www.asco.org/sites/default/files/oct_2009_-_asco_nci_core_white_paper.pdf. Accessed October 15, 2015.
4 http://www.hl7.org
5 https://en.wikipedia.org/wiki/Clinical_Document_Architecture
6 Hewitt M, Greenfield S, Stovall E. *From Cancer Patient to Cancer Survivor: Lost in Transition.* Washington, DC: The National Academies Press; 2006.
7 American Society of Clinical Oncology. Chemotherapy treatment plan and summary resources. Available from: http://www.instituteforquality.org/chemotherapy-treatment-plan-and-summaries. Accessed October 18, 2015.
8 Salz T, Oeffinger KC, McCabe MS, et al. Survivorship care plans in research and practice. *CA Cancer J Clin.* 2012;**62**:101–117.
9 HL7 CDA® R2 Implementation Guide: Clinical Oncology Treatment Plan and Summary, Release 1 Clinical Oncology Treatment Plan and Summary, DSTU Release 1 2013 [cited September 5, 2014]. http://www.hl7.org/implement/standards/product_brief.cfm?product_id=327. Accessed October 15, 2015.
10 http://www.hl7.org/implement/standards/fhir
11 http://mycourses.med.harvard.edu/ec_res/nt/6209858F-CDDD-4518-ADF8-F94DF98B5ECF/Argonaut_Project-12_Dec_2014-v2.pdf
12 http://www.healthit.gov/sites/default/files/nationwide-interoperability-roadmap-draft-version-1.0.pdf
13 Electronic Health Records (EHRs) in the Oncology Clinic: How Clinician Interaction with EHRs Can Improve Communication with the Patient http://jop.ascopubs.org/content/early/2014/07/15/JOP.2014.001385.extract.
14 McDonald CJ, Callaghan FM, Weissman A. Use of Internist's free time by ambulatory care electronic medical record systems. *JAMA Intern Med.* 2014;**174**(11):1860–1863.
15 Kuhn T, Basch P, Barr M, Yackel T. For the medical informatics committee of the American college of physicians. Clinical documentation in the 21st century:

executive summary of a policy position paper from the American college of physicians. *Ann Intern Med.* 2015;**162**:301–303.

16 Merrill M. Patients, referring docs at MD Anderson making good use of Web portal. Healthcare IT News July 6, 2010. Available from: http://www.healthcareitnews.com/news/patients-referring-docs-md-anderson-making-good-use-web-portal. Accessed March 15, 2012.

17 http://www.myopennotes.org

18 Yu PP. Knowledge bases, clinical decision support systems, and rapid learning in oncology. *J Oncol Pract.* 2015;**11**:1–4.

19 http://cancergenome.nih.gov

20 http://www.genomicsandhealth.org

21 Musen MA, Greenes RA, Middleton B: Clinical decision-support systems, in Shortliffe EH, Cimino JJ (eds): *Biomedical Informatics: Computer Applications in Health Care and Biomedicine.* London, UK, Springer London, 2014

22 http://www.hl7.org/implement/standards/product_brief.cfm?product_id=208

23 Institute of Medicine. A foundation for evidence-driven practice: a rapid learning system for cancer. Available from: http://www.nap.edu/openbook.php?record_id=12868. Accessed March 12, 2012.

24 Abernethy AP, Etheredge LM, Ganz PA, et al. Rapid-learning system for cancer care. *J Clin Oncol.* 2010;**28**:4268–4274.

25 Accelerating Progress Against Cancer: ASCO's blueprint for transforming clinical translational cancer research. November 2011. Available at http://www.cancerprogress.net/blueprint.html. Accessed March 12, 2012.

26 Sim I, Gorman P, Greenes RA, et al. Clinical decision support systems for the practice of evidence-based medicine. *J Am Med Inform Assoc.* 2001;**8**:527–534.

27 Mandl KD, Kohane IS. No small change for the health Information economy. *N Engl J Med.* 2009;**360**:1278–1281.

28 Halamka JD The rise of electronic medicine. http://www.technologyreview.com/news/425298/the-rise-of-electronic-medicine/.

29 Mandl KD. Ebola in the United States: EHRs as a public health tool at the point of care. *JAMA Published online October.* 2014;**20**. doi: 10.1001/jama.2014.15064.

30 Sinofsky S. Patience, IoT is the new electronic. http://blog.learningbyshipping.com/2015/02/02/patience-iot-is-the-new-electronic/.

31 Topol EJ. Individualized medicine from prewomb to tomb. *Cell.* 2014;**157**(1):241–253.

32 Proposed Shared Nationwide Interoperability Roadmap http://www.healthit.gov/sites/default/files/nationwide-interoperability-roadmap-draft-version-1.0.pdf.

33 Francis S, Collins FS, Varmus H. A new initiative on precision medicine. *N Engl J Med.* 2015;**372**:793–795.

Carcinogenesis

23 Chemical carcinogenesis

Lorne J. Hofseth, PhD ▪ Ainsley Weston, PhD ▪ Curtis C. Harris, MD

Overview

Human exposure to chemical carcinogens can result in cancer. What dictates this outcome is relatively predictable but highly variable. Factors governing the outcome include type of exposure, amount of exposure, time of exposure, and genetic makeup of the host (i.e., humans). The latter is comprised of variations in single nucleotides within genes (e.g., single nucleotide polymorphisms in deoxyribonucleic acid–repair genes), as well as the metabolomic, proteomic, microbiomic, transcriptomic, and epigenomic background of the individual. It is becoming increasingly clear that these endpoints can be modified by chemical carcinogens and that inflammatory load influences outcome. To this end, the past decade has seen an explosion of extremely sensitive and highly accurate technology. Linking this technology to the rapid development of bioinformatics has enabled us to begin merging the totality of lifetime exposure (exposome) with the totality of metabolomic, proteomic, microbiomic, transcriptomic, epigenomic, and other "omic" profiles. We feel optimistic that the next decade will bring the development of tools to identify an individual's weighted risk signature as a biomarker for cancer risk and develop a personalized and precise approach to cancer chemoprevention and treatment.

Human chemical carcinogenesis is a multistage process that results from carcinogen exposure; usually in the form of complex chemical mixtures, and often encountered in the environment or through our lifestyle and diet (Tables 1 and 2). A prominent example is tobacco smoke, which can cause cancers at multiple sites with the highest risk being that of lung cancer. Although most chemical carcinogens do not react directly with intracellular components, they are activated to carcinogenic and mutagenic electrophiles by metabolic processes evolutionarily designed to clear the body of toxins and to modify endogenous compounds. Electrophilic chemical species are naturally attracted to nucleophiles like deoxyribonucleic acid (DNA) and protein; and genetic damage results through covalent bonding to DNA. Once internalized, carcinogens are subject to competing processes of metabolic activation and detoxification, although some chemical species can act directly. There is considerable variation among the human population in these competing metabolic processes, as well as the capacity for repair of DNA damage and cellular growth control. This is the basis for inter-individual variation in cancer risk and is a reflection of gene–environment interactions, which embodies the concept that heritable traits modify the effects of chemical carcinogen exposure.[55,56] Such variations in constitutive metabolism, DNA repair, and cellular growth control contribute to the relative susceptibility of individual members of the population to chemical exposures. For example, only 10% of tobacco smokers develop lung cancer, albeit that tobacco use accounts for other fatal conditions, including cardiovascular disease, emphysema, and chronic obstructive pulmonary disorder (COPD). Within the conceptual framework of multistage carcinogenesis, the primary genetic change that results from a chemical–DNA interaction is termed *tumor initiation*.[13,14,57] Thus, initiated cells are irreversibly altered and are at a greater risk of malignant conversion than are normal cells. The epigenetic effects of tumor promoters facilitate the clonal expansion of the initiated cells.[58,59] Selective, clonal growth advantage causes a focus of pre-neoplastic cells to form. These cells are more vulnerable to tumorigenesis because they now present a larger, more rapidly proliferating, target population for the further action of chemical carcinogens, oncogenic viruses, and other cofactors. Additional genetic and epigenetic changes continue to accumulate.[58,59] The activation of oncogenes, and the inactivation of tumor suppressor and DNA-repair genes, leads to genomic instability or the *mutator phenotype* and an acceleration in the genetic changes taking place.[29,60,61] This scenario is followed by malignant conversion, tumor progression, and metastasis. The underlying molecular mechanisms that govern chemical carcinogenesis are becoming increasingly understood, and the insights generated are assisting in the development of better methods to investigate human cancer risk and susceptibility. The results of such studies are intended to mold strategies for prevention and intervention. Moreover, insights into the normal operations of so-called *gatekeeper* genes,[62] like the tumor suppressor *TP53*, have provided an opportunity to develop new, targeted, therapeutic approaches.

Multistage carcinogenesis

Carcinogenesis can be divided conceptually into four steps: tumor initiation, tumor promotion, malignant conversion, and tumor progression (Figure 1, Box 1). The distinction between initiation and promotion was recognized through studies involving both viruses and chemical carcinogens.[13,14,57] This distinction was formally defined in a murine skin carcinogenesis model in which mice were treated topically with a single dose of a polycyclic aromatic hydrocarbon (PAH) (i.e., initiator), followed by repeated topical doses of croton oil (i.e., promoter),[13] and this model has been expanded to a range of other rodent tissues, including bladder, colon, esophagus, liver, lung, mammary gland, stomach, and trachea.[59] During the last 65 years, the sequence of events comprising chemical carcinogenesis has been systematically dissected and the paradigm increasingly refined, and both similarities and differences between rodent and human carcinogenesis have been identified.[63] Carcinogenesis requires the malignant conversion of benign hyperplastic cells to a malignant state, and invasion and metastasis are manifestations of further genetic and epigenetic changes.[64] The study of this process in humans is necessarily indirect and uses information from lifestyle or occupational exposures to chemical carcinogens. Measures of age-dependent cancer incidence have shown, however, that the rate of tumor development is proportional to the sixth power of time, suggesting that at least four to six

Holland-Frei Cancer Medicine, Ninth Edition. Edited by Robert C. Bast Jr., Carlo M. Croce, William N. Hait, Waun Ki Hong, Donald W. Kufe, Martine Piccart-Gebhart, Raphael E. Pollock, Ralph R. Weichselbaum, Hongyang Wang, and James F. Holland.
© 2017 John Wiley & Sons, Inc. ISBN: 978-1-118-93469-2.

Table 1 Selected examples of human chemical carcinogenesis.

Organ system (specific pathology)	Chemical carcinogen	Co-carcinogen
Lung (small and nonsmall cell)	Tobacco smoke	Asbestos
	Metals: As, Be, Cd, Cr, Ni	—
	BCME	—
	Diesel exhaust	—
Pleural mesothelium	Asbestos	Tobacco smoke
Oral cavity	Smokeless tobacco	—
	Betel quid	Slaked lime [Ca(OH)$_2$]
Esophagus	Tobacco smoke	Alcohol
Nasal sinuses	Snuff	Powdered glass
	Isopropyl alcohol	—
Skin (scrotum)	Cutting oil	—
	Coal soot[a]	—
Liver (angiosarcoma)	Aflatoxin B1	HBV, HCB
	Vinyl chloride	Alcohol
Bladder	Aromatic amines (e.g., 4-ABP and benzidine)	—
	Aromatic amines from tobacco smoke[b]	—
ALL	Benzene	—
Lymphatic and hematopoietic malignancies	Ethylene oxide	—

4-ABP, 4-aminobiphenyl; ALL, acute lymphoblastic leukemia; BCME, bis-chloromethyl ether; HBV, hepatitis B virus; HCV, hepatitis C virus.
[a]Early report of occupational chemical carcinogenesis from 225 years ago.
[b]Strong circumstantial evidence.[1]
A comprehensive treatise on the evaluation of the carcinogenic risk of chemicals to humans can be found in the ongoing International Agency for Research on Cancer monograph program initiated in 1971.

independent steps are necessary.[65] Partial scheduling of specific genetic events in this process has been possible for some cancers. Examples of sequential genetic and epigenetic changes that occur with the highest probability are those found in the development of lung cancer[66] and colon cancer.[67] Recent advances in sequencing technology have allowed us to identify the genomic landscape of many tumors. In common solid tumors such as those derived from the colon, breast, brain, or pancreas, an average of 33–66 genes display subtle somatic mutations that can alter their protein products.[68] Certain tumor types display many more or many fewer mutations than average. Melanomas and lung tumors, for example, contain approximately 200 nonsynonymous mutations per tumor; a reflection of the involvement of potent mutagens [ultraviolet (UV) light and cigarette smoke, respectively] in the pathogenesis of these tumor types.[68]

Tumor initiation

Earlier concepts of tumor initiation indicated that the initial changes in chemical carcinogenesis are irreversible genetic damage. However, recent data from molecular studies of pre-neoplastic human lung and colon tissues implicate epigenetic changes as an early event in carcinogenesis. DNA methylation of promoter regions of genes can transcriptionally silence tumor suppressor genes.[69] In a broad sense, then, chemical carcinogens can be divided into genotoxic [e.g., benzo(a)pyrene or B(a)P; generally considered to act at the initiation stage] and nongenotoxic agents [e.g., 3,7,8-tetrachlorodibenzo-p-dioxin (TCDD) or 12-O-tetradecanoylphorbol-13-acetate (TPA); generally considered to act in the promotion stages]. These nongenotoxic or epigenetic agents (Figure 1) neither do not induce mutations nor do they

induce direct DNA damage in the target organ. They modulate cell growth and death and exhibit dose-response relationships between exposure and tumor formation. Although the exact mechanism(s) of action of these agents on neoplastic cell formation are yet to be determined, changes in gene expression and cell growth parameters appear to be critical, and nongenotoxic compounds exhibit temporal and threshold characteristics frequently requiring chronic treatment for carcinogenicity.

Overall, most human cancers are caused by two to eight sequential alterations that develop over the course of 20–30 years.[68] For mutations to accumulate, they must arise in cells that proliferate and survive the lifetime of the organism. A chemical carcinogen causes a genetic error by modifying the molecular structure of DNA that can lead to a mutation during DNA synthesis. Most often, this is brought about by forming an adduct between the chemical carcinogen or one of its functional groups and a nucleotide in DNA (the process by which this occurs for the major classes of chemical carcinogens is discussed in detail in "Carcinogen Metabolism"). In general, a positive correlation is found between the amount of carcinogen–DNA adducts that can be detected in animal models and the number of tumors that develop.[70,71] Thus, tumors rarely develop in tissues that do not form carcinogen–DNA adducts. Carcinogen–DNA adduct formation is central to theories of chemical carcinogenesis, and it may be a necessary, but not a sufficient, prerequisite for tumor initiation (the concept of so-called nongenotoxic carcinogens is also explored in "Carcinogen Metabolism"). DNA adduct formation that causes either the activation of a proto-oncogene or the inactivation of a tumor suppressor gene can be categorized as a tumor-initiating event (see Sections titled "Tumor progression" and "Oncogenes and tumor suppressor genes").

Tumor promotion

Tumor promotion comprises the selective clonal expansion of initiated cells. Because the accumulation rate of mutations is proportional to the rate of cell division, or at least the rate at which stem cells are replaced, clonal expansion of initiated cells, produces a larger population of cells that are at risk of further genetic changes and malignant conversion.[64,68] Tumor promoters are generally nongenotoxic, are not carcinogenic alone, and often (but not always) are able to mediate their biologic effects without metabolic activation. These agents are characterized by their ability to reduce the latency period for tumor formation after exposure of a tissue to a tumor initiator, or to increase the number of tumors formed in that tissue. In addition, they induce tumor formation in conjunction with a dose of an initiator that is too low to be carcinogenic alone. Croton oil (isolated from Croton tiglium seeds) is used widely as a tumor promoter in murine skin carcinogenesis, and the mechanism of action for its most potent constituent, TPA, which occurs via protein kinase C activation, is arguably the best understood among tumor promoters.[72] Chemicals or agents capable of both tumor initiation and promotion are known as complete carcinogens [e.g., B(a)P and 4-aminobiphenyl]. Identification of new tumor promoters in animal models has accelerated with the sophisticated development of model systems designed to assay for tumor promotion. Furthermore, ligand-binding properties can be determined in recombinant protein kinase C isozymes that are expressed in cell culture.[73] Chemicals, complex mixtures of chemicals, or other agents that have been shown to have tumor-promoting properties include dioxin, TPA, TCDD, benzoyl peroxide, macrocyclic lactones, bromomethylbenzanthracene, anthralin, phenol, saccharin, tryptophan, dichlorodiphenyltrichloroethane (DDT), phenobarbital, cigarette-smoke condensate, polychlorinated biphenyls (PCBs),

Table 2 Some landmark discoveries in chemical carcinogenesis.

Year	Event/discovery/finding	References
3000 BC	First written description of cancer (breast) in the Edwin Smith Papyrus	2
1500 BC	Egyptians treat tumors with chemicals (arsenic)	2
1620	Thomas Venner warns about immoderate use of tobacco	3, 4
1742	Hermann Boerhaave and Jean Astruc link inflammation to cancer	3, 5, 6
1775	Percival Pott describes association between soot exposure and scrotal cancer in chimney sweeps	7
1863	Rudolf Virchow: cancers tend to occur at sites of chronic inflammation	8
1879	Harting and Hesse: lung cancer is an occupational disease of miners	9
1909	First chemotherapy drug (an arsenobenzene analog, compound 606, or salvarsan) treats syphilis	10
1910	Viruses found to cause cancer	11
1932	Female hormones (estrogen) cause breast cancer in mice	12
1941	Two-stage initiation and promotion of cancers by chemical carcinogens proposed	13, 14
1950	Tobacco exposure linked to lung cancer	15, 16
1956	Nitrosamines cause cancer	17
1956	Evidence that enzymes can be activated by chemical carcinogens	18
1962, 1963	Evidence that chemical carcinogens can methylate DNA and proteins	19, 20
1964–1968	Aflatoxin B1, a fungal toxin, is carcinogenic in rats, binds to DNA and is carcinogenic in humans	21–23
1968	DNA-repair defects linked to cancer	24
1971	"Two-hit" theory of cancer causation in the Rb gene, and tumor suppressor gene discovery	25
1971	Epigenetic mechanisms for carcinogenesis proposed	26
1973	Ames assay identified to test mutagenicity of chemical carcinogens	27
1974	Evidence that chemical carcinogens are activated to form DNA adducts in human tissues	28
1974	Mutator phenotype concept identified	29
1976	Inter-individual variation in the binding of chemical carcinogens to DNA and gene–environment interactions	30
1973	Oncogene discovery	31, 32
1977	Cancer stem cells identified	33
1979	p53, the most frequently altered gene in human cancer, discovered	34, 35
1981	First quantitative estimation of the contribution of the environment and genetics to carcinogenesis	36
1982	Formal structure/model of molecular epidemiology introduced	37
1983	Single nucleotide polymorphisms can guide carcinogenesis	38
1988	Chemical carcinogens cause site-specific mutagenesis	39
1990	Sequential mutations in colon cancer introduced	40
1991	p53 identified as a tumor suppressor gene	41
1991	Identification of selective mutations in p53 (mutational hotspots) associated with specific environmental and chemical carcinogens	42, 43
2001	Draft sequence of the human genome	44, 45
2002	MicroRNA alterations in cancer	46
2002	Gene expression signatures predict prognosis	47
2005	Concept of the exposome (the entirety of exposure to which an individual is subjected, from conception to death) is introduced	48
2006	Genetic landscape of two human cancer types defined (colon and breast)	49
2006	MicroRNA signatures predict prognosis and survival	50
2006	FDA approves HPV vaccine [human papillomavirus quadrivalent (types 6, 11, 16, 18) vaccine, recombinant]	51
2011	National Research Council (United States) committee on A Framework for Developing a New Taxonomy of Disease introduces precision medicine	52
2012	Victor Velculescu: detection of chromosomal alterations in the circulation of cancer patients	53
2012	Use of integrative personal omics profile to distinguish between healthy and diseased states at an individual level	54

teleocidins, cyclamates, estrogens and other hormones, bile acids, UV light, wounding, abrasion, and other chronic irritation (i.e., saline lavage).[74]

Malignant conversion

Malignant conversion is the transformation of a pre-neoplastic cell into one that expresses the malignant phenotype. This process requires further genetic changes. The total dose of a tumor promoter is less significant than frequently repeated administrations, and if the tumor promoter is discontinued before malignant conversion has occurred, premalignant or benign lesions may regress. Tumor promotion contributes to the process of carcinogenesis by the expansion of a population of initiated cells, with a growth advantage, that will then be at risk for malignant conversion. Conversion of a fraction of these cells to malignancy will be accelerated in proportion to the rate of cell division and the quantity of dividing cells in the benign tumor or pre-neoplastic lesion. In part, these further genetic changes may result from infidelity of DNA synthesis.[75] The relatively low probability of malignant conversion can

be increased substantially by the exposure of pre-neoplastic cells to DNA damaging agents,[76] and this process may be mediated through the activation of proto-oncogenes and inactivation of tumor suppressor genes.

Box 1 Multistage carcinogenesis

Multistage carcinogenesis involves four stages:
1. *Tumor initiation*: The initial changes to normal cells that occur early in chemical carcinogenesis and involve irreversible genetic mutation(s) (genotoxic initiation) or epigenetic changes (nongenotoxic initiation) so that they are able to form tumors.
2. *Tumor promotion*: The selective clonal expansion of a population of initiated cells, causing additional genetic changes with a growth advantage that will then be at risk for malignant conversion. Tumor promoters are generally nongenotoxic, cannot drive tumorigenesis alone, and require repeat exposure over time.
3. *Malignant conversion*: The transformation of a preneoplastic cell into one that expresses a malignant phenotype. The probability of malignant conversion increases through additional genetic changes,

Multistep carcinogenesis

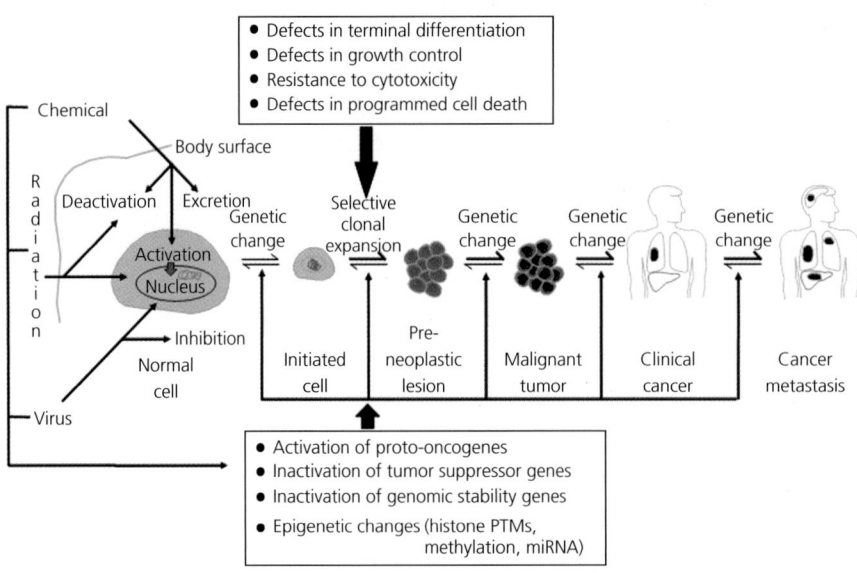

Figure 1 Multistep chemical carcinogenesis can be conceptually divided into four stages: tumor initiation, tumor promotion, malignant conversion, and tumor progression. The activation of proto-oncogenes and the inactivation of tumor suppressor genes are mutational events that result from covalent damage to DNA caused by chemical exposures. The accumulation of mutations, and not necessarily the order in which they occur, constitutes multistage carcinogenesis. During these stages, progressive epigenetic changes are also occurring due to chemical exposure.

continued exposure of preneoplastic cells to DNA damaging agents, and may be mediated through the activation of proto-oncogenes and inactivation of tumor suppressor genes.

4. *Tumor progression*: The expression of the malignant phenotype and the tendency of malignant cells to acquire more aggressive characteristics over time. A prominent characteristic of the malignant phenotype is the propensity for genomic instability and uncontrolled growth. During this process, further genetic and epigenetic changes can occur, again including the activation of proto-oncogenes and the functional loss of tumor suppressor genes.

Tumor progression

Tumor progression comprises the expression of the malignant phenotype and the tendency of malignant cells to acquire more aggressive characteristics over time. Also, metastasis may involve the ability of tumor cells to secrete proteases that allow invasion beyond the immediate primary tumor location. A prominent characteristic of the malignant phenotype is the propensity for genomic instability and uncontrolled growth.[77] During this process, further genetic and epigenetic changes can occur, again including the activation of proto-oncogenes and the functional loss of tumor suppressor genes. Frequently, proto-oncogenes are activated by two major mechanisms: in the case of the *ras* gene family, point mutations are found in highly specific regions of the gene (i.e., the 12th, 13th, 59th, or 61st codons), and members of the *myc, raf, HER2*, and *jun* multigene families can be overexpressed, sometimes involving amplification of chromosomal segments containing these genes. Some genes are overexpressed if they are translocated and become juxtaposed to a powerful promoter, for example, the relationship of *bcl-2* and immunoglobulin heavy chain gene promoter regions in B-cell malignancies. Loss of function of tumor suppressor genes usually occurs in a bimodal fashion, and most frequently involves point mutations (caused by DNA adducts, errors in DNA replication, and errors in DNA repair) in one allele and loss of the second

allele by a deletion (caused by a recombinational event, chromosomal nondisjunction, or hypermethylation). These phenomena confer to the cells a growth advantage as well as the capacity for regional invasion, and ultimately, distant metastatic spread. Despite evidence for an apparent scheduling of certain mutational events, it is the accumulation of these mutations, and not the order or the stage of tumorigenesis in which they occur, that appears to be the determining factor.[68] Recent evidence from microarray expression analysis of human cancers supports an alternative, and not mutually exclusive, mode of tumor progression. Gene expression profiles of a primary cancer and its metastases are similar, indicating the molecular progression of a primary cancer is generally retained in its metastases.[78]

Over the last decade, sequencing efforts have identified genomic landscapes of common forms of human cancer. Vogelstein and colleagues recently defined these landscapes as consisting of a small number of "mountains" (genes altered in a high percentage of tumors) and a much larger number of "hills" (genes altered infrequently).[68] Approximately 140 genes that when altered by intragenic mutations can drive tumorigenesis. A typical tumor contains two to eight of these "driver gene" mutations that control cell fate, cell survival, and genomic maintenance. Other "passenger mutations" confer no selective growth advantage. Overall, the identification of specific genes and their function in primary cancers and metastases have clinical implications in molecular diagnosis of primary cancers and targeted therapeutic strategies for personalized medicine.

Epigenetics and chemical carcinogenesis

Epigenetics describes a change in gene activity without a change in the DNA sequence.[79] Well-described mechanisms involved in epigenetics include DNA methylation and histone modification; each of which alters how genes are expressed without altering the underlying DNA sequence. Another mechanism (described in detail later) also falling under the definition of "epigenetic" is the effects of microRNA (miRNA; Figure 2, Box 2) on carcinogenesis.

Both nongenotoxic and genotoxic chemical carcinogens impact these epigenetic processes. At the cellular level, exposure to environmental factors may leave an epigenomic signature that can be exploited in discovering new biomarkers for risk assessment and cancer prevention.[80,81]

> **Box 2** Epigenetics
>
> Epigenetics describes a change in gene activity without a change in the DNA sequence. It involves changes in *DNA methylation* [hypomethylation/hypermethylation caused by carcinogens modifying methylation enzymes (e.g., DNMTs)], *histone tail modification* [acetylation, methylation, citrullination, ubiquitination, sumoylation, and phosphorylation caused by carcinogens modifying enzymes involved in such changes (e.g., HDACs)], and *small noncoding RNA's* (e.g., miRNAs caused by genetic abnormalities, modulation of biogenesis machinery, and/or epigenetic mechanisms).

DNA methylation is catalyzed by a family of DNA methyltransferases (DNMTs). In somatic mammalian cells, DNA methylation occurs at cytosine residues of CpG dinucleotides; in embryonic stem cells, DNA methylation occurs at both CpG and non-CpG sequences. DNMT expression, and therefore indirect control of DNA methylation, is controlled by DNMT3L, lymphoid-specific helicase, miRNAs, and piwi-interacting RNAs.[82] It is becoming increasingly clear that many chemical carcinogens are involved in DNA methylation. For example, the tobacco-specific carcinogen, 4-(methylnitrosoamino)-1-(3-pyridyl)-1-butanone (NNK), induces DNMT accumulation and tumor suppressor gene hypermethylation in mice and lung cancer patients.[83] As well, B(a)P and many others not only genotoxic, but also nongenotoxic chemical carcinogens have been shown to induce aberrant methylation patterns.[82,84] Several mechanisms may explain aberrant methylation patterns due to chemical carcinogens. As an example, cigarette smoke may alter DNA methylation by (1) inducing DNA damage, stimulating recruitment of DNMT1; (2) the ability of nicotine to down-regulate DNMT1 mRNA and protein expression; (3)

modulating expression and activity of DNA-binding factors, such as Sp1; and (4) inducing hypoxia, which increases HIF1α, leading to the up-regulation of methionine adenosyltransferase 2A[85] (Figure 2).

Chromatin is the complex of DNA wrapped around histone octamers, consisting of four different histones, H2A, H2B, H3, and H4. Gene expression changes with histone post-transcriptional modification (e.g., acetylation, phosphorylation, and methylation) in the *N*-terminal tail region. Enzymes that regulate histone modification include histone deacetylases (HDACs), histone acetyltransferases (HATs), and histone methyltransferases (HMTs). Chemical carcinogens can alter the activity of such enzymes. For example, challenging cells with B(a)P induces early enrichment of the transcriptionally active chromatin markers histone H3 trimethylated at lysine 4 (H3K4Me3) and histone H3 acetylated at lysine 9 (H3K9Ac), and reduces association of DNMT1 with the long interspersed nuclear element-1 (L1) promoter. These changes are followed by proteasome-dependent decreases in cellular DNMT1 expression and sustained reduction of cytosine methylation within the L1 promoter CpG island.[86] Similarly, long-term exposure of immortalized bronchial epithelial cells (HBEC-3KT) to low doses of tobacco-related carcinogens leads to oncogenic transformation, increased HDAC expression, cell-cycle independent increased DNMT1 stability, and DNA hypermethylation.[87]

miRNA's in chemical carcinogenesis

miRNA expression is regulated by a growing list of factors, including inflammatory cytokines, free radicals, and chemical carcinogens.[88–91] The specific effects of chemical carcinogens on each miRNA *in vitro* and *in vivo* have been described in detail elsewhere, so the reader is guided to that source.[91] For the purposes of this chapter, we will provide an overview of miRNAs, examples of key miRNAs affected by chemical carcinogens, and the mechanisms by which this occurs.

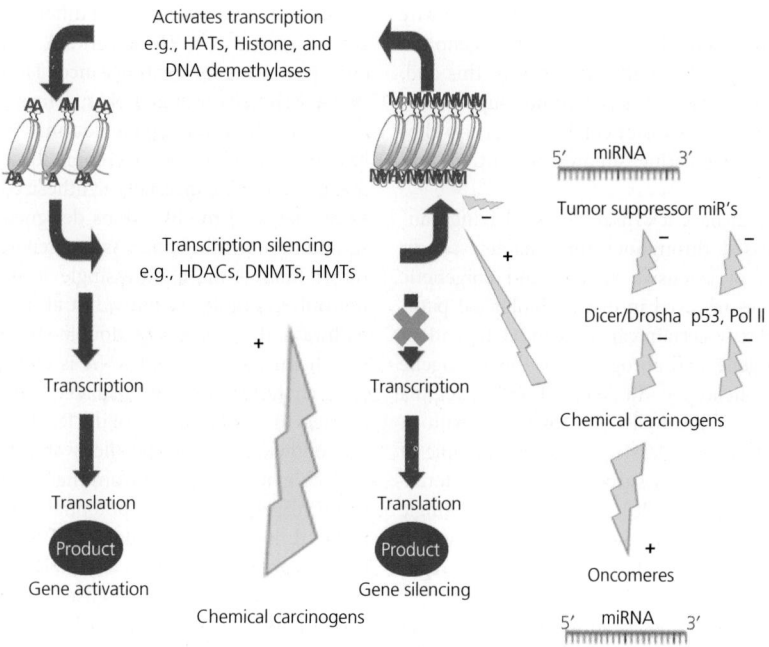

Figure 2 Epigenetic impact of chemical carcinogens. Chemical carcinogens can affect the activity of the different enzymes involved in epigenomics. Ac: acetyl; Me: methyl; DNMT: DNA methyltransferase; HAT: histone acetyltransferase; HDAC: histone deacetylase; HMT: histone methyltransferase.

miRNAs are nonprotein coding small RNAs of about 22 base pairs and regulate mRNA stability and translation into proteins.[92] miRNA genes are regulated by transcription factors including by the p53 tumor suppressor protein[93] and are involved in carcinogenesis including tumor invasion and metastasis.[94] miRNAs are produced by processing of a hairpin precursor by an enzyme called dicer, and the mature miRNA incorporates into a protein complex (the RNA-induced silencing complex—RISC), where it acts as a guide to find complementary target RNAs. Binding of RISC to the target RNA causes degradation of the target or blocks translation—in either case, preventing production of the encoded protein. The alteration of miRNA expression by chemical exposure or during inflammation potentially has enormous consequences, because of the large number of genes each miRNA regulates. Each organism encodes hundreds of miRNAs, and these affect many key biological processes, including cell proliferation, differentiation, survival, and metabolism. In the 15 or so years since miRNAs were discovered,[95–97] it has become clear that post-transcriptional control of gene expression by miRNAs provides an important and widely used level of gene regulation. In humans, it is estimated that about 60% of all protein-coding genes are regulated by a miRNA.[98,99] Because miRNAs are highly specific, potent suppressors of gene expression; and aberrant regulation of miRNA expression is associated with cancer (and many other diseases), the potential value of these small RNAs as therapeutic agents is now widely recognized.[100–104] Not surprisingly, miRNAs are also clinical biomarkers associated with diagnosis, prognosis, and therapeutic outcome of cancer.[105,106] Because miRNA levels change upon exposure to environmental and endogenous chemicals, it is possible that miRNAs can be used for biomonitoring purposes. This is supported by the understanding that miRNAs are released from the target tissues into the blood stream; and therefore, their analysis is feasible via noninvasive sampling (e.g., urine and feces).[107–109]

Oncogenic miRNAs (OncomiRs)

In 2002, the Croce group reported the first link between miRNA and the pathogenesis of cancer; specifically, miR-15a and miR-16-1 were observed to be downregulated in B-cell chronic lymphocytic leukemia (CLL) patients.[46] Since this seminal observation, many of the known miRNA genes were shown to reside in genomic regions that are commonly associated with cancer.[110] To this end, miRNAs themselves are now known to act as tumor suppressors and oncogenes (oncomiRs); and environmental carcinogens alter miRNA expression by down-regulating suppressor miRNA and up-regulating oncomiRs.

OncomiRs are miRNA that have a causal role in driving cancer phenotypes. As discussed throughout this chapter, cancer represents the summation of extensive genetic and epigenetic abnormalities found in genes involved in diverse biological pathways. Even with this complexity, certain cancers can be dependent on a single, powerful oncogene, and abrogation of this oncogene can reverse the malignant phenotype. Targeting the Philadelphia chromosome with inhibitors of the BCR-ABL kinase domain in chronic myelogenous leukemia is a classic, successful example of this approach.[111,112] Herceptin and its success in treating Her2+ breast cancer is another example.[113,114] It is also known that single oncogenes can affect miRNA expression, exemplified by Myc, which can induce the oncomiR miRNA-17/92 cluster, and negatively regulate tumor suppressor miRNA's, such as let-7 and miRNA-29.[115,116] Thus, the potential to target oncomiRs is appealing due to their capacity to control many cancer pathways. One way is to identify the exogenous and/or endogenous (e.g., free radicals) chemicals leading to an increase in oncomiR expression or imbalance of

oncomiRs. miR-21 is one key oncomiR, up-regulated in a number of human cancers.[90,117] It has been shown to be up-regulated by exposure to cancer-causing agents such as arsenite,[118] reactive oxygen species (ROS),[118] hydrogen peroxide,[119] UV irradiation,[120] TPA,[121] and nitric oxide from NOS2.[122] In addition, absence of miRNA-21 results in suppressed skin tumorigenesis induced by 7,12-dimethylbenz[a]anthracene (DMBA)/TPA. miR-21 targets include multiple tumor suppressor genes, such as phosphatase and tensin homolog (PTEN) and tropomyosin α-1 (TPM1) as well as DNA mismatch repair genes, mutS homolog 2 (MSH2) and mutS homolog 6 (MSH6).[117] Other oncomiRs, including miRNA's-17/92, -20, -106, -107, -141, -146, -155, -181, -200, -221/222, and -373, have all been shown to be a target of chemical carcinogens (e.g., BPDE, DMBA),[92,123] in that their expression is increased by these agents. This gives us initial insight into chemicals to target, as well as molecular oncomiR targets/signatures for protection against cancers associated with these chemicals.

Suppressor miRNAs

Many forms of cancer are associated with misregulation of miRNA expression and, indeed, miRNA expression profiles are now used as one way to classify tumors.[105,124–126] Often, tumor cells show a decrease in the level of certain miRNAs that function as tumor suppressors [for reviews, see refs 100, 127–130]. Each tumor suppressor miRNA is thought to regulate the expression of a broad spectrum of genes that work in different cancer pathways. Although only a subset of the direct targets of each tumor suppressor miRNA is currently known, it is clear that the overall impact of losing a tumor suppressor miRNA is to promote one or more aspects of carcinogenesis. In several cases, experiments using animal models have demonstrated that loss of a particular tumor suppressor miRNA can drive tumorigenesis. In these cases, tumorigenesis is suppressed when the missing miRNAs are added back.[129,131–133] miRNA-34a, which is a component of the p53 transcriptional network[134] and regulates cancer stem cell survival,[135,136] is a good example of this, and so far, arguably, appears to be the furthest in development for use in clinical trials.[127,136] miRNA-34a is down regulated in cancer and has been demonstrated to block the initiation and/or inhibit the growth of tumors in animal models of different kinds of cancer when levels are restored.[137–142] Thus, miRNA replacement therapy appears quite promising for treating cancer. However, as is the case for other therapies based on small RNAs, delivery of the RNA to target sites is a critical barrier to implementation.[130,133,143,144] A variety of systems have been developed to overcome these challenges. Many methods make use of commercially synthesized molecules produced with novel chemical modifications designed to improve stability.[144–146] In addition, synthetic RNAs are generally introduced as a duplex rather than as the mature single-stranded miRNA, a feature that not only promotes stability, but also triggers mammalian defense pathways that recognize double-stranded RNA. In many cases, the chemically modified RNA is conjugated to another molecule (e.g., cholesterol) or encapsulated into nanoparticles to overcome barriers to cellular uptake of the RNA.[123,141] Downsides here include the following: (1) the specificity and functionality of the modified molecule may be altered from that of the natural miRNA, resulting in decreased therapeutic potential; (2) adverse side effects can be induced, including stimulation of immune response, toxicity due to packaging components, and activation of the complement pathway; and (3) increased expense. Furthermore, delivery strategies involving expression of small RNA precursors via adenoviral- or lentiviral-based vectors are often used in animal models but are not deemed safe enough for therapies in humans. Thus, although researchers have met with some success in systemic delivery of therapeutic small RNAs, many challenges remain, including safety concerns, efficacy, and economic feasibility.

There are multiple examples of changes in (mostly decreases in) suppressor miRNA levels by chemical carcinogens. The full list has been reviewed recently, so the reader is referred to the reference.[91] Highlights include suppression of the suppressor miRNA's let-7 family and miR-34b in lungs of cigarette smoke-exposed mice. Interestingly, the expression of the let-7 family was restored 1 week after smoking cessation. However, the recovery was incomplete for a limited array of miRNAs, including miRs-34b, -345, -421, -450b, -466, and -469. Thus, it appears that miRNAs mainly behave as biomarkers of effect and that exposure to high dose, lasting for an adequate period of time, is needed to trigger the cigarette-smoke-related carcinogenesis process associated with miRNA changes.[147]

Mechanisms of chemical carcinogen-induced changes in miRNA expression

Changes in miRNA levels by environmental carcinogens appear to be reversible at low doses and short periods of exposure, but irreversible with higher doses and long periods of exposure; and that irreversible miRNA changes are predictive of the future appearance of cancer.[91,147] The mechanisms of how chemical carcinogens lead to an imbalance and changes in miRNA expression appear to involve genetic abnormalities, modulation of the biogenesis machinery, and/or epigenetic mechanisms[92,115,116] (Box 2). Genetic abnormalities include chromosomal rearrangements, genomic amplifications, deletions, and mutations.[92] This was demonstrated in the first studies identifying miRNA's in tumorigenesis. The miRNA-15/16-1 cluster was shown to be deleted in CLL, with subsequent reduced accumulation.[46] Germline mutation was also associated with reduced accumulation of this cluster.[148] The miRNA biogenesis machinery can be altered through multiple mechanism, each resulting in altered miRNA levels. For example, mutations can occur in key biogenesis enzymes (Dicer and Drosha) and/or their complexes,[149] resulting in aberrant miRNA production. Indeed, it has been shown that a series of chemical carcinogens (e.g., PAHs, heterocyclic compounds, nitrosamines, morpholine, ethylnitrosourea, benzene derivatives, hydroxyl amines, and alkenes) interfere with miRNA maturation by binding Dicer.[91,149] Although the effects of environmental chemical carcinogens on the miRNA machinery have been described in detail recently,[91] they can be summed up by three mechanisms. First, in response to DNA damage, the p53/miRNA interconnection can modify the expression of miRNA genes in the nucleus. Second, electrophilic metabolites of environmental carcinogens can bind to nucleophilic sites of miRNA precursors thus forming miRNA adducts that cannot access the catalytic pockets of Dicer in the cytoplasm. Third, metabolites of environmental carcinogens can bind to Dicer in the proximity of miRNA catalytic sites thus blocking maturation of miRNA precursors[91] (Figure 2). It remains, however, unclear to why oncomiR's are upregulated, which will be an important mechanism to delineate for a better understanding of chemical carcinogenesis and chemoprevention. To this end, there are ongoing studies identifying specific small molecule inhibitors of oncomiR biogenesis.[150]

Because miRNA expression is also altered by nongenotoxic carcinogens,[91] there are additional mechanisms modulating expression outside of the DNA damage response pathway. Epigenetic mechanisms (e.g., hypermethylation of tumor suppressor miRNA), as well as direct effects on the transcriptional machinery and post-transcriptional modifiers, play a role. For example, hypermethylation of miRNA-124a in colon cancer results in the up-regulation of the oncogene, Cdk6 kinase and

the phosphorylation of the tumor suppressor, pRb.[151] CpG island hypermethylation of additional tumor suppressor miRNAs have been shown, and the list is growing.[152-155] miRNA's have also been shown to target and alter the activity of DNMT and other enzymes involved in epigenetic modulation (HDACs and histone acetyl transferases)[156-159] (Figure 2). Carcinogens, in turn, can play an integral part in this process. For example, nickel sulfide, which is a weak mutagen but strong carcinogen, can down-regulate miRNA-152 via promoter-DNA hypermethylation.[157] Similarly, ROS inhibit miR-199a and miR-125b expression through increasing the promoter methylation of the miR-199a and miR-125b genes by DNMT1.[160]

As many miRNAs are transcribed by PolII and associated factors,[92,161,162] it stands to reason that miRNA levels are altered by an impact of environmental carcinogens on PolII and other factors with resulting altered transcriptional regulation. miR-34a and miR-34b/c, for example, are direct, conserved p53 target genes that mediate induction of apoptosis, cell-cycle arrest, and senescence by p53.[163] When p53 is mutated (often by environmental carcinogens[164]), its' transcriptional activity is compromised.[165] In a similar way, environmental carcinogens affect the activity of PolII.[166]

Overall, it is clear that chemical carcinogens alter miRNA expression. As with many biological entities, these changes occur initially due to exposure as an adaptive response to the chemical insult. Such mechanisms that miRNA work include the activation of p53, cell-cycle arrest, and apoptotic induction (e.g., by the miR-34 suppressor miRNA family). Proto-oncogene mutation ("initiation"; e.g., k-ras) can induce expression of other suppressor miR's such as the let-7 family.[167] With long-term, extensive exposure, miRNA expression changes can become irreversible. This has been shown with the miR-34 and let-7 family members where their inactivation results in the suppression of p53 and activation of k-ras.[91,168] If miRNA replacement therapy becomes mainstream, this will be a powerful tool for changing and perhaps reversing the carcinogenic process induced by chemical carcinogens. Interestingly, recent studies have found that plant miRNAs consumed by mammals are detected in mammals (including humans), have activity in mammals, and have tumor-suppressive properties.[169-171]

Gene–environment interactions and inter-individual variation

A cornerstone of human chemical carcinogenesis is the concept of gene–environment interactions (Figure 3, Box 3).[56,172] Potential inter-individual susceptibility to chemical carcinogenesis may well be defined by genetic variations in the host elements of this compound system. Functional polymorphisms in human proteins that have, or may have, a role in chemical carcinogenesis include enzymes that metabolize (i.e., activate and detoxify) xenobiotic substances, enzymes that repair DNA damage, cell surface receptors that activate the phosphorylation cascade and cell-cycle control genes (i.e., oncogenes and tumor suppressor genes that are elements of the signal transduction cascade).

Box 3 Gene–environment interactions

Genes identified that modify response to chemical carcinogens include those involved in carcinogen metabolism (e.g., p450's), DNA repair (e.g., NER), cell signaling, cell cycle, and hormonal regulation.

When chemicals or xenobiotics encounter biologic systems, they become altered by metabolic processes. This is an initial facet of

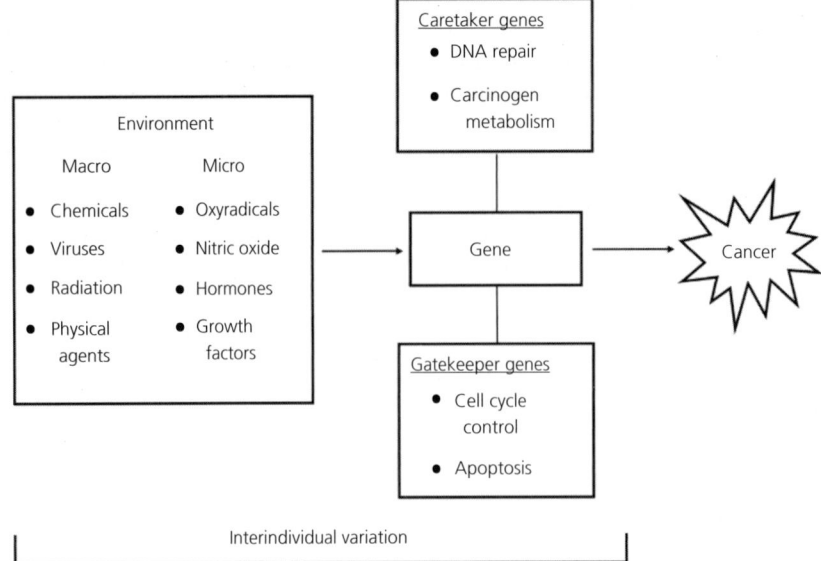

Figure 3 The concept of gene–environment interactions is multifaceted: (1) environmental chemicals are altered by the products of metabolic genes; (2) environmental chemicals disrupt the expression (induce or inhibit) of carcinogen metabolizing genes; and (3) environmental exposures cause changes (mutations) in cancer-related genes. The cancer-related genes have been classified as gatekeeper (e.g., APC) and caretaker (e.g., MSH1 and MLH1) genes. The interaction of these genes with external and internal environmental agents can lead to the derangement of regulatory pathways that maintain genetic stability and cellular proliferation.

gene–environment interaction. The inter-individual variation in carcinogen metabolism and macromolecular adduct formation arising from such processes was recognized almost 40 years ago.[30] The cytochrome P450 (CYP) multigene family is largely responsible for the metabolic activation and detoxification of many different chemical carcinogens in the human environment.[173] CYP P450s are phase I enzymes that act by adding an atom of oxygen onto the substrate; they are induced by PAHs and chlorinated hydrocarbons.[173] Phase II enzymes act on oxidized substrates and also contribute to xenobiotic metabolism. Some phase II enzymes are methyltransferases, acetyltransferases, glutathione transferases, uridine 5′-diphosphoglucuronosyl transferases, sulfotransferases, nicotinamide adenine dinucleotide (NAD)- and nicotinamide adenine dinucleotide phosphate (NADP)-dependent alcohol dehydrogenases, aldehyde, steroid dehydrogenases, quinone reductases, NADPH diaphorase, azo reductases, aldoketoreductases, transaminases, esterases, and hydrolases. The pathways of activation and detoxification are often competitive, providing yet further potential for individual differences in propensity for carcinogen metabolism to DNA damaging species. This scenario is further complicated by a second facet of gene–environment interaction that leads to enzyme induction or inhibition. In this case, environmental exposures alter gene expression, and genes responsible for carcinogen metabolism can be upregulated or repressed by certain chemical exposures.

A third facet of gene–environment interaction occurs when the chemical alters gene structure (environmentally predisposed abnormal DNA). Once a procarcinogen is metabolically activated to an ultimate carcinogenic form, it can bind covalently to cellular macromolecules, including DNA. This DNA damage can be repaired by several mechanisms.[174] Differences in rates and fidelity of DNA repair potentially influence the extent of carcinogen adduct formation (i.e., biologically effective dose) and, consequently, the total amount of genetic damage. The consequences of polymorphisms in genes controlling the cell cycle (serine/threonine kinases, transcription factors, cyclins, cyclin-dependent kinase inhibitors,

and cell surface receptors) are much less clear. However, molecular epidemiologic evidence suggests that certain common variants of these types of genes have a role in susceptibility to chemical carcinogenesis.[175] The evaluation of polymorphisms as potential biomarkers of susceptibility in the human population is discussed in Weston and Harris.[176]

Carcinogen metabolism

Inter-individual variation in cancer susceptibility, and, consequently, meaningful human cancer risk assessment, involve determination of inherited host factors as well as exposure assessment. Metabolic polymorphisms have historically been determined by the use of indicator drugs (e.g., caffeine, debrisoquine, dextromethorphan, dapsone, and isoniazid), however, these assays are being replaced by direct genetic assays. This approach has allowed the investigation of diverse host factors for which indicator drugs were not available, and it has been applied to a wide variety of cancers.[177–181] Such studies have not only made a key impact in the area of pharmacogenomics,[182,183] but genetic indicators of propensity for carcinogen activation and detoxification, DNA-repair capacity, apoptosis, and cell-cycle control are all features of molecular epidemiologic studies that are complementary to adduct studies because of the implications for a biologically effective dose after exposure.

CYP P450 polymorphisms, involved in carcinogen activation, and glutathione-S transferases, uridine diphosphate (UDP) glucuronosyltransferases, sulfotransferases, and N-acyltransferases, involved in both carcinogen activation and detoxification, could explain variations in cancer susceptibility among the human population. Evidence that absent protection of a functionally intact GSTM1 gene correlates with an increased risk of tobacco-related lung cancer.[184] Similarly, the absence of GSTM1 and GSTT1 genes increases the risk of lung cancer because of radon exposure.[185] There is a substantial reduction in risk of lung adenocarcinoma associated with genetic polymorphism in CYP2A13, the most active CYP P450 for the metabolic activation of tobacco-specific carcinogen NNK.[186] The finding that XRCC1, GSTM1, and COMT polymorphisms was strongly associated with lung cancer risk in smoking women is supportive of an interaction of repair, tobacco smoke metabolism, and estrogen metabolism in this disease and continues the controversy of an increased risk of lung cancer in women.[187] Also, UDP glucuronosyltransferases (e.g., *UGT1A1*, *UGT1A9*, and *UGT2B7*) have been implicated in cancers of the head and neck. Persons inheriting reduced activity variants of *NAT1* and *NAT2* genes, resulting in the slow acetylator phenotype, are at a greater risk of aromatic amine-induced bladder cancer. This may include persons exposed through tobacco smoke inhalation.[188,189] Over the past 25 years, there have been advances in the understanding of carcinogen metabolism, inter-individual variations, and cancer risk. A good review of the existing literature can be found elsewhere.[190]

PAHs, for example, B(a)P, were the first carcinogens to be chemically isolated.[191] They are composed of variable numbers of fused benzene rings that form from incomplete combustion of fossil fuels and vegetable matter, they are common environmental contaminants. PAHs are chemically inert, and require metabolism to exert their biologic effects.[191] This multistep process involves the following: initial epoxidation (CYP P450), hydration of the epoxide (epoxide hydrolase), and subsequent epoxidation across the olefinic bond.[173,192] The result is the ultimate carcinogenic metabolite; in the case of B(a)P it is r7, t8-dihydroxy-c9, 10 epoxy-7,8,9,10-tetrahydroxybenzo[a]pyrene (B[a]P-7,8-diol 9,10-epoxide, BPDE).[193] The biology of CYP P450 (e.g., CYP1A1) metabolism has been elucidated providing a molecular basis for inducibility and inter-individual variation, and variations in CYP levels among humans have been documented.[194] The arene ring of BPDE opens spontaneously at the tenth position, revealing a carbonium ion that can form a covalent addition product (adduct) with cellular macromolecules, including DNA. Several DNA adducts can be formed, the most abundant being at the exocyclic amino group of deoxyguanosine ([7R]-*N* 2-[10−7β,8a,9a-trihydroxy-7,8,9,10-tetrahydro-benz[a]pyrene}yl]-deoxyguanosine; BPdG). One electron oxidation has been suggested as an alternative pathway of PAH activation, here a radical cation forms at the meso position (L-region). The resulting DNA adducts at the C8 of guanine (B(a)P-6-C8Gua and BP-6-C8dGua), the N7 of guanine and adenine (B(a)P-6-N7Gua and BP-6-N7Ade) likely undergo spontaneous depurination. Firm evidence for the exfoliation of these adducts in urine has been provided.[195]

Aromatic amines are found in cigarette smoke, diesel exhaust, industrial environments, and certain cooked foods. The compound, 4-aminobiphenyl, is thought to be responsible for bladder cancer among tobacco smokers and rubber industry workers.[196] In addition, nitrated PAHs are environmental contaminants that are related to aromatic amines by nitroreduction. Aromatic amines can be converted to an aromatic amide that is catalyzed by an acetyl coenzyme A-dependent acetylation.[197] The acetylation phenotype varies among the population. Persons with the rapid acetylator phenotype are at a higher risk of colon cancer (especially in smokers),[198] whereas, those who are slow acetylators are at risk of bladder cancer.[198] This latter association may result from the fact that activation of aromatic amines by *N*-oxidation is a competing pathway for aromatic amine metabolism. The *N*-hydroxylation products when protonated (e.g., in the urinary bladder) are reactive and can cause DNA damage.

An initial activation step for both aromatic amines and amides is *N*-oxidation by CYP1A2. The reactions of *N*-hydroxyarylamines with DNA appear to be acid catalyzed, but they can be further activated by either an acetyl coenzyme A-dependent *O*-acetylase or a 3′-phosphoadenosine-5′phosphosulfate-dependent *O*-sulfotransferase. The *N*-arylhydroxamic acids arise from the acetylation of *N*-hydroxyarylamines or *N*-hydroxylation of aromatic amides; they are not electrophilic and require further activation. The predominant pathway here occurs through acetyltransferase-catalyzed rearrangement to a reactive *N*-acetoxyarylamine. Sulfotransferase catalysis forms *N*-sulfonyloxy arylamides. This complex pathway results in two major adduct types, amides (acetylated) and amines (nonacetylated).

Heterocyclic amines form in food cooking from pyrolysis (>150 °C) of amino acids, creatinine, and glucose. They have been recognized as food mutagens, shown to form DNA adducts and cause liver tumors in primates.[199] These compounds are activated by CYP1A2 and their metabolites form DNA adducts in humans. The *N*-hydroxy metabolites of heterocyclic amines like 2-amino-3-methyl-imidazo-[4,5-f]quinoline (IQ) can react directly with DNA. Enzymic *O*-esterification of *N*-hydroxy metabolites plays a key role in activating food mutagens, and because the *N*-hydroxy metabolites are good substrates for transacetylases, these chemicals may be implicated in colorectal cancer.

Aflatoxins (B1, B2, G1, and G2), metabolites of *Aspergillus flavus*, contaminate cereals, grain, and nuts. A positive correlation exists between dietary aflatoxin exposure and the incidence of liver cancer in developing countries, where grain spoilage is high. Aflatoxins B1 and G1 have an olefinic double bond at the 8,9-position that can be oxidized by several CYP P450.[173,192] This implies that the olefinic 8,9-bond is the activation site. Further support for this mechanism comes from studies of DNA adducts and the prevalence of TP53 mutations in liver cancer. In people with liver cancer from parts of China and Africa, where food spoilage caused by molds is high, G : C to T : A transversions in codon 249 are frequent.[42,43,200] This phenomenon is consistent with metabolic activation of aflatoxin B1 and the formation of depurinating carcinogen–deoxyguanosine adducts.

Carcinogenic *N*-nitrosamines are ubiquitous environmental contaminants and can be found in food, alcoholic beverages, cosmetics, cutting oils, hydraulic fluid, rubber, and tobacco.[201] Tobacco-specific *N*-nitrosamines (TSNs), for example, NNK, are not formed by pyrolysis, which accounts for the highly carcinogenic nature of snuff and chewing tobacco.[202] TSNs are not symmetric so both small alkyl adducts and large bulky adducts can be formed; for example, NNK metabolism gives rise to either a positively charged pyridyl-oxobutyl ion or a positively charged methyl ion, both of which are able to alkylate DNA.[70,203] Endogenous nitrosamines form when an amine reacts with nitrate alone or nitrite in the presence of acid. Thus, nitrite (used to cure meats) and L-cysteine, in the presence of acetaldehyde (from alcohol), form *N*-nitrosothiazolidine-4-carboxylic acid. *N*-Nitrosodimethylamine undergoes a-hydroxylation, catalyzed primarily by the alcohol inducible CYP2E1, to form an unstable a-hydroxynitrosamine. The breakdown products are formaldehyde and methyl diazohydroxide. Methyl diazohydroxide and related compounds are powerful alkylating agents that can add a small functional group at multiple sites in DNA.

Nongenotoxic carcinogens may function at the level of the microenvironment by dysregulation of hormones and growth factors, or indirectly inducing DNA damage and mutations through the action of free radicals. These chemicals are none or poorly reactive and are resistant to activation through metabolism. They are also characterized by their persistence in biological systems and consequently tend to accumulate in the food chain. However, they can stimulate oxyradical formation by at least three mechanisms: organochlorine species interact with the Ah receptor, which can lead to CYP P450 induction and associated oxyradical formation; interaction with other receptors, like interferon (IFN)-γ, can stimulate elements of the primary immune response and again generate oxyradicals; and agents like asbestos can promote oxyradical formation through interaction with ferrous metal. The resulting oxyradicals can then damage DNA. Some of the so-called "nongenotoxic" carcinogens might more appropriately be considered to be "oxyradical triggers." Indeed, chronic inflammatory states, which involve oxyradical formation, can also be cancer risk factors.[204–208]

DNA damage and repair

Another facet of inter-individual variation in risk for cancer from chemical carcinogens is inter-individual differences in the ability to repair damage from chemical carcinogens. DNA damage initiates a complex network of signaling cascades.[209] The chemical structure of DNA can be altered by a carcinogen in several ways: the formation of large bulky aromatic adducts, small alkyl adducts, oxidation, dimerization, and deamination. In addition, double- and single-strand breaks can occur. Chemical carcinogens can cause epigenetic changes, such as altering the DNA methylation status that leads to the silencing of specific gene expression.[69] A complex pattern of carcinogen–DNA adducts likely results from a variety of environmental exposures, because of the mixture of different chemical carcinogens present.

Many DNA-repair genes have been described recently, and a growing number of polymorphisms have been identified for which molecular epidemiologic studies have provided evidence that genetic variation in these attributes can be a human cancer risk factor; as well as be used to tailor cancer chemotherapy.[210,211] Typically, these types of molecular epidemiological studies initially focus on high-exposure groups such as workers, patients taking therapeutic drugs, and tobacco smokers. Several polymorphisms in DNA-repair genes have now been implicated in tobacco-related neoplasms.[212] An interesting theory developed recently is a so-called, "hide-then-hit" hypothesis. This describes the importance of DNA-repair variants in escaping checkpoint surveillance. Only cells with subtle defects in repair capacity arising from low-penetrance variants of DNA-repair genes would have the opportunity to grow and to accumulate the genetic changes needed for cancer formation, without triggering cell-cycle checkpoint surveillance.[213]

BPDE reacts with the exocyclic (N2) amino group of deoxyguanosine and resides within the minor groove of the double helix, it is typical of PAHs. This adduct, BPdG, is probably the most common, persistent adduct of B(a)P in mammalian systems, but others are possible. Adducts like BPdG are thought to induce ras gene mutations, which are common in tobacco-related lung cancers.[214,215] Aromatic amine adducts are more complex, because they have both acetylated and nonacetylated metabolic intermediates, and they form covalent bonds at the C8, N2, and sometimes O6 positions of deoxyguanosine as well as deoxyadenosine. The major adducts, however, are C8-deoxyguanosine adducts, which reside predominantly in the major groove of the DNA double helix.[216]

Aflatoxin B1 and G1 activation through hydroxylation of the olefinic 8,9-position results in adduct formation at the N7 position of deoxyguanosine. These are relatively unstable with a half-life of approximately 50 h at neutral pH; depurination products have been detected in urine.[217] The aflatoxin B1-N7-deoxyguanosine adduct also can undergo ring opening to yield two pyrimidine adducts; alternately, aflatoxin B1-8,9-dihydrodiol could result, restoring the DNA molecular structure if hydrolysis of the original adduct occurs.[218]

DNA alkylation can occur at many sites either following the metabolic activation of certain N-nitrosamines, or directly by the action of the N-alkyl ureas (N-methyl-N-nitrosourea) or the N-nitrosoguanidines. The protonated alkyl-functional groups that become available to form lesions in DNA generally attack the following nucleophilic centers: adenine (N1, N3, and N7), cytosine (N3), guanine (N2, O6, and N7), and thymine (O2, N3, and O4). Some of these lesions are known to be repaired (O6-methyldeoxyguanosine), while others are not (N7-methyldeoxyguanosine), which explains why O6-methyldeoxyguanosine is a promutagenic lesion and N7-methyldeoxyguanosine is not.[219,220]

Another potentially mutagenic cause of DNA damage is the deamination of DNA-methylated cytosine residues. 5-Methylcytosine comprises approximately 3% of deoxynucleotides. In this case, deamination at a CpG dinucleotide gives rise to a TpG mismatch. Repair of this lesion most often restores the CpG; however, repair may cause a mutation (TpA).[221] Deamination of cytosine also can generate a C to T transition if uracil glycosylation and G-T mismatch repair are inefficient.

Oxyradical damage can form thymine glycol or 8-hydroxy deoxyguanosine adducts. Exposure to organic peroxides (catechol, hydroquinone, and 4-nitroquinoline-N-oxide) leads to oxyradical damage; however, oxyradicals and hydrogen peroxide can be generated in lipid peroxidation and the catalytic cycling of some enzymes, as well as environmental sources (e.g., tobacco smoke).[204,222] Certain drugs and plasticizers can stimulate cells to produce peroxisomes, and oxyradical formation is mediated through protein kinase C when inflammatory cells are exposed to tumor promoters like phorbol esters.[223] Oxyradicals can contribute to deamination through induction of NO synthase.[224]

Maintenance of genome integrity requires mitigation of DNA damage. Thus, diminished DNA repair capacity is associated with carcinogenesis, birth defects, premature aging, and foreshortened life span. DNA-repair enzymes act at DNA damage sites caused by chemical carcinogens, and six major mechanisms are known: direct DNA repair, nucleotide excision repair, base excision (BER) repair, nonhomologous end joining (double-strand break repair), mismatch repair, and homologous recombination (HR) (postreplication repair).[225,226]

In the presence of nonlethal DNA damage, cell-cycle progression is postponed for repair mechanisms. This highly coordinated process involves multiple genes. A DNA-damage recognition sensor triggers a signal transduction cascade and downstream factors direct G1 and G2 arrest in concert with the proteins operationally responsible for the repair process. Although there are at least six discrete repair mechanisms, within five of them, there are numerous multiprotein complexes comprising all the machinery necessary to accomplish the step-by-step repair function.

Generically, DNA repair requires damage recognition, damage removal or excision, resynthesis or patch synthesis, and ligation. Recent advances have led to the cloning of more than 130 human genes involved in five of these DNA-repair pathways. A list of these genes and their specific functions was published elsewhere.[227] These genes are responsible for the fidelity of DNA repair, and when they are defective, the mutation rate increases. This is the mutator phenotype.[29,60,61] Mutations in at least 30 DNA-repair associated genes have been linked to increased cancer susceptibility or premature aging (Table 3).[227] Moreover, the role of common polymorphisms in some of these genes is associated with increased susceptibility in a gene–environment interaction scenario (this is discussed in Weston and Harris[176]). Indeed, molecular epidemiologic evidence suggests that tobacco-smoking-related lung cancer is associated with a polymorphism in the nucleotide excision repair gene, XPC (ERCC2).[228]

Direct DNA repair is affected by DNA alkyltransferases. These enzymes catalyze translocation of the alkyl moiety from an alkylated base (e.g., O6-methyldeoxyguanosine) to a cysteine residue at their active site in the absence of DNA strand scission. Thus, one molecule of the enzyme is capable of repairing one DNA alkyl lesion, in a suicide mechanism. The inactivation of this mechanism by promoter hypermethylation is associated with Kras G to A mutations in colon cancer.[229]

In DNA nucleotide excision repair, lesion recognition, precision, incision, gap filling, and ligation are required, and the so-called excinuclease complex comprises 16 or more different proteins. Large distortions caused by bulky DNA adducts (e.g., BPDE-dG and 4ABP-dC) are recognized [xeroderma pigmentosum (XPA)] and removed by endonucleases (XPF, XPG, and FEN). A patch is then constructed (pol and pol e) and the free ends are ligated.

Base excision repair also removes a DNA segment containing an adduct; however, small adducts (e.g., 3-methyladenine) are generally the target so that there is overlap with direct repair. The adduct is removed by a glycosylase (hOgg1 and UDG), an apurinic endonuclease (APE1 or HAP1) degrades a few bases on the damaged strand, and a patch is synthesized (pol β) and ligated (DNA ligases: I, II, IIIa, IIIβ, and IV).

DNA mismatches occasionally occur, because excision repair processes incorporate unmodified or conventional, but noncomplementary, Watson–Crick bases opposite each other in the DNA helix. Transition mispairs (G-T or A-C) are repaired by the mismatch repair process more efficiently than transversion mispairs (G-G, A-A, G-A, C-C, C-T, and T-T). The mechanism for correcting mispairings is similar to that for nucleotide excision repair and resynthesis described earlier, but it generally involves the excision of large pieces of the DNA containing mispairings. Because the mismatch recognition protein is required to bind simultaneously to the mismatch and an unmethylated adenine in a GATC recognition sequence, it removes the whole intervening DNA sequence. The parental template strand is then used by the polymerase to fill the gap.

Double-strand DNA breaks can occur from exposure to ionizing radiation and oxidation. Consequences of double-strand DNA breaks are the inhibition of replication and transcription, and loss of heterozygosity. Double-strand DNA break repair occurs through HR, where the joining of the free ends is mediated by a DNA-protein kinase in a process that also protects the ends from nucleolytic attack. The free ends of the DNA then undergo ligation by DNA ligase IV. Genes known to code for DNA-repair enzymes that participate in this process include XRCC4, XRCC5, XRCC6, XRCC7, HRAD51B, HRAD52, RPA, and ATM.

Postreplication repair is a damage-tolerance mechanism and it occurs in response to DNA replication on a damaged template. The DNA polymerase stops at the replication fork when DNA damage is detected on the parental strand. Alternately, the polymerase proceeds past the lesion, leaving a gap in the newly synthesized strand. The gap is filled in one of two ways: either by recombination of the homologous parent strand with the daughter strand in a process that is mediated by a helical nucleoprotein (RAD51); or when a single nucleotide gap remains, mammalian DNA polymerases insert an adenine residue. Consequently, this mechanism may lead to recombinational events as well as base-mispairing.

Persistent nonrepaired DNA damage blocks the replication machinery. Cells have evolved translesion synthesis (TLS) DNA polymerases to bypass these blocks.[230] Most of these TLS polymerases belong to the recently discovered Y family, have much lower stringency than replicative polymerases, and thus are error prone. An increased mutation frequency is an evolutionary trade-off for cellular survival.

Mutator phenotype

Cancer cells contain substantial numbers of genetic abnormalities when compared to normal cells. These abnormalities range from gross changes such as nondiploid number of chromosomes, that is, aneuploidy, and translocations or rearrangements of chromosomes, to much smaller changes in the DNA sequence including deletions, insertions, and single nucleotide substitutions. Therefore, carcinogenesis involves *errors* in (1) chromosomal segregation, (2) repair of DNA damage induced by either endogenous free radicals or environmental carcinogens, and (3) DNA replication. Loeb originally formulated the concept of the mutator phenotype in 1974[29,60] to account for the high numbers of mutations in cancer cells when compared to the rarity of mutations in normal cells. Recent advances in the molecular analysis of carcinogenesis in human cells and animal models have refined the mutator phenotype[61,231] concept that is also linked to the clonal selection theory proposed by Nowell (Figure 4).[232] Generally, the mutator phenotype hypothesis proposes that mutation rates in normal cells are insufficient to account for the large number of mutations found in cancer cells. Consequently, human tumors exhibit an elevated mutation rate that increases the likelihood of a tumor acquiring advantageous mutations. The hypothesis predicts that tumors are composed of cells harboring hundreds of thousands of mutations, as opposed to a small number of specific driver mutations, and that malignant cells within a tumor therefore constitute a highly heterogeneous population.[231]

Racial, gender, and socioeconomic disparities in chemical carcinogenesis

Genetic polymorphisms may also partially explain the increased risk of cancer-associated chemical carcinogens amongst different genders, race, and ethnicity. One of the biggest controversies surrounding this issue is the risk of lung cancer in women smokers. The initial studies finding a higher risk of lung cancer in smoking women versus smoking men[233] have been explained biologically in a number of ways. Several sources of evidence, though inconsistent, suggest that estrogens may play a role in lung cancer. Variation in risk factors and tumor characteristics between men and women has been reported in studies showing that women are more likely to have adenocarcinomas of the lung, a higher risk in never smokers, higher levels of PAH–DNA adducts, higher levels of expression of the gene encoding CYP P450 (CYP) 1A1, more frequent G : C to T : A transversions in p53, and more frequent epidermal growth factor receptor (EGFR) mutations than men.[187] Inherited genetic polymorphisms affecting activating and detoxifying enzymes could also explain a different susceptibility between the sexes to tobacco carcinogens.[234] In addition, several lifestyle and behavioral factors related to smoking habits or environmental and occupational exposures could account for some sex differences.[235] However, in recent years, differences in the susceptibility to lung cancer among smoking men and women have been called into question.[236,237]

A consistent theme is that nonsmoking women are at increased risk for lung cancer compared to nonsmoking men[237,238]; and nonsmoking women are at increased risk for lung cancer due to

Table 3 Examples of disease susceptibility and disease syndromes associated with mutations in DNA-repair genes.

Gene	Function	Pathology or cancer
Cancer susceptibility		
MMRa		
MLH1	Damage recognition	HNPCC2b, glioma
MLH2	DNA binding	HNPCC1, ovarian cancer
MSH3	—	Endometrial cancer
MSH6	Sliding clamp	Endometrial cancer, HNPCC1
PMS1	Damage recognition	HNPCC3
PMS2	Repair initiation	HNPCC4, glioblastoma
NER		
BRCA-1	Directs *p53* transcription toward DNA-repair pathways	Breast cancer, ovarian cancer
RB1	Cell-cycle restriction	Retinoblastoma, breast cancer, and progression osteosarcoma
DSB		
BRCA-2	Regulation of RAD51	Breast cancer, pancreatic cancer
HR		
RAD54	Helicase	Colon cancer, breast cancer, NHL
Other		
TP53 (DSB, NER, HR)	Cell-cycle control; exonuclease; apoptosis; DNA binding	Colon cancer, common somatic defect in human cancer in general; inherited in Li–Fraumeni syndrome and some breast cancers
hOgg1 (Various)	Glycosylase	Cancer susceptibility
Xeroderma pigmentosum (XP)		
NER		
XPD	DNA helicase	Skin and neurologic, but later onset than XPA
XPB	DNA helicase	Skin lesions
XPG	Endonuclease	Acute sun sensitivity, mild symptoms; late skin cancer
XPC (and BER)	Exonuclease	Mental retardation; skin sensitivity; microcephaly
DDB1 and *DDB2*	Binds specific DNA damage	XPE—mild skin sensitivity
XPA	Damage sensor	XPA—skin and neurologic problems: the most severe XP
XPC	Damage sensor	XPC—skin, tongue, and lip cancer
XPE	Damage sensor	XPE—neurologically normal
PRR		
POLH	Polymerase	XPV—Mild to severe skin sensitivity; neurologically normal
Other syndromes		
NER		
Cockaynes		
CSB	ATPase	Cutaneous, ocular, neurologic, and somatic abnormalities; short stature, progressive deafness, mental retardation, neurologic degeneration, early death; sometimes presents together with XPB
Juberg-Marsidi		
ATRX	Putative helicase	Thalassemia/mental retardation
SB		
Nijmegen		
NBS1	Nibrin, cell-cycle regulation	Microencephaly; mental retardation; immunodeficiency; growth retardation; radiation sensitivity; predisposition to malignancy
Ataxia-telangiectasia		
ATM	Phosphorylation	Neurologic deficiencies, manifest by inability to coordinate muscle actions; skin and corneal telangiectases. Leukemia, lymphoma, and other malignancies (breast cancer?)
MRE11 (Ataxia-like)	Exonuclease	DNA damage sensitivity; genomic instability; telomere shortening; aberrant meiosis; severe combined immunodeficiency
PRKDC	Ser/Thr kinase	SCID
Bloom's		
BLM	DNA helicase	High rate of spontaneous lymphatic and other malignancy; high rate SCE
Fanconi anemia		
FANCA-G	Protein control	Multiple congenital malformations; chromosome breaks; pancytopenia. Telomere shortening
Werner		
WRN	DNA helicase/exonuclease	Premature senility, short stature, exonuclease rapidly progressing cataracts, loss of connective tissue and muscle, premature arteriosclerosis, increase risk of malignancy
RecQ4	DNA helicase	Osteosarcoma; premature aging

Repair mechanisms: BER, base excision; DSB, double-strand break; HR, homologous recombination; MMR, mismatch; NER, nucleotide excision; PRR, postreplication; SB, strand break.
Diseases: HNPCC, hereditary nonpolyposis colon cancer; NHL, non-Hodgkin lymphoma.
Other abbreviations: SCE, sister chromatid exchange; SCID, severe combined immunodeficiency.

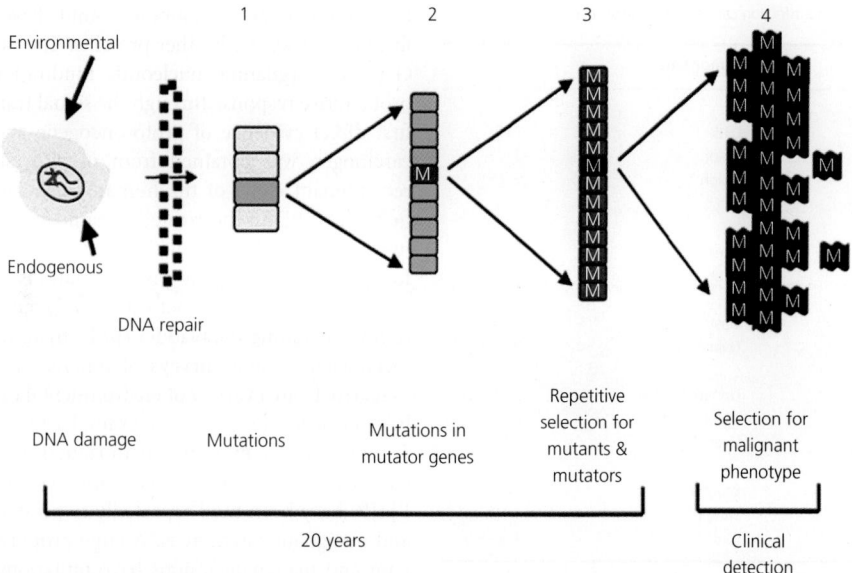

Figure 4 Mutation accumulation during tumor progression. (1) Random mutations result when DNA damage exceeds the cell's capacity for error-free DNA repair. (2) These random mutations can result in clonal expansion and mutations in mutator genes (M). (3) Repetitive rounds of selection for mutants yield coselection mutants in mutator genes. (4) From this population of mutant cancer cells, there is selection for cells that escape the host's regulatory mechanisms for the control of cell replication, invasion, and metastasis.

environmental tobacco smoke (ETS) compared to nonsmoking women not exposed to ETS.[239–244] This risk may be associated with polymorphisms. For example, in female populations, it appears that a common genetic polymorphism divides the population of never smokers into two groups of approximately equal size, one (homozygous carriers of the GSTM1 null allele) that has a statistically significant greater risk of lung cancer from ETS than the other (heterozygous or homozygous carriers of the wild-type GSTM1 allele).[240] In a similar context, genetic variants at 13q31.3 alter the expression of the glypican-5 (GPC5) gene, and down-regulation of GPC5 might contribute to the development of lung cancer in never smokers.[245,246] Other genes that have been found in never smokers and associated with lung cancer risk are LEM domain-containing protein 3 (LEMD3), transmembrane Bax inhibitor containing motif (TMBIM), ataxin 7-like 2 (ATXN7L2), Src homology 2 domain containing E (SHE), inter-α-trypsin inhibitor heavy chain H2 (ITIH2), Nudix (nucleoside diphosphate linked moiety X)-type motif 5 (NUDT5), EGFR, and echinoderm microtubule-associated protein like 4–anaplastic lymphoma kinase (EML4–ALK) fusions.[243,247,248] Similarly, α(1)ATD carriers are at a 70–100% increased risk of lung cancer.[249] Finally, as is the case for p53, the mutational profile of k-ras seems to differ greatly according to smoking status: G to T transversions are more common in ever smokers, whereas G to A transitions are seen more frequently in never smokers. K-ras and EGFR mutations are generally mutually exclusive, underlining their ordered participation in an intracellular signaling pathway, and suggesting different oncogenic mechanisms in lung cancer as a function of smoking status: tobacco carcinogens seem to be directly responsible for k-ras mutations, whereas the cause of mutations in EGFR, found particularly in never smokers, is currently not clear.

For race, it appears that compared to Caucasians, African-Americans are diagnosed earlier, have more aggressive, and consequently, have lower survival rates from breast cancers.[250,251] Racial disparities also exist in colorectal cancer.[252] Although these differences can be explained by socioeconomic differences, screening behaviors, and other behavioral differences, biological influences

can affect risk. For example, polymorphisms in nucleotide excision repair genes may modify the relationship between breast cancer and smoking in African-American women.[253] As well, the chemical carcinogen detoxifying gene, GSTM1, has a polymorphism that plays a role in the development of lung cancer and modifies the risk for smoking-related lung cancer in African-Americans.[254] Interesting recent findings highlighting gene–environment interactions indicated household income is associated with the p53 mutational frequency in patients who develop breast cancer (especially ER-negative). Furthermore, high-income patients may acquire fewer p53 mutations than other patients, suggesting that lifetime exposures associated with socio-economic status may impact breast cancer biology.[255,256]

Chronic inflammation and cancer

More than a century ago, the German pathologist, Virchow proposed that inflammation was associated with cancer.[8] Infection and inflammation significantly contribute to more than 25% of cancer cases worldwide (Table 4).[204] Free radicals, endogenous chemicals, are released during the inflammatory response. These ROS and reactive nitrogen species are generated as a physiological protective response to pathogenic microorganisms and toxic agents. During chronic inflammation (e.g., chronic viral hepatitis) and oxyradical overload conditions (e.g., hemochromatosis and inflammatory bowel diseases), these free radicals can induce genetic and epigenetic changes including somatic mutations in cancer-related genes and post-translational modifications in proteins involved in DNA repair, apoptosis, and arachidonic acid cascade (Figure 5).[8] Epigenetic transcriptional silencing of cancer-related genes including p16, Runt-related transcription factor 3 (RUNX3), and MutL homolog 1 (MLH1), by DNA methylation of their promoter regions has been associated with chronic inflammation in ulcerative colitis and Barretts esophagus.[257,258] Inflammation-mediated genetic and epigenetic alterations can also drive cancer development in the neighboring epithelium upon stromal abrogation of transforming growth factor-β signaling.[259]

Table 4 Chronic inflammation and infection can increase cancer risk.

Disease	Tumor site	Risk
Inherited		
Hemochromatosis	Liver	219
Crohn's disease	Colon	3
Ulcerative colitis	Colon	6
Acquired		
Viral		
Hepatitis B	Liver	88
Hepatitis C	Liver	30
Bacterial		
Helicobacter pylori	Gastric	11
PID	Ovary	3
Parasitic		
Schistosoma hematobium	Urinary bladder	2–14
Schistosoma japonicum	Colon	2–6
Liver fluke	Liver	14
Chemical/physical/metabolic		
Acid reflux	Esophagus	50–100
Asbestos	Lung pleural	>10
Obesity	Multiple sites	1.3–6.5

"18% of human cancers, that is, 1.6 million per year, are related to infection."—B. Stewart and P. Kleihues, World Cancer, Report, IARC Press, Lyon 2003, p. 57.
Rheumatoid arthritis is an example of a chronic inflammatory disease without a marked increased cancer risk, for example, joint sarcoma.
Oncogenic human papilloma viruses are examples of cancer-prone chronic infections without inflammation.

Finally, polymorphisms in genes involved in the production of [e.g., COX2, NOS's (NOS1, NOS2; but mostly NOS3)] or protection from (e.g., GpX, catalase, and MnSOD) free radicals also exist; can modify the effects of drugs; and increase or decrease cancer risk associated with exogenous chemical carcinogens.[260–268]

Oncogenes and tumor suppressor genes

Chronic exposures to carcinogens, accumulation of mutations, development of the mutator phenotype, and clonal selection during several decades result in cancer. Although the phenotypic traits of individual cancers are highly variable, commonly acquired capabilities include limitless replicative potential, self-sufficiency in growth signals, insensitivity to antigrowth signals, evading apoptosis, tissue invasion, sustained angiogenesis, and metastasis.[64] These phenotypic traits reflect a complex molecular circuitry of biochemical pathways and protein machines within cancer cells.[269]

The genes encoding the proteins within the cancer-associated molecular circuitry are of many functional classes and, historically, have been conceptually divided into oncogenes and tumor suppressor genes[269,270] (Box 4). Detailed descriptions of oncogenes and tumor suppressor genes are found in Chapters 4–7. The *ras* oncogene and the *TP53* tumor suppressor gene will be used as examples of molecular targets of chemical carcinogens.

Box 4 Mutational hotspots in cancer genes

Oncogenes and suppressor genes are targets of chemical carcinogens. Many genes, including K-ras and p53, have specific sequences targeted by chemical carcinogens resulting in mutational "hotspots." These mutations cause a change in expression and activity of the RNA and protein they code for.

Activated *ras* genes predominate as the family of oncogenes that are induced by chemicals in laboratory animals. Members of the *ras* gene family code for proteins of molecular weight 21,000 (p21);

these proteins are membrane bound, have GTPase activity, and form complexes with other proteins. The *ras* genes code for small G proteins (guanine nucleotide binding) that exert a powerful proliferative response through the signal transduction cascade. The first direct evidence of proto-oncogene activation by a chemical carcinogen was obtained from *in vitro* studies.[271] A wild-type recombinant clone of the human *Ha-ras* gene (pEC) was modified with BPDE. The treated plasmid was then used to transfect murine NIH-3T3 cells, with the result that the transformed cell foci contained the same point mutations (in either codon 12 or 61) known to exist in activated *ras* genes isolated from human tumors including the bladder (pEJ). In animal models of chemical carcinogenesis and surveys of different types of human tumors that arise from a variety of environmental exposures, *ras* mutations have been found.[272–275] For example, tobacco smoke can mutate *K-ras* during the molecular pathogenesis of human lung adenocarcinoma.[276] In rodents, PAHs (3-methylcholanthrene, DMBA, and B[a]P) have been used repeatedly to produce both benign tumors and malignant carcinomas. A large proportion of these premalignant and malignant lesions have mutations in either the 12th or the 61st codons. Similarly, treatment of rats with either DMBA or *N*-methyl-*N*-nitrosourea resulted in the development of mammary carcinomas containing *ras* codon 12 or 61 mutations. These types of mutations also have been observed in mouse skin after initiation with DMBA and tumor promotion with TPA. Mutations in *ras* have been found in mouse liver after treatment with vinyl carbamate, hydroxydehydroestragole, or *N*-hydroxy-2-acetylaminofluorene. The same point mutations have been found in murine thymic lymphomas after treatment with *N*-methyl-*N*-nitrosourea or γ-radiation, and in other rodent skin models after treatment with methyl methanesulfonate, α-propiolactone, dimethylcarbamyl chloride, or *N*-methyl-*N*9-nitro-*N*-nitrosoguanidine.

These data indicate that chemical carcinogens may produce site-specific mutations based, in part, on nucleoside selectivity of the ultimate carcinogen. Interestingly, noncovalent binding sites for (+)-anti-BPDE have recently been found on codons 12 and 13 of the K-ras gene.[277] Persistence of a specific mutation, however, also depends on the amino acid substitution in that the function of the mutant protein is altered to confer on the cell a selective clonal growth advantage. The types of mutations that are found in chemically activated *ras* genes cause conformational changes that alter protein binding (GTPase activating protein) in such a way that the *ras*-MAP kinase pathway is permanently activated. Data support the hypothesis that *ras* activation is associated with malignant conversion as well as tumor initiation. Transfection of activated *ras* genes into benign papillomas that did not contain a constitutively activated *ras* gene caused malignant progression.[275,278] These and other results implicate *ras* mutations in chemical carcinogenesis. Similarly, malignant transformation occurred when immortalized human bronchial epithelial cells were transfected with an activated *ras* gene.[279,280] *Ki-ras* gene mutations are also one of many changes that can arise either early or late in the development of colorectal carcinoma.[281] These findings indicate that the accumulation of mutations, and not necessarily the order in which they occur, contributes to multistage carcinogenesis. Furthermore, the stage of carcinogenesis in which each mutation occurs is not necessarily fixed. In the model for human colorectal carcinoma, *ras* mutations most often occur during malignant conversion, but can be an early event (i.e., tumor initiation), but in the rodent skin models, *ras* mutations appear to be primarily a tumor initiating event. These differences may reflect the type of exposure, both in terms of chemical class and chronic versus acute exposure, or they may be a function of tissue type.

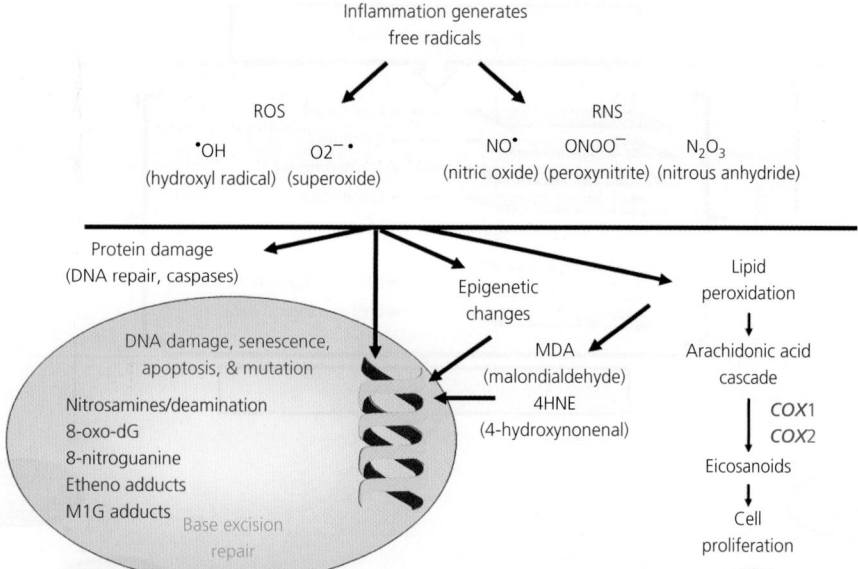

Figure 5 Several reactive oxygen species (ROS) and reactive nitrogen species (RNS) are generated during chronic inflammation. The reactive species can induce DNA damage, including point mutations in cancer-related genes, and modifications in essential cellular proteins that are involved in DNA repair, apoptosis, and cell cycle, either directly or indirectly through the activation of lipid peroxidation and generation of reactive aldehydes, for example, malondialdehyde (MDA) and 4-hydroxynonenal (4-HNE).

Table 5 Mutational spectra of *TP53* in human cancers.[a]

Carcinogen exposure	Neoplasm	Mutation
Aflatoxin B1	Hepatocellular carcinoma	Codon 249 (AGG 6 AGT)
Sunlight	Skin carcinoma	Dipyrimidine mutations (CC 6 TT) on nontranscribed DNA strand
Tobacco smoke	Lung carcinoma	G:C 6 T:A mutations on nontranscribed DNA strand (frequently codons: 157, 248, and 273)
Tobacco and alcohol	Carcinoma of the head and neck	Increased frequency p53 mutations (especially codons 157 and 248)
Radon	Lung carcinoma	Codon 249 (AGG 6 ATG)
Vinyl chloride	Hepatic angiosarcoma	A:T 6 T:A transversions
Aristolochic acid	Urothelial carcinoma	A to T transversions

[a]For reviews, see [288].

The *TP53* tumor suppressor gene is central in the response pathway to cellular stress.[282] For example, DNA damage caused by chemical carcinogens activates the p53 tumor suppressor protein by post-translational modification to transduce signals to "guard the genome"[283] by engaging cell-cycle checkpoints and enhancing DNA repair, and as a fail-safe mechanism, to cause replicative senescence or apoptotic death.[284,285] Mutations in the *TP53* gene or inactivation of its encoded protein by viral oncoproteins generally lead to a loss of these cellular defense functions. Not surprisingly, *TP53* mutations are common in human cancer.[286,287]

Molecular analysis of *TP53* can give clues to the environmental etiology of cancer (Table 5). It is implicit from the preceding text (see section titled "DNA damage and repair") that the covalent binding of activated carcinogens to DNA is not random. Therefore, the formation of a particular DNA lesion to some extent may be deduced from the resulting mutation. A dramatic example of this phenomenon is the previously mentioned *TP53* codon 249 mutation, which is detected in almost all aflatoxin-related hepatocellular carcinomas (HCC).[41,289,290] The striking nature of this association could arise by two distinct mechanisms. First, the third base in codon 249 (AGG) may be unusually susceptible to activated aflatoxin B1 mutations. As discussed earlier, aflatoxin B1-8,9-oxide causes a promutagenic lesion by covalently binding to the N7 position of deoxyguanosine. Alternately, cells bearing the codon 249 lesion may have an important selective growth advantage.

Evidence that a combination of these factors is responsible has been presented as well.[291] Another prominent example where circumstantial evidence points to specific molecular events is that of *TP53* mutations indicative of pyrimidine dimer formation in UV-light-related skin cancers.[292] In the case of tobacco smoking and lung cancer, G : C to T : A transversions indicate the formation of adducts from activated bulky carcinogens (e.g., PAHs).[41,293]

Precision medicine, molecular epidemiology, and prevention

Precision medicine is a concept developed by an *ad hoc* committee of the National Research Council in 2011.[52] The four basic premises are as follows: (1) the *Information Commons* for cancer has to be populated with a variety of –omic, phenotypic, clinical, and epidemiological data; (2) these data are integrated into a *Knowledge Network* that examines the interconnectivity of each layer of data from the Information Commons; (3) the Knowledge Network is used to develop *Taxonomic Classifiers* with the goal of improving patient diagnosis, decisions on therapeutic strategies, and health outcomes; and, finally, the knowledge is used to *guide biomedical, prevention, and clinical research* in mechanistic and observational studies (Figure 6). Precision medicine builds on the –omics revolution in molecular biology, advances in bioinformatics, tumor

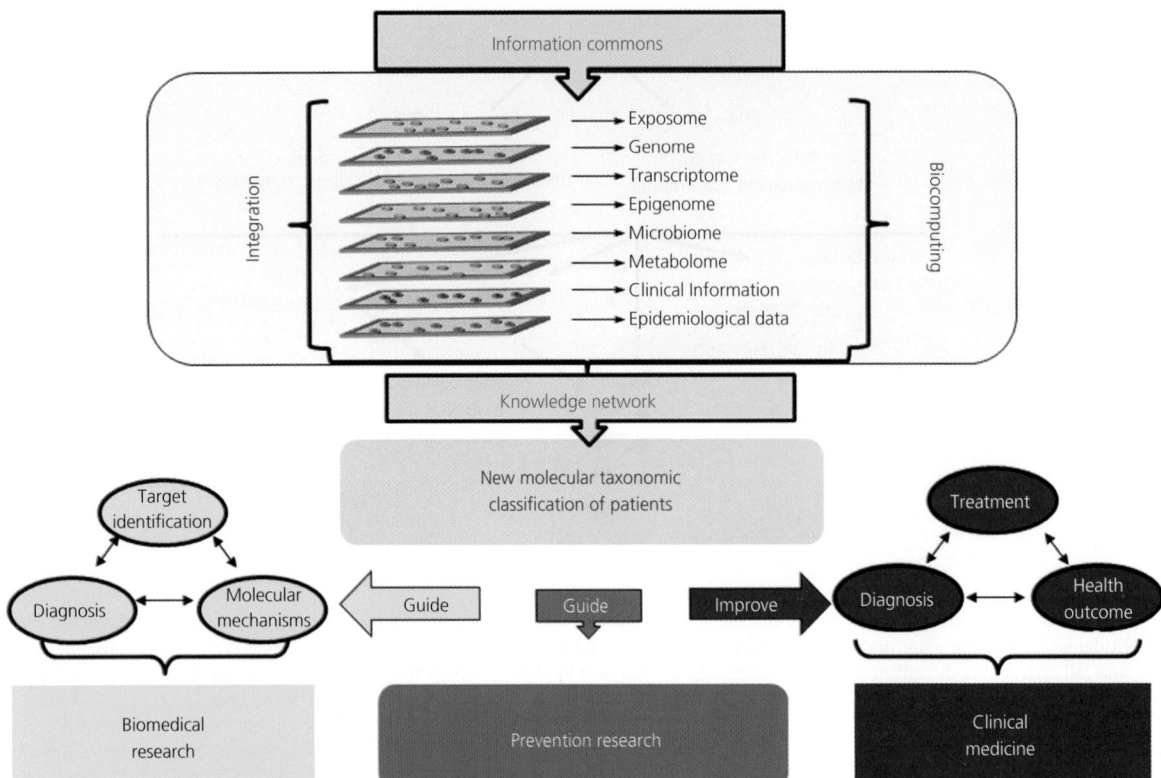

Figure 6 Precision medicine. In March 2011, at the request of the Director of the National Institutes of Health, an *ad hoc* committee of the National Research Council met to discuss the feasibility, need, scope, impact, and consequences of defining a "New Taxonomy" of human diseases based on molecular biology. The concept that developed, that of precision medicine, includes four basic premises.[52] First, the information commons for each disease type has to be populated with a variety of -omic, phenotypic, clinical, and epidemiological data. Second, these data are integrated into a knowledge network that examines the interconnectivity of each layer of data from the information commons. Third, the knowledge network is used to develop new taxonomic classifiers with the goal of improving patient diagnosis, decisions on therapeutic strategies, and health outcomes. Finally, the knowledge is used to guide biomedical and clinical research in mechanistic and observational studies. If realized, the benefits of precision medicine can be leveraged for most, if not all, disease types including cancer.

metabolism, tumor immunology, and the gene–environment concept of molecular epidemiology.

One of the biggest challenges in molecular cancer epidemiology associated with exposure to chemical carcinogens is to accurately measure exposure and then link this exposure to cancer risk. In this sense, so far, results have been disappointing. Traditionally, the paradigm, first defined by Perera and Weinstein in 1982,[37] has involved the assessment of exposure (what chemical and how much of that chemical; e.g., how much tobacco smoke or more specifically, B(a)P; BPDE; TSN), internal dose (how much of that chemical is in the body fluids, and tissues; e.g., amount of nicotine/cotinine), biological effective dose (the interaction of the chemical with biological entities; e.g., BPDE adducts), early biological response (e.g., TP53 mutation and k-ras mutation), altered structure/function (e.g., TP53 downstream functions and k-ras overexpression), and clinical disease (cancer). Intertwined with this paradigm are genetic factors and an individual's susceptibility (e.g., polymorphisms in metabolic enzymes such as p450's discussed earlier). A goal, then, of molecular cancer epidemiology is to identify biomarkers (of exposure, effect, and susceptibility) that accurately predict risk of disease. Unfortunately, to date, other than susceptibility markers [e.g., BRCA1/2 for breast cancer risk, APC (adenomatous polyposis coli) for familial colon cancer and more], few truly accurate biomarkers exist. Part of the reason is the money, man power, and time it takes to identify a biomarker, then follow that ahead in time (decades for the most part) to accurately assess cancer risk.

To this end, over the past decade, with new, highly sensitive, and sophisticated technology, this concept is evolving. The "omics" field, for example, has quickly advanced, with uses in the field of chemical carcinogen exposure and risk of cancer from that exposure. Using genetic information (genomics), biomarkers of susceptibility have been identified. In addition to such examples as BRCA1 or APC, polymorphisms in metabolic enzymes and DNA-repair pathways have been discussed. Genomics, tied in with other "omics" (adductomics, epigenomics, transcriptomics, proteomics, microbiomics, metabolomics, and cytokinomics) can be a powerful tool if properly linked to environmental chemical exposure. An evolving concept has been the "exposome".[48,294] In general, the exposome comprises every exposure to which an individual is subjected, from conception to death. Three broad categories of exposure are categorized: (1) internal exposure (metabolism, endogenous circulating hormones, body morphology, physical activity, gut microbiota, inflammation, and aging); (2) specific external exposures (radiation, infections, chemical contaminants, diet, tobacco, alcohol, occupation, and medical interventions); and (3) more general exposures/social/economic influences (education, financial status, psychological stress, and climate). Although the concept has obvious uses in epidemiological studies to establish risk factors at a population level,[294] linking numbers to and quantifying the exposome (exposomics) will be a necessary step to devise chemopreventive strategies (Figures 6 and 7).

Reconsideration of the dogma is necessary, because an extremely difficult task is to directly link a single genomic change to risk of specific types of cancer. Using genomics for somatic mutations, for example, as discussed earlier, we have identified specific k-ras and *TP53* mutational hotspots linked to specific carcinogens. The catalog of somatic mutations in cancer (COSMIC) indicates k-ras is the most frequently mutated isoform of ras isoforms and is present in 22% of all tumors analyzed compared to 8% for N-ras and 3% for H-ras and may prove to be an indicator of prognosis or a guide to treatment. The *TP53* tumor suppressor gene is mutated in most types of human cancers and it is the most commonly mutated gene yet known (e.g., mutations in *TP53* are found in approximately 50% of lung cancers).[41] Unlike *ras* gene mutations that are found in highly specific regions (codons 12, 13, 59, and 61), *TP53* mutations occur more widely. This is presumably because a positive growth advantage is conveyed only with specific ras mutations and the loss of *TP53* tumor suppressor function can occur with less specificity. However, for some malignancies, *TP53* mutations have provided clues to cancer etiology with a specific signature (hotspot) linked to specific carcinogenic exposure (Table 5).[41–43,55,286,295,296] *TP53* is further distinguished from other genetic lesions in that several possible mutant phenotypes can exist. Mutations may simply lead to the absence of *TP53*, an inactive mutant protein may exist, or the mutant might convey a growth advantage. Several studies have investigated *TP53* expression, and even though its role in prognosis has not been clearly defined, it may provide a guide to treatment options. To this end, recent advances have led to the decoding the "cancer landscape,"[68] with the identification of driver genes, classified into signaling pathways that regulate cell fate, cell survival, and genome maintenance. Such an understanding of these driver mutations will allow for the synthesis of new drugs focusing in on these molecules/pathways within a specific cancer of a specific individual to allow for specific treatment options in personalized medicine.

With the advent of microarray and other RNA detection technology [e.g., quantitative real-time PCR (polymerase chain reaction)], transcriptomics has also evolved, and transcription signatures have been identified associated with specific cancer subtypes, as well as with specific chemical carcinogen exposure. For example, papillomavirus infection is associated with the deregulation of genes involved in cell cycle; most of them E2F genes and E2F-regulated genes.[297] Genes up-regulated in samples from HCV (hepatitis C virus)-related Hepatocellular Carcinomas (HCC) have been shown to be classified in metabolic pathways, and the most represented are the aryl hydrocarbon receptor (AHR) signaling and protein ubiquitination pathways, which have been previously reported to be involved in cancer, and in particular in HCC progression. Genes up-regulated in samples from HCV-related non-HCC tissue have been shown to be classified in several pathways involved in inflammation and native/adaptive immunity and most of the overexpressed genes belonged to the antigen presentation pathway.[298]

Most studies to date investigating transcriptome changes in response to environmental exposures have relied on peripheral blood. Although details of these studies have been reviewed by Wild et al.,[294] here are a few highlights. Using peripheral blood mononuclear cells, Thomas et al. showed low levels of benzene (at or below 0.1 ppm) were observed in association with altered expression of AML pathway genes and CYP2E1. This is an important finding, because it shows that benzene alters disease-relevant pathways (AML) and genes in a dose-dependent manner, with effects apparent at doses as low as 100 ppb in air.[299] Another study showed leukemia-related chromosomal changes in hematopoietic progenitor cells from workers exposed to benzene.[300] Others have

found that telomere length was modestly, but significantly ($p = 0.03$) elevated in workers exposed to more than 31 ppm of benzene compared to controls.[301] Finally, polymorphisms in the CYP2E1 gene have been shown to be involved in benzene induction of micronuclei and may contribute to risk of cancer among exposed workers.[302]

Interestingly, many gene expression changes associated with smoking are involved in inflammatory and oxidative stress pathways. Recently, Tilley et al.[303] identified a "chronic obstructive pulmonary disease-like" small airway epithelium transcriptome signature and found xenobiotic and oxidant-related categories contained the genes displaying the greatest magnitude of change in expression levels in healthy smokers. Beane et al. showed that although large airway epithelial expression of many smoking-responsive genes is reversible upon smoking cessation, there are a number of smoking-responsive genes with persistently abnormal expression after smoking cessation. In this study, they also showed that pathways related to the metabolism of xenobiotics by CYP P450, retinol metabolism, and oxidoreductase activity were enriched among genes differentially expressed in smokers; whereas chemokine signaling pathways, cytokine–cytokine receptor interactions, and cell adhesion molecules were enriched among genes differentially expressed in smokers with lung cancer.[304] More recently, the same group showed SIRT1 activity is significantly up-regulated in cytologically normal bronchial airway epithelial cells from active smokers compared to nonsmokers.[305] Pierrou et al.[306] found significant changes in the expression of oxidant-related genes in the large airway epithelium of nonsmokers, healthy smokers, and COPD smokers, as did other studies[307,308] examining nonsmokers versus healthy smokers. Overall, transcriptomics has shown that it is possible to distinguish individual pathways associated with tobacco smoke, distinguish between individuals exposed and unexposed to tobacco smoke, and distinguish between current and past exposure to tobacco smoke. As reviewed by Wild et al.,[294] transcriptomics has also been able to identify specific signatures associated with dioxin (cell growth/ proliferation, glucose metabolism, apoptosis, and DNA replication, repair), metal fumes (inflammation, oxidative stress, phosphate metabolism, cell proliferation, and apoptosis), and diesel exhaust (inflammation and oxidative stress). In human lung tissues, a gene expression signature of 599 transcripts consistently segregated never from current smokers. Members of the CYP1 family, including CYP1A1, CYP1A2, and CYP1B1, were among the top genes up-regulated by smoking. The gene most strongly up-regulated by smoking was the aryl hydrocarbon receptor repressor (AHRR). Interestingly, six known genes were still significantly higher than never smokers after 10 years of smoking cessation (SERPIND1, AHRR, FASN, PI4K2A, ACSL5, and GANC).[309] Together, studies done with transcriptomics have demonstrated specific signatures associated with specific exposures to chemical carcinogens, suggesting potential mechanisms promoting cancer and identification of biomarkers associated with cancer risk.

The epigenome describes the totality of epigenomic changes [epigenetic marks present along the DNA and associated structures (e.g., histones) in a particular cell type]. We have already described some of the epigenetic events (mainly DNA methylation, histone modifications, and RNA-mediated gene silencing) associated with specific chemical carcinogen exposure. To this end, there have been a few studies to date attempting to link specific exposures of humans to epigenomic change. Overall, the impact of chemical carcinogens on the epigenome in human populations are limited to tobacco smoking (MTHFR and CDKN2A hypermethylation; GPR15, MSH3, NISCH, CYP1A1; RPS6KA3, ARAF, and especially AHRR hypomethylation), benzene (alu, long interspersed nucleotide elements, PTEN, ERCC3, p15, p16 hypermethylation; STAT3, MAGE-1 hypomethylation), cadmium (long interspersed nucleotide elements hypomethylation), air pollution (long interspersed nucleotide elements, tissue factor, F3, ICAM-1, and TLR-2 hypomethylation, and alu, IFN-γ, and IL-6 hypermethylation), smokey coal emissions (p16 hypermethylation), workplace exposures (iNOS hypermethylation; SATα, NBL2 hypomethylation; mgmt hypermethylation), and arsenic (alu, long interspersed nucleotide elements, RHBDF1, p16, p53 hypermethylation).[310–345] It should be pointed out that AHRR hypomethylation has been found as a common biomarker of smoking in multiple recent studies.[313,316–321,323,346] Also, importantly, recent studies suggest epigenetics is proving useful to the identification of both current and past smoking history. Past exposures can be detected and possibly even quantified based on the epigenetic footprints they leave on specific genes. Zhang et al.[347] found that coagulation factor II (thrombin) receptor-like (F2RL3) methylation intensity showed a strong association with smoking status, which persisted after controlling for potential confounding factors. Clear inverse dose-response relationships with F2RL3 methylation intensity were seen for both current intensity and lifetime pack-years of smoking. Among former smokers, F2RL3 methylation intensity increased gradually from levels close to those of current smokers for recent quitters to levels close to never smokers for long-term (>20 years) quitters. A recent study from the EPIC and NOWAC studies found 8 and 897 CpG sites differentially methylated in former and current smokers, while compared to never smokers, respectively. The eight candidate markers of former smoking showed a gradual reversion of their methylation levels from those typical of current smokers to those of never smokers. Further analyses using cumulative (over varying time windows) smoking intensities, highlighted three classes of biomarkers: short- and long-term biomarkers (measuring the effect of smoking in the past 10, and in the past 10–30 years, respectively), and lifelong biomarkers detected more than 30 years after quitting smoking.[348] Such studies show a promising ability, through epigenetics, to detect short-term to lifelong biomarkers of tobacco smoke exposure and, more generally, to potentially identify time-varying biomarkers of exposure.

Histone marks (post-translational modifications) in humans have also recently been assessed in association with chemical carcinogen exposure. Smoking is associated with a decrease in HDAC2 protein expression by 54% and activity by 47%, and concomitant enhancement of phosphorylation of Akt1 and HDAC2; workplace exposure to nickel is associated with an increase in H3K4me3 and decrease in H3K9me2; exposure to benzene is associated with reduced histone H4 and H3 acetylation and H3K4 methylation, and increased H3K9 methylation in the Topo IIα promoter; and, finally, exposure to arsenic is associated with an increased H3K4me2 and changes in global H3K9ac and H3K9me2 levels.[349–352]

In human populations, miRNA changes have been associated with exposure to cigarette smoke (40 upregulated in smokers, including miR-21, -16, -17, -29a, -221, and -223; repression of miR-15a, -199b, -125b, -218, -487, and -4423), workplace exposure (miR-21 and -222 increased in electric furnace steel plant workers post-exposure vs pre-exposure), benzene (up-regulation of miR-34a, -205, -10b, let-7d, miR-185 and -423-5p-2; down-regulation of miR-133a, -543, hsa-miR-130a, -27b, -223, -142-5p, and -320b), air pollution (up-regulation of miR-132, -143, -145, -199a*, -199b-5p, -222, -223, -25, -424, and -582-5p), and arsenic (up-regulation of miR-190, -29a, -9, and -181b; down-regulation of miR-200b).[349,353–361] Interestingly, miRNA levels have been shown to be reversed back to baseline

after cessation of smoking.[355] Overall, it is becoming increasingly clear that epigenomics is providing useful and specific biomarkers of chemical carcinogen exposure, and that these changes can be detected in humans. In addition, the observation that some changes are reversible, and some changes are not reversible allow careful monitoring of both present and past exposures and their consequences on clinical outcome.

The impact of environmental carcinogens associated with inflammatory load/cytokinomic, proteomics, metabolics, and microbiomics are still emerging. Moore et al. reviewed the use of "omic" technologies to study arsenic exposure in human populations.[362] The reader is referred to this reference for full details. In brief, though, genomic profiling has revealed long-term arsenic exposure may increase the risk of chromosome alteration prevalence in exposed bladder tissue and that chromosome 17p loss was unique to arsenic-exposed bladder cancer cases independent of p53 inactivation or aberrant protein expression. Additionally, in either human tissues or peripheral cells, arsenic has been shown in many studies to change gene expression (often involved in cell-cycle regulation, apoptosis, and DNA damage response), epigenetic events (e.g., heavily methylated promoter regions of p53 and p16), proteomic profiles (e.g., decreased levels of human b-defensin-1 and ADAM28), and metabolomic profiles.[362] In a few examples, an association with HCV and cirrhotic livers, it was recently found that there was a significant up-regulation of IL-1α, IL-1β, IL-2R, IL-6, IL-8, CXCL1, CXCL9, CXCL10, CXCL12, MIF, and β-NGF in serum compared to healthy controls.[363]

Although the concept of personalized medicine has been around for decades (and it can be argued, for centuries as medicine is given largely based on personal symptoms), we have only recently reached a tipping point with technology that has allowed us to be more precise with personalized medicine (precision medicine).[52] In the broadest sense, precision medicine is the molding of medical treatment to individual patient characteristics and moves beyond the current approach of stratifying patients into treatment groups based on phenotypic biomarkers. Now, with sensitive instrumentation and a capacity to gather large amounts of data regarding chemical carcinogens, we are poised to begin packaging, integrating, and quantifying large data sets for precise measurement of chemical carcinogen exposure. We have already discussed the exposome, which is a key first step toward this goal. Putting this exposure into numbers remains a challenge, but meeting this challenge will bring real and precise numbers that can be linked to a quantified taxonomic profile, which is a compilation of the massive data sets acquired through the different "omic" endpoints.[52] In this context, then, a precise risk signature might be realized for precision medicine and chemopreventive purposes (Box 5 and Figure 7).

Box 5 The exposome

The exposome comprises every exposure to which an individual is subjected, from conception to death. It takes into consideration the following: (1) internal exposure (metabolism, endogenous circulating hormones, body morphology, physical activity, gut microbiota, inflammation, and aging); (2) specific external exposures (radiation, infections, chemical contaminants, diet, tobacco, alcohol, occupation, and medical interventions); and (3) more general exposures/social/economic influences (education, financial status, psychological stress, and climate). Linking the exposome to metabolomic, proteomic, microbiomic, transcriptomic, and epigenomic profiles will allow us to identify an individual's risk signature as a biomarker for cancer risk and develop a precision medicine approach to cancer chemoprevention and treatment.

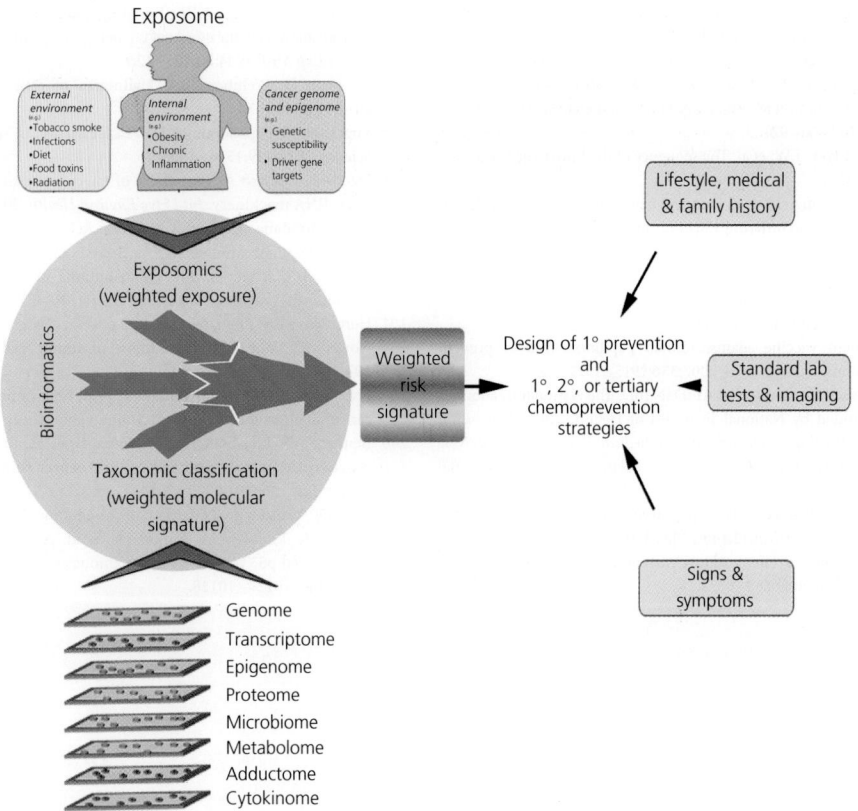

Figure 7 Connecting exposomics to toxonomics to generate a weighted risk signature for primary prevention and chemoprevention strategies. With the explosion of technology, extensive and massive data set generation over the past decade, we are in a position to use bioinformatics to merge the exposome with the various "omics" collected to generate a weighted and precise risk signature. Quantifying the internal, specific, and general external exposure of an individual or population (exposomics), then linking this to the molecular profile of an individual or population can generate a risk signature for an individual or population. Additional and continued consideration of signs/symptoms, standard lab tests, and family history will bring together a targeted primary and chemo-prevention strategy to reduce the risk of carcinogenesis in an individual or high-risk population of individuals.

Acknowledgments

We thank Glory Johnson and Karen Yarrick for their editorial assistance. This research was supported [in part] by the Intramural Research Program of the National Institutes of Health, National Cancer Institute, and Center for Cancer Research.

Key references

The complete reference list can be found on the Wiley Companion Digital Edition of this title (see inside front cover for login instructions).

2 Hajdu SI. A note from history: landmarks in history of cancer, part 1. *Cancer.* 2011;**117**:1097–1102.

3 Hajdu SI. A note from history: landmarks in history of cancer, part 2. *Cancer.* 2011;**117**:2811–2820.

5 Astruc J. *Traite de Tumeurs et des Ulceres.* Paris: P. Guillaume Cavelier; 1759.

6 Boerhaave H. *Opera Omnia Medica.* Holland: Neapoli: S. Abbate; 1742.

7 Pott P. *Cancer Scroti in Chirurgical Observations Relative to the Cataract, the Polypus of the Nose, the Cancer of the Scrotum, the Different Kinds of Ruptures, and the Mortification of the Toes and Feet.* London: Hawes, Clarke and Collins; 1775:63–65.

9 Hajdu SI. A note from history: landmarks in history of cancer, part 3. *Cancer.* 2012;**118**:1155–1168.

11 Rous P. A transmissible avian neoplasm. (sarcoma of the common fowl.). *J Exp Med.* 1910;**12**:696–705.

13 Berenblum I, Shubik P. A new, quantitative, approach to the study of the stages of chemical cartinogenesis in the mouse's skin. *Br J Cancer.* 1947;**1**:383–391.

15 Doll R, Hill AB. Smoking and carcinoma of the lung; preliminary report. *Br Med J.* 1950;**2**:739–748.

18 Conney AH, Miller EC, Miller JA. The metabolism of methylated aminoazo dyes. V. Evidence for induction of enzyme synthesis in the rat by 3-methylcholanthrene. *Cancer Res.* 1956;**16**:450–459.

21 Barnes J, Butler WH. Carcinogenic activity of aflatoxin to rats. *Nature.* 1964;**202**:1016.

22 Sporn MB, Dingman CW, Phelps HL, et al. Aflatoxin B1: binding to DNA in vitro and alteration of RNA metabolism in vivo. *Science.* 1966;**151**:1539–1541.

25 Knudson AG Jr. Mutation and cancer: statistical study of retinoblastoma. *Proc Natl Acad Sci U S A.* 1971;**68**:820–823.

27 Ames BN, Durston WE, Yamasaki E. Carcinogens are mutagens: a simple test system combining liver homogenates for activation and bacteria for detection. *Proc Natl Acad Sci U S A.* 1973;**70**:2281–2285.

28 Harris CC, Genta VM, Frank AL, et al. Carcinogenic polynuclear hydrocarbons bind to macromolecules in cultured human bronchi. *Nature.* 1974;**252**:68–69.

29 Loeb LA, Springgate CF, Battula N. Errors in DNA replication as a basis of malignant changes. *Cancer Res.* 1974;**34**:2311–2321.

30 Harris CC, Autrup H, Connor R, et al. Interindividual variation in binding of benzo[a]pyrene to DNA in cultured human bronchi. *Science.* 1976;**194**:1067–1069. 2013;**582**:768.

31 Stehelin D, Varmus HE, Bishop JM, et al. DNA related to the transforming gene(s) of avian sarcoma viruses is present in normal avian DNA. *Nature.* 1976;**260**:170–173.

32 Varmus HE, Vogt PK, Bishop JM. Integration of deoxyribonucleic acid specific for Rous sarcoma virus after infection of permissive and nonpermissive hosts. *Proc Natl Acad Sci U S A.* 1973;**70**:3067–3071.

34 Lane DP, Crawford LV. T antigen is bound to a host protein in SV40-transformed cells. *Nature.* 1979;**278**:261–263.

35 Linzer DI, Levine AJ. Characterization of a 54K dalton cellular SV40 tumor antigen present in SV40-transformed cells and uninfected embryonal carcinoma cells. *Cell.* 1979;**17**:43–52.

36 Doll R, Peto R. The causes of cancer: quantitative estimates of avoidable risks of cancer in the United States today. *J Natl Cancer Inst.* 1981;**66**:1191–1308.

37 Perera FP, Weinstein IB. Molecular epidemiology and carcinogen-DNA adduct detection: new approaches to studies of human cancer causation. *J Chronic Dis.* 1982;**35**:581–600.

41 Hollstein M, Sidransky D, Vogelstein B, et al. p53 mutations in human cancers. *Science.* 1991;**253**:49–53.

42 Hsu IC, Metcalf RA, Sun T, et al. Mutational hotspot in the p53 gene in human hepatocellular carcinomas. *Nature.* 1991;**350**:427–428.

43 Bressac B, Kew M, Wands J, et al. Selective G to T mutations of p53 gene in hepatocellular carcinoma from southern Africa. *Nature.* 1991;**350**:429–431.

44 Lander ES, Linton LM, Birren B, et al. Initial sequencing and analysis of the human genome. *Nature.* 2001;**409**:860–921.

45 Venter JC, Adams MD, Myers EW, et al. The sequence of the human genome. *Science.* 2001;**291**:1304–1351.

46 Calin GA, Dumitru CD, Shimizu M, et al. Frequent deletions and down-regulation of micro- RNA genes miR15 and miR16 at 13q14 in chronic lymphocytic leukemia. *Proc Natl Acad Sci U S A.* 2002;**99**:15524–15529.

48 Wild CP. Complementing the genome with an "exposome": the outstanding challenge of environmental exposure measurement in molecular epidemiology. *Cancer Epidemiol Biomarkers Prev.* 2005;**14**:1847–1850.

51 Group FIS. Quadrivalent vaccine against human papillomavirus to prevent high-grade cervical lesions. *N Engl J Med.* 2007;**356**:1915–1927.

52 National Research Council Committee on AFfDaNToD. The National Academies Collection: Reports funded by National Institutes of Health. *Toward Precision Medicine: Building a Knowledge Network for Biomedical Research and a New Taxonomy of Disease.* Washington (DC): National Academies Press (US) National Academy of Sciences; 2011.

54 Chen R, Mias GI, Li-Pook J, et al. Personal omics profiling reveals dynamic molecular and medical phenotypes. *Cell.* 2012;**148**:1293–1307.

55 Loeb LA, Harris CC. Advances in chemical carcinogenesis: a historical review and prospective. *Cancer Res.* 2008;**68**:6863–6872.

57 Friedewald WF, Rous P. The initiating and promoting elements in tumor production: an analysis of the effects of tar, benzpyrene, and methylcholanthrene on rabbit skin. *J Exp Med.* 1944;**80**:101–126.

64 Hanahan D, Weinberg RA. Hallmarks of cancer: the next generation. *Cell.* 2011;**144**:646–674.

68 Vogelstein B, Papadopoulos N, Velculescu VE, et al. Cancer genome landscapes. *Science.* 2013;**339**:1546–1558.

91 Izzotti A, Pulliero A. The effects of environmental chemical carcinogens on the microRNA machinery. *Int J Hyg Environ Health.* 2014;**217**:601–627.

95 Lagos-Quintana M, Rauhut R, Lendeckel W, et al. Identification of novel genes coding for small expressed RNAs. *Science.* 2001;**294**:853–858.

190 Rendic S, Guengerich FP. Contributions of human enzymes in carcinogen metabolism. *Chem Res Toxicol.* 2012;**25**:1316–1383.

191 Herenblum I. 3:4-benzpyrene from coal tar. *Nature.* 1945;**156**:601.

232 Nowell PC. The clonal evolution of tumor cell populations. *Science.* 1976;**194**:23–28.

239 Fontham ET, Correa P, Reynolds P, et al. Environmental tobacco smoke and lung cancer in nonsmoking women. A multicenter study. *JAMA.* 1994;**271**:1752–1759.

240 Bennett WP, Alavanja MC, Blomeke B, et al. Environmental tobacco smoke, genetic susceptibility, and risk of lung cancer in never-smoking women. *J Natl Cancer Inst.* 1999;**91**:2009–2014.

283 Lane DP. Cancer. p53, guardian of the genome. *Nature.* 1992;**358**:15–16.

292 Brash DE, Rudolph JA, Simon JA, et al. A role for sunlight in skin cancer: UV-induced p53 mutations in squamous cell carcinoma. *Proc Natl Acad Sci U S A.* 1991;**88**:10124–10128.

24 Endocrine and genetic bases of hormone-related cancers

Leslie Bernstein, PhD ▪ Xia Pu, PhD ▪ Jian Gu, PhD

Overview

Neoplasia of hormone-responsive tissues currently accounts for more than 30% of all newly diagnosed male cancers and almost 40% of all newly diagnosed female cancers in the United States. Given that endogenous hormones apparently affect the risk of these cancers and their overall frequency, concern exists about the effects on cancer risk if the same or closely related hormones are administered for therapeutic purposes (e.g., as contraceptives, as menopausal hormone therapy, or for the prevention of miscarriage). Depending on the timing of hormone use and the tissue-specific effects, some of these compounds will reduce risk while others increase risk of "hormone-dependent" cancers. This chapter focuses on breast, endometrial, and ovarian cancers among women and prostate cancer among men and provides a review of the epidemiologic and endocrinologic evidence for the role of hormones in cancer development. It also reviews the current status of the relationship between exogenous hormones and risk of cancers of the breast, endometrium, and ovary. In addition, it summarizes our current knowledge of genetic susceptibility to breast, endometrial, ovarian, and prostate cancers. Other less common cancers (e.g., cervical cancer, clear cell vaginal adenocarcinoma, thyroid cancer, testicular cancer, and osteosarcoma) may have a hormonal basis as well, but are not reviewed in this chapter.

Substantial and convincing bodies of experimental, clinical, and epidemiologic evidence indicate that hormones play a major role in the etiology of several human cancers. The concept that hormones can increase the incidence of neoplasia was first proposed by Bittner,[1] on the basis of experimental studies of estrogens and mammary cancer in mice. This theory has been refined into epidemiologic hypotheses related to cancers of the breast, endometrium, prostate, ovary, thyroid, bone, and testis.[2,3] The underlying mechanism proposed for these cancers is that neoplasia is the consequence of prolonged hormonal stimulation of the target organ, the normal growth and function of which is controlled by one or more steroid or polypeptide hormones. Evidence is mounting to show that the amount of hormone to which a tissue is effectively exposed is under strong genetic control.[4] Therefore, although external factors such as physical activity or exogenous hormone use may modify hormone profiles, the current evidence supports a multigenic model of cancer susceptibility.[5,6]

The major carcinogenic consequence of this hormonal exposure at the end organ is cellular proliferation, although direct carcinogenesis resulting from metabolic activation and direct DNA (deoxyribonucleic acid) binding is another potential mechanism. The emergence of a malignant phenotype depends on a series of somatic mutations that occur during cell division, but the entire sequence of genes involved in progression from normal cell to a particular malignant phenotype is not known (Figure 1). Candidate genes include those in the endocrine and growth factor pathways,[4,7,8] as well as DNA repair genes, tumor suppressor genes, and oncogenes.[9,10] Germline mutations have been described in two such tumor suppressor genes, BRCA1 and BRCA2, which are associated with susceptibility to breast and ovarian cancer.[11–14] Germline mutations in TP53 are also associated in certain kindreds with an increased risk of breast cancer.[15] However, mutations in these genes do not appear to be involved in the majority of sporadic breast cancer. Recent genome-wide association studies (GWAS) have identified many common, low-penetrance susceptibility loci for sporadic cancers.[16]

Neoplasia of hormone-responsive tissues currently accounts for more than 30% of all newly diagnosed male cancers and almost 40% of all newly diagnosed female cancers in the United States. Given that endogenous hormones apparently affect the risk of these cancers and their overall frequency, concern exists about the effects on cancer risk if the same or closely related hormones are administered for therapeutic purposes (e.g., as contraceptives, as menopausal hormone therapy, or for the prevention of miscarriage).[17] This chapter focuses on breast, endometrial, and ovarian cancers among women and prostate cancer among men and provides a review of the epidemiologic and endocrinologic evidence for the role of hormones in cancer development. It also reviews the current status of the relationship between exogenous hormones and risk of cancers of the breast, endometrium, and ovary. Other less common cancers (e.g., cervical cancer, clear cell vaginal adenocarcinoma, thyroid cancer, testicular cancer, and osteosarcoma) appear to have a hormonal basis as well, but are not reviewed here.

Breast cancer

Breast cancer is the most common cancer in women; it is expected that 232,670 new cases of invasive breast cancer and 62,570 new cases of breast carcinoma *in situ* will be diagnosed in the United States in 2014 and that 40,430 United States women will die of breast cancer.[18] A perceptible decline in breast cancer mortality has occurred since 1990,[19] resulting from greater use of mammographic screening, hormonal therapy, and therapy that targets HER2/neu.[20,21] Available evidence regarding the hormonal etiology of breast cancer is most consistent with the hypothesis that estrogen is the primary stimulant for breast cell proliferation.[2,3] The simultaneous presence of progesterone further increases the rate of proliferation.[22] This latter conclusion is based largely on the fact that breast mitotic activity peaks during the luteal phase of the menstrual cycle[23] and it is consistent with the increasing number of publications demonstrating that added progestins substantially augment the increased risk of breast cancer from estrogen therapy (ERT).[24–28]

Holland-Frei Cancer Medicine, Ninth Edition. Edited by Robert C. Bast Jr., Carlo M. Croce, William N. Hait, Waun Ki Hong, Donald W. Kufe, Martine Piccart-Gebhart, Raphael E. Pollock, Ralph R. Weichselbaum, Hongyang Wang, and James F. Holland.
© 2017 John Wiley & Sons, Inc. ISBN: 978-1-118-93469-2

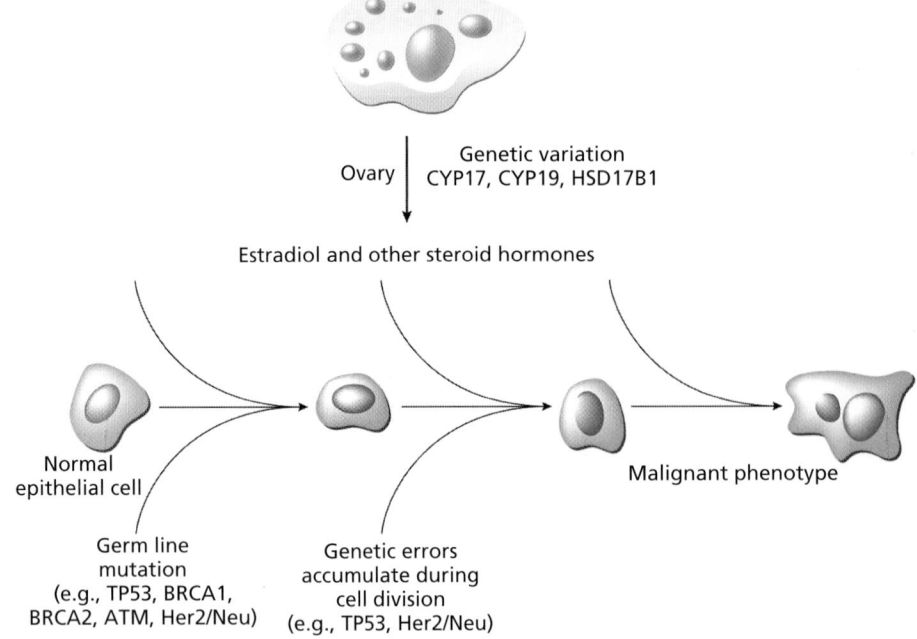

Figure 1 Estradiol and other steroid hormones (e.g., progesterone) drive breast cell proliferation, which facilitates the accumulation of random DNA copying errors in critical genes on the pathway to a malignant phenotype. Germ line mutations in relevant tumor suppressor genes accelerate the transformation to the malignant phenotype.

Table 1 A summary of established hormonal risk and protective factors for breast cancer.

Risk factors (increased exposure to estrogen and/or progesterone)
Early menarche
Late menopause
Obesity (postmenopausal women)
Hormone replacement therapy
Protective factors (reduced exposure to estrogen and/or progesterone)
Lactation
Early age at full-term pregnancy
Physical activity (exercise)

The most consistently documented, hormonally related risk factors for breast cancer are early age at menarche, late age at menopause, late age at first full-term pregnancy, and excess weight (Table 1). The age-incidence curve for breast cancer emphasizes the importance of ovulation in determining risk.[17] Cases first occur during early adulthood, and the rate of increase in incidence then rises sharply with age until the time of menopause, when it slows dramatically. The rate of increase in the postmenopausal period is approximately one-sixth the rate of increase in the premenopausal period. This age-incidence curve appears, then, to be shaped in a major way by the effects of ovarian activity. Therefore, it is critical to understand the determinants, both genetic and environmental, of the onset, regularity, and cessation of ovulation in order to continue to develop effective prevention modalities for breast cancer.

Reproductive factors

Early age at menarche is an established risk factor for breast cancer.[3] In general, risk decreases approximately 5–6% for each year that menarche is delayed, and this relationship may be further modified by the age at onset of regular ovulatory menstrual cycles. In a study of young women, Henderson et al.[29] reported that women with menarche at age 12 years or younger who experienced rapid onset of regular cycles had nearly a fourfold greater breast cancer risk than women with later menarche who experienced a long duration of irregular cycles. This is further supported by results from a study that showed that circulating estrogen and progesterone levels in daughters of women with breast cancer were higher than those of age-matched daughters of women without breast cancer.[30]

Although menarche and the onset of ovulation are to some extent genetically determined,[31] it is also critical to establish behaviors that may alter the number of ovulatory menstrual cycles a woman experiences during her reproductive years. Strenuous physical activity may delay menarche.[32] For example, in one study, the mean age at menarche of ballet dancers was 15.4 years compared to 12.5 years for control subjects. Moderate physical activity during adolescence can lead to anovulatory menstrual cycles. Girls who regularly engaged in moderate levels of physical activity (averaging at least 600 kcal of energy expended per week during a 9-month school year) were nearly three times more likely to have anovulatory menstrual cycles than were girls who were less physically active.[33] Bernstein et al.[34] have reported that lifetime patterns of leisure-time exercise activity significantly impact the breast cancer risk in young women (<40 years of age), older, postmenopausal women (55–64 years of age),[35] and African-American and Asian-American women.[36,37] Evidence continues to accumulate in support of a protective effect of physical activity on breast cancer risk with risk reductions observed in both case-control and cohort studies, although studies may vary according to the subgroups of women who benefit the most.[38–40]

Later occurrence of menopause and extended exposure to ovulatory cycles at the end of menstrual life also increase breast cancer risk. The risk of women whose natural menopause occurs before age 45 years is one-half that of women whose menopause occurs after age 55 years.[41] Artificial menopause, induced by bilateral oophorectomy or by pelvic irradiation, also markedly reduces breast cancer risk; this reduction is greater than that associated with natural menopause before age 50 years.[41–43] Following natural menopause, estrogen exposure declines gradually due to the continuing, but declining function of the ovaries and the continuing, persistent ovarian production of a small amount of testosterone.

The relationship between weight and breast cancer risk depends on menopausal status. Among postmenopausal women, a 10-kg increment in body weight results in about an 80% increase in breast cancer risk.[44] One explanation for this effect is that heavier postmenopausal women have higher circulating estrogen levels because of the conversion of an adrenal androgen, androstenedione, to estrone by aromatase present in body fat. In premenopausal women, the relationship between weight and risk is less clearly established, but if anything, the situation is the reverse of that in postmenopausal women; here, high weight is associated with reduced risk.[45] This may result from a reduction in the frequency of ovulatory menstrual cycles associated with high body weight.

Assuming ovarian activity affects breast cancer risk, case-control and cohort studies of breast cancer should find higher levels of circulating estradiol among breast cancer patients than among healthy women. Bernstein et al.[46] described the results of two concurrent case-control studies of premenopausal women in the United States (Los Angeles) and China (Shanghai). Overall, breast cancer patients had 14% higher serum estradiol concentrations, with a case-to-control excess of 17% in Chinese women and 11% in white American women, respectively. Los Angeles control women had 21% greater estradiol concentrations than did Shanghai control women, and adjustment for body weight only accounted for 25% of this difference. The results from a pooled analysis of nine prospective studies of endogenous hormones and postmenopausal breast cancer risk provide strong evidence that high estradiol concentrations are predictive of breast cancer risk, with women in the highest quintile of estradiol exposure having a twofold greater breast cancer risk than those in the lowest exposure quintile.[47]

Age at first birth

Having a first full-term pregnancy at a young age (i.e., before age 20 years) lowers a woman's breast cancer risk by about 50% relative to nulliparous women. Full-term pregnancies at later ages provide smaller increments of protection.[48] Women who have a late first full-term pregnancy (i.e., in their thirties) have greater breast cancer risk than nulliparous women have. This paradoxical cross-over effect of a late first full-term pregnancy has been repeatedly confirmed by epidemiologic studies.

The immediate effect of a full-term pregnancy on breast cancer risk is a short-term increase. Among women who have given birth within the past 3 years, breast cancer risk is nearly three times higher than that of women of the same age, parity, and age at first birth whose most recent birth occurred at least 10 years earlier.[49] On the basis of these results, it appears that a first pregnancy confers two contradictory effects on breast cancer risk: a short-term increase in risk, followed in the long term by a substantial reduction in risk.[49]

This apparent paradox has a physiologic explanation based on patterns of estrogen as well as prolactin secretion and metabolism during pregnancy. During the first trimester, the level of bioavailable estradiol rapidly rises, an effect that is more apparent during the first than in subsequent pregnancies.[50] Thus, in terms of estrogen exposure to the breast, the net effect during this early part of pregnancy is an increased risk that is equivalent to the exposure from several ovulatory cycles over a relatively short period of time.[51] At a molecular level, it is likely that the hormonal changes during pregnancy induce irreversible differentiation and apoptosis in some cells that have already accumulated one or more of the relevant somatic mutations necessary for breast cancer development. In the long run, however, this negative effect of early pregnancy on breast cancer risk can

be overridden by two beneficial hormonal consequences of completing the pregnancy. It has been reported that prolactin levels are substantially lower in parous compared to nulliparous women.[52–54] Prolactin, a polypeptide hormone, regulates lactation and appears to enhance estrogen effects on breast tissue. In addition, parous women have been reported to have lower levels of bioavailable estradiol than nulliparous women.[51]

Evidence is fairly convincing that lactation reduces the breast cancer risk of premenopausal women,[55–57] but is less consistent for postmenopausal women.[56,58] In two publications, Enger et al.[55,58] showed substantial breast cancer risk reductions, of 35% for premenopausal and 30% for postmenopausal parous women in the United States who breast fed for more than 15 months (relative to similar women who never lactated). In the United States, rates of breast feeding have varied over time; some studies may have not observed lower breast cancer risk among women who have breast fed due to the small proportion of women with a sufficient duration of lactation. Among premenopausal and postmenopausal women in Shanghai, where breast feeding often extends to more than 1 year per child, a strong dose–response effect of decreasing breast cancer risk with increasing breast feeding duration was observed.[59] The time when supplementary feedings are introduced to the infant as well as the frequency and duration of each breast feeding episode may also contribute to the inconsistent findings. Lactation may reduce breast cancer risk by reducing the total number of ovulatory menstrual cycles a woman experiences because breast feeding results in a substantial delay in reestablishing ovulation following a completed pregnancy.

Diet

Much attention has focused on dietary differences between countries, particularly fat consumption patterns, to explain both the international pattern of breast cancer occurrence and changes in rates of breast cancer following migration to high-risk from low-risk countries.[60] International breast cancer mortality and incidence rates correlate highly with per capita consumption of fat in the diet (correlation coefficient, $r = 0.93$ and $r = 0.84$, respectively).[60] As implied previously, nutrition may influence breast cancer occurrence by modifying age at menarche and body weight, but the correlation of fat consumption with international breast cancer mortality remains highly significant, even after statistical adjustment for these factors.

Although it has been theorized that fat intake in the diet may be an important contributor to breast cancer risk, many case-control studies of fat consumption and breast cancer find only small differences between cases and controls. Similarly, most of the cohort studies that have used food-frequency questionnaires to study the relationship with total fat, saturated fat, or vegetable fat have found little or no difference in breast cancer risk over a wide range of fat intake. In a meta-analysis of studies of total fat intake and breast cancer risk, the extent of increase in risk comparing women in the highest intake category with those in the lowest intake category was 14% for case-control studies (summary odds ratio (OR) $=1.14$; 95% confidence interval (CI) $= 0.99–1.32$) and 11% for cohort studies (OR $= 1.11$; 95% CI $= 0.99–1.25$).[61] The Women's Health Initiative randomized trial of more than 48,000 women tested the hypothesis that reducing intake of total fat to 20% of energy and increasing consumption of vegetables and fruit to at least five servings daily and grains to at least six servings daily would lower cancer, and particularly breast cancer, risk.[62] During 8.1 years average follow-up after randomization, the RR (relative risk) was lower in women who adhered to the diet compared to the nondietary intervention group, although the results were not quite statistically significant

(RR = 0.91; 95% CI = 0.83–1.01), but were suggestive of an impact of diet on breast cancer risk.

High-fiber diets may protect against breast cancer, perhaps because fiber reduces the intestinal reabsorption of estrogens excreted via the biliary system.[63] Assessment of fiber intake in epidemiologic studies has been problematic because of a paucity of data on the fiber content of individual foods and disagreement about the most appropriate methods of biochemical analysis to determine the different types of fiber. Case-control, but not cohort, studies have shown a consistent inverse association between dietary fiber intake and breast cancer risk.[64]

Several investigations have been undertaken to demonstrate a reduction in serum estrogen levels following dietary interventions that reduce fat or increase fiber intake.[65,66] A meta-analysis of these studies demonstrated a 7.4% average reduction in estradiol levels of premenopausal women and a 23% reduction in estradiol in post-menopausal women following trials of reduced dietary fat intake.[66] This analysis could not distinguish between a direct dietary effect on hormone levels and an indirect effect that was due to disruption of ovulatory cycles in premenopausal women; nevertheless, whatever the mechanism, such a reduction in estradiol levels is potentially very important.

Exogenous hormones

Hormone therapy and oral contraceptives are the exogenous counterparts to endogenous hormonal exposures experienced by women and therefore are of concern as potential contributors to breast cancer risk.

Oral contraceptives

The relationship between oral contraceptive use and breast cancer risk has been the topic of many review articles. A combined analysis of 54 studies that included more than 150,000 women has provided many important answers about the risk of breast cancer among users of combination oral contraceptives (COCs), which combine an estrogen and a progestin in a single pill.[67] This analysis indicates a modest increased risk of breast cancer among current (RR = 1.24) and recent (RR = 1.16) COC users. Age at first COC use modifies the association with recent use. For recent users, the risks are highest for those who began COC use before the age of 20 years. However, total duration of COCs use was not associated with increased risk of breast cancer, once recency of use was taken into account.

The pooled analysis compiled studies that mainly focused on younger women as most of these studies were conducted at a time when oral contraceptive users had not achieved their perimenopausal and postmenopausal years.[67] The Women's Contraceptive and Reproductive Experiences (Women's CARE) Study, a population-based case-control study conducted in five geographic regions of the United States,[68] involved more than 4500 newly diagnosed breast cancer patients and more than 4500 control subjects, all of whom were 35–64 years of age. This study was specifically designed to assess the impact of oral contraceptives among women who no longer used oral contraceptives. Relatively few participants in the Women's CARE Study were current oral contraceptive users; many women had stopped use at least 20 years earlier. No significant associations were observed between duration of use, estrogen dose of the formulation, age at first use, interval since last use, or use in relation to timing of pregnancy and breast cancer risk. Further, results for younger women (35–44 years) were similar to those for older women (45–64 years) who were more likely to have used earlier formulations, but were less likely to have recently used oral contraceptives.

The International Agency for Research on Cancer completed a review of all of the existing literature on COCs and breast cancer risk concluding that breast cancer risk is increased in current or recent oral contraceptive users, particularly among women under age 35 years whose first oral contraceptive use was before age 20 years.[69] The increase in risk disappeared as age at current or recent use increased and, following cessation of oral contraceptive use, any increase in risk disappeared within 10 years.

Hormone therapy

Hormone therapy has evolved over time. Originally designed to reduce the symptoms of menopause, hormone therapy gained popularity because of its efficacy in reducing the risk of osteoporosis and its purported benefits in reducing the risk of heart disease. Initially formulated as ERT, the number of women using hormone therapy increased through the mid-1970s, until concerns were raised about the carcinogenic potential of ERT on the endometrium. In the 1980s, cyclic estrogen–progestin regimens became widely recommended and prescribed to eliminate the increase in endometrial cancer associated with estrogen-alone therapy. Initially, these were prescribed as sequential regimens with estrogen given during the first 15–20 days of a 28-day cycle followed by 5–10 days when both estrogen and progestin were given. More recently, continuous combined regimens have gained favor because they reduce menstrual-like bleeding episodes and because of their ease of administration.

Most studies that have included sufficiently large numbers of women who have used ERT for extended periods of time (e.g., for more than 10 years) indicate a modest increase in breast cancer risk among exposed women, with risk increasing approximately 3% per year of use.[70] Among studies conducted in the United States, where the use of conjugated equine estrogens is the norm, it was estimated that breast cancer risk increased about 2.2% per year of use of a standard dose regimen (0.625 mg/day).

The Collaborative Group on Hormonal Factors in Breast Cancer pooled data from 51 epidemiologic studies and more than 160,000 women to assess the impact of hormone therapy on breast cancer risk.[55] Where information was available regarding type of hormone preparation used, 80% of women in these studies had used mostly estrogen-only therapy and 12% of women had used combination hormone therapy. This study showed that hormone therapy (primarily ERT) increased breast cancer risk with RRs of 1.09, 1.15, and 1.14 comparing ever users to never-users in cohort studies, population-based case-control studies, and hospital-based case-control studies, respectively. Risk was substantially elevated among women who had used hormone therapy for at least 15 years (RR = 1.58). Risk increased by 2.3% ($p = 0.0002$) for each year of use among women who had used hormone therapy within 5 years of diagnosis or an equivalent reference date (Figure 2). However, women who stopped hormone therapy use 5 or more years earlier had only a modest, nonsignificant increase in risk, regardless of duration of use.

Consistent with these estimates are the results from the Million Women Study, conducted in the United Kingdom, which recruited a cohort of women aged 50–64 years who had undergone routine mammography.[61] In this study, incidence of breast cancer was significantly greater among current users of ERT than among women who had never used hormones (RR = 1.30; 95% CI = 1.22–1.38). Risk increased with increasing duration of use among these current users, with 5–9 years of use associated with a RR of 1.32 and 10 or more years of use associated with a RR of 1.37.

The Women's Health Initiative randomized trial compared an estrogen-alone regimen to placebo among women 50–79 years

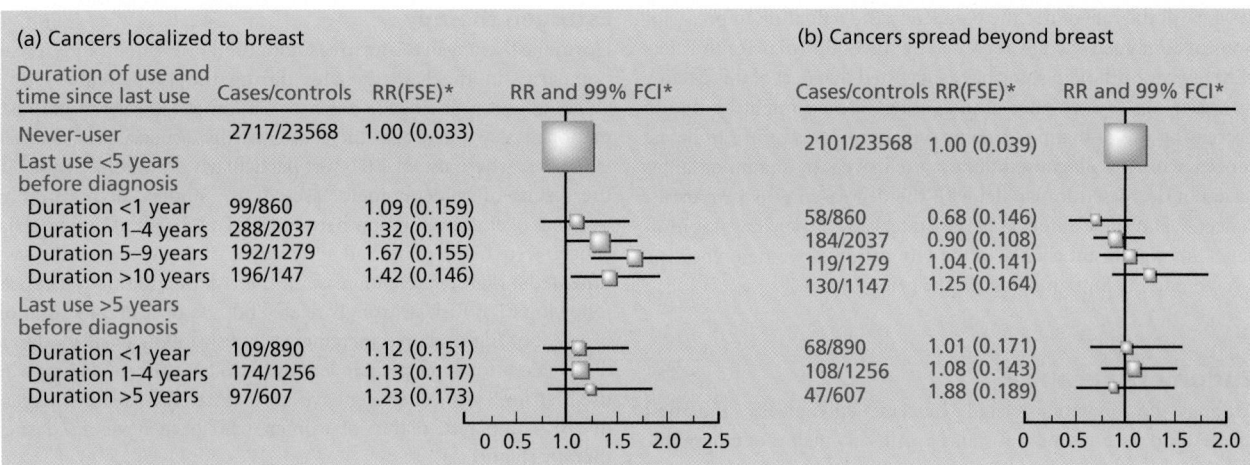

(a) Cancers localized to breast			
Duration of use and time since last use	Cases/controls	RR(FSE)*	RR and 99% FCI*
Never-user	2717/23568	1.00 (0.033)	
Last use <5 years before diagnosis			
Duration <1 year	99/860	1.09 (0.159)	
Duration 1–4 years	288/2037	1.32 (0.110)	
Duration 5–9 years	192/1279	1.67 (0.155)	
Duration >10 years	196/147	1.42 (0.146)	
Last use >5 years before diagnosis			
Duration <1 year	109/890	1.12 (0.151)	
Duration 1–4 years	174/1256	1.13 (0.117)	
Duration >5 years	97/607	1.23 (0.173)	

(b) Cancers spread beyond breast		
Cases/controls	RR(FSE)*	RR and 99% FCI*
2101/23568	1.00 (0.039)	
58/860	0.68 (0.146)	
184/2037	0.90 (0.108)	
119/1279	1.04 (0.141)	
130/1147	1.25 (0.164)	
68/890	1.01 (0.171)	
108/1256	1.08 (0.143)	
47/607	1.88 (0.189)	

Figure 2 (a,b) Relative risk of breast cancer by duration and time since last use of hormone therapy according to extent of tumor spread relative to never-users, stratified by study, age at diagnosis, time since menopause, body mass index, parity, and the age of a woman when her first child was born. "Last use within 5 years before diagnosis" includes current users. *Floated standard errors (FTEs) and floated confidence intervals (FCIs) calculated from floated variance for each category.

of age who had previously had a hysterectomy and assessed the impact of a combined estrogen plus progestin regimen versus placebo among similarly aged women who had an intact uterus. The estrogen-alone regimen consisted of 0.625 mg/day of conjugated equine estrogen,[71] and the combined regimen consisted of 0.625 mg/day of conjugated equine estrogen and 2.5 mg/day of medroxyprogesterone acetate.[27] The results for the ERT study were somewhat surprising in that, after an average follow-up of 7.1 years, the RR of breast cancer was not elevated (RR = 0.80; 95% CI = 0.62–1.04).[72] In the trial, the reduction in risk was greater and was statistically significant for ductal cancers although even in a trial this large, numbers were too small to demonstrate a difference in risk by tumor histology. In comparison to ductal tumors, risk appeared elevated for lobular cancers and the comparison of ductal to lobular cancer was of borderline statistical significance ($p = 0.054$). A similar, nonstatistically significant difference was observed by stage with risk reduced for localized cancers but not for regional cancers ($p = 0.09$).

For combined hormone therapy (CHT), the Women's Health Initiative assessed only the continuous combined regimen. Three population-based observational studies, published in 1999 and 2000, showed that CHT conferred a greater risk of breast cancer than did an estrogen-alone regimen.[24,25,73] For example, Ross et al.[25] found that the increment in risk for each 5 years of use was nearly four times greater for CHT users than for ERT users. Results from the Women's Health Initiative trial arm comparing a continuous CHT to placebo provided a risk estimate that was similar to those from these prior studies (RR = 1.24; 95% CI = 1.01–1.54).[27]

Lee et al.[74] conducted a meta-analysis of the results of studies that have evaluated the impact of CHT on breast cancer risk, separating results for use of sequential (cyclic) combined regimens from those for use of continuous combined regimens and including results from the Collaborative Group on Hormonal Factors in Breast Cancer[55] and the Women's Health Initiative.[27] Overall, users of a combined regimen had substantially elevated risk that increased 7.6% per year of use.[74] Not all studies provided data on progestin schedule. Those that did showed a small difference in risk between sequential and continuous combined regimens (increase in breast cancer risk per year of use of 8.9% and 10.3%, respectively). Notably, results from Scandinavian studies showed that continuous regimens had a greater impact on risk than sequential regimens. This

difference was not as apparent among studies from the United States or the Million Women's Study. In the United States, the total dose of progestin is comparable in continuous combined compared to sequential regimens, whereas in Scandinavia, continuous combined regimens provide a substantially higher dose of progestin. Thus, evidence is quite strong that the progestin component of combined regimens adds substantially to any increase in breast cancer risk conferred by estrogen alone and that differences in results between the United States and Scandinavia are likely due to differences in the progestin dose administered.

Recently, the Women's Health Initiative investigators published an update on health risks and benefits of CHT, examining risk following cessation of hormone therapy.[75] Risk for invasive breast cancer remained elevated after an average 2.4-years follow-up after use was stopped among women who had been randomized to the estrogen plus progestin arm of the trial evaluating combined therapy (RR = 1.27; 95% CI = 0.91–1.78), although the CI did not exclude 1.0.[75]

CHT preferentially increases the risk of lobular and ductal-lobular breast cancers, particularly those judged to have more than a 50% lobular component.[76] Among older women, ages 55–74 years, current users of combined therapy were at 2.7-fold greater risk of lobular carcinoma and 3.3-fold greater risk of ductal-lobular carcinoma compared to women who had no use of combined therapy.

Declining use of combined therapy has had a marked impact on breast cancer incidence rates in the United States and Germany.[77–79] It is important to note that rates of breast cancer in the United States began to decline before publication of the Women's Health Initiative result for combined therapy in 2002.[26] An evaluation of data from the Surveillance, Epidemiology, and End Results (SEER) registries for 1975–2003 shows a decline in invasive breast cancer from 1999 onward in all age groups of women 45 years or older, with a sharp decrease in incidence in 2002 and 2003, particularly of estrogen receptor- (ER) positive tumors, in women 59–69 years of age.[78] Data from a mammography registry in San Francisco indicate that hormone therapy prescribing peaked in 1999, then began to decline, which was amplified following publication of the Women's Health Initiative.[80] Robbins and Clarke[81] confirmed this in their analysis of breast cancer incidence across 58 counties in California, clearly demonstrating that breast cancer rates declined between 2001 and

2004, with the rate of decline paralleling the reduction in prescriptions of combined therapy recorded by the California Health Interview Survey. Although some have suggested that part of this decline in breast cancer incidence among older women might be due to decreasing use of mammographic screening, rates of *in situ* breast cancer, which is diagnosed almost exclusively by mammography, have not decreased in parallel with the decrease in invasive breast cancer,[78] and the California Health Interview Survey has not indicated any significant change in the proportion of women reporting a screening mammogram within the prior 2 years.[81]

Endometrial cancer

Among the hormone-related cancers, etiologically the best understood is endometrial cancer. All the major demographic characteristics of the disease, as well as the major nondemographic risk factors, are explicable on the basis of cumulative exposure of the endometrium to that fraction of estrogen, which is unopposed by the modifying influences of progesterone.[2,3]

Mitotic activity in the endometrium

Key and Pike[82] summarized the existing data on endometrial mitotic activity during normal menstrual cycles. Mitotic rates are low during days 1–4 of the cycle, then increase rapidly and remain stable thereafter until day 19, after which rates essentially drop to zero for the remainder of the cycle. There appears to be a lag period of about 4 days before the stimulatory effects of unopposed estrogen or the modifying influence of progesterone on endometrial mitotic activity are fully apparent.

The cellular basis for the antiestrogenic activity of progestogens on the endometrium is well understood.[2] Progestogens reduce the concentration of estradiol receptors and increase the activity of the 17-β-hydroxysteroid dehydrogenase type II enzyme, which converts estradiol to estrone,[83,84] a biologically less-potent estrogen because of its lower affinity for cellular ERs. Luteal phase progesterone causes endometrial cells to differentiate to a secretory state and progestogen withdrawal leads to cyclic sloughing of endometrial tissue.

On the basis of the concept that frequency of mitotic activity is the primary determinant of endometrial cancer risk and that such activity is controlled by cumulative exposure to unopposed estrogens, one can readily predict the most important risk factors for this disease (Table 2). Pregnancies and oral contraceptives, which expose the endometrium to constant high levels of both estrogen and progestogen, should protect against endometrial cancer development. ERT and obesity should increase the risk. All of these predicted effects have been repeatedly well documented in epidemiologic studies.[2]

Table 2 A summary of established hormonal risk and protective factors for endometrial cancer.

Risk factors (increased exposure to "unopposed" estrogen)
Estrogen replacement therapy
Obesity
Sequential oral contraceptives
Late menopause
Protective factors (decreased exposure to "unopposed" estrogen)
Pregnancy
Combination oral contraceptives

Estrogen therapy

Hormone therapy in the form of unopposed ERT gained widespread popularity in the United States during the 1960s and 1970s.[85] Concomitantly, incidence rates of endometrial cancer in postmenopausal women also increased rapidly, especially in western US states, where use of ERT was particularly common.[86] By 1975, the results of epidemiologic case-control studies, demonstrating a strong overall association between ERT and risk of endometrial cancer, were being published.[87,88] Dozens of studies have now documented a high relative increase in the risk of endometrial cancer following ERT. Risk is strongly related both to dose and to duration of use, but high relative increments in risk follow even moderate doses taken for intermediate length periods of time. Women who use ERT for 5 years or longer have approximately a 3.5-fold increase in risk compared to that of women who have never used such therapy (Figure 3a).[17]

Although use of estrogen clearly increases the incidence of aggressive endometrial cancer, the overall mortality from endometrial cancer among affected users somewhat paradoxically is much lower than among nonusers who develop endometrial cancer.[89] In fact, such women have little reduction in life span when compared to healthy women of the same age. The reasons for this are not completely known, but this phenomenon likely can be explained by the increased medical surveillance among estrogen users. Women who use ERT tend to be closely monitored because the drug frequently induces vaginal bleeding. Part of the favorable survival experience may also result from patients with estrogen-induced benign hyperplasia being misdiagnosed as having endometrial cancer. Although past users of ERT have a risk of endometrial cancer that is intermediate between that for current users of comparable duration and lifetime nonusers, risk in such women remains substantially elevated over baseline even after many years without treatment.[90]

As noted above, the newer regimens of hormone therapy typically follow one of two patterns: sequential or combined estrogen and progestin. The sequential regimen attempts to reproduce the hormonal pattern of the normal menstrual cycle, albeit at lower levels of both estrogen and progestogen. One therefore might predict that this method of hormone therapy administration would only partially offset the increased risk of endometrial cancer that is associated with unopposed ERT. Pike et al.[91] showed that if progestins are added for less than 10 days per month, the risk is only slightly reduced. However, regimens that include progestins for more than 10 days in a month, or where progestins are given continuously with estrogen, do not increase endometrial cancer risk.[91]

The Million Women Study conducted in Great Britain, which included 716,738 postmenopausal women without prior cancer or hysterectomy who were recruited between 1996 and 2001, also provides data on this issue.[74] Relative to women who had never used any hormonal therapy, endometrial cancer risk was substantially lower among women who had used continuous CHT as their most recent hormone therapy, with a RR of 0.71 (95% CI = 0.56–0.90). For women using cyclic CHT, however, risk did not differ from that of nonusers (RR = 1.05; 95% CI = 0.92–1.22). The number of cases among women taking estrogen-alone therapy was small, as, since the mid-to-late 1970s, this has rarely been given to women with an intact uterus. Among women on estrogen-alone therapy, the RR of endometrial cancer was substantially lower than prior studies had observed (RR = 1.45; 95% CI = 1.02–2.06). As expected, based on the fact that obesity increases endometrial cancer risk through an estrogen pathway causing endometrial proliferation,[82,92] the reduction in risk on CHT was greatest among obese women and the increase in risk for estrogen-alone therapy was greatest among nonobese women.

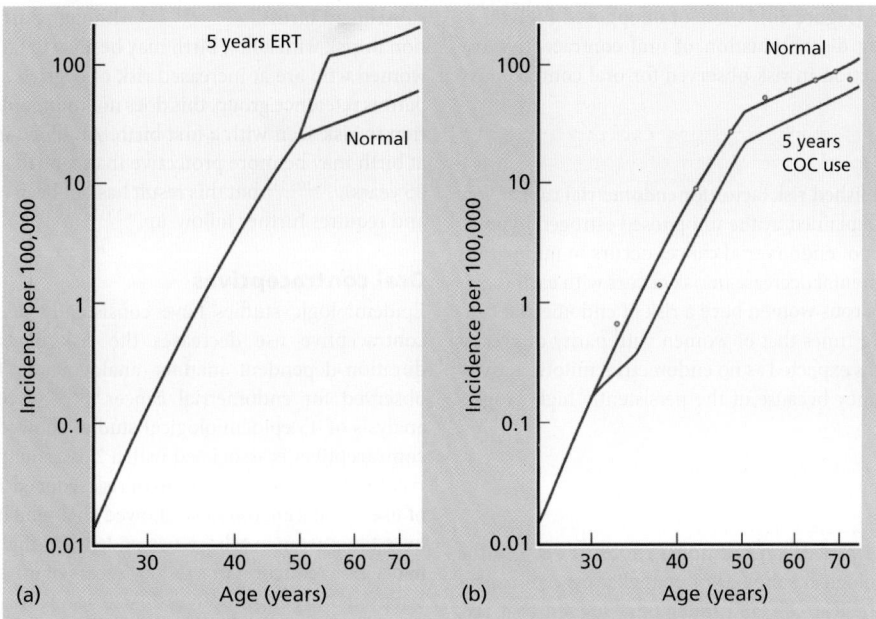

Figure 3 Age-specific incidence rates for cancers of the endometrium in women using estrogen therapy (ERT) (a) and combination oral contraceptives (COCs) (b) for 5 years. Data are from the UK Birmingham Cancer Registry for the years 1968–1972. These data largely avoid problems arising from the high hysterectomy and oophorectomy rates in the United States, which artificially distort the age-incidence curves. *Dots*, actual incidence data; solid lines marked "normal," mathematic models predicting these rates from the major known risk factors for these cancers. Source: Henderson et al. 1993.[17] Reproduced with permission from The American Association for the Advancement of Science.

The authors of the Million Women Study also provided an extensive assessment of published studies, including their own, on the impact of CHT on endometrial cancer risk.[74] Overall, they calculated a summary estimate that the RR for continuous CHT across all studies was 0.88 (95% CI = 0.75–1.03) compared to never-users. This estimate, however, was based on relatively few cases—with only 265 cases identified across six studies, including the Women's Health Initiative.[93] The estimated RR of endometrial cancer associated with use of cyclic CHT was 1.14 (95% CI = 1.01–1.28),[74] based on a total of 456 cases, from six studies, four of which overlap with the studies of continuous CHT. Overall, it appears that regimens in which estrogen and progestin are taken daily together (continuous CHT) provide a slight protection against endometrial cancer relative to the risk among women who had never used any hormonal regimen, whereas cyclic use of progestins results in a risk of endometrial cancer that is slightly higher than that of women who had never used hormone therapy.

Tamoxifen, an antiestrogen to the breast, acts as an estrogen agonist in the endometrium, and the risk of endometrial cancer is elevated by tamoxifen in a manner analogous to that of ERT.[94] Furthermore, the increase in risk is greater among women who previously used ERT and among those with high body mass.[94] The molecular basis of this agonist effect on the endometrium as opposed to the antagonist activity of tamoxifen on the breast, however, is not totally understood.

Body weight

Unlike breast cancer where high body weight is associated with lower risk among young women and higher risk among older women, high body weight leads to increased risk of endometrial cancer at all ages. Studies of postmenopausal women show at least a doubling of risk of endometrial cancer between thin and heavy women.[95,96] Adipose tissue is rich in an aromatase enzyme system that converts androstenedione to estrone. In turn, estrone can be converted directly to estradiol. In addition, protein binding of estrogens in blood is lower in obese women, so the amount of bioavailable estradiol in obese postmenopausal women is higher than would be expected from the peripheral conversion of androstenedione to estrone alone.

The explanation for the substantially increased risk of endometrial cancer with obesity in premenopausal women is less obvious.[96] Although obesity does appear to be associated with slightly increased levels of bioavailable estradiol in premenopausal women, this alone appears to be insufficient to account for such a profound effect. The more likely explanation is that obesity in premenopausal women is associated with amenorrhea and subnormal luteal phase progesterone levels, thus resulting in prolonged exposure of the endometrium to unopposed estrogen.[97]

Among postmenopausal women, obesity has become a more important factor in determining endometrial cancer risk subsequent to the declining use of CHT following publication of the Women's Health Initiative results. Results from the American Cancer Society Cancer Prevention Study II Nutrition Cohort show that the risk of endometrial cancer associated with obesity is strongly influenced by whether a women has used CHT.[98] Increasing body size, measured by body mass index (kg/m²), is associated with increasing endometrial cancer risk among postmenopausal women with no prior history of hormone therapy use but has no impact on endometrial cancer risk among women who have used CHT.[98]

Oral contraceptives

The role of estrogens as the principal cause of endometrial cancer is further supported by the markedly increased risk after a relatively short duration of use of sequential oral contraceptives, which deliver an unopposed estrogen during most of the monthly cycle.[96,99] These potent effects can be mitigated by the simultaneous administration of progestogens. A series of case-control and cohort studies has consistently demonstrated that combined oral contraceptives, which deliver estrogen and progestogen simultaneously during each day of use, decrease the risk of endometrial cancer by

11.7% per year of use (Figure 3b).[17] Use of unopposed ERT for at least 3 years following discontinuation of oral contraceptive use may counter the reduction in risk observed for oral contraceptive use.[100]

Parity

The other major, established risk factor for endometrial cancer, low parity, also is readily explained by the unopposed estrogen hypothesis.[95] The highest risk of endometrial cancer occurs in nulliparous women, and an incremental decrease in risk occurs with each increment in parity. Nulliparous women have a risk of endometrial cancer that is three to five times that of women with parity of greater than three. This effect is expected as no endometrial mitotic activity occurs during pregnancy because of the persistently high progesterone levels.

Ovarian cancer

Existing epidemiological data on hormonal exposures across the four major histopathological subtypes of epithelial ovarian cancer (serous, endometriod, clear cell, and mucinous) suggest that risk factors are consistent across all subtypes except perhaps mucinous tumors. Traditionally, the cell of origin of epithelial ovarian cancer (herein referred to as ovarian cancer) has been described as the single layer of cells lining the surface of the ovary; because these cells replicate during or after each ovulation any respite from ovulation would be protective against ovarian cancer.[101] This hypothesis, called "incessant ovulation," is supported by epidemiologic data, which consistently demonstrate that the risk of developing ovarian cancer decreases with increasing parity[102-104] and with COC use (Table 3),[104-109] both of which induce anovulation. However, emerging evidence that serous tumors of the fallopian tube and peritoneum share the same epidemiology as serous ovarian cancers has brought into question the notion that it is the actual act of ovulation and subsequent wound healing that underlies the epidemiology of the disease; instead, it may be the hormonal milieu induced as a result of parity and oral contraceptive use.[110] Further, clear evidence of an association between menopausal hormone therapy exists, suggesting that the hormonal milieu rather than ovulation itself influences risk of ovarian cancer.

As with breast and endometrial cancer, the age-incidence curve for ovarian cancer emphasizes the importance of menopause in determining risk. The age-incidence curve of ovarian cancer can be brought into line with the familiar linear log–log plot of other nonhormone-dependent epithelial tumors, if ovarian age is considered as starting at menarche, but increasing at a reduced rate (approximately 30% of normal) during periods of anovulation, including the postmenopausal years.[17]

Parity

Parity has been consistently identified as a protective factor against ovarian cancer.[102-104] After a woman's first birth, ovarian cancer risk is reduced approximately 40% with a 10% reduction associated with subsequent births.[103-105,111-113] Although part of the greater reduction in risk with a first birth may be an artifact of including infertile women who are at increased risk of ovarian cancer[114] in the nulliparous reference group, this does not fully explain the greater reduction in risk seen with a first birth. An older age (35 years or older) at birth may be more protective than a birth at a young age (under 25 years),[104,105,115] but this result has not been observed in all studies and requires further follow-up.[103,112]

Oral contraceptives

Epidemiologic studies have consistently demonstrated that oral contraceptive use decreases the risk of ovarian cancer, in a duration-dependent manner analogous to the protective effect observed for endometrial cancer.[104-109] A collaborative, pooled analysis of 45 epidemiological studies showed that any use of oral contraceptives is associated with a 27% reduction in ovarian cancer risk (95% CI = 0.70–0.76), with risk reduced 20% with each 5 years of use.[109] This analysis also showed an attenuation in risk reduction over time; women whose use ended less than 10 years previously had a 29% reduction in risk per 5 years of use, whereas women who last used oral contraceptives 20–29 years previously had only a 15% reduction per 5 years of use. Nevertheless, the reductions in risk persisted for decades. In this study, substantial statistically significant heterogeneity was observed across histopathological subtypes with no statistically significant risk reduction for mucinous tumors.

It has been hypothesized that the blocking of ovulation is the mechanism through which both parity and oral contraceptives protect against ovarian cancer; however, an alternate explanation may be the high levels of progesterone achieved through oral contraceptive use and pregnancy. The average daily exposure to progesterone during the normal menstrual cycle is approximately 3.5 ng/mL compared to 9.2 ng/mL for women taking oral contraceptives.[116,117] Likewise, pregnancy is associated with high progesterone levels. A study of female macaque monkeys showed that progestins used in oral contraceptives induce apoptosis in the ovarian epithelium, which can protect against ovarian cancer.[118] Also, *in vitro* evidence that estrogen can increase ovarian tumor cell growth exists and this effect can be blocked by progesterone.[119,120]

Hormone therapy

The epidemiologic evidence regarding hormone therapy and ovarian cancer risk has become much clearer in recent years. A detailed meta-analysis of the published literature through 2007 from population-based case-control studies[105,121-127] and cohort studies[128-132] showed that use of menopausal ERT increases ovarian cancer risk by 22% for each 5 years of use ($p < 0.0001$). These results are consistent in all but one of the publications, which showed no association.[121] Across the 13 publications showing an association, the dose–response relationship is clear.

The results with regard to menopausal estrogen–progestin therapy, while not as consistent, still provide a clear picture. The meta-analysis of population-based case-control studies,[105,121,123-126,129] cohort studies[130-132] and the Women's Health Initiative[93] show a 10% increase in ovarian cancer risk per 5 years of CHT use ($p = 0.001$). The difference in risk between estrogen-only therapy and CHT use is statistically significant ($p = 0.004$), suggesting that the addition of a progestin to ERT ameliorates the effect of the estrogen. These analyses provide further support for a protective effect of progestins on ovarian cancer risk.

It is not clear whether the effect of CHT differs depending on whether the sequential or continuous combined regimen is prescribed. Four studies shed some light on this question. The Million Women Study[131] did not find a difference in ever-use risk

Table 3 A summary of established hormonal risk and protective factors for ovarian cancer.

Risk factors (increased number of ovulations)
Late menopause
Protective factors (decreased number of ovulations)
Pregnancy
Oral contraceptives

estimates; however, no duration of use information was provided. The National Institutes of Health American Association for Retired Persons cohort study reports higher risk associated with sequential combined therapy than with continuous combined therapy, but both regimens were associated with increased risk.[130] A case-control study report from the United States shows a reduced risk of ovarian cancer associated with both types of combined therapy regimens,[126] whereas a case-control study from Sweden found that sequential combined therapy increased risk, but continuous combined therapy did not.[125] The higher dose of progestin delivered in the continuous combined versus sequential formulation in Sweden may explain the lack of association with this regimen in the Swedish study.[28] Further follow-up is needed in this area.

Given these findings for menopausal hormone therapy, the interpretation of the observations that parity and oral contraceptive use reduce risk can be viewed in a new light, specifically that the mechanism of action of these two protective factors may act by increasing exposure to progestins. This is more consistent with emerging views that the single layer of cells on the surface of the ovary may not be where ovarian cancer originates.

Prostate cancer

Prostate cancer is the most frequently diagnosed cancer in American men, with an estimated 233,000 cases expected in 2014.[18] It is also the second leading cause of cancer deaths in males, exceeded only by lung cancer, with approximately 29,480 deaths from prostate cancer occurring annually.[18] The prostate is an androgen-regulated organ with androgens considered as the major stimulus for cell division in prostatic epithelium.[7,133] Thus, androgens are strong candidates as major contributors to prostatic carcinogenesis. Until recently, only indirect evidence supported a causal role for androgens in prostate cancer development. Results from the Prostate Cancer Prevention Trial (PCPT) using an agent that reduces androgen action in the prostate provided the first direct evidence in support of an important androgen role in this process.[134] Assessing the role of androgens in prostate cancer development has been difficult in part because of a lack of easily measurable hormonal events in men as exist in women (e.g., menarche, menopause, reproductive experiences). Furthermore, use of exogenous androgens in men is relatively uncommon.

The epidemiology of prostate cancer is dominated by three observations: (1) the profound international and racial–ethnic variation in incidence and mortality, historically reported to be as much as 80-fold between the extremes of high-risk (African-Americans) and low-risk (native Japanese and Chinese) populations[135]; (2) the occurrence of occult, subclinical prostate cancer at a relatively comparable prevalence across populations[136]; and (3) the strong relationship between prostate cancer incidence and aging.[7] Prostate cancer is extremely rare before age 50 years, but it is still the most common cancer of American men, in large part because the rate of increase in prostate cancer incidence with aging is greater than for any other cancer.

Some of the indirect evidence for a role of androgens in prostate cancer development has come from comparisons of hormonal profiles of healthy men from racial–ethnic groups at high, intermediate, and low risk of prostate cancer. Although studies have not shown differences in testosterone levels between whites and African-Americans,[12,137,138] recent evidence suggests African-Americans have higher estradiol levels than whites and Latinos.[139] Asian men, while showing no evidence of low circulating testosterone levels relative to whites and African-Americans at any age, have substantially reduced levels of androstanediol

glucuronide.[140,141] This hormone reflects 5α-reductase activity (5α-reductase is the prostatic enzyme that bioactivates testosterone to dihydrotestosterone, the most biologically potent human androgen). Based on these results and the presumptive role of androgens in prostate cell proliferation, Ross et al.[140] proposed that a 5α-reductase inhibitor might be an effective chemopreventive agent for prostate cancer.

Several additional indirect lines of evidence point to a role of androgens in prostate cancer pathogenesis. Androgens are required for prostate cancer development or progression in most animal models of prostatic adenocarcinoma.[142] Prostate cancer has never been reported to occur in eunuchs or in men with genetically determined decreased 5α-reductase activity, groups with very low androgen activity and highly underdeveloped prostates.[7] Prostate cancers, at least early in their course, are almost uniformly androgen dependent, and androgen ablation therapy has been the mainstay for treating early metastatic prostate cancer for many decades.

The role of circulating androgens and prostate cancer risk has been investigated by several studies, yielding inconsistent results. A large pooled analysis of 18 prospective studies from the Endogenous Hormones and Prostate Cancer Collaborative Group found no association between the risk of prostate cancer and circulating levels of testosterone, dihydrotestosterone, dehydroepiandrosterone sulfate, androstenedione, androstanediol glucuronide, or estradiol.[143] Circulating sex hormone–binding globulin was associated with a decreased risk of prostate cancer, with a RR reduction of 14% when comparing men in the highest quintile of exposure to those in the lowest quintile. Sex hormone–binding globulin regulates circulating levels of free testosterone and estradiol and may also play a role in steroid signaling.[144] Although the majority of circulating androgens do not appear to influence prostate cancer risk, an important consideration of these studies is whether a single hormone measurement can accurately reflect the average hormone profile of an individual.

The most convincing evidence for a role of androgens in prostate cancer development comes from the PCPT.[134] In the PCPT, 18,882 healthy men aged 55 years or older, with normal range prostate-specific antigen (PSAs), were randomized to receive 5 mg daily of finasteride, a 5α-reductase inhibitor, or placebo. After 7 years, all men were designated for an end-of-trial prostate biopsy. Prostate cancer incidence in the treatment arm was reduced approximately 25%. However, paradoxically, there was a statistically significant 25% increase in high-grade prostate cancer incidence in the therapeutic arm. These disparate findings have created substantial controversy regarding the role of 5α-reductase inhibitors in prostate cancer prevention in healthy men, as well as substantial disagreement regarding the underlying cause of these curious results. It has been argued, for example, that this finding represents an artifact of disruptive morphological changes induced by finasteride in the prostate, or that the increased risk of high-grade prostate cancer is the result of detection bias due to finasteride-induced reduction in prostate volume.[145] On the other hand, others have argued that these results are more foreboding with a clear biological basis; for example, Ross et al.[146] consider that high-grade prostate cancer precursor cells, possibly with androgen receptor alterations (amplification, gene mutations) thrive in an androgen-depleted environment, that prostate cancer cells with somatic mutations of the 5α-reductase type II gene respond differently to an inhibitor than those without such changes, and that finasteride, by virtue of increased intraprostatic levels of testosterone, selectively stimulates prostate cancer precursor lesions. Understanding the true nature of these results will have enormous public health implications.

Genetic determinants

Familial risk

A family history of breast cancer is associated with an increased risk of the disease.[4] This is particularly apparent when the family history includes a woman who was affected at an early age or had bilateral disease. Whereas a two to threefold increase in the risk of the disease has been observed in first-degree relatives of women with breast cancer overall, a ninefold increase in risk has been found in the first-degree relatives of premenopausal women with bilateral breast cancer. Very high risks (i.e., fivefold or greater) also have been found in women with more than one first-degree relative with breast cancer.

Similarly, population-based case-control studies have described a two to threefold increased risk of ovarian cancer in first-degree relatives of ovarian cancer patients.[147,148] Heritability estimates for both breast and ovarian cancer are approximately 25% as estimated by a classic twin study.[149] The impact of family history on endometrial cancer risk is still controversial.[150–155] Also, unlike breast and ovarian cancer, heritability estimates from twin studies do not suggest a strong genetic component for endometrial cancer.[149]

Prostate cancer is also a highly familial disease. Men with a first-degree relative with prostate cancer have approximately a two to threefold increase in risk compared to men with no such history and this increase is observed across different racial–ethnic groups.[156] As with breast cancer, risk is elevated further when multiple first-degree relatives are affected or when affected relatives are diagnosed at relatively young ages.[157] The heritability of prostate cancer as estimated by twin studies is approximately 42%, the highest among all sporadic cancers.[149]

Genes and variants

Extraordinary success has been achieved in the past two decades to identify genetic susceptibility alleles for cancers. Genetic susceptibility alleles can be broadly categorized into high-, moderate-, and low-penetrance alleles.[5] The high-penetrance alleles typically confer a RR of ≥10 and a lifetime risk of >50%; the moderate penetrance alleles exhibit a RR of 2–9 (mostly 5 and lower) and a lifetime risk of 20–50%; and the low-penetrance alleles have a RR of <2 (mostly between 1 and 1.5) and a lifetime risk of 10–19%. The deleterious mutations of high- and moderate-penetrance genes are rare (generally 1% and lower), whereas the low-penetrance alleles are common (mostly >5%) in the general population. High-penetrance alleles, such as BRCA1 and BRCA2 for breast cancer, were identified from family-based linkage analysis and positional cloning.[11,12] The lifetime cancer risks in germline BRCA1-mutation carriers are 60–80% for breast cancer and 30–40% for ovarian cancer. For germline BRCA2-mutation carriers, the corresponding estimates are 40–50% and 10–15%, respectively.[158] A few additional high-penetrance alleles for breast cancer have been identified from familial cancer syndromes, including *TP53* mutations in Li–Fraumeni syndrome,[15] *STK11/LKB1* mutations in Peutz–Jeghers syndrome,[159] and *PTEN* mutations in PTEN hamartoma tumor syndrome.[160] The lifetime risk of endometrial cancer in hereditary nonpolyposis colorectal cancer (HNPCC or Lynch syndrome) patients reaches 40–60%, and mutations in mismatch repair genes (e.g., *MLH1, MSH2,* and *MSH6*) are responsible for Lynch syndrome and considered high-penetrance alleles for endometrial cancer.[161,162] For prostate cancer, despite two decades of effort, no consistent high-penetrance allele has yet been identified.[6]

Moderate-penetrance alleles for breast and ovarian cancers are mostly in DNA repair genes, most notably those involved in the Fanconi anemia (FA)–BRCA pathway.[163,164] These alleles were discovered by linkage analysis of DNA repair deficiency syndromes, resequencing of candidate genes, and most recently, whole exome sequencing. FA is a rare, recessive chromosome instability syndrome characterized by aplastic anemia in childhood, bone-marrow failure, and cellular sensitivity to DNA crosslinking agents.[165] To date, 15 genes have been identified as mutated in FA patients. The products of these genes interact with well-known DNA damage-response proteins, including BRCA1, ATM, and NBS1, and are involved in multiple cellular DNA repair pathways, particularly homologous recombination (HR) in repairing double-stranded breaks.[165,166] Biallelic mutations of FA genes result in FA syndrome; however, monoallelic carriers of several FA genes exhibit increased risks of breast and ovarian cancer. *BRCA2 (FANCD1)* is one of the FA genes. Interestingly, in addition to predisposing to breast and ovarian cancer, *BRCA2* is also a moderate-penetrance gene for prostate cancer: men with germline *BRCA2* mutations have a nearly fivefold higher risk of prostate cancer than men without *BRCA2* mutations.[167,168] Two other FA genes, *FANCJ/BRIP1* (a BRCA1-interating protein) and *FANCN/PALB2* (a BRCA2-interacting protein), were also demonstrated as moderate-penetrance alleles for both breast and ovarian cancers.[164,166,169–171] Besides FA genes, a number of other DNA repair and cell cycle control genes have been established as moderate-penetrance alleles for breast and ovarian cancer.[171] For example, a truncating variant (1100delC) in *CHEK2*, a cell cycle checkpoint kinase, results in an approximately twofold increase in women's breast cancer risk and a 10-fold increase in men's risk[172]; ATM mutations that cause ataxia telangiectasia in biallelic carriers are breast cancer susceptibility alleles in monoallelic carriers, with an estimated RR of 2.4[173]; deleterious mutations in *RAD51C* and *RAD51D*, two HR genes, are moderate-penetrance alleles for ovarian cancer but not breast cancer.[174,175] For endometrial cancer, germline mutations in the proof-reading domains of DNA polymerase delta (*POLD1*) gene confer a high risk.[176] For prostate cancer, a missense mutation Gly84Glu in *HOXB13*, a homeobox transcription factor involved in normal prostate development and a key determinant in response to androgens, was identified from sequencing of >200 genes of familial prostate cancers,[177] and a recent meta-analysis of 24,213 cases and 73,631 controls revealed that this mutation conferred a fourfold increased risk of prostate cancer (OR: 4.07; 95% CI = 3.05–5.45).[178]

All the high- and moderate-penetrance alleles together account for 20–25% of the familial risk of breast cancer.[179] A larger portion of the familial risk of common cancers is believed to be accounted for by common (minor allele frequency of >5% in general population), low-penetrance alleles. Association studies involving direct comparison of allele frequencies between unrelated cases and controls are the most powerful approach to identify low-penetrance alleles. Early cancer association studies starting from the mid-1990s applied a candidate gene approach, that is, selecting potential functional variants, mostly single nucleotide polymorphisms (SNPs), in genes relevant to the biology and etiology of a specific cancer. The candidate genes often encode proteins involved in hormone biosynthesis, DNA repair, cell cycle control, cell growth, apoptosis, and other critical cellular functions whose aberrations lead to carcinogenesis. However, despite the fact that hundreds of SNPs were initially reported as potential cancer susceptibility loci by candidate gene association studies, very few were convincingly replicated in larger validation studies.[180] The only convincing low-penetrance allele for breast cancer identified from candidate gene association studies was a functional SNP (Asp302His) in the caspase-8 (*CASP8*) gene: the minor allele (His allele, frequency: 13%) confers a protective effect in a per-allele dose-dependent manner (per allele OR = 0.88; 95% CI = 0.84–0.92). This result was based on an analysis of 16,423 breast cancer cases and 17,109 controls.[181] No convincing susceptibility SNPs for ovarian, endometrial, or prostate cancers have emerged from candidate gene association studies.

The advent of GWAS in 2005 has ushered in a new era of genetic association studies.[182] Leveraging high-throughput genotyping platforms that can type hundreds of thousands to millions of SNPs simultaneously, GWAS allows for an agnostic approach where no prior knowledge of gene function or SNP position is required. GWAS reveal associations between specific alleles and disease risk via a set of marker SNPs that "tag" all known common variants in the genome. As of December 2014, more than 250 publications on GWAS of cancer risks have identified hundreds of common, low-penetrance susceptibility SNPs for ~35 cancer types.[16] To date, the greatest number of susceptibility SNPs have been identified for breast cancer and for prostate cancer: over 70 breast cancer susceptibility SNPs in 28 chromosome regions and approximately 80 prostate cancer susceptibility SNPs in 47 chromosome regions identified in different racial–ethnic groups. In contrast, 20 susceptibility SNPs in nine chromosome regions have been identified for ovarian cancer, whereas only one locus at chromosome 17q12 was identified for endometrial cancer.[16] The difference in the number of GWAS-identified SNPs for different cancers can be attributed to different sample sizes (breast cancer and prostate cancer are more common and their GWAS have larger sample sizes than those of ovarian and endometrial cancer) and different genetic heritability (endometrial cancer has much lower heritability than the other three cancers). Almost all of these SNPs confer a modest risk with allelic ORs of less than 1.5. Most of these SNPs are cancer site-specific; however, there are several regions that show pleiotropic effects on multiple cancers and other traits, for instance, the *TERT-CLPTM1L* locus at 5p15.33 harbors common and distinct susceptibility SNPs for at least 10 cancers, including breast, ovarian, and prostate cancer.[183–185] Further, the 8q24 region encompassing the *MYC* oncogene is associated with at least seven malignancies including breast, ovarian, and prostate cancer.[186] The vast majority of these SNPs lie in intergenic or intronic regions and some are found within complete "gene deserts," therefore, the causal variants and culprit genes in most susceptibility regions are unknown. Nevertheless, the emerging fine mapping of the identified regions and functional studies of candidate genes have already provided significant biological insights into the etiology of specific cancers.

For breast cancer, *FGFR2* at 10q26, a tyrosine kinase receptor that is overexpressed in 5–10% of breast tumors, is the most strongly associated gene. At least three likely causal SNPs in the second intron of *FGFR2*, which can interact with the promoter of *FGFR2*, have been identified and there was evidence of allele-specific transcription factor binding for these causal SNPs.[187,188] Another strong susceptibility locus for breast cancer is *CCND1* at 11q13. A fine-mapping study identified three independent association SNPs for ER-positive breast cancer.[189] All three SNPs map to either transcriptional enhancers or silencers, which were demonstrated by chromatin conformation studies to interact with each other and with their target gene *CCND1*.[189] With regard to hormone-related biology in breast cancer etiology, two breast cancer susceptibility SNPs are near genes related to the ER pathway. The SNP rs3757318 at 6q25.1 lies ~200 kb upstream of ERα gene *ESR1*,[190] and the nearest gene to SNP rs2823093 at 21q21 is *NRIP1/RIP140*, which interacts with ERα, represses the ER signaling and inhibits its mitogenic effects.[191] Whether these two genes are the culprit genes in these two regions warrants further investigation. Other suspected susceptibility genes for breast cancer include growth

factors, oncogenes, tumor suppressors, and those involved in DNA repair, cell cycle regulation, mammary gland development, telomere maintenance, apoptosis, and tumor aggressiveness.[5] Together, the currently identified common, low-penetrance alleles explain about 14% of the familial risk of breast cancer.[192] It is estimated that more than 1000 additional breast cancer susceptibility SNPs can be identified by current GWAS platforms with larger sample sizes; however, their individual effects are very small with ORs predominantly in the range of 1.02–1.05. All these identified and yet-to-be-identified common, low-penetrance SNPs are estimated to contribute ~28% of the familial risk of breast cancer.[192]

For ovarian cancer, GWAS has identified 20 susceptibility SNPs in nine chromosome regions: 2q31, 3q25, 8q21, 8q24, 9p22.2, 10p12, 17q12, 17q21, and 19p13 in white populations[193] and two independent loci in Han Chinese.[194] The likely culprit genes in these regions include two homeobox genes *HOXD1* and *HOXD3* (both at 2q31), a poly (ADP-ribose) polymerase (PARP) gene *TiPARP* (3q25), chromatin-modifying protein 4C (*CHMP4C*) at 8q21, oncogene *MYC* (8q24), a DNA-binding zinc-finger gene *BNC2* at 9p22.2, a homeodomain-containing transcription factor *HNF1B* at 17q12, and a BRCA1-interacting gene *BABAM1/MERIT40* at 19p13. Together, these SNPs only explain about 5% of the familial risk of ovarian cancer.

For endometrial cancer, only one locus, *HNF1B* at 17q12, has been identified to date by GWAS.[195,196] SNPs at this locus are also associated with serous and clear cell ovarian cancer,[193,197] prostate cancer,[198–200] and type II diabetes.[198] *HNF1B* encodes a member of the homeodomain-containing superfamily of transcription factors and acts as a transcription activator.[201] *HNF1B* expression is altered in numerous cancers and may play a role as a tumor suppressor or oncogene depending on the tissue context. A recent fine-mapping study refined the endometrial cancer association to a single signal in intron 1 of *HNF1B* and showed that the top SNPs are located within the extended *HNF1B* promoter that contains a negative regulatory element and are associated with *HNF1B* expression in endometrial tumors.[202]

Prostate cancer is one of the most heritable cancers and GWAS have yielded the largest number of susceptibility variants for prostate cancer compared to any other cancers. All the identified susceptibility SNPs together explain about 30% of the familial risk. Similar to breast cancer, the potential culprit genes in the 47 identified prostate susceptibility loci are involved in many cellular functions, such as DNA repair, cell cycle control, telomere maintenance, cell growth, cell adhesion, and AR signaling.[6] Several regions stand out. The pleiotropic 8q24 locus is near the *MYC* oncogene and has the highest number of SNPs independently associated with prostate cancer.[6] Functional studies have shown that SNPs in this region are located within transcription enhancers and can regulate *MYC* expression through long-range interaction with *MYC*.[203,204] Another pleiotropic region 5p15 has at least four independent loci in the promoter or intronic regions of *TERT* that are associated with prostate cancer as shown by a recent fine-mapping study.[205] Furthermore, gene expression analysis of normal prostate tissue showed that one of the loci was also associated with *TERT* expression, providing a potential mechanism for predisposing to disease.[205] The 19q13 locus contains genes encoding proteins of the kallikreins (KLKs) family of serine proteases, among which PSA (encoded by *KLK3* gene) is the best known. A fine-mapping study identified a common missense coding SNP (rs17632542, Ile179Thr) in the *KLK3* gene that exhibits the most significant association with prostate cancer risk in this region.[206] This SNP is also significantly associated with serum PSA level.[207] As introduced earlier, a rare, missense mutation Gly84Glu in the *HOXB13* at 17q21 is a moderate-penetrance allele for prostate cancer. Interestingly, common SNPs in *HOXB13* are also associated with prostate cancer risk.[208] A fine mapping of this locus identified a cluster of highly correlated common SNPs situated within or closely upstream of *HOXB13*. Furthermore, these common SNPs tag the rare, partially correlated Gly84Glu mutation. This is the first report that a modest GWAS association detected through common SNPs is driven by rare causal variants with higher RRs, providing evidence for the phenomenon of synthetic association contributing to cancer susceptibility.[209] Finally, a SNP rs5919432 at the Xq12 locus is located 77 kb from AR gene, suggesting a role of AR variation in prostate cancer etiology.[210]

Despite enormous progress in the identification of high-, moderate-, and low-penetrance alleles, 50% or more of the familial risk of any specific sporadic cancer remains unexplained. Large international collaboration is needed to uncover the remainder of cancer heritability, as an extremely large sample size (>100,000 cases) is needed to identify the remaining common, low-penetrance alleles with very small effect sizes. Whole exome sequencing and whole-genome sequencing are increasingly applied in cancer association studies. Again, large sample sizes are needed to identify rare, unknown high- and moderate-penetrance alleles. In addition, other forms of susceptibility variants, such as structural changes (e.g., copy number variations), and genetic interactions (gene–gene and gene–environment interactions) may explain some of the missing heritability.[211]

Conclusions

As our understanding of the relationship between epidemiologic risk factors and the circulating levels of the relevant hormones grows, avenues for primary prevention are becoming apparent. The control of obesity has obvious implications for both endometrial cancer and postmenopausal breast cancer. More information on the relationship between childhood diet and physical activity and the onset of puberty, in conjunction with the hormonal physiology of adolescence and young adulthood may provide increasing avenues for preventing breast, ovarian, and endometrial cancer in women. Chemoprevention trials have demonstrated that tamoxifen is effective in reducing breast cancer risk among high-risk women and that raloxifene, also a selective ER modulator, and anastrozole, an aromatase inhibitor, lower breast cancer risk among high-risk postmenopausal women. Hormonal chemoprevention of ovarian and endometrial cancer is already occurring in the population as a whole through the widespread use of COCs and of endometrial cancer with increasing use of CHT. A national trial to prevent prostate cancer through use of finasteride, a 5α-reductase inhibitor, has been completed and provides convincing evidence for the role of androgens in the development of this disease. A growing knowledge of the mutations and polymorphisms in genes causing increased risk of these cancers should lead to better definition of individual susceptibility. It should then be possible to focus intervention strategies on the higher risk subgroups of the population.

Key references

The complete reference list can be found on the Wiley Companion Digital Edition of this title (see inside front cover for login instructions).

4 Henderson BE, Feigelson HS. Hormonal carcinogenesis. *Carcinogenesis.* 2000;21(3):427–433.

5 Ghoussaini M, Pharoah PD, Easton DF. Inherited genetic susceptibility to breast cancer: the beginning of the end or the end of the beginning? *Am J Pathol.* 2013;183(4):1038–1051.

6 Eeles R, Goh C, Castro E, et al. The genetic epidemiology of prostate cancer and its clinical implications. *Nat Rev Urol.* 2014;11(1):18–31.

8 Chan JM, Stampfer MJ, Giovannucci E, et al. Plasma insulin-like growth factor-I and prostate cancer risk: a prospective study. *Science.* 1998;279(5350):563–566.

11 Miki Y, Swensen J, Shattuck-Eidens D, et al. A strong candidate for the breast and ovarian cancer susceptibility gene BRCA1. *Science.* 1994;266(5182):66–71.

12 Wooster R, Bignell G, Lancaster J, et al. Identification of the breast cancer susceptibility gene BRCA2. *Nature.* 1995;378(6559):789–792.

13 Søgaard M, Kjaer SK, Gayther S. Ovarian cancer and genetic susceptibility in relation to the BRCA1 and BRCA2 genes. Occurrence, clinical importance and intervention. *Acta Obstet Gynecol Scand.* 2006;85(1):93–105.

17 Henderson BE, Ross RK, Pike MC. Hormonal chemoprevention of cancer in women. *Science.* 1993;259(5095):633–638.

22 Key TJ, Pike MC. The role of oestrogens and progestagens in the epidemiology and prevention of breast cancer. *Eur J Cancer Clin Oncol.* 1988;24(1):29–43.

25 Ross RK, Paganini-Hill A, Wan PC, et al. Effect of hormone replacement therapy on breast cancer risk: estrogen versus estrogen plus progestin. *J Natl Cancer Inst.* 2000;92(4):328–332.

27 Chlebowski RT, Hendrix SL, Langer RD, et al. Influence of estrogen plus progestin on breast cancer and mammography in healthy postmenopausal women: the Women's Health Initiative Randomized Trial. *JAMA.* 2003;289:3243–3253.

28 Lee SA, Ross RK, Pike MC. An overview of menopausal oestrogen-progestin hormone therapy and breast cancer risk. *Br J Cancer.* 2005;92(11):2049–2058.

29 Henderson BE, Pike MC, Casagrande JT. Breast cancer and the oestrogen window hypothesis. *Lancet.* 1981;2(8242):363–364.

34 Bernstein L, Henderson BE, Hanisch R, et al. Physical exercise and reduced risk of breast cancer in young women. *J Natl Cancer Inst.* 1994;86(18):1403–1408.

38 McTiernan A, Kooperberg C, White E, et al. Recreational physical activity and the risk of breast cancer in postmenopausal women: the Women's Health Initiative Cohort Study. *JAMA.* 2003;290:1331–1336.

56 Newcomb PA, Storer BE, Longnecker MP, et al. Lactation and a reduced risk of premenopausal breast cancer. *New Engl J Med.* 1994;330:81–86.

62 Prentice RL, Caan B, Chlebowski RT, et al. Low-fat dietary pattern and risk of invasive breast cancer: the Women's Health Initiative Randomized Controlled Dietary Modification Trial. *JAMA.* 2006;295(6):629–642.

67 Collaborative Group on Hormonal Factors in Breast Cancer. Breast cancer and hormonal contraceptives: collaborative reanalysis of individual data on 53,297 women with breast cancer and 100,239 women without breast cancer from 54 epidemiological studies. *Lancet.* 1996;347(9017):1713–1727.

68 Marchbanks PA, McDonald JA, Wilson HG, et al. Oral contraceptives and the risk of breast cancer. *N Engl J Med.* 2002;346:2025–2032.

71 Committee TW'sHIS. Effects of conjugated equine estrogen in postmenopausal women with hysterectomy. *JAMA.* 2004;291:1701–1712.

72 Stefanick ML, Anderson GL, Margolis KL, et al. Effects of conjugated equine estrogens on breast cancer and mammography screening in postmenopausal women with hysterectomy. *JAMA.* 2006;295(14):1647–1657.

73 Schairer C, Lubin JH, Triosi R, et al. Menopausal estrogen and estrogen-progestin replacement therapy and breast cancer risk. *JAMA.* 2000;283:485–491.

75 Heiss G, Wallace R, Anderson GL, et al. Health risks and benefits 3 years after stopping randomized treatment with estrogen and progestin. *JAMA.* 2008;299(9):1036–1045.

91 Pike MC, Peters RK, Cozen W, et al. Estrogen-progestin replacement therapy and endometrial cancer. *J Natl Cancer Inst.* 1997;89(15):1110–1116.

93 Anderson GL, Judd HL, Kaunitz AM, et al. Effect of estrogen plus progestin on gynecologic cancers and associated diagnostic procedures: the Women's Health Initiative randomized trial. *JAMA.* 2003;290:1739–1748.

94 Bernstein L, Deapen D, Cerhan JR, et al. Tamoxifen therapy for breast cancer and endometrial cancer risk. *J Natl Cancer Inst.* 1999;91(19):1654–1662.

102 Adami HO, Hsieh CC, Lambe M, et al. Parity, age at first childbirth, and risk of ovarian cancer. *Lancet.* 1994;344(8932):1250–1254.

109 Collaborative Group on Epidemiological Studies of Ovarian Cancer. Ovarian cancer and oral contraceptives: collaborative reanalysis of data from 45 epidemiological studies including 23,257 women with ovarian cancer and 87,303 controls. *The Lancet.* 2008;371:303–314.

114 Ness RB, Cramer DW, Goodman MT, et al. Infertility, fertility drugs, and ovarian cancer: a pooled analysis of case–control studies. *Am J Epidemiol.* 2002;155(3):217–224.

119 Risch HA. Hormonal etiology of epithelial ovarian cancer, with a hypothesis concerning the role of androgens and progesterone. *J Natl Cancer Inst.* 1998;90(23):1774–1786.

129 Lacey JV Jr, Mink PJ, Lubin JH, et al. Menopausal hormone replacement therapy and risk of ovarian cancer. *JAMA.* 2002;288:334–341.

130 Lacey JV Jr, Brinton LA, Leitzmann MF, et al. Menopausal hormone therapy and ovarian cancer risk in the National Institutes of Health-AARP Diet and Health Study Cohort. *J Natl Cancer Inst.* 2006;98(19):1397–1405.

131 Beral V, Bull D, Green J, et al. Ovarian cancer and hormone replacement therapy in the Million Women Study. *Lancet.* 2007;369(9574):1703–1710.

134 Thompson IM, Goodman PJ, Tangen CM, et al. The influence of finasteride on the development of prostate cancer. *New Engl J Med*. 2003;**349**:215–224.

143 Roddam AW, Allen NE, Appleby P, et al. Endogenous sex hormones and prostate cancer: a collaborative analysis of 18 prospective studies. *J Natl Cancer Inst*. 2008;**100**(**3**):170–183.

149 Lichtenstein P, Holm NV, Verkasalo PK, et al. Environmental and heritable factors in the causation of cancer—analyses of cohorts of twins from Sweden, Denmark, and Finland. *N Engl J Med*. 2000;**343**(**2**):78–85.

158 Antoniou A, Pharoah PD, Narod S, et al. Average risks of breast and ovarian cancer associated with BRCA1 or BRCA2 mutations detected in case Series unselected for family history: a combined analysis of 22 studies. *Am J Hum Genet*. 2003;**72**(**5**):1117–1130.

163 D'Andrea AD. Susceptibility pathways in Fanconi's anemia and breast cancer. *N Engl J Med*. 2010;**362**(**20**):1909–1919.

192 Michailidou K, Hall P, Gonzalez-Neira A, et al. Large-scale genotyping identifies 41 new loci associated with breast cancer risk. *Nat Genet*. 2013;**45**(**4**):353–361, 361e1-2.

208 Eeles RA, Olama AA, Benlloch S, et al. Identification of 23 new prostate cancer susceptibility loci using the iCOGS custom genotyping array. *Nat Genet*. 2013;**45**(**4**):385–391, 391e1–e2.

25 Ionizing radiation

David J. Grdina, PhD

Overview

Many experimental and epidemiologic studies have since confirmed the oncogenic effects of radiation. This chapter reviews briefly the effects of ionizing radiation on biological systems, adaptive and bystander effects, cellular and molecular mechanisms for radiation carcinogenesis, and pharmacologic countermeasures that can mitigate against these processes.

Development of radiation injury

The hazards of exposure to ionizing radiation were recognized shortly after Roentgen's discovery of the X-ray in 1895. Acute skin reactions were observed in many individuals working with early X-ray generators, and by 1902, the first radiation-induced cancer was reported arising in an ulcerated area of the skin. Within a few years, a large number of such skin cancers had been observed, and the first report of leukemia in five radiation workers appeared in 1911.[1] Figure 1 describes the interaction of ionizing radiation with biologic tissues and the development of radiation injury. The ionizing event involves the ejection of an orbital electron from a molecule, producing a positively charged or "ionized" molecule. These molecules are highly unstable and rapidly undergo chemical change. This change results in the production of free radicals. The most common products of this process are the result of the decomposition of water giving rise to both superoxide anion ($O_2{}^-$) and hydrogen peroxide (H_2O_2) and the highly reactive hydroxyl radical, which has as a result a very short life span and can diffuse only on the average about 4 nm before reacting with other molecules.[2] Reactive oxygen species (ROS) production can be amplified by intermitochondrial communication that results in a subsequent magnification of the ROS damage signal.[3] The process of "ROS-induced ROS release," or RIRR is one potential mechanism for this. Under conditions of an excessive oxygen stress burden, the increase in ROS within the mitochondria reaches a threshold that triggers the opening of either the mitochondrial permeability transition (MPT) pore or the inner membrane anion channel (IMAC), which in turn leads to the simultaneous collapse of mitochondrial membrane potential and a transient increase in ROS generation by the electron transfer chain. Release of this ROS burst into the cytosol functions as a second messenger to activate RIRR in neighboring mitochondria.[4,5] Radiation can produce a transient generation of reactive oxygen or nitrogen within minutes accompanied by a reversible depolarization of mitochondrial membrane potential.[3] Radiation damage in a single mitochondrion can be transmitted via a reversible Ca^{2+}-dependent MPT to adjacent mitochondria resulting in the amplification of ROS generation. ROS amplification and propagation resulting from such a cascade can then damage important biological targets such as DNA, the nuclear matrix, cytoplasmic transport mechanisms, and both mitochondrial and cellular membranes resulting in cell death. The ROS amplification process may also be interfered by endogenous antioxidants such as superoxide dismutases (SODs) or exogenously added antioxidants.

Principal cellular and tissue effects of radiation

Cell killing

Radiation can kill cells by apoptosis and interphase death.[6-8] Cells undergoing apoptosis usually die in interphase within a few hours of irradiation. Apoptotic cell death can be induced by exposure to relatively low doses of radiation[6] and be a significant cause of death in hematopoietic or lymphoid cells exposed to higher radiation doses.

Radiation-induced apoptosis is dependent upon both the functional activity of the p53 gene as well as p53-independent pathways[9] all of which converge on the activation of proteases called caspases.[10] It has been proposed that p53-dependent apoptosis may involve the transcriptional induction of redox-related genes with the formation of ROS, leading to cell death by oxidative stress.[11]

The second mechanism for cell killing is radiation-induced reproductive failure. The inhibition of cellular proliferation is the mechanism by which radiation kills most mammalian cells. Symptoms of acute exposure to whole-body irradiation in human beings are usually observed only following doses of 100 cGy or greater.

Mutagenesis

Studies of the induction of single-gene mutations in human cells have been limited to several genetic loci. Of particular note is the X-chromosomal gene for hypoxanthine-guanine phosphoribosyltransferase (HPRT).[12,13] The induction of mutations in human cells is a linear function of dose down to doses as low as 10 cGy, and perhaps as low as 1 cGy, and the dose-rate effect appears to be relatively small.[14,15] DNA structural analyses show that the majority of radiation-induced mutations in human cells result from large-scale genetic events involving loss of the entire active gene and often extending to other loci on the same chromosome.[16]

The major potential consequence of radiation-induced mutations in human populations is heritable genetic effects resulting from mutations induced in germinal cells. For high dose-rate exposure, the induced mutation rate per gamete generally falls in the range of 10^{-4} to 10^{-5} per cGy. The rates per locus are in the range of 10^{-7} to 10^{-8} per cGy. Protraction of exposure appears to decrease the mutation rate in rodent systems by a factor of 2 or greater. When all of the experimental data for the various genetic end points are considered, the genetic doubling dose (radiation dose necessary to

Holland-Frei Cancer Medicine, Ninth Edition. Edited by Robert C. Bast Jr., Carlo M. Croce, William N. Hait, Waun Ki Hong, Donald W. Kufe, Martine Piccart-Gebhart, Raphael E. Pollock, Ralph R. Weichselbaum, Hongyang Wang, and James F. Holland.
© 2017 John Wiley & Sons, Inc. ISBN: 978-1-118-93469-2

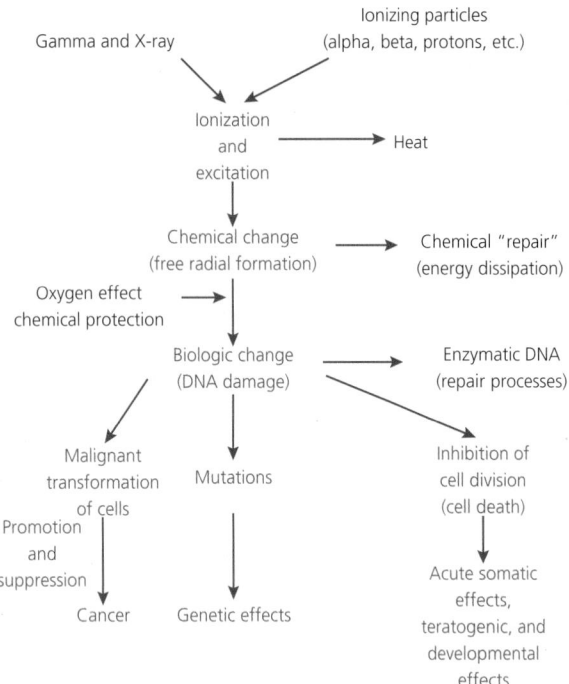

Figure 1 Development of radiation injury.

double the spontaneous mutation rate) for low dose-rate exposure appears to be in the range of 100 cGy.

Chromosomal aberrations

Radiation can induce two types of chromosomal aberrations in mammalian cells. The first have been termed "unstable" aberrations in that they are usually lethal to dividing cells. They include such changes as dicentrics, ring chromosomes, large deletions, and fragments. The frequency of such aberrations correlates well with the cytotoxic effects of radiation.

The second type has been termed "stable" aberrations. These include changes such as small deletions, reciprocal translocations, and aneuploidy changes that do not preclude the cell from dividing and proliferating. Radiation-induced reciprocal translocations may be passed on through many generations of cell replication and emerge in clonal cell populations.[17,18]

Such deletions and translocations can result in gene mutations. Specific chromosomal abnormalities are associated with specific tumor types such as the chromosome 8:14 translocation in Burkitt lymphoma. The chromosomal change can result in the activation of a specific oncogene such as a chromosome 13q14 deletion in retinoblastoma (RB).

Radiation-induced genomic instability

Radiation exposure can induce a type of transmissible genetic instability in individual cells that is transmitted to their progeny, leading to a persistent enhancement in the rate at which genetic changes arise in the descendants of the irradiated cell after many generations of replication. This is a nontargeted effect of radiation. The end points include malignant transformation, specific gene mutations, and chromosomal aberrations.

Early evidence was derived from an examination of the kinetics of radiation-induced malignant transformation of cells *in vitro*.[19,20] Transformed foci did not arise from a single, radiation-damaged cell. Rather, radiation appeared to induce a type of instability in

20–30% of the irradiated cell population; this instability enhanced the probability of the occurrence of a second, neoplastic transforming event, which is rare occurring with the frequency of $\sim 10^{-6}$. This second event occurs with a constant frequency per cell per generation and has the characteristics of a mutagenic event.[21]

This phenomenon was subsequently demonstrated in a number of experiment systems for various genetic end points.[22–25] In terms of mutagenesis, $\sim 10\%$ of clonal populations derived from single cells surviving radiation exposure showed a significant elevation in the frequency of spontaneously arising mutations compared with clonal populations derived from nonirradiated cells.[26,27] This increased mutation rate persisted for ~ 30 to 50 generations postirradiation. An enhancement of both minisatellite[28] and microsatellite[29] instability has also been observed in the progeny of irradiated cells selected for mutations at the *thymidine kinase* locus.

Transmission of chromosomal instability has been shown to occur *in vivo*,[30,31] but susceptibility to radiation-induced chromosomal instability differed significantly among different strains of mice.[32,33] A persistent increase in the rate of cell death has been shown to occur in cell populations many generations after radiation exposure.[34–36] Delayed reproductive failure has been linked to chromosomal instability[37] and malignant transformation,[38,39] and evidence presented to suggest that DNA is at least one of the critical targets in the initiation of this phenomenon.[40]

A recent novel phenomenon has been identified and coined "the delayed radioprotective effect." It is manifested by an enhanced resistance to ionizing radiation hours to days following exposure of cells to thiol-containing drugs such as *N*-acetylcysteine and captopril that have the ability to elevate intracellular antioxidant enzymes such as manganese superoxide dismutase (MnSOD).[41,42] The underlying mechanism of action responsible for this effect is the activation of the redox-sensitive nuclear transcription factor κB (NFκB) by thiol-reducing agents that subsequently results in the elevated transcription of MnSOD. The resulting 10- to 20-fold elevation of intracellular MnSOD facilitates the prevention and removal of radiation-induced oxidative damage and can enhance survival of cells by 10–30%.

Bystander effects in irradiated cell populations

It has long been thought that the cell nucleus is the target for the important biologic effects of radiation. However, recent evidence shows that targeted cytoplasmic radiation is significantly mutagenic. Damage signals may be transmitted from irradiated to nonirradiated cells in the population, leading to biologic effects in cells that received no radiation exposure,[43] for example, the "bystander" effect.

Following the exposure of monolayer cultures of cells to very low fluences of α particles, an enhanced frequency of sister chromatid exchanges (SCE) was observed in 20–40% of cells exposed to fluences by which only 1/1000 to 1/100 cells were traversed by an α particle.[44] This effect involves the secretion of cytokines or other factors by irradiated cells that leads to an upregulation of oxidative metabolism in bystander cells.[45,46] Examples of a bystander effect are presented in Figure 2. Incubation with conditioned medium from irradiated cells has cytotoxic effects on nonirradiated cells, which may be related to the release of a factor(s) into the medium.[47] An enhanced frequency of specific gene mutations[48,49] as well as chromosomal aberrations[50,51] are observed to occur in bystander cells in populations exposed to very low fluences of α particles.

DNA damage in bystander cells appears to differ from that occurring in directly irradiated cells; whereas the mutations induced in directly irradiated cells were primarily partial and total gene deletions, >90% of those arising in bystander cells were point

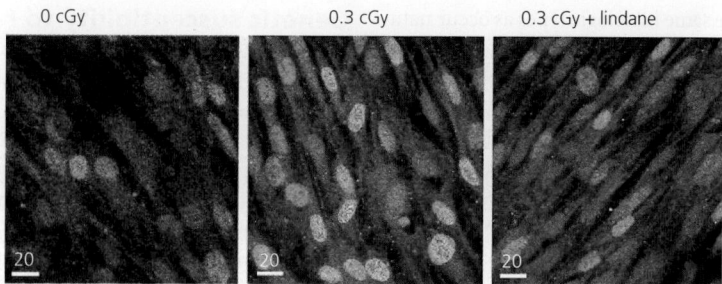

Figure 2 Bystander effect of radiation. The expression of p21^Waf1 was determined in individual cells in monolayer cultures of human diploid fibroblasts by *in situ* immunofluorescence. In cultures exposed to 0.3 cGy (<1–2% of nuclei traversed by an α particle), enhanced expression occurred in many nonirradiated cells occurring in clusters (*center panel*). The effect was suppressed by incubation with lindane, an inhibitor of gap junction-mediated intercellular communication (*right panel*).

mutations.[52] Suggesting that oxidative metabolism is upregulated in bystander cells.[45,46] Bystander effects indicate clearly that damage signals can be transmitted from irradiated to nonirradiated cells.

Adaptive responses

The original description of an adaptive response was made by investigators working with human lymphocytes in which they observed that following exposure to a very low dose of ionizing radiation in the range of 1–10 cGy cells acquired an enhanced resistance to a second but much larger dose of 2 Gy or more.[53] The expression of an adaptive response was linked to the requirement of *de novo* protein synthesis since inhibitors of protein synthesis such as cycloheximide were found to be inhibitory to this inductive effect.[54] Adaptive responses can be looked upon as the result of intercellular stress responses. The most studied such response has been identified as being mediated by MnSOD, an antioxidant enzyme localized in the mitochondria of cells, in both normal and malignant cells. As an example, it has been demonstrated that mouse skin JB6P+ epithelial cells exposed to 10 cGy exhibited an enhanced resistance to a subsequent dose of 2 Gy during which time a number of NFκB-regulated genes including MnSOD, p65, phosphorylated extracellular signal-related kinase, cyclin B1, and 14-3-3Z were elevated.[55] The importance of elevated MnSOD synthesis in the adaptive response process has been observed in cells following exposure to not only a low dose of ionizing radiation[55] but also the cytokine TNFα[56] and numerous reductive agents such as amifostine and *N*-acetylcysteine.[42,57] Treatment of cells with NFκB inhibitors and/or antisense MnSOD oligomers or siRNA MnSOD completely inhibited the adaptive response induced by these agents.[55,56] Both the radiation and cytokine-induced adaptive responses are the result of oxidative damage-initiated processes in contrast to the thiol-induced reductive response in which NFκB is activated following the reduction of cysteine residues on its p50 and p65 subunits,[58,59] a process that can be maintained in a persistent manner with chronic thiol exposure.[60]

It is now recognized that there are multiple mediators of adaptive responses, each associated with either normal and/or neoplastic cells and different radiation protocols. Under conditions of multifractionated high-dose radiation exposures, each preceded by very low imaging doses, a survivin-mediated adaptive response is expressed in tumor cells.[61] Survivin, a member of the inhibitor of apoptosis protein (IAP) group, is primarily found in neoplastic cells and has been identified as an important factor in tumor cell resistance.[62,63] Its overexpression results in elevated tumor cell resistance to radiation- and chemotherapy-induced cell killing and reduced frequencies of apoptosis.[64–66] A third adaptive response

has been identified in normal cells where lose-dose radiation exposure results in the induction of a metabolic shift from oxidative phosphorylation to aerobic glycolysis in cells and is mediated by the hypoxia-inducible factor HIF-1α.[67]

DNA damage

Track analysis studies of X-ray interactions in DNA have provided evidence for clustered damage, which results in complex DSB (double-strand break).[68] Certain types of DNA base damage such as 8-hydroxydeoxyguanosine and thymine glycols have significant potential biologic importance, but the available data suggest that such isolated base damage by itself probably plays a minor role in radiation mutagenesis. Clustered DNA damage may include abasic sites, oxidized purines, or oxidized pyrimidines.[69] The increased efficiency of DNA breaks induced by high-LET radiation appears to result primarily from their greater complexity.[70]

Cells possess a complex set of signaling pathways for recognizing such DNA damage and initiating its repair. The ATM gene is a sensor of DNA damage, which activates by phosphorylation a variety of proteins involved in cell cycle control and DNA repair. Two mechanistically distinct pathways that function in complementary ways are involved in the repair of DSB: nonhomologous end joining (NHEJ), which requires little sequence homology between the DNA ends and is error prone, and homologous recombination (HR), which uses extensive homology and is generally error-free.[71] NHEJ involves a complex of proteins, including Ku70, Ku80, the DNA-PK catalytic subunit DNA-PKcs, XRCC4, and ligase IV. The NBS1/MRE11/RAD50 complex[72] is also involved in the nucleolytic processing stages of NHEJ; this complex also contributes to HR. HR also involves a complex of proteins, notably RAD51 and other factors in the RAD50 epistasis group.[73] Strong links have been established between recombinational repair and the breast cancer susceptibility proteins BRCA1 and BRCA2,[74–76] as well as the Fanconi anemia family of proteins.[77] Un-repaired or mis-repaired DSB led primarily to large-scale genetic changes that are frequently manifested by chromosomal aberrations. However, no genetic alterations unique to radiation have been found in radiation-induced tumors.

General characteristics of radiation carcinogenesis

Ionizing radiation can induce cancer in most tissues of most species at all ages, including the fetus. It is carcinogenic to humans. It is, however, a relatively weak carcinogen and mutagen. The cancers induced by radiation are of the same histologic types as occur naturally, but the distribution of types may differ. There is a distinct latent period between exposure to radiation and the clinical appearance of a tumor.

Radiation carcinogenesis is a stochastic process; that is, the probability of the occurrence of the effect increases with dose with no threshold, but the severity of the effect is not influenced by dose. Radiation-induced cancer appears to be an all-or-none effect. The dose–response relationships for the induction of cancers in specific tissues of small animals vary with site, sex, and species.[78–80] For low LET radiation, the frequency of induced cancers generally rises with dose in the range of 0–300 cGy. In some cases, tumor incidence levels off at higher doses and may even decline. This phenomenon is thought to reflect cell killing. In the dose range up to 200–300 cGy, the dose–response curves for individual tumor types vary but generally assume a linear-quadratic to near-linear relationship. For high LET radiation, the rise in cancer incidence with dose is much steeper. The dose–response curves are approximately linear within the range of 0–20 cGy.[78,81]

The induction of carcinogenesis in experimental animals can be suppressed by treatment with certain agents that are known to inhibit radiation-induced transformation *in vitro*. An example of this includes amifostine, which is the only drug currently approved for clinical use as a radioprotector by the Food and Drug Administration.[82] As described by Kaplan–Meier plots in Figure 3, inoculation of B6CF1 hybrid mice with a single dose of 400 mg/kg of amifostine 30 min before whole-body irradiation with 2 Gy of low LET radiation significantly protected against carcinogenesis in both male and female animals. The reduction in cancer deaths due to lymphoreticular tumors by amifostine is reflected by a shift in the Kaplan–Meier survival curves for drug-treated irradiated animals to those describing the survival of nonirradiated control animals.[83–85] Causes of death due to lymphoreticular tumors that included leukemias and lymphomas were determined by both gross and microscopic analysis of individual animals by veterinarian pathologists.[83] Likewise, certain protease inhibitors have also been shown to suppress the induction of cancer in several different tumor systems.[86] It is well known that the hormonal environment is important in certain radiation-induced rodent cancers, particularly ovarian and mammary tumors.

Genetic susceptibility to radiation-induced cancer

There is little evidence to suggest that genetic factors are involved in most human cancers, but they do appear to play a role in some rare hereditary disorders that may serve as models for radiation–genetic interactions. For example, patients with hereditary RB whose somatic cells are heterozygous for the *RB* gene are at markedly increased risk for the development of radiation-induced bone sarcomas,[87] whereas patients with the nevoid basal cell carcinoma syndrome are at high risk for the development of basal cell cancers in irradiated areas. Radiation has also been associated with an enhanced incidence of early onset breast cancer. Transgenic mice heterozygous for either the p53[88] or ATM[89] tumor suppressor genes show an increased sensitivity to radiation-induced cancer; ATM and p53 heterozygosity are associated, respectively, with the human cancer-prone disorders ataxia telangiectasia and the Li–Fraumeni syndrome.

Human epidemiologic studies

There is now a large body of data on radiation-induced cancer derived from epidemiologic studies in irradiated human populations. They are derived primarily from two sources: (1) the long-term follow-up of survivors of the nuclear bombings of Hiroshima and Nagasaki[90,91] and (2) populations exposed to medical X-rays.[92,93] The results of these studies have yielded significant dose–response data for the induction of cancer in at least five tissue sites. Unfortunately, the epidemiologic studies yielding useful dose–response data generally involve relatively high-dose exposures (>10 cGy). Thus, risk estimates in the low-dose range must be derived from an extrapolation from the high-dose data. The shape of the dose–response relationship becomes of critical importance in making such extrapolations.

The observed dose–response curves from the human epidemiologic studies appear to be either linear or linear-quadratic in form (i.e., a linear component at low doses with a quadratic component at higher doses); although a threshold (dose below which there is no effect) cannot be formally excluded at very low doses.[94,95] A linear curve implies a constant risk per centigray at all doses, whereas the linear-quadratic model implies a smaller risk per centigray in

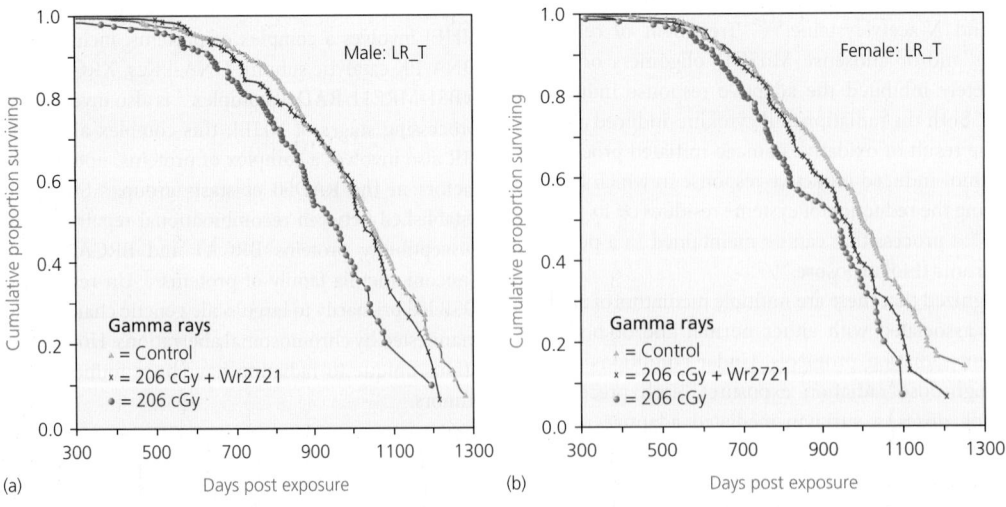

Figure 3 (a,b) Survival curves resulting from lymphoreticular cancers (LR-T), as determined by histopathological analysis of tissues taken from deceased animals that had been irradiated (206 cGy) either with or without amifostine. LR-T includes histiocytic leukemia and lymphoma, lymphocytic–lymphoblastic leukemia and lymphoma, myelogenous leukemia, undifferentiated leukemia and lymphoma, and mixed histiocytic leukemia and lymphoma.

the low-dose range. The assumption of a linear model simplifies the extrapolation from high to low doses and the corresponding estimation of risks. A final parameter of importance in determining the hazards of a given dose of radiation is the choice of risk models. For many years, risks were estimated on the basis of an absolute risk model. This model assumed that a specific number of excess cancers was induced by a given radiation dose. Radiation-induced cancers occurred in addition to the natural incidence. Increased risk could be expressed as the number of excess cancer cases (or cancer deaths) per 10^6 exposed people per year per centigray (the rate per year) or as the total number of excess cancers per 10^6 exposed people per centigray (the total risk or lifetime yield of cancers to be expected from a given radiation dose). The absolute risk model generally assumes a linear dose–response relationship, although with certain corrections it can be applied to a linear-quadratic relationship. Because the radiation exposure in Hiroshima included a small fraction of neutrons, the doses in the atom bomb survivor studies are expressed in Sieverts (Sv) rather than gray, a term that takes into account the RBE (relative biological effectiveness) of neutrons.

An analysis of the recent data from the atom bomb survivors suggests that some types of radiation-induced cancer more likely follow a relative-risk model.[90] The relative-risk model implies that radiation increases the natural incidence of cancer at all ages by a dose-dependent factor. As the excess cancer risk is proportional to the natural incidence, radiation-induced cancers would occur primarily at the times when natural tumors arose, independent of the age at irradiation. Thus, the largest cohort of radiation-induced cancers would occur in older individuals. The relative-risk model appears to fit the epidemiologic data for several solid tumors, although it does not appear to be valid for leukemia or bone and lung cancers. Risk estimates derived from the studies involving medical exposures are similar to those of the atom bomb survivors;[93,96,97] differences in the case of high-dose radiation therapy exposures can be ascribed to cell killing and the effect of dose fractionation.[92] A significantly reduced effect with fractionation for high-dose exposure was observed for lung cancer.[98] This was not the case for breast cancer, although a reduced effect was associated with low dose-rate protracted exposure.[97]

Radiation-induced secondary tumors

Radiation alone used in conventional treatment regimens may not be a very potent inducer of secondary tumors. This prediction arises from the localized nature of the exposure during clinical radiotherapy, in which the dose to normal tissues is minimized, and from the fact that ionizing radiation tends to be cytotoxic rather than mutagenic. The high radiation doses employed may thus kill potentially transformed cells in the treatment field. Exceptions may be the treatment of Hodgkin disease in which lower radiation doses are delivered to a relatively large volume of tissue, and in the use of intensity-modulated radiation therapy (IMRT). IMRT involves the use of more fields with a larger normal tissue volume exposed to lower doses.[99] It has been estimated that IMRT is likely to almost double the incidence of second malignancies compared with conventional radiotherapy from about 1% to 1.75% for patients surviving 10 years.[100] The risk may be even higher for pediatric patients.

Low-dose exposures

Sufficient data are now available from the atomic bomb survivors to allow an analysis of those survivors who received <0.5 Sv; these data are providing preliminary estimates of risk for doses as low as 5–10 cGy.[95] They indicate a statistically significant risk in this range

consistent with a linear dose–response relationship, with an upper confidence limit on any possible threshold of 6 cGy.

A careful analysis of nearly all low-dose studies indicates no significant increase in the incidence of all cancers or of cancers at specific sites. Analyses of a large number of radiation workers from the United Kingdom[101] and Canada[102] indicate that the risk estimates for leukemia and all cancers were consistent with an extrapolation from the atom bomb survivor data, providing no evidence for an unexpected increase in sensitivity at low doses such as to suggest that the current radiation protection standards might be appreciably in error.

Acknowledgments

I acknowledge the support of research grant DE-FG02-05ER64086 from the US Department of Energy (DJG) and RO1 CA132998 from the National Cancer Institute (DJG).

Key references

The complete reference list can be found on the Wiley Companion Digital Edition of this title (see inside front cover for login instructions).

1 Upton AC. Historical perspectives on radiation carcinogenesis. In: Upton AC, Albert RE, Burns FJ, Shore RE, eds. *Radiation Carcinogenesis.* New York: Elsevier; 1986:1–10.

2 Roots R, Okada S. Protection of DNA molecules of cultured mammalian cells from radiation-induced single strand scissions by various alcohols and SH compounds. *Int J Radiat Biol.* 1972;**21**:329–342.

6 Little JB. Cellular effects of ionizing radiation. I & II. *N Engl J Med.* 1968; **278**:308–315, 369–376.

12 Albertini RJ. Validated biomarker responses influence medical surveillance of individuals exposed to genotoxic agents. *Radiat Prot Dosimetry.* 2001;**97**:47–54.

23 Little JB. Radiation-induced genomic instability. *Int J Radiat Biol.* 1998;**74**: 663–671.

27 Little JB, Nagasawa H, Pfenning T, Vetrovs H. Radiation-induced genomic instability: delayed mutagenic and cytogenetic effects of X rays and alpha particles. *Radiat Res.* 1997;**148**:299–307.

33 Ponnaiya B, Cornforth MN, Ullrich RL. Radiation-induced chromosomal instability in BALB/c and C57BL/6 mice: the difference is as clear as black and white. *Radiat Res.* 1997;**147**:121–125.

34 Seymour CB, Mothersill C, Alper T. High yields of lethal mutations in somatic mammalian cells that survive ionizing radiation. *Int J Radiat Biol Relat Stud Phys Chem Med.* 1986;**50**:167–179.

35 Chang WP, Little JB. Delayed reproductive death in X-irradiated Chinese hamster ovary cells. *Int J Radiat Biol.* 1991;**60**:483–496.

39 Redpath JL, Gutierrez M. Kinetics of induction of reactive oxygen species during the post-irradiation expression of neoplastic transformation in vitro. *Int J Radiat Biol.* 2001;**77**:1081–1085.

41 Murley JS, Kataoka Y, Weydert CJ, Oberley LW, Grdina DJ. Delayed cytoprotection after enhancement of Sod2 (MnSOD) gene expression in SA-NH mouse sarcoma cells exposed to WR-1065, the active metabolite of amifostine. *Radiat Res.* 2002;**158**:101–109.

42 Murley JS, Kataoka Y, Cao D, Li JJ, Oberley LW, Grdina DJ. Delayed radioprotection by NFκB-mediated induction of Sod2 (MnSOD) in SA-NH tumor cells after exposure to clinically used thiol-containing drugs. *Radiat Res.* 2004;**162**: 536–546.

43 Little JB. Genomic instability and bystander effects: a historical perspective. *Oncogene.* 2003;**22**:6978–6987.

47 Mothersill C, Seymour CB. Cell–cell contact during gamma irradiation is not required to induce a bystander effect in normal human keratinocytes: evidence for release during irradiation of a signal controlling survival into the medium. *Radiat Res.* 1998;**149**:256–262.

50 Little JB, Nagasawa H, Li GC, Chen DJ. Involvement of the nonhomologous end joining DNA repair pathway in the bystander effect for chromosomal aberrations. *Radiat Res.* 2003;**59**:262–267.

51 Azzam EI, de Toledo SM, Gooding T, Little JB. Intercellular communication is involved in the bystander regulation of gene expression in human cells exposed to very low fluences of alpha particles. *Radiat Res.* 1998;**150**:497–504.

53 Olivieri G, Bodycote J, Wolff S. Adaptive response of human lymphocytes to low concentrations of radioactive thymidine. *Science.* 1984;**223**:594–597.

55 Fan M, Ahmed KM, Coleman MC, Spitz DR, Li JJ. Nuclear factor-kB and manganese superoxide dismutase mediate adaptive resistance in low-dose irradiated mouse skin epithelial cells. *Cancer Res.* 2007;**67**:3220–3228.

56 Murley JS, Kataoka Y, Baker LL, Diamond AL, Morgan WF, Grdina DJ. Manganese superoxide dismutase (SOD2)-mediated delayed radioprotection induced by the free thiol form of amifostine and tumor necrosis factor κB. *Radiat Res.* 2007;**167**:465–474.

57 Murley JS, Kataoka Y, Weydert CJ, Oberley LW, Grdina DJ. Delayed radioprotection by nuclear transcription factor κB-mediated induction of manganese superoxide dismutase in human microvascular endothelial cells after exposure to the free radical scavenger WR1065. *Free Radic Biol Med.* 2006;**40**:1004–1016.

58 Matthews JR, Wakasugi N, Virelizier JL, Yodoi Y, Hay RT. Thioredoxin regulates the binding activity of NF-κB by reduction of a disulphide bond involving cysteine 62. *Nucleic Acids Res.* 1992;**20**:3821–3830.

59 Murley JS, Kataoka Y, Hallahan DE, Roberts JC, Grdina DJ. Activation of NFκB and *MnSOD* gene expression by free radical scavengers in human microvascular endothelial cells. *Free Radic Biol Med.* 2001;**30**:1426–1439.

61 Grdina DJ, Murley JS, Miller RC, et al. A survivin-associated adaptive response in radiation therapy. *Cancer Res.* 2013;**73(14)**:4418–4428.

63 Marivin A, Berthelet J, Plenchette S, Dubrez L. The inhibitor of apoptosis (IAPs) in adaptive response to cellular stress. *Cells.* 2012;**1**:711–737.

64 Lu B, Mu Y, Cao C, et al. Survivin as a therapeutic target for radiation sensitization in lung cancer. *Cancer Res.* 2004;**64**:2840–2845.

67 Lall R, Ganapathy S, Yang M, et al. Low-dose radiation exposure induces a HIF-1-mediated adaptive and protective metabolic response. *Cell Death Diff.* 2014;**21**:836–844.

68 Goodhead DT. Initial events in the cellular effects of ionizing radiations: clustered damage in DNA. *Int J Radiat Biol.* 1994;**65**:7–17.

71 Jackson SP. Sensing and repairing DNA double-strand breaks. *Carcinogenesis.* 2002;**23**:687–696.

81 Ullrich RL. Tumor induction in BALB/c mice after fractionated or protracted exposures to fission-spectrum neutrons. *Radiat Res.* 1984;**97**:587–597.

82 Grdina DJ, Murley JS, Kataoka Y. Radioprotectants: current status and new directions. *Oncology.* 2002;**63**:2–10.

83 Grdina DJ, Carnes BA, Grahn D, Sigdestad CP. Protection against late effects of radiation by *S*-2-(3-aminopropylamino)-ethylphosphorothioic acid. *Cancer Res.* 1991;**51**:4125–4130.

84 Carnes BA, Grdina DJ. *In vivo* protection by the aminothiol WR-2721 against neutron-induced carcinogenesis. *Int J Radiat Biol.* 1992;**61**:567–576.

85 Grdina DJ, Carnes BA, Nagy B. Protection by WR-2721 and WR-151327 against late effects of gamma rays and neutrons. *Adv Space Res.* 1992;**12**:257–263.

88 Kemp CJ, Wheldon T, Balmain A. p53-deficient mice are extremely susceptible to radiation-induced tumorigenesis. *Nat Genet.* 1994;**8**:66–69.

93 Little MP, Weiss HA, Boice JD Jr, et al. Risks of leukemia in Japanese atomic bomb survivors, in women treated for cervical cancer, and in patients treated for ankylosing spondylitis. *Radiat Res.* 1999;**152**:280–292.

99 Goffman TE, Glatstein E. Intensity-modulated radiation therapy. *Radiat Res.* 2002;**158**:115–117.

26 Ultraviolet radiation carcinogenesis

James E. Cleaver, PhD ▪ Susana Ortiz-Urda, MD, PhD, MBA ▪ Radhika Gulhar, BA ▪ Sarah T. Arron, MD, PhD ▪ Lionel Brookes, 3rd, PhD ▪ David L. Mitchell, PhD

Overview

Skin carcinogenesis from solar ultraviolet (UV) exposure is initiated by UV photoproducts formed in the DNA of precursor cells that give rise to squamous cell carcinomas, basal cell carcinomas, and melanomas. These photoproducts consist of dimers between adjacent pyrimidines that are repaired by nucleotide excision repair (NER). Two branches of NER differ in mechanisms of damage recognition: in global genome repair (GGR), damage is recognized in nontranscribed DNA by the DDB2 and XPC proteins; in transcription-coupled repair (TCR), damage is recognized by arrest of the transcribing RNA polymerase at damaged sites. The T = C photoproduct is the predominant mutagenic product which, if unrepaired, gives rise to C to T or CC to TT mutations through replication by the low-fidelity polymerase Pol H. TCR reduces the mutation frequency in regions of transcription, in comparison to the rest of the genome subject to GGR. Deficiencies in GGR in the human disease xeroderma pigmentosum cause earlier onset and increased rates of skin cancer, which often contain UV-type mutations in genes that are rarely mutated in the general population. Deficiencies in TCR in the human disease Cockayne syndrome are associated with photosensitivity, developmental, and neurological disorders, but no cancer has been reported.

Epidemiology of skin cancer

Skin cancer frequency and age of onset

NMSCs (nonmelanoma skin cancers) are the most common cancers that occur in the United States each year,[1,2] comprising 30–40% of all cancers and have been increasing steadily for a century.[3,4] Skin cancer risks are associated with geographical location, skin type, various photosensitizing, enhancing, and protective applications and vitamin D.[4-10] There is also a possibility of greater risk when the exposure is received during childhood and adolescence.[5,11] NMSC is, therefore, one of the few human malignancies for which there is clear evidence for the initiating agent. The relationship of melanoma to sun exposure and the possible action spectrum are less clear,[12,13] but may be related to acute burns rather than accumulated dose.[5,14]

The importance of DNA as a target for ultraviolet radiation (UVR) is highlighted by the autosomal recessive disease XP (xeroderma pigmentosum). In this disease, a failure of DNA repair causes a large increase in NMSC and melanoma.[12,13] Median age for first diagnosis of NMSC in the general US population occurs after 60 years of age; in XP patients, carcinogenesis is accelerated and median age at first diagnosis is within the first decade (Figure 1).[12,13] Melanoma is also increased in XP patients, but the acceleration is less. Consequently, in XP patients, the onset of NMSC precedes melanoma, whereas in non-XP patients, melanomas generally occur earlier than NMSC.[13]

Sunlight spectrum and wavelengths responsible for skin cancer

UVR is divided into three wavelength ranges: UVA, UVB, and UVC. UVA (320–400 nm) is photocarcinogenic and involved in photoaging, but it is weakly absorbed in DNA and protein and may involve reactive oxygen species, which secondarily cause damage to DNA.[15-18] Recent evidence, however, suggests that UVA may also induce DNA damage directly in human cells.[19] UVB (290–320 nm) overlaps the upper end of the DNA and protein absorption spectra and is the range mainly responsible for skin cancer through direct photochemical damage to DNA. UVC (240–290 nm) is not present in ambient sunlight but is readily produced by low-pressure mercury sterilizing lamps (254 nm). UVC coincides with the peak of DNA absorption (260 nm) and is extensively used in experimental studies. Absorption of UVR by stratospheric ozone greatly attenuates these wavelengths, so that negligible radiation shorter than 300 nm reaches the earth's surface. Hence, although UVA and UVB light constitute a minute portion of the emitted solar wavelengths (10^{-9}), they are primarily responsible for the sun's pathological effects.

Sunlight-induced photoproducts in DNA

The absorption spectrum of DNA correlates well with photoproduct formation, lethality, and mutation.[20-24] The absorbed energy produces molecular changes, which involve single bases, interactions between adjacent and nonadjacent bases, and between DNA and proteins. The relative proportion of DNA photoproducts varies across the UV (ultraviolet) spectrum.

Dimerizations between adjacent pyrimidines are the most prevalent DNA photoproducts. Two major photoproducts are the cyclobutane pyrimidine dimer (CPD) and, at about 25% the frequency, the [6-4] pyrimidine dimer ([6-4]PD). [6-4]PDs cause a 47° helical bend in DNA, compared with 7° for CPDs. The [6-4]PD can further undergo a UVB-dependent conversion to its valence photoisomer, the Dewar pyrimidinone.[25]

The distribution of photoproducts in chromatin depends on base sequence, secondary DNA structure, and DNA–protein interactions.[24,26,27] Because cytosine more efficiently absorbs longer wavelengths of UVR than thymine, CPDs containing this base are formed more readily after UVB irradiation.[28] Cytosine CPDs and [6-4]PDs, which are preferentially induced at thymine–cytosine dipyrimidines, may play a major role in UVB (solar) mutagenesis.[29] Cytosine methylation increases the formation of CPDs by UVB, but not UVC, by 1.7-fold.[30] Methylation at PyrCG sequences in the p53 gene enhances formation of CPDs and [6-4]PDs at sites that are hotspots for mutations.[31,32] Other less common lesions include purine–purine and purine–pyrimidine photoadducts, photohydrates, and photooxidations.[33] The total yield of these photoproducts is only 3–4% of the yield of CPDs, but a minor

Holland-Frei Cancer Medicine, Ninth Edition. Edited by Robert C. Bast Jr., Carlo M. Croce, William N. Hait, Waun Ki Hong, Donald W. Kufe, Martine Piccart-Gebhart, Raphael E. Pollock, Ralph R. Weichselbaum, Hongyang Wang, and James F. Holland.
© 2017 John Wiley & Sons, Inc. ISBN: 978-1-118-93469-2

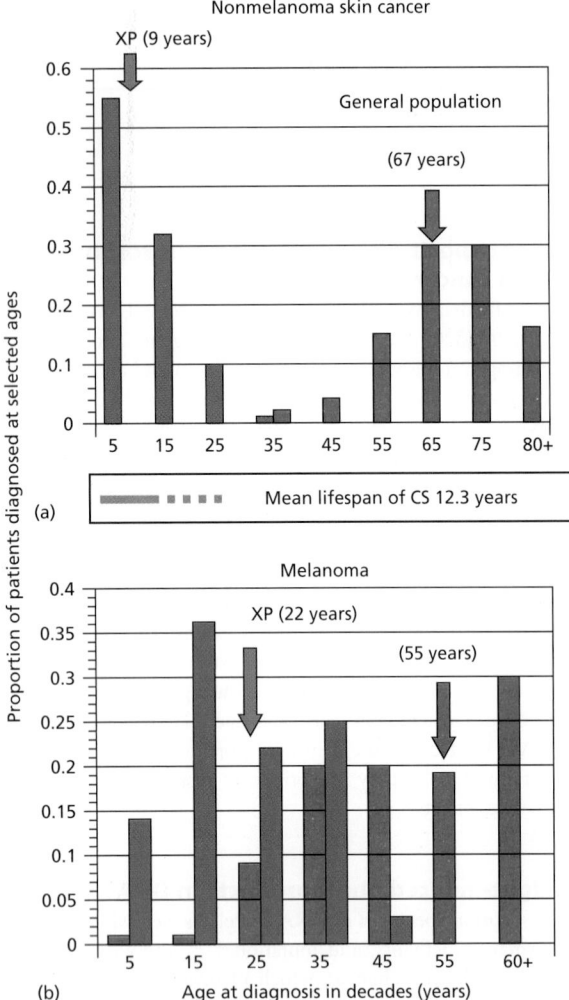

(a)

(b)

Figure 1 Diagnosis of first cancer by age and type in XP patients compared with the US general population. (a) Proportion of NMSC patients diagnosed at selected ages. (b) Proportion of melanoma patients diagnosed at selected ages. Individuals with both NMSC and melanoma were used in both panels. Ages shown are at the midpoint of each decade. XP: blue bars; general population: red bars. Colored arrows designate median ages of diagnosis for each population. The age span of Cockayne syndrome patients is also shown (orange): solid bar ends at mean age at death (12.25 years), with dashed line extending to maximum reported ages. XP and general population data redrawn from.[27] Cockayne data drawn from.[29]

biological role as premutagenic lesions at specific sites cannot be excluded.

Genetic factors in skin carcinogenesis

Recognition of UV photoproducts in DNA

The repair of UV photoproducts in DNA [nucleotide excision repair (NER)] involves sequential steps of photoproduct recognition, assembly of the excision complex, displacement of the excised fragment, and polymerization of the replacement patch.[34] The importance of NER arose from the discovery that cells from patients suffering from XP were deficient in NER.[35,36] Two major pathways of NER are known (Figure 2): transcription-coupled repair (TCR) and global genome repair (GGR), which differ in their mechanisms of damage recognition.[34,37–39] TCR removes damage more rapidly from the transcribed strands of transcriptionally

active genes, whereas GGR acts more slowly on nontranscribed regions.[40,41] The half-life of [6-4]PDs is 2–6 h, whereas for CPDs, it is 12–24 h, and much longer in rodent cells.[42,43]

GGR involves initial binding by the DDB1/DDB2(XPE) complex,[44,45] followed by recruitment of XPC/HR23B/centrin via ubiquitylation by the E3 ligase activity of DDB1/DDB2.[46–49] The XPC protein binds to the undamaged strand opposite a PD, inserting a peptide chain within the helix to displace the dimer to an extra-helical position.[50,51]

TCR is initiated by the arrest of RNA polymerase II at a damaged base, after which specific TCR factors CSA, CSB, UVSSA, and XABP, a binding partner of XPA, facilitate removal or degradation of arrested RNA polymerase II to permit access of NER proteins to damaged sites.[52,53] TCR is closely involved with the chromatin remodeling function of CSB that is a member of the SWI2/SNF2 chromatin remodeling protein family.[54,55] RNA polymerase II elongation is associated with cycles of ubiquitylation and deubiquitylation of histone H2B (H2Bub); arrest by UV damage tips the balance toward deubiquitylation and acetylation of histone H3.[56] Transcription is restored along with H2Bub after excision of the arresting photoproducts.[56]

The mechanism of nucleotide excision repair

Subsequent to damage recognition, the open helix is stabilized by XPA/RPA, which binds with a higher affinity for the [6-4]PDs than CPDs and interacts with the unwinding activity of the 10 component transcription factor TFIIH, and the 3′–5′ (XPB) and 5′–3′ (XPD) nucleases.[57,58] The opened helix is cleaved first by the ERCC1/XPF nuclease presenting a 3′OH terminus for chain elongation by the DNA Pol D, proliferating cell nuclear antigen, and single-strand binding protein.[59,60] XPG is a cryptic nuclease that cuts 3′ to the lesion after the ERCC1/XPF nuclease has cut 5′ to the CPD and polymerization.[60] A 27–29nt oligonucleotide containing the photoproduct is subsequently released and the patch is sealed by ligase I.[61]

Mutagenicity of UV photoproducts and low-fidelity DNA polymerases

Most photoproducts act as blocks to the replicative class B polymerases, Pol A, D, and E, but can be bypassed by damage-specific class Y DNA polymerases.[62–64] The class Y polymerases, Pol H, I, and K, have low fidelity due to expanded active sites, which allow the polymerases to read-through noninformative sequence information.[65] Pol H has the greatest capacity to replicate a large variety of DNA lesions,[66] and preferentially inserts adenine in the nascent strand opposite the lesion (called the "A rule").[67] Hence, Pol H replicates a thymine-containing CPD faithfully.[68–71] Pol I preferentially inserts guanines and is capable of replicating C-containing photoproducts.[72,73] Pol H or I, therefore, can insert bases opposite dipyrimidine photoproducts, but the 3′ complementary base can be mismatched by an erroneous insertion or the distortion caused by the photoproduct. Pol K or Pol Z can complete the replicative bypass by extension from the mismatched 3′ terminus.[74–76] The absence of Pol H results in increased mutagenesis in the XPV group,[77,78] but the absence of Pol Z has the converse effect of reducing mutation rates.[79]

The replication by-pass mechanism has two important implications for UV mutagenicity. First, mutations will most often occur where cytosine is a component of the photoproduct as insertion of adenine opposite thymine is a correct and nonmutagenic event. Hence, CPDs that form between two thymine bases are not mutagenic. Second, the larger distortion of [6-4]PDs is more likely to be lethal than mutagenic.

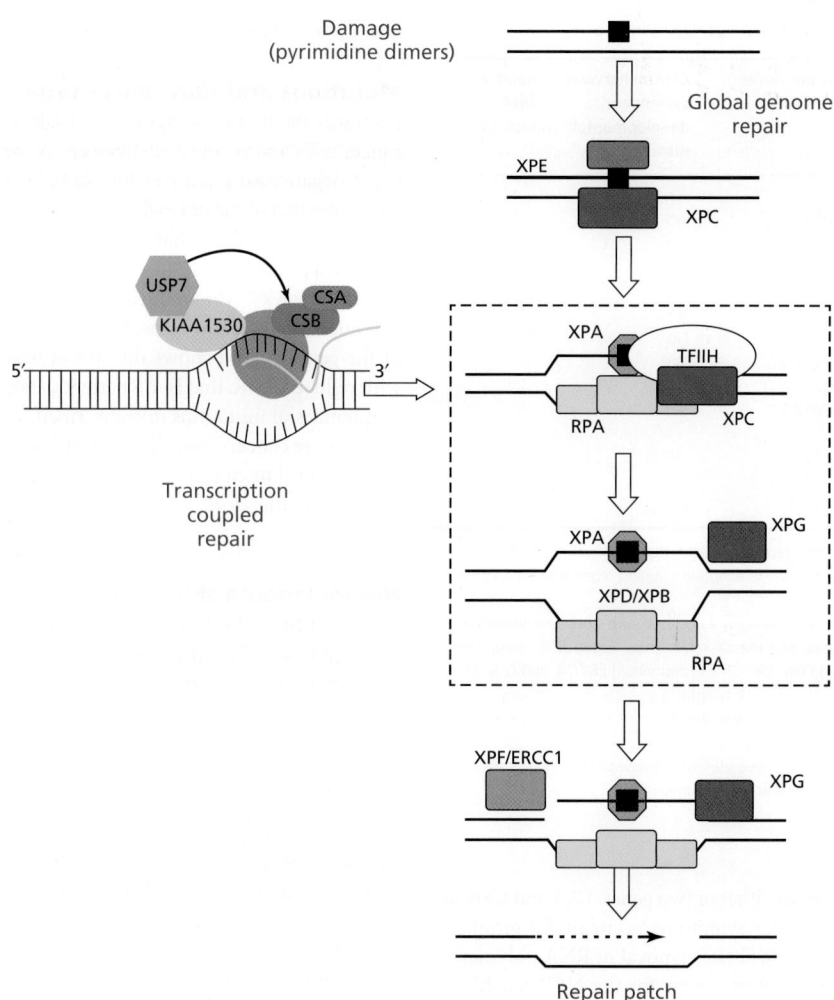

Figure 2 Biochemical steps for nucleotide excision repair of CPDs and [6-4]PDs by global genome repair or transcription-coupled repair. Initial recognition of damage by GGR involves the DDB2 and XPC gene products; initial recognition by TCR involves RNA polymerase II arrest and disengagement of the transcription complex from damage by CSA, CSB, and UVSSA. Subsequent steps involve XPA and RPA that bind to photoproducts and download the helicases XPB and XPD for local unwinding. Excision occurs when UV-specific endonucleases (XPF/ERCC1 and XPG) make incisions on the 5′ and 3′ sides. Excision and subsequent polymerization releases a 29 base oligonucleotide containing the CPD and activates the cryptic XPG endonuclease for the final cut.

Diseases of DNA repair

Xeroderma pigmentosum

XP is a rare autosomal recessive disease that occurs at a frequency of about 1 : 250,000 in the United States.[12] Affected patients (homozygotes) have sun sensitivity resulting in progressive degenerative changes of sun-exposed portions of the skin and eyes, often leading to neoplasia. Some XP patients also have progressive neurologic degeneration. Obligate heterozygotes (parents) are asymptomatic. The median age of onset of symptoms is 1–2 years of age and the median age of first diagnosis of NMSC is 9 years of age (Figure 1).[12,13] The skin rapidly takes on the appearance of that seen in individuals with many years of sun exposure. Pigmentation is patchy, and skin shows atrophy and telangiectasia with development of NMSC and melanoma. The frequency of NMSC is about 2000 times that seen in the general population <20 years of age, with an approximate 30-year reduction in lifespan. Some patients develop myelodysplasia and leukemia in later life.

Among patients who are deficient in NER, there are eight complementation groups that correspond to components of NER, XPA

through G and the exceedingly rare ERCC1.[80] An additional group, the XP variant, has mutations in the low-fidelity polymerase Pol H (Table 1). UV-damaged plasmids passaged through XP cells show increased mutagenesis due to defective repair of CPDs and nondimer photoproducts.[81] Carcinogenesis from UV damage in XP patients arises, therefore, from the loss of either NER capacity or Pol H; both lead to an increase in the amount of persistent genetic damage (mutations, gene rearrangements, deletions, and genomic instability).

Cockayne syndrome

CS (Cockayne syndrome) is an autosomal recessive disease characterized by photosensitivity, cachectic dwarfism, retinal abnormalities, microcephaly, deafness, neural defects, and retardation of growth and development after birth.[82,83] A major symptom is cerebellar degeneration and Purkinje cell loss causing difficulties in walking and balance.[84] Solar carcinogenesis is not seen in patients with CS, setting this disease apart from XP, even though their lifespan encompasses ages at which skin cancers are seen in

Table 1 Genes involved in repair of UV damage in humans.[d]

Group (gene)	Chromosome location	Central nervous system and developmental disorders	Relative DNA repair (%)[a]
Xeroderma pigmentosum			
A	9q34.1	Yes	2–5
B[b]	2q21	Yes	3–7
C	3q25	No	5–20
D[b]	19q13.2	Yes	25–50
E	11p11-12	No	50
F	16q13.1	No	18
G	13q32.3	Yes	<2
V (pol H)	6p21	No	100
ERCC1[c]	19q13.32	Yes	15
Cockayne syndrome			
A (ERCC8)	5q12.1	Yes	100[a]
B (ERCC6)	10q11.23	Yes	100[a]
UVSSA	4p16.3	No	100[a]

[a]Measurement of relative DNA repair represent mainly global genome repair. Cockayne syndrome is defective in transcription-coupled repair and has normal levels of global genome repair.

[b]Patients also exhibit symptoms commonly associated with Cockayne syndrome: dwarfism, cutaneous features, and mental retardation. Group B is designated ERCC3 and Group D is designated ERCC2, F is designated ERCC4, and G is designated ERCC5. Some patients also have symptoms of trichothiodystrophy.

[c]ERCC1 is rare and causes a neonatal fatal disorder, cerebro-oculo-facio-skeletal syndrome.

[d]Further details can be found in the web sites http://www.photobiology.info/ and http://www.cgal.icnet.uk/DNA_Repair_Genes.html.

XP (Figure 1).[82] Mutations in either of two genes, *CSA* and *CSB*, are associated with CS.[83,85] Similar symptoms occur in XP groups B, D, and G.[86] The CS proteins facilitate removal of RNA polymerase II from damaged sites permitting access for the NER machinery (Figure 2). An additional gene product UVSSA also contributes to TCR, but mutations in the *UVSSA* gene only give rise to mild photosensitivity.[87,88]

CSA and CSB proteins also contribute to the redox balance of cells by interaction with oxidative phosphorylation in the mitochondria and mitophagy.[89] Conceivably, their mitochondrial role may be more important in the developmental and neurological pathology of CS than their nuclear TCR function.[90]

Trichothiodystrophy

TTD (trichothiodystrophy) is a rare autosomal recessive disorder characterized by sulfur-deficient brittle hair that splits longitudinally into small fibers and ichthyosis. The levels of cysteine/cystine in hair proteins are 15–50% of those in normal individuals. Patients show physical and mental retardation of varying severity and often have an unusual facial appearance, with protruding ears and a receding chin. Mental abilities range from low normal to severe retardation.[91] Several categories of the disease can be recognized on the basis of UV sensitivity and DNA repair deficiences.[92,93] The most severe cases with repair deficiencies have mutations in *XPB* and *XPD*.[92] Several other TTD genes are known that are not involved in DNA repair.

Mutations in *XPD* that give rise to XP symptoms correspond to mis-sense mutations in the DNA helicase motifs, whereas those that give rise to TTD are mis-sense mutations in the RNA helicase motifs and the C-terminal end of the protein.[94] Some TTD cases do not have mutations in *XPB* or *XPD* and are due to mutations in a small 8-kDa component of TFIIH that appears to regulate the overall level of the transcription factor.[95]

Carcinogenesis

Mutations and skin cancer types

Loeb was the first to recognize the high frequency of mutations in cancer cells and invoked the concept of a mutator phenotype.[96] In triple-negative breast cancer, for example, the mutation frequency is 13.3 times that of the normal rate of 0.6 mutations per cell division.[97] NMSC and melanoma have among the highest mutation frequencies, most of which are C to T or CC to TT transitions resulting from sun exposure.[98,99] The frequency of mutations in normal and cancer genomes is reduced in transcribed regions, compared with the rest of the genome, and shows the strand bias of TCR.[97,98,100] Patients with reduced TCR, that is, CS patients, should therefore have higher frequencies of mutations in transcribed regions of the genome and hence more cancers. But they do not, unlike Cs-a or Cs-b mice that do develop skin cancer from carcinogen exposure.[101] Mutant cells in CS must, therefore, be prevented or delayed from progressing to cancers.

Nonmelanoma skin cancer

SCCs and BCCs both have UV-type mutations in genes that drive development of these tumors. Actinic keratoses, precursors to SCCs, share many mutational spectrum and global gene expression profiles.[102–104] The initiating molecular changes in SCC are UV-type mutations in p53 that result in expanding clones in the sun-exposed areas of the skin that are initially confined within the proliferating units.[105] In normal skin, 50% of SCCs have p53 mutations; in XP patients, the frequency is 90%.[106–110] Loss of p53 function causes genomic instability during DNA replication when subjected to further UV irradiation.[111–113] Many of these are likely passenger mutations that do not confer a growth advantage; mutated p53 being the more potent driver of SCC.

SCC mutations have been identified in Notch, *KNSTRN*, a kinetochore gene, *EGF, RAS, NFkb, JNK2*, and *MMP9*.[114–118] Activating mutations in *H-RAS* and *N-RAS* oncogenes at codon 61 have been associated with solar UV exposure even though they involve transversions at a TT site.[119–122]

BCCs and BCNS involve the Sonic Hedgehog pathway in which a transmembrane receptor, Patched (PTC), and the membrane protein, Smoothened (SMO), regulate signal transduction by the extracellular protein Hedgehog (HH) that binds to PTC.[123] In the general population, most UV-type BCC mutations are in the *PTC* gene or less frequently *SMO*, and rarely *HH*.[109,124–126] In XP patients, however, a significant number of mutations occur in *SMO* and *HH*.[127,128]

Melanoma

Melanomas involve a series of mutations, deletions, and amplifications (copy number changes) along the MAP kinase pathway, a phosphorylation cascade that regulates cell proliferations and differentiation.[129–135] (Figure 3). A common mutation occurs in *BRAF* (V600E), but this sequence change is not a UV type.[137,136] In contrast, 10 of 11 mutations in *BRAF* from XP melanomas were UV type and different from V600E.[136] Mutations of UV type have been identified in the promoter region of hTERT resulting in gene activation.[138,139] In addition to point mutations, melanomas have a significant frequency of translocations involving protein kinases.[140] Nevi and melanomas in XP patients are generally lentiginous and have a high incidence (53–61%) of UV-type inactivating mutations in *PTEN*.[136] These frequencies are much higher than those in *BRAF*, *NRAS*, and *KIT*, unlike the general population where *PTEN* mutations are lower.

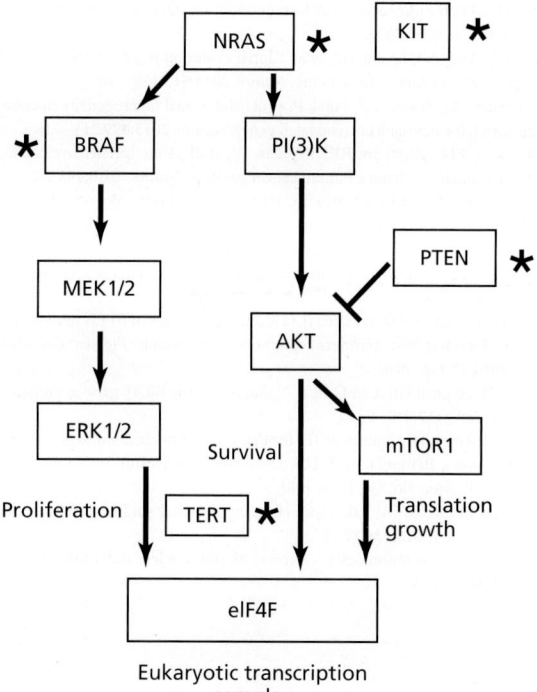

Figure 3 Pathways involved in melanoma. Proteins mutated by UV light in XP patients or the general population are designated by a star. Mutations in TERT are UV type but have yet to be reported in XP patients. Note the common *BRAF* melanoma mutation V600E is not induced by UV as it does not occur at a dipyrimidine site, but other mutations are formed by UV light in *BRAF*.[136] The most common mutated gene in XP patients is *PTEN*, in contrast to the MAPK pathway in the general population.[136]

Acknowledgments

This work was supported by the E.A. Dickson Emeritus Professorship of the University of California San Francisco (JEC) and the Simon Memorial Fund of the UCSF Academic Senate (JEC).

Summary

Skin tumors in man account for about 30% of all new cancers reported annually.[141,1] Epidemiological and laboratory studies provide evidence for a direct causal role of sunlight exposure in the induction of most forms of skin cancer,[142,5] and the high rate of skin carcinogenesis is a direct result of the high dose rate from the UV light component. Nonmelanoma skin cancers (NMSCs, basal cell, and squamous cell carcinomas) and melanomas are found on sun-exposed parts of the body (e.g., the face and trunk in men, face and legs in women), and their incidence is correlated with cumulative or acute sunlight exposure. Tumor incidence and mortality increases with occupational exposure, such as in ranchers fishermen and even flight crew members.[6,143–145] There is also an increased risk of melanoma for people using tanning parlors,[145,146] PUVA or UVA therapy,[147] or sildenafil (Viagra).[148] The use of sunscreens can also contribute to melanoma if their use results in persons staying in the sun for increased times.[149] Melanomas are additionally found on protected sites, so other factors contribute to the incidence as well as sun exposure.[12,150,151]

Human skin can be classified into types I–IV, ranging from individuals who always burn and never tan, to those who tan but never burn; skin cancer susceptibility varies accordingly.[152] The most dramatic examples of variations in human susceptibility to sunburn and skin cancer are the human genetic disorders: XP, CS, TTD, basal cell nevus syndrome (BCNS),

the porphyrias, albinism, and phenylketonuria.[12] XP, CS, and TTD involve genes with major roles in repair of UV damage to DNA. Other disorders associated with acquired sun sensitivity include polymorphous light eruption, actinic reticuloid and prurigo, solar urticaria, lupus erythematosus, and Darier's disease as well as medication and immunological status. Sunlight exposure can have an immunosuppressive effect leading to loss of antigen-presenting Langerhans cells and the appearance of dyskeratotic keratinocytes (apoptotic sunburn cells) in the upper epidermis. The erythemal response is also associated with vasodilation caused by a release of prostaglandins.[153] Immunosuppression in organ transplant and HIV patients also increases skin cancer incidence.[154]

"Mad Dogs and Englishmen Go Out in the Mid-Day Sun"—Noel Coward.

Key references

The complete reference list can be found on the Wiley Companion Digital Edition of this title (see inside front cover for login instructions).

12 Kraemer KH, Lee MM, Andrews AD, Lambert WC. The role of sunlight and DNA repair in melanoma and nonmelanoma skin cancer. The xeroderma pigmentosum paradigm. *Arch Dermatol.* 1994;**130**:1018–1021.

13 Bradford PT, Goldstein AM, Tamura DT, et al. Cancer and neurologic degeneration in xeroderma pigmentosum: long term follow-up characterises the role of DNA repair. *J Med Genet.* 2011;**48**:168–176.

25 Taylor JS, Cohrs MP. DNA, light. and Dewar pyrimidinones: the structure and significance of TpT3. *J Am Chem Soc.* 1987;**109**:2834–2835.

26 Mitchell DL, Jen J, Cleaver JE. Relative induction of cyclobutane dimers and cytosine photohydrates in DNA irradiated in vitro and in vivo with ultraviolet C and ultraviolet B light. *Photochem Photobiol.* 1991;**54**:741–746.

27 Mitchell DL, Jen J, Cleaver JE. Sequence specificity of cyclobutane pyrimidine dimers in DNA treated with solar (ultraviolet B) radiation. *Nucleic Acids Res.* 1992;**20**:225–229.

29 Mitchell DL, Cleaver JE. Photochemical alterations of cytosine account for most biological effects after ultraviolet irradiation. *Trends Photochem Photobiol.* 1990;**1**:107–119.

34 Hoeijmakers JH. Genome maintenance mechanisms for preventing cancer. *Nature.* 2001;**411**:366–374.

35 Cleaver JE. Defective repair replication in xeroderma pigmentosum. *Nature.* 1968;**218**:652–656.

36 Cleaver JE. Xeroderma pigmentosum: a human disease in which an initial stage of DNA repair is defective. *Proc Natl Acad Sci U S A.* 1969;**63**:428–435.

37 Cleaver JE, Lam ET, Revet I. Disorders of nucleotide excision repair: the genetic and molecular basis of heterogeneity. *Nat Rev Genet.* 2009;**10**: 756–768.

38 Sancar A, Lindsey-Boltz LA, Unsal-Kacmaz K, Linn S. Molecular mechanisms of mammalian DNA repair and the DNA damage checkpoints. *Annu Rev Biochem.* 2004;**73**:39–85.

40 Hanawalt PC. Transcription-coupled repair and human disease. *Science.* 1994;**266**:1957–1958.

46 Fitch ME, Nakajima S, Yasui A, Ford JM. In vivo recruitment of XPC to UV-induced cyclobutane pyrimidine dimers by the DDB2 gene product. *J Biol Chem.* 2003;**276**:46909–46910.

49 Groisman R, Polanowska J, Kuraoka I, et al. The ubiquitin ligase activity in the DDB2 and CSA complexes is differentially regulated by the COP9 signalosome in response to DNA damage. *Cell.* 2003;**113**:357–367.

50 Min JH, Pavletich NP. Recognition of DNA damage by the Rad4 nucleotide excision repair protein. *Nature.* 2007;**449**:570–575.

51 Maillard O, Solyom S, Naegeli H. An aromatic sensor with aversion to damaged strands confers versatility to DNA repair. *PLoS Biol.* 2007;**5**:e79.

52 Lindsey-Boltz LA, Sancar A. RNA poymerase: the most specific damage recognition protein in cellular responses to DNA damage. *Proc Natl Acad Sci U S A.* 2007;**104**:13213–13214.

53 Schwertman P, Lagarou A, Dekkers DHW, et al. UV-sensitive syndrome protein UVSSA recruits USP7 to regulate transcription-coupled repair. *Nat Genet.* 2012;**44**:598–602.

55 Newman JC, Bailey AD, Weiner AM. Cockayne syndrome group B protein (CSB) plays a general role in chromatin maintenance and remodeling. *Proc Natl Acad Sci U S A.* 2006;**103**:9613–9618.

56 Mao P, Meas R, Dorgan KM, Smerdon MJ. UV damage-induced RNA polymerase II stalling stimulates H2B deubiquitylation. *Proc Natl Acad Sci U S A.* 2014;**111**:12811–12816.

58 Wood RD. DNA damage recognition during nucleotide excision repair in mammalian cells. *Biochimie*. 1999;**81**:39–44.

59 Sancar A. Mechanisms of DNA excision repair. *Science*. 1994;**266**:1954–1956.

60 Fagbemi AF, Orelli B, Scharer OD. Regulation of endonuclease activity in human nucleotide excision repair. *DNA Repair*. 2011;**10**:722–729.

64 Ohmori H, Friedberg EC, Fuchs RPP, et al. The Y-family of DNA polymerases. *Mol Cell*. 2001;**8**:7–8.

65 Trincao J, Johnson RE, Escalante CR, et al. Structure of the catalytic core of S. cerevisiae DNA polymerase h: implications for translesion synthesis. *Mol Cell*. 2001;**8**:417–426.

68 Johnson RE, Prakash S, Prakash L. Efficient bypass of a thymine-thymine dimer by yeast DNA polymerase eta. *Science*. 1999;**283**:1001–1004.

82 Nance MA, Berry SA. Cockayne syndrome:review of 140 cases. *Am J Med Genet*. 1992;**42**:68–84.

87 Nakazawa Y, Sasaki K, Mitsutake N, et al. KIAA1530/UVSSA is responsible for UV-sensitive syndrome that facilitates damage-dependent processing of stalled RNA polymerase IIo in TC-NER. *Nat Genet*. 2012;**44**:586–592.

88 Zhang X, Horibata K, Saijo M, et al. Mutations in KIAA1530/UVSSA cause UV-sensitive syndrome destabilizing ERCC6 in transcription-coupled DNA repair. *Nat Genet*. 2012;**44**:593–597.

89 Scheibye-Knudsen M, Croteau DL, Bohr VA. Mitochondrial deficiency in Cockayne syndrome. *Mech Aging Dev*. 2013;**134**:275–283.

90 Cleaver JE, Brennan-Minnella AM, Swanson RA, et al. Mitochondrial reactive oxygen species are scavenged by Cockayne Syndrome B protein in human fibroblasts without nuclear DNA damage. *Proc Natl Acad Sci U S A*. 2014;**111**:13487–13492.

96 Loeb L. Mutator phenotype may be required for multistage carcinogenesis. *Cancer Res*. 1991;**51**:3075–3079.

97 Wang Y, Waters J, Leung ML, et al. Clonal evolution in breast cancer revealed by single nucleus genome sequencing. *Nature*. 2014;**512**:155–160.

98 Lawrence MS, Stojanov P, Polak P, et al. Mutational heterogeneity in cancer and the search for new cancer-associated genes. *Nature*. 2013;**499**:214–218.

99 Pleasance ED, Cheetham RK, Stephens PJ, et al. A comprehensive catalogue of somatic mutations from a human cancer genome. *Nature*. 2010;**463**:191–196.

113 Laposa RR, Huang EJ, Cleaver JE. Increased apoptosis, p53 up-regulation, and cerebellar neuronal degeneration in repair-deficient Cockayne syndrome mice. *Proc Natl Acad Sci U S A*. 2007;**104**:1389–1394.

124 Epstein EH. Basal cell carcinomas:attack of the hedgehog. *Nat Rev Cancer*. 2008;**8**:743–754.

136 Masaki T, Wang Y, DiGiovanna JJ, et al. High frequency of PTEN mutations in nevi and melanomas from xeroderma pigmentosum patients. *Pigment Cell Melanoma Res*. 2014;**27**:454–464.

137 Davies H, Bignell GR, Cox C, et al. Mutations of the BRAF gene in human cancer. *Nature*. 2002;**417**:949–954.

141 Scotto J, Fears TR, Fraumeni JF. *Incidence of Nonmelanoma Skin Cancer in the United States*. Bethesda, MD: U.S. Department of Health and Human Services, NIH Publication No. 83–2433; 1983.

151 Noonan FP, Recio JA, Takayama H, et al. Neonatal sunburn and melanoma in mice. *Nature*. 2001;**413**:271–272.

153 Kripke ML. Immunological effects of ultraviolet radiation. *J Dermatol*. 1991;**18**:429–433.

27 Inflammation and cancer

Jelena Todoric, MD, PhD ▪ Atsushi Umemura, MD, PhD ▪ Koji Taniguchi, MD, PhD ▪ Michael Karin, PhD

Overview

Epidemiological studies and experimental evidence have provided strong support to the long standing notion that chronic inflammation stimulates the development and progression of malignant neoplasms. It is now clear that pre-existing inflammation caused by persistent viral and microbial infections, autoimmune diseases, environmental irritants, and even obesity promote tumor development and may account for up to 20% of all cancer deaths. Inflammation also appears subsequent to cancer development and such "tumor-elicited inflammation" plays a key role in the malignant progression and metastatic dissemination of most cancers. Although some common anti-inflammatory drugs, such as aspirin, substantially reduce cancer risk, there is still an unmet need for the clinical development of new therapeutics that target cancer-associated inflammation.

Chronic inflammation and cancer

A potential link between inflammation and cancer was first proposed by the German pathologist, Rudolf Virchow, in the nineteenth century. Virchow supposedly detected immune cell infiltrates in solid tumors, leading him to suggest that inflammation could be a cause of tumorigenesis. Although largely forgotten for more than a century, the interest in the link between inflammation and cancer was rekindled by epidemiological studies suggesting that underlying chronic inflammation is associated with nearly 20% of cancer deaths. More recently, solid evidence has accumulated pointing to inflammation as a critical hallmark of cancer, and some of the key underlying molecular mechanisms were elucidated.[1] Furthermore, it has become clear that an inflammatory microenvironment is an important component of most cancers, including some hematopoietic malignancies, even in tumors where a direct causal relationship is yet to be established.[2] Notably, only 10% of all cancers are linked to germ line mutations, whereas the vast majority (90%) are caused by acquired somatic mutations, many of which may be caused by environmental factors that are often associated with chronic inflammation. However, in most cases, chronic inflammation caused by persistent infections (Table 1) and autoimmune disease acts as a tumor promoter.[3] One of the most notable examples is inflammatory bowel disease (IBD), such as ulcerative colitis, which greatly increases the risk of colorectal cancer (CRC).[3] Similarly, persistent *Helicobacter pylori* infection causes chronic gastritis and can lead to gastric cancer. Infections with hepatitis B virus (HBV) or hepatitis C virus (HCV) give rise to hepatitis (chronic liver inflammation), eventually culminating in liver cancer (hepatocellular carcinoma or HCC). About 85% of the current HCC cases, one of the leading causes of cancer death worldwide, are derived from chronic liver damage caused by either HBV or HCV infections.

In the past generation, obesity has become a major public health problem in most developed countries, increasing the risk of various diseases, including cancer. Obesity induces low-grade, sustained inflammation that influences many organ systems and is currently one of the most common risk factors for almost all types of cancer. Inversely, long-term use of anti-inflammatory drugs, such as aspirin or selective cyclooxygenase-2 (COX-2) inhibitors, results in a substantial reduction in the risk of cancer development. These results further underscore the importance of inflammation as one of the major causes of cancer and a driver of malignant progression and metastatic dissemination.

It is important to note that only in some types of cancer is chronic inflammation present before malignant transformation or tumor initiation, but in the majority of cancers, oncogenic and neoplastic changes induce a localized inflammatory microenvironment that further enhances tumor development and progression. Understanding the links between inflammation and cancer is essential for the development of better preventative and therapeutic strategies.

Inflammatory cells, the microenvironment, and cancer

Macrophages

Macrophages are the most abundant immune cells in the tumor microenviroment. Tumor-associated macrophages (TAMs) aquire protumorigenic properties in both primary and metastatic sites[4] and play several supportive roles in cancer development and progression. The tumor-promoting functions of TAMs affect cancer cell proliferation and survival, angiogenesis, cancer cell invasion, motility, intravasation and extravasation, as well as suppression of cytotoxic T-cell responses.[5,6] During tumor initiation/early promotion, TAMs secrete cytokines and growth factors that stimulate the proliferation and survival of initiated epithelial cells bearing oncogenic mutations.[7] It is not clear whether, at this early stage of tumor development, macrophages can eliminate abberant cells before they undergo polarization to acquire tumor-promoting properties. Two major subsets of macrophages were described: classically activated (M1) and alternatively activated (M2).[8] M1 macrophages express and secrete a variety of proinflammatory cytokines, chemokines, and effector molecules, including IL-12, IL-23, tumor necerosis factor (TNF), and iNOS, whereas M2 macrophages release anti-inflammatory mediators, such as IL-10, TGF-β, and arginase-1. During early tumor progression, several factors cause a phenotypic switch in TAM polarization to the MS phenotype, thereby providing an immunosuppressive microenvironment that is permissive for tumor growth. Exposure of macrophages to IL-4 produced by CD4+ T cells and/or cancer cells,[5,9] growth factors such as colony-stimulating factor-1 (CSF1),[10] GM-CSF,[11] and TGF-β secreted by cancer cells induces

Holland-Frei Cancer Medicine, Ninth Edition. Edited by Robert C. Bast Jr., Carlo M. Croce, William N. Hait, Waun Ki Hong, Donald W. Kufe, Martine Piccart-Gebhart, Raphael E. Pollock, Ralph R. Weichselbaum, Hongyang Wang, and James F. Holland.
© 2017 John Wiley & Sons, Inc. ISBN: 978-1-118-93469-2

Table 1 Major cancer sites and types associated with infectious agents.

Infectious agent	Cancer site and type
Helicobacter pylori	Gastric cancer
Hepatitis B viurs (HBV), hepatitis C virus (HCV)	Liver cancer
Human papillomavirus (HPV)	Cervical cancer; anogenital cancer; oropharynx cancer
Epstein–Barr virus (EBV)	Nasopharynx cancer
Schistosoma haematobium	Bladder cancer
Human immunodeficiency virus (HIV)	Non-Hodgkin lymphoma; Kaposi sarcoma; cervical cancer

As of 2008, around 16% of cancer cases worldwide are attributed to infectious agents. The most important players are *Helicobacter pylori*, HBV and HCV, and HPV.

Source: de Martel 2012.[20] Reproduced with permission of Elsevier.

the tumor-promoting M2 phenotype, but the actual origin of TAMs is still a matter of debate. Most TAMs may be derived from Ly6C$^+$ circulating monocytes,[12–14] but the classical view of the bone marrow (BM) as the major site of monocyte production has been challenged by recent studies suggesting that extramedullary hematopoiesis sustains a reservoir of tumor-infiltrating monocytes.[15] However, lineage tracing experiments demonstrated that the splenic contribution is minor and that the BM is still the major source of monocytes that give rise to TAMs, at least in some tumor models.[16] In addition to its ability to support TAM proliferation and activation, CSF1 is the major lineage regulator and a chemotactic factor for macrophages.[17] Blood vessels that provide oxygenation and nutrition dramatically increase in most tumors during malignant conversion, a process often referred to as the "angiogenic switch." TAMs that express TIE2 regulate this process mostly via production of vascular endothelial growth factor (VEGF).[18] TIE2$^+$ macrophages also promote cancer cell migration and intravasation into the circulation.[19] Furthermore, immunsuppression in the tumor bed is partially mediated by macrophages that contribute to the inhibition of cytotoxic CD8$^+$ cells, which are discussed further in the following sections (Table 1).

T and B lymphocytes

Many tumors express antigens that can be recognized by T lymphocytes, and analysis of the tumor microenviroment in a variety of solid tumors has revealed the presence of T-cell infiltrates. However, despite an active immune response in a subset of patients, including infiltration with cytotoxic CD8$^+$ T cells, tumors that progress are obviously not rejected. This indicates the existence of immunosuppressive mechanisms that counteract anticancer immunity. One such mechanism depends on accumulation of CD4$^+$Foxp3$^+$ regulatory T cells (Treg) that play a pivotal role in maintenance of immunological self-tolerance.[21] Furthermore, Treg can also produce cytokines, such as RANK ligand (RANKL) that promote tumor progression, as first demonstrated in breast cancer.[22] The CD8$^+$ T-cell response in tumors involves the participation of stress-associated or damage-associated molecular patterns (DAMP), through which tissue injury or cancer cell death can promote immunity. Production of type I interferon by CD8α$^+$ dendritic cells (DCs) also favors the activation of anticancer immunity.[23] DCs and macrophages express Major histocompatibility complex (MHC) class I molecules that present antigens to cytotoxic CD8$^+$ T cells. However, macrophages that express membrane-bound or soluble forms of histocompatibility leukocyte antigen (HLA) molecules can directly inhibit activation of natural killer (NK) cells and other T-cell subsets.[24] In addition, HLA-G

and HLA-E can inhibit NK-cell secretion of Interferon IFN-γ, an important mediator of CD8$^+$ T-cell activation.[25] Activation of the inhibitory receptors programmed cell death protein 1 (PD-1) and cytotoxic T lymphocyte antigen 4 (CTLA-4) by ligands that are expressed on either cancer cells or immune cells controls the intensity of immune response and inhibits T-cell receptor (TCR) and B-cell receptor (BCR) signaling.[26] TAMs have been shown to upregulate PD-1 ligand expression in response to hypoxia inducible factor 1α (HIF-1α) in hypoxic tumor regions, leading to T-cell suppression.[27] Furthermore, TAMs secrete a variety of cytokines and chemokines that can directly suppress T-cell activation and recruit immunosuppressive Treg cells. Th17 cells are T cells that produce the inflammatory cytokines IL-17A and IL-17F. These cells are recruited into early colon cancers and play an important role in accelerating tumor progression.[28] B lymphocytes are also present in the tumor microenvironment. In mouse models of skin cancer or squamous cell carcinoma, B cells promote tumor progression by activating cells and other myeloid cells.[29,30] In prostate cancer, newly recruited B cells promote the development of aggressive castration-resistant tumors by producing the proinflammatory cytokine lymphotoxin.[31] Tumor-infiltrating B cells can also respond to the high local concentration of TGF-β present within certain tumors and assume an immunosuppressive phenotype that prevents the activation of cytotoxic T cells.

Cancer-associated fibroblasts (CAFs)

CAFs are fibroblastic cells that reside within the tumor microenviroment. CAFs promote tumorigenesis by stimulating cancer cell proliferation, enhancing angiogenesis, and modifying the architecture of the extracellular matrix (ECM).[32–37] In normal tissues, fibroblasts prevent initiation of neoplastic growth through negative regulation of epithelial proliferation by TGF-β-mediated signaling. In contrast, CAFs show proinflammatory and tumor-promoting properties[38] and produce a wide variety of chemokines and cytokines including osteopontin (OPN), CXCL1, CXCL2, IL-6, IL1-β, CCL-5, stromal-derived factor (SDF-1α), and TNF.[39,40] In early stages of the tumorigenic process, fibroblasts "sense" changes in tissue architecture that result from increased proliferation of neighboring epithelial cells. This results in activation of proinflammatory signaling in fibroblasts.[41–43] Furthermore, the proinflammatory properties of CAFs are enhanced by mediators secreted by resident immune cells.[40] For example, B cells produce antibodies that are deposited in the tumor bed owing to small amounts of blood seeping out of leaky blood vessels and can induce secretion of IL-1 by resident immune cells. This in turn drives fibroblasts into a proinflammatory phenotype.[44,45] CAFs can also be affected by tumor hypoxia, which upregulates their ability to produce TGF-β and certain chemokines.[46] The major mechanism of tumor promotion by CAFs involves secretion of cytokines and chemokines that recruit immune cells into the tumor microenviroment and alter their function. For example, CAF-secreted CCL2 recruits macrophages to the tumor, whereas CAF-derived immunosuppressive cytokine TGF-β inhibits the function of NK and CD8$^+$ T cells[47] while inducing differentiation of Treg cells.[48] CAF-derived CXCL13 mediates recruitment of B cells into androgen-deprived prostate cancer, leading to development of castration resistance.[46]

Pro- and anti-inflammatory cytokines in cancer

Cytokines are small proteins produced and released by many types of cells, especially immune cells, and function as mediators of cell–cell communication via specific membrane receptors.[7] Cytokines are usually induced in response to inflammation and provide an important link between inflammation and cancer through cancer-intrinsic (cancer cell proliferation, survival, and invasive properties) and cancer-extrinsic (tumor microenvironment) effects (Figure 1).[49] TNF and IL-6 are the best-studied protumorigenic cytokines linking inflammation to cancer and are overexpressed in most cancers (Table 2).[50] Several transcription factors, NF-κB, signal transducer and activator of transcription 3 (STAT3), and AP-1, are the major downstream effectors of cytokine signaling and are activated in the majority of cancers, where they cooperate to regulate many cancer-related pathophysiological processes, including cell proliferation and survival, differentiation, immunity, metabolism, and metastatic behavior.[51]

Tumor necerosis factor

TNF is the founding member of a large cytokine family and major activator of inflammatory and immune responses to a variety of pathogens.[52,53] TNF is an important mediator of cachexia and several acute and chronic inflammatory diseases, such as sepsis, rheumatoid arthritis (RA), and IBD. TNF is mainly produced by macrophages, which are activated by pathogen-associated molecular patterns (PAMPs), such as lipopolysaccharide (LPS), via toll-like receptors (TLRs). TNF activates several signaling pathways by binding to TNF receptor (TNFR)1 and/or TNFR2.

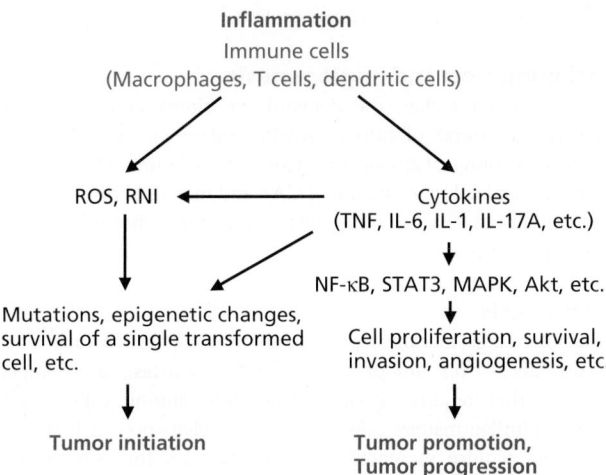

Figure 1 The role of inflammation in tumor initiation, promotion, and progression.

Table 2 Cytokines in inflammation and cancer.

Cytokine	Functions in cancer and immune cells	Pathways
TNF	Proinflammatory, cell survival or death	NF-κB, MAPK
IL-6	Proinflammatory, cell proliferation and survival	JAK/STAT3, ERK, Akt
IL-11	Tissue-protective, cell proliferation and survival	JAK/STAT3, ERK, Akt
IL-1	Proinflammatory, activates immune cells	NF-κB, MAPK
IL-17A	Proinflammatory, increases inflammation	NF-κB, MAPK
IL-12	Proinflammatory, Th1 differentiation	JAK/STAT4
IL-23	Proinflammatory, Th17 differentiation	JAK/STAT3, STAT4
IL-10	Anti-inflammatory, inhibits NF-κB	JAK/STAT3
IL-22	Tissue-protective, cell proliferation and survival	JAK/STAT3
TGF-β	Anti-inflammatory, dual role in tumorigenesis	Smad, MAPK

Activation of these pathways induces production of other inflammatory cytokines, such as IL-6 and IL-1 and, depending on cellular context, modulates cell survival and death. Elevated TNF expression promotes tumorigenesis and metastasis at multiple steps, including cellular transformation, survival, proliferation, invasion, and angiogenesis.[52,53] TNF-induced NF-κB activation enhances β-catenin activation, which leads to dedifferentiation of non-stem cells that acquire tumor-initiating capacity in a mouse model of colorectal cancer.[54] Several TNF inhibitors are clinically available and are approved for the treatment of RA and IBD. Although high doses of TNF have been used in the treatment of sarcomas of the extremities, localized production of TNF is associated with tumor promotion.

The IL-6 family of cytokines

IL-6 is another proinflammatory cytokine that activates the acute phase response characterized by expression of C-reactive protein (CRP) and serum amyloid A (SAA).[55] IL-6 is also a mediator of cancer cachexia and is one of the best-characterized protumorigenic cytokines.[56,57] The IL-6 family also includes IL-11, IL-27, IL-31, leukemia inhibitory factor (LIF), oncostatin M (OSM), ciliary neurotrophic factor (CNTF), cardiotrophin-1 (CT-1), and cardiotrophin-like cytokine (CLC), all of which control cell proliferation, survival, migration, invasion, metastasis, angiogenesis, and inflammation. IL-6 family members activate the Janus kinase (JAK)-STAT3 pathway, the Src homology 2 (SH2)-containing protein tyrosine phosphatase-2 (SHP-2)-Ras-Raf-MEK-extracellular signal-regulated kinase (ERK) pathway, and the phosphoinositide 3-kinase (PI3K)-Akt-mammalian target of rapamycin (mTOR) pathway through engagement of their unique receptor(s) that associate with the common signaling subunit gp130. Among these effectors, STAT3 is considered an oncogene and a major downstream mediator of gp130 signaling in cancer.[58,59] IL-6 and IL-11 are produced by many different types of cells, including immune cells, fibroblasts, and epithelial cells, and IL-6, IL-11, and STAT3 are highly expressed in many solid tumors. A recent report described IL-11 as the dominant IL-6 family member during gastrointestinal (GI) tumorigenesis in mice.[60] IL-6 antagonists have been approved for the treatment of RA and related diseases but need to be further evaluated in cancer.

Interleukin 1

IL-1 is another major proinflammatory and protumorigenic cytokine produced by a variety of cell types.[61] IL-1 induces fever and plays an important role in sepsis. There are two isoforms of IL-1: IL-1α and IL-1β, both of which activate NF-κB, JNK, p38, and ERK via IL-1 receptor (IL-1R) and can induce expression of other cytokines. IL-1α and IL-1β have similar functions although they are only 26% similar at the protein level. Several IL-1 antagonists have been developed and are used for the treatment of auto-inflammatory conditions. These inhibitors also need to be tested for efficacy in cancer.

Interleukin 17A

IL-17A is a member of the IL-17 family and is mainly produced by IL-17-producing T-helper (Th17) cells, γδ T cells, and innate lymphoid cells (ILCs).[62,63] IL-17A normally provides protection against extracellular bacteria and fungi and is associated with autoimmune diseases, such as psoriasis. IL-17A activates NF-κB, JNK, p38, and ERK via IL-17 receptor A (IL-17RA) in many cell types and promotes tumorigenesis, metastasis, angiogenesis, and chemotherapy resistance.[64] IL-17A induces production of many proinflammatory cytokines, including TNF, IL-6, and IL-1β, suggesting an important role of IL-17A in amplifying inflammation. IL-17A also signals within transformed enterocytes and promotes growth and progression of aberrant crypt foci in a mouse model of colorectal cancer.[64]

IL-12 and IL-23

IL-12 and IL-23 are related heterodimeric proinflammatory cytokines that share a p40 subunit, whose receptors contain a common IL-12 receptor (IL-12R) β1 subunit.[65] They are mainly produced by antigen-presenting cells and are key players in the regulation of T-cell responses. IL-12 stimulates the development of Th1 cells (typically antitumorigenic) that produce IFN-γ, whereas IL-23 promotes the development of Th17 cells (often protumorigenic) together with IL-6 and TGF-β.

IL-10 and IL-22

IL-10, the founding member of the IL-10 family, is an anti-inflammatory cytokine that activates the JAK-STAT3 pathway via IL-10 receptor 1 (IL-10R1), which is mainly expressed in immune cells.[66] IL-10 exerts its anti-inflammatory activity in part through NF-κB inhibition. IL-10 knockout mice spontaneously develop chronic colitis that resembles human IBD. In contrast, IL-22, another member of the IL-10 family of cytokines, is a proinflammatory cytokine that is produced by Th17- and IL-22-producing T-helper (Th22) cells and ILC. IL-22 also activates the JAK-STAT3 pathway via IL-22 receptor 1 (IL-22R1), which is exclusively expressed on epithelial cells and not on immune cells. IL-22 regulates innate responses related to host defense and autoimmune disease, promotes cell proliferation, survival, tissue regeneration, metastasis, and angiogenesis in a similar way to the IL-6 family of cytokines.[67]

Transforming growth factor-beta

TGF-β is the prototypical member of the TGF-β superfamily of anti-inflammatory cytokines.[68] TGF-β activates the Smad pathway and non-Smad signaling via the JNK, p38 and ERK mitogen-activated protein kinases (MAPKs), through binding to heterodimeric type I and II TGF-β receptors (TGF-RI and -RII). TGF-β also inhibits cell proliferation and regulates Treg and Th17 differentiation. TGF-β plays a dual role in the progression of cancer[69]; exerting suppressive effects in normal cells and early carcinomas, and promoting malignant progression, invasion, and metastasis in advanced tumors.

Inflammation and tumorigenesis

The tumorigenic process is composed of several steps: initiation, promotion, and metastasis. These progressive steps are accompanied by tumor angiogenesis, formation of new blood and lymph vessels that supply the growing tumor with essential nutrients and oxygen. These vessels also provide routes for metastatic dissemination. Through the release of inflammatory mediators, chronically activated TAM and CAF in the tumor microenvironment control malignant progression and tumor angiogenesis.

Tumor initiation

The initiation phase involves induction of oncogenic mutations that lead to oncogene activation and/or loss of tumor suppressors. These mutations change the behavior of normal cells to become malignant by providing them with growth and survival advantages over their neighbors. Mediators such as reactive oxygen species (ROS) and reactive nitrogen intermediates (RNI) produced by inflammatory

cells can lead to DNA damage and acquisition of oncogenic mutations. These reactive intermediates also cause genomic instability and can accelerate cell proliferation, but their over-production leads to cell death. Another mechanism through which inflammation may enhance tumor initiation is the production of growth factors and cytokines that confer a stem-cell like phenotype upon tumor progenitors or stimulate stem cell expansion, thereby enlarging the cell pool that is targeted by environmental mutagens. However, this mechanism is more akin to early tumor promotion, which is discussed in the following sections.

In most cases, a single mutation is insufficient to cause cancer and at least 4–5 mutations are needed.[70,71] Thus, tumor initiation requires continuous exposure to ROS and RNI resulting in irreversible and persistent DNA damage and accumulation of numerous mutations in dividing cells. Chronic inflammation also leads to epigenetic alterations, including DNA methylation and histone modification, that may further contribute to tumor initiation.

Tumor promotion

Tumor promotion is the process of tumor growth from a single initiated cell into a clonal population giving rise to a primary tumor. Tumor-promoting cytokines and growth factors produced by immune/inflammatory cells are central to this process. For instance, TNF and IL-6 activate AP-1, NF-κB, and STAT3 to induce genes that stimulate cell proliferation and survival. Cytokines that stimulate angiogenesis provide the growing primary tumor with blood vessels that increase oxygen and nutrient availability, altogether resulting in net tumor growth.

Inflammation and angiogenesis

As mentioned earlier, the demand for blood supply increases during the course of tumor growth. Inflammatory cells are an important source of angiogenic cytokines, including VEGF. Tumor hypoxia can lead to activation of CAF and increased production of chemokines that recruit more inflammatory and immune cells into the hypoxic tumor.[46]

Metastasis

The final stage in tumor progression is metastasis, which eventually causes over 90% of cancer deaths. Metastasis is a complex process that requires close collaboration among cancer cells, immune/inflammatory cells, and stromal elements. At first, cancer cells acquire mesenchymal characteristics through the loss of cell polarity and cell–cell adhesion, resulting in increased motility and ability to invade epithelial linings/basal membranes and enter efferent blood vessels or lymphatics.[72] This process is called epithelial-mesenchymal transition (EMT) and it is characterized by loss of E-cadherin expression. Next, cancer cells intravasate into blood vessels and lymphatics. Inflammation promotes both EMT and intravasation through production of mediators that activate NF-κB in cancer cells and increase vascular permeability, respectively. This is followed by the third step in which metastasis-initiating cells survive and travel throughout the circulation. It is estimated that only about 0.01% of cancer cells that enter the circulation will eventually survive and give rise to micrometastases.[73] Integrin-mediated attachment allows the extravasation of circulating cancer cells, and this process is governed by neutrophil-dependent upregulation of adhesion molecules.[74] Finally, single metastatic progenitors interact with immune, inflammatory, and stromal cells and start to proliferate.[75] Systemic inflammation enhances attachment of circulating cancer cells to target organs and stimulates neutrophil mobilization. Several proinflammatory cytokines present in the circulation of cancer patients upregulate expression of adhesion molecules on the endothelium or in target organs, thereby enhancing metastatic cell attachment.[2]

Inflammation-dependent cancers—examples and treatment

Colorectal cancer

IBD and colorectal cancer

IBD patients are at an elevated risk for CRC, which when present in such patients is referred to as colitis-associated cancer (CAC). Although IBD contributes to only 2–3% of all cases of CRC,[76,77] up to 20% of IBD patients develop CAC within 30 years after disease onset. In mice, CAC-like disease can be induced by combining the chemical procarcinogen azoxymethane (AOM) with the mucosal irritant dextran sulfate sodium salt (DSS), which elicits colitis-like pathology.[78] Using this model, the IL-6/IL-11-STAT3 axis and NF-κB were proven to be required for the proliferation and survival of premalignant intestinal epithelial cells and CAC development.[7,79]

Sporadic colorectal cancer and inflammation

Even sporadic CRC that does not develop as a consequence of apparent colonic inflammation exhibits extensive inflammatory infiltrates, referred to as "tumor-elicited inflammation," with high levels of cytokine expression in the tumor microenvironment.[7] Long-term intake of nonsteroidal anti-inflammatory drugs (NSAIDs), such as aspirin, that inhibit the enzymatic activity of COX-2, reduces the relative risk of sporadic CRC and hereditary CRC, suggesting that inflammation also plays an important role in spontaneous CRC development.[76] The *Adenomatous polyposis coli* (*APC*) tumor suppressor gene, encoding a negative regulator of Wnt-β catenin signaling, is the most frequently mutated gene in sporadic CRC (60%), and germ line *APC* mutations cause familial adenomatous polyposis (FAP). Accordingly, *Apc^min* mutant mice and *Apc* intestinal epithelial-specific knockout mice provide good models for sporadic CRC and FAP.[78,80,81] In these mouse models, colorectal adenomas, which develop upon loss of the normal *Apc* allele, exhibit defective expression of several epithelial barrier proteins, resulting in entry of microbial products into the tumors but not the adjacent tissue.[28] These microbial products activate macrophages associated with early adenomas to produce IL-23 and expand the population of IL-17 producing cells that drive tumor progression through activation of IL-17RA.[64]

Gut microbiota and colorectal cancer

The GI tract is the largest reservoir of commensal bacteria in the human body.[82] Commensal bacteria affect various physiological functions in the gut via host–microbe interactions, and dysbiosis of the microbiota can lead to or promote various GI diseases including IBD and CRC.[83] A correlation between gut microbiota composition and GI cancers has been investigated in experimental animal models and clinical and epidemiological studies. However, gut bacteria that trigger and promote CRC remain to be identified, although it is well known that *H. pylori* induces gastritis and gastric cancer.[76] Pathological microbes may promote intestinal tumorigenesis through chronic activation of inflammation, alteration of tumor microenvironment, induction of genotoxic responses, and metabolism. Alternatively, such pathological and tumor-promoting alterations could be caused by loss of protective or beneficial microbes.

Cancer prevention, therapy, and side effects

Conventional therapy for CRC includes surgery, chemotherapy, and radiation therapy. Given the growing body of evidence that inflammation triggers and promotes CAC and sporadic CRC, there is room for drugs that reduce inflammation in the prevention or treatment of CRC and other GI cancers. As mentioned earlier, NSAIDs and selective COX-2 inhibitors were proven effective for CRC prevention. Inhibitors of proinflammatory cytokines, such as neutralizing antibodies or decoy receptors to TNF, IL-6, IL-1, IL-17A, and IL-23 or inhibitors of cytokine signaling, including JAK, STAT3, IKK, and NF-κB, might also be useful for the treatment of CAC and spontaneous CRC.[76] However, it is unlikely that such drugs would be effective as monotherapies, and thus, they should be tested in combination with chemo- or radiotherapy. Notably, JAK inhibitors were found effective for the treatment of IBD, but their side effects include mucositis, anemia, thrombocytopenia, liver dysfunction, and infection. Importantly, mucositis is the major dose-limiting factor in cytotoxic chemotherapy, and therefore, caution should be exercised when drugs that inhibit the activity of cytokines, such as IL-6, IL-17A, and IL-23 that promote mucosal healing, are combined with chemotherapeutic agents. Some chemotherapeutics may be more amenable to such combinations, as recently shown for 5-FU in an *Apc* mutant mouse, where it was found to be much more effective in combination with an IL-17A neutralizing antibody.[64]

Another approach to control GI inflammation is to use prebiotics or probiotics, with the aim of normalizing or skewing the host microbiome to influence cancer development.[83] Several dietary compounds were found to reduce inflammation and CRC risk, including carbohydrates, fiber, unsaturated n-3 fatty acids, vitamins, minerals, and phytochemicals (resveratrol and curcumin) although the underlying molecular mechanisms are unknown.[76]

Pancreatic cancer

Inflammation and pancreatic ductal adenocarcinoma (PDAC)

Pancreatic ductal adenocarcinoma (PDAC) is an aggressive malignancy with an overall 5-year survival rate of <5%.[84] One of the major features of PDAC is remarkable desmoplasia that is composed of ECM, fibroblasts, vascular, and immune cells.[85] This cellular milieu is rich in inflammatory cytokines, growth factors and proteinases that stimulate the proliferation and survival of malignant cells.[86,87] Increased levels of proinflammatory cytokines including IL-6, IL-8, and TNF, as well as the anti-inflammatory cytokines IL-10 and TGF-β were found to correlate with cachexia and poor prognosis in PDAC patients.[88–91] The progression of early PanIN lesions into PDAC in pancreatic *KRAS*-mutated mice has been shown to depend on activation of the STAT3 pathway by JAK tyrosine kinases in response to IL-6.[92] In addition, IL-6 induces expression of VEGF in pancreatic cancer cells, thereby stimulating angiogenesis.[93] Although high-dose TNF was shown to have toxic effects on cancer cells, in the PDAC microenvironment, binding of TNF–TNFR2 results in upregulation of EGF receptor and its ligand TGF-α, leading to increased cancer cell proliferation.[94] IL-10 and TGF-β facilitate the shift from the Th1 immunophenotype, which has antitumor activity, to the Th2 immunophenotype, which has protumor activity.[95]

Anti-inflammatory strategies for PDAC therapy

Major strategies to activate antitumor immune responses that were found to be effective in highly immunogenic cancers, such as cutaneous melanoma and bladder cancer, include adoptive transfer of cancer-reactive T cells and the use of immune checkpoint inhibitors.[96] For instance, blockade of the inhibitory receptors CTLA-4 and PD-1 with specific monoclonal antibodies or depletion of Treg cells with antibodies against CD25 can result in activation of anticancer immunity.[97,98] Such strategies, so far, have not been too effective against PDAC, perhaps due to the existence of additional, yet-to-be discovered, immunosuppressive mechanisms. IL-6 monoclonal antibodies, Siltuximab and Tocilizumab, that bind to the soluble form of the IL-6 receptor are currently under evaluation in ovarian cancer patients (clinicaltrials.gov) and should be tested in PDAC as well. Ruxolitinib is a selective JAK1/JAK2 inhibitor that was approved by the FDA in 2011 for the treatment of myelofibrosis. Ruxolitinib can block STAT3 activation by IL-6 and was found to significantly improve the survival rate of a subgroup of patients with recurrent or treatment-refractory PDAC (clinicaltrial.gov). Testing whether IL-6 neutralizing antibodies or JAK inhibitors may also potentiate the activation of cytotoxic T cells targeting PDAC would be of interest.

Liver cancer

Etiology and pathogenesis

HCC is the fifth most common cancer worldwide and the third leading cause of cancer deaths. More than 90% of HCC develops in the context of chronic liver disease and persistent inflammation, with HBV or HCV infections being the main causes. Additional risk factors for HCC include fatty liver disease, aflatoxin, alcohol, and hereditary conditions such as hemochromatosis. HCC is characterized by phenotypic and molecular heterogeneity reflecting diverse pathological origin. Because of that, no clear evidence for oncogene addiction has been proved, even though hTERT, β-catenin, and *p53* gene alterations are relatively common. As HCC develops in a liver with extensive inflammation and fibrosis, the role of inflammation in HCC development is particularly important.

Therapy

Early stage HCC may be eligible for surgical resection (total or partial hepatectomy), liver transplantation, or local ablation therapy. However, 70% of HCC cases recur at 5 years after these curative therapies. If the tumor is already at advanced stages at the time of diagnosis or recurs after curative treatment, systemic chemotherapy using molecular targeted drugs is considered besides chemoembolization. However, the 5-year survival rate for HCC has remained very low (<8%).

The protein kinase inhibitor sorafenib is currently the only approved systemic drug for advanced HCC and median survival was only 2.8 months longer for patients treated with sorafenib than control group (10.7 months vs 7.9 months, respectively). Although drugs that target signaling pathways involved in HCC-tumorigenesis have been the subject of many clinical trials after the approval of sorafenib, no other drug demonstrated clear survival benefits or positive results in first-line (brivanib, sunitinib, erlotinib, and linifanib) or second-line (brivanib, everolimus) HCC therapy. Currently, clinical trials testing the MET inhibitor tivantinib and Mitogen-activated protein kinase/ERK kinase (MEK) inhibitor refametinib in RAS(+) HCC patients are ongoing. However, these drugs may be beneficial only for a subset of HCC patients because *RAS*-mutated cases represent no more than 5% of HCC patients.[99]

These failures may be due to the heterogeneous and complex molecular features of HCC, which remains a poorly understood malignancy. Liver toxicity was also seen frequently during clinical trials and is a main cause of their failure. Of note, coexistence of liver cirrhosis frequently limits treatment options for HCC patients. For instance, the rapalog everolimus did not extend overall survival compared to placebo and its use resulted in increased incidence of liver injury. Interestingly, either rapamycin treatment or hepatocyte-specific ablation of the raptor subunit of mTORC1, the molecular target for rapalogs, increased IL-6 production and activated the protumorigenic transcription factor STAT3 in a mouse model. Furthermore, loss of mTORC1 activity resulted in low-grade liver inflammation leading to enhancement of HCC development.[100]

Obesity, inflammation, and putative therapeutic options

Recently, a certain portion of HCC patients in Western countries was found not to exhibit viral infections.[101] Most of these patients are obese with manifestations of the metabolic syndrome and suffer from nonalcoholic steatohepatitis (NASH), a severe form of nonalcoholic fatty liver disease (NAFLD).[102] Indeed, obesity increases male HCC risk by up to 4.5-fold.[103] Because the prevalence of obesity has been increasing rapidly worldwide, its association with liver tumorigenesis has attracted much attention. Importantly, obesity strongly enhances HCC development in mice, allowing mechanistic studies, which revealed that obesity increases HCC risk by triggering low-grade liver inflammation associated with elevated expression of TNF and IL-6.[104] IL-6 signaling is also important to HCC development in nonobese settings, and HCC progenitor/stem cell expansion and malignant progression depend on autocrine IL-6 signaling.[105,106] In addition, obesity[107,108] and HBV/HCV infections[109] induce endoplasmic reticulum (ER) stress in hepatocytes and this may promote hepatosteatosis in humans.[110] Furthermore, ER stress contributes to NASH-like disease development and progression to HCC in mice.[111] Interestingly, HCC development in this model can be attenuated through the relief of ER stress or inhibition of TNF signaling in hepatocytes. These findings suggest that NASH and its progression to HCC may be prevented or ameliorated by anti-TNF drugs and molecules termed "chemical chaperons" that are capable of relieving ER stress.

Key references

The complete reference list can be found on the Wiley Companion Digital Edition of this title (see inside front cover for login instructions).

1 Karin M. Nuclear factor-kappaB in cancer development and progression. *Nature.* 2006;**441**(**7092**):431–436.

2 Mantovani A, Allavena P, Sica A, Balkwill F. Cancer-related inflammation. *Nature.* 2008;**454**(**7203**):436–444.

4 Biswas SK, Allavena P, Mantovani A. Tumor-associated macrophages: functional diversity, clinical significance, and open questions. *Semin Immunopathol.* 2013;**35**(**5**):585–600.

5 Coussens LM, Zitvogel L, Palucka AK. Neutralizing tumor-promoting chronic inflammation: a magic bullet? *Science.* 2013;**339**(**6117**):286–291.

6 Qian BZ, Pollard JW. Macrophage diversity enhances tumor progression and metastasis. *Cell.* 2010;**141**(**1**):39–51.

7 Grivennikov SI, Greten FR, Karin M. Immunity, inflammation, and cancer. *Cell.* 2010;**140**(**6**):883–899.

11 Su S, Liu Q, Chen J, et al. A positive feedback loop between mesenchymal-like cancer cells and macrophages is essential to breast cancer metastasis. *Cancer Cell.* 2014;**25**(**5**):605–620.

13 Franklin RA, Liao W, Sarkar A, et al. The cellular and molecular origin of tumor-associated macrophages. *Science.* 2014;**344**(**6186**):921–925.

14 Qian BZ, Li J, Zhang H, et al. CCL2 recruits inflammatory monocytes to facilitate breast-tumour metastasis. *Nature.* 2011;**475**(**7355**):222–225.

18 Lin EY, Pollard JW. Tumor-associated macrophages press the angiogenic switch in breast cancer. *Cancer Res.* 2007;**67**(**11**):5064–5066.

21 Spranger S, Spaapen RM, Zha Y, et al. Up-regulation of PD-L1, IDO, and T(regs) in the melanoma tumor microenvironment is driven by CD8(+) T cells. *Sci Transl Med.* 2013;**5**(**200**):200ra116.

22 Tan W, Zhang W, Strasner A, et al. Tumour-infiltrating regulatory T cells stimulate mammary cancer metastasis through RANKL-RANK signalling. *Nature.* 2011;**470**(**7335**):548–553.

27 Noman MZ, Desantis G, Janji B, et al. PD-L1 is a novel direct target of HIF-1alpha, and its blockade under hypoxia enhanced MDSC-mediated T cell activation. *J Exp Med.* 2014;**211**(**5**):781–790.

28 Grivennikov SI, Wang K, Mucida D, et al. Adenoma-linked barrier defects and microbial products drive IL-23/IL-17-mediated tumour growth. *Nature.* 2012;**491**(**7423**):254–258.

30 Affara NI, Ruffell B, Medler TR, et al. B cells regulate macrophage phenotype and response to chemotherapy in squamous carcinomas. *Cancer Cell.* 2014;**25**(**6**):809–821.

31 Ammirante M, Luo JL, Grivennikov S, Nedospasov S, Karin M. B-cell-derived lymphotoxin promotes castration-resistant prostate cancer. *Nature.* 2010;**464**(**7286**): 302–305.

34 Bhowmick NA, Neilson EG, Moses HL. Stromal fibroblasts in cancer initiation and progression. *Nature.* 2004;**432**(**7015**):332–337.

37 Levental KR, Yu H, Kass L, et al. Matrix crosslinking forces tumor progression by enhancing integrin signaling. *Cell.* 2009;**139**(**5**):891–906.

40 Erez N, Truitt M, Olson P, Arron ST, Hanahan D. Cancer-associated fibroblasts are activated in incipient neoplasia to orchestrate tumor-promoting inflammation in an NF-kappaB-dependent manner. *Cancer Cell.* 2010;**17**(**2**):135–147.

45 Mantovani A. La mala educación of tumor-associated macrophages: diverse pathways and new players. *Cancer Cell.* 2010;**17**(**2**):111–112.

46 Ammirante M, Shalapour S, Kang Y, Jamieson CA, Karin M. Tissue injury and hypoxia promote malignant progression of prostate cancer by inducing CXCL13 expression in tumor myofibroblasts. *Proc Natl Acad Sci U S A.* 2014;**111**(**41**):14776–14781.

48 Yang L, Pang Y, Moses HL. TGF-beta and immune cells: an important regulatory axis in the tumor microenvironment and progression. *Trends Immunol.* 2010;**31**(**6**):220–227.

49 Hanahan D, Weinberg RA. Hallmarks of cancer: the next generation. *Cell.* 2011;**144**(**5**):646–674.

53 Balkwill F. Tumour necrosis factor and cancer. *Nat Rev Cancer.* 2009;**9**(**5**):361–371.

56 Taniguchi K, Karin M. IL-6 and related cytokines as the critical lynchpins between inflammation and cancer. *Semin Immunol.* 2014;**26**(**1**):54–74.

58 Yu H, Pardoll D, Jove R. STATs in cancer inflammation and immunity: a leading role for STAT3. *Nat Rev Cancer.* 2009;**9**(**11**):798–809.

64 Wang K, Kim MK, Di Caro G, et al. Interleukin-17 receptor a signaling in transformed enterocytes promotes early colorectal tumorigenesis. *Immunity.* 2014;**41**:1052–1063.

68 Pickup M, Novitskiy S, Moses HL. The roles of TGFbeta in the tumour microenvironment. *Nat Rev Cancer.* 2013;**13**(**11**):788–799.

76 Terzic J, Grivennikov S, Karin E, Karin M. Inflammation and colon cancer. *Gastroenterology.* 2010;**138**(**6**):2101.e5–2114.e5.

79 Greten FR, Eckmann L, Greten TF, et al. IKKbeta links inflammation and tumorigenesis in a mouse model of colitis-associated cancer. *Cell.* 2004;**118**(**3**):285–296.

85 Gukovsky I, Li N, Todoric J, Gukovskaya A, Karin M. Inflammation, autophagy, and obesity: common features in the pathogenesis of pancreatitis and pancreatic cancer. *Gastroenterology.* 2013;**144**(**6**):1199.e4–1209.e4.

86 Feig C, Gopinathan A, Neesse A, Chan DS, Cook N, Tuveson DA. The pancreas cancer microenvironment. *Clin Cancer Res.* 2012;**18**(**16**):4266–4276.

92 Lesina M, Kurkowski MU, Ludes K, et al. Stat3/Socs3 activation by IL-6 transsignaling promotes progression of pancreatic intraepithelial neoplasia and development of pancreatic cancer. *Cancer Cell.* 2011;**19**(**4**):456–469.

96 Dougan M, Dranoff G. Immune therapy for cancer. *Annu Rev Immunol.* 2009;**27**:83–117.

100 Umemura A, Park EJ, Taniguchi K, et al. Liver damage, inflammation, and enhanced tumorigenesis after persistent mTORC1 inhibition. *Cell Metab.* 2014;**20**(**1**):133–144.

101 El-Serag HB. Hepatocellular carcinoma. *N Engl J Med.* 2011;**365**(**12**):1118–1127.

103 Calle EE, Teras LR, Thun MJ. Obesity and mortality. *N Engl J Med.* 2005;**353**(**20**): 2197–2199.

104 Park EJ, Lee JH, Yu GY, et al. Dietary and genetic obesity promote liver inflammation and tumorigenesis by enhancing IL-6 and TNF expression. *Cell.* 2010;**140**(**2**):197–208.

111 Nakagawa H, Umemura A, Taniguchi K, et al. ER stress cooperates with hypernutrition to trigger TNF-dependent spontaneous HCC development. *Cancer Cell.* 2014;**26**(**3**):331–343.

28 RNA tumor viruses

Robert C. Gallo, MD ▪ *Marvin S. Reitz, PhD*

Overview

Retroviruses are enveloped viruses that contain a diploid RNA genome and are defined by the presence of reverse transcriptase, a DNA polymerase that transcribes RNA into DNA, which is then inserted into the host cell chromosome. These processes often lead to the capture and/or alteration of genetic material and the transfer of information between cells, with neoplastic transformation of the infected cell being an occasional outcome of infection. Retroviruses are also associated with immunodeficiencies and with neurologic diseases, although infection is often asymptomatic. Retroviruses can also enter the germ line and be present as a part of the genetic complement of all members of a species. These viruses are called endogenous retroviruses. Although most retroviral malignancies occur as leukemia/lymphomas in nonhuman species, human T-cell leukemia virus type I (HTLV-I) causes adult T-cell leukemia/lymphoma in a minority of infected humans, as well as a neurologic disease and a variety of other pathologies. Human immunodeficiency virus type 1 (HIV-1), although not considered a tumor virus, is associated with an increased incidence of several types of tumors, especially those caused by viruses such as human papillomavirus and Epstein–Barr virus.

Retroviruses were discovered early in the twentieth century. Ellerman and Bang[1] showed the transmission of leukemia in chickens by a cell-free filtrate, and Rous[2] was similarly able to transmit sarcomas in chickens. These findings were extended to mammals by Bittner in the case of breast tumors in mice[3] and by Gross for murine leukemias.[4] Gross recognized the importance of inoculating newborn mice for development of leukemia, and in many respects, his work heralded the beginning of modern studies of retroviruses. Jarrett showed that a similar virus was responsible for leukemia in cats, which was the first demonstration of naturally transmitted leukemia in an outbred species.[5,6] Kawakami and Theilen and colleagues first showed that retroviruses could cause leukemia in primates, specifically in gibbon apes and new world monkeys.[7–9]

Biologic assays for these viruses were in use from the 1950s, but a more fundamental understanding of their life cycle was considerably advanced in the early 1970s by the discovery that they contained reverse transcriptase (RT).[10,11] This provided a far simpler, quicker, and more sensitive assay for retroviruses. Another important finding in the 1970s was that some retroviruses [e.g., Rous sarcoma virus (RSV)] contained genes for cell transformation and tumorigenesis (oncogenes) that represented captured cellular genes (proto-oncogenes).[12] This led to the identification of many similar genes and to an appreciation of their roles in cell growth and neoplastic transformation.

Despite this work and the interest it engendered, it was widely believed during the 1970s that retroviruses did not play a role in human disease and were likely not even present in the human population. Several discoveries made it clear that this was not the case. Human T-cell leukemia virus type I (HTLV-I) was the first infectious human retrovirus identified; it was discovered and shown to be a unique virus by Gallo and his colleagues.[13–16] HTLV-I was soon established as the etiologic agent of adult T-cell leukemia (ATL), a type of leukemia endemic to various locales, including southern Japan and the Caribbean.[17–21] This was quickly followed by the discovery of HTLV-II,[22] a related virus that (although widespread) has not been compellingly associated with any disease. HTLV-I was shown to be able to neoplastically transform cord blood T cells.[23]

Several years later, an epidemic of immunodeficiency and malignancies appeared within gay communities, especially in the United States. The first member of another group of human retroviruses was isolated from people with this disease, called acquired immunodeficiency syndrome (AIDS).[24] When it became possible to culture the virus on a large scale,[25] it was proven to be the etiologic agent of AIDS.[26,27] This virus, now called human immunodeficiency virus type 1 (HIV-1), has become established worldwide, and AIDS represents a current global medical and economic catastrophe. As with HTLV-I, a related virus, HIV-2, was discovered,[28] which also appears to be far less pathogenic than HIV-1.[29]

Classification

The retroviridae are a large family of viruses that have been classified using a variety of criteria,[30] originally according to their biologic effects. The subfamilies included oncoviruses, which cause leukemias or other malignancies in their hosts; lentiviruses, or "slow" viruses, which cause slow degenerative diseases; and spumaviruses, or foamy viruses, which produce a "foamy" cytopathic effect in infected cultures. The subfamilies have been divided further based on their genomic structures (Table 1). They have been historically classified on the basis of the morphology of budding and mature virions in electron micrographs (Table 2). Retroviruses can also be classified as exogenous or endogenous depending upon whether they are transmitted by infection or genetically within the germ line of a species.

Structure

Retrovirus particles are composed of a core structure or capsid, which encloses two copies of the single-stranded genomic RNA, surrounded by an envelope containing a lipid bilayer. The entire virion, or extracellular viral particle, is 100 nm in diameter. The genomic RNA is generally 8–9500 nucleotides long, and the simplest retroviruses contain three major genes (*gag*, *pol*, and *env*), all of which are contained in the virion (Figure 1). The genomic RNA contains repeat regions at both ends, called the R region. The DNA (deoxyribonucleic acid) form of the genome integrated in the host cell genome contains the R region and other regulatory

Holland-Frei Cancer Medicine, Ninth Edition. Edited by Robert C. Bast Jr., Carlo M. Croce, William N. Hait, Waun Ki Hong, Donald W. Kufe, Martine Piccart-Gebhart, Raphael E. Pollock, Ralph R. Weichselbaum, Hongyang Wang, and James F. Holland.
© 2017 John Wiley & Sons, Inc. ISBN: 978-1-118-93469-2

Table 1 Retrovirus groups.

Oncornaviruses
- Avian leukosis-sarcoma viruses (ALSV)
- Avian reticuloendotheliosis virus
- Mammalian leukemia and sarcoma viruses (mouse/cat type C viruses)

Mouse mammary tumor virus
- Primate type D viruses (Mason–Pfizer monkey virus/simian AIDS virus)
- Human T-cell leukemia virus/bovine leukemia virus/simian T-cell leukemia virus

Lentiviruses (including immunodeficiency viruses)
Spumaviruses

Table 2 Retrovirus morphology.

A-type particles
- Intracellular core formation and budding
- Intracisternal A-type particles (IAP) are products of endogenous proviruses
- Noninfectious

B-type particles (MMTV)
- Core formation occurs in the cytoplasm
- After budding at the plasma membrane, maturation to an eccentric core occurs
- Prominent surface spikes

C-type particles
- Most oncornaviruses
- Initially form electron-dense patches at the plasma membrane
- Budding at plasma membrane
- Maturation of core to yield centrally located cores
- Spikes may or may not be prominent

D-type particles
- Mason–Pfizer monkey virus, simian AIDS virus
- Intracellular nucleocapsid formation, budding at plasma membrane
- Eccentric core
- Less prominent spikes

Lentiviruses
- Visna-maedi, EIAV, CAEV, SIV, HIV, FIV, BIV
- Core formation and budding as for C-type particles
- Condensed mature core forms pyramidal shape

Spumaviruses
- IAP-like cores

---

sequences in structures called the long terminal repeat (LTR) (Figure 1). Retroviruses often become replication-defective by loss of large regions of their genomes, which are sometimes replaced by oncogenes derived from the host cell. We now describe the genome and proteins of replication-competent retroviruses.

Viral genome and gene products

Space precludes a detailed description of the retroviral genome structure and the viral proteins. Interested readers are referred to Teich et al.[30] for details. However, these are presented schematically in Figures 2 and 3.

Genomic variation

The genomic structure described earlier is representative of the simplest retroviruses; other retroviruses, especially lentiviruses and members of the HTLV group (including the related bovine

leukemia virus, BLV), contain extra genes and have a more complex genomic structure. HIV-1 encodes six regulatory proteins including a protein that activates viral RNA expression, a protein that regulates viral RNA splicing patterns, and proteins that interfere with host immune functions. The extra genes also result in a more complicated RNA splicing pattern, including multiple splicing for many of the regulatory genes. Similarly, HTLV-I encodes at least five additional proteins, including (like HIV) a protein that activates viral RNA expression and another that regulates viral RNA splicing patterns. Recently, evidence has been presented[31–33] that a protein called HTLV-I bZIP protein (HBZ) is transcribed from the 3′ LTR, translated from negative-strand viral RNA, and expressed in infected T cells and in uncultured ATL cells as a 31-kDa protein. The HBZ protein binds to cellular bZIP transcription factors including members of the CREB and Jun families[34,35] to repress Tax-mediated viral transcription and support ATL cell proliferation. At present, this appears to represent a novel genetic feature of HTLV-I. Murine mammary tumor virus (MMTV) and the spumaviruses also encode additional proteins, including those that activate viral RNA expression. Other retroviruses, especially those that are acutely transforming (such as the avian and mammalian sarcoma viruses), are generally replication-defective and have parts of their genomes deleted and replaced with captured cellular genes that confer transforming capability. These viruses require a replication-competent helper virus for transmission and replication.

Replication cycle

Space precludes a detailed description of the viral replication cycle. Details of the pertinent steps are covered in detail in Refs [36–39]. Some of the steps are presented schematically in an abbreviated form in Figures 4–6. A few important points with regard to the retroviral replication cycle should be noted. First, formation of the provirus, by the integration reaction, results in a stable genetic copy of the virus that cannot be removed from the infected cell. Infected cells can and do persist for the life of the host, and whenever the cell divides, the provirus is passed on to both daughter cells. Furthermore, when germ line cells are infected, they become part of the genome of subsequent offspring. Consequently, 5% or more of the human genome consists of proviruses from past retroviral infections. Integration, however, is not always accurate, and deletions and rearrangements can occur. Integrated proviruses can also occasionally become deleted or rearranged. Reflecting this, most endogenous proviruses are defective and not usually expressed, although expression of some does occur. It is likely, however, that this massive insertion of foreign DNA has had a profound impact on evolutionary processes. Second, after proviral formation, transcription and translation of viral gene products depend entirely on cellular factors. Thus, a retrovirus generally persists silently in quiescent cells. Activation of infected cells, such as occurs when cells of the immune system are stimulated by antigen or cells are activated by hormones, can activate viral expression, although this is modulated by the suite of transcriptional factor binding sites in the viral LTR. Also, complex retroviruses, such as HTLV and HIV, encode transcriptional activators that can profoundly affect the activity of the viral RNA polymerase promoter.[40–45]

Mechanisms of oncogenesis

Some retroviruses are acutely transforming; they are able to transform cells directly. Retroviral induction of neoplasias *in vivo* in the

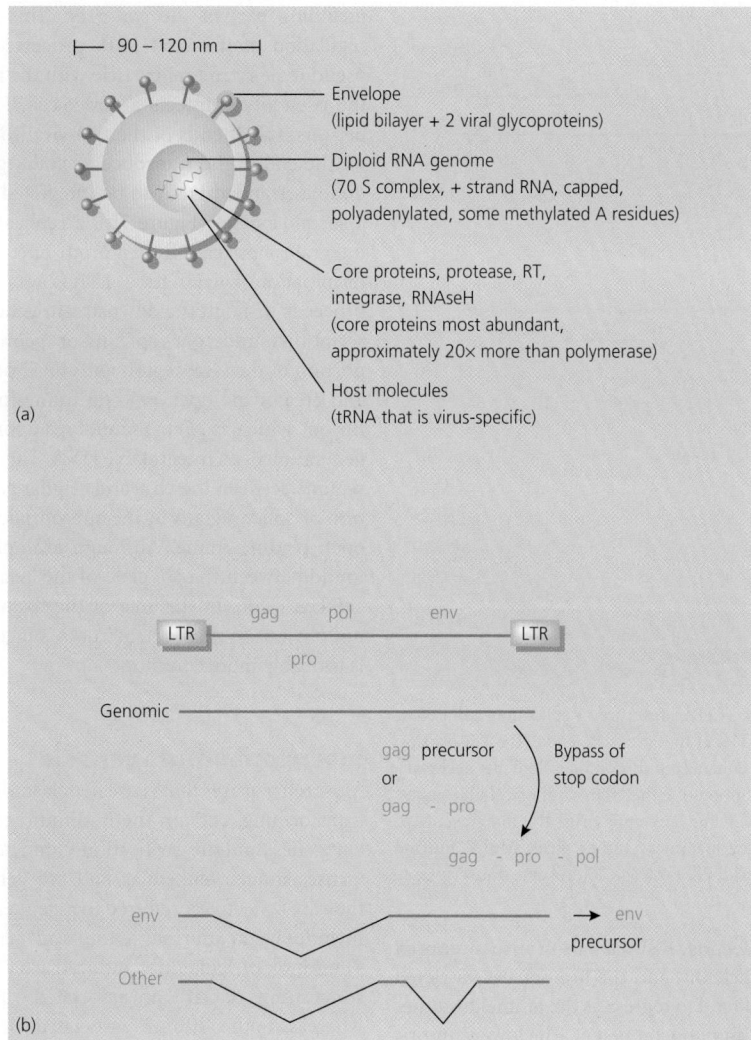

Figure 1 (a) Structure of typical retrovirus virion. (b) Structure of typical retroviral genome. All replication-competent retroviruses generate a full-length genomic ribonucleic acid (RNA) that encodes the gag and pol products and a singly spliced RNA that encodes the env product. Some retroviruses also generate smaller multiply spliced messages. *Abbreviations*: env, envelope; gag, core proteins; pol, polymerase; pro, protease.

infected host, however, involves a variety of mechanisms in addition to cell transformation by acutely transforming viruses. These are summarized in Figure 7.

Oncogene capture

Acutely transforming viruses are usually generated when a cellular proto-oncogene is captured by insertion into the viral genome during viral replication. This process usually causes genetic changes in the proto-oncogene, resulting in an oncogene, or dominant transforming gene. The same process usually also results in a replication-defective virus that requires a helper virus for its replication. The helper virus provides viral proteins to form the virion in which the RNA of the defective virus is packaged. These mixed particles are called pseudotypes.

The first discovered oncogenic virus was RSV, which was shown to be a transmissible agent causing sarcomas in chickens.[2] RSV was the first acutely transforming virus of many shown to have acquired its oncogenicity by the capture of a cellular gene, in this case *src*.[12] This was perhaps made possible in part because RSV, unlike most acutely transforming viruses, is replication competent and does not require a helper virus, thus making it simpler to study. The *src* gene

in RSV is inserted as a separate gene immediately 3′ of the other viral genes.[46,47] The transforming potential could be assigned to the viral *src* gene (v-*src*) because transformation-defective RSV was shown to have mutations specifically in v-*src* and because it conferred transforming ability to recombinant viruses that contained it.[48–50] These findings led to the recognition that normal cellular genes when modified and in the appropriate setting could cause malignant transformation.

Acutely transforming retroviruses produce tumors in susceptible hosts within days to weeks after infection. Because their transforming ability is so potent, a large fraction of infected cells become transformed; hence, the tumors that arise tend to be polyclonal. RSV infection of young chickens induces a variety of related tumor types, notably fibrosarcomas and histiocytic sarcomas. The younger the animal, the more sensitive it is to tumor formation. Tumor formation can occur within days in chicks younger than 1 month, the tumors progress rapidly, occur at many sites, and kill the animal. In the presence of an immune response, as in older chickens, the tumors tend to regress and disappear. Injection of v-*src* DNA into young birds can also induce tumors, further implicating v-*src* as causing the tumors.[51] Tumor formation with DNA is less efficient, probably reflecting the inefficiency of functional DNA uptake

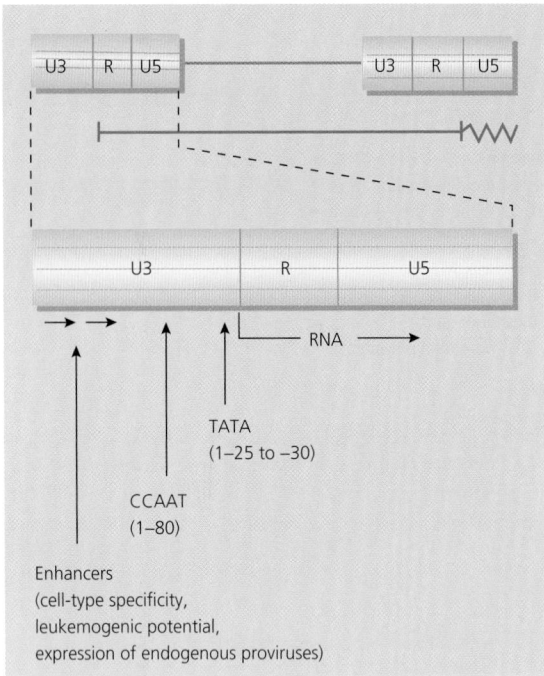

Figure 2 Long terminal repeat (LTR) structure. Replication-competent retroviruses contain identical LTRs at the 5′ and 3′ ends. The U3 portion of the 5′ LTR contains all of the enhancer and promoter elements necessary for efficient initiation of transcription of either retroviral or cellular genes. *Abbreviations*: CA, capsid; FeLV, feline leukemia virus; IN, integrase; MA, matrix protein; MMTV, Maloney mammary tumor virus; MuLV, murine leukemia virus; NC, nuclear capsid; PR, protease; RT, reverse transcriptase.

compared with retroviral infection. RSV can also cause tumors in baby rodents, although inefficiently, and the tumors are restricted to the site of inoculation and tend to regress as the animal becomes older and presumably more immunocompetent. The lower tumorigenic potential probably reflects the reduced replication rate of RSV in rodent cells.[52,53]

A more typical acutely transforming oncogene-containing retrovirus is typified by Abelson murine leukemia virus (A-MuLV). Infection of a nude mouse with a replication-competent MuLV[54,55] resulted in the replacement of most of the MuLV genes with a modified copy of the proto-oncogene c-*abl*,[56] a tyrosine kinase that is the target of the anticancer drug imatinib. Like most viral oncogenes and their cellular counterparts (summarized in Table 3), the *abl* portion of v-*abl* differs genetically from c-*abl*. The recombinant A-MuLV is unable to synthesize any of the viral genes and only codes for a fusion protein containing part of Gag and Abl (v-Abl). The presence of the amino-terminal portion of Gag on v-Abl causes it to be myristoylated and transported to the cell membrane, and this is critical for transformation by A-MuLV. The lack of functional viral genes means that A-MuLV is replication-defective and can infect and transform target cells only with the assistance of a helper virus. A-MuLV induces B-cell lymphomas in young mice, but adult animals are generally resistant to A-MuLV lymphomagenesis.[57]

Several models have been put forth for how cellular sequences are acquired by retroviral genomes, summarized in Figure 7. In one scenario (Figure 7a), a retrovirus integrates into the host cell genome just upstream from a proto-oncogene.[58] A subsequent deletion removes the 3′ portion of the provirus and the 5′ portion of the proto-oncogene, fusing the viral genome with cellular sequences and resulting in a reading frame for a fusion protein, generally

including part of the *gag* gene. This gene is transcribed under regulation of the viral LTR, processed, and co-packaged into a pseudotype retroviral particle with the helper virus genome. When the pseudotype infects a target cell, RT mediates recombination between the 3′ ends of the two viral RNAs, which places a 3′ LTR on the end of the transduced cellular gene, allowing the resultant double-stranded DNA to be integrated into the host cell DNA. In a second model (Figure 7b), a replication-competent virus again integrates upstream from a proto-oncogene. On rare occasions, the termination signal in the 3′ LTR is not recognized and transcription proceeds through the downstream gene. The large combined transcript then undergoes splicing or recombination that deletes the 3′ portion of the viral region and the 5′ portion of the cellular region and creates the open reading frame for the viral-proto-oncogene fusion, which is then pseudotyped for subsequent infection and generation of an integratable DNA. This requires either homologous regions between the viral and cellular genes to facilitate recombination or splice signals in the appropriate area for forming the fused open reading frame. Although examples of such homologies are found between the *pol* gene of the avian retrovirus MC29 and the chicken c-*myc* in the area of the fusion,[58,59] such homologies are not obvious in most retroviruses, suggesting that the first scenario is probably more common.

Insertional mutagenesis

Most retroviruses that cause neoplasms in their hosts are not acutely transforming, contain the minimum complement of *gag*, *pol*, and *env* genes, and are replication competent. Because many of these viruses induce leukemias and are genetically somewhat related, they are collectively referred to as leukemia viruses. Representatives include avian, murine, feline, and gibbon ape leukemia viruses. The kinds of leukemias induced vary with the viral strain; thus, some strains of GaLV are associated with lymphocytic leukemia,[7,60] whereas another strain is associated with myeloid leukemia.[61] Their lack of acutely transforming oncogenes means that they are not competent for direct transformation and do not transform target cells *in vitro*. The leukemias and other tumors that result from infection of the host are clonal in origin, as is evident from the insertion site of the provirus being identical in all of the neoplastic cells from a given tumor. This reflects the rarity of infection leading to malignant transformation and indicates that infection with the retrovirus preceded (and, by implication, resulted in) transformation. It also suggests that the specific insertion site is important and leads to the concept of insertional mutagenesis. In these kinds of viral neoplasias, the provirus is often found integrated in the vicinity of known cellular proto-oncogenes. The proximity of the viral LTR (or the insertion of the provirus into regulatory regions of the proto-oncogene) causes a dysregulation of its expression, leading in turn to dysregulated cell growth or differentiation. Alternatively, insertion may disrupt genes whose expression tends to prevent transformation. This mechanism of insertional mutagenesis obviously requires high levels of viral replication because integration occurs somewhat at random, and as a result, leukemia may only occur in a minority of infected animals, and latency phases (the time between infection and leukemia onset) can be quite lengthy.

Avian leukosis virus (ALV) is the prototypical simple leukemia virus. ALV is transmitted in birds both horizontally and vertically. Within several months, B-cell lymphoblasts begin to accumulate in the bursa of Fabricius.[62] With involution of the bursa, many of the enlarged follicles regress, but some tumor nodules persist and grow,

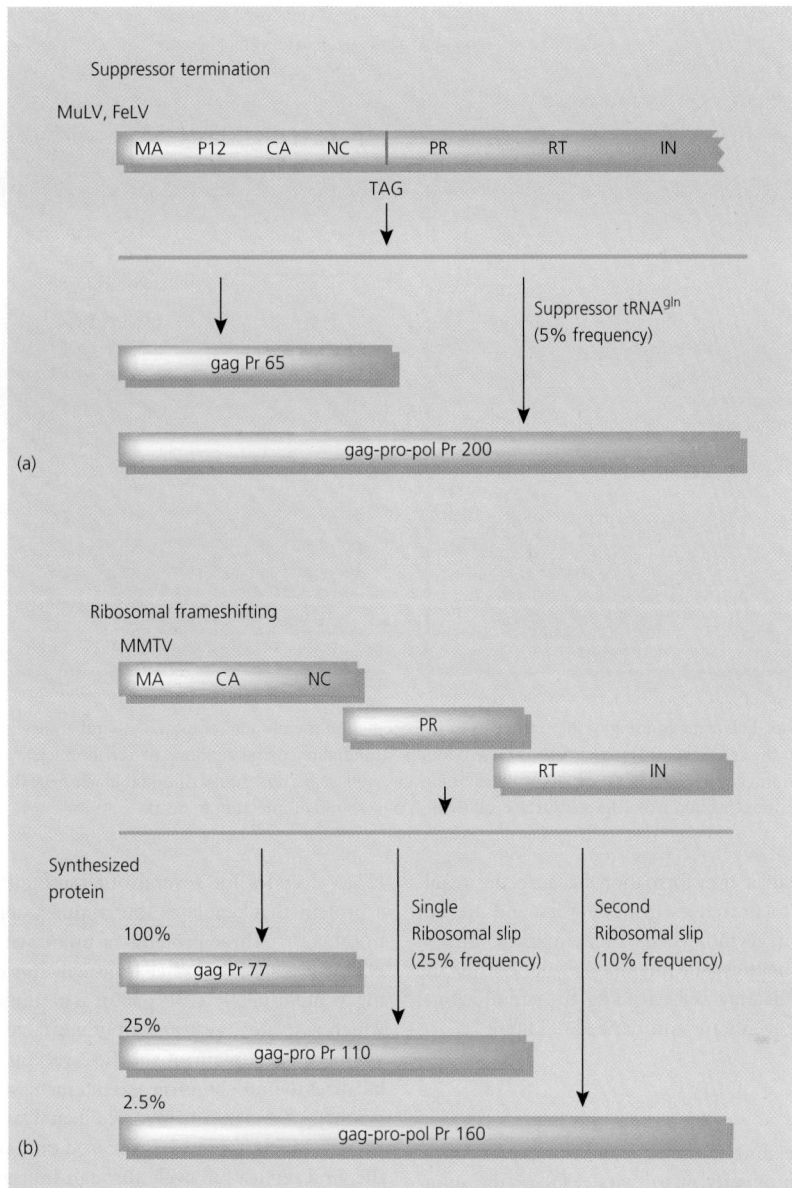

Figure 3 Alternative methods different retroviruses use to bypass the gag stop codon to generate the pro-pol products from the full-length genomic transcripts.

eventually giving rise to metastatic lymphomas. These tumors generally have a predominant provirus integrated near c-*myc*, a cellular proto-oncogene,[63-65] and c-myc RNA expression in these tumors is significantly higher than in the normal cell counterparts. Transcription is often initiated from the 3′ LTR,[66] resulting in a chimeric viral-cellular transcript, but continued expression of viral genes and viral replication is no longer needed.

Insertional mutagenesis also appears to play a critical role in MMTV and murine mammary tumors. As with ALV, MMTV can be transmitted either horizontally or vertically, and there is generally a predominant provirus in the mammary tumor cells, with similar implications. Integration was found to occur around but not within a 30-kbp sequence containing the *int*-1 proto-oncogene.[67-69] *Int*-1 expression generally only occurs in the neural tube of mid-gestational embryos and in testicular postmeiotic cells, suggesting that inappropriate expression in cells in the breast contributes to tumorigenesis by MMTV. Transgenic mice in which an int-1 transgene is regulated by the MMTV LTR

develop mammary tumors, but this is also the case when any of several other genes (including c-*myc*) are substituted for *int*-1,[70-73] suggesting that tumorigenesis simply depends on the delivery of a breast-specific promoter to dysregulate the expression of any of several proto-oncogenes.

Growth stimulation and two-step oncogenesis

The polycythemic strain of Friend murine leukemia virus (F-MuLV) represents another type of transforming replication-defective retroviruses. Unlike other viruses of these types, F-MuLV does not encode a cell-derived oncogene. An internal deletion of the *env* gene encompassing portions of the TM and SU proteins results in a nonfunctional Env, which can serve as a mimic of erythropoietin (Epo) and activate the growth of erythroid precursor cells through interaction with the Epo receptor.[74] This results in erythroleukemia and pronounced splenomegaly in infected mice,[75] which is more

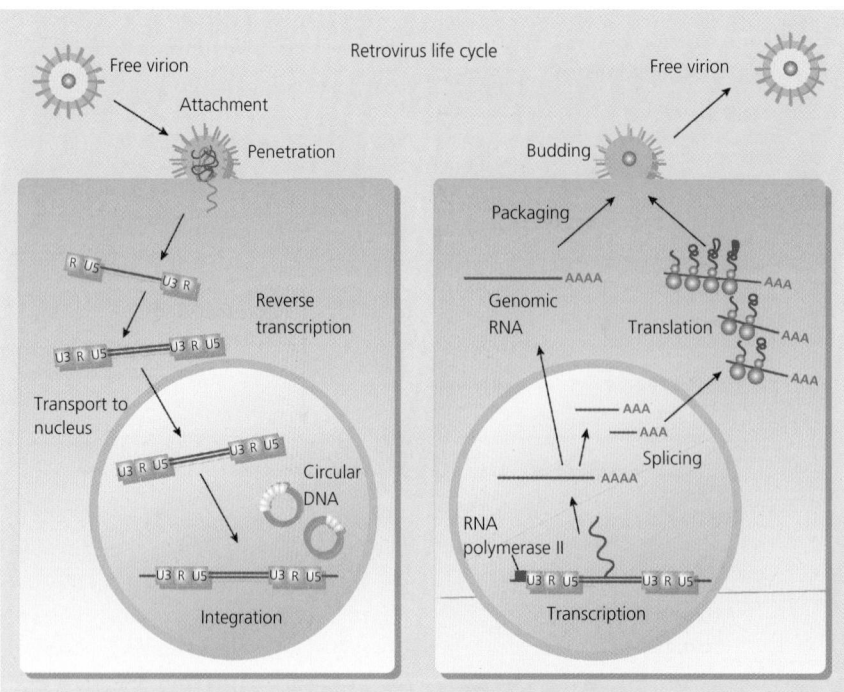

Figure 4 Life cycle of retrovirus. Following binding of the retrovirus to its specific cell membrane receptor, the viral and cellular membranes fuse, and the core virion is internalized into the cell. Reverse transcriptase-directed double-stranded retroviral genomic deoxyribonucleic acid (DNA) is then generated, followed by integrase-directed integration into host cell DNA. Retroviral transcripts using host transcriptional machinery then proceed, with the eventual formation of new retroviral virions that bud from the cell surface, allowing a new round of infection to occur.

properly a hyperplasia than a transformation because the resultant erythrocytes do not form tumors in nude mice and are not immortalized. However, if erythrocytosis is maintained, after a long latent period, subsequent genetic alterations will occasionally transform one of the replicating cells, leading to a monoclonal erythroid leukemia. These events are summarized in Figure 7c.

Transactivation

Insertional mutagenesis leading to the activation of expression of proto-oncogenes by the proximity of the viral LTR or the interruption of negative regulatory sequences by the integration event is referred to as *cis* activation. The genomes of some leukemia viruses are more complex than the simple leukemia viruses such as ALV and MuLV and contain extra genes that perform regulatory functions. The two prototypical examples are HTLV and BLV. These viruses (like the simple leukemia viruses) are replication competent, do not contain transduced proto-oncogenes in their genomes, and induce monoclonal hematopoietic malignancies only in the minority of infected hosts. However, they are like the acutely transforming viruses in that they transform cells in culture and do not appear to require a specific integration site for oncogenesis (Figure 7d). HTLV is the causative agent for ATL, a monoclonal T-cell lymphoma/leukemia with frequent cutaneous manifestations that is endemic to several areas including southern Japan and the Caribbean,[17–19,21,76] and is also the cause of a neurologic disease resembling multiple sclerosis, called tropical spastic paraparesis or HTLV-associated myelopathy.[77]

HTLV and BLV code for proteins, respectively, called Tax[41–44] and p34 Tax,[78] which activate expression by binding to the viral LTR in cooperation with transcription factors. This type of activation by a protein product rather than a DNA regulatory region is called *trans* activation, and these viral proteins are called transactivators.

HTLV-I codes for several other proteins as well, including Rex, a protein that regulates the complex splicing pattern of HTLV-I mRNAs.[79,80] Three proteins of unknown function are encoded by HTLV-I: p30(II), another transactivator that binds to CREB binding protein/p300 (CBP/p300),[81] a transcriptional factor; p12(I), which activates the transcriptional factor NFAT and binds to the cytoplasmic domain of the IL-2 receptor[82,83]; and p13(II), which localizes to mitochondria and interacts with farnesyl pyrophosphate synthetase, an enzyme involved in activation of the proto-oncogene *ras*.[84,85] Much interest has focused on Tax as it is clearly critical to the viral replication cycle through transactivation of the viral LTR and as its transactivation extends to cellular genes, including those for the IL-2 receptor, lymphotoxin, and granulocyte–macrophage stimulating factor.[86–90] The cross-transactivation of cellular genes leads to the idea that dysregulation of growth regulatory genes by Tax may play an important role in its pathogenesis.

A body of experimental evidence suggests that Tax could indeed play a role in leukemogenesis. The HTLV-I provirus in T cells transformed by HTLV-I infection or in leukemic ATL cells often has extensive deletions, but the Tax open reading frame is almost always preserved. Mice that are transgenic for Tax develop tumors, including lymphocytic leukemia, when the transgene is regulated by the viral LTR or a T-cell-specific promoter.[91–94] The T-cell lymphomas, however, differ phenotypically from ATL cells.[91,92] Tax directly transforms a rat fibroblast cell line and transforms primary rat embryo cells in cooperation with *ras in vitro*,[95,96] showing that Tax indeed has oncogenic properties. When Tax was inserted into the genome of a replication-competent but transformation-defective herpesvirus saimiri mutant, human hematopoietic cells infected *in vitro* by the chimeric virus were transformed and resembled ATL cells in morphology and cell surface phenotype,[97] suggesting that Tax is indeed important in ATL pathogenesis. It is likely that, as with F-MuLV leukemogenesis, subsequent steps are required for

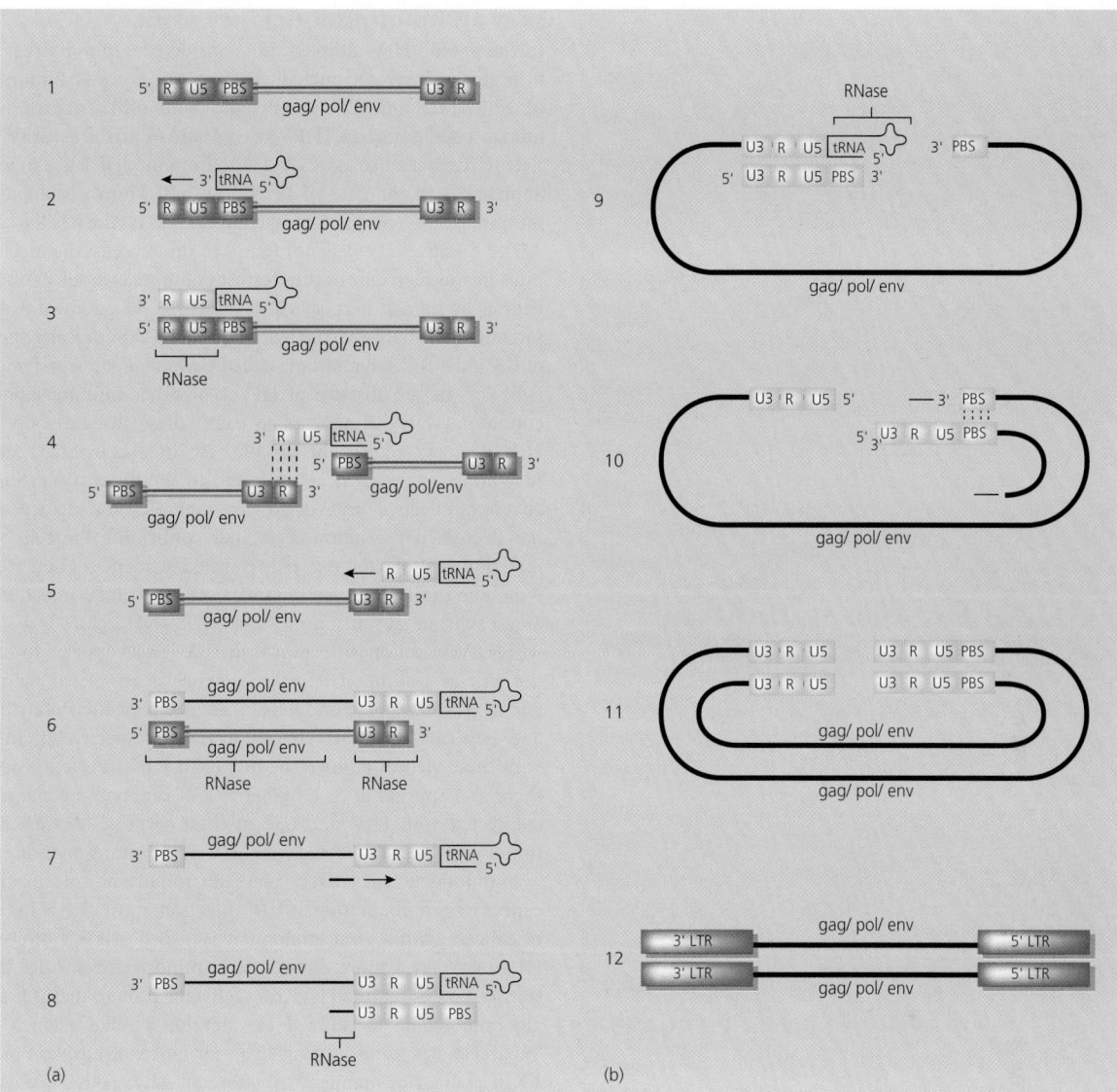

Figure 5 Reverse transcription. From a single-stranded ribonucleic acid genomic precursor (a), reverse transcriptase synthesizes a double-stranded deoxyribonucleic acid (DNA) provirus ready for integration into host cell DNA (b).

ATL to occur. The rarity of ATL as an outcome of HTLV-I infection indicates that a simple infection is not sufficient, and the lack of a common set of integration sites supports the idea that insertional mutagenesis does not play a role. Most likely, the leukemic cells do not express viral positive strand RNA until after they are cultured,[98] indicating that by the time the cells are leukemic, they no longer require viral expression and suggesting there must be subsequent genetic steps in ATL leukemogenesis.

A better understanding has emerged from the signaling pathways used by Tax for transactivation and transformation. Tax associates with members of the ATF/CREB family of transcriptional factors,[99–103] and the HTLV-I LTR has three ATF/CREB binding sites. Several cellular genes, such as serum responsive factor (SRF) and NF-κB/Rel, are transactivated by Tax through the same pathway. Tax also transactivates its LTR, as well as some cellular gene promoters such as those for IL-2 and the IL-2 receptor, directly through NF-κB.[62,104,105] This depends upon an interaction of Tax and MEKK1, which leads to phosphorylation of the NF-κB inhibitor IkB. Phosphorylation of IkB targets its removal by ubiquitination and degradation in the proteasome, which unmasks the

nuclear localization signal of NF-κB. This allows it to be transported to the nucleus, where it activates gene expression by binding to NF-κB enhancer elements present in the viral LTR. Tax also appears to directly affect the cell cycle. Tax can bind to the cell cycle inhibitor p16/INK4a and interfere with its ability to inhibit the activity of CDK4, a cyclin kinase important for G1-S progression.[106,107] Tax also mediates the phosphorylation of cyclin D3[108] and upregulates the expression of E2F[107,109] through ATF/CREB signaling, both of which likely contribute to dysregulation of the cell cycle. Cell cycle dysregulation often leads to p53-mediated apoptosis.[110] Tax also dysregulates activities of p53 required for cell cycle arrest and apoptosis,[111–113] which allows unregulated hyperproliferation and immortalization of cells expressing Tax. Tax appears to inhibit p53 functions in part by an NF-κB-dependent mechanism and in part by competing with p53 for binding to CBP/p300. Tax also has been reported to inhibit MAD1, a protein involved in G2/M transition.[114] It is interesting that Tax interferes with the p16/INK4a and p53 pathways, as alteration of these genes or their activities are quite common in naturally occurring cancers.

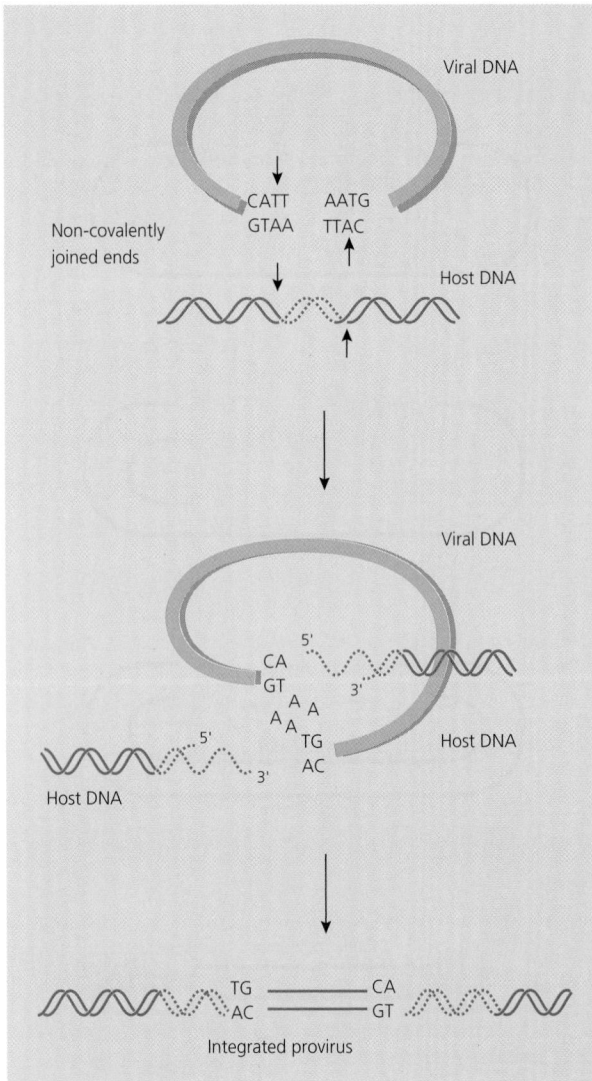

Figure 6 Integration. The newly reverse-transcribed double-stranded retroviral deoxyribonucleic acid (DNA) genome and a piece of chromosomal DNA are specifically cleaved by the retroviral integrase protein. This is accompanied by a deletion of two base pairs from the retroviral genome and a duplication of four to six base pairs from the host DNA. Following retroviral genomic insertion into the cleaved host DNA, the DNA is re-ligated.

The HBZ protein, translated from the negative strand of viral RNA, could also be a determinant of HTLV-I leukemogenesis. HBZ appears to be the only viral gene product consistently expressed in ATL cells.[115] HBZ heterodimerizes with members of the CREB and Jun families[31] and supports proliferation of ATL cells.[115] HBZ transgenic mice developed skin lesions and T-cell lymphomas resembling ATL.[116] The phenotype of Tax/HBZ double transgenic mice did not differ appreciably from HBZ single transgenic mice.[117] HBZ protein and transcripts appear to have nonoverlapping functions. HBZ mRNA supports proliferation of ATL cells in the absence of HBZ protein.[115] HBZ transcripts have splice variants called SP1, the shorter of the two, and SP2.[32] The SP1 isoform negatively regulates Tax- and c-Jun-dependent transcription. Thus, one function of HBZ protein appears to be to inhibit expression of viral proteins. Conversely, HBZ protein cooperates with JunD to upregulate expression of telomerase (hTERT).[118] To add to the complexity of regulation of viral gene expression, Tax upregulates expression of HBZ.[119]

Human immunodeficiency virus

Infection with HIV, although not considered a tumor virus, results in a greatly increased incidence of several types of tumors, most of which are linked to coinfection with other viruses such as human papillomavirus (HPV) or Epstein–Barr virus (EBV).[120,121] Retroviruses are also associated with immunodeficiency in infected animals, as in the case of FeLV. The best known example of an immunopathogenic virus is, of course, HIV-1, which is the cause of AIDS. Because HIV-1 is not found in tumor cells, the mechanism must be indirect. One of the clearest examples is its effect on pathogenesis by human herpesvirus 8 (HHV-8) [also known as Kaposi sarcoma (KS) herpesvirus (KSHV)].[122] HHV-8 is clearly the cause of KS and a B-cell lymphoma called peripheral effusion lymphoma (PEL).[123] In the absence of HIV-1 or other immunosuppressive conditions, HHV-8 appears to cause these diseases only rarely. HIV-1 infection raises the risk of these diseases by many orders of magnitude,[120,121] but it is not found in the tumor cells. Since the advent of effective viral suppressive therapies, the incidence of KS has decreased precipitously, further confirming the role of HIV infection as a cofactor. A greatly elevated incidence of non-Hodgkin lymphoma (NHL) is also seen in a setting of HIV infection,[120,121] and a substantial portion of these AIDS–NHL cases is associated with EBV infection. Infection with HIV-1 also appears to increase the risk of childhood leiomyosarcomas[121] (associated with EBV) and of cervical cancer and hepatocarcinoma (associated with HPV and hepatitis B and C virus infections, respectively). Infection with these viruses tends to be higher in HIV-infected people, but there also appears to be a higher risk of cancer in people who are coinfected with HIV and one of these viruses. As with KS, the tumor cells are not infected with HIV-1, indicating an indirect role.

Immunodeficiency likely plays an important role in elevated cancer rates in the setting of HIV infection, most clearly in the case of cancers with a viral etiology. It is also possible, however, that HIV may play a more direct role in tumorigenesis. Mice that are transgenic for Tat, the HIV transactivator protein that is functionally homologous to HTLV-I Tax, develop KS-like lesions.[124] Also, Tat accelerates tumorigenesis in a murine xenotransplant model of KS in a paracrine manner.[125] A subset of AIDS–NHL is not associated with EBV, and the reasons for its increased incidence are not clear. Some suggestive evidence has pointed to a role for HIV viral proteins, perhaps especially the p17 matrix protein. Viral proteins persist for extended time periods in lymph nodes of infected people, even in the absence of detectable viral RNA or replication.[126] HIV transgenic mice have a significantly elevated incidence of B-cell lymphoma.[127] The viral transgene, although deleted for parts of the *gag* and *pol* genes, expresses many viral proteins, including p17. Recently, p17 was shown to promote lymphangiogenesis *in vitro*, reportedly through binding to and activation of the chemokine receptors CXCR1 and 2.[128]

Endogenous retroviruses

Endogenous retroviruses are part of the normal genetic complement of species and make up an extremely large fraction (up to 5%) of various mammalian genomes. Many of these appear to have emerged after speciation, based on differences in their type and number among species. As retroviruses insert at random and as there are so many present, it is clear that they have played a profound if unclear role in evolution. It is less clear whether any endogenous retroviruses play a role in human cancer or other diseases. First, they are for the most part defective because of large deletions, although some only have a few point mutations and a

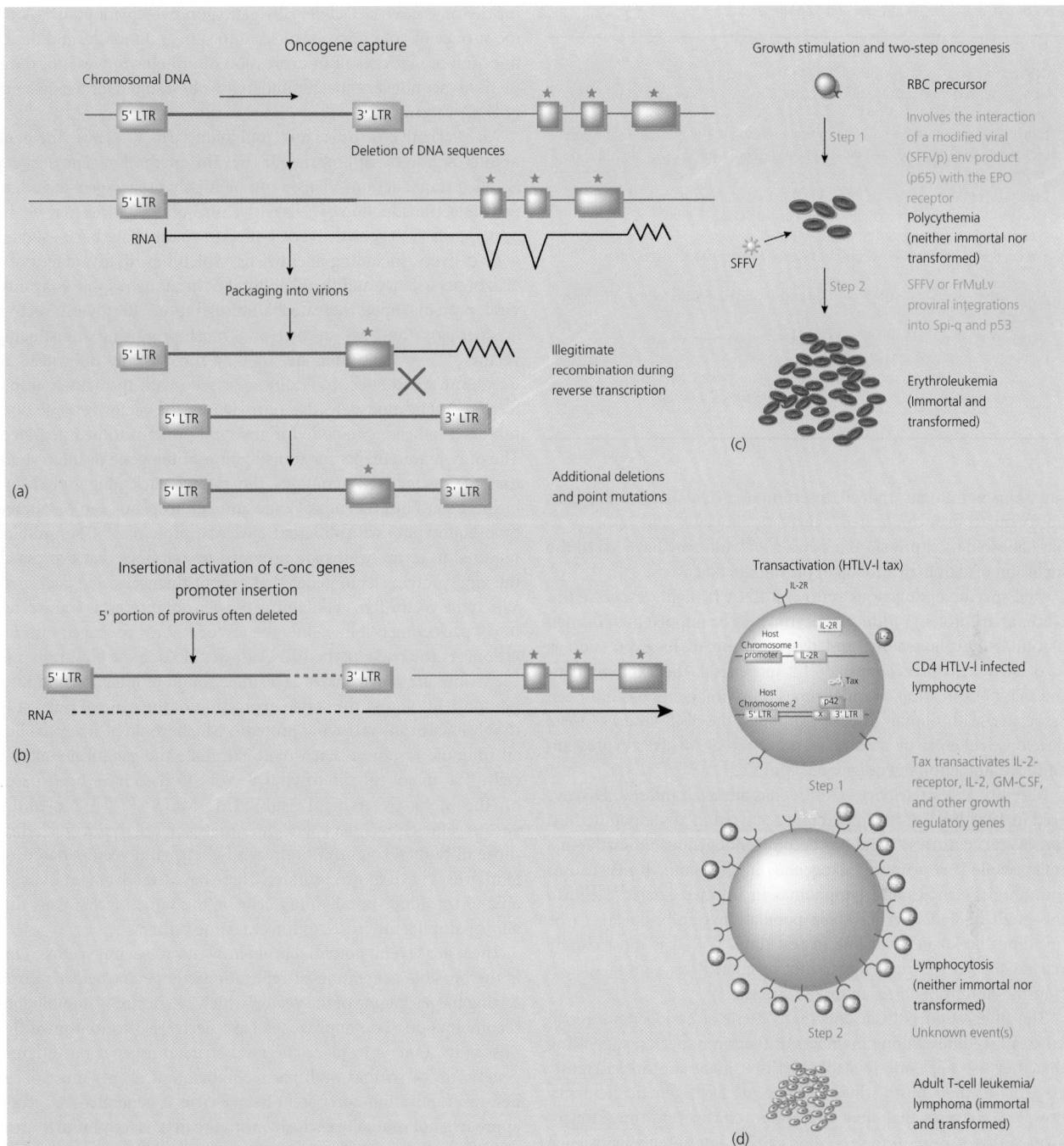

Figure 7 Four mechanisms of retrovirus-induced oncogenesis. (a) Oncogene capture. A mutated form of a cellular proto-oncogene (v-onc) is transferred (transduced) to a normal cell, thus inducing transformation (*c-oncogene). (b) Insertional activation. There is a significant increase in the rate of proto-oncogene expression secondary to LTR-directed transcriptional enhancement (*c-oncogene). (c) Growth stimulation plus two-step oncogenesis. A mutated env protein from the defective spleen focus-forming virus (SFFV) binds to the erythropoietin (EPO) receptor, causing an erythrocyte hyperplasia. This increases the target population susceptible to the actual transforming event, a retroviral insertional disruption of the Spi-I or TP53 gene. *Abbreviations*: FrMuLV, Friend murine leukemia virus. (d) Transactivation. The viral transactivating protein (tax in the case of human T-cell leukemia virus type I) causes expansion of the potential target population through transactivation of growth regulatory genes. An unknown second event then induces the actual transformation of a clone of these cells.

very few may be replication competent. Second, endogenous retroviruses are generally not expressed even at the RNA level. This may be because of mutations in the regulatory regions of their LTRs, because of their location in transcriptionally inactive areas of the chromatin, or because of methylation of promoter sequences in the LTR. When endogenous viruses are expressed as RNA, protein, or virions, it is usually in normal placentas or in teratomas, which may

reflect the presence of hormone-responsive elements in the LTRs of many endogenous retroviruses. It is possible that integration of endogenous retroviruses may result in recessive mutations. The Hr (hairless) and D (dilute brown) recessive phenotypes in mice are associated with the presence of endogenous retroviruses at the affected loci,[129–131] and reversion of the mutation is associated with proviral deletion, raising the possibility that there may be analogous

Table 3 Differences between v-onc and c-onc genes.

Often only a portion of the cellular oncogene is present in v-onc
v-onc is derived from processed mRNA, which is devoid of introns and flanking sequences
Loss of cellular control elements (promoters/repressors as well as RNA destabilizers) for some oncogenes (myc and mos) elevated level of expression in itself may be transforming
Deletions/rearrangements may affect the structure of the protein itself:
- Loss of C-terminal Tyr-containing region of c-src causes loss of phosphorylation-mediated control by host cell kinases
- v-erb B differs from EGF receptor by deletion of the extracellular domain

v-onc genes are often fused to viral sequences important for transforming function:
- gag-abl acquires a myristoylation signal for membrane localization important for transforming activity
- v-fms is the CSF-1 receptor fused to the gag gene product, the latter providing a signal sequence for placement into the cell membrane

situations in humans. Indeed, insertion of a GaLV-related provirus upstream from a duplicated pancreatic amylase gene appears to have allowed its expression in saliva[132-134] and may have led to the inclusion of starch-rich foods in the human diet.

One specific endogenous retroviral RNA is highly expressed in placenta. Its protein product, syncytin, may be important in human placental morphogenesis, and dysregulation of its expression is associated with preeclampsia.[135,136] In general, the expression or the lack of expression of endogenous retroviral genes has not been associated with human diseases, although the AKR strain of mice develops leukemia by a complex process that involves expression and recombination of endogenous MuLVs.[137-139]

Recently, koala retrovirus (KoRV) has attracted interest. Discovered in 1988,[140,141] it has apparently occurred in koala populations for several centuries[142] and has become endogenous in north Australia, while it is primarily exogenous in the south. KoRV causes immunodeficiencies and lymphomas in infected koalas[143-145] (to the point of endangering koala populations) and appears to be invading the koala germ line in real time.[144,146] It is most closely related to GaLV,[141] and apparently originated as a cross-species transmission from an Asian mouse species.[147]

The integration pattern and the content of endogenous retroviruses can differ among members of the same species, suggesting that they are not entirely stable and that many are not currently essential to their hosts. Their existence as fixed genetic elements, however, suggests that they were important at one time. Retroviruses that use the same receptor exhibit interference with each other, because infection either blocks or downregulates the cell surface expression of the receptor, rendering the cell refractory to superinfection. It may be that endogenous retroviruses provided protection by interference against pathogenic retroviruses that no longer exist and are therefore no longer important.

Retroviral vectors and gene therapy

As the understanding of the roles of specific genes in different diseases has evolved, treatment of diseases by gene therapy, or the delivery of desired genes, has become more of a possibility. One of the main obstacles has been efficient and specific delivery of a gene to the appropriate tissue and cell type. Delivery by transfection of DNA, or introduction into cells in which the membrane has been partially permeabilized by chemicals or an electrical charge, is relatively inefficient, not very specific, and not generally suitable

for delivery *in vivo*. Delivery by gene gun, which shoots DNA on the surface of gold microparticles into skin and muscle, and direct injection of DNA result in expression of proteins *in vivo*, but these methods are not very specific and may be best suited for the delivery of DNA vaccines.

An alternative is to use a recombinant virus to deliver the gene of interest into the appropriate tissue. This method of gene delivery is called transduction. Viruses can be highly tissue-specific and, in principle, transduction of cells with a recombinant virus may be the best approach to gene delivery. Different viruses have been used for gene delivery, including adenovirus, which has disadvantages of a lack of persistence and the likelihood of immune responses against viral proteins upon repeated administration. Retroviral vectors are perhaps the best studied and most promising transducing vectors.[148-151] They integrate, so they theoretically only need to be administered once. In addition, as seen with the acutely transforming replication-defective retroviruses, the vector genome does not need to be able to code for any viral proteins to be integrated. The only requirements for transduction of the gene of interest are that the vector RNA contains the proper packaging signal and has LTRs at both its ends. Tissue and cell tropisms can be altered by pseudotyping with different envelope proteins.[152] The proteins required to form virions are provided by cell lines that express all the viral proteins from genes that cannot themselves be packaged. When the vector RNA containing the gene of interest is transfected into a packaging cell line, only the vector RNA is packaged into the virion. As the pseudotyped RNA does not code for viral proteins, the virions are only capable of a single round of infection and integration. This allows the stable expression of the gene of interest in the absence of any retroviral proteins, which would be likely to elicit an immune response that would eliminate the genetically altered cells. The majority of retroviral vectors to date have been based on the Moloney strain of MuLV (Mo-MuLV).[148-151] Mo-MuLV vectors efficiently infect a wide variety of cell types, including those of human origin. More recently, retroviral vectors based on lentiviruses have shown promise. These have the advantage of being able to transduce nondividing cells by the same mechanisms that allow natural lentiviruses to infect resting cells.[153,154]

There are several potential problems with retroviral vectors. One is the possible generation of replication-competent helper viruses during the packaging of the vector, which can occur by homologous recombination. Two approaches have been used to minimize this possibility. One is to place the viral structural genes on different genetic units, so that multiple recombination events must occur before a replication-competent helper virus is generated. A second approach, not mutually exclusive with the first, is to minimize areas of homology among the units expressing the helper virus proteins and the vector by, for example, using heterologous promoters for helper virus RNA transcription. Another potential problem derives from the risk that integration in the vicinity of a proto-oncogene could lead to tumorigenesis. Although the risk appears small, it is not zero. This was the apparent reason for three of seven monkeys developing lymphomas in one gene therapy study.[155] Mo-MuLV does not replicate well in human cells, but this is not the case for other potential retroviral vectors. Minimizing integration events by rigorously excluding the presence of replication-competent helper viruses somewhat avoids this problem, but does not completely eliminate it. Indeed, treatment of young severe combined immunotherapy X1 patients with a lentiviral vector devoid of replicating helper virus appears to have resulted in insertion near the LMO2 proto-oncogene promoter followed by a leukemia-like clonal T-cell outgrowth in several of the patients.[156] Another problem is that expression is not maintained indefinitely; retroviral promoters have a tendency to become inactivated over time. A further limitation is that the genetic capacity of retroviruses is only about 8–9 kb, which restricts their ability to deliver genes to only a single gene or two.

Conclusions

The study of retroviruses has led to much of today's techniques and understanding of molecular biology. This is obviously especially true in the case of cell transformation and tumorigenesis, as many retroviruses either cause cancers or (in the case of acutely transforming viruses) capture cellular genes that have the potential to contribute to neoplastic transformation. Retroviruses were the first example of a reversal of the normal order of the flow of genetic information, that is, from RNA to DNA. The identification and elucidation of reverse transcription provided the means for cloning and characterizing mRNA, which greatly facilitated understanding gene expression and function. Furthermore, studies of the regulation of viral transcription, retroviral RNA processing, viral entry mechanisms, viral protein processing, and virion assembly have greatly increased our knowledge in the areas of transcriptional regulation, RNA splicing and translational regulation, membrane biochemistry and fusion, and protein processing and protein–protein interactions, respectively. An understanding of how retroviruses package and deliver genetic material holds promise that these viruses will be successfully used in the clinic to deliver therapeutic genes to appropriate cells and tissues in human diseases. New generations of vectors currently being developed are bringing us closer to realizing this goal.

Perhaps among the most important contributions of retroviral research to human health were the discovery of HTLV-I and HIV-1, two pathogenic human retroviruses. During the 1970s, much of the research carried out with retroviruses came under the aegis of the Virus Cancer Program (VCP) as part of President Nixon's War on Cancer. The VCP was ended because of a lack of discovery of human cancer viruses and the growing feeling that human retroviruses did not exist. Shortly thereafter, however, HTLV-I was discovered and linked to ATL. Although this discovery has not led so far to better treatment for ATL, it has led to better prevention of infection by, for example, screening blood samples and by avoiding transmission by breast-feeding, a common route of infection of babies. Ironically, the most important consequence of the VCP and retroviral research was the relatively rapid discovery and characterization of a virus not directly linked with cancer, but with immunodeficiency. HIV-1 was discovered and shown to be the cause of AIDS and a blood test was developed in a relatively short span of time, and therapies based on structural determinations of its RT and protease were developed and are being successfully used. This rapid progress would have been far slower had the means for isolating, culturing, and characterizing retroviruses not already been in place.

Key references

The complete reference list can be found on the Wiley Companion Digital Edition of this title (see inside front cover for login instructions).

4 Gross L. Neck tumors, or leukemia, developing in adult C3H mice following inoculation, in early infancy, with filtered (Berkefeld N), or centrifugated (144,000 X g). *Ak-leukemic Extracts Cancer.* 1953;**6**(5):948–958.

6 Jarrett WF, Martin WB, Crighton GW, Dalton RG, Stewart MF. Transmission experiments with leukemia (lymphosarcoma). *Nature.* 1964;**202**:566–567.

13 Kalyanaraman VS, Sarngadharan MG, Poiesz B, Ruscetti FW, Gallo RC. Immunological properties of a type C retrovirus isolated from cultured human T-lymphoma cells and comparison to other mammalian retroviruses. *J Virol.* 1981;**38**(3):906–915.

14 Poiesz BJ, Ruscetti FW, Gazdar AF, Bunn PA, Minna JD, Gallo RC. Detection and isolation of type C retrovirus particles from fresh and cultured lymphocytes of a patient with cutaneous T-cell lymphoma. *Proc Natl Acad Sci U S A.* 1980;**77**(12):7415–7419.

15 Poiesz BJ, Ruscetti FW, Reitz MS, Kalyanaraman VS, Gallo RC. Isolation of a new type C retrovirus (HTLV) in primary uncultured cells of a patient with Sezary T-cell leukaemia. *Nature.* 1981;**294**(5838):268–271.

16 Reitz MS, Poiesz BJ, Ruscetti FW, Gallo RC. Characterization and distribution of nucleic acid sequences of a novel type C retrovirus isolated from neoplastic human T lymphocytes. *Proc Natl Acad Sci U S A.* 1981;**78**(3):1887–1891.

17 Catovsky D, Greaves MF, Rose M, et al. Adult T-cell lymphoma-leukaemia in Blacks from the West Indies. *Lancet.* 1982;**1**(8273):639–643.

18 Hinuma Y, Nagata K, Hanaoka M, et al. Adult T-cell leukemia: antigen in an ATL cell line and detection of antibodies to the antigen in human sera. *Proc Natl Acad Sci U S A.* 1981;**78**(10):6476–6480.

19 Kalyanaraman VS, Sarngadharan MG, Nakao Y, Ito Y, Aoki T, Gallo RC. Natural antibodies to the structural core protein (p24) of the human T-cell leukemia (lymphoma) retrovirus found in sera of leukemia patients in Japan. *Proc Natl Acad Sci U S A.* 1982;**79**(5):1653–1657.

20 Robert-Guroff M, Ruscetti FW, Posner LE, Poiesz BJ, Gallo RC. Detection of the human T cell lymphoma virus p19 in cells of some patients with cutaneous T cell lymphoma and leukemia using a monoclonal antibody. *J Exp Med.* 1981;**154**(6):1957–1964.

21 Yoshida M, Miyoshi I, Hinuma Y. Isolation and characterization of retrovirus from cell lines of human adult T-cell leukemia and its implication in the disease. *Proc Natl Acad Sci U S A.* 1982;**79**(6):2031–2035.

22 Kalyanaraman VS, Sarngadharan MG, Robert-Guroff M, Miyoshi I, Golde D, Gallo RC. A new subtype of human T-cell leukemia virus (HTLV-II) associated with a T-cell variant of hairy cell leukemia. *Science.* 1982;**218**(4572):571–573.

24 Barre-Sinoussi F, Chermann JC, Rey F, et al. Isolation of a T-lymphotropic retrovirus from a patient at risk for acquired immune deficiency syndrome (AIDS). *Science.* 1983;**220**(4599):868–871.

25 Popovic M, Sarngadharan MG, Read E, Gallo RC. Detection, isolation, and continuous production of cytopathic retroviruses (HTLV-III) from patients with AIDS and pre-AIDS. *Science.* 1984;**224**(4648):497–500.

26 Gallo RC, Salahuddin SZ, Popovic M, et al. Frequent detection and isolation of cytopathic retroviruses (HTLV-III) from patients with AIDS and at risk for AIDS. *Science.* 1984;**224**:500–503.

27 Sarngadharan MG, Popovic M, Bruch L, Schupbach J, Gallo RC. Antibodies reactive with human T-lymphotropic retroviruses (HTLV-III) in the serum of patients with AIDS. *Science.* 1984;**224**(4648):506–508.

31 Mesnard JM, Barbeau B, Devaux C. HBZ, a new important player in the mystery of adult T-cell leukemia. *Blood.* 2006;**108**(13):3979–3982.

32 Cavanagh MH, Landry S, Audet B, et al. HTLV-I antisense transcripts initiating in the 3′LTR are alternatively spliced and polyadenylated. *Retrovirology.* 2006;**3**:15.

33 Ludwig LB, Ambrus JL Jr, Krawczyk KA, et al. Human immunodeficiency virus-type 1 LTR DNA contains an intrinsic gene producing antisense RNA and protein products. *Retrovirology.* 2006;**3**:80.

34 Gaudray G, Gachon F, Basbous J, Biard-Piechaczyk M, Devaux C, Mesnard JM. The complementary strand of the human T-cell leukemia virus type 1 RNA genome encodes a bZIP transcription factor that down-regulates viral transcription. *J Virol.* 2002;**76**(24):12813–12822.

35 Lemasson I, Lewis MR, Polakowski N, et al. Human T-cell leukemia virus type 1 (HTLV-1) bZIP protein interacts with the cellular transcription factor CREB to inhibit HTLV-1 transcription. *J Virol.* 2007;**81**(4):1543–1553.

41 Felber BK, Paskalis H, Kleinman-Ewing C, Wong-Staal F, Pavlakis GN. The pX protein of HTLV-I is a transcriptional activator of its long terminal repeats. *Science.* 1985;**229**(4714):675–679.

42 Fujisawa J, Seiki M, Kiyokawa T, Yoshida M. Functional activation of the long terminal repeat of human T-cell leukemia virus type I by a trans-acting factor. *Proc Natl Acad Sci U S A.* 1985;**82**(8):2277–2281.

44 Sodroski J, Rosen C, Goh WC, Haseltine W. A transcriptional activator protein encoded by the x-lor region of the human T-cell leukemia virus. *Science.* 1985;**228**(4706):1430–1434.

61 Kawakami TG, Kollias GV Jr, Holmberg C. Oncogenicity of gibbon type-C myelogenous leukemia virus. *Int J Cancer.* 1980;**25**(5):641–646.

62 Leung K, Nabel GJ. HTLV-1 transactivator induces interleukin-2 receptor expression through an NF-kappa B-like factor. *Nature.* 1988;**333**(6175):776–778.

64 Hayward WS, Neel BG, Astrin SM. Activation of a cellular onc gene by promoter insertion in ALV-induced lymphoid leukosis. *Nature.* 1981;**290**(5806):475–480.

65 Neel BG, Hayward WS, Robinson HL, Fang J, Astrin SM. Avian leukosis virus-induced tumors have common proviral integration sites and synthesize discrete new RNAs: oncogenesis by promoter insertion. *Cell.* 1981;**23**(2):323–334.

66 Payne GS, Bishop JM, Varmus HE. Multiple arrangements of viral DNA and an activated host oncogene in bursal lymphomas. *Nature.* 1982;**295**(5846):209–214.

67 Nusse R, Varmus HE. Many tumors induced by the mouse mammary tumor virus contain a provirus integrated in the same region of the host genome. *Cell.* 1982;**31**(**1**):99–109.

76 Robert-Guroff M, Nakao Y, Notake K, Ito Y, Sliski A, Gallo RC. Natural antibodies to human retrovirus HTLV in a cluster of Japanese patients with adult T cell leukemia. *Science.* 1982;**215**(**4535**):975–978.

89 Tschachler E, Bohnlein E, Felzmann S, Reitz MS Jr. Human T-lymphotropic virus type I tax regulates the expression of the human lymphotoxin gene. *Blood.* 1993;**81**(**1**):95–100.

91 Grossman WJ, Kimata JT, Wong FH, Zutter M, Ley TJ, Ratner L. Development of leukemia in mice transgenic for the tax gene of human T-cell leukemia virus type I. *Proc Natl Acad Sci U S A.* 1995;**92**(**4**):1057–1061.

92 Hall AP, Irvine J, Blyth K, Cameron ER, Onions DE, Campbell ME. Tumours derived from HTLV-I tax transgenic mice are characterized by enhanced levels of apoptosis and oncogene expression. *J Pathol.* 1998;**186**(**2**):209–214.

101 Suzuki T, Fujisawa JI, Toita M, Yoshida M. The trans-activator tax of human T-cell leukemia virus type 1 (HTLV-1) interacts with cAMP-responsive element (CRE) binding and CRE modulator proteins that bind to the 21-base-pair enhancer of HTLV-1. *Proc Natl Acad Sci U S A.* 1993;**90**(**2**):610–614.

120 Goedert JJ. The epidemiology of acquired immunodeficiency syndrome malignancies. *Semin Oncol.* 2000;**27**(**4**):390–401.

121 Rabkin CS. Epidemiology of AIDS-related malignancies. *Curr Opin Oncol.* 1994;**6**(**5**):492–496.

125 Guo HG, Pati S, Sadowska M, Charurat M, Reitz M. Tumorigenesis by human herpesvirus 8 vGPCR is accelerated by human immunodeficiency virus type 1 Tat. *J Virol.* 2004;**78**(**17**):9336–9342.

156 Hacein-Bey-Abina S, Von KC, Schmidt M, et al. LMO2-associated clonal T cell proliferation in two patients after gene therapy for SCID-X1. *Science.* 2003;**302**(**5644**):415–419.

29 Herpesviruses

Jeffrey I. Cohen, MD

Overview

Eight herpesviruses have been isolated from humans: two of these, Epstein–Barr virus (EBV) and Kaposi sarcoma-associated herpesvirus (KSHV), are associated with human tumors. EBV has been detected in lesions from patients with post-transplant lymphoproliferative disease, nasopharyngeal and some types of gastric carcinoma, Burkitt lymphoma, Hodgkin lymphoma, and certain other lymphoid tumors. KSHV is associated with Kaposi sarcoma, primary effusion lymphoma, and Castleman disease. Each of these viruses encodes proteins important for establishment of latency, transforming cells, and evading the immune system.

Properties of herpesviruses

Herpesviruses are enveloped DNA viruses that have the capacity to establish latent infection as well as to undergo lytic infection. The ability to establish latent infection *in vivo* and to reactivate from latency ensures a source of virus to infect previously uninfected individuals. Most adults latently harbor herpes simplex 1, varicella-zoster virus, human herpesviruses 6 and 7, and Epstein–Barr virus (EBV). Several features of herpesvirus replication are important for the maintenance of latency and for oncogenicity; EBV will serve as an example to illustrate the principles of herpesvirus infection relevant to oncogenicity.

First, viral DNA must be maintained in the cell. The EBV genome is usually maintained in latently infected B cells as a multicopy circular episome in the host cell. Second, a cell transformed by a virus must avoid immune clearance. Replication of EBV requires up to 100 viral proteins; however, latent infection of B cells with EBV results in expression of 12 or fewer genes.[1–3] This limited repertoire of gene products prevents frequent virus replication, avoiding death of the infected cell, and restricts the ability of the immune system to recognize and destroy cells latently infected with the virus. Third, specific viral proteins interact with other cell proteins or directly transactivate other cell genes to provide additional functions necessary for cell proliferation and immortalization. Several EBV proteins interact with cellular proteins to activate transcription of viral and cellular genes or to engage signal transduction pathways in the cell.

EBV: an oncogenic human herpesvirus

EBV gene expression in transformed lymphocytes

Infection of primary B cells with EBV *in vitro* results in transformation of the cells, which can then proliferate indefinitely. Eight EBV proteins and several nontranslated RNAs are expressed in latently infected B lymphocytes that have been growth transformed by EBV *in vitro* (Table 1). The EBV nuclear proteins EBNA-1, EBNA-2, EBNA-LP, EBNA-3A, EBNA-3B, and EBNA-3C comprise the EBV nuclear antigen complex. EBNA-1 binds to the oriP sequence (origin of viral DNA replication) on EBV DNA and allows the virus genome to be maintained as an episome in transformed B cells.[4] EBNA-1 also transactivates its own expression. EBNA-1 transcripts are initiated from one of four different promoters. The Cp and Wp promoters are used to express EBNA-1 in lymphoblastoid cell lines *in vitro*; the Qp promoter is used in tissues from Burkitt lymphoma, nasopharyngeal carcinoma, and Hodgkin lymphoma; and the Fp promoter is used during lytic replication.[5] EBNA-1 inhibits its own protein degradation by proteasomes[6] and limits its own translation,[7] both of which may reduce its presentation to CD8+ cytotoxic T cells; however, EBNA-1 remains a target for CD4+ cells.[8–11] EBNA-1 inhibits apoptosis induced by expression of p53.[12]

EBNA-2 transactivates expression of EBV LMP1[13] and LMP2,[14] and the cellular genes *CD21*, *CD23*, c-*myc*, and c-*fgr*.[15,16] EBNA-2 is targeted to the LMP1, LMP2, Cp EBNA, and CD23 promoters by the GTGGGAA-binding protein Jκ, and thereby activates these promoters.[17] EBNA-2 is a functional homolog of the Notch receptor, which uses Jκ to regulate gene expression during development.[18] EBNA-2 also interacts with the DNA-binding protein PU-1 to transactivate the LMP1 promoter[19] and with AUF to transactivate the EBNA Cp promoter.[20] The transactivation domain of EBNA-2 is essential for B-lymphocyte transformation.[21] This domain interacts with transcription factors TFIIB and the TATA-binding protein-associated factor TAF40.[22] EBNA-2 inhibits apoptosis mediated by Nur77.[23]

EBNA-LP interacts with and enhances the ability of EBNA-2 to transactivate LMP1 and LMP2.[24] Although EBNA-LP binds to Rb and p53 *in vitro*,[25] the significance of these interactions is uncertain. Deletion of the carboxy terminus of EBNA-LP markedly reduces the ability of the virus to transform B lymphocytes.[26]

EBNA-3A, EBNA-3B, and EBNA-3C are distantly related to each other. The EBNA-3 proteins bind to Jκ preventing it from binding DNA, thereby inhibiting transactivation by EBNA-2.[27] EBNA-3C upregulates expression of LMP1 and CD21. EBNA-3C binds to Nm23-HI, a human metastasis suppressor protein, and inhibits the protein's ability to suppress migration of Burkitt lymphoma cells.[28] EBNA-3C degrades Rb and enhances kinase activity by disrupting p27.[29,30] EBNA-3A and EBNA-3C are essential for B-lymphocyte transformation *in vitro*, while EBNA-3B is dispensable.[31,32]

LMP1 functions as a transforming oncogene in nude mice.[33] Expression of LMP1 in EBV-negative Burkitt lymphoma cells results in B-cell clumping and increased villous projections. Upregulation of bcl-2, bfl-1, and A20, and inhibition of Bax, by LMP1 in B cells protects the cells from apoptosis.[34,35] Expression of LMP1 in epithelial cells inhibits differentiation of the cells.[36]

LMP1 is a functional homolog of CD40, a member of the tumor necrosis factor receptor (TNFR) family.[37] The carboxy terminus of

Holland-Frei Cancer Medicine, Ninth Edition. Edited by Robert C. Bast Jr., Carlo M. Croce, William N. Hait, Waun Ki Hong, Donald W. Kufe, Martine Piccart-Gebhart, Raphael E. Pollock, Ralph R. Weichselbaum, Hongyang Wang, and James F. Holland.
© 2017 John Wiley & Sons, Inc. ISBN: 978-1-118-93469-2

Table 1 Selected EBV genes and their cellular homologs and activities.

Gene	Expression class	Cellular homolog	Activity
EBNA-1	Latent, lytic	None	Episome maintenance, transactivates viral genes, inhibits apoptosis
EBNA-2	Latent	Notch	Transactivates viral and cellular genes, inhibits apoptosis
EBNA-3A, B, C	Latent	None	Regulates EBNA-2 activity, transactivates cellular genes
EBNA-LP	Latent	None	Increases EBNA-2 activity
LMP1	Latent, lytic	CD40	Transactivates cellular genes, inhibits apoptosis
LMP2	Latent	None	Prevents EBV reactivation, transactivates Akt
EBERs	Latent	None	Upregulates cellular genes
BARF-1	Lytic	CSF-1R	Inhibits IFN-α
BCFR1	Lytic	IL-10	Inhibits IFN-γ and IL-12
BNLF2a	Lytic	None	Blocks antigen-specific CD8 T-cell recognition
BHRF1	Lytic	Bcl-2	Inhibits apoptosis
BALF1	Lytic	Bcl-2	Regulates BHRF1 activity
BGFL5	Lytic	None	Blocks synthesis of MHC class I and II
BILF1	Lytic	GPCR	Removes MHC class I from cell surface
BLLF3	Lytic	None	Upregulates IL-10, TNF-α, and IL-1β
BPLFI	Lytic	None	Inhibits toll-like receptor signaling
BZLF1	Lytic	None	Inhibits IFN-γ effects, inhibits function of p53, inhibits TNF-α, initiates lytic infection

LMP1 interacts with the TNFR-associated factors (TRAFs) 1, 2, 3, and 5, TRADD, RIP, and JAK3 *in vitro*.[38] LMP1 functions as a constitutively active form of CD40 resulting in activation of NF-κB, stress-activated protein kinases, STATs, adhesion molecules, the B7 co-stimulatory molecule, JNK, and B-cell proliferation.[39] LMP1 upregulates expression of intracellular adhesion molecules, Fas, CD40, and MMP-9[40] in B cells and EGF in epithelial cells.[41] LMP1 inhibits phosphorylation of Tyk2 resulting in inhibition of interferon (IFN)-α signaling.[42] LMP1 is essential for transformation of B lymphocytes by EBV.[43] Analysis of EBV-containing human lymphomas shows that LMP1 localizes with TRAF-1, TRAF-3, and that activated NF-κB is present.[44]

LMP2 is dispensable for transformation of B cells,[45] but induces a transforming phenotype in epithelial cells and promotes their motility.[46,47] LMP2 prevents lytic reactivation of EBV-infected primary B cells in response to activation of the B-cell receptor complex by cross-linking of surface immunoglobulin. LMP2 associates with the *src* family and *syk* protein-tyrosine kinases that are coupled to the B-cell receptor complex.[48] Binding of LMP2 to these proteins results in their constitutive phosphorylation, which inhibits their ability to mediate signaling for virus reactivation.[48,49] B cells from transgenic mice expressing LMP2 survive even without normal B-cell receptor signaling activity.[50] LMP2 activates β-catenin and Ras/PI3K/Akt signaling pathways in epithelial cells resulting in transformation of the cells.[51,52] LMP2 also activates mTOR and increases c-myc expression.[53]

The two EBV-encoded RNAs, EBER-1 and EBER-2, are the most abundant EBV RNAs in latently infected B cells; however, they are not required for latent or lytic EBV infection, but may contribute to B-cell transformation.[54,55] The EBERs upregulate expression of bcl-2 and IL-10[56] and interact with the double-stranded RNA-activated protein kinase, and IFN-inducible oligoadenylate synthetase.[57,58]

EBV encodes at least 44 miRNAs from the BART and BHRF1 regions of the genome; both BART and BHRF1 microRNAs downregulate cellular genes and inhibit apoptosis and enhance B-cell proliferation.[59] EBV also encodes cellular RNAs that enhance transformation.[60] Both EBV microRNAs and LMP1 are secreted from infected cells in exosomes, which may enhance tumorigenicty.[61,62]

EBV genes expressed during productive infection

Infection of epithelial cells with EBV results in productive infection, with replication of virus and lysis of infected cells. Immediate-early genes encode regulators of virus gene expression, including the BZLF1 and BRLF1 proteins, which act as switches to initiate lytic infection. The BZLF1 protein inhibits TNF-α signaling[63] and helps the virus evade T-cell responses.[64] BZLF1 protein also inhibits the expression of the IFN-γ receptor[65] and inhibits the function of p53.[66] Early genes encode proteins involved in viral DNA synthesis, while late genes encode structural proteins.

Three viral genes expressed during productive infection are functional homologs of cellular genes and are important for the survival of EBV-infected B cells.[67,68] The EBV BCRF-1 protein is homologous to IL-10 and has IL-10 activity.[69] BCRF-1 is a B-cell growth factor and inhibits IFN-γ release from activated peripheral blood mononuclear cells and secretion of IL-12 from macrophages.

The EBV BARF-1 protein acts as a soluble receptor for CSF-1.[70] BARF-1 inhibits IFN-α secretion by human monocytes. The EBV BNLF2a protein interacts with the TAP complex to block antigen-specific CD8 T-cell recognition.[71] The EBV BHRF1 protein is homologous to bcl-2 and protects cells from apoptosis.[72] EBV BALF1 is also homologous to bcl-2 and antagonizes the antiapoptotic effect of BHRF1.[73]

Clinical aspects

EBV infection is usually spread by saliva. The virus infects B cells directly, or oropharyngeal epithelial cells and then spreads to subepithelial B cells.[74] During primary infection, up to a few percent of peripheral blood B lymphocytes are infected with EBV and have the capacity to proliferate indefinitely *in vitro*. Natural killer (NK) cells, CD4 T cells, and HLA- and EBNA- or LMP-restricted cytotoxic T cells control the latently infected B lymphocytes.[8] T- and B-cell interactions release lymphokines and cytokines, giving rise to many of the clinical manifestations of acute infectious mononucleosis. After recovery, the fraction of B cells latently infected with EBV in the peripheral blood remains at 1 in 10^5 to 1 in 10^6. These lymphocytes are the primary site of EBV persistence and a source of virus for persistent infection of epithelial surfaces.

B-cell tumors that occur early after EBV infection are usually lymphoproliferative processes, in which latent virus infection in B cells is the principal cause of proliferation. In contrast, nasopharyngeal carcinoma occurs long after primary EBV infection and viral gene expression is less important to the growth of the malignant cells.

Lymphoproliferative disease

EBV is associated with B-cell lymphoproliferative disease in patients with congenital or acquired immunodeficiency. X-linked lymphoproliferative syndrome is an inherited immunodeficiency of males; most patients die of a fatal lymphoproliferative disorder or fulminant hepatitis, but some survive with hypogammaglobulinemia or develop EBV-positive lymphomas. The gene mutated in X-linked lymphoproliferative syndrome has been identified as *SAP*,[75] which encodes an SH2-containing protein that interacts with SLAM on B and T cells, and with 2B4 on NK and T cells. Anti-CD20 antibody (rituximab) has been effective in treating some patients with X-linked lymphoproliferative disease and acute EBV infection.[76] Mutations in additional cellular proteins including XIAP, ITK, CD27, MagT1, CTP synthase 1, and PI3K 110δ predispose to severe EBV infections.

EBV lymphoproliferative disease occurs in patients who are immunosuppressed as a result of transplantation or AIDS.[77–79] Risk factors for development of lymphoproliferative disease include EBV-seronegativity prior to transplant and receipt of T-cell-depleted bone marrow or antilymphocyte antibody. Lymphoproliferative lesions are most commonly seen in the lymph nodes, liver, lungs, kidney, bone marrow, or small intestine. Tumors in transplant patients are usually classified as lymphomas; some patients have hyperplastic lesions. The proliferating lymphocytes in these tumors generally do not have chromosomal translocations.

AIDS-related lymphomas may be systemic (nodal or extranodal) lymphomas or primary central nervous system lymphomas. Although most B-cell tumors in transplant recipients and central nervous system lymphomas in AIDS patients contain EBV, about 50% of other lymphomas in AIDS patients contain EBV. Tumors in patients with AIDS are usually either immunoblastic lymphomas or Burkitt lymphomas; most of the latter have c-*myc* translocations.

Tissues from transplant recipients or AIDS patients with EBV lymphoproliferative disease show expression of EBERs, EBNA-1, EBNA-2, and LMP1 (Table 2). The EBV viral load in the peripheral blood has been used to predict development of disease and to follow patients after therapy. The expression of EBV genes, which are targets for cytotoxic T cells, has important implications for therapy. Infusion of EBV-specific cytotoxic T cells, nonirradiated donor leukocytes, or HLA-matched allogeneic cytotoxic T cells have been effective in many cases for treatment of EBV lymphoproliferative disease.[80–86] Anti-CD20 antibody (rituximab) has induced remissions in some patients and has been used in some studies as pre-emptive therapy when EBV viral DNA in the blood is rising in transplant recipients at risk of lymphoproliferative disease,[87] although other studies suggest that pre-emptive therapy may be unnecessary.[88]

Burkitt lymphoma

Seroepidemiologic studies show a strong association between Burkitt lymphoma and EBV in Africa.[89,90] More than 90% of African Burkitt lymphomas are associated with EBV, whereas only approximately 20% of Burkitt lymphomas in the United States are associated with the virus. African patients with Burkitt lymphoma often have high levels of antibody to EBV antigens, and the virus can be recovered from the tissue.

Burkitt lymphomas contain chromosomal translocations that result in c-*myc* dysregulation. The most common chromosomal translocation, t(8;14), places a portion of the c-*myc* oncogene adjacent to an immunoglobulin heavy chain gene. Less common translocations involve the c-*myc* oncogene and the κ or λ immunoglobulin light chain genes t(2;8) and t(8;22), respectively. These translocations result in high constitutive expression of c-*myc*. New approaches to treating Burkitt lymphoma based on inhibition of c-myc are in development.[91]

EBV-associated endemic Burkitt lymphoma is thought to develop in steps. First, EBV infection may expand the pool of differentiating and proliferating B cells. Second, chronic endemic malaria may cause T-cell suppression and B-cell proliferation. Third, enhanced proliferation of differentiating B cells may favor the chance occurrence of a reciprocal c-*myc* (t[8;14] or t[8;22]) translocation placing c-*myc* partially under the control of immunoglobulin-related transcriptional enhancers, with development of a monoclonal tumor.

Nasopharyngeal carcinoma

The nonkeratinizing nasopharyngeal carcinomas are uniformly associated with EBV. Patients with nasopharyngeal carcinoma have high levels of antibodies to EBV antigens. A prospective study of Taiwanese men showed that those with IgA antibodies to EBV viral capsid antigen (VCA) and anti-EBV deoxyribonuclease antibodies had an increased risk for developing nasopharyngeal carcinoma when compared to men without these antibodies.[92] These antibodies are useful in screening patients for early detection of nasopharyngeal carcinoma and are prognostic for patients after treatment. Another study showed that quantifying the level of EBV DNA in plasma of patients with advanced nasopharyngeal carcinoma was useful for monitoring patients and predicting outcomes.[93] Nasopharyngeal carcinoma tissue contains EBV genomes in every cell. These tumors are monoclonal with regard to EBV infection, indicating that EBV infection precedes malignant cell outgrowth at the cellular level. Unlike Burkitt lymphoma, the association of EBV with nasopharyngeal carcinoma is uniform and universal. Infusions of EBV-specific cytotoxic T cells resulted in remissions in some patients with refractory nasopharyngeal carcinoma.[94]

Hodgkin lymphoma

Persons with a history of infectious mononucleosis are at a greater risk of developing Hodgkin lymphoma.[95] Patients with Hodgkin lymphoma generally have higher titers of antibody to EBV VCA than does the general population. Tissues from ~40% to 60% of patients with Hodgkin lymphoma contain EBV genomes. Cases of Hodgkin lymphoma in patients with HIV or from developing countries are more likely to contain EBV genomes than persons without HIV or from developed countries.[96] The EBV genome is monoclonal and present in Reed–Sternberg cells. EBV is more often associated with aggressive subtypes (especially mixed cellularity) of Hodgkin lymphoma. Tumors from patients with EBV+ Hodgkin lymphoma and some from patients with lymphoproliferative disease arise from postgerminal center cells.[97] Infusion of cytotoxic T cells generated from 11 patients with relapsed Hodgkin lymphoma and measurable disease resulted in complete remissions in two patients, partial remission in one patient, stable disease in five patients, and no response in three patients.[98] Infusion of arginine butyrate and ganciclovir to induce EBV thymidine kinase

Table 2 Diseases associated with EBV latent gene expression.

Disease	BARTs	EBERs	EBNA-1	EBNA-2	LMP1	LMP2
Burkitt lymphoma	+	+	+	−	−	−
Nasopharyngeal carcinoma	+	+	+	−	+	+
Hodgkin lymphoma	+	+	+	−	+	+
Peripheral T-cell lymphoma	+	+	+	−	+	+
Lymphoproliferative disease	+	+	+	+	+	+

expression with phosphorylation of ganciclovir and induction of apoptosis resulted in antitumor responses in some patients with EBV B-cell malignancies.[99]

Other tumors associated with EBV

EBV has also been detected in non-Hodgkin's lymphomas. EBV-positive diffuse large B-cell lymphoma has a poorer prognosis than EBV-negative lymphoma.[100] Treatment of patients with EBV+ non-Hodgkin's lymphoma in remission with autologous antigen-presenting cells transduced with LMP2 resulted in increased frequencies of LMP2-specific cytotoxic T cells and tumor responses in several patients with relapsed disease.[101] EBV DNA and latency proteins have been detected in tissues from patients with peripheral T-cell lymphomas.[102] EBV DNA has also been detected in central nervous system lymphomas from patients with no underlying immunodeficiency, T cells in patients with virus-associated hemophagocytic syndrome, nasal T-cell lymphoma, carcinoma of the palatine tonsil, laryngeal carcinoma, and angioimmunoblastic T-cell lymphoma. EBV DNA and nuclear antigens have been detected in thymic carcinomas and in B-cell lesions from patients with lymphomatoid granulomatosis.

EBV DNA has been found in leiomyosarcomas in AIDS patients,[103] and viral RNA and EBNA-2 have been detected in smooth muscle tumors in organ transplant recipients.[104] About 7% of primary gastric carcinomas are EBV+, especially in undifferentiated lymphoepithelioma-like carcinomas.

KSHV and malignancies

In 1994, Chang et al.[105] detected sequences of a new human herpesvirus, Kaposi-sarcoma-associated herpesvirus (KSHV) in Kaposi sarcoma tissues from patients with AIDS. KSHV is present in B cells in asymptomatic persons. B-cell lines derived from primary effusion lymphomas maintain KSHV in a latent state and can be induced to undergo lytic virus replication by the addition of phorbol ester or butyrate. Infection of dermal microvascular endothelial cells *in vitro* with KSHV results in transformation of the cells with maintenance of long-term infection. The cells become spindle-shaped and show loss of contact inhibition with anchorage-independent growth.[106] Although KSHV transforms bone-marrow-derived endothelial cells, virus is present in only a small fraction of the cells.[107]

Viral proteins

Several KSHV proteins are important for transformation, establishing latency, and modulating the immune response to the virus.[108–110] KSHV encodes a large number of cellular homologs (Table 3) that have been grouped into different classes, depending on when they are expressed in primary effusion lymphoma cell lines.[111] Expression of the KSHV K1 gene in rodent fibroblasts results in transformation of the cells.[112] The K1 protein induces tyrosine phosphorylation in cells[113] and activates the Akt signaling pathway.[114] The K1 protein inhibits apoptosis[115] and results in constitutive calcium-dependent signal activation in B cells.[116]

The KSHV K2 gene encodes an IL-6 homolog (vIL-6). IL-6 is a B-cell growth factor and acts as an autocrine growth factor for lymphoid tumors resulting in proliferation.[117] vIL-6 prevents death of IL-6-dependent B9 cells *in vitro*,[118] promotes hematopoiesis, and induces VEGF to promote angiogenesis.[119] The K3 [modulator of immune recognition 1 (MIR1)] and K5 (MIR2) proteins induce rapid endocytosis of MHC (major histocompatibility complex) class I molecules and IFN-γ receptor 1 from the surface of cells

by ubiquitination of these proteins.[120–122] The K5 protein also downregulates ICAM-1 and B7.2, which results in inhibition of NK-cell-mediated cytotoxicity,[123] and removes CD31 from the surface of endothelial cells.[124]

The KSHV K4, K4.1, and K6 genes encode three chemokines: the viral macrophage inflammatory proteins (MIP)-II, -III, and -I, respectively. vMIP-I inhibits replication of HIV strains dependent on CCR5.[118] vMIP-I and vMIP-III are chemokine receptor agonists for CCR8[125] and CCR4,[126] respectively, while vMIP-II is a broad-spectrum chemokine receptor antagonist. vMIP-II is a chemoattractant for eosinophils,[127] binds to both CC and CXC chemokines, and blocks calcium mobilization induced by chemokines.[128]

The KSHV K9, K11.1, and K10.5 proteins are referred to as viral IFN regulatory factor (vIRF)-1, -2, and -3, respectively. Each of these proteins inhibits virus-mediated activation of the IFN-α promoter.[129] vIRF1 inhibits MHC-1 transcription and surface expression.[130] vIRF1 and vIRF3 inhibit p53-mediated apoptosis[131,132] and transform NIH 3T3 cells.[133] vIRF3 (also called LANA2) protects cells from p53-induced apoptosis.[134,135] KSHV ORF45 blocks the activity of IRF7 and inhibits the activation of IFN-α and -β.[136]

The KSHV K12 locus encodes several proteins termed kaposins. Kaposin A induces transformation of cells.[137] Kaposin B increases expression of cytokines by activating MAP-kinase-associated protein kinase 2 and inhibiting the degradation of cytokine mRNA.[138,139] The KSHV K14 protein, a homolog of the cellular OX2 protein, stimulates monocytes to produce proinflammatory cytokines such as TNF-α, IL-1β, and IL-6.[140] KSHV ORF4 protein inhibits the complement system.[141] KSHV ORF16 encodes a homolog of bcl-2 and inhibits bax-induced apoptosis.[142] The ORF71 gene encodes a homolog of cellular FLIP that blocks apoptosis. ORF71 binds to Atg3 and protects cells from autophagy. KSHV ORF71 activates NF-κB, promotes tumor growth, and is required for survival of KSHV-infected lymphoma cells.[143–147] KSHV ORF72 encodes a cyclin D homolog that binds to and activates cdk6 and phosphorylates p27, and stimulates cell-cycle progression in normally quiescent fibroblasts.[148,149] The viral cyclin protein phosphorylates and thereby inactivates Rb.[150]

KSHV ORF73 encodes LANA1 that localizes with viral DNA episomes and tethers them to chromosomes during cell division.[151] KSHV LANA1 is required for persistence of the episome in dividing cells and transactivates its own promoter. In addition, LANA1 inhibits the activity of both p53 and Rb,[152,153] upregulates expression and stabilizes β-catenin,[154] upregulates and activates survivin,[155] induces nuclear accumulation of HIF,[156] and activates c-myc.[157] Expression of LANA in transgenic mice results in development of lymphomas.[158] LANA inhibits TGF-β signaling.[159] KSHV ORF74 encodes a G-protein-coupled receptor that is homologous to the cellular IL-8 receptor; unlike the latter protein, however, the KSHV receptor is constitutively active and induces cellular proliferation.[160] ORF74 protein induces angiogenesis,[161] activates the Akt signaling pathway,[162] and induces proliferation and vascular permeability of endothelial cells.[163–165] ORF74 activates NF-κB and JNK, and upregulates IL-1, IL-8, TNF-α, and FGF, and inhibits viral lytic gene expression.[166]

KSHV K15 encodes the latency-associated membrane protein (LAMP) and interacts with TRAFs 1, 2, and 3.[167] K15 suppresses tyrosine phosphorylation and intracellular calcium mobilization, inhibiting B-cell receptor signaling.[168] KSHV encodes several microRNAs located between K12 and ORF71 or within K12 that are expressed during latency and detected in patient plasma.[169] These microRNAs are important for NF-κB activation and blocking

Table 3 Selected KSHV genes and their cellular homologs and activities.

Gene	Expression class	Cellular homolog	Activity
K1	II	ITAM motif	Transformation, activates signaling pathways
K2	II	IL-6	B-cell growth factor, angiogenesis, hematopoiesis
K3	III	None	Reduces surface MHC class I
K4	II	MIP-1α	Chemokine receptor antagonist; angiogenesis; chemotaxis
K4.1	II	MIP-1α	Chemokine receptor agonist; angiogenesis; chemotaxis
K5	II	None	Inhibits NK-cell activity; reduces surface MHC class I; increases monocyte proliferation
K6	II	MIP-1α	Chemokine receptor agonist; angiogenesis; chemotaxis
K8	III	None	Inhibits p53
K9	II	IRF	Represses IFN activity, transformation, inhibits p53
K10.5 (LANA-2)	II	IRF	Represses IFN activity; inhibits apoptosis; inhibits p53
K11.1	I	IRF	Represses IFN activity
K12 (Kaposin A)	II	None	Transformation
K12 (Kaposin B)	II	None	Increases cytokine mRNA stability
K14	II	OX-2	Induces proinflammatory cytokines
K15 (LAMP)	III	None	Binds TRAFs, inhibits B-cell receptor signaling
ORF4	II	CR2	Complement-binding protein
ORF16	II/III	Bcl-2	Inhibits apoptosis
ORF45	III	None	Inhibits IRF7
ORF50	III	None	Increases CD21 and CD23 expression, degrades IRF7
ORF63	III	NLR proteins	Inhibits NLRP1
ORF71	I	FLIP	Inhibits apoptosis; activates NF-κB
ORF72	I	Cyclin D	Cell-cycle progression, inhibits Rb
ORF73 (LANA-1)	I	None	Episome maintenance, inhibits p53 and Rb
ORF74	II	GPCR	Angiogenesis, transformation, and proliferation

Expression class I = latent gene, expressed in uninduced primary effusion lymphoma cells, not induced by phorbol ester; class II = expressed in uninduced cells, induced by TPA; class III = lytic gene, expressed only after induction by TPA (includes many structural proteins and DNA replication enzymes). FLIP = FLICE inhibitory protein; GPCR = G-protein-coupled receptor; IRF = interferon regulatory factor; ITAM = immunoreceptor tyrosine-based activation motif; MHC = major histocompatibility complex; MIP = macrophage inflammatory protein; NK = natural killer; Rb = retinoblastoma protein; TRAFs = TNFR-associated factors.

cell-cycle arrest of latently infected cells.[109,170] KSHV microRNAs also target cellular genes.[171]

Clinical aspects

Seroprevalence rates for KSHV vary from <5% in normal blood donors in the United States or United Kingdom to 30–35% in HIV-positive homosexual men.[172] Antibody to KSHV is more common in African and Mediterranean populations. At least 85% of patients with Kaposi sarcoma have antibodies to KSHV.[173] The prevalence of Kaposi sarcoma is lower in women than in men, and HIV-seropositive women have a much lower incidence of antibody to KSHV than do seropositive men. KSHV seropositivity in HIV-positive homosexual men is predictive of subsequent development of Kaposi sarcoma.[174] Levels of KSHV DNA are higher in patients with active Kaposi sarcoma or multicentric Castleman disease, than in those in remission, and are also elevated in patients with primary effusion lymphoma.[175] The virus is not thought to be pathogenic in most healthy individuals and can persist in a latent phase for life; however, in immunocompromised persons, it is strongly associated with Kaposi sarcoma. Thus, although infection with KSHV appears to be required for development of Kaposi sarcoma, it is probably not sufficient by itself and other cofactors, such as HIV and impaired cellular immunity, are important. KSHV is thought to be sexually transmitted in homosexual men[172] and has been associated with sexual transmission and intravenous drug use in women.[176] In endemic populations (e.g., Africa), KSHV may be transmitted vertically from mother to child and between siblings. KSHV has been transmitted by renal allografts.[177,178]

Kaposi sarcoma

KSHV has been found in nearly all biopsies of classic Kaposi sarcoma, African endemic Kaposi sarcoma, Kaposi sarcoma in HIV-seronegative transplant recipients and homosexual men, and Kaposi sarcoma in patients with AIDS.[179,180] KSHV is present in

Table 4 Diseases associated with KSHV gene expression.

Gene	Kaposi sarcoma	Primary effusion lymphoma	Castleman disease
LANA (ORF73)	+	+	+
K12 (Kaposin)	+	+	−
ORF72 (v-cyclin)	+	+	−
ORF71 (v-FLIP)	+	+	+
ORF74 (GPCR)	+	−	−
K10.5 (vIRF3)	−	+	+
K9 (vIRF1)	−	−	+
K2 (vIL-6)	−	±	+

the endothelial and spindle cells of the tumor, but not in normal endothelium.[181] Most of the tumor cells are latently infected with the virus, but 1–5% of the spindle cells in HIV-positive Kaposi sarcoma show lytic KSHV infection. Kaposi sarcoma can be polyclonal, oligoclonal, or monoclonal. KSHV is also present in the peripheral blood mononuclear cells of approximately 50% of patients with Kaposi sarcoma, and its presence is predictive of development of the malignancy.[172] KSHV has also been detected in the saliva of patients with Kaposi sarcoma, and, infrequently, in semen. Several KSHV proteins are expressed in Kaposi's tissues (Table 4). Foscarnet and ganciclovir reportedly reduce the frequency of new Kaposi sarcoma lesions in some, but not all, studies.[182,183] Cidofovir had no effect on treatment of established lesions.[184] In contrast, HIV protease inhibitors have been reported to induce regression of Kaposi sarcoma lesions.[185] IL-12, in combination with liposomal doxorubicin, resulted in tumor responses in AIDS patients with Kaposi sarcoma receiving HAART; responses were maintained with IL-12 therapy.[186] Sirolimus,[187] imatinib,[188] bevacizumab,[189] and paclitaxel[190] have all been reported to have activity against Kaposi sarcoma.

Primary effusion lymphoma

KSHV has also been found in primary effusion lymphomas in patients with AIDS.[180,181,191] These body-cavity-based lymphomas of B-cell lineage are located in the pleural, peritoneal, or pericardial space and usually contain EBV as well as KHSV genomes. Some KSHV-positive lymphomas have been found in patients without AIDS.

Multicentric Castleman disease

KSHV has also been detected in biopsies from some patients with multicentric Castleman disease, especially in the variant known as the plasma cell type.[180,181,192–194] This disease is usually polyclonal and presents as generalized lymphadenopathy, fever, and hypergammaglobulinemia. Symptoms are thought to be due to increased levels of IL-6 and vIL-6.[195] KSHV is detected more frequently in biopsies from HIV-positive patients than in biopsies from those patients without HIV. KSHV is present in the immunoblastic B cells of the mantle zone of the lesions. Zidovudine plus valganciclovir showed activity in some patients with KSHV-associated Castleman disease.[196]

Summary

- Two herpesviruses, Epstein–Barr virus (EBV) and Kaposi sarcoma-associated herpesvirus (KSHV), are associated with human tumors.
- EBV is associated with Burkitt lymphoma, Hodgkin and non-Hodgkin lymphoma, post-transplant lymphoproliferative disease, T-cell lymphoma, nasopharyngeal carcinoma, and certain types of gastric carcinoma.
- EBV transformed B cells and EBV post-transplant lymphoproliferative lesions express EBNA-1, -2, -3s, and -LP and LMP1 and LMP2 and RNAs including EBERs and BARTs in culture. Burkitt lymphomas express only EBNA-1, EBERs, and BARTs. Hodgkin lymphomas and nasopharyngeal carcinomas express EBNA-1, LMP1, LMP2, EBERs, and BARTs.
- EBV EBNA-1 is important for maintaining the viral episome during replication of the cells. EBNA-2 transactivates several virus and cellular promoters and is a functional homolog of the Notch receptor. EBNA-3's regulate the activity of EBNA-2 and also transactivate viral genes. LMP1 is a functional homolog of CD40 and binds to TNFR-associated factors to upregulate NF-κB, STATs, JNK, and stress-activated protein kinases.
- KSHV is associated with primary effusion lymphoma, Kaposi sarcoma, and Castleman disease.
- Each of the three KSHV-associated tumors express LANA (ORF73) and v-FLIP (ORF71). Other KSHV proteins, including Kaposin (K12), v-cyclin (ORF72), a G-protein-coupled receptor (GPCR, ORF74), v-IRF3 (K10.5), v-IRF1 (K9), and v-IL-6 (K2) are expressed in some, both not all virus-associated malignancies.
- LANA maintains the viral episome during replication and inhibits the activity of Rb and p53. KSHV v-FLIP is a homolog of cellular FLIP and inhibits apoptosis and activates NF-κB. Kaposin increases the activity of cytokines, v-cyclin inhibits Rb and helps virus-infected cells to progress through the cell cycle, and the viral GPCR contributes to proliferation of KSHV-infected cells. v-IRF1 and v-IRF3 inhibit the activity of interferon and p53, while v-IL-6 functions as a B-cell growth factor.

Key references

The complete reference list can be found on the Wiley Companion Digital Edition of this title (see inside front cover for login instructions).

1 Longnecker R, Kieff E, Cohen JI. Epstein-Barr virus. In: Knipe DM, Howley PM, Cohen JI, Griffith DE, Lamb RA, Martin MA, Racaniello V, Roizman B, eds. *Fields Virology*. Philadelphia: Lippincott Williams & Wilkins; 2013:1898–1959.

2 Thorley-Lawson DA, Gross A. Persistence of the Epstein-Barr virus and the origins of associated lymphomas. *N Engl J Med*. 2004;**350**:1328–1337.

3 Price AM, Luftig MA. Dynamic Epstein-Barr virus gene expression on the path to B-cell transformation. *Adv Virus Res*. 2014;**88**:279–313.

8 Hislop AD, Taylor GS, Sauce D, Rickinson AB. Cellular responses to viral infection in humans: lessons from Epstein-Barr virus. *Annu Rev Immunol*. 2007;**25**:587–617.

37 Uchida J, Yasui T, Takaoka-Shichijo Y, et al. Mimicry of CD40 signals by Epstein-Barr virus LMP-1 in B lymphocyte responses. *Science*. 1999;**286**:300–303.

59 Klinke O, Feederle R, Delecluse HJ. Genetics of Epstein-Barr virus microRNAs. *Semin Cancer Biol*. 2014;**26**:52–59.

62 Meckes DG Jr, Gunawardena HP, Dekroon RM, et al. Modulation of B-cell exosome proteins by gamma herpesvirus infection. *Proc Natl Acad Sci U S A*. 2013;**110**:E2925–E2933.

67 Horst D, Verweij MC, Davison AJ, Ressing ME, Wiertz EJ. Viral evasion of T cell immunity: ancient mechanisms offering new applications. *Curr Opin Immunol*. 2011;**23**:96–103.

74 Cohen JI. Epstein-Barr virus infection. *N Engl J Med*. 2000;**343**:481–492.

76 Milone MC, Tsai DE, Hodinka RL. Treatment of primary Epstein-Barr virus infection in patients with X-linked lymphoproliferative disease using B-cell-directed therapy. *Blood*. 2005;**105**:994–996.

85 Leen AM, Bollard CM, Mendizabal AM, et al. Multicenter study of banked third-party virus-specific T cells to treat severe viral infections after hematopoietic stem cell transplantation. *Blood*. 2013;**121**:5113–5123.

86 Bollard CM, Rooney CM, Heslop HE. T-cell therapy in the treatment of post-transplant lymphoproliferative disease. *Nat Rev Clin Oncol*. 2012;**9**:510–519.

89 Grömminger S, Mautner J, Bornkamm GW. Burkitt lymphoma: the role of Epstein-Barr virus revisited. *Br J Haematol*. 2012;**156**:719–729.

91 Schmitz R, Young RM, Ceribelli M, et al. Burkitt lymphoma pathogenesis and therapeutic targets from structural and functional genomics. *Nature*. 2012;**490**:116–120.

92 Chien Y-C, Chen J-Y, Liu M-Y, et al. Serological markers of Epstein-Barr virus infection and nasopharyngeal carcinoma in Taiwanese men. *N Engl J Med*. 2001;**345**:1877–1882.

93 Lin JC, Wang WY, Chen KY, et al. Quantification of plasma Epstein-Barr virus DNA in patients with advanced nasopharyngeal carcinoma. *N Engl J Med*. 2004;**350**:2461–2470.

94 Louis CU, Straathof K, Bollard CM, et al. Adoptive transfer of EBV-specific T cells results in sustained clinical responses in patients with locoregional nasopharyngeal carcinoma. *J Immunother*. 2010;**33**:983–990.

95 Hjalgrim H, Askling J, Rostgaard K, et al. Characteristics of Hodgkin's lymphoma after infectious mononucleosis. *N Engl J Med*. 2003;**349**:1324–1332.

98 Bollard CM, Gottschalk S, Torrano V, et al. Sustained complete responses in patients with lymphoma receiving autologous cytotoxic T lymphocytes targeting Epstein-Barr virus latent membrane proteins. *J Clin Oncol*. 2014;**32**:798–808.

99 Perrine SP, Hermine O, Small T, et al. A phase 1/2 trial of arginine butyrate and ganciclovir in patients with Epstein-Barr virus-associated lymphoid malignancies. *Blood*. 2007;**109**:2571–2578.

101 Bollard CM, Gottschalk S, Torrano V, et al. Sustained complete responses in patients with lymphoma receiving autologous cytotoxic T lymphocytes targeting Epstein-Barr virus latent membrane proteins. *J Clin Oncol*. 2014;**32**:798–808.

105 Chang Y, Cesarman E, Pessin MS, et al. Identification of herpesvirus-like DNA sequences in AIDS-associated Kaposi's sarcoma. *Science*. 1994;**266**:1865–1869.

108 Damania B, Cesarman E. Kaposi's sarcoma-associated herpesvirus. In: Knipe DM, Howley PM, Cohen JI, Griffith DE, Lamb RA, Martin MA, Racaniello V, Roizman B, eds. *Fields Virology*. Philadelphia: Lippincott Williams & Wilkins; 2013:2080–2128.

109 Giffin L, Damania B. KSHV: pathways to tumorigenesis and persistent infection. *Adv Virus Res*. 2014;**88**:111–159.

110 Cesarman E. How do viruses trick B cells into becoming lymphomas? *Curr Opin Hematol*. 2014;**21**:358–368.

117 Chatterjee M, Osborne J, Bestetti G, et al. Viral IL-6-induced cell proliferation and immune evasion of interferon activity. *Science*. 2002;**298**:1432–1435.

118 Moore PS, Bashoff C, Weiss RA, Chang Y. Molecular mimicry of human cytokine and cytokine response path-way genes by KSHV. *Science*. 1996;**274**:1739–1744.

127 Bashoff C, Endo Y, Collins PD, et al. Angiogenic and HIV-inhibitory functions of KSHV-encoded chemokines. *Science*. 1997;**278**:290–294.

150 Chang Y, Moore PS, Talbot SJ, et al. Cyclin encoded by KS herpesvirus. *Nature*. 1996;**382**:410.

152 Friborg J, Kong W, Hottiger MO, et al. p53 inhibition by the LANA protein of KSHV protects against cell death. *Nature*. 1999;**402**:889–894.

155 Lu J, Jha HC, Verma SC, Sun Z, et al. Kaposi's sarcoma-associated herpesvirus-encoded LANA contributes to viral latent replication by activating phosphorylation of survivin. *J Virol*. 2014;**88**:4204–4217.

160 Arvanitakis L, Geras-Raaka E, Varma A, et al. Human herpesvirus KSHV encodes a constitutively active G-protein–coupled receptor linked to cell proliferation. *Nature*. 1997;**385**:347–350.

169 Chugh PE, Sin SH, Ozgur S, et al. Systemically circulating viral and tumor-derived microRNAs in KSHV-associated malignancies. *PLoS Pathog*. 2013;**9**:e1003484.

172 Martin JN, Ganem DE, Osmond DH, et al. Sexual transmission and the natural history of human herpesvirus 8 infection. *N Engl J Med*. 1998;**338**:948–954.

174 Gao SJ, Kingsley L, Hoover DR, et al. Seroconversion of antibodies to Kaposi's sarcoma-associated herpesvirus related latent nuclear antigens prior to onset of Kaposi's sarcoma. *N Engl J Med*. 1996;**335**:233–241.

180 Sullivan RJ, Pantanowitz L, Casper C, Stebbing J, Dezube BJ. HIV/AIDS: epidemiology, pathophysiology, and treatment of Kaposi sarcoma-associated herpesvirus disease: Kaposi sarcoma, primary effusion lymphoma, and multicentric Castleman disease. *Clin Infect Dis*. 2008;**47**:1209–1215.

186 Little RF, Aleman K, Kumar P. Phase 2 study of pegylated liposomal doxorubicin in combination with interleukin-12 for AIDS-related Kaposi sarcoma. *Blood*. 2007;**110**:4165–4171.

187 Stallone G, Schena A, Infante B, et al. Sirolimus for Kaposi's sarcoma in renal-transplant recipients. *N Engl J Med*. 2005;**352**:1317–1323.

194 Uldrick TS, Polizzotto MN, Yarchoan R. Recent advances in Kaposi sarcoma herpesvirus-associated multicentric Castleman disease. *Curr Opin Oncol*. 2012 Sep;**24(5)**:495–505.

195 Polizzotto MN, Uldrick TS, Wang V, et al. Human and viral interleukin-6 and other cytokines in Kaposi sarcoma herpesvirus-associated multicentric Castleman disease. *Blood*. 2013;**122**:4189–4198.

196 Uldrick TS, Polizzotto MN, Aleman K, et al. High-dose zidovudine plus valganciclovir for Kaposi sarcoma herpesvirus-associated multicentric Castleman disease: a pilot study of virus-activated cytotoxic therapy. *Blood*. 2011;**117**:6977–6986.

30 Papillomaviruses and cervical neoplasia

Michael F. Herfs, PhD ▪ Martin C. Chang, MD, PhD, FCAP, FRCPC ▪ Christopher P. Crum, MD, FRCP

Overview

The field of HPV continues to move forward with new insights into pathogenesis, refined screening approaches using HPV testing, and the evolution of vaccines to include a wider range of HPV types covered. The squamocolumnar junction has been more precisely characterized, and its potential as a target for prevention in women beyond optimal age for vaccination is being discussed. HPV testing is assuming a major role in screening women over age 30, to the expense of the Papanicolaou smear, which will be largely limited to women between age 20 and 30, with reduction or elimination of cervical screening for women under age 20. For prevention of cervical neoplasia, the expansion of the range of HPV types targeted is now a reality, with new broader spectrum vaccines (such as 9-valent vaccines) being introduced.

The causal relationship between human papillomaviruses (HPVs) and cervical neoplasia is an accepted fact, and this virus has been the focus of strategies designed to elucidate mechanisms of virus-induced tumorigenesis, to improve the diagnosis and screening of uterine cervical neoplasms, and to exploit the host immune response to prevent these diseases. Technological advances have dictated both the tempo and the direction of this research, which began with descriptive and experimental pathology, progressed to molecular biology, and finally involved molecular immunology in efforts both to implicate the virus directly in producing neoplasia and to unravel the mechanisms of host response and prevention with vaccines.

Definitions, HPV-target cells, and mechanisms of infection and transformation

Definitions

Genital "infections" are best defined by the presence of clinically or colposcopically identifiable flat or raised lesions that contain papillomaviral deoxyribonucleic acid (DNA), the prototype of which is genital warts. In this instance, infectious virus is likely to be identified within the epithelium (Figure 1). More recently, the term infection has been expanded to include HPV-related precancerous lesions, or even cancers—the term being used loosely to denote the presence of viral DNA. However, integrated viral DNA rather than virions is more likely to be identified in advanced lesions (Figure 2).[1] As is detailed subsequently (see the section titled "Risk Factors"), HPV DNA may be associated with no visible abnormality; active, clinically, or morphologically conspicuous infection; and advanced neoplasia (Tables 1 and 2). The hallmark of significant HPV infection is a morphologic transformation of the target tissue. This is not synonymous with the term transformation as classically

applied to changes in cultured cells produced after introduction of HPV nucleic acids. Rather, it defines the morphologic alterations that can be most consistently associated with the presence of HPV nucleic acids. Depending on host factors and HPV type involved in the infection, it may be defined as a low- or high-grade genital precancer, either of which is distinct from the normal epithelium (Figures 1 and 2).

HPV-target cells and mechanism of infection

The cells initially infected by HPV have traditionally been presumed to be in the basal layer of the squamous epithelium lining the ectocervix and the region of the cervix where the columnar epithelium has been replaced by squamous mucosa (transformation zone). According to this theory, it is presumed that the virus gains access to the basal proliferating epithelial cells through microtraumas or abrasions in the stratified mucosa that expose these latter cells to virion particles.[5] In support of this hypothesis is the demonstration of HPV DNA and ribonucleic acids in basal cells and the observation that experimental infection of the squamous mucosa by pseudovirions is enhanced by disturbing the epithelial surface (and hence exposing the basal cells) before exposure.[6] Although basal keratinocyte infection is likely to result in productive infections and subsequent (pre)neoplastic lesions developing in the outer part of the cervix and other mucosal sites (vagina, vulva), this hypothesis is inconsistent with the long-term observation that about 90% of cervical (pre)cancer develops specifically in the squamocolumnar junction (SCJ).[7] For several years, this specific microenvironment has been speculated to contain multipotent cells that by virtue of their biology or location render them uniquely vulnerable to HPV infection. A discrete population of residual embryonic (Müllerian) cells has been recently discovered in the cervical SCJ.[8] In addition to being involved in adult cervical remodeling (metaplasia, hyperplasia),[9] these SCJ cells are proposed to be targeted by HPV and are thus the progenitors to cervical neoplasia. In this model, the basal keratinocytes are still susceptible to HPV, but less so relative to the SCJ cells.

Whatever the cell initially infected by HPV, host cell entry of HPV is initiated by binding of the mature viral capsid to heparan sulfate proteoglycans on the basement membrane. Then, a cleavage of the HPV minor capsid protein L2 at a furin (convertase) consensus site induces a capsid conformation change allowing HPV capsid endocytosis.[10] Endocytic pathways and HPV cellular receptor are, however, still controversial and several candidates such as α 6 integrin have been proposed.[11]

Mechanisms of neoplastic transformation

The mechanism by which HPV infection produces neoplastic transformation has been progressively elucidated and consists of at least four components (Figure 3).[12] The first is the direct effects of the viral oncoproteins on the cell cycle, mediated via interactions

Holland-Frei Cancer Medicine, Ninth Edition. Edited by Robert C. Bast Jr., Carlo M. Croce, William N. Hait, Waun Ki Hong, Donald W. Kufe, Martine Piccart-Gebhart, Raphael E. Pollock, Ralph R. Weichselbaum, Hongyang Wang, and James F. Holland.
© 2017 John Wiley & Sons, Inc. ISBN: 978-1-118-93469-2

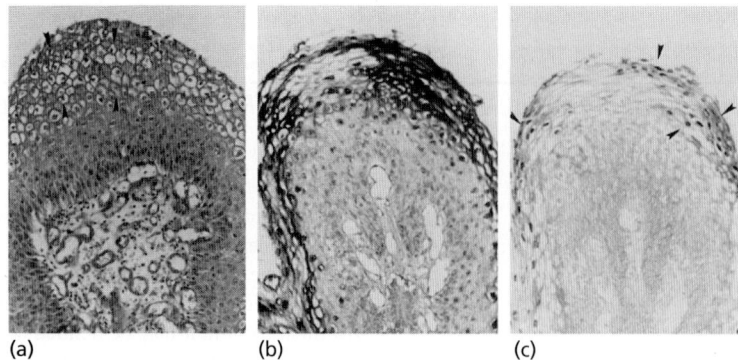

(a)   (b)   (c)

Figure 1 Histopathology of a classic human papillomavirus (HPV) infection (condyloma) of the cervix associated with low-risk HPV types (HPV type 6 or 11). (a) Morphologic features of HPV infection include nuclear atypia in the superficial epithelial cells with prominent cytoplasmic halos (*arrowheads*). The lower cell layers contain minimal cytologic atypia. (b) Appearance following *in situ* hybridization with a biotin-labeled mixed deoxyribonucleic acid (DNA) probe containing HPV types 6 and 11 (VIRATYPE, Life Technologies, Gaithersburg, MD). The dark staining in the superficial cell nuclei and cytoplasm represents viral DNA and ribonucleic acid produced during viral replication. (c) An immunoperoxidase stain for HPV capsid proteins, highlighting several dark-staining nuclei in the superficial epithelium (*arrowheads*).

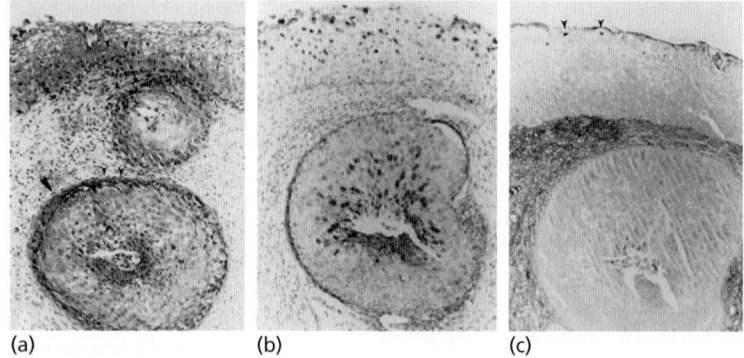

(a)   (b)   (c)

Figure 2 Histopathology of cervical intraepithelial neoplasm associated with high-risk human papillomavirus (HPV) types (i.e., 16, 31, 33, and 35). (a) Lesion involving the superficial and crypt (gland) epithelium (*large arrowhead*). Koilocytotic atypia is present (upper right), but, in addition, nuclear atypia is conspicuous in the lower cell layers (*small arrows*). (b) Appearance following *in situ* hybridization with a mixed probe containing HPV types 31, 33, and 35. Note the similar distribution of staining as in Figure 1b. (c) In contrast to Figure 1c, capsid proteins are infrequently identified by immunostaining, with rare positive nuclei observed (*arrowheads*).

Table 1 Definitions.

HPV, human papillomavirus
CIN, cervical intraepithelial neoplasia, synonymous with papillomavirus-related squamous intraepithelial lesions. Low-grade CIN (CIN I) is synonymous with flat or exophytic condyloma and exhibits nuclear atypia, principally in the upper epithelial layers. High-grade CIN (CIN II or III) is characterized by atypia in all epithelial layers. HPV-related lesion includes HPV infections such as condylomata and also any lesion associated with papillomaviruses, including high-grade CIN and various invasive carcinomas
Occult or latent HPV, defined as the presence of HPV DNA in the absence of morphologic evidence of HPV infection (i.e., no lesion is present)
High-risk HPV, HPV with documented association with cancer (this is not an assessment of cancer risk and will vary between high-risk HPVs)
Low-risk HPV, HPV with no association with cancer
VLP, viral-like particle; pertains to papillomavirus-like particles generated *in vitro*

Table 2 Genital HPVs and relationship to disease.

HPV(s)	Associated diseases
16	More than 50% of high-grade CIN and carcinomas (both squamous and adenocarcinoma)
18	10% of squamous carcinomas, 50% of adenocarcinomas and adenocarcinomas *in situ*, and 90% of neuroendocrine carcinomas
31, 45	5–10% of CIN, squamous carcinomas
33, 39, 51, 52, 55, 56, 58, 59, 68	Less than 3% (each) of CIN, squamous carcinomas
6, 11, 40, 42, 53, 54, 57, 66, 84	Low-risk HPVs, essentially never detected in carcinoma
61, 62, 64, 67, 69–72, 81, cp6108, iso39	Insufficient data to ascertain risk

Source: Adapted from Refs 2–4.

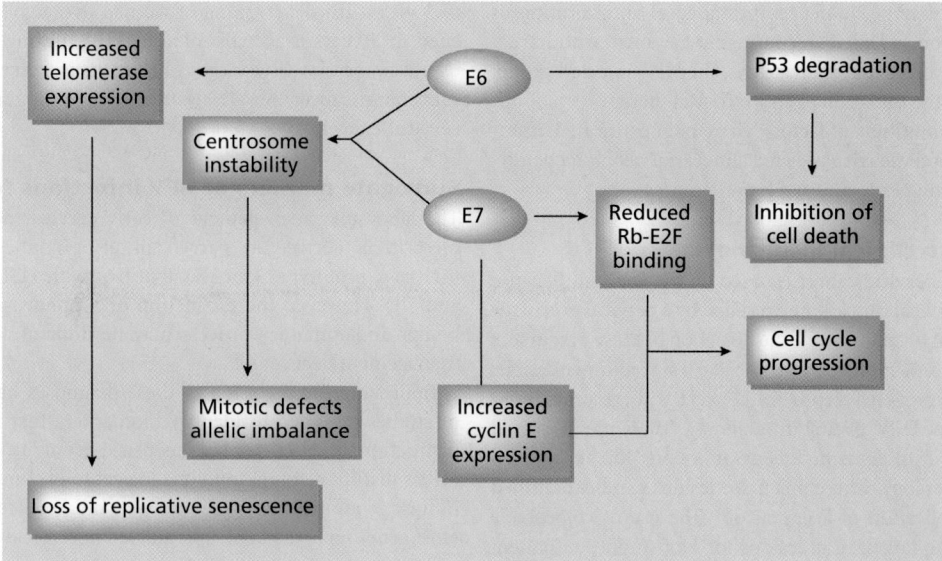

Figure 3 Schematic of potential mechanisms of human papillomavirus-related neoplastic transformation.

between E6 and E7 oncoproteins of cancer-associated (high-risk) HPVs and the tp53 and Rb proteins, respectively (Figure 3). A direct influence of these oncoproteins on other cell-cycle regulators, such as cyclin E, has also been demonstrated.[13] Compensatory elevation in expression of the cyclin-dependent kinase inhibitor p16 results from the above disturbances.[14,15] The second effect is also mediated via viral oncoproteins and consists of abnormalities in centrosome duplication, leading to genomic instability, subsequently reflected in progressive allelic imbalance.[2,16] The latter include alterations in 3p and specific amplifications at 3q25–27.[17,18] The third component is mediated via E6 and consists of telomerase upregulation and a disruption of normal replicative senescence.[19] These events occur ultimately as a function of expression of viral oncoproteins (E6 and E7). A fourth mechanism is the inactivation of tumor suppressor genes by methylation.[20] For example, the epigenetic repression of E-cadherin by E7 protein has been shown to increase the migratory properties of HPV-infected cells.[21]

HPV and human genital neoplasia

Risk factors

HPV infection is ubiquitous in the young, sexually active population, peaks in the early reproductive years, is often transient, and becomes increasingly less prevalent with increasing age.[22,23] However, persistent infection by the same HPV type is strongly associated with the risk of a current or subsequent cervical neoplasm.[24] At least 30 HPV types are associated with cervical neoplasia, with a broad gradient of risk imposed by these HPV types. Types 6 and 11 are prototypical "low-risk" HPVs associated with genital warts (condylomata).[25,26] In contrast, type 16 is the prototypical "high-risk" HPV, present in more than 50% of cervical carcinomas.[27] HPV 18 predominates in glandular and neuroendocrine carcinomas.[28,29] However, all of these HPVs may be found in women with normal cytology. A variety of other HPVs are associated with cancer at a lower frequency. Currently, these "intermediate-risk" and the high-risk types are combined into a single category. The presence of any HPV, high- or low-risk, does not exclude the subsequent emergence of another HPV infection of different risk, meaning that infection with one virus may serve

as a surrogate marker for subsequent infection by a high-risk HPV. Predictably, most HPVs detected in women with normal Pap smears have some association with cancer risk, albeit low.[3]

If a woman is found to harbor a high-risk HPV in her genital tract, what is her risk of developing a high-grade squamous intraepithelial lesion (HSIL)? In general, approximately 15% of reproductive-age women will score positive for high-risk HPVs. The risk of HSIL ranges from less than 5% to over 80%, depending on whether the Pap smear is normal, contains a minor or nondiagnostic atypia (atypical squamous cells of undetermined significance [ASCUS]), or is HSIL. Repeated detection of the same HPV type—even in the presence of a normal Pap smear—increases the risk to nearly 20%.[30] There is a strong theoretic basis for assuming that intratypical sequence variants influence outcome following infections by HPV 16.[31] However, the use of this information in patient management awaits greater consistency in study design and outcome and a clearer understanding of the mechanisms influencing the relationship between intratypical variants and the risk of developing high-grade cervical intraepithelial neoplasia (CIN) or cancer.

Young, sexually active women are at greatest risk of HPV infection and preinvasive cervical neoplasia, and this risk drops significantly with increasing age. As many as 39% of adolescents may score positive at a single visit.[22] The index of HPV detection drops further with the approach of menopause, presumably signifying a long-standing and effective immune response to the virus that follows the onset of sexual activity and exposure to HPVs in early life.[23,24]

The risk of anogenital neoplasia or HPV infection in immunosuppressed individuals is well documented, particularly in transplantation patients.[32] Human immunodeficiency virus (HIV) infection has been the most intensively studied. The risk of HPV positivity and persistent positivity is increased in women who are HIV positive.[33] Furthermore, persistence was 1.9 (95% confidence interval [CI] 1.5–2.3) times greater if the subject had a CD4 cell count <200 cells/μL (vs >500 cells/μL) in one study.[33] The risk of a subsequent squamous intraepithelial lesion is significantly higher in HIV-infected women.[34] The proportion of advanced precursor lesions is not significantly higher, but the risk of lesion persistence is.[34,35] The risk of invasive carcinoma in HIV-infected women is controversial but may be influenced by the level and duration of immunosuppression.[36] This is in contrast to gay men, who have a high risk of anal cancer that is greatest in the HIV-infected group, particularly since the initiation of antiretroviral therapy.[37]

In summary, a multitude of factors, virus and host related, influence the risk of papillomavirus-related anogenital neoplasia before, during, and following exposure and lesion progression.

Applications to clinical medicine

The prevention of cervical cancer is based on the Pap test. Because the majority of cervical cancers are preceded by a cervical precursor (CIN) lesion, often by many years, the detection of these precursors is fundamental to cancer prevention. The Pap test recommendations have undergone revision recently, in concert with recommendations for the use of HPV testing in screening. These are discussed together in the next segment. Precursor lesions are recognized clinically on colposcopy, where precursor lesions can be identified following the application of acetic acid.[38] The use of colposcopy has maximized the targeting of lesions for biopsy, and outpatient removal is the usual approach, including cryotherapy, laser, and, recently, loop electrical excision.[39] The latter procedures target the entire transformation zone, removing the lesion and replacing the process of chronic repair with a brief period of re-epithelialization. Recurrence after removal or ablation is linked to either inadequate excision or infection by another HPV following therapy. The former is increased when margins are positive. Infection with new HPV types appears to explain why many "recurrences" following ablation for high-grade precursors are low grade in nature. Reinfection with the same HPV type is uncommon except in immunosuppressed women. The potential significance of these findings in cancer prevention is discussed at the end of this chapter.

HPV testing in management of the abnormal Pap smear and primary screening

HPV testing has emerged as a viable management tool for a subset of women with abnormal cervical cytology. Because HPV is so strongly linked to cervical neoplasia and because high-risk HPV types predominate in the cervix, a substantial proportion of women with a cytologic diagnosis of low- or high-grade precancerous changes will score positive. For this reason, HPV testing is of limited value in this population. However, women with nondiagnostic squamous atypias (ASCUS) present a management dilemma in which the clinician must decide between colposcopy and Pap smear follow-up.

HPV testing offers the additional opportunity to triage the patient into colposcopy and follow-up groups by immediately testing the cytologic sample, which is possible with the newer liquid-based technologies. Newer generations of HPV testing, such as the Hybrid Capture II test, are extremely sensitive and will detect more than 95% of women with histologically proven preinvasive disease.[40] If HPV negative, women with ASCUS have a <1% risk of high-grade CIN, in contrast to a 20% risk if they are HPV positive.[40] Similar results have been seen with the management of abnormal glandular cells on the smear.[41] Recently, the test has been approved as an adjunct to the Pap smear for screening women over age 30. The basis for this approach lies in the high negative predictive value of both a normal smear and negative HPV assay, which may permit a longer cytology screening interval. Recently, the American Cancer Society and United States Preventative Task Force have made the following recommendations that will impact on reimbursement. First screening of women under age 21 and over age 65 will not be recommended unless there is a history of cervical neoplasia. Second, screening interval of women age 21–65 will be lengthened

to 3 years. Third, screening of women over age 30 can be lengthened to 5 years if accompanied by HPV testing (see http://www.uspreventiveservicestaskforce.org/uspstf/uspscerv.htm, http://www.cancer.org/Cancer/news/News/new-screening-guidelines-for-cervical-cancer).[42]

Surrogate markers of HPV infections for diagnosis

The laboratory management of early cervical neoplasia is based on criteria derived in part from prior studies correlating the high-risk prototypes (such as type 16) with HSIL (CIN grades II and III). However, the distinction of a preinvasive lesion from a benign inflammatory process may be difficult and can influence management decisions.

Improving the precision of these diagnoses has been the focus of studies designed to identify biomarkers that may simplify the distinction of HPV-related neoplasia from its mimics. Because HPVs disrupt cell function, it is logical to presume that alterations in host genes may serve as "surrogate markers" for HPV infection. Host genes reported to be upregulated in cervical neoplasia include telomerase, p16ink4, cyclin E, Ki-67, MN, and others.[14] Some of these, such as Ki-67, cyclin E, and p16ink4, have practical value in triaging histologic abnormalities.[14,15] The lower anogenital tract task force has recently recommended p16 staining as an adjunct to histologic evaluation, a positive test being continuous horizontal linear (or block) staining.[43] The most appropriate use of this biomarker is to solidify a CIN2 or CIN3 diagnosis on histologic exam by inferring the presence of a carcinogenic HPV. However, because up to 70% of CIN1 lesions will stain positive for this marker, p16 immunostaining cannot be used in a vacuum to make a diagnosis of CIN2 or CIN3.[44] Moreover, strong p16 staining is no guarantee of lesion progression; up to 67% of histologically verified CIN2 lesions will regress in 3 years.[45]

Clinical management

Management of HPV-related cervical neoplasms continues to be defined and redefined, in step with the methods used for lesion removal. Most women with low- or high-grade CIN on Pap smear or an atypical smear that is HPV positive will be referred to colposcopic examination. Of those who have a negative examination or a low-grade CIN on biopsy, 10–13% will develop a biopsy-proven high-grade CIN within 2 years. Many practitioners will follow patients with low-grade abnormalities and negative colposcopy by repeat cytology in 6–12 months, with attention to this risk.

Biopsy-proven high-grade CIN is typically managed by the loop electrical excision procedure or cone biopsy. Thus, the outcome of a given case will be dependent on the application of the histologic criteria for distinguishing low- from high-grade squamous intraepithelial lesions.[44] Long-term follow-up of all women with cervical abnormalities, treated or otherwise, customarily includes Pap smear evaluations but may eventually include periodic HPV testing as well.

Prevention

Efforts to elucidate the immune response to HPV have evolved from studies of fusion proteins and linear epitopes to the production in vitro of virus-like particles (VLPs) (Figure 4).[45–48] VLPs are produced by expressing the entire late region of papillomaviruses in eukaryotic systems, contain the conformational epitopes operative in generating host immunity, and can be used to study (or generate) host immunity.[49,50] This avenue of investigation was the most promising because it offered the advantage of intact particles that were highly immunogenic. Recent large-scale trials have validated the merits of VLP vaccination, demonstrating high efficacy for both preventing infection and lesions attributed to the HPV type(s)

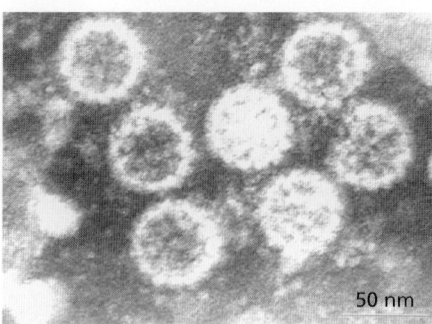

Figure 4 Electron micrograph depicting papillomavirus-like particles generated *in vitro*. Source: Courtesy of Ian Frazer, MD, Princess Alexandra Hospital, Queensland, Australia.

targeted in the vaccine.[51,52] Trials are ongoing that test multivalent vaccines containing not only HPV 16 but also HPVs 18, 6, and 11 (the latter two target genital warts). These trials have shown a high efficacy (95% or higher) for preventing both cervical and genital infection by the HPV types targeted in women who have not been exposed.[53] Predictably, efficacies in women who have been exposed are lower, and the overall reduction in HPV-related disease is under 20%.[54] However, vaccine efficacy against nonvaccine types has been recorded to be 27% and cross protection against specific types such as 31, 45, and 52 has been reported. Thus, the benefit obtained by the vaccination with HPV 16 and 18 is substantial.[55] Moreover, more broad-based vaccines employing HPV L2 are under investigation.[56] The value of these newer more broadly inclusive vaccines will hopefully address the regional variations in prevalence of certain HPV types.

The strong association between the squamocolumnar junction and cervical carcinoma and the discovery of a putative cell of origin in this site have raised the possibility that prophylactic ablation of this small region might significantly reduce the risk of cervical cancer. The yearly incidence of cervical cancer worldwide exceeds that of vaginal/vulvar carcinoma by nearly 20-fold, further evidence of the potential influence of the SC junction on cancer risk.[57] Anecdotes, studies of HPV infection following cryoablation, and topographic recurrence patterns and differences in CIN grade following SC junction excision or ablation have all pointed to the possibility of a profound change in precancer risk imposed by removal of the SC junction. Whether this information can be translated into a viable cancer prevention program is unclear and awaits further study.[58]

Key references

The complete reference list can be found on the Wiley Companion Digital Edition of this title (see inside front cover for login instructions).

1 Cullen AP, Reid R, Campion M, Lorincz AT. Analysis of the physical state of different human papillomavirus DNAs in intraepithelial and invasive cervical neoplasm. *J Virol.* 1991;**65**:606–612.

3 Koutsky LA, Holmes KK, Critchlow CW, et al. A cohort study of the risk of cervical intraepithelial neoplasia grade 2 or 3 in relation to papillomavirus infection. *N Engl J Med.* 1992;**327**:1272–1278.

4 FUTURE II Study Group. Quadrivalent vaccine against human papillomavirus to prevent high-grade cervical lesions. *N Engl J Med.* 2007;**356**:1925–1927.

7 (a) Marsh M. Original site of cervical carcinoma; topographical relationship of carcinoma of the cervix to the external os and to the squamocolumnar junction. *Obstet Gynecol.* 1956;**7**:444–452; (b) Richart RM. Cervical intraepithelial neoplasia. *Pathol Annu.* 1973;**8**:301–328.

8 Herfs M, Yamamoto Y, Laury A, et al. A discrete population of squamocolumnar junction cells implicated in the pathogenesis of cervical cancer. *Proc Natl Acad Sci U S A.* 2012;**109**:10516–10521.

9 Herfs M, Vargas SO, Yamamoto Y, et al. A novel blueprint for 'top down' differentiation defines the cervical squamocolumnar junction during development, reproductive life, and neoplasia. *J Pathol.* 2013;**229**:460–468.

10 Kines RC, Thompson CD, Lowy DR, Schiller JT, Day PM. The initial steps leading to papillomavirus infection occur on the basement membrane prior to cell surface binding. *Proc Natl Acad Sci U S A.* 2009;**106**:20458–20463.

13 Kreider JW, Howett MK, Wolfe SA, et al. Morphologic transformation in vivo of human uterine cervix with papillomavirus from condylomata acuminata. *Nature.* 1985;**317**:639.

14 Keating JT, Cviko A, Riethdorf S, et al. Ki-67, cyclin E, and p16INK4 are complementary surrogate biomarkers for human papilloma virus-related cervical neoplasia. *Am J Surg Pathol.* 2001;**25**:884–891.

15 Sano T, Masuda N, Oyama T, Nakajima T. Overexpression of p16 and p14ARF is associated with human papillomavirus infection in cervical squamous cell carcinoma and dysplasia. *Pathol Int.* 2002;**52**:375–383.

18 Rader JS, Gerhard DS, OíSullivan MJ, et al. Cervical intraepithelial neoplasia III shows frequent allelic loss in 3p and 6p. *Genes Chromosomes Cancer.* 1998;**22**:57–65.

19 Klingelhutz AJ, Foster SA, McDougall JK. Telomerase activation by the E6 gene product of human papillomavirus type 16. *Nature.* 1996;**380**:79–82.

22 Rosenfeld WD, Rose E, Vermund SH, et al. Follow-up evaluation of cervicovaginal human papillomavirus infection in adolescents. *J Pediatr.* 1992;**121**:307–311.

24 Bory JP, Cucherousset J, Lorenzato M, et al. Recurrent human papillomavirus infection detected with the hybrid capture II assay selects women with normal cervical smears at risk for developing high grade cervical lesions: a longitudinal study of 3091 women. *Int J Cancer.* 2002;**102**:519–525.

25 de Villiers EM, Gissmann L, zur Hausen H. Molecular cloning of viral DNA from human genital warts. *J Virol.* 1981;**40**:932–935.

26 Gissmann L, Wolnik L, Ikenberg H, et al. Human papillomavirus types 6 and 11 DNA sequences in genital and laryngeal papillomas and in some cervical cancers. *Proc Natl Acad Sci U S A.* 1983;**80**:560–563.

27 Durst M, Gissmann L, Ikenberg H, zur Hausen H. A papillomavirus DNA from a cervical carcinoma and its prevalence in cancer biopsy samples from different geographic regions. *Proc Natl Acad Sci U S A.* 1983;**80**:3812.

29 Stoler MH, Walker AN, Mills SE. Small cell neuroendocrine carcinoma of the cervix: a human papillomavirus type 18 associated cervix cancer. *Lab Invest.* 1989;**60**:92A.

32 Fairley CK, Sheil AG, McNeil JJ, et al. The risk of ano-genital malignancies in dialysis and transplant patients. *Clin Nephrol.* 1994;**41**:101–105.

33 Ahdieh L, Klein RS, Burk R, et al. Prevalence, incidence, and type-specific persistence of human papillomavirus in human immunodeficiency virus (HIV)-positive and HIV-negative women. *J Infect Dis.* 2001;**184**:682–690.

35 La Ruche G, Leroy V, Mensah-Ado I, et al. Short-term follow up of cervical squamous intraepithelial lesions associated with HIV and human papillomavirus infections in Africa. *Int J STD AIDS.* 1999;**10**:363–368.

36 Parkin DM, Wabinga H, Nambooze S, Wabwire-Mangen F. AIDS-related cancers in Africa: maturation of the epidemic in Uganda. *AIDS.* 1999;**13**:2563–2570.

38 Richart RM. Current concepts in obstetrics and gynecology: the patient with an abnormal Pap smearóscreening techniques and management [review]. *N Engl J Med.* 1980;**302**:332–334.

40 Solomon D, Schiffman M, Tarone R. Comparison of three management strategies for patients with atypical squamous cells of undetermined significance: baseline results from a randomized trial. *J Natl Cancer Inst.* 2001;**93**:293–299.

42 Hoyer H, Scheungraber C, Kuehne-Heid R, et al. Cumulative 5-year diagnoses of CIN2, CIN3 or cervical cancer after concurrent high-risk HPV and cytology testing in a primary screening setting. *Int J Cancer.* 2005;**116(1)**:136–143.

44 Crum CP. Our wages of CIN. *Obstet Gynecol.* 2012;**120**:1261–1262.

45 Moscicki AB, Ma Y, Wibbelsman C, et al. Rate of and risks for regression of cervical intraepithelial neoplasia 2 in adolescents and young women. *Obstet Gynecol.* 2010;**116**:1373–1380.

47 Zhou J, Sun XY, Stenzel DJ, Frazer IH. Expression of vaccinia recombinant HPV 16 L1 and L2 ORF proteins in epithelial cells is sufficient for assembly of HPV virionlike particles. *Virology.* 1991;**185**:251–257.

50 Rose RC, Bonnez W, Reichman RC, Garcea RL. Expression of human papillomavirus type 11 L1 protein in insect cells: in vivo and in vitro assembly of viruslike particles. *J Virol.* 1993;**67**:1936–1944.

51 Kirnbauer R, Booy F, Cheng N, et al. Papillomavirus L1 major capsid protein self-assembles into virus-like particles that are highly immunogenic. *Proc Natl Acad Sci U S A.* 1992;**89(24)**:12180–12184.

52 Ghim SJ, Jenson AB, Schlegel R. HPV-1 L1 protein expressed in cos cells displays conformational epitopes found on intact virions. *Virology*. 1992;**190**(**1**): 548–552.

53 Koutsky LA, Ault KA, Wheeler CM, et al. Proof of Principle Study Investigators. A controlled trial of a human papillomavirus type 16 vaccine. *N Engl J Med*. 2002;**347**:1645–1651.

54 Harper DM, Franco EL, Wheeler C, et al. GlaxoSmithKline HPV Vaccine Study Group. Efficacy of a bivalent L1 virus-like particle vaccine in prevention of infection with human papillomavirus types 16 and 18 in young women: a randomised controlled trial. *Lancet*. 2004;**364**:1757–1765.

57 Chaturvedi AK. Beyond cervical cancer: burden of other HPV-related cancers among men and women. *J Adolesc Health*. 2010;**46**(**4 Suppl**):S20–S26.

58 Herfs M, Somja J, Howitt BE, et al. Unique recurrence patterns of cervical intraepithelial neoplasia after excision of the squamocolumnar junction. *Int J Cancer*. 2015;**136**:1043–1052.

31 Hepatitis viruses and hepatoma

Hongyang Wang, MD ▪ Guangwen Cao, MD, PhD ▪ Jing Fu, MD, PhD ▪ Guishuai Lv, MD

Overview

Hepatitis is an inflammation of the liver, occurring as the result of a viral infection or the exposure of liver to toxic substances such as alcohol or aflatoxin B. Hepatitis viruses are the most common cause of hepatitis in the world, of which HBV and HCV can cause persistent liver infection, frequently resulting in chronic hepatitis, liver cirrhosis, and eventually hepatocellular carcinoma (HCC). HBV belongs to the genus *Orthohepadnavirus* of the *Hepadnaviridae* with a circular incomplete double-stranded DNA genome, containing four overlapping open reading frames (ORFs) that encode the surface envelope protein (HBsAg), the core protein (HBcAg and HBeAg), a polymerase, and a multifunctional nonstructural protein termed X (HBx), respectively. HBV genotypes and subgenotypes have distinct geographical distributions. In East Asia, HBV genotypes B and C are endemic. Accordingly, any differences in its global incidence may be explained by differences in the HCV and HBV prevalence. It has been estimated that 57% of cirrhosis is attributable to either HBV (30%) or HCV (27%) and 78% of HCC is attributable to HBV (53%) or HCV (25%). In China, up to 80% of HCC cases are attributable to HBV, and approximately 20% of HCC patients test positive for HCV-RNA. Besides the oncogenic function of HBV-encoding protein, the HBV infection-induced virus or host DNA mutation has been found contribution for HCC development. Unlike to HBV, HCV belongs to the genus *Hepacivirus* of the Flaviviridae family, with a single-stranded positive-sense RNA genome. There is no host genome integration, nor does HCV contain any known oncogenes. The major mechanisms of HCV-induced hepatocarcinogenesis include the oncogenic effect of HCV viral proteins, steatosis and insulin resistance, chronic inflammation and fibrosis, oxidative stress, and chromosomal instability. This chapter exclusively focuses on hepatitis and hepatoma caused mainly by HBV and HCV infection, discussing epidemiologic considerations, construction and genotype, role of virus in performing HCC, and early diagnosis and prophylaxis. Still, viruses that selectively infect endemic host predispose patients to malignant hepatoma, to some extent, placing a burden on the healthcare worldwide. Therefore, an upturn in morbidity of hepatitis and hepatoma will be of great importance in public health.

Hepatitis and hepatoma

Liver diseases, including hepatitis B virus (HBV) and hepatitis C virus (HCV) infections, alcoholic liver disease (ALD), nonalcoholic fatty liver disease (NAFLD) and associated cirrhosis, and HCC, are major causes of illness and death worldwide.[1] Liver disease causes serious public health problems because of its high prevalence worldwide and poor long-term clinical outcome, including premature deaths from liver decompensation, cirrhosis, and HCC. Among liver diseases, hepatitis and HCC harm to people's health seriously due to the disease susceptibility, cryptobiosis, and refractoriness, respectively.[1]

Human hepatitis viruses

Human viruses that selectively infect human hepatocytes and cause liver diseases are termed as human hepatitis viruses including hepatitis A virus (HAV, HBV, HCV, hepatitis D virus (HDV), and hepatitis E virus (HEV). Through fecal-to-mouth transmission, HAV or HEV causes temporary hepatic infection, varying from an asymptomatic infection to a fulminant disease. HAV, a single-stranded RNA virus, is a major cause of acute viral hepatitis worldwide. It occasionally causes an acute liver failure. HEV, a single-stranded, non-enveloped RNA virus, is endemic in several Asian and African countries. Pregnant women and patients with pre-existing chronic liver diseases are at a high risk of fulminant liver failure upon HEV infection.[2] HBV (alone or co-infected with HDV or super-infected with HDV) and HCV can cause persistent liver infection, frequently resulting in chronic hepatitis, liver cirrhosis, and eventually HCC.

Hepatitis B virus

HBV belongs to the genus *Orthohepadnavirus* of the *Hepadnaviridae* with a circular incomplete double-stranded DNA genome of about 3.2 kb in length. HBV genome contains four overlapping ORFs that encode the surface envelope protein (HBsAg), the core protein (HBcAg and HBeAg), a polymerase, and a multifunctional nonstructural (NS) protein termed X (HBx). The PreS region that consists of PreS1 (nt.2848-3204) and PreS2 (nt.3205-154) domains overlaps a region encoding the polymerase gene (P gene). The enhancer II (EnhII; nt.1636-1744) and basic core promoter (BCP; nt.1751-1769) regions overlap with the X gene (nt.1374-1835). HBV genome contains two viral enhancers that regulate transcription of the HBV promoters, including the BCP that controls the transcription of the pre-core and core regions. Following the entry into hepatocytes, HBV enters the nuclei of hepatocytes. HBV genome forms a relaxed circular DNA that is converted into covalently closed circular DNA (cccDNA) in the nuclei. The cccDNA transcribes all viral RNAs including pregenomic (pg) RNA as a replicative RNA intermediate. The pgRNA, viral core, and polymerase proteins are assembled into the nucleocapsid in the cytoplasm and then the pgRNA is converted into an HBV DNA by viral polymerase. Approximately 10^{11} viral particles are released into the circulation of the individuals with chronic HBV infection per day, and HBV particles are cleared from the plasma with a half-life of approximately 1.2 day. During viral replication, the partially double-stranded HBV DNA is generated from an intermediate RNA via reverse transcription activity of the viral polymerase. HBV reverse transcriptase lacks proofreading capacity, resulting in mutation rates of 1.5×10^{-5} to 5×10^{-5} nucleotide substitutions/site/year in HBV-infected subjects at their HBeAg-positive stage.[3,4] However, owing to the extreme overlapping ORFs, HBV genome evolution is constrained to maintain essential protein functions required for viral replication.[5] This plasticity of HBV

Holland-Frei Cancer Medicine, Ninth Edition. Edited by Robert C. Bast Jr., Carlo M. Croce, William N. Hait, Waun Ki Hong, Donald W. Kufe, Martine Piccart-Gebhart, Raphael E. Pollock, Ralph R. Weichselbaum, Hongyang Wang, and James F. Holland.
© 2017 John Wiley & Sons, Inc. ISBN: 978-1-118-93469-2

genome allows the generation of viral mutants that can occur under the pressures of immune selection.

Eight genotypes (genotypes A–H) have been determined according to a sequence divergence >8% in the entire HBV genome or a sequence divergence >4% in the S region. Genotypes have further been classified into subgenotypes if the divergence in whole nucleotide sequence is between 4% and 8%. Subgenotypes 1–5 of genotype A, subgenotypes 1–8 of genotype B, subgenotypes 1–8 of genotype C, and subgenotypes 1–7 of genotype D have been recently nominated. HBV genotypes and subgenotypes have distinct geographical distributions.[3,6,7] HBV genotypes A1, A3, A4, and A5 are endemic in Africa, especially in West Africa, whereas genotype A2 is endemic in Europe. Genotypes B and C are endemic in Asia. Of HBV genotypes B and C, subgenotypes B2 and C2 are endemic in most parts of Asia. Subgenotype C4 is encountered in Aborigines from Australia and frequently termed as the Australian aboriginal strain. Subgenotypes B3–B8, C1, C3, and C5–C8 are present in Indonesia and the Philippines. Genotype D is endemic in the entire Old World including Northern Africa, Northern and South Asia, the Mediterranean area, and most European countries. Subgenotype D1 is predominant in Moslem ethnicity. Subgenotype D2 is endemic in Russia and the Baltic region. Subgenotypes D4 and D6 are endemic in Oceania and Indonesia, respectively. HBV genotype E is endemic in Western and Central Africa. HBV genotypes F, G, and H are endemic in Middle and Southern America. HBV genotype and subgenotype correlate not only with the clinical outcomes but also with the response to interferon-α treatment.[7,8] In East Asia where HBV genotypes B and C are endemic, genotype B is more apt to cause acute infection in young people and to be more easily cleared than genotype C, whereas genotype C leads to higher persistence following an acute course and is more apt to cause cirrhosis and HCC than genotype B.[8–11] Thus, HBV genotyping is not only important in reconstructing the evolutionary history of HBV and humans but also helpful in indicating clinical outcomes of HBV infection and responses to antiviral treatments.

Chronic HBV infection frequently occurs in individuals infected perinatally or during early childhood, when the immune system is immature. HBV infection in adults is mostly asymptomatic or experiences an acute course. Invasive medical procedures, household contact with HBV carriers, body care and beauty treatments, and lack of HBV vaccination are the major risk factors of acute hepatitis B in adults. About 8.5% of adult patients with acute hepatitis B in mainland China will develop a chronic infection.[9] HBV genotype C (vs genotype B) and genotype D (vs other HBV genotypes) are more apt to cause persistent infection following an acute course.[9,11] Genetic polymorphisms of human leukocyte antigen (HLA) in the *HLA-DP* and *HLA-DQ* regions contribute to immune imbalance (such as Th1/Th2 cells or Th17/Treg cells, neutrophil/lymphocyte, neutrophil/CD8+ T cell, and Th1/Th2 cytokines balances) upon HBV infection, resulting in HBV persistence and possible chronic liver inflammation.[12–14] Allelic frequencies of the *HLA-DP* polymorphisms differ greatly among races. According to the NCBI database (http://www.ncbi.nlm.nih.gov/projects/SNP/), the *HLA-DP* (or *HLA-DQ*) alleles that facilitate chronic HBV infection are the major allele in the Asian population,[13,14] whereas they are the variant alleles in the European population. This might be one of the reasons why HBV persistence is more frequent in Asians than in Europeans. These *HLA-II* genetic polymorphisms may predispose the host to maintaining chronic HBV infection, facilitate the immune selection of the disease-related HBV mutants, and affect the risks of cirrhosis and HCC contributed by the HBV mutations.

Hepatitis B virus and hepatocellular carcinoma

In general, without efficient treatment, all types of chronic hepatitis will finally progress into ESLDs (end-stage liver diseases), such as cirrhosis and HCC. Most ESLD displays a poor clinical outcome. HCC is a major cause of cancer mortality worldwide, and any differences in its global incidence may be explained by differences in the HCV and HBV prevalence.[1] In 2013, the World Health Organization reported that primary liver cancer caused 745,517 deaths worldwide and that HCC represented the major histological type of these liver cancers.[15] In another comprehensive review of global mortality, deaths from HCV-related HCC were estimated at 195,700 in 2010. In China, HCC is the second leading cause of cancer mortality, and its annual death rate was 24.15 per 100,000 persons in 2009.[16] Approximately 383,203 persons die from liver cancer every year in China, which accounts for 51% of the deaths from liver cancer worldwide.[16] Up to 80% of HCC cases in China are attributable to HBV, and approximately 20% of HCC patients test positive for HCV-RNA.[17]

Epidemiologic considerations

Approximately 2 billion people have ever been exposed to HBV worldwide. Of those, 350 million people are chronically infected with HBV. It has been estimated that 57% of cirrhosis is attributable to either HBV (30%) or HCV (27%) and 78% of HCC is attributable to HBV (53%) or HCV (25%).[18] A prospective study conducted in Taiwan has proved that the cumulative lifetime (age 30–75 years) incidences of HCC for men and women positive for both HBsAg and antibodies against HCV are 38.35% and 27.40%; for those positive for HBsAg only, 27.38% and 7.99%; and for those positive for neither, 1.55% and 1.03%, respectively.[19] Prospective epidemiological studies have proved that male gender, increasing age, cirrhosis, high viral load, HBeAg positivity, HBV genotype C (vs genotype B), low albumin, alanine aminotransferase (ALT) elevation, and viral mutation A1762T/G1764A independently increase HCC risk in chronic HBV-infected patients.[11,19–23] HBV demonstrates "mutation–selection–adaptation," a viral evolutionary process involved in hepatocarcinogenesis. During this process, especially during HBeAg seroconversion, HBV accumulates HCC-risk mutations, predominantly in the core promoter and preS regions of HBV genome.[24–26] A1762T/G1764A can predict HCC prospectively, possibly because this mutation is earlier generated during the evolutionary process.[27] These demographic, clinical, and viral factors harvested before HCC occurrence should be prognostic and even predictive for HCC in HBV-infected patients.

Role of HBV mutations in HCC development

Insufficient immune responses elicited by HBV antigens select the HCC-related HBV mutations during long-term evolutionary process. Only the HBV strains/variants best adapted to the immune system will survive and thrive in liver. Genetic predispositions of HLA-II antigens and other inflammatory factors such as NF-κB and STAT3 may contribute to immune imbalance upon HBV infection, leading to persistent infection and chronic inflammation in liver, which facilitate the generation of the HCC-risk HBV mutations.[13,28,29] Inflammatory factors promote HBV mutations, at least partially, via activating cytidine deaminases.[5]

Host somatic mutations

Cytidine deaminases and their analogs, whose expressions and activities can be activated by proinflammatory cytokines generated during the inflammation, not only promote HBV mutagenesis but also facilitate somatic mutations.[5] Important HCC-related somatic mutations are found in critical genes such as RNA editing genes (*ADAR1, ADAR2, KHDRBS2,* and *RTL1*), chromatin remodeling genes (*ARID1A, ARID1B,* and *ARID2*), DNA-binding genes (*HOXA1*), growth factor signaling pathway genes (*CDH8, CDK14, CNTN2, ERRFI1, RPS6KA3, P62,* and *PROKR2*), transcriptional regulation genes (*AXIN1, CCNG1, CTNNB1, IRF2, NFE2L2, PARP4, PAX5, ST18, TP53, TRRAP,* and *ZNF717*), cell structure modification genes (*FLNA* and *VCAM1*), epigenetic modification genes (*MLL3*), and JAK/STAT pathway genes (*JAK1* and *JAK2*).[30] These somatic mutations should affect major signaling pathways, which can serve as therapeutic targets for HCC aggressiveness.

The roles of HBV-encoding proteins

(1) Excess production of the HBV envelope proteins, or truncated forms of the middle (preS2/S) and large (preS1/preS2/S) envelope protein, can activate cellular signal transduction pathways or endoplasmic reticulum (ER) stress pathways, induce cell proliferation by upregulating cyclin A expression, and activate c-Raf-1 and extracellular regulated kinase (ERK) signaling to stimulate cell proliferation. Accumulation of the S proteins in the ER can activate the unfolded protein response and cause oxidative stress. Epidermal growth factor receptor (EGFR) overexpression, which occurs in 40–70% of human HCCs, has been linked with tumorigenesis.[31] Aberrant activation of Raf-MEKERK and PI3K-Akt pathways driven by EGFR is commonly observed and implicated in the tumor growth and progression of many human cancer types, including HCC.[32] Moreover, activation of EGFR signaling pathways via the high expression of either its cognate ligands or itself is strongly associated with the poor prognosis of HCC. (2) HBx serves as a transactivator of several cellular signaling pathways including Wnt that contributes to HBV-related HCC and also interacts with tumor suppressor adenomatous polyposis coli (APC) to activate Wnt/β-catenin signaling. HBx promotes the invasive ability and metastatic potential of HCC. For example, as recently reported, using HBx transgenic mice and human HBV-related HCC specimens demonstrates that expression of HBx promotes expansion and tumorigenicity of HPCs (hepatic progenitor cells) that contribute to HBx-mediated tumor formation in a diethyldithiocarbamate (DDC)-induced mouse model. These studies shed novel light on the notorious role of HBx in the relationship between chronic hepatitis infection and liver cancer.[33] Carboxylic acid-terminal truncated HBx protein (Ct-HBx), a common form of HBV DNA integrated into the host genome, can enhance HCC cell invasiveness and metastasis in a manner that is more potent than that evoked by full-length HBx. HBV genome integration in the promoter of the human telomerase reverse transcriptase (TERT) locus is frequently observed in a high clonal proportion, which correlates with increased TERT expression.[5] Whether the preference of integration into specific host genomic loci and characteristics of the inserted fragments endow HBV integration a greater potential to drive oncogenic transformation remains to be elucidated.

Early diagnosis and prophylaxis of HCC

Across all countries, 5-year overall survival of HCC is approximately 10%. This dismal outcome is due partly to the lack of an effective method for timely diagnosis, which leads to only 30–40% of patients with HCC being suitable for potentially curative treatments at the time of diagnosis. α-Fetoprotein (AFP) has been used as biomarker for diagnosis of HCC, but its sensitivity is low (25–65%) at the commonly used cutoff of 20 ng/mL, particularly in detection of early-stage HCC.[34] In addition, many patients with non-malignant chronic liver disease have raised AFP concentrations in serum, including 15–58% of patients with acute-on-chronic

hepatitis and 11–47% with liver cirrhosis.[34] Therefore, novel and reliable diagnostic biomarkers to complement AFP are urgently needed to improve clinical outcomes.

Glypican-3 (GPC3) is a heparan sulfate glycoprotein that is highly expressed in approximately 70% of HCC cases[35] but poorly expressed in pre-neoplastic lesions and in normal liver tissue.[36] GPC3 is considered a biomarker for HCC diagnosis, and multiple studies have demonstrated that GPC3 is an attractive liver cancer-specific target.[37] Furthermore, GPC3 is one of the most promising markers according to preclinical exploratory studies.[38] GPC3 kit has been pathologically utilized to diagnose and classify HCC, especially in antidiastole of liver tumor between carcinoid and malignancy, thereby providing a promising therapeutic intervention for GPC3-positive HCC.[37] As it has diagnostic value to cure patients individually and the ability to avoid over-treatment on benign lesion, GPC3 kit has been expectedly approved by China Food and Drug Administration (CFDA) with a forthcoming popularized application in clinic. Dickkopf-1 (DKK1), a secretory antagonist of the canonical Wnt signaling pathway, is overexpressed in HCC tissue but is not detectable in corresponding non-cancerous liver tissue. A large-scale multicenter study shows that DKK1 could complement measurement of AFP in the diagnosis of HCC and improve identification of patients with AFP-negative HCC and distinguish HCC from non-malignant chronic liver diseases.[38] A plasma microRNA panels (plasma miR-122, miR-192, miR-21, miR-223, miR-26a, miR-27a, and miR-801) are potential circulating markers for diagnosing HCC with a large number of participants that ranges HCC from healthy, CHB, and cirrhosis with a high degree of accuracy. The microRNA panel with the seven microRNAs from the multivariate logistic regression model demonstrates high accuracy in the diagnosis of HCC, especially for patients with early BCLC stages (0 and A) who can benefit from the optimal therapy.[39]

Importantly, receptor-binding region of pre-S1 can specifically interact with sodium taurocholate cotransporting polypeptide (NTCP), a multiple transmembrane transporter predominantly expressed in the liver using near zero distance photo-cross-linking and tandem affinity purification. It is demonstrated that NTCP is a functional receptor for HBV and HDV; therefore, it is of great significance for the therapy of HBV infection and HBV-related HCC in the near future.[40]

HBV vaccination is effective for those without HBV infection. However, for 350 million HBV carriers worldwide, antiviral treatment is effective for those chronically infected with HBV, respectively. Active inflammation stimulated by HBV replication is indispensible for HBV-induced hepatocarcinogenesis. HCC occurs much less in inactive HBV carriers than in active chronic hepatitis B patients even if the patients are treated with antiviral treatment with oral nucleos(t)ide analogs.[41] Standard antiviral treatments with IFN-α and/or nucleos(t)ide analogs can greatly decrease hepatic inflammation and improve liver function, thus significantly reducing HCC occurrence in HBV-infected subjects and increasing the survival of the patients who received curative surgery.[41–43] Furthermore, the available research suggests that the miR-26 expression status of such patients is associated with survival and response to adjuvant therapy with IFN-α, meanwhile the expression patterns of microRNAs in liver tissue differ between men and women with HCC.[44] It should be noted that the result involves Chinese patients with a high rate of HBV positivity. HBV replication is the driving force of HCC evolution in inflammatory microenvironment. As approximately 30% of male and 10% of female HBV carriers may develop HCC in their lifetime, it is important to identify the HBV-infected subjects who are more likely to develop HCC and need the cost-effective antiviral treatment and regular screening for early HCC. However, antiviral treatment is effective in normalizing liver function, decreasing HBV–HCC recurrence, and improving postoperative survival. In the RCT (randomized controlled trial) of Eastern Hepatobiliary Surgery Hospital in China, nucleotide/nucleoside analog (NA) significantly decreased HCC recurrence and HCC-related death. Patients who received antiviral treatment had significantly decreased early recurrence and improved liver function 6 months after surgery compared with the controls ($P < 0.001$). Those with recovered liver function had a higher 2-year recurrence-free survival (RFS) rate than those without. Furthermore, Ct-HBx expression in adjacent hepatic tissues significantly predicts an unfavorable RFS in the antiviral group.[43]

Surgical resection is still the first-line treatment for HCC patients with well-preserved liver function worldwide, but the rate of postoperative recurrence at 5 years is as high as 70%. Some prognostic factors indicating that postoperative recurrence of HCC can be detected in removed tumor tissues, adjacent liver tissues, and peripheral blood. In tumors, high ratios of neutrophil-to-CD8[+] T cell and Treg-to-CD8[+] T cell, high expression of pro-angiogenic factors such as hypoxia-inducible factor-1-α and cell growth/survival factors such as CD24, and activation of inflammatory signaling pathways such as Wnt/β-catenin, NF-κB, and STAT3 predict early recurrence. In peritumoral hepatic tissues, high HBV DNA, HBV mutations, high densities of macrophages, activated stellates and mast cells, high expression of macrophage colony-stimulating factor/its receptor and placental growth factor, Th1/Th2-like cytokine shift, inflammation-related signature, and activation of carcinogenesis-related pathways predict late recurrence. In preoperative peripheral blood, high HBV DNA and the genotypes and HBV mutations, high neutrophil-to-lymphocyte ratio and high concentrations of macrophage migration inhibitory factor and osteopontin predict poor prognosis.[45] As a chemotherapeutic agent, at least working in part by the targeted inhibition of the hyperactivated ERK pathway, which is associated with postoperative liver regeneration, sorafenib is the first and only systemic therapy to significantly prolong the survival of HCC patients with advanced-stage disease until now. Recently, it has been proved that use of sorafenib after surgical resection for early-stage HCC was a promising approach for preventing recurrence and improving postoperative outcomes. Thus, sorafenib is currently used as a standard treatment for patients with HCC in spite of its shortcoming in specificity.[46]

As the population infected with HBV is increasing, inflammation-driven HCC formation has made early diagnosis and timely treatment more important. Even though targeting kinase addiction is an effective strategy for cancers, EGFR inhibitors have shown disappointing clinical results. A crucial rule of EGFR signaling in Kupffer cells or macrophages during inflammation-driven HCC formation is reported.[40] EGFR is required in liver macrophages to transcriptionally induce interleukin-6, which triggers hepatocyte proliferation and HCC. Importantly, the presence of EGFR-positive liver macrophages in HCC patients is associated with poor survival.[47] This study demonstrates that a tumor-promoting mechanism for EGFR in non-tumor cells, which could lead to more effective precision medicine strategies EGFR-positive Kupffer cells, might constitute a future prognostic marker and could potentially represent a target for HCC therapy.

Hepatitis C virus

HCV is the genus *Hepacivirus* of the Flaviviridae family. It is a small enveloped virus with a single-stranded, positive-sense RNA genome of 9.6 kb. It circulates as a highly lipidated viral particle. There are six known major genotypes and many more subtypes of HCV. This genetic variability promotes viral persistence, generates viral escape mutants from the immune system, and produces resistance to antiviral therapy.

Once the virus enters the cell, the viral RNA genome is uncoated and translated within the cytoplasm into a single, long polypeptide of 3011 amino acids.[48] The cleavage of the HCV polypeptide, mediated by host and viral proteases, yields 10 viral proteins. These are subclassified as structural proteins (C, E1, and E2) and NS proteins (p7, NS2, NS3, NS4A, NS4B, NS5A, and NS5B). The structural proteins serve the assembly of progeny virions and comprise two envelope glycoproteins (E1 and E2) and a nucleocapsid protein (core protein).[49,50] Core protein not only essential for virus particle assembly but also possesses several regulatory functions, including cellular transcription, virus-induced transformation, and signal transduction.[51] The NS proteins are responsible for executing viral replication and propagation.[52,53] HCV genome undergoes rapid mutation in a hypervariable region coding for the envelope proteins to escape immune surveillance. Most HCV-infected subjects develop chronic infection and eventually liver cirrhosis.

More than 185 million people were estimated to be HCV-specific antibody positive, representing 2.8% of the world's population in 2005. However, there are marked differences in HCV prevalence among different countries and regional age and risk groups, ranging from 0.1% to 5%. The most affected regions are Central and East Asia and North Africa. In the United States, it is estimated that 3.9 million individuals (or 1.8% of the general population) are infected with HCV. China has been considered a relatively high endemic area for HCV infection in the past. The prevalence of anti-HCV was estimated to average 3.2% in the general population, according to a national epidemiological survey carried out in most regions of China in 1992, with blood or blood product transfusion as the major route of infection. Since 1993, mandatory screening for anti-HCV and other precautions to prevent bloodborne disease transmission have been implemented extensively. New cases of HCV infection have declined dramatically. As shown by a recent national survey in 2006, the prevalence of anti-HCV is only 0.43% in China.[54]

HCV genotypes also display substantial differences worldwide.[1] HCV variants are classified into six genotypes. HCV-1b is the commonest one worldwide and more prevalent in patients with HCC than in those with cirrhosis and chronic hepatitis. In the United States, genotype 1a predominates, whereas the predominant genotype in Europe and China is 1b. In China, genotype 1b accounts for 68.4%, followed by 2a at 19.5%.[55] Interestingly, subtype 1b strains are more likely to be associated with transmission by blood transfusion and medical procedures, whereas subtype 6a strains are more likely to be linked to intravenous drug use (IDU) and sexual transmissions.[56] This genotypic difference in HCV between Western countries and China may be, to some extent, associated with each population's responsiveness to Peg-IFN-a and ribavirin (RBV) treatment.[57] In addition, single-nucleotide polymorphisms near the interleukin (IL)-28B gene region have also been found to be associated with the treatment efficacy of Peg-IFN-a/RBV in HCV-infected patients.[58] The frequency of the rs12979860 C allele is higher in Chinese HCV patients than in Caucasian patients. Evaluation of a large cohort of Chinese HCV patients showed that the major HCV genotype is 1b (approximately 60–70%) and the predominant host IL28b genotype of rs12979860 is CC (84%).[59] These data suggest that the global differences in the IL28B allele frequency and HCV genotypes may explain the better response to Peg-IFN-a/RBV therapy observed in Chinese patients.

Hepatitis C virus and hepatocellular carcinoma

There are 130–150 million individuals chronically infected with HCV worldwide.[60] Only a minority of those infected spontaneously clear the virus; most HCV-infected subjects, about 55–85% of persons, develop chronic HCV infection and are at increased risk of developing cirrhosis and HCC.[61-63] Of subjects with chronic HCV infection, the risk of liver cirrhosis is 15–30% within 20 years. Elevated HCV loads significantly increase HCC risk. HCV infection is estimated to increase the risk of HCC up to 17-fold.[64] The average time from HCV infection to the onset of cirrhosis is 13–25 years, and the time to onset of HCC is 17–32 years.[65] Annual incidence of HCC in HCV-infected subjects with cirrhosis is approximately 3–5%.[66] In addition, successful clearance of HCV infection reduces overall liver-related mortality and HCC incidence, suggesting a causal role of HCV.[67]

HCV is an RNA virus with an exclusively cytoplasmic life cycle. Unlike in HBV infection, there is no host genome integration, nor does HCV contain any known oncogenes. The mechanisms of HCV-induced hepatocarcinogenesis are intricate and several of them have been identified, including the oncogenic effect of HCV viral proteins, steatosis and insulin resistance, chronic inflammation and fibrosis, oxidative stress, and chromosomal instability. In experimental animal models, it has been reported that HCV-encoded proteins, core, E2, NS3, and NS5A, are directly involved in the tumorigenic process through interaction with a number of host factors and signaling pathways that affect cell survival, proliferation, migration, and transformation.[68-71] The HCV core protein can also influence or interact with several molecules that play important role in fatty acid transport and catabolism.[72-74] The HCV-associated hepatic steatosis, insulin resistance, and oxidative stress could lead to chronic liver inflammation, apoptosis, and fibrogenesis. These mechanisms are central to the development of liver cirrhosis and HCC in patients with chronic HCV.

Prevention and treatment

As there is no vaccine for hepatitis C, the primary prevention of HCV infection mainly depends on reducing the risk of exposure to the virus in higher risk populations. Among HCV-infected persons, about 15–45% of them spontaneously clear the virus within 6 months without any treatment. When treatment is necessary, the current standard treatment for hepatitis C is antiviral therapy with a combination of interferon and RBV, which are effective against all the genotypes of HCV. Effective treatment with interferon-based regimens has been available for many years, and achievement of sustained virologic response (SVR) to antiviral therapy is associated with improved morbidity and mortality.[75,76] In addition, with the rapid development of oral directly acting antiviral agents (DAAs), IFN-free therapeutic regimens for chronic HCV infection are becoming a reality, and they appear to be much more effective, safer, and better tolerated than interferon-based therapies. DAAs therapies also simplify HCV treatment by significantly decreasing monitoring requirements and by increasing cure rates.

It is anticipated that 12-week courses of interferon-free regimens with SVR rates of 90% or higher will soon be available to most HCV patients in whom cirrhosis has not yet developed.[77,78] Experience with interferon-free DAA regimens in patients with cirrhosis is limited, and available data indicate that SVR rates are lower with some regimens.[79] Therefore, early diagnosis and referral for treatment are important.

Key references

The complete reference list can be found on the Wiley Companion Digital Edition of this title (see inside front cover for login instructions).

1 Wang FS, Fan JG, Zhang Z, Gao B, Wang HY. The global burden of liver disease: the major impact of China. *Hepatology*. 2014;**60**(6):2099–2108.

2 Wedemeyer H, Pischke S, Manns MP. Pathogenesis and treatment of hepatitis e virus infection. *Gastroenterology*. 2012;**142**(4):1388–1397.e1.

4 Orito E, Mizokami M, Ina Y, et al. Host-independent evolution and a genetic classification of the hepadnavirus family based on nucleotide sequences. *Proc Natl Acad Sci U S A*. 1989;**86**(18):7059–7062.

6 Yin J, Zhang H, He Y, et al. Distribution and hepatocellular carcinoma-related viral properties of hepatitis B virus genotypes in Mainland China: a community-based study. *Cancer Epidemiol Biomarkers Prev*. 2010;**19**(3):777–786.

8 Wai CT, Chu CJ, Hussain M, Lok AS. HBV genotype B is associated with better response to interferon therapy in HBeAg(+) chronic hepatitis than genotype C. *Hepatology*. 2002;**36**:1425–1430.

9 Zhang HW, Yin JH, Li YT et al. Risk factors for acute hepatitis B and its progression to chronic hepatitis in Shanghai, China. *Gut*. 2008;**57**(12):1713–1720.

11 Chan HL, Tse CH, Mo F, et al. High viral load and hepatitis B virus subgenotype ce are associated with increased risk of hepatocellular carcinoma. *J Clin Oncol*. 2008;**26**(2):177–182.

12 Kamatani Y, Wattanapokayakit S, Ochi H et al. A genome-wide association study identifies variants in the HLA-DP locus associated with chronic hepatitis B in Asians. *Nat Genet*. 2009;**41**(5):591–595.

15 Globocan. *Estimated Incidence, Mortality and Prevalence Worldwide in 2012* (2012), http://globocan.iarc.fr/Pages/fact_sheets_cancer.aspx (accessed 12 October 2015).

18 Perz JF, Armstrong GL, Farrington LA, Hutin YJ, Bell BP The contributions of hepatitis B virus and hepatitis C virus infections to cirrhosis and primary liver cancer worldwide. *J Hepatol*. 2006;**45**(4):529–538.

19 Huang YT, Jen CL, Yang HI, et al. Lifetime risk and sex difference of hepatocellular carcinoma among patients with chronic hepatitis B and C. *J Clin Oncol*. 2011;**29**(27):3643–3650.

20 Wong VW, Chan SL, Mo F, et al. Clinical scoring system to predict hepatocellular carcinoma in chronic hepatitis B carriers. *J Clin Oncol*. 2010;**28**:1660–1665.

21 Lee MH, Yang HI, Liu J, et al. Prediction models of long-term cirrhosis and hepatocellular carcinoma risk in chronic hepatitis B patients: risk scores integrating host and virus profiles. *Hepatology*. 2013;**58**:546–554.

22 Yuen MF, Tanaka Y, Fong DY, et al. Independent risk factors and predictive score for the development of hepatocellular carcinoma in chronic hepatitis B. *J Hepatol*. 2009;**50**:80–88.

27 Li Z, Xie Z, Ni H, et al. Mother-to-child transmission of hepatitis B virus: evolution of hepatocellular carcinoma-related viral mutations in the post-immunization era. *J Clin Virol*. 2014;**61**(1):47–54.

29 Zhang Q, Ji XW, Hou XM, et al. Effect of functional nuclear factor-kappaB genetic polymorphisms on hepatitis B virus persistence and their interactions with viral mutations on the risk of hepatocellular carcinoma. *Ann Oncol*. 2014;**25**(12):2413–2419.

30 Ji X, Zhang Q, Du Y, et al. Somatic mutations, viral integration and epigenetic modification in the evolution of hepatitis B virus-induced hepatocellular carcinoma. *Curr Genomics*. 2014;**15**(6):1–12.

31 Buckley AF, Burgart LJ, Sahai V, Kakar S. Epidermal growth factor receptor expression and gene copy number in conventional hepatocellular carcinoma. *Am J Clin Pathol*. 2008;**129**:245–251.

33 Wang C, Yang W, Yan HX, et al. Hepatitis B virus X (HBx) induces tumorigenicity of hepatic progenitor cells in 3,5-diethoxycarbonyl-1,4-dihydrocollidine-treated HBx transgenic mice. *Hepatology*. 2012;**55**(1):108–120.

34 Gao H, Li K, Tu H, et al. Development of T cells redirected to glypican-3 for the treatment of hepatocellular carcinoma. *Clin Cancer Res*. 2014;**20**:6418–6428.

35 Marrero JA, Lok ASF. Newer markers for hepatocellular carcinoma. *Gastroenterology*. 2004;**127**:S113–S119.

36 Shen Q, Fan J, Yang XR, et al. Serum DKK1 as a protein biomarker for the diagnosis of hepatocellular carcinoma: a large-scale, multicentre study. *Lancet Oncol*. 2012;**13**(8):817–826.

37 Zhao J, Yu L, Gao X, et al. Plasma microRNA panel to diagnose hepatitis B virus-related hepatocellular carcinoma. *J Clin Oncol*. 2011;**29**(36):4781–4788.

38 Nakatsura T, Yoshitake Y, Senju S, et al. Glypican-3, overexpressed specifically in human hepatocellular carcinoma, is a novel tumor marker. *Biochem Biophys Res Commun*. 2003;**306**(1):16–25.

40 Yan H, Zhong G, Xu G, Li W, et al. Sodium taurocholate cotransporting polypeptide is a functional receptor for human hepatitis B and D virus. *Elife*. 2012;**1**:e00049.

41 Cho JY, Paik YH, Sohn W, et al. Patients with chronic hepatitis B treated with oral antiviral therapy retain a higher risk for HCC compared with patients with inactive stage disease. *Gut*. 2014;**63**(12):1943–1950.

42 Papatheodoridis GV, Lampertico P, Manolakopoulos S, Lok A. Incidence of hepatocellular carcinoma in chronic hepatitis B patients receiving nucleos(t)ide therapy: a systematic review. *J Hepatol*. 2010;**53**:348–356.

43 Yin J, Li N, Han Y, et al. Effect of antiviral treatment with nucleotide/nucleoside analogs on postoperative prognosis of hepatitis B virus-related hepatocellular carcinoma: a two-stage longitudinal clinical study. *J Clin Oncol*. 2013;**31**:3647–3655.

44 Ji J, Shi J, Budhu A, et al. MicroRNA expression, survival, and response to interferon in liver cancer. *N Engl J Med*. 2009;**361**(**15**):1437–1447.

45 Chen L, Zhang Q, Chang W, Du Y, Zhang H, Cao G. Viral and host inflammation-related factors that can predict the prognosis of hepatocellular carcinoma. *Eur J Cancer*. 2012;**48**(**13**):1977–1987.

47 Lanaya H, Natarajan A, Komposch K, et al. EGFR has a tumour-promoting role in liver macrophages during hepatocellular carcinoma formation. *Nat Cell Biol*. 2014;**16**(**10**):972–981, 1–7.

49 Fusco DN, Chung RT. Novel therapies for hepatitis C: insights from the structure of the virus. *Annu Rev Med*. 2012;**63**:373–387.

54 Chen YS, Li L, Cui FQ, et al. A seroepidemiological study on hepatitis C in China. *Zhonghua Liu Xing Bing Xue Za Zhi*. 2011;**32**:888–891.

57 Ghany MG, Liang TJ. Current and future therapies for hepatitis C virus infection. *N Engl J Med*. 2013;**368**:1907–1917.

60 WHO (World Health Organization). *Hepatitis C*. Rep. 164. Geneva: WHO; 2014. http://www.who.int/mediacentre/factsheets/fs164/en/.

67 Hino K, Okita K. Interferon therapy as chemoprevention of hepatocarcinogenesis in patients with chronic hepatitis C. *J Antimicrob Chemother*. 2004;**53**: 19–22.

77 Zeuzem S, Jacobson IM, Baykal T, et al. Retreatment of HCV with ABT-450/r-ombitasvir and dasabuvir with ribavirin. *N Engl J Med*. 2014;**370**(**17**):1604–1614.

78 Feld JJ, Kowdley KV, Coakley E, et al. Treatment of HCV with ABT-450/rombitasvir and dasabuvir with ribavirin. *N Engl J Med*. 2014;**370**(**17**):1594–1603.

79 Afdhal N, Reddy KR, Nelson DR, et al. Ledipasvir and sofosbuvir for previously treated HCV genotype 1 infection. *N Engl J Med*. 2014;**370**(**16**):1483–1493.

32 Parasites

Mervat Z. El Azzouni, MD, PhD ▪ Radwa G. Diab, MD, MBBCH, PhD

Overview

Many parasites were studied for a possible role in oncogenesis. *Schistosoma haematobium* was proved to play an important role in developing urinary bladder cancer. Other *Schistosoma* species, *Schistosoma japonicum* is classified as a colorectal carcinogen especially in the Far East. Other helminths *Clonorchis* and *Opisthorchis* are proved to induce hepatobiliary cancer. In Africa, a strong correlation between Ebstein–Barr virus infection and Burkitt lymphoma is present, with an evident enhancing role for *Plasmodium falciparum*. Chronic inflammation was incriminated to be the most accepted mechanism for parasite-induced cancer; however, the roles of certain carcinogens, oncogenes, DNA mutations, and others were all approved as mechanisms enhancing carcinogenesis in parasitic infections. Strikingly, despite the above-mentioned data, it seemed that certain parasites can modulate the host immune response in a manner that could lead to cancer regression or prevention. This is in the prospect of revaluation of the clinical importance of infectious agents; an issue that requires future concern.

The intensity of parasitic infection frequently correlates with its prevalence.[1] Thus, when relatively uncommon neoplasms are noted with undue frequency in countries with a high prevalence of parasitic diseases, the question of the role of parasites arises. In this respect, the two most intriguing examples are probably the relationships of schistosomiasis to bladder cancer (BC) and that of malaria to Burkitt lymphoma (BL). Classic references have been presented before.[2]

Schistosomiasis and cancer of the bladder

Schistosoma haematobium was first incriminated for a potential role in induction of urinary BC in Egypt in 1911 by Fergusson[3]; an issue that was finally confirmed by the International Agency of Research on Cancer (IARC) in 1994; which reported the parasite as a carcinogen.[4] Bilharzial bladder cancer (BBC) is theoretically a preventable malignancy if nationwide preventive strategies, including snail control and mass treatment campaigns, and screening projects could be adopted.[5]

Epidemiologic aspects

The highest incidence rates of BC are found in the countries of Europe, North America, and Northern Africa.[6] Smoking and occupational exposure are the major risk factors in Western countries; however, the morbidity and mortality due to BC have declined over the past decade owing to changing the habits of cigarette smoking.[7] Chronic infection with *S. haematobium* in developing countries, particularly Africa and the Middle East, accounts for about 50% of the total burden,[8] with Egyptian males having the highest mortality rates (16.3/100,000).[9] The association between *S. haematobium* infection and BC is far greater than that for any other parasitic infection,[10] and it was classified as group 1 carcinogen.[11] Association between *S. haematobium* and BC was initially established through case-controlled studies and close correlation of the incidence of BC with the prevalence of parasite. Clinically, the evidence of association was based on the presence of parasite eggs and *Schistosoma*-induced histopathological changes in cases of BC.[12]

Urinary BC is morphologically heterogeneous. More than 90% of the cancers are of the transitional cell carcinoma type (TCC),[13] as in case of BC associated with smoking and occupational hazards.[14] In Africa, squamous cell carcinoma (SCC) of the bladder is greatly overrepresented among the fellaheen of Egypt and the Africans of Mozambique, Zimbabwe, and Zambia (formerly Rhodesia), where *S. haematobium* is endemic.[15-17] However, a shift toward TCC subtype was observed in developing countries owing to shift in risk factors with increased urbanization and industrialization.[7] In Egypt, following the construction of the High Dam in the 1960s that led to changes in the water flow with direct impact on the intermediate snail host, *S. haematobium* was gradually replaced by *Schistosma mansoni* that causes intestinal rather than urinary disease.[18] Furthermore, effective oral treatment campaigns in Egypt since 1977 resulted in significant decrease in urinary schistosomiasis.[19] Strikingly, despite the large decline in *S. haematobium* infection in Egypt, BC continues to be the most common cancer among males. This is because the decline in BBC is being offset by increase in smoking-associated BC.[20] This is evidenced by the shift in the incidence of SCC in Egypt from 78% in the 1980s to 27% in 2005 with a shift to TCC.[21] Another retrospective study was conducted in Egypt, from 2001 to 2010, on two groups: group 1 included 1002 patients from 2001 to 2005 and group 2 included 930 patients from 2006 to 2010. The authors found that the incidence of BBC decreased from 80% in group 1 to 50% in group 2. Besides, a significant increase in TCC from 20% to 66% was observed with a significant decrease in SCC from 73% to 25% by comparing the two groups.[22] Hamed et al.[23] suggested another cause for the general decline in BBC in Egyptian governorates. Tendency toward warming, with high temperature exceeding 45°C, and increased number of hot days all over the year are incriminated in damaging the effectiveness of the snail host and hence schistosomal transmission.

The association of BC with schistosomal infection seems to become stronger with long standing and more severe infection.[24] In Egypt, this association is directly related to the extent of perennial irrigation through canals, which creates a constant risk of reinfection, and inversely related to control measures and availability of safe and effective therapy.[25] Children of school age are especially at risk because of their daily contact with infected water in rural areas.[26] Besides, it was noted that in endemic areas in Iraq, Coastal Kenya, Ghana, Malawi, Mozmbique, Zambia, and

Holland-Frei Cancer Medicine, Ninth Edition. Edited by Robert C. Bast Jr., Carlo M. Croce, William N. Hait, Waun Ki Hong, Donald W. Kufe, Martine Piccart-Gebhart, Raphael E. Pollock, Ralph R. Weichselbaum, Hongyang Wang, and James F. Holland.
© 2017 John Wiley & Sons, Inc. ISBN: 978-1-118-93469-2

Zimbabwe, a high association between *S. haematobium* and BC is present, whereas it was absent in Nigeria and areas in Southern Africa and Saudi Arabia with moderate to high prevalence of *S. haematobium*.[27] Typically, schistosomiasis is a disease affecting agricultural communities, particularly those dependent upon irrigation to support their agriculture. The problem became much more significant in the nineteenth century, when the combination of new irrigation projects and population increases led to a higher probability of exposure to the parasite.[28]

Geographical distribution of *S. haematobium* seems to play an important role in determining the susceptible groups as regards their age and gender. The peak incidence of BC in schistosomiasis-nonendemic areas is in the sixth and seventh decades of life.[29] In Egypt, Sudan, Iraq, Zambia, Malawi, and Zimbabwe, the mean age of the highest incidence of BC is between 40 and 49 years.[10] The male : female ratio of BBC incidence in *Schistosoma*-endemic countries is in average 5 : 1,[30] and this could be explained by prolonged contact with infected waters during agricultural activities in rural areas, which are normally done by men rather than women.[5] Recent observation showed that the relative frequency of BBC was increasing among females during the period 1995–2005 in Egypt. This was explained by increasing migration of male farmers from the Nile Valley and Delta to the Urban and Frontier governorates seeking for jobs. Therefore, the females were expected to take place of their husbands in agricultural work and thus their exposure risk to infection was increased.[23] Another study found that females were more affected by BBC (51.4%) compared to the males in the western part of Tanzania on the shores of Lake Victoria in the period 2000–2010.[31]

Variability in criteria for diagnosing urinary schistosomiasis influences the epidemiological rates for BBC. Ruling out a diagnosis of schistosomiasis because of the absence of ova in the centrifuged urine specimen would be unrealistic in many cases of contracted bladder owing to bilharzial fibrosis, in which the dense scar tissue precludes shedding of ova from the submucosa.[25] Thus, by expanding the criteria for diagnosis of bilharzial bladder to include recent imaging and molecular techniques with high sensitivity and specificity, the epidemiological rates for BBC are expected to be more accurate.

Progression of bilharzial bladder cancer

BC cells require the acquisition of certain properties before being able to grow rapidly, invade, and metastasize.[5]

Chronic infection leads to trapping of *Schistosoma* eggs in the bladder wall. Proliferation of cells in the bladder mucosa results from constant irritation and inflammation.[12] This mucosal damage increases the frequency of urinary tract infection.[32] Besides, activated macrophages induced at the sites of inflammation are implicated in the generation of carcinogenic *N*-nitrosamines and reactive oxygen radicals.[33] Mucosal fibrosis and dysuria associating chronic inflammation and bacterial infection lead to urinary stasis that, in turn, allows prolonged contact of urothelium with these carcinogens.[34]

Nitrate-reducing bacterial species accompanying urinary schistosmiasis can mediate the *N*-nitrosation of amines[10] with the liberation of *N*-nitroso compounds.[35] At the molecular level, these compounds are implicated in tumorigenic alkylation of specific bases and DNA sequences,[36–38] leading to mutations in oncogenes, tumor suppressor genes, and genes for cell cycle control.[5] Molecular events associating BBC include the activation of H-ras gene,[39] inactivation of *p53*,[40] and inactivation of retinoblastoma (Rb) gene.[41] In 2010, Botelho et al.[42] suggested that the parasite extract had

carcinogenic ability through oncogenic mutation of the K-ras gene. The frequency of *p53* mutations varies with the different grades of BBC.[43] For BBC in Egypt,[44] it was reported that about 86% had *p53* mutations in exons 5, 6, 8, and 10 and that the in activation of *p53* ranged from 0% to 38% at the early stage of the disease, as opposed to 33–86% in the advanced tumor stage.[43] On the other hand, habitual smoking in a group of Japanese BC patients did not increase the frequency of *p53* mutations, but caused unusual AT : GC mutation patterns.[44] Mutations observed in *p53* gene mostly involve transitions at CpG dinucleotides, which are in excess in cases of BBC. These transitions are explained by the effect of nitric oxide produced by the inflammatory response to *Schistosoma* eggs. Nitric oxide, released during the inflammatory response, can cause such mutations directly by deamination of 5-methylcytosine or indirectly via its capacity to form endogenous *N*-nitroso compounds leading to DNA alkylation.[45] Over representation of the protein encoded by the *MDM2* gene found in the majority of the studied cases may account for the frequent inactivation of the *p53* gene observed in BBC, and hence the accumulation of DNA damage and the aggressive clinical course.[46]

Cancer development is closely related to uncontrolled cell cycles.[47] Deletions and mutations in the gene coding for p16[INK4], a cyclin-dependent kinase (CDK) inhibitor, were found in 53% of BBC.[48] Moreover, deletions in chromosome 9, where the CDKN2 gene is located, were found in 92% of SCC in Egypt.[49]

Human papilloma virus

The possibility of association between HPV and BBC remained open for long.[50] A study done by Khaled et al.[51] showed that the virus was present in 23 out of 40 cases of BC. Recently, a study using the Mass ARRAY technology showed all BBC blood-tested samples to be associated with HPV-16 DNA.[52]

Metabolic observations during schistosomiasis

In the study of BBC, the metabolism of tryptophan along the formylkynurenine pathway leading to nicotinic acid has elicited considerable interest.[53] The justification for this interest originally stemmed from industrial oncology; however, epidemiologic support is also derived from the high prevalence of classic pellagra that used to be observed in Egypt but not in other parts of Africa where SCC is infrequently reported despite endemic schistosomiasis. In pellagra, exaggeration of the pathway from tryptophan to nicotinic acid occurs, producing larger amounts of tryptophan intermediates along the formylkynurenine pathway.[25]

Our understanding of the role played by *Schistosoma* infection in disturbed tryptophan metabolism is complicated by geographic variations of dietary habits. In fact, serotonin metabolites such as 5-hydroxyindoleacetic acid, which are excreted in large amounts by plantain-eating Africans, are low in Africans on other diets.[54] Similar differences attributable to dietary habits have been found between bilharzial patients in Mozambique and South Africa. Egyptian peasants are not plantain eaters but subsist mostly on beans, lentils, and rice. Those with bilharzial cancer metabolize tryptophan into 3-hydroxyanthranilic acid, anthranilic acid, 5-hydroxyindoleacetic acid, and kynurenine. The excretion of these metabolites is enhanced by a loading dose of tryptophan. Therefore, schistosomiasis should not be considered the only causal factor in the associated excretion of abnormal tryptophan metabolites because, with or without cancer, urinary schistosomiasis is almost universally accompanied by urinary tract infection. The bacterial flora may, thus, contribute to a spurious accumulation of some metabolites of tryptophan.[25]

Potentially carcinogenic metabolites of tryptophan, which may be the true oncogenic agent in the presence of bilharzial bladder inflammation, are principally determined by hepatic metabolic patterns. Factors that bear on this are coincident infestation of the liver by S. mansoni, pyridoxine deficiency, and chronic protein starvation. In the presence of advanced abnormalities in any of these factors, certain amounts of potential carcinogenic metabolites might be formed owing to lack of hepatic enzymes or cofactors.[55,56] The hepatic drug-metabolizing capacity of mice infected with S. mansoni is markedly reduced.[57] The mutagen-inactivating potential of S. japonicum-infected mouse liver is similarly reduced,[58] which results in longer persistence of the mutagen in the host body.[59] It seems likely that the carcinogen dose is a determining factor in the aggressiveness of a bladder tumor, and that a low-grade carcinoma can be converted into a high-grade one if exposed continuously to low doses of N-nitroso compounds. This would explain, at least in part, the overrepresentation of deeply invasive SCC in the bilharzial urinary bladder.[60]

Apoptosis in schistosomal bladder cancer

One negative impact of the several cytogenetic changes that happen in the course of chronic schistosomiais is decreasing cell apoptosis and thus enhanced oncogenesis.[12] In 2009, Botelho et al.[61] showed that cells exposed to S. haematobium total antigen (worm extract) were found to divide faster than those not exposed to the antigen, and died much less. This was explained by increased level of Bcl-2, which is one gene that can contribute to oncogenesis by suppressing apoptosis.[5] The overexpression of the Bcl-2 gene in BBC patients was found to be upregulated in SCC but not TCC.[62]

Pathology of benign and preneoplastic schistosomal bladder lesions

An intense, delayed-sensitivity reaction is elicited by viable Schistosoma eggs plugging the vesical venules leading to tubercules, nodules, or polyps. In bilharzial cystitis, the papilloma, covered as it is by one or two layers of flattened cells, which merge with the transitional epithelium at its base, is essentially a granuloma and not a precancerous lesion. With recurrent inflammation and fibrosis, some transitional epithelial cells become sequestered in the vesical submucosa and acquire a globular arrangement around a central cavity. When they open into the bladder cavity, the cystic formations become pseudoglandular. These structures, as part of cystitis glandularis, are at times precancerous; an adenocarcinoma may arise from the columnar epithelium, into which their lining has differentiated. In patients with schistosomiasis, squamous metaplasia is frequently encountered because it is a common concomitant of chronic inflammation. This type of metaplasia is a nearly consistent precursor of BC, and for this reason, leukoplakia acquires clinical importance as a precancerous condition.[25]

Site of origin

In patients in Western countries, BC frequently arises in the trigone; in patients in Egypt, it usually develops in areas remote from the ureters, mostly in the anterior and posterior bladder walls. This peculiarity tends to strengthen its association with schistosomal infection because the scanty or altogether absent submucosal tissue of the trigone discourages significant deposition of ova.[25]

Histologic classification

Significant changes in the pathological types of schistosomiasis-associated bladder tumors have been found over the past decades.[10] Comparing the periods 1962–1967 and 1987–1992, there was a decrease in the incidence of nodular tumors (83.4% to 58.7%) and of SCC (65.8% to 54.0%) but an increase in the incidence of papillary tumors (4.3% to 34.8%) and TCC (31.0% to 42.0%).[63–65] Similar results were proved by comparing the periods 2001–2005 and 2006–2010 as was fore-mentioned.[22] The extent of Schistosoma infection apparently plays a significant role in the induction of different types of carcinoma; SCC is usually associated with moderate and/or high worm burdens, whereas TCC occurs more commonly in areas associated with lower degrees of infection[63–65] (Figure 1). Adenocarcinoma of the bilharzial bladder is particularly aggressive owing to its proneness to develop gross chromosomal aberrations combined with high cell proliferation.[66] Another rare, though distinct, variant of SCC is verrucous carcinoma of the bilharzial bladder (Figure 2). Despite reports to the contrary, a large proportion develop into invasive SCC, with which they share the same adverse prognosis.[67]

Experimental data for BBC

In a number of nonhuman primates, infection with S. haematobium resulted in epithelial proliferation, squamous metaplasia, and TCC of the urinary bladder.[68] These types of carcinoma were morphologically similar to those observed in human bladders,[69] and such observations suggest that there is an association between S. haematobium and BC. These early experimental observations were important because eggs of S. haematobium, lyophilized worms, and urine from bilharzia patients have not been found to be carcinogenic to mice.[70,71] However, 2-acetyl-aminofluorene appears to promote

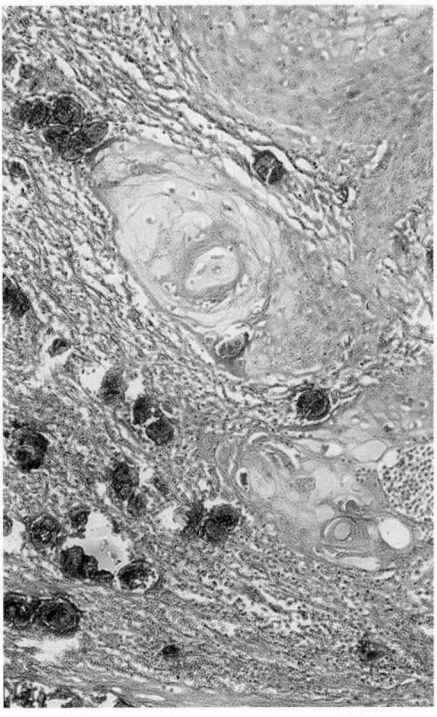

Figure 1 Bilharzial bladder cancer. Infiltrating, well-differentiated squamous cell carcinoma with adjacent calcified S. hematobium eggs (H&E ×100). Source: Courtesy of Drs M.R. Mahran and M. El-Baz, Mansoura University, Egypt.

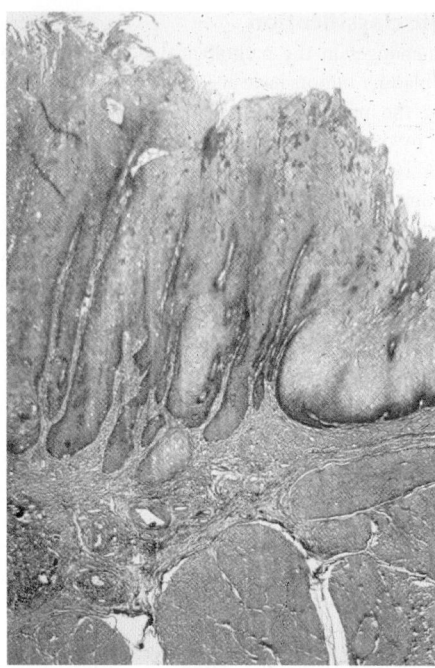

Figure 2 Verrucous carcinoma (noninvasive) of bladder with superficial filamentous elongated surface projections (H&E ×40). Source: Courtesy of Drs M.R. Mahran and M. El-Baz, Mansoura University, Egypt.

malignant and benign bladder neoplasms of mice infested with schistosomes more often than does either agent alone.[72] Cancer development was thought to have been accelerated by schistosomal infection, presumably acting as a late-stage cocarcinogen by virtue of its direct proliferative effect on the urothelium.[73]

Schistosomiasis and cancer of other sites

Large intestine
Intestinal infestation with *S. japonicum* in Asia is considered a significant contributory factor to the development of colorectal cancer (CRC). Female *S. japonicum* lays a very large number of eggs (2000 per day per pair of worms), whereas *S. mansoni*'s eggs are considerably less numerous and, thus, cause fewer pathologic problems.[74] In Shanghai, patients with intestinal schistosomiasis and cancer of the large intestine are, on average, 6 years younger than patients with spontaneous intestinal cancer. Furthermore, the male-to-female ratio of schistosomal CRC is consistently higher than in nonschistosomal cancer.[75,76] Recently, Madbouly et al.[76] studied the *S. mansoni*-associated CRC and showed that it has distinctive pathological features often similar to those of colitis-induced carcinoma. The parasitism is strongly associated with microsatellite instability, which is a sign of defective DNA repair,[77] which in turn affects normal colonocyte homeostasis resulting in malignant growth.[78] Another study showed that *S. mansoni*-associated colorectal tumors are characterized by Bcl-2 overexpression and less apoptotic activity than ordinary colorectal tumors.[79]

The liver
A study of liver cancer and its association with a previous diagnosis of schistosomiasis was performed in rural Sichuan, China. Previous schistosomal infection was found to be significantly associated with liver cancer and that a fraction of the disease (27%) was attributable

to schistosomiasis among hepatitis-negative population.[80] Experimental data showed remnants of schistosomal eggs in the severe granulomatous reaction present within a well-differentiated hepatocellular carcinoma that had developed in a hepatitis-B and -C, seronegative chimpanzee.[81]

Lymphoma
The association between schistosomiasis and lymphomas is far less reported.[82] Occurrence of an isolated, primary T-cell lymphoma of the bladder may represent an unusual immune response to schistosomiasis.[83] Discrete case reports of lymphoma in patients with hepatosplenic and chronic intestinal infections with *S. mansoni* and *S. japonicum* have been known. Types detected were histiocytic lymphoma[84] and large B-cell lymphoma;[82,85,86] where lymphoma cells proliferated around egg emboli and adult worms.[86]

Other organs
Immunohistochemical studies confirmed invasive SCC of the prostate in three prostatic schistosomiasis patients coming from a population where prostatic cancer is uncommon.[87] Mazigo et al.[88] reported three cases of adenocarcinoma of the prostate gland associated with *S. haematobium* in Tanzania.

A case report of a 34-year-old white woman was suspected for genital cervical schistosomiasis. A cervical smear showed cytologic changes suggesting dysplasia and *S. haematobium* eggs inside the chorion surrounded by granulomatous inflammation. The patient showed marvelous response to praziquantel, and all clinical and histopathological changes were relieved. It was concluded that cervical schistosmiasis should be considered a curable cause of dysplasia. It was postulated that schistosomiasis of the cervix might play an additional role in HPV-induced cervical dysplasia and cancer.[89]

Evaluation of carcinogenicity of schistosomiasis
According to accepted international criteria, infection with *S. haematobium* is carcinogenic to humans (group 1); infection with *S. mansoni* is not classifiable as to its carcinogenicity to humans (group 3); and infection with *S. japonicum* is possibly carcinogenic to humans (group 2B).[90]

East Asian distomiasis

Liver and pancreas
Clonorchiasis and opisthorchiasis are caused by chronic infection of the human liver flukes in the biliary tree. The three species of flukes *Clonorchis sinensis*, *Opisthorchis viverrini*, and *Opisthorchis felineus* are closely related trematodes that have similar life cycles and they cause the same pathophysiology to the biliary tract.[91] Globally, nearly 35 million people are infected with *C. sinensis*, with approximately 15 million being in China.[92] Clonorchiasis is predominantly endemic in China, the Republic of Korea, Vietnam, and a part of Russia.[93] A similar species, *O. viverrini*, causes distomiasis in Thailand. Cholangiocarcinoma (CCA) is a cancer of the bile ducts that is considered the most severe complication of liver fluke infection. Exceptionally high incidence of CCA in Thailand and Korea is strongly related with the high prevalence of opisthorchiasis and clonorchiasis[91]; hence, *C. sinensis* and *O. viverrini* have been classified as "carcinogenic to humans" (Group 1) by the IARC in 2009.[94,95] However, infection with *O. felineus* is not classifiable as to

its carcinogenicity to humans (group 3).[94–96] The highest recorded incidence of CCA in the world is present in North-eastern Thailand, where 70–90% of the population are infected with *O. viverrini*. In Korea, where infestation with *C. sinensis* is widely prevalent, CCA accounts for more than 20% of liver cancers.

Intraductal papillary neoplasm of the bile duct is known to be a premalignant condition often associated with mucin over-production. There have been a few recent articles revealing that the disease was related with *C. sinensis* infection. Suh et al.[97] reported that 5 of 16 (31%) of intraductal papillary tumors of the bile duct were associated with *C. sinensis* infection. Jang et al.[98] reported that when CCA was associated with *C. sinensis* infection, intraductal papillary neoplasm was much more common than the usual adenocarcinoma.

Human infection results from eating raw or undercooked parasitized freshwater fish. In humans, the ingested parasites excyst in the duodenum and ascend the bile ducts and canaliculi, where they mature, causing biliary epithelial hyperplasia and fibrosis. Promotors of carcinogenesis as nitroso compounds are incriminated. In the Far East, nitrosamines are commonly found in traditional Chinese preserved foods such as salted fish, dried shrimp, and sausage.[99] Precursors of nitroso compounds have been identified in the body fluid of men infested with *O. viverrini*.[100] Pancreatic ducts may also be infected with *C. sinensis*; this frequently results in squamous metaplasia and mucous gland hyperplasia.

Malaria

The geographic distribution of BL in the classic malarial belt initially suggested the possible role of an arthropod vector in oncogenesis.[101,102] BL is a highly aggressive B-cell non-Hodgkin's lymphoma and is the fastest growing human tumor.[103] Two major epidemiological clues to the pathogenesis of BL are early infection by Epstein–Barr virus (EBV) and the geographical association with malaria. Both agents cause B-cell hyperplasia, which is almost certainly an essential component of lymphomagenesis in BL. Recent figures suggest that the incidence in children in equatorial Africa is similar to that of acute lymphoblastic lymphoma (ALL) in high-income countries—probably of the order of 3–6 per 100,000 in children aged 0–14 per year, accounting for 30–50% of all childhood cancers in equatorial Africa. This correlates with the high frequency and intensity of malaria in young children.[104] Incidence figures from other parts of the world, though limited, are considerably lower than those in equatorial Africa.[105] These data give the disease its name in Africa, endemic Burkitt lymphoma (eBL).

The possibility that drugs taken for malaria prophylaxis could have contributed to the development of BL[106,107] was considered unlikely because no increase (and indeed a decrease) in eBL was observed in the Malagasy Republic[108] and in Imesi, West Africa,[109] where intensive antimalarial prophylaxis was practiced. Interestingly, recent studies showed that chloroquine could play a role in cancer prevention.[110,111] Within endemic areas, the peak incidence of BL follows closely the incidence of severe *Plasmodium falciparum* malaria, and malarial prophylaxis reduces the incidence of the lymphoma.[108,109]

Of considerable interest are studies on the frequency of sickle-cell trait in eBL patients and controls. Persons with sickle trait are protected against the lethal effect of overwhelming *P. falciparum* malaria in early childhood and from the intense reticuloendothelial stimulation that sometimes progresses to hyper-reactive malarial splenomegaly.[112] Sickle cells exposed to low oxygen tension do not support the growth of parasites *in vitro*. A similar phenomenon

may explain why children with the sickle-cell trait have a lower *P. falciparum* parasitemia. As a result, a lower mortality rate, lower IgM levels, and reduced lymphoproliferation (as measured by spleen size) are found among individuals with hemoglobin AS genotype. However, most studies attempting to relate eBL to AS hemoglobinopathy have failed to reach statistical significance.[113,114] Other hemoglobinopathies, such as hereditary ovalocytosis, also protect against malaria. If eBL turns out to be underrepresented in populations where both ovalocytosis is prevalent, as in Papua, New Guinea,[115] such information would provide strong supporting evidence for malaria as a cofactor in the genesis of eBL.[113]

One way of explaining the observation that the malaria patient harboring a multitude of parasite-derived antigens becomes a host susceptible to eBL is the suggestion that malaria patients produce so many nonspecific and "useless" antibodies that they are unable to recognize and respond to the threat posed by a small clone of malignant lymphoid cells.[116]

Malaria and EBV

More significant are the epidemiologic observations that have linked eBL to the potentiating effect of malaria on EBV infection.[117] Endemic BL is only found in areas where malaria is holoendemic or hyperendemic; and within these areas, it is absent in malaria-free pockets, such as urban centers. Vigorous cellular and serologic responses occur during malarial infection.[118] This renders the plausible argument that persistent reticuloendothelial stimulation experienced among malarial populations conditions the EBV-infected African patient to develop a neoplasm rather than a self-limited disease, such as infectious mononucleosis.[119] The potentiation effect adopted by malaria to induce BL is B-cell hyperplasia. A cystein-rich-inter-domain-region1alpha (CIDR1a) of the *Plasmodium falciparum* erythrocyte membrane protein 1 (PfEMP1) is expressed on the surface of infected erythrocytes. This protein was shown to cause an increase in the number of circulating B cells carrying the EBV in acute malaria.[120,121] This was explained by two mechanisms; first, the protein stimulates B memory cell replication, including the B-cell compartment where EBV resides.[122] Second, CIDR1a can induce virus production from infected B cells, which in turn leads to infection of other B cells.[122–124] Acute malaria, which increases B-cell proliferation, also impairs EBV-specific T-cell responses.[101,113,125] This results in a larger pool of EBV-infected cells with increased likelihood for chromosomal translocation and lymphomagenesis.[126] Chattopadhyay et al.[127] defined a malaria-associated aberration localized to the EBV-specific CD8+ T-cell compartment.

African children with eBL develop autoantibodies, the elevated titers of which show no linear correlation with EBV titers for viral capsid antigen (VCA) or EBNA[128] suggesting that a factor independent of EBV causes an immunologic imbalance and autoantibody production. The notion that this could be due to malaria is supported by the observation that Caucasians suffering from acute *P. falciparum* malaria develop autoantibodies,[129,130] and *in vitro* experiments that demonstrated that normal human lymphocytes can produce autoantibodies as a response to malarial antigens.[131]

Chromosomal aberrations and lymphomagenesis

Overexpression of *c-myc* appears to be central to the pathogenesis of typical and atypical BL. Although *c-myc* translocation occurs in all cases of BL, differences are seen in the translocation patterns in the endemic and sporadic varieties of the disease. Typically, sporadic BL has translocations involving sequences within or immediately 5′ to *myc* on chromosome 8 and sequences within or near the immunoglobulin heavy chain S region on chromosome

14. In contrast, eBL tends to be characterized by a translocation involving sequences on chromosome 8 further upstream from *myc* and sequences within or near the JH region on chromosome 14.[131] A mechanism by which malaria can directly produce chromosomal translocations associated with BL is the interaction with toll-like receptors (TLRs),[104] which are stimulated in malaria infection by certain agonists such as haemozoin and CpG-enriched DNA, and, in turn, activate the adaptive immune system. This is explained by their ability to induce activation-induced cytidine deaminase (AID) in B cells, an enzyme that induces hyper-variable region mutations and class switch recombination as well as activating B lymphocytes.[132–134]

Recent evidences

Several studies demonstrated the relationship between several parasites and oncogenesis, for example, the relation between cryptosporidiosis and intestinal cancer.[135,136] The study done by Certad et al.[135] was the first to record that a human-derived *Cryptosporidium parvum* isolate can induce cancer in mice. Another protozoan *Trichomonas vaginalis* was incriminated. Although the latter has a possible role in cancer of the cervix, its role in prostatic cancer is still arguable.[137] Neurocysticercosis was also incriminated in hematological malignancies.[138] Parasite-induced immunomodulation, DNA damage, and nitric oxide release due to chronic inflammation were the mechanisms proposed.[139] The relationship of the nematode *Strongyloides stercoralis* to hepatobiliary cancer[140] and Kaposi sarcoma[141] was studied, as well as the role of *Toxoplasma gondii* in brain cancer[142,143] and lymphoma.[144] These parasites and others were incriminated in cancer development; however, clues are not yet sufficient to include them in the IARC roster.[137]

In view of recent revaluation of the role of parasites, it was found that infectious agents and their products can orchestrate a wide range of host immune responses, through which they may positively or negatively modulate cancer development and/or progression. Interestingly, certain types of pathogens, including parasites, can decrease the risk of tumorigenesis or lead to cancer regression.[145] *Trypanosoma cruzi* was found to decrease the incidence of experimentally induced rodent colon cancer.[146] The nematode *Trichuris suis* was investigated clinically and experimentally for its ability to alleviate diseases, such as inflammatory bowel disease (ulcerative colitis, Crohn disease), multiple sclerosis, and allergy.[147,148] The applicability of this to cancer pathology, and more specifically to tumors of the gastrointestinal system, is a question open to future investigations.[145]

Summary

When uncommon neoplasms are noted with undue frequency in countries with a high prevalence of parasitic diseases, parasites become incriminated. Many parasites were studied for a possible role in oncogenesis; however, not all of them were registered as true carcinogens by the IARC. Chronic inflammation, immunomodulation, overexpression of certain carcinogens, DNA mutations, and suppression of apoptosis are the frequent well-common mechanisms for parasite-induced oncogenesis. Besides, concomitant presence of other infectious agents is proved to be an enhancing factor in many situations. Epidemiological, cytogenetic, and animal studies were used to prove the relationship between parasites and cancer. In this view, *S. haematobium* was proved to play an important role in developing urinary BC due to chronic irritation by submucosal egg deposition, constant high levels of *N*-nitroso compounds that lead

to DNA mutations, suppression of apoptosis, and, hence, histopathological changes in the urinary epithelium. Human papilloma virus is still suspected to play an assistant role in this sequence. Other *Schistosoma* species *S. japonicum* is classified as a colorectal carcinogen especially in the Far East. Other helminthes *Clonorchis* and *Opisthorchis* are proved to induce hepatobiliary cancer. In Africa, a strong correlation between BL and EBV infection is present, with an evident enhancing role for *P. falciparum*. These and more can be viewed as possible human carcinogens in respect of chronic inflammatory process associating several parasitic infections. However, strong evidences, especially cytogenetic, are usually required. Strikingly, despite the above-mentioned data, it seemed that certain parasites can modulate the host immune response in a manner that could lead to cancer regression or prevention. This is in the prospect of revaluation of the clinical importance of infectious agents; an issue that requires future concern.

Key references

The complete reference list can be found on the Wiley Companion Digital Edition of this title (see inside front cover for login instructions).

7 Ploeg M, Aben KK, Kiemeney LA. The present and future burden of urinary bladder cancer in the world. *World J Urol.* 2009;**27**:289–293.

11 International Agency of Research on Cancer. Infection with schistosomes (*Schistosoma haematobium, Schistosoma mansoni* and *Schistosoma japonicum*). *IARC Monogr Eval Carcinog Risks Hum.* 1994;**61**:45–119.

12 Zaghloul MS. Bladder cancer and schistosomiasis. *J Egypt Natl Canc Inst.* 2012;**24**:151–159.

21 Felix AS, Soliman AS, Khaled H, et al. The changing patterns of bladder cancer in Egypt over the past 26 years. *Cancer Causes Control.* 2008;**19**(4):421–429.

22 Salem HK, Mahfouz S. Changing patterns (age, incidence, and pathologic types) of Schistosoma-associated bladder cancer in Egypt in the past decade. *Urology.* 2012;**79**(2):379–383.

23 Hamed MA, Ahmed SA, Hussein AS, El Feel A. Time series trend of bilharzial bladder cancer in Egypt and its relation to climate change: a study from 1995–2005. *IJPCR.* 2014;**6**(1):46–53.

27 Bustinduy AL, King CH. Helminthic infections: schistosomiasis. In: Farrar J, Hotez P, Junghanss T, Kang G, Lalloo D, White N, eds. *Manson's Tropical Diseases*, 23rd ed. Philadelphia, PA: Elsevier/Saunders; 2014:698–725.

29 La Vecchia C, Nagri B, D'Avanzo B, Savoldelli R, Franceshi S. Genital and urinary tract diseases and bladder cancer. *Cancer Res.* 1991;**51**:629–631.

34 Zaghloul MS, Gouda I. Bladder cancer and schistosomiasis: is there a difference for the association. In: Canda AE, ed. Bladder Cancer from Basic Science to Robotic Surgery. Croatia: In Tech open publisher, Rajeko; 2012:195–218.

36 O'Brien PJ. Radical formation during the peroxidase-catalised metabolism of carcinogens and xenobiotics. The reactivity of these radicals with GSH, DNA and unsaturated fatty lipid. *Free Radical Biol. Med.* 1988;**4**:216–226.

42 Botelho MC, Machado JC, de Costa JM. Schistosoma hematobium and bladder cancer. *Virulence.* 2010;**1**(2):84–87.

45 Lozano JC, Nakazawa H, Cros MP, Cabral R, Yamasaki H. G:T mutations in p53 and H-ras genes in esophageal papillomas induced by N-nitroso methyl benzyamine in two strains of rats. *Mol Carcinog.* 1994;**9**:33–39.

46 Osman I, Scher HI, Zhang ZF, et al. Alterations affecting the p53 control pathway in bilharzial-related bladder cancer. *Clin Cancer Res.* 1997;**3**:531–536.

50 Chung KT. The etiology of bladder cancer and its prevention. *J Cancer Sci Ther.* 2013;**5**(10):346–361.

52 Yang H, Yang K, Khafagi A, et al. Sensitive detection of human papilloma virus in cervical, head/neck, and schistosomiasis-associated bladder malignancies. *Proc Natl Acad Sci.* 2005;**102**(21):7683–7688.

59 Aji T, Matsuoka H, Ishii A, et al. Retention of a mutagen, 3 amino-1-methyl-5 H-pyrido[4,3,6] indole (Trp P2) in the liver of mice infected with S. japonicum. *Mutat Res.* 1994;**305**:265.

62 Chaudhary KS, Lu KS, Abel PD, et al. Expression of Bcl-2 and p53 oncoproteins in schistosomiasis-associated transitional and squamous cell carcinoma of the urinary bladder. *Br J Urol.* 1997;**79**:78–84.

66 Shabaan AA, Elbaz AE, Tribukait B. Primary nonurachal adenocarcinoma in the bilharzial urinary bladder: deoxyribonucleic acid flow cytometric and morphologic characterization in 93 cases. *Urology.* 1998;**51**:469.

76 Madbouly KM, Senagore AJ, Mukerjee A, et al. Colorectal cancer in a population with endemic Schistosoma mansoni: is this an at-risk population? *Int J Colorectal Dis.* 2007;**22**(2):175–181.

77 Soliman AS, Bondy ML, El-Badawy SA, et al. Contrasting molecular pathology of colorectal carcinoma in Egyptian and Western patients. *Br J Cancer.* 2001;**85**(7):1037–1046.

78 Itzkowitz SH, Yio X. Inflammation and cancer IV. Colorectal cancer in inflammatory bowel disease: the role of inflammation. *Am J Physiol Gastrointest Liver Physiol.* 2004;**287**(1):G7–17.

79 Zalata KR, Nasif WA, Ming SC, et al. p53,Bcl-2 and C-Myc expressions in colorectal carcinoma associated with schistosomiasis in Egypt. *Cell Oncol.* 2005;**27**(4):245–253.

80 Qiu DC, Hubbard AE, Zhong B, Zhang Y, Spear RC. A matched, case–control study of the association between Schistosoma japonicum and liver and colon cancers, in rural China. *Ann Trop Med Parasitol.* 2005;**99**(1):47–52.

88 Mazigo HD, Zinga M, Heukelbach J, Rambau P. Case series of adenocarcinoma of the prostate associated with Schistosoma haematobium infection in Tanzania. *J Global Infect Dis.* 2010;**2**(3):307–309.

89 Dzeing-Ella A, Mechaï F, Consigny PH, Zerat L, et al. Case report: cervical Schistosomiasis as a risk factor of cervical uterine dysplasia in a traveler. *Am J Trop Med Hyg.* 2009;**81**(4):549–550.

91 Lim JH. Liver Flukes: the Malady Neglected. *Korean J Radiol.* 2011;**12**(3):269–279.

93 Qian MB, Chen YD, Liang S, Yang GJ, Zhou XN. The global epidemiology of clonorchiasis and its relation with cholangiocarcinoma. *Infect Dis Poverty.* 2012;**1**:4. http://www.idpjournal.com/content/1/1/4.

94 Bouvard V, Baan R, Straif K, et al. WHO international agency for research on cancer monograph working group: a review of human carcinogens—part B: biological agents. *Lancet Oncol.* 2009;**10**:321–322.

99 Schwartz DA. Cholangiocarcinoma associated with liver fluke infection: a preventable source of morbidity in Asian immigrants. *Am J Gastroenterol.* 1986;**81**(1):76–79.

103 De Leval L, Hasserjan RP. Diffuse large B-cell lymphomas and Burkitt lymphoma. *Hematol Oncol Clin North Am.* 2009;**23**:791–827.

110 Maclean KH, Dorsey FC, Cleveland JL, Kastan MB. Targeting lysosomal degradation induces p53-dependent cell death and prevents cancer in mouse models of lymphogenesis. *J Clin Invest.* 2008;**118**:79–88.

111 Dang CV. Antimalarial therapy prevents Myc-induced lymphoma. *J Clin Invest.* 2008;**118**(1):15–17.

112 Morrow RH, Sever JL, Henderson BE. Antibody levels to infectious agents other than Epstein-Barr virus in Burkitt's lymphoma patients. *Cancer Res.* 1974; **34**:1212.

113 Whittle HC, Brown J, Marsh K, et al. T-cell control of Epstein-Barr virus-infected B-cells is lost during P falciparum malaria. *Nature.* 1984;**312**:449.

119 O'Conor GT. Persistent immunologic stimulation as a factor in oncogenesis with special reference to Burkitt's tumor. *Am J Med.* 1970;**48**:279.

120 Moormann AM, Chelimo K, Sumba OP, Cynthia JB, Chelimo K. Exposure to holoendemic malaria results in elevated Epstein–Barr virus loads in children. *J Infect Dis.* 2005;**19**:1233–1238.

125 Mulama D, Chelimo K, Collins O, Jura W, Otieno J, et al. EBNA-1 specific effector T cell deletion associated with holoendemic malaria exposure in the etiology of endemic Burkitt's lymphoma (P3063). *J Immunol.* 2013;**190**:187.7.

135 Certad G, Benamrouz S, Guyot K, et al. Fulminant cryptosporidiosis after near-drowning: a human Cryptosporidium parvum strain implicated in invasive gastrointestinal adenocarcinoma and cholangiocarcinoma in an experimental model. *Appl Environ Microbiol.* 2012;**78**(6):1746–1751.

141 Lin CJ, Katongole-Mbidde E, Byekwaso T, Orem J, Rabkin CS, Mbulaiteye SM. Intestinal parasites in Kaposi Sarcoma patients in Uganda: indication of shared risk factors or etiologic association. *Am J Trop Med Hyg.* 2008;**78**(3): 409–412.

143 Thomas F, Lafferty KD, Brodeur J, et al. Incidence of adult brain cancers is higher in countries where the protozoan parasite Toxoplasma gondii is common. *Biol Lett.* 2012;**8**(1):101–103.

Epidemiology, Prevention and Detection

33 The burden of cancer worldwide: current and future perspectives

Jacques Ferlay, MSc, ME ▪ *Christopher P. Wild, PhD* ▪ *Freddie Bray, PhD*

Overview

Cancer, once seen as a problem only of high-income countries, is now a leading global cause of death responsible for one in three premature deaths from non-communicable diseases. The global trend is set to continue over the next decades through population and lifestyle changes, part of an ongoing demographic and epidemiologic transition that will see the 14 million new cancer cases and 8 million cancer deaths estimated worldwide in 2012 rise by 55% by 2030. This chapter has three main aims. The first is to portray the marked diversity in the scale and profile of cancer in different regions of the world. Secondly, we point to the transitional nature of cancer incidence, showing that the rising incidence rates and shifting profiles of common cancers are linked to societal and economic change. Thirdly, present inequities are highlighted in countries undergoing transition, where a rising cancer incidence and mortality burden is often matched by limited data for planning purposes and an absence of operational national cancer plans. We conclude by discussing the means to improve data in resource-constrained settings for cancer control action through the planning and development of population-based cancer registries.

Introduction

Cancer, once seen as a problem of the industrialized world and high-income countries, is now a leading cause of morbidity and mortality in the majority of countries of the world. Mortality statistics from the World Health Organization (WHO) for 2011 reveal that cancer is of greater frequency as a cause of death than either ischemic heart disease or stroke, or chronic obstructive pulmonary disease and lower respiratory infections combined. The disease now constitutes one in four NCD (non-communicable disease)-related deaths overall and one in three-related NCD deaths below the age of 70. The global trend is set to intensify over the next two or three decades as population and lifestyle changes, part of an ongoing demographic and epidemiologic transition, continue to take hold. The 14 million new cancer cases and 8 million cancer deaths estimated worldwide in 2012 is projected to rise by 55% by 2030.

The impact will be greatest in the so-called developing world and countries undergoing rapid social and economic changes. An increasingly disproportionate burden of cancer will therefore fall in Africa, Asia, and Latin America, putting strain on lower-resource countries in these regions already ill-equipped at present to deal with the need for cancer services for an increasing number of cancer patients.

This chapter has three primary aims. The first is to highlight, using such global statistics, the marked diversity of cancer in terms of its scale and the range of frequent cancer forms observed in different regions of the world. Seen at the country level, 20 different

cancer types rank within the five most frequent causes of cancer incidence or mortality by sex, and we briefly review and elucidate the cancer-specific patterns. Secondly, we point to the transitional nature of the cancer burden from a temporal perspective, showing that the rising incidence and shifting profiles of cancer are linked to societal and economic changes within countries and utilize trends in the human development index (HDI) as a national proxy for such changes. Thirdly, we link the estimation and interpretation back to the express purpose of these descriptive results, to advocate for, and support the implementation of cancer control actions. We underline the present inequities seen in countries under transition where the rising cancer burden is often matched by a lack of data fit for cancer control purposes and an absence of operational national cancer plans. We discuss the means to improve the cancer data in resource-constrained settings to inform planning through the development of population-based cancer registries (PBCR). We conclude by stressing the need to implement prevention strategies alongside those of cancer treatment, management, and palliative care and integrate these into NCD plans.

Following this introduction, the next section reviews the definitions of the key indicators for cancer, the available data sources, and the methods of estimation used to derive cancer incidence, mortality, and prevalence at the national level and the global estimates within GLOBOCAN. The third section examines the key aspects of the cancer burden by development level and the patterns of the eight most frequent cancers worldwide, briefly noting the major causes for the variations observed. The fourth section focuses on human development and the extent to which socioeconomic transitions are changing the scale and profile of cancer worldwide. The final section links these findings to the equitable delivery of national cancer control policies to avert the increasing burden. We discuss the overwhelming need for better data for cancer planning in resource-constrained settings, as an integral part of global cancer control strategies. The descriptive epidemiology contained in this chapter provides strong support for prioritizing primary and secondary preventions, as an essential means to ameliorate the rising future cancer burden.

Definitions, data sources, and methods

The International Agency for Research on Cancer (IARC) is recognized as a definitive reference source for global cancer information; in addition, over the past 40 years, the Agency has prepared updated estimates of the worldwide burden from cancer. Beginning in 1975 with broad estimates of numbers of new cases for 12 common types of cancer in different areas of the world,[1] IARC now provides detailed country-specific estimates of incidence, mortality, and prevalence, by sex and age group for 27 types of cancer through the GLOBOCAN series.[2] An emphasis has been consistently placed on directly estimating the magnitude of cancer using locally recorded

Holland-Frei Cancer Medicine, Ninth Edition. Edited by Robert C. Bast Jr., Carlo M. Croce, William N. Hait, Waun Ki Hong, Donald W. Kufe, Martine Piccart-Gebhart, Raphael E. Pollock, Ralph R. Weichselbaum, Hongyang Wang, and James F. Holland.
© 2017 John Wiley & Sons, Inc. ISBN: 978-1-118-93469-2

data at the country level, either from PBCR (new cancer cases) or from vital registration systems (cancer deaths), wherever the source information is available. Methods of estimation are refined with every iteration of GLOBOCAN as the quality and availability of the data increases. The latest release contains estimates for the year 2012,[2] with online facilities for the tabulation and graphical description of the full dataset for 184 countries and 30 world regions by sex (http://globocan.iarc.fr). In the following discussion, we define the core measures of incidence, mortality, and prevalence used in this chapter and the underlying data sources that build up the global profile of cancer.

Incidence, the number of new cases occurring, can be expressed as an absolute number of cases per unit time (commonly in years), as a rate per 100,000 person-time, or as a cumulative risk (expressed as a percentage) of developing a cancer up to a certain age (commonly up to 75 years), assuming an absence of competing causes of death. Incidence data are produced by PBCR, which routinely and systematically collect information on all new cases of cancer within a defined population. PBCR may cover entire national populations but more often cover smaller, subnational areas, and particularly in less developed countries, only major urban areas (cities). Less than one-quarter of the world population is covered by population-based cancer registries currently, with sparse registration in Asia (8% of the total population) and in Africa (11%).[3] When considering data of high quality [e.g., datasets included in the latest volume (X) of the *Cancer Incidence in Five Continents* (CI5) series,[4,5]] these percentages are lower, and only 14% of the world population is covered with cancer registries that match the CI5 inclusion criteria. Presently, about one in every three (mainly higher-income) countries have high-quality PBCR. While the information from some registries in lower resource settings does not currently meet the quality standards of CI5, it is still of unique importance as a relatively unbiased source of data for cancer control purposes (see section titled "Integrating Population-Based Cancer Registries"). PBCR may also produce survival statistics by following up the vital status of registered cancer patients. Survival represents the probability that an individual with cancer will not die from it and can be used to estimate mortality from incidence in the absence of mortality data and vice versa.

Mortality is the number of deaths occurring and, as with incidence, is expressed in terms of numbers of deaths, or as a rate or cumulative risk. Mortality is the product of incidence and the *case fatality* (the inverse of survival). Mortality statistics are collected and made available by the WHO. Their advantages are national coverage and long-term availability, although for some countries, coverage of the population is incomplete, so that the mortality rates produced are implausibly low, while in others, the reliability of cause of death information is questionable. By 2003, around one-third of the world population was covered by mortality statistics,[6] although less than half of the countries producing data currently report statistics of high quality to WHO. While almost all European and American countries have comprehensive death registration systems, most African and Asian countries (including the populous countries of Nigeria, India, Indonesia, and Pakistan) do not. The mortality data used to estimate the burden of cancer in China is available from a sample survey based on the "disease surveillance points" project covering around 6% of the total Chinese population. These statistics are considered nationally representative given the samples include both urban and rural areas.

Prevalence measures the absolute number (or relative proportion) of individuals alive in the population at a particular point in time and affected by the disease. Although incidence and mortality are considered the key measurements of cancer burden, prevalence is an important supplementary indicator for developing strategies for service provision. Unlike incidence and mortality, however, there is no clear definition of cancer prevalence. Total (or complete) prevalence is the number of persons in a defined population alive at a given time who have had cancer diagnosed at some time in the past, even if this was many years ago, and the person is cured. Beyond measures of numbers of persons living with cancer, prevalence is usually of greater utility for planning purposes to consider only those persons requiring some form of cancer services and by partitioning prevalence into defined phases of cancer care. Therefore, cancer prevalence is generally presented as the number of persons still alive after a given number of years following diagnosis.[7] We use 5-year prevalence in this chapter and define it as the number of persons alive at the end of 2012 who had been diagnosed with cancer in the previous 5 years, a surrogate for care requirements (diagnosis, initial treatment, and follow-up) before the point of cure; this may be less useful for cancer survivors who require some form of care beyond 5 years, such as for female breast cancer where the disease remains a chronic condition affecting average prognosis decades after initial diagnosis.[8]

The global incidence, mortality, and prevalence estimates in GLOBOCAN are built up from within-country data sources considered the most recent and reliable in a given country. The methods used in the estimation process have been described in detail in various reports[2,7,9] and are summarized in Table 1.

Global cancer diversity

The burden of cancer worldwide

Table 2 presents the estimated number of new cases and deaths by sex, together with the risk of developing the disease before the age of 75 years, for 27 major cancers and for all cancers combined (excluding non-melanoma skin cancers) for the year 2012. Figure 1 shows the distribution of cancer incidence and mortality together with 5-year prevalence by continent and region/country. There were over 14 million new cancer cases in 2012, 8.2 million cancer deaths, and more than 32 million persons living with cancer (within 5 years of their diagnosis). Around half of the incidence burden occurs within Asia and almost a quarter (22%) in China and a further 7% in India. A further one-quarter of the burden resides in Europe with the remainder divided between the Americas and Africa, with 1% in Oceania. The relative proportions of cancer-related deaths are higher in Asia and Africa and lower in Europe and North America reflecting the frequency of cancer types associated with a poorer prognosis, as well as lower survival for certain frequent cancers treatable at early stages.

Lung cancer remains the most common cancer worldwide, both in terms of numbers of new cases (1.8 million) and deaths (1.6 million deaths). Breast cancer is the second most common cancer overall (1.7 million cases) but ranks fifth as a cause of cancer death (522,000 deaths) reflecting a more favorable average prognosis. These two neoplasms are followed, in terms of incidence, by colorectal cancer (1.4 million cases, 694,000 deaths), prostate cancer (1.1 million cases, 307,000 deaths), and stomach cancer (952,000 cases, 723,000 deaths). These five cancers represent almost half the global incidence burden in 2012.

Around 32.5 million people were alive and living with a cancer diagnosed in the previous 5 years at the end of 2012 (Table 2). By far, the most prevalent cancer (in both sexes) is female breast cancer (Figure 2), with an estimated 6.3 million women living with the disease. The second most prevalent cancer is prostate affecting

Table 1 Data quality and methods of estimation for the year 2012: status of 184 countries presented in GLOBOCAN.

		Status	Number of countries
Mortality			
	Data quality		
	1	Vital registration	95
	2	Incomplete or sample vital registration	2
	3	Other sources (cancer registries, verbal autopsy surveys, etc.)	7
	4	No data	80
	Methods		
	1	Rates projected/applied to 2012	95
	2	Estimated as the weighted average of regional rates	1
	3	Estimated from national incidence estimates and modeled survival	85
	4	The rates are those of neighboring countries or registries in the same area	3
			184
Incidence			
	Data quality		
	1	High-quality national data or high-quality regional	67
	2	National data (rates)	24
	3	Regional data (rates)	18
	4	Frequency data	13
	5	No data	62
	Methods		
	1	Rates projected/applied to 2012	58
	2	Estimated from national mortality estimates using modeled incidence mortality ratios	22
	3	Estimated from national mortality estimates using modeled survival	32
	4	Estimated as the weighted average of the local rate(s)	27
	5	Age/sex-specific rates for "all cancers" were partitioned using data on relative frequency of different cancers	12
	6	The rates are those of neighboring countries or registries in the same area	33
			184
Prevalence			
	Methods		
	1	Estimated from national incidence estimates and country-specific survival	32
	2	Estimated from national incidence estimates and pooled regional survival	152
			184

Source: GLOBOCAN 2012.

3.9 million men, closely followed by colorectal cancer (3.5 million). Prevalence reflects the integration of incidence and prognosis, and lung cancer, the most frequent cancer globally but one associated with a poor prognosis, has a 5-year prevalence (1.9 million) rather close to the annual mortality figure, ranking in fourth place.

Patterns of cancer by level of development
In the following discussion, we use four levels of HDI, (low, medium, high, and very high) as a proxy for social and economic development (Ref. 10; http://hdr.undp.org/en). HDI is a composite measure of life expectancy at birth, access to education, and income [GDP (gross domestic product) per capita]. While HDI is highly correlated with GNI (gross national income), HDI additionally provides an indication as to how income is spent in a country, at least in the areas of health and education (Figure 3a).

Figure 3b–e draws attention to the diverse cancer incidence and mortality profiles globally and according to broad levels of HDI. The relative frequency of different cancers is determined by key reproductive and lifestyle determinants of cancer and the availability of health services including early detection and clinical interventions driven by the level of resources and extent of inequalities in individual countries, and thus, the degree of societal and economic transition. In regions with either high or very high HDI levels (Figure 3c), breast, lung, colorectal, and prostate cancer explain half the overall cancer incidence burden, with stomach cancer in fifth; this is a common "top five" profile in many high-income countries, and because of the relative contribution of these geographic areas to the burden worldwide (56%), it is equivalent to the world profile for incidence (Figure 3b); it is also worth noting that

pancreatic cancer, a tumor associated with a very dismal prognosis, now lies in fifth place as a cause of cancer deaths in high and very high HDI countries. In low HDI (Figure 3e) and medium HDI (Figure 3d) regions, esophageal, stomach, liver, and cervical cancer remain common cancers. The profile in medium HDI settings is not dissimilar to that of China, which, given its population size (1.35 billion inhabitants), comprises two-fifths of the medium HDI burden. In low HDI settings including many Eastern African and other sub-Saharan African countries, there is a residual burden from cancer associated with the HIV/AIDS (human immunodeficiency virus infection and acquired immune deficiency syndrome) epidemic, including Kaposi sarcoma, an HIV-associated cancer caused by human herpes virus-8; rates are however declining due to a decline in HIV prevalence and an increasing availability of highly active antiretroviral therapy.[11–13]

Figure 4a and b shows the global distribution of the estimated risk of dying from cancer (before the age of 75 years) in men and women. High risks of cancer mortality in men are seen in Europe and the Americas (Figure 4a), and mortality is also elevated in a number of Central and Eastern Asian countries including Kazakhstan and China, where lung cancer is the most frequent cause of male cancer incidence and mortality (Figure 5a). In women, there are substantive mortality risks in Eastern and Southern Africa, where the burden from both cervical cancer and breast cancer is high in many countries in these regions.

Patterns for eight major cancer types
A brief description of the global patterns of the eight most common cancers globally follows.

Table 2 Estimated cancer incidence, mortality, and prevalence by cancer site and sex, worldwide 2012.

Cancer site	Incidence						Mortality						Prevalence		
	Both sexes		Male		Female		Both sexes		Male		Female		Numbers (×1000)		
	Cases (×1000)	Cumulative risk (0–74)	Cases (×1000)	Cumulative risk (0–74)	Cases (×1000)	Cumulative risk (0–74)	Deaths (×1000)	Cumulative risk (0–74)	Deaths (×1000)	Cumulative risk (0–74)	Deaths (×1000)	Cumulative risk (0–74)	Both sexes	Male	Female
Lip, oral cavity	300	0.5	199	0.6	101	0.3	145	0.2	98	0.3	47	0.1	702	467	235
Nasopharynx	87	0.1	61	0.2	26	0.1	51	0.1	36	0.1	15	0.0	229	162	67
Other pharynx	142	0.2	115	0.4	27	0.1	96	0.2	78	0.3	19	0.1	310	251	59
Esophagus	456	0.7	323	1.1	133	0.4	400	0.6	281	0.9	119	0.3	465	337	128
Stomach	952	1.4	631	2.0	320	0.8	723	1.0	469	1.4	254	0.6	1538	1031	507
Colon and rectum	1361	2.0	746	2.4	614	1.6	694	0.9	374	1.0	320	0.7	3543	1953	1590
Liver	782	1.1	554	1.7	228	0.6	746	1.0	521	1.6	224	0.6	633	453	180
Gallbladder	178	0.2	77	0.2	101	0.3	143	0.2	60	0.2	82	0.2	205	90	115
Pancreas	338	0.5	178	0.6	160	0.4	330	0.4	174	0.5	157	0.4	211	114	97
Larynx	157	0.3	138	0.5	19	0.1	83	0.1	73	0.2	10	0.0	442	389	53
Lung	1825	2.7	1242	3.9	583	1.6	1590	2.2	1099	3.3	491	1.2	1893	1267	626
Melanoma of skin	232	0.3	121	0.4	111	0.3	55	0.1	31	0.1	24	0.1	870	453	417
Kaposi sarcoma	44	0.1	29	0.1	15	0.0	27	0.0	17	0.1	10	0.0	80	55	25
Breast	1677	4.6	—	—	1677	4.6	522	1.4	—	—	522	1.4	6255	—	6255
Cervix uteri	528	1.4	—	—	528	1.4	266	0.8	—	—	266	0.8	1547	—	1547
Corpus uteri	320	1.0	—	—	320	1.0	76	0.2	—	—	76	0.2	1217	—	1217
Ovary	239	0.7	—	—	239	0.7	152	0.4	—	—	152	0.4	587	—	587
Prostate	1112	3.8	1112	3.8	—	—	307	0.6	307	0.6	—	—	3924	3924	—
Testis	55	0.1	55	0.1	—	—	10	0.0	10	0.0	—	—	215	215	—
Kidney	338	0.5	214	0.7	124	0.3	143	0.2	91	0.3	53	0.1	907	581	326
Bladder	430	0.6	330	1.0	99	0.2	165	0.2	123	0.3	42	0.1	1319	1018	301
Brain, nervous system	256	0.3	140	0.4	117	0.3	189	0.3	106	0.3	83	0.2	343	190	153
Thyroid	298	0.4	68	0.2	230	0.6	40	0.1	13	0.0	27	0.1	1206	271	935
Hodgkin lymphoma	66	0.1	39	0.1	27	0.1	25	0.0	15	0.0	10	0.0	188	108	80
Non-Hodgkin lymphoma	386	0.5	218	0.6	168	0.4	200	0.3	115	0.3	84	0.2	832	463	369
Multiple myeloma	114	0.2	62	0.2	52	0.2	80	0.1	43	0.1	37	0.1	229	125	104
Leukemia	352	0.4	201	0.5	151	0.4	265	0.3	151	0.4	114	0.3	501	285	216
All cancers excluding non-melanoma skin cancer	14090	18.5	7427	21	6663	16.4	8201	10.5	4653	12.7	3548	8.4	32544	15362	17182

Source: GLOBOCAN 2012.

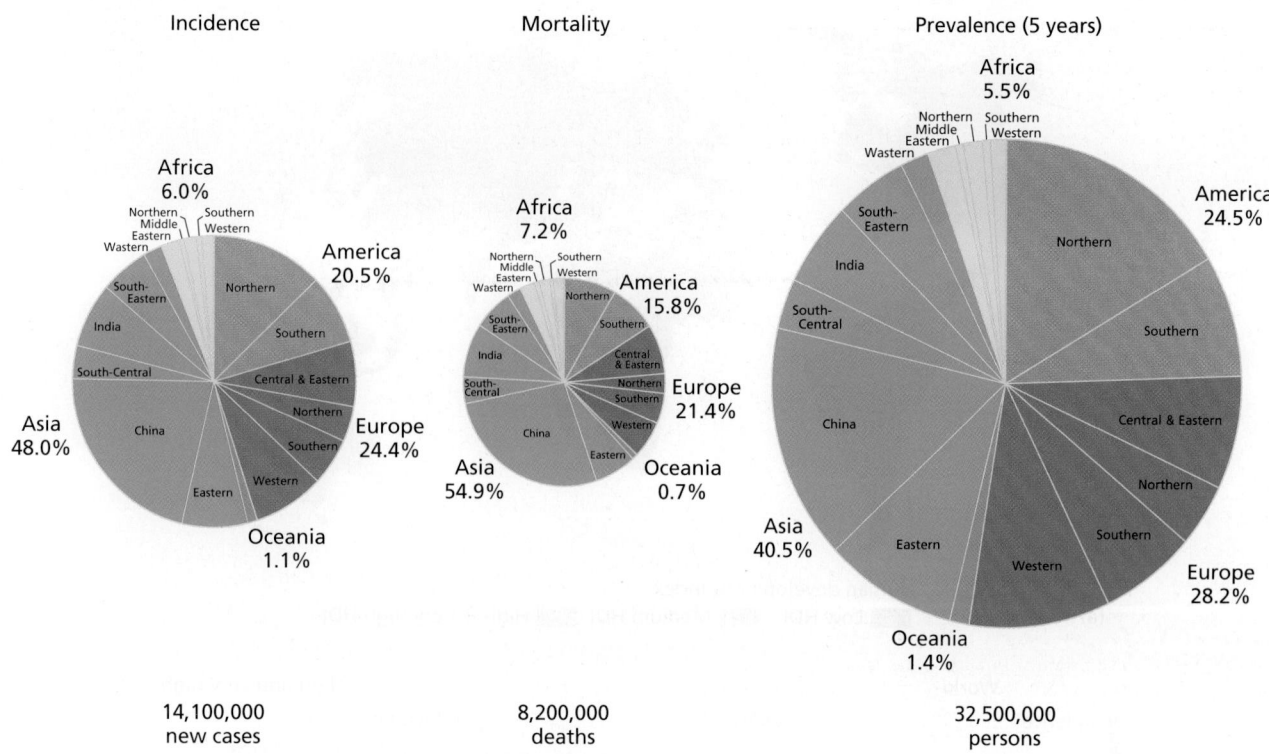

Figure 1 Global burden of cancer in 2012: estimated incidence, mortality, and 5-year prevalence by continent. Source: GLOBOCAN 2012.

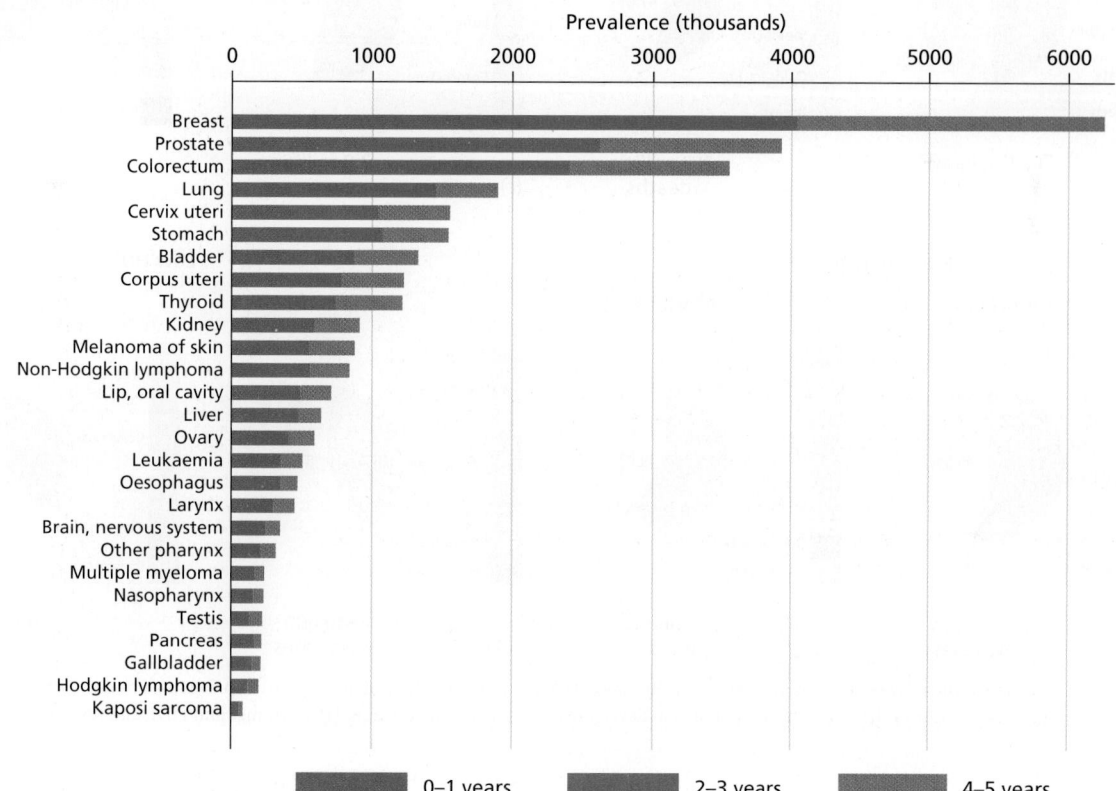

Figure 2 Bar chart of global 5-year cancer prevalence (millions) by cancer site; stacked bars denote prevalence among patients alive at end-2012 diagnosed in 2012, 2010–2011, and 2008–2009, respectively; for example, <1 year, 2–3, and 4–5 years after diagnosis. Both sexes and ages 15 years and above, sorted by magnitude of prevalence. Source: GLOBOCAN 2012.

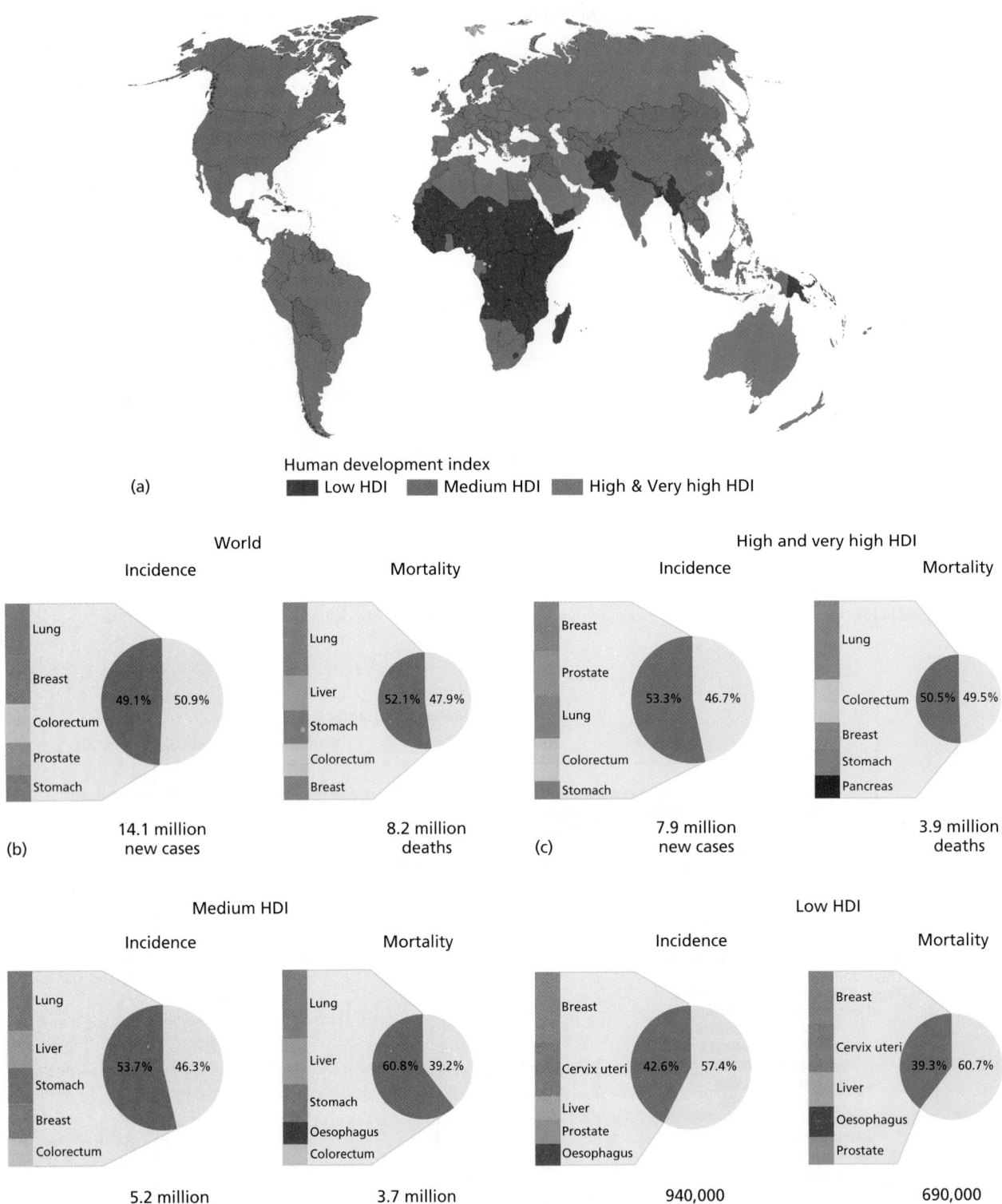

Figure 3 (a) Map depicting three levels of the human development index (HDI) in 2012; pie charts depicting. (b) Top five most frequent cancers in terms of incidence and mortality 2012 worldwide and by level of human development: (c) high and very high HDI, (d) medium HDI, and (e) low HDI. Source: GLOBOCAN 2012.

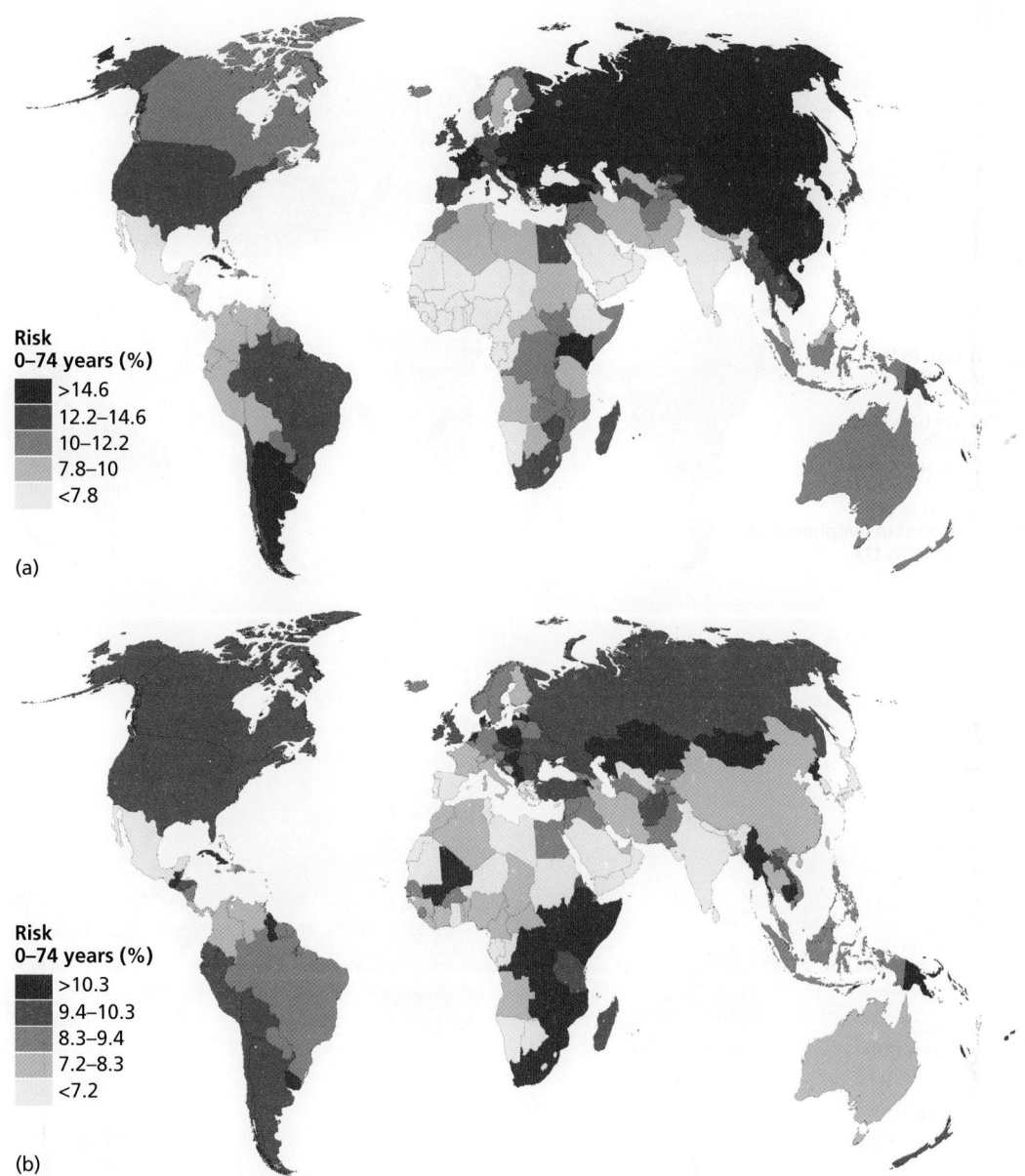

Figure 4 Maps depicting the global distribution of the cumulative risk (%) of dying from cancer (before the age of 75 years) in (a) men and (b) women in 2012. Source: GLOBOCAN 2012.

Lung

Lung cancer remains the most frequent cancer worldwide. There were more than 1.8 million new cases (13% of total cancer incidence) and almost 1.6 million deaths (20% of total cancer mortality). More than one-third of all newly diagnosed cases occurred in China. Lung cancer is the leading cause of cancer incidence in 38 countries in men (Figure 5a), but it is the leading cause of cancer mortality in men (89 countries) and the most common cause of cancer death in women in 26 countries. Owing to a high and rather stable case fatality rate, patterns and trends for mortality rates are similar to those for incidence rates, irrespective of level of resource within a given country. Recent trends in lung cancer reflect the evolution of the smoking epidemic,[14] and in men, incidence rates have peaked and begun to decline in a number of highly developed countries at a late stage of the epidemic, while rates continue to rise among women. Only in a few countries (in Northern Europe, Australia, and the United States), where the epidemic is most advanced and smoking prevalence has been

declining for several decades are there recent peaks or downward turns in female incidence rates. The prevalence of smoking in men has however increased sharply in many middle income countries, including China and Indonesia.[15] The future burden of lung cancer and other smoking-related cancers will largely depend on future sex-specific smoking patterns, including the smoking duration, the extent of cessation, and the types of tobacco smoked.[16]

Breast

Breast cancer is by far the most frequently diagnosed cancer and cause of cancer death among women. There were an estimated 1.7 million new cases (25% of all cancers in women) and 0.5 million cancer deaths (15% of all cancer deaths in women). Breast cancer is the most common cancer diagnosis in women in 140 countries (Figure 5) and the most frequent cause of cancer mortality in 101. About 42% of the estimated new cases and 34% of the cancer deaths occurred in Europe and North America. Mortality rates vary approximately 2.5-fold worldwide, with the case fatality rate

(a)

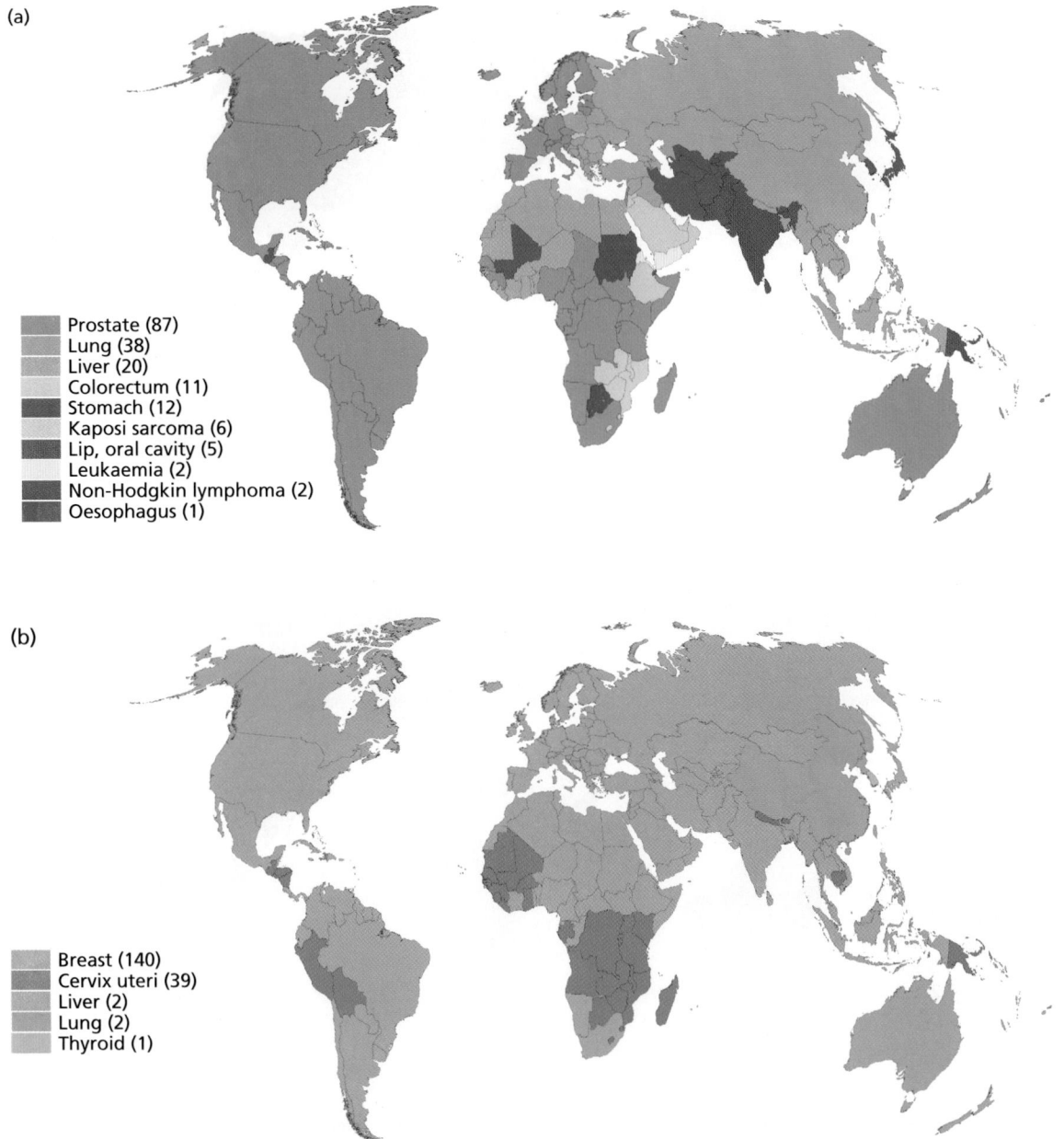

Prostate (87)
Lung (38)
Liver (20)
Colorectum (11)
Stomach (12)
Kaposi sarcoma (6)
Lip, oral cavity (5)
Leukaemia (2)
Non-Hodgkin lymphoma (2)
Oesophagus (1)

(b)

Breast (140)
Cervix uteri (39)
Liver (2)
Lung (2)
Thyroid (1)

Figure 5 Maps depicting the most frequently occurring form of cancer in 2012 in 184 countries in (a) males and (b) females. Source: GLOBOCAN 2012.

higher in lesser developed countries. While incidence has been generally increasing in most areas of the world (Figure 6a), breast cancer has peaked and declined over the past decade or so in a number of highly developed countries, part-linked to the impact of national screening and in some, to a population-wide reduction in the prevalence of HRT (hormone replacement therapy) use. Mortality rates have been declining in a number of highly developed countries since the late 1980s and early 1990s, a result of a combination of earlier diagnosis and treatment including a number of breakthroughs in effective therapeutics.

Prostate

Globally, prostate cancer is the second most frequently diagnosed cancer and the fifth most common cause of cancer death among men, with an estimated 1.1 million new cases (15% of all cancers in men) and 0.3 million cancer deaths (7% of all cancer deaths in men). In 2012, 60% of the estimated new cases but only 41% of the

cancer deaths occurred in Europe and North America. Mortality rates are highest in countries and areas with predominantly black populations—in the Caribbean and in parts of sub-Saharan Africa—but mortality rates are also high in certain northern European countries, such as the Nordic countries. Incidence rates of prostate cancer vary more than 25-fold worldwide. The highest rates are in Australia and New Zealand, Northern and Western Europe, and North America. Prostate cancer is the most frequent type of cancer among men in 87 countries worldwide in 2012, largely in countries that have attained high or very high levels of human development, but also in several countries in Central and Southern Africa (Figure 5a). Incidence rates increased dramatically in the late-1980s in North America and the Nordic countries as prostate-specific antigen (PSA) testing became available; a similar pattern developed in many of the highest-resource countries during the 1990s (Figure 6b). Incidence rates have leveled off in some of these countries but continue to uniformly increase in countries transitioning toward higher levels of human development.

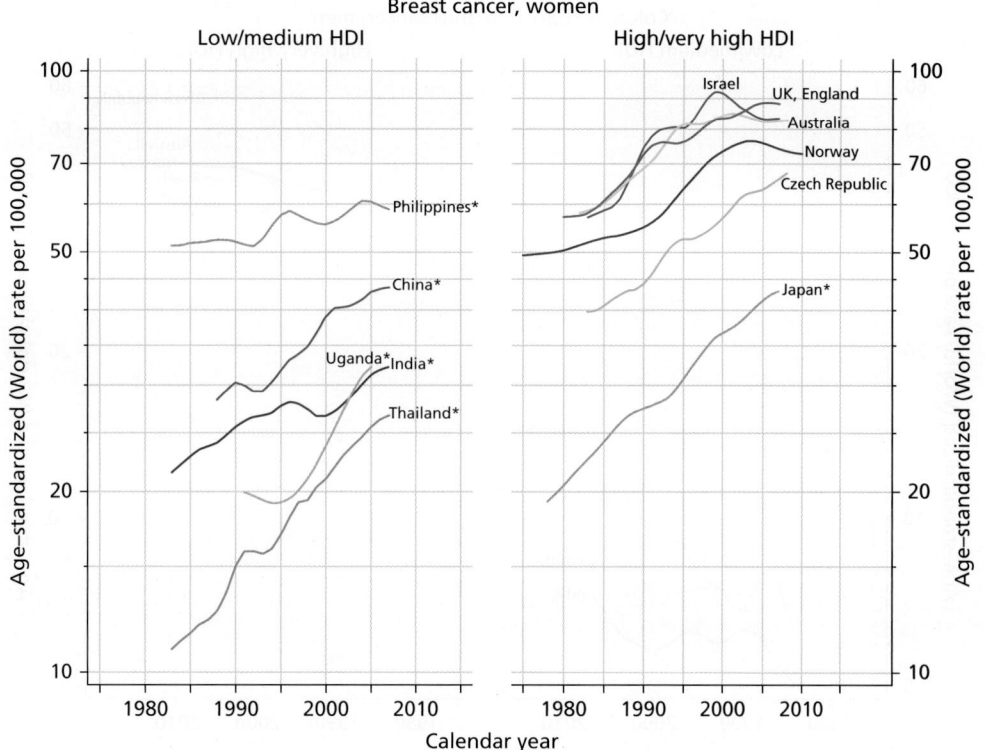

National data except*: China (Hong-Kong and Shangai), India (Chennai and Mumbay), Philippines (Manila),
Japan (Miyagi, Nagasaki and Osaka), Thailand (Chiang Mai), Uganda (Kampala)

(a)

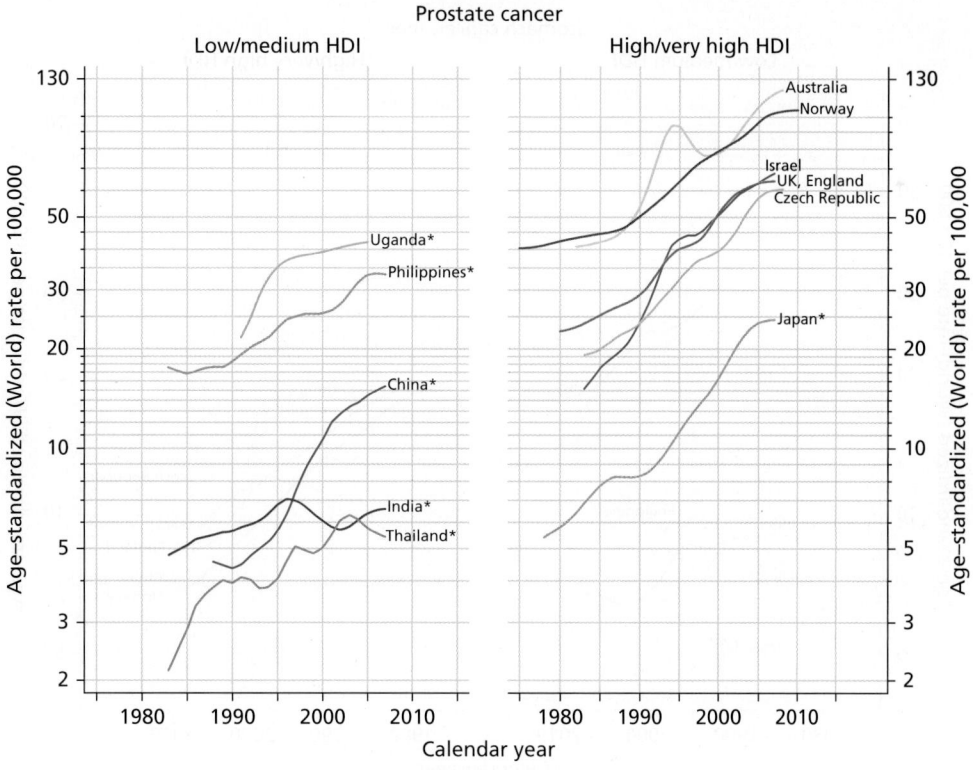

National data except*: China (Hong-Kong and Shangai), India (Chennai and Mumbay), Philippines (Manila),
Japan (Miyagi, Nagasaki and Osaka), Thailand (Chiang Mai), Uganda (Kampala)

(b)

Figure 6 Time trends in incidence of cancer of (a) female breast, (b) prostate, (c) colorectum (males), (d) stomach (males), and (e) cervix. Rates are smoothed using lowess regression. Source: Cancer Incidence in Five Continents.

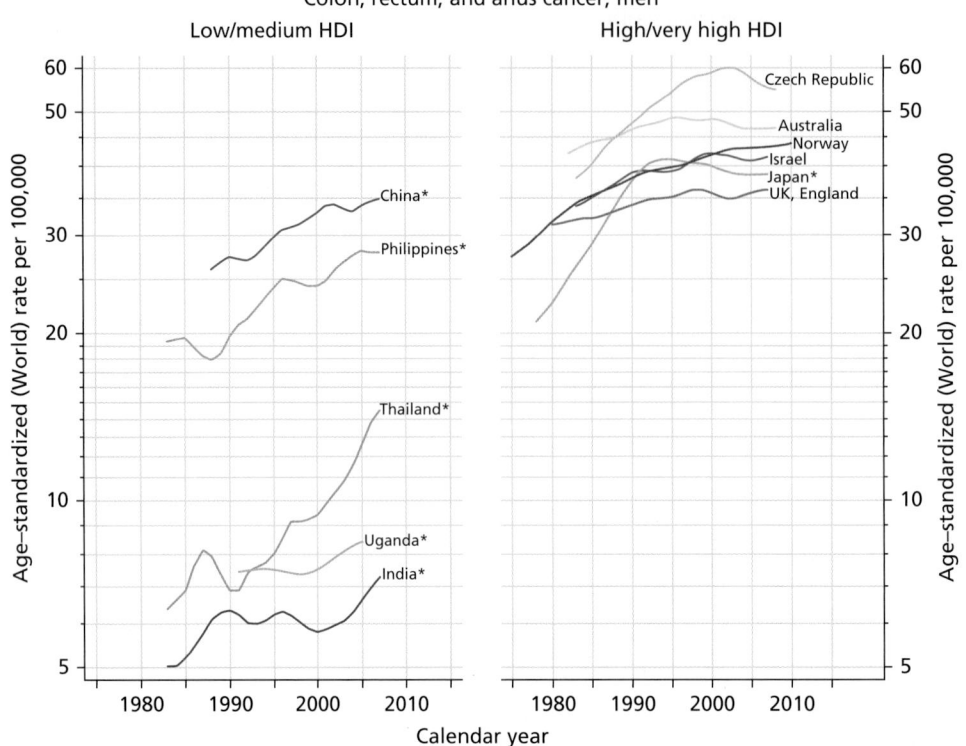

(c)

National data except*: China (Hong-Kong and Shangai), India (Chennai and Mumbay), Philippines (Manila), Japan (Miyagi, Nagasaki and Osaka), Thailand (Chiang Mai), Uganda (Kampala)

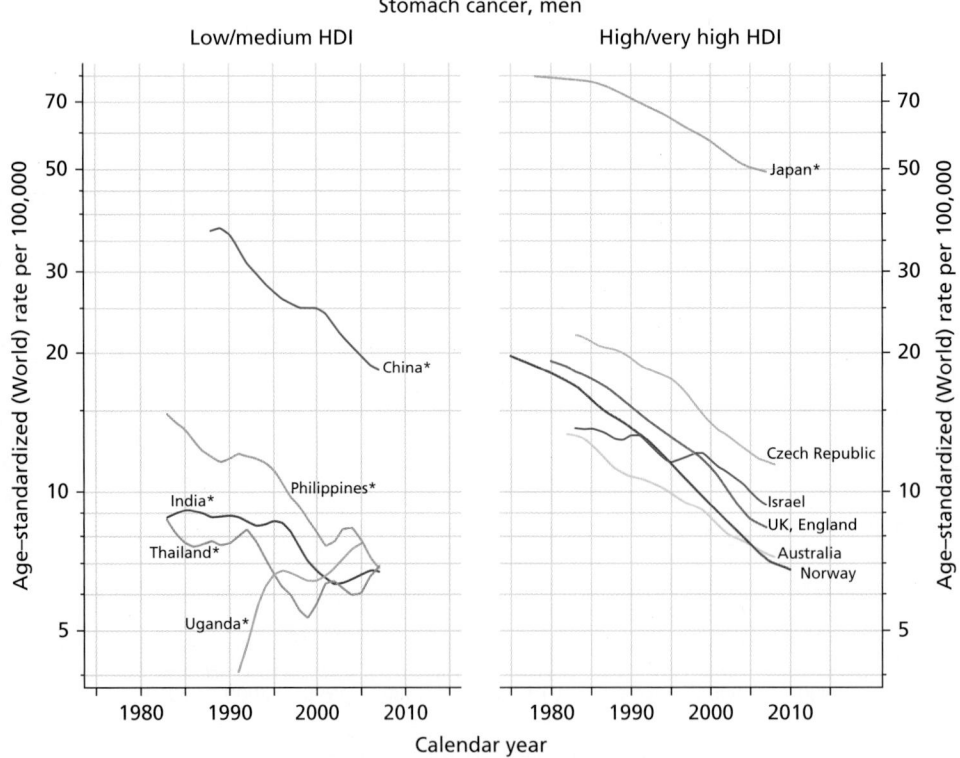

(d)

National data except*: China (Hong-Kong and Shangai), India (Chennai and Mumbay), Philippines (Manila), Japan (Miyagi, Nagasaki and Osaka), Thailand (Chiang Mai), Uganda (Kampala)

Figure 6 (*Continued*)

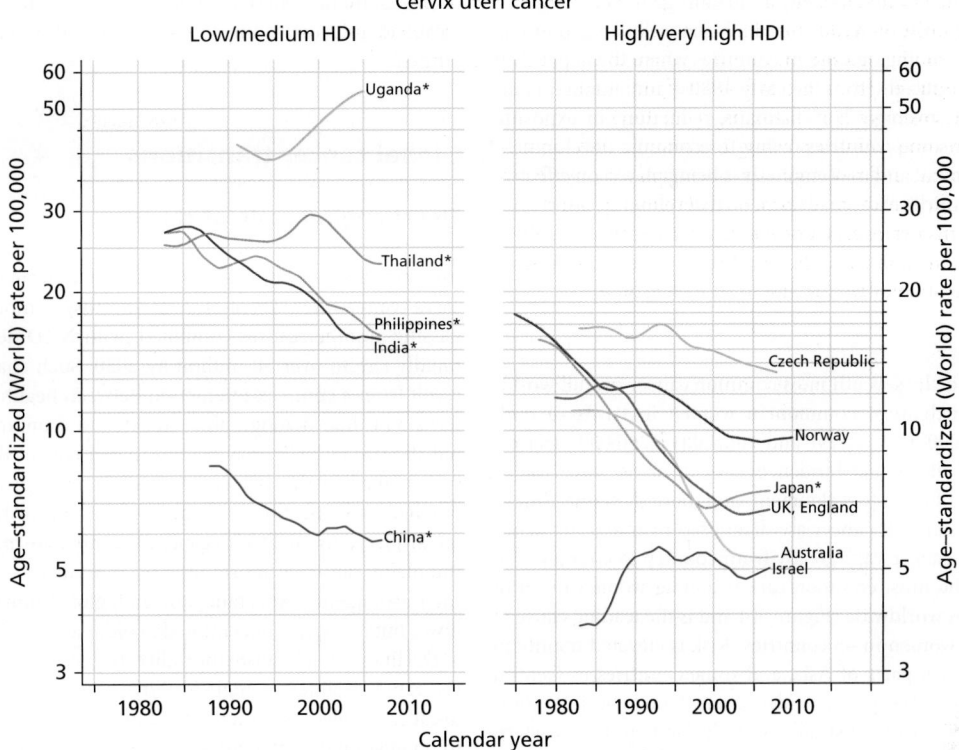

Cervix uteri cancer

(e)

National data except *: China (Hong-Kong and Shangai), India (Chennai and Mumbay), Philippines (Manila), Japan (Miyagi, Nagasaki and Osaka), Thailand (Chiang Mai), Uganda (Kampala)

Figure 6 (*Continued*)

Colon and rectum

Colorectal cancer represents almost 10% of the global cancer incidence burden and is the third most common cancer in men (an estimated 746,000 cases) and the second most common in women (614,000 cases). The disease is the fourth most common cause of death from cancer worldwide, with an estimated 694,000 deaths. Almost two-thirds of new cases occur in countries with high or very high levels of human development, with half of these occurring in Europe and the Americas. Colorectal cancer is now a common cancer in countries that have attained high levels of human development, and elevated incidence rates are seen in men in Eastern Europe (Slovakia, Hungary, and the Czech Republic) and in the Republic of Korea; incidence rates in women tend to rank second to breast cancer in countries where cervical cancer has been historically low such as in the Eastern Mediterranean region. Incidence varies 10-fold between countries worldwide, in both sexes, and rates tend to be relatively low in most African countries. As with incidence, mortality rates are lower in women than in men, except in the Caribbean. The scale of the colorectal cancer incidence and its temporal development are key markers of human development transitions in a given country. Incidence is increasing in many countries transitioning toward higher levels of development, whereas trends appear to be stabilizing or declining in countries that have attained the highest levels of human development (Figure 6c).

Stomach

Stomach cancer is the fifth most common cancer worldwide, with an estimated 952,000 new cases (7% of total cancer incidence) and 723,000 deaths (9% of total cancer mortality). Almost three quarters of the new cases occurred in Asia, and more than two-fifths occurred in China. There is a 10-fold international variation in

stomach cancer incidence; rates in men are approximately double those observed in women. The highest age-standardized incidence rates are in Eastern Asia and in Central and Eastern Europe. Incidence rates remain relatively low in Africa and North America. Over the past 50 years, incidence and mortality rates of stomach cancer have been uniformly decreasing in almost all countries (Figure 6d). This may be related to changing prevalence of Helicobacter pylori infection, a major risk factor for gastric cancer and for which trials are underway to inform the best public health approach to prevention.[17] Overall rates largely comprise the non-cardia type of gastric cancer: rates of gastric cardia cancer have, in contrast, been stable or have been increasing in recent two to three decades in the same populations.

Liver

Liver cancer represents 6% and 9% of the global cancer incidence and mortality burden, respectively. With an estimated 746,000 deaths, liver cancer is the second most common cause of death from cancer worldwide. Liver cancer is the fifth most common cancer in men (554,000 new cases, 8% of the total) and the ninth most common in women (228,000 cases, 3% of the total). Almost three quarters of the new cases occur in areas with low and medium human development; more than half of the global incidence and mortality is in China. Given the high fatality of liver cancer (overall mortality-to-incidence ratio, 0.95), the geographical patterns and trends for mortality are very similar to those observed for incidence. By far, the highest age-standardized incidence rate is seen in Mongolia. There are elevated incidence rates in East and South-East Asia, Africa, and Melanesia. Incidence rates tend to be lower in most highly developed regions. A higher prevalence of chronic infection with hepatitis B is one of the explanations for high incidence in lower resource countries as is widespread dietary exposure to aflatoxins, which occurs in many of the same geographic regions. There is the promise of reductions in hepatocellular carcinoma incidence in the coming decades in countries where the hepatitis B vaccine was introduced (from the early-1980s) and attained complete population coverage. For aflatoxins, reductions in exposure are occurring in some countries owing to economic development (e.g., parts of China), and new emphasis is being placed on effective interventions at the level of small farmers in developing countries.[18] There are concerns regarding a possible rise of liver cancer resulting from increasing infection with the hepatitis C virus, alongside the rising prevalence of obesity rates, and misuse of alcohol.[19]

Cervix uteri

Cervical cancer is the seventh most common cancer overall worldwide and is fourth most common in women in terms of both incidence (528,000 new cases) and mortality (266,000 deaths). Almost 70% of the global burden occurs in areas with low or medium levels of human development, and more than one-fifth of all new cases of cervical cancer are diagnosed in India. Incidence rates of cervical cancer vary greatly from country to country. The disease is still the most common cancer among women in 39 of the 184 countries worldwide (Figure 5b) and is the leading cause of cancer death in women in 45 countries. Risk is elevated mainly in sub-Saharan Africa, parts of Asia, and some countries in Central and South America. The lowest incidence rates tend to be in Western Europe, North America, Australia, New Zealand, and the eastern Mediterranean. Over the past 30 years, cervical cancer incidence rates have declined in many countries with notable exceptions (Figure 6e). This trend reflects changing societal factors linked to economic progress in countries in transition but in highly resourced countries reductions have been hastened by the implementation of effective screening programs. In contrast, however, there is little evidence for declines in incidence in recent years in Uganda, whereas rates are also increasing in several Eastern European and Central Asian countries. Recent changes in sexual behavior have led to an increase in the risk of infection with high-risk human papillomavirus types and, consequently, to increasing incidence rates in the absence of effective screening programs.[20]

Esophagus

Esophageal cancer is the eighth most common cancer worldwide, with an estimated 456,000 new cases (3% of all cancers) and 0.4 million cancer deaths (5% of all cancer deaths). About 73% of all new cases occurred in countries at low or medium levels of human development, and 49% of all new cases occurred in China. Incidence and mortality rates are elevated in Central and East Asia as well as in Eastern Africa. Incidence rates tend to be relatively low in Western Africa and some Latin American countries. While alcohol and tobacco are common causes of esophageal cancer in high income countries, these risk factors explain far less of the burden in the high incidence, low- and middle-income countries. Incidence varies 15-fold between countries worldwide in men and almost 20-fold in women. Incidence and mortality rates are 2–4 times as high in men as in women. Owing to the high fatality rate, mortality rates are close to incidence rates, whereas trends are variable, reflecting the changing prevalence and distribution of the underlying risk factors for esophageal cancer and its main histological subtypes (adenocarcinoma and squamous cell carcinoma). A recent study[21] providing global estimates of esophageal cancer incidence by histology suggested a high concentration of adenocarcinoma in high-income countries, with men at greater risk and a link to increasing obesity rates. An increasing tendency to classify cancers located at the gastro-esophageal junction as

adenocarcinoma (rather than gastric cardia cancer) may also have had a distortive impact on the overall trends and the cancer burden.

Global cancer transitions

The changing scale of cancer

NCDs were responsible for 36 million deaths in 2011 (with cancer, cardiovascular diseases, diabetes, and chronic respiratory diseases comprising 82% of all NCD deaths), a mortality figure surpassing all other causes combined, with NCD deaths expected to rapidly rise to over 50 million by 2030. Such changes in societies result from a complex interaction between health and disease patterns and their demographic, social, and economic determinants, but the rise of NCD may be considered part of the epidemiologic transition.[22] In this late stage of the transition, malnutrition and pandemics of infection (e.g., through the control of TB and malaria) are displaced by NCD—"degenerative and man-made diseases"—as the major causes of morbidity and mortality as societies increase their average life expectancy; overall, global mortality is generally lower but becomes concentrated at older ages.

Declines in all-cause mortality trigger fertility declines, and the rapid declines in high fertility rates projected over the next decades coupled with increasing longevity are the key contributors to population growth and population ageing worldwide. The global population of 7 billion in 2012 will reach 8.3 billion by 2030.[23] The population expansion is expected to be particularly dramatic in rapidly transitioning countries currently classified as low and medium HDI countries; as population aging is much less advanced, many are poised to enter a period of rapid increases in this parameter. Such demographic transitions are the major drivers of the increasing global cancer burden, assuming that incidence rates remain unchanged: when rates are allowed to vary and trends in major cancers are incorporated into projections, further increases in the future burden are expected. This is particularly so in countries in transition where the most rapid increasing incidence in major cancers is observed. In any case, the changes in population structure and those in the underlying rates contribute to the rise in a ratio of $4:1^9$; the demographic component alone translates to a predicted global burden of almost 19 million new cases of cancer in 2025 and 21.6 million cases by 2030, compared with the estimated 14.1 million cases in 2012 (Figure 7). The proportional growth in population and corresponding number of future cancer cases are inversely related to current level of development, with the biggest relative increases seen in low HDI areas. Medium HDI countries will experience the greatest absolute population growth and thus the greatest absolute increase in the future cancer burden in 2025. Increases of 60–70% in the cancer incidence are forecast in Latin America, Asia, and Africa by 2030.

The changing profile of cancer

Cancer has emerged as one of major causes of death in human populations, and the lowering of death rates of degenerative diseases among the aged, such as cerebrovascular disease and stroke, signify that cancer is also one of the major barriers to a longer average life expectancy. The disease burden is changing in its profile as well as scale as countries transit towards higher levels of human development, and the disease has transitional hallmarks as noted earlier: cancers associated with infection (e.g., cervical and stomach cancer above) have, from a global perspective, been surpassed by cancers more associated with affluence (e.g., breast, colorectal, and prostate

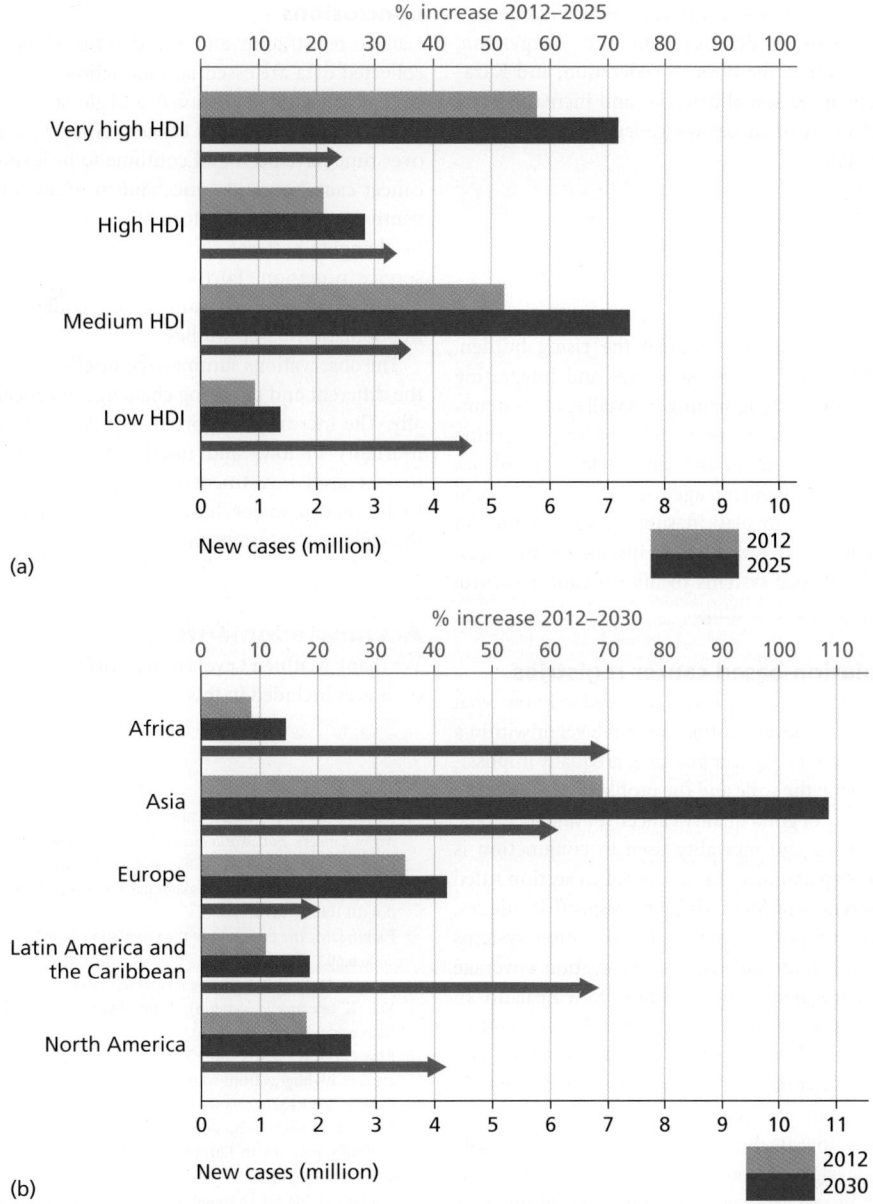

Figure 7 Bar charts depicting (a) the percentage increase in cancer incidence 2012–2025 by HDI and (b) the percentage increase in cancer incidence 2012–2030 in five world regions. Source: GLOBOCAN 2012.

cancer). For colorectal cancer in particular, the rapid increases in countries that have attained medium or higher levels of human development are indicative of a westernization effect: a changing population prevalence of a number of reproductive, dietary, metabolic and hormonal risk factors—toward levels more akin to those more commonly observed in the west—and a corresponding increase in risk of the disease.[24]

Kuwait, a highly resourced country that has scored highest of all Arab countries in the HDI, now has a similar cancer profile to many countries in the west (personal communication, Dr. Amani Elbasmy), with high frequencies of breast, prostate, and colorectal cancer (similar to Australian registries despite an overall rate three times lower) and a rising and increasing relative importance of certain types of cancer—leukemia and non-Hodgkin lymphoma, and in 10th place in men, testicular cancer—for which there remains only limited understanding of the respective causative factors.[25]

It has been noted that the basic models of Omran's epidemiological transition fail to grasp the global nature and therefore

heterogeneity of the mortality transition and that "there are probably as many models as there are societies."[26] For cancer, the description of a *cancer transition* and indeed the disease as purely non-communicable is an over simplification, particularly as it fails to address the importance of infection as an important and persistent cause of cancer.[27] It has been estimated that around one-third of all cancers in Sub-Saharan Africa are caused by infectious agents including cancers of the cervix, liver, stomach, bladder, and Kaposi sarcoma.[28] While rapid increases in the incidence of breast, prostate and colorectal cancer are observed in high-quality cancer registries in Kampala, Uganda, and among Harare blacks in Zimbabwe,[12,13] corresponding rates of cervical cancer also show increases in incidence. In low HDI Eastern Africa, infection- and poverty-related cancers are the major forms diagnosed. In Blantyre, Malawi, cervical cancer, Kaposi sarcoma, non-Hodgkin lymphoma, and esophageal cancer are ahead of female breast cancer as the top five incidence cancers. In high and very high HDI Eastern Europe and Central Asia, many countries have observed increasing cervical cancer mortality rates in young women. In the absence of effective screening programs, trends in Belarus, Tajikistan, Kyrgyzstan, Armenia, Azerbaijan, Ukraine, the Russian Federation, and Kazakhstan are linked to changing sexual behavior and increasing risk of persistent HPV infection in successive generations of women born around 1940–1950.[29]

Using descriptive epidemiology to inform cancer control policy

Clearly, a step-change in investment in the control of cancer and other major NCD is necessary to stem the rising burden. In developing national cancer control strategies and integrating these into NCD planning, strengthening surveillance systems, including population-based cancer registries and implementing population-level primary prevention and early detection policies are critical aspects, and development agencies and international partners have a distinct role to play in supporting activities in resource-challenged countries. We close by discussing the need to enhance cancer surveillance systems to inform cancer control action, notably in lower resource settings.

Integrating population-based cancer registries

In order to plan and evaluate health services, we need to know what is happening at a population level—at the national level or within a province or a substantial sector. Cancer planning is equally impossible without first identifying the scale and the profile of cancer in the community. While the use of good quality cancer surveillance data, including cancer incidence and mortality used in conjunction is ideal, for many developing countries (as discussed in section titled "Definitions, Data Sources, and Methods"), the respective sources, population-based cancer registries and vital registration systems are very limited in availability, quality, and population coverage outside of Europe, North America, and Australia/New Zealand. In particular, PBCR are feasible to implement even in lower resource settings, and guidance for planning and developing such registries is available.[30] It is of acute concern that currently only 67 (mainly high-income) countries are equipped with high-quality PBCR, whereas in 62 (mainly low-income) countries, no reliable data are available. Many developing countries endure the very same obstacles facing other health services including a lack of financial resources and expertise.

The political recognition of NCD has changed however recently and world leaders agreed in 2011 to a roadmap to address the global burden, including a time-bound commitment to establish policies for the prevention and control of NCDs by 2013, and the adoption of nine global targets for 2025 (including a 25% reduction in premature mortality from NCDs). Importantly, all countries agreed to collect cancer incidence data as one of 25 indicators to monitor progress, and the IARC-led *Global Initiative for Cancer Registry Development (GICR)* partnership (http://gicr.iarc.fr) aims to support this high-level commitment by aiding and accelerating the availability of PBCRs for national cancer control purposes. The key instrument through which the ambitions are realized is the formation of six IARC Regional Hubs for Cancer Registration in Africa, Asia, Latin America, the Caribbean, and the Pacific Islands, which provide localized programs of training, support, and advocacy to targeted countries within defined regions. A key medium-term aim of IARC and GICR is to support 50 countries in resource-challenged settings in providing measurable improvements in cancer surveillance for cancer control action by 2018, via the planning and development of PBCR.

Conclusions

Cancer registration and the descriptive epidemiology using the collected data are essential foundations for evidence-based cancer control at a national, regional, and global level. The markedly different rates and patterns of cancer across the world, and their trends over time have been and continue to be a source of hypotheses on cancer causation and a mechanism to measure the impact of preventive interventions. Information on the burden of the disease and its changing patterns should also underpin the planning of health service provision. Furthermore, cancer registries make valuable research partners, for example, in the identification of cancer cases in population-based studies.

The observations summarized briefly in this chapter demonstrate the different and changing challenge of cancer control internationally. The increased importance of cancer as a cause of premature mortality in low- and middle-income countries must translate to increased investment in cancer control if this disease is not to become a major barrier to sustainable human development throughout the twenty-first century.

Acknowledgments
We thank Mathieu Laversanne, IARC, for development of a number of figures included in this chapter.

References

1 Parkin DM, Stjernsward J, Muir CS. Estimates of the worldwide frequency of twelve major cancers. *Bull World Health Organ.* 1984;**62**:163–182.
2 Ferlay J, Soerjomataram I, Dikshit R, et al. Cancer incidence and mortality worldwide: sources, methods and major patterns in GLOBOCAN 2012. *Int J Cancer.* 2014. doi: 10.1002/ijc.29210.
3 Parkin DM. The evolution of the population-based cancer registry. *Nat Rev Cancer.* 2006;**6**:603–612.
4 Forman D, Bray F, Brewster DH, et al. (eds). *Cancer Incidence in Five Continents.* Vol. X (electronic version). Lyon: IARC; 2013. Available at: http://ci5.iarc.fr (accessed 2 December 2013).
5 Bray F, Ferlay J, Laversanne M, et al. Cancer incidence in five continents: inclusion criteria, highlights from volume X and the global status of cancer registration. *Int J Cancer.* 2015;**137**(9):2060–2071.
6 Ferlay J, Steliarova-Foucher E, Lortet-Tieulent J, et al. Cancer incidence and mortality patterns in Europe: estimates for 40 countries in 2012. *Eur J Cancer.* 2013;**49**:1374–1403.
7 Mathers C, Ma Fat D, Inoue M, et al. Counting the dead and what they died from: an assessment of the global status of cause of death data. *Bull World Health Organ.* 2005;**83**:171–177.
8 Bray F, Ren JS, Masuyer E, Ferlay J. Estimates of global cancer prevalence for 27 sites in the adult population in 2008. *Int J Cancer.* 2013;**132**:1133–1145.
9 Bray F, Jemal A, Grey N, Ferlay J, Forman D. Global cancer transitions according to the human development index (2008-2030): a population-based study. *Lancet Oncol.* 2012;**13**:790–801.
10 United Nations Development Programme. *Human Development Report.* 2013, http://hdr.undp.org/en (accessed 12 February 2013).
11 Chaabna K, Bray F, Wabinga HR, et al. Kaposi sarcoma trends in Uganda and Zimbabwe: a sustained decline in incidence? *Int J Cancer.* 2013;**133**(5):1197–1203.
12 Chokunonga E, Borok MZ, Chirenje ZM, Nyakabau AM, Parkin DM. Trends in the incidence of cancer in the black population of Harare, Zimbabwe 1991–2010. *Int J Cancer.* 2013;**133**:721–729.
13 Wabinga HR, Nambooze S, Amulen PM, Okello C, Mbus L, Parkin DM. Trends in the incidence of cancer in Kampala, Uganda 1991–2010. *Int J Cancer.* 2014;**135**(2):432–439. doi: 10.1002/ijc.28661
14 Lopez A. Changes in tobacco consumption and lung cancer risk: evidence from national statistics. In: Hakama M, Beral V, Cullen V, Parkin DM, eds. *Evaluating Effectiveness of Primary Prevention of Cancer.* Lyon: IARC Scientific Publications No. 103; 1990:133–149.
15 Jha P. Avoidable global cancer deaths and total deaths from smoking. *Nat Rev Cancer.* 2009;**9**(9):655–664. doi: 10.1038/nrc2703. Epub 2009 Aug 20. Review. PubMed PMID: 19693096.
16 Thun M, Peto R, Boreham J, Lopez AD. Stages of the cigarette epidemic on entering its second century. *Tob Control.* 2012;**21**(2):96–101.

17 Herrero R, Parsonnet J, Greenberg ER. Prevention of gastric cancer. *JAMA*. 2014;**312**(**12**):1197–1198. doi: 10.1001/jama.2014.10498. PubMed PMID: 25247512.

18 International Agency for Research on Cancer. Pitt JI, Wild CP, Baan RA, Gelderblom WCA, Miller JD, Riley RT, Wu F, eds. *Improving Public Health through Mycotoxin Control*. Lyon, France: IARC Scientific Publication, No 158.; 2012.

19 McGlynn KA, London WT. The global epidemiology of hepatocellular carcinoma: present and future. *Clin Liver Dis*. 2011;**15**:223–243, vii–x.

20 Vaccarella S, Lortet-Tieulent J, Plummer M, Franceschi S, Bray F. Worldwide trends in cervical cancer incidence: impact of screening against changes in disease risk factors. *Eur J Cancer*. 2013;**49**(**15**):3262–3273.

21 Arnold M, Soerjomataram I, Ferlay J, Forman D. Global incidence of esophageal cancer by histological subtype in 2012. *Gut*. 2014;**64**:381–387.

22 Omran AR. The epidemiologic transition. A theory of the epidemiology of population change. *Milbank Mem Fund Q*. 1971;**49**:509–538.

23 United Nations Population Division. *World Population Prospects, the 2010 Revision*. 2010, New York: United Nations, http://esa.un.org/wpp/index.htm (accessed 12 October 2015).

24 Bray F. Transitions in human development and the global cancer burden. In: Wild CP, Stewart B, eds. *World Cancer Report 2014*. Lyon, France: International Agency for Research on Cancer; 2014.

25 Maule M, Merletti F. Cancer transition and priorities for cancer control. *Lancet Oncol*. 2012;**13**(**8**):745–746. doi: 10.1016/S1470-2045(12)70268-1. PubMed PMID: 22846827.

26 Caldwell JC. Population health in transition. *Bull World Health Organ*. 2001;**79**(**2**):159–160.

27 Gersten O, Wilmoth JR. The cancer transition in Japan since 1951. *Demogr Res*. 2002;**7**:271–306.

28 De Martel C, Ferlay J, Franceschi S, et al. Global burden of cancers attributable to infections in 2008: a review and synthetic analysis. *Lancet Oncol*. 2012;**13**:607–615.

29 Bray F, Lortet-Tieulent J, Znaor A, Brotons M, Poljak M, Arbyn M. Patterns and trends in human papillomavirus-related diseases in Central and Eastern Europe and Central Asia. *Vaccine*. 2013;**31**(**Suppl 7**):H32–H45.

30 Bray F, Znaor A, Cueva P, et al. *Planning and Developing Population-Based Cancer Registration in Low- and Middle-Income Settings*. Lyon, France: International Agency for Research on Cancer; 2014. IARC Technical Publication No. 43.

34 Cancer epidemiology

Xifeng Wu, MD, PhD ▪ Xia Pu, PhD ▪ Stephanie C. Melkonian, PhD ▪ Margaret R. Spitz, MD, MPH

Overview

According to the World Health Organization (WHO) there are over 14 million new cancer cases per year worldwide. As the epidemiologic transition continues, we see increases in cancer incidence in developing nations with more than 50% of all new cancers occurring in low- and middle-income countries. This chapter will review cancer disparities in developed and developing nations, as well as traditional and emerging risk factors, particularly tobacco smoking and factors related to energy balance. It will also summarize the novel and emerging wealth of genomic, epigenomic, metabolomic, and transcriptomic information for the prediction of cancer risk and outcomes.

Descriptive cancer statistics

Global cancer statistics

According to the World Health Organization (WHO), there are over 14 million new cancer cases and 8 million cancer-related deaths per year worldwide.[1] The top 10 commonly diagnosed cancers worldwide are lung (13%), breast (11.9%), colorectal (9.7%), prostate (8%), stomach (6.8%), liver (5.5%), cervical (3.7%), esophageal (3.2%), and bladder (3%) cancers, and non-Hodgkin lymphoma (2.7%).[1] The most frequently diagnosed cancers differ between men and women; lung (16.7%), prostate (15%), colorectal (10%), stomach (8.5%), and liver (7.5%) cancers are the most commonly diagnosed cancers in men, whereas breast (25.2%), colorectal (9.2%), lung (8.8%), cervical (8%), and endometrial (5%) cancers are the most common cancers in women (excluding nonmelanoma skin cancers) worldwide.[1] It has been suggested that if the recent trends in cancer incidence continue, then the burden of cancer will increase to 23.6 million new cases each year by 2030. In 2013, there were an estimated 8.2 million deaths from cancer in the world—4.7 million (57%) in males and 3.5 million (43%) in females, giving a male to female ratio of 10 : 8.[1]

US cancer statistics

In 2014, there were over 1.6 million new cancer cases in the United States with nearly 600,000 cancer-related deaths.[2] According to Surveillance, Epidemiology, and End Results (SEER) program data, the top incident cancers in the United States excluding non-melanoma skin cancers) are cancers of the prostate (27%), lung (14%), colorectum (8%), bladder (6.6%), melanoma of the skin (5.1%), kidney (4.6%), non-Hodgkin lymphoma (4.5%), oral cavity (3.5%), leukemia (3.5%), and pancreas (2.8%) in men and cancers of the breast (29%), lung (13%) colorectum (8%), endometrium

Supported by the Center for Translational and Public Health Genomics, The University of Texas MD Anderson Cancer Center.

(6.5%), thyroid (5.9%), melanoma (4%), non-Hodgkin's lymphoma (4%), kidney (3.1%), pancreas (2.8%), and ovary (2.7%) in women.[3] The overall cancer incidence rate is 529.4 per 100,000 in men and 411.3 per 100,000 in women; however, the rates have been decreasing in recent years due to rapid declines in colorectal, prostate, and lung cancers, largely due to improvements in primary prevention and screening.[3] However, incidence rates for cancers such as melanoma of the skin, esophageal adenocarcinoma; cancers of the thyroid, liver, kidney, anus, and pancreas; and human papillomavirus-positive oropharyngeal cancers are increasing.[4] Although the overall cancer death rate rose for a good portion of the twentieth century, there has been a steady decline in cancer death rates over the past 20 years (from 215.1 deaths per 100,000 population in 1991 to 171.8 per 100,000 deaths per 100,000 population in 2010).[2,3]

Rates of cancer incidence and mortality also vary significantly by ethnicity, race, and socioeconomic status (SES). These variations, both in the United States and worldwide, contribute to a growing concern regarding cancer health disparities.

Cancer health disparities

Cancer health disparities represent differences in cancer incidence, prevalence, and mortality among different populations based on factors such as race, ethnicity, poverty, SES, inadequate education, lack of access to care, and various behavioral, environmental, lifestyle, and occupational exposures.[5-7] The elimination of disparities in the burden of cancer is a primary concern worldwide.

Variation in cancer incidence and mortality by race and ethnicity in the United States

Cancer incidence and death rates vary fairly dramatically between racial and ethnic groups in the United States (broadly defined as non-Hispanic White, Black, Asian American/Pacific Islander, American Indian/Alaska native, and Hispanic). Cancer incidence rates are highest among African-American (AA) men (554.5 per 100,000 population) followed by whites (499.7 per 100,000), Hispanics (393.5 per 100,000), Asian/Pacific Islanders (310.1 per 100,000), and American Indian/Alaska natives (293.5 per 100,000) (Figure 1a).[4] AA men also have the highest cancer death rates (253.9 per 100,000), nearly double those of Asian Americans (131.1 per 100,000), who have the lowest out of the five racial/ethnic groups (Figure 2a).[2,4] Cancer incidence and death rates are higher among black men than white men for almost every cancer site, except for kidney cancer.[4,8]

Among women, cancer incidence rates are highest among whites (414.8 per 100,000 population), followed by AA (393.8 per 100,000), Hispanics (324.2 per 100,000), Asian/Pacific Islanders (279.8 per 100,000), and American Indian/Alaska natives (261.0 per 100,000) women (Figure 1b). Black women have the highest cancer death

Holland-Frei Cancer Medicine, Ninth Edition. Edited by Robert C. Bast Jr., Carlo M. Croce, William N. Hait, Waun Ki Hong, Donald W. Kufe, Martine Piccart-Gebhart, Raphael E. Pollock, Ralph R. Weichselbaum, Hongyang Wang, and James F. Holland.

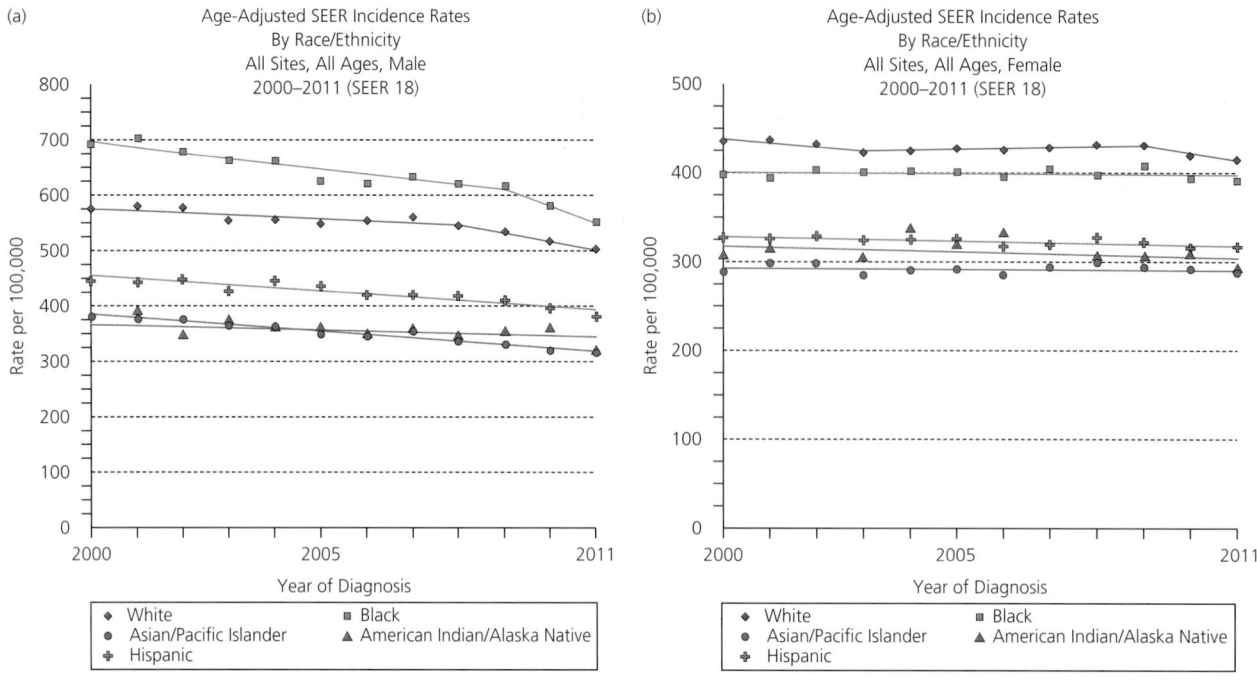

Figure 1 (a,b) Incidence rates for all cancers combined by race/ethnicity and sex, United States, 1999–2011. Source: Data from/generated at http://seer.cancer.gov/faststats/selections.php?series=race.

rates (166.2 per 100,000) versus Asian/Pacific Islanders (91.1 per 100,000) (Figure 2b). Overall, cancer incidence and death rates are lower among Asian Americans/Pacific Islanders, American Indians/Alaska natives, and Hispanics than whites for all cancer sites combined and for the four most common cancer sites.[3] However, cancers associated with infectious agents (uterine cervix, stomach, and liver) are generally more common in nonwhite populations. Asian Americans/Pacific Islanders having the highest incidence of stomach and liver cancer and Hispanics with the highest incidence of cervical cancer.[9]

In developed nations such as the United States, lower SES groups tend to have poorer access to care and resources for cancer prevention, detection, and control, resulting in a disproportionate burden of cancer in poorer communities.[5,7,9] Although there is commonly an overlap between minority status and lower SES, it has been noted that even after taking into account factors related to SES, minority populations and medically underserved groups tend to be differentially burdened by cancer incidence and mortality.[9] These groups tend to enter the healthcare system with later-stage disease, which negatively impacts cancer morbidity and mortality in those populations.[7,9]

Cancer disparities in developing nations

Cancer is often overlooked as a major source of disease burden in developing nations where infectious disease and perinatal and maternal mortality are primary health concerns.[6] However, large declines in mortality have been observed and are expected to continue for all the principal communicable diseases (with the exception of HIV/AIDS) and noncommunicable diseases such as cancer are projected to increase over the next 30 years.[6,7,10,11] More than 50% of all new cancers and two-thirds of annual cancer mortality worldwide occur in low- and middle-income countries.[1,11] The cancer burden in these countries disproportionately affects the poor, who are more likely to use tobacco, have poorer diets, have higher exposure to sunlight and other occupational exposures, and are at higher risk for infection-related cancers and have limited access to care.[12]

Although higher income countries have long-term survival rates for cancer upwards of 60%, these rates are closer to 20% for developing nations. Likely due to the lack of infrastructure, and available channels for early detection, approximately 70% of cancers diagnosed in developing nations are diagnosed in a late stage.[1,12] Incidence of infection-related cancers, such as cervical cancer and hepatocellular cancer, remain high in low- and middle-income countries.[1,7] However, as these nations become more industrialized and modifiable risk factors such as sedentary lifestyle and Westernized diets become more prominent, cancers more prevalent in Western nations, such as breast and colorectal cancer, will also become more common.[7]

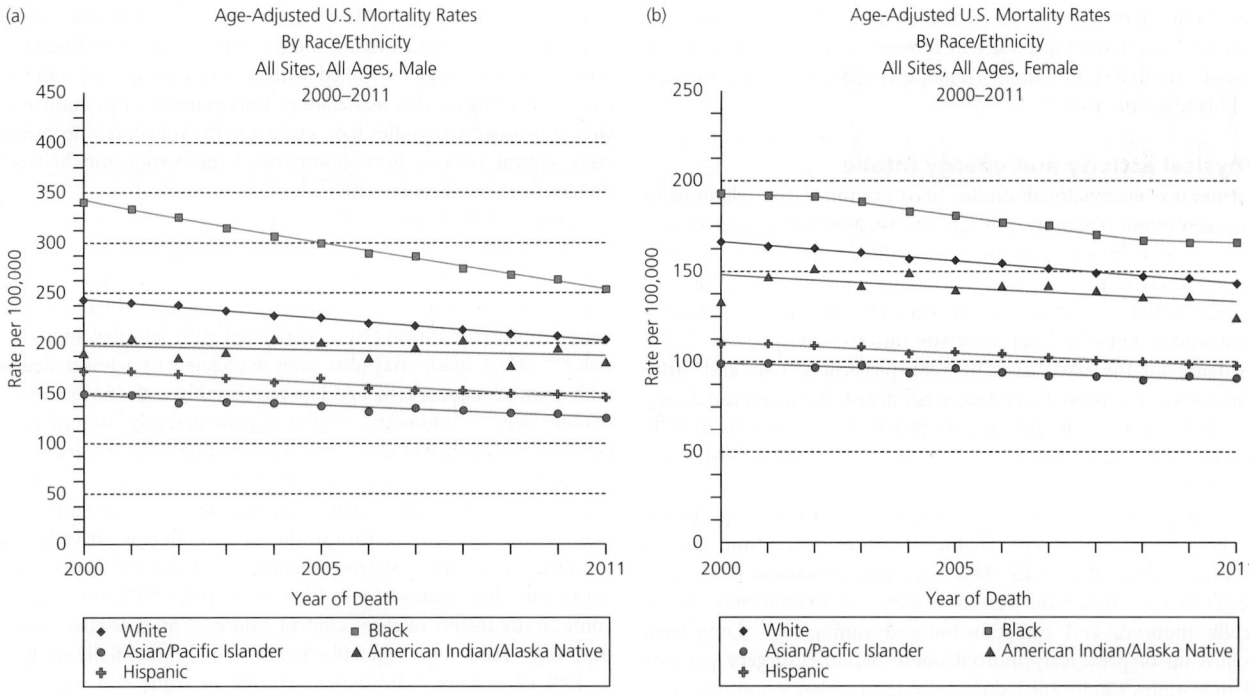

(a) Age-Adjusted U.S. Mortality Rates
By Race/Ethnicity
All Sites, All Ages, Male
2000–2011

(b) Age-Adjusted U.S. Mortality Rates
By Race/Ethnicity
All Sites, All Ages, Female
2000–2011

Cancer sites include invasive cases only unless otherwise noted.
Rates for American Indian/Alaska native are based on the CHSDA (Contract Health Service Delivery Area) counties.
Hispanics and non-Hispanics are not mutually exclusive from whites, blacks, Asian/Pacific Islanders, and American
Indians/Alaska natives.
Mortality source: US Mortality Files, National Center for Health Statistics, CDC.
Rates are per 100,000 and are age-adjusted to the 2000 US standard population (19 age groups–Census P25-1130).
Regression lines are calculated using the Joinpoint Regression Program Version 4.1.0, April 2014,
National Cancer Institute.

Figure 2 (a,b) Death rates for all cancers combined by race/ethnicity and sex, United States, 1999–2011. Source: Data from/generated at http://seer.cancer.gov/faststats/selections.php?series=race.

Emerging cancer risk factors

Although factors such as genetic susceptibility and family history play an important role in cancer etiology, they only explain part of the variance observed in cancer risk across different populations and subgroups. For example, evidence suggests that in the United States, for those individuals who do not use tobacco, the most important modifiable determinants of cancer risk are associated with energy balance—the integrated effects of diet, physical activity, and genetics on body weight over an individual's lifetime.[13,14] Together these factors contribute to approximately one-third of preventable cancers each year, equal to the number of preventable cancers due to smoking, and are responsible for the same number of cancer-related deaths.[15,16] The carcinogens in different cancer etiologic risk factors may cause specific molecular (e.g., nucleic acids and protein) defects that eventually lead to cancer development.

Energy balance

Obesity: According to the WHO, the rates of obesity have doubled worldwide since 1980.[17] Globally, between 1980 and 2008, obesity prevalence rose from 4.8% to 9.8% in men and from 7.9% to 13.8% in women.[17,18] The WHO estimates that by 2008, more than 1.4 billion adults over the age of 20 were overweight, and of these overweight adults, nearly 500 million were obese.[17] The United States has the highest prevalence of obesity. More than one-third (34.9%) of adults are considered obese with rates of obesity varying

drastically by racial and socioeconomic subgroups.[19] For example, non-Hispanic blacks have the highest age-adjusted rates of obesity (47.8%), followed by Hispanics (42.5%). Obesity and cancer may be linked via mechanisms related to insulin and insulin-like growth factors, sex steroid levels, and the adipocyte-derived cytokines, or adipokines.[20-22] Adipose tissue has in recent years been recognized as an active and major endocrine and metabolic organ, important in regulation of energy balance and lipid metabolism through the release of peptide hormones such as leptin, adiponectin, and the cytokine TNFα. Depending on the cancer site and population in question, population attributable fractions due to obesity range from 14% for colorectal cancer (CRC) and over 50% for endometrial cancer.[23] The heritability of body weight is high, estimated to range between 40% and 70%.[24-26] Studies have suggested that genetic variation, particularly in genes such as *FTO*, *MC4R*, and *TMEM18*, plays a major role in determining interindividual differences in susceptibility or resistance to the obesogenic environment.[27]

Once considered to be a concern only in high-income westernized nations, obesity has become a major contributor to the global burden of disease.[18] Over the next two decades, some of the largest proportional increases in the number of adults classified as overweight or obese are expected to occur in low- to middle-income nations including South Asia, East Africa, Southeast Asia, West Africa, and the Caribbean.[18,28] The rapid increase in rates of obesity in developing nations has been driven by urbanization and economic growth, which continue to fuel dramatic changes in living and labor environments as well as diet and lifestyle.[18,28] Studies to date indicate a role for obesity in several cancers including colon, breast, endometrium, kidney (renal cell), gastric cardia, pancreas, gallbladder, and liver.[20]

Physical activity and energy intake

Numerous observational studies have examined the relationship between physical activity and cancer risk at various cancer sites.[29] The most definitive epidemiologic evidence for the association between physical activity and cancer risk exists for CRC.[30] Studies suggest a risk reduction of approximately 30% when comparing individuals with the highest versus lowest activity levels.[30] The evidence for the association between physical activity and other cancers such as prostate, endometrial, breast, lung, and renal cancers is less consistent and suggests that these associations may be jointly impacted by factors such as body mass index (BMI) and family history.[31]

Total caloric intake, or energy intake, has also been proposed to be a major cancer risk factor.[32] Early evidence from animal models suggest that a 15–53% reduction in caloric intake can result in a 20–62% reduction in incidence of spontaneous, chemically induced, and radiation-induced tumors.[32–34] Long-term follow-up of previously morbid obese bariatric surgery patients demonstrates significant reduction in the incidence and mortality of cancer, especially those related to obesity.[35] Although it currently remains unclear if this reduction in incidence is due to the profound metabolic changes related to weight loss, this evidence is supported by well-known pathophysiological consequences of obesity including chronic inflammation and hormonal changes.[35] Caloric restriction-mediated benefits on cancer are thought to involve metabolic adaptations including decreased production of growth factors and anabolic hormones, decreased reactive oxygen species production, decreased levels of inflammatory cytokines, and the potential impact on cellular processes including apoptosis and DNA repair.[32]

Recent epidemiologic evidence has suggested that high total caloric intake is associated with increased cancer risks, particularly for CRC.[36] For example, a large population-based case–control study of CRC concluded that total energy intake was associated with an approximately 56% increased risk of cancer for those in the highest versus lowest category of total energy intake. Similarly, a familial study of breast cancer risk identified a nearly 60% increased risk associated with high versus low caloric intake.[37] Other case–control studies of prostate cancer and kidney cancer have also suggested that high caloric intake is associated with increased cancer risks.[38,39] However, measures of total caloric intake in epidemiologic studies are often prone to recall bias and misclassification due to the use of self-reported data, and findings regarding energy intake and physical activity have been inconsistent.[38,39]

Metabolic, hormonal, and growth factor alterations that affect the regulation and expression of genes involved in DNA repair, cell proliferation, and apoptosis have been associated with increased food consumption and decreased physical activity.[40] Regular physical activity and caloric restriction have been shown to significantly lower levels of insulin and insulin-like growth factors.[41] Physical activity may play a role in cancer etiology through changes in endogenous sexual and metabolic hormone levels and growth factors, decreasing obesity and central adiposity and by potentially impacting immune function and response.[40]

Diet

Dietary factors are believed to account for nearly one-third of all cancers in Western countries.[42] Early studies linking diet to cancer etiology observed that dietary intake patterns and cancer rates varied by populations around the world, suggesting that these dietary patterns may be linked with cancer etiology. In order to further investigate this association, hundreds of case–control as well as prospective studies have evaluated the role of diet in cancer risk. Several reviews have summarized the association between dietary intake and cancer risk.[42–45]

Briefly, dietary factors such as meat intake, dietary fat consumption, and fruit and vegetable intake have all been studied extensively with regard to cancer risk. A meta-analysis suggested that high red meat intakes were associated with 28–35% increased risk of CRC, whereas processed meats were associated with 20–40% increased risk.[46,47] Meat intake has also been associated to a lesser degree with stomach cancer risk, and less consistently with cancers of the bladder, breast, endometrium, glioma, pancreas, prostate, and renal cell.[46] Case–control studies have suggested up to a 35% increased risk of breast cancer associated with high dietary fat intake; however, prospective studies, which are less prone to the sources of bias common in case–control studies (i.e., recall bias), have largely found no association between dietary fat intake and cancer risk, suggesting that methodological biases are potentially the cause of some of the results of case–control studies.[48] Studies also suggest that high fruit and vegetable intake could potentially prevent 5–12% of cancers.[49] Substances present in fruits and vegetables may have anticarcinogenic effects—these include dithiolthiones, isothiocyanates, indole-3-carbinol, allium compounds, isoflavones, protease inhibitors, saponins, phytosterols, inositol hexaphosphate, vitamin C, D-limonene, lutein, folic acid, β carotene, lycopene, selenium, vitamin E, flavonoids, and dietary fiber.[50] These substances have been shown to play a role in estrogen metabolism, protecting DNA from oxidative damage, DNA methylation, and cell proliferation.[51]

Electronic cigarettes (E-cigarettes)

E-cigarette use, also called "vaping," employs battery-powered devices that deliver nicotine-containing vapor rather than inhaled smoke of traditional cigarettes.[52] E-cigarettes constitute a growing market with around $2.2 billion estimated in 2014.[53] E-cigarettes are controversial in their role as a smoking cessation aid and in tobacco harm reduction as a substitute for traditional cigarettes. There is evidence that the convenient features of e-cigarettes make it more difficult to quit compared with traditional cigarettes.[52] The US Food and Drug Administration (FDA) reported that e-cigarettes contained many dangerous chemicals that are carcinogenic.[54] In April 2014, FDA announced its intention to regulate e-cigarette devices to make them subject to the established regulation terms of tobacco products.[53] It remains to be seen what the long-term adverse effects of e-cigarette use are.

Genetic susceptibility

Although cancer is mainly caused by environmental exposures, genetic susceptibility also plays an important role.[55] Susceptibility genes are categorized as rare high penetrant variants [odds ratio (OR)] > 10, moderate penetrant variants (OR = 2–5), or common low penetrant variants (OR = 1.2–1.5). The known hereditary cancers are uncommon and are usually associated with highly penetrant genes. For example, germline mutations in BRAC1 and BRCA2 genes are responsible for the majority of hereditary breast/ovarian cancer syndromes and can also increase the risk of several other cancers, such as prostate and pancreas cancers.[56] The MLH1 and MLH2 genes cause the majority of hereditary non-polyposis colorectal cancer (HNPCC) cases.[57] Children with two copies of mutated *RB1* genes are at 90% risk of developing pediatric retinoblastoma.[58]

Although the penetrance for these inherited cancer syndromes is high, they only represent a very small portion of all cancer cases. The majority of cancers are sporadic, attributed to a large number of common, low-penetrance genes. Historically, the candidate gene approach only identified a handful of true cancer susceptibility loci, such as *GSTM1* and *NAT2* for bladder cancer and *CASP* for breast cancer.[59-61] The problems associated with such studies included low throughput of platforms, limited study size and power, nonreproducibility of gene–environmental interactions, and, above all, the failure to pick functional variants to evaluate. The explosion of genome-wide association studies (GWAS) in recent years has revolutionized studies of genetic susceptibility. To date, there are over 250 publications on GWAS of cancer risks that have identified hundreds of single nucleotide polymorphisms (SNPs) as genetic susceptibility variants for 35 cancer sites, including 95 SNPs in 48 regions for prostate cancer, 81 SNPs in 28 regions for breast cancer, and 17 SNPs in 12 regions for lung cancer (a catalog of published GWAS is available at http://www.genome.gov/gwastudies). These genetic variants are often located in gene deserts and intergenic regions. However, some identified susceptibility genes have provided important biological insights into the etiology of cancers, such as the lung cancer susceptibility loci at chromosome 15q25.1 containing nicotinic acetylcholine receptor genes,[62-64] breast cancer susceptibility loci at 6q25.1 containing estrogen receptor 1 gene,[65,66] and multiple prostate cancer susceptibility loci containing androgen-receptor-binding regions.[67] In addition to these specific cancer susceptibility regions, many "hot-spot" regions have been found to harbor susceptibility loci for multiple cancers. For example, the chromosome 8q24 region flanking the oncogene *MYC* harbors susceptibility loci for five cancers, including breast, colorectal, bladder, prostate, and ovarian cancers. Chromosome 5p15.33, which maps to the *TERT-CLPTM1L* region, harbors susceptibility loci for at least six cancers, including melanoma, basal cell carcinoma, glioma, lung, bladder, breast, prostate, pancreas, and testicular cancers. A third region chromosome 11q13 contains susceptibility loci for at least four cancers, including prostate, kidney, colorectal, and breast cancer. The major signal mapped in this region is an intergenic region near *TPCN2* and *MYEOV*.[68,69]

Despite the success of the GWAS approach in identifying cancer susceptibility loci, each region only confers a small OR for cancer risk, and the clinical application of these low-penetrance loci is unclear. The biological mechanisms underlying these GWAS hits are largely unknown. Future studies are warranted to decipher gene–environment interactions, explore the functional relevance of the hot spots identified, and pinpoint the biological mechanisms of these loci.

Emerging methods and technologies

The rapid technological advancement over the past decade has had a tremendous impact on the practice of cancer epidemiology. In particular, various "omics" technologies are changing the landscape of epidemiologic research at an unprecedented pace. In addition to genomics, epigenomics, transcriptomics, proteomics, and metabolomics are all being applied to cancer epidemiological research. However, there has been limited success to date applying these technologies in cancer epidemiology due to study design and confounding issues. Unlike inherited genetic variations that are a stable trait, molecular features at the epigenetic, RNA, protein, and metabolite level are influenced by environmental exposures, pathological status, sample collection and processing,

and technical reproducibility. With proper study design (e.g., prospective, longitudinal study), standardized data collection, well-controlled sample collection and processing procedures, and maturing technology, these "omics" approaches have the potential to identify novel biomarkers for cancer risk and outcome in cancer epidemiology research.

Next-generation sequencing (NGS)

The success of GWAS in identifying genetic susceptibility loci has benefited from advances in genomic technology, and the human genome and HapMap projects. GWAS have been fruitful in identifying new genetic susceptibility loci; however, GWAS only test common alleles and GWAS hits so far only explain a small fraction of the heritability of cancer.[70] Next-generation sequencing (NGS) (e.g., exome or whole genome sequencing) has facilitated the effort to identify the missing hereditability of cancer. There have been success stories in using NGS in cancer association studies. The identification of a germline mutation in *PALB2* as a familial pancreatic cancer susceptibility gene was among the early efforts in the application of NGS in cancer gene discovery.[71] The *POLE* and *POLD1* germline variations, which result in a defective protein, have been identified by NGS as high-penetrance susceptibility genes for colorectal adenomas and carcinomas, improving our understanding of the etiology of these diseases.[72] Earlier this year, NGS found a significant enrichment of novel and rare germline variants in *JMJD1C*, which codes for a histone demethylase and is a coactivator of the androgen receptor, among patients with intracranial germ cell tumors (IGCTs), suggesting *JMJD1C* as a susceptibility gene for this rare brain tumor.[73] Most recently, germline mutations in *POT1*, encoding one member of the telomere shelterin complex, have been identified by NGS as predisposing people to familial melanoma and glioma.[74,75]

Epigenome-wide association study (EWAS)

Epigenetic changes refer to changes that may modulate gene expression without affecting DNA sequence. The epigenome sits at the interface between the dynamic external environment and the static human genome. There is extensive interindividual variation in the epigenome. Epigenome-wide association study (EWAS) generally refers to the study of genome-wide epigenetic profiles and represents a novel tool to understand disease etiology and predict treatment response and clinical outcome.[76] For example, a prospective breast cancer EWAS study identified a blood methylation signature as having higher predictive power for breast cancer risk than eight GWAS-identified SNPs combined.[77] Likewise, a genome-wide methylation analysis found methylation signatures to be a robust predictor for estrogen receptor subtype and patients' clinical outcome.[78] Although the epigenome has the advantage of capturing a dynamic picture of cancer processes resulting from the interplay between inherited and environmental factors, there are specific challenges in conducting EWAS studies—including sample selection and handling, meticulous exposure phenotyping, sample size, and population selection. Therefore, the results should be interpreted with caution, as epigenetic changes could be either causal or consequential for a specific phenotype. MicroRNAs (miRNAs) are another important epigenetic modifier that regulate a third of human genes post-transcriptionally.[79] Evidence supports the role of miRNAs in many cellular processes critical in carcinogenesis, such as cell proliferation, differentiation, and cell death. MiRNAome is the profile of global miRNAs in the genome. Considering the complex regulation network of miRNA-target genes, the comprehensive analysis of microRNAome could provide insight into cancer etiology, treatment effects, and potential therapeutic molecules.[79,80]

The microbiome

Chronic infections contribute to carcinogenesis, with approximately 16% of the global cancer burden being directly attributable to infectious agents. The mechanism through which pathogens, such as viruses, promote cancer has also been well described. For example, *Helicobacter pylori* and hepatitis C virus (HCV) promote cancer development through epithelial injury and inflammation. Recent evidence also suggests, however, that cancer initiation and progression may not be attributable simply to one pathogen, but also potentially to global changes in our microbiome.[81]

Microorganisms make up only 1–2% of the mass of the body of a healthy human, but microbial cells are estimated to outnumber human cells by 10 to 1, and the number of microbial genes (i.e., the microbiome) is suggested to outnumber human genes by 100 to 1.[82,83] Since metabolic processes coded in the human genome are integrated with those of the associated microbiome, NGS technologies have enabled researchers to explore the bacterial microbiome and the role it plays in metabolism and inflammation, two factors involved in carcinogenesis. The 16S rRNA gene, present in all microbes, is a useful tool for characterizing microbial community structure.[83] Early animal models have linked alterations in the microbiota to carcinogenesis, particularly colorectal carcinogenesis. Tumor promoting effects of the microbiota in cancer have been largely attributed to dysbiosis, or the microbial imbalance on or inside the body, rather than infections with specific pathogens. Interindividual variability in the microbiome is influenced by a variety of factors including host physiology, pathobiology, environment, and lifestyle (diet) and behavioral factors, and microbial community structure in turn has been shown to impact important risk factors for cancer including obesity.[83–85] This area of research is still novel and the complex relationship between the microbiota and the host in respect to carcinogenesis is just now starting to be described.[86–88] Future work in this area will provide critical contributions for diagnostic, preventative, and therapeutic approaches.[81]

Other omic and digital epidemiology

Cancer is a complex disease contributed by many environmental and host factors along with their interactions. Therefore, to study those interacting factors as a whole instead of separate individual parts is critical to discovering the causal pathways. "Interactome" is a new term that refers to the characterization of a whole network of interactions among different factors (usually biological molecules) in a cell or organism contributing to a condition or disease.[89] The network is usually depicted by graphs of interconnecting lines. As an example, the interactome for *Notch2* has found a novel tumor suppressor gene *WWP2* as it serves as a negative regulator for *Notch2*,[90] which could not be discovered by traditional candidate gene approaches. In addition, genome–environment wide interaction studies (GEWIS) could address the joint effect and interactions between genetic and environmental factors.[91] An exploratory GEWIS for CRC uncovered an SNP that had significant interaction with being overweight to increase CRC risk.[92]

Advances in "digital epidemiology" developed based on communication technology devices, imaging, advanced statistical methods, and bioinformatics tools have also contributed to the advances in cancer epidemiology.[93] Traditionally, epidemiological data were collected by personal interview, which is costly and time consuming. With the advancement in digital technology, these data can now be collected using mobile phones and Internet. The digital revolution provides resources for timely computer-based data mining. At the same time, sophisticated statistical and bioinformatics tools are fundamental to analyzing the vast amount of data to draw meaningful conclusions. Unfortunately, many epidemiologists are not equipped with the training to design, conduct, and analyze these data-driven, complex, and expensive high-resolution studies, and team studies and new educational approaches are now being recognized as urgently needed.

Perspective and future direction

In the past, cancer epidemiologists have been too focused on etiologic research and are now being urged to broaden their perspective across the entire translational spectrum.[94] Khoury et al.[95] have summarized a roadmap for translational epidemiology as it impacts every step in translation research. Spitz et al.[96,97] proposed the concept of "integrative epidemiology," which expanded the boundary of epidemiology to include a cohesive integration of traditional epidemiological study design with advanced analytic and data-mining tools, to integrate and analyze information from multiple sources, and to examine influence on a wide spectrum of endpoints, from risk assessment to outcomes and treatment effects. These analytical methods for cancer epidemiology require multilevel approaches. Taplin et al.[98] have proposed a model for multilevel analysis across the cancer continuum based on the assumption that multiple levels of contextual influence affect behaviors through interdependent interactions. Lynch and Rebbeck extended this approach to a "Multilevel Biologic and Social Integrative Construct" (MBASIC) framework to integrate macroenvironment and individual factors with biology to explore multifactorial relationships and to guide study design and statistical or mechanistic models to study these relationships.[99]

The core implication in cancer epidemiology is knowledge integration, the process of integrating information and accelerating the translation and application of research findings. The process includes three key processes: knowledge management, synthesis, and translation.

Validated risk prediction models that employ such data synthesis and knowledge integration approaches could improve the outcomes of screening efforts and have substantial public health implication. Further, risk prediction tools could be incorporated into the design of smaller, more powerful, and "smarter" prevention trials. The development of risk prediction modeling is based on stringent statistical approaches incorporating information from a wide spectrum of risk factors. By quantifying risk at the individual level, the model provides evidence-based criteria for designing and subject recruitment in cancer surveillance and intervention programs.[100] For breast cancer, the multivariable statistical Gail model is the paradigm that estimates a woman's absolute risk of breast cancer given her current age, age at menarche, age at first live birth, family history of breast cancer, and number of previous breast biopsies. This model has been extended to include more comprehensive exposure and genetic and phenotypic variations.[101–103] Several studies have added additional breast cancer risk factors, such as BMI, breast density, and nutrition into the model, and provided modest improvement in the discriminative ability.[104–107] Tammemagi et al.[108] developed a lung cancer risk prediction model with an AUC of 0.8 using the large data set of the Prostate, Lung, Colorectal, Ovarian (PLCO) cancer screening trial and further showed that using their risk prediction model was more sensitive than the National Lung Screening Trial (NLST) criteria for lung cancer detection. Wen et al.[109] developed a series of models for hepatocellular carcinoma that incorporated variables of hepatitis B virus (HBV) and HCV infections as well as a panel of serum biomarkers.

Risk modeling holds great potential as the most efficient tool to implement results from cancer epidemiology studies; however, challenges still exist regarding the generally low-prediction discriminatory ability of the published models, which mostly have an AUC of around 0.55–0.70.[100] There have been continued efforts to improve prediction ability, for example, methylation profiling of DNA has increased AUC of a breast cancer risk model by 9.8%,[77] and a DNA repair assay could improve AUC of a bladder cancer risk model by 10%.[110] The major challenge associated with risk modeling, especially when using high-throughput data and intermediate biomarker data, is model validation. Collaboration is essential to provide external validation to evaluate the utility and generalization of models developed.

Summary

Lam et al.[94] have outlined four driving forces that are impacting translational cancer epidemiology in the twenty-first century: increasingly large-scale collaborative and team science, emerging novel genomic technology and application into large-scale epidemiology studies, multilevel data analysis and interventions, and the increasing complex analytical techniques to enable effective knowledge integration of large multilevel data. All of these features have allowed cancer epidemiology to evolve rapidly and become a comprehensive research "tool science" for knowledge integration at all aspects of the cancer continuum with the aim to ultimately bridge the gap from discovery to translation.

Key references

The complete reference list can be found on the Wiley Companion Digital Edition of this title (see inside front cover for login instructions).

3 Siegel R, Ma J, Zou Z, et al. Cancer statistics, 2014. *CA Cancer J Clin.* 2014;**64**(1):9–29.

7 Jones LA, Chilton JA, Hajek RA, et al. Between and within: international perspectives on cancer and health disparities. *J Clin Oncol.* 2006;**24**(14):2204–2208.

9 Ward E, Jemal A, Cokkinides V, et al. Cancer disparities by race/ethnicity and socioeconomic status. *CA Cancer J Clin.* 2004;**54**(2):78–93.

10 Kamangar F, Dores GM, Anderson WF. Patterns of cancer incidence, mortality, and prevalence across five continents: defining priorities to reduce cancer disparities in different geographic regions of the world. *J Clin Oncol.* 2006;**24**(14):2137–2150.

18 Malik VS, Willett WC, Hu FB. Global obesity: trends, risk factors and policy implications. *Nat Rev Endocrinol.* 2013;**9**(1):13–27.

22 Park J, Morley TS, Kim M, et al. Obesity and cancer—mechanisms underlying tumour progression and recurrence. *Nat Rev Endocrinol.* 2014;**10**(8):455–465.

23 Calle EE, Kaaks R. Overweight, obesity and cancer: epidemiological evidence and proposed mechanisms. *Nat Rev Cancer.* 2004;**4**(8):579–591.

24 Stunkard AJ, Foch TT, Hrubec Z. A twin study of human obesity. *JAMA.* 1986;**256**(1):51–54.

29 Kushi LH, Doyle C, McCullough M, et al. American Cancer Society Guidelines on nutrition and physical activity for cancer prevention: reducing the risk of cancer with healthy food choices and physical activity. *CA Cancer J Clin.* 2012;**62**(1):30–67.

31 McTiernan A. Mechanisms linking physical activity with cancer. *Nat Rev Cancer.* 2008;**8**(3):205–211.

33 Tannenbaum A, Silverstone H. The influence of the degree of caloric restriction on the formation of skin tumors and hepatomas in mice. *Cancer Res.* 1949;**9**(12):724–727.

45 Key TJ, Allen NE, Spencer EA, et al. The effect of diet on risk of cancer. *Lancet.* 2002;**360**(9336):861–868.

52 Electronic cigarettes (e-cigarettes). *CA: Cancer J Clin.* 2014;**64**(3):169–170.

53 Cobb NK, Abrams DB. The FDA, e-cigarettes, and the demise of combusted tobacco. *N Engl J Med.* 2014;**371**(16):1469–1471.

55 Lichtenstein P, Holm NV, Verkasalo PK, et al. Environmental and heritable factors in the causation of cancer—analyses of cohorts of twins from Sweden, Denmark, and Finland. *N Engl J Med.* 2000;**343**(2):78–85.

56 Lindor NM, McMaster ML, Lindor CJ, et al. Concise handbook of familial cancer susceptibility syndromes—second edition. *J Natl Cancer Inst Monogr.* 2008;(**38**):1–93. doi: 10.1093/jncimonographs/lgn001.

58 Gallie BL. Retinoblastoma gene mutations in human cancer. *N Engl J Med.* 1994;**330**(11):786–787.

59 Dong LM, Potter JD, White E, et al. Genetic susceptibility to cancer: the role of polymorphisms in candidate genes. *JAMA.* 2008;**299**(20):2423–2436.

62 Amos CI, Wu X, Broderick P, et al. Genome-wide association scan of tag SNPs identifies a susceptibility locus for lung cancer at 15q25.1. *Nat Genet.* 2008;**40**(5):616–622.

65 Zheng W, Long J, Gao YT, et al. Genome-wide association study identifies a new breast cancer susceptibility locus at 6q25.1. *Nat Genet.* 2009;**41**(3):324–328.

66 Garcia-Closas M, Couch FJ, Lindstrom S, et al. Genome-wide association studies identify four ER negative-specific breast cancer risk loci. *Nat Genet.* 2013;**45**(4):392–398, 398e1-2.

68 Chung CC, Chanock SJ. Current status of genome-wide association studies in cancer. *Hum Genet.* 2011. doi: 10.1007/s00439-011-1030-9.

71 Jones S, Hruban RH, Kamiyama M, et al. Exomic sequencing identifies PALB2 as a pancreatic cancer susceptibility gene. *Science.* 2009;**324**(5924):217.

76 Rakyan VK, Down TA, Balding DJ, et al. Epigenome-wide association studies for common human diseases. *Nat Rev Genet.* 2011;**12**(8):529–541.

79 Berindan-Neagoe I, Monroig PC, Pasculli B, et al. MicroRNAome genome: a treasure for cancer diagnosis and therapy. *CA: Cancer J Clin.* 2014. doi: 10.3322/caac.21244:n/a-n/a.

81 Schwabe RF, Jobin C. The microbiome and cancer. *Nat Rev Cancer.* 2013;**13**(11): 800–812.

84 Ley RE, Turnbaugh PJ, Klein S, et al. Microbial ecology: human gut microbes associated with obesity. *Nature.* 2006;**444**(7122):1022–1023.

85 Tilg H, Kaser A. Gut microbiome, obesity, and metabolic dysfunction. *J Clin Invest.* 2011;**121**(6):2126–2132.

86 Ahn J, Sinha R, Pei Z, et al. Human gut microbiome and risk for colorectal cancer. *J Natl Cancer Inst.* 2013;**105**(24):1907–1911.

89 Vidal M, Cusick ME, Barabasi AL. Interactome networks and human disease. *Cell.* 2011;**144**(6):986–998.

91 Thomas D. Gene–environment-wide association studies: emerging approaches. *Nat Rev Genet.* 2010;**11**(4):259–272.

94 Lam TK, Spitz M, Schully SD, et al. "Drivers" of translational cancer epidemiology in the 21st century: needs and opportunities. *Cancer Epidemiol Biomarkers Prev.* 2013;**22**(2):181–188.

95 Khoury MJ, Gwinn M, Ioannidis JPA. The emergence of translational epidemiology: from scientific discovery to population health impact. *Am J Epidemiol.* 2010;**172**(5):517–524.

96 Spitz MR, Caporaso NE, Sellers TA. Integrative cancer epidemiology—the next generation. *Cancer Discov.* 2012;**2**(12):1087–1090.

97 Spitz MR, Wu X, Mills G. Integrative epidemiology: from risk assessment to outcome prediction. *J Clin Oncol.* 2005;**23**(2):267–275.

100 Pu X, Ye Y, Wu X. Development and validation of risk models and molecular diagnostics to permit personalized management of cancer. *Cancer.* 2014;**120**(1):11–19.

103 Gail MH. Value of adding single-nucleotide polymorphism genotypes to a breast cancer risk model. *J Natl Cancer Inst.* 2009;**101**(13):959–963.

109 Wen CP, Lin J, Yang YC, et al. Hepatocellular carcinoma risk prediction model for the general population: the predictive power of transaminases. *J Natl Cancer Inst.* 2012;**104**(20):1599–1611.

110 Wu X, Lin J, Grossman HB, et al. Projecting individualized probabilities of developing bladder cancer in white individuals. *J Clin Oncol.* 2007;**25**(31):4974–4981.

35 Behavioral approaches to cancer prevention

Errol J. Philip, PhD ▪ *Jamie S. Ostroff, PhD*

Overview

Certain health behaviors increase the risk of being diagnosed with cancer. It has been estimated that 35% of cancer deaths throughout the world could be avoided through adoption of health promoting behaviors. This chapter summarizes research on the effects of behavioral risk factors on cancer incidence and behavioral interventions for cancer prevention. Several behavioral risk factors—tobacco use, unhealthy diet, sedentary lifestyle and obesity, sun and UV exposure—have all been associated with cancer etiology, and clinical recommendations for health promoting behavior change interventions have been developed. Physician recommendations and delivery of health promotion counseling are essential for effective dissemination of cancer prevention efforts.

Tobacco use

Tobacco use remains the leading preventable cause of morbidity and mortality. In the United States, tobacco use is responsible for nearly one in five deaths or roughly 480,000 early deaths each year (*US Surgeon General Report 2014*). Tobacco use accounts for at least 30% of all cancer deaths, causing 87% of lung cancer deaths in men and 70% of lung cancer deaths in women. (Source: *Cancer Facts & Figures 2014*.) In addition to lung cancer, cigarette smoking also increases the risk for cancers of the oral cavity, larynx, pharynx, esophagus, stomach, liver, pancreas, kidney, bladder, cervix, colon/rectum, and acute myeloid leukemia. (Source: *Cancer Facts & Figures 2014*.) Secondhand smoke exposure is also considered a risk factor for lung cancer with about 3400 nonsmoking adults dying each year of lung cancer as a result of breathing secondhand smoke. (Sources: *Cancer Facts & Figures 2014*; SGR, 2014.) Cigar smoking causes cancers of the lung, mouth, throat, larynx, and esophagus. (Source: *CDC, Consumption of Cigarettes and Combustible Tobacco—United States, 2000–2011, 2012*.) Smokeless tobacco products increase the risk of developing cancer of the mouth and throat, esophagus, and pancreas.

Although cigarette use has declined dramatically since the release of the first US Surgeon General's Report on Smoking and Health in 1964, 18.1% of all adults or more than 42 million American adults currently smoke cigarettes. (Source: *CDC, Current cigarette smoking among adults—United States, 2005–2012, 2014*.) In 2012, approximately 20.5% of men and 15.8% of women were considered to be current cigarette smokers. African Americans, Native Americans, individuals with lower income, lower education, sexual minorities, and those with comorbid substance abuse and mental illness are more likely to be current smokers. Fortunately, daily consumption of cigarettes has declined with about 22% of smokers reporting nondaily smoking. (Source: *CDC, Current cigarette smoking among adults—United States, 2005–2012, 2014*.)

Fortunately, there have also been noteworthy declines in youth smoking. In 1997, nearly half (48%) of male high school students

and more than one-third (36%) of female students reported using some form of tobacco—cigarettes, cigars, or smokeless tobacco—in the past month. In 2012, tobacco use declined to 23% for male students and 18% for female students. (Sources: *Cancer Facts & Figures 2010*; CDC, *Tobacco Product Use Among Middle and High School Students—United States, 2011 and 2012, 2013*.) On the other hand, there are growing concerns about the increasing use of electronic cigarettes, hookah, and other noncigarette tobacco products.[1,2]

Tobacco cessation in health care settings

Most recently updated in 2008 and representing current best practices, the US Public Health Service Treating Tobacco Use and Dependence Clinical Practice Guideline (PHS Guideline)[3] recommends that evidence-based tobacco treatment be delivered to all smokers in health care settings.

Brief counseling

The PHS Guideline recommends the use of a brief counseling method. As shown in Table 1, physicians are encouraged to: ask, assess, advise, assist, and arrange. Health care providers are encouraged to *ask* their patients about their smoking status at every encounter. Once current smokers are identified, clinicians should *assess* readiness to quit to inform the tobacco treatment plan. Clinicians should strongly advise their patients against smoking, personalizing the cancer and other risks of persistent smoking and the benefits of cessation in relation to their patients' disease and treatment. The next A, *assist*, involves providing education, addressing barriers to quitting such as concerns about coping, suggesting behavioral strategies that may help them overcome these barriers, developing a quit plan, and prescribing pharmacotherapy as needed. For patients who are reluctant to quit, clinicians should provide motivational counseling in an effort to encourage them to cut down or reduce their daily cigarette consumption. Finally, clinicians are encouraged to *arrange* follow-up support such as referring smokers to other resources such as Quitlines or onsite tobacco treatment specialists.

Pharmacotherapy

The guidelines strongly recommend use of pharmacotherapy along with counseling in order to optimize cessation outcomes. There are several safe and effective medications indicated for smoking cessation: nicotine replacement therapies (NRT) (patch, gum, lozenge, nasal spray, and inhaler), bupropion (Wellbutrin), and varenicline (Chantix). Refer to Table 2 for list of cessation medications, dose, duration, potential contraindications, and side effects. Combination and extended use pharmacotherapy have been shown to enhance effectiveness of tobacco dependence treatment. More research is needed to identify methods for personalizing treatments, including the tailoring of interventions to the smoker's readiness to quit, sociocultural factors, gender, age, and health status. Neuroscience

Holland-Frei Cancer Medicine, Ninth Edition. Edited by Robert C. Bast Jr., Carlo M. Croce, William N. Hait, Waun Ki Hong, Donald W. Kufe, Martine Piccart-Gebhart, Raphael E. Pollock, Ralph R. Weichselbaum, Hongyang Wang, and James F. Holland.
© 2017 John Wiley & Sons, Inc. ISBN: 978-1-118-93469-2

Table 1 The "5 A's" model for treating tobacco use and dependence.

Ask about tobacco use	Identify and document tobacco use status for every patient at every visit (*Strategy A1*)
Advise to quit	In a clear, strong, and personalized manner, urge every tobacco user to quit (*Strategy A2*)
Assess willingness to make a quit attempt	Is the tobacco user willing to make a quit attempt at this time? (*Strategy A3*)
Assist in quit attempt	For the patient willing to make a quit attempt, offer medication and provide or refer for counseling or additional treatment to help the patient quit (*Strategy A4*)
	For patients unwilling to quit at the time, provide interventions designed to increase future quit attempts (*Strategies B1 and B2*)
Arrange follow-up	For the patient willing to make a quit attempt, arrange for follow-up contacts, beginning within the first week after the quit date (*Strategy A5*)
	For patients unwilling to make a quit attempt at the time, address tobacco dependence and willingness to quit at the next clinic visit

research focusing on the genetic basis of nicotine addiction may also lead to the development of precision interventions for high-risk groups.

Currently, there is much debate and little data as to whether e-cigarettes will facilitate or impede smoking cessation and reduction of known hazards of traditional cigarettes and other combustible tobacco products.[4] The American Society of Clinical Oncology and the American Association of Cancer Research have recently published a literature summary and policy statement[5] about electronic cigarettes. Oncologists should advise smokers to quit smoking traditional cigarettes, encourage use of FDA (Food and Drug Administration)-approved cessation medications, refer patients for tobacco cessation counseling, and provide education about the potential risks and lack of known benefits of e-cigarette use with regard to long-term cessation.

Prevention of tobacco use

Preventing tobacco-related cancers requires the development and implementation of effective multipronged tobacco prevention programs. In the most recent Best Practices for Comprehensive Tobacco Control Programs,[6] the Centers for Disease Control and Prevention (CDC) recommends statewide programs that combine community-based interventions that focus on (1) preventing initiation of tobacco use among youth and young adults through tobacco control policies (i.e., taxation, tobacco-free laws), (2) promoting quitting among adults and youth, (3) eliminating exposure to secondhand smoke, and (4) identifying and eliminating tobacco-related disparities among population groups. Tobacco prevention programs should also consider targeting those children with highest biological susceptibility and sociocultural factors that increase the risk for initiating regular smoking.

Secondary and tertiary cancer prevention

An emerging body of evidence demonstrates that for individuals diagnosed with cancer, smoking is also associated with several adverse outcomes such as increased complications from surgery, increased treatment-related toxicity, decreased treatment effectiveness, poorer quality of life, increased risk of recurrence, increased risk of second primary tumors, increased noncancer-related comorbidity and mortality, and decreased survival.[7–9] Despite these risks, at least 15.1% of all adult cancer survivors report current cigarette smoking.[10] Continued tobacco use after diagnosis and resumption of smoking after initial quit attempt should be

seen as a modifiable clinical problem. In fact, there is a growing consensus among oncology leadership organizations that tobacco use assessment and treatment should be treated as a quality of care metric.[11–14] Unfortunately, a recent survey of practicing oncologists showed that oncologists provide quitting advice to only 25% of their patients[15] and that only half of National Cancer Institute-designated Comprehensive Cancer Centers offer any type of tobacco treatment program.[16] These survey findings highlight the need to identify and address barriers to tobacco treatment delivery in cancer care. Barriers to addressing tobacco use include patient factors (shame, helplessness, addiction), physician barriers (lack of training and referral options, beliefs about patients' lack of interest or ability to quit), and systems levels factors (inadequate identification of smokers, costs) that impede the delivery of effective tobacco programs.[17] Further research examining patient, provider, and systems-level strategies for engagement and retention of smokers into evidence-based tobacco treatment is needed.

Energy balance: diet, physical activity, and body weight

Energy balance represents the nexus of diet, physical activity, and body weight and has been shown to be a significant contributor to the global burden of cancer. Although research is ongoing concerning the mechanisms by which these factors relate to cancer and cancer outcomes, there is strong evidence to support an association between energy balance and cancer development and progression.

Obesity and dietary factors are estimated to account of nearly 35% of cancer cases in the United States. Strong evidence exists regarding an association between excess weight and an increased risk of many common cancer types, as well as emerging evidence of a link to poorer disease outcomes. The greatest consistency in research examining diet and cancer has been established in regard to broader dietary patterns, with prudent plant-based diets that limit meat and dairy intake generally associated with reduced cancer risk. Engagement in physical activity has been consistently shown to confer a protective effect across common cancer types.

This expansive literature has provided a foundation for lifestyle-based cancer prevention and control guidelines that all patients and survivors should be encouraged to adopt. These include consuming a healthy diet, maintaining or achieving a normal weight, and engaging in regular physical activity, all of which are key components to both cancer prevention and the pursuit of long-term health among those diagnosed with cancer.

Excess weight remains a critical modifiable risk factors linked to cancer risk in the United States,[18,19] with further contributions from physical inactivity and dietary factors. These three interrelated factors, collectively referred to as energy balance, represent primary targets of investigation and intervention in cancer prevention and control. An extensive body of research exists concerning components of energy balance and their association with increased risk of primary and secondary cancers, treatment complications, impaired quality of life, and poorer disease outcomes.[20]

Lifestyle behavior guidelines have been published by national organizations targeting cancer prevention and control. The American Cancer Society notes the importance of maintaining a healthy weight, adopting a healthy diet and engaging in regular exercise.[21,22] These recommendations are summarized in Table 3. Importantly, the broad nature of these recommendations align with disease prevention guidelines beyond cancer, and adhering

Table 2 Tobacco treatment pharmacotherapy guidelines.

Pharmacotherapy	Dosage	Duration	Availability	Precautions/ contraindications	Adverse effects	Patient education
• Nicotine Patch NicoDerm CQ® Habitrol®	*If smoking 11 cig/day or >:* • 21 mg/24 h • 14 mg/24 h • 7 mg/24 h *If smoking 10 cig/day or <:* • 14 mg/24 h • 7 mg/24 h	• 6 weeks • 2 weeks • 2 weeks • 6 weeks • 2 weeks	• Over the counter (OTC) • Medicaid reimbursement by prescription only	• Uncontrolled hypertension	• Skin irritation ° Redness ° Swelling ° Itching • Disruption in sleep ° Nightmares ° Vivid dreams	• Instruct patient to rotate patch site daily • Instruct patient to remove patch prior to bedtime if sleep is disrupted and bothersome
• Nicotine Polacrilex Gum Nicorette Gum®	• *2 mg* if smoking 24 or less cigarettes per day • *4 mg* if smoking 25 or more cigarettes per day • Do not exceed 24 pieces of gum/24 h	• Up to 12 weeks	• Over the counter • Medicaid reimbursement by prescription only	• Poor dentation • Xerostomia	• Hiccups • Upset stomach • Jaw ache	• Chew gum on a fixed schedule • "Chew and Park" each piece of gum for 30 min • Avoid eating/ drinking anything except water 15 min before and during chewing
• Nicotine Lozenge Commit®	• *2 mg* if smoking the first cigarette *more than* 30 min after waking up • *4 mg* if smoking the first cigarette *within* 30 min after waking up • Do not use more than 20 lozenges/24 h	• Up to 12 weeks	• Over the counter • Medicaid reimbursement by prescription only	• Xerostomia	• Local irritation to mouth and throat • Upset stomach	• Avoid eating/ drinking anything except water 15 min before and during when using a lozenge • Each lozenge will take 20–30 min to dissolve
• Nicotine Inhalation System Nicotrol Inhaler®	• 6–16 cartridges/day	• Up to 6 months	• Prescription only		• Local irritation to mouth and throat • Upset stomach	• Each cartridge will take 80–100 inhalations over 20 min • Instruct patient to puff on inhalers like a cigar. Absorption is in the buccal mucosa
• Nicotine Nasal Spray Nicotrol NS®	• *0.5 mg*/inhalation/ nostril 1–2 times/h or PRN dosing	• Up to 12 weeks	• Prescription only	• Sinus infections	• Nose/eye/ upper respiratory irritation	
• Bupropion Zyban® Wellbutrin SR®	• 150 mg daily × 3 days *Then* • 150 mg BID	• 12 weeks	• Prescription only	• History of seizures • History of eating disorders • Bulimia • Anorexia	• Insomnia • Dry mouth • Restlessness • Dizziness	• Overlap with smoking for 1–2 weeks • Does not need to be tapered off
• Varenicline Chantix®	• Days 1–3: 0.5 mg daily *Then* • Days 4–7: 0.5 mg BID *Then* • Days 8–end of treatment: 1 mg BID	• 12 weeks • If the patient has quit smoking, may be given another 12 weeks of treatment to prevent relapse	• Prescription only	• Kidney problems or undergoing dialysis • Pregnant or planning of getting pregnant • Breast feeding	• Mild nausea • Sleep problems • Headaches	• Take medication with a full glass of water after you eat a meal • Allow 8 h between each dose • Take this medication a few hours before bedtime to avoid restlessness

Table 3 ACS adult guidelines for energy balance for cancer prevention and control.

Achieve and maintain healthy weight	• Balance energy intake and expenditure through portion control, an emphasis on a plant-based diet and the limiting of high caloric foods and beverages
Engage in regular physical activity	• Engage in 150 min of moderate activity (e.g., brisk walking) or 75 min of vigorous activity (e.g., jogging) per week and limit sedentary activity
Maintain a healthy diet	• Emphasize a plant-based diet that includes whole grains and 2.5 cups of fruits and vegetables per day, while limiting intake of processed and red meats • Alcohol consumption should be limited to two standard drinks per day for men and one standard drink for women

to such advice will serve to also reduce risk of other chronic conditions such as cardiovascular disease, diabetes, and hypertension. Unfortunately, despite a variety of efforts to raise awareness of lifestyle-based recommendations and increase adoption, adherence among the general population and cancer survivors alike remains low.[23,24] Recent calls have been made to promote the use of the term energy balance in clinical practice and oncology,[25] thus reinforcing the interdependent nature of diet, exercise, and weight, and in turn lessen the potential for patients to focus on such factors in isolation.

A recent study of nearly 112,000 nonsmoking individuals examined the association between adherence to ACS health guidelines and disease outcomes across 14 years of follow-up. The authors reported that greater adherence to health recommendations were associated with reduced risk of both cancer and all-cause mortality.[26] The next section will provide an overview of current research findings concerning the relationship between energy balance and cancer. While acknowledging the synergistic and interrelated nature of diet, weight, and physical activity, each will be addressed separately with focus given to the four most common cancers diagnosed in the United States.

Diet and cancer

Breast cancer

The potential association between diet and breast cancer has received extensive empirical attention over the past three decades. The WCRF (World Cancer Research Fund) reported that based on observational studies, certain dietary patterns that include a high intake of fruit and vegetables, along with consumption of poultry, fish, and low-fat dairy products,[27] are associated with reduced disease risk. Similar findings were reported by Brennan et al. in a 2010[28] systematic review and meta-analysis of 39 case-control and cohort studies examining various dietary patterns. Despite its primary role among prudent dietary patterns, little evidence exists supporting the isolated protective effect of fruit and vegetable intake alone.[29] The Women's Health Initiative Trial sought to establish whether reduced fat intake could impact cancer risk in a randomized clinical trial involving nearly 50,000 postmenopausal women. Reduction in fat intake was associated with only a marginal reduction in disease risk, and no difference in invasive breast cancer cases during the 8-year follow-up period.[30] Finally, evidence suggests that alcohol consumption may increase risk of breast cancer in a dose–response manner for both pre and postmenopausal

women,[27,29] while a recent meta-analysis suggested that there currently exists no evidence linking red meat consumption with breast cancer risk across the lifespan.[31]

Prostate cancer

As the literature examining the relationship between diet and prostate cancer has matured, recent studies have suggested that this association may differ based on the aggressiveness of the disease. In their systematic review, Ma and Chapman[32] proposed that further work is needed to account for this potential influence, and that there is not yet sufficiently rigorous evidence to provide firm recommendations on the role of diet in prostate cancer. Despite this, there exists suggestive evidence of a protective effect of vegetable and soy consumption, and an increased risk of disease associated with dairy products. Kirsh et al.[33] reported that men who had a high intake of cruciferous vegetables (e.g., cabbage, broccoli) had a decreased risk of aggressive prostate cancer. Dairy consumption may lead to a possible increased risk of prostate cancer,[27] with a further analysis of the PLCO trial, and nearly 30,000 men establishing a modest increase in the risk of nonaggressive cancers among those reporting a higher intake of dairy products.[34] There was no association established between dairy intake and more aggressive forms of disease.

Colorectal cancer

Considerable effort has been devoted to examine the potential impact of nutrition on the development and progression of colorectal cancer. A number of recent international reports and meta-analyses noted convincing evidence of an increased risk of colon, colorectal, and rectal cancer associated with the consumption of red meat and processed meat products.[27,35] These recent studies, including an updated meta-analysis,[36] noted a dose–response relationship between meat consumption and cancer risk, including a 21% increased risk with 50 g/day consumed and a 29% increased risk with 100 g/day consumed.[35] For comparative purposes, the recommended serving size for a portion of lean meat is approximately 85 g.

The relationship between fiber and disease risk has also received considerable attention; however, despite plausible biological mechanisms, early reports found little evidence of an association between fiber consumption and colorectal cancer.[37–39] More recent studies have, however, noted a relationship.[40,41] A systematic review of 25 prospective studies reported a dose–response relationship between cereal fiber and whole grains and a reduced risk of colorectal cancer.[42] The authors reported a statistically significant 10% decrease in cancer risk with 10 g of daily fiber intake. The recommended daily intake of fiber for adults is 25 g.

Alcohol consumption has also been associated with increased risk of colorectal cancer.[35] In a review of 103 cohort studies, Huxley found that those reporting the highest levels of alcohol consumption had a 60% increased risk of colorectal cancer compared to non- or light drinkers. This relationship was particularly prominent among male participants.[43] Chung et al.[44] conducted a systematic review and reported inconsistent results concerning the relationship between calcium and vitamin D and colorectal cancer. Importantly, while evidence is evolving and currently suggests that increased calcium intake could reduce risk of colorectal cancer; this benefit must be weighed against potential increase in prostate cancer risk. At present, there exist no recommendations to increase calcium intake as a means of reducing cancer risk.

Lung cancer

The WRCF/AICR (American Institute for Cancer Research) report established that higher rates of fruit and vegetable consumption is consistently associated with reduced risk of lung cancer among both smokers and nonsmoking populations.[27] The report notes, however, that despite this consistency, the protective effect of a healthy diet is minimal compared to risk associated with tobacco use.

Obesity and cancer

Obesity rates have increased dramatically over the past 30 years, with over 35% of US adults now considered obese.[45] A 2003 report estimated 14–20% of all cancer deaths to be attributable to excess weight,[46] and in combination with the dietary intake, accounts for nearly one in three cancers and may soon overtake tobacco as the primary modifiable risk factor in cancer.[27,47] The unprecedented increase in weight of the general population, along with the increased risk of cancer associated with excess weight, means that an estimated 10 of the 14 million survivors are overweight or obese.[48–50] A report published by the WCRF/AICR, along with an updated review by Renehan in 2008, noted evidence of a link between excess body weight and many common types of cancer.[27,51] These include colon, kidney, pancreatic cancer, and esophageal adenocarcinoma among both sexes, as well as thyroid cancer for men and gallbladder, endometrial, ovarian, and postmenopausal breast cancers among women.

Breast and Prostate Cancer

Excess body weight and weight gain in adulthood have both been consistently associated with risk of breast cancer.[52,53] A further meta-analysis by Vrieling et al.[54] noted a stronger association between weight gain and estrogen-/progesterone-positive breast cancers. The impact of obesity on prostate cancer appears to be moderated by disease severity, and thus, more recent studies have emphasized the importance of examining this relationship in greater detail. Obese weight status has been associated with greater risk of being diagnosed with advanced disease,[55] increased risk of recurrence,[56] and poorer prognosis.[57] In contrast, Wright et al.[58] reported an inverse association between BMI (body mass index) and risk of early stage disease among a large population of men enrolled in the National Institutes of Health–AARP Diet and Health Study. This complex relationship is believed to be partly due to challenges inherent to screening and diagnosis among obese men, however, research continues.

Colorectal cancer and other notable findings

The majority of studies have supported a positive association between weight and risk of colorectal cancer, most strongly among men,[35,46] including a recent meta-analysis over 56 observational studies.[59] Norat et al.[35] noted that this association was more consistent among studies that examined measures of body fat distribution beyond BMI, with excess weight in the abdominal region most predictive of increased cancer risk.

Endometrial cancer remains the most consistent cancer linked to excess weight, with an estimated 60% of new cases attributable to obesity.[60] Obese women are 2–3.5 times more likely to be diagnosed with this form of cancer,[61] including a large-scale European study that followed one million women for nearly 40 years reporting obese women to be 2.5 times more likely to be diagnosed with cancer of the uterine corpus compared to those of normal weight.[62]

Physical activity and cancer

Engagement in physical activity remains an important component of health recommendations and has been associated with reduced risk across a number of common cancer types.[22]

Breast and prostate cancer

The association between physical activity and breast cancer risk has been extensively researched and deemed convincing.[63] This has included a review of more than 70 observational reports that established an absolute risk reduction of between 20% and 30% in breast cancer risk when comparing those who were most active to those who are least active.[61,64] In a systematic review and meta-analysis of over 40 reports, including over two million men and nearly 90,000 cases of cancer, Liu et al.[65] reported an 10% overall risk reduction in prostate cancer associated with engagement in physical activity.

Colorectal and lung cancer

The relationship between physical activity and colorectal cancer has also received considerable empirical attention. A 2009 meta-analysis by Wolin et al.[66] examined over 50 studies and reported on overall reduction in risk of 24%, with greater risk reduction reported in case-control studies. Similar findings were reported by Harris and Thune in relation to colon cancer, including evidence of a dose–response relationship between physical activity engagement and cancer risk among both genders.[67,68] No evidence of a relationship was established, however, among seven studies of rectal cancer.

In a review of predominantly cohort studies, Emaus and Thune[69] reported a 23% reduction in lung cancer risk among those engaged in physical activity, with a greater rate of 38% once again reported among case-control studies. A further meta-analysis reported similar results, although risk reduction varied based on intensity of activity, with moderate engagement associated with a 13% reduction in risk and rigorous activity associated with 30% reduction in risk.[70] A recent systematic review noted the need for ongoing research in this arena, particularly among women, with 10 studies reporting an inverse association between physical activity and lung cancer and nearly as many reporting a null association.[71]

Energy balance and cancer survivorship

As survival rates across many common cancers have increased; emerging research has begun to address the role of lifestyle in cancer prognosis and survivorship. Research and clinical programs in this domain have sought to build upon the noted potential for a cancer diagnosis to act as a teachable moment,[72] and to thus seize upon a period in which patients and survivors may be motivated to enact lifestyle changes.[73–75] In a systematic review of physical activity and cancer survival, authors reported, among 27 published studies, there was sufficient evidence supporting an association between physical activity and a reduction in all-cause mortality, as well as breast and colon-specific cancer mortality.[76] In a review by Davies et al.,[77] a healthy or prudent diet pattern low in fat and high in fiber may be broadly associated with a reduced risk of cancer recurrence and progression; however, further research is needed. This is particularly true in regard to establishing whether the protective effects of a healthy diet and/or physical activity may be due to their promotion of a healthy body weight. Finally, Parekh et al.[78] reported in a systematic review of the literature pertaining to breast, colon, and prostate cancer that the majority of studies suggest a negative effect of excess weight on cancer survival outcomes. However, the authors noted that breast cancer is overrepresented in this literature, and that many studies examining obesity and cancer survival were not initially designed to examine such outcomes. In light of these emerging findings, the American Society of Clinical Oncology has created a toolkit to help oncologists counsel their patients about the importance of weight management for cancer survivors.[79]

Promoting behavioral change in diet and physical activity

Although some individuals may require more intensive intervention, a recommendation from a health care provider can play an important role in promoting energy balance and lifestyle change.[20] Evidence-based behavioral lifestyle programs exist for those individuals who require more support. These 6–12-month programs usually adopt a group-based format and include dietary counseling and caloric reduction, along with promotion of physical activity engagement. Such programs routinely result in weight loss of 5–10% of initial body weight[80] and can provide clinically relevant improvements in many disease markers with plausible downstream benefits for reducing cancer risk.[81,82] Maintenance of weight loss remains a challenge and providers should remain supportive of patients seeking to adopt changes.[83] Evidence pertaining to the impact of behavior change on cancer-related outcomes is growing, with evidence suggesting that bariatric surgery results in reduced cancer risk[84] and that changes in diet and physical activity behavior change can improve biological markers among survivors.[85]

Risk behaviors for skin cancer

Skin cancers are commonly divided into melanoma and non-melanoma skin cancers. Melanoma is less common but more aggressive than other types of skin cancer, affecting some 68,000 Americans each year.[86] Exposure to ultraviolet radiation (UVR) from the sun or from indoor tanning devices is a significant risk factor for skin cancer,[87] and there are well-established behavioral strategies for skin cancer prevention. These recommendations,[88] include nonuse of artificial tanning beds and limiting unprotected exposure to the sun—especially strong midday sunlight—whenever possible. When exposure to sunlight is not avoidable, individuals should be advised to apply a broad spectrum sunscreen (i.e., effective against both UVA (ultraviolet A) and UVB (ultraviolet B) radiation with a sun protection factor (SPF) of 30 or greater) very liberally, approximately 30 min before going out into the sunlight and then reapplying every 2 h or after any exposure to water. Most importantly, individuals should be advised that sunscreens offer only *partial* protection from UVR and should best be used in combination with avoiding exposure to strong sunlight and wearing sun protective clothing (i.e., hats, long-sleeved garments).

Unfortunately, only 30% of US adults routinely report using sunscreen and/or sun protective clothing.[89] Remarkably, surveys show that even cancer survivors do not consistently protect themselves from UV light, especially younger survivors who are most likely to be exposed to UVR.[50,90,91]

Summary

The importance of reducing behavioral risks on cancer prevention is well established.[92] Healthy People 2020[93] goals emphasize health promoting behavior change efforts such as not smoking, maintaining a healthy weight, eating a low-fat, high-fiber diet, being physically active, and limiting UVR exposure.

Key references

The complete reference list can be found on the Wiley Companion Digital Edition of this title (see inside front cover for login instructions).

3 Fiore M, Jaén C, Baker T, et al. Treating tobacco use and dependence: 2008 update U.S. Public Health Service Clinical Practice Guideline executive summary. *Respir Care.* 2008;**53**(9):1217–1222.

5 Brandon TH, Goniewicz ML, Hanna NH, et al. Electronic nicotine delivery systems: a policy statement from the American Association for Cancer Research and the American Society of Clinical Oncology. *J Clin Oncol.* 2015;**33**(8):952–963.

6 Centers for Disease Control and Prevention. Best Practices for Comprehensive Tobacco Control Programs-2014. Atlanta: U.S. Department of Health and Human Services, Centers for Disease Control and Precention, National Center for Chronic Disease Prevention and Health Promotion, Office on Smoking and Health, 2014.

10 Underwood JM, Townsend JS, Stewart SL, et al. Surveillance of demographic characteristics and health behaviors among adult cancer survivors—behavioral risk factor surveillance system, United States, 2009. *Morb Mortal Wkly Rep Surveill Summ.* 2012;**61**(Suppl 1):1–23.

18 Danaei G, Vander Hoorn S, Lopez AD, Murray CJ, Ezzati M. Causes of cancer in the world: comparative risk assessment of nine behavioural and environmental risk factors. *Lancet.* 2005;**366**(9499):1784–1793.

21 Rock CL, Doyle C, Demark-Wahnefried W, et al. Nutrition and physical activity guidelines for cancer survivors. *CA J Clin.* 2012;**62**(4):243–274.

22 Kushi LH, Doyle C, McCullough M, et al. American Cancer Society Guidelines on nutrition and physical activity for cancer prevention: reducing the risk of cancer with healthy food choices and physical activity. *CA Cancer J Clin.* 2012;**62**(1):30–67.

23 Blanchard CM, Courneya KS, Stein K. Cancer survivors' adherence to lifestyle behavior recommendations and associations with health-related quality of life: results from the American Cancer Society's SCS-II. *J Clin Oncol.* 2008;**26**(13):2198–2204.

26 McCullough ML, Patel AV, Kushi LH, et al. Following cancer prevention guidelines reduces risk of cancer, cardiovascular disease, and all-cause mortality. *Cancer Epidemiol Biomarkers Prev.* 2011;**20**(6):1089–1097.

28 Brennan SF, Cantwell MM, Cardwell CR, Velentzis LS, Woodside JV. Dietary patterns and breast cancer risk: a systematic review and meta-analysis. *Am J Clin Nutr.* 2010;**91**(5):1294–1302.

30 Prentice RL, Caan B, Chlebowski RT, et al. Low-fat dietary pattern and risk of invasive breast cancer: the Women's Health Initiative Randomized Controlled Dietary Modification Trial. *JAMA.* 2006;**295**(6):629–642.

31 Alexander DD, Morimoto LM, Mink PJ, Cushing CA. A review and meta-analysis of red and processed meat consumption and breast cancer. *Nutr Res Rev.* 2010;**23**(2):349–365.

32 Ma RW, Chapman K. A systematic review of the effect of diet in prostate cancer prevention and treatment. *J Hum Nutr Diet.* 2009;**22**(3):187–199; quiz 200–2.

33 Kirsh VA, Peters U, Mayne ST, et al. Prospective study of fruit and vegetable intake and risk of prostate cancer. *J Natl Cancer Inst.* 2007;**99**(15):1200–1209.

36 Chan DS, Lau R, Aune D, Vieira R, Greenwood DC, Kampman E, et al. Red and processed meat and colorectal cancer incidence: meta-analysis of prospective studies. *PLoS One.* 2011;**6**(6):e20456.

37 Schatzkin A, Lanza E, Corle D, et al. Lack of effect of a low-fat, high-fiber diet on the recurrence of colorectal adenomas. Polyp prevention trial study group. *N Engl J Med.* 2000;**342**(16):1149–1155.

38 Park Y, Hunter DJ, Spiegelman D, et al. Dietary fiber intake and risk of colorectal cancer: a pooled analysis of prospective cohort studies. *JAMA.* 2005;**294**(22):2849–2857.

41 Bingham SA, Day NE, Luben R, et al. Dietary fibre in food and protection against colorectal cancer in the European Prospective Investigation into Cancer and Nutrition (EPIC): an observational study. *Lancet.* 2003;**361**(9368):1496–1501.

42 Aune D, Chan DS, Lau R, et al. Dietary fibre, whole grains, and risk of colorectal cancer: systematic review and dose–response meta-analysis of prospective studies. *BMJ.* 2011;**343**:d6617.

43 Huxley RR, Ansary-Moghaddam A, Clifton P, Czernichow S, Parr CL, Woodward M. The impact of dietary and lifestyle risk factors on risk of colorectal cancer: a quantitative overview of the epidemiological evidence. *Int J Cancer.* 2009;**125**(1):171–180.

46 Calle EE, Rodriguez C, Walker-Thurmond K, Thun MJ. Overweight, obesity, and mortality from cancer in a prospectively studied cohort of U.S. adults. *N Engl J Med.* 2003;**348**(17):1625–1638.

48 Howlader N, Noone AM, Krapcho M, et al. *SEER Cancer Statistics Review, 1975–2008.* Bethesda, MD: National Cancer Institute; 2011.

50 Coups EJ, Ostroff JS. A population-based estimate of the prevalence of behavioral risk factors among adult cancer survivors and noncancer controls. *Prev Med.* 2005;**40**(6):702–711.

51 Renehan AG, Tyson M, Egger M, Heller RF, Zwahlen M. Body-mass index and incidence of cancer: a systematic review and meta-analysis of prospective observational studies. *Lancet.* 2008;**371**(9612):569–578.

52 Michels KB, Mohllajee AP, Roset-Bahmanyar E, Beehler GP, Moysich KB. Diet and breast cancer: a review of the prospective observational studies. *Cancer*. 2007;**109**(Suppl 12):2712–2749.

54 Vrieling A, Buck K, Kaaks R, Chang-Claude J. Adult weight gain in relation to breast cancer risk by estrogen and progesterone receptor status: a meta-analysis. *Breast Cancer Res Treat*. 2010;**123**(3):641–649.

55 Cao Y, Ma J. Body mass index, prostate cancer-specific mortality, and biochemical recurrence: a systematic review and meta-analysis. *Cancer Prev Res*. 2011;**4**(4):486–501.

58 Wright ME, Chang SC, Schatzkin A, et al. Prospective study of adiposity and weight change in relation to prostate cancer incidence and mortality. *Cancer*. 2007;**109**(4):675–684.

59 Ning Y, Wang L, Giovannucci EL. A quantitative analysis of body mass index and colorectal cancer: findings from 56 observational studies. *Obes Rev*. 2010;**11**(1):19–30.

60 Calle EE, Kaaks R. Overweight, obesity and cancer: epidemiological evidence and proposed mechanisms. *Nat Rev Cancer*. 2004;**4**(8):579–591.

64 Friedenreich CM. Physical activity and breast cancer: review of the epidemiologic evidence and biologic mechanisms. *Recent Results Cancer Res*. 2011;**188**: 125–139.

65 Liu Y, Hu F, Li D, et al. Does physical activity reduce the risk of prostate cancer? A systematic review and meta-analysis. *Eur Urol*. 2011;**60**(5):1029–1044.

66 Wolin KY, Yan Y, Colditz GA, Lee IM. Physical activity and colon cancer prevention: a meta-analysis. *Br J Cancer*. 2009;**100**(4):611–616.

67 Harriss DJ, Atkinson G, Batterham A, et al. Lifestyle factors and colorectal cancer risk (2): a systematic review and meta-analysis of associations with leisure-time physical activity. *Colorectal Dis*. 2009;**11**(7):689–701.

70 Tardon A, Lee WJ, Delgado-Rodriguez M, et al. Leisure-time physical activity and lung cancer: a meta-analysis. *Cancer Cause Contr*. 2005;**16**(4):389–397.

72 Demark-Wahnefried W, Aziz NM, Rowland JH, Pinto BM. Riding the crest of the teachable moment: promoting long-term health after the diagnosis of cancer. *J Clin Oncol*. 2005;**23**(24):5814–5830.

76 Ballard-Barbash R, Friedenreich CM, Courneya KS, Siddiqi SM, McTiernan A, Alfano CM. Physical activity, biomarkers, and disease outcomes in cancer survivors: a systematic review. *J Natl Cancer Inst*. 2012;**104**(11):815–840.

79 American Society for Clinical Oncology. Obesity and Cancer Toolkit Alexandria, VA: American Society for Clinical Oncology; 2015 [3/1/2015]. Available from: http://www.asco.org/practice-research/obesity-and-cancer.

85 Rock CL, Byers TE, Colditz GA, et al. Reducing breast cancer recurrence with weight loss, a vanguard trial: the Exercise and Nutrition to Enhance Recovery and Good Health for You (ENERGY) Trial. *Contemp Clin Trials*. 2013;**34**(2): 282–295.

91 Tercyak KP, Donze JR, Prahlad S, Mosher RB, Shad AT. Multiple behavioral risk factors among adolescent survivors of childhood cancer in the Survivor Health and Resilience Education (SHARE) program. *Pediatr Blood Cancer*. 2006;**47**(6):825–830.

36 Diet and nutrition in the etiology and prevention of cancer

Steven K. Clinton, MD, PhD ▪ Elizabeth M. Grainger, PhD, RD ▪ Edward L. Giovannucci, MD, ScD

Overview

Associations between nutrients, foods, dietary patterns, and cancer risk have been the source of substantial scientific inquiry as improved tools to assess dietary exposures and cancer outcomes have emerged for different populations around the globe. Research includes observational studies, epidemiologic cohort studies, and some human intervention trials that are supported by mechanistic laboratory investigations. These efforts strongly implicate dietary patterns as a major risk factor in the global cancer burden and have resulted in the formulation of dietary guidelines for prevention of cancer by several public health organizations. The dietary recommendations, which also include maintaining a healthy weight and participating in regular physical activity, are interrelated and are intended to guide the development of behavior patterns regarding diet orchestration and exercise that are consistent with reducing the risk of cancer. Those undergoing cancer treatment with diverse therapeutic interventions require personalized consultations with nutrition professionals, such as registered dietitians, in order to maintain optimal health while reducing toxicity and enhancing efficacy of therapy. Increasingly, the role of diet and physical activity in cancer survivorship is being addressed, and the future will likely include more specific survivorship guidelines, personalized for individuals, that reduce the risk of cancer recurrence, lower the long-term consequences of cancer therapy, and promote health and quality of life.

Over the past two centuries, improvements in food production, processing, storage, and distribution have led to major changes in diet composition throughout the world. During this period, life expectancy also dramatically increased within economically developed nations because of a combination of factors, including public health measures, improved occupational safety, and major reductions in nutrient deficiency syndromes. As the populations age, there has been a shift in the major causes of morbidity and mortality toward chronic diseases, such as cancer and cardiovascular disease. In the United States, recent decades are characterized by an increasingly sedentary population with an epidemic of obesity, a trend that is emerging worldwide. Although nutritional deficiencies still plague subpopulations in developed nations such as the poor, the aged, alcoholics, and the chronically ill, we now recognize that the affluent dietary pattern contributes to the pathogenesis of many chronic diseases, including cancer, that afflict the vast majority of the population. Efforts to understand the often complex etiologies of various cancers have led to laboratory, clinical, and epidemiologic studies that strongly implicate specific nutrients and certain dietary patterns in human carcinogenesis.

It is important to establish a conceptual framework for organizing data regarding diet, nutrition, and cancer that will help readers provide guidance to the public and patients. We arbitrarily divide the topic into the realms of prevention, therapy, and survivorship. Organizations such as the National Cancer Institute, the American Cancer Society (ACS), the World Health Organization, and the American Institute for Cancer Research/Word Cancer Research Fund have published recommendations defining achievable dietary and nutritional goals for the populations that may help reduce the overall cancer burden through primary prevention (Table 1). These goals are evidence-based and increasingly utilize a systematic review process. Some individuals, particularly those deemed to be at higher risk of specific types of cancer as a result of environmental exposures, family history, or the presence of premalignant conditions, are more readily pursuing dietary and lifestyle interventions that may be tailored to lower their chances of developing a specific cancer. Patients actively undergoing cancer therapy represent another group profoundly interested in the role of dietary and nutritional interventions to enhance the efficacy of treatment while reducing the frequency and severity of side effects. These issues are diverse and best addressed in the medical clinics with a therapeutic team that includes registered dietitians (RD). Finally, as cancers are detected earlier and treatment interventions become more successful, the number of cancer survivors is increasing rapidly. Those completing cancer therapy are seeking guidance regarding diet and lifestyle interventions that will lower their risk of recurrence (secondary prevention) and reduce the severity of long-term complications of their cancer treatment, including therapy-related second malignancies and long-term organ dysfunction. Thus, those involved in cancer therapy and management of long-term health are ever more being asked to provide evidence-based guidance in an area where scientific studies are few. Thus, vulnerable survivors frequently fall prey to purveyors of alternative diet- or nutrient-based interventions marketed in the absence of scientific data regarding efficacy and safety. Although this chapter focuses upon prevention, we briefly review the therapeutic and survivorship phases and provide information that will assist in counseling individuals and groups interested in dietary and nutritional interventions.

The vast majority of research conducted in the field of diet, nutrition, and cancer focuses on etiology and prevention. Thus, this chapter emphasizes the public health model and focuses on the interventions that may reduce the overall cancer burden of large populations. We then consider the evidence for prevention of the most commonly occurring cancers involving specific organs. Rather than detailing the complex, often incomplete, and occasionally contradictory literature concerning the role of dietary components in the etiology of specific cancers, this chapter provides a general guide with an emphasis on the major emerging concepts in the area. We conclude with a brief overview of the role of diet and nutrition to enhance therapy and survivorship.

Holland-Frei Cancer Medicine, Ninth Edition. Edited by Robert C. Bast Jr., Carlo M. Croce, William N. Hait, Waun Ki Hong, Donald W. Kufe, Martine Piccart-Gebhart, Raphael E. Pollock, Ralph R. Weichselbaum, Hongyang Wang, and James F. Holland.
© 2017 John Wiley & Sons, Inc. ISBN: 978-1-118-93469-2

Table 1 Guidelines for nutrition and cancer prevention.

	American Institute of Cancer Research[1]	American Heart Association and the American College of Cardiology[2,3]	Dietary Guidelines for Americans[4] [a]	American Cancer Society[5]
Body weight	Ensure that body weight through childhood and adolescent growth is toward the lower end of normal BMI by age 21 Maintain body weight within the normal range from age 21 on Avoid weight gain	For individuals who are overweight, participation in a professionally-guided lifestyle program (>6 mo duration) promoting a lower-calorie diet is advised Medical team should use NHLBI body mass index (BMI) tables to stratify risk and define interventions	Prevent and/or reduce overweight and obesity through improved eating and physical activity Control calorie intake. For people who are overweight, consume fewer calories from foods and beverages Maintain appropriate calorie balance during each stage of life	Achieve and maintain a healthy weight throughout life Be as lean as possible throughout life without being underweight Avoid excess weight gain at all ages Engage in regular physical activity while limiting high calorie foods and beverages
Physical activity	Be moderately physically active for at least 30 min each day As fitness improves, aim for at least 60 min of moderate activity or 30 min of vigorous activity every day Limit sedentary habits	Engage in 2 h and 30 min/wk of moderate intensity or 75 min/wk of vigorous-intensity aerobic physical activity To reduce weight, 150 min/wk of aerobic physical activity. Higher levels (200–300 min/wk) are recommended to maintain weight loss and prevent regain	Increase physical activity and reduce time spent in sedentary behaviors	Adopt a physically active lifestyle Adults: engage in at least 150 min of moderate intensity or 75 min of vigorous intensity activity each week Limit sedentary behavior such as sitting, lying down, watching television, or other screen-based entertainment
Plant-based diet	Eat at least five servings (at least 400 g) of a variety of nonstarchy vegetables and fruits each day Eat relatively unprocessed cereals and legumes with every meal Limit refined starchy foods	Consume a dietary pattern that emphasizes intake of vegetables, fruits, and whole grains and includes low-fat dairy products, poultry, fish, legumes, nontropical vegetable oils, and nuts		Consume a healthy diet with an emphasis on plant foods
Vegetable and fruit	Eat at least five servings (at least 400 g) of a variety of nonstarchy vegetables and fruits each day	Consume a dietary pattern that emphasizes intake of vegetables and fruits	Increase fruit and vegetable intake Eat a variety of vegetables, especially dark-green, red, and orange vegetables, beans and peas	Eat at least 2.5 cups of vegetables and fruits each day
Breads, grains, and cereals	Eat relatively unprocessed cereals and legumes with every meal Limit refined starchy foods	Consume a plant-based dietary pattern that includes whole grains	Consume at least half of all grains as whole grains Increase whole grain intake by replacing refined grains with whole grains	Choose whole grains instead of refined grain products
Animal products	People who choose to eat red meat should consume less than 500 g (18 oz) per week, very little if any to be processed meat	Consume a dietary pattern that includes low-fat dairy products, poultry, and fish; limit intake of red meat	Choose a variety of protein foods, which include seafood, lean meat and poultry, and eggs Increase intake of fat-free or low-fat milk and milk products	Limit consumption of processed meats and red meat
Dietary fat	Consume energy-dense foods sparingly Consume "fast foods" sparingly, if at all	Reduce percent of calories from saturated fat Aim for a dietary pattern that achieves 5–6% of calories from saturated fat Reduce percent of calories from *trans*-fat	Consume less than 10% of calories from saturated fat Consume less than 300 mg per day of cholesterol Keep *trans*-fatty acid consumption as low as possible	
Processed foods and refined sugar	Avoid salt-preserved, salted, or salty foods; preserve without using salt Avoid sugary drinks	Limit intake of sweets and sugar-sweetened beverages	Reduce the intake of calories from added sugars	
Salt and sodium	Avoid salt-preserved, salted, or salty foods; preserve without using salt Limit consumption of processed foods with added salt to ensure an intake of less than 6 g (2.4 g sodium) per day	Consume no more than 2400 mg of sodium per day Further reduction of sodium intake to 1500 mg/day can result in even greater reduction in blood pressure	Reduce daily sodium intake to less than 2300 mg. Certain populations of people, including African Americans, persons with diabetes or chronic kidney, disease and all adults 51 years of age and older, should reduce sodium to 1500 mg per day	

Table 1 *(Continued)*

	American Institute of Cancer Research[1]	**American Heart Association and the American College of Cardiology**[2,3]	**Dietary Guidelines for Americans**[4] [a]	**American Cancer Society**[5]
Alcohol	If alcoholic drinks are consumed, limit consumption to no more than two drinks a day for men and one drink a day for women		If alcohol is consumed, it should be consumed in moderation—up to 1 drink/day for women and up to 2 drinks/day for men	If you drink alcoholic beverages, limit consumption Drink no more than 1 drink per day for women and 2 per day for men
Miscellaneous	Dietary supplements are not recommended for cancer prevention Unless otherwise advised, cancer survivors should aim to follow the recommendations for diet, healthy weight, and physical activity		Select an eating pattern that meets nutrient needs over time at an appropriate calorie level	Increase access to affordable, healthful foods in communities, worksites, and schools

[a]Updated Dietary Guidelines for Americans are scheduled for release in 2016, and will be accessed at http://health.gov/dietaryguidelines/.

Methodologic issues in diet, nutrition, and cancer studies

It is valuable to briefly consider how evidence-based dietary recommendations are established. The unbiased detection and quantification of risks that are associated with variations in diet and nutrient intake would ideally be achieved through randomized and prospective trials. Unfortunately, the enormous costs of long-term nutrition studies and the scientific difficulties in controlling or measuring dietary patterns and nutrient intake limit their feasibility. Therefore, current nutritional guidelines for disease prevention are based on the integration of information derived from a variety of different epidemiologic approaches and laboratory investigations, and, thus, most guidelines are developed by expert committees convened by organizations such as the National Cancer Institute, the ACS, the American Institute of Cancer Research (AICR)/World Cancer Research Fund (WCRF), and the World Health Organization, among others.[1,2,5,6] The evidence derived from epidemiologic studies, clinical investigations, and laboratory studies is reviewed and discussed relative to criteria of causality, defined as a specific occurrence or outcome that is consistently preceded by a known set of circumstances or conditions. In nutritional sciences, clear representations of causality have been the demonstration of single-nutrient deficiency syndromes and their complete reversal by exposure to the nutrient. For example, the lack of fruits and vegetables in the diet leads to scurvy, which is readily reversed by vitamin C. Unfortunately, relationships between diet and cancer are much more complex than simple nutrient-deficiency syndromes. To establish causality, conclusions about the occurrence of an event and its etiologic factors are based on consensus criteria. These criteria have evolved over many years and include consistency, strength of association, biologic gradient, temporality, specificity, biologic plausibility, biologic mechanism, coherence, and experimental evidence.[7] Precisely quantitating risk due to a dietary variable has been difficult, because the etiologies of most cancers are multifactorial, and the interactions are poorly understood. Human cancers show striking variations based on factors such as age, sex, race, socioeconomic status, and host genetics, as well as many environmental, occupational, and lifestyle variables. The potential for complex interactions between these factors and diet is enormous, and this emphasizes the difficulties in demonstrating causal associations with the same clarity as is demonstrable for high-risk environmental exposures, such as the impact of cigarette smoking on lung cancer.

Assessment of the human diet

Nutritional epidemiology poses some unique obstacles in that food is a universal exposure, in stark contrast to many cancer-causing environmental exposures, such as cigarette smoke. Table 2 details the strengths and limitations of various types of study designs used in nutrition research. The outcomes of interest in epidemiology include nutrients, nonnutrient bioactive components, and dietary patterns. Nutrients are components where known deficiency syndromes have been characterized. These include the energy-supplying macronutrients, which are lipids, carbohydrates, and proteins, and the various constituents, such as essential fatty acids and amino acids, as well as micronutrient vitamins and minerals. Nonnutrient components include thousands of potential bioactives, particularly rich in fruits and vegetables, such as fiber, polyphenols, and carotenoids. Currently, strategies to define dietary patterns, such as a Mediterannean-style, vegetarian, or affluent dietary pattern may provide greater insight into combined effects of multiple variables; nevertheless, standardized definitions and statistical approaches to assessing dietary patterns are lacking.

The critical limiting feature of most human studies is the imprecision of quantifying dietary intake. Estimating the usual intake of foods or nutrients, as well as accounting for intraindividual variation over time, is a critical area of research.[8–10] An estimate of human nutrient intake is derived from a two-step process. First, interviews, questionnaires, or food diaries must determine the amounts and types of foods that are consumed.[11] This information is then used to calculate nutrient intake if an accurate database has been established that quantifies the amount of each nutrient contained in the foods consumed by the population under investigation. Each step can be associated with significant error and contributes to the challenges in defining nutrient and cancer associations. The human diet is a complex array of foods that exhibits significant day-to-day and seasonal variations. The complexity of diet also differs widely among populations, cultures, and geographic areas. This often requires the development of different assessment methods for each population or subgroup. Future progress will depend, in part, on identifying biomarkers of nutrient exposure. Development of valid and reliable biomarkers of nutrient intake offers the promise of improved precision in epidemiologic studies

Table 2 Types of studies used to assess diet and disease relationships.

Study type	Methods	Strengths	Limitations
Ecologic/correlational studies	The unit of observation is a population defined by a discriminator location (Japan vs United States, northern vs southern latitudes). Mortality or incidence among groups is compared with estimates of nutrient or food intake	Large differences in cancer incidence and dietary patterns are often identified, and hypotheses can be generated	There are often many diet and lifestyle differences between populations; therefore, correlations between disease incidence, and dietary factors are confounded by known or unknown variables Cancer incidence data and diet patterns may not be similarly quantitated among nations
Case–control studies	Individuals experiencing a disease are identified, and a similar group of matched subjects without the disease are identified. Information about past diet and nutrients is obtained from both the cases and controls for comparison	Studies can be conducted over a relatively short period of time	Selection bias can occur if a non-representative control group is selected Recall bias can occur when subjects with a disease alter their perceptions and recall of past dietary habits. This often occurs when participants are familiar with a particular diet/disease hypothesis
Prospective/cohort studies	A study population is identified and diet patterns assessed. The population is followed over time for disease outcome and changes in exposure to dietary risk factors	Dietary intake can be monitored periodically over time Diet assessment does not rely on long-term memory and is less affected by recall bias Biochemical measures can be obtained periodically	Long periods of time may be necessary for a disease to be diagnosed, so cohort studies often require many years of follow-up A large number of subjects are required to compensate for subjects who drop out, subjects lost to follow-up, and/or the possibility that the frequency of the outcome of interest is low Long term, large prospective studies are expensive
Randomized controlled trials	Individuals are screened, and, based on specific characteristics; a proper target population is identified and randomized to a control arm (standard of care) or an intervention arm. The subjects are followed for disease outcome or other biomarkers	Especially useful for testing compounds (vitamins and minerals) that can be incorporated into pills or capsules and provided in a double-blind manner over a period of years	Difficult to implement for many nutrition and cancer hypotheses (weight loss, exercise, dietary fat, fiber, fruits, and vegetables), because trials of dietary change cannot be blinded Manipulation of single dietary components in large-scale intervention studies is difficult, because foods are complex and contain many compounds Compliance with food changes may be difficult to determine Randomized, controlled trials can take a long time to complete and can be very expensive

because of reduced misclassification of participants according to intake estimates.[12] Finally, for many of the bioactive compounds in foods that may impact cancer risk, including the vast array of non-nutrient phytochemicals derived from plants, our ability to estimate exposure remains a challenge, as databases regarding content in foods often do not exist.[13]

Laboratory models

The effects of nutrients or food components and their interactions on carcinogenesis can be rigorously tested in a growing array of animal models. Although the information derived from animal models must be extrapolated to humans with caution, the literature does provide important evidence for the biologic plausibility of relationships suggested by epidemiologic studies. The nutrient requirements of most laboratory animals have been precisely defined, and purified ingredients can be used to formulate diets for cancer studies. The rapid emergence of new animal models based on transgenic and knockout technology has provided new opportunities to examine interactions between specific genetic targets and dietary variables.[14]

Public health guidelines for cancer prevention

We begin this section with a synthesis of public health dietary guidelines for cancer prevention and health published by several organizations, including the AICR/WCRF, ACS, and The American Heart Association (AHA).[1,2,3,5] The public health approach is a preventive strategy to decrease the overall disease incidence by reducing the adverse dietary habits of the entire population. Implementation of dietary recommendations requires cooperation among the media, food industry, public health workers, medical practitioners, educators, and government agencies.[1] To

achieve success, dietary recommendations must be clear, as well as feasible and have minimal risk, low cost to society, and the potential to benefit the population.[1] In addition, economic issues relative to the food and agricultural industry are factors that may influence decisions, particularly by government agencies, to define nutritional guidelines. Past efforts have been successful in the area of nutrition. For example, iron fortification of cereals benefits a large number of children and adult women through prevention of anemia, while risk is limited to a small number of individuals with hemochromatosis. The current evidence-based dietary recommendations can be made with a reasonable degree of certainty with the likelihood of minimal risk and the potential for significant public health benefits.[1,6,15–17] Table 1 summarizes the current population-based dietary recommendations that together may lower the risk of chronic diseases, including cancer.[1,4,5] In early 2016, a revision of Dietary Guidelines for America will be published by the National Institutes of Health and should be examined by those interested in disease-prevention strategies.

Public health guidelines for nutrition and cancer prevention

Maintain a healthy weight

Increasingly, studies document that sedentary behavior, weight gain, overweight, and obesity are major risk factors for human cancer.[1–3,5,18–23] Women with a body mass index (BMI) of >25 kg/m^2 and men with a BMI > 27 kg/m^2 should make weight loss a priority. Weight loss of just 5–10% is associated with improved health and can reduce the incidence or severity of several cancers.[20–23] Weight loss is best achieved by reducing total calorie consumption and increasing calorie expenditure to create a negative energy balance, resulting in a modest, but consistent weight loss over time. Maximum weight loss of 1–2 pounds per week is appropriate for most people. Rapid weight loss achieved through fad diets does not encourage individuals to establish healthy eating and physical activity patterns, and weight loss is typically not maintained with these regimens.[3] It is increasingly clear that maintaining a healthy weight throughout life may be one of the most critical approaches to protect against many common malignancies.[1,2,5,18]

Participate in physical activity daily and moderate-to-vigorous intensity exercise several days each week

The energy expenditure associated with physical activity is a critical component of maintaining a healthy body weight and preventing adult weight gain, which is associated with risk of several types of cancer.[1,5,24] Additionally, a combination of daily physical activity and regular bouts of moderate-to-vigorous intensity exercise has been shown in many studies to reduce cancer risk independent of weight and diet.[25–27] Physical activity should be incorporated into activities of daily living in combination with regular moderate-to-vigorous intensity exercise on most days of the week. There is general agreement that a minimum of 150 min/week of moderate intensity activity or 75 min/week of vigorous physical activity is recommended.[1,5,28]

Consume a plant-based diet that is rich in fruits, vegetables, and a variety of whole grains and cereals

Several hundred studies have examined the relationships between fruit and vegetable intake and cancer risk.[1] The vast majority suggests a significant protective effect of a plant-based diet relative to cancer risk at many sites. Fruits and vegetables not only contain a diverse array of vitamins, minerals, fiber, and phytochemicals, but they are lower in caloric density than most other foods. A variety of nonstarchy fruits and vegetables should be included at every meal with a goal of consuming at least five servings (or at least 400–600 g) of fruits and vegetables per day. Additionally, emphasis should be placed on consumption of beans and legumes, which provide protein, fiber, B vitamins, and iron, as well as whole grain breads, cereals, and pastas, which provide fiber, B vitamins, and a vast array of phytochemicals. As a plant-based diet is compatible with modest lean meat consumption, it should not be interpreted as a vegetarian dietary pattern.

Minimize consumption of energy-dense foods and sugary drinks

This recommendation has emerged as vital to the overall prevention of weight gain and obesity. Diets that are rich in processed foods are typically high in refined sugars and/or fats that contribute excess calories to the diet and do not provide a concentrated source of vitamins, minerals, and bioactive phytochemicals. Consumption of processed foods with added sugars has significantly increased in recent decades and currently contributes over 15% of total calorie consumption.[29,30] The majority of this increase comes from the consumption of sugary beverages, especially soda.[1] Drinks containing added sugars have been associated with an increased risk of overweight and obesity in children, adolescents, and adults. The consumption of sugary beverages should be minimized.

For people who enjoy red meat, moderate portion sizes and reduced intake of highly processed red meats are advisable

Populations consuming plant-based diets are often found to exhibit lower risk for various diseases, including some types of cancer;

however, a specific role for meat in promoting cancer, independent of other variables, is not causally established. In addition, meat is an important source of many nutrients, such as protein, iron, and vitamin B12. Thus, modest meat consumption of 18 ounces or less of red meat (beef, lamb, and pork) per week likely does not significantly contribute to an overall significant increase in cancer risk, especially if meat does not displace consumption of fruits, vegetables, and whole grains. The impact of different cooking methods, which lead to the production of carcinogens on cancer, continues to be examined.[31] Modest exposure to meats cooked for long periods of time and over flames is prudent.[32] Historically, populations consuming diets rich in various forms of processed meat, including smoked, cured, or salted meats, have experienced greater risk of various cancers; therefore, limiting consumption of these meat products is advised.[1,33] For those choosing meat, it is sensible to select a variety of sources, including fresh chicken, fish, and turkey.[1]

Alcohol, if consumed at all, should be limited

The risks and potential benefits of modest alcohol consumption remain a subject of debate. Although the health effects of alcohol or specific types of alcoholic beverages is an active area of research, chronic consumption of alcohol is strongly associated with cancers of the oropharynx, larynx, esophagus, and breast (both pre- and postmenopausal).[1,5] Smoking tobacco acts synergistically with alcohol in the pathogenesis of oral and upper aerodigestive cancers. Significant consumption of alcoholic beverages also contributes to liver cancer and perhaps colon cancer.[1] Even a moderate amount of daily alcohol consumption may slightly, but significantly, increase the risk of breast cancer.[1,34] Because there is some evidence that alcohol in moderation may reduce the risk of heart disease, individuals need to consider their personal health history and risk profile when deciding whether or not to consume alcohol. For those who choose to drink, alcohol intake should be limited to one drink per day for women and two drinks per day for men.[1,2,5]

Optimal food preservation, processing, and preparation

Salt is vital for human health, but adequate amounts are achieved at levels much lower than those typically found in the American diet.[35] Salt-preserved foods are associated with gastric cancer, a major malignancy worldwide, particularly in developing nations. Although relationships remain uncertain, diets high in salt-rich processed meats are associated with risk of several cancers and, consequently, should be consumed in moderation.[1,36] Meat that is cooked at very high temperatures, grilled, and charred favors the formation of certain types of chemical carcinogens and should be consumed in moderation.[1] Microbial contamination of the food supply is a major problem globally. Most critically, the contamination of grains and legumes with fungal aflatoxins contributes significantly to the risk of liver cancer, and public heath approaches by government agencies to limit exposures are necessary.

Dietary supplements are probably unnecessary in the context of a healthy diet

An increasing proportion of the American population consumes some type of self-prescribed nutrient or dietary supplement on a regular basis. The public increasingly perceives heavily marketed supplements and alternative medications as an important form of self-therapy for the prevention and treatment of many ailments, including cancer.[1,24] Multivitamin and mineral supplements are usually inexpensive, easy to consume, obtained without a prescription, and relatively free of side effects when taken at the dosages approximating the recommended dietary allowance (RDA). There has been very little evidence in support of routine dietary supplements for population-wide cancer prevention.[5,37] Although it is clear that Americans can achieve adequate nutrient intake by consuming a diverse diet based on the above recommendations, a standard multivitamin/mineral supplement providing the RDA may be beneficial to some and entails minimal risk. Increasingly, supplements that contain high concentrations of specific nutrients combined with other components, such as herbals, extracts, and concentrates, are being aggressively marketed. Consumers should be aware that regulations regarding implied health claims and requirements that products contain the stated ingredients and have demonstrated safety and efficacy are minimal, and the buyer should maintain skepticism and caution. The Office of Dietary Supplements of the National Institutes of Health provides web-based information for interested consumers.

Summary of research efforts focusing on specific cancers

It is unlikely that any food, nutrient, or dietary pattern will influence all cancers uniformly.[1,5,24] Thus, in reviewing the relationships between nutrition and cancer risk, it is important to examine the data for each tissue or organ separately. It is clear that research will continue to improve our ability to identify individuals at high risk of specific cancers based on genetic tests, family history, exposure to carcinogenic agents, and the presence of premalignant conditions. A future goal is to provide tailored dietary recommendations and chemopreventive strategies for individuals at risk. Additional research will define unique preventive strategies for various cancers. The following is a brief summary of the current understanding of relationships between diet, nutrition, and the risk of specific, commonly occurring cancers. For additional information, please refer to Table 3.

Colon and rectum

Colorectal cancer is the third most common cancer worldwide and the third leading cause of cancer death in the United States.[1,38]

Table 3 World Cancer Research Fund (WCRF)/American Institute for Cancer Research (AICR) Guidelines.

AMERICAN INSTITUTE FOR CANCER RESEARCH / WORLD CANCER RESEARCH FUND
SUMMARY OF STRONG EVIDENCE ON DIET, NUTRITION, PHYSICAL ACTIVITY AND PREVENTION OF CANCER

Legend:
- ↓↓ Convincing decreased risk
- ↓ Probable decreased risk
- ↑↑ Convincing increased risk
- ↑ Probable increased risk
- • Substantial effect on risk unlikely

	Mouth, Pharynx, Larynx (2007)	Nasopharynx (2007)	Esophagus (2007)	Lung (2007)	Stomach (2007)	Pancreas (2007)	Gallbladder (2007)	Liver (2007)	Colorectum (2011)	Breast Premenopause (2010)	Breast Postmenopause (2010)	Ovary (2014)	Endometrium (2013)	Prostate (2014)	Kidney (2007)	Skin (2007)
Foods containing dietary fiber									↓↓							
Aflatoxins								↑↑								
Non-starchy vegetables¹	↓		↓		↓											
Allium vegetables					↓											
Garlic									↓							
Fruits²	↓		↓	↓	↓											
Red meat									↑↑							
Processed meat									↑↑							
Cantonese-style salted fish		↑														
Diets high in calcium³									↓							
Salt, salted and salty foods					↑											
Glycemic load													↑			
Arsenic in drinking water				↑↑												↑
Maté		↑														
Alcoholic drinks⁴	↑↑	↑↑						↑	↑⁴ ↑↑⁴	↑↑	↑↑				•	
Coffee						•							↓		•	
Beta-carotene⁵				↑↑										•		•
Physical activity⁶									↓↓		↓		↓			
Body fatness⁷			↑↑			↑↑	↑		↑↑	↓	↑↑	↑	↑↑	↑	↑↑	
Adult attained height						↑			↑↑	↑	↑↑	↑↑		↑		
Greater birth weight										↑						
Lactation										↓↓	↓↓					

¹Includes evidence on foods containing carotenoids for mouth, pharynx, larynx; foods containing beta-carotene for esophagus; foods containing vitamin C for esophagus.

²Includes eveidence on foods containing carotenoids for mouth, pharynx, larynx and lung; foods containing beta-carotene for esophagus; foods containing vitamin C for esophagus

³Evidence is from milk and studies using supplements for colorectum

⁴Convincing increased risk for men and probable increased risk for women for colorectum. Evidence applies to adverse effect for kidney

⁵Evidence derived from studies using supplements for lung

⁶Convincing increased risk for colon not rectum

⁷Probable increased risk for advanced not non-advanced prostate cancer

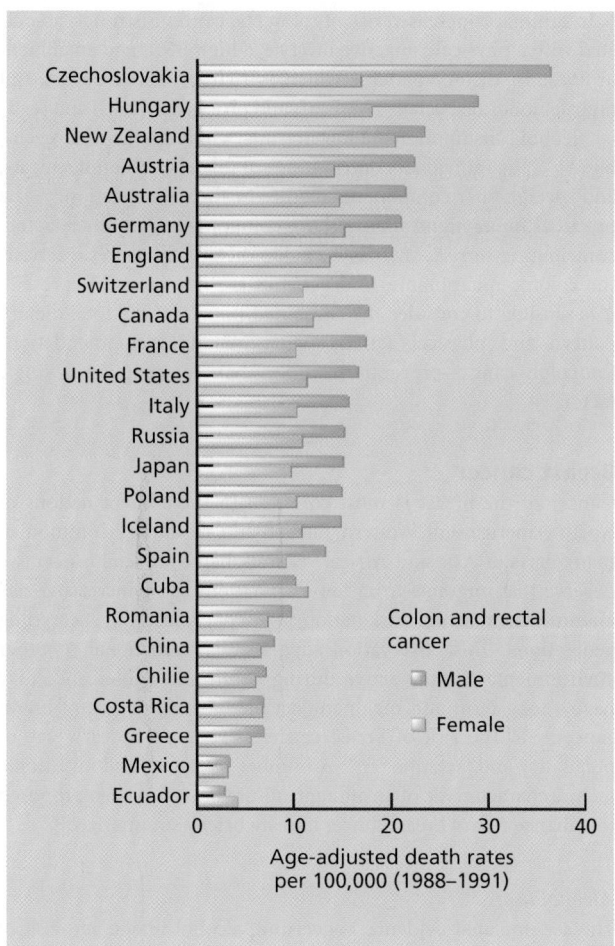

Figure 1 Age-adjusted death rates per 100,000 population from colon and rectal cancer in selected countries. Source: Data from Boring 1994.[39]

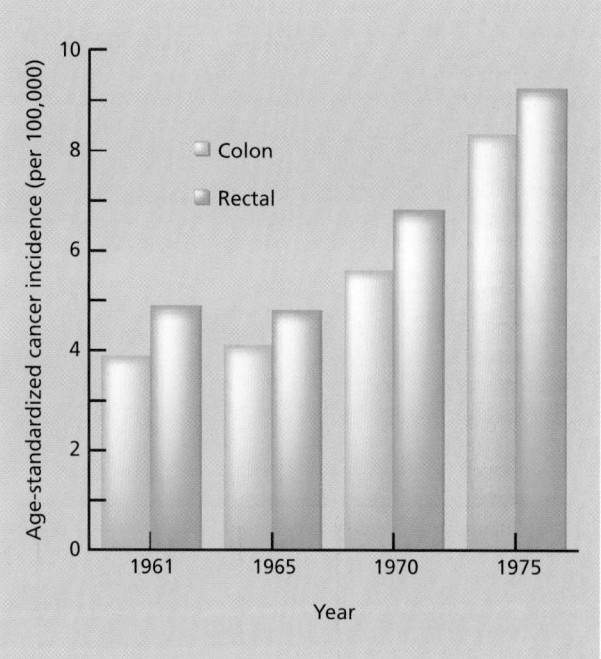

Figure 2 Age-standardized colon and rectal cancer incidence per 100,000 men in Japan from 1960 to 1977.

Genetic factors and premalignant conditions are being characterized that will define high-risk groups for chemoprevention and diet-intervention studies, which show promise in preclinical testing. The international variation in colorectal cancer is large (Figure 1). Although screening differences may account for some of the international variation, it is unlikely to account for the greater than 10-fold variations that are observed between nations.[1] The lower rates in Asian nations suggest that cultural and lifestyle variables, rather than industrialization, are the critical factors.[1,40,41] Dramatic increases in incidence among Japanese and Chinese migrants to the United States[42] clearly indicate that international variations primarily result from environmental influences rather than genetic background.[43,44] Examination of time trends in colorectal cancer incidence, particularly in Japan since the 1940s, strongly suggests major contributions from diet and lifestyle factors associated with the Westernization of cultures (Figure 2).[1]

Energy balance, body mass, and physical activity
Energy intake, physical activity, and various measures of body size or obesity are all intimately related and associated with colon cancer risk. It is difficult to quantitate or ascertain the role of each component without considering them as a group. A convincing inverse association between physical activity and risk of colon cancer has been consistently reported.[1,45–47] Several studies have found an association between BMI or adiposity and elevated risk of colon cancer.[1,44,48–50] The associations between obesity and

inactivity with risk of colon cancer have been observed in several countries (United States, China, Sweden, and Japan), among men and women, and for both occupational and recreational activities.[1] Obesity is also associated with risk of colon adenoma.[51] Some evidence suggests that height (perhaps a proxy of the net energy intake during childhood and adolescence) is related also to a higher risk of colon cancer.[52–54] Studies in rodent models of colon carcinogenesis have reported enhanced tumorigenesis with greater *ad libitum* intake[55] and reduced risk with restricted intake.[56] Overall, the evidence is convincing that physical activity, appropriate energy balance, and maintaining the ideal BMI will decrease the risk of colon cancer.[1,47]

Dietary pattern
In general, a Western dietary pattern that is rich in red and processed meat, high in fat, and low in fruits, vegetables, and fiber is associated with an increased risk of colon cancer.[1,57,58] The relationship between total fat intake, fat saturation, or different sources of fat and risk of colon cancer remains an active area of research, but definitive conclusions regarding fat *per se* are not yet possible.[1,5,42,59–62] For example, Figure 3 illustrates a population-based case–control study suggesting that dietary fat accounts for 60% of colorectal cancer risk among Chinese migrants to the United States. Other cohort studies report that fat from red meats rather than total fat may increase colon cancer risk.[50,61,63–65] Dietary consumption of processed meats, which not only contain fat but also may contain suspected procarcinogens, have emerged as a convincing risk factor for colon cancer.[1,47,66,67] Thus, moderation in consumption of red meats and processed meats should be considered for those at risk of colorectal cancer. Efforts are underway examining complex dietary patterns, such as the Mediterranean-style diet, rather than single variables, with emerging data supporting benefits of a healthy dietary pattern.[68,69]

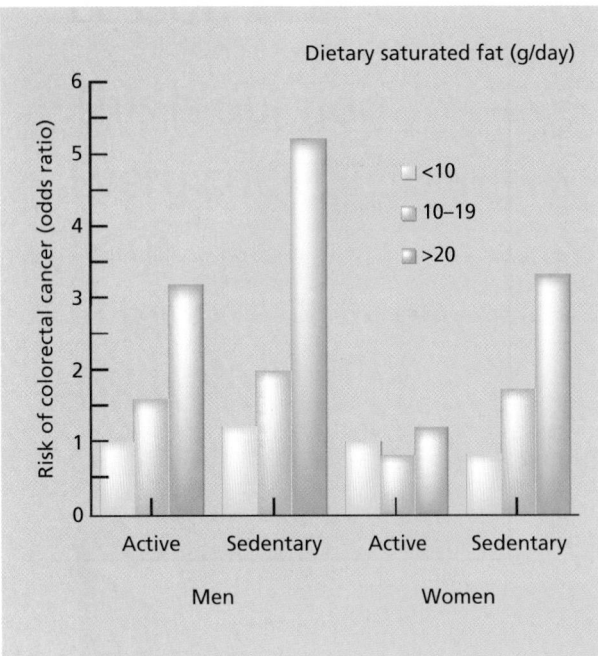

Figure 3 The risk of colorectal cancer in Chinese migrants to the United States according to dietary fat intake and level of physical activity.[42]

Fruits, vegetables, and fiber
Dietary patterns rich in plant products, particularly grains and vegetables, are often associated with a lower risk of colon cancer, and many have postulated that the fiber content is one major mediating factor.[1,15,26,59,61,70–73] The chemistry of dietary fiber is exceptionally complex, and, unfortunately, the quantitative and qualitative assessment of fiber intake in human epidemiologic studies is very difficult. However, the majority of studies suggest that a diet rich in diverse fiber-containing foods may be beneficial. The large European Prospective Investigation into Cancer (EPIC) study involving over 500,000 men and women reported a 13% reduction in colon cancer risk for each 10 g/day increase in dietary fiber derived from cereals, fruit, or vegetables.[74,75] A few intervention trials have evaluated interventions focusing upon specific types of dietary fiber and colon cancer risk, and, to date, the results are equivocal.[76–80] A specific role for any one type or class of fruits, vegetables, or grains has not been established; yet, a diverse plant-based dietary pattern is an advisable strategy.

Alcohol
A positive association between alcohol intake and risk of colon cancer is consistent among many ecologic, cohort, and population-based case–control studies.[1,5,47,81–83] Alcohol is also related to higher risk of colorectal adenoma.[1,5,47] Overall, the impact is related more to total alcohol intake rather than to the source of alcohol.[1,5] Studies suggest that the elevated risk associated with alcohol occurs predominantly in the rectum or distal colon.[65] Recent studies indicate that high intakes of folate or methionine, both of which are crucial for normal methyl-group metabolism and, particularly, deoxyribonucleic acid (DNA) methylation, appears to mitigate the influence of alcohol.[81] This suggests that alcohol, which has a well-known adverse effect on methyl-group metabolism, increases the risk of colorectal cancer via this mechanism; however, the role of folate during various stages of carcinogenesis remains to be clearly defined.[84]

In summary, increased risk of colorectal cancer is strongly associated with a physically inactive lifestyle, a high BMI, and an affluent or Western dietary pattern, which is rich in simple sugars and high-fat foods (especially red meats and processed meats) and regular alcohol consumption but low in fruits, whole-grains, and vegetables.[1,5,47] The individual contributions of folate, methionine, meats, and specific fiber components require further investigation.[1,5] The potential interactions among these components and other factors contributing to risk, such as early life dietary exposures, exercise, the colonic microbiome, and genetics are numerous. At present, it is sensible to consider the combined impact of the total dietary pattern and physical activity when making recommendations for colon cancer prevention, rather than focusing on a single factor.

Breast cancer
Cancer of the breast is most common in the affluent nations of North America and Western Europe and much less common in many parts of Asia and Africa,[1,5,38] and, like colorectal cancer, we observe that migrants from low-risk nations show increasing risk after moving to a high-risk nation,[1,5,38,43] particularly in succeeding generations. This observation suggests that nutritional or other environmental factors active during youth and adolescence may have a long term and major impact on subsequent risk of breast cancer.[1,5,38] The risk of breast cancer is reduced by early age of pregnancy and lactation.[1,23,85] A number of dietary and nutritional factors characteristic of an affluent culture have also been proposed to enhance risk of breast cancer and are briefly summarized.[1,5]

Alcohol use
The accumulated evidence concerning alcohol intake and risk of breast cancer shows a positive and convincing association.[1,5,23] The relative risk (RR) from the consumption of one typical serving of beer, wine, or liquor (~12 g of ethanol) per day is estimated to be 1.4, whereas three drinks per day approximately doubles the risk. Recent analyses have reported a linear relationship between breast cancer risk and each 10 g increase in daily alcohol consumption, even across different estrogen/progesterone hormone subtypes.[34,86]

Energy balance, weight, and obesity
Evidence is accumulating that body fatness, adult weight gain, and a lack of physical activity are important risk factors for breast cancer.[1,5,23,87,88] The role of energy intake as a stimulator of mammary carcinogenesis has been well-established by rodent studies using diet or energy restriction[89,90] and regression analysis of *ad libitum* feeding.[55,91] Overall, higher levels of adult physical activity seem to be associated with a modest protection (~25% risk reduction) against breast cancer risk, and the protective effect may also be independent of BMI or weight gain as an adult.[88,92–94] However, the precise relationships between energy intake, energy expenditure, anthropometrics, and risk of breast cancer must be examined for different critical periods in a woman's life cycle. The effects of these factors may vary during adolescence, the reproductive years, and the postmenopausal period.

Dietary fat
The controversy concerning the contribution of dietary fat concentrations or sources, independent of energy intake, to risk of breast cancer can best be appreciated through examination of the representative data presented in Figure 4. Geographic studies show

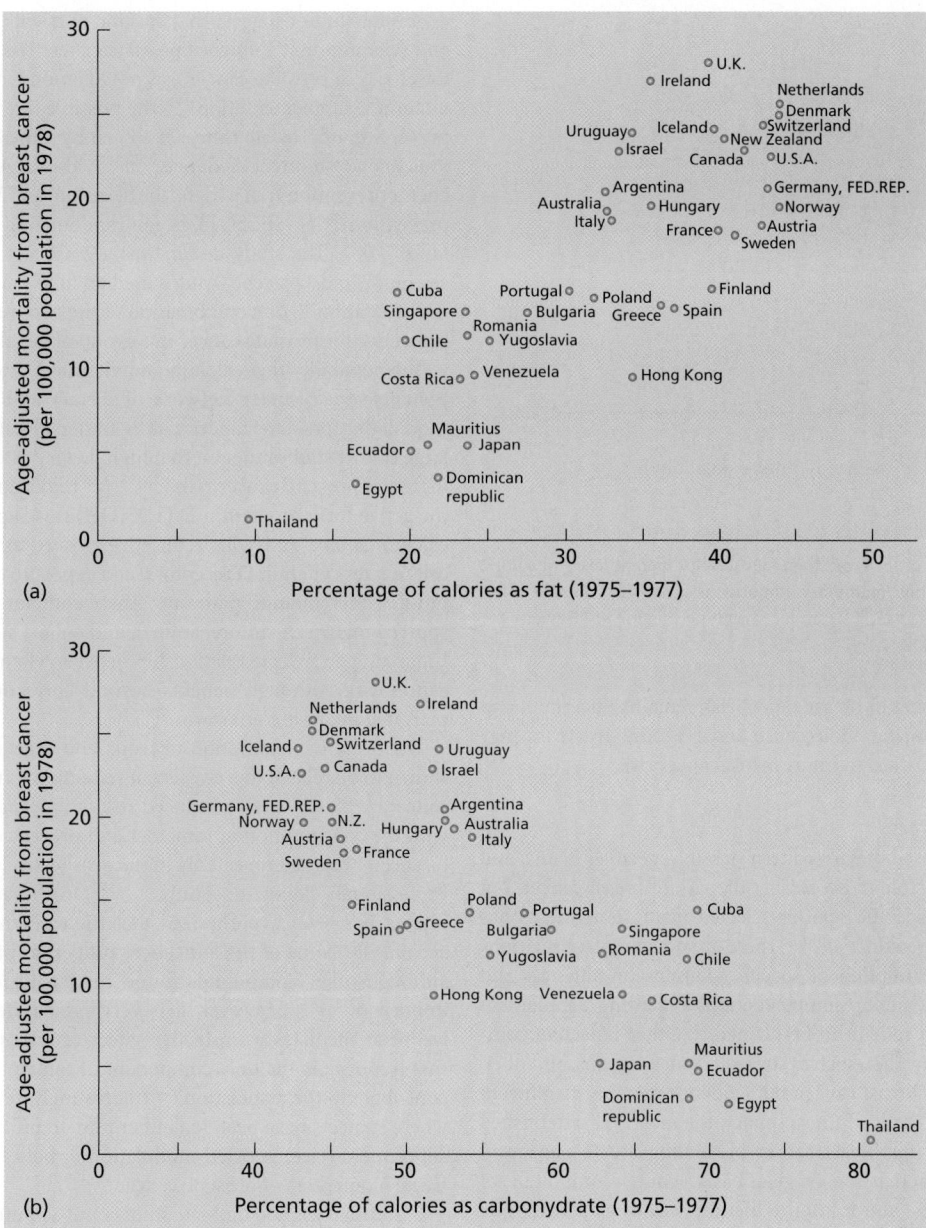

Figure 4 International correlation of (a) estimated dietary fat intake (percentage of calories as fat) and (b) estimated carbohydrate intake (percentage of calories as carbohydrate) and age-adjusted breast-cancer mortality. Source: Carroll 1991.[95] Reproduced with permission of Springer.

strong correlations between national rates of breast cancer and the estimated per capita fat consumption.[60,96] There are wide international variations in breast cancer rates as well as per capita fat consumption, or the percentage of calories derived from fat. Breast cancer rates have been observed to increase significantly in populations migrating from low-risk areas, such as Japan, where diets were traditionally low in fat, to high-risk areas, such as the United States, where populations consume diets rich in fat.[43,97] Time–trend studies also support a dietary fat and breast cancer association. Within Japan, estimates of per capita daily fat intake have risen over the decades following World War II. During this period, breast cancer mortality increased in Japan by >30%. These examples illustrate that correlation does not prove cause and effect, and many investigators argue that fat intake may be an indicator of some other unidentified combination of diet and environmental components that are the truly critical risk factors. The relationship between fat intake and risk of breast cancer has been examined in many case–control

and cohort studies with inconsistent results.[98–101] Although the epidemiologic data have not provided definitive results concerning dietary fat and breast cancer, accumulated evidence from >100 animal studies using chemical carcinogens, hormones, irradiation, or viruses to induce breast cancer indicate that, as a single variable, fat enhances mammary carcinogenesis (Figure 5).[1,55,91,102] One randomized intervention study of women who had been treated for breast cancer suggested a 24% risk reduction in breast cancer recurrence among women who were able to reduce their dietary fat consumption to ~33 g/day (vs 51 g/day for the control group).[103] Although not statistically significant, similar trends were observed in the very large, randomized Women's Health Initiative study.[98] The large EPIC study followed over 33,000 women for 11.5 years and found diets high in total and saturated fat to be associated with a significantly increased risk of ER(+)PR(+) disease but not with ER(−)PR(−) breast cancer.[104] Overall, the possibility that achievable reductions in fat intake during adulthood will cause an

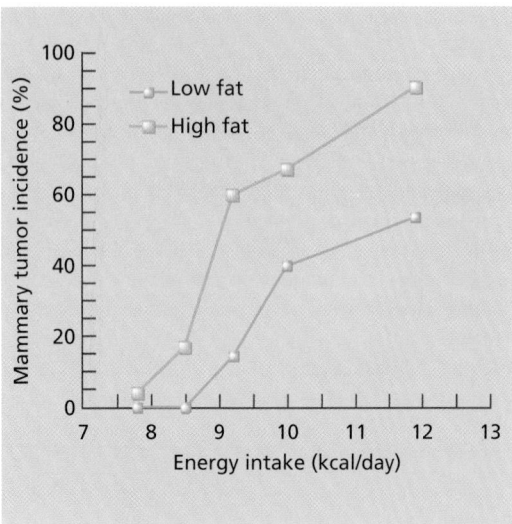

Figure 5 The effects of low- and high-fat diets at different levels of caloric intake on spontaneous mammary tumorigenesis in C3H female mice. Source: Tannenbaum 1945.[90] Reproduced with permission of Elsevier.

appreciable reduction in breast-cancer risk remains uncertain, and dietary patterns during adolescence and reproductive years may prove to be more critical to future breast cancer risk.[1]

Other dietary factors

Overall, a plant-based dietary pattern rich in vegetables, fruits, and grains may have a role in decreasing the risk of breast cancer, but a conclusive and specific role for selected plant components has not been demonstrated.[1,5,23,101,105] There are no consistent relationships for the consumption of specific vitamins or minerals and breast-cancer risk, and recommendations regarding supplement use for prevention remain to be defined.[1,5] Other bioactive compounds found in the diet, such as soy isoflavones, lignans, and fiber, may play a role in breast cancer, but evidence remains insufficient for recommendations.[1,5,101] In summary, the most well-established recommendations for breast cancer prevention are to engage in vigorous physical activity on a regular basis, avoid or limit intake of alcoholic beverages, and minimize lifetime weight gain and body fatness through physical activity and energy restriction.

Prostate cancer

Cancer of the prostate is one of the most frequently diagnosed malignancies in American men, and it is especially common among the African-American population.[1,38] Prostate cancer is a disease of aging men, and the international distribution of prostate cancer is similar to that of colon and breast cancer; therefore, it correlates with affluent dietary patterns.[1,106] Relationships between diet and prostate cancer are not clearly defined, and specific recommendations to prevent the disease remain speculative. A role for weight gain and obesity resulting from excess energy intake and a lack of physical activity is accumulating in human studies and is clearly demonstrated in rodent studies.[1,18,106–109] The evidence is most clear for the increase in the risk of advanced prostate cancer.[22] International and intracountry correlational studies suggest associations between prostate cancer mortality and the per capita intake of total fat.[1,106] Similarly, several analytic epidemiologic studies and case–control studies have reported associations between prostate cancer and total fat or the consumption of foods high in fat, particularly saturated fats from animal products.[1,106–108,110,111]

Several studies suggest that specific nutrients such as vitamin E and selenium may influence prostate cancer risk.[112] A significantly lower risk of prostate cancer was noted among men randomized to vitamin E supplementation.[112] The possible role of selenium in the prevention of prostate cancer has been hypothesized based on various lines of indirect evidence.[1,113–116] The largest prostate cancer chemoprevention trial to date, the Selenium and Vitamin E Chemoprevention Trial (SELECT), began randomizing 33,000 men in the fall of 2001. The study design was a 2×2 factorial of vitamin E, selenium, and a placebo. After a median follow-up of 5.4 years, selenium, vitamin E, or a combination of the two were not found to be protective for prostate cancer in a group of healthy men.[117]

The possibility that calcium and vitamin D are interacting components of a complex network of dietary and endocrine factors modulating prostate cancer risk is under investigation.[118] Several large cohort studies suggest that high dietary calcium consumption increases prostate cancer risk.[1,22,118–122] Endogenous production of the active form of vitamin D (1,25(OH)2) is suppressed with high calcium intake and with reduced exposure to sunlight. Prostate cells express vitamin D receptors, and exposure to a ligand tends to induce differentiation pathways. These complex relationships have spurred many cell culture, animal, and cohort studies, with several suggesting an inverse relationship between vitamin D and prostate cancer risk, although benefits beyond correction of deficient or marginal intake are unknown.[123–126]

The overall consumption of fruits and vegetables has not been shown to be related to a consistent reduction in the risk of prostate cancer.[1,22,106] However, a reduced risk of prostate cancer associated with the consumption of tomatoes and processed tomato products has been observed repeatedly in the prospectively evaluated Health Professional's Follow-up Study.[127–131] On the basis of these findings, it has been hypothesized that the carotenoid lycopene may account for some of the anticancer properties of tomato products, although other compounds found in tomato foods may also be important.[131–137] However, it is very premature to conclude that lycopene mediates a protective effect against prostate cancer or that lycopene is the only component of tomato products that may contribute to the association.[138] Interestingly, several interventions where subjects have been fed either tomato products or a lycopene supplement have reported modulation of both blood and prostate tissue biomarkers of prostate cancer.[135,139–141]

In summary, epidemiologic studies and a limited number of laboratory investigations suggest a role for an affluent dietary pattern in prostate cancer risk. Rates of prostate cancer are higher in nations consuming an affluent dietary pattern coupled with obesity and a sedentary lifestyle, although the contributions of specific components are not well-defined and are being actively investigated.

Lung cancer

Lung cancer is currently the most common worldwide malignancy and the leading cause of cancer-related death.[1] Cigarette smoking accounts for the vast majority of cases, and incidence rates continue to climb in parallel with the globalization of cigarette manufacturing, marketing, and advertising.[1] Certain occupational exposures, such as asbestos or radiation, may act synergistically with cigarette smoking to increase the risk.[1] Compared with the role of tobacco, the potential contribution of diet and nutrition is relatively modest. However, an inverse relationship between the greater intake of fruits and vegetables and lower risk of lung cancer has been a frequent finding in human nutritional epidemiology.[1,142–144] Many hypothesized that β-carotene found in fruits and vegetables or vitamin A derived from cleavage of β-carotene may be the critical active agents in these foods.[1,145] However, two randomized controlled intervention trials in high-risk populations found no reduction, and perhaps an increase, in the incidence of lung cancer among male smokers after several years of supplementation with β-carotene at 20 or 30 mg/day.[146] A recent study of over 72,000 Chinese women reported that, among women who were exposed to side-stream smoke, dietary intake of foods rich in tocopherols was inversely related to lung-cancer incidence. In contrast, supplemental vitamin E significantly increased risk of total lung cancers and, in particular, lung adenocarcinoma.[147] These reports emphasize that protective benefits of diets rich in fruits and vegetables probably involve many interacting components and will not be reproduced by providing a single agent.[1,148] Overall, elimination of cigarette smoking and occupational risk factors will have the greatest impact on decreasing the incidence of lung cancer. Among high-risk individuals, the frequent consumption of a diverse array of fruits, vegetables, and other plant foods may provide some degree of protection against lung cancer.

Oral cavity, larynx, and oropharynx cancers

Like lung cancer, cancers of the oral cavity and the larynx are strongly related to the use of tobacco products.[1,2,24] Case–control studies completed over several decades have documented associations between the consumption of alcoholic beverages and cancers of these tissues. A dose–response relationship of alcohol and oral cancer, independent of tobacco usage, has been observed in a number of studies (Figure 6).[150,151] Additional evidence is derived from studies of populations who exhibit increased risk, such as alcoholics. Seventh-Day Adventists and Mormons in the United States, who refrain from alcohol and have a much lower risk.[152,153] It is of interest that feeding pure alcohol as part of a nutritionally sound diet does not produce oral cancers in experimental animals. The extent that this represents biochemical differences between man and rodents, the lack of a direct carcinogenic effect of ethanol, the presence of carcinogens in alcoholic beverages consumed by man, the passive inhalation of ambient tobacco smoke in the places where ethanol is consumed, or the importance of other interacting carcinogens and nutritional deficits must be further evaluated.

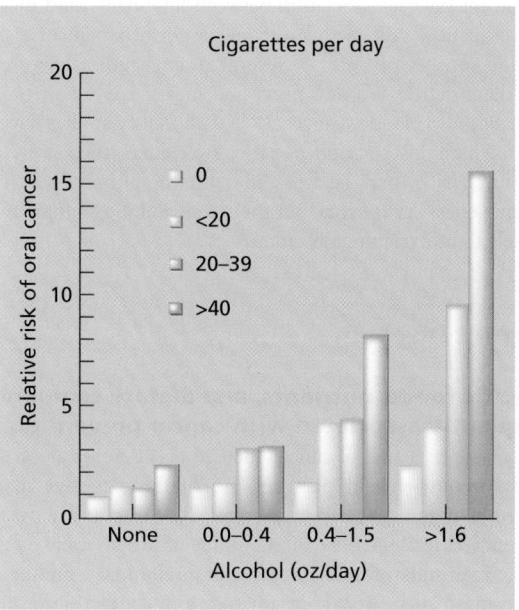

Figure 6 The interactions between alcohol intake and cigarette smoking on the relative risk of oral cancer. Source: Rothman 1972.[149] Reproduced with permission of Elsevier.

Both epidemiologic and laboratory studies provide convincing evidence supporting a protective role for diets rich in fruits and vegetables.[1,49,154] In addition, clinical and laboratory investigation has suggested that vitamin A and analogs or metabolites, as well as certain carotenoids, may serve as inhibitors of carcinogenesis in the oral and respiratory epithelia.[155] In summary, tobacco products are major contributors to cancers of the mouth and pharynx, especially in conjunction with the consumption of alcoholic beverages.[1] Further efforts to better define the roles of vitamin A and derivatives, other phytochemicals, and a diverse plant-based diet for prevention in high-risk groups are warranted.

Esophageal cancer

Squamous cell cancer of the esophagus is the eighth most common cancer worldwide and varies several hundredfold between nations and between geographic regions within nations.[1,154] In most developed nations, correlational analyses and case–control studies indicate that the major risk factors are ethanol and cigarette smoking for squamous-type esophageal cancer.[1] Risk increases in proportion to the amount of alcohol consumed.[1,156,157] A number of studies show an alcohol dose–response relationship after controlling for cigarette smoking, although the two factors may show a significant additive effect.[1] Increasing consumption of alcohol generally is associated with the marginal intake of many nutrients, which is thought to predispose individuals to greater risk. For example, alcohol may interact with folate, vitamin B12, and methyl group metabolism to modulate risk.[158] A number of studies suggest an inverse relationship between risk of esophageal cancer and consumption of fresh fruits and vegetables.[1,143,159] In certain parts of Asia where alcohol consumption does not explain the high risk for esophageal cancer, there may be a relationship between esophageal cancer and the indigenous diet, which is low in fresh fruits, vegetables, and animal products, and the estimated intakes of vitamin A, vitamin C, riboflavin, zinc, and several trace elements, such as molybdenum, frequently are cited as being low, as well.[1,160,161] In summary, cigarette smoking and alcohol consumption are the most important etiologic factors. The possibility that marginal intakes of one or more nutrients may contribute to risk in affluent populations has been suggested but not firmly established. The most important protective dietary intervention is a dietary pattern characterized by frequent consumption of fruits and vegetables.[1]

Adenocarcinoma of the esophagus and gastric cardia

The incidence of adenocarcinoma of the distal esophagus and gastric cardia has been increasing rapidly over the past two decades in the United States and Western Europe.[162] Among white men, adenocarcinoma of the distal esophagus has increased >350% since the mid-1970s.[163] Current or past cigarette smoking may be one of the contributing factors.[163,164] However, one of the most consistent observations has been a positive association between risk and BMI and/or abdominal obesity.[165–168] As the prevalence of obesity has increased in the United States, a parallel trend is observed in the incidence of adenocarcinoma of the esophagus and gastric cardia.[169] The mechanism remains under investigation; however, it has been speculated that obesity may predispose to gastroesophageal reflux disease. Other nutritional factors that have been investigated relative to the increased adenocarcinoma risk include dietary patterns characterized as rich in animal sources of fat, low in fiber, and low in fruits and vegetables.[170,171] Additional efforts are needed to clarify the risk factors in addition to obesity that are responsible for the dramatic increases in the incidence of adenocarcinoma of the esophagus and to devise effective intervention strategies.

Stomach cancer

Gastric cancer is the fourth most common cancer worldwide.[39] The incidence varies dramatically among countries and is highest in parts of Asia (e.g., Japan) and South America. A dramatic decrease in the incidence of stomach cancer in many affluent nations has been documented over the past century. In the United States, the current rate is among the lowest in the world, whereas, in 1930, gastric cancer was the most frequently diagnosed malignancy in Americans. In recent years, investigators have identified a divergent incidence pattern for cancers of the gastric cardia and distal stomach, which suggests different etiologies. Adenocarcinoma of the cardia is typically grouped etiologically with those arising from the metaplastic distal esophagus, which show a similar histology and may share risk factors. Convincing evidence for specific foods and nutrients is lacking. However, several variables under study are considered to be likely related, including: (1) the protective role of diets rich in fruit and vegetables[172,173]; (2) the protective effects of modern food processing and storage, thereby reducing spoilage; (3) the increased risk due to high exposure to foods with salt curing, pickling, and nitrates for preservation[174]; (4) the role of *Helicobacter pylori* infection and interactions with dietary factors[175–177]; (5) identification of natural carcinogens or precursors, such as nitrates, found in foods[178]; (6) the production of carcinogens during food storage and preparation; and (7) the synthesis of carcinogens from dietary precursors, such as nitrates, in the acid environment of the stomach.[1,164,175,176]

Liver cancer

Primary hepatocellular carcinoma is less common in the United States and Northern Europe. In contrast, it is one of the most frequent types of cancer in the developing nations of sub-Saharan Africa and Asia and is now ranked as the sixth most common cancer worldwide.[1] Hepatitis B and C infections appear to be the major etiologic factors in many high-risk areas, where the carrier state imparts an increased risk of ~200-fold.[179] Contamination of foods with carcinogenic fungal products, such as certain aflatoxins, also likely contribute to risk in some populations.[1] Aflatoxins are found in geographic areas where food processing and storage are not optimal. Groups with high aflatoxin exposure often have high rates of hepatitis B infection, parasitic infections, and nutritional deficiencies, which may interact to determine risk. In low-risk nations, obesity, overweight, the syndrome of nonalcoholic steato-hepatitis (NASH), and the consumption of alcohol are relevant dietary factors in the pathogenesis of liver cancer.[1,59,72,180,181] The data also suggest that risk factors may act in an additive or synergistic manner.[182] It has been hypothesized that liver cancer primarily occurs in those whose cumulative experiences with alcohol, viral hepatitis, and toxin exposure lead to cirrhosis. Increasingly, coffee intake is associated with a decreased risk, and there is limited evidence that consumption of fish and regular physical activity may also reduce the risk of liver cancer.[183–186]

Pancreatic cancer

Pancreatic cancer is frequently detected at an advanced stage and, thus, is highly lethal. Cigarette smoking has been firmly established as one etiologic factor.[24,187] The risk of smoking at least a pack per day is approximately fourfold, compared with that of nonsmokers.[1] There is limited evidence that diets rich in red and processed meats, alcohol, fructose-containing foods, and saturated fat may increase pancreatic-cancer risk.[188] Body fatness and excess energy intake are positively associated with pancreatic-cancer risk,[1,188,189] and are consistently supported by studies in animal models.[190]

Endometrial cancer

In general, endometrial cancer shows an international distribution similar to that of other cancers of affluence, such as breast, colon, and prostate cancers. Evidence for association between endometrial cancer and excess energy intake, lack of physical activity, obesity, and high glycemic load continues to accumulate.[1,18,20,97,108,187] Coffee consumption has emerged as a protective factor in the development of endometrial cancer, with several studies suggesting a 7–8% reduction in risk for each cup consumed on a daily basis.[20,191] A role for fruits and vegetables in decreasing the risk of endometrial cancer is suggested by some studies.[1,192] At the present time, the most appropriate guidance is to avoid obesity through reduced energy consumption and regular physical exercise coupled with a dietary pattern rich in fruits, vegetables, and grains.

Ovarian cancer

There is considerable international and geographic variation in the incidence and mortality rates of ovarian cancer. The disease is more common in nations exhibiting Western culture, especially among the higher socioeconomic groups.[1,187] At present, no conclusive role for dietary components in the pathogenesis of ovarian cancer has been established although there is increasing evidence that body fatness enhances risk and limited evidence that lactation may decrease risk.[21] Additional studies are needed, particularly in conjunction with known risk factors of low parity and specific inherited genetic abnormalities.[1]

Bladder cancer

Bladder cancer is more frequent in industrialized nations, especially among smokers and those in urban areas and of lower socioeconomic status.[1,59,143,193,194] The majority of epidemiologic and case–control studies support the hypothesis that the frequent consumption of fruits and vegetables will reduce risk.[1,143,193,195] A diet rich in cruciferous vegetables, such as broccoli, but not other classes of fruits and vegetables, has been associated with a reduced bladder cancer risk in both smokers and nonsmokers.[195] The role of fluid intake in bladder cancer risk has frequently been proposed.[1,196] The prospective evaluation of fluid intake found a significant inverse association between total daily fluid intake and bladder-cancer risk, with no evidence for a benefit or risk from specific sources of fluid.[196] Several recent studies have reported that diets rich in red and processed meats may be an important contributor to bladder cancer.[197–199] Laboratory studies have found that the high doses of non-nutritive sweeteners, such as cyclamates and saccharine, may be weak initiators or promoters of bladder carcinogenesis in rodents, but their contribution to human cancer is likely to be exceptionally small.[1]

Current research

Specific foods, nutrients, and dietary components frequently associated with cancer prevention

Many people at risk of cancer focus their attention upon specific foods or nutrients in part because of the extensive marketing of products and publicity generated by the popular press. This tendency is facilitated by the news media when science reporters publicize results of single studies or preliminary findings, often confusing readers with contradictory and conflicting results. The following section briefly summarizes data regarding selected food components or nutrients and might assist the medical practitioner in responding to specific inquiries from individuals.

Vitamins

Vitamin A

Vitamin A is essential for the normal growth and development of epithelial tissues. Vitamin A deficiency is common in many parts of the developing world, but is extremely rare in Americans. Vitamin A is provided in the diet as retinol and its esters, primarily from milk and organ meats, and as β-carotene and a few other provitamin A carotenoids in yellow and leafy green vegetables. A protective effect of consuming foods rich in vitamin A has been hypothesized for several types of cancer.[1,5,143] However, there is no clear evidence that vitamin A supplementation will decrease the risk of cancer in populations or individuals consuming a healthy diet. Although many studies in laboratory models indicate that vitamin A deficiency increases the susceptibility of tissues to chemical carcinogenesis, these observations do not support the concept that a lower risk will be observed by excessive supplementation in persons with adequate vitamin A status. The use of vitamin A and synthetic retinoids as pharmacologic agents in chemoprevention trials to determine their efficacy in specific high-risk populations is an important area of translational research.[200]

Vitamin D

Vitamin D is a hormone-like nutrient obtained through the diet, and it is endogenously produced with exposure to sunlight. Evidence has accumulated that suggests an important role of vitamin D in several cancer subtypes including colon, prostate, breast, among others, though clear dose–response relationships and a benefit beyond the recommended daily allowances remains uncertain.[1,119] Recent studies indicate that a vitamin D deficiency may be much more common than previously recognized and may contribute to cancer risk.[201] Cancer cells derived from many human tumors express the receptor for 1,25-dihydroxy vitamin D3 and respond to this agent *in vitro*, but the pathophysiologic significance in human cancer remains to be determined, particularly, beyond dosages considered adequate to correct risk of deficiency.[5,202]

Vitamin E

Vitamin E is a family of eight compounds that are collectively referred to as *tocopherols*. Vegetable oil, eggs, and whole grains are the major sources of dietary vitamin E. The antioxidant and free-radical scavenger properties of vitamin E suggest a possible role in the inhibition of carcinogenesis.[202,203] However, few rodent, epidemiologic, or intervention studies provide strong evidence to support the consumption of vitamin E supplements, particularly beyond the requirement, to prevent cancer.[1,204]

Vitamin C

Vitamin C, which includes ascorbic acid and dehydroascorbic acid, functions as a water-soluble antioxidant and a component of several enzymatic reactions in intermediary metabolism. Citrus fruits, leafy vegetables, tomatoes, and potatoes are rich sources of vitamin C. Despite a large volume of publications, very little evidence supports a critical role of dietary vitamin C in the etiology of most human cancers, although several studies suggest that diets rich in foods containing vitamin C may be cancer protective.[5] Supplement studies, although few in number, have failed to show a reduced risk of cancer.[205] Some provocative evidence concerns the ability of vitamin C to inhibit the formation of carcinogenic nitrosamines, which ultimately may reduce the incidence of cancers that are thought to be associated with nitrosamines, such as gastric cancer.[206] At present, there is no evidence to suggest that consumption of vitamin C supplements at levels higher than the typical amount achieved in a well-balanced diet containing ample fresh fruits and vegetables is useful for the prevention or treatment of human cancer.[1,5]

Folate

Folate is an essential, water-soluble B vitamin required for the normal metabolism of amino acids, methyl groups, and nucleotides. It is found in many vegetables, fruits, beans, and whole grains, and folic acid is also found in fortified grain products in the United States.[207] Folate plays a role in the methylation of DNA, which may be critical for the normal regulation of gene expression and tissue differentiation. Epidemiologic and laboratory studies are beginning to accumulate evidence suggesting that insufficient folate may relate to the risk of several malignancies, particularly colon and breast cancers.[208] Cancer risk may also be higher among persons who consume alcohol regularly with a low-folate diet.[5,16,111,209] However, caution should be advised, as folate is critical for DNA metabolism and cell proliferation, and the potential for high folate to enhance cancer progression has been raised.[84,210]

Minerals

Calcium

Calcium is hypothesized to reduce the risk of colon cancer but enhance the risk of prostate cancer.[1,5] For example, several prospective cohort studies have found that those who develop colon cancer had a significantly lower intake of calcium and vitamin D.[1,5,211] Calcium supplementation of 1.2 g/day reduced the proliferative rate of colonic cells in patients who are considered to be at an increased risk of colon cancer.[47,212] Several clinical trials to determine the effects of calcium supplementation on polyp formation are currently ongoing with initial reports suggesting a modest benefit. Conversely, calcium from dietary sources and from supplements has been demonstrated in several prospective studies to be associated with an increased risk of prostate cancer,[118,121,213] particularly cancers with more aggressive characteristics. At this time, it is appropriate to target calcium intake at RDA levels from a variety of food sources. The RDA is currently 1000 mg/day for those aged 19–50 years and 1200 mg/day for people older than 50 years of age.

Selenium

Selenium is a mineral required in the diet at very small concentrations with an RDA of 55 μg/day for both men and women. Grains, cereals, seafood, and meat are good sources of selenium. Selenium is an essential constituent of glutathione peroxidase, and it participates in the destruction of hydrogen peroxide and organic hydroperoxides, using reducing equivalents from glutathione. Selenium, thus, participates in cellular and tissue defense against oxidative damage. A major obstacle for epidemiologic studies is that estimates of dietary selenium intake are unreliable, especially in the developed nations where foods are extensively processed and shipped for long distances, because the selenium content of food is very sensitive to soil concentrations. An inverse association between the selenium levels in forage crops from different geographic areas or tissue selenium and mortality rates from certain cancers has been suggested.[1,5,113] A landmark human intervention trial reported that selenium supplements might reduce the risk of lung, colon, and prostate cancers.[113] However, larger randomized controlled trials are required to confirm and expand upon these findings. Overall, individuals choosing to consume a selenium supplement should be advised to consume the requirement of 55 μg/day and not more than 200 μg/day because there is a narrow margin between safe and potentially toxic dosages.[1,5]

Foods and food components

Soy products

People living in countries such as Japan and China, where soy foods are regularly consumed, have a much lower risk of cancers of the breast, colon, and prostate than do people living in the United States where soy foods are not commonly consumed. However, many other variables in addition to soy undoubtedly contribute to the geographic variations. Soy foods contain several components, including soy protein, isoflavones, lignans, and saponins, which have been investigated for their anticancer effects in laboratory models.[214,215] Although many studies are currently underway, there is no convincing evidence demonstrating that the use of soy supplements, soy extracts, pure soy concentrates, or other soy components currently marketed will significantly impact human cancer risk. Some concerns have been raised about the risks and benefits of soy consumption relative to breast or endometrial cancer. Several soy isoflavones have a chemical structure similar to estrogen and may bind to the estrogen receptor and act as weak estrogen. It is plausible that high amounts of phytoestrogens may actually increase cell proliferation, although this remains controversial. At this time, it is probably best for women at high risk of breast cancer to avoid concentrated isoflavone supplements, but it is unlikely that moderate amounts of soy foods, as part of a plant-based diet, will increase cancer risk.[37,216–220]

β-Carotene

Foods rich in β-carotene, including many fruits and vegetables, are associated with a lower risk of cancer. However, recent intervention trials with pharmacologic doses of β-carotene clearly question the hypothesis that the benefits of a plant-based diet can be produced through β-carotene supplements. Two large intervention studies of β-carotene, utilizing doses beyond that achieved from dietary sources, demonstrated a higher risk of lung cancer in smokers.[146,221] Although β-carotene is a potential antioxidant and source of vitamin A, supplements should be discouraged for cancer prevention, and diets rich in carotenoids should be encouraged.

Lycopene

The bright red color of tomato products is caused by the non-provitamin carotenoid lycopene. Interest in lycopene has emerged, because many studies demonstrate that the consumption of tomato products is associated with a lower risk of several cancers, particularly prostate cancer.[129,130,133] The recent WCRF/AICR Continuous Update Project report concluded that the relationship between lycopene and prostate cancer is too limited to draw a conclusion.[1,22] However, at the present time, it is sensible to consume tomatoes and tomato products as one component of a carotenoid-rich dietary pattern based on fruit and vegetable intake.

Omega-3 fatty acids, fish oil, and olive oil

Diets rich in total fat have a high caloric density and may contribute to excess energy intake and obesity. Thus, most healthy dietary patterns are slightly lower in total fat than the current American pattern. However, differing types of lipids also may have varying impacts upon cancer. Fish is a rich source of omega-3 fatty acids that can influence cell biology through a number of mechanisms, including modulation in the production of bioactive lipids such as prostaglandins and leukotrienes. Animal models suggest some inhibition of specific cancers, such as prostate and breast.[222] Olive oil has generated interest because of its lack of association with cancers in studies, where total lipids, saturated fats, and other measures of lipid intake demonstrate positive associations. Like other lipids, olive oil contributes to caloric intake and risk of obesity but can be used in certain recipes to replace other types of lipid that may have a greater association with cancer and cardiovascular disease. Overall, definitive data regarding lipid sources or fatty-acid profiles and human cancer risk do not exist; it is yet under study, and specific recommendations are not possible at this time.[1,5]

Organic and natural foods

Government regulators will continue to evaluate information and provide updated standards and recommendations to consumers regarding expectations when the term "organic" is used in food labeling. In general, the term refers to foods grown without the use of synthesized pesticides or herbicides, and it has been expanded to include non-genetically manipulated foods. At the present time, there are very few studies suggesting that consuming organic foods will substantially lower cancer risk when compared to the same foods produced by standard farming practices.[1,5] One notable prospective study evaluating intake of organic foods and cancer risk in over 600,000 women followed for 9.3 years found that consumption of organic foods was not associated with total cancer incidence or cancer subtype incidence, with the exception of non-Hodgkin lymphoma.[223]

Pesticides, herbicides, and environmental contaminants in food

Residues of pesticides and herbicides are found in low concentrations in fruits and vegetables. Overall, studies have not clearly defined cancer risks associated with exposure to the modern agents at low concentrations, and the preponderance of data supports the recommendation that fruits and vegetables should be consumed at greater concentrations. Additional concerns relate to the accumulation of some environmental toxins in meats, including fish, but without definitive evidence of a cancer risk. Certainly, exposures to high concentrations of these compounds through industrial and agricultural exposures are associated with toxicity and raise concerns about cancer risk. Most importantly, regulatory agencies must continue to monitor agents and ensure safety at expected exposure levels in the food supply.[1,5]

Artificial sweeteners (aspartame and saccharin)

Artificial sweeteners are the basis of many low-calorie foods currently marketed. No links between aspartame and human cancer have been identified. Saccharin has been shown to slightly enhance the risk of bladder cancer in rodent studies when provided concentrations that would greatly exceed that consumed by humans. Human epidemiologic studies have not identified saccharin or aspartame consumption as a risk factor for human cancer.[1,5]

Sugar

Highly refined simple sugars provide calories but without the nutrients associated with whole foods. Diets containing large amounts of simple sugars are frequently nutrient-poor and might also contribute to promoting obesity and hormonal changes that could potentially increase cancer risk. However, sugars *per se* are not carcinogens, and a diet with a modest amount of sweets should not be a concern in the context of a healthy dietary pattern.[1,5]

Tea

Clinical investigations of green and black teas are currently underway to determine whether these products may have anticancer properties in humans to support data derived from laboratory studies. Thus far, tea has not been shown to lower the risk of any human cancer, but important studies are underway.[1,5]

Survivorship: diet and nutritional guidance during and following cancer treatment

Although the focus of this chapter is diet and nutrition in the etiology and prevention of cancer, we briefly introduce the emerging field of diet and nutrition during cancer survivorship. "Survivorship" is now accepted as beginning at the time of cancer diagnosis and continuing throughout the life of the individual. Diet and nutrition may have a role in several components of cancer survivorship, including (1) enhancing the benefits of treatment and reducing the frequency or severity of acute treatment-related toxicities; (2) promoting recovery during the immediate post-treatment phase; (3) supporting of patients suffering from cancer cachexia and during terminal phases of incurable or advanced cancers; and (4) promoting long-term survivorship by reducing the chance of recurrent disease, secondary prevention of cancer, and reducing the frequency and severity of late complications of therapy and enhancing overall health and longevity. At current rates, >1.2 million Americans are diagnosed with cancer each year, and >10 million are categorized as survivors. The need for scientifically based recommendations is now acute and has not kept pace with the desire of patients or survivors to obtain information on diet and nutrition. The ACS recently published a review of the field, summarizing the state of nutrition and physical activity research and providing guidelines for communicating with survivors (Table 4).[37]

Diet and nutrition represents, for many cancer patients, an opportunity to counteract the profound sense of loss of control that accompanies cancer treatment. Quality of life is improved when patients feel that they are active participants in the course of their care. Unfortunately, scientific evidence to help a patient choose optimal diet and nutritional information is insufficient in most areas. Cancer survivors are faced with a bewildering array of sources of dietary information, ranging from well-intended family and friends to alternative healthcare providers and those marketing products or selling publications touting dietary approaches. Coupled with the limited training and knowledge of nutrition by many health-care providers, including physicians and nurses, a survivor is frequently confused or easily misled. Although definitive and detailed guidelines are not possible at the present, the following provides a framework for communicating with patients and directing future survivorship research.

Table 4 Public health guidelines for cancer survivorship.

	American Cancer Society[37]	National Comprehensive Cancer Network[224]
Body weight	Achieve and maintain a healthy weight (BMI between 18.5 and 25 kg/m^2). After cancer treatment, weight gain or loss should be managed with a combination of diet, physical activity, and behavioral strategies	Maintain a healthy weight. Weight gain and being overweight during cancer treatment and survivorship may increase risk of recurrence and lower odds for survival
Physical activity	Engage in regular physical activity. Avoid inactivity and return to normal daily activities as soon as possible following diagnosis. Aim to exercise at least 150 min/wk. Include strength training at least 2 days/wk	Engage in at least 30 min of moderate-intensity activity on 5 days/wk or more, or at least 20 min of vigorous-intensity activity on 3 days or more. In addition, perform strength training at least 2 days/wk
Plant-based diet	Achieve a dietary pattern that is high in vegetables, fruits, and whole grains	Aim for a variety of foods. Create a balanced plate that is one-half cooked or raw vegetables, one-fourth lean protein (chicken, fish, lean meat, or dairy), and one-fourth whole grains
Vegetable and fruit	Few studies exist that evaluate fruit, vegetables, and cancer recurrence or survival. Consistent with the *2010 Dietary Guidelines for Americans*, cancer survivors should consume at least 2–3 cups of vegetables and 1.5–2 cups of fruits each day for health benefits	Eat a minimum of five servings of fruits and vegetables per day. Use plant-based seasonings, such as herbs and spices
Breads, grains, and cereals	Choose whole grains instead of refined grain products. Eat plenty of high-fiber foods	Choose whole grains. Opt for high-fiber breads and cereals. Avoid refined foods and those high in sugar
Animal products	Limit intake of processed and red meats. Avoid cooking these and other high-fat sources of protein at high temperatures	Choose lean protein such as fish, poultry, and tofu. Limit red meat and processed meats Eat fatty fish at least twice a week. Choose low-fat dairy products. Select skim milk, low fat yogurt, and reduced fat cheeses
Dietary fat	Limit the intake of foods and beverages high in fat and with added sugar to promote healthy weight control	Eat fatty fish, such as salmon, sardines, and canned tuna, at least twice a week. Walnuts, canola oil, and flaxseeds are additional sources of heart healthy omega-3 fats
Processed foods and refined sugar	Limit the intake of foods and beverages high in fat and with added sugar to promote healthy weight control	Avoid refined foods and those high in sugar
Salt and sodium		
Alcohol	Alcoholic drinks (up to one or two drinks per day for women and men, respectively) can lower the risk of heart disease, but higher levels may increase the risk of specific cancers. It is important for the health care provider to tailor advice on alcohol consumption to the individual survivor	Limit alcohol consumption. Alcohol has been linked to cancer risk. Men should have no more than two drinks per day and women no more than one drink per day
Supplements	Before supplements are prescribed or taken, all attempts should be made to obtain needed nutrients through dietary sources. Supplements should be considered only if a nutrient deficiency is biochemically or clinically demonstrated	A healthy dietary pattern, not supplements, is the ideal strategy for adequate vitamin and mineral intake. There is no evidence that dietary supplements alone provide the same anticancer benefits as a healthy dietary pattern. Some high-dose supplements may actually increase cancer risk

Active treatment phase

Cancer treatment often includes surgery, radiation, chemotherapy, or biologic treatments, as well as combinations of approaches as multimodality interventions are established for a greater number of clinical scenarios. The key to guiding a patient undergoing therapy is to individualize the nutritional support. The care team should monitor individual needs through assessment of body weight, lean body mass, and the presence of eating or digestive impairments. Treatments for some cancers may compromise nutritional status as a result of impairment of food intake, digestion, absorption, and metabolism of nutrients. For example, loss of appetite, nausea, vomiting, altered taste and smell perception, constipation, and diarrhea may transiently occur. Individually tailored interventions to nutritionally support a patient during these periods will enhance quality of life. In some patients, maintaining adequate energy intake is an obstacle, and specific commercially prepared and tested nutritional products can easily be incorporated into a diet plan. Early referrals of patients at high risk for nutritional complications to a RD can prevent the development of more severe malnutrition that may limit the ability of the medical team to provide the optimal treatment intensity.[37]

The use of nutritional supplements during cancer therapy is controversial, and few studies have been conducted to provide detailed guidance. For example, vitamin supplements with high doses of antioxidants (vitamins C or E, selenium, etc.) during chemotherapy or radiation therapy are considered by some clinicians to potentially reduce the efficacy of treatments that may depend on oxidative stress in the cancer cell as the mechanism of action. However, others suggest that antioxidant supplements may provide a benefit to patients by limiting damage to normal tissues, such as bone marrow. In general, it is judicious for clinicians to advise patients undergoing chemotherapy or radiation therapy to limit antioxidants to levels that do not exceed the RDAs and avoid other products that contain herbals or extracts enriched in antioxidant components. Folic acid is one nutrient where large dosages exceeding the RDA could influence the outcome of chemotherapy with agents such as methotrexate or 5-fluorouracil (5-FU) that target metabolic pathways involving folate. Daily supplements containing folate above the RDA should be discouraged for these patients.[37]

Recovery following treatment

The days and weeks following completion of intensive treatment are points in the cancer care continuum where many patients explore dietary and nutritional interventions to enhance survivorship. During this period, the frequency of contact with health-care providers lessens, and the patient is concerned about the efficacy of treatment and recovery from therapy. Diet and physical activity should be a component of the treatment plan with the goal of restoring muscle mass and functional status. Health-care providers must continue to question patients regarding supplements and alternative medical treatments and provide counseling as needed. Continuing individualized nutritional evaluation will identify those with more serious long-term nutritional complications of therapy, such as dysphagia, malabsorption, and bowel changes common in those treated for cancers of the oral pharynx, esophagus, stomach, pancreas, bowel, and others. A focus on energy balance and ensuring adequate intake of essential nutrients is critical. For example, gastric surgery or resection of the terminal ileum may lead to a vitamin B12 deficiency unless parenteral administration is initiated.[37] Consultation with a RD can provide each individual with a risk assessment and personalized counseling.

Advanced cancer

In general, progressive cancer is associated with a loss of appetite, and, if a patient does not succumb quickly to a complication of the disease or co-morbid condition, progressive weight loss and other features of malnutrition will become evident. Unfortunately, many families and caretakers have the impression that reversal of the nutritional deficits will significantly prolong life. In reality, the failure to control the growth of the cancer, rather than malnutrition, is the critical issue. Frequently, the patient and caregivers experience conflict based on loss of appetite and food consumption. The medical team should be alert in order to identify conflicts centering on food, help establish understanding, and provide guidance to families. In the setting of advanced disease, dietary and nutritional interventions can contribute to a sense of well-being and quality of life. Dietitians and the medical team can assist the patient in altering food choices and eating patterns and help maintain nutritional status in the setting of advanced disease often complicated by pain-control issues and the resulting constipation caused by narcotic analgesics. Some medications can be coupled with limited physical activity to enhance appetite and improve bowel function. In some cases, additional nutritional support may be indicated.[37]

Prevention of cancer recurrences and long-term complication of therapy

The patient who achieves a complete remission from cancer is concerned about the reappearance of the primary cancer. Additionally, survivors of certain cancers are at greater risk of second primaries. Indeed, survivors of oral or lung cancer may experience a ~10% chance of a second tobacco-related primary cancer yearly. Many cancer survivors are also at risk for cancers of other sites, which are often related to treatment; for instance, patients cured of testis cancer via treatment with etoposide-based chemotherapy are at a higher risk for secondary leukemia, and survivors of adolescent lymphoma treated with mediastinal radiation have a higher risk of secondary breast cancer. Very little research has been undertaken to establish optimal dietary patterns to prevent recurrent disease or second primaries at the same or different sites. In general, most experts will focus on the dietary recommendations summarized at the beginning of this chapter and by various groups for the prevention of cancer.[1,5,37]

As the population of cancer survivors expands and physicians continue to monitor them over longer periods, long-term complications of treatments that are potential targets of dietary interventions are becoming apparent. For example, premature menopause in women treated with chemotherapy for breast cancer may contribute to accelerated osteoporosis[225] that may require alterations in dietary calcium and physical activity. Mediastinal radiation in young adults and children may contribute to premature coronary atherosclerosis. Medical caregivers should emphasize early interventions with dietary and exercise patterns that will maintain healthy blood cholesterol and triglyceride profiles. Although very little research concerning diet and nutrition has been accumulated to provide clear guidance to cancer survivors thus far, we anticipate that future efforts in this area will expand rapidly as a result of patient demands and the response of the National Institutes of Health through their support of survivorship research.

Key references

The complete reference list can be found on the Wiley Companion Digital Edition of this title (see inside front cover for login instructions).

1 World Cancer Research Fund. *Food, Nutrition and the Prevention of Cancer: A Global Perspective*. Washington, DC: American Institute for Cancer Research; 2007.

2 Eckel RH, Jakicic JM, Ard JD, et al. AHA/ACC guideline on lifestyle management to reduce cardiovascular risk: a report of the American College of Cardiology/American Heart Association Task Force on Practice Guidelines. *J Am Coll Cardiol*. 2013;**63(25 Pt B)**:2960–2984.

3 American College of Cardiology/American Heart Association Task Force on Practice Guidelines. Based on a systematic review from the The Obesity Expert Panel. Executive summary: Guidelines (2013) for the management of overweight and obesity in adults: a report of the American College of Cardiology/American Heart Association Task Force on Practice Guidelines and the Obesity Society published by the Obesity Society and American College of Cardiology/American Heart Association Task Force on Practice Guidelines. Based on a systematic review from the The Obesity Expert Panel, 2013. *Obesity (Silver Spring)*. 2013;**22(Suppl 2)**:S5–S39.

4 U.S. Department of Agriculture and U.S. Department of Health and Human Services. *Dietary Guidelines for Americans, 2010*. Washington, DC: US Government Printing Office; 2010.

5 Kushi LH, Doyle C, McCullough M, et al. American Cancer Society Guidelines on nutrition and physical activity for cancer prevention: reducing the risk of cancer with healthy food choices and physical activity. *CA Cancer J Clin*. 2012;**62(1)**:30–67.

7 Weed DL, Greenwald P, Kramer BS (eds). *In Cancer Prevention and Control*. New York: Marcel Dekker, Inc; 1995:385–402.

10 Willett W. *Nutritional Epidemiology*, 3rd. ed. New York: Oxford University Press; 2012.

12 Colditz GA, Willet WC. Epidemiologic approaches to the study of diet and cancer. In: Alfin-Slater RB, Kritchevsky D, eds. *Human Nutrition: A Comprehensive Treatise*. New York: Plenum; 1991:1–51.

15 National Academy of Sciences Committee on Diet and Health Food and Nutrition Board N.R.C. Commission on Life Sciences, ed. *Diet and Health: Implications for Reducing Risk of Chronic Disease*. Rockville, MD: Academy Press; 1989.

18 Calle EE, Rodriguez C, Walker-Thurmond K, Thun MJ. Overweight, obesity, and mortality from cancer in a prospectively studies cohort of U.S. adults. *N Engl J Med*. 2003;**348(17)**:1625–1638.

20 World Cancer Research Fund/American Institute for Cancer Research, *Continuous Update Project Report. Food, Nutrition, Physical Activity, and the Prevention of Endometrial Cancer*. 2013.

21 World Cancer Research Fund / American Institute for Cancer Research, *Continuous Update Project Report. Food, Nutrition, Physical Activity, and the Prevention of Ovarian Cancer*. 2014.

22 World Cancer Research Fund / American Institute for Cancer Research, *Continuous Update Project Report. Food, Nutrition, Physical Activity, and the Prevention of Prostate Cancer*. 2014.

23 World Cancer Research Fund / American Institute for Cancer Research, *Continuous Update Project Report. Food, Nutrition, Physical Activity, and the Prevention of Breast Cancer*. 2010.

24 Eyre H, Kahn R, Robertson RM. Preventing cancer, cardiovascular disease, and diabetes. A common agenda for the American Cancer Society, the American Diabetes Association, and the American Heart Association. *Stroke*. 2004;**35**:1999–2010.

28 United States Department of Health and Human Services. *Physical Activity Guidelines for Americans*. Rockville, MD: United States Department of Health and Human Services; 2008.

34 Smith-Warner SA, Spiegelman D, Yaun SS, et al. Alcohol and breast cancer in women: a pooled analysis of cohort studies. *JAMA*. 1998;**279(7)**: 535–540.

37 Rock CL, Doyle C, Demark-Wahnefried W, et al. Nutrition and physical activity guidelines for cancer survivors. *CA Cancer J Clin*. 2012;**62(4)**:243–274.

43 Haenszel W. Cancer mortality among the foreign-born in the United States. *J Natl Cancer Inst*. 1961;**26**:37.

47 World Cancer Research Fund/American Institute for Cancer Research, *Continuous Update Project Report. Food, Nutrition, Physical Activity, and the Prevention of Colorectal Cancer*. 2011.

59 Armstrong B, Doll R. Environmental factors and cancer incidence and mortality in different countries, with special reference to dietary practices. *Int J Cancer*. 1975;**15(4)**:617–631.

62 Willett WC, Hunter DJ, Stampfer MJ, et al. Dietary fat and fiber in relation to risk of breast cancer. An 8-year follow-up. *JAMA*. 1992;**268(15)**:2037–2044.

69 Romaguera D, Vergnaud AC, Peeters PH, et al. Is concordance with World Cancer Research Fund/American Institute for Cancer Research guidelines for cancer prevention related to subsequent risk of cancer? Results from the EPIC study. *Am J Clin Nutr*. 2012;**96(1)**:150–163.

85 Colditz GA, Bohlke K. Priorities for the primary prevention of breast cancer. *CA Cancer J Clin*. 2014;**64(3)**:186–194.

90 Tannenbaum A. The dependence of tumor formation on the composition of the calorie-restricted diet as well as on the degree of restriction. *Cancer Res*. 1945;**5**:616.

100 Holmes MD, Hunter DJ, Colditz GA, et al. Association of dietary intake of fat and fatty acids with risk of breast cancer. *JAMA*. 1999;**281**:914–920.

103 Chlebowski RT, Blackburn GL, Elashoff C, et al. Dietary fat reduction in postmenopausal women with primary breast cancer: phase III Women's Intervention Nutrition Study (WINS). *J Clin Oncol*. 2005;**23(16S)**:3S (ASCO conference proceedings abstract).

131 Zu K, Mucci L, Rosner BA, et al. Dietary lycopene, angiogenesis, and prostate cancer: a prospective study in the prostate-specific antigen era. *J Natl Cancer Inst*. 2014;**106(2)**:djt430.

146 Omenn GS, Goodman GE, Thornquist MD, et al. Risk factors for lung cancer and for intervention effects in CARET, the Beta-Carotene and Retinol Efficacy Trial. *J Natl Cancer Inst*. 1996;**88(21)**:1550–1559.

168 Steffen A, Huerta JM, Weiderpass E, et al. General and abdominal obesity and risk of esophageal and gastric adenocarcinoma in the European Prospective Investigation into Cancer and Nutrition (EPIC). *Int J Cancer*. 2015;**137(3)**:646–657.

183 Arem H, Moore SC, Park Y, et al. Physical activity and cancer-specific mortality in the NIH-AARP Diet and Health Study cohort. *Int J Cancer*. 2014;**135(2)**:423–431.

188 World Cancer Research Fund/American Institute for Cancer Research, *Continuous Update Project Report. Food, Nutrition, Physical Activity, and the Prevention of Pancreatic Cancer*. 2012.

195 Michaud DS, Spiegelman D, Clinton SK, Rimm EB, Willett WC, Giovannucci EL. Fruit and vegetable intake and incidence of bladder cancer in a male prospective cohort. *J Natl Cancer Inst*. 1999;**91(7)**:605–613.

208 de Batlle J, Ferrari P, Chajes V, et al. Dietary folate intake and breast cancer risk: European prospective investigation into cancer and nutrition. *J Natl Cancer Inst*. 2015;**107(1)**:367.

210 Mason JB. Folate consumption and cancer risk: a confirmation and some reassurance, but we're not out of the woods quite yet. *Am J Clin Nutr*. 2011;**94(4)**:965–966.

219 Shu XO, Zheng Y, Cai H, et al. Soy food intake and breast cancer survival. *JAMA*. 2009;**302(22)**: 2437–2443.

220 Guha N, Kwan ML, Quesenberry CP Jr, Weltzien EK, Castillo AL, Caan BJ. Soy isoflavones and risk of cancer recurrence in a cohort of breast cancer survivors: the Life After Cancer Epidemiology study. *Breast Cancer Res Treat*. 2009;**118(2)**:395–405.

221 The Alpha-Tocopherol Beta-Carotene Cancer Prevention Study Group. The effect of vitamin E and beta carotene on the incidence of lung cancer and other cancers in male smokers. *N Engl J Med*. 1994;**330(15)**:1029–1035.

223 Bradbury KE, Balkwill A, Spencer EA, et al. Organic food consumption and the incidence of cancer in a large prospective study of women in the United Kingdom. *Br J Cancer*. 2014;**110(9)**:2321–2326.

224 National Comprehensive Cancer Network. Nutrition for Cancer Survivors. 2015. Available from: http://www.nccn.org/patients/resources/life_after_cancer/nutrition.aspx

37 Chemoprevention of cancer

William N. William, Jr., MD ▪ Waun Ki Hong, MD ▪ Scott M. Lippman, MD

Overview

The field of cancer chemoprevention is underpinned by two phenomena of neoplasia: field carcinogenesis and multistep carcinogenesis. Accurate cancer risk models are critical to chemoprevention and may accelerate drug development in this setting. The Food and Drug Administration has approved several chemoprevention strategies. This chapter describes completed chemoprevention clinical trials focused on the four major cancer sites in the Western world (lung, colon and rectum, prostate, and breast), as well as site-agnostic chemoprevention studies. The contributions of vaccines to cancer prevention are also discussed.

Biology of chemoprevention

The field of cancer chemoprevention is underpinned by two phenomena of neoplasia: (1) field carcinogenesis, which is the multifocal development of intraepithelial neoplasia (IEN, or precancer) or the clonal spread of one or more IENs, and (2) multistep carcinogenesis, which is driven by genetic instability and accumulates progressive genetic and epigenetic changes.[1-4] These processes spur evasion of apoptosis, strong replicative potential, and sustained angiogenesis leading to IEN and cancer development. Multistep carcinogenesis allows chemopreventive interventions at step(s) of neoplasia that precede invasive cancer. Drugs developed for cancer therapy can be examined for cancer chemoprevention because of important commonalities—including genetic and epigenetic abnormalities, loss of cellular control, and certain phenotypic characteristics—between cancer and multistep IEN.[5] Field carcinogenesis makes approaches such as systemic agents attractive for controlling the neoplastic results of diffuse exposure to carcinogens throughout an epithelial field. The FDA has approved several treatments for IEN.

Cancer risk modeling

Accurate cancer risk models are critical to chemoprevention. Models based on clinical/demographic factors have been developed for breast cancer risk (Gail model) and lung cancer risk (Spitz model), and established identifiers of increased risk include precursor clinical/histologic lesions.[6,7] These risk models and lesions are useful on a population-wide basis but are less helpful in identifying individual or personalized risk. Recent work showed that clinical lung cancer risk models integrating genomics (somatic gene-expression arrays and host DNA-repair capacity) and metabolomics assessed risk more accurately than did the clinical models alone.[8-10] Barrett's esophagus is a well-established but modest predictor of absolute esophageal cancer risk, whereas a striking model incorporating certain loss of heterozygosity (LOH) and DNA-content profiles with Barrett's distinguished between populations with a high (79% in 6 years) and low (0% in over 6 years) esophageal cancer risk.[11] In

oral leukoplakia, LOH at specific loci in chromosomes 3p and/or 9p confers a substantially increased risk of oral cancer (vs oral leukoplakia without such LOH)[12-14] especially in patients with a previously treated oral cancer,[15] and this marker was used as a selection criterion in the first and only personalized, molecularly based, randomized oral cancer chemoprevention trial completed till date—the Erlotinib Prevention of Oral Cancer study.[16,17] A high cancer risk is associated with a specific cyclin D1 genotype (adenine/guanine single-nucleotide polymorphism at position 870 of exon 4 of the cyclin D1 gene)[18] in patients with dysplastic oral and/or laryngeal premalignant lesions. Recent work has shown that high cyclin D1 protein expression plus the high-risk cyclin D1 genotype further increased the cancer risk of laryngeal dysplasia patients.[19] As such, selection of high-risk individuals for chemoprevention based on cancer risk modeling is considered a key factor to increase the therapeutic index of any given intervention, leading to successful drug development in this area.

Chemoprevention trials

This section describes completed chemoprevention clinical trials focused on the four major cancer sites in the Western world (lung, colon and rectum, prostate, and breast), as well as site-agnostic chemoprevention studies. The contributions of vaccines to cancer prevention are also discussed.

The lung

Premalignancy

Clinical and translational chemoprevention trials, including five negative randomized trials of retinoids in smokers with metaplasia, have had little to no effect in reversing lung premalignancy.[20] Despite the general negative results, encouraging phase IIb data have emerged from studies of 9-*cis*-retinoic acid modulation of RAR-β and Ki-6,[21,22] myo-inositol modulation of the PI3 kinase gene-expression pathway,[23] budesonide modulation of computed tomography-detected peripheral nodules,[24] and anethole dithiolthione[25] and iloprost[26] modulation of bronchial dysplasia.

Prevention of primary lung cancer

The *National Cancer Institute*-sponsored Alpha-Tocopherol, Beta-Carotene (ATBC) Cancer Prevention Study was a phase III trial of α-tocopherol and β-carotene to prevent primary lung cancer. The ATBC study involved 29,133 male smokers between 50 and 69 years of age who had smoked an average of one pack of cigarettes a day for approximately 36 years.[27] This trial's 2 × 2 factorial design called for α-tocopherol (50 mg/day) and β-carotene (20 mg/day) to be given in a randomized, double-blind, placebo-controlled fashion. The factorial design allowed the study scientists to assess the individual effects of each agent. Significant increases in lung

Holland-Frei Cancer Medicine, Ninth Edition. Edited by Robert C. Bast Jr., Carlo M. Croce, William N. Hait, Waun Ki Hong, Donald W. Kufe, Martine Piccart-Gebhart, Raphael E. Pollock, Ralph R. Weichselbaum, Hongyang Wang, and James F. Holland.
© 2017 John Wiley & Sons, Inc. ISBN: 978-1-118-93469-2

cancer incidence (18% increase, $p = 0.01$) and total mortality (8%, $p = 0.02$) occurred in the β-carotene-treated subjects after 6.1 years' median follow-up. α-Tocopherol had no significant impact on the lung cancer mortality rate, and there was no evidence of an interaction between α-tocopherol and β-carotene.[28]

The Beta-Carotene and Retinol Efficacy Trial (CARET) tested the combination of β-carotene (30 mg/day) plus retinyl palmitate (25,000 IU/day) in 17,000 smokers and asbestos workers.[29] It confirmed the major finding of the ATBC study with its primary finding that the β-carotene combination increased lung cancer risk in this high-risk population. There was no evidence from either the ATBC study or the CARET that β-carotene increased lung cancer risk in nonsmokers, or former or moderate (<1 pack a day) smokers.

SPT prevention

Two large-scale phase III retinoid trials have been completed in the setting of second primary tumor (SPT) prevention: one in Europe (investigating retinyl palmitate and/or N-acetyl-L-cysteine)[31] and the other in the United States (investigating low-dose 13cRA).[32] Neither demonstrated a reduction in SPT in the population overall. Selenium also failed to prevent SPTs compared with placebo in a RCT of 1151 patients with resected stage I nonsmall cell lung cancers.[33]

Colon and rectum

Colorectal trial designs have primarily employed the intermediate end points of adenomatous polyp development and response and hyperproliferation markers.

Sulindac and celecoxib can effectively treat (but not prevent) adenomas in individuals with familial adenomatous polyposis (FAP).[34,35] High-dose celecoxib (800 mg/day) reduced large-bowel polyposis by 28% and duodenal polyposis, which is difficult to resect, by 14% (vs placebo).[36] These studies led to the interim FDA approval of celecoxib as an adjunct to endoscopic and surgical treatment of FAP patients. However, the labeled indication for polyp management in FAP patients was withdrawn due to challenges in conducting confirmatory trials in this high-risk setting. Calcium (1200 mg/day) reduced the risk of sporadic adenomas by 15% overall[37] and even more in later-stage disease (vs placebo). The CAPP-1 and CAPP-2 trials examined aspirin (600 mg q.d.) in subjects with the hereditary colorectal cancer (CRC) syndromes of FAP and Lynch syndrome, respectively. CAPP-1 identified a nonsignificant reduction (23%) in polyp count and a trend toward reduced largest polyp size within the aspirin-treated group, after a median of 17 months of intervention. CAPP-2 found a significant reduction in risk of CRC (59%) only in subjects completing at least 2 years of intervention after a mean of 55.7 months of follow-up.[38,39]

Four RCTs have tested the efficacy of aspirin in preventing sporadic adenomas, showing significant reductions in recurrent adenomas among patients treated for 1 or more years.[40–43] There was no protective effect of aspirin on CRC risk in men and women in the Physician's Health Study and Women's Health Study (WHS). However, after an overall follow-up time of 18 years, recent results from the WHS indicate a significantly reduced risk for CRC in healthy women.[44] Recent pooled analyses of the British Doctors Aspirin Trial and the UK Transient Ischaemic Attack Aspirin Trial found that aspirin was associated with a significant 26% reduction in CRC risk. The effect was greatest with at least 5 years treatment and did not appear for at least 10 years.[45] The latter results are consistent with a recent, very large cohort study involving over 47,000 men from the Health Professionals Follow-up Study, which found a significant dose- and duration-related reduction in CRC risk.[46]

Three RCTs assessed coxibs (vs placebo) in preventing sporadic adenomas in patients with a prior history of colorectal polyps. The Adenomatous Polyp Prevention on Vioxx (APPROVe) trial tested rofecoxib, and various doses of celecoxib were tested in the APC and Prevention of Colorectal Sporadic Adenomatous Polyps (PreSAP) trials. Interim cardiovascular event rates were unexpectedly higher in APPROVe and APC but not PreSAP.[47–49] The relevant data and safety monitoring committees stopped all three RCTs early because of these safety issues, despite significant activity against colorectal adenomas, and rofecoxib was withdrawn from the world market by the manufacturer. In APPROVe (2587 randomized subjects), rofecoxib reduced adenomas by 24%.[50] In the APC (2035 randomized patients), adenoma rates were significantly different at 37.5% (celecoxib, 400 mg twice daily), 43% (celecoxib, 200 mg twice daily), and 60% (placebo) ($p < 0.001$)[51]; serious cardiovascular adverse event rates significantly increased in a dose-dependent manner. The PreSAP trial with 1561 randomized patients found incidences of adenomas of 33.6% (celecoxib, 400 mg once daily) and 49.3% (placebo) ($p < 0.001$).[47] The risk of cardiovascular events did not increase in the PreSAP trial. In a recent extension analysis of APC patients, it appeared that the serious cardiovascular event rate wore off 2 years after stopping the drug and that a repression of adenomas persisted (albeit diminished), particularly for advanced adenomas. Results of a recent pooled analysis of the major celecoxib placebo-controlled trials (double-blind and planned follow-up of at least 3 years in nonarthritis disease settings) suggested that there was no increase in serious cardiovascular events at any studied dose (up to 400 mg b.i.d.) in people with a low-baseline cardiovascular risk (about 15–20% of people on these trials). These results strongly suggest that low-baseline cardiovascular risk can improve risk-benefit and help in selecting patients for future COX-2-specific NSAID (nonsteroidal anti-inflammatory drug) trials.[52]

Trials of vitamins and diet (low-fat, high fruits and vegetables and fiber) for reducing colorectal adenoma risk have had largely negative results.[53,54] Calcium reduced adenoma risk by a modest statistically significant 19%,[37] which persisted in long-term follow-up.[55] Two RCTs of folate showed no reduction in adenoma risk with a 0.5- or 1-mg/day dose; a subset analysis of one study suggested that folate (1 mg/day) may even increase the risk of advanced or multiple adenomas.[43,56]

Preclinical studies of low doses of DFMO and sulindac supported an RCT of combined oral DFMO (500 mg) and sulindac (150 mg; vs placebo) for 36 months in 375 patients with a history of resected (≥3 mm) adenomas [stratified by use of low-dose aspirin (81 mg) at baseline and clinical adenoma site].[57] Colorectal adenoma recurrence rates were as follows: one or more adenomas—41.1% placebo versus 12.3% (combination; relative risk (RR) 0.30; 95% confidence interval (CI), 0.18–0.49; $p < 0.001$); one or more advanced adenomas—8.5% (placebo) versus 0.7% (combination; RR 0.085; 95% CI, 0.011–0.65; $p < 0.001$); multiple adenomas—13.2% (placebo) versus 0.7% (combination; RR 0.055; 95% CI, 0.0074–0.41; $p < 0.001$). Combination chemoprevention has been long believed to have great potential for enhancing the activity and reducing the toxicity of active single agents, a belief that is reinforced by the landmark advance of this combination trial.

The breast

Based on highly significant positive results of the Breast Cancer Prevention Trial (BCPT), the selective estrogen-receptor modulator (SERM) tamoxifen became the first chemopreventive agent to earn FDA approval. Conducted by the National Surgical Adjuvant Breast and Bowel Project (NSABP), the BCPT compared tamoxifen with placebo in preventing breast cancer in 13,388 women at high-risk of this disease.[58] The major high-risk eligibility criteria were age >60 years and history of lobular carcinoma *in situ* (LCIS), or women from 35 to 59 years old with 5-year breast cancer risk of 1.66% based on the Gail model. The actual overall average, 5-year baseline, breast cancer risk was 3.2%. At a median follow-up of 55 months, primary invasive breast cancer findings for the tamoxifen and placebo groups were 89 versus 175, respectively, for a 49% relative reduction ($p < 0.00001$). The relative breast cancer risk reduction was similar for all age and risk groups and was limited to ER (estrogen-receptor)-positive tumors. Tamoxifen nonsignificantly reduced overall and breast cancer mortality. Beneficial secondary findings included 19% fewer fractures in the tamoxifen group. Secondary adverse findings associated with tamoxifen were increased endometrial cancers, vascular events, and cataracts.

Although the BCPT successfully completed testing its primary hypothesis, it also raised several key unresolved issues, such as effects on mortality, optimal tamoxifen duration, generalizability of results, and the issue of prevention versus treatment. The FDA subsequently approved tamoxifen for breast cancer risk reduction in high-risk women. The FDA recommendation is 20 mg/day for 5 years for high-risk women and warns of tamoxifen-associated risks. The FDA also approved tamoxifen for reducing the incidence of contralateral breast cancers, based on consistent secondary adjuvant data.[59]

The NSABP B-24 study tested 5 years of tamoxifen (20 mg/day) versus placebo after resection and radiation in 1804 patients with ductal carcinoma *in situ* (DCIS).[60] At a median follow-up of 74 months, 5-year incidences of all breast cancer events (invasive and noninvasive) were 8.2% and 13.4% in the tamoxifen and placebo groups, respectively, representing a 43% relative risk reduction ($p = 0.0009$). The cumulative incidence at 5 years of all invasive breast cancer events in the tamoxifen group was 4.1% versus 7.2% in the placebo group ($p = 0.004$). The FDA approved tamoxifen for risk reduction in the setting of locally treated (resection and radiation) breast DCIS.

The International Breast Cancer Intervention Study (IBIS-I) randomized 7410 women and showed a 32% reduction in breast cancer risk with tamoxifen.[60] The positive results in this trial and the BCPT (the two stronger RCTs in this setting) were limited to ER-positive cancers. A report of the long-term follow-up of IBIS-I suggests that the beneficial tamoxifen effects on breast cancer risk reduction persist for at least 10 years, but most side effects resolve after the 5-year treatment period, including all serious adverse events (e.g., thrombotic events and endometrial cancer).[61] These long-term findings have important implications for the risk/benefit profile of tamoxifen for prevention.

The Study of Tamoxifen and Raloxifene (STAR) tested the SERM raloxifene against its fellow SERM tamoxifen for better efficacy and lesser toxicity in breast cancer prevention.[62] A total of 19,747 postmenopausal women with an increased risk of breast cancer were randomized to tamoxifen (20 mg/day) or raloxifene (60 mg/day) for 5 years. On long-term follow-up, raloxifene had slightly higher rates of invasive breast cancer (RR 1.24; 95% CI, 1.05–1.47), but produced fewer cases of uterine cancer than tamoxifen (RR 0.55; 95% CI, 0.36–0.83). Furthermore, the risks of thromboembolic events and cataracts were statistically significantly lower with raloxifene than with tamoxifen. Tamoxifen and raloxifene had similar effects in reducing noninvasive breast cancer.[63] Raloxifene was approved by the FDA for invasive breast cancer risk reduction in postmenopausal women at a high such risk or with osteoporosis.

Following these seminal trials, the chemopreventive effect of third-generation SERMs was investigated. The Postmenopausal Evaluation and Risk-Reduction with Lasofoxifene Trial studied the effects of lasofoxifene in postmenopausal women with low bone mineral density (BMD),[64,65] showing a 79% reduction of invasive breast cancer and an 83% reduction in ER-positive breast cancer. A similar phase III prevention trial, known as the Generations Trial, reported a 56% decrease in invasive breast cancers in postmenopausal women with low BMD treated with arzoxifene.[66,67] These trials found that both lasofoxifene and arzoxifene reduce the risk of nonvertebral and vertebral fractures; however, these third-generation SERMs, like raloxifene and tamoxifen, still increase the risk of venous thromboembolic events.

A recent meta-analysis that included all nine of the large-scale phase III SERM prevention trials[68] found that both overall and ER-positive breast cancer incidence is decreased by SERMs, and that DCIS incidence is decreased by all SERMs analyzed except raloxifene.

Based largely on results of the Anastrozole, Tamoxifen Alone or in Combination (ATAC) trial,[69] there has been great interest in aromatase inhibitors for breast cancer prevention in postmenopausal women. The Mammary Prevention 3 trial randomized 4560 postmenopausal high-risk women to receive 25 mg of exemestane or placebo for 5 years. There was a 65% reduction in the annual incidence of invasive breast cancer in favor of exemestane (hazard ratio (HR) 0.35; 95% CI, 0.18–0.70). There were no differences between the groups in bone fractures, cardiovascular events, or other cancers.[70] The IBIS-II trial evaluated anastrozole 1 mg daily versus placebo for 5 years in 3864 high-risk postmenopausal women and also demonstrated a reduction in the incidence in invasive breast cancer in favor of the aromatase inhibitor (HR 0.47; 95% CI, 0.32–0.68). Anastrozole also reduced the incidence of skin, gynecologic, gastrointestinal, and other cancers. More aches and pains, joint stiffness, vasomotor symptoms, dry eyes, and hypertension were seen in the anastrozole group, but there was no statistical significant difference in the incidence of fractures between the arms.[71] To date, no agent has proven efficacy in the prevention of ER-negative breast cancer, although a number of drugs are under investigation.

The prostate

Prostate carcinogenesis is an androgen-driven process, and a large-scale RCT, the Prostate Cancer Prevention Trial (PCPT), tested finasteride (5 mg/day), which inhibits 5-α-reductase from converting testosterone into the more potent androgen dihydrotestosterone, versus placebo for 7 years in 18,882 men 55 years of age or older who had normal digital rectal exam (DRE) and prostate-specific antigen (PSA) level. Finasteride not only reduced the 7-year prostate cancer prevalence by 24.8%[72] but also appeared to increase high-grade disease—6.4% (finasteride) versus 5.1% (placebo). Finasteride also reduced the risk of high-grade prostatic IEN.[73] PCPT analyses also indicated a reduction in benign prostatic hypertrophy symptoms and an increase in sexual side effects, although a recent detailed analysis found that the effect of finasteride on sexual functioning was minimal.[74] Secondary PCPT findings indicated a high risk of prostate cancer, including high-grade disease, among men with normal PSA levels[75] and differences in PSA screening performance in men taking or not taking finasteride.[76,77] The adverse high-grade disease finding has sharply limited public interest in finasteride for prostate cancer prevention, and another major concern is that intensive PSA/DRE screening and early detection of prostate cancer in the PCPT could mean that finasteride may have prevented clinically "insignificant" more than "significant" prostate cancer. Several analyses, however, challenge these concerns.[77–83] A recent long-term (18-year) follow-up report attempted to address the significance of the high-grade finding (e.g., finasteride-driven artifact vs new finasteride-induced high-grade cancers) and found no significant between-group difference in the rates of overall survival or survival after the diagnosis of prostate cancer.[84]

The Reduction by Dutasteride of Prostate Cancer Events study compared dutasteride 0.5 mg/day versus placebo in 8231 men 50–75 years of age, with a PSA level between 2.5 and 10 ng/mL and a negative prostate biopsy within 6 months. Participants underwent ultrasound-guided biopsies at years 2 and 4 of treatment. There was a 22.8% relative risk reduction in prostate cancer favoring dutasteride (95% CI, 15.2–29.8; $p < 0.001$). There were 29 and 19 cancers with Gleason scores of 8–10 in the dutasteride and placebo groups, respectively ($p = 0.15$) over years 1 through 4; however, during years 3 and 4, there were 12 tumors with Gleason scores of 8–10 in the dutasteride group, and only 1 in the placebo group ($p = 0.003$). Acute urinary retention was less frequent, but the composite end point of cardiac failure as well as erectile dysfunction and loss of libido was more common in the dutasteride group.[85]

Another very large RCT, the Selenium and Vitamin E Cancer Prevention Trial (SELECT), recently discontinued supplements and reported results demonstrating that selenium or vitamin E, alone or in combination, did not prevent prostate cancer at the doses and formulations used in a heterogeneous population of 35,533 relatively healthy men. A harmful trend for increased risk of prostate cancer in the vitamin E arm ($p = 0.06$; RR 1.13; 99% CI, 0.195–1.35)[86] became statistically significant on further follow-up.[87] A recent follow-on analysis of SELECT investigated whether selenium or vitamin E might benefit men with low-baseline selenium. Contrary to this hypothesis, there was no evidence of benefit of the intervention in the low-baseline selenium group; in fact, vitamin E supplementation actually increased the risk of total prostate cancer by 63% in men with low-baseline toenail selenium, and this effect was even stronger for high grade.[88]

Vaccines

The proof of principle of vaccinating against infection-related cancer was provided in Taiwan, where vaccinating children against hepatitis B has dramatically reduced the incidence and the mortality of liver cancer.[89]

HPV infection is an established major risk factor for cervical cancer, and molecular targeting through immunization against infections related to neoplasia is a very successful way to prevent early steps of host cell damage that otherwise can lead to cancer. The landmark advances of cancer chemoprevention are the relatively recent RCTs of HPV vaccines to prevent HPV infection in girls and young women and subsequent FDA approval of HPV vaccination in this setting.

The placebo-controlled (phase III) trial, Females United to Unilaterally Reduce Endo/Ectocervical Disease (FUTURE) I, evaluated the role of quadrivalent vaccine against HPV types 6, 11, 16, and 18 in preventing anogenital diseases in women aged 16–24 years. The co-primary composite end points were the incidence of genital warts, vulvar or vaginal IEN, or cancer and the incidence of cervical IEN, adenocarcinoma *in situ*, or cancer associated with HPV types 6, 11, 16, or 18 in a per-protocol susceptible population of women without virologic evidence of HPV infection. The vaccine efficacy was 100% for each of the co-primary end points.[90] Similarly, the FUTURE II study found that the quadrivalent vaccine reduced the risk of the primary composite end point [cervical IEN (grades 2 and 3), adenocarcinoma *in situ*, or cancer-related to HPV types 16 or 18]

by 98% in women between ages 15 and 26 years with no virologic evidence of HPV types 16 or 18.[91] Another phase III trial tested a bivalent (HPV types 16 and 18) vaccine in 18,644 girls and women aged 15–25 years. The primary end point, grade 2 cervical IEN associated with HPV types 16 or 18, was reduced by 90% in women with no evidence of prior HPV infection.[92] In a community-based, randomized, control trial in young women aged 18–25 years, the bivalent vaccine has been demonstrated to have high efficacy against HPV types 16 or 18 persistent infection and partial cross-protection against HPV types 31, 33, and 45.[93]

In males, the quadrivalent HPV vaccine has also been shown to reduce HPV infections and development of related external genital lesions,[94] as well as anal IEN.[95] Oral HPV infections are also reduced by HPV vaccination in women (bivalent vaccine), but it is unknown whether this will eventually translate into prevention of HPV-related head and neck squamous cell carcinomas.[96] HPV vaccines have not been shown to accelerate HPV clearance and so are unlikely to prevent cancer in already infected patients.[97]

Overall cancer

Two important large US trials have tested the ability of β-carotene to reduce overall cancer incidence. The Physicians' Health Study (PHS) was a 12-year test of β-carotene effects on overall cancer incidence.[98] β-Carotene produced no significant differences in overall incidence of cancer (including lung cancer). Only 11% of this population were current smokers. Similar β-carotene results of the Women's Health Study were reported.[99] Recently, the results of the PHS II were reported. This large-scale ($N = 14,641$ men), randomized, placebo-controlled study demonstrated that daily low-dose multivitamin led to a statistically significant reduction in the incidence of total cancer compared with placebo (17.0 and 18.3 events, respectively, per 1000 person-years; HR 0.92, 95% CI, 0.86–0.998; $p = 0.04$), primarily in individuals with a prior cancer history. There were no reductions in the incidence of site-specific cancers.[100] The clinical significance of this modest effect is yet to be determined.

Conclusions

Clinical cancer chemoprevention has matured with the FDA approvals of several agents to prevent cancer or to treat or prevent IEN, most recently raloxifene is used for preventing invasive breast cancer in high-risk women and HPV vaccine is used for anogenital cancer prevention. The current list of FDA-approved agents for cancer prevention includes diclofenac, Photofrin [in conjunction with photodynamic therapy (PDT)], tamoxifen, hepatitis B vaccine, bacillus Calmette–Guerin, valrubicin, masoprocol, 5-FU, aminolevulinic acid (with PDT), and HPV vaccine. Personalized approaches to identify patients most likely to benefit and least likely to be harmed by particular interventions are evolving from continued study of aspirin and celecoxib in colorectal neoplasia. One of the most promising current directions of cancer chemoprevention is combined agents. The concept that combinations can increase the ratio of benefit (activity) to risk (toxicity) for effective single agents received strong support from the stunning colorectal adenoma results of the DFMO-sulindac trial discussed earlier. Based on this trial, chemopreventive combinations may be at the threshold of becoming a standard clinical reality, and other active combinations should be moved into clinical trials.[101]

Summary

Cancer chemoprevention is beginning to add impressive data to the long list of advances resulting from cancer therapy. There have been several exciting developments in clinical chemoprevention, including, for example, the US Food and Drug Administration (FDA) approval of tamoxifen for reducing the risk of preinvasive and invasive breast cancer in the late 1990s, followed by subsequent FDA approvals of raloxifene for reducing the risk of invasive breast cancer and of human papillomavirus (HPV) vaccine for reducing cervical neoplasia risk. More recently, aromatase inhibitors have been shown to prevent breast cancers in postmenopausal women, with a favorable side effect profile. A randomized controlled trial (RCT) of combined sulindac and difluoromethylornithine (DFMO) achieved an extraordinary 70% reduction in colorectal adenomas (>90% in advanced adenomas) highlighting the chemoprevention focus on combined agents and signaling, perhaps the near realization of this approach in standard clinical practice.

Key references

The complete reference list can be found on the Wiley Companion Digital Edition of this title (see inside front cover for login instructions).

6 Gail MH, Brinton LA, Byar DP, et al. Projecting individualized probabilities of developing breast cancer for white females who are being examined annually. *J Natl Cancer Inst*. 1989;**81**:1879–1886.

27 The Alpha-Tocopherol, Beta Carotene Cancer Prevention Study Group. The effect of vitamin E and beta carotene on the incidence of lung cancer and other cancers in male smokers. *N Engl J Med*. 1994;**330**:1029–1035.

29 Omenn GS, Goodman GE, Thornquist MD, et al. Effects of a combination of beta carotene and vitamin A on lung cancer and cardiovascular disease. *N Engl J Med*. 1996;**334**:1150–1155.

35 Steinbach G, Lynch PM, Phillips RK, et al. The effect of celecoxib, a cyclooxygenase-2 inhibitor, in familial adenomatous polyposis. *N Engl J Med*. 2000;**342**:1946–1952.

41 Baron JA, Cole BF, Sandler RS, et al. A randomized trial of aspirin to prevent colorectal adenomas. *N Engl J Med*. 2003;**348**:891–899.

45 Flossmann E, Rothwell PM, British Doctors Aspirin Trial, et al. Effect of aspirin on long-term risk of colorectal cancer: consistent evidence from randomised and observational studies. *Lancet*. 2007;**369**:1603–1613.

47 Arber N, Eagle CJ, Spicak J, et al. Celecoxib for the prevention of colorectal adenomatous polyps. *N Engl J Med*. 2006;**355**:885–895.

48 Bresalier RS, Sandler RS, Quan H, et al. Cardiovascular events associated with rofecoxib in a colorectal adenoma chemoprevention trial. *N Engl J Med*. 2005;**352**:1092–1102.

49 Solomon SD, McMurray JJ, Pfeffer MA, et al. Cardiovascular risk associated with celecoxib in a clinical trial for colorectal adenoma prevention. *N Engl J Med*. 2005;**352**:1071–1080.

50 Baron JA, Sandler RS, Bresalier RS, et al. A randomized trial of rofecoxib for the chemoprevention of colorectal adenomas. *Gastroenterology*. 2006;**131**:1674–1682.

51 Bertagnolli MM, Eagle CJ, Zauber AG, et al. Celecoxib for the prevention of sporadic colorectal adenomas. *N Engl J Med*. 2006;**355**:873–884.

57 Meyskens FL Jr, McLaren CE, Pelot D, et al. Difluoromethylornithine plus sulindac for the prevention of sporadic colorectal adenomas: a randomized placebo-controlled, double-blind trial. *Cancer Prev Res (Phila)*. 2008;**1**:32–38.

58 Fisher B, Costantino JP, Wickerham DL, et al. Tamoxifen for prevention of breast cancer: report of the National Surgical Adjuvant Breast and Bowel Project P-1 Study. *J Natl Cancer Inst*. 1998;**90**:1371–1388.

60 Cuzick J, Forbes J, Edwards R, et al. First results from the International Breast Cancer Intervention Study (IBIS-I): a randomised prevention trial. *Lancet*. 2002;**360**:817–824.

62 Vogel VG, Costantino JP, Wickerham DL, et al. Effects of tamoxifen vs raloxifene on the risk of developing invasive breast cancer and other disease outcomes: the NSABP Study of Tamoxifen and Raloxifene (STAR) P-2 trial. *JAMA*. 2006;**295**:2727–2741.

70 Goss PE, Ingle JN, Ales-Martinez JE, et al. Exemestane for breast-cancer prevention in postmenopausal women. *N Engl J Med*. 2011;**364**:2381–2391.

71 Cuzick J, Sestak I, Forbes JF, et al. Anastrozole for prevention of breast cancer in high-risk postmenopausal women (IBIS-II): an international, double-blind, randomised placebo-controlled trial. *Lancet*. 2014;**383**:1041–1048.

72 Thompson IM, Goodman PJ, Tangen CM, et al. The influence of finasteride on the development of prostate cancer. *N Engl J Med*. 2003;**349**:215–224.

84 Thompson IM Jr, Goodman PJ, Tangen CM, et al. Long-term survival of participants in the prostate cancer prevention trial. *N Engl J Med*. 2013;**369**:603–610.

85 Andriole GL, Bostwick DG, Brawley OW, et al. Effect of dutasteride on the risk of prostate cancer. *N Engl J Med*. 2010;**362**:1192–1202.

89 Chiang CJ, Yang YW, You SL, et al. Thirty-year outcomes of the national hepatitis B immunization program in Taiwan. *JAMA*. 2013;**310**:974–976.

90 Garland SM, Hernandez-Avila M, Wheeler CM, et al. Quadrivalent vaccine against human papillomavirus to prevent anogenital diseases. *N Engl J Med*. 2007;**356**:1928–1943.

91 Group FIS. Quadrivalent vaccine against human papillomavirus to prevent high-grade cervical lesions. *N Engl J Med*. 2007;**356**:1915–1927.

92 Paavonen J, Jenkins D, Bosch FX, et al. Efficacy of a prophylactic adjuvanted bivalent L1 virus-like-particle vaccine against infection with human papillomavirus types 16 and 18 in young women: an interim analysis of a phase III double-blind, randomised controlled trial. *Lancet*. 2007;**369**:2161–2170.

94 Giuliano AR, Palefsky JM, Goldstone S, et al. Efficacy of quadrivalent HPV vaccine against HPV Infection and disease in males. *N Engl J Med*. 2011;**364**:401–411.

95 Palefsky JM, Giuliano AR, Goldstone S, et al. HPV vaccine against anal HPV infection and anal intraepithelial neoplasia. *N Engl J Med*. 2011;**365**:1576–1585.

100 Gaziano JM, Sesso HD, Christen WG, et al. Multivitamins in the prevention of cancer in men: the Physicians' Health Study II randomized controlled trial. *JAMA*. 2012;**308**:1871–1880.

38 Cancer screening and early detection

Otis W. Brawley, MD, MACP

Overview

Cancer screening is an intervention to find cancer at an early stage. The primary goal of screening is to reduce the mortality from the disease being screened for. Secondary is to successfully treat the disease with the least morbidity. In order for screening to be effective, the disease must have a phase in its natural history in which the disease is localized and therapeutic interventions can successfully stop disease progression. The natural history of some cancers is such that screening is not effective. One can best assess a disease as screenable and a screening intervention as useful through a prospective randomized in which people at risk for the cancer are enrolled and randomized to the screening intervention, which is administered on a regular basis or not to get the screening intervention. People who are diagnosed with the disease on both arms should have access to adequate treatment. Over time, the death rate from those who were to be screened is compared to those who were not to be screened. Of note, assessment should be by intention to screen. A successful screening test reduces the death rate. Assessment through a prospective randomized trial is important as some screening tests have been associated with an increase in overall and 5-year survival rate without a decrease in mortality or risk of death. Indeed, the benefit and risk of a screening test is important in determining whether a screening test should be recommended or used.

Cancer screening is a means of early detection of malignancy in an asymptomatic individual at risk for a disease. A positive test indicates that disease may be present and additional "diagnostic" testing is necessary to confirm the presence and extent of disease. In a symptomatic person, the same test is often considered "diagnostic" rather than screening.[1]

The purpose of screening is not simply to find disease, but to reduce the incidence of advanced disease, and find disease at a point in its natural history where treatment will prevent death. In clinical study, prevention of death is demonstrated by reduction in cancer mortality rates.[2] Some screening tests decrease morbidity associated with treatment and/or improve quality of life. Some screening efforts now focus on identifying and treating precursor lesions to prevent malignancy.

Key criteria for screening

Cancer screening is most effective and efficient if performed for diseases with high prevalence and significant population impact. The *sojourn time* is the period in which an occult tumor can be detected by screening before metastasis or the onset of symptoms.[2] For successful screening, the sojourn time should be sufficiently long to allow periodic screening to detect cancer in the target population before disease has spread; treatment of disease should have greater benefit when given before compared to after symptom onset; and the screening test should meet acceptable levels of accuracy and cost.[1]

Evaluation of early detection programs

Evaluation of a screening test should assess whether the test finds cancer, truly increases survival time, and whether subjects have a lower risk of dying from the disease as a result of screening. Evaluations of screening tests outside the context of a rigorous research design are subject to many biases that can invalidate the conclusions drawn.

Potential biases in the evaluation of screening

Lead-time bias: The time from an occult condition being detected by screening and the moment that condition would have become known through development of symptoms is known as the *lead time*. There is always a bias toward better survival in a screened group because screening moves the point of diagnosis earlier. True lead time bias occurs when earlier detection only advances the time of a patient's diagnosis, without prolonging life (Figure 1). Because of the effect of lead-time bias, an increase in survival or improved 5-year survival rates cannot be used alone to assess a screening test.

Length bias is the bias toward detection of less-threatening cancers (Figure 2). Cancers that grow more slowly and have a long sojourn time are more likely to be detected in screening. Faster growing, more aggressive, cancers with a short sojourn time are more apt to escape detection and be diagnosed due to symptoms in between scheduled screens. A cohort of cancer patients with screen-detected tumors will have a higher proportion of slow growing tumors compared to a population diagnosed without screening, and thus will appear to have better survival.

Overdiagnosis is the concept that some tumors fulfill all histologic criteria of malignancy, but are not destined to cause death and would not have become known to the patient without screening (Figure 3).[3] Overdiagnosis is an extreme example of length bias. There are two kinds of overdiagnosis. First is the disease that histologically is indistinguishable from precancer or cancer but has no biological propensity to progress.[4] This is common among screen-detected premalignant lesions of the uterine cervix and cancers of the prostate and thyroid.[5] Second are tumors that can be lethal, but not in the specific patient because she/he would have died from another cause during the sojourn time.[4] A persistently higher incidence rate within a population can be due to lead-time or the introduction of unscreened cohorts into a screening program and overdiagnosis.

Selection bias is the concept that individuals who participate in screening may differ from those who do not, that is, they may be more health conscious, more likely to control risk factors, more disease aware, more adherent to treatment, and generally live healthier lives.[6] Selection bias can give the appearance of better screening outcomes than expected and may even limit the

Holland-Frei Cancer Medicine, Ninth Edition. Edited by Robert C. Bast Jr., Carlo M. Croce, William N. Hait, Waun Ki Hong, Donald W. Kufe, Martine Piccart-Gebhart, Raphael E. Pollock, Ralph R. Weichselbaum, Hongyang Wang, and James F. Holland.
© 2017 John Wiley & Sons, Inc. ISBN: 978-1-118-93469-2

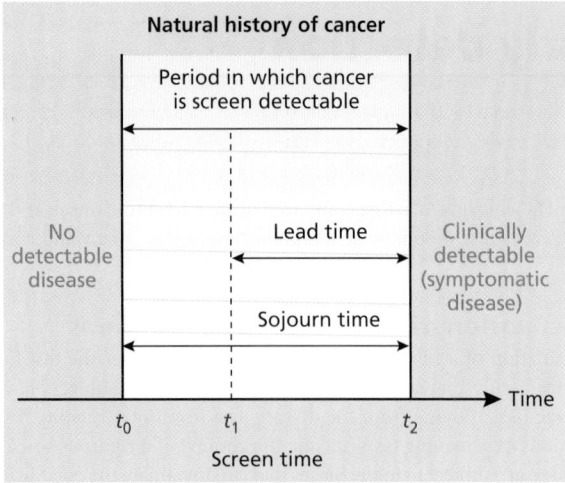

Figure 1 The natural history of cancer. In this figure, $t_2 - t_0$ is the duration of the preclinical screen-detectable period, known as the "sojourn time"; $t_2 - t_1$ is the amount of time by which the diagnosis is advanced by screening, known as the "lead time." Under the assumption of an exponential distribution of sojourn time, the expected lead time of an individual screen-detected case is equal to the mean of the distribution of the sojourn time.

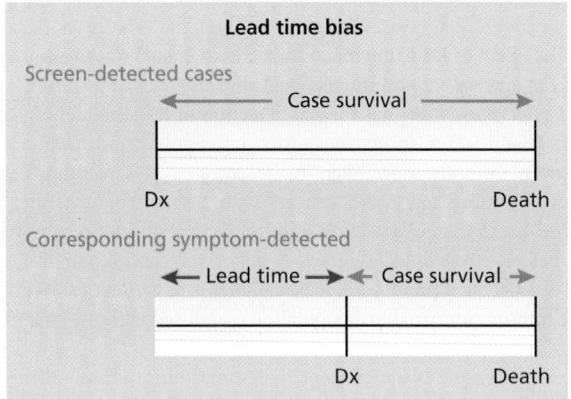

Figure 2 Lead-time bias. In this figure, Dx is the time of diagnosis. Note that the screen-detected cases and the cases diagnosed with symptoms each die at the same time, but the survival time looks greater in the screen-detected case because of lead-time bias.

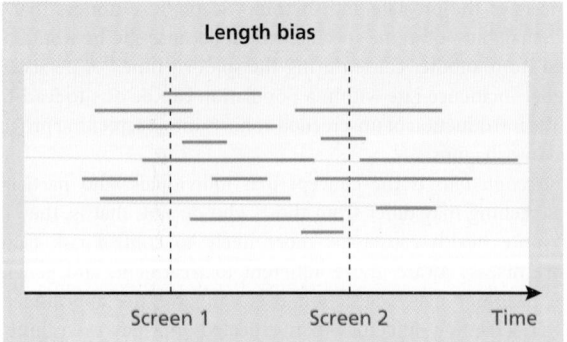

Figure 3 Length bias. In this figure, the horizontal lines represent the sojourn times of individual tumors detected in a screening program. The two screening examinations detect six out of eight long sojourn time tumors, but only two out of six short sojourn time tumors.

Table 1 Measures of screening performance.

	Disease	Status
Screening test results	Yes	No
Positive	a	b
Negative	c	d

Sensitivity = $a/(a + c)$; specificity = $d/(b + d)$; positive predictive value (PPV) = $a/(a + b)$; negative predictive value (NPV) = $c/(c + d)$.

generalizability of results of studies designed to overcome the influence of selection bias. For example, current and former smokers who entered the National Lung Screening Trial (NLST) had substantially less emphysema, cardiac disease, and diabetes compared to a representative sample of Americans.[6]

A unique form of selection bias can occur in a randomized trial in which subjects in the intervention arm are consented, while those in the control arm are not aware they are being followed in the study. Less-healthy individuals in the intervention arm may refuse participation, while those in the control arm cannot.[7]

Characteristics of a screening test

Sensitivity and Specificity: Sensitivity or the positive rate is the probability of a positive result when applied to a person who truly has the disease. Specificity or the true negative rate is the probability of a negative result in a person who does not have the disease (Table 1). Both high sensitivity and high specificity are desirable in a screening test. Unfortunately, they tend to be negatively correlated. While tests with high sensitivity succeed at detecting most occult disease, a test with low specificity will lead to many false positives and additional workup.

Positive and negative predictive values: The positive predictive value (PPV) is the probability that a subject with a positive screening result actually has the disease (Table 1). The negative predictive value (NPV) is the probability that a subject who screens negative is truly free of disease and provides some quantification of the reassurance value of a negative test. It is arguably more important to have a high NPV, as this will mean that few disease subjects are missed and potentially have delayed diagnosis and treatment.

Efficacy versus effectiveness: Screening studies usually assess the *efficacy* of an intervention, that is, whether the test saves lives among the population enrolled in the trial. An additional question is the *effectiveness* of the intervention when it is widely used. A few large clinical trials come close to assessing effectiveness, although these studies may be influenced by healthy volunteer effects due to the consent process.[1] Ultimately, the effectiveness of a screening intervention should be assessed through program evaluation in "real-world" situations rather than experimental studies, in order to consider factors such as provider experience, improvements in screening technology over time, acceptability to the population, and cost effectiveness.

Research designs to evaluate a screening intervention

Descriptive studies are the easiest screening studies to perform and often provide the first evidence that screening may contribute to disease control. These are uncontrolled observations based on the experience of physicians, clinics, or cancer registries. Descriptive studies can yield useful information, but provide the weakest evidence owing to inherent biases and cannot establish efficacy because of the absence of a control group.

Case–control studies are typically retrospective studies comparing a group of patients (cases) who have an outcome of interest (disease, death, interval cancer, etc.) with a group of patients (controls) who do not, in order to examine factors that may have contributed to the outcome.[8] Cases and controls are matched for key characteristics, such as age, gender, and socioeconomic status. Case–control studies are generally inexpensive and provide evidence more quickly than prospective studies.[8] These studies are challenging owing to the need to avoid biases, and results can be easily confounded by uncontrolled factors.

Prospective randomized clinical trials (RCTs) are the most rigorous assessment of screening, in that they typically compare disease-specific mortality in a group randomized to receive a screening invitation with a group that receives usual care. The distorting effects of self-selection and other biases are minimized through randomization. The mortality endpoint is not subject to the effects of lead-time, length bias, or overdiagnosis. RCTs should be analyzed by intention-to-treat (ITT), meaning end results are based on comparisons between invited and uninvited groups rather than screened and unscreened groups. Analysis that includes only those who are screened interjects bias.

The large sample size required, the expense, and the long duration has limited the number of prospective RCTs conducted. Some have argued that all-cause mortality is preferred to disease-specific mortality as the primary endpoint, as it avoids potential biases in allocation of cause of death and avoids failure to measure other causes of death that may be an outcome of diagnostic and treatment interventions. The greater size and cost of an RCT measuring all-cause mortality makes them highly impractical.[9]

A number of medical and professional organizations review the scientific literature and develop screening recommendations or guidelines.[5] The US Preventive Services Task Force (USPSTF) is known for using a very conservative process designed to minimize the influence of conflicts of interest, financial, intellectual, and emotional.[10] These recommendations are available at www.uspreventiveservicestaskforce.org. The American Cancer Society (ACS) also publishes guidelines (Table 2). A number of medical specialty societies publish guidelines or screening recommendations for specific their disease.

Organized versus opportunistic screening: Screening can be offered in a regimented program in which subjects are tracked for compliance with screening recommendations and quality of screening is measured through systematic audit. This is how screening is done in many European countries. In the United States, most screening is opportunistic, with limited tracking of compliance or quality. Some American mammography facilities do meet high world-class standards. In the United States and Europe, there are very few broad standards for screening in other diseases.

Breast cancer screening

Among women worldwide, breast cancer is the most commonly diagnosed cancer and the leading cause of cancer death. In the United States, the median age at diagnosis is 61, and the median age of death is 68.[11]

Screening methods for breast cancer

Mammography is an X-ray examination of the breasts that produces high-quality craniocaudal (CC) and mediolateral oblique (MLO) images of each breast with minimum X-ray dose. Evidence suggests that digital imaging allows for more accurate interpretation, improved diagnosis in women with dense breasts, and equivalence to traditional film mammography for postmenopausal women.[12]

The rate of abnormal interpretations is higher for first screening (5–10%) than for later mammograms. Most abnormalities are resolved through additional imaging with other mammographic views or by ultrasonography. Abnormalities that cannot be resolved are biopsied with ultrasonographic or radiographically directed fine needle aspiration, core needle biopsy, or surgical excision.

Nine RCTs of breast cancer screening have been published to date (Table 3). The trials vary in the age range of women enrolled, the screening tests used [mammography alone or with clinical breast examination (CBE)], the screening intervals, and even the years of follow-up. All RCTs were started and most completed before the modern era of adjuvant chemotherapy, and several before the advent of hormonal therapy. Screening and diagnostic equipment have also improved.[13] Experts try to take these limitations and flaws into account by considering nonrandomized studies and mathematical models.[14,15] There is consensus that a well-run screening program has the potential to reduce risk of breast cancer-specific death.[8]

There has been tremendous debate about whether screening of normal risk women should begin at age 40 or 50.[13] The dispute is based largely on the lack of clear evidence from RCTs that mammography screening for women aged 40–49 years is effective. Some studies show a statistically significant advantage to screening women in their forties and others do not.[16] The most recent RCT is the AGE Study, in which some patients may have received modern adjuvant therapy.[17] In all, 53,884 women aged 39–41 years were invited to screening. The control group was unaware of their participation and received "usual medical care." With 10.7 years of follow-up, there was a statistically nonsignificant 17% lower relative risk of breast cancer death in the screening versus control group (RR = 0.83, 0.66–1.04).[17]

The USPSTF meta-analysis of large RCTs (Table 4), including AGE, concluded a 15% relative risk reduction in mortality (RR = 0.85, 95% CI, 0.75–0.96) for women aged 40–49 invited to 2–9 rounds of screening after 11–20 years of follow-up.[18] This translates into 1904 women being invited to screening to prevent or delay one breast cancer death.[19] More than half of these women are estimated to have a false-positive scan during the 10 years of screening. Changing the screening interval to every 2 years marginally decreases the number of lives saved while nearly halving the false positive rate.[20]

The higher prevalence of mammographic density among women in their forties compared to their fifties complicates interpretation of mammogram in the younger group. Studies show that the accuracy, sensitivity, and specificity of a given mammogram vary by radiologist, but in general improve with increasing patient age.[21,22] Among women screened regularly, interval cancers are more prevalent in women aged 40–49 years.[23]

CBE and breast self-examination (BSE): A competent CBE involves physical palpation of the breast by a trained healthcare provider in small segments, from the nipple to the periphery of the breast, including the axilla.[24] In some settings (especially in developing countries), this may be the only method of breast cancer screening available.[18]

No RCT has adequately evaluated CBE as a single screening modality. A small proportion of palpable masses are not seen on mammography, leading to screening guidelines that include routine CBE, ideally just before mammography. Some data suggest that CBE contributes very little in a setting of high adherence with regularly scheduled high-quality mammography.[18]

BSE has appeal as a screening test because it is simple, convenient, and noninvasive. The "monthly BSE" was once widely advocated.[25] However, two prospective RCTs have reported a lack

Table 2 American Cancer Society screening guidelines for the early detection of cancer in average-risk asymptomatic people.

Cancer site population test or procedure frequency			
Breast	Women, ages 40–44	Mammography	All women should become familiar with the potential benefits, limitations, and harms associated with breast cancer screening. Women should have the opportunity to begin annual mammographic screening between the ages of 40 and 44 years
	Women, ages 45–54	Mammography	Women with an average risk of breast cancer should undergo annual screening mammography starting at age 45 years
	Women, ages 55+	Mammography	Women who are 55 years and older should be screened every 2 years but may choose to continue annual screening
Mammography			
Cervix	Women, ages 21–65	Pap test & HPV DNA test	Cervical cancer screening should begin at age 21. For women ages 21–29, screening should be done every 3 years with conventional or liquid-based Pap tests. For women ages 30–65, screening should be done every 5 years with both the HPV test and the Pap test (preferred), or every 3 years with the Pap test alone (acceptable). Women ages 65+ who have had ≥3 consecutive negative Pap tests or ≥2 consecutive negative HPV and Pap tests within the past 10 years, with the most recent test occurring within 5 years, and women who have had a total hysterectomy should stop cervical cancer screening. Women should not be screened annually by any method at any age
Colorectal	Men and women, ages 50+	Fecal occult blood test (FOBT) with at least 50% test sensitivity for cancer, or fecal immunochemical test (FIT) with at least 50% test sensitivity for cancer, *or*	Annual, starting at age 50. Testing at home with adherence to manufacturer's recommendation for collection techniques and number of samples is recommended. FOBT with the single stool sample collected on the clinician's fingertip during a digital rectal examination is not recommended. Guaiac-based toilet bowl FOBT tests also are not recommended. In comparison with guaiac-based tests for the detection of occult blood, immunochemical tests are more patient-friendly, and are likely to be equal or better in sensitivity and specificity. There is no justification for repeating FOBT in response to an initial positive finding
		Stool DNA test, *or*	Every 3 years, starting at age 50
		Flexible sigmoidoscopy (FSIG), *or*	Every 5 years, starting at age 50. FSIG can be performed alone, or consideration can be given to combining FSIG performed every 5 years with a highly sensitive gFOBT or FIT performed annually
		Double-contrast barium enema (DCBE), *or*	Every 5 years, starting at age 50
		Colonoscopy	Every 10 years, starting at age 50
		CT colonography	Every 5 years, starting at age 50
Endometrial	Women, at menopause		At the time of menopause, women at average risk should be informed about risks and symptoms of endometrial cancer and strongly encouraged to report any unexpected bleeding or spotting to their physicians
Lung	Current or former smokers aged 55–74 in good health with at least a 30 pack-year history	Low-dose helical CT (LDCT)	Clinicians with access to high-volume, high-quality lung cancer screening and treatment centers should initiate a discussion about lung cancer screening with apparently healthy patients aged 55–74 who have at least a 30 pack-year smoking history, and who currently smoke or have quit within the past 15 years. A process of informed and shared decision making with a clinician related to the potential benefits, limitations, and harms associated with screening for lung cancer with LDCT should occur before any decision is made to initiate lung cancer screening. Smoking cessation counseling remains a high priority for clinical attention in discussions with current smokers, who should be informed of their continuing risk of lung cancer. Screening should not be viewed as an alternative to smoking cessation
Prostate	Men, ages 50+	Digital rectal examination (DRE) and prostate-specific antigen test (PSA)	Men who have at least a 10-year life expectancy should have an opportunity to make an informed decision with their health care provider about whether to be screened for prostate cancer, after receiving information about the potential benefits, risks, and uncertainties associated with prostate cancer screening. Prostate cancer screening should not occur without an informed decision-making process
Cancer-related checkup	Men and women, ages 20+		On the occasion of a periodic health examination, the cancer-related checkup should include examination for cancers of the thyroid, testicles, ovaries, lymph nodes, oral cavity, and skin, as well as health counseling about tobacco, sun exposure, diet and nutrition, risk factors, sexual practices, and environmental and occupational exposures

Table 3 Breast cancer screening randomized trials.

Study	Randomization	Sample size	Intervention	Follow up	Finding
Health Insurance Plan, United States 1963[a]	Individual	60,565–60,857	MMG and CBE for 3 years	18 years	RR 0.77 (0.61–0.97)
Malmo, Sweden 1976[b,c]	Individual	42,283	Two-view MMG every 18–24 months × 5	12 years	RR 0.81 (95% CI, 0.62–1.07)
Ostergotland (County E of Two-County Trial) Sweden 1977[d,e]	Geographic cluster	38,405–39,034 study / 37,145–37,936 control	Three single-view MMG / Every 2 years women-50 / Every 33 months women 50+	12 years	RR 0.82 (95% CI, 0.64–1.05) Ostergotland
Kopparberg (County W of Two-County Trial) Sweden 1977[d,e]	Geographic cluster	38,562–39,051 intervention / 18,478–18,846 control	Three single-view MMG / Every 2 years women-50 / Every 33 months women 50+	12 years	RR 0.68 (95% CI, 0.52–0.89)
Edinburgh, United Kingdom[f]	Cluster by physician practice	23,266 study / 21,904 control	Initially, two-view MMG and CBE / Then annual CBE with single-view MMG years 3, 5, and 7	10 years	RR 0.84 (95% CI, 0.63–1.12)
NBSS-1, Canada 1980[g]	Individual	25,214 study (100% screened after entry CBE) / 25,216 control	Annual two-view MMG and CBE for 4–5 years	13 years	RR 0.97 (95% CI, 0.74–1.27)
NBSS-2, Canada 1980[h]	Individual	19,711 study (100% screened after entry CBE) / 19,694 control	Annual two-view MMG and CBE	11–16 years (mean 13 years)	RR 1.02 (95% CI, 0.78–1.33)
Stockholm, Sweden 1981[i]	Cluster by birth date	Declined from 40,318 to 38,525 intervention group / Rose from 19,943 to 20,978 control group	Single view MMG every 28 months × 2	8 years	RR 0.80 (95% CI, 0.53–1.22)
Gothenberg, Sweden 1982[j]	Complex	21,650 invited / 29,961 control	Initial two-view MMG. Then single-view MMG every 18 months × 4. Single read first three rounds, then double-read	12–14 years	RR 0.79 (95% CI, 0.58–1.08)
AGE Trial[k]	Individuals	160,921 (53,884 invited; 106,956 not invited)	Invited group aged 48 and younger offered annual screening by MMG (double-view first screen, then single mediolateral oblique view thereafter); 68% accepted screening on the first screen an 69% and 70% were reinvited (81% attended at least one screen).	10.7 years	RR 0.83 (95% CI, 0.66–1.04)

a Shapiro S, Venet W, Strax P, Venet L, Roeser R. Ten- to fourteen-year effect of screening on breast cancer mortality. J Natl Cancer Inst 1982;69:349–55.

b Andersson I, Aspegren K, Janzon L, et al. Mammographic screening and mortality from breast cancer: the Malmo mammographic screening trial. Bmj 1988;297:943–8.

c Nystrom L, Andersson I, Bjurstam N, Frisell J, Nordenskjold B, Rutqvist LE. Long-term effects of mammography screening: updated overview of the Swedish randomised trials. Lancet 2002;359:909–19.

d Tabar L, Fagerberg G, Duffy SW, Day NE, Gad A, Grontoft O. Update of the Swedish two-county program of mammographic screening for breast cancer. Radiologic clinics of North America 1992;30:187–210.

e Tabar L, Fagerberg G, Duffy SW, Day NE. The Swedish two county trial of mammographic screening for breast cancer: recent results and calculation of benefit. Journal of epidemiology and community health 1989;43:107–14.

f Roberts MM, Alexander FE, Anderson TJ, et al. Edinburgh trial of screening for breast cancer: mortality at seven years. Lancet 1990;335:241–6.

g Miller AB, To T, Baines CJ, Wall C. The Canadian National Breast Screening Study-1: breast cancer mortality after 11 to 16 years of follow-up. A randomized screening trial of mammography in women age 40 to 49 years. Ann Intern Med 2002;137:305–12.

h Miller AB, Baines CJ, To T, Wall C. Canadian National Breast Screening Study: 2. Breast cancer detection and death rates among women aged 50 to 59 years. CMAJ : Canadian Medical Association journal = journal de l'Association medicale canadienne 1992;147:1477–88.

i Frisell J, Eklund G, Hellstrom L, Lidbrink E, Rutqvist LE, Somell A. Randomized study of mammography screening—preliminary report on mortality in the Stockholm trial. Breast Cancer Res Treat 1991;18:49–56.

j Bjurstam N, Bjorneld L, Warwick J, et al. The Gothenburg Breast Screening Trial. Cancer 2003;97:2387–96.

k Moss SM, Cuckle H, Evans A, et al. Effect of mammographic screening from age 40 years on breast cancer mortality at 10 years' follow-up: a randomised controlled trial. Lancet 2006;368:2053–60.

Table 4 Pooled RRs for breast cancer mortality from mammography screening trials for all ages.

Age (years)	Trials included, n	RR for breast cancer mortality (95% CrI)	NNI to prevent 1 breast cancer death (95% CrI)
39–49	8[a]	0.85 (0.75–0.96)	1904 (929–6378)
50–59	6[b]	0.86 (0.75–0.99)	1339 (322–7455)
60–69	2[c]	0.68 (0.54–0.87)	377 (230–1050)
70–74	1[d]	1.12 (0.73–1.72)	Not available

CrI, credible interval; NNI, number needed to invite to screening; RR, relative risk.

[a]Health Insurance Plan of Greater New York,[f] Canadian National Breast Screening Study-1,[g] Stockholm,[e] Malmö,[e] Swedish Two-County trial (two trials),[e,j] Gothenburg trial,[i] and Age trial.[h]

[b]Canadian National Breast Screening Study-1,[g] Stockholm,[e] Malmö,[e] Swedish Two-County trial (2 trials),[1,31] and Gothenburg trial.[i]

[c]Malmö[e] and Swedish Two-County trial (Östergötland).[e]

[d]Swedish Two-County trial (Östergötland).[e]

[e]Nyström L, Andersson I, Bjurstam N, Frisell J, Nordenskjöld B, Rutqvist LE. Long-term effects of mammography screening: updated overview of the Swedish randomised trials. *Lancet* 2002;359:909–19.

[f]Habbema JD, van Oortmarssen GJ, van Putten DJ, Lubbe JT, van der Maas PJ. Age-specific reduction in breast cancer mortality by screening: an analysis of the results of the Health Insurance Plan of Greater New York study. *J Natl Cancer Inst*. 1986;77:317–20.

[g]Miller AB, To T, Baines CJ, Wall C. The Canadian National Breast Screening Study-1: breast cancer mortality after 11 to 16 years of follow-up. A randomized screening trial of mammography in women age 40 to 49 years. *Ann Intern Med* 2002;137:305–12.

[h]Moss SM, Cuckle H, Evans A, Johns L, Waller M, Bobrow L; Trial Management Group. Effect of mammographic screening from age 40 years on breast cancer mortality at 10 years' follow-up: a randomised controlled trial. *Lancet* 2006;368:2053–60.

[i]Bjurstam N, Björneld L, Warwick J, Sala E, Duffy SW, Nyström L, et al. The Gothenburg Breast Screening Trial. *Cancer* 2003;97:2387–96.

[j]Tabar L, Fagerberg G, Chen HH, Duffy SW, Smart CR, Gad A, et al. Efficacy of breast cancer screening by age. New results from the Swedish Two-County Trial. *Cancer*. 1995;75:2507–17.

Source: Taken from **The Breast Cancer Evidence Review: An Update for the U.S. Preventive Services Task Force.** *Heidi D. Nelson, MD, MPH; Kari Tyne, MD; Arpana Naik, MD; Christina Bougatsos, BS; Benjamin K. Chan, MS; and Linda Humphrey, MD, MPH.* www.uspreventiveservicestaskforce.org/Page/SupportingDoc/breast-cancer-screening/final-evidence-summary9.

of evidence of efficacy and even some evidence of harm, although both studies have some methodological issues.[26,27] Monthly BSE promotion distracts from the importance of mammography, can provide false reassurance, can heighten anxiety about breast cancer, and create false positives. Today, no professional organization in the United States or Europe encourages monthly BSE, instead advocating "breast awareness" and consulting a healthcare provider if a possible abnormality is found.[25,28]

Evaluation of the effectiveness of screening

While the RCTs of breast cancer screening suggest a benefit, estimating the effectiveness of routine screening programs in the community is not straightforward. The United States has had a 35% decline in age-adjusted mortality from 1989 to 2011. Mathematical modeling estimates that screening and improvements in breast cancer therapy, especially hormonal therapy, are each responsible for about half of the mortality decline.[29]

The harms of breast cancer screening

Every screening test has some associated harms. Slightly more than half of women screened in a 10-year period will have a false positive requiring at least additional imaging.[30,31] Surveys show about a quarter of these women still suffered distress and anxiety 3 months after cancer was ruled out.[32] False negatives lead to a false sense of security. Overdiagnosis estimates in breast cancer screening range from 0% to 54% of cancers diagnosed with the aid of mammography, with most estimates suggesting overdiagnosis is 10–30%.[14,33]

Mammography screening has also caused a dramatic rise in the diagnosis of ductal carcinoma *in situ* (DCIS). Previously a rare, incidental finding after mastectomy, there are now >70,000 cases diagnosed annually in the US Study which has yet to show that early detection and treatment of DCIS reduces mortality. It is believed that most DCIS lesions do not progress to invasive cancer,[15,34] and there is increasing interest in its overtreatment.[35] Renaming DCIS has been suggested to remove the word carcinoma.[36] In the future, genomic medicine may allow us to distinguish the tumors (in situ and true cancer) that need aggressive therapy from those that should be observed.

New technologies

Digital breast tomosynthesis (DBT) and 3D mammography are newer technologies that appear to offer increased sensitivity and a reduction in recall rates.[37]

Magnetic resonance imaging (MRI) is more sensitive but less specific than mammography in detecting breast cancer.[38] Initial MRI is associated with a very high number of false positive results, which is reduced with subsequent studies. MRI has found a niche in screening women with significant breast density and women who may be at elevated risk due to mutations in breast cancer susceptibility genes.

Ultrasound imaging has been used for many years as a diagnostic. The limitations of mammography in screening the dense breast have led to ongoing interest in using ultrasound for primary screening or as an adjunct to mammography.[39,40]

In 2003, the American College of Radiology Imaging Network (ACRIN) initiated a multicenter trial in women at increased risk for breast cancer due to family history and significant breast density.[41,42] The breast cancer detection rate was increased by 4.2 cancers per 1000 women screened with mammography and ultrasound versus mammography alone (11.8 vs 7.6 per 1000). However, the false-positive and negative biopsy rates were also very high. While a significant improvement was seen in the diagnostic yield of small, node-negative cancers in this higher-risk population, it is unclear that it will save additional lives and questions remain about the potential for screening ultrasound.[40] Routine ultrasound screening is not advocated at this time.

An interesting technology that is gaining use is 3D automated breast ultrasound. It offers more standardized imaging compared to conventional ultrasound and can be performed by a technologist instead of a radiologist. It is still used as a diagnostic, but there is interest in using it as an initial screening test with mammography and CBE.

Screening recommendations

As of 2015, the ACS guideline recommends that all women become familiar with the potential benefits, limitations, and harms associated with breast cancer screening. Women with an average risk of breast cancer should undergo regular screening mammography starting at age 45 years. Women who are aged 45–54 years should be screened annually. Women who are 55 years and older should be screened every 2 years but may choose to continue annual screening. Women should have the opportunity to begin annual screening between the ages of 40 and 44 years. Women should continue screening as long as their overall health is good and they have a life expectancy of 10 years or more. Beginning in 2015, the ACS does not recommend clinical breast examination for breast cancer screening among women at any age with an average risk of breast cancer. The ACS guideline applies to women who have access to mammographic screening.

The 2009 USPSTF recommendation is women aged 50–75 years have a mammogram every 1–2 years.[43] USPTF did not recommend CBE, citing the lack of study to show it beneficial. The Task Force recommends against "routine" mammographic screening for women aged 40–49 years, instead advising this decision be made following physician–patient discussion including individual risks and concerns.

As of December 2014, the USPSTF, the American College of Physicians, and the Canadian Task Force on the Periodic Health Examination recommend routine screening beginning at age 50.[44] An advisory committee on cancer prevention in the European Union recommends that screening be offered to women aged 50–69 years in an organized screening program.[45]

On the basis of the accumulation of data, but no RCTs, the ACS now recommends that women at very high risk of breast cancer begin annual mammography and MRI at age 30, or perhaps earlier if she and her physician believe it is prudent.[38] It is impossible to perform a prospective RCT in this population. High risk is defined as having a known mutation of *BRCA1* or *BRCA2*, 20–25% or greater lifetime risk based on family history, a high-risk genetic syndrome, such as Li-Fraumeni syndrome or Cowden disease, or having received high-dose mantle radiation to the chest.[22]

Colorectal cancer

Worldwide, colorectal cancer is the third most commonly diagnosed cancer in men and the second in women and accounts for 8% of all deaths. In the United States, colorectal cancer is the third most commonly diagnosed cancer and the third leading cause of cancer death among men and women. While most cases are diagnosed among individuals aged 60–80 years, there is increasing concern about colorectal cancer in those aged 40–50 years.[11]

The goal of colorectal screening is both the detection of early-stage adenocarcinomas and the detection and removal of adenomatous polyps, given the significant evidence that adenomatous polyps are precancerous lesions. Colorectal polyps are common in adults over age 50. One-half to two-thirds of all colorectal polyps are adenomatous, which can progress to cancer, although the majority never will. It is estimated that it takes 10 years for an adenomatous polyp <1 cm to become an invasive lesion.[46] Other polyps, including incidental hyperplastic polyps and mucosal tags, are not significant in the development of colorectal cancer.[47]

Screening methods for colorectal cancer

Evidence suggests that a number of tests, applied in a program of regular surveillance, have the potential to reduce deaths from colorectal cancer. They include:

1. *Fecal occult blood tests (FOBTs)* aim to discover occult blood in stool, which is often caused by polyps (especially >2 cm). Common FOBTs include *guaiac-based tests (gFOBTs)* and *fecal immunochemical tests (FITs)*.

   The *gFOBT* detects blood in the stool through the pseudoperoxidase activity of heme. This test requires diet modification, as it can react positively with red meat, cruciferous vegetables, and some fruits. Rehydration of gFOBT not only improves sensitivity but also increases the false-positive rate.[48] The gFOBT can be done in the physician office but it is preferred that patients collect the specimen at home for processing in a laboratory. Any positive stool blood test requires follow-up diagnostic colonoscopy.

   Limitations of gFOBT have led to a decrease in usage but some high-sensitivity tests are still available. The gFOBT performed with stool collected during a digital rectal examination (DRE) is not recommended.

   The *FIT* reacts to human globin. FIT is not reactive to diet as gFOBT is, and will not react to digested human blood from upper gastrointestinal bleeding. The fecal hemoglobin threshold can be set to balance sensitivity and specificity based on individual risk or programmatic requirements. FITs are usually processed in a laboratory. Sensitivity declines with delay in sample processing. Even a 5-day delay is significant.[49]

   In 1000 ambulatory patients (with and without symptoms of colorectal cancer), the sensitivity for cancer with three FIT samples with a hemoglobin threshold of 75 ng/mL was 94.1%, and specificity was 87.5%. In a screening study with one FIT evaluation of stool followed by colonoscopy, FIT had higher sensitivity for detection of advanced neoplasms in patients taking low dose aspirin compared to those not taking aspirin. There was a minor decrease in specificity.[50]

   In a systematic review of gFOBT and FIT, there was no clear evidence for superiority of either test.[51] Bleeding from cancers or large polyps may be intermittent. Generally, FIT requires two tests over a week or so and gFOBT requires three. In practice, FIT is replacing gFOBT.

2. *Stool DNA (sDNA)* testing detects relatively well-defined DNA markers associated with colorectal neoplasia in cells exfoliated by colorectal polyps and malignancies into the colonic lumen. Available sDNA tests focus on >21 separate point mutations in the K-*RAS* oncogene, a probe for BAT-26 (a marker of microsatellite instability), and a marker of DNA integrity analysis (DIA) to achieve high sensitivity.[52] As with stool blood testing, any positive stool blood or DNA test must be followed up with colonoscopy to rule out the presence of polyps or cancer.

3. *Flexible sigmoidoscopy (FSIG)* with a 60 cm scope is a relatively simple procedure, requires minimal preparation, and allows for examination of about half of the average colon.[53] Generally, the test is performed without sedation. The presence of polyps in the distal bowel signals an elevated risk for polyps or cancer in the proximal bowel. If FSIG is positive, the patient is referred for colonoscopy.

   Quality indicators for FSIG have been published and emphasize appropriate training, satisfactory examination rates to >40 cm, expected adenoma detection rates based on age and gender, and ability to biopsy suspected adenomas.

4. *Barium enema* is an X-ray examination of the bowel that derives contrast from barium (single-contrast study) or the combination of barium and instilled air (double-contrast barium enema study, DCBE). DCBE is more sensitive than single-contrast study for both malignancies and polyps. If the patient has a positive test, the next step is a colonoscopy.[54]

Evidence for the efficacy of DCBE is largely indirect, based on its performance in detecting small malignant lesions and polyps and on the known benefits of early detection and polypectomy for reducing mortality. The proportion of examinations in which adenomatous polyps identified by colonoscopy were also detected by DCBE was significantly influenced by lesion size. Among all currently recommended screening tests, barium enema is the least utilized.

5. *Colonoscopy* has a unique advantage among colorectal cancer screening tests in that direct visualization of the entire bowel is possible, with >90% of examinations terminating at the cecum, and clinically significant adenomas can be identified and removed during the examination.[24,55] Colonoscopy is done in an outpatient setting predominantly. While conscious sedation is standard, some patients receive general anesthesia. Proper bowel preparation is critical to ensure that the bowel is clean.

The examination is more complicated than sigmoidoscopy with higher risk of complications due mostly to sedation, biopsy, or polypectomy. Blood loss can be seen with polyps of any size but is more common when removing large polyps or polyps in the proximal colon. Risk of bowel perforation increases with age and is higher in individuals with diverticular disease. Perforation occurs in about 1 in 500 Medicare beneficiaries and 1 in 1000 patients overall.

In 1256 adults rescreened about 5 years after a negative colonoscopy, no cancers were detected, but 201 (16%) adults had one or more adenomas, of which 16 were advanced.[56] The findings support the conclusion that the 5-year risk of colorectal cancer is extremely low among those with a normal colonoscopy.

In a study of 35,000 asymptomatic patients in Manitoba who had undergone negative colonoscopy and were followed for 10 years, reductions in the expected colorectal cancer incidence of 45% at 5 years and 72% at 10 years were observed.[57] These findings suggest some detection failures during the initial apparently normal colonoscopy.

The long duration of reduced risk of colorectal cancer after colonoscopy depends on quality of the examination and complete removal of polyps. Quality assurance recommendations emphasize training and experience, proper risk assessment and documentation, complete examination to the cecum with adequate mucosal visualization and bowel preparation, ability to detect and remove polyps safely, documentation of polypoid lesions and removal, timely and appropriate management of adverse events, appropriate follow-up of histopathology findings, appropriate recommendation for surveillance or repeat screening based on published guidelines, and continuous assessment and evaluation of performance, with corrective action when necessary.

6. *CT colonography* or virtual colonoscopy is an imaging procedure that computationally combines multiple helical CT scans to create two- or three-dimensional images of the colon interior. These images can be rotated for different views and even combined for a complete, "virtual" view.[54]

Evaluations of CT colonography have typically involved CT examination followed by optical colonoscopy, with the colonoscopist blinded to the CT results. Although early results with 2D imaging were disappointing, recent back-to-back evaluations of CT colonography using faster scanners, updated 3D luminal displays, and oral stool tagging with digital subtraction have demonstrated sensitivities for large adenomas equivalent to colonoscopy. Using these advances, one study of back-to-back CT and optical colonoscopy in asymptomatic adults reported 94% sensitivity for large adenomas, with per-patient sensitivity for adenomas ≥6 mm of 89%.[58]

In a collaborative ACRIN/NCI trial,[59] CT colonography detected 90% of patients with large (≥10 mm) adenomas and cancers, with 86% specificity and 84% per-polyp sensitivity. Thirty large lesions were detected by CT colonography that were not detected by optical colonoscopy. Five of 18 lesions ≥10 mm were confirmed by colonoscopy as true positives. Although the sensitivity of CT colonography is lower for lesions ≤6 mm, generally, these lesions are regarded as clinically insignificant. For lesions of ≥1 cm in size, CT colonography has performance very similar to optical colonoscopy.[58]

CT colonography requires the same full bowel preparation and restricted diet as optical colonoscopy, and as an "imaging-only" evaluation, patients with polyps ≥6 mm in size must be referred to therapeutic colonoscopy and polypectomy.[59]

Colorectal screening trials

The initial evidence that colorectal screening saves lives was based on studies showing that gFOBT found lesions at earlier stages than cases diagnosed with symptoms. This led to prospective trials in Europe and the United States evaluating the efficacy of FOBT. In the Minnesota trial, 46,551 asymptomatic participants aged 50–80 years were randomized to invitation to annual screening, biennial screening, or usual care.[60] Participants with positive gFOBT received colonoscopy. The 13-year cumulative mortality was 5.33, 8.33, and 8.83 per 1000 in the annual screening, biennial screening, and usual care (control) groups, respectively. After 18 years of follow-up, both annual and biennial gFOBT were associated with a statistically significant reduction in deaths and with a 20% and 18% reduction in cancer incidence, respectively.[48] Cancer prevention was attributed to detection and removal of adenomatous polyps. Similar results with gFOBT every 2 years have been observed in two other trials.[61]

Sigmoidoscopy. In the early 1990s, two case–control studies evaluating the efficacy of screening sigmoidoscopy reported a 70% or more reduction in risk of colorectal cancer death.[62,63] Five sigmoidoscopy screening RCTs have reported incidence and mortality results. In meta-analysis, there was a 28% relative risk reduction in colorectal cancer mortality (RR = 0.72, 95% CI, 0.65–0.80). Incidence was reduced by 18% (RR = 0.82, 95% CI, 0.73–0.91). Left-sided cancer was reduced by 33% (RR = 0.67, 95% CI, 0.59–0.76).[64,65]

Combined stool blood testing and FSIG every 5 years is superior to FOBT or FSIG alone. FOBT provides some surveillance in the proximal colon (outside the reach of FSIG), and FSIG has higher sensitivity and specificity than FOBT in the distal colon. In an RCT in asymptomatic individuals aged ≥40 years, there were fewer colorectal cancer deaths in patients receiving annual FOBT and sigmoidoscopy than in those receiving sigmoidoscopy alone (0.36 vs 0.63 per 1000; P = 0.53) after 5–11 years of follow-up.[64] On the basis of modeling, USPSTF concluded that combining FSIG every 5 years with high-sensitivity FOBT every 3 years is approximately equivalent in terms of life years gained to colonoscopy every 10 years.[65]

Colonoscopy. No prospective RCTs with mortality endpoints have been conducted to evaluate whether colonoscopy screening prevents colorectal cancer death. That more than 40% of those receiving annual FOBT in the Minnesota trial ultimately received at least one colonoscopy is perhaps the strongest evidence of efficacy. In addition, several case–control studies suggest that screening with colonoscopy and polypectomy has significant impact on colorectal cancer incidence and by extension, mortality.[66,67]

Screening recommendations

As given in Table 2, the ACS recommendations for average-risk individuals include seven options for regular surveillance for colorectal cancer beginning at age 50,[68,69] including annual high-sensitivity FOBT (gFOBT or FIT); sDNA (interval unknown); FSIG every 5 years, annual high-sensitivity gFOBT or FIT and FSIG every 5 years after initial screening with both tests; total colonic examination with DCBE every 5 years; or total colonic examination with colonoscopy every 10 years. In reality, most adults who undergo screening have stool testing with gFOBT or FIT or colonoscopy. In clinics where endoscopists are experienced and perform complete examination on well-prepared patients with scope insertion >40 cm, a 10-year interval between screening FSIG may be justified. Annual DRE is no longer recommended, owing to low sensitivity, but DRE should be done before FSIG or colonoscopy. While there is strong consensus among US organizations about the value of colorectal cancer screening in adults ≥50 years of age, the USPSTF states that, currently, there is insufficient evidence to recommend for or against CT colonography or sDNA.

Guidelines for higher-risk individuals recommend earlier onset of surveillance and more thorough examinations of the colon (Table 5). Higher-risk individuals include those with family history of adenomatous polyps or colorectal cancer, FAP, or hereditary nonpolyposis colorectal cancer (HNPCC), or a history of inflamma.[70]

Cervical cancer

Cervical cancer is the third most commonly diagnosed cancer in women and fourth leading cause of cancer death worldwide,[11] and is still the leading cause of cancer death among women in some areas of Africa and Asia. A dramatic decline in mortality due to improvements in both treatment and early detection has occurred, particularly in the United States and western Europe, where the mortality rate in 1980 was >70% lower than in 1930.[71]

The improvement in early detection was due to the Pap test or smear, developed by Dr. George Papanicolaou in the 1920s. In many western countries, it gained widespread adoption in the late 1940s to 1950s.[72] The Pap test diagnoses early cancers and precursor lesions [dysplasia or cervical intraepithelial neoplasia (CIN)], for which a variety of treatment options are available. The diagnosis of treatable precursor lesions is considerably more common than the diagnosis of invasive disease, and screening has caused a drop in cervical cancer incidence far more dramatic than the decline in mortality.[73]

Screening and diagnostic methods

In many respects, the Pap test is extremely low tech.[69] It involves the collection of exfoliating epithelial cells from the cervical squamocolumnar junction or transformation zone. Both the ectocervix and endocervix are sampled. Two samples are applied to one side of a glass slide and quickly fixed to prevent air-drying. The slide is stained and examined under a microscope by a cytotechnologist. Although simple to conduct, its accuracy is highly dependent on obtaining a high-quality specimen, good slide preparation, expert microscopic examination, and interpretation.[69]

The Pap smear has a significant error rate. Sampling error is estimated to account for about two-thirds of false-negative tests and errors in interpretation for the remaining third. Pap smear screening is estimated to have specificity of 98% and sensitivity of 51%.[74] The NCI's Bethesda System (Table 6), released in 1988, provides " … a uniform format for cytopathology reports. It is

Table 5 Guidelines for screening and surveillance for early detection of colorectal polyps and cancer for individuals at greater than average risk.

Risk category and description	Recommendation	Age to begin	Screening interval and recommendation
Moderate risk			
People with single, small (<1 cm) adenomatous polyps	Colonoscopy	At the initial polyp diagnosis	TCE within 3 years after initial polyp removal; if normal, follow recommendations for average-risk individuals
People with large (≥1 cm) or multiple adenomatous polyps of any size	Colonoscopy	At time of initial polyp diagnosis	TCE within 3 years after initial polyp removal; if normal TCE every 5 years
Personal history of curative-intent resection of colorectal cancer	TCE[a]	Within 1 year after resection	If normal, TCE in 3 years; If second TCE is normal, TCE in 5 years
Colorectal cancer or adenomatous polyps, in first-degree relative younger than age 60 or in two or more first-degree relatives of any ages	TCE[a]	40 years, or 10 years before the youngest case in the family, whichever is earlier	Every 5 years
Colorectal cancer in other relatives (not first degree)	Follow recommendations for age-risk individuals	—	—
High risk			
Family history of FAP	Early surveillance with endoscopy, counseling to consider genetic testing, and referral for specialty care	Puberty	If genetic test is positive or polyposis is confirmed, consider colectomy; otherwise, continue endoscopy every 1–2 years
Family history of HNPCC	Colonoscopy and counseling to consider genetic testing	21 years	If untested, or if genetic test is positive, colonoscopy every 2 years until age 40; after age 40, colonoscopy every year
Inflammatory bowel disease	Colonoscopy with biopsies for dysplasia	8 years after the start of pancolitis; 12–15 years after the start of left-sided colitis	Colonoscopy every 1–2 years

Abbreviations: FAP, familial adenomatous polyposis; HNPCC, hereditary nonpolyposis colorectal cancer; TCE, total colon examination.
[a]TCE includes either colonoscopy, DCBE, or CT colonography. CT colonography or DCBE should be added to the colonoscopy examination in those instances when the entire colon cannot be visualized by colonoscopy.

Table 6 Bethesda System 2001.

Specimen type	Indicate conventional smear (Pap smear) versus liquid-based versus other
Specimen adequacy	
Satisfactory for evaluation	Describe presence or absence of endocervical/transformation zone component and any other quality indicators, for example, partially obscuring blood and inflammation
Unsatisfactory for evaluation	Specimen rejected/not processed (specify reason), or specimen processed and examined, but unsatisfactory for evaluation of epithelial abnormality because of (specify reason)
General categorization (optional)	Negative for intraepithelial lesion or malignancy
	Epithelial cell abnormality: see interpretation/result (specify "squamous" or "glandular" as appropriate)
	Other: see interpretation/result (e.g., endometrial cells in a woman >40 years of age)
Automated review	If case examined by automated device, specify device and result
Ancillary testing	Provide a brief description of the test methods and report the result so that it is easily understood by the clinician
Interpretation/result negative for intraepithelial lesion or malignancy	When there is no cellular evidence of neoplasia, state this in the general categorization above and/or in the interpretation/result section of the report, whether or not there are organisms or other non-neoplastic findings)
Organisms	Trichomonas vaginalis
	Fungal organisms morphologically consistent with Candida spp.
	Shift in flora suggestive of bacterial vaginosis
	Bacteria morphologically consistent with Actinomyces spp.
	Cellular changes consistent with herpes simplex virus
Other non-neoplastic findings	Reactive cellular changes associated with inflammation (includes typical repair) radiation intrauterine contraceptive device (IUD)
(Optional to report; list not inclusive)	Glandular cells status post hysterectomy
	Atrophy
Other	Endometrial cells (in a woman ≥ 40 years of age) (specify if "negative for squamous intraepithelial lesion")
Epithelial cell abnormalities	
Squamous cell	Atypical squamous cells of undetermined significance (ASC-US) cannot exclude HSIL (ASC-H)
	Low grade squamous intraepithelial lesion (LSIL) encompassing: HPV/mild dysplasia/CIN 1
	High grade squamous intraepithelial lesion (HSIL) encompassing: moderate and severe dysplasia, CIS/CIN 2 and CIN 3 with features suspicious for invasion (if invasion is suspected)
	Squamous cell carcinoma
Glandular cell	Atypical
	Endocervical cells (NOS or specify in comments)
	Endometrial cells (NOS or specify in comments)
	Glandular cells (NOS or specify in comments)
	Endocervical cells, favor neoplastic
	Glandular cells, favor neoplastic
	Endocervical adenocarcinoma in situ
	Adenocarcinoma
	Endocervical
	Endometrial
	Extrauterine
	Not otherwise specified
Other malignant neoplasms	Specify
Educational notes and suggestions (optional)	Suggestions should be concise and consistent with clinical follow-up guidelines published by professional organizations (references to relevant publications may be included)

intended to communicate clinically relevant information using standardized terminology."[75]

Clinical studies of efficacy

Screening with the Pap smear is comparatively inexpensive and is widely accepted, although no RCTs of its efficacy have been conducted. Perhaps the most widely cited evidence for its effect on mortality is the long-term decline in cervical cancer death rate in the United States coincident with the introduction of the Pap smear.[25] Death rates had begun to decline before widespread use of the test, owing to factors such as an increase in the hysterectomy rate and improved treatment of cervical cancer. However, the decline in incidence and mortality was so significant that improvements in treatment could not account for all of it. Furthermore, from the 1950s to 1970s, cervical cancer mortality remained comparatively unchanged in Norway, a late adapter to cervical screening, whereas it dropped by more than 70% in Iceland, an early adapter.[71] Numerous case–control studies also show a benefit from cervical cancer screening. The majority of American women diagnosed with cervical cancer today have no history of cervical screening in the 5 years before diagnosis; compelling evidence that screening reduces incidence.[76,77]

Precursor lesions usually take years to progress to cancer such that it is safe to screen normal risk women every 3 years.[78] Overdiagnosis and overtreatment is a significant concern as observational studies show that untreated lesions such as atypical squamous cells of undetermined significance (ASCUS) often regress.[79] Strategies of triage, observation, and repeat testing are being used to avoid overtreatment.[80]

New technologies

Liquid-based cytology uses specimen collection techniques similar to the conventional Pap smear. It is equally dependent on collecting an adequate sample, but the sample is suspended in a fixative solution, dispersed, filtered, and distributed on a glass slide to achieve a monolayer of cells. Computer-aided diagnosis of liquid-based cytology is common, and abnormal smears are reviewed by a cytotechnologist.[81]

Accuracy is increased because there are fewer artifacts (blood, mucus, etc.) and because cells are not overlapping. Studies have shown liquid-based cytology to have higher sensitivity in populations with lower prevalence of cytologic abnormalities.[81] Reviews applying rigorous evidence-based criteria found no significant advantage in sensitivity or specificity for liquid-based over conventional Pap testing. The number of inadequate specimens is considerably reduced, however, with liquid-based cytology.

There is a strong association between persistent infection with certain subtypes of human papilloma virus (HPV) and cervical cancer.[82] The ability to test for HPV DNA or HPV RNA has allowed for better diagnosis of cervical dysplasia. Increasingly, HPV testing is used as a cotest to triage women with abnormal cytologic tests [ASCUS and atypical glandular cells of undetermined significance (AGUS)]. There is also movement toward HPV screening tests replacing the Pap smear in women aged ≥30 years.[83] A prospective randomized trial in India demonstrated that HPV testing detects high grade cervical dysplasia and early cervical cancer and treatment leads to a decrease in mortality.[84] The US Food and Drug Administration (FDA) has approved an HPV DNA test that can be used alone for primary screening. This screen is not used among women in their 20s because an active and transient HPV infection is common among women under 30. HPV testing may represent a lower resource-intense strategy for screening.[85]

Screening recommendations

In 2012, the ACS, the American Society for Colposcopy and Cervical Pathology (ASCCP), and the American Society for Clinical Pathology (ASCP) issued joint guidelines for cervical cancer screening based on a systematic and collaborative review of evidence among 25 professional organizations.[86] Similar recommendations were released in 2012 by the USPSTF.[85] While these new recommendations still endorse more aggressive screening than in many European countries, they specify a more rational, cost-effective approach than earlier guidelines. However, many American clinicians are hesitant to embrace less frequent cervical cancer screening, despite good evidence that overscreening is wasteful of resources and contributes to potential harms.[78]

The screening guidelines specifically recommend:

- Women under age 21 years should not be screened regardless of their age of sexual initiation.
- Women aged 21–29 years should receive cytology screening (conventional smears or liquid-based cytology) every 3 years. HPV testing should not be used for women in this age group (but can be used as a reflex test for women diagnosed with ASCUS). For women aged 30–65 years, the preferred approach is to be screened every 5 years with the combination of HPV testing and cytology (co-testing). It is also acceptable for women to continue to be screened every 3 years with cytology alone.
- Women should discontinue screening after age 65 if they have had 3 consecutive negative cytology tests or 2 consecutive negative co-tests within the previous 10-year period, with the most recent test occurring within the last 5 years.
- Women at any age should NOT be screened annually by any screening method.

These recommendations were developed for women at average risk and do not apply to women with a history of cervical cancer; who were exposed to diethylstilbestrol while *in utero*; and who are immunocompromised due to medical therapy, or infected with the human immunodeficiency virus (HIV). Women who have had their cervix removed should not be screened, unless they have a history of CIN2 or a more severe cervical disease. Women with a history of CIN2 or more severe diagnosis should follow screening recommendations for women aged 30–65 for at least 20 years after definitive treatment, even if screening extends beyond age 65 years. Recommended screening practices should not change based on HPV vaccination status.

Prostate cancer

Worldwide, prostate cancer is the second most common cancer diagnosed and the sixth most common cause of cancer death among men.[11] Incidence and mortality rates vary considerably. Among American males, prostate cancer is the most commonly diagnosed nonskin cancer, and the second leading cause of cancer death. Mortality rates are higher in men of African ancestry, in Caucasian men in the Americas, and in Scandinavia. Rates are lowest in Asia.

A subset of prostate cancers is aggressive and poses a significant risk of death. Unfortunately, they often do not produce symptoms until locally advanced or metastatic. Prostate cancer among older men is more often slow growing or indolent. Efforts to distinguish clinically significant versus nonsignificant localized prostate cancer have included pathologic grading and genomic testing.[87]

Screening and diagnostic methods

DRE aims to find hard nodular areas that sometimes indicate the presence of prostate cancer. There are three principal limitations of DRE: the test is highly operator-dependent, the majority of palpable cancers are not early cancers, and many clinically important cancers are located in regions of the prostate inaccessible to palpation. DRE is often recommended as a screening component because it can detect prostate cancers missed by other tests; may predict high-grade disease; is a low-cost procedure; and can detect other abnormalities such as benign prostatic hyperplasia. Even with the above, in the early phases of the European Randomized Study of Prostate Cancer, DRE appeared to have limited value as a stand-alone test even though between one-quarter and one-third of all prostate cancers were detected by DRE in the normal PSA range (<4.0 ng/mL).[88]

Prostate-specific antigen (PSA) is a glycoprotein secreted by the epithelial component of the prostate. Progression of prostate cancer is correlated with a rise in serum PSA. Serum PSA measurement was first used to monitor metastatic disease in the early 1980s. By 1992, it gained high patient acceptance and became a widely used screening test in the United States. Unfortunately, its operating characteristics were determined far later.[89] Today, we know that serum PSA can be elevated in a variety of conditions besides cancer, such as benign prostatic hyperplasia, inflammation, and following trauma to the gland. PSA screening both finds and misses a lot of cancer. Whether PSA screening results in a decline in mortality rate is one of the most pressing questions in cancer medicine today.[90]

Accumulating evidence supports the efficacy (vs effectiveness) of PSA testing, alone or in combination with DRE, in finding localized disease.[88,91] Approximately, one in four men aged ≥50 years with PSA >4 ng/dL has cancer after prostate biopsy. Reducing the cutoff makes the test more sensitive but reduces specificity.

The Prostate Cancer Prevention Trial (PCPT) randomized more than 19,000 men aged ≥55 years with initial PSA of 3.0 ng/mL to finasteride or placebo.[92] Subjects were screened every year for 7 years (eight total screens) with serum PSA and DRE, and 14% were diagnosed with prostate cancer. Among men with normal PSAs and DREs, an additional 14% were diagnosed with prostate cancer based on end of study biopsy.[92] The fact that more than 25% of men completing PCPT were diagnosed with prostate cancer suggests some overdiagnosis. PCPT also showed that a PSA cutoff of 4 ng/mL as an upper limit of normal or a 1 ng/mL increase in 1 year missed essentially as much cancer as it found. There is no natural cut point for PSA screening. Indeed, there were men diagnosed with prostate cancer with serum PSA <0.6 ng/mL.[89]

Transrectal ultrasonography (TRUS) uses a small rectal probe placed against the prostate to image the entire gland. Unfortunately, cancer within the prostate has no unique and reliably assessed ultrasonic signature. TRUS as a sole screening modality has poor sensitivity and specificity. It can be used to accurately measure gland dimensions and volume and to direct prostate needle biopsies.

Endorectal MRI is not used in screening but has an evolving role in diagnostic evaluation of the prostate and following men with confirmed disease.[93]

Clinical trials of prostate cancer treatment

In a study started before the PSA era, 767 men with localized prostate cancer were followed expectantly. A small proportion died of prostate cancer, suggesting significant overdiagnosis. After 20 years of follow-up, 4–7%, 6–11%, and 18–30% of men with Gleason 2–4, 5, and 6 disease, respectively, had died of prostate cancer.[87] This raises the question whether treatment of localized or locally advanced prostate cancer is beneficial or saves lives. Prospective RCTs published in the late 1990s were the first to demonstrate a positive treatment effect for men with locally advanced disease. These studies demonstrated an advantage to radiation and hormonal therapy over radiation therapy alone.[94,95]

In 2002, the Scandinavian Prostate Cancer Group-4 study (SPCG-4) was the first to show that treatment of localized disease saved lives. They randomized 695 men with clinically localized prostate cancer to radical prostatectomy or watchful waiting, with hormonal therapy if symptoms dictated. At median follow-up of 12.8 years, 14.6% of the prostatectomy group had died versus 20.7% of the watchful waiting group (RR = 0.75, P = 0.007). The number needed to treat to prevent one death was 15. Less than 15% of participants had PSA-detected disease.[96] One would predict that the NNT in a screened population would be much higher.

The Prostate Intervention Versus Observation Trial (PIVOT) randomized 731 men with PSA screen-detected disease to radical prostatectomy or watchful waiting.[97] At median follow-up of 12 years, prostatectomy was associated with a statistically insignificant 2.9% absolute and 2.6% prostate cancer-specific reduction in mortality. Subgroup analyses suggested a small, but statistically significant, mortality benefit for men diagnosed with PSA >10 ng/mL and for those with intermediate- and high-risk disease.[97]

Taken together, the SPCG-4 and PIVOT studies suggest that our therapeutic interventions save lives in a minority of those diagnosed, and that a substantial proportion of men diagnosed with prostate cancer are overdiagnosed and do not need treatment. Substantial efforts are being made to identify these patients.

The effects of prostate cancer screening

Prostate cancer screening rates increased dramatically after FDA approval of PSA for following diagnosed disease in 1989. The FDA has since approved PSA for diagnosis of suspected disease but not for screening. The simplicity of a blood test enabled mass PSA screening at health fairs and community events and American prostate cancer incidence rates went up.

Prostate cancer mortality rates were rising for 20 years before the approval of PSA testing. Rates peaked in 1993, and since, the United States has experienced a 40% decline in age-adjusted prostate cancer death rates.[98] How much of the decline is due to screening is unknown. Etzioni and Feuer[99] argued that declining mortality within the first decade of widespread PSA testing is unlikely to be entirely due to PSA testing, given the long natural history of prostate cancer. Prostate cancer mortality rates have declined in 21

countries.[100] Screening is common in the United States and very few other countries.

Possible explanations for the decline in prostate cancer mortality seen in all countries are (1) a shift in the tendency to classify prostate cancer as the underlying cause of death and (2) significant improvements in prostate cancer treatment at all stages.[101] Supporting the first theory, the World Health Organization (WHO) algorithm for adjudicating cause of death was changed as mortality rates began to rise in the late 1970s and reverted back to the older algorithm in 1991 about the time when prostate cancer mortality began declining.[102] Supporting the second theory is the fact that prostate cancer is overwhelmingly a disease of older men. Even a 2- to 3-month increase in median survival due to more effective treatment could cause a decline in prostate cancer mortality as competing causes of death become more significant. Others have speculated that aggressive use of newer hormonal therapies may have increased cardiovascular deaths and thereby prevented prostate deaths.[103] All three could contribute to the decline in prostate cancer death rates in the United States in addition to the possibility that screening could have a positive effect.

Epidemiological studies show a significant decrease in the incidence of distant disease at diagnosis by the year 2000. On the basis of the assumption that screening results in a shift from distant to local/regional disease, modeling efforts within the NCI's Cancer Intervention Surveillance Modeling Network (CISNET) estimate 45–70% of the observed prostate cancer mortality decline in the United States could plausibly be attributed to screening-induced stage shifts.[99]

Ultimately, the strongest assessment of screening efficacy requires long-term large prospective RCTs with a mortality endpoint. Five studies have been reported, all of which are judged to have some limitations. The two trials considered of higher quality are the multicenter US NCI Prostate, Lung, Colorectal, and Ovarian trial (PLCO) and the multicenter European Randomized Study of Prostate Cancer (ERSPC).[88,91]

The PLCO was initiated in 1992.[91] Nearly 77,000 men aged 55–74 years were randomized to annual PSA testing for 6 years or usual care. At 13 years of follow-up, a statistically insignificant increase in prostate cancer mortality was observed among men randomized to annual screening (RR = 1.09, 95% CI, 0.87–1.36).[91] A limitation of this trial was the high rate of PSA testing in the control arm, which reduced statistical power. Rather than screening versus no screening, PLCO is best viewed as comparing routine to opportunistic screening.

The ERSPC was initiated in 1991,[88] with seven countries eventually reporting results. Prostate cancer-specific mortality was not reduced by screening in the initial analysis of 182,160 men, aged 50–74 years, but significantly decreased in a subset of men aged 55–69 years. A 21% relative reduction of prostate cancer death (RR = 0.79, 95% CI, 0.68–0.91) was observed after median follow-up of 11 years and maintained at 13 years. The number of men needed to be diagnosed and treated to prevent one prostate cancer death was 37 after 11 years and 27 after 13 years.[104–106]

Applying the ERPC findings to an American population would suggest that for every 200 men diagnosed through screening, about 8 lives would be saved after 13 years; about 1 in 200 men treated with radical prostatectomy dies as a result of surgery. The remaining 191 men would experience the negative effects of diagnosis and treatment but their prostate cancer destiny would not be changed. In comparison, after 13 years, 32 men would have died of prostate cancer. It is unknown how many of the 159 remaining would die of prostate cancer in the future.

The ERSPC trial would have been negative if not for the Swedish component. Screening was very effective in Sweden, marginally effective in the Netherlands, and showed a statistically insignificant trend toward benefit in four countries. The Finnish component of ERSPC was the largest and did not show benefit at 12 years.[107] Screening may have been more effective in Sweden because of the higher risk of prostate cancer death or because the randomization scheme in Sweden might have created a "healthy volunteer" selection bias among those in the screening arm that is not seen in the control group. Those who were screened were consented, while those in the control arm did not know they were in a clinical trial.[101]

Screening recommendations

A number of professional organizations in the United States, Europe, and Canada have issued prostate cancer screening guidelines. All acknowledge legitimate concerns regarding the risk–benefit ratio of screening. There is general agreement that screening should be done only in the context of fully informed consent with a decision between a man and his physician.[108–110] All recommend against mass screening in public places. The investigators of ERSPC also concluded that data do not support widespread screening.[106]

The ACS 2010 guidelines state that the balance of benefits and harms related to prostate cancer early detection are uncertain and the existing evidence is insufficient to support a recommendation for or against routine PSA screening.[109] The ACS calls for discussion and shared decision making within the physician–patient relationship.

The USPSTF 2012 guideline recommends against the *routine* use of PSA screening on the basis of its conclusion that there is moderate certainty that the harms of PSA testing outweigh the benefits.[10] The task force acknowledged that some men will continue to request screening and some physicians will continue to offer it. Similar to the ACS and AUA, they state that screening under such circumstances should respect an informed patient's preferences.[10]

In 2013, the AUA conducted a systematic review of over 300 studies and updated its guideline.[110] It concluded that the greatest benefit of screening appears to be in men aged 55–69 years although "the quality of evidence for benefits associated with screening was moderate, whereas the quality of the evidence for harm was high." The AUA places primacy on shared decision making versus physician judgments about the balance of benefits and harms at the population level even for men aged 55–69 years.[111] The committee recommends screening every 2 years instead of every year. They recommend *against* screening men <40 years of age, average-risk men aged 40–54 years, most men >70 years of age, and men with a life expectancy of <10–15 years. They recommend that screening decisions be individualized for higher risk men aged 40–54 years and men >70 years of age in excellent health.

The author believes that men should be informed of the potential benefits of screening and the documented harms associated with screening, especially the risk of overdiagnosis. Observation is appropriate for many. The decision to screen should include a commitment not to rush into aggressive therapy, if diagnosed.

Lung cancer

Worldwide, as in the United States, lung cancer is the most commonly diagnosed nonskin cancer and the leading cause of cancer death in men and second leading cause of cancer death in women.[11,19]

Screening and diagnostic methods

Chest X-ray screening was first advocated in the early 1950s, and by 1960, several lung cancer screening campaigns began. The Mayo Lung Project (MLP), initiated in 1971, enrolled more than 9200 male smokers and randomized them to chest X-ray and sputum cytology every 4 months or every year, for 6 years. Follow-up continues to this day.[112,113] After 13 and 20 years of follow-up, the intensively screened arm had an increased number of lung cancers diagnosed and a significant increase in disease-specific survival.[113,114] Lung-cancer mortality was not reduced, demonstrating that screening can increase survival rates without decreasing mortality. An estimated 18% of cancers diagnosed in the intensive group were judged to be overdiagnosis of cancer in one study.[115] Three other large, randomized studies of chest X-ray and sputum cytology using different screening schedules confirmed the findings of the MLP.[116,117]

These chest X-ray studies had important limitations, that is, they did not randomize to an unscreened control group, and they used 1960s to 1970s X-ray and treatment technology. Whether lung cancer screening was effective was readdressed in the US PLCO.[118] Participants were randomized to annual posteroanterior view chest radiograph for 4 years or usual care (without screening). With a median of 12 years of follow-up, PLCO found no mortality advantage to chest X-ray screening.[119]

Spiral computed tomography (CT) is more sensitive than chest X-ray in detecting small lung nodules. Low-dose computed tomography (LDCT) uses an average 1.5 mSv of radiation to perform a lung scan in 15 s. This led to the launch of the NLST in 2002.[120] Approximately 53,000 persons at high risk for lung cancer were randomized to three annual LDCT scans or single-view postero-anterior chest X-rays. With median follow-up of 6.5 years, there was a 20% relative reduction in lung cancer mortality (95% CI, 6.8–26.7; $P = 0.004$) compared to the chest X-ray arm.[120] This corresponds to lung cancer death rates of 247 and 309 per 100,000 person-years, respectively. There was a 6.7% decrease in death from any cause in the LDCT group (95% CI, 1.2–13.6; $P = 0.02$), a rare finding in a prospective RCT. Screening prevented the greatest number of lung cancer deaths among participants who were at highest risk and very few deaths among those at lowest risk. These findings provide empirical support for risk-based screening.[121]

LDCT screening is clearly promising but has limitations. In NLST, 96.4% of positive findings were false.[120] Positive results require additional diagnostic procedures, mostly conventional CT scans, but in some cases, needle biopsy, bronchoscopy, mediastinoscopy, or thoracotomy, which are associated with anxiety, expense, and complications (e.g., pneumo- or hemothorax after lung biopsy). The NLST reported 16 deaths within 60 days of an invasive diagnostic procedure; whether the procedure was causative is unknown. Of these participants, 6 did not have cancer. There is increasing interest in evaluation algorithms to decrease the number of invasive diagnostic procedures.[122,123]

Other harms from screening include the theoretical potential for radiation-induced cancers resulting from LDCT and overdiagnosis. Overdiagnosis was estimated to be 18.5% (95% CI, 5.4–30.6%) in NLST.[124] Interestingly, this is very similar to the MLP.[112] Overdiagnosis is impossible to prove in the living, but in one autopsy study, one-sixth of all lung cancers found had not been diagnosed before death.[125] Some believe that NLST needs longer follow-up to make an accurate overdiagnosis estimate.

Screening recommendations

The ACS, the American College of Chest Physicians (AACP), and the American Society of Clinical Oncology (ASCO) recommend that clinicians discuss lung cancer screening with patients who would have qualified for the NLST: aged 55–74 years, ≥30 pack-year smoking history, currently smoke or have quit within the past 15 years, relatively good health.

This discussion should include the benefits, uncertainties, and harms associated with LDCT screening for lung cancer. Adults who choose to be screened should enter an organized screening program at an institution with expertise in LDCT and access to a multidisciplinary team skilled in the evaluation, diagnosis, and treatment of abnormal lung lesions. If a high-quality program is not available, the risks of harm associated with screening may be greater than the benefits.[70,126] Recommendations state an annual LDCT should be performed as long as subjects would benefit from treatment if diagnosed. All screening guidelines also stress that current smokers should be offered help with smoking cessation.

Testicular cancer

Testicular cancer is relatively uncommon[11] and its treatment is often successful. Over 70% of patients with metastatic disease have prolonged complete remissions.

Screening and diagnostic methods

Most diagnoses are made through the patient or physician recognizing an abnormality in the scrotum. Suspicious masses are evaluated further through ultrasonography and biopsy.

While self-palpation of the testes is simple, available data suggest that it is of low specificity and predictive value, and would be done infrequently if advocated.[127] Self-examinations result in false alarms that burden the healthcare system and can be costly. A useful intervention may be health education to encourage men to seek medical care if they notice a lump or nodule or any change in the size, shape, or consistency of the testes. Patient delay after becoming aware of a testicular abnormality is clearly associated with poorer survival.

Screening recommendations

No organization recommends routine screening for testicular cancer in average-risk men. The American Academy of Family Physicians recommends palpation of testicles for men aged 13–39 years at higher risk due to a history of cryptorchidism, orchiopexy, or testicular atrophy.[127]

Hepatocellular cancer

Hepatocellular cancer (HCC) is the fourth most common cancer worldwide.[128] Age-standardized incidence rates are 40-fold higher in China compared to North America. Rates are rising in the United States.[11]

Chronic hepatitis B and C are major risk factors. Other risk factors include alcoholic cirrhosis, hemochromatosis, alpha-L-antitrypsin deficiency, glycogen storage disease, porphyria cutanea tarda, tyrosinemia, and Wilson disease.[128] In parts of Africa, the high incidence of HCC may be related to ingestion of aflatoxin-contaminated foods.

Currently, four types of tumor markers are being used or studied as screening tests: oncofetal antigens and glycoprotein antigens, enzymes and isoenzymes, genes, and cytokines.[129] Serum AFP, a fetal-specific glycoprotein antigen, is the most widely used. In high-risk populations, sensitivity of 39–97%, specificity of 76–95%,

and PPV of 9–32% have been reported. AFP is not specific for HCC. It rises due to hepatitis, pregnancy, and germ cell tumors.[128]

Ultrasound and CT imaging have been studied as adjuncts to AFP.[130] These tests have limited sensitivity and specificity. A prospective randomized study in China using AFP and US found HCC mortality was lower in the screened group [83.2 vs 131.5 per 100,000 with a mortality rate ratio of 0.63 (95% CI: 0.41–0.98)]. The results from this study have differed in various publications and it is unclear that this was an intention to screen analysis.[131,132]

Screening recommendations

Screening is not advocated among the general population and its benefit among those with HCC risk factors is questioned.

Endometrial cancer

Endometrial cancer is the most commonly diagnosed gynecologic malignancy among women in the United States and western Europe[11] where approximately one in four endometrial cancers is advanced at the time of diagnosis.

Screening and diagnostic methods

The efficacy of screening for endometrial cancer has never been evaluated in a prospective RCT. Occasionally, the Pap test identifies endometrial abnormalities, but it is insensitive and should not be used for endometrial cancer screening. Endometrial biopsy is the gold standard screening test. More recently, interest in transvaginal ultrasound (TVU) screening has increased.[133] Two well-designed studies of endometrial screening with TVU and biopsy have reported disappointing results and significant harms, including some cases of uterine perforation.

Screening recommendations

At this time, no organization recommends routine screening for endometrial cancer in average-risk women. The ACS recommends women be informed of the risk and symptoms of endometrial cancer at the time of menopause and strongly encouraged to report unexpected bleeding or spotting to their physician.[134]

The ACS recommends a risk-based approach for women at high risk for endometrial cancer.[69] High risk includes women known to carry HNPCC-associated mutations (Lynch syndrome), women likely to be a mutation carrier based on relatives known to be mutation carriers, and women from families appearing to have an autosomal dominant predisposition to colon cancer in the absence of genetic testing results.[269] Women known or suspected to have Lynch syndrome should be offered endometrial screening annually beginning at age 35 following discussion of benefits, risks, and limitations of testing.[84]

Ovarian cancer

Ovarian cancer has the highest mortality rate of all gynecologic cancers and accounts for 6% of all cancer deaths among women in the United States.[11] Recent science shows that many so-called ovarian cancers actually are primary fallopian tube cancers. A few start as primary abdominal wall tumors. Most women are diagnosed with "ovarian cancer" after symptoms develop, and only 19% have disease truly localized to the ovary.[19]

Screening and diagnostic methods

Pelvic examination has low sensitivity and specificity for the detection of ovarian cancer and thus cannot be recommended alone as a screening method. However, recent studies suggest that a more favorable diagnosis may be possible if early symptoms are evaluated.

CA-125 is the most extensively studied ovarian cancer serum marker. It is a tumor-associated antigen, mainly used for surveillance after surgical removal of an epithelial ovarian cancer. The currently available assay, CA-125 II, utilizes both OC125 and MC11 antibodies.[135] CA-125 levels >30–35 U/mL are considered abnormal. Although CA-125 is elevated in the majority of advanced ovarian cancers, only half of early ovarian cancers yield a positive test. Moreover, CA-125 levels can be elevated in noncancerous diseases of the ovaries[136] and influenced by the presence of other cancers, a history of hormone use, and current smoking.

Ultrasonography: Abdominal ultrasonography has been used in ovarian cancer screening with poor results, owing to low specificity.[137] TVU is capable of detecting small masses but is poor at indicating malignancy. Color Doppler ultrasonography was believed to hold promise for differentiating benign from malignant masses, but studies have not shown that it improves diagnostic accuracy. Current data are insufficient to support TVU or other imaging modalities as stand-alone screening tools in average-risk asymptomatic women.[138]

Combination CA-125 and ultrasound: Nonrandomized cohort studies and pilot RCTs in average- and high-risk women have shown the limited sensitivity of CA-125 or ultrasound (abdominal or transvaginal) alone at an acceptable level of specificity and the poor predictive value of a positive test. High specificity is especially important because laparoscopy and/or laparotomy is required to rule out the presence of ovarian cancer when screening is positive. Multimodal approaches that combine CA-125, ROC CA-125 algorithms, and imaging have been evaluated in prospective RCTs. The PLCO is a prospective RCT. It recruited 78,237 women aged 55–74. A total of 39,115 were randomized to ovarian cancer screening with baseline CA-125 and TVU tests, followed by three additional annual rounds of TVU and five of CA-125. There were 2.1 versus 2.6 ovarian cancer deaths per 10,000 women-years in the screened versus control group (RR = 1.18, 95% CI, 0.82–1.71).

Several studies targeting women at high risk for ovarian cancer are also underway.[138] The United Kingdom Collaborative Trial of Ovarian Cancer Screening (UKCTOCS)[139,140] randomized 200,000 average risk, postmenopausal women aged 50–74 years to usual care (*n* = 100,000); annual multimodal screening with serum CA-125 followed by CA-125 and ultrasound (*n* = 50,000); or annual ultrasound screening with repeat ultrasound in 6–8 weeks (*n* = 50,000) for 7 years. The primary endpoint is ovarian cancer mortality screening using multiple modalities reduced overall average mortality by 20% (RR = 0.80, 95% CI, 0.60–0.98).

Serum proteomic pattern recognition algorithms are being developed to identify a key subset of peptides that discriminate ovarian cancer cases from control subjects. The potential for either a stand-alone or adjunctive proteomic test for ovarian cancer screening is regarded as promising but remains unrealized.

Screening recommendations

No major guideline-making organization recommends ovarian cancer screening in average-risk women, and the USPSTF specifically recommends against it.[141] In 1994, a NIH Consensus Panel concluded that a comprehensive family history should be taken from all women, and women with two or more first-degree relatives with a history of ovarian cancer should be offered counseling by a gynecologic oncologist (or other qualified specialist) as these women have a 3% chance of being positive for an ovarian cancer hereditary syndrome.[142] Women with known hereditary ovarian

cancer syndrome, such as mutations on *BRCA1* and *BRCA2*, including breast-ovarian cancer syndrome, site-specific ovarian cancer syndrome, and HNPCC, should receive annual recto-vaginal pelvic examinations, CA-125 determinations, and TVU until childbearing is completed or at least until age 35, at which time prophylactic bilateral oophorectomy is recommended. Women with these hereditary syndromes are estimated to represent only 0.05% of the female population and have a 40% estimated lifetime risk of ovarian cancer.

Melanoma and nonmelanoma skin cancer

Skin cancers, together, are the most common cancers diagnosed worldwide and in the United States. They account for nearly half of all malignancies.[11] The most common are basal cell and squamous cell skin cancer, which are referred to as nonmelanoma skin cancer (NMSC). NMSC is highly curable, although significant morbidity can result from delayed diagnosis and treatment. Melanoma, however, is a significant cause of cancer death. In the United States, melanoma accounts for 2% of all skin cancer cases but the vast majority of skin cancer deaths.

Screening and diagnostic methods

Interest in screening for melanoma has increased in recent years because mortality rates are increasing. Screening involves a visual skin examination, by a clinician or self-examination. A 2- to 3-min total examination of the skin is preferable because skin cancers often occur at anatomic sites that are not directly exposed to sunlight. Skin examinations by a healthcare provider are uncommon in the United States but are more common among dermatologists than primary care physicians. Basal cell skin cancer may appear as a flat growth or a small, raised pink or red translucent shiny area that may bleed following a minor injury. Squamous cell skin cancer may appear as a growing lump, often with a rough surface, or as a flat, reddish patch that grows slowly. Signs of melanoma include changes over time in size, shape, or color of a mole or other skin lesion. This is summarized as an ABCD algorithm that emphasizes asymmetry [A] of the lesion, uneven borders [B], changes in color [C], and changes in diameter [D]. A Cochrane Review endorsed the addition of an "E" category—"evolving"—to emphasize the importance of change over time in the lesion. However, it appears most dermatologists rely on the overall pattern of appearance (ugly duckling sign) versus a stepwise assessment of features.

Case–control studies have suggested that increased awareness of melanoma and its symptoms leads to earlier presentation and thinner lesions at presentation.[143] High-risk patients routinely screened by dermatologists have thinner lesions at diagnosis than among historical or population-based controls.

The American Academy of Dermatology program of skin cancer screening has examined >600,000 people of various risk categories since 1985.[144] In addition to detecting >35,000 NMSCs, melanomas diagnosed by screening were more likely than historical controls to be <1.5 mm. Skin cancer screening may be more effective if targeted to high-risk persons such as Caucasian patients aged >20 years with atypical mole syndrome or congenital melanocytic nevi, patients with specific phenotypic traits, or patients with a history of NMSC.[144]

No RCT has assessed whether skin cancer screening decreases mortality. Some large observational studies suggest its efficacy. A Scottish campaign to promote melanoma awareness and early presentation appears to be associated with a decline in mortality. The Skin Cancer Research to Provide Evidence for Effectiveness of Screening (SCREEN) Project launched an intensive screening program among 360,000 participants in one area of Germany.[145,146]

Although there were many false positives, melanoma incidence was raised by 16% in men and 38% in women in a 2-year period of time and returned to baseline after conclusion of the intervention period. Five years after the end of the intervention period, melanoma death rates were half that of the rest of Germany[147,148] A community-based, randomized population trial of self-examination versus clinician skin examination is underway in Australia, with a primary outcome of melanoma mortality after 15 years of follow-up.[69,149]

Screening recommendations

The ACS recommends skin examination during periodic preventive health examinations.[69] The American College of Preventive Medicine recommends periodic total cutaneous examinations for high-risk populations, including those with Caucasian race, fair complexion, presence of pigmented lesions (dysplastic or atypical nevus), several large nondysplastic nevi, many small nevi, moderate freckling, or familial dysplastic nevus syndrome.

The USPSTF recommends people, especially high-risk individuals, be alert to skin abnormalities.[149] The Taskforce concluded that evidence was insufficient to recommend for or against routine screening using total-body skin examination for the early detection of cutaneous melanoma, basal cell cancer, or squamous cell skin cancer.

Oral cancer

Oral cancer is more common in men than in women.[11] Approximately one-third of oral cancers are diagnosed at a localized stage.[150]

Screening and diagnostic methods

Oral cancer is generally accessible to physical examination by the patient and healthcare providers, especially the dentist. Screening can be made more efficient by inspecting high-risk sites where 90% of squamous cell cancers arise: floor of mouth, ventrolateral aspect of the tongue, and soft-palate complex. Leukoplakia and erythroplastic lesions are the earliest and most serious signs of squamous cell carcinoma.[151] Although new technological approaches to screening are being evaluated, such as toluidine blue, brush cytology, tissue reflectance, and autofluorescence, none has been shown to be reliably superior to conventional oral examination.

Using a cluster-RCT design, high-risk men and women aged ≥35 years in Kerala, India were randomized to three rounds of oral visual inspection by trained health workers at 3-year intervals.[152] There were 21% fewer oral cancer deaths in the 96,517 participants in the intervention group compared with the control group (RR = 0.79, 95% CI, 0.51–1.22), which rose to 34% fewer among tobacco and alcohol users.

While some have advocated oral cavity inspection as part of every physical examination in dental and physician offices, the absence of a general recommendation results in this occurring infrequently. Ironically, those at highest risk for oral cancer (smokers and heavy alcohol drinkers) are less likely to see a physician or dentist than those at lower risk. Common symptoms leading to diagnostic evaluation include sores on the lip or mouth, oral bleeding, persistent white or red patches in the mouth or on the gums, oral swelling and/or pain, sore throat, and difficulty swallowing.

Conclusion

In the near term, the greatest potential for reducing deaths from cancer is through early detection and appropriate treatment. Complete

benefit of early detection strategies remains unfulfilled globally due to limitations in access, insufficient resources, uneven quality, and lack of organized systems. Screening opportunistically rather than systematically is inefficient at both the individual and population level. A comprehensive system of early detection and intervention can lead potentially to high levels of participation, provide the readiness to implement any new early detection technology that could improve disease control, and ensure that all program elements are highly competent, interrelated, and interdependent. A systematic approach has the potential not only to increase quality but also to reduce the volume of small errors that contribute to incremental erosion of efficiency, as well as the volume of gross failures that result in death when mortality is avoidable. While many practical barriers must be overcome to establish true population-based screening programs, a system of organized screening holds the greatest potential to realize the benefits of reducing the incidence rate of advanced cancers and, subsequently, avoiding premature mortality.

Key references

The complete reference list can be found on the Wiley Companion Digital Edition of this title (see inside front cover for login instructions).

1 Croswell JM, Ransohoff DF, Kramer BS. Principles of cancer screening: lessons from history and study design issues. *Semin Oncol.* 2010;**37**:202–215.

3 Welch HG, Black WC. Overdiagnosis in cancer. *J Natl Cancer Inst.* 2010;**102**:605–613.

4 Baker SG, Prorok PC, Kramer BS. Lead time and overdiagnosis. *J Natl Cancer Inst.* 2014;**106**:109.

8 Marmot MG, Altman DG, Cameron DA, Dewar JA, Thompson SG, Wilcox M. The benefits and harms of breast cancer screening: an independent review. *Br J Cancer.* 2013;**108**:2205–2240.

10 Moyer VA. Screening for prostate cancer: U.S. preventive services task force recommendation statement. *Ann Intern Med.* 2012;**157**:120–134.

16 Nelson HD, Zakher B, Cantor A, et al. Risk factors for breast cancer for women aged 40 to 49 years: a systematic review and meta-analysis. *Ann Intern Med.* 2012;**156**:635–648. doi: 10.7326/0003-4819-156-9-201205010-00006.

18 U.S. Preventive Services Task Force. Screening for breast cancer: U.S. Preventive Services Task Force recommendation statement. *Ann Intern Med.* 2009;**151**:716–726, W-236.

20 Mandelblatt J, van Ravesteyn N, Schechter C, et al. Which strategies reduce breast cancer mortality most? Collaborative modeling of optimal screening, treatment, and obesity prevention. *Cancer.* 2013;**119**:2541–2548.

21 Harris R, Yeatts J, Kinsinger L. Breast cancer screening for women ages 50 to 69 years a systematic review of observational evidence. *Prev Med.* 2011;**53**:108–114.

25 Smith RA, Manassaram-Baptiste D, Brooks D, et al. Cancer screening in the United States, 2014: a review of current American Cancer Society guidelines and current issues in cancer screening. *CA Cancer J Clin.* 2014;**64**:30–51.

29 Berry DA, Cronin KA, Plevritis SK, et al. Effect of screening and adjuvant therapy on mortality from breast cancer. *N Engl J Med.* 2005;**353**:1784–1792.

36 Esserman LJ, Thompson IM Jr, Reid B. Overdiagnosis and overtreatment in cancer: an opportunity for improvement. *JAMA.* 2013;**310**:797–798.

38 Saslow D, Boates C, Burke W, et al. American Cancer Society guidelines for breast screening with MRI as an adjunct to mammography. *CA Cancer J Clin.* 2007;**57**:90–104. Available on line at http://caonline.amcancersoc.org.

47 Shaukat A, Mongin SJ, Geisser MS, et al. Long-term mortality after screening for colorectal cancer. *N Engl J Med.* 2013;**369**:1106–1114.

48 Mandel JS, Church TR, Bond JH, et al. The effect of fecal occult-blood screening on the incidence of colorectal cancer. *N Engl J Med.* 2000;**343**:1603–1607.

51 Burch JA, Soares-Weiser K, St John DJ, et al. Diagnostic accuracy of faecal occult blood tests used in screening for colorectal cancer: a systematic review. *J Med Screen.* 2007;**14**:132–137.

52 Imperiale TF, Ransohoff DF, Itzkowitz SH, et al. Multitarget stool DNA testing for colorectal-cancer screening. *N Engl J Med.* 2014;**370**:1287–1297.

60 Mandel JS, Bond JH, Church TR, et al. Reducing mortality from colorectal cancer by screening for fecal occult blood. Minnesota Colon Cancer Control Study [published erratum appears in N Engl J Med 1993 26;329(9):672]. *N Engl J Med.* 1993;**328**:1365–1371.

68 Levin B, Lieberman DA, McFarland B, et al. Screening and surveillance for the early detection of colorectal cancer and adenomatous polyps, 2008: a joint guideline from the American Cancer Society, the US Multi-Society Task Force

on Colorectal Cancer, and the American College of Radiology. *CA Cancer J Clin.* 2008;**58**:130–160.

73 Janerich DT, Hadjimichael O, Schwartz PE, et al. The screening histories of women with invasive cervical cancer, Connecticut. *Am J Public Health.* 1995;**85**:791–794.

74 Kulasingam SL, Havrilesky L, Ghebre R, Myers ER. *U.S. Preventive Services Task Force Evidence Syntheses, Formerly Systematic Evidence Reviews. Screening for Cervical Cancer: A Decision Analysis for the US Preventive Services Task Force.* Rockville, MD: Agency for Healthcare Research and Quality (US); 2011.

75 Solomon D, Davey D, Kurman R, et al. The 2001 Bethesda System: terminology for reporting results of cervical cytology. *JAMA.* 2002;**287**:2114–2119.

84 Sankaranarayanan R, Nene BM, Shastri SS, et al. HPV screening for cervical cancer in rural India. *N Engl J Med.* 2009;**360**:1385–1394.

85 Moyer VA. Screening for cervical cancer: U.S. Preventive Services Task Force recommendation statement. *Ann Intern Med.* 2012;**156**:880–891, W312.

86 Saslow D, Solomon D, Lawson HW, et al. American Cancer Society, American Society for Colposcopy and Cervical Pathology, and American Society for Clinical Pathology screening guidelines for the prevention and early detection of cervical cancer. *CA Cancer J Clin.* 2012;**62**:147–172.

87 Albertsen PC, Hanley JA, Fine J. 20-year outcomes following conservative management of clinically localized prostate cancer. *JAMA.* 2005;**293**:2095–2101.

88 Schroder FH, Hugosson J, Roobol MJ, et al. Screening and prostate-cancer mortality in a randomized European study. *N Engl J Med.* 2009;**360**:1320–1328.

89 Thompson IM, Ankerst DP, Chi C, et al. Operating characteristics of prostate-specific antigen in men with an initial PSA level of 3.0 ng/ml or lower. *JAMA.* 2005;**294**:66–70.

91 Andriole GL, Crawford ED, Grubb RL 3rd, et al. Mortality results from a randomized prostate-cancer screening trial. *N Engl J Med.* 2009;**360**:1310–1319.

97 Wilt TJ, Brawer MK, Jones KM, et al. Radical prostatectomy versus observation for localized prostate cancer. *N Engl J Med.* 2012;**367**:203–213.

106 Schroder FH, Hugosson J, Roobol MJ, et al. Screening and prostate cancer mortality: results of the European Randomised Study of Screening for Prostate Cancer (ERSPC) at 13 years of follow-up. *Lancet.* 2014;**384**:2027–2035.

107 Kilpelainen TP, Tammela TL, Malila N, et al. Prostate cancer mortality in the Finnish randomized screening trial. *J Natl Cancer Inst.* 2013;**105**:719–725.

110 Carter HB, Albertsen PC, Barry MJ, et al. Early detection of prostate cancer: AUA guideline. *J Urol.* 2013;**190**:419–426.

115 Marcus PM. Estimating overdiagnosis in lung cancer screening. *JAMA Intern Med.* 2014;**174**:1198.

120 Aberle DR, Berg CD, Black WC, et al. The National Lung Screening Trial: overview and study design. *Radiology.* 2011;**258**:243–253.

126 Bach PB, Mirkin JN, Oliver TK, et al. Benefits and harms of CT screening for lung cancer: a systematic review. *JAMA.* 2012;**307**:2418–2429.

131 Zhang BH, Yang BH, Tang ZY. Randomized controlled trial of screening for hepatocellular carcinoma. *J Cancer Res Clin Oncol.* 2004;**130**:417–422.

140 Goff BA, Mandel LS, Drescher CW, et al. Development of an ovarian cancer symptom index: possibilities for earlier detection. *Cancer.* 2007;**109**:221–227.

141 Moyer VA. Screening for ovarian cancer: U.S. Preventive Services Task Force reaffirmation recommendation statement. *Ann Intern Med.* 2012;**157**:900–904. doi: 10.7326/0003-4819-157-11-201212040-00539.

144 Geller AC, Zhang Z, Sober AJ, et al. The first 15 years of the American Academy of Dermatology skin cancer screening programs: 1985–1999. *J Am Acad Dermatol.* 2003;**48**:34–41.

Clinical Disciplines

39 Nexgen pathology: predicting clinical course and targeting disease causation

Carlos Cordon-Cardo, MD, PhD ▪ Adolfo Firpo-Betancourt, MD, MPA

Overview

Pathology is a bridging discipline involving basic and clinical biomedical sciences. This context includes both descriptive and mechanistic approaches, with the goals of understanding the anatomical changes and underlying molecular events involved in disease-related processes. Neoplastic disorders are a focal point for the further development of this chapter. The two main objectives of pathology are to define disease causation [from "Pathos" (Greek) "Disease"] and categorize disease states to render clinical diagnostic services. A modern academic Department of Pathology encompasses education activities, including teaching students, training residents and fellows, and mentoring faculty; and hospital-based clinical services usually under three divisions, comprising anatomic pathology (surgical pathology, cytology, and autopsy services); clinical pathology (embodying a variety of laboratory services from blood bank and coagulation to chemistry and microbiology, among others); and molecular pathology (commonly housing somatic genetics, cytogenomics, and flow cytometry). During the past two decades, we have witnessed the transition from descriptive analysis of tissue histology and analyte variables that categorized patients and broad disease stages to more objective and quantitative multidimensional studies aimed at defining individual patient signatures. More traditional population and cohort-based classifications are turning into patient-specific profiles that optimize treatment efficacy and outcome: from diagnostic and prognostic approaches that group patients into disease categories to the development of a more precise, predictive, and individualized patient assessment (Table 1). Such an integrated care model drives selection of evidence-based treatment protocols to optimize clinical outcome, engendering a cost-effective and personalized healthcare. Disease classification and assistance in selection of therapy is the focus of this "patient-centric" pathology approach, expanding into monitoring of therapy (such as assessing therapeutic index and mutational load through tumor genotypes) and managing high-risk patients through early diagnosis of their disease condition (Figure 1). The ultimate goals are to move from treating symptomatology to treating disease causation once origin of the disease is better understood and to move from a fee-for-service to population-based accountable healthcare management.

From anatomic and clinical pathology to molecular and predictive integrated diagnostics

The origins and the academic establishment of pathology can be traced to the sixteenth to seventeenth centuries in Italy, where physicians systematically performed autopsies to further elucidate diseases suffered by their patients. It is in the writings of Benivieni (1443–1502) and Morgagni (1682–1771) that we find the first clinicopathological correlations, based on meticulous autopsy studies. This descriptive, gross anatomic approach was supplanted by the French and English "tissue pathology" schools, represented by Bichat (1771–1802) and eventually by the German school of "cellular pathology," led by Muller (1801–1858) and Virchow (1821–1902).[1] The cell was defined as the unit of life and the target for most diseases, being further expressed by histopathological alterations in the tissue of origin (Figure 2).[2] Biochemical, immunological, and genetic discoveries brought scientific knowledge into clinical medicine, and a new armamentarium of technologies during the mid-to-late 1900s. An upsurge of innovative approaches, from DNA amplification and mutation-identification platforms to automated clinical chemistry appeared in the late twentieth century. Molecular pathology evolved from these investigations, integrating histology with immunohistochemical (IHC) and genetic technologies to render phenotype/genotype correlations, thus establishing individualized patient assessment (Figure 3).[3,4]

The role of the pathologist has changed over the years. Traditionally, the main task of the pathologist was the evaluation of patients through morphologic analyses of human tissues and analysis of certain chemicals and biomolecules in body fluids. The diagnosis of cancer involves the analysis of tissue samples and body fluids for features that correlate with malignant transformation and tumor progression. Tissue specimens, cells, and fluids (e.g., blood, urine, and effusions) are obtained through several procedures, including surgical biopsy, endoscopic biopsy, core or aspirational needle biopsy, venipuncture, spinal tap, scraping of tissue surfaces, and collection of exfoliative cells from urine or sputum. The acquired tissue or cell specimens are subjected to a series of analytic modalities for diagnostic purposes. Light microscopy, assessing morphological features of the procured specimens, was utilized almost as the sole approach for many years and remains the standard diagnostic method to which all novel methods need to be compared. The use of enzyme histochemistry and electron microscopy expanded the primary microanatomical evaluation to include biochemical and subcellular structural features. More recently, cytogenetics, analysis of DNA content, molecular genetic assays, and IHC studies have been added as valuable adjuncts to light microscopy in cancer diagnosis, expanding to an in-depth genotype–phenotype characterization. These methods, particularly IHC, have enhanced significantly our ability to define the lines of differentiation of human tumors. The inclusion of these technologies with more recent high throughput, such as next generation DNA sequencing platforms and RNA expression arrays among others, constitutes the basis for molecular pathology, and has added valuable information to the current classification schemes.[5] The main goal now is to integrate the data that emanate from this multidimensional arsenal of technologies and translate it into knowledge and to manage such knowledge in order to better manage our patients and community of individuals at high risk for developing certain diseases.

Holland-Frei Cancer Medicine, Ninth Edition. Edited by Robert C. Bast Jr., Carlo M. Croce, William N. Hait, Waun Ki Hong, Donald W. Kufe, Martine Piccart-Gebhart, Raphael E. Pollock, Ralph R. Weichselbaum, Hongyang Wang, and James F. Holland.
© 2017 John Wiley & Sons, Inc. ISBN: 978-1-118-93469-2

Table 1 Evolution of pathology from diagnostic to integrated predictive platforms.

	Classical pathology	Molecular and systems pathology
Diagnosis and staging	Descriptive analysis of clinical variables, tissue histology, and biomarkers to categorize patients into broad disease stages; no predictive value to inform treatment selection	Objective, quantitative multidimensional analysis of clinical variables, tissue morphometrics, and molecular tumor signatures to define individual patient tumor phenotype and genotype
Prognostic evaluation	Traditional population and cohort-based classification used to deduce disease progression and likelihood of treatment response; nonspecific	Patient-specific characteristics and molecular tumor profiles are used to predict drug sensitivity and radiation response, thus optimizing treatment efficacy and outcome
Treatment selection	Group management approach that stratifies patients into disease categories, assigning therapies on predetermined population-based protocols instead of being patient specific	Personalized and integrated care model drives selection of evidence-based treatment protocol to optimize clinical outcome; patient-tailored treatments improve survival and quality of life
	Diagnostic and prognostic approach that "groups" patients into disease categories	*Precise, predictive, and cost effective; individualized patient management*

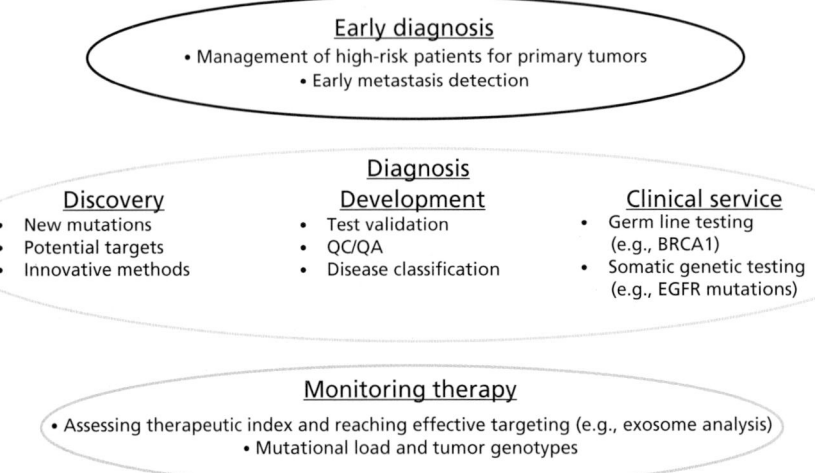

Figure 1 Integrated approach to disease management: translating data into knowledge.

Molecular pathology

Molecular pathology studies the origins and pathogenesis of disease at the biochemical, immunological, and genetic levels. Cancer is a clonal disease driven primarily by genetic mutations and epigenetic derangements.[6,7] This means that any given tumor originates in a single cell (clonality) that has been primed by specific molecular triggers (tumorigenesis). Such a cell accepts genetic manipulation, does not activate pathways of cell death or immune surveillance, and progresses toward invasion and metastatic spread, the ultimate malignant phenotype. Even though several tumors have their origin in viral infections (oncoviruses) in which certain viral proteins (oncoproteins) enhance proliferation and abolish apoptotic responses, such as the case of certain human papilloma virus subtypes, most cancers can be defined as diseases driven by either inherited or somatic mutations. In this regard, pathology differs from medical genetics, in which the main objective is to determine the abnormalities associated with inherited disorders carried as germ-line mutations. Molecular pathology of cancer aims to identify and understand the aberrations involved in the development and progression of neoplastic diseases. Clinically relevant objectives include (1) establishing a definitive diagnosis and classification of tumors, based on the recognition of complex profiles (fingerprints) or unique molecular alterations that occur in specific tumor types; (2) providing early detection of tumor cells using sensitive molecular techniques, thus anticipating therapeutic intervention; (3) rendering prognostic information of clinical relevance, through the

assessment of molecular predictors of outcome; and (4) assisting in the selection of individualized treatment regimens, thereby gaining specificity and avoiding unnecessary drug toxicity. Companion diagnostic tools are designed to guide targeted clinical trials and personalized oncological treatments. The clinical services rendered also include the analysis of minimal residual disease and evidence of early relapse usually driven by new resistant clones of cancer cells. Protocols based on molecular markers have been proven to increase the chances for cure by opting for the right management approach and improve the quality of life of patients with cancer.

Molecular pathology also serves as a bridge between clinical and basic biomedical sciences. The translational aspects of research in molecular pathology are bidirectional, involving both the active transfer of relevant observations that are the result of the analysis of primary tumors and clinicopathological correlations to basic laboratory studies and the effective transfer of laboratory findings into clinical analyses and protocols. Molecular pathology thus facilitates the transfer of biological discoveries into diagnostic, prognostic, and therapeutic applications.

The use of molecular techniques has led to remarkable progress in our understanding of cell growth, differentiation, maintenance of genomic integrity, and programmed cell death, these being key pathways in tumor development and progression.[3-5] Certain biological markers, such as alterations of TP53 tumor suppressor gene, correlate with tumor behavior when detected in specific tumor types.[8] Similarly, prospective clinical analyses utilizing

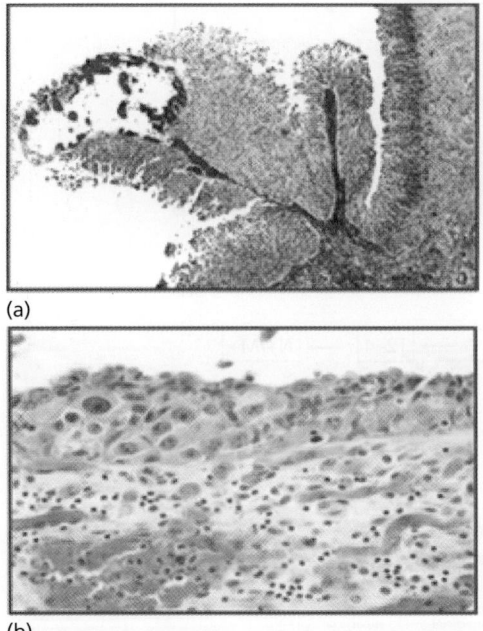

(a)

(b)

Figure 2 (a, b) Cellular profiling. The microscope became the innovative device that allowed Dr. Rudolf Virchow (1821–1902) to describe the cell as the unit of life and main target of disease. Disease classification based on histogenesis was developed. Hematoxylin and eosin (H&E) of bladder cancer histological sections; upper microphotograph illustrating a papillary noninvasive transitional cell carcinoma; lower microphotograph illustrating a transitional cell carcinoma *in situ* of the urinary bladder.

well-characterized cohorts of patients and properly selected normal and tumor paired samples are needed to better delineate the role of mutations occurring in these genes, as they impact on patients affected with cancer. Discrepancies of reported results aimed at the identification of gene mutations and altered patterns of gene

expression in primary tumors can be explained by the use of different probes and methods. Critical caveats include the presence of viable tumor, the extent of necrosis, normal-to-tumor cell ratio, and the stage and grade of the lesion being studied. Distinct methods are often available to detect a given marker, differing in specificity, sensitivity, speed, and cost, as well as appropriateness for particular clinical situations. The application of the full spectrum of molecular methods to evaluate tissue specimens and the potential availability of therapeutic agents aimed at specific molecular targets have led to changes in the established patterns of tissue procurement, processing, and tissue banking. Protocols should be implemented and constantly updated to guarantee that samples are handled in a way that will allow optimal application of molecular testing. In daily practice, this means that part of a specimen should be set aside prospectively for advanced diagnostics whenever possible. Adding predictive assays to our diagnostic and prognostic tools will enhance our ability to design effective treatment regimens.

Bladder cancer as a model of molecular pathology classification

Bladder cancer is the fifth most commonly diagnosed noncutaneous solid malignancy and the second most frequently diagnosed genitourinary tumor after prostate cancer.[9–11] Prevalence of bladder cancer is 6 times higher in developed compared to developing countries. As it is characterized by frequent recurrences, bladder cancer represents one of the most costly malignancies to health care systems owing to the requirement for intensive surveillance with cystoscopies and urinary cytologies, as well as frequent tumor resections under anesthesia.[9–11] Clinically, most patients with bladder cancer present with dysuria and hematuria.[12] After cystoscopy and biopsy evaluation, two distinct superficial (noninvasive) type lesions have been described: low-grade neoplasms, which are always

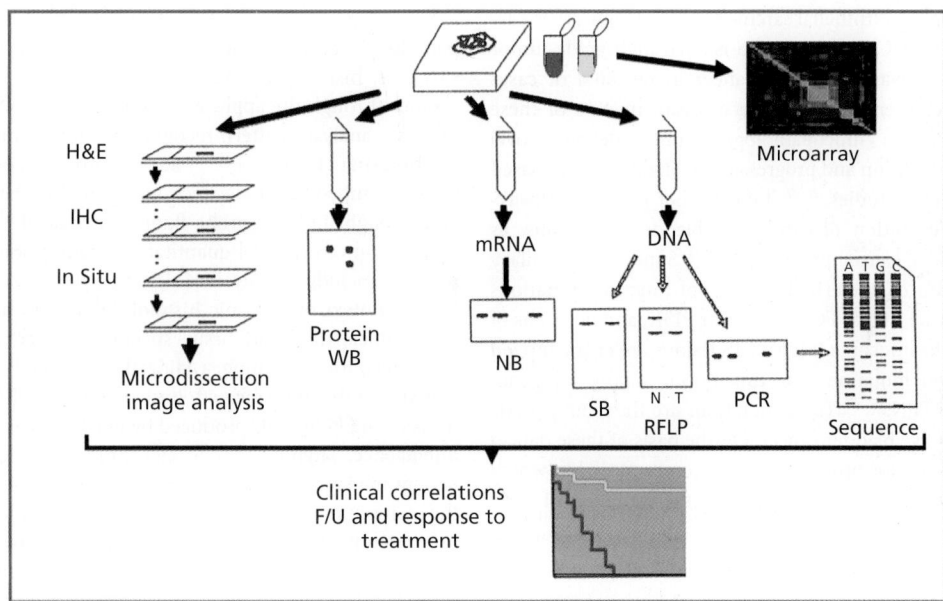

Figure 3 Molecular pathology. Integration of histological, immunochemical, and genetic approaches defines the nature of molecular profiling. Phenotype and genotype are integrated using low- and high-throughput technologies, including histology, protein studies, and nucleic acid analyses. The use of microarray technologies allows the interrogation of multiple analytes on a single assay. H&E: hematoxylin and eosin stain; IHC: immunohistochemistry; WB: western blot; NB: northern blot; SB: southern blot; PCR: polymerase chain reaction; RFLP: restriction fragment length polymorphism; F/U: follow-up.

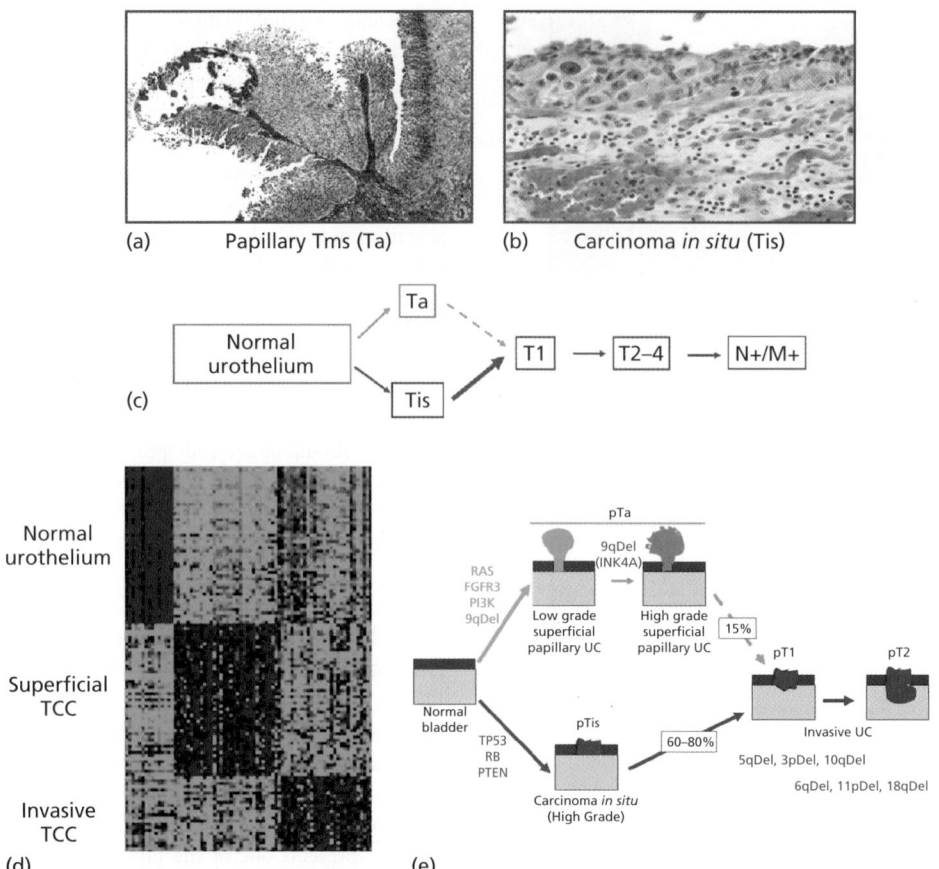

Figure 4 (a–e) A molecular approach to disease classification: bladder cancer as a model. Bladder tumors present as initial clinical entities as either papillary noninvasive (Ta) tumors that tend to recur but not to progress to invasion, or noninvasive dysplastic carcinoma *in situ* (Tis) lesions that tend to invade and progress to a clinical aggressive disease and, ultimately, metastasis spread. Multiple technologies, including expression profiling, reveal also a two-stage molecular classification, namely superficial and invasive bladder cancer. Superficial papillary bladder tumors are characterized by mutations affecting oncogenes (e.g., H-RAS, FGFR3, and PI3K), and/or chromosome 9 (9q) deletions; while carcinoma *in situ* tumors are characterized by mutations affecting tumor suppressor genes (e.g., p53, RB, and PTEN).

papillary (Ta low-grade urothelial carcinomas), and high-grade carcinoma *in situ* (Tis or CIS) lesions. CIS is a flat high-grade tumor that progresses to invasive bladder cancer in 60–80% of cases within 5 years, representing the cause of death in 40% of these patients.[13–15] These two clinicopathological entities define a novel model for tumor initiation and progression of bladder cancer based on molecular genetic studies.[16–22] Two distinct genetic pathways characterize the evolution of early-stage bladder neoplasms, as well as later bladder cancer progression.[23,24] Superficial papillary bladder tumors are characterized by gain-of-function mutations affecting oncogenes H-RAS, FGFR3, and/or PI3K, and deletions of the long arm of chromosome 9 (9q). CIS lesions are characterized by loss-of-function mutations affecting tumor suppressor genes p53, RB, and/or PTEN.[25–40] These mutations are the main genetic precursors of invasive bladder cancer. On the basis of these data, a model for bladder tumor progression has been proposed in which two separate genetic pathways characterize the evolution of early bladder neoplasms (Figure 4).

Systems pathology and predictive oncology

Most diagnostic platforms are based on unidimensional tools, extracting morphological or biomarker information based usually on a particular technology. Systems pathology represents a novel, comprehensive approach to personalized medicine. "Systems pathology" can be defined as the platform that integrates clinical variables, histological and cellular features, as well as molecular profiles through the application of novel technologies in the areas of image analysis, pattern recognition, and quantitative biomarker multiplexing (Figure 5).[41–46] Such approach, from formalin-fixed paraffin-embedded tissue sections stained by hematoxylin–eosin and through antibody/probe-fluorescence-labeled analytes, enables conduction of cell-level quantitative imaging studies. Tumor phenotypes, including analysis of signaling pathways, can be evaluated in the context of dynamic histological studies using the patient's own clinical data and tissue specimens to construct a baseline characterization defining a clinical risk state.[42,44] The data generated can be transformed into actionable clinical options for decision-making tools produced by machine learning and artificial intelligence. Highly accurate algorithms of predictive nature for patient management can be generated to improve outcomes. After the computations are complete, the end result often renders a user-friendly report providing an individualized prediction for the patient's probability of experiencing a specific outcome over time. For example, in the case of prostate cancer, this can include predictions of the time to disease recurrence and of clinical failure after radical prostatectomy.[45,46] The systems pathology approach can be further illustrated using prostate cancer as a model. The diagnosis and staging of prostate cancer has become increasingly

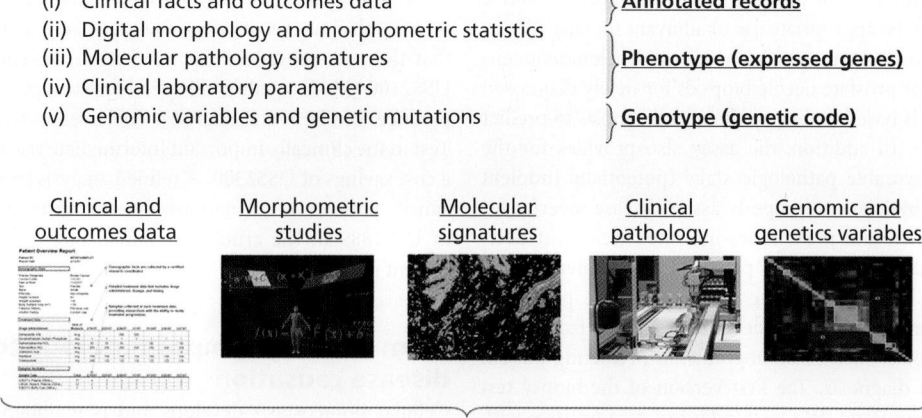

(i)   Clinical facts and outcomes data   } **Annotated records**
(ii) Digital morphology and morphometric statistics
(iii) Molecular pathology signatures   } **Phenotype (expressed genes)**
(iv) Clinical laboratory parameters
(v)   Genomic variables and genetic mutations   } **Genotype (genetic code)**

| Clinical and outcomes data | Morphometric studies | Molecular signatures | Clinical pathology | Genomic and genetics variables |

Algorithm-based platform for the accurate diagnosis and better management of cancer patients, founded on tests of higher precision that render more efficient patient care.

Figure 5 Systems pathology. A novel diagnostic and predictive oncology platform integrating phenotype and genotype using artificial intelligence and algorithms.

problematic in recent years. As a result of widespread screening, the incidence of late-stage disease has declined dramatically. Furthermore, earlier diagnoses have led to a compression of clinical assessments, whereby approximately 85% of diagnosed patients are categorized as low or intermediate risk, categories where current risk stratification tools (e.g., Gleason score) are less well correlated with outcomes.[47–51] Given the current homogeneity in initial clinical impression, traditional diagnostics have left physicians without a reliable method of determining who will go on to develop life-threatening disease and who has indolent disease that will not exhibit symptoms or limit longevity. Part of the stratification problem rests with the limitations of the currently available tests. Prostate-specific antigen (PSA) is neither a very sensitive nor a very specific indicator for the presence of prostate cancer. PSA is also not very good at predicting clinically significant disease for the majority of patients. With earlier detection, significant problems arise surrounding the current Gleason grading systems that are subjective and lack reproducibility, specifically for diagnosing dominant high-grade Gleason 4 disease. Multiple prognostic features can be discordant when reviewed as a group. For example, a patient can have a high PSA but a "low-risk" Gleason score (e.g., six or less). In addition, a large subjective component exists in defining surgical margin status. There is a significant clinical need to incorporate additional quantitative, objective measures that are derived from the analysis of an individual

patient's tissue specimen to provide a personalized prediction of risk (Figure 6).

The first version of a precision pathology platform was aimed at risk evaluation after surgical removal of the prostate gland affected by prostatic carcinoma.[45,46,52] This "Post-Prostatectomy" assay uses prostatectomy tissue to predict which patients are likely to have either disease progression, which reflects on the aggressive nature of the disease, or biochemical recurrence (through PSA detection and rising PSA) within 5 years after surgery. Such an assay assists physicians to properly assess the risk of disease progression postradical prostatectomy by identifying a baseline objective phenotype that can be used to guide potential future treatment. The assay was developed using a cohort of 758 patients from Memorial Sloan-Kettering Cancer Center, New York. The predictive models in this assay outperformed independent clinical factors and other common postsurgical risk factors such as positive surgical margins, extracapsular extension, as well as integrative nomograms in predicting patient progression postsurgery. The postoperative assay added significant biometric information to standard of care features with improved risk stratification accuracy [hazard ratio (HR) 11.4, concordance index (CI) 0.84, $P < 0.0001$]. After radical prostatectomy, the postprostatectomy assay yields a personalized risk assessment report that (1) provides more information on the risk of serious disease progression for patients experiencing a biochemical recurrence; (2) predicts serious disease progression and

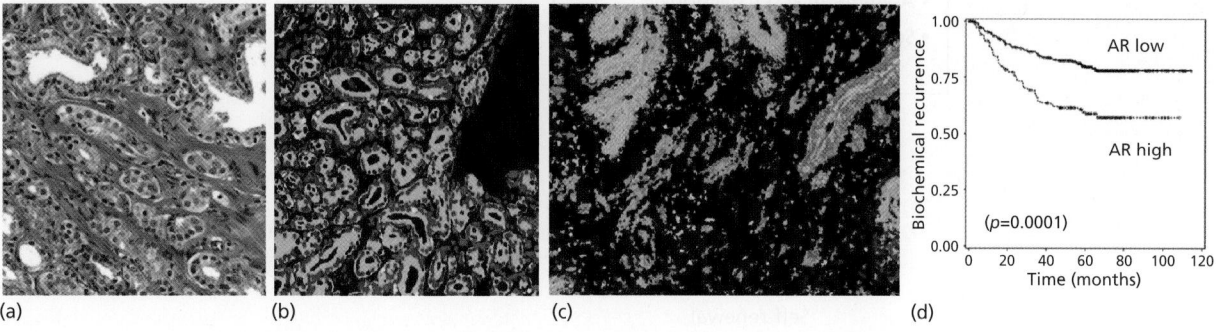

Figure 6 (a–d) An integrated system approach for outcome prediction: prostate cancer as a model. Digital conversion of hematoxylin and eosin stain tissue sections (a) into morphometric images that allows quantification of microanatomical features (e.g., number of glands) (b). Protein multiplexing using antibodies to clinical relevant biomarkers (e.g., androgen receptor or AR, proliferation index by Ki67 analysis) (c) allows quantitation of biological markers and stratification of patients in clinically significant groups, such as prostate cancer patients with low versus high AR levels.

PSA recurrence at the time of surgery; and (3) supports objective decision making on the appropriate use of adjuvant therapy.[45,46,52]

Following the prostatectomy model, a second development centered on an assay for prostate needle biopsies for newly diagnosed patients.[53] The test is based on biopsy tissue at diagnosis to predict disease progression. In addition, the assay also provides for the recognition of a favorable pathologic stage (potentially indolent disease). It helps physicians to properly assess disease severity for newly diagnosed men and make more-informed treatment decisions. The test was developed on 1027 patients from an international multi-institutional cohort of leading institutions. The predictive models in this assay outperform independent clinical factors and other integrative tools, such as nomograms, in predicting patient risk at the time of diagnosis. The first version of the biopsy test added important biometric data to standard of care features with significant risk stratification accuracy (HR 3.47, CI 0.73, $P < 0.001$). This test allows the treating physician to apply appropriate treatment paradigms to individual patients. At diagnosis, the biopsy test provides physicians with objective, actionable information that adds significantly to the clinical information currently used to assess risk. In this context, it can assist the urologist in (1) predicting disease progression after definitive treatment (e.g., prostatectomy); (2) making objective, informed treatment decisions; (3) identifying high-risk patients presenting as lower risk; (4) re-classifying clinically ambiguous intermediate-risk patients as either high or low risk; (5) helping to alleviate some of the anxiety of the unknown for patients. For patients who proceed to radiotherapy, the initial biopsy sample and associated Gleason score will be the only "tissue view" of their disease. There will never be the opportunity to evaluate the resected prostate. The assay provides an additional and unique window on the status of the prostate and associated tumor. Of note, exploratory validation of the assay in a small cohort treated by radiotherapy yielded strong results. In addition, low-risk patients considering active surveillance/watchful waiting can use the biopsy results to determine if they should avoid this conservative regimen and instead proceed with treatment. Of particular significance are the promising results of the assay in a preliminary active surveillance population. Briefly, a well-characterized cohort ($n = 181$) of men enrolled in an active surveillance program was studied using the Needle Biopsy assay and found that the integrated analytics successfully predicted time to treatment (e.g., exit from active surveillance) with a CI of 0.65 and HR of 3.6 ($P < 0.0001$).

As a corollary of the above-referred studies and developments, pharmacoeconomic analyses were performed revealing that the post-prostatectomy test had a cost-effectiveness ratio of US\$2100/QALY (quality-adjusted life years) compared with clinical practice. Similarly, an initial cost-effectiveness analysis of the Biopsy Test in the clinically important intermediate risk population yielded a cost savings of US\$2300. A refined analysis based on 233 prostate cancer patients of 23 nationwide urologists yielded cost savings of US\$1889 in the crucial combined intermediate and high-risk patient population.[54–56]

From treating symptomatology to treating disease causation

Cellular homeostasis develops and is maintained by the coordinated balance of four critical programs: proliferation (cell-cycle division), differentiation, senescence, and cell death (apoptosis).[4,7] Tissue renewal has been postulated to be regulated by a balance of these programs guided by a tissue-specific stem cell compartment.[57–62] Many characteristic properties have been attributed to stem cells. There are two cardinal features: (1) stem cells are capable of self-renewal, producing new stem cells through cell division and (2) stem cells are multipotent progenitors that can give rise to differentiated transient amplifying cells through asymmetrical cell division. Of course, these cells also display an undifferentiated phenotype (Figure 7).

Cancer is a term used to define a group of diseases characterized by unregulated cell proliferation, aberrant differentiation, and defective apoptosis. Two major hypotheses regarding tumor initiation have been postulated: the "stochastic model" which predicts that every neoplastic cell can generate an entirely new tumor; and the "cancer stem cell (CSC) model" which proposes that tumor cells exist in a hierarchical state and that only a few stem cells possess tumor-initiating potential (Figure 8).[58–62] Regarding the latter model, all neoplastic diseases may have in common an initial transforming event that is manifold in nature (e.g., viral infection, chemical carcinogens, and spontaneous mutation) that impacts this unique somatic tissue cell, the so-called adult stem cell. These transforming events are believed to generate a CSC that is responsible for tumor initiation and the hierarchical organization of cancer. Supporting this hypothesis is the fact that cancer is a clonal disease, meaning that it develops as the progeny evolves from a single cell.

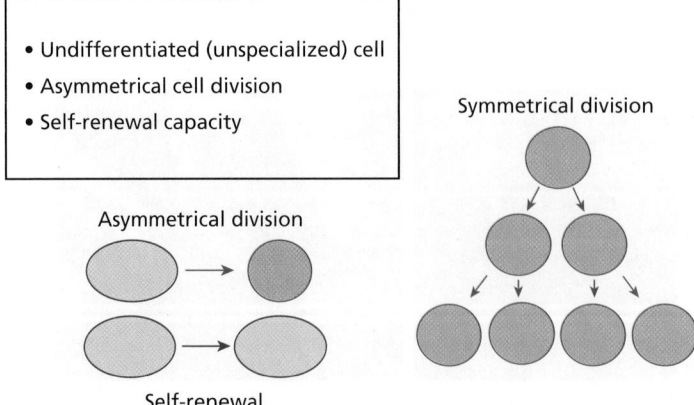

Figure 7 Characteristics of stem cells versus differentiated cells. Essential characteristics of stem cells include an undifferentiated phenotype, asymmetrical cell division, and self-renewal capacity. Differentiated cells divide through symmetrical division, also known as mitosis. The originating cell after completion of asymmetrical cell division or self-renewal persists and continues its physiological functions; while the originating cell in mitosis disappears through nuclear division and cytokinesis producing two identical daughter cells.

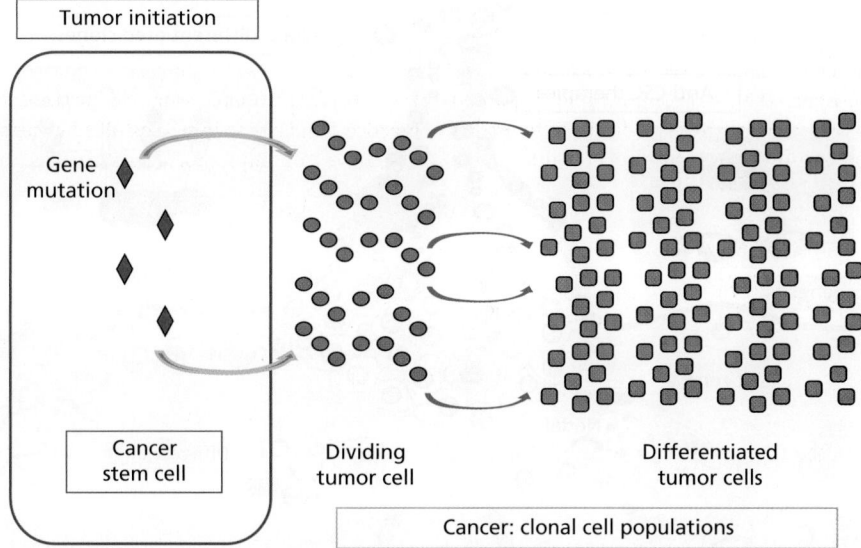

Figure 8 Cancer stem cell model of tumorigenesis and tumor progression. It is our working hypothesis that neoplastic transformation initiates in a somatic tissue stem cell capable of sustaining genetic manipulation, based on down-regulated apoptotic programs and an HLA-negative phenotype that favors escaping immune surveillance. This transformed cancer stem cell undergoes self-renewal as well as asymmetrical cell division, producing differentiated clones that rapidly expand, creating heterogeneous populations of differentiated tumor cells.

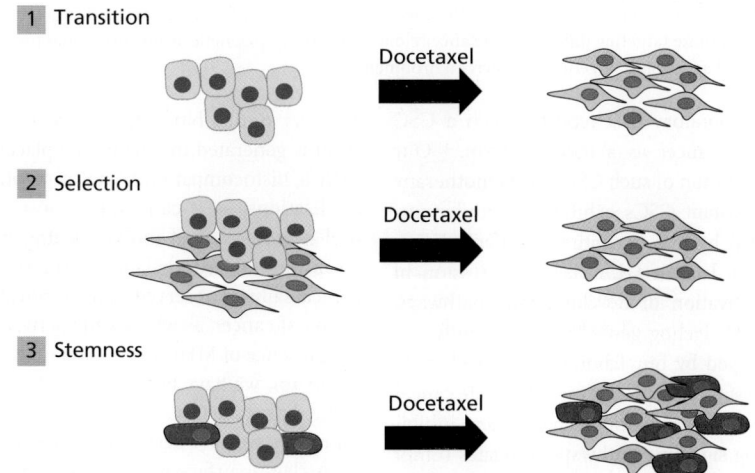

Figure 9 Cancer stem cell and chemotherapy resistance. Different models have been postulated to address chemoresistance. The transition model proposes that a state transition develops whereby sensitive tumor changes into a resistant clonogenic neoplasm. The selection model follows a Darwinian hypothesis and proposes that heterogeneous subpopulations exist in the primary, untreated tumor and that while sensitive clones die, resistant clones survive and expand. The stemness model proposes that cancer stem cells represent a small subpopulation of the tumor and that such cancer stem cells are nonresponsive to most conventional agents, and while sensitive cells die, the cancer stem cell compartment expands through self-renewal and new resistant clones to the agent are generated through asymmetrical cell division.

The CSC hypothesis posits that in addition to CSC, tumors comprise a small population of transit amplifying clonogens and large sets of differentiated malignant cells (Figure 9).[62] CSCs, like their normal stem cell counterparts, are characterized by a specific set of properties that include an undifferentiated phenotype capable of displaying asymmetrical cell division, resulting in self-renewal and production of differentiated clonogens, thus contributing to tumor heterogeneity. In addition, CSCs have been postulated to be refractory to most standard chemotherapy treatments, although such treatments frequently result in eradication of the fastest dividing cells, an early tumor response, but not in CSC depletion.[62] Such a model could explain why standard human cancer chemotherapy frequently results in initial tumor shrinkage, although most cancers eventually recur owing to regeneration by surviving CSCs.

It is important to define and differentiate "resistance" versus "nonresponse" phenotypes. Resistance in the context of chemotherapeutic resistance is an acquired phenomenon after overcoming the sensitivity state. However, nonresponse is a *de novo* phenomenon that does not imply a preceding responder phenotype. CSC expresses high levels of export pumps of the multidrug resistance protein (MRP), including the multidrug resistance 1 (MDR1) or P-glycoprotein. In addition, the mechanism by which asymmetrical division proceeds is not well defined, but there is documented *in vitro* evidence that asymmetrical division occurs even in the presence of certain conventional mitotic inhibitors, such as taxanes. Taken together, these mechanisms can confer a nonresponding phenotype to CSC enabling survival despite exposure to certain chemotherapeutic agents. These viable CSC then produce resistant clones that eventually preclude successful

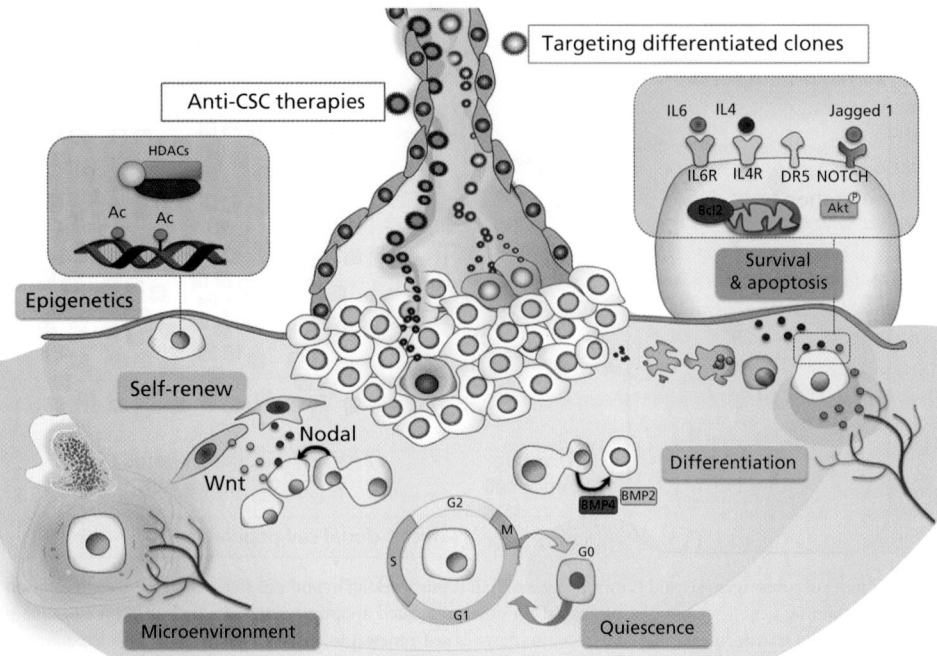

Figure 10 A working model for targeting symptomatology and causation. This model postulates that in order to eradicate cancer two different subpopulations need to be targeted: the differentiated tumor clones and the cancer stem cells. This figure illustrates distinct approaches to combine anticancer stem cell (anti-CSC) therapies with those targeting differentiated cancer clones, including epigenetic agents that could turn an undifferentiated clone into a differentiated clone, as well as novel agents and targeting the microenvironment.

treatment (Figure 9). Our laboratory first reported such a CSC subpopulation using prostate cancer as a model system.[63] Our study also revealed the contribution of such CSCs to chemotherapy resistance. These therapy-resistant CSCs exhibit an undifferentiated phenotype characterized by loss of epithelial differentiation markers (e.g., cytokeratins[18]), lack of HLA class I expression in the cell membrane, and activation of developmental pathways, programmed by Notch and Hedgehog genes.[63,64] Importantly, the experimental models developed by our laboratory enabled us to isolate and identify for the first time CSCs in clinical prostate cancer tissues and to elucidate a novel therapeutic strategy where inhibition of Notch and Hedgehog signaling pathways abrogates tumor relapse after conventional therapy using patient-derived tumor xenografts in an immunodeficient murine model. More recently, through the interrogation of public patient-derived data sets with the gene expression profiles of chemotherapy-resistant CSC models, we found that the transcription factor GATA2 regulates an IGF2-driven polykinase program that contributes to chemotherapy resistance and tumorigenicity in lethal prostate cancer.[65] Notably, in this study, we generated for the first time patient-derived xenografts from circulating tumor cells that facilitated the preclinical validation of a promising new treatment combination (docetaxel or cabazitaxel plus a dual IGF1R/INSR inhibitor) for prostate cancer. The initial prostate cancer translational model has been extended to other cancers, including breast and colon carcinomas, as well as gliomas and sarcomas.

The fact that these CSC generically exhibit a negative histocompatibility signature is consistent with our previous report that single cells and clusters of human tumor cells that lacked HLA class I expression, correlated with aggressive behavior locally and metastatic capacity.[64] Furthermore, an HLA-negative phenotype is also shared by embryonic stem cells. Human preimplantation embryos are reported to be HLA class I and class II negative. This phenomenon precludes rejection because of expression of paternal

antigens, until a blood-tissue barrier develops, which in this situation is generated in part by the placenta. In the context of CSCs, such a histocompatibility negative phenotype has major clinical implications, as it can explain host mutation permissiveness, as well as tumor spread and metastatogenic capabilities, as CSC could escape immune surveillance. Furthermore, it may be linked to some clinical failures observed in the innovative immunotherapeutic targeting of cancer, as when using activated T lymphocytes for which the presence of MHC expression on the target cells is critical.

In sum, we have been able to identify and characterize a newly defined prostate CSC in human cancer cell lines and tissue samples. Moreover, we have been able to isolate this population of cells using HLA class I surface marker and demonstrated its tumor initiating capacity. Further, we show that similar CSC populations are present in human breast, colon, lung, and bladder carcinomas, as well as in human sarcomas and glioblastomas, a fact that gives further universality to the findings. The discovery of this human CSC has important clinical implications in diagnostic and predictive laboratory assays, as well as for development of novel therapeutic strategies targeting both the CSC and the differentiated clones (Figure 10).

References

1 Virchow R. *Cellular Pathology*. London: John Churchill; 1860.

2 Rosai J. *Guiding the Surgeon's Hand, The History of American Surgical Pathology*. Washington, D.C.: American Registry of Pathology; 1997.

3 Cordon-Cardo C. Applications of molecular diagnostics: solid tumor genetics can determine clinical treatment protocols. *Mod Pathol*. 2001;**14**:254–257.

4 Cordon-Cardo C. Mutation of cell cycle regulators: biological and clinical implications for human neoplasias. *Am J Pathol*. 1995;**147**:545–560.

5 Donovan MJ, Cordon-Cardo C. Predicting high-risk disease using tissue biomarkers. *Curr Opin Urol*. 2013;**23**:245–251.

6 Clark WH. Tumour progression and the nature of cancer. *Br J Cancer*. 1991;**64**:631–644.

7 Hanahan D, Weinberg RA. The hallmarks of cancer. *Cell*. 2000;**100**:57–70.

8 Vousden KH, Prives C. Blinded by the light: the growing complexity of p53. *Cell*. 2009;**137**:413–431.

9 Ferlay J, Soerjomataram I, Ervik M, et al. *Cancer Incidence and Mortality Worldwide: IARC CancerBase No. 11*. International Agency for Research on Cancer: Lyon, France; 2013.

10 Siegel R, Ma J, Zou Z, Jemal A. Cancer statistics, 2014. *CA Cancer J Clin*. 2014;**64**:9–29.

11 Ye F, Wang L, Castillo-Martin M, et al. Biomarkers for bladder cancer management: present and future. *Am J Clin Exp Urol*. 2014;**2**:1–14.

12 Holmang S, Hedelin H, Anderstrom C, Johansson SL. The relationship among multiple recurrences, progression and prognosis of patients with stages Ta and T1 transitional cell cancer of the bladder followed for at least 20 years. *J Urol*. 1995;**153**:1823–1826.

13 Botteman MF, Pashos CL, Redaelli A, Laskin B, Hauser R. The health economics of bladder cancer: a comprehensive review of the published literature. *Pharmacoeconomics*. 2003;**21**:1315–1330.

14 Cordon-Cardo C, Cote RJ, Sauter G. Genetic and molecular markers of urothelial premalignancy and malignancy. *Scand J Urol Nephrol*. 2000;**34(Suppl. 205)**:82–93.

15 Eble JN, Sauter G, Epstein JI, Sesterhenn IA. *WHO Classification of Tumors: Pathology and Genetics of Tumours of the Urinary System and Male Genital Organs*. Lyon: IARC Press; 2004.

16 Presti JC, Reuter VE, Galan T, Fair WR, Cordon-Cardo C. Molecular genetic alterations in superficial and locally advanced human bladder cancer. *Cancer Res*. 1991;**51**:5405–5409.

17 Dalbagni G, Presti J, Reuter V, Fair WR, Cordon-Cardo C. Genetic alterations in bladder cancer. *Lancet*. 1993;**324**:469–471.

18 Dalbagni G, Cordon-Cardo C, Reuter V, Fair WR. Tumor suppressor gene alterations in bladder carcinoma: translational correlates to clinical practice. *Surg Oncol Clin N Am*. 1995;**4**:231–240.

19 Sanchez-Carbayo M, Socci N, Charytonowicz E, Prystowski M, Childs G, Cordon-Cardo C. Molecular profiling of bladder cancer using cDNA microarrays: defining histogenesis and biological phenotypes. *Cancer Res*. 2002;**62**:6973–6980.

20 Sanchez-Carbayo M, Socci ND, Lozano JJ, Haab BB, Cordon-Cardo C. Profiling bladder cancer using targeted antibody arrays. *Am J Pathol*. 2006;**168**:93–103.

21 Sanchez-Carbayo M, Socci ND, Lozano JJ, Saint F, Cordon-Cardo C. Defining molecular profiles of poor outcome in patients with invasive bladder cancer using oligonucleotide microarrays. *J Clin Oncol*. 2006;**24**:778–789.

22 Jia AY, Castillo-Martin M, Domingo-Domenech J, et al. A common MicroRNA signature consisting of miR-133a, miR-139-3p, and miR-142-3p clusters bladder carcinoma in situ with normal umbrella cells. *Am J Pathol*. 2013;**182**:1171–1179.

23 Sanchez-Carbayo M, Cordon-Cardo C. Molecular alterations associated with bladder cancer progression. *Semin Oncol*. 2007;**34**:75–84.

24 Castillo-Martin M, Domingo-Domenech J, Karni-Schmidt O, Matos T, Cordon-Cardo C. Molecular pathways of urothelial development and bladder tumorigenesis. *Urol Oncol*. 2010;**28**:401–408.

25 Fradet Y, Cordon-Cardo C, Thomson T, et al. Cell surface antigens of human bladder cancer defined by mouse monoclonal antibodies. *Proc Natl Acad Sci USA*. 1984;**81**:224–228.

26 Fradet Y, Cordon-Cardo C, Whitmore WF, Melamed MR, Old LJ. Cell surface antigens of human bladder tumors: definition of tumor subsets by monoclonal antibodies and correlation with growth characteristics. *Cancer Res*. 1986;**46**:5183–5188.

27 Cordon-Cardo C, Wartinger D, Petrylak D, et al. Altered expression of the retinoblastoma gene product as predictor of outcome in bladder cancer. *J Natl Cancer Inst*. 1992;**84**:1251–1256.

28 Sarkis A, Dalbagni G, Cordon-Cardo C, et al. Detection of p53 mutations in superficial (T1) bladder carcinomas as a marker of disease progression. *J Natl Cancer Inst*. 1993;**85**:53–59.

29 Orlow I, Lianes P, Lacombe L, Dalbagni G, Reuter VE, Cordon-Cardo C. Chromosome 9 deletions and microsatellite alterations in human bladder tumors. *Cancer Res*. 1994;**54**:2848–2851.

30 Sarkis AS, Dalbagni G, Cordon-Cardo C, et al. Association of p53 nuclear overexpression and tumor progression in carcinoma in situ of the bladder. *J Urol*. 1994;**152**:388–392.

31 Lianes P, Orlow I, Zhang ZZ, et al. Altered patterns of MDM2 and TP53 expression in human bladder cancer. *J Natl Cancer Inst*. 1994;**86**:1325–1330.

32 Gruis NA, Weaver-Feldhaus J, Liu Q, et al. Genetic evidence in melanoma and bladder cancers that p16 and p53 function in separate pathways of tumor suppression. *Am J Pathol*. 1995;**146**:1199–1206.

33 Orlow I, Lacombe L, Hannon GJ, et al. Deletion of the p16 and p15 genes in human bladder tumors. *J Natl Cancer Inst*. 1995;**87**:1524–1529.

34 Cordon-Cardo C, Zhang ZF, Dalbagni G, et al. Cooperative effects of p53 and pRB alterations in primary superficial bladder tumors. *Cancer Res*. 1997;**57**:1217–1221.

35 Orlow I, LaRue H, Osman I, et al. Deletions of the INK4A gene in superficial bladder tumors: association with recurrence. *Am J Pathol*. 1999;**155**:105–113.

36 Mo L, Zheng X, Huang HY, et al. Hyperactivation of Ha-ras oncogene, but not Ink4a/Arf deficiency, triggers bladder tumorigenesis. *J Clin Invest*. 2007;**117**:314–325.

37 Puzio-Kuter SA, Castillo-Martin M, Shen TH, et al. Inactivation of p53 and Pten promotes invasive bladder cancer. *Genes Dev*. 2009;**23**:675–680.

38 Karni-Schmidt O, Castillo-Martin M, HuaiShen T, et al. Distinct expression profiles of p63 variants during urothelial development and bladder cancer progression. *Am J Pathol*. 2011;**178**:1350–1360.

39 Jia AY, Castillo-Martin M, Bonal DM, Sánchez-Carbayo M, Silva JM, Cordon-Cardo C. MicroRNA-126 inhibits invasion in bladder cancer via regulation of ADAM9. *Br J Cancer*. 2014;**110**:2945–2954.

40 Gaya JM, López-Martínez JM, Karni-Schmidt O, et al. ΔNp63 expression is a protective factor of progression in clinical high grade T1 bladder cancer. *J Urol*. 2015;**193**:1144–1150.

41 Donovan MJ, Costa J, Cordon-Cardo C. Systems pathology: a paradigm shift in the practice of diagnostic and predictive pathology. *Cancer*. 2009;**115**:3078–3084.

42 Capodieci P, Donovan M, Buchinsky H, et al. Gene expression profiling in single cells within tissues. *Nat Methods*. 2005;**2**:663–665.

43 Saidi O, Cordon-Cardo C, Costa J. Technology insights: will systems pathology replace the pathologist? *Nat Clin Pract Urol*. 2007;**4**:39–45.

44 Donovan MJ, Cordon-Cardo C. Genomic analysis in active surveillance: predicting high-risk disease using tissue biomarkers. *Curr Opin Urol*. 2014;**24**:303–310.

45 Cordon-Cardo C, Kotsianti A, Verbel D, et al. Improved prediction of prostate cancer recurrence through systems pathology. *J Clin Invest*. 2007;**117**:1876–1883.

46 Donovan MJ, Hamann S, Clayton M, et al. A systems pathology approach for the prediction of prostate cancer progression after radical prostatectomy. *J Clin Oncol*. 2008;**26**:3923–3929.

47 Shariat S, Roehrborn C. Using biopsy to detect prostate cancer. *Rev Urol*. 2008;**10**:262–280.

48 Rosario D, Lane JA, Metcalfe C. Short term outcomes of prostate biopsy in men tested for cancer by prostate specific antigen: prospective evaluation within ProtecT study. *BMJ*. 2012;**344**:d7894.

49 Gonzalez CM, Averch T, Boyd LA. *AUA/SUNA White Paper on the Incidence, Prevention and Treatment of Complications Related to Prostate Needle Biopsy*. Linthicum, Maryland: American Urological Association; 2012.

50 Yaskiv O, George AK, Fakhoury M, et al. Improving detection of clinically significant prostate cancer: MRI/TRUS fusion-guided prostate biopsy. *J Urol*. 2014;**191**:1749–1754.

51 Miyake H, Fujisawa M. Prognostic prediction following radical prostatectomy for prostate cancer using conventional as well as molecular biological approaches. *Int J Urol*. 2013;**20**:301–311.

52 Donovan MJ, Khan FM, Powell D, et al. Postoperative systems models more accurately predict risk of significant disease progression than standard risk groups and a 10-year postoperative nomogram: potential impact on the receipt of adjuvant therapy after surgery. *BJU Int*. 2012;**109**:40–45.

53 Donovan MJ, Khan FM, Fernandez G, et al. Personalized prediction of tumor response and cancer progression on prostate needle biopsy. *J Urol*. 2009;**182**:125–132.

54 Zubek VB, Konski A. Cost effectiveness of risk-prediction tools in selecting patients for immediate post-prostatectomy treatment. *Mol Diagn Ther*. 2009;**13(1)**:31–47.

55 Zubek VB, Khan FM. *Cost-Minimization Analysis of Biopsy-based Risk Stratification Tools in Intermediate-risk Prostate Cancer Patients*. 15th Annual Meeting of ISPOR (International Society for Pharmacoeconomics and Outcomes Research). May, 2010.

56 Zubek VB, Khan FM, Karvir H. *Cost-Minimization Analysis of Biopsy-Based Risk Stratification Tools in Intermediate and High Risk Prostate Cancer Patients Based on Results from Physician Case Studies*. 16th Annual Meeting of ISPOR (International Society for Pharmacoeconomics and Outcomes Research). May, 2011.

57 Cordon-Cardo C. Cancer Stem Cells. *Ann Oncol*. 2010;**21**:93–94.

58 Dick JE. Stem cell concepts renew cancer research. *Blood*. 2008;**112**:4793–4807.

59 Magee JA, Piskounova E, Morrison SJ. Cancer stem cells: impact, heterogeneity, and uncertainty. *Cancer Cell*. 2012;**21**:283–296.

60 Valent P, Bonnet D, De Maria R, et al. Cancer stem cell definitions and terminology: the devil is in the details. *Nat Rev Cancer*. 2012;**12**:767–775.

61 Visvader JE, Lindeman GJ. Cancer stem cells: current status and evolving complexities. *Cell Stem Cell*. 2012;**10**:717–728.

62 Vidal SJ, Rodriguez-Bravo V, Galsky M, Cordon-Cardo C, Domingo-Domenech J. Targeting cancer stem cells to suppress acquired chemotherapy resistance. *Oncogene*. 2014;**33**:4451–4463.

63 Domingo-Domenech J, Vidal SJ, Rodriguez-Bravo V, et al. Suppression of acquired Docetaxel resistance in prostate cancer through depletion of Notch and Hedgehog dependent tumor initiating cells. *Cancer Cell*. 2012;**22**:373–388.

64 Cordon-Cardo C, Fuks Z, Eisenbach L, Feldman M. Expression of HLA-A,B,C antigens on primary and metastatic tumor cell populations of human carcinomas. *Cancer Res*. 1991;**51**:6372–6380.

65 Vidal SJ, Rodriguez-Bravo V, Quinn SA, et al. A targetable GATA2-IGF2 axis confers aggressiveness in lethal prostate cancer. *Cancer Cell*. 2015;**27**:223–239.

40 Molecular diagnostics in cancer

Roshni D. Kalachand, MBBCh, MD ▪ Bryan T. Hennessy, MD ▪ Robert C. Bast Jr., MD ▪ Gordon B. Mills, MD, PhD

Overview

Molecular diagnostics refers to the use of molecular alterations that are associated with cancers to facilitate detection, diagnosis, monitoring, and/or treatment. Molecular biomarkers have often been studied in cancer tissue but potentially can be assayed in readily available patient samples (saliva, sputum, blood, urine, and feces), thereby minimizing the need for invasive biopsies. Traditional blood biomarkers—CEA (carcinoembryonic antigen), PSA (prostate specific antigen), hCG (human chorionic gonadotropin), AFP (alpha-fetoprotein), CA125 and CA15-3—have been used to monitor response to treatment and to detect disease recurrence. Their clinical utility often depends on the availability of effective treatment for residual or recurrent disease. Early detection requires biomarkers with high sensitivity to detect preclinical and ideally premetastatic disease, as well as high specificity to permit efficient, cost-effective screening. Two-stage strategies are often most promising where rising biomarkers trigger imaging or results of imaging are combined with biomarkers to improve positive predictive value. Cancer-specific genomic aberrations have been identified which guide therapy and predict outcomes in subgroups of patients. Trastuzumab has dramatically altered the outcomes of patients with *HER2* amplified breast cancers, as have EGFR (epidermal growth factor receptor) inhibitors in the treatment of metastatic *EGFR* mutation positive non-small-cell lung cancer. As single driver gene aberrations frequently are not sufficient to predict therapeutic responses, gene signatures and multimarker panels incorporating DNA, RNA, and/or protein aberrations are being evaluated as potential effective biomarkers. A panel of multiple biomarkers (Onco-Type Dx®) has proven useful in predicting the need for chemotherapy in addition to hormonal therapy in hormone receptor-positive breast cancer. As targeted therapies are becoming a reality, so is the predictable emergence of resistance to these therapies, often occurring through gene amplification, secondary mutations, or reactivation of signaling mechanisms downstream from the targeted molecular aberration. The search for molecular biomarkers, the so-called companion diagnostics, predictive of first-line therapy resistance and second-line therapy response, is now inherent to targeted drug development. However, these emerging integrative technologies have yet to benefit the majority of patients with cancer. Interpretation of the extensive number of aberrations identified by high-throughput technologies, availability of adequate high-quality tissue, cost, and clinical validation remain significant challenges to developing and implementing effective biomarkers. Strategic use of bioinformatics, international collaboration, development of prospectively collected clinically annotated biobanks containing fresh frozen tissue, and clinical validation in large prospective data sets key to bringing useful molecular biomarkers into clinical practice.

Introduction

Molecular diagnostics involves the use of molecular biomarkers (Box 1) to detect, diagnose, or monitor cancer, as well as to estimate patient prognosis or to predict therapeutic interventions likely to benefit the patient. Ultimately, the development of molecular diagnostics is expected to facilitate the individualization of cancer treatment with the goal of maximizing treatment benefit for individual cancer patients, while minimizing toxicity. Important progress has already been made in developing and applying molecular diagnostics to clinical management. This chapter provides an overview of the current status of molecular diagnostics for cancer. It will also review potential approaches to the integration of biomarker-driven approaches into the future development of individualized cancer therapies, as well as new techniques and likely problems and hurdles that will need to be addressed and overcome.

> **Box 1** Cancer biomarkers
>
> A cancer biomarker includes any characteristic of tumor cells, stroma, normal tissues, or body fluids that aid in detecting, diagnosing, monitoring, defining prognosis, or predicting response or toxicity from treatment. Thus biomarkers include alterations in DNA, RNA, protein, carbohydrate, lipid, or metabolites as well as biophysical characteristics of tumor cells, the tumor microenvironment, or the host genome and response. Pathologic examination and imaging techniques have provided conventional tumor histologic and staging information that have guided patient management to date. However, these approaches do not consider the full inter- and intratumoral heterogeneity of cancers at the molecular level. Individualization of screening, prevention, and treatment should be substantially improved by considering the profile of multiple molecular biomarkers across different platforms.

Molecular biomarkers for screening and early detection of cancer

Early detection implies the diagnosis of cancer at its earliest stage of development. It is essential that early diagnosis occur at a stage of tumor development where cure can be achieved with currently available therapy. Screening strategies generally require high sensitivity and specificity. Early detection could be facilitated by identifying individuals at high risk for developing specific cancers, decreasing the hurdle of specificity by assessing higher risk individuals.[1-4] Screening is a term used for approaches that facilitate detection of tumors at an early curable stage. Effective cancer screening strategies must be cost effective, acceptable to patients and associated with limited morbidity from both the intervention and from false positive results. As screening of the entire population is seldom practicable, guidelines for patient risk assessment are often necessary to appropriately target approaches to prevent and diagnose cancer early. As our understanding of cancer's molecular heterogeneity advances, novel criteria can be added to the conventional criteria that describe an ideal screening biomarker (Box 2). Thus, as most cancer treatments are effective in only a minority of cancer patients, future useful screening

Holland-Frei Cancer Medicine, Ninth Edition. Edited by Robert C. Bast Jr., Carlo M. Croce, William N. Hait, Waun Ki Hong, Donald W. Kufe, Martine Piccart-Gebhart, Raphael E. Pollock, Ralph R. Weichselbaum, Hongyang Wang, and James F. Holland.
© 2017 John Wiley & Sons, Inc. ISBN: 978-1-118-93469-2

biomarkers could also guide appropriate therapies in individual patients.

Emerging radiologic and endoscopic techniques afford increasingly more sensitive noninvasive procedures for early detection of small tumors. Despite some controversy, low-dose computed tomography appears to detect early lung cancer and decrease lung cancer-related mortality in people at high risk from cigarette smoking, in contrast to routine chest films.[5] Similarly, the addition of annual bilateral breast magnetic resonance imaging to annual mammography as an early breast cancer detection strategy for *BRCA1/2* gene mutation carriers could decrease the use of bilateral prophylactic mastectomies to reduce the risk of breast cancer in these patients.[6,7] In colon cancer, the ability of colonoscopy to visualize small lesions throughout the entire colon has made this the screening method of choice over double contrast barium enemas. Nonetheless, such tools depend on a tumor's anatomical features for detection, whereas molecular markers could identify cancer at an early and perhaps premalignant stage, before anatomical detection. Moreover, biomarkers can be detected in bodily fluids (urine, feces, and blood), avoiding potential patient discomfort from endoscopy preparation as well as potentially harmful ionizing radiation from radiologic imaging.

Screening is generally applied to those populations where there is conclusive evidence of an associated survival benefit and, to assure cost effectiveness, where the cancer is a common cause of mortality. As an example, although controversial, most regulatory agencies in the United States recommend annual mammography for women aged 40 years and older.[8] Alternatively, risk assessment can be used to stratify select patients to screening or, if the risk is high enough, prevention. This way, the exposure of large numbers of individuals to false positive screening tests and unnecessary biopsies is avoided while maintaining a high cancer detection rate in at-risk patients. Currently, risk assessment is based largely on patient-specific factors, including age, family history, and social factors (e.g., tobacco use), as is the case in lung cancer screening. However, some molecular markers, such as mutations in cancer predisposition genes (e.g.,

BRCA1, BRCA2, and p53), have demonstrated utility in the identification of at-risk populations.

Molecular biomarkers in current clinical practice for screening, prevention and early detection

Prostate cancer

Prostate-specific antigen (PSA) is normally present in the blood at very low levels ranging between 0 and 4.0 ng/mL. Increased PSA levels can be associated with an underlying prostate cancer. Serum PSA measurement for prostate cancer screening is controversial, despite widespread use.[9] Up to 15% of prostate cancers can occur in the absence of an elevated PSA. PSA levels can be elevated due to prostate infection, irritation, benign prostatic hypertrophy, or recent ejaculation. Thus, PSA is not an adequately sensitive or specific marker for prostate cancer screening. PSA screening can lead to a high rate of unnecessary biopsies, over-diagnosis and overtreatment, resulting in morbidity. Both prostatectomy and radiotherapy can be associated with impotence and incontinence. Patients diagnosed with less aggressive (Gleason score < 7) prostate cancer can survive decades with their cancer, often dying from comorbid diseases. PSA screening in men over the age of 50 years can confer up to a 20% decrease in prostate-cancer-specific mortality, although this may or may not translate into a decrease in overall mortality, judging from large multicenter trials.[10,11] In the past, PSA screening has been recommended for men older than 50 years with an expected life expectancy of 10 years or more, following discussion with the patient about screening-associated risks.[12] The United States Preventive Health Task Force now recommends against using PSA for screening.[13] The American Urological Association (AUA) has more nuanced age-dependent guidelines.[14] The AUA recommends against PSA screening for men under age 40. Between age 40 and 54, PSA screening is recommended only for African-American men or men with a positive family history conferring increased risk. For men ages 55–69, the benefits of preventing prostate cancer mortality in one man for every 1000 men screened over a decade must be weighed against the known harms associated with screening and treatment. PSA screening is not recommended for men over 70 years.

Most PSA in the blood is bound to serum proteins. A small amount is not, and is called free PSA, an isoform of which, [-2]proPSA, is highly associated with prostate cancer. The combination of PSA, free PSA, and [-2]proPSA in a single score, the Prostate Health Index (PHI), shows increased sensitivity over PSA screening alone in men with PSA levels between 4 and 10 ng/mL but has not been widely adopted as a prostate cancer screening tool.[15]

Ovarian cancer

The relatively low prevalence of ovarian cancer—1 : 2500 in the United States—means that strategies for early ovarian cancer detection must have relatively high sensitivity (>75%) for preclinical disease and an extremely high specificity (99.6%) to attain a positive predictive value of at least 10%, that is, 10 operations for each case of ovarian cancer detected. Serum CA125 has received the most attention but lacks the sensitivity or specificity to function as a stand-alone screening test. Two-stage screening strategies promise to be more effective, where increasing levels of serum biomarkers over time prompt transvaginal sonography (TVS) to detect lesions that require laparotomy. With annual determination of CA125 in women at average risk for ovarian cancer, a computer algorithm has been developed to determine deviations from each woman's own baseline. If CA125 increases significantly, TVS is performed and if imaging is abnormal, laparotomy is undertaken. If the CA125 is unchanged, a woman returns in 1 year and if CA125 is mildly elevated, biomarker levels are obtained in 3 months. On the basis of this strategy, a study of more than 5000 healthy postmenopausal women coordinated by MD Anderson, performed 18 operations to detect 2 borderline and 10 invasive cancers with 75% in stage I or II.[16] No more than three operations were required to detect each cancer. A much larger randomized trial involving 200,000 in the United Kingdom is powered to test the impact of this strategy on survival and mortality. Data from the first 2 years of accrual suggest that a two-stage strategy could increase the fraction of disease detected in early stage.[17] Using deviations from each woman's baseline, rather than a single cutoff for CA125 alone, doubled the number of ovarian cancer cases detected.[18] Outcome of the study will be reported in the near future and could change practice, if positive. As only 80% of ovarian cancers express CA125, other markers will be required for early detection of all ovarian cancers. The development of technologies that measure multiple serum markers simultaneously, linked to the creation of statistical methods that enhance sensitivity without sacrificing specificity, hold great promise.

Cervical cancer

The establishment of national cervical cancer screening programs involving the detection and treatment of the premalignant stage of cervical intra-epithelial neoplasia (CIN) through cervical Pap smear cytology has reduced incidence and mortality from cervical cancer by 80%. Isolated Pap smears have false negative rates of 20–40%, which are partly overcome by regular screening (every 3 years). The human papilloma virus (HPV), in particular strains 16 and 18, is critical to cervical carcinogenesis. Testing for HPV DNA in cervical smears increases the cervical cancer detection by 30% over cytology-based screening and could lengthen the screening interval to 5 years.[19] Incorporation of HPV-based screening into guidelines is being considered. Importantly, however, the Pap smear and HPV DNA function as primary screens that are followed by visual and pathologic evaluation through colposcopy as a secondary screen.

Individuals at elevated risk

Specific guidelines exist for patients with strong family histories of cancer, particularly for carriers of genomic biomarkers of high cancer risk. When the cancer risk associated with the specific (usually hereditary) biomarker is high enough, recommendations focus on prevention rather than early detection. As prevention strategies generally impact quality of life to a greater degree than does screening, the identification of inherited mutations associated with a very high cancer risk necessitates patient education and careful shared decision making. Furthermore, hereditary biomarkers testing has significant implications for family members. Prophylactic surgery and chemoprevention are particularly effective risk reduction techniques that are reserved for people at highest risk. Prophylactic oophorectomy and/or mastectomy has the greatest protective effect for *BRCA1/BRCA2* mutation carriers, reducing the risk of ovarian cancer and breast cancer by more than 90%.[20,21] However, some patients prefer mammography, MRI, or other screening approaches to delay surgical intervention either for personal preference or to allow childbearing. There are many factors (e.g., ethics and cost) to consider in discussing options for early detection and prevention with very high-risk patients, and this area of medicine is a rapidly evolving specialty.[22–24]

Breast and ovarian cancer

In families with a significant history of breast and/or ovarian cancer, key cancer risk biomarkers (usually hereditary mutations) can now be identified in a minority of cases, using clinical prediction models (e.g., BRCAPRO model).[25] Such models can be useful in guiding specific molecular tests that further stratify risk and guide subsequent screening or prevention. Inherited mutations in *BRCA1* and *BRCA2* account for 5–10% and 10–15% of all breast cancers and ovarian cancers, respectively.[26,27] Furthermore, approximately 15% of patients with triple negative breast cancers or with high-grade serous ovarian cancer will carry deleterious germ line mutations in BRCA1/2 in the absence of a significant family history. Moreover, *BRCA1/2* mutations guide therapy in ovarian cancer, as outlined in the following section. Approximately 12% of women at high-risk do not carry *BRCA1/2* mutations and are estimated to have another cancer predisposing genomic alteration,[28] suggesting a need for improved testing approaches that identify additional risk biomarkers. Less well-studied breast cancer susceptibility genes include *CHEK2, ATM, RAD51C, BRIP1, PALB2, NBS1, LKB1, PTEN, p53, XRCC1*, and *STK11*, but these are not commonly assessed due to the rarity of inherited mutations.[29–32] Recently, these genes have been integrated into multiplex sequencing assays, both providing more information and greater challenges in patient decision making for genes associated with a lower frequency of cancer development.

Colon cancer

Familial adenomatous polyposis (FAP) and hereditary non-polyposis colon cancer (HNPCC) predispose to early-onset familial/hereditary colon cancer. They are characterized by germ line mutations in the adenomatous polyposis coli (*APC*) and DNA mismatch repair genes, respectively. In HNPCC, routine tumor molecular screening using antibodies to mismatch repair proteins has superseded clinical risk models to guide screening (e.g., revised Bethesda guidelines). Tumor molecular screening, however, results in excessive genetic testing for HNPCC, as 10–15% of cases represent sporadic disease.[33] Combining the clinical risk prediction models with tumor molecular screening, or testing the tumor for molecular markers of sporadic disease (*MLH1* promoter methylation and/or *BRAF* V600E gene mutation) could improve screening for HNPCC while maintaining high detection rates.[34] Management guidelines entail surgical cancer prevention (colectomy) with FAP and intensive colonoscopic screening with HNPCC.

In a recent study, fecal hemoglobin detection was combined with fecal DNA tests for mutant K-Ras, aberrant *NDRG4* and *BMP3* methylation and B-actin.[35] When compared to a standard fecal immmunohistochemical test (FIT) in 9989 evaluable participants at average risk, the composite Cologuard® test demonstrated greater sensitivity for detecting colorectal cancer (92.3% vs 73.8%, $P = 0.002$), greater sensitivity for detecting advanced precancerous lesions (42.4% vs 23.8%, $P < 0.001$), a higher rate of detection of high-grade dysplastic polyps (69.2% vs 46.2%, $P = 0.004$), and greater detection of serrated sessile polyps measuring 1 cm or more (42.4% and 5.1%, $P < 0.001$). Specificity, however, was somewhat lower with DNA testing than with FIT (86.6% vs 94.9%). On the basis of these results, the test was approved in 2014 by the United States FDA for individuals greater than 50 years of age.

Future approaches to early detection and screening

While current approaches to early detection have impacted mortality from certain forms of malignancy such as cervical cancer, low sensitivity, unnecessary use of invasive diagnostic procedures due to false positives, and overdiagnosis/treatment remain significant issues. Moreover, many tumor types, such as ovarian and pancreatic cancer, do not benefit from these approaches. Patients continue to present with advanced disease and thus have poor outcomes. Elevation of circulating tumor biomarkers may require a substantial tumor volume. Autoantibodies could be evoked by small volumes of cancer at an earlier interval. Novel molecular screening techniques, including circulating DNA, RNA, and exosomes, have the potential to complement current protein-based screening markers and revolutionize early cancer detection, while facilitating accurate risk assessment and individual treatment planning.

Current molecular biomarkers for predicting outcomes and therapy responsiveness

Although molecular biomarkers that predict outcomes in cancer patients are useful, greater clinical utility lies in biomarkers that predict benefit from specific cancer therapies. There is considerable overlap between both types, as those biomarkers that predict benefit for particular patients from specific cancer therapies will predict improved outcomes.

Breast cancer

Hormone receptors (HR)

Hormone receptors (HR)-positive breast cancer comprises approximately 70% of all breast cancers and is marked by the expression of estrogen receptor (ER) alpha and/or progesterone receptor (PR). The HR biomarkers identify breast tumors that are sensitive to growth inhibition by antihormonal treatments, including ER partial agonists/antagonists (e.g., tamoxifen), ER downregulators (e.g., fulvestrant), and aromatase inhibitors (e.g., letrozole).[36,37] In clinical practice, HR protein expression is assessed routinely in all breast cancers using immunohistochemistry. Despite 5 years of adjuvant antihormonal therapy, however, a significant fraction of women with early stage HR-positive breast cancer relapse, and the majority of women with metastatic HR-positive breast cancer, develop resistance to antihormonal manipulation. Thus, in the United States, over 25,000 women with HR-positive breast tumors die each year, more annual deaths than are caused by all other types of breast cancer combined.

Multiparameter gene expression profiles

Our ability to predict the likelihood of cure for patients with HR-positive breast cancer after treatment with antihormonal drugs has improved dramatically. *Oncotype Dx* (Table 1), based on the expression of 21 genes, predicts the benefit for individual node-negative HR-positive breast tumor patients from adjuvant tamoxifen and selects patients for cytotoxic chemotherapy based on features associated with tamoxifen resistance.[38] However, despite this approach's clinical utility, this and similar assays such as PAM50 and Mammoprint do not increase our understanding of antihormone resistance mechanisms in HR-positive breast cancer beyond the known roles of tumor grade, HER2, and HR levels.[36,38,39] The phosphatidylinositol-3-kinase (PI3K)/AKT/mTOR and mitogen-activated protein kinase (MAPK) pathways are major mediators of the effects of membrane receptor tyrosine kinases (RTKs) such as HER2 and mediate resistance to antihormonal therapies.[40] The mTOR inhibitor everolimus improves progression-free survival for approximately 60% of women with HR-positive breast cancers resistant to antihormonal therapies.[41] A predictive molecular biomarker of response to this drug is lacking however.

HER2

The oncogene encoding *HER2* is amplified and the protein overexpressed in 15–20% of invasive breast cancers. *HER2* overexpression dictates an aggressive breast tumor phenotype and poor prognosis.[42] Combining trastuzumab (Herceptin), a recombinant humanized monoclonal antibody targeting *HER2*, with cytotoxic chemotherapy to treat patients with metastatic and early stage *HER2* oncogene-amplified breast cancer, has resulted in increased response rates and improved survival.[43] Thus, *HER2* is a biomarker for breast tumor responsiveness to trastuzumab and other *HER2*-targeted therapies (e.g., pertuzumab, lapatinib, and TDM1).[44] More recently, HER2 has been validated also as a biomarker predictive of response to trastuzumab-based chemotherapy in 15–20% of advanced gastric cancer patients with HER2-driven oncogenesis.[45]

A significant fraction of *HER2*-amplified breast and gastric cancers do not respond initially to trastuzumab or acquire resistance to trastuzumab. This could be mediated by a cleaved form of *HER2* that does not bind trastuzumab (p95-HER2), by upregulation of

Table 1 The panel of 21 genes in *Oncotype Dx* and their subdivision based on function.

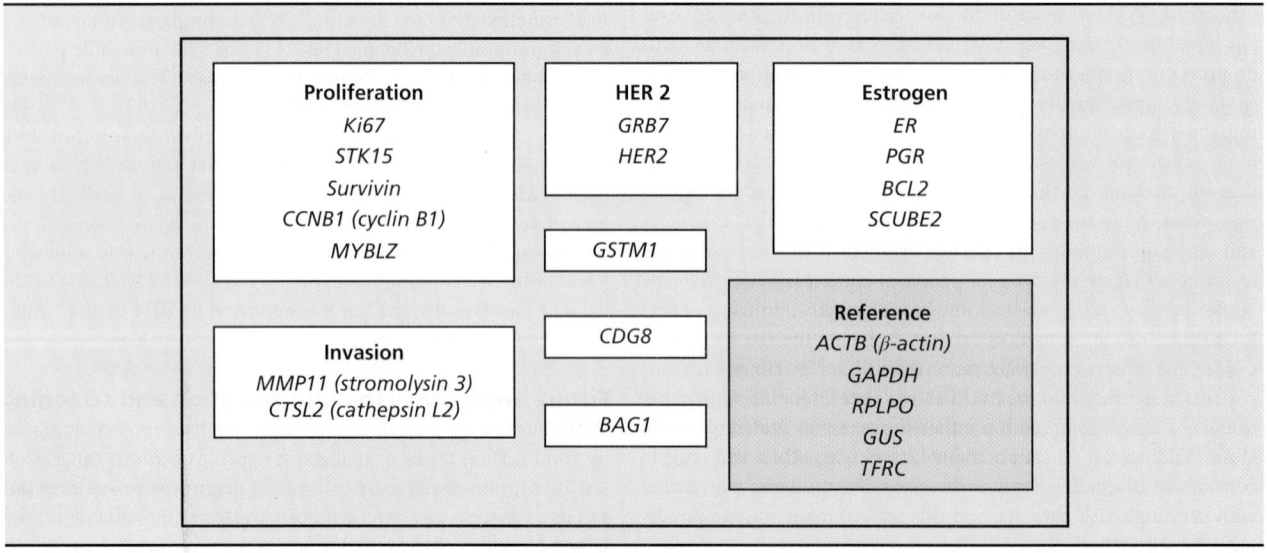

Proliferation	HER 2	Estrogen
Ki67	GRB7	ER
STK15	HER2	PGR
Survivin		BCL2
CCNB1 (cyclin B1)		SCUBE2
MYBLZ	GSTM1	
		Reference
	CDG8	ACTB (β-actin)
Invasion		GAPDH
MMP11 (stromolysin 3)		RPLPO
CTSL2 (cathepsin L2)	BAG1	GUS
		TFRC

other membrane RTKs such as IGF1R or MET or by upregulation of the PI3K/AKT pathway.[46–49] The latter can occur through inactivating mutations of PTEN (a negative PI3K/AKT regulator), PTEN loss, or by PIK3CA mutations, the oncogene that encodes the p110α subunit of PI3K.[50] Indeed, PI3K pathway activation and mutations in PIK3CA and PTEN are negative prognostic markers in HER2-positive breast cancers treated with anti-HER2 targeted therapies.[51]

A panel of the American Society of Clinical Oncology (ASCO) thus recommended that *HER2* status should be determined for all invasive breast cancers.[52] This panel has proposed a testing algorithm that relies on accurate, reproducible assay performance, including newly available types of bright-field *in situ* hybridization (ISH), and has specified elements to reliably reduce assay variation (e.g., specimen handling, assay exclusion, and reporting criteria). This emphasizes the need for quality control and validation approaches for all predictive markers, both in terms of reliability and clinical utility.

Ovarian cancer: BRCA1/2

Approximately 20% of high-grade serous ovarian cancers have an underlying inherited or somatic *BRCA1/2* mutation, rendering them deficient in homologous recombination, a pathway essential for repairing double-stranded DNA breaks.[53] These tumors rely on alternative DNA repair mechanisms such as base excision repair, to which the PARP enzyme is key. Inhibitors of PARP exploit vulnerability of *BRCA1/2*-mutated ovarian cancers to DNA damage. In a randomized phase II trial, the PARP inhibitor olaparib increased progression-free survival by 82% as compared to placebo when used as maintenance therapy in platinum-sensitive recurrent *BRCA1/2*-mutated ovarian tumors.[54] Olaparib has now been approved for use with this indication, with approvals for other PARP inhibitors and other uses expected imminently. Resistance mechanisms include function-restoring *BRCA1/2* mutations, loss of 53BP1 (a protein involved in an alternative DNA repair mechanism), and upregulation of the PI3K/AKT/mTOR pathway.[55] The combination of olaparib and BKM120, a PI3K inhibitor, has shown activity in early clinical studies of high-grade serous ovarian and triple negative breast cancer.[56]

Lung cancer

Epidermal growth factor receptor

The reversible EGFR (epidermal growth factor receptor) tyrosine kinase inhibitors (TKIs) gefitinib and erlotinib and irreversible pan-HER TKI afatinib and dacomitinib provide effective therapies in approximately 10–30% of patients with non-small-cell lung cancer, whose tumors harbor activating EGFR mutations, the common ones being located on exon 19 and 21.[57–60] Female nonsmokers of Asian origin with adenocarcinoma represent the typical phenotype, although EGFR mutations are also observed in men and former smokers. While first line treatment with dacomitinib in EGFR-mutant lung cancers has been associated with an impressive progression-free survival (18.2 months), and afatinib shows greatest efficacy in exon 19 mutations, the benefit of one TKI over another has yet to be established.

Multiple acquired resistance mechanisms to EGFR inhibitors, including secondary mutation in *EGFR* (T790M) and MET amplification,[61] limit the efficacy of EGFR-targeted therapy. New EGFR TKIs have shown promise in treating or preventing resistance in phase I/II studies and are being evaluated in larger clinical trials,[62] with the hope that they will translate into effective therapies for patients with lung cancer.

ALK and ROS-1

Two targetable chromosomal gene rearrangements leading to oncogenic gene fusions guide novel therapies in advanced adenocarcinoma of the lung.[63,64] ALK (anaplastic lymphoma kinase) and ROS-1 gene translocations are present in 4–6% and 1–2% of advanced lung adenocarcinomas, respectively, rendering them markedly sensitive to the ALK, ROS-1, and MET inhibitor, crizotinib. The short period between the identification of these targets and crizotinib's approval engenders excitement for an evolution away from the prolonged time period traditionally required for drug discovery and implementation. Crizotinib is associated with response rates of over 70% and a median progression-free survival of 11 and 19 months for ALK and ROS-1 rearranged tumors, respectively. Gene overexpression, bypass mechanisms, and secondary mutations commonly cause acquired resistance, though unlike EGFR-mutated non-small-cell lung cancer, multiple mutation types are observed in a single tumor at disease progression. Strategies to overcome acquired resistance involving second-generation ALK inhibitors such as ceritinib show promise in early clinical trials.[65]

On the basis of these results, routine molecular testing is recommended for EGFR and ALK in all advanced stage lung adenocarcinomas (or lung tumors with an adenocarcinoma component), regardless of clinical characteristics. Tumors that do not contain an adenocarcinoma component perhaps due to a sampling error but are suspected as such due to clinical characteristics (young, never smoker) may also be tested.[66]

Colon cancer

Microsatellite instability

Current guidelines recommend adjuvant 5-fluorouracil-based chemotherapy in stage II colon cancer in "high-risk" patients, defined by the presence of high-grade tumors with lymphovascular space invasion, evidence of tumor perforation, and/or less than 12 nodes extracted at surgery. Approximately 11% of stage II colon cancers have a deficiency in mismatch DNA repair, manifested as microsatellite instability.[67] Such tumors have good outcomes in the absence of adjuvant chemotherapy. Therefore, guidelines advise routine immunohistochemical testing of stage II colon cancers for mismatch repair proteins, the absence of which obviates the need for adjuvant chemotherapy.

KRAS, BRAF, and NRAS

KRAS is a proto-oncogene downstream of EGFR that initiates signaling through the Ras-Raf-MAPK pathway. Approximately 60% of metastatic colorectal cancers have the favorable wild type *KRAS* profile, predicting sensitivity to the anti-EGFR monoclonal antibodies, cetuximab and panitumumab. KRAS mutations, found mainly at codons 12 and 13 of exon 2, predict resistance to these therapies, as do the rarer *NRAS* mutations.[68–71] Downstream *BRAF* mutations occur in about 5–9% of cases and correlate with poor prognosis, although their reported lack of benefit from EGFR inhibitors remains uncertain.

Gastrointestinal stromal tumors (GIST): KIT and PDGFRA

GIST (gastrointestinal stromal tumor) is associated with primary activating mutations in the *KIT* (80% of GISTs) or platelet-derived growth factor receptor A (*PDGFRA*; 5–10% of *GISTs*) genes that result in constitutive RTK activation.[72] Imatinib (Gleevec), which inhibits both KIT and PDGFRA, results in clinical benefit in approximately 85% of patients with unresectable or metastatic disease, with a median progression-free survival of 20–24 months, although patients with exon 11 mutations fare better than exon 9 mutations. In the latter case, a higher dose of imatinib confers a greater benefit. The mechanisms of acquired resistance to imatinib are heterogeneous, involving mostly the emergence of secondary mutations in *KIT* exons 13, 14, or 17. In patients with imatinib-resistant *GIST*, novel kinase inhibitors, such as sunitinib, nilotinib, dasatinib, and regorafenib, can inhibit the mutant protein's function and restore antitumor activity.

Melanoma

BRAF

About half of all melanomas carry the *BRAF* V600E gene mutation, leading to constitutive downstream activation of the MAPK pathway engendering sensitivity to BRAF inhibitors (e.g., vemurafenib and dabrafenib).[73,74] Clinically, the duration of response to these drugs is short, with progression occurring at a median of 6–7 months. Novel approaches to overcome resistance resulting from compensatory overactivation of the MAPK pathway involve the upfront combination of BRAF and MEK inhibitors (such as trametinib), which increases the efficacy and decreases the toxicity of therapy.[75]

NRAS

MEK inhibitors will likely play a significant role in treating *NRAS*-mutated melanoma, which involves approximately 15–20% of all melanomas and dictates a particularly aggressive biology. Interestingly, MEK inhibitors may demonstrate activity in combination with immune therapies.[76]

KIT

A small number (3%) of *BRAF/NRAS*-negative melanomas carry *KIT* proto-oncogene mutations, particularly in mucosal and acral melanomas. Targeted therapies with imatinib or sunitinib are viable therapeutic options that can provide durable responses, with evidence of nilotinib activity at progression post imatinib therapy.[77,78]

Chronic myeloid leukemia (CML)

Bcr-Abl translocation

Most chronic myeloid leukemia (CML) cases are driven by constitutive activation of the Abl kinase as a result of the breakpoint cluster region (Bcr) to the Abl kinase translocation (Philadelphia chromosome). Imatinib targeted therapy, which inhibits the kinase activity of Abl, has markedly improved the outlook for patients with CML. However, imatinib resistance can emerge despite initial benefit. Furthermore, efficacy of imatinib is limited in advanced "blast-crisis" CML.[79] Resistance is due predominantly to novel mutations in the Abl kinase domain, interfering with drug binding. Thus, new Abl kinase inhibitors (AKIs) were developed, among which nilotinib, dasatinib, and bosutinib gained regulatory approval. Unfortunately, all available AKIs exhibit inactivity to certain kinase domain mutations, the cross-resistant *Bcr-Abl* (*T315I*) mutant being the most common. The third-generation AKI ponatinib demonstrates clinical benefit in *Bcr-Abl* (*T315I*) mutant CML and some other multidrug-resistant mutations. However, cardiovascular toxicity concerns, potentially related to the choice of a high-drug dose during clinical development, precluded regulatory approval. Trials investigating dose-optimized ponatinib are underway.[80]

Lymphoma

CD20 and other biomarkers

Biomarker-targeted therapeuties have impacted significantly the treatment of non-Hodgkin lymphoma (NHL).[81,82] The development of the chimeric anti-CD20 antibody rituximab heralded a new era in NHL treatment approaches. Rituximab is now standard monotherapy for front-line treatment of follicular lymphoma and is used in conjunction with chemotherapy for other CD20-positive B-cell lymphomas. The subsequent development and approval of radio-immunoconjugates of rituximab (^{90}Y-ibritumomab tiuxetan and ^{131}I-tositumomab) has improved outcomes further.

Clinical evaluation of antibodies has been based largely on knowledge of antigen expression on the lymphoma cells' surface, leading to the development of antibodies against CD22 (e.g., unconjugated epratuzumab), CD80 (galiximab), CD52 (alemtuzumab), CD2 (siplizumab), CD40 (SGN-40), and CD30.[83] The anti-CD30 antibody brentuximab has been conjugated with a drug, vedotin, to target cytotoxic drug delivery to CD30-positive Hodgkin's or anaplastic large cell lymphoma, producing significant clinical benefit with acceptable toxicity. It was approved for use recently in relapsed Hodgkin's lymphoma following autologous stem cell transplant and relapsed anaplastic large cell lymphoma. Currently, it is being investigated for use upfront with chemotherapy.

Oropharyngeal cancer (OPC)

Human papilloma virus

The epidemiology of oropharyngeal cancer (OPC) has changed over the last two decades with studies reporting the presence of HPV p16 subtype in 60–70% of all OPC in western countries. Molecular tumor testing is easily done using p16 immunohistochemistry, which has a high concordance with HPV FISH. Retrospective analyses of large clinical trials demonstrate superior response rates and survival with chemoradiotherapy in HPV-related OPCs, as compared to HPV-negative OPCs.[84] Therefore, HPV is an important stratification tool for future therapeutic investigations in OPCs and may dictate a different therapeutic approach. Suggestions that HPV-associated OPCs may benefit from less intensive chemoradiotherapy require further evaluation.

Molecular biomarkers for monitoring of cancer

A number of circulating biomarkers are used for monitoring of cancer response to therapy and/or for the early detection of recurrent disease in cancer patients.

Alpha-fetoprotein (AFP) and human chorionic gonadotropin (hCG)

Many germ cell tumors [most male testicular cancers, gestational trophoblastic disease (choriocarcinoma), and rare ovarian cancers] produce circulating tumor markers [AFP (alpha-fetoprotein), hCG (human chorionic gonadotropin), lactate dehydrogenase (LDH)].[67] These biomarkers are useful in diagnosing, staging, monitoring therapeutic response, and detecting early tumor recurrence. As recurrent germ cell tumors can be cured with cytotoxic chemotherapy, particularly when the recurrence is detected early, increasing tumor marker levels during patient follow-up are an indication for initiating salvage therapy, despite absence of evident disease. The markers' half-lives must be considered when evaluating therapeutic responses.

AFP is a glycoprotein normally produced by the fetal yolk sac, liver, and gastrointestinal tract but not by normal adult tissues. It is re-expressed in germ cell tumors, including yolk sac tumors and embryonal carcinomas. hCG is a glycoprotein produced by syncytiotrophoblastic cells consisting of two subunits, α and β. The α-subunit is common to three pituitary trophic hormones: FSH, LH, and TSH; the β-subunit makes hCG enzymatically and immunologically distinct. Assays measure only the β subunit (β-hCG). In males, it is highly specific for testicular cancer, in particular choriocarcinoma cells and 5–10% of pure seminomas. LDH reflects "tumor burden," growth rate, and cellular proliferation and has independent prognostic significance. LDH is increased in about 80% of advanced seminomas and about 60% of advanced nonseminomatous germ cell tumors. The LDH isoenzyme 1 seems to be more specific and sensitive for germ cell tumors than isoenzymes 2–5.[85]

CA125

CA125 is a mucinous transmembrane glycoprotein product of the MUC16 gene that ranges up to 5 mD. CA125 is best known as an ovarian cancer marker, though elevations in endometrial, fallopian tube, lung, breast, and gastrointestinal cancers, as well as relatively benign conditions including endometriosis, are observed. CA125, when used alone on a single occasion, is not sensitive or specific enough for ovarian cancer screening.[86] Moreover, 20% of ovarian cancers do not produce elevated CA125 levels. However, serum CA125 is very useful for following treatment response, for predicting post-therapy prognosis, and for detecting recurrence in women with ovarian cancer. During first-line platinum-based ovarian cancer chemotherapy, CA125 levels should be followed regularly (e.g., every 3 weeks). The CA125 level at nadir, 3-month normalization of CA125 and CA125 half-life are strong predictors of progression-free and overall survival times.[87–89] The failure of serum CA125 normalization after initial treatment with surgery and platinum-based chemotherapy is a particularly ominous indication of poor prognosis in women with ovarian cancer.

In women in clinical remission following previously treated ovarian cancer, the National Comprehensive Cancer Network (NCCN) (www.nccn.org) recommends evaluation of serum CA125 level at each follow-up visit if the CA125 level was elevated at the initial diagnosis. After a documented CA125 elevation, the median time to clinical disease relapse is over 4 months, although increases within the normal range can produce much longer lead times. One large, randomized study in the United Kingdom concluded a lack of overall survival benefit when women with recurrent disease were treated at the time of CA125 elevation, although only 25% of women on the control and experimental arms were treated promptly with optimal combination chemotherapy.[90] At a minimum, earlier recurrence detection with CA125 provides time to receive known and novel agents, given the relatively short interval between symptomatic recurrence and death. With such controversy, however, using CA125 to monitor recurrence should be discussed with each patient.

CA15-3 and CA27.29

CA15-3 and CA 27.29 are well-characterized assays that detect circulating MUC1 antigen in peripheral blood.[91] Several studies support the prognostic relevance of this circulating marker in early stage breast cancer though monitoring MUC1-based serum markers has demonstrated utility in making treatment decisions.[92,93] ASCO regards available data as insufficient to recommend using CA15-3 or CA 27.29 for breast cancer screening, diagnosis, staging, or for monitoring patients for recurrence, as conclusive evidence

that early detection of recurrence improves survival is lacking.[91] Although present data cannot recommend the use of CA15-3 or CA 27.29 alone for monitoring treatment response, rising CA15-3 or CA27.29 may be used to indicate treatment failure in the absence of readily measurable disease. However, caution should be used when interpreting a rising CA27.29 or CA15-3 level during the first 4–6 weeks of a new therapy, as spurious early rises may occur. These recommendations apply also when monitoring metastatic colon cancer with CEA (carcinoembryonic antigen).

CA19-9

Carbohydrate antigen 19-9 is elevated primarily in the serum of patients with gastrointestinal tract carcinomas. The greatest utility of serum CA19-9 is in monitoring treatment response in pancreatic cancer. For patients with locally advanced or metastatic pancreatic cancer undergoing active therapy, ASCO recommends measurement of serum CA19-9 levels every 1–3 months.[94] Serial CA19-9 elevations suggest progressive disease in the face of treatment, but confirmatory studies (e.g., CT scanning) should be sought before a therapy change is initiated.

Carcinoembryonic antigen (CEA)

CEA is a cell adhesion glycoprotein.[95] It is produced during fetal development and is not usually present in healthy adults' blood, although levels are raised in heavy smokers. Serum CEA may be elevated in patients with colorectal, gastric, pancreatic, lung, breast, and medullary thyroid carcinomas. ASCO has developed clinical practice guidelines to monitor serum CEA levels in patients with colorectal cancer, in whom serum CEA should be ordered preoperatively, if it would assist in staging and surgical planning. Postoperative CEA levels should be performed every 3 months, for patients with stages II and III colorectal cancer, for at least 3 years if the patient is a potential candidate for surgery (e.g., liver resection) or chemotherapy for metastatic disease. CEA is also the marker of choice for monitoring systemic therapy response in metastatic colorectal cancer.

Prostate specific antigen

Measuring serum PSA is important in men with an established diagnosis of prostate cancer. The rate of PSA rise can predict prostate cancer prognosis. Men with prostate cancer whose PSA level increased by more than 2.0 ng/mL during the year before the diagnosis of prostate cancer have a higher risk of death from prostate cancer after radical prostatectomy. PSA level along with clinical stage and Gleason tumor grade are components of most nomograms and predictive models used for prostate cancer risk assessment.[96] Further, serum PSA provides an indicator of disease response to treatment.

For prostate cancer patients treated initially with curative intent, serum PSA level should be assessed every 6–12 months for 5 years and annually thereafter. A rising PSA level indicates biochemical failure and often precedes a clinically detectable recurrence by several years. As biochemical failure may represent an isolated local recurrence, identifying those patients is important as they may be candidates for salvage therapy.

Novel molecular biomarkers and platforms for their detection

Malignant tumors are characterized by multiple molecular anomalies responsible for the behavior of individual cancers. The driving aberrations can be in the germ line genome or may occur in a somatic or acquired manner in the cancer genome and/or proteome. Novel cancer biomarkers may be detectable not only in the tumor or its microenvironment but also in the circulation, either as circulating tumor cells (CTCs) or as circulating nucleotides, proteins, or metabolites.

Novel high-throughput molecular technologies that comprehensively characterize the cancer genome and proteome are creating many new possibilities for the identification of biomarkers and, in particular, the development of multimarker (e.g., multigene) panels that integrate information across many markers. Many of the earlier high-throughput approaches such as gene methylation analysis, gene microarrays, comparative genomic hybridization, mass spectrometry/spectroscopy, and bead-based analysis methods are being replaced by next generation sequencing. Gene expression profiles have been explored extensively to identify good and poor prognosis subsets of various human tumors.[97] Currently, the ability of methylation analysis to detect early cancer cell DNA methylation aberrations is being investigated. The high-throughput reverse phase protein lysate array (RPPA) proteomic technology allows concurrent analysis of the expression and activation of multiple specific kinases and other proteins.[98–102] This platform is particularly suited to investigate kinase signaling in cancer and the molecular effects of novel agents (e.g., TKIs) during treatment and in high-risk tissue during chemoprevention (Figure 1). Emerging mass spectrometry approaches such as MRM (multiple reaction monitoring) and SWATH could provide additional information on candidate genes when high-quality antibodies are not available, and mass spectrometry is particularly useful for biomarker discovery. Together, genomic and proteomic platforms provide information that can be incorporated to develop meta-signatures reflecting global DNA, RNA, and protein abnormalities. These may be capable of outperforming data derived from a single technology examining only one of these platforms.[103] For example, proteomic studies can augment genomic panels by providing information

on posttranslational modifications and on proteins' relative levels and activation. As such, data sets, systems for effective data management, integrated analysis of pathways, and "meta-analysis" are critical components of successful development of molecular markers.[104–106]

Novel germ line biomarkers

The germ line genome likely contains an underexplored trove of novel cancer risk biomarkers as well as biomarkers for toxicity and efficacy of specific anticancer treatments. For example, germ line polymorphisms have been associated with toxicity and efficacy of the *EGFR* inhibitor erlotinib in lung cancer.[107] Recent large-scale studies of the germ line genome have also begun to uncover a large set of cancer susceptibility markers, many with low penetrance, thereby improving our ability to predict high cancer risk as well as response to therapy utilizing novel germ line biomarkers.[108–110]

Tissue-specific biomarkers of high risk and for early detection of cancer

Early malignant change may be an indicator of high cancer risk in specific tissues. With availability of less invasive ways to obtain cells likely to be at risk of or to harbor early neoplastic change in tissue at risk of cancer (e.g., in sputum, bronchial washings, blood, feces, urine, or nipple aspirate), the study of tissue markers for screening of carcinogenesis risk and of early malignant transformation becomes more feasible. To date, the cost, invasiveness, lack of large prospective outcome validation studies, and absence of standardized guidelines has confined most of these potentially useful approaches to small clinical studies.

Although screening to detect lung cancer at an early stage using routine cytological examination of sputum did not decrease cancer-specific mortality, the application of molecular detection methods to sputum and bronchial washings is now being studied in an attempt to detect molecular changes associated with premalignant and early malignant bronchial epithelial cells.[111] For

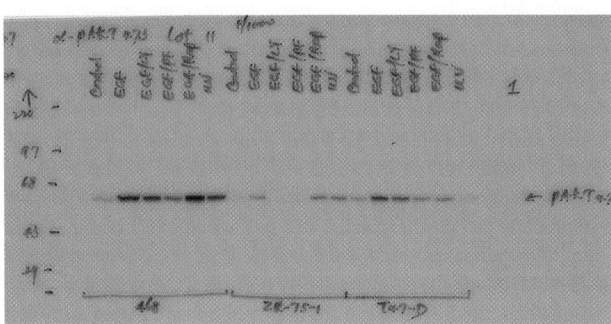
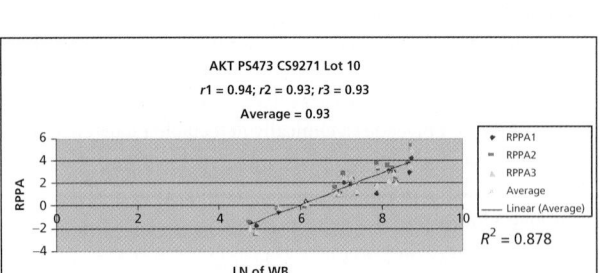
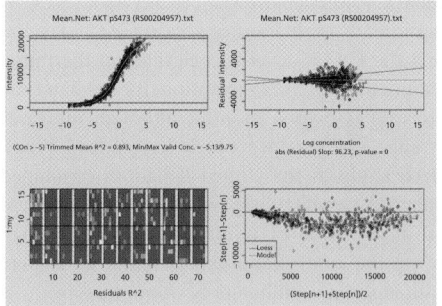
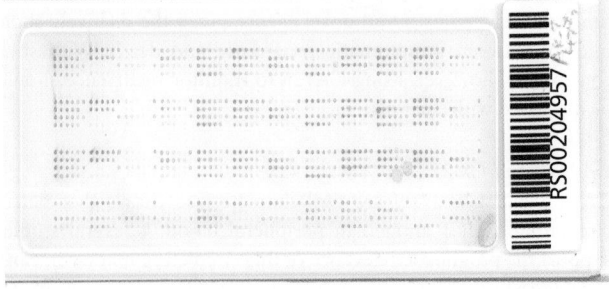

Figure 1 Validation of antibodies for reverse phase protein lysate arrays (RPPAs). Protein lysates from cell lines have been serially diluted on a nitrocellulose-coated slide followed by probing with monospecific antibodies to phosphorylated Akt and signal detection and amplification. Serial dilution curves are used for quantification purposes. Comparisons to western blotting are demonstrated with an *r* value of 0.878. Quantification and quality control of staining are represented in the upper right panel.

example, FISH with locus-specific probes to chromosomal regions 5p15, 7p12 (EGFR), 8q24 (C-Myc), and the centromere of chromosome 6 may improve significantly the sensitivity for detection of malignancy in sputum and bronchial washing specimens.[112]

Cancer-specific biomarkers

As discussed earlier, progress has been made in identifying single biomarkers and multimarker panels (e.g., *Oncotype Dx*) to predict responses and overcome resistance to targeted therapy. However, progress in this regard has been more limited in other cancer types. Emerging basket clinical trials may address this deficiency in part. Basket trials are based on the observation that common molecular aberrations occur across different cancer types. These trials evaluate the role of targeted therapies against specific molecular aberration(s), regardless of cancer type, within the same trial.[113]

In the future, pharmacodynamic biomarkers of early drug activity must also be defined in preclinical tumor models and then confirmed in patient samples to assure that patients are receiving a biologically relevant dose of the drug. In this regard, optimal target inhibition by the drug in the tumor may be a more important endpoint than maximum tolerated dose of the drug. However, whether optimal drug activity is dependent on maximal target inhibition, area under the curve, or trough values is not known for most drugs. Precepts derived from Systems Biology such as sensitivity analysis may provide guidelines regarding the optimal inhibition pattern required. This approach may optimize drug efficacy, decrease toxicity, in particular off-target toxicity, and facilitate early identification of nonresponders for triage to alternative therapies. For example, perifosine-induced inhibition of AKT in the tumor correlates remarkably well with tumor growth inhibition using multiple dosing schedules of perifosine. Furthermore, the integrated assessment of the activation status of multiple PI3K/AKT pathway members in the tumor soon after initiation of therapies, using proteomics assays such as RPPA, may prove superior to single markers for prediction of tumor response to PI3K pathway inhibitors.

Serum and urine biomarkers

Novel serum biomarkers have potential utility in cancer screening, in prediction of tumor responsiveness to specific therapies, and in monitoring tumor responses to therapy. As discussed earlier, while conventional serum cancer biomarkers are used routinely for cancer monitoring, their application to screening is limited by suboptimal sensitivity and specificity.[114–116] Specificity can be improved by monitoring increases in individual marker levels over time, but marker panels will almost certainly be required to increase sensitivity for screening. The conventional concept concerning the screening utility of serum biomarkers is that their detection should trigger clinical assessment by imaging and biopsy or increased surveillance if appropriate. Alternatively, novel serum markers might be used following screening by other means to increase the specificity of the latter approach. Thus, a novel biomarker may allow definition of an equivocal mammographic lesion as appropriate for serial monitoring or immediate biopsy.

Mass spectrometry-based unbiased approaches to identify novel serum biomarkers from the proteome or metabolome present in blood or urine have the potential to identify biomarker panels that could identify tumors from an early stage of development. Ovarian cancer has been the subject of several such studies because of diagnosis in advanced stages, poor patient outcomes, and the absence of a well-established screening method. Two general approaches have been utilized: identification of distinctive signatures and discovery of discrete markers that might be assembled into panels. However,

Table 2 Sensitivity, specificity, and positive predictive value of urine cytology, bladder tumor antigen (BTA) immunoassay, nuclear matrix protein-22 (NMP22) detection, ImmunoCyt, and urine FISH for early detection of bladder cancer.

	Sensitivity (%)	Specificity (%)	PPV (%)
PSA	72	93	25
Urine cytology	48–73	48–100	48–69
BTA	53	77	63
NMP22	71	66	21
ImmunoCyt	78–81	74–100	26
FISH	69–71	78–95	68

Note: Serum prostate-specific antigen (PSA) in prostate cancer screening is shown only as a point of reference. ImmunoCyt is currently approved by the US Food and Drug Administration for the monitoring of recurrent bladder cancer. ImmunoCyt uses a cocktail of three monoclonal antibodies to detect bladder cancer cells in the urine. One antibody is directed against a high-molecular-weight form of glycosylated carcinoembryonic antigen, 19A211. The other two antibodies, LDQ10 and M344, are directed against mucins that are specific for bladder cancer and are labeled with fluorescein.
Source: Hu 2007. Reproduced with permission of Oxford University Press.

none of the mass spectrometry-based approaches have validated in large prospectively based sample sets.[117]

In the urine, the sensitivity of FISH or of cytokeratin (e.g., keratin 19, 20) detection using IHC or reverse transcriptase (RT)-polymerase chain reaction (PCR) may be higher than that of conventional cytology for bladder and urothelial cancer screening.[118] A commercial kit (UroVysion) containing hybridization probes for chromosomes 3, 7, 9p21, and 17 is used for FISH analysis of urine. The sensitivity and specificity associated with this analysis were 60% and 82.6%, respectively, for detection of bladder cancer. In contrast, the sensitivity and specificity associated with urine cytology were 24.1% and 90.5%, respectively. Thus, a FISH assay for chromosomes 3, 7, 9, and 17 may have a higher sensitivity than cytology and a similar specificity for the detection of urothelial cancers. Table 2 summarizes the various approaches that have been investigated as potential tools to facilitate bladder cancer screening.[119]

Circulating tumor cells

CTCs have potential utility in cancer screening, target identification, response prediction, and in monitoring response to treatment. Indeed, the predictive and prognostic utility of CTCs and, more recently, circulating tumor DNA have already been demonstrated in metastatic breast cancer.[120,121] Initial studies of the utility of CTCs in breast cancer screening are proceeding.[122] In ovarian cancer, peripheral blood CTC-specific *p53* sequences are detectable in some FIGO stage III/IV ovarian cancer patients, suggesting that this approach may be useful as a building block toward early detection.[123]

The use of CTCs to study molecular biomarkers is limited currently to gene expression signatures because of the need for substrate amplification. However, CTCs have the potential to replace invasive tumor biopsies with "liquid" biopsies and facilitate early access to the tumor genome and proteome for molecular biomarkers predictive of therapy response and resistance, as demonstrated in lung and prostate cancers.[124,125] A major challenge is the difficulty in harvesting CTCs and exploring molecular markers in a limited number of cells. Methods of CTCs enrichment are being explored and include the enhanced density gradient system.[126] Currently, we are investigating novel methods of DNA and protein extraction to allow detection of mutations and protein expression/activation changes in CTCs, the latter utilizing RPPA.[127,128]

Circulating nucleotides

DNA, RNA, microRNA, and proteins are released from tumor cells and can be found in the circulation. Circulating biomarkers have the potential to reflect processes occurring across all tumor sites in the body that cannot be detected by analysis of the primary tumor and/or metastatic sites. Thus, there is great excitement in the potential for "liquid" biopsies to provide information not accessible from tumor biopsies. Moreover, they would obviate the need for tumor biopsy and, in particular, repeat tumor biopsies to determine tumor response and molecular evolution following therapy. Tumors can release large amounts of nucleotides into the circulation with up to 20% of circulating DNA being derived from a patient tumor. Thus, any aberration such as mutation, rearrangement, increased copy number, increased microRNA, or RNA level could be detected in the circulation, as is the case with *KRAS* and *p53* mutations. However, the amount of DNA in the circulation and the ability to detect tumor-related aberrations varies markedly across tumor types. Nevertheless, commercial tests based on circulating DNA are becoming available.

Challenges in validation of novel molecular biomarkers

The novel unbiased technologies being used to profile the cancer genome or proteome to define new biomarker panels are susceptible to challenges in reproducibility that can be attributed to the simultaneous assay of many gene or protein markers with a limited number of cancer specimens. The large number of potential biomarker combinations introduces a significant likelihood that uncovered associations are simply the result of chance. A rigorous train, test, and validation approach to novel biomarker studies is critical to impact patient management meaningfully. Most studies presenting novel biomarker panels have not impacted patient management to date, either because they did not contend with this multiple parameter problem or because they did not adopt sufficiently robust statistical approaches to validation. The importance of bioinformatic and biostatistical support for the development of novel molecular diagnostics cannot be overemphasized.

Rigorous validation of molecular marker panels in large numbers of well-documented cases is required to test their clinical utility before adoption for routine use in patient management. The applicability of several preliminary panels is still being validated.[129,130] A major hindrance to designing novel molecular studies for biomarker discovery and validation is the frequent lack of availability of adequately preserved and annotated tissue or blood samples in large numbers to correlate with outcome using emerging technologies. In particular, novel high-throughput approaches are often limited in their utility to fresh frozen specimens (paraffin-embedded samples are more plentiful). Thus, a popular model for biomarker development involves discovery using novel high-throughput profiling technologies (e.g., transcriptional profiling) in frozen tissue, followed by validation using moderate-throughput technologies (e.g., RT-PCR) applied to paraffin-embedded tissue. The specific tissue type in which a molecular marker will be validated for clinical use is critical to define.[131,132] Novel comprehensive approaches to biomarker discovery using proteome- or genome-wide expression profiling have now redefined ways tumor banks collect and store tumor samples, with a major emphasis placed on fresh frozen specimens.[133,134]

Presently, it is not possible to apply all available investigative technologies to every person, or even every patient at high risk for the development of cancer. Putting cost issues aside, one challenge is to obtain adequate material from biopsy, cellular or serum specimens. Indeed, several hundred nanograms are required for comprehensive analysis of genomic *DNA* or *RNA*, but the amount of DNA and RNA available from a fine needle aspirate is in picograms. Furthermore, biopsies frequently have relatively low tumor content, thereby complicating analysis. In the case of CTCs and circulating nucleotides, the DNA and RNA yield can be even smaller. Amplification by PCR can increase mRNA yield, but PCR-generated errors are not uncommon. Approaches to contend with low amounts of protein are minimal. As noted earlier, MRM and other mass spectrometry approaches may complement antibody-based approaches. Currently, we are exploring "barcoding" antibodies with DNA sequences to allow use of amplification approaches that have been applied to DNA detection. These major difficulties need to be addressed to facilitate the routine application of novel molecular technologies to cancer diagnostics.

Recommendations

The effective discovery of novel cancer biomarkers requires the integration of multiple critical factors, including collaborative studies, availability of appropriate human tissue sample sets, standardized reagents and technologies for analyzing, identifying and quantitating candidate biomarkers in tissue and fluid, mouse models of disease, integrated bioinformatics platforms, and implementation of automation, all of which were key to achieving the Human Genome Project, for example. Standard operating procedures (SOPs) regarding tumor specimen biobanking, specimen processing and quality control, validation, performance, and interpretation of analytical assays should be developed at a national or, ideally, international level, to allay concerns regarding potentially unreliable study results and permit accurate pooling and comparison of cross-study results. The American Association for Cancer Research (AACR), the Food and Drug Administration (FDA), the National Cancer Institute (NCI) Cancer Biomarker Collaborative, and the European Group on Tumour Markers have defined these key procedures for effective biomarker development. These strategies can be facilitated by the creation of national biospecimen repositories such as the Cancer Human Biobank, which retrieves highly clinically annotated tumor specimens across centers in the United States and processes them according to SOPs before being made available for analysis.

As biomarker discovery programs characterize tissues using high-throughput genomic, transcriptional and proteomic approaches, the development of adequate and centralized computational infrastructure is critical to allow storage, utilization, and integration of the vast and heterogeneous data derived from novel "omics" technologies. Such a computational resource should be easily accessible to all investigators, protect confidentiality, and avoid duplication of efforts. These resources should facilitate data mining, retrieval, and automated analysis, thus facilitating data integration across molecular platforms and between data sets, and the association of specific aberrations with clinical endpoints. Currency should be maintained as novel "omics" technologies are introduced and upgraded. Access should foster novel biostatistical approaches that further our ability to select clinically useful cancer biomarkers. Approaches are being implemented to facilitate sample and data sharing across the community, given that the amount of data available far exceeds the ability of any group to adequately mine and interpret it. The Biospecimen and Biorepositories Research Branch of the NCI provides effective tools and resources to establish high-quality biobanking. A significant number of online data repositories, such as The Cancer Genome Atlas Portal and The Clinical Proteomic

Tumor Analysis Consortium, are now publicly available, thereby facilitating the interrogation of biomarkers by different research groups.

The selection of novel biomarkers from data derived using novel high-throughput technologies needs careful consideration, to discern chance associations from true biological relationships. False biomarker discovery can result from selection bias, overfitting, intrapatient correlation, multiplicity, multiple clinical endpoints, and intrapatient correlation, which must be eliminated from research designs using accurate statistical methods and study designs including sample sizes that enable markers meeting prespecified performance characteristics for well-defined clinical applications to be identified. New biomarkers should be validated before potential introduction into clinical management by measuring the biomarker's impact on costs and carefully chosen clinical outcomes in a prospective, randomized study.[135] However, study costs and regulatory and healthcare market constraints often make such clinical trials impractical. Improved study designs involving restrospective samples, such as the ProBE method, have been developed as alternatives. Alternatively, retrospective analysis of archived prospectively collected samples, or pooled analyses of published and unpublished cohorts with a systematic review can also provide a high level of evidence, as long as specific requirements ensuring high quality within these study designs are met. Moreover, researchers and policymakers turn to simulation modeling to predict the effects of new biomarkers on outcomes. The latter approach can optimize sensitivity, specificity, and cost in addition to identifying leverage points where more definitive biomarkers may be needed. This approach has already been used to assess the cost effectiveness of flexible sigmoidoscopy for colorectal cancer screening.

A Committee on Developing Biomarker-Based Tools for Cancer Screening, Diagnosis, and Treatment of the Institute of Medicine of the National Academies has produced a formal set of recommendations for development of biomarker-based tools for cancer (Box 3).

Box 3 Summary of recommendations to develop biomarker-based tools for cancer

Methods, tools, and resources needed to discover and develop biomarkers
1. Federal agencies should develop an organized, comprehensive approach to biomarker discovery and foster development of novel technologies.
2. Industry and other funders should establish international consortia to generate and share precompetitive biomarker data.
3. Funders should place a major emphasis on developing pathway biomarkers to broaden applicability.
4. Funders should sponsor demonstration projects to develop biomarkers that can predict efficacy and safety in patients for drugs already on the market.
5. Government agencies and other funders should sustain support for high-quality biorepositories of prospectively collected samples.
6. Biomarkers should be developed and validated with high negative predictive value for prediction of response to targeted therapies, particularly those with high cost.

Guidelines, standards, oversight, and incentives needed for biomarker development
7. Government agencies and other stakeholders should develop a transparent process to create well-defined consensus standards and guidelines for biomarker development, qualification, validation, and use.
8. The FDA and industry should work together to facilitate the codevelopment and approval of diagnostic-therapeutic combinations.
9. The FDA should clearly delineate and standardize its oversight of biomarker tests used in clinical decision making.
10. The Centers for Medicare and Medicaid Services should develop a specialty area for molecular diagnostics under the CLIA.

Methods and processes needed for clinical evaluation and sdoption
11. The Centers for Medicare & Medicaid Services should revise and modernize its coding and pricing system for diagnostic tests.
12. The Centers for Medicare and Medicaid Services, as well as other payors, should develop criteria for conditional coverage of new biomarker tests.

As a component of conditional coverage, procedures for high-quality population-based assessments of efficacy and cost effectiveness of biomarker tests should be established.

Source: From the Institute of Medicine of the National Academies.

Conclusion

In summary, significant progress has been made in the development of molecular diagnostics in certain forms of cancer such as breast cancer. Recent molecular studies have revealed the biologic heterogeneity and complexity of cancer and this necessitates the application of more global studies of the cancer genome and proteome to identify novel biomarkers that facilitate further advances in the understanding, treatment and early detection of cancer. Indeed, the application of high-throughput technologies is already advancing significantly the ability to predict responsiveness to specific cancer treatments. Improving understanding of the molecular heterogeneity of cancer along with rapid improvements in molecular technologies that can profile this heterogeneity has revealed possibilities for the development of molecular diagnostics in cancer. Eventually, these approaches will not only advance our ability to diagnose cancer at an early stage but will also allow simultaneous profiling of molecular targets that will facilitate individualization of patient care. Achievement of these goals necessitates overcoming many challenges that presently preclude successful application of both traditional and novel molecular technologies to cancer diagnostics. As high-throughput technologies acquire an increasing foothold in the development of novel molecular cancer diagnostics, the establishment of robust collaborations and bioinformatics approaches to high-throughput data storage, integration, analysis and validation will be critical.

Key references

The complete reference list can be found on the Wiley Companion Digital Edition of this title (see inside front cover for login instructions).

1 Fisher B, Costantino JP, Wickerham DL, et al. Tamoxifen for the prevention of breast cancer: current status of the National Surgical Adjuvant Breast and Bowel Project P-1 study. *J Natl Cancer Inst.* 2005;**97**:1652–1662.
2 Barrett-Connor EL, Mosca L, Collins P, et al. Effects of raloxifene on cardiovascular evenets and breast cancer in postmenopausal women. *N Engl J Med.* 2006;**355**:125–137.
5 The National Lung Screening Trial Team. Reduced lung-cancer mortality with low-dose computed tomographic screening. *N Engl J Med.* 2011;**365**:395–409.
6 Kriege M, Brekelmans CT, Boetes C, et al. Efficacy of MRI and mammography for breast cancer screening in women with a familial or genetic predisposition. *N Engl J Med.* 2004;**351**:427–437.
10 Schroder FH, Hugosson J, Roobol MJ, et al. Screening and prostate-cancer mortality in a randomized European study. *N Engl J Med.* 2009;**360**(**13**):1320–1328.
11 Andriole GL, Crawford ED, Grubb RL 3rd, et al. Mortality results from a randomized prostate-cancer screening trial. *N Engl J Med.* 2009;**360**:1310–1319.
12 Basch E, Oliver TK, Vickers A, et al. Screening for prostate cancer with prostate-specific antigen testing: American Society of Clinical Oncology Provisional Clinical Opinion. *J Clin Oncol.* 2012;**30**(**24**):3020–3025.
13 Moyer VA, on behalf of the U.S. Preventive Services Task Force. Screening for prostate cancer: U.S. Preventive Services Task Force recommendation statement. *Ann Int Med.* 2012;**157**:120–134.

14 Carter HB, Albertsen PC, Barry MJ, et al. *Early Detection of Prostate Cancer: AUA Guideline*. Linthicum, MD: American Urological Association Education and Research, Inc.; 2013.

16 Lu KH, Skates S, Hernandez MA, et al. A 2-stage ovarian cancer screening strategy using the Risk of Ovarian Cancer Algorithm (ROCA) identifies early-stage incident cancers and demonstrates high positive predictive value. *Cancer*. 2013;**119**(**19**):3454–3461.

17 Menon U, Gentry-Maharaj A, Hallet R. Sensitivity and specificity of multimodal and ultrasound screening for ovarian cancer, and stage distribution of detected cancers: results of the prevalence screen of the UK Collaborative Trial of Ovarian Cancer Screening (UKCTOCS). *Lancet Oncol*. 2009;**10**(**4**):327–340.

18 Menon U, Ryan A, Kalsi J, Gentry-Maharaj A, et al. Risk algorithm using serial biomarker measurements doubles the number of screen-detected cancers compared with a single-threshold rule in the United Kingdom Collaborative Trial of Ovarian Cancer Screening. *J Clin Oncol*. 2015;**33**(**18**):2062–2071.

19 Ronco G, Dillner J, Elfström KM. Efficacy of HPV-based screening for prevention of invasive cervical cancer: follow-up of four European randomised controlled trials. *Lancet*. 2014;**383**(**9916**):524–532.

27 Bolton KL, Chenevix-Trench G, Goh C. Association between BRCA1 and BRCA2 mutations and survival in women with invasive epithelial ovariancancer. *JAMA*. 2012;**307**(**4**):382–390.

32 Couch FJ, Hart SN, Sharma P, et al. Inherited mutations in 17 breast cancer susceptibility genes among a large triple-negative breast cancercohort unselected for family history of breast cancer. *J Clin Oncol*. 2015;**33**(**4**):304–311.

33 Pérez-Carbonell L, Ruiz-Ponte C, Guarinos C. Comparison between universal molecular screening for Lynch syndrome and revised Bethesda guidelines in a large population-based cohort of patients with colorectal cancer. *Gut*. 2012;**61**(**6**):865–872.

38 Paik S, Shak S, Tang G, et al. A multigene assay to predict recurrence of tamoxifen-treated, node-negative breast cancer. *N Engl J Med*. 2004;**351**:2817–2826.

42 Slamon DJ, Clark GM, Wong SG, et al. Human breast cancer: correlation of relapse and survival with amplification of the HER-2/neu oncogene. *Science*. 1987;**235**:177–182.

51 Majewski IJ, Nuciforo P, Mittempergher L, et al. PIK3CA mutations are associated with decreased benefit to neoadjuvant human epidermal growth factor receptor 2-targeted therapies in breast cancer. *J Clin Oncol*. 2015;**33**(**12**):1334–1339.

52 Wolff AC, Hammond EH, Hicks DG. Recommendations for human epidermal growth factor receptor 2 testing in breast cancer: American Society of Clinical Oncology/College of American Pathologists Clinical Practice Guideline Update. *J Clin Oncol*. 2013;**31**(**31**):3997–4013.

53 Hennessy BT, Timms KM, Carey MS. Somatic mutations in BRCA1 and BRCA2 could expand the number of patients that benefit from poly (ADP ribose) polymerase inhibitors in ovarian cancer. *J Clin Oncol*. 2010;**28**(**22**):3570–3576.

56 Matulonis UA, Wolff G, Barry W, et al. *Phase I of Oral BKM120 or BYL719 and Olaparib for High-Grade Serous Ovarian Cancer or Triple-Negative Breast Cancer: Final Results of the BKM120 Plus Olaparib Cohort*. Proceedings of the 106th Annual Meeting of the American Association for Cancer Research; 2015 April 18–22; Philadelphia, PA. Philadelphia (PA): AACR; 2015. Abstract nr CT324.

57 Rosell R, Carcereny E, Gervais R. Erlotinib versus standard chemotherapy as first-line treatment for European patients with advanced EGFR mutation-positive non-small-cell lung cancer (EURTAC): a multicentre, open-label, randomised phase 3 trial. *Lancet Oncol*. 2012;**13**(**3**):239–246.

58 Fukuoka M, Wu YL, Thongprasert S. Biomarker analyses and final overall survival results from a phase III, randomized, open-label, first-line study of gefitinib versus carboplatin/paclitaxel in clinically selected patients with advanced non-small-cell lung cancer in Asia (IPASS). *J Clin Oncol*. 2011;**29**(**21**):2866–2874.

59 Yang JC, Wu YL, Schuler M. Afatinib versus cisplatin-based chemotherapy for EGFR mutation-positive lung adenocarcinoma (LUX-Lung 3 and LUX-Lung 6): analysis of overall survival data from two randomised, phase 3 trials. *Lancet Oncol*. 2015;**16**(**2**):141–151.

60 Jänne PA, Ou S-HI, Kim D-W, et al. Dacomitinib as first-line treatment in patients with clinically or molecularly selected advanced non-small-cell lung cancer: a multicentre, open-label, phase 2 trial. *Lancet Oncol*. 2014;**15**(**13**):1433–1441.

63 Shaw AT, Kim DW, Nakagawa K. Crizotinib versus chemotherapy in advanced ALK-positive lung cancer. *N Engl J Med*. 2013;**368**(**25**):2385–2394.

64 Shaw AT, Ou SH, Bang YJ. Crizotinib in ROS-1 rearranged non-small cell lung cancer. *N Engl J Med*. 2014;**371**(**21**):1963–1971.

65 Shaw AT, Kim DW, Mehra R. Cetirinib in ALK-rearranged non-small cell lung cancer. *N Engl J Med*. 2014;**370**(**13**):1189–1197.

66 Leighl NB, Rekhtman N, Biermann WA. Molecular testing for selection of patients with lung cancer for epidermal growth factor receptor and anaplastic lymphoma kinase tyrosine kinase inhibitors: American Society of Clinical Oncology endorsement of the College of American Pathologists/International Society for the Study of Lung Cancer/Association of Molecular Pathologists guideline. *J Clin Oncol*. 2014;**32**(**32**):3673–3679. doi: 10.1200/JCO.2014.57.3055.

68 Douillard JY, Oliner KS, Siena S, et al. Panitumumab-FOLFOX4 treatment and RAS mutations in colorectal cancer. *N Engl J Med*. 2013;**369**:1023–1034.

70 Van Cutsem E, Köhne CH, Láng I, et al. Cetuximab plus irinotecan, fluorouracil, and leucovorin as first-line treatment for metastatic colorectal cancer: updated analysis of overall survival according to tumor KRAS and BRAF mutation status. *J Clin Oncol*. 2011;**29**(**15**):2011–2019.

72 Cioffi A, Maki RG. GI stromal tumors: 15 years of lessons from a rare cancer. *J Clin Oncol*. 2015;**33**(**16**):1849–1854. doi: JCO.2014.59.7344.

73 Chapman PB, Hauschild A, Robert C, et al. Improved survival with vemurafenib in melanoma with BRAF V600E mutation. *N Engl J Med*. 2011;**364**:2507–2516.

74 Hauschild A, Grob JJ, Demidov LV, et al. Dabrafenib in BRAF-mutated metastatic melanoma: a multicentre, open-label, phase 3 randomised controlled trial. *Lancet*. 2012;**380**:358–365.

75 Long GV, Stroyakovskiy D, Gogas H, et al. Combined BRAF and MEK inhibition versus BRAF inhibition alone in melanoma. *N Engl J Med*. 2013;**371**:1877–1888.

76 Johnson DB, Puzanov I. Treatment of NRAS-mutant melanoma. *Curr Treat Options Oncol*. 2015;**16**(**4**):15.

77 Hodi FS, Corless CL, Giobbie-Hurder A, et al. Imatinib for melanomas harboring mutationally activated or amplified KIT arising on mucosal, acral, and chronically sun-damaged skin. *J Clin Oncol*. 2013;**31**(**26**):3182–3190.

90 Rustin G, van der Burg M, Griffin C. Early versus delayed treatment of relapsed ovarian cancer (MRC OV05/EORTC55955): a randomised trial. *Lancet*. 2010;**376**(**9747**):1155–1163.

91 Harris L, Fritsche H, Mennel R, et al. American Society of Clinical Oncology. American Society of Clinical Oncology 2007 update of recommendations for the use of tumor markers in breast cancer. *J Clin Oncol*. 2007;**25**(**33**): 5287–5312.

94 Locker GY, Hamilton S, Harris J, et al. American Society of Clinical Oncology 2006 update of recommendations for the use of tumor markers in gastrointestinal cancer. *J Clin Oncol*. 2006;**24**:5313–5327.

100 Stemke-Hale K, Gonzalez-Angulo AM, Lluch A, et al. An integrative genomic and proteomic analysis of PIK3CA, PTEN, and AKT mutations in breast cancer. *Cancer Res*. 2008;**68**:6084–6091.

102 Hennessy BT, Lu Y, Poradosu E, et al. Quantified pathway inhibition as a pharmacodynamic marker facilitating optimal targeted therapy dosing: proof of principle with the AKT inhibitor perifosine. *Clin Cancer Res*. 2007;**13**:7421–7431.

113 Sleijfer S, Bogaerts J, Siu LL. Designing transformative clinical trials in the cancer genome era. *J Clin Oncol*. 2013;**31**(**15**):1834–1841.

120 Cristofanilli M, Budd GT, Ellis MJ, et al. Circulating tumor cells, disease progression, and survival in metastatic breast cancer. *N Engl J Med*. 2004;**351**: 781–791.

121 Dawson SJ, Tsui DW, Murtaza M, et al. Analysis of circulating tumor DNA to monitor metastatic breast cancer. *N Engl J Med*. 2013;**368**:1199–1209.

127 Becker FF, Wang XB, Huang Y, et al. Separation of human breast cancer cells from blood by differential dielectric affinity. *Proc Natl Acad Sci U S A*. 1995;**92**:60–864.

132 Segal E, Friedman N, Kaminski N, Regev A, Koller D. From signatures to models: understanding cancer using microarrays. *Nat Genetics*. 2005;**37**(**suppl**):S38–S45.

135 Hartwell L, Mankoff D, Paulovich A, Ramsey S, Swisher E. Cancer biomarkers: a systems approach. *Nat Biotechnol*. 2006;**24**:905–908.

41 Principles of imaging

Lawrence H. Schwartz, MD

Overview

Imaging is an indispensable component of clinical oncology. Computed tomography (CT) is usually more informative than plain X-rays. Metabolic imaging with ^{18}F-fluorodeoxyglucose is best combined with anatomical verification by CT. Evolving studies of function linking magnetic resonance to CT imaging is another advance for precision assessment. Targeting specific molecules with labeled agents is an evolving sector. Invasive procedures performed under radiologic imaging have substantially displaced open surgery, with benefits to patients in comfort, time and costs.

Imaging plays a major and fundamental role in every aspect of oncology. Radiological studies provide invaluable information about tumor detection, characterization, staging, and therapeutic response monitoring. Increasingly, imaging in oncology is being used both as a prognostic biomarker and as a predictive biomarker, either alone or in combination with other tissue and serum biomarkers. Screening examinations such as mammography, low-dose CT for lung cancer, and virtual colonoscopy are other examples of the use of imaging in oncology. Finally, image-guided intervention has evolved significantly over the past few years and has tremendous potential for minimizing the invasiveness of many cancer therapies.

Cross-sectional imaging studies, including computed tomography (CT) and positron emission tomography (PET) scans using ionizing radiation as well as nonionizing magnetic resonance (MR) imaging, are the mainstay of care in the oncology patient and typically complement more traditional radiographs. While conventional radiological studies such as plain diagnostic X-ray examination films are easy to perform, deliver a low-dose of radiation, and are relatively inexpensive, their utility in the care of cancer patients is limited.

The type and frequency of radiological evaluation of the cancer patient depend on the tumor, the stage of the disease, and the specific clinical indication for the scan. There is a wide spectrum of indications that include screening, workup of the symptomatic patient, further evaluation of an abnormality found on another imaging study, assessing response or progression of a patient's disease after a therapy or intervention, and evaluating complications of therapy. Before every radiology study is ordered, it is imperative to understand the clinical scenario, what information is needed, whether the test can provide the necessary evidence, and, importantly, what can and will be done with the results to change the treatment of the patient and potentially the patient's outcome.

Integration of imaging with other diagnostic tools, including genomic and proteomic assays, is enabling complementary information to be obtained for the cancer patient. However, there is growing need for these imaging studies to provide more information that simple anatomic visualization and localization of tumors. Contemporary oncology requires that imaging studies visualize basic molecular events that would increase our understanding of malignancies and eventually influence clinical practice.

The growth of a molecular imaging began in the early 1990s, with the use of PET imaging and the glucose analog probe, [^{18}F]-2-fluoro-2-deoxy-D-glucose (FDG). Over the past several years, FDG-PET imaging has become one of the most important tools to evaluate cancer patients for characterization of primary tumors and their metastases as well as for monitoring treatment response to cancer therapy. PET images are less detailed anatomically and create the potential for fusion of morphologic, detailed anatomic information from a CT scan with a PET scan. Hybrid, dual PET/CT scanners as well as PET/MRI provide combination imaging, which is of higher diagnostic value than separate PET, CT, or MRI scans in many cancers and clinical indications. As a move toward molecular imaging continues, the development of new targets, techniques, and tumor-specific imaging probes should provide more accurate diagnostic information. The use of PET imaging and other molecular imaging techniques has increased along with MRI to evaluate cell metabolism, cell proliferation, hypoxia, apoptosis, receptor expression, gene expression, angiogenesis, and signal transduction. In the future, molecular imaging may be able to address many current unresolved diagnostic issues in oncology. Although the technology is undergoing dramatic expansion, the radiologic community has a responsibility to study new molecular imaging techniques carefully to determine if they are truly useful and cost effective. The ability to create ever more spectacular images does not necessarily improve patient management and outcomes.

Hypothesis-driven, evidence-based studies are essential if noninvasive anatomic and molecular imaging is to have an impact on patient care. Because imaging is a fundamental part of diagnostic evaluation, understanding the utility of particular tests will guide a more efficient patient evaluation. This section's collection of chapters provides an overview of imaging principles, with a focus on the cancer patient. Imaging plays a central role in clinical management, and the information presented here provides general guidelines for using radiologic studies in everyday clinical practice.

Further reading

Apolo AB, Pandit-Taskar N, Morris MJ. Novel tracers and their development for the imaging of metastatic prostate cancer. *J Nucl Med.* 2008;**49**:2031–2041.

Boss DS, Olmos RV, Sinaasappel M, Beijnen JH, Schellens JH. Application of PET/CT in the development of novel anticancer drugs. *Oncologist.* 2008;**13**(1):25–38.

Czernin J, Ta L, Herrmann K. Does PET/MR imaging improve cancer assessments? Literature evidence from more than 900 patients. *J Nucl Med.* 2014;**55**(Supplement 2):59S–62S.

Farwell MD, Pryma DA, Mankoff DA. PET/CT imaging in cancer: current applications and future directions. *Cancer.* 2014;**120**(22):3433–45.

Fleming IN, Manavaki R, Blower PJ, et al. Imaging tumour hypoxia with positron emission tomography. *Br J Cancer.* 2015;**112**(2):238–250.

Holland-Frei Cancer Medicine, Ninth Edition. Edited by Robert C. Bast Jr., Carlo M. Croce, William N. Hait, Waun Ki Hong, Donald W. Kufe, Martine Piccart-Gebhart, Raphael E. Pollock, Ralph R. Weichselbaum, Hongyang Wang, and James F. Holland.
© 2017 John Wiley & Sons, Inc. ISBN: 978-1-118-93469-2

Gerstner ER, Sorensen AG, Jain RK, Batchelor TT. Advances in neuroimaging techniques for the evaluation of tumor growth, vascular permeability, and angiogenesis in gliomas. *Curr Opin Neurol.* 2008;**21**(**6**):728–735.

Heron DE, Andrade RS, Beriwal S, Smith RP, et al. PET-CT in radiation oncology: the impact on diagnosis, treatment planning, and assessment of treatment response. *Am J Clin Oncol.* 2008;**31**(**4**):352–362.

Iagaru A, Mittra E, Minamimoto R, et al. Simultaneous whole-body time-of-flight 18F-FDG PET/MRI: a pilot study comparing SUVmax with PET/CT and assessment of MR image quality. *Clin Nucl Med.* 2015 Jan;**40**(**1**):1–8.

Kim JH, Choi SH, Ryoo I, et al. Prognosis prediction of measurable enhancing lesion after completion of standard concomitant chemoradiotherapy and adjuvant temozolomide in glioblastoma patients: application of dynamic susceptibility contrast perfusion and diffusion-weighted imaging. *PLoS One.* 2014;**9**(**11**):e113587.

Kuehl H, Veit P, Rosenbaum SJ, Bockisch A, Antoch G. Can PET/CT replace separate diagnostic CT for cancer imaging? Optimizing CT protocols for imaging cancers of the chest and abdomen. *J Nucl Med.* 2007;**48**(**suppl 1**):45S–57S.

Kundra V, Silverman PM, Matin SF, Choi H. Imaging in oncology from the University of Texas M. D. Anderson Cancer Center: diagnosis, staging, and surveillance of prostate cancer. *AJR Am J Roentgenol.* 2007;**189**(**4**):830–844.

Malviya G, Nayak TK. PET imaging to monitor cancer therapy. *Curr Pharm Biotechnol.* 2013;**14**(**7**):669–682.

Schaefer JF, Schlemmer HP. Total-body MR-imaging in oncology. *Eur Radiol.* 2006;**16**(**9**):2000–2015.

Tanvetyanon T, Eikman EA, Sommers E, Robinson L, Boulware D, Bepler G. Response by PET scan versus CT scan to predict survival after neoadjuvant chemotherapy for resectable non-small cell lung cancer. *JCO.* 2008;**26**:4610–4616.

Veit P, Ruehm S, Kuehl H, et al. Lymph node staging with dual-modality PET/CT: enhancing the diagnostic accuracy in oncology. *Eur J Radiol.* 2006;**58**(**3**):383–389.

Wirth A, Foo M, Seymour JF, Macmanus MP, Hicks RJ. Impact of [18f] fluorodeoxyglucose positron emission tomography on staging and management of early-stage follicular non-hodgkin lymphoma. *Int J Radiat Oncol Biol Phys.* 2008;**71**(**1**):213–219.

Wong TZ, Paulson EK, Nelson RC, Patz EF Jr, Coleman RE. Practical approach to diagnostic CT combined with PET. *AJR Am J Roentgenol.* 2007;**188**(**3**):622–629.

Zhao B, Schwartz LH, Larson SM. Imaging surrogates of tumor response to therapy: anatomic and functional biomarkers. *J Nucl Med.* 2009;**50**(**2**):239–249.

42 Interventional radiology for the cancer patient

Judy U. Ahrar, MD ■ *Michael J. Wallace, MD* ■ *Rony Avritscher, MD*

Overview

In the past decades, there has been a substantial expansion in the use of image-guided procedures for diagnosing and treating various types of cancer. Percutaneous biopsy is usually the first step in obtaining a definitive diagnosis and aids in the development of the treatment plan. Patients with primary or metastatic disease involving the liver are candidates for a wide range of image-guided interventions such as hepatic arterial embolization procedures, liver tumor ablation, and portal vein embolization. Cancer patients also benefit from a variety of palliative image-guided interventions, such as vena cava filter placement, biliary drainage and stent placement, and renal artery embolization, to name a few. Interventional radiology offers a multitude of minimally invasive procedures that are a key component in the management of cancer patients.

In the past decades, there has been a substantial expansion in the use of image-guided procedures for diagnosing and treating various types of cancer. There are several reasons for this increased use. Advances in cancer diagnosis and novel medical and surgical therapies have led to increased survival in this patient population. Owing to the prevalence of imaging, more patients now present with primary or metastatic disease confined to an organ and, consequently, are more likely to benefit from locoregional therapies than from systemic treatment. Thus, a neoplasm can be defined using standard imaging modalities, and then minimally invasive percutaneous techniques can be used to establish the diagnosis and provide locoregional or palliative therapies to treat the cancer patient. Recent improvements in catheter/device technology, embolic agents and chemotherapy drugs, and delivery systems are associated with improved patient outcome and have sparked renewed interest in these approaches. In this chapter, we discuss hepatic vascular interventions, genitourinary interventions, thoracic interventions, several forms of palliative therapeutic procedures, and some additional image-guided procedures (vena cava filter placement, biopsy, and intratumoral gene therapy).

Hepatic vascular interventions

The liver has long occupied center stage in interventional oncology, the practice of interventional radiology specific to the oncology patient. Hepatic interventions for diagnosis and treatment are popular for a number of reasons, among them being that this organ is a common site of metastatic disease and can be accessed easily percutaneously. However, the key feature that makes liver tumors particularly amenable to catheter-delivered therapies stems from the unique nature of their blood supply. Hepatic tumors derive most of their blood supply from the hepatic artery, whereas normal hepatic parenchyma derives most of its supply from the portal venous system. This unique arrangement allows the interventional oncologist to treat hepatic lesions while sparing the surrounding normal liver.

Arterial infusion therapy

The goal of arterial infusion is to achieve better tumor response by delivering chemotherapeutic agents directly into the artery that supplies the neoplasm. The rationale behind arterial infusion therapy is based on the first-pass effect, which occurs when a drug is given directly into the tissue that metabolizes it. The first-pass effect, compared with systemic administration, can lead to a several-fold increase in the drug concentration within the affected organ and, at the same time, a reduction in systemic concentration. Therefore, regional drug delivery is seen as a method of overcoming the limitations of the maximum-tolerated dose.[1]

Arterial infusion therapy has been used primarily for the treatment of metastatic colorectal cancer confined to the liver. A meta-analysis by Mocellin et al. [2] summarized the results of 10 randomized controlled trials that compared hepatic arterial infusion (HAI) with systemic chemotherapy. Although the study revealed better tumor response to fluoropyrimidine-based HAI than systemic fluoropyrimidine therapy, tumor response rates for modern systemic chemotherapy regimens using a combination of fluorouracil with oxaliplatin or irinotecan were similar or superior to those for HAI. Moreover, the meta-analysis showed no survival benefit associated with fluoropyrimidine-based HAI therapy. Further studies of the use of HAI for the delivery of novel anticancer agents will be instrumental in determining the role of this approach in future locoregional cancer therapy.

Arterial embolization

The aim of transcatheter hepatic arterial embolization is to completely or partially occlude the arterial supply to the tumor. The rationale is that such occlusion will cause tumor ischemia, which in turn will lead to growth arrest and necrosis. After hepatic arterial embolization, collateral hepatic circulation comes into play immediately. This collateral circulation should be traced and occluded if it supplies the neoplasm. The more central the occlusion, the more abundant is the collateral flow. Therefore, to maximize ischemia, the most effective embolization should result in distal terminal vessel occlusion. Peripheral (segmental and subsegmental) vascular embolization is best accomplished with coaxial catheters and small particles.

Many different embolic agents have been used with success for hepatic embolization. The most common agents include absorbable gelatin sponge particles and powder, polyvinyl alcohol foam granules, fibrin glue, *n*-butyl cyanoacrylate, ethiodized oil, microspheres, and absolute alcohol. Gelatin sponge segments or stainless steel coils are used for central occlusion and not often used for tumor embolotherapy.

Holland-Frei Cancer Medicine, Ninth Edition. Edited by Robert C. Bast Jr., Carlo M. Croce, William N. Hait, Waun Ki Hong, Donald W. Kufe, Martine Piccart-Gebhart, Raphael E. Pollock, Ralph R. Weichselbaum, Hongyang Wang, and James F. Holland.
© 2017 John Wiley & Sons, Inc. ISBN: 978-1-118-93469-2

The most common complication after hepatic arterial embolization is postembolization syndrome. This syndrome consists of fever, nausea, fatigue, and elevated white blood cell count and liver function tests. These symptoms are usually self-limited. Complications resulting from nontarget embolization include cholecystitis, pancreatitis, and gastrointestinal ulcers. Hepatic embolization may also lead to liver necrosis, hepatic abscess, and liver failure. Failure to recognize intrahepatic arteriovenous shunts during embolization may cause embolic material to reach the pulmonary circulation, which can in turn lead to respiratory failure. The complications of hepatic embolization in 284 patients who underwent 410 embolizations over a 10-year period were analyzed by Hemingway and Allison.[3] Minor complications occurred in 16% of patients, serious complications in 6.6%, and death in 2%.

Arterial chemoembolization

Arterial chemoembolization consists of intra-arterial delivery of a combination of chemotherapy drugs and an embolic agent into a liver tumor. The rationale behind chemoembolization is based on the theory that tumor ischemia caused by embolization of the dominant arterial supply has a synergistic effect with the chemotherapeutic drugs. This technique has been the mainstay of interventional radiology since it was introduced by Yamada in 1977.[4] The introduction of iodized oil, an iodinated ester derived from poppy-seed oil, advanced this technique significantly. Iodized oil is well suited for chemoembolization because of its preferential tumor uptake by hepatocellular carcinoma (HCC) and certain hepatic metastases; it acts simultaneously as an embolic agent and a vehicle for the chemotherapeutic agent.[5,6] These findings are explained partially by the concept of enhanced permeability and retention suggested by Maeda et al.[7] Newly formed tumor vessels are more permeable. This increased permeability coupled with a lack of lymphatics in the neoplasm results in retention of molecules of higher molecular weight within the tumor interstitium for a more prolonged period. This retention may explain, in part, the accumulation of iodized oil or the increase in concentration of polymer conjugates of chemotherapeutic agents in neoplasms.

There are many different chemoembolization protocols. The most commonly used chemotherapy agent is doxorubicin, which is combined with cisplatin and mitomycin C. Subsequently, these chemotherapeutic agents are mixed with iodized oil and infused slowly into the hepatic artery branch that feeds the tumor. Drug-eluting beads, which are microspheres loaded with chemotherapy agents (doxorubicin and irinotecan), have recently come into common use for chemoembolization. Additional embolization with gelatin sponge or particles can be performed to enhance tumor ischemia. The proximal arterial supply to the tumor should be preserved because increased response is observed with repeated procedures.

Transcatheter arterial chemoembolization has been used to treat unresectable HCC, cholangiocarcinomas, and hepatic metastases and has been used in conjunction with liver resection or tumor ablation or as a bridge to liver transplant. Two randomized clinical trials[8,9] showed a survival advantage when chemoembolization was performed in selected HCC patients. Recent advances in chemotherapy agents and embolic material suggest future potential for this technique. Incorporation of antiangiogenic agents into the mixture to be delivered to the tumor is being investigated.[10,11] Moreover, advances in technology now allow intraprocedural acquisition of cross-sectional images using C-arm cone-beam computed tomography (Figure 1). This technique enables more selective embolization as multiplanar and three-dimensional images are

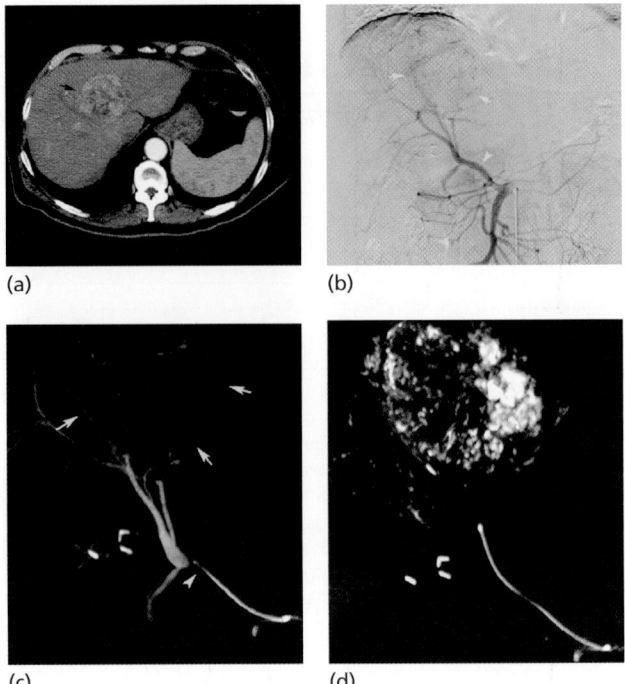

(a)   (b)

(c)   (d)

Figure 1 Transcatheter arterial chemoembolization performed in a 71-year-old man with unresectable hepatocellular carcinoma. (a) Contrast-enhanced CT scan obtained before chemoembolization shows a large, solitary, hypervascular mass in segment IV of the liver (arrow). (b) Anteroposterior digital subtraction angiography (DSA) of the abdomen shows a replaced right hepatic artery arising from the proximal superior mesenteric artery (arrowhead). This vessel supplies the hypervascular tumor in the left liver (arrows). (c) C-arm cone-beam CT images obtained during the procedure show tip of 3-French catheter in the distal replaced right hepatic artery (arrowhead) confirming origin of vascular supply to the hepatocellular carcinoma (arrows). (d) C-arm cone-beam CT images obtained after chemoembolization demonstrate retention of iodized oil throughout the lesion.

used to understand the arterial anatomy and assess completeness of embolization.[12]

Hepatic intra-arterial brachytherapy

Radioembolization with yttrium-90 (^{90}Y) microspheres is a technique in which particles incorporating the isotope ^{90}Y are infused through a catheter directly into the hepatic arteries. Yttrium-90 is a beta emitter with a short half-life. The concept is similar to chemoembolization in that the injected particles are distributed selectively into the tumor arterial bed. This distribution is possible because the arterial blood flow within the tumor is several times greater than the flow in the surrounding liver parenchyma. Consequently, a much higher amount of radiation can be delivered to the lesion than with external-beam radiation, and at the same time, the potential for radiation-induced hepatitis is reduced.

TheraSphere beads (MDS Nordion, Ottawa, Canada) are FDA approved for neoadjuvant treatment of unresectable HCC in patients with portal vein thrombosis or as a bridge to transplantation. SIR-Spheres (Sirtex Medical, Lane Cove, Australia) with concomitant use of floxuridine is approved for the treatment of colorectal cancer metastatic to the liver. Knowledge of the vascular anatomic variants in the celiac axis and superior mesenteric artery is critical to administering this therapy safely to avoid nontarget embolization of the radioactive microspheres, which can have devastating consequences. Multiple studies have demonstrated the safety of radioembolization with yttrium-90 for the treatment of unresectable HCC and metastatic colorectal cancer.[13-15]

Local tissue ablation

Image-guided tumor ablation of focal hepatic malignancies can be accomplished using chemical agents or thermal energy. Chemical ablation options include direct intratumoral percutaneous ethanol injection (PEI) and ablation using hot water or saline, acetic acid, or chemotherapeutic agents that induce tumor cell death. Thermal ablation options include high-energy radiofrequency (RF), interstitial laser photocoagulation, microwave, cryotherapy, and high-intensity focused ultrasound that causes coagulation necrosis. These procedures can be performed under imaging guidance by interventional radiologists or surgeons in the operating suite.

Ethanol is the most commonly used agent for chemical tumor ablation worldwide.[16] Once ethanol is injected into the tumor, it causes cytoplasmic dehydration, denaturation of cellular proteins, and small-vessel thrombosis.[17] PEI is well established for the treatment of HCC, but it is much less successful in the treatment of hepatic metastases; in metastases, thermal ablation methods are more promising. This distinction appears to stem from the way in which ethanol disseminates within the different tumors. The distribution of ethanol tends to be uniform in soft lesions surrounded by hardened cirrhotic liver parenchyma, as is the case in HCC. However, when the surrounding parenchyma is softer than the tumor, as is often the case with metastases, ethanol distribution is less uniform and the treatment is less effective. Ebara et al.[18] reported on 20 years of experience with PEI for HCC lesions ≤3 cm in a total of 270 patients. The local recurrence rate at 3 years was 10%, with overall 3- and 5-year survival rates of 81% and 60%, respectively.

Livraghi et al.[19] studied RF ablation versus PEI in the treatment of small HCCs (≤3 cm in diameter). Complete necrosis was achieved in 47 of 52 tumors (90%) in an average of 1.2 sessions per tumor with RF ablation and 48 of 60 tumors (80%) in an average of 4.8 sessions per tumor with PEI. One major complication (hemothorax) and four minor complications (bleeding, hemobilia, pleural effusion, and cholecystitis) occurred with RF ablation, although there was none with PEI. Lencioni et al.[20] reported treatment of HCC with either RF ablation or PEI in a randomized series of 102 patients with hepatic cirrhosis. Although there was no overall difference in 1- and 2-year survival, there was a significant difference in 1- and 2-year local recurrence-free survival (98% for RF ablation vs 83% for PEI at 1 year and 96% vs 62% at 2 years). The study was limited to patients with either a single HCC ≤5 cm in diameter or a maximum of three HCCs ≤3 cm in diameter. However, up to 25% of the lesions in Ebara and colleagues' study[18] of PEI could not have been treated by RF ablation because of anatomic considerations, which emphasizes that there is still a role for PEI in small tumors despite results that overall favor RF ablation. Thermal ablation for hepatic metastases from colorectal cancer has also been reported to improve survival. Median survival time after thermal ablation was increased to 39 months from 21 to 25 months in a study reported by Gillams and Lees.[21]

Portal vein embolization

Successful resection of the liver depends on the function of the residual hepatic parenchyma. When the portal vein is occluded, hepatocyte growth factors (hepatopoietin A, insulin, and glucagon) are shunted into the liver segments supplied by nonembolized vessels.[22] The result is atrophy of the segments supplied by the occluded vessels and hypertrophy of the other areas of the liver. Thus, portal vein

embolization (PVE) is used preoperatively to induce liver hypertrophy in potential surgical candidates with anticipated marginal future liver remnant (FLR) volumes (Figure 2).

PVE is performed if the FLR is estimated to be <20% of the estimated total liver volume (TLV) in patients without underlying liver disease, <30% of TLV in patients with underlying severe liver injury, and <40% of TLV in patients with cirrhosis.[23] For embolizations performed before extended right hepatectomy, modification of the preoperative embolization to include segment IV may optimize liver hypertrophy. The range of reported mean absolute FLR increase for PVE in general was 46–70%, depending on the particle type used for embolization. PVE results in hepatocyte apoptosis, so the postembolization syndrome associated with transarterial embolization and necrosis does not occur. Madoff et al.[24] reported on 44 patients who underwent PVE before major liver surgery. None of the patients developed liver failure after the resection.

Fibrin glue, gelatin sponge, thrombin, particles, coils, and absolute ethanol all have been used for PVE. In the United States, a combination of particles and embolization coils is the most common embolic agent.

Retrospective studies and meta-analysis suggest improved surgical outcomes after PVE.[23,25] For this reason, PVE before a major hepatectomy is now considered the standard of care in many comprehensive hepatobiliary centers worldwide.

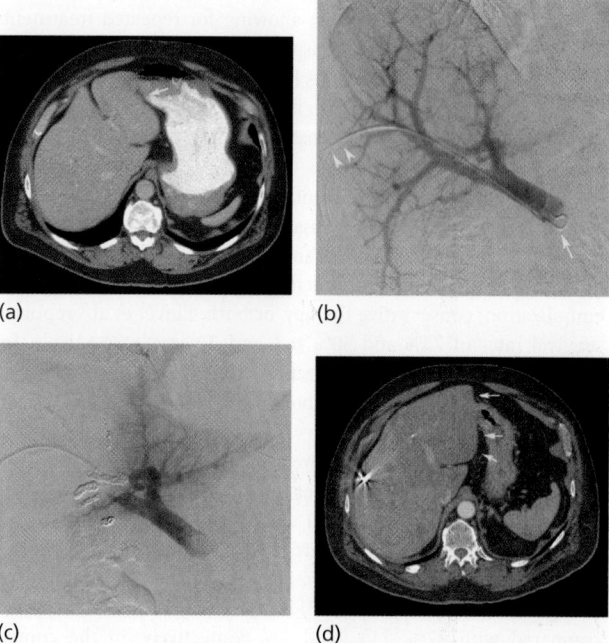

(a)   (b)

(c)   (d)

Figure 2 Transhepatic ipsilateral right portal vein embolization (PVE) extended to segment IV using Tris-acryl particles and coils performed in a 52-year-old man with rectal cancer metastatic to the liver. (a) CT scan obtained before PVE shows marginal future liver remnant (FLR) [FLR-to-TELV (total estimated liver volume) ratio = 17%] (arrows). (b) Anteroposterior DSA portogram shows a 6-French vascular sheath in a right portal vein branch (arrowheads) and a 5-French flush catheter within the main portal vein (arrow). (c) Final DSA portogram shows occlusion of the portal vein branches to segments IV through VIII with continued patency of the vein supplying the left lateral liver. (d) CT scan obtained 1 month after right PVE extended to segment IV shows substantial FLR hypertrophy (FLR-to-TELV ratio = 27%) (arrows). The degree of hypertrophy is 10%.

Considerations in hepatocellular carcinoma

HCC is the fifth most prevalent type of cancer and the third most common cause of cancer death in the world.[26] This disease is common worldwide because of its strong association with underlying liver cirrhosis and hepatitis. Surgical removal of the tumor is the only potentially curative treatment. However, curative resection is possible only in 20–30% of patients.[27] Recurrence rates after surgical resection are high because of dissemination of primary disease, undetected hepatic micrometastases, or metachronous lesions. Five-year survival after partial hepatic resection is approximately 50%.[28] For patients with cirrhosis and unresectable disease, liver transplantation can potentially cure both the underlying liver disease and the tumor. Intra-arterial therapies (embolization, chemoembolization, and radioembolization) and ablative techniques are viable alternatives in patients who are not candidates for partial hepatectomy or transplantation. Systemic chemotherapy for HCC has been disappointing because of the low response rates. In recent times, sorafenib, a multikinase inhibitor with antiangiogenic, proapoptotic, and Raf kinase-inhibitory activity, has been shown to be well tolerated; it is the first agent to demonstrate a statistically significant improvement in overall survival for patients with advanced HCC.[29]

Local etiologic factors have to be evaluated when considering locoregional therapy because HCC in western countries is often different from the typical HCC treated by interventional radiologists in Japan and the far east.[30] Nodular HCC is seen in fewer than 25% of western patients but is seen in approximately 75% of patients in Japan. For patients with early to intermediate disease, ablative techniques are appealing, as the damage to the surrounding liver parenchyma is minimized, allowing for repeated treatments and serving as a bridge to transplantation. The current literature supports the use of percutaneous RF ablation in patients with HCC and either a single lesion <5 cm in diameter or up to three lesions <3 cm in diameter if partial hepatic resection or transplantation is not available.[31]

Chemoembolization is currently used for noncurative therapy for nonsurgical patients with large or multifocal HCC that has not spread extrahepatically. Two randomized studies have reported more favorable results for chemoembolization than for bland embolization, conservative therapy, or both. Llovet et al.[9] reported survival rates of 75% and 50% at 1 and 2 years, respectively, for 37 patients assigned to embolization alone, 82% and 63% for 40 patients assigned to chemoembolization, and 63% and 27% for 35 patients assigned to conservative treatment. The study was stopped early because of the proven survival benefit. Another study by Lo et al.[8] demonstrated a benefit in survival for patients with unresectable HCC treated with chemoembolization (iodized oil, cisplatin, and gelfoam) compared with a control group treated with symptomatic therapy only. Survival in the chemoembolization group was 57% at 1 year, 31% at 2 years, and 26% at 3 years, compared with 32%, 11%, and 3%, respectively, in the control group. Radioembolization with yttrium-90 is FDA approved for neoadjuvant treatment of unresectable HCC in patients with portal vein thrombosis or as a bridge to transplantation, but randomized studies are needed to establish a wider role.

Considerations in hepatic metastases

Colorectal metastases

The liver is often the first and only site of metastasis from colon cancer. Many of these patients will die of their liver disease, thus local control can affect patient outcome positively. Although surgical resection is the first line of treatment for liver metastases, the majority of patients are not surgical candidates because of extent of disease or presence of medical comorbidities. Novel systemic chemotherapy agents are now available, which have been shown to effect significant improvement in patient survival.[32] In addition, local tissue ablation can be offered to patients who are not surgical candidates because of the presence of medical comorbidities or to patients with bilobar disease that can be treated with a combination of ablation and surgery. Recent series of patients with up to five lesions, each measuring ≤5 cm, showed 5-year survival ranges of 24–44%.[33,34] PVE may also be employed to increase the number of patients who can be converted into surgical candidates.[23] Palliative treatment can be offered in the form of arterial infusion therapy and radioembolization. The role of novel chemotherapy agents combined with arterial infusion is being investigated as an alternative viable palliative therapy. Radioembolization with SIR-Spheres (resin microspheres) and concomitant use of floxuridine are approved for the treatment of colorectal cancer metastatic to the liver.

Neuroendocrine metastases

Hepatic artery embolization or chemoembolization is indicated for patients with multiple nonresectable, hormonally active tumors. The goal of treatment is to reduce tumor bulk and hormone secretion. The 5-year postembolization survival range is 50–60%, with symptomatic and biochemical response ranges of 40–80% and 50–60%, respectively.[35] Moertel et al.[36] reported their 10-year experience in 111 patients with neuroendocrine hepatic metastases, usually hypervascular, who received vascular occlusion therapy by a variety of methods. As many as 71 patients received subsequent alternating chemotherapy regimens (dacarbazine combined with doxorubicin, alternating with streptozotocin combined with 5-fluorouracil). Response rates of 60% with vascular occlusion alone and 80% with sequential therapy of vascular occlusion and chemotherapy were observed. Median survival times of 37 and 49 months were experienced in patients with islet cell carcinoma and carcinoid hepatic metastases, respectively. For the symptomatic treatment of hormonally active liver metastases, the use of repeated embolizations is preferred.

The best results for metastatic disease of the liver treated with hepatic artery embolization have been observed in patients with neuroendocrine tumors metastatic to the liver. Sequential and periodic embolization is required for effective palliation. Gupta et al.[37] have reported on 81 patients with carcinoid syndrome who were treated with either bland embolization or chemoembolization. Imaging was available for evaluation of a response in 69 patients. Partial response occurred in 67% of the patients, stable disease in 16%, and progression of tumor in 8.7%. The median response duration was 17 months in those patients with a partial response. A reduction of tumor-related symptoms occurred in 63%, with a median progression-free survival of 19 months and a median overall survival time of 31 months. In a subsequent study by Gupta et al.,[38] these 69 patients with carcinoid tumors were compared with 54 patients who had islet cell tumors with metastases to the liver. Patients with carcinoid tumors had a higher response rate and a longer progression-free survival than did patients with islet cell tumors (67% vs 35% and 23 months vs 16 months). Although chemoembolization, compared with bland embolization, did not prove to be beneficial for survival in patients with carcinoid tumors, it did result in improved overall survival and improved response (32 months vs 18 months and 50% vs 25%) in patients treated for islet cell tumors.

RF ablation can be used to palliate symptoms associated with metastatic neuroendocrine tumors. In a series by Berber et al.,[39] RF ablation provided complete symptomatic relief in 63% of 222 patients and partial relief in 95%. Radioembolization is another minimally invasive alternative to palliating a large burden of hepatic metastases from neuroendocrine tumors.

Other hepatic metastases

Other types of hepatic metastases are usually not as well suited for locoregional therapy as the tumor is likely widespread by the time of liver involvement. However, occasionally, certain types of hepatic metastases are amenable to local treatment because of the indolent nature of the primary disease. Such hepatic metastases that can sometimes be treated by chemoembolization include ocular melanoma, leiomyosarcoma, breast carcinoma, and renal cell carcinoma. In a group of 30 patients with metastatic ocular melanoma, chemoembolization with cisplatin produced a response rate of 46% and a median survival period of 11 months.[40] The longest survival was 5 years from the initial chemoembolization. In the past, such patients lived for 2–6 months after presentation with hepatic metastases. Additional studies have been reported using HAI of carboplatin-based chemotherapy and fotemustine, with response rates of 38% and 40%, respectively.[40] Hepatic artery immunoembolization has also been reported with variable responses. A group of 14 patients with leiomyosarcoma metastatic to the liver were treated with chemoembolization every 4 weeks with cisplatin and polyvinyl alcohol foam granules 150–250 μm in size, followed by vinblastine infusion.[41] The response rate was 70%, and responses lasted 4–19 months (median, 9 months). This rate compared well with the response rate of 15% obtained after systemic therapy with ifosfamide with doxorubicin. Of note, these are not common tumors and most are treated on protocol studies. At MD Anderson, our approach to chemoembolization of hepatic metastases is similar to our approach to HCC; that is, a hypervascular tumor is more likely to benefit from the treatment than a hypovascular tumor. The goal of treatment, whether it is to provide symptomatic relief or to prolong survival, must be weighed against the risk of complications.

Genitourinary interventions

Renal arterial embolization

Renal artery embolization for renal cell carcinoma may be performed preoperatively to decrease operative blood loss in patients with extensive local disease. A study by Zielinski et al.[42] showed a survival benefit to preoperative embolization, although previous studies have not demonstrated this advantage. Embolization of renal carcinoma can be performed for palliative relief of symptoms in patients with extensive local tumor or as a cytoreductive measure when patients are not candidates for surgery.[43] Renal artery embolization has been used in the management of congestive heart failure caused by arteriovenous shunting through the renal carcinoma and for hypertension, hypercalcemia, polycythemia, and hemorrhage caused by the renal neoplasm. Selective segmental embolization is especially necessary and effective in patients with impaired renal function or solitary kidney.

Renal ablation

Thermal ablation plays an increasingly important role in the management of renal cell carcinoma. Although nephrectomy remains the gold standard for treatment of renal cell carcinoma, RF ablation is increasingly a viable alternative (Figure 3). RF ablation for the treatment of renal tumors is minimally invasive with a low morbidity rate.[44] Patients who are candidates for renal RF ablation include those with high surgical risk secondary to medical comorbidities; patients with a solitary kidney or multifocal disease, who are not candidates for nephron-sparing surgery; and patients who do not wish to undergo surgery. Patients with hereditary syndromes, such as von Hippel–Lindau disease, are at high risk for multiple renal neoplasms over their lifetimes. These patients may be treated repeatedly with RF ablation, in an effort to preserve normal renal parenchyma adjacent to the tumors.

Gervais et al.[45,46] demonstrated that tumor size and location are related directly to ablation effectiveness. Exophytic lesions can be ablated more effectively because of surrounding fat, the presence of which makes lesions easier to target and provides heat insulation during ablation. Complete necrosis was achieved in 90% of tumors measuring <4.0 cm. Larger or central tumors may not be amenable to complete ablation and may require multiple ablations or, in some cases, multiple treatment sessions. This owes in part to the proximity of medullary tumors to the renal hilar vessels resulting in an increased heat-sink effect, which affects ablation efficacy by lowering intralesional temperatures. A medullary tumor location also increases the risk of procedure-related complications. The most common complication of renal RF ablation is hemorrhage. This complication was observed in 5% of the patients in the series of 100 lesions treated by Gervais et al.[45,46] Hemorrhage can occur into the collecting system requiring stent placement for ureteral obstruction, or it can be confined to the subcapsular space.

Ahrar et al.[44] described their experience with 29 patients with 30 renal tumors who underwent percutaneous RF ablation. The lesions had a mean largest diameter of 3.5 ± 0.24 cm. The primary

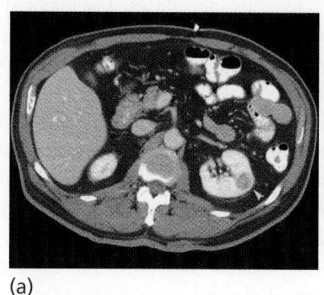 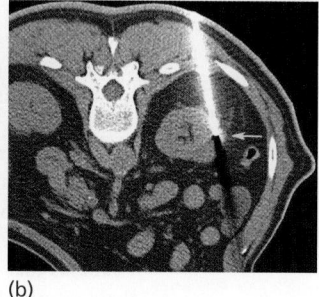 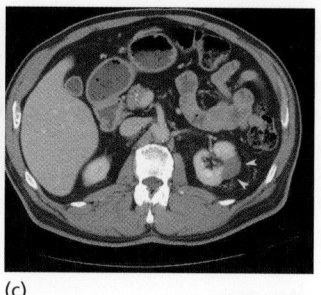

(a)   (b)   (c)

Figure 3 Percutaneous radiofrequency (RF) ablation performed in a 62-year-old man with biopsy-proven renal cell carcinoma. (a) Contrast-enhanced CT image obtained before RF ablation shows an enhancing mass in the left kidney (arrowhead). (b) CT image obtained with patient in prone position at RF ablation shows single needle electrode in tumor (arrow). (c) Contrast-enhanced CT image obtained after RF ablation shows no residual enhancement in the treated kidney (arrowheads).

tumor was completely ablated in 96% of patients. Mean and median follow-up intervals were 10 and 7 months, respectively. Major complications were observed in 12% of the patients, including gross hematuria and urinary obstruction in three patients. All hemorrhagic complications were treated successfully. One patient had persistent weakness of the anterior abdominal wall. None of the patients in the study showed significant degradation of renal function after treatment.

Thoracic interventions

Lung ablation

Thermal ablation can be used to treat primary and metastatic lung cancers. Lung ablation is optimal for patients with early lung cancer, where complete ablation with curative intent can be attempted. In patients with large tumor burden, ablation may provide palliation of tumor-related symptoms.[47] Lung ablation is offered primarily to patients with lung cancer who are not operative candidates as well as to patients with pulmonary metastases.

Simon et al.[48] reported a series of 153 patients with 189 primary or metastatic inoperable lung cancers treated with percutaneous pulmonary RF ablation. The overall 1-, 2-, 3-, 4-, and 5-year survival rates, respectively, for stage I non-small-cell lung cancer were 78%, 57%, 36%, 27%, and 27%; rates for colorectal pulmonary metastasis were 87%, 78%, 57%, 57%, and 57%. The incidence of pneumothorax was 28.4%. Postablation pneumothorax may be treated conservatively if the patient remains asymptomatic. In the patients with symptoms or progressively enlarging pneumothorax, placement of a chest drain is necessary. In the series by Simon et al.,[48] procedure-related 30-day mortality rate was 2.6%.

Pleural effusion is also a common complication after lung ablation. In their series of 60 patients, de Baere et al.[49] reported a minor pleural effusion in 9% of patients immediately after treatment and on 60% of CT scans obtained 24–48 h after treatment. Postprocedure hemoptysis was observed in 10% of the patients. The hemoptysis started 1–9 days after the ablation and lasted 2–13 days. These complications did not require any treatment.

Lung chemoembolization

Lung chemoembolization can be used for the treatment of a multitude of lung tumors. The purpose of lung chemoembolization is to deliver chemotherapeutic agents to the tumor while blocking its blood supply. This is accomplished by simultaneously injecting embolic material and the chemotherapy into the pulmonary artery branches that supply the tumor. The embolization increases the chemotherapy dwell time within the lesion by slowing agent washout.

In 2005, Vogl et al.[50] examined transpulmonary chemoembolization with mitomycin C combined with iodized oil as an option for treatment of unresectable lung metastases in 23 patients. This study demonstrated that transpulmonary chemoembolization was feasible and well tolerated. No major complications were observed; 35% of patients had a partial response, 26% had stable tumor size, and 39% showed progression of disease.

Palliative therapy

Percutaneous biliary drainage

Pancreatic carcinoma, cholangiocarcinoma, and ampullary carcinoma are the primary neoplasms that produce intrinsic biliary obstruction, whereas lymphadenopathy, HCC, and hepatic metastasis can produce extrinsic compression. Nonsurgical palliation of malignant biliary obstruction may be accomplished either endoscopically or percutaneously. The percutaneous methods include drainage by insertion of external or internal–external percutaneous biliary catheters.

The aims of palliative therapy are to provide relief of jaundice and pruritus as well as associated cholangitis and, most important, to prepare patients for anticancer therapy. Neither the endoscopic nor the percutaneous approach has an advantage with regard to influencing survival, and the choice of technique is often a team decision based on the available local expertise.

Internal drainage via endoscopy is preferable because of the inconvenience of an external catheter and the potential for pain at the tube entry site, bile leakage around the catheter, and sepsis from skin organisms. The percutaneous approach has the advantage of allowing prompt access to the biliary tree. Regardless of the approach, partial or complete jaundice relief can be achieved in 73–100% of treated patients.[51]

Percutaneous biliary stenting

Speer et al.[52] described 70 patients with malignant biliary obstruction who were randomized to undergo percutaneous versus endoscopic biliary stent placement. The success rate in relieving jaundice was 81% for endoscopically placed stents compared with 61% for the percutaneously placed stents. The complication rate was 19% versus 67%, in favor of the endoscopic approach. In addition, the 30-day mortality rate in the two groups was 15% for endoscopic stents versus 33% for the percutaneous method.

Cholangitis, hemorrhage, and bile leakage are the most common complications of stent placement. The incidence of cholangitis is lower in patients treated with a metallic stent than in patients treated with a plastic stent.[53] Plastic stents are also more prone to migration and remain patent on average for only 3–4 months.[53] Self-expanding metallic stents have longer patency but are more expensive. Metallic stents may be dislodged by balloon dilation immediately after deployment, but the incidence of spontaneous migration over the long term is negligible. These uncovered metallic stents cannot be removed. Despite advances in stent technology, occlusion secondary to tumor ingrowth or overgrowth remains a complex issue.

Musculoskeletal ablation

The majority of patients with breast, prostate, and lung cancer show evidence of bone metastases at the time of death. These lesions are often accompanied by pain and occasional fractures, which can dramatically decrease the quality of life of this patient population.[54] External-beam radiation therapy is the gold standard for localized pain secondary to osseous metastases. The majority of the patients will experience symptomatic relief after radiation therapy. However, in a substantial minority of patients, radiation therapy provides suboptimal response and durability of relief.[55]

Patients are candidates for ablative therapy of painful metastases when a patient reports moderate or severe musculoskeletal pain, the patient's pain is focal in nature and correlates with abnormality evident with radiological imaging, and the painful metastatic lesion is accessible to percutaneous treatment.[56]

Lesions that are amenable to ablative therapy are typically osteolytic or mixed osteolytic and osteoblastic in nature or otherwise composed of soft tissue. RF ablation and cryoablation are safe and effective treatments for the palliation of painful metastatic lesions that are refractory to standard therapies. Importantly, the quality of life for these patients is improved with this therapy. Goetz et al.[57] reported on 43 patients with painful bone metastases treated with RF ablation. As many as 95% of the patients experienced symptomatic relief that was considered clinically significant with decrease of opioid usage. A single ablative treatment is effective in most patients and appears to provide a long duration of pain relief.

Miscellaneous

Vena cava filter placement

Cancer patients experience an increased incidence of thrombosis and pulmonary embolism (PE). The percutaneous placement of a vena cava filter is the optimal therapeutic approach for patients with PE, who have a contraindication to anticoagulant therapy or who develop recurrent emboli despite adequate anticoagulant administration. There are numerous filters currently in use, including devices that are retrievable and MRI compatible.

Wallace et al.[58] reported on the experience of vena cava filter placement in 308 patients with venous thromboembolic disease in the setting of malignancy. Median survival times were 145 and 207 days for 267 patients with solid tumors and 41 patients with liquid tumors, respectively. Patients with metastatic or disseminated disease were 3.7 times as likely to die as those with local disease, and patients with deep venous thrombosis and a history of hemorrhage were twice as likely to die as those with deep venous thrombosis and no history of hemorrhage. Major complications included pulmonary emboli, new caval thrombus, retroperitoneal hemorrhage, and incorrect filter deployment.

Prophylactic placement of retrievable IVC filters in the perioperative period has also become common practice. The current indications are for patients who have a history of thromboembolic disease and must come off therapy for planned surgery or patients who will be at high risk for developing clots in the immediate postoperative period. Once patients are eligible for systemic anticoagulation therapy, then IVC filter retrieval should be scheduled.

Stent placement for venous stenosis

Vena caval syndrome is most frequently the result of intrinsic or extrinsic malignant disease.[59] In this syndrome, neoplasms, by their extension and localization or by causing mediastinal, retroperitoneal, and pelvic lymphadenopathy, create stenosis and obstruction by extrinsic compression of the vena cava. The complications of radiation therapy and chemotherapy for this syndrome include mediastinal fibrosis and thrombophlebitis.[59]

Superior vena cava syndrome symptoms have been grouped into four classes: (1) central nervous system symptoms, including headache, blurred vision, and cognitive dysfunction; (2) laryngopharyngeal edema, producing dyspnea and hoarseness; (3) nasal or facial edema; and (4) other signs of venous congestion and dilatation.[60] In addition to the stenosis or obstruction, there is frequently thrombosis complicating the mediastinal compression or intraluminal invasion by the tumor. Parish et al.[61] reported an average survival time of 7 months after the diagnosis of malignant superior vena cava obstruction. Vascular stents can effectively palliate symptoms of malignant vena cava stenosis in 68–80% of patients.[59]

Biopsy

Percutaneous biopsy has been traditionally a cost-effective modality to diagnose the patient with cancer. Almost all tissues, including the myocardium, are accessible to percutaneous biopsy. Various needles (11–25 gauge) as well as biopsy forceps are efficient in obtaining representative specimens. Biopsy guns are available to automate the procedure. However, a negative biopsy result does not exclude the possibility of malignancy; it may represent merely an error in sampling. Most biopsies of lesions in adults are scheduled electively on an outpatient basis.

Guidance by CT is usually adequate for biopsy of the lung or mediastinum.[62] The reported accuracy of percutaneous transthoracic needle biopsy in patients with lung cancer and pulmonary metastases is 90–98%,[63] whereas the diagnostic yield for local pulmonary infection in immunocompromised patients is 73%.[64] Serious complications of lung and mediastinal biopsies include systemic air embolization, hemorrhage, pericardial tamponade, seeding of malignant cells into the needle track, and empyema. The incidence of pneumothorax, when using CT guidance, is approximately 22–45%.[65,66] In a study described by Cox et al.,[67] when biopsies were done under CT guidance, smaller lesions (<2 cm) and the presence of emphysema correlated strongly with the occurrence of pneumothorax.

Abdominal biopsies guided by ultrasonography, CT, and MRI yielded adequate diagnostic material for cytologic analysis in 84–95% of patients. When a 20- to 23-gauge needle is used, biopsies of the liver, pancreas, kidney, adrenal gland, spleen, and ovary, among other organs, are performed with a sensitivity of 86%, a specificity of 98%, and an accuracy of 90%. The overall complication rate in a study of 63,180 biopsies was 0.16%. Seeding of malignant cells along the needle track occurred in 0.05% of patients.[68-70]

The diagnostic accuracy of percutaneous skeletal biopsy is on average 80%. The overall diagnostic accuracy of 78% was reported in a series of 178 patients with primary skeletal tumors who underwent percutaneous needle biopsy.[71] The procedure was more accurate for malignant neoplasms (83%) than benign tumors (64%).

Transjugular intrahepatic portosystemic shunt placement

The formation of a transjugular intrahepatic portosystemic shunt (TIPS), by placing a metallic stent between the hepatic and portal venous systems, is an accepted means of decreasing certain sequelae associated with portal hypertension. Indications include gastrointestinal variceal bleeding, ascites, portal gastropathy, hepatic hydrothorax, and Budd–Chiari syndrome. Cancer patients with hepatic disease may be candidates for this procedure. Wallace et al.[72] have described 38 patients with malignancy and hepatic disease treated with TIPS placement. Technical success was achieved in 97% of patients. Recurrent variceal hemorrhage occurred in only 1 of 19 patients (5%), and ascites or hydrothorax resolved or significantly improved in 9 of 12 patients (75%). Intimal hyperplasia and occlusion of the TIPS stent is the most feared postprocedural complication. The 1-year patency rate for TIPS is reported at 25–66%.[73] Development of covered stents to prevent stenosis has shown dramatic promise, with two studies demonstrating identical 1-year primary patency of 84%.[74,75]

Key references

The complete reference list can be found on the Wiley Companion Digital Edition of this title (see inside front cover for login instructions).

1 Collins JM. Pharmacologic rationale for regional drug delivery. *J Clin Oncol.* 1984;2(5):498–504.
2 Mocellin S, Pilati P, Lise M, Nitti D. Meta-analysis of hepatic arterial infusion for unresectable liver metastases from colorectal cancer: the end of an era? *J Clin Oncol.* 2007;25(35):5649–5654.
3 Hemingway AP, Allison DJ. Complications of embolization: analysis of 410 procedures. *Radiology.* 1988;166(3):669–672.

4 Yamada R, Nakatsuka H, Nakamura K, et al. Hepatic artery embolization in 32 patients with unresectable hepatoma. *Osaka City Med J*. 1980;**26**(2):81–96.

5 Nakakuma K, Tashiro S, Hiraoka T, et al. Studies on anticancer treatment with an oily anticancer drug injected into the ligated feeding hepatic artery for liver cancer. *Cancer*. 1983;**52**(12):2193–2200.

8 Lo CM, Ngan H, Tso WK, et al. Randomized controlled trial of transarterial lipiodol chemoembolization for unresectable hepatocellular carcinoma. *Hepatology*. 2002;**35**(5):1164–1171.

9 Llovet JM, Real MI, Montana X, et al. Arterial embolisation or chemoembolisation versus symptomatic treatment in patients with unresectable hepatocellular carcinoma: a randomised controlled trial. *Lancet*. 2002;**359**(9319):1734–1739.

10 Liapi E, Georgiades CC, Hong K, Geschwind JF. Transcatheter arterial chemoembolization: current technique and future promise. *Tech Vasc Interv Radiol*. 2007;**10**(1):2–11.

11 Yoshizawa H, Nishino S, Shiomori K, Natsugoe S, Aiko T, Kitamura Y. Surface morphology control of polylactide microspheres enclosing irinotecan hydrochloride. *Int J Pharm*. 2005;**296**(1–2):112–116.

12 Wallace MJ, Murthy R, Kamat PP, et al. Impact of C-arm CT on hepatic arterial interventions for hepatic malignancies. *J Vasc Interv Radiol*. 2007;**18**(12):1500–1507.

13 Geschwind JF, Salem R, Carr BI, et al. Yttrium-90 microspheres for the treatment of hepatocellular carcinoma. *Gastroenterology*. 2004;**127**(5 Suppl):S194–S205.

14 Salem R, Lewandowski RJ, Atassi B, et al. Treatment of unresectable hepatocellular carcinoma with use of ^{90}Y microspheres (TheraSphere): safety, tumor response, and survival. *J Vasc Interv Radiol*. 2005;**16**(12):1627–1639.

15 Stubbs RS, Cannan RJ, Mitchell AW. Selective internal radiation therapy (SIRT) with ^{90}Yttrium microspheres for extensive colorectal liver metastases. *Hepatogastroenterology*. 2001;**48**(38):333–337.

16 Livraghi T, Giorgio A, Marin G, et al. Hepatocellular carcinoma and cirrhosis in 746 patients: long-term results of percutaneous ethanol injection. *Radiology*. 1995;**197**(1):101–108.

18 Ebara M, Okabe S, Kita K, et al. Percutaneous ethanol injection for small hepatocellular carcinoma: therapeutic efficacy based on 20-year observation. *J Hepatol*. 2005;**43**(3):458–464.

19 Livraghi T, Goldberg SN, Lazzaroni S, Meloni F, Solbiati L, Gazelle GS. Small hepatocellular carcinoma: treatment with radio-frequency ablation versus ethanol injection. *Radiology*. 1999;**210**(3):655–661.

20 Lencioni RA, Allgaier HP, Cioni D, et al. Small hepatocellular carcinoma in cirrhosis: randomized comparison of radio-frequency thermal ablation versus percutaneous ethanol injection. *Radiology*. 2003;**228**(1):235–240.

21 Gillams AR, Lees WR. Survival after percutaneous, image-guided, thermal ablation of hepatic metastases from colorectal cancer. *Dis Colon Rectum*. 2000;**43**(5):656–661.

22 Yokoyama Y, Nagino M, Nimura Y. Mechanisms of hepatic regeneration following portal vein embolization and partial hepatectomy: a review. *World J Surg*. 2007;**31**(2):367–374.

24 Madoff DC, Abdalla EK, Gupta S, et al. Transhepatic ipsilateral right portal vein embolization extended to segment IV: improving hypertrophy and resection outcomes with spherical particles and coils. *J Vasc Interv Radiol*. 2005;**16**(2 Pt 1):215–225.

25 Abulkhir A, Limongelli P, Healey AJ, et al. Preoperative portal vein embolization for major liver resection: a meta-analysis. *Ann Surg*. 2008;**247**(1):49–57.

27 Yamada R, Kishi K, Sato M, et al. Transcatheter arterial chemoembolization (TACE) in the treatment of unresectable liver cancer. *World J Surg*. 1995;**19**(6):795–800.

28 Bruix J, Sherman M. Management of hepatocellular carcinoma. *Hepatology*. 2005;**42**(5):1208–1236.

31 Chen MS, Li JQ, Zheng Y, et al. A prospective randomized trial comparing percutaneous local ablative therapy and partial hepatectomy for small hepatocellular carcinoma. *Ann Surg*. 2006;**243**(3):321–328.

32 Goldberg RM, Sargent DJ, Morton RF, et al. A randomized controlled trial of fluorouracil plus leucovorin, irinotecan, and oxaliplatin combinations in patients with previously untreated metastatic colorectal cancer. *J Clin Oncol*. 2004;**22**(1):23–30.

33 Lencioni R, Crocetti L, Cioni D, Della Pina C, Bartolozzi C. Percutaneous radiofrequency ablation of hepatic colorectal metastases: technique, indications, results, and new promises. *Invest Radiol*. 2004;**39**(11):689–697.

34 Gillams AR, Lees WR. Radio-frequency ablation of colorectal liver metastases in 167 patients. *Eur Radiol*. 2004;**14**(12):2261–2267.

35 Ramage JK, Davies AH, Ardill J, et al. Guidelines for the management of gastroenteropancreatic neuroendocrine (including carcinoid) tumours. *Gut*. 2005;**54**(Suppl 4):iv1–iv16.

36 Moertel CG, Johnson CM, McKusick MA, et al. The management of patients with advanced carcinoid tumors and islet cell carcinomas. *Ann Intern Med*. 1994;**120**(4):302–309.

37 Gupta S, Yao JC, Ahrar K, et al. Hepatic artery embolization and chemoembolization for treatment of patients with metastatic carcinoid tumors: the M.D. Anderson experience. *Cancer J*. 2003;**9**(4):261–267.

38 Gupta S, Johnson MM, Murthy R, et al. Hepatic arterial embolization and chemoembolization for the treatment of patients with metastatic neuroendocrine tumors: variables affecting response rates and survival. *Cancer*. 2005;**104**(8):1590–1602.

44 Ahrar K, Matin S, Wood CG, et al. Percutaneous radiofrequency ablation of renal tumors: technique, complications, and outcomes. *J Vasc Interv Radiol*. 2005;**16**(5):679–688.

45 Gervais DA, McGovern FJ, Arellano RS, McDougal WS, Mueller PR. Radiofrequency ablation of renal cell carcinoma: part 1, Indications, results, and role in patient management over a 6-year period and ablation of 100 tumors. *Am J Roentgenol*. 2005;**185**(1):64–71.

46 Gervais DA, Arellano RS, McGovern FJ, McDougal WS, Mueller PR. Radiofrequency ablation of renal cell carcinoma: part 2, lessons learned with ablation of 100 tumors. *Am J Roentgenol*. 2005;**185**(1):72–80.

48 Simon CJ, Dupuy DE, DiPetrillo TA, et al. Pulmonary radiofrequency ablation: long-term safety and efficacy in 153 patients. *Radiology*. 2007;**243**(1):268–275.

49 de Baere T, Palussiere J, Auperin A, et al. Midterm local efficacy and survival after radiofrequency ablation of lung tumors with minimum follow-up of 1 year: prospective evaluation. *Radiology*. 2006;**240**(2):587–596.

50 Vogl TJ, Wetter A, Lindemayr S, Zangos S. Treatment of unresectable lung metastases with transpulmonary chemoembolization: preliminary experience. *Radiology*. 2005;**234**(3):917–922.

52 Speer AG, Cotton PB, Russell RC, et al. Randomised trial of endoscopic versus percutaneous stent insertion in malignant obstructive jaundice. *Lancet*. 1987;**2**(8550):57–62.

56 Callstrom MR, Charboneau JW. Image-guided palliation of painful metastases using percutaneous ablation. *Tech Vasc Interv Radiol*. 2007;**10**(2):120–131.

57 Goetz MP, Callstrom MR, Charboneau JW, et al. Percutaneous image-guided radiofrequency ablation of painful metastases involving bone: a multicenter study. *J Clin Oncol*. 2004;**22**(2):300–306.

58 Wallace MJ, Jean JL, Gupta S, et al. Use of inferior vena caval filters and survival in patients with malignancy. *Cancer*. 2004;**101**(8):1902–1907.

59 Carrasco CH, Charnsangavej C, Wright KC, Wallace S, Gianturco C. Use of the Gianturco self-expanding stent in stenoses of the superior and inferior venae cavae. *J Vasc Interv Radiol*. 1992;**3**(2):409–419.

60 Kee ST, Kinoshita L, Razavi MK, Nyman UR, Semba CP, Dake MD. Superior vena cava syndrome: treatment with catheter-directed thrombolysis and endovascular stent placement. *Radiology*. 1998;**206**(1):187–193.

62 Gupta S, Seaberg K, Wallace MJ, et al. Imaging-guided percutaneous biopsy of mediastinal lesions: different approaches and anatomic considerations. *Radiographics*. 2005;**25**(3):763–786; discussion 86–88.

63 Westcott J. Lung biopsy. In: Dondelinger RF, Rossi P, Kurdziel JC, Wallace S, eds. *Interventional Radiology*. Stuttgart: Thieme; 1990:9–17.

66 Kazerooni EA, Lim FT, Mikhail A, Martinez FJ. Risk of pneumothorax in CT-guided transthoracic needle aspiration biopsy of the lung. *Radiology*. 1996;**198**(2):371–375.

67 Cox JE, Chiles C, McManus CM, Aquino SL, Choplin RH. Transthoracic needle aspiration biopsy: variables that affect risk of pneumothorax. *Radiology*. 1999;**212**(1):165–168.

69 Stewart CJ, Coldewey J, Stewart IS. Comparison of fine needle aspiration cytology and needle core biopsy in the diagnosis of radiologically detected abdominal lesions. *J Clin Pathol*. 2002;**55**(2):93–97.

71 Ayala AG, Zornosa J. Primary bone tumors: percutaneous needle biopsy. Radiologic-pathologic study of 222 biopsies. *Radiology*. 1983;**149**(3):675–679.

72 Wallace MJ, Madoff DC, Ahrar K, Warneke CL. Transjugular intrahepatic portosystemic shunts: experience in the oncology setting. *Cancer*. 2004;**101**(2):337–345.

43 Principles of surgical oncology

Mark Bloomston, MD, FACS ▪ Kenneth K. Tanabe, MD, FACS ▪ Raphael E. Pollock, MD, PhD, FACS ▪ Donald L. Morton, MD, FACS (deceased)[†]

Overview

The discipline of surgical oncology describes a surgical super specialty to which a board certification process is now attached in the United States. A cognitive as well as technical surgical focus, the surgical oncologist is an oncology specialist who uses surgery as his or her mainstay therapeutic modality in treating tumor problems. As such, the surgical oncologist has a thorough grounding in the natural history of solid malignancy, extensive experience in tumor biopsy and staging approaches, the knowledge needed to orchestrate a multidisciplinary solid tumor treatment program, and the commitment, via vigorous personal participation, in the many relevant research opportunities by which we will advance comprehensive care of the cancer patient.

In spite of significant advances in various systemic approaches to the care of the cancer patient, surgical therapy remains the mainstay of treatment for most solid malignancies and plays a role in various components of the cancer care continuum, from prevention to diagnosis, curative therapy, survival prolongation, and palliation. To be maximally effective, the cancer surgeon must function as a member of the oncology team and is frequently the first oncology specialist that a patient will consult. The cancer surgeon is commonly charged with the responsibility to establish a tissue diagnosis for a suspicious lesion; this may require either an operative procedure or an image-directed or other biopsy approach. The cancer surgeon will usually bear the responsibility for communicating the biopsy findings to the patient, completing the procedures needed to stage the cancer, and initiating subsequent interaction between the patient and other members of the multimodality oncology team. Because of these responsibilities, it is most often the cancer surgeon

†This chapter is dedicated in memoriam of Dr. Donald Lee Morton, one of the giants of Surgical Oncology who had direct and indirect impacts on the career of three other current chapter authors. In honor and recognition of Dr. Morton's coeditor contribution to many editions of *Cancer Medicine*, we have chosen to maintain his position as the senior author of this chapter as well. Born into less than propitious circumstances in rural West Virginia during the Great Depression, Dr. Morton was a graduate of the University of California, Berkeley, and the University of California, San Francisco, from which he received his MD degree. An initial period of time in the Surgery Branch at the National Cancer Institute was followed by a 20-year stint at the University of California, Los Angeles. This was followed by his role as the founding President of the John Wayne Cancer Institute, an institutional affiliation maintained in multiple capacities, until his death from lymphoma in 2014.

Dr. Morton was the consummate academic surgical oncologist, maintaining a vigorous clinical practice as well as laboratory and clinical trials presence throughout his career. His formal and informal mentorship of so many young surgical oncologists and immunologists worldwide is a remarkably leveraged legacy. His contributions to immunomodulatory therapies on behalf of melanoma patients as well as his development of sentinel node approaches for melanoma and carcinoma of the breast have revolutionized our treatment of these diseases, and comprise an enduring contribution of transcendent magnitude.

who initially explains to the patient the sequence and rationale of the various treatment components that will be used to manage the specific malignancy. To be maximally effective, the cancer surgeon must therefore be aware of the different therapeutic options, the natural history of a given malignancy, and how these factors will be integrated into a well-conceived and appropriate multimodality treatment algorithm. It is also usually the surgical oncologist's responsibility to provide initial information about prognosis and to make decisions about follow-up care and surveillance to detect tumor recurrence. In these aspects, the surgical oncologist is unlike almost any other surgical specialist in that the commitment to a given patient is for both the acute and the long-term components of the patient's disease process.

Over the years, the practice of surgical oncology has come full circle. Originally, surgeons attempted to treat cancer conservatively by removing only the gross lesion. Unfortunately, this led to extremely high rates of local recurrence and subsequent patient mortality. In the late nineteenth century, surgeons began to undertake radical en bloc resections and amputations to treat patients with malignant disease. These techniques yielded improved results, but the procedures were often mutilating. With the advent of other complementary and effective treatment modalities, notably radiation therapy in the 1920s and chemotherapy after the 1940s, the orientation of surgical resection is once again becoming conservative with a focus on organ preservation and restoring the comorbid state when possible.

Adjuvant chemotherapy, alone or in combination with radiation therapy, has improved disease free survival and prolonged quality of life for patients who have been rendered free of gross disease by surgery but who still have a high likelihood of recurrence as a consequence of microscopic residual metastases. Randomized clinical trials have demonstrated the benefit of adjuvant chemotherapy in a variety of tumors, including breast cancer, colorectal cancer, pancreatic cancer, osteosarcoma, testicular cancer, ovarian cancer, and certain lung cancers.

Surgery is most effective in the treatment of apparently locoregionally confined primary disease. The principles of surgical resection include en bloc resection of the primary tumor that attempts to encompass gross and microscopic tumor in all contiguous and adjacent anatomic locations. For some tumor types, concomitant resection of regional lymph nodes comprises an important component of the initial surgical management. In many cases, when disease is diagnosed and removed at an early stage, resection is the single therapeutic modality, often associated with a high rate of long-term success. Intuitively, it appears logical that surgery should have little role in disease management once a neoplasm has spread from the primary location to a distant site. However, surgical therapy is being applied with increasing frequency for metastatic disease as well. Prolonged survival can be seen in selected patients following resection of various metastatic

Holland-Frei Cancer Medicine, Ninth Edition. Edited by Robert C. Bast Jr., Carlo M. Croce, William N. Hait, Waun Ki Hong, Donald W. Kufe, Martine Piccart-Gebhart, Raphael E. Pollock, Ralph R. Weichselbaum, Hongyang Wang, and James F. Holland.
© 2017 John Wiley & Sons, Inc. ISBN: 978-1-118-93469-2

sites, including in the liver, lung, or brain. In particular, complete resection of hepatic colorectal metastases results in 5-year survival rates in excess of 50% in most contemporary series. As more active systemic cytotoxic and targeted therapies are prolonging survival in patients with various tumor types, resection or ablation of residual metastatic sites are being utilized with increasing frequency.

Surgery operates by zero-order kinetics, in which 100% of excised cells are destroyed. In contrast, chemotherapy and radiation therapy operate by first-order kinetics, where only a fraction of tumor cells are killed by each treatment. It is for this reason that these therapies can be considered complementary. Surgical resection reduces the tumor burden, which hopefully increases the efficacy of nonsurgical adjuvant therapies intended to eliminate microscopic residual disease, thereby decreasing the risk of recurrence and prolonging survival.

During the past several decades, a significant reduction has been seen in the morbidity and mortality associated with many complex cancer operations. These results, in part, can be attributed to improvements in surgical technique, patient selection, and regionalization to high-volume centers. For example, both perioperative risk and long-term survival after pancreaticoduodenectomy have been shown to be strongly influenced by hospital volume.[1] In addition, trends toward more limited cancer resections are being seen with comparable of improved oncologic outcome. Specifically, breast-conserving surgery has become an alternative to mastectomy in patients with breast carcinoma, limb salvage is often possible in patients with bone and soft-tissue sarcomas, and sphincter function and sexual potency can frequently be preserved for patients with rectal cancer. Because surgery is increasingly combined with other treatment modalities, it is essential that most patients with solid neoplasms have their treatment planned by a multidisciplinary team, which includes radiation and medical oncologists as well as surgical oncologists. To retain a primary role in the management of the cancer patient, the successful surgical oncologist must be able to coordinate and integrate the efforts of the entire oncologic team while maintaining a patient-centered focus on dignity and quality of life.

The history of surgical oncology

Oncology (from the Greek words onkos, meaning mass or tumor, and logos, meaning study) is the study of neoplastic diseases. Early authors suggested that certain families, races, and working classes were predisposed to neoplastic transformations. In 1862, Edwin Smith, an American Egyptologist, discovered the apparently earliest recordings of the surgical treatment of cancer.[2] Written in Egypt circa 1600 BC, this treatise was based on teachings possibly dating back to 3000 BC. The Egyptian author advised surgeons to contend with tumors that might be cured by surgery but not to treat those lesions that might be fatal.

Hippocrates (460–375 BC) was the first to describe the clinical symptoms associated with cancer. He advised against treating terminal patients, who would enjoy a better quality of life without surgical intervention.[3] He also coined the terms carcinoma (crab legs tumor) and sarcoma (fleshy mass). In the second century ad, Galen published his classification of tumors, describing cancer as a systemic disease caused by an excess of black bile.[4] Galen cautioned that as a systemic disease, cancer was not amenable to cure by surgery, which was often promptly followed by patient death. This strong admonition against surgery for cancer persisted for more than 1500 years until eighteenth-century pathologists discovered that cancer often grew locally before spreading to other anatomic sites. Before the advent of safe general anesthetics, surgery was used primarily to manage trauma or severe infectious problems such as abscess drainage. In that era, cancer surgery consisted primarily of amputation or cauterization of surface tumors of the trunk or extremities. Patients were usually unwilling to submit to the pain of tumor surgery, when there was little likelihood of improved survival.

During the eighteenth and nineteenth centuries, advances in anatomic pathology led to an increase in autopsies, which in turn resulted in a better understanding of human anatomy and physiology. The early work of Morgagni, Le Dran, and Da Salva established that there was an initial period of local tumor growth before distant dissemination. This led to the understanding that not all tumors spread systemically and that certain malignancies cause death solely by local invasive growth. Percival Pott (1714–1788) was the first to describe a specific etiologic factor associated with cancer development. In 1775, Pott demonstrated a high incidence of cancer of the scrotum in chimney sweeps who had reached puberty and recommended wide local resection for cure. In 1829, the French Surgeon Joseph Recamier (1774–1852) first described the complicated process of tumor dissemination. The first recorded elective tumor resection was performed in 1809 by Ephraim McDowell, an American surgeon. He successfully removed a 22-pound ovarian tumor from a patient, who subsequently survived 30 years. McDowell's work, which included 12 more ovarian resections, stimulated greater interest in elective surgery for cancer patients.

Surgeons were initially hindered by the extreme discomfort that patients experienced during surgical procedures as well as the lack of agents that could reduce the incidence of infection. Crawford Long (1815–1878) was the first to use ether for general anesthesia in 1842, but it was the reported work of John Collins Warren (1778–1856) and William T.G. Morton (1819–1868) that brought the potential of anesthesia to public attention. The surgical procedure in Warren's first published account of ether anesthesia (1846) was the elective removal of a tongue carcinoma for which submaxillary gland resection and partial glossectomy were performed. Warren was also responsible for the first American-authored textbook of tumor surgery, *Surgical Observations on Tumors*, published in 1838. Joseph Lister (1827–1912) was the first to report the successful use of antisepsis during elective surgery. In 1867, Lister applied Pasteur's concept that bacteria caused infection, when he introduced the use of carbolic acid as an antiseptic agent in conjunction with heat sterilization of surgical instruments. Lister is also credited with the introduction of absorbable ligatures as well as the placement of drainage tubes to control secretions and dead space in surgical wounds.

Even with the advent of antisepsis and general anesthesia, surgical oncology in the second half of the nineteenth and early twentieth centuries was still associated with high mortality rates. Cancer was rarely diagnosed in the early stages; consequently, few patients were considered candidates for curative surgery. Those surgeons who did attempt surgical excision of malignant lesions were hindered by rudimentary anesthesia, which was also independently associated with high patient mortality. Antibiotics were not yet available, and surgical instruments were crude. The importance of the microscope to evaluate frozen tissues for surgical margins was not yet appreciated, and surgeons had great faith in their own unaided gross visual assessment of the tumor perimeter. However, several important developments in this era led to rapid advancements in surgical oncology. Emphasizing meticulous surgical technique, gentle tissue handling, and applications of Listerian principles, pioneers such as Albert Theodore Billroth (first gastrectomy, laryngectomy, and esophagectomy), William Stewart Halsted (en bloc resection, radical mastectomy), and many other more contemporary

Table 1 Landmark advances in surgical oncology.

Year	Event	Surgeon
1775	Etiologic basis of cancer	Percival Pott
1809	Elective oophorectomy	Ephraim McDowell
1829	Metastatic process	Joseph Recamier
1846	Ether as anesthesia	John Collins Warren
1867	Carbolic acid as antisepsis	Joseph Lister
1873	Laryngectomy	Albert Theodore Billroth
1878	Resection of rectal tumor	Richard von Volkman
1880	Esophagectomy	Albert Theodore Billroth
1881	Gastrectomy	Albert Theodore Billroth
1890	Radical mastectomy	William Stewart Halsted
1896	Oophorectomy for breast cancer	G.T. Beatson
1904	Radical prostatectomy	Hugh H. Young
1906	Radical hysterectomy	Ernest Wertheim
1908	Abdominoperineal resection	W. Ernest Miles
1909	Thyroid surgery (Nobel Prize)	Theodore Emil Kocher
1910	Craniotomy	Harvey Cushing
1912	Cordotomy for the treatment of pain	E. Martin
1913	Thoracic esophagectomy	Franz Torek
1927	Resection of pulmonary metastases	George Divis
1933	Pneumonectomy	Evarts Graham
1935	Pancreaticoduodenectomy	Allen O. Whipple
1945	Adrenalectomy for prostate cancer	Charles B. Huggins
1957	Isolated limb perfusion	Oliver Creech
1958	Organization of National Adjuvant Breast and Bowel Project (NSABP) to conduct prospective randomized trials	Bernard Fisher
1965	Hormonal therapy of cancer	Charles Huggins
1971	Free tissue transfer with microvascular anastomosis	Harry Buncke

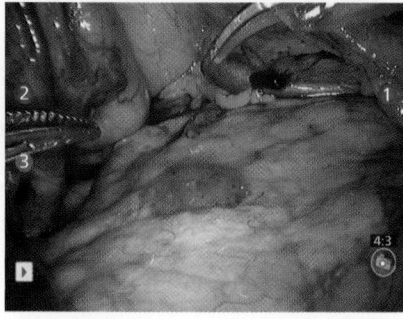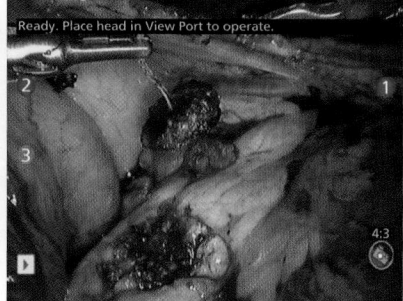

Figure 1 Robotic enucleation of insulinoma in the body of the pancreas.

surgeons defined and advanced the boundaries of surgical oncology (Table 1).[3]

Ongoing innovations to advance effective surgical primary tumor control have improved surgical outcomes and quality of life. Advances in microvascular surgery now permit the free transfer of complex autologous tissues, such as free jejunal grafts to reconstitute the upper aerodigestive system or osteomyocutaneous flaps to reconstruct extremities and other mobile body parts such as the jaw. Automatic stapling devices as well as laparoscopic/robotic instrumentation coupled with high-resolution optics have remarkably advanced minimally invasive cancer surgery resulting in less-morbid procedures that require significantly less patient discomfort and recuperation time (Figure 1). The rapid deployment of robotic technologies is changing traditional surgical interventional approaches. Among the potential advantages, robotic surgery is performed as a direct extension of the operator's prehensile hand replete with multiplanar articulating robotic "wrists," thereby avoiding the crossed rigid armature impediments of laparoscopic surgical maneuvers. Optoelectronic visualization systems incorporated into robotic display enables the appearance of three-dimensional surgical fields with supra-normal visual acuity. Gating the displayed

images coupled with the ability to scale up or down discrete surgical actions (e.g., suture placement and cannulation) enables damping out of tremor effects while facilitating operations performed on moving anatomic structures, especially on the microscopic level. Robotic procedures can be performed over great distances between the robot and console display systems, which will facilitate telesurgical applications in the future. The development of molecular radiologic probes for imaging tumor cellular components possessing more ominous genetic character portends a future in which interventional onco-radiologists and minimally invasive surgical oncologists will work together in the operating room to laser capture micro-dissect these less favorable tumor subsections, perhaps in conjunction with intraoperative navigation systems and various visual interfaces such as direct retinal display systems.

Improvements in preoperative optimization of comorbid disease and advances in perioperative critical care have made it possible to safely undertake increasingly complicated surgical procedures. A more sophisticated awareness of the patterns of tumor spread has also resulted in increasing opportunities for less-invasive surgical approaches. One example is the use of lymphatic mapping and sentinel node biopsy instead of formal lymphadenectomy in early-stage melanoma and breast carcinoma. In other cases, this better understanding of recurrence risk has led to more, not less, extensive surgical resections. An example of this includes the selected use of total hepatectomy and orthotopic liver transplantation for early-stage hepatocellular carcinoma.

Surgical oncology in the modern era

Surgical oncologists are surgeons who devote most of their time to the study and treatment of malignant neoplastic disease. They must possess the necessary knowledge, skills, and clinical experience to perform both the standard and extraordinary surgical procedures required for patients with cancer. Surgical oncologists must be able to diagnose tumors accurately and differentiate aggressive neoplastic lesions from benign reactive processes. In addition, surgical oncologists should have a firm understanding of radiation oncology, medical oncology, and diagnostic and interventional radiology. They must also be capable of organizing interdisciplinary studies of cancer. Surgical oncologists should also be trained in pathology because they will be called on to excise appropriate tumor samples for pathologists and make decisions about adequacy of surgical margins. Surgical oncologists should have a shared role with medical oncologists as the "primary care physicians" of cancer treatment. Almost all cancer patients will initially be managed by one of these two specialists, who will bear the ultimate responsibility for coordinating appropriate multimodality care for the individual patient.

Given the complexity of contemporary multidisciplinary approaches to the cancer patient, cancer centers have developed facilities to provide the needed planning expertise, clinical care, patient support services, and access points to clinical trials. Comprehensive cancer centers are often affiliated with academic medical institutions and offer the complete spectrum of oncology therapies, clinical trials, rehabilitation, and social services as well as basic and translational research programs to move new knowledge from the laboratory bench to the patient bedside. In this contemporary understanding of the continuum of care of the cancer patient, the role of the surgical oncologist is taking on an ever-increasing importance.

Surgical oncology is more of a cognitive than a technical surgical specialty. With the exception of a small cluster of index operations, such as pancreaticoduodenectomy, limb salvage, retroperitoneal sarcoma surgery, isolated limb perfusion, and complex liver resection, most of the surgical procedures that are performed by surgical oncologists are similar to those performed by surgeons who are not oncologically trained. What frequently differentiates these two types of surgeons is not mere knowledge about *how* to do a specific operation but an awareness of how and *when* to do that operation; that is, the cognitive knowledge of contemporary multimodality cancer care. A broad knowledge of cancer in its presenting and recurring forms as well as an awareness of the mechanisms driving tumor proliferation and dissemination is an integral part of the special cognitive database of the surgical oncologist.

As cancer management continues to march forward in the age of genomics, proteomics, and metabolomics, there is an ever-increasing need to study human tumor tissue. At a minimum, the surgical oncologist can contribute to cancer science by helping to secure access to these precious tissues. In reality, the surgical oncologist can do much more than passively provide tumor tissue access. An unparalleled understanding of the pathophysiology of solid tumors coupled with intimate knowledge of anatomy and the workflow in the operating room and pathology department places the cancer surgeon in the central role of organizing, maintaining, optimizing, and overseeing effective tissue procurement and tumor

banking; thus making the surgical oncologist a vital member of a translational science team. In addition, the cancer surgeon, working with pathologists and researchers, has the opportunity to provide meaningful clinical information, which can be used to annotate archival tissue repositories and aid in the creation of tissue microarrays. These are valuable tools whose utility can range from explorative, hypothesis-generating retrospective studies to confirmation of specific laboratory findings.

As part of the larger surgical community, the surgical oncologist is a critical conduit for the dissemination of cancer information to colleagues in general surgery and other surgical specialties. This individual makes academic presentations at large surgical meetings, directs hospital-based tumor boards, and consults on behalf of individual cancer patients. Because of their leading role in the initial diagnosis of cancer, it is not surprising that surgical oncologists are also frequently in leadership roles in cancer prevention and screening programs. Nationally based multimodality clinical trial groups also depend on surgical oncology expertise in helping with trial design; establishing the criteria of surgical quality control; educating trial participants regarding standards of surgical care (including indications for procedures); assuring safe acquisition of research grade tumor and autologous normal tissues for correlative studies, and assisting in accurate data collection, analysis, and presentation of trial results.

Multidisciplinary management

Multidisciplinary management of solid tumors requires surgeons to play a key role in decisions concerning sequencing of treatment modalities. For example, a patient with rectal cancer and resectable liver metastases may ultimately be treated with a liver resection, rectal resection, rectal radiation therapy, and systemic chemotherapy. Traditionally, the sequence for these treatments was preoperative chemoradiation therapy, followed by rectal resection (e.g., abdominoperineal resection or low anterior resection), subsequent liver resection, and then adjuvant chemotherapy—an aggressive approach but one that produces long-term survival in a subset of patients. However, in recognition that the greatest risk for mortality in these patients comes from systemic relapse, there is a more recent trend toward starting with chemotherapy, rather than leaving it to the end. Another benefit of this approach is that the nature of response to neoadjuvant treatment serves as an important prognostic marker. Moreover, tumor shrinkage may lead to a less difficult liver resection or rectal resection. While liver and bowel operations were rarely performed simultaneously, these are now more commonly performed together based on data showing safety of this approach in select patients. More often, in cases in which the two operations are performed separately, liver resection is now often performed first. The basis for this approach is that while preoperative chemotherapy rarely has any adverse impact on colon or rectal operations, accumulation of chemotherapy treatments is known to increase the risk of chemotherapy-induced liver pathology leading to complications from liver surgery. Use of short course adjuvant radiation therapy such as 25 Gy in five fractions followed by surgery 1 week later rather than the traditional 5-week course of radiation shortens the time required for trimodality treatment and reduces the length of time off of chemotherapy. Fundamental principles that influence the sequence of multimodality treatment apply to most other solid tumors as well, and are requisite knowledge for surgical oncologists.

Pediatric oncologists pioneered the use of combined modality therapy (radiation in combination with chemotherapy and surgery) as effective management of childhood neoplasms. Control of localized retinoblastoma in children has been dramatically increased using multimodality therapy. The cure rate for patients with Wilms tumor is 75% and if surgical therapy is followed by chemotherapy and, in some cases, radiation, by an increase of 40% over operation alone. Embryonal rhabdomyosarcoma responds best to combinations of radiation, chemotherapy, and operation. Until recently, the effectiveness of multimodality therapy was only occasionally demonstrable for adult neoplasms. A striking example is the approach to skeletal and soft-tissue sarcomas. Surgical therapy, the accepted method for local management of most skeletal and soft-tissue sarcomas of the extremities, is associated with frequent treatment failure if used alone. In the past, approximately 50% of patients with soft-tissue sarcomas and 80% of those with bone sarcomas eventually succumbed to distant metastases, even after amputation of the extremity bearing the primary tumor. Consequently, multimodality treatment regimens were developed to improve these results. Preoperative chemotherapy with intra-arterial doxorubicin followed by radiation resulted in extensive tumor cell necrosis in as many as 75% of patients.[4] The effectiveness of this preoperative therapy permitted local resection of the sarcoma and salvage of a viable functional extremity. Local recurrence rates were as low as with amputation, and long-term results were functionally and psychologically superior. In addition, there was no decrease in overall or disease-free survival rates. Multimodality therapy is also effective for other solid malignancies, including colorectal cancer. Specifically, clinical trials have demonstrated improved efficacy and higher sphincter-preservation rates with the use of neoadjuvant chemoradiation therapy for stage II or III rectal cancer. Multimodality therapy has also been demonstrated to improve resectability rates and long-term survival in patients with hepatic colorectal metastases.[5]

Unlike surgery and radiation therapy, systemic therapies, such as chemotherapy, immunotherapy, and hormonal therapy, are treatments that can kill tumor cells that have already metastasized to distant sites. These systemic modalities have a greater chance of cure in patients with minimal (or even subclinical) tumor burden as compared with those patients with clinically evident disease. Consequently, surgery and radiation therapy may be useful in decreasing a given patient's tumor burden thereby maximizing the impact of subsequent systemic approaches. Whether the goals of therapy should be cure or palliation depends on the stage of a specific cancer. If the cancer is localized without evidence of spread, it may be possible to eradicate the cancer and cure the patient. When the cancer has spread beyond the possibility of cure, the goal is to control symptoms and maintain maximum activity and quality of life for as long as possible. Patients are generally judged incurable if they have distant metastases or evidence of extensive local infiltration of critical structures adjacent to tumor. However, some patients are potentially curable even though they have distant metastases. Specifically, patients with solitary hepatic or pulmonary metastases may still be curable by resection, and patients with disseminated germ cell or gastrointestinal stromal tumor may still be cured using systemic therapy alone. Histologic proof of distant metastases should be obtained before the patient is deemed incurable. Occasionally, an exploratory operation may be necessary to determine the histology of ambiguous lesions in the lungs or liver. In rare situations, the clinical situation may point so overwhelmingly to distant metastases that the patient may be considered incurable without biopsy. For each anatomic site, there are certain local criteria that place the patient unequivocally in an incurable status, whereas other anatomic constraints may imply a poor prognosis but are not an absolute indication of incurability per se. In equivocal situations where extensive studies fail to demonstrate metastatic or incurable local extension, the patient deserves the benefit of the doubt and should be treated for cure.

The selection of therapeutic modalities depends not only on the type and extent of cancer but also on the patient's general condition and the presence of any comorbid conditions. For example, surgery may be contraindicated in a patient who has significant emphysema or liver failure. A patient with preexisting diabetes will be much more susceptible to the toxic effects of hormonal therapy with corticosteroids. Renal disease may increase the toxicity of some of the chemotherapeutic agents, such as cisplatin or ifosfamide. Extensive staging procedures may indicate that a tumor is localized to a primary site and/or regional lymph nodes and hence potentially curable by locoregional therapy. However, approximately 60% of localized malignant tumors ultimately recur, suggesting that many such patients must have had subclinical metastases at the time of initial diagnosis. The probability of cure may be improved if systemic approaches are coupled with local treatment. Chemotherapeutic drugs must be given when the number of tumor cells is low enough to permit their destruction at doses that can be tolerated by the patient. The opportunity for cure is most likely during the early stage of disease or immediately after surgery when the tumor burden has been minimized. Adjuvant chemotherapy has remarkably improved surgical results in some malignancies, primarily because of cytocidal effects on clinically undetectable malignant cells outside the operative field. Neoadjuvant chemotherapy that is initiated before local and regional treatments also can affect micro-metastatic distant disease while significantly cytoreducing the primary tumor.

Classically, surgical extirpation has been first in the sequence of therapies for resectable solid malignancies, but increasing evidence suggests that it may be more effective when used later in the treatment plan, particularly in more advanced tumors. Chemotherapy and radiation therapy both work by first-order kinetics. However, because of tumor cell heterogeneity, it can be anticipated that resistant clones of viable neoplastic cells may persist in the primary tumor after these therapies. Such clonal heterogeneity is more likely in large tumors that are both poorly perfused by chemotherapeutic agents and are also relatively hypoxic and therefore resistant to radiation therapy. Because surgery works by zero-order kinetics, it effectively removes the local residual primary tumor cells that are resistant to these other modalities.

From a practical management standpoint, the use of chemotherapy before surgical therapy can provide useful prognostic information regarding response to therapy. Presence of response to neoadjuvant therapy can aid in the planning of additional postoperative adjuvant chemotherapy. In addition, earlier administration of systemic therapy addresses the potential occult micro-metastatic disease. In some cases, preoperative therapy (or "conversion" therapy) can be used to downsize a tumor from an unresectable to resectable status (Figure 2).

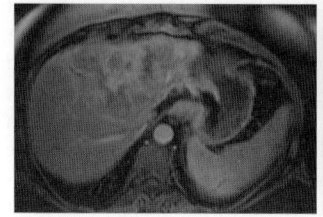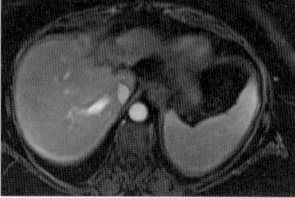

Figure 2 Previously unresectable (involvement of all three hepatic veins) intrahepatic cholangiocarcinoma downstaged using neoadjuvant gemcitabine and cisplatin.

Components of surgical management in the care of the cancer patient

Surgical prevention

As the role of genetic mutations that pre-dispose to subsequent cancer development expands, one can anticipate that prophylactic surgery will be extended to encompass some of these conditions. In such cases, it is imperative that the surgical oncologist become intimately knowledgeable about the indications, limitations, and ethical considerations regarding genetic counseling, if only because it will be the responsibility of the surgeon to alert other family members at risk and arrange for appropriate testing. The above emerging indications are being added to an already established role for prophylactic surgery in the prevention of predisposing malignancies, including ulcerative colitis with dysplasia, familial adenomatous polyposis, multiple endocrine neoplasia syndromes, and hereditary breast cancer. Assessing the risk–benefit ratio of prophylactic surgery is critical but frequently inexact. The future advent of inexpensive and reliable genetic screening technologies, coupled with emerging insights derived from the new field of molecular epidemiology, should bring more definitive understanding of prophylactic surgery benefits in populations at risk.

Biopsy and diagnosis

The diagnosis of solid tumors depends on locating and performing a biopsy of the lesion. The findings from biopsy specimens will be used to determine the histology and/or grade of a tumor, which is a prerequisite for planning definitive therapy. Significant therapeutic errors have been made when biopsy confirmation of malignancy was not obtained before treatment. Even when biopsy reports from another hospital are available, the slides of the previous biopsy must be obtained and reviewed before the institution of therapy. This is essential because all too often an erroneous interpretation may have been made in the initial pathology assessment.

Surgeons play a key role in the initial diagnosis for many solid tumors, including the decision on whether and how to biopsy a mass. In the case of a clinically suspicious breast mass combined with an abnormal mammogram, core biopsy rather than excisional biopsy is often appropriate as a strategy to limit the number of surgical procedures and allow for multidisciplinary planning and possibly neoadjuvant therapy. Conversely, in a patient with chronic viral hepatitis, and an arterially enhancing mass with imaging features suggestive of a resectable hepatocellular carcinoma, needle biopsy is typically not indicated if resection represents the most appropriate treatment pathway. Proper approaches to biopsy of a cutaneous pigmented lesion for possible melanoma requires understanding of the importance of proper intraoperative tissue manipulations to avoid compromising tumor thickness measurements by leaving a positive deep margin and understanding the difficulty in clinically following an atypical nevus that has only been partially biopsied; complete excisional biopsy is appropriate in most circumstances. The strategy for biopsy of masses suspicious for soft tissue sarcomas involves thoughtful planning to obtain sufficient tissue for histologic study, minimize disruption and potential seeding of tissue planes and allow for needle biopsy tracks to be placed within fields used for adjuvant or neoadjuvant radiation therapy. The strategy for biopsy of very small lesions causing obstruction of the common bile duct typically integrates understanding of the relatively high likelihood of false-negative results and the observation that the most curable lesions are the smallest and most difficult from which to attain a true-positive result. Resection is commonly performed in such circumstances even in the absence of a positive biopsy. And because diagnosis of distant metastases

will often change overall management, surgeons commonly decide on how to achieve a tissue diagnosis at distant sites with minimal morbidity and high sensitivity. Fundamental principles that influence approaches to biopsy are requisite knowledge for surgical oncologists.

Biopsy is easiest when the tumor is near the surface or involves an orifice that can be examined with appropriate visualizing instruments, such as the bronchoscope, colonoscope, or cystoscope. Carcinomas of the breast, tongue, or rectum can be seen or palpated and a portion can be excised for definitive diagnosis. In contrast, deep-seated lesions may grow to quite a large size before causing symptoms. Ultrasonography, computed tomography (CT), and magnetic resonance imaging (MRI) are all useful techniques for localizing such lesions at the time of invasive biopsy. However, although image-directed needle biopsy may be useful in some patients, exploratory surgery is occasionally required to obtain a definitive biopsy that establishes the exact histologic diagnosis. In some cases, tissue samples larger than that which is obtained by percutaneous biopsy may be required for tumor characterization, such as lymphoma, necessitating surgical biopsy. Fortunately, such procedures can now be frequently performed on an outpatient basis using minimally invasive technology such as laparoscopic surgical approaches.

Three methods are commonly used to biopsy suspicious lesions: needle biopsy (fine needle aspiration (FNA) or core), open incisional, or excisional biopsy. Regardless of the method used, the pathologic interpretation of the tumor mass will be valid only if a representative section of tumor is obtained. The surgical oncologist must be aware that a sampling error can occur with needle and incisional biopsies where only small portions of the total tumor mass are submitted for pathologic examination. It is the surgeon's task to provide adequate tissue for diagnosis. Orientation of the specimen, as may be necessary, is also the responsibility of the surgeon. It is axiomatic that adequate tissue can provide the basis for diagnosis by an adequate pathologist, whereas inadequate tissue will be insufficient for diagnosis by an adequate or inadequate pathologist.

FNA is a cytologic technique in which cells are aspirated from a tumor using a needle and syringe. The technique can be performed using image-directed guidance and is particularly helpful in the diagnosis of relatively inaccessible lesions such as deep visceral tumors. Because the aspirate consists of disaggregated cells rather than intact tissue, diagnosis of malignancy usually depends on detection of abnormal intracellular features, such as nuclear pleomorphism; thus, the margin of error is higher than with other biopsy techniques. In addition, because of the lack of intact tumor architecture, FNA cannot distinguish invasive from noninvasive malignancy. Negative results do not rule out malignancy. Depending on the clinical context, such as distinguishing carcinoma *in situ* from an infiltrating malignancy, other types of biopsy may be more appropriate.

Core biopsy is the simplest method of histologic (as opposed to cytologic) diagnosis and may be useful for biopsy of subcutaneous masses and muscular masses as well as some internal organs, such as liver, kidney, and pancreas. The added benefit is that this method is inexpensive and causes minimal disturbance of the surrounding tissue. Cutting-core biopsies are performed with a large-bore needle such as the Vim Silverman or Tru-Cut appliance. This technique retrieves a small piece of intact tumor tissue, which allows the pathologist to study the invasive relationship between cancer cells and the surrounding microenvironment. The danger of implanting tumor cells in a needle track during biopsy is extremely small. This risk can be avoided altogether if the needle track is positioned so that it can be excised en bloc at the time of the definitive surgical procedure. Needle biopsy may be less appropriate if the specimen is small, which increases the likelihood of the needle missing the lesion or the biopsy not being representative of the entire tumor. Consequently, a needle biopsy report that is negative for malignant disease should be viewed with skepticism if it is inconsistent with the clinical presentation and should be followed by incisional or excisional biopsy.

Incisional biopsy for pathologic examination involves removal of a small portion of the tumor mass. It is best performed in circumstances where the incisional wound can be totally excised in continuity with the definitive surgical resection in the event that any tumor cells are spilled at the time of biopsy. Incisional biopsy is indicated for deeper subcutaneous or intramuscular tumor masses when initial needle biopsy fails to establish a diagnosis. An incisional biopsy is also appropriate when a tumor is so large that complete local excision would violate wide tissue planes and impair a subsequent wide local resection for curative purposes. If possible, an incisional biopsy should retrieve a deep section of tumor as well as a margin of normal tissue. Incisional biopsies suffer from the same disadvantages as needle biopsies in that the removed portion may not be representative of the entire tumor. Consequently, a negative biopsy does not preclude the possibility of cancer in the residual mass.

Excisional biopsy completely removes the mass of interest. It is used for small, discrete masses that are generally <3 cm in diameter, where complete removal will not interfere with a subsequent wider excision that may be required for definitive local control. Excisional biopsy allows the pathologist to examine the entire lesion. However, this method is contraindicated in large tumor masses because the biopsy procedure could scatter tumor cells throughout a large surgical field that would need to be widely and totally encompassed by the ultimate surgical resection. For this reason, excisional biopsy is usually contraindicated for skeletal and soft tissue masses when the diagnosis of sarcoma is being entertained. The excisional method is also used for polypoid lesions of the colon, for thyroid and breast nodules, lymph nodes, for small skin lesions, and when the pathologist cannot make a definitive diagnosis from tissue removed by incisional biopsy. An unbiopsied mass is also surgically removed when the suspicious character of the lesion, the need for its removal (whatever the diagnosis), and the nonmutilating nature of the operation render such an approach feasible. Examples of such procedures include subtotal thyroidectomy for thyroid nodules after an inconclusive FNA and a right hemicolectomy for a cecal mass that might be either inflammatory or neoplastic. In the latter instance, colonoscopic biopsy is informative only if positive for neoplasm. Surgeons should always mark the excisional biopsy margins with sutures or metal clips so that if removal is incomplete and further excision is needed the positive margin can be accurately identified *in situ*.

Orientation of biopsy incisions is also extremely important. Ill-conceived incisions can unnecessarily open up additional tissue planes, necessitating subsequent wider radiotherapy fields or more extensive ultimate surgical resections. For example, tumors of the extremities are best biopsied using incisions that run parallel to the long axis of that limb. This facilitates a definitive en bloc resection that encompasses the biopsy track (Figure 3). Biopsy incisions should be closed using meticulous hemostasis because a hematoma can lead to dissemination of tumor cells with contamination of tissue planes. Instruments, gloves, gowns, and drapes should be discarded and replaced with unused substitutes if the definitive surgical resection immediately follows the biopsy procedure.

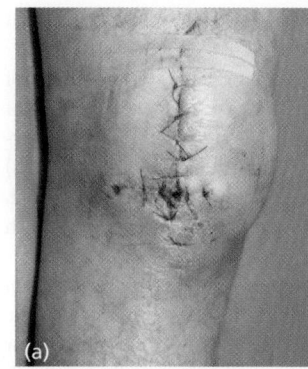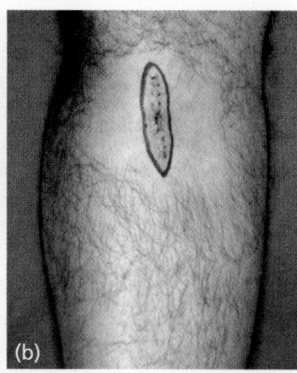

Figure 3 Appropriate and inappropriate biopsy incisions. (a) A patient with a cruciate-shaped biopsy scar overlying the patellar tendon that contained a synovial sarcoma. Note the erythema in this infected incision. This ill-conceived biopsy scar would have required a wide-field soft tissue and osseous composite resection to encompass all of the violated tissue planes. Unfortunately, tumor was *intruded* into the joint space at the time of this biopsy, and this patient ultimately required an above-knee amputation to treat this small, otherwise limb-salvageable sarcoma. (b) An appropriately oriented incisional biopsy scar in the lower extremity. Note the alignment of the scar parallel with the long axis of the extremity and the meticulous placement of small biopsy wound sutures. The entire scar could be excised at surgery (blue ellipse) with minimal concomitant normal tissue sacrifice.

Lymph nodes should be carefully selected for biopsy. Axillary nodes may be preferable to groin nodes if both are enlarged because of a decreased likelihood of postoperative infection. Other caveats are also noteworthy. For example, lymph node specimens preserved in formaldehyde cannot be analyzed for cytogenetics or flow cytometric immunophenotyping. The laboratory work-up for lymphoma usually requires unfixed sterile tissue. Cervical lymph nodes should not be biopsied until a careful search for a primary tumor has been made using nasopharyngoscopy, esophagoscopy, and bronchoscopy because enlargement of the upper cervical nodes by metastases is usually caused by laryngeal, oropharyngeal, and nasopharyngeal primary neoplasms. In contrast, supraclavicular nodes are more frequently enlarged as a result of metastases from primary tumors of the thoracic or abdominal cavities or breast.

The tumor specimen may be prepared for pathologic examination by either frozen or permanent sections. Frozen sections are made at the time of biopsy, and pathologic diagnosis can typically be obtained within 10 min. Frozen sections are used when the diagnosis is required to assess resectability at the time of major surgery or to check tumor margins intraoperatively. Frozen-section biopsy-proven carcinomatosis may mandate abandoning a procedure with a curative intent in favor of a palliative approach. Occasionally, mediastinoscopy, laparoscopy (peritoneoscopy), thoracoscopy, exploratory thoracotomy, or even laparotomy is necessary to obtain adequate representative tissue samples for microscopic examination to confirm diagnosis or tumor stage.

Staging

Tumor staging is a system used to describe the anatomic extent of a specific malignant process in an individual patient. Staging systems cluster relevant prognostic factors about the primary tumor, such as size, grade, and location, as well as information about dissemination to regional sites, such as lymph nodes or distant metastatic sites. Accurately staging a cancer is essential in designing an appropriate therapeutic program and advising on prognosis. Without accurate staging, it is impossible to meaningfully compare the results of therapies administered in different centers. New forms of therapy can be appropriately evaluated only by comparing the impact of current therapy of neoplasms of equivalent stage.

The recognized importance of staging has led to a variety of international and national attempts to standardize the staging of the patient with cancer. To date, no single system has been universally accepted. The American Joint Committee on Cancer (AJCC) has recommended a staging system ranging from stage I (small, localized malignancy) to stage IV (distant metastatic spread).[6] Both the AJCC and the Union Internationale Contre Cancer (International Union Against Cancer, UICC) have adopted a shared TNM system that defines a cancer in terms of the primary tumor (T), the presence or absence of nodal metastases (N), and the presence or absence of distant metastases (M). Increasing numerals after the T, such as T1, T2, T3, or T4, indicate lesions of increasing size or depth of penetration that are usually associated with a poorer prognosis. The absence of nodal metastasis is designated as N0, the presence of nodal metastasis is N1, and for more extensive nodal involvement, additional numbers may be used. Finally, distant metastases are indicated by adding the numeral 1 following M for metastases, or the numeral 0 signifying their absence. Thus, a small lesion that has neither spread to regional nodes nor metastasized to distant sites would be designated as T1 N0 M0. A larger lesion that involved regional nodes but not distant sites might be identified as T2 N1 M0. A large neoplasm associated with both regional and distant metastases would be designated T3 N1 M1. For some tumor types, such as soft tissue sarcoma, a G for grade of malignancy is added. High-grade tumors are less differentiated and tend to metastasize more readily.

The TNM system has four chronologic classifications. The clinical classification (cTNM or TNM) represents the extent of the disease before first definitive treatment as determined from physical examination, imaging studies, endoscopy, biopsy, surgical exploration, and any other relevant findings. The pathologic classification (pTNM) incorporates the additional information available at the time of surgery or derived from pathologic examination of a completely resected specimen. This is especially useful in planning adjuvant therapy. A *y* prefix may be added to denote pathologic staging after initial systemic or radiation therapy has been performed (ypTNM). The retreatment classification (rTNM) is used to stage a cancer that has recurred after a disease-free interval; it includes clinical and/or pathologic evidence of recurrence. Finally, the autopsy classification (aTNM) is based on postmortem examination.

Patterns of tumor spread

In general, a malignant tumor may spread (1) by direct extension into surrounding structures, (2) via the lymphatics, (3) by hematogenous spread, or (4) by implantation in serous cavities. However, many cancers spread by more than one route, and an orderly course of metastasis is not predictably certain. For example, patients with breast cancer or melanoma can manifest distant metastatic disease in the lungs, liver, or skeleton without ever developing evidence of lymph node metastases. Table 2 summarizes the metastatic patterns of various human tumors.

Cancer cells may also spread by direct extension through tissue spaces and planes. Some neoplasms, such as soft tissue sarcomas and adenocarcinomas of the stomach or esophagus, may extend for a considerable distance (10–15 cm) along tissue planes beyond the palpable tumor mass. Other neoplasms, such as a basal cell carcinoma of skin, rarely extend for more than a few millimeters beyond the visible margin. Even though most central nervous system (CNS) tumors infrequently metastasize, they may penetrate nearby brain

Table 2 Patterns of neoplastic spread for common human malignancies.

Neoplasms	Hematogenous	Lymphatic	Local infiltration (expressed as local recurrence)
Adenocarcinoma			
Breast	++++	+++	++
Endometrium	+	++	+
Ovary	++	+++	++++
Stomach	++++	++++	+++
Pancreas	++++	++++	+++
Colon	+++	+++	+
Kidney	++	++	++
Prostate	+++	+++	+++
Liver	+	+	++++
Epidermal carcinoma			
Lung	++++	+++	++
Oropharynx	++	+++	+++
Larynx	+	+++	++
Cervix	+	++++	+++
Transitional cell carcinoma			
Bladder	++	+++	++++
Cutaneous neoplasm			
Squamous cell carcinoma	+	++	+
Melanoma	+++	+++	++
Basal cell carcinoma	0	0	+
Sarcoma			
Bone	++++	+	+
Soft tissue	++++	+	+++
Brain neoplasm	0	0	++++

Key: Does not occur; 0, <1%; +, 1–5%; ++, 15– +++0%; 3, 30%; and ++++, 50%.

tissue, and their location can cause death by interfering with vital CNS functions.

Tumor cells can readily enter the lymphatics and extend through these channels by permeation or embolization to regional lymph nodes. Permeation is the growth of a colony of tumor cells along the course of the lymphatic vessel. This commonly occurs in the skin lymphatics in carcinoma of the breast and in the perineural lymphatics in carcinoma of the prostate. Lymphatic involvement is extremely common in malignant epithelial neoplasms of all types, except basal cell carcinoma of the skin, which metastasizes to regional lymphatics in <0.1% of cases, or mesenchymal neoplasms, such as sarcomas, which metastasize to lymph nodes in only 2–5% of cases.

Spread along the lymphatics by embolization to regional or distant lymph nodes is of great clinical importance. Tumor cells travel within local lymphatics and can spread to proximal nodal basins via the collateral lymphatic channels. Lymph node metastases are first confined to the subcapsular space; at this stage, the node is not enlarged and may appear grossly normal. Gradually, the tumor cells permeate the sinusoids and replace the nodal parenchyma, changing the shape and texture of the node. There is little direct spread from node to node because the nodal capsule is not penetrated until a late stage. However, when an involved lymph node is more than 3 cm in diameter, tumor has usually extended beyond the capsule into the perinodal fat.

Lymph from the abdominal organs and lower extremities drains into the cisterna chyli and then into the thoracic duct, which finally opens into the left jugular vein. Using this route, tumor cells can pass freely from the lymphatic system into the bloodstream. Oncologists originally believed that solid neoplasms first involved regional lymph nodes and then spread into the bloodstream by drainage into the thoracic duct and then to other parts of the body. An alternative explanation now favored by most oncologists assumes that the presence of cancer cells in regional lymph nodes indicates an unfavorable host–tumor relationship and the concomitant high likelihood of distant metastases.

Cancer cells may reach the bloodstream either through the thoracic duct or by direct invasion of blood vessels. Capillaries offer no resistance to tumor cell transgression. Small veins are frequently invaded, whereas thicker-walled arteries are rarely violated. Veins frequently form a plexus extending to the subendothelial regions, which provide a portal of entry through the thin vein wall. When the vascular endothelium is destroyed, a thrombus can form that is quickly invaded by tumor. This combination of thrombus and tumor may detach to form large tumor emboli. Vascular invasion is common in both carcinomas and sarcomas and is associated with a poor prognosis. Some types of neoplasms have a remarkable tendency to grow as a solid column along the course of veins. For example, renal cell carcinoma can grow into the renal vein and up the inferior vena cava extending to the right atrium. In this situation, a spectacular en bloc removal requiring cardiopulmonary bypass may still result in long-term survival or even cure.

Tumor cells occasionally gain entrance to serous cavities by growing through the wall of an organ. Many tumor cells can grow in suspension without a supporting matrix and may widely spread within the peritoneal cavity or attach to serous surfaces. Thus, widespread peritoneal seeding is common with gastrointestinal and ovarian cancers. Similarly, malignant gliomas may spread widely within the CNS via the cerebrospinal fluid.

Although much is known about the routes of tumor spread, the mechanisms underlying this process remain unclear. Some cancers are metastatic at the time of clinical discovery, whereas others of the same type and in the same organ tissue may remain localized for years. Metastases may dominate the presenting clinical picture although the primary tumor remains latent and asymptomatic or even undetectable. For example, cerebral metastases from silent cancers in the bronchus or the breast are often mistaken for primary benign CNS neoplasms.

Preoperative preparation

Preparation of a patient for surgical cancer therapy is important in order to minimize perioperative complications, hasten recovery to premorbid state of health, and avoid delay in possible initiation of postoperative adjuvant therapy. Every effort should be made to correct nutritional deficiencies if present, restore depleted blood volume, and correct electrolyte imbalances before extensive surgical procedures. Total parenteral nutrition (TPN) can be used to prepare the extremely malnourished patient for a major operation, although reconstitution is a slow process, and TPN may chiefly serve to interrupt further deterioration by restoring positive nitrogen balance. Surgical morbidity and mortality following extensive cancer operations will predictably be problematic if critical physiologic and biochemical deficiencies are not corrected in advance.

Determining the risk inherent in a given operation is a complicated and inexact assessment based on a number of factors. The physical status of the patient, including cardiopulmonary reserve, comorbid conditions, debility inherent to a specific operation, hepatic and renal function, and the intent of surgical procedure (curative vs palliative), are all pertinent to this assessment. The technical complexity of an operation, the type of anesthetic used, and the relative experience of the involved health care personnel can all impact on the complications of a procedure. Various schema for risk assessment, such as the five-level physical status classification of the American Society of Anesthesiologists (Table 3) and the Eastern Cooperative Oncology Group Five-Step Performance Scale (Table 4), may be useful in assessing the appropriateness of

Table 3 American Society of Anesthesiologists: Physical status classification.

Class	Description
P-1	A normal healthy patient
P-2	A patient with mild systemic disease
P-3	A patient with severe systemic disease
P-4	A patient with severe systemic disease that is a constant threat to life
P-5	A moribund patient who is not expected to survive without the operation
P-6	A declared brain-dead patient whose organs are being removed for donor purposes

Source: Saklad 1941.[7] Reproduced with permission of Wolters Kluwer.

Table 4 Eastern Cooperative Oncology Group: Performance scale and corresponding Karnofsky rating.

Grade	Description
0	Fully active, able to carry on all predisease activities without restriction (Karnofsky 100)
1	Restricted in physically strenuous activity but ambulatory and able to carry out work of a light or sedentary nature, for example, light housework/office work (Karnofsky 80–90)
2	Ambulatory and capable of all self-care but unable to carry out any work activities; up and about more than 50% of waking hours (Karnofsky 60–70)
3	Capable of limited self-care; confined to bed or chair 50% or more of waking hours (Karnofsky 40–50)
4	Completely disabled; cannot carry on any self-care; totally confined to bed or chair (Karnofsky 30 or less)

Source: Adapted from Etzioni 2003.[15] Reproduced with permission of Springer.

a given operation for a specific patient. More recently, it has been the introduction of the American College of Surgeons surgical risk calculator (www.riskcalculator.facs.org), which takes into account 21 patient characteristics that can be entered online and used to predict any of the nine possible procedure-specific outcomes including death, any complication, severe complications, and surgical site infection among others. The calculator was developed based on data obtained from over 1.4 million operations at 393 hospitals participating in the ACS NSQIP project between 2009 and 2012.[8]

Operative mortality is defined as mortality that occurs within 30 days of an operative procedure. In cancer patients, the underlying disease is a major determinant of operative mortality. Although it is true that comparable operations are usually more morbid in the geriatric age group as compared with other adults, advanced age per se should not disqualify a patient from a potentially curative surgical procedure. Because of their high-risk nature, decisions about the indications for palliative surgical procedures are particularly difficult. For example, palliative surgery for extensive metastatic disease or symptomatic intestinal obstruction secondary to carcinomatosis has a 20–30% perioperative mortality. In such circumstances, the risk–benefit ratio and ultimate surgical objectives must be defined as clearly as possible and accepted by patient, family, and surgeon.

Preoperative chemotherapy and or radiation therapy is being administered with increasing frequency in patients undergoing cancer operations. In some cases, these therapies can be associated with increased perioperative complications. For example, the antivascular endothelial growth factor antibody bevacizumab is associated with increased risk of wound healing complications when administered within several weeks before surgery.[9] As this targeted therapy has a 21-day half-life, discontinuation of bevacizumab is recommended at least 6–8 weeks before elective surgery.

Operative considerations

Once a decision has been made to proceed with surgical therapy, the operative procedure itself must be carefully planned for the specific surgical patient. It is essential to realize that the best (and often the only) opportunity for cure is with the first resection, at the time of initial tissue plane, lymphatic, and blood vessel potential exposure to tumor cells that may be dislodged within the operative field. A subsequent recurrence may be difficult to distinguish from the normal postsurgical inflammatory reaction and scarring.

The principle of the "no touch technique" has maintained some traction in the surgical lore. This opinion is based on the theoretical concept that direct contact with and manipulation of the tumor during resection can lead to an increased risk in local implantation and embolization of tumor cells. Although little clinical evidence exists to support this principle, there may be some validity to this concept with respect to tumors that extend directly into the vascular system, such as hepatocellular or renal tumors with extension to the large veins or vena cava. Although not definitively proved to be detrimental, the general tenet of avoidance of forceful handling of the tumor and care to avoid any tumor disruption during surgical resection is sound technique. Similarly, every attempt should be made to extirpate a tumor with meticulous attention to detail while avoiding excessive blood loss or operative time. Although the need for contiguous multivisceral resection may, by its nature, result in prolonged operation with high blood loss, familiarity and experience with such complicated operations such as major hepatectomy, pancreatectomy, and retroperitoneal tumor removal potentially minimizes operative morbidity and maximizes oncologic benefit

Types of cancer operations

Wide local resection with removal of an adequate margin of normal peritumoral tissue may be adequate treatment of low-grade neoplasms that very rarely metastasize to regional nodes or widely infiltrate adjacent tissues. Basal cell carcinomas and mixed tumors of the parotid gland are examples of such tumors. In contrast, neoplasms that spread widely by infiltration into adjacent tissues, such as soft tissue sarcomas and esophageal and gastric carcinomas, must be excised with a wide margin of normal tissue. This wide tissue margin between the line of excision and the tumor mass may also act as a protective barrier against intraoperative tumor cell traversal into severed lymphatics and vessels. Tumor cells may have been implanted in the incision when an incisional biopsy alone had been previously performed. To encompass potentially contaminated tissues, it is extremely important to remove a wide segment of skin and underlying muscle, fat, and fascia beyond the limits of the original incision.

Malignant neoplasms are usually not truly encapsulated. The tumor is commonly encased by a pseudocapsule comprising a compression zone of normal tissue interspersed with neoplastic cells. This pseudoencapsulation offers a great temptation for simple enucleation in that the tumor may be easily dislodged from its bed. However, this approach must be resisted because microscopic extensions of tumor from the primary through the pseudocapsule will be left behind after simple enucleation, dooming the patient to a local recurrence. Ideally, the surgeon should operate through normal tissues at all times and never encounter or even directly visualize the neoplasm during its removal. Dissection should proceed with meticulous care to avoid tumor cell spillage. Many neoplasms metastasize via the lymphatics, and operations have been designed to remove the primary neoplasm and draining regional lymph nodes in continuity with all intervening tissues. Circumstances favor this type of operative approach when the

lymph nodes draining the neoplasm lie adjacent to the tumor bed or when there is a single avenue of lymphatic drainage that can be removed without sacrificing vital structures. It is important to avoid cutting across involved lymphatic channels, which markedly increases the possibility of local recurrence.

At the present time, it is generally agreed that en bloc regional lymph node dissection is indicated for clinically demonstrable nodal involvement with metastatic tumor. However, in many cases, the tumor has already spread beyond regional nodes. Although the cure rates following resection in such circumstances may be quite low (20–50%), undue pessimism should not prevent such patients from receiving appropriate surgical treatment. En bloc removal of the involved lymph nodes may offer the only chance for cure and can at least provide significant palliative local control. Regional lymph node involvement should therefore not be viewed as a contraindication to surgery but as a possible indication for adjuvant therapies, such as radiation or chemotherapy.

The routine dissection of regional nodes in close proximity to the primary malignancy is recommended for most cancer types even when these structures are not clinically involved with tumor. This recommendation is based on the high rate of locoregional recurrence following surgical resection when multiple lymph nodes are microscopically involved and the high error rate when palpation alone is used to assess possible lymph node involvement with tumor. Microscopic tumor dissemination to regional lymph nodes can be detected in 20–40% of clinically node-negative carcinomas and melanomas.

The extent of lymph node dissection remains controversial. Sentinel lymphadenectomy is now a well-established technique for detection of early nodal disease in selected tumor types. First introduced by Morton et al.[10] for melanoma, it is now being applied as well for the management of breast carcinoma[11] and other neoplasms.[12] Initially, the technique relied on the injection of a vital blue dye at the tumor site and visual tracking of this dye along the lymphatics draining to the nodal basin, sentinel node mapping has been facilitated by adding a radiolabeled isotope to the dye and monitoring its path using a handheld gamma probe. Sentinel lymphadenectomy is a low-morbidity procedure that accurately stages the regional lymph nodes and identifies the 60–80% of melanoma and breast cancer patients who do not require complete lymphadenectomy.

Advances in surgical technique, anesthesia, and supportive care (blood transfusion, antibiotics, and fluid and electrolyte management) permit the more radical, extensive, and lengthy operative procedures to be done more safely. Such procedures offer a chance for a cure that cannot be achieved by other means and are justified in selected situations, if there is no evidence of distant metastases. For example, some slow-growing primary tumors may reach an enormous size and widely infiltrate locally without metastasizing to distant sites. Supra-radical operative procedures should be considered for these extensive and nearly inoperable tumors because the occasional patient is cured. However, such operations should be undertaken only by experienced surgeons who can select those patients most likely to benefit. As an example of carefully indicated radical surgery, pelvic exenteration is a well-conceived operation capable of curing patients with radiation-treated recurrent cancer of the cervix and certain well differentiated and locally extensive adenocarcinomas of the rectum. This operation removes all pelvic organs (bladder, uterus, and rectum) and soft tissues within the pelvis. Bowel function is restored with colostomy. Urinary tract drainage is established by anastomosis of the ureters into a segment of the bowel (ileum or sigmoid colon). The 5-year relapse-free survival is 25% when pelvic exenteration is used to manage these problems. It is also imperative that the surgical oncologist be willing to accept responsibility for helping to optimize the postoperative emotional and psychological rehabilitation of the patient before embarking on extensive resections, such as hemipelvectomy, forequarter amputation, mutilating operations for head and neck carcinomas, or total pelvic exenteration.

Although logic might suggest that once a neoplasm has metastasized to a distant site, it is no longer curable by surgical resection, experience shows otherwise. The removal of metastatic deposits within the liver, lung, or other sites can occasionally result in long-term cure. In others, often with favorable biology and good response to systemic chemotherapy, metastatectomy can significantly prolong survival beyond that of chemotherapy alone, not infrequently turning advanced disease into a chronic condition. Before undertaking resection, an extensive work-up should be performed to rule out metastatic spread to other body sites outside of the proposed operative field.

Some patients with liver-only metastases may benefit from surgical resection, particularly when of colorectal origin. Advances in preoperative evaluation, surgical technique, and systemic therapies have all contributed to an increasingly aggressive approach to such patients. Although in the past, resectability was defined by the number, size, and distribution of hepatic metastases, more recently, resectability is defined by the capability to resect all disease with negative margins (R0) and have a sufficient functional remnant liver, regardless of the tumor number. Even patients with limited and resectable extrahepatic disease combined with liver metastases may be candidates for surgical therapy provided all disease can be safely removed. Moreover, when not initially optimally resectable, approaches to (1) reduce tumor size with preoperative chemotherapy, (2) expand the remnant liver with preoperative portal vein embolization or staged liver resections, or (3) application of thermal ablative approaches combined with resection, all can contribute to increasing the number of patients eligible for surgical therapy of liver metastases with curative intent. Even with increasingly aggressive approaches, contemporary series are reporting 5-year survival rates following complete resection in excess of 50%.[13]

Surgical procedures are sometimes indicated to palliate symptoms without attempting to cure the patient, thereby prolonging a useful and comfortable life. A palliative operation may be justified to relieve pain, hemorrhage, obstruction, or infection when it can be done without untoward risk to the patient. Palliative surgery may also be applicable when there are no better nonsurgical means of palliation or when the procedure will improve the quality of life, even if it does not result in prolonged survival. In contrast, surgery that only prolongs a miserable existence is not of benefit to the patient. Examples of indicated palliative surgical procedures include (1) colostomy, enteroenterostomy, or gastrojejunostomy to relieve intestinal obstruction; (2) cordotomy or celiac block to control pain; (3) hepaticojejunostomy to relieve biliary obstruction and pruritis; (4) amputation for intractably painful tumors of the extremities; (5) simple mastectomy for carcinoma of the breast, when the tumor is infected, large, ulcerated, and locally resectable (even in the presence of distant metastases); and (6) resection of obstructing colon cancer in the presence of disseminated metastatic disease. Surgery for residual disease is a special application of palliative surgery. In some patients, extensive yet isolated local spread of malignancy precludes gross total resection of all disease. In these patients, cytoreductive surgery may be of benefit, such as biologically indolent disease or that which is producing local or hormonal symptoms such as metastatic neuroendocrine tumors.

Problems with exsanguinating hemorrhage, perforated viscus, abscess formation, or impending obstruction of a hollow viscus, such as gastrointestinal organs, critical blood vessels, or respiratory structures, are sometimes amenable to emergency surgical intervention. Emergency surgery may also be indicated to decompress tumors that are invading the CNS or that are destroying critical neurologic components by exerting pressure in closed spaces. The cancer patient being evaluated for emergency surgery may be neutropenic or thrombocytopenic as a consequence of recent myelosuppressive chemotherapy. Sometimes, a potential catastrophe can be avoided by operating on such patients expectantly just after they have gone through the nadir of their most recent myelosuppressive chemotherapy. Because of the high risks involved, each patient and the patient's family must be made aware of the dangers and benefits of the proposed surgery, as well as of other potentially effective treatments that might be available if the patient survives this emergency operation.

Reconstructive surgery after tumor resection has remarkably improved the quality of life for many cancer patients. The routine application of microvascular anastomotic techniques has enabled the free transfer of composite grafts containing skin, muscle, and/or bone to surgically created bodily defects. Breast reconstruction after mastectomy, tissue transfers as part of extremity surgery for sarcoma or mandible reconstruction, and aerodigestive reconstruction using jejunal-free grafts are examples of these dramatic improvements in the combined surgical management of complex cancer problems. In the future, applications of the new discipline of tissue engineering will remarkably extend the reconstructive armamentarium. Using these approaches in the future, it may be possible to custom-grow nerve, fat, muscle, bone cartilage, or other body components as replacements for tissues that will need to be resected as part of a composite cancer procedure.[14]

Cancer/surgical quality control

Constant and ongoing assessment of personal and institutional outcomes provides opportunity to improve systems that can result in safer operations and identify new markers or therapies that can improve oncology outcomes. Oncologists, particularly surgeons, are well positioned to develop databases that can be used to identify etiologic factors for cancer development, predictors of surgical complications, markers of cancer outcomes, and potential changes in management schemes. Such comprehensive data sets can be combined across institutions to provide insight for uncommon cancers and/or procedures. When combined to create annotated tumor banks, these become very powerful tools that can be used to identify potential targets for drug discovery in addition to process improvement. The American College of Surgeons Commission on Cancer provides a forum by which more than 1500 associated institutions monitor quality of cancer care. Through this accreditation mechanism, institutions are required to have state-of-the-art clinical cancer services, cancer committee leadership, cancer conferences for care planning and provider education, quality improvement program in part through compliance with accepted cancer treatment guidelines (e.g., NCCN), and a comprehensive cancer registry to monitor quality of care. The surgical oncologist is well suited to lead these efforts.

The future of surgical oncology

Within the next decade, cancer is predicted to replace cardiovascular disease as the leading cause of death among Americans. The aging of the population will generate an enormous growth in demand for oncological procedures. By 2020, the number of patients undergoing oncological procedures is projected to increase by 24–51% (Table 5).[15] If a shortage of surgeons performing these

Table 5 Projected numbers of surgical oncological procedures: 2010–2020.

Variable	2000[a]	2010[b]	2020[b]	Increase (2000–2020)
Breast (diagnostic)	364,800	416,100 (14.1%)	464,100 (27.2%)	99,300
Breast (excisions)	392,700	440,200 (12.1%)	485,600 (23.7%)	92,900
Outpatient total	757,500	856,300 (13.0%)	949,700 (25.4%)	192,200
Breast (mastectomy)	90,400	106,000 (17.3%)	123,700 (36.8%)	33,300
Colon resection	96,300	113,700 (18.1%)	141,100 (46.5%)	44,800
Rectal resection	27,800	33,300 (19.7%)	40,900 (47.0%)	13,100
Stomach resection	9400	11,100 (17.6%)	13,700 (45.1%)	4300
Pancreas resection	3900	4700 (19.7%)	5800 (47.4%)	1900
Esophageal resection	1400	1700 (24.0%)	2100 (51.2%)	700
Inpatient total	229,200	270,500 (18.0%)	327,100 (42.7%)	97,900

[a]Figures listed for inpatient procedures in 2000 are the numbers of procedures performed that year, based on NIS 2000. Figures for outpatient procedures (breast diagnostic and breast excisions) represent projections based on data from the NSAS 1996.
[b]Figures listed for 2010 and 2020 are projections; percentages listed indicate percent growth relative to the year 2000.
Source: Adapted from Etzioni 2003.[15] Reproduced with permission of Springer.

procedures does occur, the result will inevitably be decreased access to care. To prevent this from happening, the ability of surgeons to cope with an increased burden of work needs to be critically evaluated and improved. Given that there are no more than approximately 50 surgical oncologists produced yearly in the United States, it is clear that the traditional surgical oncology educational roles in academic medical centers as well as in the larger health care community will continue and perhaps come under increasing pressure to expand.

As multimodality care grows in complexity and chemotherapy/radiotherapy move more prominently into the neoadjuvant position, surgical oncologists will have to become increasingly involved in clinical trial design. To be effective in this arena, understanding the natural history of specific malignancies will require an expanded knowledge base about the mutated genes and their cognate proteins that drive solid-tumor proliferation and metastasis. Surgical oncologists will have to become more knowledgeable about these factors, both during training and as a lifelong commitment to self-education.

An important effort to strengthen the position of surgical oncology in medical community has been establishing board certification in surgical oncology, beginning in 2014. The past half-century has seen the unprecedented evolution of surgical specialties into their current status as discrete disciplines, with specialized knowledge, techniques, anatomic challenges, and diseases of focus. This is especially true in surgical oncology, which has attracted many owing to its strong allure as a combination of the technical and the cognitive. There is an emerging understanding that the surgical oncologist has specialized knowledge that is not acquired in general surgical training: knowledge of the natural history of malignant disease, knowledge of the multidisciplinary care for the cancer patient, and, certainly, knowledge of how to perform some very unusual and technically demanding oncological operative procedures. These factors, coupled with an awareness of the rapidly increasing manpower need, have led to creating a board certification mechanism for surgical oncology. Entitled board certification in *complex general surgical oncology*, the assessment process includes both a written and oral examination component. Eligibility to sit for these examinations is limited to graduates of American Council of Graduate medical Education (ACGME) accredited surgical oncology fellowship programs, meaning that graduates of such

fellowship program that were not ACGME accredited at the time of an individual fellowship graduation renders such individuals ineligible for *complex general surgical oncology* board certification. This stipulation effectively limits the annual total number of board eligible candidates, yet has resulted in a doubling of the fellowship applicant pool in the United States over the past several years. Board certification will strengthen the position and impact of surgical oncologists practicing in the community and academic environments and might also aid in the development of comparable certification mechanisms in other countries, leading to enhanced cancer care worldwide.

References

1 Birkmeyer JD, Warshaw AL, Finlayson SR, et al. Relationship between hospital volume and late survival after pancreaticoduodenectomy. *Surgery*. 1999;**126**:178–183.
2 Breasted JH. *The Edwin Smith Surgical Papyrus*. Chicago: University of Chicago Press; 1930.
3 Hill GJ II., Historic milestones in cancer surgery. *Semin Oncol*. 1979;**6**:409–427.
4 Antman KA, Eilber FR, Shiu MH. Soft tissue sarcomas: current trends in diagnosis and management. *Curr Prob Cancer*. 1989;**13**:339–367.
5 Choti MA, Sitzmann JV, Tiburi MF, et al. Trends in long-term survival following liver resection for hepatic colorectal metastases. *Ann Surg*. 2002;**235**:759–766.
6 Edge SB, Byrd DR, Compton CC, et al. (eds). *American Joint Committee on Cancer (AJCC) Cancer Staging Manual*, 7th ed. New York: Springer-Verlag; 2010.
7 Saklad M. Grading of patients for surgical procedures. *Anesthesiology*. 1941;**2**:281.
8 Bilimoria KY, Liu Y, Paruch JL, et al. Development and evaluation of the universal ACS NSQIP surgical risk calculator: a decision aid and informed consent tool for patients and surgeons. *J Am Chem Soc*. 2012;**217**:833–842.
9 Scappaticci FA, Fehrenbacher L, Cartwright T, et al. Surgical wound healing complications in metastatic colorectal cancer patients treated with bevacizumab. *J Surg Oncol*. 2005;**91**:173–180.
10 Morton DL, Wen D-R, Wong JH, et al. Technical details of intraoperative lymphatic mapping for melanoma. *Arch Surg*. 1992;**127**:392–399.
11 Giuliano AE, Kirgan DM, Guenther JM, Morton DL. Lymphatic mapping and sentinel lymphadenectomy for breast cancer. *Ann Surg*. 1994;**220**:391–398.
12 Koch WM, Choti MA, Civelek AC, Eisele DW, Saunders JR. Gamma probe-directed biopsy of the sentinel node in oral squamous cell carcinoma. *Arch Otolaryngol Head Neck Surg*. 1998;**124**:455–459.
13 Pawlik TM, Scoggins CR, Zorzi D, et al. Effect of surgical margin status on survival and site of recurrence after hepatic resection for colorectal metastases. *Ann Surg*. 2005;**241**:715–722.
14 Patrick CW Jr, Mikos AG, McIntire LV. *Frontiers in Tissue Engineering*. New York: Pergamon Press; 1998.
15 Etzioni DA, Liu JH, Maggard MA, O'Connell JB, Ko CY. Workload projections for surgical oncology: will we need more surgeons? *Ann Surg Oncol*. 2003;**10**:1112–1117.

44 Principles of radiation oncology

Philip P. Connell, MD ▪ *Ralph R. Weichselbaum, MD*

Overview

In recent decades, we have witnessed major technologic advances that have influenced how radiotherapy is delivered to cancer patients. Simultaneously, our understanding of the underlying basic biology that governs radiation effects in human cells and tissues has grown rapidly. Here, we summarize some of these key advances and place them into the context of the evolving paradigms that shape cancer therapeutics more generally. Key biologic topics covered in this chapter involve the molecular responses of cells to DNA damage by ionizing radiation, including the repair of DNA damage, cell cycle arrest and death, cellular signaling, and the influence of tumor-initiating cells (tumor stem cells) on post-treatment outcomes. As radiation generates an inflammatory microenvironment in tumors, drugs that modulate immune functions also represent a potential therapeutic opportunity. We also describe newer biology-based technologies that can accurately predict the intrinsic sensitivity of cells to radiation, and pharmacologic agents that can modulate this radiation sensitivity. Finally, this chapter reviews the major physics-based technologic innovations that have improved the accuracy and utility of clinical radiotherapy. Despite these advances, several unmet challenges continue to limit the impact of radiotherapy, and these remaining hurdles should be the factors that guide future innovations of our field.

Introduction

The medical specialty of radiation oncology began shortly after the discovery of X-rays and their effects on tissue in 1895.[1] This first consisted of single large radiation exposures, using low-energy cathode ray tubes or radium-filled glass tubes positioned in close proximity to tumors. Technological developments between 1920 and 1950 improved the beam output and levels of deliverable energy. This was important because low energy (200–500 kV) X-rays used in these early periods had poor penetration into tissue, resulting in burned skin. The development of cobalt-60 units and linear accelerators in the 1950s to deliver "supervoltage" radiation energies (≥ 1 MeV) was a major advance, because these higher energy photons could penetrate more deeply into tissue. Another important advance was the use of fractionated therapy, in which treatment is divided into multiple small doses rather than one large dose. This enabled better tolerance of normal tissues to radiation. Additional improvements in treatment delivery technology, imaging, and cancer biology over subsequent decades have advanced the field of radiation oncology closer to the idealized goal of maximizing local cancer control while minimizing normal tissue toxicity.

General principles of radiotherapy in cancer treatment

Cancers tend to grow locally and spread systemically via lymphatic or hematogenous routes. Therefore, successful cure often requires therapies that are targeted toward all sites of involvement. The three major modalities of oncological therapy—surgery, radiotherapy, and chemotherapy—can be used alone or combined to address all sites. Surgery and radiotherapy are generally used to address local–regional areas of cancer risk. By its nature, surgery can be both therapeutic and diagnostic, as tumor removal provides tissue for histologic examination. Radiotherapy alone can sometimes offer a noninvasive alternative to surgery, with the possibility for organ preservation. In the adjuvant therapy setting, radiotherapy can be used before surgery to render tumor more resectable or to treat microscopic residual disease after surgery is completed. By contrast to these local therapies, chemotherapy can be used to address metastatic disease or to reduce the risk of potential micrometastasis. Chemotherapy can also act as a radiosensitizer, thereby increasing local tumor control provided by radiotherapy. The optimal use of these three modalities is tailored to the tumor type, anatomic location, stage of cancer, and other patient factors. Each modality carries a different set of risks that need to be balanced against one another to provide the optimal risk-benefit ratio for each individual patient.

Most clinical radiation regimens consist of fractionated therapy, in which treatment is divided into multiple small doses [expressed in units of Gray (Gy)] rather than one large dose. A common course of modern radiotherapy can average 6–8 weeks of treatment, with 5–6 daily treatments per week. The concept of fractionation is based on early empiric clinical observations that small daily radiation exposures can induce death in cancerous cells while allowing for normal tissue recovery. Radiobiologists have proposed various mechanistic explanations for this effect, but our understanding of this process continues to evolve. For example, the ability of normal tissue to repopulate itself with healthy cells represents one important component of normal tissue tolerance.

The impact of radiotherapy at the tissue level is commonly represented graphically by a sigmoid-shaped curve, as a function of increasing radiation dose on the *x*-axis (Figure 1). Ideally, the sigmoidal curve that describes tumor control probability is situated to the left of the curve that depicts normal tissue toxicity. The amount of separation between these two curves defines the therapeutic window, which describes the dose range wherein treatment may successfully eradicate tumor while maintaining normal tissue tolerance. These curves imply that for any given tissue, there exists a dose threshold above or below which incremental changes in dose yield little additional impact. However, within the steep portion of each curve, small changes in dose may yield large differences in terms

Holland-Frei Cancer Medicine, Ninth Edition. Edited by Robert C. Bast Jr., Carlo M. Croce, William N. Hait, Waun Ki Hong, Donald W. Kufe, Martine Piccart-Gebhart, Raphael E. Pollock, Ralph R. Weichselbaum, Hongyang Wang, and James F. Holland.
© 2017 John Wiley & Sons, Inc. ISBN: 978-1-118-93469-2

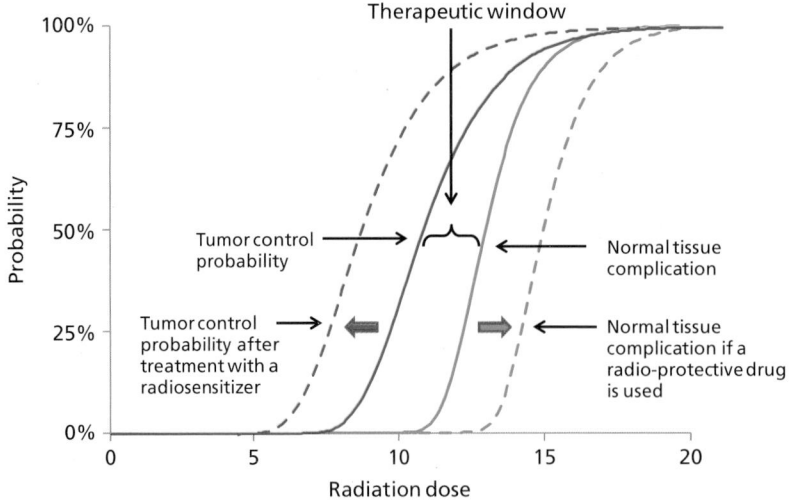

Figure 1 **Effects of radiotherapy at the tissue level are graphically represented.** The solid sigmoid-shaped curves denote idealized probability of tumor control and normal tissue complication risk. The dashed curves denote these same predicted effects following administration of drugs that modulate radiation sensitivity.

of clinical impact. For any clinical situation there exists a unique relationship between the dose–response curves representing tumor kill and surrounding normal tissue toxicity, and these vary widely for different clinical circumstances. One should note that the curves in Figure 1 describe an idealized case, and in reality the relationship in sensitivity of actual tumors versus adjacent normal tissues is usually far more complex.

Biologic impact of radiation therapy

Radiation effects in cells and tissues

The molecular responses to radiotherapy in cells
One Gy leads to the formation of about 10^5 ionization events per cell, which yields approximately 1000–2000 single-stranded DNA breaks (SSBs) and about 40 double-stranded DNA breaks (DSBs) per nucleus. This DNA damage elicits the activation of a growing list of non-DNA repair/checkpoint-related mechanisms that mediate important cellular responses.[2] Radiation-induced DSBs are generally thought to represent the principal lethal events occurring at doses relevant to clinical radiotherapy. This damage elicits numerous cellular responses including DNA damage recognition, transduction of the signal resulting in cell cycle checkpoint activation, induction and coordination of stress response genes, DNA repair, and/or activation of the apoptotic cascade (Figure 2). The MRN protein complex (Mre11, Rad 50, and Nbs1) and ataxia telangiectasia-mutated (ATM) protein are central sensors of DNA damage, and these proteins accumulate at DSBs rapidly. ATM, the related protein ataxia telangiectasia, and RAD3-related (ATR) are members of the PI-3 kinase family, which have central roles in recognizing DNA damage and initiating responses. ATM and ATR appear to perform partially overlapping functions; however, ATM preferentially recognizes DSBs, while ATR preferentially senses replication-blocking DNA lesions. They both phosphorylate downstream targets that modulate pathways that invoke cell cycle checkpoints, apoptosis, senescence, autophagy, and DNA repair. The chromatin protein histone H2AX is one such phosphorylation target, and its activation leads to chromatin structure becoming less condensed and receptive to the recruitment of repair proteins.

Because H2AX phosphorylation is easily visible with fluorescent microscopic methods, it has become a commonly used marker of DSB formation and repair. Phosphorylated H2AX is centrally important to radiation response because it promotes the recruitment of other sensor/effector proteins including 53BP1, MDC1, and BRCA1.

Repair of DSBs in cells
Homologous recombination (HR) and nonhomologous end joining (NHEJ) are the dominant pathways that repair of DSBs. Both pathways act following the recruitment of the sensor/effector proteins, as previously reviewed.[2] In HR, cells identify a stretch of homologous DNA and replicate the missing genetic information from this homologous DNA template.[3] By comparison, the NHEJ pathway processes the broken DNA ends and religates them, sometimes using a region of microhomology.[4] The NHEJ pathway is considered the dominant pathway for repairing radiation-induced DSBs during G0/G1. The generally accepted model involves the binding and processing of DNA ends by Ku70/80, Artemis, and DNA–PKcs complexes. The DSB is subsequently religated by the Ligase IV/XRCC4 complex.[5] Because NHEJ sometimes requires processing of the DSB ends before religation, repair by this pathway has the potential to be error prone. HR, by comparison, is a generally error-free mode of DSB repair because the repair template is an undamaged sister chromatid. HR requires the action of many proteins including the key recombinase RAD51 and additional factors that promote its assembly on DNA, including BRCA2, RAD52, and the RAD51 paralogs.[3] In addition to this DSB repair function, HR proteins promote tolerance of replication-blocking lesions (like damage by interstrand DNA cross-linkers) and collapsed replication forks. The ability of some common chemotherapeutic agents to act as radiosensitizers may result from their interference with these pathways.

Radiation-induced cell-cycle arrest and death
Cell-cycle arrest in G1 and G2 following radiation exposure was described by early pioneers like Hartwell, Nurse, and Hunt.[2] Activated ATM and ATR lead to the phosphorylation of key downstream effector kinases such as Chk1 and Chk2. Following activation, Chk1 and Chk2 phosphorylate the phosphatase

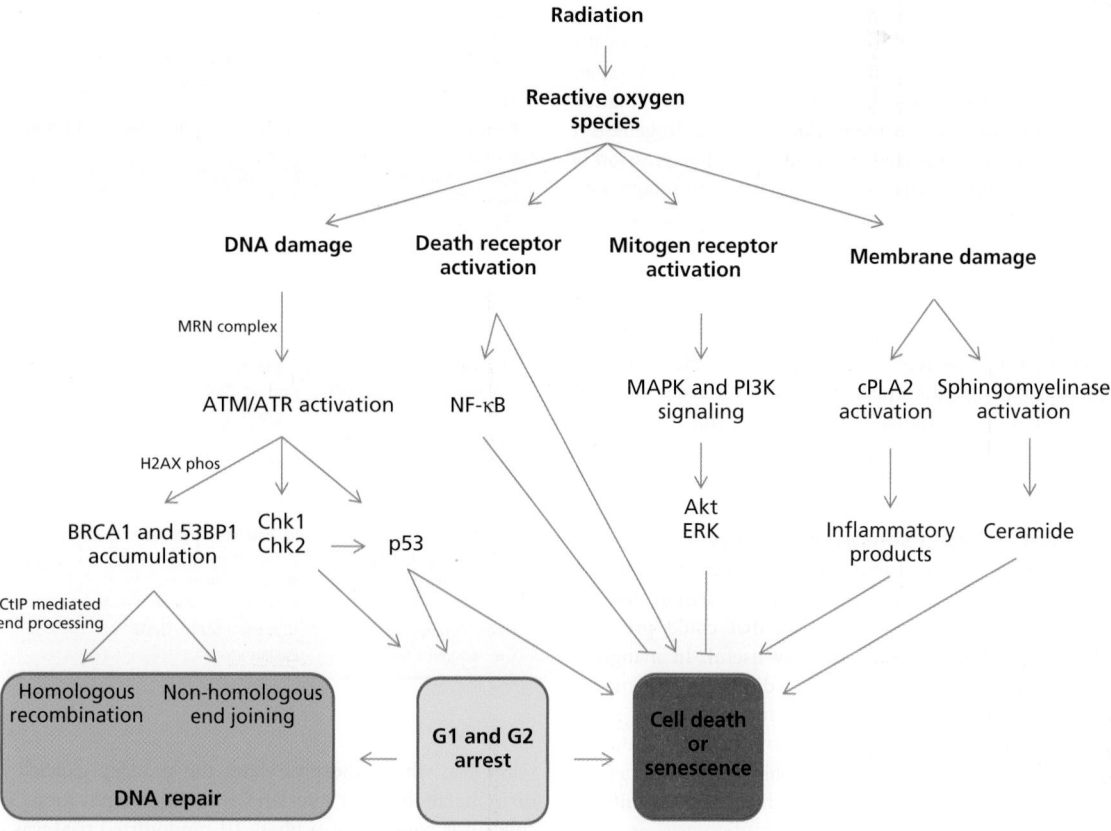

Figure 2 An overview is displayed for molecular responses that occur after radiation exposure.

CDC25A, which in turn becomes degraded. As a result of this, CDC25A is unable to dephosphorylate and activate CDK2. The net result is cell-cycle arrest. Importantly, Chk2 also phosphorylates p53, leading to p21-mediated cell-cycle arrest. These damaged cells subsequently face a critical period, particularly if radiation damage is not completely repaired.[6] Damaged cells may progress unrepaired into mitotic catastrophe. Alternatively, cells may simply lose proliferative capacity by undergoing senescence. Radiation-induced senescence is associated with the activation of the p16/RB and p53/p21 tumor suppressors. Alternatively, cells may undergo apoptotic death, which classically involves p53-dependent activation of the caspase cascade. Additionally, apoptotic death can occur via radiation-induced activation of cell surface "death receptors" (receptors of TNF, Fas, or TRAIL). Paradoxically, these death receptors can also generate cyto-protective effects in some situations by activating transcription factor nuclear factor kappa B (NFκB) to oppose apoptosis.

Major pathways involved in cellular signaling following radiation

Irradiation of tissue leads to the formation of radical oxygen species (ROS), which interact with many cellular contents including DNA. These ROSs, including superoxide and hydroxyl radicals, can deplete cellular stores of antioxidants such as glutathione,[7] creating cellular stresses that stimulate a complex set of signaling cascades.[8] For example, pathways normally used by cells to respond to mitogens are activated, which in turn promote survival, antiapoptotic responses, and transcriptional changes. The net effect can be variable and cell-type dependent, but this generally includes activation of cell surface receptors like the ErbB family that includes epidermal growth factor receptor (EGFR),

which consequently activates other downstream pathways like the mitogen-activated protein kinase (MAPK) superfamily of cascades (ERK, JNK, and p38) and the phosphatidyl inositol 3 kinase (PI3K) pathways.[2] These pathways tend to promote antiapoptotic signals via Akt and Erk signaling. Radiation can also trigger autocrine mechanisms, including the release of transforming growth factor alpha (TGFα), which binds and activates EGFR.[8] Additional proinflammatory cytokines like tumor necrosis factor-alpha (TNF-α) and interleukin-6[9] are also released, and these contribute to the bystander effect—a phenomenon where adjacent nonirradiated cells exhibit similar responses (described in detail in Dr. Grdina's chapter on Ionizing Radiation). Finally, radiation induces the breakdown of membrane-based sphingomyelin into ceramide, which is proapoptotic, independent of DNA damage.[10] Similarly, radiation activates cytosolic phospholipase A2 (cPLA2), an enzyme that recognizes phospholipids on the cell membrane and degrades them into inflammatory products such as arachidonic acid and eventually eicosanoids. For example, lysophosphatidylcholine (LPC) is a product of cPLA2 that leads to activation of Akt and enhanced cell death.[11]

Tumor-initiating cells (tumor stem cells) in irradiated tumors and normal tissues

Despite some disagreements surrounding the nomenclature and basic biology of "tumor stem cells," there clearly exists a population of tumor cells that exhibit an exclusive ability for self-renewal and differentiation into the heterogeneous lineages that promote tumor maintenance.[12-14] These studies predict that targeting cancer stem cells may improve therapeutic outcomes. Interestingly, radiation of tumor cell populations is known to enrich cells expressing putative markers of "stemness," suggesting that tumor stem cells are treatment resistant. For example, radiation leads to the enrichment of glial cancer stem cells that exhibit preferential activation of the DNA damage checkpoint responses and increased DNA repair capacity.[15] The underlying mechanisms that mediate this radiation resistance remain unclear; however, aldehyde dehydrogenase 1 (ALDH1) may represent a partial explanation. High expression of ALDH1 protein in tumor cells confers a survival advantage, perhaps due to aldehyde-catabolizing activity. ALDH1 is also known to cooperate with Fanconi anemia-associated DNA repair genes. This suggests that ALDH1 activity might play a role in repairing adducts on DNA,[16] thereby promoting radioresistance in stem cell clones. Another interesting feature of cancer stem cells is their propensity to repair DSBs using HR repair,[17] suggesting that HR inhibitors might represent a therapeutic strategy for depleting cancer stem cell reservoirs in tumors. Additionally, salinomycin and thioridazine are compounds developed to target cancer stem cells[18,19]; however, they have not yet been tested clinically with radiotherapy.

Development of radio sensitizing drugs

Tumors are frequently located immediately adjacent to radiosensitive normal tissues, which limits the level of radiation that can be safely administered. Therefore, a drug that could preferentially radiosensitize tumors would be very useful. In malignant gliomas, for example, lethality occurs as a direct consequence of local tumor recurrence after treatment: a tumor-selective sensitizer might increase tumor curability. By contrast, some tumors such as prostate cancers are already curable with radiotherapy; however, this requires very high doses, which carry significant toxicity. In such situations, a tumor-specific radiosensitizer might allow for dose de-escalation and reduction of side effects. Standard chemotherapeutic agents remain the most commonly used for increasing the local efficacy of radiotherapy. We recently published a review that details the progress of newer strategies of targeted radiosensitizers.[2] An exhaustive discussion of these novel drugs is not possible in this chapter; however, various classes of agents are shown in Table 1. Many of these agents target proteins that sense radiation injury and coordinate the cellular responses, while others take advantage of the hypoxic or abnormal redox environments that exist in tumors. The ultimate success of any of these drugs will depend on their ability to improve the therapeutic index of radiation (see illustration of this concept in Figure 1). Unfortunately, the development of truly tumor-selective radiosensitizers has proved elusive.

Radiotherapy in combination with gene therapy

Extensive preclinical work and some limited clinical trials have combined gene therapy with radiotherapy, using replication-defective viruses to deliver radiosensitizing prodrugs, cytokines, tumor suppressor genes, and immune-activating compounds. For example, TNFerade (Ad.Egr-TNF11D) is a replication-defective adenoviral vector comprised of radio- and chemo-inducible elements from the Egr-1 promoter upstream to cDNA encoding TNF-α, which acts as a direct radiosensitizer and immune activator. This makes use of radiation-inducible Egr-1 promoter elements, such that TNF-α is specifically secreted within the radiotherapy target volume.[20] Early-phase clinical trials with TNFerade have demonstrated impressive tumor response rates in patients with soft tissue sarcomas, as well as carcinomas of the esophagus, head and neck region, and rectum.[21] However, a randomized phase III trial in pancreatic cancer failed to improve survival, although there was a trend to improve survival in early stage tumors.[22]

Other trials have employed enzyme/prodrug strategies such as virus-directed expression of herpes simplex virus thymidine kinase

Table 1 Drug candidates that may serve in modulating radiation effects.

Level (target)	Radiation sensitizer or protector
Reactive oxygen species	
Radicals	Amifostine, pyridoxamine, UROD RNAi
DNA damage response	
DSB recognition	Mirin, ATM/ATR inhibitors (e.g., KU-55933), DT01
HR repair	RS-1, RI-1, modulators of RAD51 expression
NHEJ repair	DNA-PK inhibitors (e.g., NU7441, Salvicine)
PARP	Veliparib, olaparib
Chromatin organization	
HDAC	Vorinostat, belinostat, panobinostat
Cellular response	
Cell cycle arrest	Chk1/Chk2 inhibitors, CDK4/6 inhibitors
Mitogen signaling	Cetuximab
Pro-death signaling	Pifithrin, GSK-3β inhibitors, anticeramide, cytochrome c peroxidase inhibitors
Tumor microenvironment	
Inflammatory products	Statins
Hypoxia	Carbogen, efaproxiral, tirapazamine, MGd, EZN-2968
Tumor stem cells	Salinomycin, thioridazine, HR inhibitors
Effects at tissue level	
Angiogenesis	Bevacizumab
Immune effects	Anti-CTLA-4, anti-PD-1, IL-2 + SBRT
Gene therapy	NFerade, HSV-tk, G207
Cell repopulation	Palifermin

(HSV-tk), which phosphorylates the prodrug ganciclovir into a toxic metabolite that interferes with DNA replication. While this concept is compelling, a phase III randomized trial was unable to show improved survival for glioblastoma multiforme.[23] Related strategies have combined HSV-tk with an additional "suicide gene" such as cytosine deaminase, which converts the pro-drug 5-fluorocytosine into 5-FU.[24] This strategy combined with prostate radiotherapy has yet to demonstrate efficacy in phase II–III trials. Finally, oncolytic viruses have been combined with radiotherapy, to exploit the concept that some viruses can cooperate with radiotherapy by preferentially infecting and lysing cancer cells. For example, a replication-competent herpes simplex virus I (HSV-1) has been delivered with radiotherapy in malignant gliomas and in locally advanced head and neck cancer.[25] Similarly, a reovirus was recently combined with palliative radiotherapy in a phase I trial.[26]

Immune modulation in combination with radiotherapy

Radiation generates an inflammatory microenvironment in tumors, whereby damaged cells increase antigen presentation and immune recognition. These effects include an elevation of major histocompatibility complex class I (MHC-I) expression, changes in antigenic peptide repertoire, decreases in regulatory T cells, and upregulation in cytokines and adhesion molecules that recruit and activate CD8+ cytotoxic T lymphocytes and dendritic cells.[2] Radiation also leads to a depletion of immunosuppressive processes.[27,28] This immune-modulating activity may allow for therapeutic combinations of radiotherapy and immunotherapy.[29] This approach has been investigated with prostate cancer, using standard radiotherapy combined with gene therapy-based vaccine that encodes PSA.[30] Most of the PSA "vaccinated" patients developed increases in PSA-targeted T cells. Other related strategies have investigated different vaccines, intratumoral injection of immature dendritic cells, or adoptive immunotherapy via infusion with expanded tumor-infiltrating lymphocytes. These trials commonly demonstrate impressive induction of immune responses. As an example, metastatic melanoma or kidney cancers treated with high-dose IL-2 and stereotactic body radiotherapy showed impressive outcomes, compared with historical controls treated with high-dose IL-2 alone.[31] A related strategy involves combinations of radiotherapy with antagonists of cytotoxic T-lymphocyte-associated antigen 4 (CTLA-4) or programmed death 1 (PD-1), which are used by tumor cells to evade the immune system.[32]

Hyperthermia in combination with radiotherapy

Localized heat delivery can be administered to patients using external devises that produce microwave, ultrasound, or radiofrequency (RF) sources of energy. Lab-based experiments show that temperatures above 41°C kill cells, and that small increments above 42.5°C generate steep increases in lethality.[33] Heat-induced death is most pronounced when cells are in S-phase, which is consistent with the proposed mechanism involving the denaturation of proteins.[34] Combinations of hyperthermia and radiation generate a greater than additive lethal effect,[35] which may represent the denaturation of proteins required for radiation-induced DNA damage. This apparent synergy does not, however, translate to the clinical setting, where the two modalities appear to be only additive or independent. Several randomized clinical trials have tested combinations of radiation ± hyperthermia, and the results are conflicting. Additionally, a clinical limitation of hyperthermia is the technical difficulty of delivering homogenous doses of heat to deep-seated anatomic locations. As such, skin and breast cancers remain among the most common uses for this modality.

Protection of normal tissues from radiation injury

Acute side effects of radiotherapy in normal tissues are principally caused by damage to rapidly proliferating cell renewal systems, whereas late side effects are generally related to vascular damage, fibrosis, and poor repopulation of normal tissue components by healthy cells. Radiation also generates mutations that can induce secondary cancers, especially in the pediatric patient population. Therefore, efforts are underway to generate radioprotective drugs that minimize this problem. "Radioprotectors" are classified as drugs given prophylactically before radiation exposure, whereas radiation "mitigators" are administered during or after radiation exposure. Finally, "therapeutic agents" are a third class of drugs that modulate normal tissue healing after radiation exposure. The major challenge in generating such drugs is that they must not also protect tumor cells from radiation-induced death.[2] An exhaustive discussion of these novel drugs is not possible due to space limitations; however, some classes of agents are shown in Table 1. Sulfhydryl-containing compounds such as amifostine act as ROS-scavenging agents, thereby absorbing the ROS generated by radiation.[36] Amifostine is the only such drug to obtain FDA (Food and Drug Administration) approval, and it remains the best studied of this class.[37] Widespread use of amifostine has been limited due to fears that it protects tumors; however, there is little evidence suggesting that this occurs in clinically relevant situations.[38] More recent programs have focused on nonthiol agents, such as drugs that affect cell cycle distribution or radiation-induced apoptosis.[39–43] Finally, therapeutic agents are those that reduce endothelial cell damage, inflammatory cascades, and tissue ischemia.[44,45] Various growth factors have been used in this context to promote normal cell proliferation. One such example is keratinocyte growth factor (palifermin), which reduces mucositis during chemoradiotherapy for locally advanced head and neck cancer.[46]

Molecular classifiers capable of predicting radiotherapy outcomes

Genomic analysis methods are increasingly utilized to classify malignancies and to predict clinical outcomes, based on genetic and epigenetic tumor characteristics. This has helped fuel a vision of personalized medicine, wherein individualized treatment courses are tailored to specific molecularly defined patient and tumor characteristics. Our discussion herein will focus only on systems that predict responsiveness to radiotherapy. The radiosensitivity index (RSI) is one such method, which used the mRNA levels of 10 genes to predict radiosensitivity within a collection of human cancer cell lines.[47] It was been clinically validated in five independent clinical data sets, which include rectal, esophageal, head and neck, and breast cancers treated with chemoradiation or radiotherapy alone.[48] A competing method that we developed, called the interferon-related damage signature (IRDS), successfully predicted the efficacy of adjuvant chemotherapy and local–regional control after radiation.[49] Additionally, we recently reported a new method to quantify the efficiency of DNA repair pathways in the context of cancer therapy.[50] The recombination proficiency score (RPS) is calculated based on the expression levels for four genes involved in DNA repair pathway preference (Rif1, PARI, RAD51, and Ku80), such that high expression of these genes yields a low RPS. We validated the RPS system clinically in patients with breast and nonsmall-cell lung carcinomas (NSCLCs). Tumors with low RPS were associated with adverse features, suggesting that HR suppression contributes to the genomic instability that fuels malignant progression. This adverse prognosis associated with low RPS was diminished if NSCLC patients received adjuvant platinum-based chemotherapy, suggesting that HR suppression and associated sensitivity to platinum-based drugs counteract the adverse prognosis associated with low RPS. We are currently testing whether this system can similarly predict the radiosensitivity of tumors. An alternative approach for predicting radiosensitivity is to look for genetic alterations with comparative genomic hybridization arrays or next-generation sequencing,[51,52] which are rapidly evolving methods that will presumably revolutionize these types of approaches in coming years.

Physical and clinical aspects of modern radiotherapy

A large majority of radiation treatments consist of external-beam radiotherapy (XRT), which involves the use of a linear accelerator to generate high-energy (6–20 MV) photons. Less commonly, XRT consists of particle beams, comprised of electrons, protons, carbon ions, or neutrons. To accomplish treatment, patients are generally immobilized daily on a fixed treatment table, and beams are directed toward the patient's tumor from multiple angles. Each linear accelerator is attached to a "gantry," which can be rotated around the treatment table. As an alternative to XRT, treatment can also be delivered by placing radioactive sources proximal to tumors (termed brachytherapy). Using various combinations of these modalities, a wide array of radiotherapeutic approaches are possible (outlined in Table 2). In some circumstances, advanced specialized versions of these modalities can provide better therapeutic ratios. The ultimate selection of a particular modality depends on several factors, including predicted tumor radio-responsiveness, susceptibility of adjacent normal tissue to radiation injury, and nonradiotherapeutic alternatives for a given cancer type.

Table 2 Different classes of radiation therapy and clinical examples of their use.

	Fractionated XRT with photons 3D-CRT, IMRT	Ablative methods of XRT SRS, SBRT	XRT with particle beams Proton or carbon ion beam therapy	Brachytherapy Intracavitary or interstitial
Common indications	Many	Brain metastases Early-stage lung cancer Oligo-metastatic disease	Pediatric malignancies Uveal melanoma chordoma	Prostate cancer Cervical cancer
Illustrations	An anal cancer was treated with different types of X-ray-based XRT The yellow shaded area denotes the target volume, which includes the anus/rectum and the draining lymph nodes. The pelvic bones and bladder represent the adjacent normal tissues in this situation The IMRT-based plan conforms to the shape of the target more closely, thereby exposing less normal tissue to treatment 3D-CRT: 45 Gy at 1.8 Gy/fx IMRT: 45 Gy at 1.8 Gy/fx	These treatments involve specialized approaches that enable delivery of ablative doses, using a single or a few[1–5] large fractions Numerous intersecting beams chosen generate very conformal plans that markedly reduce normal tissue exposure SRS for brain metastasis: 18 Gy delivered in a single fraction SBRT for lung cancer: 12 Gy/fraction delivered over 5 fractions	Proton beam therapy generates specific dose distributions in tissue XRT is used to treat the craniospinal axis of a child with medulloblastoma. The proton-based treatment results in less exposure to normal tissues located anterior to the spinal column Photons protons Craniospinal radiation: 36 Gy at 1.8 Gy/fraction	Radioactive sources are positioned within or near a target volume. This limits exposure to surrounding tissue. This represent a common and effective treatment for prostate cancer, wherein permanent seeds placed from a perineal approach using real-time imaging via trans-rectal ultrasound A plain film X-ray shows small seeds throughout the prostate (contrast media fills the bladder) Implant dosimetry: 145 Gy
Distinguishing features	These treatments are among the most widely used forms of radiotherapy	Advanced targeting enables steep dose gradients, which allow for tolerance of large fraction sizes. This relies heavily on precise immobilization and imaging	Requires a specialized and expensive cyclotron facility. In some clinical settings, proton-based treatment may reduce toxic risks of XRT	Results in very low exposure to adjacent normal tissue. Anatomic barriers limit brachytherapy to only a small subset of cancer types

XRT, external beam radiotherapy; 3D-CRT, three-dimensional conformal radiotherapy; IMRT, intensity-modulated radiation therapy; SBRT, stereotactic body radiation therapy; SRS, stereotactic radiosurgery.

3D-conformal RT, intensity-modulated radiation therapy, and imaged-guided radiation therapy

In recent decades, the use of axial imaging coupled with three-dimensional (3D) treatment planning software has significantly improved the quality of radiotherapy. Additionally, the ability to shape radiation beams with automated devices has enabled many technologic advances. Beam shaping is now generally accomplished with multileaf collimators (MLCs), which are small metallic robotically controlled blocks located in the head of the linear accelerator. This hardware-based innovation combined with treatment optimizing software packages has yielded a process now generally referred to as three-dimensional conformal radiotherapy (3D-CRT). Dosimetrists, physicists, and physicians collaborate to generate optimized 3D-CRT treatment plans, such that plans are both conformal (i.e., high doses "wrap" closely around the target volume) and homogeneous (i.e., little dose variability occurs within the target). Compared to older methods, 3D-CRT allows for more effective coverage of tumors, while better protecting adjacent normal organs.

Intensity-modulated radiation therapy (IMRT) is another commonly utilized method of XRT. Like 3D-CRT, IMRT utilizes multiple intersecting X-ray beams to "cross-fire" a target volume. In IMRT, the intensity of each beam is modulated in a grid pattern to provide more conformal distributions of doses. IMRT planning software utilizes iterative algorithms to optimize treatment, based on user-defined goals of tumor coverage and normal tissue sparing. This high degree of conformality is particularly useful for treating irregularly shaped tumors that lie in close proximity to critical structures.[53] The widespread use of IMRT in recent years has simultaneously enabled dose escalation to tumors and reduced toxicity. For example, IMRT is standardly used in the organ-sparing treatment of head and neck cancers, thereby allowing for protection of salivary glands and a resulting reduction in xerostomia.[54] IMRT also enables the ability to differentially dose various parts of a tumor, using methods termed dose painting or simultaneous integrated boost.[55]

While these advances provide better radiotherapy plans, the actual treatment delivered to patients depends highly on the ability to reproducibly deliver the plan daily. Variability in daily patient positioning and internal organ motion (such as respiratory motion) can undermine the accuracy of this treatment delivery. Recent advancements termed image-guided radiation therapy (IGRT) have addressed these challenges. Linear accelerators are now commonly equipped with "onboard" imaging devices, which provide real-time (or nearly real time) diagnostic imaging with kilovolt X-rays or cone-beam CT (computed tomography) scans. In some situations, anatomic structures are implanted with radio-opaque "fiducial" markers used to fine-tune patient positioning.[56] Other commercially available packages can account for physiologic motion such as respiratory motion. As IGRT methods can reduce the magnitude of positioning setup error, they enable the use of smaller treatment volumes that require smaller margins to account for positional error.[2]

Ablative radiotherapy methods using large fraction sizes

These improvements in treatment accuracy have enabled a paradigm shift in recent years, favoring shorter treatment courses that utilize higher daily doses of radiation (termed hypofractionated RT). This reduction in overall treatment time offers predicted benefits, in part by counteracting the proliferation of tumor cell clones (termed accelerated repopulation) that occurs during prolonged courses of XRT.[57] Single-fraction stereotactic radiosurgery (SRS) represents an extreme version of hypofractionated RT used to ablate brain tumors.[58] Fractionated stereotactic body radiation therapy (SBRT) is a similar method for treating extra-cranial targets, and it typically consists of either a single dose or a small number of large-sized fractions.[59] SRS and SBRT both rely on the previously discussed methods for improved accuracy of radiation planning and delivery, which in turn enable the use of smaller target volumes. These modalities have proven safe and effective for select situations. For example, high local control rates with a single treatment of 20 Gy for small brain metastases, or 20 Gy × 3 for liver metastases, have been shown to result in local control rates of >80–85%. Early-stage NSCLCs can also be effectively treated with short courses (3–5 fractions of 12–20 Gy) of SBRT.[60] However, the best uses of SBRT remain to be completely defined. Multiple factors including tumor volume and the nature of adjacent normal tissue play critical roles in determining whether SBRT or fractionated XRT is most appropriate for a specific clinical situation.[61,62]

Brachytherapy

Brachytherapy is a method where radioactive sources are placed in close proximity to tumors. This can potentially outperform external beam RT for specific clinical situations. By varying the strength, location, and exposure time of the radioactive sources, it is possible to achieve highly conformal and dose-intense radiation distributions within tumors. Simultaneously, this can result in relatively low exposures to adjacent normal organs. Radioactive source placement can be interstitial, such that "seeds" are placed directly into the target tissue. Alternatively, sources can be placed in a cavity (e.g., a body cavity or lumen) that is adjacent to target tissue (termed intracavitary brachytherapy). In some situations, brachytherapy offers major dosimetric advantages. However, brachytherapy is not used as commonly as XRT because only a few clinical situations exhibit a well-defined target anatomy that can be safely accessed with radioactive sources. Given this practical limitation, cancers of the cervix, prostate, breast, and skin are the most common sites treated with brachytherapy. In prostate cancer, for example, brachytherapy may be superior to dose-escalated XRT for select clinical situations.[63] However, many anatomic locations are less well suited for brachytherapy because the therapeutic ratio for XRT exceeds that of brachytherapy. Additionally, brachytherapy carries potential risk for increased morbidity if sources are misplaced or migrate after placement.[64]

Particle beam therapy

Particle therapy is a form of XRT in which beams of particles are delivered rather than photons, and this can consist of electrons, protons, carbon ions, or neutrons.[65] The use of proton beam therapy in particular has grown in recent years and deserves special attention. As proton beams pass through tissue, most of their energy is deposited immediately before the particle comes to rest.

This deposition occurs at a specific depth in tissue (termed the Bragg peak), which can be manipulated by varying the energy of the photon beam. The clinical implication is that proton beams can be used to minimize radiation exposure to normal tissues situated adjacent to the target volume, especially for tissues situated more deeply than the tumor. In some situations this can translate to reduced treatment complications, so proton use has rapidly grown in pediatric diseases—particularly in pediatric brain tumors, where reductions in normal brain exposure can reduce neurocognitive sequela of XRT. Moreover, tumors located near the spine, such as chordomas or para-spinal chondrosarcomas, represent a well-defined indication for proton beam therapy, as it allows these relatively radioresistant tumors to be aggressively treated while respecting the radiation tolerance of the surrounding normal tissues.[66]

Some types of particle beams also generate relative biologic effectiveness (RBE) per unit of energy deposited. For example, the RBE of protons is 1–1.2 times that of photons, whereas for neutrons or carbon ions, the RBE can be 4–10 times that of photons. Further research is necessary to determine whether these RBE differences will translate into better, or possibly worse, therapeutic indices relative to photon-based therapy. As a practical issue, the facilities that generate proton or carbon ion beams are expensive to build, and they require significantly more physical space and highly trained staff.

Conclusions and future directions in radiotherapy

In recent decades, we have witnessed massive technologic changes that have influenced how radiotherapy is delivered to cancer patients. Simultaneously, there has been major growth in our understanding of the basic biology that governs radiation effects in human cells and tissues. However several unmet challenges continue to limit the impact of radiotherapy, and these remaining hurdles should be factors that guide the development of our field in the coming decades.[2] One such issue is that inherent cellular radioresistance still prevents local control in many tumor types. In tumors such as glioblastoma, for example, the probability of local tumor control remains miserably poor, despite the use of advanced radiotherapy technologies and very high doses of radiotherapy. Avenues to overcome this resistance will require continued growth in our understanding of the underlying biological problems. We will also need a better arsenal of drugs that can specifically sensitize tumor cells or protect normal tissues. Finally, more individualized approaches will be needed in future radiotherapy. Currently, the decision to deliver radiation and the key parameters of radiation (e.g., dose and volume) are standardized based on the stage of disease at presentation. As molecular predictors of radiation sensitivity become more accurate and accessible in the community setting, more personalized information can be used to guide management based on patients' individual biology.

Key references

The complete reference list can be found on the Wiley Companion Digital Edition of this title (see inside front cover for login instructions).

1 Connell PP, Hellman S. Advances in radiotherapy and implications for the next century: a historical perspective. *Cancer Res.* 2009;**69**(**2**):383–392.

2 Liauw SL, Connell PP, Weichselbaum RR. New paradigms and future challenges in radiation oncology: an update of biological targets and technology. *Sci Transl Med.* 2013;**5**(**173**):173sr2.

4 Thompson LH, Schild D. Recombinational DNA repair and human disease. *Mutat Res.* 2002;**509**(1–2):49–78.

6 Eriksson D, Stigbrand T. Radiation-induced cell death mechanisms. *Tumour Biol.* 2010;**31**(4):363–372.

8 Dent P, Yacoub A, Contessa J, et al. Stress and radiation-induced activation of multiple intracellular signaling pathways. *Radiat Res.* 2003;**159**(3):283–300.

10 Kolesnick R, Fuks Z. Radiation and ceramide-induced apoptosis. *Oncogene.* 2003;**22**(37):5897–5906.

15 Bao S, Wu Q, McLendon RE, et al. Glioma stem cells promote radioresistance by preferential activation of the DNA damage response. *Nature.* 2006;**444**(7120):756–760.

17 Al-Assar O, Mantoni T, Lunardi S, Kingham G, Helleday T, Brunner TB. Breast cancer stem-like cells show dominant homologous recombination due to a larger S-G2 fraction. *Cancer Biol Ther.* 2011;**11**(12):1028–1035.

20 Hallahan DE, Mauceri HJ, Seung LP, et al. Spatial and temporal control of gene therapy using ionizing radiation. *Nat Med.* 1995;**1**(8):786–791.

21 Weichselbaum RR, Kufe D. Translation of the radio- and chemo-inducible TNFerade vector to the treatment of human cancers. *Cancer Gene Ther.* 2009;**16**(8):609–619.

22 Herman JM, Wild AT, Wang H, et al. Randomized phase III multi-institutional study of TNFerade biologic with fluorouracil and radiotherapy for locally advanced pancreatic cancer: final results. *J Clin Oncol.* 2013;**31**(7):886–894.

29 Kamrava M, Bernstein MB, Camphausen K, Hodge JW. Combining radiation, immunotherapy, and antiangiogenesis agents in the management of cancer: the Three Musketeers or just another quixotic combination? *Mol Biosyst.* 2009;**5**(11):1262–1270.

31 Seung SK, Curti BD, Crittenden M, et al. Phase 1 study of stereotactic body radiotherapy and interleukin-2—tumor and immunological responses. *Sci Transl Med.* 2012;**4**(137):137ra74.

33 Dewey WC, Hopwood LE, Sapareto SA, Gerweck LE. Cellular responses to combinations of hyperthermia and radiation. *Radiology.* 1977;**123**(2):463–474.

35 Sapareto SA, Hopwood LE, Dewey WC. Combined effects of X irradiation and hyperthermia on CHO cells for various temperatures and orders of application. *Radiat Res.* 1978;**73**(2):221–233.

36 Yuhas JM, Yurconic M, Kligerman MM, West G, Peterson DF. Combined use of radioprotective and radiosensitizing drugs in experimental radiotherapy. *Radiat Res.* 1977;**70**(2):433–443.

37 Brizel DM, Wasserman TH, Henke M, et al. Phase III randomized trial of amifostine as a radioprotector in head and neck cancer. *J Clin Oncol.* 2000;**18**(19):3339–3345.

46 Le QT, Kim HE, Schneider CJ, et al. Palifermin reduces severe mucositis in definitive chemoradiotherapy of locally advanced head and neck cancer: a randomized, placebo-controlled study. *J Clin Oncol.* 2011;**29**(20):2808–2814.

49 Weichselbaum RR, Ishwaran H, Yoon T, et al. An interferon-related gene signature for DNA damage resistance is a predictive marker for chemotherapy and radiation for breast cancer. *Proc Natl Acad Sci U S A.* 2008;**105**(47):18490–18495.

50 Pitroda SP, Pashtan IM, Logan HL, et al. DNA repair pathway gene expression score correlates with repair proficiency and tumor sensitivity to chemotherapy. *Sci Transl Med.* 2014;**6**(229):229ra42.

53 Bortfeld T. IMRT: a review and preview. *Phys Med Biol.* 2006;**51**(13):R363–R379.

54 Lin A, Kim HM, Terrell JE, Dawson LA, Ship JA, Eisbruch A. Quality of life after parotid-sparing IMRT for head-and-neck cancer: a prospective longitudinal study. *Int J Radiat Oncol Biol Phys.* 2003;**57**(1):61–70.

55 de Arruda FF, Puri DR, Zhung J, et al. Intensity-modulated radiation therapy for the treatment of oropharyngeal carcinoma: the Memorial Sloan-Kettering Cancer Center experience. *Int J Radiat Oncol Biol Phys.* 2006;**64**(2):363–373.

56 Shirato H, Harada T, Harabayashi T, et al. Feasibility of insertion/implantation of 2.0-mm-diameter gold internal fiducial markers for precise setup and real-time tumor tracking in radiotherapy. *Int J Radiat Oncol Biol Phys.* 2003;**56**(1):240–247.

57 Schmidt-Ullrich RK, Contessa JN, Dent P, et al. Molecular mechanisms of radiation-induced accelerated repopulation. *Radiat Oncol Investig.* 1999;**7**(6):321–330.

58 Leksell L. The stereotaxic method and radiosurgery of the brain. *Acta Chir Scand.* 1951;**102**(4):316–319.

59 Potters L, Kavanagh B, Galvin JM, et al. American Society for Therapeutic Radiology and Oncology (ASTRO) and American College of Radiology (ACR) practice guideline for the performance of stereotactic body radiation therapy. *Int J Radiat Oncol Biol Phys.* 2010;**76**(2):326–332.

60 Grills IS, Mangona VS, Welsh R, et al. Outcomes after stereotactic lung radiotherapy or wedge resection for stage I non-small-cell lung cancer. *J Clin Oncol.* 2010;**28**(6):928–935.

61 Hoyer M, Roed H, Sengelov L, et al. Phase-II study on stereotactic radiotherapy of locally advanced pancreatic carcinoma. *Radiother Oncol.* 2005;**76**(1):48–53.

62 Timmerman R, McGarry R, Yiannoutsos C, et al. Excessive toxicity when treating central tumors in a phase II study of stereotactic body radiation therapy for medically inoperable early-stage lung cancer. *J Clin Oncol.* 2006;**24**(30):4833–4839.

63 Jabbari S, Weinberg VK, Shinohara K, et al. Equivalent biochemical control and improved prostate-specific antigen nadir after permanent prostate seed implant brachytherapy versus high-dose three-dimensional conformal radiotherapy and high-dose conformal proton beam radiotherapy boost. *Int J Radiat Oncol Biol Phys.* 2010;**76**(1):36–42.

64 Bogdanich W. *At V.A. Hospital, a Rogue Cancer Unit.* 2009, New York City: The New York Times; June 20 [cited 2012 September 29], http://www.nytimes.com/2009/06/21/health/21radiation.html?_r=0. (accessed 12 October 2015)

65 Durante M, Loeffler JS. Charged particles in radiation oncology. *Nat Rev Clin Oncol.* 2010;**7**(1):37–43.

66 Schulz-Ertner D, Tsujii H. Particle radiation therapy using proton and heavier ion beams. *J Clin Oncol.* 2007;**25**(8):953–964.

45 Principles of medical oncology

William N. Hait, MD, PhD ▪ James F. Holland, MD, ScD (hc) ▪ Emil Frei III, MD (deceased) ▪ Donald W. Kufe, MD ▪ Robert C. Bast Jr., MD ▪ Waun Ki Hong, MD, DMSc (Hon)

Overview

The practice of medical oncology is evolving more rapidly than any field in medicine. The uncovering of the molecular basis of the numerous malignancies and their subtypes created a seemingly bewildering collection of new information that confronts the practicing physician. Since the principles that underlie the practice of this subspecialty, by definition, should remain constant, they can provide the scaffolding on which new information can be attached. To that end, this chapter attempts to define those immutable areas that apply to the care of the oncology patient, and through their understanding the massive amount of new information presented in this text can be organized.

Medical oncology evolved from a subspecialty of internal medicine whose hallmark was the ability to diagnose cancer and to safely administer dangerous drugs to the branch of medicine most directly linked to modern molecular biology; today, it heralds in the era of personalized medicine. A medical oncologist understands the biologic basis of malignant transformation and applies this knowledge to the prevention, early detection, and treatment of cancer patients. An individual with cancer should be viewed in the context of the etiology, pathogenesis, pathology, genetics, immunology, and biochemistry of the neoplastic process and humanistically as a person struggling with a terrifying disease.

Training of medical oncologists originated in cancer institutes, divisions of hematology, and departments of pharmacology. The American Board of Internal Medicine established the subspecialty as a separate discipline in 1971.[1] Medical oncologists and hematologists have overlapping interests in neoplastic diseases of the hematopoietic tissues and share historic interests in training subspecialists in both fields. However, because each discipline became more complex, individual training programs have become the preferred approach.

In this chapter, we introduce the subspecialty by attempting to define a set of principles that underlie the practice of medical oncology.

Principles

Certain principles underlie the practice of medical oncology and are listed in Table 1. These tenets, although not mathematically derived or subject to rigorous validation, should nonetheless serve the purpose of providing both the uninitiated young practitioner and the seasoned veteran with a perspective gleaned from the several vantage points of the authors.

The treatment of cancer is multidisciplinary, requiring consultation with knowledgeable colleagues in related subspecialties

The practice of medical oncology is dependent on highly productive interactions with cognate disciplines, particularly surgical oncology, radiation oncology, urology, orthopedic surgery, radiology, and pathology. Multiple other interactions occur with nursing oncology, psycho-oncology, neuro-oncology, gynecologic oncology, rehabilitation medicine, and, for young patients, pediatric oncology. Infectious diseases and more recently autoimmune diseases are common complications of cancers and their treatments, forming a natural alliance with specialists in infectious diseases and rheumatology. Today, with the gratifying number of long-term survivors, the medical oncologist must work closely with primary care physicians for follow-up surveillance and psychologists and psychiatrists, who may be required to address the existential complexities of survivorship and the sequelae of treatment.

The medical oncologist is often involved in the final decisions concerning management and is frequently the final common pathway through which decisions are implemented. The timing of surgery and radiotherapy, the decision whether to take a curative or a palliative approach, and the decision whether watchful waiting is the appropriate course, or whether vigorous action is necessary are often entrusted to the medical oncologist.

Most patients have a relationship with other physicians before being diagnosed with cancer; a family physician or internist who referred the patient to a medical oncologist and other specialists may already have been involved with the patient before the recognition of a neoplastic disease. Medical oncologists must recognize their interest and continuing role in the management of patients with multisystem disease and communicate with them effectively. In the absence of such consultants, however, the medical oncologist must also attend to all aspects of internal medicine. This book contains detailed descriptions of various diseases; the modalities used in their treatment; the pharmacologic, immunologic, neurologic, psychological, biochemical, epidemiologic, and the modern emphasis on molecular biologic aspects of cancers; and the complications that cancers cause. Oncologic emergencies, rehabilitation, and the oncologist's relationship to medical informatics and to government are also presented. Familiarity with these topics constitutes a foundation for medical oncology from which the principles derive.

The suspicion of cancer is based on clinical acumen; the diagnosis on examination of tissue

Oncologists must be highly competent internists to diagnose, exclude, and treat cancer. Many diseases can mimic the signs and symptoms of cancer, but the medical oncologist must not miss a nonmalignant cause. Conversely, the internist and the medical

Holland-Frei Cancer Medicine, Ninth Edition. Edited by Robert C. Bast Jr., Carlo M. Croce, William N. Hait, Waun Ki Hong, Donald W. Kufe, Martine Piccart-Gebhart, Raphael E. Pollock, Ralph R. Weichselbaum, Hongyang Wang, and James F. Holland.
© 2017 John Wiley & Sons, Inc. ISBN: 978-1-118-93469-2

Table 1 Principles of medical oncology .

The treatment of cancer is multidisciplinary, requiring consultation with knowledgeable colleagues in related subspecialties
The suspicion of cancer is based on clinical acumen and the diagnosis on examination of tissue
Prevention is more effective than treatment
The medical treatment of cancer patients is based on a clear understanding of the mechanism of drug action, potential for harmful side effects, mechanisms of drug resistance, and the principles of therapeutics
Early stage cancers are more curable than late-stage cancers; the first treatment is more effective than the next
The best treatment is often found through participation in clinical trials
Cancer surveillance must be based on validated assumptions
Oncologic care is for life

oncologist must remember that cancer, like syphilis in the past, is the "great masquerader" and, thus, must be considered in every differential diagnosis.[2] A medical oncologist must understand the pathophysiology of cancer, the genetic predispositions, the existence of molecular subtypes, and the basic pharmacology that is the bedrock of effective cancer treatment. All cancers are not the same, and all patients with a given type of cancer do not behave in a similar manner. Increasingly, cancers are being segmented into a variety of distinct molecular entities, each with subtle and not so subtle differences in prognosis and treatment. As the more precise classification of leukemias and lymphomas led to improvements in treatment in the past, the use of powerful diagnostic tests is identifying subsets of solid tumors that respond differently to treatment are leading to improvements in treatment today.

When new syndromes appear in a patient who once had cancer, such as pulmonary insufficiency, meningoencephalopathy, or inexplicable pain, it is indispensable to establish by objective criteria that cancer is the proximate cause. Cancer patients are not protected from other symptomatic noncancerous diseases, such as pulmonary fibrosis and central nervous system disorders, or painful conditions, such as a herniated disk. No symptom should be attributed to cancer without persuasive evidence. Yet cancer must be suspected every time.

To ascribe a finding to cancer requires proof. Modern medical oncologists will need to both understand the histologic appearance of malignant and premalignant lesions and be able to understand the interpretation of complex profiles of nucleic acid sequences (DNA and RNA), gene transcription and protein translation, as well as chromosomal abnormalities to properly diagnose and manage their patients. These advances will lead to an even greater number of individuals who know that they are at risk of developing cancer, living with a diagnosis of cancer, or putatively cured of cancer but are concerned about recurrence due to the presence of minimal residual disease. It is an exceptional case when a medical oncologist can consider treatment without a firm diagnosis. Certain oncologic emergencies, such as spinal cord compression or superior vena cava syndrome, were once considered exceptions, but with modern imaging and biopsy techniques, a tissue diagnosis can usually be made rapidly and safely. Cytologic diagnoses may provide sufficient information in the presence of unambiguous clinical syndromes, but cytology of the bronchus, stomach, cervix, and body fluids has produced sufficient numbers of false-positive identifications to show that corroborating evidence is essential. The use of circulating tumor cells and free tumor DNA can aid in diagnosis and monitoring of patients, but as yet these surrogates have not been fully validated. Highly specific biochemical and molecular markers may be helpful when clinical and radiologic findings are characteristic and when a major intracavitary (cranial, thoracic, or abdominal) biopsy procedure would constitute an ominously serious event for a

particular patient. It is always preferable to have histologic evidence whenever possible.

The management of cancer patients requires an understanding of the genetics, biology, and pharmacology of neoplasia and the psychosocial impact of a cancer predisposition or diagnosis on patient and physician

The practice of medical oncology requires wisdom, sensitivity, and resourcefulness. For the patient in whom relatively asymptomatic findings lead to a diagnosis of cancer, it is useful to consider that the day before the discovery, the patient was living with cancer. It is a source of some encouragement to patients to know that a diagnosis of cancer does not lead immediately or inevitably to death. The medical oncologist may be able to stress the long-term evolution of a cancer, the several stages that intervene between the carcinogenic stimulus, genetic mutations, selection of cells with a survival advantage, and the appearance of an autonomous neoplasm. Because this process usually takes years and often decades, it is of value to place the neoplastic process in perspective (vide infra). This is particularly important when a patient is being urged to make an immediate decision regarding surgery, radiation, or chemotherapy. When one considers that, on average, it will take more than 5 years for a malignant cell to undergo the requisite 30 doublings to achieve a 1 cm mass (one billion cells) required for most diagnoses, an additional week or two to gather information and opinions is unlikely to have a negative impact on the ultimate course of the disease. In contrast, the situation with certain malignancies such as acute myelogenous leukemia requires immediate action as the diagnosis is made when the near-fatal 10^{12} malignant cells exist.

Increasingly, individuals are recognized to harbor genetic predispositions to cancer owing to subtle genomic and epigenomic alterations. The oncologist must combine an understanding of the impact of these changes on the probability of being diagnosed with cancer and weigh the risks and benefits of medical intervention while being sensitive to the emotional impact that this knowledge has on individuals and their families. In some, cancer or the prevention of cancer may become a chronic process requiring ongoing treatment analogous to the management of diabetes or hypertension. Similarly, oncologists must recognize environmental exposures that increase the risk of cancer and attempt intervention to mitigate that risk.

The medical oncologist must distinguish between a neoplasm in which a chance for cure exists versus one that is currently incurable (precurable). Most cancers are curable if detected early, and most cancers are incurable if detected late. Whereas the former is likely to be driven by few genomic alterations and confined to one or two critical pathways, the latter is likely to harbor multiple changes in several pathways that make successful treatment less likely. The medical oncologist must therefore appreciate the importance of prevention, screening, and early detection and must actively educate colleagues and patients.

Advances in our understanding of cancer biology encourage the belief that one day all cancers will be prevented or cured. It is axiomatic that the day before the first metastatic choriocarcinoma was cured with high-dose methotrexate,[3,4] metastatic cancer, in general, was considered incurable by most observers. Similar considerations apply to every neoplastic disease that is now curable (Table 2). Other neoplasms are currently not cured by medicines alone but require participation of surgery or radiotherapy as an intrinsic part of the therapeutic process (Table 3).

Patients are often influenced by their present state of subjective well-being. It is the responsibility of an oncologist to recognize the

Table 2 Cancers curable with chemotherapy.

Choriocarcinoma
Acute lymphocytic leukemia of childhood
Burkitt's lymphoma
Hodgkin's disease
Acute promyelocytic leukemia
Large follicular center cell lymphoma
Embryonal carcinoma of testis
Hairy cell leukemia

Table 3 Cancers subcurable with chemotherapy[a]

With regional therapy
Wilms' tumor
Osteosarcoma
Ewing's sarcoma
Embryonal rhabdomyosarcoma
Adenocarcinoma of breast
Small cell carcinoma of lung
Squamous cell carcinoma of upper aerodigestive tract[b]
Adenocarcinoma of ovary
Thymoma without regional therapy
Acute lymphocytic leukemia of adulthood
Acute myeloid leukemia
Lymphomas, some subsets

[a] By definition, <50% curable with chemotherapy alone; cure rates obtained with chemotherapy plus regional therapy are significantly superior to those with regional therapy alone (i.e., chemotherapeutic cure of micrometastatic disease only).

[b] Cure rates <50% in most series.

often pernicious behavior of cancer in its potential for recurrence and metastasis. In this context, the medical oncologist must interact directly with the patient and family, as well as with the medical record, films, slides, and other critical raw data. It is important to understand how patients make choices so as to present information in a way that does not bias an eventual decision. In addition, there is an opportunity to alter behaviors of patients and their families at the time of a cancer evaluation.[5] For example, following a "scare" that a lung nodule could have been malignant may be the best time to treat nicotine addiction in the patient and in members of the family. The diagnosis of cancer constitutes a serious emotional burden that may distort ordinary reason. By firsthand intimacy with the diagnosis, the extent of the disease, and the patient's attitudes and infirmities, the medical oncologist can make rational recommendations to the patient and to the other physicians involved.

Explanations of disease, anticipated therapies, randomized protocols, and unknowns must be tailored to the intellectual and emotional levels of the particular patient. It is never permissible to lie, but it may be prudent not to deposit all of the truth at once on a patient who cannot accept the full details and ramifications of diagnosis and management. "Your patient has no more right to all the truth you know than to all the medicine in your saddle-bags" was a humane and ethical tenet advanced by Oliver Wendell Holmes more than a century ago.[6] It is dishonest to twist facts or to deny specific features, such as the existence of metastases. It is also wrong to deny a patient an opportunity to make final dispositions with respect to self, family, religion, the law, and business by falsely stating that a disease is benign or cured. Families who assert that the patient must not know because the patient could not stand it are usually twice wrong: the patient often knows already or may be more distraught by being excluded from knowing, and the patient ordinarily incorporates the information into his or her life equation indistinguishably

from other patients. A reading of Tolstoy's masterful *The Death of Ivan Ilyich* should convince any doubting oncologist about the terror of uncertainty and the value of direct and honest, yet humane, interactions with the patient. When a patient asks, "There is hope, isn't there?" the oncologist can always be positive. Hope is a uniquely human characteristic that sustains the will to continue, and all oncologists and all patients do hope for a better outcome.

The treatment of patients with life-threatening disease can take its toll on providers of care. A sense of frustration can affect anyone who encounters barriers to successful completion of an important task. This is particularly true of intellectual tasks and invisible barriers. When the barrier is a lethal disease about which the oncologist can do little that is effective, the frustration can be all consuming. Oncologists who encounter several instances of recrudescent or refractory disease in a short time (especially if punctuated by the deaths of young or favorite patients, uninterrupted by counterbalancing compensatory successes) may well experience frustration, a sense of inadequacy, and depression. Frequent repetition of this cyclic phenomenon may lead to burnout.

The medical oncologist knows that many of today's cancers are not yet curable. To the extent that the medical oncologist can be involved, actually and conceptually, in the solution to these complex mysteries, the frustration is lessened. Cancer research, whether at the basic or the clinical level, is held in high esteem by our fellow citizens. Group identity, "being one of the team," helps offset the self-deprecation when human tragedies mount despite one's best efforts. The camaraderie of other oncologists helps because they battle the same enemy with the same primitive weapons. Another oncologist can understand the trauma and the distress; it is an encounter on familiar terrain.

The appreciation that the horizon is distant, and that oncologists are all working intently to see beyond it, puts present frustration in a more appropriate perspective. Involvement in the systematized academic pursuit, whether in an academic setting, a medical school outreach, an oncology society, or a local collaborative group, provides the security of collegial support. A sound mind in a sound body implies rest, exercise, nutrition, and enjoyment. To ensure the last, the first three are prerequisites. Avocation and vacation are a portion of good mental health, included in the terms rest and exercise.

Finally, all oncologists can benefit from the vast array of continuing medical education programs given at academic medical centers, on the World Wide Web, at national meetings such as the American Association for Cancer Research and the American Society of Clinical Oncology, the American Society of Hematology, and through textbooks such as *Cancer Medicine*.

Prevention is more effective than treatment

The seminal work of Dr. Bert Vogelstein of John Hopkins Medical School demonstrated that as a normal epithelium transforms through dysplasia, anaplasia, and, eventually, neoplasia, that there is a progressive increase in genomic alterations, a process that may take many years.[7] Similarly, as chronic myelogenous leukemia progresses from the chronic phase, through the accelerated phase to blast crisis, more chromosomal and genetic abnormalities are acquired. Exposure to environmental carcinogens, most commonly through tobacco use owing to nicotine addiction, accelerates the oncogenic process most prominently in the bronchial mucosa. These nucleic acid changes can activate complex signaling pathways that favor cell viability and inactivate pathways that normally balance uncontrolled growth through mechanisms of cell death. Not surprisingly, many of these molecular changes impart resistance to cancer treatment. It follows that the earlier a cancer is diagnosed and treated, the more effective the treatment. Furthermore, the oncogenic process provides substantial time for interventions that could prevent the formation of cancer in susceptible individuals, so-called disease interception.

Inhibition of cyclooxygenases within the intestinal epithelium with nonsteroidal anti-inflammatory drugs prevented many cases of colorectal cancer.[8,9] Hepatitis B vaccines dramatically reduced the incidence of hepatoma, once the Eastern world's most common malignancy, by preventing the chronic inflammation and cellular damage produced by chronic hepatitis.[10] New curative treatments for hepatitis C should also decrease the burden of hepatocellular carcinoma.[11] Retinoic acid can decrease the appearance of second malignancies in heavy smokers[12]; tamoxifen and raloxifene can prevent breast cancer in patients at substantial risk.[13] Minor surgical interventions, such as colonic polypectomy[14] and loop electrosurgical procedure for carcinoma in situ of the cervix,[15] can prevent colon and cervical cancer, respectively.

Increasingly, the medical oncologist will be called on to decide whether medical or surgical prevention is indicated in individuals without cancer but for whom cancer is a significant risk. This will ultimately extend to subtle genetic abnormalities, such as single nucleotide polymorphisms and circulating biomarkers. In addition, the use of preventive drugs will require long-term monitoring if used each day for years. Currently, the medical oncologist is asked to decide who should receive tamoxifen for prevention of breast cancer, retinoids for prevention of head and neck cancer, and oral contraceptives for prevention of ovarian cancer. Medical oncologists frequently advise patients regarding the benefits of prophylactic oophorectomy and mastectomy in patients with *BRCA1* and *BRCA2* mutations. Similarly, oncologists must be aware that the hepatitis B vaccine will prevent hepatoma, and a vaccine against human papillomavirus will prevent many cases of cancer of the uterine cervix.[16] The oncologist must take a leading role in treating addiction to nicotine in all of its manifestations and must educate physicians and the public on the importance of early detection through appropriate screening.

Medical oncologists should counsel patients and families about good nutrition and healthy sexual practices as well as screening tests available for some cancer types. Several chapters of this treatise deal with prevention and early detection, and numerous publications that deal with these topics are available for distribution to patients and families from the National Cancer Institute (NCI) and the American Cancer Society (ACS). The NCI Cancer Information Service (800-4-CANCER) and the ACS National Cancer Information Center (800-ACS-2345) will send available publications free of charge and publish this information on their web sites.

Cancer therapeutics is evolving

The origins of cancer chemotherapy began with the observation that mustard derivatives such as mechlorethamine could treat patients with lymphoma, evolved through targeting biochemical pathways involved in DNA synthesis (antimetabolites) and microtubule function (vinca alkaloids and taxanes), through combination chemotherapy to the era of targeted therapies. These new medications are likely to be less toxic than traditional cancer chemotherapy drugs that most commonly target DNA or microtubules. The proper use of the new-targeted therapies will require an understanding of the molecular pathways responsible for malignancy in general and possibly in each individual's tumor. Recent examples include imatinib to inhibit the transforming oncogenic protein in chronic-phase chronic myelogenous leukemia (*Bcr-Abl*)[17]; gefitinib

to effectively treat patients with nonsmall cell lung cancer by targeting those individuals whose tumors harbor activating mutations in the epidermal growth factor receptor (EGFR)[18]; erlotinib to extend survival in patients with nonsmall cell lung cancer[19]; trastuzumab to treat metastatic breast cancer in patients whose cancers have amplification of the HER2/neu oncogene[20]; cetuximab to treat colorectal cancers by targeting the EGFR[21]; bevacizumab to treat colorectal cancer by targeting the vascular endothelial growth factor receptor and blocking angiogenesis,[22] and venurafinib to inhibit mutant bRAF in patients with melanoma.[23]

Today, we are in the modern era of immuno-oncology, which began with the pioneering work of Dr. Steve Rosenberg at the NCI who demonstrated that certain T-cell subsets could be harnessed to treat refractory melanoma and renal cell carcinoma.[24] Today, with the advent of immune check point inhibitors (e.g., ipilimumab), the medical oncologist is faced with a new set of therapeutic challenges based on autoimmune side effects that require additional skills to manage.

In addition, one must appreciate the importance of drug resistance and recognize it when it occurs. When choosing treatment for recurrent disease, one should consider the likely cross-resistance to several natural products owing to the multidrug resistance phenotype mediated by the adenosine triphosphate–binding cassette family transporters [(e.g., P-glycoprotein, MRPs (multidrug resistance proteins)], the low probability of response to drugs of the same drug class (e.g., taxanes), or sequential hormonal therapies when selecting drugs with the same mechanism of action (e.g., aromatase inhibitors). Furthermore, the medical oncologist be familiar with mutations within drug targets that lead to either sensitivity or resistance to a given class of drug, for example, EGFR inhibitors, bRAF inhibitors, abl inhibitors, and inhibitors of BTK (Bruton's tyrosine kinase) to name a few.

Treatment of cancer patients includes the use of drugs for host support. The effects of the tumor and its products on the structure and function of the patient's normal tissues, as well as the mind and emotions, define an understanding of the disease process and of the patient in whom it takes place. It is not sufficient to order a therapy with the appropriate dose and schedule. There must be a broad understanding of and attention to potential toxicities, which represent the drug's effects on normal tissues. A medical oncologist should understand the interaction of the administered drug with target molecules present in normal tissues and the potential for drug–drug interactions to avoid unnecessary toxicities.

The availability of effective antibiotics and the use of platelet transfusions were intrinsic to early cures of the acute leukemias. Colony-stimulating factors (filgrastim and sargramostim) have significantly altered the prospect of drug-induced granulocytopenia, and recombinant erythropoietin can diminish drug-induced anemia. Means to ameliorate thrombocytopenia, other than with platelet transfusions, are now available.

The use of cytokines to collect circulating hematopoietic progenitor (CD34) cells enabled the convenient collection of marrow-repopulating precursors, allowing autologous stem cell transfusions to substitute for autologous marrow transfusion. New antibiotics make granulocytopenia less ominous, and oral prophylaxis with antibiotics and antifungal agents has decreased hospital admissions. These assets allow chemotherapy to be given more safely at the intended dose and schedule without delay or dose reduction.

The availability of highly effective antiemetics makes cancer chemotherapy less dreaded than in the past. The emergence of psycho-oncology as a widely appreciated discipline has also made it possible for patients to strengthen their resolve to undertake approaches aimed at cure or to accept the unlikelihood of cure with greater serenity.

Intravenous medications that may be toxic to the venous wall, and vesicant if extravasated, require the use of central venous access. When venipuncture is difficult because of anatomy or obesity, repeated needle sticks and much time are wasted in attempting peripheral cannulation. Needle phobia is a perverse part of being under treatment; establishing permanent venous access can largely obviate it.

Most patients with cancer are over the age of 60 and are receiving treatment for comorbid conditions. Therefore, care must be taken when prescribing treatments that could have dire drug interactions, leading to untoward side effects. No modern physician should be without ready access to the Internet for a compendium of drug interactions, drug descriptions, and appropriate methods of monitoring for efficacy and toxicity. A medical oncologist benefits from using an electronic medical record system that saves time and prevents errors through online calculation of dosing and electronic ordering. These systems also allow the creation of databases that can be queried for identification of trends and unexpected results.

Therapies that are totally appropriate for someone whose disease might be cured by judicious application of surgery, radiotherapy, and/or chemotherapy might be totally inappropriate when applied to another person with widely metastatic disease for whom no known cure exists. Therapy with curative intent may be toxic but of relatively short duration. On the one hand, conservatism aims at saving a life, not avoiding toxicity; on the other hand, treatment for palliative purposes would not ordinarily condone similar risks and iatrogenic effects that diminish the quality of life, even temporarily. The same is true for therapies aimed at cancer prevention because these may be taken by asymptomatic individuals for prolonged periods of time. The recent experiences with high-dose cyclooxygenase II inhibitors over long periods, which caused increased cardiovascular side effects in patients participating in one of two cancer prevention studies, resulted in serious consequences for the pharmaceutical manufacturers.[25]

Certain principles govern the application of therapies, no matter what the disease. These were enunciated more than a half-century ago by Robert F. Loeb, Bard Professor of Medicine at Columbia University's College of Physicians and Surgeons. These simple rules have profundity and nearly universal applicability but must be tempered, however, by an understanding of the neoplastic process.

The first law is if what you are doing is "doing good," keep doing it. It is implicit that a physician measures the effects of any intervention on both the tumor and the host. However, the lessons learned from the treatment of acute lymphocytic leukemia of childhood are noteworthy. For example, vincristine plus prednisone is an excellent induction treatment, but in 1968, a question was raised: why not keep administering this highly active induction regimen rather than shifting to antimetabolite management? A cohort of children who were induced into remission by vincristine and prednisone were randomized to continue the induction treatment or shift to the antimetabolite. They rapidly became resistant and relapsed, whereas those who were shifted to the antimetabolite experienced long-term sustained remissions and cures (Cancer and Leukemia Group B, unpublished data). Thus, the first law of therapeutics does not always apply to cancer for which sequential treatment regimens may have special importance. Much of curative oncology relates to the biology of the unseen tumor (minimal residual disease), for which the current clinical status may not be informative. The first law seems more applicable to clinically recognizable disease.

The second law of therapeutics states that if what you are doing is not "doing good," stop doing it. Most therapeutic regimens have little chance of success if after 8 weeks of treatment they have failed to elicit therapeutic benefit. It is, nonetheless, advantageous to undertake a second month of treatment in most instances because a well-documented early increase in tumor diameter on radiographic examinations or increased pain can, indeed, be followed by tumor regression, notably for certain forms of hormonal therapy as well as immunotherapy. Before stopping treatment, corroborating information should be sought by direct measurements, biomarkers that include circulating tumor cells and circulating tumor DNA may aid in the decision to stop an ineffective treatment. Increased bony uptake of radionuclides can be a sign of bone healing, even of a previously unsuspected lesion, and is not a suitable end point. The appearance of a new metastatic deposit or the continued growth of a previously documented tumor despite treatment speaks against continuing that regimen.

Hippocrates' admonition, *Primum non nocere* (first do no harm), is also subject to careful cautious consideration in oncology.[26] Thus, the second law of therapeutics does not extend to toxic effects unless they are life-threatening or profoundly disabling. With many of the therapeutic agents available today, complete avoidance of toxicity would doom many patients to death from their neoplasm. Some patients can obtain cure, and more can achieve meaningful remission by accepting the transient effect of intensive therapy that kills tumor cells and normal cells alike. The patient almost always recovers, but the less resilient tumor may not. To treat a population of patients at so low a dose that it would avoid toxic harm to any patient would surely exact a higher price in depriving others of adequate doses to achieve maximum benefit. Curative and subcurative cancer chemotherapy as well as newer immunotherapies, as we know it today, are often toxic but rarely fatal. Attempts to abrogate toxicity for all by reducing the dose of an established regimen might compromise benefit for the majority.[27,28] Dose adjustment for an individual may be necessary and prudent but must always be considered with respect to other means of mitigating toxicity without dose reduction.

The third law of therapeutics—"if you do not know what to do, do nothing"—counsels against uninformed action. In many circumstances, a rush to judgment or, worse, a rush to do something, anything, can be disastrous. Aside from oncologic emergencies and certain forms of leukemia, there is rarely an occasion when observing the evolution of symptoms and findings or seeking consultation with another individual for a fresh viewpoint is contraindicated because of time pressure. In the presence of pain, one should not delay pain relief, but other therapy may be delayed to build an informed formulation. In the presence of a differential diagnosis that includes diseases other than cancer, particularly infections, one must be certain that delay does not risk mortality or morbidity from the other possible disorders. Thus, the time invested for observation and consultation should not be extravagant. In circumstances where the benefits of existing treatment are poor or unknown, clinical trials should be a first consideration.

The fourth law of therapeutics is "never make the treatment worse than the disease." This relates to total life equation: the price the oncologist knows the patient may be obliged to pay in present side effects to attain future real effects. Often, the patient's vision is foreshortened because today's symptoms caused by drug toxicity can be more severe than the original complaints related to the cancer. The medical oncologist must ascertain the patient's attitude toward quality of life versus duration of life. It is a medical oncologist's responsibility to counsel the patient concerning this weighty topic. With the rapid appearance of new oncology products and numerous new types of treatments available through clinical trials, it is becoming increasingly difficult to distinguish therapy with curative intent from a palliative orientation, except in the extreme situations of newly diagnosed, low-stage and grade disease versus palliative care for the terminally ill. In all cases, the proper goal is maximal life at maximal quality. For some patients, the toxic effects of treatment outweigh the value of possible extension of life. This perception is often related directly to age. Pain and disability from cancer may temper the desirability of certain therapies, which offer only temporary and partial relief. It is not a kindness to defer death only transiently by rescuing a dying patient back to a raft of suffering. Heroic efforts are justified only when a meaningful therapeutic option exists.

It is inappropriate for the medical oncologist to substitute professional judgment for a patient's ardent wishes when the patient strives to accomplish something that is a reasonable therapeutic goal. The medical oncologist must serve as a bastion of reality, however, advising the patient of what is possible and of what is likely. In the course of doing this, the laws of therapeutics and of humanity always include hope.

Finally, the medical oncologist must remember that patients do not fail treatments; rather, treatments fail patients. The careless use of the former, inadvertently implies a disrespect for the patient and a lack understanding of the extremely fragile state of patients whose disease is unresponsive to treatment.

Early stage cancers are more curable than late-stage cancers; the first treatment is more effective than the next

As no method of prevention is likely to be completely effective, medical oncologists must recommend appropriate tests to detect cancer at its earliest possible stage. They include mammography, colonoscopy, occult blood in the feces, digital rectal examination of the prostate, Papanicolaou smears, and examination of the skin and body orifices for signs of premalignancy, such as leukoplakia and dysplastic nevi. Soon, a variety of validated biomarkers will likely be available to identify early cancer or the presence of premalignancies, for example, ductal carcinoma *in situ*, prostatic intraepithelial neoplasia, colonic polyps, and cervical dysplasia. As described earlier, progression of cancer leads to the acquisition of changes in the host and the cancer genome that select for cell survival over cell death. Many of these changes allow tumor cells to exist in harsh environments characterized by hypoxia and a low pH. These same changes produce tumor cells that are increasingly resistant to cancer therapies.

Cancer cells that emerge following initial treatment often represent clones of cells with intrinsic resistance or cells in which the treatment has selected for drug resistance mechanisms. For example, treatment of patients with adenocarcinoma of the lung who progress after initial response to inhibitors of EGFR may acquire a mutation that renders these kinase inhibitors ineffective.[29] This reality places a premium on getting it right the first time so that medical oncologists and their team must be certain that they have all of the requisite information at hand to allow the best choice for initial treatment. For example, treating a breast cancer patient without knowledge of the status of estrogen and progesterone receptors and the *HER2/neu* oncogene correctly measured, or subtyping nonsmall cell lung cancers in terms of EGFR, alk, and other genomic alterations would likely compromise initial treatment. Similarly, embarking on the treatment of acute myelogenous leukemia without full genotyping and phenotyping risks making the wrong choice for initial treatment. Furthermore, resistance to imatinib is associated with both P-glycoprotein and specific mutations in the *BCR*:*ABL* gene. These changes are defined, and new drugs are available to overcome these forms of resistance.

Finally, the proper approach to patients with lung cancer and melanoma requires molecular characterization to select the proper treatment.

The advantage of treating early stage patients has proved so persuasive that the profession and patients have accepted the technique of postsurgical or adjuvant chemotherapy, acknowledging that this entails treating some if not the majority of patients whose risk of relapse is already zero. Adjuvant therapy after surgery has been demonstrated to be curative in several diseases for which surgery alone has low cure rates and where chemotherapy alone cannot cure metastatic disease. Breast cancer, Wilms tumor, and osteosarcoma are the prime examples. In many diseases, there is evidence of prolonged disease-free survival and of longer survival, such as stage II and III breast cancer,[30,31] stage III ovarian cancer,[32] and stage III colon cancer.[33] Recent evidence suggests that transcriptional profiling of breast cancer specimens may help identify patients for whom adjuvant therapy is unnecessary.[34]

Because adjuvant treatment is aimed at micrometastatic disease remote from the primary tumor, exploration of chemotherapy before surgery (neoadjuvant) has been undertaken in a few types of cancer. In addition to earlier exposure of the micrometastases, this approach has two other beneficial characteristics. First, regression of the primary lesion predicts that the micrometastases will also likely be sensitive.[35] Second, regression of the primary tumor may make primary surgery unnecessary or less debilitating or disfiguring, allowing curative radiotherapy, as in some head and neck cancers and as shown in a large series of patients with breast cancer.[36] In other instances, surgery after chemotherapy may be technically easier, although not always less radical, because there is no certainty that every cell has been eradicated at the original boundaries. Induction or concurrent chemotherapy may also significantly enhance the effectiveness of radiotherapy for other tumors, such as anal carcinoma, thereby decreasing the need for surgery.

In the past, treatment of recurrent disease was too often empiric. The response to these subsequent treatments predictably diminishes over time. For example, a breast cancer patient whose tumor strongly expresses the estrogen and progesterone receptor has more than a 50% chance of responding to first-line hormonal therapy, with a likely duration of response of approximately 18 months.[37] On relapse, that same patient's probability of response to second-line therapy is cut in half, as is the likely duration of response.[38] Today, the use of dynamic monitoring of circulating tumor cells, circulating tumor DNA, and re-biopsy with genomic analysis promises to help select the most appropriate treatment for the relapsed patient.

The best treatment is often found through participation in clinical trials

The most common and lethal cancers, including metastatic lung, colon, and breast, are often incurable by approved treatments. Furthermore, most approved treatments have significant risks of side effects and produce limited prolongation of life. Yet, under these circumstances, most patients receive standard rather than experimental therapies. For many, the best choice of treatment may be available only through clinical trials.

Patients are increasingly involved in decisions regarding the choice of therapy, having been empowered by information widely available through the Internet. Patients with cancer are often apprehensive that they may not receive the best treatment and will challenge us with appropriately tough questions before moving ahead. The medical oncologist can speak with greater authority when a deliberate comparison is being made because the goal of such studies is toward improvement on the standard, not toward finding treatments that are equally good.

A number of ethical issues are abrogated by the certainty that a specific patient's disease is not currently curable. For metastatic disease for which no cure is known, it is not only ethical but also important that a systematically designed investigation of new treatments through participation in clinical trials be undertaken early in the course of the patient's disease. This allows assessment of a drug's activity before toxicity arises from conventional therapies that might limit dosing. Conventional therapies might also elicit resistance of one or another kind or immune system depression, which might foreclose the opportunity to recognize the activity of the candidate compound.

For diseases with an especially unfavorable outlook and rare therapeutic success, delays in introducing candidate compounds to ensure that they carry little or no risk of toxicity are an unwise investment of resources and time, let alone the patient's short-lived opportunity for possible benefit. The outcome of unsuccessfully treated cancer is more ominous than the hazards of clinical investigation.

Patients should be made aware of clinical trials as part of the initial discussions regarding treatment. Too often patients are not aware of clinical trials and discover this option through friends or the Internet rather than through their physicians. A trial of candidate phase II agents prior to conventional chemotherapy for metastatic breast cancer has been conducted without significant compromise in response to the established regimen.[39] Today, therapies aimed at validated molecular targets may enter the clinic once proof-of-principle is obtained in cell lines and safety and efficacy are confirmed in animal models. Major differences in pharmacokinetics exist between mouse and man, and the ultimate test remains the carefully designed, meticulously conducted clinical trial. The testing of new, targeted therapies is likely to change how we view early trials of anticancer drugs. For example, the phase I trial of imatinib did not reach a maximum tolerated dose. Rather, the dose was determined based on "maximum biological dose," that is, the dose in which the target enzyme was maximally inhibited.[40] Similarly, dynamic imaging techniques, such as positron emission tomography, predict the responsiveness to imatinib in patients with gastrointestinal stromal tumors well before changes occur in tumor size.[41] Finally, several newer agents are showing promising activity in very early phase studies, further compelling patients and their physicians to participate in properly designed studies.

Therefore, until the day arrives when all cancers are preventable or curable, enrollment of patients in clinical trials will be the hallmark of the practice of the best medical oncologists. No cancer is so well treated that an improvement in outcome or therapeutic approach cannot readily be imagined. Thus, research is imperative.

An individual in practice cannot devote the same time and energy to clinical research as one who serves full time on the faculty of a university, research institute, or hospital. However, the private practitioner has an opportunity to participate in clinical trials through cooperative groups or in collaboration with cancer centers; this opportunity should not be wasted. Every oncologist should participate in clinical research during his or her training, and the oncologist's office should include the capacity to perform clinical research. It is the responsibility of the medical oncologist to discuss clinical trials with patients in a way that does not bias an ultimate decision. There is much reason to anticipate that progress would be more rapid if clinical research were accepted as an integral part of the practice of medical oncology, as it is in pediatric oncology. The technology exists in medical informatics for community oncologists to ally themselves with their alma mater

or other academic centers to participate in diagnostic, preventive, and therapeutic research trials using the computer, electronic mail, and fax as expedient tools. Those oncologists who have so heavy a workload that it prevents their devoting the necessary time to participate in clinical research risk depriving their patients of access to research advances. Clinical investigation should serve as the bridge to fundamental science and the excitement generated by the new molecular biologic understanding of cancer as a malignant tissue.[42]

Cancer surveillance must be based on validated assumptions
Following completion of curative therapy and attainment of a complete remission or following adjuvant therapy, surveillance for early signs of recurrence is based on the logical assumption that the earlier a recurrence is detected, the better the outcome of a therapeutic intervention. Although true in principle, in practice, this is rarely the case. There are several reasons for this illogical result, including the possibilities that surveillance tests are insensitive or nonspecific or that further treatment options are ineffective. Over testing of patients at low risk of recurrence increases the probability of a false-positive result and the attendant morbidity, psychological or physical, associated with attempting to make a definitive diagnosis. In contrast, under testing in patients at risk of recurrence of a form of cancer for which effective salvage therapy is available (e.g., germ cell tumors, large cell lymphoma, Hodgkin disease, osteosarcoma, breast cancer, prostate cancer) is inexcusable. Thus, the oncologist must be aware of the predictive value of surveillance tests (tumor markers and imaging studies) in the context of specific malignancies and apply them accordingly.

Standards for quantifying diagnostic tests used frequently in surveillance have been adopted in most parts of the world [Système Internationale (SI) units], except the United States. It is impossible to read an international medical journal without being thoroughly familiar with SI units. They are presented in Table 4 so that readers can have ready access to a source for translation from the old nomenclature, characteristically American, which pervades this treatise.

Oncologic care is for life
The relationship of a medical oncologist with patients is intimate and should not end once therapies aimed at controlling the spread of cancer are no longer effective. The medical oncologist must be skilled in the principles and practice of palliative care and collaborate actively with specialists in symptom control, for example, neurologists, psychiatrists, and hospice staff. No greater feeling of abandonment can occur than when a patient is abruptly released from care by an oncologist who fails to recognize this lifelong responsibility.

It is, however, also the responsibility of the medical oncologist to address end-of-life planning with the patient and the family. Advice regarding living wills, power of attorney, and resuscitation falls squarely within the purview of the medical oncologist. This responsibility is highlighted in states that require that do not resuscitate (DNR) orders be written on patient charts prior to death. In the absence of such orders, when a nurse finds a patient apparently dead, she must, by law, initiate emergency calls for resuscitative efforts.

When death comes from cancer as the expected final event of a gradual deterioration of vital forces, resuscitative efforts do not succeed. When we are unable to keep someone alive, the likelihood of bringing him or her back to meaningful life is infinitesimal. Resuscitative efforts should be applied to patients with cancer

Table 4 Representative Système International units for laboratory tests of importance in oncology.

Component	Present reference interval	Present unit	Conversion factor	Intervals	Unit symbols
Albumin	4.0–6.0	g/dL	10.0	40–60	g/L
α-Fetoprotein, radioimmunoassay	0–20	ng/mL	1.00	0–20	g/L
Bilirubin					
Total	0.1–1.0	mg/dL	17.10	2–18	μmol/L
Conjugated	0–0.2	mg/dL	17.10	0–4	mol/L
Calcium	8.8–10.3	mg/dL	0.2495	2.20–2.58	μmmol/L
Cholesterol	<200+	mg/dL	0.02586	<5.20	μmmol/L
Cortisol	4–19	g/dL	27.59	110–520	nmol/L
Creatinine	0.6–1.2	mg/dL	88.40	50–110	mol/L
Fibrinogen	200–400	mg/dL	0.01	2.0–4.0	g/L
Glucose	70–110	mg/dL	0.05551	3.9*6.1	μmmol/L
Hemoglobin					
Male	14.0–18.0	g/dL	10.0	140–180	g/L
Female	11.5–15.5	g/dL	10.0	115–155	g/L
Immunoglobulins					
IgG	500–1200	mg/dL	0.01	5.00–12.00	g/L
IgA	50–350	mg/dL	0.01	0.50–3.50	g/L
IgM	30–230	mg/dL	0.01	0.30–2.30	g/L
IgD	<6	mg/dL	10	<360	mg/L
IgE	20–1000	ng/mL	1.00	20–1000	g/L
Iron	80–180	g/dL	0.1791	14–32	μmol/L
Iron-binding capacity	250–460	g/dL	0.1791	45–82	μmol/L
Lipoproteins					
Low-density lipoproteins (LDL), as cholesterol	50–190	mg/dL	0.02586	1.30–490	mmol/L
High-density lipoproteins (HDL), as cholesterol	30–70	mg/dL	0.02586	0.80–1.80	mmol/L
Magnesium	1.8–3.0	mg/dL	0.4114	0.80–1.20	mmol/L
	1.6–2.4	mEq/L	0.500	—	—
Metanephrines (as normetanephrine)	0–2.0	mg/24 h	5.458	0–11.0	μmol/day
Osmolality	280–300	mOsm/kg	1.00	280–300	nmol/kg
Phosphate (as inorganic P)	2.5–5.0	mg/dL	0.3229	0.80–1.60	mmol/L
Potassium	3.5–5.0	mEq/L	1.00	3.5–5.0	mmol/L
Protein, total	6–8	g/dL	10.0	60–80	g/L
Serotonin	8–21	g/dL	0.05675	0.45–1.20	mol/L
Thyroxine, free (T$_4$)	0.8–2.8	ng/dL	12.87	10–36	pmol/L
Triiodothyronine (T$_3$)	75–220	ng/dL	0.01536	1.2–3.4	nmol/L
Urate (as uric acid)	2.0–6.0	mg/dL	59.48	120–360	μmol/L
Urea nitrogen	8–18	mg/dL	0.3570	3.0–6.5	mmol/L
Vanillylmandelic acid	<6.8	mg/24 h	5.046	<35	μmol/day

who were not expected to die because reversible phenomena, such as pulmonary emboli, cardiac arrhythmias, aspiration, and similar events, can provoke unexpected death in a patient with a neoplasm, just as in any other hospitalized or ambulatory patient. Many patients, particularly the elderly and those apprised of the progress of their disease, can discuss the decision not to resuscitate with equanimity and, indeed, with a certain personal satisfaction of avoiding the fruitless anguish that such a procedure entails for the surviving family. Most patients sign living wills or appoint a health care proxy if these possibilities are presented to them.

Because of the legal implications involved, where particular religious scruples obtain or where families have emotionally uncontrolled members who cannot accept the anticipated death of a loved one, the medical oncologist should spend considerable time planning for an eventual death. DNR forms are a technique of documentation and constitute further evidence that society has moved medicine onto a new plateau of accountability.

The medical oncologist should make known his or her intentions concerning the advisability of resuscitative efforts for each particular patient in advance to forestall unnecessary trauma to the patient, family, and staff; to forestall litigation; and to settle in advance any serious disagreements with the patient or family. An impasse might occasion a medical oncologist to find a suitable substitute physician if there is irresolvable conflict concerning the plans surrounding an anticipated death.

DNR orders do not imply that there be diminution of effort to control or palliate the disease before death. However, if good judgment indicates that continued efforts are fruitless and can only inflict suffering, with no prospect of benefit, discontinuation of active therapy should always be accompanied by DNR orders.

Summary

The medical oncologist stands at the crossroads of modern molecular biology and medical practice and often serves as the final common pathway for the application of cancer research to patients. A complex corpus of information is available that expands rapidly, both deeper into the nature of the cancer process and wider into new approaches that provide demonstrated effectiveness in therapy, prevention, or support.

The increasing appreciation that oncogenes and tumor suppressors act through usurpation of normal autocrine and paracrine signaling pathways and that cancer is in reality not merely a disease of cancer cells but of a cast of supporting characters that form a malignant tissue (blood vessels, fibroblasts, smooth muscle cells, macrophages, lymphocytes, etc.) provides a variety of new targets for therapy. The realization that malignant transformation is a multistep process of accumulation of genetic abnormalities over long periods of time gives impetus for the design of rational preventive strategies and guidance to target patients at highest risk. These pathways have already led to effective targeted therapies that are less toxic than traditional cancer chemotherapy. Thus, the tide of fundamental discovery is washing away many of the unknowns. It is axiomatic that certain cancers can be cured today without knowing the intimate nature of neoplasia. How better the day, perhaps soon upon us, when we are more confident that we know what we are doing!

Clinical accomplishments have similarly been exceptionally productive in the 60 years since the first cancer was cured with drugs.[3] A large assortment of drugs has since been provided. A new array of genetically engineered drugs support host function, and others that are still early in their development are on the way. Imaging technologies will continue to revolutionize the ability to detect, stage, treat, and monitor cancers. Biochemical markers of tumor behavior will provide increasing diagnostic and monitoring capacity and may offer new targets for therapy.

There is probably no cancer in which some progress in diagnosis or therapy has not been achieved in the last decade. Similar achievements for cancer prevention are materializing. Oncologists must assume greater responsibility for health preservation. Much could be accomplished by applying what is already known about lifestyle, diet, and exercise. Medical facts without political action were slow to change the tax on health that tobacco levies. A concerted effort within most states has begun, but a federal role in managing the tobacco plague has been thwarted.

The horizon has never been closer. Although still distant, there are enough promising paths to follow that one of them may prove considerably faster than even reasonable optimism would suppose. The information that serves as our foundation, its rate of accrual, its revelations, and the demonstrated success of translating science to clinical applications augur well for the future of medical oncology and for cancer patients.

References

1 Kennedy BJ, Calabresi P, Carbone PP, et al. Training program in medical oncology. *Ann Intern Med.* 1973;**78**:127–130.
2 Holland J. The diseases that cancer causes. *J Chron Dis.* 1963;**16**:635.
3 Hertz R, Li MC, Spencer DB. Effect of methotrexate therapy upon choriocarcinoma and chorioadenoma. *Proc Soc Exp Biol Med.* 1956;**93**:361–366.
4 Holland JF. Methotrexate therapy of metastatic choriocarcinoma. *Am J Obstet Gynecol.* 1958;**75**:195–199.
5 Mitka M. "Teachable moments" provide a means for physicians to lower alcohol abuse. *JAMA.* 1998;**279**:1767–1768.
6 Holmes O. Medical Essays, 1842–1882. New York, NY: Houghton, Mifflin and Company; 1891.
7 Vogelstein B, Fearon ER, Hamilton SR, et al. Genetic alterations during colorectal-tumor development. *N Engl J Med.* 1988;**319**:525–532.
8 Thun MJ, Namboodiri MM, Heath CW Jr. Aspirin use and reduced risk of fatal colon cancer. *N Engl J Med.* 1991;**325**:1593–1596.
9 Koehne CH, Dubois RN. COX-2 inhibition and colorectal cancer. *Semin Oncol.* 2004;**31**:12–21.
10 O'Brien TR, Kirk G, Zhang M. Hepatocellular carcinoma: paradigm of preventive oncology. *Cancer J.* 2004;**10**:67–73.
11 Lawitz E, Lawitz MS, Lawitz R, et al. Simeprevir plus sofosbuvir, with or without ribavirin, to treat chronic infection with hepatitis C virus genotype 1 in non-responders to pegylated interferon and ribavirin and treatment-naive patients: the COSMOS randomised study. *Lancet.* 2014;**384**(9956):1756–1765.
12 Hong WK, Lippman SM, Itri LM, et al. Prevention of second primary tumors with isotretinoin in squamous-cell carcinoma of the head and neck. *N Engl J Med.* 1990;**323**:795–801.
13 Vogel VG, Costantino JP, Wickerham DL, et al. Effects of tamoxifen vs raloxifene on the risk of developing invasive breast cancer and other disease outcomes: the NSABP Study of Tamoxifen and Raloxifene (STAR) P-2 trial. *JAMA.* 2006;**295**:2727–2741.
14 Thiis-Evensen E, Hoff GS, Sauar J, et al. Population-based surveillance by colonos-copy: effect on the incidence of colorectal cancer. Telemark Polyp Study I. *Scand J Gastroenterol.* 1999;**34**:414–420.
15 Boardman LA, Steinhoff MM, Shackelton R, et al. A randomized trial of the Fischer cone biopsy excisor and loop electrosurgical excision procedure. *Obstet Gynecol.* 2004;**104**:745–750.
16 Koutsky LA, Ault KA, Wheeler CM, et al. A controlled trial of a human papillomavirus type 16 vaccine. *N Engl J Med.* 2002;**347**:1645–1651.
17 Druker BJ, Talpaz M, Resta DJ, et al. Efficacy and safety of a specific inhibitor of the BCR-ABL tyrosine kinase in chronic myeloid leukemia. *N Engl J Med.* 2001;**344**:1031–1037.
18 Lynch TJ, Bell DW, Sordella R, et al. Activating mutations in the epidermal growth factor receptor underlying responsiveness of non-small-cell lung cancer to gefitinib. *N Engl J Med.* 2004;**350**:2129–2139.
19 US Food and Drug Administration, 2004. Available at: www.fda.gov division.
20 Slamon DJ, Leyland-Jones B, Shak S, et al. Use of chemotherapy plus a monoclonal antibody against HER2 for metastatic breast cancer that overexpresses HER2. *N Engl J Med.* 2001;**344**:783–792.
21 Cunningham D, Humblet Y, Siena S, et al. Cetuximab monotherapy and cetuximab plus irinotecan in irinotecanrefractory metastatic colorectal cancer. *N Engl J Med.* 2004;**351**:337–345.
22 Hurwitz H, Fehrenbacher L, Novotny W, et al. Bevacizumab plus irinotecan, fluorouracil, and leucovorin for metastatic colorectal cancer. *N Engl J Med.* 2004;**350**:2335–2342.
23 Sosman JA, Kim KB, Schuchter L, et al. Survival in BRAF V600-mutant advanced melanoma treated with vemurafenib. *N Engl J Med.* 2012;**366**:707–714.
24 Rosenberg SA, Yang JC, Restifo NP. Cancer immunotherapy: moving beyond current vaccines. *Nat Med.* 2004;**10**(9):909–915.
25 Masters BA, Kaufman M. Painful withdrawal for makers of Vioxx: pulling of arthritis drug raises questions on marketing, safety risks. *Washington Post.* 2004; Sect. A:1, 8.
26 Holland JF. Ethics for a clinical investigator. Non primum non nocere. *Am J Med.* 1979;**66**:554–555.
27 Frei E III. Combination cancer therapy: presidential address. *Cancer Res.* 1972;**32**:2593–2607.
28 Frei E III, Canellos GP. Dose: a critical factor in cancer chemotherapy. *Am J Med.* 1980;**69**:585–594.
29 Kobayashi S, Boggon TJ, Dayaram T, et al. EGFR mutation and resistance of non-small-cell lung cancer to gefitinib. *N Engl J Med.* 2005;**352**:786–792.
30 Early Breast Cancer Trialists' Collaborative Group. Systemic treatment of early breast cancer by hormonal, cytotoxic, or immune therapy. 133 randomised trials involving 31,000 recurrences and 24,000 deaths among 75,000 women. *Lancet.* 1992;**339**:71–85.
31 Perloff M, Norton L, Korzun AH, et al. Postsurgical adjuvant chemotherapy of stage II breast carcinoma with or without crossover to a non-cross-resistant regimen: a Cancer and Leukemia Group B study. *J Clin Oncol.* 1996;**14**:1589–1598.
32 McGuire WP, Hoskins WJ, Brady MF, et al. Cyclophosphamide and cisplatin compared with paclitaxel and cisplatin in patients with stage III and stage IV ovarian cancer. *N Engl J Med.* 1996;**334**:1–6.
33 Moertel CG, Fleming TR, Macdonald JS, et al. Levamisole and fluorouracil for adjuvant therapy of resected colon carcinoma. *N Engl J Med.* 1990;**322**:352–358.
34 Paik S, Shak S, Tang G, et al. A multigene assay to predict recurrence of tamoxifen treated, node-negative breast cancer. *N Engl J Med.* 2004;**351**:2817–2826.
35 Rosen G, Caparros B, Huvos AG, et al. Preoperative chemotherapy for osteogenic sarcoma: selection of postoperative adjuvant chemotherapy based on the response of the primary tumor to preoperative chemotherapy. *Cancer.* 1982;**49**:1221–1230.
36 Jacquillat C, Weil M, Baillet F, et al. Results of neoadjuvant chemotherapy and radiation therapy in the breast-conserving treatment of 250 patients with all stages of infiltrative breast cancer. *Cancer.* 1990;**66**:119–129.
37 Sawka CA, Pritchard KI, Shelley W, et al. A randomized crossover trial of tamoxifen versus ovarian ablation for metastatic breast cancer in premenopausal women: a report of the National Cancer Institute of Canada Clinical Trials Group (NCIC CTG) trial MA.1. *Breast Cancer Res Treat.* 1997;**44**:211–215.
38 Robertson JF, Osborne CK, Howell A, et al. Fulvestrant versus anastrozole for the treatment of advanced breast carcinoma in postmenopausal women: a prospective combined analysis of two multicenter trials. *Cancer.* 2003;**98**:229–238.
39 Costanza ME, Weiss RB, Henderson IC, et al. Safety and efficacy of using a single agent or a phase II agent before instituting standard combination chemotherapy in previously untreated metastatic breast cancer patients: report of a randomized study—Cancer and Leukemia Group B 8642. *J Clin Oncol.* 1999;**17**:1397–1406.
40 Druker BJ, Sawyers CL, Kantarjian H, et al. Activity of a specific inhibitor of the BCR-ABL tyrosine kinase in the blast crisis of chronic myeloid leukemia and acute lymphoblastic leukemia with the Philadelphia chromosome. *N Engl J Med.* 2001;**344**:1038–1042.
41 Demetri GD, von Mehren M, Blanke CD, et al. Efficacy and safety of imatinib mesylate in advanced gastrointestinal stromal tumors. *N Engl J Med.* 2002;**347**:472–480.
42 Weinberg RA. The biology of cancer. In: *Garland Science.* New York, NY: Taylor and Francis Group, LLC; 2007.

46 Palliative care and pain management

Cardinale B. Smith, MD, MSCR

Overview

Palliative care is an essential component of comprehensive cancer care. Palliative care is given concurrently with other disease-modifying, life-prolonging, and curative therapy. Palliative medicine specialists focus on helping patients and their families with a variety of care needs including symptom control, psychosocial support, physician–patient communication, addressing care goals in relation to the patient's condition, prognosis, values, and preferences, as well as with transitions in care. Cancer patients often experience significant symptom distress either from the illness itself or from the associated treatments. The beneficial effects of palliative care have been well documented. When integrated into early oncologic care, palliative care is associated with a significant improvement in quality of life, depression, and survival. As such, palliative care should be given throughout the trajectory of cancer care whether during early stage disease in which the focus is on cure or in more advanced disease when the focus is on maximizing quality of life. Currently, national and international organizations have clinical guidelines that recommend palliative care be routinely integrated into comprehensive cancer care.

provisional opinion recommending incorporation of palliative care *"for any patient with metastatic cancer and/or high symptom burden."*[4] In 2013, The Institute of Medicine's report, Delivering High-Quality Cancer Care, recommended that cancer care teams *"place primary emphasis on palliative care, psychosocial support and timely referral to hospice for end of life care."*[5]

There are several core components involved in providing quality palliative care for oncology patients. These include the following:

- Whole patient assessment
- Effective communication
- Advanced care planning
- Symptom management
- Care at the end of life
- Grief and bereavement support

Palliative care

Palliative care is medical care focused on the relief of suffering and support for the best possible quality of life for patients and their families facing serious, life-threatening illness.[1] It aims to identify and address the physical, psychological, and practical burdens of illness and is provided as an extra layer of support for seriously ill patients. Palliative care is delivered simultaneously with all appropriate curative and life-prolonging interventions. Palliative care specialists provide assessment and treatment of pain and other symptoms; employ communication skills with patients, families, and colleagues; support complex medical decision making and goal setting based on identifying and respecting patient wishes and goals; promote medically informed care coordination, continuity, and practical support for patients, family caregivers, and professional colleagues across health care settings and through the trajectory of an illness. Palliative care in cancer patients should begin at the time of diagnosis. The emphasis of care will vary over the course of illness, with anticancer therapy provided concomitantly with supportive care and symptom management.

Several randomized studies have demonstrated a benefit of incorporating early palliative care into standard oncologic care.[2,3] In these studies, palliative care has been shown to improve mood, quality of life, and potentially survival among patients with advanced cancer. As such, oncology guidelines now recommend the routine integration of palliative care into routine oncologic care. In 2012, the American Society for Clinical Oncology (ASCO) issued a

Whole patient assessment

The whole patient assessment is guided by the National Comprehensive Cancer Network (NCCN) guidelines and core elements of palliative care as detailed in the National Quality Forum and involves evaluating all aspects of the impact of cancer and its treatments on the patient and family.[6] In addition to routine medical history, patient assessment explores the patients' social and community support, impact of the cancer diagnosis and treatment on patients' quality of life, spiritual and social well-being, as well as patients' expectations of therapy and goals of care. The whole patient assessment improves patient–physician communication and assists the physician in understanding potential barriers to patient adherence with treatment plans. This assessment is optimized by utilization of the interdisciplinary team to attend to all medical and psychosocial aspects of diagnosis, treatment, and to assist with patient and family distress.

Communication

Effective communication is an important component of the oncologist–patient relationship and assists in providing the highest quality cancer care. In an ASCO survey conducted in 1998, approximately 60% of respondents indicated that they broke bad news to patients from 5 to 20 times per month. Despite these challenges, <10% of respondents received formal training in breaking bad news.[7] Similarly, in a survey conducted at the 2004 ASCO meeting, oncology fellows reported being more likely to have observation and feedback on bone marrow biopsies than on goals of care

Holland-Frei Cancer Medicine, Ninth Edition. Edited by Robert C. Bast Jr., Carlo M. Croce, William N. Hait, Waun Ki Hong, Donald W. Kufe, Martine Piccart-Gebhart, Raphael E. Pollock, Ralph R. Weichselbaum, Hongyang Wang, and James F. Holland.
© 2017 John Wiley & Sons, Inc. ISBN: 978-1-118-93469-2

Table 1 Protocol for breaking bad news and addressing goals of care.

Recommendation	Comments
Create the proper setting	• Prior to the meeting determine the most appropriate participants (family members and other health care providers) • Allow adequate time • Determine what to say prior to the meeting
Clarify what the patient and family already know	• "What have you been told about your medical situation so far?" • This allows you to correct any misinformation and tailor the conversation based on their prior knowledge
Explore hopes and expectations of patient and family	• Allows you to distinguish between attainable and unattainable goals
Suggest realistic goals	• Suggest attainable goals based on the present clinical scenario and how they can best be achieved • Review appropriateness of disease-modifying treatments • Try to explain using simple language why unrealistic goals cannot be met
Use empathic responses	• Very important to allow silence and to listen • Let patient and family express emotions • Once emotions are expressed use a connector such as "I can see how upsetting this is to you"
Make a plan and follow through	• Summarize the plan to ensure that your interpretation of the conversation and decisions is in concordance with patient and family and how the plan of care will meet their goals • Make a plan for continued follow-up • Inform the patient and family how to contact you if they have further questions or concerns • Continue to review and revise the plan as needed

Source: Data from Refs [13] and [14].

Table 2 Palliative care Internet resources.

• www.capc.org: Center to Advance Palliative Care: Educational-based content to learn primary palliative care skills. Technical assistance for clinicians and hospitals seeking to establish or strengthen a palliative care program
• www.vitaltalk.org: Website to help providers learn communication skills
• www.epeconline.net: Education on Palliative and End of Life Care (EPEC): Comprehensive curriculum covering fundamentals of palliative medicine; free downloadable power point and teaching guides
• www.palliativedrugs.com: Extensive information on pharmacologic symptom management
• www.aahpm.org: American Academy of Hospice and Palliative Medicine: Physician membership organization; board review courses, publications
• www.hms.harvard.edu/cdi/pallcare: Center for Palliative Care at Harvard Medical School: Faculty development courses, other educational programs
• www.nationalconsensusproject.org: National Consensus Project for Quality Palliative Care: Clinical practice guidelines
• http://endoflife.stanford.edu/: Joint project of the US Veterans Administration and SUMMIT, Stanford University Medical School. Curriculum covering fundamentals of palliative medicine

discussions.[8] This lack of training can have a negative impact on cancer patients and providers. Poor communication skills have been associated with decreased patient participation in decision making,[9] missed opportunities to respond empathically to patient concerns, ignored patient wishes to discuss health-related quality of life issues, and an increased likelihood of receiving anticancer treatment at the end of life.[10] Alternatively, effective communication has been shown to influence desirable outcomes such as patient satisfaction, adherence with treatments, decreased patient distress, and reduces physician burnout.[11,12]

There are existing protocols to help deliver bad news and address goals of care (Table 1).[13,14] These protocols can be applied to most situations including a new diagnosis of cancer, cancer recurrence, progression of disease, and transition to hospice. This communication process attempts to achieve four main goals: gathering information from the patient to elicit readiness to hear the news; providing information in accordance with the patient's needs and desires; reducing the emotional impact and isolation experienced by the recipient of the bad news; and developing a treatment plan that aligns with patient preferences. When communicating with patients and families, it is important to use open-ended questions such as "What are your hopes and fears?" and "What is important in your life?"[14] It is important to avoid language with unintended consequences such as "There is nothing more we can do for you" and "Do you want everything done for you?"[14] Instead, try saying "We will do everything to give you the best quality of life" or

"We will manage your symptoms very aggressively." Additionally, it is important to avoid jargon or euphemisms, and instead use plain, simple language. Once the goals of care are established, it becomes much easier to construct a plan of care centered on those preferences. There are currently training programs that are offered to train oncologists in these specific skills, a list if available resources can be found in Table 2.

Advance care planning

Once the patients' goals of care are established, they should be documented in the form of advance directives. Advance directives consist of two main components: the health care proxy or durable power of attorney for health care and treatment directives.[15] A commonly used comprehensive advance directive is the medical orders for life-sustaining treatment (MOLST) or physician orders for life-sustaining treatment (POLST) and is currently in use or under development in over 40 states.[16] POLST is appropriate for people with cancer and a prognosis measured in 1–2 years. It specifically addresses medical decisions and options that are likely to arise in the near future, including cardiopulmonary resuscitation, antibiotics for infections, artificial food and fluids, and whether or not the patient would want to be re-hospitalized. Additionally, it can be transported across care settings. POLST appears to be associated with better receipt of medical care reflecting patient treatment preferences (decreased hospitalization and life-sustaining treatments) when compared to traditional practices, improved surrogate understanding of patient goals and preferences and an improved prevalence, clarity, and specificity of preferences documented.[17-19] It is important for every cancer patient to have advance directives to help avoid confusion and conflict, to prepare for future medical care, and to ensure that patients' wishes will be followed.

Symptom management

Patients with cancer experience many physical and psychosocial symptoms either as a consequence of therapy or as a result of the disease itself. The essential components of symptom management include (1) routine and repeated formal assessment, (2) expertise in prescribing medications, including the safe use of opioid analgesics, adjuvant approaches to pain management, and management of a wide range of other common and distressing symptoms and syndromes, and (3) skillful management of treatment side effects. Currently, there is no gold standard for symptom assessment in palliative care. Although several tools exist, the most commonly used is the Edmonton Symptom Assessment System, which consists of nine visual analog scales or numerical rating scales that evaluate a combination of the most common physical and psychological symptoms.[20] The most common symptom experienced by cancer patients is pain.[21] The most frequent nonpain symptoms are constipation, nausea and vomiting, anorexia/cachexia, dyspnea, delirium, and anxiety.[21] The management of some of these symptoms will be discussed in the following sections.

Pain

The International Association for the Study of Pain defines pain as "an unpleasant sensory and emotional experience associated with actual or potential tissue damage or described in terms of such damage."[22] Although the cause of the pain and the type of injury vary, the constellation of complex neurophysiologic phenomena of pain includes two broad categories, nociceptive pain, which include both somatic and visceral pain, and neuropathic pain.[23] Somatic pain is characterized as well localized, intermittent, or constant and is described as aching, gnawing, throbbing, or cramping (e.g., bone metastases). Visceral pain is mediated by discrete nociceptors in the cardiovascular, respiratory, gastrointestinal (GI), and genitourinary systems. It is usually described as deep, squeezing, or colicky and is commonly referred to cutaneous sites, which may be tender. Neuropathic pain is clinically described as a burning, tingling, or numb sensation with paroxysms of shock-like pain. Cancer history should include description of the pain complaint, including the patient's description of pain and intensity; its quality, exacerbating, relieving factors, and its radiation if any; its exact onset and temporal pattern. Impact of pain on the activities of daily living, sleep, mood, and affect should be assessed.

The guiding principles of a therapeutic strategy for cancer pain should include (1) detailed assessment of the patient's pain, (2) making a pain diagnosis, (3) understanding the goals of care and the patient's preferences, (4) developing and implementing the best therapeutic and diagnostic strategy, (5) continual reassessment of the degree of pain and analgesia, and (6) expertise to provide alternative therapeutic strategies. Of greatest importance, no patient should be inadequately evaluated because of patient's experiencing "too much pain." A series of algorithms have been developed for the management of cancer pain.[24,25] The World Health Organization Cancer Pain and Palliative Care Program advocates a three-step approach, which advocates starting with nonopioid analgesia [e.g., nonsteroidal, anti-inflammatory drugs (NSAIDs)] and then

titrating up to low- then high-potency opioids.[23] Similarly, NCCN pain management guidelines provide an algorithm of a stepwise approach to the treatment of mild, moderate, and severe pain and strategy of rapid but safe opioid titration to provide analgesia.[26] General guidelines of cancer pain treatment are listed in Table 3. Management of cancer pain can be divided into pharmacologic approaches, interventional approaches, and psychological management.

Pharmacological approaches are the most commonly used method for managing cancer pain. The brief outline of pharmacologic approach is detailed in Table 4. The selection of the right analgesic to maximize pain relief and minimize adverse effects begins with the use of nonopioids for mild pain. In patients with moderate pain that is not controlled with nonopioids such as acetaminophen, NSAIDs, and adjuvant medications (WHO step 1), the so-called weak opioid agonists (codeine, hydrocodone, and tramadol) alone or in combination are prescribed (step 2). In patients with severe pain, a strong opioid (morphine, hydromorphone, fentanyl, methadone, oxycodone, oxymorphone, or levorphanol) is the drug of choice (step 3). At all levels, certain NSAIDs and adjuvant drugs may be used for specific indications. A number of opioid analgesics is available for clinical use and are listed in Table 4.

Selection of the opioids should be based on patient's analgesic history, renal and hepatic function (Table 5), side effects, and severity of pain. Short-acting opioids are usually used for opioid titration and as needed (PRN, pro re nata) for breakthrough pain. After an effective stable 24-h opioid requirement is established, a switch to a long-acting formulation should be considered. Long-acting opioids allow patients to achieve more consistent blood levels, reduce pain recurrence, improve compliance, and reduce the iatrogenic dependence. Rescue medications equivalent to 10% of the standing 24-h dose should also be made available to patients.[27,28] Overall, opioid dose, route, and titration schedule should be tailored to the patient's medical needs, treatment goals, and side-effect profile. There is no minimum or maximum dose. The opioid dose needs to be titrated to maintain the patient's desired balance between pain relief and opioid-related side effects.

Interventional approaches can be divided into six major types: (1) trigger-point injections, (2) peripheral nerve blocks, (3) autonomic nerve blocks, (4) epidural and intrathecal infusions, (5) surgical approaches, and (6) neurostimulatory approaches. The techniques for each of these procedures are outside the scope of this chapter, but have been described in detail elsewhere.[29]

Psychological management of cancer pain includes the use of psychotherapeutic, cognitive-behavioral, and psychopharmacologic interventions. These techniques are most useful in three clinical situations: (1) in the management of patients with intermittent predictable pain (such as pain associated with procedures), (2) in the management of incident pain (e.g., in the patient with pain on movement), and (3) in the management of chronic cancer pain.[30,31]

Constipation

Constipation is defined as the infrequent and difficult passage of hard stool. It is a common cause of morbidity in the palliative care setting and affects more than 95% of patients who are treated with opioids for cancer-related pain.[15] The two most common etiologies are related to the side effects of opioids and the effects of progressive disease. Severe constipation can lead to bowel obstruction and perforation and can be a cause of severe morbidity. In patients who are neutropenic, severe constipation can lead to bacterial transfer across the colon, resulting in bacteremia and potentially sepsis. The Rome

Table 3 Guidelines for the use of analgesic drugs in cancer pain management.

Start with a specific drug for a specific type of pain
1. Clarify the patient's pain, its nature, site, duration, and intensity, and the degree of pain relief from prior nonopioid and opioid drug use
2. Complete a careful medical and neurologic history and examination. Assess the potential role of radiotherapy, surgery, and/or chemotherapy in pain control
3. Assess the psychological factors contributing to the pain complaint and understand the meaning of the pain for the patient
4. Choose the route of administration to fit the needs of the individual patient
i. Choose the oral route as the simplest approach
ii. Consider the buccal or rectal routes for patients who cannot tolerate oral drugs and refuse parenteral routes. Start intravenous intermittent boluses or continuous infusions in patients requiring rapid escalation of opioids for pain control
iii. Use intermittent boluses or continuous subcutaneous infusions for patients without venous access or in patients at home
iv. Choose the epidural or intrathecal route in patients who develop limiting side effects from systemic opioids
v. Use PCA pumps for selected patients in hospital and at home
5. Know the pharmacology of the available opioid drugs. Titrate the dose to the individual needs of the patient
i. Start with a dose that is at least equivalent or slightly greater than the equianalgesic dose of the previous analgesic used
ii. Order the medication on a regular basis (oral–every 3–4 h, intravenous–every 15–60 min as needed)
iii. Instruct the patient to take the medication on a PRN basis if the patient is opioid naive
iv. Order "rescue medication" equivalent to 10% of the standing 24-h dose to begin with on a PRN basis
v. Inform the patient of options in taking the medication and request that he or she report side effects of excessive sedation or confusion. Monitor the side effects closely
6. Use a combination of drugs to provide additive analgesia to reduce side effects or to control other symptoms
i. Know the various adjuvant drugs that provide additive analgesia, for example, anticonvulsants, corticosteroids
ii. Use neurostimulants to reduce sedative effects, for example, caffeine, dextroamphetamine, methylphenidate, modafinil
iii. Use antidepressant, anticonvulsant, and other analgesics to manage neuropathic pain
7. Anticipate and treat side effects
i. Watch for respiratory depression and use naloxone if needed (in diluted doses to prevent acute withdrawal)
ii. Counteract sedation with neurostimulants
iii. Use antiemetics to suppress the emetic effect of opioids
iv. Define an individualized bowel regimen to prevent and manage constipation
v. Treat myoclonus by switching to an alternative analgesic, or suppress it with anxiolytic drugs
8. Watch for the development of tolerance
i. Distinguish tolerance from progression of tumor
ii. Recognize that there is no limit to tolerance
iii. Switch to an alternative opioid if the dose of the current opioid cannot be escalated
iv. Consider opioid rotation if one or more intractable side effects are noted

Abbreviations: PCA, patient-controlled analgesia; PRN, pro re nata (according as circumstances may require).

Table 4 Opioid analgesics commonly used for moderate to severe pain narcotic agonists.

	Parenteral (mg)	Oral (mg)	Conversion factor (IV to PO)	Comments
Morphine	10	30	1 : 3	Standard of comparison for opioid analgesics; lower dose for aged patients
Hydromorphone	1.5	7.5	1 : 5	Slightly shorter-acting
Fentanyl	25 µg = 1 mg morphine IV	—	—	Short half-life; transdermal and transmucosal preparations available
Codeine	130	200	1 : 1.5	Often used in combination with nonopioid analgesics; biotransformed, part, to morphine
Oxycodone	—	20	–	Also in combination with nonopioid analgesics that limit dose escalation
Oxymorphone	1	10	1 : 10	Not available orally
Methadone[a]	—	—	—	—

[a]Methadone has a complex pharmacokinetic and pharmacodynamic profile that makes equianalgesic dosing particularly difficult. Consult with an experienced clinician before initiating or adjusting the dose of methadone.

criteria defines constipation as the presence of two or more of the following symptoms[32]:

- Straining at least 25% of the time
- Hard stools at least 25% of the time
- Incomplete evacuation at least 25% of the time
- ≤2 bowel movements per week.

Assessment of constipation should involve a history of the patient's bowel pattern, fluid intake, recent dietary changes, review of current medications, and a thorough physical examination, including a rectal exam—with caution in patients with neutropenia. In addition, abdominal radiography can be performed to look for the presence of stool if the diagnosis remains unclear.

Constipation can be managed with nonpharmacologic measures as well as pharmacologic interventions. Nonpharmacologic measures include increasing fluid intake if possible and regular toileting as colonic activity is highest early in the morning, after walking, and 30 min after meals. Pharmacologic interventions for the management of constipation may be administered orally or rectally and are summarized in Table 6. There is no single correct management approach to laxative prescribing. Initial regimens often include a stimulant, such as senna, given once or twice per day and titrated according to response. Stool-softening agents, such as docusate, are commonly prescribed, but they have not been shown to be efficacious in this setting.[33] Whichever bowel regimen is initiated should be individualized and titrated to response. It is important to note

Table 5 Guidelines for opioids in kidney and liver disease.

	Kidney disease[a]		Liver disease	
	Renal failure	Dialysis	Stable cirrhosis	Severe disease
Morphine	Do not use	Do not use Not dialyzed	Caution ↓ dose ↓ frequency[b]	Do not use
Oxycodone	Caution ↓ dose ↓ frequency[b]	Caution	Caution ↓ dose ↓ frequency[b]	Caution ↓ dose ↓ frequency[b]
Hydromorphone	Preferred ↓ dose ↓ frequency[b]	Preferred Not dialyzed, but minimal toxicity	Caution ↓ dose ↓ frequency[b]	Caution ↓ dose ↓ frequency[b]
Fentanyl	Preferred	Preferred Not dialyzed, but minimal toxicity	Preferred	Preferred
Codeine	Do not use	Do not use	Do not use	Do not use
Methadone[c]	Preferred—with consultation only	Preferred—with consultation only. Not dialyzed, but minimal toxicity	Preferred—with consultation only	Preferred—with consultation only

[a] Avoid sustained release oral opioids and fentanyl patches in kidney disease. Note that even the "safest" opioids are not dialyzable.
[b] ↓ dose means reduce dose by 25–50%. ↓ frequency means reduce standing orders for short-acting opioids from q4h to q6h.
[c] Consult with an experienced clinician before initiating or adjusting the dose of methadone.

that the best treatment of constipation is prevention. A prophylactic bowel regimen should be initiated at the time opioids are initially prescribed and should be continued for as long as the patient remains on opioids.

Nausea and vomiting

Nausea and vomiting are reported to affect between 40% and 70% of patients with cancer.[34] Nausea and vomiting can cause substantial psychological distress for patients and families and impact overall quality of life.[35] Nausea is subjective and is defined as an unpleasant sensation of the need to vomit and can be associated with autonomic symptoms, including pallor, cold sweats, tachycardia, and diarrhea. Vomiting is the forceful discharge of gastric contents via the mouth resulting from the contraction of the abdominal musculature and diaphragm. The pathophysiology of nausea and vomiting is complex and involves four pathways (chemoreceptor trigger zone, cortex, peripheral pathways in the GI tract, and vestibular system), which when stimulated can induce nausea and vomiting.[36,37]

The etiology of nausea and vomiting are varied, but it is important to determine the exact cause in order to select targeted and effective treatment. The most common etiologies in patients with cancer are chemotherapy-induced nausea and vomiting (CINV) and opioid-induced, bowel obstruction and constipation. Once the likely etiology of nausea and vomiting is identified, directed therapy can begin. There are guidelines for the prevention and treatment of CINV in patients on antineoplastic therapy.[38] The most commonly used approach is based on identifying the etiology and administering the most potent antagonist targeted toward the implicated receptors. This strategy has been shown to be effective in up to 80–90% of patients. Some practitioners recommend starting an empirical antiemetic regimen, typically with a dopamine antagonist, regardless of the presumed etiology.[39–41] No direct comparisons currently exist between mechanism-based and empirical therapy.

Therapy should consist of nonpharmacologic and pharmacologic measures aimed at alleviating the cause of the symptoms. Nonpharmacologic measures include avoiding strong smells or other nausea triggers, eating small, frequent meals, limiting oral intake during periods of extreme emesis,[42] relaxation techniques,[43] acupuncture, and acupressure.[44] Progressive muscle relaxation and guided mental imagery during periods of chemotherapy have also shown beneficial effects.[45] The most commonly used antiemetics worldwide are metoclopramide, dexamethasone, haloperidol, hyoscine butylbromide, and cyclizine. Antiemetics are available in the form of pills,

orally dissolvable tablets, intravenous infusion, rectal suppositories, and subcutaneous infusions. Thought should be given to selection of the appropriate route of administration of the antiemetic to ensure maximum efficacy. A list of antiemetics, routes of administration, and their properties can be found in Table 7.

Anorexia/cachexia syndrome (ACS)

ACS (anorexia/cachexia syndrome) is characterized by disproportionate and excessive loss of lean body mass. ACS may occur in up to 80% of patients with advanced cancer.[46] ACS is usually a marker of disease progression. In a multicenter retrospective review of 3047 cancer patients enrolled on clinical trials from the Eastern Cooperative Oncology Group, weight loss of more than 5% of premorbid weight prior to the initiation of chemotherapy was predictive of early mortality.[47] Weight loss was independent of disease stage, tumor histology, and patient performance status in its predictive value.[47]

Management of this syndrome should first focus on trying to treat any of the contributing secondary causes. Because anorexia is a prevalent and distressing symptom suffered by most cancer patients, the basis of pharmacologic treatment has focused on alleviating this symptom. The two classes of drugs that have been shown to be effective in phase III clinical trials are corticosteroids and progestational agents.[48,49] These drugs do not appear to improve survival, but may improve quality of life. Corticosteroids, usually in the form of dexamethasone at a dose of 4 mg/day (although doses of 2–20 mg/day can be used), has been shown to alleviate cancer anorexia on a short-term basis. This finding has been replicated by other studies and both prednisolone and methylprednisolone have been shown to be effective.[50] As the duration of appetite stimulation is short lived, and the side effects increase over time, it is most useful for patients with a life expectancy of <6 weeks. Megestrol acetate has been shown to result in dose-dependent improvements in appetite, which usually occur in about 1 week. Improvement in overall well-being has been demonstrated in more than 60% of patients starting at doses of 160 mg/day. The optimal dosing for weight gain appears to be between 480 and 800 mg/day. Effects are seen after several weeks in only 25% of patients.[51] It is important to start at a lower dose and titrate upwards as adverse events are dose related. Adverse events include deep vein thrombosis, especially in those concomitantly on chemotherapy, edema, hyperglycemia, and elevated liver enzymes. Cannabinoids, in its synthetic form of dronabinol, may have some limited effects on improving appetite,

Table 6 Laxatives commonly used to treat constipation.

Class of drug	Preparation	Starting dose	Mechanism of action	Comments
Oral				
Lubricant	Mineral oil	5–10 mL/day	Lubricates stool surface, allows easier passage	Adverse effects include lipoid pneumonia, leakage of oily fecal material. 255 paraffin and magnesium hydroxide considered safest
Bulk-forming agents	Methycellulose, bran, psyllium	Bran 8 g daily Others 3–4 g daily	Increases stool bulk, stimulating peristalsis	Good for mild constipation. Caution as needs to be taken with at least 200–300 mL of water. May precipitate obstruction in a debilitated patient by forming a viscous mass May cause flatulence and bloating
Osmotic (poorly absorbed sugars)	Lactulose	15–30 mL daily	Retention of water in the lumen via osmotic effects	Sweet taste that may not be well tolerated. Bloating, abdominal cramping, and flatulence are common
Saline	Magnesium hydroxide Sodium bisphosphonate	2.4–4.8 g daily	High osmolarity compounds causes retention of water in the lumen throughout the entire gut. Directly stimulates peristalsis	Strong cathartic. Mostly used as a bowel prep for endoscopic procedures. May alter fluid and electrolyte imbalance. Caution in patients with heart failure or renal insufficiency
Anthraquinones	Senna	Max 100 mg/day	Direct stimulation of myenteric plexus causing induction of peristalsis	Often combined with docusate. May cause abdominal cramping. Do not use if obstruction is suspected
Polyphenolic	Bisacodyl	10 mg daily	Stimulates secretion and motility of small intestine and colon	May cause abdominal cramping
Rectal				
Lubricant	Mineral oil enema	One enema	Used as retention enema to allow evacuation or manual removal of impacted stool	Efficacy is dependent on ability to retain the oil
Osmotic	Glycerin	One suppository	Softens stools via osmosis	
Saline	Sodium phosphate	One enema or suppository	Releases bound water from feces. May stimulate rectal or distal colonic peristalsis	May alter fluid and electrolyte balance. Caution in patients with heart failure or renal insufficiency
Polyphenolic	Bisacodyl	10 mg suppository	Promotes colonic peristalsis	Activity depends on bisacodyl reaching the rectal wall
Subcutaneous				
Peripheral opioid receptor antagonist	Methylnaltrexone	<38 kg:0.15 mg/kg 38 to <62 kg: 8 mg 62–114 kg: 12 mg >114 kg: 0.15 mg/kg (round up)	Selectively blocks opioid binding at the mu receptor, in the GI tract	Only for opioid-induced constipation

but it does not contribute to significant weight gain. In a randomized trial comparing dronabinol to megestrol acetate, significantly more patients had improvement in appetite and weight gain with megestrol acetate.[52] Combined therapy with both megestrol acetate and dronabinol had no benefit beyond that obtained with megestrol acetate alone. Adverse events with dronabinol include sedation, confusion, and perceptual disturbances.

Dyspnea

Dyspnea is the awareness of an uncomfortable or unpleasant sensation of breathing. The prevalence of dyspnea varies greatly and ranges from 21% to 79% depending on primary disease site, stage of disease, and location of metastasis.[53] The sensation of dyspnea is a subjective experience with numerous etiologies. The presence of tachypnea and hypoxia does not adequately reflect the severity of symptoms felt by the patient.[54] It is not uncommon that patients with moderate to severe tachypnea will not complain of dyspnea. In contrast, patients who are not tachypneic may report severe dyspnea. It is therefore of utmost importance that assessment be based on patient report. The goal of treatment is symptomatic relief of the patient's expression of dyspnea, rather than the correction of objective variables (tachypnea and low oxygen saturation).

The most common modalities used to treat dyspnea include oxygen therapy and opioids. Three randomized controlled crossover studies have evaluated the use of oxygen (4 or 5 L/min) versus air in advanced cancer patients with dyspnea. Two of these studies evaluated patients with hypoxemia on room air and found that oxygen therapy was more beneficial.[55,56] The third evaluated non-hypoxemic cancer patients and found that there was no difference between oxygen therapy and air in reducing the intensity of dyspnea.[57] Opioids are the pharmacologic treatment of choice in the management of dyspnea. Several randomized controlled trials in cancer patients with dyspnea have demonstrated their benefit. In opioid-naive patients, a starting dose of morphine sulfate 2.5–5 mg orally or its equivalent intravenously every 4 h can be effective. In those patients already on opioid therapy, an increase of 25% in the baseline dose may provide relief.[58]

The terminal phase

Death is a natural process that will occur for every patient. About 10% of people will die suddenly and unexpectedly, while the other 90% die after a period of illness with gradual deterioration until an active dying phase occurs signifying the end of life.[5] There are "two roads to death,"[59] the usual road that occurs in most patients and

Table 7 Antiemetics commonly used to treat nausea and vomiting.

Receptor site of action	Drug name	Dosage/route	Adverse effects
Dopamine antagonists (D$_2$)	Chlorpromazine	10–25 mg PO every 4–6 h, 25–50 mg IM every 3–4 h	Dystonia, akathisia, sedation, and postural hypotension
	Haldol	10–20 mg PO, IV/SQ before meals and at bedtime or every 6 h	Dystonia and akathisia
	Metoclopramide	10–20 mg PO every 6 h, 5–10 mg IV every 6 h or 25 mg rectally every 6 h	Dystonia, akathisia, abdominal cramping in obstruction
	Prochlorperazine	5–10 mg PO every 6–8 h or 25 mg rectally every 12 h	Dystonia, akathisia, and sedation
	Olanzapine	5–10 mg PO once daily for up to 5 days	
Histamine antagonists (H$_1$)	Cyclizine	25–50 mg PO/SQ or rectally every 8 h	Dry mouth, sedation, skin irritation at SQ sites may occur
	Diphenhydramine	25–50 mg PO/IV/SQ every 4–8 h	Sedation, dry mouth, and urinary retention
	Promethazine (also has activity on D$_2$ and ACH)	12.5–25 mg PO, IV/IM rectal every 4–6 h	Dry mouth, dystonia, akathisia, and sedation
Acetylcholine antagonists (ACH)	Glycopyrrolate	0.2 mg IV/SQ every 4–6 h	Dry mouth, blurred vision, confusion, urinary retention, ileus
	Hycosamine	0.125–0.25 mg PO/SL every 4 h or 0.25–0.5 mg IV/SQ every 4 h	Dry mouth, blurred vision, confusion, urinary retention, ileus
	Scopolamine	0.1–0.4 mg IV/SQ every 4 h or 1.5 mg transdermal patch every 72 h	Dry mouth, blurred vision, confusion, urinary retention, ileus
Serotonin antagonists (5HT$_3$)	Dolasetron	100 mg PO daily	Headache, diarrhea
	Granisetron	2 mg PO daily or daily	Headache, constipation, weakness
	Ondansetron	4–8 mg PO/IV or dissolvable tablet IV every 4–8 h (max 32 mg/day)	Headache, constipation, weakness
	Palonosetron	0.25 mg IV prior to start of chemotherapy[a]	Headache, constipation
Substance P antagonist	Aprepitant	125 mg PO on day 1 of chemotherapy 80 mg PO on days 2 and 3[a]	Headache
	Fosaprepitant	150 mg IV day 1 of chemotherapy	Headache, infusion site pain
Other Corticosteroids	Dexamethasone	10–20 mg PO/IV each treatment day	Hyperglycemia, GI bleeding, insomnia, psychosis
Cannabinoids	Dronabinol	2–20 mg PO daily in divided doses	Dizziness, euphoria in the young and dysphoria in the elderly, paranoid reaction, somnolence
Benzodiazepines	Lorazepam[b]		
Somatostatin analog	Octreotide	0.5–2 mg PO/IV every 4–6 h	Sedation, respiratory depression
		100 mcg every 8–12 h IV/SQ or 100 mcg/h as continuous IV infusion	Bradycardia, headache, malaise, hyperglycemia

[a]Have not been shown to be effective in terminating nausea or vomiting once it occurs and should not be used for this purpose.
[b]Best used for anticipatory nausea and vomiting.

presents as decreasing level of consciousness that leads to coma and death, and the difficult road. The difficult road is marked by terminal delirium, which can manifest as restlessness, confusion, and agitation; it can be a source of great distress for patients, family, and loved ones.[59] The most common symptoms reported by families in the last week of life are fatigue, dyspnea, and dry mouth, while the most distressing are fatigue, dyspnea, and pain.[60] The Clinical Practice Guidelines for Quality Palliative Care emphasize that families should be educated regarding the signs and symptoms of approaching death in a manner that is developmentally, age, and culturally appropriate.[6] While patients and families may still be focused on glucose or blood pressure control, such preventive measures must be taken into the context of the patients' life expectancy. Discontinuation of such medications often involves a detailed discussion about the risks and adverse effects outweighing the probable lack of benefit. The least invasive rate of medication administration should be attempted initially using the most invasive route only when absolutely necessary. A variety of physiologic changes occur in the last hours to days of life and the following is a summary of the most common changes that occur[61,62]:

1. *Weakness and fatigue*. Weakness and fatigue usually increase as the patient is approaching death. Patients will begin to spend all

of their time in bed and will be less interested in participating in usual activities, including visiting with others.

2. *Decreased oral intake*. Most dying patients lose their appetite and stop drinking. Many caregivers interpret this as a patient "giving up" or "starving to death." It is important to explain to patients and their family members that there is a decreased need for food and drink during this phase. There is some evidence suggesting that prolonged anorexia is not uncomfortable. One study found that 97% of dying patients who stopped eating experienced no hunger or hunger only initially.[63] It has been proposed that terminal anorexia induces a ketosis that contributes to a sense of well-being and diminished discomfort and may in fact be beneficial to dying patients.[61,64] Two meta-analyses of studies of both parenteral[65] and enteral[66] nutrition in patients with metastatic cancer found that neither therapy resulted in an improvement in morbidity or mortality and actually resulted in an increased total complication rate. The evidence with respect to hydration in dying patients is less straightforward with many differing expert opinions.[61,67–69] Some studies suggest that parenteral hydration prevents and treats some cases of terminal delirium,[67,68,70] and others correlate dehydration with adverse symptoms such as thirst.[69,71,72] Still others believe that the data does not support a

Table 8 Pharmacologic therapy of delirium.

Drug name	Dosage/route	Comments
Haloperidol	0.5–5 mg PO/IV/IM/SC every 6–12 h	Most commonly used agent. Can prolong QT interval
Chlorpromazine	12.5–50 mg PO/IV/IM every 8–12 h	Has similar efficacy to haloperidol, but more sedating, anticholinergic and hypotensive effects
Lorazepam	0.5–2 mg PO/SL/IV every 4–8 h and titrate as needed	Most commonly used as a second agent in combination with haloperidol. Can also be used as a continuous infusion for refractory cases where deep sedation is needed. May worsen delirium in the elderly. Caution with liver failure
Risperidone	Start at 0.5–1 mg/day PO and titrate up to 4–6 mg/day	In one study shown to have no differences in side effects when compared to haloperidol. Limited use as only available in oral route
Olanzapine	5 mg PO qhs and titrated to effect (max 20 mg/day)	Risk factors for a poor response to olanzapine in cancer patients are: ° Age >70 ° History of dementia ° CNS metastases ° Hypoxia ° Hypoactive delirium
Midazolam	1 mg/h IV and titrated to effect	Most commonly used for refractory cases where sedation is needed

correlation between dehydration and symptoms and that rehydration does not improve patient comfort.[63,70] A randomized control trial of advanced cancer patients within weeks of death demonstrated no improvement in symptoms, quality of life, or survival when compared to placebo.[73] It is important that each individual patient be evaluated to determine the risk benefit ratio. Attention should be placed on minimizing the sense of thirst and maintaining patient comfort even when dehydration is present, with oral hygiene. This can be achieved by using lollipop sponges dipped in cold fluids such as water, a lemon-flavored drink or sorbet.

3. *Delirium.* While reversible factors may be identified in up to half of cases, terminal delirium management typically focuses on symptom control with medications.[72] Treatment should be aimed at the symptoms of delirium while simultaneously attempting to treat reversible causes. Although delirium is most often associated with the last hours to days of life, in some episodes it may be reversible with therapeutic intervention.[72,74] Neuroleptic agents are the mainstay of pharmacologic treatment as they are effective in both hypoactive and hyperactive delirium. Of these agents, haloperidol is the agent of choice as it has lower sedating properties, less anticholinergic and cardiovascular effects. The pharmacologic agents commonly used in the management of delirium can be found in Table 8.

Grief and bereavement

Bereavement is the state of loss as a consequence of death.[75] Grief is defined as the emotional response to loss and mourning, and often refers to social expressions associated with loss.[75] Several types of grief exist: anticipatory grief, uncomplicated grief, and complicated grief. Anticipatory grief refers to the mourning that occurs in patients and families prior to death and is a way to facilitate

the adjustment to bereavement. Uncomplicated grief is the most common type of grief reaction and is socially perceived as normal. Complicated grief involves the persistence of grief reactions over a long period of time and is characterized by an inability to return to the pre-loss level of functioning.[76] Palliative care provides grief and bereavement services to patients and their caregivers before, during, and after death to help promote healthy grieving.

Both hospice and palliative care have been shown to provide effective pre-loss interventions for preventing complicated bereavement. These interventions are associated with a reduced risk of major depressive disorder in caregivers.[77] The multidisciplinary palliative care team including physicians, social workers, nurses, psychologists, and chaplains performs a psychosocial assessment of the patient and caregiver in order to identify those that may be high risk for complicated grief. The palliative care team can provide basic practical help before death such as assisting with advanced directives, assistance with financial matters, and encouraging individual medical care of the caregiver as well as providing assistance after death by offering counseling or referral to other support services.

Hospice

Hospice is a philosophy of care. The goal of hospice is to focus on maintaining the best quality of life rather than length of life in patients who have a life expectancy of 6 months or less. It is different from palliative care in that palliative care is given simultaneously with other curative and life-prolonging therapies. Hospice services have been available in the United States since 1974 and have been funded by Medicare as part of the Medicare hospice benefit since 1982.[78]

Hospice is the only Medicare benefit that includes medications, durable medical equipment, and continuous around-the-clock access to care and support. Bereavement services are also offered to family members after a patient's death. The Medicare hospice benefit covers all care related to the cancer diagnosis. The patient can still receive Medicare benefits for the treatment of other illnesses.

Most hospice care is delivered at home. It is also provided in other settings such as inpatient hospice facilities, nursing homes, assisted living facilities, and hospitals. It is estimated that approximately 45% of all people who died in the United States in 2011 were under the care of a hospice program and of all patients enrolled, 38% had a diagnosis of cancer.[79] In a study comparing survival of hospice to nonhospice patients, hospice care prolonged the lives of some terminally ill cancer patients.[80] The mean survival period was significantly longer for hospice patients with lung cancer (39 days longer) and pancreatic cancer (21 days), while marginally significant for colon cancer (33 days).[80]

Summary

Palliative care is patient- and family-centered interdisciplinary care that focuses on relieving suffering and providing the best quality of life for patients undergoing curative and life-prolonging treatments as well as for patients in whom cancer specific treatments are no longer available. It is estimated that 35% of patients with cancer will die from their disease.[81] Increasing attention has been given to improvements in quality of life issues in oncology, for patients undergoing chemotherapy, patients at the end of life as well as cancer survivors. Prevalence of symptoms during cancer treatment can be substantial. Palliative care is an integral part of comprehensive cancer care. Palliative care is most effective when initiated at the time of diagnosis allowing for patients to be followed through the trajectory of illness. The oncologist plays a key role in discussing treatment options, curative or palliative, from the outset of the diagnosis. Assessing the patients' goals is equally as important. Patients should be made aware that receiving anticancer treatments does not preclude them from access to palliative care services. Increasing the emphasis on palliative care in oncology should improve patient outcomes and can diminish some of the oncologist's stress of caring for patients with serious and life-threatening illness.

Palliative care has experienced a rapid growth in the last two decades in response to the increasing number of patients living with serious illness, an increased demand for high-quality symptom control, desire for improved coordination of care across settings and increased need for advance care planning. The number of palliative care programs within hospital settings has increased by 138% since 2000.[82] Expansion of palliative medicine education is supported by the Liaison Committee on Medical Education, which has mandated medical school education in palliative medicine, and the ACGME (accreditation council for graduate medical education), which requires oncology fellow training in palliative medicine. There is a plethora of Internet-based resources that provide physicians in practice with access to further information and education on palliative care (Table 2).

Key references

The complete reference list can be found on the Wiley Companion Digital Edition of this title (see inside front cover for login instructions).

1 Morrison RS, Meier DE. Clinical practice. Palliative care. *N Engl J Med.* 2004;**350**(25):2582–2590.
2 Temel JS, Greer JA, Muzikansky A, et al. Early palliative care for patients with metastatic non-small-cell lung cancer. *N Engl J Med.* 2010;**363**(8):733–742.
3 Bakitas M, Lyons KD, Hegel MT, et al. Effects of a palliative care intervention on clinical outcomes in patients with advanced cancer: the Project ENABLE II randomized controlled trial. *JAMA.* 2009;**302**(7):741–749.
4 Shih YC, Ganz PA, Aberle D, et al. Delivering high-quality and affordable care throughout the cancer care continuum. *J Clin Oncol.* 2013;**31**(32):4151–4157.
5 Field MJ, Cassel CK. *Approching Death: Improving Care at the End of Life.* Institute of Medicine: Washington, DC; 1997.
6 National Consensus Project for Quality Palliative Care. Clinical Practice Guidelines for quality palliative care, executive summary. *J Palliat Med.* 2004;**7**(5):611–627.
8 Buss MK, Lessen DS, Sullivan AM, Von Roenn J, Arnold RM, Block SD. A study of oncology fellows' training in end-of-life care. *J Support Oncol.* 2007;**5**(5):237–242.
9 Beach WA, Easter DW, Good JS, Pigeron E. Disclosing and responding to cancer "fears" during oncology interviews. *Soc Sci Med.* 2005;**60**(4):893–910.
10 Detmar SB, Muller MJ, Wever LD, Schornagel JH, Aaronson NK. The patient-physician relationship. Patient-physician communication during outpatient palliative treatment visits: an observational study. *JAMA.* 2001;**285**(10):1351–1357.
11 Baile WF, Aaron J. Patient-physician communication in oncology: past, present, and future. *Curr Opin Oncol.* 2005;**17**(4):331–335.
12 Zachariae R, Pedersen CG, Jensen AB, Ehrnrooth E, Rossen PB, von der Maase H. Association of perceived physician communication style with patient satisfaction, distress, cancer-related self-efficacy, and perceived control over the disease. *Br J Cancer.* 2003;**88**(5):658–665.
13 Baile WF, Buckman R, Lenzi R, Glober G, Beale EA, Kudelka AP. SPIKES-A six-step protocol for delivering bad news: application to the patient with cancer. *Oncologist.* 2000;**5**(4):302–311.
19 Hammes BJ, Rooney BL, Gundrum JD. A comparative, retrospective, observational study of the prevalence, availability, and specificity of advance care plans in a county that implemented an advance care planning microsystem. *J Am Geriatr Soc.* 2010;**58**(7):1249–1255.

20 Bruera E, Kuehn N, Miller MJ, Selmser P, Macmillan K. The Edmonton Symptom Assessment System (ESAS): a simple method for the assessment of palliative care patients. *J Palliat Care.* 1991;**7**(2):6–9.
22 International Association for the Study of Pain. http://www.iasp-pain.org/AM/Template.cfm?Section=Pain_Defi … isplay.cfm&ContentID=1728, accessed 23 November, 2010.
24 Du Pen SL, Du Pen AR, Polissar N, et al. Implementing guidelines for cancer pain management: results of a randomized controlled clinical trial. *J Clin Oncol.* 1999;**17**(1):361–370.
25 Moulin DE, Clark AJ, Gilron I, et al. Pharmacological management of chronic neuropathic pain—consensus statement and guidelines from the Canadian Pain Society. *Pain Res Manag.* 2007;**127**(1):13–21.
26 Levy MH, Adolph MD, Back A, et al. Palliative care. *J Natl Compr Cancer Netw.* 2012;**10**(10):1284–1309.
28 Davies AN, Dickman A, Reid C, Stevens A-M, Zeppetella G. The management of cancer-related breakthrough pain: recommendations of a task group of the Science Committee of the Association for Palliative Medicine of Great Britain and Ireland. *Eur J Pain.* 2009;**13**(4):331–338.
29 Miguel R. Interventional treatment of cancer pain: the fourth step in the World Health Organization analgesic ladder? *Cancer Control.* 2000;**7**(2):149–156.
33 Hawley PH, Byeon JJ. A comparison of sennosides-based bowel protocols with and without docusate in hospitalized patients with cancer. *J Palliat Med.* 2008;**11**(4):575–581.
36 Wood GJ, Shega JW, Lynch B, Von Roenn JH. Management of intractable nausea and vomiting in patients at the end of life: "I was feeling nauseous all of the time … nothing was working". *JAMA.* 2007;**298**(10):1196–1207.
38 (NCCN) NCCN. Antiemesis. NCCN Clinical Practice Guidelines in Oncology. Version 1.2013; http://www.nccn.org/professionals/physician_gls/pdf/antiemesis.pdf (accessed 28 January 2013).
39 Stephenson J, Davies A. An assessment of aetiology-based guidelines for the management of nausea and vomiting in patients with advanced cancer. *Support Care Cancer.* 2006;**14**(4):348–353.
41 Bruera E, Belzile M, Neumann C, Harsanyi Z, Babul N, Darke A. A double-blind, crossover study of controlled-release metoclopramide and placebo for the chronic nausea and dyspepsia of advanced cancer. *J Pain Symptom Manage.* 2000;**19**(6):427–435.
49 Servaes P, Verhagen C, Bleijenberg G. Fatigue in cancer patients during and after treatment: prevalence, correlates and interventions. *Eur J Cancer.* 2002;**38**(1):27–43.
51 Loprinzi CL, Michalak JC, Schaid DJ, et al. Phase III evaluation of four doses of megestrol acetate as therapy for patients with cancer anorexia and/or cachexia. *J Clin Oncol.* 1993;**11**(4):762–767.
57 Bruera E, Sweeney C, Willey J, et al. A randomized controlled trial of supplemental oxygen versus air in cancer patients with dyspnea. *Palliat Med.* 2003;**17**(8):659–663.
63 McCann RM, Hall WJ, Groth-Juncker A. Comfort care for terminally ill patients. The appropriate use of nutrition and hydration. *JAMA.* 1994;**272**(16):1263–1266.
64 Musgrave CF, Bartal N, Opstad J. The sensation of thirst in dying patients receiving i.v. hydration. *J Palliat Care.* 1995;**11**(4):17–21.
65 Koretz RL, Lipman TO, Klein S, American Gastroenterological Association. AGA technical review on parenteral nutrition. *Gastroenterology.* 2001;**121**(4):970–1001.
66 Koretz RL, Avenell A, Lipman TO, Braunschweig CL, Milne AC. Does enteral nutrition affect clinical outcome? A systematic review of the randomized trials. *Am J Gastroenterol.* 2007;**102**(2):412–429; quiz 468.
73 Bruera E, Hui D, Dalal S, et al. Parenteral hydration in patients with advanced cancer: a multicenter, double-blind, placebo-controlled randomized trial. *J Clin Oncol.* 2013;**31**(1):111–118.
79 National Hospice and Palliative Care Organization. NHPCO's Facts and Figures Hospice Care in America. http://www.nhpco.org/sites/default/files/public/Statistics_Research/2012_Facts_Figures.pdf, accessed January 2015; 2012.
80 Connor SR, Pyenson B, Fitch K, Spence C, Iwasaki K. Comparing hospice and non-hospice patient survival among patients who die within a three-year window. *J Pain Symptom Manage.* 2007;**33**(3):238–246.
81 Siegel RL, Miller KD, Jemal A. Cancer statistics, 2015. *CA Cancer J Clin.* 2015;**65**(1):5–29.
82 Center to Advance Pallaitive Care. *Public Opinion Research on Palliative Care: A Report Based on Reseach by Public Opinion Strategies*; 2011.

47 Principles of psycho-oncology

Jimmie C. Holland, MD ■ Talia W. Wiesel, PhD

Overview

This chapter provides oncologists with the present state of the art in psycho-oncology, a subspecialty that has evolved over the past 30 years. The basic treatment, particularly pharmacologic, is outlined for anxiety, depression, and delirium, as well as the psychotherapeutic interventions which are based on evidence. The field has come of age since it received the Institute of Medicine blessing in 2008 stating that quality cancer care must integrate the psychosocial domain in routine care. This was given a strong boost from the American College of Surgeons Commission on Cancer which made screening for distress a quality standard for accreditation in 2015, requiring that all cancer centers have in place—or in development—an on-site program to identify and triage patients who are distressed. This has resulted in a strong effort to develop routine screening of all new patients to assure that they are recognized early and treated appropriately. Implementation of programs is in progress across the country with assistance available from the American Psychosocial Oncology Society (APOS) which has organized training, consultation, and ongoing mentoring for cancer staff. Indeed, thanks to these changes in national policy related to cancer, it is a different experience for patients today to cope with cancer. Attention has turned to providing patient-centered care which encompasses care of the whole person.

Psychiatric terms seem poorly descriptive of the emotional responses of cancer patients who are finding ways of coping with an overwhelming but "real" reality. Words such as courage and strength often appear more appropriate

J.C. Holland, Cancer Medicine, 1973, p. 992

Introduction

The above quote appeared in the first edition of Cancer Medicine in 1973. Over the past 40 years, the human aspects of cancer care have not changed in terms of patients' emotions. However, there is now a range of interventions to make the journey more tolerable. Part of this remarkable change relates to contributions from psycho-oncology. These changes were made possible by, first, the development of assessment tools, which quantitatively measured subjective symptoms that were previously considered unmeasurable. Second, these tools permitted conduct of clinical trials, which resulted in evidence-based interventions. These were integrated in the first NCCN Clinical Practice Guidelines in Oncology (NCCN Guidelines®) for Distress Management, in the late 1990s.[1] The third event was the first policy statement noting this body of work by the Institute of Medicine in its report in 2008, Care of the Whole Patient, which stated that the psychosocial domain must be integrated into routine care.[2] This was carried to an even higher policy level by the American College of Surgeons Commission on Cancer, which, in 2015, required accredited cancer centers to have a program in place to identify and refer distressed patients for appropriate care.[3] This has led to efforts by psycho-oncologists to help the multidisciplinary teams at cancer centers implement this new policy.[4,5] Patients in the future should be identified earlier in the course of illness by these routine screening programs. However, the new procedure places a bigger burden on oncologists in busy practices to assure that patients with identified distress are treated by the primary team or referred for more specialized psychosocial care. Figure 1 presents the NCCN Guideline® for evaluation and treatment suggesting that all new patients be screened for distress.[6] Figure 2 shows the NCCN single question recommended for identifying distressed patients in busy clinics. Patients and oncologists have found asking the question, "How is your distress level on a scale of 0 to10" to be acceptable, brief, and nonstigmatizing. Called the Distress Thermometer, it is widely utilized internationally, containing the scale and a Problem List to identify frequent causes of distress. Validation studies have found that a score of 4 or more should prompt a second evaluation by a team member to determine the nature of the distress and if the patient should be referred to mental health, social work, or chaplaincy.

This chapter outlines the basic information an oncologist needs for rapid assessment and management of the most common psychiatric complications.[7]

Clinical management

Vulnerable patients

Patients who are most vulnerable to distress are those with[8]:
- Prior psychiatric disorder (depression and substance abuse)
- Cognitive problems
- Language or communication problems
- Comorbid medical illnesses
- Social problems (family, financial, and living alone)
- Spiritual or religious concerns.

Points of increased vulnerability to distress for patients with cancer[8]
- Finding a symptoms suspicious of cancer
- Learning the cancer diagnosis
- Waiting for biopsy and genomic testing of tumor tissue to determine mutations to guide targeted treatment
- Awaiting initial treatment
- Transitions in treatment
- Finish of curative treatment
- Transition from curative to palliative care
- Advanced cancer and end of life
- Fears of recurrence during survivorship.

Holland-Frei Cancer Medicine, Ninth Edition. Edited by Robert C. Bast Jr., Carlo M. Croce, William N. Hait, Waun Ki Hong, Donald W. Kufe, Martine Piccart-Gebhart, Raphael E. Pollock, Ralph R. Weichselbaum, Hongyang Wang, and James F. Holland.
© 2017 John Wiley & Sons, Inc. ISBN: 978-1-118-93469-2

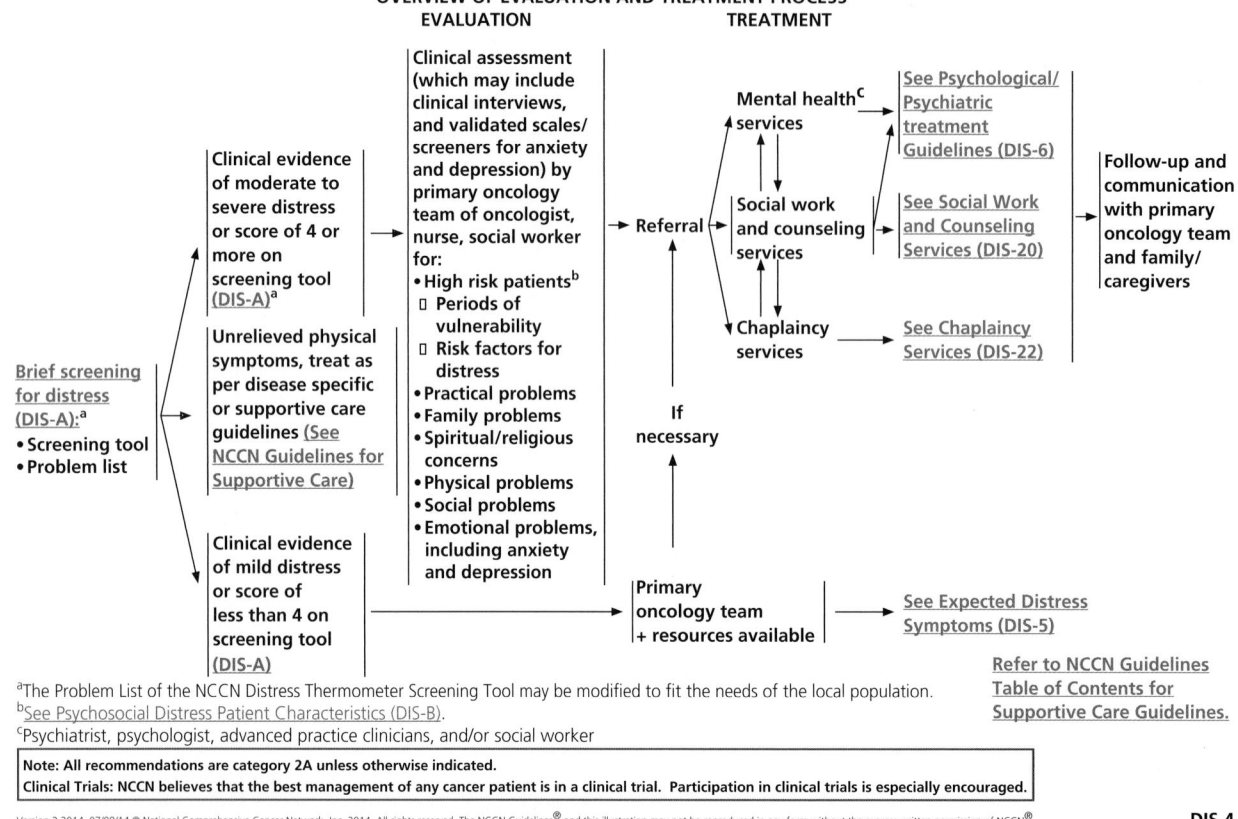

Figure 1 NCCN Guideline®. Source: Reproduced with permission from the NCCN Clinical Practice Guidelines in Oncology (NCCN Guidelines®) for Distress Management V.2.2014. © 2014 National Comprehensive Cancer Network, Inc. All rights reserved. The NCCN Guidelines® and illustrations herein may not be reproduced in any form for any purpose without the express written permission of the NCCN. To view the most recent and complete version of the NCCN Guidelines, go online to NCCN.org. NATIONAL COMPREHENSIVE CANCER NETWORK®, NCCN®, NCCN GUIDELINES®, and all other NCCN Content are trademarks owned by the National Comprehensive Cancer Network, Inc.

Among these patients, most are managed well by the primary oncology team. Situational anxiety, sadness, insomnia, fatigue, fears, and concerns are common and respond to reassurance and medication. However, some patients experience more difficulty coping and have significant distress that requires more aggressive interventions. Management of the most commonly occurring psychiatric disorders is outlined below for anxiety, depression, suicidal risk, delirium, and personality disorders.

Anxiety disorders

Anxiety occurs as a reaction to the threat of illness, but it also occurs from a range of metabolic states and medications, requiring a careful clinical review of these issues. It may occur with panic attacks (tachycardia and hyperventilation) and depressive symptoms. Treatment may be psychological by psychotherapy, particularly cognitive–behavioral approaches; relaxation and meditation are useful, as well as online interventions. If anxiety persists or is severe, several medications are useful. Table 1 outlines the most commonly used drugs. However, olanzapine, an antipsychotic, is also often used off label to treat severe anxiety with good result.

Table 1 Pharmacological treatment of anxiety.

Drug	Starting dose	Maintenance dose
Selective serotonin reuptake inhibitors		
Escitalopram (Lexapro®)	10–20 mg	10–20 mg/day PO
Fluoxetine (Prozac®)	10–20 mg qAM	20–60 mg/day PO
Citalopram (Celexa®)	10–20 mg	10–20 mg/day PO
Benzodiazepines		
Alprazolam (Xanax®)	0.25–1.0 mg	PO q 6–24 h
Clonazepam (Klonopin®)	0.5–2.0 mg	PO q 6–24 h
Diazepam (Valium®)	2–10 mg	PO/IV q 6–24 h
Lorazepam (Ativan®)	0.5–2.0 mg	PO/IM/IVP/IVPB q 4–12 h

Abbreviations: IM, intramuscular; IVP, IV push; IVPB, IV piggyback; PO, oral.
Data from *Psycho-Oncology: A Quick Reference on the Psychosocial Dimensions of Cancer Symptom Management.*[7]

Depressive disorders and suicidal risk

Depressive disorders

Sadness is part of the normal response to cancer; however, more significant symptoms are lack of pleasure (anhedonia), hopelessness, and despair. They often contribute to stopping or delaying

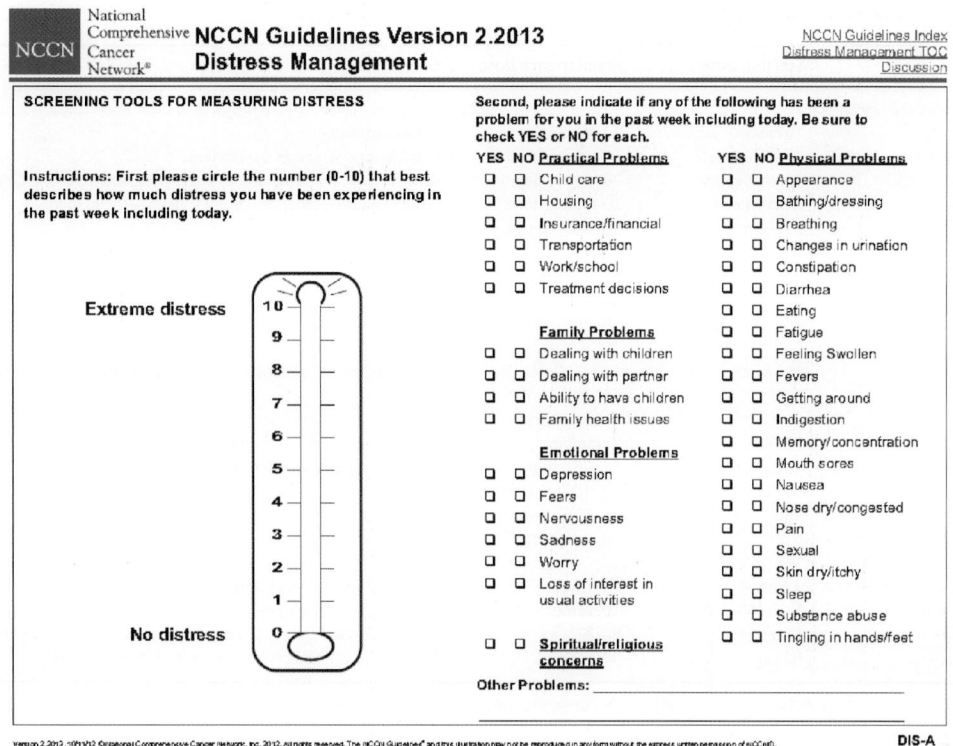

Figure 2 NCCN Distress Thermometer. Source: Reproduced with permission from the NCCN Clinical Practice Guidelines in Oncology (NCCN Guidelines®) for Distress Management V.2.2014. © 2014 National Comprehensive Cancer Network, Inc. All rights reserved. The NCCN Guidelines® and illustrations herein may not be reproduced in any form for any purpose without the express written permission of the NCCN. To view the most recent and complete version of the NCCN Guidelines, go online to NCCN.org. NATIONAL COMPREHENSIVE CANCER NETWORK®, NCCN®, NCCN GUIDELINES®, and all other NCCN Content are trademarks owned by the National Comprehensive Cancer Network, Inc.

treatment, and thereby, contribute to a poorer outcome. These symptoms may be accompanied by insomnia, fatigue, and anorexia, all of which must be differentiated from cancer-related causes. The symptoms may be psychological in origin, but drug side effects, metabolic abnormalities, and paraneoplastic disorders also cause depression.

Treatment may be psychological alone, using supportive and cognitive psychotherapy approaches, as well as behavioral interventions of relaxation and meditation. If the symptoms persist or are severe, a combined psychological and medication approach is useful. Table 2 outlines the medications, which are recommended, including psychostimulants, which are increasingly used for patients with fatigue and poor concentration.

Suicidal risk

Many patients comment "If things get bad enough, I will kill myself." Few rarely come to that point. It seems to represent a way to emotionally maintain control over the disease. However, any suicidal threat must be taken seriously and evaluated. Thoughts about it must be explored. Questions to open the discussion may be, "Have you felt like you did not want to live anymore?" There is greater concern if the person outlines a plan. Those at the highest risk of suicide are patients with

- Prior psychiatric or suicide attempt history
- Severe uncontrolled pain
- Advanced disease
- Mild delirium (interfering with rational judgment)
- Alcohol and substance use.

Recognizing patients at higher risk for suicide[8]

- Initial diagnosis of advanced disease
- Risk of suicide is highest within the first month and remains high for 6 months
- Lung cancer has the highest suicide rates followed by head and neck, stomach, pancreas, and colon
- Anticipation of debilitating or deforming surgery
- Patients with depression, hopelessness, or guilt for being a burden
- Severe pain that is constant and poorly controlled.

It is important in evaluating suicide risk to treat it as a possible psychiatric emergency. The person should not be left alone until the level of risk is fully assessed. If risk is high, referral to a safe environment may be necessary. However, this is often difficult in a patient with advanced cancer, and every effort should be made to maintain the patient in the same environment, controlling any physical symptoms, particularly pain. Consultation with a mental health professional may be needed, with full involvement of family to continue surveillance at home.

Delirium

Delirium is common in hospitalized patients, particularly in the postoperative state, and among older people who may have underlying mild cognitive impairment. It is often under-recognized and undertreated as it occurs commonly with fever, drugs, metabolic disturbances, central nervous system metastases, and paraneoplastic disorders. The classic symptoms are acute onset with fluctuating attention and confusion and either psychomotor slowing or agitation. Misperceptions (illusions) of the environment are common as are visual or auditory hallucinations, usually paranoid

Table 2 Selected antidepressants to treat depression in cancer patients.

Drug	Starting dose	Maintenance dose	Comments
Selective serotonin reuptake inhibitors			
Citalopram (Celexa®)	10 mg/day	20–40 mg/day	Soltabs available
Escitalopram (Lexapro®)	5–10 mg/day	10–20 mg/day	Possible nausea, sexual dysfunction
Fluoxetine (Prozac®)	10–20 mg/day	20–60 mg/day	Long half-life; possible nausea, sexual dysfunction; strong CYP450-2 D6 inhibitor
Paroxetine (Paxil®)	20 mg/day	20–60 mg/day	Possible nausea, sedation, strong CYP450-2D6 inhibitor
Sertraline (Zoloft®)	25–50 mg/day	50–150 mg/day	Possible nausea
Tricyclic antidepressants			
Amitriptyline (Elavil®)	25–50 mg qhs	50–200 mg/day	Maximal sedation; anticholinergic effects; useful for neuropathic pain
Desipramine (Norpramin®)	25–50 mg/day	50–200 mg/day	Modest sedation; anticholinergic
Nortriptyline (Pamelor®)	25–50 mg qhs	50–200 mg/day	Moderate sedation; useful for neuropathic pain
Other agents			
Bupropion (Wellbutrin®)	100 mg/day	100–400 mg/ day 450 mg/day XL; 400 mg/day SR	Activating; sexual dysfunction; seizure risk in predisposed patients
Duloxetine (Cymbalta®)	20–40 mg/day	60 mg/day	Possible nausea, dry mouth; may be useful for neuropathic pain
Mirtazapine (Remeron®)	15 mg qhs	15–45 mg qhs	Sedating, variable appetite-stimulant, antiemetic effects
Desvenlafaxine (Pristiq®)	50 mg daily	50–100 mg daily	Nausea
Venlafaxine (Effexor®)	18.75–37.5 mg/ day	75–225 mg/day; XR once daily	May be used for neuropathic pain, hot flashes, nausea
Psychostimulants			
Dextroamphetamine (Dexedrine®)	2.5 mg BID	5-30 mg	Possible blood pressure/cardiac complications
Methylphenidate (Ritalin®)	5 mg BID	10-60 mg	Agitation, anxiety, nausea
Modafinil (Provigil®)	50 mg BID	50-200 mg	Activating, nausea, cardiac side effects; usually well tolerated
Armodafinil (Nuvigil®)	50 mg	50–200 mg	Morning only; headache, nausea, dizziness, dry mouth

Data from *Psycho-Oncology: A Quick Reference on the Psychosocial Dimensions of Cancer Symptom Management.*[7]

in nature. Medications that control these symptoms are antipsychotics, benzodiazepines, and short-acting anesthetics that are used primarily in intensive care units. The patient must be placed in a safe environment, which may include use of physical restraints to prevent self-harm from pulling out catheters and tubes. Constant observation initially is important, best in an intensive care unit or in a quiet room with familiar figures, including family members, who can reassure and reorient the patient to the environment. See Table 3 for drugs that are commonly utilized.

Personality disorders

Patients with personality disorders are difficult because there is no distinct psychiatric disorder *per se* to treat, and the oncologist must deal with the unusual ideas and behaviors of the patient that can impact treatment. There are several personality types that are most difficult during cancer treatment.

Paranoid disorder. These patients are suspicious, quickly take offense, and can be argumentative and angry with oncology team members.

Borderline disorder. These patients act out their emotions and may make suicide attempts, have wide mood swings, and often challenge the team with demands that cannot be met. It is necessary to set boundaries and alert *all* team members about the treatment plan.

Histrionic disorder. These patients tend to dramatize symptoms. They express intense emotions that can be difficult to manage. They are suggestible and may be sexually provocative. Awareness of these qualities is important.

Narcissistic disorder. The patient is self-centered, is entitled, expects to be treated as "special," is arrogant, and seems to care little for the problems of others.

Obsessive compulsive. These patients are concerned with minute details about illness and treatment and are demanding of self and others. They lack flexibility and may have compulsive rituals.

Table 3 Selected medications for management of delirium in cancer patients.

Antipsychotics		
Haloperidol[a] (Haldol®)	0.5–5 mg q 30 min–12 h PO, IM, IV	
Chlorpromazine[a] (Thorazine®)	25–100 mg q 4–12 h PO, IM, IV	
Risperidone (Risperdal®)	0.5–2 mg q 12 h PO	
Olanzapine (Zyprexa®)	2.5–5 mg q 12–24 h PO, IM	
Quetiapine (Seroquel®)	12.5–50 mg q 12 h PO	
Benzodiazepines		
Lorazepam[a] (Ativan®)	0.5–2 mg q 1–4 h PO, IM, IV	Only in the setting of alcohol withdrawal delirium
Midazolam[a] (Versed®)	0.003 mg/kg/h titrate to effect IV (per anesthesiologist)	
Anesthetics		
Propofol[a] (Diprivan®)	0.5 mg/kg/h titrate to effect IV	Rapid onset of sedation and recovery
Alpha agonists		
Dexmedetomidine (Precedex®)	1 mcg/kg over 10 min followed by continuous infusion 0.2–0.7 mcg/kg/h	Rapid onset sedation and recovery; no effect on cognition
Intensive care setting: Propofol and dexmedetomidine provide rapid onset of sedation and recovery		

[a]May be administered by continuous infusion usually in the intensive care setting.
Data from *Psycho-Oncology: A Quick Reference on the Psychosocial Dimensions of Cancer Symptom Management.*[7]

Dependent disorder. These are patients who lack self-confidence, need frequent reassurance, and have trouble making decisions. These traits interfere with treatment and often require greater time for emotional support.

The primary issue for the oncologist is to be aware of these characteristics in patients and not to respond personally to their quirks but recognize that they are part of a personality pattern. An oncology team does well to discuss those patients with severe disorders and share the emotional stress. Unfortunately, they are often angered by suggestion of a psychiatric referral and will refuse it.

Psychosocial interventions

A number of clinical trials have given an evidence base for several nonpharmacologic psychosocial interventions.[5,9]

Psychotherapies in cancer care

Cognitive therapies

While supportive psychotherapy is at the heart of relating to all patients, several cognitive-based therapies have shown efficacy. Cognitive-behavioral therapy (CBT) is widely used for anxiety and depressive symptoms[10] as well as post-traumatic stress disorder (PTSD). It is a short-term therapy that addresses the current issues of coping with illness and assists the patient to perceive fears and concerns in a more constructive way. Problem-solving therapy encourages seeing illness in a new way, being optimistic, planning with family and patient to address the challenges together. Interpersonal psychotherapy concentrates on the changed relationships caused by illness and explores ways to relate to the altered roles. These therapies can be learned rapidly by psycho-oncology clinicians. There are also therapies now that are developed for special problems, such as grief. Others are directed for use at a particular stage of illness or age, particularly therapies developed for adolescents, young adults, and older patients. Dignity therapy and mindfulness-based therapy address the issues at the end of life, providing a comforting perspective.

Behavioral interventions

Behavioral interventions have also proven of value in cancer patients. Progressive muscle relaxation (PMR) exercises, guided by a person or a tape, are helpful for insomnia and anxiety, and once learned, they can be applied by the patient when needed. Mindfulness-based stress reduction/meditation has been studied and is widely practiced, coming from the eastern Buddhist tradition. It is learned in individual or group sessions and is best applied as a daily practice, which has a calming effect on anxiety. Similarly, guided imagery has a soothing effect. Physical exercise, on a daily basis, as illness will allow, is highly recommended today throughout treatment and as a health habit for survivors. It has both mental and physical benefits.

Group and online therapies

Groups for psychosocial support have proven their value over many years. They are most effective when they bring together patients who are coping with the same cancer. The sharing of experience is highly beneficial and supportive. Today, virtual groups are common, and they too have proven efficacious by telephone and online. Less research has been done on these newer approaches, but they are increasingly used with far less cost and likely will become more popular. Helplines are part of advocacy organizations' services, such as Cancer Care and Cancer Support Community. All have web sites with reliable information and directories of mental health clinicians who accept referrals. Helplines for specific sites of cancer also provide a telephone "buddy" who matches the situation of the person calling for help. Excellent resources for information about psychological support are CancerCare 1800-813-HOPE (4673) (www.cancercare.org) and Cancer Support Community (CSC) 1-888-793-9355 (www.cancersupportcommunity.org).

Today, patients have access to a range of psychological supports that vary from free online telephone counseling to individual therapy sessions based on fee for service. Insurance for psychiatric and psychological visits is not yet on parity with medical coverage, but there is optimism that this may be achieved in the near future. There is a shortage of mental health professionals trained in psycho-oncology to meet the present clinical need, in part because reimbursement is so low.

Complementary therapies

Today, there is a range of interventions that patients may choose from which fit their lifestyle best. Art therapy is a very good way to express emotions. Music and dance therapies are available and also provide support. Writing and guided reading are both therapeutic. Most cancer centers have integrative therapies available for patients so that they can choose the complementary therapy they want, which includes acupuncture, nutritional advice, and psychological and behavioral interventions.

Burnout in oncology

Caring for patients with cancer demands time and emotional resources of the oncologist and the team. When the stress is severe or prolonged, it is called burnout syndrome. Surveys suggest that it affects approximately one-third of medical oncologists[11-17] and may be higher for radiation oncologists.[18-20] The syndrome was first described by Freudenberger[21] in 1974. It comprised symptoms in three areas: emotional exhaustion, depersonalization (reduced capacity for empathy), and a sense of low achievement.[22] The syndrome has professional and personal consequences for the physician. It impairs clinical judgment, which can lead to medical error.[23,24] Similarly, risk of suicide is greater.

A national study of 7000 physicians revealed a slightly lower prevalence of burnout for medical oncologists (37.9%) than other internal medicine physicians (48.8%).[25] They more often experienced depression. However, they more often said that they would repeat their choice of medical oncology if given the chance.

The causes of burnout are related to prolonged heavy work schedules, increased demands, and conflicts between work and personal life. Oncologists work a median of 63 h/week, compared to the average physician 50-h work week.[26] Malpractice suits increase the risk of burnout. Medical oncologists carry the highest risk among nonsurgical specialties.[27]

Burnout is preventable and treatable, but it requires being alert to its diagnosis responds to early intervention. Prospective studies suggest that training oncologists through self-awareness techniques and mindfulness-based meditation results in improved empathy and less depression.[28,29] Physical exercise is useful for both its physical and mental effects. Studies are investigating teaching resilience in medical school curricula.[30,31] Physicians who note a high level of positive meaning in their work, who have a reasonable work–life balance, and who focus on clear priorities are less vulnerable to burnout.[32,33] There is also an advantage in working in an environment where referral for family or social problems is encouraged. Many physicians blame their distress on work when, in fact, they are suffering from serious unacknowledged problems in marriage and home life.

Summary

The person who is treated for cancer today experiences a far more psychologically supportive environment than 40 years ago. Society is better educated about cancer, which has reduced fears and stigma. The successes of cancer therapies have resulted in 14 million survivors. Today, patients have access to a more empathic primary oncology clinic team whom they come to know well and rely on. In addition, there are often social work and mental health resources available, as well as dietitians, rehabilitation medicine, and complementary therapies. Patients with significant distress are increasingly being identified earlier in their course of treatment through routine screening and are referred to counselors. As compared to the situation in 1973, as described in the first edition of Cancer Medicine, the 40 years has produced a remarkable increase in concern about patients' well-being during cancer treatment. Psycho-oncology has had a role in this change through the development of a science of its own, which has resulted in a range of evidence-based psychological, behavioral, and pharmacologic interventions. The challenge today is to implement the psychosocial domain into routine care so that no patients who are distressed go untreated.

References

1 Holland JC, Benedeti C, Breitbart W, et al. Update: NCCN practice Guidelines for the management of psychosocial distress Version 1.2000. *Oncology*. 1999;**11(11A)**:459–507 © 1999 National Comprehensive Cancer Network.

2 Institute of Medicine. *Cancer Care for the Whole Patient: Meeting Psychosocial Health Needs*. Washington, DC: The National Academies Press; 2008.

3 Jacobsen PB, Wagner L. A new quality standard: the integration of psychosocial care into routine cancer care. *J Clin Onc*. 2012;**30**:1154–1159.

4 Pirl WF, Fann JR, Greer JA, et al. Recommendations for the implementation of distress screening programs in cancer centers: Report from the American Psychosocial Oncology Society (APOS), Association of Oncology Social Work (AOSW), and Oncology Nursing Society (ONS) joint task force. *Cancer*. 2014;**120**:2946–2954.

5 Holland JC, Breitbart WS, Jacobsen PB, Loscalzo MJ, McCorkle R, Butow PN. *Psycho-Oncology*, 3rd ed. New York, NY: Oxford University Press; 2015.

6 Holland JC, et al., NCCN Clinical Practice Guidelines in Oncology (NCCN Guidelines®) Distress Management Version 2. © 2014 National Comprehensive Cancer Network, Inc. Available at NCCN.org (accessed 1 February 2015); 2014.

7 Holland JC, Golant M, Greenberg DB, et al. *Psycho-Oncology: A Quick Reference on the Psychosocial Dimensions of Cancer Symptom Management*; New York, NY: Oxford University Press; 2015.

8 Holland JC, Weiss Wiesel T, Nelson CJ, Roth AJ, Alici Y. *Geriatric Psycho-Oncology: A Quick Reference on the Psychosocial Dimensions of Cancer Symptom Management*. New York, NY: Oxford University Press; 2015.

9 Golant M, Loscalzo M, Walsh M. *Psychological Non-pharmacological Interventions. Psycho-Oncology: A Quick Reference on the Psychosocial Dimensions of Cancer Symptom Management*, 2nd ed. New York, NY: Oxford University Press; 2015.

10 Watson M, Kissane D. *Handbook of Psychotherapy in Cancer Care*. Wiley; 2011.

11 Ramirez AJ, Graham J, Richards MA, et al. Burnout and psychiatric disorder among cancer clinicians. *Br J Cancer*. 1995;**71**:1263–1269.

12 Shanafelt T, Dyrbye L. Oncologist burnout: causes, consequences, and responses. *J Clin Oncol*. 2012;**30**:1235–1241.

13 Allegra CJ, Hall R, Yothers G. Prevalence of burnout in the U.S. Oncology community: results of a 2003 survey. *J Oncol Pract*. 2005;**1**:140–147.

14 Whippen DA, Canellos GP. Burnout syndrome in the practice of oncology: results of a random survey of 1,000 oncologists. *J Clin Oncol*. 1991;**9**:1916–1920.

15 Arigoni F, Bovier PA, Mermillod B, Waltz P, Sappino AP. Prevalence of burnout among Swiss cancer clinicians, paediatricians and general practitioners: who are most at risk? *Support Care Cancer*. 2009;**17**:75–81.

16 Grunfeld E, Whelan TJ, Zitzelsberger L, Willan AR, Montesanto B, Evans WK. Cancer care workers in Ontario: prevalence of burnout, job stress and job satisfaction. *CMAJ*. 2000;**163**:166–169.

17 Grunfeld E, Zitzelsberger L, Coristine M, Whelan TJ, Aspelund F, Evans WK. Job stress and job satisfaction of cancer care workers. *Psychooncology*. 2005;**14**: 61–69.

18 Dyrbye LN, Shanafelt TD. Physician burnout: a potential threat to successful health care reform. *JAMA*. 2011;**305**:2009–2010.

19 Kuerer HM, Eberlein TJ, Pollock RE, et al. Career satisfaction, practice patterns and burnout among surgical oncologists: report on the quality of life of members of the Society of Surgical Oncology. *Ann Surg Oncol*. 2007;**14**:3043–3053.

20 Balch CM, Shanafelt TD, Sloan J, Satele DV, Kuerer HM. Burnout and career satisfaction among surgical oncologists compared with other surgical specialties. *Ann Surg Oncol*. 2011;**18**:16–25.

21 Freudenberger HJ. Staff burnout. *J Soc Issues*. 1974;**30**:159–165.

22 Cherniss C. *Staff Burnout: Job Stress in Human Services*. Beverly Hill: Sage Publications; 1980.

23 Shanafelt TD, Balch CM, Dyrbye L, et al. Special report: suicidal ideation among American surgeons. *Arch Surg*. 2011;**146**:54–62.

24 Dyrbye LN, Thomas MR, Massie FS, et al. Burnout and suicidal ideation among U.S. medical students. *Ann Intern Med*. 2008;**149**:334–341.

25 Shanafelt TD, Boone S, Tan L, et al. Burnout and satisfaction with work-life balance among US physicians relative to the general US population. *Arch Intern Med*. 2012;**172**:1377–1385.

26 Wetterneck TB, Linzer M, McMurray JE, et al. Worklife and satisfaction of general internists. *Arch Intern Med*. 2002;**162**:649–656.

27 Jena AB, Seabury S, Lakdawalla D, Chandra A. Malpractice risk according to physician specialty. *N Engl J Med*. 2011;**365**:629–636.

28 Krasner MS, Epstein RM, Beckman H, et al. Association of an educational program in mindful communication with burnout, empathy, and attitudes among primary care physicians. *JAMA*. 2009;**302**:1284–1293.

29 Epstein RM. Mindful practice. *JAMA*. 1999;**282**:833–839.

30 Epstein RM, Krasner MS. Physician resilience: what it means, why it matters, and how to promote it. *Acad Med J Assoc Am Med Coll*. 2013;**88**:301–303.

31 Dyrbye LN, Power DV, Massie FS, et al. Factors associated with resilience to and recovery from burnout: a prospective, multi-institutional study of US medical students. *Med Educ*. 2010;**44**:1016–1026.

32 Shanafelt T, Chung H, White H, Lyckholm LJ. Shaping your career to maximize personal satisfaction in the practice of oncology. *J Clin Oncol Off J Am Soc Clin Oncol*. 2006;**24**:4020–4026.

33 Shanafelt TD, Novotny P, Johnson ME, et al. The well-being and personal wellness promotion strategies of medical oncologists in the North Central Cancer Treatment Group. *Oncology*. 2005;**68**:23–32.

48 Principles of cancer rehabilitation medicine

Michael D. Stubblefield, MD ▪ David C. Thomas, MD, MHPE ▪ Kristjan T. Ragnarsson, MD

Overview

Many of the more than 14 million cancer survivors in the United States suffer from complications of disease and treatments such as surgery, chemotherapy, and radiotherapy. Restoring and maintaining the cancer survivors' function and quality of life often requires specialized rehabilitative services. The cancer rehabilitation specialist is dedicated to the identification, evaluation, and rehabilitation of neuromuscular, musculoskeletal, pain, and functional disorders associated with cancer and its treatment. This discusses the principles and practice of rehabilitation in this challenging group of patients.

Introduction

The cancer rehabilitation specialist focuses on the identification, evaluation, and rehabilitation of neuromuscular, musculoskeletal, pain, and functional disorders associated with cancer and its treatment emphasizing the restoration and maintenance of function and quality of life. There are now more than 14 million cancer survivors in the Unites States.[1] This number is expected to grow to more than 18 million by 2020.[2] Many of these patients have complications of disease and treatment that are often compounded by medical comorbidities that require specialized rehabilitative services. This chapter discusses the role of the rehabilitation medicine specialist in restoring and maintaining function and quality of life to select groups of cancer survivors including those with cancer of the brain, head and neck, breast, and those with spinal cord dysfunction (SCD).

The rehabilitation team

Organized cancer rehabilitation programs can significantly improve a patient's physical function and community reintegration.[3-6] An integral part of such programs is an interdisciplinary cancer rehabilitation and adaptation team. The exact composition of the team varies considerably, depending on the program's philosophy and size, the type of institution, and the range of disabilities encountered. Ideally, the team should be led by a physiatrist. The team members and their roles are described in Table 1.

Cancer of the brain

Brain damage may result from primary tumors of the brain, metastases, or treatments such as surgery, radiation, and chemotherapy. The symptoms and resulting disability vary extensively, but are often similar to those seen after a stroke (Table 2). Functional recovery in patients with brain tumors is equivalent to that of patients with acute stroke.[7] The deficits are determined by the location and size of the brain lesion, but their variability demands individual evaluation and treatment planning. All patients with brain cancer and impaired function in mobility and activities of daily living (ADL) should be referred for rehabilitation with a goal of helping them become independent in these two areas. The length of stay in an inpatient rehabilitation facility for patients with a brain tumor is generally shorter than for patients with traumatic brain injury and stroke.[8,9] Simple instructions, training by therapists, and provision of assistive devices may help the patient to quickly regain greater or even total independence. When life expectancy appears to be good and deficits are more profound, a comprehensive inpatient rehabilitation program may be the best option. Strengthening of weak muscles, stretching of tight joints and muscles along with skills training can be very effective in order to restore mobility and self-care functions. Reduction of spasticity with thorough frequent stretching of all joints, appropriate medications, and targeted use of botulinum toxin injections can be very helpful. Impaired balance and abnormal gait may be related to muscle weakness, fatigue, spasticity, proprioceptive loss, as well as diminished vision and cognition. All of these increase the risk of falling. Such risk may be decreased by muscle strengthening and aerobic exercises, balance and gait training using proper mobility aids (canes, crutches, walkers), wearing proper shoes and orthoses, modification of the home and workplace environment, reducing use of sedating drugs, and so on. Control of pain is important as well as elimination of joint contractures. Various visual deficits, including double vision and field deficits, need to be addressed, often by the use of alternating eye patches or special prism glasses. Speech disorders, such as dysarthria and aphasia, with impaired communication skills need to be evaluated and properly managed, often by introducing alternative communication methods such writing, typing, sign language, and pictures.

Neuropsychological changes of varying degrees are associated with cancer affecting the cerebral hemispheres and may include reduced memory, judgment, visual perception, and so on. Careful evaluation of such deficits, followed by education of the patient and the family of the impact of such changes, is fundamental. Neuropsychological remediation and compensation strategies, such as provision of a "memory book," may be helpful as well.

Spinal cord dysfunction

Primary tumors of the spine are uncommon, the most frequent being multiple myeloma. Metastases are much more common and are found in 5% of all cancer patients at autopsy.[10] The most common cause of SCD is metastatic epidural compression.[11] SCD may also be iatrogenic resulting from radiation, chemotherapy, or surgical intervention. The most common initial symptom of a spinal tumor is pain. Neurologic dysfunction of varying degree may develop either suddenly or gradually depending on the cancer's

Holland-Frei Cancer Medicine, Ninth Edition. Edited by Robert C. Bast Jr., Carlo M. Croce, William N. Hait, Waun Ki Hong, Donald W. Kufe, Martine Piccart-Gebhart, Raphael E. Pollock, Ralph R. Weichselbaum, Hongyang Wang, and James F. Holland.
© 2017 John Wiley & Sons, Inc. ISBN: 978-1-118-93469-2

Table 1 Interdisciplinary cancer rehabilitation team.

Team member	Role
Caregiver(s)	Participates as source of support for the patient as well as developing a relationship with the team as an extension of the patient
Chaplain	Evaluates and assists with the spiritual needs of the patient and caregivers
Nutritionist	Evaluates the patient's nutritional condition, assesses the additional metabolic demands that the cancer places on the body, and recommends the optimal diet with respect to specific clinical condition, caloric intake, food ingredients of choice, optimal consistency for easy swallowing, and the individual's tastes
Occupational therapist	Evaluates and develops a plan with a focus on the upper extremities range of motion and strength as well as training in self-care activities
Patient	Participates as an active member of the team in decisions regarding all aspects of treatment
Physical therapist	Evaluates and develops a plan to improve joint range of motion, strengthen muscles, increase stamina with a focus on improving functional skills such as bed mobility, transfers, wheelchair locomotion, and ambulation with or without assistive devices
Physician (physiatrist)	Leads the rehabilitation team to establish realistic goals and prescribe an appropriate rehabilitation program including a plan for preventive, restorative, supportive, and palliative therapies
Prosthetist–orthotist	Evaluate and fabricate artificial limbs (prostheses) or special braces (orthoses) according to the patient's needs
Psychologist	Assesses the patient's cognition and behavior, including intelligence, personality, personal history, motivation, and reaction to the illness, and assists the patient and the caregivers in developing a plan for coping with the medical illness
Recreational therapist	Offers various activities to each patient to meet their individual needs such as art and/or music therapy, attending events, and other social activities important to the patient
Rehabilitation nurse	Evaluates the patient's specific nursing needs and determines a plan including education of the patient and caregivers
Speech-language pathologist	Evaluates and provides therapy for impaired oral communication and works closely with the occupational therapist and nutritionist in the assessment and care of swallowing disorders
Social worker	Evaluates and plans for the psychosocial aspects of the patients treatment especially with respect to discharge planning, facilitating a smooth transition to the community, ensuring continuity of care, and securing appropriate follow-up services after discharge
Vocational counselor	Evaluate needs of patients who may potentially return to work and assist with planning re-entry to the workforce

Table 2 Rehabilitation problems associated with cancer of the brain.

- Paralysis
- Spasticity
- Joint contractures
- Pain
- Sensory deficits
- Visual field deficits
- Diplopia
- Aphasia
- Dysarthria
- Dysphagia
- Ataxia
- Cognitive and behavioral deficits
- Visual perceptual deficits
- Psychosocial vocational deficits

Table 3 Conditions associated with spinal cord dysfunction.

- Loss of motor power
- Loss of sensation
- Pressure sores
- Urinary dysfunction
- Bowel dysfunction
- Sexual dysfunction
- Pain
- Spasticity
- Autonomic dysreflexia
- Joint contractures
- Heterotopic ossification
- Circulatory disturbances
- Orthostatic hypotension
- Edema
- Deep vein thrombophlebitis
- Respiratory insufficiency
- Metabolic disturbances
- Hormone imbalance
- Psychological problems
- Social problems
- Vocational problems

growth and location. The neurologic level refers to the most caudal segment with normal sensory and motor function bilaterally. Below that level, the neurologic deficits are classified by using the American Spinal Injury Association(ASIA) impairment scale.[12] The neurologic level and degree of complications caused by a lesion will help predict the functional prognosis. Prognosis for life varies with cancer type. The median survival for spinal metastases is 7.7 months, worse for those with colon and lung cancer, but better for those with sarcoma, prostate, kidney, and breast cancer.[13]

Most spinal metastases are managed nonsurgically. When neurologic deficits occur rapidly, surgical decompression and/or radiotherapy is generally indicated. Spinal metastases and primary tumors may result in spinal instability, which should be managed with surgical stabilization.[14] The rehabilitation of cancer patients with SCD depends on assessment of their neurologic, oncologic, medical, pain, and social support status.[11] SCD with profound paralysis and sensory loss, along with bladder and bowel dysfunction, requires specialized medical and nursing care, followed by comprehensive rehabilitation addressing each of the associated

conditions (Table 3). Prevention of urinary tract complications, pressure ulcers, deep vein thrombosis/pulmonary embolism, joint contractures, and other complications must be addressed immediately with implementation of intermittent bladder catheterizations, prophylactic anticoagulation, proper bed positioning, and turning at least every 2 h, range of motion exercises, bowel evacuation routine, and focused emotional support. Physical and occupational therapists aim to restore mobility and self-care skills. Ambulation with assistive devices may be possible for many patients with incomplete lower level SCD, but those with neurologically complete thoracic or cervical level SCD will require a manual or powered wheelchair. Persons with incomplete SCD may benefit from ambulation training, which includes body weight support, that is, overhead suspension. Those with complete thoracic level SCD will require orthoses to stabilize their knees and ankles. Many with low lumbar level SCD may benefit from ankle-foot orthoses to compensate for ankle muscle weakness, such as a foot drop, in addition to using crutches or walkers for ambulation.

Recent development of robotic exoskeleton electrically powered devices, with a variety of controlled mechanisms, holds promise to enable people with complete paraplegia to regain a degree of independent and functional ambulation.[15] As soon as deemed medically and functionally appropriate, the patient with SCD is discharged with necessary assistive devices, nursing supplies, personal assistance, and instruction for subsequent medical care.

Cancer of the head and neck

Contemporary multimodal treatment of head and neck cancer (HNC) can involve surgery and/or intensity-modulated radiation therapy (IMRT) with or without platinum-based chemotherapy. Surgery often involves resection of the primary tumor as well as neck dissection historically classified as radical [removal of all lymph nodes, spinal accessory nerve (SAN), sternocleidomastoid (SCM) muscle, internal jugular vein (IJV)], modified radical (removes all lymph nodes but spares one or more of the SAN, SCM, IJV), or selective (preserves one or more lymph node level normally removed in a radical neck dissection).[16]

In general, the more extensive neck dissections result in more severe shoulder dysfunction, pain, and reduced quality of life.[17] Although resection or damage to the SAN is a major cause, this morbidity, damage to other key structures, including the cervical root branches and cervical plexus, also plays an important role.[18-20] Perturbation of scapulothoracic motion from trapezius weakness (compromised SAN) and rotator cuff (RTC) weakness (compromised root branches) can lead to musculoskeletal shoulder disorders such as RTC tendonitis and adhesive capsulitis.[21] Damage to the cervical plexus and its branches, as well as the cervical root branches, can cause neuropathic pain.[20]

Radiation can damage any structure in the radiation field including nerve, muscle, tendon, ligament, blood vessel, lymphatic, and bone.[22] Late effects of radiation in HNC include radiculopathy, cervical and/or brachial plexopathy, and mononeuropathies of the cranial and other nerves located within the radiation field. Late effects of radiation include dysphagia, dysarthria, xerostomia, trismus, dropped head syndrome, cervical dystonia, shoulder dysfunction, neck and/or shoulder pain, and multiple other adverse sequelae.[23-26] The combination of surgery and radiation likely has additive morbidity.

The treatment of late effects in HNC survivors varies depending on the specific issues. Physical therapy is the primary modality for most disorders. In two prospective randomized trials, progressive resistance training (PRT) for HNC cancer patients with SAN neurapraxia/neurectomy and shoulder dysfunction was shown to be more effective than standard physical therapy in terms of improving shoulder pain, range of motion, and disability.[27,28] Nociceptive pain (RTC tendonitis, adhesive capsulitis) not responsive to physical therapy may require nonsteroidal anti-inflammatory drugs (NSAIDs) or opioid analgesics. Shoulder injection may be beneficial in some patients but generally only produces transient effect in the face of chronic neuromuscular dysfunction. Neuropathic pain and muscle spasm should initially be treated with nerve stabilizing agents (gabapentin, pregabalin, duloxetine, tricyclic antidepressants).[22] HNC can cause dysphagia, if it affects the structure and function of the mouth, throat, and/or esophagus. Impaired swallowing can lead to complications, such as aspiration pneumonia and malnutrition. Rehabilitation first involves a comprehensive evaluation, which begins with bedside swallow tests using liquids and food

of different consistencies, proceeding as needed to video fluorography and endoscopy of the pharynx, larynx, and esophagus. Training to improve swallowing involves strengthening exercises for weak muscles, identification of optimal head and neck positions for swallowing, careful feeding of liquids and foods of different viscosities, providing intraoral devices and adaptive bottles, cups, plates, and utensils and sometimes by undergoing specific surgical procedures.

Cancer of the breast

Treatment of breast cancer may include lumpectomy, mastectomy, sentinel lymph node biopsy, and axillary lymph node dissection with or without radiation and chemotherapy.[29] There are multiple potential complications of breast cancer and its treatment that benefit from rehabilitative intervention resulting primarily from effects of disease and surgery, radiotherapy, chemotherapy, and other agents used in its treatment.

The incidence of lymphedema varies from 6% to 28%.[30] Mastectomy, extent of axillary lymph node dissection, radiotherapy, and positive lymph nodes increase the risk of developing lymphedema.[31] Treatment options for lymphedema include comprehensive physical therapy, low-level laser therapy (LLLT), pharmacotherapy, and surgery.[32] Comprehensive physical therapy (including complete decongestive therapy) may include manual lymphatic drainage (MLD), progressive exercise, low-stretch compression bandaging, fitting of appropriate gradient compression garments, and education regarding skin care and other aspects of lymphedema management.

Upper body pain and dysfunction in breast cancer survivors is caused by a variety of disorders (Table 4).[33] The rehabilitation of these disorders varies greatly, but often involves physical therapy and medications such as NSAIDs, opioids, nerve stabilizers, and occasionally injection (i.e., intra-articular corticosteroids for RTC tendonitis).[33] Women who choose mastectomy often request reconstructive breast surgery with filler implants made of materials, such as saline solution, silicone gel, or compound substances. Others prefer to use external breast prostheses, made either of silicone or light weight foam or fiber fill. These come in various sizes and consistencies, but all require wearing custom fit bras and garments for optimal cosmesis.

Cancer of the limbs

Primary malignant tumors of the limbs require surgical treatment. The exact type of surgery depends on the tumors location, size, type, grade, and stage as well as on the age and general health of the patient. The main goal is to remove the tumor by an excision with wide margins through a site well clear of any malignancy or by radical removal of the entire bone or the compartment afflicted by the tumor. A subsequent surgical goal is to reconstruct the resulting defect for optimal function and cosmesis. Although limb amputation has been practiced for centuries, in recent years, limb salvage by extended local or regional excision and reconstruction has become the principal goal and is now the chosen surgical intervention in approximately 90% of cases. The survival and disease-free survival after both types of surgical approaches are similar and have been greatly improved in recent years by consequent use of chemotherapy, radiation, or both.

Metastases to bones are more common than primary bone tumors, but usually metastases affect the spine rather than limbs. Bone tumors often present initially with localized pain or with a pathologic fracture. Pathologic fractures require internal fixation

Table 4 Upper body pain disorders in breast cancer survivors

Musculoskeletal

    Postsurgical pain
    Rotator cuff disease
    Bicipital tendonitis
    Adhesive capsulitis
    Bony metastases
    Epicondylitis
    De Quervain's tenosynovitis
    Arthralgias
    Arthritis

Neuromuscular

    Cervical radiculopathy
        Leptomeningeal disease
    Brachial plexopathy
    Polyneuropathy
        Chemotherapy-induced peripheral neuropathy
        Diabetic peripheral neuropathy
    Mononeuropathy
        Dorsal scapular (rhomboids C5)
        Suprascapular (supraspinatus and infraspinatus C5–C6)
        Long thoracic (serratus anterior (C5–C6–C7)
        Lateral pectoral (pectoralis major and minor (C5 to T1)
        Medial pectoral (pectoralis major and minor (C5 to T1)
        Thoracodorsal (latissimus dorsi C6–C7–C8)
        Median
            Carpal tunnel syndrome
        Ulnar
            Cubital tunnel
        Guyon canal
        Radial
        Radial groove
    Postmastectomy pain syndrome
        Intercostobrachial neuralgia
    Complex regional pain syndrome

Lymphovascular

    Lymphedema
    Axillary web syndrome
    Deep vein thrombosis
    Post-thrombotic syndrome

Integumentary

    Cellulitis
    Radiation dermatitis

Source: Stubblefield and Keole 2014 [33]. Reproduced with permission from Elsevier.

combined with the use of methyl methacrylate, which may relieve pain, restore early mobility, ease nursing care, and provide psychological reassurance.

Regardless of whether amputation or limb sparing surgery is planned, preoperative rehabilitation should start immediately after the diagnosis of limb cancer is established. This will include discussing the surgery and the anticipated postoperative course, establishing realistic expectations, and offering peer counseling by a successfully rehabilitated amputee. Simultaneously, appropriate physical exercise program should begin with strengthening exercises for all four limbs and trunk, as well as ambulation training with nonweight bearing on the affected lower limb.

Local resection of the tumor with limb sparing reconstruction results in disease-free survival equal to that for amputation, but more important in better function, cosmesis, and emotional adjustment. The goal is to remove the active tumor, while saving adjacent nerves, tendons, and vessels. The cancerous bone may be replaced by transplanting a fresh frozen cadaveric bone allograft or

an autograft or by installing a synthetic metallic prosthetic implant. Alternatively after removal of the bone tumor, the limb may be placed in an external fixation device which maintains distraction between the bone ends and allows new bone growth by periodically adjusting the pins and fixators frame. This method is often preferred for growing children and adolescents. It will ultimately fill the gap between bone ends and result in the appropriate bone length and solid healing. Rehabilitation following lower limb sparing surgery is lengthy, intense, and crucial for success. It involves strengthening exercises for the uninvolved limbs on the first postoperative day, but the intensity of strengthening exercises and the amount of weight bearing on the affected limb depend on the exact limb reconstruction and the postoperative course. For most, long-term outcomes are excellent with complete self-sufficiency and ability to ambulate without assistive devices.

Limb amputation for cancer may be the preferred surgical intervention for large tumors that involve nerve and vessels, and thus make limb salvage impossible. Although maximum preservation of limb length compatible with eradication of the cancer is desirable, certain amputation levels will make it easier to fit a prosthesis to the residual limb. Thus, amputations through the hind foot, distal tibia, or the femoral supracondylar region are best avoided. Optimally, 12–18 cm of the tibia should be preserved for below knee amputations and at least similar femoral length and above knee amputations. Postoperatively, physical and occupational therapy should begin within 2 days, for muscle strengthening, joint mobilization, and ambulation training with a walker, crutches, and ultimately with prosthesis and a cane. All the lower limb prostheses require a custom-molded plastic socket for the residual limb with an inside silicone liner for comfort and often layers of socks to accommodate a shrinking residual limb. Attached to the socket of a below knee prosthesis is a shank and ankle foot mechanism, but an above knee prosthesis would also have a knee joint mechanism. The prosthetic knee joint and ankle foot mechanisms vary greatly in design from the most basic to those with microprocessor control and battery power source. Accordingly, the function provided and cost differs significantly.

Cancer of an upper limb can be treated with limb salvage surgery, although a proximal location may involve nerves and vessels and require shoulder disarticulation or even interscapular-thoracic amputation. A variety of prostheses are available for cosmesis or functional use depending on the individual's condition, abilities, and desires.

Conclusion

Management of cancer appropriately focuses on prevention, early diagnosis, and cure, but following effective treatment, many cancer patients experience neuromuscular, musculoskeletal, pain, and functional disorders that result in physical disability or handicap. As the prognosis for cancer improves, it becomes more important to ensure that all cancer patients regain maximum function in the broadest sense to ensure return to all former roles. Multidisciplinary rehabilitation, therefore, is an integral part of the total management of the cancer patient. The exact functional deficits need to be identified for each patient and proper rehabilitation interventions started promptly or at the same time as other treatments.

References

1 Siegel R, Ma J, Zou Z, Jemal A. Cancer statistics, 2014. *CA Cancer J Clin.* 2014;**64**(1):9–29.

2 Mariotto AB, Yabroff KR, Shao Y, Feuer EJ, Brown ML. Projections of the cost of cancer care in the United States: 2010–2020. *J Natl Cancer Inst*. 2011;**103**(2):117–128.

3 Cole RP, Scialla SJ, Bednarz L. Functional recovery in cancer rehabilitation. *Arch Phys Med Rehabil*. 2000;**81**(5):623–627.

4 Franklin DJ. Cancer rehabilitation: challenges, approaches, and new directions. *Phys Med Rehabil Clin N Am*. 2007;**18**(4):899–924, viii.

5 Hinterbuchner C. Rehabilitation of physical disability in cancer. *N Y State J Med*. 1978;**78**(7):1066–1069.

6 Harvey RF, Jellinek HM, Habeck RV. Cancer rehabilitation. An analysis of 36 program approaches. *JAMA*. 1982;**247**(15):2127–2131.

7 Geler-Kulcu D, Gulsen G, Buyukbaba E, Ozkan D. Functional recovery of patients with brain tumor or acute stroke after rehabilitation: a comparative study. *J Clin Neurosci*. 2009;**16**(1):74–78.

8 Greenberg E, Treger I, Ring H. Rehabilitation outcomes in patients with brain tumors and acute stroke - Comparative study of inpatient rehabilitation. *Am J Phys Med Rehab*. 2006;**85**(7):568–573.

9 O'Dell MW, Barr K, Spanier D, Warnick RE. Functional outcome of inpatient rehabilitation in persons with brain tumors. *Arch Phys Med Rehab*. 1998;**79**(12):1530–1534.

10 Parsch D, Mikut R, Abel R. Postacute management of patients with spinal cord injury due to metastatic tumour disease: survival and efficacy of rehabilitation. *Spinal Cord*. 2003;**41**(4):205–210.

11 Stubblefield MD, Bilsky MH. Barriers to rehabilitation of the neurosurgical spine cancer patient. *J Surg Oncol*. 2007;**95**(5):419–426.

12 International standards for neurological classification of spinal cord injury, revised 2002. Chicago, IL: American Spinal Injury Association; 2002.

13 Wang JC, Boland P, Mitra N, et al. Single-stage posterolateral transpedicular approach for resection of epidural metastatic spine tumors involving the vertebral body with circumferential reconstruction: results in 140 patients. Invited submission from the Joint Section Meeting on Disorders of the Spine and Peripheral Nerves, March 2004. *J Neurosurg Spine*. 2004;**1**(3):287–298.

14 Fourney DR, Frangou EM, Ryken TC, et al. Spinal instability neoplastic score: an analysis of reliability and validity from the spine oncology study group. *J Clin Oncol*. 2011;**29**(22):3072–3077.

15 Chen G, Chan CK, Guo Z, Yu H. A review of lower extremity assistive robotic exoskeletons in rehabilitation therapy. *Crit Rev Biomed Eng*. 2013;**41**(4–5):343–363.

16 Inoue H, Nibu K, Saito M, et al. Quality of life after neck dissection. Archives of otolaryngology—head & neck surgery. 2006;**132**(6):662–666.

17 Kuntz AL, Weymuller EA Jr. Impact of neck dissection on quality of life. *Laryngoscope*. 1999;**109**(8):1334–1338.

18 Umeda M, Shigeta T, Takahashi H, et al. Shoulder mobility after spinal accessory nerve-sparing modified radical neck dissection in oral cancer patients. *Oral Surg Oral Med Oral Pathol Oral Radiol Endod*. 2010;**109**(6):820–824.

19 Roh JL, Yoon YH, Kim SY, Park CI. Cervical sensory preservation during neck dissection. *Oral Oncol*. 2007;**43**(5):491–498.

20 Dilber M, Kasapoglu F, Erisen L, Basut O, Tezel I. The relationship between shoulder pain and damage to the cervical plexus following neck dissection. *Eur Arc Otorhinolaryngol*. 2007;**264**(11):1333–1338.

21 Stubblefield MD. Cancer rehabilitation. *Semin Oncol*. 2011;**38**(3):386–393.

22 Stubblefield MD. Radiation fibrosis syndrome: neuromuscular and musculoskeletal complications in cancer survivors. *PM R*. 2011;**3**(11):1041–1054.

23 Rong X, Tang Y, Chen M, Lu K, Peng Y. Radiation-induced cranial neuropathy in patients with nasopharyngeal carcinoma. A follow-up study. *Strahlenther Onkol*. 2012;**188**(3):282–286.

24 Tuan JK, Ha TC, Ong WS, et al. Late toxicities after conventional radiation therapy alone for nasopharyngeal carcinoma. *Radiother Oncol*. 2012;**104**(3):305–311.

25 Chen AM, Hall WH, Li J, et al. Brachial plexus-associated neuropathy after high-dose radiation therapy for head-and-neck cancer. *Int J Radiat Oncol Biol Phys*. 2012;**84**(1):165–169.

26 Smillie I, Ellul D, Townsley R, et al. Head drop syndrome secondary to multimodality treatments for head and neck cancer. *Laryngoscope*. 2013;**123**(4):938–941.

27 McNeely ML, Parliament M, Courneya KS, et al. A pilot study of a randomized controlled trial to evaluate the effects of progressive resistance exercise training on shoulder dysfunction caused by spinal accessory neurapraxia/neurectomy in head and neck cancer survivors. *Head Neck*. 2004;**26**(6):518–530.

28 McNeely ML, Parliament MB, Seikaly H, et al. Effect of exercise on upper extremity pain and dysfunction in head and neck cancer survivors—a randomized controlled trial. *Cancer*. 2008;**113**(1):214–222.

29 NCCN Clinical Practice Guidelines in Oncology (NCCN Guidelines) Breast Cancer. Available from: http://www.nccn.org/professionals/physician_gls/pdf/breast.pdf, accessed 9 May 2014.

30 DiSipio T, Rye S, Newman B, Hayes S. Incidence of unilateral arm lymphoedema after breast cancer: a systematic review and meta-analysis. *Lancet Oncol*. 2013;**14**(6):500–515.

31 Tsai RJ, Dennis LK, Lynch CF, Snetselaar LG, Zamba GK, Scott-Conner C. The risk of developing arm lymphedema among breast cancer survivors: a meta-analysis of treatment factors. *Ann Surg Oncol*. 2009;**16**(7):1959–1972.

32 Paskett ED, Dean JA, Oliveri JM, Harrop JP. Cancer-related lymphedema risk factors, diagnosis, treatment, and impact: a review. *J Clin Oncol*. 2012;**30**(30):3726–3733.

33 Stubblefield MD, Keole N. Upper body pain and functional disorders in patients with breast cancer. *PM&R*. 2014;**6**(2):170–183.

49 Integrative oncology in cancer care

Gabriel Lopez, MD ▪ Richard T. Lee, MD ▪ Alejandro Chaoul, PhD ▪ M. Kay Garcia, DrPH, MSN, LAc ▪ Lorenzo Cohen, PhD

Overview

Integrative medicine seeks to merge conventional medicine and complementary therapies in a manner that is comprehensive, personalized, evidence based, and safe. Integrative oncology is the term used to describe the application of integrative medicine to cancer care. The field of integrative oncology is a constantly evolving set of disciplines. This chapter reviews the role of integrative medicine in cancer care with an emphasis on effective communication, an overview of the evidence, integrative-based resources to guide health care providers and patients, and presents a model of how to effectively incorporate integrative medicine within cancer care. Existing research suggests that the majority of cancer patients desire communication with their physicians about integrative medicine. It is the healthcare professional's responsibility to ask patients about their use of complementary medicines and to provide evidence-based advice to guide patients in this evolving area. Key findings in the areas of mind-body practices, massage, and acupuncture are presented. Mind-body practices help to improve mood, sleep quality, physical functioning, and overall well-being. Massage is helpful at relieving pain, anxiety, and increasing relaxation. Acupuncture has the greatest evidence to support its use in managing symptoms such as chemotherapy-induced nausea, vomiting, and pain; initial research suggests benefit in providing relief for radiation-induced xerostomia and other symptoms. Many authoritative resources now exist to help guide patients' appropriate use of complementary therapies, allowing the medical team to follow evidence-based guidelines.

Introduction

Integrative medicine seeks to combine conventional medicine with the safest and most effective complementary therapies. Although applying the concept of integrative medicine to cancer care is still relatively new, a number of comprehensive cancer centers in the United States are trying to put this concept into practice under the term *integrative oncology*. As a result of growing interest in integrative oncology, the National Cancer Institute formed the Office of Cancer Complementary and Alternative Medicine, the American Cancer Society dedicated a portion of its web site to assessment of complementary therapies, the Consortium of Academic Health Centers for Integrative Medicine (CAHCIM) formed an oncology working group, and the Society for Integrative Oncology (SIO) was formed. This chapter reviews the role of integrative medicine in cancer care with an emphasis on effective communication, an overview of the evidence, integrative-based resources to guide health care providers and patients, and an example of how to effectively incorporate integrative medicine within cancer care.

Definitions

Complementary and alternative medicine (CAM) has been defined by the National Center for Complementary and Integrative Health (NCCIH) (formerly the National Center for Complementary and Alternative Medicine) and major US surveys as " ... diverse medical and healthcare systems, practices, and products that are not presently considered to be part of conventional medicine."[1] Although evidence may exist for some of these modalities, it may not be sufficient to bring them into the realm of *conventional* medicine, and other CAM modalities may have no support for their use. *Alternative* medicine is the use of a nonconventional treatment modality in place of conventional medicine whether or not there is evidence for its efficacy. *Complementary* medicine, on the other hand, is making use of a CAM modality in combination with conventional medicine whether or not evidence exists for its efficacy. Several different types of specialty health care providers offer CAM therapies and these may include physicians, nurses, physical therapists, psychologists, acupuncturists, and massage therapists who are operating within the guidelines of their licenses or accrediting organizations. Practitioners of all disciplines should be knowledgeable and aware of all treatment options and open to communication with other types of practitioners.

Integrative medicine seeks to merge conventional medicine and complementary therapies in a manner that is comprehensive, personalized, evidence based, and safe. CAHCIM has defined integrative medicine as "the practice of medicine that reaffirms the importance of the relationship between practitioner and patient, focuses on the whole person, is informed by evidence, and makes use of all appropriate therapeutic approaches, healthcare professionals and disciplines to achieve optimal health and healing."[2] The application of integrative medicine to cancer care has come into practice under the term *integrative oncology*. The terms CAM and CIM are often used interchangeably; however, when the term CAM is used, it includes treatment that could be considered alternative and used in place of conventional care; the term CIM would not include alternative treatment approaches.

Utilization

The World Health Organization (WHO) estimates that up to 80% of people in developing countries rely on nonconventional traditional medicines for their primary health care.[3] People in more developed countries also seek out complementary medicine and practices. A 2007 survey by the US Centers for Disease Control found that 38% of adults had used CAM therapies during the past 12 months[4]; results from the 2012 survey are upcoming.

Holland-Frei Cancer Medicine, Ninth Edition. Edited by Robert C. Bast Jr., Carlo M. Croce, William N. Hait, Waun Ki Hong, Donald W. Kufe, Martine Piccart-Gebhart, Raphael E. Pollock, Ralph R. Weichselbaum, Hongyang Wang, and James F. Holland.
© 2017 John Wiley & Sons, Inc. ISBN: 978-1-118-93469-2

Among patients and families touched by cancer, the use of CAM is higher than in the general population. An estimated 48–69% of US patients with cancer use CAM therapies and percentages increase if spiritual practices are included.[5] CAM therapies are used by up to 69% of cancer patients, with increased use in those with advanced cancers.[5,6]

In most cases, people who use CAM are not disappointed or dissatisfied with conventional medicine but want to do everything possible to regain health and to improve quality of life (QOL), reduce side effects, stimulate immunity, or prevent new cancers or recurrences.[5,7] Whether or not patients use CAM therapies to treat cancer or its effects, they may use them to treat other chronic conditions such as arthritis, heart disease, diabetes, and chronic pain.

Communication

Research indicates that neither adult nor pediatric patients receive sufficient information or discuss CAM therapies with physicians, pharmacists, nurses, or CAM practitioners.[8] It is estimated that 38–60% of patients with cancer are taking complementary medicines without informing any member of their healthcare team.[6,7] Most patients do not bring up the topic of CAM because no one asks; thus patients may believe that it is unimportant. This lack of discussion is of grave concern because herbs and supplements may have direct toxicity or interact with cancer treatments. Patients are commonly unaware of the differences between the United States Food and Drug Administration (FDA)-approved medications (which require evidence of efficacy, safety, and quality control manufacturing) and supplements, which are governed not by the FDA but by the Dietary Supplement Health and Education Act (DSHEA) of 1994. Supplements under this legislation are exempt from the same scrutiny the FDA imposes on medications; furthermore, these supplements are not intended to treat, prevent, or cure diseases. The common belief by patients is that "natural" means safe needs to be addressed with education as some herbs and supplements have been associated with multiple drug interactions, as well as increased cancer risk and organ toxicity.[9,10]

Existing research suggests that the majority of cancer patients desire communication with their physicians about CAM.[11] There is general agreement within the oncology community that in order to provide optimal patient care, oncologists must not only be aware of CAM use but also be willing and able to discuss all therapeutic approaches with their patients. It is the healthcare professional's responsibility to ask patients about their use of complementary medicines, and the discussion should ideally take place before the patient starts using a complementary treatment—whether it is a nutritional supplement, mind-body therapy, or other CAM approach.

A number of strategies can be used to increase the chance of a worthwhile dialogue. One approach is to include the topic of CAM as part of a new patient assessment. For example, when asking about medications, physicians should inquire about everything the patient ingests—including over-the-counter products, vitamins, minerals, herbs, and even the patient's diet. Physicians may consider having the patients bring in the actual bottles of herbs and supplements for evaluation. When asking about a patient's past medical history, physicians may ask about all other healthcare professionals involved in the patient's care to learn if the patients have visited with CAM practitioners such as naturopaths or chiropractors. If the issue of CAM arises, clinicians need to develop an empathic communication strategy that addresses the patient's needs while maintaining an understanding of the current state of the science.[12] In other words, this strategy needs to be balanced between clinical objectivity and

bonding with the patient so that it can benefit both the patient and the healthcare provider. The physician who is receptive to patient inquiries is able to establish an environment in which a patient feels comfortable to bring up the topic of CAM therapies. Part of this strategy should be an open attitude combined with a willingness to review evidence-based references and consult with other health care professionals. Patients need reliable information on CAM from reliable resources, as well as adequate time to discuss this information with their oncologists.[13]

The evidence

The field of integrative oncology is a constantly evolving set of disciplines. There has been a dramatic increase in research in integrative oncology. In the following section, we list some of the key findings to date in integrative oncology in the main areas of CAM where there is sufficient evidence to recommend the therapies: mind-body practices, massage, and acupuncture. Although there is ongoing research in many other areas such as healing touch, homeopathy, natural products, and special diets, there is insufficient evidence to recommend these at this point in time.

Mind-body practices

The belief that what we think and feel can influence our health and healing dates back thousands of years. The importance of the role of the mind, emotions, and behaviors in health and well-being is central to traditional Chinese, Tibetan, Greek, and Ayurvedic medicines and other medical traditions of the world.

The health-damaging effects of chronic stress are well documented in the medical literature. Research shows that chronic stress affects almost every biological system in our bodies.[14] Unmanaged chronic stress can speed the aging process through telomere shortening,[15] increasing the risk for heart disease,[16] sleeping difficulties,[17] digestive problems,[18] and even depression.[19] Research has shown that stress can also decrease compliance with health-screening behaviors and treatment.[20] Moreover, it can also cause patients to forego healthy eating and exercise habits that help prevent cancer and other disease.

With regard to cancer, there is little convincing evidence that chronic stress affects cancer initiation; however, there is extensive evidence that chronic stress can promote cancer growth and progression.[21,22] The underlying mechanisms for such effects are complex and involve chronic activation of the sympathetic nervous system (SNS) and the HPA axis.[23] Sustained elevations from these pathways (e.g., norepinephrine and cortisol) can result in diverse effects including stimulation of cancer invasion, angiogenesis, inflammation and immune dysregulation, reduced anoikis, and even reduced efficacy of chemotherapy drugs.[24] The underlying signaling pathways offer opportunities for designing new therapeutic approaches for disrupting the effects of stress biology on cancer biology and include both behavioral and pharmacological (e.g., beta-blockers) approaches.

The clinical significance of stress-related biological changes and the changes in the tumor micro-environment has not been widely studied. However, these changes may be significant enough to affect not only the immediate health of the patient but also the course of the disease and thus the future health of the patient. It is, therefore, prudent to suggest that patients engage in some type of practice to reduce stress in their lives.

Mind-body practices are defined as a variety of techniques designed to enhance the mind's capacity to affect bodily function and symptoms. Mind-body techniques include relaxation, hypnosis, visual imagery, meditation, biofeedback, yoga, tai chi, qigong, and other movement-based therapies, cognitive-behavioral therapies, group support, autogenic training, and spirituality as well as expressive arts therapies such as art, music, or dance. As research continues, the treatments that are found beneficial will hopefully become integrated into conventional medical care.

Research has shown that after being diagnosed with cancer, patients try to bring about positive changes in their lifestyles, indicating a tendency to take control of their health care.[25] Techniques of stress management that have proven helpful include progressive muscle relaxation, diaphragmatic breathing, guided imagery, and social support. Participating in stress management programs before treatment has enabled patients to tolerate therapy with fewer reported side effects. Supportive expressive group therapy has also been found to be useful for patients with cancer. Although there is some data to support the use of expressive art therapies such as music therapy,[26] art therapy,[27] and expressive writing[28] and journaling to improve QOL, the number of trials is limited and they typically have small sample sizes and often no control groups. Psychosocial interventions have been shown to specifically reduce anxiety, depression, and mood disturbance in cancer patients and assist their coping skills.[29]

Newell et al.[30] reviewed psychological therapies for cancer patients and concluded that interventions involving self-practice and hypnosis for managing nausea and vomiting could be recommended but that further research was suggested to examine the benefits of relaxation training and guided imagery. Ernst et al.[31] examined the change in the state of the evidence for mind-body therapies for various medical conditions between 2000 and 2005 and found that there is now maximal evidence for the use of relaxation techniques for anxiety, hypertension, insomnia, and nausea due to chemotherapy. The beneficial effects of hypnosis, and especially self-hypnosis, is further supported by more recent research as hypnosis was found beneficial for reducing distress and discomfort during difficult medical procedures.[32] An NIH Technology Assessment Panel found strong evidence for hypnosis in alleviating cancer-related pain.[33] Hypnosis effectively treats anticipatory nausea in pediatric and adult cancer patients, reduces postoperative nausea and vomiting, and improves adjustment to invasive medical procedures, and when combined with cognitive behavioral therapy (CBT), hypnosis leads to reduced fatigue in women with breast cancer at the end of radiotherapy and 1 and 6 months later.[34]

Research examining yoga, tai chi, and meditation, including mindfulness-based stress reduction (MBSR), incorporated into cancer care suggests that these mind-body practices help to improve aspects of QOL including improved mood, sleep quality, physical functioning, and overall well-being of patients undergoing treatment and cancer survivors.[35]

The meditation practice that has been researched the most is MBSR. The larger randomized controlled trials (RCTs) of meditation published in the past few years have used some form of MBSR for women with breast cancer. MBSR has been found to reduce self-reported levels of anxiety and depression and improve sleep quality; it has reduced the long-term emotional and physical adverse effects of medical treatments, including endocrine treatment; and resulted in a significant reduction in mood disturbance and symptoms of stress. A cancer-specific version of MBSR called mindfulness-based cancer recovery (MBCR) found that breast cancer survivors scoring 4 or greater in the distress thermometer had lower symptoms of stress and improved QOL.[36] In addition, both MBCR and a supportive expressive therapy group resulted in more normative diurnal cortisol profiles than a control group.

The more movement-based mind-body practices such as Indian-based yoga, Tibetan yoga, and Chinese tai chi/qigong typically combine physical postures or movements, breathing techniques, and meditation with the goal to enhance health and well-being. Indian-based yoga ("yoga" is Sanskrit for "to yoke" or "join"), one of the most widely practiced Eastern traditions in Western cultures, focuses on the union of mind and body or the harmonic synchronization of body, breath, and mind. Yoga has increasingly gained popularity in the cancer setting. In fact, several systematic reviews and meta-analyses indicate the QOL benefits associated with practicing yoga in cancer patients and survivors.[37,38] Research demonstrates that yoga is useful for treating sleep disturbances[39] and fatigue.[40] Yoga has also been found to reduce inflammatory signaling and stress hormone regulation,[41] which plays a role in behavioral symptoms such as fatigue after breast cancer treatment.[42] Thus, yoga may actually impact biological pathways beyond patients' perceptions of QOL and symptoms. Although most yoga research has been conducted in women with early-stage breast cancer, efforts are underway to extend these findings to women with advanced breast cancer and survivors of lung cancer and caregivers.[43]

Less research has examined the effects of *tai chi/qigong* in oncology.[44] Encouraging advances are evident and *tai chi/qigong* has been found to reduce fatigue and distress, improve peripheral circulatory status and functional aerobic capacity, and lead to less postoperative humoral and cellular immunity dysregulation.

Massage

Massage has shown promise for relief of cancer and cancer treatment-related symptoms. As a manipulative touch-based therapy, massage can benefit cancer patients when performed by therapists who have an awareness of the special needs of cancer patients.[45] A massage therapist with special training in oncology massage is the best equipped to safely deliver the massage. Risk of bruising, bleeding, or injury can be minimized by careful application of pressure, avoiding massage into the deep tissue or bone in selected patients. Areas that have recently had surgery or radiation should be avoided. In patients with extremities subject to lymphedema, therapists will need to adjust their technique to maximize safety. Patients may benefit from formal lymphedema therapy as part of a physical therapy program.[46]

Research to date suggests that massage is helpful at relieving pain, anxiety, fatigue, distress, and increasing relaxation.[47,48] Benefit on mood and pain relief is limited to the more immediate effect of massage, with no current studies demonstrating long-term relief.[49,50] Anecdotal and case report evidence has suggested benefit of massage for the relief of chemotherapy-induced peripheral neuropathy. A massage to the feet, hands, and head can provide therapeutic benefit as these areas are especially sensitive to tactile stimulation and can result in relaxation and increased well-being. Massage provided by caregivers may offer a unique opportunity for interaction between patient and caregiver that can help enhance well-being of both.[51] In addition to symptomatic relief, studies have also demonstrated systemic effects of massage, with the decreases in cortisol levels resulting from a massage intervention.[52] More research is needed to better understand massage mechanisms and treatment protocols (ideal massage-type, dosing) to better define the role of massage therapy in cancer symptom management.

Acupuncture

Acupuncture is a treatment modality that is part of traditional Chinese medicine (TCM). It has been practiced in China for thousands of years and is used in at least 78 countries throughout the

Table 1 Recommended web sites for evidence-based resources.

Organization/web site (alphabetical order)	Address/URL
Cochrane Review Organization	www.cochrane.org
Memorial Sloan-Kettering Cancer Center	www.mskcc.org/cancer-care/integrative-medicine/about-herbs
Natural Medicines Comprehensive Database	www.naturaldatabase.com/
Natural Standard	www.naturalstandard.com/
NCI Office of Cancer Complementary and Alternative Medicine (OCCAM)	www.cancer.gov/cam
University of Texas MD Anderson Cancer Center Integrative Medicine Program	www.mdanderson.org/integrativemed

world. According to TCM theory, the placement of acupuncture needles, heat, or pressure at specific body points can help regulate the flow of Qi (vital energy) within the body. The most common form of acupuncture involves the placement of solid, sterile, stainless steel needles into various sites on the body that are believed to have reduced bioelectrical resistance and increased conductance. The needles may be stimulated manually or a mild electrical current may be applied directly to the needles after insertion. Stainless steel or gold (semi-permanent) needles, or "studs," are also sometimes placed at points on the ears and left in place for 3–5 days.

The strongest evidence supporting the use of acupuncture in cancer care is for symptom management. Studies have shown that acupuncture is helpful to control nausea and vomiting from multiple causes (i.e., chemotherapy-induced nausea and vomiting (CINV), postoperative nausea and vomiting, and pregnancy),[53,54] and although there is good evidence for the use of acupuncture to control pain, there is still limited research in a cancer setting. In a large individual patient-level data meta-analysis of 29 trials involving noncancer patients ($N = 14,597$) with chronic pain, significantly better pain control was found in favor of real acupuncture compared to no acupuncture (50% vs 30%, $P < 0.001$) as well as real acupuncture compared to sham acupuncture, though to a lesser degree (50% vs 42.5, $P < 0.001$).

For the management of other treatment- or cancer-related symptoms, the evidence is not as strong as that for pain and nausea; however, initial research suggests that acupuncture may help reduce the severity of radiation-induced xerostomia with a lasting benefit.[55,56] There is also some evidence to suggest that acupuncture may be useful in treating or helping to manage symptoms such as constipation, loss of appetite, peripheral neuropathy, hot flushes, fatigue, insomnia and sleep disorders, dyspnea, anxiety/depression, and leukopenia, but the quality of research for these indications remains weak and further studies are needed.[57] When performed correctly, acupuncture has been shown to be a safe, minimally invasive procedure with very few side effects. The side effects most commonly reported are fainting, bruising, and mild discomfort. Infection is a potential risk, but very uncommon when treatment is provided by a qualified acupuncturist. Treatments should only be performed by a health care professional with an appropriate license and experience.

The mechanisms of acupuncture are not well understood, but for symptoms such as CINV and pain, there is clear evidence to support its use. Although data are still lacking for other symptom control, as a cost-effective treatment option with minimal associated risks, acupuncture may be a helpful addition to cancer care for patients suffering from uncontrolled treatment-related side effects or for those in whom conventional treatment approaches have failed.

Educational resources

Comprehensive reviews can quickly become outdated, and the ease of Internet publishing has fostered the growth of comprehensive scientific review organizations that provide electronic access to their reviews. We outline websites of organizations providing reliable information for providers and patients (Table 1).

The American Cancer Society (ACS) and National Cancer Institute (NCI) Office of Cancer Complementary and Alternative Medicine (OCCAM) provide valuable educational resources for patients and the general public on complementary therapies. Natural Medicines Comprehensive Database provides evidence-based reviews of complementary therapies. The Cochrane Review Organization, founded in 1993 as an international nonprofit independent organization, provides systematic reviews that include complementary therapies.

Natural Standard is part of a multidisciplinary, multi-institutional initiative dedicated to the review of complementary and alternative therapies. It follows a similar process to build in-depth evidence and consensus-based analysis of scientific data in addition to historic and folkloric perspectives. The integrative medicine service at the Memorial Sloan-Kettering Cancer Center provides evidence-based reviews as part of their "About Herbs, Botanicals & Other Products" Internet resource. The integrative medicine program at the University of Texas MD Anderson Cancer Center offers an Internet resource for patients and providers to learn more about the evidence-based role of Integrative Medicine in cancer care.

Integrative oncology in clinical practice

Integrative oncology has the ability to enhance the care provided for cancer patients by incorporating additional treatment options that lead to improved health, symptom management, and QOL. Most major medical centers now offer some complementary medicine treatment modalities alongside the conventional care.[58] In order to create comprehensive integrative cancer care, these types of therapies must be delivered in a manner that does not just avoid potential interactions but works to create synergy with ongoing treatment. To do so, the integrative oncology approach must incorporate principles of being evidence based, personalized, and safe.

The Integrative Medicine Center at MD Anderson Cancer Center is one example. The center utilizes a bio-psychosocial model of healthcare (Figure 1) as a clinical framework to guide the implementation of services to patients throughout the cancer continuum (prevention, treatment, and survivorship), and some services are also provided for caregivers. The clinical services are provided to address specific medical conditions such as pain or anxiety or the appropriate use of herbs and supplements and not available to patients as part of a spa service. The center provides patient care on an individual bases as well as in groups. Patients may receive inpatient and outpatient physician consultation, acupuncture, massage, mind-body therapy such as meditation, and music therapy. Physical therapy for exercise counseling, a dietician for nutrition counseling, and a psychologist for mood management and behavioral counseling are also available for all patients. Patients may also

Integrative medicine center model

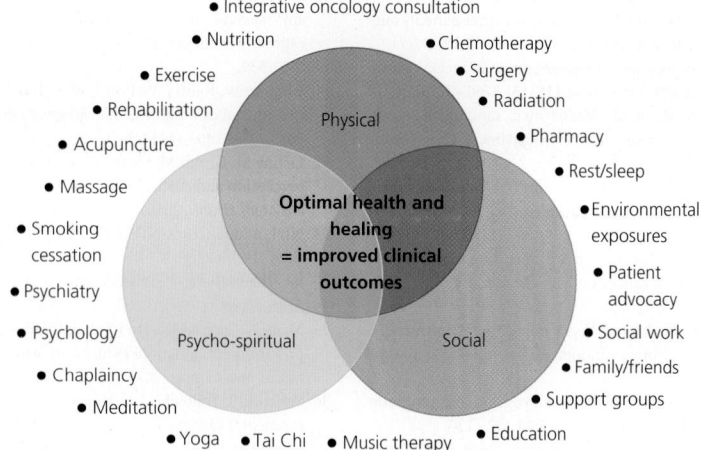

Figure 1 Integrative medicine center model. Based on the bio-psychosocial model of health care, our center functions within a framework of cancer care delivery.

attend free group classes such as meditation, yoga, tai chi/qigong, music therapy, exercise, and cooking classes. All staff members meet on weekly bases to discuss challenging new patients and to help coordinate care. Clinical notes are available in the electronic health record. As part of routine care, patients complete validated instruments on symptoms and QOL and are included as part of a broader clinical research initiative to understand the clinical impact of the clinical services provided. The integrative medicine center works collaboratively with similar supportive services such as palliative medicine, psychiatry, pain center, and rehabilitation services. Most referrals come from these service areas as well as from primary oncologists.

Conclusion

Integrative oncology is a rapidly expanding discipline that holds tremendous promise for additional treatment options and more effective symptom control. An integrative approach also provides patients with a more personalized system of care for meeting their needs. The majority of patients either are using complementary medicines or want to know about them, so it is incumbent on the conventional medical system to provide appropriate education and clinical services. The clinical model for integrative care requires a patient-centered approach with attention to patient concerns and enhanced communication skills. In addition, it is essential that conventional and nonconventional practitioners work together in developing an integrative model. In this way, cancer patients will be receiving the best medical care making use of all appropriate treatment modalities.

Key references

The complete reference list can be found on the Wiley Companion Digital Edition of this title (see inside front cover for login instructions).

1 NCCAM. National Center for Complementary/Alternative Medicine of the National Institutes of Health. What is complementary and alternative medicine? (2015) http://nccam.nih.gov/health/whatiscam/ (accessed January 15, 2015).

4 Barnes PM, Bloom B, Nahin R. CDC National Health Statistics Report #12. Complementary and Alternative Medicine Use Among Adults and Children: United States, 2007. December 10, 2008.

5 Richardson MA, Sanders T, Palmer JL, Greisinger A, Singletary SE. Complementary/alternative medicine use in a comprehensive cancer center and the implications for oncology. *J Clin Oncol.* 2000;**18**(**13**):2505–2514.

6 Navo MA, Phan J, Vaughan C, et al. An assessment of the utilization of complementary and alternative medication in women with gynecologic or breast malignancies. *J Clin Oncol.* 2004;**22**(**4**):671–677.

9 Ulbricht C, Chao W, Costa D, Rusie-Seamon E, Weissner W, Woods J. Clinical evidence of herb-drug interactions: a systematic review by the natural standard research collaboration. *Curr Drug Metab.* 2008;**9**(**10**):1063–1120.

11 Verhoef MJ, White MA, Doll R. Cancer patients' expectations of the role of family physicians in communication about complementary therapies. *Cancer Prev Control.* 1999;**3**(**3**):181–187.

14 Chrousos GP, Gold PW. The concepts of stress and stress system disorders. Overview of physical and behavioral homeostasis. *JAMA.* 1992;**267**(**9**):1244–1252.

15 Epel ES, Blackburn EH, Lin J, et al. Accelerated telomere shortening in response to life stress. *Proc Natl Acad Sci U S A.* 2004;**101**(**49**):17312–17315.

19 Hammen C. Stress and depression. *Annu Rev Clin Psychol.* 2005;**1**:293–319.

20 Prasad SM, Eggener SE, Lipsitz SR, Irwin MR, Ganz PA, Hu JC. Effect of depression on diagnosis, treatment, and mortality of men with clinically localized prostate cancer. *J Clin Oncol.* 2014;**32**(**23**):2471–2478.

21 Lutgendorf SK, Sood AK, Antoni MH. Host factors and cancer progression: biobehavioral signaling pathways and interventions. *J Clin Oncol.* 2010;**28**(**26**):4094–4099.

22 Lutgendorf SK, Sood AK, Anderson B, et al. Social support, psychological distress, and natural killer cell activity in ovarian cancer. *J Clin Oncol.* 2005;**23**(**28**):7105–7113.

23 Lutgendorf SK, Sood AK. Biobehavioral factors and cancer progression: physiological pathways and mechanisms. *Psychosom Med.* 2011;**73**(**9**):724–730.

24 Thaker PH, Han LY, Kamat AA, et al. Chronic stress promotes tumor growth and angiogenesis in a mouse model of ovarian carcinoma. *Nat Med.* 2006;**12**(**8**):939–944.

26 Archie P, Bruera E, Cohen L. Music-based interventions in palliative cancer care: a review of quantitative studies and neurobiological literature. *Support Care Cancer.* 2013;**21**(**9**):2609–2624.

29 Devine EC, Westlake SK. The effects of psychoeducational care provided to adults with cancer: meta-analysis of 116 studies. *Oncol Nurs Forum.* 1995;**22**(**9**):1369–1381.

30 Newell SA, Sanson-Fisher W, Savolainen NJ. Systematic review of psychological therapies for cancer patients: Overview and recommendations for future research. *J Natl Cancer Inst.* 2002;**94**(**8**):558–584.

31 Ernst E, Pittler MH, Wider B, Boddy K. Mind-body therapies: are the trial data getting stronger? *Altern Ther Health Med.* 2007;**13**(**5**):62–64.

33 NIH Technology Assessment Panel. Integration of behavioral and relaxation approaches into the treatment of chronic pain and insomnia. NIH Technology Assessment Panel on Integration of Behavioral and Relaxation Approaches into the Treatment of Chronic Pain and Insomnia. *JAMA.* 1996;**276**:313–318.

34 Montgomery GH, David D, Kangas M, et al. Randomized controlled trial of a cognitive-behavioral therapy plus hypnosis intervention to control fatigue in patients undergoing radiotherapy for breast cancer. *J Clin Oncol.* 2014;**32**(**6**):557–563.

35 Chaoul A, Milbury K, Sood AK, Prinsloo S, Cohen L, et al. Mind-body practices in cancer care. *Curr Oncol Rep.* 2014;**16**:417.

36 Carlson LE, Doll R, Stephen J, et al. Randomized controlled trial of mindfulness-based cancer recovery versus supportive expressive group therapy for distressed survivors of breast cancer. *J Clin Oncol*. 2013;**31**(25):3119–3126.

37 Cramer H, Lange S, Klose P, Paul A, Dobos G. Yoga for breast cancer patients and survivors: a systematic review and meta-analysis. *BMC Cancer*. 2012;**12**:412.

38 Bower JE, Garet D, Sternlieb B, et al. Yoga for persistent fatigue in breast cancer survivors: a randomized controlled trial. *Cancer*. 2012;**118**(15):3766–3775.

39 Mustian KM, Sprod LK, Janelsins M, et al. Multicenter, randomized controlled trial of yoga for sleep quality among cancer survivors. *J Clin Oncol*. 2013;**31**(26):3233–3241.

40 Bower JE, Greendale G, Crosswell AD, et al. Yoga reduces inflammatory signaling in fatigued breast cancer survivors: a randomized controlled trial. *Psychoneuroendocrinology*. 2014;**43**:20–29.

41 Chandwani KD, Perkins G, Nagendra HR, Raghuram NV, et al. Randomized, controlled trial of yoga in women with breast cancer undergoing radiotherapy. *J Clin Oncol*. 2014;**32**(10):1058–1065.

42 Kiecolt-Glaser JK, Bennett JM, Andridge R, et al. Yoga's impact on inflammation, mood, and fatigue in breast cancer survivors: a randomized controlled trial. *J Clin Oncol*. 2014;**32**(10):1040–1049.

43 Milbury K, Chaoul A, Engle R, et al. Couple-based Tibetan yoga program for lung cancer patients and their caregivers. *Psychooncology*. 2015;**24**:117–120.

45 Collinge W, MacDonald G, Walton T. Massage in supportive cancer care. *Semin Oncol Nurs*. 2012;**28**(1):45–54.

46 Torres Lacomba M, Yuste Sanchez MJ, Zapico Goni A, et al. Effectiveness of early physiotherapy to prevent lymphoedema after surgery for breast cancer: randomised single blinded, clinical trial. *BMJ*. 2010;**340**:b5396.

48 Russell NC, Sumler S-S, Beinhorn CM, Frenkel M. Role of massage therapy in cancer care. *J Altern Complement Med*. 2008;**14**(2):209–214.

49 Wilkinson SM, Love SB, Westcombe AM, et al. Effectiveness of aromatherapy massage in the management of anxiety and depression in patients with cancer: a multicenter randomized controlled trial. *J Clin Oncol*. 2007;**25**(5):532–539.

51 Collinge W, Kahn J, Walton T, et al. Touch, Caring, and Cancer: randomized controlled trial of a multimedia caregiver education program. *Support Care Cancer*. 2013;**21**(5):1405–1414.

52 Listing M, Krohn M, Liezmann C, et al. The efficacy of classical massage on stress perception and cortisol following primary treatment of breast cancer. *Arch Womens Ment Health*. 2010;**13**:165–173.

53 NIH. Acupuncture. NIH Consensus Statement. 1997;**15**(5):1–34.

54 Ezzo J, Vickers A, Richardson MA, et al. Acupuncture-point stimulation for chemotherapy-induced nausea and vomiting. *J Clin Oncol*. 2005;**23**(28):7188–7198.

55 Meng Z, Garcia MK, Hu C, et al. Randomized controlled trial of acupuncture for prevention of radiation-induced xerostomia among patients with nasopharyngeal carcinoma. *Cancer*. 2012;**118**:3337–3344.

56 Simcock R, Fallowfield L, Monson K, et al. ARIX: a randomised trial of acupuncture v oral care sessions in patients with chronic xerostomia following treatment of head and neck cancer. *Ann Oncol*. 2013;**24**:776–783.

57 Garcia MK, McQuade J, Haddad R, et al. Systematic review of acupuncture in cancer care: a synthesis of the evidence. *J Clin Oncol*. 2013;**31**(7):952–960.

50 Health services research

Michaela A. Dinan, PhD ▪ Bradford R. Hirsch, MD, MBA ▪ Amy Abernethy, MD, PhD

Overview

Health services research (HSR) describes a diverse group of research strategies and fields that seek to evaluate the impact of health care on patients and populations and has been a critical component of understanding the use, outcomes, and costs associated with oncology care since its inception over 100 years ago. In modern times, physicians and researchers often tout "bench to bedside" innovations as the goal of biomedical research. However, patients, physicians, and health care systems in the real world are subjected to a host of factors that impact patient care before, during, and after an intervention occurs at the bedside. Although HSR is a complex and evolving concept, a basic understanding of the key principles of HSR is needed to accurately assess, quantify, and optimize the real-world impact of progress in oncology today and in the future.

Introduction—what is health services research?

Health services research (HSR) comprises a diverse group of research strategies and fields that seek to evaluate the impact of health care on patients and populations. While the focus of the included disciplines may differ, there are similarities which allow us to group them together under the umbrella of HSR. In each case the same basic methodology applies: A treatment or intervention is examined in the context of an outcome of interest in order to better understand and guide clinical practice.

According to the Institute of Medicine (IOM), HSR focuses on the investigation of three major aspects of health care including (1) access to care, (2) the quality of care, and (3) the cost of health care in order to inform health care consumers about their best options for medical treatment and/or prevention.[1] The IOM has also developed a list of the major issues that health services researchers are studying today (Table 1).

HSR is truly a multidisciplinary field. Health services researchers, biostatisticians, economists, and clinicians are all examples of critical and necessary players in the HSR arena. In oncology, the clinical expertise of medical, surgical, and radiation oncologists as well as pathologists and radiologist are all needed to develop clinically relevant questions that will lead to improvements in patient care. Close collaboration between methodologists and clinicians is essential to ensure both the scientific validity and clinical significance of HSR studies.

The goals of HSR in oncology are many. While some research focuses on the investigation of diagnostics and treatments to prolong survival, other seeks to improve quality of life (QOL), inform decision making, improve access to care, ensure guideline concordant care, or examine the economic impact of care for cancer patients. In addition to the wide range of these and other potential outcomes, HSR in oncology has several stakeholders with vested interests in the results including patients and their families, physicians and other medical staff, additional providers and payers of health care, industry, and policy makers that must be considered in any effort to make advances in oncology.

The significance of health services research in cancer

HSR in oncology is the principal means by which we frame the scope of cancer and attempt to improve cancer care delivery in the real world. Discoveries made in the controlled environments of laboratories and clinical trials may or may not translate when taken out of the context of a select group of trial participants and applied to the larger population of patients. That is to say, most clinical trials are focused on the *efficacy* of a specified intervention or the ability of an intervention to provide benefit under tightly controlled circumstances. In contrast, HSR focuses on the *effectiveness* of these interventions, which describes the ability of an intervention to provide benefit under real-world conditions. The goal of HSR is to improve the effectiveness of interventions as they are disseminated into broader, more diverse populations and promote the health of all members of the population.

HSR in oncology has been used to provide estimates of the scope of cancer on a national scale and as a prediction of how it will change in the future. For example, HSR using the population-based Surveillance, Epidemiology, and End Results (SEER) registry provides the estimate that in 2014, there were an estimated 1,665,540 patients newly diagnosed with cancer and 585,720 people who died from their cancer. As the U.S. population continues to age, this number is expected to increase. For example, in 2010, the total direct estimated cost of cancer care in the United States was $124.5 billion. After only reflecting demographic changes, by 2020, this cost has been projected to increase to $157.8 billion.[2] These costs will likely be much higher in reality due to the adoption of expensive innovative therapies, the widespread diffusion of advanced technologies without supporting evidence, inappropriate use (either over or under) of existing treatments, and patient demands and unrealistic expectations are additional areas of concern. HSR provides a framework to consider how to mitigate the impact of this surge in need on current medical resources and infrastructure.

Disciplines within health services research

In practice, HSR is often separated into multiple distinct fields of discipline—health economics, epidemiology, qualitative research, implementation research. The distinctions have developed over time based on the data requirements, methodologies, and expertise needed to answer questions meaningfully. Despite these potential differences, there is considerable overlap and a common goal of inferring causality and informing practice. Outcomes research

Holland-Frei Cancer Medicine, Ninth Edition. Edited by Robert C. Bast Jr., Carlo M. Croce, William N. Hait, Waun Ki Hong, Donald W. Kufe, Martine Piccart-Gebhart, Raphael E. Pollock, Ralph R. Weichselbaum, Hongyang Wang, and James F. Holland.
© 2017 John Wiley & Sons, Inc. ISBN: 978-1-118-93469-2

Table 1 IOM list of major health services research topics.

- Health services organization and financing
- Access to health care
- Behaviors of practitioners, patients, and health care consumers
- Quality of care
- Clinical outcomes research
- Health care decision-making and informatics
- Health professions workforce

revolves around the identification of a treatment or exposure of interest and a relevant outcome (i.e., the impact of a new treatment on survival). Health economists focus on health care costs and resource utilization, epidemiologists on naturally occurring exposures and patterns, and health services researchers on questions that examine exposures or treatments within the health care system—either directly or indirectly.

An overview of health services research study designs

HSR can be conducted with a variety of different study designs. They may analyze primary data (collected prospectively as part of a clinical study) or secondary data (collected for some other purpose, such as for hospital billing, and are then repurposed). Clinical trial study designs are more familiar, where a specific intervention is imposed on a study group. Randomized Clinical Trials (RCTs) are considered the gold standard of clinical research because the intervention or exposure of interest is randomly designated across study participants. RCTs are often blinded, where the physician is not aware of a subjects assignment to a given study arm, or even double blinded, where neither the physician nor the subject is aware of the assignment. These design elements help to avoid any biases that may occur by ensuring the random distribution of interventions across subjects.

Observational analyses do not assign interventions among subjects and are most often retrospective in nature. Instead, researchers examine the relationship between exposures or events of interest that occurred and the associated effects or outcomes. The studies can be descriptive or analytic in their design. Descriptive studies include case reports or case series, ecologic studies, and cross-sectional studies, while analytic studies include longitudinal cohort and case–control studies. Descriptive analyses are used to generate hypotheses, whereas analytic analyses are used to test specific hypotheses about the association between a specific exposure and outcome.

Types of secondary data sources relevant to HSR in oncology

A common understanding among health services researchers is that the study is only as good as the data. There are limitations to every data source so health services researchers must use multiple approaches to be able to address a question of interest. Primary data quality will depend largely on the instrument design and any logistic constraints involved in data collection. Secondary data are often limited by the purpose for which they were originally collected. Billing data (aka claims data), are collected as documentation of services provided and payments received; studies using these data must account for the inherent limitations when designing an analytic plan.

There are a few commonly encountered types of oncology databases available for secondary analyses in HSR which include clinical registries, administrative datasets, clinical trial databases, and more recently an increasing body of data from aggregated electronic medical records (EMRs) (described later in the chapter). A thorough understanding of the strengths and limitations of the dataset is critical for one to conduct a valid analysis (Table 2). Clinical registries may collect relevant data on patients with an incident cancer diagnosis within a specific population, health care system, network, or region. Strengths of clinical registries include high-quality short-term exposure and outcome data, clinically rich data specific to a disease of interest, collection of potential confounders, and the potential for large sample sizes. The principal weakness of registry data are a lack of randomization to key exposures of interest, poor intermediate and long-term follow-up and outcomes, and lack of data regarding unrelated disease states such as cardiovascular disease.

Administrative datasets consist of information that is routinely collected within the operations of a given health care entity, such as an insurer (i.e, Medicare), integrated health care systems (i.e., Veterans Affairs Hospitals), or large health care organizations (i.e., Kaiser Permanente). The strength of administrative data lie in their broad coverage of tens or even hundreds of millions of lives, the efficiency of data availability, and the long-term follow-up available through the use of patient identifiers. In addition, administrative data are representative of the population at large, while data collected within a clinical trial are clinically rich but limited to a carefully pre-selected, smaller population because of cost and scientific considerations. The weaknesses of administrative data stem from their collection for purposes of billing and tracking health care resource utilization, often limiting the granularity of available information. Information such as dates of claims and types of procedures performed are highly accurate. However, information that is not critical to billing, such as cancer stage, are not always captured.

Different types of data can be linked together to help offset limitations of any single data set. For example, registry and clinical trial data, which often suffer from a lack of long-term follow-up and incompleteness can be supplemented with administrative claims data (such as Medicare) to augment the available follow-up and survival data.

Data is universally important across all study designs but the type of data is highly specific to the type of study being conducted. Further discussion of specific datasets and approaches will be presented subsequently in the context of different methdologies. However, two cancer-specific registries, SEER and the National Cancer Data Base (NCDB) that are particularly important to know as they play central roles in HSR in oncology are worth describing in detail.

Surveillance, Epidemiology, and End Results

The SEER tumor registry program collects detailed clinical and pathological information on 28% of cancer patients in the United States, aggregating it from participating registries that are representative of the national patient population. Limitations of these data include a lack of detailed information on treatments, providers, and cost. To address these needs, linkages were pursued to generate a richer set of variables. This resulted in a collaboration between the National Cancer Institute (NCI) and the Centers for Medicare and Medicaid Services (CMS) to make a SEER-Medicare dataset available that adds Medicare administrative data and health care claims. As CMS provides health insurance to over 97% of Americans aged 65 and older, this allows a detailed assessment of health care utilization and costs among SEER patients. The SEER-Medicare

Table 2 Strengths and weaknesses of commonly encountered large secondary databases.

Data Source	Examples	Strengths	Weaknesses
Disease registries	SEER NCDB EMR data-generated	• high-quality short-term exposure and outcome data • clinically rich • collection of potential confounders • large sample sizes across a broad population	• lack of randomization to key exposure • poor long-term follow-up • lack of data for unrelated disease states
Administrative data	CMS (Medicare) VA (Veterans Affairs) Kaiser Permanente	• broad coverage of the population • efficiency of data collection • long-term follow-up availability of patient-specific identifiers that can be linked to additional data sources	• lack of randomization to key exposure • inaccurately recorded data • limited clinical details
Clinical trials	Collaborative group studies Industry trials Institutional trials	• clinically rich data • random assignment of key exposures	• pre-selected population and smaller sample sizes • loss to follow-up

data have been used to examine cancer care quality around issues of racial disparities, physician and hospital characteristics, screening, treatment choices (i.e, surgery, chemotherapy, radiation), complications, costs, and mortality.[3] While powerful, a core limitation of the SEER-Medicare dataset is that it only includes those 65 years of age and older.

National Cancer Data Base (NCDB)

Another oncology-specific dataset which is widely used is the NCDB which is a joint project of the American Cancer Society and the American College of Surgeons' Commission on Cancer (CoC). The NCDB was established in 1989 as a nationwide, hospital-based, comprehensive clinical surveillance data set. The NCDB obtains data from more than 1,500 CoC-accredited facilities which captures 30 million patient records and 70% of all newly diagnosed cancer cases.[4] The key strength of the NCDB is its sheer size and capture of the majority of cancers diagnosed within the United States. It is well posed to study nationwide patterns of care, adoption of novel surgical procedures, and the approach to rare cancers. As a surgical data set, it contains excellent data on the details of a patient's surgery and survival. However, some aspects of the data are not reliably coded; there are limited details regarding chemotherapy, radiation or noncancer related health; and there is no information on relapse, recurrence, or subsequent treatments.

Statistical analyses in health services research

An in depth review of statistics is well beyond the scope of this chapter, so we will focus on commonly used techniques that encompass the vast majority of HSR. In HSR, statistical analyses are used to analyze data from a population of interest in order to either describe or learn something (i.e., make an inference) about the general state of affairs in that population. Descriptive statistics simply describe or summarize a set of data, by providing means, frequencies, counts, plots, or other depictions. Inferential or analytic statistics use more complex methodologies to attempt to draw generalizable inferences from a set of data, such as whether or not two groups differ from one another by more than what would reasonably be expected by chance.

Multivariable versus univariate analyses

In HSR, one of the most common distinctions made in practice is the use of statistics to investigate single variables vs. multiple variables. Single variable or "univariate" analyses are used to summarize or describe the properties of a single variable, such as what

percent of a population has ever smoked. Multivariable or multivariate analyses (in practice these are used interchangeably) are more complex and seek to explain the relationship between a single variable of interest and multiple other variables at the same time.

Often univariate versus multivariable analyses are referred to as "unadjusted" and "adjusted," as the multivariable approach "adjusts" for potential confounding by control variables. Such control variables might include clinically relevant variables associated with the outcome of interest such as age, stage, or grade and *must* include any variables that might be associated with both the exposure and outcome of interest in order to fully control for potential confounding. In a study that performs both "unadjusted" and "adjusted" analyses, the results from the adjusted (or multivariable) analyses are more likely to reflect the true relationship of interest, as these models have at least attempted to adjust for factors that might otherwise explain the observed relationship. Variables are often inter-related in HSR and a failure to account for these relationships can result in erroneous conclusions. The key question that HSR seeks to answer is often how a certain treatment, condition, or exposure impacts a specific outcome of interest after controlling for all other relevant factors.

Multivariable analyses

One of the most widely used methods in multivariable analysis in HSR is that of multivariable regression analysis. The term "regression" was original coined in the late 1800s by Francis Galton to describe the tendency of tall or short pea plants (outliers) to produce offspring that were more similar to or "regressed" towards the overall population height.[5] In its simplest form, this is essentially drawing a simple straight line through a plot of two variables that shows the mean or average of one variable as a function of the other. Significant mathematical and computational progress since has allowed for the routine use of far more complicated models that are able to predict the value of a so-called "dependent" variable whose value is predicted *depending* on the values of multiple "independent" variables. Such models come in many forms and have been refined and developed to be able to predict, model, or describe any combination of different variable types. Most often in HSR, continuous data are modeled using linear regression, dichotomous data using logistic regression (from its use of binary logic values, i.e., zero or one to describe the dependent variable), and survival data using cox proportional hazard models (survival variables include an event such as death or relapse vs. no death or relapse combined with the time to that event). Linear regressions will predict the mean value of the dependent variable as a function of each independent variable (i.e., average weight as a function of sex and height), logistic regressions will estimate odds ratios (OR) associated with a particular exposure, and cox proportional hazards models yield hazard ratios (HR). Other frequently used multivariable statistical analyses include variations of the χ^2 test (chi-squared), such as the Cochran–Mantel–Haenszel test,[6,7] which essentially performs the χ^2 test for an association between two categorical variables while controlling for other potentially confounding variables.

One of the benefits of multivariable regression is the ability to capture "interaction effects," or an interaction between two independent or explanatory variables on the dependent variable of interest. Interaction effects can capture cases where a variable might only impact the outcome of treatment within a subset of patients. For example, a meta-analysis of three randomized controlled trials in nonsmall cell lung cancer found a significant interaction between squamous tumor histology, receipt of pemetrexed, and a lack of treatment response.[8] This meta-analysis confirmed that the drug pemetrexed is associated with improved outcomes, but only in patients with nonsquamous cell histology. As a result, pemetrexed is now the drug of choice in nonsquamous NSCLC.

Bias and confounders

Perhaps the single most important concept in HSR is the idea of bias or confounding. A confounder is anything that confuses, obscures, or otherwise mixes the effect of the characteristic of interest with others. The word "confound" comes from the latin for "pour together,"[9] and so literally describes a situation where the observed association is mixed or confused by a confounder. An example of confounding can be demonstrated using a hypothetical retrospective study of patients with metastatic disease, in which patients who have less aggressive disease and receive surgery for their metastatic disease are observed to live longer. In this case, the observed association of surgery with prolonged survival is being confused with, or "confounded" by, the association of nonaggressive disease with both surgery and survival.

Bias is also used to describe confounding, but can be more descriptive by additionally specifying the direction of the observed erroneous association. Bias is a related term from the old French biais, meaning "slant,"[9] and describes the situation where the observed association is biased, or unfairly slanted, to yield either a false positive (can bias the estimate of an association upward or downward) or false negative (biased towards the null hypothesis) association between two variables.

One specific example of bias in the HSR oncology literature comes from analyses of survival in patients with nonsmall cell lung cancer (NSCLC). Several studies had observed that receipt of PET scans are associated with improved survival, and erroneously concluded that receipt of PET *improves* survival. However, upon closer examination, we know that PET scans are generally administered to patients with early stage disease who are candidates for curative surgery and definitive treatment. The use of PET scans is not indicated for patients with obvious advanced or metastatic disease. In this case, one would say that the association of PET with survival is confounded by selection bias, or selective administration of PET scans to patients with less advanced disease. Another way to describe this would be to say that the association of PET with survival is being confounded by selective administration of PET to lower risk patients.[10,11]

There are several commonly encountered types of bias that are important in the accurate interpretation of observational HSR studies. *Omitted variable bias* is one of the principal forms of bias in observational studies and is nearly always present to some extent in

HSR. It will occur in any situation where (1) a variable exists that is associated with both the outcome and exposure of interest and (2) is omitted as a control. For example, in the PET-NSCLC scenario, disease stage was correlated with both PET and survival, but was not included in the model.

Selection bias is used to describe when a group or exposure is not randomly applied to patients, or in the example case above, where PET scans were *selectively* applied to patients with less advanced disease. *Recall bias* refers to the situation where one population is more likely to recall an event than another. For example, patients with a rare form of cancer might be more likely to recall exposure to any number of environmental stimuli that have been forgotten or would have been overlooked by patients without cancer who had the identical exposure. Bias due to *loss to follow-up* can occur if patients who remain in the study are systematically different from those who do not. *Nonresponse bias* can be seen in self-reported surveys, where survey participants are often more likely to express stronger beliefs than that held by the overall target study population. *Misclassification bias* refers to the case where either the exposure or outcome of interest is misclassified. Lastly, *interviewer bias* can occur when the interviewer knows which exposure or treatment a patient has had, and probes more deeply than they otherwise would have in patients without that exposure.

Minimizing confounders and bias

There are several potential methods that can be used to minimize confounders. Several of these methods can only be implemented during the design phase of a study, and it is therefore key to involve a statistician or HSR methodologist early on in the design of any study, when the full set of all options are available. For example, RCTs will often stratify by key variables known to influence the outcome of interest in order to ensure that they will not wind up with an unbalanced treatment and control group in the final analysis. Multivariable regression analyses are commonly used to help adjust or control for potential confounders. However, a key limitation of such attempts is that variables that are not or cannot be observed cannot be controlled. There are nearly always such unobservable factors at play to some extent in most observational HSR studies, which is why any observed associations should not be reported as causal without further confirmation.

Commonly used methods that are used to mitigate the impact of bias include matching, stratification, subgroup analysis, and instrumental variable analysis.

Matching is the process whereby the characteristics between two groups are matched as closely as possible, in order to create populations that are similar in all respects. The quality of the match can be indirectly assessed by checking to make sure that observable variables that were not used to match patients appear to be similar between groups.

When there are many factors that may differ between two populations, exact matching on all factors is not possible. A calculated *propensity score* may be used to predict the likelihood (or propensity) to receive the treatment or exposure of interest.[12] Patients can then either be matched directly or stratified by their propensity to assess the exposure or treatment of interest, thereby mitigating important differences between study groups.

Related to matching approaches is the idea of *stratification or subgroup analysis*, which respectively control for, or limit analysis to, a specific subgroup of selected patients in which outcomes are predicted to be similar (i.e. stage, age, performance status).

The above approaches all have in common are that they identify potential confounders and attempt to correct or adjust for them. In contrast, an approach called *instrumental variable (IV)* analysis is meant to minimize bias by avoiding confounders all together. In the IV approach, researchers attempt to identify a so-called "instrument," or proxy that is strongly associated with the exposure of interest, but that is not associated with the outcome of interest through confounding. For example, distance to the nearest facility with PET scanners might predict the likelihood of undergoing a PET scan (the exposure of interest), but should not otherwise be directly associated with stage or survival (outcomes) except through the exposure of interest (PET). Strong "instruments" can be difficult to identify and often are unavailable.

It is important to realize that none of the above methods will completely eliminate bias in real-world HSR analyses. As such, the ability to mitigate, and test for, residual bias is paramount in conducting accurately interpreting observational HSR.

Internal and external validity

Internal validity refers to whether or not observed findings are likely to be reflective of the examined population. In other words, interval validity describes whether the observed findings can be believed within the patients that were analyzed in the study. Any and all studies must have internal validity in order to allow for clinically meaningful interpretation. Common threats to interval validity include selection bias, differential follow-up, recall bias, confounding, misclassification, investigator or interviewer bias, or any systematic differences between control and treatment groups that are associated with the exposure of interest.

External validity refers to whether the associations observed within the confines of the population studied can be generalized to patients outside (external to) the study sample. Not all studies will be externally valid to the same extent. For example, many RCTs are limited to young patients with few comorbidities. The benefit seen in RCTs may not extend to older, sicker, or heavily pretreated patients who were not included in the study.

Different outcomes methods

Meta-analyses and systematic reviews

Systematic reviews are thorough, systematized reviews of the literature on a specific question in HSR and often take place as the preliminary step within a meta-analysis. Meta-analysis describes a statistical technique for combining data from multiple studies in order to try and provide a more precise estimate of the true impact of an intervention or exposure. In order for such studies to be valid, meta-analyses should first perform a quality systemic review of the existing literature, incorporate all relevant data, and check for evidence of heterogeneity in reported studies in order to assess whether or not there is evidence of a potential bias in the field to only publish positive associations. Major findings should be confirmed via the use of sensitivity analyses that ensure that observed estimates are robust to reasonable variations in the analysis. Systematic reviews and meta-analysis are often considered a principal component of the evidence development process, and are particularly important in supporting the generalizability and understanding of clinical effectiveness.

Randomized controlled trials

RCTs have long been considered to produce the highest level of evidence among individual trials. In an RCT, patients are randomly assigned to either a control (placebo or standard of care) arm or an experimental arm. Such trials have been used in countless assessments of therapeutic benefit of medications, behavioral interventions, screening studies, and chemoprevention studies. Although such trials represent the pinnacle of evidence development and have a number of strengths, it is critical for care providers and researchers to have a thorough understanding of both the benefits and limitations of such studies so that they are able to accurately interpret and incorporate their findings in guiding clinical practice and future HSR studies.

The key strength of the RCT is its ability to ensure that a treatment was assigned at random, which serves as the single most reliable method to remove potential sources of bias. This allows the closest ability we have to study what we truly want to understand—the "counterfactual condition." Counterfactual means literally "against the facts" and describes a "what-if" situation. What we really want to know is "what if" the same patient was exposed to treatment A versus treatment B? If we could go back in time and administer a different treatment to the same patient, would it have changed their outcome? This is obviously not possible. However, through the use of RCTs, we are able to randomly assign treatment so that we can indirectly infer, on average, what would have been the impact had a patient received treatment A versus treatment B. Again, the potential for bias introduced by confounders in observational studies is the principal weakness of observational studies and the ability to avoid confounded treatment assignment is the fundamental strength of RCTs.

Potential limitations of randomized controlled trials

RCTs are not able to address many questions in HSR. Perhaps the most significant reason is that RCTs are often impossible to conduct because of ethical concerns about a lack of equipoise, or equal validity of both proposed treatment strategies. Because of this, there is often only a limited period during which equipoise of two proposed management strategies exists. A classic example of this is the comparison of radical prostatectomy to radiation therapy in the definitive management of localized prostate cancer. In most cases, a patient's provider and the patient themselves are generally unwilling to randomly assign such substantially different treatments. Numerous RCTs attempting to compare the two strategies have resulted in limited accrual, leading to concerns about sample sizes and external validity.[13] In the United Kingdom, only 1 of 20 patients enrolled on such a study consented to randomization.[14]

Even when adequate equipoise exists to enroll meaningful numbers of patients into RCTs, there are additional limitations. Caution should always be taken whenever interpreting a "negative study" to make sure that the study was adequately powered to answer the question being asked.

Another key limitation of RCTs is that such studies are often applied to a selected group of patients that lack external validity. Patients who are eligible for clinical trials are heavily screened and reflect a group of patients whose outcomes are often superior to those seen in the community. An example of difficulties with external validity comes from a high-quality and well-known meta-analysis of the benefit of chemotherapy in localized breast cancer.[15] Despite the inclusion of 194 trials, few patients were over the age of 69, which leaves the benefit of chemotherapy unclear in women over 70.

The process of study design, enrollment, follow-up and analysis of RCTs can take decades or longer before results are known. The studies can be outdated before they are completed, particularly in areas of cancer care where practice is changing rapidly and the natural disease history is relatively indolent or protracted such as in localized breast or prostate cancer. RCTs cannot assess how the general population is treated, examine the extent to which risks and benefits seen in controlled settings match those observed in actual practice, or characterize adoption, utilization, costs, or factors associated with the use of an intervention in real-world practice. Although RCTs remain a critical component in creating high-level evidence of the efficacy of experimental treatments, observational studies must be used as a complement in order to provide a full and balanced perspective of the true impact and effectiveness of proposed treatment strategies.

Observational studies

Observational studies do not assign or alter any factor of interest as, by definition, they cannot control which patients receive a given exposure or treatment. They are performed on the various data sources described previously—administrative claims data, disease registries, data collected within large health organizations (i.e., Veterans Affairs), and as secondary analyses of clinical trial data. SEER, the population-based registry outlined earlier that now covers 28% of the US population, and the NCDB, the hospital-based registry of more than 1,500 CoC-accredited facilities that captures 70% of newly diagnosed cancer cases nationally, are excellent examples.[4] The Nationwide Inpatient Sample (NIS) is another example, as it contains discharge data from 44 states since 2012, representing 20% of all community hospitals.[16] Large administrative claims data bases, such as Medicare claims and those curated by large private insurers, are also routinely linked to provide additional data such as death, treatment, patient surveys, or other factors of interest. This results in large, comprehensive samples of current practice within the United States.

The potential for bias or confounding is the primary limitation of observational studies, and a host of advanced statistical methods discussed earlier have been developed to help combat and mitigate potential biases in order to avoid invalid conclusions. Despite this fundamental weakness, observational studies continue to play an important and critical role in much of HSR that cannot be addressed by RCTs. Perhaps the single most important risk factor for developing cancer in the modern era, smoking, has never been examined within a RCT, but has been firmly established by countless observational studies across numerous cancer types.

There are several principal strengths of observational studies. They examine real-world practice in the community, as opposed to that limited to major academic or cancer trial centers, and provide a representation of the actual use and outcomes associated with an intervention as it is used in practice. Compared to interventional studies, observational studies have the additional benefits of significantly reduced costs, large sample sizes, the potential to observe extended follow-up, and often the statistical power necessary to detect heterogeneous treatment effects or risks among rare patient subgroups.

Types of observational studies

Observational studies can be primarily classified as descriptive or analytic. The focus of analytic studies is similar to that of randomized trials, where the goal is to assess whether or not a causal relationship exists between an exposure or treatment and the outcome of interest. Such studies seek to test a specific hypothesis, for example one might hypothesize that patients undergoing surgery at a high-volume center have superior outcomes compared to those treated at lower volume centers. In contrast, descriptive studies characterize a particular set of patient characteristics or outcomes and can be used to generate hypotheses to be tested in future studies.

The two most common examples of analytic observational studies are case–control and cohort studies. Case–control studies are often used in cancer HSR to assess the association between environmental exposures such as smoking, genotype, geography, drugs, diet, or toxins and the likelihood of developing cancer (the outcome). Such studies identify patients with the outcome of interests (cases, i.e., cancer) and match them to patients who did not experience the outcome (controls, i.e., no cancer). Interviews or surveys are then often conducted to obtain additional information from both sets of patients. The strength of such studies is that they can be used to analyze factors that might predispose people to rare cancers that would otherwise be difficult to evaluate. The primary challenge of these studies is often identifying controls that are otherwise similar to the cases except for the exposure of interest and ensuring that recall bias among controls does not over-report exposures compared to the control cases.

In contrast to case–control studies, cohort studies select a group of patients based on their exposure and then follow them forward over time. Cohort studies are called as such because they first define the specific cohorts of interest—that is exposure and nonexposure—before examining outcomes. There are numerous examples of cohort studies in HSR, which include analyses of clinical trials, registries, and other retrospective or prospective databases. These studies are often used to characterize the adoption and costs of emerging medical technology such as advanced imaging and PET scans[17] or Intensity Modulated Radiation Therapy (IMRT) in the treatment of prostate cancer.[18]

Prospective analyses consist of data collected with the intention of analyzing it for a given purpose. In contrast, retrospective analyses utilize data that have already been collected for a different reason, often leveraging administrative claims used to bill insurance companies or general cancer registries that include treatment data. Although a distinction is often made between prospective and retrospective analyses, the methods and approaches used to analyze the data are similar. However, prospective analyses, especially those for which a detailed analysis plan is created prior to collecting and viewing the data, are less likely to lead to extensive subgroup analyses or other approaches that may identify spurious associations due to chance and extensive data manipulation. The strengths of observational cohort studies include the ability to examine rare exposures over prolonged periods of time, such as the impact of atomic bomb radiation exposure on the risk of developing leukemia and other cancers decades later. In contemporary HSR, cohort studies are perhaps the most commonly used observational study approach and are used to compare the impact of a particular treatment on patient outcomes. For example, given the difficulties of conducting large RCTs of prostatectomy versus radiation in prostate cancer, many cohort studies have compared outcomes following treatment with these two modalities (Sun 2014).

Descriptive studies include ecologic studies, cross-sectional studies, and case reports or case series. Unlike analytic studies, such studies are not designed to test hypotheses, but rather to generate hypotheses that may be tested in later studies. Ecologic studies describe situations where the exposure and outcomes occur at the individual-level, but are measured at the population level.[19] For example, ecologic studies of many cancers have been used to demonstrate changes in the risk of specific cancers such as breast or prostate between the US and other countries, presumably due to cultural, environmental, lifestyle, or dietary differences in exposures.[20] Such studies, while hypothesis generating, suffer from the primary weakness that they cannot confirm individual-level associations between exposures and outcomes.

In contrast to *ecologic studies*, cross-sectional studies are used to observe individuals at a single snapshot in time, and can characterize the association of exposures and outcomes among those patients.

However, the primary limitation of these studies is that they cannot be used to draw causal inferences, as it is not possible to distinguish whether such an association represents the exposure causing the outcome or the outcome causing the exposure.

Lastly, *case reports or case series* describe detailed exposures and outcomes of a small number of patients. Such studies have often heralded the potential for extraordinary therapeutic efficacy of novel treatment strategies. A contemporary example of a high impact case report comes from the case of combining novel immune checkpoint inhibitors with radiation, where radiation to a single site of disease was observed to induce complete systemic resolution of all sites of disease in a patient with metastatic melanoma. The effect was attributed to a radiation-induced stimulation of a systemic immune response.[21]

Common limitations of most retrospectively performed analyses include a lack of personal risk factors, detailed performance status, and other factors that might influence or more accurately characterize the exposure or outcome of interest that would have been collected had the analysis plan been known at the time of data collection. The quality of analyses performed on any data set will vary widely depending on the quality of the data. Key to the internal validity of any study is the reliability of key exposures, outcomes, and potential confounders contained within the data. In administrative claims data, for example, claim dates and procedural codes are typically heavily audited and highly reliable, since this information is used to determine payment information. However, the reliability of a diagnosis of constipation or some other minor complication that does not impact payment might be missed in a large proportion of patients. Therefore, familiarity with the data being analyzed is paramount to performing a well-conducted study.

Modeling

Modeling studies in HSR refer to the creation of algorithms to describe complex associations and relationships between exposures, outcomes, and confounders.[22] Modeling can play a particularly important role in guiding the design of policies, guidelines, treatment approaches, or reimbursement that would otherwise be too time consuming, costly, and complicated to analyze using direct interventional or conventional observational approaches. Modeling also provides a means of exploring relationships among data which cannot be directly observed or feasibly obtained in practice, such as those involving costs or long term outcomes. Models used in HSR often examine the impact of various decision algorithms, new interventions, policies, or patient factors on associated outcomes or costs. The studies often use metrics such as health adjusted life-years (QUALYs) to objectively provide an indication of the balance between overall quantify and QOL for cancer patients. Cost-effectiveness analyses often report incremental cost effectiveness ratios (ICERs), which describe the relative cost and gains of alternative management strategies or exposures.

An example in the cancer literature comes from several analyses of the impact of Oncotype DX testing in breast cancer. Use of the Oncotype DX test, which predicts the benefit associated with receipt of chemotherapy, has been previously shown to change physician recommendations to prescribe less overall chemotherapy. Modeling studies of Oncotype DX testing have been used to perform cost-effectiveness analyses and have predicted that the use of the assay has the potential to be cost-saving.[23] The advantage of modeling is that various factors and their relative impact on outcomes of interest can be dissected—for example, one could adjust estimates of cost savings from Oncotype DX testing depending on the utilization strategy, the age of the population, and the cost of chemotherapy. The obvious disadvantage of modeling is that many assumptions must be made that may impact the findings.

Quality of care

The IOM has defined quality of care as "the degree to which health care services for individuals and populations increase the likelihood of desired health outcomes and are consistent with current professional knowledge," and then later extended the definition to encompass "care that incorporates respect for patients' values and preferences."[24,25] It is underappreciated that, despite substantial improvements in available treatments and technology, the main determinants of patient health outcomes, quality of care, and overall costs are related to variability in clinical practice[26,27] and the failure of patients to receive basic care.[28]

One such example comes from studies of surgery at high-volume centers. For over thirty years it has been consistently observed that centers with higher volume, or total number of cases performed, are often associated with improved outcomes.[29] Twenty years after this was initially observed, this was confirmed in a meta-analysis showing that in 123 of 128 studies included, lower hospital mortality was observed in high-volume centers across 40 different procedures.[30] The risk of receiving a procedure a low-volume center was highest for complicated procedures such as esophagectomy and pancreatectomy, where differences in 30-day mortality approach 5–10%.[31] However, it is important to note that such studies are observational in nature, vary in their definition of "high volume," and may be significantly biased by case selection of patients willing to travel to higher volume centers. Quality of care may also vary by geographic region owing to differences in regional treatment patterns, patient populations, available oncology specialists, or other factors. For example, rates of laparoscopic colectomy[32] and end of life care[33] vary widely by geography.

The quality metrics used to describe the structure, process, and outcomes of care were proposed by Dr. Donabedian in 1950 and continue to be used to this day.[1] Structure describes the context in which care is provided and its associated financial and personnel resources. Examples might include institutional characteristics such as provider expertise, accreditation, and case volume. Processes consist of patient and provider activities in the diagnosis and treatment of an illness and are often defined in terms of guidelines issued by national organizations such as the National Comprehensive Cancer Network (NCCN) or American Society of Clinical Oncology (ASCO). Outcomes describe the patient's health post treatment and are defined in terms such as overall survival, disease-specific survival, objective response rates, time to progression, and toxicity. The use of outcomes in formal metrics is often debated in oncology due to variations in case-mix, disease-severity, and other potential confounders that might be outside an institution's control. Increasingly, methods are used to overcome this limitation.

Despite the potential for each of these to impact the quality of care, there are inherent challenges in using outcomes and structure-based endpoints to define quality in a way that can incentivize health care providers and systems to improve care. For example, outcomes may be significantly impacted by the case-mix seen by an institution. Efforts to "cherry-pick" or otherwise select patients may be effective at increasing profits, but not improve care. Structure-based endpoints may not be appropriate as a one size fits all solution depending on the total case volume, case mix, amount of resources, or rural versus urban location. As a result, assessments of health quality in both HSR and in practical use are dominated by procedural measures. As an example, the majority of Healthcare Effectiveness Data and Information Set (HEDIS) measures currently used to assess health care performance across a wide variety of settings relies almost entirely on procedure-based definitions of quality such as the use of cancer screening, immunizations, or specific treatments for disease.[34] Procedures can be underused, overused, or misused. In practice, underuse is often most easily studied in the setting where current guidelines recommend a specific procedure and whether or not patients received the recommended standard of care can be examined. Overuse and misuse, however, are challenging to prove, since guidelines tend to be less likely to describe situations where a specific test should not be performed under any circumstances. For example, although a PET scan may not be indicated for all patients with breast or colorectal cancer, a borderline CT scan or other equivocal study would be a reasonable indication to perform a PET. Such nuances can be difficult to describe systematically within many retrospective data sets. Lastly, misuse can be similarly difficult to confirm in the absence of detailed treatment records, which typically are not available in larger retrospective studies.

HSR 2.0

HSR has advanced quickly over the last two decades due in part to the rapid progress made in computational power and the ability to generate, store, link, analyze, and interpret large datasets. Until 1970, it would often take up to 24 hours to run a single regression analysis using the electromechanical desk calculators of the day.[35] Advances in personal computing, the internet, and now mobile devices, provide a previously unparalleled opportunity to fully capture and analyze health services from the patient, provider, and health system perspectives. The IOM has formally acknowledged the idea of a learning health system (LHS), defined as an organization in which "science, informatics, incentives, and culture are aligned for continuous improvement and innovation—with best practices seamlessly embedded in the delivery process and new knowledge captured as an integral by-product of the delivery experience."[36] The idea behind the LHS is to provide rapid learning personalized health care, in which patient care naturally feeds back information on patient outcomes to help guide future management decisions.[37] Although the idea of the LHS is becoming increasingly more common, "use cases" describing their effective implementation to assess patient outcomes and recommend future areas for research are only beginning to emerge. For example, an LHS approach is being used to evaluate the role of biologics in pediatric crohn's patients.[38]

EMRs are foundational to a learning health system, as they provide a digital footprint of each patient's story. Multiple patient cases are aggregated to generate streams of continuously updating information. To the effect that data in the EMR can be codified to a common standard, then EMR data can approximate registry data. In order to solve this, information in structured data feeds (e.g., laboratory data) needs to be harmonized and normalized to a single common data model; information trapped in unstructured documents (e.g., PDFs of clinical notes, pathology reports) must be transferred to a codifiable digital standards. Multiple groups are focused on solving this problem in cancer.

The potential contributors to LHS and related efforts are broad, spanning organizations such as traditional health organizations, government entities, and genomics companies. HSR will benefit from real-world data obtained in real time through the linking of EMRs to numerous external databases. The potential to incorporate decisions support into routine care, leveraging patient specific data in areas such as genomics, treatment history, and predicted outcomes will require knowledge of how to manage such data

from technical, medicolegal, ethical, and practical perspectives. In the face of rising health care costs and inefficiencies, oncology workshops focused on the delivery of affordable care have proposed the use of LHS to provide a potential solution to help economize health services and clinical research.[39]

Outcomes and endpoints

Although HSR can encompass any outcome or endpoint associated with patient care, there are a number of types of outcomes and endpoints that form the bulk of current HSR including QOL, cost, quality, access, patterns of care, and CER.

Patient reported outcomes

Patient reported outcomes (PROs) are generated by questions posed to patients regarding their symptoms and other concerns, as opposed to being documented by physicians or other members of the health care team.

Widespread internet access and advances in computational technology now provide the opportunity to engage with patients and collect longitudinal PROs, which has grown dramatically over the past few years. As a result, the collection and utilization of PROs has emerged as a distinct area of study with networks of researchers dedicated to its implementation. In support of this, researchers with expertise in the collection and utilization of PROs often collaborate with QOL researchers to efficiently achieve their research goals. For the purpose of the discussion, we will only briefly mention QOL as a subset of PRO research, noting that it in fact composes a large portion of PRO research but will be described in more detail in the next section.

The use of PROs in HSR has several strengths including efficient collection, improved accuracy as to the patient's experience when compared to physician-reported measures, and the ability to use them to predict objective clinical outcomes such as survival, patient satisfaction, and general health.[40] PRO measures can be either generic or disease-specific, each of which have their respective advantages and weaknesses.[41] Advantages of general PRO tools include wider generalizability across disease types and a larger body of literature to support both their validity and association with traditional objective endpoints.

Although a large number of PROs have been used in the literature, there are several PRO measures that have been specifically evaluated in oncology and are worth brief mention here and include the EORTC QOL Questionnaire (EORTC QLQ-C30), Functional Assessment of Cancer Therapy (FACT), MD Anderson Symptom Inventory (MDASI), PRO version of the Common Terminology Criteria for Adverse Events (PRO-CTCAE), and PRO Measurement Information System (PROMIS).[40] Efforts to validate, standardize, and compare PROs have greatly improved the quality of PRO measures, which are now used routinely in clinical trial design and the approval of new drug applications submitted to the FDA.

A recent advance in the LHS field has been the incorporation of the patient's voice using PROs. In particular, the capture of electronic PROs (ePROs) over conventional PROs are numerous, and include reduced cost, increased efficiency of delivery and completion for both patients and providers, and the ability to use computer adaptive testing (CAT) to further economize and personalize the data gathered from these interactions. Through this cycle, these data can then be used to help inform clinical care, provide decision support, and educate patients and clinicians in real-time at the point of care.

Quality of life

Measures of QOL are numerous and complex, each containing specific domains or areas of interest (i.e., fatigue, urinary symptoms, medical events), with each domain including multiple items. Key measures of the utility of specific QOL instruments include their reliability, internal consistency, reproducibility between interviewers, and validity (content and construct). The short form—36 item (SF-36) is an example of a questionnaire that has been used in hundreds of studies and disease types with a large body of literature supporting its reliability and applicability. Alternatively, disease-specific measures provide a more targeted assessment of key factors relevant to a particular patient population. For example, for patients with prostate cancer, urologic and sexual QOL metrics should be directly assessed through disease-specific tools such as the International Index of Erectile Function (IIEF) and American Urologic Association (AUA). Choosing the best measures of QOL requires a thorough understanding of the most relevant symptoms and outcomes to a specific patient population.[40] QOL research can also be used to derive utilities, or quantitative measures of QOL. Such utilities can be used to adjust survival analyses to represent both quantity and QOL.

QOL measures have a number of limitations, including the fact that they often contain a large number of domains and items, with many potential permutations of measures, dysfunctions and symptoms, impeding efforts at standardization, and validation. QOL measures may also not hold the same value for all patients. For example, elderly patients may not be as concerned with sexual function and previously disabled patients may have a different baseline level of functionality that precedes their diagnosis. Lastly, as with any data, missing data or failure of patients to complete questionnaires may occur due to fatigue, apathy, decline in mental function, or overall decline in health. Such declines are notorious in palliative care settings, where non-participation may be strongly associated with declining patient overall performance status and can result in reporting bias.

Costs

As described previously in this chapter, the cost of cancer in the US is increasing rapidly due to the aging of the population and the adoption, and increased use, of expensive emerging medical technologies. Efforts to accurately quantify current costs, understand factors driving costs, and model the impact of alternative strategies are a critical component of HSR. Such analyses may examine overall costs, cost-effectiveness, cost-utility, cost-benefits, and help provide a uniform framework and set universal thresholds to objectively and rationally inform policy, reimbursement, payer, provider, and patient decisions.

Even the most basic cost analyses are more complex and nuanced than one might initially expect. Patients undergoing the same treatment, at the same institution, for the same condition, may pay vastly different amounts for the same service (e.g., owing to different insurance). Because of the nature of health care and its perception as a right (i.e., emergency care), "customers" cannot be turned away for certain services. The means by which hospitals and medical facilities balance the costs of those who can pay versus those who cannot set the stage for a widely variable, often obscure, pricing system in which the physician often is not able to know the cost of the treatment they are prescribing. This is in stark contrast to other consumer services in which charges are known in advance and discussed upfront by service providers such as is done by mechanics and veterinarians.

As a result, the method and perspective used to estimate costs of medical care must be carefully specified and can include payments made by the insurer (payer perspective), out of pocket payments by the patient (patient perspective), total payments, total charges, lost wages due to lost productivity, and the additional burden placed on family members or other caregivers (societal perspective). Many interventions may alter subsequent management strategies and outcomes, which may impact overall costs via these "indirect costs." Of all these metrics, hospital listed charges vary the most widely, are the least reliable indicators of true cost, and are rarely used since most patients pay a lower price as negotiated by their insurance company. Marginal costs indicate the additional cost of a change in treatment strategies or additional services and are often used to examine the incremental impact of changes in treatment strategies. Because of the complexity of calculating health care costs, and the potential variation in the cost for a given service, close attention should be paid to the details and underlying assumptions of any cost estimates.

Bundled episodes of care

Many payers no longer operate using an a-la-carte, fee for service system where each service or good is associated with a payment. Inpatient costs are increasingly bundled and rates of reimbursements set by a Diagnosis Related Group (DRG) code which consists of a single lump sum that is paid to hospitals to cover all care administered during a hospitalization. These DRG codes are based on estimates of how much an admission should reasonably cost given the reason for the admission and potential complicating factors. Similarly, surgical procedures are often bundled, where a single reimbursement is expected to cover the surgery and all associated follow-up care, including complications within a predetermined timeframe. These systems are designed to incentivize providers and hospitals to provide efficient care and minimize complications.

Cost-effectiveness analysis

There are several types of cost analyses beyond simple summations that provide objective data with which patient, providers, payers, and policy makers can make informed decisions. Commonly analyses include cost-effectiveness analyses and modeling (described previously in this chapter). A cost-effectiveness analysis has been defined by the National Institute for Health and Clinical Excellence (NICE) as an economic study design in which consequences of different interventions are measured using a single outcome (i.e., life-years gained, deaths avoided, cases detected). Alternative interventions are then compared in terms of cost per unit of effectiveness.[42] This key metric is referred to as the incremental cost-effectiveness ratio (ICER). Whether or not a specific intervention is considered "cost-effective" depends on the available resources and willingness to pay of the target population. A classic analysis of over 500 life-saving interventions suggested that the median cost per life year saved was approximately $42,000 per life year saved[43] (in 1995 dollars), providing a rough benchmark of the relative willingness of the American public to pay. In contrast, global health initiatives, vaccinations, and the treatment of malaria are highly cost-effective at less than $100 per life year saved. A screening colonoscopy every 10 years beginning at age 50 costs roughly $11,000 per year of life saved.[44] The World Health Organization recommends considering cost-effectiveness in terms of gross domestic product (GDP) per capita.[45] Using this schema, interventions are considered highly cost-effective (less than GDP per capita); cost-effective (between one and three times GDP per capita); and not cost-effective (more than three times GDP per capita). For the United States (2012 GDP per capita) this would equate to <$50,000, $50,000–$150,000, and >$150,000, respectively. In the end, cost-effectiveness analyses are often phrased in terms of currently accepted ICERs. For example, if a given health system is already paying for interventions that cost $60,000 per QALY, it would make logical sense for them to cover a novel intervention with an ICER <$60,000. In current US practice interventions, ICERs of <$50,000 are generally considered cost-effective. Such analyses provide a detailed and objective framework with which patients, providers, and policy makers can make rational tradeoffs in costs, care, and outcomes.

Comparative effectiveness research

According to the Agency for Healthcare Research and Quality (AHRQ), CER is "designed to inform health care decisions by providing evidence on the effectiveness, benefits, and harms of different treatment options."[46] The term "comparative effectiveness" was coined roughly 25 years ago and was originally used to describe research to "help patients, family, and caregivers make more informed decisions with providers."[47] In practice, the use of CER is used to describe studies (often observational) that attempt to compare the benefits of two interventions or management strategies. The 2010 Patient Protection and Affordable Care Act (PPACA) established the Patient-Centered Outcomes Research Institute (PCORI) to fund and conduct research to determine the effectiveness of various medical services. PCORI explicitly emphasized the incorporation of costs and cost-effectiveness into studies.[48] As a result, the use of CER has evolved over recent years to include a greater focus on cost and cost-effectiveness.

CER is not a specific analysis technique or approach but a re-framing of existing observational study methodologies to focus on the comparison of potential treatment strategies. Most CER studies are simply cohort-based studies, described previously in this chapter, with an emphasis on attempting to simulate an RCT comparing two treatment arms with the goal of performing causal inference. At the end of the day, the key challenge in CER studies, much like other observational studies, is the mitigation of potential bias and confounding.

Key references

The complete reference list can be found on the Wiley Companion Digital Edition of this title (see inside front cover for login instructions).

1 Donabedian A. Evaluating the quality of medical care. 1966. *Milbank Q.* 2005;**83**(4):691–729.

2 Mariotto AB, Yabroff KR, Shao Y, Feuer EJ, Brown ML. Projections of the cost of cancer care in the United States: 2010–2020. *J Natl Cancer Inst.* 2011;**103**(2):117–128. Epub 2011 Jan 2012.

3 Warren JL, Klabunde CN, Schrag D, Bach PB, Riley GF. Overview of the SEER-Medicare data: content, research applications, and generalizability to the United States elderly population. *Med Care.* Aug 2002;**40**(8 **Suppl**):IV-3–IV-18.

5 Pearson K. *The Life, Letters and Labors of Francis Galton.* London: Cambridge University Press; 1930.

7 Mantel N, Haenszel W. Statistical aspects of the analysis of data from retrospective studies of disease. *J Natl Cancer Inst.* Apr 1959;**22**(4):719–748.

8 Scagliotti G, Brodowicz T, Shepherd FA, et al. Treatment-by-histology interaction analyses in three phase III trials show superiority of pemetrexed in nonsquamous non-small cell lung cancer. *J Thorac Oncol: official publication of the International Association for the Study of Lung Cancer.* Jan 2011;**6**(1):64–70.

10 Dinan MA, Curtis LH, Carpenter WR, et al. Stage migration, selection bias, and survival associated with the adoption of positron emission tomography among medicare beneficiaries with non-small-cell lung cancer, 1998–2003. *J Clin Oncol.* Aug 1 2012;**30**(22):2725–2730.

11 Chee KG, Nguyen DV, Brown M, Gandara DR, Wun T, Lara PN Jr. Positron emission tomography and improved survival in patients with lung cancer: the Will Rogers phenomenon revisited. *Arch Intern Med.* Jul 28 2008;**168**(14):1541–1549.

12 D'Agostino RB Jr. Propensity score methods for bias reduction in the comparison of a treatment to a non-randomized control group. *Stat Med.* 1998;**17**(19):2265–2281.

13 Penson DF. An update on randomized clinical trials in localized and locoregional prostate cancer. *Urol Oncol.* Jul-Aug 2005;**23**(4):280–288.

14 O'Reilly P, Martin L, Collins G. Few patients with prostate cancer are willing to be randomised to treatment. *BMJ.* Jun 5 1999;**318**(7197):1556.

15 Early Breast Cancer Trialists Group. Effects of chemotherapy and hormonal therapy for early breast cancer on recurrence and 15-year survival: an overview of the randomised trials. *Lancet.* May 14–20 2005;**365**(9472):1687–1717.

16 AHRQ. Health Care Utilization Project: Overview of the National (Nationwide) Inpatient Sample (NIS). 2015; http://www.hcup-us.ahrq.gov/nisoverview.jsp.

17 Dinan MA, Curtis LH, Hammill BG, et al. Changes in the use and costs of diagnostic imaging among Medicare beneficiaries with cancer, 1999–2006. *JAMA.* Apr 28 2010;**303**(16):1625–1631.

18 Dinan MA, Robinson TJ, Zagar TM, et al. Changes in initial treatment for prostate cancer among Medicare beneficiaries, 1999–2007. *Int J Radiat Oncol Biol Phys.* Apr 1 2012;**82**(5):e781–e786.

20 Buell P. Changing incidence of breast cancer in Japanese-American women. *J Natl Cancer Inst.* Nov 1973;**51**(5):1479–1483.

21 Postow MA, Callahan MK, Barker CA, et al. Immunologic correlates of the abscopal effect in a patient with melanoma. *N Engl J Med.* Mar 8 2012;**366**(10):925–931.

22 Ringel JS, Eibner C, Girosi F, Cordova A, McGlynn EA. Modeling health care policy alternatives. *Health Serv Res.* Oct 2010;**45**(5 Pt 2):1541–1558.

23 Vanderlaan BF, Broder MS, Chang EY, Oratz R, Bentley TG. Cost-effectiveness of 21-gene assay in node-positive, early-stage breast cancer. *Am J Manag Care.* 2011;**17**(7):455–464.

25 IOM. *Crossing the Quality Chasm: A New Health System for the 21st Century.* Washington, DC: National Academy Press; 2001.

27 Fisher ES, Wennberg DE, Stukel TA, Gottlieb DJ, Lucas FL, Pinder EL. The implications of regional variations in Medicare spending. Part 1: the content, quality, and accessibility of care. *Ann Intern Med.* Feb 18 2003;**138**(4):273–287.

28 McGlynn EA, Asch SM, Adams J, et al. The quality of health care delivered to adults in the United States. *N Engl J Med.* Jun 26 2003;**348**(26):2635–2645.

29 Luft HS, Bunker JP, Enthoven AC. Should operations be regionalized? The empirical relation between surgical volume and mortality. *N Engl J Med.* Dec 20 1979;**301**(25):1364–1369.

30 Dudley RA, Johansen KL, Brand R, Rennie DJ, Milstein A. Selective referral to high-volume hospitals: estimating potentially avoidable deaths. *JAMA.* Mar 1 2000;**283**(9):1159–1166.

31 Begg CB, Cramer LD, Hoskins WJ, Brennan MF. Impact of hospital volume on operative mortality for major cancer surgery. *JAMA.* Nov 25 1998;**280**(20):1747–1751.

32 Reames BN, Sheetz KH, Waits SA, Dimick JB, Regenbogen SE. Geographic variation in use of laparoscopic colectomy for colon cancer. *J Clin Oncol.* Nov 10 2014;**32**(32):3667–3672.

33 Morden NE, Chang CH, Jacobson JO, et al. End-of-life care for Medicare beneficiaries with cancer is highly intensive overall and varies widely. *Health Aff (Millwood).* Apr 2012;**31**(4):786–796.

34 Havrilesky LJ, Moorman PG, Lowery WJ, et al. Oral contraceptive pills as primary prevention for ovarian cancer: a systematic review and meta-analysis. *Obstet Gynecol.* Jul 2013;**122**(1):139–147.

35 Ramcharan R. Regressions: Why Are Economists Obsessed with Them? *Finance & Development.* 2006;**43**(1). http://www.imf.org/external/pubs/ft/fandd/2006/03/basics.htm

36 IOM. *Roundtable on value & science-driven health care.* 2014.

37 Abernethy AP, Etheredge LM, Ganz PA, et al. Rapid-learning system for cancer care. *J Clin Oncol.* Sep 20 2010;**28**(27):4268–4274.

38 Abernethy AP. Demonstrating the learning health system through practical use cases. *Pediatrics.* Jul 2014;**134**(1):171–172.

39 Shih YC, Ganz PA, Aberle D, et al. Delivering high-quality and affordable care throughout the cancer care continuum. *J Clin Oncol.* Nov 10 2013;**31**(32):4151–4157.

40 Basch E, Abernethy AP, Mullins CD, et al. Recommendations for incorporating patient-reported outcomes into clinical comparative effectiveness research in adult oncology. *J Clin Oncol.* Dec 1 2012;**30**(34):4249–4255.

41 Dinan MA, Compton KL, Dhillon JK, et al. Use of patient-reported outcomes in randomized, double-blind, placebo-controlled clinical trials. *Med Care.* Apr 2011;**49**(4):415–419.

43 Tengs TO, Adams ME, Pliskin JS, et al. Five-hundred life-saving interventions and their cost-effectiveness. *Risk Anal: an official publication of the Society for Risk Analysis.* Jun 1995;**15**(3):369–390.

44 Sonnenberg A, Delco F. Cost-effectiveness of a single colonoscopy in screening for colorectal cancer. *Arch Intern Med.* Jan 28 2002;**162**(2):163–168.

45 WHO. World Health Organization. Cost effectiveness and strategic planning (WHO-CHOICE) 2015; http://www.who.int/choice/costs/CER_thresholds/en/.

47 Comparative effectiveness: its origin, evolution, and influence on health care. *J Oncol Pract.* Mar 2009;**5**(2):80–82.

48 Kinney ED. Comparative effectiveness research under the Patient Protection and Affordable Care Act: can new bottles accommodate old wine? *Am J Law Med.* 2011;**37**(4):522–566.

PART 7

Individualized Treatment

51 Personalized medicine in oncology drug development

Nicholas C. Dracopoli, PhD ▪ Iqbal Grewal, PhD, DSc, FRCPath ▪ Chris H. Takimoto, MD, PhD, FACP ▪ Peter F. Lebowitz, MD, PhD

Overview

The concept of personalized medicine in oncology drug development is no longer an aspiration; it is now, in large measure, the accepted paradigm of how oncology drugs should be developed. In modern oncology drug development, determining which molecularly characterized tumors will benefit the most from a drug is a critical part of the development plan. In addition, another important personalized medicine approach is emerging whereby a therapeutic is specific to an individual patient. Examples of this individualized therapeutic approach include engineering of autologous immune cells with reinfusion into the patient or cancer vaccines that are specific to an individual tumor.

A growing number of successful examples have demonstrated that the personalized medicine approach via biomarker selection can provide more benefit to patients and more rapid approval of drugs. The benefits of a personalized medicine strategy in oncology drug development are multiple and include an increased probability of overall success, smaller Phase 3 registration trials, and the potential for enhanced clinical benefits for patients. In a recent review, Falconi and colleagues examined the outcome of 676 Phase 1, 2, and 3 clinical trials of novel therapeutics for non-small cell lung cancer conducted from 1998 to 2012.[1] Overall, the cumulative success rate, as defined by the advancement to the next stage of clinical testing or to approval, was only 11%. However, when a biomarker was utilized for patient selection, the cumulative success rate increased by nearly sixfold to 62%. Thus, there is strong objective evidence for predictive biomarkers to enhance the probability of success in drug development. Using specific genetic and/or protein markers, a number of important drugs have been developed and approved in specific populations. This approach represents a paradigm shift that has proved so powerful that it is now a standard.

Introduction

The growing armamentarium of biomarker tools will allow a further expansion of the personalized drug development approach. It will also increase complexity across development and this will come with challenges. While precision medicine is now a reality, the successes have generally been where the companion diagnostic is the same as the target of the drug. As the science advances, efforts will need to be expanded in a few areas of personalized medicine to realize further gains. Some examples include

1. Multiplex biomarker panels as diagnostics. With few exceptions, most successful personalized medicine programs in oncology have measured a single gene or protein. As multiplexed approaches become mainstream with the analysis of thousands of datapoints, diagnostics using full panels will begin to emerge. This may require different clinical development strategies with the identification of a biomarker panel in early clinical trials and confirmation in registration studies.

   Some successful examples of multiplex diagnostics include transcriptional profiling efforts. Using this approach, a gene expression pattern is identified for responders versus nonresponders. This profile is then prospectively applied to a validation set of samples to determine the predictive value, sensitivity, and specificity of the test. Of the profiles in clinical use, such as Oncotype Dx (Genomic Health, Redwood City, California), MammaPrint (Agendia BV, Amsterdam, the Netherlands), and H/I (AvariaDX, Carlsbad, California), these tests are better at identifying the patients unlikely to benefit from treatment than the potential responders.

2. Immuno-oncology personalized medicine. While analysis of cancer cells has formed the mainstay of personalized medicine, it is becoming increasingly clear that other components of a tumor, such as immune cells and stromal cells, are critical biologic mediators that can now be manipulated for therapeutic benefit. As new therapies target these microenvironment cells, new technologies for profiling are being developed. The complexity of measuring multiple markers in multiple cell types presents challenges in the development of novel immunotherapy.

3. Personalized therapeutics. These include engineered autologous cells and individual tumor antigen approaches and are discussed in detail below.

Thus, while personalized medicine has finally become a reality in oncology drug development, it is becoming a far more complex proposition as we address more complex mechanisms and biology. In this chapter, we try to cover some of the key issues that are critical to understand in order to achieve further successes.

Role of biomarkers and companion diagnostics in personalized medicine

Types of biomarkers

Biomarkers and their associated diagnostics are critical components of most personalized drug development efforts. Biomarkers can be classified into several types as shown in Table 1. These include predictive, prognostic, and surrogate end points. All of these biomarker types contribute in critical ways to drug development, but we typically think of predictive biomarkers as being the driving force in personalized medicine. These are used to identify patients within a population who have a higher probability of responding to treatment than the "all-comer" population. The symbiotic development of molecular profiling technologies and the completion of the human genome sequence created new opportunities for the comprehensive discovery of markers to help predict drug efficacy or reduce risk of drug toxicity.

Holland-Frei Cancer Medicine, Ninth Edition. Edited by Robert C. Bast Jr., Carlo M. Croce, William N. Hait, Waun Ki Hong, Donald W. Kufe, Martine Piccart-Gebhart, Raphael E. Pollock, Ralph R. Weichselbaum, Hongyang Wang, and James F. Holland.
© 2017 John Wiley & Sons, Inc. ISBN: 978-1-118-93469-2

Table 1 Types of Biomarkers and Diagnostics

Marker	Function	Test
PD/MOA	• Determine whether a drug hits the target and has impact on the biological pathway • Evaluate mechanism of action (MOA) • PK/PD correlations and determine dose and schedule • Determine biologically effective dose	• Research test used during drug development • Not developed as companion diagnostic
Predictive	• Identify patients most likely to respond, or are least likely to suffer an adverse event when treated with a drug	• Companion diagnostic test (e.g., herceptin, EGFR)
Resistance	• Identify mechanisms driving acquired drug resistance	• Mutation analyses (e.g., Bcr-Abl mutation in imatinib treated CML)
Prognostic	• Predict course of disease independent of any specific treatment modality	• Approved tests (e.g., CellSearch, Mammaprint)
Surrogate	• Approved registrational end points	• Commercial diagnostic tests (e.g., LDL, HbA1c, viral load, blood pressure)

Today, an enormous number of biomarkers have been described, but most lack sufficient characterization necessary for clinical application. In October 2014, the GOBIOM database (www.gvkbio.com) lists more than 45,000 biomarkers. In effect, this is the equivalent of two biomarkers for every gene in the human genome! This suggests that the term biomarker is being greatly overused as we simply do not have this many useful biomarkers to support all different research applications. The vast majority of these biomarkers are poorly characterized and cannot be used effectively in research or clinical applications without considerable efforts to develop analytically valid assays as well as correlative data to confirm their role as a biomarker of a biological process.

Biomarkers have diverse uses throughout the drug development process as readouts for mechanism of action (MOA), pharmacodynamics (PDs), prognosis, response prediction, drug resistance, and surrogate markers (Table 1). Perhaps the most common use is as MOA markers to confirm the drug is hitting the expected target and having the desired downstream effect, often by measuring protein phosphorylation in members of the downstream signaling pathway. PD biomarkers are widely employed with pharmacokinetic (PK) analyses to determine a biologically effective dose and define the dose for the first Phase 2 efficacy studies. Prognostic markers are developed to determine the likely course of disease in the absence of any specific pharmaceutical intervention and have been widely used in some oncology indications to predict the likelihood of disease recurrence after resection of the primary tumor (e.g., Mammaprint and Oncotype Dx). Predictive biomarker tests are used to predict response to a specific treatment and are discussed in detail below. Increasingly, biomarker strategies are being used to detect and follow emergent resistance to therapy and considerable success has been achieved for the class of tyrosine kinase inhibitors to predict resistance to therapy.

Successes and challenges with companion diagnostics

As a testament to the successes of personalized drug development in oncology, as of January 2015, a total of 20 companion diagnostic tests have been approved by the FDA and are broadly used today in the treatment of cancer patients.[2] These 20 tests are described in Table 2. Several important factors emerge upon close examination of the approved companion diagnostics in this table. Firstly, all the tests are simple and measure the status of the drug target or, for Kirsten-Ras (KRAS), a resistance pathway downstream of the drug target.[3,4] Each test is a single analyte test that measures the

somatic genetic changes that activate the drug target including gene amplification (HER2, KIT), mutation (KRAS, epidermal growth factor receptor (EGFR), BRAF) or translocation (ALK). Secondly, all of the approved companion diagnostics in oncology are for signal transduction inhibitors with driver mutations in the target or downstream pathways. In contrast, there are no FDA-approved companion diagnostics for other drug mechanisms including cytotoxic drugs, epigenetic modulators, or immuno-oncology therapies. Why is it that we have been successful in developing companion diagnostics for signal transduction inhibitors but not for other important oncology drug targets? The answer is mainly that these driver mutations are the target (or closely related to the target) of the drugs being developed. Consequently, it is possible to quickly test the hypothesis that proliferation and metastasis of a tumor are driven by somatic abnormality detected in the drug target and that only those patients with such a somatic aberration will respond to inhibition of this target. This hypothesis can begin to be confirmed or refuted in clinical studies as soon as an efficacious dose is established in Phase 1 studies. In contrast, if samples have to be collected in Phase 2 for molecular profiling in order to develop a hypothesis, the development of a predictive marker becomes much more difficult. In this scenario, a stepwise approach must be taken which includes biomarker hypothesis generation, hypothesis testing and validation, and, finally, diagnostic development.

One recent example of this complexity is seen with the development of immuno-oncology agents. Checkpoint inhibitors like anti-PD-1 antibodies have demonstrated significant survival benefits and are the vanguard of a new wave of immune modulators.[5] These new drugs function by inhibiting immune checkpoints and preventing the tumor from evading the host immune system. However, early clinical data show that measuring the expression of the target checkpoints is quite complex as a predictive biomarker. While the response rate can be improved by—three to four times with high expression of PDL1 when using a PD1 inhibitor, it is also true that tumors without detectable expression respond to the drug. Consequently, simply testing for the expression of the checkpoint target may be insufficient as a predictive marker for this new type of drug and we may have to develop new molecular profiles to predict response to these important immune-modulating drugs.

In addition to the FDA-approved companion diagnostics for oncology drugs, there are many more tests being used for research and clinical applications in Clinical Laboratory Improvement Amendment (CLIA) and College of American Pathology (CAP) accredited laboratories. These tests vary from single-analyte tests to

Table 2 List of approved FDA companion diagnostics in October 2014.

TEST	Manufacturer	Drug(s)	Method	Analyte
therascreen KRAS RGQ PCR Kit	Qiagen	Erbitux (cetuximab)	PCR	KRAS
—	—	Vectibix (panitumumab)	—	—
EGFR PharmDx Kit	DAKO	Erbitux (cetuximab)	IHC	EGFR
—	—	Vectibix (panitumumab)	—	—
therascreen EGFR RGQ PCR Kit	Qiagen	Gilotrif (afatanib)	PCR	EGFR
C-KIT PharmDx	DAKO	Gleevec (imatinib mesylate)	IHC	KIT
INFORM HER-2/NEU	Ventana Medical Systems	Herceptin (trastuzumab)	FISH	HER2
PATHVISION HER-2 DNA Probe kit	Abbott Molecular	Herceptin (trastuzumab)	FISH	HER2
PATHWAY ANTI-HER-2/NEU (4B5)	Ventana Medical Systems	Herceptin (trastuzumab)	IHC	HER2
INSITE HER-2/NEU Kit	Biogenex Laboratories	Herceptin (trastuzumab)	IHC	HER2
SPOT-Light HER2 CISH Kit	Life Technologies	Herceptin (trastuzumab)	CISH	HER2
Bond Oracle HER2 IHC System	Leica Biosystems	Herceptin (trastuzumab)	IHC	HER2
HER2 CISH PharmDx Kit	Dako Denmark A/S	Herceptin (trastuzumab)	CISH	HER2
INFORM HER2 DUAL ISH DNA Probe Cocktail	Ventana Medical Systems	Herceptin (trastuzumab)	CISH	HER2
HERCEPTEST	Dako Denmark A/S	Herceptin (trastuzumab)	IHC	HER2
—	—	Perjeta (pertuzumab)	—	—
—	—	Kadcyla (ado-trastuzumab emtansine)	—	—
HER2 FISH PharmDx Kit	Dako Denmark A/S	Herceptin (trastuzumab)	FISH	HER2
—	—	Perjeta (pertuzumab)	—	—
—	—	Kadcyla (ado-trastuzumab emtansine)	—	—
THxID BRAF Kit	bioMerieux	Mekinist (trametinib)	PCR	BRAF
—	—	Tafinlar (dabrafenib)	—	—
cobas EGFR mutation test	Roche Molecular Systems	Tarceva (erlotinib)	PCR	EGFR
VYSIS ALK Break Apart FISH Probe Kit	Abbott Molecular	Xalkori (crizotinib)	FISH	ALK
COBAS 4800 BRAF V600 mutation test	Roche Molecular Systems	Zelboraf (vemurafenib)	PCR	BRAF
BRACAnalysis CDx™	Myriad Genetic Laboratories, Inc.	Lynparza™ (olaparib)	PCR	BRCA1/2
Ferriscan	Resonance Health Analysis Services Pty Ltd	Exjade (deferasirox)	MRI	Liver iron

Source: Data from http://www.fda.gov/MedicalDevices/ProductsandMedicalProcedures/InVitroDiagnostics/ucm301431.htm.

complex molecular profiles. Some have highly validated analytical performance and strong evidence of clinical utility, while other tests are much less well characterized. Recently, many laboratories have developed sequencing panels to screen for canonical cancer mutations in 30–300 genes. These panels are mostly used for research purposes and increasingly for screening cancer patients for enrollment into targeted clinical studies. Perhaps the best known of these tests is FoundationOne, provided by Foundation Medicine Inc. This test sequences 230 cancer genes in formalin-fixed paraffin-embedded tissue (FFPET) to identify somatic mutations. This information is analyzed and may be used by physicians to direct patients to appropriate clinical trials with targeted agents or, sometimes, off-label treatment with approved agents.

Strategies for companion diagnostic development

Companion diagnostic (CDx) development—preclinical approach

The first step in the CDx development is the formulation of the predictive biomarker hypothesis. Ideally, this begins at the same time a new therapeutic agent or target is identified. The predictive biomarker hypothesis outlines a strategy for identifying and testing assays that can prospectively predict drug sensitivity or resistance. Beginning at the earliest stages of drug discovery, this hypothesis should incorporate a thorough understanding of target biology and the drug's proposed MOA. The resulting output is a series of candidate predictive biomarker assays that will undergo rigorous preclinical and clinical evaluation testing their value as CDx tests. Candidate biomarkers may predict either drug sensitivity or resistance. In either case, the CDx co-development strategy is similar.

As discussed above, in some programs, the predictive biomarker hypothesis is inherently defined by the drug target. For example, a

program targeting a tumor resistance mutation might use the presence of that mutation as a predictive biomarker to select patients for early clinical trial evaluation to demonstrate rapid proof of concept. This approach has been utilized in the development of the second generation of EGFR inhibitors that target the T790M resistance mutation in NSCLC patients.[6] In other situations, a predictive biomarker might simply be high expression of the drug target such as HER2/Neu expression in breast cancer patients optimally treated with trastuzumab.[7] Most of the currently approved oncology CDx assays measure a single gene or protein directly related to the drug's molecular target.

The specific characteristics of the proposed predictive biomarker test can influence its clinical validation. For example, a biomarker with a binary readout, such as the presence or absence of a mutation, is the simplest to evaluate in clinical trials because of the lack of ambiguity about what constitutes a positive test. In contrast, a continuous variable, such as intensity of immunohistochemical staining or the degree of gene amplification or copy number, is more complex because of the need to establish a threshold for test positivity in actual clinical studies. Even more complicated are multivariate tests, such as microarray signatures or composite parameters derived from a variety of different tests. In general, as these predictive biomarkers grow more sophisticated, the burden to conduct more highly powered clinical trials for clinical validation also increases.

If the drug MOA is not well characterized, then the predictive biomarker hypothesis may be difficult to formulate and an exploratory approach may be warranted. For example, the potency of a new therapeutic across a panel of molecularly characterized tumor cell lines can be explored and used to identify molecular signatures, or, ideally, individual gene alterations, that strongly associate with drug sensitivity or resistance. To date, complex gene signatures associated with drug sensitivity have not been useful as companion diagnostics; however, this approach might still be valuable as a tool for biomarker discovery. The prevalence of any newly identified candidate predictive biomarkers can be ascertained in archived tumor tissues to explore potential clinical relevance. Ultimately, the exploratory predictive biomarker hypothesis should yield a series of promising candidate assays for further evaluation in the clinic.

Once a series of potential candidate predictive biomarkers are identified, the strength of the predictive biomarker hypothesis should be evaluated. The predictive potential of the associated candidate biomarkers can be explored in preclinical experiments conducted in relevant *in vitro* cell lines and *in vivo* tumor models. The presence of the predictive biomarker should strongly correlate with drug sensitivity over a series of tumor models. Confirmatory findings in patient-derived xenografts would further support the clinical relevance of the candidate predictive biomarker. The strength of the predictive biomarker hypothesis could substantially impact the choice of patient populations studied. If the predictive biomarker potential is highly compelling, then treatment in early trials might be restricted to biomarker-positive patients as a rapid proof-of-concept strategy. However, if the biomarker correlation is more tenuous, then treating both biomarker-positive and biomarker-negative patients early in clinical development is warranted.

A final preclinical step in CDx development is the preparation of qualified laboratory assays suitable for application to clinical trials. Ideal tests should be simple, robust, sensitive, and possess a rapid turnaround if used for patient screening. Analysis of circulating tumor cells, plasma proteins, or tests performed on formalin-fixed, paraffin-embedded tumor archival tissues are more advantageous than tests that require fresh tumor biopsies. Prototype assays for several different predictive biomarker candidates may be used for exploratory evaluation in preclinical experiments and for non-screening studies in patients enrolled in early clinical studies.[8] However, complete analytical validation will be required for full CDx testing, ideally prior to the initiation of pivotal later stage trials. Careful coordination between the clinical study team and the translational research personnel handling predictive biomarker logistics is essential to ensure consistent sample processing, shipping, and turnaround of test results.

CDx development in early clinical trials

The procedures required to develop a drug therapeutic are well characterized, but the steps required for CDx validation are often less well appreciated. In the past, predictive biomarkers were explored retrospectively by conducting *post hoc* analyses on clinical trial data for hypothesis generation.[9] However, this slow, linear way of thinking is outdated and remains at odds with the requirement to develop CDx tests rapidly alongside new therapeutics. In the modern era, proactive co-development plans are essential.

Development of a CDx can strongly influence the design of traditional first-in-human Phase 1 oncology studies. These trials are traditionally performed in cancer patients and their classic endpoints include dose selection, PKs, toxicity profiles, and the determination of the maximum tolerated dose. Phase 1 trials also frequently incorporate PD biomarker endpoints such as receptor occupancy, or target inhibition, to assess target engagement and downstream pathway modulation. These PD assays can assist in the selection of a recommended Phase 2 dose; however, they are generally not used as companion diagnostics, and their use is limited to early development trials. A traditional solid tumor Phase 1 oncology study will accrue patients with a variety of advanced tumor types,

independent of their biomarker status, to ensure rapid determination of toxicity profiles, collect PKs data, and establish firm dosing recommendations.

Increasingly, Phase 1 oncology trials are incorporating early assessment of drug activity in expansion cohorts opened immediately after dose selection. This attempt to establish rapid proof of concept in a defined population has diminished the role of standalone Phase 2a efficacy trials in many current drug development programs.[10,11] However, it has fueled a corresponding increase in Phase 1 trial size and complexity. A critical early decision is whether to limit enrollment in these expansion cohorts to biomarker-positive patients or to include an all-comer, biomarker agnostic approach. If the biomarker hypothesis is compelling and biomarker-negative patients are not expected to benefit from treatment, there is good rationale to limit accrual to biomarker-positive patients. A popular Phase 1 strategy is to enroll unselected patients during dose escalation but to restrict expansion cohort accrual to biomarker-positive patients. This type of enrichment approach provides an early opportunity to observe an efficacy signal in the proof-of-concept population deemed most likely to respond to the investigational treatment. A disadvantage is that many patients will have to be screened if the prevalence of the predictive biomarker is low, and this can further increase the study complexity. Alternatively, if an all-comer or biomarker-stratified approach is used in the Phase 1 expansion, then the retrospective determination of the predictive biomarker status in all patients should be mandatory.

Even if a biomarker enrichment strategy is employed, the exploratory nature of these early trials should enforce a measure of clinical equipoise. Overly strict assumptions about the utility of the candidate predictive biomarkers must be avoided until sufficient supportive clinical data are collected. In CDx development, biomarker misspecification is not unusual, and the initial candidate predictive biomarker may be superseded by new markers identified in these exploratory clinical trials. For example, the first Phase 1 trials of the kinase inhibitor, crizotinib, initially focused on patients with tumors harboring cMET alterations because this was the major discovery target for the drug. However, crizotinib is also a potent ALK tyrosine kinase inhibitor; and in Phase 1 trials, the EML4/ALK translocation was identified as a definitive companion diagnostic for further lung cancer development.[12]

CDx development in later stage clinical trials

Prior to the initiation of pivotal registration trials, the predictive biomarker assay should undergo full analytical validation. Ideally, only one validated version of the assay conducted at a central laboratory should be employed in Phase 2b or Phase 3 trials.[8] If two versions of the CDx assay are used in clinical validation, then a bridging diagnostic study will be necessary. Because later stage trials will require large numbers of patients and study centers, the uniform implementation of the CDx across a wide geographical area presents additional logistical challenges. These factors have to be carefully considered when the program transitions into later stages of development because of the shift in focus from biomarker exploration to validation of a full-fledged companion diagnostic.

The design of late-stage CDx development clinical trials will heavily depend on the clinical data collected to date regarding the proposed CDx. If the predictive biomarker test is unambiguous and little or no activity is still anticipated in biomarker negative patients, then a pure enrichment strategy can be pursued (Figure 1). This approach focuses solely on biomarker-positive patients and relatively conventional Phase 2b and Phase 3 study designs can be considered. However, if meaningful drug activity may still occur in biomarker-negative

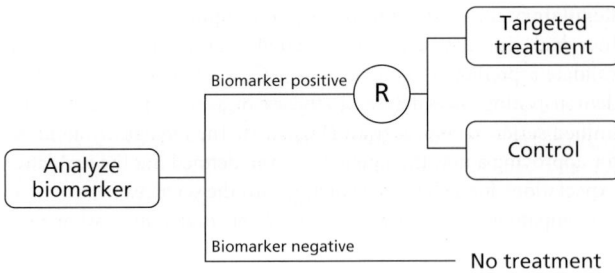

Figure 1 Targeted enrichment design.

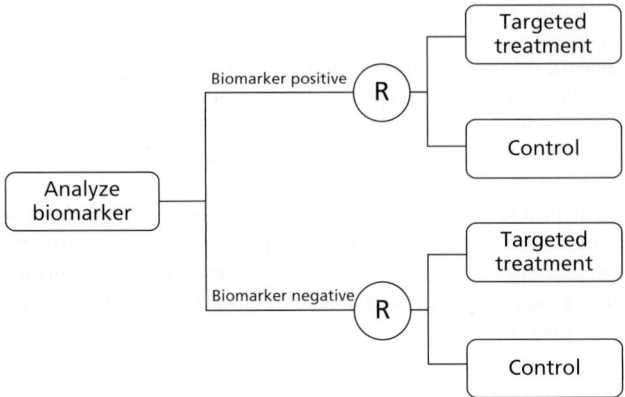

Figure 2 Biomarker stratification design. R = Randomized.

patients, then a biomarker-stratified study design that includes both biomarker-positive and biomarker-negative patients should be considered (Figure 2). The study design options for biomarker-stratified randomized trials are quite large and this is a rapidly growing area of clinical research. Some general illustrative examples of both enrichment and biomarker-stratified clinical trial designs are discussed in the following sections.

Enrichment study designs

In a pure enrichment strategy, randomized studies are conducted only in biomarker-positive patients and study designs remain relatively conventional (Figure 1).[13] If the biomarker strongly predicts treatment effect, the resulting randomized trial will be smaller than a corresponding unselected patient trial due to the larger clinical benefit anticipated in patients with tumors with reduced molecular heterogeneity. The efficiency of an enrichment design over an all-comer treatment approach depends on the prevalence of the predictive biomarker and the effectiveness of the treatment in the biomarker-negative patients. When the biomarker is present in less than half of the potential patients and the treatment effect is minimal in the marker-negative population, the enrichment design will randomize substantially fewer patients than an unselected trial.[9,13] However, depending on the prevalence of the predictive biomarker, many patients may need to be screened to identify sufficient biomarker-positive patients.

A disadvantage of the pure enrichment strategy for CDx development is that the negative predictive value of the biomarker is unknown because these patients are excluded from the study. There is at least one example of a CDx approved with a novel therapeutic that later failed to demonstrate medical or clinical utility. The original approval of the anti-EGFR antibody, cetuximab, for patients with metastatic colorectal cancer, included a CDx test using immunohistochemistry to document EGFR expression. However, later trials demonstrated that cetuximab was equally as

effective in EGFR-negative and EGFR-positive patients[14] consistent with a lack of medical utility for the CDx. As a consequence, a successful enrichment strategy registration program may require additional testing in biomarker-negative patients as a post-approval commitment. Nonetheless, the enrichment clinical trial designs remain popular and there are many successful oncology CDx co-development programs that have utilized this approach. Prominent recent examples include the approval of the registration of vemorafenib in melanoma patients with V600E BRAF mutations[15] and crizotinib in NSCLC patients with EML4/ALK translocations.[12]

Biomarker-stratified designs

If the predictive biomarker test characteristics are unambiguous but the question of clinical validation remains, then a biomarker-stratified trial design that enrolls both biomarker-positive and biomarker-negative patients should be considered. In the simplest form, the treatment effect is examined by randomizing both biomarker groups to receive experimental or control treatment (Figure 2).[9] The need for prestratification by biomarker status will depend on the prevalence of the biomarker in the study population. When appropriately powered, this study design provides the most information about the treatment effect and the biomarker's predictive and prognostic power. However, it is relatively inefficient because of the need to examine sufficient numbers of patients in the both biomarker subgroups. Numerous modifications of this approach have been proposed using different statistical analysis plans to enhance efficiency.[9,13] Some examples include the sequential accrual design that starts enrolling biomarker-positive patients with expansion to biomarker-negative patients only after an initial treatment effect is observed.[9] Another alternative, called the "fall-back" design, starts by treating all comers followed by a narrower focus on biomarker-positive patients only if the overall results lack statistical significance.[16] Detailed descriptions of these and other biomarker-stratified study designs are beyond the scope of this discussion but are described thoroughly by Simon and colleagues.[9,13,16]

Because choice of biomarker study designs in later development may be difficult, Freidlin and colleagues proposed a novel Phase 2 strategy to guide decision making for further co-development trials.[17] For situations where a well-defined predictive biomarker exists, the following strategy can help choose between enrichment and biomarker-stratified study designs. Briefly, the outcome of the Phase 2 trial is used to recommend one of four different options for the Phase 3 CDx trial. First is to perform a randomized Phase 3 study enrolling only biomarker-positive patients using an enrichment design because the drug is active and the diagnostic defines the sole treatment population. Second is to implement a randomized biomarker-stratified design, because the treatment is active in both marker-positive and marker-negative patients but the biomarker has some power to predict clinical outcomes. Third is to enroll all patients regardless of biomarker status because the drug is broadly active and the biomarker lacks clinical validity. Finally, the fourth option is to not proceed to Phase 3 and to halt all further development because the drug lacks efficacy in any population.

Using Freidlin's Phase 2 strategy, patients are randomly assigned to experimental and control treatments and the predictive biomarker status is determined.[17] The treatment effect is assessed first in the biomarker-positive population and later, depending on the results, in the overall population or the biomarker-negative subgroup. The decision algorithm for this approach is outlined by Freidlin, with the resulting output being a recommended Phase 3 strategy. In this example, the hazard ratio for progression-free survival is used to assess the treatment effect, although it can adapt to a variety of Phase 2 endpoints. This approach nicely highlights the decisions that drug development scientists face when designing a CDx development program. However, a potential disadvantage of this biomarker Phase 2 trial is that it can be large and complex, and it may recommend an additional large and complex CDx Phase 3 trial.

If questions persist about the predictive biomarker at the end of Phase 2, it may still be possible to discover or refine an existing diagnostic during Phase 3 trials. Several innovative adaptive Phase 3 study designs have been proposed to explore and adjust new predictive biomarkers while simultaneously evaluating therapeutic efficacy. For example, the biomarker-adaptive threshold design can select the optimal cut-point for test positivity for a continuous or graded predictive biomarker in Phase 3 trials.[18] This has utility if the biomarker threshold for positivity has not been determined at the start of the pivotal trial, and it preserves statistical power to detect an overall broad treatment effect. A more generalized variation on this approach, called the adaptive biomarker design, can analyze the predictive power of several different predefined binary biomarkers simultaneously, allowing for the selection of one that has the greatest correlation with clinical outcome.[13,18]

If no candidate predictive biomarker exists at the end of Phase 2 but gene expression profiling can be conducted in Phase 3 patients, Freidlin and colleagues proposed a novel adaptive signature design that prospectively defines a predictive biomarker signature and validates its correlation with therapeutic efficacy in the same pivotal Phase 3 trial.[19] In this study design, a predictive biomarker signature is developed in a training subset and validated in separate, mutually exclusive patient subgroup while preserving statistical power to evaluate the overall treatment effect. In simulation tests, the adaptive signature design reduced the chance of rejecting an active treatment when the fraction of sensitive patients is low; however, when the treatment is broadly active, it still detects an overall treatment effect similar to a conventional trial. Freidlin et al. recently published a more statistically robust version of this approach called the cross-validated adaptive signature design that utilizes the full patient population for signature development and validation.[20] One of the stated goals of the adaptive signature design is to allow pharmaceutical companies to invest in pharmacogenomic biomarkers for patient selection without compromising the opportunity for broader indications where supported by Phase 3 data.[19] Performing biomarker discovery and validation in a single trial is an attractive concept, but, at present, no approved CDx has used this approach. Thus, this remains a promising but, at present, theoretical option for future CDx development.

Regulatory considerations in CDx development

In a dual drug-diagnostic co-development program, the goal is to validate a predictive biomarker as a CDx while at the same time demonstrating the safety and efficacy of a novel therapeutic in a unified series of clinical trials (Figure 3). The regulatory standards for approving a new therapeutic are well defined but the regulatory expectations for a CDx are evolving with the science.

Companion diagnostic tests have been under increasing regulatory scrutiny because of the recognition that their misuse could potentially harm patients. For example, a false-positive diagnostic result might expose a cancer patient to a toxic treatment with minimal chance of benefit, while a false-negative test could deprive a patient of a possibly efficacious therapy. In order to be labeled a companion diagnostic, a predictive biomarker must demonstrate analytical validity, clinical validity, and medical utility. Analytical validity requires the technical demonstration of robustness and reproducibility under relevant laboratory conditions.[13,21,22] If a gold standard reference test exists, then formal accuracy parameters, such as specificity and sensitivity, should also be determined. Analytical validation is predominantly a laboratory-based exercise that can be performed on clinical specimens from stored tissue banks; however, the demonstration of clinical validity and medical utility require appropriately designed clinical trials. Clinical validity is defined by the correlation of the predictive biomarker with a specific clinical end point or treatment effect.[13,21,22] For example, a specific gene translocation might predict objective responses to a novel therapeutic. Finally, and most importantly, medical or clinical utility is achieved by showing that the use of the biomarker improves clinical outcomes.[13,21,22]

In 2004, the FDA released a document entitled "Drug-Diagnostic Co-Development Concept Paper" that addressed the challenges of coordinated development of a therapeutic drug and diagnostic product.[21] Further, FDA guidance on this and related topics has been released;[23] however, as described by Fridlyand et al., many strategic dilemmas remain when designing and implementing CDx co-development programs.[22]

Personalized immunotherapeutics

Recent advances in tumor immunology have offered strong scientific basis for advancing personalized immunotherapy. This is a rapidly expanding area of drug development where immune-based treatments can be tailored to a single patient or novel immune-based predictive biomarkers can be used to select patients who are most likely to benefit from specific treatments. The latter approach

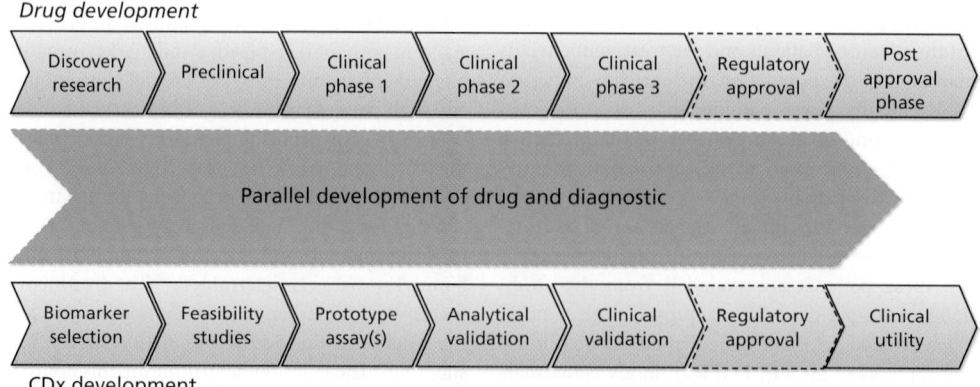

Figure 3 The drug-diagnostic co-development model showing the drug development process and the parallel companion (CDx) process striving for an aligned regulator co-approval at the end of Phase 3. Source: Olsen 2014.[8] Used under CC BY (http://creativecommons.org/licenses/by/3.0/)

is very similar to the personalized medicine approaches discussed in previous sections. The former approach, personalized immunotherapeutics, involves the production of a specific therapeutic for a specific patient. The technical and logistical hurdles for personalized immunotherapeutics are significant but the potential to dramatically impact disease outcomes is compelling.

Tumor immunology has burgeoned as a field thanks to many exciting discoveries that have uncovered how tumors evade the body's immune system and clinical studies which test new therapeutics that exploit the immune dynamics of tumors.[24] Approval of new immunotherapies such as cancer vaccines for prostate cancer and monoclonal antibodies targeting the immune checkpoints for melanoma has provided the human proof of concept that the immune system can successfully eliminate tumors and eradicate cancer.[24-26] Investigations of complex interactions between the host immune response against tumors and tumor immune evasion mechanisms have now become an intensely studied area of research. However, tumors are also diverse in nature, displaying distinct characteristics in different patients, and they may use various methods to subvert the immune system. The complex nature of interactions of tumor cells with the host immune system and unique attributes of individual patients suggest that personalized methods to leverage the body's own immune system may offer the most promising therapy for patients.

Recently, the field of tumor immunology has been growing, with innovative therapeutic advances on many fronts. The most popular immunotherapy strategy is specific T-cell activation, which has been fairly successful in initial experiments. Other therapeutics like cancer vaccines have had mixed results, proving effective against some cancers but not against all others.[27] One new technology that has been receiving attention is T-cell reprogramming, which utilizes genetic modifications to program the body's own immune cells against tumors. This approach involves *ex vivo* modification of autologous T cells with reinfusion into the patient. Furthermore, new methods of molecular analytics such as immunophenotyping allow for the collection of patient data, which can be used and applied to make personalized immunotherapies. In this respect, intensive research in patient-specific genomic and molecular analyses and the application of this information to develop personalized immunotherapies to selectively treat patients' cancers are being aggressively pursued.[28]

Identification of genetic alterations for finding unique antigens

Cancer cells undergo high rates of mutations and other epigenetic alterations that, in theory, should make them recognizable by the immune system. Understanding the nature of these alterations and translating this into useful information could be used to engineer personalized immunotherapies. Various technologies are now available for genome-wide DNA and RNA sequencing, deciphering epigenetic regulation, and identifying transcript variation within the tumor cells that can be used to profile the tumors within a given patient. Patient-specific T-cell epitope discovery and immunophenotyping of patient biopsies and other tumor samples could be used to identify protein mutations in cancer cells. By defining unique protein sequences that harbor epitopes recognizable to the immune system, researchers may be able to create a personalized vaccine to treat patients with recurrent cancers. Thus, identification of epitopes specific to individuals may help develop tailored therapies that maximize effectiveness based on the biology of a patient.

Genetic profiling of tumors is also applicable to T-cell reprogramming, since it allows for discovery of distinct T-cell-binding antigens and the development of personalized T-cell-based immunotherapies. Genetic methods can be applied to T-cell programming in two ways. First, genome sequencing of tumor cells may reveal mutations that occurred in cell-surface receptors, which would allow for the selection of a target antigen and reprogramming of the T cells against that antigen. Considering intratumor heterogeneity, it may be necessary to select multiple mutant antigens. Second, as tumor cells are known to change over time, they may lose initial antigens or gain new cell-surface mutations. Thus, tumors have to be carefully monitored for any changes in the selected antigens. The whole process would have to be repeated over time to account for future mutations and to select new target antigens, in the case that the therapy does not wipe out all of the cancer cells. Monitoring cancer cells as well as antitumor immune response is a key to the success of T-cell programming against specific antigens.

To validate the therapeutic utility of unique tumor-specific antigens and develop methods for monitoring specific antitumor T-cell response, studies in animals that have yielded useful information have been conducted and these could be applied to develop human therapeutics.[29] An approach combining whole-exome and transcriptome sequencing analysis with mass spectrometry was used to identify neo-epitope-containing peptides in murine tumor models. Vaccination of mice with these peptides generated strong antitumor T-cell responses, confirming the therapeutic potential of this approach. These studies open the door for developing personalized vaccines and PD monitoring of antitumor T-cell responses in cancer patients.

Personalized vaccines using individualized tumor specific antigens

Cancer vaccines that activate the immune system have shown some promise in animal models, but they have not been as successful in human trials.[30] Cancer vaccines should theoretically work by activating host-adaptive immune response against tumor-associated antigens that are contained within the vaccines. In order for this to happen, a given antigen must be taken up by antigen-presenting cells such as dendritic cells (DCs). The DC then must process the antigen, display the processed antigen on its surface in the form of a complex with the human leukocyte antigen (HLA) molecule, and migrate to the lymph node where it can present the antigen/HLA complex to T cells. This process activates the T cells which may then enter the circulation and migrate to the tumor, orchestrating an immune response to kill tumor cells. One key feature of a successful vaccine is an antigen that can be processed with a peptide fragment so that it can bind appropriately to HLA molecules.

New research methods are now being employed to discover which tumor-derived antigens may serve as good tumor antigens for efficient recognition by the immune system. Sophisticated tools that predict binding of a given peptide to a number of different HLA alleles, such as NetMHC, could be used to determine how strongly the immune system recognizes a change in the cancer.[31] In this method, each peptide is assigned a score based on the affinity to HLAs to determine if the host immune system has the potential to recognize changes in the cancer. However, high recognition does not necessarily correlate to strong vaccine potential. To further improve the chances of generating a strong immune response, experiments could be conducted to determine which epitopes are involved in the host antitumor response. By comparing NetMHC scores of different peptides, those with the strongest immunogenic activity could be selected. This method can be used to select peptides using patient data to create personalized vaccines.[31]

Idiotype-based vaccines

Tumor-specific immunity can also be induced by immunizing patients with unique antigenic determinants that are displayed on hematological malignancies. For example, in the case of B-cell malignancies, tumors usually arise from a single clone that expresses an immunoglobulin (Ig) molecule with a unique amino acid sequence in the variable regions of Ig called the idiotype (Id). Thus, for a given patient, the Id can be considered as tumor-associated antigens and could serve as very specific target antigens for vaccination.[32] Tumor-specific Id containing Ig from B-cell lymphomas have been successfully prepared by creating a cell line that secretes the tumor-derived Igs. These Igs can then be purified and used for vaccine preparation.[33]

Although, vaccination with Id-based vaccines has shown success in the clinic, progress in this area is very limited.[34] The biggest challenge is that tumor cells from each patient express unique Ids, and a vaccine needs to be patient specific and catered for an individual patient. In addition, there are the logistical issues of sequencing patients' Ids and then preparing vaccines for each individual patient and the Id. Nevertheless, clinical trials with custom-made monoclonal antibodies against tumor-associated Ids have been conducted and have shown remarkable efficacy, leading to long-term remission in many patients.[34] Some patients treated with this approach have become refractory to the treatment due to mutations in the Id that prevent anti-Id antibody binding.

Since the Ids are derived from self-proteins, many of the Id-based vaccines do not induce a good immune response. Because of this, studies have been conducted to improve the immunogenicity of vaccines by combining these antigens with DCs to promote the uptake and presentation of the antigen to the immune system. This approach has shown some promise by inducing both humoral and cellular responses. For example, a clinical trial using Id-pulsed DCs was conducted in B-cell lymphoma patients, where 8/10 patients showed efficacy as measured by T-cell proliferative anti-Id responses.[35]

Use of patient-specific tumor-infiltrating lymphocytes (TILs)

As discussed earlier, tumor cells harbor many genetic mutations and other alterations that give rise to neo-epitopes that may serve as novel antigens to induce an antitumor T-cell response.[36] It has been found that many immunogenic tumors have high rates of mutation and are often infiltrated by T lymphocytes that possess the ability to recognize antigens expressed by the tumor cells.[37] The presence of tumor-infiltrating lymphocytes (TILs) is thought to mediate a critical role in the efficacy of adoptive cell therapy and other forms of immunotherapies in melanoma patients.[38-40] Based on this notion, adoptive cell therapy using patient's own TILs has been tried in melanoma patients. In this therapeutic approach, TILs are collected from patients, expanded in the laboratory, and produced in large quantities in order to infuse back into the patient. While this type of personalized therapy has shown success in melanoma patients, it remains to be seen if similar successes can be achieved against epithelial cancers.[41] Epithelial cancers usually contain fewer mutations than melanoma, which may make them less immunogenic.[42] Some progress in this field is being made, such as the mapping of the mutant antigens in human epithelial tumors, but strategies to exploit this newfound information for developing effective therapies still remains an open question despite some promising case reports with TILs in epithelial tumors.[43]

DC-based personalized immunotherapy by using tumor cells as an immunogen

Despite the identification of unique tumor-associated mutant peptides, a relatively small number of these critical mutations are actually seen by the immune system because they may not be presented by DCs. In order to be presented by DCs, the specific epitope must bind HLA and this does not occur for all peptides. This limitation usually restricts the induction of a broad repertoire of tumor-specific T-cell clones, thereby leading to potential tumor escape. Thus, personalized tumor-derived vaccines that overcome this limitation are desirable. In this respect, whole dead tumor preparations that may contain large numbers of known and unknown antigens can be used to facilitate the induction of a polyclonal T-cell response against tumor cells.[44,45] Thus, loading of DCs with whole tumors could offer the distinct advantage of presenting all of the antigenic components of the tumor to T cells, compared with loading the DCs with just a few peptides. In addition, this approach offers a truly personalized therapy as it would be specific to a patient's own tumors. The general approach of this immune therapy is clearly appealing; however, many questions still remain unanswered. For example, it is not clear whether dead tumor cells in the form of apoptotic cells, necrotic cells, or whole lysates are better sources of antigens for pulsing DCs.[46-48] Another approach is to use amplified tumor-derived RNA to generate tumor antigens.[49] Clinical trials using whole-tumor cell preparations to pulse DCs have resulted in efficient antitumor immunity as well as clinical responses. Durable complete responses have been reported in advanced melanoma patients after treatment with autologous tumor cell-pulsed DC vaccine.[45] Clinical benefits have also been observed with tumor cell lysate-pulsed DC vaccination in renal cell carcinoma patients as well as in clinical trials using DC-based therapy in prostate cancer patients.[50]

Conclusions

Cancers are highly heterogeneous and vary from patient to patient, which makes personalized therapeutics a highly compelling approach. It is thus anticipated that personalized immunotherapy will play a critical role in harnessing the power and precision of the immune system to mount antitumor immune responses. However, this approach will require novel technologies and extensive research. Although considerable progress has been made, many questions still remain unanswered: How do we identify and prioritize antigens? How can we selectively activate the immune response and avoid toxicity? What are the best approaches to immune profiling? What is the feasibility of autologous therapeutics requiring processing of cells and antigens for each patient? There is no doubt that the future research in personalized therapy will take the center stage to answer these questions in the coming years and offer personalized immunotherapy for improving outcomes for the cancer patients.

Key references

The complete reference list can be found on the Wiley Companion Digital Edition of this title (see inside front cover for login instructions).

1 Falconi A, Lopes G, Parker JL. Biomarkers and receptor targeted therapies reduce clinical trial risk in non-small-cell lung cancer. *J Thorac Oncol.* 2014;**9**(2):163–169.

2 Food and Drug Administration (2014), *List of Cleared or Approved Companion Diagnostic Devices,* http://www.fda.gov/MedicalDevices/ProductsandMedical Procedures/InVitroDiagnostics/ucm301431.htm (accessed 23 December 2014).

3 Lièvre A, Bachet JB, Le Corre D, et al. KRAS mutation status is predictive of response to cetuximab therapy in colorectal cancer. *Cancer Res.* 2006;**66**(8):3992–3995.

doi: 10.1158/0008-5472.CAN-06-0191 DOI:10.1158%2F0008-5472.CAN-06-0191. PMID 16618717.

4 Pao W, Wang TY, Riely GJ, et al. KRAS mutations and primary resistance of lung adenocarcinomas to gefitinib or erlotinib. *PLoS Med*. 2005;**2**(**1**):e17.

5 Herbst RS. A study of MPDL3280A, an engineered PD-L1 antibody in patients with locally advanced or metastatic tumors. *J Clin Oncol*. 2013. (suppl; abstr 3000).

6 Yu HA, Riely GJ, Lovly CM. Therapeutic strategies utilized in the setting of acquired resistance to EGFR tyrosine kinase inhibitors. *Clin Cancer Res*. 2014;**20**:5898–5907.

7 Fornier M, Risio M, Van Poznak C, Seidman A. HER2 testing and correlation with efficacy of trastuzumab therapy. *Oncology* (Williston Park). 2002;**16**(**10**):1340-8–1351-2; discussion 1352, 1355-8.

8 Olsen D, Jorgensen JT. Companion diagnostics for targeted cancer drugs - clinical and regulatory aspects. *Front Oncol*. 2014;**4**:105.

9 Simon R. Drug-diagnostics co-development in oncology. *Front Oncol*. 2013;**3**:315.

10 Dahlberg SE, Shapiro GI, Clark JW, Johnson BE. Evaluation of statistical designs in phase I expansion cohorts: the Dana-Farber/Harvard Cancer Center experience. *J Natl Cancer Inst*. 2014;**106**(**7**).

11 Manji A, Brana I, Amir E, et al. Evolution of clinical trial design in early drug development: systematic review of expansion cohort use in single-agent phase I cancer trials. *J Clin Oncol*. 2013;**31**(**33**):4260–4267.

12 Kwak EL, Bang YJ, Camidge DR, et al. Anaplastic lymphoma kinase inhibition in non-small-cell lung cancer. *N Engl J Med*. 2010;**363**(**18**):1693–1703.

13 Simon R. Clinical trial designs for evaluating the medical utility of prognostic and predictive biomarkers in oncology. *Per Med*. 2010;**7**(**1**):33–47.

14 Chung CH, Mirakhur B, Chan E, et al. Cetuximab-induced anaphylaxis and IgE specific for galactose-alpha-1,3-galactose. *N Engl J Med*. 2008;**358**(**11**):1109–1117.

15 Chapman PB, Hauschild A, Robert C, et al. Improved survival with vemurafenib in melanoma with BRAF V600E mutation. *N Engl J Med*. 2011;**364**(**26**):2507–2516.

16 Simon R, Wang SJ. Use of genomic signatures in therapeutics development in oncology and other diseases. *Pharmacogenomics J*. 2006;**6**(**3**):166–173.

17 Freidlin B, McShane LM, Polley MY, Korn EL. Randomized phase II trial designs with biomarkers. *J Clin Oncol*. 2012;**30**(**26**):3304–3309.

18 Jiang W, Freidlin B, Simon R. Biomarker-adaptive threshold design: a procedure for evaluating treatment with possible biomarker-defined subset effect. *J Natl Cancer Inst*. 2007;**99**(**13**):1036–1043.

19 Freidlin B, Simon R. Adaptive signature design: an adaptive clinical trial design for generating and prospectively testing a gene expression signature for sensitive patients. *Clin Cancer Res*. 2005;**11**(**21**):7872–7878.

20 Freidlin B, Jiang W, Simon R. The cross-validated adaptive signature design. *Clin Cancer Res*. 2010;**16**(**2**):691–698.

22 Fridlyand J, Simon RM, Walrath JC, et al. Considerations for the successful co-development of targeted cancer therapies and companion diagnostics. *Nat Rev Drug Discov*. 2013;**12**(**10**):743–755.

25 Kantoff PW, Higano CS, Shore ND, et al. Sipuleucel-T immunotherapy for castration-resistant prostate cancer. *N Engl J Med*. 2010;**363**:411–422.

26 Hodi FS, O'Day SJ, McDermott DF, et al. Improved survival with ipilimumab in patients with metastatic melanoma. *N Engl J Med*. 2010;**363**:711–723.

27 Melero I, Gaudernack G, Gerritsen W, et al. Therapeutic vaccines for cancer: an overview of clinical trials. *Nat Rev Clin Oncol*. 2014;**11**:509–524.

28 Noguchi M, Sasada T, Itoh K. Personalized peptide vaccination: a new approach for advanced cancer as therapeutic cancer vaccine. *Cancer Immunol Immunother*. 2013;**62**:919–929.

29 Yadav M, Jhunjhunwala S, Phung QT, et al. Predicting immunogenic tumour mutations by combining mass spectrometry and exome sequencing. *Nature*. 2014;**515**:572–576.

30 Palena C, Abrams SI, Schlom J, Hodge JW. Cancer vaccines: preclinical studies and novel strategies. *Adv Cancer Res*. 2006;**95**:115–145.

31 Duan F, Duitama J, Seesi SA, et al. Genomic and bioinformatic profiling of mutational neoepitopes reveals new rules to predict anticancer immunogenicity. *J Exp Med*. 2014;**211**:2231–2248.

32 Muraro E, Martorelli D, Dolcetti R. Successes, failures and new perspectives of idiotypic vaccination for B-cell non-Hodgkin lymphomas. *Hum Vaccin Immunother*. 2013;**9**:1078–1083.

34 Meeker T, Lowder J, Cleary ML, et al. Emergence of idiotype variants during treatment of B-cell lymphoma with anti-idiotype antibodies. *N Engl J Med*. 1985;**312**:1658–1665.

35 Timmerman JM, Czerwinski DK, Davis TA, et al. Idiotype-pulsed dendritic cell vaccination for B cell lymphoma: clinical and immune responses in 35 patients. *Blood*. 2002;**99**:1517–1526.

36 Vogelstein B, Papadopoulos N, Velculescu VE, Zhou S, Diaz LA, Kinzler KW. Cancer genome landscapes. *Science*. 2013;**339**:1546–1558.

37 Robbins RF, Lu YC, El-Gamil M, et al. Mining exomic sequencing data to identify mutated antigens recognized by adoptively transferred tumor-reactive T cells. *Nat Med*. 2013;**19**:747–752.

38 van Rooij N, van Buuren MM, Philips D, et al. Tumor exome analysis reveals neoantigen-specific T-cell reactivity in an ipilimumab-responsive melanoma. *J Clin Oncol*. 2013;**31**:e439–e442.

41 Wedén S, Klemp M, Gladhaug IP, et al. Long-term follow-up of patients with resected pancreatic cancer following vaccination against mutant K-ras. *Int J Cancer*. 2011;**128**:1120–1128.

42 Tran E, Turcotte S, Gros A, et al. Cancer immunotherapy based on mutation-specific CD4+ T cells in a patient with epithelial cancer. *Science*. 2014;**344**:641–645.

43 Turcotte S, Gros A, Hogan K, et al. Phenotype and function of T cells infiltrating visceral metastases from gastrointestinal cancers and melanoma: implications for adoptive cell transfer therapy. *J Immunol*. 2013;**191**:2217–2225.

44 de Gruijl TD, van den Eertwegh AJM, Pinedo HM, Scheper RJ. Whole-cell cancer vaccination: from autologous to allogeneic tumor- and dendritic cell-based vaccines. *Cancer Immunol Immunother*. 2008;**57**:1569–1577.

45 O'Rourke MG, Johnson M, Lanagan C, et al. Durable complete clinical responses in a Phase I/II trial using an autologous melanoma cell/dendritic cell vaccine. *Cancer Immunol Immunother*. 2003;**52**:387–395.

46 Sauter B, Albert ML, Francisco L, Larsson M, Somersan S, Bhardwaj N. Consequences of cell death: exposure to necrotic tumor cells, but not primary tissue cells or apoptotic cells, induces the maturation of immunostimulatory dendritic cells. *J Exp Med*. 2000;**191**:423–434.

47 Jarnjak-Jankovic S, Pettersen RD, Saeboe-Larssen S, Wesenberg F, Olafsen MRK, Gaudernack G. Preclinical evaluation of autologous dendritic cells transfected with mRNA or loaded with apoptotic cells for immunotherapy of high-risk neuroblastoma. *Cancer Gene Ther*. 2005;**12**:699–707.

49 Muller MR, Grunebach F, Nencioni A, Brossart P. Transfection of dendritic cells with RNA induces CD4- and CD8-mediated T cell immunity against breast carcinomas and reveals the immunodominance of presented T cell epitopes. *J Immunol*. 2003;**170**:5892–5896.

50 Holtl L, Zelle-Rieser C, Gander H, et al. Immunotherapy of metastatic renal cell carcinoma with tumor lysate-pulsed autologous dendritic cells. *Clin Cancer Res*. 2008;**8**:3369–3376.

PART 8

Chemotherapy

Preclinical and early clinical development of chemotherapeutic drugs, mechanism-based agents and biologics

52

Axel-R. Hanauske, MD, PhD, MBA ▪ *Daniel D. Von Hoff, MD, FACP*

Overview

Over the past 10 years, the approach to drug development has changed considerably. Owing to the enormous increase in insights into the molecular biology of cancer cells, a largely empirical approach has been mostly abandoned and replaced with a biology-driven, hypothesis-based, and translational approach. Notwithstanding this dramatic development, the hierarchical sequence of clinical drug-development trials basically remained unchanged and is divided into three phases. This chapter provides an overview of the various steps of early clinical development with milestones of the drug-development process, the role of the National Cancer Institute, and the switch to mechanism-based drug development. It outlines challenges in the clinical development of these new agents and provides a fundamental understanding of the complexity involved in early clinical drug development.

While the overall age-adjusted cancer death rates have been declining in most countries over the past decade, there remains a great need for development of new agents for treatment of patients with advanced cancer. There is also a perceived need for developing new agents that will be used to treat patients with "early cancer" (either before evidence of metastatic disease or at the state referred to as intraepithelial neoplasia).[1,2] This latter approach for treating early cancer, referred to in the past as chemoprevention, represents a new concept that could have an enormous impact on the disease.

In this chapter, we describe the fundamentals of development of new agents from discovery through the initial safety (Phase I) clinical trials. Along the way, we discuss a few studies that illustrate new methodologies introduced into drug development in recent years. This chapter largely concentrates on the development of new chemical entities and not on the development of biologic agents, although some of the principles outlined here also apply to the development of those agents.

As an overview, Figure 1 describes the classic stages in the development of a new agent. Using this basic process, there have been well over 150 new agents developed for treatment of patients with a variety of malignancies as well as for treatment of early cancer. Although this is an impressive list of agents available to treat patients with a variety of cancers, it is—in light of the biological diversity of the various types of cancer—obvious that we still need major additions to our armamentarium. Table A1 details all of the anticancer agents that are approved by the Federal Drug Administration and their official approved indications. We provide that table because, as noted below, as new strategies are being developed for the proper testing of new agents, one has to be cognizant of the agents that are

already approved for a specific indication. One must also be aware as to whether a new agent should be developed alone or in combination in a "front-line" setting or in a salvage or palliative setting. Table A1, together with Figures 1 and 2, helps to understand how to design pivotal clinical trials that will lead to approval by regulatory agencies and, most importantly, make an active and safe new drug available for patients.

Evolution of the discovery process

Clinical observation in the discovery process

As this chapter is being written, the process for discovery is changing rapidly. Initial anticancer drug discovery was based on important observations by clinicians and preclinical scientists. An example of such observations, where many feel the field of chemotherapy of cancer began, was the observation by Adair and Bogg in 1931 that troops in World War I exposed to sulfur mustard developed lymphoid and bone marrow hypoplasia.[3] They then used this very toxic agent to treat a number of patients with cancer with sulfur mustard. The agent had a limited effect. Further studies of the related nitrogen mustard (of World War II) demonstrated more substantial antitumor effects, particularly in patients with lymphoma.[4,5]

Another classic example of an astute observation by clinicians was when Farber and colleagues noticed that young patients with leukemia who were treated with liver extracts or folic acid had worsening of their leukemia.[6] They then treated the patients with folic acid antagonists and described the antileukemic activity of these antagonists.

Histocytotoxic effects and physiologic observations

Just like the observation that mustard gases cause hypoplasia of lymph nodes, spleen, and bone marrow (with subsequent clinical activity of nitrogen mustard and other alkylating agents in patients with lymphoma), there have been a number of other correlations between specific histocytotoxicity (toxicity to a particular type of tissue) and clinical activity of an agent. One of the best examples is the finding that the agent streptozocin caused destruction of the islet cells in animals (leading to diabetes).[7] Streptozocin was tried and found to have clinical activity in patients with insulinomas (a histocytotoxic effect).[8]

In early animal toxicology studies, cisplatin caused hypoplasia of the testes and ovaries in animals and was subsequently found to have substantial activity in patients with testicular or ovarian cancer.[9–11]

As an example of a physiologic observation leading to the development of a series of new anticancer agents, the physiologic

Holland-Frei Cancer Medicine, Ninth Edition. Edited by Robert C. Bast Jr., Carlo M. Croce, William N. Hait, Waun Ki Hong, Donald W. Kufe, Martine Piccart-Gebhart, Raphael E. Pollock, Ralph R. Weichselbaum, Hongyang Wang, and James F. Holland.
© 2017 John Wiley & Sons, Inc. ISBN: 978-1-118-93469-2

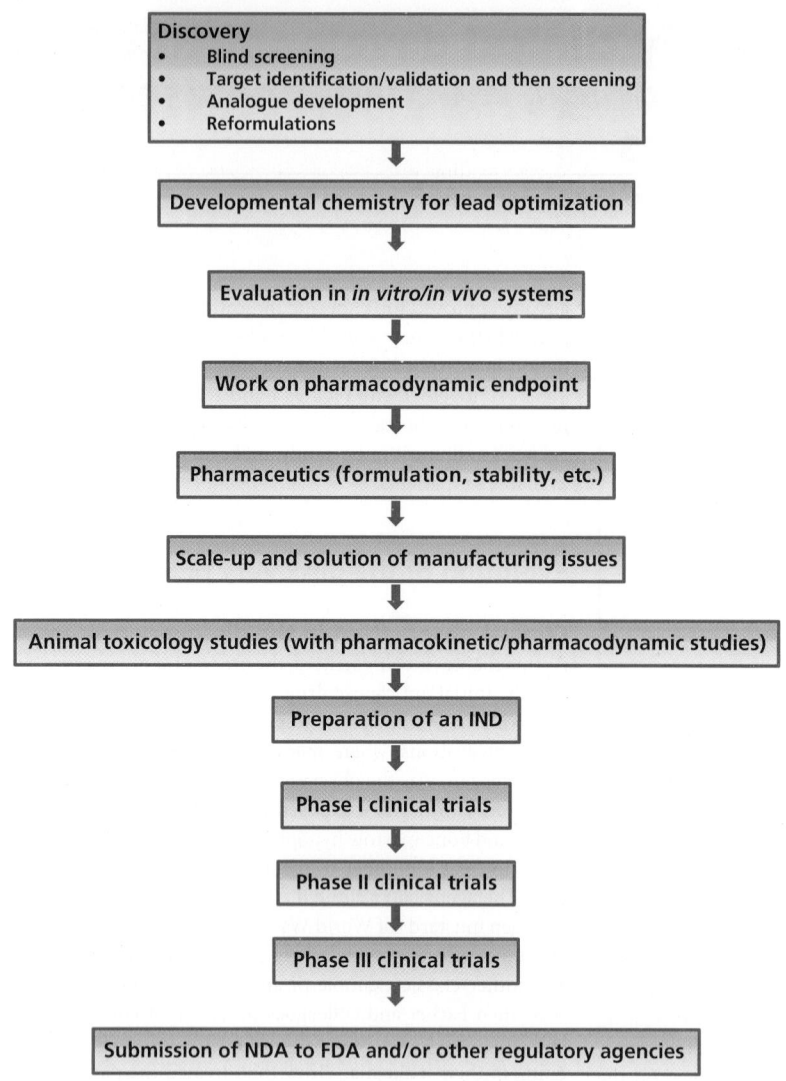

Figure 1 The stages in development of a new anticancer agent.

FDA: US Food and Drug Administration
IND: Investigational New Drug
NDA: New Drug Application

observation that rat hepatomas incorporated more uracil than the surrounding normal liver led to the Heidelberger group synthesizing the 5-fluoropyrimidines.[12,13] The observations by Elion and Hitchings, who surmised (based on the presumption that nucleic acids were in control of cell growth) that purine and pyrimidine analogs would be useful in treatment of cancers, certainly led to the development of 6-mercaptopurine, 6-thioguanine, and many other useful anticancer agents.[14–16] Although there is still clearly room for important clinical, toxicological, and physiologic observation, these observations will probably not dominate future drug discovery. However, readers are encouraged to keep their eyes open to clinical, histocytotoxic, and physiologic observations as described above as serendipity has been historically pivotal in successful drug development.

Early and continuing role of the National Cancer Institute drug-discovery program in the drug-discovery process

In the early 1960s, the US National Cancer Institute (NCI) began a major leadership role in the discovery and development of new anticancer agents. This was critical at that time because industry felt that investment in this area would not be feasible financially and

that the risks were high. The NCI began its leadership by establishing the National Service Center (NSC), which served as a clearinghouse (and a bank of compounds) for all compounds for all chemists, biologists, and other interested investigators. Compounds could be submitted to the NSC, assigned an NSC number (e.g., NSC 3101139 for mitoxantrone), and tested in a series of *in vitro* and *in vivo* preclinical models. Agents that passed certain hurdles of *in vitro* and *in vivo* antitumor activity were considered by a body at the NCI called the "Decision Network" for bringing them into toxicology studies and eventually into clinical trials.

The very early efforts of the NCI used the KB squamous cancer cell line, originally obtained from a patient with a carcinoma of the mouth, to screen a large numbers of compounds. Compounds that were active against that cell line were further evaluated *in vivo* in the two murine leukemias called P388 and L1210.[17,18] These *in vitro* and *in vivo* screens did lead to compounds with clinical activity against leukemia and lymphoma (e.g., vinca alkaloids and nitrosoureas). Finding agents with antitumor activity against solid tumors was much less successful.[18] In 1975, the NCI revisited their evaluation process to include *in vivo* evaluation of compounds against solid tumors (both autologous animal tumors and human tumors growing as xenografts in nude mice). A very important

Table 1 The most predictive animal models: The National Cancer Institute Experience 1978–1982.

Reasonably predictive[a]	Not predictive at all
P388 leukemia (mouse)	Lewis lung
L1210 leukemia (mouse)	CD8 (breast)
Bl6 melanoma (mouse)	Co38 (colon)
MX-I mammary[b]	LXI[b] (lung)
	CXI[b] (colon)

[a]Especially with regression of established tumors.
[b]Xenografts.
Source: Adapted from Staquet 1983.

retrospective analysis of that big experiment was conducted by Staquet and colleagues.[19] The results of their analyses are detailed in Table 1.

As can be seen in the table, the P388 and L1210 mouse leukemias continued to be predictive for activity of new agents in the clinic, as did the B16 mouse melanoma solid tumor autologous model growing in immunocompetent mice. The only human tumor xenograft that appeared to be predictive for clinical antitumor activity was the MX I mammary tumor xenograft growing in nude mice. The predictivity of these models was not tumor specific but rather *in vivo* activity in those systems predicted, in general, for clinical activity.[18] Also of importance in the report by Staquet and colleagues was the finding that actual regression of established tumors in these models and the percentage of animals surviving for ≥ 45 days were even stronger predictors of eventual clinical efficacy of the agents.[19]

In 2001, Johnson et al.[20] reported on the relationship between drug activity in NCI preclinical *in vitro* and *in vivo* models and clinical activity of a new agent. It is of interest that of 39 agents for which there were both xenograft and Phase II clinical data available, clinical activity in at least some Phase II trials was observed if there was activity in at least one-third of the xenograft models tested. Of particular note was that if there was preclinical activity in one-third or more of the xenografts tested, there was a 45% chance that the compound would have clinical activity. In that same study, only nonsmall-cell lung cancer (NSCLC) xenografts were predictive for the clinical activity against the same histology (e.g., nonsmall-cell lung cancer). Thus, although these *in vivo* evaluations systems are often maligned, when a systematic large-scale evaluation of them was examined, some models appeared to be reasonable predictors (although not tumor-specific predictors) for activity in the clinic.

Of additional note in Table 1 is the finding that several models were judged as not predictive at all for clinical activity. Some of the models, such as the Lewis lung model, continue to be used to justify bringing many new agents into clinical trials (particularly new agents, such as angiogenesis inhibitors). It is important that investigators who are contemplating bringing new agents into the clinic based on preclinical activity only in the Lewis lung, CD8, Co38, LXI, or CX1 models are mindful of the extensive prior experience demonstrating them not to be predictive for clinical activity.

To be most successful, however, it is important to remember the parameter Staquet and colleagues used for evidence of activity in the clinic (to make the correlation with the preclinical models): tumor shrinkage. Thus, their findings might not be applicable to the newer generations of more cytostatic agents (rather than the cytotoxic agents being evaluated in the 1960s–1980s).

The NCI made a further revision in their evaluation strategy in 1985 when they placed a large series of 60 human tumor cell lines in place for screening purposes.[18,21–25] They have attempted to make this a more tumor-type-oriented approval with inclusion of breast, lung, colon, kidney, brain, ovary, prostate, and melanoma human tumor lines.[18,22,23] At the time of introduction of this concept into the drug evaluation process, there was a great deal of discussion in the research community on how these cell lines were selected. Many investigators felt that cell lines with too rapid a doubling time were selected and did not represent the more slowly dividing solid tumors. However, this 60-cell-line screening panel is the system that is currently in place. More can be learned about the 60-cell-line success by visiting the website of the NCI at http://dtp.nci.nih.gov/branches/btb/ivclsp.html. Agents that are deemed active in the cell-line screens (based on criteria outlined in Refs 18 and 23 and based on other criteria, such as disease-specific activity) are then evaluated in the traditional *in vivo* models to determine their therapeutic index. If they are found active, they are moved forward into preclinical toxicology studies (see below).[24,25]

The true predictivity of the NCI-60-cell-line panel is as yet unknown as there are no published analyses as to the true predictivity of this approach for antitumor activity in the clinic. However, many excellent analyses of the results from the NCI-60-cell lines have led to some very provocative and useful research tools.

As an initial example of a unique use of results from the 60-cell-line screening, Paull and colleagues described a method (which they dubbed the COMPARE program) in which a compound evaluated in the 60-cell-line screen is used as a seed and the COMPARE program is used to detect the compounds that have similar patterns (or fingerprints) of activity against the 60-cell lines.[26] A correlation coefficient is then calculated to describe the closeness of other agents to the pattern of activity of the seed compound. It appears that if two compounds have similar correlation coefficients, this will predict for comparable mechanisms of action of the compounds or even the existence of a similar intracellular target, as described by Weinstein and colleagues.[27] If the correlation coefficient of a new, active compound is low compared with the compounds evaluated in the NCI screen, it might substantially increase interest in the new compound as it is very likely to have a new (unique) mechanism of action.

Of additional importance and of great interest to the cancer research community is that the NCI-60-cell lines continue to be characterized for presence or absence of specific targets (kinases, telomerase, mismatch repair proteins, and receptors).[28–30] Most recently, this cell-line panel underwent complete whole exome sequencing, and genetic alterations that may affect protein function were identified in 6% of all genes.[31] The precise molecular characterization of these lines is certain to help the evaluation not only of novel compounds but has also been reported to identify gene signatures that are indicative of radiation responsiveness.[32]

Historically, other preclinical models explored by the NCI for evaluating compounds that deserve mention were models put in place to evaluate agents against tumors taken directly from patients. There were two systems including the *in vitro* human tumor cloning assay (HTCA) and the *in vivo* subrenal capsule system (SRC). Although initial correlations were promising between agents detected as active in these assays and having subsequent antitumor activity in the clinic, the assays were deemed logistically too difficult to use as an up-front screen to evaluate the vast array of compounds.[33–36]

More recently, methods have been established to grow tumor tissue that is directly taken from patients or is taken from adequately stored tumor banks directly in diabetic and severely immune-compromised mice (NOD-SCID mice). This results in patient-derived xenografts (PDX, also termed "xenopatients") that more accurately reflect the pathologic and molecular characteristics of the original patients' tumors.[37–41] While these models may still not be feasible for routine clinical use in personalized medicine, they do provide another progress in the early drug-development process and may help identify sensitive tumor types and molecular patterns of resistance. They are specifically useful in the development of mechanism-based therapeutics.[42] With the advent of immunotherapeutic therapies (e.g., anti-CTLA-4, anti-PD1, and anti-PD-L1 monoclonal antibodies), preclinical mouse models using allografts into immunocompetent mice will be more often used.[43]

As whole exome sequencing of patients' tumors becomes affordable, attempts have been published to generate mouse models that resemble the same combination of abnormalities as detected in the individual patient. These "avatar" models are then treated with anticancer agents, and the patient would receive the drug that is active in the model.[44]

Mechanistically based ("targeted") drug discovery and evaluation

With the explosion of molecular techniques and knowledge of cell biology, there is now an incredible array of new methods for discovery of potential targets present in tumor cells versus normal cells.

One spectacular example of a mechanistically based approach to therapy was the development of imatinib, which has substantial activity against chronic myelogenous leukemia and against gastrointestinal stromal sarcomas. To put the timeline for development of imatinib into perspective, the basic biology ground work for the discovery and development of imatinib actually began with the discovery of the Philadelphia chromosome in chronic myeloid leukemias (CMLs) in 1960.[45] This was actually the first consistent chromosomal abnormality discovered in any type of cancer. The abnormality is a translocation involving chromosomes 9 and 22.[46] Work done in 1990–1993 documented that the translocation caused the *ABL* gene on the chromosome 9 (a nonreceptor tyrosine kinase) to move next to the *BCR* (breakpoint cluster region) gene on 22. This translocation codes the BCR-ABL protein, which is a 210-kDa transforming tyrosine kinase constitutively expressed and responsible for about 95% of patients with CML.[47,48] This abnormal tyrosine kinase does not exist in normal cells of the patients; therefore, it was an excellent target for development of an agent with activity against CML.

Screening was conducted to find compounds with specific activity against the BCR-ABL tyrosine kinase, and the agent (CGP57148, aka STI 571, imatinib) was found to be the most selective inhibitor of the kinase by targeting the adenosine triphosphate-binding site (ATP-pocket) of the enzyme.[49] The agent was tested *in vitro* and *in vivo* and found to be selectively toxic to BCR-ABL-positive cells.[49–51] Phase I and II trials in 1999 and 2000 documented that dramatic activity of imatinib against CML, particularly in the chronic phase of the disease.[52,53] As noted above, this impressive example of drug development really spanned nearly 40 years from identification of the target until documentation of clinical activity of a compound against the disease (only 10 years if one starts counting from the time of discovery of the target, the p210 BCR-ABL tyrosine kinase). Of note is that additional work has shown that imatinib also has substantial activity against several other neoplastic diseases such as gastrointestinal stromal sarcomas, which possess abnormalities in the KIT oncogene and has received regulatory approvals for a total of nine different indications (Table A1).

Although not in the scope of this chapter, a variety of other targeted therapeutics has also demonstrated substantial clinical antitumor activities (antiestrogens, antiandrogens, aromatase inhibitors, and monoclonal antibodies to CD20, CD52, HER-2/*neu*,

etc.). However, at the time of the writing of this chapter, there were also some disappointments in the area of targeting. For example, the farnesyl transferase inhibitors that have been developed to target tumors with mutations in *ras* have not shown activity against pancreatic cancer, even though they have clear clinical activity against breast cancer and acute leukemias, where *ras* mutations are not thought to be critical to the development or progression of either disease.[54–56] Another example of difficulties with targeting is the finding that despite the upregulation of the epidermal growth factor receptor (EGFR) in a number of malignancies, the activities of small-molecule inhibitors of the EGFR kinase or monoclonal antibodies to the EGFR do not appear to correlate with the increased expression of EGFR (at least by currently available methods of measuring the receptor or its kinase).[57] These findings, however, should not discourage the search for useful applications either within hematology/oncology or outside of malignant diseases. As an example, recent publications indicate a beneficial effect of farnesyl transferase inhibitors in Hutchinson–Gilford progeria.[58,59]

Clearly, there is a great deal of work to do if targeted therapy is to succeed in major tumor types. In a recent piece of work, Druker and Lydon[60] outlined the lessons learned for the development of imatinib. These lessons provide guidelines for thinking about improved mechanism-based approaches, including the following:

1. Identification of an appropriate target molecule for drug development. The identification of the BCR-ABL tyrosine kinase as the kinase to cause CML (i.e., a single molecular defect as a target) was important. The kinase was a "disease gene." For success, one probably should have a target that is critical to the disease process.
2. Availability of a validated surrogate endpoint that can be easily measured in patients to ensure that the new agent is indeed interfering with the desired target and has the desired effects. For CML, this is the Philadelphia chromosome, which is monitored in blood cells (and by blood counts).
3. Improvements in techniques important for drug designs (e.g., crystallography and molecular modeling) to optimize the selectivity (specificity) of compounds.

There is no question that with improvements in our understanding of the wiring of the cell there will be continuing efforts at developing mechanism-based agents.[60–65] However, given the terrific amount of work and substantial resources necessary to clinically develop a new agent, it is very critical that targets are selected wisely.[66] In addition, it has become clear that the biologic role of a target identified may not be static throughout the clinical course of a patient. Thus, early drug development has led to the insight that repeat biopsies are necessary to understand sensitivity and resistance mechanisms. Conducting pre- and post-treatment biopsies remains a challenge in the clinic and may not be possible in all tumor types.

In addition to targeting the tumor cells, it is now clear that targeting the environment of tumor cells is taking on a whole new importance. The exciting area of angiogenesis has given all clinicians a sense of optimism, given the finding that the monoclonal antibody bevacizumab, directed against VEGF-A, has substantially improved the survival (when combined with chemotherapy) of patients with colorectal cancer, non-small-cell lung cancer, and possibly breast cancer.[67–69] It is clear that the agent also has single-agent activity against renal cell and ovarian cancers.[70,71] While bevacizumab is neutralizing the ligand to the VEGF receptor 2, recently ramucirumab—another monoclonal antibody—has created much interest because it binds to the extracellular domain and blocks the VEGF receptor 2 directly. Conceptually, this would impede binding of all ligands and not only of VEGF-A to the receptor.[72,73] Small molecules that target VEGF and PDGF pathways (to alter the angiogenic process) such as sunitinib (SU 1248) or regorafenib (BAY 73-4506) are also demonstrating substantial clinical antitumor activity. Research inspired by the successful development of antiangiogenic compounds has also led to the very important insight that not only is tumor angiogenesis induced and sustained through a network of signaling pathways, but that autocrine and paracrine loops of angiogenic factors may also play a pivotal role in determining the cancer stem cell pool size.[74] Despite these impressive advances and the new mechanism of action, the new agents affecting the tumor environment still require the steps of drug development as outlined in this chapter. One of the biggest challenges for antiangiogenic compounds is the identification of a predictive biomarker, which is sufficiently robust to select patients for treatment decisions.

As early clinical trial designs move toward molecularly characterized tumors, the development of biomarkers remains a challenge for several reasons[75]:

- Lack of comprehensive understanding of the tumor biology or the mechanism of action of the candidate drug;
- Lack of a reliable, reproducible, sufficiently sensitive, or specific methods to measure the candidate biomarker molecule(s);
- Lack of statistical power that the observation made in early-phase studies can be carried over into larger studies (Phase II or Phase III).

For an example see Refs 76, 77.

Because of these complexities, drugs that reach Phase I often lack relevant, clinically meaningful pharmacodynamic markers. The validation of biomarkers in Phase I would require a conceptual redesign of Phase I trials with enrichment of target-carrying patients during the dose-escalation phase or at least during subsequent expansion cohorts that need to be large enough to allow for sound biostatistics in patient populations specifically expressing the candidate biomarker or biomarker profile, adaptive trial designs that allow learning during ongoing trials, and randomized dose-refining Phase II trials (Figure 2).[78,79] Even in the presence of a robust and predictive PD marker, it may be wise to continue dose escalation until a maximally tolerated dose (MTD) is reached so that a good understanding of the dose range can be generated in consideration of both acute and delayed toxicities. On the basis of statistical simulations, Hoering and colleagues have proposed a Phase I/II hybrid trial design that includes an initial traditional dose escalation, which is subsequently followed by a modified, single arm Phase II part that includes both dose and schedule optimization and efficacy testing. The authors hypothesize that this will be helpful in determining the best dose to move into large, randomized studies.[80]

Special aspects developing protein-engineered compounds

Protein-engineered compounds like monoclonal antibodies, peptides, peptibodies, or fusion proteins are developed against soluble peptide ligands or membrane-bound receptors. During Phase I studies, these compounds may not deliver DLTs or MTDs. Absolute doses exceeding 20 mg/kg may also raise the concern of nonspecific, protein-related toxicities when treatment is to be administered over a long time. As the production of monoclonal antibodies may occur in virally transformed cells, the residual viral load—despite all efforts to remove the viruses—may also be a concern if very high protein doses are administered for long periods. For these reasons, the choice of doses and schedules for later development in Phase II or Phase III studies often rests on a "biologically effective dose (BED)" or "biologically active dose (BAD)." This dose schedule may be derived from PK observations in animal models. As an example, the minimum plasma concentration of the monoclonal antibody that resulted in xenograft responses in mice may be used, and doses in Phase I trials that result in the respective or higher plasma concentrations may be carried forward into later Phase II or Phase III trials. However, this approach carries a significant risk for a dose and schedule in patients that have suboptimal efficacy and require subsequent refinement after Phase III trials have been completed and analyzed. The reasons are that animal models may not be predictive and may require species-specific antibodies/engineered proteins, which are different from those used in human trials. The development of protein-engineered drugs like monoclonal antibodies thus will profoundly benefit from robust and *predictive* PK/PD modeling and the application of a reliable biomarker as early in the process of preclinical and clinical studies as possible. Without a PK/PD model, a biomarker, an MTD, and unequivocally drug-related DLTs, the choice of a dose and schedule for subsequent trials means flying blindly even if the compound has encouraging early clinical activity. It carries the risk for losing a potentially active compound and for very late dose/schedule optimization studies that impact on life-cycle management. Encore studies in tumor types, which had shown a negative or marginally positive result in completed Phase III trials, may be ethically debatable. This creates the challenge to use the Phase I setting and add expansion cohorts to optimize dosing and scheduling in order to achieve maximum target blockade and provide an early proof of concept in humans. Such an approach may also include intrapatient dose escalations although these should be considered in individual cases and with appropriate care.

Of specific interest is the development of immunotherapeutic antibodies. In general, compounds in clinical use and development have a negative effect on cells, for example, by shutting

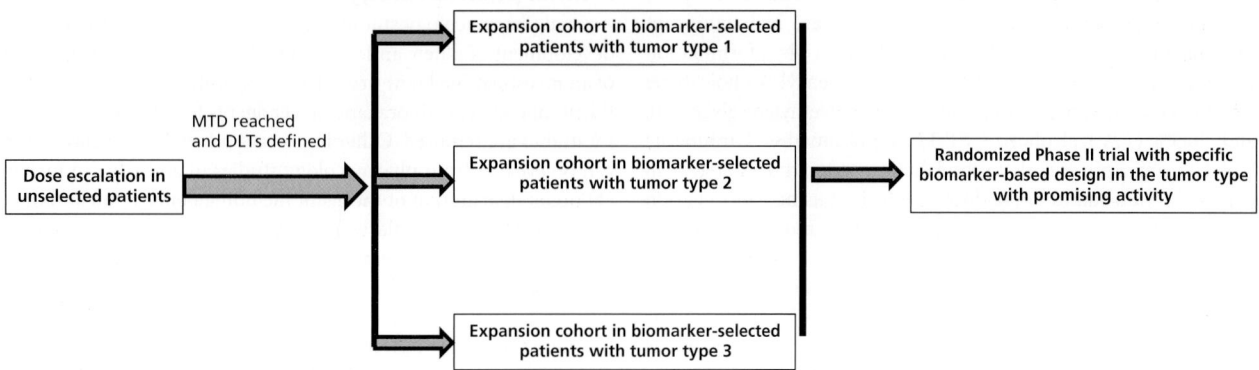

Figure 2 An example of an early phase trial design with targeted agents and patient enrichment.

down metabolic or reproductive pathways or blocking receptors or downstream phosphorylation events. In contrast, the blockage of immune checkpoint receptors/ligands by immunotherapeutic antibodies *reactivates* the immune system. Thus, the activity of these new compounds is not directly on the tumor but on the immune system. Early-phase trials of this type of agents need to involve assays to determine the cellular immune response, awareness of delayed tumor shrinkage including the potential for initial increase in tumor lesions, and awareness of novel toxicities (e.g., hypophysitis, thyroiditis, and autoimmune-like states due to overactivation of the immune system), which may require immunosuppressive therapies.[81–83]

Sources of compounds to evaluate against targets

There is no question that the most rational way to develop a new agent against a target is to understand the crystal structure of that target (at least for nonbiologic agents) and rationally design an agent to interact with that target.[60,61,66] However, for a vast majority of these targets, there is not a crystal structure identified. Fortunately, there can usually be a method developed to aid in identifying inhibitors of targets using molecular screening.[84] Therefore, it is necessary for a drug-development team to have access to major libraries of compounds to use against their target with a high-throughput system. The NCI has always been a key resource for libraries of compounds, including natural products.[85] The NCI has made the NCI Diversity Library (http://dtp.nci.nih.gov/branches/dscb/diversity_explanation.html) available to investigators. In addition, there are a number of additional libraries available for investigator use (e.g., http://htbc.stanford.edu/compounds.html; http://www.chemdiv.com, etc.)

Preparation of agents for clinical trials

Formulation

Pharmaceutics or the formulation of a compound for preclinical pharmacology, toxicology, and clinical trials is an often overlooked but very important aspect of drug development. It is very desirable to have the best formulation in place that one plans to use in clinical trials before proceeding with animal pharmacology and toxicology.[86]

Difficult formulations have often led to prolonged development programs that have occasionally caused such difficulties that development of the compound was nearly discontinued. This was certainly the case with paclitaxel, which requires for solubilization a difficult cremaphor-containing combination that may result in idiosyncratic reactions in some patients.[87] A multitude of other anticancer agents (in addition to paclitaxel) have had significant formulation problems, including etoposide (solved by a formulation using 20 mg etoposide, 2 mg citric acid, 30 mg benzyl alcohol, 80 mg modified polysorbate 80/Tween 80, 650 mg polyethylene glycol300, and 30.5% (V/V) alcohol), CPT-11 (topoisomerase I inhibitor) (solved using a prodrug that is broken down by carboxylesterase in patients' serum and tumors), docetaxel (solved using a formulation of polysorbate 80), and several others. If one requires an exotic formulation for intravenous use, there may be a major delay in the start of clinical trials. In general, only formulations that have already been used in patients should be used to formulate a new agent. Recently, there have been some important advances in the area of formulation. As an example, the packaging of paclitaxel into specially prepared albumin particles (called "nab-technology") has

changed the characteristics of paclitaxel and has led to impressive activity of nab-paclitaxel in breast, non-small-cell lung cancer, and pancreas cancer.[88–90]

Another major question that frequently arises in the formulation process is whether an oral route of administration would be preferable over an intravenous route. In general, for cytotoxic agents, there is a worry that there is a much greater chance for wide variability in the gastrointestinal absorption of agents. This variability could lead to unpredictable and potentially serious side effects in some patients and not in others. In addition, patient compliance with oral drug intake has been questioned, particularly if these drugs can cause nausea or vomiting. Therefore, in general, if an agent can be formulated for both intravenous and oral use, it is deemed preferable to develop the intravenous formulation first. This allows one to carefully determine the pharmacology of the compound in a situation in which absorption is not an issue. An exception to this is when the compound has great schedule dependency in its preclinical activity work-up. In that situation, an oral formulation may be more desirable.[91] Moreover, if the drug is predicted to be taken repeatedly (e.g., daily) for a prolonged period of time, development of an oral application may be advantageous.

Development of an assay for a pharmacodynamic endpoint (surrogate marker)

The development of anticancer agents had been for the most part empiric. More specifically, there had not been a prior emphasis on ensuring that the new agent actually affected the target it was designed to hit. With more mechanism-based drug design, it has been recommended to try to have some assay in place to determine whether the agent is having the desired effect on the target (i.e., a pharmacodynamic endpoint). As it is plausible to assume that any compound exerts a variety of biological effects, such an assay—of course—may not reflect the totality of a drug's biochemical or clinical effects.

This area is becoming critically important. As an example, Hidalgo and colleagues have measured phosphorylation of the EGFR in skin biopsies in patients receiving EGFR antagonists.[92] Moreover, the likelihood to respond to pemetrexed has been linked to the expression level of thymidylate synthase and mrp-4, and the antitumor activity of the serine-threonine kinase inhibitor enzastaurin has been correlated with the expression of GSK-3ß.[93,94] It is extremely important that these surrogate markers accompany mechanism-based drug development. Without these markers, their development will be confusing, and it will not be known whether it was an inappropriate target or whether the new agent just did not affect the target (for pharmacokinetic and a variety of other possible reasons) if the compound failed.

Animal pharmacology

Animal pharmacology studies have rarely been a major part of the development of a new anticancer agent [at least in the preparation of an investigational new drug (IND) application]. The exception to this is, of course, with oral anticancer agents for which bioavailability studies are required. Other important pieces of information that can be learned from pharmacology studies in animals can include (1) organ distribution of the agent including penetration and dwell time in tumors (particularly useful for compounds that are formulated in liposomes or are new compounds formulated in nanoparticles encapsulated in albumin) and (2) penetration into the central nervous system or other sanctuaries.[95,96]

One other very powerful piece of information that can be gleaned from animal pharmacology was described by Collins and colleagues.[97] This often forgotten piece of work demonstrated that there was a direct relationship between the concentration × time ($C \times T$) product at the LD$_{10}$ in mice and the $C \times T$ product at the MTD in patients.[97] Essentially (based on a milligram per square meter basis), the $C \times T$ in mouse is equal to $C \times T$ in humans. This important relationship appears to hold up across most animal species and can be used as a target for dose escalation in Phase I trials with a new agent in patients (see below). Work by others has confirmed the relationship and has documented how that relationship can be used to determine which serum concentrations of agents will be achieved in patients (and should therefore be used in *in vitro* model systems).[98,99]

Animal toxicology

These studies are a critical part of any drug-development program. In general, the models used for toxicology studies to date (mouse, rat, or beagle dog, used because of a biliary system closer to human) have given an excellent safety record for the development of new anticancer agents (e.g., there essentially have been no catastrophes in the initial Phase I clinical trials in patients). One area in which one must be a bit more careful is in the area of nucleosides and antimetabolites. As an example, the starting dose for fludarabine phosphate was too high and substantial bone marrow toxicity was noted in the first dose level in patients presumably owing to the fact that fludarabine requires activation by deoxycytidine kinase and the levels of this enzyme are much higher in human cancer cells than they are in mouse and canine marrow cells.[100,101] Pemetrexed (MTA, LY231514), a multitargeted enzyme inhibitor approved for the treatment of patients with mesothelioma and non-small-cell lung cancer, had a similar problem, but with worse toxicities in animals than in patients.[102] Therefore, investigators should be alert about the possibility of discordance between animals and humans when examining results of animal toxicity studies with nucleoside analogs or other antimetabolites. This is particularly important when anticancer agents are studied in very innovative formulations like nanoparticles.[103]

As noted above, the usual animal species required for formal toxicology studies is either a mouse or a rat plus the beagle dog.[104] For monoclonal antibodies and other biologics, a primate model is frequently required. An excellent review of toxicity requirements by the US Food and Drug Administration (FDA) has been published by DeGeorge et al.[104] In Europe, there is a movement to use only two murine species (mouse and rat) as a toxicology package necessary to begin a Phase I trial in patients.[105] However, if the tolerable doses in those species (based on a milligram per square meter basis) are widely divergent, additional toxicology studies in the dog are a necessity before beginning the Phase I clinical trial in patients.

In general, the animal models used are reliable in predicting certain types of organ toxicities (such as myelosuppression).[106,107] However, the dog has been noted to be somewhat overpredictive for renal, hepatic, and gastrointestinal toxicities.[108] Neurologic, pancreatic, dermatologic, and pulmonary toxicities are generally not well predicted by the murine and canine models. The models are imperfect in predicting other organ toxicities, and, occasionally, toxicities are noted in one species (e.g., a murine species) but do not occur in another (e.g., the dog). This is often attributable to a difference in metabolism of the agent between the species. If unacceptable toxicities are noted in mice, one should still strongly consider going into dogs or primates as they may not exhibit toxicities reported in murine models. This has been done for a few compounds that were cardiotoxic in the mouse toxicology

program, but the dog correctly predicted that no serious cardiac toxicity would be noted in patients.[109]

As will be outlined below, the animal toxicology package is most critical to help define the starting doses in patients beginning with the Phase I trial of the agent.

Preparation of an IND (investigational new drug) application

Before a clinical trial can begin in the United States and most other countries, it is necessary to prepare an IND application and to submit this document to a regulatory agency (e.g., the FDA). The necessary components of the IND are outlined in Table 2.

The clinical trial can proceed with a new agent if 30 days go by after filing the IND package and there is no comment by the FDA. Of course, if the FDA requires additional information before the 30-day waiting period expires, that information must be supplied and approved before the first Phase I trial can proceed.

Early clinical trials

Phase 0 clinical trials

Phase 0 trials are designed to be conducted before regular Phase I trials. Conceptually, they have been proposed to inform later Phase I trials regarding pharmacokinetic/pharmacodynamic relationships, starting dose, and other parameters. Phase 0 trials have short durations (usually just one course), and use doses far below the subsequent starting dose for Phase I. The regulatory requirements have been laid out in an FDA guidance paper on an abbreviated IND published in January 2006 and are considerably easier than requirements for a full IND document. Owing to ethical considerations (no therapeutic benefit), failure to accelerate drug development and increase in resource consumption, this trial design has been largely abandoned.[110–115]

Table 2 Investigational New Drug (IND) application.

1. Cover sheet—Form 1571
   - (a) Name, address, and telephone number of sponsor, etc.
   - (b) Phase of clinical investigation
   - (c) Commitment not to begin clinical investigation until an IND is in effect
   - (d) IRB commitment
   - (e) Commitment to follow all regulation requirements
   - (f) Name and title of person responsible for monitoring
   - (g) Name and title of person responsible for safety
   - (h) Any transfer obligations, e.g., Clinical Research Organization
   - (i) Signature of sponsor
2. Table of contents
3. Introductory statement and general investigational plan
4. Reserved for FDA
5. Investigator's brochure
6. Protocols
7. CMC information
8. Pharmacology and toxicology information
9. Previous human experience with the investigational drug
10. Additional information

CMC, chemistry, manufacturing, and control; FDA, US Food and Drug Administration; IND, investigational new drug.

More details can be found at the FDA website: http://www.fda.gov/drugs/develop mentapprovalprocess/howdrugsaredevelopedandapproved/approvalapplications/ investigationalnewdrugindapplication/default.htm.

Phase I clinical trials

This is the first trial of a new agent in patients (or in normal volunteers). Several excellent reviews have been written on Phase I trial methodologies.[116-118] The objectives of the first Phase I trial in humans differ as to whether the agent is first given to patients or is first given to normal volunteers.

Phase I trial in normal volunteers versus patients

There is always some interest in conducting initial Phase I clinical trials of new anticancer agents in normal volunteers rather than in patients. The number one reason cited for this approach is that the normal volunteers have normal organ function not impaired by malignancy and by prior treatment of their malignancy as in the case in patients. In addition, normal volunteers would not normally be on other concomitant medications (usually an average of 10 for patients on a Phase I trial), which could complicate the pharmacokinetics and the side effect profile of a new agent.[119] However, clinicians caring for patients with cancer often view the conduct of the initial Phase I trial in normal volunteers as a waste of precious time and a step that delays the administration of a promising agent to the very people who need it: patients with advanced cancer. Nevertheless, with the development of many new cytostatic rather than cytotoxic agents that are noncarcinogenic, there is more and more interest in first trying the new agents in normal volunteers—just as is done in other areas of drug development such as cardiology.

For a new agent to even be considered for administration to a normal volunteer, it, of course, must be demonstrated to be noncarcinogenic and nonmutagenic in the appropriate preclinical systems. Then an initial trial in normal volunteers can begin.

The objectives of the initial clinical trial of a new anticancer agent performed in normal volunteers are more limited than if the initial clinical trial is performed in patients with advanced cancer. The objectives include the following:

1. To determine the clinical pharmacology of a *single dose* of the agent when given at the starting dose (and perhaps at one additional dose level, to ensure linear kinetics for the agent). This clinical pharmacology information would include peak plasma levels, half-lives of the agent, and the area under the curve (AUC) for the agent. In addition, some pharmacodynamic data could be collected, for example, whether the agent hits a target in a particular normal tissue (such as white blood cells).
2. To determine the clinical pharmacology of multiple daily doses (usually not to exceed 5–7 days) of the new agent at the starting dose (and perhaps at one additional dose level) to ensure that no accumulation of the agent occurs. The clinical pharmacology of the agent would include peak plasma levels, trough levels, half-lives of the agent, AUC for the agent, and steady-state plasma levels. In addition, some pharmacodynamic data could also be collected, for example, whether the agent was hitting a target in a particular normal tissue (such as white blood cells, buccal mucosal cells, saliva, hair, and fingernails).
3. To determine if there are any *side effects* noted for these low doses of the agent in these volunteers. This is usually done by having placebo controls. This can be done by either a balanced randomization (one normal volunteer receives placebo for every one normal volunteer receiving the new agent) or by an unbalanced randomization (one normal volunteer receiving the placebo for every two or more normal volunteers receiving the new agent).

The thought using the normal volunteer approach for the initial trials of a new agent is that the pharmacokinetic data obtained will provide clean, important information with less variability (vs the variability in patients with advanced cancer). It is felt that this solid information might actually shorten the Phase I clinical trials for the new agent in patients and indeed allow patients with advanced cancer to receive more effective doses and schedules of the new agent, which would give them a better chance of benefitting from treatment. There can, however, be problems with taking a new cytostatic agent—even at low doses—into a normal volunteer population. There has been a recent instance in which a cytostatic agent was taken into normal volunteers and at low doses of daily administration caused a very severe cutaneous reaction (which had not been seen with the single dose). Although not life threatening, it was cosmetically severe and actually delayed the administration of the agent to patients. In summary, the administration of new anticancer agents to normal volunteers remains somewhat controversial in oncology drug-development circles.

The objectives for a Phase I trial in patients with advanced malignancies include the following:

1. To determine the maximum tolerated dose (MTD) of the drug. The MTD is the dose recommended for subsequent Phase II trials of the new agent.
2. To define the qualitative and quantitative toxicities of the new agent. In traditional Phase I trials this is described by grading of toxicities according to internationally accepted tables and by observing dose-limiting toxicities (DLTs). These tables are regularly updated and are published under http://ctep.cancer.gov/protocolDevelopment/electronic_applications/ctc.htm. The dose at which DLTs are seen has recently been referred to as "NTD" or nontolerated dose.
3. To obtain robust information on the clinical pharmacology of the new agent. The need for this important aspect has been recently re-emphasized.[120]
4. To obtain pharmacodynamic information on the new agent (e.g., does a specific plasma concentration of the new agent interact with/modulate a particular target). These studies can be done using tissue samples (normal and tumor), peripheral blood cells, skin biopsies, effusions, serum proteins, buccal mucosal cells, or new imaging techniques.
5. To document early evidence of antitumor activity (e.g., objective responses, tumor marker decline, and clinical benefit).

Selection of schedule and route for a Phase I trial

The schedules most commonly explored in Phase I trials include (1) single dose repeated every 3 or 4 weeks, (2) daily × 5 administration repeated every 3 or 4 weeks, (3) weekly × 4 repeated every 6 weeks, (4) weekly × 3 repeated every 4 weeks, (5) 120 h continuous infusion, and (6) daily × 21 every 28 days. Of course, as more information (e.g., pharmacokinetic/pharmacodynamic information) becomes available on the new agent, it may become necessary to explore other schedules. The choice of what schedule to use (e.g., the choice between a bolus vs a more frequent, e.g., daily × 5 or daily × 21 schedule) is most frequently based on (1) the schedule-dependency for antitumor activity in the preclinical models, (2) the pharmacokinetics of the agent in the preclinical model (and eventually from data in patients), and (3) very importantly, the mechanism of action and preclinical data regarding the mechanism of action (e.g., dwell time for a drug to be "on target" to have an effect). The reader is cautioned that decisions on schedule based on the most active schedule in the preclinical animal models need to take into account the fact that animal tumors have a more rapid doubling time and a much higher growth fraction than do most types of human cancers (other than leukemias or aggressive lymphomas).

As far as the route is concerned, the tried and true method for development of new agents (even if an oral route is possible with the new agent) was to proceed with the first Phase I trial by the intravenous route. This intravenous trial could then be followed by the oral Phase I trial. This has classically been done because (1) there is certainty of delivery of the agent with the intravenous route (many patients with cancer may have abnormalities of their gastrointestinal tracts, they may have low-grade nausea from other medications (e.g., pain medication), or swallowing might be difficult for them and compliance may be an issue); (2) with the intravenous route, there is no question that the drug is delivered with a chance for the greatest peak plasma levels of the agent; and (3) having the correct intravenous dose first and then proceeding with the oral Phase I trial of the agent allows one to assess the bioavailability of the oral form of the agent.

With the introduction of new cytostatic agents, which tend to have more schedule dependence, it is becoming more and more common to only develop the oral form of the agent (e.g., tamoxifen, capecitabine, imatinib, and vemurafenib). With the oral form of the agent, there is more room for creativity in schedules (e.g., daily $\times$ 5, 2 days off; daily $\times$ 5; and daily $\times$ 42). However, one must remember that the schedules used for the Phase I trial cannot be greatly different than the schedules used in the animal toxicology package and should be manageable in a more uncontrolled clinical setting after approval of the new agent. With better diagnostic tools, pharmacogenetic variability of patients is garnering increasing awareness. Pharmacogenetic variability may be important for differences in clinical activity and toxicities and thus may need to be considered when dose and schedule of a mechanistically based agent are chosen.[121]

Calculation of the starting dose for a Phase I trial

The criteria for calculation of a starting dose include using either one-tenth the LD10 (or MTD) in the mouse or rat or one-third or one-sixth of the toxic dose low (TDL) in the dog. The TDL is defined as the lowest dose that produces a toxic effect and usually a dose that, if doubled, causes no lethality. The decision to use the murine model or the dog to guide the starting dose considers which dose will give the lower or more conservative starting dose on the schedule planned for later use.[122]

Because animal toxicology studies frequently give data on a milligram per kilogram basis, it is critical to scale all doses between animals and humans using a milligram per square meter basis.[123,124] Table 3 details the conversion factor suggested by Freireich et al.[123] for milligram per kilogram in an animal species to a milligram per square meter scale.

To demonstrate of how one would calculate the starting dose for a new agent, we could use the example of the development of the topoisomerase I inhibitor CPT-11.[125] In animal toxicology studies with CPT-11, the most sensitive animal species was the mouse using a weekly schedule. For CPT-11, the MTD in the mouse given

CPT-11 on the weekly schedule was 70 mg/kg. Using the conversion factor of 3 (Table 3), the MTD in the mouse on a milligram per square meter level would be 70 mg/kg $\times$ 3 = 210 mg/m^2. Then, the starting dose in humans using the mouse information would be one-tenth of the MTD in mouse or one-tenth of 210 or 21 mg/m^2 given weekly. If the dog had been the most sensitive animal species to CPT-1 I, we would have used that dog toxicology information to determine our starting dose for CPT-11.

Methods for dose escalation

Dose-escalation methodologies are used to determine the DLTs, which in turn define the MTD. Side effects are used to titrate further dose increases and it is assumed that there is a monotone relationship among dose, toxicity, and activity.

The method used for dose escalation in Phase I trials has classically been the *modified Fibonacci* search scheme.[118,126] However, as can be seen in Table 4, there are now several methods for escalation of dose in Phase I trials that can be used.[127–133] Most of these other methods of dose escalation were developed to try to minimize the number of patients receiving very low, ineffective doses of a new agent and to try to improve the ethics of the situation.[134,136,137] The modified Fibonacci search scheme is the most often used method of dose escalation. However, it can result in the highest number of patients receiving ineffective doses, largely because while the initial dose escalations are substantial, there is eventually a tapering off of the percent dose escalation to just 33% escalations at each subsequent dose level. Table 5 details a classic modified Fibonacci dose-escalation scheme. The real benefit of starting a Phase I clinical trial with a new agent using the modified Fibonacci scheme is that it has a superb record of safety. It is particularly the preferred method when one has an agent that has a steep dose–toxicity curve in the animal toxicology studies with the new agent.

Along with the modified Fibonacci method cohort sizing usually follows a 3 + 3 design for each dose level. This must be done carefully. In general, the first patient (patient l) at a new dose level

Table 3 Conversion factor for changing milligram per kilogram to milligram per square meter for starting dose in humans.

Animal model	Appropriate conversion factor for converting mg/kg mg/m^2
Mouse	3
Rat	6
Monkey	12
Dog	20
Human	37

Source: Adapted from Freireich 1966.

Table 4 Methods for dose escalation in Phase I trials.

Method	Proposed by
Modified Fibonacci	Hansen[126]
Doubling method	Gottlieb[127]
	Freireich (personal communication)
Pharmacologically guided	Collins[97]
2 × AUC method	Evans[128]
Geometric mean + extended factor of 2	Erlichmann[129]
Continual reassessment	O'Quigley[130,131]
(and modified continual reassessment)	Faries[132]
Accelerated titration design	Simon[133]
Selection by patient method	Freedman[134,135]

Table 5 Modified Fibonacci dose-escalation scheme in Phase I trials.

Dose level	Dose	Increase above preceding dose (%)
1	N	Starting dose
2	2 N	100
3	3,3 N	67
4	5 N	50
5	7 N	40
6	12 N	33
7	16 N	33
And so on	—	—

is entered into the study and observed for 3 weeks. If no toxicities are noted in patient 1, patient 2 on the same dose level is then entered and observed for at least 2 weeks (note that, by that time, patient 1 will be well into his/her second course). If no toxicities are noted in patient 2, patient 3 can be entered after patient 2 is observed for 2 weeks. Although there is always pressure from many quarters to enter patients more quickly into a Phase I trial, following this methodology provides the highest degree of safety possible and provides added protection in cases in which the new agent (or its metabolites) has a particularly long half-life or a new agent has nonlinear kinetics. One must also be careful and probably use the modified Fibonacci method when one is dealing with an agent that is a prodrug (as is CPT-11), and limited information is available on the active metabolite.

If no DLT (see definition below) is reached at a dose level, the dose is escalated for the next cohort of patients. If only one of the three patients at a particular dose level is noted to have a DLT, then up to three more patients can be entered onto that dose level. If two or more patients of three or six patients are noted to have DLTs, then one has exceeded the MTD of the drug. Then, additional patients are entered on the preceding dose level to ensure that one has a correct MTD—the dose to be taken into Phase II trials with the new agent. It is very important to note that there is no real scientific basis for the three patients per dose level used in standard Phase I trials.[138] The major rationale for the 3 + 3 cohort size design per dose level is that, to date, it has provided a good safety record for Phase I trials, allows for a more thorough pharmacokinetic and possibly also pharmacodynamic evaluation at lower dose levels, is straightforward to use, is generally accepted by Institutional Review Boards, and comes at no model-related additional cost. In a recent literature review, which retrospectively analyzed 1235 Phase I trials, the 3 + 3 cohort size approach has been found to be by far the most frequently used approach despite concerns that the 3 + 3 cohort sizing may be inferior compared to more complicated model-based cohort sizing.[139,140]

The next dose-escalation method outlined in Table 4 is the *doubling method.* This was proposed to try to minimize the number of patients entered at ineffective dose levels. This method provides a more rapid dose escalation. Theoretically, it could lead to overshooting the dose with attendant severe toxicities (although one cannot find any examples of problems in the literature). This doubling method of dose escalation (n, $2n$, $4n$, $8n$, $16n$ …) is probably now one of the most commonly used methods of dose escalation in Phase I trials at least at low doses of the agent that do not cause toxicities.

Another method for dose escalation introduced by Simon et al.[133] that also uses one patient per dose level is the *accelerated titration* design. They introduced two designs (design I and II). With design I, cohorts of one patient per dose level are treated with 40% escalations between dose levels. With the first DLT, there is an expansion of the cohort to a total of three new patients. With design II, there is only one patient per dose level, but there are dose escalations of 100% between levels, and with the first DLT, the level is also expanded to three new patients. Then, escalation proceeds by 40% increments. On both designs I and II, intrapatient dose escalation is allowed if patients had grade 0 or 1 toxicity on the prior course.

Another Phase I dose-escalation methodology that is now used very infrequently is the method proposed in 1990 by Collins et al.[97] This method is also known as the *pharmacologically guided dose-escalation* method. The method is based on an important piece of work showing that the area under the C × T plasma disappearance curve (AUC) at the LD 10 (or MTD) in the mouse is equal to the AUC at the MTD in humans. Basically, that finding provides

the investigators with a target AUC. In practice, at each dose level, an AUC is determined for patients receiving that dose of the new agent. The AUC at that level is then used to determine what the next dose escalation will be (if the agent has linear kinetics). Use of this method for pharmacologically guided dose escalation requires real-time pharmacokinetics, which is sometimes problematic in a clinical situation. However, it can lead to more aggressive dose escalations. There have been some suggested improvements in the methodology, which have been implemented by some Phase I clinical trials groups.[141,142]

The most aggressive concept introduced to try to minimize the number of patients receiving ineffective doses of a new agent is the *continual reassessment method* proposed by O'Quigley and colleagues in 1990. This model has been repeatedly commented on and has been modified by other authors.[130–132,143–145] In this modified continual reassessment method (MCRM), a group of clinicians estimates the lower and upper dose limits where clinical toxicities might be noted (based on animal toxicology data). A Bayesian approach is then used to construct a dose–toxicity curve. The Phase I trial is started at one-tenth of the LD 10 or MTD in the mouse or at one-third or one-sixth of the TDL in the dog. However, the difference is that only one patient is entered at the first dose level. After the appropriate amount of follow-up (usually 2–3 weeks), it is judged whether the patient had toxicities (≥grade 1). If not, then the dose–toxicities curve is consulted to determine the next dose escalation. Dose escalation usually can proceed by doubling the dose as long as the dose is below the estimated MTD (on the dose–toxicity curve). The CRM/MCRM methods have now been in use for some time. There have been a few reviews of the results of trials conducted using modifications of the continual reassessment method.[141,146,147] In general, the MCRM does not seem to decrease the time it takes to complete a Phase I trial, nor does it actually substantially decrease the number of patients entered into the Phase I trial. It does require quick and complete availability of toxicity information before the next patient is treated. It does shorten the time it takes to get to a dose that is close to the MTD for the study, and the MCRM helps decrease the number of patients who receive a potentially ineffective (<80% of the MTD) dose in the context of a Phase I study (see response rate information below) but consequently may also increase the number of patients treated at toxic doses. One potential issue with the CRM approach also is when toxicities occur late and thus cannot be captured during the dose-determining process. This is important as a recent review on early studies with mechanism-based compounds found that 57% of grade ≥3 toxicities occurred after the completion of the first course of treatment.[148] This observation together with the observation that long-lasting, low-grade toxicities after treatment with mechanism-based agents may also define a "DLT" has been corroborated by international retrospective analyses.[149,150] Modifications of the CRM may be helpful taking these important aspects in consideration, but it is unclear whether they are generally useful.[151] Iasonos and O'Quigley have recently analyzed the published performance of adaptive dose-finding studies including various modifications of the originally proposed continual reassessment method.[152] The authors concluded that adaptive designs in Phase I trials are at least safe and can be adjusted to various clinical situations in Phase I.

Bayesian Phase I trial designs have been developed for combination Phase I studies with mechanism-based novel compounds but have not yet been broadly used clinically for this purpose. These mathematical methods also pay attention to the time-to-onset of toxicities.[153,154]

Another frequent issue in selection of patients for a Phase I trial is whether only patients with a certain disease should be entered into the study (e.g., only patients with prostate cancer). Interestingly, this is not frequently done, but will probably be done more frequently as more targeted disease-specific agents are brought into Phase I trials. Until that is done, it is likely that most Phase I trials, particularly with cytotoxic agents, will continue to allow entry of patients with a variety of malignancies.

Definitions of MTD and DLTs

The classic definition of an *MTD* is the highest dose that causes one or less of six patients to have DLT. This MTD is the dose that is generally recommended as the dose to be used in single-agent Phase II trials. However, there have been different definitions of the MTD used by the European research groups and it is important to carefully review the MTD definition before working with a new agent.

The definition of a *DLT* is grade ≥ 3 nonhematologic or grade 4 hematologic (e.g., absolute neutrophil count $<500/\mu L$) toxicities according to the NCI Common Toxicity Criteria for Adverse Events (NCI CTCAE) found at the following website: http://ctep.cancer.gov/protocolDevelopment/electronic_applications/ctc.htm.

There are frequent discussions as to whether Phase I trials should always see to define the MTD and DLTs. This question is becoming increasingly asked in clinical trials with agents that are mechanism based (e.g., monoclonal antibodies and kinase inhibitors). Rather than defining an MTD, there is an increasing emphasis (using pharmacodynamic measurements) on defining a BED. Of note is that often the BED and the MTD are actually quite close to each other. In addition, caution is urged at stopping the Phase I trial at the BED. The Phase I trials with imatinib may have stopped too early if only the BED was used. There is new evidence that one mechanism of resistance of CML cells to imatinib may be attributable to low-dose exposure. It would be nice to know whether higher doses of imatinib could be used to kill these clones of tumor cells.

Selection criteria for patients for Phase I trials

Table 6 details the traditionally used selection criteria for inclusion in a Phase I trial. These are offered as guidelines only. As Phase I clinical trials theoretically could pose a risk to patients, efforts have been made to generate additional scoring systems or measurements that could predict the prognosis of patients who are candidates for Phase I inclusion more precisely than traditional eligibility criteria.[155–158] These systems are refined with new information on cancer biology and, as an example, a study by Olmos and colleagues concluded that the number of circulating tumor cells—together with albumin, lactate dehydrogenase, and the number of metastatic sites—could be used to better predict the prognosis of Phase I candidate patients.[159] Similar efforts have been undertaken to predict which patients may develop serious drug-related toxicities, and these patients may be excluded from entering a Phase I trial.[160,161] These efforts are directed to detect which patient may have benefit from study participation but also ensure that the agent receives adequate evaluation in a patient population with adequate life expectancy. On the flip side of this approach there is discussion whether Phase I trials are biased to include patients who are not representative of the population treated after marketing authorization has occurred. In fact, even if the final recommended Phase II dose is used in and confirmed by subsequent Phase III trials, "real world" use after approval shows that dose and schedule modifications are frequent.[162] These modifications are usually driven by concerns about toxicities, but one must keep in mind that a reduced dose may also lead to reduced clinical benefit.

A few points of the traditional exclusion criteria are also worthy a discussion. First, an important question is whether older patients should participate in Phase I trials. Of note is the study by Bowen et al.,[163] which indicated that a patient's chronologic age did not impact on the toxicities experienced in Phase I trials of a new agent. In contrast to these findings, Schwandt et al.[164] found in their retrospective analysis of more than 500 patients older than 70 years in fact a slightly increased likelihood for toxicities, but the authors

Table 6 Common selection criteria for entry of patients into a Phase I trial.

1. Age ≥ 18 years
2. Pathologically confirmed diagnosis of any malignant solid tumor
3. Measurable disease not required
4. Life expectancy ≥ 12 weeks
5. Karnofsky Performance Status of $\geq 70\%$ (ECOG ≤ 2)
6. Adequate organ function:
   (a) Neutrophils $\geq 1500/\mu L$, hemoglobin ≥ 9 g/dL
   (b) Platelets $\geq 100,000/\mu L$
   (c) Serum bilirubin with normal limits
   (d) SGOT $\leq 3 \times$ ULN (except if owing to disease, then $\leq 5 \times$ ULN is acceptable)
   (e) Serum creatinine within normal limits and calculated creatinine clearance ≥ 60 mL/min
   (f) No atrial or ventricular arrhythmias requiring control by medication; no ischemic event experienced within the preceding 6 months
   (g) No history of seizure disorder requiring active therapy; no clinical evidence of malignancy of the central nervous system

7. Must have exhausted all therapy, which has a better chance of working for the patients (including investigational therapy) or must be in a situation for which there is no standard therapy
8. Must not have received any chemotherapy within 4 weeks before entry (6 weeks for mitomycin-C or nitrosoureas) with complete recovery from toxic effects of that therapy
9. Patients must not be receiving any concomitant radiation therapy
10. Patients must have recovered from the reversible toxicities of prior therapy
11. Female patients must be of nonchild-bearing potential or nonlactating and using adequate contraception with a negative pregnancy test at study entry and before each course of therapy
12. Male patients must also be using adequate contraception
13. No other serious concurrent medical illness or active infection should be present that would jeopardize the ability of the patient to receive (with reasonable safety) the chemotherapy outlined in the protocol
14. An effort must be made to minimize concomitant medications to those necessary for pain control, patient comfort, or life-threatening problems
15. Patients must sign an informed consent form. The patient must be aware of the neoplastic nature of his/her disease and willingly consent after being informed of the procedure to be followed, the experimental nature of the therapy, alternatives, potential benefits, side effects, risks, and discomforts

SGOT, serum glutamic-oxaloacetic transaminase; ULN, upper limits of normal.

concluded that this risk remained within the acceptable range in Phase I trials. Both studies concluded that age alone is no criterion to exclude a patient from participating in a Phase I trial.

Second, one of the most interesting new questions that is arising in the Phase I trial arena (because of the development of more targeted agents) is whether only patients whose tumors exhibit the particular target should be entered into the Phase I trial. This would seem to make sense because if the patient's tumor has the target (e.g., estrogen receptor or *HER2/neu*, CD20 or CD52 positivity, or the BCR-ABL rearrangement or mutated c-kit), the patients should be more likely to respond to the new agent. A strong plea has been made to only include target-carrying patients at least in Phase II trials.[165] It is fairly clear that the presence of the target in the patient's tumor should be a criterion for entry into the study if the agent is *certain* to work only on tumors that possess the target and if one is certain that the mechanism of action for the new agent is only against that particular target. In addition, one must be certain that the assay used to measure that particular target is accurate and reproducible. In this context, archival tissues or blood samples are unlikely to yield relevant information at later stages of the tumor evolution as tumors change their molecular characteristics during the clinical course.[166] When these criteria are met, the limitation of the patient population to those expressing the target can be very effective as has been shown by a Phase I trial with ceritinib in non-small-cell lung cancer patients carrying the EML-ALK translocation.[167] The selection of patients for entry on a new agent trial based on the presence of the target in their tumors thus is a strategy that will become more a standard as we can better pinpoint the precise mechanism(s) of action of new agents. Until then, the need to select patients based on the presence of a specific target either in peripheral tissues or tumor biopsies is a bit uncertain for many compounds in the area of Phase I trials.

Third, a frequent issue in selection of patients for a Phase I trial is whether only patients with a certain disease should be entered into the study (e.g., only patients with prostate cancer). Interestingly, this is not frequently done but will probably be done more frequently as more targeted disease-specific agents are brought into Phase I trials.

While traditionally Phase I studies only served as lead-ins for larger randomized trials, the recent progress in the development of mechanistically based agents has allowed a new—though still experimental—regulatory approach to drug approval. In 2012, FDA has issued a new guidance that one can obtain "Breakthrough Designation" based on limited data with a mechanism-based compound (http://www.fda.gov/downloads/drugs/guidancecomplianceregulatoryinformation/guidances/ucm358301.pdf).[168,169] This is a promising new model for drug development and has been used for two anticancer drugs (obinutuzumab and ibrutinib) and one noncancer agent in 2013 and, at the writing of this chapter, for five anticancer compounds (ofatumumab, ceritinib, idelalisib, ibrutinib, and pembrolizumab) and one noncancer agent in 2014 (Table A1). Ceritinib was approved through this process based on Phase I data only.[120,167] Approvals based on Breakthrough Designation are, however, preliminary approvals, and follow-up trials will be mandated by the FDA to confirm the benefit-risk ratio for patients.

Combination of agents in Phase I trials

Ethics are more straightforward in the conduct of Phase I trials, which combine a new agent with an already approved agent. In this setting, the patient will at least receive one agent with proven clinical activity (usually an approved small molecule). Novel anticancer agents may also be combined with traditional radiation therapy in a Phase I setting.[170] There is an increasing amount of clinical trial activity in this area with initial experience at least with monoclonal antibodies (e.g., trastuzumab, rituximab, and cetuximab) demonstrating increased clinical activity when used in combination with standard chemotherapeutic agents. On the other hand, there are also examples with small molecules in which the add-on strategy has not validated the initial enthusiasm at least in unselected patient populations.[171] Nevertheless, this remains an area of active exploration with the recent addition of mechanism-based agents such as signal transduction inhibitors used in combination with standard chemotherapeutic agents. General guidelines include the fact that the standard agent should generally be administered at the dose and schedule that are usually used (e.g., used at their approved dose and schedule) if at all possible. This improves acceptance by investigators and patients of the study design. Sequencing of the agents should be worked out in preclinical models (if at all possible), although the predictive value of these models is not established. By starting with the recommended/acceptable dose of the standard agent, one can then start escalation of the new agent with a fixed dose of the standard agent. In general, the starting dose for the new agent would be 25% of the MTD (or BED where applicable) for the new agent alone (if there are no overlapping toxicities with the standard agent). Depending on what is seen at that initial level, the next dose levels of the new agent would be 50% of its MTD, 75% of its MTD, and then 100% of its MTD (if possible). There are also some sophisticated models that have been reported to provide additional rationales for the dose escalations used in combination Phase I studies.[172]

With specific focus on early studies involving mechanism-based agents, Yap et al.[173] have recently nicely summarized a number of trial designs based on the basic concepts of reversal of resistance, sequencing of drugs, addition of a novel drug to a backbone treatment, alternating drugs, and pulsed schedules. There is thus a multitude of combination opportunities to address vertical resistance or horizontal resistance by alternative pathways and the decision which combination to use for drug development must be made on sound understanding of tumor biology.[174] Independent of which approach is ultimately applied, one should always be mindful that mechanism-based agents may have unexpected toxicities when combined, but one should never allow to compromise on dose in such a way that both agents are administered at suboptimal doses or target inhibition.[175,176] Most recently, the Clinical Trial Design Task Force of the NCI Investigational Drug Steering Committee has published the following set of recommendations: how to rationally choose combinations for Phase I testing[177]:

- the new combination should have a clear pharmacologic or biologic rationale and hypotheses explained in the protocol
- it should be described in the protocol how the combination will translate into clinical benefit and what the next steps in development of the combination will be beyond Phase I
- the design of the study should address DLT, potential for PK interactions contributing to toxicities, and a hypothesis for the mechanistic basis of such interaction.

Are Phase I clinical trials therapeutic?

Phase I trials have sometime been considered as nontherapeutic, that is, without therapeutic intent or benefit to the patient. This connotation needs to be corrected because several studies have been documenting that, indeed, conventional responses (complete and partial responses) can be seen in patients with advanced malignancies who are participating in single-agent Phase I trials of a new agent.[178–182] The reported response rates range from 5% to 7% (with about 1% complete response rate). However, there are also examples of considerably higher response rates, particularly in Phase I combination trials.[52,183–186] Most responses are noted in a range of 80–120% of the MTD for the agent. Roberts and colleagues reviewed 213 studies (6474 cancer patients) published in peer-reviewed journals.[187] They noted an overall response rate of 3.8%. Of note is that they found that response rates have decreased over the 12-year study period (6.2% in 1991–1994 vs 2.5% 1999–2002). During the observation period, toxic death rates also declined from 1.1% (1991–1994) to 0.06% (1999–2002). From these data, the authors concluded that the ratio of risk to benefit probably has improved. In an analysis of 24 Phase I studies, Jain et al. found a correlation between RECIST-based response and overall survival of patients.[188] This finding also supports the value of using response as an outcome measure in Phase I trials. For head and neck cancer, a study by Garrido-Laguna suggested that the progression-free survival of patients entered in Phase I studies is similar to the progression-free survival of their last treatment with an FDA-approved agent.[157] Of interest is whether the category of stable disease will become an increasingly used measure of interest (particularly stable disease lasting ≥4 months). There is interest in this category of nonprogressing patients, and it is likely to be increasingly used as a criterion used to determine whether a new agent exhibits some antitumor effect in a Phase I setting.[189] However, the use of WHO or RECIST criteria practically dichotomizes patient response (no response vs response) based on more or less arbitrary thresholds. Even if a more granular categoric grouping is used (CR, PR, SD, and PD), this approach may miss beneficial effects of smaller than threshold tumor shrinkage. Using tumor shrinkage as a continuous variable instead provides more granular information on antitumor activity, and thus is increasingly used alone or in combination with functional imaging procedures to assess biologic activity of novel compounds studied in early clinical trials.[165,186,188,190] Many other attempts to detect early signs of anticancer activity have been published. They include immune elements of tumor response, functional imaging procedures that measure tumor metabolism or perfusion, and tumor growth rate calculations.[167,191–195] A yet experimental approach is to measure time to tumor growth (TTG) as a relatively fast endpoint to determine clinical activity. This endpoint has been proposed based on a modeling of two large randomized Phase III studies in colorectal cancer by Claret and colleagues, and while it is still experimental and not validated for the Phase I setting, it is a potentially valuable additional tool to identify drug activity in early clinical development phases.[196,197]

Another method that is gaining interest to determine whether a new agent is having some antitumor activity is the concept of using patients as their own controls.[198] In this method, one uses the time a patient who is about to enter a new agent Phase I trial has been on their prior therapeutic regimen as a comparator to the time the patient is on trial without progressive disease. If the patient remains on the new Phase I agent for a period of time (period B) longer than he/she was on a prior therapy, the agent is judged to have had some impact on the natural history of the patient's tumor. If 30% of patients on the Phase I trial (who are at or near the MTD) have a period B that is longer than period A, the agent may be a promising one. This method is becoming increasingly used by clinicians in the Phase I trial arena.

Issues regarding Phase I trials in general

There is more and more being written about the ethics of patient participation in Phase I trials.[134,199–203] In recent publications it was noted that instead of the often-quoted perception by many that patients were motivated by altruism, the motivation for patients participating in Phase I trials included the following[186,203–206]:

1. Hope for improvement in their condition (high motivation)
2. Pressure exerted by relatives and friends (high motivation)
3. They felt they had no choice (high motivation)
4. Advice or trust of physicians (low motivation)
5. Altruism (low motivation)

These findings again emphasize how important it is for the patient to have all of the facts from the clinical development team so that they can take an informed decision as to whether to participate in a Phase I trial.[207] Several studies have found, however, that quite often important information on prognosis, supportive care, and the experimental nature of early clinical studies are either missed by clinicians or misunderstood by patients, and thus "therapeutic misconceptions" are a real risk for the physician–patient interaction.[208–210] In this context, a study by Berger et al. is of interest, which reports that the length of the consent documents in Oncology trials in Norway has doubled between 1987 and 2007.[211] This observation is certainly also directionally true for the United States. It is not necessarily a reflection of biologic complexity, but rather the result of an increasingly complex legal and administrative bureaucratic environment. For studies that include additional biopsies or biomarkers, often several separate informed consent forms need to be signed by the patient. Despite these complex formalities, several studies demonstrated that participation of a patient in a Phase I trial increased a patient's level of hope and appetite, which are both measures for quality of life.[212,213] Particularly, younger patients may also be interested to understand whether there could be a potential conflict of interest by the physician/institution offering participation in clinical trials.[214]

Learning from failures is an important part of early-phase drug development. A salient example at the writing of this chapter is the tremendous effort that went into the development of agents that disrupt the insulin-like growth factor pathway (IGF-receptor inhibitors). This concept has been taken back to the drawing board, and some of the following aspects may have contributed to the clinical failure of monoclonal antibodies to the IGF receptor: suboptimal PK and PD behavior, patient selection, absence of predictive and robust biomarkers, tumor choice based on nonpredictive cell-line data, lack of clear driver mutations in cancer, IGF copy number retrieved from biobase data, and misinterpretation of elevated IGF serum concentrations, which may have been bystander effects related to tumor hypoxia. In this context, an interesting analysis by Camaccho and colleagues found that only about two-thirds of Phase I trials presented at an annual meeting of the American Society of Clinical Oncology were subsequently actually published as article.[215] This is unfortunate as patients dedicate their time, health, and hope to these trials and it should thus be expected that the results of the treatment will be shared with the medical community in an appropriately detailed manner.

As already stated at the beginning of this chapter, the change in the types of compounds coming up for early-phase studies is remarkable. Several types of compounds can be identified: (1) chemotherapeutic agents with no "off-target" effects, (2) mechanism-based agents that—at high doses—may have significant and usually toxic "off-target" effects, (3) mechanism-based biologic compounds that have no further effect beyond a maximum, and (4) immunotherapy compounds for which not only toxicity but also traditional efficacy endpoints in early-phase studies may not be adequate. In today's Phase I era, it has become important to tailor the methodology of early-phase clinical evaluations to the type of compound or otherwise risk misleading results.

Future technologies likely to impact on Phase I trials

Over the past 10 years, the development of new agents has shifted from classic cytotoxic agents to molecularly mechanism-based compounds. However, the initial hopes of a faster and more efficient drug-development process have not been consistently met, and the early phase as well late phase development has often been slow, more complicated, and more expensive. New trial designs that incorporate predictive and robust biomarkers, pharmacokinetics, and pharmacodynamics are needed. In some cases of multitargeted agents, a biomarker signature may be necessary.[216]

In addition, the rapid advances in functional imaging (e.g. dynamic magnetic resonance imaging, positron emission tomography, and single-photon emission computed tomography) are likely to dramatically impact on the Phase I clinical trial both by helping investigators assess pharmacodynamic endpoints and perhaps assess early evidence of an antitumor effect.

Recent reports on the use of proteomics on serum (with distinct patterns of proteins predicting for presence of disease) represent new patterns of tumor markers that will certainly become useful for detecting early effects of new agents.[217,218]

The above and other new technologies should help the Phase I investigator determine early whether a particular new agent is helping that particular patient and improve the prospect for gain for patients who are willing to participate in Phase I trials with new agents.

Summary

Since the early beginnings of systematic anticancer therapy in the 1930s, more than 150 drugs have been identified to be active against cancer and have been approved by the US Food and Drug Administration. Despite this tremendous effort, cancer remains one of the biggest health care burdens, and only a minority of metastatic cancers can be cured. Along with the development of anticancer agents, methods have been established to standardize the development process itself and to provide objective assessments of the benefit a new drug may deliver. The past 10 years have seen a particularly dramatic acceleration of our understanding of the molecular biology and wiring of cancer cells, and this has greatly impacted on the understanding of how new drugs that target specific molecular processes should be developed. At the writing of this chapter, the efforts to develop such mechanism-based agents has largely replaced the more traditional development of chemotherapy directed against general features of cell growth. Nevertheless, it must not be forgotten, how important the initial, serendipity-based observations were and that these observations have led to the National Cancer Institute's extensive efforts to identify potential candidates for clinical drug discovery and preclinical assays to predict clinical activity. This was the beginning of what is now called "personalized" medicine—yet at that time without fundamental understanding of the complexity of mutational events. The identification of imatinib as active agent against chronic myelogenous leukemia provided a milestone in the new era of drug development and has inspired an intensive search for more drugable targets and subsequent drug development. Despite the tremendous progress in the early development of mechanism-based drugs, the clinical methodology has been largely unchanged and is divided into three phases based on different endpoints (Phase I, Phase II, and Phase III). The increasing understanding of how to best develop mechanism-based agents is in the process of mending some of the clinical development phases with new Phase I designs based on Bayesian approaches becoming more popular. Mechanism-based drugs also have toxicities that may differ from those caused by traditional chemotherapy, and this needs to be considered. Their use would also only make sense if the tumor expresses the targeted molecular abnormality. Given the biologic drift a tumor may undergo

during initial treatment, repetitive biopsies may become mandatory for treatment decisions/decisions to include a patient into a specific trial. As we are heading into this new and exciting era of anticancer therapy, new technologies like imaging techniques, proteinomics, and metabolomics will add to our understanding how it will be possible to develop more active and tolerable drugs.

Appendix

See Table A1 *FDA-approved anticancer agents, their primary mechanisms of action, and their indications* can be found on Vital Source version of this title, see inside front cover.

Appendix Table A1 should appear in online only not for print.

Key references

The complete reference list can be found on the Wiley Companion Digital Edition of this title (see inside front cover for login instructions).

4 Goodman LS, Wintrobe MM, Damashek W, Goodman MJ, Gilman A. Nitrogen Mustard Therapy – Use of methyl-bis (β-chlorethyl)amine hydrochloride and tris (β-chloroethyl)amine hydrochloride for Hodgkin's disease, lymphosarcoma, leukemia and certain allied and miscellaneous disorders. *JAMA.* 1946;**132**:126–132.

6 Farber S, Diamond LK, Mercer RD, Sylvester RF Jr, Wolff JA. Temporary remissions in acute leukemia in children produced by folic acid antagonist 4-aminopteroyl-glutamaic acid (aminopterin). *N Engl J Med.* 1948;**238**:787–793.

15 Elion GB, Hitchings GH, Vanderwerff H. Antagonists of nucleic acid derivatives. VI. Purines. *J Biol Chem.* 1951;**192**:505–518.

16 Elion GB. Nobel Lecture. The purine path to chemotherapy. *Biosci Rep.* 1989;**9**:509–529.

19 Staquet MJ, Byar DP, Green SB, Rozencweig M. Clinical predictivity of transplantable tumor systems in the selection of new drugs for solid tumors: rationale for a three-stage strategy. *Cancer Treat Rep.* 1983;**67**:753–765.

23 Grever MR, Schepartz SA, Chabner BA. The National Cancer Institute: cancer drug discovery and development program. *Semin Oncol.* 1992;**19**:622–638.

37 Seol HS, Kang H, Lee SI, et al. Development and characterization of a colon PDX model that reproduces drug responsiveness and the mutation profiles of its original tumor. *Cancer Lett.* 2014;**345**:56–64.

38 Julien S, Merino-Trigo A, Lacroix L, et al. Characterization of a large panel of patient-derived tumor xenografts representing the clinical heterogeneity of human colorectal cancer. *Clin Cancer Res.* 2012;**18**:5314–5328.

43 Das TM, Pryer NK, Singh M. Mouse tumour models to guide drug development and identify resistance mechanisms. *J Pathol.* 2014;**232**:103–111.

45 Nowell PS, Hungerford DA. A minute chromosome in human granulocytic leukemia. *Science.* 1960;**132**:1497.

52 Druker BJ, Talpaz M, Resta DJ, et al. Efficacy and safety of a specific inhibitor of the BCR-ABL tyrosine kinase in chronic myeloid leukemia. *N Engl J Med.* 2001;**344**:1031–1037.

63 Hanahan D, Weinberg RA. The hallmarks of cancer. *Cell.* 2000;**100**:57–70.

65 Hanahan D, Weinberg RA. Hallmarks of cancer: the next generation. *Cell.* 2011;**144**:646–674.

74 Goel HL, Mercurio AM. VEGF targets the tumour cell. *Nat Rev Cancer.* 2013;**13**:871–882.

78 Hollebecque A, Postel-Vinay S, Verweij J, et al. Modifying phase I methodology to facilitate enrolment of molecularly selected patients. *Eur J Cancer.* 2013;**49**:1515–1520.

81 Hoos A, Eggermont AM, Janetzki S, et al. Improved endpoints for cancer immunotherapy trials. *J Natl Cancer Inst.* 2010;**102**:1388–1397.

82 Wolchok JD, Hoos A, O'Day S, et al. Guidelines for the evaluation of immune therapy activity in solid tumors: immune-related response criteria. *Clin Cancer Res.* 2009;**15**:7412–7420.

104 DeGeorge JJ, Ahn CH, Andrews PA, et al. Regulatory considerations for preclinical development of anticancer drugs. *Cancer Chemother Pharmacol.* 1998;**41**:173–185.

116 Eisenhauer EA, O'Dwyer PJ, Christian M, Humphrey JS. Phase I clinical trial design in cancer drug development. *J Clin Oncol.* 2000;**18**:684–692.

118 Von Hoff DD, Kuhn J, Clark GM. Design and conduct of Phase I trials. In: Staquet M, Sylvester R, Buyse M, eds. *EORTC.* Oxford: Oxford University Press; 1984:210–220.

121 Deenen MJ, Cats A, Beijnen JH, Schellens JH. Part 2: pharmacogenetic variability in drug transport and phase I anticancer drug metabolism. *Oncologist*. 2011;**16**:820–834.

130 O'Quigley J, Pepe M, Fisher L. Continual reassessment method: a practical design for Phase I clinical trials in cancer. *Biometrics*. 1990;**46**:33–48.

132 Faries D. Practical modifications of the continual reassessment method for phase I cancer clinical trials. *J Biopharm Stat*. 1994;**4**:147–164.

136 Ratain MJ, Mick R, Schilsky RL, Siegler M. Statistical and ethical issues in the design and conduct of Phase I and II clinical trials of new anticancer agents [see comments]. *J Natl Cancer Inst*. 1993;**85**:1637–1643.

139 Rogatko A, Schoeneck D, Jonas W, Tighiouart M, Khuri FR, Porter A. Translation of innovative designs into phase I trials. *J Clin Oncol*. 2007;**25**:4982–4986.

143 Piantadosi S, Fisher JD, Grossman S. Practical implementation of a modified continual reassessment method for dose-finding trials. *Cancer Chemother Pharmacol*. 1998;**41**:429–436.

148 Postel-Vinay S, Gomez-Roca C, Molife LR, et al. Phase I trials of molecularly targeted agents: should we pay more attention to late toxicities? *J Clin Oncol*. 2011;**29**:1728–1735.

149 Postel-Vinay S, Collette L, Paoletti X, et al. Towards new methods for the determination of dose limiting toxicities and the assessment of the recommended dose for further studies of molecularly targeted agents – Dose-Limiting Toxicity and Toxicity Assessment Recommendation Group for Early Trials of Targeted therapies, an European Organisation for Research and Treatment of Cancer-led study. *Eur J Cancer*. 2014;**50**:2040–2049.

150 Paoletti X, Le TC, Verweij J, et al. Defining dose-limiting toxicity for phase 1 trials of molecularly targeted agents: results of a DLT-TARGETT international survey. *Eur J Cancer*. 2014;**50**:2050–2056.

151 Liu S, Yin G, Yuan Y. Bayesian data augmentation dose finding with continual reassessment method and delayed toxicity. *Ann Appl Stat*. 2013;**7**:1837–2457.

153 Tighiouart M, Liu Y, Rogatko A. Escalation with overdose control using time to toxicity for cancer phase I clinical trials. *PLoS One*. 2014;**9**:e93070.

160 Hyman DM, Eaton AA, Gounder MM, et al. Nomogram to predict cycle-one serious drug-related toxicity in phase I oncology trials. *J Clin Oncol*. 2014;**32**:519–526.

168 Darrow JJ, Avorn J, Kesselheim AS. New FDA breakthrough-drug category – implications for patients. *N Engl J Med*. 2014;**371**:89–90.

169 Darrow JJ, Avorn J, Kesselheim AS. New FDA breakthrough-drug category – implications for patients. *N Engl J Med*. 2014;**370**:1252–1258.

173 Yap TA, Omlin A, de Bono JS. Development of therapeutic combinations targeting major cancer signaling pathways. *J Clin Oncol*. 2013;**31**:1592–1605.

176 Hu-Lieskovan S, Robert L, Homet MB, Ribas A. Combining targeted therapy with immunotherapy in BRAF-mutant melanoma: promise and challenges. *J Clin Oncol*. 2014;**32**:2248–2254.

177 Paller CJ, Bradbury PA, Ivy SP, et al. Design of Phase I combination trials: recommendations of the Clinical Trial Design Task Force of the NCI Investigational Drug Steering Committee. *Clin Cancer Res*. 2014;**20**:4210–4217.

178 Von Hoff DD, Turner J. Response rates, duration of response, and dose response effects in phase I studies of antineoplastics. *Invest New Drugs*. 1991;**9**:115–122.

181 Jones RL, Olmos D, Thway K, et al. Clinical benefit of early phase clinical trial participation for advanced sarcoma patients. *Cancer Chemother Pharmacol*. 2011;**68**:423–429.

184 Thödtmann R, Depenbrock H, Dumez H, et al. Clinical and pharmacokinetic Phase I study of Multitargeted antifolate (LY231514) in combination with cisplatin. *J Clin Oncol*. 1999;**17**:3009–3016.

53 Tumor growth kinetics

Elizabeth Comen, MD ■ *Teresa A. Gilewski, MD* ■ *Larry Norton, MD*

Overview

Kinetics is the study of movement and changes in magnitude over time. Kinetics is a central concept in oncology; cancer progression reflects changes in cancer cell numbers, metastatic sites, and tumor mass as a function of time. It is the purpose of this chapter to illustrate both the practical applications and theoretical implications of one aspect of kinetics—tumor growth kinetics. Just as time and space are inextricably linked so too are growth kinetics and the tumor's microenvironment. Here we review the kinetics of cellular proliferation and population growth, finding a theoretical basis for improved practices in cancer chemotherapy.

Introduction

Kinetics is the study of movement or, more generally, changes in magnitude—size, shape, distance, velocity, or indeed anything quantifiable—over time. As a science, therefore, kinetics should be considered central to oncology. Cancer is, after all, all about changes in cancer cell numbers, sites of involvement, and tumor mass sizes as a function of time. Morbidity and mortality from cancer is a consequence of such changes, as measured by recurrence-free, progression-free, and overall survival (OS) times. Moreover, at the molecular level, cancer is not a static process, but involves aberrations in gene integrity, copy number and expression, post-translational modification, and RNA and protein production and degradation that are time dependent. Failure to analyze and interpret cancer biology with regard to changes over time, therefore, may miss the essences of phenomena and thereby lead to misinterpretations, both conceptual and clinical.

The purpose of this chapter is to use recent results in cancer research to illustrate both the practical applications and theoretical implications of one aspect of kinetics—tumor growth kinetics, the study of changes in cell number and over time tumor mass—for cancer medicine. In evaluating carcinogenesis within a time-dependent fashion, it is critical to understand the relevance of the space in which cancer cells change over time. Specifically, cancer–stromal interactions uniquely influence cancer growth. Just as time and space are inextricably linked so are growth kinetics and the tumor's microenvironment. Here, we offer novel insights into how a multitude of cancer processes are best understood by evaluating not simply a kinetic framework but also how the stroma mediates cancer growth.

Some mysteries in cancer medicine

The study of cancer reveals many enigmas, sets of observations that are both true and seemingly incompatible. Identifying enigmas thereby indicates weakness in theories, creating opportunities for progress by hypothesis-testing experimentation. We will examine some of these and then seek their elucidation using kinetic science.

Polygenetic etiology of cancer

As our first example, let us consider the observation that cancer cells manifest myriad changes in gene morphology and copy numbers. This is consistent with the theory that malignancy results from accumulated abnormalities in diverse, somewhat independent genomic processes, the *polygenetic* concept of cancer. The functionalities associated with such changes include self-sufficiency in growth signals, insensitivity to antigrowth and pro-apoptotic signals, and the abilities to invade, to form metastases, to induce angiogenesis, and to replicate without limit. Yet how is this theory compatible with the equally well-documented observation that carcinomas *in situ*, which are clinically benign in that they do not metastasize and rarely grow to large sizes, are usually as aberrant genetically as the malignancies they spawn?

The concept of a polygenetic etiology of malignancy presents another mystery, which concerns the strong statistical association of histologic grade, tumor size, and propensity for traveling to regional (largely nodal) and distant sites. These traits are so commonly grouped together that we may forget that they are manifestations of distinct biologic processes: morphogenesis, regulation of mitosis apoptosis, and metastasis, respectively. Indeed, metastatic behavior presents many thought-provoking enigmas. Toward the end of the nineteenth century, Halsted used the prevailing mechanics of his time to hypothesize that the malignant spread of primary breast cancer could be halted by the meticulous removal of a whole breast containing the tumor in contiguity with the ipsilateral axillary contents. The idea behind the radical mastectomy was that cancer cells gain access to the rest of the body by invading lymphatic channels in the breast, channels that then traverse the axilla before connecting with the systemic circulation.

Many observations would seem to support Halsted's contention. Radical mastectomies did indeed cure some individuals, almost all of whom would have died of metastatic cancer had their breast cancers been left intact—a fact proven by observational studies in the nineteenth century. Also, lymphatic invasion is a powerful prognostic variable. Most compelling is the modern observation that sentinel lymph node mapping confirms a common flow pattern from the breast for lymph and cancer cells. Yet how would one invoke Halsted's theory to explain how some patients with uninvolved axillary lymph nodes at the time of radical local surgery still develop distant metastases?

Molecular classification versus cancer stem cell concept

Another enigma concerns the classification of tumors by RNA expression profiling. It is unquestionably true that tumors differ in

Holland-Frei Cancer Medicine, Ninth Edition. Edited by Robert C. Bast Jr., Carlo M. Croce, William N. Hait, Waun Ki Hong, Donald W. Kufe, Martine Piccart-Gebhart, Raphael E. Pollock, Ralph R. Weichselbaum, Hongyang Wang, and James F. Holland.
© 2017 John Wiley & Sons, Inc. ISBN: 978-1-118-93469-2

their patterns of gene expression, and that these differences correlate with clinically meaningful endpoints such as disease-free and OS and benefit from chemotherapy.[1] Hence, testing a small anatomic sample of a cancerous mass is informative regarding the behavior of the whole cancer, as if all of the cells in the cancer carry the critical information. Yet how can we reconcile this observation with the popular, experimentally derived hypothesis that it is only a tiny minority of cancer cells—"cancer stem cells" or tumor-initiating cells—within the mass that have the capacity to form new tumors?

Cancer as a local versus systemic disease

It is well known that breast cancer is often a systemic disease early in its life-history; this is underscored by the fact that systemic adjuvant therapies like hormonal treatments and chemotherapy improve cancer-free and OS. But how is this compatible with the equally venerable observation that better local control, as by radiation therapy to the remaining breast tissue following breast-conserving surgery, improves survival? Indeed, it seems that for every four cases of local recurrence prevented by radiation therapy, one patient is saved from distant metastases and subsequent death. If the disease is metastatic early, why should local control make any difference at all? Part of the answer may be found in the observation that on detailed histopathological analysis, breast cancer cells are commonly found centimeters away from the clear margins of excised primary tumors. But this raises new questions. How did these cells get there, and what is the relationship between such cells and distant metastases?

Gompertzian growth

Another enigma concerns growth patterns. It has been shown that the growth pattern of breast cancer cannot be explained by simple exponential or linear kinetics, but must follow an S-shaped curve intermediate between these two extremes (Figure 1).[2] The evidence is not only from direct clinical observations but also from logical inferences based on clinical observations. For example, based on retrospective analyses of preexisting mammograms after the clinical diagnosis of breast cancer, it has been estimated that an average tumor may take 2 years to grow in size from one cell to 10^9 or 10^{10} cells. This number of cells corresponds to a tumor volume of $1-10\,cm^3$ if all of the cells were packed tightly together, which for the sake of this argument is a rational size range for the diagnosis of a primary mass.

Now let us consider what would happen should cancers grow in a linear pattern. This means that growth would be from one cell to two cells, then three cells, the four cells, and so on in equal units of time. By this pattern, if it took a tumor 2 years to grow from one cell to this size range (10^9 or 10^{10} cells), it would take another 2 years for it to double in size to $2-20\,cm^3$ and yet another 2 years to triple in size to $3-30\,cm^3$. This is clearly an unrealistically slow growth for an untreated primary cancer. Hence, it is extremely unlikely that cancers grow linearly.

Nor is exponential kinetics applicable to real-life examples. An exponential growth pattern involves constant doubling times. That is, if it takes a week for one cell to divide into two cells, by exponential kinetics, it would take another week for those two cells to become four, an additional week for those four to divide into eight, and so on. Many decades ago, Howard Skipper and colleagues used exponential kinetics to explain the growth and response to therapy of a murine leukemia, laying the groundwork for much of the experimental and clinical chemotherapy to follow. But does exponential kinetics apply to human disease? Let us turn again to the case of a primary breast cancer growing from one cell to 10^9 or 10^{10} cells over 2 years. Were it to have grown exponentially to this point and continue to grow exponentially thereafter the mass would double in size every $22-24$ days, which means that it would reach a size of $4-40\,cm^3$ in <7 weeks from diagnosis. This is an explosive growth rate that is just incompatible with general medical experience. Hence, exponential kinetics cannot apply. Yet, mitosis does produce two cells from one, so early malignant growth at the few-cell stage must be approximately exponential. This is truly an enigma.

The only way to resolve this mystery is to hypothesize that although growth may start in an exponential fashion, there is a progressive deviation toward slower growth as the tumor becomes larger. Of the infinite number of possible decremented exponential curves, one type has been shown to accurately fit actual tumor growth curves.[3] This type was defined by Benjamin Gompertz in 1825 and has since been one of the most utilized mathematical formulas in all of biomathematics. It is illustrated in Figure 1 on two different scales of size: arithmetic and logarithmic. The "S" shape is apparent on the arithmetic scale, but on the logarithmic scales, the relative growth rate is seen to be continuously decreasing as the mass grows larger. As will be discussed in depth later, Gompertzian kinetics have proven very useful in designing improved regimens of anticancer chemotherapy, not only in breast cancer—where it was first explored—but also in malignant lymphoma, childhood sarcoma, and other malignant diseases. But if Gompertzian growth kinetics is ubiquitous in nature, what is its (necessarily ubiquitous) etiology?

In this chapter, we will explore these issues—carcinogenesis, the behavior of tumor-initiating cells, pathohistologic grading, and patterns of metastatic spread—using the framework provided by

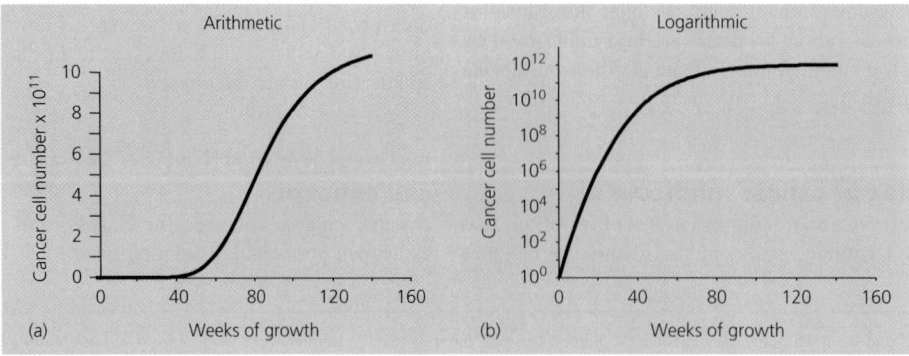

Figure 1 (a,b) Gompertzian growth on two scales.

the science of kinetics. We will examine the fundamentals of cell proliferation as a cause of tumor growth and the development of cellular heterogeneity. We will seek in modem molecular science an etiology of Gompertzian growth. We will also illustrate the clinical relevance of growth kinetics in practical cancer medicine with a focus on the therapeutic implications of Gompertzian growth on the dose scheduling of anticancer drugs. We will identify new areas for kinetic research that have implications for prognostication, choice of therapies, the discovery of new therapeutic targets, and the design of prevention strategies.

The kinetics of cellular proliferation

The study of how cancer cells divide provides some insight into these enigmas, but presents mysteries of its own, the contemplation of which may provide further illumination. As tumors are comprised of cancer cells with their supporting stroma, it is reasonable to start a discussion of tumor kinetics by considering the proliferative kinetics of cancer cells.

Assessing growth parameters

Mitosis, or cell division, is the basic biologic process that results in an increase in somatic cell numbers over time. The term *growth* applies to the increasing volume of a cellular population and is measured in units of volume (cubic centimeters) or weight (milligrams). Growth is largely the consequence of increasing numbers of cells but also can be influenced by the increasing size of the individual cells, edema, and changes in the context of the extracellular matrix, hemorrhage, and infiltration by host cells, such as leukocytes. The term *proliferation*, in contrast, applies specifically to an increase in the number of cells, which is measured as cell number as a function of time. Cells divide by progressing through a sequence of steps that are collectively called the mitotic or "cell" cycle.

It is important for the student of cell kinetics to understand the methods for assessing cell cycle phases because—as in all areas of science—concepts are inextricably confounded with their means of quantification.[4] At the simplest level, metaphase cells may be counted on a microscope slide. This *mitotic index* is a rough estimate of the percent of cells in M phase. Experimentally, the mitotic index can be improved by a now seldom used method called the stathmokinetic technique, in which a mitotic poison is applied at a known time before counting. The proliferative activity of a tissue may also be estimated by examining microscopic slides after immunohistologic staining for the Ki-67 protein, present in all proliferating cells and absent in nonproliferating cells. Although Ki-67 staining is now mostly used, historically the most productive technique is the thymidine labeling index (TLI). Here, viable cells are exposed briefly *in vitro* to a radiolabeled precursor of DNA. The most common thymidine label is tritium, but carbon 14 has also been used. The percentage of tumor cells with autoradiographic grains over their nuclei estimates the fraction of cells that were in S phase during the period of thymidine exposure.

Except for the stathmokinetic technique, all of the above are static assays, providing a snapshot rather than a movie of proliferation.[5] Nevertheless, the snapshot is of a concept called the *growth fraction*, the proportion of the cancerous mass that is actually involved in proliferation. Previously, the growth fraction of human leukemias was assessed by the use of the TLI *in vivo*, now no longer permissible.

A kinetic extension of the TLI is the percentage of labeled mitoses curve. This technique counts, as a function of time after exposure, the number of M phases that contain radioactive label.

This measures the cells currently in M phase that had been in S phase during the exposure to radioisotope. Hence, it is the only technique that actually measures cell cycle durations. Kinetic autoradiographic techniques of this type were used decades ago to divide the cell cycle into four phases: the synthesis of DNA occurs mostly in the S phase and the actual division of the parent cell into two daughters during the M phase; the time gap between cell division and DNA synthesis is gap number 1, or G1, and the time gap between DNA synthesis and cell division is gap number 2, or G2. Although the term *mitosis* is often used to refer to the M phase, the adjective *mitotic* properly refers to all cells that are engaged in any portion of the whole process of self-replication: G1, S, G2, and M phases. This distinguishes mitotic cells from cells that do not divide within a defined period of observation, called G0 cells. The M phase is the least variable in length, lasting about 1 h in most mammalian cells. The G2 phase is usually 3 h in length. The total duration of the cell cycle varies considerably, but the average in human cancer is between 2 and 4 days. Most of this variability is accounted for my variability in the length of the G1 phase. The long mitotic cycle in adult humans is in marked contrast with the cell cycle duration in *Drosophila*, which may take minutes, or with that of mammalian embryos, which may take only hours.

In G1 phase, a normal mammalian somatic cell contains a diploid number of chromosomes and hence diploid (2N) DNA content. During the S phase, a cell's DNA content should increase from 2N to 4N. (A very small number of so-called S0 cells may stop synthesizing DNA before completing the S phase, and rarely a cell can rest in the G2 phase and not proceed into M phase.) G0 cells tend to be smaller than G1 phase cells and have lower RNA and protein conten ts. The variations in cellular DNA content during the proliferative cycle can be exploited analytically by a collection of automated methods called *flow cytometry*. In fluorescence-activated cell sorting, a suspension of individual cells is automatically counted by being allocated into bins by DNA content, RNA content, cell size, antibody (such as Ki-67) label, uptake of bromodeoxyuridine and/or tritiated thymidine during the S phase, or combinations of such markers. This can be performed on fresh tissue—leukemias, tumor cells in effusions or ascites, enzymatically dispersed solid tumors—or on cells recovered from paraffin-embedded specimens. By measuring DNA content per cell, flow cytometry can also identify cells with abnormal amounts of DNA in the G0–G1 peak, termed *aneuploid*. The S-phase fraction may be impossible to measure in the presence of marked aneuploidy, one limitation of this method.

Growth fraction, death fraction, tumor size, and therapeutic response

Using the previous techniques, it has been determined that 2–20% of cells in a typical cancer are in the S phase at any point in time. Because the S phase occupies one-quarter to one-half of the cell cycle, the growth fraction is usually 4–80%, with an average of <20%. For a given tissue, malignant or benign, the length of the cell cycle *in vivo* is fairly constant in spite of variations in the number of cycling cells in that population. However, subtle changes in cycle kinetics have been seen in cancers in laboratory animals that are allowed to grow large and phase lengths can shift significantly as cells are cultured *in vitro*. This is in addition to changes in the growth fraction itself during tumor growth: one of the most robust, and mysterious, observations in tumor growth kinetics is that the growth fraction decreases with increasing tumor size. Is this the etiology or the consequence of Gompertzian growth? We will further discuss this later.

It is relevant in this regard that the rate of decrease in the growth fraction as the mass gets larger is slower for malignant than for benign tissues. But this is one of the few quantitative differences between malignant and benign tissues in cytokinetic terms. Some normal tissues, such as bone marrow and alimentary mucosa, have larger growth fractions and shorter mitotic cycle times than many cancers, even cancers of those tissues. This is the second major enigma presented by cytokinetic data. Although the growth fraction of a malignancy may be no greater than that of normal tissues from which it sprang, within a given histologic type of cancer, both a high S-phase fraction and the presence of aneuploidy are frequently associated with a growth rate that is relatively more rapid. This rapid growth suggests a malignant behavior that is relatively more aggressive, and often portends a poorer therapeutic response. These observations amplify rather than solve the enigma mentioned earlier of the association between histologic grade, tumor size, and metastatic behavior.

A partial answer may perhaps be found in the important companion concept to the concept of the growth fraction: the *death fraction* or *cell-loss fraction*. This is simply the proportion of the cellular mass that is lost by cell death per unit of time. The cell-loss fraction is hard to estimate from actual measurements since apoptosis—a common path of cell death—can leave few anatomic traces. It is usually inferred by comparing the expected growth rate (calculated from the measured growth fraction) with the actual growth rate. The impact of a high cell-loss fraction can be considerable. For example, basal cell epitheliomas of the skin grow slowly in spite of demonstrating a large number of metaphase figures. The importance of cell loss, however, goes beyond its impact on growth rate. Each mitotic cycle carries with it a finite probability of mutation. A tumor with a higher cell loss rate takes more mitotic cycles to double in size than a tumor with a lower cell loss rate. Thus, the rate of cell loss relates directly to the rate of mutations toward biologic properties of clinical importance.

Indeed, high rates of cell turnover are implicated in carcinogenesis itself. Elevated levels of thyroid-stimulating hormone predispose to thyroid cancer. Chronic thermal injury with compensatory hyperplasia and hyperplasia secondary to solar damage lead to skin cancer. Hyperproliferation of the bone marrow in dysmyelopoiesis and in chronic granulocytic leukemia is a likely contributor to the development of acute leukemia. Hyperproliferation of benign colonic and breast epithelium is clearly associated with neoplastic transformation. Indeed, chemical carcinogenesis requires a growth promoter. It is even possible—based on studies of Hodgkin's lymphoma and gastrointestinal cancer—that the hyperproliferation of residual cancer cells in compensation for cell death secondary to antineoplastic drug treatment may predispose to the development of drug resistance.

But the concept of the cell-loss fraction is not free of its own enigmas. Chemotherapy is thought to shrink cancers by damaging cancer cells and thus inducing them to undergo apoptosis. Mitotic cells, especially those in S phase, are thought to be especially vulnerable to this process, and indeed a great deal of experimental evidence supports this hypothesis. However, if the growth fraction of a typical tumor is <20%, meaning that the S phase fraction is 5–10%, and if the spontaneous cell-loss fraction is already greater than zero even in the absence of chemotherapy, how does chemotherapy increase the cell-loss fraction further so that cytoreductions of more than 90% are routine? Furthermore, attempts to increase chemotherapy effects by recruiting breast cancer cells into S phase by the use of estradiol have not yielded the expected large therapeutic benefits.

Another enigma concerns the effect of chemotherapy on normal host tissues. Chemotherapy is certainly toxic to rapidly dividing bone marrow, alimentary mucosa, and hair follicles. Yet, these tissues usually recover from the impact of chemotherapy. Some cancers, however, that are growing no more rapidly than these normal tissues may experience cytoreductions from which they never recover, that is, acute leukemias, malignant lymphomas, choriocarcinomas, and germ cell cancers may be cured by chemotherapy regimens that do not eradicate the patient's normal tissues that have comparable growth kinetics.

Hence, the study of cellular proliferation raises as many questions as answers. Why does the growth fraction decrease with population size, but less so in cancer than in normal tissues? How are the growth and cell-loss fractions related to histologic grade, tumor size, and metastatic potential? How does chemotherapy work given that so few cells, even in virulent cancers, are mitotic at the time of treatment? To approach an answer to these enigmas, we need to expand our focus from the kinetic behavior of cells to the kinetic behavior of cellular populations.

The kinetics of chemotherapy response

We have already critically examined tumor growth and have concluded that the Gompertzian curve or patterns of growth closely approximating Gompertzian curves are the only tenable ways to explain clinical observations. Nevertheless, some concepts derived from non-Gompertzian laboratory models are useful and merit discussion. Foremost in this regard is the body of work associated with Howard Skipper and colleagues at the Southern Research Institute.[6] The experimental leukemia they studied grows exponentially and regresses exponentially in response to effective treatment. This means that the percentage of cells killed is always the same regardless of the tumor size at the time of treatment. When graphed on a logarithmic scale of cell number versus an arithmetic scale of time, it would appear that the amount of cell death caused by the treatment is always the same in terms of logarithmic displacement: a log-kill of one means that 90% of the cells were killed, a log-kill of two means that 99% of the cells were killed, and so on. If a given dose of a given drug reduces 10^6 cells to 10^5 cells, the same therapy applied against 10^4 cells will result in 10^3 survivors.

The second seminal observation associated with these scientists is that for many drugs, the log-kill increases with increasing dose. Hence, it requires higher drug dosages to eradicate larger-sized transplanted tumors. Moreover, if two or more drugs are used, the log-kills are multiplicative: if drug A at a certain dose level causes a log-kill of one and drug B at a certain dose level also causes a log-kill of one, then the combination of A plus B, each given at the same dose levels as when they were used as single agents, would cause a log-kill of two.

The third observation recalled the Nobel Prize winning work of Max Delbrück and Salvador Luria concerning mutations toward resistance to destruction.[7] Although Delbrück and Luria worked on bacterial resistance to viral infection, Skipper and colleagues evaluated resistance to chemotherapy, based on Lloyd Law's demonstration of the applicability of the Delbrück–Luria model to this setting.[8] The concept is that genetic alterations for survival traits arise in the absence of selection pressure, rather than being in response to selection pressure. In fact, the concept is similar to Darwin's evolutionary theory of natural selection, but applied at the cellular rather than the organism level. A new way of stating this observation is as follows: if in one mitosis a bacterium or mammalian cell mutates toward a given property with small probability x, the probability of the unit not developing that property in one mitosis is $1 - x$. In y mitoses, the probability of no mutations occurring is $(1 - x)^y$. If each mitosis produces two viable cells (no cell loss), it takes $N - 1$ mitoses for one cell to grow into N cells. Hence, the probability of not finding any one unit with that property in N cells is $\exp[(N - 1)^* \ln(1 - x)]$, which is a very small number. Adding cell loss into the model, which increases the number of mitoses necessary to reach N cells, would make the probability of no mutations occurring even smaller. Hence, mutations toward drug resistance must be common in a clinical cancer, which has been shown in many experiments over many decades. The same mathematics would explain why aneuploidy, as a manifestation of genetic change, is so strongly associated with high cell turnover. It might also explain the positive association of primary tumor size with the probability of metastatic spread due to cells that mutated toward that property.

On the basis of this evolutionary model, some theoreticians suggested that when two equally active chemotherapy regimens were available, if they could not be given together at full dose levels, they should be strictly alternated so as to kill cells as quickly as possible before they had a chance to mutate toward drug resistance.[9] Others argued that mutations had more likely occurred before diagnosis, so it was more important to achieve as high cell-kill as possible in each of the subpopulations of cells already present at the time of diagnosis.[10-12] Although the former model argues that adjuvant treatment must be instituted as early as possible in the growth history of a cancer to be effective, many trials have failed to find an advantage to preoperative chemotherapy for primary breast cancer, which is more consistent with the latter model. Indeed, both points of view may be argued convincingly on theoretical grounds, but experimental evidence including large prospective clinical trials has strongly favored the latter. The latter model is also concordant with the observation that many cancers—malignant lymphomas, acute leukemias, and breast cancers specifically—that are not cured by chemotherapy often still retain sensitivity to the same chemotherapy when it is applied at a later time.[13] Hence, all chemotherapeutic failure cannot be attributed to permanent drug resistance, but rather the persistence of cells that were not eradicated. A tumor may relapse because some of its cells, relatively but not absolutely insensitive to the agents applied, are not exposed to enough drug for a long time to be eradicated.[14] This is analogous to a bacterial infection relapsing because an insufficient dose intensity of an antibiotic is applied, even though the microorganisms are sensitive *in vitro*. In both infection and neoplasia, however, prolonged or repeated episodes of low-dose therapy can give rise to absolute resistance by the selection of cells that are biochemically resistant to treatment.

Can manipulations of dose level or schedule overcome this problem? As mentioned earlier, the strict alternation of agents or combinations of agents has not proven useful in this regard. Dose level escalations of a moderate degree have improved results

in many common cancers including primary and metastatic breast cancer, childhood acute lymphoblastic leukemia, and adult germ cell tumors. Yet, results do not indicate a strictly rising dose–response relationship. For example, doses of cyclophosphamide over $600\,\mathrm{mg/m^2}$ do not improve results in the adjuvant chemotherapy of breast cancer, nor do doses of doxorubicin over $60\,\mathrm{mg/m^2}$. Neither has massive dose level escalation requiring autologous bone marrow rescue proven to be an advantageous strategy.

Yet, schedule alterations are feasible and have provided some improvement in results. The principles established by Skipper and colleagues in the exponentially growing murine leukemia have been translated into the Gompertzian setting.[15] The implications are illustrated in Figures 2 and 3, which are computer simulations of the mathematical model produced by this translation. In Figure 2a, a tumor comprised of cells sensitive to therapy is shown to be growing in a Gompertzian fashion. In response to each administration of treatment, indicated by the arrows, the tumor volume shrinks because of the induced log-kill and then regrows partially before the next administration for the first three cycles of treatment. After the fourth dose of chemotherapy, the cancer is left untreated, eventually reaching 10^{10} cells, a clinically appreciable number, at the time indicated (dashed line) and continuing to grow thereafter. Figure 2b illustrates what would happen if the same tumor were treated with the same four cycles of chemotherapy, but with a shorter intertreatment interval. As there is less time for the tumor to regrow between cycles, the cancer cell number is smaller for each successive treatment after the first. It has been determined empirically that for Gompertzian populations, the log-kill is proportional to the relative rate of growth at the time of treatment. Clearly, this may be because a greater percentage of the cells may be in S phase and hence vulnerable. Because—in Gompertzian growth—the relative rate of growth is more rapid for smaller populations compared with larger populations, the log-kill is greater for smaller populations as well. When, after the fourth dose of chemotherapy, the tumor grows in an unimpeded fashion, it is shown to take longer to reach 10^{10} cells (having started its regrowth at a smaller size), which translates to improved prognosis for the patient. Indeed, prospective, randomized clinical trials in primary breast cancer, then malignant lymphoma, then childhood Ewing's-family sarcoma have confirmed that the more frequent administration of chemotherapy improves OS time as predicted by this simulation.[16-19] The administration of CHOP chemotherapy for lymphoma each 14 days (as permitted by the use of granulocyte colony stimulating factor, G-CSF) rather than each 21 days, as was the old standard, is now widely used.[18]

Figure 3 extends this analysis to the case of a tumor that has developed heterogeneity in drug sensitivity before the time of initiation of therapy. This is illustrated by two growth curves, one black and one red, but the total tumor volume would be the sum of the

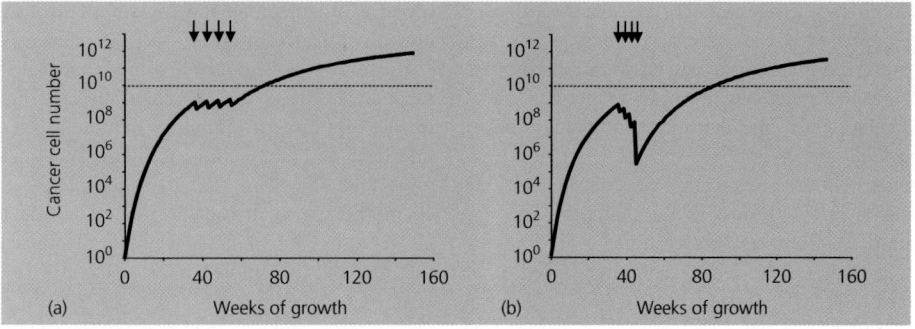

Figure 2 (a,b) Impact of dose density.

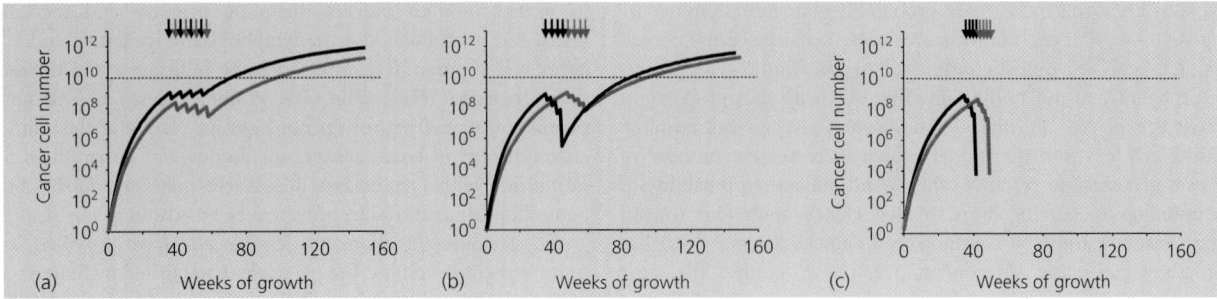

Figure 3 (a–c) Impact of sequential dose density.

two as the "black" cells and the "red" cells would be admixed in the tumor mass. The "black" cells are sensitive to the therapy symbolized by the black arrows, but are resistant to the therapy symbolized by the red arrows. In a parallel fashion, the "red" cells are sensitive to the therapy symbolized by the red arrows, but are resistant to the therapy symbolized by the black arrows. In Figure 3a, the black and red therapies are given in an alternating manner. In Figure 3b, the same therapies are given in sequence. It is clear that the log-kill from the sequential approach is greater in the "black" cancer cell population and not inferior in the "red" cells. Hence, the overall cytoreduction is greater—which results in a better prognosis for the patient—shown by increased time to 10^{10} cells. The reason for the greater log-kill is the increased density of the black treatment, as in Figure 2b. In the adjuvant chemotherapy of breast cancer, the first use of doxorubicin—now a standard drug in this setting—was in such a sequential fashion.[20] The advantages of this approach have been shown in a prospective, randomized adjuvant chemotherapy trial conducted by the National Cancer Institute in Milan, Italy.[21] The administration of four cycles of doxorubicin followed by eight cycles of the three-drug combination CMF (cyclophosphamide, methotrexate, and 5-fluorouracil) was superior in disease-free and OS to a regimen giving the same drugs for the same number of cycles but in an alternating fashion. Similarly, the Breast International Group (Study 02-98) has published that taxane added benefit to doxorubicin only when used sequentially, not when used simultaneously at somewhat reduced dose levels.[22] (Both arms were followed by identical courses of CMF, which does not impact the conclusion that sequential therapy was superior to combination therapy.)

Figure 3c takes this concept further by reducing the intertreatment time for both the black and red therapies. Here, the log-kill is much greater that regrowth may be precluded. This is the treatment plan tested in the breast cancer adjuvant setting by the North American Breast Intergroup in a trial (c9741) coordinated by the Cancer and Leukemia Group B. The use of G-CSF allowed for 14-day cycles of doxorubicin plus cyclophosphamide for four cycles followed sequentially by four 14-day cycles of paclitaxel. Compared with the same chemotherapy given each 21 days, the dose-denser regimen not only improved disease-free and OS, but was less toxic by virtue of preserved granulocyte counts and perhaps other effects.[16] More recently, in a systematic review and meta-analysis of 10 randomized controlled trials, dose-dense chemotherapy demonstrated improved overall and disease-free survival, particularly in hormone-receptor-negative breast cancers.[17] Specifically, in three of trials (3337 patients in total), dose-dense chemotherapy was compared to standard chemotherapy with similar chemotherapy agents. In these three studies, dose-dense chemotherapy led to an improved OS [hazard ratio (HR) of death = 0.84, 95% confidence interval (CI) = 0.72–0.98, P = 0.03] and as well as disease-free survival (HR of recurrence or death = 0.83, 95% CI = 0.73–0.94,

$P = 0.005$) when compared to alternative schedules. In seven other trials (8652 patients in total), dose-dense chemotherapy was compared to standard regimens with a variety of different chemotherapy agents and dosages. In this mixed group, dose-dense chemotherapy continued to demonstrate improved OS and disease-free survival (HR of death = 0.85, 95% CI = 0.75 to 0.96, P = 0.01 and HR of recurrence or death = 0.81, 95% CI = 0.73 to 0.88, P < 0.001, respectively).[17] Figure 4 compares HRs for patients who received dose-dense chemotherapy versus those who received conventional chemotherapy.[17]

The concepts illustrated in Figure 3b are relevant to modern combinations of chemotherapy with biological agents. The use of a prolonged, continuous treatment that inhibits cancer growth but does not interfere with the ability of Figure 5 simulates chemotherapy to kill cancer cells. In Figure 5a, the growth-inhibitory treatment (cross-hatched box) is started after the chemotherapy is completed. In Figure 5b, the treatment is given simultaneously with the red chemotherapy. It is clear that the plan in Figure 5b is superior in time-to-10^{10}-cells for two reasons. The first is that the "black" cells, which are not sensitive to the red therapy, are inhibited earlier in their regrowth. The second is that because the growth of the "red" cells is inhibited by the growth-inhibitory therapy, there is less regrowth between cycles of therapy, so fewer cells are present with each cycle after the first, meaning greater log-kill (as in Figure 3c). This may explain the efficacy of the HER2-modulating drug trastuzumab in adjuvant chemotherapy of HER2 over-expressing mode-positive primary breast cancer. In this trial (9831), coordinated for the North American Breast Intergroup by the North-Central Cancer Treatment Group, all patients received doxorubicin plus cyclophosphamide followed by weekly paclitaxel. The patients wh o received a year of continuous trastuzumab starting with the paclitaxel experienced fewer recurrences of breast cancer than those who started their trastuzumab after the paclitaxel was completed.[23] To build on these results, investigators at Memorial Sloan-Kettering Cancer Center have completed a phase II study proving the tolerability of a dose-dense chemotherapy regimen, following the concept in Figure 3c, with a year of trastuzumab starting simultaneously with the paclitaxel portion of the treatment.

However, it must not be assumed that growth-inhibitory therapy must always be given with chemotherapy. Figure 6 illustrates the impact of a growth-inhibitory treatment (cross-hatched box) that interferes with the action of chemotherapy. In Figure 6a, this is given after the chemotherapy is completed and because it has no chemotherapy to disrupt, it yields identical results to Figure 5a. However, in Figure 6b, it is seen that the impact of the treatment on the "red" cells is complex. Because the growth-inhibitory treatment is started earlier on the "red" cells than in Figure 5a, there is a greater effect. But also the impact of the chemotherapy, symbolized by the red arrows, is reduced, which is disadvantageous. The net

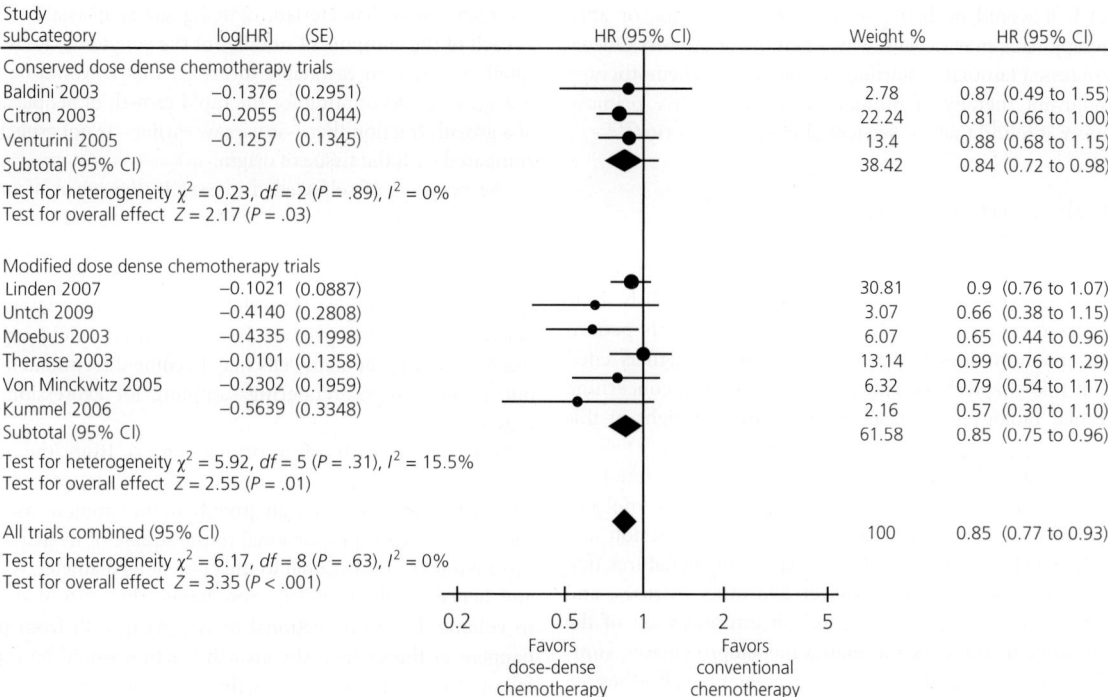

Figure 4 Forest plot of HR comparing OS in patients who received dose-dense versus conventional chemotherapy. Source: Bonilla et al. 2010.[17] Reproduced with permission from Oxford University Press.

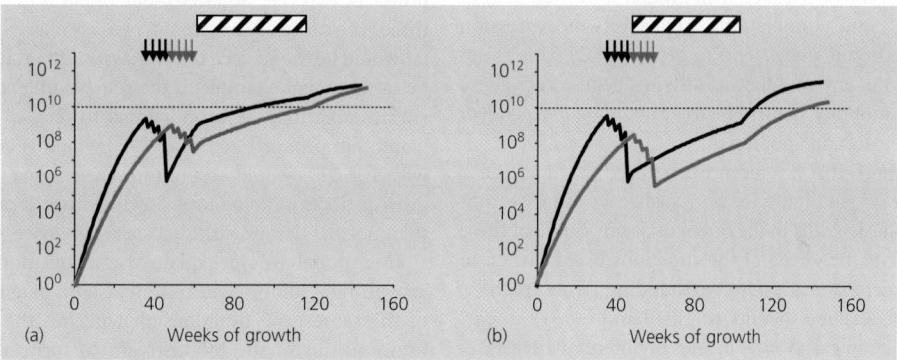

Figure 5 (a,b) Impact of growth-inhibitory therapy (that does not inhibit chemotherapy).

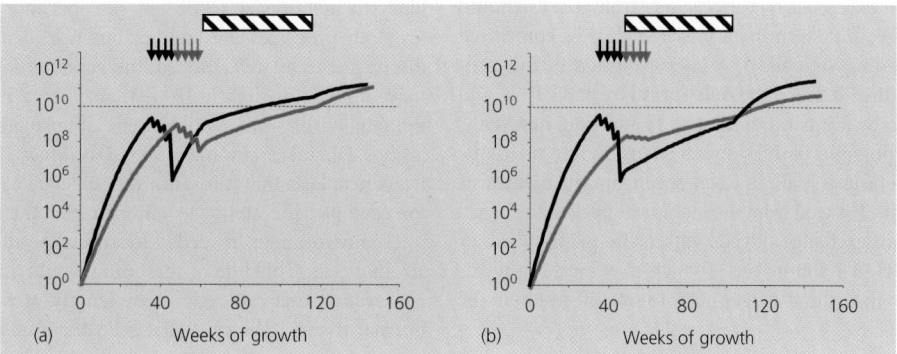

Figure 6 (a,b) Impact of growth-inhibitory therapy (that inhibits chemotherapy).

effect—as measured by the time to 10^{10} cells—is neutral in this simulation. Should the growth-inhibitory drug be better at slowing growth or less interfering with chemotherapy, the net effect would be beneficial to the patient as concerns the "red" cancer cells. But if the drug is less growth-inhibitory or more potent at interfering with

chemotherapy, then the net effect would not be beneficial. The other factor in this complex equation is the effect of earlier institution of the growth-inhibitory drug on the "black" cells. Hence, when one is dealing with a drug that might not only slow growth but also interfere with the action of chemotherapy, it would be difficult to predict if it would be better to use the drug during or after chemotherapy. This may explain why when the Southwest Oncology Group tested tamoxifen starting during or after chemotherapy for the adjuvant therapy of hormone-receptor positive primary breast cancer, it found that the sequential plan was superior.[24]

The etiology of Gompertzian growth

That malignant cellular populations follow Gompertzian growth curves and that such curves are useful in predicting or explaining therapeutic response to anticancer therapy are established by the examples previously. But what is the etiology of this pattern of growth and how does that relate to the other enigmas cited throughout this chapter? An emerging body of work concerning the molecular biology of metastases may provide insight in this regard.

One of the cardinal features of cancer cells is their abnormal mobility. This is manifested on both the phenotypic and molecular levels. Oncogenes often co-deregulate both cell adhesion and mitosis. There exist several sets of gene expression signatures that predict poor prognosis in breast cancer and other diseases, and many of the implicated gene products concern alteration of the microenvironment. These include matrix metalloproteinases, stimulators of angiogenesis, and molecules that influence cell adhesion, shape, and spatial orientation. Laboratory models of metastasis frequently involve genes of these functional classes. Indeed, a poor-prognosis signature in human breast cancer has been created that totally excludes genes associated with proliferation. Yet, in both the laboratory and clinic, tumors with high levels of expression of environment-modifying genes tend to grow rapidly. This raises the question: how do environment-modifying genes, and genes associated with cell mobility, contribute to growth rate *independent* of aberrations in mitosis and apoptosis?

A working hypothesis that has recently proposed this question is illustrated in Figure 7.[25] In Figure 7a, we visualize a primary tumor as a collection of cohesive cells in the organ of origin. Some of these cells have the capacity, by virtue of the functions listed earlier, to move, either by direct extension into surrounding tissue (path A) or into blood vessels in their vicinity (paths B and C). We understand that these cells can extravasate in sites of potential metastases (path B), but why cannot they also travel back to the primary site (path C), with preference for locations close to the primary mass where growth factors secreted by cancer and stromal cells should be in abundance? We may term path C *self-seeding* as contrasted with the distant seeding via path B. A later evolution of this process is shown in Figure 7b. Here, the cells spread by paths A, B, and C above have grown by mitosis into masses. In addition, new paths of seeding are now possible: path D, direct extension into the tissue surrounding the metastasis; path E, a self-seed from the metastasis to the metastasis; path F, a seed from the metastasis back to the organ of origin; path G, an exchange of cells within the primary tumor location; and path H, a systemic seed (which may locate in a distant site or return to the primary organ) from a satellite lesion in the primary organ.

Although data confirming the existence of these pathways are still accumulating, the implications regarding tumor growth kinetics are so compelling as to merit careful consideration. In Figure 7b, it is apparent that the tumor mass is not a discrete, organized entity but rather a collection or conglomerate of smaller masses. Each, being independent, may induce its own blood supply, perhaps by attraction of marrow-derived circulating endothelial cell precursors as well as cytokine-rich leukocytes. This would explain not only the abundance of vessels in many cancers but the architectural

disorganization characteristic of malignant anaplasia. Furthermore, as each of the component nodules of the conglomerate is relatively small, it is not unreasonable to expect that it would be relatively fast-growing, accounting for the rapid growth of neoplasia in spite of a growth fraction that—as we saw earlier—is not especially large compared with the tissue of origin.

The presence of self-seeded masses in the organ of origin (the progeny of path C in Figure 7a) that can then send seeds back into circulation (path H, Figure 7b) would explain why it is necessary to irradiate residual "normal" tissue in organs after the "clean" excision of primary lesions from those organs. The exchange of seeds between sites in the primary lesion (path G) would explain how tumor-initiating or stem cells may become disseminated throughout a tumor mass, rendering sampling for expression profiling practical.

Moreover, growth of a primary mass from the outside-in (self-seeding) as well as the inside-out (mitosis) provides a ready explanation for Gompertzian growth. In the simplest case, a sphere, the surface area is proportional to the square of its diameter while the volume is proportional to the cube of its diameter. As the mass and hence its diameter (d) grow larger, the ratio of surface area to volume drops proportional to $1/d$. As growth from outside-in happens at the surface, the growth fraction would be expected to fall proportional to $1/d$. That is, the relative growth rate would fall as the mass grew large, which is exactly what is seen in Gompertzian growth. Now cancerous masses are not perfect spheres, so the surface area would not be proportional to the diameter raised to a power of two (i.e., squared), but rather a power between two and three. The more aggressive the process of seeding, the more irregular would be the surface of the mass, and the closer the power would be to three. For example, if the self-seeding is very prominent, the surface area may be proportional to $d^{2.9}$, so the growth fraction would fall proportional to $d^{2.9}/d^3$, which is very slowly compared with $1/d$. This would account for the enigma, cited earlier, that the growth fraction falls more slowly with increasing population size than normal tissues with surface areas closer to a proportion of d^2.

This model would explain the association between anaplasia, growth rate, tumor size, and metastatic potential as follows: many of the same gene functions that permit the movement of a cell into and out of the bloodstream to form a self-seed should be involved in the formation of distant metastases. Hence, cancers that are more likely to involve regional lymph nodes are more likely to metastasize to distant sites because the genetic tool kits for both processes are similar, but not identical, accounting for discrepancies as well. Indeed, the genetic tool kit for preneoplasia may differ only slightly from that of invasive cancer, explaining the enigma of similar polygenetic abnormalities in both types of lesions. Ductal carcinoma *in situ* of the breast, for example, may be a frank neoplasia that is just not very efficient at self-seeding, lacking, for example, the ability to enter or exit the circulation, alter the microenvironment in seeded locations, or attract marrow-derived stromal cells. This line of reasoning would also explain the earlier observation that cell cycle phase lengths are similar in cancer and normal tissues. The cells that seed the component masses of the primary-site conglomerate may be quite normal except for the fact that they are abnormally re-located because of their abnormal mobility. In this regard, a primary breast cancer could be thought of as a contiguous collection of dozens to thousands of embryonic breasts, each within itself close to normal.

The growth by seeding depends to such a large degree on supporting stroma, including or particularly marrow-derived cells that contribute to angiogenesis and matrix formation, would seem to make cancers vulnerable to interventions that attack these

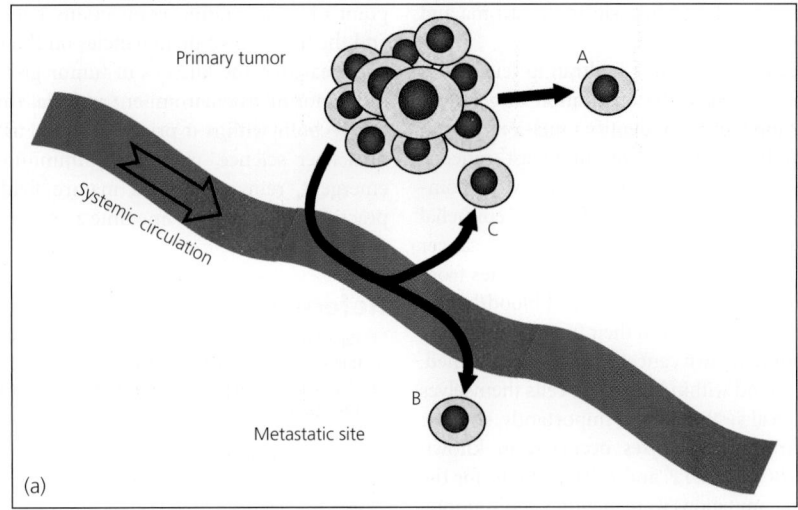

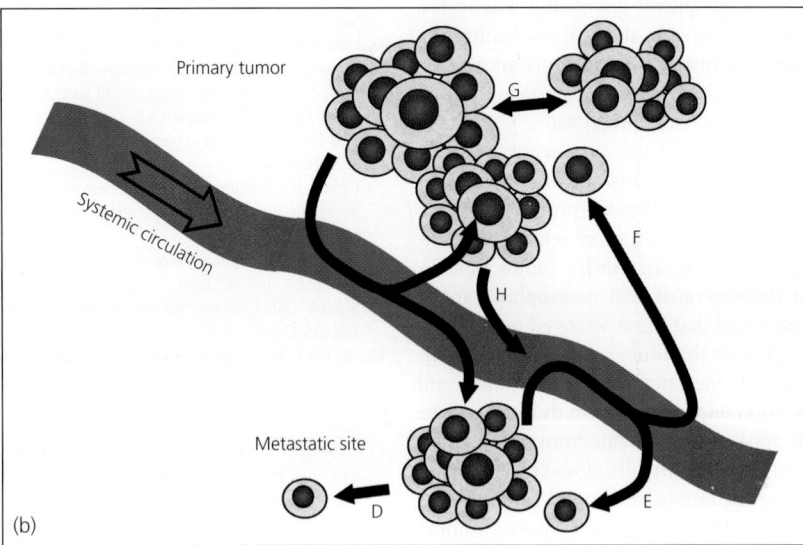

Figure 7 (a) Patterns of seeding—early. (b) Patterns of seeding—later.

component in addition to the cancer cells themselves. This might explain how chemotherapy—which has profound effects on bone marrow—can be so effective against tumor in which five or fewer percent of the cells are in S phase. How the self-seeding model relates to the very controversial but provocative concept of tumor dormancy and the impact of surgical debulking on such dormancy is a topic of active interest.[26]

The interrelationship of tumor self-seeding and tumor microenvironment

The self-seeding model, as described previously, depends not only on the inherent mobility of cancer cells, but equally on the noncancerous cells, which allow circulating tumor cells to migrate to and survive in distant sites. Ultimately, the tumor microenvironment or "soil" inextricably influences the capacity of cancer cells to grow and thrive. The tumor microenvironment is a complex mix of stromal cells, extracellular matrix, vasculature, and other supportive cells. Each of these factors may uniquely mediate tumor growth and metastasis. Most notably, the recognition that some of these noncancerous cells include the immune system has sparked increasing interest in developing immunotherapies for cancer patients.

Since the late nineteenth century, when Rudolf Virchow first recognized the presence of leukocytes within tumors, immunotherapy has remained largely an elusive strategy to treat cancer. More recently, burgeoning evidence across multiple solid tumors points toward a critical interplay between solid tumors and immune regulating cells. Experimental models suggest that the innate immune system is essential to primary tumor growth and routing metastasis, working in concert to either inhibit or promote growth, invasion, and spread.[27] Indeed, tumor-infiltrating lymphocytes, peritumor lymphoid structures, and their associated molecular signatures may have prognostic relevance. Three recent studies noted a potential relationship between levels of tumor-infiltrating lymphocytes and breast cancer prognosis.[28–30] It also appears that tumor-infiltrating stromal and immune cells may function quite differently than those in the circulation or in the noncancerous tissue.[31,32] For example, disseminated tumor cells found in the bone marrow of newly diagnosed breast cancer patients predict an overall poor prognosis, but not all of the patients with cancer cells found in their bone marrow will develop fulminant bone metastasis.[33] More recently, two unique studies suggest a novel role that leukocytes may play in mediating tumor growth and spread. These studies suggest that improving cancer outcomes will come from treating not only the cancer cells but key immune regulator both within the stroma and circulation.

First, the evolving evidence that tumor-infiltrating leukocytes may influence tumor behavior led to the application of genomic profiling techniques, commonly used to identify mutations within tumor cells, to tumor-infiltrating leukocytes in breast cancers. Mutations found in the tumor-infiltrating leukocytes were compared to the mutations found in circulating leukocytes, epithelial cells (buccal swab), as well as those found in the breast cancer cells themselves. In 20 patients, tumor-infiltrating leukocytes from breast cancer samples were matched to 20 peripheral blood/buccal swab samples. In 8 of the 20 patients, within their tumor-infiltrating lymphocytes only, mutations in known cancer genes were identified. These mutations were not found within the tumor cells themselves or the peripheral blood/buccal swab samples. Importantly, somatic mutations in tumor-infiltrating leukocytes occurred in known leukemia genes, including *BCOR*, *TET2*, and *EZH2*.[34] Thus, for the first time, somatic oncogenic mutations were identified only among tumor-infiltrating leukocytes in breast cancer samples and not in germline epithelial samples or peripheral circulating leukocytes. Notably, from a morphologic standpoint, these tumor-infiltrating leukocytes appeared entirely "normal." Investigations are underway to assess the functional role these mutated tumor-infiltrating leukocytes may have in tumor growth and progression.

Second, neutrophils, most often associated with their role against infections, appear to have a polarizing function in response to cancer. Specifically, neutrophils can act either in a protumorigenic[35] or in a antimetastatic[36] manner depending on relative concentrations of select cytokines. In murine mammary tumor models, for example, it has been demonstrated that neutrophils can be activated by a primary tumor and that these activated neutrophils can inhibit metastatic seeding to the lung.[36] In metastatic sites, varying cytokine levels appear to mediate neutrophil function, and in turn either growth inhibition or progression. In this respect, the tumor microenvironment appears to modulate immune function depending on the relative milieu. In newly diagnosed breast cancer patients with no evidence of metastasis, neutrophil function was explored. Women with newly diagnosed primary breast tumors who were undergoing either a lumpectomy or mastectomy had peripheral neutrophils purified from their circulation at the time of their surgery. These neutrophils were compared to neutrophils purified from the circulation of healthy volunteers with no evidence of cancer. *In vitro* assays demonstrated that the neutrophils from breast cancer patients were cytotoxic to select breast cancer cell lines as opposed to neutrophils obtained healthy women.[36] These experiments suggest that women with intact primary breast tumors activated neutrophils are capable of killing cancer cells in laboratory models. Neutrophils from women with no history of cancer did not share this capacity. Ongoing research will assess whether efforts to stimulate neutrophils in breast cancer patients will improve outcomes. Increasingly, research points to the impact of interactions between cancer cells and hematopoietic cells, both infiltrating and in the circulation, on cancer pathogenesis and therapeutic response. Modeling cancer growth patterns will undoubtedly need to incorporate the integral role of the tumor microenvironment in order improve clinical outcomes.

Conclusion

In this chapter, we have reviewed the kinetics of cellular proliferation and population growth, finding a theoretical basis for improved practices in cancer chemotherapy. Moreover, we have examined various clinical and laboratory-derived enigmas from a kinetic point of view, finding connections between molecular oncology and the behavior of malignancies on the macroscopic scale. Lastly, it is clear that the kinetics of tumor growth may be connected to the tumor microenvironment and that this microenvironment can evolve both within a primary tumor as well as metastatic sites. This later science, particularly immuno-oncology, is young but emergent, reinvigorating a mature field that has demonstrated practical worth at the same time as it promises future advances.

References

1 van't Veer LJ, Paik S, Hayes DF. Gene expression profiling of breast cancer: a new tumor marker. *J Clin Oncol.* 2005;**8**:1631–1635.

2 Norton LA. Gompertzian model of human breast cancer growth. *Cancer Res.* 1988;**48**:7067.

3 Laird AK. Dynamics of growth in tumors and normal organisms. *Monogr Natl Cancer Inst.* 1969;**30**:15.

4 Steel GG. Autoradiographic analysis of the cell cycle. Howard and Pelc to the present day. *Int J Radiat Biol.* 1986;**49**:227.

5 Frei E III, Whang J, Scoggins RB, et al. The stathmokinetic effect of vincristine. *Cancer Res.* 1964;**18**–25.

6 Skipper HE, Schabel FM Jr, Wilcox WS. Experimental evaluation of potential anti-cancer agents XIII. On the criteria and kinetics associated with "curability" of experimental leukemia. *Cancer Chemother Rep.* 1964;**35**:1.

7 Luria SE, Delbruck M. Mutations of bacteria from virus sensitivity to virus resistance. *Genetics.* 1943;**28**:491.

8 Law LW. Origin of resistance of leukaemic cells to folic acid antagonists. *Nature.* 1952;**169**:628.

9 Goldie JH, Coldman AJ. A mathematic model for relating the drug sensitivity of tumors to their spontaneous mutation rate. *Cancer Treat Rep.* 1979;**63**:1727.

10 Shapiro DM, Fugmann RA. A role for chemotherapy as an adjunct to surgery. *Cancer Res.* 1957;**17**:1098.

11 Schabel FM. Concepts for the systemic treatment of micrometastases. *Cancer.* 1975;**35**:15.

12 Norton L. Implications of kinetic heterogeneity in clinical oncology. *Semin Oncol.* 1985;**12**:231.

13 DeVita VT. The relationship between tumor mass and resistance to treatment of cancer. *Cancer.* 1983;**51**:1209.

14 Holland JF. Clinical studies of unmaintained remissions in acute lymphocytic leukemia. In: *The Proliferation and Spread of Neoplastic Cells. 21st Annual Symposium on Fundamental Cancer Research 1967.* Baltimore, MD: Williams & Wilkins; **1968**:453–462.

15 Norton L, Simon R. Tumor size, sensitivity to therapy, and the design of treatment schedules. *Cancer Treat Rep.* 1977;**61**:1307.

16 Citron ML, Berry DA, Cirrincione C, et al. Randomized trial of dose-dense versus conventionally scheduled and sequential versus concurrent combination chemotherapy as postoperative adjuvant treatment of node-positive primary breast cancer: first report of Intergroup Trial C9741/Cancer and Leukemia Group B Trial 9741. *J Clin Oncol.* 2003;**21**:1431–1439.

17 Bonilla L, Ben-Aharon I, Vidal L, Gafter-Gvili A, Leibovici L, Stemmer SM. Dose-dense chemotherapy in nonmetastatic breast cancer: a systematic review and meta-analysis of randomized controlled trials. *J Natl Cancer Inst.* 2010;**102(24)**:1845–1854.

18 Held G, Schubert J, Reiser M, et al. Dose-intensified treatment of advanced-stage diffuse large B-cell lymphomas. *Semin Hematol.* 2006;**43(4)**:221–229.

19 Womer RB, West DC, Krailo MD, et al. Randomized comparison of every-two-week vs every-three-week chemotherapy in Ewing sarcoma family tumors. *J Clin Oncol.* 2008;**26(Suppl. 15)**:10504.

20 Perloff M, Norton L, Korzun AH, et al. Postsurgical adjuvant chemotherapy of stage II breast carcinoma with or without crossover to a non-cross-resistant regimen: a Cancer and Leukemia Group B study. *J Clin Oncol.* 1996;**14(5)**:1589–1598.

21 Bonadonna G, Zambetti M, Moliterni A, et al. Clinical relevance of different sequencing of doxorubicin and cyclophosphamide, methotrexate, and Fluorouracil in operable breast cancer. *J Clin Oncol.* 2004;**22(9)**:1614–1620.

22 Francis P, Crown J, Di Leo A, et al. Adjuvant chemotherapy with sequential or concurrent anthracycline and docetaxel: Breast International Group 02–98 randomized trial. *J Natl Cancer Inst.* 2008;**100(2)**:121–133.

23 Baselga J, Perez EA, Pienkowski T, Bell R. Adjuvant trastuzumab: a milestone in the treatment of HER2-positive early breast cancer. *Oncologist.* 2006;**11(Suppl. 1)**:4–12.

24 Albain KS, Green SJ, Ravdin PM, et al. Adjuvant chemohormonal therapy for primary breast cancer should be sequential instead of concurrent: initial results from Intergroup trial 0100 (SWOG-8814). *Proc Am Soc Clin Oncol.* 2002;**21**; abstr 143.

25 Norton L, Massagué J. Is cancer a disease of self-seeding? *Nat Med*. 2006;**12**: 875–878.

26 Demicheli R, Miceli R, Moliterni A, et al. Breast cancer recurrence dynamics following adjuvant CMF is consistent with tumor dormancy and mastectomy-driven acceleration of the metastatic process. *Ann Oncol*. 2005;**16**(**9**):1449–1457.

27 Grivennikov SI, Greten FR, Karin M. Immunity, inflammation, and cancer. *Cell*. 2010;**140**(**6**):883–99.

28 Mohammed ZM, et al. The relationship between lymphocyte subsets and clinico-pathological determinants of survival in patients with primary operable invasive ductal breast cancer. *Br J Cancer*. 2013;**109**(**6**):1676–84.

29 Loi S, et al. Prognostic and predictive value of tumor-infiltrating lymphocytes in a phase III randomized adjuvant breast cancer trial in node-positive breast cancer comparing the addition of docetaxel to doxorubicin with doxorubicin-based chemotherapy: BIG 02–98. *J Clin Oncol*. 2013;**31**(**7**):860–7.

30 Adams S, et al. Prognostic value of tumor-infiltrating lymphocytes in triple-negative breast cancers from two phase III randomized adjuvant breast cancer trials: ECOG 2197 and ECOG 1199. *J Clin Oncol*. 2014;**32**(**27**):2959–2966.

31 Orimo A, Weinberg RA. Stromal fibroblasts in cancer: a novel tumor-promoting cell type. *Cell Cycle*. 2006;**5**(**15**):1597–601.

32 Li HJ, et al. Cancer-stimulated mesenchymal stem cells create a carcinoma stem cell niche via prostaglandin E2 signaling. *Cancer Discov*. 2012;**2**(**9**):840–855.

33 Braun S, Vogl FD, Naume B, et al. A pooled analysis of bone marrow micrometastasis in breast cancer. *N Engl J Med*. 2005;**353**(**8**):793–802.

34 Comen E, Kleppe M, Wen H, et al. Somatic leukemogenic mutations associated with infiltrating white blood cells in breast cancer patients. San Antonio Breast Cancer Symposium. PD1-4; 2014.

35 Fridlender ZG, Sun J, Kim S, et al. Polarization of tumor-associated neutrophil phenotype by TGF-beta: "N1" versus "N2" TAN. *Cancer Cell*. 2009;**16**(**3**):183–194.

36 Granot Z, Henke E, Comen EA, et al. Tumor entrained neutrophils inhibit seeding in the premetastatic lung. *Cancer Cell*. 2011;**20**(**3**):300–314.

54 Principles of dose, schedule, and combination therapy

William N. Hait, MD, PhD ▪ *Joseph P. Eder, MD*

Overview

The discovery and development of oncology drugs are complex and associated with a high failure rate. For example, the chance of a new drug that enters clinical trial has an approximately ten percent chance of achieving regulatory approval and ultimately becoming available for patients. Determining the proper dose and schedule of a drug are arguably the two most important determinants of both safety and efficacy, the primary determinants of regulatory approval. Understanding how to best estimate the proper dose and schedule for the many types of therapeutic agents now widely available and in development is a critical skill for those in the drug discovery and development field. This area of expertise has been made more complex with the addition of biological agents such as monoclonal antibodies, alternative protein scaffolds, and vaccines to that of hormones and small molecule platforms. In this chapter, we review the basic principles that underlie the appropriate selection of dose and schedule with a major focus on cytotoxic chemotherapy. In addition, we discuss the many variables that can underlie the dose-response relationship including characteristics of the tumor, the tumor microenvironment, the host including enzymes of drug metabolism and mechanisms of drug clearance. Finally, we review the clinical trial designs that have been successfully used to properly select dose and schedule for oncology drugs.

Introduction

The identification of novel, clinically active agents has been central to progress in cancer chemotherapy. Table 1 presents examples of new agents and of cellular pathways and targets being explored for new therapeutic targets. Dose is a significant determinant of the antitumor activity and toxicology for the established, "classical" cytotoxic chemotherapeutic agents.[1] These agents are DNA damaging agents, directly or indirectly, or inhibitors of cell division, and a quantitative relationship between target interaction and cell lethality is unknown. High-dose chemotherapy (4–10 times the baseline dose), made possible by hematopoietic stem cell transplantation, has proved curative for selected hematologic neoplasms. The FDA is quite explicit in the centrality of the dose–response relationship of any agent for any purpose "Exposure-response information is at the heart of any determination of the safety and effectiveness of drugs. That is, a drug can be determined to be safe and effective only when the relationship of beneficial and adverse effects to a defined exposure is known."[2]

The effect of dose for biologically therapeutic agents such as the interferons, interleukins, monoclonal antibodies, hormones, and for molecularly targeted tyrosine kinase inhibitors is complicated, and there is not the same unequivocal evidence for a dose–response effect with these agents. Contemporary targeted agents have a much more specific relationship to the extent of target interaction, such as receptor occupancy (RO) for monoclonal antibodies or extent of phosphorylation inhibition for kinase inhibitors (proof of mechanism) and a measured pharmacodynamics effect (proof of principle), such as phosphorylation inhibition expected to correlate with clinical efficacy in the proper molecularly selected patient segment (proof of concept) than dose alone implies, although in clinical medicine this is the surrogate used.

The schedule of drug administration may be important to the therapeutic index independent of dose. Cytokinetic studies related to drug schedule have led to the improved use of agents such as cytosine arabinoside (cytarabine, ara-C) in both experimental and clinical leukemia (see the section titled "Cytokinetics of bone marrow").[3,4] Most of the molecularly targeted agents, whether small molecules or monoclonal antibodies, are dosed to provide a continuous effect, which markedly changes the clinical toxicity profile.

Combination chemotherapy has been crucial in the development of curative regimens for hematologic malignancies, pediatric solid tumors, testicular cancer, and ovarian cancer and for the adjuvant regimens for breast, lung, and bowel cancer, and for osteosarcomas.[5,6] The rationale for combination chemotherapy is discussed under the various topical headlines. The principal rationales include (1) the empiric: almost all therapy that has proven curative in the clinic involves the use of agents in combination (Table 2); (2) the fact that genetic instability results in tumor cell heterogeneity, which manifests as drug resistance in cancer therapy[6–8]; and (3) signal transduction inhibitors molecularly targeted to specific cancer driver mutations, with the possible exception of imatinib in some patients with chronic myelogenous leukemia (CML),[9] invariably induce resistance that can be circumvented by either combining a second agent (dabrafenib and trametinib in melanoma)[10] or using second-generation agent with a broader spectrum of targets specific for the mutations conferring resistance which develop (ceritinib in EML4/ALK mutant NSCLC)[11,12] to have significant therapeutic benefit. Although dose and combination chemotherapy are generally considered separately, they have an important and complex relationship.[13,14] There is an impressive increase in the number of putative molecular targets for cancer treatment in development (Table 1). A major clinical research challenge will be not only to maximize the effectiveness of individual agents but also to integrate drugs into optimal combination strategies.

Dose

In controlled experimental systems, such as established tumor cell lines in culture, the relationship between dose and tumor cytotoxicity may be close to linear-log (i.e., exponential).[15] For example, a linear increase in the dose of selected chemotherapeutic agents causes a log reduction of MCF7 human breast cancer cells in culture.[16] When the dose is expressed as multiples of the IC_{90}

Holland-Frei Cancer Medicine, Ninth Edition. Edited by Robert C. Bast Jr., Carlo M. Croce, William N. Hait, Waun Ki Hong, Donald W. Kufe, Martine Piccart-Gebhart, Raphael E. Pollock, Ralph R. Weichselbaum, Hongyang Wang, and James F. Holland.
© 2017 John Wiley & Sons, Inc. ISBN: 978-1-118-93469-2

Table 1 Molecular targets for cancer treatment.

The cell cycle
• Cyclin-dependent kinases, cyclins, cyclin-dependent kinase inhibitors, and mitotic tubule-associated proteins

Differentiation
• Retinoid and vitamin D nuclear steroid receptors

Apoptosis
• BCL2, NF-kB, TP53, TNFSF10, and FAS

Angiogenesis
• KDR, the endothelial integrins, and PDGFRB

Signaling cell surface receptors
• Insulin-like growth factor receptor (IGF), ERBB family of receptors, and KIT

Metastasis
• Matrix metalloproteinases and chemokine receptors

Intracellular signaling elements
• BCR-ABL1, ras, raf, MADD, PI3 kinase, m-TOR, src, protein kinase C, focal adhesion kinase (PTK2: protein tyrosine kinase 2), anaplastic lymphoma kinase (ALK), the STAT family of proteins, and the MAP family of protein kinases

Nuclear transcription factors
• For example, steroid hormone No. 4

Potential targets
• Telomerase
• DNA methylation (human DNA methyltransferase [MeTase]), proteasome 20S, farnesyltransferase, histone deacetylase, and hsp90 (chaperone protein)

Cell surface antigens
• For example, CD20

(i.e., the dose or concentration that reduces the number of tumor cells by 90%), a very good response in terms of tumor regression in a patient is obtained. The estimated total tumor burden for patients with clinically evident cancer is $5 \times 10^{11} \pm 10^{1}$ (11 ± 1 logs). Thus, a dose that produces a good partial remission (e.g., 50–90% tumor regression) produces at most a 1-log reduction, which is <10% of the "exponential iceberg." Numerous factors influence the dose effect. They are presented in the subsections that follow.[17,18]

Factors influencing the dose effect

Class of antineoplastic agent

The ideal therapeutic agent would maintain a linear relationship between dose and log tumor cell reduction (log-TCR) down through multiple logs of tumor cell death. Ionizing radiation comes closest to this ideal. As a group, alkylating agents maintained dose/log-TCR superior to the other chemotherapeutic agents. DNA damaging alkylating agents exhibit major activity during the S and M periods of the cell cycle, but unlike other chemotherapeutic agents, they maintain activity throughout the cell cycle. Although comparative studies demonstrate a dose effect in chemotherapy-sensitive tumors such as the leukemias

and lymphomas, the effect of dose is less evident in solid tumors, particularly those tumors of epithelial origin.[19,20] Purine- and pyrimidine-targeted antimetabolites are active mainly in proliferating cells, and therefore pharmacokinetic resistance occurs that is overcome less by increasing dose than by increasing the duration of exposure, allowing more cells to enter the proliferative compartment. This also applies to the DNA-damaging topoisomerase I and II directed agents and microtubule-interacting agents, where the target must be encountered in the setting of DNA synthesis or mitotic spindle assembly to produce antineoplastic cytotoxicity.[21,22]

Agents directed at hormone receptors, growth factor receptors and intracellular kinase signaling targets have a different relationship as once receptor/kinase interactions are saturated, further dose increases will produce no further effect.[23] Hence, these agents are analogous to antimetabolites in that dose escalation once saturation levels of drug are achieved produces no further benefit. Higher doses of imatinib in chronic phase or accelerated phase CML with a suboptimal response to standard dose can benefit a subgroup of patients, but the percentage is low and the duration of response brief.[24,25]

Tumor factors

Intrinsic tumor cell sensitivity

The more sensitive the tumor is to a given agent, the steeper the dose effect. Thus, if a unit dose produces a 0.5 log-TCR, then doubling that dose may produce up to a 1.0 log tumor cell kill—which clinically represents only a partial remission. In a chemotherapy-sensitive tumor, where a unit dose produces a 3 log-TCR, doubling the dose may produce up to a 6 log-TCR, depending on the degree of tumor cell heterogeneity and drug resistance (see the section titled "Drug resistance"). A 6 log-TCR would produce a major clinical achievement in terms of complete response, duration of complete response, and, most important, an approach to tumor cure or eradication. Thus, for patients with a metastatic common epithelial tumor, such as breast cancer, the most that can be achieved with standard single-agent chemotherapy is a partial response (<1 log-TCR) in about 30% of patients. Combinations result in higher partial response rates and a low (10–20%) complete response rate. Alternatively, combination chemotherapy regimens in patients with chemotherapy-sensitive tumors (e.g., non-Hodgkin's lymphoma, Hodgkin's disease, and germ cell tumors) may achieve multi-log-TCR as a result of combination chemotherapy.[26]

Tumor burden

Tumor burden is a consistent adverse prognostic factor for response to chemotherapy. This finding was first demonstrated for transplanted tumors in mice; in these animals, macroscopic (i.e., palpable) tumors often respond minimally to chemotherapy. The

Table 2 Number of agents and curative treatment for childhood acute lymphoblastic leukemia (ALL).

	Number of chemotherapeutic agents							
	1	2	3	4	5	6	7	8
Year	1948	1954	1956	1960	1965	1974	1985	1988
Agent	Methotrexate	MP	Prednisone	Vincristine	Methotrexate[a]	Adriamycin	Asparagine	ara-C
CR (%)	20–40	40–92	80–95	>95	>95	>95	>95	>95
Cure (%)	0	0	0	15	5–35	55	75	80

[a]Intrathecal methotrexate.
Abbreviations: CR, complete response; MP, 6-mercaptopurine.

same tumor, at a microscopic tumor burden size, may be much more responsive and potentially curable.[26,27]

These observations in mice are consistent with the parallel observation that adjuvant cancer treatment can be curative for patients with breast cancer but not for those with overt metastatic breast cancer. Postulates for the delay in growth of microscopic metastases include a balanced rate of cell loss (i.e., apoptosis) and cell production and inability to support tumor neovascularization (angiogenesis). Resistant microscopic tumor may persist in most long-term survivors, an observation that has major implications for therapeutic strategy (see the section titled "Cytokinetics of the tumor—The growth fraction").

The study of microscopic metastases in patients may become increasingly possible with molecular techniques for detection and characterization of minimal residual tumor.[26] The kinetics of microscopic disease can be inferred from adjuvant chemotherapy studies (see the section titled "Adjuvant chemotherapy").

Drug resistance

In the laboratory, drug resistance is usually produced by "selection pressure"—that is, by exposing target cells to progressively increasing concentrations of the selecting agent. Drug resistance is usually expressed as the concentration of drug that is required to produce 50% inhibition in a colony or growth assay (IC_{50}) for the resistant cell line, divided by the concentration required (IC_{50}) for the parent sensitive cell line. For a detailed presentation of drug resistance, see the section titled "Combination chemotherapy" and **Chapter 62**.

Cytokinetics of the tumor—The growth fraction

The growth fraction (GF) of the tumor and the dose of cell cycle-specific agents have a major effect on the log-TCR of tumor cells. The generation time of cycling (i.e., mitotically active) cells is much shorter than the volume doubling time.[28–32] Thus, many cells within tumors are dying or "noncycling"—that is, in G_0/G_1. The GF of a tumor is the ratio of the cycling cells to the total number of tumor cells.

For the common epithelial solid tumors, the GF is often <5%.[33,34] A solid tumor with a GF of 5% would be minimally responsive to cell cycle-specific agents and variably sensitive to other chemotherapeutic agents. Repetitive treatments, however, might "recruit" cells into cycle by allowing dormant, noncycling cells access to necessary growth conditions and thus enabling them to be more effective. Prolonged exposure to cell cycle-specific agents might be effective in low—GF tumors. In contrast, a high-GF tumor such as Burkitt's lymphoma might have a multilog response with the same treatment or even the same dose over a shorter period.[1] A recent challenge to the long-standing clonal evolution model of cancer evokes specific cancer progenitor cells (CPCs) as responsible for the continued proliferation of a tumor. By this model, self-renewing CPCs give rise to all progenitor and differentiated cells within a tumor but remain a small proportion of all tumor cells.[35] CPCs, as with normal tissue stem cells, are extremely resistant to chemotherapy and radiotherapy.[36] The difference between curative therapeutic regimens and those that are only palliative may be attributable to the relative sensitivities of CPCs and the progenitor and differentiated cancer cells incapable of self-renewal. Identification of therapeutic targets within the CPC population should offer significant opportunities for more effective therapies.

Tumor hypoxia

Hypoxia commonly occurs in both experimental and clinical solid tumors, a condition presumably resulting from inadequate angiogenesis and high metabolic activity (oxygen consumption). Oxygen distribution within tumors is heterogeneous and even a small fraction of hypoxic cells can profoundly affect chemotherapy responsiveness. The farther cells are from blood vessels, the lower the concentration of chemotherapeutic agents in those cells. Cellular proliferation decreases as a function of distance from blood vessels, with a significant fraction of nonproliferating cells conferring kinetic resistance to cell cycle-specific agents. Certain cancer chemotherapy agents require oxygen as an intermediate in toxicity or metabolism.[37] Finally, hypoxia produces altered gene expression. Hypoxia-inducible factor 1 (*HIF1*) stops proliferation and prevents apoptosis in the hypoxic fraction of cells by increasing angiogenesis. Hypoxia increases the production of hepatocytes growth factor (*HGF*) and its receptor *MET*, with a further increase in angiogenesis, and increased incidence of metastasis and drug resistance.[38,39] There may be increased expression of adenosine triphosphate-binding cassette (ABC) proteins such as p-glycoprotein (PgP) that may confer resistance to chemotherapeutic agents. Hypoxia also selects for *TP53* mutants with a reduced apoptotic response to DNA damage or cell cycle arrest targeted agents.[40] Exploiting hypoxia as a target in cancer therapy with bioreductive alkylating agents such as mitomycin C and the nitroimidazoles, which can serve as electron acceptors in lieu of oxygen, has been tried in numerous clinical circumstances with no or minimal benefit.[41,42] Impaired chemosensitivity is not universal, and in selected cell lines (i.e., renal), some drugs appear even less effective in normoxia than hypoxia.[43] Radiotherapy in particular requires molecular oxygen for cytotoxicity.[44]

Oncogene addiction-growth factor signaling

The maintenance of the transformed state results in significant metabolic and genetic stress on cancer cells. Maintaining viability under these conditions requires positive anti-apoptotic signaling factors and interfering with these survival pathways can result in tumor cell lethality. In particular, mutant oncogenes such as *BCR-ABL* in CML, or mutant growth factor receptors such as *EGFR* (*ERBB1*) in lung cancer, *BRAF* in melanoma, and *CKIT* in gastrointestinal stromal tumors (GIST) provide essential survival signals and interruption of these pathways produces significant clinical benefit in affected patient. The emergence of diagnostic molecular testing enables identification of patients and permits selection of appropriate therapy.

Host factors

Cytokinetics of bone marrow

Because of the bone marrow's proliferative activity and relative lack of DNA repair capacity, myelosuppression is dose limiting for many chemotherapeutic agents. Exploiting the cytokinetic difference between marrow and tumor has been a basis for the construction of selected clinical strategies.[4,28]

Normal marrow recovers within 1–2 weeks after cytarabine, with little cumulative myelosuppression. For many patients, recovery of acute myelogenous leukemia (AML) cells as compared with normal marrow cells between courses of cytarabine is incomplete. AML cells *in vitro* are less susceptible to growth factors such as G- and GM-CSF than are the cells of the normal marrow.[45] Thus, when marrow CSFs increase in homeostatic response to cytarabine-induced myelosuppression, the interval recovery of normal marrow may be more rapid than that demonstrated by the AML cells, a factor that should, with successive dosing, result in a cumulative effect—the therapeutic advantage.

Similar changes occur in other proliferative tissues, including the gastrointestinal tract, where drugs cause mitotic arrest with loss of epithelial surface cells, including cells involved in the adsorption of fluids. This requires a recovery period just as the marrow does.[46]

Pharmacokinetics
Pharmacokinetic factors commonly affect the dose–response curve. If an inactivating enzyme for the drug becomes saturated, both toxicity and antitumor effect may increase disproportionately, an effect observed with certain dose schedules of 5-fluorouracil (5-FU) for example.[47,48]

The opposite effect may occur if a drug activation system becomes saturated. Ifosfamide, a prodrug, is activated by the cytochrome P450, oxygen-dependent, drug-metabolizing enzymes in the liver to the biologically active 4-hydroxyl derivative. The 3-day conventional dose of ifosfamide is higher (1200 to 2400 mg/m^2 daily) than that for cyclophosphamide (600 mg/m^2) because the rate of P450 activation of ifosfamide is relatively slow. With increasing doses of cyclophosphamide, a constant fractional conversion to active 4-hydroxyl cyclophosphamide occurs. However, for ifosfamide, once the P450 enzyme system becomes saturated, a decreasing proportion of ifosfamide is converted into the active form, with a consequent loss of antitumor effect at higher doses.[37]

Clinical trials and the dose effect

Dose selection in patients
Clearance determines the total drug exposure (area under the curve of concentration multiplied by time [AUC]), and AUC in mice correlates with toxicity in that species. This relationship of AUC with drug exposure and toxicity also holds true in humans and can be predicted from mouse data.[49] The process for initial dose selection in phase I clinical trials is detailed in **Chapter 44**. In most circumstances, the dose is determined in phase I trials and in other situations is individualized to the body surface area (BSA), weight or exposure (AUC) of the patient.

The Dubois BSA formula is useful in allometric scaling of drug-dose selection between species. The expectation was that similar adjustments would reduce the variability in clearance between patients and is often used in determining the initial dose in first time in human (FTIH) trials. BSA may be helpful in selecting the dose of cytotoxic agents in childhood leukemia and was subsequently incorporated into standard usage.[50,51] Recent reviews of the literature and individual institutional experience can find no significant correlation between BSA and clearance variability with investigational or commonly used anticancer drugs except for paclitaxel, oral busulfan, and possibly temozolomide.[52,53]

BSA may correlate with glomerular filtration rate, blood volume, and basal metabolic rate.[52] However, the variability in drug clearance introduced by these factors is small (<25%) compared with that induced by hepatic metabolic enzymes, and there is no correlation between BSA and metabolic activity.[52]

Cytochrome P450 3A4 (family 3, subfamily A, and polypeptide 4) is the most prevalent metabolic enzyme in humans and is responsible for more than 55% of drug metabolic clearance.[54] Recent studies utilizing noncancer drugs as indicators of *CYP3A4* metabolic activity, such as midazolam clearance,[55] suggest potential clinical utility with agents that are metabolized by this pathway—for example,

docetaxel.[56] Enzymatic pathways are responsible for the clearance of 5-FU and 6-mercaptopurine (6-MP) and for glucuronidation via *UGT1A1* for clearance of SN-38, the active product of irinotecan (see individual chapters). Each of these enzymes has a significant incidence of polymorphisms that affect drug disposition and correlate with toxicity. Persons with the UGT1A1*28 homozygous 7/7 genotype have a reduced capacity for glucuronidation as the major metabolic pathway of SN-38 and higher drug exposure (AUC). Several studies have confirmed a significant correlation among the SN-38 exposure, 1A1*28 genotype, and severe neutropenia and diarrhea.[57] Pharmacogenetic profiling offers the prospect of individualized dose selection in the future and is a frequent component in early clinical drug development. These DNA-based tests are not commercially available yet and have no clinical role at the present time.

Glomerular filtration rate as estimated from serum creatinine does correlate with toxicity for topotecan, etoposide, and carboplatin. Indeed, calculated AUC from serum creatinine (Calvert formula) is now used to dose carboplatin.[51] At present, these alternatives (except for carboplatin AUC dosing) remain under investigation, and BSA-based dosing remains the standard of clinical practice for classical chemotherapy agents.

All the molecularly targeted tyrosine kinase inhibitors approved for clinical use as well as the many more in clinical development are administered as a flat dose with no adjustment for weight or BSA. Dose selection of monoclonal antibodies used in cancer medicine also does not follow a classical dose escalation to toxicity. RO of a surface glycoprotein target is a quantitative measure of an appropriate dose of agents directed at surface proteins (i.e., anti PD 1 immune checkpoint agents) or depletion of a circulating protein (VEGF (vascular endothelial growth factor) and bevacizumab).

Real-time pharmacokinetics and patient safety
Pharmacokinetic studies provide important information regarding the dose effect. Such studies indicate substantial variation in serum drug levels and in the AUC per given dose. For methotrexate and 6-MP in acute leukemia and for high-dose busulfan and carmustine bis-chloroethylnitrosourea (BCNU) in the transplant setting, the AUC level of drug or its active metabolites (or both) correlates with toxicity and therapeutic effect.[58-61]

Plasma levels of methotrexate used in high doses (>1 gm/m^2) in selected settings of ALL or DLBCL are clinically tested and are used to determine the duration and dose of leucovorin rescue in these patients.[62] Substantial variation in the AUC per given dose of paclitaxel was also observed in patients with solid tumors. Real-time adjustment of dose on subsequent days significantly reduced mucositis requiring morphine administration and decreased the duration of hospital stay.[63]

Dose effect in sensitive tumors
Few clinical studies have included dose intensity as an independent, randomized variable. In a Cancer and Leukemia Group B (CALGB) study, 596 patients with AML were randomized to receive four 5-day courses of cytarabine at one of three dose schedules: (1) 100 mg/m^2 daily (standard arm), (2) 400 mg/m^2 by continuous infusion, or (3) 3 g/m^2 in a 3-h infusion every 12 h (twice daily) on days 1, 3, and 5[3]. For patients 60 years of age or younger, the probability of remaining in continuous complete remission after 4 years was 24% in the 100 mg/m^2 group; 29% in the 400 mg/m^2 group; and 44% in the 3 g/m^2 group ($p = 0.002$), indicating a better response with increased dose. Elderly patients were less responsive. In acute lymphocytic leukemia (ALL), the dose rate of maintenance chemotherapy had a major impact on the duration of response.[64]

Similarly, in studies of combination chemotherapy in small cell lung cancer, the dose effect was significant, albeit with outmoded therapy.[65]

Increased doses of anthracycline combined with standard dose cytarabine in the initial therapy of patients with AML resulted in an increase in CR rate and PFS (progression free survival) in both young and elderly patients.[66]

Dose–response effects are less well studied in the new kinase inhibitors, which tend to be dosed at the maximum tolerated daily dose, leaving little opportunity for significant increases. Increasing doses of imatinib in patients with chronic phase or accelerated phase CML and in GIST show an increase in response rate in a subgroup of patients. In cases where resistance to imatinib is due to increased metabolic clearance, increased activity of PgP or amplification of the BCR-ABL gene, this might be expected although responses were seen even in patients with mutations in the BCR-ABL kinase itself.[24,25,67,68]

In treating individual patients, dose is a key factor if cure is possible. Thus, for leukemias, lymphomas, testicular cancer, childhood solid tumors, and conventional-dose adjuvant treatment of breast cancer, dose should not be compromised even at the risk of significant toxicity. For more resistant tumors, where palliation is the goal, dose should be adjusted primarily on the basis of toxicity.

Peripheral blood stem cell and marrow transplantation

Allogeneic bone marrow transplantation produces disease-free survival plateaus (i.e., cures) in patients with acute and chronic leukemias and lymphomas, but because of the effect of graft versus leukemia, the component contributed by dose cannot be independently evaluated.

The most compelling evidence regarding dose–response is in high-dose, autologous stem cell rescue studies in patients with relapsed lymphoma.[69,70] Alkylating agents and total body radiotherapy-based regimens are commonly used because their dose-limiting toxicity is myelosuppression. Depending on the agent, dose can be escalated between 3 and 20 times baseline before nonmyelosuppressive toxicity becomes dose limiting. Given the considerable overlap of AUCs for serum levels of drugs at dose escalations of 2–4 times baseline, the escalations possible with stem cell support allow better comparisons of the effect of dose. High-dose therapy with autologous stem cell rescue produces high complete response rates and cures in non-Hodgkin's lymphoma and testicular cancer.[70,71] However, because toxicity can be lethal, high-dose therapy should be limited to specialized centers.[72]

Adjuvant chemotherapy

Randomized studies
Cytokinetics provides an experimental basis for many therapeutic designs. A brief review of the related history follows.

Skipper et al.[15] established the fundamental exponential relationship between drug treatment and surviving tumor fractions. It is the fractional TCR that is constant for a given dose and drug. Although this exponential relationship is modified by other factors, such as drug resistance and microenvironment, it remains the fundamental tenet of cytokinetics and chemotherapy. Norton and Simon[73] applied Gompertzian theory and analysis to treatment during remission and demonstrated the potentially greater effectiveness of late intensification. Goldie and Coldman[74] introduced the mutation-to-resistance theory, relating tumor burden and inherent mutation rate to potential for cure. Hryniuk and colleagues found a significant dose–response effect not only in the leukemias and

lymphomas but also in the relatively less chemosensitive tumors, such as breast cancer.[75–77]

The adjuvant setting, where the tumor burden is microscopic, should be ideal for demonstrating a dose effect. There, many factors that could reduce tumor cytotoxicity (tumor size, decreased and abnormal vascularity, low GF, hypoxia, and increased tumor heterogeneity) and contribute to chemotherapy resistance are less evident in the microscopic tumor (adjuvant) setting. Combination chemotherapy with cyclophosphamide, methotrexate, and 5-FU (CMF) or with cyclophosphamide, doxorubicin (Adriamycin), and 5-FU (CAF), which produces only transient partial and a few complete responses in metastatic breast cancer, reduces relapse and mortality rates by 20–30% in the adjuvant breast cancer setting.[78] Similar effects are seen in colon cancer.[79]

Attempts to improve disease-free survival by increasing the adjuvant chemotherapy dose in breast cancer have produced mixed results. The first statistically robust positive study was conducted by the CALGB.[19] Patients with node-positive breast cancer were randomized to one of three CAF regimens. The high-dose arm involved four courses of CAF at doses of 600 cyclophosphamide, 60 doxorubicin, and 600 mg/m^2 5-FU every 3–4 weeks; in the low-dose arm, the doses were 300, 30, and 300 mg/m^2, respectively. A 10% difference in the relapse-free curve developed by 2 years and persisted through 10 years. That result represents an approximately 20% reduction in mortality. The dose effect was seen most prominently in the 20% of patients whose tumors overexpressed ERBB2 (HER2/neu). For tumors without ERBB2 overexpression, no significant dose effect was seen.[20,80,81] This subset effect would not have been identified in the absence of the molecular marker.

Two other studies conducted by the National Surgical Adjuvant Breast and Bowel Project (NSABP) failed to show that a 2 or 4 times increase in the dose of cyclophosphamide alone affected response in terms of relapse or survival in adjuvant breast cancer.[80,81] Thus, in the comparative study of CAF, the dose of doxorubicin was probably important; however, in another study of adjuvant breast cancer, patients randomized to three doses of doxorubicin[82] (60, 75, and 90 mg/m^2, all given with the standard dose of cyclophosphamide) showed no difference in disease-free or overall survival (OS). The 60 mg/m^2 is probably a threshold dose, above which no further benefit accrues.

The basis for the seemingly discordant results of dose in major clinical trials has been the subject of preclinical and mechanism-of-action studies, but it remains unexplained. It can be speculated how often in the analysis of large comparative studies an important effect has been missed within a subset not known to exist at the time. That possibility is an important limitation in the interpretation of negative studies.

Dose-dense chemotherapy
The concept behind dose-dense chemotherapy is to increase the intensity of drug administration by shortening the interval between treatments without increasing the total dose of drug administered. This increase is accomplished by escalating the dose or the number of cycles in a given period of time. The use of neutrophil-colony-stimulating factors is an essential requirement for dose-dense therapy. Interim reports on the CALGB 9741 study, the use of dose-dense therapy with cyclophosphamide, doxorubicin, and paclitaxel in adjuvant breast cancer, either concurrently or sequentially in 2-week as opposed to the standard 3-week cycles significantly reduced the annual risk of recurrence or death. The DFS (risk ratio [RR] = 0.74, $P = 0.10$) and OS (RR = 0.69, $P = 0.013$) were prolonged in the dose-dense arms. There was no difference in either DFS or OS between sequential and concurrent therapy.

There was no interaction between dose-density and sequence. This preliminary report supported the concept of dose-dense intensification as a means to enhance chemotherapy efficacy, albeit at a cost of increased toxicity.[82] Definitive randomized trials have not confirmed these initial reports, although not all the studies are completed.[83]

Summary

In the clinic, the effect of dose correlates generally with the basic chemosensitivity of the tumor. Thus, Burkitt's lymphoma, ALL, and testicular cancer are all highly sensitive and highly responsive to dose intensity, including achievement of cure. On the other hand, relatively insensitive tumors such as gastrointestinal and lung cancers respond poorly to chemotherapy and are not significantly affected by dose. There are clearly unknown factors at work in the human cancer patient, which continue to defy simple explanation, among them the complex milieu of the inherent genetic background in the particular cell type and patient in which cancer arises, the effect of somatic and nontransformed stromal cells, the emerging role of cancer stem cells and other unappreciated factors not accounted for by the reductionist *in vitro* and *in vivo* models on which cancer researchers depend.

Schedule of drug administration

Schedule effects of individual agents

Cytarabine

Skipper and colleagues performed elegant, quantitative studies of L1210 mouse leukemia using the prototype cell-cycle phase-specific agent cytarabine.[4,15] Cytarabine was shown to produce optimal therapeutic effects when given in courses of appropriate duration and with intervals that allowed for recovery of normal bone marrow. Extrapolating their work to human AML, the investigators gave patients repeated courses of a continuous infusion for 5–7 days separated by 2–3 weeks for recovery. In patients with AML, this schedule produced a 30–40% complete response rate as compared with 10% for other schedules, such as daily intravenous administration.[4,84,85] The addition of daunorubicin to cytarabine further increased the complete response rate and has become the backbone for remission induction therapy for the treatment of AML in adults for more than four decades (for details, see the section titled "Cytokinetics of bone marrow").

Gemcitabine

The dose-limiting toxicity of gemcitabine, a nucleoside analog structurally related to cytarabine, is myelosuppression.[86,87] Unlike cytarabine, gemcitabine has activity in solid tumors, particularly in pancreatic, breast, and non-small-cell lung cancer. Weekly or biweekly bolus treatments are well tolerated, with toxicity largely limited to the marrow. Clinically and in experimental animals, gemcitabine given by continuous infusion necessitates a marked reduction in dose, particularly because of myelosuppression but also because of gastrointestinal toxicity and, in some circumstances, hypotension.[87]

Methotrexate

Intermittent methotrexate (5-day bolus courses every 3–4 weeks), developed by Li and colleagues for gestational choriocarcinoma, proved to be curative.[88] Goldin et al.[89] demonstrated in L1210 mouse leukemia that intermittent methotrexate was superior to continuous (daily) methotrexate. In a randomized, comparative study of patients with ALL in complete remission, intermittent methotrexate was significantly superior to daily therapy.[90] This empiric observation is consistent with subsequent findings by Schimke et al.,[91] indicating that continuous exposure to methotrexate *in vitro* produces drug resistance more consistently than does intermittent methotrexate. Moreover, with continuous administration, resistance results from gene amplification as compared with a transport defect following intermittent methotrexate.[91,92] The kinetics of bone marrow recovery and mucosal cell replacement, important in cytarabine scheduling, may be important clinical determinants of scheduling with methotrexate as well.

Fluoropyrimidines

In clinical studies, 5-FU is commonly administered in daily pulse doses of 350–450 mg/m² for 5 days. Using that schedule, myelosuppression is dose limiting. Twice that dose can be delivered by continuous infusion over 5 days, in which case mucositis and diarrhea become dose limiting.[93]

Fluorodeoxyuridine (FUDR) is much more toxic when delivered by continuous infusion than by intermittent bolus dosing. For example, daily doses in the range 30–50 mg/m² produce toxicity. The biochemical basis for the schedule difference is speculative. Continuous-infusion FUDR may have a greater effect on DNA synthesis; other schedules have a relatively greater effect on host tissue ribonucleic acid (RNA) and RNA synthesis.[93] Data regarding the effect of these differences in schedule on the therapeutic index are few. (Modulation with leucovorin is discussed later in this chapter.) Longer durations of systemic administration currently are under study.[94]

Capecitabine is an oral prodrug of 5-FU. It has allowed protracted administration with opportunities for increased effectiveness and simplicity of administration. It has not fully supplanted intravenous 5-FU in all indications, as in the FOLFOX regimen for colorectal and gastric cancer.[95]

Thus, mechanisms of action, resistance, and cross-resistance for 5-FU appear to differ depending on the analog chosen and the schedule of administration, among other factors.[96]

Alkylating agents

The alkylating agents are a heterogeneous group of compounds that have in common interaction with DNA. That interaction leads to malignant transformation of mammalian cells in culture and to carcinogenesis in patients. The cytotoxic action of these agents is produced by the addition of an alkyl (CH3) group and/or intra- and interstrand linkages that impair or prevent DNA replication directly or produce lethal double-stranded breaks if not fully repaired by DNA damage repair mechanisms, which are frequently defective in transformed cells. This mutagenic interaction also explains its teratogenic and carcinogenic potential.

The alkylating agents are of equal potency in terms of antitumor effect. The difference is primarily host toxicity. This variation in toxicity is particularly true for the dichloroplatinum group of compounds, which closely resemble X-radiation in terms of antitumor effect. They are substantially different in toxicity depending on the nature of the trans-adducts. Most experimental data regarding alkylating agents suggest that they are schedule independent: that is, the antitumor and host effects are dose-related, independent of schedule.[97] (See the sections titled "Pharmacokinetics" and "Adjuvant chemotherapy" for discussions of specific aspects of cyclophosphamide and ifosfamide.)

Anthracyclines

Cardiotoxicity is an important delayed toxicity of anthracyclines. In experimental studies, peak concentrations produced more cardiotoxicity for an equivalent dose than did lower concentrations achieved by continuous-infusion schedules. Weiss and Manthel[98] first demonstrated that weekly doxorubicin administration produced less cardiotoxicity per total dose administered than did standard triweekly regimens. Legha and colleagues demonstrated that a 4-day, continuous infusion of doxorubicin every 3 weeks is less cardiotoxic than bolus injections, an observation confirmed in randomized studies.[99–101] Infusion approaches allow a 30–50% increase in total cumulative dose before cardiotoxicity develops. In experimental and preliminary clinical studies, liposomal doxorubicin may be less cardiotoxic than doxorubicin.[102,103] The use of the cardioprotective agent dexrazoxane is current clinical practice in selected settings.[104]

Etoposide

An inhibitor of topoisomerase II that produces DNA double-strand breaks, etoposide is selectively active against cells in cycle. Etoposide is commonly used in combination chemotherapy of solid tumors, particularly with cisplatin. Preclinical studies showed that etoposide must be present both during and immediately following cisplatin to achieve optimal effect, consistent with a possible interaction with cisplatin involving inhibition of DNA repair. In small cell lung cancer, the optimal etoposide dose schedule of five daily doses every 3–4 weeks is consistent with the discussion earlier in this chapter of marrow and tumor cytokinetics and response to cell cycle-specific agents.[105]

Tubulin binders

Although the *Vinca* alkaloids vincristine and vinblastine are cell cycle-specific, no schedule appears superior to standard weekly dosing.[106] On the basis of limited data, the same is true for vinorelbine. Paclitaxel schedule considerations have been dominated by acute histamine-like toxicity, probably related to the vehicle (Cremophor EL); this toxicity is relieved by antihistamines and corticosteroids. Practical and economic considerations favoring outpatient use have resulted in 1- to 3-h intravenous infusions, although some randomized trials suggest an advantage for infusions that are even longer.[107]

Weekly infusions are superior to intermittent administration in breast and ovarian cancer.[108,109] Myelosuppression correlates with the duration of plasma concentrations of paclitaxel above the threshold of 0.1 mol/L.[107] Neutropenia appears to be related more to schedule than to dose, although neuropathy appears dose related.[110]

General use of intermittent dosing

For most chemotherapeutic agents that directly or indirectly target DNA or the mitotic spindle used alone or in combination, intermittent courses (e.g., four 5-day courses every 3–4 weeks) are generally superior to other schedules such as continuous (i.e., daily) dosing. Such is the case for cyclophosphamide and methotrexate in Burkitt's lymphoma, methotrexate and actinomycin D in choriocarcinoma, melphalan in myeloma, cytarabine in AML, and methotrexate in ALL.[111] It is also true for combination regimens for Hodgkin's disease, ALL, and childhood solid tumors.[106,111,112] In experimental and clinical studies alike, intermittent intensive treatment for rapidly proliferating tumors is superior. The reason may be recruitment of resting G_0/G_1 cells into active cycle. Continuous

treatment may be superior for more indolent, low-GF tumors, but more definitive studies are needed.[113]

Advances in supportive care now allow a novel approach to intermittent intensive chemotherapy. Neutrophil colony stimulating factors in dose-dense adjuvant breast cancer therapy[114] or leukapheresis following marrow recovery from chemotherapy and treatment with G-CSF allow the harvest of sufficient peripheral blood circulating stem cells to rescue as many as four courses of moderately intensive chemotherapy.[115]

Continuous administration

Protracted infusions (6 weeks) of 5-FU combined with local radiotherapy in adjuvant rectal cancer demonstrated both a lower local recurrence rate in the irradiated field and a reduced incidence of metastatic relapse.[116] Capecitabine is an orally absorbable agent that undergoes biotransformation to 5-FU. Prolonged administration over 14 days of capecitabine as a single agent, repeated at 21-day intervals, shows a response rate that is superior to that of intravenous 5-FU and leucovorin, although no survival benefit accrues.[117,118] Capecitabine is also active in refractory breast cancer as monotherapy or in combination. The role of continuous fluoropyrimidine administration with capecitabine is being explored in combination chemotherapy and with radiation. The treatment interruption every 3 weeks does seem to significantly reduce dose-limiting hand-foot syndrome toxicity with capecitabine.

Targeted kinase inhibitors

For reasons related to the mechanism of action, continuous oral administration of many new targeted therapies such as imatinib in CML and GIST is the current clinical schedule.[113,119] The continued suppression of proliferative growth factor signals and interruption of survival pathway signals in tumor cells or the tumor vascular network appears necessary in the clinic and in preclinical models. One clinical trial of a randomized discontinuation of the multitargeted tyrosine kinase inhibitor sorafenib in renal cell cancer patients with stable disease demonstrated a significant PFS advantage at 6 months for patients who continued to receive sorafenib versus placebo, which supports the preclinical modeling in the clinic.[120] For other agents such as the multi-kinase inhibitor sunitinib, intermittent schedules are used because of better tolerance, similar to the DNA damaging agents and mitotic spindle inhibitors.[121]

Combination chemotherapy

Rationale

The most compelling rationales for combination chemotherapy are (1) tumor cell heterogeneity and its implication for drug resistance and (2) the success of combination chemotherapy in the clinic. In practical clinical terms, the selection of specific combinations in particular types of cancer depends on the individual activity of the agents in the target cancer type and the absence of overlapping toxicities. The agents with the highest single-agent activity are preferred, particularly agents that produce complete responses (if any such agents exist), with different mechanisms of action to address the theoretical heterogeneity issue.

Combination chemotherapy in the clinic

Ample clinical precedent exists for using multiple agents. An example is the treatment of ALL in children, where multiple active agents have been identified. A direct correlation is seen between the number of agents used and the cure rate (Table 2). In fact, essentially

Table 3 Cancer chemotherapy—number of agents required for cure by tumor type.

Tumor	Number of agents required for cure	Adjuvant or neoadjuvant	Number of agents required for cure
Acute lymphoblastic leukemia (children)	4–7	Wilms tumor	2–3
Gestational choriocarcinoma[a]		Embryonal rhabdomyosarcoma	2–3
Early	1–3	Osteogenic sarcoma	3
Advanced	2–4	Soft tissue sarcoma	3
Acute myeloid leukemia	3+	Ovarian cancer	3–4
Testicular cancer	3	Breast cancer	2–4
Burkitt lymphoma[b]	1–4	Colorectal cancer	2
Hodgkin disease	4–5	Non-small-cell lung carcinoma, stage IIIA	2
Diffuse histiocytic lymphoma	4–5	Small-cell lung carcinoma, limited	2–4

[a]One agent is curative, but a higher cure rate results with two or more agents.
[b]One agent cures state 1 African Burkitt lymphoma, but two or more agents are better.

all curative chemotherapy involves combinations of two and usually three or more agents (Table 3).Curative combinations need not incorporate each agent at each dosing encounter; for example, the sequential use of taxanes after doxorubicin and cyclophosphamide in breast cancer or in pediatric soft tissue cancers, but within a patients total treatment course. Normal tissue tolerance often limits the number of agents that can be administered at one time).

Current studies have demonstrated evidence for synergy or an additive effect between established DNA/mitotic spindle targeted chemotherapeutic agents and agents representing other classes. Molecularly targeted agents, whether monoclonal antibodies or small molecules, have been combined with cytotoxic agents as well as other targeted agents. Trastuzumab, a monoclonal antibody to *ERBB2*, is synergistic with doxorubicin and paclitaxel. *ERBB2* is present on the cancer cell surface in 25% of patients with breast cancer, and benefit is restricted to only those patients with amplification of the *ERBB2* gene.[122] Toxicities may be substantial, however. Trastuzumab in combination with doxorubicin increased cardiac toxicity. A lesser risk of cardiac toxicity exists when trastuzumab is included in paclitaxel combinations. The addition of a complement-fixing monoclonal antibody, rituximab, to cyclophosphamide, hydroxydaunomycin/doxorubicin, vincristine sulfate, and prednisone chemotherapy in non-Hodgkin's lymphoma increases response without an increase in toxicity. The addition of the mTOR inhibitor everolimus to an aromatase inhibitor (AI) markedly prolongs the PFS in estrogen receptor-dependent metastatic breast cancer.[123] The addition of the CDK 4/6 inhibitor palbociclib to an AI increases the PFS in ER positive breast cancer.[124] This compatibility of new and old is not to be assumed, as combinations of cytotoxic chemotherapy with both erlotinib and gefitinib fail to produce significant benefit in lung cancer.[125]

The combination of multiple targets in a single molecule can be incorporated into novel molecularly targeted agents. Certainly, multiple targets within a single small molecule, such as VEGFR and PDGFR, in the angiogenesis pathways produce greater clinical benefit than targeting either alone, as the success, limited as it may be, of single agent sorafenib and sunitinib demonstrates *viz-a-viz* single agent, including bevacizumab and many failed compounds limited to VEGFR2 alone.[12]

Multiple agents can be directed at a single target protein or to sequential proteins in a single pathway essential to the neoplastic process. Combining the monoclonal antibodies trastuzumab and pertuzumab, which bind to different epitopes of the ERBB2 receptor, produces unprecedented OS in ERBB2-expressing metastatic breast cancer.[126] Sequential inhibition of BRAF and MEK in BRAF[V600E] melanoma produces greater response rates, PFS and

OS.[10] All-trans-retinoic acid and arsenic trioxide interact with the PML protein in acute progranulocytic leukemia cells with resultant differentiation and durable remission.[127]

Technology has reached a point where a monoclonal antibody can be conjugated to a small molecule to deliver therapy in a highly selective manner, such as the T-DMI conjugate of trastuzumab and auristatin in breast cancer or radioactive yttrium to anti CD30 in Hodgkin's lymphoma.[128,129]

Tumor cell heterogeneity and drug resistance

Tumors are clonal in origin, but the increasing DNA instability that accompanies the onset of neoplasia leads to increased variation in the daughter cells, called "clonal evolution" to tumor cell heterogeneity. This evolution is associated with selection for progeny with greater survival capacity, which is evident as higher proliferative capacity, resistance to apoptosis, greater metastatic or invasive potential, reduced dependence on normal cellular growth factors, and angiogenesis.[130] Heterogeneity among tumor cells increases the number and diversity of potential target sites for chemotherapy and the need to combine therapeutic agents.

Initially, resistance was thought to be limited to the selecting agent (mono-drug resistance). The recognition of multidrug resistance required a reexamination of this rationale for combination chemotherapy.[131] The ABC family of transport proteins such as (ABCB1, PgP), the multidrug resistance proteins (ABCC1), and the breast cancer-related protein (ABCG2) confer multidrug resistance that relates almost exclusively to natural products. Prolonged exposure to low doses of substrate drugs such as doxorubicin may overcome resistance mediated by these transport proteins.[132] However, glutathione transferase, DNA repair capacity, and topoisomerase II alterations also may be associated with multidrug resistance.[133]

Recent studies of multicellular drug resistance indicate an altered set point for apoptosis.[134] Differences between *in vitro* and *in vivo* drug resistance are modifying the approach to combination chemotherapy.[135] Although prolonged drug exposure results in stable, resistant cell lines, acute exposure may induce short-term, reversible resistance. How the short-term resistance relates mechanistically to the long-term, presumably genetic, resistance is under study.

The advent of molecular profiling of patient tumors as a clinical means of treatment selection continues to emphasize the heterogeneity that exists within a single tumor at a single point in time and also the variability that occurs over time in a single tumor and the heterogeneity that exists in a single point in time in different metastases in the same patient. New treatment algorithms are being developed to address this complex problem (*see* **Chapter 41** for a more detailed discussion).

Cytokinetics

The discovery that solid tumors contain a large number of potentially clonogenic cells in G_1 or G_0—presumably because of tumor hypoxia and a low GF—provided a basis for combination chemotherapy.[27,28,33] Thus, cell cycle-specific agents were employed to kill mitotically active cells, and non-cell cycle-specific agents (e.g., alkylating agents) were added to damage the noncycling tumor cells. The use of repeated cycles allows normal tissues to recover, so that dose need not be compromised, and G_0/G_1 tumor cells can be recruited into the proliferating fraction by increased availability of nutrients, oxygen, and vascular access.

Synchronization

Synchronization of tumor or normal cells *in vitro* and *in vivo* with drugs that inhibit DNA synthesis or that arrest cells in mitosis can be achieved. Experimentally, the most impressive synchronization has been achieved with hormonal agents that affect tumor but not essential normal cells.

Some degree of tumor-cell synchrony follows this hormonal manipulation in experimental studies but the heterogeneity of human tumors with regard to the time course of recruitment and synchronization has limited this approach, and it remains investigational.[136,137]

Modulation

Agents that are nontoxic may still improve the therapeutic index of an established chemotherapeutic agent, either by reducing normal-tissue toxicity—as leucovorin does for methotrexate, for example—or by preferentially enhancing antitumor efficacy—as 5-FU and leucovorin do in metastatic and adjuvant colon cancer studies.[138-144]

Biochemically, the product of 5-FU, fluorodeoxyuridine monophosphate (FdUMP), binds to the substrate site of thymidylate synthase (TS), thus inhibiting DNA synthesis and, therefore, cellular replication. The stability and duration of this inhibition directly relate to a third agent, 5, 10-methylenetetrahydrofolate, which is a metabolic product of leucovorin that also binds to TS, producing the so-called ternary complex (FdUMP—TS—5,10-methylenetetrahydrofolate). In preclinical systems, *in vitro* and *in vivo* alike, leucovorin favorably modulated the therapeutic index of 5-FU. A number of clinical trials comparing 5-FU to 5-FU with leucovorin indicated an advantage for 5-FU/leucovorin in patients with metastatic colorectal cancer at a cost of only moderately increased mucositis and diarrhea. The combination of 5-FU with leucovorin improved survival rates in two separate studies in metastatic and adjuvant colon cancers.[143,144]

Bevacizumab (Avastin) is a monoclonal antibody that depletes serum VEGF. VEGF is an essential mitogenic and antiapoptotic factor for endothelial cells (*see* **Chapter 11**). Signaling through the VEGF receptor 2 (KDR) and platelet-derived growth factor receptor beta (PDGFRB) acts to increase endothelial cell permeability, which results in increased interstitial fluid pressure (IFP) within tumors. In colon, breast, lung, head and neck, cervix, and skin carcinomas, the IFP is significantly higher than in normal tissues.[145-148] Increased tumor IFP acts as a barrier for tumor transvascular transport; reduction of tumor IFP, or modulation of microvascular pressure, increases the transvascular transport of tumor-targeting antibodies or low-molecular-weight tracer compounds.[149,150] Growing evidence indicates that the PDGFRB and KDR tyrosine kinases play a crucial role in increased tumor IFP. That makes them candidate targets for pharmacologic intervention for tumor interstitial hypertension[151-154] and for a novel, possibly general, combination strategy that will enhance the therapeutic effects of standard chemotherapeutics. Bevacizumab reduces the IFP in patients with advanced colorectal cancer and increases the uptake of gadolinium in the tumors. Combined with irinotecan, 5-FU, and leucovorin, bevacizumab produces a significant prolongation of survival in patients with metastatic colorectal cancer.[155] This modulation of IFP occurs only within tumors and provides a selective increase in drug levels to the tumor without increasing host toxicity, as was noted in both of the latter two studies. Those findings offer a general treatment strategy for solid tumors of any type.

Bevacizumab (and similar agents) combined with cytotoxic chemotherapy has shown improvements in PFS and OS in many—though not all—types of cancer. Given the many mechanisms of VEGF action, it is uncertain which mechanism(s) mediates this effect. That VEGF-targeted therapy is more effective in combination, concurrent or sequential, than as a single agent denotes it as a modulator in most clinical circumstances.

Implications of drug resistance

Tumor cell heterogeneity in response to the potentially cytotoxic and antiproliferative effects of cancer chemotherapeutic agents has been the stimulus for a current novel approach to combination chemotherapy. Avoiding therapeutic resistance has been from the beginning a major rationale for combination chemotherapy.

Initial observations about resistance involved reduced drug levels at the site of action because of increased efflux, alteration or amplification of the target, and cellular inactivation. Recent investigations have focused on mechanisms of drug sensitivity or resistance operative after interaction of the drug and its target receptor, including apoptosis (programmed cell death). The cell damage caused by various chemotherapeutic agents has the common property of triggering the apoptosis cascade in an active process that requires energy, enzymes, and cytostructure for completion.[156] In addition to apoptosis, under certain circumstances, cells undergo necrotic cell death owing to drug-induced depletion of ATP.[157] Finally, autophagy, a highly conserved process of cell survival under conditions of nutrient and or oxygen deprivation can lead to a previously unappreciated form of drug resistance following treatment with cytotoxic drugs, hormonal agents, and radiation.[158] Drug resistance must always be viewed in the context of therapeutic index. Resistance fundamentally means that there exists no selective cancer cytotoxicity in relation to toxicity in the cancer-bearing host. This may be present at the outset or become apparent only during therapy. This narrow or lack of therapeutic index is present in most cancer therapeutic agents.

Reversal of drug resistance

Another approach to modulation involves reversal of drug resistance, the most studied of which is multidrug resistance mediated by PgP. Verapamil and several other lipid-soluble heterocyclic drugs, including cyclosporine analogs, can inhibit PgP and thus reduce the efflux of a number of natural antitumor products (doxorubicin, vincristine, taxanes, and others) from the cell, thereby increasing cytotoxicity. PgP is increased in B-cell tumors, AML, sarcoma, and tumors previously treated with drugs that led to multidrug resistance.[159] This approach has not yet produced significant clinical benefit in clinical trials or practice.

Molecular biology/targeted therapy

Implications for dose and schedule

The level of optimism among researchers has increased substantially as a result of recent "proof of concept" regarding the clinical effectiveness of more-targeted therapies. Evidence for unique molecular targets in cancer cells (e.g., fusion genes, mutations, and recombinations) and on their surfaces has led to synthesis of small molecules and monoclonal antibodies with a target specificity achieved only rarely in cancer therapeutics.[160-162]

Table 1 presents a sampling of combinations of molecules and biochemical pathways that are currently being evaluated as targets for selective antitumor agents. The magnitude of such activity and the number of active agents in preclinical systems offer remarkable opportunities for the use of agents in combination. The cumulative effect of these agents on a molecular level suggests an interaction that may result from the diversity of target interaction and a sequential or simultaneous attack on critical cell behavior.

Another important area of diversity relates to anticipated toxicity. Thus, as compared with classical chemotherapy agents, where dose-delineating toxicity usually relates to proliferating tissues and is relatively uniform, the molecular biologic agents will almost certainly express toxicity that varies from agent to agent and that largely differs from the classical antitumor agents. Molecular agents are under extensive study not only for their antitumor properties but also most particularly for their interaction with each other and other established antitumor agents.

Experimental models of combination therapy

The classical antitumor agents are limited largely to those that directly or indirectly produce DNA damage; the products of the molecular biology era markedly extend the diversity of target mechanisms. Indeed, using experimental models, a number of interesting preclinical experiments have demonstrated an additive or synergistic effect. The literature on preclinical models and computer analysis has been reviewed by Rideout and Chou.[163]

The future of combination chemotherapy will be influenced substantially by the number of these compounds and their interactions. The strategy of combining drugs whose mechanisms of action vary has been successful, even in the curative treatment of hematologic, childhood, and embryonal neoplasms.

The terms "additive" and "synergistic" are commonly used in the clinic but are not well defined. In considering these terms, selectivity for the tumor as compared to the host—the *therapeutic index*—is key. If two agents with additive therapeutic effect have a differing dose-limiting toxicity, so that the toxicity is nonadditive, the overall antitumor effect should be described as additive. When the effects are greater than "additive," the term "synergism" may be appropriate.

Table 4 presents the properties and comparisons of combination chemotherapy and combined modality therapy. Incorporation of many more classes of agents will force more efficient experimental designs. Such designs may include, for example, a rolling phase II/phase III study design. Increasingly, quantitative molecular markers and "real-time" pharmacology will be integrated operationally into clinical studies. The effectiveness of such related approaches should improve the efficiency and effectiveness of clinical trials.

Oncogenes and tumor-suppressor genes may operate by modifying or exploiting abnormalities in the cell cycle, by interfering with growth factors, angiogenesis, and DNA repair. Identification of the specific genes or gene pathways in a particular patient by tumor profiling will allow identification of the precise agents most likely to be effective in that patient, with the goal of personalizing cancer therapy.

An integrated approach to cancer chemotherapy

More than a half-century has elapsed since cancer chemotherapy began. The chemotherapy agents now in use originated as biologically targeted therapy. Hitchings and Elion developed specific inhibitors of purine synthesis such as 6-MP and 6-TG; Heidelberger targeted RNA synthesis with 5-FU; and Farber targeted the reduced folate pathway with aminopterin. These innovations not only provided the groundwork for cancer treatment but also became tools for discovery of the basic workings of transformed cancer cells.

Natural products such as the *Vinca* alkaloids, anthracyclines, and taxanes were selected specifically for activity against cancer proliferation. These agents were combined with other classes of agents—for example, hormones, alkylating agents, and irradiation—which are active against proliferating cells. The optimal use of the new agents requires their integration into increasingly complex combinations so that a greater therapeutic index results. The same is true for the current classical chemotherapeutic agents, which largely inhibit proliferation.

Molecular biology particularly has expanded the number of classes. Thus, hormones, immunotoxins, and inhibitors of invasion and metastasis are available in addition to the classical antiproliferation and DNA damaging compounds. Receptors and kinases of unique structure and quantity, capable of targeting with specific molecular agents, continue to be discovered and the pathways activated in cancer further elucidated.

Table 4 Combination chemotherapy versus holotherapy.

Combination	Chemotherapy	Holotherapy
Diversity of agents	Drawn from one class, antiproliferative	Drawn from all classes[a]
Number of agents	2–5	4–12+
Toxicity	Bone marrow and gastrointestinal (steep dose); cardiac, neuralgic, and pulmonary	Major diversity, including that relative to dose and toxicity; toxicity commonly nonadditive; limited, greater selection
Experimental design of clinical trials	Rigid, establishment	Flexible, innovative, semi-Bayesian; patient participation
Endpoints	Classical; R, dR, DFS, OS	MRT
Integration with basic science	Limited	Extensive, operational; PK, PD; targets

[a]Chemotherapy, immunotherapy, endocrinology, antiangiogenesis, antimatrix, gene therapy, and control of cell cycle (anticyclins [*CDK* family], transcriptional control, and antisense).

Abbreviations: DFS, disease-free survival; dR, duration of response; MRT, microbeam radiation therapy; OS, overall survival; PD, pharmacodynamics; PK, pharmacokinetics; R, response (partial or complete).

Table 5 Therapeutic interaction between agents of different classes.

Agent	Cancer acted on
Chemotherapy + other systemic agent	
Chemo + immunotherapy	
Cisplatin + herceptin	Breast cancer
Taxol + herceptin	Breast cancer
CHOP + rituximab	Lymphoma
Chemotherapy → MRT → recovery of immunity → vaccine	
Minitransplant chemotherapy followed by allogeneic armed lymphocyte	
Chemotherapy + hormonal therapy	
Vincristine + prednisone	Acute lymphocytic leukemia
Chemotherapy + tamoxifen	Breast cancer
Chemotherapy + differentiation agent	
Daunorubicin + ATRA	Acute progranulocytic leukemia
Chemotherapy + antiangiogenesis	
IFL + bevacizumab	Colorectal cancer

Abbreviations: ATRA, all-*trans*-retinoic acid; IFL, irinotecan/5-fluorouracil/leucovorin; MRT, microbeam radiation therapy.

It has become readily apparent that the vast majority of cancers will be treated successfully only with combinations of agents chosen for the highest possible individual activity against a specific type of cancer. Ideally, such drugs will have different dose-limiting toxicities. Empiricism was an essential component in the development of contemporary cancer therapy, but rational drug discovery, analog development, preclinical modeling, precise pathologic diagnosis, careful staging of disease, and clinical trial design are the foundation for the measure of success known today.

The breakthroughs in molecular biology have presented the cancer therapist with enormous opportunities and challenges. On the basis of these breakthroughs, a molecular diagnosis will be able to not only determine where and how cancer originates but also the processes that are essential to its survival. The specific processes that initiate and propagate cancer have become the targets of unprecedented rational drug development (Table 1). Pharmaceutical technology provides not only small molecules but also monoclonal antibodies, immunoconjugates, ribozymes, antisense RNA, and recombinant viruses.

The therapy of cancer now has the potential to combine agents with even more mechanisms of action to confront the heterogeneity of cancer with a wider array of therapeutics. Some of these combinations are now the standard of care, as improvements in response and survival demonstrate (Table 4). The challenges to be overcome include (1) clinical development of cytostatic agents without the expectation of significant acute toxicity; (2) combining of classes of targeted agents (Table 5) both molecular and biologic, with regard to dose and schedule; and (3) selection of the appropriate types of cancer and individual patients for a specific therapy.

With molecular biology playing an increasing role, the clinical and laboratory sciences that address the therapy of cancer will continue to accelerate toward cancer control.

Key references

The complete reference list can be found on the Wiley Companion Digital Edition of this title (see inside front cover for login instructions).

1 Frei E 3rd, Canellos GP. Dose: a critical factor in cancer chemotherapy. *Am J Med*. 1980;**69**(4):585–594.

4 Skipper HE, Schabel FM Jr, Wilcox WS. Experimental evaluation of potential anticancer agents. XXI. Scheduling of arabinosylcytosine to take advantage of its S-phase specificity against leukemia cells. *Cancer Chemother Rep*. 1967;**51**(3):125–165.

10 Robert C, Karaszewska B, Schachter J, et al. Improved overall survival in melanoma with combined dabrafenib and trametinib. *N Engl J Med*. 2015;**372**(1):30–39.

14 Hryniuk W, Frei E 3rd, Wright FA. A single scale for comparing dose-intensity of all chemotherapy regimens in breast cancer: summation dose-intensity. *J Clin Oncol*. 1998;**16**(9):3137–3147.

16 Frei E 3rd, Cucchi CA, Rosowsky A, et al. Alkylating agent resistance: in vitro studies with human cell lines. *Proc Natl Acad Sci U S A*. 1985;**82**(7):2158–2162.

19 Wood WC, Budman DR, Korzun AH, et al. Dose and dose intensity of adjuvant chemotherapy for stage II, node-positive breast carcinoma. *N Engl J Med*. 1994;**330**(18):1253–1259.

23 Dowsett M. Clinical development of aromatase inhibitors for the treatment of breast and prostate cancer. *J Steroid Biochem Mol Biol*. 1990;**37**(6):1037–1041.

24 Zonder JA, Pemberton P, Brandt H, Mohamed AN, Schiffer CA. The effect of dose increase of imatinib mesylate in patients with chronic or accelerated phase chronic myelogenous leukemia with inadequate hematologic or cytogenetic response to initial treatment. *Clin Cancer Res*. 2003;**9**(6):2092–2097.

27 Norton L, Simon R, Brereton HD, Bogden AE. Predicting the course of Gompertzian growth. *Nature*. 1976;**264**(5586):542–545.

32 Tannock I. Cell kinetics and chemotherapy: a critical review. *Cancer Treat Rep*. 1978;**62**(8):1117–1133.

36 Visvader JE, Lindeman GJ. Cancer stem cells in solid tumours: accumulating evidence and unresolved questions. *Nat Rev Cancer*. 2008;**8**(10):755–768.

39 Engelman JA, Janne PA. Mechanisms of acquired resistance to epidermal growth factor receptor tyrosine kinase inhibitors in non-small cell lung cancer. *Clin Cancer Res*. 2008;**14**(10):2895–2899.

40 Achison M, Hupp TR. Hypoxia attenuates the p53 response to cellular damage. *Oncogene*. 2003;**22**(22):3431–3440.

49 Baker SD, Verweij J, Rowinsky EK, et al. Role of body surface area in dosing of investigational anticancer agents in adults, 1991–2001. *J Natl Cancer Inst*. 2002;**94**(24):1883–1888.

51 Jodrell DI, Egorin MJ, Canetta RM, et al. Relationships between carboplatin exposure and tumor response and toxicity in patients with ovarian cancer. *J Clin Oncol*. 1992;**10**(4):520–528.

55 Dresser GK, Spence JD, Bailey DG. Pharmacokinetic-pharmacodynamic consequences and clinical relevance of cytochrome P450 3A4 inhibition. *Clin Pharmacokinet*. 2000;**38**(1):41–57.

58 Evans WE, Crom WR, Abromowitch M, et al. Clinical pharmacodynamics of high-dose methotrexate in acute lymphocytic leukemia. Identification of a relation between concentration and effect. *N Engl J Med*. 1986;**314**(8):471–477.

64 Pinkel D, Hernandez K, Borella L, et al. Drug dosage and remission duration in childhood lymphocytic leukemia. *Cancer*. 1971;**27**(2):247–256.

73 Norton L, Simon R. The Norton-Simon hypothesis revisited. *Cancer Treat Rep*. 1986;**70**(1):163–169.

78 Early Breast Cancer Trialists' Collaborative Group. Polychemotherapy for early breast cancer: an overview of the randomised trials. *Lancet*. 1998;**352**(9132):930–942.

82 Citron ML, Berry DA, Cirrincione C, et al. Randomized trial of dose-dense versus conventionally scheduled and sequential versus concurrent combination chemotherapy as postoperative adjuvant treatment of node-positive primary breast cancer: first report of Intergroup Trial C9741/Cancer and Leukemia Group B Trial 9741. *J Clin Oncol*. 2003;**21**(8):1431–1439.

83 Swain SM, Tang G, Geyer CE Jr, et al. Definitive results of a phase III adjuvant trial comparing three chemotherapy regimens in women with operable, node-positive breast cancer: the NSABP B-38 trial. *J Clin Oncol*. 2013;**31**(26):3197–3204.

90 Frei E 3rd, Karon M, Levin RH, et al. The effectiveness of combinations of antileukemic agents in inducing and maintaining remission in children with acute leukemia. *Blood*. 1965;**26**(5):642–656.

97 Teicher BA, Holden SA, Eder JP, Brann TW, Jones SM, Frei E 3rd. Influence of schedule on alkylating agent cytotoxicity in vitro and in vivo. *Cancer Res*. 1989;**49**(21):5994–5998.

100 Smith LA, Cornelius VR, Plummer CJ, et al. Cardiotoxicity of anthracycline agents for the treatment of cancer: systematic review and meta-analysis of randomised controlled trials. *BMC Cancer*. 2010;**10**:337.

109 Pignata S, Scambia G, Katsaros D, et al. Carboplatin plus paclitaxel once a week versus every 3 weeks in patients with advanced ovarian cancer (MITO-7): a randomised, multicentre, open-label, phase 3 trial. *Lancet Oncol*. 2014;**15**(4):396–405.

112 Devita VT Jr, Serpick AA, Carbone PP. Combination chemotherapy in the treatment of advanced Hodgkin's disease. *Ann Intern Med*. 1970;**73**(6):881–895.

113 Heinrich MC, Corless CL, Demetri GD, et al. Kinase mutations and imatinib response in patients with metastatic gastrointestinal stromal tumor. *J Clin Oncol*. 2003;**21**(23):4342–4349.

121 Motzer RJ, Hutson TE, Olsen MR, et al. Randomized phase II trial of sunitinib on an intermittent versus continuous dosing schedule as first-line therapy for advanced renal cell carcinoma. *J Clin Oncol.* 2012;**30**(**12**): 1371–1377.

122 Slamon D, Eiermann W, Robert N, et al. Adjuvant trastuzumab in HER2-positive breast cancer. *N Engl J Med.* 2011;**365**(**14**):1273–1283.

129 Francisco JA, Cerveny CG, Meyer DL, et al. cAC10-vcMMAE, an anti-CD30-monomethyl auristatin E conjugate with potent and selective antitumor activity. *Blood.* 2003;**102**(**4**):1458–1465.

131 Gottesman MM, Ling V. The molecular basis of multidrug resistance in cancer: the early years of P-glycoprotein research. *FEBS Lett.* 2006;**580**(**4**): 998–1009.

147 Less JR, Posner MC, Boucher Y, Borochovitz D, Wolmark N, Jain RK. Interstitial hypertension in human breast and colorectal tumors. *Cancer Res.* 1992;**52**(**22**):6371–6374.

151 Ferrara N, Gerber HP, LeCouter J. The biology of VEGF and its receptors. *Nat Med.* 2003;**9**(**6**):669–676.

154 Willett CG, Boucher Y, di Tomaso E, et al. Direct evidence that the VEGF-specific antibody bevacizumab has antivascular effects in human rectal cancer. *Nat Med.* 2004;**10**(**2**):145–147.

158 Hait WN, Jin S, Yang JM. A matter of life or death (or both): understanding autophagy in cancer. *Clin Cancer Res.* 2006;**12**(**7 Pt 1**):1961–1965.

160 Druker BJ, Lydon NB. Lessons learned from the development of an abl tyrosine kinase inhibitor for chronic myelogenous leukemia. *J Clin Invest.* 2000;**105**(**1**):3–7.

55 Pharmacology

Manish R. Sharma, MD ■ Mark J. Ratain, MD

Overview

The biology and clinical indications relevant to systemic anticancer therapies are covered extensively in other chapters in this book. In this chapter, we will focus on the principles of clinical pharmacology as they apply to systemic anticancer therapies and will attempt to illustrate how an understanding of clinical pharmacokinetics and pharmacodynamics can optimize the therapeutic index of these agents. The United States Food and Drug Administration (FDA) conducts a question-based clinical pharmacology and biopharmaceutics review for each approved drug (http://www.fda.gov/downloads/AboutFDA/ReportsManualsForms/Staff PoliciesandProcedures/ucm073007.pdf). Their reviews are publicly available on the FDA website (http://www.accessdata.fda.gov/scripts/cder/drugsatfda/) by searching for the drug name, and often include details that are not included in the product label. We will use their standard questions to introduce the principles of clinical pharmacology and will highlight examples that illustrate these principles.

General attributes of the drug

What are the highlights of the chemistry and physical-chemical properties of the drug substance and the formulation of the drug product as they relate to clinical pharmacology and biopharmaceutics review?

The FDA introduced the biopharmaceutics classification system (BCS) in 2000 (http://www.fda.gov/downloads/Drugs/Guidances/ucm070246.pdf) to establish the criteria that could be used to qualify a new molecular entity for a waiver of *in vivo* bioequivalence studies. The concept, initially developed by Amidon et al.,[1] was that *in vivo* performance could be predicted from *in vitro* measurements of permeability and solubility. BCS class 1 drugs (high permeability/high solubility) are eligible for a waiver of *in vivo* bioequivalence studies. The Biopharmaceutics Drug Disposition Classification System (BDDCS) was subsequently proposed by Wu and Benet[2] and based on the hypothesis that high permeability-rate compounds are readily reabsorbed from the potential unchanged excretion routes (urine and bile) and therefore are primarily eliminated through metabolism. Many oral kinase inhibitors that have been developed as anticancer therapies are high permeability/low solubility compounds that are BCS and BDDCS class 2. These drugs are susceptible to food effects on intestinal absorption; drug–drug interactions related to efflux transporters in the gut, uptake/efflux transporters in the liver, or metabolism; and pharmacogenetic variants that impact transporters or metabolism.[3]

What are the proposed mechanism(s) of action and therapeutic indication(s)?

There are three major types of anticancer therapies: cytotoxics, biologics, and small molecule non-cytotoxics. Classes of each type of therapy, examples of drugs within each class, and their presumed mechanisms of action are shown in Table 1 and covered extensively in other chapters. It is noteworthy that the mechanism of action of a kinase inhibitor may be unclear even after a drug has demonstrated efficacy in a therapeutic indication. For example, regorafenib inhibits multiple tyrosine kinases with relatively high affinity, but the mechanism by which it prolongs survival in chemotherapy-refractory metastatic colorectal cancer (presumed to be related to inhibition of angiogenesis) remains elusive.[4]

What are the proposed dosage(s) and route(s) of administration?

Potential routes of administration for cancer therapies are intravenous, oral, intravascular, intracavitary, subcutaneous, or intramuscular. The optimal route of administration depends on a number of factors. By definition, drugs administered by the intravenous route are 100% available in the blood. For oral drugs, the fraction of an administered dose of drug that reaches systemic circulation is referred to as its bioavailability. Alternatively, it is the ratio of the plasma area under the concentration–time curve (AUC) after oral administration to the plasma AUC after intravenous administration of the same dose. Bioavailability is influenced by both absorption and the first-pass effect, which is the reduction in available drug due to metabolism in the gastrointestinal tract and liver before an orally administered dose reaches systemic circulation. Oral drugs are convenient and theoretically should be less expensive, but are plagued by inconsistent bioavailability both within and between patients.[5] Factors influencing the bioavailability of oral drugs include adherence, release of the drug from its formulation, stability in the gastrointestinal tract, factors influencing dissolution and rate of absorption (including coadministration with food), metabolism in the intestinal wall or liver before systemic circulation, and concurrent medications (impacting absorption or metabolism).[6] Intravascular or intracavitary administration of drugs may be employed to achieve a higher drug concentration in the vicinity of the tumor.[7–9] Finally, subcutaneous formulations often deliver comparable exposure to intravenous administration, as demonstrated with trastuzumab in breast cancer.[10]

Holland-Frei Cancer Medicine, Ninth Edition. Edited by Robert C. Bast Jr., Carlo M. Croce, William N. Hait, Waun Ki Hong, Donald W. Kufe, Martine Piccart-Gebhart, Raphael E. Pollock, Ralph R. Weichselbaum, Hongyang Wang, and James F. Holland.
© 2017 John Wiley & Sons, Inc. ISBN: 978-1-118-93469-2

Table 1 Anticancer therapies and their mechanisms of action.

(a) Cytotoxics		
Class of drugs	**Example drug(s)**	**Target/mechanism of action**
Alkylating agents	Cyclophosphamide	Cross-linking of DNA
Platinum agents	Cisplatin, carboplatin, oxaliplatin	Cross-linking of DNA
Antibiotics	Doxorubicin	Inhibits topoisomerase II; stabilizes topoisomerase II-DNA complex
Antimetabolites	Antifolates: methotrexate	Interference with the incorporation of nucleotides into DNA
	Pyrimidine analogs: 5-fluorouracil	
	Purine analogs: 6-mercaptopurine	
Tubulin-binding agents	Taxanes: paclitaxel	Enhance or inhibit tubulin polymerization
	Vinca alkaloids: vincristine	
	eribulin, ixabepilone	
Camptothecins	Irinotecan	Stabilizes topoisomerase I DNA to induce DNA strand breaks
(b) Biologics		
Class of drugs	**Example drug(s)**	**Target/mechanism of action**
Monoclonal antibodies	Anti-CD20: rituximab	Binding to cell surface receptor or ligand to block signal transduction and enhance antibody-dependent cellular cytotoxicity
	Anti-HER2: trastuzumab	
	Anti-EGFR: cetuximab, panitumumab	
	Anti-PD-1: pembrolizumab, nivolumab	
	Anti-VEGF: bevacizumab	
Antibody-drug conjugates	Trastuzumab emtansine	Binds to HER2 to deliver a tubulin-binding agent to cells
Protein-based	Ziv-aflibercept	Binds to VEGF-A, -B, -C
Cytokines	IL-2, interferon-alpha	Immune system activation
Autologous cellular immunotherapy	Sipuleucel-T	Sensitizes the immune system to prostate cancer antigens
(c) Small molecule non-cyotoxics		
Target/mechanism of action	**Example drug(s)**	
EGFR inhibitor	Erlotinib, afatinib	
HER2 inhibitor	Lapatinib	
ALK inhibitor	Crizotinib, ceritinib	
VEGFR2 inhibitor	Sorafenib, sunitinib, pazopanib	
BRAF inhibitor	Vemurafenib, dabrafenib	
MEK inhibitor	Trametinib	
mTOR inhibitor	Everolimus, temsirolimus	
BCR-ABL inhibitor	Imatinib, nilotinib	
KIT inhibitor	Imatinib, sunitinib, regorafenib	
PARP inhibitor	Olaparib	
ER antagonist	Tamoxifen, fulvestrant	
Aromatase inhibitor	Anastrazole, letrozole, exemestane	
AR antagonist	Flutamide, bicalutamide, enzalutamide	
CYP17A1 inhibitor	Abiraterone	
Proteasome inhibitor	Bortezomib, carfilzomib	
Bruton's tyrosine kinase inhibitor	Ibrutinib	

This is intended to be an illustrative rather than a comprehensive list.

General clinical pharmacology

What are the design features of the clinical pharmacology and clinical studies used to support dosing or claims?

The optimal dosing strategy for an anticancer therapy is the one that maximizes efficacy, minimizes severe toxicity, and minimizes pharmacokinetic variability between patients. With few exceptions, cytotoxic therapies are typically dosed by body surface area for historical reasons, even though height and weight are only two of the many variables that influence pharmacokinetic variability.[11] Biologics have typically been dosed by weight, while small molecule non-cytotoxics have typically been assigned a fixed dose for all patients. Because it was assumed that a higher dose of a drug would lead to greater efficacy, traditional phase I trials sought to determine the maximum tolerated dose (MTD), defined as the dose immediately below that which caused a prespecified rate of dose-limiting toxicity in a dose-escalation design.[12]

It is increasingly recognized that the conventional paradigm for dosing of anticancer therapy is suboptimal for two reasons. First, it does not evaluate the sources of interpatient variability in response and/or toxicity, and as such does not

facilitate individualized dosing. Second, many biologics and small molecule non-cytotoxics may achieve maximum efficacy at a dose lower than the MTD because of either saturable bioavailability or a saturable effect on the targeted signaling pathway.[13,14] A number of recently approved anticancer therapies have required evaluation of alternative doses in postmarketing trials, whereas the ideal approach would be to conduct randomized dose-comparison studies with pharmacokinetic sampling and exposure-response analyses in the premarketing setting.[15]

What is the basis for selecting the response endpoints (i.e., clinical or surrogate endpoints) or biomarkers (collectively called pharmacodynamics) and how are they measured in clinical pharmacology and clinical studies?

The conventional response endpoints in trials of anticancer therapy are overall survival (OS), progression-free survival (PFS; defined as time to death or disease progression, whichever comes first), or objective response rate, with response defined as ≥30% reduction in the sum of the longest diameters of target lesions as defined by the response evaluation criteria in solid tumors (RECIST).[16] Although there are a number of limitations to RECIST as a method for evaluating drug effect, it remains the most commonly used approach.[17] Recommendations from the National Cancer Institute's Investigational Drug Steering Committee (IDSC) exist regarding the selection of endpoints for phase II trials of anticancer therapies and regarding the use of biomarkers in early clinical trials of novel anticancer therapies.[18,19]

Are the active moieties in the plasma (or other biological fluid) appropriately identified and measured to assess pharmacokinetic parameters and exposure–response relationships?

Many anticancer therapies require activation before they are able to have their anticancer effect, with an activation process involving chemical or enzymatic reactions in normal or tumor tissues. In most cases, the activation process happens intracellularly, such that the active moieties cannot be measured in the plasma. Cisplatin, for example, undergoes a chemical reaction with water molecules intracellularly, resulting in the generation of a positively charged aquated species that attacks nucleophilic sites on DNA.[20] Antimetabolites such as gemcitabine, 5-fluorouracil, and methotrexate undergo intracellular phosphorylation, phosphoribosylation, and polyglutamylation, respectively, to have and/or maximize their effects.[21–23] On the other hand, some anticancer therapies are activated primarily in the liver, such that active moieties can and should be measured in the plasma in order to explore valid exposure–response relationships. One example is the topoisomerase-interacting agent irinotecan, which is converted by liver carboxylesterase into SN-38, an active moiety that is released into the systemic circulation and exposure to which predicts severe toxicity from irinotecan.[24]

Exposure–response

What are the characteristics of the exposure–response relationships for efficacy?

The results of treatment with an anticancer therapy depend on both pharmacokinetics and pharmacodynamics. Pharmacokinetics refers to the relationship between dose and concentration, whereas pharmacodynamics refers to the relationship between concentration (or exposure) and "response," with response broadly defined as any measurable effect of the drug related to efficacy, toxicity, or neither. Exposure–response relationships help to define the target exposure range at which the drug is effective without causing severe toxicity (often referred to as the therapeutic index). Many anticancer therapies have a narrow therapeutic index.

In general, any drug may be considered to have a maximal effect and a median dose (the dose required for 50% of the maximal effect). Wagner proposed a generalized sigmoidal model of drug effect (Figure 1), based on the hypothesis that all drug effects require an initial interaction with a receptor.[25] Pharmacodynamic models are generally different for agents that only work during certain phases of the cell cycle (phase-specific agents) compared with agents that work during any phase of the cell cycle (nonphase-specific agents). For nonphase-specific agents, such as cyclophosphamide and other alkylating agents, a simple log-linear model can be used as follows:

$$\text{Survival fraction} = \text{No. of treated cells/No. of control cells} = e^{-KC}$$
(1)

This model has a steep exposure–response curve, as the effect continues to increase proportionally as the concentration (C) increases. For any K (in Equation 1), an increase in C by $2.3/K$ will result in a 1-log increase in antitumor effect (Figure 2a).[26,27]

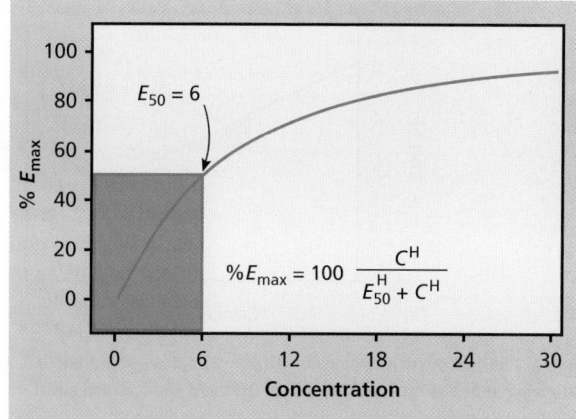

Figure 1 Example of E_{max} model as proposed by Wagner. The maximum effect is 100%, and a concentration of six results in 50% effect. The exponent H, also known as the Hill constant, determines the shape of the curve and is usually between 1 and 2.

For phase-specific agents, such as the antimetabolites, the exposure–response relationships are much more complicated. By definition, some cells are out of phase and therefore not sensitive (or relatively insensitive) to the effects of the drug during the period of drug exposure. This cannot be overcome by increasing the dose, but can potentially be overcome by increasing the duration of drug exposure.[28] The result is the appearance of a plateau in the exposure–response curve (Figure 2b). To further complicate matters, plasma concentrations may be an inadequate predictor of clinical effect for those agents that undergo intracellular anabolism to active metabolites, as is the case for cytarabine and many other antimetabolites.[29]

Trastuzumab emtansine (T-DM1), an antibody-drug conjugate consisting of a recombinant humanized monoclonal antibody targeting the extracellular domain of HER2 linked to a microtubule-stabilizing agent, is a recent example of a drug for which the exposure–response relationship for efficacy has been well studied. In the case of T-DM1 for the treatment of HER2-positive metastatic breast cancer, higher trough concentrations on day 21 of cycle 1 are associated with improved OS and PFS after adjusting for baseline risk factors. In fact, patients with exposures below the median level had OS and PFS comparable to the active control arm of lapatinib plus capecitabine, suggesting that dose escalation might improve efficacy for this subset of patients.[30] Relationships between exposure and efficacy have also been found for a number of other anticancer therapies that are summarized with references in Table 2. Although still controversial, therapeutic drug monitoring has been suggested for many kinase inhibitors on the basis of these exposure–efficacy relationships.[43]

What are the characteristics of the exposure–response relationships for safety?

Exposure–response relationships for safety are analogous to those for efficacy, except that the phenotypes of interest are potentially severe toxicities of the drug rather than efficacy measures. Many historical examples with cytotoxic therapies highlight the value of elucidating such relationships. The relationship between toxicity subsequent to high-dose methotrexate and that of delayed methotrexate clearance has led to the routine use of therapeutic drug monitoring of plasma methotrexate concentrations to guide leucovorin dosing.[44] The relationship between paclitaxel and neutropenia (generalizable to other cytotoxic therapies) is

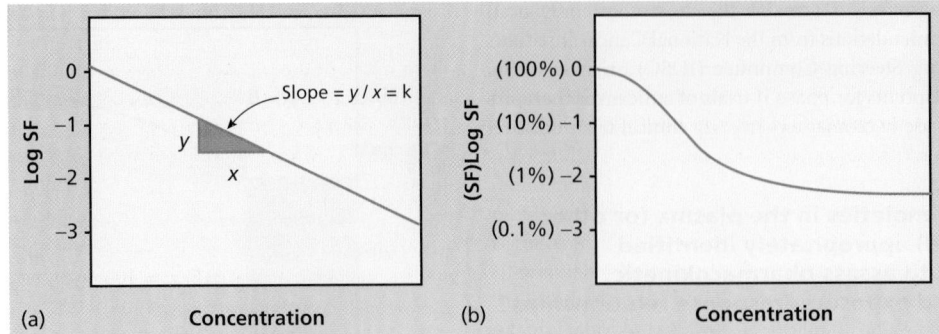

Figure 2 Pharmacodynamic plots for drugs with (a) nonsaturable and (b) saturable effects. In the simplest pharmacodynamic model (a), there is a linear relationship between dose and log kill. In (b) there is a maximal effect, resulting in a plateau in the dose-response curve. *Abbreviation:* SF, survival fraction.

Table 2 Anticancer therapies (in alphabetical order) for which a relationship between exposure and efficacy has been established, including the disease context and reference.

Drug	Disease	References
Axitinib	Renal cell carcinoma	Rini et al.[31]
Busulfan	Allogeneic bone marrow transplantation	Bleyzac et al.[32]
Carboplatin	Ovarian cancer	Jodrell et al.[33]
Dasatinib	Chronic myeloid leukemia	Wang et al.[34]
Erlotinib	Non-small cell lung cancer	Tiseo et al.[35]
5-Fluorouracil	Head and neck cancer	Milano et al.[36]
Imatinib	Chronic myeloid leukemia gastrointestinal stromal tumor (GIST)	Larson et al.[37] Demetri et al.[38]
Methotrexate	Acute lymphoblastic leukemia	Evans et al.[39]
Omacetaxine	Chronic myeloid leukemia	FDA review[a]
Pazopanib	Renal cell carcinoma	Suttle et al.[40]
Sunitinib	Renal cell carcinoma, GIST	Houk et al.[41]
Trastuzumab	Gastric/gastroesophageal cancer	Cosson et al.[42]
Trastuzumab emtansine	HER2-positive breast cancer	Wang et al.[30]
Vemurafenib	Melanoma	FDA review[b]

This is intended to be an illustrative rather than a comprehensive list.

[a] http://www.accessdata.fda.gov/drugsatfda_docs/nda/2012/203585Orig1s000ClinPharmR.pdf

[b] http://www.accessdata.fda.gov/drugsatfda_docs/nda/2011/202429Orig1s000ClinPharmR.pdf

best described using nonlinear models that allow for an indirect effect of plasma concentration on bone marrow suppression, and these types of models have informed the optimization of the dose and schedule for many drugs.[45,46] Another example of a drug with a very well-characterized exposure–response relationship for safety is carboplatin, an analogue of cisplatin. Unlike cisplatin, the dose-limiting toxicity of carboplatin is thrombocytopenia, which is a function of drug dose, renal function, pretreatment platelet count, and prior therapy.[47] The platelet nadir produced by a dose of carboplatin is related to the carboplatin clearance, which is directly proportional to creatinine clearance. Thus, patients at high risk of severe thrombocytopenia following carboplatin therapy can be identified prospectively, and the drug doses can be modified by monitoring creatinine clearance. Although many attempts have been made to avoid severe toxicities of cytotoxic therapies by monitoring plasma drug concentrations during treatment, these attempts have generally not led to changes in clinical practice.

Vemurafenib, an oral small molecule inhibitor of the BRAF kinase harboring the V600E or V600K mutations in patients with metastatic melanoma, provides a more recent example of a drug with a well-established exposure–response relationship for safety in addition to an exposure–response relationship for efficacy. (Of note, although the FDA label indicates that the drug may be administered with or without food, exposure is increased when the drug is taken with food.) When exposure is measured by trough concentration at steady state, there is an increased probability of squamous cell carcinoma (SCC; a well-known, treatment-related adverse effect)

with increasing exposure in a logistic regression model ($p < 0.0001$) (http://www.accessdata.fda.gov/drugsatfda_docs/nda/2011/202429 Orig1s000ClinPharmR.pdf). Despite this clear relationship, dose reductions for SCC events are not recommended because the survival benefits outweigh this safety risk.

Does this drug prolong the QT or QTc interval?

Many drugs prolong the QT interval by delaying depolarization and repolarization of the ventricles in the heart. The QT interval is corrected for the heart rate by one of two accepted formulas to calculate the heart-rate corrected QT (QTc) interval. QTc prolongation is associated with a higher incidence of ventricular tachyarrhythmias (particularly torsade de pointes) that can potentially lead to sudden cardiac death. As an increased risk of sudden cardiac death is a major safety issue, FDA and other regulatory authorities require that sponsors adequately assess this risk during clinical development of a new drug. In 2005, international guidelines were developed to guide the design and data interpretation of thorough QT studies, and these guidelines were circulated by FDA in a Guidance to Industry (Guidance for Industry: E14 Clinical Evaluation of QT/QTc Interval Prolongation and Proarrhythmic Potential for Non-Antiarrhythmic Drugs. FDA, October 2005). In this guidance document, FDA recommends that the ΔΔQTc (change in QTc compared to baseline, corrected for placebo effect) be used as the endpoint for thorough QT studies, and that the upper bound of the one-sided 95% CI (identical to the upper bound of a two-sided 90% CI) of the largest time-matched mean effect of the drug on the QTc interval should exclude 10 ms in order to conclude that there is no significant safety risk related to QTc prolongation.

Nilotinib is an oral small molecule inhibitor of BCR-ABL and other kinases that is used in the treatment of chronic myeloid leukemia (CML). A thorough QT study in healthy volunteers, in accordance with the E14 guidance, was conducted and demonstrated a clear relationship between steady-state concentration and $\Delta\Delta$QTc, while concentrations in that study were lower than concentrations that can be expected with the approved therapeutic dose in cancer patients (http://www.accessdata.fda.gov/drugsatfda_docs/nda/2007/022068s000_ClinPharmR.pdf). As a result, it is recommended that the drug not be used in patients with hypokalemia, hypomagnesemia, or long QT syndrome who would be at especially high risk for QTc prolongation leading to sudden cardiac death. Furthermore, the FDA required that the sponsor initiate a Risk Evaluation and Mitigation Strategy (REMS) to "minimize the risk of QT prolongation and its potential cardiac sequelae" (http://www.accessdata.fda.gov/drugsatfda_docs/label/2010/022068s001rems.pdf). As part of the REMS and also in a "black box" warning on the drug label, prescribers and patients are cautioned to avoid concomitant use of drugs known to prolong the QT interval as well as CYP3A4 inhibitors and food, both of which are expected to substantially increase exposure to the drug. ECG (electrocardiogram) monitoring is recommended at baseline, 1 week after starting therapy, and periodically thereafter, including after any dose adjustments (Tasigna prescribing information, http://www.accessdata.fda.gov/drugsatfda_docs/label/2007/022068lbl.pdf).

Is the dose and dosing regimen selected by the sponsor consistent with the known relationship among dose, concentration, and response, and are there any unresolved dosing or administration issues?

While the dose and schedule for most anticancer therapies are selected on the basis of dose–concentration–response relationship, there are some for which there are unresolved dosing issues. One example is omacetaxine, a protein synthesis inhibitor that is approved for use in CML after resistance and/or intolerance of two or more tyrosine kinase inhibitors. Although the drug is labeled to be prescribed at an induction and maintenance dose of 1.25 mg/m² because this is the dose that was used in the pivotal study, the reviewers found no evidence of a correlation between clearance of the drug and BSA. As a result, BSA-based dosing results in lower concentrations in patients with smaller body size, such as women, which was associated with a decrease in efficacy (http://www.accessdata.fda.gov/drugsatfda_docs/nda/2012/203585Orig1s000ClinPharmR.pdf). Another example is cabazitaxel, a microtubule-stabilizing agent that is approved for use in hormone-refractory metastatic prostate cancer after previous therapy with docetaxel. In a phase II trial in advanced breast cancer, the initial dose was 20 mg/m² every 3 weeks, and dose escalation to 25 mg/m² was allowed if no grade > 2 toxicity was observed in cycle 1. Even though only 21 of 71 patients could be escalated in cycle 2, the sponsor chose 25 mg/m² every 3 weeks as the dose for the pivotal phase III trial in prostate cancer. On the basis of the available data, there is no clear exposure–response relationship for efficacy but there is a relationship between AUC and probability of grade 3+ neutropenia, suggesting that some patients could avoid the need for dose reduction and growth factor support by starting at a lower initial dose (http://www.accessdata.fda.gov/drugsatfda_docs/nda/2010/201023s000ClinPharmR.pdf). Finally, correct dosing can often be an issue when a drug is studied in a new disease and gets approved for

a new indication. In the case of trastuzumab, the approved dose for breast cancer was used in the randomized phase III trial that demonstrated the efficacy of trastuzumab in combination with chemotherapy compared to chemotherapy alone for metastatic HER2-positive gastric/gastroesophageal junction (GEJ) cancer.[48] Subsequently, a case report and review of pharmacokinetic data from the sponsor have suggested that clearance of the drug is ~70% higher in patients with gastric cancer than in those with breast cancer.[49] One possible explanation is that patients with metastatic gastric cancer have higher tumor burden and higher levels of circulating HER2 extracellular domains, resulting in higher clearance of the drug. Another possibility is that patients with gastric cancer may have lower albumin concentrations, leading to higher clearance of the drug. Standard dose versus higher dose trastuzumab is currently being explored in a randomized phase III trial in patients with HER2-positive metastatic gastric/GEJ cancer (HELOISE study; NCT01450696).

What are the pharmacokinetic characteristics of the drug and its major metabolite?

What are the single-dose and multiple-dose pharmacokinetic parameters?

Pharmacokinetics is the study of drug absorption, distribution, metabolism, and excretion. A fundamental concept in pharmacokinetics is drug clearance, that is, elimination of the drug from the body, analogous to the concept of creatinine clearance. In clinical practice, clearance of a drug is rarely measured directly but is calculated as either of the following:

$$\text{Clearance} = \text{Dose}/\text{AUC} \tag{2}$$

$$\text{Clearance} = \text{Infusion rate}/C_{ss} \tag{3}$$

The AUC represents the total drug exposure integrated over time and is an important parameter for both pharmacokinetic and pharmacodynamic analyses. As indicated in Equation 2, the clearance is simply the ratio of the dose to the AUC, so that the higher the AUC for a given dose is, the lower will be the clearance. If a drug is administered by continuous infusion and a steady state is achieved, the clearance can be estimated from a single measurement of the plasma drug concentration (C_{ss}) as in Equation 3.

Clearance can conceptually be considered to be a function of both distribution and elimination. In the simplest pharmacokinetic model,

$$\text{Clearance} = VK \tag{4}$$

where V is the volume of distribution and K is the elimination constant. V is the volume of fluid in which the dose is initially diluted, and thus the higher the V is, the lower will be the initial concentration. K is the elimination constant, which is inversely proportional to the half-life, the period of time that must elapse to reach a 50% decrease in plasma concentration. When the half-life is short, K is high and plasma concentrations decline rapidly. Thus, both a high V and a high K result in high clearance and relatively low plasma concentrations.

In most phase I trials of anticancer therapy, pharmacokinetic sampling is done at multiple time points after the first dose of drug administration and is repeated again after multiple doses of drug administration, the latter of which may or may not correspond to steady state. For single-dose sampling, parameters that are presented typically include the maximum concentration observed

(C_{max}), the time at maximum concentration (T_{max}), AUC, V, clearance, and the half-life. For multiple-dose sampling, parameters are generally the same except for the potential addition of the minimum concentration (C_{min}) before a dose. Pharmacokinetic parameters can be described by one of two methods. The first is noncompartmental analysis, a two-step process in which parameters such as C_{max} and AUC are estimated for each patient and summary statistics are calculated for the population. Noncompartmental analysis can be done quickly and does not require special software. The second is population pharmacokinetic modeling, a one-step process in which parameters are estimated for the population of patients by developing a nonlinear mixed effects model with one or more compartments. Population pharmacokinetic modeling has several advantages: (1) it can be done with sparse (fewer time points) sampling data; (2) it is less susceptible to missing data; and (3) it can easily include covariates that minimize the between patient variability. A disadvantage is that it requires special software and training.[50] The interested reader is likely to benefit from hands on experience with such software. Several caveats need to be emphasized for the casual reader. The validity of pharmacokinetic modeling depends to a large extent on the quality of the data that are used to develop the model. Thus, drug infusions must be precisely timed, a sufficient number of plasma samples must be drawn, the samples must be obtained on schedule, and analytic methods must be sensitive and specific. The data must be properly weighted to avoid bias due to the increased probability of analytic errors at drug concentrations near the detection limit of the assay. Results obtained using a specific model should be compared with those using noncompartmental analysis. Extrapolation of models outside the known time points must be done with great caution.

What are the characteristics of drug absorption?
Variability in absorption is a major source of interpatient variability in pharmacokinetics. The rate and extent of drug absorption depends on its solubility and permeability across the mucosal lining of the intestine. In pharmacokinetic models, absorption is typically estimated by a first-order rate constant, K_a. Absorption may be saturable, meaning that higher doses do not lead to higher exposure above a certain threshold dose. BCS class 1 drugs with high permeability/high solubility are absorbed quickly and extensively, whereas drugs in BCS classes 2–4 have variable absorption and may be influenced by a number of factors. For example, many small molecule tyrosine kinase inhibitors have their absorption limited by membrane efflux transporters such as P-glycoprotein (also known as ABCB1), breast cancer resistance protein (ABCG2), and members of the multi-drug resistance protein family (ABCC family), the same transporters that may be overexpressed in cancer cells as a resistance mechanism.[51] Prandial conditions are also very important, as a number of oral anticancer therapies have enhanced absorption leading to increased exposure (and potentially increased toxicity) when coadministered with food, particularly a high-fat meal. Examples include erlotinib, lapatinib, nilotinib, pazopanib, vemurafenib, and abiraterone, the last of which can have a 10-fold increase in AUC with a high fat meal (compared to an overnight fast).[52–54] These oral anticancer therapies are generally labeled to be taken fasting despite the fact that exposure is increased with food, in contrast to the typical approach for noncancer therapies; theoretically increasing the risks of the drug if patient adherence to labeling is suboptimal.[53,55] Finally, a number of oral anticancer therapies are weak bases that have pH-dependent solubility and may have their absorption decreased by concomitant use of proton-pump inhibitors or other acid-reducing agents that are frequently prescribed and/or used over-the-counter. Examples of therapies with

clinically significant decreases in exposure when coadministered with acid-reducing agents include dasatinib, erlotinib, gefitinib, and nilotinib.[56] When these kinase inhibitors are prescribed, patients should be instructed to abstain from the use of acid-reducing agents that might compromise the efficacy of these drugs.

What are the characteristics of drug distribution?
In pharmacokinetic models, there is a volume of distribution for each compartment in the model. Distribution is impacted by a number of factors, most notably water solubility and protein binding. Hydrophilic compounds, such as methotrexate, can distribute into fluid collections (such as pleural effusions or ascites) and significantly delay clearance of the drug from the central (plasma) compartment.[57] On the other hand, pegylated liposomal doxorubicin is an example of a drug that has been engineered to be hydrophobic. Compared to free doxorubicin, its volume of distribution is very small and is mostly restricted to the intravascular compartment because the tight junctions of endothelial cells in blood vessels prevent extravasation of the liposomes, a fact that likely explains its reduced cardiotoxicity.[58] Protein binding is very important because only unbound drug can reach the target site and be eliminated. Vismodegib is an example of a drug that has high-affinity reversible binding to alpha-1-acid glycoprotein (AAG) and albumin, resulting in plasma levels of unbound drug that are <1% of total drug levels and contributing to low clearance of the drug. AAG levels account for approximately 70% of the pharmacokinetic variability between patients, suggesting that this is the single most important factor influencing the pharamacokinetics of the drug.[59] Concomitant drugs or disease states (e.g., hypoproteinemia) might increase the fraction of unbound drug but the clinical significance of this remains unclear for vismodegib and most other drugs.[60]

Does the mass balance study suggest renal or hepatic as the major route of elimination?
Mass balance studies involve the administration of radiolabeled drug to humans. Radioactivity is measured at different time points in the blood, urine, and feces, in order to understand to what extent hepatic metabolism, biliary excretion, and urinary excretion are contributing to elimination. The biological specimens are also used to identify and quantify the parent drug and its metabolites.[61] FDA guidance recommends that any metabolite whose exposure exceeds 10% of the parent AUC at steady state should be evaluated in a preclinical animal model for toxicology (http://www.fda.gov/OHRMS/DOCKETS/98fr/FDA-2008-D-0065-GDL.pdf).

There are many examples of anticancer therapies that are eliminated primarily by renal or hepatic routes. Carboplatin and methotrexate are examples of drugs that are predominantly excreted unchanged in the kidney. This is relevant to carboplatin dosing, which is calculated by a simple formula based on renal function, as shown in Equation 5.[62]

$$\text{Dose(mg)} = (\text{Target AUC}) \times (\text{GFR} + 25) \qquad (5)$$

As for methotrexate, its urinary excretion can result in precipitation in renal tubules and resulting nephrotoxicity. It has been shown that nephrotoxicity and other toxicities can be prevented after the administration of high-dose methotrexate by urinary alkalinization, as the drug is significantly more soluble at a higher pH.[63,64] On the other hand, all of the taxanes (including paclitaxel, nab-paclitaxel, docetaxel, and cabazitaxel) undergo extensive hepatic metabolism and biliary excretion, resulting in the need for dose adjustment in patients with hepatic dysfunction.[65] Well-conducted organ dysfunction studies are necessary to guide selection of the most appropriate dose/schedule of anticancer therapies in patients with compromised renal and/or hepatic function. Ideally, these would be done before marketing the drug, but imatinib and sorafenib are examples for which these studies were done in the post-marketing setting.[66,67]

What are the characteristics of drug metabolism?

If it is determined by a mass balance study that a drug undergoes significant metabolism, then a number of follow-up questions need to be addressed. The hepatic extraction ratio, which varies between 0 and 1, is roughly a measure of the liver's efficiency for eliminating drug from the systemic circulation during a single pass through the liver. Drugs with a low (<0.3) extraction ratio will not have their clearance influenced by hepatic blood flow but will have their clearance correlated with plasma protein binding. On the other hand, drugs with a high (>0.7) extraction ratio will have their clearance correlated with hepatic blood flow but will not have their clearance influenced by plasma protein binding. The concept of using floxuridine rather than 5-FU for the hepatic arterial infusion of chemotherapy for liver metastases is based on the fact that floxuridine has a higher hepatic extraction ratio, allowing high doses to be administered locally to the tumors without excessive systemic toxicity.[68] The enzymes responsible for metabolism fall into one of three phases of metabolism: modification (phase I), conjugation (phase II), or excretion (phase III). Phase I reactions include oxidation, reduction, and hydrolysis, and are typically catalyzed by cytochrome P450 enzymes that are abundant in liver microsomes. In phase II reactions, the activated metabolites of phase I reactions are conjugated with charged species to make them more hydrophilic. Finally, in phase III reactions, members of the ATP-binding cassette (ABC) family of transporters remove phase II products to the extracellular medium. For example, irinotecan is first activated by carboxylesterase (phase I) to its active metabolite SN-38 and by CYP3A4 to the inactive metabolite aminopentane carboxylic (APC) acid. SN-38 is then glucuronidated by UDP glucuronosyltransferase 1 polypeptide A1 (UGT1A1; phase II) to SN-38-glucuronide (SN-38-G). SN-38-G is excreted into bile by the ABCC2 transporter (phase III).[69] In the case of irinotecan, the parent drug and these three metabolites (APC, SN-38, and SN-38-G) accounted for 93% of the mean radiochemical AUC in the mass balance study, indicating that these are the metabolic enzymes of interest.[70] Enzymes responsible for drug metabolism are often first identified using *in vitro* studies in human liver microsomes or human hepatocytes, followed by *in vivo* studies in animals and finally *in vivo* studies in humans. Liquid chromatography-mass spectrometry (LC-MS) technology is now widely used to identify and measure metabolites in drug metabolism studies.[71]

What are the characteristics of drug excretion?

The characteristics of drug excretion include not only whether the drug is eliminated primarily by biliary or renal excretion but the specific metabolites that are eliminated and the transporters that are involved in their excretion. While excretion is straightforward in some cases, in other cases, it can be quite complicated. Irinotecan again serves as an instructive example. After SN-38-G is excreted in bile, intestinal bacteria such as *Escherichia coli* can convert the compound back to the active metabolite SN-38 by producing the enzyme β-glucuronidase, and this SN-38 can be reabsorbed and returned to the liver in a phenomenon known as enterohepatic recirculation.[69] In fact, a pharmacokinetic model for SN-38 after irinotecan dosing required inclusion of enterohepatic recirculation

in order to accurately describe the observed data.[72] Cisplatin provides another example of complicated excretion, as it is known to be both actively secreted and reabsorbed in the renal tubules.[73,74]

On the basis of pharmacokinetic parameters, what is the degree of linearity or nonlinearity in the dose–concentration relationship?

The key feature of a linear pharmacokinetic model is that

$$dC/dt = -KC \tag{6}$$

This indicates that the instantaneous rate of change in drug concentration depends only on the current concentration. The clearance and half-life will remain constant no matter how high the concentration is. One implication of this principle is that the AUC is not affected by changes in drug schedule. For example, the AUC after a 60 mg/m^2 bolus dose of doxorubicin equals the total AUC for 3 daily (or weekly) bolus doses of 20 mg/m^2, which equals the AUC for the same dose administered as a 96-h infusion. A second implication is that the AUC is proportional to the dose. Thus, if one measures the AUC for a 60 mg/m^2 dose, one can estimate the AUC for a 90 mg/m^2 dose in the same patient as being 50% greater. A simple graph of dose versus AUC in a dose-ranging study can be used to determine whether or not a drug has linear pharmacokinetics.

The simplest linear pharmacokinetic model, shown graphically in Figure 3, is

$$C(t) = \frac{\text{Dose}}{V}(e^{-kt}) \tag{7}$$

This model assumes that the drug is administered as an instantaneous bolus and that complete distribution of the drug is also instantaneous. These assumptions are often not valid. If the drug is administered as a slow bolus or infusion, the model must be corrected for the infusion duration (T). During the administration of the drug, the concentration is increasing:

$$C(t) = \frac{\text{Dose}}{VKT}(1 - e^{-kt}) \tag{8}$$

After the infusion is terminated, the drug concentration decays at the same rate as if it had been administered as an instantaneous bolus. Thus, if T represents the infusion time, then the post-infusion drug concentrations can be represented as

$$C'(t) = C(T)e^{-k(t-T)} \tag{9}$$

Often, the pharmacokinetic data are more complex than those shown in Figure 3 and may be optimally fitted to a multi-compartment model, usually two or three compartments (Figure 4). It must be emphasized that the compartments are theoretical and do not necessarily correlate with any anatomic space or physiologic process.

The presence of nonlinear pharmacokinetics implies that some aspect of the pharmacokinetic behavior of the drug is saturable. The mathematics of nonlinear models is beyond the scope of this chapter, but the principles are very relevant to several anticancer agents.[75,76] In contrast to the administration schedule of drugs with linear pharmacokinetics, alteration of the administration schedule of drugs that display nonlinear kinetics may markedly affect the AUC and potentially alter clinical effects.

Nonlinear pharmacokinetic behavior commonly occurs when there is saturation of a major metabolic or transport pathway. This results in decreased clearance at higher doses, with a greater than proportional increase in the AUC. The AUC will also increase if the

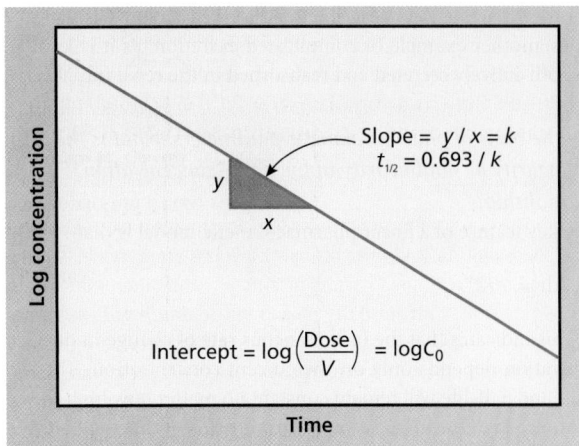

Figure 3 Concentration-time plot for 1-compartment linear pharmacokinetic model. C_0 represents the initial concentration, assuming instantaneous administration and distribution. The half-life is $\log_e(2)/k$. *Abbreviation: V*, volume of distribution.

infusion duration is shortened because of slower clearance at the higher peak plasma concentrations. This is clearly the case for 5-FU, probably because of saturation of its conversion to dihydrofluorouracil by the enzyme dihydropyrimidine dehydrogenase.[77-79] As 5-FU is used on a variety of schedules, its nonlinear pharmacokinetic behavior may be one factor in its highly schedule-dependent effects. Paclitaxel has also been demonstrated to have nonlinear pharmacokinetics, owing to its formulation.[80-82] Thus, the AUC is higher, for a fixed dose, when administered by a shorter (3-h vs 24-h) infusion schedule, although this does not result in enhanced toxicity.[83]

The opposite situation arises when a drug's absorption from the gastrointestinal tract (or renal tubular reabsorption) is saturable. In this case, an increase in dose results in a less than proportional increase in the AUC. Gastrointestinal absorption of drugs that resemble natural compounds is frequently mediated by active transport processes that display saturable kinetics. Folate analogues such as methotrexate or leucovorin and amino acid analogues such as melphalan are examples of drugs with saturable absorption.[84-86] Cisplatin appears to have nonlinear pharmacokinetics owing to the saturation of its renal tubular reabsorption.[74,87] Free plasma platinum is increased by 42% when the drug is given as a 24-h continuous infusion, rather than as a 20-min infusion.[87]

How do the pharmacokinetic parameters change with time following chronic dosing?

Steady state occurs when the rate of drug administration is equal to the rate of drug elimination. The accumulation ratio relates the exposure (measured by C_{max}, AUC, or C_{min}) at steady state to the exposure after a single dose, and is inversely related to the dosing interval. Although this ratio can be predicted using single-dose pharmacokinetic parameters, it is more accurate to measure the ratio directly using observed data. For drugs with one compartment pharmacokinetics, the time to steady state is directly proportional to the half-life and is independent of the dose and dosing interval. In practice, steady state is generally assumed to be reached in 4–5 half lives. The plasma concentration at steady state (C_p^{ss}) can be estimated as,

$$C_p^{ss} = S \times F \times D/\text{CL} \times \tau \tag{10}$$

where S is the salt factor, F is the bioavailability, D is the dose, CL is clearance, and τ is the dosing interval. Nonadherence to medication can decrease the C_p^{ss} over time, whereas drug–drug interactions and prandial conditions can either increase or decrease the C_p^{ss} over time. There are specific examples of anticancer therapies that are susceptible to changes in C_p^{ss} over time. For example, cyclophosphamide autoinduction of CYP450 enzymes involved in its metabolism resulted in an approximate doubling of CL by the end of a 96-h infusion.[88] Although the mechanism remains unclear, a prospective study in patients with gastrointestinal stomal tumors demonstrated that imatinib exposure decreased by approximately 30% over the first 90 days of therapy before stabilizing.[89] Therapeutic drug monitoring is a consideration in the case of drugs such as imatinib with an established exposure–response relationship and changes in exposure over time with chronic dosing.

What is the inter- and intra-subject variability of pharmacokinetic parameters in volunteers and patients, and what are the major causes of variability?

Interpatient variability of pharmacokinetic parameters is potentially of great importance for optimizing anticancer therapy. The extent of variability in a parameter is usually presented as a coefficient of variation (ratio of standard deviation to the mean). It can be estimated by noncompartmental methods or by a population pharmacokinetic model. Owing to variability in bioavailability, oral agents generally have higher pharmacokinetic variability than intravenous agents.

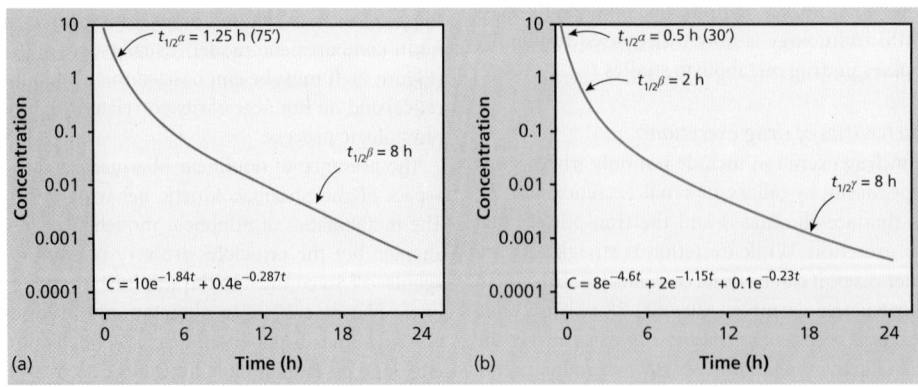

Figure 4 Concentration-time plots for representative 2-compartment (a) and 3-compartment (b) linear pharmacokinetic models. The two curves are very similar, with $C_0 \sim 10$ for both models. Note that for each "compartment" there is one term, and the corresponding half-life equals $t^{1/2} \log_e(2)/k^n$, where k^n is the nth term.

Table 3 Potential sources of interpatient pharmacokinetic variability in cancer patients.

Factors affecting absorption
Nausea/vomiting[a]
Prior surgery, radiotherapy, and/or chemotherapy
Concurrent antiemetics affecting gut motility (e.g., metoclopramide)[a]
Patient adherence[a]
Genetic differences in intestinal drug metabolizing and/or drug transport enzymes
Concomitant medications[a]
Prandial state (for drugs with a significant food effect)[a]
Factors affecting distribution
Weight loss[a]
Obesity
Decreased body fat (lipophilic drugs)[a]
Pleural effusions or ascites (methotrexate)[a]
Factors affecting elimination (metabolism and/or excretion)
Hepatic dysfunction[a]
Renal dysfunction[a]
Genetic differences in drug metabolizing and/or drug transport enzymes
Hypoalbuminemia (for biologics)[a]
Concomitant medications[a]
Factors affecting protein binding
Hypoalbuminemia[a]
Concomitant medications[a]

[a]Potential source of intrapatient pharmacokinetic variability.

For example, in a study of etoposide, the coefficient of variation of the AUC for oral versus intravenous drug was 58% and 28%, respectively.[90]

Table 3 lists the potential sources of interpatient pharmacokinetic variability in cancer patients, many of which are also potential sources of intrapatient pharmacokinetic variability. In a population pharmacokinetic model, the variables in Table 3 can be explored as covariates and included in the model if their inclusion significantly reduces interpatient variability and improves the overall model fit to the observed data. Concomitant medications can explain variability by affecting absorption, elimination, and protein binding. Symptoms that are more commonly encountered in patients than in volunteers, such as nausea/vomiting and weight loss, can contribute to variability in the therapeutic setting. Hypoalbuminemia is commonly encountered in cancer patients and can potentially lead to higher clearance of biologics. For example, a population pharmacokinetic model of trastuzumab in patients with advanced gastric or GEJ cancer found that decreasing serum albumin levels were associated with increased clearance of the drug.[42] Similarly, estimates of bevacizumab clearance in patients with advanced gastric cancer using a previously established population pharmacokinetic model (developed using data from patients with other cancers) were used to demonstrate that clearance of the drug is faster in patients with lower albumin.[91] Prandial state can have a significant impact on both interpatient and intrapatient pharmacokinetic variability. A population pharmacokinetic model of abiraterone demonstrated that higher fat content of food taken with abiraterone decreased its bioavailability, while patients with metastatic castrate-resistant prostate cancer (compared with healthy subjects) had lower clearance of the drug.[92]

Intrapatient pharmacokinetic variability is much more difficult to estimate because it requires repeated pharmacokinetic sampling in the same subjects at later time points. For example, oncologists are commonly faced with the clinical situation of increasing myelosuppression after repetitive dosing. This is generally assumed to be due to the cumulative effects of chemotherapy, making the patient more sensitive to subsequent doses. However, it is also possible that the patient's clearance of the drug(s) may have decreased, resulting in increased drug exposure. Changes in organ function are a major

source of intrasubject pharmacokinetic variability. Renal function may change because of progressive disease (ureteral obstruction), complications of therapy (volume depletion), or as a direct toxic effect of therapy (cisplatin). Similarly, renal function may improve over time, reducing the actual drug exposure. Hepatic function may also change, producing changes in drug clearance that may result in the appearance of increased toxicity over time.

Intrinsic factors

What intrinsic factors (age, gender, race, weight, height, disease, genetic polymorphism, pregnancy, and organ dysfunction) influence exposure and/or response, and what is the impact of any differences in exposure on efficacy or safety responses? On the basis of what is known about exposure–response relationships and their variability and the groups studied, healthy volunteers versus patients versus specific populations, what dosage regimen adjustments, if any, are recommended for each of these groups?

As intrinsic patient factors can influence exposure to an anti-cancer therapy, dose adjustments and/or recommendations to avoid using the drug in certain populations may be necessary if the impact on exposure is significant enough to also impact efficacy or safety responses. For example, 6-mercaptopurine is a drug that is commonly used in the treatment of pediatric acute lymphoblastic leukemia. 6-mercaptopurine, along with its prodrug azathioprine and the purine analog 6-thioguanine, is metabolized primarily by thiopurine S-methyltransferase (TMPT). The *TPMT* gene is subject to a number of polymorphisms that decrease the activity of TMPT, the first of which was identified in 1995.[93] Other polymorphisms have been identified since and there are substantial ethnic differences in the frequencies of these rare variants, but three polymorphisms account for more than 90% of inactivating alleles. As individuals who inherit two inactive *TPMT* alleles (<1% of the population) universally experience severe myelosuppression and a high proportion of those who inherit one inactive allele (~3–14% of the population) experience moderate to severe myelosuppression; the Clinical Pharmacogenetics Implementation Consortium has published guidelines that recommend dose reductions in these patients.[94] Similarly, patients treated with irinotecan who are homozygous for the *UGT1A1*28 polymorphism have higher exposure to SN-38 and are at higher risk for severe neutropenia, suggesting that a dose reduction is necessary in these patients.[24]

In other cases, dose adjustments and/or recommendations to avoid use of the drug may be unnecessary even when such recommendations have made it into the drug label. This is illustrated by the recommended dose reduction for capecitabine in the setting of renal impairment (Xeloda prescribing information, http://www.accessdata.fda.gov/drugsatfda_docs/label/2005/020896s016lbl.pdf). In an editorial regarding this recommendation,[95] Ratain noted that the recommended 25% reduction was for patients with a creatinine clearance of 31–50 mL/min as estimated by the Cockcroft–Gault formula, which has been criticized as inaccurate.[96] This formula estimates a lower creatinine clearance for women and individuals with increased serum creatinine, low weight, and increased age. Furthermore, this definition of renal impairment is not adjusted for BSA. As a result, it is possible that a small woman would receive a dose reduction and a large man would not, even though their BSA-normalized creatinine clearances were the same.

Extrinsic factors

What extrinsic factors (drugs, herbal products, diet, smoking, and alcohol use) influence dose–exposure and/or—response and what is the impact of any differences in exposure on response? On the basis of what is known about exposure–response relationships and their variability, what dosage regimen adjustments, if any, do you recommend for each of these factors?

Drug–drug interactions can compromise efficacy or safety by decreasing or increasing exposure to a drug, respectively, with impact on the associated response. Prescription and over-the-counter drugs are often used concomitantly with anticancer therapy, sometimes without the oncologist being aware of such use. Common mechanisms for drug–drug interactions are induction or inhibition of CYP450 enzymes, and inhibition of the P-glycoprotein transporter. For example, a drug–drug interaction with potential therapeutic implications is that of tamoxifen and selective serotonin reuptake inhibitor (SSRI) antidepressants. Paroxetine, an SSRI that is commonly prescribed for depression or for hot flashes associated with tamoxifen therapy, is a strong inhibitor of the CYP2D6 enzyme that converts tamoxifen into its active metabolite endoxifen.[97] In a prospective clinical trial, 12 women with breast cancer who were taking adjuvant tamoxifen underwent pharmacokinetic sampling before and after 4 weeks of paroxetine coadministration. Endoxifen concentrations decreased by 64% in subjects who were homozygous for the wild-type CYP2D6 allele, but only by 24% in women with a variant CYP2D6 genotype.[98] Similar results were reported in a prospective study of 80 women taking tamoxifen, approximately 30% of whom were taking various SSRIs, after a period of 4 months.[99] Although the precise clinical implications of a decrease in endoxifen concentrations are still under investigation,[100] these data have resulted in recommendations to avoid SSRIs that are potent CYP2D6 inhibitors (such as paroxetine and fluoxetine) in patients treated with tamoxifen owing to concerns about compromising efficacy.[101] The drug label warns prescribers to weigh the benefits for treating vasomotor symptoms against the potential risk of reduced effectiveness of tamoxifen (Brisdelle prescribing information, http://www.accessdata.fda.gov/drugsatfda_docs/label/2013/204516 s000lbl.pdf).

Although anticancer drugs are often administered in combination, there have been relatively few studies to explore the potential pharmacokinetic and/or pharmacodynamic interactions between drugs. For example, with the combination of paclitaxel and cisplatin, an important regimen for ovarian cancer, cisplatin reduces paclitaxel clearance if given first.[102] On the other hand, paclitaxel and carboplatin do not have a pharmacokinetic interaction, but it has been observed that paclitaxel mitigates the thrombocytopenia caused by carboplatin,[103] and a mechanism has been proposed that explains this phenomenon at the level of the megakaryocyte.[104] Another issue with combination therapy is that drugs may be labeled to be coadministered without considering whether they are matched with regard to prandial conditions. For example, capecitabine and lapatinib are used together in the treatment of metastatic breast cancer. Capecitabine is labeled to be taken twice daily with food, whereas lapatinib (which has a significant increase in exposure with food) is labeled to be taken once daily fasting.[105] When possible, it makes sense to match prandial conditions for colabeled drugs, in order to maximize patient adherence to the prescribed dose and schedule for both drugs.

Besides drugs, many other extrinsic factors can influence exposure and response to anticancer therapies. An excellent example is the induction of CYP1A1/1A2 by cigarette smoking and the impact of this factor on exposure to erlotinib in patients with lung cancer. A dose-escalation study of erlotinib in current smokers demonstrated that the MTD was 300 mg daily, and that steady-state trough plasma concentrations and incidence of rash and diarrhea in patients treated at this dose were similar to those in former or never smokers receiving 150 mg daily in previous studies.[106] St. John's wort (*Hypericum perforatum*), a herbal antidepressant commonly used by cancer patients, is a known ligand for the pregnane X receptor (PXR) that can induce the transcription of PXR-regulated genes such as CYP3A and UGTs.[107–110] Concomitant administration of St. John's wort has been demonstrated to significantly decrease exposure to irinotecan, imatinib, and docetaxel.[111–113] The opposite is true for grapefruit juice, which is a potent inhibitor of CYP3A4 and has been demonstrated to increase exposure to sirolimus with the implication that it would likely do the same for other anticancer therapies that are CYP3A4 substrates.[114]

General biopharmaceutics

On the basis of the biopharmaceutics classification system (BCS) principles, in what class is this drug and formulation? What solubility, permeability, and dissolution data support this classification?

As discussed at the beginning of this chapter, the BCS predicts the *in vivo* performance of drugs on the basis of *in vitro* measurements of permeability and solubility, whereas the BDDCS predicts drug disposition and drug–drug interactions in the intestine and liver.[3] BCS class 1 drugs have high solubility and high permeability with rapid dissolution, suggesting that an *in vivo* bioequivalence study is not necessary because they will be absorbed quickly and completely. BCS class 2 drugs have low solubility and high permeability, and many kinase inhibitors fall into this class. BCS class 3 drugs have high solubility and low permeability, whereas BCS class 4 drugs have low solubility and low permeability. BDDCS class 1 drugs have high solubility with transporter effects that are minimal in the gut and liver, implying that they are predominantly eliminated by metabolism. As P-glycoprotein efflux is not a major method of elimination for BDDCS class 1 drugs, these drugs tend to overcome the blood–brain barrier and have good distribution into the brain. BDDCS class 2 drugs have low solubility with efflux transporter effects predominating in the gut and both uptake and efflux transporters affecting the liver. BDDCS class 3 drugs have high solubility with absorptive transporter effects predominating.

What is the effect of food on the bioavailability (BA) of the drug from the dosage form? What dosing recommendation should be made, if any, regarding administration of the product in relation to meals or meal types?

In general, high-fat meals have little to no effect on the extent of absorption of BDDCS class 1 drugs, increase exposure to BDDCS class 2 drugs (such as many kinase inhibitors), and decrease exposure for BDDCS class 3 drugs.[3] Food may affect pharmacokinetics by any number of mechanisms, including delaying gastric emptying, stimulating bile flow, changing the pH of the gastrointestinal tract, increasing splanchnic blood flow, changing intestinal metabolism of a drug, and physically/chemically interacting with the drug or dosage form.[90] In food effect studies, the FDA recommends reporting the ratio of geometric means between groups for exposure parameters such as C_{max} and AUC, along with 90% confidence intervals. Bioequivalence in the fed state is successfully demonstrated if the 90% CI is contained within the range 80–125% while ratios outside of that range would establish a significant food effect (FDA Guidance for Industry entitled "Food Effect Biovailability and Fed Bioequivalence Studies," 2002).

Small molecule non-cytotoxics that have been demonstrated to have an increase in exposure with food include erlotinib, lapatinib, nilotinib, pazopanib, vemurafenib, and abiraterone.[52–54] A recent example of another FDA-approved drug with a significant food effect is ceritinib, the second-generation ALK inhibitor that has demonstrated efficacy in ALK-rearranged non-small cell lung cancer.[115] Ceritinib is a BCS class 4 compound that is a substrate for the apical efflux transporter, P-glycoprotein. In the FDA New Drug Application leading to accelerated approval, the sponsor relied upon pharmacokinetic data for a single 500 mg dose in healthy subjects under fasting, low-fat, or high-fat prandial conditions. The FDA used a pharmacokinetic model to predict the effect of food after multiple doses of ceritinib 750 mg daily and 600 mg daily. At steady state, the model predicted that food increases ceritinib C_{max} and AUC by 68% and 67%, respectively, and that 600 mg daily with food yields comparable exposure to 750 mg daily fasting (http://www.accessdata.fda.gov/drugsatfda_docs/nda/2014/205755 Orig1s000ClinPharmR.pdf). The drug was labeled to be taken fasting at a dose of 750 mg daily because this is the dose that was used in the pivotal trial. FDA has issued a post-marketing requirement to evaluate 450 mg daily with food versus 750 mg daily fasting in patients, and one can presume that evidence of noninferiority of the lower dose would result in a label change.

Conclusions

As illustrated earlier, there are examples from all classes of anticancer therapies that illustrate how an understanding of clinical pharmacology can enhance the therapeutic use of these agents. As the goal is to maximize efficacy while maintaining tolerability, the oncologist needs to understand the basic relationship between dose and exposure (pharmacokinetics), as well as exposure and response (pharmacodynamics) for the population as a whole. The oncologist also needs to understand how and why a certain patient might have a different response than an average patient, and why drug effects may vary over time (interpatient and intrapatient variability). When questions arise, the drug label is a reasonable place to start, but the question-based FDA clinical pharmacology and biopharmaceutics review provides more detailed answers that may be missing from the label. As many new observations about the clinical pharmacology of anticancer therapies are made after drugs are marketed, a current review of the literature is always recommended as well.

Acknowledgments

The authors would like to thank William K. Plunkett Jr., PhD for his contributions to this chapter in previous editions of this book. Some of the key concepts and content from the last edition were carried forward into the current version.

Key references

The complete reference list can be found on the Wiley Companion Digital Edition of this title (see inside front cover for login instructions).

3 Benet LZ. The role of BCS (biopharmaceutics classification system) and BDDCS (biopharmaceutics drug disposition classification system) in drug development. *J Pharm Sci.* 2013;**102**(1):34–42.

6 Stuurman FE, Nuijen B, Beijnen JH, Schellens JH. Oral anticancer drugs: mechanisms of low bioavailability and strategies for improvement. *Clin Pharmacokinet.* 2013;**52**(6):399–414.

11 Bins S, Ratain MJ, Mathijssen RH. Conventional dosing of anticancer agents: precisely wrong or just inaccurate? *Clin Pharmacol Ther.* 2014;**95**(4):361–364.

18 Seymour L, Ivy SP, Sargent D, et al. The design of phase II clinical trials testing cancer therapeutics: consensus recommendations from the clinical trial design task force of the national cancer institute investigational drug steering committee. *Clin Cancer Res Off J Am Assoc Cancer Res.* 2010;**16**(6):1764–1769.

19 Dancey JE, Dobbin KK, Groshen S, et al. Guidelines for the development and incorporation of biomarker studies in early clinical trials of novel agents. *Clin Cancer Res Off J Am Assoc Cancer Res.* 2010;**16**(6):1745–1755.

24 Ramchandani RP, Wang Y, Booth BP, et al. The role of SN-38 exposure, UGT1A1*28 polymorphism, and baseline bilirubin level in predicting severe irinotecan toxicity. *J Clin Pharmacol.* 2007;**47**(1):78–86.

25 Wagner JG. Kinetics of pharmacologic response. I. Proposed relationships between response and drug concentration in the intact animal and man. *J Theor Biol.* 1968;**20**(2):173–201.

26 Jusko WJ. A pharmacodynamic model for cell-cycle specific chemotherapeutic agents. *J Pharmacokinet Biopharm.* 1973;**1**:175–200.

28 Skipper HE, Schabel FM Jr, Mellett LB, et al. Implications of biochemical, cytokinetic, pharmacologic, and toxicologic relationships in the design of optimal therapeutic schedules. *Cancer Chemother Reports Part 1.* 1970;**54**(6):431–450.

30 Wang J, Song P, Schrieber S, et al. Exposure-response relationship of T-DM1: insight into dose optimization for patients with HER2-positive metastatic breast cancer. *Clin Pharmacol Ther.* 2014;**95**(5):558–564.

31 Rini BI, Garrett M, Poland B, et al. Axitinib in metastatic renal cell carcinoma: results of a pharmacokinetic and pharmacodynamic analysis. *J Clin Pharmacol.* 2013;**53**(5):491–504.

33 Jodrell DI, Egorin MJ, Canetta RM, et al. Relationships between carboplatin exposure and tumor response and toxicity in patients with ovarian cancer. *J Clin Oncol Off J Am Soc Clin Oncol.* 1992;**10**(4):520–528.

34 Wang X, Roy A, Hochhaus A, Kantarjian HM, Chen TT, Shah NP. Differential effects of dosing regimen on the safety and efficacy of dasatinib: retrospective exposure-response analysis of a phase III study. *Clin Pharmacol Adv Appl.* 2013;**5**:85–97.

35 Tiseo M, Andreoli R, Gelsomino F, et al. Correlation between erlotinib pharmacokinetics, cutaneous toxicity and clinical outcomes in patients with advanced non-small cell lung cancer (NSCLC). *Lung Cancer.* 2014;**83**(2):265–271.

38 Demetri GD, Wang Y, Wehrle E, et al. Imatinib plasma levels are correlated with clinical benefit in patients with unresectable/metastatic gastrointestinal stromal tumors. *J Clin Oncol Off J Am Soc Clin Oncol.* 2009;**27**(19):3141–3147.

39 Evans WE, Relling MV, Rodman JH, Crom WR, Boyett JM, Pui CH. Conventional compared with individualized chemotherapy for childhood acute lymphoblastic leukemia. *N Engl J Med.* 1998;**338**(8):499–505.

40 Suttle AB, Ball HA, Molimard M, et al. Relationships between pazopanib exposure and clinical safety and efficacy in patients with advanced renal cell carcinoma. *Br J Cancer.* 2014;**111**(12):2383.

42 Cosson VF, Ng VW, Lehle M, Lum BL. Population pharmacokinetics and exposure-response analyses of trastuzumab in patients with advanced gastric or gastroesophageal junction cancer. *Cancer Chemother Pharmacol.* 2014;**73**(4):737–747.

43 Yu H, Steeghs N, Nijenhuis CM, Schellens JH, Beijnen JH, Huitema AD. Practical guidelines for therapeutic drug monitoring of anticancer tyrosine kinase inhibitors: focus on the pharmacokinetic targets. *Clin Pharmacokinet.* 2014;**53**(4):305–325.

45 Karlsson MO, Molnar V, Bergh J, Freijs A, Larsson R. A general model for time-dissociated pharmacokinetic-pharmacodynamic relationship exemplified by paclitaxel myelosuppression. *Clin Pharmacol Ther.* 1998;**63**(1):11–25.

46 Minami H, Sasaki Y, Saijo N, et al. Indirect-response model for the time course of leukopenia with anticancer drugs. *Clin Pharmacol Ther.* 1998;**64**(5):511–521.

47 Egorin MJ, Van Echo DA, Tipping SJ, et al. Pharmacokinetics and dosage reduction of cis-diammine(1,1-cyclobutanedicarboxylato)platinum in patients with impaired renal function. *Cancer Res.* 1984;**44**(11):5432–5438.

50 Mould DR, Upton RN. Basic concepts in population modeling, simulation, and model-based drug development-part 2: introduction to pharmacokinetic modeling methods. *CPT: Pharmacometr Syst Pharmacol.* 2013;**2**:e38.

51 Deng J, Shao J, Markowitz JS, An G. ABC transporters in multi-drug resistance and ADME-Tox of small molecule tyrosine kinase inhibitors. *Pharm Res.* 2014;**31**(9):2237–2255.

53 Szmulewitz RZ, Ratain MJ. Playing Russian roulette with tyrosine kinase inhibitors. *Clin Pharmacol Ther.* 2013;**93**(3):242–244.

56 Budha NR, Frymoyer A, Smelick GS, et al. Drug absorption interactions between oral targeted anticancer agents and PPIs: is pH-dependent solubility the Achilles heel of targeted therapy? *Clin Pharmacol Ther.* 2012;**92**(2):203–213.

57 Evans WE, Pratt CB. Effect of pleural effusion on high-dose methotrexate kinetics. *Clin Pharmacol Ther.* 1978;**23**(1):68–72.

60 Benet LZ, Hoener BA. Changes in plasma protein binding have little clinical relevance. *Clin Pharmacol Ther*. 2002;71(3):115–121.

61 Penner N, Klunk LJ, Prakash C. Human radiolabeled mass balance studies: objectives, utilities and limitations. *Biopharm Drug Dispos*. 2009;30(4):185–203.

62 Calvert AH, Newell DR, Gumbrell LA, et al. Carboplatin dosage: prospective evaluation of a simple formula based on renal function. *J Clin Oncol Off J Am Soc Clin Oncol*. 1989;7(11):1748–1756.

64 Relling MV, Fairclough D, Ayers D, et al. Patient characteristics associated with high-risk methotrexate concentrations and toxicity. *J Clin Oncol Off J Am Soc Clin Oncol*. 1994;12(8):1667–1672.

66 Miller AA, Murry DJ, Owzar K, et al. Phase I and pharmacokinetic study of sorafenib in patients with hepatic or renal dysfunction: CALGB 60301. *J Clin Oncol Off J Am Soc Clin Oncol*. 2009;27(11):1800–1805.

72 Rosner GL, Panetta JC, Innocenti F, Ratain MJ. Pharmacogenetic pathway analysis of irinotecan. *Clin Pharmacol Ther*. 2008;84(3):393–402.

73 Reece PA, Stafford I, Davy M, Freeman S. Disposition of unchanged cisplatin in patients with ovarian cancer. *Clin Pharmacol Ther*. 1987;42(3):320–325.

75 Wagner JG, Szpunar GJ, Ferry JJ. A nonlinear physiologic pharmacokinetic model: I. Steady-state. *J Pharmacokinet Biopharm*. 1985;13(1):73–92.

77 Collins JM, Dedrick RL, King FG, Speyer JL, Myers CE. Nonlinear pharmacokinetic models for 5-fluorouracil in man: intravenous and intraperitoneal routes. *Clin Pharmacol Ther*. 1980;28(2):235–246.

80 Gianni L, Kearns CM, Giani A, et al. Nonlinear pharmacokinetics and metabolism of paclitaxel and its pharmacokinetic/pharmacodynamic relationships in humans. *J Clin Oncol Off J Am Soc Clin Oncol*. 1995;13(1):180–190.

90 Singh BN, Malhotra BK. Effects of food on the clinical pharmacokinetics of anticancer agents: underlying mechanisms and implications for oral chemotherapy. *Clin Pharmacokinet*. 2004;43(15):1127–1156.

91 Han K, Jin J, Maia M, Lowe J, Sersch MA, Allison DE. Lower exposure and faster clearance of bevacizumab in gastric cancer and the impact of patient variables: analysis of individual data from AVAGAST phase III trial. *AAPS J*. 2014;16(5):1056–1063.

94 Relling MV, Gardner EE, Sandborn WJ, et al. Clinical Pharmacogenetics Implementation Consortium guidelines for thiopurine methyltransferase genotype and thiopurine dosing. *Clin Pharmacol Ther*. 2011;89(3):387–391.

98 Stearns V, Johnson MD, Rae JM, et al. Active tamoxifen metabolite plasma concentrations after coadministration of tamoxifen and the selective serotonin reuptake inhibitor paroxetine. *J Natl Cancer Inst*. 2003;95(23):1758–1764.

103 Calvert AH. A review of the pharmacokinetics and pharmacodynamics of combination carboplatin/paclitaxel. *Semin Oncol*. 1997;24(1 Suppl 2):S2-85–S2-90.

106 Hughes AN, O'Brien ME, Petty WJ, et al. Overcoming CYP1A1/1A2 mediated induction of metabolism by escalating erlotinib dose in current smokers. *J Clin Oncol Off J Am Soc Clin Oncol*. 2009;27(8):1220–1226.

107 Moore LB, Goodwin B, Jones SA, et al. St John's wort induces hepatic drug metabolism through activation of the pregnane X receptor. *Proc Natl Acad Sci U S A*. 2000;97(13):7500–7502.

114 Cohen EE, Wu K, Hartford C, et al. Phase I studies of sirolimus alone or in combination with pharmacokinetic modulators in advanced cancer patients. *Clin Cancer Res Off J Am Assoc Cancer Res*. 2012;18(17):4785–4793.

56 Folate antagonists

Peter D. Cole, MD ▪ Lisa Figueiredo, MD ▪ Joseph R. Bertino, MD

Overview

Folic acid antagonists (antifols) are cytotoxic drugs used as antineoplastic, antimicrobial, anti-inflammatory, and immune-suppressive agents. While several folate antagonists have been developed, methotrexate (4-amino-4-deoxy-10-*N*-methyl-pteroylglutamic acid; MTX) is the antifol with the most extensive history and widest spectrum of use. MTX remains an essential drug in curative chemotherapy regimens used to treat patients with acute lymphoblastic leukemia, osteosarcoma, and choriocarcinoma and is an important agent in the therapy of patients with lymphoma, breast cancer, bladder cancer, and head and neck cancer. In addition, it is used for patients with nonmalignant diseases such as rheumatoid arthritis, psoriasis, autoimmune diseases, and graft versus host disease. This chapter will review the clinical use of and the metabolism of MTX and discuss structurally related folate antagonists that have been developed to overcome resistance or have alternate intracellular targets.

Historical overview

In the early 1940s, the combined observations that patients with acute leukemia often have serum folate deficiency and that the bone marrow megaloblasts of folate-deficient patients morphologically resemble leukemic blasts prompted some investigators to postulate that leukemia might be a result of a deficiency of this B vitamin. However, it rapidly became apparent that administration of folic acid to patients with leukemia was not only ineffective but often accelerated the course of the disease.[1] Thus, efforts to treat these leukemias turned to pharmacologically mimicking folate deficiency using folate analogs with effects antagonistic to those of the vitamin. Aminopterin (4-amino-4-deoxy PGA; AMT; Figure 1) was the first of these analogs to produce temporary remissions in 5 of 16 patients with acute leukemia.[2] This report was a landmark in cancer chemotherapy, as the first successful example of the power of rational drug design leading to an effective antineoplastic agent.

Since the initial study indicating the usefulness of AMT in the treatment of acute leukemia of childhood, there has been sustained interest in folate antagonists. Although known to be less potent, 4-amino-4-deoxy-10-*N*-methyl-pteroylglutamic acid (MTX) supplanted AMT in the clinic in the early 1950s because the toxicity caused by AMT was greater and less predictable.[3-5] Newer antifols, rationally designed analogs of folate or MTX, have been synthesized either in an effort to overcome cellular resistance to MTX or to target alternative folate-dependent processes. This chapter will discuss two, pralatrexate and pemetrexed, which recently received FDA approval for oncologic indications.

Mechanisms of action of MTX

Folate antagonists function in several ways: by competing with folates for uptake into cells, by inhibiting the formation of folate coenzymes, or by inhibiting one or more reactions that are mediated by folate coenzymes. Thus far, the clinically important anti-neoplastic folate analogs appear to work primarily by inhibiting dihydrofolate reductase (DHFR) or thymidylate synthase (TS). The prototypic DHFR inhibitor is a 4-amino-substituted pterin compound, such as MTX or AMT (Figure 1). Substitution of an amino group for the 4-hydroxy moiety results in a folate analog with a several thousand-fold increase in affinity for DHFR. The K_i of MTX for DHFR is below 10^{-10} *M*, well below the micromolar K_m of the natural substrate, dihydrofolate. By stoichiometrically inhibiting DHFR at slightly acidic pH, MTX blocks the cell's ability to replenish a supply of reduced folates necessary for *de novo* thymidylate synthesis (Figure 2).[6] In rapidly dividing cells, the inhibition of thymidylate biosynthesis leads to a decrease in thymidine triphosphate pools, a decrease in DNA synthesis, and eventually cell death.[7]

Intracellular metabolism of classical antifols such as MTX to polyglutamate species significantly impacts their function and mechanisms of cytotoxicity.[8] Folylpolyglutamate synthetase (FPGS) adds glutamate residues in γ-carboxyl linkage to both folate coenzymes and classical folate antagonists (those with a glutamate moiety). This addition of up to seven or eight additional glutamate molecules serves to add mass and negative charge, markedly reducing efflux and increasing total intracellular accumulation at steady state.[9] Both quantitative differences in FPGS expression and qualitative differences in FPGS function[10] exist between neoplastic and non-neoplastic tissues, which may explain some of the selectivity of antifolates for neoplastic cells.[11] A relative lack of FPGS may explain the observation that a cell population with a large number of G_0 cells would be less affected by the same concentration and time of exposure to MTX than a population with more actively dividing cells.

MTX polyglutamates are more potent inhibitors of DHFR than the parent compound because they bind as tightly to DHFR as MTX but dissociate less rapidly.[12] In addition, MTX polyglutamates are potent inhibitors of other folate-requiring enzymes, including TS[13] and two of the rate-limiting steps of *de novo* purine synthesis: glycinamide ribonucleotide (GAR) and aminoimidazole carboxamide ribonucleotide (AICAR) transformylases.[14] These two enzymes are potently inhibited by DHF-polyglutamates and 10-formyl-DHF polyglutamates, which increase after MTX inhibits DHFR.[15] As a result, inhibition of *de novo* purine synthesis may be at least as relevant as DHFR inhibition to the cytotoxic effects of MTX in cancer cells[16] and for the anti-inflammatory action of MTX in patients with rheumatologic diseases.[17,18]

Other possible mechanisms by which MTX exerts antineoplastic or anti-inflammatory action are worth mentioning. First, by inhibiting folate-dependent methionine biosynthesis, MTX causes

Holland-Frei Cancer Medicine, Ninth Edition. Edited by Robert C. Bast Jr., Carlo M. Croce, William N. Hait, Waun Ki Hong, Donald W. Kufe, Martine Piccart-Gebhart, Raphael E. Pollock, Ralph R. Weichselbaum, Hongyang Wang, and James F. Holland.
© 2017 John Wiley & Sons, Inc. ISBN: 978-1-118-93469-2

625

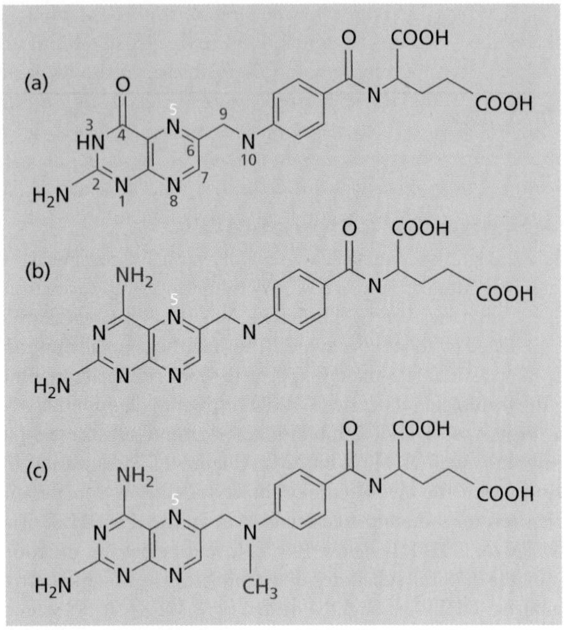

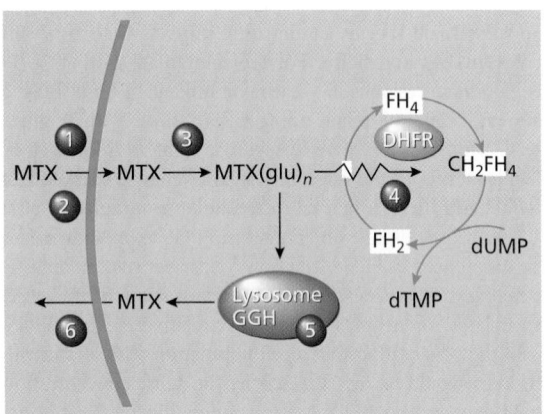

Figure 1 Structure of folic acid and structurally related classical antifols, AMT and MTX. (a) Folic acid (pteroylglutamic acid; PGA). (b) Aminopterin (4-amino-PGA). (c) Methotrexate (4-amino-*N*-10-methyl PGA).

Figure 2 Primary site of action of MTX and MTX(glu)$_n$. MTX enters cells by either the reduced folate carrier (1) or the membrane folate-binding protein (2). MTX is then metabolized by the cytosolic enzyme folylpolyglutamate synthetase (3) to MTX(glu)$_n$, a potent inhibitor of dihydrofolate reductase (DHFR) (4). MTX(glu)$_n$ can be hydrolyzed to MTX by the lysosomal enzyme γ-glutamyl hydrolase (GGH) (5). *Abbreviations*: CH$_2$FH$_4$, N$_5$, N10-methylene tetrahydrofolate; dTMP, deoxythymidine monophosphate; dUMP, deoxyuridine monophosphate/deoxyuridylate; FH$_2$, dihydrofolate; FH$_4$, tetrahydrofolate; MTX, methotrexate; MTX(glu)$_n$, MTX polyglutamates.

intracellular concentrations of homocysteine (Hcy) to increase, resulting in a secondary increase in *S*-adenosyl-homocysteine (SAH), a potent inhibitor of many folate-dependent methylation reactions. MTX exposure, therefore, can block membrane localization of ras,[19] a member of a family of critical signal transduction proteins constitutively activated in a number of human cancers. Second, the anti-inflammatory effects of MTX and some component of its antineoplastic activity may be due to its ability to inhibit endothelial cell proliferation at low concentrations.[20] Preclinical data confirm that low-dose methotrexate can inhibit the growth of

microscopic metastatic disease through its antiangiogenic properties.[21] In addition to the mechanisms mentioned earlier, rapidly proliferating cancer cells overexpress enzymes of the mitochondrial and glycine-serine pathway, and this phenotype is a recently appreciated determinant of methotrexate sensitivity.[22]

Pharmacokinetics of MTX

MTX is one of few anticancer agents for which pharmacokinetic data are routinely used in clinical practice to modulate the balance between efficacy and toxicity.[23] Retrospective analysis of children with acute lymphoblastic leukemia (ALL) shows that lower MTX clearance[24] and higher MTX concentrations[25] are associated with lower risk of relapse. Even more intriguing are data from a prospective randomized trial in patients with ALL comparing dosing by body surface area with individualized dosing based on pharmacokinetic data, which showed significantly improved complete continuous remission rates in the individualized therapy arm.[26] It is possible, however, that these results are protocol specific, as others have found that pharmacologically guided treatment intensification led to inferior outcomes for some subpopulations.[27]

Absorption

Following oral administration, peak plasma concentrations occur 1–5 h after a dose of 15–30 mg/m^2. Absorption can be relatively poor and unpredictable,[28,29] affected by food, nonabsorbable antibiotics, bile salts, and a shortened intestine transit time. Thus, it is suggested that the drug be taken on an empty stomach with clear liquids. Nevertheless, at a dose and schedule of 25 mg/m^2, given orally every 6 h for four doses, plasma MTX concentration >0.5 μ*M* was seen in more than 85% of pediatric patients with ALL, indicating the reliability of this oral regimen.[30]

Distribution

After intravenous (IV) administration of MTX, the initial volume of distribution (V_d) is approximately 0.18 L/kg of body weight. The initial distribution phase has a $t_{1/2}$ of 30–45 min; the beta $t_{1/2}$ is 3–4 h. Steady-state V_d is between 0.4 and 0.8 L/kg.[31]

After high doses of MTX (>3 g/m^2), peak serum concentrations in the range 10^{-4} to 10^{-3} *M* are achieved.[32] At these concentrations, transmembrane transport is saturated, limiting further influx of MTX to passive diffusion. Uptake of reduced folates, including leucovorin (LV), is inhibited as well. Studies of MTX metabolism in lymphoblasts *in vitro* have also shown that too high an extracellular concentration of drug can impede metabolism of MTX to a polyglutamate.[33]

MTX binding to plasma proteins, especially to albumin, is approximately 50%.[34,35] The 7-hydroxy metabolite of MTX is 90% bound to plasma proteins, but apparently does not interfere with MTX binding to plasma proteins at clinically observed concentrations. The highest tissue-to-plasma concentrations found in humans are in the liver and kidney, followed by the gastrointestinal tract. Prolonged plasma levels after high-dose MTX infusions in humans have been attributed to decreased transit rate secondary to gastrointestinal obstruction.

Because of the blood–brain barrier and efflux mechanisms that actively remove MTX from the CNS,[36] cerebrospinal fluid (CSF) MTX concentrations are approximately 1% of those in the plasma; therefore, cytocidal concentrations are not obtained in the CSF after conventional doses but only with doses of 500 mg/m^2 and higher.[37] After high-dose systemic MTX administration, lumbar CSF and ventricular CSF concentrations were similar. HDMTX may be able to replace intrathecal drug for the treatment of patients with nonleukemic leptomeningeal disease.[38] However, a recent meta-analysis of CNS-directed therapy for children with ALL concluded that efforts to increase CSF penetration using HDMTX have not produced the desired result of lowering the rate of CNS relapse in this population.[39]

As MTX is accumulated poorly into the CSF, even small doses of LV given orally can increase CSF folates significantly. This systemic rescue, especially if given too early after MTX, may rescue leukemic cells in the CSF compartment.[40]

When injected into an indwelling ventricular catheter, MTX reaches reproducible therapeutic drug concentrations ($>10^{-6}$ M) for at least 48 h.[41] In contrast, when MTX is given by the lumbar route into the CSF, it distributes unreliably into the ventricles. An improved dose schedule utilizing the administration of multiple small doses of intrathecal MTX has been suggested.[42] Following intrathecal administration, MTX slowly exits into the systemic circulation with a $t_{1/2}$ of 8–10 h.[36] Systemic toxicity can be observed if multiple doses of intrathecal MTX are administered without LV rescue. The pharmacology of intrathecal MTX and the amount of intraventricular MTX may be altered by overt meningeal leukemia and the position of the patient at the time of lumbar puncture.[43] The clinical observation that irradiation followed by MTX treatment may predispose patients to neurotoxicity may be a consequence of the effect of radiation therapy on the blood–brain barrier.[44]

Patients with pleural or peritoneal effusions may be at increased risk for developing toxicity to HD-MTX as a result of "third spacing" or MTX trapping in the infusion and slow release leading to sustained MTX concentrations in serum.[45] In these circumstances, higher LV doses and prolonged LV rescue may be necessary, until the serum level of MTX decreases to $<0.05 \times 10^{-6}$ M.

Metabolism

The major metabolite of MTX, produced by the action of hepatic aldehyde oxidase, is 7-hydroxy MTX (7-OH MTX) (Figure 3), which is only 1% as potent an inhibitor of DHFR as MTX.[46] It

is also less water soluble than MTX and may contribute to renal toxicity after high doses.[47]

A second, less important pathway of metabolism of MTX occurs in the intestine. MTX is hydrolyzed by bacteria to the pteroate (4-deoxy-4-amino-N10-methyl pteroic acid; dAMPA) and glutamic acid (Figure 3).[48] dAMPA, like 7-OH MTX, is also a relatively inactive metabolite with approximately 1/200th the affinity of MTX for DHFR. dAMPA excretion in the urine accounts for <5% of the dose administered.

The third metabolic product of MTX is MTX polyglutamate. As discussed earlier, MTX polyglutamates are at least as potent inhibitors of DHFR as is MTX and have a slower rate of disassociation from DHFR.[12] MTX polyglutamates are not found in plasma or urine because of the abundant activity of γ-glutamyl hydrolase(s) (GGH) in plasma that convert folyl- and MTX-polyglutamates to monoglutamates. Similar to MTX, 7-OH MTX is also polyglutamylated intracellularly, and retention of these polyglutamate forms could contribute to MTX cytotoxicity.[49]

Compliance with oral MTX regimens can be monitored by measuring MTX-polyglutamate concentrations within circulating erythrocytes red blood cells (RBCs).[50–52] Nucleated RBC precursors within the bone marrow will accumulate and metabolize circulating MTX. The resulting MTX polyglutamates will remain within the mature RBC throughout its lifespan,[53] while unmetabolized MTX will gradually efflux.[54]

Excretion

The majority of administered MTX (and its metabolites 7-OH MTX and DAMPA) is excreted unchanged in the urine.[55,56] Because of active secretion in the proximal tubules, renal clearance of MTX can exceed creatinine clearance.[57] There is wide inter-patient variability in MTX clearance, which does not correlate perfectly with renal function.[58] MTX excretion is reported to be inversely related to age as plasma clearance of renal eliminated drugs is closely correlated with maturation of kidney function. Children tend to exhibit more rapid MTX clearance than adults, and a general trend toward

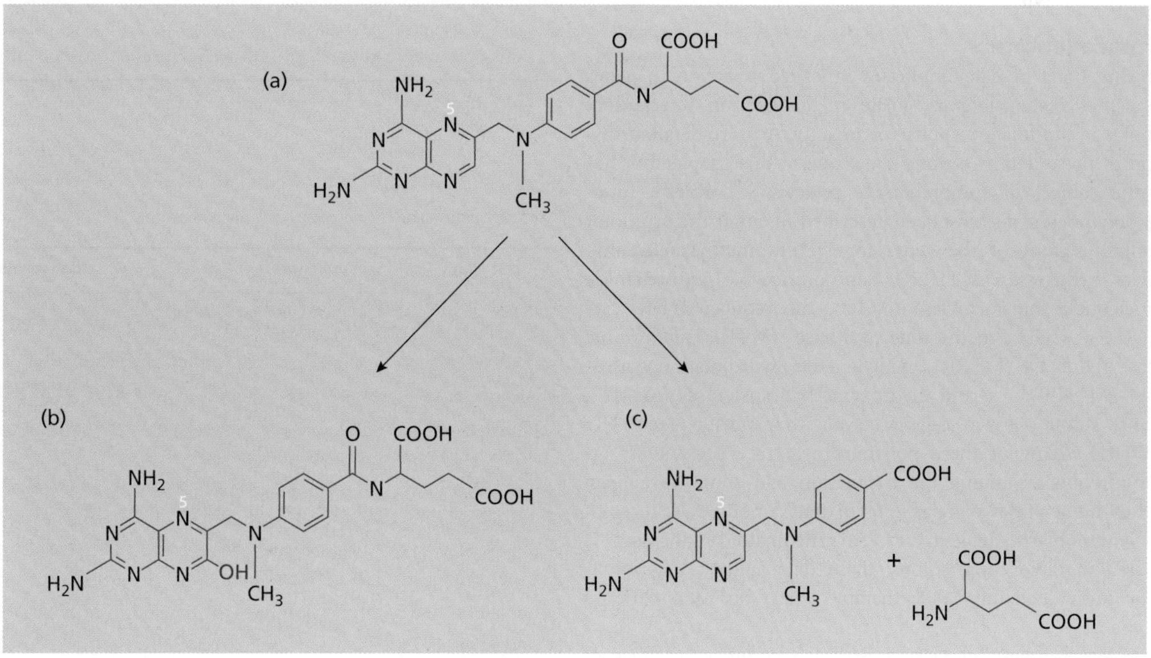

Figure 3 Catabolism of MTX. MTX (a) can be converted in the liver to 7-OH MTX (b). In addition, enteric bacteria will cleave the molecule to dAMPA plus glutamate (c).

decreasing clearance with increasing age has been observed.[59] MTX excretion through organic acid transporters can be inhibited by probenecid or competitively blocked by other weak organic acids, such as aspirin or penicillin G. MTX elimination is increased by drugs that block distal tubular reabsorption, such as folic acid, some cephalosporins, and sulfamethoxazole.

Less than 10% of MTX is typically recovered in the feces.[60] Following IV administration of doses of 30–80 mg/m², 0.4–20% of the administered dose is excreted through the canalicular multiorganic acid transporter (cMOAT; ABCC2; MRP2) into the bile. Using a knock-out mouse model (ABCC2$^{-/-}$; ABCG2$^{-/-}$), it was shown that both transporters play overlapping roles in the elimination of MTX and 7-OH-MTX. Many polymorphisms and mutations of these transporters have been identified, leading to differences in expression and activity, affecting systemic MTX exposure. Consequently, patients with mutations or heterozygous polymorphisms in ABCC2 and/or ABCG2 might be at increased risk for MTX toxicity.[61]

Drug interactions

Several drugs used in cancer patients, including antibiotics, may alter the renal excretion of MTX, increasing toxicity or decreasing efficacy. Deleterious and even fatal reactions have been reported between MTX and nonsteroidal anti-inflammatory drugs, in particular with naproxen and ketoprofen.[62,63] This increased toxicity may be due to decreased renal elimination, possibly as a result of competition for renal secretion.[57] Other commonly used organic drugs may also potentiate MTX toxicity, such as phenylbutazone, salicylate, and probenecid.[64,65] Probenecid increased the efficacy of MTX in tumor-bearing mice, but it has not been used clinically with this goal in mind.[66]

Increased toxicity was also reported when trimethoprim, the antibacterial agent, was used together with MTX. Presumably, this antifolate, with only weak binding affinity to mammalian DHFR, lowers folate stores, especially in patients with subclinical folate deficiency, making marrow cells more susceptible to MTX-induced toxicity.[67] Alcohol should also be avoided in patients receiving MTX because of the risk of hepatic fibrosis and cirrhosis.

Pharmacogenomics

A growing body of data implicates inherited variation in genes for enzymes responsible for folate metabolism in interpatient variability in antifolate response or toxicity. A more detailed discussion of these data is beyond the scope of this chapter but has been the subject of comprehensive reviews.[68–71] Briefly, functional polymorphisms have been described in either the promoter or coding regions of the genes for DHFR, methylenetetrahydrofolate reductase (MTHFR), aminoimidazole carboxamide ribonucleotide transformylase (ATIC), the reduced folate carrier (RFC), GGH, methionine synthase (MTR), methionine synthase reductase (MTRR), methylenetetrahydrofolate dehydrogenase (MTHFD), serine hydroxymethyltransferase (SHMT), TS, and solute carrier organic anion transporter gene 1B1 (SLCO1B1). Many of these polymorphisms are present at significant frequency among the population and some have been linked to higher rates of relapse or toxicity among patients with acute lymphoblastic leukemia[72–77] or rheumatoid arthritis.[78] If replicated in larger populations, these data suggest the potential for individualizing MTX therapy, based on each patient's genotype.

Gene–environment interactions may also modulate the effects of genotypic variation on toxicity. To focus on one relevant example, some of the observed variation in serum homocysteine (a marker of functional folate deficiency) is explained by two common functional polymorphisms in the MTHFR gene, C677T and A1298C, but only under conditions of decreased intake of dietary folate.[79,80] Adequate dietary folate in countries with mandated folate supplementation could erase the effects of genetic polymorphisms.

Clinical application

Clinical dosage schedules

MTX has been administered on a variety of dosage schedules since its introduction into the clinic more than six decades ago (Table 1). In a trial of MTX in patients with head and neck cancer treated with 50, 500, or 5000 mg/m² with LV "rescue," a trend of dose responsiveness was seen (5 of 24, 5 of 16, 9 of 18, respectively). Some responses were noted with the 5000 mg/m² dose regimen in patients who did not respond at lower doses.[81] The importance of dose scheduling was emphasized by an experimental study showing that resistance to high-dose pulse MTX may not extend to continuous low-dose exposure.[82] Determining the optimum dose schedule of MTX is complicated by the use of the drug in combination therapy (Table 2). Sequencing appears to be important when MTX is used with 5-fluorouracil (5-FU), with L-asparaginase, and probably with cytosine arabinoside and 6-mercaptopurine or 6-thioguanine. Table 2 summarizes the use of some common drug combinations that include MTX, along with sequence specificity.

Table 1 Dosage schedules commonly used for methotrexate (MTX).

Schedule and dose	Use/comments
Oral	
Weekly or biweekly (15–25 mg in single or divided doses)	Mainly for nonmalignant conditions, such as psoriasis or rheumatoid arthritis
Weekly or biweekly (20–30 mg/m²)	Maintenance therapy for ALL
Parenteral	
Pulse weekly (30–60 mg/m²)	Choriocarcinoma, ALL
Intermediate dose (120–500 mg/m² weekly)	ALL, NHL; requires LV rescue, 10–15 mg/m² q 6 h × 6–8 doses
High dose (500–12,000 mg/m² weekly or every other week)	Osteosarcoma, ALL, neoplastic meningitis; requires LV rescue

Abbreviations: ALL, acute lymphoblastic leukemia; LV, leucovorin; NHL, non-Hodgkin lymphoma.

Table 2 Combination chemotherapy with methotrexate (MTX).

Used with	Schedule notes	Result	Comments
5-FU	MTX must precede 5-FU by 24 h	Synergistic	
Anthracyclines		Additive	
Bleomycin		Additive	Mucosal toxicity is increased
Corticosteroids	Used together	Synergistic	Used in ALL
Cyclophosphamide	Used together	Additive	
Cytarabine	Used together	Additive or synergistic	
L-asparaginase	If MTX precedes l-asparaginase by 24 h	Synergistic	Used in ALL, AML
	If used simultaneously	Antagonistic	
Vinca alkaloids		Additive	

Abbreviations: ALL, acute lymphoblastic leukemia; AML, acute myelogenous leukemia; 5-FU, 5-fl uorouracil.

Current uses for MTX in the treatment of neoplastic disease

Acute lymphoblastic leukemia

MTX is a component of nearly all multiagent therapeutic regimens for patients with acute lymphoblastic leukemia post-remission, and some protocols include MTX in remission induction. In addition to systemic use, MTX is administered intrathecally for the treatment of meningeal leukemia and for prophylaxis against CNS relapse.

During the intensive, early post-remission phases, MTX can be administered orally or parenterally. Parenteral administration at intermediate dose ($100-500$ mg/m^2/dose) or high dose (≥ 1000 mg/m^2) has been incorporated in some protocols to increase accumulation of MTX-polyglutamates by blast cells,[83] to overcome mechanisms of resistance and to increase penetration into protected sites including the CNS and testes.[84] While the ability of HD-MTX to prevent CNS relapse is not clearly proven,[39] the rate of isolated testicular relapse does appear to have decreased with the addition of intermediate or HD-MTX.[85] Randomized trials comparing escalating IV doses with oral MTX showed a significant improvement in 5-year event-free survival (EFS) in those patients randomly assigned to the IV MTX-based interim maintenance compared with the oral MTX-based arm.[86–89] However, in some studies, the increase in EFS came at the expense of increased hematologic and neurologic toxicity.[90–93]

During later maintenance phases, most current protocols rely on prolonged weekly administration of MTX at low doses ($20-50$ mg/m^2/dose) in combination with daily mercaptopurine. Early studies showed that twice-weekly therapy (20 mg/m^2) was superior to continuous daily oral administration for treatment during remission.[94] The effectiveness of an oral divided dose ($25-30$ mg/m^2 given every 6 h for 4–6 doses weekly) has also been shown.[30]

Acute myelogenous leukemia

MTX has limited value in the current treatment of patients with acute nonlymphocytic leukemia. Complete remissions can be seen in approximately one quarter of adults with AML treated with MTX-containing regimens: prednisone, Oncovin, methotrexate, and Purinethol (POMP)[95] or MTX with L-asparaginase (the "Capizzi Regimen").[96,97] High-dose regimens with LV rescue have a transient but rapid effect on the peripheral blood count without producing marrow remissions in the large majority of these patients.[98] The lack of efficacy of MTX in this disease has been attributed to poor intracellular retention of the drug caused by a lack of polyglutamylation and an increase of the target enzyme DHFR following treatment.[99]

Lymphoma

On the basis of the phase II studies that indicated that moderate to high doses of MTX (200 mg/m^2 to 3 gm/m^2) with LV rescue could produce transient regressions in patients with large cell lymphoma, MTX with LV rescue has been added to combination regimens for intermediate- and high-grade lymphomas. In some regimens (e.g., M-BACOD), MTX is used with LV during the leukopenic phase of drug treatment, as the MTX/LV combination has little marrow toxicity.[100] On the basis of the experimental studies showing that MTX and cytosine arabinoside produce additive and possibly synergistic effects,[101] this combination has also been utilized in regimens to treat this disease (e.g., COMLA; cyclophosphamide, vincristine, MTX, cytosine arabinoside, and LV). Similarly, following documentation of responses to therapy including MTX,[102,103] among patients with Burkitt's lymphoma, high-dose MTX with LV rescue has been added to CVAD, cytarabine and intrathecal therapy as well as to other combination chemotherapy regimens[104–106] for patients with Burkitt's lymphoma.

Most treatment regimens for patients with primary CNS lymphoma include high-dose MTX, as conventional radiation doses may lead to neurotoxicity. In a retrospective review of 226 patients with primary CNS lymphoma, those patients treated with regimens that included HDMTX followed by radiotherapy had an improved survival, with no higher risk of late neurotoxicity.[107]

Choriocarcinoma

Choriocarcinoma is unique in that single-drug treatment with either MTX or actinomycin D produces a substantial number of cures.[108] The basis for the unusual sensitivity of this tumor to MTX is not entirely clear, but choriocarcinoma cells may accumulate and retain this drug effectively by synthesizing long-chain polyglutamates. The JAR (human choriocarcinoma) cell line was shown to have active-receptor coupled uptake (potocytosis) of folates and antifolates.[109] Current programs for the treatment of this malignancy utilize MTX in combination with other drugs, especially for "poor risk" or relapsed patients.[110]

Breast cancer

MTX as a single agent causes regressions of breast cancer in approximately 30% of patients. When used with fluorouracil, sequential use of MTX followed by 5-FU improved response rates to 50% and improves disease-free survival when used as adjuvant therapy.[111] The adjuvant use of cyclophosphamide, MTX and 5-FU cyclophosphamide methotrexate fluorouracil (CMF) also significantly reduces the risk of relapse,[112] may allow more conservative surgery among women with localized disease when used as neoadjuvant therapy,[113] and has a role in the treatment of patients with inoperable, advanced disease.[114] The combination of MTX, 5-FU with vinorelbine (VMF) instead of cyclophosphamide, has also shown activity among women with advanced breast cancer.[115] An additional advantage of this combination is the diminution of long-term toxicity (infertility, carcinogenesis) compared to regimens containing alkylating agents. Finally, it is interesting to note that low-dose oral MTX (2.5 mg BID $\times$ 2 days/week) with daily oral cyclophosphamide has shown activity among heavily pretreated women with advanced metastatic breast cancer.[116]

Gastrointestinal cancer

Antifolates have limited effectiveness in the treatment of gastrointestinal malignancies. The role of MTX in the treatment of these diseases is mainly to modulate, and possibly improve, the effectiveness of 5-FU. By inhibiting purine synthesis, MTX pretreatment increases phosphoribosyl pyrophosphate, a precursor necessary for 5-FU nucleotide formation.[117] Data from recent trials using high-dose MTX followed by LV/5-FU in patients with colon cancer highlight the need for a 7- to 24-h interval between MTX and 5-FU administration.[118] However, a randomized phase III study comparing 5-FU plus MTX to standard, continuous infusion of 5-FU demonstrated increased toxicity among those treated with MTX, and no difference in overall survival between the two arms. On the basis of these findings, 5-FU remains the standard of care for advanced gastric cancer.[119–121]

Genitourinary cancer

MTX alone (100 mg/m^2), or in high doses (≥ 500 mg/m^2) with LV rescue, is active in the treatment of advanced bladder cancer. The response rate reported (approximately 30%) is similar to the response rate of the other most active single drug, cisplatin. Combinations of drugs including MTX with cisplatin, vinblastine, and doxorubicin (M-VAC) have resulted in a substantial number of long-term clinical remissions.[122] A meta-analysis of randomized trials found that neoadjuvant treatment with MTX-containing regimens conferred a survival advantage.[123]

Head and neck cancer

MTX is an active agent for the treatment of patients with advanced carcinoma of the head and neck region. High-dose MTX regimens with LV rescue appear to improve response rates from 30% to 50%, but remission duration and survival are not improved.[124] MTX has also been used with 5-FU in this disease, with response rates as high as 60%.[125,126] The sequence and timing of drug administration have not been shown to affect the response rate, although different patterns of toxicity were observed.

Lung cancer

MTX as a single agent in conventional doses, or in high doses with LV rescue, has only marginal activity in non-small-cell lung cancer (NSCLC). This drug does have limited activity in small cell lung cancer and has been used in combination regimens to treat that disease. Pralatrexate, a nonclassical antifolate discussed later in further detail, has been shown to have activity for patients with previously treated NSCLC.[127]

Osteogenic sarcoma

Osteosarcoma responds poorly to conventional doses of methotrexate. However, high-dose methotrexate has been one of the mainstays of treatment since its introduction in the 1970s.[128] Randomized trials of pre- and post-definitive treatment demonstrated the beneficial effect of chemotherapy that includes high-dose MTX with LV rescue.[129] Different studies investigated whether MTX peak concentration and area under concentration–time curve (AUC) are significant prognostic factors of osteosarcoma.[130] Controversy remains as to whether there is correlation between MTX exposure and outcome.[131] A recent study analyzed the relation between MTX pharmacokinetics, toxicity and survival in children with osteosarcoma. Although there was no correlation between survival and peak concentration or AUC, the 48-h MTX concentration had significant correlation to survival, confirming that systemic MTX exposure was a significant prognostic factor of treatment outcome.[132]

Neoplastic meningitis

Intrathecal MTX is often a component of therapy for patients with solid-tumor neoplastic meningitis. High-dose IV MTX ($8\,g/m^2$) given as the sole treatment with LV rescue may be a reasonable alternative,[38] as therapeutic antineoplastic concentrations of MTX can be achieved more easily in the presence of neoplastic meningitis.[133]

Adverse effects

Hematologic toxicity

Expression of many folate-dependent enzymes targeted by MTX are cell-cycle specific, consistent with their role in DNA synthesis. Tissues that are self-renewing, with a higher S-phase fraction, are therefore at highest risk for damage by the folate antagonists. Bone marrow progenitor cells of all lineages are affected by MTX, but neutropenia usually predominates, with a nadir 10 days after drug administration and recovery typically between days 14 and 21. The effects on the marrow are dose related, but there is considerable

variability among patients. Genetic variants,[71,134,135] subclinical folate deficiency, impaired renal function, a damaged marrow owing to previous radiation therapy, chemotherapy, or infection, and the use of trimethoprim-sulfamethoxazole for *Pneumocystis carinii* prophylaxis may predispose patients to hematologic (and gastrointestinal) toxicity. Young patients usually tolerate MTX better than older individuals, a fact presumably related to clearance of the drug by the kidneys. The administration of LV can prevent or lessen MTX toxicity and allows larger doses of the antifolate to be administered.

Gastrointestinal toxicity

Nausea and vomiting, even with high doses of MTX, are usually mild to moderate. In contrast, mucositis is a common side effect of MTX treatment. Mucositis usually manifests 3–5 days following exposure to the drug. This is an early sign of MTX toxicity and the drug should be discontinued when it occurs. More severe gastrointestinal toxicity is manifest by diarrhea, which may progress to severe bloody diarrhea. When this occurs in association with neutropenia, patients are at high risk of typhlitis, sepsis, and death. These severe side effects generally occur in a setting of renal damage, usually a consequence of high doses of MTX ($\geq 500\,mg/m^2/dose$), but may also occur in patients treated with conventional doses. MTX blood levels and serum creatinine levels should be followed, and appropriate doses of LV administered, along with supportive measures (see the following discussion).

Renal toxicity

Renal toxicity occurs occasionally following high-dose regimens of MTX and is rare during treatment with lower doses. When it occurs, renal toxicity leads to delayed MTX clearance and subsequently to severe marrow and gastrointestinal toxicity, which can be fatal, especially in adults.[136] This toxicity is believed to be due to precipitation of MTX and its less soluble metabolite 7-OH MTX (Figure 3) in the tubules, as well as to a possible direct effect of this drug on the renal tubule.[47] The use of vigorous hydration, often with osmotic diuresis and alkalinization of urine to increase solubility of MTX and 7-OH MTX, has markedly ameliorated this problem. Occasional patients, even with this regimen (Table 3), exhibit renal impairment; therefore, careful monitoring of MTX and creatinine serum levels is essential. For those patients who have markedly delayed clearance of MTX secondary to acute renal dysfunction, increasing the dose and rate of LV administration has been the routine therapeutic maneuver to counteract the consequences of prolonged exposure to high MTX levels.[137]

Methylxanthines, such as caffeine or aminophylline, may be useful in the setting of delayed MTX clearance. MTX administration

Table 3 Supportive care for high-dose methotrexate (MTX) treatment.

Pretreatment hydration and alkalinization
8–12 h before treatment, patients should receive $1.5\,L/m^2$ of saline or 5% glucose with 100 mEq HCO_3 and 20 mEq KCl/L. Continue hydration until urine pH is 7.0 or greater before MTX administration
Monitoring
MTX levels should be monitored at 24 h after completion of MTX infusion. Serum creatinine should be measured pretreatment, at 24, and at 48 h
Additional LV rescue
Required for an MTX level $>10^{-6}\,M$ at 24 h. Increase LV dose to $100\,mg/m^2$ q 6 h for levels above $10^{-6}\,M$ and $200\,mg/m^2$ q 6 h for levels above $5 \times 10^{-6}\,M$. Monitor MTX levels daily and continue LV until plasma MTX concentration is $<10^{-8}\,M$

Abbreviation: LV, leucovorin.

has been shown to increase serum adenosine concentrations, which will decrease glomerular filtration rate.[17] Adenosine receptor competitive antagonists, such as the methylxanthines, may therefore act as a specific diuretic to increase MTX elimination.[138]

Extremely high levels of MTX ($>10^{-3}$ M) are difficult to rescue, even with high doses of LV.[139] Removal of MTX by peritoneal dialysis or hemodialysis is ineffective because the drug is extensively protein bound. Charcoal hemoperfusion columns have been used successfully in a small number of patients, but its efficacy is limited by rebounds in MTX levels.[140] Extracorporeal methods of methotrexate removal such as high-flux hemodialysis and hemodiafiltration have had variable efficacy, but both are highly invasive procedures that have resulted in only transient and small decreases in MTX levels, necessitating their combined or repeated daily use to lower MTX concentration effectively.[141,142] Oral charcoal and cholestyramine have also been used to bind MTX in the gut, thus limiting enterohepatic recirculation and toxicity.[143] Thymidine (1–3 g/m^2/day) is also capable of rescuing patients from MTX toxicity, but this metabolite is not generally available.[144] A recombinant form of bacterial carboxypeptidase, glucarpidase [carboxypeptidase-G$_2$ (CPDG$_2$)], an enzyme that hydrolytically cleaves the peptide bond in MTX resulting in glutamate and dAMPA (Figure 3), has been reported to reduce systemic MTX concentrations rapidly by >95% within 1 h of administration[145,146] When given in combination within 96 h after the start of the MTX infusion in addition to LV, carboxypeptidase G2 is highly effective in patients at high risk for developing life-threatening MTX toxicity after IV[146–148] or intrathecal administration.[149] While most studies are reported in the adult population, a recent retrospective review in pediatric patients showed similar results.[150]

Hepatotoxicity

Chronic low-dose weekly MTX treatment for patients with psoriasis, rheumatoid arthritis, or ALL has been associated with portal fibrosis, and in some patients, with frank cirrhosis.[151] Among cancer patients, acute elevations of liver enzymes commonly occur within days after treatment with MTX, but rapidly return to normal, and do not appear to predict chronic liver toxicity, even when elevated to 10–20 times the upper limit of normal.[152,153] Concurrent administration of dexamethasone may increase MTX-induced hepatotoxicity.[154] Alcohol and other hepatotoxic drugs should be avoided in these patient populations.

Central nervous system toxicity

Intrathecal MTX and IV administration of high-dose MTX have been associated with acute neurotoxicity, ranging from mild to severe. In cases of inadvertent overdosing (>100 mg intrathecally), fatalities have been reported. Greater understanding of the pathophysiology of MTX-induced neurotoxicity is now beginning to lead to therapeutic interventions to prevent or treat this complication of therapy.

The most common immediate side effect of intrathecal MTX administration, manifest by severe headache, fever, meningismus, vomiting, and CSF pleocytosis, is thought to be caused by a chemical arachnoiditis, or perhaps by the release of adenosine, which is a potent autocoid in the CNS.[155] This effect of adenosine has been ameliorated by systemic administration of low doses of methylxanthines, such as aminophylline and theophylline, which act as competitive antagonists at adenosine receptors.[138] Dosage adjustment or switching to cytosine arabinoside may be required if these symptoms persist. Acute toxicity occurring several days after high-dose systemic MTX treatment manifests with headache,

paresis, aphasia, or seizures. It is usually transient, resolving within 2–3 days.[156]

Subacute neurotoxicity (7–14 days after administration) has been observed in 5–18% of patients receiving intrathecal MTX and/or IV high-dose MTX. At its most severe, it presents with motor paralysis of the extremities, cranial nerve palsies, seizures, and even coma. While the pathogenesis of subacute antifolate-induced neurotoxicity is likely multifactorial, disruption to homocysteine homeostasis may play a pivotal role. By inhibiting remethylation to methionine, MTX leads to increased amounts of homocysteine in the plasma and CSF of patients.[157] Homocysteine may cause neurotoxicity through induction of oxidative damage to neuronal tissue and vascular endothelium.[158,159] In addition, homocysteine and its metabolites are excitotoxic amino acids (glutamate analog) that activate the N-methyl-D-aspartate (NMDA) class of glutamate receptors. Subacute neurotoxicity of MTX may be ameliorated by an antagonist of the NMDA receptor, such as dextromethorphan or memantine.[160–162]

Delayed MTX-induced neurotoxicity may be associated with chronic demyelinating encephalopathy in as many as 80% of children with acute lymphoblastic leukemia, and the magnitude of the radiographic changes seems to correlate with dose and number of doses of IV MTX.[92,93] Computed tomography scans show cortical thinning, ventricular enlargement, and diffuse intracerebral calcifications. Although most commonly attributed to the combination of cranial radiation with intrathecal MTX, encephalopathy has been reported in patients treated only with high-dose IV MTX. The pathogenesis of delayed neurotoxicity may be a result of impairing folate-dependent methylation of components of the myelin sheath.[163]

In patients who receive an MTX overdose intrathecally (>100 mg), immediate CSF removal with ventriculolumbar perfusion is indicated.[164] Intrathecal use of carboxypeptidase G2 was shown to decrease mortality in animals given a lethal dose of MTX intrathecally and may be the preferred treatment for this complication.[165] Intrathecal or systemic LV is not indicated in these cases, as it is unlikely that this toxicity is attributable to inhibition of DHFR.

Pulmonary toxicity

Although uncommon, pulmonary toxicity due to MTX has been noted in patients treated chronically with low-dose oral MTX.[166] The clinical picture usually consists of cough, dyspnea, fever, and hypoxemia. Chest radiograph findings are nonspecific but may show patchy interstitial infiltrates. *P. carinii* must be ruled out, especially in patients also receiving steroids. Histologic examinations show diffuse interstitial lymphocytic infiltrates, giant cells, and noncaseating granulomas. In some patients, a peripheral eosinophilia is observed, raising the possibility that this is an allergic pneumonitis. The process may progress to fibrosis and discontinuing MTX while the pulmonary toxicity is reversible is important. Some patients have been retreated without recurrence of the problem.

Skin toxicity

Skin toxicity to MTX occurs in 5–10% of patients. It manifests as an erythematous rash, characteristically noted on the neck and upper trunk. The rash may be pruritic and relatively insignificant and usually lasts for several days. A cutaneous vasculitis after intermediate-dose MTX has also been reported.[167] In the setting of severe systemic MTX toxicity following HD-MTX or overdose, the skin manifestations may progress to severe bullous formation and desquamation.[168]

Teratogenic and mutagenic effects

Folate deficiency alters gene expression by causing hypomethylation of DNA and increases DNA strand breaks by causing mis-incorporation of uracil instead of thymine. Consequently, folate deficiency can directly influence carcinogenesis.[169] MTX is known to be a potent abortifacient, especially if administered during the first trimester of pregnancy. Nevertheless, there is no direct evidence that MTX has any mutagenic or carcinogenic effects.

Miscellaneous toxicity

Osteoporosis has been reported with chronic low-dose MTX administration[170] and may result from direct inhibition of osteoblastic differentiation.[171] Fever, seizures, radiation recall, phototoxicity, and anaphylactoid reactions have been reported with high-dose administration. Pleuritic and left-upper-quadrant pain, presumably attributable to splenic capsule inflammation, has been reported with a moderately high-dose regimen. An acute hemolytic anemia due to an IgG-3 antibody that reacts with erythrocytes only in the presence of MTX has been described.[172]

Resistance to antifolates

Although the development of effective chemotherapeutic regimens including MTX has improved significantly the therapy of a number of different malignancies, achieving prolonged disease-free survival is still difficult even in chemotherapy-sensitive diseases. The efficacy of MTX, as with other antineoplastic agents, is limited ultimately by either inherent resistance or resistance acquired during the course of therapy. Distinct categories of resistance mechanisms have been described: (1) decreased accumulation due to impaired transport into the cell, (2) decreased accumulation of polyglutamate forms, owing to either decreased polyglutamate formation or increased removal of glutamate residues, (3) an increase in DHFR, (4) altered or mutated DHFR that binds MTX less avidly than the normal enzyme. In addition, because both DHFR and FPGS activities fluctuate with cell cycle, dysregulation of cell cycle genes may have a profound effect on antimetabolite resistance.

Intrinsic resistance to MTX

Intrinsic sensitivity to antifolates has been shown to relate to expression of mitochondrial enzymes.[22] Driven by *myc* activation, enzymes related to the cellular metabolism of serine, folate, and glycine are upregulated in many tumor types. This differential expression leads to selective sensitivity to folate antagonists relative to normal tissues.

Impaired ability to transport MTX into cells through the RFC results in intrinsic resistance in many tumor types. The vast majority of mechanisms of impaired antifolate transport involve quantitative and/or qualitative alterations at the RFC level. This includes mutations in RFC that alter its transport activity, RFC silencing via promoter methylation and 3′-UTR alterations, RFC silencing via loss of function of transcriptional regulators, and alterations in gene copy number of RFC in antifolate-resistant cells.[173] Decreased expression of RFC mRNA has been documented by quantitative reverse transcription polymerase chain reaction (RT-PCR) in osteosarcoma samples at initial biopsy.[174] In other tumors, decreased expression can result from aberrant methylation in the promoter region.[175,176]

Mutations in the RFC gene corresponding to altered transport function have been documented both in resistant cell lines[177] and in leukemic blasts at diagnosis.[178] Single nucleotide polymorphisms (SNPs) in the gene for RFC can result in proteins with a decreased affinity for antifolates, while maintaining sufficient affinity for folate to allow continued cell growth. Other known polymorphisms selectively increase affinity for folates and increase the intracellular folate pool. However, in one analysis of 246 pediatric leukemia patient samples, only three were found to have potentially functional RFC polymorphisms, suggesting that they do not appear to play a major role in intrinsic MTX resistance in this population.[179]

Polyglutamylation enhances cellular retention of classical antifolates. Therefore, loss of FPGS activity can confer relative resistance. Differing ability to form long-chain MTX polyglutamates to some degree explains the relative intrinsic resistance of AML to MTX, compared with ALL.[180,181] Similarly, tumor cells from patients with soft tissue sarcomas intrinsically resistant to MTX have a low capacity to form long-chain MTX polyglutamates.[182,183] Higher MTX-polyglutamate accumulation in B-lineage ALL blasts as compared to T-lineage blasts may be explained by the finding of higher FPGS activity in B-lineage blasts.[184,185] The possibility that different isoforms (splice variants) of FPGS are expressed in different tissues is supported by the finding of differences in FPGS affinity for MTX between AML and ALL cell lines and blast samples,[186] between resistant and sensitive sarcoma cell lines,[187] and by differences between FPGS isolated from L1210 cells and murine liver in degree of inhibition by long-chain folylpolyglutamates.[10]

Increased expression of the target enzyme DHFR, a well-described mechanism of acquired MTX resistance, may also confer intrinsic resistance. A polymorphism in the 3′ untranslated region that decreases binding of an inhibitory micro-RNA species (miR-24) leads to increased DHFR expression without prior MTX exposure.[188] Although this SNP was initially described as existing in 11–16% of a Japanese cohort,[189] the prevalence of this SNP may be much lower in other populations.[190]

Lack of the retinoblastoma protein, frequently deleted or altered in many tumor types, may play a role in intrinsic MTX resistance. In the absence of retinoblastoma protein, levels of the transcription factor E2F increase, resulting in an increase in transcription of several genes involved in DNA replication, including DHFR.[191]

Overexpression of *p*-glycoprotein does not confer resistance to MTX. However, MTX is a substrate for the related proteins, multidrug resistance proteins 1–5 (ABCC1–5)[192,193] and the breast cancer resistance protein (ABCG2).[194] ABCC5[193] and ABCG2[195] are able to transport both MTX and MTX-diglutamate. Overexpression of these proteins produces MTX resistance *in vitro*[193,196,197] and may affect the response to therapy among patients with leukemia.[198,199] To what degree these proteins contribute to clinically relevant intrinsic resistance to MTX in other diseases is not clear.

Acquired resistance to MTX

Four predominant mechanisms of acquired resistance to MTX have been described in experimental tumors and clinical samples: an increase in DHFR activity due to amplification of this gene; altered binding of MTX to DHFR due to DHFR mutations; decreased influx of MTX through the RFC; or to a decrease of long-chain polyglutamate formation.

At the point of entry into the cell, either mutations or deletions in the RFC could result in decreased uptake of MTX and MTX resistance. Although polymorphisms in the gene for RFC do not seem to be a common mechanism of intrinsic resistance among patients with leukemia,[179] decreased transport of MTX through the RFC has been shown to be a common mechanism of acquired resistance to MTX in leukemic blasts from patients with relapsed ALL.[200]

Exposure to MTX leads to a rapid increase in DHFR protein, as DHFR bound to MTX will not bind to its own mRNA and inhibit further translation.[201] Unstable or reversible resistance due to gene amplification has also been associated with the presence of "double minute" chromosomes containing the DHFR amplicon,[202] while high-level stable resistance has been associated with an abnormal banding region, often referred to as a homogeneously staining region.[203–207] Point mutations in DHFR in several cell lines, including human cells, have been detected that cause a change in the binding of MTX to the enzyme and have usually involved amino acids that bind to the inhibitor by hydrophobic interaction.[208]

Although defects in polyglutamylation have been described in several MTX-resistant cell lines,[209] the resistance of these cells has usually been found to be attributable to a combination of mechanisms. Increased hydrolysis of MTX polyglutamates can result from increased transport of MTX-polyglutamates into the lysosome[210] or increased levels of GGH activity.[183,211] Recent studies have provided ample evidence that epigenetic regulation and SNPs in the promoter and coding region of GGH can affect GGH expression and, therefore, responsiveness to antifolate therapy.[212–214] However, forced overexpression of GGH in cancer cell lines does not confer resistance to short exposure to MTX.[215]

Strategies to overcome resistance to MTX using new (or older) antifols

The rational design of new folate antagonists is driven by an increasing understanding of the molecular basis of normal folate physiology, of MTX cytotoxicity and MTX resistance, and is guided by crystallographic data from the target enzymes.[208] Newer antifolates have been designed to have one or more of the following properties: increased transport into the cell by either increased affinity for the RFC or independence of the RFC, independence of polyglutamylation or increased polyglutamylation by virtue of increased affinity for FPGS, increased inhibition of DHFR or TS, or increased inhibition of enzymes responsible for purine synthesis.

Aminopterin (AMT), an older antifol

Preclinical and clinical data support reevaluating an antifol older than MTX, 4-amino-pteroyl-glutamic acid (AMT; Figure 1), the first antifolate to produce remissions among patients with leukemia.[2] AMT has several advantages over MTX, including 20–40 times greater clinical potency,[216] more efficient conversion (higher $V_{max}:K_m$ ratio) by FPGS to polyglutamates[217] leading to greater accumulation by patients' leukemic blasts *in vitro*,[218] and complete oral bioavailability.[219] Twenty-seven percent of children with refractory ALL had clinically significant responses to oral AMT in a phase II trial,[220] and a phase IIb trial demonstrated that AMT can be substituted safely for MTX without excessive toxicity[134] in multiagent therapy for children with newly diagnosed ALL at high risk of relapse. Recent preclinical data suggest that AMT may benefit patients with atopic dermatitis.[221]

Pralatrexate, a second-generation DHFR inhibitor

Similar to MTX, pralatrexate (10-propargyl-10-deazaaminopterin; PDX; Figure 4) competitively inhibits DHFR, limiting thymidine synthesis and cell division. PDX was designed to have high affinity for the RFC and FPGS, leading to enhanced and selective intracellular internalization and retention in tumor cells.[222] Consequently, PDX exhibits a 14-fold greater rate of influx[223] and more potent inhibition of tumor growth when compared to MTX.[224]

Pralatrexate is given via IV administration. The total systemic exposure (AUC) and maximum plasma concentration (C_{max}) increase proportionally with dose. The terminal elimination $t_{1/2}$ of PDX is 12–18 h. Approximately one-third of an IV dose is excreted

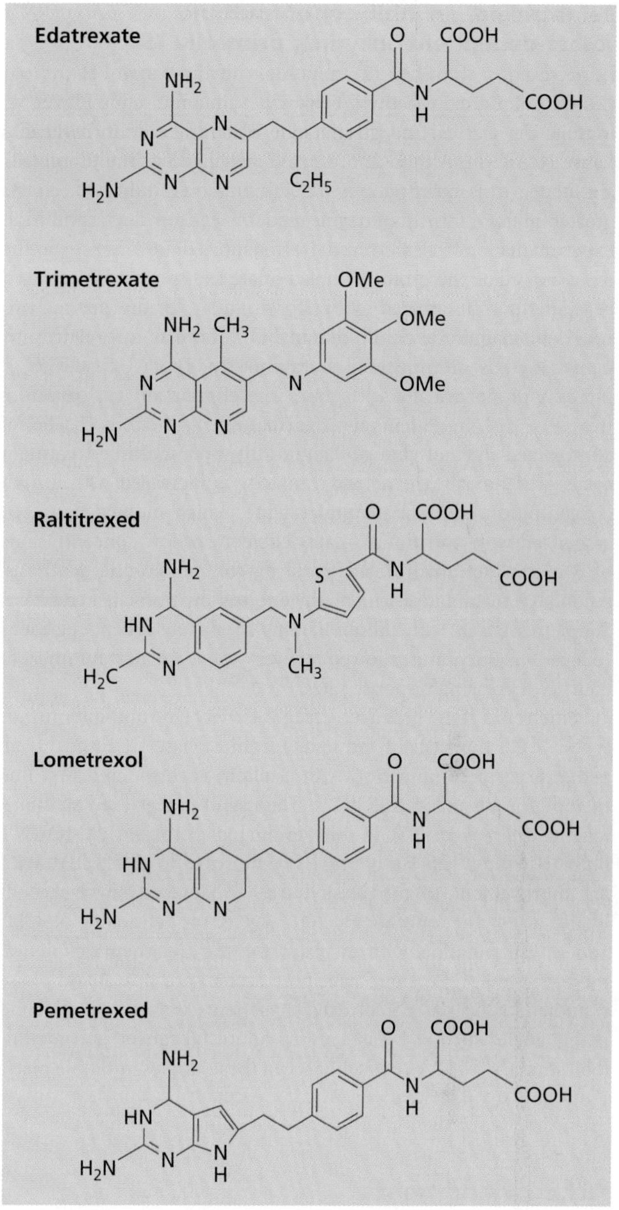

Figure 4 Novel folate antagonists of clinical interest.

unchanged in urine, and clearance decreases with decreasing creatinine clearance. The PK of PDX does not change significantly over multiple treatment cycles.[225]

Preclinical studies of PDX in combination with gemcitabine[226] and bortezomib[227] led to clinical trials of these combinations for patients with lymphoma. The overall response rate among those with T-cell lymphomas was significantly higher than those with B-cell lymphoma, suggesting a possible selectivity of the T-cell malignancies.[228] PROPEL (pralatrexate in relapsed or refractory peripheral T-cell lymphoma) was a prospective study looking at relapsed or refractory PTCL. It included 115 patients, most of whom had been heavily pretreated. An overall response rate of 29% was reported, and based on this finding, the FDA approved the use of PDX for treatment of relapsed and refractory T-cell lymphoma.[229] PDX has also been shown to have high activity with acceptable toxicity in patients with NSCLC[127] and relapsed or refractory cutaneous T-cell lymphoma.[230] A recent study using both *in vitro* and *in vivo* models demonstrated the protective effect of LV on PDX toxicity.[231]

Pemetrexed, an inhibitor of multiple folate-dependent enzymes, primarily TS

Pemetrexed (N-[4-[2-(2-amino-3,4-dihydro-4-oxo-7H-pyrrolo [2,3-d]pyrimidin-5-yl)ethyl] benzoyl]-ʟ-glutamic acid; Figure 4) inhibits TS, DHFR, and glycinamide ribonucleotide formyltransferase (GARFT). Although promoted initially as a "multitargeted" antifolate, it is primarily a TS inhibitor, as indicated by its greater affinity for this enzyme and by end-product inhibition experiments.[232,233] Pemetrexed is transported into cells via the RFC, as well as the proton-coupled folate transporter. Pemetrexed is rapidly polyglutamated by FPGS, with a K_m for the enzyme two orders of magnitude below that of MTX. Similar to pralatrexate, pemetrexed is administered intravenously. The AUC and C_{max} increase proportionally with dose. The elimination $t_{1/2}$ of pemetrexed is 3.5 h in patients with normal renal function. The PK of pemetrexed did not change significantly over multiple treatment cycles.[234] Clinically, pemetrexed toxicity is increased with a high concentration of plasma homocysteine, which in turn has been associated with nutritional folate deficiency or low concentrations of 5-methyl tetrahydrofolate required for methionine synthesis, secondary to mutations in methylene tetrahydrofolate reductase. Supplementation with these vitamins in all subsequent regimens reduced toxicity and allowed delivery of a greater number of courses, increasing response rates.[235]

Pemetrexed has broad-spectrum activity in multiple tumor types.[236] On the basis of the results from a phase III clinical trial, pemetrexed in combination with cisplatin is considered first-line therapy for advanced NSCLC.[237] The use of pemetrexed as maintenance therapy in NSCLC was evaluated in the PARAMOUNT phase III study. This study proved pemetrexed to be effective with an improvement in progression free and overall survival.[238] It is also used as monotherapy for relapsed or refractory NSCLC and in combination with cisplatin for the treatment of pleural mesothelioma.[235,239] There have been several preclinical and phase I studies looking at pemetrexed in patients with advanced solid malignancies such as breast cancer, colorectal cancer, and medulloblastoma.[240–242] As a consequence of these studies, multiple phase II studies are underway.

Acknowledgments

Barton A. Kamen, MD, PhD, an author of previous versions of this chapter, died in 2012 after a battle with cancer. Bart was a respected clinician, clinical researcher, teacher, and basic scientist with a legacy of many significant contributions to the (anti)folate field, including the identification of the folate-binding protein and description of its defining characteristics.

Key references

The complete reference list can be found on the Wiley Companion Digital Edition of this title (see inside front cover for login instructions).

1 Farber S, Cutler EC, Hawkins JW, Hartwell Harrison J, Converse Peirce E, Lenz GG. Action of pteroylglutamic conjugates on man. *Science.* 1947;**106**:619–621.

2 Farber S, Diamond L, Mercer RD, Sylvester RF Jr, Wolff JA. Temporary remissions in acute leukemia in children produced by folic acid antagonist, 4-aminopteroyl-glutamic acid (aminopterin). *N Engl J Med.* 1948;**238**:787.

6 Osborne MJ, Freeman MB, Huennekens FM. Inhibition of dihydrofolic reductase by aminopterin and amethopterin. *Proc Soc Exp Biol Med.* 1958;**97**:429–431.

8 Chabner BA, Allegra CJ, Curt GA, et al. Polyglutamation of methotrexate. Is methotrexate a prodrug? *J Clin Invest.* 1985;**76**(3):907–912.

16 Allegra CJ, Hoang K, Yeh GC, Drake JC, Baram J. Evidence for direct inhibition of de novo purine synthesis in human MCF-7 breast cells as a principal mode of metabolic inhibition by methotrexate. *J Biol Chem.* 1987;**262**(28):13520–13526.

17 Cronstein BN, Naime D, Ostad E. The antiinflammatory mechanism of methotrexate. Increased adenosine release at inflamed sites diminishes leukocyte accumulation in an in vivo model of inflammation. *J Clin Invest.* 1993;**92**(6):2675–2682.

22 Vazquez A, Tedeschi PM, Bertino JR. Overexpression of the mitochondrial folate and glycine-serine pathway: a new determinant of methotrexate selectivity in tumors. *Cancer Res.* 2013;**73**(2):478–482.

23 Stoller RG, Hande KR, Jacobs SA, Rosenberg SA, Chabner BA. Use of plasma pharmacokinetics to predict and prevent methotrexate toxicity. *N Engl J Med.* 1977;**297**(12):630–634.

26 Evans WE, Relling MV, Rodman JH, Crom WR, Boyett JM, Pui CH. Conventional compared with individualized chemotherapy for childhood acute lymphoblastic leukemia. *N Engl J Med.* 1998;**338**(8):499–505.

30 Winick N, Shuster JJ, Bowman WP, et al. Intensive oral methotrexate protects against lymphoid marrow relapse in childhood B-precursor acute lymphoblastic leukemia. *J Clin Oncol.* 1996;**14**(10):2803–2811.

31 Huffman DH, Wan SH, Azarnoff DL, Hogstraten B. Pharmacokinetics of methotrexate. *Clin Pharmacol Ther.* 1973;**14**(4):572–579.

40 Thyss A, Milano G, Etienne MC, et al. Evidence for CSF accumulation of 5-methyltetrahydrofolate during repeated courses of methotrexate plus folinic acid rescue. *Br J Cancer.* 1989;**59**(4):627–630.

81 Woods RL, Fox RM, Tattersall MH. Methotrexate treatment of squamous-cell head and neck cancers: dose–response evaluation. *Br Med J (Clin Res Ed).* 1981;**282**(6264):600–602.

82 Pizzorno G, Mini E, Coronnello M, et al. Impaired polyglutamylation of methotrexate as a cause of resistance in CCRF-CEM cells after short-term, high-dose treatment with this drug. *Cancer Res.* 1988;**48**(8):2149–2155.

89 Matloub Y, Bostrom BC, Hunger SP, et al. Escalating intravenous methotrexate improves event-free survival in children with standard-risk acute lymphoblastic leukemia: a report from the Children's Oncology Group. *Blood.* 2011;**118**(2):243–251.

90 Mahoney DH Jr, Shuster JJ, Nitschke R, et al. Acute neurotoxicity in children with B-precursor acute lymphoid leukemia: an association with intermediate-dose intravenous methotrexate and intrathecal triple therapy—a Pediatric Oncology Group study. *J Clin Oncol.* 1998;**16**(5):1712–1722.

101 Edelstein M, Vietti T, Valeriote F. The enhanced cytotoxicity of combinations of 1-beta-D-arabinofuranosylcytosine and methotrexate. *Cancer Res.* 1975;**35**(6):1555–1558.

107 Blay JY, Conroy T, Chevreau C, et al. High-dose methotrexate for the treatment of primary cerebral lymphomas: analysis of survival and late neurologic toxicity in a retrospective series. *J Clin Oncol.* 1998;**16**(3):864–871.

108 Hammond CB, Hertz R, Ross GT, Lipsett MB, Odell WD. Primary chemotherapy for nonmetastatic gestational trophoblastic neoplasms. *Am J Obstet Gynecol.* 1967;**98**(1):71–78.

112 Bonadonna G, Moliterni A, Zambetti M, et al. 30 years' follow up of randomised studies of adjuvant CMF in operable breast cancer: cohort study. *BMJ.* 2005;**330**(7485):217.

125 Coates AS, Tattersall MH, Swanson C, Hedley D, Fox RM, Raghavan D. Combination therapy with methotrexate and 5-fluorouracil: a prospective randomized clinical trial of order of administration. *J Clin Oncol.* 1984;**2**(7):756–761.

128 Jaffe N, Frei E 3rd, Traggis D, Bishop Y. Adjuvant methotrexate and citrovorum-factor treatment of osteogenic sarcoma. *N Engl J Med.* 1974;**291**(19):994–997.

134 Cole PD, Drachtman RA, Masterson M, et al. Phase 2B trial of aminopterin in multiagent therapy for children with newly diagnosed acute lymphoblastic leukemia. *Cancer Chemother Pharmacol.* 2008;**62**(1):65–75.

138 Bernini JC, Fort DW, Griener JC, Kane BJ, Chappell WB, Kamen BA. Aminophylline for methotrexate-induced neurotoxicity. *Lancet.* 1995;**345**(8949):544–547.

146 Buchen S, Ngampolo D, Melton RG, et al. Carboxypeptidase G2 rescue in patients with methotrexate intoxication and renal failure. *Br J Cancer.* 2005;**92**(3):480–487.

157 Cole PD, Beckwith KA, Vijayanathan V, Roychowdhury S, Smith A, Kamen BA. CSF folate homeostasis during therapy for acute lymphoblastic leukemia. *Pediatr Neurol.* 2009;**40**(1):35–42.

160 Drachtman RA, Cole PD, Golden CB, et al. Dextromethorphan is effective in the treatment of subacute methotrexate neurotoxicity. *Pediatr Hematol Oncol.* 2002;**19**(5):319–327.

165 Adamson PC, Balis FM, McCully CL, et al. Rescue of experimental intrathecal methotrexate overdose with carboxypeptidase-G2. *J Clin Oncol.* 1991;**9**(4):670–674.

177 Zhao R, Assaraf YG, Goldman ID. A mutated murine reduced folate carrier (RFC1) with increased affinity for folic acid, decreased affinity for methotrexate, and an obligatory anion requirement for transport function. *J Biol Chem.* 1998;**273**(30):19065–19071.

178 Jansen G, Mauritz R, Drori S, et al. A structurally altered human reduced folate carrier with increased folic acid transport mediates a novel mechanism of antifolate resistance. *J Biol Chem.* 1998;**273**(46):30189–30198.

188 Mishra PJ, Humeniuk R, Longo-Sorbello GS, et al. A miR-24 microRNA binding-site polymorphism in dihydrofolate reductase gene leads to methotrexate resistance. *Proc Natl Acad Sci U S A.* 2007;**104**(**33**):13513–13518.

200 Gorlick R, Goker E, Trippett T, Waltham M, Banerjee D, and Bertino JR. Intrinsic and acquired resistance to methotrexate in acute leukemia. *N Engl J Med.* 1996;**335**(**14**):1041–1048.

201 Ercikan-Abali EA, Banerjee D, Waltham MC, Skacel N, Scotto KW, and Bertino JR. Dihydrofolate reductase protein inhibits its own translation by binding to dihydrofolate reductase mRNA sequences within the coding region. *Biochemistry.* 1997;**36**(**40**):12317–12322.

202 Alt FW, Kellems RE, Bertino JR, and Schimke RT. Selective multiplication of dihydrofolate reductase genes in methotrexate-resistant variants of cultured murine cells. *J Biol Chem.* 1978;**253**(**5**):1357–1370.

208 Schweitzer BI, Dicker AP, Bertino JR. Dihydrofolate reductase as a therapeutic target. *FASEB J.* 1990;**4**(**8**):2441–2452.

209 Pizzorno G, Chang YM, McGuire JJ, Bertino JR. Inherent resistance of human squamous carcinoma cell lines to methotrexate as a result of decreased polyglutamylation of this drug. *Cancer Res.* 1989;**49**(**19**):5275–5280.

222 Marchi E, Mangone M, Zullo K, O'Connor OA. Pralatrexate pharmacology and clinical development. *Clin Cancer Res.* 2013;**19**(**24**):6657–6661.

229 O'Connor OA, Pro B, Pinter-Brown L, et al. Pralatrexate in patients with relapsed or refractory peripheral T-cell lymphoma: results from the pivotal PROPEL study. *J Clin Oncol.* 2011;**29**(**9**):1182–1189.

232 Chattopadhyay S, Moran RG, Goldman ID. Pemetrexed: biochemical and cellular pharmacology, mechanisms, and clinical applications. *Mol Cancer Ther.* 2007;**6**(**2**):404–417.

238 Paz-Ares LG, de Marinis F, Dediu M, et al. PARAMOUNT: final overall survival results of the phase III study of maintenance pemetrexed versus placebo immediately after induction treatment with pemetrexed plus cisplatin for advanced non-squamous non-small-cell lung cancer. *J Clin Oncol.* 2013;**31**(**23**):2895–2902.

239 Vogelzang NJ, Rusthoven JJ, Symanowski J, et al. Phase III study of pemetrexed in combination with cisplatin versus cisplatin alone in patients with malignant pleural mesothelioma. *J Clin Oncol.* 2003;**21**(**14**):2636–2644.

242 Morfouace M, Shelat A, Jacus M, et al. Pemetrexed and gemcitabine as combination therapy for the treatment of Group3 medulloblastoma. *Cancer Cell.* 2014;**25**(**4**):516–529.

57 Pyrimidine and purine antimetabolites

Robert B. Diasio, MD

Overview

The development of pyrimidine and purine antimetabolite drugs has been based on the rationale that nucleic acids are critical to cell replication and, therefore, the pyrimidine and purine bases (and their nucleosides) that are the "building blocks" necessary to synthesize nucleic acids are themselves potential sites for designing drugs that could be effective in inhibiting nucleic acid synthesis, whether that be in bacteria, viruses, or tumor cells. In this chapter, the various antimetabolites or analogs of uracil/thymine, cytidine/deoxycytidine, hypoxanthine/guanine, and adenosine that are currently used in the management of cancer are presented and reviewed with regard to metabolism, mechanism of action, clinical pharmacology, clinical activity, and toxicity.

The development of pyrimidine and purine antimetabolite drugs has been based on the rationale that nucleic acids are critical to cell replication and, therefore, the pyrimidine and purine bases (and their nucleosides) that are the "building blocks" necessary to synthesize nucleic acids are themselves potential sites for designing drugs that could be effective in inhibiting nucleic acid synthesis, whether that be in bacteria, viruses, or tumor cells. Recognizing that neoplastic cells (e.g., leukemic cells) often reproduce rapidly compared to their normal counterparts (e.g., lymphocytes or granulocytes), there is further logic for designing drugs similar to the pyrimidine or purine base or nucleoside precursors in the hope that they might disrupt nucleic acid synthesis. The term "antimetabolite" refers to the ability of synthetic pyrimidines and purines to mimic the structure of the naturally occurring pyrimidine and purine bases (or nucleoside metabolites) and, therefore, to enter biochemical pathways similar to their natural counterparts. However, the slight molecular differences in the antimetabolite analogs can result in interference with the synthesis of DNA and RNA. The resultant disruption in naturally occurring nucleic acid synthesis may occur in several ways. Thus, the pyrimidine or purine antimetabolites might compete with the naturally occurring counterpart for an enzyme that is critical in the nucleic acid synthesis pathway, thereby disturbing the pools of natural pyrimidine and purine nucleotides needed to synthesize DNA or RNA. Alternatively, the pyrimidine of purine may be incorporated directly into DNA or RNA resulting in the formation of a dysfunctional nucleic acid or possibly resulting in nucleic acid fragmentation as the DNA or RNA seeks to correct the abnormality.[1]

Pyrimidine antimetabolites

Potential pyrimidine antimetabolite cancer chemotherapy drugs might include structural modifications of the naturally occurring pyrimidine bases uracil, cytosine, or thymine or their ribose or deoxyribose nucleosides (Figure 1a). While thymine antimetabolites, such as azidothymidine (AZT), are effective in the treatment of viral infections, they are not as useful as uracil and cytosine antimetabolites in the treatment of cancer.

Uracil antimetabolites

Over the years, there have been several uracil antimetabolites that have shown potential activity in the treatment of various malignancies. The only uracil antimetabolites that remain actively used today in the United States are the 5-fluorouracil (5-FU) drugs (Figure 1), including the parent drug 5-FU, its deoxyribose nucleoside, 5-fluorodeoyxuridine (Floxuridine, FUdR or FdUrd) that is used occasionally today with hepatic arterial infusion, and the prodrug of 5-FU, capecitabine. In other parts of the world, particularly Asia, there has been widespread use of other 5-FU prodrugs (e.g., UFT, S-1), but in the United States, capecitabine is the only one presently approved.[2]

5-Fluoruracil (5-FU)

5-FU is one of the first rationally synthesized antineoplastic agents.[3] The stimulus for developing this antimetabolite derives from the observation that rapidly growing tumor cells require an exogenous source of uracil for growth (beyond what can be provided by the endogenous natural synthetic pathway forming uracil from orotic acid). Exogenously formed uracil can be converted into deoxyuridylate (dUMP), which in turn, in the presence of 5,10 methylene tetrahydrofolate, can form thymidylate required for DNA synthesis, from donation of a methyl group to the fifth position of the uracil (Figures 1 and 2). 5-FU is a close analog of uracil with fluorine effectively substituting for hydrogen at the fifth position of uracil due to similar conformation, including a similar van der Waals radius. As can be seen in Figure 2, this allows 5-FU to enter the biochemical pathways used naturally by uracil.

Metabolism

Following administration into the circulation, 5-FU may undergo glomerular filtration as a small molecule and pass directly into the urine or enter the anabolic and catabolic pathways, depending on the tissues, efficiently substituting for uracil and uracil-derived metabolites as substrates for its various enzymatic steps. Approximately 85% of the 5-FU that enters the circulation is destined for catabolism, with 10–15% being excreted through the urine and 1–3% being available for anabolism. Dihydropyrimidine dehydrogenase (DPD), the initial step in uracil catabolism, is the major rate-limiting step in the overall metabolism of 5-FU and is the major determinant of 5-FU available for anabolism.[4] Most 5-FU will be anabolized to the ribonucleotide form by conversion through orotate phosphoribosyltransferase in the presence of PRPP or via the sequential action of uridine phosphorylase and

Holland-Frei Cancer Medicine, Ninth Edition. Edited by Robert C. Bast Jr., Carlo M. Croce, William N. Hait, Waun Ki Hong, Donald W. Kufe, Martine Piccart-Gebhart, Raphael E. Pollock, Ralph R. Weichselbaum, Hongyang Wang, and James F. Holland.
© 2017 John Wiley & Sons, Inc. ISBN: 978-1-118-93469-2

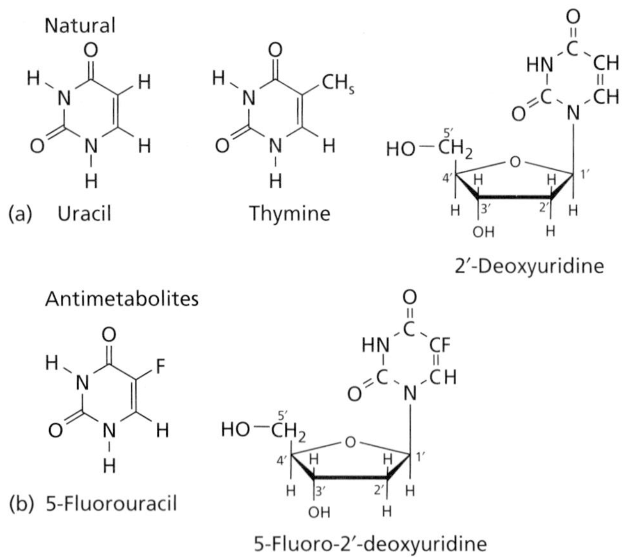

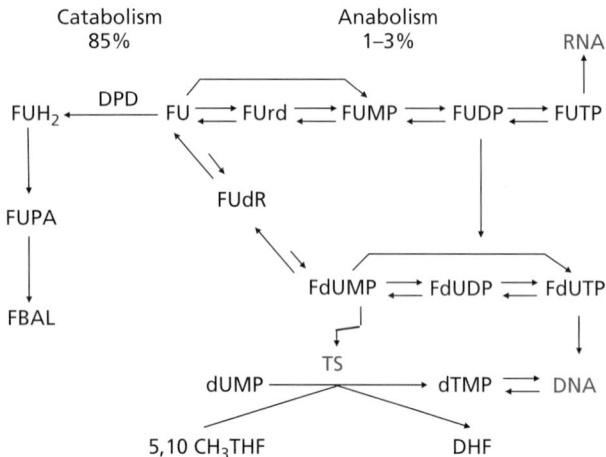

Figure 1 Uracil/thymine antimetabolites. (a) Natural occurring pyrimidine bases uracil and thymine together with the uracil deoxyribonucleoside (2′-deoxyuridine). (b) Antimetabolites 5-fluorouracil and 5-fluoro-2′deoxyuridine developed from structural modifications of uracil and 2′-deoxyuridine.

Figure 2 Metabolism and sites of action of 5-fluorouracil. The catabolic (to left of FU) and the anabolic (to right of FU) pathways that 5-FU may enter. Approximately 85% of administered 5-FU is catabolized via the rate-limiting enzymatic step (*DPD*) to dihydrofluorouracil (FUH_2) and then to fluoroureidopropionic acid (FUPA) and finally 2-fluoro-β-alanine (FBAL) with only 1–3% being anabolized (the rest being excreted into the urine). 5-FU is anabolized to nucleosides and then nucleotides as shown (these metabolites and the enzymatic steps are described in more detail in Refs 2, 3). The three primary sites of action are shown and include (1) inhibition of thymidylate synthase (TS) by the 5-fluoro-2′-deoxyuridylate (FdUMP) in the presence of 5,10 methylene tetrahydrofolate ($5,10 \, CH_3THF$); (2) incorporation of 5-fluoro uridylate triphosphate (FUTP) into RNA; and (3) incorporation of 5-fluoro-2′-deoxyuridylate triphosphate (FdUTP) into DNA, which in turn is removed by uracil glycosylase causing DNA fragmentation.

uridine kinase. Less likely is the formation of the deoxyribonucleotide 5-fluoro-2′-deoxyuridine monophosphate (FdUMP) via the sequential action of deoxyuridine phosphorylase (dUrdase) and deoxyuridine (or thymidine) kinase as the activity of dUrdase favors conversion to the base rather than the reverse reaction. Formation of the 5-FU nucleotides (in particular FdUMP, FUTP, and FdUTP) is critical to the activity of 5-FU (see the following

discussion). More information about the individual metabolic steps is provided elsewhere.[2,3]

Resistance to 5-FU theoretically can be secondary to any barrier to the formation of the 5-FU nucleotides critical to the potential mechanisms of action.[5] Thus, this could include inhibition of uptake of 5-FU into the cell, any enzymatic limitation of conversion of 5-FU to the nucleoside and then to the nucleotide. Thus, reduced uridine phosphorylase/kinase or orotate phosphoribosyltransferase could result in decreased levels of 5-FU nucleotides.

One aspect of 5-FU metabolism and pharmacology that is somewhat different from other agents is the concept of "biochemical modulation," in which the activity of 5-FU at an important enzymatic step or a critical site of action is influenced by the addition of an important chemical or precursor to a critical metabolite.[6] The best example of this is the use of leucovorin (folinic acid) that is often administered with 5-FU to increase the likelihood of adequate amounts of 5,10 methylene tetrahydrofolate being available to insure combination with FdUMP and thymidylate synthase (TS) to form a ternary complex capable of inhibiting DNA synthesis.

Mechanism of action

5-FU is thought to derive its anticancer activity from the effect of its nucleotide metabolites at three different sites (Figure 2). Inhibition of the enzyme TS by FdUMP (which actually has an affinity for TS greater than that of the natural substrate dUMP) in the presence of 5,10-methylene tetrahydrofolate inhibits the formation of thymidylate (TMP), which is critical for DNA synthesis. This has long been thought to be the primary mechanism by which fluoropyrimidine drugs work.[5] A second possible mechanism is the incorporation of the 5-FU ribonucleotide fluoro uridylate triphosphate (FUTP) into RNA in place of the natural uracil ribonucleotide UTP. This form of RNA may also be important owing to its effect on small RNAs.[2] The third mechanism is somewhat similar to the second with incorporation of the 5-FU deoxyribonucleotide FdUTP into DNA in place of the natural thymidylate nucleotide TTP. In this latter setting, however, it is the excision and repair of DNA containing FdUTP by uracil glycosylase resulting in DNA fragmentation that is thought to contribute to cytotoxicity.[3]

Clinical pharmacology

5-FU is typically administered as either an intravenous bolus or an intravenous infusion. Following administration as an intravenous bolus, 5-FU is rapidly cleared following first pass through the liver where it is rapidly catabolized with more than 85% of the administered dose being inactivated by initial degradation to dihydrofluorouracil (FUH_2).[3] The half-life of 5-FU in this setting is typically approximately 13 ± 7 min with the clearance being approximately 600 ± 200 mL/min/m^2.[4] Administering 5-FU by continuous infusion over 5 days or as a protracted multiday infusion by ambulatory pump, leads to a predicted, relatively constant but low level of 5-FU.[2]

Variability in the efficiency of catabolism exists with the main determinant being DPD, the rate-limiting step in 5-FU catabolism. In a small (<5%) but significant part of the population, genetic variants in the gene coding for DPD (*DPYD*) can result in decreased DPD activity that can shift more 5-FU into the anabolic pathway and in turn result in increased toxicity.[7,8]

Clinical use and indications

5-FU continues to be widely used to treat several common malignancies, including colorectal cancer and certain forms of skin cancer and breast cancer. It remains the major component of both adjuvant and advanced colorectal cancer regimens typically being administered with other drugs.[2]

Toxicities

Toxicities from 5-FU vary depending on dose and schedule of administration. Acute toxicities associated with intravenous bolus administration include myelosuppression, mucositis, and diarrhea. Prolonged exposure to 5-FU from continuous infusion may result in palmar-plantar erythrodysesthesia (hand-foot syndrome).[2,3]

Other 5-FU drugs

Over the past 60 years, there have been many additional 5-FU analogs synthesized. Most of these have been prodrugs of 5-FU.

5-Fluorodeoxyuridine

Background

5-Fluorodeoxyuridine (FdUrd, FUDR), the deoxyuridine of 5-FU, was synthesized about the same time as 5-FU in the late 1950s. Today it has relatively limited use. Its structure is shown in Figure 1.

Metabolism

FdUrd can function as a prodrug of 5-FU, being converted by deoxyuridine or thymidine phosphorylase into 5-FU. However, because it is a very good substrate for deoxyuridine or thymidine kinase, it is more likely rapidly directly converted into FdUMP, one of the primary active metabolites of 5-FU.

Mechanism of action

Formation of FdUMP can, in the presence of 5,10 methylene tetrahydrofolate, form an irreversible ternary complex with TS thereby blocking DNA synthesis. As most administered FdUrd will be metabolized directly to FdUMP, FdUrd is a relatively pure S-phase inhibitor.[9]

Clinical pharmacology

Today, when FdUrd is used, it is mainly as a continuous hepatic arterial infusion through an implantable pump.[10]

Clinical activity

FdUrd is utilized mainly in the treatment of hepatocellular cancer and colorectal cancer metastases to the liver.

Toxicities

With prolonged hepatic arterial infusion, the major toxicities are hepatic and include biliary sclerosis and occasional elevation of transaminases.[2,3]

Capecitabine

Background

There have been many attempts to develop an oral 5-FU drug that could not only provide a more convenient way of receiving 5-FU but also mimic the desirable effects of a 5-FU infusion.[11] Capecitabine is the only oral 5-FU prodrug FDA approved in the United States, although other oral forms of 5-FU are available in Asia and Europe.

Metabolism

Capecitabine is converted into 5-FU by the sequential action of three enzymes: (1) hepatic carboxylesterase, which initially hydrolyzes the drug to 5′-deoxy-5-fluorocytidine; (2) cytidine deaminase, which in turn deaminates this derivative to 5′-deoxy-5-fluorouridine (5′-dFUrd); and (3) finally, thymidine phosphorylase, which converts 5′-dFUrd into 5-FU (Figure 3). Because tumor tissue often

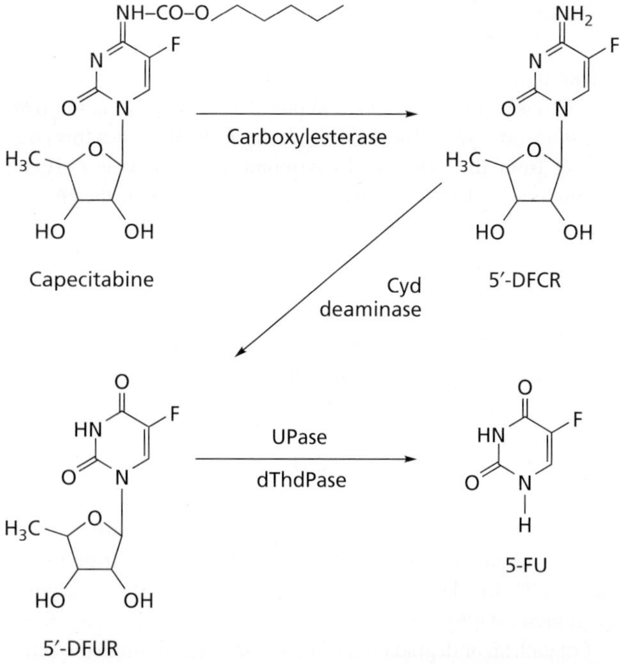

Figure 3 Structure and activation of capecitabine. The prodrug capecitabine is converted into 5-FU by three enzymatic steps carboxylesterase, cytidine deaminase, and uridine (or thymidine) phosphorylase. Intermediate metabolites include 5′-deoxyfluorocytidine (5′dFCR) and 5′-deoxyfluorouridine (5′dFUR).

has a higher activity of thymidine phosphorylase compared to most normal tissues, there is a potential selective benefit and in turn an improved therapeutic index.

Mechanism of action

Following conversion into 5-FU, the mechanism of action is identical with that of 5-FU (see above).

Clinical pharmacology

Capecitabine provides an alternative, more patient-friendly way of administering 5-FU to produce the effects of a 5-FU protracted infusion.

Clinical activity

Capecitabine has a similar spectrum of activity as 5-FU and is typically used in the treatment of colorectal and breast cancer.

Toxicities

The toxicities of Capecitabine are similar to those of 5-FU infusion with palmar-plantar erythrodysesthesia being the major toxicity seen with continuous Capecitabine use. Of interest has been a difference in the dose tolerance of Capecitabine in European versus American populations. It remains unclear what the basis for this is although external factors such as folate levels may contribute.[12]

Cytosine antimetabolites

Cytosine antimetabolites with clinical anticancer activity have been mainly nucleosides, where the major structural modification has been in the sugar part of the molecule and not the base. Currently, there are four cytosine antimetabolites used clinically. These include cytosine arabinoside (ara-C), 5-azacytidine (and the related decitabine), and gemcitabine (Figure 4).

Cytosine arabinoside

Background

Ara-C was identified as a natural product following isolation from *Cryptotethya crypta*. The arabinoside sugar differentiates this compound from the cytosine deoxyribonucleoside that is normally a component of DNA in that the 2′-OH group is in the *cis* configuration relative to the *N*-glycosyl bond between the cytosine and the sugar (Figure 4).[13] Today, ara-C is prepared synthetically for commercial use. Its effectiveness in cancer chemotherapy led to the synthesis of other arabinoside compounds, such as the purine antimetabolites 2-fluoro-ara-adenosine monophosphate and nelarabine (see the following discussion).

Metabolism

Following uptake into cells through nucleoside transporters, ara-C must first be converted into ara-C monophosphate (ara-CMP) by the action of deoxycytidine kinase and then further phosphorylated to the diphosphate (ara-CDP) and triphosphate (ara-CTP), the latter which is critical for cytostatic activity[14] (Figure 5).

Catabolism or degradation of ara-C can occur through the action of either cytidine deaminase, converting ara-C to ara-U, which is inactive, or deoxycytidylate deaminase, converting ara-CMP to ara-UMP, which is also inactive. Increased deamination is a basis for increased resistance as is decreased transport into the cell or any other potential mechanism for decreased anabolism to the active metabolite ara-CTP.

Mechanism of action

The mechanism of action of ara-C is thought to occur at several potential sites. Thus, ara-CTP is a potent inhibitor of DNA polymerases α, β, γ resulting in inhibition of DNA synthesis, elongation, and repair. An alternative mechanism of action occurs following incorporation of ara-CTP into DNA where it can terminate DNA elongation acting as a DNA chain terminator.[15]

Clinical pharmacology

The bioavailability of ara-C is poor with extensive deamination occurring in the gastrointestinal tract. This has necessitated intravenous administration typically by continuous infusion. Ara-C undergoes metabolism to ara-U within the plasma, liver, and various peripheral tissues with >80% excreted into the urine as ara-U. Ara-C can also cross the blood–brain barrier and enter the cerebrospinal fluid.

Clinical activity

Ara-C is an effective anti-leukemic agent, often used as the standard induction regimen for acute myelogenous leukemia (AML). It also has activity in acute lymphocytic leukemia (ALL) and chronic myelogenous leukemia (CML), as well as other hematologic malignancies such as non-Hodgkin's lymphoma. Of interest, the drug has essentially no activity in nonhematologic solid tumors.

Toxicities

Toxicities vary depending on both dose and schedule. As one might predict, one of the most prominent toxicities is myelosuppression. This is seen with standard 7-day regimens with peak myelosuppression at 7–14 days and is particularly prominent with the use of high doses ($2–3\,\text{g/m}^2$). Accompanying the myelosuppression are other hematologic toxicities in particular thrombocytopenia. Other toxicities include gastrointestinal manifestations such as nausea, anorexia, and vomiting as well as diarrhea, mucositis, and abdominal pain at times with pancreatitis and finally cerebellar toxicities at high doses.

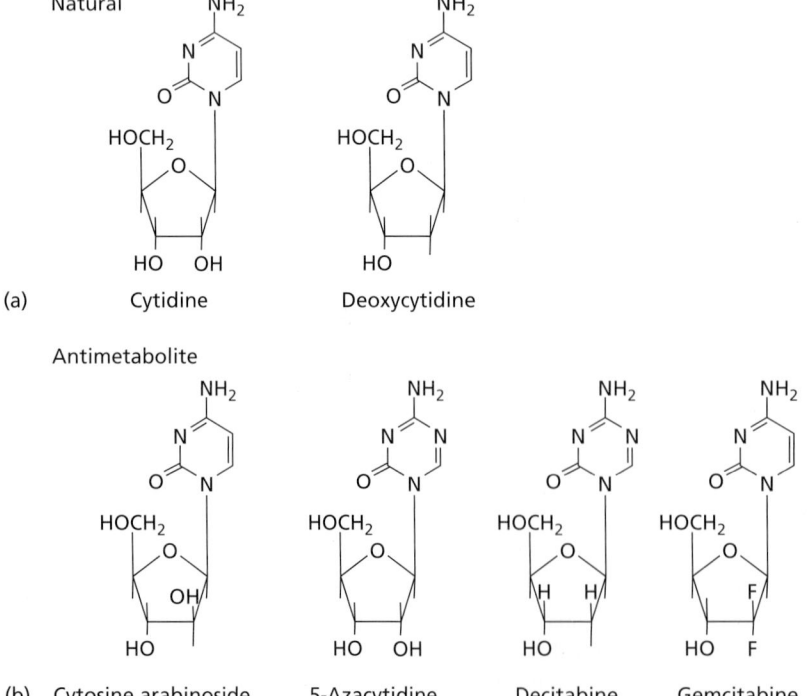

Figure 4 Cytidine/deoxycytidine antimetabolites. (a) Natural occurring cytosine nucleosides cytidine and deoxycytidine. (b) Antimetabolites cytosine arabinoside, 5-azacytidine, decitabine, and gemcitabine developed from structural modifications of the sugar of the cytosine nucleosides.

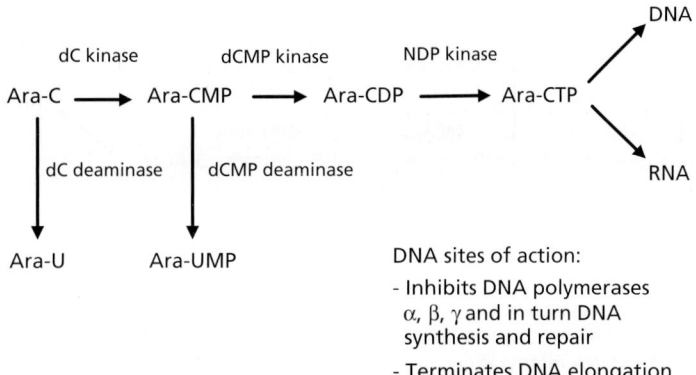

Figure 5 Metabolism and sites of action of ara-C. The metabolic pathway used by ara-C. Ara-C is activated to ara-CTP by the sequential action of three kinases: deoxycytidine kinase (*dC kinase*), deoxycytidine monophosphate kinase (*dCMP kinase*), and nucleotide diphosphate kinase (*NDP kinase*). Ara-C is inactivated by both cytidine deaminase (*CdR deaminase*) and deoxycytidine monophosphate deaminase (*dCMP deaminase*). Also listed are the sites of action of ara-C.

5-Azacytidine and decitabine

Background

5-Azacytidine represents an attempt to improve on the success of ara-C in treating leukemias. Of particular interest was identifying cytidine analogs that did not require activation by deoxycytidine kinase, the enzyme with decreased or absent activity in many ara-C-resistant tumors. A number of analogs were synthesized, in particular ribonucleosides, where structural changes had been made in the pyrimidine ring that still allowed the compound to be anabolized by uridine–cytidine kinase.[13] The most active of these was 5-azacytidine, which was also later identified occurring naturally in fungal cultures (Figure 4). 5-Azacytidine was shown to be toxic to both bacterial and mammalian cells. A related drug is decitabine (Figure 4).

Cellular uptake and metabolism

5-Azacytidine utilizes the equilabrative nucleoside transporter to enter human cells. Once within the cell, it is anabolized by utilizing the uridine–cytidine pathway to form 5-azacytidine monophosphate. This is converted into 5-azacytidine triphosphate by the sequential action of deoxycytidine monophosphate kinase and deoxycytidine diphosphate kinase (Figure 6). Decitabine's cellular uptake and metabolism are similar.

Resistance to 5-azacytidine might occur through several mechanisms. Thus, a deficient or altered nucleoside transporter on the cell surface could inhibit cellular uptake and in turn result in relative resistance. Endogenous levels of uridine and/or cytidine can compete with 5-azacytidine for phosphorylation resulting in less activity. Similarly decreased or absent expression of uridine–cytidine kinase could produce resistance. The presence of increased activity of catabolizing enzymes (e.g., cytidine deaminase) could result in the formation of 5-azauridine, which lacks cell toxicity.[13]

Mechanism of action

5-Azacytidine triphosphate is the critical metabolite. There are several suggested sites of action. The 5-azacytidine triphosphate first competes with naturally occurring CTP for incorporation into RNA. 5-Azacytidine triphosphate that gets incorporated into RNA can produce several detrimental effects on RNA processing and function including inhibition of ribosomal 328S and 18S formation, alteration of acceptor function of transfer RNA, disruption of polyribosomal assembly, and resultant inhibition of protein synthesis.[9] In addition, 5-azacytidine triphosphate can be incorporated into DNA, leading to the inhibition of DNA methylation following replication of DNA.[13] It is the latter effect that makes this drug particularly interesting to the study of epigenetic effects secondary to methylation. Decitabine has a similar mechanism of action. This includes demethylation or interference with the methylation of DNA. As a result, normal function to the tumor suppressor genes is restored, enabling control over cell growth. As a typical antimetabolite decitabine can also be incorporated into nucleic acid, interacting with a number of potential targets to produce a direct cytotoxic effect that causes death of rapidly dividing cancer cells.

Clinical pharmacology

5-Azacytidine is administered via intravenous infusion and undergoes rapid deamination to 5-azauridine. Plasma clearance is often lower in women and the elderly, and caution should therefore be used in these groups.

Clinical activity

With both 5-azacytidine and decitabine, clinical activity has been observed in both AML and myelodysplasia.[16] As noted earlier, 5-azacytidine's inhibitory effect on DNA methylation is of particular interest in that it enables a mechanism clinically and experimentally to increase expression of epigenetically suppressed genes.

Toxicities

Similar to other members of this antimetabolite group, the major dose-limiting toxic manifestation for both 5-azacytidine and decitabine is myelosuppression in particular neutropenia as well as thrombocytopenia. Nausea and vomiting occur particularly with bolus administration. Other toxicities observed particularly with high dose 5-azacytidine include hepatocellular abnormalities, hyperbilirubinemia, muscle tenderness and weakness, CNS toxicity with lethargy, confusion, and even coma.[17] Because of these latter toxicities, one should use caution in administering these drugs in the presence of hepatic failure or altered mental status.

Gemcitabine

Background

Gemcitabine is a synthetic nucleoside analog in which two fluorines have been substituted for the hydrogens in deoxycytidine.[13] The structure of gemcitabine is shown in Figure 4.

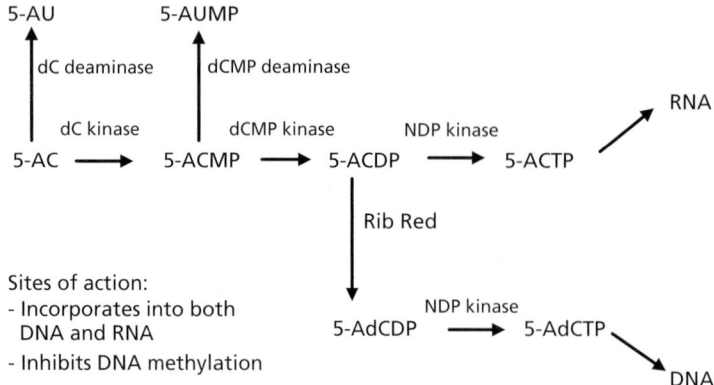

Figure 6 Metabolism and sites of action of 5-azacytidine. The metabolic pathway used by 5-AC. 5-AC is initially activated by the sequential action of deoxy-cytidine kinase (*dC kinase*) and deoxycytidine monophosphate kinase (*dCMP kinase*) to 5-ACDP. This can then be converted into 5-ACTP by nucleotide diphosphate kinase (*NDP kinase*) or into 5-AdCDP by the action of ribonucleotide reductase (*Rib Red*). 5-AdCDP can then be converted into 5-AdCTP by *NDP kinase*. 5-AC is inactivated by both cytidine deaminase (*dC deaminase*) and deoxycytidine monophosphate deaminase (*dCMP deaminase*). Also listed are the sites of action of 5-AC.

Cellular uptake and metabolism

Similar to other antimetabolites, gemcitabine utilizes the cell's nucleoside transporter to enter human cells. Once within the cell, it must be anabolized utilizing the cell's natural deoxycytidine pathways to form the gemcitabine triphosphate to achieve activity; it is inactive as the parent drug (Figure 7).[18]

There are several theoretical sites of resistance to gemcitabine. Thus, a deficient or altered nucleoside transporter can inhibit the cellular uptake of gemcitabine and result in relative resistance.[13] Metabolically, resistance can occur through both decreased activity of critical anabolizing enzymes (e.g., deoxycytidine kinase) or increased activity of catabolizing enzymes (e.g., cytidine deaminase or deoxycytidylate deaminase).

Mechanism of action

Gemcitabine triphosphate is the critical metabolite. There are several suggested sites of action. The most important is thought to be chain termination and inhibition of DNA synthesis and function following incorporation into DNA.[19] Gemcitabine triphosphate is also thought to directly inhibit DNA polymerases α, β, γ and can result in chain termination and inhibition of DNA synthesis and also DNA repair. Lastly, gemcitabine triphosphate is capable of inhibiting ribonucleotide reductase, further contributing to inhibition of DNA synthesis by depleting critically needed deoxyribonucleotide pools.

Clinical pharmacology

Gemcitabine is typically administered via intravenous infusion because of rapid deamination to 2′,2′-difluoro-2′-deoxyuridine (dFdU). Plasma clearance is often lower in women and the elderly, and caution should therefore be used in these groups.

Clinical activity

Although it has structural similarity and shares an identical site of action with ara-C, gemcitabine has a much broader spectrum of clinical activity including several solid tumors for example, pancreatic, lung (small cell and non-small cell), ovarian, bladder, and breast cancers as well as in hematologic malignancies, for example, both Hodgkin's and non-Hodgkin's lymphoma.

Toxicities

The major dose-limiting toxicity is myelosuppression with both neutropenia and to a somewhat lesser extent thrombocytopenia. When infusions are increased beyond 30 min, hematologic toxicity

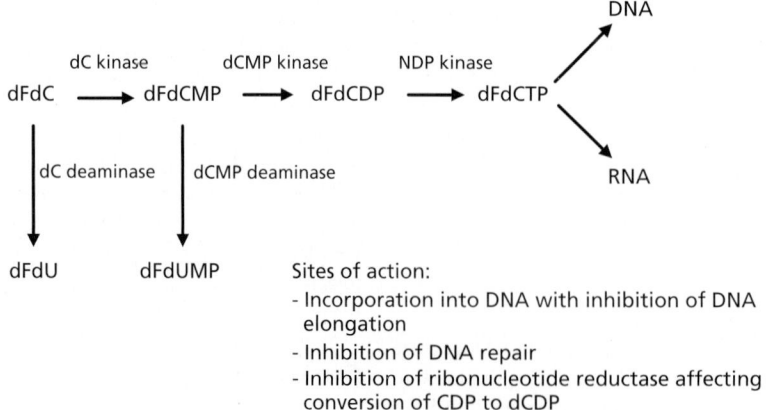

Figure 7 Metabolism and sites of action of gemcitabine (dFdC). The metabolic pathway used by gemcitabine (dFdC). Initially, dFdC must be activated to dFdCTP by the sequential action of three kinases: deoxycytidine kinase (*dC kinase*), deoxycytidine monophosphate kinase (*dCMP kinase*), and nucleotide diphosphate kinase (*NDP kinase*). Similar to ara-C, dFdC is inactivated by both cytidine deaminase (*dC deaminase*) and deoxycytidine monophosphate deaminase (*dCMP deaminase*). Also shown are the sites of action of dFdC.

tends to be more severe. Other frequently observed toxicities include flu-like symptoms including fever, headaches, myalgias, and arthralgias.

Purine antimetabolites

Purine antimetabolite cancer chemotherapy drugs include structural modifications of the naturally occurring purine bases, guanine and adenine, or their ribose or deoxyribose nucleosides. As with the pyrimidine antimetabolites, the structural changes can be in either the base or the sugar.[20]

Guanine antimetabolites

Two guanine antimetabolites, 6-mercaptopurine (6-MP) and 6-thioguanine (6-TG), have shown potential anticancer activity. Both were synthesized more than six decades ago but continue to be used today. While not having significant anticancer activity (and therefore not discussed here), azathioprine, a pro-drug of 6-MP that results in slow release of 6-MP is an effective immunosuppressant that has been widely used in organ transplantation, inflammatory bowel disease (e.g., Crohn's), and rheumatologic diseases.

6-Mercaptopurine

Background

The structure of 6-MP is closely related to the naturally occurring purine base hypoxanthine (Figure 8a); a thiol group substituting for the hydroxyl group at the sixth position. As is characteristic of other antimetabolites, 6-MP can enter the anabolic and catabolic pathways used by the natural occurring metabolites, in this case hypoxanthine.

Metabolism

Following uptake into cells, 6-MP can be immediately anabolized by hypoxanthine guanine phosphoribosyltransferase (HGPRT) to 6-thioinosine monophosphate (TIMP). TIMP can be further anabolized to the triphosphate and then be incorporated into DNA. The metabolism of 6-MP is shown in Figure 9.

Resistance can result from decreased availability of TIMP from either decreased anabolism or increased catabolism primarily mediated by phosphatases.

Mechanism of action

TIMP is thought to be the active metabolite deriving its mechanism of action through inhibiting *de novo* purine biosynthesis leading to a disturbance in the size of the natural purine nucleotide pools needed for nucleic acid synthesis (Figure 9).

Clinical pharmacology

6-MP is administered orally (typically $90 \, mg/m^2$), although its absorption can be erratic with variation in peak concentrations and peak times. 6-MP has minimal binding to serum proteins with the half-life of free drug being in 20–45 min range.[21]

6-MP is metabolized by xanthine oxidase. Because other drugs used in the oncologic setting such as allopurinol also utilize this same enzyme in its metabolism, this can lead to a potential serious drug interaction accompanied by increased toxicity (in effect more active 6-MP metabolite present). Therefore, with concomitant use, the dose of 6-MP is typically reduced 50–75%.[22]

Another important clinical pharmacologic finding with 6-MP use is pharmacogenetic. Thus, because there is variability in the expression of thiopurine methyltransferase (TPMT) in the general population owing to variants within the TPMT gene, the metabolism and hence the availability of active drug may vary. It is possible now to screen for these TPMT variants before 6-MP administration and thereby avoid toxicity.[23]

Clinical activity

Although introduced clinically more than 50 years ago, 6-MP continues to have a clinical role in the management of ALL, particularly in children. 6-MP lacks efficacy in solid tumors. Because of its immunosuppressive effects, it has also been used for nononcologic diseases (e.g., Crohn's disease).

Toxicities

The primary toxicity with 6-MP is myelosuppresion. Other toxicities include gastrointestinal, in particular anorexia, nausea, vomiting,

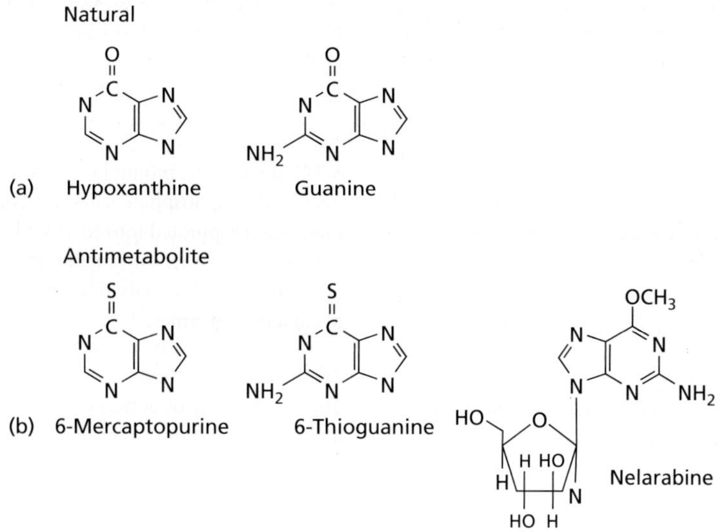

Figure 8 Hypoxanthine/guanine antimetabolites. (a) Natural occurring purine bases hypoxanthine and guanine. (b) Antimetabolites 6-mercaptopurine and 6-thioguanine developed from structural modifications of hypoxanthine and guanine as well as nelarabine a pro-drug of the dexoyguanosine antimetabolite 9-β-D-arabinofuranosylguanine (ara-G).

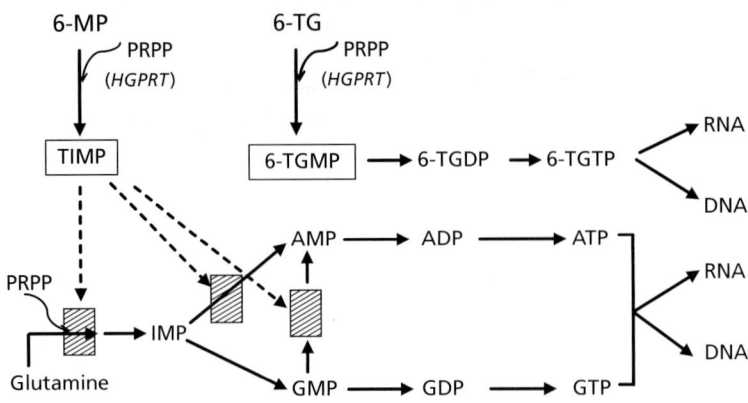

Figure 9 Metabolism and sites of action of 6-mercaptopurine (6-MP) and 6-thioguanine (6-TG). 6-MP is converted into 6-thioinosine monophosphate (TIMP) and 6-TG is converted into 6-thioguanine ribonucleotide monophosphate (6-TGMP) by hypoxanthine guanine phosphoribosyltransferase (*HGPRT*) in the presence of PRPP. TIMP is active by inhibiting *de novo* purine biosynthesis at three steps: (1) inhibiting formation of inosine monophosphate (IMP) from glutamine and PRPP, (2) inhibiting conversion of IMP into AMP, and (3) inhibiting conversion of GMP into AMP. Through the sequential activation of nucleotide kinases, 6-TGMP can be eventually converted into the ribonucleotide diphosphate (6-TGDP) and then ribonucleotide triphosphate (6-TGTP). 6-TGTP is active following incorporation into both RNA and DNA, resulting in a disturbance of nucleic acid function.

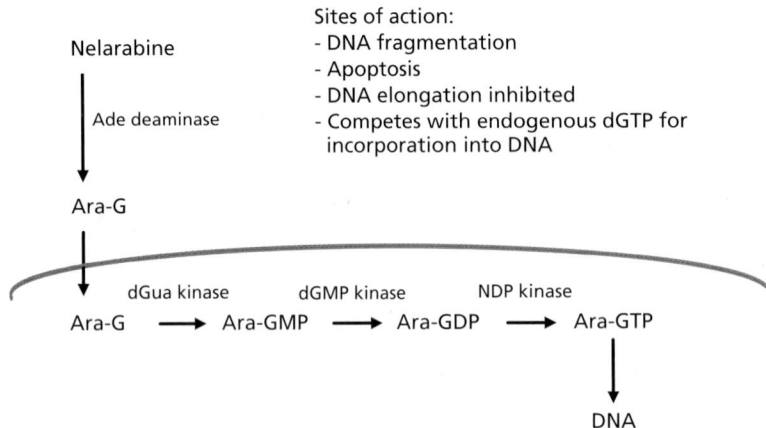

Figure 10 Metabolism and sites of action of nelarabine. Nelarabine is a prodrug that following intravenous administration is undergoes O-demethylation in the blood by adenosine deaminase (*Ade deaminase*) to Ara-G. Ara-G then transported into cells by nucleoside transporters where it is converted by deoxyguanosine kinases (*dGua kinase*) into the monophosphate, ara-GMP, and then through the sequential action of nucleotide kinases, dGMP kinase and NDP kinase, to the active metabolite ara-GTP. Also shown are the sites of action ara-GTP.

and diarrhea. Hepatotoxicity may also be seen. For this reason, concomitant use of hepatotoxic agents should be avoided. Finally, 6-MP, like its prodrug azathioprine, can produce immunosuppression, and with this an increased risk of infections.

6-Thioguanine

Background
6-TG, like 6-MP, is one of the original purine antimetabolites, first synthesized in the 1950s. It too belongs to the family of guanine antimetabolites. Its structure is shown in Figure 8.

Metabolism
Following uptake into cells, 6-TG is anabolized utilizing the endogenous enzymes in the guanine pathway as shown in Figure 9. 6-TG differs from 6-MP in that it is converted directly into

6-TG nucleotide monophosphate and then subsequently to the nucleotide diphosphate and nucleotide triphosphate, which can then be incorporated into RNA and DNA.

Similar to other antimetabolites, resistance may occur from either decreased activity of anabolic enzymes or increased activity of catabolic enzymes.[20]

Mechanism of action
The mechanism of action of 6-TG is thought to be secondary to its incorporation into both RNA and DNA where it interferes with nucleic acid synthesis and function.[24]

Clinical pharmacology
6-TG is typically administered orally. Its oral bioavailability is variable with peak levels occurring 2–4 h after dosing. Its metabolism differs from that of 6-MP in that it is not metabolized by xanthine

oxidase. Therefore, no drug interactions occur with concomitant administration of allopurinol, and unlike 6-MP, the dose of 6-TG need not be reduced to avoid toxicity.

6-TG, however like 6-MP, is a substrate for TPMT and therefore in the presence of decreased expression secondary to genetic variability in the TPMT gene expression, one must be adjust for dose in affected individuals. TPMT deficiency is common enough (approximately 10% of all patients) that TPMT screening is recommended before drug administration.[23]

Clinical activity
6-TG is active in AML, where it is sometimes used for remission induction and maintenance therapy. 6-TG is also used in ALL.

Toxicities
Myelosuppression is the major toxicity. Other toxicities include stomatitis and gastrointestinal toxicities in particular anorexia, nausea/vomiting, and diarrhea. Hepatotoxicity may also be seen in a significant percentage of patients, in particular cholestatic jaundice and occasionally transaminase elevations. For this reason, concomitant use of hepatotoxic agents should be avoided. Finally, like 6-MP, 6-TG is also associated with immunosuppression with an increased risk of infections.

Nelarabine

Background
Nelarabine is a prodrug of the deoxyguanosine antimetabolite 9-β-D-arabinofuranosylguanine (ara-G), which is cytotoxic. It is one of the newer purine antimetabolites that was developed for use in patients resistant to fludarabine (see the following discussion). Its structure is shown in Figure 8.

Metabolism
As a prodrug, Nelarabine must first be converted into ara-G[25] by adenosine deaminase (ADA)-mediated demethylation. Once transported into the tumor cells by nucleoside transporters, ara-G is anabolized to the ribonucleotide triphosphate (ara-GTP), which is the active metabolite. It utilizes the same enzymes used by naturally occurring purines in the purine anabolic pathway (Figure 10). Similar to other antimetabolites, the activity of catabolic enzymes may contribute to relative resistance.

Mechanism of action
Ara-GTP is active following incorporation into DNA where it can result in DNA fragmentation and apoptosis. Similar to other antimetabolites, ara-GTP competes with the naturally occurring deoxyguanosine triphosphate (dGTP) for incorporation into DNA. Following incorporation at the 3′ end of the elongating DNA, further incorporation into DNA is inhibited resulting in apoptosis and cellular death. Other mechanisms of action cannot be ruled out but remain unclear at present.[26]

Clinical pharmacology
Nelarabine is a soluble prodrug typically administered by 2–3 h intravenous infusion. Neither nelarabine nor ara-G is significantly bound by plasma proteins and is eliminated through the kidney.[27]

Clinical activity
Nelarabine was approved by FDA in 2005 for use in patients with T-cell acute leukemia or T-cell lymphoblastic lymphoma, who were unresponsive to previous chemotherapy or relapsed after at least two chemotherapy regimens.[28]

Toxicities
Common toxicities include malaise, fever, nausea, and myelosuppression. Serious (Grades 3 and 4) neurologic toxicities occur in 10–15% of patients and may include both central nervous system side effects, for example, obtundation, seizures, and encephalopathy, and peripheral neuropathy.

Adenosine antimetabolites
The adenosine analogs represent the other major class of purine antimetabolites. In contrast to the guanine antimetabolites that depend on structural modification within the purine base, the adenosine antimetabolites rely on changes within the sugar portion of the molecule. This structural change results in decreased effectiveness of ADA. Halogen substitution at the second position of the deoxyadenosine with fluorine in fludarabine and chlorine in cladribine also contributes to the desired effect. Currently, there are several adenosine antimetabolites approved for clinical use (Figure 11). These include fludarabine, cladribine, and clofarabine. A fourth adenosine-like analog, pentostatin (Deoxycoformycin), is a naturally, occurring purine analog that was first identified in fermentation broths of *Streptomyces antibioticus*. Its structure is similar to the transitional form of adenosine in the ADA reaction. It is one of the most effective inhibitors of ADA and more details are covered elsewhere.[20]

Fludarabine

Background
Fludarabine, also known as 9-β-D-arabinosyl-2-fluoroadenine monophosphate or F-ara-AMP, has a structure that is shown in Figure 11.

Metabolism
Following intravenous administration, it is rapidly dephosphorylated to F-ara A (Figure 12). This can then cross into cells using the nucleoside transporters. Within the cells in the presence of ATP and deoxycytidine kinase, it is converted back into a nucleotide monophosphate and then sequentially converted into F-ara-ATP.[29]

Mechanism of action
F-ara-ATP is the active metabolite responsible for the mechanism of action. This results from competition with the natural metabolite deoxyadenosine triphosphate (dATP).

Clinical pharmacology
F-ara-AMP must be administered by the intravenous route. Peak concentrations are observed after 3–4 h. It is excreted into the urine with almost 25% of the administered drug being eliminated unchanged.

Clinical activity
This purine antimetabolite is active in chronic lymphocytic leukemia where it was first approved. It also has activity in several other hematologic malignancies including prolymphocytic leukemia, indolent non-Hodgkin's lymphoma, cutaneous T-cell lymphoma, mantle cell lymphoma, and Waldenstrom macroglobulinemia. Fludarabine has essentially no activity in nonhematologic solid tumors.[30]

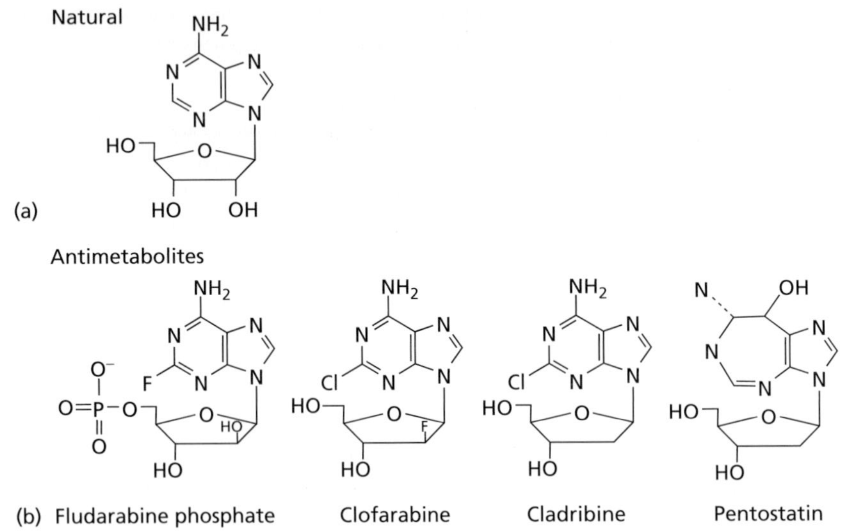

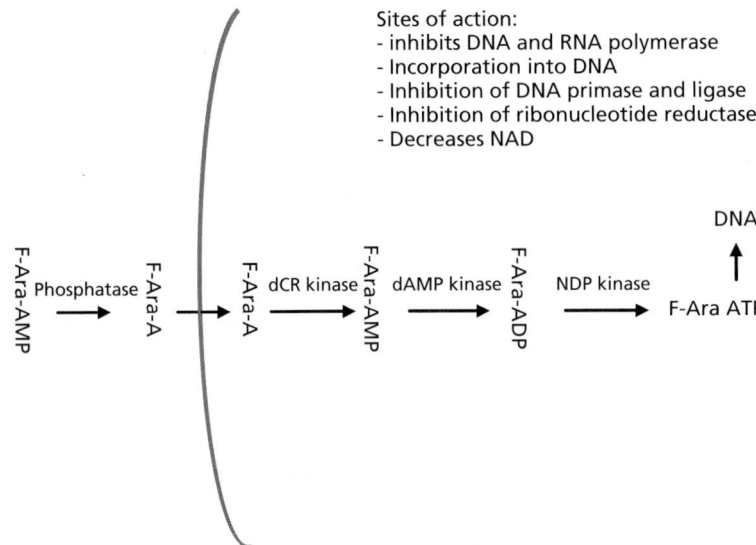

Figure 11 Adenosine antimetabolites. (a) The natural occurring purine base adenosine. (b) The antimetabolites fludarabine monophosphate, cladribine, and clofarabine developed from structural modifications of adenosine. In addition (although not discussed in this chapter), pentostatin, an adenosine analog first isolated from fermentation broths of *Streptomyces antibioticus*, is shown for comparison as it corresponds to the transitional form of adenosine in the adenosine deaminase reaction.

Figure 12 Metabolism and sites of action of fludarabine (FAraAMP). Following intravenous administration, FAraAMP is dephosphorylated in the blood by ubiquitous phosphatases to FAra-A. FAra-A is then transported into cells by nucleoside transporters where it is reconverted by deoxycytidine kinase (*dCR kinase*) into the monophosphate, FAra-AMP, and then through the action of nucleotide kinases (*dAMP kinase and NDP kinase*) converted into the active metabolite FAra-ATP. Listed are the sites of action for FAra-ATP.

Toxicities

The two major side effects limiting F-ara-AMP in the clinic are myelosuppression and immunosuppression. The myelosuppression is often lymphocytopenia and thrombocytopenia. Fever is often seen with myelosuppression. Immunosuppression is primarily T-cell mediated with much less effect on B-cells. Lymphocyte counts, in particular CD4 cells, are often depressed after F-ara-MP and may take more than a year to recover. The combined effect of myelosuppression and immunosuppression may result in an increased risk for opportunistic infections such as *Candida albicans*, *Pneumocystis carinii*, or viral *infections with varicella-zoster*. Prophylactic antibiotic coverage for *P. carinii* is often recommended with trimethoprim sulfamethoxazole the drug of choice to be coadministered with F-ara-AMP. Other less frequent toxicities include anorexia, nausea, vomiting, diarrhea, abdominal pain and at times

increased salivation, and parageusia (metallic taste), skin rash, and stomatitis.[20] Laboratory abnormalities include transient elevations of hepatic enzymes as well as evidence of renal dysfunction.

Cladribine

Background

Cladribine is a purine deoxyadenosine analog. Its structure is shown in Figure 11.

Metabolism

Following entry into the cell using the cell's nucleoside transporters, cladribine is anabolized via deoxycytidine kinase (dC kinase) to cladribine monophosphate eventually being converted into cladribine triphosphate, the active metabolite[31,32] (Figure 13).

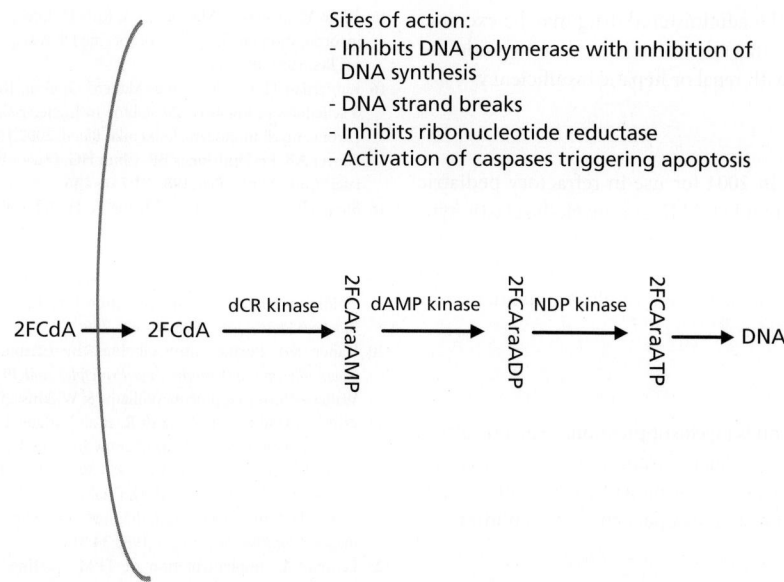

Sites of action:
- Inhibits DNA polymerase with inhibition of DNA synthesis
- DNA strand breaks
- Inhibits ribonucleotide reductase
- Activation of caspases triggering apoptosis

2FCdA → 2FCdA —dCR kinase→ 2FCAraAMP —dAMP kinase→ 2FCAraADP —NDP kinase→ 2FCAraATP → DNA

Figure 13 Metabolism and sites of action of cladribine. Following intravenous administration, cladribine is transported into cells by nucleoside transporters where it is reconverted by deoxycytidine kinase (*dCR kinase*) into the monophosphate, 2CFAra-AMP, and then through the action of nucleotide kinases (*dAMP kinase and NDP kinase*) to the active metabolite 2CFAra-ATP. Also listed are the sites of action ara-2CFAra-ATP.

Altered metabolism of cladribine can contribute to resistance, in particular decreased activity of dC kinase, a critical step in the anabolism of this drug. Similarly, increased expression of catabolic enzymes, in particular 5′-nucleotidase, may contribute to resistance.

Mechanism of action
The active metabolite cladribine triphosphate competes with naturally occurring dATP for incorporation into DNA where it can cause termination of chain elongation. There can also be inhibition of DNA synthesis and repair due to an imbalance in critical deoxyribonucleotide pools as well as inhibition of ribonucleotide reductase.

Clinical pharmacology
Cladribine can be administered orally. The drug is primarily excreted via the kidney with approximately 50% cleared into the urine, with as much as 25% unchanged. The drug can cross the blood–brain barrier into the cerebrospinal fluid.

Clinical activity
Cladribine was initially approved by the FDA for treatment of hairy cell leukemia and remains the drug of choice for that disease. Its response rate is 60% or greater for treatment of hairy cell leukemia with both primary and relapsed disease. The drug also has activity in low-grade lymphoproliferative diseases. It has potential activity for patients with CLL and non-Hodgkin's lymphoma.[33,34]

Toxicities
Myelosuppresion is the primary dose-limiting toxicity at standard doses with both thrombocytopenia and neutropenia. Other toxicities include nausea, vomiting and diarrhea, and neurotoxicity. Cladribine can also cause immunosuppression with decreased lymphocyte counts particularly CD-4 positive cells. These depressed counts may take years to recover after finishing treatment. The decreased CD-4 counts predispose patients to developing opportunistic infections.

Clofarabine

Background
Clofarabine was synthesized to develop a potentially more effective adenine analog than fludarabine and cladribine (Figure 11). This 2-halo-2′-halodeoxyarabinofuranosyl adenine analog has the 2-chloroadenine aglycone that conveys resistance to inactivation by ADA. It also is thought to benefit from the fluorine in the 2′ position of the sugar in the arabinosyl configuration that potentially contributes to its DNA inhibition. The fluorine substituted at the C-2′ position is thought to inhibit the effect of purine nucleoside phosphorylase (PNP) (phosphorolysis) in contrast to what typically occurs with fludarabine and cladribine.[20]

Metabolism
Following uptake into tumor cells, clofarabine must be anabolized to a triphosphate, which is the active metabolite. Its chemistry potentially contributes to decreased catabolism and hence increased effectiveness. Clofarabine is actually a better substrate for deoxycytidine kinase than fludarabine or cladribine.[35]

Resistance can result from perturbation of metabolism due to either decreased anabolism or increased catabolism.

Mechanism of action
Several possible sites of action include inhibition of DNA synthesis due to chain termination following incorporation into DNA; inhibition of DNA synthesis by inhibiting DNA polymerases α, β, and γ, which in turn interferes with DNA chain elongation and synthesis and repair of DNA. DNA synthesis is further inhibited by depletion of intracellular deoxyribonucleotide pools through inhibition of ribonucleotide reductase.[36,37]

Clinical pharmacology
Clofarabine is typically administered as an intravenous infusion at doses between 2 and 40 mg/m² over 5 days. Half-life is approximately 5 h with plasma concentrations as high as 2.5 μM being achievable, although there is interpatient variability. It is

estimated that 50–60% of the administered drug may be excreted unchanged into the urine. Currently, there is no data to guide use of this drug in individuals with renal or hepatic insufficiency.

Clinical activity

FDA approved clofarabine in 2004 for use in refractory pediatric ALL. It has also been used in adult AML and myelodysplastic syndrome. Of particular clinical interest is the combined use of clofarabine with ara-C with increased response being reported without increased toxicity. This is thought to be a result of potentiation by increasing ara-C concentrations.[38–40]

Toxicities

The major toxic manifestation is myelosuppression, which results in an increased risk for infection. Hepatic transaminase elevation has also been noted in as many as 25% of patients. Other side effects include anorexia, nausea, and skin rash particularly in children.

References

1 Chabner BA. General principles of cancer chemotherapy. In: Brunton LL, Chabner BA, Knollmann BC, eds. *Goodman & Gilman's the Pharmacological Basis of Therapeutics*, 12th ed. New York: McGraw-Hill; 2011.

2 Grem JL, Chabner BA, Ryan DR. 5-Fluoropyrimidines. In: Chabner BA, Longo DL, eds. *Cancer Chemotherapy and Biotherapy; Principles and Practice*, 5th ed. Philadelphia, PA: Walters Kluwer Lippincott Williams & Wilkins; 2011.

3 Diasio RB, Harris BE. Clinical pharmacology of 5-fluorouracil. *Clin Pharmacokinet.* 1989;**4**:215–237.

4 Heggie GD, Sommadossi JP, Cross DS, Huster WJ, Diasio RB. Clinical pharmacokinetics of 5-fluorouracil and its metabolites in plasma, urine, and bile. *Cancer Res.* 1987;**478**:2203–2206.

5 Wilson PM, Danenberg PV, Johnston PG, Lenz HJ, Ladner RD. Standing the test of time: targeting thymidylate biosynthesis in cancer therapy. *Nat Rev Clin Oncol.* 2014;**11**:282–298.

6 Anderson N, Lokich J, Bern M, Wallach S, Moore C, Williams D. A phase I clinical trial of combined fluoropyrimidines with leucovorin in a 14-day infusion. Demonstration of biochemical modulation. *Cancer.* 1989;**63**:233–237.

7 Diasio RB, Beavers TL, Carpenter JT. Familial deficiency of dihydropyrimidine dehydrogenase. Biochemical basis for familial pyrimidemia and severe 5-fluorouracilinduced toxicity. *J Clin Invest.* 1988;**81**:47–51.

8 Chong CR, Zirkelbach JF, Diasio RB, Chabner BA. Pharmacogenetics. In: Chabner BA, Longo DL, eds. *Cancer Chemotherapy and Biotherapy; Principles and Practice*, 5th ed. Philadelphia, PA: Walters Kluwer Lippincott Williams & Wilkins; 2011.

9 Veselý J. Mode of action and effects of 5-azacytidine and of its derivatives in eukaryotic cells. *Pharmacol Ther.* 1985;**28**:227–235.

10 Kemeny NE, Schwartz L, Gönen M, et al. Treating primary liver cancer with hepatic arterial infusion of floxuridine and dexamethasone: does the addition of systemic bevacizumab improve results? *Oncology.* 2011;**80**:153–159.

11 de Bono JS, Twelves CJ. The oral fluorinated pyrimidines. *Invest New Drugs.* 2001;**19**:41–59.

12 Midgley R, Kerr DJ. Capecitabine: have we got the dose right? *Nat Clin Pract Oncol.* 2009;**6**:17–24.

13 Chabner BA, Glass J. Cytidine analogues. In: Chabner BA, Longo DL, eds. *Cancer Chemotherapy and Biotherapy; Principles and Practice*, 5th ed. Philadelphia, PA: Walters Kluwer Lippincott Williams & Wilkins; 2011.

14 Chou TC, Arlin Z, Clarkson BD, Phillips FS. Metabolism of 1-D-arabinofuranosylcytosine in human leukemic cells. *Cancer Res.* 1977;**37**:3561–3570.

15 Ohno Y, Spriggs D, Matsukage A, Kufe D. Effects of 1-d-arabinofuranosylcytosine incorporation on elongation of specific DNA sequences by DNA polymerase. *Cancer Res.* 1988;**48**:1494–1498.

16 Kantarjian H, Oki Y, Garcia-Manero G, et al. Results of a randomized study of 3 schedules of low-dose decitabine in higher-risk myelodysplastic syndrome and chronic myelomonocytic leukemia. *Blood.* 2007;**109**:52–57.

17 Glover AB, Leyland-Jones BR, Chun HG, Davies B, Hoth DF. Azacitidine: 10 years later. *Cancer Treat Rep.* 1987;**71**:737–746.

18 Shewach DS, Hahn TM, Chang E, Hertel LW, Lawrence TS. Metabolism of 2′,2′-difluoro-2-deoxycytidine and radiation sensitization of human colon carcinoma cells. *Cancer Res.* 1994;**54**:3218–3223.

19 Ruiz van Haperen VW, Veerman G, Vermorken JB, Peters GJ. 2′,2′-Difluorodeoxycytidine (gemcitabine) incorporation into RNA and DNA of tumour cell lines. *Biochem Pharmacol.* 1993;**46**:762–766.

20 Hande KR. Purine antimetabolites. In: Chabner BA, Longo DL, eds. *Cancer Chemotherapy and Biotherapy; Principles and Practice*, 5th ed. Philadelphia, PA: Walters Kluwer Lippincott Williams & Wilkins; 2011.

21 Zimm S, Collins JM, Riccardi R, et al. Variable bioavailability of oral mercaptopurine: is maintenance chemotherapy in acute lymphoblastic leukemia being optimally delivered? *N Engl J Med.* 1983;**308**:1005–1009.

22 Zimm S, Collins JM, O'Neill D, Chabner BA, Poplack DG. Inhibition of first-pass metabolism in cancer chemotherapy: interaction of 6-mercaptopurine and allopurinol. *Clin Pharmacol Ther.* 1983;**34**:810–817.

23 Lennard L. Implementation of TPMT testing. *Br J Clin Pharmacol.* 2014;**77**:704–714.

24 Karran P, Attard N. Thiopurines in current medical practice: molecular mechanisms and contributions to therapy-related cancer. *Nat Rev Cancer.* 2008;**8**:24–36.

25 Nelson JA, Carpenter JW, Rose LM, Adamson DJ. Mechanisms of action of 6-thioguanine, 6-mercaptopurine and 8-azaguanine. *Cancer Res.* 1975;**35**:2872–2878.

26 Gandhi V, Keating MJ, Bate G, Kirkpatrick P. Nelarabine. *Nat Rev Drug Discov.* 2006;**5**:17–18.

27 Sanford M, Lyseng-Williamson KA. Nelarabine. *Drugs.* 2008;**68**:439–447.

28 Cohen MH, Johnson JR, Justice R, Pazdur R. FDA drug approval summary: nelarabine (Arranon) for the treatment of T-cell lymphoblastic leukemia/lymphoma. *Oncologist.* 2008;**13**:709–714.

29 Gandhi V, Plunkett W. Cellular and clinical pharmacology of fludarabine. *Clin Pharmacokinet.* 2002;**41**:93–103.

30 Montillo M, Ricci F, Tedeschi A. Role of fludarabine in hematological malignances. *Expert Rev Anticancer Ther.* 2006;**6**:1141–1161.

31 Griffig J, Koob R, Blakley RL. Mechanisms of inhibition of DNA synthesis by 2-chlorodeoxyadenosine in human lymphoblastic cells. *Cancer Res.* 1989;**49**:6923–6928.

32 Fukuda Y, Schuetz JD. ABC transporters and their role in nucleoside and nucleotide drug resistance. *Biochem Pharmacol.* 2012;**83**:1073–1083.

33 Grever MR, Lozanski G. Modern strategies for hairy cell leukemia. *J Clin Oncol.* 2011;**29**:583–590.

34 Sigal DS, Miller HJ, Schram ED, Saven A. Beyond hairy cell: the activity of cladribine in other hematologic malignancies. *Blood.* 2010;**116**:2884–2896.

35 Zhenchuk A, Lotfi K, Juliusson G, Albertioni F. Mechanisms of anti-cancer action and pharmacology of clofarabine. *Biochem Pharmacol.* 2009;**78**:1351–1359.

36 Nagai S, Takenaka K, Nachagari D, et al. Deoxycytidine kinase modulates the impact of the ABC transporter ABCG2 on clofarabine cytotoxicity. *Cancer Res.* 2011;**71**:1781–1791. PMID: 21245102.

37 Aye Y, Stubbe J. Clofarabine 5′-di and -triphosphates inhibit human ribonucleotide reductase by altering the quaternary structure of its large subunit. *Proc Natl Acad Sci U S A.* 2011;**108**:9815–9820.

38 Ghanem H, Kantarjian H, Ohanian M, Jabbour E. The role of clofarabine in acute myeloid leukemia. *Leuk Lymphoma.* 2013;**54**:688–698.

39 Bryan J, Kantarjian H, Prescott H, Jabbour E. Clofarabine in the treatment of myelodysplastic syndromes. *Expert Opin Investig Drugs.* 2014;**23**:255–263.

40 Wiernik PH. Optimal therapy for adult patients with acute myeloid leukemia in first complete remission. *Curr Treat Options Oncol.* 2014;**15**:171–186.

58 Alkylating agents and platinum antitumor compounds

Zahid H. Siddik, PhD

Overview

Alkylating agents and platinum-based compounds are highly potent antitumor drugs used in the treatment of a variety of cancers. These drugs target DNA (deoxyribonucleic acid) but require activation by spontaneous or metabolic transformation to induce formation of DNA monofunctional adducts and interstrand and intrastrand crosslinks. As a result of this damage, the DNA unwinds and/or bends, and such distortions are then recognized by specialized DNA damage recognition proteins to activate checkpoints, which arrest the cell cycle to allow cells time to repair the damage and survive. If the DNA damage is extensive and repair cannot be completed, then cells activate p53-dependent or independent apoptosis (programmed cell death) to affect antitumor drug response. As activated species from alkylating agents and platinum compounds are not tumor-selective, they will also interact with DNA and other endogenous macromolecules in normal cells to induce severe side effects; at times the toxicity can be irreversible and cumulative and, thereby, presents a dose-limiting barrier. Another limitation is that genetic changes in tumors that are either intrinsic or acquired can inhibit apoptosis and induce resistance to alkylating and platinating drugs. Resistance mechanisms may be observed in the form of reduced drug accumulation, increased drug inactivation, increased DNA repair, failure of DNA damage recognition system to recognize the damage, and aberrant apoptotic signal transduction pathways. Rational strategies to circumvent resistance mechanisms are, therefore, needed desperately to enhance patient care.

Introduction

Hallmarks of cancer include sustained proliferative signaling and replicative immortality as biological features that contribute to uncontrolled increase in tumor mass.[1,2] These characteristics are consistent with absence of feedback or inhibitory control on DNA (deoxyribonucleic acid) replication and the cell cycle that is commonly found in tumor cells. It is not surprising, therefore, that therapeutics targeting or covalently interacting with DNA to inhibit DNA replication and, thereby, cellular proliferation, have been the mainstay for clinically managing patients with cancer. Such therapeutics are broadly known as DNA alkylating agents and include platinum-based antitumor compounds. These agents form monofunctional and/or bifunctional adducts, with bifunctional adducts existing in several forms, including interstrand and intrastrand DNA crosslinks (Figure 1).

The foundation for alkylating agents as therapeutics dates back to the 1914–1918 Great War when poison gases, such as chlorine or the fatally vesicant sulfur mustard gas, were used indiscriminately against enemy soldiers in chemical warfare. The sulfur mustard (Figure 2) was first used by the Germany military in 1917 against British, Canadian, and French soldiers near the town of Ypres,

Belgium. During autopsy of dead soldiers, it was noted that mustard gas was highly myelosuppressive and produced lymphoid aplasia.[3] Thus, the notion that such agents could combat uncontrolled growth of cancers was conceptualized, but the high toxicity and reactivity of mustard gas precluded its clinical application. Efforts in early 1940s at Yale University by Goodman and Gilman[4,5] eventually resulted in the less-reactive and less-toxic nitrogen mustard, mechlorethamine or mustine (Figure 2), as the first agent to be tested in antitumor clinical trials in lymphoma patients, and its demonstrated activity firmly laid the foundation for modern cancer chemotherapy. Its activity also spawned the development of more effective and less-toxic alkylating agents, and some of these remain part of the present-day clinical anticancer armamentarium. Apart from the nitrogen mustards, several structural classes of alkylating agents are also of considerable interest, including the aziridines, hexitol epoxides, alkyl sulfonates, nitrosoureas, and the triazines/hydrazines, and these, together with the platinum-containing antitumor drugs, form the basis of this article.

General mechanisms of cytotoxicity

Alkylating agents and platinum antitumor compounds can transform to highly reactive species that indiscriminately form strong chemical bonds with endogenous macromolecules having electron-rich (nucleophilic) centers, such as nitrogen and sulfur atoms. The macromolecules can be peptides, proteins, or nucleic acids, but the interaction with DNA is the basis for their potent cytotoxic effects. Interactions with DNA can be monofunctional, when only a single alkylating or platinating reaction is permissible, or bifunctional, when covalent bonds are formed at nucleophilic centers of two different bases on DNA to induce crosslinks or adducts. Moreover, such crosslinks, formed predominantly through the N7 position of guanine, can be interstrand (between opposite DNA strands; induced preferentially by alkylating agents) or intrastrand (on the same DNA strand; induced preferentially by platinum drugs) (Figure 1).

Although the chance interaction between alkylating agents and DNA can be influenced by a number of factors, such as formation, detoxification, and nuclear access of the active alkylating moiety, the actual interaction with DNA is site specific. The N7 site of guanine, for instance, is electron rich and facilitates preferential covalent interaction with the positively charged alkylating species. The interaction is further facilitated by the nucleotide sequence, that is, interstrand GG crosslinks with nitrogen mustards are favored when guanine is in the 5′-GC-3′ or 5′-GXC-3′ sequence (where X = any nucleotide) in both DNA strands.[6,7] On the other hand, N2-guanine in the 5′-CG-3′ sequence (cytosine preceded by guanine) is preferred for crosslinking by mitomycin C owing to its orientation in the minor groove of DNA.[8] Alkylation at O6-guanine and N3-cytosine can also occur.

Holland-Frei Cancer Medicine, Ninth Edition. Edited by Robert C. Bast Jr., Carlo M. Croce, William N. Hait, Waun Ki Hong, Donald W. Kufe, Martine Piccart-Gebhart, Raphael E. Pollock, Ralph R. Weichselbaum, Hongyang Wang, and James F. Holland.
© 2017 John Wiley & Sons, Inc. ISBN: 978-1-118-93469-2

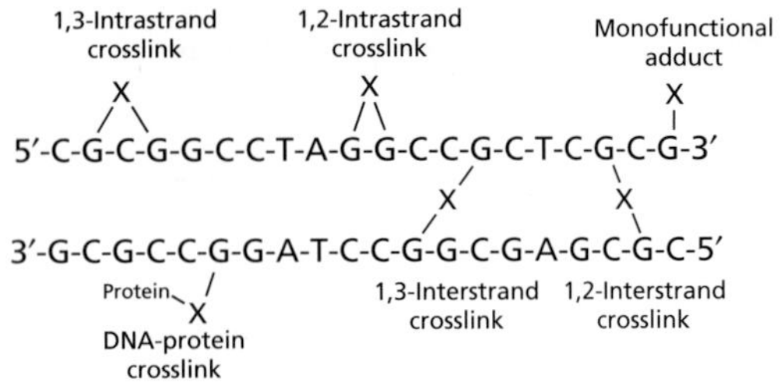

Figure 1 Monofunctional DNA adducts and interstrand and intrastrand crosslinks induced by DNA damaging agents (X = alkyl or platinum species).

The critical nature of N7-diguanyl crosslinks in the cytotoxicity of alkylating agents was established in early 1960s.[6,9] Although interstrand crosslinks may be envisioned as preventing separation of DNA strands during replication of the genome to induce cytotoxicity, this is by no means certain; it is clear that monofunctional, interstrand, and intrastrand adducts all have cellular effects, including inhibition of DNA synthesis, cell cycle arrest and apoptosis; however, the bifunctional drugs have greater potency than monofunctional agents. These cellular effects are the net result of specific distortions and unwinding in DNA induced by the alkylating or platinating drug and resultant coordinated assembly of distinct proteins at the DNA damage site to activate a number of signal transduction pathways. The final cellular effect is dependent on the concentration of the drug and, thereby, the extent of DNA damage; low level of DNA damage induces cell cycle arrest to permit DNA repair and cell survival, whereas extensive DNA damage overwhelms the capacity of the repair machinery and activates apoptosis. These events occur in both tumor and normal cells, and the small difference in relative tolerance to DNA damage between normal and tumor cells makes side effects of therapy inevitable that prevent administration of larger doses.

Alkylating agents

Bifunctional alkylating agents

Nitrogen mustards

Soon after the initial report of clinical activity of mechlorethamine in 1946,[4,5] many nitrogen mustards were evaluated for their antitumor potential through structure–activity relationships. Of the handful that advanced to clinical trials, a few were approved by the FDA and are still in use today. In addition to mechlorethamine, these include cyclophosphamide, ifosfamide, melphalan, chlorambucil, and bendamustine, which are shown in Figure 2. Also shown in this figure is 4-hydroperoxycyclophosphamide, which is the prodrug form of active 4-hydroxycyclophosphamide.

The sequence of events and specificity of the reaction between nitrogen mustards and DNA have been well described by Colvin et al.[10] The bis-chloroethyl group of these agents is critically important for the predominant alkylation of N7-guanine in DNA, although alkylation can occur but infrequently at O6-guanine and at N3- and N7-adenine. The alkylation is sequence specific and requires guanine in the 5′-GXC-3′ sequence (where X = any nucleotide). For interaction, the chloroethyl moiety cyclizes to form the highly reactive aziridinium ion intermediate that reacts readily with electron-rich sites, as shown with N7-guanine in Figure 3. It is possible that the aziridinium ion may first rearrange to the reactive carbonium ion intermediate for the alkylation reaction, but this remains uncertain. As there are two chloroethyl groups present, this results in sequential bifunctional alkylation to crosslink DNA. As indicated above, interstrand crosslinks are preferred by nitrogen mustards, with 1,3-crosslinks being the favored interaction. However, DNA–DNA intrastrand, DNA–protein, and DNA–glutathione crosslinks are also formed, but lack cytotoxic potential. Interstrand DNA crosslinks are the critical lesions, and according to Roberts et al.,[11] bifunctional interstrand DNA

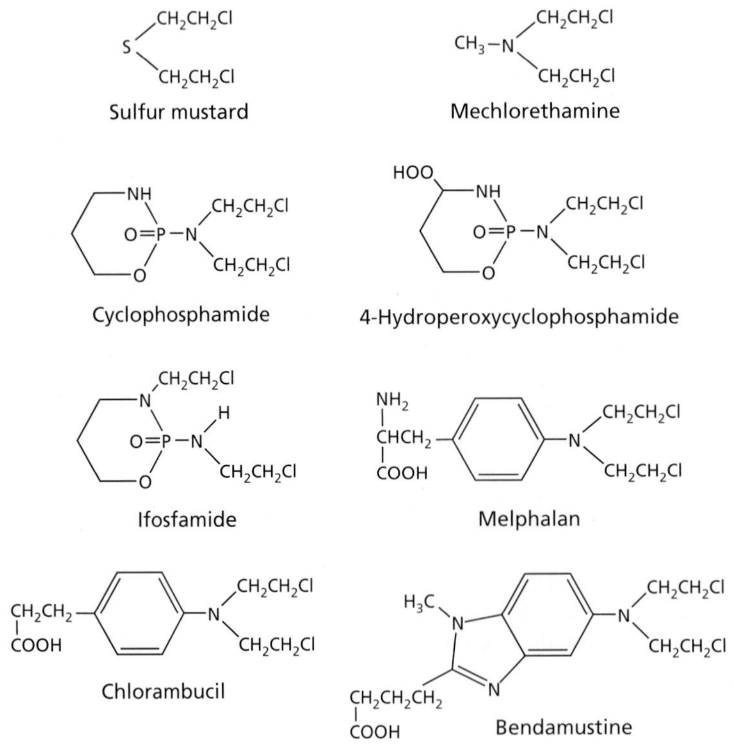

Figure 2 Structures of sulfur and nitrogen mustards.

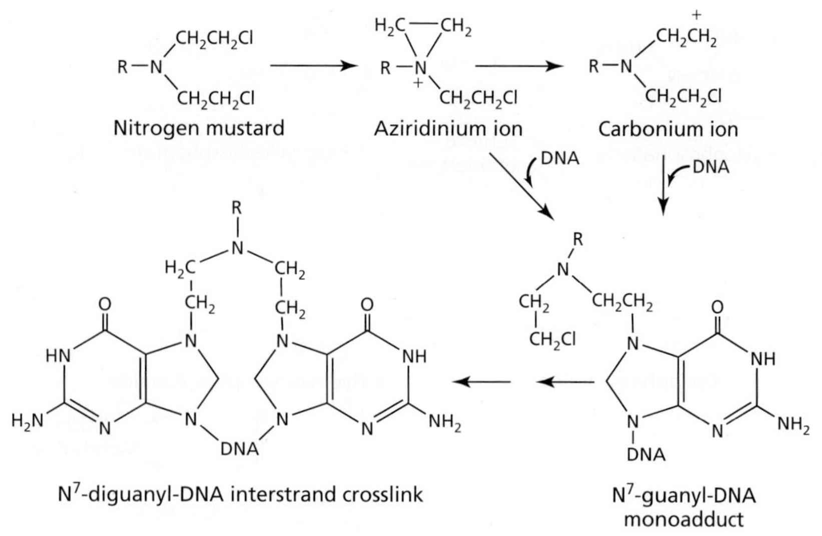

Figure 3 DNA alkylation by nitrogen mustard to form interstrand crosslink.

crosslinks are about 100-fold more effective at killing cells than monofunctional DNA adducts.

All nitrogen mustards are neutral and must be activated to interact with DNA target sites. Mechlorethamine, for instance, is activated spontaneously at physiological pH, but the rapid rate of activation is a major cause of much of the unwanted side effects. Chemical modification of the molecule, however, has played a crucial role not only to stabilize nitrogen mustard congeners, but also to influence their physicochemical properties that regulate transport, distribution, and reactivity of the molecule in order to enhance clinical utility.[12] Cyclophosphamide, which has an oxazaphosphorine ring, was selected from over a 1000 oxazaphosphorine candidates, and its chemical inertness and dependence on metabolic activation were considered as desirable characteristics.[13,14] The primary site for this activation is the liver, where the P450-mediated mixed function oxidase reaction initiates a complex series of chemical transformation events[15–18] that is depicted in part in Figure 4. The 4-hydroxycyclophosphamide is the most significant metabolite, which is relatively nonpolar and can readily distribute throughout the body, including tumor cells. This metabolite can be formed directly from the prodrug 4-hydroperoxycyclophosphamide (Figure 2), which has demonstrated utility in purging tumor cells in bone marrow aspirates of patients undergoing autologous bone marrow transplant.[19] At physiologic pH, a small amount of the 4-hydroxycyclophosphamide exists in equilibrium with aldophosphamide, which is relatively unstable and spontaneously decomposes to form the highly reactive phosphoramide mustard and then nornitrogen mustard.

An important by-product of the metabolism of cyclophosphamide, resulting from the conversion of aldophosphamide to phosphoramide mustard (Figure 4), is acrolein,[18] which induces hemorrhagic cystitis as a serious side effect,[20] but whether it has antitumor activity is of interest. Although a study with the model compound didechloro-4-hydroperoxycyclophosphamide indicated that the spontaneously released acrolein lacked cytotoxicity,[21] other studies have demonstrated that acrolein indeed has antitumor and carcinogenic activities but is inactivated by O6-alkylguanine-alkyltransferase.[22–24] Aldehyde dehydrogenase can also play a significant role in moderating activity by converting aldophosphamide to the inactive carboxyphosphamide metabolite, which accounts for about 80% of the cyclophosphamide dose excreted in the urine. Not surprisingly, this enzyme can confer

resistance to cyclophosphamide in tumor cells when ectopically overexpressed.[25] Thus, high levels of aldehyde dehydrogenase in the liver, early hematopoietic cells, and intestinal stem and mucosal absorptive cells are consistent with reduced hepatic, gastrointestinal (GI), and hematopoietic toxicities associated with cyclophosphamide as compared to other alkylating agents. Urinary excretion of metabolites can be compromised at high doses of cyclophosphamide by an antidiuretic effect owing to sodium loss and water reabsorption by renal tubules, with resultant edema.[26] The electrolyte imbalance may also contribute to the reported dose-limiting and fatal cardiotoxicity of high-dose chemotherapy.[27] This limitation has been recognized and doses are now monitored clinically to prevent this lesion from becoming serious.

Ifosfamide (Figure 2) is a structural isomer of cyclophosphamide that is important in the treatment of testicular cancer and sarcomas. Like cyclophosphamide, it also requires activation by hepatic mixed function oxidase,[13] but the low rate of metabolic activation by 4-hydroxylation and conversion to the corresponding active isophosphoramide mustard decreases its potency approximately fourfold.[28,29] On the other hand, increase in the dose to compensate for the lower potency leads to a greater cumulative production of acrolein, which increases the incidence of urothelial toxicity that requires concurrent administration of the thiol-based mesna to inactivate the toxic by-product. Renal and bladder toxicity, as well as neurotoxicity, of ifosfamide have also been ascribed to the formation of chloroacetaldehyde,[30] the product of oxidation of the chloroethyl side chain (Figure 4) that is generated in greater quantities with ifosfamide than with cyclophosphamide (∼50% vs ∼10% of the dose). The primary metabolite of ifosfamide, aldoifosfamide, is also a substrate for aldehyde dehydrogenase, and this is consistent with low toxicity of the drug to the bone marrow and the GI tract due, as mentioned previously with cyclophosphamide, to the presence of high levels of the enzyme in these organs.

Melphalan, chlorambucil, and bendamustine do not have the oxazaphosphorine ring of cyclophosphamide and ifosfamide in their structure, and so do not require metabolic activation, although metabolism of these agents does occur in the liver, but only for its disposition. These agents instead have an unsaturated electron-withdrawing aromatic ring (Figure 2) that moderates activation of the bis-chloroethyl group and formation of the aziridinium ion in order to minimize side effects. Owing to its phenylalanine-based structure, melphalan can be transported

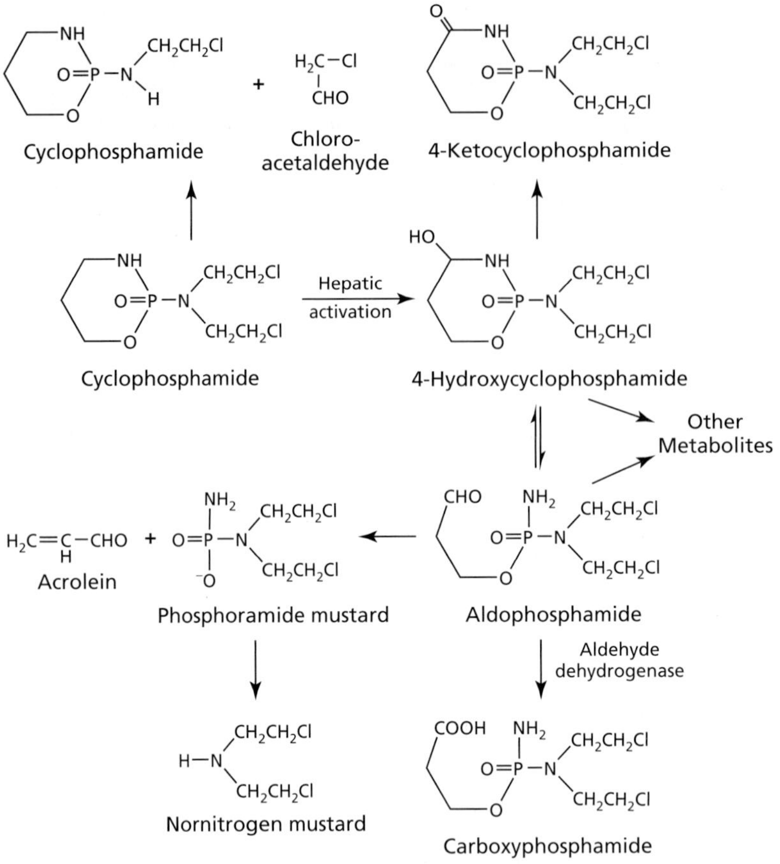

Figure 4 Metabolic activation and inactivation of cyclophosphamide.

actively into cells and across the blood–brain barrier.[31–33] These nitrogen mustards have found important applications against several cancers: melphalan against multiple myeloma, breast cancer, and ovarian carcinoma[34]; chlorambucil against ovarian cancer, chronic lymphocytic leukemia (CLL), and Hodgkin's and non-Hodgkin's lymphoma[35–37]; and bendamustine against CLL and lymphomas.[38] Owing to its improved tolerance, bendamustine is reported to be more cost-effective as a therapeutic drug than the structurally similar chlorambucil.[39]

Aziridines
Also known as ethyleneimines, the aziridines alkylate through the three-membered heterocyclic aziridine ring. Aziridine family of drugs includes thiotepa (*N,N′,N″*-triethylenethiophosphoramide), mitomycin C, and triethylenemelamine, which are shown in Figure 5. Also shown is hexamethylmelamine, which is similar to triethylenemelamine, but lacks the classical aziridine ring. Of these, thiotepa and mitomycin C are of clinical interest for a number of diseases, including refractory osteosarcoma and bladder cancer, respectively.[40,41] High-dose thiotepa has also been used in drug combination regimens with[42] or without[43] autologous stem cell support for breast cancer. Hexamethylmelamine, on the other hand, has found application in salvage therapy for recurrent ovarian cancer.[44]

The aziridine ring in the chemical structure of thiotepa is not charged, which makes it less reactive with electron-rich centers in RNA (ribonucleic acid), DNA, protein, and thiols (such as glutathione) than the structurally similar aziridinium ring formed with nitrogen mustards. In DNA, thiotepa alkylates sites in all four nucleotides, particularly at O2-cytosine, N1-thymine, N1-,

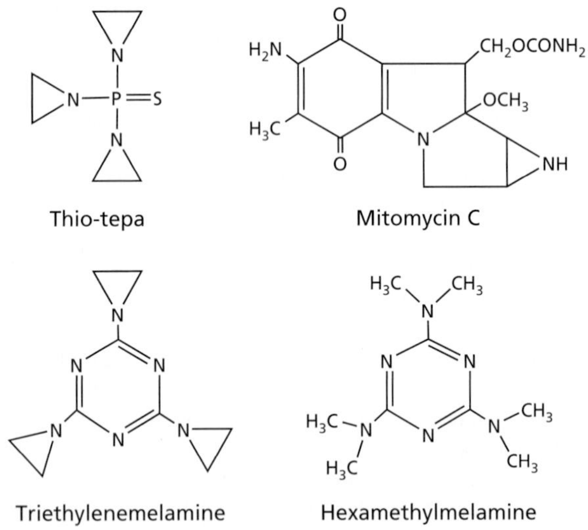

Figure 5 Chemical structures of aziridines and hexamethylmelamine.

N2-, and N7-adenine, and N1-, N7-, and O6-guanine.[45] However, N7-guanine remains the preferential target, as with other alkylating agents, and results in guanine–guanine (GG) and adenine–guanine (AG) interstrand crosslinks, primarily 1,2-crosslinks.[46] These crosslinks are formed sequentially; the first reaction at N7-guanine leads to the monofunctional adduct, and the second reaction with a nearby guanine results in the crosslink, as shown by pathway A in Figure 6. Crosslinking may also proceed via metabolism of thiotepa to tepa (sulfur replaced by oxygen), followed by opening

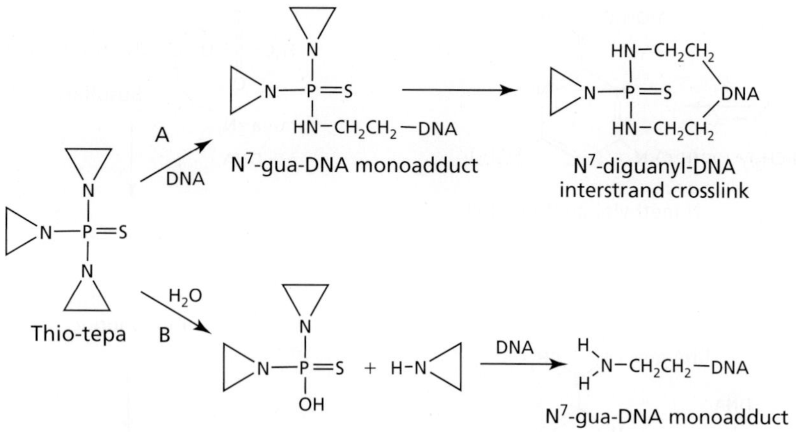

Figure 6 Metabolism and interaction of thiotepa with DNA to form interstrand crosslinks (pathway A) or monofunctional adducts (pathway B).

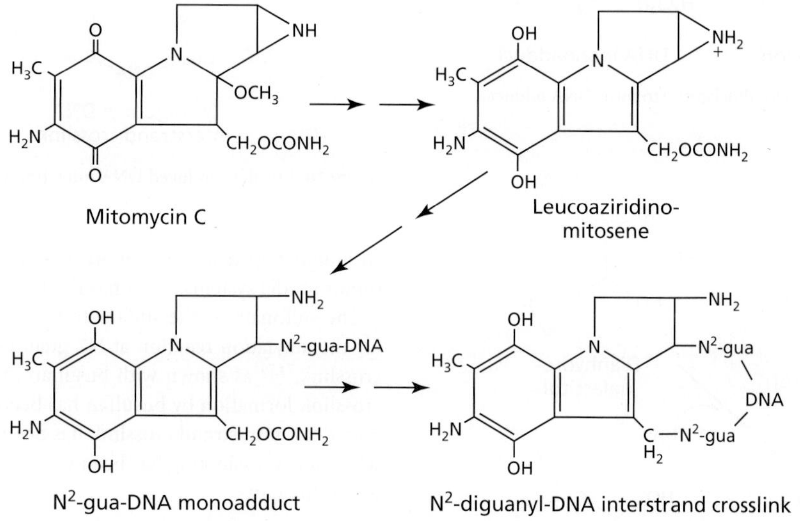

Figure 7 DNA interstrand crosslinks induced by mitomycin C.

of the aziridine ring and conversion to the chloroethyl-containing crosslinking species, as found in nitrogen mustards.[47] Alternatively, the aziridine ring is cleaved to mediate alkylation of N7-guanine and forms a monofunctional DNA adduct (Figure 6, pathway B), which induces DNA single-strand breaks and then cell death.[48,49]

Unlike thiotepa, interaction of mitomycin C with DNA requires metabolic reduction to leucoaziridinomitosene for the formation of the monofunctional adduct.[50] Spontaneous intramolecular rearrangement and elimination of the carbamate group at C10 of mitomycin C results in a second alkylation reaction with the opposite strand of DNA to induce cytotoxic 1,2-GG interstrand crosslink lesions (Figure 7). Interestingly, alkylation at the N2-guanine site of DNA is preferred by mitomycin C, particularly if guanine is present in the 5′-purine-CG-pyridine-3′ sequence in both strands of the duplex.[8]

On the basis of the presence of the aziridine ring in the triethylenemelamine structure, alkylation by this agent likely occurs in the same manner as that described for thiotepa. However, with hexamethylmelamine, metabolic activation in the liver is required.[51,52] The metabolism generates a carbinolamine intermediate, N-methylol-pentamethylmelamine, which rearranges to the reactive iminium ion as the species responsible for alkylation of guanine in DNA (Figure 8). As hexamethylmelamine metabolism can also result in the dicarbinolamine product

N,N′-dimethylol-tetramethylmelamine,[53] bifunctional interstrand DNA crosslink is the likely outcome, particularly as the tricarbinolamine-based prodrug of hexamethylmelamine, trimelamol, readily forms such crosslinks.[54] It is noteworthy that trimelamol has been investigated in clinical trials,[55] but the development did not continue, owing likely to limited clinical activity[56] and/or drug formulation/stability issues.[57]

Hexitol epoxides

The di-epoxide 1,2:5,6-dianhydrogalactitol (DAG) and its prodrug 1,2-dibromodulcitol (DBD), like the aziridines, also alkylate via a strained tricyclic ring (Figure 9). Chemical interaction between DAG and DNA results in alkylation at N7-guanine,[58] a site commonly preferred by several other alkylating agents. In cell-free, cellular, and in vivo rodent systems, N7-monoguanyl and N7-diguanyl derivatives are detected as two major products that represent monofunctional and interstrand crosslinked DNA adducts, respectively.[58–61]

Both DBD and DAG have shown antitumor properties that were similar to alkylating agents in some experimental antitumor models, but different in others. Lack of cross-resistance with DAG, for instance, was observed in a nitrosourea (BCNU)-resistant L1210 leukemia model.[62] Of the two hexitols, DAG has greater chemical stability and better preclinical antitumor activity profile.[63,64] Nevertheless, both DBD and DAG entered clinical trials in 1970s and

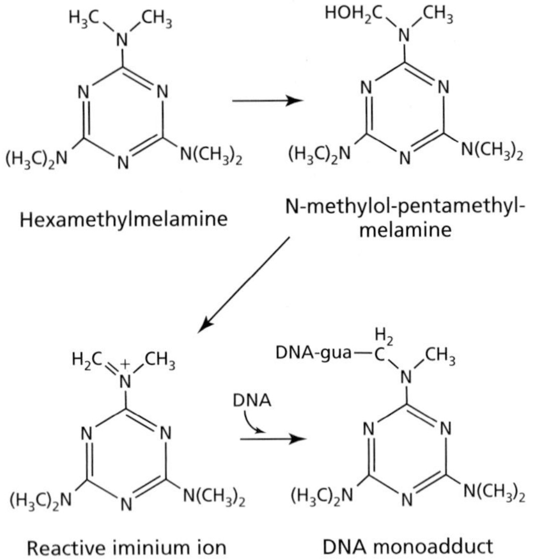

Figure 8 Activation of hexamethylmelamine to form DNA adducts.

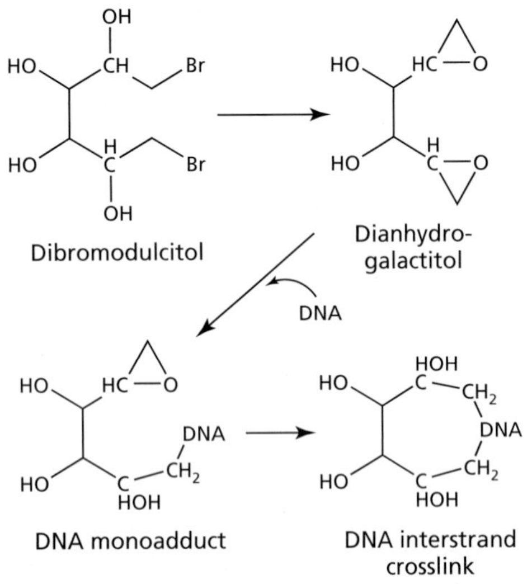

Figure 9 Conversion of dibromodulcitol to dianhydrogalactitol to form intertrand crosslinks.

demonstrated some activity in GI and lung cancer.[65,66] Interestingly, these hexitols cross the blood–brain barrier in patients,[67–69] and follow-up clinical trials found a 44% response rate with DAG in brain cancer.[66] DAG was recently granted orphan designation in the United States and Europe for brain cancer, and clinical trials are currently underway in the United States (ClinicalTrials.gov Identifier: NCT01478178). In China, however, it has been marketed for the treatment of chronic myelogenous leukemia (CML) and lung cancer for over 20 years.

Alkyl sulfonates
Busulfan and the analog hepsulfam are the best known alkyl sulfonates, which are symmetrical and have either two sulfonates (busulfan) or sulfamates (hepsulfam) separated by a linear alkyl chain. Busulfan was approved in 1999 as a standard of care for CML, but its clinical application subsequently diminished by first the introduction of the less-toxic hydroxyurea and then by the targeted therapeutic Gleevec. However, busulfan is still used in the allogeneic stem cell or bone marrow transplantation setting.[70,71]

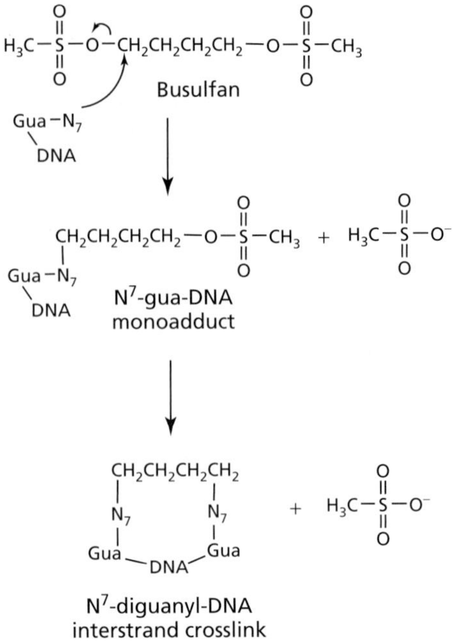

Figure 10 Busulfan-induced DNA interstrand crosslinks.

Although hepsulfam was more potent than busulfan in human tumor model systems,[72,73] it has not been effective in clinical trials.

The sulfonate or the sulfamate is the critical group responsible for the alkylation reaction at N7-guanine to form GG interstrand crosslink,[74,75] as shown with busulfan in Figure 10. However, this crosslink formation by busulfan has been disputed[76] and the alternative GA intrastrand crosslink has been proposed.[77] Significantly, where any crosslinking has been reported, this has been correlated to cytotoxicity.

Nitrosoureas
Much of the structure–activity understanding, and the basis for clinical development of 2-chloroethylnitrosoureas (CENUs) as derivatives of urea, came from the work of Montgomery and his colleagues.[78–80] With the ability to cross the blood–brain barrier, four analogs entered the clinic,[81,82] and these are shown in Figure 11. BCNU (Carmustine) and CCNU (Lomustine) are effective against several types of cancers, including glioma, glioblastoma

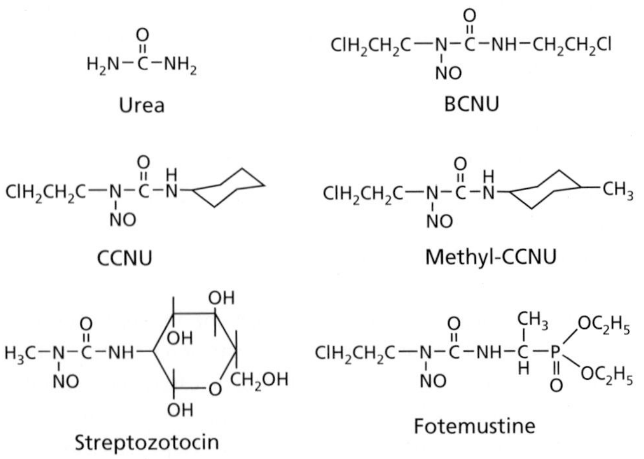

Figure 11 Chemical structures of urea and selected chloroethylnitrosourea derivatives.

multiforme, GI tumors, breast, and multiple myeloma, with strep- tozotocin (Zanosar) effective against cancers of the pancreatic islet cell, owing primarily to its uptake via the glucose transport protein GLUT2 that is present at relatively high levels in these cells.[83] Absence of any advantage over other nitrosoureas has halted the use of methyl-CCNU (Semustine). The limitation in clinical utility of nitrosoureas is ascribed to their severe side effects, including hematopoietic and renal toxicities, with streptozotocin in particular demonstrating substantial toxicity to β cells of the normal pan- creatic islets owing to the GLUT2 transporter.[84] The development of novel nitrosoureas, therefore, continues, and a third generation analog, fotemustine (Muphoran) (Figure 11), has shown activity in brain cancer and metastatic melanoma, with or without brain involvement, and has received approval in Australia, Brazil, China, and Europe, but not as yet in the United States.[85,86]

It is widely acknowledged that CENUs as bifunctional DNA interstrand crosslinkers are unstable, as exemplified by a short half-life of about 50 min for BCNU[82]; the several products of decomposition are shown in Figure 12. An unusual feature of

some CENUs is that they can generate isocyanate, which carbomy- lates the ε-amino group of lysine in proteins, including histone and other nuclear proteins, but there is disagreement whether the carbomylated-protein contributes to cytotoxicity.[79,87,88] A second unusual feature is that CENUs can alkylate at O6-guanine in DNA, likely through formation of the 2-chloroethyl diazene hydroxide and the analogous 2-hydroxyethyl diazene hydrox- ide species (Figure 12).[81,82] Rearrangement of these species to carbonium ions leads to alkylation at the O6-site of guanine to form monoadducts.[89] The O6-alkylation reaction is considered important as upregulation of O6-alkylguanine-DNA alkyltrans- ferase, which repairs the O6-adduct, increases resistance and, conversely, inhibition of this enzyme with O6-benzylguanine sen- sitizes tumor cells to nitrosoureas.[89-91] However, adducts from N7-alkylation of guanine (Figure 12) are normally the predominant species, particularly where this purine is in the middle of a GGG sequence.[92] These DNA monoadducts form rapidly (often within an hour), but then slowly convert to the cytotoxic N7-diguanyl interstrand crosslink that may take up to 8 h.[82] It is noteworthy

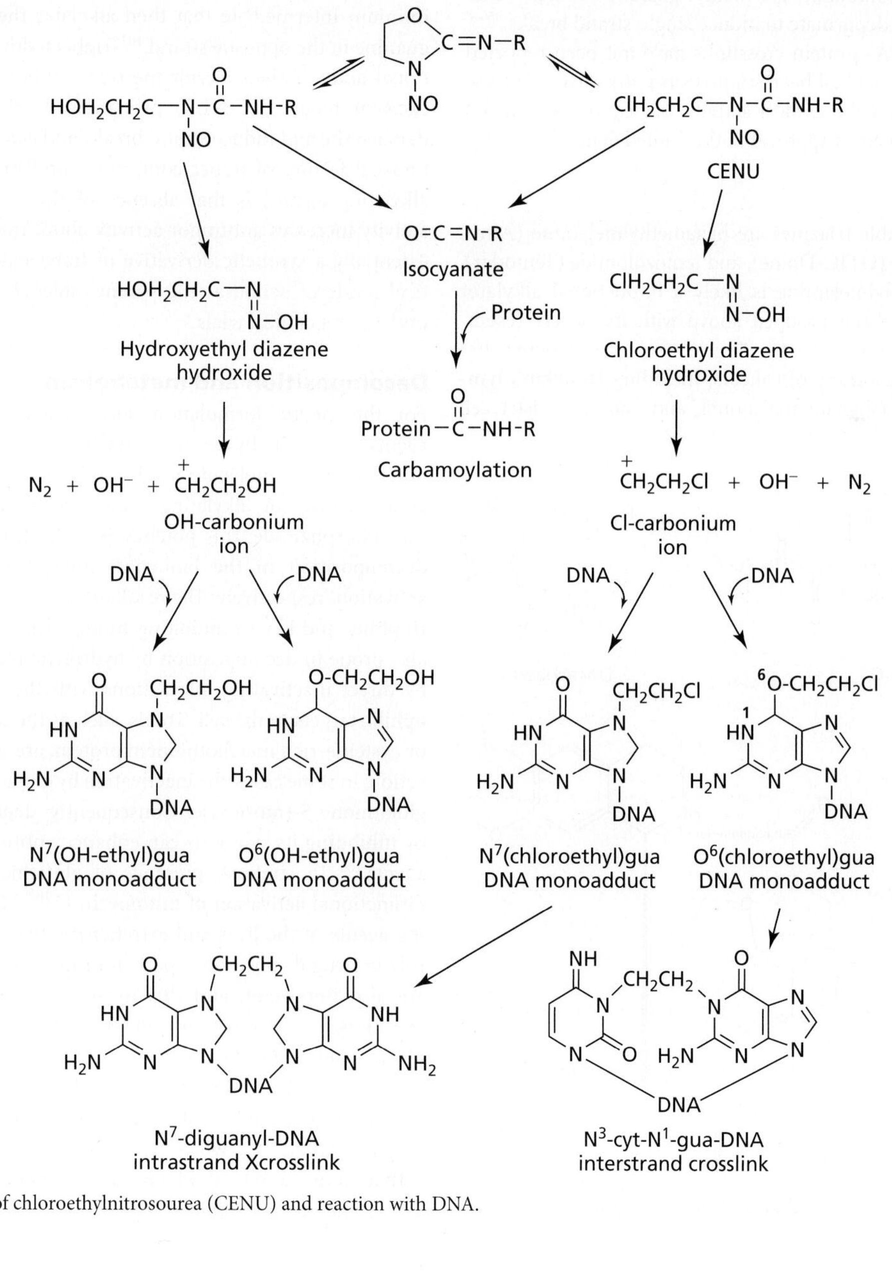

Figure 12 Activation of chloroethylnitrosourea (CENU) and reaction with DNA.

that N3-cytosine–N1-guanyl crosslinks are also formed through cyclization of the O6-chloroethyl-guanine monoadduct to the O6,N1-ethanoguanine pentacyclic intermediate, which reacts with N3-site of cytosine and becomes crosslinked to the N1-site of guanine following opening and rearrangement of the ethanoguanine ring.[82,93,94] There is also a proposal from steric considerations that only the CG crosslink of CENUs is interstrand, with the similarly cytotoxic GG adduct being intrastrand.[89]

Monofunctional alkylating agents

Structures of some monoalkylators discussed below are shown in Figure 13.

Hydrazines

More than 400 hydrazine compounds have been tested preclinically, but only procarbazine has received clinical approval for the treatment of cancers, specifically Hodgkin's lymphoma, lung cancer, and melanoma. Its activation is poorly understood, but metabolic oxidation to azoxy-procarbazine is an important step. This metabolite rearranges to a reactive methyl diazonium intermediate that forms O6- and predominantly N7-methyl-guanine adducts, which then spontaneously depurinate to induce single-strand breaks.[95–97] DNA–DNA or DNA–protein crosslinks have not been reported. Another hydrazine that had been studied since the early 1970s was hydrazine sulfate, but the clinical activity was equivocal, and the compound never received approval in the United States.

Triazines

The most recognizable triazines are hexamethylmelamine (Altretamine), dacarazine (DTIC-Dome), and temozolomide (Temodar). Of these, hexamethylmelamine is likely a bifunctional alkylator and, therefore, has been grouped above with its closely resembling trimethylmelamine under "aziridines." Dacarbazine has been used against a variety of cancers, including Hodgkin's lymphoma, sarcoma, malignant melanoma, and pancreatic islet cell

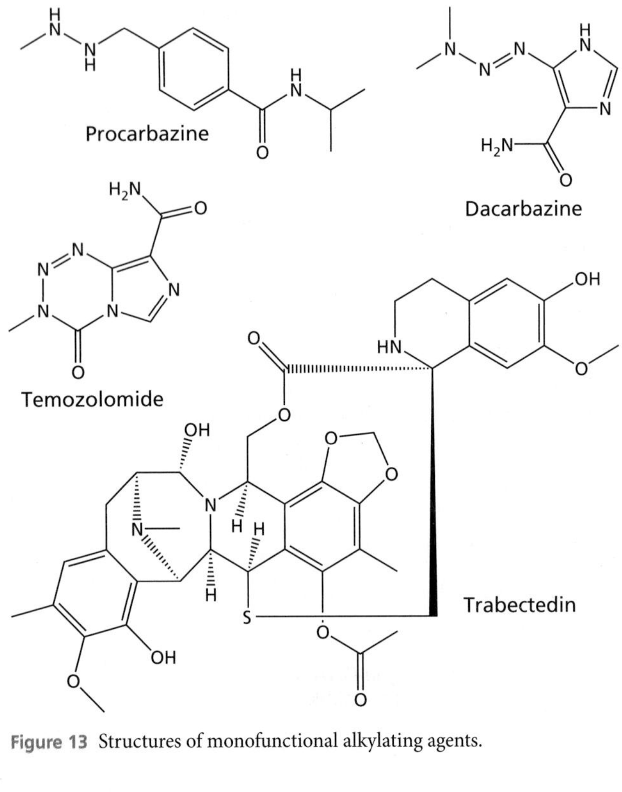

Figure 13 Structures of monofunctional alkylating agents.

carcinoma. Temozolomide is an imidazotetrazine derivative of dacarbazine that is particularly active against astrocytoma, as well as melanoma. Triazines methylate O6- and N7-guanine,[98] but, like the hydrazines, require metabolic activation for cytotoxic alkylation and DNA single-strand breaks. For dacarbazine, hepatic activation to [methyl-triazenyl]-imidazole-carboxamide (MTIC) generates the reactive DNA-methylating methyldiazonium ion.[99] Temozolomide, in contrast, functions as a prodrug of MTIC and spontaneously generates the reactive species.[100]

Isoquinoline alkaloids

The two naturally occurring tetrahydroisoquinoline alkaloids of interest are trabectedin (ecteinascidin-743, Yondelis) and Zalypsis. Trabectedin is the first marine-derived antitumor agent to be approved in Europe, Russia, and South Korea for cancer treatment, specifically advanced soft tissue sarcoma and platinum-resistant ovarian cancer.[101] Its approval in the United States, however, is pending. The drug initially binds noncovalently to TCG, CGG, AGC, or GGC sequence of one strand in the DNA minor groove, where dehydration of the carbinolamine group generates the iminium intermediate that then alkylates the unusual N2-site of guanine in the opposite strand.[102] Trabectedin-induced monofunctional adducts then recruit the transcriptionally coupled nuclear excision repair (TC-NER) protein Rad13/ERCC5 to the DNA damage site and induce strand breaks and cell death. An additional unusual feature of trabectedin, not found in several bifunctional alkylating agents, is that absence of the p53 tumor suppressor activity increases antitumor activity about threefold.[103] Zalypsis is essentially a synthetic derivative of trabectedin that has an identical mode of action as the parent molecule.[104,105] It is presently undergoing clinical trials.

Decomposition and metabolism

For therapeutic formulation and medical handling, alkylating agents must initially be in an inactive state to preserve maximal potency of the molecule until administered to patients. As discussed above for alkylating agents, such as temozolomide and cyclophosphamide, this potency is realized through spontaneous decomposition in the biological milieu or through metabolic activation, respectively. The resultant active species are strong electrophiles and key to inhibiting tumor growth, but are themselves also prone to decomposition by hydrolytic reactions with water or by direct inactivating interactions with the abundance of nucleophilic targets in the cell. Thiols, such as the tripeptide glutathione or cysteine-rich metallothionein protein, are major targets of interaction; in some cases, the inactivation by glutathione is facilitated by glutathione S-transferase. Consequently, depletion of glutathione by inhibiting its synthesis can enhance antitumor activity of these agents.[106] In contrast, presence of glutathione is important for bifunctional activation of mitomycin C.[107] Metabolism of alkylating agents in the liver and extrahepatic tissues also plays a major role in drug disposition. Apart from hyroxylation, other reactions are also important, and this includes dechlorination and denitrosation, as observed with nitrosoureas.[87] As noted earlier, high levels of aldehyde dehydrogenase in the GI and hematopoietic cells can protect cells by detoxifying metabolites of cyclophosphamide. Moreover, metabolism can be influenced by other agents, such as phenobarbital,[108,109] which can increase microsomal enzymatic activity and the rate at which the active species and the inactive metabolites are generated and disposed of.

Resistance to alkylating agents

A major clinical limitation of alkylating agents is resistance of tumor cells. This resistance can be intrinsic that arises during tumor development or it can be acquired by tumor cells via drug selection pressures. In many tumors, presence of a single resistance mechanism is rare, but multiple mechanisms abound, as has been reported for melphalan[110] and temozolomide.[111] Thus, any effort to induce antitumor response in refractory cancers will require circumventing multiple mechanisms of resistance, and this makes the task more challenging. However, knowledge of individual mechanisms may allow identification of weakness in the signaling network within tumor cells that may be exploited for synthetic lethality approaches.[112] Alternatively, identifying a resistance mechanism that, if circumvented, will provide a dominant trigger for apoptosis and over-ride remaining resistance mechanisms may have potential also.

In general terms, resistance of tumor cells can be due to (1) reduced intracellular drug concentration, (2) increased cellular inactivation, (3) enhanced DNA repair, and (4) downregulation of apoptotic signaling. Reduced uptake in resistant cells has been observed with melphalan owing to downregulation of the L-type amino acid transporter.[110,113] However, most alkylating agents rely on diffusion for cell entry and are not affected by transporters. Resistance to alkylating agents can occur from increased inactivation due to elevated levels of thiol-containing compounds or thiol-related enzymes, such as glutathione, metallothionein, γ-glutamylcysteine synthase (involved in glutathione synthesis), and glutathione S-transferase (increases drug conjugation with glutathione).[114–118] Increased inactivation can also occur by elevated levels of aldehyde dehydrogenase, which readily detoxicates cyclophosphamide and related alkylating agents.[119,120]

Alkylating agents target DNA, and persistence of DNA adducts correlates with cytotoxicity. In resistant tumor cells, these adducts are repaired efficiently. As discussed above, one repair mechanism involves the enzyme O6-alkylguanine-alkyltransferase, which reverses the initial alkylation of O6-guanine in DNA and prevents the formation of interstrand crosslinks. Thus, upregulation of this alkyltransferase increases resistance in cancers, as observed in human glioma cells resistant to BCNU.[121] In contrast, the cytotoxic effects of O6-alkylguanine adducts (O6-methyl ≫ O6-ethyl) are facilitated by the mismatch repair (MMR) pathway[122] and, conversely, resistance to the methyl-alkylator temozolomide arises when defects in the MMR pathway are present.[123] Repair of crosslinks also occurs by the nucleotide excision repair (NER) and the alternative nonhomologous end-joining (NHEJ) pathways. Thus, increased repair by the NER and NHEJ system in human tumor cells induces resistance to cyclophosphamide, melphalan, and chlorambucil.[124–127] In contrast, and as noted above, the activity of the monofunctional alkylating agent trabectedin is in fact enhanced by the participation of NER protein Rad13/ERCC5.[102]

Adduct formation and interstrand crosslinks kill cells by apoptosis, which has been demonstrated for a number of alkylating agents, including cyclophosphamide and temozolomide.[128,129] DNA damage activates a complex set of signal transduction pathways that converge on the apoptotic machinery to induce cell death. Specifically, alkylation of nucleotide bases induces unwinding and bending of DNA, and the resultant conformational changes in DNA are sensed by specialized recognition proteins that transduce DNA damage signals. This results in transcriptional activation of specific genes that finally activate caspases, which carry out the apoptotic cell death program. As a large number of proteins are involved, such as ATR, Chk1, Chk2, p53, Bak, and Bax, apoptosis

can be inhibited if any critical step of the apoptotic cell death program becomes disrupted, and this leads to resistance to alkylating agents. As an example, loss of p53 function through mutation or other means leads to temozolomide resistance.[111,130] Resistance to this agent has also been noted in stem-like glioblastoma cells by overexpression of Mdm2 protein, which inhibits p53 by increasing its proteosomal degradation.[131] On the other hand, overexpressed Bcl-2 protein in some cancers binds to Bax and, thereby, blocks the caspase-9/caspase-3 cascade to inhibit cyclophosphamide-induced apoptosis.[128] Alternatively, resistance to cyclophosphamide, chlorambucil, and temozolomide in human B cell CLL and U87MG glioblastoma cells can occur when Bax expression is low.[132,133]

Although drug resistance to alkylating agents in tumor cells can often be observed in both tissue culture and in rodent models, this is not always the case. In a classical example, EMT-6 murine mammary tumors that developed resistance to cyclophosphamide by directly injecting tumor-bearing mice with the drug did not display this resistance when cells from these tumors were exposed to this agent in vitro.[134] This demonstrates that some mechanisms of resistance to alkylating agents, such as the influence of TGF-β (transforming growth factor-beta) growth factor, poor tumor perfusion, changes in intracellular pH, and the tumor microenvironment, may only operate in vivo.[135–137]

Clinical pharmacology

The pharmacokinetics (PK) of a drug dictates its pharmacodynamics (PD), and this PK–PD relationship is integral to understanding the basis for drug activity and toxicity and designing regimens that maximize activity against cancer and minimize side effects. The pharmacology of alkylating agents has been studied for over six decades, but it was clear as early as 1952 that an ideal alkylating agent should be administered in an inactive form and converted into an active form in patient's tumor.[12,138] The essential knowledge on the clinical pharmacology of these agents of interest is summarized below.

Cyclophosphamide

A systemic dose of 50–75 mg/kg cyclophosphamide produces plasma levels of up to 400 μmol/L of the intact drug, which then decays with a half-life of 3–10 h.[139–141] Peak plasma concentration of 50–100 μmol/L phosphoramide mustard metabolite was also observed at about 3 h. Interestingly, the AUC of this and the 4-hydroxy-cyclophosphamide metabolite were similar after intravenous and oral administration, and this indicated both routes to be therapeutically effective. However, there is considerable variation in the PK of the drug among patients, but this is likely due to a prior dose of cyclophosphamide autoinducing its own metabolism or to administration of metabolism-inducing drugs, such as phenobarbital.[109,142,143] At conventional doses, however, variations in PK do not significantly affect its toxicity or therapeutic effects.[144] One explanation for this is that the final AUC for the active metabolites is unaffected, which is supported by the demonstration that cyclophosphamide given iv over 90 min yields 4-hydroxycyclophosphamide AUC of 105–110 μmol/L that is similar to an AUC when the dose is infused over 4 days.[145] Although high-dose therapy is an attractive approach in bone marrow transplantation regimens, the benefits can be limited by saturable PK.[146] Urinary excretion of cyclosphosphamide, predominantly as inactive metabolites, is the main route of excretion and accounts for about 60–70% of the dose.[147,148] Renal function does not appear to correlate with the toxicity of cyclophosphamide, and this supports drug clearance of active metabolites being determined by spontaneous decomposition, and not renal excretion.

Ifosfamide

The clinical PK data on ifosfamide is limited, but appears to be similar to that of cyclophosphamide. However, levels of the active 4-hydroxy metabolite from ifosfamide are lower than from cyclophosphamide.[149-151] As with cyclophosphamide, ifosfamide is orally bioavailable and can autoinduce its own metabolism.[141,152] Although such similarities may make the choice between these two agents difficult, the potential for larger interpatient variation in metabolism of the side chain and the impact of concomitantly administered drugs altering the metabolic pathway may limit the utility of ifosfamide more than that of cyclophosphamide.[153-155]

Melphalan

An iv dose of 0.6 mg/kg results in peak melphalan plasma levels of 4–13 μmol/L, which then decays biexponentially, with a rapid α-phase half-life ($T^1/_2α$) of 8 min and a relatively slower β-phase half-life ($T^1/_2β$) of 1.8 h.[156,157] At this dose, the mean AUC of 8 μmol h/L of melphalan was achieved and 24-h urinary excretion of melphalan was about 13% of the dose. Similar plasma PK has been observed following high-dose iv melphalan, and as spontaneous degradation of melphalan plays a major role in drug elimination, renal insufficiency was reported not to impact drug clearance.[158] Another study, however, has demonstrated that renal insufficiency reduces drug clearance and increases myelosuppression, which disappears with dose reduction.[159] Melphalan has good oral bioavailability, and conventional doses of 0.15–0.25 mg/kg melphalan given orally resulted in peak plasma levels of up to 0.2–0.6 μmol/L by 1–2 h, which decayed with a half-life of 0.6–3 h.[160] However, absorption after oral dosing can vary, with food reducing drug absorption and high doses subject to saturable absorption kinetics.[161-163]

Chlorambucil

An oral dose of 0.6 mg/kg chlorambucil produced peak plasma levels of 2–6 μmol/L of the intact drug an hour later and 2–4 μmol/L of the metabolite phenylacetic acid mustard by 2–4 h.[157] The β-phase half-life of the parent compound was 92 min, with that of the metabolite being 145 min. In another study, PK analysis of an oral daily dose of 0.8–0.9 mg/kg over 4 days indicated that the AUC of about 10 μmol h/L of chlorambucil on day 1 decreased 17% by day 4, with further progressive decreases noted with each 4-week treatment cycle.[164] This suggests that chlorambucil, as with cyclophosphamide and ifosfamide, may also be subject to autoinduction of its metabolism and excretion, although an alternative possibility is that repeat dosing reduces absorption from the gut. A two- to fourfold inter- and intraindividual variation in the PK of oral chlorambucil has also been reported.[165] Interestingly, plasma AUC of the drug or its metabolite phenylacetic acid mustard was unaffected by food intake.[166]

Bendamustine

A bolus iv dose of 5 mg/kg bendamustine was eliminated rapidly from the plasma, with $T^1/_2α$ of about 10 min and $T^1/_2β$ of 36 min, and a resultant AUC of about 28 μmol h/L.[167] The oral bioavailability is good and in the range 0.25–0.94 (mean, 0.57). The drug is metabolized by hepatic mixed function oxidases to N-demethyl- and γ-hydroxy-bendamustine as major metabolites.[168] Glutathione conjugates of the metabolites are also known, and an additional metabolite, dihydroxy-bendamustine, has been observed in patients plasma after an iv dose.[169] Total excretion of the drug accounts for 76% of the iv dose, with similar amounts appearing in the urine and the feces. Only about 5% of the dose was recovered as unchanged

parent drug, and this indicates that bendamustine is extensively metabolized.

Thiotepa

Administration of thiotepa at 12 mg/m² iv resulted in peak plasma levels of about 5 μmol/L for the parent drug, which then decayed biphasically with a $T^1/_2α$ of 8 min and a $T^1/_2β$ of 2 h, and resulting in an AUC of about 9 μmol h/L.[170] The peak concentration of the metabolite tepa of about 1 μmol/L was reached 2 h after drug administration and persisted in the plasma longer than thiotepa. Urinary excretion accounted for about 30% of the dose in 24 h, with 1.5% as unchanged drug and the majority (∼24% of dose) representing unknown, but reactive, species. Thus, the biotransformation of thiotepa is extensive. In a 4-day continuous iv infusion study using high doses (up to 900 mg/m²), peak plasma levels of thiotepa were reached during the first day, but then declined progressively by about 30% over the next 3 days.[171] The high dose also produced corresponding high plasma AUC values of up to 600 μmol h/L. Thiotepa has also been given intraperitoneally, with absorption occurring rapidly and resulting in plasma levels that were similar to those observed after iv administration.[172] However, the AUC of the drug in the peritoneum was over fourfold higher than in the plasma, and provides a strong rationale for intraperitoneal drug administration to increase drug exposure to cancers confined to this region.

Nitrosoureas

The PK of BCNU has been studied after iv infusion of 60–170 mg/m², which produced peak plasma concentrations of about 5 μmol/L that then decayed biphasically with a $T^1/_2α$ of 6 min and a $T^1/_2β$ of 68 min.[173] PK of high-dose BCNU (300–750 mg/m²), when normalized to a constant dose of 1 g/m², demonstrated a peak plasma level as ultrafilterable BCNU of 7.8 μmol/L and a mean AUC of 9 μmol h/L.[174] This represents only 23% of the total plasma BCNU that is bioavailable for alkylation function. The PK study of CCNU given orally at a dose of 130 mg/m² to patients failed to detect the parent compound in the plasma, likely due to rapid conversion to trans-4-hydroxy CCNU and cis-4-hydroxy CCNU.[175] These two metabolites reached peak levels of 3 μmol/L by 2–4 h after administration. The half-life for the plasma clearance of hydroxy-CCNU metabolites was about 1–3 h.

Busulfan

The insolubility of busulfan in aqueous solutions requires the drug to be used largely as an oral preparation. At an oral dose of 1 mg/kg, absorption is highly variable, as seen in the wide range for peak plasma levels of 1–10 μmol/L, AUC of 10–85 μmol h/L, and plasma elimination half-lives of 1–7 h.[176] However, in young children (2 months to 3.6 years), the peak plasma concentrations are lower (1–5 μmol/L), the mean elimination time was 34% faster than in adults, and the AUC consistently about threefold lower than in adults.[177] Since 2002, busulfan has been available as an iv-formulated Busulfex, which is now widely used, particularly as it is well tolerated and provides more consistent dose-dependent linear PK.[178] Thus, at 0.8 mg/kg busulfan given iv as Busulfex, peak plasma concentration of about 15 μmol/L is achieved, that then declines with a half-life of about 3 h, resulting in a mean AUC of about 80 μmol h/L.

Temozolomide

An oral dose of 150 mg/m² temozolomide was absorbed rapidly, with peak plasma levels of 40 μmol/L observed within an hour and an AUC of 116 µmol h/L.[179,180] Elimination from the plasma was rapid, with a half-life of about 1.8 h. Food intake reduced absorption and, thereby, peak concentration by 32% and AUC by 9%, and delayed time to reach peak concentration to 2.3 h. Temozolomide infused iv over 90 min gave peak drug levels of 38 µmol/L and an AUC of 127 µmol h/L, which are similar to those after oral administration and consistent with rapid and complete absorption of the drug from the gut. About 38–39% of temozolomide dose is excreted over 7 days, with the majority (37.7%) in the urine and the remainder (0.8%) in the feces. Of the dose in the urine, only about 6% is unchanged temozolomide.

Trabectedin

The maximally tolerated dose (MTD) of trabectedin when administered either as a 1 or 3 h iv infusion for 3 consecutive weeks every 4 weeks was about 0.6 mg/m^2,[181] which indicates that this agent has high potency. The plasma concentrations and AUC of trabectedin increase linearly with dose. At the MTD, the 1-h infusion resulted in a mean peak concentration of 15 nmol/L, mean AUC of 43 nmol h/L, and terminal phase plasma $T^1/_2$ of about 4 days. In comparison, the 3-h infusion gave corresponding values of 8 nmol/L, 31 nmol h/L, and 2 days, respectively. As a 24-h infusion every 21 days, the MTD was 1.5 mg/m^2, but a significant increase in total body clearance was noted between the first and fifth course of treatment.[182] The MTD on course one gave a peak concentration of 2.4 nmol/L, AUC of 74 nmol h/L, and terminal plasma $T^1/_2$ of about 4 days. This AUC value when adjusted for dose is consistent with that obtained with the shorter 1 or 3 h infusion. Biotransformation of trabectedin occurs in the liver, and several metabolites are excreted in the urine and feces of patients.[183]

Adverse effects

Given that alkylating agents target DNA, normal tissues have the potential to be impacted by treatment with these drugs, particularly those having a high proliferation rate. However, unwanted toxicities may arise in any tissue owing to several reasons, including tissue-specific increases in accumulation of active drug and/or toxic metabolite. Owing to their narrow therapeutic index, each alkylating agent will likely induce several side effects, some that are mild but others that become dose-limiting and attenuate clinical utility.

Hematopoietic toxicity, particularly affecting granulocytes and platelets, is the most common dose-limiting toxicity associated with alkylating agents. However, this is reversible, as has been demonstrated with temozolomide.[180] Interestingly, cyclophosphamide and ifosfamide are less myelosuppressive, and this is likely due to the presence of aldehyde dehydrogenase, which inactivates the aldophosphamide metabolite in hematopoietic stem cells and early granulocytes. In cases of severe hematopoietic toxicities with other alkylating agents, counter measures available to stimulate recovery include granulocyte-macrophage colony-stimulating factor (GM-CSF) and granulocyte colony-stimulating factor (G-CSF). These protective measures also allow dose intensification for increased antitumor response. However, use of these protective agents is not without additional complications.[184] As DNA alkylation of normal hematopoietic cells is also increased in high-dose therapy, secondary leukemia is a serious side effect in up to 10% of the patients. Similarly, with DNA as a target, alkylating agents are high-risk teratogens, particularly in the first trimester of pregnancy.[185]

The GI tract expresses aldehyde dehydrogenase to protect itself from toxic effects of cyclophosphamide and ifosfamide. However, other alkylating agents target the rapidly proliferating cells in the GI tract to induce side effects, particularly in high-dose regimens. For instance, high doses of melphalan and thiotepa induce stomatitis, esophagitis, and diarrhea. Nausea and vomiting, which involve the GI tract, are mediated in part by a CNS (central nervous system) effect, which may be due to the high lipophilicity of the drugs and their ability to cross the blood–brain barrier. Fortunately, nausea and vomiting can be controlled with antiemetics, including dopamine and serotonin antagonists[186] in conjunction with improved guidelines.[187,188]

The use of busulfan, and to a limited extent melphalan, cyclophosphamide, and chlorambucil, has been associated with pulmonary damage,[189] which may manifest as nonproductive cough and dyspnea, possibly progressing to pulmonary insufficiency and eventual death. Busulfan-induced pulmonary toxicity can occur rapidly, as early as 6 weeks after initiating therapy, and impacting 3–43% of the patients, depending on the therapeutic protocol and inclusion of high-dose therapy. Hepatotoxicity also can be induced by high-dose therapy, and fatal veno-occlusive disease syndrome following bone marrow transplantation, characterized in part by hepatomegaly, has been observed in up to 25% of patients receiving cyclophosphamide and busulfan.[190,191] Mild and transient hepatotoxicity has been reported at standard doses of melphalan, busulfan, chlorambucil, and trabectedin. The more serious cirrhosis, fibrosis, and cholestasis have also been implicated. Nitrosoureas are also hepatotoxins, with BCNU in particular associated with liver abnormalities in up to 26% of patients that are usually reversible, but have proved to be fatal in a few cases.[190]

Gonadal damage is a serious side effect of alkylating agents, such as cyclophosphamide, chlorambucil, melphalan, busulfan, mechlorethamine, CCNU, and BCNU, but reverses in most cases over a period of a few years.[192] Procarbazine-containing regimens, on the other hand, render permanent infertility in the majority of men being treated for lymphomas. In women, procarbazine and cyclophosphamide induce ovarian failure and transient amenorrhea.[193] Significantly, women older than 25 years are at a higher risk of ovarian failure, and those older than 30 years have a 12-fold greater risk of menstrual irregularities.

Although hematopoietic and GI toxicities are mild with cyclophosphamide and ifosfamide, hemorrhagic cystitis of the bladder is serious.[194] Busulfan, thiotepa, and temozolomide have also been implicated in this side effect. However, use of thiols, such as mesna to inactivate metabolites, and adequate hydration, to force their urinary excretion, have provided some protection. Toxicity to the kidney is also a serious side effect of therapy, particularly with nitrosoureas. In a study using six courses of therapy with 200 mg/m^2 BCNU or methyl-CCNU, renal impairment was common, as evidenced by elevation in blood urea nitrogen or serum creatinine.[195] In some patients, renal damage manifested as tubular atrophy, interstitial fibrosis, and glomerular sclerosis.

Cardiotoxicity can also be a serious side effect induced by cyclophosphamide, ifosfamide, and busulfan, and has known to be fatal in the case of high-dose cyclophosphamide.[196–198] Pathological findings indicated endothelial injury and hemorrhagic myopericarditis as specific drug-induced cardiotoxic effects. In contrast, neurotoxicity as a serious complication is not common at standard doses of busulfan or BCNU, but becomes severe only at high iv doses or when administered at a standard dose by the intracarotid route.[199–201]

Alkylating agents can induce severe alopecia as a side effect, and this is seen particularly with cyclophosphamide, ifosfamide, and busulfan.[202] This side effect is exacerbated by inclusion of vincristine or doxorubicin in drug-combination protocols. The toxicity may be due to the penetration of lipophilic metabolites into the hair follicles,[203] but it is usually reversible. Other minor toxicities associated with alkylating agents and observed on rare occasions include allergic reactions and transient antidiuretic effects.

Platinum antitumor compounds

The most recognizable platinum antitumor compound is cisplatin (cis-diamminedichloroplatinum(II)), which is a neutral, square planar inorganic complex with two labile chloro and two stable ammine ligands in a cis-configuration. This chemical geometry is important, as the analogous trans-geometry in transplatin (Figure 14) renders the molecule about 20-fold less cytotoxic. However, there are some exceptions to the low potency associated with the trans-geometry.[204] Cisplatin was first described in 1844 as Peyrone's salt, but its cytotoxic activity was not discovered until 1969 when a serendipitous observation was made by the Rosenberg group that passing direct current via platinum electrodes immersed in a culture of *Escherichia coli* prevented cell division, but the bacteria continued to grow as filaments. Detailed examination led to the discovery that the electrodes had reacted with nutrients in the culture medium to form several products, including cisplatin, that potently arrested cell division in *E. coli*. Cisplatin was selected for eventual development as an antitumor agent, and it received approval for clinical use in 1978 by the US Food and Drug Administration (FDA).[205]

Basis for cisplatin analog development

Since its FDA approval, cisplatin has been extensively used in the treatment of several cancers, including testicular, ovarian, head and neck, bladder, and cervical cancers.[206] The cure rate for testicular cancer, in particular, increased from 10% to 85% with inclusion of cisplatin as part of the therapeutic regimen. Although cisplatin is stable and easy to handle, it demonstrated some major clinical limitations. For this reason, hundreds of platinum molecules were synthesized to identify alternative platinum congeners with improved toxicity profiles and a broader spectrum of activity. In the 20 year span between 1979 and 1999, 23 platinum drugs entered clinical trials, but none since, with a majority failing to demonstrate clinical activity.[207] Some of these molecules are shown in Figure 14,

which includes carboplatin and oxaliplatin as the only other platinum compounds to have received FDA approval. Cisplatin and similar square planar analogs have the central platinum(II) in a divalent state, but others, such as the octahedral ormaplatin, have the tetravalent platinum(IV) atom.

A major drawback of cisplatin that was apparent early was its irreversible and cumulative toxicities to the kidneys and the peripheral nerves. The dose-limiting nephrotoxicity, however, became the driver of a search for a safer platinum analog. An examination of some 300 analogs by the Harrap group led to the selection of carboplatin for clinical trials in early 1980s.[208] This analog has a bidentate cyclobutanedicarboxylate ligand that replaces the two chloro-atoms (Figure 14), and this was sufficient to obviate not only nephrotoxicity, but also peripheral neuropathy. On the basis of the clinical activity, however, carboplatin is similar to cisplatin and, therefore, cancers refractory to cisplatin are fully cross-resistant to carboplatin.[209,210] This renewed an interest in identifying an analog that lacked the cross-resistance characteristic, and required modification of the ammine ligand. Several such analogs entered clinical trials, including ormaplatin and oxaliplatin, which have the bidentate 1,2-diaminocyclohexane (DACH) moiety, and picoplatin, which has one ammine group substituted by methylpyridine (Figure 14), but only oxaliplatin has demonstrated significant activity in specific refractory cancers.[208] In contrast to others, satraplatin, which also has one ammine substituted with a monoaminocyclohexane group, was tested clinically as an oral formulation, and although it has demonstrated some activity,[211] its future, like that of picoplatin, remains unclear.[207]

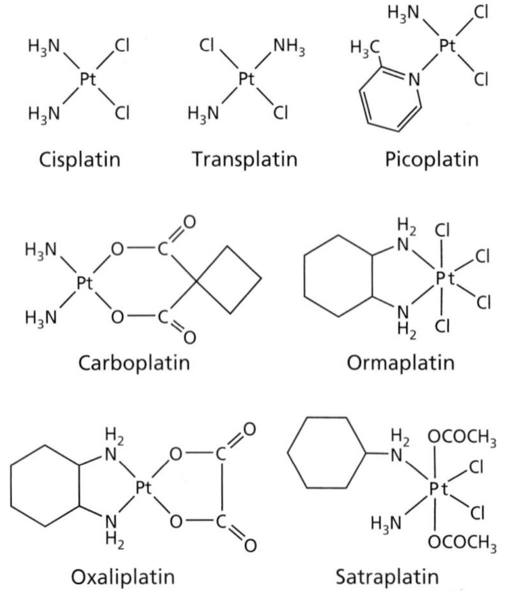

Basis for activity of platinum compounds

Although cisplatin, carboplatin, and oxaliplatin are considered chemically inert, they are, nevertheless, clinically active. For activity, the neutral platinum molecules are transformed spontaneously to reactive species in an aqueous or biological environment. This entails displacement of the chloro (in cisplatin) or the dicarboxylato ligand (in carboplatin and oxaliplatin) with water molecules, as exemplified in Figure 15 with cisplatin.[212,213] The resulting species exist in equilibrium in an aqueous solution, but in a biological environment, the equilibrium is not established as the chloro-monoaquo species reacts immediately with nucleophilic sites in biomolecules. In carboplatin, the bidentate cyclobutane-dicarboxylic acid (CBDCA) ligand slows the aquation reaction and this in turn reduces drug potency that requires the clinical dose to be fourfold greater than that of cisplatin.[214] The bidentate oxalate group of oxaliplatin, on the other hand, is relatively more labile, and its potency is comparable to that of cisplatin. The platinum(IV) compounds, such as satraplatin, are stable in an aqueous environment, and their reduction to platinum(II) species

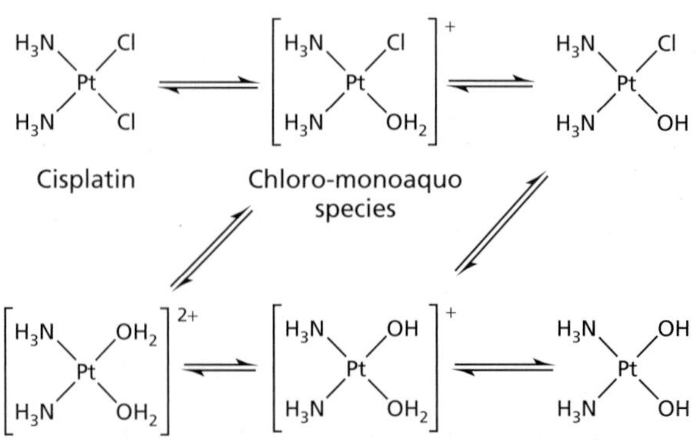

Figure 14 Structures of cisplatin and selected analogs.

Figure 15 Aquation of cisplatin to active platinating species.

is a prerequisite for aquation reactions. Surprisingly, ormaplatin is highly reactive and binds rapidly to plasma proteins,[215] and this indicates that the nature of the equatorial ligands in Pt(IV) compounds dictates the rate of reduction and activation of the molecule (Cl ≫ acetate).

Interaction of platinum drugs with DNA

Several studies have established that DNA is the primary cytotoxic target of platinum drugs.[216] As platinum drugs react immediately with endogenous macromolecules upon activation, it is likely that the drug enters the nucleus in an intact neutral form and becomes aquated in situ for interaction with DNA, primarily at N7-site of guanine. Platinum drugs form both interstrand and intrastrand crosslinks in various configurations (Figure 1). As with nitrogen mustards, interstrand crosslinks are readily formed when guanine is in the 5′-GC-3′ sequence.[217]

Cisplatin-induced interstrand crosslinks have biological effects, such as cytotoxicity and inhibition of transcriptional activity of DNA-dependent RNA polymerases,[218,219] but available evidence suggests that intrastrand adducts are the more potent cytotoxic lesions. This is consistent with the inability of weakly active transplatin to form intrastrand adducts.[219] Moreover, 85–90% of adducts formed by cisplatin are 1,2-intrastrand AG and GG crosslinks, with 1,3-intrastrand GXG crosslinks (where X = any

nucleotide), interstrand GG-crosslinks, and monofunctional adducts, each representing 2–6%. The low level of interstrand crosslinks may also be due to their unstable nature, and they slowly convert to the stable intrastrand adduct.[217,220] DNA–protein crosslinks and monofunctional adducts are also formed but are not considered cytotoxic based on the fact that they are formed extensively by transplatin[221] or they fail to inhibit DNA-dependent RNA polymerases.[222,223]

The ability of DACH-containing platinum compounds, such as oxaliplatin, to circumvent cisplatin resistance has drawn considerable attention.[224] Interestingly, the profile of monoadducts and interstrand and intrastrand diadducts formed by the analogous model drug DACH-sulfato-platinum(II) was essentially similar to those found with cisplatin.[225] Thus, circumvention of cisplatin resistance must be due to the subtle chemical difference in the DNA adduct formed between oxaliplatin versus cisplatin (Figure 16). As cisplatin and carboplatin form identical bifunctional adducts, this explains why their cytotoxic profiles are similar.

DNA-damage signals and cell death

Only a few crosslinks by cisplatin are sufficient to inhibit DNA replication, and this conveys the high potency of the drug.[226] Thus, crosslinks provide the basic understanding for cell death with platinum drugs. However, differences in activity between cisplatin

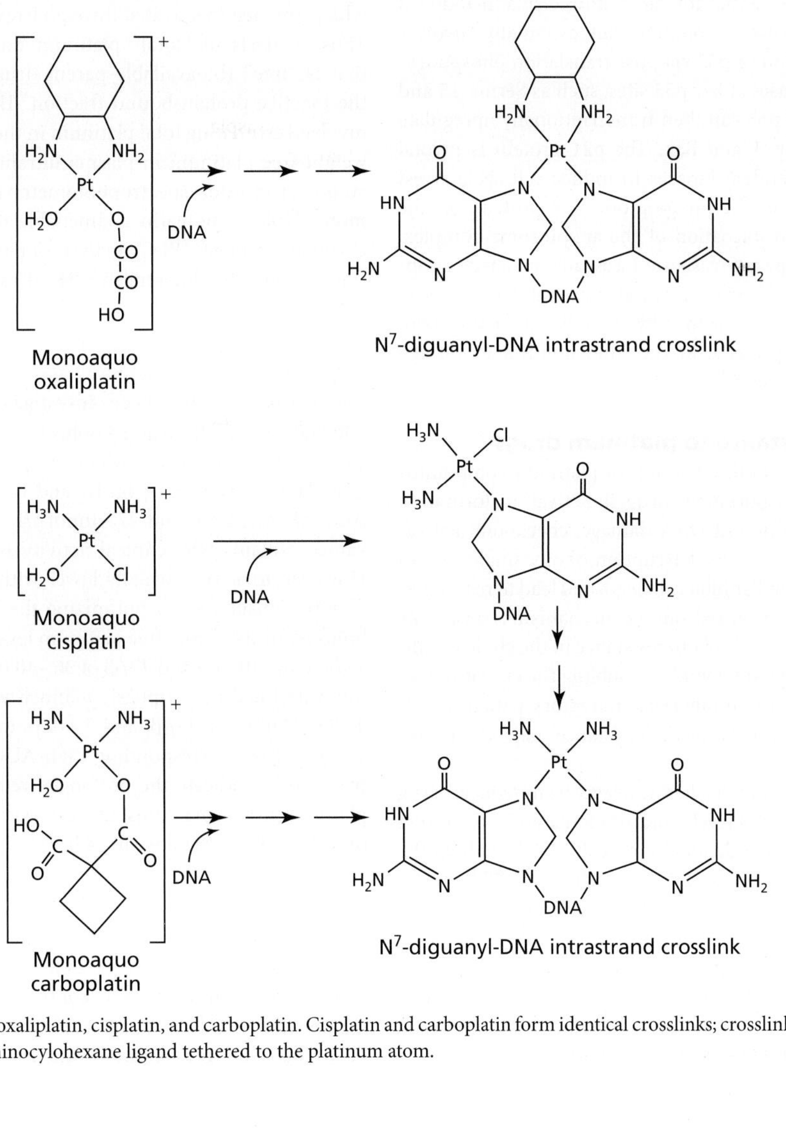

Monoaquo oxaliplatin

N⁷-diguanyl-DNA intrastrand crosslink

Monoaquo cisplatin

Monoaquo carboplatin

N⁷-diguanyl-DNA intrastrand crosslink

Figure 16 DNA crosslinks of oxaliplatin, cisplatin, and carboplatin. Cisplatin and carboplatin form identical crosslinks; crosslink of oxaliplatin is structurally different by virtue of the diaminocylohexane ligand tethered to the platinum atom.

and oxaliplatin in cisplatin-resistant cells warrant additional discussion. Both intrastrand and interstrand adducts induce the DNA to unwind and bend at the site of DNA damage. For instance, cisplatin intrastrand crosslink unwinds DNA by 13°–23° and bends it by 32°–34°,[227] whereas interstrand crosslinks unwind the double helix by 79°, with bends of 45°.[217,228] Interstrand crosslinks formed by oxaliplatin, on the other hand, induce unwinding by 82° and bending by 61°. Such differences in DNA conformation induced by distinct platinum drugs are recognized differentially by DNA damage sensor proteins; for instance, the nonhistone chromosomal protein HMGB1 and MMR proteins hMLH1, hMSH2, and hMSH6 recognize GG crosslinks of cisplatin but not those of satraplatin or the clinically active oxaliplatin.[228–230] In this respect, loss of MMR proteins leads to cisplatin resistance but not oxaliplatin resistance.[230,231] Similarly, HMGB1 fails to recognize interstrand crosslinks of the poorly active transplatin.[232] Thus, recognition by independent proteins of oxaliplatin-induced local DNA distortions results in propagation of distinct signaling that bypasses the block in cisplatin-induced signaling and enables oxaliplatin to activate DNA damage checkpoints and circumvent cisplatin resistance. However, identity of proteins that specifically recognize oxaliplatin adducts is not known.

DNA damage checkpoints activate several kinases, such as ATR, Chk1, and Chk2, which function in an orchestrated manner to activate target proteins for cellular effects. A critical target protein in this regard is the tumor suppressor p53, which is a transcription factor that is essential for facilitating cisplatin-induced cytotoxicity.[233] The process is complex, but essentially involves stabilization and activation of p53 via post-translation phosphorylation by checkpoint kinases at key p53 sites, such as Serine-15 and Serine-20. The activated p53 can then transcriptionally upregulate gene targets, including p21 and Bax. The p21 protein is pivotal in inhibiting cyclin-dependent kinases to induce cell cycle arrest by cisplatin.[234] Increase in the proapoptotic Bax protein, on the hand, eventually leads to formation of the apoptosome complex, which activates the caspase-9/caspase-3 cascade to affect apoptotic cell death.[235] The p53 protein can also activate apoptosis in a transcription-independent manner by directly interacting with pro- and antiapoptotic proteins in the mitochondria to tilt the balance in favor of apoptosis.[233]

Mechanism of resistance to platinum drugs

As discussed earlier, the mode of action of platinum compounds involves intracellular transport of the drug, its activation, formation of DNA adducts, recognition of DNA damage, checkpoint activation, and induction of apoptosis. Disruption of any single step in this coordinated process will inhibit cell death and lead to resistance, which may be intrinsic or acquired, but the mechanism is invariably multifactorial.[236] The level of cisplatin resistance in the clinic is difficult to define, but it is at least twofold as doubling the cisplatin dose induces antitumor response in otherwise refractory patients.[237,238] It is likely that in some tumor cells the resistance may be substantially greater.[233,236]

Resistance can occur at the biochemical level from reduced drug accumulation, increased thiol levels, and/or increased DNA adduct repair in tumor cells that individually or collectively reduce the level or persistence of cytotoxic DNA crosslinks.[239,240] Reduced accumulation of cisplatin by 20–70% has been documented and these can be due to altered levels of transporter proteins involved in influx (e.g., lower Ctr1 expression) or efflux (e.g., increased ATP7A, ATP7B, or ATP11B expression).[236,241,242] Resistance due to thiols can occur following elevation in levels of metallothionein and/or glutathione, or in expression of enzymes involved in their

biosynthesis, such as glutathione-associated γ-glutamylcysteine synthetase, or in catalyzing their inactivating conjugation with the platinum drug, such as glutathione S-transferase that has been observed in head and neck cancer patients.[236,243] Enhanced removal of adducts by DNA repair to affect resistance by a factor of up to twofold is frequently encountered, and this has been correlated to increased expression of repair genes, such as the NER gene ERCC1 in ovarian cancer patients.[244]

Before repair of crosslink adducts can be initiated, the DNA lesion has to be first recognized. Thus, downregulation of MMR proteins can prevent recognition of DNA damage; specifically, hMLH1, hMSH2, and hMSH6 can become mutated or silenced by promoter hypermethylation.[236] Molecular mechanisms of resistance can also occur through defects in checkpoint proteins, as exemplified by mutation or silencing of Chk2 in nonsmall cell lung cancer patients that likely impedes stabilization and activation of p53 and, thereby, apoptosis.[245] This p53-dependent apoptosis can also be inhibited by other factors, including upregulation of Bcl-2 protein, inhibitors of apoptosis protein, and Her-2/neu, PI3K/Akt, and Ras/MAPK pathways.[236] The p53 itself can become mutated, and this probably has the greatest impact in inducing cisplatin resistance.[233,246]

Clinical pharmacology

The PK of cisplatin or oxaliplatin as the intact molecule is complicated by its rapid and spontaneous transformation to active species, which are then inactivated through irreversible binding to proteins. Thus, analysis of "total" platinum does not reveal the fraction that is "free" (bioavailable parent drug and active species) from the inactive protein-bound fraction. Therefore, PK in plasma has involved estimating total platinum in the plasma and low molecular weight free platinum in plasma ultrafiltrates, usually by flameless atomic absorption spectrophotometry (FAAS).[215,247] However, the more stable carboplatin is amenable to high-performance liquid chromatography (HPLC) analysis of parent drug in the ultrafiltrate fraction, but the difference in PK of carboplatin using HPLC and FAAS is minimal.[248,249]

Cisplatin

The plasma PK has been investigated at a standard dose of 100 mg/m² cisplatin using a bolus (4–15 min infusion) or a 3- and 24-h infusion schedule, which, respectively, gave peak levels as free platinum species of 44, 10, and 1.4 μmol/L and corresponding AUC of 24.7, 27.4, and 27.8 μmol h/L.[250] Similarity in these AUC values explains why clinical activity is independent of schedule. However, toxicity is usually lower with longer infusions, and this may be considered for optimizing the therapeutic schedule. After bolus administration, free platinum levels decline biphasically, with $T^1/_2\alpha$ of 6–10 min and $T^1/_2\beta$ of 36–40 min.[215,251] Total plasma platinum declined in a triphasic manner, with half-lives of 13 min for $T^1/_2\alpha$, 43 min for $T^1/_2\beta$, and 5.4 days for terminal $T^1/_2\gamma$. This long $T^1/_2\gamma$ and the corresponding high AUC of 908 μmol h/L for total platinum[247] indicate the prolonged retention of covalently bound platinum in plasma. Thus, urinary excretion is low, accounting for only 28–33% of the dose in 24 h.[215,252]

Oxaliplatin

As with cisplatin, covalent interaction with plasma proteins and urinary excretion of 37% in 24 h of a standard 130 mg/m² dose given as a 2-h infusion also contribute to the rapid clearance of oxaliplatin.[215] Peak plasma concentration at this schedule was 6.2 μmol/L for free platinum and 18.5 μmol/L for total platinum on cycle 5. The threefold difference between free and total peak concentration may be due to accumulation of protein-bound platinum from previous cycles of treatment. Nevertheless, the AUC values of 61 and 1062 µmol h/L for free and total platinum compare reasonably with those with cisplatin.[215,247] The free plasma platinum decays triexponentially, with a $T^1/_2\alpha$ of 17 min, a $T^1/_2\beta$ of 16 h, and a $T^1/_2\gamma$ of about 270 h.

Carboplatin

The low reactivity of carboplatin results in high urinary excretion of about 77% of the dose in 24 h, with most (41%) as intact carboplatin drug.[215,249] Peak total platinum concentration of 251 µmol/L was observed after a dose of 550 mg/m^2, and this likely represents intact drug based on slow reaction kinetics of carboplatin with plasma proteins[247] and similar $T^1/_2\alpha$ and/or $T^1/_2\beta$ values for total and free platinum and for intact drug.[215,247] As free platinum, the drug decays biphasically, with $T^1/_2\alpha$ of 23 min and $T^1/_2\beta$ of 2 h. Total platinum, however, decayed triphasically, with a similar $T^1/_2\alpha$ of 22 min and $T^1/_2\beta$ of 1.9 h, and a prolonged $T^1/_2\gamma$ of 5.8 days. The AUC for total and free platinum and for intact carboplatin were 1385, 506, and 456 µmol h/L, respectively, and this supports intact carboplatin as the major component of the plasma "free" drug fraction.

Adverse effects

The dose-limiting complication with cisplatin is the cumulative and irreversible nephrotoxicity, which manifests as a decrease in the glomerular filtration rate and is characterized by focal acute tubular necrosis, dilatation of convoluted tubules, and formation of casts.[253,254] Serum electrolyte imbalance also occurs, including hypomagnesemia, in over 50% of the patients.[255] The cause may be due to active tubular transport of cisplatin that increases tubular drug concentration.[256] However, hydration and forced diuresis may reduce the severity and/or incidence of kidney damage. Nephrotoxicity is rare with oxaliplatin and carboplatin, which are cleared by glomerular filtration only.[215,257] On the basis of this, the Calvert formula was devised to individualize carboplatin dosing based on renal function and this is now in standard use.[257]

Cumulative ototoxicity has also been a significant problem with cisplatin, usually in the form of tinnitus and hearing loss, with young children being more susceptible.[258] High-frequency hearing loss is often the first sign, progressing to involve the middle frequencies at doses in excess of 100 mg/m^2, and finally resulting in total loss of hearing in about 50% of patients receiving cumulative doses greater than 400 mg/m^2.[259] Radiation treatment in combination therapy exacerbates the toxicity. The incidence of ototoxicity with carboplatin or oxaliplatin, however, is low and this may be due to reduced cochlear drug accumulation in contrast to cisplatin.[260-262]

Peripheral neuropathy has been described for all three drugs.[261] With cisplatin, it is more frequent, cumulative, and irreversible, involving mainly sensory neuropathy in up to 50% of the patients receiving cumulative doses in excess of 300 mg/m^2. Tingling paresthesia, weakness, tremors, and loss of taste are usually encountered, and seizures have also been described. Neurotoxicity is particularly severe following intra-arterial administration of cisplatin in head and neck patients. Peripheral neuropathy with oxaliplatin is dose limiting and can be acute or chronic, but symptoms of the chronic form improve after treatment stops and resolves completely over a period of 6–8 months in 40% of the cases. Carboplatin is the least neurotoxic, affecting only 4–6% of the patients. For chemoprotection of peripheral neuropathy, several strategies have been devised, including the use of thiol compounds and vitamin E.[261]

Cisplatin is considered one of the most emetic antitumor agents. This drug at doses >50 mg/m^2 has a 90% risk of inducing emesis, with lower doses associated with reduced risk (30–90%).[263] In comparison, carboplatin and oxaliplatin pose only moderate risks at therapeutic doses. Antiemetics have been developed to provide relief from this side effect, and include the dopamine antagonist metoclopramide and the serotonin receptor antagonists, such as ondansetron, granisetron, and dolasetron.

Myelosuppression is associated with the use of the platinum drugs, but the effects are usually reversible. Cisplatin-induced hematological toxicity is manifested as leucopenia, whereas carboplatin induces thrombocytopenia as its dose-limiting toxicity, which may be severe enough to cause internal bleeding. Neutropenia and thrombocytopenia have been reported with oxaliplatin. Pulmonary toxicity, hepatotoxicity, alopecia, and/or allergic reactions are among several other side effects that may also be observed with these platinum drugs.

Acknowledgments

The research support from the US Public Health Service grants CA160687 to ZHS and Support Grant CA16672 to MD Anderson Cancer Center awarded by the National Cancer Institute, and in part from the Megan McBride Franz Endowed Research Fund, is gratefully acknowledged.

Key references

The complete reference list can be found on the Wiley Companion Digital Edition of this title (see inside front cover for login instructions).

2 Hanahan D, Weinberg RA. Hallmarks of cancer: the next generation. *Cell.* 2011;**144**:646–674.

12 Brock N. Oxazaphosphorine cytostatics: past-present-future. Seventh Cain Memorial Award lecture. *Cancer Res.* 1989;**49**:1–7.

14 Brock N. The history of the oxazaphosphorine cytostatics. *Cancer.* 1996;**78**:542–547.

20 Emadi A, Jones RJ, Brodsky RA. Cyclophosphamide and cancer: golden anniversary. *Nat Rev Clin Oncol.* 2009;**6**:638–647.

21 Flowers JL, Ludeman SM, Gamcsik MP, et al. Evidence for a role of chloroethylaziridine in the cytotoxicity of cyclophosphamide. *Cancer Chemother Pharmacol.* 2000;**45**:335–344.

25 Magni M, Shammah S, Schiro R, et al. Induction of cyclophosphamide-resistance by aldehyde-dehydrogenase gene transfer. *Blood.* 1996;**87**:1097–1103.

28 Colvin M. The comparative pharmacology of cyclophosphamide and ifosfamide. *Semin Oncol.* 1982;**9**:2–7.

38 Tageja N, Nagi J. Bendamustine: something old, something new. *Cancer Chemother Pharmacol.* 2010;**66**:413–423.

49 Musser SM, Pan SS, Egorin MJ, et al. Alkylation of DNA with aziridine produced during the hydrolysis of N,N',N''-triethylenethiophosphoramide. *Chem Res Toxicol.* 1992;**5**:95–99.

51 Ames MM, Sanders ME, Tiede WS. Role of N-methylolpentamethylmelamine in the metabolic activation of hexamethylmelamine. *Cancer Res.* 1983;**43**:500–504.

56 Judson IR, Calvert AH, Gore ME, et al. Phase II trial of trimelamol in refractory ovarian cancer. *Br J Cancer.* 1991;**63**:311–313.

59 Institoris E. In vivo study on alkylation site in DNA by the bifunctional dianhydrogalactitol. *Chem Biol Interact.* 1981;**35**:207–216.

71 Hassan M. The role of busulfan in bone marrow transplantation. *Med Oncol.* 1999;**16**:166–176.

74 Bedford P, Fox BW. DNA-DNA interstrand crosslinking by dimethanesulphonic acid esters. Correlation with cytotoxicity and antitumour activity in the Yoshida lymphosarcoma model and relationship to chain length. *Biochem Pharmacol.* 1983;**32**:2297–2301.

78 Schabel FM Jr. Nitrosoureas: a review of experimental antitumor activity. *Cancer Treat Rep.* 1976;**60**:665–698.

82 Gnewuch CT, Sosnovsky G. A critical appraisal of the evolution of N-nitrosoureas as anticancer drugs. *Chem Rev.* 1997;**97**:829–1014.

87 Lemoine A, Lucas C, Ings RM. Metabolism of the chloroethylnitrosoureas. *Xenobiotica.* 1991;**21**:775–791.

92 Hartley JA, Gibson NW, Kohn KW, Mattes WB. DNA sequence selectivity of guanine-N7 alkylation by three antitumor chloroethylating agents. *Cancer Res.* 1986;**46**:1943–1947.

96 Tweedie DJ, Erikson JM, Prough RA. Metabolism of hydrazine anti-cancer agents. *Pharmacol Ther*. 1987;**34**:111–127.

101 D'Incalci M, Badri N, Galmarini CM, Allavena P. Trabectedin, a drug acting on both cancer cells and the tumour microenvironment. *Br J Cancer*. 2014;**111**:646–650.

106 Hamilton TC, Winker MA, Louie KG, et al. Augmentation of adriamycin, melphalan, and cisplatin cytotoxicity in drug-resistant and -sensitive human ovarian carcinoma cell lines by buthionine sulfoximine mediated glutathione depletion. *Biochem Pharmacol*. 1985;**34**:2583–2586.

108 Cohen JL, Jao JY. Enzymatic basis of cyclophosphamide activation by hepatic microsomes of the rat. *J Pharmacol Exp Ther*. 1970;**174**:206–210.

122 Hickman MJ, Samson LD. Role of DNA mismatch repair and p53 in signaling induction of apoptosis by alkylating agents. *Proc Natl Acad Sci U S A*. 1999;**96**:10764–10769.

125 Torres-Garcia SJ, Cousineau L, Caplan S, Panasci L. Correlation of resistance to nitrogen mustards in chronic lymphocytic leukemia with enhanced removal of melphalan-induced DNA cross-links. *Biochem Pharmacol*. 1989;**38**: 3122–3123.

132 Bosanquet AG, Sturm I, Wieder T, et al. Bax expression correlates with cellular drug sensitivity to doxorubicin, cyclophosphamide and chlorambucil but not fludarabine, cladribine or corticosteroids in B cell chronic lymphocytic leukemia. *Leukemia*. 2002;**16**:1035–1044.

135 Teicher BA, Holden SA, Ara G, Chen G. Transforming growth factor-beta in in vivo resistance. *Cancer Chemother Pharmacol*. 1996;**37**:601–609.

148 Wagner T, Heydrich D, Jork T, et al. Comparative study on human pharmacokinetics of activated ifosfamide and cyclophosphamide by a modified fluorometric test. *J Cancer Res Clin Oncol*. 1981;**100**:95–104.

157 Alberts DS, Chang SY, Chen HS, et al. Comparative pharmacokinetics of chlorambucil and melphalan in man. *Recent Results Cancer Res*. 1980;**74**: 124–131.

180 Agarwala SS, Kirkwood JM. Temozolomide, a novel alkylating agent with activity in the central nervous system, may improve the treatment of advanced metastatic melanoma. *Oncologist*. 2000;**5**:144–151.

182 van Kesteren C, Cvitkovic E, Taamma A, et al. Pharmacokinetics and pharmacodynamics of the novel marine-derived anticancer agent ecteinascidin 743 in a phase I dose-finding study. *Clin Cancer Res*. 2000;**6**:4725–4732.

195 Schacht RG, Feiner HD, Gallo GR, et al. Nephrotoxicity of nitrosoureas. *Cancer*. 1981;**48**:1328–1334.

206 Prestayko AW, D'Aoust JC, Issell BF, Crooke ST. Cisplatin (cis-diamminedichloroplatinum II). *Cancer Treat Rev*. 1979;**6**:17–39.

207 Wheate NJ, Walker S, Craig GE, Oun R. The status of platinum anticancer drugs in the clinic and in clinical trials. *Dalton Trans*. 2010;**39**:8113–8127.

215 Graham MA, Lockwood GF, Greenslade D, et al. Clinical pharmacokinetics of oxaliplatin: a critical review. *Clin Cancer Res*. 2000;**6**:1205–1218.

217 Malinge JM, Giraud-Panis MJ, Leng M. Interstrand cross-links of cisplatin induce striking distortions in DNA. *J Inorg Biochem*. 1999;**77**:23–29.

227 Bellon SF, Coleman JH, Lippard SJ. DNA unwinding produced by site-specific intrastrand cross-links of the antitumor drug cis-diamminedichloroplatinum(II). *Biochemistry*. 1991;**30**:8026–8035.

232 Kasparkova J, Brabec V. Recognition of DNA interstrand cross-links of cis-diamminedichloroplatinum(II) and its trans isomer by DNA-binding proteins. *Biochemistry*. 1995;**34**:12379–12387.

233 Martinez-Rivera M, Siddik ZH. Resistance and gain-of-resistance phenotypes in cancers harboring wild-type p53. *Biochem Pharmacol*. 2012;**83**:1049–1062.

257 Calvert AH, Newell DR, Gumbrell LA, et al. Carboplatin dosage: prospective evaluation of a simple formula based on renal function. *J Clin Oncol*. 1989;**7**:1748–1756.

262 Hellberg V, Wallin I, Eriksson S, et al. Cisplatin and oxaliplatin toxicity: importance of cochlear kinetics as a determinant for ototoxicity. *J Natl Cancer Inst*. 2009;**101**:37–47.

59 DNA topoisomerase targeting drugs

Anish Thomas, MBBS, MD ▪ Susan Bates, MD ▪ William D. Figg Sr, Pharm D ▪ Yves Pommier, MD, PhD

Overview

DNA topoisomerase targeting drugs are widely used in the treatment of multiple cancers. These drugs act by generating topoisomerase-linked DNA breaks and by blocking the religation of the cleavage complexes. Although topoisomerase targeting drugs have a wide spectrum of activity, structural, pharmacokinetic, and pharmacodynamic characteristics somewhat limit their efficacy and safety. To circumvent these limitations and to further exploit its activity, newer inhibitors- including novel formulations and those that achieve targeted delivery- are being developed. Recently described mechanisms that underlie cellular sensitivity to these agents will enable us to predict the activity of topoisomerase targeting drugs and to precisely select patients who are most likely to benefit. Understanding the genetic variants in drug metabolizing enzymes, transporters, and other proteins that influence the pharmacology of these drugs will allow for further individualizing the use of these drugs.

Introduction

The human genome consists of long double-stranded and helical DNA polymers (46 chromosomes) densely packaged in the cell nucleus (~1.8 m of DNA squeezed in a nucleus almost 1 million times smaller in diameter). Relaxing DNA supercoiling by topoisomerases is obligatory when the two genomic strands separate for transcription and replication, because the nucleosomal structure of chromatin constrains and generates DNA supercoiling. Moreover, Type II topoisomerases are required at mitosis for the even distribution of the genome between daughter cells following replication. Thus, topoisomerases are ubiquitous and essential for all organisms as they prevent and resolve DNA and RNA entanglements and resolve DNA supercoiling during transcription and replication.

Topoisomerases were named historically with the first topoisomerase being Topo I in *Escherichia coli*[1] and Top1 in mouse.[2] Notably, most of the anticancer and antibacterial agents, which are highly specific for their topoisomerase targets, are integral to the anticancer chemotherapeutic armamentarium and were discovered independently and before the term topoisomerase was even coined.

Topoisomerase biology

Human cells contain six topoisomerase genes, with three of the encoded enzymes targeted by anticancer drugs: Top1, Top2α, and Top2β (Table 1).[3–5]

The type of topoisomerase-mediated DNA break is specific of each topoisomerase (Figure 1; Table 1). These catalytic intermediates are referred to as cleavage complexes (Figure 1b, e). The reverse religation reaction is carried out by the attack of the ribose hydroxyl ends toward the tyrosyl-DNA bond.

Top1 (and Top1mt) covalently attaches to the 3′-end of the break, whereas the other topoisomerases (Top2α and β and Top3α and β) attach to the 5′-end of the break Topoisomerases act by cutting and religating the DNA backbone without assistance of nucleases and ligases. Top1 and Top1mt cleave and religate one strand of DNA duplex, whereas Top2α and β cleave and religate both strands with a four base-pair staggered cut (Figure 1). The DNA cutting-religation mechanism is common to all topoisomerases and utilizes an enzyme catalytic tyrosine residue acting as nucleophile and becoming covalently attached to the end of the broken DNA. The polarity of the attachment to the 3′- versus the 5′-ends of the DNA Top3α and β has the opposite polarity, with covalent attachment to the 5′-end of the breaks (Table 1; Figure 1b, e). Topoisomerases are biochemically distinct. Top1 and Top1mt act as monomers in the absence of nucleotide or metal cofactors, whereas Top2α and β act as dimers, requiring ATP and Mg^{2+} for catalysis. Top3α and β also require Mg^{2+} but function as monomers without ATP. Notably, the DNA substrates differ for Top3 enzymes. Both Top1 and Top2 process double-stranded DNA, whereas the Top3 substrates need to be single-stranded nucleic acids (DNA for Top3α and RNA for Top3β).

Mechanisms of action

Common mechanism of action and molecular pharmacology of topoisomerase inhibitors: trapping the topoisomerase cleavage complexes by interfacial inhibition

Topoisomerase cleavage complexes are normally highly reversible and therefore transient and hardly detectable in the absence of the topoisomerase inhibitor. This is because the religation of the cleavage complexes is driven by the realignment of the broken ends, which itself is determined by two basic structural features of double-stranded DNA: (1) the stacking of adjacent bases by π–π interactions within each strand, and (2) the pairing of bases across the opposite strands by hydrogen bond interactions (duplex DNA can be viewed as a "powerful molecular zipper").

The clinical topoisomerase inhibitors act by generating topoisomerase-linked DNA breaks as they block the religation of the cleavage complexes when a single drug molecule tightly binds at the interface of the topoisomerase-DNA cleavage complex. The selectivity and strength of the drug binding is established by (1) the stacking of the drug with the bases flanking the cleavage site and (2) a network of hydrogen bonds with the topoisomerase (Figure 2). As the drug is bound within the cleavage site, it prevents DNA religation by misaligning the DNA end, which is normally required to attack the phosphotyrosyl bond. This mode of binding led to the concept of "interfacial inhibition," which applies not only to protein–DNA interfaces but also to protein–protein interfaces, as

Holland-Frei Cancer Medicine, Ninth Edition. Edited by Robert C. Bast Jr., Carlo M. Croce, William N. Hait, Waun Ki Hong, Donald W. Kufe, Martine Piccart-Gebhart, Raphael E. Pollock, Ralph R. Weichselbaum, Hongyang Wang, and James F. Holland.
© 2017 John Wiley & Sons, Inc. ISBN: 978-1-118-93469-2

Table 1 Characteristics of topoisomerases.

Genes	Chromosome	Proteins	Drugs	Mechanism	Polarity[a]	Main functions
TOP1	20q12-q13.1	**Top1** 100 kDa monomer	**Camptothecins** **Indenos**	Swivelling Rotation	3'-Y	Nuclear supercoiling relaxation
TOP1MT	8q24.3	**Top1mt** 70 kDa monomer	None			Mitochondrial supercoiling relaxation
TOP2A	17q21-q22	**Top2α** 170 kDa dimer	**Anthracyclines,** **Anthracediones** **Epipodophyllotoxins**	Strand passage ATPase	5'-PY	Decatenation/replication
TOP2B	3p24	**Top2β** 180 kDa dimer				Transcription
TOP3A	17p12-p11.2	**Top3α** 100 kDa monomer	None	Strand passage	5'-PY	DNA replication with BLM[b]
TOP3B	22q11.22	**Top3β** 100 kDa monomer				RNA topoisomerase

[a]Covalent linkage between the catalytic tyrosine and the end of the broken DNA.
[b]Bloom syndrome, RecQ helicase.

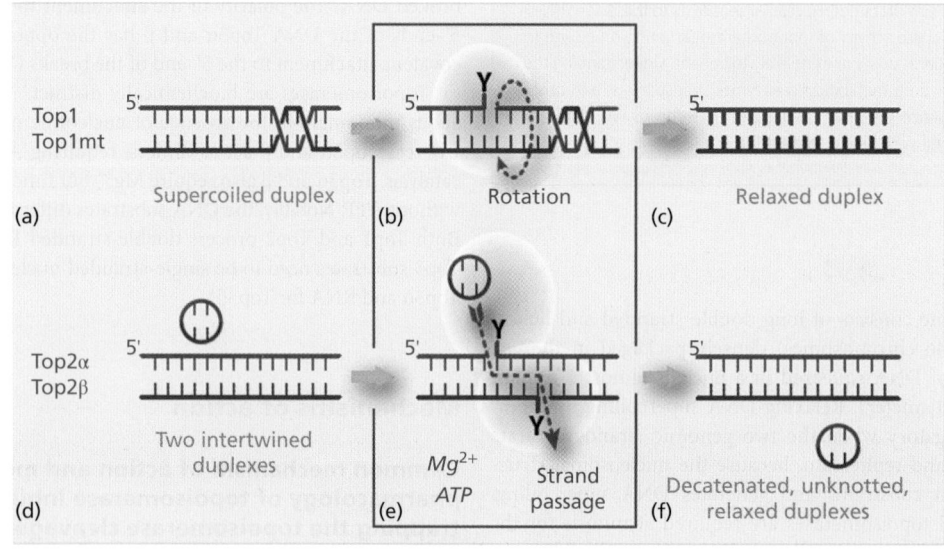

Cleavage complexes

Figure 1 Topoisomerase molecular mechanisms. (a–c) Topoisomerases I (Top1 for nuclear DNA and Top1mt for mitochondrial DNA) relax supercoiled DNA (a) by reversibly cleaving one DNA strand, forming a covalent bond between the enzyme catalytic tyrosine and the 3'-end of the nicked DNA (the Top1 cleavage complex: Top1cc; b). This reaction allows the swiveling of the broken strand around the intact strand. Rapid religation allows the dissociation of Top1 (c). (d–f) Topoisomerases II act on two DNA duplexes. They act as homodimers, cleaving both strands by forming a covalent bond between their catalytic tyrosine and the 5'-end of the DNA break (Top2cc; e). This reaction allows the passage of the intact duplex through the Top2 homodimer (red dotted arrow; e). Top2 inhibitors trap the Top2cc and prevent the normal religation (f). Topoisomerase cleavage complexes (b and d) are the targets of topoisomerase inhibitors.

in the case of tubulin and mTOR inhibitors.[6] Crystal structures of drug-bound cleavage complexes have firmly established this mechanism for both Top1- and Top2-targeted drugs.[6] The structural characteristics of each drug (differences in chemical scaffold and arrangement of hydrogen-bond donors and acceptors) (Figure 3) accounts for the selectivity of each drug for Top1 versus Top2 cleavage complexes, and for the differential DNA sequence selectivity and genomic targeting for different topoisomerase inhibitors within each class.[5,7]

It is key to understand that the cytotoxicity of topoisomerase inhibitors is due to the trapping of topoisomerase cleavage complexes as separate from the associated topoisomerase catalytic inhibition. Except in molecularly defined settings, it is the topoisomerase cleavage complexes (the DNA breaks and associated topoisomerase-DNA covalent complexes) that kill cancer cells. This sets apart topoisomerase inhibitors from classical enzyme inhibitors such as antifolates. Indeed, knocking out Top1 renders

yeast cells totally immune to camptothecin[8] and reduction of enzyme levels renders cancer cells drug resistant.[3,5] Also, mutations of TOP1 and TOP2 that render cells insensitive to the trapping of topoisomerase cleavage complexes confer high resistance to Top1 or Top2 inhibitors. Conversely, amplification of TOP2A, which is on the same locus as HER2, contributes to the selectivity and activity of doxorubicin in breast cancers with amplification at this locus.

The outcome of topoisomerase trapping is determined first by the ability of the cell to repair the cleavage complexes, and then by two common pathways: the apoptotic and the cell cycle checkpoint pathways. Topoisomerase repair pathways are specific to Top1 or Top2 and are discussed in the paragraphs that follow. Defects in pro-apoptotic molecules and excess of anti-apoptotic molecules, which are commonly associated with cancers, confer global resistance to topoisomerase inhibitors, as well as to other anticancer agents. Systematic analyses of cell lines with specific DNA repair alterations revealed that cells deficient in DNA double-strand break

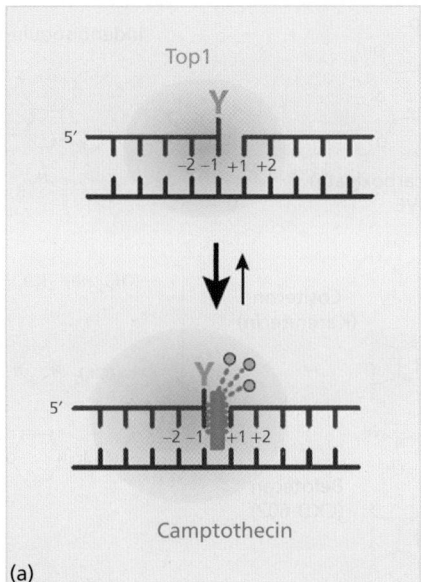

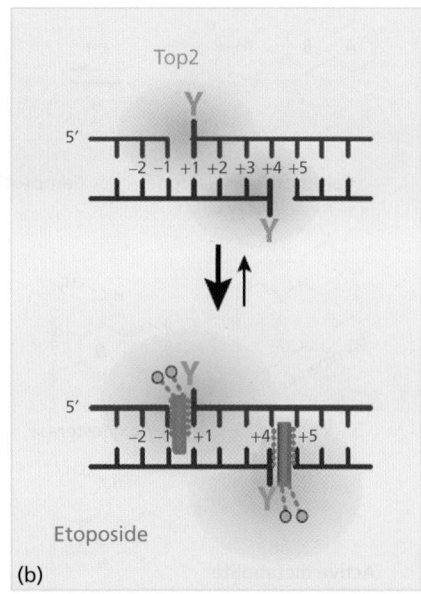

Figure 2 Trapping of topoisomerase cleavage complexes by interfacial inhibition. (a) Binding of camptothecin and non-camptothecin Top1 inhibitors (green rectangle) at the cleavage site generated by the Top1. A single-drug molecule binds reversibly to the Top1cc by stacking against the bases flanking the cleavage site (intercalation) and by a network of hydrogen bonds with Top1 (orange circles and dashed green lines). (b) Same for etoposide with a single-drug molecule (green) intercalated in the cleavage site formed by each Top2 monomer. Hydrogen bonds with Top2 are shown as orange circles and dashed green lines.

repair may be selectively sensitive to topoisomerase inhibitors.[9] Genomic analyses recently uncovered a previously unsuspected common pathway that determines cellular sensitivity to both Top1 and Top2 inhibitors (and also other DNA damaging agents, including cisplatin and carboplatin). This novel pathway is centered on the gene SLFN11 (Schlafen 11).[10,11] This finding could be viewed as a paradigm for discovering genomic determinants and signatures to predict response to topoisomerase inhibitors and staging of patients who are most likely to respond to topoisomerase inhibitors.

Molecular pathways specific for cancer cell killing and DNA repair by Top1 inhibitors

Top1cc-targeted drugs (topotecan, irinotecan, and indenoisoquinoline derivatives) kill cancer cells primarily by replication collisions. Indeed, Top1cc's by themselves are not cytotoxic as they remain reversible even in the presence of drugs that increase their persistence.[12] Top1cc's damage DNA by replication and transcription fork collisions. This explains why cytotoxicity is directly related to drug exposure and why arresting DNA replication protects cells from camptothecin.[4] Collisions arise from the fact that the drugs, by slowing down the nicking-closing activity of Top1, uncouple the Top1 from the polymerases and helicases, leading polymerases to collide into Top1cc. Such collisions have two consequences. They generate double-strand breaks (replication and transcription run-off) and irreversible Top1-DNA adducts, known as cleavage complexes. The replication double-strand breaks are repaired by homologous recombination, which explains the hypersensitivity of BRCA-deficient cancer cells to Top1cc-targeted drugs.[9] The Top1-covalent complexes can be removed by two pathways, the excision pathway involving tyrosyl-DNA-phosphodiesterase 1 (TDP1) and the endonuclease pathway involving 3′-flap endonucleases such as XPF-ERCC1.[13] It is also possible that drug-trapped Top1cc directly generate DNA double-strand breaks when they are within 10 base pairs on opposite strands of the DNA duplex or when they occur next to a preexisting single-strand break on the opposite strand.[14] Finally, it is not excluded that topological defects

contribute to the cytotoxicity of Top1cc-targeted drugs (accumulation of supercoils[15]) and formation of alternative structures such as R-loops[16] and reversed replication forks.[17]

Molecular pathways specific for cancer cell killing and DNA repair by Top2 inhibitors

Contrary to Top1 inhibitors, Top2 inhibitors can kill cancer cells independently of DNA replication fork collisions. The collision mechanism in the case of Top2cc-targeted drugs involves transcription and proteolysis of both Top2 and RNA polymerase II, leading to DNA double-strand breaks by disruption of the Top2 dimer. Alternatively, the Top2 homodimer interface could be disjoined by mechanical tension. It is important to note that 90% of Top2cc trapped by etoposide are not concerted and therefore consist in single-strand breaks, which is different from doxorubicin, which produces a majority of Top2-mediated DNA double-strand breaks.[4,5] Finally, it is not excluded that topological defects resulting from Top2 sequestration by the drug-induced cleavage complexes could contribute to the cytotoxicity of Top2cc-targeted drugs. Such topological defects would include persistent DNA knots and catenanes, potentially leading to chromosome breaks during mitosis. Top2 covalent complexes are removed by TDP2[13] in conjunction with the end-joining pathway [Ku, DNA-dependent protein kinase (DNA-PK), ligase IV, and XRCC4].[9,18]

The anticancer activity of intercalating Top2 inhibitors (anthracyclines and anthracenediones) extends beyond the trapping of Top2 cleavage complexes

Some Top2 inhibitors are also potent DNA intercalating agents; this is the case of the anthracyclines (Figure 3c) and mitoxantrone (Figure 3e). Consequently, anthracyclines and mitoxantrone affect Top2cc in two ways: at low drug concentrations, they trap Top2cc, whereas at higher concentrations (>5 μM), high levels of intercalation outside of the Top2cc suppress the binding of Top2 to DNA and thereby inhibit the formation of Top2cc. As a result, the

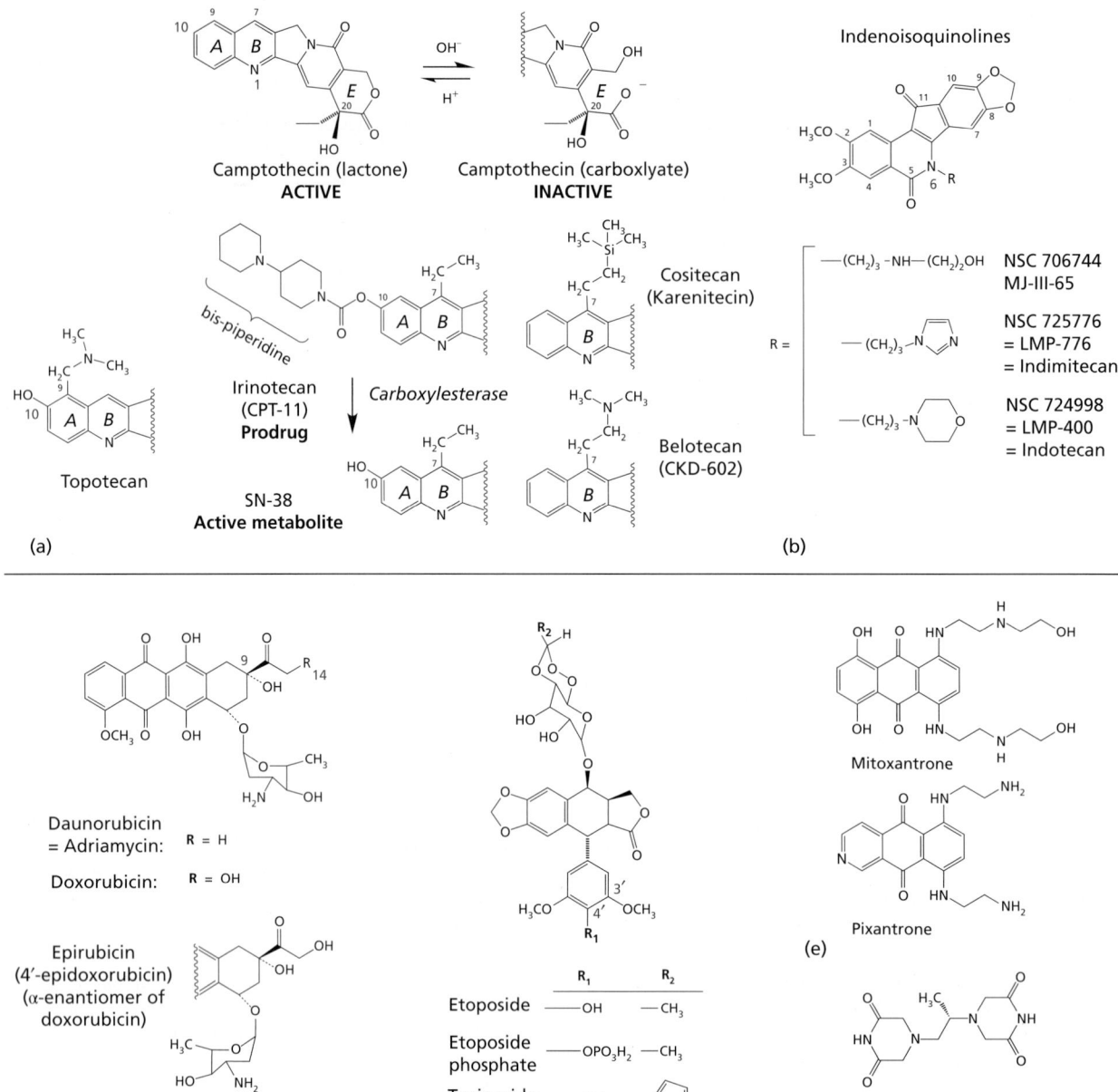

Figure 3 Clinical topoisomerase inhibitors. (a) Camptothecin derivatives are instable at physiological pH, with formation of a carboxylate derivative within minutes. Irinotecan is a prodrug, which needs to be converted to SN-38 to trap Top1cc. (b) Non-camptothecin indenoisoquinoline derivatives in clinical trials. (c) Anthracycline derivatives. (d) Demethylepipodophyllotoxin derivatives. (e) Mitoxantrone. (f) Dexrazoxane, which acts as a catalytic inhibitor of Top2.

concentration-response curve of doxorubicin is "bell-shaped."[4,19] Intercalation of anthracylines also destabilizes chromatin structure with nucleosome eviction.[20] Another property of the anthracyclines is the generation of oxygen radicals due to their quinone structure.[21]

Topoisomerase I inhibitors

Topotecan

Camptothecin and its derivatives were found to have a high degree of *in vitro* antitumor activity in the 1960s, which was then confirmed in early clinical trials.[22–24] Clinical development was limited by unpredictable toxicities, including severe myelosuppression and

diarrhea, and an incomplete understanding of the mechanism of antitumor activity. Topotecan has since been shown to be a specific inhibitor of the nuclear enzyme Top1[25] Following this, topotecan has been developed for a number of clinical indications (Table 2).

Clinical pharmacology

Topotecan (9-dimethylaminomethyl-10-hydroxycamptothecin) (Figure 3a) is a semisynthetic analog of camptothecin, an alkaloid derived from the oriental tree *Camptotheca acuminata*. The side chain at the 9-position of the A-ring (Figure 3a), provides water solubility. Lactone topotecan, the active form of the drug, is unstable as it is rapidly and reversibly converted to the open-ring carboxylate in a pH-dependent reaction[12] (Figure 3a). At neutral pH, the open-ring form predominates.[26]

Table 2 DNA topoisomerase targeting drugs.

Drug class	Drugs	Year of FDA approval	Approved indication
Camptothecin	Irinotecan	1996	Colorectal cancer
	Topotecan	1996	Cervical cancer, ovarian cancer, small cell lung cancer
Anthracycline	Doxorubicin	1974	Breast cancer, acute lymphoblastic leukemia, acute myeloid leukemia, Wilms tumor, neuroblastoma, soft tissue and bone sarcomas, ovarian cancer, transitional cell bladder carcinoma, thyroid carcinoma, gastric carcinoma, Hodgkin lymphoma, non-Hodgkin lymphoma, bronchogenic carcinoma
	Pegylated liposomal doxorubicin	1999	AIDS-related Kaposi sarcoma, multiple myeloma, ovarian cancer
	Daunorubicin	1979	Acute lymphocytic leukemia, acute myeloid leukemia
	Idarubicin	1990	Acute myeloid leukemia
Anthraquinone	Mitoxantrone	1987	Acute nonlymphocytic leukemias, advanced hormone-refractory prostate cancer
Podophyllotoxin	Etoposide	1984	Small cell lung cancer, testicular cancer
	Teniposide	1992	Acute lymphoblastic leukemia

Topotecan pharmacokinetics fit a two-compartment model with a terminal half-life of 2–3 h. The plasma concentrations increase linearly with increasing doses, but do not show evidence of accumulation on the 30-min infusion X 5-day schedule.[27] Binding of topotecan to plasma proteins is about 35%.[27]

Topotecan lactone is widely distributed, with a steady-state mean volume of distribution of 75 L/m^2. Topotecan is predominantly eliminated in the urine after its conversion to the carboxylate species. Although large interindividual variability exists, about 30% of the administered dose is excreted unchanged in urine.[27]

Renal dysfunction decreases topotecan plasma clearance, such that mild dysfunction (creatinine clearance 40–60 mL/min) and moderate dysfunction (creatinine clearance 20–39 mL/min), lead to reductions to 67% and 34% of normal values, respectively.[28] Dose adjustments are therefore recommended in case of renal impairment. Liver impairment does not influence topotecan clearance and doses do not need to be adjusted for patients with hepatic dysfunction.[29]

Although the typical route of administration is IV, an oral formulation is available. The oral formulation of topotecan was aimed at maintaining sufficiently prolonged drug exposures, which are known to produce highest antitumor efficacy *in vitro* and *in vivo*,[12] without the need for infusion pumps.[30] The approved oral dose is 2.3 mg/m^2 once daily for 5 consecutive days repeated every 21 days. The oral bioavailability of topotecan is approximately 35%.[27] The low bioavailability may be caused by hydrolysis of topotecan lactone in the gut, yielding the poorly absorbed open-ring form. Oral topotecan has shown clinical activity comparable to the IV dose in small cell lung cancer (SCLC).[31]

Clinical use
Topotecan monotherapy is approved in the United States and Europe for patients with metastatic ovarian cancer patients after failure of initial or subsequent chemotherapy, and in patients with relapsed SCLC. It is also approved in combination with cisplatin for recurrent or resistant (stage IVB) cervical cancer.[32]

Topotecan has shown clinical activity in other tumor types, including pediatric medulloblastoma,[33] non-SCLC,[34] myelodysplastic syndrome, chronic myelomonocytic leukemia,[35] Ewing's sarcoma,[36] rhabdomyosarcoma,[37] and multiple myeloma.[38] In addition to the combination with cisplatin approved in cervical cancer, combinations of Top1 inhibitors with other antitumor agents have been pursued. Synergistic and additive combinations have been observed in preclinical models, including with histone deacetylase

inhibitors and PARP inhibitors, and a number of drug combination strategies have been investigated in patients.[39,40] Topotecan diffuses to the spinal fluid and can be considered for treating brain metastases.[41]

Schedule of administration
Various schedules of topotecan have been evaluated in phase I studies. The FDA (Food and Drug Administration)-recommended dose of topotecan in recurrent ovarian cancer and SCLC is 1.5 mg/m^2 by IV infusion over 30 min on days 1 to 5 of a 21-day cycle.

Despite the high incidence of grade 3 or 4 myelosuppression associated with this dose and schedule of topotecan, it remains the standard of care. To mitigate this toxicity, multiple dose and schedule variations have been evaluated in phase I and II trials.[42,43] In ovarian cancer, weekly topotecan (4 mg/m^2/week administered on days 1, 8, and 15) has been reported to have efficacy comparable to the standard schedule, but with less toxicity.[43] The weekly schedule has not been directly compared with the 5-day schedule in SCLC.[31] In cervical cancer, topotecan is approved in combination with cisplatin. In this setting, the recommended dose of topotecan is 0.75 mg/m^2 IV over 30 min on days 1, 2, and 3 with cisplatin 50 mg/m^2 IV on day 1 repeated every 21 days.[44]

Toxicity
The dose-limiting toxicity of topotecan is bone marrow suppression, primarily neutropenia, but thrombocytopenia and anemia may also occur. At a dose of 1.5 mg/m^2/day for 5 days, topotecan produces an 80% to 90% decrease in white blood cell count at nadir after the first cycle of therapy. The degree of neutropenia has been correlated with the area under the curve (AUC) of the intact lactone or total drug concentrations.[45] Topotecan should not be administered to patients with baseline neutrophils <1500/mm^3 or platelets <100,000/mm^3.

As discussed above, renal dysfunction decreases topotecan clearance and increases toxicity. Additional factors associated with greater hematologic toxicity include advance age and prior therapy, including platinum administration (especially carboplatin), radiation therapy.[46] In high-risk patients receiving topotecan for 5 consecutive days, the incidence of severe myelosuppression may be mitigated by reduction of the topotecan dose to 1.0 or 1.25 mg/m^2/day. Hematopoietic growth factors, transfusions, and schedule adjustments may also help manage myelosuppression. Alternative schedules of 3-day, weekly dosing or oral administration are associated with less myelosuppression.[47]

Other toxicities of topotecan less common than bone marrow suppression include rash, fever, fatigue, nausea and vomiting, mucositis, and elevated serum transaminases.[48] Most nonhematological side effects are generally manageable. Diarrhea is uncommon with IV administration, but has been reported with oral topotecan. Rare, but life-threatening nonhematologic toxicities includes interstitial lung disease and neutropenic colitis.

Irinotecan

Irinotecan is a potent water-soluble camptothecin derivative.

Clinical pharmacology

Irinotecan (CPT-11) is the prodrug of the potent 7-ethyl-10-hydroxy analog of camptothecin (SN-38) (Figure 3a).[45] It contains a bispiperidine substituent at C-10, to confer water solubility for parenteral administration. Irinotecan undergoes extensive metabolic conversion by esterases to its active metabolite SN-38 (Figure 3a). Irinotecan prodrug is activated by carboxylesterases to SN-38, the biologically active compound. This explains why irinotecan is orders of magnitude less active than SN-38 in *in vitro* cytotoxicity assays.[49,50]

Irinotecan peak plasma concentration and AUC increase proportionally with the administered dose, suggestive of linear pharmacokinetics. The plasma AUC of SN-38 is only 2% to 8% of irinotecan, indicating that only a small fraction of irinotecan is converted to SN-38, its active form. Both irinotecan and SN-38 exist in the active lactone form and the inactive carboxylate form. Similar to topotecan, both forms are in a pH-dependent equilibrium.[12]

Irinotecan plasma concentrations decline in a multiexponential manner after IV infusion. The mean terminal elimination half-life of irinotecan is 6 to 12 h and that of SN-38 10 to 20 h, both much longer than that of topotecan. The relatively large percentage of the lactone form of both irinotecan and SN-38, which persists in plasma after drug administration, is attributable to the preferential binding of the lactone forms to albumin.[26] SN-38 is 95% bound to plasma proteins compared to approximately 50% for irinotecan.[45]

Unlike topotecan, irinotecan elimination occurs predominantly by biliary excretion.[45] Renal excretion of SN-38 and irinotecan represents only a fraction of the administered dose. The 1A1 isoform of uridine 5′-diphospho-glucuronosyl transferase (UGT1A1; encoded by the *UGT1A1* gene) mediates glucuronidation of SN-38 to the inactive metabolite SN-38G (see section titled "Pharmacogenomics"). There is wide interpatient variability in UGT1A1 enzyme activity related to UGT1A1 gene polymorphisms.[51,52] In addition, polymorphisms of this enzyme are associated with conditions causing familial hyperbilirubinemia such as Crigler–Najjar syndromes and Gilbert's disease.[53] UGT1A1 polymorphisms can significantly alter the metabolism of irinotecan and thereby impact its toxicity in individual patients, and dose reduction is recommended for patients bearing particular variants of UGT1A1. Irinotecan is also inactivated by CYP3A4-mediated oxidative metabolism.[54] The impact of polymorphic variants is discussed in more detail in the subsequent sections.

Clinical use

Irinotecan is approved in the United States and Europe for first-line therapy in combination with 5-fluorouracil and leucovorin for metastatic colorectal cancers. It is also approved for metastatic colorectal cancer in patients whose disease has recurred or progressed following fluorouracil-based therapy.[49,55]

Irinotecan monotherapy or combinations with other agents have shown clinical activity in diverse tumor types, including extensive-stage SCLC,[56] squamous cell carcinoma of the cervix,[57] recurrent glioblastoma,[58] gastric cancer, esophageal cancer,[59] non-SCLC,[60] pancreatic cancer,[61] rhabdomyosarcoma,[62] and ovarian cancer.[63]

Schedule of administration

Monotherapy with irinotecan is usually administered at 125 mg/m^2 IV infusion over 90 min on days 1, 8, 15, and 22 followed by 2-week rest (6-week treatment cycles). An alternative dosing regimen is 350 mg/m^2 given as a 60-min IV infusion once every 3 weeks. In patients with 5-fluorouracil-refractory, metastatic colorectal cancer, the weekly and once every 3-week schedule demonstrated similar efficacy and quality of life. The regimen of once every 3 weeks was associated with a significantly lower incidence of severe diarrhea.[64]

In combination with 5-fluorouracil and leucovorin, irinotecan is used at 125 mg/m^2 IV infusion over 90 min on days 1, 8, 15, and 22 (6-week treatment cycles). An alternative dosing regimen is 180 mg/m^2 over 90 min on days 1, 15, and 29 (6-week treatment cycles).

Toxicity

Diarrhea and myelosuppression are the most concerning toxicities of irinotecan. Late-onset diarrhea occurs more than 24 h after irinotecan. When prolonged, it can lead to life-threatening dehydration and electrolyte imbalance.[65] Grade 3 or 4 late-onset diarrhea occurs in about a third of patients receiving weekly dosing. The median time to the onset of late diarrhea was 5 days with 3-week dosing and 11 days with weekly dosing.[49,55] Free intestinal luminal SN-38, either from bile or SN-38G deconjugation is responsible for late-onset diarrhea. SN-38 induces direct mucosal damage with resultant water and electrolyte malabsorption and mucous hypersecretion.[66] Late diarrhea should be treated without delay with loperamide, and fluid and electrolytes as needed. Antibiotic therapy is warranted if the patient develops ileus, fever, or severe neutropenia. Predisposing factors for late-onset diarrhea include increasing age, poor performance status, and prior abdominopelvic radiotherapy.[67] A reduced starting dose should be considered in patients with risk factors. Treatment-related diarrhea should have fully resolved before initiating the next course of treatment. Dose reductions are recommended for grades 3 and 4 diarrhea. Various measures to reduce its severity have been studied, but none have an established role in practice.[68] In 2005, the FDA approved a diagnostic test for the UGT1A1 variant allele *28, which has been associated with reduced expression leading to impaired clearance and increased toxicity.[69] However, other variant alleles that impair expression of the enzyme are also known and impact clearance of drugs requiring glucuronidation (discussed in greater detail below).

Less commonly, irinotecan can also cause early-onset diarrhea during or within 24 h of the infusion. It is usually transient and only infrequently severe. It is attributed to a cholinergic syndrome mediated by anticholinesterase activity of irinotecan.[70] This cholinergic syndrome tends to occur at higher irinotecan dose levels at peak irinotecan plasma levels. Other cholinergic symptoms including abdominal cramping, rhinitis, tearing, and increased salivation may occur. The mean duration of symptoms is 30 min and usually responds rapidly to atropine.

Other common toxicities observed with irinotecan are nausea, vomiting, abdominal pain, constipation, anorexia, asthenia, fever, decrease in body weight, and alopecia. Rare, but life-threatening nonhematological toxicities include interstitial lung disease and hypersensitivity reactions. Risk factors for pulmonary toxicity include preexisting lung disease, use of pulmonary toxic medications, radiation, and use of colony-stimulating factors. Patients with risk factors should be monitored for respiratory symptoms while on irinotecan and for several weeks after treatment.[71]

Camptothecin analogs and non-camptothecin Top1 inhibitors

As discussed above, camptothecin derivatives have several well-established limitations. They are inactivated within minutes at physiological pH by lactone E ring opening (Figure 3a). This results in a loss of antitumor activity since the lactone form is essential for antitumor activity. Other limitations include fast reversal of the trapped DNA-Top1 cleavage complex following drug removal and drug resistance mediated by ATP-binding cassette (ABC) transporters.[12]

Several newer derivatives of camptothecin currently in clinical development aim to mitigate some of the shortcomings of camptothecins and their derivatives (Table 3). Camptothecin analogs, derived from modifications to the parent drug, have been an area of active research.[72] Belotecan hydrochloride, a water-soluble camptothecin analog is in clinical development for SCLC and ovarian cancer.[73] Cositecan (Karenitecin) (Figure 3a) is an orally active, highly lipophilic, semisynthetic camptothecin, under development for ovarian cancer. Due to its lipophilicity, cositecan exhibits enhanced tissue penetration and bioavailability compared to water-soluble camptothecins and are less sensitive to drug resistance.

Several approaches have been taken to stabilize the lactone ring of camptothecins without interfering with their antitumor activity.[19] Indenoisoquinolines are non-camptothecin inhibitors of Top1, but with better chemical stability, producing stable DNA-Top1 cleavage complexes. They also have a preference for unique DNA cleavage sites, compared with their camptothecin counterparts and have demonstrated activity against camptothecin-resistant cell lines and produce DNA protein cross-links, which are resistant to reversal. They also show less or no resistance to cells overexpressing the ABC transporters, ATP-binding cassette subfamily G member 2 (ABCG2), and multidrug resistance (MDR)-1.[74] Other approaches to address E-ring instability include the conversion of the E ring to a five-membered ring, which completely stabilizes the drug.[75]

Targeted delivery of Top1 inhibitors

Several approaches are being explored to improve the targeted delivery, and tumor localization of camptothecins. Broadly they involve (1) liposomal or nanoparticle formulation to increase plasma half-life and tumor localization, (2) antibody conjugation

for targeted delivery, and (3) conjugation to agents to improve pharmacokinetic properties and exposure.

Liposomal/nanoparticle formulations

Liposomes are microscopic phospholipid spheres with an aqueous core.[76] Due to their biphasic character, they can act as carriers for both lipophilic and hydrophilic drugs; hydrophilic drugs tend to be entrapped in the core, whereas the hydrophobic ones are entrapped within the lipid bilayers. Stable liposomal encapsulation of camptothecin minimizes its conversion to the inactive carboxylate form by reducing the direct exposure of the drug to physiologic pH and prolonging the residence time of the lactone active drug. PEGylation increases the size and molecular weight of conjugated biomolecules.[77] PEGylated molecules show increased half-life, decreased plasma clearance, and different biodistribution compared with non-PEGylated counterparts. PEGylation of liposomes further improves the stability and circulation time. Polymeric nanoparticles are drug carriers that are designed to have defined size and surface properties to favor drug deposition and retention in tumors.[78] These formulations are thought to improve the "passive" targeting of tumors, through a process known as the enhanced permeation retention effect, wherein macromolecules penetrate and are trapped in tumor tissue due to the abnormally leaky vasculature of tumors.[79]

MM-398 (nal-IRI) is a nanoliposomal encapsulation of irinotecan sucrosofate. In preclinical studies, MM-398 improved the pharmacokinetics and tumor biodistribution of both irinotecan and SN-38 when compared with the free form of the drug, with less accumulation in organs responsible for dose-limiting toxicities.[80] MM-398 has shown clinical activity in combination with 5-fluorouracil and leucovorin in metastatic pancreatic cancer patients who have previously received gemcitabine-based therapy.[81]

CRLX101 is a nanoparticle therapeutic comprised of camptothecin covalently conjugated to a linear, cyclodextrin-polyethylene glycol copolymer.[72] CRLX101 self-assembles in solution into nanoparticles with solubility increases of over 1000-fold compared with the parent drug camptothecin. CRLX101 is currently being evaluated in patients with renal, ovarian, and rectal cancers.

Antibody drug conjugates

Antibody drug conjugates (ADCs) generated by conjugating camptothecins to monoclonal antibodies are being investigated to facilitate targeted drug delivery to tumors. Sacituzumab govitecan is a humanized antibody against trophoblast cell-surface antigen

Table 3 Investigational Top1 inhibitors in clinical development.

	Drugs/drug class	Comments
Camptothecin analogs	Belotecan	Water-soluble camptothecin analog
	Cositecan	Lipophilic, semisynthetic camptothecin
	Lipotecan	Lactone ring modified to increase antitumor potency
	Simmitecan	Ester prodrug of the Top1 inhibitor chimmitecan
Targeted camptothecin delivery	*Liposomal/nanoparticle/PEGylated formulations*	
	MM-398 Onivyde	Nanoliposomal formulation of irinotecan
	CPX-1	Liposome-encapsulated formulation of Irinotecan and floxuridine
	Firtecan pegol	Pegylated formulation of SN-38
	CRLX101	Cyclodextrin-based polymer conjugate of camptothecin
	Antibody-drug conjugates	
	Sacituzumab govitecan	Antibody drug conjugate [antibody that binds to trophoblast cell-surface antigen (TROP-2) and SN-38]
	Camptothecin conjugates	
	HA-irinotecan	Irinotecan complexed with hyaluronic acid
	Etirinotecan pegol (NKTR-102)	Irinotecan bound to polyethylene glycol core by a biodegradable linker
Non-camptothecin Top1 inhibitors	Indenoisoquinoline derivatives	Chemical stability, stable DNA-TOP1 trapping, no affected by drug efflux pumps

(TROP-2) conjugated by a pH-sensitive linker to SN-38.[82] TROP-2 is a type I transmembrane, calcium-transducing, protein expressed by many epithelial cancers, but with limited normal tissue expression. The antibody internalizes selectively into cancer cells following binding to TROP-2 encoded by the *TACSTD2* gene. Sacituzumab govitecan is being investigated in triple-negative breast cancer and SCLC.

Camptothecin conjugates
Etirinotecan pegol is a long-acting topoisomerase-I inhibitor that consists of irinotecan conjugated to a polyethylene glycol core by a biodegradable linker. The linker slowly hydrolyses *in vivo* to form SN38, the active moiety. The drug is designed to provide prolonged continuous exposure to SN38 while reducing the toxicities associated with excessively high irinotecan and SN38 plasma concentrations. Etirinotecan pegol at a dose of 145 mg/m² administered IV every 21 days is being studied in a phase III trial in women with advanced breast cancer.[83] Hyaluronic acid-irinotecan is an IV formulation of irinotecan conjugated with hyaluronic acid.[84] Hyaluronic acid selectively binds cancer cells via CD44, thereby enhancing membrane fluidity and potentially reducing side effects.

Top2 inhibitors
Top2 targeting drugs used in clinic can be divided into intercalating and non-intercalating poisons. The intercalators are chemically diverse, and include doxorubicin and other anthracyclines, and anthracenediones (Figure 3c, e). Non-intercalating Top2 poisons include the epipodophyllotoxins, etoposide and teniposide (Figure 3d; Table 2).

Anthracyclines
Anthracycline antibiotics, originally isolated from fermentation products of *Streptomyces peucetius*, were shown to have antineoplastic activity decades ago, before topoisomerase enzymes were identified. It was not until 1984 that the anthracyclines were found to inhibit Top2.[85] Doxorubicin, also known as adriamycin and daunorubicin, represent first-generation anthracyclines; epirubicin and idarubicin are second-generation compounds aimed at reducing cardiotoxicity and drug efflux by ABC transporters. Anthracyclines have wide-ranging activity against human cancers and are used extensively in the curative, adjuvant, and palliative settings, both as single agents and in combination regimens.

Doxorubicin is the most commonly used anthracycline (Figure 3c). The anthracycline ring is lipophilic, but the presence of abundant hydroxyl groups adjacent to the amino sugar produces an amphoteric molecule. Doxorubicin binds to cell membranes, including cardiolipin as well as plasma proteins. Daunomycin differs from doxorubicin by a single hydroxyl group on carbon-14 (Figure 3c), but has a distinct spectrum of antitumor activity. Idarubicin is a semisynthetic derivative of daunomycin (4-demethoxy daunorubicin) without the 4-methoxy group (Figure 3c). Epirubicin is an epimer of doxorubicin: the C4' hydroxyl group on the amino sugar is in the equatorial rather than in the axial position which increases its lipophilicity. None of these analogs have stronger antitumor efficacy than the original two anthracyclines, but they tend to limit the toxicity of doxorubicin and daunorubicin.[86]

Clinical pharmacology
Doxorubicin displays linear pharmacokinetics and exhibits a triphasic disposition after IV injection. The initial half-life is very short, approximately 5 min, suggesting rapid tissue uptake. The second phase of approximately 10 h represents its metabolism and the slow final phase of 24 to 48 h, the gradual release of doxorubicin from multiple sites of binding including the DNA.[87] Doxorubicin and its major metabolite, doxorubicinol, are substantially bound to plasma proteins, about 50% to 90%.[88] Doxorubicin does not cross the blood-brain barrier.

Plasma clearance of doxorubicin is predominantly by metabolism and biliary excretion. The drug is extensively metabolized in the liver by aldo-keto reductase, to yield the dihydrodiol derivative doxorubicinol, which retains antitumor activity, and by the NADPH-dependent cytochrome P450 reductase to cleave the glycosidic bond and release aglycone metabolites.[89] The clearance of doxorubicin and doxorubicinol are reduced in patients with impaired hepatic function.[90] Renal clearance is quantitatively unimportant, and dose modification is not required in renal failure.

Liposome encapsulation of doxorubicin has been successfully used as a strategy to reduce toxicity without losing efficacy.[91] Pegylated liposomal doxorubicin is a liposomal formulation of doxorubicin, which compared with unencapsulated doxorubicin has a long half-life and delayed uptake by the reticuloendothelial system due to the attachment of polyethylene glycol polymers to a lipid anchor and stable retention of the drug as a result of liposomal entrapment via an ammonium sulfate chemical gradient.[92] The pharmacokinetic profile of this drug is characterized by an extended circulation time and a reduced volume of distribution, which promotes tumor uptake.

Clinical use
Doxorubicin is utilized in multiple human cancer types. It is FDA approved for adjuvant chemotherapy following resection of primary breast cancer for patients with axillary lymph node invasion. Doxorubicin is also used for the treatment of acute lymphoblastic and myeloblastic leukemias, and in combination regimens for non-Hodgkin's and Hodgkin's lymphoma. Doxorubicin has activity in many solid tumors including breast, ovarian, bladder, thyroid, gastric and lung cancers, soft tissue and bone sarcomas. Pegylated liposomal doxorubicin is used in treatment of AIDS-related Kaposi sarcoma after failure of or intolerance to prior systemic therapy and in multiple myeloma as a component of combination therapy.[93,94] It is also used in the treatment of progressive or recurrent ovarian cancer after platinum-based treatment.[95]

Epirubicin has a spectrum of activity very similar to doxorubicin, but with lower toxicity.[96] Epirubicin is used as a component of adjuvant therapy for primary breast cancer and for esophageal and gastric cancers, and soft tissue and uterine sarcomas.[97]

Daunomycin (Figure 3c) is used mostly as part of an induction regimen in acute lymphocytic leukemia and acute myeloid leukemia. It is also active in pediatric solid tumors, but has little activity against adult solid tumors. Idarubicin is used predominantly in the treatment of acute myeloid and lymphoid leukemia.[98]

Schedule of administration
Single-agent doxorubicin is administered IV at 60 to 75 mg/m² every 21 days. In combination therapy, it is administered at 40 to 75 mg/m² every 21 to 28 days. Daunorubicin is given IV at 30 to 60 mg/m² daily for 3 days. Idarubicin is given IV at 12 mg/m² daily for 3 days. Epirubicin is given IV at 100 to 120 mg/m² by bolus injection every 3 weeks. Pegylated liposomal doxorubicin is administered IV at 20 mg/m² every 21 days for AIDS-related Kaposi sarcoma and 50 mg/m² once every 28 days in ovarian cancer.

Toxicity

All anthracyclines produce cardiac damage that can result in serious and even life-threatening complications.[99,100] It is the major dose-limiting toxicity of prolonged treatment with doxorubicin. Cardiac toxicity is more common with doxorubicin and daunorubicin than with epirubicin or idarubicin.[96] Cardiac toxicity manifests acutely with electrocardiographic abnormalities, including ST-T elevations and arrhythmias and can occur at any time from initiation of treatment to several weeks afterward. Cardiomyopathy, a manifestation of chronic cardiotoxicity, may also occur early, within 1 year of termination of the treatment, or be delayed beyond 1 year after treatment.

Doxorubicin-associated cardiomyopathy and congestive heart failure are dose dependent. Risk increases proportionally to the total accumulated dose in a nonlinear fashion (1–5% up to 550 mg/m^2, 30% at 600 mg/m^2, and 50% at 1 g/m^2 or higher) with marked interindividual variation.[101] The frequency of these complications is unacceptably high when the cumulative dose of the drug exceeds 550 mg/m^2 of body-surface area.[102] The mode of administration plays an important role in cumulative cardiotoxicity and bolus administration appears to be involved.[103] Continuous infusion regimens have been studied in an effort to reduce cardiotoxicity. Infusion over 48 or 96 h has been studied, demonstrating a shift in the side effect profile, with less nausea and vomiting and cardiotoxicity to enhanced mucositis,[104] but allowing dosing above conventional limits. Despite evident advantages, the difficulty of administering a continuous infusion schedule meant that this approach has not had significant uptake in the community.

The cardiotoxicity of doxorubicin had been attributed to redox cycling and reactive oxygen species (ROS) generation; however, ROS scavengers have failed to prevent this toxicity.[102,105] More recent data implicate Top2β[106] Top2α is overexpressed in tumors and represents the molecular basis of doxorubicin antitumor activity, whereas Top2β is expressed by cardiomyocytes and non-replicating cells.[13,107] Multiple lines of evidence indicate the role of Top2β in contributing to the development of doxorubicin-induced cardiomyopathy. Top2β-doxorubicin-DNA ternary cleavage complex can induce DNA double-strand breaks leading to cell death in cardiomyocytes. TOP2β-deleted mouse embryonic fibroblasts have been shown to be resistant to doxorubicin-induced cell death.[108] Recent studies also indicate that the mitochondrial topoisomerase, Top1mt, counteracts the cytotoxicity of doxorubicin by enabling mitochondrial DNA replication and maintaining functional oxidative phosphorylation.[107]

Several factors increase the risk for anthracycline cardiotoxicity. The strongest predictor is cumulative drug dose.[109] Age at the time of drug exposure, concomitant administration of other cardiotoxic drugs, radiation to the chest, and preexisting cardiovascular disease are other risk factors. A number of approaches have been taken to decrease the risk of cardiotoxicity while maintaining efficacy. These include alternate schedules of drug administration, modifications of the anthracycline molecule, and adjunctive treatment with beta-adrenergic blockers or dexrazoxane.[108] Recent evidence implicates Top1mt mutations, which exist as normal SNPs (single nucleotide polymorphisms), as potential determinants of the cardiotoxicity of doxorubicin.[107]

Dexrazoxane (Figure 3f) is an ethylenediaminetetraacetic acid (EDTA)-like chelator that prevents anthracycline damage by binding to iron released from intracellular storage secondary to lipid peroxidation.[110] Breast cancer patients treated with dexrazoxane experienced fewer cardiac events compared with those treated with anthracycline only.[111] Dexrazoxane is approved in the United States and Europe for patients with advanced or metastatic breast cancer who have already received 300 mg/m^2 of doxorubicin or 540 mg/m^2 of epirubicin. However, concerns exist regarding the possibility of lower response to chemotherapy and more myelosuppression with dexrazoxane use.[112] Dexrazoxane is therefore not recommended for routine use in breast cancer with doxorubicin-based chemotherapy. Continued cardiac monitoring is recommended in patients receiving doxorubicin.[113]

Other toxicities of anthracyclines include myelosuppression, mucositis, and alopecia, nausea, vomiting, diarrhea, and increased skin pigmentation. Myelosuppression is the acute dose-limiting toxicity. After bolus dose, the white blood cell count begins to fall in 7 days. The count reaches a nadir at 10 to 14 days and recovers 1 to 2 weeks later. Thrombocytopenia and anemia are less severe. Erythema at the injection site (flare reaction) is benign, in contrast to extravasation, which can lead to serious local complications such as severe necrosis of surrounding tissues. Inflammation at sites of previous radiation (radiation recall) can lead to unanticipated complications, including pericarditis, pleural effusion, and skin rash. The incidence of nausea and vomiting, and alopecia, are less with epirubicin than with doxorubicin.[96]

The toxicity profile of pegylated liposomal doxorubicin is characterized by mucosal and cutaneous toxicities, mild myelosuppression, and decreased cardiotoxicity compared with doxorubicin and minimal alopecia. Palmar-plantar erythrodysesthesia is the most common grade 3 or 4 toxicity observed, frequently at the second or third cycle, and occurs at a higher frequency than with patients receiving conventional doxorubicin.[114] The mucocutaneous toxicities are dose limiting. The pathophysiology of palmar-plantar erythrodysesthesia is not well understood. It has been hypothesized that following the local trauma, pegylated liposomal doxorubicin may extravasate via the eccrine glands from the deeper microcapillaries in the hands and feet where its accumulation is facilitated by the hydrophilic coating of the liposomes.[115] Reduced cardiotoxicity of pegylated liposomal doxorubicin allows a larger cumulative dose than that of doxorubicin. Acute hypersensitivity reaction may occur usually with the first infusion.[116]

Newer anthracyclines

Although anthracyclines have wide spectrum of activity, structural, pharmacokinetic, and pharmacodynamic characteristics somewhat limit their efficacy and safety. To circumvent these limitations and to further exploit its activity, newer anthracyclines and anthracycline conjugates have been developed.

Amrubicin is a completely synthetic anthracycline with a structure similar to doxorubicin and potent Top2 inhibitory activity that is available only in Japan, where it is approved for use in non-SCLC and SCLC.[117] Amrubicin itself has a weak antitumor effect and needs to be converted to its active form, amrubicinol, to be effective.[118] In preclinical studies, amrubicin caused almost no cardiotoxicity. The lower cardiotoxicity of amrubicin has been attributed to lower levels of accumulation and metabolic advantages over doxorubicin.[119] In second-line treatment of SCLC, although it was associated with better response rates, amrubicin did not improve survival compared with topotecan.[120] In first-line SCLC, amrubicin plus cisplatin was inferior to irinotecan plus amrubicin.[121]

Anthracenediones

Mitoxantrone (Figure 3e) is a potent inhibitor of Top2 derived in part from an early hypothesis that the cardiotoxicity of the anthracyclines might depend on the presence of an amino sugar.[122] Since the aglycones of the cardiac glycosides have less cardiotoxic potency than the parent compounds, it was thought that a polycyclic aromatic molecule that intercalates with DNA, but which does not have an amino sugar might be an effective antitumor agent without cardiotoxicity. The antitumor spectrum of mitoxantrone is limited compared to that of doxorubicin. Mitoxantrone is used in the initial treatment of acute nonlymphocytic leukemias and is active in advanced castrate-resistant prostate cancer and breast cancer. The dose-limiting toxicity of mitoxantrone is leucopenia in patients with solid tumors, whereas stomatitis may be dose limiting in patients with leukemia. Other adverse effects are usually of mild or moderate severity. Cardiac effects, particularly congestive heart failure, may be of concern, especially in patients previously treated with anthracyclines, mediastinal irradiation or patients with cardiovascular disease.

Pixantrone (Figure 3e) is an aza-anthracenedione with structural similarity to mitoxantrone. In preclinical models, compared with doxorubicin, pixantrone showed enhanced activity and decreased cardiotoxicity with decreased free radical formation.[123] Single-agent salvage therapy with pixantrone has received conditional marketing authorization in the European Union for the treatment of patients with multiply relapsed or refractory aggressive non-Hodgkin's B-cell lymphoma.[124] The recommended dose of pixantrone is 50 mg/m^2 administered on days 1, 8, and 15 of each 28-day cycle for up to six cycles. The most common side effects with pixantrone are bone marrow suppression (particularly of the neutrophil lineage) nausea, vomiting, and asthenia. It is not approved for use in the United States.

Epipodophyllotoxins

Podophyllotoxin is a natural product isolated from *Podophyllum peltatum* and *Podophyllum emodi*.[125] Although the anticancer activity of podophyllotoxin and selected derivatives were known in the 1940s, the prohibitive toxicity of podophyllin precluded further development. Demethylepipodophyllotoxin Top2 inhibitors are podophyllotoxin derivatives, which resulted from efforts to identify agents that retained antineoplastic activity, but had less toxicity.

Etoposide

Etoposide (VP-16) (Figure 3d) was the first agent to be recognized as a Top2 inhibiting anticancer drug.[126] As with several other topoisomerase inhibitors, the appreciation of its clinical activity and approval preceded the understanding of its mechanism of action and pharmacology.

Clinical pharmacology

Etoposide is not water soluble, which presents difficulties for rapid administration and drug hypersensitivity reactions related to the vehicles utilized as solubilisers. Etoposide phosphate, a water-soluble ester of etoposide at concentrations up to 20 mg/mL, is a result of efforts to overcome this issue and has been approved for IV use by the FDA.[127] The water solubility of etoposide phosphate also alleviates the risk of drug precipitation during IV administration. *In vivo* etoposide phosphate is rapidly converted to the active moiety, etoposide, by dephosphorylation. The pharmacokinetic profile, toxicity, and clinical activity of etoposide phosphate are similar to that of etoposide.

Etoposide exhibits a biphasic pharmacokinetics with a distribution half-life of about 1.5 h and terminal elimination half-life ranging from 4 to 11 h. There is a linear relationship between the AUC and peak plasma concentrations achieved following IV administration.[128] cerebrospinal fluid (CSF) concentrations of etoposide, albeit

lower than in extracerebral tumors and in plasma, may exceed minimum cytotoxic levels and may be useful in central nervous system (CNS)-directed therapy.[129]

Etoposide is highly bound to plasma proteins with an average free plasma fraction of 6%. Since free drug is biologically active, conditions that decrease protein binding increase the pharmacological effect of the drug.[130] Etoposide clearance is modestly decreased in patients with renal failure, and dose modification is recommended in patients with moderate renal impairment. Biliary excretion represents a minor route of elimination and clearance is not affected in patients with hepatic obstruction.[131]

Although the typical route of administration is IV, an oral formulation of etoposide is available.[132] Bioavailability of oral etoposide is widely variable both within and between patients as compared to the IV route and ranges from 40% to 75%. Oral bioavailability also varies with drug dose and is better at lower doses.[133] Despite its limitations, oral etoposide allows long-term drug administration and is approved by the FDA.

Clinical use

Etoposide is approved for use in combination with other agents in refractory testicular tumors and in first-line treatment of SCLC. Etoposide has also shown clinical activity in other tumor types, including non-Hodgkin's lymphomas, leukemias, Kaposi sarcoma, neuroblastoma, and soft-tissue sarcomas. It is also an important component of preparatory regimens given prior to bone marrow and peripheral stem-cell rescue.

Schedule of administration

Etoposide is administered in combination with other agents at a dose of 80–120 mg/m^2 IV on days 1–3 every 21 to 28 days in SCLC. The typical doses for testicular cancer are 50 to 100 mg/m^2/day for days 1 to 5 or 100 mg/m^2/day on days 1, 3, and 5 repeated every 21 to 28 days.

The duration of exposure to etoposide is an important determinant of activity, with many studies indicating that prolonged administration maximizes activity.[134,135] In SCLC, the 3–5 day schedule has greater efficacy than single-day administration.[135,136] To determine whether administration schedules longer than a standard 3- to 5-day treatment might further improve the therapeutic index of etoposide, prolonged oral dose regimens were developed. However, in phase III trials, patients with SCLC who were treated with 21 days of oral etoposide did not have any improvement in response rates or survival over those receiving the drug for 3–5 days.[137]

Toxicity

Myelosuppression is the major dose-limiting toxicity of etoposide, IV or orally. Granulocyte and platelet nadirs occur 7 to 14 days and 9 to 16 days, respectively, after drug administration. Bone marrow recovery is usually complete by day 20. Other possible toxicities include allergic or other infusion reactions, which manifests as fever, bronchospasm, and hypotension. Toxicities associated with oral etoposide include nausea, vomiting, and mucositis.

Teniposide

Teniposide (VM-16) (Figure 3d) an etoposide analog is a semisynthetic derivative of podophyllotoxin. Teniposide differs from etoposide by its sugar ring. Although it was isolated and evaluated in patients before etoposide, early concerns about hypersensitivity reactions and use at low doses led to slower development of this drug.[132] *In vitro*, teniposide is more potent than etoposide in killing cancer cells possibly related to its better cellular uptake.[138–140]

A greater fraction of teniposide is protein bound relative to etoposide,[141] and renal function is less relevant to teniposide clearance.[142] Myelosuppression is the dose-limiting toxicity for teniposide. It can also produce hypersensitivity reactions. Teniposide is approved for the treatment of refractory childhood acute lymphocytic leukemia. Few studies have directly the activity of these two agents.

Therapy-related secondary acute leukemia (t-AML)

One of the major complications of Top2 inhibitors, especially etoposide and mitoxanthrone, is acute secondary leukemia, occurring in approximately 5% of patients. Therapy-related acute myelocytic leukemias (t-AML) are characterized by their relatively rapid onset (they can occur only a few months after therapy) and the presence of recurrent balanced translocations involving the mixed lineage leukemia (MLL) locus on 11q23 and over 50 partner genes.[143] The proposed molecular mechanism is by the disjoining of two drug-trapped Top2 cleavage complexes on different chromosomes in relationship with transcription collisions and illegitimate religation.[144] Top2β has been implicated in the generation of these disjoined cleavage complexes.[144,145]

Pharmacogenomics

Genetic variants in drug metabolizing enzymes, transporters, and other proteins have been shown to influence the pharmacology of topoisomerase inhibitors including irinotecan and doxorubicin. An understanding of these genetic variants will allow for individualized dosing of each drug, with the aim of increasing therapeutic efficacy and minimizing toxicity.

Irinotecan

UDP-glucuronosyl transferase 1A

Several enzymes and drug transporters are involved in the elimination of irinotecan. Variations in irinotecan dosing are affected by genetic polymorphisms in the *UGT1A*, *CYP3A*, and *ABC* gene families. Several allelic variants of these genes alter functional activity, thereby contributing to interindividual differences in irinotecan metabolism and predisposing patients to variable toxicity.

SNPs have been described in the promoter and coding regions of the *UGT1A1* gene, which significantly impact irinotecan metabolism and toxicity.[146,147] The variants are described as alleles denoted by the * symbol followed by a number. While there are over 113 gene variants, only several variants have been described to influence irinotecan pharmacodynamics (*6, *27, *28, *36, *37, *60, *93). This chapter focuses on *28 and *6 variants, which are clinically relevant with supporting studies. Clearance of SN-38 via this pathway contributes to interindividual variability in irinotecan-induced toxicity that is associated with a variant allele in the proximal promoter region of *UGT1A1* (*UGT1A1*28*). The *UGT1A1*28* (rs8175347, also referred to as the UGT1A1 7/7 genotype) allele has a seventh dinucleotide repeat in the TATA box of the promoter region, while the wildtype *UGT1A1*1* allele has six repeats, resulting in reduced rates of transcription, protein expression, and enzyme activity. The frequency of *UGT1A1*28* in the Caucasian and African American populations is 0.26–0.31 and 0.42–0.56, respectively.[148,149] Patients with the UGT1A1*28 homozygous variant have significantly higher systemic exposure to SN-38 and lower plasma SN-38G/SN-38 ratio than *1/*1 patients and commonly develop dose limiting severe diarrhea or neutropenia.[52,150–153] The *UGT1A1*6* polymorphism is characterized by a single-nucleotide substitution in exon 1 of *UGT1A1*, resulting in decreased expression and increased toxicity similar to *UGT1A1*28*. The *UGT1A1*6* (rs4148323) variant occurs at a higher frequency in Asians (frequency of 0.13–0.25)[154] and was associated with irinotecan-related diarrhea and neutropenia in Asians.[150,155,156]

The concept of *UGT1A1* genotype–directed dosing of irinotecan has been evaluated in patients receiving single-agent irinotecan in an every-2-week regimen[157] or an every-3-week regimen[158] or in combination therapy involving irinotecan with fluorouracil,[159,160] capecitabine,[161] or capecitabine and oxaliplatin.[162] Despite differences in patient population and regimens, the general consensus with these studies is that patients with the *28/*28 genotype are at the highest risk of irinotecan-related toxicity and require a dose reduction of up to 40%. Since 2005, the US Food and Drug Administration has recommended a reduction of the initial irinotecan dose (by at least one level) for individuals who are *UGT1A1*28* homozygous variant because they are at increased risk for neutropenia.

Numerous meta-analyses have evaluated the association of *28/*28 genotype to the risk of toxicity as a function of irinotecan dose. Hoskins et al.[51] ($n = 821$) showed that severe hematotoxicity was significantly higher in *28*/28 patients for both high/intermediate doses. Hu et al.[163] ($n = 1998$) demonstrated the risk of grade 3–4 neutropenia is significantly increased in *28/*28 patients, and the risk is higher for high doses compared to intermediate or low doses. A recent meta-analysis of 16 colorectal cancer studies ($n = 2328$), revealed that regardless of irinotecan dose neutropenia grade 3–4 occurred more frequently in patients with *28/*28 as compared to *1/*1 (OR = 4.79, 95% CI = 3.28 to 7.01, $p < 0.00001$) or *1/*28 (OR = 3.44, 95% CI = 2.45 to 4.82, $p < 0.00001$).[164]

Studies of irinotecan pharmacogenetics have mainly focused on the association of *UGT1A1*28* allele to irinotecan-related toxicity. The clinical utility of *UGT1A1*28* genotyping for preemptive dose reductions depends on whether *UGT1A1*28* also affects treatment efficacy and studies to date have been contradictory. A recent meta-analysis found no difference between the *UGT1A1*28* genotypes (homozygous, heterozygous, or wild type) and patient survival related to irinotecan therapy and included data for overall ($n = 1524$ patients) and progression-free survival ($n = 1494$ patients).[165] Therefore, while genotyping for *28 was shown to be cost-effective, clinical utility was classified as unclear.[166,167] Clinical implementation remains to be determined since studies to date on whether *28 affects treatment efficacy have been contradictory and since most episodes of severe toxicity (neutropenia or diarrhea) are managed by dose reduction in subsequent cycles.

In addition to *UGT1A1*, variants in the *UGT1A7* and *UGT1A9* genes are also involved in interpatient irinotecan-related toxicity differences. *UGT1A7* is primarily involved in extrahepatic metabolism (located in the intestine) and is responsible for detoxifying SN-38, whereas *UGT1A9* is necessary for conjugation of SN-38 to SN-38G in the liver.[168] *UGT1A7*2, UGT1A7*3*, or *UGT1A7*4*, polymorphisms may result in altered irinotecan metabolism and related toxicity.[169–172] Patients homozygous for *UGT1A9*1* have been reported to have more severe diarrhea than *UGT1A9*9* or *UGT1A9*22* carriers.[172,173]

Together, these studies suggest that clinical outcome is likely the result of complex combined signature of the haplotypes involving key genomic variations in UGT metabolic detoxification (*UGT1A1*, *UGT1A7*, and *UGT1A9*) pathways.[168,171]

CYP3A and drug transporters

The *CYP3A4* and *CYP3A5* genes are crucial for oxidative metabolism of irinotecan to inactive metabolites APC and NPC.

In vitro studies have shown variants (*CYP3A4* 16* or *CYP3A4*18* or *CYP3A5*3*) with decreased activity, resulting in reduced rates of oxidative metabolism and hence less APC and NPC metabolite production.[173,174] However, correlations between these genetic variants with irinotecan treatment outcome remain to be elucidated.

Elimination of irinotecan is also dependent on the ABC drug transporters, present on the bile canalicular membrane that facilitates the secretion of irinotecan and its metabolites.[175] Specific polymorphisms of ABCB1 and ABCC2 can influence irinotecan drug disposition and tumor response.[176] While the *ABCC2*2* haplotype is associated with lower rates of irinotecan-induced diarrhea,[177] patients with *ABCC2* (rs3740066) and *ABCG2* (rs2231137) variants experience greater rates of grade 3 diarrhea.[173,178,179] A pharmacogenomic profile of irinotecan-induced gastrointestinal toxicity using the novel drug-metabolizing enzyme and transporter (DMET) microarray genotyping platform identified three additional SNPs mapping to the *ABCG1*, *ABCC5*, and *OATP1B1/SLCO1B1* transporter genes in colorectal cancer patients.[180] Moreover, a recent study demonstrated that *OATP1B1* and tumor *OATP1B3* modulated exposure, toxicity, and survival after irinotecan-based chemotherapy.[181]

Doxorubicin

Genetic polymorphisms exist in genes that mediate the metabolism, transport, and pharmacological actions of doxorubicin, but the clinical significance of these variants and their impact on doxorubicin efficacy and toxicity has only been evaluated in recent years. Doxorubicin is characterized by substantial interindividual variations in pharmacokinetic parameters[182] and cumulative dose is the most significant risk factor for doxorubicin-induced cardiotoxicity.

The major metabolite of doxorubicin is 13-C alcohol, doxorubicinol; metabolized by enzymes carbonyl reductase 1 (CBR1), CBR3 and aldo-keto reductase 1C3 (AKR1C3). Functional SNPs have been characterized in CBR1, CBR3, and AKR1C3. Two SNPs (rs1143663 and rs9024) in *CBR1* that have a functional impact on CBR1 activity[183] or expression have been described.[184] To date, there are limited studies investigating the influence of genetic polymorphisms in the *CBR1* gene and no association was seen in a population of patients with breast cancer.[185] However, patients who were heterozygous for rs9024 and another *CBR1* variant with which it is in linkage disequilibrium (LD) had a lower clearance of doxorubicin.[186]

Two common SNPs in CBR3 G730A (rs1056892) and G11A (rs8133052) in LD were shown to have reduced catalytic efficiency compared with wild type *in vitro*.[187] It has been suggested that the wild-type *CBR3* G730A allele, which exhibits higher activity and increased expression, is associated with the risk of anthracycline-related congestive heart failure among childhood cancer survivors.[188] Higher CBR3 expression was found in tumor tissues from Asian patients with breast cancer, with the variant being associated with higher doxorubicinol AUC.[185] In the same cohort, the G11A minor allele was associated with greater hematotoxicity and efficacy in addition to an influence on doxorubicin pharmacokinetics (PK) and CBR expression.[185] Voon et al.[189] also showed that the G11A minor allele correlated with lower doxorubicinol AUC and longer overall survival. However, other studies in breast cancer patients showed no effect of these variants on doxorubicin PK[186] or survival.[190]

An *in vitro* study has demonstrated that two nonsynonymous SNPs in exon 5 of the aldo-keto reductase 1C3 (AKR1C3) gene 508 C>T (rs35575889) and 538 C>T (rs34186955) encode enzymes that significantly reduced doxorubicin metabolism compared with wild type.[191] In a clinical study of Asian patients with breast cancer,

the above 2 SNPs were not identified; however, two intronic variants IVS4−212 C>G (rs1937840) and IVS4+218 G>A (rs1937841) were detected. The AKR1C3 IVS4-212 GG allele was associated with greater hematological toxicity and longer overall and progression-free survival after doxorubicin-based therapy.[189]

Several transporters have been shown to be involved in transporting doxorubicin including ABCB1, ABCC1, ABCC2, ABCG2, RALBP1, and SLC22A16. Doxorubicin is a substrate for ABCB1 and doxorubicin efflux mediated by ABCB1 can lead to decreased efficacy in laboratory and animal models. Inhibition of ABCB1 may lead to increased doxorubicin-induced toxicity. Three high-frequency *ABCB1* polymorphisms, 1236C>T (rs1128503), 2677G>A/T (rs2032582), and 3435C>T (rs1045642) have been proposed to alter pharmacokinetics of substrate drugs, but there has been some controversy in the literature, with both positive and negative studies. This is likely due to different patient populations, other covariants, and individual substrate drug. One small study in Asian patients noted impaired doxorubicin pharmacokinetics, resulting in significantly increased exposure levels and reduced clearance; however, the study involved only a small number of patients.[192] Moreover, while the 2677A allele was associated with a shorter overall and progression-free survival in breast cancer patients treated with adjuvant doxorubicin and cyclophosphamide, the C1236T, G2677T, and C3435T SNPs had no effect on survival.[193] In Asian patients with breast cancer on a doxorubicin-based regimen, *ABCB1* G2677T/A was associated with drug clearance and platelet toxicity, and *ABCB1* IVS26+59 T>G was associated with overall survival.[189] The 3435T allele was significantly correlated with a prolonged progression-free survival in multiple myeloma patients treated with doxorubicin and bortezomib, consistent with the hypothesized loss of function or expression.[194] Other studies have found no impact of ABCB1 genotypes in response to doxorubicin.[195] An additional *ABCB1* G1199T/A (rs2229109) variant found in European populations, not in LD with the other three, is less well studied clinically, but has been shown to have a functional impact on doxorubicin efflux and toxicity.[196] Given the inconsistencies in studies across populations, the functional significance of *ABCB1* SNPs on the disposition of doxorubicin remains controversial.

ABCG2-mediated resistance to doxorubicin is dependent on an acquired mutation (R482T/G).[197] In a clinical study of breast cancer patients, no significant influences on doxorubicin pharmacokinetic parameters were observed in relation to the *ABCG2* 421C>A polymorphism,[192] which has been previously demonstrated to have less ATPase activity than wildtype.[198] Expression of other ABC family members, including ABCB5, ABCB8, ABCC5, and RALBP1, also confers resistance to doxorubicin; however, the clinical implications remain unknown.

The organic cation exporter SLC22A16 transports doxorubicin into the cell. Homozygotes of the *SLC22A16* A146G (rs714368) may have a higher AUC for doxorubicin[199] and carriers of the same minor allele, and other SLC22A16 SNPs (T312C and T755C variants) in LD, are less likely to have a dose delay during adjuvant doxorubicin and cyclophosphamide therapy for breast cancer.[193] A higher incidence of dose delay, indicative of increased toxicity, was seen in SLC22A16 T1226C (rs12210538) carriers.[193]

In a study of pharmacogenomic predictors of anthracycline-induced cardiotoxicity involving SNPs of 82 genes from 1697 patients, 3.2% of whom developed the toxicity acutely or chronically, five significant associations were identified and the polymorphisms were located in genes of the NAD(P)H oxidase complex (CYBA rs4673, NCF4 rs1883112, and RAC2 rs13058338), and doxorubicin transporters (ABCC1 rs45511401, ABCC2 rs8187694 and rs8187710).[200] Rossi et al.[201] also showed CYBA rs4673 and NCF4 rs1883112 being associated with toxicity in lymphoma patients treated with doxorubicin-containing chemotherapy. Polymorphisms in genes that reduce ROS may result in increased efficacy or toxicity following doxorubicin treatment and may include variants of superoxide dismutase II (SOD2), glutathione S-transferases (GSTs), or NAD(P)H:quinone oxidoreductase 1 (NQO1). Furthermore, pharmacogenetic studies have evaluated gene copy number for *ERBB2* and *TOP2A* as predictors of response to doxorubicin with contradictory results.[202–204]

Daunorubicin, epirubicin, etoposide

Limited data are available on pharmacogenomics of daunorubicin, epirubicin, or etoposide. A pharmacogenomics study of daunorubicin in children using the DMET platform found associations between *FMO3* and *GSTP1* haplotypes with daunorubicin PK that could potentially affect efficacy and toxicity.[205] The major inactivation pathway for epirubicin and epirubicinol is glucuronidation catalyzed by uridine diphosphate-glucuronosyltransferase 2B7 (UGT2B7). Breast cancer patients with the *UGT2B7* 802 C>T homozygous minor allele may benefit most from adjuvant epirubicin-based chemotherapy.[206] In a pharmacogenetic study of adjuvant breast cancer treatment with cyclophosphamide, epirubicin, and 5-fluorouracil, an NQO2 exonic SNP was associated with a higher exposure to epirubicinol relative to epirubicin. Other polymorphic variants of NQO1, CBR, UGT enzymes, and transporters had no influence on epirubicin or its metabolite.[207] Finally, 63 genetic variants that contribute to etoposide-induced cytotoxicity were identified through a whole-genome association study using data generated on the HapMap cell lines.[208]

Perspectives

Topoisomerase inhibitors represent a basic component of the anticancer armamentarium. Four points are relevant to their future use: (1) novel formulations and targeted delivery approaches (exemplified by liposomes and antibody conjugates) may enable the selective targeting of tumors while limiting dose-limiting toxicities; (2) detailed understanding of the chemical limitation of the drugs (chemical instability of the camptothecins and redox reactions of the anthracyclines) and molecular mechanism of toxicities should enable the design of novel topoisomerase inhibitors, such as the non-camptothecin Top1 inhibitors (indenoisoquinoline LMP derivatives) and Top2α-specific inhibitors that would avoid serious toxicities related to Top2β inhibition (cardiac toxicity of the anthracyclines and secondary leukemia induced by the epipodophyllotoxins); (3) better understanding of the molecular basis of sensitivity will allow better choice of combinations of anticancer agents.[10,11] To date, combinations have been developed empirically, but going forward a better understanding of genomics and epigenomics will allow development of rational combination therapies. (4) Finally, it remains critically important to predict the activity of topoisomerase inhibitors and precisely select patients based on modern technology such as tumor genomic signatures.[10,11,209] These agents, while identified before the era of personalized medicine, do have specific cellular targets, and it is important to understand them as such. It is important to identify the molecular basis of sensitivity and resistance so that in the future, strategies can be developed for making optimal therapeutic choices.

References

1 Wang JC. Interaction between DNA and an *Escherichia coli* protein omega. *J Mol Biol*. 1971;**55**(3):523–533.

2 Champoux JJ, Dulbecco R. An activity from mammalian cells that untwists superhelical DNA—a possible swivel for DNA replication (polyoma-ethidium bromide-mouse-embryo cells-dye binding assay). *Proc Natl Acad Sci U S A*. 1972;**69**:143–146.

3 Pommier Y. *DNA Topoisomerases and Cancer*. New York, Dordrecht, Heidelberg, London: Springer & Humana Press; 2012.

4 Pommier Y. Drugging topoisomerases: lessons and challenges. *ACS Chem Biol*. 2013;**8**(1):82–95.

5 Gheeya J, Johansson P, Chen QR, et al. Expression profiling identifies epoxy anthraquinone derivative as a DNA topoisomerase inhibitor. *Cancer Lett*. 2010;**293**(1):124–131.

6 Pommier Y, Marchand C. Interfacial inhibitors: targeting macromolecular complexes. *Nat Rev Drug Discov*. 2012;**11**(1):25–36.

7 Capranico G, Binaschi M. DNA sequence selectivity of topoisomerases and topoisomerase poisons. *Biochim Biophys Acta*. 1998;**1400**:185–194.

8 Nitiss J, Wang JC. DNA topoisomerase-targeting antitumor drugs can be studied in yeast. *Proc Natl Acad Sci U S A*. 1988;**85**:7501–7505.

9 Maede Y, Shimizu H, Fukushima T, et al. Differential and common DNA repair pathways for topoisomerase I- and II-targeted drugs in a genetic DT40 repair cell screen panel. *Mol Cancer Ther*. 2014;**13**(1):214–220.

10 Zoppoli G, Regairaz M, Leo E, et al. Putative DNA/RNA helicase Schlafen-11 (SLFN11) sensitizes cancer cells to DNA-damaging agents. *Proc Natl Acad Sci U S A*. 2012;**109**(37):15030–15035.

11 Barretina J, Caponigro G, Stransky N, et al. The Cancer Cell Line Encyclopedia enables predictive modelling of anticancer drug sensitivity. *Nature*. 2012;**483**(7391):603–607.

12 Pommier Y. Topoisomerase I inhibitors: camptothecins and beyond. *Nat Rev Cancer*. 2006;**6**(10):789–802.

13 Zhang H, Zhang YW, Yasukawa T, Dalla Rosa I, Khiati S, Pommier Y. Increased negative supercoiling of mtDNA in TOP1mt knockout mice and presence of topoisomerases IIalpha and IIbeta in vertebrate mitochondria. *Nucleic Acids Res*. 2014;**42**(11):7259–7267.

14 Pommier Y, Jenkins J, Kohlhagen G, Leteurtre F. DNA recombinase activity of eukaryotic DNA topoisomerase I; effects of camptothecin and other inhibitors. *Mutat Res*. 1995;**337**(2):135–145.

15 Koster DA, Palle K, Bot ES, Bjornsti MA, Dekker NH. Antitumour drugs impede DNA uncoiling by topoisomerase I. *Nature*. 2007;**448**(7150):213–217.

16 Sordet O, Redon CE, Guirouilh-Barbat J, et al. Ataxia telangiectasia mutated activation by transcription- and topoisomerase I-induced DNA double-strand breaks. *EMBO Rep*. 2009;**10**(8):887–893.

17 Ray Chaudhuri A, Hashimoto Y, Herrador R, et al. Topoisomerase I poisoning results in PARP-mediated replication fork reversal. *Nat Struct Mol Biol*. 2012;**19**:417–423.

18 Gomez-Herreros F, Romero-Granados R, Zeng Z, et al. TDP2-dependent non-homologous end-joining protects against topoisomerase II-induced DNA breaks and genome instability in cells and in vivo. *PLoS Genet*. 2013;**9**(3):e1003226.

19 Pommier Y, Leo E, Zhang H, Marchand C. DNA topoisomerases and their poisoning by anticancer and antibacterial drugs. *Chem Biol*. 2010;**17**(5):421–433.

20 Pang B, Qiao X, Janssen L, et al. Drug-induced histone eviction from open chromatin contributes to the chemotherapeutic effects of doxorubicin. *Nat Commun*. 2013;**4**:1908.

21 Doroshow JH. Effect of anthracycline antibiotics on oxygen radical formation in rat heart. *Cancer Res*. 1983;**43**(2):460–472.

22 Gottlieb JA, Guarino AM, Call JB, Oliverio VT, Block JB. Preliminary pharmacologic and clinical evaluation of camptothecin sodium (NSC-100880). *Cancer Chemother Rep*. 1970;**54**(6):461–470.

23 Moertel CG, Schutt AJ, Reitemeier RJ, Hahn RG. Phase II study of camptothecin (NSC-100880) in the treatment of advanced gastrointestinal cancer. *Cancer Chemother Rep*. 1972;**56**(1):95–101.

24 Muggia FM, Creaven PJ, Hansen HH, Cohen MH, Selawry OS. Phase I clinical trial of weekly and daily treatment with camptothecin (NSC-100880): correlation with preclinical studies. *Cancer Chemother Rep*. 1972;**56**(4):515–521.

25 Hsiang YH, Liu LF. Identification of mammalian DNA topoisomerase-I as an intracellular target of the anticancer drug camptothecin. *Cancer Res*. 1988;**48**(7):1722–1726.

26 Burke TG, Munshi CB, Mi Z, Jiang Y. The important role of albumin in determining the relative human blood stabilities of the camptothecin anticancer drugs. *J Pharm Sci*. 1995;**84**(4):518–519.

27 Herben VMM, Huinink WWTB, Beijnen JH. Clinical pharmacokinetics of topotecan. *Clin Pharmacokinet*. 1996;**31**(2):85–102.

28 O'Reilly S, Rowinsky EK, Slichenmyer W, et al. Phase I and pharmacologic study of topotecan in patients with impaired renal function. *J Clin Oncol*. 1996;**14**(12):3062–3073.

29 O'Reilly S, Rowinsky E, Slichenmyer W, et al. Phase I and pharmacologic studies of topotecan in patients with impaired hepatic function. *J Natl Cancer Inst.* 1996;**88(12)**:817–824.

30 Gerrits CJH, Schellens JHM, Burris H, et al. A comparison of clinical pharmacodynamics of different administration schedules of oral topotecan (hycamtin). *Clin Cancer Res.* 1999;**5(1)**:69–75.

31 Eckardt JR, von Pawel J, Pujol JL, et al. Phase III study of oral compared with intravenous topotecan as second-line therapy in small-cell lung cancer. *J Clin Oncol.* 2007;**25(15)**:2086–2092.

32 GlaxoSmithKline. *HYCAMTIN- Topotecan Hydrochloride for Injection Package Insert.* Research Triangle Park, NC: GlaxoSmithKline; 2015.

33 Stewart CF, Iacono LC, Chintagumpala M, et al. Results of a phase II upfront window of pharmacokinetically guided topotecan in high-risk medulloblastoma and supratentorial primitive neuroectodermal tumor. *J Clin Oncol.* 2004;**22(16)**:3357–3365.

34 Joppert MG, Garfield DH, Gregurich MA, et al. A phase II multicenter study of combined topotecan and gemcitabine as first line chemotherapy for advanced non-small cell lung cancer. *Lung Cancer.* 2003;**39(2)**:215–219.

35 Beran M, Estey E, O'Brien S, et al. Topotecan and cytarabine is an active combination regimen in myelodysplastic syndromes and chronic myelomonocytic leukemia. *J Clin Oncol.* 1999;**17(9)**:2819–2830.

36 Hunold A, Weddeling N, Paulussen M, Ranft A, Liebscher C, Jurgens H. Topotecan and cyclophosphamide in patients with refractory or relapsed Ewing tumors. *Pediatr Blood Cancer.* 2006;**47(6)**:795–800.

37 Walterhouse DO, Lyden ER, Breitfeld PP, Qualman SJ, Wharam MD, Meyer WH. Efficacy of topotecan and cyclophosphamide given in a phase II window trial in children with newly diagnosed metastatic rhabdomyosarcoma: a children's oncology group study. *J Clin Oncol.* 2004;**22(8)**:1398–1403.

38 Kraut EH, Crowley JJ, Wade JL, et al. Evaluation of topotecan in resistant and relapsing multiple myeloma: a Southwest Oncology Group Study. *J Clin Oncol.* 1998;**16(2)**:589–592.

39 Bruzzese F, Rocco M, Castelli S, Di Gennaro E, Desideri A, Budillon A. Synergistic antitumor effect between vorinostat and topotecan in small cell lung cancer cells is mediated by generation of reactive oxygen species and DNA damage-induced apoptosis. *Mol Cancer Ther.* 2009;**8(11)**:3075–3087.

40 Kummar S, Chen A, Ji JP, et al. Phase I Study of PARP Inhibitor ABT-888 in Combination with Topotecan in Adults with Refractory Solid Tumors and Lymphomas. *Cancer Res.* 2011;**71(17)**:5626–5634.

60 Agents targeting microtubules and mitotic processes

Eric K. Rowinsky, MD

Overview

The treatment of many diseases owes much to the importance of medicines derived from natural sources, and the treatment of malignant disease is no exception. Billions of years of evolutionary pressure have resulted in the natural selection of plants, fungi, and microorganisms capable of producing potent and specific toxins. After several plant-derived compounds and other natural products, many of which targeted the mitotic processes, demonstrated prominent anticancer activity in the 1950s and 1960s, the microtubule was recognized as a subcellular target of major strategic importance.

The first widely used class of antimicrotubule agents, the plant-derived vinca alkaloids, had been the mainstay of both palliative and curative regimens for treating malignancies for several decades. The addition of the plant-derived taxanes, which possess a unique mechanism of action and anticancer spectra, to our therapeutic arsenal several decades later resulted in renewed interest in the microtubule and mitotic processes as targets for which to develop cancer therapeutics, as well as in the identification of other natural products to treat cancers. More recently, several plant- and marine-derived compounds as well as synthetic agents with yet even more distinctive disruptive actions on microtubules and other mitotic constituents have been identified. These include the analogs of the epothilones and halichondrin B, which were isolated from soil-dwelling myxobacterium and marine sponges, respectively. They also include potent antimicrotubule agents, such as analogs of maytansine and dolastatin, which are components of antibody-drug conjugates. This chapter focuses on the microtubule as a target for therapeutic development and antimicrotubule agents that comprise our therapeutic armamentarium.

Introduction

The treatment of many diseases owes much to the importance of medicines that have been derived from natural sources, and the treatment of malignant disease is no exception. In essence, billions of years of evolutionary pressure have resulted in the natural selection of plants, fungi, and microorganisms that are capable of producing highly potent and specific toxins. After several plant-derived compounds and other natural products, many of which were noted to suspend cell division in mitosis by affecting the mitotic spindle, demonstrated prominent anticancer activity in patients with advanced malignancies in the 1950s and 1960s, the microtubule was recognized as a subcellular target of major strategic importance.

The first widely used class of antimicrotubule agents, the plant-derived vinca alkaloids, had been the mainstay of both palliative and curative regimens for treating malignancies for

several decades. The addition of the plant-derived taxanes, which possess a unique mechanism of action and anticancer spectra, to our therapeutic arsenal several decades later resulted in renewed interest in the microtubule and mitotic processes as targets for which to develop cancer therapeutics, as well as in the identification of other natural products to treat cancers. More recently, several plant- and marine-derived compounds as well as synthetic agents with yet even more distinctive disruptive actions on microtubules and other mitotic constituents (e.g., mitotic kinesins and kinases) have been identified and added to our therapeutic arsenal. These include the analogs of the epothilones (e.g., ixabepilone) and halichondrin B (e.g., eribulin), which were isolated from soil-dwelling myxobacterium and marine sponges, respectively. They also include the highly potent antimicrotubule agents, such as analogs of maytansine and dolastatin, which are components of antibody-drug conjugates (ADCs) that utilize monoclonal antibodies (mAbs) to deliver them selectively cancer cells that express the mAb targets. This chapter focuses on the microtubule as a target for therapeutic development and antimicrotubule agents that comprise our therapeutic armamentarium, particularly the vinca alkaloids and taxanes, as well as several classes of promising antimicrotubule agents undergoing clinical evaluation.

Microtubules as strategic targets against cancer

Microtubules are highly regulated and integral components of the cellular cytoskeleton that can be disrupted by various natural products (e.g., vinca alkaloids, taxanes, epothilones, halichondrins, others), as well as an increasingly number of synthetic compounds.[1-6] Microtubules, together with microfilaments and intermediate filaments, form the cytoskeleton and maintain cell structure. Although the most important functions of microtubules in proliferative cells are through their actions as components of the cytoskeleton and mitotic spindle apparatus, which pulls apart chromosomes and is vital to cell division, they are involved in many other critical functions throughout the cell cycle, including intracellular transport of vesicles and organelles, trafficking of proteins including many oncoproteins, locomotion, adhesion, and anchorage of subcellular organelles and receptors.[1-8] The cytoskeleton, particularly microtubules, also influences gene expression and signal transduction, and vice versa; however, the mechanisms involved in these interactions are not well understood. The specific expression of transcription factors in concert with drug-mediated depolymerization of microtubules has been well described and such has provided information on the differential expression of specific genes.[9] Lastly, the state of the cytoskeleton mediates cellular response via the action of various growth factors.[9] Antimicrotubule agents disrupt these functions.[1-9]

Holland-Frei Cancer Medicine, Ninth Edition. Edited by Robert C. Bast Jr., Carlo M. Croce, William N. Hait, Waun Ki Hong, Donald W. Kufe, Martine Piccart-Gebhart, Raphael E. Pollock, Ralph R. Weichselbaum, Hongyang Wang, and James F. Holland.
© 2017 John Wiley & Sons, Inc. ISBN: 978-1-118-93469-2

Microtubule structure and dynamics

Microtubules are dimeric structures made up of two globular subunits, α-tubulin and β-tubulin monomers, each of which consists of approximately 450 amino acids with a molecular weight of 50 kD.[10] The α/β-tubulin dimers assemble into microtubules by forming linear protofilaments. Typically, microtubules are formed by the parallel association of 13 protofilaments, although microtubules composed of fewer or more protofilaments have been observed *in vitro*. Microtubules have distinct polarity, which is conferred by the unique alignment of the protofilaments. The protofilaments form a cylindrical wall around a hollow core; tubulin polymerizes end to end, with the α-tubulin subunit of one dimer in contact with the β-tubulin subunit of the next, as shown in Figure 1. Therefore, one end of a protofilament will have the α-tubulin subunits exposed, while the other end will have the β-tubulin subunits exposed. These ends are designated the minus and plus ends, respectively. The protofilaments align parallel to one another with the same polarity, so, in a microtubule, there is one end, the plus end, with only β-tubulin subunits exposed, while the other end, the minus end, has only α-tubulin subunits exposed. At the plus end, there is guanosine triphosphate (GTP) binding, rapid assembly, and net elongation, whereas assembly is slow and net shortening occurs at the minus end. The unique functions of microtubules are related to their polymerization dynamics, involving a dynamic equilibrium between an intracellular pool of α/β-tubulin dimers and microtubule polymers, and simultaneous release of the α/β-tubulin dimers into the soluble tubulin pool. Tubulin polymerization occurs by a nucleation–elongation mechanism, in which the slow formation of a short microtubule "nucleus" is followed by rapid elongation of the microtubule at its ends by the reversible, noncovalent addition of α/β-tubulin dimers. The dynamic equilibrium between free α/β-tubulin dimers and the microtubule occurs simultaneously at both ends of the microtubule.[1-7] Each tubulin molecule is associated with two molecules of GTP. The nucleoside bound to α-tubulin, at the N site, is nonexchangeable, whereas the one bound to β-tubulin, at the E site, can be exchanged with free guanosine diphosphate (GDP). The assembly process utilizes energy provided by the hydrolysis of GTP.

Tubulin binds GTP with high affinity, and as tubulin-GTP is added to the ends of growing microtubules, GTP is gradually hydrolyzed to GDP and Pi.[11] The Pi ultimately dissociates, leaving a microtubule core that consists of tubulin bound to GDP. The GDP nucleotide remains nonexchangeable until the tubulin subunit dissociates from the microtubule. Although tubulin polymerization and dissociation, and consequently microtubule elongation and shortening, occur simultaneously at each end of the microtubule, the net changes in length at the more kinetically dynamic plus end are much larger over time than those at the minus end. If the polymerization reaction is followed *in vitro*, an initial lag phase is noted, after which microtubules form rapidly until a plateau phase is reached. In the intact cell, the minus ends of the microtubule are anchored at each of the two microtubule-organizing centers (MTOCs), whereas the plus end is free in the cytoplasm radiating toward the cell periphery. The centrosome, the principal MTOC of most cells, is the nidus for mitotic spindles; however, the Golgi apparatus can also serve as a platform for the nucleation of microtubules.[12] Because nucleation from the centrosome is inherently symmetrical, Golgi-associated microtubule nucleation permits formation of an asymmetrical microtubule network. In interphase, the MTOC organizes the microtubules that provides polarity to the cytoplasm and is involved in the trafficking of proteins, including several oncoproteins.[8]

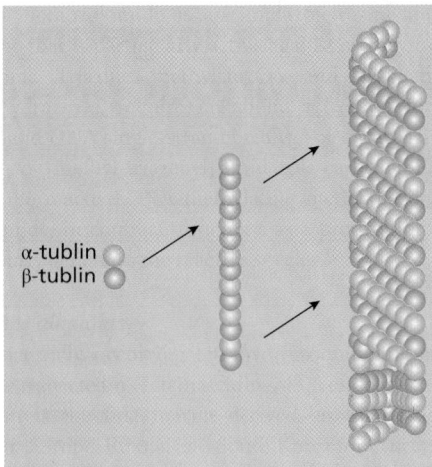

Figure 1 Schematic model of the α/β-tubulin dimer with the monomers represented by shades of gray and white. The dimers associate linearly to form protofilaments that then in turn associate laterally to form the hollow cylindrical wall of the microtubule. Protofilaments can twist slowly around the microtubule axis, although these shown here are in parallel as in microtubules containing 13 protofilaments. Throughout most of the microtubule, lateral contacts involve α–α and β–β monomer interactions. Monomers of each type thus are in contact along a shallow spiral path around the microtubule.

Treadmilling and dynamic instability

Two principal processes govern microtubule dynamics in live cells.[1-15] The first, known as *treadmilling*, is the net growth at one end of the microtubule and the net shortening at the opposite end.[8]

Mitotic spindle formation and chromosomal segregation during the anaphase stage of mitosis, among other microtubule processes, occur by treadmilling. The second dynamic process, termed *dynamic instability*, occurs when the plus ends of microtubules switch spontaneously between states of slow sustained growth and rapid shortening.[11,13-15] Dynamic instability is dependent on a cycle of GTP hydrolysis and exchange. Mechanistically, the GTP cap model, in which a cap on the ends of the microtubule, consisting of GTP or GDP with associated nonexchangeable Pi, stabilizes the microtubule, thus allowing growth at the plus end, likely explains the process of dynamic instability. In essence, the switch between growth and shortening depends on the end conformation of the microtubule where growing ends are stabilized by a layer of GTP-tubulin subunits (GTP cap), whereas shortening ends have lost their GTP, allowing terminal GDP-tubulin dimers to dissociate from the microtubule lattice.[16]

Microtubules and mitosis

At the onset of mitosis, the interphase array of microtubules, which are attached to the MTOC, disassemble and are replaced by a new population of spindle microtubules that are much more dynamic.[2,13,17,18] Contained within the MTOC is another type of tubulin, γ-tubulin, which associates with other proteins to form a lock washer-like structure called the γ-tubulin ring complex. This complex acts as a template for α/β-tubulin dimers to begin polymerization; it caps the negative end, while microtubule growth occurs at the free positive end.[19] A recently identified protein complex called augmin is critical for MTOC-dependent, spindle-based microtubule generation as it interacts with the γ-tubulin ring complex to increase microtubule density around the mitotic spindle origin.[20] As the spindle-shaped array of newly assembled microtubules is organized, the nuclear envelope breaks down and releases the newly condensed chromosomes, and the centrosomes, which were duplicated before mitosis, separate into the poles of the forming mitotic spindle. The rate of dynamic instability is accelerated during mitosis, resulting in the formation and attachment of the mitotic spindles to the chromosomes. In most cells, mitosis progresses rapidly, and the highly dynamic microtubules that comprise the mitotic spindle render them sensitive to antimicrotubule agents that disrupt polymerization dynamics.[3,13]

Dynamic instability and treadmilling are vital to the assembly and function of the mitotic spindle, and the high dynamicity of the microtubules that comprise the mitotic spindle is required for the precise alignment of the chromosomes and their attachment to the mitotic spindle during metaphase, as well as chromosome separation during anaphase. Dynamic instability and treadmilling enable the microtubules of the mitotic spindle to make vast growing and shortening excursions, often termed search and capture, essentially probing the cytoplasm, until their positive ends become attached to a chromosome at its kinetochore. If even a single chromosome is unable to achieve a bipolar attachment to the spindle, perhaps because of drug-induced suppression of microtubule dynamics, the cell will not traverse beyond a prometaphase/metaphase-like state and instead will undergo apoptosis due to a complex series of processes involving the spindle assembly checkpoint.[21,22] Although mitotic spindles can assemble even in the presence of low concentrations of antimicrotubule agents, mitosis cannot progress beyond the mitotic checkpoint at the metaphase/anaphase transition.[13,17,22] Such perturbations in mitotic spindle dynamics may delay cell-cycle progression at critical mitotic checkpoints, ultimately triggering apoptosis through a complicated interplay of checkpoint and mitotic kinases.[7,13,17,22] In the unperturbed normal state, oscillations of the duplicated chromosomes, dynamic instability, and treadmilling, in which there is addition of tubulin to the spindle at the kinetochore and loss of tubulin at the spindle poles, exert considerable tension on the chromosomes in metaphase and facilitate progression to anaphase. In anaphase, microtubules attached to the chromosomes undergo shortening, while another subpopulation of microtubules, called interpolar microtubules, lengthen, resulting in polar movement of the chromosomes. Suppression of spindle-microtubule treadmilling and dynamic instability by antimicrotubule agents reduce spindle tension and impede progression from metaphase to anaphase, thereby triggering cell death.[3-5,13,17,18,23,24] A similar process of positive-end capping activity for interphase microtubules, which is mediated by formins, the adenomatous polyposis coli protein, and EB1, has also been described.

Regulating microtubule dynamics and functional diversity

The net direction of the dynamic equilibrium between the intracellular pool of tubulin and the microtubule polymer is influenced by several factors that regulate the critical concentration of tubulin required for polymerization, including the GTP/GDP ratio, the ionic microenvironment, cell-cycle modulators, and various microtubule-associated proteins (MAPs) and regulatory proteins.[1,4,5,25,26] MAPs are partly responsible for the functional diversity of microtubules in different tissues and are directly and indirectly being targeted for therapeutic development against cancer.[26] The major classes of MAPs include those that favor microtubule polymerization such as the tau proteins (molecular weights, 40–60 kD) and the high molecular weight (200–300 kD) proteins MAP1, MAPc (an adenosine triphosphatase [ATPase]), MAP2, MAP4, and XMAP215.[4,25-27] Other regulatory proteins include

stathmin, XKCM1, XKIF2, and katanin, all of which favor depolymerization.[27] MAPs generally possess two binding domains, one of which binds to microtubules and facilitates the initial nucleation step of tubulin polymerization and a second that links microtubules to other cellular constituents. Still, other MAPs, such as the dyneins (GTPases) and kinesins (ATPases), function as microtubule motor proteins, transmitting chemical energy to mechanical force and moving various solutes and subcellular organelles along the microtubule.[1,4,5,25-27] Motor proteins play key roles in mitosis, premeiotic events, and organelle transport and are being evaluated as targets for anticancer therapeutic development (see section titled "Targeting Mitotic Motor Proteins and Kinases").[28,29]

In addition to MAPs, the functional diversity of microtubules in various tissues is, in part, conferred by differences in tubulin isotypes and posttranslational modifications. There are at least six isotypes of α-tubulin and β-tubulin each in human cells, which are distinguished by different C-terminal amino acid sequences and encoded by a large multigene family that has been highly conserved throughout evolution.[4,30-33] Analysis of tubulin isotype expression in various tissues has demonstrated a complex, albeit highly conserved, pattern of isotype distribution, suggesting functional specificity.[1,4,5,25-27] Both forms of tubulin also undergo various posttranslational modifications, including phosphorylation, detyrosylation, polyglycylation, delta 2 tubulin formation, acetylation, and polyglutamylation, by microtubule-bound enzymes.[34,35] Posttranslational modifications confer stability to the microtubule polymer, as well as structural and functional diversity.[34,35] Most modifications are rapidly reversed by soluble enzymes when microtubule depolymerization occurs. Posttranslational modifications generally occur on the C-terminal region of α-tubulin. This region, which is rich in negatively charged glutamate, forms relatively unstructured tails that project out from the microtubule and contact motor proteins. Therefore, posttranslational modifications appear to regulate the interactions of motor proteins with microtubules.

Vinca alkaloids: Introduction and indications

The vinca alkaloids are naturally occurring or semisynthetic nitrogenous bases extracted from the pink periwinkle plant *Catharanthus roseus* G. Don. The early medicinal uses of this plant led to screening these compounds for their hypoglycemic activity, which was ultimately of minor importance compared to their cytotoxic effects. Many vinca alkaloids have been extensively evaluated, but only vincristine (VCR), vinblastine (VBL), and vinorelbine (VRL) are approved for use in the United States and elsewhere, whereas vinflunine (VFL) and vindesine (VDS) are approved for use in some regions. VCR sulfate liposomal injection is also available for use in the United States and elsewhere.

The vinca alkaloids have dimeric structures composed of two basic multiringed units (Figure 2), an indole nucleus (catharanthine), and a dihydroindole nucleus (vindoline), joined together with other complex systems.[36-38] Structurally, VCR and VBL are identical except for a single substitution on the vindoline nucleus, where VCR and VBL possess formyl and methyl groups, respectively. Although this minor difference does not fundamentally alter the mechanisms and tubulin-binding properties of these agents, the anticancer and toxicologic profiles of VCR and VBL differ significantly.[4,36-41]

VCR is used more commonly to treat pediatric malignancies, which is due, in part, to a generally greater level of intrinsic sensitivity of pediatric malignancies to VCR and better tolerance of therapeutic VCR doses in children. In both children and adults,

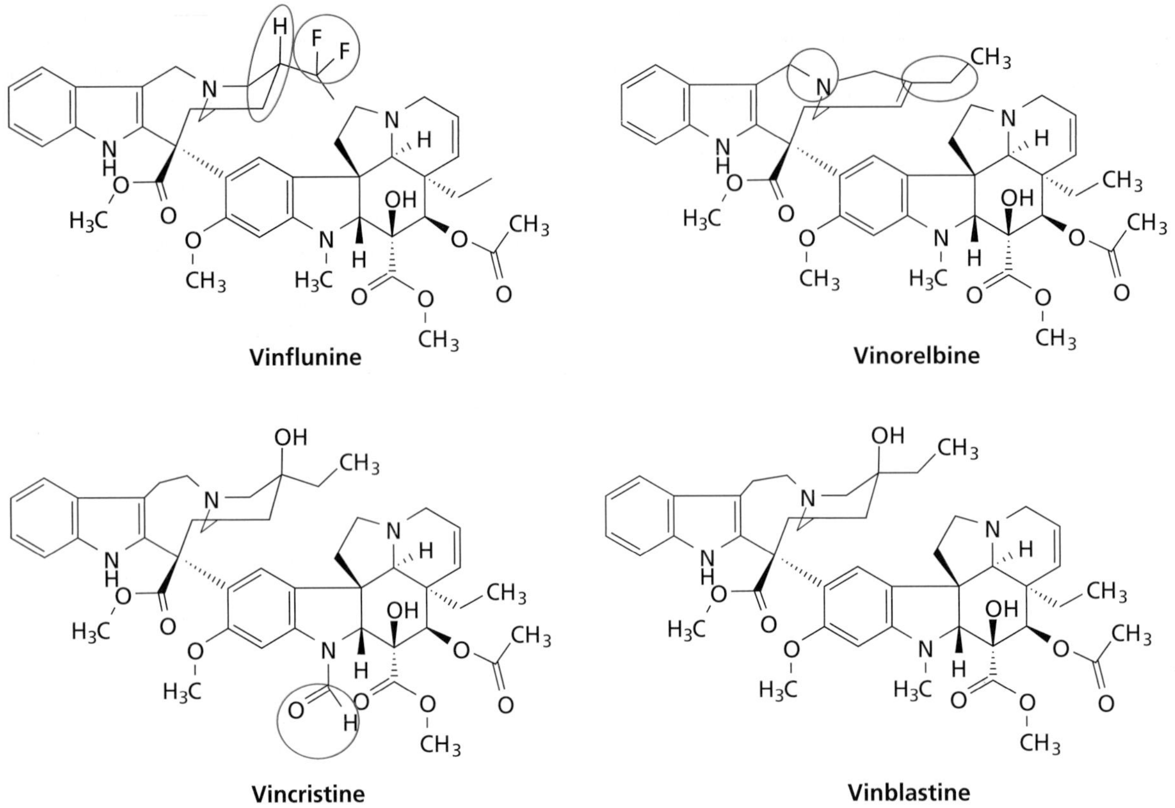

Figure 2 Chemical structures of the vinca alkaloids. Structural modifications with vinblastine as the reference are circled.

however, VCR is an essential component of the chemotherapy regimens used to treat acute lymphocytic leukemia (ALL), lymphoid blast crisis of chronic myeloid leukemia (CML), and both Hodgkin and non-Hodgkin lymphoma. VCR also plays a role in some multimodality therapies of Wilms' tumor, Ewing's sarcoma, neuroblastoma, and rhabdomyosarcoma and is occasionally used in treating multiple myeloma, particularly as a component of the VAD (VCR, doxorubicin, and doxorubicin) regimen, recurrent small cell lung cancer, and sarcoma of both soft tissue and bone. The agent has also been used as a component of a combination regimen, known as PCV (procarbazine, lomustine, and VCR), which is used in early and advanced settings of anaplastic oligoastrocytoma and oligodendroglioma.[42] More for a historical sense, indicating a wide range of utility, VCR and VCR-laden platelet transfusions have been effective in refractory autoimmune thrombocytopenia; VCR has been effective in treating both nonmalignant and immunologically mediated disorders such as autoimmune hemolytic anemia, hemolytic uremic syndrome, thrombotic thrombocytopenia purpura, and steroid-dependent nephritic syndrome.[38–40,43]

VBL has been a mainstay component of chemotherapy for germ cell malignances and some types of advanced lymphoma.[38] For many years, a regimen termed PVB, consisting of cisplatin, VBL, and bleomycin, was a standard therapy for germ cell carcinoma; however, VBL has largely been replaced by etoposide in this setting because of the more favorable toxicity profile of the cisplatin–etoposide regimen. For Hodgkin's lymphoma, VBL is often used in combination with doxorubicin, bleomycin, vinblastine, and dacarbazine (ABVD).[38] This regimen has been either administered alone, alternated with nitrogen mustard, VCR, procarbazine, and prednisone (MOPP), which is noncross-resistant to ABVD, or used as a hybrid (MOPP/ABV) that includes both VCR and VBL, which has also been extensively studied. Anticancer

activity has been observed with VBL as a single agent or in combination with other anticancer drugs in patients with advanced and/or relapsed carcinoma of the breast, bladder, and lung, as well as Kaposi's sarcoma, choriocarcinoma, terminal phase of CML, cutaneous T-cell lymphoma, and histiocytosis X.[38] Infusions of VBL or VBL-laden platelets have been effective in some cases of refractory autoimmune thrombocytopenia because of its avidity to platelets.[38,43] VBL has also been used alone or in combination with other agents to treat Kaposi's sarcoma and bladder, breast, and some types of malignancies of the central nervous system.[38,44–48]

The semisynthetic VBL derivative vinorelbine (5'-norhydro-VBL; VRL), which is structurally modified on its catharanthine nucleus, resulting in much greater lipophilicity as compared with the other vinca alkaloids, is approved in the United States for treating nonsmall cell lung cancer as either a single agent or in combination with cisplatin and has been registered elsewhere to treat patients with advanced breast cancer. The agent has also demonstrated clinical activity in advanced ovarian carcinoma and lymphoma, but a unique role in treatment of these cancers has not been defined. VRL has also been shown to confer favorable therapeutic indices to patients with advanced breast and lung cancers who are elderly and/or have diminished performance abilities.[4,38,44–48]

Several other vinca alkaloids or reformulated versions of older vinca alkaloids are available for treating relevant malignancies worldwide. One widely studied vinca alkaloid, vindesine (desacetyl-VBL caroxyamide), a semisynthetic derivative and human metabolite of VBL, was introduced in the 1970s and several regions outside the United States. In some reports, response rates in nonsmall cell lung cancer with combinations of VDS and cisplatin or mitomycin appear to be superior to those achieved with standard combinations or with either agent alone.[38,40,41] In addition, anticancer activity has been seen in ALL, blast crisis of CML, malignant melanoma, various pediatric solid neoplasm, and advanced renal, breast, and esophageal carcinoma. In addition, VFL, which is a bifluorinated vinca alkaloid, has shown notable clinical activity in bladder, breast, lung, and other cancers.[4,38,44–52] In Europe, VFL is approved as a treatment option for patients with advanced urothelial cancer who have failed a prior platinum-containing regimen.[52] Lastly, a sphingomyelin- and cholesterol-based liposomal nanoparticle formulation of VCR (vinCRIStine sulfate LIPOSOME injection (VSLI)) is registered in the United States for the treatment of adult patients with Philadelphia chromosome-negative ALL whose disease has progressed following at least two prior therapies.[53,54] Although the liposomal formulation permits delivery of higher VCR doses, has a longer circulatory time, and delivers greater amounts of active VCR to target tissues compared to standard VCR, the overall clinical benefits of the new formulation of VCR over standard VCR are not known.

Mechanism of action

The vinca alkaloids principally induce cytotoxicity by disrupting microtubule function, particularly that of microtubules that comprise the mitotic spindle apparatus, leading to metaphase arrest and cell death.[2–7,36–38,55–59] However, they are capable of many other biochemical activities that may or may not be related to their effects on microtubules, including inhibiting synthesis of proteins and nucleic acids, elevating oxidized glutathione, altering lipid metabolism and membrane lipids, elevating cyclic adenosine monophosphate (cAMP), and inhibiting calcium–calmodulin-regulated cAMP phosphodiesterase.[38] Many effects that do not involve microtubule disruption occur only after treatment with superphysicological concentrations that are not readily attained *in vivo*, whereas nanomolar concentrations, which are readily achievable in following drug administration in clinical practice, induce typical antimicrotubule effects. The vinca alkaloids also disrupt the structural integrity of platelets and other cells, which are rich in tubulin. In addition to mitotic disruption, the vinca alkaloids and other antimicrotubule agents perturb cells in nonmitotic cell-cycle phases, which is not surprising because microtubules are involved in many nonmitotic functions.[38,57–59] The vinca alkaloids bind rapidly and reversibly to sites on tubulin (called the vinca domain), which are distinct from those of the taxanes, colchicine, podophyllotoxin, and GTP but similar to those of maytansine and several other plant alkaloids.

The vinca alkaloids appear to bind to two binding sites with different affinities.[2,4,6,7,10,37,38,51,55–57,60,65] Binding of the vinca alkaloids to high-affinity sites (Kd, 1–2 μmol), which are at the ends of microtubules, is responsible for the potent suppression of tubulin exchange at low concentrations (<1 μmol). At low vinca alkaloid concentrations, processes dependent on microtubule dynamics (treadmilling and dynamic instability) are disrupted, but microtubule mass is not affected. The overall result is a potent mitotic block at the metaphase/anaphase boundary. Binding of vinca alkaloids to low-affinity sites (Kd, 0.25–3.0 mmol) along the sides of microtubules appears to result in reduced microtubule mass due to tubulin depolymerization and the splaying of microtubules into spiral aggregates or spiral protofilaments that form paracrystals, ultimately leading to microtubule disintegration. These effects occur at high drug concentrations (>1–2 μmol) by a self-propagated mechanism, initially involving drug binding to a limited number of sites, which progressively weakens the lateral interactions between the protofilaments, thereby exposing new sites and augmentation of the process.

The vinca alkaloids induce a potent block in mitosis at the metaphase/anaphase transition.[2,4,66] Following nuclear envelop breakdown, the vinca alkaloids block mitotic spindle formation and reduce the tension at the kinetochores of the chromosomes. Although chromosomes may condense, they remain scattered in the cells. The chromosomes separate along their lengths but still remain attached at their centromeres.[2,4,9,13,18,24,58,59,67] Mitotic progress is delayed in a metaphase-like state, with chromosomes "stuck" at the spindle poles, unable to move to the spindle equator. The cell-cycle signal to the anaphase-promoting complex, which is required for the cell to transition from metaphase to anaphase, is blocked, and apoptotic cell death ensues. Cell-cycle progression in the absence of anaphase or cytokinesis may occur, resulting in chromatin decondensation and formation of multilobed nuclei.[2,4,13,24] Disruption of dynamics without depolymerization of the microtubules that constitute the mitotic spindle ultimately induces apoptosis that involves expression of proapoptotic genes and both activation and inactivation of proapoptotic and antiapoptotic proteins, respectively (see section titled "Vinca Alkaloids, Mechanism of Action" and "Vinca Alkaloids, Mechanisms of Resistance" and "Taxanes, Mechanisms of Action, and Resistance").[2,4,9,13,18,21,23,51,67–72] Induction of apoptosis, however, is not dependent on the presence of an intact TP53 checkpoint. The loss of p21, a protein that controls entry into mitosis at the G_2/M checkpoint, sensitizes tumor cells to both vinca alkaloids and taxanes, possibly by hastening entry of drug-damaged cells into mitosis.[23,68–70]

The relationships between microtubule depolymerization caused by the vinca alkaloids and their resultant effects on cell proliferation, mitotic arrest, and mitotic spindle disruption have been characterized in a series of studies whose results indicate that cell growth inhibition is directly related to metaphase arrest.[18] The inhibition of proliferation and blockage of cells in metaphase at the lowest effective drug concentration occur with little or no microtubule depolymerization or disorganization of the mitotic spindle apparatus. With increasing drug concentrations, the organization of microtubules and chromosomes in arrested mitotic spindles breaks down in a manner similar to most antimicrotubule drugs, regardless of the underlying mechanism.[2–4,13,14]

In addition to their direct cytotoxic effects on tumor cells, the vinca alkaloids as well as the maytansinoids, taxanes, and various other antimicrotubule agents confer anticancer effects by inhibiting processes associated with malignant angiogenesis with surprising potency.[73] These antiangiogenic effects are most likely caused by drug-induced microtubule perturbations in vascular endothelial cells; however, the relative contribution of these effects to the clinical anticancer activity is unclear.

The reasons for the disparate sensitivity of various tissues and tumors to the vinca alkaloids are multifactorial. One possible explanation is the differential sensitivity of tissues with varying tubulin isotype composition, which may affect intracellular drug accumulation and drug binding to tubulin.[4,33,74–75] In addition, differences in the type and concentration of MAPs and posttranslational tubulin modifications, which may influence drug interactions with tubulin, as well as variability in cellular permeability and retention, may affect the formation and stability of complexes formed between the vinca alkaloids and tubulin. Palmitoylation, a posttranslational tubulin modification, is directly inhibited by the vinca alkaloids, and depalmitoylation of tubulin may not only be a mechanism of action, but may also relate to drug sensitivity.[76] Other putative factors include differences in tubulin isotypes (see sections titled "Vinca Alkaloids, Mechanisms of Resistance" and "Taxanes, Mechanisms of Resistance"), GTP content, rates of GTP hydrolysis, and cellular permeability.[74,77–81]

Mechanisms of resistance

In most preclinical models, resistance to the vinca alkaloids develops rapidly and is associated with decreased drug accumulation and retention. At least two types of mechanisms of resistance have been characterized. The first typifies the "classic" pleiotropic or multidrug-resistant (MDR) phenotype that can be either primary or acquired. Although many proteins that mediate MDR have been characterized, the most well known are the ATP-binding cassette (ABC) transporters that belong to the largest known transporter gene family and translocate a wide range of substrates across cellular compartments.[82,83] These intracellular and extracellular membrane-spanning proteins, which transport both endobiotics and xenobiotics, confer resistance to the vinca alkaloids and other structurally bulky natural products. The best characterized ABC transporters are the permeability glycoproteins (Pgp) or the MDR-encoded gene product MDR1 (ABC subfamily B1) and the multidrug resistance protein (MRP; ABC subfamily C2).[82]

MDR1 is a 170-kDa Pgp energy-dependent transmembrane pump that regulates the efflux of a wide range of bulky hydrophobic substances.[82] The protein is constitutively overexpressed in various normal tissues, which include renal tubule epithelium, colonic mucosa, and adrenal medulla, as well as tumors derived from tissues that constitutively overexpress Pgp. Pgp, an ATPase, functions to bind and extrude the vinca alkaloids from the tumor cell in a process that requires energy in the form of ATP. The MDR phenotype also confers varying degrees of cross-resistance to other structurally bulky natural products such as the taxanes, anthracyclines, epipodophyllotoxins, and colchicine. The specific Pgp associated with vinca alkaloid resistance shows slight antigenic and amino acid sequence differences and a different amino acid map after digestion than does Pgp from cells selected for resistance to colchicines or taxanes.[84–87] In fact, two forms of the protein have been demonstrated to be produced by a single clone of VCR-resistant cells, and these forms undergo posttranslational N-glycosylation and phosphorylation, which lead to further structural diversity and may explain the greater degree of resistance for the specific agent used compared with the resistance of other drugs conferred by MDR and may also account for the variable patterns of resistance among MDR cells. The composition of membrane gangliosides in cancer cells resistant to the vinca alkaloids has also been shown to differ from that of wild-type cells. The clinical ramifications of these resistance mechanisms are not known. In one study in childhood ALL, however, VCR resistance measured *in vitro* did not correlate with Pgp overexpression.[88]

MRP1, a 190-kD membrane-spanning protein that shares 15% amino acid homology with MDR1, also confers resistance to the vinca alkaloids *in vitro*.[39,82,83,89–92] MRP1 expression is found in many tumors and has been associated with the MDR phenotype in cancers of the lung, colon, breast, bladder, and prostate, as well as leukemia. MRP1 transports glutathione conjugates of alkylating agents and several xenobiotics such as etoposide and doxorubicin but confers resistance only to the latter agents. MRP1 confers resistance to the vinca alkaloids and methotrexate.[39,82,83,89–92] Although other ABC transporters have been identified and several confer cellular resistance to the vinca alkaloids *in vitro*, their roles in conferring inherent or acquired drug resistance in the clinic are less clear than those of MDR1 and MRP1.

Drug resistance conferred by MDR1 and MRP *in vitro* is reversible after treatment with agents that have distinctly different structural and functional characteristics, such as the calcium channel blockers, calmodulin inhibitors, detergents, progestational and antiestrogenic agents, antibiotics, antihypertensives, antiarrhythmics, antimalarials, and immunosuppressives, which has been a source of clinical interest.[39,82,93,94] Those reversal agents bind directly to Pgp, thereby blocking the efflux of the cytotoxic drugs and increasing intracellular drug concentrations. However, clinical studies of resistance modulation have been confounded by the fact that MDR modulators, particularly MDR1 reversal agents, also enhance drug uptake in normal cells, decrease biliary elimination and drug clearance, and lead to enhanced toxicity.[39,82,93,94] Overall, clinical strategies aimed at reversing resistance to the vinca alkaloids with pharmacologic modulators of both MDR1 and MRP have been disappointing, most likely owing to the fact that the MDR1 expression is associated with overexpression of a large number of resistance proteins.[82]

Structural and functional alterations in α- and β-tubulins due to either genetic mutations, posttranslational modifications, or differential expression of tubulin isotypes, particularly the ßIII-tubulin isotype, have been identified in tumor cells with resistance to the vinca alkaloids and taxanes in both preclinical and clinical studies.[95–106] These studies suggest that the ßIII-tubulin isotype could be both a prognostic and a predictive determinant of clinical benefit. Expression of ßII-tubulin, which appears to depend on TP53 suppressor function, may also relate to vinca alkaloid resistance.[107]

Increased expression of MAPs, particularly MAP4, has also been associated with vinca alkaloid resistance.[75] This alteration, as well as alterations in α- and β-tubulin, promotes resistance to agents that inhibit microtubule assembly by enhancing microtubule stability, possibly by promoting longitudinal inter- and intradimer interactions and/or lateral interactions between protofilaments. Furthermore, these "hyperstable" microtubules are collaterally sensitive to the taxanes (see sections titled "Taxanes, Mechanisms of Resistance"). Although such tubulin modifications have been demonstrated repeatedly in tumor cells that are continuously exposed to the vinca alkaloids *in vitro*, the relevance of "hyperstable tubulin" caused by alterations in tubulins or MAPs is not known.

Variability in cellular permeation and retention may also influence the formation and stability of vinca alkaloid-tubulin complexes.[51,79,108–114] The vinca alkaloids are rapidly taken up into cells and then accumulate intracellularly, with intracellular to extracellular concentration ratios as high as 5- to 500-fold, depending on the cell type.[80,81] In murine leukemia cells, the intracellular concentrations of VCR are 5- to 20-fold higher than the extracellular concentrations, and ratios ranging from 150- to 500-fold have been reported with other vinca alkaloids.[81,108,115] There are also marked differences in cellular uptake and retention between the vinca alkaloids, the latter of which may relate to potency and the duration of drug action. For example, VRL is more rapidly taken up and metabolized than other vinca alkaloids in isolated human hepatocytes,[116] and the greater potency of VCR during exposures of short duration compared with VBL was related to the greater cellular retention of VCR in another model system. A key determinant of drug accumulation and retention is lipophilicity. The differences in the catharanthine ring of VRL render it a more lipophilic agent and increase its retention in tissues, which may explain why it is more effective at disrupting the microtubules of the mitotic spindles compared with axonal microtubules.[114] The differential effects of the vinca alkaloids on axonal microtubules due to variable cellular retention and lipophilicity may explain why VRL treatment results in less neurotoxicity than other vinca alkaloids. The mechanisms responsible for the intracellular accumulation of the vinca alkaloids and other agents that bind to tubulin are not fully known, but may relate to their tubulin-binding properties and several other factors. Differential drug uptake among different tumor types may also relate to tubulin isotype expression, differential uptake and efflux, and intracellular reservoirs for drug accumulation. Lastly, pharmacokinetic differences related to the formulation vehicle appear to influence tissue uptake. For VSLI, liposomal entrapment appears to be associated with increased circulating time and tumor permeability in preclinical studies.[53] Increased tumor uptake of VCR following administration of VSLI may be due, in part, to the enhanced permeability and retention effect conferred by the liposomal formulation.

Pharmacology

Cellular pharmacology

Temperature-independent nonsaturable mechanisms, analogous to simple diffusion, are responsible for most transport of the vinca alkaloids, and temperature-dependent saturable processes are less important.[117] Although drug concentration and duration of treatment are determinants of drug accumulation and cytotoxicity, the duration of drug exposure above a critical threshold concentration is perhaps the most important pharmacologic determinant of cytotoxicity.[80] Cytotoxicity is directly related to the extracellular concentration of drug when the duration of treatment is kept constant; for prolonged exposure to VCR, the concentration yielding 50% inhibition lies in the range of 1–5 nmol/L.[118]

Clinical pharmacology

The clinical pharmacology of the vinca alkaloids, which were largely studied decades ago, largely reflects the fact that sensitive, specific, and reliable analytic assays capable of measuring the minute plasma concentrations resulting from the administration of milligram quantity doses were not available. Early results may have been confounded by the use of radiolabeled drugs and assay methods. The vinca alkaloids, particularly VCR and VBL, undergo spontaneous degradation, forming degradative products that can be separated using high-pressure liquid chromatography (HPLC). Radiolabeled compounds coupled to HPLC improved separation of the various chemical moieties. Radioimmunoassay (RIA) and enzyme-linked immunosorbent assay (ELISA) methods can measure drug concentrations in the picomolar range; however, these methods cannot distinguish between the parent compounds and related derivatives and, therefore, may not provide sufficient quantitative information about degradation products and metabolites. To meet the challenge, more refined RIA and ELISA methods using mAbs with considerably greater sensitivity and specificity have been developed. Furthermore, recent technical advances in extraction and detection methodologies have increased the sensitivity and specificity of chromatographic methods, particularly tandem mass spectroscopy in conjunction with HPLC. Table 1 summarizes the pharmacokinetic characteristics of the vinca alkaloids, which generally exhibit triphasic clearance in human plasma following intravenous administration as a brief infusion. Except for VSLI, the pharmacokinetic behavior of these agents is typified by large volumes of distribution (Vd), high early clearance rates, long terminal half-lives, extensive hepatic metabolism, and biliary/fecal elimination. The relatively short α and ß phases, which are likely a result of rapid distribution and uptake and binding to tubulin in peripheral tissues and formed blood elements, are similar for all vinca alkaloids. However, the terminal (γ) phase, which is relatively long because of the avid tissue sequestration and slow release of drug, has been reported to vary by approximately fourfold.

Vincristine (VCR)

VCR is rapidly distributed to from the circulatory to the peripheral compartment following administration. There is extensive binding to both plasma proteins and formed blood elements, particularly platelets, which contain large quantities of tubulin. This served as the rationale for using VCR-laden platelets to treat disorders of platelet consumption such as refractory thrombocytopenia.[38,43] In contrast, penetration of VCR and all other vinca alkaloids across the blood–brain barrier is poor, probably because of the molecule's large size and high substrate affinity for ABC transporter pumps that maintain the integrity of the blood–brain barrier. Following administration of conventional doses ($1.4\,mg/m^2$), given as a brief intravenous infusion, peak plasma levels approach $0.4\,\mu mol$.[38,117,119–124] Total VCR clearance is slow, which reflects avid tissue binding and slow release, and terminal half-life ($t_{1/2}$) values in the range of 23–85 h have been reported.[38,117,119–124] VCR is metabolized and excreted primarily by the hepatobiliary system. Seventy-two hours after the administration of radiolabeled VCR, approximately 12% and 70% of the radioactivity are recovered in the urine (50% of which consists of metabolites) and feces (40% of which consists of metabolites), respectively.[38,117,119–126] As many as 11 metabolites have been detected in humans and other species.[113] The nature of the VCR metabolites identified to date, such as 4-deacetyl-VCR and N-deformyl-VCR, which have been isolated from human bile, and 4′-deoxy-3′-hydroxyVCR and 3′,4′-epoxy-VCR N-oxide following incubation of VCR with bile, indicates that the agent is principally metabolized by hepatic cytochrome P450 CYP3A.[38,117,119–127] There has been conflicting, albeit sparse, evidence that peak plasma concentration and systemic exposure are the principal pharmacologic determinants of neurotoxicity.[127]

Vinblastine (VBL)

The pharmacologic behavior of VBL is similar to that of VCR. Following rapid intravenous injection of VBL at standard doses, peak plasma drug concentrations are approximately $0.4\,\mu mol/L$.[38,117,128] Tissue distribution is also extensive. Like VCR, binding of VBL to plasma proteins and formed elements of blood is considerable. Furthermore, distribution is rapid with $t_{1/2}$ values of approximately 4 min and 1.6 h for α and ß phases, respectively. Terminal half-life values ranging from 20 to 24 h have been reported. Like VCR, VBL disposition is principally through the hepatobiliary system. The principal mode of VBL disposition is hepatic metabolism and biliary excretion. Fecal excretion of the parent compound is low, indicating that metabolism is substantial. The cytochrome P450 CYP3A isoform appears to be principally responsible for its biotransformation.[116] At least one metabolite, 4-deacetyl-VBL, or VDS, which appears to be as active as the parent compound, has been identified in humans, and small quantities have been detected in both urine and feces.

Vinorelbine (VRL)

The pharmacologic behavior of VRL is similar to those of the other vinca alkaloids, and plasma concentrations decline in a biexponential or triexponential manner. Immediately after intravenous administration, plasma concentrations decline rapidly followed by much slower elimination phases ($t_{1/2}$, 18–49 h).[38,46,47,129,130] Plasma protein binding has been reported to range from 80% to 91%, with binding primarily to α_1-acid glycoprotein, albumin, and lipoproteins. VRL is widely distributed with extensive sequestration in virtually all tissues, except the brain and testes. The drug is also extensively bound to platelets. The wide distribution of VRL may reflect the agent's lipophilicity, which is among the highest of the vinca alkaloids. Tissue to plasma ratios range from

Table 1 Vinca alkaloids: comparative pharmacokinetic and toxicologic characteristics.

	Vincristine	Vinblastine	Vindesine	Vinorelbine	Vinflunine	Vincristine sulfate liposome injection
Standard adult dose range (mg/m^2)	1–2 (weekly)	6–8 (weekly)	3–4 (weekly)	15–30 (weekly)	320 (every 3 weeks)	2.25 (weekly)
Pharmacokinetic behavior	Triphasic	Triphasic	Triphasic	Triphasic	Multiphasic	Biphasic
Plasma half-lives						
α(min)	<5	<5	<5	<5	—	—
β(min)	50–155	53–99	55–99	49–168	—	—
γ(h)	23–85	20–64	20–24	18–49	40	7.66^a
Clearance (L/h/kg)	0.16	0.74	0.25	0.4–1.29	0.64	0.35 (L/h)
Primary route	Hepatic metabolism and biliary elimination	Hepatic metabolism and biliary elimination	Hepatic metabolism and biliary elimination	Hepatic metabolism and biliary elimination	Hepatic metabolism and biliary elimination (≈66%); renal (≈33%)	Hepatic metabolism and biliary elimination
Principal toxicity	Neurotoxicity	Neutropenia	Neutropenia	Neutropenia	Neutropenia	Neutropenia
Other common toxicities	Constipation, SIADH	Alopecia neurotoxicity, mucositis	Alopecia, neurotoxicity	Neurotoxicity vomiting, constipation, mucositis	Neurotoxicity, myalgia, fatigue, anorexia, constipation, nausea/vomiting, anemia, injection site, thrombocytopenia, hyponatremia	Neurotoxicity, thrombocytopenia, anemia

^{a}Represents noncompartmental half-live value.
SIADH, syndrome of inappropriate antidiuretic hormone secretion.

20 to 80, although VRL concentrations in human lung have been reported to be 300-fold greater than plasma concentrations and 3.4–13.8-fold higher than lung concentrations achieved with VDS and VCR, respectively. Hepatic metabolism and biliary excretion of metabolites and VRL are the principal modes of drug disposition.[38,46,47,129–132] Approximately 33–80% of the administered dose of VRL is excreted into the feces, whereas urinary excretion represents only 16–30% of total drug disposition, the majority of which is metabolized. Cytochrome P450 isoform CYP3A is principally involved in biotransformation in humans.[46–48,132–137] The principal metabolites appear to be 4-O-deacetyl-VRL, 3,6-epoxy-VRL, and several hydroxy-VRL isomers. Most metabolites are inactive. Although 4-O-deacetyl-VRL may be as active as VRL, this finding is of minor importance since concentrations are minute.

The total body clearance of VRL (1.2 L/h/kg) and mean $t_{1/2}$ values of approximately 26 h were found to be the same in elderly and younger patients with normal hepatic function in one study. Clearance has been found to be adversely affected in patients who have liver metastases that involve more than 75% of the organ; clearance can be predicted in such patients by the monoethylglycinexylidide clearance test, which assesses CYP3A4 function.[137] Dexamethasone has also been used as a probe of CYP3A metabolism in the assessment of VRL pharmacokinetics.[131] Although VRL clearance is not accurately predicted by bilirubin concentrations in serum, markedly elevated levels have been associated with significant reductions in clearance in the few patients studied. VRL is active when given orally. In animals, 100% of radioactivity is absorbed after the ingestion of tritium-labeled VRL. The bioavailability of the parent compound in human studies is 43% and 27% for the powder-filled and liquid-filled capsules, respectively; the bioavailability of the gel-filled capsule was negligibly affected by food.[129,138,139] C_{max} values are achieved within 1–2 h after ingestion, and interindividual variability is moderate.

Vinflunine (VFL)

The pharmacokinetics of VFL have been demonstrated to be linear at clinically relevant doses (30 mg/m^2 to 400 mg/m^2).[49,50] VFL undergoes multiexponential decay following intravenous administration, with a rapid initial distribution phase. Similar to other vinca alkaloids, the Vd of its terminal phase is large (2.42 L or 35 L/kg), indicating wide distribution to a large tubulin-rich tissue compartment.[49,50] Total clearance is large (43.9 L/h, 0.640 L/h/kg), reflecting its initial rapid distribution and binding to tubulin-rich tissues. Its terminal $t_{1/2}$ is approximately 40 h, reflecting its slow clearance from the peripheral compartment. VFL is moderately bound to human plasma proteins (67.2%). Protein binding is nonsaturable in the range of clinically achievable VFL concentrations and mainly involves high-density lipoproteins and serum albumin; binding to α_1-acid glycoprotein and to platelets is negligible (<5%). Two-thirds of VFL is disposed of via hepatic metabolism and biliary excretion, whereas renal excretion accounts for one-third of administered drug.[140,141] Except for the principal metabolite, 4-O-deacetyl-VFL (DVFL) that is formed via multiple esterases, hepatic metabolism is mediated through CYP3A4. DVFL has comparable activity to the parent compound and a terminal $t_{1/2}$ of about 120 days. VFL has not been demonstrated to inhibit nor induce CYP3A4 nor other CYP metabolism enzymes in *in vitro studies*; however, coadministration of ketoconazole resulted in 30% and 50% increases in exposures to VFL and DVFL, respectively. Despite VFL's extensive liver metabolism and excretion, the pharmacokinetics of both VFL and DVFL were similar among 25 patients with varying degrees of liver dysfunction in one study. Nevertheless, dose adjustments for hepatic dysfunction are recommended (see section titled "Administration, Dose, and Schedule").[142] Since VFL clearance has been shown to be significantly decreased in patients ≥80 years old as compared to a control group of younger patients <70 years, dose reductions are recommended for elderly patients (≥75 years (see section titled "Administration, Dose and Schedule").

Vincristine sulfate liposome injection (VSLI)

The pharmacokinetics of VCR following administration of VSLI are typified by much slower clearance rates from the central compartment compared to VCR administered in a conventional nonliposomal formulation.[53] The lipid composition and the approximate 100 ηm mean particle size of the VSLI liposome contribute to low protein binding that result in a longer circulation time for the nanoparticle.[53] *In vitro* protein binding assays demonstrated negligible levels of human plasma proteins absorbed to VSLI. Approximately 18–39% of encapsulated VCR was released at 24 h *in vitro* using human plasma. These characteristics are likely responsible for preferential accumulation of VSLI accumulation in tumors and tissues of the macrophage phagocytic system (e.g., lymph nodes, bone marrow, spleen, and liver), possibly due to the larger microvascular fenestrations in those tissues, as well as enhanced permeability and retention.[143] In studies of mice with implanted human tumor xenografts, significantly faster accumulation of drug occurred in tumors than in nontumor tissues after a single dose of VSLI.[144] The interstitial amounts of drug were approximately 70-fold higher in tumor tissues compared to nontumor tissues at 1 h and remained higher at 48 h. Combined, these distribution data are consistent with VSLI exiting the systemic circulation, accumulating at the site of tumors where they act as a reservoir for the release of localized VCR to enhance the anticancer activity.

In human subjects receiving treated with VSLI 2.25 mg/m^2, mean plasma clearance was determined to be 345 mL/h.[53] Peak plasma concentration (C_{max}) values averaged 1220 ng/mL, whereas values for the elimination $t_{1/2}$ averaged 7.66 h, and mean values for total and steady-state Vd were 3.57 and 2.91 L, respectively. Following intravenous administration of VSLI, fecal and urinary excretion over 96 h accounted for 69% and <8% of administered drug.

Drug interactions

The vinca alkaloids, particularly VCR and VBL, enhance methotrexate accumulation in tumor cells *in vitro*, an effect mediated by a vinca alkaloid-induced blockade of drug efflux; however, the minimal VCR concentrations required to achieve this effect (0.1 µmol/L) are attained transiently *in vivo*.[145–147] The vinca alkaloids also inhibit the cellular influx and cytotoxicity of the epipodophyllotoxins *in vitro*, but the clinical ramifications of this effect are unknown.[148] L-Asparaginase may reduce the hepatic clearance of the vinca alkaloids, particularly VCR, which may result in increased toxicity. To minimize the possibility of this interaction, it is recommended that VCR be given 12–24 h before L-asparaginase. A pharmacokinetic interaction between VFL and pegylated liposomal doxorubicin was observed, resulting in a 15–30% apparent increase and a two to threefold decrease in VFL and doxorubicin exposure, respectively, whereas for doxorubicinol, the concentrations of the metabolite were not affected. According to an *in vitro* study, such changes could be related to adsorption of VFL on the liposomes and a modified blood distribution of both compounds. Therefore, caution should be exercised when this type of combination is used. A possible interaction between VFL and the taxanes, paclitaxel and docetaxel, which are CYP3A substrates, has been suggested based on the results of an *in vitro* study.

Treatment with the vinca alkaloids has precipitated seizures associated with subtherapeutic plasma phenytoin concentrations, most likely due to the induction of CYP3A-mediated clearance of phenytoin.[149–152] Reduced plasma phenytoin levels have been noted from 1 to 10 days after treatment with both VCR and VBL. Administration of the any of the vinca alkaloids with erythromycin, itraconazole, ketoconazole, ritonavir, ketoconazole, grapefruit juice, and other pharmacologic inhibitors of CYP3A may lead to severe toxicity due to reduced hepatic metabolism.[41,152,153] Drugs that induce CYP3A4, such as rifampin, and *Hypericum perforatum* (St. John's wort) should be avoided since they may accelerate the clearance of vinca alkaloids and increase drug exposure.[50] Concomitantly administered drugs, such as pentobarbital and H2-histamine

antagonists, may also influence VCR clearance by modulating hepatic cytochrome P450 metabolic processes.[152,154] It is important to be cognizant that concurrent use of the 3′-azido-3′-deoxythymidine (AZT) and the vinca alkaloids, such as in patients with Kaposi's sarcoma and acquired immune deficiency syndrome, may result in reduced metabolism of AZT since the vinca alkaloids inhibit glucuronidation of AZT to its 5′-O-glucuronide metabolite.[155] Based on a report of a constellation of severe toxicities, including syndrome of inappropriate antidiuretic hormone secretion (SIADH), bilateral cranial nerve palsies, peripheral neuropathy, cranial nerve palsies, heart failure, and cardiovascular effects following VCR treatment in children with ALL who had been receiving treatment with nifedipine and itraconazole, it is possible that these medications may enhance the neurologic and cardiovascular effects of the vinca alkaloids.[154] Lastly, the significant interindividual and intraindividual variability of VCR pharmacokinetics in children has been attributed to the variable induction of P450 metabolism due to concurrent use of P450-inducing corticosteroids.[150,151]

Mitomycin C combined with the vinca alkaloids has been associated with pulmonary toxicity (see sections titled "Toxicity, Miscellaneous").

Toxicity

The principal toxicities of the vinca alkaloids differ despite their structural and pharmacologic similarities. Neurotoxicity is the predominant toxicity of VCR, whereas myelosuppression predominates with VBL, VDS, VRL, VFL, and VSLI. However, peripheral neurotoxicity is noted after cumulative treatment with VBL, VDS, VRL, VFL, and VSL and in patients who are inherently susceptible.

Neurotoxicity

Although the vinca alkaloids are similar from a structural standpoint, their toxicologic profiles differ significantly. All of the vinca alkaloids induce a characteristic peripheral neurotoxicity, but VCR is most potent in this regard. The neurotoxicity is principally characterized by a peripheral, symmetric mixed sensory motor and autonomic polyneuropathy.[37,38,41,48,156–160] The primary pathologic effects are axonal degeneration and decreased axonal transport, most likely caused by a drug-induced perturbation of microtubule function. At onset, only symmetric sensory impairment and paresthesia in a length-dependent manner, initially in the distal extremities, are often encountered. Neuritic pain and loss of deep tendon reflexes may develop with continued treatment, which may be followed by foot drop, wrist drop, motor dysfunction, ataxia, and paralysis. Back, bone, and limb pains may occur. Electrophysiologic studies typically reveal normal nerve conduction velocities; however, diminished amplitude of sensory and motor nerve action potentials and prolonged distal latencies, resembling axonal degeneration, may be noted.[156–160] Rarely, cranial nerves are affected, resulting in hoarseness, diplopia, jaw pain, facial palsies, and laryngeal paralysis.[38,161,162] The uptake of VCR into the brain is low, and the central nervous system effects, such as confusion, mental status changes, depression, hallucinations, agitation, insomnia, seizures, coma, SIADH, and visual disturbances, may occur in rare situations.[38,48,163–165] Auditory effects, possibly secondary to disruption of the medial olivocochlear bundle, have also been reported. Acute, severe autonomic neurotoxicity is uncommon but may arise as a consequence of high-dose therapy (>2 mg/m^2) or in patients with diminished drug clearance because of altered hepatic function.[38,158–160,164–169] Toxic manifestations of autonomic neurotoxicity include constipation, abdominal cramps, paralytic ileus, urinary retention, orthostatic hypotension, and hypertension.[38,156–159,166–169] Acute neurotoxic manifestations resembling Guillain–Barré syndrome have also been reported.[160] In adults treated with VCR, the neurotoxic effects may begin with cumulative doses as little as 5–6 mg, and manifestations may be cumulative doses of 15–20 mg. Neurotoxic manifestations are generally cumulative and resolve slowly after treatment, often requiring many years. Neurotoxicity occasionally worsens for a short time following treatment.[170] Although it has been remarked that children are less susceptible to neurotoxicity than adults and that the elderly are particularly prone, these apparent age-related differences may, in fact, be caused by previously inaccurate dose calculation using body weight in children and adults and using body surface area in infants. In infants, VCR doses are calculated now according to body weight, which may be more accurate from a pharmacologic standpoint because of ubiquitous tissue distribution. Patients with antecedent neurologic disorders, such as Charcot–Marie–Tooth disease, hereditary and sensory neuropathy type 1, Guillain–Barré syndrome, and childhood poliomyelitis, are highly predisposed to neurotoxicity.[171–173] VCR treatment in patients with hepatic dysfunction or obstructive liver disease is associated with an increased risk of developing neuropathy because of impaired drug metabolism and delayed biliary excretion.[174,175] An inherited polymorphism in the promoter region of CEP72, which encodes a centrosomal protein involved in microtubule formation, was associated with increased risk and severity of VCR-related peripheral neuropathy.[176] If replicated in additional populations, this finding may provide a basis for safer dosing of this widely prescribed anticancer agent.

The only known effective intervention for vinca alkaloid neurotoxicity is discontinuing treatment or reduction of the dose or frequency of drug administration.[166,176,177] Although several antidotes, including thiamine, vitamin B12, folinic acid, pyridoxine, and neuroactive agents (e.g., sedatives, tranquilizers, anticonvulsants), have been used, these treatments have not been undoubtedly shown to be consistently effective.[38,127,178–180] Folinic acid protects mice against otherwise lethal doses of the vinca alkaloids, and there are anecdotal reports of its successful use following VCR overdosage in man; however, prospective studies have never been performed. Suggested dosages for folinic acid for the treatment of overdosage are 15 mg every 3 h for 24 h and then every 6 h for at least 48 h.[38] There have been promising results with other neuroprotective agents. In one randomized double-blind trial, coadministration of glutamic acid and VCR appeared to reduce neurotoxicity.[180] An adrenocorticotropin analog (ORG 2766) also demonstrated protection against VCR-induced neuropathy in an animal model and in a double-blind, placebo-controlled pilot study in patients.[38] Several other agents, including nerve growth factor, insulin growth factor-1, and amifostine, appear to alter the course of neurotoxicity in experimental models, but there is no definitive evidence that these agents may be effective in the clinic. Severe neurotoxicity is observed less frequently with VBL, VDS, VRL, and VFL, as compared with VCR.[114,181] VRL has a lower affinity for axonal microtubules than either VCR or VBL, which seems to be confirmed by clinical observations.[36,38,48,114,181] Characteristic vinca alkaloid neurotoxicity occurs with VSLI, but the agent has largely been evaluated in patients who have previously received VCR, and the relative neurotoxic effects of VCR and VSLI have not been studied.

Myelosuppression

Neutropenia is the principal dose-limiting toxicity of VBL, VDS, VRL, and VFL. It is also common with VSLI. Thrombocytopenia and anemia are usually less common and less severe. The onset of neutropenia is usually 7–11 days after treatment, and recovery is generally by days 14–21. Myelosuppression is not typically cumulative. Although VCR is rarely associated with hematologic toxicity, severe myelosuppression has been observed in situations, resulting in increased drug exposure, such as following inadvertent overdose, and hepatic insufficiency.

Gastrointestinal

Gastrointestinal toxicities, aside from those caused by autonomic dysfunction, may also occur.[37,38,41,48,127,182,183] Gastrointestinal autonomic dysfunction, as manifested by bloating, constipation, and abdominal pain, occurs most commonly with VCR, high doses of the other vinca alkaloids, or settings associated with high drug exposure (e.g., hepatic dysfunction, overdosages). An initial manifestation of autonomic dysfunction due to slow intestinal transit may be impaction of stool in the upper colon. An empty rectum may be noted on digital examination, or an abdominal radiograph may be useful in diagnosing this condition, which may be responsive to high enemas and laxatives. A routine prophylactic regimen to prevent constipation is therefore recommended for all patients receiving VCR. Severe autonomic toxicity may lead to paralytic ileus, intestinal necrosis, and even intestinal perforation. The ileus, which may mimic a "surgical abdomen," usually resolves slowly with conservative measures after termination of treatment. Patients who receive high dosages of VCR or have hepatic dysfunction may be especially prone to develop severe gastrointestinal complications due to autonomic neurotoxicity. Although success with drugs used prophylactically to minimize toxicity, including lactulose, cerulein, metoclopramide, and a cholecystokinin analog (sincalide), has been reported anecdotally, these agents also may alter the pharmacokinetic behavior of the vinca alkaloids by affecting biliary excretion and/or enterohepatic recirculation, which may ultimately result in increased drug clearance.[38]

Mucositis, stomatitis, and pharyngitis occur more frequently with VBL than VCR, but not uncommon with VFL, VRL, and VDS. Nausea, vomiting, and diarrhea may also occur to a lesser extent. Asymptomatic and brief elevations in serum levels of hepatic transaminases and alkaline phosphatase have been noted. Pancreatitis has also been reported rarely with VRL.[182]

Miscellaneous

All vinca alkaloids should be considered potent vesicants and may cause profound tissue damage if extravasation occurs. This warning should apply to VSLI as there is no evidence that the formulation protects against tissue damage if extravasation occurs. If extravasation is suspected, treatment should be discontinued immediately and aspiration of any residual drug remaining in the tissues should be attempted.[38,184–189] In experimental studies, cold packs have been shown to increase toxicity, while heat appears to limit damage. The application of local heat immediately for 1 h four times daily for 3–5 days and the injection of hyaluronidase, 150–1500 units (15 units/mL in 6 mL of 0.9% sodium chloride solution) subcutaneously, through 6 clockwise injections in a circumferential manner using a 25-gauge needle and changing the needle with each injection) into surrounding tissues are the treatment of choice in minimizing both discomfort and latent cellulitis.[187–189] The use of leucovorin, diphenhydramine, hydrocortisone, isoproterenol, sodium bicarbonate, and vitamin A cream has been ineffective in animal models.[185] An immediate surgical consultation to consider early debridement is recommended. Discomfort and signs of phlebitis may also occur along the course of an injected vein, with resultant sclerosis, but phlebitis may be minimized if the vein is adequately flushed after treatment.

Mild and reversible alopecia occurs in approximately 10% and 20% of patients treated with VRL and VCR, respectively. Acute cardiac ischemia, chest pains without evidence of ischemia, fever without an obvious source, Raynaud's phenomenon, and palmar–plantar erythrodysesthesia (hand–foot syndrome) have also been reported.[190–192] Respiratory reactions, characterized by dyspnea, is noted in approximately 5% of patients, particularly when the vinca alkaloids are combined with mitomycin C.[193,194] The onset of pulmonary toxicity may be acute, with bronchospasm and dyspnea as the predominant manifestations, resembling an allergic reaction. The second type of toxicity is a subacute reversible reaction associated with cough and dyspnea and occasionally with interstitial infiltrates. It typically occurs within 1 h of treatment. Corticosteroids may be beneficial in severe cases, and several patients have been re-treated without complications. There is no clear evidence that implicates VRL as a cause of chronic pulmonary toxicity.

All vinca alkaloids have been implicated in causing SIADH, and patients receiving vigorous hydration are particularly prone to severe hyponatremia due to SIADH.[36–38,48,127] Plasma levels of antidiuretic hormone, which generally remit within 3 days' posttreatment, have been noted. Hyponatremia generally responds to fluid restriction. VBL may cause photosensitivity reactions, possibly due to corneal irritation, and muscular effects.[195] The inadvertent intrathecal administration of the vinca alkaloids causes an ascending myeloencephalopathy that is usually fatal. Reports of immediate cerebrospinal fluid withdrawal and lavage with Ringer's lactate solution supplemented with fresh frozen plasma (15 mL/L) at a rate of 55 mL/h for 24 h have provided encouraging results, with two affected patients surviving with paraplegia, albeit intact cerebral function.[196] To prevent this error, intrathecal methotrexate and intravenous VCR setting should not be administered in close temporal proximity, and the drugs should not be delivered together to staff.[197] Hepatic transaminase elevations have also been reported, particularly with VSLI.

Administration, dose, and schedule

It is recommended that the vinca alkaloids be administered by rapid intravenous injection. Inadequate flushing following treatment may increase the risk of phlebitis and injection site reactions, and, therefore, the catheter should not be removed before the vein is flushed. VCR is commonly administered to children weighing more than 10 kg as a bolus intravenous injection at a dosage of 1.5–2.0 mg/m² weekly, although 0.05–0.65 mg/kg weekly is commonly used in smaller children. For adults, the conventional weekly dose is 1.4–2.0 mg/m². A restriction of the absolute dose of VCR to 2.0–2.5 mg in children and 2.0 mg in adults, which is often referred to as "capping," has been generally adopted based on early reports of gastrointestinal toxicity (autonomic neuropathy) in patients treated at higher doses. However, there is little factual evidence to support this practice, and available evidence suggests that it should be reconsidered, particularly in light of the wide interpatient variability in pharmacokinetic behavior and tolerance. There is significant interpatient variability in the clearance of VCR (up to 11-fold), and some patients are able to tolerate much higher doses with little or no toxicity. Moreover, the safety and efficacy of treatment regimens that do not employ capping at 2.0 mg have been documented in adults.[198] In any case, doses should not be reduced for mild peripheral neurotoxicity, particularly if VCR is being used in a potentially curative setting. Instead, doses should be modified for manifestations of more serious neurotoxicity, including severe symptomatic sensory changes, motor and cranial nerve deficits,

and ileus, until toxicity resolves. In clearly palliative situations, dose reductions, lengthening dosing intervals, or selecting an alternative agent may be justified in the event of moderate neurotoxicity. A routine regimen to prevent serious consequences of severe autonomic toxicity, particularly constipation, is also recommended.

The recommended dose of VSLI is 2.25 mg/m² intravenously every 7 days. VSLI is prepared by mixing three components from a kit supplied by the manufacturer, which includes VCR sulfate, sodium phosphate, and sphingomyelin/cholesterol liposome injection. Following the manufacturer's procedure, VSLI should appear as a white to off-white, translucent suspension, essentially free of visible foreign matter and aggregates, comprised of sphingomyelin/cholesterol liposomes, with an approximate liposome mean diameter of 100 nm. Greater than 95% of the drug is encapsulated in the liposome. The procedure results in a solution that is diluted with either 5% dextrose injection or 0.9% sodium chloride injection to a final volume of 100 mL that is infused intravenously over 1 h.

The most common VBL schedule in chemotherapy regimens is a rapid intravenous injection at a dose of 6 mg/m² weekly. Approved weekly dosing recommendations are 2.5 and 3.7 mg/m² for children and adults, respectively, followed by gradual escalation in increments of 1.8 and 1.25 mg/m² weekly based on hematologic tolerance. It is recommended that weekly VBL doses of 18.5 mg/m² in adults and 12.5 mg/m² in children not be exceeded as a single agent; however, these doses are much higher than most patients can tolerate because of myelosuppression, even on less frequent administration schedules. Because the severity of leukopenia that may occur with identical VBL doses varies widely, VBL should probably not be given more frequently than once each week. Five-day continuous infusions of VBL have been used at dosages ranging from 1.5 to 2.0 mg/m² per day, which achieves biologically relevant plasma concentrations of approximately 2.0 nmol/L, but the overall advantages of using protracted infusions for a drug that is widely distributed and avidly bound to peripheral tissues are unclear.

VRL is usually administered at a dosage of 30 mg/m² on a weekly or biweekly schedule as a 6–10-min intravenous injection through a side-arm port into a running infusion (alternatively, a slow bolus injection followed by flushing the vein with 5% dextrose or 0.9% sodium chloride solutions) or as a short infusion over 20 min. It appears that more rapid infusions are associated with less local venous toxicity. Oral dosages of 80–100 mg/m² given weekly are generally well tolerated, but an acceptable oral formulation has not been approved. Other dosing schedules that have been evaluated include chronic oral administration of low doses, intermittent high doses, and prolonged intravenous infusion schedules.

The recommended dose of VLF is 320 mg/m² as a 20-min intravenous infusion every 3 weeks. A reduced dose of 280 mg/m² is recommended for patients with World Health Organization or Eastern Cooperative Oncology Group performance status of 1 or 0 and a history of pelvic irradiation. In the absence of hematological toxicity in the first cycle causing treatment delay or dose reduction, the dose should be increased to 320 mg/m² for the subsequent cycles.

Because of their remarkable vesicant properties, the vinca alkaloids should not be administered intramuscularly, subcutaneously, intravesically, or intraperitoneally. Direct intrathecal injection of VCR and other vinca alkaloids inadvertently has induced a severe myeloencephalopathy characterized by ascending motor and sensory neuropathies, encephalopathy, and death (see sections titled "Toxicity, Neurotoxicity").

Although specific dosing guidelines for patients with hepatic dysfunction have not been thoroughly formulated, the major role of the liver in the disposition of the vinca alkaloids implies that dose modifications should be considered for patients with hepatic dysfunction, particularly hepatic excretory dysfunction. For VCR, VRL, VDS, and VBL, a 50% dose reduction is often recommended for patients with total bilirubin levels between 1.5 and 3.0 mg/dL (50% dose reduction for bilirubin levels between 2.0 and 3.0 mg/dL is recommended for VRL), as well as at least a 75% dose reduction for plasma total bilirubin levels above 3.0 mg/dL. Dosing guidelines for patients with hepatic dysfunction have not been formulated, and therefore conservative measures, perhaps similar to the afore-mentioned guidelines for nonencapsulated vinca alkaloids, may be prudent since hepatic metabolism and biliary excretion are the principal processes involved with the disposition of VSLI. However, the pharmacokinetics of VSLI were evaluated in patients with moderate hepatic dysfunction (Child–Pugh B) and the dose-adjusted maximum plasma concentration and exposure were comparable to those with normal hepatic function.[49] The recommended doses of VFL are 250 and 200 mg/m^2 given once every 3 weeks for patients with mild (Child–Pugh grade A) and moderate (Child–Pugh grade B) liver impairment, respectively, as defined further in the prescribing information.

Dose reduction for renal impairment is not indicated for any of the vinca alkaloids except for VFL in which the recommended starting doses are 280 and 250 mg/m^2 every 3 weeks for patients with moderate (creatinine clearance rate between 40 and 60 mL/min) and severe (creatinine clearance rate between 20 and 40 mL/min) renal impairment, respectively.[53]

VFL dose reductions are also recommended for elderly patients since drug clearance relates to age. In patients whose ages are between 75 and 80 years and for patients whose age exceeds 80 years, the recommended dose is 280 and 250 mg/m^2 every 3 weeks, respectively.[53]

Taxanes: Introduction and indications

Although the taxanes affect microtubules, their principal mechanisms of action, pharmacology, clinical indications, and toxicities substantially differ from those of the vinca alkaloids. Interest in the taxanes began in 1963, when a crude extract of the bark of the Pacific yew tree, *Taxus brevifolia*, demonstrated notable anticancer activity in preclinical studies. In 1971, Wall and colleagues identified paclitaxel as the active constituent of the bark extract; however, the limited supply of its primary source that was exclusively derived from the Pacific yew tree, the difficulties inherent in large-scale isolation, extraction, and preparation of bulk compound, and its poor aqueous solubility delayed its development.[199] Interest was maintained after characterization of its novel mechanism of action and the availability of an adequate supply for requisite preclinical and limited clinical studies. The early search for taxanes derived from more abundant and renewable resources led to the semisynthesis of docetaxel by the addition of a side chain to 10-deacetylbaccatin III, an inactive taxane precursor found in the needles and other components of more abundant yew species.[200] The supply of paclitaxel is no longer preclusive due to the development of commercially feasible semisynthetic processes. A wide variety of taxane analogs, as well as paclitaxel formulations, have been evaluated. The most recent to be broadly registered is protein-bound paclitaxel particles for injection (PBPPI), sometimes called "nab-paclitaxel" or nanoparticle albumin-bound paclitaxel, which is an albumin-bound formulation of paclitaxel.[201]

Figure 3 shows the structures of paclitaxel, docetaxel, and cabazitaxel, which are complex esters consisting of a 15-member taxane ring system linked to an unusual 4-member oxetane ring. The taxane rings of both paclitaxel and docetaxel, but not 10-deacetylbaccatin III, are linked to an ester side chain attached to the C-13 position of the ring, which is essential for antimicrotubule activity.[202] The structures of paclitaxel and docetaxel differ in substitutions at the C-10 taxane ring position and on the ester side chain attached at C-13, which render docetaxel slightly more water soluble and potent than paclitaxel. However, the clinical ramifications of these differences are not entirely clear. Another more recent addition to the therapeutic armamentarium is cabazitaxel, a dimethoxy derivative of docetaxel that is partially synthesized into a single diastereomer from 10-deacetylbaccatin III.[203] Cabazitaxel is more potent and has lower substrate affinity for Pgp and other transmembrane drug efflux pumps than docetaxel, which, in part, explain its notable activity in docetaxel-resistant cancers.[204]

Clinical indications

Paclitaxel initially received regulatory approval in the United States and elsewhere for the treatment of patients with ovarian cancer after failure of first-line or subsequent chemotherapy. Its use in combination with a platinum compound as primary induction therapy in suboptimally debulked stages III or IV ovarian cancer has demonstrated a survival advantage over preexisting standard therapy in randomized phase III studies.[205] In the United States, paclitaxel is also indicated for treatment of patients with metastatic breast cancer after failure of combination chemotherapy for metastatic disease or at relapse within 6 months of adjuvant chemotherapy, with prior therapy that includes an anthracycline.[206] Paclitaxel is also indicated for the adjuvant treatment of node-positive breast cancer administered sequentially to standard doxorubicin-containing combination chemotherapy. In the clinical trial, there was an overall favorable effect on disease-free and overall survival in the total population of patients with both hormone receptor-positive and hormone receptor-negative tumors, but the benefit has been irrefutably demonstrated only in patients with hormone receptor-negative cancers.[207–209] Compelling results have been noted following treatment of patients with both metastatic breast cancer and high-risk early-stage breast cancer with alternative taxane-containing regimens, particularly "dose-dense" and weekly regimens; however, these efficacy results should not be generalized to other indications and/or other taxanes.[210,211] Weekly administration schedules using paclitaxel and other taxanes have been associated with lower incidences of some adverse effects, particularly myelosuppression, compared to less frequent dosing schedules.

Various therapeutics received regulatory approval as components of paclitaxel-based combination regimens. The combination of gemcitabine and paclitaxel demonstrated superior survival to paclitaxel alone in the first-line treatment of metastatic breast cancer, and gemcitabine received regulatory approval for use with paclitaxel in this setting. Similarly, the combination of trastuzumab and paclitaxel is indicated in the first-line treatment of women with HER-2-amplified metastatic breast cancer.[212] Paclitaxel is also indicated for adjuvant treatment of HER-2-amplified lymph node positive or negative (hormone receptor negative or with at least one high-risk feature) as part of a regimen consisting of doxorubicin, cyclophosphamide, and trastuzumab.[213,214] Paclitaxel has also received regulatory approval in the United States for second-line treatment of Kaposi's sarcoma associated with the acquired immunodeficiency syndrome and in combination with cisplatin as primary treatment advanced stage IIIB and stage IV nonsmall cell lung cancer patients who are not candidates for radiation therapy or

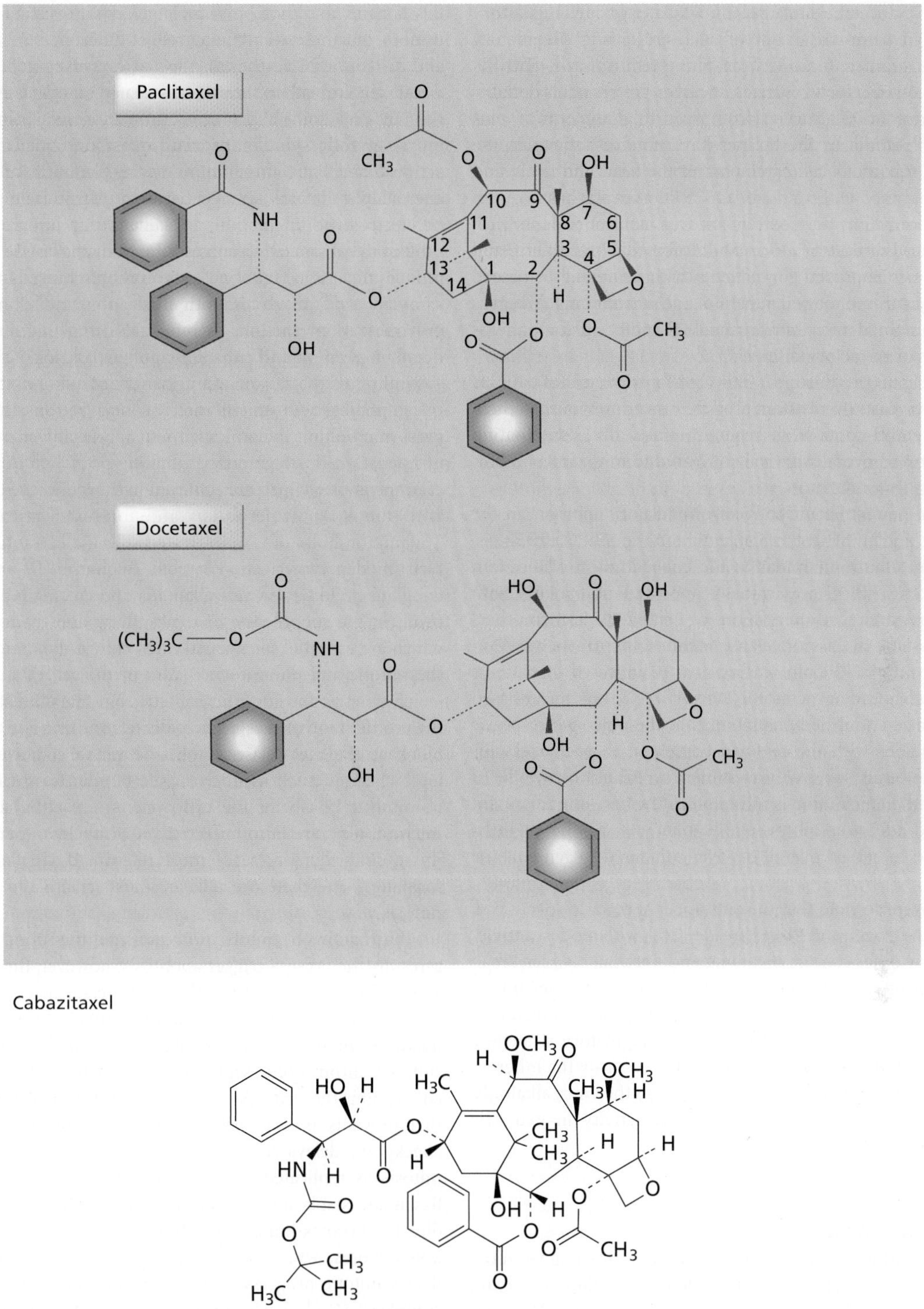

Figure 3 Chemical structures of the taxane: paclitaxel, docetaxel, and cabazitaxel.

potentially curative surgery.[215,216] Bevacizumab, in combination with paclitaxel and carboplatin, is approved for the treatment of stage IIIB and IV nonsquamous nonsmall cell lung cancer.[217]

Docetaxel initially received regulatory approval in the United States and elsewhere for patients with metastatic or locally advanced breast cancer after failure of anthracycline-based chemotherapy, which was later broadened to a more general indication following chemotherapy failure.[200] Subsequently, the combination of capecitabine and docetaxel demonstrated superior overall

survival over docetaxel alone after failure of an anthracycline in patients with locally advanced or metastatic breast cancer, and capecitabine as a component of this doublet received regulatory approval.[218] Regulatory approval has also been granted for docetaxel combined with cyclophosphamide and doxorubicin as adjuvant treatment for locally advanced breast cancer.[219] In nonsmall cell lung cancer, docetaxel initially is approved for treatment of unresectable locally advanced or metastatic disease after demonstrating increased survival after failure of cisplatin-based therapy, and the combination of docetaxel and cisplatin was later granted regulatory approval as first-line treatment of such patients.[220] Regulatory approval was granted for docetaxel plus prednisone in patients with hormone-refractory prostate cancer as the regimen demonstrated superior overall survival compared to mitoxantrone plus prednisone.[221] Similarly, the taxanes have notable activity in the treatment of squamous cell carcinoma of the head and neck, and docetaxel combined with cisplatin and 5-fluorouracil has received regulatory approval in the neoadjuvant treatment of patients with locally advanced disease.[222] Docetaxel combined with cisplatin and 5-fluorouracil is approved for patients with untreated advanced gastric and gastroesophageal junction adenocarcinoma, whereas paclitaxel combined with ramucirumab is indicated for patients with relapsed or refractory disease.[223,224]

Cabazitaxel plus prednisone is indicated for treatment of patients with metastatic castrate-resistant prostate cancer previously treated with a docetaxel-containing regimen since the combination showed improved overall survival compared to mitoxantrone plus prednisone in this indication.[225]

PBPPI, the newest taxane to receive regulatory approval in the United States and elsewhere, is a formulation of paclitaxel in 3–4% human serum albumin, similar to the concentration of albumin in the blood.[201] PBPPI was initially approved in patients with metastatic breast cancer after failure of combination chemotherapy for metastatic disease or relapse within 6 months of adjuvant chemotherapy.[226] PBPPI plus carboplatin is indicated in patients with locally advanced or metastatic nonsmall cell lung cancer based on a randomized trial demonstrating that the objective response rates were higher with the regimen compared to paclitaxel plus carboplatin; overall survival was similar.[227] Additionally, PBPPI combined with gemcitabine is indicated in the first-line treatment of metastatic adenocarcinoma of the pancreas, as the regimen demonstrated increased overall survival compared to gemcitabine alone.[201]

It is important to note that the anticancer spectra for paclitaxel, docetaxel, cabazitaxel, and PBPPI are identical, with modest activity noted in many other cancers including endometrial, bladder, small cell lung, and germ cell carcinoma, lymphoma, and melanoma. Differences in clinical efficacy endpoints and regulatory indications between these taxanes may reflect different regulatory strategies, study designs, and dose schedules and not necessarily the inherent superiority of any specific taxane. In contrast to the vinca alkaloids, the taxanes do not seem to have relevant activity in pediatric malignancies.

Mechanisms of action

The binding site for paclitaxel on microtubules is different from the binding sites for exchangeable GTP, colchicine, podophyllotoxin, and the vinca alkaloids. Paclitaxel binds to the N-terminal 31 amino acids of the β-tubulin subunit of tubulin polymers; however, other sites may be involved.[199,228–234] Paclitaxel binds in a pocket that is lined by several hydrophobic residues on the luminal side of the microtubule wall, roughly in the middle of the monomer along the protofilament direction.[3–7,199,234,235] Docetaxel, which most likely shares the same binding site as paclitaxel, appears to have a 1.9-fold higher affinity for the site, and the tubulin assembly process induced by docetaxel proceeds with a critical protein concentration that is 2.1-fold lower than that of paclitaxel.[233,236–240] However, it is not clear whether these differences translate into increased therapeutic indices for docetaxel in the clinic since higher potency may result in more severe toxicity at identical drug concentrations. Nevertheless, the results of both preclinical and clinical studies indicate that

the taxanes may not be completely cross-resistant in individual tumors, but these results may reflect differences in delivered dose and schedule. Nevertheless, the anticancer spectra of paclitaxel, docetaxel, and other taxanes are nearly identical. Although both the vinca alkaloids and taxanes produce similar disruptive effects on the mitotic spindle apparatus, their principal mechanisms of action differ. Following binding to the β-tubulin subunit, the taxanes stabilize lateral contacts between microtubule protofilaments by electrostatic interactions.[7] In effect, this interaction alters the tubulin rate dissociation constants at both ends of the microtubules, reduces the critical tubulin concentration required for microtubule assembly, and promotes both nucleation and elongation of the polymerization reaction, thereby stabilizing microtubules against depolymerization and enhancing polymerization.[2–7,55,239–245]

Binding of the taxanes to polymerized tubulin strengthens the microtubule. At substoichiometric concentrations, the taxanes suppress microtubule dynamics without appreciably increasing the rate of formation of polymerized tubulin.[2–7,55,239–245] At much higher concentrations, which are achieved in the clinic, the taxanes induce both tubulin polymerization and increased microtubule mass. The microtubules of taxane-treated cells are extraordinarily stable, resisting depolymerization by cold, calcium, GTP, and depolymerizing agents like the vinca alkaloids and colchicine. These actions result in the suppression of treadmilling and dynamic instability, which are essential for normal microtubule dynamics during both the mitotic and nonmitotic phases of the cell cycle.[2,3,13,17,20] Both stoichiometric and substoichiometric binding of the taxanes inhibit the proliferation of cells, principally by inducing a sustained mitotic block at the metaphase/anaphase boundary; however, morphologic changes, such as microtubule bundle formation during the nonmitotic phases of the cell cycle, suggest that the interphase microtubules are also affected. Nevertheless, perturbations in microtubule dynamics are most relevant during mitotic spindle formation, and therefore cells are most sensitive to the taxanes in mitosis.

Perturbations of mitotic processes and the induction of mitotic arrest by the taxanes trigger apoptosis; however, the precise mechanisms by which these perturbations result in cell death are not entirely clear. Nevertheless, the disruptive effects of the taxanes on the formation of functional mitotic spindle, which is responsible for chromosome segregation, ultimately activates the mitotic checkpoint, the principal cell-cycle control mechanism in mitosis that prevents missegregation of the chromosomes. The mitotic checkpoint delays separation of the chromosomes, which enter mitosis as replicated pairs of sister chromatids, until each pair has made stable attachments to both poles of the mitotic spindle. The taxanes impede attachment of the mitotic spindle to the kinetochores, which activate a signal transduction cascade that delays mitotic progression by inhibiting the anaphase-promoting complex.[22,246–248] Paclitaxel-treated cells ultimately enter anaphase and undergo mitosis, but the presence of unattached kinetochores result in the division of chromosomes in multiple directions; chromosome segregation is random due to multipolar division followed by partial cytokinesis failure. The resultant daughter cells are aneuploid, and a portion of these cells die, presumably due to loss of one or more essential chromosomes.

Microtubule perturbations induced by the taxanes trigger a delay in the mitotic checkpoint, which ultimately results in cell death via the intrinsic pathway of apoptosis.[22,75,244–262] This process involves various regulatory constituents such as the tumor suppressor gene TP53, inhibitors of cyclin-dependent kinases (e.g., p21/Waf-1), and regulators of other protein kinases.[244,245,262] As a consequence, cells are arrested in G_2/M, after which time they either undergo apoptosis or traverse through G_2/M and ultimately divide.[248,259] The apoptotic initiating events include activation of the proapoptotic molecules Bax and Bad, as well as inactivation of the antiapoptotic regulators Bcl-2 and BclxL.[248,259-261] Various kinases have been implicated in the inactivation of Bcl-2 induced by the taxanes and other antimicrotubule agents, including Jun N-terminal kinase and its proapoptotic effectors (e.g., Bim, c-Raf, extracellular signal-regulated kinase 1 and 2, apoptosis signal-regulated kinase, cyclin-dependent kinase 1 (CDK-1), cAMP-dependent protein kinase A, and protein kinase C).[69,250,260-264] Inactivation of Bcl-2 family members and activation of proapoptotic molecules stimulate the intrinsic pathway of apoptosis and downstream effector caspases.[257,259] The taxanes may also induce cell death independent of caspase activation.[241,265]

The taxanes also perturb interphase microtubules in nonproliferating cells as manifested by the formation of microtubule bundles.[248] Paclitaxel has been reported to induce transcription factors and enzymes that mediate proliferation, apoptosis, and inflammation.[252,262,266,267] The taxanes also enhance the effects of ionizing radiation *in vitro* and *in vivo*, most likely by inhibiting cell-cycle progression in G_2/M, which is the most radiosensitive phase of the cell cycle.[268-272] In addition, the taxanes inhibit angiogenesis at concentrations below those that induce cytotoxicity, but the contribution of these antiangiogenic effects to the anticancer effects of the taxanes is not entirely clear.[258,273,274]

Similar to the vinca alkaloids, the taxanes induce many other cellular effects that may or may not relate to their disruptive effects on microtubule dynamics. Although the taxanes primarily block cell-cycle traverse in the mitotic phases, the agents prevent G_0- to S-phase transition.[260,275] Explanations that have been proposed to account for the nonmitotic actions of the taxanes include disruptive effects on tubulin in the cell membrane, the interphase cytoskeleton, and microtubules that are involved in growth factor signaling and vascular endothelial growth factor expression through reactive oxygen species production and/or hypoxia inducible factor-1α.[38,276,277]

The taxanes perturb nonmalignant, as well as malignant, tissues. These effects are mediated, at least, in part, by disrupting microtubule dynamics. Paclitaxel inhibits relevant morphologic and biochemical processes in human neutrophils, including chemotaxis, migration, spreading, polarization, hydrogen peroxide generation, and killing of phagocytized microorganisms.[38] Paclitaxel also antagonizes the effects of microtubule-disrupting drugs on lymphocyte function and cAMP metabolism and inhibits the proliferation of stimulated human lymphocytes. Paclitaxel mimics the effects of endotoxic bacterial lipopolysaccharide on macrophages, which results in a rapid decrement in tumor necrosis factor-α (TNF-α) receptors and TNF-α release.[261,266,267] The agent also induces expression of the gene for TNF-α, but these activities are not related to paclitaxel's disruptive effects on microtubule assembly, which suggests that cytokine activation, in part, confers the anticancer activities of the taxanes.[266] In addition, paclitaxel inhibits chorioretinal fibroblast proliferation and contractility in models of proliferative retinopathy, as well as neointimal smooth muscle cell proliferation after cardiac and peripheral vascular angioplasty.[278,279] Cardiac and femoropopliteal arterial stents coated with paclitaxel to prevent restenosis from proliferation of neointimal tissue received regulatory approval in the United States and elsewhere.[280,281] Finally, paclitaxel inhibits secretory functions in many specialized cells, such as insulin secretion in isolated rat islets of Langerhans, protein secretion in rat hepatocytes, and the nicotinic receptor-stimulated release of catecholamines from chromaffin cells of the adrenal medulla.[38]

Although PBPPI likely affects the microtubules' malignant and nonmalignant tissues similar to conventional formulations of paclitaxel, the binding of paclitaxel to albumin in PBPPI increases accumulation of paclitaxel molecules in tumor tissue. Albumin has several characteristics that make it an attractive drug vehicle for cancer drugs. It is a natural carrier of endogenous hydrophobic molecules that are bound in a reversible noncovalent manner and facilitates endothelial transcytosis of protein-bound and unbound plasma constituents principally by binding to a 60-kDa glycoprotein (gp60) cell surface receptor. Following binding of albumin to gp60, the complex then interacts with caveolin-1, an intracellular protein, with subsequent formation of transcytotic vesicles (caveolae) that transport the complex to the intracellular compartment. Osteonectin, which is also known as secreted protein acidic and rich in cysteine (SPARC), also binds albumin because of a sequence homology with gp60.[201,282-284] Similar to caveolin-1, SPARC is expressed in several malignancies, including breast, lung, and prostate cancer, as well as by the stroma of these and others, which may account for the intratumoral accumulation of albumin, as well as the accumulation of albumin-bound drugs like PBPPI.[201,282-284] However, SPARC expression in tumor and/or stroma has yet to be definitely shown to predict for the anticancer activities of PBPPI.[201,282-286]

PBPPI, which was developed as an alternate paclitaxel formulation to polyoxyethylated castor oil, is an albumin-bound, 130-ηm particle formulation of paclitaxel, free from any solvent. It is used as a colloidal suspension derived from the lyophilized formulation of paclitaxel and human serum albumin. Human serum albumin stabilizes the drug particle at an average size of 130 ηm to prevent capillary obstruction, and the lack of a solvent requires no particular premedication nor infusion system.[201,282-284] Further, preclinical studies conducted in athymic mice with human tumor xenografts have shown that PBPPI delivers higher paclitaxel concentrations to tumor cells, resulting in greater anticancer activity than equivalent doses of paclitaxel in polyoxyethylated castor oil. SPARC-albumin interactions may also be responsible for more rapid systemic distribution and clearance of paclitaxel than poloxyethylated castor oil formulations.

Mechanisms of resistance

Two general types of mechanisms of acquired taxane resistance have been described in cells made resistant by prolonged drug treatment at low concentrations. The best characterized mechanism is the MDR phenotype, which can be mediated by several ABC multidrug transporter family members. The most important ABC transporter with respect to conferring taxane resistance is the 170-kDa Pgp efflux pump or the MDR1-encoded gene product MDR1 (ABC subfamily B1; ABCB1) and MDR2 (ABC subfamily ABCB4) (see sections titled "Vinca Alkaloids, Introduction and Indications" and "Vinca Alkaloids, Mechanisms of Resistance").[83,86,87,233,287,288] In addition, low-level taxane resistance appears to be conferred by the bile salt export pump (BSEP) (also known as ABCC11).[293,294] Unlike the vinca alkaloids, ABCC1 (MRP1) and ABCC2 (MRP2) do not appear to be involved in transporting the taxanes.[289-292] In murine systems, the particular species of Pgp found in paclitaxel-resistant cells is similar, but not identical, to that found in VBL and colchicine-resistant cells derived from the same parental line.[92,287,288] These cells are cross-resistant with many other natural products, and resistance to both paclitaxel and docetaxel conferred by MDR can be reversed by many classes of membrane-active drugs, including the calcium channel blockers, tamoxifen, cyclosporine A, and antiarrhythmic agents.[287,291-294]

Even the principal component of the formulations of paclitaxel and docetaxel—polyoxyethylated castor oil and polysorbate-80, respectively—can reverse taxane resistance; however, whereas the plasma concentrations of polyoxyethylated castor oil achieved with paclitaxel are sufficient to reverse MDR, sufficient modulatory concentrations of polysorbate-80 are not achieved with docetaxel in the clinic.[291,292] In general, strategies aimed at reversing resistance to taxanes and other MDR substrates in the clinic have not been successful, but most have involved MDR modulators that reduce taxane clearance and increase toxicity (e.g., verapamil, cyclosporine A), thereby confounding the interpretation of the inherent effects of these agents on MDR modulation. However, MDR and/or MRP modulators that do not affect taxane clearance and toxicity do not appear to enhance anticancer activity.[293,294]

Although the potency of cabazitaxel is similar to that of docetaxel in cancer cell lines and human tumor xenografts sensitive to docetaxel, cabazitaxel retains relevant activity in docetaxel-resistant cancer cell lines and human tumor xenografts that possess the MDR phenotype, which is due to the lower substrate affinity for Pgp. Resistance ratios range from 1.8 to 10 for cabazitaxel compared with 4.8–59 for docetaxel.[203,204] The extent to which the differences in Pgp substrate affinity account for cabazitaxel activity following failure of docetaxel in castrate-resistant prostate cancer is not known.

Similar to the vinca alkaloids, several human cell lines rendered taxane resistant by treatment with high drug concentrations for protracted periods have structurally altered α- and β-tubulins and an impaired ability to polymerize tubulin dimers into microtubules (see sections titled "Vinca Alkaloids, Introduction and Indications" and "Vinca Alkaloids, Mechanisms of Resistance").[106,107,295–307] These cells lack normal microtubules in their interpolar mitotic spindles and have an inherently slow rate of microtubule assembly when grown in the absence of drug. The continuous presence of the taxanes is required for microtubule assembly to proceed. Furthermore, these mutants are also collaterally sensitive to the vinca alkaloids. In some experimental systems, paclitaxel-resistant cells had mutated β-tubulin alleles, predominately involving β1-tubulin, with mutations involving the putative taxane binding sites; specifically, leucines at positions 215, 217, and 228 were mutated to histidine, arginine, or phenylalanine.[297,299,300,306] Low-level expression resulted in drug resistance, whereas high-level expression of these mutations caused impairment of microtubule assembly, cell-cycle arrest, and failure to proliferate, all of which were reversed by incubation with paclitaxel. Even though mutations of tubulin isotype genes, gene amplifications, and isotype switching have been reported in taxane-resistant cell lines, there is little indication that mechanisms are clinically relevant and, if they do occur, they are likely to be rare events.[306] In a study that examined paclitaxel-naive and paclitaxel-resistant samples from nonsmall cell lung cancer and ovarian cancer, ovarian cancer xenografts, and ovarian cancer cell lines, no βI-tubulin mutations were identified.[306] However, silent polymorphisms in exon 1 of βI-tubulin were detected at a very low frequency, suggesting that the polymorphisms are not relevant.[306]

Alterations in tubulin content, tubulin isotype profiles, and tubulin polymerization dynamics confer resistance to the taxanes in preclinical studies, and available evidence indicates that these mechanisms may explain variability responsiveness to the taxanes in the clinic.[306] As previously discussed, there are multiple α- and β-tubulin isotypes that are encoded by different genes that are located on different chromosomes and that have tissue- and cell-specific expression patterns. These tubulin isotypes can undergo posttranslational modifications, which can alter the interaction of microtubules with MAPs and change their function.

Predictive molecular modeling, which has been used to examine how the affinity of tubulin-binding agents for different β-tubulin isotypes varies, may explain differential sensitivity. For example, paclitaxel is thought to diffuse through nanopores in the microtubule to reach its binding site on the interior-facing lumen of the microtubule. It has been predicted that this movement is mediated by the formation of a hydrogen bond that involves serine 275 in all β-tubulin isotypes, except βII- and βVI-tubulin.[306] Paclitaxel-resistant tumors have been shown to have high levels of class I, III, and IVa isotypes of β-tubulin.[20,100–107,295–306,308,309] High intratumoral levels of the ßIII-tubulin isotype, which is a minor component of cellular β-tubulin, increases dynamic instability, and impedes microtubule assembly, have been identified in cell lines with acquired taxane resistance, as well as in taxane-resistant tumors sampled from patients.[100–106,298–307,310–322] The absence of ßIII-tubulin is associated with more rapid rates of microtubule assembly *in vitro*, whereas overexpression is associated with a decreased rate of microtubule assembly.[316]

The differential functional aspects of the various tubulin isotypes have not been fully elucidated, and the many posttranslational modifications that tubulins undergo add another layer of complexity. Pro- and antiapoptotic proteins, including the TP53 and Bcl2, are tethered or transported by microtubules. The induction of apoptosis by antimicrotubule agents is mediated through the intrinsic apoptotic pathway, principally by Bcl2 family members.[23,306,317,318] The proapoptotic protein Bim is tethered to microtubules, and, after treatment with paclitaxel, Bim translocates from microtubules to mitochondria.[306,319] Cancer cell lines with high Bim expression are more susceptible to the cytotoxic effects of the taxanes than cells with low expression. How differential expression of β-tubulin isotypes or posttranslational modifications affect the ability of antimicrotubule agents to bind, transport, and release of factors that induce apoptosis is not entirely clear; however, the expression of specific β-tubulin isotypes and MAPs has been related to drug resistance in a range of cancers, including lung, ovarian, breast, and prostate cancers.[20,100–107,295–306,308,309]

Aberrant proliferative signaling may contribute to taxane resistance by raising the cell's threshold for taxane-induced apoptosis. Insulin-like growth factor-1, for example, appears to protect responsive breast cancer cell lines from the cytotoxic effects of the anthracyclines and taxanes, possibly by activating the phosphatidylinositol 3-kinase pathway and inducing inactivation of antiapoptotic factors.[320] Other mediators that may influence the cell's threshold for drug-induced apoptosis include TP53, HER-2, aurora 2-kinase, survivin, and BRAC1. The centromere-associated serine/threonine kinase, aurora 2-kinase, which is involved in centrosome, biopolar spindle formation, and chromosomal kinetochore attachment to the mitotic spindle separation (see section titled "Targeting Mitotic Motor Proteins and Kinases"), appears to override the mitotic assembly checkpoint and induce taxane resistance.[21,22,306,] Also, overexpression of survivin, a member of the inhibitor of apoptosis family of proteins, inhibits caspase activity and apoptosis induced by antimicrotubule agents. The disruption of the tumor suppressor gene, BRAC1, which maintains genomic stability through DNA repair and appears to be involved in hereditary breast and ovarian cancers, appears to play a role in conferring resistance to paclitaxel, and the inducible expression of BRAC1 may enhance apoptosis induced by paclitaxel.[306,321] The mutational loss of the TP53 tumor suppressor does not appear to confer resistance to microtubule-polymerizing agents in contrast to DNA-disruptive agents.[306]

MAPs play a role in resistance by impeding apoptosis following treatment with the taxanes and other antimicrotubule agents.

For example, tau and MAP2, which are principally expressed in neuronal tissues, as well as the principal nonneuronal MAP, MAP4, bind to and stabilizes microtubules against depolymerization.[28–28] Tau expression relates to paclitaxel resistance in breast cancer, which seems to be through steric hindrance as tau masks the outer microtubule wall and limits access of paclitaxel to the inner luminal surface of the microtubule.[316,322] MAP4 confers microtubule stability, and induction of TP53 leads to decreased MAP4, resulting in reduced sensitivity to paclitaxel, albeit increased sensitivity to VBL.[323,324]

The microtubule-sequestering protein stathmin, which is overexpressed in several hematologic and solid malignancies, is a major cytosolic phosphoprotein that regulates the mitotic spindle by binding to tubulin heterodimers and inducing microtubule destabilization. Overexpression of stathmin decreases breast cancer cell sensitivity to paclitaxel and VBL.[306] High stathmin expression has also been associated with an unfavorable prognosis in patients with epithelial ovarian cancer treated with paclitaxel and cisplatin.[295,306] Finally, alterations in other cytoskeletal components, particularly reduced γ-actin and regulators of γ-actin, have been related to resistance to antimicrotubule agents.[306]

Transfection of cells with HER-2, a member of the epidermal growth factor receptor family that is amplified in approximately 30% of breast cancers, increases taxane resistance, and high expression of HER-2 relates to taxane resistance *in vitro*.[325,326] Overexpression of HER-2 can also inhibit CDK1 by either inducing p21, which participates in the G2/M checkpoint and contributes to resistance to apoptosis induced by antimicrotubule agents, or directly phosphorylating (inactivating) CDK1, which may block taxane-mediated entry into mitosis and apoptosis. Consistent with this relationship, downregulation of HER-2 by the anti-HER-2 antibody trastuzumab sensitizes breast cancer cells to the taxanes, and the combination of trastuzumab and either paclitaxel or docetaxel is associated with increased survival compared with the taxanes alone.[325,326] Nevertheless, the presence of amplified HER-2 does not adversely influence response to first-line paclitaxel-containing chemotherapy.[212] In one study, the expression and/or amplification of HER-2 related to benefit is derived from the addition of paclitaxel after adjuvant treatment with doxorubicin plus cyclophosphamide in lymph node-positive breast cancer regardless of estrogen-receptor status, whereas women with HER-2-negative disease derived little, if any, benefit.[212]

Clinical pharmacology

General

The taxanes are most commonly administered intravenously at every 3-week intervals at dosages ranging from 175 to 225 mg/m² over 3 h (paclitaxel), 75 to 100 mg/m² over 1 h (docetaxel), 260 mg/m² over 30–40 min (PBPPI), or 25 mg/m² (cabazitaxel), but other schedules, particularly weekly schedules, are commonly used (see section titled "Administration, Dose, and Schedule"). PBPPI is registered at a dose of either 100 or 125 mg/m² on days 1, 8, and 15 of an every 21- or 28-day schedule, respectively, for treating patients with nonsmall cell lung cancer (with carboplatin) or pancreatic cancer (with gemcitabine) in the first-line metastatic setting. For the most part, the oral bioavailability of the taxanes is poor and erratic, which is due, in part, to the constitutive overexpression of Pgp and P-450 metabolizing capability of enterocytes and/or first-pass metabolism. As shown in Table 2, the taxanes share the following pharmacologic characteristics: large Vd, rapid and avid binding to all tissues except for the unperturbed central

nervous system, long terminal half-lives and substantial hepatic metabolism, biliary excretion, and fecal elimination. Cabazitaxel differs in some respects, particularly its ability to penetrate the blood–brain barrier, which may be explained by its reduced substrate affinity for Pgp.

Paclitaxel

Paclitaxel's pharmacokinetic behavior is nonlinear or pseudononlinear.[292,327–329] Nonlinear behavior is more apparent with shorter infusions that result in higher plasma paclitaxel concentrations and more effective saturation of both drug elimination and tissue distribution processes. Both saturable distribution and elimination processes are, in part, responsible for paclitaxel's nonlinear behavior, with tissue distribution becoming effectively saturated at lower drug concentrations (achieved with paclitaxel dosages of <175 mg/m² over 3 h) as compared with elimination processes that are saturated at higher concentrations (achieved with paclitaxel dosages >175 mg/m² over 3 h). A potential ramification of true nonlinearity is that dose escalation may result in a disproportionate increase in drug exposure and toxicity, whereas dose reduction may result in a disproportionate reduction in drug exposure. However, the range of effective doses is relatively broad. Further, the use of shorter infusion schedules also results in higher plasma concentrations of paclitaxel's polyoxyethylated castor oil vehicle, which may simulate nonlinearity (pseudononlinearity) by binding paclitaxel and inhibiting drug distribution and clearance.[330,331]

The pharmacologic behavior of paclitaxel in plasma has been modeled as either triphasic or biphasic. The initial rapid decline represents distribution to the peripheral compartment and elimination of the drug. The later phase is due, in part, to a relatively slow efflux of paclitaxel from the peripheral compartment. Its Vd is much larger than the volume of total body water, indicating extensive drug binding to plasma proteins or other tissue elements, most likely tubulin, which is ubiquitous. Plasma protein binding is reversible and ranges from 89% to 98%.[292] Albumin and α1-acid glycoprotein contribute nearly equally to drug binding with a minor contribution from lipoproteins.[332–334] None of the drugs that are commonly administered with paclitaxel, including ranitidine, dexamethasone, diphenhydramine, doxorubicin, 5-fluorouracil, and cisplatin, significantly alter protein binding.[334] Drug binding to tubulin-rich platelets is extensive and saturable, and animal distribution studies with radiolabeled paclitaxel indicate extensive uptake and retention by virtually all tissues except for normal sanctuary sites such as the brain and testes, possibly due to xenobiotic efflux pumps in these tissues.[335,336]

Clearance is closely related to body surface area, providing a rationale for dosing based on this parameter. In humans, peak plasma concentrations achieved with 3- to 96-h schedules (more than 0.05–10 μmol/L) and drug concentrations in third-space fluid collections such as ascites (>0.1 μmol/L), are capable of inducing relevant biologic effects *in vitro*, but drug penetration into the unperturbed central nervous system is negligible.[292,337,338] The principal mode of paclitaxel disposition is hepatic metabolism and biliary excretion. The liver metabolizes and excretes both paclitaxel and paclitaxel metabolites into the bile, which is eliminated in the feces.[292,336,339–344] In rats treated with radiolabeled paclitaxel, 98% of radioactivity is recovered from feces collected for 6 days, and approximately 71% of an administered dose of paclitaxel is excreted in the feces over 5 days as either parent compound or metabolites in humans, with 6α-hydroxypaclitaxel being the largest component, accounting for 26% of the dose; unmetabolized paclitaxel accounts for only 5% of the dose. Renal clearance of paclitaxel and metabolites may account for up to 14% of the administered

Table 2 Taxanes: comparative pharmacokinetic and toxicologic characteristics.

Parameter	Paclitaxel	PBPPI	Docetaxel	Cabazitaxel
Standard adult dose				
Range (mg/m²/3 week)	175–225 (3-h infusion)	260 (30-min infusion)	75–100 (1-h infusion)	25 (1-h infusion)
(mg/m²/week)	80	100–125 (× 3 weeks every 4 weeks)[b]	30–36	
Pharmacokinetic behavior (clinically relevant doses)	Triphasic	Biphasic	Triphasic	Triphasic
Dose-proportional pharmacokinetics	Saturable taxane elimination and distribution; pseudononlinearity due to vehicle	Dose proportional to 360 mg/m²	Dose proportional to 115 mg/m²	Dose proportional to 30 mg/m²
Plasma half-life (terminal phase)	10–20 h	27 h	10–20 h	95 h
Clearance	20–25 L/h[a]	15 L/h/m²	36 L/h	48.5 L/h
Primary route	Hepatic metabolism and biliary elimination	Hepatic metabolism and biliary elimination	Hepatic metabolism and biliary elimination	Hepatic metabolism and biliary elimination
Principal toxicity	Neutropenia	Neutropenia	Neutropenia	Neutropenia
Other toxicities	Alopecia, neurotoxicity, myalgia, arthralgia, hypersensitivity reactions, asthenia	Alopecia, neurotoxicity, arthralgia, hypersensitivity reactions, nausea, vomiting, diarrhea, skin	Alopecia, skin and nail toxicity, asthenia, myalgia, arthralgia, fluid retention, neurotoxicity, hypersensitivity reactions	Diarrhea, fatigue, asthenia, nausea, vomiting, neurotoxicity, constipation, alopecia, skin and nail toxicity, hypersensitivity reactions, arthralgia

[a] 175 mg/m² over 3 h (dose schedule).

[b] 100 or 125 mg/m²/weekly × 3 weeks every 4 weeks combined with gemcitabine (pancreatic cancer) or carboplatin (nonsmall cell lung cancer), respectively.

dose.[292] In humans, cytochrome P450 mixed-function oxidases are responsible for the bulk of drug disposition, specifically the isoenzymes CYP2C8 and CYP3A4, which metabolize paclitaxel to 6α-hydroxypaclitaxel and another hydroxylated metabolite, both of which are much less active than paclitaxel *in vivo*, possibly due to their greater polarity which precludes intracellular uptake.[292,336,339–342] There is considerable interindividual variability in paclitaxel metabolism that can be attributed to pharmacogenetic differences in P450 metabolism and concurrent medications that alter metabolism.[292,341–344]

Pharmacodynamic analyses demonstrate that drug exposure relates to the principal toxicities of paclitaxel, the most important and consistent of which is the relationship between neutropenia and the duration of drug exposure above biologically relevant plasma concentrations ranging from 0.05 to 0.1 µmol/L.[292,345] A prospective analysis of pharmacokinetic determinants of outcome in several hundred patients with advanced nonsmall cell lung cancer treated with the combination of cisplatin and paclitaxel at either 135 or 250 mg/m² over 24 h demonstrated that the magnitude of the steady-state plasma paclitaxel concentration relates to neither objective response, disease-free survival, nor overall survival.[345]

Docetaxel

The pharmacokinetics of docetaxel (1-h schedule) in plasma are similar to that of paclitaxel. Docetaxel is cleared from plasma in a triphasic manner and linear at doses of 115 mg/m² or less.[200,346–351] The distribution phases are rapid (α- and β-phase $t_{1/2}$ values of 4 and 36 min, respectively), and the terminal half-life is long ($t_{1/2\gamma}$ range, 11.1 to 18.5 h in one study) for the same reasons as discussed earlier for paclitaxel. In one population study, plasma concentration data revealed triphasic pharmacokinetics and the following pharmacokinetic parameters: $t_{1/2\gamma}$ of 12.4 h, clearance of 21 L/h/m², and steady-state Vd of 74 L/m².[200,346–351] The most important determinants of docetaxel clearance were body surface area, hepatic function, and plasma α1-acid glycoprotein concentration, whereas age and plasma albumin level had significant, albeit minor, influences on clearance. Like paclitaxel, plasma protein binding is high (>80–97%), and binding is primarily to α1-acid glycoprotein, albumin, and lipoproteins.[352,353] Like paclitaxel,

docetaxel is widely distributed to peripheral tissues and released slowly, but the agent does not enter "sanctuary sites" laden with Pgp efflux pump barriers such as the unperturbed central nervous system. In both dogs and mice treated with radiolabeled drug, fecal excretion accounts for 70–80% of total radioactivity, whereas urinary excretion accounts for 10% or less. In limited human studies in which cancer patients were administered radiolabeled docetaxel, about 6% and 75% of the administered radioactivity was excreted in the urine and feces, respectively, over 7 days. Approximately 80% of radioactivity excreted in the feces occurs during the first 48 h as one major and three minor metabolites, with very small amounts (<8%) consisting of unchanged docetaxel. The hepatic cytochrome P450 mixed-function oxidases, particularly CYP3A, the activity of which, in adults, is represented by the combined activities of CYP3A4, CYP3A5, CYP3A7, and CYP3A43, is responsible for most of docetaxel's metabolism.[354–356] In contrast to paclitaxel, the C-13 side chain, instead of the taxane ring, is metabolized.[354–357] These metabolites are much less active than docetaxel.

The principal pharmacokinetic determinants of toxicity, particularly neutropenia, are drug exposure and the time that plasma concentrations exceed biologically relevant concentrations.[351] A population pharmacodynamic analysis of determinants of outcome in phase II trials of docetaxel revealed that the most important determinants of the time to progression in patients with metastatic breast cancer are the pretreatment plasma concentration of α1-acid glycoprotein, number of prior chemotherapy regimens, and number of disease sites, whereas both drug exposure and the pretreatment plasma concentration of α1-acid glycoprotein were positive determinants of time to progression in patients with advanced lung cancer.[347,349] Conversely, the pretreatment plasma level of α1-acid glycoprotein was negatively, albeit significantly, related to the probability of experiencing severe neutropenia and febrile neutropenia. Docetaxel clearance has also been related to CYP3A4 activity, as assessed by the [¹⁴C-*N*-methyl]erythromycin breath test.[355]

PBPPI

In clinical studies that evaluated the administration of PBPPI at doses ranging from 80 to 360 mg/m², paclitaxel pharmacokinetics were dose proportional and independent of infusion duration in the range of 30–180 min.[285,286,358,359] Clearance was 43% faster and the Vd was 53% higher for PBPPI than for paclitaxel formulated in polyoxyethylated castor oil, and there were no appreciable differences in terminal $t_{1/2}$. At the recommended dose of 260 mg/m^2 for patients with advanced breast cancer, total clearance averaged 15 L/h/m^2, and the Vd averaged 632 L/m^2, which suggests extensive extravascular distribution and/or tissue binding of paclitaxel following administration of PBPPI. About 89–98% of paclitaxel is protein bound *in vitro*. In a within-patient comparison study, the fraction of unbound paclitaxel in plasma was significantly higher with PBPPI (6.2%) than with solvent-based paclitaxel (2.3%), possibly contributing to higher exposure to unbound paclitaxel with PBBPI compared with solvent-based paclitaxel, when the total exposure is comparable.[358,359] As expected, PBBPI and solvent-based paclitaxel have similar metabolic profiles. Fecal and urinary excretion accounts for approximately 20% and 4% of the total dose of PBBPI administered. In a study that examined plasma pharmacokinetics and partitioning of radiolabeled paclitaxel from PBBPI and a polyoxyethylated paclitaxel formulation into red blood cells and tumor tissue for 24 h following tail vein injection of 20 mg/kg paclitaxel in an MX-1 human breast cancer xenograft, the distribution of PBPPI was rapid and extensive, as manifested by a fivefold larger Vd and much lower C_{max} and area under the concentration–time curve (AUC) values compared with a polyoxyethylated castor oil formulation.[285,358,359] Furthermore, PBBPI demonstrated a significantly lower plasma/blood ratio of paclitaxel across all time points and distributed more effectively into MX-1 tumors. Tumor AUC values of paclitaxel were 1.6-fold higher, on average, with PBBPI, and terminal half-life values for PBBPI were significantly longer than from the polyoxyethylated castor oil formulation (17.1 vs. 4.0 h). The prolonged half-life of PBPPI could be attributed to red blood cell penetration and temporary storage of paclitaxel for PBBPI releasing paclitaxel as plasma levels decrease.

Cabazitaxel

In clinical studies in which cabazitaxel has been administered at doses of 10–30 mg/m^2, plasma disposition is triphasic and dose proportional.[203,360,361] Similar to paclitaxel and docetaxel, the distribution of the agent from the central compartment is rapid, while elimination from the peripheral compartment is slow, most likely due to extensive tissue distribution and avid binding to tubulin; α-, β-, and γ-phase $t_{1/2}$ values averaged 4.4 min, 1.6 h, and 95 h, respectively, in a population pharmacokinetic study; cabazitaxel had a plasma clearance of 48.5 L/h.[203,360,361] Cabazitaxel is equally distributed between blood and plasma, and its Vd is large, averaging 2.64 L/m^2 at steady state. The binding of cabazitaxel to human serum proteins, mainly almumin and lipoproteins, ranges from 89% to 92% *in vitro*.

Cabazitaxel is extensively metabolized in the liver (>95%), mainly by the CYP3A4 and CYP3A5 isoenzyme (80–90%) and to a lesser extent by CYP2C8.[361] Cabazitaxel is the principal circulating moiety in human plasma, but seven metabolites have also been detected, three of which are active and formed by *O*-demethylation, with the main one accounting for 5% of cabazitaxel exposure. Approximately 20 metabolites of cabazitaxel are excreted into human urine and feces. Following administration of radiolabeled cabazitaxel, approximately 80% of the administered dose was eliminated within 2 weeks, with 76% and 3.7% excreted as cabazitaxel and metabolites in the feces and urine, respectively.

Drug interactions

Both sequence-dependent pharmacokinetic and toxicologic interactions between taxanes and several other chemotherapy agents have been noted.[362] The most prominent sequence-dependent effects relate to the platinum compound and the taxanes, particularly with protracted taxane administration schedules. Sequence dependence has been principally noted with paclitaxel, which most likely relates to the fact that docetaxel has been evaluated on a shorter (e.g., 1-h) schedule. The sequence of cisplatin followed by paclitaxel (24-h schedule) induces more profound neutropenia than the reverse sequence, which is explained by a 33% reduction in the clearance of paclitaxel following cisplatin.[363,364] The less toxic sequence, paclitaxel before cisplatin, was demonstrated to induce more cytotoxicity *in vitro*, and therefore it was selected for clinical development.[364] Treatment with paclitaxel on either a 3-h or 24-h schedule followed by carboplatin results in equivalent neutropenia and less thrombocytopenia as compared with carboplatin as a single agent, which is not explained by pharmacokinetic interactions.[365,366] Both mucositis and neutropenia are more severe when paclitaxel on a 24-h schedule is administered before doxorubicin, as compared with the reverse sequence, which is most likely caused by an approximately 32% reduction in the clearance of doxorubicin and doxorubicinol when the agent is administered after paclitaxel.[367–369] Neither sequence-dependent pharmacologic nor toxicologic interactions between doxorubicin and paclitaxel on a shorter (3-h) schedule have been noted; however, the doxorubicin clearance is reduced with both sequences, and the combination of paclitaxel (3-h schedule) and doxorubicin (bolus infusion) produces a much higher rate of congestive cardiotoxicity than would have been expected from an equivalent cumulative doxorubicin dose given without paclitaxel (see section titled "Toxicity").[367,368] Although similar decrements in the clearance of epirubicin and its metabolites have been noted in studies of paclitaxel combined with epirubicin, an increased incidence of cardiotoxicity has not been observed.[370] The precise etiology for these interactions is unclear. The pharmacokinetic interactions may not be of any sufficient magnitude to account for the enhanced cardiotoxicity of the combination, and there are experimental data indicating that paclitaxel enhances the metabolism of doxorubicin to cardiotoxic metabolites, such as doxorubicinol, in cardiomyocytes. Docetaxel does not appear to influence doxorubicin pharmacokinetics, but, like paclitaxel, docetaxel can enhance the metabolism of doxorubicin to toxic species in the human heart.[371] Competition for hepatic or biliary Pgp transport of the anthracyclines with paclitaxel or its polyoxyethylated castor oil vehicle, or both, is an alternate explanation.[291,362,367] Similar effects have not been noted with docetaxel, which is not formulated in polyoxyethylated castor oil. Hematologic toxicity has been more profound with the sequence of cyclophosphamide before paclitaxel (24-h schedule) than with the reverse sequence.[372] Sequence-dependent cytotoxic effects have been reported when the taxanes are combined with 5-fluorouracil, etoposide, cytosine arabinoside, fludarabine, and flavopiridol, among other agents *in vitro*.[362] In human tumor xenografts, both paclitaxel and docetaxel induce thymidine phosphorylase activity, which may increase the metabolic activation of the oral fluoropyrimidine prodrug capecitabine.[373,374]

Interactions between the taxanes and other classes of drugs, particularly those dependent on cytochrome P450-dependent metabolism, have been noted as well.[374] Strong inducers of cytochrome P450 mixed-function oxidases, such as the anticonvulsants phenytoin and phenobarbital, accelerate the metabolism of the taxanes in microsomal systems, as well as in both children and adults who are concurrently receiving treatment with these anticonvulsants, as manifested by rapid drug clearance and tolerance of higher taxane doses.[292,336,340,342,362,367,368,375–378] There is preclinical evidence to suggest that docetaxel has a reduced propensity to cause drug interactions that may entail hepatic CYP3A4 induction.[344] Conversely, many types of agents that inhibit cytochrome P450 mixed-function oxidases, especially CYP3A4, such as orphenadrine, erythromycin, cimetidine, testosterone, ketoconazole, fluconazole, midazolam, polyoxyethylated castor oil, and corticosteroids, interfere with the metabolism of paclitaxel (in both albumin and solvent formulations), docetaxel, and cabazitaxel in human microsomes *in vitro*. Besides the potent inhibitors of CYP3A4 listed earlier, other well-established inhibitors and inducers of CYP3A, including grapefruit juice and herbal products (e.g., St. John's wort and *Echinacea*), may potentially induce pharmacokinetic interactions with the taxanes. Although there has been concern that the use of different H2-receptor antagonists with variable cytochrome P450 inhibitory activities as components of premedication regimens may differentially affect drug clearance and hence toxicity, neither toxicologic nor pharmacologic differences between the agents were noted in a randomized clinical trial.[379] A review of early clinical trial results with docetaxel has not demonstrated significant alterations in docetaxel clearance by corticosteroids. In addition, interactions between warfarin and the taxanes, possibly due to protein-binding displacement effects, have been reported.[380] The incidence of congestive heart failure has also been higher in breast cancer patients treated with the combination of trastuzumab and paclitaxel than with paclitaxel alone, but the explanation for this observation has not been determined.[381–383]

Preclinical studies indicate that PBPPI and paclitaxel formulated in polyoxyethylated castor oil are likely to have similar drug interactions.[286,359] The protein binding of paclitaxel in PBPPI is not affected by cimetidine, ranitidine, nor dexamethasone *in vitro*. Although paclitaxel metabolism is inhibited by many agents, including ketoconazole, verapamil, diazepam, quinidine, dexamethasone, cyclosporine, teniposide, etoposide, and VCR, the concentrations used in these studies exceed those achieved in the clinic. Testosterone, 17α-ethinyl estradiol, retinoic acid, and quercetin, a specific inhibitor of CYP2C8, also inhibited the formation of the principal metabolite, 6α-hydroxypaclitaxel, *in vitro*. Similar to paclitaxel in polyoxyethylated castor oil, paclitaxel pharmacokinetics following PBPPI administration may be altered as a result of interactions with compounds that are substrates, inducers, or inhibitors of CYP2C8 and/or CYP3A4.

Toxicity

General

Myelosuppression is the principal toxicity of the taxanes. However, despite similar structures, these agents possess modest differences in their toxicity spectra.

Paclitaxel

Neutropenia is the principal toxicity of paclitaxel.[384] The onset is usually on days 8–10, and recovery typically occurs by days 15–21. The main clinical determinant for the severity of neutropenia is the extent of prior myelosuppressive therapy; however, neutropenia is typically noncumulative, and the duration of severe neutropenia even in heavily pretreated patients is generally brief. Pharmacokinetic parameters of paclitaxel in plasma that reflect drug exposure, particularly the duration that plasma concentrations are maintained above biologically relevant levels (0.05–0.10 μmol/L;

see section titled "Clinical Pharmacology"), relate to the severity of neutropenia, which may explain why neutropenia is more severe with longer infusion schedules.[385,386] Paclitaxel distributes widely and avidly even following treatment on short schedules, and therefore protracted schedules do not seem to confer superior anticancer activity. At paclitaxel dosages exceeding 175 mg/m^2 on a 24-h schedule and 225 mg/m^2 on a 3-h schedule, neutrophil counts typically decrease to below 500/μL for fewer than 5 days in most courses, even in untreated patients. Even patients who have received extensive prior therapy can usually tolerate paclitaxel dosages in the range of 175–200 mg/m^2 administered over 3 or 24 h. More frequent schedules, particularly weekly treatment with 80–100 mg/m^2, have resulted in less severe neutropenia than single-dosing schedules (see section titled "Administration, Dose, and Schedule"). Severe thrombocytopenia and anemia are unusual, except in heavily pretreated patients with diminished hematopoietic stem cell capacity. The incidence of major hypersensitivity reactions (HSRs) in early phase I trials approached 30%, but the incidence is approximately 1–3% following the advent and broad adoption of effective prophylaxis.[377–393]

Most major reactions are characterized by dyspnea with bronchospasm, urticaria, and hypotension, which typically occur within the first 10 min after the first, and less frequently after the second, treatment. Major HSRs generally resolve completely after stopping treatment and occasionally after treatment with antihistamines, fluids, and vasopressors. Patients who have major reactions have been rechallenged successfully after receiving high doses of corticosteroids, but this approach is not always successful.[384,387–390] Patients who have experienced paclitaxel-related HSRs have also received other taxanes, such as docetaxel uneventfully.[394] Less severe manifestations of hypersensitivity phenomena, such as flushing and rashes, have been noted in as many as 40% of patients, and it is particularly important to note that minor HSRs do not portend the development of major reactions. The HSRs are most likely caused by a nonimmunologically mediated release of histamine or histamine-like substances in the polyoxyethylated castor oil vehicle, but the taxane moiety may also be contributory.[384,393] In some cases, complement activation has been demonstrated.[394] Although the incidence of major HSRs is reduced with lower administration rates and longer infusion durations, the rates of major reactions are low on both 3- and 24-h schedules when patients are premedicated with corticosteroids and both H1- and H2-histamine antagonists (see section titled "Administration, Dose, and Schedule"). In an assessment of the relative safety of two different paclitaxel schedules (24 h vs. 3 h), the rates of major reactions were low and similar (2.1% vs. 1.0%) in patients receiving paclitaxel for 3 or 24 h, respectively, with premedication.[384,395]

A peripheral neuropathy dominated by sensory manifestations, such as numbness and paresthesia, in a glove-and-stocking distribution is the principal neurotoxic effect of paclitaxel.[384,396,397] There is often symmetric distal loss of sensation carried by both large (proprioception, vibration) and small (temperature, pinprick) fibers. Symptoms may begin as soon as 24–72 h after treatment with higher doses (≥250 mg/m^2), but usually occur only after multiple courses at 135–250 mg/m^2 every 3 weeks or 80–100 mg/m^2 weekly, and are cumulative thereafter. Severe neurotoxicity precludes chronic treatment with paclitaxel at dosages above 250 mg/m^2 over 3 h or 24 h, but severe neurotoxicity is uncommon at conventional doses (<200 mg/m^2) of paclitaxel alone even in patients who previously received other neurotoxic agents such as cisplatin. Patients treated with paclitaxel over shorter (e.g., 3-h) schedules may be more prone to the neurotoxicity compared with those treated with longer (e.g., 24- or 96-h) schedules, which argues that peak concentration may be a principal pharmacologic determinant of neurotoxicity. Neurotoxicity is particularly common and severe in patients receiving paclitaxel as a 3-h infusion combined with cisplatin. The distal, symmetric, length-dependent neurologic deficits suggest that paclitaxel causes a sensory and motor axonal loss similar to the dying back neuropathies that may have their origin in the cell body or in axonal transport, but a few patients have the simultaneous onset of symptoms in the arms and legs, involvement of the face (perioral numbness), the predominance of large fiber loss, and diffuse areflexia, suggestive of a neuronopathy. Both types of neuropathy depend on the dose of paclitaxel or its combination with cisplatin.[364,398] Motor and autonomic dysfunction may also occur, especially at high doses and in patients with preexisting neuropathies caused by diabetes mellitus and alcoholism. Although the administration of amifostine, glutamate, pyridoxine, sulfhydryl group scavenger drugs, and anticonvulsants reduces the neurotoxic effects of paclitaxel in some experimental models, anecdotal reports, or insufficiently powered randomized trials, there is no convincing evidence that any specific measure effectively ameliorates existing manifestations or prevents development or worsening of neurotoxicity.[398–400]

Optic nerve disturbances, characterized by scintillating scotomata, may also occur.[401] Acute encephalopathy, which can progress to coma and death, has been reported following treatment with high doses (>600 mg/m^2).[402] A transient acute encephalopathy following paclitaxel treatment in patients who receive prior cranial irradiation is rare.[403]

Paclitaxel may produce transient myalgia without physical or biochemical evidence of myositis. Myalgia is typically experienced 2–5 days after treatment with doses above 170 mg/m^2.[384,404] A constellation of muscular and neuropathic effects often precludes continuous treatment with paclitaxel administered on a weekly schedule, requiring the institution of rest periods. In general, nonsteroidal anti-inflammatory agents are effective at palliating or preventing symptoms, and the use of narcotics prophylactically on days 2–5 posttreatment may be useful in previously affected patients. Antihistamines have been anecdotally reported to prevent acute myalgia. Treatment with corticosteroids, specifically prednisone 10 mg twice daily for 5 days beginning 24 h after treatment, has been reported to be effective at reducing myalgia and arthralgia, and gabapentin, glutamate, and antihistamines may be useful for management or prevention.

In the early studies, where routine cardiac monitoring was performed because of the high rate of major HSRs, paclitaxel was noted to cause cardiac rhythm disturbances, an overwhelming majority of which was not associated with symptoms or sequelae; therefore, the clinical relevance of these effects is not known.[384,405] The most common rhythm disturbance is transient bradycardia. The cumulative experience to date suggests that isolated asymptomatic bradycardia without hemodynamic effects is not an indication for discontinuing paclitaxel. More important bradyarrhythmias, including Mobitz type 1 (Wenckebach syndrome), Mobitz type 2, and third-degree heart block, have been noted, but the incidence in a large National Cancer Institute database was only 0.1%.[406] Most documented episodes have been asymptomatic. Because such events were noted in patients enrolled in early trials that required continuous cardiac monitoring, second- and third-degree heart blocks are likely underreported because cardiac monitoring is not usually performed. Interestingly, reports of similar disturbances in both animals and humans who ingested various species of yew plants and related taxanes affecting cardiac automaticity and conduction suggest that the bradyarrhythmias are caused by paclitaxel. Myocardial infarction, cardiac ischemia, atrial arrhythmias, and

ventricular tachycardia have been noted, but whether there is a causal relationship between paclitaxel and these events is uncertain. There is no evidence that chronic, long-term treatment with paclitaxel causes progressive cardiac dysfunction. Routine cardiac monitoring during therapy is not necessary, but is recommended for those patients who may not be able to tolerate bradyarrhythmias, such as those with atrioventricular conduction disturbances or ventricular dysfunction. Although patients with a wide range of cardiac abnormalities and cardiac histories were broadly and empirically restricted from participating in early clinical trials, paclitaxel treatment has been reported to be well tolerated in a small series of gynecologic cancer patients with major cardiac risk factors.[357] On the other hand, repetitive treatment of patients with the combined regimen of paclitaxel on a 3-h schedule and doxorubicin as a brief infusion is associated with a higher frequency of congestive cardiotoxicity than would be expected to occur with the same cumulative doxorubicin dose given without paclitaxel (see section titled "Drug Interactions"). In one study in previously untreated women with advanced breast cancer treated with escalating doses of paclitaxel as a 3-h infusion and doxorubicin 60 mg/m^2 to a cumulative dose of 480 mg/m^2, which would be predicted to result in a less than 5% incidence of cardiotoxicity in patients treated with doxorubicin alone, the incidence of congestive cardiotoxicity was approximately 25%.[367] However, the incidence of cardiotoxicity was <5% when similar patients received identical schedules of paclitaxel and doxorubicin, but the cumulative doxorubicin dose did not exceed 360 mg/m^2.[407,408] Both experimental and early clinical results suggest that deferoxamine may reduce the cardiotoxicity of the doxorubicin–paclitaxel combination.[407,408] The incidence of congestive heart failure was also significantly higher in breast cancer patients treated with the combination of trastuzumab and paclitaxel than in those treated with paclitaxel alone in a randomized phase III trial; consequently, careful monitoring of patients receiving this combination is warranted.[212–214]

Gastrointestinal toxicities, including nausea, vomiting, and diarrhea, are uncommon. Higher paclitaxel doses may cause mucositis, especially in patients with leukemia who may be more prone to mucosal barrier breakdown or in patients receiving protracted infusions. Rare cases of neutropenic enterocolitis and gastrointestinal necrosis have been noted, particularly in patients given high doses of paclitaxel in combination with doxorubicin or cyclophosphamide.[409,410] Severe hepatotoxicity and pancreatitis have also been noted, but these events are rare. Acute bilateral pneumonitis occurs in <1% of patients treated on a 3-h schedule in one series, and both interstitial and parenchymal pulmonary toxicities have been reported, but clinically significant pulmonary effects are uncommon.[391,411]

Paclitaxel also induces reversible alopecia of the scalp, but all body hair is usually lost with cumulative therapy. Alopecia appears to be dose related and occurs only following repetitive treatment with weekly administration. Although the agent is often not considered a vesicant, extravasation of large volumes can cause moderate soft tissue injury. Inflammation at the injection site and along the course of an injected vein can occur.[412] Nail disorders have been noted, particularly in patients treated on weekly schedules. Radiation recall reactions have been reported. Taxane-induced taste alterations are common.

Docetaxel

Similar to paclitaxel, neutropenia is the principal toxicity of docetaxel.[200,413,414] At dosages ranging from 75 to 100 mg/m^2 administered as a 1-h infusion, neutrophil counts usually decrease to below 500/μL. The onset of neutropenia is usually noted on day 8 and complete resolution typically occurs by days 15–21. Neutropenia is significantly less when low doses are administered frequently, such as on a weekly schedule (see section titled "Administration, Dose, and Schedule"). The most important determinant of neutropenia is the extent of prior therapy, but α1-acid glycoprotein and the duration of drug exposure above biologically relevant concentrations appear to be important determinants (see section titled "Clinical Pharmacology"). Significant effects on platelets and red blood cells are uncommon.

Even though docetaxel is not formulated in polyoxyethylated castor oil, HSRs have been reported in approximately 31% of patients receiving docetaxel without premedications, but most are not severe.[200,413,414] Nevertheless, major reactions, characterized by dyspnea, bronchospasm, and hypotension, particularly during the first two courses and within minutes after the start of treatment, have been reported. Manifestations generally resolve within 15 min after cessation of treatment, and docetaxel is usually able to be reinstituted without consequences, occasionally after treatment with an H1-histamine antagonist. Both the incidence and severity of HSRs appear to be reduced significantly by premedication with corticosteroids and both H1- and H2-histamine antagonists (see section titled "Administration, Dose, and Schedule"). Like paclitaxel, patients who experience major HSRs have been re-treated successfully after resolution of symptoms and following treatment with corticosteroids and Hl-histamine antagonists. Although patients who have experienced HSRs following paclitaxel treatment have been re-treated successfully with docetaxel, this strategy has not been studied in a rigorous fashion.

In early studies, a unique fluid retention syndrome, characterized by edema, weight gain, and third-space fluid collection (e.g., pericardial, pleural, ascites), has been noted in patients treated with multiple courses of docetaxel.[200,413–416] Fluid retention did not appear to be related to hypoalbuminemia or cardiac, renal, or hepatic dysfunction, but to increased capillary permeability. Capillary filtration studies revealed a two-stage process with progressive congestion of the interstitial space by proteins and water, starting between the second and fourth course that progressed to insufficient lymphatic drainage. In early studies in which prophylactic medication was not used, fluid retention was not usually significant at cumulative docetaxel doses below 400 mg/m², however, the incidence and severity of fluid retention increased sharply at cumulative doses exceeding 400 mg/m² and often resulted in the delay or termination of treatment. Prophylactic treatment with corticosteroids with or without H1- and H2-histamine antagonists reduces the incidence of fluid retention and increases the number of courses and cumulative docetaxel dose before the onset of this toxicity (see section titled "Administration, Dose, and Schedule").[415] In fact, drug-induced fluid retention has been uncommon following the broad adoption of corticosteroid premedication. Fluid retention resolves slowly after docetaxel is stopped, with complete resolution occurring several months after treatment in patients with severe toxicity. Aggressive and early treatment with progressively more potent diuretics, starting with potassium-sparing diuretics, has been successfully used to manage fluid retention. The incidence of fluid retention appears to be lower in studies that used lower doses (60–75 mg/m²) during each course, but this may be a result of the administration of lower overall cumulative doses, and the effects of lower doses on anticancer activity are unknown.

Although both neurosensory and neuromuscular effects due to docetaxel are similar to paclitaxel, they are less common and appear to be less severe compared with paclitaxel.[200,397,413,414,417] In a phase III trial, patients with advanced ovarian carcinoma receiving first-line treatment with docetaxel and carboplatin experienced less severe neurotoxicity than did those receiving treatment with paclitaxel and carboplatin.[417,418] Mild to moderate peripheral neurotoxicity is observed in approximately 40% of previously untreated patients. Previous treatment with platinating agents appears to increase the likelihood of developing neurotoxicity. The neurotoxicity is qualitatively similar to that of paclitaxel, with sensory effects predominating.[364,396–400] Patients typically complain of paresthesia and numbness, but peripheral motor disturbances may also occur. Severe toxicity is unusual following repetitive treatment with docetaxel doses <100 mg/m², except in patients with antecedent disorders such as alcohol abuse.

Although cardiovascular effects, including angina, arrhythmia, conduction disturbances, congestive heart failure, hypertension, and hypotension, have been noted rarely in the pretreatment period, there is no convincing evidence that directly links docetaxel to these events. Stomatitis appears to occur more frequently with docetaxel than paclitaxel, particularly with prolonged infusions that are used rarely. Nausea, vomiting, and diarrhea have also been observed infrequently, and severe manifestations are rare.

Phlebitis along the course of the infused veins and local inflammation at the injection site are occasionally noted; however, severe tissue damage following drug extravasation is not generally observed. Transient arthralgia and myalgia without inflammatory manifestations are occasionally noted within days following treatment. Malaise, often referred to as asthenia, has been a prominent complaint in patients who have been treated with large cumulative doses, particularly when docetaxel is administered on a continuous weekly schedule.[419]

Skin toxicity may occur in as many as 50–75% of patients;[364,420] however, premedication may reduce the overall incidence of this toxicity. An erythematous pruritic maculopapular rash that affects the forearms, hands, and/or feet is typical. Desquamation of the hands and feet, which is a component of a more general palmar–plantar erythrodysesthesia syndrome that may respond to pyridoxine or cooling, and onychodystrophy characterized by brown discoloration, ridging, onycholysis, soreness, and brittleness and loss of the nail plate have been reported.[318,420] Skin and nail changes appear to be most prominent in patients treated frequently with low doses (i.e., weekly schedules). Excessive lacrimation, occasionally due to canalicular stenosis, may also occur.[421] Other rare events that may or may not be related to docetaxel itself include confusion, erythema multiforme, neutropenic enterocolitis, hepatitis, ileus, interstitial pneumonia, seizures, pulmonary fibrosis, hepatitis, radiation recall, and visual disturbances.

PBPPI

The toxicity profile of PBPPI is similar to that of paclitaxel, with neutropenia as the principal dose-limiting toxicity.[201,283–286,358,359] Most other paclitaxel-related toxicities have also been observed with PBPPI. The rate of HSRs, particularly major reactions, is less with PBPPI than that of paclitaxel formulated in polyoxyethylated castor oil. A premedication regimen to prevent HSRs is not recommended since the rate of HSRs, particularly major reactions, is less with PBPPI than that of paclitaxel formulated in polyoxyethylated castor oil. In randomized studies in patients with either advanced breast or nonsmall cell lung cancer treated with either PBPPI- or paclitaxel-based regimens, toxicity profiles are similar. Neutropenia and neurotoxicity are the principal toxicities of PBPPI. Other relatively common adverse effects include arthralgia, myalgia, asthenia, fatigue, mucositis, and diarrhea. Additional toxicities, most of which are noted with other taxane formulations, include increased lacrimation, conjunctivitis, radiation recall, Stevens–Johnson syndrome, toxic epidermal necrolysis, photosensitivity reactions, and palmar–plantar erythrodysesthesia in patients previously treated with capecitabine.

Cabazitaxel

The adverse effects seen with cabazitaxel are very similar, both qualitatively and quantitatively, to those noted with docetaxel.[203,225,359,360] The most common toxicity is neutropenia, which, like the other taxanes previously discussed, is noncumulative and brief. In the phase III randomized pivotal trial of cabazitaxel plus prednisone versus mitoxantrone plus prednisone in men with castrate-resistant prostate cancer who had received prior treatment with docetaxel, 82% of the patients experienced grade 3–4 neutropenia, 8% experienced neutropenic fever, and several patients experienced fatal adverse infectious events. Severe anemia (11%) and thrombocytopenia (4%) were far less common.[225] Common nonhematologic toxicities were mainly gastrointestinal in nature: diarrhea (47%, all grades), nausea (34%), vomiting (22%), and constipation (20%). Importantly, in this population of patients who previously received docetaxel, severe (grade 3–4) peripheral neuropathy was noted in <1% of patients. Other common adverse effects, without attribution to disease or drug, included fatigue (37%), asthenia (20%), and hematuria (17%), with the most commonly reported nonhematologic grade 3–4 adverse events being diarrhea (6%), fatigue (5%), and asthenia (5%). Anaphylaxis and severe HSRs (dyspnea requiring bronchodilators, hypotension requiring treatment, syncope, or bradycardia) occurred in <4% of patients. Routine premedication, including histamine H1 and H2 receptor antagonists and corticosteroid (see section titled "Administration, Dose and Schedule"), is recommended 30 min prior to reduce this even further. Myalgia, arthralgia, stomatitis, mucositis, and peripheral edema were seen rarely and were mild in severity (grade 1–2). Alopecia occurred in 33% of patients. Nausea, vomiting, and severe diarrhea, at times, may occur. Death related to diarrhea and electrolyte imbalance occurred in the randomized clinical trial.[225] Other gastrointestinal toxicities, including hemorrhage, perforation, ileus, enterocolitis, gastritis, intestinal obstruction, and persistent constipation, have been reported in patients treated with cabazitaxel. Abdominal pain and tenderness, fever, persistent constipation, diarrhea, and with or without neutropenia may be early manifestations of serious gastrointestinal toxicity and should be evaluated and treated promptly. Cabazitaxel treatment delay or discontinuation may be necessary. Transaminitis has been noted rarely.

Administration, dose, and schedule

Paclitaxel

Discerning the optimal dose and schedule for the taxanes, principally paclitaxel, has been a major focus of many evaluations over the last decade. The collective results of these efforts indicate that paclitaxel has prominent anticancer activity on multiple schedules and, although no particular schedule is superior from an efficacy standpoint across all tumor types, a weekly schedule was demonstrated to be superior to an every-3-week schedule in the adjuvant treatment of breast cancer.[422,423] As a rule, however, toxicity profiles are schedule dependent. The earliest clinical studies of paclitaxel were limited to the 24-h schedule, largely as a consequence of an apparent increased rate of severe HSRs on shorter schedules, but the development of effective premedication regimens led to evaluation of a broad range of dosing schedules. Although paclitaxel 135 mg/m^2 on a 24-h schedule was initially approved for patients with refractory and recurrent ovarian cancer, regulatory approval

was later obtained for paclitaxel 175 mg/m^2 on a 3-h schedule in these and other indications. In patients with advanced breast and ovarian cancer, the collective results of randomized studies indicate that response rates have occasionally been higher with more protracted (24–96-h) infusion schedules, but other indices of efficacy do not appear to relate to infusion duration. The extensive distribution of the taxanes to peripheral tissues, as well as the avid and protracted tissue binding of these agents, may explain the lack of substantial differences in anticancer activity between short and more protracted administration schedules despite substantial differences *in vitro*.[385,424,425] There has also been considerable interest in intermittent schedules, particularly those in which paclitaxel is administered as a 1-h infusion weekly, which results in substantially less myelosuppression than every-3-week schedules.[422–424,426,427] Furthermore, there have been reports of impressive and superior activity of weekly compared with every-3-week schedules in several disease settings, particularly in treatment of both early-stage (adjuvant) and advanced breast cancer patients.[210,422,423] However, there is no convincing evidence that weekly treatment results in relevant activity in tumors unresponsive to the taxanes on less intermittent schedules. The weekly schedule may also be advantageous for patients who are at high risk of developing severe myelosuppression, but it seems to confer a higher incidence of neuromuscular effects.

Paclitaxel is indicated and generally administered at a dosage of 175 mg/m^2 over 3 h or, less frequently, 135–175 mg/m^2 over 24 h every 3 weeks. Several randomized trials in patients with advanced lung, head and neck, and ovarian cancers have consistently failed to show that paclitaxel dosages above 135–175 mg/m^2 on a 24-h schedule are superior to conventional doses.[385,424,428] Nearly identical results have been obtained in a phase III study in patients with metastatic breast cancer, in which greater efficacy was not observed in patients treated with paclitaxel dosages above 175 mg/m^2 on a 3-h schedule.[429] The following dosages have been recommended on less conventional schedules: 200 mg/m^2 over 1 h as either a single dose or 3 divided doses every 3 weeks, 140 mg/m^2 over 96 h every 3 weeks, and 80–100 mg/m^2 weekly or weekly for 3 weeks every 4 weeks. The most common schedules evaluated in patients with Kaposi's sarcoma associated with the acquired immunodeficiency syndrome are paclitaxel 135 mg/m^2 over 3 h or 24 h every 3 weeks and 100 mg/m^2 every 2 weeks.[215] Paclitaxel has also been administered into the pleural and peritoneal cavities. Biologically relevant plasma concentrations have been achieved with intraperitoneal administration, and concentrations in the peritoneal cavity are several orders of magnitude higher than plasma concentrations. The following premedication regimen is recommended to prevent major HSRs: dexamethasone 20 mg orally or intravenously, 12 and 6 h before treatment; an H1-histamine antagonist (such as diphenhydramine, 50 mg intravenously) 30 min before treatment; and an H2-histamine antagonist (such as cimetidine, 300 mg; famotidine, 20 mg; or ranitidine, 150 mg intravenously) 30 min before treatment. A single dose of a corticosteroid (dexamethasone 20 mg intravenously) administered 30 min before treatment also appears to confer effective prophylaxis of major HSRs.

Hepatic metabolism and biliary excretion are the principal modes of drug disposition of paclitaxel, and dose modifications are required for patients with hepatic dysfunction. Prospective study results suggest that patients with moderate to severe elevations in serum concentrations of hepatocellular enzymes and/or bilirubin are more predisposed to severe toxicity than patients without hepatic dysfunction. It is therefore recommended that paclitaxel doses be reduced by at least 50% in patients with moderate hepatic dysfunction.[430] It is recommended that doses of paclitaxel on a

3-h schedule be reduced from 175 to 135 mg/m^2 for elevations of hepatic transaminases up to 10 times the upper limit of normal (ULN) and bilirubin to 1.26–2.0 times the ULN. For further elevations of bilirubin up to 5.0 times along with transaminase elevations up to 10 times the ULN, paclitaxel 90 mg/m^2 is recommended. Dose recommendations have not been formulated for more transaminitis and/or hepatic excretory dysfunction. Since renal disposition contributes minimally to overall clearance (5–10%), patients with severe renal dysfunction do not appear to require dose modification.[292,431] Based on the pharmacologic behavior, particularly the wide distributive properties of the taxanes, dose modifications are not required solely for peripheral edema and third-space fluid collections.

Contact of the paclitaxel-polyoxyethylated castor oil formulation with plasticized polyvinyl chloride (PVC) equipment or devices must be avoided because of the risk of patient exposures to plasticizers, especially the extractable plasticizer di-(2-ethylhexyl)phthalate (DEHP), that may be leached from PVC infusion bags or sets. Paclitaxel solutions should be diluted and stored in glass or polypropylene bottles or suitable plastic bags (polypropylene or polyolefin) and administered through non-PVC administration sets such as those that are polyethylene lined. Paclitaxel should be administered through an in-line filter with a microporous membrane not >0.22 μm.

Docetaxel

Docetaxel is indicated at a dosage range of 60–100 mg/m^2 (1-h intravenous infusion) in advanced breast cancer and 75 mg/m^2 as either a single agent or combined with other agents in all other indications. It should be noted that most clinical evaluations focused on docetaxel doses at the higher end of this range (75–100 mg/m^2) and relatively scant data are available for patients treated with docetaxel (60 mg/m^2).[200] Although some untreated or minimally pretreated patients generally tolerate docetaxel at a dose of 100 mg/m^2, which is the only approved dose in select indications in many regions, 75 mg/m^2 appears to be more reasonable from a toxicologic perspective in more heavily re-treated patients.[432] Like paclitaxel, docetaxel has also been administered as a 1-h infusion weekly, but a clear efficacy benefit of a weekly schedule over the conventional every-3-week frequency has not been established.[210,418] Additionally, hematologic toxicity is less with the more frequent weekly schedule. Both cumulative asthenia and neurotoxicity are the principal toxicities of docetaxel administered weekly, precluding treatment with dosages exceeding 36 mg/m^2/week. Despite the use of a polysorbate-80 formulation instead of polyoxyethylated castor oil, which is used to formulate paclitaxel, a relatively high rate of HSRs and profound fluid retention in patients who did not receive premedication has led to the use of several effective premedication regimens, the most popular of which is dexamethasone 8 mg orally twice daily for 3 days starting 1 day before docetaxel, with or without both H1- and H2-histamine antagonists given 30 min before docetaxel.[413,414] For patients with metastatic prostate cancer, given the concurrent use of prednisone, the recommended dose of dexamethasone is 8 mg orally at 8, 3, and 1 h prior to docetaxel. Administration of docetaxel without corticosteroids is not recommended, even in patients who do not develop HSRs, because drug-related fluid retention, which is a chronic toxicity, requires drug discontinuation.[414,415]

A retrospective review of docetaxel pharmacokinetics in patients without hyperbilirubinemia demonstrated that docetaxel clearance is reduced by approximately 25% in patients with elevations in serum concentrations of both hepatic transaminases (1.5-fold or greater) and alkaline phosphatase (2.5-fold or greater), regardless of whether the elevations are a result of hepatic metastases.[346–349,433] Therefore, dose reductions by at least 25% have been recommended for such individuals. Although more substantial reductions may be required in patients who have moderate or severe hepatic excretory dysfunction (hyperbilirubinemia), the near exclusive role of the liver in drug disposal has resulted in the manufacturer's recommendation that docetaxel not be administered to subjects with transaminase elevations exceeding 1.5 times the ULN concomitant with an alkaline phosphatase elevation exceeding 2.5-fold, or an elevated bilirubin value. Similar to paclitaxel (see sections titled "Paclitaxel, Administration, Dose, and Schedule"), there is no rationale for dose modification solely for renal deficiency and/or third-space fluid accumulation. Also similar to the case with paclitaxel (see sections titled "Paclitaxel, Administration, Dose, and Schedule"), contact with plasticized PVC equipment or devices is not recommended. In order to minimize patient exposure to the plasticizer DEHP, which may be leached, bottles (glass or polypropylene) or plastic bags (polypropylene or polyolefin) should be used for preparation and storage, and docetaxel should be administered through polyethylene-lined administration sets.

PBPPI

PBPPI received initially regulatory approval in the United States for the treatment of patients with metastatic breast cancer after failure of combination chemotherapy for metastatic disease or relapse within 6 months of adjuvant chemotherapy.[226] The recommended dosage schedule for this indication is 260 mg/m^2 as a 30-min intravenous infusion; however, notable anticancer activity has been observed on various other schedules, particularly doses in the range of 100–150 mg/m^2 administered as a 30-min intravenous infusion weekly for 3 out of every 4 weeks, similar to the paclitaxel and docetaxel. PBPPI was soon after registered in the United States and elsewhere as first-line treatment of patients with locally advanced or metastatic pancreatic cancer or nonsmall cell lung cancer as a 30–40-min intravenous infusion weekly for 3 weeks every 28 days at doses of either 125 or 100 mg/m^2, respectively, with carboplatin or gemcitabine.[200,227] No premedication to prevent HSRs or edema is recommended prior to administration. The use of specialized DEHP-free (i.e., PVC-free) solution containers and administration are not necessary, and the use of an in-line filter is not recommended. The most appropriate doses for patients with hepatic insufficiency (bilirubin, 1.5 > mg/dL) and renal insufficiency are not known; however, similar to the case with other taxanes, renal disposition is likely negligible. The manufacturer recommends dose reduction from 260 to 200 mg/m^2 or 100 to 80 mg/m^2 for patients with advanced or metastatic breast cancer or nonsmall cell lung cancer, respectively, with moderate or severe hepatic dysfunction as defined by bilirubin elevations that do not exceed five times the ULN with or without transaminase elevations that do not exceed 10 times the ULN. PBPPI is not recommended for pancreatic cancer patients with bilirubin exceeding 1.5 times the ULN. Dose reduction is not necessary for patients with transaminase elevations below 10 times the ULN as long as bilirubin values do not exceed 1.5-fold. The manufacturer does not recommend PBPPI in patients whose bilirubin exceeds 5 times the ULN. It is recommended that patients who experience severe neutropenia and/or thrombocytopenia during PBPPI treatment should have their treatment discontinued until sufficient recovery, followed by dose reduction in subsequent treatments. In cases of severe sensory neuropathy, it is recommended that treatment be discontinued until resolution to mild or moderate manifestations followed by a dose reduction for all subsequent courses. For patients with pancreatic cancer receiving treatment with PBPPI plus gemcitabine, PBPPI treatment is withheld in the event of grade 3 mucositis or diarrhea and resumed at a lower dose following toxicity resolution to grade 1 or less. Lastly, dose reduction of PBPPI is recommended in the event of grade 2 or 3 cutaneous toxicity in patients treated with PBPPI plus gemcitabine, with discontinuation of treatment if the toxicity persists.

Cabazitaxel

Cabazitaxel is indicated for treatment of patients with metastatic castrate-resistant prostate cancer previously treated with a docetaxel-containing treatment regimen.[203,225,360,361] It is specifically indicated at a dose of 25 mg/m^2 as a 60-min infusion administered every 3 weeks in combination with oral prednisone 10 mg daily throughout treatment. Alternate schedules have not been fully evaluated. The following intravenous premedication regimen is recommended at least 30 min prior to each dose of cabazitaxel to reduce the risk and/or severity of HSRs: diphenhydramine 25 mg or an equivalent H1-histamine antagonist, dexamethasone 8 mg or an equivalent steroid, and an H2-histamine antagonist such as ranitidine 50 mg or equivalent. Antiemetic prophylaxis is recommended and can be given orally or intravenously as needed. Like docetaxel, cabazitaxel is formulated in polysorbate-80 and is diluted with ethanol followed by dilution in either 0.9% sodium chloride solution or 5% dextrose solution. Due to the potential for polysorbate-80 to leach plasticizers, neither PVC infusion containers nor polyurethane infusion sets should be used to prepare or administer cabazitaxel. An in-line filter of 0.22 μm nominal pore size (also referred to as 0.2 μm) should be used during administration.

No dedicated hepatic impairment trial for cabazitaxel has been conducted, and therefore no dosing recommendations have been formulated for patients with either hepatic dysfunction or renal impairment. Although docetaxel and cabazitaxel have similar modes of clearance and it may seem reasonable to modify doses similar to docetaxel, the manufacturer does not officially recommend that cabazitaxel be given to patients with hepatic impairment. Based on population pharmacokinetic data, there were no significant differences in clearance in patients with mild to moderate (30 mL/min ≤ creatinine clearance), and dose reduction for such subjects is not warranted. However, caution should be used in patients with severe renal impairment (creatinine clearance < 30 mL/min) and patients with end-stage renal diseases. Similar to paclitaxel, docetaxel, and PBPPI, cabazitaxel doses should be modified and/or treatment held for relevant degrees of neutropenia, diarrhea, and/or peripheral neuropathy. For example, a dose reduction to 20 mg/m^2 is warranted if the patient experienced grade ≥3 neutropenia lasting at least 7 days despite appropriate medication including growth factors following treatment at the 30 mg/m^2 dose level. For patients developing grade ≥3 diarrhea or persistent diarrhea despite appropriate medication, fluid, and electrolyte replacement or grade 2 peripheral neuropathy, cabazitaxel treatment should be held until improvement or resolution followed by dose reduction to 20 mg/m^2. Cabazitaxel should not be administered to patients who have developed peripheral neuropathy of grade 3 severity.

Other natural products that enhance tubulin polymerization

The success of the taxanes has led to efforts to identify other agents that confer cytotoxicity by enhancing tubulin polymerization, yielding several leads over the last two decades, the most relevant of which have been the epothilones. The epothilones are polyketide macrolactones which were initially isolated from the soil-dwelling myxobacterium *Sorangium cellulosum*. Other natural products that enhance tubulin polymerization include discodermolide (isolated from the Caribbean marine sponge *Discodermia dissoluta*), eleutherobin (isolated from the soft coral *Eleutherobia* sp.) and laulimalide (isolated from the marine sponge *Cacospongia mycofijiensis*), peloruside A (isolated from a New Zealand marine sponge *Mycale hentscheli*), the taccalonolides (plant-derived natural steroids), and sarcodictyins (isolated from the Mediterranean stoloniferan coral *Sarcodictyon roseum*). Some of these compounds compete with paclitaxel for binding to microtubules and appear to bind at or near the taxane site (epothilones, discodermolide, eleutherobins, and sarcodictyins), but others, such as laulimalide and peloruside A, seem to bind to unique sites on microtubules.[2–7,237,316] Eleutherobin, epothilones A and B, and discodermolide competitively inhibit paclitaxel binding to microtubules, and a common pharmacophore that may enable the development of hybrid constructs with more desirable biological characteristics was identified.[237,240,316] Interestingly, discodermolide and paclitaxel demonstrate synergistic cytotoxicity *in vitro*, suggesting that their tubulin binding sites and microtubule effects are not identical.[433] However, unforeseen pulmonary toxicity has been seen in early clinical studies of XAA296, a completely synthetic discodermolide.[434] Most of the aforementioned agents, particularly epothilone B, discodermolide, and the taccalonolides, possess either low-level or no substrate affinity for ABC transporters, and others retain various degrees of activity against taxane-resistant cells *in vitro* including βIII-tubulin-expressing malignancies (epothilone B, taccalonolides). Although clinical implications of these characteristics are not entirely clear, the epothilones have demonstrated clinically relevant activity in patients who have been previously treated with taxanes, some of whom are clearly taxane resistant. Of the nontaxane tubulin-polymerizing agents, the epothilones are the furthest along in development, and one epothilone B analog, ixabepilone, has been registered for treating patients with advanced breast cancer who no longer benefit from paclitaxel.

Ixabepilone and the epothilones

The epothilones A and B (patupilone) are 16-member polyketide macrolides with nearly identical structures, except that epothilone B has an additional methyl group at the C-12 position. *In vitro* studies in tumor cell lines have shown that epothilone B is more active than epothilone A. Both epothilones A and B have greater potency than paclitaxel or docetaxel *in vitro*, with mean inhibitory concentration (IC$_{50}$) values in the low nanomolar range.[435,436] A semisynthetic derivative of epothilone B, ixabepilone (azaepothilone B), was synthesized by converting the lactone of epothilone B to a lactam (Figure 4). This structural modification resulted in improved solubility, low plasma protein binding, and higher metabolic stability than its precursor. The distinct mechanism of binding of the epothilones, particularly epothilone B analogs, to β-tubulin may contribute, at least in part, to their increased potency and broader spectrum of activity than the taxanes, as well as their ability to stabilize yeast microtubules.[437] The promising activities of epothilones A and B led to further modifications of the macrolactone ring, generating deoxyepothilone B (epothilone D), which possess a similar range of anticancer activity as epothilones A and B.

Lxabepilone

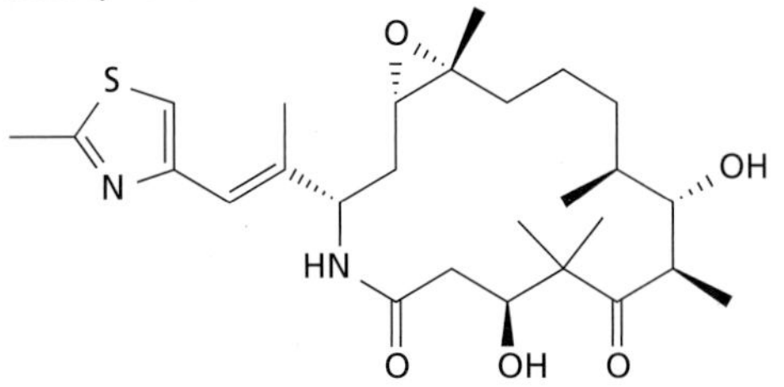

Eribulin

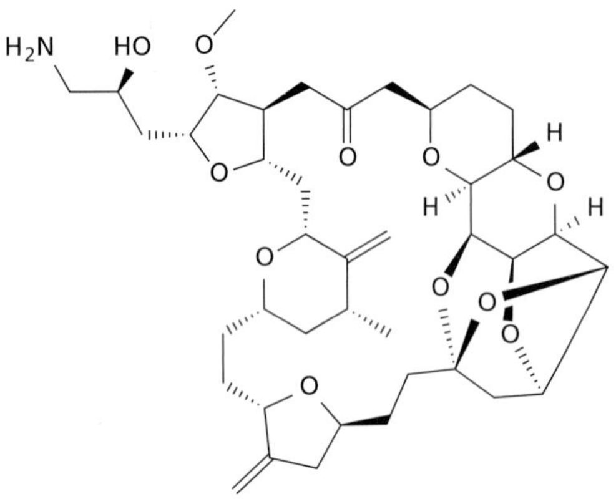

Figure 4 Chemical structures of ixabepilone and eribulin.

Clinical indications

Ixabepilone is registered as a single agent for treating patients with metastatic or locally advanced breast cancer after failure of a taxane, anthracycline, and capecitabine, whereas the combination of ixabepilone and capecitabine is indicated after failure of an anthracycline and a taxane.[438] Both ixabepilone and other epothilones, especially epothilone B, have demonstrated anticancer activity in various other malignancies, mainly those that are sensitive to taxanes such as nonsmall cell lung, prostate, and ovarian cancers.[439,440]

Mechanism of action

Like the natural epothilones A and B, ixabepilone stabilizes microtubules and induces apoptosis.[433,436,440,441] Ixabepilone exhibits prominent activity against human and murine tumor xenografts and is active against paclitaxel-resistant cell lines and tumors, including those with elevated expression of Pgp and/or ßIII- or ßIV-tubulin isotypes.[433,435,436,440,441] Both epothilones A and B and their relevant analogs competitively inhibit binding of paclitaxel to tubulin polymers *in vitro*, inferring that the binding sites of the epothilones and taxanes may overlap.[435–437] They also have similar binding affinities. In fact, the epothilones and taxanes possess a common pharmacophore for microtubule binding.[237,240] Epothilones A and B promote tubulin polymerization *in vitro* with kinetics similar to paclitaxel, but epothilone B appears to be a more potent inducer than both epothilone A and paclitaxel. Similar to the taxanes, the epothilones also induce tubulin polymerization in the absence of GTP and/or MAPs, resulting in microtubules that are long, rigid, and resistant to destabilization by cold temperature, and calcium, resulting in enhanced microtubule stability and microtubule bundling.[237,435–437,439–446] Furthermore, the epothilones induce formation of abnormal mitotic spindles, resulting in cell-cycle arrest in G_2/M. At low concentrations, however, epothilone B does not induce mitotic arrest, but transforms proliferating cells into large aneuploid cells, which undergo apoptotic cell death in G_1. Thus, protracted mitotic arrest may not be essential for apoptotic cell death.[446]

Despite the mechanistic similarities of the epothilones and taxanes, studies using electron crystallography have shown that epothilones interact with β-tubulin through unique and independent molecular interactions, possibly resulting in the ability of these agents to disrupt various βIII- and βIV-tubulins and other tubulin isotypes that are less susceptible to the taxanes.[446] Additionally, various mutations in β-tubulin that confer resistance to taxanes do not significantly alter the cytotoxicity of epothilones A and B, but the clinical relevance of tubulin mutations is not entirely clear.[296]

An important feature of the epothilones, of which ixabepilone has been studied most, appears to be the mechanism in which cell death is induced following the induction of microtubule perturbations. Whereas taxane-induced apoptosis is conveyed by a mitochondrial-mediated pathway involving cytochrome C release and activation of Apaf-1 and caspase-9, ixabepilone-induced apoptosis involves activation of caspase-3 and caspase-8.[447–450] In paclitaxel-refractory ovarian cancer cells, ixabepilone was shown to induce p53-dependent induction of the p53 upregulated modulator of apoptosis (PUMA), leading to activation of caspase-2, the death effector Bax, and apoptosis.[451,452]

Mechanisms of resistance

In contrast to the taxanes and vinca alkaloids, overexpression of the transporters Pgp and MRP1 minimally affects the cytotoxicity of the epothilones as they are weak substrates for these transporters.[2,3,240,433,437,440,441,446] Epothilones A and B possess strong antiproliferative activity in human cancer cells with high expression of Pgp (ABCB1), which are resistant to paclitaxel, and tumor samples obtained from patients with tumors responsive to ixabepilone showed significant expression of both MDR1 and MRP1, also suggesting that these proteins may not confer resistance, at least at a relevant level, to the epothilones in the clinic.[453,454] The epothilone B analog ixabepilone is not a substrate for the breast cancer resistance protein (BCRP) *in vitro*.

In preclinical systems, cancer cells with several distinct types of β-tubulin mutations, such as several βI-tubulin mutations that are critical for microtubule stabilization, appear to be resistant to the epothilones, but the clinical implications of these observations are unknown.[296] Preclinical reports have also suggested additional mechanisms of resistance such as α-tubulin mutations, altered expression of tubulin isotypes, and altered MAP structure and function.[433,435,440,443,454]

Clinical pharmacology

Ixabepilone exhibits dose-proportional pharmacokinetics in the range of 15–57 mg/m^2 (Table 3).[435,440,454] Following administration of a single 40 mg/m^2 dose, the mean C_{max} was 252 ng/mL (coefficient of variation, 56%), and the terminal phase $t_{1/2}$ averaged 52 h. Therefore, no drug accumulation is expected if the agent is administered every 3 weeks. Similar to the taxanes and vinca alkaloids, ixabepilone's Vd at steady state is large, with mean values exceeding 1000 L. Binding to human serum proteins ranges from 67% to 77% *in vitro*, and the blood-to-plasma concentration ratios in human blood range from 0.65 to 0.85. The principal mode of systemic elimination of ixabepilone is hepatic metabolism. Following intravenous administration of radiolabeled ixabepilone, approximately 86% of the dose is eliminated within 7 days; fecal and urinary

Table 3 Ixapebilone and eribulin: comparative pharmacokinetic and toxicologic characteristics.

Parameter	Ixabepilone	Eribulin
Standard adult dose (mg/m^2/3 week)	40 (3-h infusion); Should be capped at 2.2 mg/m^2 for body surface area exceeding this value	—
Standard adult dose (mg/m^2/week)	16 ($\times$ 3 every 4 weeks)	1.4 ($\times$ 2 every 3 weeks) or 1.4 ($\times$ 3 every 4 weeks) as a 2–5-min infusion
Pharmacokinetic behavior (clinically relevant doses)	Multiexponential	Biexponential
Dose proportional in range (mg/m^2)	15–57	0.25–4.0
Plasma half-life (terminal phase)	52 h	40 h
Clearance	36–40 L/h	1.15–2.42 L/h
Primary route	Hepatic metabolism and biliary elimination	Hepatic metabolism and biliary elimination
Principal toxicity	Neurotoxicity, neutropenia	Neutropenia
Other toxicities	Hypersensitivity reactions, anemia, thrombocytopenia	Neurotoxicity, fatigue, thrombocytopenia, anemia, fatigue

elimination, principally of inactive metabolites, accounts for 65% and 21% of the dose, respectively. The parent compound accounts for approximately 1.6% and 5.6% of the dose in feces and urine, respectively. The principal metabolic pathway *in vitro* is oxidative metabolism via CYP3A4. More than 30 inactive metabolites have been identified in human urine and feces, but no single metabolite accounts for more than 6% of the administered dose.

Drug interactions

In vitro studies using human liver microsomes have indicated that clinically relevant concentrations of ixabepilone do not affect the activities of CYP3A4, CYP1A2, CYP2A6, CYP2B6, CYP2C8, CYP2C9, CYP2C19, or CYP2D6 and therefore would likely not affect the pharmacokinetics and metabolism of drugs that are substrates of these enzymes.[435,440,454] However, coadministration of ixabepilone with ketoconazole, a potent CYP3A4 inhibitor, increased ixabepilone AUC values by 79%, on average, compared to ixabepilone alone. With regard to ketoconazole and similar potent inhibitors of CYP3A4, if alternative treatment cannot be administered, a dose adjustment should be considered, and patients should be monitored for toxicity. Since the effect of mild or moderate CYP3A4 inhibitors (e.g., erythromycin, fluconazole, or verapamil) on exposure to ixabepilone has not been studied in the clinic, caution should be exercised if such agents must be administered during ixabepilone treatment. Coadministration of rifampin, a potent inducer of CYP3A4 metabolism, reduced ixabepilone AUC by 43% compared to ixabepilone alone, and it would be expected that other potent CYP3A4 inducers, such as dexamethasone, phenytoin, carbamazepine, rifampin, rifabutin, and phenobarbital, may do the same, thereby possibly leading to subtherapeutic ixabepilone concentrations; therefore, agents with no or low CYP3A4 induction potential should be considered for coadministration with ixabepilone. St. John's wort may decrease ixabepilone plasma concentrations unpredictably and should be avoided. If patients must be coadministered with a strong CYP3A4 inducer, a gradual dose adjustment may be considered. In studies involving cancer patients who received ixabepilone (40 mg/m^2) in combination with capecitabine (1000 mg/m^2), the effects of ixabepilone on the C_{max} and AUC values of capecitabine and 5-fluorouracil, and vice versa, were modest and not apparently relevant.

Ixabepilone does not inhibit CYP enzymes at relevant clinical concentrations and is not expected to appreciably alter the plasma concentrations of other drugs. To this point, ixabepilone C_{max} values decreased by 19%, capecitabine C_{max} values decreased by 27%, and 5-fluorouracil AUC increased by 14%, compared to ixabepilone or capecitabine administered individually in patients who were treated with ixabepilone (40 mg/m^2) in combination with capecitabine (1000 mg/m^2). Based on clinical efficacy data that supports a unique role for the combination, the interaction is not clinically relevant.

Toxicity

Peripheral neurotoxicity is the most common serious toxicity observed with ixabepilone as both monotherapy and combined with capecitabine, as summarized in Table 3.[435,439,440,454,455] A burning sensation, hyperesthesia, hypoesthesia, paresthesia, and other manifestations of neuropathic pain are common symptoms. Approximately 63% and 67% of breast cancer patients who had prior taxane-based treatment develop peripheral neurotoxicity after treatment with ixabepilone alone and combined with capecitabine, respectively; however, more severe (grades 3 and 4) toxicity was noted in 14% and 23%, respectively. In heavily pretreated patients, neuropathy occurs early, with about 75% of new-onset or worsening neuropathy occurring during the first three cycles and the most serious manifestations experienced after four cycles. Although prior exposure to neurotoxic drugs does not seem to predispose to neuropathy based on a large retrospective analysis of clinical trial data, it should be noted that patients with neuropathy of at least moderate severity were excluded from entry of early studies. Patients who have hepatic insufficiency and diabetes mellitus are at increased risk of developing severe neuropathy (see section titled "Administration, Dose, and Schedule"). In clinical trials, peripheral neuropathy was managed using dose reduction, dose delay, and treatment discontinuation (see section titled "Administration, Dose, and Schedule"). After treatment discontinuation and/or dose reduction, manifestations resolve rapidly relative to the taxanes, vinca alkaloids, and eribulin, with median times of 4–6 weeks for resolution of severe manifestation to grade 1 severity, with almost all grade 3–4 events resolving to this level within 12 weeks after onset.

Dose-dependent myelosuppression, principally neutropenia, is common with ixabepilone treatment. Effects on platelets and red blood cells are less common. Grade 4 neutropenia (<500 cells/μL) occurred in 36% of patients treated with ixabepilone in combination with capecitabine and in 23% of patients treated with monotherapy; however, febrile neutropenia and infection with neutropenia have been reported in 5% and 6% of patients treated with ixabepilone in combination with capecitabine, respectively, and 3% and 5% of patients treated with ixabepilone alone. Myelo-suppression does not generally worsen with successive treatment, suggesting that hematopoietic progenitor cells are not significantly affected. Dose reduction is recommended for patients experiencing severe neutropenia, and dose modification is recommended for patients with moderate hepatic dysfunction (see section titled "Administration, Dose, and Schedule"). Since ixabepilone is formulated in polyoxyethylated castor oil, severe HSRs, largely secondary to this diluent, are noted. Manifestations of hypersensitivity include flushing, rash, dyspnea, and bronchospasm. For this reason, it is recommended that patients receive premedication with H1- and H2-histamine antagonists approximately 1 h before treatment (see section titled "Administration, Dose, and Schedule"). In the case of severe HSRs, treatment should be stopped, and aggressive supportive treatment (e.g., epinephrine, corticosteroids) started. In clinical studies, approximately 1% of patients have experienced severe reactions despite various premedication regimens. There have been reports of successful re-treatment of patients who had experienced prior reactions following the addition of a corticosteroid (e.g., dexamethasone 20 mg intravenously 30 min before or orally 60 min before) and H1- and H2-histamine antagonists and extension of the infusion time.

Patients treated with ixabepilone have experienced cognitive dysfunction, lethargy, and discoordinated movements in the peritreatment period, possibly due to the ethanol in the diluent. Myalgia and arthralgia have been noted in the peritreatment period. Various cardiac disturbances, including myocardial infarction, supraventricular arrhythmia, left ventricular dysfunction, angina pectoris, atrial flutter, cardiomyopathy, and myocardial ischemia, have been observed, but these occurrences have not been directly attributed to ixabepilone. Ileus, colitis, impaired gastric emptying, esophagitis, dysphagia, gastritis, gastrointestinal hemorrhage, hepatic insufficiency, erythema multiforme, muscle spasms, trismus, and renal failure have also been reported on rare occasion.

Administration, dose, and schedule

The recommended dosage of ixabepilone is 40 mg/m^2 intravenously over 3 h every 3 weeks.[436,440,454,455] Because of the lack of dosing data for patients whose body surface area exceeds 2.2 m^2, the doses for such individuals should be calculated based on a cap of 2.2 m^2. Although a range of intermittent dosing schedules have been evaluated, particularly 16 mg/m^2 weekly for 3 weeks every 4 weeks, most efficacy data relate to the 3-h-every-3-week dosing schedule, and superior efficacy has not been demonstrated on more intermittent schedules to date. Ixabepilone is intended for intravenous use only after constitution with the supplied diluent, which is a nonpyrogenic solution of 52.8% (w/v) purified polyoxyethylated castor oil and 39.8% (w/v) dehydrated alcohol, USP, and after further dilution with Lactated Ringer's Injection, USP, or 0.9% sodium chloride injection, USP (pH adjusted between 6.0 and 9.0 with Sodium Bicarbonate, USP, prior to addition of the constituted ixabepilone solution). To minimize the chance of occurrence of major HSRs, all patients should be premedicated approximately 1 h before treatment with both an H1-histamine antagonist (e.g., diphenhydramine 50 mg orally or equivalent) and an H2-histamine antagonist (e.g., ranitidine 150–300 mg orally or equivalent). For patients who experience an HSR, premedication with corticosteroids (e.g., dexamethasone 20 mg intravenously, 30 min before infusion or orally, 60 min before treatment), in addition to pretreatment with H1- and H2-histamine antagonists, is recommended.

Dose modification and/or treatment delay is recommended for patients who develop clinically relevant grades of neuropathy and/or myelosuppression. Dose reduction by 20% is recommended for patients who develop neuropathic manifestations of grade 2 severity lasting at least 7 days or of grade 3 severity lasting less than 7 days. Discontinuation of treatment is recommended for more protracted grade 3 neuropathy or any grade 4 toxicity. Dose reduction by 20% is also recommended for patients who experience a neutrophil count <500/μL lasting at least 7 days and/or associated with fever, a platelet count <25,000/μL, or a platelet count <50,000/μL with bleeding. A similar dose reduction (20%) is recommended for patients who experience other types of grade 3 (severe) toxicities, except fatigue, palmar–plantar erythrodysesthesia, and/or arthralgia/myalgia. Drug discontinuation is recommended for any grade 4 (i.e., disabling) nonhematologic toxicity. In a study of ixabepilone in patients with mild to severe hepatic impairment, ixabepilone AUC values increased by 22% in patients with bilirubin values ranging from >1 to 1.5 times the ULN or AST values exceeding the ULN with bilirubin <1.5 times the ULN, whereas AUC values increased by 30% in patients with bilirubin elevations ranging from 1.5 to 3 times the ULN and any AST level and increased by 81% in patients with bilirubin values exceeding 3 times the ULN with any AST level. Doses of 10 and 20 mg/m^2 as monotherapy were tolerated in a small number of patients with severe hepatic impairment (bilirubin >3 times the ULN). It is recommended that the dose of ixabepilone as monotherapy be reduced to 32 mg/m^2 in patients with AST or ALT elevations up to 10 times the ULN and bilirubin up to 1.5 times the ULN. For patients with AST or ALT elevations up to 10 times the ULN and bilirubin ranging from 1.5 to 3.0 times the ULN, ixabepilone monotherapy doses should be reduced to 20 mg/m^2. If tolerated, the dose can be increased up to but not exceeding 30 mg/m^2 in subsequent cycles. Use of ixabepilone is not recommended in patients with severe hepatic dysfunction defined as ALT or AST values exceeding 10 times the ULN or bilirubin exceeding 3 times the ULN. Treatment with ixabepilone combined with capecitabine is not recommended for patients who have AST, ALT, and/or bilirubin levels exceeding the ULN. A standard dose of ixabepilone (40 mg/m^2) is recommended for patients who have AST and ALT <2.5 times the ULN and normal bilirubin values.

Ixabepilone is minimally excreted by the kidney; however, the agent has not been evaluated in patients with creatinine >1.5 times ULN. In a population pharmacokinetic analysis of ixabepilone as monotherapy, the pharmacokinetics of ixabepilone were not affected by mild or moderate renal insufficiency (creatinine clearance >30 mL/min). The regimen of ixabepilone combined with capecitabine has not been evaluated in patients with creatinine clearance values below 50 mL/min. The use of concomitant strong CYP3A4 inhibitors (e.g., ketoconazole, itraconazole, clarithromycin, atazanavir, nefazodone, saquinavir, telithromycin, ritonavir, amprenavir, indinavir, nelfinavir, delavirdine, or voriconazole) should be avoided (see section titled "Drug Interactions"). Grapefruit juice may also impede metabolic clearance and should be avoided. Based on pharmacokinetic studies, if a strong CYP3A4 inhibitor must be coadministered, dose reduction to 20 mg/m^2, which should adjust the ixabepilone AUC to that observed without inhibitors, should be considered. If the strong inhibitor is discontinued, a 1-week washout period is recommended before the ixabepilone dose is increased to the indicated dose.

Eribulin mesylate and natural products that enhance tubulin depolymerization

Several other natural and semisynthetic agents that bind to either the vinca or colchicine binding domains of tubulin are approved or under evaluation. Eribulin mesylate, a macrocyclic ketone analog of the marine natural product halichondrin B (Figure 4) originally isolated from the marine sponge *Halichondria okadai,* is perhaps the most relevant since the agent has been registered worldwide to treat women with advanced breast cancer after failure of anthracyclines and taxanes. Eribulin mesylate and other halichondrin B analogs bind to tubulin and inhibit tubulin polymerization, disrupt mitotic spindle formation and centromere dynamics, induce mitotic arrest followed by apoptosis, and possess growth inhibitory properties in the subnanomolar range and marked anticancer activity in preclinical studies.[456-458] Synthetic forms of hemiasterlin (HTI-286 and E7974), which is a natural product derived from marine sponges, are also in clinical development.[459] Hemiasterlin and its analogs bind to the vinca domain on tubulin, disrupt normal microtubule dynamics, and depolymerize microtubules at stoichiometric concentrations. They are much weaker substrate for Pgp than the vinca alkaloids and taxanes and have prominent anticancer activity in human tumor xenografts, including those that express Pgp.[460,461] The hemiasterlins are also cross-resistant with the vinca alkaloids and other agents that bind to the vinca binding site of tubulin but minimally cross-resistant with the taxanes, epothilones, and colchicine. In preclinical studies, resistance appears to be at least partially mediated by α-tubulin mutations and/or an ABC drug pump distinct from Pgp, ABCG2, MRP1, or MRP3.[460,461]

Among other potent natural products that enhance tubulin polymerization are the dolastatins, which constitute a series of oligopeptides isolated from the sea hare, *Dolabella auricularia.* The dolastatins inhibit binding (noncompetitively) of vinca alkaloids to tubulin, tubulin polymerization, and tubulin-dependent GTP hydrolysis.[462] They also stabilize the colchicine binding activity of tubulin and possess cytotoxic activity in the picomolar to low nanomolar range.[462] Auristatin, a potent dolastatin-10 analog, has been incorporated into several ADCs, including brentuximab vedotin that targets CD-30 (see section titled "Antibody-Drug Conjugates Carrying Antimicrotubule Drug Payloads")

Most efforts targeting the tumor vasculature involve inhibition of the development of malignant angiogenesis, but several antimicrotubule agents rapidly shut down existing tumor vasculature by inhibiting tubulin function in vascular endothelial cells.[463,464] Since the late 1990s, the combretastatins and *N*-acetylcolchicinol-*O*-phosphate which resemble colchicine and bind to the colchicine domain on tubulin have undergone extensive clinical development as antivascular agents in a wide range of cancers; however, they have yet to demonstrate favorable therapeutic indices.

Eribulin mesylate

In 1986, Hirata and Uemura extracted halichondrin B, a large polyether macrolide, from a rare marine Japanese sponge, *H. okadai.* Based on its potent anticancer activity in preclinical models, it was further evaluated against other known antimicrotubule and cytotoxic drugs.[458] Although the antiproliferative effects of halichondrin B were similar to other antimicrotubule agents, its mechanism of action was distinct.[458] However, despite its impressive anticancer activity in preclinical studies, sufficient quantities of its natural source were not available. More than one decade later, however, structural activity studies indicated that the antimicrotubule activity of halichondrin B was conferred by its macrocyclic

lactone C1–C38 moiety and a completely synthetic and structurally simplified derivative with retained high potency of its parent compound, eribulin mesylate, was developed.

Clinical indications

Eribulin mesylate has demonstrated clinical activity in various solid malignancies, but it is registered worldwide for treating patients with metastatic breast cancer who have previously received at least two chemotherapeutic regimens for the treatment of metastatic disease. The agent demonstrated improved overall survival over a group of other relevant anticancer agents, including taxanes, capecitabine, gemcitabine, and VRL, but the study was not sufficiently powered to gauge the superiority of eribulin mesylate compared to any specific single agent in the group.[465] In addition, eribulin mesylate has recently demonstrated superior overall survival over dacarbazine in patients with soft tissue sarcoma who had received at least two prior chemotherapy regimens, and has been approved for the treatment of patients with unresectable liposarcoma who have received a prior anthracycline containing regimen. Notable activity has been noted in patients with advanced cancers of the head and neck, bladder, prostate, ovary, pancreas, and lung.[458]

Mechanism of action

The mechanisms by which eribulin exerts its effects differ from those of other microtubule-depolymerizing agents. Eribulin mesylate binds with high affinity to the plus ends of microtubules to a maximum of 15 sites per microtubule and suppresses dynamic instability. The binding site of eribulin differs from that of taxanes and vinca alkaloids, which is thought to be responsible for eribulin's activity against some cancer cells with MDR or β-tubulin mutations.[456-458] It is a noncompetitive inhibitor of VBL binding and binds to β-tubulin at a slightly different site than the vinca alkaloids. Like the vinca alkaloids, eribulin inhibits tubulin polymerization and suppresses the microtubule growth phase. In contrast to the vinca alkaloids, however, eribulin does not affect shortening.[456-458,466,467] Referred to as having an "end-poisoning" mechanism, eribulin mesylate either binds directly to microtubule ends or induces tubulin aggregates, which compete with soluble tubulin for addition to the growing ends of microtubules. By doing so, eribulin disrupts mitotic spindle assembly, blocking cell-cycle traverse in G$_2$/M. Prolonged G$_2$/M blockade and incomplete repair of relevant perturbations at the mitotic checkpoint are followed by followed by apoptosis, as evidenced by phosphorylation of Bcl-2, cytochrome C release from mitochondria activation of caspase-3 and caspase-9, and cleavage of PARP.[466] Eribulin mesylate is relatively stable on or near tubulin surfaces, which enables it to be retained in tumor cells for longer periods than other halichondrin B analogs.

While both eribulin and the vinca alkaloids inhibit nucleotide exchange on β-tubulin, as well as cross-linking between β-tubulin residues, the polymer structures formed by these agents differ. Vinca alkaloids create a large, stable structure that inhibits microtubules, whereas both halichondrin B and eribulin form smaller, unstable tubulin polymers. In addition to inhibiting microtubule growth, eribulin sequesters tubules into globular aggregates, which differ from the ring or spiral aggregates seen with vinca alkaloids. Further, in contrast to the vinca alkaloids, eribulin does not cause splaying of microtubule ends or heterodimer linking of α- and β-tubulin. Eribulin's unique mechanism is thought to be important for its clinical activity in patients who have been previously treated with other types of antimicrotubule drugs.

Mechanism of resistance

The mechanisms of cellular resistance to eribulin are not entirely known; however, since eribulin disrupts microtubule dynamics and blocks cell-cycle traverse in G_2/M, cycling cells are most susceptible to its actions.[458–462,466,467] Nevertheless, the relative drug susceptibility of microtubules involved in mitotic spindle dynamics and interphase functions is not known. Like the vinca alkaloids and taxanes, resistance to eribulin appears to be conferred by MDR1; however, the clinical relevance of this phenomenon is not known. In general, eribulin demonstrates greater efficacy than the taxanes and vinca alkaloids against a wide range of human tumors in preclinical studies. It has also induced relevant degrees of inhibition in taxane-resistant human ovarian cancer cells harboring β-tubulin mutations and tumors that express relatively high concentrations of the βIII-tubulin isotype.[458–462,467]

Clinical pharmacology

Eribulin mesylate exhibits dose-proportional pharmacokinetics in the dose range of 0.25–4.0 mg/m² (Table 3). When administered intravenously, plasma disposition is biexponential with a rapid and initial distribution phase followed by a slow elimination phase. Eribulin's elimination $t_{1/2}$ averages 40 h; estimates of its Vd range from 43 to 114 L/m², and systemic clearance ranges from 1.15 to 2.42 L/h/m² over the aforementioned dose range. The plasma protein binding of eribulin mesylate ranges from 49% to 65% at concentrations of 100–1000 ng/mL.[458,467] Drug exposure achieved with multiple dosing is comparable to that following a single dose. No drug accumulation is observed with weekly administration.

Unmetabolized eribulin is the major circulating species following administration of radiolabeled eribulin mesylate to cancer patients. Eribulin is excreted unchanged in the feces, and metabolite concentrations represent <0.6% of parent compound, confirming that metabolism is negligible. The liver disposes of parent compound and four minor CYP3A4-generated monooxygenated metabolites. A small amount of eribulin (≈9%) is renally excreted as parent compound.

Drug interactions

Eribulin mesylate shows no induction potential for CYP1A, CYP2C9, CYP2C19, or CYP3A in primary human hepatocytles.[458,467] It inhibits CYP3A4 activity in liver microsomes, but not enough to substantially increase the plasma concentrations of CYP3A4 substrates. No significant inhibition of CYP1A2, CYP2C9, CYP2C19, CYP2D6, or CYP2E1 has been detected with eribulin concentrations as high as 5 μmol/L in human microsomes. Drug interaction studies *in vitro* indicate that eribulin does not significantly affect the metabolism or plasma concentrations of drugs that are substrates of these CYP enzymes. Eribulin is a low-affinity substrate and a weak inhibitor of the drug efflux transporter Pgp.

As predicted by *in vitro* studies, the results of clinical studies to date indicate that eribulin presents a negligible potential, if any, for drug–drug interactions with both CYP3A4 inhibitors and inducers.[467] Relevant pharmacokinetic interactions were not observed when eribulin was administered with a ketoconazole, a strong CYP3A4 and a Pgp inhibitor, or rifampin, a strong CYP3A4 inducer.

Toxicity

The most common adverse reactions reported in patients receiving eribulin was neutropenia, with 57% of 503 heavily treated breast cancer patients treated with eribulin 1.4 mg/m² on days 1 and 8 of a 21-day cycle experiencing neutrophil count nadirs of 1000/uL or less in a pivotal trial.[458,465,467] Febrile neutropenia occurred in 5% of patients. Dose reduction or drug discontinuation due to neutropenia was required in 12% and <1% of patients, respectively; granulocyte-colony stimulating factor was used in 19% of patients. The mean time to neutrophil nadir was 13 days, and the mean time to recovery from severe neutropenia (<500/μL) was 8 days. Grade 3 or greater thrombocytopenia and anemia occurred in <1% and 2% of patients, respectively. Other common adverse events in the eribulin group included fatigue (54%), alopecia (45%), and peripheral neuropathy (35%; 8% grade 3 or 4). The neuropathy is predominately sensory but motor effects do occur. Approximately 5% of patients discontinued eribulin primarily due to peripheral neuropathy, the incidence of which was similar to that in the taxane subgroup. The incidence of severe (grade 3 or 4) neuropathy was similar in patients with and without a preexisting mild to moderate neuropathy. A recent randomized phase II study showed no significant difference in the incidence and severity of neuropathy between eribulin and ixabepilone; however, the neuropathy induced by ixabepilone reversed more rapidly.[467] Higher incidences of severe toxicities were observed in Japanese patients treated with eribulin 1.4 mg/m² administered as a brief intravenous infusion on days 1 and 8 of a 21-day cycle.[467] In an uncontrolled open-label electrocardiographic study involving 26 patients, QT prolongation was observed on day 8 irrespective of eribulin concentrations, with no QT prolongation observed on day 1. Therefore, electrocardiographic monitoring and restrictions are recommended in patients possibly susceptible to the effects of electrocardiographic disturbances (see sections "Eribulin Mesylate and Natural Products that Enhance Tubulin Depolymerization" and "Administration, Dose, and Schedule").

Among patients with grade 0 or 1 hepatic transaminase elevation pretreatment, approximately 18% of eribulin-treated patients experience at least grade 2 transaminase elevations. Other adverse events, albeit rarely severe, reported in patients treated with eribulin, albeit rarely severe, include stomatitis, diarrhea, constipation, nausea, vomiting, anorexia, myalgia, arthralgia, increased lacrimation, weight loss, fever, anemia, and headache.

Administration, dose, and schedule

Eribulin mesylate is indicated at a dose of 1.4 mg/m² intravenously over 2–5 min on days 1 and 8 of a 21-day cycle for patients with metastatic breast cancer. It has also been administered at a dose of 1.4 mg/m² on days 1, 8, and 15 of a 28-day cycle. A head-to-head comparison of the two dosing schedules in patients with metastatic breast cancer showed that the 21-day regimen is associated with a slightly, albeit not significantly, higher response rate.[458,467] Each vial contains 1 mg of eribulin mesylate as a 0.50 mg/mL colorless, sterile solution for injection in a 5:95 ratio of ethanol to water. The required amount of eribulin should be withdrawn from the vial and mixed with 100 mL of 0.9% Sodium Chloride Injection, USP. Dextrose should not be used for dilution or administration. Pretreatment with corticosteroids or antihistamines is not required since its water solubility negates the requirement for a lipophilic vehicle such as polysorbate-80 or polyoxyethylated castor oil, which may result in HSRs.

Lower starting doses of eribulin mesylate, 1.1 and 0.7 mg/m², are recommended for patients with mild (Child–Pugh A) and moderate (Child–Pugh B) hepatic impairment, respectively.[458,467] The agent has not been evaluated in patients with severe hepatic insufficiency. For patients with moderate or severe renal impairment (creatinine clearance, 15–49 mL/min), the recommended starting dose is 1.1 mg/m². Eribulin should not be administered on day 8 of a day 1–8 every-21-day schedule, if neutrophil and/or platelet counts are <1000 and <75,000/μL, respectively, and/or in the event of grade 3–4 nonhematologic toxicity. The day 8 dose can be delayed for a maximum of 1 week. The dose should be omitted if the toxicities do not resolve or improve to at least grade 2 severity by day 15. If toxicities resolve or improve to at least grade 2 severity by day 15, eribulin may be administered at a dose of 1.1 mg/m², and the next cycle should be initiated no sooner than 2 weeks later. A second dose reduction to 0.7 mg/m² is recommended in the event of similar toxicity. The dose of eribulin should not be re-escalated after it has been reduced.

Electrocardiographic monitoring is recommended in patient with congestive heart failure, bradyarrhythmias, and electrolyte abnormalities and in those receiving drugs known to prolong the QT interval. Hypokalemia or hypomagnesemia should be corrected prior to treatment, and electrolytes should be monitored periodically during treatment. Eribulin should not be administered in patients with congenitally long QT syndrome.

Targeting mitotic motor proteins and kinases

Although tubulin is the most abundant protein component of the mitotic spindle apparatus, several other proteins, such as mitotic kinesins, centrosomal proteins, and mitotic kinases, play key roles in the mechanics of mitosis and cell-cycle progression through the pre-mitotic checkpoint. Over the last decade, many of these subcellular constituents have been evaluated as targets for therapeutics against cancer.

Mitotic kinesins

Kinesins are motor proteins that convert energy released by the hydrolysis of ATP into mechanical force for movement of cargo (e.g., organelles, constituents) along microtubules and the intracellular organization of the mitotic spindle, and other microtubule-containing structures.[28,29,468,469]

The mitotic kinesins function exclusively in mitosis in proliferating cells.[28,29,468–470] During mitosis, different, highly specialized mitotic kinesins play critical roles in various aspects of mitotic spindle formation, including establishment of spindle bipolarity, spindle pole organization, chromosome alignment and segregation, and regulation of microtubule dynamics. The establishment of mitotic spindle bipolarity is among the earliest events in spindle assembly, and it requires the function of a specific kinesin motor protein KSP, also known as Eg5, which has no known role other than in mitosis. The expression profiles of KSP mRNA in normal tissues are consistent with preferential expression of KSP in proliferating cells relative to normal adjacent tissue and postmitotic neurons. As essential elements in mitotic spindle assembly and function, KSP and mitotic kinesins provide attractive targets for intervention into the cell cycle.

Several KSP inhibitors have been evaluated as anticancer therapeutics over the past decade. One of the first, ispinesib, a polycyclic, nitrogen-containing heterocycle and allosteric inhibitor of KSP motor domain ATPase with a Ki of 12 nM and a potent KSP inhibitor, potently induces mitotic arrest in both solid and hematologic malignancies in preclinical models.[28,29,468–470] Similar to various other KSP inhibitors that have entered clinical evaluations, ispinesib is 10,000-fold more selective for KSP relative to

other members of the kinesin superfamily and blocks assembly of a functional mitotic spindle, thereby causing cell-cycle arrest in mitosis and subsequent cell death.[470] In tumor-bearing mice, ispinesib and several other KSP inhibitors have exhibited anti-cancer activity comparable to or exceeding that of the taxanes and induced formation of monopolar mitotic figures identical to those produced in cultured cells. KSP inhibitors have been shown to be effective on both taxane-sensitive and taxane-resistant cells, which either have multidrug resistance product Pgp overexpression or acquired β-tubulin mutations. Interestingly, the combination of KSP inhibitors with taxanes produce an antagonistic effect on mitotic arrest and cell death, indicating that the combination of an KSP inhibitor with a taxane may not be useful. Although highly specific KSP inhibitors have demonstrated anticancer activity in both solid and hematologic malignancies, including breast cancer, lymphoma, and multiple myeloma, toxicity in tissues with high proliferative rates, namely, neutropenia, has been significant at clinically relevant doses, thereby requiring the use of granulocyte colony-stimulating factors. A unique clinical role for KSP inhibitors has not yet been clearly elucidated.

The mitotic centromere-associated kinesin (MCAK), a member of the kinesin-13 family that regulates microtubule dynamics by removing tubulin subunits from the polymer end, is another potential target for therapeutic development.[471] The depolymerizing activity of MCAK plays pivotal roles in spindle formation, correcting erroneous attachments of microtubule–kinetochore and chromosome movement. Thus, the accurate regulation of MCAK by mitotic kinases, Aurora-A and Aurora-B, polo-like kinase-1, and CDK1 is important for ensuring the faithful segregation of chromosomes in mitosis and for safeguarding chromosome stability. There are increasing data indicating that MCAK is aberrantly regulated in cancer cells, thereby contributing to tumorigenesis, invasiveness, metastasis, and drug resistance, most probably due to increased chromosomal instability and remodeling of the microtubule cytoskeleton in cancer cells. Most interestingly, recent observations suggest that MCAK could be a novel molecular target for cancer therapy, as a new cancer antigen or as a mitotic regulator.

The centromere-associated protein E (CENP-E) is another type of mitotic kinesin. CENP-E associates with the kinetochores and plays an essential role in chromosome movement in early mitosis and integrates mitotic spindle mechanics with regulators of the mitotic checkpoint, thereby facilitating cell-cycle transition from metaphase to anaphase.[472] Inhibition of CENP-E induces cell-cycle arrest during cell duplication, leading to subsequent apoptosis or cell death. In preclinical studies, GSK-923295 demonstrated a broad spectrum of activity against a range of human tumor xenografts grown in nude mice, including models of colon, breast, ovarian, lung, and other tumors.[469]

Mitotic kinases

Mitotic kinases, particularly the aurora and polo-like kinases, are being evaluated for anticancer therapeutic development.[473] The aurora kinases, which encompass three principal family members known as Aurora-A, Aurora-B, and Aurora-C, regulate chromosome segregation and cytokinesis during mitosis. Aberrant expression and activity of these kinases that may lead to aneuploidy and tumorigenesis occur in many types of human cancer. Aurora-A and Aurora-B kinases have distinct roles in mitosis. Aurora-A kinase, which is typically found in the pericentrosomal region, recruits important components to the mitotic spindle, such as γ-tubulin, while the mitotic spindle is formed from the daughter centrosomes. Aurora-B kinase is localized to the interphase chromosomes proximal to the centromere, and as chromosome condensation occurs at the start of mitosis, both Aurora-A and Aurora-B kinases share responsibility for phosphorylating histone H3. Both kinases also have distinct roles in the function of the contractile ring that participates in the formation of two daughter cells. Aurora-C kinase has a highly specialized, albeit as of yet undetermined, role in mitosis, but it appears to complement Aurora-B kinase, and the expression of all three aurora kinases are increased in several types of cancers. Highly potent and both selective and nonselective small-molecule inhibitors of Aurora-A and Aurora-B kinases, which block cell-cycle progression and induce apoptosis in experimental models of human cancer, are undergoing clinical development. Neutropenia is their principal toxicity, and although anticancer activity has been observed, largely in hematologic malignancies, a unique clinical role for these agents has not yet been demonstrated, most likely due to the narrow therapeutic index of potential susceptible malignancies and hematopoietic cells.[473]

Like the aurora family of kinases, the polo-like kinases, NIMA-related kinases, and other families of mitotic kinase participate in the centrosome cycle and modulate spindle function, while Bub1, BubR1, and Mps1 kinases regulate the spindle assembly checkpoint.[474,475] Family members, like polo-like kinase-1, are also involved in the regulation of key steps during cell division, DNA damage repair pathways, apoptosis, and the progression of the cell cycle. At least one family member, polo-like kinase-3, is a multifunctional stress response protein that responds to signals induced by DNA damage and/or mitotic spindle disruption. After demonstrating broad-spectrum anticancer activity in preclinical studies against both solid and hematologic malignancies, small-molecule inhibitors of polo-like kinase are in clinical development.[474,475] Similar to the mitotic kinesins and aurora kinases in clinical development, unique roles in cancer therapeutics have not been discerned, possibly due to the emergence of hematologic toxicity, principally neutropenia, at relevant dose levels.

Antibody-drug conjugates carrying antimicrotubule drug payloads

Antibody therapies offer many advantages over cytotoxic agents, the main one being the specificity of each mAb for its target antigen.[476,477] Since their discovery in the early 1970s, mAbs have been evaluated as therapeutic agents and have enjoyed considerable success in recent years. However, mAbs also have their disadvantages, including poor inherent cytotoxicity and suboptimal penetration into malignancies. Combining mAbs with potent cytotoxic agents, however, may provide the best of both worlds—the specificity of a mAb for tumors and the potency of the agent for cytotoxicity. ADCs utilize the exquisite specificity of a mAb for its antigen to selectively deliver a highly toxic drug to the cancer cell, thereby increasing the selectivity and therapeutic window of any potent cytotoxic that is utilized as the ADC's payload. The design of an ADC relies on the proper selection of a tumor-specific antigen that is accessible for antibody binding and delivery to its target. The rationale for ADCs lies in the specificity of antigen expression by cancer cells, which permits drug delivery to target tissues with relative sparing of healthy tissues that express little to no antigen. Likewise, the level of expression of the target antigen on tumor cells determines drug delivery as well as effect on normal tissues. If a target antigen is not expressed at high levels on tumor cells, ADC uptake will be low, which will limit cytotoxicity and lead to accumulation of drug extracellularly and nonspecific toxicity to normal cells. Since antimicrotubule agents act intracellularly, it is crucial that the target antigen transports the ADC intracellularly.

If the antigen does not internalize, the drug will not achieve sufficiently adequate concentration to cause cytotoxicity, and the ADC may ultimate expose normal cells to toxic effects. It is also crucial that the antigen be expressed homogeneously among cancer cells that constitute the tumor. Additionally, the target antigen must be easily accessible from the blood. Lastly, the payload must be highly potent because only minute quantities are administered. The maytansinoids and dolastatins, which are highly potent inhibitors of microtubule assembly, have been the principal payloads incorporated into ADCs that are registered in the United States and elsewhere.[476–479]

The discovery of maytansine, a benzoansamacrolide that was first isolated from the bark of the Ethiopian shrub *Maytenus ovatus* in the early 1970s, as well as maytansine analogs, generated much interest as they were demonstrated to be 100- to 1000-fold more potent than the vinca alkaloids and other antimicrotubule agents. However, systemic administration resulted in an unacceptably high incidence of adverse gastrointestinal effects, peripheral neuropathy, and hematologic toxicity.[480,481] Maytansine bind to tubulin at a site overlapping the vinca alkaloid binding site but differs from the colchicine binding site. Both the vinca alkaloids and maytansinoids bind to the β-tubulin subunit. The structure–activity relationship of maytansinoids for tubulin binding correlates well with their activity *in vitro*; this and the absence of other primary effects suggest that mitotic inhibition represents the main mechanism of anticancer action of the maytansinoids. It has been suggested that maytansine acts by binding to key sulfhydryl groups of tubulin.[480] Maytansinoids have a high affinity for tubulin located at the ends of microtubules yet lower affinity to sites distributed throughout the microtubules. The suppression of microtubule dynamics results in cell-cycle arrest in G_2/M, ultimately resulting in cell death by apoptosis. The high potency of the maytansinoids makes them ideal candidates for conjugation to antibodies. Two maytansine derivatives—emtansine (also referred to as DM1 (Figure 5a) and ravtansine (also referred to as DM4 [Figure 5b])—have been widely used in combination with irreversible and reversible linkers. Trastuzumab-emtansine was the first ADC registered; it is indicated for woman with metastatic breast cancer progressing on trastuzumab (*see **Chapter 108***). The cytotoxic effects of trastuzumab-emtansine likely vary depending on the intracellular concentration of DM1 accumulated in cancer cells, high intracellular levels resulting in rapid apoptosis, and somewhat lower levels in impaired cellular trafficking and mitotic catastrophe, while the lowest levels lead to poor response to T-DM1.[481] Primary resistance of HER-2-amplifed advanced breast cancer to trastuzumab-emtansine appears to be relatively infrequent, but most patients treated with trastuzumab-emtansine develop acquired drug resistance. The mechanisms of resistance are incompletely understood, but mechanisms limiting the binding of trastuzumab to cancer cells may be involved. The cytotoxic effect of trastuzumab-emtansine may be impaired by inefficient internalization or enhanced recycling of the HER-2-ADC complex in cancer cells or impaired lysosomal degradation of trastuzumab or intracellular trafficking of HER2. The effect of trastuzumab-emtansine may also be compromised by MDR proteins that pump DM1 out of cancer cells.

Dolastatin and many of its synthetic derivatives have been evaluated in a wide range of clinical trials, but these agents have not shown appreciable anticancer activity and/or favorable therapeutic indices (see section titled "Eribulin Mesylate and Natural Products That Enhance Tubulin Depolymerization"). However, the ADC brentuximab vedotin, which is composed of the dolastatin analog monomethyl auristatin E (MMAE) covalently linked to CD30, a type II transmembrane protein belonging to the TNF

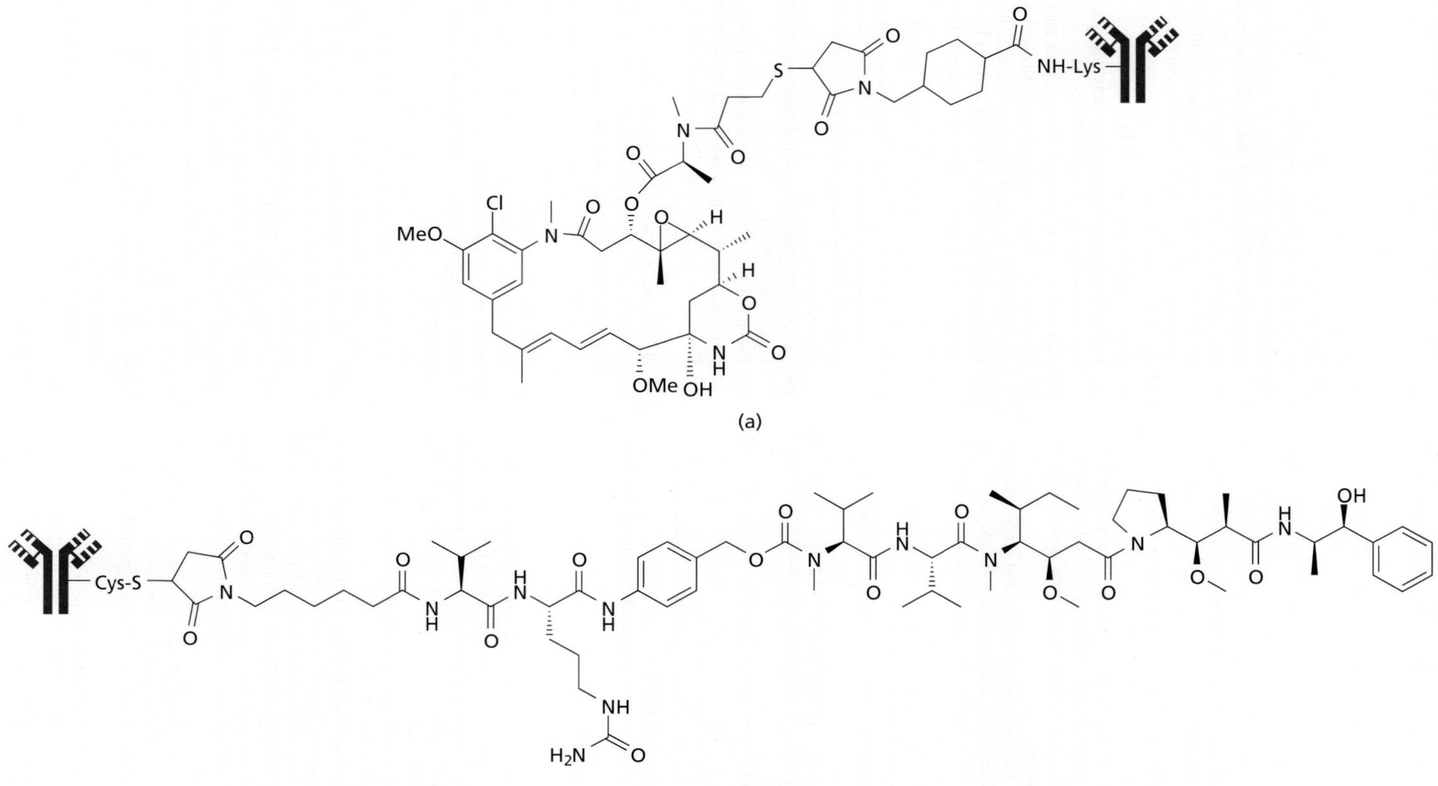

Figure 5 Representations of the ADCs trastuzumab emtansine (a) and brentuximab vedotin (b) with chemical structures of their cytotoxic payloads emtansine (DM1) and monomethyl auristatin E, respectively.

family, has received regulatory approval for patients with relapsed refractory Hodgkin's lymphoma and anaplastic large cell lymphoma (*see **Chapter 64***). Brentuximab vedotin's toxic payload MMAE is stably attached to the antibody with only 2% release following a 10-day incubation in human plasma, but selectively cleaved by lysosomal enzymes, presumably cathepsin B, after CD30 receptor-mediated internalization.[480] In addition to the requirement for CD30 expression, multiple factors such as internalization, intracellular trafficking, or enzymatic cleavage and undoubtedly factors related to the MMAE determine tumor cell sensitivity *in vitro*.

Key references

The complete reference list can be found on the Wiley Companion Digital Edition of this title (see inside front cover for login instructions).

2   Jordan MA, Wilson L. Microtubules as a target for anticancer drugs. *Nat Rev Cancer*. 2004;**4**:253.

13   Wilson L, Panda D, Jordan MA. Modulation of microtubule dynamics by drugs: a paradigm for the actions of cellular regulators. *Cell Struct Funct*. 1999;**24**:329.

29   Vale RD, Milligan RA. The way things move: looking under the hood of molecular motor proteins. *Science*. 2000;**288**:88.

38   Rowinsky EK, Donehower RC. The clinical pharmacology and use of antimicrotubule agents in cancer chemotherapeutics. *Pharmacol Ther*. 1992;**52**:35.

61   Himes RH. Interactions of the Catharanthus (vinca) alkaloids with tubulin and microtubules. *Pharmacol Ther*. 1991;**51**:256.

82   Lockhart A, Tirona G, Kim B. Pharmacogenetics of ATP binding cassette transporters in cancer and chemotherapy. *Mol Ther*. 2003;**2**:685.

158   Quasthoff S, Hartung HP. Chemotherapy-induced peripheral neuropathy. *J Neurol*. 2002;**249**:9.

175   Diouf B, Crews KR, Lew G, et al. Association of an inherited genetic variant with vincristine-related peripheral neuropathy in children with acute lymphoblastic leukemia. *JAMA*. 2015;**313**:815.

199   Rowinsky EK, Donehower RC. Drug therapy: paclitaxel (Taxol). *N Engl J Med*. 1995;**332**:1004.

200   Cortes JE, Pazdur R. Docetaxel. *J Clin Oncol*. 1995;**13**:2643.

201   Ma WW, Hidalgo M. The winning formulation: the development of paclitaxel in pancreatic cancer. *Clin Cancer Res*. 2013;**19**:5572.

203   Villanueva C, Bazan F, Kim S, et al. Cabazitaxel: a novel microtubule inhibitor. *Drugs*. 2011;**71**:125.

205   McGuire WP, Hoskins WJ, Brady MF, et al. Cyclophosphamide and cisplatin compared with paclitaxel and cisplatin in patients with stage III and IV ovarian cancer. *N Engl J Med*. 1996;**334**:1.

207   Citron ML, Berry DA, Cirrincione C, et al. Randomized trial of dose-dense versus conventionally scheduled and sequential versus concurrent combination chemotherapy as postoperative adjuvant treatment of node-positive primary breast cancer: first report of Intergroup Trial C9741/Cancer and Leukemia Group B Trial 9741. *J Clin Oncol*. 2003;**21**:1432.

210   Sparano JA, Wang M, Martino S, et al. Weekly paclitaxel in the adjuvant treatment of breast cancer. *N Engl J Med*. 2008;**358**:1663.

216   Bonomi P, Kim K, Fariclough D, et al. Comparison of survival and quality of life in advanced nonsmall cell lung cancer patients treated with two dose levels of paclitaxel combined with cisplatin versus etoposide with cisplatin: results from an Eastern Cooperative Oncology Group trial. *J Clin Oncol*. 2000;**18**:623.

219   Martin M, Pienkowski T, Mackey J, et al. Breast cancer international research group 001 investigators. Adjuvant docetaxel for node-positive breast cancer. *N Engl J Med*. 2005;**352**:2302.

220   Fossella F, Pereira JR, von Pawel J, et al. Randomized, multinational, phase III study of docetaxel plus platinum combinations versus vinorelbine plus cisplatin for advanced nonsmall-cell lung cancer: the TAX 326 study group. *J Clin Oncol*. 2003;**21**:3016.

221   Tannock IF, de Wit R, Berry WR, et al. Docetaxel plus prednisone or mitoxantrone plus prednisone for advanced prostate cancer. *N Engl J Med*. 2004;**351**:1502.

222   Posner MR, Hershock DM, Blajman CR, et al. TAX 324 study group. Cisplatin and fluorouracil alone or with docetaxel in head and neck cancer. *N Engl J Med*. 2007;**357**:1705.

224   Van Cutsem E, Moiseyenko VM, Tjulandin S, et al. Phase III study of docetaxel and cisplatin plus fluorouracil compared with cisplatin and fluorouracil as first-line therapy for advanced gastric cancer: a report of the V325 Study Group. *J Clin Oncol*. 2006;**24**:4991.

225   de Bono JS, Oudard S, Ozguroglu M, et al. Prednisone plus cabazitaxel or mitoxantrone for metastatic castration-resistant prostate cancer progressing after docetaxel treatment: a randomised open-label trial. *Lancet*. 2010;**376**:1147.

226   Gradishar WJ, Tjulandin S, Davidson N, et al. Phase III trial of nanoparticle albumin-bound paclitaxel compared with polyethylated castor oil-based paclitaxel in women with breast cancer. *J Clin Oncol*. 2005;**23**:7794.

227   Socinski MA, Bondarenko I, Karaseva NA, et al. Weekly nab-paclitaxel in combination with carboplatin versus solvent-based paclitaxel plus carboplatin as first-line therapy in patients with advanced nonsmall-cell lung cancer: final results of a phase III trial. *J Clin Oncol*. 2012;**30**:2055.

228   Manfredi JJ, Parness J, Horwitz SB. Taxol binds to cellular microtubules. *J Cell Biol*. 1982;**94**:688.

229   Schiff PB, Fant J, Horwitz SB. Promotion of microtubule assembly in vitro by taxol. *Nature*. 1979;**22**:665.

230   Horwitz SB, Cohen D, Rao S, et al. Taxol: mechanisms of action and resistance. *J Natl Cancer Inst Monogr*. 1993;**15**:55.

235   Jordan A, Hadfield JA, Lawrence NJ, McGowan AT. Tubulin as a target for anticancer drugs which interact with the mitotic spindle. *Med Res Rev*. 1998;**18**:259.

237   Giannakakou P, Gussio R, Nogales E, et al. A common pharmacophore for epothilone and taxanes: molecular basis for drug resistance conferred by tubulin mutations in human cancer cells. *Proc Natl Acad Sci U S A*. 2000;**97**:2904.

239   Ringel I, Horwitz SB. Studies with RP56976 (Taxotere): a semisynthetic analogue of taxol. *J Natl Cancer Inst*. 1991;**83**:288.

243   Jordan MA. Kamath K How do microtubule-targeted drugs work? An overview. *Curr Cancer Drug Targets*. 2007;**7**:730.

248   Weaver BA. How taxol/paclitaxel kills cancer cells. *Mol Biol Cell*. 2014;**25**:2677.

252   Dumontet C, Sikic B. Mechanism of action and resistance to antitubulin agents: microtubule dynamics, drug transport, and cell death. *J Clin Oncol*. 1999;**17**:1061.

265   Rowinsky EK, Donehower RC, Jones RJ, Tucker RW. Microtubule changes and cytotoxicity in leukemic cell lines treated with taxol. *Cancer Res*. 1988;**48**:4093.

282   Desei N. Nanoparticle albumin bound (nab) technology: targeting tumors through the endothelial gp60 receptor and SPARC. *Nanomedicine*. 2007;**3**:339.

286   Desai N, Trieu V, Yao Z, et al. Increased anticancer activity, intratumor paclitaxel concentrations, and endothelial cell transport of cremophor-free, albumin-bound paclitaxel, ABI-007, compared with cremophor-based paclitaxel. *Clin Cancer Res*. 2006;**12**:1317.

306   Kavallaris M. Microtubules and resistance to tubulin-binding agents. *Nat Rev Cancer*. 2010;**10**:194.

347   Bruno R, Hille D, Riva A, et al. Population pharmacokinetic/pharmacodynamics of docetaxel in phase II studies in patients with cancer. *J Clin Oncol*. 1998;**16**:186.

395   Eisenhower E, ten Bokkel HW, Swenerton KD, et al. European-Canadian randomized trial of Taxol in relapsed ovarian cancer: high vs low dose and long vs short infusion. *J Clin Oncol*. 1994;**12**:2654.

396   Rowinsky EK, Chaudhry V, Cornblath DR, Donehower RC. The neurotoxicity of taxol. *Monogr Natl Cancer Inst*. 1993;**15**:107.

415   Piccart MJ, Klijn J, Paridaens R, et al. Corticosteroids significantly delay the onset of docetaxel-induced fluid retention: final results of a randomized study of the European organization for research and treatment of cancer, investigational drug branch for breast cancer. *J Clin Oncol*. 1997;**15**:149.

435   Bollag DM, McQueney PA, Zhu J, et al. Epothilones, a new class of microtubule-stabilizing agents with a taxol-like mechanism of action. *Cancer Res*. 1995;**55**:2325.

437   Bode CJ, Gupta ML Jr, Reiff EA, Suprenant KA, Georg GI, Himes RH. Epothilone and paclitaxel: unexpected differences in promoting the assembly and stabilization of yeast microtubules. *Biochemistry*. 2002;**41**:3870.

438   Lechleider RJ, Kaminskas E, Jiang X, et al. Ixabepilone in combination with capecitabine and as monotherapy for treatment of advanced breast cancer refractory to previous chemotherapies. *Clin Cancer Res*. 2008;**14**:4378.

443   Goodin S, Kane MP, Rubin EH. Epothilones: mechanism of action and biologic activity. *J Clin Oncol*. 2004;**22**:2015.

456   Dybdal-Hargreaves NF, Risinger AL, Mooberry SL. Eribulin mesylate: mechanism of action of a unique microtubule-targeting agent. *Clin Cancer Res*. 2015;**21**:2445.

458   Jain S, Vahdat LT. Eribulin mesylate. *Clin Cancer Res*. 2011;**17**:6615.

463   Tozer GM, Kanthou C, Baguley BC. Disrupting tumour blood vessels. *Nat Rev Cancer*. 2005;**5**:423.

473   Goldenson B, Crispino JD. The aurora kinases in cell cycle and leukemia. *Oncogene*. 2015;**34**:537.

474   Archambault V, Lépine G, Kachaner D. Understanding the polo kinase machine. *Oncogene*. 2015;**10**:1038.

477   Iyer U, Kadambi VJ. Antibody drug conjugates—Trojan horses in the war on cancer. *J Pharmacol Toxicol Methods*. 2011;**64**:207.

478   Klute K, Nackos E, Tasaki S, et al. Microtubule inhibitor-based antibody-drug conjugates for cancer therapy. *Onco Targets Ther*. 2014;**7**:2227.

480   Chari RV, Martell BA, Gross JL, et al. Immunoconjugates containing novel maytansinoids: promising anticancer drugs. *Cancer Res*. 1992;**52**:127.

61 Endocrine therapy for hormone receptor-positive breast cancer

Aman U. Buzdar, MD, FACP ▪ Shaheenah Dawood, MD, MBBch, FACP, FRCP, MPH, CPH ▪ Harold A. Harvey, MD ▪ Virgil Craig Jordan, OBE, PhD, DSc, FMedSci

Overview

The importance of the reproductive endocrine system in breast cancer treatment began to be appreciated at the turn of nineteenth century. It was around this time that it was realized that approximately one-third of premenopausal women with advanced breast cancer would respond to oophorectomy. However, it was only when the estrogen receptor (ER) was discovered that it was possible to fully appreciate the mechanisms underlying the activity of ovarian ablation and other associated treatments for breast cancer such as ovarian irradiation, adrenalectomy, and hypophysectomy. Research into both the estrogen and progesterone pathways not only provided a deeper understanding of the underlying mechanism of the carcinogenic pathway involved in the development of breast cancer but also allowed identification of potential targets for therapeutic intervention.

This chapter discusses recent advances in the molecular biology and physiology underlying the estrogen and progesterone receptor (PR) pathways and potential targets for intervention. In addition it examines and compares the pharmacology and efficacy of the different endocrine agents used in the management of both early and advanced stage breast cancer.

Biology of progestin production and action

Progestins are involved in the regulation of development and differentiation, proliferation, apoptosis, and metabolism in many target tissues with broad implications in neoplasia. In addition progestins serve as precursors to the estrogens, androgens, and adrenocortical steroids. Some of the progestin effects on target tissues are mediated by transcription, whereas other effects are more rapid and do not involve direct transcriptional effects. Progestins (Figure 1) include the naturally occurring hormone progesterone, 17α-acetoxyprogesterone derivatives in the pregnane series, 19-nortestosterone derivatives (estranes), and norgestrel and related compounds in the gonane series. In humans progesterone is the most important progestin.

Synthesis and sites of production

Progesterone is produced early in the scheme of the synthetic pathway involving the conversion of cholesterol to androgens, progestins, and estrogens. After menopause, in the absence of hormone replacement, the adrenal gland becomes the principal source of progestins (through the conversion of pregnenolone) as well as other sex steroids. In the premenopausal woman, progesterone is principally derived from the corpus luteum of the ovary, but in pregnancy after the eighth week of gestation, placental progesterone production greatly exceeds ovarian-derived progesterone. The placental trophoblast is the dominant cell responsible for progesterone production by the placenta. The development of

a secretory endometrium in which the blastocyst can implant requires progesterone. Progesterone levels of 25 ng/mL are usual in the luteal phase of the menstrual cycle, whereas levels up to 150 ng/mL are seen in late pregnancy.

Mechanism of action

Progesterone functions in RNA transcription regulation through a complex series of interactions that is initiated by binding of the hormone to its cognate receptor. There are two isoforms of the progesterone receptor (PR) known as PR-A and PR-B that have distinct biological activities. PR-B has been shown to mediate the stimulatory activities of progesterone, while PR-A functions to inhibit the action of PR-B as well as other steroid receptors.[1–3] Both isoforms are encoded by a single gene, and their ratios vary in reproductive tissues as a consequence of developmental status, hormonal levels, and tissue type. Both isoforms of PR contain AF-1 and AF-2 transactivation domains with PR-B also containing an additional AF-3 domain which functions to contribute to its cell- and promoter-specific activity. The ligand for both isoforms of PR is identical.

In the absence of the hormone, PR is found in the nucleus in an inactive monomeric state associated with a complex of heat shock proteins (HSP -90, 70, 60, and 40) and is transcriptionally inactive.[4,5] Binding of progesterone to PR results in the dissociation of the heat shock proteins leading to the formation of receptor-ligand homodimers that remain localized in the nucleus and bind to highly selective progesterone response elements (PREs) located on target genes.[6] It is important to note that target cells must distinguish not only progesterone from other steroids, present in small amounts, but also progesterone from other hydrophobic molecules that are frequently found in 100-fold or greater excess. Such a high degree of discrimination is limited to differentiated cells that possess PR proteins and activatable PREs in their genome.[6,7] The next step in the process is the transcriptional activation by PR, which results from the interaction with a number of coactivators including steroid receptor coactivator 1 (SRC-I), transcription intermediary factor 2, and retinoic acid coactivator 3, among others.[6–9] The SRC-1 interacts with the N-terminal AF-1 and the C-terminal AF-2 of the PR. This serves to emphasize that SRC-1 function to synergize the ligand-independent amino terminal AF-1 with the ligand-responsive carboxyl terminal AF-2 of the PR. The PR-coactivator complex then interacts further with additional proteins that have histone acetylase activity that causes chromatin remodeling serving to increase accessibility of transcriptional proteins to the promoter target.[8]

Physiologic actions

Progestins are involved in a number of benign physiologic changes ranging from differentiated secretory activity to edematous changes

Holland-Frei Cancer Medicine, Ninth Edition. Edited by Robert C. Bast Jr., Carlo M. Croce, William N. Hait, Waun Ki Hong, Donald W. Kufe, Martine Piccart-Gebhart, Raphael E. Pollock, Ralph R. Weichselbaum, Hongyang Wang, and James F. Holland.
© 2017 John Wiley & Sons, Inc. ISBN: 978-1-118-93469-2

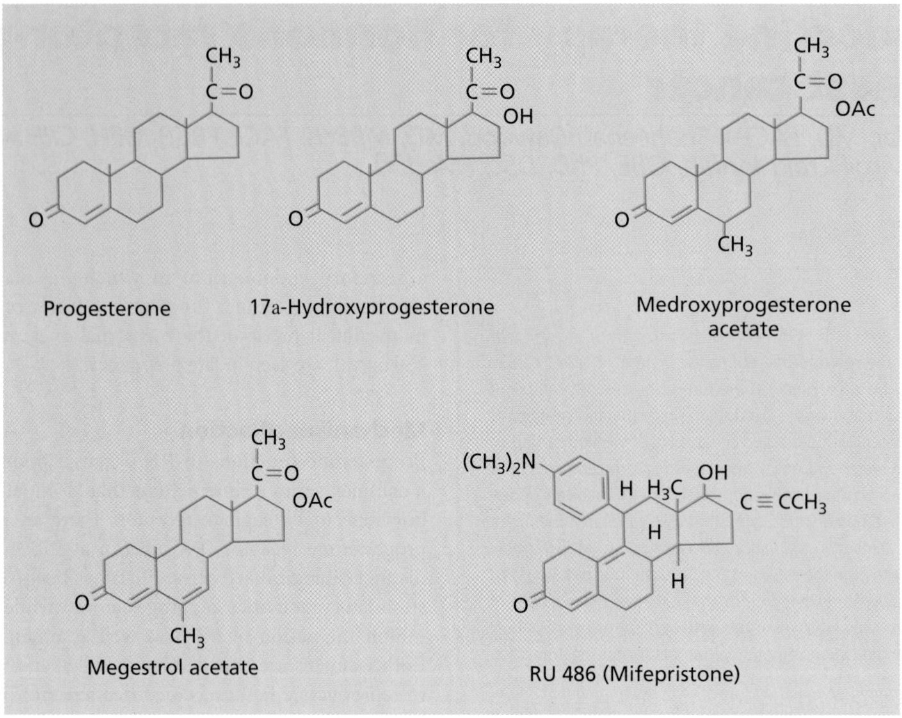

Figure 1 Structure of progesterone, 17α-hydroxyprogesterone, and synthetic progestins.

in stromal tissues of the breast. They also have implications on neoplastic processes being associated with both a decreased risk of endometrial neoplasms and a slightly increased risk of breast neoplasms when used in conjunction with estrogen replacement for menopause. Progestins have a critical role in the support of the products of conception: the differentiation of the endometrium and the promotion of the secretory phase of the endometrium; the maturation and cornification of the vaginal mucosal epithelium; the suppression of ovulation; the inhibition of gonadotropin release; the proliferation of breast epithelium and the induction of secretory activity in breast epithelium; and a natriuretic effect on the kidneys. A number of these biologic effects of progesterone are seen only in concert with priming of the target tissues with estrogen, whereas other effects appear to be interrelated with the actions of other steroid hormones, peptide hormones, and/or growth factors. Possible interactions between progesterone, estrogen, and growth factors must be taken into account when constructing treatment strategies.

Synthetic progestins

Synthetic progestins are derivatives of the steroid structure of either progesterone or testosterone. The synthetic progestins most often encountered include 17-hydroxyprogesterone, medroxyprogesterone (Provera), medroxyprogesterone acetate (MPA), megestrol acetate (MA) (Megace), norethindrone, norethindrone enanthate, norethindrone acetate, norethynodrel, norgestrel, desogestrel, and gestodene. The two most widely used synthetic progestins are MPA and MA, which differ only by a single bond at C6–C7. MPA can be administered as either an oral or intramuscular (IM) preparation, while MA is administered as an oral preparation.

Synthetic progestins are used most frequently in contraception, in conjunction with estrogen in postmenopausal hormone replacement therapy (HRT) and in endocrine treatment of uterine and breast cancer. In postmenopausal HRT, progestins are added to estrogen replacement principally to minimize the risk of uterine cancer associated with estrogen-only therapy, although the effects of adding progestins to estrogen on the risk of breast cancer have become of increasing concern.[10] In premenopausal women, progestins and antiprogestins are used predominantly in contraceptive preparations.[11] Progestins are often used alone in selected women with climacteric symptoms who are advised not to take estrogens.

Metastatic breast cancers

Progestins and PR have been studied extensively in cancerous human breast tissue. Patients whose tumors are PR positive have a higher probability of responding to endocrine therapy (not necessarily progestins) and in most series show a somewhat better prognosis with respect to both survival and disease-free interval.[12] Both MPA and MA have been shown to produce similar reductions in serum estrogen levels and produce responses of approximately 30% in patients with metastatic breast cancer.[13] The principal progestin used for metastatic breast cancer has been MA. The response of metastatic breast cancer to MA is predicted not only by the presence of ER (estrogen receptor) and/or PR but also by the observation of an objective response to previous hormonal therapy. Randomized studies have shown comparable efficacy of progestins to tamoxifen, aminoglutethemide, and aromatase inhibitors in the second and subsequent lines of treatment of metastatic breast cancer.[13,14] Currently progestin therapy for hormone receptor-positive metastatic breast cancer is used principally after disease progression has been observed following use of selective ER modulators (e.g., tamoxifen) and aromatase inhibitors. As such a trial of progestins is commonly used as the third or subsequent line of therapy in patients with hormone receptor-positive metastatic breast cancer (Figure 2).

Treatment of uterine cancer

Progestins are also used in the treatment of endometrial carcinoma.[15] When diagnosed, adenocarcinoma of the uterus is cured

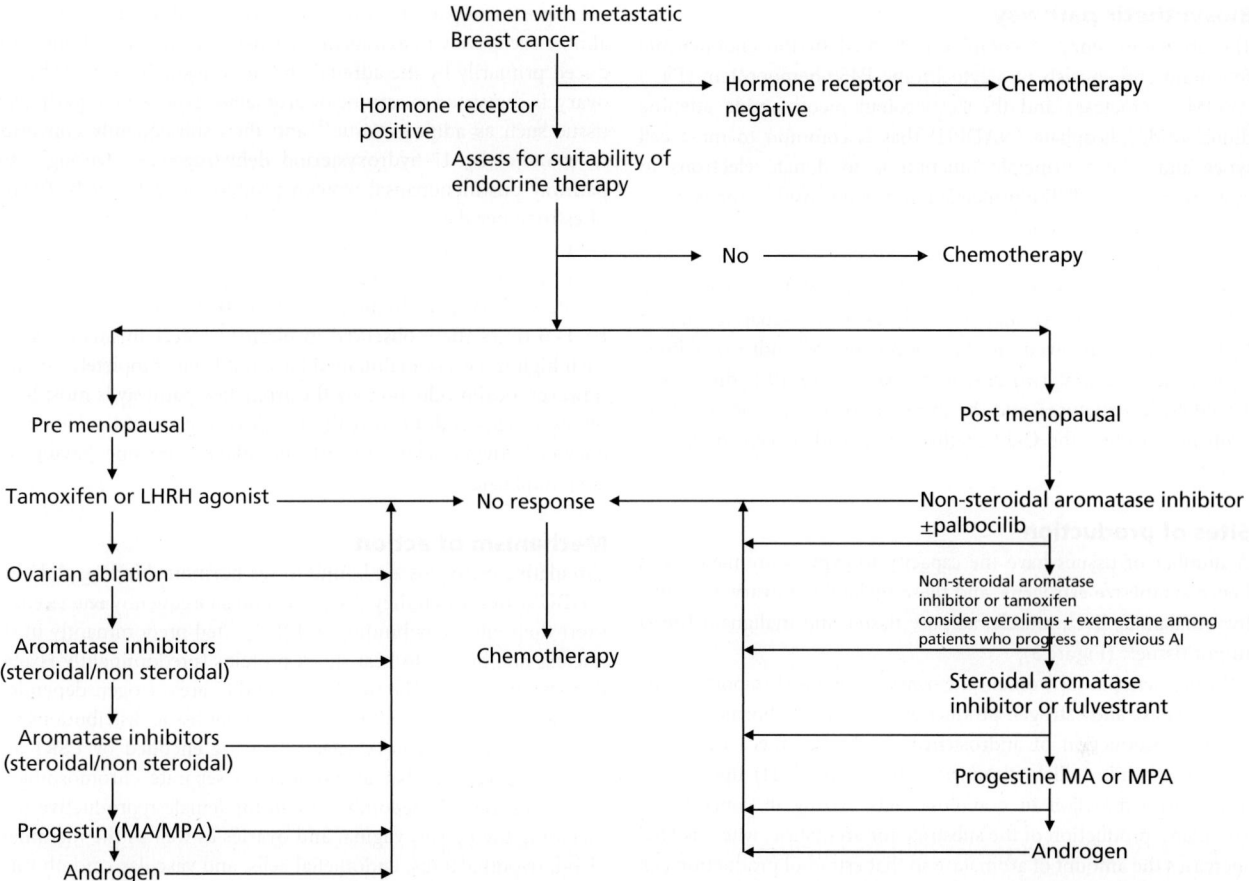

Figure 2 Algorithm for endocrine therapy among women with metastatic breast cancer.

by local therapy in 80% of cases. In the event of recurrence, exoge-nous progestin is an effective treatment in a significant fraction of cases: more than 30% of patients with recurrent disease demon-strate an objective response to exogenous progestins. ER and PR can be measured in these tumors, and the presence of these recep-tors correlates with differentiation of the tumor, prognosis for the patient, and response to progestins. The duration of response is not predicted by the presence of a receptor and varies from months to years. Tumors that lack ER and PR respond objectively to progestins in fewer than 10% of cases.[15]

Side effects and dosing of progestin

The most common adverse effect of progestin is weight gain, which occurs as a result of increased appetite and fluid retention. Its appetite-stimulating effect has frequently been used to treat cancer-induced cachexia. Other reported side effects include hot flashes, sweating, vaginal bleeding, nausea, dyspnea, thromboem-bolism, and rare cardiovascular events such as heart failure. Various dosing regimens of MA and MPA have been studied with a possible dose–response effect observed. The recommended dose of MA is 160 mg/day and that of MPA is at least 400–500 mg/day.[16]

Antiprogestins

Antiprogestins have wide and varied therapeutic applications including uses as contraceptives, to induce labor or to treat breast cancer, endometriosis, uterine leiomyomas, and meningiomas.[17] The oldest and most widely used antiprogestin is RU 38486 or mifepristone that is a derivative of the 19-norprogestin norethin-drone containing a dimethyl-aminophenol substituent at the 11β-position.[11,18] This compound is effectively absorbed orally and appears to bind with PR with high affinity and to effect altered coregulatory protein interaction after binding. It has been shown to have both antagonist and some agonist activity and is thus considered to be a PR modulator. Together with prostaglandins it is used for the termination of early pregnancy.[18]

Biology of estrogen production and action

A number of naturally occurring endogenous estrogens are produced in women with the most potent for both ER α- and β-mediated actions being estradiol followed by estrone and estriol. All three contain a phenolic A ring with a hydroxyl group at carbon 3 and a β-OH or ketone in position 17 of ring D with the phenolic A ring being the principle structural feature responsible for their selective high-affinity binding to both ERs.

The principle role of naturally occurring estrogens is to modulate cell growth by causing an increase in stimulatory growth factors [e.g., transforming growth factor-alpha (TGF-α)] and a decrease in inhibitory growth factors (e.g., TGF-β).[19] These growth factors are thought to initiate or prevent progress through the cell cycle by interaction with their respective membrane receptors, with the reg-ulatory mechanism functioning as an autocrine loop. There are also paracrine (cell–cell) influences of growth factors [e.g., insulin-like growth factor 1 (IGF-1)] that can play a role in modulating the replication of epithelial cells.

Biosynthetic pathway

The aromatase enzyme complex is located in the endoplasmic reticulum and consists of a cytochrome P450 hemoprotein (P450 AROM, aromatase) and the flavoprotein nicotinamide adenine dinucleotide phosphate (NADPH) that is common to most cell types and whose principle function is to donate electrons to cytochrome P450.[20] The principle enzyme involved in the conversion of androstenedione to estrone in the estrogen biosynthetic pathway is aromatase, a product of the CYP 19 gene that encodes a polypeptide of 503 amino acids with a molecular weight of 55 kilodaltons (KDa). Aromatase catalyzes three separate steroid hydroxylations involved in the conversion of androstenedione to estrone. The first two reactions give rise to 19-hydroxy and 19-aldehyde structures, and the third, although still controversial, probably involves the C-19 methyl group with release of formic acid.[21]

Sites of production

A number of tissues have the capacity to express aromatase and hence synthesize estrogens, and these include the ovary, placenta, hypothalamus, liver, muscle, adipose tissue, and malignant breast tumor tissue[22] (Figure 3).

In premenopausal women, the ovary is the most important site of aromatase and estrogen production. Luteinizing hormone (LH) controls production of androstenedione by the theca cell compartment, while follicle stimulating hormone (FSH) upregulates aromatase expression in granulose cells. Acting in concert, LH stimulates production of the substrate for aromatase, whereas FSH increases the amount of aromatase so that estradiol production can increase by 8- to 10-fold at the time of ovulation.

In postmenopausal women estrogen production takes place almost exclusively in extraglandular tissue. Androstenedione, produced primarily by the adrenal and, to a negligible extent, by the ovary, is converted to estrone by aromatase expressed in peripheral tissue such as adipose tissue[23] and then subsequently converted to estradiol by 17-hydroxysteriod dehydrogenase. Through this pathway postmenopausal women produce approximately 100 mg of estrone per day, with higher levels observed in obese women.[24] A fraction of estrone is also converted to estradiol to produce circulating plasma concentrations of approximately 10–20 pg/mL.

Estradiol levels in human breast tumor tissue are estimated to be 4–6 times these observed in plasma.[25] Mechanisms by which such high levels are maintained have not been completely defined; however local production via the aromatase pathway is most likely involved with additional pathways involving steroid sulfatase, an enzyme known to hydrolyze estrone sulfate to estrone, having also been implicated.[26]

Mechanism of action

Circulating estrogens are bound to sex hormone binding globulins (SHBG) from which they dissociate and subsequently enter cells to exert their effects by binding to ERs located predominantly in the nucleus and bound to heat shock proteins (predominantly Hsp90) that stabilize them. The two ERs α- and β- are estrogen-dependent nuclear transcription factors, with different tissue distributions and transcriptional regulatory effects that are encoded by ESR1 and ESR2, respectively, that are located on separate chromosomes.[27] ER α is expressed predominantly in the female reproductive tract including the uterus, vagina, and ovaries as well as the mammary gland, hypothalamus, endothelial cells, and vascular smooth muscles. ER β expression is found mainly in the prostate and ovaries

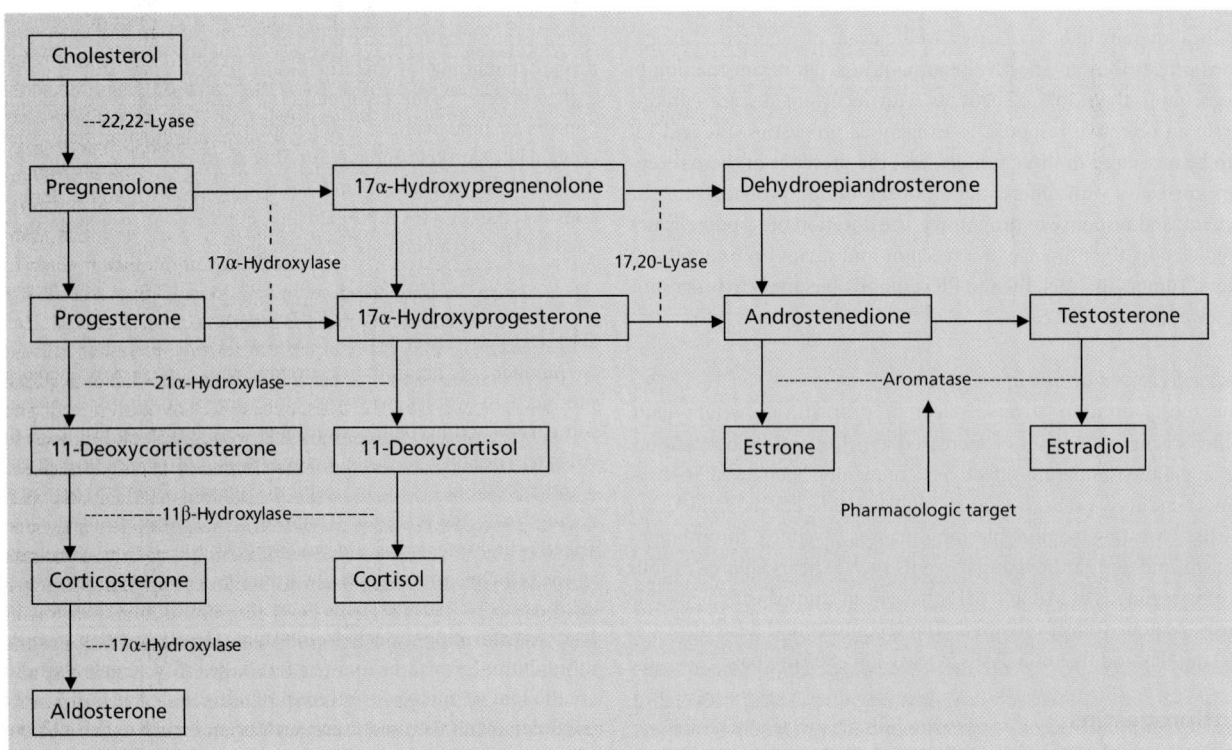

Figure 3 Sources of estrogen in postmenopausal women. The adrenal gland secretes androstenedione (A), which enters plasma and then tissue. Extraglandular and breast tumor tissues contain the enzymes necessary to convert A to estrone (E1) and to estradiol (E2) or to estrone sulfate (E1S). These steroids circulate in the plasma at levels indicated within the brackets and are expressed as picogram per milliliter.

with lower expression exhibited in the lung, brain, bone, and blood vessels. Coexpression of both ER α and β receptors are found in several tissues, the most notable being the mammary tissue where they form either homo- or heterodimers.

Binding of estrogen to the ERs results in a conformational change in the receptor leading to the release of ER from the stabilizing proteins. The estrogen–ER homodimeric complex then binds to a specific sequence of nucleotides called estrogen response elements (EREs) that are located in the promoter region of various genes. This binding interaction also involves a number of nuclear proteins, coregulators, as well as other components of the transcription machinery. Thus the genomic effects of estrogen are mainly the result of proteins synthesized from the regulation of transcription of a responsive gene. Two main modalities of treatment have been developed to treat estrogen-responsive breast cancers that either target preventing its production or inhibiting its interaction with ERs.

Carcinogenic effects

The major concern with the use of synthetic estrogens either alone or as a part of the preparation of oral contraceptives has been the development of cancer. Studies that reported the link between the intake of diethylstilbestrol (a synthetic estrogen) during the first trimester of pregnancy and the incidence of clear cell vaginal and cervical adenocarcinoma in later life of the offspring exposed in utero established for the first time that developmental exposure to estrogens was associated with an increase in human cancer.[28,29] Studies have also shown that unopposed estrogen as part of the HRT in postmenopausal women increased the risk of endometrial cancer by 5- to 15-fold[30] with the increased risk prevented by the addition of a progestin.[31]

The relation of breast cancer risk and HRT in postmenopausal women has also been reported by two large trials. The Women's Health Initiative (WHI) was a large prospective trial that randomized women to either placebo or HRT. The investigators reported an increase in total risk of breast cancer of 24% among women who took an estrogen–progestin combination and a decrease of 23% among women without a uterus who took estrogen only compared to women who took placebo.[10,32] In the extended poststopping phases of the WHI trials, the investigators further reported that some elevation in the risk of breast cancer risk still persisted in the cumulative follow-up period [HR 1.28, 95% CI (confidence interval) 1.11–1.48].[33] The Million Women Study (MWS) was a large cohort study that reported an increased relative risk (RR) of invasive breast cancer among women who did and did not take HRT.[34] Among women who took an estrogen–progestin combination, the increased RR of invasive breast cancer was 2 and that for women who took estrogen alone was reported as 1.3.

Epidemiological studies have also linked high levels of natural estrogens to the development of cancer. High levels of natural estrogens are observed in women who are overweight. Among postmenopausal women who had never received HRT in the WHI, those who were heavier (body mass index >31.1) had an elevated risk of breast cancer compared to slimmer women (body mass index <22.6) (RR = 2.52; 95% CI = 1.62–3.93).[32] High levels of natural estrogens were also found to be associated with breast cancer risk in a case-cohort study involving women who had never received exogenous estrogens.[35] The investigators reported that compared to women with the lowest levels of circulating estradiol, those with the highest levels (> or = 6.83 pmol/L or 1.9 pg/mL) had a RR of 3.6 (95% CI, 1.3–10.0).

Bone mineral density has also been shown to be a surrogate marker of estrogen exposure. A high endogenous estrogen concentration has been reported to be associated with greater bone mineral density in elderly women.[36] Postmenopausal women with higher bone mineral densities have also been shown to have a higher incidence of breast cancer.[37] Such studies serve to indicate the potential benefit of circulating estrogens as a surrogate marker of breast cancer risk. However its reliability as a surrogate marker is controversial due to the low baseline levels observed among postmenopausal women and the timing of circulating estrogen level measurement with relation to the menstrual cycle being important in premenopausal women. Regardless, enough evidence exists connecting estrogens to the development of hormone-responsive breast cancer that has spawned a number of prevention trials that have used agents targeted either at blocking the production of estrogens or its interaction with its receptor.

Selective estrogen receptor modulators and antiestrogens

The first indication of the role of hormones in the development of breast cancer occurred more than a century ago when in 1896, Beatson observed that remission could be induced by removal of the ovaries in a subset of breast cancer patients.[38] Although not originally understood the observed effects occurred as a result of eliminating the primary source of estrogen in premenopausal women. This was confirmed in preclinical studies that demonstrated estradiol to promote proliferation of ER-positive breast cancer cells in culture[39] and numerous epidemiological studies that have linked estrogens to breast cancer risk.[32–37] With the realization of the important role estrogen played in the development and progression of breast cancer, two groups of drugs were developed to counteract the action of estrogens. The first group essentially prevented the interaction of estrogen to its receptor and included the selective estrogen receptor modulators (SERMs) and antiestrogens. SERMs including tamoxifen, raloxifene, and toremifene display unusual tissue-selective pharmacology having estrogen agonist properties in some tissues (bone, liver, and cardiovascular system), estrogen antagonist properties in other tissues (brain and breast), and mixed agonist/antagonist estrogen properties in the uterus. The antiestrogens which include fulvestrant are distinguished from SERMs in that they are uniformly estrogen antagonists. The second group of drugs blocks the production of estrogen by blocking the action of the aromatase enzyme and is known as aromatase inhibitors. In this section we will review the various SERMs and antiestrogens used in clinical practice for the treatment and prevention of hormone receptor-positive breast cancers (Figure 4).

Tamoxifen

Mode of action

Tamoxifen is a nonsteroidal triphenylethylene compound that exerts its effects by competitively inhibiting the binding of estradiol to ER thereby negating the stimulatory effects of estrogen causing the cell to be held at the G1 phase of the replication cycle.[40] Tamoxifen is an estrogen antagonist in the breast and an estrogen agonist in the endometrium and bone, and it is this balance in biological properties that is key to the current strategies for the use of tamoxifen.

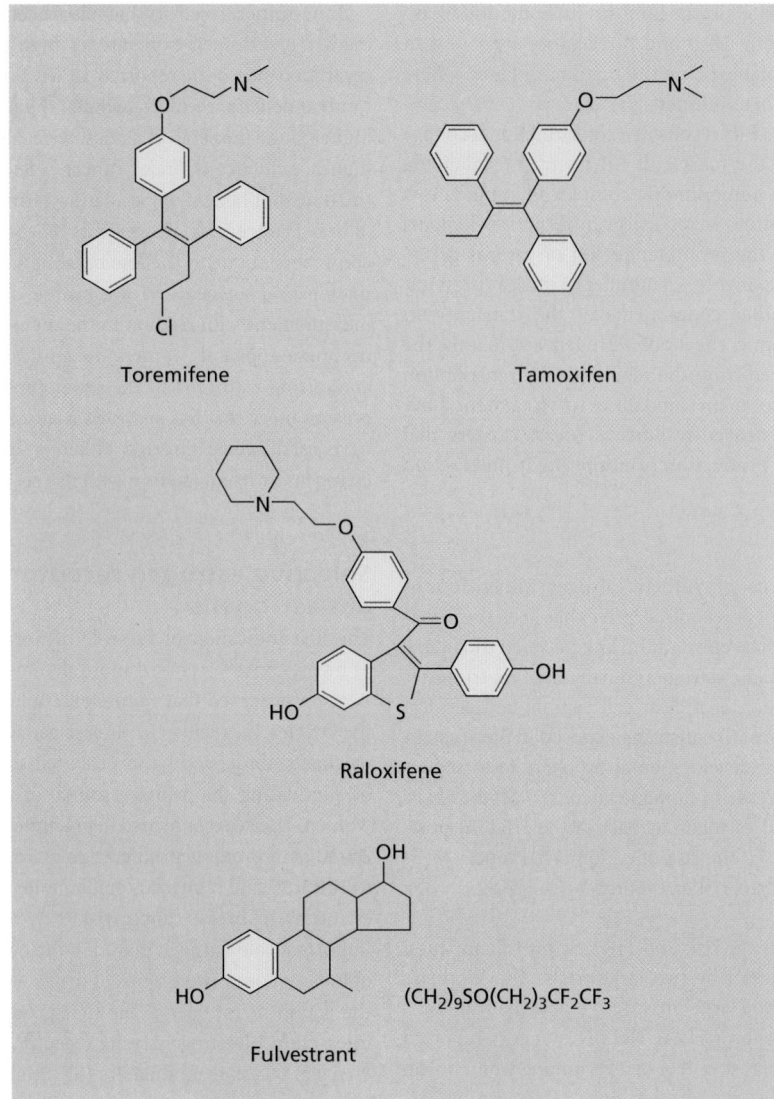

Figure 4 Structure of selective estrogen receptor modulators (SERMs) and antiestrogens.

Clinical pharmacology

The high therapeutic index of tamoxifen has permitted wide variations in dosage with schedules and dosage of treatment varying depending on the country and its initial clinical trials that evaluated efficacy of this drug. Schedules of 10 mg twice daily or 20 mg once daily are recommended in the United States, although 10 mg three times daily and 20 mg twice daily have been used in other countries.

Tamoxifen is administered orally and is rapidly absorbed, achieving steady state serum levels within 4–6 weeks. It is metabolized in the liver by the cytochrome P450 isoform CYP2D6 and CYP3A4 into *N*-desmethyltamoxifen (major metabolite) and 4-hydroxytamoxifen (minor metabolite); both of which have the potential to be further metabolized to 4-hydroxy-*N*-desmethyltamoxifen (minor metabolite endoxifen) which have 30–100 times more affinity to the ER compared to tamoxifen itself.[41] Tamoxifen has a long serum half-life of 7 days, and the metabolite *N*-desmethyltamoxifen has an even longer half-life of 14 days.[42] These long serum half-lives are probably why a withdrawal response has not been routinely documented when tamoxifen therapy is discontinued. Currently no clinical cases of teratogenesis have been documented with tamoxifen. As the potential for

teratogenicity is unclear, it is as such not recommended in pregnant women. Furthermore tamoxifen is known to cause ovarian stimulation in premenopausal women with ovulatory cycles, and thus women taking tamoxifen who are at risk of getting pregnant should be counseled about various contraceptive options.[43]

Tamoxifen in advanced breast cancer

Tamoxifen is an endocrine option for metastatic disease in postmenopausal women and those with ER-positive disease are more likely to benefit from this therapy.[44] More recent data suggests that aromatase inhibitors are a better option as first-line treatment for this cohort of patients so long as resistance to the drug has not developed. This will be discussed in further detail in the section of "Aromatase inhibitors."

Tamoxifen is an option for first-line endocrine therapy in premenopausal women with advanced breast cancer. A meta-analysis of individual patient data from four studies has demonstrated that tamoxifen produces a response rate and overall survival (OS) similar to what is seen after oophorectomy.[45] However, with the development of effective luteinizing hormone-releasing hormone (LHRH) agonists such as goserelin (Zoladex), which acts to reduce ovarian steroidogenesis by preventing LH release from the pituitary gland, the combination of LHRH agonist and tamoxifen has become established as an effective therapeutic option, and the combination of which in meta-analysis has been shown to significantly improve progression free and OS compared to LHRH agonist alone.[46] Hence recent guidelines have suggested that the use of LHRH agonists and tamoxifen alone or in combination are appropriate therapeutic options for premenopausal women with advanced metastatic hormone receptor-positive disease[47] (Figure 3).

Tamoxifen in the adjuvant setting

Many randomized trials have addressed the question of tamoxifen efficacy in the adjuvant setting among women with early-stage breast cancer. An overview and meta-analysis of the results from 145,000 women with early-stage breast cancer who were randomized to 194 trials of adjuvant systemic therapy (chemotherapy and/or hormonal therapy) were recently updated by the Early Breast Cancer Trialists' Collaborative Group (EBCTCG).[48] The EBCTCG reported that 5 years of adjuvant tamoxifen among women with ER-positive disease resulted in reduction in the annual breast cancer death rate by 31% regardless of age, PR status, menopausal status, or use of chemotherapy with benefit persisting up to 15 years of follow-up. In this report 1 year of tamoxifen conferred little benefit, 5 years of tamoxifen was significantly more effective than 2 years, with long-term follow-up still required for assessing the benefit of more than 5 years of adjuvant tamoxifen treatment. A number of prospective trials have looked at the efficacy of tamoxifen beyond 5 years in the adjuvant setting (Table 1).[49–53] The B-14 trial, a National Surgical Adjuvant Breast and Bowel Project (NSABP) trial, in which women with lymph node-negative ER-positive disease still in remission after receiving 5 years of tamoxifen were randomized to receive either placebo or more prolonged therapy with tamoxifen, did not show any advantage from prolonged tamoxifen treatment after 7 years of follow-up.[49] Indeed longer duration of tamoxifen use was associated with shorter disease-free survival (DFS) compared to the group who had stopped taking tamoxifen after 5 years (78% vs 82%, $p = 0.03$). Recently long-term follow-up data of two large phase III trials that randomized women with early-stage breast cancer who had completed 5 years of tamoxifen to either another 5 years tamoxifen or stopping endocrine therapy have been reported.[50,51] In the Adjuvant Tamoxifen: Longer Against Shorter (ATLAS) trial, 12894 women with early breast cancer were enrolled.[50] Among the 6846 women who had ER-positive disease, the investigators reported a significant reduction in the risk of breast cancer recurrence ($p = 0.002$), breast cancer mortality ($p = 0.01$), and overall mortality ($p = 0.01$) favoring patients who were randomized to receive 10 years of tamoxifen. The investigators

further reported that between years 5 and 14 of follow-up, 10 years of tamoxifen resulted in an absolute reduction in risk of breast cancer recurrence and mortality of 3.7% and 2.8%, respectively. However, between years 5 and 14 of follow-up, there was also an increased cumulative risk of endometrial cancer among patients allocated to 10 years of tamoxifen (3.1% vs 1.6%) which was associated with an absolute mortality increase of 0.2%. In the Adjuvant Tamoxifen Treatment Offer More (aTTom) trial, 6953 women with early breast cancer were enrolled.[51] Similar to the ATLAS trial, the investigators reported reductions in breast cancer recurrence, breast cancer specific mortality, and overall mortality favoring patients who received 10 years of tamoxifen. The investigators observed that continuing tamoxifen beyond 5 years reduced breast cancer recurrence beginning year 7 and breast cancer mortality after year 10. In view of the evidence from these two clinical trials, current guidelines recommend consideration of 10 years of adjuvant tamoxifen.[47] This should be considered after full discussion about potential associated increase in associated side effects.

Tamoxifen and chemotherapy

The latest update of the EBCTCG revealed that addition of anthracycline-based polychemotherapy regimens was reported to be associated with annual reduction of mortality of 38% and 20% among women aged <50 years and 50–69 years, respectively.[48] The question however is whether the addition of an endocrine agent such as tamoxifen could further add to this benefit among women with ER-positive breast tumors. In the EBCTCG among 3330 women with ER-positive or ER-unknown tumors, 28.1% of women who received only chemotherapy experienced a recurrence compared to 17.5% who received chemotherapy and 5 years of tamoxifen, with the difference being statistically significant.[48] Similarly, among women with ER-positive or ER-unknown breast tumors, for those who were less than 50 years of age and received chemotherapy and tamoxifen, the EBCTCG reported a recurrence rate ratio of 0.64 (SE = 0.08) and annual breast cancer mortality ratio of 0.65 (SE = 0.10) compared to those who received tamoxifen alone. In addition similar trends were observed among women in the 50–69 years age group. Therefore chemotherapy alone is not enough among women with ER-positive tumors with the data clear that the addition of tamoxifen is important. The EBCTCG also explored the question about the sequence of chemotherapy and tamoxifen. Among women 50–69 years of age, a recurrence rate ratio and annual breast cancer mortality rate ratio of 0.80 (SE = 0.03) and 0.90 (SE = 0.03) was reported, respectively, among women treated with chemotherapy and tamoxifen compared to those who received tamoxifen alone. A recurrence rate ratio and annual breast cancer mortality rate ratio of 0.77 (SE = 0.08) and

Table 1 Efficacy data from trials comparing continuing tamoxifen beyond five years and stopping it.

Trial	Intervention	Risk of recurrence	Breast cancer specific mortality	Disease-free survival	Overall survival
ECOG[53] (1996)	Continue vs stop	15% vs 25% ($p = 0.014$ among ER + patients)	8% vs 8.6%	85% vs 73% ($p = 0.10$)	86% vs 89% ($p = 0.81$ among ER+ patients)
NSABP-14[49] (2001)	Continue vs stop	NR	NR	78% vs 82% ($p = 0.03$)	91% vs 94% ($p = 0.07$)
Scottish cancer trials breast group[52] (2001)	Continue vs stop	5.2% vs 7.1%	23% vs 15%	54% vs 61% ($p = 0.15$)	59.5% vs 68% ($p = 0.12$)
ATLAS[50] (2012)	Continue vs stop	RR = 0.81 (premenopausal) RR = 0.85 (postmenopausal)	12.2% vs 15% ($p = 0.01$) during years 5–14 RR = 0.75 ($p = 0.002$) after year 10	NR	NR
aTTom[51] (2013)	Continue vs stop	28% vs 32% ($p = 0.003$)	RR = 0.75 ($p = 0.007$) after year 10	NR	24.5 % vs 26.1% ($p = 0.1$)

0.80 (SE = 0.10) was reported, respectively, among women treated with chemotherapy followed by tamoxifen compared to those who received tamoxifen alone.[48] The question about sequence of therapy was also explored by the Southwest Oncology Study Group (SWOG) 8814 study that reported improved disease-free and OS outcomes when tamoxifen was given sequentially following CAF (cyclophosphamide, doxorubicin, and 5-fluorouracil) compared with concurrent administration or tamoxifen alone.[54] Taken together the data are suggestive that the sequential hormonal therapy with chemotherapy may be a better a better option.

Prevention of breast cancer
Observations that long-term tamoxifen therapy reduced the incidence and risk of contralateral breast cancer in women with early-stage breast cancer fueled interest in exploring the effect of tamoxifen in preventing the occurrence of breast cancer. An overview of the main outcomes from the five main breast cancer prevention trials, covering more than 28,000 patients, has shown that tamoxifen produced a 38% reduction in breast cancer incidence ($p < 0.0001$).[55] There was no effect on ER-negative disease ($p = 0.21$), but ER-positive cancers were reduced by 48% ($p < 0.0001$). However, endometrial cancer rates were increased (consensus RR 2.4; $p = 0.0005$) in patients receiving preventive tamoxifen, as were venous thromboembolic events (relative risk 1.9; $p < 0.0001$). Thus when considering using tamoxifen as a preventive agent, it will be important to balance the risks of developing complications to that of developing breast cancer, and as such the unrestricted use of tamoxifen among young women of reproductive age should be used with caution. An exception to this is when tamoxifen is used for the reduction of breast cancer risk in high-risk women, for which it is the first medicine to be approved by the US Food and Drug Administration. Thus use of tamoxifen in preventive setting should be individualized to a woman's risk of developing breast cancer. As such, women with a prior history of ductal carcinoma *in situ*, lobular carcinoma *in situ*, atypical hyperplasia, or those with a deleterious mutation of BRCA 1 or 2 are considered to be at higher risk of developing breast cancer and represent an ideal cohort to target where benefit outweighs risk of adverse events associated with tamoxifen.[56–58] The side effects associated with tamoxifen meant that it was important to evaluate the action of other agents such as aromatase inhibitors in the preventive setting. The results of studies evaluating aromatase inhibitors as preventive agents will be discussed under the section titled "Aromatase inhibitors."

Raloxifene

Raloxifene is a benzothiophene second-generation SERM that is FDA approved for the treatment and prevention of osteoporosis and for the reduction of risk of invasive breast carcinoma in postmenopausal women with either osteoporosis or who are at high risk for invasive breast cancer, respectively.[59–62] This agent has no significant antitumor activity in the metastatic setting and as such is not approved for the treatment of advanced metastatic breast cancer. Four large prospective trials have reported on the efficacy of raloxifene as a chemopreventive agent for breast cancer. The Multiple Outcomes of Raloxifene Evaluation (MORE) trial that randomized 7705 postmenopausal women with osteoporosis to receive either raloxifene or placebo, whose primary end point was development of a fracture, was the first major trial to suggest raloxifene as a potential agent for chemoprevention of breast cancer.[59] In this trial, following 4 years of treatment, raloxifene reduced the risk of ER-positive invasive breast cancer by 84% (RR 0.16, 95% CI 0.09, 0.30). The Continuing Outcomes Relevant to Evista

(CORE) trial was an extension of the MORE trial to examine the effect of 4 additional years of raloxifene therapy on the incidence of invasive breast cancer in women enrolled in MORE who agreed to continue on the trial.[60] Combining the 8 years of follow-up of both the MORE and CORE trials, the investigators reported that the incidences of invasive breast cancer overall and ER-positive invasive breast cancer were reduced by 66% (HR = 0.34; 95% CI = 0.22 – 0.50) and 76% (HR = 0.24; 95% CI = 0.15 – 0.40), respectively, in the raloxifene group compared with the placebo group. The goal of the Raloxifene Use for the Heart (RUTH) trial was to investigate the effect of raloxifene on the incidence of coronary events and breast cancer in 10,101 postmenopausal women.[61] The investigators found reductions in breast cancer similar in size to that seen for tamoxifen in other studies. The NSABP P-2 trial is a prospective, double-blinded, randomized clinical trial that compared the efficacy and safety of tamoxifen with raloxifene on the risk of developing invasive breast cancer in a cohort of 19,747 postmenopausal women.[62] The investigators reported similar efficacy of tamoxifen compared to raloxifene in reducing the risk of invasive breast cancer (RR = 1.02; 95% CI 0.82 – 1.28). In terms of side effects, compared to tamoxifen, raloxifene had fewer gynecological and thromboembolic events. Interestingly raloxifene reduced the risk of invasive breast cancer but had no effect on the incidence of ductal carcinoma *in situ*.

Lasofoxifene

Lasofoxifene is a third-generation nonsteroidal SERM that has been shown to selectively bind to both ER α- and β with a high affinity and a median inhibitor concentration that is 10-fold higher than reported for raloxifene and tamoxifen. Furthermore it has demonstrated improved oral bioavailability when compared to other SERMs due to its increased resistance to intestinal wall glucuronidation.[63] Among postmenopausal women lasofoxifene has been shown to decrease bone loss, bone resorption, and low density lipoprotein (LDL) cholesterol. In a prospective randomized clinical trial, 8556 postmenopausal women who had a bone mineral density T score of −2.5 or less were randomly assigned to receive lasofoxifene or placebo for 5 years.[64] The investigators reported that compared to placebo, use of lasofoxifene among postmenopausal women with osteoporosis was associated with a reduced risk of ER-positive breast cancer, coronary heart disease, stroke, and nonvertebral and vertebral fractures. However it was also reported to be associated with an increased risk of venous thromboembolic events.

Toremifene

Toremifene (Fareston) is a structural derivative of tamoxifen with similar antiestrogenic and estrogenic properties demonstrated in laboratory animals. In general, toremifene is highly protein bound, which could explain its long serum half-life. Toremifene is less potent than tamoxifen, and, consequently, clinical studies have evaluated doses of toremifene up to 240 mg/day. Toremifene is cross-resistant with tamoxifen, but clinical trials have shown that it exhibits a similar efficacy and side effect profile to tamoxifen and so may be used as an alternative to treat advanced breast cancer.[65,66] At this time there is insufficient data to recommend its use in the adjuvant setting.

Trilostane

Trilostane (Modrenal) is an antiadrenal drug that is usually used for short-term adrenal suppression in the treatment of Cushing's syndrome. However, trilostane's ability to modify the binding of estrogen to the ER has prompted interest in its potential to block breast tumor cell proliferation. A meta-analysis of several small studies investigating the use of trilostane in postmenopausal women with advanced breast cancer reported clinical benefit with this agent, and further trials are needed to evaluate its worth as an endocrine therapy for advanced breast cancer.[67]

Fulvestrant

Fulvestrant (Faslodex) is an antiestrogen with no agonist properties and unlike tamoxifen has the following mechanism of action: it binds, blocks, and increases degradation of ER protein, leading to an inhibition of estrogen signaling through the ER together with dramatic loss of cellular ER levels and is also associated with a significant reduction in PgR expression.[68,69] A prospective combined analysis of two phase III trials comparing fulvestrant (250 mg IM injection once monthly) to anastrozole in a cohort of postmenopausal women with advanced breast cancer who had progressed on prior tamoxifen therapy indicated that, after a median follow-up of 15.1 months, fulvestrant was at least as effective as anastrozole [median times to progression (TTP) were 5.5 months vs 4.1 months] with a similar and acceptable adverse event profile.[70] Subsequently fulvestrant (at a dose of 250 mg IM) as first-line treatment of advanced breast cancer was compared to tamoxifen among postmenopausal women (whose tumors were either hormone receptor positive or hormone receptor unknown) in a randomized clinical trial.[71] At a median follow-up of 14.5 months in the overall population, noninferiority of fulvestrant compared to tamoxifen could not be demonstrated. In a preplanned subgroup analysis focusing on the cohort of patients with hormone receptor-positive disease, fulvestrant was observed to have a similar efficacy to tamoxifen. In the setting of a phase III, randomized clinical trial fulvestrant (at a dose of 250 mg IM) has also been compared to exemestane for the treatment of postmenopausal women with hormone receptor-positive advanced breast cancer who had progressed or recurred on a nonsteroidal aromatase inhibitor.[72] In this study overall response rate (7.4% vs 6.7%; $p = 0.736$) and time to treatment progression (3.7 months in both groups) were similar between the fulvestrant and exemestane groups suggesting that fulvestrant was no more effective than a steroidal aromatase inhibitor among women who had progressed on a nonsteroidal aromatase inhibitor. Since fulvestrant can take 3–6 months to reach steady state plasma levels at the 250 mg/month dose (previously approved dosing schedule), clinical trials have evaluated the standard dosing regimen to a loading dosing schedule. In a phase III double-blinded multicenter study, postmenopausal women with ER-positive advanced breast cancer who had progressed on prior endocrine therapy were assigned to receive IM monthly fulvestrant at a dose of 500 mg or 250 mg.[73] The investigators reported a significantly longer DFS with the 500 mg dosing schedule (HR 0.8, 95% CI 0.68–0.94, $p = 0.006$) with no associated increase in toxicity. Based on these results fulvestrant is approved at a dose of 500 mg a month for the treatment of hormone receptor-positive metastatic breast cancer in postmenopausal who had progressed on prior antiestrogen therapy. As the 500 mg dosing schedule was found to be superior to the 250 mg dosing schedule, trials are underway investigating whether the use of the new approved dose of fulvestrant is superior to aromatase inhibitors in the treatment of advanced hormone receptor-positive breast cancer in the first-line setting. In an open-labeled randomized phase II trial, postmenopausal women with advanced breast cancer were randomized in the first-line setting to either 500 mg of fulvestrant or anastrozole.[74] The investigators reported a significantly longer time to progression of disease with fulvestrant compared to anastrozole. Updated results of this analysis have recently been presented with

the investigators further reporting a significant improvement in OS with 500 mg of fulvestrant compared to anastrozole.[75] Phase III trials are currently ongoing to confirm these results (FALCON trial).

Side effects of SERMs and antiestrogens

Side effects related to the SERMs and antiestrogens develop mainly as a result of the blockade of the stimulatory function of estrogen on a variety of tissues. The most frequent side effects encountered are hot flashes, night sweats, and vaginal dryness similar to that seen in women undergoing menopause. Other less frequent but important side effects pertain to the bone, blood vessels, and carcinogenic effects.

Osteoporosis

Estrogen is important in maintaining bone health in premenopausal women with HRT and is often recommended to prevent the development of osteoporosis in postmenopausal women. Long-term administration of an antiestrogen has the potential to cause premature osteoporosis in premenopausal women. However due to the partial estrogen agonist function of SERMs, clinical studies have shown tamoxifen therapy to not be associated with a reduction of bone density,[76] and raloxifene is an approved treatment for osteoporosis.[69]

Coronary heart disease

Estrogen lowers LDL cholesterol levels and raises high-density lipoprotein (HDL) cholesterol levels, and thus prolonged administration of an antiestrogen could produce a population at risk of premature coronary heart disease. However, the estrogen-like effects of tamoxifen have been shown to lower the circulating levels of cholesterol in female patients[77,78] with clinical studies reporting tamoxifen to be associated with either a significant or trend in reduction of risk of coronary heart disease.[79] Raloxifene has also been shown to reduce serum cholesterol levels[80]: however it has not been shown in a large randomized clinical trial to reduce the risk of coronary heart disease.[61]

Thromboembolism

A number of studies have demonstrated an association between the use of tamoxifen and subsequent thromboembolic episodes in both the treatment and preventive setting.[55,81] This is comparable with increases noted with HRT or raloxifene[81] Patients with a known history of thromboembolic disorders should be carefully evaluated before a decision is made to use long-term tamoxifen therapy.

Endometrial tumors

Research has demonstrated that increases in endometrial thickness, hyperplasia, and fibroids may follow treatment with tamoxifen.[82] Endometrial thickening is associated with the stromal component of the uterus rather than the epithelial component.[83] Clinical trials evaluating the efficacy of tamoxifen in the treatment and prevention of breast cancer have demonstrated an increased risk of endometrial tumors including carcinomas and to a smaller extent sarcomas.[84,85] Endometrial carcinoma that develops on tamoxifen therapy is not of high grade and as such is not associated with poor prognosis, while endometrial sarcomas are generally associated with a poorer prognosis, seemingly because of less favorable histology and higher stage.[86] Thus when monitoring patients on tamoxifen treatment, all cases of persistent vaginal bleeding should be followed up with a gynecological examination and an endometrial biopsy. It is important to note that this increased risk is restricted to postmenopausal women with premenopausal women not at risk of an increase in endometrial cancer. When raloxifene was directly compared to tamoxifen in the prevention of breast cancer (STAR trial), 36 cases of endometrial cancer were observed in the tamoxifen group compared to 23 cases in the raloxifene group (RR, 0.62; 95% CI, 0.35–1.08).[62] In the ATLAS and aTTom trials that evaluated the efficacy of 5 years of tamoxifen to 10 years of tamoxifen in the adjuvant setting, the investigators reported that longer duration of tamoxifen was associated with increased incidence of endometrial cancer and associated increase risk of mortality from endometrial cancer.[50,51] The risk associated with tamoxifen usage appears confined to the duration of its administration. In the randomized International Breast Cancer Intervention Study (IBIS-I) (a prevention study that randomized patients to tamoxifen vs placebo), the rates of side effects pertaining to tamoxifen including deep vein thrombosis, pulmonary embolism, and endometrial cancer was higher in the tamoxifen arm of the study compared to the placebo arm during the active treatment period of the study but not in the subsequent years posttamoxifen treatment.[87]

Other side effects

Antiestrogens and SERMs have also been associated with ophthalmic side effects such as cataracts and retinal changes.[88,89] Preclinical studies have also demonstrated tamoxifen to cause carcinogenesis in the liver; however an increase in human hepatocellular carcinoma has not been demonstrated.[90]

Aromatase inhibitors

In contrast to SERMs and antiestrogens, aromatase inhibitors work by blocking the enzyme complex responsible for the final step in estrogen biosynthetic pathway and is thereby essentially preventing the production of the ER substrate. Moreover, unlike tamoxifen, aromatase inhibitors have no partial estrogen agonist function. Despite the ovaries being a rich source of aromatase, aromatase inhibitors are unable to sufficiently suppress ovarian estrogen production to postmenopausal levels which may be due to compensatory rise in gonadotrophins which maintains adequate estrogen production, despite the presence of the inhibitor. In contrast aromatase inhibitors have been shown to adequately suppress estrogen production in postmenopausal women.

Aromatase inhibitors are classified into first, second, and third-generation aromatase inhibitors according to the specificity and potency with which they inhibit the aromatase enzyme (Table 2). They are further subclassified according to their mechanism of action into steroidal (irreversible, type I) and nonsteroidal (reversible, type II) inhibitors. Type 1 inhibitors, including formestane and exemestane, function by irreversibly inhibiting the aromatase enzyme by covalently binding to it, resulting in permanent inactivation that persists even after discontinuation of the drug until the peripheral tissues synthesize new enzymes. Type II inhibitors, including anastrozole, letrozole, and fadrozole, in contrast bind reversibly to the active site of the aromatase enzyme and prevent product formation only as long as the inhibitor occupies the catalytic site. In this section we will focus on the newer third-generation aromatase inhibitors letrozole, anastrozole, and exemestane that are routinely used in clinical practice today. These aromatase inhibitors have challenged tamoxifen as the gold standard and are now the preferred first-line treatment of postmenopausal women with hormone-responsive breast cancer in either the early or advanced setting, whenever there is a moderate or high risk of relapse.

First generation

Aminoglutethimide, a derivative of the sedative agent glutethimide, was initially introduced as an inhibitor of cytochrome P450 N-mediated steroid hydroxylations.[91] The effects of this compound, however, are rather nonspecific, because the drug affects a number of hydroxylation steps in the metabolic conversion of cholesterol to active steroid products, and, overall, the use of aminoglutethimide plus glucocorticoid in women with breast cancer produces results similar to those expected from other forms of endocrine therapy. Side effects observed with standard doses of aminoglutethimide (1000 mg/day) include drug rash, fever, and lethargy.[91] With the development of more selective second and third-generation aromatase inhibitors, aminoglutethimide is now rarely used for the treatment of breast cancer

Second generation

The two second-generation aromatase inhibitors on the market are fadrozole and formestane. Fadrozole (4-[5,6,7,8-tetrahydroimidazo-(1,5-a)-pyridin-5yl] benzonitrile), a type II inhibitor, is a highly potent inhibitor of aromatase. Two large multicenter phase III trials have compared fadrozole with MA in patients who had received only tamoxifen as prior hormone therapy. No significant differences were observed between the two treatment arms of the trials with respect to time to treatment progression, overall response rate, response duration, or OS.[92] When compared to tamoxifen as a first-line treatment among postmenopausal women with advanced breast cancer, similar efficacy was observed between the two agents with fadrozole having a better tolerability profile.[93] Fadrozole has also been compared to letrozole in a double-blind randomized trial in the advanced breast cancer setting with letrozole having superior efficacy to fadrozole in this setting.[94] Toxicity attributed to fadrozole is mild and consists mainly of nausea, anorexia, fatigue, and hot flashes. Fadrozole represents a major improvement over aminoglutethimide, and the drug is approved in Japan for the treatment of patients with breast cancer.

Formestane (4-hydroxyandrostenedione, Lentaron), a type I inhibitor, is given by IM injection and is thus associated with in-site reactions. It has been tested in clinical trials as second-line treatment for postmenopausal women with metastatic disease and demonstrated similar efficacy to MA among those who had progressed on tamoxifen[95] with clinical benefit also demonstrated in patients who have progressed on nonsteroidal aromatase inhibitors.[96]

Third generation

Third-generation aromatase inhibitors have now become the standard treatment for postmenopausal women with either advanced or early-stage hormone-responsive breast cancer having demonstrated superior efficacy and tolerability compared to tamoxifen. Third-generation aromatase inhibitors include exemestane, letrozole, and anastrozole.

Exemestane (6-methylene-androsta-1,4-diene-3,17-dione, Aromasin), a type I aromatase inhibitor, is an oral analogue of the natural substrate androstenedione. It is rapidly absorbed from the gastrointestinal tract, reaching maximum plasma levels after 2 h and has been shown to lower estrogen levels more effectively than formestane. Single-dose administration of 25 mg/day exemestane inhibits aromatase activity by 97.9% and lowers plasma estrone and estradiol levels by about 90%.[97] The FDA-approved dosing regimen for exemestane is 25 mg once daily as an oral preparation.

Table 2 Structure and classification of representative aromatase inhibitors.

Generation		Steroidal irreversible type I inhibitors	Nonsteroidal reversible type II inhibitors
First generation			Aminoglutethimide
Aminoglutethimide	Rogletimide		
Second generation		Formestane	Fadrozole
Lentaron	Exemestane		
Fadrozole			
Third generation		Exemestane	Anastrozole
			Letrozole
			Vorozole
Letrozole	Arimidex	Vorozole	

Compounds are shown in approximate order of increasing specificity and potency of aromatase inhibition.

Anastrozole (Arimidex), a type II inhibitor, is a potent and selective benzotriazole derivative absorbed rapidly after oral administration with peak concentration achieved after 2 h and steady state after 7 days and has an elimination half-life in humans of approximately 32.2 h.[98] Anastrozole at doses of 1 or 10 mg administered once daily for 28 days has been shown to reduce total body aromatization by 96.7% and 98.1%, respectively.[98] The FDA-approved dosing regimen of anastrozole is 1 mg orally once a day.

Letrozole (4,4′-[(1H-1,2,4-triazol-1-yl) methylene] bis-benzonitrile, Femara), a type II inhibitor, is a highly potent inhibitor of aromatase *in vitro* and *in vivo* and is associated with greater suppression of estrogen plasma levels than is achieved with other aromatase inhibitors.[99] When administered orally to adult female rats at a dose of 1 mg/L/day for 14 days, letrozole decreased

uterine weight to that observed after a surgical ovariectomy.[99] Clinical studies in normal healthy volunteers, as well as phase I trials in postmenopausal women with advanced breast cancer, showed that letrozole in a dose as little as 0.25 mg/day PO caused maximal suppression of plasma and urinary estrogens.[100] The FDA-approved and recommended dosing regimen for letrozole is 2.5 mg orally once a day.

Vorozole (R83842; R76713; 6-[(S)4-Chlorophenyl]-1H-1,2,4-triazol-1-ylmethyl]-1-methyl-1H-benzotriazole), another specific type II aromatase inhibitor, has shown little toxicity in animal studies. However, despite results from a phase III study that have demonstrated the clinical efficacy of vorozole in postmenopausal women with metastatic disease,[101] this drug has been withdrawn from further clinical development.

Treatment of metastatic breast cancer

Preclinical studies have shown aromatase inhibitors to be effective after initial treatment with tamoxifen.[102] Following demonstrated efficacy in phase II trials, a number of phase III trials have evaluated the efficacy of third-generation aromatase (letrozole, anastrozole, and exemestane) inhibitors as a second-line agent compared to MA in the treatment of postmenopausal women with metastatic breast cancer who had previously been treated with tamoxifen (Table 3). In a cohort of 769 postmenopausal women with metastatic breast cancer, exemestane produced a statistically significant increase in median duration of overall clinical benefit (60.1 vs 49 weeks, $p = 0.025$), median time to tumor progression and median survival compared to MA.[103] In a similar cohort of 764 women from two pivotal phase III trials, patients randomized to either anastrozole (1 mg/day PO) or anastrozole (10 mg/day PO) had estimated hazards of progression of 0.97 (97.5% CI 0.75–1.24) and 0.92 (97.5% CI, 0.71–1.19), respectively, compared to patients receiving MA.[104] No statistically significant dose–response differences were observed between the 1 mg/day and 10 mg/day dosage. With subsequent follow-up 2-year survival was 56.1% for the group of patients receiving anastrozole (1 mg/day), compared with 46.3% for patients treated with MA.[105] Similarly the efficacy of letrozole was evaluated in a pivotal trial of 555 postmenopausal women with metastatic breast cancer that had progressed on tamoxifen.[106] Letrozole (2.5 mg/day) yielded overall response rates of 36% and 35%, respectively, compared with 27% and 33% for letrozole (0.5 mg/day) and 32% for MA, respectively. The median duration of response for letrozole (2.5 mg/day) was 33 months, compared with 18 months for both MA and letrozole 0.5 mg/day. A trend in time to tumor progression and survival that favored letrozole 2.5 mg/day was also observed.[106]

Following the success of third-generation aromatase inhibitors in the second-line treatment of postmenopausal women with metastatic breast cancer, focus shifted to first-line treatment directly comparing these agents with tamoxifen (Table 4). In a phase II study comparing exemestane (25 mg/day) with tamoxifen (20 mg/day) as first-line treatment for metastatic disease, patients receiving exemestane had better objective response rates (complete response plus partial response) and median duration of response compared to tamoxifen.[107] The study was subsequently extended into a phase III trial where exemestane was reported to be well tolerated and was associated with a significantly longer progression-free survival compared with tamoxifen (10.9 months vs 6.7 months, respectively).[108] In a combined analysis of two pivotal phase III trials that involved 1021 postmenopausal women with metastatic breast cancer, first-line treatment of anastrozole at a dose of 1 mg/day was compared to tamoxifen.[109] At a median follow-up of 18.5 months for patients with hormone receptor-positive tumors (59.8% of patients), median time to progression was significantly superior in the group receiving anastrozole compared to those receiving tamoxifen (10.7 months vs 6.4 months, $p = 0.022$). Similarly a large, multicenter, double-blind, first-line phase III clinical trial in 907 postmenopausal women with locally advanced or metastatic breast cancer compared letrozole (2.5 mg/day) with tamoxifen (20 mg/day).[110] At a median follow-up of 32 months, time to progression (median, 9.4 months vs 6.0 months, respectively; $p < 0.0001$), time to treatment failure (median, 9 months vs 5.7 months, respectively; $p < 0.0001$), and overall objective response rate (32% vs 21%, respectively; $p = 0.0002$) were all reported to be significantly superior in the group receiving letrozole compared to tamoxifen. Median OS was 34 months for letrozole and 30 months for tamoxifen. It is clear from the data presented that aromatase inhibitors, in particular third-generation inhibitors, have demonstrated superior efficacy to tamoxifen among women with advanced breast cancer. However currently there is no evidence to

Table 3 Combined data from phase III trials comparing anastrozole, letrozole, and exemestane with megestrol acetate in postmenopausal women previously treated with tamoxifen.

	Combined data		Initial trial		Second trial		Initial trial	
	Anastrozole	Megestrol acetate	Letrozole	Megestrol acetate	Letrozole	Megestrol acetate	Exemestane	Megestrol acetate
Number of patients	263	253	174	189	199	201	366	403
Objective response[a] (%)	12.6	12.2	23.6	16.4	16.1	14.9	15	12
Clinical benefit[b] (%)	42.2	40.3	34.5	31.7	26.7	23.4	37	35
Progression (%)	57.4	59.3	53.4	56.1	51.3	50.7	48	53
Median TTP (months)	5	5	5.6	5.5	3	3	5	5
Median duration of benefit (months)	18.3	15.7	33	18	17.5	15.4	15	12
Median survival (months)	28.7	21.5	25.3	21.5	28.6	26.2	NA	28

[a]Objective response = complete response + partial response.
[b]Clinical benefit = complete response + partial response + stable disease for ≥ 6 months.
Abbreviations: NA, not available; TTP, time to progression.

Table 4 Efficacy data from trials comparing anastrozole, letrozole, and exemestane with tamoxifen in the first-line treatment of postmenopausal women with metastatic breast cancer.

	Phase 2 studies				Phase 3 studies			
	Letrozole	Tamoxifen	Exemestane	Tamoxifen	Anastrozole[a]	Tamoxifen[a]	Anastrozole[b]	Tamoxifen[b]
Number of patients	453	454	61	59	170	182	340	453
Objective response (%)	30	20[c]	41	14	21	17	33	30
Clinical benefit (%)	49	38[c]	56	42	59	46[c]	56	56
TTP (months)	9	6[c]	9	5	11	6[c]	8	8
TTF (months)	6	6[c]	NR	NR	8	5	6	6

[a]North American Study.
[b]European Study.
[c]Difference is statistically significant.
Abbreviations: Nonprotocol analysis; NR, not recorded.

prove superiority of one aromatase inhibitor over another in this setting.

With the demonstrated efficacy of third-generation aromatase inhibitors among patients with metastatic breast cancer in the first-line setting, research focus shifted to investigating methods to improve on the efficacy. One method was to combine aromatase inhibitors with the antiestrogen fulvestrant. The mechanism of action of aromatase inhibitors is to ultimately result in a low-estrogen environment, and fulvestrant has been shown in preclinical models to work well in such an environment.[111] Furthermore the combination of fulvestrant and an aromatase inhibitor has been shown in preclinical models to delay the development of resistance by downregulating several signaling molecules that are known to be associated with the development of resistance.[112] Three randomized clinical trials have compared the combination of fulvestrant and an aromatase inhibitor to single-agent aromatase inhibitor among postmenopausal women with metastatic hormone receptor-positive disease.[113–115] The monthly dosing schedule of 250 mg was used for fulvestrant in these trials. In a phase III open-labeled randomized trial [Fulvestrant and Anastrozole Combination Therapy (FACT)], patients at first relapse after their primary disease were randomized to either fulvestrant and anastrozole or single-agent anastrozole.[113] The investigators observed no clinical benefit with the addition of fulvestrant for both time to progression (10.8 months vs 10.2 months, $p = 0.91$) and median OS (37.8 months vs 38.2 months, $p = 1.00$). In a cohort of patients who had progressed on a nonsteroidal aromatase inhibitor, the authors observed that the efficacy of fulvestrant and anastrozole was similar to either single-agent fulvestrant or exemestane. In a phase III trial conducted by SWOG, women with previously untreated breast cancer were randomized to receive either a combination of fulvestrant and anastrozole or single-agent anastrozole.[114] The authors reported a significantly improved progression-free survival (15 months vs 13.5 months, $p = 0.007$) favoring the combination arm. In a multicenter, randomized placebo-controlled phase III trial [Study of Faslodex with or without concomitant Arimidex vs exemestane following progression on nonsteroidal Aromatase inhibitors (SoFEA)], women who had relapsed or progressed with metastatic disease on a nonsteroidal aromatase inhibitor were randomized to receive either a combination of fulvestrant and anastrozole or fulvestrant and placebo or single-agent exemestane.[115] There is no doubt that the three trials were different in terms of the types of patients enrolled which could explain the differing results observed. For example, in the FACT trial three quarters of the cohort had received prior treatment with aromatase inhibitor, and in the SoFEA trial, patients had to have progressed on a nonsteroidal aromatase inhibitor to be eligible for the entry into the study. This is in contrast to the cohort enrolled in the SWOG trial where the majority of patients did not receive a prior aromatase inhibitor. However with the variable results observed and the fact that fulvestrant was used at a dose that is now considered to be suboptimal, no definitive conclusions regarding combination therapy between fulvestrant and aromatase inhibitors can be made at this time. As of now current guidelines indicate that among postmenopausal women with hormone receptor-positive metastatic breast cancer, aromatase inhibitors remain the preferred first-line treatment with a sequencing strategy of various available endocrine agents preferred[47] (Figure 2).

Adjuvant studies

With the efficacy of third-generation aromatase inhibitors proved in the treatment of postmenopausal women with hormone-responsive metastatic breast cancer, focus then shifted to proving their efficacy in the adjuvant treatment of early-stage breast cancer. With the recognized increased risk of endometrial carcinoma and thromboembolic events associated with the use of tamoxifen, an alternative was the use of aromatase inhibitors.. Adjuvant studies evaluating third-generation aromatase inhibitors have explored their efficacy both as upfront adjuvant treatment and following a course of adjuvant tamoxifen (Table 5; Figure 5). The following section will review results of the major adjuvant trials.

Upfront treatment of early disease in postmenopausal women
The Arimidex, Tamoxifen, Alone or in Combination (ATAC) trial is a randomized, double-blind study of 9366 postmenopausal women with early-stage breast cancer that was designed to compare the efficacy and tolerability of 5 years of treatment with tamoxifen with that of anastrozole versus the combination of anastrozole and tamoxifen.[116] A planned analysis at a median follow-up of 33 months resulted in the combination arm being discontinued due to lack of superior efficacy or tolerability to tamoxifen alone. The primary end point for this study was DFS and secondary end points were time to recurrence (TTR), incidence of new contralateral breast cancer, time to distant recurrence (TTDR), and OS. At a median follow-up of 120 months among women with hormone receptor-positive, DFS was significantly superior in the anastrozole group compared to tamoxifen (HR = 0.86, 95% CI 0.78–0.95, $p = 0.003$) as were TTR, TTDR, and incidence of contralateral breast cancer. There was no significant difference in the overall mortality between the two groups (HR = 0.95, 95% CI 0.84–1.06, $p = 0.7$).[117]

The Breast International Group (BIG) 1-98 trial randomized 8028 postmenopausal women with hormone receptor-positive breast cancer. BIG 1-98 included two primary adjuvant arms comparing 5 years of letrozole with 5 years of tamoxifen and two sequential

Table 5 Efficacy data from studies of aromatase inhibitors in the adjuvant treatment of postmenopausal women with early breast cancer.

Trial	Drugs	Median follow-up (months)	Disease-free survival (95% CI or p value)
Initial treatment			
ATAC	5 Years of anastrozole vs 5 years of tamoxifen	120	0.86 (0.78–0.95)
BIG 1-98	5 Years of letrozole vs 5 years of tamoxifen	8.7 years	0.86 (0.78–0.96)
Posttamoxifen			
MA 17	5 Years of tamoxifen followed by either 5 years of letrozole or placebo	30	0.58 (0.45–0.76)
IES	2–3 Years of tamoxifen followed by either exemestane or tamoxifen for a total of 5 years	55.7	0.76 (0.66–0.88)
NSABP B-33	5 Years of tamoxifen followed by either 5 years of exemestane or placebo	30	0.68 ($p = 0.07$)
ITA	2–3 Years of tamoxifen followed by either anastrozole or tamoxifen for a total of 5 years	64	0.56 (0.35–0.63)
ABCSG trial 6a	5 Years of tamoxifen followed by either 3 years of anastrozole or placebo	62.3	0.62[a] (0.40–0.96)

[a]Risk of recurrence.

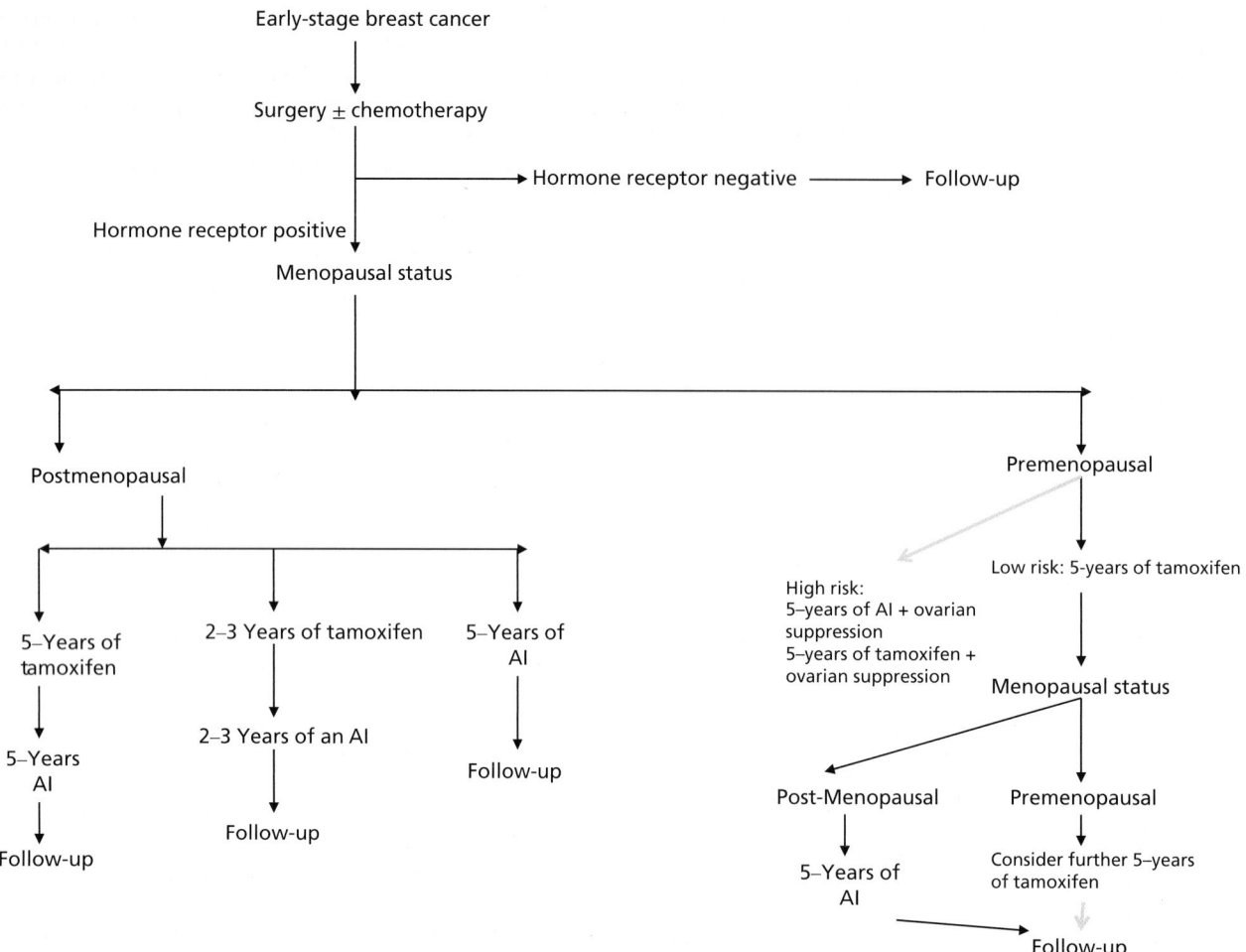

Figure 5 Algorithm for endocrine therapy among women with nonmetastatic breast cancer.

treatment arms comparing 2 years of letrozole followed by 3 years of tamoxifen and 2 years of tamoxifen followed by 3 years of letrozole.[118] The primary end point was DFI. At a median follow-up of 8.7 years from randomization, women who received letrozole monotherapy had a significantly improved DFI (HR 0.86, 95% CI 0.78–0.96) and OS (HR 0.87, 95% CI 0.77–0.999) compared to the cohort who received tamoxifen monotherapy.[119]

Postamoxifen treatment in postmenopausal women (switching strategy)
The second issue to be explored was the sequential use of a third-generation aromatase inhibitor following a period of adjuvant treatment of tamoxifen among postmenopausal women with early-stage breast cancer, a method commonly referred to as a switching strategy. The MA 17 trial was a randomized, double-blind, extended adjuvant, placebo-controlled trial in 5187 postmenopausal women who had received 5 years of adjuvant treatment with tamoxifen with.[120] Due to superior efficacy observed in the letrozole group compared to the placebo group at the first interim analysis, the study was prematurely terminated. In an updated analysis, at a median follow-up of 30 months, the letrozole group had a significantly longer DFS compared to the placebo group (HR = 0.58, 95% CI 0.45–0.76; $p < 0.001$).[121] Letrozole was found to be well tolerated and was associated with a lower incidence of vaginal bleeding and an increase in low-grade hot flashes, arthritis, arthralgia, and myalgia, compared with placebo. After premature

termination of the study, the group who were in the placebo of arm of the trial was offered letrozole. Women who elected to take letrozole did so at a median of 2.8 years from completion of tamoxifen treatment with a recent update reporting improved DFS among those who elected to take letrozole compared to those who did not.[122] In an exploratory analysis after statistical adjustment for crossover effect, the investigators reported that at a median follow-up of 64 months, extended adjuvant letrozole continued to superior to placebo for both DFS and OS.[123] The investigators further noted that although extended adjuvant letrozole after 5 years of tamoxifen was beneficial to women who were either pre- or postmenopausal at initial diagnosis, prognostic impact appeared to be greater among women who were initially premenopausal.[124]

The Intergroup Exemestane Study (IES) examined the efficacy and safety of exemestane therapy after 2–3 years of adjuvant tamoxifen therapy. The trial enrolled 4742 patients who were randomly assigned to continue with tamoxifen or to switch to exemestane for the remainder of the 5-year treatment period. At a median follow-up of 30.6 months, the data indicate that switching to exemestane was associated with a significant improvement in DFS compared with continuing with tamoxifen (HR = 0.68, 95% CI 0.56–0.82; $p < 0.001$).[125] At a median follow-up of 55.7 months, switching to exemestane resulted in a 24% improvement in DFS (HR = 0.76, 95% CI 0.66–0.88, $p = 0.0001$) and a 15% improvement in OS (HR = 0.85, 95% CI 0.71–1.02, $p = 0.08$) as compared to the tamoxifen group.[126] The NSABP B-33 trial, similar to the IES trial, is a randomized trial that evaluated 5 years of exemestane to 5 years of placebo following the completion of 5-years of tamoxifen.[127] Due to the results of the MA 17 study, the NASBP B-33 study was terminated early and was unblinded. Despite a premature closure and crossover of patients, a statistically significant 4-year DFS was observed among the original cohort who received exemestane compared to the placebo group (91% vs 89%; HR = 0.68; $p = 0.07$).[127]

The adjuvant tamoxifen and exemestane in early breast cancer (TEAM) trial was a phase III study; the aim of which was to compare exemestane monotherapy upfront to sequential treatment of exemestane following completion of 5 years of tamoxifen.[128] Over 9000 patients were recruited on this trial. The investigators noted no significant difference in the 5 year DFS between the two treatment strategies (hazard ratio 0.97, 95% CI 0.88–1.08; $p = 0.60$) and concluded that exemestane either upfront or after a course of tamoxifen were both appropriate options for postmenopausal women with early-stage breast cancer.

Several smaller trials have also looked at the issue of sequential aromatase inhibitors. The Italian Tamoxifen Anastrozole (ITA) and Arimidex Nolvadex 95/Austrian Breast Cancer Study Group 8 (ARNO 95/ABCSG 8) have shown that switching to anastrozole after 2–3 years of tamoxifen significantly reduced the risk of recurrence.[129,130] In the ABCSG trial 6a postmenopausal women were randomized to either anastrozole or placebo following 5 years of adjuvant tamoxifen therapy.[131] At a median follow-up of 62.3 months, women in the anastrozole group had a 38% risk reduction in recurrence compared to placebo (HR = 0.62; 95% CI = 0.40–0.96, $p = 0.031$).

When putting all the aforementioned trials together, it is clear that among postmenopausal women with hormone receptor-positive breast cancer, the adjuvant use of an aromatase inhibitor either upfront or as sequential treatment following tamoxifen is superior compared to using to tamoxifen alone. Both strategies are recommended and incorporate in a number of international guidelines.

Aromatase inhibitors in premenopausal women

From the data summarized earlier, it is clear that aromatase inhibitors are superior to tamoxifen in the adjuvant setting. Due to their mechanism of action, aromatase inhibitors can only be used among women who are postmenopausal. Tamoxifen has to date been the only agent recommended for use in the adjuvant setting among premenopausal women with hormone receptor-positive breast cancer. The therapeutic value of suppression of ovarian estrogen production among premenopausal women who receive tamoxifen has been uncertain.[132] Provocative data has also been published, suggesting that ovarian suppression occurring secondary to chemotherapy (i.e., developing an amenorrhea state) is associated with a reduced risk of relapse which led to guidelines for management of breast cancer among young women recommending that the addition of GnRH analogues with tamoxifen be discussed on an individualized basis.[133,134] We know that the actual use of ovarian ablation has not resulted in improved outcome despite an observed trend for benefit in terms of recurrence and DFS in premenopausal women <40. However keeping in mind that the majority of these studies have not compared ovarian ablation with tamoxifen included in both arms, it was unclear whether the benefit from ovarian ablation is superior to tamoxifen alone.

As such in 2003 the International Breast Cancer Study Group (IBCSG) launched two phase III randomized clinical trials that focused on premenopausal women with early-stage hormone receptor-positive breast cancer [Suppression of Ovarian Function

Trial (SOFT), Tamoxifen and Exemestane Trial (TEXT)] that were designed to determine whether adjuvant aromatase inhibitors improved DFS compared to tamoxifen and to determine the value of ovarian suppression.[135,136] The TEXT randomized premenopausal women with early-stage breast cancer to either 5 years of exemestane and ovarian suppression or 5 years of tamoxifen and ovarian suppression. The SOFT randomized premenopausal women with early-stage breast cancer to either 5 years of tamoxifen alone, tamoxifen and ovarian suppression, or exemestane and ovarian suppression. In a preplanned combined analysis of data derived from TEXT and SOFT, the investigators observed that at a median follow-up of 68 months, 5-year DFS was significantly improved among premenopausal women treated with exemestane and ovarian suppression compared to those treated with tamoxifen and ovarian suppression (91.1% vs 87.3%, HR 0.72, 95% CI 0.60–0.85, $p < 0.001$).[133] This was however associated with a higher incidence of grade 3 or 4 adverse events among women receiving exemestane (30.6% vs 29.4%).[135] The SOFT randomized over 3000 premenopausal women with hormone receptor-positive early-stage breast cancer to either tamoxifen alone, tamoxifen and ovarian suppression, or exemestane and ovarian suppression with the underlying goal of trying to determine the value of ovarian suppression in this cohort of patients.[136] The investigators reported that at a median follow-up of 67 months in the overall study population, the addition of ovarian suppression to tamoxifen did not significantly improve 5-year DFS compared to tamoxifen alone (86.6% vs 84.7%, $p = 0.10$) on univariate analysis. In the multivariable model after adjusting for covariates, the combination of ovarian suppression and tamoxifen resulted in a 22% reduction in the RR of breast cancer recurrence, a second invasive cancer or death ($p = 0.03$) compared to tamoxifen alone. The authors further observed that among premenopausal women who are at sufficiently high risk of recurrence to receive chemotherapy, the 5-year rate of freedom from breast cancer was 78% among women receiving tamoxifen alone, 82.5% among those receiving tamoxifen and ovarian suppression (when comparing to tamoxifen alone HR 0.78; 95% CI 0.60–1.02), and 85.7% among those receiving exemestane and ovarian suppression (when comparing to tamoxifen alone HR 0.65; 95% CI 0.49–0.87). The investigators reported an increasing rate of nonadherence to ovarian suppression with increasing year from initiation of treatment. Side effects reported to be associated more frequently with ovarian suppression included hot flashes, insomnia, depression, vaginal dryness, musculoskeletal symptoms, hypertension, and glucose intolerance. Rate of osteoporosis was also higher among women receiving ovarian suppression. In a third randomized phase III trial (Austrian Breast and Colorectal Cancer Study Group (ABCSG)-12), 1803 premenopausal women who undergone surgery for stage I or II hormone receptor-positive breast cancer were randomized to either anastrozole and ovarian suppression or tamoxifen with ovarian suppression with or with zoledronic acid.[137] The primary end point of this study was DFS with RFS and OS being secondary end points. At a median follow-up of 94.4 months, the investigators reported no significant difference in DFS between the tamoxifen and anastrozole groups although a higher risk of death was observed among group of patients receiving anastrozole and ovarian suppression compared to the group receiving tamoxifen and ovarian suppression (HR = 1.63; 95% CI, 1.05–1.45; $p = 0.030$). Interestingly the addition of zoledronic acid was observed to be associated with improved DFS. Multiple reasons have been hypothesized to account for the discordant results between the ABCSG-12 and that observed with the TEXT and SOFT; the most important of which is statistical power with the TEXT/SOFT having higher statistical power to answer the question regarding the role of ovarian suppression and aromatase inhibitors in the premenopausal setting. Longer-term follow-up of the TEXT and SOFT will be vital in determining long-term efficacy as well as defining associated toxicity in this young population of patients.

Based on the evidence presented earlier, the author recommends that aromatase inhibitors be offered upfront as adjuvant therapy among postmenopausal women with hormone receptor-positive early-stage breast cancer. Current guidelines of adjuvant endocrine therapy for postmenopausal women recommend an aromatase inhibitor as either initial therapy or after an initial period of treatment with tamoxifen[138] with the decision based on the risks and benefits of each agent for an individual patient. Using an aromatase inhibitor beyond 5 years is currently not recommended, and ongoing clinical trials will answer the question of the clinical utility of this method. Among premenopausal women the story is a little more complex. The use of 10 years of tamoxifen or the use of ovarian suppression and aromatase inhibitors have both been included in the updated guidelines, and use of either should be based on individual risk assessment and a thorough discussion regarding associated side effects.[47] Longer-term follow-up of the adjuvant trials described earlier are awaited to better define long-term efficacy results, side effect profile, and delineate duration of required treatment for an aromatase inhibitor used in the adjuvant setting.

Neoadjuvant studies

Neoadjuvant treatment is intended to downstage a tumor before primary locoregional therapy with surgery, thus allowing breast-conserving surgery in a greater number of patients or making surgery possible in cases that were considered inoperable. As the third-generation aromatase inhibitors have demonstrated efficacy in the treatment of advanced and early disease, it is important to examine the benefits these agents may bring to the preoperative setting.

Compared to neoadjuvant chemotherapy trials, the neoadjuvant studies exploring the effect of endocrine therapy in the treatment of breast cancer are much smaller. Several trials have compared neoadjuvant tamoxifen to a third-generation aromatase inhibitor among postmenopausal women with hormone receptor-positive breast cancer.[139–143] The Immediate Preoperative Arimidex, Tamoxifen, or Combined with Tamoxifen (IMPACT) trial compared 3 months of preoperative anastrozole with tamoxifen or a combination of both in 330 postmenopausal women with hormone receptor-positive breast cancer.[139] No difference in overall response was noted in three groups (37% vs 36% vs 39%). However among the 124 women considered to require a mastectomy at baseline, 46% treated with anastrozole were considered to be candidates for breast-conserving surgery by their surgeon, compared with 22% receiving tamoxifen ($p = 0.03$).[139] Similarly the PReOperative Arimidex Compared with Tamoxifen (PROACT) trial that randomized 451 postmenopausal women to either 3 months of neoadjuvant anastrozole or tamoxifen with or without chemotherapy reported that among the hormone therapy-only group of patients, feasible surgery at baseline improved in 43.0% of patients receiving anastrozole compared to 30.8% receiving tamoxifen ($p = 0.04$).[140]

In the P024 study where 337 postmenopausal women were randomly assigned to either 4 months of neoadjuvant letrozole or tamoxifen, overall response rate (55% vs 36%, $p < 0.001$) and rate of breast-conserving surgery (45% vs 35%, $p = 0.022$) were significantly superior in the letrozole arm of the study.[138] In addition in the P024 study differences in response rates between letrozole and tamoxifen were most marked in the subgroup that was positive for ErbB-1 and/or ErbB-2 (88% vs 21%, $p = 0.0004$); however this part

of the study was largely underpowered.[142] In a small randomized study of 151 patients, exemestane was also reported to be more effective than tamoxifen in neoadjuvant setting for both clinical overall response (76.3% vs 40%; $p = 0.05$) and breast-conserving surgery (exemestane 36.8% vs tamoxifen 20%; $p = 0.05$).[140]

In the ACOSOG Z1031 phase II trial, the three aromatase inhibitors were compared in the preoperative setting. Over three hundred postmenopausal women with clinical stage II to III breast cancer were enrolled with the primary end point being clinical response.[144] The clinical response among patients receiving exemestane, letrozole, and anastrozole was 62.9%, 74.8%, and 69.1%, respectively. No differences in surgical outcome, Preoperative Endocrine Prognostic Index (PEPI) score, or Ki67 suppression were detected (secondary end points of the study).

At present time, outside the context of a clinical trial, neoadjuvant endocrine therapy with aromatase inhibitors are recommended for postmenopausal patients who are not believed to be candidates for preoperative chemotherapy because of associated existing comorbidity.[145] Several questions still remain to be addressed by future clinical trials including the appropriate duration of neoadjuvant endocrine therapy.

Chemoprevention of breast cancer

As discussed earlier the side effect profile of tamoxifen restricts its use in the prevention of breast cancer. Furthermore trials looking at tamoxifen and raloxifene in the prevention setting reduced the incidence of ER-positive breast cancers by about 50%, and thus looking for an agent that would reduce the incidence further is important. Aromatase inhibitors, with their proven efficacy in the treatment of hormone receptor-positive breast cancers, are a viable option. In the ATAC trial[117] at a median follow-up of 100 months, it was observed that the incidence of hormone receptor-positive contralateral breast cancers was significantly lower in the anastrozole group compared to the tamoxifen group (HR 0.60, 95% CI 0.42–0.85, $p = 0.004$). Similarly in the BIG 1-98 trial,[118,119] fewer cases of contralateral breast cancer were identified in the letrozole group than in the tamoxifen group (16 cases vs 27 cases). In the IES study[126] at a median follow-up of 55.7 months, 17 cases of contralateral breast cancer were observed in the exemestane group compared to 35 cases in the tamoxifen group with the time to development of ER-positive contralateral breast cancer significantly reduced in the exemestane group compared to the tamoxifen group (HR = 0.56, 95% CI 0.33–0.98, $p = 0.04$).

These trials indicated that third-generation aromatase inhibitors reduce the incidence of contralateral breast cancer by approximately 40%–50% above and beyond that observed by tamoxifen. By extrapolation this would imply that on their own these aromatase inhibitors would reduce the incidence of ER-positive contralateral breast cancer by approximately 70%–80%.[142] With such impressive results large randomized clinical trials were designed to look at the use of aromatase inhibitors in the setting of primary prevention.[147,148] In a phase III trial, 4560 postmenopausal women who were at moderately increased risk of developing breast cancer were randomized to receive exemestane or placebo.[147] The authors reported that at a median follow-up of 35 months, invasive breast cancer was detected in 11 women in the exemestane cohort compared to 32 cases of invasive breast cancer in the placebo cohort. The use of exemestane in this cohort of women translated into a 65% relative reduction in the annual incidence of invasive breast cancer compared to placebo (HR 0.35, 95%CI 0.18–0.70, $p = 0.002$). Minimal quality of life differences were observed between the two groups with no significant difference observed between the two groups in terms of skeletal fractures, other cancers, treatment-related deaths, and cardiovascular events. In a second phase III trial (IBIS-II), 1920 postmenopausal women at high risk of developing breast cancer were randomized to either anastrozole or placebo for 5 years.[148] At a median follow-up of 5 years, breast cancer was detected among 40 women in the anastrozole cohort and 85 women in the placebo cohort (HR 0.47, 95% CI 0.32–0.68, $p < 0.0001$). The cumulative incidence of all breast cancers after 7 years of follow-up was 2.8% in the anastrozole group and 5.6% in the placebo group. Considering the data described and the better side effect profile compared to tamoxifen current guidelines recommend considering the use of aromatase inhibitors among postmenopausal women who are at moderate to high risk of developing breast cancer.[47]

Side effects

Bone disease
As discussed earlier estrogen deprivation is associated with an increased risk of developing osteoporosis and is more so in women with breast cancer.[149] While tamoxifen, through its estrogen agonist function on the bone, has been shown to have a beneficial effect on bone health,[76] all three third-generation aromatase inhibitors appear to increase bone loss. In the 120-month analysis of the ATAC trial, fracture rates were significantly higher in the anastrozole group compared to the group receiving tamoxifen (451 fractures vs 351 fractures, HR 1.33, 95% CI 1.15–1.55; $p < 0.0001$); however the fracture rate was not significantly different between the anastrozole and tamoxifen groups after completion of 5-year treatment (110 vs 112, OR 0.98, 95% CI 0.74–1.30, $p = 0.9$).[117]

In the BIG 1-98 trial at a median follow-up of 60.3 months, 9.3% of patients in the letrozole group experienced a fracture compared to 6.5% of patients in the tamoxifen group with the wrist being the most common site of fracture.[150] Similar observations were also made in the IES trial where at a median follow-up of 55.7 months, a significantly increased fracture rate of 7% was observed in the exemestane group compared to 5% in the tamoxifen group (odds ratio = 1.45, 95% CI 1.13–1.87; $p = 0.003$).[151] One method of preventing or reversing bone loss associated with aromatase inhibitors would be to use bisphosphonates. In the integrated analysis of two randomized Zometa-Femara Adjuvant Synergy Trials (Z-FAST and ZO-FAST), 1667 patients that were receiving adjuvant letrozole received either upfront zoledronic acid or received it only when bone mineral density decreased to below −2.[152] At 12-month follow-up, the upfront group had lumbar spine bone mineral density that was 5.2% higher than the group of patients who received delayed zoledronic acid. Longer follow-up will be needed to confirm these results.

Cardiovascular disease
Postmenopausal women with breast cancer may be at a higher risk of cardiovascular events due to their age, menopausal status, associated comorbid conditions, and exposure to chemotherapeutic agents used in the treatment of breast cancer. As described earlier, tamoxifen, through its estrogen agonist function, has been shown to have a lipid-lowering effect that has translated into modest reductions in cardiovascular events.[79] Anastrozole has not been shown to appreciably alter lipid profiles,[153,154] and in the adjuvant setting myocardial infarctions experienced by women taking anastrozole was similar compared to the group taking tamoxifen.[117] In the BIG 1-98 trial at a median follow-up of 51 months, women in the letrozole group experienced significantly higher low-grade cholesterol elevation and cardiovascular events (other than ischemic heart disease and cardiac failure) compared to women in the tamoxifen group.[119] The higher low-grade cholesterol elevation in the letrozole group relative to that of patients in the tamoxifen group may be a reflection of the lipid-lowering effect of tamoxifen as mentioned earlier. Studies with exemestane have shown that apart from a modest drop in HDL cholesterol,[155] exemestane has no appreciable effect on lipid levels. In the IES study, at a median follow-up of 55.7 months, among all patients the incidence of cardiovascular events (excluding thromboembolic events) did not seem to differ between the exemestane and tamoxifen groups with approximately 1.3% of exemestane-treated patients experiencing a myocardial infarction compared to 0.8% of tamoxifen-treated patients ($p = 0.08$). Although longer follow-up will be required to assess the cardiovascular effects of the clinically used third-generation aromatase inhibitors, women with breast cancer are in general at higher risk of developing a cardiovascular event due to a multitude of factors and as such should monitored and managed appropriately.

Other adverse events
Another important side effect of aromatase inhibitors is the development of arthralgia which can significantly impact quality of life. For example, the incidence of arthralgia associated with the use of letrozole in the BIG 1-198 trial was 20.3% compared to the 12.3% observed among women taking tamoxifen ($p < 0.001$).[119] The COMPliance and Arthralgia in Clinical Therapy (COMPACT) trial was an open-label trail; the primary end point of which was to look at arthralgia compliance.[156] Nearly two thousand postmenopausal women received upfront anastrozole. The investigators noted that compliance with anastrozole gradually decreased over time with a significant association observed between arthralgia mean scores and noncompliance. Other side effects commonly associated with aromatase inhibitors include vaginal dryness and dyspareunia. Although treatment with aromatase inhibitors increases the risk of vasomotor symptoms and vaginal bleeding/discharge, large trials have shown that the incidence of these events are lower compared to that experienced on tamoxifen treatment.[116-130] Furthermore these trials also reported that the incidence of thromboembolic events and endometrial carcinoma were also lower in women taking an aromatase inhibitor compared to those taking tamoxifen.

Resistance to endocrine therapy
We have certainly come a long way in the management of women with hormone receptor-positive breast cancer in both the adjuvant and metastatic setting. However although endocrine therapy is effective in the metastatic setting, only 30% of patients with hormone receptor-positive breast cancer have an objective response with approximately only 50% gaining clinical benefit from endocrine therapy.[157] In clinical practice, the sequential use of hormonal agents can produce long-term palliation of hormone-dependent metastatic breast cancer. Eventually, however, the problem of hormone resistance is encountered. In the adjuvant setting clinical trials have demonstrated that approximately fifty percent of patients with hormone receptor-positive breast cancer benefit from endocrine therapy, while the rest develop either a primary or acquired resistance. Several patterns of resistance are commonly encountered in clinical practice. A primary resistance describes a scenario whereby a tumor is inherently resistant to ER targeting despite ER expression. An acquired resistance describes a situation where an ER-positive tumor initially responds and then progresses on endocrine therapy. Agent-selective resistance describes a scenario where the ER-positive tumor is resistant to a specific endocrine agent.

The mechanisms by which tumors become resistant to hormones, in general, are only partially understood.[158] Refractoriness to therapy with aromatase inhibitors is related not to the failure of these agents to suppress estradiol levels but rather because of alterations in other cellular components, such as the growth factor receptor pathways.[159] Some of the mechanisms of endocrine resistance include activation of the cell surface growth factor receptors [including epidermal growth factor receptor, human epidermal growth factor receptor 2 (HER2), and IGF-1 receptor] and downstream elements of the receptor tyrosine kinases (including phosphatidylinositol 3-kinase (PI3K), AKT, and mammalian target of rapamycin (mTOR)]. Activation or dysregulation of any of these pathways ultimately results in ligand-independent activation of the ER-signaling pathways that results in these pathways becoming resistant to endocrine agents used in the clinic. With an increased understanding of the mechanisms of resistance, selective targeted inhibitors have been introduced which when used in combination with endocrine therapy can overcome resistance.

Targeting the HER2 pathway

The HER2 is known to be over expressed or amplified in approximately one-fifth of patients with newly diagnosed breast cancer and is typically associated with a poor prognostic outcome. The introduction of a number of anti-HER2 agents (e.g., trastuzumab, lapatinib, pertuzumab, and TDM-1) has effectively altered the natural history of this breast tumor subtype. Preclinical evidence indicates that crosstalk between the HER2 and ER pathways results in resistance to established endocrine therapies.[160–162] Based on this evidence a number of clinical trials investigated the combination of an anti-HER2 agent and endocrine therapy with the underlying hypothesis that the combination would be superior to endocrine therapy alone. The TANDEM trial was a phase III study that randomized postmenopausal women with hormone receptor-positive/HER2-positive metastatic breast cancer to either a combination of trastuzumab and anastrozole or anastrozole alone.[163] The investigators noted that the combination was associated with a statistically significant although clinically modest improvement in progression-free survival (HR 0.63; 95% CI, 0.47–0.84; median PFS, 4.8 months vs 2.4 months; $p = 0.0016$) although there was no difference in OS between the two groups. In a second trial where postmenopausal women with hormone receptor-positive/HER2-positive breast cancer were randomized to receive lapatinib and letrozole or letrozole alone, the investigators observed that the addition of lapatinib to letrozole significantly reduced the risk of disease progression compared to letrozole alone (HR 0.71; 95% CI 0.53–0.96; $p = 0.019$, median PFS 8.2 months vs 3.0 months).[164]

Targeting the PI3Kinase pathway

The PI3K pathway is known to modulate cell growth, proliferation, and survival with mTOR being a signal transduction kinase in this pathway. mTOR exists in two multiprotein complexes. mTORC1 consists of mTOR that is associated with a regulatory protein of mTOR (raptor) and is located downstream of AKT, while mTORC2 is associated with rapamycin-insensitive companion of mTOR (rictor) and it phosphorylates AKT. Pathway PI3K activation results in phosphorylation of AKT which in turn leads to phosphorylation of mTORC1 and its effectors [4E binding protein 1 (4E-BP-1) that enhances cell proliferation, survival, and angiogenesis and S6 kinase 1 (S6K1) that regulate cell growth]. Preclinical evidence has shown that activation of the PI3K pathway is associated with endocrine therapy resistance with S6K1 being responsible for phosphorylating the activating domain of ERs.[165,166]

A number of studies also indicated that inhibition of mTOR reversed endocrine resistance especially when mTOR inhibitors were combined with endocrine therapy.[167,168] Such evidence led to the development of a number of mTOR inhibitors that were investigated in combination with endocrine therapy in clinical trials. In a phase III (HORIZON) trial, that tested the clinical efficacy of the mTOR inhibitor temsirolimus, 1112 patients with hormone receptor-positive metastatic breast cancer who had not received a prior aromatase inhibitors were randomized to receive either letrozole or letrozole combined with temsirolimus. This study was closed for futility when it was observed that the combination of letrozole and temsirolimus was highly unlikely to demonstrate an improvement in PFS over letrozole alone.[169] Everolimus (rapamycin analogue that inhibits mTORC1 kinase) was tested in the phase III Breast Cancer Trial of Oral Everolimus 2 (BOLERO-2) trial where patients with hormone receptor-positive metastatic breast cancer who had progressed on a prior nonsteroidal aromatase inhibitor were randomized to receive either everolimus and exemestane or exemestane alone.[170] To enroll in the study patients had to have disease that was previously refractory to either letrozole or anastrozole, and this was defined as recurrence during or within 12 months of completion of adjuvant treatment or in the case of metastatic disease, patients had to have experienced progression of disease either during treatment or within 1 month of ending treatment. In this population of patients who were resistant to nonsteroidal aromatase inhibitors, the investigators demonstrated a statistically significant improvement in median PFS of 4.6 months ($p < 0.0001$) in the combination arm. However this improvement did not translate into a significant improvement in the secondary end point of OS (31 months vs 26.6 months, $p = 0.14$). The addition of everolimus to exemestane increased toxicities including stomatitis (grade 3 8% vs 1 %), pneumonitis (grade 3, 3% vs 0%), liver dysfunction, and hyperglycemia. A third trial [tamoxifen plus everolimus (TAMRAD)] was a randomized phase II trial that evaluated the combination of everolimus and tamoxifen compared to tamoxifen alone among 111 women who had been previously treated with an aromatase inhibitor.[171] The primary end point of the TAMRAD study was clinical benefit rate at 6 months which was found to be significantly improved among patients receiving tamoxifen and everolimus compared to tamoxifen alone (61% vs 42%). By restricting enrollment to patients who had progressed on a prior aromatase inhibitor, the BOLERO-2 and TAMRAD trials are likely selected for patients whose tumors were being driven by the PI3K/AKT/mTOR pathways which would explain the discordant results observed compared to the HORIZON study. At present the combination of everolimus and exemestane has been recommended for use among patients whose disease has progressed on a prior aromatase inhibitor.[47] Since the addition of everolimus is associated with unique and significant toxicities, a thorough discussion with the patient is important prior to commencing treatment.

Targeting the CDK 4/6 pathway

The cyclin-dependent kinases (CDKs) together with regulatory proteins cyclins have a critical role in the controlled progression through the cell cycle. Alterations in the genes controlling the cell cycle are potential targets for treatment with CDK-targeted agents being the most attractive.[172] CDK4/6 and cyclin D regulate the phosphorylation of pRb (retinoblastoma) which when hyperphosphorylated results in the release of transcription factors that allow cells to transition from the GI to the S phase of the cycle.[173] Palbociclib (PD-0332991) is a selective, reversible small molecule inhibitor of CDK 4/6 which in preclinical studies of human breast cancer cell lines has been shown to have potent activity in the ER-positive and

HER2-amplified subtypes.[174] In these subtypes it was found to result in blockade of pRb hyperphosphorylation that ultimately resulted in cycle arrest in GI phase. Synergistic growth inhibitor effect was seen with the combination of tamoxifen and palbociclib in a model with acquired tamoxifen resistance. In a single arm phase II trial of 36 patients with heavily pretreated metastatic breast cancer that was positive for Rb protein expression, single-agent palbociclib showed activity in some patients with hormone receptor-positive breast cancer.[175] Associated grade 3/4 toxicities included transient neutropenia and thrombocytopenia. In a randomized open-label phase II PALOMA trial, 165 postmenopausal women with hormone receptor-positive and HER2-negative metastatic breast cancer who had not received treatment for their advanced disease were randomized to receive letrozole or letrozole and palbociclib.[176] The addition of palbociclib to letrozole was noted to improve progression-free survival from 10.2 to 20.2 months (HR 0.488, 95% CI 0.319–0.718, $p = 0.0004$). Grade 3/4 neutropenia (54% vs 1%) and fatigue (4% vs 1%) were reported with higher frequency in the palbociclib/letrozole group compared to the single-agent letrozole group. Based on these results the FDA granted accelerated approval for palbociclib in combination with letrozole as a first-line treatment among patients with hormone receptor-positive metastatic breast cancer. Recently the results of the PALOMA-3 trial, that randomized over 500 patients with hormone receptor-positive and HER2-negative metastatic breast cancer who had either relapsed or progressed during endocrine therapy to either fulvestrant alone or in combination with palbociclib, were published.[177] This phase III trial included premenopausal and perimenopausal patients who receive goserelin. The investigators reported a significant improvement in the progression-free survival (9.2 months vs 3.8 months, $p < 0.001$) with the addition of palbociclib to fulvestrant.

GnRH analogues and ovarian function preservation

With the improvement in prognostic outcome associated with adjuvant chemotherapy among younger premenopausal women with early-stage breast cancer, the issue of premature menopause and infertility associated with chemotherapy has become an important one. Among women who receive chemotherapy those younger than age 35 years, the long-term incidence of amenorrhea is at approximately 10%, while it is approximately 50% among women between the ages of 35 and 40 years and can be up to 85% among those above age 40 years.[178] Infertility associated with premature ovarian failure can impact treatment decisions in almost 30% of younger women with breast cancer.[179] Currently there are no standards for fertility preservation among premenopausal women who receive chemotherapy. The 2013 guidelines from the American Society of Clinical Oncology (ASCO) on fertility preservation recommend that a thorough discussion on the risks of infertility with chemotherapy and/or radiation therapy be discussed upfront before commencing treatment with the issue of trying to preserve fertility be addressed as early possible.[180] Recommended options for fertility preservation among women of reproductive age include embryo and oocyte cryopreservation and ovarian transposition in the case of pelvic radiation therapy. The use of GnRH analogues concurrently with chemotherapy has also been explored as a method of ovarian function preservation. Ovarian function preservation with GnRH analogues has been postulated to occur via several mechanisms including interruption of FSH secretion, decrease in utero-ovarian perfusion, and protection of undifferentiated germline stem cells.[181] Data from a number of animal and human models have suggested that temporary ovarian

suppression associated with use of GnRH analogues may preserve ovarian function.[181–185] However clinical data regarding the use of GnRH analogues for ovarian function preservation has been conflicting. In the ZOladex Rescue of Ovarian Function (ZORO) trial that randomized 60 women with ER-negative breast cancer who were scheduled to receive chemotherapy with an anthracycline and taxane to either chemotherapy alone or chemotherapy in combination with goserelin, the investigators found no statistical difference in resumption of ovarian function between the two arms of the study.[185] Similarly in the Ovarian Protection Trial in Premenopausal Breast Cancer Patients (OPTION) trial that randomized 227 patients to chemotherapy alone or in combination with goserelin, no difference in ovarian protection between the two groups was noted.[186] In contrast a number of studies have noted a benefit with the use of GnRH analogues. In the phase III PROMISE-GIM6 trial that randomized 281 premenopausal women with early-stage breast cancer to either chemotherapy alone or chemotherapy and the GnRH analogue triptorelin, the investigators observed a 17% absolute reduction in the occurrence of early menopause.[187] Recently the long-term results of this trial were reported.[188] The investigators noted that at a median follow-up of 7.3 years, there was no difference in 5-year DFS (83.7% with chemotherapy alone vs 80.5% with chemotherapy in combination with triptorelin, $p = 0.519$). Four pregnancies were noted in the chemotherapy alone groups, and 8 pregnancies occurred in the group who received chemotherapy and triptorelin (OR 1.84; 95% CI 0.54–6.27, $p = 0.39$). In the IBCSG-/SWOG-coordinated phase III trial (POEMS), premenopausal women with hormone receptor-negative breast cancer were randomized to either receive chemotherapy alone or in combination with goserelin.[189] The primary end point was 2-year primary ovarian failure. Two year ovarian failure rate was 22% in the chemotherapy alone arm and 8% in the chemotherapy and goserelin arm of the trial (OR = 0.30, 95% CI 0.10–0.87, $p = 0.03$). Thirteen pregnancies were noted in the chemotherapy alone arm, and 22 pregnancies were noted in the chemotherapy in combination with goserelin arm (OR = 2.22, 95% CI 1.00–4.92, $p = 0.05$). Limitations of this study included the fact that it did not reach its target accrual (416 target accrual, 214 randomized and reported), missing end point data for 38% of patients, and the data was not stratified for disease risk factors (HER2, nodal status, and stage of disease). The 2013 ASCO guidelines currently do not recommend the use of GnRH analogues as a method of fertility preservation noting that there is insufficient evidence regarding its effectiveness in ovarian function preservation.[180] The authors of this chapter recommend that the issue of fertility preservation be discussed as early as possible and that all methods be discussed including the pros and cons of each.

Conclusion

In summary a number of endocrine agents are now available for the management of both early and advanced stage hormone response breast cancer, each unique in its mechanism of action targeting different points in the ER and PR pathways. Tamoxifen has been ubiquitous as the frontline therapy for the treatment of all stages of breast cancer and remains the central choice for the treatment of premenopausal women. Emerging data suggests that the use of aromatase inhibitors with ovarian function suppression among premenopausal women with early-stage breast cancer who are at high risk of recurrence may be associated with improved prognostic outcome. Among postmenopausal women the introduction of the noncross-resistant aromatase inhibitors has changed recommendations being now at the forefront of treatment of both early and advanced staged breast cancers. However several questions regarding the use of aromatase inhibitors still remain including duration of use in the adjuvant setting and sequence of use with tamoxifen. Moreover among the three third-generation aromatase inhibitors, there are no head to head comparisons to support the superiority of one aromatase inhibitor over another. Furthermore the use of aromatase inhibitors are not without side effects with various methods available (e.g., use of zoledronic acid, denosumab) for preventing bone loss which can have a significant impact on quality of life. We have also come a long way in understanding mechanisms underlying the development of endocrine resistance with agents such as everolimus now approved for use in combination aromatase inhibitors. Progestins including MA and MPA are useful agents to try when resistance to tamoxifen and aromatase inhibitors has developed.

Lastly, as more antihormonal therapies become available and our understanding of the molecular pathways underpinning resistance increases, it is essential that the optimal sequence of endocrine agents be established in the treatment of breast cancer. This may prolong the time during which endocrine therapies can be used, so postponing the time when cytotoxic chemotherapy becomes a necessary option.

Key references

The complete reference list can be found on the Wiley Companion Digital Edition of this title (see inside front cover for login instructions).

45 Crump M, Sawka CA, DeBoer G, et al. An individual patient-based meta-analysis of tamoxifen versus ovarian ablation as first line endocrine therapy for premenopausal women with metastatic breast cancer. *Breast Cancer Res Treat.* 1997;**44**(3):201–210.

46 Klijn JG, Blamey RW, Boccardo F, et al. Combined tamoxifen and luteinizing hormone-releasing hormone (LHRH) agonist versus LHRH agonist alone in premenopausal advanced breast cancer: a meta-analysis of four randomized trials. *J Clin Oncol.* 2001;**19**(2):343–353.

48 Early Breast Cancer Trialists' Collaborative Group (EBCTCG). Effects of chemotherapy and hormonal therapy for early breast cancer on recurrence and 15-year survival: an overview of the randomised trials. *Lancet.* 2005;**365**(9472):1687–1717.

49 Fisher B, Dignam J, Bryant J, Wolmark N. Five versus more than five years of tamoxifen for lymph node-negative breast cancer: updated findings from the National Surgical Adjuvant Breast and Bowel Project B-14 randomized trial. *J Natl Cancer Inst.* 2001;**93**(9):684–690.

50 Davies C, Pan H, Godwin J, Gray R, Arriagada R, et al. Long-term effects of continuing adjuvant tamoxifen to 10 years versus stopping at 5 years after diagnosis of oestrogen receptor-positive breast cancer: ATLAS, a randomised trial. *Lancet.* 2013;**381**(9869):805–816.

51 Gray RG, Rea D, Handley D, Bowden SJ, Perry P. aTTom: long-term effects of continuing adjuvant tamoxifen to 10 years versus stopping at 5 years in 6,953 women with early breast cancer. *J Clin Oncol.* 2013;**31** (suppl; abstr 5):2013.

54 Albain KS, Barlow WE, Ravdin PM, et al. Adjuvant chemotherapy and timing of tamoxifen in postmenopausal patients with endocrine-responsive, node-positive breast cancer: a phase 3, open-label, randomised controlled trial. *Lancet.* 2009;**374**(9707):2055–2063.

56 Fisher B, Costantino JP, Wickerham DL, et al. Tamoxifen for prevention of breast cancer: Report of the National Surgical Adjuvant Breast and Bowel Project P-1 Study. *J Natl Cancer Inst.* 1998;**90**:1371–1388.

62 Vogel VG, Costantino JP, Wickerham DL, et al. Effects of tamoxifen vs raloxifene on the risk of developing invasive breast cancer and other disease outcomes: The NSABP Study of Tamoxifen and Raloxifene (STAR) P-2 trial. *JAMA.* 2006;**295**:2727–2741.

72 Chia S, Gradishar W, Mauriac L, et al. Double-blind, randomized placebo controlled trial of fulvestrant compared with exemestane after prior non-steroidal aromatase inhibitor therapy in postmenopausal women with hormone receptor-positive, advanced breast cancer: results from EFECT. *J Clin Oncol.* 2008;**26**(10):1664–1670.

73 Di Leo A, Jerusalem G, Petruzelka L, et al. Results of the CONFIRM phase III trial comparing fulvestrant 250 mg with fulvestrant 500 mg in postmenopausal women with estrogen receptor-positive advanced breast cancer. *J Clin Oncol.* 2010;**28**(30):4594–4600.

75 Ellis MJ, Llombart-Cussac A, Feltl D, et al. Fulvestrant 500 mg versus anastrozole 1 mg for the first-line treatment of advanced breast cancer: overall survival analysis from the phase II first study. *J Clin Oncol.* 2015;**33**(32):3781–7. doi: 10.1200/JCO.2015.61.5831

87 Cuzick J, Forbes JF, Sestak I, et al. Long-term results of tamoxifen prophylaxis for breast cancer – 96-month follow-up of the randomized IBIS-I trial. *J Natl Cancer Inst.* 2007;**99**(4):272–282.

113 Bergh J, Jönsson PE, Lidbrink EK, et al. J FACT: an open-label randomized phase III study of fulvestrant and anastrozole in combination compared with anastrozole alone as first-line therapy for patients with receptor-positive postmenopausal breast cancer. *Clin Oncol.* 2012;**30**(16):1919–1925.

114 Mehta RS, Barlow WE, Albain KS, et al. Combination anastrozole and fulvestrant in metastatic breast cancer. *N Engl J Med.* 2012;**367**(5):435–444.

115 Johnston SR, Kilburn LS, Ellis P, et al. Fulvestrant plus anastrozole or placebo versus exemestane alone after progression on non-steroidal aromatase inhibitors in postmenopausal patients with hormone-receptor-positive locally advanced or metastatic breast cancer (SoFEA): a composite, multicentre, phase 3 randomised trial. *Lancet Oncol.* 2013;**14**(10):989–998.

117 Cuzick J, Sestak I, Baum M, et al. Effect of anastrozole and tamoxifen as adjuvant treatment for early-stage breast cancer: 10-year analysis of the ATAC trial. *Lancet Oncol.* 2010;**11**(12):1135–1141.

119 Regan MM, Neven P, Giobbie-Hurder A, et al. Assessment of letrozole and tamoxifen alone and in sequence for postmenopausal women with steroid hormone receptor-positive breast cancer: the BIG 1-98 randomised clinical trial at 8·1 years median follow-up. *Lancet Oncol.* 2011;**12**(12):1101–1108.

120 Goss PE, Ingle JN, Martino S, et al. A randomized trial of letrozole in postmenopausal women after five years of tamoxifen therapy for early-stage breast cancer. *N Engl J Med.* 2003;**349**(19):1793–1802.

125 Coombes RC, Hall E, Gibson LJ, et al. A randomized trial of exemestane after two to three years of tamoxifen therapy in postmenopausal women with primary breast cancer. *N Engl J Med.* 2004;**350**(11):1081–1092.

127 Mamounas EP, Jeong JH, Wickerham DL, et al. Benefit from exemestane as extended adjuvant therapy after 5 years of adjuvant tamoxifen: intention-to-treat analysis of the National Surgical Adjuvant Breast and Bowel Project B-33 trial. *J Clin Oncol.* 2008;**26**(12):1965–1971.

128 van de Velde CJ, Rea D, Seynaeve C, et al. Adjuvant tamoxifen and exemestane in early breast cancer (TEAM): a randomised phase 3 trial. *Lancet.* 2011;**377**(9762):321–331. doi: 10.1016/S0140-6736(10)62312-4.

135 Pagani O, Regan MM, Walley BA, et al. Adjuvant exemestane with ovarian suppression in premenopausal breast cancer. *N Engl J Med.* 2014;**371**(2):107–118.

136 Francis PA, Regan MM, Fleming GF, et al. Adjuvant Ovarian Suppression in Premenopausal Breast Cancer. *N Engl J Med.* 2014;**372**(5):436–446.

137 Gnant M, Mlineritsch B, Stoeger H, et al. Zoledronic acid combined with adjuvant endocrine therapy of tamoxifen versus anastrozol plus ovarian function suppression in premenopausal early breast cancer: final analysis of the Austrian Breast and Colorectal Cancer Study Group Trial 12. *Ann Oncol.* 2015;**26**(2):313–320.

148 Cuzick J, Sestak I, Forbes JF, et al. Anastrozole for prevention of breast cancer in high-risk postmenopausal women (IBIS-II): an international, double-blind, randomised placebo-controlled trial. *Lancet.* 2014;**383**(9922):1041–1048.

156 Hadji P, Jackisch C, Bolten W, et al. COMPliance and Arthralgia in Clinical Therapy: the COMPACT trial, assessing the incidence of arthralgia, and compliance within the first year of adjuvant anastrozole therapy. *Ann Oncol.* 2014;**25**(2):372–377.

176 Finn RS, Crown JP, Lang I, et al. The cyclin-dependent kinase 4/6 inhibitor palbociclib in combination with letrozole versus letrozole alone as first-line treatment of oestrogen receptor-positive, HER2-negative, advanced breast cancer (PALOMA-1/TRIO-18): a randomised phase 2 study. *Lancet Oncol.* 2015;**16**(1):25–35. pii: S1470-2045(14)71159-3.

177 Turner NC, Ro J, André F, et al. Palbociclib in Hormone-Receptor-Positive Advanced Breast Cancer. *N Engl J Med.* 2015;**373**(3):209–219. doi: 10.1056/NEJMoa1505270.

185 Gerber B, von Minckwitz G, Stehle H, et al. Effect of luteinizing hormone- releasing hormone agonist on ovarian function after modern adjuvant breast cancer chemotherapy. The GBG 37 ZORO study. *J Clin Oncol.* 2011;**29**:2334–2341.

186 Leonard RC, Adamson D, Anderson R, et al. The OPTION trial of adjuvant ovarian protection by goserelin in adjuvant chemotherapy for early breast cancer. *J Clin Oncol.* 2010;**28**(suppl):15S.

188 Lambertini M, Boni L, Michelotti A, et al. Long-term outcome results of the phase III PROMISE-GIM6 study evaluating the role of LHRH analog (LHRHa) during chemotherapy (CT) as a strategy to reduce ovarian failure in early breast cancer (BC) patients. *J Clin Oncol.* 2014;**32**(suppl 26: abstr 105).

189 Moore HCF, Unger JM, Phillips K-A, et al. Phase III trial (Prevention of Early Menopause Study [POEMS]-SWOG S0230) of LHRH analog during chemotherapy (CT) to reduce ovarian failure in early-stage, hormone receptor-negative breast cancer: an international Intergroup trial of SWOG, IBCSG, ECOG, and CALGB (Alliance). *J Clin Oncol.* 2014;**32**:5s (suppl; abstr LBA505).

62 Drug resistance and its clinical circumvention

Jeffrey A. Moscow, MD ■ *Kenneth H. Cowan, MD, PhD* ■ *Branimir I. Sikic, MD*

Overview

Tumors initially sensitive to chemotherapeutic agents frequently develop resistance to them, resulting in the familiar clinical pattern of initial response, followed by a recurrence that no longer responds to therapy. Laboratory and clinical investigations have identified a plethora of drug-resistance mechanisms, some that are particular to an individual agent and others that are generalizable across classes of agents. These mechanisms include altered cellular accumulation and detoxification of drugs, mutation of the drug target, change in expression of the drug target, and activation of alternative signaling pathways. The identification of drug-resistance mechanisms has led to strategies to overcome resistance and improved clinical outcomes.

Systemic therapy with cytotoxic drugs or targeted agents is the basis for most of the effective treatments of disseminated cancers. Additionally, adjuvant chemotherapy can offer a significant survival advantage to selected patients, following the treatment of localized disease with surgery or radiotherapy, presumably by eliminating undetected, minimal, or microscopic residual tumor. However, the responses of tumors to chemotherapeutic regimens vary, and failures are frequent owing to the emergence of drug resistance.

The phenomenon of clinical drug resistance has prompted studies to clarify mechanisms of drug action and to identify mechanisms of antineoplastic resistance. It is expected that through such information, drug resistance may be circumvented by rational design of new noncross-resistant agents, by novel delivery or combinations of known drugs, and by the development of other treatments that might augment the activity of or reverse resistance to known antineoplastics. While earlier mechanisms of drug resistance were identified experimentally by generation of resistant cell lines, recent advances in genomic technology have allowed the direct determination of resistance mechanisms present in clinically resistant tumors.

General mechanisms of resistance to single agents

Experimental selection of drug resistance by repeated exposure to single antineoplastic agents will generally result in cross-resistance to some related agents of the same drug class. This phenomenon is explained based on shared drug transport carriers, drug metabolizing pathways, and intracellular cytotoxic targets of these structurally and biochemically similar compounds.

Generally, the resistant cells retain sensitivity to drugs of different classes with alternative mechanisms of cytotoxic action. Thus, cells selected for resistance to alkylating agents or antifolates will usually remain sensitive to unrelated drugs, such as anthracyclines. Exceptions include emergence of cross-resistance to multiple, apparently structurally and functionally unrelated drugs, to which the patient or cancer cells were never exposed during the initial drug treatment. Despite apparent differences in their presumed sites of action within cells, the drugs associated with multidrug-resistance (MDR) phenotypes frequently share common metabolic pathways or efflux transport systems.

In this section, the processes related to drug resistance will be described. A more comprehensive discussion of selected mechanisms of resistance to specific classes of drugs will be discussed in subsequent sections.

Decreased drug accumulation

Decreased intracellular levels of cytotoxic agents is one of the most common mechanisms of drug resistance. As polar, water-soluble drugs cannot penetrate the lipid bilayer of the cell membrane and require specific mechanisms of cell entry, resistance to these drugs is readily mediated by downregulation of drug uptake mechanisms in tumor cells. For example, antifolates such as methotrexate require specific transporters to gain intracellular access, including high-affinity folate receptors, the reduced folate carrier (SLC19A1), and the proton-coupled folate transporter (SLC46A1) and downregulation of these mechanisms of uptake has been described as causes of methotrexate resistance.[1] For hydrophobic, nonpolar drugs that can easily diffuse across the cell membrane, decreased intracellular drug concentrations can be achieved by increasing the activities of drug efflux pumps. For example, overexpression of the P-glycoprotein (*MDR1/ABCB*1) drug efflux pump is an important example of this mechanism of resistance.[2]

Altered drug metabolism

Decreased drug activation, increased drug inactivation, or alterations in necessary cofactors can also confer resistance to selected antineoplastic agents. For example, decreased conversion of nucleobase analogs to their cytotoxic nucleoside and nucleotide derivatives by alterations in specific kinases and phosphoribosyl transferase salvage enzymes can lead to resistance to these anticancer drugs.[3] Another example associated with resistance is decreased levels of carboxyesterase—an activity necessary to convert a topoisomerase I inhibitor, CPT-11, to its active metabolite, SN-38.[4]

On the other hand, enhanced inactivation of pyrimidine and purine analogs by increased expression of deaminases is linked to resistance toward these agents.[5] Finally, alterations in cofactor levels can also modify drug toxicity. For example, optimal formation of inhibitory complexes between 5-fluorodeoxyuridine

Holland-Frei Cancer Medicine, Ninth Edition. Edited by Robert C. Bast Jr., Carlo M. Croce, William N. Hait, Waun Ki Hong, Donald W. Kufe, Martine Piccart-Gebhart, Raphael E. Pollock, Ralph R. Weichselbaum, Hongyang Wang, and James F. Holland.
© 2017 John Wiley & Sons, Inc. ISBN: 978-1-118-93469-2

monophosphate (FdUMP) and its target enzyme, thymidylate synthase, require the cofactor 5,10-methylene tetrahydrofolate.[6] Alterations in the intracellular levels of this cofactor can lead to resistance to fluoropyrimidines.

Increased repair or cellular tolerance to drug-induced damage

Cells contain multiple complex systems involved in the repair of damage to membranes and deoxyribonucleic acid (DNA), and changes in these repair processes can influence drug sensitivity. For example, resistance to cisplatin, a drug whose cytotoxic action involves intrastrand DNA crosslinkages, is associated with increased DNA repair. Conversely, defects in mismatch repair (MMR) are associated with tolerance to cisplatin-induced DNA damage. In this form of platinum resistance, the repair system is apparently unable to recognize platinum-DNA adducts and fails to activate the normal, appropriate programmed cell death response.

Increased rate of detoxification

The manner in which cells metabolize cancer drugs and other xenobiotics is often described as involving three phases of detoxification. Although none of these phases are obligatory steps in the metabolism of every drug, the concept represents a useful framework with which to view cellular detoxification mechanisms. Alterations in any of these three phases can influence the sensitivity or resistance to a particular drug or xenobiotic toxin. Phase 1 drug metabolism is mediated by cytochrome P-450 mixed-function oxidases. Generally, the drug or xenobiotic is rendered into a more electrophilic, reactive intermediate—a process that may enhance toxicity. These metabolites may then be converted to a less-reactive, presumably less-toxic form in phase 2 reactions, which include the formation of drug/xenobiotic conjugations with glutathione (GSH), glucuronic acid, or sulfate—reactions that are catalyzed by multiple isozymes, each of glutathione S-transferases (GSTs), uridine diphosphate (UDP)-glucuronosyl transferases, and sulfatases, respectively. Phase 3 detoxification consists of export of the parent drug/xenobiotic or its metabolites by energy-dependent transmembrane efflux pumps, including MRP (ABCC) family members as described above.

Altered drug targets

Qualitative changes in the enzyme targets of antineoplastic drugs can compromise drug efficacy and have been associated with resistance to targeted agents, especially tyrosine kinase inhibitors (TKIs). These mutations that are acquired through selective pressure often occur in locations that alter the binding site of the TKI. Similarly, other direct targets of enzyme inhibitors develop mutations that overcome resistance to cytotoxic chemotherapy agents, including dihydrofolate reductase (DHFR) resistance to methotrexate, thymidylate synthase resistance to fluoropyrmidines, and topoisomerases I and II resistance to camptothecins.

Altered gene expression

Increased or decreased expression of target enzymes can also lead to drug resistance. These alterations may result from changes that occur at any point along the pathways of gene expression and regulation, including DNA deletion or amplification, altered transcriptional or post-transcriptional control of ribonucleic acid (RNA) levels, and altered post-translational modifications of proteins. In addition, the same molecular mechanisms that lead to oncogenesis can also lead to drug resistance through altered expression of drug targets. Increased expression of DHFR is a mechanism

of resistance to methotrexate, while decreased expression of topoisomerase I is a mechanism of resistance to camptothecins.

Activation of alternative signaling pathways

Resistance to targeted agents such as TKIs can be mediated by activation of alternative signaling pathways that provide continued growth stimulation signaling despite successful inhibition of a primary oncogenic event. Activations of several bypass track-signaling pathways have been found in lung cancer patients treated with inhibitors of mutant EGFR and ALK.[7] These alternative pathways include amplification of *MET*, increased HGF expression, *PIK3CA* mutation, *BRAF* mutation, and *HER2* amplification. The alternative resistance pathways can be identified, and patients treated with relevant inhibitors. In melanomas treated with inhibitors of mutant BRAFV600, mechanisms of resistance include *BRAF* amplification, increased activity of A-RAF and C-RAF, mutations of *NRAS* and *MEK1*, and loss of *NF1*.[8] One strategy for overcoming drug resistance to BRAF inhibitors is concurrent inhibition of more than one kinase in the RAF–MEK–ERK pathway. This strategy was successfully tested in a randomized clinical trial in BRAF-mutated metastatic melanomas of the BRAF inhibitor vemurafenib alone versus vemurafenib plus the MEK inhibitor cobimetinib.[9] The combination resulted in a median progression free survival of 9.9 months and remission rate of 68%, compared to 6.2 months and 45% for vemurafenib alone.

KEY POINTS

Mechanisms of resistance to single agents

- Decreased drug accumulation
- Altered drug metabolism
- Increased DNA repair
- Increased detoxification
- Mutation of drug target
- Altered drug target expression

General mechanisms of resistance to multiple agents

Transport-mediated multiple drug resistance (MDR)

De novo and acquired cross-resistance to multiple antineoplastic agents can result from increased expression of a host of promiscuous drug efflux pumps known as ATP-binding cassette (ABC) proteins (Table 1). ABC proteins constitute a large family of 48 transport proteins organized into seven subfamilies, ABCA–ABCG. Of these, at least three have been directly shown to cause MDR, namely MDR1/P-glycoprotein (ABCB1), multidrug resistance-associated protein 1 (MRP1), (ABCC1), and BCRP/MXR/ABC-P (ABCG2). Classic MDR associated with resistance to drugs listed in Table 2 is mediated by P-glycoprotein (MDR1 or ABCB1). A similar but distinct MDR phenotype was attributed to the energy-dependent drug efflux activities of multidrug-resistance protein (MRP) family members, including MRP1 or ABCC1.[10]

The genetic basis of acquired MDR has been studied by whole genome sequencing of tumor samples from high grade, serous ovarian cancers. The sequencing disclosed acquired mutations associated with increased expression of the *ABCB1* multidrug transporter gene in approximately 8% of patients with recurrent

Table 1 ABC transporters associated with multidrug resistance (MDR).

- P-Glycoprotein/MDR 1/ABCB1-mediated classic MDR
- MRP family member-mediated MDR (currently at least three members, MRP1, 2, and 3 in ABCC1, ABCC2, and ABCC3 implicated in MDR drug efflux and detoxification)
- BCRP (ABCG2)-mediated MDR (putative ABC half-transporter implicated in mitoxantrone and anthracycline resistance)

Table 2 Cross-resistance pattern of classic (P-glycoprotein-mediated) MDR.

Class	Drug
Anthracyclines	Doxorubicin
	Daunorubicin
	Mitoxantrone
Antibiotics	Actinomycin D
	Plicamycin
Antimicrotubule drugs	Vincristine
	Vinblastine
	Colchicine
Epipodophyllotoxins	Etoposide
	Tenoposide

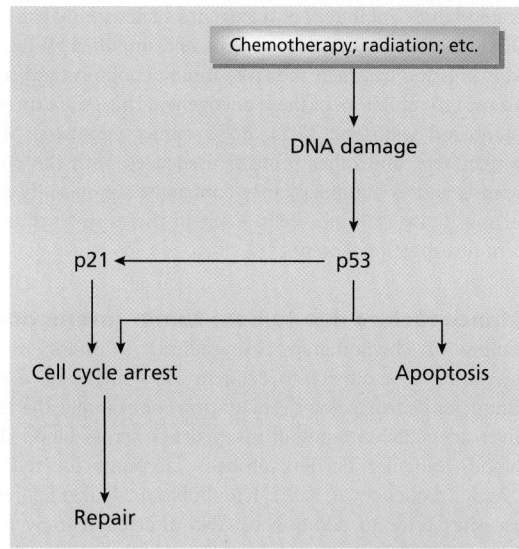

Figure 1 Alternative cellular responses to cancer therapeutic stress.

disease after chemotherapy.[11] These patients had all been treated with taxanes and/or doxorubicin, which are substrates for the P-glycoprotein transporter. The mutations included fusions at the *ABCB1* promoter and translocations in the 5′ region of the gene.

Inhibition of P-glycoprotein during exposure of cancer cells to taxanes such as cabazitaxel has revealed other, alternative mechanisms of resistance to taxanes.[12] These alternate mechanisms of resistance include induction of an epithelial to mesenchymal transition (EMT) and increased dynamic instability of microtubules by overexpression of the TUBB3 isoform of beta tubulin.

Another overlapping but discrete MDR phenotype is associated with increased expression of the recently isolated putative efflux transporter, breast cancer resistance protein (BCRP or ABCG2).[13] MDR has also been described in association with overexpression of the lung resistance protein (LRP). The mechanism of LRP-associated resistance is unclear, and whether LRP alone is sufficient to confer resistance is unknown. It is speculated that as a major vault protein, LRP is involved in nucleocytoplasmic transport and may be able to prevent entry of drugs into the nucleus.[14]

Multidrug resistance related to suppression of cell death pathways

Although chemotherapeutic drugs initiate cytotoxicity through their interactions with a variety of molecular targets, cancer drugs affect cell death, at least partially, via downstream events that converge upon pathways mediating type 1 (apoptotic) or type 2 (autophagic) programmed cell death or apoptosis. Apoptosis refers to an orderly cellular death program with predictable molecular and morphologic changes, including nuclear pyknosis and fragmentation, internucleosomal endonucleolytic DNA fragmentation, formation of cytoplasmic apoptotic bodies, and plasma membrane changes, such as transposition of phosphatidylserine to the extracellular surface.[15,16] Autophagy is a pathway for bulk degradation of subcellular constituents that occurs in response to stresses such as nutrient deprivation.[17] It involves the creation of autophagosomes/autolysozymes, and can be inhibited by PI3 kinase inhibitors such as 3-methyladenosine and wortmannin.

Although apoptosis may be either TP53-dependent or -independent, frequently the cellular response to DNA damage is regulated by TP53.[18] As shown in a simplified diagram (Figure 1), cancer

therapy-induced DNA damage is sensed by TP53 by incompletely understood mechanisms. Depending on the particular cell type and damage, TP53 expression may then initiate one of two possible pathways: apoptosis or a process of cell-cycle arrest and repair. In cells where the apoptotic pathway dominates, changes that cause dysfunction or deletion of TP53 are likely to result in reduced apoptosis in response to DNA damage, leading to relative resistance and cell survival with damage.

Other components of cell death-signaling pathways include: the mitogen-activated protein kinase (MAPK)-signaling cascades, which are involved in the regulation of cellular response to exogenous factors, including geno- and cytotoxic cancer treatments; the extracellular stimulus-regulated kinase (ERK1/2) pathway, which is implicated in the proliferative response to growth factors; and the p38 and stress-activated/c-Jun N-terminal protein kinase (SAPK/JNK) pathway. Modulation of these interacting pathways can have a profound effect on whether a cancer cell responds to cytotoxic challenge by activation of apoptosis or by cell-cycle arrest and repair, leading to resistance to treatment.[19]

Although their mechanism(s) of action is incompletely known, the balance of expressed antiapoptotic family members (Bcl-2 and Bcl-XL) and proapoptotic family members (Bax, Bak, Bad, and Bid) can influence the relative sensitivity of cells to toxic stressors.[20] Indeed, increased Bcl-2 and its antiapoptotic homologs are associated with increased resistance of lymphoid cells to the cytotoxic effects of corticosteroids, radiation, and DNA damage from chemotherapeutic drugs.[21,22] It has been proposed that increased levels of antiapoptotic proteins Bcl-2 or Bcl-XL may result in reduced sensitivity to DNA-damaging cancer drugs—a resistance phenotype characterized by cell survival and increased tolerance to DNA damage and genomic instability. This genomic instability may lead to further mutations activating additional resistance mechanisms and conferring more aggressive tumor behavior.[20] Although the role of Bcl-2 family proteins and the multidomain proapoptotic members of this family in the development of type 1 (apoptotic) programmed cell death has been extensively characterized, recent studies indicate that these proteins also control type 2 (autophagy) and nonapoptotic programmed cell death.[23]

The members of the BCL2 family also play important roles in resistance to targeted therapies.[24] BIM and PUMA are both proapoptotic BCL2 family members whose expression is induced by targeted kinase inhibitors of oncogenes such as mutated EGFR and BRAF, the BCR-ABL fusion protein, and amplified HER2. Loss of BIM expression has been shown to inhibit apoptosis and results in resistance to inhibitors of these oncogenes. Thus, the expression of mutant and wild-type TP53, Bcl-2 family members, MAPK family members, and other proteins associated with the control of apoptosis and/or autophagy may contribute significantly to the clinical sensitivity of tumor cells. Each of these proteins are the targets of investigational agents.[20,25]

Resistance factors due to host-tumor interactions

The failure of chemotherapy to eradicate a tumor in vivo despite exquisite sensitivity to drug in vitro might be a result of anatomic or pharmacologic sanctuaries. For example, the failure to deliver adequate amounts of many drugs across blood–brain and blood–testicular barriers probably accounts for the relatively high frequency of acute lymphoblastic leukemia relapse at these sites prior to addition of CNS-directed therapy to the treatment plans.[26] In large solid tumors, chemotherapeutic failures are frequently attributed to decreased drug delivery to a tumor that has overgrown its vascular supply. Additionally, development of acidosis and hypoxia in poorly perfused areas of large tumors may interfere with the cytotoxicity of some drugs. Altered prodrug activation by liver or other normal tissues may profoundly influence the efficacy of drugs such as cyclophosphamide.

Studies by Teicher and Herman[27] suggest that tumor–host interactions may influence drug pharmacokinetics and tumor resistance in unexpected ways. In this study, tumor cells selected for cyclophosphamide and cisplatin resistance in vivo were normally sensitive to drugs in vitro. When the tumor cells were reimplanted into nude mice, in vivo drug resistance was restored. These results suggest that resistant tumors may harbor cellular resistance factors that are operative only in conjunction with host factors and, therefore, mediate resistance by altered drug pharmacokinetics in vivo only. If this novel host-dependent mechanism of tumor resistance proves common, these results would provide one explanation for the failure of conventional in vitro testing to predict clinical responsiveness in all cases.

Cancer stem cells and drug resistance

The concept of cancer stem cells (CSCs) developed from observations that individual malignant cells within a cancer differ in their capacity to form tumors. These CSCs, or "tumor initiating cells" form a few to less than 1% of the population, have the property of plasticity or ability to change between tumorigenic and nontumorigenic states, and are a significant factor in the drug resistance of cancers.[28] Relapsed cancers are enriched in CSCs, and this subpopulation is known to express high levels of multidrug transporters as well as other drug-resistance genes. At the same time, CSCs offer new targets for cancer therapy, including inhibition of the Notch, Wnt, and Hedgehog pathways.

Genetic basis of acquired drug resistance and tumor heterogeneity

High resolution, deep sequencing of individual cancer genomes has revealed intratumoral heterogeneity of many cancers.[29] These data support a branched evolutionary model of tumor growth, with many competing clones differing in growth rates, metastatic potential, and sensitivity to various drugs. There are many implications for anticancer drug resistance that arise from this model. The dominant clone of a cancer derived from a drug-resistant normal tissue, such as colon or kidney, usually reflects the intrinsic resistance of the normal cells from which the cancer is derived. For cancers where the dominant clone is sensitive to a particular drug, the chances are high that drug-resistant minor clones are present at the time of cancer diagnosis. The oncogenic mutations that cause a cancer can contribute to drug sensitivity, by driving cell replication and increasing cancers' vulnerability to chemotherapy drugs that kill proliferating cells. However, acquired resistance to an anticancer therapy after remission results from resistant clones, some of which may have been present before treatment and some that may have developed during therapy. The emergence of drug resistance is reflected in the disappearance of drug-sensitive clones and overgrowth of resistant clones, an example of Darwinian "survival of the fittest" within cancer populations.[30] Heterogeneity in drug-resistance mechanisms and the nature of these mechanisms is also increasingly evident from comparisons of DNA sequences of sequential specimens from individual patients, as well as the evolution of resistance among different patients.[31]

Deep sequencing is also disclosing differences in genomic instability and apparent rates of mutation among cancers. The factors underlying these differences in genomic instability are not well understood, except for the subset of cancers that have MMR deficiencies. MMR deficiency is associated with a high rate of point mutations, and this may actually lead to more favorable outcomes for immunotherapies that enhance antitumor immunity via immune checkpoint controls (e.g., CTLA4, PD-1, and PDL-1).[30] In addition to mutational load, sequencing of melanoma specimens has identified a neo-antigen landscape that was strongly associated with a good response to CTLA-4 blockade by ipilumumab or tremelimumab.[32]

Both whole genome and targeted genomic sequencing can disclose "actionable mutations" such as BRAFV600E or HER2 amplification that can guide selection of specific targeted drugs, a concept that is being tested in several clinical trials, such as NCI-MATCH (NCT02465060), TRACERx (NCT01888601), DARWIN (NCT02183883), and BATTLE-2 (NCT01248247). Moreover, subclones may be detected that predict eventual failure of a particular therapy, and inform the selection of a noncross-resistant drug active against those subclones.[30] The so-called "liquid biopsies" analyzing the circulating free tumor DNA in blood can also detect targetable mutations and the presence of drug-resistant mutations in cancer patients.

In summary, the concept that tumor masses and their metastases were composed of genetically identical clones has given way to a model that pictures each tumor as a tree-like structure with tumor stem cells at the center and multiple evolving clones branching out from the trunk. Therefore, a tumor becomes a heterogeneous collection of related but not identical cells, both in the primary mass and in distant metastases. Selection pressures such as prior therapy can shape the characteristics of the overall tumor cell population in a patient, and spatially separated clones can develop different mechanisms of resistance. This picture of a tumor with its own organism-like qualities has emerged from studies that have performed deep sequencing on multiple biopsies from primary tumor masses and their metastases. The heterogeneity of a tumor extends to both genetic and epigenetic diversity. Thus, strategies to overcome drug resistance must take into account the diversity of mechanisms of resistance to any agent because distinct populations of cells within a patient may harbor different resistance mechanisms.

Potential clinical application of strategies to avert or overcome drug resistance

Approaches to overcome chemotherapeutic failures include efforts to prevent the emergence of drug resistance (Table 3). An appreciation of factors that induce resistance mechanisms may lead to the choice of more efficacious treatment regimens. Classically, aggressive combination chemotherapy with noncross-reacting drugs have been developed to eliminate tumor cells rapidly enough to prevent the selection of tumor cell clones with multiple resistance. Another approach is to develop therapies aimed at reversing or circumventing clinical drug resistance.

Reversal of ABC transporter-mediated resistance

Although preclinical studies in murine models showed efficacy of P-glycoprotein inhibitors, most clinical studies involving the use of MDR-reversing agents in the treatment of solid human tumors have been disappointing, and despite the plethora of MDR-reversing agents identified in hundreds of preclinical studies, none have evolved into clinically useful agents. Clinical trials of MDR-reversing agents encountered significant obstacles, including (1) increased toxicity of the chemotherapy agents caused profound effects on the pharmacokinetics and pharmacodynamics of MDR1-reversing agents on the cytotoxic drugs associated with MDR, (2) the toxicity of some of the early MDR1-reversing agents themselves, such as verapamil, prevented adequate exposure to them; (3) lack of screening of patients for *MDR1/ABCB1* expression in tumors; (4) involvement of other transporters and other mechanisms of resistance at the time of recurrence; and (5) lack of understanding of how MDR1 polymorphisms affect susceptibility to MDR1 inhibition.[2] While P-glycoprotein and other ABC transporters may play important roles in tumor biology and drug resistance, no pharmacologic strategy has emerged that can improve clinical outcomes by inhibiting the activity of these transporters once clinical drug resistance has been established.

Table 3 Approaches to overcome or circumvent drug resistance.

Prevention	Aggressive multiple-agent therapy
	Appreciation of factors that induce resistance mechanism
	Concurrent blockade of a resistance pathway
Circumvention	Drug-screening programs and rational drug design
	Circumvention of drug uptake defects
	Dose escalation
	Drugs that use alternative transport mechanisms
	Agents that reverse increased efflux
	Cofactors that augment drug activation or efficacy
	Inhibition of drug inactivation
	Novel treatment modalities
	Immunotherapy
	Inhibit alternative signaling pathways
	Enhance apoptotic pathways
	Noncross-resistant analogs against the same target

Reversal of resistance to nucleoside analogs

While cellular accumulation of lipophilic cytotoxic agents that are substrates for ABC transporters can be limited by upregulation of these transporters, the problem is reversed for hydrophilic nucleoside analogs that depend on specific transporters for cellular uptake. So, in contrast to MDR, where the problem is reversing the activity of an efflux pump, overcoming resistance to nucleoside analogs can involve strategies to increase cellular uptake. This can include making nucleoside analog prodrugs that are more lipophilic, so they can more easily diffuse across the cell membrane; using nanoparticle delivery systems to bypass nucleoside transporters; and even gene therapy to increase expression of nucleoside transporters in tumors.[33,34]

Resistance to targeted agents

BCR/ABL

The first approved kinase inhibitor was imatinib, with remarkable activity against chronic myeloid leukemia (CML), a disease driven by the BCR/ABL fusion mutation. Imatinib and BCR/ABL have become a paradigm of an important class of resistance mechanisms to kinase inhibitors, point mutations directly affecting drug binding or changing the conformation of the BCR/ABL protein to reduce drug binding.[35,36] More than 100 such point mutations have been found in resistant CML specimens. Deep sequencing of the *BCR/ABL* fusion gene in CML specimens has enabled the identification of emerging resistant clones, and even the detection of such clones early in the course of imatinib treatment. Genomic instability, increased by the perturbation of several DNA repair pathways by BCR/ABL, contributes to the high frequency of imatinib-resistant point mutations.[36] Remarkably, the FDA has approved several new kinase inhibitors that are active against imatinib-resistant BCR/ABL, including dasatinib, nilotinib, bosutinib and ponatinib.

EGFR

Agents directed at the Epidermal Growth Factor Receptor, EGFR, fall into two categories. Antibodies directed at EGFR are approved for use in colon cancer and in head and neck cancers, malignancies where tumor cells are dependent on signaling of WT EGFR, while small molecule TKIs of EGFR are indicated in the treatment of nonsmall-cell lung cancer (NSCLC) with activating mutations of EGFR. Resistance develops to both anti-EGFR antibodies and TKIs, and the mechanisms have predictable similarities and differences. Resistance can develop through mutation of EGFR, but the resistance mutations occur at different sites depending on the agent: for first-generation EGFR TKIs such as erlotinib and gefitinib, the major resistance mutation is T790M, which affects the ATP-binding domain targeted by these agents; while resistance to the anti-EGFR antibody cetuximab occurs at several sites that alter the binding epitope of the antibody, including S492R, S464L, G465R, and I491M.[11]

Resistance to both types of EGFR-inhibitory agents can occur through activation of bypass-signaling pathways, which continue to activate the same downstream effectors, such as activation of HER2, a tyrosine kinase receptor belonging to the same family as EGFR, as well as MET. Moreover, resistance to both anti-EGFR TKIs and antibodies has been ascribed to histologic transformation of the tumor, often described as an EMT, which is marked by the loss of the pan-epithelial marker E-cadherin, increased expression of the mesenchymal-associated antigens vimentin and fibronectin, and loss of sensitivity toward EGFR-directed agents. An unexpected mechanism of resistance to mutant EGFR inhibitors in lung cancers was the transformation from nonsmall cell to small cell lung cancers in 14% of cases.[37]

It is not known why individual tumors develop different mechanisms of resistance or why one bypass pathway is activated in one tumor and not in another. However, one difference between NSCLC and colon cancer is that the activating EGFR mutation in NSCLC appears to be a driver mutation in that disease, so resistance mutations of EGFR play a more prominent role, whereas EGFR signaling is one of many signaling pathways upregulated in colon cancers, so activation of bypass signaling occurs more frequently in that context.

Strategies to overcome resistance to EGFR-targeted agents fall into four categories. First, for NSCLC, new agents are under development that are more active against mutated EGFR, including both activating mutations and the T790M resistance mutations, that promise to increase the therapeutic index of these agents as well as diminish the possibility of the development of resistance mutations. Two third-generation EGFR inhibitors have been shown to be effective in the common, drug-resistant T790M mutation. These are rociletinib (CO-1686)[38] and AZD9291.[39]

Second, dual inhibition of EGFR by combining an anti-EGFR TKI with an anti-EGFR antibody, testing the hypothesis that this approach more completely suppresses EGFR signaling, is in clinical testing. Third, several inhibitors of bypass signaling, such as inhibitors of MET and MEK, have been combined with anti-EGFR therapies. Finally, agents that might inhibit EMT, such as histone deacetylase inhibitors, have also been combined with EGFR inhibitors to both prevent and reverse resistance.

ALK

A genomic rearrangement of the anaplastic lymphoma kinase (ALK) gene is the second most common oncogenic mutation in lung adenocarcinomas (after EGFR). Crizotinib was the first FDA-approved ALK kinase inhibitor, but resistance to crizotinib invariably develops and includes point mutations of ALK as well as activation of bypass-signaling pathways.[40] The FDA has approved ceritinib as a second-generation ALK inhibitor that overcomes some of the resistance mechanisms to crizotinib.[41,42] In crizotinib-resistant patients, ceritinib produced a remission rate of 56%, with a median progression-free survival of 7 months.[42]

BRAF

Approximately 50% of malignant melanomas are caused by an activating mutation of the BRAF gene, most commonly the V600E mutation. The FDA has approved two kinase inhibitors, vemurafenib and dabrafenib, that inhibit this V600E mutant BRAF. However, resistance to these kinase inhibitors occurs in almost all cases, including NRAS and MEK1 mutations, BRAF amplification, loss of NF1, and other MAPK pathway alterations.[8] As previously noted, concurrent inhibition of both mutated BRAF and MEK has been a successful strategy to delay resistance to BRAF inhibitors in melanomas.[9]

Activating BRAF mutations occur in a small percentage of other cancer types, including 10% of colorectal cancers. Resistance mechanisms to BRAF inhibitors in colorectal cancers are predominantly alterations in MAPK pathway genes that produce sustained MAPK pathway activity, including amplifications of KRAS and BRAF, and MEK1 mutation.[43]

Bruton's tyrosine kinase (BTK)

Ibrutinib is an irreversible binder of Bruton's tyrosine kinase (BTK), which is an enzyme crucial for B-cell development and survival.

Inhibition of BTK by ibrutinib is clinically effective in many B-cell malignancies, including mantle cell lymphoma and chronic lymphocytic leukemia. Mechanisms of resistance to ibrutinib include mutation C481S in the BTK gene at the drug-binding cysteine residue and mutations of PLCγ2 that result in autonomous B-cell receptor activity.[44]

Conclusion and future directions

The diversity of mechanisms of antineoplastic drug resistance, combined with the biologic heterogeneity of tumors, presents a formidable therapeutic challenge. Nevertheless, the identification of the drug-resistance mechanisms has led to useful approaches to overcoming clinical drug resistance and improving therapeutic outcomes. These approaches include the design of novel drugs that are less likely to share resistance mechanisms and the development of combination therapies that target resistance pathways. Despite these efforts, many tumors will remain refractory to conventional and targeted chemotherapeutic agents.

References

1 Matherly LH, Wilson MR, Hou Z. The major facilitative folate transporters solute carrier 19A1 and solute carrier 46A1: biology and role in antifolate chemotherapy of cancer. *Drug Metab Dispos.* 2014;**42**(4):632–649.

2 Amiri-Kordestani L, Basseville A, Kurdziel K, Fojo AT, Bates SE. Targeting MDR in breast and lung cancer: discriminating its potential importance from the failure of drug resistance reversal studies. *Drug Resist Updat.* 2012;**15**(1-2):50–61.

3 Drahovsky D, Kreis W. Studies on drug resistance. II. Kinase patterns in P815 neoplasms sensitive and resistant to 1-beta-D-arabinofuranosylcytosine. *Biochem Pharmacol.* 1970;**19**(3):940–944.

4 Haaz MC, Rivory LP, Riche C, Robert J. The transformation of irinotecan (CPT-11) to its active metabolite SN-38 by human liver microsomes. Differential hydrolysis for the lactone and carboxylate forms. *Naunyn Schmiedeberg's Arch Pharmacol.* 1997;**356**(2):257–262.

5 Hunt SW 3rd, Hoffee PA. Amplification of adenosine deaminase gene sequences in deoxycoformycin-resistant rat hepatoma cells. *J Biol Chem.* 1983;**258**(21):13185–13192.

6 Houghton JA, Maroda SJ Jr, Phillips JO, Houghton PJ. Biochemical determinants of responsiveness to 5-fluorouracil and its derivatives in xenografts of human colorectal adenocarcinomas in mice. *Cancer Res.* 1981;**41**(1):144–149.

7 Camidge DR, Pao W, Sequist LV. Acquired resistance to TKIs in solid tumours: learning from lung cancer. *Nat Rev Clin Oncol.* 2014;**11**(8):473–481.

8 Van Allen EM, Wagle N, Sucker A, et al. The genetic landscape of clinical resistance to RAF inhibition in metastatic melanoma. *Cancer Discov.* 2014;**4**(1):94–109.

9 Larkin J, Ascierto PA, Dreno B, et al. Combined vemurafenib and cobimetinib in BRAF-mutated melanoma. *N Engl J Med.* 2014;**371**(20):1867–1876.

10 Cole SP. Multidrug resistance protein 1 (MRP1, ABCC1), a "multitasking" ATP-binding cassette (ABC) transporter. *J Biol Chem.* 2014;**289**(45):30880–30888.

11 Arena S, Bellosillo B, Siravegna G, et al. Emergence of Multiple EGFR Extracellular Mutations during Cetuximab Treatment in Colorectal Cancer. *Clin Cancer Res.* 2015;**21**(9):2157–2166.

12 Duran GE, Wang YC, Francisco EB, et al. Mechanisms of resistance to cabazitaxel. *Mol Cancer Ther.* 2015;**14**(1):193–201.

13 Ishikawa T, Nakagawa H. Human ABC transporter ABCG2 in cancer chemotherapy and pharmacogenomics. *J Exp Ther Oncol.* 2009;**8**(1):5–24.

14 Slovak ML, Ho JP, Cole SP, et al. The LRP gene encoding a major vault protein associated with drug resistance maps proximal to MRP on chromosome 16: evidence that chromosome breakage plays a key role in MRP or LRP gene amplification. *Cancer Res.* 1995;**55**(19):4214–4219.

15 Adams JM, Cory S. Bcl-2-regulated apoptosis: mechanism and therapeutic potential. *Curr Opin Immunol.* 2007;**19**(5):488–496.

16 Hanahan D, Weinberg RA. Hallmarks of cancer: the next generation. *Cell.* 2011;**144**(5):646–674.

17 Levine B, Kroemer G. Autophagy in the pathogenesis of disease. *Cell.* 2008;**132**(1):27–42.

18 Vousden KH, Lu X. Live or let die: the cell's response to p53. *Nat Rev Cancer.* 2002;**2**(8):594–604.

19 Abrams SL, Steelman LS, Shelton JG, et al. The Raf/MEK/ERK pathway can govern drug resistance, apoptosis and sensitivity to targeted therapy. *Cell Cycle.* 2010;**9**(9):1781–1791.

20 Thomas S, Quinn BA, Das SK, et al. Targeting the Bcl-2 family for cancer therapy. *Expert Opin Ther Targets*. 2013;**17**(1):61–75.

21 Herr I, Debatin KM. Cellular stress response and apoptosis in cancer therapy. *Blood*. 2001;**98**(9):2603–2614.

22 Stahnke K, Fulda S, Friesen C, Strauss G, Debatin KM. Activation of apoptosis pathways in peripheral blood lymphocytes by in vivo chemotherapy. *Blood*. 2001;**98**(10):3066–3073.

23 Levine B, Sinha S, Kroemer G. Bcl-2 family members: dual regulators of apoptosis and autophagy. *Autophagy*. 2008;**4**(5):600–606.

24 Hata AN, Engelman JA, Faber AC. The BCL2 family: key mediators of the apoptotic response to targeted anticancer therapeutics. *Cancer Discov*. 2015;**5**(5):475–487.

25 Mohell N, Alfredsson J, Fransson A, et al. APR-246 overcomes resistance to cisplatin and doxorubicin in ovarian cancer cells. *Cell Death Dis*. 2015;**6**:e1794.

26 Poplack DG, Reaman G. Acute lymphoblastic leukemia in childhood. *Pediatr Clin N Am*. 1988;**35**(4):903–932.

27 Teicher BA, Herman TS, Holden SA, et al. Tumor resistance to alkylating agents conferred by mechanisms operative only in vivo. *Science*. 1990;**247**(**4949 Pt 1**):1457–1461.

28 Mertins SD. Cancer stem cells: a systems biology view of their role in prognosis and therapy. *Anti-Cancer Drugs*. 2014;**25**(4):353–367.

29 Swanton C. Intratumor heterogeneity: evolution through space and time. *Cancer Res*. 2012;**72**(19):4875–4882.

30 Jamal-Hanjani M, Quezada SA, Larkin J, Swanton C. Translational implications of tumor heterogeneity. *Clin Cancer Res*. 2015;**21**(6):1258–1266.

31 Patch AM, Christie EL, Etemadmoghadam D, et al. Whole-genome characterization of chemoresistant ovarian cancer. *Nature*. 2015;**521**(7553):489–494.

32 Snyder A, Makarov V, Merghoub T, et al. Genetic basis for clinical response to CTLA-4 blockade in melanoma. *N Engl J Med*. 2014;**371**(23):2189–2199.

33 Adema AD, Bijnsdorp IV, Sandvold ML, Verheul HM, Peters GJ. Innovations and opportunities to improve conventional (deoxy)nucleoside and fluoropyrimidine analogs in cancer. *Curr Med Chem*. 2009;**16**(35):4632–4643.

34 Hung SW, Mody HR, Govindarajan R. Overcoming nucleoside analog chemoresistance of pancreatic cancer: a therapeutic challenge. *Cancer Lett*. 2012;**320**(2):138–149.

35 Jabbour EJ, Cortes JE, Kantarjian HM. Resistance to tyrosine kinase inhibition therapy for chronic myelogenous leukemia: a clinical perspective and emerging treatment options. *Clin Lymphoma Myeloma Leuk*. 2013;**13**(5):515–529.

36 Lamontanara AJ, Gencer EB, Kuzyk O, Hantschel O. Mechanisms of resistance to BCR-ABL and other kinase inhibitors. *Biochim Biophys Acta*. 2013;**1834**(7):1449–1459.

37 Sequist LV, Waltman BA, Dias-Santagata D, et al. Genotypic and histological evolution of lung cancers acquiring resistance to EGFR inhibitors. *Sci Transl Med*. 2011;**3**(75):75ra26.

38 Sequist LV, Soria JC, Goldman JW, et al. Rociletinib in EGFR-mutated non-small-cell lung cancer. *N Engl J Med*. 2015;**372**(18):1700–1709.

39 Janne PA, Yang JC, Kim DW, et al. AZD9291 in EGFR inhibitor-resistant non-small-cell lung cancer. *N Engl J Med*. 2015;**372**(18):1689–1699.

40 Wilson FH, Johannessen CM, Piccioni F, et al. A functional landscape of resistance to ALK inhibition in lung cancer. *Cancer Cell*. 2015;**27**(3):397–408.

41 Friboulet L, Li N, Katayama R, et al. The ALK inhibitor ceritinib overcomes crizotinib resistance in non-small cell lung cancer. *Cancer Discov*. 2014;**4**(6):662–673.

42 Shaw AT, Kim DW, Mehra R, et al. Ceritinib in ALK-rearranged non-small-cell lung cancer. *N Engl J Med*. 2014;**370**(13):1189–1197.

43 Ahronian LG, Sennott EM, Van Allen EM, et al. Clinical acquired resistance to RAF inhibitor combinations in BRAF-mutant colorectal cancer through MAPK pathway alterations. *Cancer Discov*. 2015;**5**(4):358–367.

44 Woyach JA, Furman RR, Liu TM, et al. Resistance mechanisms for the Bruton's tyrosine kinase inhibitor ibrutinib. *N Engl J Med*. 2014;**370**(24):2286–2294.

Biological and Gene Therapy

PART 9

Biological and Gene Therapy

63 Cytokines, interferons, and hematopoietic growth factors

Suhendan Ekmekcioglu, PhD ▪ Elizabeth A. Grimm, PhD

Overview

Cytokines are important mediators of immune responses and produced by almost every cell in the body. Growth stimulatory or inhibitory cytokines could be subclassified as interleukins (ILs), lymphokines, monokines, chemokines, and hematopoietic growth factors. In cancer, certain cytokines act directly on the growth, differentiation, or survival of endothelial cells, whereas others act by attracting inflammatory cell types affecting angiogenesis or by inducing secondary cytokines or other mediators regulating angiogenesis. Proinflammatory and chemotactic cytokines influence the tumor environment and control the quantity and nature of infiltrating hematopoietic effector cells, with inhibiting or enhancing effects on tumor growth. The important role of cytokines in regulating immune responses may permit an effective immune response against the tumors or suppress the function of antigen-presenting cells (APC).

The understanding of cytokines has now emerged as complex picture of interacting stimulatory and inhibitory factors. Many of the molecules that govern this process have been cloned and have entered clinical trials. It is now clear that regulatory cytokines are characteristically pleiotropic and, at the same time, exhibit significant functional redundancy.

The biologic characterization of the known clinically relevant ILs, interferons and selected growth factors, the rationale for their use in therapy for patients with cancer, and the accumulated clinical experience represent the subjects of this chapter.

Cytokines, a diverse family of signaling molecules, are important mediators of immune responses and produced by almost every cell in the body, including various cancer cells. In general, some cytokines are growth stimulatory and others are inhibitory. Cytokines with clinical relevance to cancer include those subclassified further as interleukins (ILs), monokines, chemokines, and hematopoietic growth factors. IL designates any soluble protein or glycoprotein product of leukocytes that regulates the responses of other leukocytes. ILs produce their effects primarily through paracrine interactions. In cancer, certain cytokines act directly on the growth, differentiation, or survival of endothelial cells, whereas others act by attracting inflammatory cell types affecting angiogenesis or by inducing secondary cytokines or other mediators regulating angiogenesis. Proinflammatory and chemotactic cytokines influence the tumor environment and control the quantity and nature of infiltrating hematopoietic effector cells, with inhibiting or enhancing effects on tumor growth. The important role of cytokines in regulating immune responses may permit an effective immune response against the tumors or suppress the function of APC. Presuming antigens exist on tumor cells, various immunostimulatory cytokines, and particularly ILs, are now administered to patients in an attempt to initiate, augment, or otherwise stimulate a weak or previously

nonexistent antitumor immune response. In addition to immune response stimulation, some ILs have been used to stimulate the growth and differentiation of various subpopulations of blood cells after chemotherapy or bone marrow transplantation (BMT) in a restorative role.

It is now clear that the pleiotropic nature of many cytokines allows them to influence virtually all organ systems (Figure 1). Cytokines may have their own private receptor but may also share a "public" receptor with other cytokines (Tables 1 and 2).

The biologic characterization of selected ILs (those for which we discuss a role in cancer), interferons (IFNs) and selected growth factors, the rationale for their use in therapy for patients with cancer, and the accumulated clinical experience represent the subjects of this chapter.

Interleukins

Interleukin-1

IL-1 (IL-1α and IL-1β) is the prototypic pleiotropic cytokine and influences nearly every cell type.[1,2] Because IL-1 is a highly inflammatory cytokine, the margin between salutary effects and serious toxicity in humans is exceedingly narrow. Compounds that attenuate the production and/or activity of IL-1 are therefore being explored in clinical trials.

Biologic effects of IL-1

IL-1 can increase the expression of itself as well as many other cytokines (including IL-1RA), cytokine receptors (including IL-2, IL-3, IL-5, granulocyte macrophage-colony-stimulating factor [GM-CSF], and c-kit), inflammatory mediators (such as cyclooxygenase and inducible nitric oxide synthase), hepatic acute-phase reactants, growth factors, clotting factors, neuropeptides, lipid-related genes, extracellular matrix molecules, and oncogenes (e.g., *c-jun, cabl, c-fms, c-myc,* and *c-fos*).[1] Data suggest that an inflammatory component is present in the microenvironment of most neoplastic tissues, including those not causally related to an obvious inflammatory process. Thus, as a proinflammatory cytokine, IL-1 may also be a major proangiogenic stimulus of both physiological and pathological angiogeneses.

The IL-1 family has been implicated in the function and the dysfunction of virtually every human organ system. Indeed, increased IL-1 production has been reported in patients with infections (viral, bacterial, fungal, and parasitic), intravascular coagulation, cancer (both solid tumors and hematologic malignancies), Alzheimer's disease, autoimmune disorders, trauma, ischemic diseases, pancreatitis, graft-versus-host disease, transplant rejection, and in healthy subjects after exercise.[1]

It has been suggested that the balance between IL-1 and its naturally occurring antagonists is most relevant to illness.[3] This balance

Holland-Frei Cancer Medicine, Ninth Edition. Edited by Robert C. Bast Jr., Carlo M. Croce, William N. Hait, Waun Ki Hong, Donald W. Kufe, Martine Piccart-Gebhart, Raphael E. Pollock, Ralph R. Weichselbaum, Hongyang Wang, and James F. Holland.
© 2017 John Wiley & Sons, Inc. ISBN: 978-1-118-93469-2

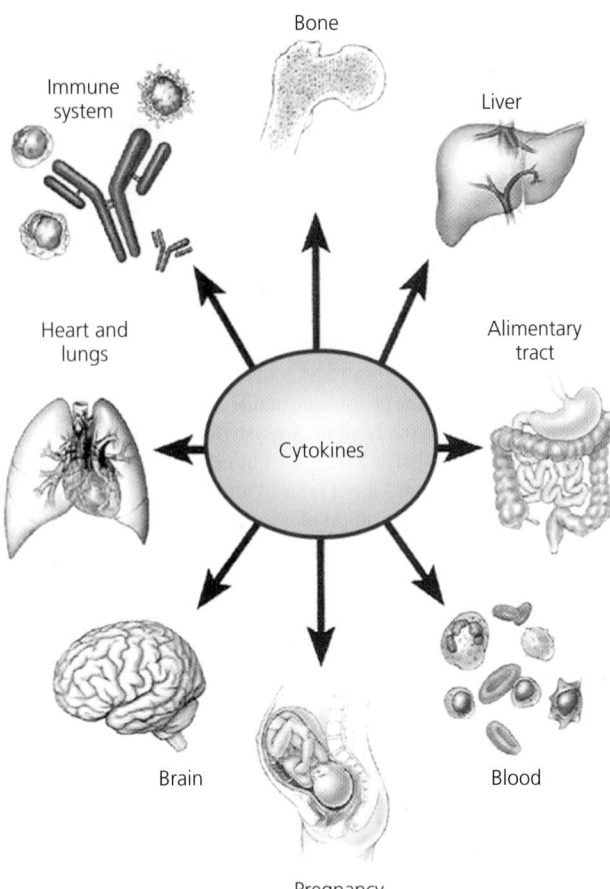

Figure 1 In addition to their effects on hematopoiesis and immunocompetence, "hematopoietic" growth factors influence multiple organ systems, including (but not limited to) bone remodeling, cardiorespiratory function, hepatic function, and the gastrointestinal tract.

may be altered in different ways, depending on the disease. In AML, IL-10 is spontaneously expressed, but IL-1RA gene expression is suppressed even when stimulated with GM-CSF.[4,5] CML patients with advanced disease and poor survival have suppressed IL-1RA accompanied by high IL-1β.[6] In AML and CML patients, IL-1β acts as an autocrine growth factor; exposure to molecules that decrease the activity of IL-1 suppresses leukemic proliferation.[7,8] Constitutive production of IL-lα, IL-1β, and/or IL-1RA in solid tumors (melanomas, hepatoblastoma, sarcomas, squamous cell carcinomas, transitional cell cancers, and ovarian carcinomas) has

been described and may, in some cases, contribute to metastatic potential. However, the relationship between IL-1 and tumor growth is complex.

IL-1 in the clinic

IL-lα and IL-1β have both been administered in clinical cancer trials.[1] In general, the acute toxicities of both isoforms were greater after intravenous than subcutaneous injection. Subcutaneous injection was associated with significant local pain, erythema, and swelling. Dose-related chills and fever were observed in nearly all patients, and even a 1 ng/kg dose was pyrogenic. Nearly all patients receiving intravenous IL-1 at doses of 100 ng/kg or greater were experienced significant hypotension, probably because of induction of nitric oxide.

IL-1 infusion into humans significantly increased circulating IL-6 levels and resulted in a rise in leukocyte counts, even at doses as low as 1 or 2 ng/kg. Increases in platelets, peripheral monocyte count, and phorbol-induced superoxide production were also observed in patients with normal marrow reserves. In contrast to the results in patients with good marrow function, patients with aplastic anemia treated with five daily doses of IL-lα (30–100 ng/kg) had no increases in peripheral blood counts or bone marrow cellularity.[9] However, after chemotherapy, two doses of IL-10 significantly shortened the duration of neutropenia,[10] and IL-lα (5 days) significantly reduced thrombocytopenia.[11] Overall, the benefits of IL-1 therapy were compromised by its toxicity.

Interleukin-2

Originally described as a T-cell growth factor, the function of IL-2 extends beyond lymphocyte activation and population expansion, although T cells still appear to be its major target.[12]

Biologic activities of IL-2

IL-2 primarily acts as a T-cell growth factor, but B cells, natural killer (NK) cells, and lymphokine-activated killer (LAK) cells are also responsive to this cytokine. Following binding of IL-2 with the trimeric receptor complex, internalization occurs and cell-cycle progression is induced in association with the expression of a defined series of genes.[13] A second functional response occurs through the IL-2β, dimeric receptor, also known as the intermediate affinity dimeric complex (kDa, 10^{-9}), and involves the differentiation of several subclasses of lymphocytes into LAK cells.[14] This response occurs in patients with cancer who receive IL-2[15,16] and was originally considered to be a critical part of the anticancer effect of IL-2.

Table 1 Types of hematopoietic growth factor receptors.

Type	Characteristics	Receptor examples
Type I cytokine receptor	Does not possess intrinsic kinase activity. Receptor acts as docking site for adaptor molecules, which leads to phosphorylation of cellular substrates	IL-1, IL-2, IL-3, IL-4, IL-5, IL-6, IL-7, IL-9, IL-13, IL-18, IL-21, GM-CSF, G-CSF, EPO, TPO, and leukemia inhibitory factor
Type II cytokine receptor	Contains extracellular fibronectin III type domain	Interferon and IL-10
Receptors with tyrosine kinase domains (type III)	Large extracellular immunoglobulin-like domain, single transmembrane spinning region, and a cytoplasmic tyrosine kinase domain(s)	fms (M-CSF receptor), FLT-3, c-kit (SCF receptor), and PDGFR
Chemokine receptor	Seven transmembrane spanning G protein-linked regions	IL-8
Tumor necrosis factor family	Cysteine-rich repeats in the extracellular domain, and cytoplasmic 80 amino acid "death domain"	Tumor necrosis factor and Fas

Abbreviations: EPO, erythropoietin; G-CSF, granulocyte colony-stimulating factor; GM-CSF, granulocyte macrophage colony-stimulating factor; IL, interleukin; M-CSF, macrophage colony-stimulating factor; SCF, stem cell factor; TPO, thrombopoietin.

Table 2 Interleukins.

	Chromosomal location	Receptors	Selected biologic activities
IL-1	2q13	IL-1RI and IL-1RII	Promotes acute-phase response. IL-1 acts on nearly every organ system. Induces production of multiple cytokines Upregulates cell-surface cytokine expression Synergizes with other cytokines to stimulate hematopoietic progenitor proliferation Influences immune regulation Modulates endocrine function Affects bone formation IL-1R acts as a cofactor in neural transmission
IL-2	4q26-q27	$\alpha\beta\gamma$ heterotrimeric complex	Induces proliferation and activation of T cells, B cells, and NK cells
IL-3	5q31	IL-3 receptor (heterodimer of IL-3-specific α subunit and β subunit)	Stimulation of multilineage hematopoietic progenitors, especially when used in combination with other cytokines (SCF, IL-1, IL-6, G-CSF, GM-CSF, EPO, and TPO)
IL-4 and IL-13	5q31	Type I IL-4 receptor (IL-4Rα and IL-2 receptor γc chain subunits) transduces IL-4 Type II IL-4 receptor (IL-4Rα and the IL-13 Rα1 subunits) transduces IL-4 and IL-13 IL-4Rα and IL-13 Rα2 complex or two IL-13 Rα transduce IL-13	IL-4 and IL-13 are involved in allergic reaction (induce switch to IgE)
IL-5	5q31	Consists of IL-5Rα (IL-5-specific) and a β subunit β subunit is common to IL-3 and GM-CSF complexes	Regulates production, function, survival, and migration of eosinophils Enhances basophil number and function
IL-6	7p21	IL-6Rα together with gp130	B- and T-cell development and function Thrombopoiesis Acute-phase protein synthesis Inhibition of hepatic albumin excretion Osteoclastic bone resorption Neural differentiation
IL-7	8q12-q13	Composed of IL-7Rα (CD127) and the common γc chain subunits	Critical for T- and B-cell development
IL-8	4q12-q13	IL-8Rα and IL-8Rβ exist	Potent chemoattractant agent for a variety of leukocytes, especially neutrophils Suppresses colony formation of immature myeloid progenitors Increases keratinocyte and endothelial cell proliferation
IL-9	5q31.1	IL-9 receptor	Supports clonogenic maturation of erythroid progenitors Acts as a mast cell differentiation factor Protects lymphomas from apoptosis Cooperates with IL-4 in B-cell responses Enhances neuronal differentiation
IL-10	1q31-q32	IL-10 receptor interferon receptors	Inhibits cytokine synthesis by Th1 cells and monocytes/macrophages Stimulates B-cell proliferation Involved in transformation of B cells by Epstein–Barr virus and tumor necrosis factor (TNF) receptors
IL-11	19q13.3-q13.4	IL-11Rα and gp 130 subunits gp 130 = CD130 on 5q11 IL-6, oncostatin M, and leukemia inhibitory factor also use gp130 subunit	Best known as a thrombopoietic factor Stimulates multilineage progenitors, erythropoiesis, myelopoiesis, and lymphopoiesis Decreases mucositis in animal models Stimulates osteoclast development Inhibits adipogenesis Stimulates proliferation of neuronal cells
IL-12	IL-12A:3p12-q13.2 IL-12B:5q31.1-q33.1	IL-12Rβ1 and IL-12Rβ2 chains are related to gp 130	Proinflammatory cytokine important in resistance to infections Th1 development Stimulatory and inhibitory effects on hematopoiesis
IL-15	4q31	High-affinity receptor requires IL-2Rβ and γ chains and IL-15 Rα chain	Triggers proliferation and immunoglobulin production in preactivated B cells Number of CD8$^+$ memory T cells may be controlled by balance of IL-15 (stimulatory) and IL-12 (inhibitory) Stimulates proliferation of NK cells and activated CD4$^+$ or CD8$^+$ T cells Facilitates the induction of LAK cells and CTLs Stimulates mast cell proliferation Promotes proliferation of hairy-cell leukemia and chronic lymphocytic leukemia cells
IL-16	15q26.1	Requires CD4 for biologic activities Tetraspanin CD9	Chemoattractant for CD4$^+$ cells (T cells, monocytes, and eosinophils) May be involved in asthma and in granulomatous inflammation Has antiviral effects on HIV-1

(continued overleaf)

Table 2 *(Continued)*

	Chromosomal location	Receptors	Selected biologic activities
IL-17	2q31	IL-17 receptor	May mediate, in part, T-cell contribution to inflammation
			Stimulates epithelial, endothelial, fibroblastic, and macrophage cells to express a variety of inflammatory cytokines
			Promotes the capacity of fibroblasts to sustain hematopoietic progenitor growth
			Promotes differentiation of dendritic cell progenitors
			May be involved in the pathogenesis of rheumatoid arthritis and graft rejection
IL-18	11q22.2–q22.3	IL-18 receptor	Promotes production of IFN-γ and TNF
			Targets are T cells, NK cells, and macrophages
			Promotes Th1 responses to virus
IL-19	1q32	IL-20RI and IL-20R2	Induces IL-6 and TNF-α
IL-20	1q32	IL-20R1 and IL-20R2	Induction of genes involved in inflammation such as TNF-α, MRP14, and MCP-1
IL-21	4q26–27	IL-21 receptor	Mainly regulates T-cell proliferation and differentiation
			Regulates cell-mediated immunity and the clearance of tumors
IL-22	12q14	IL-22R1 and IL-10R2	Upregulates the production of acute-phase reactants
			Induces the production of ROS in resting B cells
IL-23	12q13	IL-12Rb1 and IL-23R	A unique function of IL-23 is the preferential induction of proliferation of the memory subset of T cells
IL-24	1q32	IL-20R1 and IL-20R2	Induces IL-6, TNF-a, IL-1b, IL-12, and GM-CSF
		IL-22R1 and IL-20R2	Functionally it has opposite effects with IL-10
			Infection with Ad-IL24 results in downregulation of Bcl-2 and Bcl-XL (antiapoptotic proteins) and upregulation of Bax and Bak (proapoptotic proteins) in cancer cells
IL-25	14q11	IL-17BR	IL-25 induces IL-4, IL-5, and IL-13 gene expression and protein production
IL-26	12q14	IL-20R1 and IL-10R2	Immune-protective role against viral infection
IL-27	12q13	TCCR/WSX-1 and GP130	Early Th1 initiation
			Synergizes with IL-12 in inducing IFN-γ production by T cells and NK cells
IL-28A, 28B, and 29	19q13	IL-28R1 and IL-10R2	Antiviral activities
IL-31	12q24	IL-31 receptor A and oncostatin M receptor	Responsible for promoting the dermatitis and epithelial responses that characterize allergic and nonallergic diseases
IL-32	16p13.3	Proteinase 3	Induces other proinflammatory cytokines and chemokines such as TNF-α, IL-1β, IL-6, and IL-8
			Induces IκB degradation
			Phosphorylates p38 MAPK signaling pathway
IL-33	9p24.1	ST2	Activates NF-κB and MAP kinases
			Drives production of Th2-associated cytokines from in vitro polarized Th2 cells
			Induces the expression of IL-4, IL-5, and IL-13
			Leads to severe pathologic changes in mucosal organs
IL-35	19p13.3	IL-12Rβ2 and gp130	Contributes Treg suppressor activity
			Induces IL-10 and IFN-g serum levels
			Reduces induction of IL-17
IL-36	IL36A;2q12-q14.1	IL-1Rrp2 and IL-1RAcP	Activates NF-κB and MAP kinases
	IL36B;2q14		Plays important role in skin biology
	IL36G:2q12-q21		Involved in the initiation and regulation of immune responses
	IL36RN:2q14		
IL-37	2q12-q14.1	IL-18R	Regulates inflammatory responses
IL-38	2q13	IL36R	Reduces IL-36g-induced IL-8 production

IL-2 in the clinic

IL-2 has had a profound impact on the development of cancer immunotherapy. The administration of IL-2 and the adoptive transfer of antitumor T cells grown in IL-2 represented the first effective immunotherapies for cancer in humans.[17] Since 1992, numerous clinical trials using high-dose IL-2 (HD IL-2) have delivered a remarkably consistent 7% complete response rate in two advanced cancer types, renal cell carcinoma (RCC) and malignant melanoma.[18–22] Many of these complete responses have been durable beyond 10 years. HD IL-2 likely enhances the immune response against cancer cells. Its anticancer activity is strongly related to its ability to act as a growth factor for T lymphocytes, its capacity to stimulate antigen-independent NK cells and LAK cells, and its ability to increase lymphocytes at the site of malignancy. The significant adverse effects of HD IL-2 are largely a result of severe vasodilation and capillary leak syndrome, and include hypotension, arrhythmias, and liver and renal toxicities. Its administration requires an inpatient intensive care-like setting, thus it is recommended in patients with few comorbidities and an excellent performance status. There is a 1–2% risk of mortality with

IL-2, which highlights the importance of choosing a well-suited patient for this treatment modality.[23]

Historically, HD IL-2 was first used in a combinational biochemotherapy (BCT) setting, usually involving cisplatin, vinblastine, and dacarbazine (CVD) or cisplatin, vinblastine, and temozolomide (CVT), plus the biologic agents IFN α and IL-2. However, a modest increase in survival came with a substantial increase in toxicity.[24] More recently, as drugs such as ipilimumab demonstrate durable responses, the role of HD IL-2 as a single agent is becoming more controversial. One rational approach is to combine the two approved immunotherapies for stage IV melanoma, ipilimumab and IL-2. No data are currently available regarding the correct sequencing of immunotherapies. Some melanoma experts believe that IL-2 is best used very early on in therapy when subjects have more limited disease (M1a disease) and good performance status. A small study has indicated that there may be a higher response rate (47%) in patients with NRAS-mutant melanoma, but further validation of this finding is needed.[25] A 2005 study in 36 patients with advanced melanoma who received a combination of ipilimumab (0.1–3 mg/kg every 3 weeks) and IL-2 demonstrated an overall response rate of 22%.[26] Studies evaluating the role of ipilimumab with adoptive cell therapy are ongoing. Another approach to extend or enhance the efficacy of HD IL-2 or ipilimumab therapy is to combine immunotherapy with BRAF inhibitors for treatment of patients with BRAFV600-mutant advanced melanoma.[27] Preclinical studies showed an increase in melanoma antigen expression and the number of tumor-infiltrating lymphocytes in tumor biopsies after BRAF inhibitor therapy, which correlated with a reduction in tumor size and an increase in necrosis.[28,29] Current efforts are examining tumor biopsies from patients receiving vemurafenib to assess the mechanisms and kinetics of T-cell accumulation within tumors and characterize the specificity and function of immune infiltrating cells to design more successful combination treatments of BRAF inhibitor and immunotherapy regimens.

Interleukin-3

IL-3 was first described as a T-cell product involved in the pathogenesis of Moloney leukemia virus-induced T-cell lymphomas.[30] This molecule is of interest because of its ability to stimulate multilineage hematopoietic progenitors both *in vitro* and *in vivo*.[30-37]

Biologic properties of IL-3

In vitro, IL-3, in combination with other cytokines, such as stem cell factor (SCF), IL-6, IL-1, GM-CSF, GM-CSF, erythropoietin (EPO), or thrombopoietin (TPO), induces the proliferation of colony-forming unit (CFU)-GM, CFU-Eo, CFU-Baso, BFU-E, and CFU-GEMM in semisolid medium and stimulates the proliferation of purified CD34+ cells in suspension culture.[31] Indeed, IL-3 is combined with other cytokines, in particular SCF, IL-6, IL-1, FL, G-CSF (granulocyte colony-stimulating factor), and/or EPO, in almost all protocols to expand hematopoietic stem and progenitor cells *in vitro*.

IL-3 in the clinic

IL-3 has been used in a variety of clinical trials; peripheral blood stem cell mobilization, postchemotherapy and transplantation, and bone marrow failure states. The majority of studies show only modest effects of IL-3 by itself but significant salutary effects in conjunction with other growth factors. For instance, in mobilization studies, treatment with IL-3 did not mobilize by itself but significantly potentiated G-CSF-induced yield of all progenitor cell types used to restore hematopoiesis after high-dose chemotherapy. After transplantation, the combination of IL-3 and GM-CSF proved more efficient to support bone marrow engraftment than IL-3 or GM-CSF alone. The combination of IL-3 and GM-CSF was more efficient than G-CSF for supporting platelet recovery but was of similar benefit for the reconstitution of myelopoiesis. Following chemotherapy, IL-3 was found to attenuate neutropenia and/or thrombocytopenia in some but not all clinical studies.

Interleukin-4 and interleukin-13

IL-4 and IL-13 are closely related.[38-40] They share biologic and immunoregulatory functions on B cells, monocytes, dendritic cells, and fibroblasts. Both IL-4 and IL-13 genes are located in the same vicinity on chromosome 5. The major regulatory sequences in the IL-4 and IL-13 promoters are identical, thus explaining their restricted expression pattern in activated T cells and mast cells. Furthermore, the IL-4 and IL-13 receptors are multimeric and share at least one common chain—IL-4RA. This, together with similarities in IL-4 and IL-13 signal transduction, explains the striking overlap of biologic properties between these two cytokines. The inability of IL-13 to regulate T-cell differentiation due to a lack of IL-13 receptors on T lymphocytes, however, represents a major difference between these cytokines. Therefore, despite the impact redundancy of these two molecules, regulatory mechanisms are in place to guarantee their distinct functions.

Biologic activities of IL-4 and IL-13

IL-13 elicits many, but not all, of the biologic actions of IL-4. IL-4 is, however, distinguished from IL-13 by its T-cell growth factor activity and its ability to drive differentiation of Th0 precursors toward the Th2 lineage. Th2 cells secrete IL-4 and IL-5 and lead to a preferential stimulation of humoral immunity. In contrast, Th1 cells, which produce IL-2 and IFN-γ, lead to a preferential stimulation of cellular immunity.

IL-4 and IL-13 possess potent antitumor activity *in vivo* in mice.[41] They can inhibit the proliferation of some human cancer cell lines *in vitro* and *in vivo* in nude mice. A similar antiproliferative effect of IL-13 on human breast cancer cells has been described. Moreover, a chimeric protein composed of IL-13 and a truncated form of *Pseudomonas* exotoxin A exhibits specific cytotoxic activity toward human RCC but not against normal hemopoietic cells.[42]

Clinical trials of IL-4

Despite the preclinical promise of IL-4, to date, clinical trials in humans demonstrated that although the molecule is safe and nontoxic, only sporadic antitumor activity is observed in a variety of cancers, including melanoma, lung cancer, and AIDS-related Kaposi's sarcoma.[43-45]

Interleukin-6

IL-6 was first cloned in 1986.[46] It is a typical cytokine, exhibiting functional pleiotropy and redundancy. IL-6 is involved in the immune response, inflammation, and hematopoiesis. IL-6 is a 21- to 30-kDa glycoprotein of 212 amino acids that binds to a specific receptor that requires the same 130-kDa membrane glycoprotein for mediation of signal transduction, as has been described for several cytokines, including IL-2.[47,48]

Biologic activities of IL-6

IL-6 affects the hypothalamic-pituitary axis, bone resorption, and both the humoral and cellular arms of the immune system[49-53] and is a potent and essential factor for the normal development and function of both B and T lymphocytes.[54] IL-6 is also involved in the differentiation of myeloid leukemic cell lines into macrophages, megakaryocyte maturation, neural differentiation, and osteoclast development. As a major inducer of acute-phase protein synthesis in hepatocytes,[55] this cytokine may play a role in the pathogenesis of sepsis.

IL-6 acts as a growth factor for myeloma/plasmacytoma, keratinocytes, mesangial cells, RCC, and Kaposi sarcoma and promotes the growth of hematopoietic stem cells. On the other hand, IL-6 inhibits the growth of myeloid leukemic cell lines and certain carcinoma cell lines. Significant correlations between serum IL-6 activity and serum levels of acute-phase proteins have been demonstrated in a variety of inflammatory conditions. IL-6 has been implicated as a mediator of B symptoms in lymphoma.[56] Elevated serum IL-6 levels have also been associated with an adverse prognosis in both Hodgkin lymphoma and non-Hodgkin lymphoma (NHL).[57-60] In diffuse large-cell lymphoma, IL-6 levels were found to be the single most important independent prognostic factor selected in multivariate analysis for predicting complete remission rate and relapse-free survival.[58] IL-6 levels may also be exploitable as a prognostic factor in RCC and multiple myeloma (MM), and high levels are observed in prostate and ovarian cancers. IL-6 probably also plays an etiologic role in the systemic manifestations of the lymphoproliferative disorder Castleman's disease.[61] High IL-6 levels are also an adverse prognostic factor in pancreatic cancer.[62]

IL-6 in the clinic

In patients undergoing chemotherapy or autologous transplantation, IL-6 has minimal to no platelet-enhancing activity at tolerable doses. Toxicity includes fever and anemia.[63–65] IL-6 has also been tested as an antitumor agent in melanoma and RCC. Response rates have been low (<15%).[55] Because high levels of IL-6 correlate with an adverse outcome in many cancers and function as an autocrine/paracrine growth factor in some tumors, clinical studies of an IL-6 inhibitor may be worthwhile.

IL-6 is one of the most ubiquitously deregulated cytokines in cancer, and increased levels of IL-6 have been observed in virtually every tumor studied. Preclinical and translational findings support a role for IL-6 in diverse malignancies, including breast, lung, colorectal, ovarian, prostate, pancreatic cancers, MM, glioma, melanoma, RCC, leukemia, lymphoma, and Castleman's disease, and provide a biologic rationale for targeted therapeutic investigations. Various compounds antagonize IL-6 production, including corticosteroids, nonsteroidal anti-inflammatory agents, estrogens, and cytokines. Targeted biologic therapies include IL-6 conjugated toxins and monoclonal antibodies directed against IL-6 and its receptor. As an example, a chimeric murine antihuman IL-6 antibody, CNTO 328, has been used in a phase 1 trial in subjects with B-cell NHL, MM, and Castleman's disease.[66] The treatment resulted in tumor response and disease control, especially in Castleman's disease, where striking responses have been seen.[67]

Interleukin-7

IL-7 was identified and cloned on the basis of its ability to induce proliferation of B-cell progenitors in the absence of stromal cells.[68–76] It is now known that this cytokine is secreted by stromal cells in the bone marrow and thymus and is irreplaceable in the development of both B and T cells.[69–71] Indeed, the nonredundant nature of IL-7 is underscored by the observation that ablation of IL-7 or parts of the IL-7 receptor in gene knockout mice ineluctably leads to a major defect in lymphocyte development.

Biologic activities of IL-7/IL-7 receptor

While most single cytokine knockout mice show relatively normal B- and T-cell compartments, indicating that many cytokine functions are redundant, IL-7-deficient mice present with striking lymphocyte depletion in both the thymus and bone marrow. Collectively, these genetic experiments identify clearly distinct *in vivo* roles for various lymphoid factors. IL-2 and IL-4 function by influencing mature lymphocyte populations during immune responses, whereas IL-7 plays a singularly dominant role for the production and expansion of lymphocytes. The upregulation of IL-7R occurs at the stage of the clonogenic common lymphoid progenitor that can give rise to all lymphoid lineages at a single-cell level.[74] There are at least three principal means by which IL-7R-mediated signals act in lymphocyte development: enhancement of proliferation, triggering of lineage-specific developmental programs, and maintenance of viability of appropriately selected cells.

High IL-7 levels are found in states of T-cell depletion and may, therefore, play a role in promoting T-cell expansion.[75] High levels of IL-7 are also found in CLL and Burkitt lymphoma, and transgenic mice overexpressing the IL-7 gene show dramatic changes in lymphocyte development, which, in some instances, can result in the formation of lymphoid tumors.[76]

Interleukin-8

IL-8 was first identified in 1987 as a potent, proinflammatory chemokine that induces trafficking of neutrophils across the vascular wall (chemotaxis).[77] This molecule belongs to a chemokine superfamily whose members include neutrophil-activating peptide-2, platelet factor-4, growth-related cytokine (GRO), and IFN-inducible protein-10, all of which are responsible for the directional migration of various cells.[78] IL-8 receptor demonstrates strong homology to a gene encoded by human herpesvirus-8 (HHV-8).[79,80]

Biologic activity of IL-8

The chemotactic agents generated by inflammatory stimuli recruit circulating leukocytes, in particular neutrophils, for defensive purposes and direct them to injury sites. Among the neutrophil-affecting chemokines, IL-8 is one of the most potent.[81] On exposure to a chemokine, neutrophils are activated, and within seconds, their shapes change. The process of shape change is crucial. It is modulated by perturbations of cellular integrins and the actin cytoskeleton. The activation and upregulation of integrins also permits the adherence of neutrophils to the endothelial cells of the vessel wall, to allow for subsequent migration into the tissues. Leukocytes follow the IL-8 concentration gradient and accumulate at the location of elevated concentration. These processes play a fundamental role in the host defense as activated leukocytes act to kill and engulf invading bacteria at the site of injury.

IL-8 can induce tumor growth, an effect attributed to its angiogenic activity. On the one hand, the administration of anti-IL-8 to SCID mice bearing xenografts of IL-8-expressing human lung cancer has been shown to have beneficial effects.[82] On the other hand, antitumor effects of IL-8 have also been reported. Of interest in this regard is the fact that increased levels of IL-8 have been discerned in lung carcinomas and in melanomas. IL-8 may be a growth factor for pancreatic cancer and for melanoma.[78] In melanomas, IL-8 levels correlate with the growth and metastatic potential of the tumor cells, and exposure of the cells to IFN (an agent with known antitumor activity in melanoma) decreases IL-8 levels and cancer cell proliferation.[83] Blocking IL-8 or IL-8R has been suggested as a therapeutic strategy.[78]

Interleukin-9

Human IL-9 was initially identified and cloned as a mitogenic factor for a human megakaryoblastic leukemia. Subsequently, IL-9 targets were found to encompass a wide range of cells.[84,85]

Biologic activities of IL-9

Cellular elements responsive to IL-9 include erythroid progenitors, human T cells, B cells, fetal thymocytes, thymic lymphomas, and immature neuronal cell lines.[84]

IL-9 can support the clonogenic maturation of erythroid progenitors in the presence of EPO. In contrast, granulocyte or macrophage colony formation (CFU-GM, CFU-G, or CFU-M) is usually not influenced by IL-9. IL-9 is more effective on fetal than adult progenitors and in cells that are activated. In addition to its proliferative activity, IL-9 also seems to be a potent regulator of mast cell effector molecules.

There is an interesting paradox between the unresponsiveness of normal T cells to IL-9 and the potent activity of this molecule on lymphoma cells. This contrast is illustrated by the observation that murine T cells acquire the ability to respond to IL-9 after a long period of *in vitro* culture, while they simultaneously acquire characteristics of tumor cell lines. Observations made with transgenic mice also demonstrate the oncogenic potential of dysregulated IL-9 production as 5–10% of mice that overexpress this cytokine develop lymphoblastic lymphomas.[85] In line with these data, constitutive IL-9 production by human Hodgkin lymphomas and large-cell anaplastic lymphomas has now been clearly documented.[84] Even so, the pathophysiologic role of IL-9 remains elusive.

Interleukin-10

IL-10 is a pleiotropic cytokine discovered in 1989 as an activity produced by murine type 2 helper T cells (Th2).[86,87] It was initially designated as cytokine synthesis inhibitory factor because of its ability to inhibit the production of certain cytokines.[88] Of interest, IL-10 exhibits strong DNA and amino acid sequence homology to an open reading frame—BCRF1—in the Epstein–Barr virus (EBV) genome.[88] Indeed, the BCRF1 protein product displays many of the biologic properties of cellular IL-10 and has, therefore, been termed viral IL-10.

Biologic activities of IL-10

IL-10 inhibits the synthesis of Th1-derived cytokines, including IL-2, IFN-γ, GM-CSF, and lymphotoxin and of monocyte-derived IL-1α and β, IL-6, IL-8, TNF-α, GM-CSF, and G-CSF. Exogenous IL-10 can also suppress expression of IL-10.[87] At the same time, IL-10 induces the synthesis of the IL-1 receptor antagonist by macrophages. IL-10 also suppresses the CD28 costimulatory pathway and hence acts as a decisive mechanism in determining if a T cell will contribute to an immune response or become anergic.

From the molecular standpoint, IL-10 suppresses cytokine expression at a transcriptional and posttranscriptional level.[89] Both these mechanisms appear to require new protein synthesis. At a cellular level, Th1 cytokines synthesis inhibition is mediated indirectly through the effect of IL-10 on APC, as suppression occurs when macrophages, but not B cells, are used as APC.[90]

In the presence of monocytes/macrophages, IL-10 inhibits proliferation of resting T cells, including Th0, Th1, and Th2 CD4+ T-cell clones. This inhibition can only be partially reversed by high concentrations of IL-2, suggesting that the reduced proliferation is only partially a reflection of reduced IL-2 production. IL-10 can also enhance the cytotoxic activity of CD8+ T cells. All these effects support an important role of IL-10 in regulating inflammatory responses. In contrast to the inhibitory effects on other lineages, IL-10 has a stimulatory effect on B cells and mast cells.[91] For instance, IL-10 strongly stimulates proliferation and differentiation of activated B cells.

The role of IL-10 in cancer should be considered within the frame of a highly complex biological puzzle. It is known that IL-10 can have pleiotropic effects on adaptive and innate immunity cell mediators. Although several studies show that IL-10 can actively mediate immune suppression, some experimental models describe relatively opposite conclusions. Recent data on the relationship between IL-10 and anticancer immunity support an effective immune attack against malignant cells, which challenges the common belief that IL-10 acts as an immunosuppressive factor promoting tumor immune escape.

Interleukin-11

Originally characterized as a thrombopoietic factor, IL-11 is now known to be expressed and have activity in a multitude of other systems, including the gut, testes, and the central nervous system.[92,93] Clinically, this cytokine has been approved by the FDA for amelioration of chemotherapy-induced thrombocytopenia.

Biologic activities of IL-11

IL-11 was originally isolated from cells derived from the hematopoietic microenvironment and may act as a paracrine or autocrine growth factor in this environment. IL-11 acts synergistically with other early- and late-acting growth factors, including IL-3, IL-4, IL-7, IL-12, IL-13, SCF, FLT-3 ligand, and GM-CSF, to stimulate various stages and lineages of hematopoiesis.[92] The synergistic effects of IL-11 and TPO on multilineage cells may be mediated in part by SCF/c-kit interactions.

IL-11 acts synergistically with IL-3, TPO, or SCF to stimulate various stages of megakaryocytopoiesis and thrombopoiesis.[94,95] IL-11, alone or in combination with other cytokines (IL-3, SCF, or EPO), can stimulate multiple stages of erythropoiesis. IL-11 also modulates the differentiation and maturation of myeloid progenitor cells. IL-11 in combination with SCF stimulates myeloid colony formation. The combination of IL-11 with IL-13 or IL-14 can reduce the proportion of granulocytes and blasts in myeloid colonies, with a concomitant increase in macrophages. IL-11 in combination with SCF or IL-4 effectively supports the generation of B cells in primary cultures. IL-11 and IL-4 can also reverse the inhibitory effect of IL-3 on early B-lymphocyte development. The promotion of B-cell differentiation may be mediated by T cells.

IL-11 acts as a synergistic factor with IL-3, GM-CSF, and SCF to stimulate proliferation of human primary leukemia cells, myeloid leukemia cell lines, megakaryoblastic cell lines, and erythroleukemic cell lines and to stimulate leukemic blast colony formation. IL-11 mRNA expression in leukemic cells and inhibition of leukemic cell growth by IL-11 antisense oligonucleotides suggest that IL-11 may function as an autocrine growth factor in leukemic cell lines.[96] Although IL-11 stimulates the proliferation of murine plasmacytoma cells and murine hybridoma cells, the effect of IL-11 on the growth of human myeloma/plasmacytoma cells is controversial.[92]

Clinical use of IL-11

IL-11 was the second IL to receive FDA approval. It is indicated for the secondary prevention of chemotherapy-induced thrombocytopenia and for the reduction of the need for platelet transfusion in patients with nonmyeloid malignancies.

Interleukin-12

IL-12 was first identified as an NK-cell stimulatory factor.[97] Subsequently, it was demonstrated that IL-12 is crucial to the development of Th1 cells.[98] Indeed, there appears to be a common pathway leading from the innate immune response to adaptive immunity; intracellular pathogens stimulate macrophages to produce IL-12, which then promotes the development of Th1 cells from a naïve cell population. This pathway may be exploitable in the design of novel immunotherapies and vaccines.

Biologic activities of IL-12 and role in human disease

IL-12 is a potent proinflammatory molecule, which is essential for resistance to bacterial, fungal, and parasitic infections. It is produced within a few hours of infection, activates NK cells, and, through its ability to induce IFN-γ production, enhances the phagocytic and bactericidal activities of phagocytic cells and their ability to release proinflammatory cytokines, including IL-12 itself. IL-12 is also a key immunoregulatory molecule, especially of Th1 responses. It is produced during the early phases of infection and inflammation and sets the stage for the ensuing antigen-specific immune response, favoring the differentiation and function of Th1 T cells, while inhibiting the differentiation of Th2 T cells. IL-12 does not induce proliferation of resting peripheral blood T cells or NK cells; it does potentiate the proliferation of T cells induced by various mitogens and has a direct proliferative effect on preactivated T and NK cells.

IL-12 synergizes with other hematopoietic factors to promote survival and proliferation of early multipotent hematopoietic progenitor cells and lineage-committed precursor cells.[99] Although *in vitro* IL-12 has mostly stimulatory effects on hematopoiesis, *in vivo* IL-12 treatment results in decreased bone marrow hematopoiesis and both transient anemia and neutropenia, an effect mediated by IFN-γ.

IL-12 in the clinic

IL-12 has potential for exploitation in allergy and as an adjuvant for infectious disease therapy.[100] In addition, the ability of IL-12 to revert existing states of tolerance or anergy makes it a candidate for use in the composition of vaccines for infectious agents or tumors. Phase 1 clinical trials have been started in the past few years in oncology, as well as in the setting of HIV infection and chronic hepatitides B and C. To date, administration of IL-12 to patients with chronic hepatitis C does not appear advantageous.[101] What is more worrisome is that in cancer patients treated with high doses of IL-12, acute hematopoietic, hepatic, and gastrointestinal toxicities were observed and several deaths were reported. In long-term treatments, toxicity was mostly pulmonary. It has been suggested that some of the severe toxicity of IL-12 can be attenuated if a single injection is administered 1 to 2 weeks before initiating daily dosing.[102]

Interleukin-15

IL-15 shares biologic activities with IL-2.[103]

Biologic activities of IL-15

Similar to IL-2, IL-15 is able to trigger both proliferation of and immunoglobulin production by normal B lymphocytes. These biologic functions may be acquired, however, only when B cells have been preactivated *in vitro* with polyclonal mitogens or when they are cultured in association with other stimuli. IL-15 also stimulates the proliferation of NK cells and activated CD4+ and CD8+ T cells and facilitates the induction of cytolytic effector cells (such as LAK cells). Finally, the numbers of CD8+ memory T cells are maintained in animals by a balance between the stimulatory effect of IL-15 and the suppressive effects of IL-12.[104]

IL-15 responsiveness distinguishes malignant B cells from normal B lymphocytes. In contrast to normal B lymphocytes, which require preactivation in order to proliferate in response to IL-15, leukemic cells from patients with chronic B-cell malignancies proliferate in response to IL-15 regardless of *in vitro* preactivation, which is mainly related to the presence of the β and γ chains of the IL-2R system on the malignant B lymphocytes.[103] Even so, IL-15 cannot be considered an autocrine factor in these leukemias, as it is not produced by the leukemic cells themselves. Rather, the major reservoir of IL-15 in these patients is from cells belonging to the monocyte/macrophage lineage.[103]

Interleukin-17

Human IL-17 has 72% overall sequence identity at the amino acid level with open reading frame 13 of herpesvirus Saimiri (HVS).[105]

Biologic activities of IL-17

Although limited in number, studies suggest that IL-17 may be a soluble factor by which T cells induce or contribute to inflammation.[106] IL-17 can also stimulate epithelial, endothelial, and fibroblastic cells, and macrophages to express a variety of cytokines,[99] which appear to be cell specific. For instance, fibroblast cells produce IL-1, G-CSF, IFN-γ, IL-6, and IL-8 in response to IL-17, whereas macrophages produce TNF-α, IL-1β, IL-1Rα, IL-6, IL-10, and IL-12.[107]

IL-17 also exhibits indirect hematopoietic activity by enhancing the capacity of fibroblasts to sustain the proliferation of CD34+ hematopoietic progenitors and their differentiation into neutrophils.[108,106] IL-17 can also promote the maturation of dendritic cell progenitors.[109] Because IL-17 acts to differentiate early dendritic cells, it has been implicated in host T-cell allostimulation and graft rejection.[109]

Interleukin-18

IL-18 (IFN-inducing factor) was first described as a serum activity that induced IFN-γ production in mouse spleen cells.[110] IL-18 has a molecular weight of 18–19 kDa and has homology to IL-1.[111,112] Like IL-1β, IL-18 is initially synthesized as an inactive precursor molecule (pro-IL-18) lacking a signal peptide and is cleaved by ICE to yield an active molecule.[113,114]

Biologic activities of IL-18

T lymphocytes, NK cells, and macrophages are primary targets for IL-18. For example, IL-18 directly stimulates production of tumor necrosis factor (TNF) in human blood CD4+ T lymphocytes and NK cells and plays an important role in promoting a long-lasting Th1 lymphocyte response to viral antigens. IL-18 does not appear to be an endogenous pyrogen but may nevertheless contribute to inflammation and fever because it is a potent inducer of TNF, chemokines, and IFN.[115] In the case of IFN-γ induction, IL-18 acts as a costimulant with mitogens or IL-2. Indeed, mice deficient in ICE, the molecule that cleaves pro-IL-18 to its mature form, fail to produce IFN-γ in response to endotoxin.

Interleukin-21

IL-21, a cytokine most closely related to IL-2 and IL-15, is involved in the proliferation and maturation of NK-cell populations from bone marrow, as well as in the proliferation of mature B-cell and T-cell populations.[116] IL-21 has been implicated in the activation of innate immune responses and in the Th1 response. IL-21 also plays a critical role in regulating immunoglobulin production of B cells.[117]

Interleukin-24

IL-24 was originally named melanoma differentiation-associated gene-7 (*mda-7*) when it was discovered in 1995. It was identified by subtractive hybridization after the treatment of melanoma cells with IFN-β and mezerein, which caused their terminal differentiation and growth arrest.[118] In 2001, it was discovered that *mda-7* encodes a secreted protein that exhibits significant homology to IL-10. This molecule was officially designated as IL-24.[119] Human IL-24 is secreted by activated peripheral blood mononuclear cells and is the ligand for two heterodimeric receptors, IL-22R1/IL-20R2 and IL-20R1/IL-20R2.[120] IL-24 also acts as a tumor-suppressor gene and the protein product was found to be constitutively expressed by melanocytes, nevus cells, and some primary melanomas but not metastatic lesions of melanoma.[121,122] This is possibly the first example of a tumor-suppressor gene exhibiting immune stimulatory properties.[123]

Biologic activities of IL-24
IL-24 has a number of interesting and unique properties, including direct cancer-killing activity, potent bystander antitumor activity, immune-modulating activity, and antiangiogenic properties. As an antitumor agent, *mda-7/IL-24* is truly unique, displaying selective antitumor activity in cancer cells and having the capacity to utilize diverse signaling pathways in mediating tumor cell death.

IL-24 in the clinic
On the basis of its remarkable attributes and effective antitumor therapy in animal models, this cytokine has taken the important step of entering the clinic. In a phase 1 clinical trial, intratumoral injection of adenovirus-administered *mda-7/IL-24* (INGN 241) was safe, elicited tumor-regulatory and immune-activating processes and provided clinically significant activity.[124,125]

Interleukin-26
Subtraction hybridization coupled with representational differential analysis identified IL-26/AK155 as a gene upregulated in human T cells following infection with vesicular stomatitis virus (VSV), human cytomegalovirus (HCMV), and herpes simplex virus type 1 (HSV-1).[126] It has the capacity to transform these cells in culture. The IL-26 protein has 24.7% amino acid identity and 47% amino acid similarity with human IL-10. Structural analysis revealed that IL-26 contains six helices with four highly conserved cysteine residues, which are assumed to be relevant for dimer formation as is the case with IL-10. It was determined that IL-26 mRNA is specifically overexpressed by T cells after HVS transformation.

Interleukin-27
In 2002, Pflanz et al.[127] described a new heterodimeric cytokine, related to IL-12. This cytokine was designated IL-27. It acts together with IL-12 to trigger IFN-γ production by naïve CD4+ T cells. They also identified IL-27 as the ligand for TCCR/WSX-1, a novel member of the class I cytokine receptor family shown to be important for Th1 development.[128] Studies revealed that IL-27 has the ability to induce tumor-specific antitumor activity and protective immunity and that the antitumor activity is mediated mainly through CD8+ T cells, and IFN-γ.[129]

Interleukin-28 and interleukin-29
The IL-28 family has been identified from the human genomic sequence, designated IL-28A, IL-28B, and IL-29. These molecules were originally described as distantly related to type I IFNs and the IL-10 family. IL-28 and IL-29 are induced by viral infection and show antiviral activity. Moreover, IL-28 and IL-29 interact with a heterodimeric class II cytokine receptor that consists of IL-10Rβ and an orphan class II receptor chain, designated IL-28Rα. Now, they are subclassified as type III IFNs and seem to be promising candidates for the development of alternatives to type I IFNs, as suggested by their potent antiviral and antitumor properties. Given the fact that IL-28/29 primarily influence epithelial cells, melanocytes and tumor cells derived thereof, as well as hepatocytes, there are several potential therapeutic fields in which these cytokines could be applied, including as antitumor therapy for carcinoma and melanoma.[130]

Interleukin-31
IL-31 has been identified as a four-helix bundle cytokine that is preferentially produced by T helper type 2 cells. IL-31 signals through a receptor composed of IL-31 receptor A and oncostatin M receptor. Expression of IL-31 receptor A and oncostatin M receptor mRNA is induced in activated monocytes, whereas epithelial cells expressed both mRNAs constitutively. More specifically, the data indicate that IL-31 may be involved in promoting the dermatitis and epithelial responses that characterize allergic and nonallergic diseases.[131]

Interleukin-35
IL-35 represents a new member of the heterodimeric IL-12 cytokine family. IL-35 is a novel inhibitory cytokine that is produced by Treg cells and contributes to their suppressive activity. Moreover, ectopic expression of IL-35 confers regulatory activity on naive T cells, whereas recombinant IL-35 suppresses T-cell proliferation. Because IL-35 may be secreted exclusively by Treg cells and other cell populations with regulatory potential, it represents a novel potential target for the therapeutic manipulation of Treg activity to treat cancer and autoimmune diseases.[132]

Interleukin-37
Since the discovery of IL-1 in 1977, the IL-1 family of cytokines list is continually evolving.[133] IL-37 was originally defined as IL-1 family member 7 (IL-1F7) and transcripts are detected in lymph nodes, thymus, bone marrow, lung, testis, uterus, and placenta.[134] TGF-β and several Toll-like receptor (TLR) ligands induce production of high levels of IL-37 by PBMCs; proinflammatory cytokines such as IL-18, IFN-γ, IL-1β, and TNF moderately increase IL-37 levels.[135] In addition, expression of IL-37 in monocytic cells has been shown to reduce several intracellular kinases important for transducing proinflammatory signals, such as focal adhesion kinase (FAK), STAT1, p38 MAPK, and c-jun. Therefore, IL-37 is considered one of the many key modulators of inflammation.

Interferons
The IFNs are a large family of multifunctional secreted proteins involved in antiviral defense, cell growth regulation, and immune activation. There are three types of IFNs; types I (IFNα, β), II (IFNγ), and III (IFNλ). Each IFN type has sequence similarity, signals via specific cell-surface receptor complexes (Table 3), and mediates its effect by activating multiple signaling pathways, including the JAK-STAT pathway, among others. JAK-STAT signaling events lead to the activation of transcription factor complexes and homo- or heterodimerized STAT molecules, and their subsequent binding to IFN-stimulated response element (ISRE), γ-activated sequence (GAS), and STAT-binding sites in promoters of IFN-regulated genes (IRG), resulting in the transcriptional activation of those IRGs.[136]

The genes that encode type I, II, and III IFNs are clustered on chromosomes 9, 12, and 19, respectively, in humans. Cellular action follows binding to a relatively small number of high-affinity receptors. Regulatory proteins then transcriptionally regulate gene expression resulting in production of proteins that are not expressed constitutively or only at low levels. The products of these IFN-stimulated genes (ISGs) underlie the pleiotropic biologic effects: virus inhibition, immunomodulation, inhibition of cell

Table 3 Interferons (IFN).

Type		Stimuli	Receptors	Signaling molecules
Type I IFNs	IFN α IFN β	• Viruses • Other microorganisms	IFNAR: IFNAR1–IFNAR2	• JAK1 and TYK2 • STAT1–STAT2–IRF9 complexes • STAT1–STAT1 complexes
Type II IFN	IFN γ	• Antigen–MHC complexes • Activating NK-cell ligands • IL-12 plus IL-18 • TLRs	IFNGR: IFNGR1–IFNGR2	• JAK1 and JAK2 • STAT1–STAT1 complexes
Type III IFN	IFN λ	• Viruses • Other microorganisms	IL10R2 and IFNLR1	• JAK1 and TYK2 • STAT1–STAT2–IRF9 complexes • STAT2–STAT2 complexes

proliferation, alterations in differentiation, increased apoptosis, and angiogenesis inhibition. However, which of the specific ISG products result in the various biologic and therapeutic effects remains undefined, as do the specific cellular mechanism(s) of antitumor action. Antitumor effects result from either a direct effect on viability and proliferation or antigenic expression of tumor cells, or an effect on modulation of immune effector or endothelial cell populations. IFNs regulate gene expression, modulate expression of proteins on the cell surface, and induce synthesis of new enzymes. Alterations in gene expression result in modulation of receptors for other cytokines, concentration of regulatory proteins on the surface of immune effector cells, and activities of enzymes that control cellular growth and function. On a cellular basis, these effects translate into alterations of the state of differentiation, rate of proliferation and death, and functional activity of many cell types. Induced proteins and their products can be identified on cells and in serum of treated patients. Their measurement or the quantitation of immune effector cell function can be used to define biologically active molecules, doses, schedules, and routes of administration.

Antitumor effects in humans

Both natural and recombinant IFNs have shown definite antitumor activity in patients with various malignancies. Clinically beneficial therapeutic activity of IFN-α2 as a single agent has been demonstrated in more than a dozen malignancies. The unique molecular and cellular effects of IFNs also complement the mechanisms of actions of other therapies. Most gene and biologic response modulatory effects peak at 24–48 h, which contrasts with maximal serum levels of minutes to hours after intravenous or subcutaneous administration.[137–139] After intravenous bolus administration, the $t^1/_2\alpha$ of IFN-α2 is short (<60 min); mean terminal half-life is 4–5 h with no serum levels measurable at 12 h. After intramuscular or subcutaneous administration, peak levels are 3–8 h.[137] The pharmacologic hallmark of IFN-β is virtual absence of serum levels with subcutaneous or intramuscular administration; yet, biologic response modulatory and therapeutic effects occur.[139] Pegylated IFNs have markedly different kinetics than do unmodified IFNs.[140–142] Once-weekly administration has resulted in measurable serum levels of IFN-α2 at 7 days—in excess of that required for gene induction and cellular effects *in vitro*. Pegylated IFN-α2 has resulted in tumor responses in metastatic renal carcinoma, CML, and melanoma.[142,143]

Hematologic malignancies

In CML, IFN-α2 resulted in sustained therapeutic response in a majority (>75%) of newly diagnosed patients in early clinical studies.[144,145] Complete cytogenetic remissions were noted in a

minority of patients and the rate was higher in younger patients. However, owing to the considerable side effects from IFN, many clinicians chose to stop therapy if cytogenetic improvement was not seen after approximately 1 year of treatment. Before the development of the tyrosine kinase inhibitors (TKIs), IFNs were the treatment of choice for most patients with CML. With the development of imatinib mesylate and the increased toxicity of IFN compared with TKIs, it has been used much less commonly for the treatment of CML. More recently, combinational therapies, such as IFN plus imatinib, have produced long-term remissions in patients with CML in clinical trials and have become the standard therapy for patients with newly diagnosed CML in chronic phase. The French SPIRIT trial demonstrated higher rates of molecular response using the combination of imatinib and peg-IFN compared with IFN alone,[146] but another study failed to demonstrate an improvement in progression-free survival.[147] Therefore, additional clinical data are necessary before this combination can be recommended.

IFN-γ has been used as therapy in CML and demonstrated varying degrees of cytogenetic improvement[148] but failed to show any effect in subsequent studies and hence, it is not recommended for treatment of CML.

Solid tumors

Response rates for metastatic melanoma in patients who received IFN-α2 as a single agent have approximated 15%, comparable to cytotoxic agents used alone.[149–152] Suggestions of response durability set IFN apart from DTIC as a therapy for metastatic melanoma. When combined with chemotherapy and IL-2, response rates can exceed 45% but with increased toxicity and with no marked prolongation in progression-free survival or overall survival.[24,152–156] Increase in disease-free survival with an impact on overall survival has, however, emerged in some trials from the use of IFN-α2 as an adjuvant to surgery for melanoma for patients at high risk for disease recurrence (stage IIb or stage III).[143,157–160] Analysis of quality-of-life adjusted survival in the adjuvant setting has also identified an advantage for the use of IFN-α2.[161] Thus, IFN-α2 has become a standard of care for patients with stage IIb or stage III melanoma in the United States, a use supported by meta-analyses.[161,162] A large European trial that used pegylated IFN-α2 for longer duration has confirmed benefit on disease-free survival in high-risk primary patients.[163] Pegylation has resulted in responses in metastatic melanoma leading to an innovative trial design of long-duration treatment with dose adjusted for fatigue and anorexia with confirmed increase in disease-free survival.[143,160,164]

IFN has been extensively used in the treatment of RCC. Response rates from 4% to 26% have been reported in trials of IFN-α2 in metastatic RCC, with a mean response of 15% in a cumulative summary of several trials.[165] Subsequent efforts have been made to evaluate IFN together with other biological response modifiers including IL-2 or in combination with chemotherapeutic agents, in particular 5-fluorouracil (5-FU). The combination of IFN-α and IL-2 has been extensively investigated in patients with metastatic RCC. Phase I and II trials have demonstrated response rates of approximately 20%, with 5% CR.[166] In two randomized trials comparing IFN-α alone or in combination with other treatments, a statistically significant increase in survival resulted.[167,168] Other randomized trials have suggested survival prolongations that may be greatest for patients who have nephrectomies despite the presence of metastases and who then receive IFN-α.[169,170] In summary, as numerous studies have failed to show a survival advantage for patients with metastatic RCC receiving combination cytokine therapy, it cannot be recommended as standard treatment. Other solid tumors, such as ovarian, bladder, and basal cell carcinomas, have responded to IFN-α administered regionally, particularly in patients with lesser tumor bulk.[171–173]

The shared gene induction profile of type I and type III IFNs has led to investigations of the potential role of type III IFN in cancer therapy. The hope is that type III IFN will be effective against responsive cancer cells while showing fewer side effects than type I IFN owing to the restricted distribution of the receptor.[174] The favorable side effect profile of type III over type I IFN was recently demonstrated in a phase I study of the effect of type III IFN against HCV. While some of the patients treated with type I IFN developed neutropenia or anemia, patients treated with type III IFN remained symptom free.[175] The data suggest that type III IFN can play a positive role in cancer therapy with few or no side effects, yet it is still in its infancy.

Hematopoiesis and the role of growth factors

Through a series of well-orchestrated divisions, hematopoietic stem cells give rise to all blood cells. Functionally, these early progenitors are capable of self-renewal as well as proliferation and differentiation. The development, homeostasis, trafficking, and response capacity of the hematopoietic system are tightly regulated by a complex communications network that is mediated by intercellular signals. These signals are triggered by direct cell-to-cell or cell-to-matrix contact or by the release of soluble cytokine mediators.

The identification and cloning of hematopoietic growth factors have revolutionized hematology practice. Raising white blood cell counts in neutropenic patients was unimaginable until the advent of G-CSF and GM-CSF. Today, growth factors are routinely used to alleviate neutropenia and, to a lesser extent, thrombocytopenia and anemia after chemotherapy. They can also help mobilize stem cells for transplantation, reverse cytopenias in a variety of nonmalignant illnesses, and may have the potential to mobilize the immune system against infection or cancer.

Erythropoietin

EPO is the major hormone regulator of erythropoiesis. It has an established role in the treatment of anemia associated with a variety of illnesses (Table 4).

Biologic activities of EPO

EPO provides a proliferative signal to early erythroid progenitors [burst-forming unit erythroid (BFU-E)] and a differentiation signal to a later erythroid precursor [colony-forming unit erythroid (CFU-E)]. EPO can also promote megakaryocyte differentiation, B-cell proliferation, and endothelial cell chemotaxis.

EPO in malignancy

High levels of endogenous EPO are often found in patients with anemia due to cancer, especially hematologic malignancies. In contrast, in many patients with anemia, even anemia due to cancer, there is a relative deficiency in endogenous EPO. In other words, although the levels of this molecule are elevated, they are not as high as they should be for the degree of anemia. Certain cases of familial erythrocytosis have been attributed to the presence of EPO-hypersensitive cells. This heightened EPO response results from the formation of a truncated EPO receptor, which is missing a negative regulatory domain.[176]

Table 4 Hematopoietic growth factors.

	Chromosomal location	Receptors	Selected biologic activities
EPO	7q21	EPO receptor	Promotes the proliferation, differentiation, and survival of erythroid precursors
GM-CSF	5q31.1	Type I receptor with α (CD116) and β (CDw131) subunits	Stimulates growth of multilineage progenitors, BFU-E, granulocyte, macrophage, and eosinophil colonies
			Induces migration and proliferation of vascular endothelial cells
			Activates mature phagocytes (neutrophils, macrophages, and eosinophils)
G-CSF	17q11.2-q12	G-CSF receptor (CD114)	Regulates production and function of neutrophils
M-CSF	1p21-p13	Fms (CD115)	Influences most aspects of monocyte/macrophage development and function
			Stimulates hematopoiesis
			Induces osteoclast production
			Helps maintain pregnancies
			Lowers cholesterol levels
			Affects microglial function
SCF	12q22-12q24	c-kit (CD117)	Promotes hematopoiesis at multiple levels
			Influences primordial germ cell and melanocyte migration during embryonic life
			Affects immunoregulatory cells (B and T cells, mast cells, NK cells, and dendritic cells)
			Influences hematopoietic cell adhesive properties
TPO	3q27-q28	Mpl (CD110)	Major regulator of platelet production
			Acts in synergy with EPO to stimulate growth of erythroid progenitors
			Acts in synergy with IL-3 and SCF to stimulate proliferation and prolong survival of hematopoietic stem cells

EPO in the clinic

EPO is most useful in those anemias where there is an absolute or a relative deficiency in endogenous EPO levels. First used successfully as replacement therapy to correct the anemia associated with chronic renal failure, EPO is also effective in increasing hemoglobin in some patients with both solid tumors and hematologic malignancies as well as in those with a variety of other conditions.[177]

EPO has generally been used for patients with significant anemia, i.e., hemoglobin <10 g/dL. The US FDA suggests that EPO should be used conservatively to avoid transfusion but not to normalize hemoglobin levels. In the case of cancer, however, not all patients respond, and those with the highest levels of endogenous EPO are probably less likely to benefit.

Granulocyte macrophage colony-stimulating factor

GM-CSF was the first CSF to enter clinical trials. It has now been approved in many countries for treatment of neutropenia after chemotherapy or transplantation, for treatment of graft failure, and for peripheral blood stem cell mobilization.

Major biologic activities of GM-CSF

GM-CSF stimulates proliferation of multilineage progenitors and the growth of BFU-E, granulocyte, macrophage, and eosinophil colonies. GM-CSF also enhances the functional activity of most phagocytes, including neutrophils, macrophages, and eosinophils.

GM-CSF in malignancy

Autocrine expression of GM-CSF in myeloid leukemia cells and cell lines has been proposed to play a role in neoplasia.[178] Autonomous production of GM-CSF (or G-CSF) by the tumor has also been implicated as one possible pathophysiologic mechanism underlying leukemoid reactions in cancer patients.[179] In addition, the presence of GM-CSF biologic activity in synovial fluid from patients with rheumatoid arthritis suggests that it may enhance the tissue destruction associated with this disorder.

GM-CSF has been shown to be safe and effective in the treatment of patients with acute myelogenous leukemia (AML) who are undergoing induction therapy. This molecule shortens the neutropenic period and decreases the rate of serious infections in older individuals. GM-CSF is also indicated for accelerating myeloid reconstitution after allogeneic BMTs. It also enhances survival in patients who experience engraftment failure or delay after allogeneic or autologous transplantation. Finally, peripheral blood stem cells mobilized in the presence of GM-CSF yield significantly higher colony counts than those mobilized without this molecule and, after transplantation, recipients of GM-CSF-mobilized progenitors have quicker neutrophil, platelet, and red blood cell recovery and shorter hospital stays.

Granulocyte colony-stimulating factor

G-CSF has revolutionized the treatment of neutropenia and its sequelae (infection). It has been used worldwide and has been found to be remarkably effective and virtually devoid of side effects.[180,181]

Biologic activities of G-CSF

G-CSF is a relatively specific stimulator of the growth and differentiation of hematopoietic progenitor cells committed to the neutrophil lineage. It also protects neutrophils from apoptosis and enhances their function. Finally, G-CSF moves mature neutrophils from the marrow into the circulation.

G-CSF in human disease

In healthy persons, mean ± SD G-CSF levels are 25 ± 19.7 pg/mL. G-CSF levels increase by 30-fold in infection and by 10,000-fold in septic shock.[182] Some patients with solid tumors present with significantly increased leukocyte counts. In several of these individuals, elevated serum levels of G-CSF (or GM-CSF) have been demonstrated and probably account for the rise in white blood cell count.[179] Presumably, G-CSF (or GM-CSF) is produced by the tumor itself.

Point mutations in the gene for the G-CSF receptor have been described in patients with AML, which evolved from severe congenital neutropenia. These mutations truncate the C-terminal cytoplasmic region of the G-CSF receptor and hence are presumed to disrupt the maturation signal of the receptor.[183]

Studies of G-CSF as an adjunct to standard-dose cytotoxic chemotherapy for solid tumors and lymphomas demonstrate that the duration of neutropenia, the number of days of hospitalization, and the number of days of antibiotic treatment are reduced significantly during G-CSF cycles. Placebo-controlled studies in patients with small-cell lung cancer showed a clinically significant protective effect of G-CSF against febrile neutropenia.[184] After high-dose chemotherapy, recovery from neutropenia and its associated complications is more rapid when patients receive G-CSF. These studies suggest that the dose intensity of nonmyeloablative chemotherapy can be increased with G-CSF support. In the transplantation setting, the administration of G-CSF results in reductions in neutropenia and infection.[185] G-CSF also mobilizes autologous peripheral blood progenitor cells; these cells are used to accelerate hematopoietic recovery in patients who have received myeloablative or myelosuppressive chemotherapy.[186]

A new form of G-CSF has been developed; a conjugate of G-CSF and monomethoxypolyethylene glycol. Pegylated G-CSF has a prolonged half-life because of its reduced renal clearance. Serum clearance is directly related to neutrophil number. As a result, only a single SC dose of pegylated G-CSF (Neulasta) is required after chemotherapy. On the basis of the results of randomized, blinded trials, this molecule is indicated to decrease the incidence of infection in patients with nonmyeloid malignancies receiving myelosuppressive chemotherapy with a significant incidence of febrile neutropenia.[187]

Macrophage colony-stimulating factor

Although macrophage colony-stimulating factor (M-CSF) is known to affect a variety of organ systems, its cardinal effect remains its ability to influence most aspects of monocyte/macrophage development and function.

Biologic activities of M-CSF

M-CSF stimulates differentiation of progenitor cells to mature monocytes and prolongs the survival of monocytes. It enhances cytotoxicity, superoxide production, phagocytosis, chemotaxis, and secondary cytokine production (G-CSF, IL-6, and IL-8) in monocytes and macrophages. In addition to stimulation of hematopoiesis, M-CSF also promotes differentiation and proliferation of osteoclast progenitor cells and has profound effects on lipid metabolism.

M-CSF in malignancy

M-CSF is intricately involved in atherosclerosis, but information about its role remains contradictory. For instance, M-CSF administration lowers cholesterol levels. Paradoxically, it appears that an absence of M-CSF protects against atherosclerosis even in the presence of hyperlipidemia.[188] M-CSF and Fms are expressed in the brain. This cytokine induces microglial proliferation, activation, and survival.

In malignancy, mutations in Fms (the M-CSF receptor) have been reported at codon 969 in about 10% of cases of human myeloid malignancies (including myelodysplasia and AML).

M-CSF in the clinic
In a large-scale study, it has been shown that the administration of M-CSF to AML patients after consolidation chemotherapies shortens the periods of neutropenia and thrombocytopenia after chemotherapy and reduces the incidence and shortens the duration of febrile neutropenia.[189] Similar benefits have been reported after chemotherapy or BMT. M-CSF can elevate neutrophil counts in children with chronic neutropenia. Finally, preliminary results in uncontrolled trials suggest that this molecule may improve outcome after fungal infections.[190]

Stem cell factor
SCF is also known as kit ligand, mast cell growth factor, or steel factor. It functions as a hematopoietic cytokine that triggers its biologic effect by binding to c-kit (the SCF receptor).[191]

Biologic activities of SCF
SCF is constitutively produced by marrow stromal elements. It is now well established that SCF acts on hematopoietic stem cells and, in some lineages, mature cells.

SCF synergizes with other cytokines (including EPO and IL-3) to support the direct colony growth of BFU-E, CFU-GM, and CFU-granulocyte/erythroid/macrophage/megakaryocyte in semisolid media, and current data suggest that SCF can act on a more primitive cell (pre-CFU-C) capable of generating the direct colony-forming cells. SCF can also promote progenitor cell survival, accelerate stem cell entry into cell cycle, and function as a chemotactic and chemokinetic factor for these cells. Synergistic proliferative effects on megakaryocytic progenitor cells are observed when SCF is combined with TPO or IL-3.[192] SCF is also involved in processes of cell adhesion and trafficking. SCF induces progenitor cell adhesion to fibronectin, a process that may involve alteration of integrin avidity through an inside–out signal initiated in response to c-kit receptor kinase activation after ligand binding. Alternatively, it is possible that the transmembrane form of SCF displayed on fibroblasts binds directly to the c-kit receptor on the surface of hematopoietic cells and, thus, helps to anchor the hematopoietic cells in the microenvironment.[192]

The effects of SCF when combined with G-CSF are even more pronounced.[193] Phase 1 clinical studies show that treatment with SCF increases the numbers of progenitor cells of many types (including BFU-E, CFU-GM, CFUMeg, and CFU-GEMM) in the marrow.[194]

SCF and c-kit in malignancy
The concentration of SCF in normal human serum is, on average, 3.3 ng/mL. Serum SCF levels are not elevated in patients with aplastic anemia, myelodysplasia, chronic anemia, or after marrow ablative therapy.[192] Thus, the level of SCF in the circulation, unlike the level of EPO, is not inversely related to the hematocrit.

Alterations in the local distribution of SCF within the skin have been implicated in the pathogenesis of cutaneous mastocytosis.[192] Point mutations in the c-kit receptor cytoplasmic domain have been identified in murine and human mast cell lines and in hematopoietic

cells from patients with mast cell disorders.[192] Activating mutations in kit characterize a type of leiomyosarcoma known as gastrointestinal stromal tumors.

Neoplastic human hematopoietic cells can also display the c-kit receptor. Receptor density is highest in erythroleukemia cell lines, which may express up to 50,000 to 100,000 c-kit receptors per cell. Solid tumor cell lines and a variety of fresh human tumor tissues also express c-kit receptor protein.[192]

SCF in the clinic
Clinical trials of SCF in a number of situations have been undertaken. SCF factor seems to be reasonably well tolerated, with the predominant side effects being transient local erythema and long-lasting hyperpigmentation at injection sites. The most worrisome toxicity is a mast cell effect resulting in allergic-like reactions characterized by urticaria, with or without respiratory symptoms.[192] The side effects of SCF, including the allergic phenomenon, appear to be dose dependent.

Of special interest is the role of mutations in the SCF receptor (kit) in gastrointestinal stromal tumors. These mutations activate the kinase enzymatic activity of kit. A kinase inhibitor targeted against kit (STI571 or imatinib mesylate) has been found to be dramatically effective in these notoriously chemotherapy-resistant tumors.[195]

Thrombopoietin
The humoral basis of megakaryocyte and platelet production has been more enigmatic than that of other lineages. Factors that have now been implicated in at least some aspects of thrombocyte development include IL-3, IL-6, IL-9, IL-11, G-CSF, GM-CSF, SCF, leukemia-inhibiting factor, and TPO. The latter molecule is believed to be of paramount importance in the physiologic regulation of platelet production. Unfortunately, however, compared with the striking effects of the granulopoietic factors in neutropenic patients, the use of the thrombopoietic molecules in the clinic setting has met with less success.

Biologic properties of TPO
TPO participates in hematopoiesis in general, in addition to thrombopoiesis, as supported by experiments demonstrating that genetic elimination of TPO or its receptor causes a 65–95% reduction in the numbers of transplantable stem cells. The survival of TPO in the circulation is longer than that of other hematopoietic growth factors (half-life = 30 h).

TPO in malignancy
High serum levels of TPO have been found in patients with autosomal dominant hereditary thrombocythemia.[196] Overproduction has been attributed to a splice donor mutation in the gene for TPO, which leads to a shortened 5′-untranslated region that is more efficiently translated than its normal counterpart.[196] Because platelets themselves regulate the level of circulating TPO, high levels of TPO are also found in patients with bone marrow failure states. Homozygous elimination of c-mpl (TPO receptor) results in congenital amegakaryocytic thrombocytopenia.

TPO in the clinic
Two forms of TPO have entered clinical trials[197,198]: TPO (the full-length polypeptide) and PEG-conjugated recombinant human megakaryocyte growth and development factor (PEG-rHuMGDF).

Because its biologic action is prolonged, parenteral administration of TPO for 7–10 days results in increased platelet production

6–16 days later.[199] Results of clinical trials of PEG-rHuMGDF or recombinant human TPO in patients with cancer who were receiving chemotherapy, albeit with regimens that produce only moderate thrombocytopenia, suggest that platelet counts return to baseline significantly faster and the nadir platelet counts are higher.[200,201] However, the effectiveness of these molecules in accelerating platelet recovery after myeloablative therapy has not been impressive.[202] Furthermore, in patients with delayed platelet recovery after peripheral blood stem cell or BMT, recombinant human TPO did not significantly raise platelet counts in most patients.[203]

Future perspectives

The inchoate understanding of cytokines of some decades ago has now emerged as a complex picture of interacting stimulatory and inhibitory factors. Many of the molecules that govern this process have been cloned and have entered clinical trials. It is now clear that regulatory cytokines are characteristically pleiotropic and, at the same time, exhibit significant functional redundancy.

The history of medicine is replete with examples that show how innovative technologies improve clinical outcomes. The genetic engineering techniques that permitted the rapid cloning of newly identified cytokines and their translation into clinical therapies in hematology and oncology are an exciting example of this phenomenon.[204] However, it should be remembered that many, if not most, cytokines and their respective natural inhibitors are ubiquitously expressed and have myriad biologic properties that influence virtually every organ system (Figure 1). It is already apparent that these molecules may also be effective in allergic and inflammatory conditions. Furthermore, the emerging understanding of their role and the availability of recombinant molecules for therapeutics suggests that the clinical role of these agents will continue to grow and may ultimately impact most fields of medicine.

Acknowledgment

This chapter combined and updated from the earlier chapters, called "Interferons" and "Cytokines and Hematopoietic Growth Factors", in the prior edition of Cancer Medicine. In this earlier edition, these chapters were written by the authors, Dr. Ernest C. Borden (Interferons) and in collaboration with Dr. Razelle Kurzrock (Cytokines and Hematopoietic Growth Factors), whose prior contributions provided important basis of this update.

Key references

The complete reference list can be found on the Wiley Companion Digital Edition of this title (see inside front cover for login instructions).

1 Dinarello CA. Interleukin-1, interleukin-1 receptors and interleukin-1 receptor antagonist. *Int Rev Immunol.* 1998;**16**:457–499.

14 Grimm EA, Owen-Schaub LB, Loudon WG, et al. Lymphokine-activated killer cells. Induction and function. *Ann N Y Acad Sci.* 1988;**532**:380–386.

17 Rosenberg SA. IL-2: the first effective immunotherapy for human cancer. *J Immunol.* 2014;**192**:5451–5458.

21 Prieto PA, Yang JC, Sherry RM, et al. CTLA-4 blockade with ipilimumab: long-term follow-up of 177 patients with metastatic melanoma. *Clin Cancer Res.* 2012;**18**:2039–2047.

23 Saranga-Perry V, Ambe C, Zager JS, et al. Recent developments in the medical and surgical treatment of melanoma. *CA Cancer J Clin.* 2014;**64**:171–185.

27 Ribas A, Flaherty KT. BRAF targeted therapy changes the treatment paradigm in melanoma. *Nat Rev Clin Oncol.* 2011;**8**:426–433.

28 Frederick DT, Piris A, Cogdill AP, et al. BRAF inhibition is associated with enhanced melanoma antigen expression and a more favorable tumor

microenvironment in patients with metastatic melanoma. *Clin Cancer Res.* 2013;**19**:1225–1231.

37 Kurzrock R, Talpaz M, Estrov Z, et al. Phase I study of recombinant human interleukin-3 in patients with bone marrow failure. *J Clin Oncol.* 1991;**9**:1241–1250.

56 Kurzrock R, Redman J, Cabanillas F, et al. Serum interleukin 6 levels are elevated in lymphoma patients and correlate with survival in advanced Hodgkin's disease and with B symptoms. *Cancer Res.* 1993;**53**:2118–2122.

62 Ebrahimi B, Tucker SL, Li D, et al. Cytokines in pancreatic carcinoma: correlation with phenotypic characteristics and prognosis. *Cancer.* 2004;**101**:2727–2736.

66 Blade J, de Larrea CF, Rosinol L. Incorporating monoclonal antibodies into the therapy of multiple myeloma. *J Clin Oncol.* 2012;**30**:1904–1906.

90 Akdis CA, Blaser K. Mechanisms of interleukin-10-mediated immune suppression. *Immunology.* 2001;**103**:131–136.

100 Trinchieri G. Interleukin-12: a cytokine at the interface of inflammation and immunity. *Adv Immunol.* 1998;**70**:83–243.

104 Ku CC, Murakami M, Sakamoto A, et al. Control of homeostasis of CD8+ memory T cells by opposing cytokines. *Science.* 2000;**288**:675–678.

116 Parrish-Novak J, Dillon SR, Nelson A, et al. Interleukin 21 and its receptor are involved in NK cell expansion and regulation of lymphocyte function. *Nature.* 2000;**408**:57–63.

119 Caudell EG, Mumm JB, Poindexter N, et al. The protein product of the tumor suppressor gene, melanoma differentiation-associated gene 7, exhibits immunostimulatory activity and is designated IL-24. *J Immunol.* 2002;**168**:6041–6046.

121 Ekmekcioglu S, Ellerhorst J, Mhashilkar AM, et al. Down-regulated melanoma differentiation associated gene (mda-7) expression in human melanomas. *Int J Cancer.* 2001;**94**:54–59.

128 Chen Q, Ghilardi N, Wang H, et al. Development of Th1-type immune responses requires the type I cytokine receptor TCCR. *Nature.* 2000;**407**:916–920.

130 Witte K, Witte E, Sabat R, et al. IL-28A, IL-28B, and IL-29: promising cytokines with type I interferon-like properties. *Cytokine Growth Factor Rev.* 2010;**21**:237–251.

133 Dinarello C, Arend W, Sims J, et al. IL-1 family nomenclature. *Nat Immunol.* 2010;**11**:973.

135 Nold MF, Nold-Petry CA, Zepp JA, et al. IL-37 is a fundamental inhibitor of innate immunity. *Nat Immunol.* 2010;**11**:1014–1022.

141 Talpaz M, O'Brien S, Rose E, et al. Phase 1 study of polyethylene glycol formulation of interferon alpha-2B (Schering 54031) in Philadelphia chromosome-positive chronic myelogenous leukemia. *Blood.* 2001;**98**:1708–1713.

146 Preudhomme C, Guilhot J, Nicolini FE, et al. Imatinib plus peginterferon alfa-2a in chronic myeloid leukemia. *N Engl J Med.* 2010;**363**:2511–2521.

148 Kurzrock R, Talpaz M, Kantarjian H, et al. Therapy of chronic myelogenous leukemia with recombinant interferon-gamma. *Blood.* 1987;**70**:943–947.

154 Ridolfi R, Chiarion-Sileni V, Guida M, et al. Cisplatin, dacarbazine with or without subcutaneous interleukin-2, and interferon alpha-2b in advanced melanoma outpatients: results from an Italian multicenter phase III randomized clinical trial. *J Clin Oncol.* 2002;**20**:1600–1607.

158 Kirkwood JM, Manola J, Ibrahim J, et al. A pooled analysis of eastern cooperative oncology group and intergroup trials of adjuvant high-dose interferon for melanoma. *Clin Cancer Res.* 2004;**10**:1670–1677.

169 Mickisch GH, Garin A, van Poppel H, et al. Radical nephrectomy plus interferon-alfa-based immunotherapy compared with interferon alfa alone in metastatic renal-cell carcinoma: a randomised trial. *Lancet.* 2001;**358**:966–970.

170 Flanigan RC, Salmon SE, Blumenstein BA, et al. Nephrectomy followed by interferon alfa-2b compared with interferon alfa-2b alone for metastatic renal-cell cancer. *N Engl J Med.* 2001;**345**:1655–1659.

174 Hamming OG, Gad HH, Paludan S, Hartmann R. Lambda interferons: new cytokines with old functions. *Pharmaceuticals.* 2010;**3**:795–809.

175 Miller DM, Klucher KM, Freeman JA, et al. Interferon lambda as a potential new therapeutic for hepatitis C. *Ann N Y Acad Sci.* 2009;**1182**:80–87.

177 Adamson JW. Epoetin alfa: into the new millennium. *Semin Oncol.* 1998;**25**:76–79.

182 Hubel K, Dale DC, Liles WC. Therapeutic use of cytokines to modulate phagocyte function for the treatment of infectious diseases: current status of granulocyte colony-stimulating factor, granulocyte-macrophage colony-stimulating factor, macrophage colony-stimulating factor, and interferon-gamma. *J Infect Dis.* 2002;**185**:1490–1501.

192 Broudy VC. Stem cell factor and hematopoiesis. *Blood.* 1997;**90**:1345–1364.

195 Demetri GD, von Mehren M, Blanke CD, et al. Efficacy and safety of imatinib mesylate in advanced gastrointestinal stromal tumors. *N Engl J Med.* 2002;**347**:472–480.

197 Kaushansky K, Drachman JG. The molecular and cellular biology of thrombopoietin: the primary regulator of platelet production. *Oncogene.* 2002;**21**:3359–3367.

64 Monoclonal serotherapy

Robert C. Bast Jr., MD ▪ *Michael R. Zalutsky, PhD, MA* ▪ *Arthur E. Frankel, MD*

Overview

Monoclonal antibodies have impacted significantly the care of patients with cancer. Some 22 monoclonal antibodies, cytotoxic drug conjugates, radionuclide conjugates, and targeted toxins have been approved by the US FDA for the treatment of a dozen different malignancies, although three of these biologicals are no longer marketed. Useful monoclonal antibodies have targeted proteins on the cancer cell surface most frequently (CD20 by rituximab and HER2 by trastuzumab and pertuzumab), inhibiting growth, inducing apoptosis, and enhancing chemotherapy, but some have targeted cytokines (IL-6 by siltuximab), growth factors [vascular endothelial growth factor (VEGF) by beva-cizumab], and growth factor receptors (VEGFR2 by ramucirumab) that can affect endothelial cells in tumor vessels, or have altered the immune response by neutralizing checkpoint inhibitors (CTLA4 by ipilimumab and PD1 by nivolumab or pembrolizumab). In the case of trastuzumab and pertuzumab, binding of the two antibodies to different sites on HER2 cell surface receptors has produced greater antitumor activity than either alone. Enhanced cancer cell killing has also been achieved by conjugation of antibodies with cytotoxic drugs (emtansine to anti-HER2 trastuzumab and vedotin to anti-CD30 brentuximab) or radionuclide conjugates (^{90}Y to anti-CD20 ibritumomab tiuxetan) permitting effective treatment for patients who had failed therapy with unconjugated antibodies. There are several barriers to effective therapy with monoclonal antibodies including antigen specificity, antigenic modulation, heterogeneity of antigen expression, effective delivery of antibodies to cancer cells, potency of effector mechanisms, and response to foreign globulin. The latter problem has been circumvented with the use of chimeric constructs, humanization of murine antibodies, and developing genetically engineered mice with the ability to develop fully human antibodies. Use of unconjugated antibodies is likely to improve as our knowledge of tumor biology and immunology grows, identifying targets such as OX-40 ligand. Use of smaller molecularly engineered binding constructs may improve pharmacokinetics and pharmacodynamics of serotherapy. Combinations of antibodies may be required to compensate for antigenic heterogeneity. Development of antibody drug conjugates will require the identification of monoclonal reagents that target tumor initiating stem cells. Pretargeting and the use of α-emitters are promising approaches to improving antibody-radionuclide conjugates. Development of targeted toxins must be further explored.

Introduction

Following the initial report of Kohler and Milstein,[1] monoclonal antibody technology exerted a prompt and substantial impact on laboratory investigation. Over the past four decades, the availability of monoclonal reagents has permitted the development of novel markers for *in vitro* applications, including monitoring response to treatment, detecting malignant cells histochemically, identifying subsets of patients with particularly favorable or unfavorable prognoses, and distinguishing some tumors of unknown origin. Application of monoclonal antibodies for the *in vivo* treatment of human cancer has been more gradual, but serotherapy with monoclonal antibodies and their conjugates now has an established role in the management of a dozen hematopoietic and solid cancers.[2-5]

By 2015, the United States Food and Drug Administration (FDA) has approved 43 unconjugated monoclonal antibodies, drug conjugates, and radionuclide conjugates for therapeutic indications, including transplant rejection, coronary thrombosis, respiratory syncytial virus and anthrax infections, rheumatoid arthritis, systemic lupus erythematosus, paroxysmal nocturnal hemoglobinuria, macular degeneration, inflammatory bowel disease, psoriasis, asthma, and cancer.[6,7] Twenty-one of the 43 have been approved for the treatment of different cancers, as has one targeted toxin (Table 1). Three previously approved antibodies with anticancer activity have been withdrawn from the market. Unmodified monoclonal antibodies contribute to the care of patients with acute lymphoblastic and chronic lymphocytic leukemias (CLLs), Hodgkin and non-Hodgkin lymphomas (NHLs), Castleman disease, neuroblastoma, HER2-amplified breast cancer, non-small-cell lung cancer (NSCLC), head and neck cancer, renal cell cancer (RCC), colorectal cancer, and gastric cancer. With the general availability of these agents, it appears that monoclonal serotherapy has a well-established role in clinical oncology.

In an attempt to exert greater antitumor activity *in vivo*, monoclonal antibodies have been linked to cytotoxic drugs, radionuclides, and immunotoxins. Extensive preclinical and clinical studies have now been performed with each type of immunoconjugate, with several approved by the FDA for the treatment of different cancers.[8] This chapter considers the current use as well as some of the challenges and additional opportunities for the further clinical application of monoclonal reagents, drug conjugates, radionuclide conjugates, and targeted toxins for the treatment of patients with cancer.

Serotherapy for leukemia and lymphoma with unmodified monoclonal antibodies

With rare exceptions, murine monoclonal antibodies raised against human neoplasms recognize tumor-associated antigens, which are also expressed by normal adult or fetal tissues. Some antigens, however, are expressed by only a small number of normal cells that may not be essential to a patient's well-being. Unconjugated monoclonal antibodies have contributed significantly to the care of patients with lymphoma[3] and leukemia.[9,10]

Holland-Frei Cancer Medicine, Ninth Edition. Edited by Robert C. Bast Jr., Carlo M. Croce, William N. Hait, Waun Ki Hong, Donald W. Kufe, Martine Piccart-Gebhart, Raphael E. Pollock, Ralph R. Weichselbaum, Hongyang Wang, and James F. Holland.
© 2017 John Wiley & Sons, Inc. ISBN: 978-1-118-93469-2

Table 1 Monoclonal antibodies, radionuclide conjugates, and targeted toxins approved in the United States for treatment of cancer[7].

Antibody	Product name	FDA approved	Type	Antigenic target	Indication
Rituximab	Rituxan	1997	Chimeric	CD20	Relapsed or refractory follicular and low-grade non-Hodgkin lymphoma
Trastuzumab	Herceptin	1998	Humanized	HER-2	Metastatic breast cancers that overexpress HER-2
Denileukindefitox	Ontak	1999	Humanized	CD25	Cutaneous T-cell leukemia
Gemtuzumab	Mylotarg	2000[a]	Humanized ADC	CD33	Relapsed acute myelogenous leukemia in elderly patients
Alemtuzumab	Campath	2001[a]	Humanized	CD52	B-cell chronic lymphocytic leukemia
[90]Y-ibritumomab tiuxetan	Zevalin	2002	Murine ARC	CD20	Relapsed or refractory follicular and low-grade non-Hodgkin lymphomas in elderly patients and rituximab-resistant disease
[131]I-tostuzumab	Bexxar	2003[a]	Murine ARC	CD20	Relapsed or refractory follicular and low-grade non-Hodgkin lymphomas in elderly patients and rituximab-resistant disease
Cetuximab	Erbitux	2004 2006	Chimeric	EGFR	Metastatic colorectal cancer with irinotecan Head and neck cancers with radiotherapy
Bevacizumab	Avastin	2004 2006 2008 2009 2009 2014	Humanized	VEGF	Metastatic colorectal cancer Non-small cell lung cancer Advanced breast cancer[a] Renal Cell Glioblastoma Ovarian

[a]Withdrawn from the market.

Source: http://www.antibodysociety.org/news/approved_mabs.php. Reproduced with permission of the Antibody Society.

Anti-idiotypic antibodies

In the early 1980s, Levy and colleagues prepared tumor-specific murine monoclonal antibodies against the unique idiotypes associated with cell surface membrane immunoglobulin present on human B-cell lymphomas, but expressed by a very small subset of normal B cells.[11,12] Treatment of 18 lymphoma patients with anti-idiotypic antibodies alone produced an objective response rate of 67% with little toxicity, and one patient remained in complete remission for 72 months and survived for >17 years.[6] In subsequent trials, anti-idiotypic antibodies were combined with interferon (IFN)-α, chlorambucil, or interleukin (IL)-2. Most of the antibodies that produced responses *in vivo* were of the murine immunoglobulin G1 (IgG1) isotype, which is generally least efficient in fixing complement or participating in antibody-dependent cell-mediated cytotoxicity (ADCC). Anti-idiotypic antibodies that bind to the B-cell receptor complex appear to induce apoptosis (programmed cell death) by delivering a death signal. In a fraction of patients treated with anti-idiotypic antibodies, recurrence of lymphoma is associated with loss of the relevant antigen from the cancer cells. Genes encoding the cell surface membrane immunoglobulin continue to undergo point mutations, resulting in the loss of idiotypic determinants.[13] Use of anti-idiotypic antibodies has provided critical proof of concept, but widespread application has been hindered by the logistic challenge of developing reagents for each patient.

Anti-CD20 antibodies

Rituximab (Rituxan®)

Monoclonal antibodies against B cell differentiation antigens expressed by malignant cells from different patients have been used to treat NHL, as well as acute and chronic leukemias. One useful target is CD20, a 35-kDa phosphoprotein calcium channel expressed on the surface of all normal B cells and in 80% of NHLs but not on other normal tissues. Antibodies specific for different epitopes on CD-20 are classified as type I antibodies

that translocate CD20 into detergent-insoluble lipid rafts in the cell membrane facilitating complement-dependent cytotoxicity (CDC) and type II antibodies that do not induce lipid rafts and facilitate ADCC by Fcγ receptor-bearing natural killer (NK) cells and macrophages.[3] Repeated weekly administration of the type I chimeric mouse/human IgG1 anti-CD20 antibody rituximab produced a 48–50% response rate in patients with relapsed low-grade follicular NHL, with a median time to progression of 10.2–13.2 months.[14,15] In 37 newly diagnosed patients, treatment with rituximab produced an overall response rate (ORR) of 72%, with 36% complete responses and median time to disease progression of 2.2 years.[16] Consequently, rituximab was used initially to treat patients with relapsed or refractory indolent follicular NHL. Use was extended to treat newly diagnosed low-grade NHL patients with rituximab alone or in combination with chemotherapy as well as for maintenance therapy.[17] Rituximab has also contributed to the care of patients with diffuse large B cell NHL, CLL and autoimmune diseases.

Follicular and indolent NHL

Since regulatory approval by the US FDA in 1997 for the treatment of patients with recurrent or refractory follicular or indolent NHL, indications have been extended to provide 8 rather than 4 weekly courses and to retreat patients who had responded previously.[18] After relapse, retreatment with a similar course of rituximab produced an overall response rate of 38% in 60 patients, with 10% complete remissions. Median time to progression exceeded 15 months.[19] Combination of rituximab with cyclophosphamide, doxorubicin, vincristine, and prednisone (CHOP) chemotherapy (R-CHOP) in 40 patients with low-grade follicular lymphoma, some of whom had been treated previously, resulted in an overall response of 100%, with 58% complete remissions and 42% partial remissions. Median time to progression exceeded 40.5 months.[20] In a meta-analysis of 7 trials with 1943 patients with follicular lymphoma, other indolent lymphomas, and the more aggressive mantle cell lymphoma, the addition of rituximab to chemotherapy improved overall survival (OS), although the statistical significance was higher with indolent lymphomas than with the mantle cell histotype.[21] The addition of rituximab to cyclophosphamide, vincristine, and prednisone (CVP) chemotherapy prolonged time to progression in patients with newly diagnosed follicular NHL, resulting in FDA approval in 2006 for use of rituximab in first-line therapy.[22] Maintenance therapy with rituximab has prolonged progression-free survival (PFS) in four randomized trials, while OS has been extended in some but not all studies.[23] In 2011, the US FDA approved rituximab for maintenance therapy based on a randomized comparison of rituximab (up to 12 8-week cycles) to no maintenance therapy in 1018 patients with high tumor burden follicular NHL who had complete or partial response to rituximab plus one of three chemotherapy regimens. Maintenance rituximab reduced the risk of a PFS event by 46% ($P < 0.0001$). At 3 years, PFS in the rituximab maintenance group was 74.9% versus 57.6% in the observation group ($P < 0.0001$).[24]

Diffuse large B-cell NHL

More aggressive diffuse large B-cell lymphoma (DLBCL) has been less responsive to rituximab alone. Among 54 patients with disease in relapse, the overall response rate to 8 cycles of rituximab was 31%, including 9% complete remissions with a median time to progression in responders of 8 or more months.[25] Subsequently, 399 elderly patients with more aggressive DLBCL were randomized to receive R-CHOP or CHOP alone. A complete response rate of 76% was observed with the combination, compared with 60% with CHOP alone.[26] Event-free survival ($P < 0.005$) and OS ($P < 0.01$) were prolonged significantly by the addition of rituximab. Similar results were obtained in two confirmatory trials,[27,28] both in young and elderly individuals, resulting in FDA approval in 2006 for use of R-CHOP in DLBCL, and providing the first improvement in the systemic treatment of DLBCL in two decades. In a recent meta-analysis of 7 trials involving 1470 patients with relapsed or refractory DLBCL, maintenance therapy with rituximab provided numerically improved PFS and OS, but the differences were not statistically significant, whereas incorporation of rituximab in salvage therapy led to statistically significantly better OS ($P = 0.02$) and PFS ($P < 0.05$) than rituximab-free regimens.[29] However, the rate of infection-related adverse events was higher with rituximab treatment (RR = 1.37; $P = 0.001$).

CLL and Waldenstrom macroglobulinemia

Treatment with rituximab, alone or in combination with fludarabine, has been extended to CLL.[30] In early studies, only a very modest response rate (15%) was observed with low standard doses of rituximab, possibly related to the lower concentration of CD20 on the CLL cell surface (8–15,000 vs 90,000 sites/cell) and to the shedding of soluble CD20, creating an "antigenic sink."[31,32] Treatment with higher doses of rituximab or thrice weekly administration achieved an overall response rate of 46%, with an even higher response rate in previously untreated patients.[31] A Cancer and Leukemia Group B (CALGB) trial of fludarabine and rituximab in 42 patients with CLL yielded a 100% response rate, with 48% of patients achieving complete remission.[33] On the basis of the two randomized phase III studies where the addition of rituximab to fludarabine and cyclophosphamide extended PFS by 10–19 months in previously treated and untreated patients with CLL,[34,35] the US FDA approved rituximab in combination with fludarabine and cyclophosphamide in 2010. Rituximab has also been used with alkylating agents to treat Waldenstrom macroglobulinemia. One study reported a 74% response rate and

67% 2-year PFS with a combination of rituximab, dexamethasone, and cyclophosphamide.[36]

Autoimmune disease

Depletion of B lymphocytes has contributed to the management of autoimmune diseases. Rituximab has been approved in combination with methotrexate for the treatment of rheumatoid arthritis that has failed anti-tumor necrosis factor (TNF) therapy, as well as for treatment of granulomatosis polyangiitis (Wegener's granulomatosis) and microscopic polyangiitis (MPA) with glucocorticoids.[37]

Toxicity

Rituximab therapy is generally well tolerated. Most side effects are infusion related and occur within the first few hours of treatment. Adverse events generally last minutes to hours and include chills, fever, nausea, vomiting, fatigue, headache, pruritus, and the sensation of throat swelling.[38] Although side effects are experienced by up to 77% of patients, they are severe in only 10%.[39] Normal B-lymphocyte counts can decrease to zero after initial infusion; recovery begins by 6 months and is generally complete by 9–12 months. As CD20 is not expressed on mature plasma cells, immunoglobulin levels are maintained, and intercurrent infections requiring hospitalization occurred in only 2% of patients during 1-year follow-up. Following FDA approval in 1997 and before 2002, >125,000 patients were treated with rituximab in the United States. Among these individuals, only eight deaths were associated with treatment related to the development of infusion reactions, paraneoplastic pemphigus, Stevens-Johnson syndrome, and toxic epidermal necrolysis.[40] More than 120 cases of interstitial lung disease have been reported, generally when rituximab has been given with chemotherapy, but associated with monotherapy in 25%.[41] In recent years, rituximab treatment has been linked to reactivation of hepatitis B virus (HBV) in HBsAg-negative/HBcAb-positive patients. In one meta-analysis of 578 patients across 15 studies, the risk of reactivation was estimated at 6.3%,[42] suggesting that patients should be tested and antiviral prophylaxis given to patients with evidence of previous HBV infection who are receiving rituximab.

Mechanism of action and resistance

The mechanism(s) by which rituximab kills leukemia and lymphoma cells is not completely understood but probably involves ADCC, CDC, and the direct effect of CD20 ligation.[43] In cancer cells, cross-linking CD20 can induce cell cycle arrest, inhibit DNA synthesis, activate caspases, and induce apoptosis.[33] Sensitization to chemotherapy may relate to inhibiting the constitutive activation of AKT, thus downregulating the antiapoptotic protein Bcl-XL.[44] NK cells, macrophages, and polymorphonuclear leukocytes can be important effectors for ADCC,[33] and a correlation has been observed in some studies, between clinical response to rituximab and the presence of specific allelic polymorphisms in the FcγRIIIa and FcγRIIa receptors for IgG that are required to mediate ADCC.[45] Individual NK cells are capable of "serial killing" of multiple lymphoma cells, particularly in the presence of rituximab that creates a "cap" at one pole of the cancer cell containing CD20, ICAM-1, and the microtubule-organizing center that enhances sensitivity to NK killing.[3,46] The response to rituximab is impaired in mice genetically deficient in C1q that lack the first component of the CDC pathway but that have intact ADCC.[47] Clinical resistance to rituximab treatment rarely involves loss of CD20 expression but can be associated with upregulation of complement resistance proteins CD55 and CD59.[48] Interestingly, different patterns of gene expression have been observed in lymphoma cells obtained before treatment from responders and nonresponders to rituximab.[49]

Gene expression in tumors that failed to respond resembled that in normal lymphoid tissues and exhibited higher expression of genes encoding certain complement components and genes involved in cytokine, T cell, and TNF signaling.

Ofatumumab (Arzerra®)

Ofatumumab (Arzerra®) is a type I human anti-CD20 IgG1 that binds to an epitope distinct from that recognized by rituximab with greater avidity and slower off-rates facilitating both CDC and ADCC. Ofatumumab was approved by the US FDA in 2009 for treatment of CLL based on a multicenter, randomized, open-label trial comparing ofatumumab in combination with chlorambucil to single agent chlorambucil.[50] The trial enrolled 447 patients for whom fludarabine-based therapy was considered inappropriate by the investigator for reasons that included advanced age (median 69 years) or presence of comorbidities (72% with two or more comorbidities). Median PFS was 22.4 months for patients receiving ofatumumab in combination with chlorambucil compared to 13.1 months for patients receiving single-agent chlorambucil ($P < 0.001$).

Toxicity

The most common (>5%) adverse reactions with ofatumumab in combination with chlorambucil were infusion reactions, neutropenia, asthenia, headache, leukopenia, herpes simplex, lower respiratory tract infection, arthralgia, and upper abdominal pain. Overall, 67% of patients who received ofatumumab experienced one or more episodes of infusion reaction and 10% experienced a grade 3 or greater infusion reaction.

Obinutuzumab (Gazyva®)

Obinutuzumab (Gazyva®) is a type II humanized anti-CD20 IgG1 that acts predominantly through ADCC and has been glycoengineered to enhance binding to FcγR on effector cells.[3] Binding of obinutuzumab to CD20 can initiate intracellular signaling, reorganizing actin fibers, increasing lysozomal membrane permeability, and producing nonapoptotic cell death.[51] Obinutuzumab was approved by the US FDA in 2013 for treatment of CLL based on a randomized open-label multicenter trial comparing chlorambucil alone and in combination with obinutuzumab in 781 previously untreated participants who were elderly or had comorbidities.[52] Patients receiving obinutuzumab in combination with chlorambucil demonstrated a significant improvement in average PFS of 26.7 months compared to 11.1 months with chlorambucil alone.

Toxicity

The most common side effects in participants receiving obinutuzumab in combination with chlorambucil were infusion-related reactions, neutropenia, thrombocytopenia, anemia, musculoskeletal pain, and fever. Obinutuzumab was approved with a boxed warning regarding HBV reactivation observed with other anti-CD20 antibodies and rare cases of progressive multifocal leukoencephalopathy identified in participants on other trials of obinutuzumab.

Chlorambucil in combination with either obinutuzumab or ofatumumab provides an alternative for elderly CLL patients with comorbidities who are unlikely to tolerate fludarabine-based therapy.[10]

Antibodies against other lymphocyte-associated cell surface proteins

Over the past three decades, clinical trials have been conducted to evaluate antibodies against CD22, CD23, CD40, CD74, and CD80 in patients with different B cell-derived cancers.[23] In early studies of CD10-positive acute lymphoblastic leukemia (ALL), anti-CD10 antibody-induced prompt modulation of the common ALL antigen, preventing effective therapy.[53] Intravenous infusion of anti-CD5 also produced antigenic modulation and only transient, partial regression in a fraction of patients with T-cell leukemia/lymphoma and CLL.[54] In one of the first studies of serotherapy with monoclonal reagents, a serum-blocking factor was demonstrated that prevented binding of the monoclonal antibody to circulating lymphosarcoma cells, consistent with the presence of shed tumor antigen.[55]

Antibodies against IL-6

Castleman disease is a lymphoproliferative disorder caused by release of IL-6 or other cytokines that can be localized to a single lymph node group or can be multicentric. Cytokine release can be stimulated by HHV-8 infection, but a fraction of Castleman disease cases are HHV-8 negative and the source of IL-6 has not been well defined.

Siltuximab (Sylvant®)

Siltuximab (Sylvant®) was approved by the US FDA and the EU in 2014 for treatment of HIV-negative, HHV-8-negative multicentric Castleman disease. Approval was based on an international, multicenter, randomized (2 : 1), phase 2 study comparing intravenous infusions of siltuximab and best supportive care (BSC) in 53 patients to placebo and BSC in 26 patients.[56] Siltuximab produced a greater fraction of durable (18 weeks) tumor and symptomatic responses (34% vs 0%; $P = 0.0012$), tumor responses (38% vs 4%; $P < 0.05$), median time-to-treatment failure (>422 days vs 134 days; $P < 0.05$), and increased hemoglobin (36% vs 0%; $p < 0.05$) relative to placebo controls. Despite success in the management of Castleman disease, siltuximab has failed to demonstrate clinical activity against other malignancies where IL-6 signaling is thought to be important, including multiple myeloma, RCC, and prostate cancer.[57]

Toxicity

Common adverse reactions (>10% compared to placebo) during treatment with siltuximab include pruritus, increased weight, rash, hyperuricemia, and upper respiratory tract infections. Consequently, siltuximab provides an excellent example of a targeted therapy against a cytokine that drives a rare, but debilitating lymphoproliferative disease.

Serotherapy for solid tumors with unmodified monoclonal antibodies

The HER family of transmembrane tyrosine kinase growth factor receptors has provided targets for serotherapy in solid tumors. As outlined in *Chapter 107*, interaction of peptide growth factor ligands with HER family receptors triggers signaling through the Ras-mitogen-activated protein kinase (MAPK) pathway and the phosphatidylinositol 3-kinase (PI3K) pathways, enhancing cell cycle progression, proliferation, and survival in normal cells and cancer cells. Of the four HER family receptors, most attention has been given to HER-1 (epidermal growth factor receptor or EGFR) and to HER-2.

Anti-EGFR antibodies

Several monoclonal antibodies have been prepared against the extracellular domain of the 170-kDa EGFR that is overexpressed in a number of carcinomas, including NSCLC, head and neck cancers, pancreatic cancer, and colorectal cancers.

Cetuximab (Erbitux®)

Cetuximab (Erbitux®) is a chimeric IgG1 monoclonal antibody that blocks the ligand-binding site of EGFR, preventing receptor activation, inducing internalization, and downregulating receptor levels. In experimental systems, treatment of human cancer cells with cetuximab produces cell-cycle arrest in G0–G1, induces p21, directs hypophosphorylation of Rb, inhibits proliferation, and blocks the production of angiogenic factors such as vascular endothelial growth factor (VEGF).[58] In addition, treatment with cetuximab potentiates the activity of doxorubicin, paclitaxel, topotecan, and irinotecan as well as radiation therapy in nude mouse heterografts of human cancer. Potentiation of cytotoxic chemotherapy and radiation therapy may relate to inhibition of MAPK and PI3K with induction of BAX, activation of caspase 8, and downregulation of BCL-2 and NFκB, rendering cancer cells more sensitive to apoptotic stimuli.[59] In addition, cetuximab can induce ADCC in the presence of peripheral blood mononuclear cells. Very little EFGR expression is required to mediate cancer cell death from ADCC.[60] As in the case of rituximab, FcγR polymorphisms correlated with PFS after treatment with cetuximab, consistent with the importance of ADCC as a mechanism of cancer cell killing.[61]

Colorectal cancer

Weekly treatment with cetuximab alone produced partial remissions in 9% of 57 patients with chemotherapy-refractory colorectal cancer.[62] In two larger trials, a combination of irinotecan and cetuximab was used to treat a total of 450 patients with documented metastases from EGFR-positive colorectal cancer who had received irinotecan previously.[63] A combination of cetuximab and irinotecan produced a partial response in 17–23% compared with 11% of patients retreated with irinotecan alone. In one study, PFS, but not OS, was prolonged significantly from 1.1 to 4.1 months with the combination. In a subsequent phase III study, 1289 patients with recurrent EGFR expressing colorectal cancer who had been treated previously with first-line fluorouracil- and oxaliplatin-containing regimens were randomized to cetuximab plus irinotecan or irinotecan alone. Cetuximab improved disease-free survival significantly, but not OS, possibly related to cross-over in 47% of patients.[64] Interestingly, the level of EGFR expression has not correlated with response to cetuximab-based therapy. Consistent with this observation, 4 of 16 previously treated patients (25%) with EGFR immunohistologically negative cancers responded to a combination of cetuximab and irinotecan.[60] Consequently, patients should not be excluded from treatment based on immunohistochemical evaluation of EGFR. In 2004, the US FDA provided accelerated approval for cetuximab in combination with irinotecan to treat patients with irinotecan-resistant colorectal cancer. In 2007, regular approval was given, based on a trial where 572 patients with advanced EGFR-positive colorectal cancers that had failed oxaliplatin- and irinotecan-based regimens were randomized to BSC with or without cetuximab until progression. Cetuximab improved OS from 4.6 to 6.1 months ($P = 0.0048$).[65] Approval was given also for use of cetuximab as a single agent to treat colorectal cancer that had failed oxaliplatin- and irinotecan-based regimens.

Similar to clinical results with small molecule inhibitors and other monoclonal antibodies reactive with EGFR, responses to cetuximab are rare in cancers with *KRAS* mutations.[66] In retrospect, exclusion of patients with *KRAS* mutations affected the outcome substantially of the CRYSTAL trial where 1217 previously untreated patients with metastatic colorectal cancer were randomized to FOLFIRI alone or in combination with cetuximab, irrespective of *KRAS* mutation status.[67,68] Addition of cetuximab prolonged median PFS from 8.1 to 8.9 months ($P = 0.036$) and did not affect OS. When cancers were tested for KRAS mutations, the addition of cetuximab to FOLFIRI increased OS (19.5–23.5 months), PFS (8.1–9.5 months), and ORR (39% vs 57%) in patients with *KRAS* wild-type tumors. In patients with *K-RAS* mutant cancers, no improvement in OS, PFS, or ORR was associated with the addition of cetuximab to FOLFIRI. Supportive data were found in two other randomized trials where only patients with KRAS wild-type cancers benefitted,[69,70] resulting in approval in 2012 for cetuximab in combination with FOLFIRI for previously untreated patients with colorectal cancer.

Head and neck cancer

Cetuximab has also been approved for use in squamous cell carcinoma of the head and neck (SCCHN). In a pivotal multinational, phase III study, 424 patients with locally advanced head and neck cancers were randomized to high-dose radiotherapy or to a combination of radiotherapy with cetuximab.[71] The addition of cetuximab increased the duration of locoregional control from 15 to 24 months and increased OS from 29 to 49 months. When cetuximab was administered to patients with recurrent SCCHN who had progressed on platinum-based therapy, response rates of 10–13% were observed over three prospective trials ($n = 103$) with disease control rates of 46–56%.[72] The median time to disease progression ranged between 2.2 and 2.8 months, and the median OS ranged between 5.2 and 6.1 months.

Cetuximab has also improved the efficacy of platinum-based chemotherapy for SCCHN. Approval by the US FDA in 2011 was based on a multicenter trial in 442 patients with locoregionally recurrent or metastatic head and neck cancer who were randomly assigned to receive cisplatin (or carboplatin) with 5-FU with or without cetuximab.[73] Significant improvements were seen in OS (10.1 months vs 7.4 months; $P = 0.34$), PFS (5.5 months vs 3.3 months; $P < 0.0001$), and objective response rates (35.6% vs 19.5%; $P = 0.0001$) in patients receiving cetuximab plus chemotherapy.

Toxicity

Side effects in a majority of patients included an acneiform rash, predominantly on the face and upper torso (Figure 1), and a composite syndrome of asthenia, fatigue, and malaise or lethargy. Treatment with minocycline can reduce the severity of the acneiform rash.[74] Meta-analysis has found that the intensity of the rash correlates with OS, PFS, and ORR.[75] Hypomagnesemia results from the direct effect of cetuximab on EGFR in distal renal tubules, producing magnesium wasting.[76] A small minority of patients have experienced severe anaphylactic reactions, often on the initial infusion of cetuximab, related to a preexisting IgE antibody against galactose–α-1,3-galactose oligosaccharide found on the Fab portion of the cetuximab heavy chain.[77]

Panitumumab (Vectibix®)

Panitumumab (Vectibix®) is a fully humanized IgG2 anti-EGFR antibody that was given accelerated approval by the US FDA in 2006 based on a trial in 463 patients with EGFR-positive colorectal cancer resistant to standard drugs who were randomized to single-agent antibody therapy or BSC. Treatment with panitumumab produced an objective response of 10% compared to 0% in the BSC

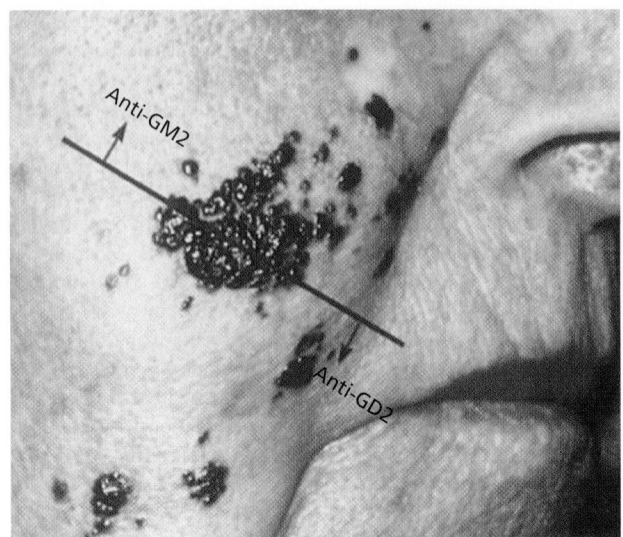

Figure 1 Recurrent melanoma, unresponsive to radiotherapy, before immunotherapy with intralesional injections of human monoclonal antibody to GM2 or GD2.

control group and extended mean PFS from 60 to 96 days.[78] As with cetuximab, responses were limited to patients with wild-type nonmutated *KRAS*.[79] Interestingly, in a recent meta-analysis, neither panitumumab nor cetuximab improved OS, PFS, or ORR in patients with *HRAS* wild type but *BRAF* mutant colorectal cancer, suggesting that sequencing *BRAF* might also identify patients who would not benefit from anti-EGFR treatment.[80] Approval of the antibody by the EU for use in colorectal cancer occurred in 2007. In previously untreated recurrent colorectal cancer, attempts to add panitumumab to bevacizumab plus FOLFOX-4 or FOLFIRI were discontinued when interim analysis of >1000 patients showed a statistically significant advantage in the control arm without panitumumab.[81]

Toxicity
A similar spectrum of side effects has been observed with panitumumab and cetuximab. Acneiform rash and hypomagnesemia have been most notable.[81] To date, fewer allergic reactions have been observed with panitumumab than with cetuximab.

Anti-HER-2 antibodies
Approximately 20–30% of breast cancers overexpress the 185-kDa tyrosine kinase growth factor receptor c-erbB2 (HER-2).[82] While HER-2 lacks a functioning ligand-binding domain, it is the preferred dimerization partner for the other HER family members including EGFR, HER-3, and HER-4.[83] Overexpression of HER-2 by breast cancer cells is associated with poor prognosis, particularly in node-positive disease, as well as with resistance to paclitaxel, CMF, and tamoxifen; however, it is associated with an improved response to doxorubicin.[84,85] Resistance to systemic therapy, increased risk of recurrence, and shortened survival reflect the biological consequences of HER-2 overexpression, including increased proliferation, increased cell survival, increased invasion and metastasis, and increased angiogenesis. Monoclonal antibodies directed against the extracellular domain of this receptor can inhibit growth of cancer cells that overexpress HER-2.[86,87] In addition, treatment with anti-HER-2 antibodies can increase the susceptibility of cancer cells to platinum compounds, taxanes,

doxorubicin, and 4-hydroperoxy-cyclophosphamide.[88,89] Interestingly, binding of anti-HER-2 antibodies to HER-2 receptors in the juxtamembrane region[90] can activate the tyrosine kinase[87] but may prevent ligand-driven interaction of HER-2 with HER-3 to activate the PI3 kinase pathway, decreasing the antiapoptotic activity of phospho-AKT.[87,91,92] Antibodies have been developed that bind to different sites on the HER-2 molecule.

Trastuzumab (*Herceptin®*)
Trastuzumab (Herceptin®) is a humanized IgG1 antibody that binds to subdomain 4 of the extracellular domain of the HER-2 receptor preventing homodimerization to other HER-2 receptors and downregulating HER-2 receptor levels. *In vivo*, inhibition of proangiogenic factors and mediation of ADCC may also play a role. Trastuzumab has received FDA approval for treatment of metastatic breast cancer, early breast cancer, gastric cancer, and gastro-esophageal junction (GEJ) cancer.

Breast cancer
In early clinical studies, trastuzumab produced objective regression of recurrent breast carcinoma in 12–15% of 269 heavily pretreated women.[93,94] Although cisplatin has demonstrated marginal activity against breast cancer in previous studies, a combination of cisplatin and trastuzumab produced an objective clinical response in 24% of 37 patients, with median duration of 8.4 months.[95] A critical international multi-institutional study was performed in 469 women with recurrent breast cancer.[96] Patients who had not previously received adjuvant therapy with doxorubicin were randomized to doxorubicin (or epirubicin) and cyclophosphamide, with or without trastuzumab. Women who had received adjuvant doxorubicin were randomized to paclitaxel with or without trastuzumab. The addition of trastuzumab to chemotherapy was associated with longer time to disease progression (median 7.4 months vs 4.6 months; $P < 0.001$), higher objective response rate (50% vs 32%; $P < 0.001$), longer duration of response (median 9.1 months vs 6.1 months; $P < 0.001$), and longer survival (median 25.1 months vs 20.3 months; $P = 0.01$). This study resulted in the approval of trastuzumab by the US FDA in 1998 and the EU in 2000 for the treatment of recurrent HER-2-overexpressing breast cancers. Subsequently, six large, multicenter adjuvant trials were undertaken (reviewed in Breast Cancer Neoplasms) to test whether the addition of trastuzumab improved the ability of chemotherapy to prevent recurrence of primary HER-2-positive breast cancer. Interim analysis in five of the six trials demonstrated sufficiently dramatic improvement in disease-free survival to terminate the clinical studies and to recommend use of trastuzumab in this setting.[97–99] Addition of trastuzumab produced a 46–58% reduction in risk of recurrence, associated with an absolute reduction of 8–12% at 3 years in the 5 positive trials. Similarly, mortality was reduced 33–59%, producing an absolute decrease of 2–6% at 3 years.

On the basis of the results of two of these trials (NSABP B31 and NCCTGN9831) including 3752 women, the FDA granted approval in 2006 for the addition of trastuzumab to cyclophosphamide, doxorubicin, and paclitaxel for adjuvant therapy of women with HER-2-overexpressed cancer.

Trastuzumab enhances the response rate to several other cytotoxic agents used to treat breast cancer, including vinorelbine, gemcitabine, and platinum compounds.[100–104] A randomized trial in 81 patients with metastatic HER-2-positive breast cancer who had not received chemotherapy for recurrent disease demonstrated a 51% response rate to vinorelbine and trastuzumab compared to a 40% response rate with paclitaxel and trastuzumab.[105] In most studies, only those breast cancers with strong expression of HER-2, driven by gene amplification, responded to the antibody alone or to a combination of antibody with chemotherapy. Immunohistochemistry can provide an initial screen for HER-2 overexpression, but 2+ to 3+ reactions should be confirmed with the more reliable fluorescence *in situ* hybridization assay.[106] HER-2 gene amplification can be acquired as breast cancers progress, arguing for repeated testing for HER-2 overexpression.[107] Because only a fraction of patients responds, overexpression of HER-2 is necessary, but not sufficient reason to ensure response to trastuzumab. Lack of response to trastuzumab correlated with lack of expression of the PTEN phosphatase, the enzyme that removes phosphate groups from PI3 and interrupts signaling through AKT.[108] Treatment with trastuzumab increased PTEN membrane localization and phosphatase activity by reducing PTEN tyrosine phosphorylation through inhibition of Src that could no longer dock on the HER-2 receptor.

Gastric and GEJ cancers

In 2010, the FDA granted approval for trastuzumab in combination with cisplatin and a fluoropyrimidine (either capecitabine or 5-fluorouracil) for the treatment of patients with HER-2-overexpressing metastatic gastric or GEJ carcinomas who had not received prior treatment for metastatic disease. The approval was based on results of a single international multicenter open-label randomized clinical trial, BO18255 (ToGA trial), which enrolled 594 patients with locally advanced or metastatic HER2-overexpressing adenocarcinoma of the stomach or GEJ.[109] Patients were randomly assigned to receive trastuzumab plus chemotherapy or chemotherapy alone. The trial was closed after the second interim analysis, when the addition of trastuzumab was associated with improved median survival (13.5 months vs 11.0 months; $P = 0.0038$). An updated survival analysis demonstrated a persistent advantage to trastuzumab (13.1 vs 11.7) with the greatest benefit seen in HER-2 overexpressing cancers.

Toxicity

Treatment with trastuzumab is well tolerated and is associated with low-grade fever, chills, and fatigue that, generally, are observed with the first administration. In many studies, trastuzumab has been administered weekly, but it has been administered every 3 weeks at higher dosage with acceptable toxicity and trough levels.[110] When trastuzumab has been combined with doxorubicin or paclitaxel, increased cardiotoxicity has been observed. In the pivotal trial that demonstrated the efficacy of trastuzumab in recurrent breast cancer, American Heart Association class III and IV cardiac dysfunction occurred in 27% of the group given trastuzumab with anthracycline and cyclophosphamide compared to 8% of the group given anthracycline and cyclophosphamide alone.[111] A similar degree of cardiac dysfunction was observed in 13% of patients who received paclitaxel and trastuzumab compared with 1% who received paclitaxel alone. Long-term treatment of 218 breast cancer patients with trastuzumab-based therapy for at least 1 year was associated with an 11% incidence of class III cardiac dysfunction.[112] In the six adjuvant trials where trastuzumab was given sequentially or concurrently with paclitaxel or carboplatin, but not doxorubicin, class III/IV cardiac dysfunction was observed in 0.5–4.1%.[98,99] Cardiac dysfunction generally responds to discontinuing trastuzumab and providing medical management. Thus, the benefits of trastuzumab for recurrent disease or adjuvant treatment generally outweigh the risks in patients with normal baseline cardiac function. The mechanism for trastuzumab-induced cardiac dysfunction remains obscure. Only low levels of HER-2 are found on cardiac myocytes, but trastuzumab can localize to the myocardium, and the ligand heregulin that binds to HER-2-HER-3 and HER-2-HER-4 dimers

appears critical to the fetal development and survival of cardiac tissue under apoptotic stress.[113] Use of less cardiotoxic anthracyclines in combination with trastuzumab offers one alternative. A neoadjuvant trial has been reported where concurrent epirubicin, paclitaxel, and trastuzumab produced a significantly higher pathological complete response (pCR) rate than did chemotherapy alone (67% vs 25%) without development of clinically evident congestive heart failure.[114]

Pertuzumab (*Perjeta®*)

Pertuzumab (Perjeta®) is an IgG1-humanized monoclonal antibody that binds to the dimerization domain of HER-2 at a site distinct from trastuzumab, preventing ligand-driven dimerization of HER-2 with multiple HER family members.[115,116] Use of pertuzumab in combination with trastuzumab synergistically inhibited survival of a breast cancer cell line that overexpressed HER-2 associated with increased apoptosis and blockade of signaling through AKT but not through MAPK.[117] Pertuzumab was approved by the US FDA in 2012 and by the EU in 2013 for treatment of HER-2 amplified breast cancer based on a single clinical trial, Cleopatra, involving 808 patients with HER2-positive metastatic breast cancer who were randomly assigned to receive pertuzumab, trastuzumab and docetaxel, or trastuzumab and docetaxel with a placebo.[118] Patients receiving pertuzumab had a median PFS of 18.7 months versus 12.4 months in the placebo group. With further follow-up, the addition of pertuzumab to trastuzumab and docetaxel increased OS by 15.7 months from 40.8 to 56.5 months ($P < 0.001$) and improved PFS by 6.3 months.[119]

In 2013, pertuzumab became the first FDA-approved drug for the neoadjuvant treatment of breast cancer in patients with HER-2-positive, locally advanced, inflammatory, or early-stage breast cancer (>2 cm in diameter or with positive lymph nodes) who are at high risk for recurrence and death. Pertuzumab was approved for use in combination with trastuzumab and other chemotherapy before surgery and, depending on the treatment regimen used, can be followed by chemotherapy after surgery. Following surgery, patients should continue to receive trastuzumab to complete 1 year of treatment. Pertuzumab's accelerated approval for neoadjuvant treatment was based on a study designed to measure pCR in accordance with a new FDA advisory that this could be used as a surrogate endpoint. In the NeoSphere study, 417 participants were randomly assigned to receive one of four neoadjuvant treatment regimens: trastuzumab plus docetaxel, pertuzumab plus trastuzumab and docetaxel, pertuzumab plus trastuzumab, or pertuzumab plus docetaxel.[120] About 39% of participants who received pertuzumab plus trastuzumab and docetaxel achieved pCR, compared to 21% who received trastuzumab plus docetaxel. The confirmatory trial for this accelerated approval is being conducted in participants with HER2-positive breast cancer who have had prior breast cancer surgery and are at high risk of having their cancer return. More than 4800 participants are enrolled in this trial, which will provide further data on efficacy, safety, and long-term outcomes. Results are expected in 2016.

Toxicity

The most common side effects reported in participants receiving pertuzumab plus trastuzumab and paclitaxel or docetaxel were hair loss, diarrhea, nausea, and neutropenia. Other significant side effects included decreased cardiac function, infusion-related reactions, hypersensitivity reactions, and anaphylaxis. There is a black box warning for cardiac failure and fetal damage.

Antiganglioside antibodies

GD2 is a disialoganglioside expressed on neuroblastomas and melanomas as well as on normal neurons, melanocytes, and pain fibers. Expression on cancer cells is relatively uniform and GD2 is not lost from the cell surface after treatment with monoclonal antibodies.[121]

Dinutuximab *(Unituxin®)*

Dinutuximab (Unituxin®) is a chimeric anti-GD2 IgG1 antibody that was approved by the US FDA in 2015 for treatment of newly diagnosed pediatric patients with high-risk neuroblastoma who have achieved at least a partial response to first-line multiagent, multimodality therapy. Addition of dinutuximab improved outcomes for patients who received maintenance therapy with granulocyte-macrophage colony-stimulating factor (GM-CSF), IL-2, and 13-cis-retinoic acid (RA).[122] The pivotal COG trial randomized 226 patients to either dinutuximab/RA or RA alone for six cycles of treatment. An improvement in event-free survival (EFS) (HR 0.57; $P = 0.01$, log-rank test) was demonstrated during follow-up and the trial terminated. At that time, the median EFS was not reached [3.4 years, NR, in the dinutuximab/RA arm, and 1.9 years (1.3, NR) in the RA arm]. An analysis of OS conducted 3 years later documented an improvement in OS in the dinutuximab/RA arm compared to the RA arm (HR 0.58), although median OS had not yet been reached in either arm.

Toxicity

The most common (>25%) adverse drug reactions in the dinutuximab/RA group were pain, pyrexia, thrombocytopenia, infusion reactions, hypotension, hyponatremia, increased alanine aminotransferase, anemia, vomiting, diarrhea, hypokalemia, capillary leak syndrome, neutropenia, urticaria, hypoalbuminemia, increased aspartate aminotransferase, and hypocalcemia. The most common (>5%) serious adverse reactions in the dinutuximab/RA group were infections, infusion reactions, hypokalemia, hypotension, pain, fever, and capillary leak syndrome.

Antivascular therapy

Angiogenesis is critical for normal fetal growth and wound healing but is also required for tumor growth and metastasis.[123] Novel approaches to inhibiting angiogenesis have exploited the presence of antigens displayed on tumor-associated endothelium or the proangiogenic factors produced by tumor cells.

Bevacizumab *(Avastin®)*

Bevacizumab (Avastin®) is a humanized IgG1 that binds to the proangiogenic VEGF-A that has also been characterized as vascular permeability factor (VPF). Blockade of VEGF/VPF can inhibit tumor-driven angiogenesis in xenografts.[124] Expression of VEGF/VPF has correlated with formation of ascites in mice with ovarian cancer xenograft models.[125] Treatment with bevacizumab can completely inhibit ascites formation.[126] In addition, cancer cells themselves can express VEGF receptors. Autocrine stimulation with VEGF can enhance proliferation and resistance to chemotherapy. Bevacizumab has received FDA approval for treatment of colorectal cancer (2004, 2006, and 2013), NSCLC (2006), breast cancer (2008; withdrawn 2011), RCC (2009), glioblastoma (2009), cervical cancer (2014), and ovarian cancer (2014), but its place in oncologic practice is still being defined.[127]

Colorectal cancer

In patients with previously untreated metastatic colorectal carcinoma, the addition of bevacizumab to irinotecan, fluorouracil, and leucovorin increased the overall response rate (34.8–44.8%) and significantly prolonged median PFS (7.4–10.4 months) and median OS (15.6–20.3 months).[128] This trial led to the initial FDA approval in 2004 of bevacizumab for use with chemotherapy for first-line therapy of colorectal cancer. Two subsequent randomized phase 2 trials have demonstrated improved response rate, PFS, and OS when bevacizumab was added to 5-FU and leucovorin.[129–131] In phase 3 studies where bevacizumab has been added to more effective first-line regimens, including FOLFOX-4 and XELOX, response rate, and OS were not significantly improved.[132,133] A number of combinations of bevacizumab and multiple drug combinations have provided similar results in noninferiority studies.[134] In second-line therapy, however, addition of a higher dose of bevacizumab to FOLFOX-4 significantly increased response rate (9–23%), PFS (4.7–7.3 months), and OS (10.8–12.9 months) in bevacizumab-naive patients, leading to the approval of bevacizumab for second-line therapy in 2006.[135] In patients with metastatic colorectal cancer who had progressed on bevacizumab in combination with irinotecan-based chemotherapy or oxyplatin-based regimens, continued use of bevacizumab in combination with the complementary chemotherapy regimen improved OS (11.2 months vs 9.8 months; $P = 0.0062$) and PFS (5.7 months vs 4.0 months; $P < 0.0001$), leading to approval for continued use of bevacizumab in second-line therapy.[136]

Non-small-cell lung cancer

In previously untreated metastatic NSCLC, three phase III trials have studied the addition of bevacizumab to carboplatin/paclitaxel,[137,138] or to gemcitabine/cisplatin.[139] Significant increases have been observed in response rates (range 14–28.1%) with a more modest increase in PFS (0.6–2.7 months) or OS (0.5–2.0 months).[134]

Breast cancer

Addition of bevacizumab to paclitaxel in first-line treatment of patients with recurrent metastatic breast cancer significantly increased response rate (21–37%) and PFS (5.9–11.8 months).[140] A modest, but significant, increase in PFS (8.0–8.8 months) was observed when bevacizumab was added to docetaxel.[141] In second-line therapy, the addition of bevacizumab to capecitabine significantly increased the response rate (9–20%) but not PFS (4.2–4.9 months) or OS (14.5–15.1 months).[142] Given the limited effect of bevacizumab in confirmatory trials, approval of the drug was withdrawn for breast cancer.

Renal cell cancers

A majority of sporadic RCCs exhibit inactivation of the von Hippel Lindau (VHL) gene with consequent overexpression of VEGF.[143] In a randomized phase 2 trial that compared two doses of bevacizumab (3 or 10 mg/kg every 2 weeks) with placebo in previously treated patients with RCC, a significant prolongation of PFS was observed when high-dose bevacizumab was compared with placebo (2.5–4.8 months, $P < 0.01$).[144] IFN-α is a standard initial therapy for RCC with a modest response rate and a survival advantage demonstrated in randomized trials. Two phase 3 trials have compared treatment with IFN-α and bevacizumab to IFN-α alone in previously untreated patients with RCC.[145,146] PFS was increased significantly from 5.2–5.4 to 8.5–10.2 months.

Glioblastoma multiforme (GBM)

Bevacizumab demonstrated activity against GBM (glioblastoma multiforme) in two single-armed trials, AVF3708g and NCI 06-C-0064E, where monotherapy produced a 20–25% response rate lasting a median of 3.9–4.2 months in a total of 141 patients who had relapsed after surgery, radiotherapy, and temozolomide.[147] This prompted accelerated FDA approval for use in this setting. A recent double-blind, randomized trial evaluated whether the addition of bevacizumab to radiotherapy and temozolomide would improve outcomes in 637 patients with newly diagnosed GBM.[148] Addition of bevacizumab increased PFS from 7.3 to 10.7 months ($P = 0.007$), but did not affect OS.

Ovarian cancer

In heavily pretreated patients with recurrent ovarian cancer, administration of bevacizumab, alone[149,150] or in combination with daily oral low-dose cyclophosphamide to provide "metronomic" therapy,[151] has produced response rates of 16–24% with PFS of 4.4–7.2 months. Stabilization of disease for 6 months has been observed in approximately 40% of ovarian cancer patients. Four randomized studies have been performed evaluating the addition of bevacizumab to standard chemotherapy for front-line treatment (GOG 218[152] and ICON7[153]) and for recurrent "platinum sensitive" (OCEANS[154]) and "platinum resistant" (AURELIA[155]) disease.[156] PFS was improved in these studies by 3.8 months ($P < 0.001$), 1.7 months ($P = 0.001$), 3.3 months ($P = 0.001$), and 4.0 months ($P < 0.0001$), respectively. OS was not improved in any of the studies, but subsets of patients in GOG 218 and ICON7 with poor prognosis appeared to benefit. Lack of impact on OS overall and similar enhancement of PFS in first-line and recurrent disease has raised the question of whether treatment with bevacizumab should be delayed until disease recurrence.[156] Approval for use of bevacizumab in combination with chemotherapy for recurrent disease was granted based on the Aurelia trial.

Cervical cancer

Addition of bevacizumab to a combination of carboplatin with paclitaxel or topotecan increased OS by 3.7 months (from 13.3 to 17.0 months, $P = 0.004$) and increased the rate of response from 36% to 88% ($P = 0.008$) in a randomized trial including 452 women with recurrent, persistent, or metastatic cervical cancer.[157]

Toxicity

In patients with NSCLC, RCC, colorectal, breast, cervical, and ovarian cancer, bevacizumab administration has been well tolerated by the majority. Grade 3 hypertension has been observed in approximately 20% of patients. While hypertension has been readily managed in most cases, malignant hypertension and fatal hemorrhagic stroke have been observed, arguing for aggressive monitoring and management of blood pressure. Significant proteinuria occurs in <5% of cases. Nasal bleeding has been observed. Greater risk for delayed wound healing and bleeding has been observed when bevacizumab was administered within 60 days of surgery.[158] In patients with NSCLC, major hemoptysis was associated with 4 deaths among 35 patients in one early trial. Life-threatening hemoptysis occurred most frequently in elderly males with squamous cell histology, tumor necrosis, and cavitation, as well as disease close to major vessels. Patients with these characteristics have been excluded from many trials. Thromboembolic events have been observed in 5–7.4% of participants on randomized trials in ovarian cancer.[156] Arterial thromboembolism has been observed in 2% of patients in large phase 3 trials across disease sites. In heavily pretreated patients with ovarian cancer, perforation

of the bowel has been observed in 5–7% of cases, generally in the setting of partial small bowel obstruction and treatment response in lesions that involve the bowel wall. Bowel perforation has occurred in 2.6–3% of ovarian cancer patients on front-line adjuvant trials[156] and in only 1% of colorectal cancer patients when bevacizumab was administered with FOLFOX.[135]

Ramucirumab (Cyramza®)

Ramucirumab (Cyramza®) is a human IgG1 monoclonal antibody that binds to the human VEGFR2 and prevents interaction with VEGF ligands. Ramucirumab has been approved by the US FDA for treatment of gastric and GEJ cancers (2014), lung cancer (2014), and colon cancer (2015).

Gastric and GEJ cancers

Ramucirumab can be used for treatment of fluoropyrimidine-resistant or platinum-resistant gastric or GEJ cancer as a single agent or with paclitaxel. Approval of ramucirumab as a single agent was based on a multinational, randomized double-blind trial in 655 patients with previously treated advanced or metastatic disease who were randomized (2 : 1) to ramucirumab or placebo plus BSC. Addition of ramucirumab to paclitaxel significantly improved OS (9.6 months vs 7.4 months, $P = 0.017$) and PFS (4.4 months vs 2.9 months, $P < 0.001$).[159]

Lung cancer

Ramucirumab in combination with docetaxel was approved for treatment of metastatic NSCLC that had progressed on platinum-containing regimens or anti-EGFR or anti-ALK targeted therapy. Approval of ramucirumab in combination with docetaxel was based on a double-blind, placebo-controlled clinical trial that enrolled 1253 patients with previously treated metastatic NSCLC.[160] Addition of ramucirumab to docetaxel significantly increased OS (10.5 months vs 9.1 months; $P = 0.024$) and PFS ($P < 0.001$).

Colorectal cancer

Ramucirumab can be used in combination with FOLFIRI for the treatment of patients with metastatic colorectal cancer whose disease has progressed on a first-line bevacizumab-, oxaliplatin- and, fluoropyrimidine-containing regimen. This approval is based on the results of a randomized, double-blind, multinational trial enrolling 1072 patients who were randomly allocated to receive FOLFIRI plus placebo or FOLFIRI plus ramucirumab.[161] Addition of ramucirumab to FOLFIRI improved OS (13.3 months vs 11.7 months; $P = 0.023$) and PFS (5.7 months vs 4.5 months; $P < 0.001$).

Toxicity

Ramucirumab treatment can be associated with fatigue, weakness, hypertension, hyponatremia, diarrhea, and nose bleeds. When combined with paclitaxel or docetaxel, neutropenia, febrile neutropenia, and anemia have been observed. Other rare, but important risks described in product labeling include hemorrhage, arterial thromboembolic events, infusion-related reactions, gastrointestinal obstruction, gastrointestinal perforation, impaired wound healing, clinical deterioration in patients with cirrhosis, and reversible posterior leukoencephalopathy. Hypothyroidism has been observed in patients with colorectal cancer.

Immune checkpoint inhibitors

Anti-CTLA4

Anti-CTLA4 monoclonal antibodies have been used to intervene in immunoregulation. CD4+CD25+ T regulatory (Treg) cells express cytotoxic T-lymphocyte antigen 4 (CTLA4). The presence of Treg cells in tumor tissue has been associated with a poor prognosis in several human cancers and their elimination can potentiate antitumor responses in preclinical models. In addition, effective activation of tumor immunity can be blocked by the interaction of CD80/86 on antigen-presenting cells with CTLA4 on T lymphocytes. Inhibiting this interaction with anti-CTLA4 antibody could enhance tumor-specific immunity.[162]

Ipilimumab (Yervoy®)

Ipilimumab (Yervoy®) is a fully human IgG1 monoclonal antibody that reacts with CTLA4 and was approved for use by the US FDA and the EU in 2011 based on a single international study of 676 patients with melanoma who had stopped responding to other FDA approved or commonly used treatments for melanoma and were randomized to ipilimumab, ipilimumab plus a gp100 vaccine, or vaccine alone. Those who received the combination of ipilimumab plus vaccine or ipilimumab alone lived an average of about 10 months, while those who received only the experimental vaccine lived an average of 6.5 months. Administration of ipilimumab as a single agent has produced a 7–15% objective response rate in human melanomas and RCC.[163,164] Greater activity might be anticipated using these reagents to augment the effects of specific tumor vaccines. Among 1861 patients, median OS was 11.4 months, which included 254 patients with at least 3 years of survival follow-up. The survival curve began to plateau around year 3. Three-year survival rates were 22%, 26%, and 20% for all patients, treatment-naïve patients, and previously treated patients, respectively.[165] In an adjuvant study, 951 patients with completely resected stage III melanoma were randomized to ipilimumab or placebo. Median recurrence-free survival was prolonged by ipilimumab (26.1 months vs 17.1 months; $P = 0.0013$). Five (1%) patients died of drug-related events in the ipilimumab group.[166] Response to CTLA4 blockade correlates with mutational load, neo-antigens, and expression of cytolytic markers.[167,168]

Toxicity

Common side effects that can result from autoimmune reactions associated with ipilimumab use include fatigue, diarrhea, skin rash, uveitis, hypophysitis, endocrine deficiencies, and inflammation of the intestines (colitis) and hepatitis.[164] Severe to fatal autoimmune reactions were seen in 12.9% of patients treated with ipilimumab. When severe side effects occurred, ipilimumab was stopped and corticosteroid treatment was started. Not all patients responded to this treatment. Patients who did respond, in some cases, did not see any improvement for several weeks.

Anti-PD1

Anti-PD1 antibodies target T cell associated PD1, a second regulator of T-cell immunity, preventing interaction with the PD-L1 and PD-L2 ligands on cancer cells and macrophages. Blocking this interaction, releases inhibition of immune responses, including those to cancer cells.[169]

Pembrolizumab (Keytruda®)

Pembrolizumab (Keytruda®), a humanized IgG4 that targets PD1 and prevents interaction with PD-L1 and PD-L2, was approved by the US FDA in 2014 for the treatment of melanoma that had progressed on ipilimumab but had not yet been treated with BRAF inhibitors. Approval was based on the results of a multicenter, open-label, randomized, dose-comparative, activity-estimating cohort including 173 patients with unresectable or metastatic melanoma who were randomized to receive 2 mg/kg ($n = 89$) or 10 mg/kg ($n = 84$) of pembrolizumab intravenously once every 3 weeks until disease progression or unacceptable toxicity. The ORR was 24% in the 2 mg/kg arm, consisting of one complete response and 20 partial responses. Among the 21 patients with an objective response, 3 (14%) had disease progression at 2.8, 2.9, and 8.2 months after initial response. The remaining 18 patients (86%) have ongoing responses, ranging from 1.4+ to 8.5+ months; 8 patients had ongoing responses of 6 months or longer. Similar ORR results were observed in the 10 mg/kg arm. In an extended randomized phase II trial, 6-month PFS was 34% in the 2 mg/kg arm, 38% in the 10 mg/kg arm, and 16% in a group receiving chemotherapy of the investigators' choice.[170] Pembrolizumab every 2 or 5 weeks has been compared to ipilimumab in a randomized trial with 834 patients. Six month PFS was 47.3% for pembrolizumab every 2 weeks, 46.4% for pembrolizumab every 3 weeks, and 26.5% for ipilimumab ($P < 0.001$).[171]

Toxicity

The most common (>20%) adverse reactions among patients receiving pembrolizumab 2 mg/kg every 3 weeks were fatigue, cough, nausea, pruritus, rash, decreased appetite, constipation, arthralgia, and diarrhea. The most frequent ($\geq$2%) serious adverse drug reactions observed with pembrolizumab were renal failure, dyspnea, pneumonia, and cellulitis. Additional clinically significant immune-mediated adverse reactions included pneumonitis, colitis, hypophysitis, hyperthyroidism, hypothyroidism, nephritis, and hepatitis.

Nivolumab (Opdivo®)

Nivolumab (Opdivo®), a human IgG4 anti-PD1 antibody, was approved by the FDA in 2014 for the treatment of previously-treated unresectable or metastatic melanoma that had failed ipilimumab and BRAF inhibitors. Approval was based on a single arm trial including 120 participants with a 32% objective response rate where approximately one-third of responders remained in remission for 6 months or more. When nivolumab was compared to dacarbazine in 418 previously untreated patients with BRAF wild-type melanoma, nivolumab produced >1 year OS (72.9% vs 42%, $P < 0.001$), PFS (5.1 months vs 2.2 months, $P < 0.001$), and objective response rate (40% vs 13.9%, $P < 0.001$).[172] In patients who had progressed on anti-CTLA4, nivolumab improved objective response rate compared to the investigators' choice of chemotherapy (37.7% vs 10.6%).[173]

Non-small-cell lung cancer

FDA approval was obtained in 2013 for nivolumab to treat patients with NSCLC who had failed platinum-based therapy based on a randomized trial where patients with metastatic squamous NSCLC who had experienced disease progression during or after one prior platinum-based chemotherapy regimen were assigned to nivolumab (135) or docetaxel (137).[174] Nivolumab demonstrated a statistically significant improvement in OS as compared with docetaxel (9.2 months vs 6 months; $P = 0.00025$). Approval was supported by a single-arm, multinational, multicenter trial in patients with metastatic squamous NSCLC who had progressed after receiving a platinum-based therapy and at least one additional systemic regimen. Patients ($n = 117$) who received nivolumab exhibited an ORR of 15%. All were partial responses, but 10 of the 17 responding patients (59%) had response durations of 6 months or longer.

Toxicity

The most common (>30%) adverse reactions among the 117 patients receiving nivolumab in the above single-arm trial were fatigue, dyspnea, musculoskeletal pain, decreased appetite, and cough. The most frequent grade 3 and 4 adverse drug reactions observed in at least 5% of patients treated with nivolumab were dyspnea, fatigue, and musculoskeletal pain. Clinically significant immune-mediated adverse reactions included pneumonitis, colitis, hepatitis, nephritis/renal dysfunction, hypothyroidism, and hyperthyroidism.

Combined nivolumab and Ipilimumab

A combination of nivolumab and ipilimumab improved objective response rate when compared to ipilimumab alone (61% vs 11%; $P < 0.001$) in 142 previously untreated melanoma patients with BRAF wild type cancer. Complete responses were observed in 22% of patients receiving the combination and 0% in patients receiving ipilimumab alone. PFS was prolonged in the combination arm ($P < 0.001$). Similar results were observed in patients with BRAF mutant melanomas.[175] A second randomized phase III study compared nivolumab plus ipilimumab to ipilimumab or nivolumab monotherapy in previously untreated stage III or stage IV melanoma. PFS was 11.5, 2.9, and 6.9 months, respectively ($P < 0.001$ for the combination). Grade 3–4 treatment-related adverse events occurred in 55% of patients in the combination arm compared to 27.3% in the ipilimumab arm.[176]

Bispecific antibodies

Immunoglobulins can be engineered to contain binding sites with two different specificities. The same can be done with smaller single-chain variable fragments (scFv) that contain the relevant binding sites and have better tissue penetrance. Bispecific constructs with one scFv fragment that recognizes a determinant found only on B cells with a second scFv fragment that binds to a determinant found only on T cells can enhance contact between cytotoxic T cells and malignant B cells, encouraging immunologic cancer cell killing.

Blinatumomab (Blincyto®)

Blinatumomab (Blincyto®) is a bispecific antibody with scFv fragments that bind to the CD3 T-cell determinant and the CD19 B cell determinant that is expressed on ALL cells. Blinatumomab was approved by the US FDA in 2014 for the treatment of ALL refractory to conventional therapy based on a study involving 185 adults with Philadelphia chromosome-negative relapsed or refractory precursor B-cell ALL. All participants were treated with blinatumomab for at least 4 weeks via infusion, producing CR in 32% for 6.7 months.[177]

Toxicity

Blinatumomab carries a boxed warning that some clinical trial participants had experienced cytokine-release syndrome at the start of the first treatment and experienced a short period of encephalopathy. The most common side effects seen in blinatumomab-treated participants were fever, headache, peripheral edema, febrile neutropenia, nausea, hypokalaemia, fatigue, constipation, diarrhea, and tremor.

Barriers to treatment with unmodified monoclonal antibodies

Antigen specificity

Few, if any, monoclonal antibodies react only with tumor cells and fail to react with normal tissues. The remarkable efficacy and modest toxicity of anti-idiotypic antibodies reflect, at least in part, their limited reactivity with the vast majority of human B cells. The toxicity of Campath-1, now withdrawn from the market, reflects reactivity with normal lymphocytes and monocytes. To treat cancers in some organs, such as ovary or thyroid, tissue-specific antibodies rather than tumor-specific antibodies may suffice because all normal tissue is removed during primary therapy.

Antigenic modulation

Antigens that modulate and are shed into the circulation, such as CD10 in ALL, have generally proven to be poor targets for serotherapy. An exception to this generalization has been observed with trastuzumab treatment of breast cancers that overexpress HER-2. The extracellular domain of HER-2 is cleaved and has been used as a marker for receptor overexpression.

Heterogeneity of antigen expression

Heterogeneity has been observed in antigen expression within and between cancers from different individuals. Cells that lack antigen expression cannot be targeted effectively. With unconjugated antibodies that lack "bystander" activity, a combination of several reagents may be required to target all cells. In the case of different breast cancers, a combination of five monoclonal reagents can target >90% of cells in >90% of cancers from different individuals.[178]

Effective delivery of antibody to tumor cells

Most attempts to develop effective serotherapy have utilized IgG antibodies with an Mr of 150 kDa. In contrast, most conventional cytotoxic drugs have a mass of <1 kDa. Consequently, monoclonal antibodies have slower kinetics of distribution and less tissue penetration than do conventional drugs.[179] For example, intravenous injection of an IgG2a murine monoclonal antibody against a 250-kDa melanoma-associated chondroitin sulfate proteoglycan core protein resulted in selective localization of antibody in metastatic nodules of malignant melanoma.[180] The greater the amount of antibody administered, the greater was the accumulation of murine immunoglobulin that could be demonstrated immunohistochemically in biopsied material. Even after the infusion of 500 mg of antibody, complete saturation of antigenic sites was not achieved in all patients, consistent with limited access of antibody to tumor cells outside the vascular compartment. Successful tumor localization of an antibody depends on several factors. The ability of monoclonal antibodies to reach tumor cells can be limited by abnormal vascularity, elevated interstitial pressure, and relatively large distances for transport of immunoglobulins through the interstitium.[181,182] Disordered tumor vessels permit greater leakage of albumin and other plasma proteins into the interstitial space around cancer cells. Blockage of lymphatic outflow by tumor cells prevents clearance of interstitial protein, increasing oncotic pressure, and fluid accumulation. Increased interstitial pressure impedes effective translocation of antibody. Biodistribution studies indicate that distance from blood vessels is an important factor affecting antigen recognition and binding. The central areas of bulky disease not only have increased fluid pressure but also are poorly perfused, making these regions less accessible to antibodies.[183] In addition, large tumor masses can act as antigenic sinks, decreasing drug delivery to other tumor sites.[184] Modeling studies led Juweid and colleagues to formulate the hypothesis of the binding-site barrier, which postulated that antibody molecules could be prevented from penetrating tumors by the very fact of their successful binding to peritumoral antigen.[185] Subsequent experimental studies have supported this hypothesis. Intracavitary therapy has been used in an attempt to improve access of antibody to tumor cells, but antibody generally penetrates only a few millimeters beneath the serosal surface.

Immune response to foreign immunoglobulin

Substantial effort has been expended on the development of human monoclonal antibodies that should be less immunogenic, but their titer, specificity, isotype, and affinity continue to limit the clinical utility of these reagents.[186-188] Because a large number of antibodies used clinically are derived from mice, they can induce the development of human antimouse antibodies (HAMAs). The presence of HAMAs can prevent effective delivery of murine monoclonal antibodies to tumor cells, particularly when multiple doses must be administered to obtain optimal antitumor activity. Genetic manipulation of murine monoclonal antibodies has been used to generate less immunogenic reagents. Chimeric (60% human) and humanized (95% human) antibodies have been engineered to retain the murine antigen-binding complementarity regions in association with human framework regions.[186] Although the immunogenicity of such antibodies can be reduced substantially and HAMA responses can be limited, their injection can still evoke an anti-idiotypic response. The availability of antibodies derived entirely from humans, isolated from combinatorial libraries using the process of phage display, has revolutionized therapeutic strategies.[188] Transgenic genetically engineered mice have also been created with human immunoglobulin genes that can produce fully human antibodies. Unlike murine antibodies, human or humanized antibodies that contain the human Fc antibody portion trigger ADCC and CDC. An array of novel affinity maturation techniques such as bacterial cell surface scFv display and cell-free ribosome display is emerging to isolate rare high-affinity clones.[189] Genetic engineering has also been used to produce single-chain antigen-binding proteins that may have more favorable pharmacokinetic properties than intact immunoglobulin or Fab fragments.[190]

Potency of effector mechanisms

To the extent that unmodified monoclonal antibodies inhibit tumor growth, several mechanisms may be important for antitumor activity, including direct growth inhibition, induction of apoptosis, inhibition of angiogenesis, CDC, and ADCC, in addition to possible intervention in the specific immunoregulatory network of the host. Antibodies that react with EGFR or HER-2 can inhibit the growth of tumor cells *ex vivo* in the absence of complement components or host effector cells.[87,191] Antibodies that block EGF binding to the EGFR, such as cetuximab, affect growth more readily than do antibodies that bind to other sites on the receptor. Inhibition of ligand binding appears important for the inhibition of anchorage-dependent, but not anchorage-independent, growth. Antibodies have been described that produce apoptosis in some lymphoid cell lines, activated T cells, and certain carcinoma cell lines.[192] Murine antibodies of the IgM, IgG2a, and IgG3 isotypes can fix human complement but often rather poorly. The rat monoclonal antibody, Campath-1G, is an important exception to this generalization in that the antibody can mediate lysis of human cells

that bear the appropriate antigen in the presence of human complement components.[193] Murine antibodies of IgG3, IgG2a, and IgG2b have been reported to mediate ADCC in which large granular lymphocytes (LGLs), monocytes, macrophages, or polymorphonuclear leukocytes are bound to tumor cells through Fc receptors after antibody has bound to specific antigenic determinants on the tumor cell surface. IgG3 appears to be particularly important for ADCC with LGLs, whereas IgG2a may interact more effectively with human monocytes.[194] In some instances, arming mononuclear leukocytes with antibody before interaction with tumor targets has been possible. *In vivo*, ADCC may be compromised in cancer patients owing to a paucity of appropriate effector cells or to the presence of circulating immune complexes that occupy or downregulate Fc receptors. Antibodies that react against GD3 on melanoma cells can also bind to GD3 on the surface of T cells, enhancing their cytotoxic and proliferative responses.[195] Hybrid antibodies have been generated with one binding site for T-cell-associated antigens and one binding site for tumor-associated antigens.[196] Such hybrid antibodies enhance tumor cell killing by IL-2-activated T cells, possibly by encouraging contact between effector cells and tumor targets.[197]

Serotherapy with monoclonal antibody drug conjugates (ADCs)

Murine monoclonal antibodies have been coupled to a variety of conventional cytotoxic agents, including antifolates, anthracyclines, vinca alkyloids, and alkylating agents. Prepolymerization of some drugs, such as doxorubicin, before conjugation can achieve higher ratios of drug to antibody. Drugs can be bound to the amino side chains of lysine residues, provided that the most reactive residues are not found in the antigen-binding site. Linkage of drugs to antibody through the carbohydrate moieties of the murine immunoglobulin has provided site-specific conjugation that generally does not impair antibody binding.[198,199]

One concern raised by some investigators is based on the observation that many cell surface antigens have fewer than 10^5 copies per cell. Release of $1-3 \times 10^6$ drug molecules at the cell surface might or might not be sufficient to eliminate tumor. Another concern relates to the ability of large immunoglobulin carrier complexes to translocate across tumor capillaries. In preclinical studies, however, drug-monoclonal antibody conjugates proved substantially more effective than did the free drug. Only some of these conjugates are more potent, but many are less toxic, providing an improved therapeutic index. Therapeutic advantage may relate to different rates or patterns of drug uptake when linked with monoclonal reagents. In some instances, novel linkages have been devised that would release drug at low pH or only in the presence of lysosomal proteases.

Gemtuzumab ozogamicin (Mylotarg®)

Calicheamicin has been conjugated with an anti-CD33 antibody.[200] CD33 is a 67-kDa glycoprotein expressed on the surface of >90% of AMLs and on early myeloid progenitor cells but not on normal pluripotent stem cells. Gemtuzumab ozogamicin, a conjugate of humanized anti-CD33 antibody and the cytotoxic antibiotic calicheamycin, is rapidly internalized by myeloblasts and induces apoptosis.[201] Three multicenter trials evaluated gemtuzumab ozogamicin in 142 patients with CD33 + AML in first relapse, administering two doses of 9 mg/m² on days 1 and 15 by 2-h intravenous infusion.[202] Complete remission, with or without full platelet recovery, was observed in 30% of patients.

Toxicity

Because CD33 is expressed on hematopoietic precursors, grade 3 or 4 neutropenia and thrombocytopenia were observed in 99% of 101 patients age 60 years or above. Infections (27%) and mucositis (4%) were observed less frequently.[203] Veno-occlusive disease occurred in 14 of 119 patients (12%) who received gemtuzumab ozogamicin-based regimens, including 5 patients who had not undergone stem cell transplantation previously.[204] Despite these toxicities, gemtuzumab ozogamyycin was given accelerated approval by the FDA in 2000. The confirmatory trial was stopped in 2004 owing to lack of benefit at interim analysis, and the conjugate was voluntarily withdrawn from the market in 2010. Recent meta-analysis indicated that while gemtuzumab ozogamicin improved PFS, it did not improve OS.[205]

Brentuximab vedotin *(Adcetris®)*

Brentuximab vedotin (Adcetris®), a conjugate of an anti-CD30 chimeric IgG1 antibody and 3–5 units of vedotin (monomethethyl auristatin E), a small molecule inhibitor of mitosis, was granted accelerated approval by the US FDA in 2011 and the EU in 2012 for treatment of relapsed Hodgkin lymphoma (HL) and anaplastic large cell lymphoma (ALCL). The effectiveness of brentuximab vedotin in patients with HL was evaluated in a single clinical trial involving 102 patients where 73% of patients achieved either a complete or partial response to the treatment for an average of 6.7 months. The effectiveness of brentuximab vedotin in patients with systemic ALCL was evaluated in a single-arm clinical trial in 58 patients where 86% experienced either a complete or partial response on average for 12.6 months.[206] Regular approval was based on a randomized, double-blind, placebo-controlled, post-human stem cell transplant (HSCT), phase III clinical trial in 329 patients with classical HL at high risk of relapse or progression based on pretransplant factors.[85] Following an auto-HSCT, patients were randomized to brentuximab vedotin or placebo once every 3 weeks for a maximum of 16 cycles. The median PFS in the brentuximab vedotin arm was 42.9 months compared to 24.1 months in the placebo arm ($P = 0.001$).

Toxicity

The most common adverse reactions (>20%) in patients treated with brentuximab vedotin were neutropenia, peripheral sensory and motor neuropathy, thrombocytopenia, anemia, upper respiratory tract infection, fatigue, nausea, and diarrhea. Twenty-five percentage of patients reported serious adverse reactions. The most common serious adverse reactions were pneumonia, pyrexia, vomiting, nausea, hepatotoxicity, and peripheral sensory neuropathy. In the registration trial, adverse reactions led to discontinuation of treatment in 32%.

Ado-trastuzumab-emtansine *(TDM-1; Kadcyla®)*

Ado-trastuzumab-emtansine (TDM-1; Kadcyla®) is a conjugate of the humanized anti-HER-2 humanized IgG1 antibody trastuzumab and a 148 D cytotoxic drug emtansine (DM1) that binds to tubulin. The conjugate was approved by the US FDA and the EU in 2013 for treatment of recurrent HER-2-amplified breast cancer based on a randomized, multicenter, open-label trial enrolling 991 patients who had failed prior taxane and trastuzumab-based therapy before enrollment. Patients were randomly allocated to receive intravenous ado-trastuzumab emtansine or oral lapatinib and capecitabine. Ado-trastuzumab emtansine produced greater PFS (9.4 months vs 6.4 months, $P < 0.0001$) and OS (30.9 months vs 25.1 months, $P = 0.0006$) compared to lapatinib and capecitabine.[207]

Toxicity

The most common adverse reactions observed in patients receiving ado-trastuzumab emtansine are fatigue, nausea, musculoskeletal pain, thrombocytopenia, headache, transaminasemia, anemia, and constipation. The most common (>2%) grade 3–4 adverse reactions were thrombocytopenia, transaminasemia, anemia, hypokalemia, peripheral neuropathy, and fatigue. The most common adverse events leading to ado-trastuzumab emtansine withdrawal were thrombocytopenia and transaminasemia. Serious hepatobiliary disorders, including at least two fatal cases of severe drug-induced liver injury and associated hepatic encephalopathy, have been reported in clinical trials with ado-trastuzumab emtansine. Other significant adverse reactions include left ventricular dysfunction, interstitial lung disease, and infusion-associated reactions.

Radioimmunotherapy of cancer

Radioimmunotherapy (RIT) is a method of cancer treatment that involves the selective delivery of a radionuclide emitting cytotoxic radiation to tumor cells via an antibody or antibody fragment. While the concept of antibody-based targeting of radionuclides to cancer cells has long been appreciated, this approach did not become practical until the development of monoclonal reagents, which has permitted more specific targeting and the large-scale production of conjugates for clinical trials. With external beam therapy, only a limited area of the body is irradiated, with the dimensions defined to match the known limits of tumor location. While conventional radiotherapy can be effective for localized disease, diffuse cancers generally are difficult to treat because of normal tissue toxicity concerns and because metastatic disease beyond the margins of the radiation field escape treatment. With RIT, if the targeted antigen or receptor is also present on metastases, in principle, they can also be treated, even if their presence is unknown at the time of treatment.

Perhaps the largest impediment to the acceptance of RIT is fear of radioactive materials among physicians and patients, which can be ameliorated by better education. On the other hand, RIT offers several important advantages compared with other antibody-based strategies discussed in this chapter. First, the antibody can be labeled with a small dose of either the therapeutic radionuclide or an analogous radionuclide and then the pharmacokinetics of the RIT agent can be determined in individual patients by nuclear medicine imaging. This information can then be used to select patients most likely to benefit from RIT and determine patient-specific radioactivity levels required to deliver the desired radiation dose to tumor.[208] Second, unlike ADCs (antibody drug conjugates) and immunotoxins that kill only the targeted cell, the cytotoxic effects of radionuclides, summarized in a review,[209] can extend beyond the targeted cell and include self-irradiation, crossfire irradiation, and a bystander effect. Crossfire occurs because the range of most therapeutic radiation is multicellular, while the bystander effect can kill neighboring cells not directly traversed by radiation by a mechanism not fully understood.[210,211] Both can result in the destruction of adjacent cells not taking up the labeled antibody, helping to compensate for heterogeneities in antibody delivery, target molecule expression, or both.

Role of the radionuclide

An advantage of RIT is the potential to match the range of action of the radionuclide to the need to balance normal toxicity constraints and the desire to maximize homogeneity of tumor dose deposition for a given clinical application. Other factors that must be considered in the selection of radionuclides for RIT include (1) compatibility of physical half-life with antibody pharmacokinetics, (2) existence of labeling chemistry that provides acceptable stability, and (3) commercial availability of the radionuclide in a form suitable for clinical use. The characteristics of the radionuclides that have been most widely investigated for RIT and other targeted radiotherapy approaches have been discussed in a review.[212] The vast majority of RIT studies have utilized radionuclides decaying by the emission of β particles or α particles, which have tissue ranges of 1–10 mm and 50–90 μm, respectively. Recently, radionuclides that emit subcellular range (<1 keV) Auger electrons, originally thought to be cytotoxic only when localized in close proximity to the cell nucleus, have been evaluated.[213] However, at least one study suggests that Auger electron emitters may also be effective when delivered by noninternalizing antibodies.[214]

β emitters

Most clinical RIT trials and the only two FDA-approved RIT products involve radionuclides that decay by the emission of β particles. The cytotoxic effects of radiation agents depend largely on their linear energy transfer (LET), which is the amount of energy they deposit over a given distance. β Particles have an LET of approximately 0.2 keV/μm, are considered sparsely ionizing radiation, and produce mostly single-stranded DNA lesions that are readily repairable.[207] Given their path length in tissue, β emissions are most appropriate for treating tumors >0.5 cm because under these circumstances, most of their decay energy will be absorbed by the tumor and not neighboring normal tissues. Shorter-range β emitters such as ^{131}I, ^{177}Lu, and [67]Cu might be better in minimum residual disease settings because a greater fraction of their decay energy would be deposited within small tumor cell clusters. Conversely, more energetic, longer-range β emitters such as ^{90}Y and [186]Re could destroy larger tumor deposits and eliminate tumor cells that escape direct targeting owing to lack of antigen expression or poor vascularity.

α Emitters

α Particles generally have higher energies than β particles and exhibit very short path lengths (<100 μm) in tissue. α Particles have an LET of about 100 keV/μm, are densely ionizing, and produce clusters of DNA damage, including double-strand DNA breaks, which are difficult to repair.[207] Moreover, the cytotoxic effectiveness of α particles is largely independent of dose rate and oxygenation, offering the possibility of treating hypoxic tumor regions. Because of their short range, α emitters may be most effective in RIT directed against blood–borne tumor cells, micrometastatic disease, and cancer cells on the surface of cavities, such as ovarian carcinoma and neoplastic meningitis. α-Particle-emitting radionuclides that have been most widely investigated for use in RIT include 61-min [212]Bi, 46-min [213]Bi, 7.2-h [211]At, 10-day [225]Ac, and most recently, 18.7-day [227]Th.[215,216] The half-lives of [212]Bi and [213]Bi are so short that they complicate the logistics of antibody radiolabeling and patient management. The much longer half-lives of [225]Ac and [227]Th, while advantageous in terms of convenience and commercialization potential, are challenging from a radiochemistry perspective because strategies must be devised to maintain a stable link between the radionuclide and the antibody over a multi-week time course. This is complicated further by the need to trap multiple α-emitting daughter radionuclides with diverse chemistries in the tumor and avoid dose-limiting toxicities to normal tissues. For these reasons, the most widely used α emitter for labeling antibodies has been

[211]At.[217] Clinical RIT trials with α emitters will be described in a later section of this chapter.

Radioimmunotherapy of lymphoma

Hematological malignancies, particularly lymphomas, are attractive targets for RIT because of their inherent radiosensitivity. The only two RIT agents that have FDA approval are indicated for relapsed or refractory low-grade B-cell NHL (Table 2). These are ^{90}Y-ibritumomab tiuxetan and ^{131}I-tositumomab, which received clearance in 2002 and 2003, respectively. Both target the CD20 cell surface antigen that is expressed not only on about 95% of B-cell lymphoma but also on normal B cells. For this reason, an essential part of the treatment protocol is the administration of a relatively large dose of cold antibody in order to saturate normal B cell–binding sites before administration of the radiolabeled antibody. Standard protocols and other practical aspects for the use of these RIT agents have been described.[218,219]

[90]Y-ibritumomab tiuxetan (Zevalin®)

[90]Y-ibritumomab tiuxetan (Zevalin®) consists of the anti-CD20 murine monoclonal antibody parent of the chimeric antibody rituximab covalently linked to ^{90}Y via the MX-DTPA (tiuxetan) chelate. Initially, imaging the patient with ibritumomab labeled with another radiometal, ^{111}In, was performed to document acceptable antibody biodistribution before treatment with [90]Y.[220] A number of early studies demonstrated significantly enhanced therapeutic effectiveness for ^{90}Y-ibritumomab tiuxetan RIT compared with rituximab immunotherapy in patients with recurrent follicular lymphoma. In a randomized trial comparing ^{90}Y-ibritumomab tiuxetan and rituximab treatment in 143 patients with relapsed lymphoma, ^{90}Y-ibritumomab tiuxetan produced an 80% response rate compared with 56% with rituximab ($P = 0.002$).[221] Treatment of 54 patients with rituximab-refractory follicular NHL with ^{90}Y-ibritumomab tiuxetan resulted in an overall response rate of 74%, with 15% achieving complete remission.[222] Extended follow-up of 211 patients documented long-term responses of >12 months in 37% of patients with a median time to progression

Table 2 Approved radioimmunotherapy treatments for non-Hodgkin lymphoma.

Property	^{90}Y-Ibritumomab Tiuxetan	^{131}I-Tositumomab
Product name	Zevalin	Bexxar
Antibody for labeling	Ibritumomab	Tositumomab
Form	Murine IgG1	Murine IgG2a
Antibody for blocking	Chimeric rituximab	Murine tositumomab
Dose	250 mg/m²	450 mg
Therapy radionuclide	Yttrium-90 (^{90}Y)	Iodine-131 (^{131}I)
Half-life	2.7 days	8.1 days
Maximum beta energy	2.28 MeV	0.61 MeV
Maximum tissue range	11.3 mm	2.3 mm
γ Ray emission	No	Yes
Labeling method	Bifunctional chelate (tiuxetan)	Electrophilic radiohalogenation
Imaging radionuclide	Indium-111 (^{111}In)	Iodine-131 (^{131}I)
Role of imaging	Demonstrate acceptable biodistribution	Determine whole-body clearance kinetics
Patient-specific dosimetry	No	Yes
Administered activity	20–30 mCi	50–200 mCi
Parameter for dosing	mCi per kg body weight	Calculated whole-body dosimetry
Benchmark if platelets >150,000/mm³	0.4 mCi/kg	75 cGy
Benchmark if platelets 100,000–149,000/mm³	0.3 mCi/kg	65 cGy

in the long-term responder group of 29.3 months.[223] More recent trials have evaluated the therapeutic potential of ^{90}Y-ibritumomab tiuxetan in combination with high-dose chemotherapy protocols,[224] as consolidation after induction therapy, including in other forms of B-cell lymphoma,[225–228] and as a front-line monotherapy in patients with follicular lymphoma[229,230] with significant improvements in PFS and OS observed in most studies.

^{131}I-tositumomab (Bexxar®)

Clinical procedures with ^{131}I-tositumomab are similar to those for ^{90}Y-ibritumomab tiuxetan except that in order to minimize thyroid radiation dose resultant from dehalogenation of the radioiodinated antibody, a thyroid protective dose of potassium iodide (or Lugols solution) is administered before treatment.[231] In addition, injection of a 5 mCi dosimetry dose of ^{131}I-tositumomab is performed to determine the whole-body clearance rate in order to calculate total body dose—the antibody is then labeled with the ^{131}I activity estimated to yield a total body dose of 65 or 75 cGy, depending on whether the platelet count is above or below 150,000/mm^3. Objective response rates of 47–68% and complete response rates of 20–38% following ^{131}I-tositumomab treatment were reported in a long-term analysis of 250 heavily pretreated patients with indolent lymphoma.[232] For complete responders, the median duration of response after the last qualifying chemotherapy was 6.1 months, whereas the median duration of response after RIT was >47 months. These results were similar to those obtained with the chimeric anti-CD20 antibody rituximab when labeled with ^{131}I.[233] With regard to long-term follow-up, 6 of 12 patients with relapsed indolent lymphoma treated with ^{131}I-tositumomab remained disease free for a mean of 9.8 years after RIT.[234] RIT with ^{131}I-tositumomab at myeloablative doses followed by autologous stem cell infusion in relapsed/refractory NHL patients resulted in an overall response rate of 87% and median PFS of 47.5 months and OS of 101.5 months.[235] Finally, two recent phase III studies have shown similarly encouraging responses for single doses of ^{131}I-tositumomab and multiple doses of rituximab when combined with BEAM and CHOP chemotherapy for the treatment of relapsed DLBCL[236] and previously untreated follicular NHL,[237] respectively.

Despite the compelling response data obtained with Zevalin and Bexxar, neither RIT agent has become the standard first-line treatment for patients with lymphoma. Because of poor sales, Glaxo-SmithKline stopped selling Bexxar in February 2014, and there is speculation that Zevalin (Spectrum Pharmaceuticals) could suffer a similar fate. This situation can be attributed to a number of factors. Current regulations require radioactive drugs to be administered by nuclear medicine or radiation oncology staff, not by the oncologists who are responsible for the care of NHL patients. This results in a financial disincentive for oncologists who are paid to administer chemotherapy and rituximab but not RIT agents. Moreover, RIT is performed in the hospital setting, not in an outpatient facility, and performance of the low-radiation dose imaging study to determine patient-specific dosing complicates scheduling of other procedures. Finally, with these RIT treatments, there is a risk of developing secondary malignancies, leukemia, and myelodysplasia,[238] although in these heavily pretreated populations, other drugs likely contribute to these adverse effects.

Radioimmunotherapy of solid tumors

The successful treatment of solid tumors with RIT has been much more difficult to achieve owing to a number of factors, not the least of which is their lower sensitivity to radiation. With external beam radiation, doses as low as 4 Gy can be effective in lymphoma while

with solid tumors including breast, lung, prostate, colorectal, and pancreatic carcinoma as well as glioblastoma, clinical responses generally require doses ranging from 50 to 80 Gy.[239] That apoptosis is the predominant mechanism in cell killing in NHL, but not solid tumors, plays a role in their differential response to radiation.[207] Other barriers to effective treatment of solid tumors by RIT include accessibility of large intact antibodies in the face of tumor interstitial pressure and heterogeneous blood flow, and tumor hypoxia. The results of trials in patients with solid tumors have been summarized in two recent reviews,[240,241] and, in general, variable tumor responses were observed that were less impressive than those seen in hematological malignancies. Some of the most encouraging results have been obtained in minimum residual disease settings, which minimize the deleterious effects of heterogeneous dose deposition and are difficult to treat by conventional approaches. Examples of promising work are the treatment of colorectal cancer, prostate cancer, and brain tumors after surgical debulking.

Colorectal cancer

In a phase II study, the therapeutic efficacy of ^{131}I-labetuzumab, a humanized anticarcinoembryonic antigen (CEA) monoclonal antibody, was evaluated as an adjuvant treatment after salvage resection of liver metastases in patients with colorectal cancer.[242] Iodine-131 was utilized as the radiolabel because the relatively short range of its β-particles was considered a good match for the dimensions of micrometastatic disease. Twenty-three patients received 40–60 mCi/m^2 ^{131}I-labetuzumab and 19 were evaluated for response in comparison to a contemporaneous control group that did not receive RIT. At a median follow-up of 91 months, the median survival in patients receiving RIT was 58 months, compared with 31 months for the control group, with a 5-year survival of 42.1%.

Prostate cancer

J591 is a humanized monoclonal antibody specific for the extracellular domain of prostate-specific membrane antigen (PSMA) that has been labeled with ^{90}Y[243] and ^{177}Lu[244] and evaluated in phase I studies as a targeted radiotherapeutic in patients with metastatic castrate-resistant prostate cancer. The ^{177}Lu-labeled version was selected for phase II evaluation based on its lower β particle energy, resulting in less bone marrow toxicity and its emission of a γ ray that permits imaging.[245] A total of 47 patients were treated with 65 or 70 mCi/m^2 ^{177}Lu-J591; the lower dose resulted in 30% PSA declines in 13.3% of patients and a median survival of 11.9 months, while at the maximum tolerated dose, 30% PSA declines occurred in 46.9% of patients with a median survival of 21.8 months. Gamma camera imaging of ^{177}Lu activity distribution revealed that metastatic sites were targeted in 93.6% of patients.

Brain tumors

Because brain tumors in adults rarely metastasize outside the cranium, locoregional approaches for RIT can be utilized, where the labeled antibody is injected directly into a surgically created tumor resection cavity. More than 300 brain tumor patients have been treated to date with radiolabeled antibodies that bind to tenascin-C, an extracellular matrix glycoprotein that is overexpressed in >90% of GBM biopsies, with the level of expression increasing with advancing tumor grade.[246] Encouraging responses were obtained in a series of phase I and II trials with ^{131}I-labeled antitenascin 81C6 antibody in patients with both recurrent and newly diagnosed GBM. These were performed on a fixed radioactivity basis, as mandated by the FDA. In the most recent trial, the efficacy of ^{131}I-labeled 81C6 administered at the ^{131}I dose required to deliver an average radiation dose of 44 Gy to the 2-cm surgically created resection cavity was investigated.[247] The 44 Gy benchmark was based on analysis of prior fixed activity level protocols that demonstrated that this dose provided maximum tumor control without accompanying radionecrosis. Median OS in these newly diagnosed patients (16 GBM, 5 anaplastic astrocytoma) was 97 and 91 weeks for all patients and GBM patients, respectively.

Strategies for improved radioimmunotherapy

Particularly for the treatment of patients with solid tumors, improving RIT therapeutic outcomes will require the development of more sophisticated strategies both in terms of the antibody-based delivery vehicle and the nature of the radionuclide. A variety of enzymatically and genetically derived antibody fragments of varying size have been evaluated[248,249] with the goal of seeking the best balance between better tumor penetration and more rapid normal tissue clearance, achievable with smaller constructs and longer tumor residence time, generally better with intact IgG antibodies. Tumor vasculature plays an important role in that it provides an impediment to homogeneous antibody delivery, which might be overcome through the use of vascular disruptive agents such as combretastatin.[250] On the other hand, tumor vasculature provides an intriguing target for RIT, because damaging tumor blood vessels could increase the efficiency and homogeneity of treatment.[251] Two approaches for improving RIT that have received particular attention are pretargeting and α-particle-emitting radionuclides.

In pretargeting, the antibody is administered first, and after a delay period to achieve sufficient uptake in the tumor and normal tissue clearance, a radiolabeled lower molecular-weight compound is injected. By shifting the label from the antibody to a smaller molecule, enhanced tumor-to-normal tissue ratios and tumor radiation dose can be achieved.[252] Initial approaches used antibody-streptavidin conjugates followed by radiolabeled biotin, with or without an intermediate clearing agent[253]; however, immunogenicity and interference by endogenous biotin were confounding factors. A second pretargeting tactic that has also entered the stage of clinical investigation involves the use of bispecific antibodies that bind to a tumor-associated molecular target as well as to a small molecule or peptide containing a radiometal-chelate complex.[254] The feasibility of this approach has been evaluated in patients with recurrent medullary thyroid carcinoma.[255] Patients first received a bispecific anti-CEA antibody and then after 4 days, ^{131}I-labeled peptide bearing two hapten groups. Median OS was 110 months, significantly longer than that observed in untreated patients (61 months).

The most attractive feature of *α-particle-emitting radionuclides* for RIT is their markedly increased potency compared with other types of radiation. Studies in cell culture have demonstrated that human tumor cells can be killed after only a few α particles traverse a cell.[256] Furthermore, the cytotoxicity of α particles is nearly independent of dose rate, oxygen concentration, and cell-cycle stage.[207] While the conceptual advantages of α particles for RIT were known for a long time, practical investigation in patients required developments in radionuclide production, protein-labeling chemistry, and radiation dosimetry.

The first RIT clinical trial with an α-particle-emitting radionuclide involved *[213]Bi-labeled HuM195*, a humanized antibody reactive with the CD33 antigen that is overexpressed on human leukemia cells.[257] A phase I trial was conducted in 18 patients with relapsed and refractory AML or chronic myelomonocytic leukemia. Because of the 46-min half-life of [213]Bi, the labeled antibody was administered in multiple doses (3–7) in order to achieve the desired administered activity levels (602–3515 MBq). Absorbed dose ratios

between potential tumor sites (bone marrow, liver, and spleen) and whole body were about 1000 times higher than seen previously when this antibody was labeled with β emitters. Large leukemia volume reductions were achieved in many patients; however, no complete remissions were observed. A follow-up phase I/II trial evaluating the efficacy of [213]Bi-labeled HuM195 after partial cytoreductive chemotherapy with cytarabine reported complete remissions and partial responses in 6 of 25 patients. A phase I trial has recently been initiated of HuM195 labeled with the 10-day half-life α particle emitter [225]Ac.[258]

A phase 1 trial has been reported in which the pharmacokinetics and response to *[211]At-labeled chimeric 81C6 antitenascin* monoclonal antibody was evaluated in recurrent glioma patients after administration into surgically created tumor resection cavities.[259] The patient population consisted of 14 patients with GBM, 3 with anaplastic astrocytoma and 1 with anaplastic oligodendroglioma. Serial gamma camera imaging and blood counting demonstrated that the [211]At-labeled immunoconjugate was stable *in vivo* with $96.7 \pm 3.6\%$ of the decays occurring in the resection cavity. The median survival in patients with recurrent GBM was 54 weeks, markedly better than that obtained with conventional treatment (31 weeks). The survival of two of these recurrent GBM patients for 150 and 151 weeks is particularly encouraging and a clinical trial is planned with [211]At-labeled 81C6 antibody in newly diagnosedGBMpatients.

Therapy with targeted toxins

Targeted toxins are hybrid protein drugs that contain cell-binding domains and toxin domains. The cell-binding domain delivers the drug to the cell surface. After processing and/or internalization, the toxin domain triggers cell death. The toxins may create pores (proaerolysin) or catalytically inactivate cytosolic protein synthesis (diphtheria toxin, Pseudomonas exotoxin, or saporin). In some cases, specificity is provided by protease-specific cleavage sequences added to the toxin. A major challenge in the construction of targeted toxins is to identify target receptors or proteases that permit cell selective killing. Most of the agents consist of a single polypeptide, although several compounds have separate cell binding and effector/toxin peptides. Targeted toxins were designed to be clinically useful in patients with malignancies or other cell disorders that are resistant to standard cytotoxic or pathway inhibitor agents. None of the targeted toxins is absolutely tumor-specific, different side effects are observed dependent upon the binding or activation specificity and the particular toxin. While the synthesis and scaleup of such complex protein compounds are challenging, several agents have shown excellent clinical benefit with mild-moderate side effects in a range of human cancers and other chronic diseases. We will address only agents that are either approved or in middle-late stage clinical testing in humans. Pharmacokinetics, immune response, toxicities, and response are described for each—although many share common pharmacologic and toxicologic properties.

Targeted toxins for leukemia and lymphoma

Denileukin diftitox

Diphtheria toxin is a 58-kDa Mr protein with three domains. An *N*-terminal domain catalyzes ADP-ribosylation of elongation factor-2 (EF-2) that inactivates cellular protein synthesis leading to cell death. The middle domain is a hydrophobic domain, facilitating transfer of the catalytic domain to the cell cytosol. The *C*-terminal domain is a beta sheet-rich region that causes cell binding. Denileukin diftitox replaces the normal cell-binding domain with human IL-2. In the pivotal phase 3 study, patients with IB to IVA cutaneous T-cell lymphoma (CTCL) received 9 or 18 µg/kg/day IVC drug for 5 days every 3 weeks for up to 8 cycles.[260] The drug half-life was 30 min, and the side effects included an acute cytokine reaction (fever, chills, nausea, vomiting, myalgias, arthralgias, chest pain, and back pain), transient liver enzyme abnormalities (transaminasemia), and a vascular leak syndrome (hypotension, hypoalbuminemia, dyspnea, and edema). Most patients developed an immune response to the agent, but this did not correlate with toxicities or response. More responses were noted at 18 µg/kg versus 9 µg/kg. Clinical responses were seen in 30% of patients including 20% with partial responses and 10% with complete responses lasting a median of 6 months. In later follow-up, there were a number of patients with maintained responses over 2 years.[261] On the basis of these results, denileukin diftitox was approved for refractory CTCL. Denileukin diftitox also yields responses in T-cell NHL (48% response), CLL (27%), B-cell NHL (25%) and in isolated case reports in systemic mastocytosis, extranodal NK/T-cell lymphoma, peripheral T-cell lymphoma, subcutaneous panniculitis-like T-cell lymphoma, and adult T-cell leukemia.[262–269] Further, rare toxicities of thyrotoxicosis and vision loss have been reported.[270,271] Combination of denileukin diftitox with other agents such as cytotoxic drugs, rituximab, bexarotene, or electron beam radiation may enhance responses.[272,273] Currently, denileukin diftitox is not available for use owing to manufacturing problems.

Moxetumomab pasudotox

Pseudomonas exotoxin is a 68-kDa Mr polypeptide with an *N*-terminal cell-binding domain followed by an amphipathic helix-containing translocation domain and a *C*-terminal ADP-ribosylation domain. Pseudomonas exotoxin was altered to eliminate normal tissue binding by deleting amino acid residues 1–252 and 365–380; a disulfide-stabilized anti-CD22 Fv was fused to the 38-kDa Mr modified toxin (PE38). Then hot-spot mutagenesis was used to increase the affinity of the molecule. A threonine-histidine-tryptophan replaced serine-serine-tyrosine in the antigen-binding site of the heavy chain. Administration of moxetumomab pasudotox to 28 patients with hairy cell leukemia at doses of 5–30 µg/kg every other day 3 times for 1–16 cycles yielded no dose-limiting toxicities.[274] Side effects included grade 2 hemolytic uremic syndrome, hypoalbuminemia, transaminasemia, edema, headaches, hypotension, nausea, and fatigue. Only 5% of patients developed neutralizing antibodies beyond cycle 1. The overall response rate was 86% with 46% complete remissions. Median disease-free survival time exceeded 2 years. Moxetumomab pasudotox also produced remissions in ALL patients.

SL-401

The catalytic and translocation domains of diphtheria toxin were fused via a Met-His linker to human IL-3. SL-401 was administered IV over 15 min every other day for up to 6 doses to 45 patients with poor-risk, relapsed, or refractory acute myeloid leukemia or myelodysplasia.[275] Half-life was 30 min and peak levels were dose dependent. An interpatient dose escalation schema was used with doses from 4 to 12.5 µg/kg/dose. Dose-limiting toxicity was not observed, but side effects included transient transaminasemia, hypoalbuminemia, fever, chills, nausea, and vomiting. Antifusion protein antibodies occurred between day 15 and day 30 in most patients. Responses included one complete remission lasting 8 months and two partial remissions of 3 and 4 months duration. Separately, SL401 was given as 12.5 µg/kg IV over 15 min daily for

up to 5 doses to 11 patients with blastic plasmacytoid dendritic cell neoplasm.[276] Seven of the nine evaluable patients (78%) had major responses including five complete remissions and two partial remissions. The median duration of response was 5 months but 2 patients remain in remission for >2 years.

DT2219

The catalytic and translocation domain of diphtheria toxin was fused with bispecific scFv of antibodies targeting human CD19 and human CD22 to produce DT2219 that was administered as 2-h IV infusions every other day for 4 total doses from 0.5 to 80 µg/kg/day to 25 patients with mature or precursor B-cell lymphoid malignancies expressing CD19 and/or CD22.[277] Drug half-life was 1–2 h. Neutralizing antibodies developed in 30% of patients after 1 week. Dose-limiting toxicity was vascular leak syndrome. Other side effects included transient weight gain, edema, hypoalbuminemia, fever, fatigue, and transaminasemia. Maximal tolerated dose exceeds 80 µg/kg. Two patients achieved partial remissions lasting 2+ and 8+ months.

Resimmune

The catalytic and translocation domains of diphtheria toxin were fused to two single-chain antibody fragments reactive with an acidic loop on the extracellular domain of CD3ε. Resimmune was given as 15-min IV infusions twice daily for up to 4 days at doses of 2.5–11.25 µg/kg in an interpatient dose escalation to patients with CD3-positive lymphomas.[278] Dose-limiting toxicities were EBV reactivation and vascular leak syndrome. The maximal tolerated dose was 7.5 µg/kg. Other common adverse events were fever, chills, hypophosphatemia, and transaminasemia. Among 25 CTCL patients, there were 9 responses for a response rate of 36%. Median complete remission duration exceeds 5 years.

Targeted toxins for solid malignant and benign tumors

PRX302

The furin cleavage site of proaerolysin was modified to a prostate-specific antigen-selective cleavage site. Proaerolysin is a channel-forming bacterial protoxin that binds to ubiquitous cell surface receptors. The recombinant-modified proaerolysin, PRX302, was administered interstitially to 24 patients with locally recurrent prostate cancer after primary radiotherapy failure and to 92 patients with benign prostatic hyperplasia (BPH).[279,280] The drug was well tolerated in each study with only mild, transient local discomfort, and irritative urinary symptoms occurring in the first few days. Doses ranged from 0.03 to 3 µg/g tissue for prostate cancer and 0.6 µg/g tissue for BPH. Delivery was by a single ultrasound-guided transperineal intraprostatic injection. PSA decreased in 63% of prostate cancer patients, and prostatic symptoms improved in BPH patients. Median response duration in the BPH patients exceeded 1 year.

SS1P

The binding site-deleted Pseudomonas exotoxin PE38 fragment used to construct moxetumomab pasudotox was fused to an antimesothelin disulfide-stabilized Fv to create the recombinant immunotoxin, SS1P. SS1P was given as a 30-min IV infusion every other day for 3–6 doses to 34 patients with advanced mesothelioma, ovarian cancer, and pancreatic cancer at doses of 18–45 µg/kg/dose.[281] Dose-limiting toxicities were urticaria, vascular leak syndrome, and pleuritis. The maximal tolerated dose was 45 µg/kg on a three-dose schedule. There were 4/33 minor responses, and 19/33 stable disease. In a separate study, 24 patients with mesothelioma, ovarian cancer, or pancreatic carcinoma received 4–25 µg/kg/day SS1P by continuous infusion for 10 days.[282] The maximal tolerated dose was 25 µg/kg/day, and the dose-limiting toxicity was vascular leak syndrome. Immunogenicity was observed in 75 patients. Constant plasma levels of SS1P were maintained for 10 days with a median peak level of 153 ng/mL. One patient showed a partial response. Dramatic antimesothelioma activity for SS1P has been observed when combined with pentostatin plus cyclophosphamide or premetrexed plus cisplatin.[283,284] In the former case, 3/10 patients had major tumor responses. In the latter case, 12/20 patients exhibited partial remissions.

IL13-PE

IL13-PE is a recombinant cytotoxic consisting of human IL-13 fused to a truncated form of Pseudomonas exotoxin. Eight patients with metastatic adrenocortical carcinoma received 1 or 2 µg/kg of IL13-PE IV.[285] The mean peak serum concentration was 21 ng/mL and the half-life was 30 min. Five out of eight patients developed neutralizing antibodies within 14–28 days. Toxicities were thrombocytopenia and renal insufficiency. One patient showed stable disease.

Targeted toxins for cancer-associated illness

SP-SAP

The neuropeptide substance P was chemically conjugated to recombinant saporin. SP-SAP has been given to cancer patients with refractory pain in the lower half of the body.[286] A single intrathecal dose was administered via lumbar puncture over 2 min. To date, patients have received 1–16 µg. Dose escalation is proceeding, but transient pain reductions and reductions in opioid use have been observed.

Targeted toxins: conclusions

Toxicities appear predictable with targeted toxins. In cases where the receptor/antigen recognized by the targeted toxin is present on normal tissues, side effects related to the damaged normal tissue are observed. SS1P binds normal pleural surface mesothelin and yields pleuritis. Other toxicities are independent of ligand binding and are mediated by binding hepatocyte, vascular endothelia, and macrophage protein receptors. The nonspecific update of targeted toxins by these normal tissues produces transaminasemia, vascular leak syndrome, and acute infusion reactions. Prophylactic corticosteroids may ameliorate some of these toxicities.

Most of the targeted toxins have circulating half-lives of 30–120 min. Clearance occurs in the kidney and liver. Penetration of these drugs to extravascular sites is limited owing to their large size. Thus, higher response rates are seen in hematologic neoplasms with more accessible malignant cells. Immunogenicity of the targeted toxins has impacted pharmacokinetics and retreatment response rates in some of the studies.

Response rates are excellent for some of these agents—particularly in the setting of cytotoxic drug-resistant disease. The catastrophic death induced by toxins may trigger immune activation and be partly responsible for the long duration of remissions. Combinations of targeted toxins with other therapeutics with non-cross-resistant mechanisms of action and nonoverlapping toxicities offer additional hopes for clinical benefit.[287,288] Thus, the field retains an important niche in the anticancer drug armamentarium.

Key references

The complete reference list can be found on the Wiley Companion Digital Edition of this title (see inside front cover for login instructions).

1 Kohler G, Milstein C. Continuous cultures of fused cells secreting antibody of pre-defined specificity. *Nature.* 1975;**256**:495–497.

3 Teo EC, Chew Y, Phipps C. A review of monoclonal antibody therapies in lymphoma. *Crit Rev Oncol Hematol.* 2016;**97**:72–84.

6 Levy R. Karnofsky lecture: immunotherapy of lymphoma. *J Clin Oncol.* 1999;**17**:7–12.

7 Reichart, JM. http://www.antibodysociety.org/news/approved_mabs.php (accessed 11 December 2015).

11 Miller RA, Maloney DG, Warnke R, Levy R. Treatment of B-cell lymphoma with monoclonal anti-idiotype antibody. *N Engl J Med.* 1982;**306**:517–522.

23 Cheson BD, Leonard JP. Monoclonal antibody therapy for B-cell non-Hodgkin's lymphoma. *N Engl J Med.* 2008;**359**:613–626.

26 Coiffier B, Lepage E, Briere' E, et al. CHOP chemotherapy plus rituximab compared with CHOP alone in elderly patients with diffuse large B-cell lymphoma. *N Engl J Med.* 2002;**346**:235–242.

35 Robak T, Dmoszynska A, Solal-Celigny A, et al. Rituximab plus fludarabine and cyclophosphamide prolongs progression-free survival compared with fludarabine and cyclophosphamide alone in previously treated chronic lymphocytic leukemia. *J Clin Oncol.* 2010;**28**:1756–1765.

36 Dimopoulos MA, Anagnostopoulos A, Kyrtsonis MC, et al. Primary treatment of Waldenstrom macroglobulinemia with dexamethasone, rituximab, and cyclophosphamide. *J Clin Oncol.* 2007;**25**:3344–3349.

42 Mozessohn L, Chan KKW, Feld J, Hicks LK. Hepatitis B reactivation in HBsAg-negative/HBcAb-positive patients receiving rituximab for lymphoma: a meta-analysis. *J Viral Hepat.* 2015;**22**:842–849.

50 Hillmen P, Robak T, Janssens A, et al. Ofatumumab + chlorambucil versus chlorambucil alone in patients with untreated chronic lymphocytic leukemia (CLL): results of the phase III study complement 1 (OMB110911). *Blood.* 2013;**122**(21):528a.

52 Goede V, Fischer K, Busch R, et al. Obinutuzumab plus chlorambucil in patients with CLL and coexisting conditions. *N Engl J Med.* 2014;**370**:1101–1110.

56 Van Rhee F, Wong R, Nikhil M, et al. Siltuximab for multi-centric Castleman's disease: a randomised, double-blind, placebo-controlled trial. *Lancet Oncol.* 2014;**15**:966–974.

63 Cunningham D, Humblet Y, Siena S, et al. Cetuximab monoclonal and cetuximab plus irinotecan in irinotecan refractory metastatic colorectal cancer. *N Engl J Med.* 2004;**351**:337–345.

65 Jonker DJ, O'Callaghan CJ, Carpetis CS, et al. Cetuximab for treatment of colorectal cancer. *N Engl J Med.* 2007;**357**:2040–2048.

68 Van Cutsem E, Köhne CH, Láng I, et al. Cetuximab plus irinotecan, fluorouracil, and leucovorin as first-line treatment for metastatic colorectal cancer: updated analysis of overall survival according to tumor KRAS and BRAF mutation status. *J Clin Oncol.* 2011;**29**:2011–2019.

71 Bonner JA, Harari PM, Giralt J, et al. Radiotherapy plus cetuximab for squamous-cell carcinoma of the head and neck. *N Engl J Med.* 2006;**354**:567–578.

73 Vermorken JB, Mesia R, Rivera F. Platinum-based chemotherapy and cetuximab in head and neck cancer. *N Engl J Med.* 2008;**359**:1116–1127.

78 Giusti RM, Shastri K, Pilaro AM, et al. US food and drug administration approval: panitumumab for epidermal growth factor receptor-expressing metastatic colorectal carcinoma with progression following fluoropyrimidine, oxaliplatin, and irinotecan containing chemotherapy regimens. *Clin Cancer Res.* 2008;**14**:1296–1302.

82 Slamon DJ, Godolphin W, Jones LA, et al. Studies of the HER-2/neu protooncogene in human breast and ovarian cancer. *Science.* 1989;**244**:707–712.

85 http://investor.seattlegenetics.com/phoenix.zhtml?c=124860&p=irol-newsArticle&ID=2080061 (accessed 11 December 2015).

96 Slamon DJ, Leyland-Jones B, Shak S, et al. Use of chemotherapy plus a monoclonal antibody against HER2 for metastatic breast cancer that overexpresses HER2. *N Engl J Med.* 2001;**344**:783–792.

109 Bang YJ, Van Cutsem E, Feyereislova A. Trastuzumab in combination with chemotherapy versus chemotherapy alone for treatment of HER-2 positive advanced gastric or gastro-esophageal junction cancer (ToGA): a phase 3, open label, randomized controlled trial. *Lancet.* 2010;**376**:687–697.

119 Swain SM, Baselga J, Kim S-B, et al. Pertuzumab, trastuzumab and docetaxel in HER-2 positive metastatic breast cancer. *N Engl J Med.* 2015;**372**:724–734.

122 Yu AL, Gilman L, Oskaynak MF, et al. Anti-GD2 antibody with GM-CSF, interleukin-2, and isotretinoin for neuroblastoma. *N Engl J Med.* 2010;**363**:1324–1334.

128 Hurwitz H, Fehrenbacher L, Novotny W, et al. Bevacizumab plus irinotecan, fluorouracil, and leucovorin for metastatic colorectal cancer. *N Engl J Med.* 2004;**350**:2335–2342.

137 Sandler A, Gray R, Perry M, et al. Paclitaxel-carboplatin alone or with bevacizumab for non-small cell lung cancer. *N Engl J Med.* 2006;**355**:2542–2550.

144 Yang JC, Haworth L, Sherry RM, et al. A randomized trial of bevacizumab, an anti-vascular endothelial growth factor antibody, for metastatic renal cancer. *N Engl J Med*. 2003;**349**:427–434.

148 Gilbert MR, Dignam JJ, Armstrong TS, et al. A randomized trial of bevacizumab for newly diagnosed glioblastoma. *N Engl J Med*. 2014;**370**:699–708.

152 Burger RA, Brady MF, Bookman MA, et al. Gynecologic Oncology Group. Incorporation of bevacizumab in the primary treatment of ovarian cancer. *N Engl J Med*. 2011;**365**:2473–2483.

155 Pujade-Lauraine E, Hilpert F, Weber B, et al. Bevacizumab combined with chemotherapy for platinum-resistant recurrent ovarian cancer: the AURELIA open-label randomized phase III trial. *J Clin Oncol*. 2014;**32**:1302–1308.

156 Monk BJ, Pujade-Loraine E, Burger RA. Integrating bevacizumab into the management of epithelial ovarian cancer: the controversy of front-line versus recurrent disease. *Ann Oncol*. 2013;**24**(**supplement 10**):53–58.

159 Wilke H, Muro K, Van Cutsem E, et al. Ramucirumab plus paclitaxel versus placebo plus paclitaxel in patients with previously treated advanced gastric or gastro-oesophageal junction adenocarcinoma (RAINBOW): a double-blind, randomised phase 3 trial. *Lancet Oncol*. 2014;**15**:1224–1235.

165 Schadendorf D, Hodi FS, Rovert C, et al. Pooled analysis of long-term survival data from phase II and phase III trials of ipilimumab in unresectable or metastatic melanoma. *J Clin Oncol*. 2015;**33**:1889–1894.

167 Snyder A, Makarov V, Merghoub T, et al. Genetic basis for clinical response to CTLA-4 blockade in melanoma. *N Engl J Med*. 2014;**4**:2189–2199.

172 Robert C, Long GV, Brady B, et al. Nivolumab in previously untreated melanoma without BRAF mutation. *N Engl J Med*. 2015;**372**:320–330.

175 Postow MA, Chesney J, Pavlick A, et al. Nivolumab and ipilimumab in untreated melanoma. *N Engl J Med*. 2015;**372**:2006–2017.

176 Larkin J, Chiarion-Sileni V, Gonzalez R, et al. Combined nivolumab and ipilimumab in untreated melanoma. *N Engl J Med*. 2015;**373**:23–34.

177 Przepiorka D, Ko CW, Deisseroth A, et al. FDA approval: Blinatumomab. *Clin Cancer Res*. 2015;**21**:403555–403559.

202 Sievers EL, Larson RA, Stadtmauer EA, et al. Efficacy and safety of gemtuzumab ozogamicin in patients with CD33-positive acute myeloid leukemia in first relapse. *J Clin Oncol*. 2001;**19**:3244–3254.

207 Amiri-Kordestani L, Blumenthal GM, Xu QC, et al. FDA approval: ado-trastuzumab emtansine for the treatment of patients with HER2-positive metastatic breast cancer. *Clin Cancer Res*. 2014;**20**:4436–4441.

208 Sgorous G, Hobbs RF. Dosimetry for radiopharmaceutical therapy. *Semin Nucl Med*. 2014;**44**:172–178.

209 Pouget JP, Navarro-Teulon I, Bardies M, et al. Clinical radioimmunotherapy—the role of radiobiology. *Nat Rev Clin Oncol*. 2011;**8**:720–734.

211 Prise KM, O'Sullivan JM. Radiation-induced bystander signaling in cancer therapy. *Nat Rev Cancer*. 2009;**9**:351–360.

215 Huclier-Markai S, Alliot C, Varenot N, Cutler CS, Barbet J. Alpha-emitters for immuno-therapy: a review of recent developments from chemistry to clinics. *Curr Top Med Chem*. 2012;**12**:2642–2654.

218 Macklis RM, Pohlman B. Radioimmunotherapy for non-Hodgkin's lymphoma: a review for radiation oncologists. *Int J Radiat Oncol Biol Phys*. 2006;**66**:833–841.

233 Leahy MF, Turner JH. Radioimmunotherapy of relapsed indolent non-Hodgkin lymphoma with 131I-rituximab in routine clinical practice: 10-year single-institution experience of 142 consecutive patients. *Blood*. 2011;**117**:45–52.

248 Steiner M, Neri D. Antibody-radionuclide conjugates for cancer therapy: hisorical considerations and new trends. *Clin Cancer Res*. 2011;**17**:6406–6416.

259 Zalutsky MR, Reardon DA, Akabani G, et al. Clinical experience with alpha-particle emitting 211At: treatment of recurrent brain tumor patients with 211At-labeled chimeric antitenascin monoclonal antibody 81C6. *J Nucl Med*. 2008;**49**:30–38.

260 Olsen E, Duvic M, Frankel AE, et al. Pivotal phase III trial of two dose levels of denileukin diftitox for the treatment of cutaneous T-cell lymphoma. *J Clin Oncol*. 2001;**19**:376–388.

262 Dang NH, Hagemeister FB, Pro B, et al. Phase II study of denileukin diftitox for relapsed/refractory B-cell non-Hodgkin's lymphoma. *J Clin Oncol*. 2004;**22**:4095–4102.

274 Kreitman RJ, Tallman MS, Robak T, et al. Phase I trial of anti-CD22 recombinant immunotoxin moxetumomab pasudotox (CAT-8015 or HA22) in patients with hairy cell leukemia. *J Clin Oncol*. 2012;**30**:1822–1828.

276 Frankel AE, Woo JH, Ahn C, et al. Activity of SL-401, a targeted therapy directed to interleukin-3 receptor, in blastic plasmacytoid dendritic cell neoplasm patients. *Blood*. 2014;**124**:385–392.

281 Hassan R, Bullock S, Premkumar A, et al. Phase I study of SS1P, a recombinant anti-mesothelin immunotoxin given as a bolus IV infusion to patients with mesothelin-expressing mesothelioma, ovarian, and pancreatic cancers. *Clin Cancer Res*. 2007;**13**:5144–5149.

65 Vaccines and immunostimulants

Jeffery Schlom, PhD ▪ *James L. Gulley, MD, PhD, FACP* ▪ *James W. Hodge, PhD, MBA*

Overview

The U.S. Food and Drug Administration approvals of the prostate cancer therapeutic vaccine sipuleucel-T, the checkpoint inhibitor anti-CTLA-4 and anti-PD-L1/PD-1 monoclonal antibodies, along with the results of recent clinical studies involving cancer vaccines and other immunotherapeutics, have placed immunotherapy into the mainstream of the management of many cancer types. This chapter reviews the various cancer vaccine platforms now under clinical evaluation, the range of potential tumor-associated antigen vaccine targets, and the use of cancer vaccines in combination with so-called nonimmune standard-of-care therapies as well as other immunotherapeutics. The distinction in the clinical evaluation of cancer vaccines versus more conventional cytotoxic therapies is also discussed.

The U.S. Food and Drug Administration (FDA) approvals of (1) the prostate cancer therapeutic vaccine sipuleucel-T, (2) anti-CTLA-4 monoclonal antibody (MAb) ipilimumab for metastatic melanoma, and (3) the MAbs directed against the programmed death ligand 1 (PD-L1)/PD-1 immunosuppressive axis for the therapy of metastatic melanoma and lung carcinoma, along with the results of recent clinical studies involving immunotherapeutics, have placed immunotherapy into the mainstream of the management of many cancer types.

This chapter reviews the various cancer vaccine platforms now under clinical evaluation, the range of potential tumor-associated antigen (TAA) vaccine targets, and the use of cancer vaccines with so-called nonimmune standard-of-care therapies as well as other immunotherapeutics. The distinction in the clinical evaluation of cancer vaccines versus more conventional cytotoxic therapies is also discussed.

Targets for vaccine therapy

Many potential TAA targets for cancer immunotherapy have been identified. Targets of vaccine therapy need not be cell-surface proteins. When a molecule is a target for vaccine therapy, the activated T cells induced by vaccination recognize complexes of tumor antigen peptide and major histocompatibility complex (MHC) molecules on the cell surface. TAA vaccine targets can be grouped into several major categories (Table 1).

Tumor-specific antigens

Tumor-specific antigens (TSAs) comprise gene products that are uniquely expressed in tumors, such as point-mutated *ras* oncogenes, p53 mutations, and products of ribonucleic acid (RNA) splice variants and gene translocations. Three mutations at codon 12 represent the vast majority of *ras* mutations, which are found in approximately 20% to 30% of some human tumors.[1] Although the *ras* protein is not found on the cell surface, one can envision vaccine therapy directed against peptide–MHC complexes on the cell surface. Indeed, there have been clinical trials in pancreatic carcinoma that target *ras*.[2,3] B-cell lymphomas overexpress a single immunoglobulin (Ig) variant on their cell surface; therefore, each B-cell lymphoma displays a unique target for immunotherapy.[4–6] The gene products of RNA splice variants and deoxyribonucleic acid (DNA) translocations also represent unique fusion proteins that can be specific targets for immunotherapy, including c-erb-B2 RNA splice variants and the bcr/abl product of DNA translocation of chronic myelogenous leukemia.

Several viruses are associated with the etiology of some cancers. An excellent example of this is the connection between human papillomavirus (HPV) and cervical cancer. This has led to FDA approval of the HPV vaccine for prevention of cervical cancer.[7]

Tumor-associated antigens

TAAs can be categorized into three major groups: oncofetal antigens, oncogene products, and tissue-lineage antigens (Table 1). Oncofetal antigens, normally found during fetal development, are greatly downregulated after birth. This class of antigens, which includes prostate-specific membrane antigen (PSMA), carcinoembryonic antigen (CEA), and the cancer mucin MUC-1, are often overexpressed in tumors compared with normal tissues. The MUC-1 TAA is overexpressed in the majority of human carcinomas and several hematologic malignancies. Much attention has been paid to the hypoglycosylated variable number of tandem repeats (VNTR) region of the N-terminus of MUC-1 as a vaccine target. While previous studies have described MUC-1 as a tumor-associated tissue differentiation antigen, studies have now determined that the C-terminus of MUC1 is an oncoprotein, and its expression is an indication of poor prognosis in numerous tumor types.[8]

Oncogene and suppressor gene products, such as nonmutated HER2/*neu* and p53, are analogous to oncofetal antigens in that they can be overexpressed in tumors and may be expressed in some fetal and normal tissues. Similarly, telomerase, an enzyme important in cellular replication and chromosomal stability, is overexpressed in malignant cells as compared with most normal cells. Epitopes derived from human telomerase have been reported and presumably may be overexpressed by neoplastic cells.[9]

Tissue-lineage antigens such as prostate-specific antigen (PSA) and the melanocyte antigens MART-1/Melan A, tyrosinase, gp100, and TRP-1/gp75 are usually expressed in a tumor of a given type and the normal tissue from which it is derived. Tissue-lineage antigens are potentially useful targets for immunotherapy if the normal organ/tissue in which they are expressed is not essential, such as the prostate, breast, or melanocyte.

Holland-Frei Cancer Medicine, Ninth Edition. Edited by Robert C. Bast Jr., Carlo M. Croce, William N. Hait, Waun Ki Hong, Donald W. Kufe, Martine Piccart-Gebhart, Raphael E. Pollock, Ralph R. Weichselbaum, Hongyang Wang, and James F. Holland.
© 2017 John Wiley & Sons, Inc. ISBN: 978-1-118-93469-2

Table 1 Spectrum of current and potential therapeutic cancer vaccine targets.

Target type	Examples
Tumor-associated antigens	
Oncofetal antigen	CEA, MUC-1
Stem cell/EMT	Brachyury, SOX-2, OCT-4, TERT, CD44^high/CD24^lo, CD133+
Oncogene	MUC-1 C terminus, p53, EGFR, HER2/neu, WT1
Cancer—testes	MAGE-A3, BAGE, SEREX-defined, NY-ESO, survivin
Tissue lineage	PAP, PSA, gp100, tyrosinase, glioma antigen
Glycopeptides	STn-KLH
Anti-angiogenic	VEGF-R
Tumor-specific antigens	
Oncogene	point mutated: ras, B-raf, frame shift mutations, undefined unique tumor mutations
Viral	HPV, HCV
B-cell lymphoma	Anti-id

BAGE, B melanoma antigen; CEA, carcinoembryonic antigen; EMT, epithelial–mesenchymal transition; gp100, glycoprotein 100; HCV, hepatitis C virus; HPV, human papillomavirus; MAGE-A3, melanoma-associated antigen-A3; MUC-1, mucin 1; NY-ESO, New York esophageal carcinoma antigen 1; OCT-4, octamer-binding transcription factor 4; PAP, prostatic acid phosphatase; PSA, prostate-specific antigen; SOX-2, (sex-determining region Y)-box-2; STn-KLH, sialyl-Tn-keyhole limpet hemocyanin; TERT, telomerase reverse transcriptase; VEGF-R, vascular endothelial growth factor receptor; WT-1, wild-type 1.

Antigens associated with driving EMT, the metastatic process and drug resistance

The most provocative potential targets for vaccine therapy are those molecules associated with cancer "stem cells" and/or the epithelial-mesenchymal transition (EMT) process, both of which are associated with drug resistance. Drivers of EMT are also associated with tumor cell extravasation and intravasation to the metastatic site. Recent studies have described the plasticity of the so-called cancer stem cells and the similarities between cells undergoing EMT and the acquisition of "stemness" characteristics.[10] Gene products associated with EMT and cancer "stemness" are SOX-2, OCT-4, and carcinoma cells with the phenotype CD44^high/CD24^lo, and/or are CD133+.[11–15] Each of these gene products is currently being evaluated for immunogenicity in terms of generating human T-cell responses *in vitro*, but some also have a relatively broad range of expression in some normal adult tissues. The T-box transcription factor brachyury has recently been identified as a major driver of EMT.[16] It has been shown to be selectively expressed on both primary and metastatic lesions of several carcinoma types. Vaccines that have the ability to generate human T cells capable of lysing a range of human carcinoma cells have been developed.[17] Vaccines are currently in clinical trials to target gene products associated with EMT and cancer cells with "stemness" characteristics.[18–20]

Types of vaccines

Numerous vaccine-delivery platforms have been analyzed in experimental models and many of these are now being evaluated in the clinic (Table 2). Each of these platforms has advantages and disadvantages. Some of these modalities may eventually prove to be most beneficial when used in combination or in tandem.

Whole-tumor-cell vaccines

The major advantage of using whole-tumor-cell vaccines is that tumor-cell-mutated TSAs and TAAs, some identified and most as yet undefined, may be present in the vaccine preparation. The two types of whole-tumor-cell vaccine platforms being examined

clinically are (1) autologous (i.e., manipulating the tumor from a patient into a vaccine for that patient) and (2) allogeneic, in which tumor cells from other patients, usually from established tumor cell lines, are used. Preparing an autologous tumor cell vaccine requires an enormous amount of effort, as fresh tumor needs to be obtained at surgery and prepared in a similar manner for each patient. Due to the considerable variability of tumors among patients, and costs associated with custom vaccine production, most current whole-tumor-cell vaccine approaches have centered on the use of allogeneic cell lines and cell banks.[21–26] Moreover, the cell lines used in the preparations can be infected with vectors that express cytokine genes such as granulocyte-macrophage colony-stimulating factor (GM-CSF)[27] or other immunostimulatory transgenes[28] to enhance the immunogenicity of the tumor cell. Studies employing tumor cell lines transfected to express GM-CSF have met with some success in treating pancreatic cancer and other tumor types.[24–27,29,30]

Direct injection of cytokine genes or costimulatory molecule genes into tumor (in situ autologous whole tumor cell vaccines)

Two signals are required for the efficient activation of T cells. The first signal is mediated through a peptide–MHC complex on the cell surface of the antigen-presenting cell (APC), which binds to the T-cell receptor (TCR) on the surface of the T cell. The second signal involves the interaction of a T-cell costimulatory molecule on the surface of the APC with its ligand on the surface of the T cell. To date, the most studied of the T-cell costimulatory molecules is B7-1, which interacts with two ligands on the T-cell surface: CD28 for upregulation of T-cell function and CTLA-4 for downregulation of T-cell function. Numerous preclinical studies show that the addition of B7-1 to a weakly immunogenic tumor will make it more immunogenic.[28] This phenomenon has also occurred when other costimulatory molecules, such as intercellular adhesion molecule (ICAM)-1 and lymphocyte function-associated antigen (LFA)-3, have been added to tumors. Thus, one can envision the direct injection of a vector expressing one or more costimulatory molecules into a tumor mass to induce an antitumor immune response. The advantage of this direct-injection approach is that the "vaccine" is the patient's own tumor, which may express unique mutated TSAs or TAAs. In clinical studies, vaccinia- and avipox-based recombinants expressing the B7-1 costimulatory molecule have been directly injected into melanoma or carcinoma lesions.[31] A clinical study has been reported with interesting findings in which recombinant vectors containing a triad of costimulatory molecules (B7-1, ICAM-1, and LFA-3; designated TRICOM) were directly injected into melanoma tumor lesions.[32,33] Cytokines can also be introduced into the tumor mass using vectors as delivery vehicles, as in the case of a recombinant vaccinia virus expressing GM-CSF directly injected into melanoma lesions.[34]

Peptides

Most peptides used to induce an immune response are from TSAs or TAAs and are approximately 8 to 11 amino acids in length. These peptides can bind with the appropriate class of the MHC molecule on the APC surface. These MHC-restricted responses are thus effective only if the appropriate MHC allele is present in a patient. The most studied MHC restriction element in the human population is the MHC class I allele, human leukocyte antigen (HLA)–A2, which is found in approximately 50% of the Caucasian population.

Using peptides as immunogens has some advantages: (1) preparation is relatively easy and affordable; (2) because the immunogen is extremely well-defined, the immune response can be analyzed

Table 2 Spectrum of current vaccine platforms in phase II/III clinical studies.

Vaccine platform	Example	Cancer type
Peptides/proteins		
Peptide	gp100, MUC-1, HER2/neu	Melanoma, lung
Protein	MAGE-A3, NY-ESO	Melanoma
Antibody	Anti-idiotype	Lymphoma
Glycoproteins	sTn-KLH	Melanoma
Recombinant vectors		
Adenoviruses	Adeno-CEA, alpha-CEA	Carcinoma
Poxvirus	Vaccinia virus, MVA, fowlpox, (PROSTVAC)	Prostate
Saccharomyces cerevisiae (yeast)	Yeast-CEA	Pancreatic
Listeria	Listeria-mesothelin	Pancreatic
Tumor cells		
Allogeneic	GVAX (+ GM-CSF)	Pancreatic
Dendritic cell/autologous tumor cell fusions		Myeloma
Autologous	Adeno-CD40L, colon (BCG)	Chronic lymphocytic leukemia, colon, melanoma
Dendritic cells/APCs		
Dendritic cell–peptide	Glioma peptides	Glioma, melanoma
Dendritic cells–vector infected	rV, rF-CEA-MUC1-TRICOM (Panvac-DC)	Colorectal
APC-protein	Sipuleucel-T (PAP-GM-CSF)	Prostate

APC, antigen-presenting cell; BCG, Bacillus Calmette–Guerin adjuvant; CD40L, CD40 ligand; CEA, carcinoembryonic antigen; gp100, glycoprotein 100; GM-CSF, granulocyte macrophage colony-stimulating factor; MAGE-A3, melanoma-associated antigen 3; MUC-1, mucin 1; NY-ESO, New York esophageal carcinoma antigen 1; PAP, prostatic acid phosphatase; PSA, prostate-specific antigen; rF, recombinant fowlpox; rV, recombinant vaccinia; STn-KLH, sialyl-Tn-keyhole limpet hemocyanin.

in several ways and quantitated; and (3) peptides can be modified to be more immunogenic in the form of peptide agonists. The same property that makes a peptide vaccine attractive—its specificity—can also be a disadvantage. For example, a CTL (cytotoxic T-lymphocyte) epitope peptide may induce a CTL response that is short lived because of the lack of help provided by helper peptides. Moreover, peptides are useful only in the vaccination of patients who have that specific allele. Some peptide vaccines under study include HPV,[35] ras,[36,37] HER-2/neu,[38] MAGE,[39] MART-1, tyrosinase,[40] gp100,[41,42] CEA,[43] MUC-1,[44] and PSMA[45,46] among others.[47]

Agonist peptides
Peptide agonists fall into two general categories. In the first category, amino acids of the peptide that bind to the MHC are modified. More vigorous MHC binding (i.e., higher affinity for the MHC molecule) often leads to the generation of a more vigorous T-cell response. Examples of this are the alterations in the brachyury, gp100 melanoma, and MUC-1 peptides.[8,41,48] The second category of agonist has been termed a TCR agonist. In this case, an amino acid of the peptide that interacts with the TCR on the T cell is modified; this can also result in a more vigorous induction of the T-cell response. An example of this is the generation of the TCR agonist for CEA.[49]

Anti-idiotypes
The idiotypic network is involved in the control of immune regulation. B-cell lymphomas present unique Igs on their cell surface, which make exquisite targets for immunotherapy. For this malignancy, anti-idiotype (Id) MAb vaccines have been quite successful clinically.[4,5,50–55] But the specificity inherent in these vaccine strategies is both an advantage and a disadvantage; different B-cell lymphomas will display unique Ids on their cell surface, making their preparation for each patient labor intensive.[56]

Vectors
Vectors are among the more flexible means of vaccine delivery. Several major platforms of both viral and bacterial vectors are now in

use in the clinic (Table 2). Each vector category and type has its own potential advantages and disadvantages. Review articles have been published on the potential merits of these vectors.[57–63] In general, the advantage of a vector-based vaccine is that (1) multiple genes (including genes for costimulatory molecules and cytokines) can be inserted into some types of vectors; (2) the relative cost of production is low compared to the preparation and purification of proteins or whole-tumor-cell vaccines; (3) many vectors have the ability to infect professional APCs so that the antigens they express can be processed; and (4) viral and bacterial vectors are composed of prokaryotic proteins that act as natural vaccine adjuvants in stimulating the host immune response. The disadvantage of some, but not all, vectors is the development of host-induced immunity to the vector itself, thus limiting its continued use.

Viral vectors
One of the most studied groups of vaccine vectors is the poxvirus group. Vaccinia virus, which was derived from a benign pox disease in cows, has been administered to more than 1 billion people and is responsible for the worldwide eradication of smallpox.[64] As a result, smallpox vaccinations in the United States and most Western countries were halted approximately 40 years ago. However, most cancer patients are older than 40 and, therefore, have some level of pre-existing immunity to vaccinia virus. For this reason, recombinant vaccinia viruses cannot be given multiple times in vaccine protocols. The poxvirus family contains the replication-incompetent modified vaccinia Ankara (MVA), a derivative of vaccinia virus.[57] MVA is thought of as a safer alternative to the smallpox vaccine because it can infect mammalian cells but cannot replicate.[65] Other replication-defective members of the poxvirus family are the avipox vectors (fowlpox and canarypox/ALVAC).[58] These avipox vectors infect human cells and express their transgenes for 2 to 3 weeks before cell death; they are incapable of reinfecting cells. Clinical studies have shown that avipox-based CEA vectors can be given to patients numerous times with a resulting increase in CEA-specific T-cell responses.[47,66] Preclinical and clinical studies[47,67–69] show that optimal use of recombinant vaccinia or MVA may be to prime the immune response, followed by boost vaccinations with other

vectors such as replication-defective pox vectors, peptides, or DNA. Advantages of using vaccinia virus or the replication-incompetent MVA avipox are (1) large amounts of foreign DNA can be inserted into the vector and (2) proteins expressed in poxviruses are more immunogenic than the native protein, which is most likely a result of the inflammatory responses triggered against highly immunogenic poxvirus proteins. Several clinical trials with recombinant poxviruses containing TAAs such as CEA, MUC-1, PSA, and HPV have been completed and others are ongoing.

Adenovirus has also been proposed as a vector in recombinant vaccine design because its viral genome can be altered to accept foreign genes that are stably integrated. To produce recombinant adenovectors, endogenous viral DNA sequences are typically deleted from replication-competent regions, which results in an attenuated form of the virus with potentially improved safety. A new viral vector gene delivery platform, adenovirus serotype-5 (Ad5) [E1-, E2b-],[70–79] has been described. The platform consists of a replication-defective Ad5 in which portions of the early 1 (E1), early 2 (E2b), and early 3 (E3) gene regions have been deleted; the deletions have been reported to result in a dramatic decrease of late gene expression, which results in a marked reduction in host inflammatory responses and anti-Ad host responses. Human cells transfected with these adenovirus constructs were shown to express the encoded transgene(s) for prolonged times *in vivo* compared to other adeno vector platforms. In a Phase I/II clinical trial, cohorts of patients with metastatic colorectal cancer (mCRC) were vaccinated with escalating doses of the Adeno platform carrying a gene for CEA. CEA-directed T-cell responses were induced and patients exhibited evidence of a favorable survival probability.[80]

Yeast and bacterial vectors

One advantage of recombinant *Saccharomyces cerevisiae* as a vaccine vehicle is its lack of toxicity. Besides being inherently nonpathogenic, this particular species of yeast can be heat killed before administration and has been shown to be safe in humans in several clinical trials, with maximum tolerated dose not reached.[63,81,82] *S. cerevisiae* can be easily engineered to express one or more antigens in large quantities, can be propagated and purified rapidly, and is very stable.[83] In addition, recombinant yeast has been shown to induce a robust host immune response to non-self-antigens.[19,63,83–86]

Bacterial vectors, such as *Salmonella*[87,88] and *Listeria*,[62] have the advantage of tropism for professional APCs, such as macrophages. While these vectors are potentially virulent in humans, several attenuated strains have been developed for human use. From a clinical perspective, both recombinant *Salmonella* and recombinant *Listeria monocytogenes*-based vectors may be administered orally.

Plasmid DNA

Polynucleotide vaccines are easy to prepare, but the mode of action of these vectors in inducing an immune response is not fully understood because most studies have involved intramuscular inoculations, and it is not known how antigens get to professional APCs. Many preclinical and clinical studies using infectious disease agents and cancer antigens have been carried out with DNA vectors.[89–92]

Dendritic cell vaccines

The dendritic cell (DC) is considered the most potent APC and, therefore, one of the most attractive means of immunization.[93,94] DCs can be employed by (1) loading with a peptide, protein, or anti-Id Ab, (2) infecting with a viral vector, (3) loading with apoptotic bodies from tumor cells, or (4) fusing with a tumor cell.[95–98]

The major disadvantages of this approach are the great cost and effort involved. Large amounts of peripheral blood mononuclear cells (PBMCs) must be obtained from patients via leukapheresis. The PBMCs must then be cultured for several days in the presence of cytokines such as GM-CSF, IL-4, and/or TNF-α, and then reinfused into the patient. This must be done for each patient. A successful strategy, approved by the FDA, involves immunization with autologous DCs loaded *ex vivo* with a recombinant fusion protein consisting of the tumor antigen prostatic acid phosphatase (PAP) linked to GM-CSF for patients with metastatic prostate cancer, as is discussed below.

Combination of vaccines

Although each of the various methods of immunization described has advantages and disadvantages, the most effective immunization protocol may involve priming with one type of immunogen and boosting with another. This method may be advantageous because (1) two different arms of the immune system may be enhanced by using two different modalities (i.e., CD4+ and then CD8+ T cells); (2) one methodology may be more effective in priming naive cells while another modality may be more effective in enhancing memory cell function; and (3) some of the most effective methods of immunization, like the use of recombinant vaccinia virus or adenoviruses, can be used only a limited number of times because of host anti-vector responses. These vectors may be most effective when used as priming agents, followed by boosts with other agents. Numerous preclinical and clinical studies demonstrate the advantages of diversified prime-and-boost protocols.[47,66,67,99–103]

Non-specific immune stimulants

TAAs and TSAs are, by definition, weak immunogens because tumors develop, persist, and grow in the presence of an intact immune system. Conventional adjuvants such as incomplete Freund's adjuvant (IFA) will allow the immunogen to be maintained at the injection site (the so-called depot effect) so that infiltrating APCs and effector cells can initiate a more vigorous immune response. Immunostimulants also work by crossing membrane barriers. In this case, proteins must be taken up by professional APCs and presented in the context of MHC molecules for effective presentation to the immune system. Adjuvants with lipophilic components and liposomes[104] facilitate this process.

Microbial products such as those present in certain adjuvants (i.e., IFA), bacillus Calmette–Guerin adjuvant (BCG), and even viral vectors also are potent activators of DCs, partly because they contain agonists of toll-like receptors (TLRs). TLRs are expressed by DCs and other innate immune cell types and comprise a family of approximately 10 to 15 receptors.[105,106] Activation of DC via their TLRs augments expression of adhesion, chemokine, and chemokine receptor molecules, which, in turn, regulate cellular trafficking to sites of inflammation and pathogenic encounters. Thus, the biological consequences of TLR engagement lead to inflammation, characterized by the recruitment of key immune and nonimmune effector cells to mediate pathogen destruction. In regard to TLR agonists, CpG motifs constitute the most studied of these sequences.[107–110]

In addition, certain cytokines and chemokines have been shown to enhance the level of APC and/or effector cell function either locally or systemically. For example, GM-CSF has been reported to enhance antigen-specific T-cell responses, delayed-type hypersensitivity reactions, and antitumor responses.[111–120] Clinical studies using GM-CSF along with protein immunogens have shown an enhancement of the antigen-specific immune response.[50,121] Flt-3L administration has been shown to enhance the number of DCs systemically, both in animal models and clinically.[122,123] Finally, several cytokines and chemokines have been shown to play a critical role in enhancing T-cell function.[124–128] The most studied of these is IL-2.[129,130] When used as a single agent, IL-2 has been shown to have antitumor effects in melanoma and renal cell carcinoma (RCC) patients[129,131] and, as recently reported, to enhance the effectiveness of melanoma-based peptide vaccines.[41] Other cytokines, such as IL-7, IL-12, and IL-15, have been shown to enhance T-cell responses and antitumor activity in experimental models and may have more potential clinical utility than IL-2.[125,132–134]

One strategy for improving the safety of proinflammatory cytokines, such as IL-2 and IL-12, is to direct their delivery to tumors via fusion to a tumor-targeting antibody. Such antibody-cytokine fusion proteins, or "immunocytokines," have previously demonstrated the ability to enhance antitumor immunity in preclinical models.[135] To maximize immunocytokine tolerability, the antibody selected as a vehicle must bind specifically to an antigen found in tumors. A tumor-targeted IL-12 immunocytokine, called NHS-IL12, was engineered by genetically fusing two human IL-12 heterodimers to the C-termini of the heavy chains of the NHS76 antibody. NHS-IL12 was superior to recombinant IL-12 when evaluated as an antitumor agent in three murine tumor models. In preclinical studies combining NHS-IL12 treatment with a cancer vaccine, radiation, or chemotherapy resulted in greater antitumor effects than each individual therapy alone.[136]

Vaccine clinical trials

Below is a representative description of prior and ongoing vaccine clinical trials.

Prostate cancer

PAP, which is expressed on over 95% of prostate cancer cells, has been used as a target of the vaccine sipuleucel-T, also called Provenge® (PAP-GM-CSF-pulsed APCs). After early clinical trials of the sipuleucel-T vaccine demonstrated safety, larger trials were conducted in asymptomatic or minimally symptomatic metastatic castration-resistant prostate cancer (mCRPC). A Phase III trial[137] was conducted with overall survival (OS) as the endpoint, enrolling more than 500 patients. No change in time to progression (TTP) was seen, but OS was improved in the vaccine arm (25.8 months vs 21.7 months; $p = 0.032$). In April 2010, the FDA approved sipuleucel-T for the treatment of minimal or nonsymptomatic mCRPC. A second prostate cancer vaccine has also been evaluated in this same prostate cancer population. This "off-the-shelf" platform (PROSTVAC) consists of a recombinant vaccinia prime and multiple fowlpox booster vaccinations. Each vector contains transgenes for PSA and three costimulatory molecules (B7-1, ICAM-1 and LFA-3, designated TRICOM).[138,139] A randomized placebo-controlled 43-center Phase II trial enrolled 125 minimally symptomatic mCRPC patients.[140] Similar to the experience with sipuleucel-T, PROSTVAC did not alter TTP, yet improved median OS relative to placebo (control vector), 25.1 versus 16.6 months. Patients receiving PROSTVAC also had a 44% reduction in death rate compared to the control cohort ($p = 0.0061$).[140] The median OS in a second single-arm Phase II study[141] was 26.6 months, similar to the larger PROSTVAC randomized trial. A global Phase III placebo-controlled trial of PROSTVAC in patients with minimally symptomatic prostate cancer ($n = 1298$) has now completed accrual. The endpoint is OS.

A recent review[142] analyzed the immune impact induced by PROSTVAC (PSA-TRICOM) in prostate cancer patients. Of 104 patients tested for T-cell responses, 57% demonstrated an increase in PSA-specific T cells 4 weeks after vaccine, and 68% of patients mounted post-vaccine immune responses to TAAs not present in the vaccine (antigen spreading/antigen cascade). Measurements of systemic immune response to PSA may underestimate the true therapeutic immune response (as this does not account for cells that have trafficked to the tumor) and does not include antigen spreading/antigen cascade (as described below). Furthermore, although the entire PSA gene is the vaccine, only one epitope of PSA is evaluated in the T-cell responses. Because this vaccine is directed at generating a cellular/Th1 immune response, less than 0.6% of patients tested had evidence of PSA antibody induction following vaccine. Active surveillance is becoming an increasingly utilized approach in men diagnosed with "low-risk" prostate cancer. A randomized, multicenter, placebo-controlled study of PROSTVAC vaccination versus active surveillance in patients with newly diagnosed clinically localized prostate cancer is under way. The endpoints of this study will be the changes in immune infiltrate and tumor extent at the 12-month biopsy versus initial biopsy.

GVAX, a GM-CSF-secreting vaccine, is an admixture of two prostate cancer cell lines that have been transduced with a replication-defective retrovirus for GM-CSF expression. In two separate multicenter Phase II trials, patients with asymptomatic CRPC given GVAX had a median survival of 26.2–35.0 months.[24,143] By estimating predicted survival based on a commonly used nomogram,[144] patients in both trials exceeded anticipated survival by > 6 months.[145]

Nineteen HLA-A2-positive patients with rising PSA without detectable metastatic disease or local recurrence received a vaccine containing 11 HLA-A*0201-restricted and two HLA class II synthetic peptides derived from prostate carcinoma tumor antigens subcutaneous (s.c.) for 18 months or until PSA progression. PSA doubling time of 4/19 patients (21%) increased from 4.9 to 25.8 months during vaccination.[146] A Phase II adenovirus/PSA vaccine trial was conducted in patients with recurrent or hormone refractory prostate cancer. The majority of the patients demonstrated anti-PSA T-cell responses above pre-injection levels. Sixty-four percent of the patients demonstrated an increase in PSA doubling time.[147] Clinical trials have also been carried out using peptide-pulsed DCs loaded with peptides of human PSMA,[148–150] as well as DCs transfected with PSA tumor RNA.[151] In these studies, antigen-specific immune responses have been observed and some decreases in serum PSA have also been noted.

Melanoma

The vast majority of vaccine clinical trials have been conducted in patients with melanoma because (1) interferon (IFN) and IL-2 have both shown clinical responses in melanoma; (2) melanoma lesions often are readily accessible and thus can be studied for immune infiltrate and cells from melanoma lesions can be grown in culture to obtain both tumor cells and tumor-infiltrating lymphocytes (TILs); and (3) numerous melanoma-associated antigens have been identified.

Clinical trials have been conducted using various peptides derived from melanoma-associated antigens, including tyrosinase, MART-1, gp100, Melan-A (a modified gp100 epitope[152]), and members of the MAGE family.[152–157] Vaccination-induced immune responses as well as clinical benefits were reported. Newer approaches have combined these peptides with GM-CSF emulsified in Montanide ISA-51.[158] Another peptide approach is vaccination with autologous tumor-derived heat shock protein/peptide complexes.[159] Immune responses and clinical responses have also been observed using melanoma peptide vaccination in conjunction with anti-CTLA-4,[160] melanoma peptide-pulsed DCs,[94,154] tumor RNA-transfected DCs,[161] and intratumoral administration of autologous DCs.[162] A randomized Phase III study showed no benefit using an autologous peptide-pulsed DC vaccine compared to dacarbazine in first-line treatment of patients with metastatic melanoma.[163]

A randomized Phase III trial was conducted involving 185 patients with stage IV or locally advanced stage III cutaneous melanoma, expression of HLA*A0201, and suitability for high-dose IL-2 therapy. Patients were randomly assigned to receive IL-2 alone or gp100 plus IFA, followed by IL-2. The vaccine–IL-2 group, as compared with the IL-2-only group, had a significant improvement in overall clinical response (16% vs 6%, $p = 0.03$).The median OS was also longer in the vaccine–IL-2 group than in the IL-2-only group (17.8 months vs 11.1 months; $p = 0.06$).[164] In a multicenter randomized trial, 175 patients with stage IV melanoma were enrolled into four treatment groups. Best clinical response was partial response in 7/148 evaluable patients (4.7%) without significant difference among study arms.[165] In another trial, three HLA class I peptides were administered in a factorial 2×2 design: peptide vaccine alone, or combined with GM-CSF, or combined with IFN-α2b, or combined with both. At a median follow-up of 25.4 months, the median OS of patients with vaccine immune response was significantly longer than that of patients with no immune response (21.3 months vs 13.4 months; $p = 0.046$).[166]

Vitespen is an autologous, tumor-derived heat shock protein gp96 peptide vaccine. Patients ($n = 322$) with stage IV melanoma were randomly assigned 2:1 to receive vitespen or physician's choice of a treatment. OS in the vitespen arm was statistically indistinguishable from that in the physician's choice arm.[167] A randomized trial provided evidence that a DC vaccine is associated with longer survival compared with a tumor cell vaccine, and is consistent with previous data suggesting a survival benefit from this patient-specific immunotherapy.[168] A Phase II trial of a DC vaccine for metastatic melanoma patients with mainly the HLA-A24 genotype was investigated; OS analysis revealed a significant survival prolongation effect in patients receiving the DC vaccine.[169] Studies were also carried out to detect a pretreatment gene expression signature predictive of response to MAGE-A3 vaccine in patients with metastatic melanoma. An expression signature was associated with the patient's clinical response.[170] A Phase II trial investigated a peptide vaccination against survivin, a protein crucial for the survival of tumor cells, in patients with treatment-refractory stage IV metastatic melanoma. Survivin-specific T-cell reactivities strongly correlated with tumor response and patient survival.[171]

Several clinical studies have employed autologous melanoma cells as vaccine. Clinical responses were observed when these melanoma-cell vaccines were preceded by cyclophosphamide.[172,173] Clinical responses were also observed when autologous melanoma cells were transduced with GM-CSF and given as vaccine.[174,175] In addition, intratumoral administration of recombinant vaccinia encoding GM-CSF in patients with cutaneous melanoma has been reported to induce antitumor immune responses.[31,32,176] Several randomized Phase II trials have been carried out using either autologous[177,178] or allogeneic[179,180] melanoma vaccine in patients with resected melanoma. In these trials, there is evidence of improved disease-free survival (DFS) in the vaccine arm versus control or no-treatment groups. Recent research indicates that immunization with hybrids of tumor cells and APCs can induce protective immunity and rejection of established tumors in various rodent models.[95,181,182] Novel clinical trial strategies incorporating DC-based vaccines have recently been

reported.[183–185] Purified hybrids from the fusion of DCs and tumor cells (dendritomas) have been shown to be safe and to induce both immunological and clinical responses when combined with low-dose IL-2.[184]

T-VEC is an intralesional oncolytic immunotherapy comprising an HSV-type 1 engineered to make GM-CSF. In the randomized Phase III trial, 436 patients with stage IIIB-IV melanoma were randomized 2:1 to receive intralesional T-VEC versus s.c. GM-CSF. T-VEC significantly improved the proportion of patients with duration of response ≥ 6 months (16% vs 2%) and an overall response rate (26% vs 6%) versus s.c. GM-CSF. Many patients remained in remission with a median follow-up of over 18.4 months.[186,187]

Colorectal carcinoma

A prospective randomized-controlled Phase III clinical trial was carried out in 254 patients with stage II and stage III colon cancer using autologous tumor cell vaccine with BCG postsurgery. A 5.3-year median follow-up showed 40 recurrences in the control group and 25 in the vaccine group. The vaccine showed a statistically significant recurrence-free survival (RFS) in patients with surgically resected stage II colon cancer, but not stage III colon cancer.[188] Further follow-up demonstrated a significant survival benefit in the vaccine arm over surgery alone.[189]

Several clinical trials have been conducted employing CEA-based vaccines. Results of vaccination in patients with recombinant vaccinia virus,[69] recombinant avipox virus,[66,190,191] or a prime with recombinant vaccinia (rV)-CEA and multiple boosts with avipox-CEA[47] have demonstrated the generation of CEA-specific immune responses in patients with advanced gastrointestinal (GI) carcinomas and other CEA-expressing carcinomas. A trial using both vaccinia- and avipox-CEA vaccines containing TRI-COM has suggested improved survival in patients receiving the prime-and-boost regimen plus GM-CSF; 40% had stable disease (SDs) for at least 4 months.[47,79,192,193] In a multicenter Phase II study, colorectal cancer patients received PANVAC vaccine (rV-, rF-CEA-MUC1-TRICOM) post-metastasectomy for liver and lung metastases.[192] Patients received either PANVAC or PANVAC-infected DCs and there was no statistical difference in clinical outcome in the two arms. Vaccinated patients ($n = 74$) were compared to a contemporary "control" (not randomized) group of colorectal cancer patients ($n = 161$) undergoing metastasectomy and receiving standard-of-care therapies. Both this control group and the PANVAC-vaccinated groups had similar prognostic characteristics and TTP for both groups was virtually identical with a median TTP of approximately 24 months.[20,192] However, the OS of PANVAC-vaccinated patients was 95% at 2 years and 90% at 40 months, compared to the contemporary control group with an OS of 75% at 2 years, and 47% at 40 months. The OS values of the control group are similar to 3–5 year survival data in this population from five other clinical studies.[194–199] This is yet another example (as seen with ipilimumab, sipuleucel-T, and PROSTVAC) of no increase in TTP versus control with an increase in OS.

CEA peptide-pulsed DCs have also been employed in clinical studies using a modified CEA agonist peptide.[200] Two of 12 patients with advanced colorectal cancers experienced tumor regression, one patient had a mixed response, and two had SD. Clinical responses correlated with the expansion of CEA-specific T cells. Twenty-six patients who had undergone resection of colorectal metastases were treated with intranodal injections of an autologous tumor lysate- and control protein-pulsed DC vaccine. Patients were randomized to receive DCs that had either been activated or not activated with CD40L. All patients were followed up for a minimum of 5.5 years. Patients with evidence of a vaccine-induced, tumor-specific T-cell-proliferative or IFN-γ response 1 week after vaccination had a markedly better RFS at 5 years (63% vs 18%, $p = 0.037$) than nonresponders.[201]

Clinical studies have also been carried out using anti-Id antibodies directed against anti-CEA MAbs. These studies have demonstrated the induction of immune responses,[202,203] slowed disease progression, and prolonged survival.[204] MVA containing the gene for an oncofetal antigen found on many tumors (5T4) has been tested in a variety of cancers (TroVax, Oxford, UK). In a trial of 22 patients with mCRC, immune responses appeared to correlate with disease control, which was seen up to 18 months in patients with immune responses.[205–207]

Pancreatic carcinoma
Allogeneic whole-tumor-cell vaccines modified to secrete GM-CSF have also been employed in patients with pancreatic cancer. Evidence of vaccine-induced immune responses were observed as measured by delayed-type hypersensitivity.[25,208] A 60-patient Phase II study of the same vaccine in the adjuvant setting showed that post-chemotherapy induction of mesothelin-specific CD8 cells correlated with progression-free survival.[209] The median OS was about 26 months compared with 21 months for chemotherapy alone in this same patient population at the same institution.[210] GVAX and CRS-207 are cancer vaccines that have been evaluated in pancreatic ductal adenocarcinoma (PDA). GVAX is composed of two irradiated GM-CSF-secreting allogeneic PDA cell lines administered 24 h after treatment with low-dose cyclophosphamide (Cy) to inhibit regulatory T cells. CRS-207 is recombinant live-attenuated, double-deleted *Listeria monocytogenes*, engineered to express mesothelin. GVAX induces T cells against a broad array of PDA antigens, and mesothelin-specific T-cell responses have been shown to correlate with survival. Mesothelin is a TAA overexpressed in most PDAs. In a prior study, patients with previously treated advanced PDA who received Cy/GVAX had better induction of mesothelin-specific CD8+ T cells than those treated with GVAX alone. Median survival was 4.3 and 2.3 months, respectively. Previously treated patients with metastatic pancreatic adenocarcinoma were randomly assigned at a ratio of 2 : 1 to two doses of Cy/GVAX followed by four doses of CRS-207 or Cy/GVAX alone. In a pre-specified per-protocol analysis of patients who received at least three doses (two doses of Cy/GVAX plus one of CRS-207 or three of Cy/GVAX), OS was 9.7 months versus 4.6 months. Enhanced mesothelin-specific CD8+ T-cell responses were associated with longer OS, regardless of treatment arm.[211]

Breast cancer
Sialyl-Tn (STn) is a glycopeptide contained in carcinoma-associated mucin. Patients were randomized to receive vaccine [STn coupled to keyhole limpet hemocyanin (KLH)] with or without cyclophosphamide. Patients treated with vaccine and cyclophosphamide were reported to have lived significantly longer[212] than those treated with the same vaccine without cyclophosphamide. In addition, STn KLH vaccine has been administered to breast and ovarian cancer patients after an autologous stem cell transplant following high-dose chemotherapy. Vaccinated patients appeared more likely to survive and less likely to relapse, but further studies are required.[213] A multicenter, double-blinded, randomized Phase III trial of STn conjugated to KLH vaccine was completed in 1028 women with metastatic breast cancer who had nonprogressive disease or no evidence of disease after first-line chemotherapy. The women treated with concomitant endocrine therapy and STn-KLH had longer TTP and OS than the control group of women who received KLH alone. Moreover, of the women who received endocrine therapy, those

who had a median or greater antibody response to the STn-KLH vaccine had significantly longer median OS than those who had a below-median antibody response.[214]

Several clinical trials have been carried out using MUC-1 as a target, including the use of MUC-1 peptides,[215–217] recombinant vaccinia virus encoding MUC-1 and IL-2,[218] MVA expressing human MUC-1,[219] and mannan–MUC-1 fusion protein.[220,221] In studies carried out with the HER2/*neu* peptides with or without GM-CSF, patients with breast cancer were able to generate HER2-specific immune responses.[222–224] A Phase I/II clinical trial was carried out vaccinating breast cancer patients with E75, an HLA-A2/A3-restricted HER2/neu peptide, and GM-CSF. The 24-month analysis DFS was 94.3% in the vaccinated group and 86.8% in the control group ($p = .08$). In subset analyses, patients who benefited most from vaccination had lymph-node-positive, HER2 IHC 1+-2+, or grade 1 or 2 tumors and were optimally dosed.[225] Fusion-cell (DCs and tumor cells) vaccination of patients with metastatic breast and renal cancer was shown to induce both immunological and clinical responses.[226] An anti-Id antibody that mimics the human milk-fat globule antigen has also been utilized as a breast cancer vaccine in conjunction with autologous stem cell transplantation (ASCT). In that study, the 3-year OS rate was 48%, whereas the progression-free survival rate was 32%.[227] A HER2 peptide-based vaccine (nelipepimut-S) has been tested in a Phase II trial of 195 patients with localized breast cancer at high risk of recurrence. HLA-A2-/A3-positive patients received vaccine with GM-CSF and those that were not HLA-A2 or -A3 positive were controls. The 5-year DFS was 89.7% in vaccinated patients versus 80.2% in nonvaccinated patients. The 5-year DFS was 94.5% in optimally dosed patients. A Phase III study has been initiated.[228]

Lung cancer
Three Phase III studies in patients with non–small cell lung cancer (NSCLC) failed to meet their primary endpoints. A MAGE-A3 peptide-based vaccine was evaluated in stages IB, 2 and 3A tumor-resected NSCLC patients whose tumors expressed the MAGE-A3 gene.[229,230] The L-BLP25 vaccine consists of a peptide of the tandem repeat region of the MUC-1 gene. A Phase III trial employing this vaccine after chemoradiation in patients with unresectable stage 3 NSCLC did not meet its primary endpoint of increased OS.[231] Lucanix is a vaccine composed of four TGF-β2 antisense modified, irradiated allogeneic NSCLC cell lines. In a Phase III trial in stages IIIA, IIIB, and IV, for those NSCLC patients who did not progress after front-line chemotherapy, a considerable increase in OS was not observed in the vaccine arm; however, the time elapsed between randomization and the end of front-line chemotherapy had a significant impact on survival ($p = 0.002$).[232,233] Other vaccines in patients with NSCLC are also being evaluated. A modified vaccinia virus (MVA) encoding the MUC-1 and IL-2 genes was assessed in combination with first-line chemotherapy in patients ($n = 74$) with advanced NSCLC. Six-month PFS was 43.2% in the vaccine plus chemotherapy group versus 31.5% in the chemotherapy-alone group.[234] A Phase II study of a telomerase peptide vaccine in NSCLC patients ($n = 23$) after chemoradiation has also been evaluated.[235] Immune responders recorded a median PFS of 371 days versus 182 days for nonresponders.

Ovarian/cervical cancer
Clinical findings have also been reported in patients with advanced ovarian cancer using a vaccine consisting of an MAb directed against the tumor antigen CA125.[236] A Phase II study examining an anti-idiotypic antibody vaccine that functionally imitated the CA125 antigen reported survival benefit; median OS of the

vaccine group was 19.4 months versus 4.9 months for the control group.[237]

The purpose of another Phase II single-arm clinical trial was to evaluate whether pretreatment with low-dose cyclophosphamide improves immunogenicity of a p53-synthetic long peptide vaccine in patients with recurrent ovarian cancer. SD was observed in 20.0% (2/10) of patients.[238] Two independent consecutive studies were conducted of combinatorial immunotherapy comprising DC-based autologous whole-tumor-antigen vaccination in combination with anti-angiogenesis therapy. Thirty-one patients had recurrent progressive stage III and IV ovarian cancer. Vaccination was well tolerated and elicited tumor-specific T-cell responses against various ovarian tumor antigens in both studies, and a clinical benefit of 65% correlated with the immune response with some experiencing prolonged PFS.[239] A Phase II clinical trial of recombinant vaccinia-NY-ESO-1 (rV-NY-ESO-1) followed by booster vaccinations with recombinant fowlpox-NY-ESO-1 (rF-NY-ESO-1) in 22 epithelial ovarian cancer (EOC) patients with advanced disease who were at high risk for recurrence/progression was conducted. Median PFS was 21 months, and median OS was 48 months. CD8[+] T cells derived from vaccinated patients were shown to lyse NY-ESO-1-expressing tumor targets. These data provide preliminary evidence of clinically meaningful benefit for diversified prime and boost recombinant poxviral-based vaccines in ovarian cancer.[240]

Studies were undertaken to determine the toxicity, safety, and immunogenicity of a human papillomavirus 16 (HPV16) E6 and E7 long peptide vaccine administered to end-stage cervical cancer patients. The HPV16 E6 and E7 long peptide-based vaccine was well tolerated and capable of inducing a broad IFN-γ-associated T-cell response even in end-stage cervical cancer patients.[241] Vulvar intraepithelial neoplasia is a chronic disorder caused by high-risk types of HPV, most commonly HPV type 16 (HPV-16). Twenty women with HPV-16-positive, grade 3 vulvar intraepithelial neoplasia were vaccinated with a mix of long peptides from the HPV-16 viral oncoproteins E6 and E7.[242] One-half of a group of 20 patients with HPV16-induced vulvar intraepithelial neoplasia grade 3 displayed a complete regression after therapeutic vaccination. There was a strong correlation between a defined set of vaccine-prompted specific immune responses and the clinical efficacy of therapeutic vaccination.[243]

Leukemia/lymphoma

The variable regions of B-cell receptor Igs on lymphomas are excellent targets for vaccines. These Ids have now been used successfully in the treatment of B-cell lymphomas.[50,244–247] An Id protein vaccine was used in 25 patients after a chemotherapy-induced second complete clinical remission in follicular lymphoma (FL). After vaccination, tumor-specific humoral or cellular immune responses were found in 20 of 25 patients.[246] All of the responders with enough follow-up maintained a second CR longer than the first CR, whereas the five patients who did not mount an immune response had a second CR that was, as expected, shorter than the first CR. Vaccination with hybridoma-derived autologous tumor Ig Id conjugated to KLH and administered with GM-CSF induces FL-specific immune responses. A double-blind multicenter controlled Phase III trial of this vaccine was conducted. Of 234 patients enrolled, 177 (81%) achieved CR/CRu after chemotherapy and were randomly assigned. For the 177 randomly assigned patients, median DFS between Id-vaccine and control arms was 23.0 months versus 20.6 months, respectively (p = 0.256). For patients who received Id vaccine, median DFS after randomization was 44.2 months for Id-vaccine arm versus 30.6 months for control

arm. Vaccination with patient-specific hybridoma-derived Id vaccine after chemotherapy-induced CR/CRu may prolong DFS in patients with FL.[248]

A multiple myeloma vaccine has been developed whereby patient-derived tumor cells are fused with autologous DCs, creating a hybridoma that stimulates a broad antitumor response. A Phase II trial was conducted in which patients underwent vaccination following ASCT to target minimal residual disease. Seventy-eight percent of patients achieved a best response of CR or PR and 47% achieved a CR/near CR (nCR). Remarkably, 24% of patients who achieved a partial response following transplant were converted to CR/nCR after vaccination and at more than 3 months post transplant, consistent with a vaccine-mediated effect on residual disease. The post-transplant period for patients with multiple myeloma provides a unique platform for cellular immunotherapy in which vaccination with DC/myeloma fusions resulted in the marked expansion of myeloma-specific T cells and cytoreduction of minimal residual disease.[249] Clinical responses have also been observed using Id vaccine in patients with multiple myeloma.[52,250]

For patients with chronic myelogenous leukemia, vaccination with bcr-abl oncogene breakpoint fusion peptides has generated specific immune responses.[251] A study investigated the immunogenicity of Wilms tumor gene product 1 (WT1)-peptide vaccination in WT1-expressing acute myeloid leukemia (AML). Vaccination consisted of GM-CSF and WT1 peptide and KLH. AML patients (n = 17) received a median of 11 vaccinations. Objective responses in AML patients were 10 SDs including four SDs with more than 50% blast reduction and two with hematologic improvement. An additional four patients had clinical benefit after initial progression, including one complete remission and three SDs.[252] A Phase I/II trial investigated the effect of autologous DC vaccination in 10 patients with AML. Two patients in partial remission after chemotherapy were brought into complete remission after intradermal administration of full-length WT1 mRNA-electroporated DCs. In these two patients and three other patients who were in complete remission, the AML-associated tumor marker returned to normal after DC vaccination, compatible with the induction of molecular remission. Clinical responses were correlated with vaccine-associated increases in WT1-specific CD8[+] T cell frequencies.[253]

Other tumor types

Intravesical BCG has been used successfully in the treatment of bladder cancer, implicating immune mechanisms.[254] Intravesical administration of wild-type vaccinia virus has now been shown to be safe, and three of four patients treated were disease free at 4-year follow-up.[255] The response of renal carcinoma to high-dose IL-2 and IFN-alpha also implicates immune mechanisms in therapeutic responses.[256] An autologous RCC tumor-cell vaccine that was genetically modified to overexpress B7-1 to provide costimulation to tumor-reactive T cells was employed.[257] In this single-arm Phase II study, 66 patients enrolled and 39 received at least one dose of vaccine and low-dose IL-2. Best responses were CR (3%), PR (5%), SD (64%), and PD (28%). A *post hoc* analysis suggested that lymphocytic infiltration of the vaccine site determined by biopsy directly correlated with survival (28.4 months versus 17.8 months, p = 0.045). A Phase I trial was conducted to evaluate the feasibility, safety, and efficacy of a DC-based vaccination in patients (n = 21) with metastatic RCC. Autologous mature DCs were pulsed with HLA-A2-binding MUC1 peptides. In six patients, regression of the metastatic sites was induced after vaccinations with three patients achieving an objective response (one complete response, two partial responses, two mixed responses, and one SD). An additional four patients were stable during the treatment for up to 14 months.[258]

Vaccination of pediatric solid tumor patients with tumor-lysate-pulsed DCs has been shown to expand specific T cells and mediated some tumor regression.[259] In addition to DC fusion vaccination of patients with metastatic breast and renal cancer, clinical trials have examined vaccination of glioma patients with DC/glioma fusions.[226,260] Early clinical trials in patients with primary brain tumors have shown immune responses and objective responses with DC vaccines,[261] autologous formalin-fixed[262] or TGF-β-modified[263] whole-tumor-cell vaccines. A pilot study of s.c. vaccinations with glioma-associated antigen (GAA) epitope peptides in HLA-A2-positive children with newly diagnosed brainstem gliomas (BSGs) and high-grade gliomas (HGGs) was undertaken. Twenty-six children were enrolled, 14 with newly diagnosed BSGs treated with irradiation and 12 with newly diagnosed BSGs or HGGs treated with irradiation and concurrent chemotherapy. Five children had symptomatic pseudoprogression, which responded to dexamethasone and was associated with prolonged survival. Only two patients had progressive disease during the first two vaccine courses; 19 had SD, two had partial responses, one had a minor response, and two had prolonged disease-free status after surgery.[264]

Considerations in the analysis of vaccine clinical trial results

It has now been demonstrated that appropriate vaccine delivery systems and vaccine strategies can elicit immune responses to TAAs in patients with a range of cancers and, in some cases, can mediate prolonged survival, prolonged disease-free interval, drops in serum tumor markers, and/or regression of metastatic disease. Patients with advanced cancers are perhaps the least appropriate population to demonstrate the efficacy of a cancer vaccine; thus, future clinical trials should be carried out in patients with less or with low tumor burden metastatic disease or earlier in the disease process. Optimal use of vaccines should occur immediately prior to, during, or immediately following adjuvant therapy. Several such studies are ongoing. The overall goal is the use of vaccine regimens in combination with front-line cancer therapies, thereby reducing the interval between disease diagnosis and the initiation of vaccine; this would bring the use of cancer vaccines closer to their original intention—use in patients with minimal disease.

Combination therapies

There are numerous ways in which vaccine therapy can be used in combination with the so-called non-immune-based therapies (Table 3) as well as with other immunotherapies. One of the major advantages of cancer vaccines is their reduced toxicity. One of the conventional thoughts now being reevaluated is that cancer vaccines cannot be used in combination with chemotherapy or radiation therapy. One should not confuse the potential reduced efficacy of a vaccine given to patients who have failed multiple rounds of prior chemotherapy versus administration of vaccine with or prior to chemotherapy. Preclinical studies, and now several clinical studies, have shown that patients can mount an immune response to a cancer vaccine when given in combination with certain cytotoxic drugs, hormones, or local radiation of tumor. Studies have shown that when tumor cells are exposed to sublethal doses of radiation or certain chemotherapeutic agents, the phenotype of tumor cells is actually modulated to make them more susceptible to T-cell-mediated killing (Figure 1). Indeed, the era of the use of therapeutic cancer vaccines in combination with other

Table 3 Vaccines in combination with other therapeutic modalities.

Modality	Mechanism of action to enhance vaccine efficacy
Radiation	Alteration in tumor cell phenotype
Chemotherapy	"Immunologic" tumor cell death
	Alteration in tumor cell phenotype
	Enriched effector: regulator cell ratios
Hormonal therapy	Thymic regeneration and induction of naive T cells
	Alteration of tumor cell phenotype
Small-molecule-targeted therapeutics	Modulate tumor microenvironment
	Alteration in tumor cell phenotype
Monoclonal antibodies	Enhanced antibody-dependent cell-mediated cytotoxicity
	Immune checkpoint modulation
Imids[a] (lenalidomide)	Stimulate T-cell proliferation

[a]Imids are a novel class of immunomodulators.

immunotherapeutics as well as the so-called nonimmune conventional cancer therapeutics is still in its early stage of development and full clinical potential.

Vaccination plus other immunotherapies

The recent clinical studies employing MAbs directed against the checkpoint inhibitor PD-L1/PD-1 immune suppressive axis have placed cancer immunotherapy into consideration as a mainstream component of cancer therapy. Results with checkpoint inhibitors have been most impressive in the treatment of the majority of patients with metastatic melanoma and subsets of patients with lung carcinoma.[266–271] The use of the PD-L1/PD-1 checkpoint inhibitors has also shown some activity in a minority of patients with other tumor types (e.g., bladder cancer) and extremely low levels of activity in other cancers such as colorectal and prostate cancer. The major correlate of clinical response in virtually all of these studies with the PD-L1/PD-1 checkpoint inhibitors is the presence of T cells in the tumor. It would appear that these TILs are inducing PD-L1 on tumor cells and consequently becoming anergized, thus recapitulating the process of the body's defense against autoimmunity. The administration of an anti-PD-L1/PD-1 agent would "release the brakes" on T cells by reducing or eliminating this immunosuppressive phenomenon, leading to the activation of the TILs and subsequent tumor cell destruction (Figure 2). One potential reason for the lack of success of some tumor vaccine trials could be due to this upregulation of PD-L1 on tumor cells in response to the presence of TILs. It would thus appear that the use of a therapeutic vaccine prior to or at the same time as the use of an anti-PD-L1/PD-1 agent would induce the presence of T cells in the tumor, which would subsequently be activated by inhibiting the PD-L1 expression on the tumor, leading to tumor cell lysis (Figure 2). Carefully controlled randomized clinical studies will be required to validate this hypothesis.

Preclinical studies have shown that vaccine plus checkpoint inhibition can act synergistically. The addition of anti-CTLA4 MAb to CEA-TRICOM vaccination was shown to increase the avidity of T-cell responses, resulting in enhanced antitumor activity of the vaccine.[138,272] When used in combination with GVAX vaccine, blockade of both PD-1 and CTLA-4 resulted in reversal of CD8+ TIL dysfunction and enhanced antitumor activity.[273]

In a Phase I clinical study,[274] 30 metastatic prostate cancer patients received PROSTVAC vaccine in combination with increasing doses of ipilimumab (anti-CTLA4). Fifty-eight percent of patients had PSA declines. While this trial was not randomized, median OS for patients receiving the combination was 34.4 months compared to 26.3 months for patients receiving PROSTVAC

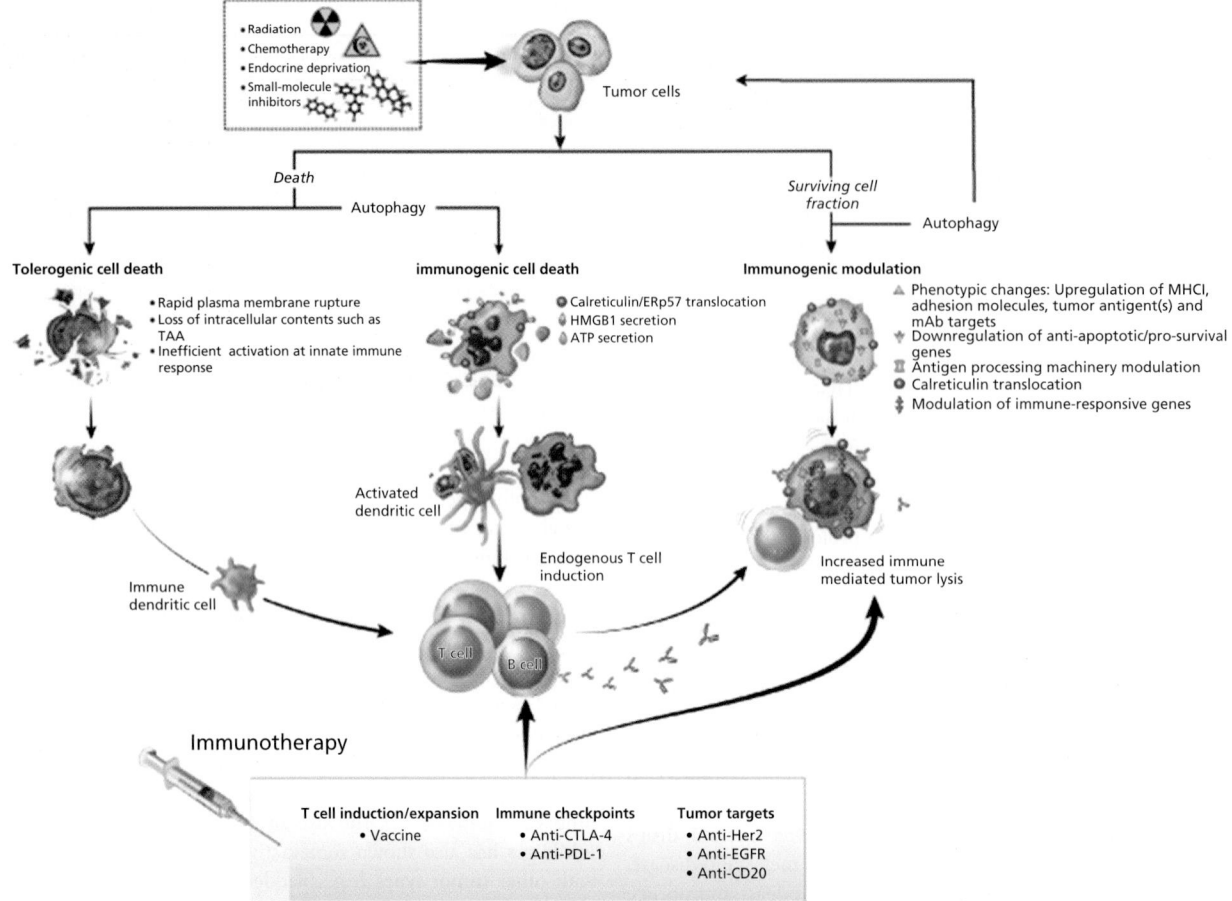

Figure 1 Multiple immunogenic consequences of radiation therapy, chemotherapy, endocrine deprivation, or small-molecule inhibitors that can be harnessed to promote synergy with immunotherapeutic regimens. These immunogenic consequences of anticancer therapy, ranging from immunogenic cell death to immunogenic modulation, can be exploited to achieve optimal synergy with therapeutic cancer vaccines. Source: Adapted from Ref. 265.

alone in another trial (Halabi-predicted survival[144] was similar for patients in both trials at about 18 months). A recently completed trial in mCRPC patients using ipilimumab plus radiation showed a median OS of 17.3 months. Also, no additional toxicity above that observed with ipilimumab alone was seen in the vaccine plus ipilimumab-treated patients. In another study, a DNA/peptide vaccine induced T-cell responses in melanoma patients that were "boosted" following CTLA-4 blockade.[275] CTLA-4 MAb was also infused into nine previously immunized advanced cancer patients[276]; evidence of increased tumor immunity was seen in some melanoma and metastatic ovarian cancer patients.

There are also several ways in which vaccine and MAbs can be used in combination. These include (1) the use of therapeutic antibodies such as herceptin or rituxan in combination with vaccine, in which each acts independently, (2) the use of antitumor antibody cytokine fusion proteins such as antitumor antibody/IL-12 to enhance T-cell activity at the site of tumor,[277–281] and (3) the use of MAbs or fusion proteins directed against regulatory T cells.[282–284] Vaccines can also be employed in combination with adoptive transfer of antigen-specific T cells. In preclinical studies, point-mutated ras-specific T cells were adoptively transferred into immunodepleted hosts. Donor antigen-specific T-cell responses were greatest in recipient mice that received peptide boosts (with or without IL-2). These results indicate that a vaccine administration after T-cell transfer was more obligatory than exogenous IL-2 to sustain adoptively transferred T cells.[285]

Immunogenic cell death and immunogenic modulation

Certain cancer therapeutic regimens have the ability to trigger cancer cell death, which leads to stimulating endogenous immune responses against the tumor; this is termed "immunogenic cell death" (Figure 1).[286–293] The cardinal signs of immunogenic cell death are (1) calreticulin exposure on the surface of dying cells, (2) the release of high-mobility group box 1 (HMGB1), (3) the release of ATP and, most importantly, (4) cell death.[289] Each of these molecules acts on DCs to facilitate the presentation of tumor antigens to the immune system.[287] Calreticulin, a chaperone and calcium regulator, when exposed on the surface of a dying cell, serves as a phagocytic signal to DCs.[291,294] When HMGB1, a non-histone chromatin-binding protein, is released from dying cells, it engages TLR-4 on DCs, leading to DC maturation.[289] The secretion of ATP by dying cells binds receptors on DCs, further supporting T-cell activation.[288] In addition, tumor cells that survive therapy have been shown to alter their biology to render them more sensitive to immune mediated killing; this phenomenon is termed "immunogenic modulation" (Figure 1).[295–302] Immunogenic modulation encompasses a spectrum of molecular alterations in the biology of the cancer cell that independently or collectively make the tumor more amenable to CTL-mediated destruction. These include (1) downregulation of anti-apoptotic/survival genes,[297,298,303] (2) modulation of antigen-processing machinery (APM) components,[299,302] and (3) calreticulin translocation to the cell surface of the tumor (Figure 1).[265,299] One can envision that

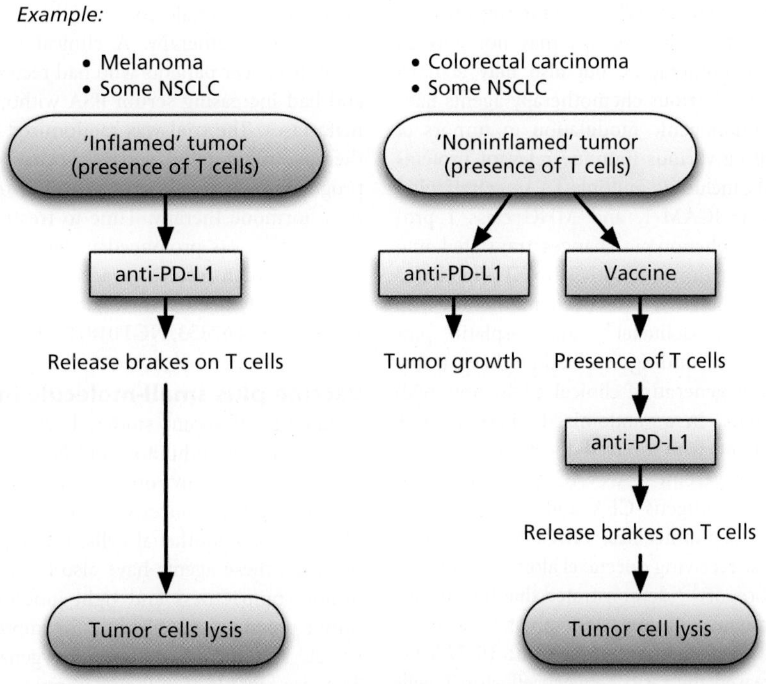

Example:

Figure 2 Working model for understanding T-cell-inflamed versus noninflamed tumor microenvironments with implications for vaccine therapy. The potential reasons for lack of spontaneous immune responses against a subset of tumors despite T-cell infiltration include failed immune activation (a) by extrinsic inhibition by PD-L1/PD-1 interactions. This local inhibition may be overcome by blockade with anti-PD-L1/PD-1 checkpoint inhibitor monoclonal antibodies, yielding clinical benefit. Other tumor types, termed "noninflamed," typically do not respond to PD-L1 inhibition due to lack of potential infiltrating responding T cells. This model suggests that these tumors may be converted to an "inflamed" T-cell-infiltrated phenotype by vaccine regimens (b). These T cells may then be further activated by PD-L1/PD-1 blockade.

these immunogenic consequences of anticancer therapy, ranging from immunogenic cell death to immunogenic modulation, can thus be harnessed to achieve optimal synergy with therapeutic cancer vaccines and other immunotherapy regimens, thereby maximizing the clinical benefit for patients receiving combination therapies.

Vaccine plus radiation

Radiation therapy is standard-of-care for multiple malignancies, aimed at direct tumor destruction. However, systemic disease, treatment resistance, or the need for sublethal dosing to minimize normal tissue toxicity, often translates into surviving tumor cell populations and disease progression.[304,305] Radiation can induce a continuum of immunogenic alterations in dying and/or surviving tumor cells (Figure 1). Lethal irradiation has been reported to induce immunogenic cell death.[306] Although immune responses in cancer patients receiving radiation alone are often weak and rarely translate into protective immunity, the immunogenic effects of radiation therapy can be exploited to promote synergistic clinical benefit for patients receiving combination regimens with immunotherapy.[304,305,307] It has been demonstrated that the use of relatively low doses of external beam radiation, insufficient to kill tumors, induces immunogenic modulation, altering those tumor cells to render them more susceptible to T-cell-mediated lysis. Cell-surface expression of MHC class I molecules and calreticulin on tumors was increased in a radiation-dose-dependent manner, ultimately rendering tumor cells more susceptible to T-cell-mediated killing.[265,298,302] It has been demonstrated in preclinical studies that radiation combined with a cancer vaccine elicits greater tumor antigen-specific CD8+ T-cell responses and/or reduction in tumor burden than either modality alone.[298,308–310] Importantly, the induction of CD8+ T cells specific for multiple

TAAs not encoded by the vaccine was observed after the combination therapy (antigen cascade). This polyclonal T-cell response functionally mediated the regression of TAA-negative metastases at distal s.c. or pulmonary sites.[310]

These findings have translated into promising clinical findings for patients receiving radiation therapy plus immunotherapy.[304,305,307,311,312] A Phase I study evaluated the combination of radiation therapy plus injection of an autologous DC vaccine in 14 patients with advanced-stage/metastatic hepatoma.[311] Patients received a single fraction of radiation followed by two intratumoral injections of autologous immature DCs. This combination resulted in tumor-specific immune responses in 7/10 assessable patients, and six patients had objective clinical responses. Utilizing poxviral vaccines, patients in a randomized Phase II study with localized prostate cancer who were treated with radiation and a poxviral-based vaccine had a significant increase in PSA-specific T-cell responses compared to patients receiving radiation alone.[312] In a multicenter Phase II study, patients with mCRPC ($n = 44$) were randomized to receive ^{153}Sm-EDTMP (Quadramet®, an FDA-approved radiopharmaceutical targeting bone metastasis) alone or in combination with PSA-TRICOM vaccine. TTP significantly improved ($p = 0.03$) with combination therapy (3.7 months) compared to ^{153}Sm-EDTMP alone (1.7 months).[313] In addition, several ongoing clinical trials are investigating this combination strategy,[314] including a Phase II study of sipuleucel-T plus radiation therapy,[62] a Phase II study of sipuleucel-T plus stereotactic ablative body radiation,[63] and a pilot study of sipuleucel-T plus high-dose single-fraction radiation[64] in hormone-refractory prostate cancer.

Vaccine plus chemotherapy

If cancer vaccines are to be used early in the disease process, they would most likely need to be used in combination with certain chemotherapeutic regimens. While counterintuitive, it has recently been shown that vaccine therapy may not only be compatible with certain chemotherapies, but also may actually be synergistic (Figure 1).[296,315] Various chemotherapy agents have been shown to induce immunogenic modulation in tumors of diverse origin by upregulating various immune-relevant proteins on the surface of cancer cells, including multiple TAAs, calreticulin, adhesion molecules such as ICAM-1, and MHC class I proteins.[295,298–300,303,316,317] These phenotypic changes translated into increased murine and/or human tumor sensitivity to CTL-mediated lysis *in vitro* after exposure to sublethal doses of chemotherapy with cisplatin/5-FU[317] docetaxel,[299] paclitaxel[299] and cisplatin plus vinorelbine.[317] These preclinical findings and others have translated into various hypothesis-generating clinical trials, now with encouraging preliminary data. In a randomized Phase II trial, metastatic breast cancer patients who received docetaxel combined with the therapeutic cancer vaccine PANVAC (poxvirus-based vaccine encoding the tumor antigens CEA and MUC-1, along with three T-cell costimulatory molecules; TRICOM) attained a superior PFS relative to those receiving docetaxel alone (6.6 months vs 3.8 months).[318] A recent report[319] demonstrated that the administration of docetaxel to patients with metastatic prostate or breast cancer, as well as that of cisplatin plus vinorelbine to NSCLC patients, significantly increased the ratio between effector T cells and Tregs and reduced the immunosuppressive activity of the latter in the majority of patients. These studies provide the rationale for the selective use of active immunotherapy regimens in combination with specific standard-of-care therapies to achieve the most beneficial clinical outcome among carcinoma patients. Several things are important in considering the use of chemotherapy with vaccine: (1) the combined use of vaccine and chemotherapy early in the disease process should not be confused with the use of vaccines following multiple regimens of different chemotherapeutic agents in the advanced disease setting, where the immune system would most likely be impaired, (2) not all chemotherapeutic agents will be compatible with vaccine, and (3) dose scheduling of vaccine when used with chemotherapy may be extremely important. Obviously, future studies will be required to optimize the combined use of vaccine and chemotherapy. A recent review on combining antineoplastic drugs with tumor vaccines has been published.[320]

Vaccine plus hormone therapy

The use of vaccines with anti-androgen therapy represents an intriguing possibility for the treatment of prostate cancer. It has previously been shown that androgen-ablative therapy induces T-cell infiltration in the prostate. T-cell infiltration was readily apparent after 1 to 3 weeks of therapy.[321] The immunogenic modulation potential of androgen deprivation has been described with a second-generation androgen-receptor antagonist (ARA), enzalutamide, using the murine TRAMP model of prostate carcinoma.[322] *In vitro* exposure of TRAMP-C2 prostate tumor cells to enzalutamide significantly enhanced cell-surface expression of Fas and MHC class I, consequently improving their sensitivity to immune-mediated lysis. These immunomodulatory properties of enzalutamide were exploited upon combination with a therapeutic cancer vaccine targeting a transcription factor associated with the metastatic process. Combination treatment significantly increased antigen-specific T-cell proliferation and OS compared to the levels observed in mice receiving no treatment or enzalutamide alone. In addition, enzalutamide or abiraterone, an inhibitor of androgen biogenesis, were both able to render androgen receptor positive LNCaP human prostate tumor cells more sensitive to T-cell-mediated lysis.[316] Findings from these and other studies

provided a rationale for the use of ADT in combination with active immunotherapy. A clinical trial has been conducted in prostate cancer patients who had received prior hormonal therapy and had increasing serum PSA without radiographic evidence of metastases. The trial was randomized for a second-line hormone therapy (nilutamide) versus vaccine with a crossover at disease progression so that each arm would receive combination vaccine plus hormone therapy. Time to treatment failure and survival at 4+ years[323] was prolonged in patients initially receiving vaccine alone and then receiving vaccine plus nilutamide. Further studies are obviously needed to validate such observations and are under way (NCT01867333, NCT01875250).

Vaccine plus small-molecule inhibitors

A number of recent studies have indicated that antiangiogenic tyrosine kinase inhibitors (TKIs) target multiple components of the tumor microenvironment and are an ideal class of agents for synergizing with cancer vaccines.[324] TKIs are well known to modulate tumor endothelial cells, leading to vascular normalization; however, these agents have also been recently shown to decrease tumor compactness and tight junctions, thereby reducing solid tumor pressure and allowing for improved perfusion of collapsed vessels and increased tumor oxygenation.[325] In addition, select TKIs are capable of inducing immunogenic modulation (Figure 1). The alteration of the immune landscape, direct modification of tumor cells, and improved vascular perfusion lead to improved antitumor efficacy when antiangiogenic TKIs are combined with immunotherapy. These data support the clinical combination of multitargeted antiangiogenic TKIs, including, but not limited to, cabozantinib,[326] sunitinib,[325,327–329] and sorafenib,[325] as well as to other antiangiogenic therapies, such as the anti-VEGF antibody bevacizumab, with cancer vaccines for improved treatment of solid tumors.

Dose scheduling of vaccine with other therapies

Arguably the most unique feature of cancer vaccine therapy is a vaccine's ability to initiate a dynamic process of host immune responses that can be exploited in subsequent therapies (Table 4). In a Phase I study, patients with advanced-stage progressive cancer received a vaccine directed against cytochrome *P*4501B1. Most patients who developed immunity to vaccine but required salvage therapy on progression showed marked responses to their next treatment regimen; most of these responses lasted >1 year.[331] In another study in patients with extensive-stage small cell lung cancer,[332] a high rate of objective clinical responses to chemotherapy immediately followed vaccine therapy. These clinical responses were also closely associated with induction or augmentation of immune response to vaccine.

Three randomized clinical trials in prostate cancer provided further evidence of this phenomenon. In the first trial, patients with metastatic CRPC were randomized to receive vaccine alone or vaccine plus weekly docetaxel.[333] Patients on the vaccine-alone arm were allowed to cross over to receive docetaxel at time of progression. After vaccine, median PFS on docetaxel was 6.1 months compared with a PFS of 3.7 months with the same docetaxel regimen and patient population at the same institution. Similar findings were observed using the sipuleucel vaccine.[334] In a randomized multicenter study, patients in both the vaccine and placebo arms received docetaxel at progression. There was a statistically significant ($p = 0.023$) increase in OS with docetaxel in patients who had prior vaccine versus placebo.

In a Phase II trial,[335] patients with nonmetastatic CRPC and rising serum PSA were randomized to receive either vaccine or

Table 4 Therapeutic vaccines versus conventional therapy.

	Therapeutic vaccines	Conventional therapy
Target	Immune system	Tumor or its microenvironment
Pharmacodynamics	Delayed (adaptable, may get better over time)	Often immediate action
Memory response	Yes	No
Tumor evolution/new mutations	New immunogenic targets	Resistance to therapy
Limitations	Requires adequate immune system function (both systemically and at tumor site)	Toxicity

Source: Adapted from Ref. 330.

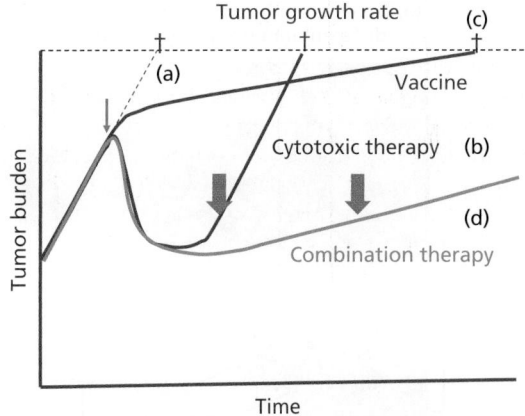

Figure 3 Tumor growth rates in patients with metastatic prostate cancer, from four trials with chemotherapy and one with PROSTVAC (PSA-TRICOM) (adapted from data in Refs 337–339). (a) Tumor growth rate with no therapy. (b, blue line) Chemotherapy-induced initial tumor reduction, but tumor growth rate at cessation of therapy due to toxicity or drug resistance was similar to pretreatment tumor growth rate. (c, red line) PROSTVAC vaccine reduced tumor growth rate following therapy. Thus, patients who received vaccine showed little if any tumor reduction (and virtually no increase in time to progression), but showed an increase in overall survival. (d, green line) Predictions of enhanced overall survival for patients treated with both vaccine and cytotoxic therapy. Combination therapy couples the reduced tumor burden from cytotoxic therapy with the reduced growth rate from immunotherapy, culminating in both objective clinical responses and increased overall survival. This phenomenon could potentially be further enhanced if vaccine were initiated earlier in the disease process or in patients with low tumor burden. Arrows indicate the initiation of treatment; crosses indicate time of death from cancer. Source: Adapted from Gulley 2011[338] and Madan 2010.[339]

nilutamide, an ARA. After 6 months, patients with rising PSA were allowed to cross over to a combination of both therapies. Median time to treatment failure was similar in the vaccine and ARA arms. However, for patients who received vaccine first and then received vaccine plus ARA, time to treatment failure was 13.9 months from the initiation of ARA and the time to treatment failure from the initiation of any therapy was 25.9 months. Of the initial randomized population, for those patients who first received nilutamide alone or nilutamide and then vaccine, 5-year OS was 38% versus a median OS of 59% for patients who first received vaccine alone or nilutamide plus vaccine.[336]

With traditional cytotoxic agents, it is widely believed that improved TTP is a prerequisite for improved OS. A recent study[337] evaluated tumor regression and growth rates in four chemotherapy trials and one vaccine trial in patients with mCRPC. Cytotoxic agents affect the tumor only during the period of administration; soon after the drug is discontinued, due to drug resistance or toxicity, antitumor activity ceases and the growth rate of the tumor increases (Figure 3). The mechanism of action and kinetics of clinical response with vaccine therapy appears to be quite different (Table 4).[337] Therapeutic vaccines do not directly target the tumor, but rather target the immune system. Immune responses often take time to develop and can potentially be enhanced by continued booster vaccinations; any resulting tumor-cell lysis can lead to cross-priming of additional TAAs, thus broadening the immune repertoire via a phenomenon known as antigen cascade or epitope spreading (Figure 4). This broader, and perhaps more relevant, immune response may also take some time to develop. Although a vaccine may not induce any significant reduction in tumor burden, vaccines as monotherapy have the potential to apply antitumor activity over a long period of time, resulting in a slower tumor growth rate (Figure 3). This deceleration in growth rate may continue for months or years and, more importantly, through subsequent therapies. This process can thus lead to clinically significant improved OS, often with little or no difference in TTP and a low rate of or lack of objective response[340]; thus, treating patients with lower tumor burden with vaccine may result in far better outcomes. It is hypothesized that the combined use of vaccine and cytotoxic therapy may result in both tumor regression (via the cytotoxic therapy) and reduced tumor growth rate (via vaccine therapy) (Figure 3).[337,338] Early clinical trials with vaccine may thus well have been terminated prematurely with the observance of tumor progression before sufficient vaccine boosts could be administered. This phenomenon has actually led to modifications in how vaccine clinical trials are now designed and to "new immune response criteria" for immunotherapy.[341]

Mechanisms involved in vaccine activity

Recent studies have shown that a range of effector cells can be involved in antitumor effects. In most preclinical studies, the CD8+ CTL is involved in antitumor effects and the CD4+ helper T cell is important for supplying help via cytokines to further activate the CTL. Other effector cells, however, can be involved, including macrophages and natural killer (NK) cells, and studies have also shown that in certain cases the generation of antitumor antibodies can mediate antitumor effects via antibody-dependent cell-mediated cytotoxicity.[342] T-cell activation has been shown to be a complex phenomenon involving the interaction of the peptide–MHC complex on the APC with the TCR on the T cell; for weak antigens such as TAAs, however, accessory molecules are necessary for efficient T-cell activation. These have been termed T-cell costimulatory molecules. At this time, over a dozen such costimulatory molecules have been identified. Costimulatory molecules are found on professional APCs, such as DCs, but are not found on the vast majority of solid tumors. It has also recently been shown that combinations of these costimulatory molecules act synergistically to further enhance T-cell activation.[139] Recent studies have also shown that it is not necessarily the quantity of T cells generated that is essential, but their quality, or avidity.[138,343,344] This is measured by the ability of different populations of T cells to actually kill targets. It has recently been shown that the use of vaccines with T-cell costimulation and certain cytokines can actually enhance T-cell avidity.[138]

Several different types of regulatory T cells have now been identified.[345–348] The evolutionary reason for their existence is most likely to reduce autoimmune phenomena. Since TAAs for the most part are self-antigens, regulatory T cells appear to have a major role in reducing immune responses to TAAs. Several types of regulatory T

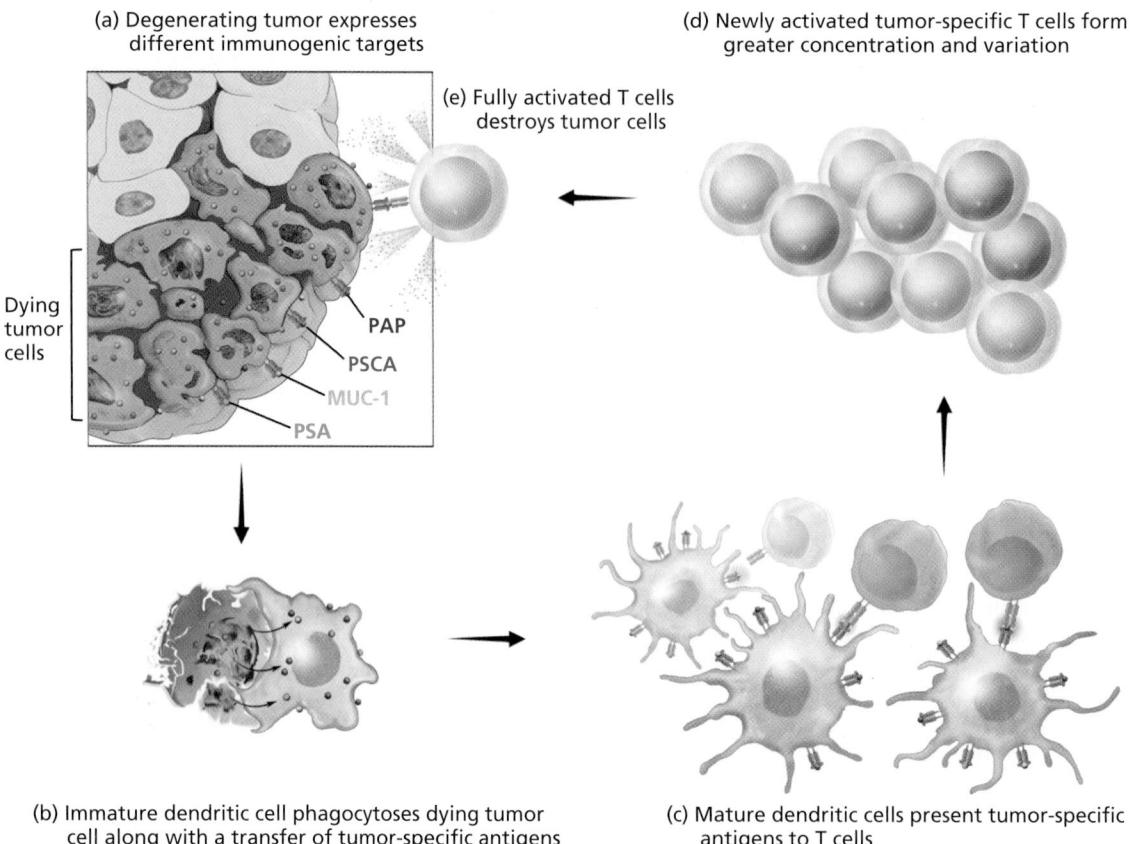

(a) Degenerating tumor expresses different immunogenic targets

Dying tumor cells

PAP
PSCA
MUC-1
PSA

(e) Fully activated T cells destroys tumor cells

(d) Newly activated tumor-specific T cells form in greater concentration and variation

(b) Immature dendritic cell phagocytoses dying tumor cell along with a transfer of tumor-specific antigens

(c) Mature dendritic cells present tumor-specific antigens to T cells

Figure 4 Antigen cascade. Multiple antigens are released from dying tumor cells that can activate an immune response. (a) Cancer therapy induces death of cancer cells. (b) As these tumor cells die, they release a range of tumor protein antigens (including mutated proteins) that are taken up by scavenger cells called antigen-presenting cells. (c) These antigen-presenting cells then travel to regional lymph nodes where they present these multiple antigens to T cells, initiating or potentiating an antitumor immune response. (d) Activated polyclonal tumor-specific T cells can then traffic to areas of tumor to participate in immune-mediated tumor killing, destroying more cancer cells and further potentiating the cascade.

cells that have now been identified are CD4+CD25+FoxP3+ (Tregs), immature macrophages, and CD4+ NKT+ cells.[347,348] Studies are ongoing employing reagents that can potentially reduce the activity of these regulatory T cells, including the fusion protein Ontak,[349] cyclophosphamide,[212,221,350] and anti-CD25 Abs.[351,352] The inhibition of these cells will most likely be a part of cancer vaccine therapy in the future.

Antigen cascade

The phenomenon of antigen cascade (Figure 4) is now evolving as an important facet in the evaluation of cancer vaccines. This was first defined using the term epitope spreading, in which a given peptide was used as a vaccine and the host immune response post vaccination was not only directed to that epitope, but also to other epitopes of the same tumor antigen.[308,352,353] This phenomenon has now been expanded using the term antigen cascade, in which a given antigen is used as a vaccine and the host immune response post vaccination is not only directed against the antigen in the vaccine but also to other antigens in the tumor. The explanation for these phenomena is that as a consequence of some tumor-cell destruction induced by the vaccine, APCs will engulf tumor fragments and then cross-present those tumor fragments to T cells, thus initiating the antigen cascade phenomenon. It has also been shown that 1/8 prostate cancer patients receiving radiation developed antibodies to an array of TAAs, while 15/33 patients receiving PROSTVAC plus radiation developed such antibodies.[354,355] Antigen cascade has now been observed in preclinical models[356] and

several trials have shown that antigen cascade correlated with antitumor activity.[142,357–361] This phenomenon of antigen cascade is also a mechanism by which the host will direct an immune response to the many mutated gene products in the tumor. Some studies have also suggested improved clinical outcomes for patients who demonstrated a broadened immune response to epitopes not found in the vaccine.[359,362–364]

Immune monitoring

One is always asked for immune correlates of patient benefit in therapeutic cancer vaccine clinical studies. See Ref. 365 for an excellent review. The extreme complexity of the human immune system, the genetic diversity of the human population, and the diversity among cancer patients in terms of type and stage of disease make this a truly daunting task. In addition to the analysis of antigen-specific CD4 and CD8 immune cell subsets, numerous other immune subsets may play an important and/or interdependent role in patient responses; these include regulatory T cells and myeloid-derived suppressor cells as examples. Over 130 different human immune cell subsets have now been identified. Soluble factors produced by tumors or in the tumor microenvironment can also influence immune responses; these include, among others, TGF-β, IL-8, VEGF, IFN-γ, TNF, CD40L, and sCD27. Confounding factors other than those mentioned above include number and type of prior therapies, age and sex of the patient, and size of tumor lesions. Differences in immune cells in the periphery versus different locations within the tumor are of extreme importance. These types of data are more easily obtained in melanoma patients, but biopsies of metastatic lesions are not as easily obtained in most patients with solid tumors.

Newer techniques are currently being employed to investigate patients' immune responses; these include, among others, gene chip RNA arrays of tumor and peripheral blood samples, analysis of changes in TCR clones pre- versus post vaccination, and changes in over 100 immune cell subsets via multilaser FACS analyses. In addition, analyses of numerous immune cell subsets of patients prior to therapy are emerging as a valuable tool in determining which patients are more likely to benefit from vaccine therapy.[318,366]

Paradigm shifts

The evaluation of cancer vaccines in clinical trials may well necessitate new paradigms.[20,315] Cancer vaccines and cytotoxic drugs act differently in terms of mode of action dynamics, as well as limitations (Table 4, Figure 3). Cytotoxic drugs either kill or do not kill tumor cells. Lack of efficacy is due to either drug resistance by tumor cells, inadequate amounts of drug delivered to the tumor, and/or drug-induced toxicity in the host. Thus, if a patient's disease is progressing on a cytotoxic drug, that drug is immediately withdrawn. The use of a cancer vaccine involves the initiation of a dynamic process in which the patient's own immune system is activated. It is clear from decades of preclinical studies, and now clinical trials, that to maximize the host immune response, one must not only give a primary vaccination but also multiple booster vaccinations over a period of weeks or months to further enhance the level of the immune response. Multiple vaccinations are especially important because factors that will blunt the immune response may be given off by the tumor. Thus, it is not unusual to see disease progression following early vaccinations, only to see disease stabilization or a reduction in tumor burden following multiple vaccinations. Thus, the paradigm of "drug withdrawal upon progression" should be revisited with the use of cancer vaccines.

Clinical trials with a new drug are traditionally evaluated in patients with advanced tumors (many times with a large tumor burden) who have failed prior cytotoxic therapies. Objective clinical responses are evaluated by RECIST criteria, looking for a sustained ≥ 30% reduction in the sum of the longest diameter of target lesions. The scenario is all too familiar where antitumor activity is observed with cytotoxic agents or small-molecule targeted therapies via a reduction of tumor burden by RECIST criteria, but no statistical difference in survival is seen. Unfortunately, there is still a "paradigm paralysis" by some who hold on to this paradigm for the evaluation of immunotherapy agents as the only means of evaluation of efficacy.

Since generation of an immune response to a vaccine is a dynamic process in which T cells can be continually generated upon booster vaccines, a more appropriate endpoint for evaluation should be TTP and, more importantly, survival. Since only a finite amount of T cells can be generated by a vaccine, it may be inappropriate to evaluate a cancer vaccine by its ability to drastically reduce a large tumor burden; this is especially true in patients whose immune system has been compromised due to numerous rounds of prior chemotherapy. A more appropriate setting would be the evaluation of cancer vaccines earlier in the disease setting (e.g., neoadjuvant or adjuvant setting), or in metastatic patients with a small tumor burden. This should particularly be considered in light of the relatively low level of toxicity seen in the use of cancer vaccines.

Summary

The U.S. Food and Drug Administration approvals of (1) the prostate cancer therapeutic vaccine sipuleucel-T, (2) anti-CTLA-4 monoclonal antibody (MAb) ipilimumab, and (3) the MAbs directed against the programmed death ligand 1 (PD-L1)/PD-1 immunosuppressive axis, along with the results of recent clinical studies involving cancer vaccines and other immunotherapeutics, have placed immunotherapy into the mainstream of the management of many cancer types. Many potential TAA targets and vaccine platforms for cancer immunotherapy have been identified. The evaluation of cancer vaccines in clinical trials may well necessitate new paradigms. Cancer vaccines and cytotoxic drugs act differently in terms of mode of action and dynamics. Cytotoxic drugs either kill or do not kill tumor cells; lack of efficacy is due to drug resistance by tumor cells, inadequate amounts of drug delivered to the tumor, and/or drug-induced toxicity in the host. The use of a cancer vaccine involves the initiation of a dynamic process in which the patient's own immune system is activated. Thus, it is not unusual to see disease progression following early vaccinations, only to see disease stabilization or a reduction in tumor burden following multiple vaccinations. Thus, the paradigm of "drug withdrawal upon early progression" should be revisited with the use of cancer vaccines. Preclinical studies, and now several clinical studies, have shown that patients can mount an immune response to a cancer vaccine when given in combination with certain cytotoxic drugs, hormones, or local radiation of tumor. Studies have shown that when tumor cells are exposed to sublethal doses of radiation, certain chemotherapeutic agents, hormone manipulating therapeutics or small-molecule targeted therapeutics, the phenotype of tumor cells is actually modulated to make them more susceptible to vaccine-mediated T-cell-mediated killing. It would also appear that the use of a therapeutic vaccine prior to or at the same time as the use of an anti-PD-L1/PD-1 agent would induce the presence of T cells in the tumor, which would subsequently be activated by inhibiting the PD-L1 expression on tumor, leading to tumor cell lysis.

Acknowledgments

The authors gratefully acknowledge the assistance of Debra Weingarten in the preparation of this chapter.

Key references

The complete reference list can be found on the Wiley Companion Digital Edition of this title (see inside front cover for login instructions).

7 The Future II Study Group. Quadrivalent vaccine against human papillomavirus to prevent high-grade cervical lesions. *N Eng J Med.* 2007;**356**:1915–1927.

10 Polyak K, Weinberg RA. Transitions between epithelial and mesenchymal states: acquisition of malignant and stem cell traits. *Nat Rev Cancer.* 2009;**9**:265–273.

17 Palena C, Polev DE, Tsang KY, et al. The human T-box mesodermal transcription factor Brachyury is a candidate target for T-cell-mediated cancer immunotherapy. *Clin Cancer Res.* 2007;**13**:2471–2478.

20 Schlom J. Therapeutic cancer vaccines: current status and moving forward. *J Natl Cancer Inst.* 2012;**104**:599–613.

25 Jaffee EM, Hruban RH, Biedrzycki B, et al. Novel allogeneic granulocyte-macrophage colony-stimulating factor-secreting tumor vaccine for pancreatic cancer: a phase I trial of safety and immune activation. *J Clin Oncol.* 2001;**19**:145–156.

38 Disis ML, Grabstein KH, Sleath PR, et al. Generation of immunity to the HER-2/neu oncogenic protein in patients with breast and ovarian cancer using a peptide-based vaccine. *Clin Cancer Res.* 1999;**5**:1289–1297.

50 Bendandi M, Gocke CD, Kobrin CB, et al. Complete molecular remissions induced by patient-specific vaccination plus granulocyte-monocyte colony-stimulating factor against lymphoma. *Nat Med.* 1999;**5**:1171–1177.

51 Kwak LW, Campbell MJ, Czerwinski DK, et al. Induction of immune responses in patients with B-cell lymphoma against the surface-immunoglobulin idiotype expressed by their tumors. *N Engl J Med.* 1992;**327**:1209–1215.

98 Kugler A, Stuhler G, Walden P, et al. Regression of human metastatic renal cell carcinoma after vaccination with tumor cell-dendritic cell hybrids. *Nat Med.* 2000;**6**:332–336.

115 Dranoff G. GM-CSF-based cancer vaccines. *Immunol Rev*. 2002;**188**:147–154.

132 Waldmann TA, Dubois S, Tagaya Y. Contrasting roles of IL-2 and IL-15 in the life and death of lymphocytes: implications for immunotherapy. *Immunity*. 2001;**14**:105–110.

136 Fallon J, Tighe R, Kradjian G, et al. The immunocytokine NHS-IL12 as a potential cancer therapeutic. *Oncotarget*. 2014;**5**:1869–1884.

137 Kantoff PW, Higano CS, Shore ND, et al. Sipuleucel-T immunotherapy for castration-resistant prostate cancer. *N Eng J Med*. 2010;**363**:411–422.

138 Hodge JW, Chakraborty M, Kudo-Saito C, et al. Multiple costimulatory modalities enhance CTL avidity. *J Immunol*. 2005;**174**:5994–6004.

140 Kantoff PW, Schuetz TJ, Blumenstein BA, et al. Overall survival analysis of a phase II randomized controlled trial of a Poxviral-based PSA-targeted immunotherapy in metastatic castration-resistant prostate cancer. *J Clin Oncol*. 2010;**28**:1099–1105.

142 Gulley JL, Madan RA, Tsang KY, et al. Immune impact induced by PROSTVAC (PSA-TRICOM), a therapeutic vaccine for prostate cancer. *Cancer Immunol Res*. 2014;**2**:133–141.

158 Markovic SN, Suman VJ, Ingle JN, et al. Peptide vaccination of patients with metastatic melanoma: improved clinical outcome in patients demonstrating effective immunization. *Am J Clin Oncol*. 2006;**29**:352–360.

166 Kirkwood JM, Lee S, Moschos SJ, et al. Immunogenicity and antitumor effects of vaccination with peptide vaccine+/-granulocyte-monocyte colony-stimulating factor and/or IFN-alpha2b in advanced metastatic melanoma: Eastern Cooperative Oncology Group Phase II Trial E1696. *Clin Cancer Res*. 2009;**15**: 1443–1451.

167 Testori A. Phase III comparison of vitespen, an autologous tumor-derived heat shock protein gp96 peptide complex vaccine, with physician's choice of treatment for stage IV melanoma: the C-100-21 Study Group. *J Clin Oncol*. 2008;**26**: 955–962.

170 Ulloa-Montoya F. Predictive gene signature in MAGE-A3 antigen-specific cancer immunotherapy. *J Clin Oncol*. 2013;**31**:2388–2395.

181 Rosenblatt J, Kufe D, Avigan D. Dendritic cell fusion vaccines for cancer immunotherapy. *Expert Opin Biol Ther*. 2005;**5**:703–715.

186 Andtbacka RHI, Kaufman HL, Collichio F, et al. Talimogene laherparepvec improves durable response rate in patients with advanced melanoma. *J Clin Oncol*. 2015;**33**:2780–2788.

192 Morse MA, Niedzwiecki D, Marshall JL, et al. A randomized phase II study of immunization with dendritic cells modified with poxvectors encoding CEA and MUC1 compared with the same poxvectors plus GM-CSF for resected metastatic colorectal cancer. *Ann Surg*. 2013;**258**:879–886.

211 Le DT, Wang-Gillam A, Picozzi V, et al. Safety and survival with GVAX pancreas prime and Listeria monocytogenes-expressing mesothelin (CRS-207) boost vaccines for metastatic pancreatic cancer. *J Clin Oncol*. 2015;**33**:1325–1333.

222 Disis ML, Gooley TA, Rinn K, et al. Generation of T-cell immunity to the HER-2/neu protein after active immunization with HER-2/neu peptide-based vaccines. *J Clin Oncol*. 2002;**20**:2624–2632.

225 Mittendorf EA. Clinical trial results of the HER-2/neu (E75) vaccine to prevent breast cancer recurrence in high-risk patients: from US Military Cancer Institute Clinical Trials Group Study I-01 and I-02. *Cancer*. 2012;**118**:2594–2602.

226 Avigan D, Vasir B, Gong J, et al. Fusion cell vaccination of patients with metastatic breast and renal cancer induces immunological and clinical responses. *Clin Cancer Res*. 2004;**10**:4699–4708.

248 Schuster SJ, Neelapu SS, Gause BL, et al. Vaccination with patient-specific tumor-derived antigen in first remission improves disease-free survival in follicular lymphoma. *J Clin Oncol*. 2011;**29**:2787–2794.

253 Van Tendeloo VF. Induction of complete and molecular remissions in acute myeloid leukemia by Wilms' tumor 1 antigen-targeted dendritic cell vaccination. *Proc Natl Acad Sci U S A*. 2010;**107**:13824–13829.

264 Pollack IF, Jakacki RI, Butterfield LH, et al. Antigen-specific immune responses and clinical outcome after vaccination with glioma-associated antigen peptides and polyinosinic-polycytidylic acid stabilized by lysine and carboxymethylcellulose in children with newly diagnosed malignant brainstem and nonbrainstem gliomas. *J Clin Oncol*. 2014;**32**:2050–2058.

269 Pardoll DM. The blockade of immune checkpoints in cancer immunotherapy. *Nat Rev Cancer*. 2012;**12**:252–264.

273 Duraiswamy J, Kaluza KM, Freeman GJ, et al. Dual blockade of PD-1 and CTLA-4 combined with tumor vaccine effectively restores T-cell rejection function in tumors. *Cancer Res*. 2013;**73**:3591–3603.

274 Madan RA, Mohebtash M, Arlen PM, et al. Ipilimumab and a poxviral vaccine targeting prostate-specific antigen in metastatic castration-resistant prostate cancer: a phase 1 dose-escalation trial. *Lancet Oncol*. 2012;**13**:501–508.

298 Hodge JW, Ardiani A, Farsaci B, et al. The tipping point for combination therapy: cancer vaccines with radiation, chemotherapy, or targeted small molecule inhibitors. *Semin Oncol*. 2012;**39**:323–339.

305 Formenti SC, Demaria S. Combining radiotherapy and cancer immunotherapy: a paradigm shift. *J Natl Cancer Inst*. 2013;**105**:256–265.

306 Kroemer G, Galluzzi L, Kepp O, et al. Immunogenic cell death in cancer therapy. *Annu Rev Immunol*. 2013;**31**:51–72.

337 Stein WD, Gulley JL, Schlom J, et al. Tumor regression and growth rates determined in five intramural NCI prostate cancer trials: the growth rate constant as an indicator of therapeutic efficacy. *Clin Cancer Res*. 2011;**17**:907–917.

353 Ribas A, Timmerman JM, Butterfield LH, et al. Determinant spreading and tumor responses after peptide-based cancer immunotherapy. *Trends Immunol*. 2003;**24**:58–61.

365 Butterfield LH. Cancer vaccines. *BMJ*. 2015;**350**:h988.

66 Cell-based cancer immunotherapy

Krina K. Patel, MD ▪ *Judy S. Moyes, MA (Cantab), MB, BChir, FRCPC, FRCPCH* ▪ *Laurence J. Cooper, MD, PhD*

Overview

For decades, scientists have applied cell-based immunotherapies for treatment of cancers. The successful administration of polyclonal populations of donor-derived or autologous T cells is based in part on defining the precise cellular effectors and identifying tumor-associated antigens (TAAs) that can be targeted to safely achieve an antitumor effect without engendering on-target, but off-tissue toxicity, such as manifested by graft-versus-host-disease (GvHD). The adoptive transfer of T cells can reconstitute or enhance resident immunity, which is in contrast to the apparent limitations associated with vaccine-based strategies in recipients whose endogenous immune system may fail to respond to immunogen. Other cytolytic circulating lymphocyte populations can be harnessed for infusion. These include allogeneic NK cells that may mediate an antitumor effect without *a priori* defining the TAA and perhaps without the risk of GvHD. In some cases, a TAA can be identified, for example, the B-lineage TAA CD19, but host immune tolerance prevents the emergence of an effective immune response. Genetic engineering has been combined with T-cell therapy to generate antigen-specific cells *ex vivo*, through the enforced expression of chimeric antigen receptors (CARs). The adoptive transfer of CD19-specific CAR⁺ T cells has shown promise in initial clinical trials for successful disease control in patients with B-cell malignancies resistant to conventional therapeutic modalities. Here, we describe the current status of cell-based immunotherapy for cancer.

Introduction

Allogeneic hematopoietic stem-cell transplantation (HSCT) can be considered as the first effective form of cellular-based therapy for hematologic malignancies. Successful outcome for patients undergoing allogeneic-HSCT is directly linked to the emergence of a graft-versus-tumor (GvT)-effect mediated by donor-derived immune cells. The relevant cellular immune components of the allograft include T cells, natural killer (NK) cells, and B cells that are recognized as potential effectors of the GvT-effect. The observation that engrafted T cells can eliminate residual tumor cells led to the use of donor leukocyte infusions (DLI) to treat a subset of relapsed leukemias, which provided direct evidence for a GvT reaction.[1] While cytotoxic T cells are the primary mediators of the GvT effect, unfortunately, they also are closely associated with development of graft-versus-host-disease (GvHD)[2] as major and minor histocompatability antigens can be shared between malignant and normal cells. In practical terms, DLI and allogeneic HSCT are limited by GvHD offsetting the benefits of the GvT effect.

For several decades, scientists have applied cell-based immunotherapy for cancer. The successful administration of polyclonal populations of donor-derived or autologous T cells is based in part on defining the precise cellular effectors and identifying

tumor-associated antigens (TAAs) that can be targeted to safely achieve an antitumor effect without engendering on-target, but off-tissue toxicity, such as manifested by GvHD. The adoptive transfer of T cells can enhance resident immunity, which is in contrast to the limitations associated with vaccine-based strategies in patients whose endogenous immune system may fail to respond to an immunogen.[3,4] Other lymphocyte populations can be harnessed for infusion. These include allogeneic NK cells that may mediate an anti-tumor effect without *a priori* defining the TAA and without the risk of GvHD.[5–7] In some cases, a TAA can be identified, for example, CD19, but tolerance prevents the emergence of an effective immune response. Genetic engineering has been combined with T-cell therapy to generate antigen-specific cells *ex vivo*, through the enforced expression of chimeric antigen receptors (CARs). Indeed, the adoptive transfer of CD19-specific CAR⁺ T cells has shown promise in initial clinical trials for successful disease control in patients with B-cell malignancies resistant to conventional therapeutic modalities, as summarized in Table 1. In this chapter, we will describe the current status of cell-based immunotherapy for cancer.

Generation of cellular therapy products

T cells

The immune system of the patient with cancer can be manipulated through the administration of lymphocytes as well as immunomodulatory approaches aimed at enhancing the endogenous T cells' adaptive ability to kill tumor cells. Both of these approaches have led to antitumor effects. Clinical trials infusing antibodies to break checkpoint blockade against CTLA4 and the PD-1/PDL-1 axis lead to activation of an endogenous antitumor immune response and have reported significant long-lasting responses.[13–15] Analysis of biopsy samples reveals that by blocking the PD-1/PDL-1 axis, the antitumor effect is correlated with the baseline density and location of T cells in metastatic melanomas.[16,17] For some tumors, there may not be sufficient quality or quantity of infiltrating T cells in the tumor microenvironment. These tumor types may be targeted by an exogenous source of *ex vivo* expanded effector cells. Thus, adoptive cellular therapy (ACT) has emerged as a highly effective modality capable of eliciting sustained clinical responses for some hematologic malignancies as well as solid tumors as described in Table 2.

In general terms, five forms of T cells have been manipulated for human application. These are (1) lymphokine-activated killer (LAK) cells; (2) cytokine-induced killer (CIK) cells; (3) tumor-infiltrating lymphocyte (TIL) using lymphocytes expanded from a tumor biopsy; (4) antigen-specific T cells based on identification and/or selection of endogenous and typically circulating T cells; and (5) genetically engineered T cells that express a TAA-specific T-cell receptor (TCR) or CAR.

Holland-Frei Cancer Medicine, Ninth Edition. Edited by Robert C. Bast Jr., Carlo M. Croce, William N. Hait, Waun Ki Hong, Donald W. Kufe, Martine Piccart-Gebhart, Raphael E. Pollock, Ralph R. Weichselbaum, Hongyang Wang, and James F. Holland.
© 2017 John Wiley & Sons, Inc. ISBN: 978-1-118-93469-2

Table 1 Selected CD19 CAR T-cell trials.

Type of CAR	Costimulatory domain	Cancer type	Outcomes	Total number of patients	Toxicities	References
Lentivirus	4-1BB	ALL	27 CR	30	Severe CRS	Maude et al.[8]
Gammaretrovirus	CD28	ALL, NHL	14 CR	19	Severe CRS	Lee et al.[9]
Gammaretrovirus	CD28	ALL	14 CR	16	Severe CRS	Davila et al.[10]
Gammaretrovirus	CD28	DLBCL, indolent lymphoma, CLL	8 CR, 4 PR, 1 SD, and 2 were not evaluable	15	Neurologic, delirium	Kochenderfer et al.[11]
Lentivirus	4-1BB	CLL	3 CR, 5 PR, and 6 no response	14	Fever	Porter et al.[12]

ALL, acute lymphoblastic leukemia; NHL, non-Hodgkin lymphoma; DLBCL, diffuse large B-cell lymphoma; CLL, chronic lymphocytic leukemia; CR, complete remission; PR, partial response; SD, stable disease; CRS, cytokine-release syndrome.

Table 2 Selected cellular therapy trials for solid tumors.

Cancer type	Type of ACT	Target antigen	Outcomes	Total number of patients	Toxicities	References
Melanoma	TCR	MART-1; gp-100	8 PR; 1 CR	36	Skin, eyes, and ear	Johnson et al.[18] and Morgan et al.[19]
Melanoma, synovial sarcoma, and esophageal cancer	TCR	MAGE-A3	1 CR, 4 PR, 4 no response, and 2 deaths	9	Recognized MAGE-A12 expressed in the brain and led to neurotoxicity: 3 patients with mental status changes, 2 of whom went into comas and subsequently died	Morgan et al.[20]
Melanoma, high-risk multiple myeloma	TCR	MAGE-A3	Both patients developed fever, progressive hypoxia, and hypotension and expired 4–5 days after infusion	2	Crossreacted with Titin protein on cardiac myocytes which led to heart failure and death	Linette et al.[21]
Synovial sarcoma; melanoma	TCR	NY-ESO-1	2 CR; 7 PR	17	None	Robbins et al.[22]
Renal cell carcinoma	1st gen CAR	CAIX	No objective responses	11	Hepatotoxicity	Lamers et al.[23,24]
Colorectal cancer	TCR	CEA	1 PR	—	Colitis	Ma et al.[25]
Colorectal cancer	3rd gen CAR	ErbB2	1 death	1	Fatal lung toxicity and organ failure from recognition of normal lung ErbB2 expression	Morgan et al.[26]
Ovarian cancer	1st gen CAR	αFR	No objective responses	14	IL-2 related	Kershaw et al.[27]
Neuroblastoma	1st gen CAR	GD2	3 CR	19	Pain	Pule et al.[28] and Louis et al.[29]

Infusion of LAK cells, produced from peripheral blood after culturing with high doses of interleukin-2, was one of the first applications of ACT.[30] Unfortunately, high dose IL-2 led to terminal differentiation and inability to recycle effector function. Furthermore, the positive responses seen in early clinical trials with LAK cells could have been the result of the IL-2 coinfusion.[31] However, the clinical data associated with LAK cells led to the development of TIL, which have antitumor activity, especially for patients with melanoma. CIK cells are a heterogeneous subset of *ex vivo* expanded T-lymphocytes that present a mixed T-NK phenotype and are endowed with major histocompatibility complex (MHC)-unrestricted antitumor activity[32]; antitumor cytotoxic activity is represented by surface markers for both T cells ($CD3^+TCR$ $\alpha^+\beta^+$) and natural killer T (NKT) cells ($CD3^+CD56^+$).[33] T cells that express a TCR composed of αβ heterodimers are the most prevalent T-cell population in peripheral blood; thus, they have been the most widely studied for ACT. Both effector ($CD8^+$) and helper ($CD4^+$) T cells have been evaluated for ACT as bulk populations, antigen-specific clones, or subsequent to genetic modification to express TAA-specific receptors.

Tumor infiltrating lymphocytes (TILs)

Animal studies demonstrated that TIL were significantly more effective than LAK cells in eliminating tumors,[34] prompting clinical trials infusing *in vitro* expanded TIL for patients with metastatic melanoma.[35,36] These trials were begun at the NIH and are now being undertaken worldwide.[37–39] These clinical data reveal that subsets of the inoculum recognize TAAs that can be identified as mutated epitopes based on whole-exon sequencing of tumor samples.[40,41]

Rosenberg and colleagues at the Surgery Branch of the National Cancer Institute (NCI) pioneered and standardized methods for TIL expansion for ACT.[42] First, during the pre-expansion phase, surgically excised tumor specimens were digested and cultured in single-cell suspensions with media containing IL-2, examined for growth and reactivity, and then selected for further expansion and characterization. Early studies showed promising results[35] with remarkable objective response rates of about 50% in metastatic melanoma. Inopportunely, only a subset of patients who were initially enrolled in most of these trials actually underwent infusion of TIL.[43] The lack of an available tumor for surgical harvest, difficulty to isolate and grow TIL from harvested tumor, or inability to show robust, specific effector function of isolated TIL were all reasons that have confined this treatment strategy to academic centers skilled in the generation of this type of cellular product. Toxicities such as hypotension, arrhythmias, and vascular leak syndrome were attributed to the high doses of recombinant IL-2, which was coinfused to improve TIL persistence. The judicious selection of recipients for TIL therapy and management of patients receiving high-dose IL-2 has improved outcomes in subsequent trials. Specifically, those patients who achieved complete remissions (approximately 1/5 of all patients treated) remained disease-free 3 years or greater after treatment.[44] Furthermore, it appears that IL-2 at high doses may not be needed, which will likely broaden the application of this therapy.[45,46]

In efforts to improve the outcome of TIL therapy, a lymphodepletion regimen was added before TIL transfer.[47–49] Lymphodepletion is thought to enhance the persistence of T lymphocytes by providing a pro-proliferative environment through elimination of cytokine sinks (which leads to increased availability of prosurvival cytokines, e.g., IL-7 and IL-15), myeloid-derived suppressor cells and T regulatory cells.[50] The addition of lymphodepletion led to the engraftment of TIL and improved the clinical responses. As a consequence though, the loss of a normal immune defense system led to increased rates of opportunistic infections.

The degree of lymphodepletion appears to impact the antitumor response. Non-myeloablative lymphodepletion regimens with cyclophosphamide and fludarabine achieved response rates reaching 51%.[51,52] When total body irradiation (TBI) was included at doses that required rescue of hematopoiesis with autologous hematopoietic cell transplantation, the overall response rate increased to 70% with complete remission (CR) of 40%; however, the increased intensity of the conditioning regimen was associated with more serious adverse toxicities including febrile neutropenia, infections, and thrombotic microangiopathy.[44,48]

A limitation of using TIL has been patient attrition owing to disease progression or overall clinical decline while waiting for TIL to meet release criteria for administration. Thus, strategies are being developed to decrease the time in culture from TIL collection to infusion.[53] In a recent trial, shortening of the pre-expansion phase allowed TIL to be produced within 28 days which led to a 74% enrollment. These "younger TIL" may also have improved therapeutic benefit as they contain T cells that are not terminally differentiated and avoid replication senescence.[54] Approaches using activation and propagation cells (AaPC) as irradiated feeders to numerically expand TILs are also emerging.[55] These feeder cells may thus help broaden the number of patients who can benefit from TILs and enable tumor-specific T cells to be generated without the need to harvest tumor.

As knowledge about immunotherapy grows rapidly, the number of current clinical trials employing TIL therapy also increases. These include comparing lymphodepleting regimens (NCT01807182; Fred Hutchinson Cancer Center), combination immunotherapy with CTLA-4 (NCT01701674; Moffitt Cancer Center) or PD-1/PDL-1 axis blockade or vaccines (NCT00338377; MD Anderson Cancer Center), and evaluating TIL efficacy in tumor types other than melanoma (NCT01174121; National Cancer Institute).

Peripheral blood T cells

TAA-specific T cells can be collected from peripheral blood using MHC multimers containing peptide epitopes. These are complexed to a fluorescent reagent to stain circulating T cells. The desired population of autologous effector cells can then be sorted, activated, and expanded *in vitro* and infused into the patient to induce tumor regression and long-term immunoprotection.[45,56] The prevalence of TAA-specific effector T cells in peripheral blood can be rare (on the order of 0.2%); however, some studies in melanoma have reported T cells specific for melanocyte antigens such as gp100, tyrosinase, and MART-1 at frequencies reaching 2%.[57] This *in vitro* study also suggested that even though systemic TAA-specific T-cell responses can develop *de novo* in cancer patients, antigen-specific unresponsiveness may explain why such cells are unable to control tumor growth. Therefore, activation of the TCR in the presence of costimulatory molecules, followed by cytokine-induced expansion, is needed to enrich the TAA-specific effector T cells.[58] TCR engagement is mediated by the peptide–MHC complex that presents the antigen to the T cell.

The very low frequency of T cells recognizing commonly expressed antigens limits the applicability of this approach. To overcome this instability, Pollack et al.[59] tested the strategy combining IL-21 modulation during *in vitro* stimulation with tetramer-guided cell sorting to generate TAA specific cytotoxic T lymphocytes. T cells stained with the TAA NY-ESO-1 tetramer were enriched from frequencies as low as 0.4% to >90% after single pass through a clinical grade sorter. NY-ESO-1-specific T cells were generated from all patients included in the study and the final products expanded on average 1200-fold were oligoclonal and contained 67–97% CD8+, tetramer+ T cells with a memory phenotype that recognized endogenous NY-ESO-1.

Peripheral blood dendritic cells

Autologous dendritic cells (DCs), a class of professional antigen-presenting cells, are used to selectively propagate autologous T cells by coculture *in vitro*. To obtain DCs, monocytes from peripheral blood are cultured in IL-4 and granulocyte-macrophage colony-stimulating factor (GM-CSF) to dedifferentiate into immature DCs. These immature DCs can then be loaded with tumor antigen or lysate and cultured in cytokines to mediate maturation and upregulation of costimulatory ligands such as CD80 and CD86. Alternatively, the use of peptide to pulse mature DCs generates high-affinity CD8+ and CD4+ T cells recognizing only a single antigenic epitope. Artificial antigen-presenting cells (aAPCs) have also been developed as an alternative to DCs, derived from the human erythroleukemia cell line, K562. These cells express HLA (human leukocyte antigen) C alleles and no other classical HLA class I or II molecules and can be genetically modified to express TAA, HLA, and costimulatory molecules to optimize generation of the antigen-specific T-cells.[55,60]

Both TIL and antigen-specific T-cell therapy provide complementary strategies for the treatment of patients with solid tumor malignancies and represent promising prospects in the development of ACT as a treatment modality. They not only provide effective treatment for patients but also supply a rich source of data for immunobiological discovery.

Genetically engineered T cells

With advancements in immunology and gene transfer, T-cell function has been enhanced by altering receptor specificity and signaling functions that control ability to recycle antigen-dependent effector functions.[61] A justification for genetic retargeting of T cells is that the endogenous TAA-specific T-cell repertoire undergoes immune-mediated tolerance rendering these cells unable to either recognize or effectively respond to malignant cells. Two types of genetically modified T cells are in current clinical trials for oncology based on redirecting specificity through enforced expression of defined TCRs or CARs.

Efficient gene transfer into T cells is necessary to generate both TCR and CAR cellular products. γ-Retroviral and lentiviral transduction techniques rely on the propensity of these viruses to integrate permanently into the host genome. GMP (good manufacturing practice)-grade viral vector production is a costly, time-consuming, and specialized technique. Despite early concerns about insertional mutagenesis, decades of experience with transduction of primary T cells have failed to show any examples of this theoretical complication.[62] Nonviral gene transfer is an alternative and relatively cheaper approach. The most commonly used approaches are transposon/transposase systems such as Sleeping Beauty. This system results in sustained expression of CAR on T cells, and anti-CD19 transposon CAR T cells are in early-phase clinical trials.[63] Another novel approach is the electroporation of T lymphocytes with *in vitro* transcribed RNA.[64] This leads to high, but transient, expression of the CAR. With the exception of the mRNA electroporation technique, gene transfer into T cells is typically carried out at the beginning of a period of *in vitro* culture and stimulation. This system leads to more efficient transduction and a greatly expanded number of T cells for subsequent adoptive transfer.

T-cell receptors (TCRs)

The rationale for engrafting high-affinity TCRs is that the endogenous repertoire for TCRs is generally of low affinity when targeting self-TAAs. The assumption is that as such low-affinity TCR chains are unable to control malignancy, increasing the affinity will initiate an effective antitumor response.[65] Indeed, there is precedent based on animal studies.[66] There are three general approaches to increasing the affinity of TCRs (1) *in silico* changes to antigen-binding domains, especially CDR3[67]; (2) using combination platforms such as the XPRESIDENT technology that uses mass spectrometry, gene expression profiling, literature-based functional assessment, *in vitro* human T-cell assays, and bioinformatics to select the most appropriate tumor-associated peptides[68]; and (3) CARs that recognize peptide in context of restricting HLA molecules.[69,70] The TCR is composed of a complex of six polypeptide chains (α, β, γ, δ, ε, and ζ), which connect on the cell surface as part of the immunological synapse to initiate a T-cell activation signal. The α and β chains comprise a heterodimer to form the primary binding domain of the TCR, which recognize intracellularly processed peptides presented on the surface of target cells by classical HLA class I and II molecules. Other constituents of the immunological synapse such as costimulatory and adhesion molecules increase the strength and quality of the TCR-HLA-peptide engagement leading to a fully competent T-cell activation event, defined at a minimum as (1) serial killing, (2) sustained proliferation, (3) T_c1 cytokine production, and (4) protection from activation-induced cell death (AICD). The genetic modification of T cells to enforce expression of TCR has been translated from the bench[71] to the bedside. Initial clinical efforts adoptively transferred autologous T cells that had been rendered specific for melanoma.[19] The clinical responses were inferior to recipients of (nongenetically modified) TIL. However, these data established the proof-of-principle that T cells could be engineered to target TAAs and provided justification for targeting tumors other than melanoma. They also provided a glimpse of the future as T cells expressing high-affinity TCRs participated in on-target and off-tissue recognition of normal melanin expressing cells in the inner ear and retina.[18]

The broad human application of T cells genetically modified to express TAA-specific TCR faces two significant challenges. The first is the unwanted mispairing between the introduced $\alpha\beta$ TCR and endogenous $\alpha\beta$ TCR, which could (1) reduce the number of appropriately paired chains that can recognize HLA-peptide and (2) generate TCR heterodimers that have not undergone thymic selection and tolerance, which could lead to deleterious recognition of normal structures. This has been demonstrated in the mouse[72,73] but has not led to clinical compromise in human trials. Table 3 provides a current list of approaches to eliminate mispairing between introduced and endogenous TCR. The second problem is associated with the affinity of the engrafted TCR. Methods to increase affinity are also not subject to thymic selection and tolerance mechanisms, which, when coupled with an incomplete understanding of their specificity, exposes the recipient to on target but off-tissue side effects. Most approaches currently rely on targeting nonmutated self-antigens, the most promising of which may be gene products from the cancer testis family of genes.[22] An affinity-enhanced NY ESO-1-specific and HLA-A2-restricted TCR was tested in patients with melanoma and synovial cell sarcoma and no serious toxicity was seen.[22] However, the adoptive transfer of autologous T cells expressing an affinity-enhanced[21] HLA-A1-restricted MAGE A3-specific TCR led to lethal cardiac toxicity in two patients owing to off-target recognition of Titin. In another trial,[20] in which autologous T cells with affinity-enhanced TCR recognizing MAGE A3 in the context of HLA-A2 were infused in patients with melanoma, significant neurotoxicity from a cross-reactive antigen MAGE A12 present on brain cells occurred; specifically, three patients experienced mental status changes and two lapsed into comas and died. Systemic administration of corticosteroids did not help to reverse the toxicities. While these events illustrate the potency that engineered autologous T cells can display, they highlight the urgent need for improved preclinical systems to uncover off-target adverse events before initiation of clinical trials.

Although TCR-based ACT approaches have great potential, they do have inherent limitations. The HLA-restricted specificity of engineered TCR limits the number of potential patients to those expressing the relevant HLA allele recognized by the T cells. In addition, because tumors often downregulate HLA alleles and interrupt proteasomal processing pathways, antigen escape variants and lack of complete remissions are relevant.

Chimeric antigen receptors (CARs)

Prototypical CARs combine an extracellular single-chain variable fragment (scFv) of an antibody with a transmembrane (TM) domain and intracellular signaling domains derived from molecules involved in T-cell signaling complex. Typically, clinically appealing

Table 3 Methods typically used to eliminate mispairing between introduced and endogenous alpha/beta TCR.

Various methods to facilitate introduced $\alpha\beta$ TCR pairing	References
Use of full or partial mouse TCR α and β	Cohen et al.,[74] Sommermeyer and Uckert,[75] and Cohen et al.[76]
Addition of another disulfide bond within constant region	Kuball et al.[77] and Cohen et al.[78]
Use of Knob-into-hole configuration	Voss et al.[79]
Application of short hairpin RNAs (shRNAs) against TCR$\alpha\beta$ constant regions to suppress endogenous TCR$\alpha\beta$ expression	Okamoto et al.[80,81]
Introduction of zinc finger nucleases (ZFNs) or other artificial nucleases to completely disrupt endogenous TCR$\alpha\beta$ expression at genomic level	Provasi et al.,[82] Poirot, et al.,[83] Torikai et al.[84]

CARs use the signaling motif from the CD3-ζ chain in combination with signaling domains from molecules involved in T-cell activation or costimulation.[85,86] As the scFv domain binds directly to target cell surface epitopes, CARs can bypass the need for MHC-restricted antigen presentation and, therefore, are immune to tumor escape mechanisms related to HLA downregulation. CARs can overcome T-cell triggering limitations related to epitope density, as the scFv can have a high affinity for the TAA. Multigeneration CARs have been developed which have a combination of signaling domains attached to the cytosolic activation domain. These CAR species are designed to provide a fully competent T-cell activation event in the tumor microenvironment. It appears that CARs that are capable of signaling in addition to the phosphorylation of the immunoreceptor tyrosine-based activation motif (ITAM) in CD3-ζ have improved *in vivo* persistence[87] and thus antitumor effects. Two second-generation CARs have resulted in dramatic antitumor effects in patients with CD19[+] malignancies. CAR[+] T cells with the chimeric CD137 signaling domain (i.e., 4-1BB) have resulted in dramatic antitumor effects in patients with acute and chronic B-cell leukemias.[88–90] In addition, CAR[+] T cells with chimeric CD28 signaling domain have potent antitumor effects in patients with B-cell leukemias and lymphomas.[9,10,91] Patients with B-lineage acute lymphoblastic leukemia (ALL) that is refractory to conventional therapy have had high response rates with more than 90% achieving a CR.[8] The sustained antitumor effect associated with these two CAR designs appears to be related to two events: the *in vivo* proliferation of genetically modified T cells, and whether the patient relapses with leukemic blasts that have lost expression of CD19.

The clinical data targeting acute versus chronic CD19[+] leukemias have revealed differences in the ability of autologous CAR[+] T cells to eliminate these hematologic malignancies. The targeting of ALL with CD19-specific CARs activated through CD28 or CD137 appears to achieve superior rates of remission when compared to these same two CAR designs targeting chronic lymphocytic leukemia (CLL). These clinical data underscore the need to understand the microenvironment in which genetically modified T cells operate as well as nongenetically modified T cells in their ability to participate in a fully competent T-cell activation event.

CAR T cells targeting CD19 with a CD28 signaling domain have shown significant effects in patients with ALL[63]; however, the outcomes for CLL patients with this CAR have been modest.[92] Unlike the CARs with 4-1BB, these CARs with CD28 have not displayed long-term engraftment or persistence. Second-generation CD28-based CARs have shown improved survival over first-generation CD3ζ CAR T cells, but the average survival of CAR T cells in patients with ALL treated at the Memorial Sloan Kettering Cancer Center was approximately 28 days.[10] A phase I trial at NCI also demonstrated loss of persistence of CD19 CAR with CD28 signaling domain by 28 days in the majority of patients.[9] However, both trials showed significant responses with maximum expansion of CAR T cells occurring within the first 14 days of infusion, which coincided with the disappearance of peripheral blasts in those patients with a positive response. Remarkably, most patients had regeneration of nonmalignant B cells by day 28, contrary to those patients on trials who had long-lived persistence of CD19 CAR T cells and sustained B-cell aplasia. The short duration of engraftment has made it more appealing to use as a bridge to transplant. Third-generation CARs, such as the CD20-specific CAR T cell with CD28 and 4-1BB costimulatory domains, have also shown early potential but need further evaluation.[93] Recently, Long et al. identified that 4-1BB diminishes exhaustion in persistently stimulated CAR T cells, implying a basis for its improved

persistence in patients compared to those CAR T cells with CD28 signaling which likely augments exhaustion. They are conducting essential ongoing studies to elucidate potential pathways involved in CAR T-cell exhaustion.[94] Time will tell whether CAR T cells will replace the need for allogeneic stem cell transplantation, or if they will serve as a bridge to transplantation or as a form of consolidation therapy. It is not yet known if every tumor cell is eradicated in patients in remission, or if there are dormant tumor cells that are controlled by the long-term persistence of CAR T cells. Likely, different CAR designs may be needed for varying levels of "bioburden" of tumor cells.

Multiple early phase clinical trials have also highlighted the potential toxicities for CAR T-cell therapies. On-target, but off-tumor, toxicities are a consequence of varying levels of expression of the targeted tumor-associated antigen in normal tissues. Redirected T cells can be highly potent and toxic to normal tissues that express low levels of the targeted antigen. This can be extremely detrimental as described in 2006 by the Erasmus University in Rotterdam.[95] Here, patients infused with T cells modified with a CAR specific for carbonic anhydrase 9, which is physiologically expressed on bile duct epithelial cells, had significant levels of cholestasis. The severity of on-target, but off-tumor toxicities is dependent on whether the tissues expressing the targeted antigen are essential for survival, and if the injuries are manageable by other means. For example, in clinical trials investigating T cells modified with a CD19-specific CAR, the resulting profound B-cell aplasia post-therapy has been managed successfully by gamma-globulin replacement.[89] Conversely, low-level ERBB2 expression on lung epithelia may have led to fatal lung toxicity in a patient with colon cancer who received a high dose of third-generation CAR-modified T cells after intensive lymphodepletion, as reported by the NCI in Bethesda.[26] Baylor College of Medicine (BCM) is targeting ERBB2 in patients with glioblastoma multiforme; thus far, significant toxicities with lower doses of second-generation CAR-modified T cells without lymphodepletion have not been reported. When developing CARs/TCRs, analyzing in detail the target antigen expression on normal tissues and verifying normal cells' susceptibility to being killed by the genetically targeted T cells is critical. *In vitro* experiments will not always accurately predict these important data as the targeted antigen could be expressed only at certain stages of differentiation (i.e., CD123) or could be altered by environmental signals (i.e., CD44v6). Therefore, *in vivo* experiments in appropriate preclinical models should be considered.

The most severe toxicity observed in patients treated with CAR-modified T cells has been the cytokine-release syndrome (CRS), which manifests as a rapid immune reaction driven by the massive release of a large group of cytokines, including IFN-gamma and IL-6.[96] The high levels of IFN-gamma result from a robust effector function of CAR-modified T cells, while increase in IL-6 is likely a consequence of a macrophage activation syndrome (MAS). In different trials, patients infused with second-generation CD19-specific CAR T cells developed a clinical picture resembling MAS (fever, hypotension, and hemophagocytic syndrome). Furthermore, because administration of the IL-6 receptor antagonist mAb tocilizumab leads to improvement in patients with this clinical picture,[96] it is believed that abnormal activation of macrophages may be the driving force behind CRS. A range of precautions has been proposed for mitigating the risk of life-threatening CRS, including splitting the initial dose of CAR-modified T cells over 3 days, strict monitoring of vital parameters during the first hours after infusion, early detection of clinical and laboratory signs heralding the syndrome such as C reactive protein (CRP),[97] and therapeutic interventions, including high-dose corticosteroids and tocilizumab. Although these measures have been variously effective, CRS remains a matter of serious concern for the overall safety of CAR-modified T cells. However, CRS may also serve as a biomarker indicating that the T-cell therapy is working. Interestingly, not all trials have reported CRS; disease status at time of infusion as well as type of CAR being infused may be variables influencing the risk for CRS.

The type of T-cell subset that is engineered for adoptive immunotherapy is associated with various clinical outcomes.[56] Initially, effector T cells (Teff) were postulated to be superior cellular substrate for adoptive immunotherapy because of their high cytotoxic ability. However, early clinical trials demonstrated that highly differentiated, tumor-specific Teff CD8+ T cells engrafted inadequately, were less capable of tumor killing compared with heterogeneous populations of TIL and had inferior clinical outcomes when infused in patients compared to those infused with less differentiated cell products. Animal studies have revealed that transfer of less differentiated T-cell populations has resulted in better *in vivo* expansion, persistence, and antitumor activity.[98] In nonhuman primates, the transfer of Teff CD8+ T cells derived from central memory T cells (Tcm), as opposed to effector memory-derived T cells, demonstrated long-term *in vivo* persistence and reacquired memory T-cell properties.[87] Continuing along this line of reasoning, Teff cells derived from the naive T-cell subset (Tn) have been shown to possess greater antitumor activity and enhanced *in vivo* persistence than transferred Tcm-derived Teff.[99] Recently, a stem cell memory T-cell subset (Tscm) has been newly identified and is described to be a long-lived memory T cell that has the capability of self-renewal, as well as multipotent capacity to derive all other T-cell memory subsets.[100] *In vivo* experiments demonstrated that Tscm were superior in antitumor response in comparison to all other T-cell memory subsets,[100] whereas recent clinical observations have indicated that expansion of CAR-modified T cells in patients was correlated solely with the frequency of a subset characterized to be closely related to Tscm,[51] putatively making this the ideal T-cell subset for cellular engineering.

With a shifting paradigm focusing on utilizing lesser differentiated T-cell subsets and preserving their memory characteristics, several avenues are being investigated to manufacture the best quality T-cell product for adoptive transfer. One main approach has been to modify the culture conditions by selection of choice cytokines, and their combination, from the common gamma chain cytokine receptor family. Interleukin-7 (IL-7), IL-15, and IL-21 have emerged as key factors in the generation of desired Tcm and Tscm subsets[51,101–103] Delving into the details of pathway signal transduction, accumulating evidence illustrates the importance of several pathways in dictating T-cell differentiation based on the strength of stimulation. Activation of the phosphatidylinositol 3-kinase (PI3K)/Akt pathway and mammalian target of rapamycin complex 1 (mTORC1) results in induction of T-cell differentiation programs in a progressive manner, and the use of AKT and mTOR inhibitors has been shown to enhance the generation of memory T cells,[104–107] whereas activating Wnt signaling can enhance memory CD8+ T-cell formation including the Tscm subset.[108] While these pathways tie into nutrient sensing and signal integration, more specific details have emerged recently on the effects of T-cell metabolism on memory formation. Enhancing CD8 T-cell memory can be achieved by accentuating fatty acid oxidation in T cells or inhibiting glycolytic metabolism.[107,109,110] The generation of such T cells with preserved memory characteristics is of great value and implementation in culture methods for clinical manufacture of such T cells is critical in the continued efforts to enhance T-cell quality for improved therapeutic potential.

Gamma delta T cells (γδ T cells)

Gamma delta T cells (CD3+TCR γ+δ+) are a distinct population of T cells, although they represent only a minority of T cells in peripheral blood (1–5%). This specialized group of T cells recognizes an extensive range of targets in an MHC-unrestricted approach and manifests lytic activity and proinflammatory cytokine secretion. A better recovery of γδ T lymphocytes after unmanipulated allogeneic bone marrow transplantation has been associated with an increased probability of leukemia-free survival, without an augmented risk of GvHD.[111] Aminobisphosphonates, for example, zoledronic acid, resulted in *in vivo* propagation of γδ T cells, and the use of aminobisphosphonates has been translated into laboratory practice to grow γδ T cells *ex vivo*[112]; however, only the Vγ9Vδ2 T-cell subset expands out with this approach. Recent advances using immobilized antigens, agonistic monoclonal antibodies (mAbs), tumor-derived aAPC, or combinations of activating mAbs and aAPC have been successful in expanding γδ T cells with oligoclonal or polyclonal TCR repertoires.[113,114] These cells are being tested for ACT,[115,116] as both unmodified cells following *ex vivo* expansion[117] and postgenetic engineering using CARs, as described earlier.[118]

NK cells

Approximately 10% of peripheral blood lymphocytes are NK cells,[119] typically defined as CD56+ CD3−, which are the primary cytotoxic component of the innate immune system. Having both cytotoxic and regulatory activity, NK cells recognize virus-infected or malignant cells that express danger signals (stress ligands and antibodies) and/or lack class I MHC[120] and are potent mediators of antibody-dependent cell cytotoxicity (ADCC).[121] NK cells have been used in various ACT applications, and most commonly with peripheral blood NK cells from donor sources that have been collected and activated.[122] Many *ex vivo* expansion protocols have been developed to increase both number and function of adoptively transferred NK cells.[123–126] In addition to antitumor activity when delivered as ACT in nontransplant settings,[127–132] NK cells may have potential for moderating infection and GvHD in the HSCT setting.[133–137]

NKT cells

Smaller lymphocyte subsets, phenotypically in-between typical NK and T cells, have been tested for ACT. These NKT cells (CD3+CD56+), Invariant natural killer T cell (iNKT) cells (CD3+CD56+Va24-Ja18), and CIK cells (CD3+CD56+) are effector lymphocyte subpopulations with potential advantages. NKT cells modulate immune responses against malignant cells and stimulate effector cell functioning. Furthermore, NKT cells traffic to solid tumors in response to chemokines produced by tumor cells and tumor-associated macrophages (TAMs),[138,139] colocalize with TAMs and can kill or inhibit these growth-promoting cells[140] in a CD1d-dependent manner.[141] Heczey et al.[142] have shown in a mouse model that GD2-specific CAR renders NKT cells cytotoxic against neuroblastoma cells and results in potent *in vivo* antitumor activity without graft-versus-host disease. iNKT cells recognize a distinctive glycolipid molecule (αGalCer) in the context of the CD1d molecule, which can specifically expand them *ex vivo* as well as *in vivo*. Other NKT cell subsets have been delineated but have not been developed yet for ACT.

Regulatory T cells

Naturally occurring regulatory T cells (Treg) have potential for prevention of GvHD.[143,144] Novel methods of Treg expansion to generate clinically relevant numbers have been discovered recently.[145,146] Furthermore, in a xenogeneic model of GvHD, prophylactic injection of third-party, cord blood (CB)-derived, *ex vivo* expanded Treg led to the prevention of GvHD that translated into improved GvHD score, decreased circulating inflammatory cytokines and significantly superior overall survival.[147] Early clinical trials for prevention and treatment of GvHD by infusing regulatory T cells are currently under investigation. Several early clinical trials are being conducted to assess the effect on GvHD of infusing regulatory T cells following hematopoietic stem cell transplantation[148] and also the infusion of Treg in type I diabetes[149] (NCT01210664).

Dendritic cells

Sipuleucel-T is a type of autologous cellular immunotherapy that stimulates an immune response against the antigen prostatic acid phosphatase (PAP) expressed in most prostate cancer tissues and is FDA (Food and Drug Administration) approved for the treatment of metastatic hormone-refractory prostate cancer (HRPC) in patients who are asymptomatic or minimally symptomatic. Peripheral blood is collected from the patient via leukopheresis, from which peripheral blood mononuclear cells (PBMCs) are isolated. Antigen presenting cell (APC) precursors, consisting of CD54-positive cells that include DCs, are isolated from the PBMCs. The APCs are then activated *in vitro* with a recombinant human fusion protein, PAP-GM-CSF, and cultured for 40 h. The final product is reinfused into the patient, inducing T-cell immunity to tumors that express PAP. Full treatment included three infusions with two weeks between successive infusions.

Sipuleucel-T showed overall survival benefit to patients in three double-blind randomized phase III clinical trials: D9901, D9902a,[150] and IMPACT.[151] The IMPACT trial served as the basis for licensing approval of sipuleucel-T by the FDA. This trial enrolled 512 patients (randomized in a 2:1 ratio) with asymptomatic or minimally symptomatic metastatic HRPC. The median survival time for patients receiving sipuleucel-T was 25.8 months compared to 21.7 months for placebo-treated patients ($P = 0.032$).

Sipuleucel-T was predicted to become a blockbuster. Unfortunately, Dendreon, the company which invented this innovative treatment, filed for bankruptcy in November 2014. Sales were hampered by the drug's high cost of $93,000 for a course of treatment, the complexity of customizing the therapy for each patient, and competition from new oral therapies for prostate cancer that were recently FDA approved.

Off-the-shelf (OTS) therapy

To eliminate the need for patient-specific products for ACT and, therefore, decrease the time needed to generate cellular therapy, efforts have been focused on generating "universal donor T cells" by the use of artificial nucleases to eliminate the expression of the endogenous TCRs, for example, zinc finger nucleases (ZFNs)[84,152] or transcription activator-like effector nucleases (TALENs).[153] Furthermore, reducing the allo-recognition of engineered T cells will lead potentially to an OTS (off-the-shelf) therapy by generating universal allogeneic TAA-specific T cells from one donor that may be administered to multiple recipients.

Cord blood

Umbilical CB is increasingly used to restore hematopoiesis in patients undergoing hematopoietic stem cell transplantation who lack a suitable HLA-matched donor. CB offers the advantage of lower incidence of graft-versus-host disease compared with bone marrow or mobilized peripheral blood. CB transplantation is limited by low cell doses and delays in neutrophil and platelet engraftment; however, CB progenitors expanded *ex vivo* before

transplantation provide more rapid hematopoietic and immune reconstitution as well as less engraftment failure compared with unmanipulated CB. Infusion of expanded CB products is safe and associated with a low likelihood of severe reactions. Recent studies demonstrate that *ex vivo* fucosylation of CB can enhance engraftment in murine models, and *ex vivo* treatment of CB with fucosyltransferase (FT) VI before transplantation is currently under clinical evaluation.[154–157]

CB also provides a source of cells for cellular therapy. Virus infections after stem cell transplantation are among the most common causes of death, especially after cord blood transplantation (CBT) where the CB does not contain appreciable numbers of virus-experienced T cells that can protect the recipient from infection. Hanley et al. developed a strategy to generate autologous CB T cells specific for CMV (cytomegalovirus) and adenovirus. On the basis of this approach, a clinical trial led by Bollard et al. has been testing the use of CB-derived multivirus-specific T cells targeting EBV, CMV, and adenovirus for the prevention and treatment of viral infections after transplantation.[158]

As described previously, NK cells and Tregs can also be expanded from CB for use as cellular therapy. Resting CB NK cells are reported to have significantly less cytotoxicity compared with peripheral blood NK cells. However, after cytokine stimulation, the cytotoxicity of CB NK cells can be rapidly increased to levels comparable to peripheral blood NK cells. Brunstein et al. expanded Tregs obtained from a third party CB unit and infused them into 23 patients undergoing double CBT. No severe Treg-related acute toxicities were observed and incidence of GvHD was decreased.[159] Further studies indicate a higher incidence of viral infections in the first 30 days post Treg infusion; however, there were no adverse long-term effects.[160]

Safety

In case of adverse events, a safety mechanism which would allow the rapid elimination of the infused cells is required for adoptively transferred cells, especially those that have been manipulated genetically. One such mechanism involves using an inducible safety switch that is based on the fusion of human caspase 9 to a modified human FK-binding protein, allowing conditional dimerization.[161] When exposed to a synthetic dimerizing drug, the inducible caspase 9 (iCasp9) becomes activated and leads to the rapid death of cells expressing this construct. At the 2014 annual meeting of the American Society of Hematology, Bonini et al.[162] presented their preliminary data from a phase III trial evaluating T cells genetically modified to express the HSV-TK suicide gene. In the phase II study, they showed that these cells can safely induce early immune reconstitution when given after a T-cell depleted haploidentical transplant and can be killed with a dose of ganciclovir if graft versus host occurs.[163]

Conclusion

The potential of cellular therapy as an effective anticancer treatment is being realized, and as a result, immunotherapy was celebrated as the 2013 Science Breakthrough of the Year.[164] ACT utilizing engineered T cells has illustrated impressive effectiveness in clinical studies by attaining complete and deep responses in patients with treatment refractory disease. Major hurdles include incomplete understanding of TAA and the need for safer TAAs. Currently, hundreds of patients are being treated per year at individual academic centers. With ACT now being commercialized, the infrastructure to provide access to tens-of-thousands of patients across the United States and around the world is still needed.[165]

Acknowledgments

The authors would like to thank Drs. Dean Lee, Hiroki Torikai, Lenka Hurton, and George McNamara for their contributions to this chapter.

Key references

The complete reference list can be found on the Wiley Companion Digital Edition of this title (see inside front cover for login instructions).

2 Weiden PL et al. Antileukemic effect of graft-versus-host disease in human recipients of allogeneic-marrow grafts. *N Engl J Med.* 1979;**300(19)**:1068–1073.

3 Rapoport AP et al. Restoration of immunity in lymphopenic individuals with cancer by vaccination and adoptive T-cell transfer. *Nat Med.* 2005;**11(11)**:1230–1237.

4 Walter EA et al. Reconstitution of cellular immunity against cytomegalovirus in recipients of allogeneic bone marrow by transfer of T-cell clones from the donor. *N Engl J Med.* 1995;**333(16)**:1038–1044.

5 Ruggeri L et al. Effectiveness of donor natural killer cell alloreactivity in mismatched hematopoietic transplants. *Science.* 2002;**295(5562)**:2097–2100.

8 Maude SL et al. Chimeric antigen receptor T cells for sustained remissions in leukemia. *N Engl J Med.* 2014;**371(16)**:1507–1517.

9 Lee DW et al. T cells expressing CD19 chimeric antigen receptors for acute lymphoblastic leukaemia in children and young adults: a phase 1 dose-escalation trial. *Lancet.* 2014;**385**:517–528.

10 Davila ML et al. Efficacy and toxicity management of 19-28z CAR T cell therapy in B cell acute lymphoblastic leukemia. *Sci Transl Med.* 2014;**6(224)**:224ra25.

19 Morgan RA et al. Cancer regression in patients after transfer of genetically engineered lymphocytes. *Science.* 2006;**314(5796)**:126–129.

21 Linette GP et al. Cardiovascular toxicity and titin cross-reactivity of affinity-enhanced T cells in myeloma and melanoma. *Blood.* 2013;**122(6)**:863–871.

22 Robbins PF et al. Tumor regression in patients with metastatic synovial cell sarcoma and melanoma using genetically engineered lymphocytes reactive with NY-ESO-1. *J Clin Oncol.* 2011;**29(7)**:917–924.

30 Rosenberg SA et al. Observations on the systemic administration of autologous lymphokine-activated killer cells and recombinant interleukin-2 to patients with metastatic cancer. *N Engl J Med.* 1985;**313(23)**:1485–1492.

35 Rosenberg SA et al. Use of tumor-infiltrating lymphocytes and interleukin-2 in the immunotherapy of patients with metastatic melanoma. A preliminary report. *N Engl J Med.* 1988;**319(25)**:1676–1680.

36 Schwartzentruber DJ et al. In vitro predictors of therapeutic response in melanoma patients receiving tumor-infiltrating lymphocytes and interleukin-2. *J Clin Oncol.* 1994;**12(7)**:1475–1483.

40 Robbins PF et al. Mining exomic sequencing data to identify mutated antigens recognized by adoptively transferred tumor-reactive T cells. *Nat Med.* 2013;**19(6)**:747–752.

41 Tran E et al. Cancer immunotherapy based on mutation-specific CD4+ T cells in a patient with epithelial cancer. *Science.* 2014;**344(6184)**:641–645.

45 Yee C et al. Adoptive T cell therapy using antigen-specific CD8+ T cell clones for the treatment of patients with metastatic melanoma: in vivo persistence, migration, and antitumor effect of transferred T cells. *Proc Natl Acad Sci U S A.* 2002;**99(25)**:16168–16173.

48 Dudley ME et al. Adoptive cell therapy for patients with metastatic melanoma: evaluation of intensive myeloablative chemoradiation preparative regimens. *J Clin Oncol.* 2008;**26(32)**:5233–5239.

49 Rosenberg SA, Spiess P, Lafreniere R. A new approach to the adoptive immunotherapy of cancer with tumor-infiltrating lymphocytes. *Science.* 1986;**233(4770)**:1318–1321.

56 Hunder NN et al. Treatment of metastatic melanoma with autologous CD4+ T cells against NY-ESO-1. *N Engl J Med.* 2008;**358(25)**:2698–2703.

57 Lee PP et al. Characterization of circulating T cells specific for tumor-associated antigens in melanoma patients. *Nat Med.* 1999;**5(6)**:677–685.

60 Huls MH et al. Clinical application of Sleeping Beauty and artificial antigen presenting cells to genetically modify T cells from peripheral and umbilical cord blood. *J Vis Exp.* 2013;**72**:e50070.

62 Scholler J et al. Decade-long safety and function of retroviral-modified chimeric antigen receptor T cells. *Sci Transl Med.* 2012;**4(132)**:132ra53.

70 Hwu P et al. In vivo antitumor activity of T cells redirected with chimeric antibody/T-cell receptor genes. *Cancer Res.* 1995;**55(15)**:3369–3373.

80 Okamoto S et al. Improved expression and reactivity of transduced tumor-specific TCRs in human lymphocytes by specific silencing of endogenous TCR. *Cancer Res.* 2009;**69(23)**:9003–9011.

82 Provasi E et al. Editing T cell specificity towards leukemia by zinc finger nucleases and lentiviral gene transfer. *Nat Med.* 2012;**18(5)**:807–815.

84 Torikai H et al. A foundation for universal T-cell based immunotherapy: T cells engineered to express a CD19-specific chimeric-antigen-receptor and eliminate expression of endogenous TCR. *Blood.* 2012;**119(24)**:5697–5705.

87 Xu Y et al. Closely related T-memory stem cells correlate with in vivo expansion of CAR.CD19-T cells and are preserved by IL-7 and IL-15. *Blood.* 2014;**123(24)**:3750–3759.

89 Grupp SA et al. Chimeric antigen receptor-modified T cells for acute lymphoid leukemia. *N Engl J Med.* 2013;**368(16)**:1509–1518.

90 Porter DL et al. Chimeric antigen receptor-modified T cells in chronic lymphoid leukemia. *N Engl J Med.* 2011;**365(8)**:725–733.

94 Long AH et al. 4-1BB costimulation ameliorates T cell exhaustion induced by tonic signaling of chimeric antigen receptors. *Nat Med.* 2015;**21(6)**:581–590.

96 Maude SL et al. Managing cytokine release syndrome associated with novel T cell-engaging therapies. *Cancer J.* 2014;**20(2)**:119–122.

97 Lee DW et al. Current concepts in the diagnosis and management of cytokine release syndrome. *Blood.* 2014;**124(2)**:188–195.

100 Gattinoni L et al. A human memory T cell subset with stem cell-like properties. *Nat Med.* 2011;**17(10)**:1290–1297.

107 Gattinoni L, Klebanoff CA, Restifo NP. Pharmacologic induction of CD8+ T cell memory: better living through chemistry. *Sci Transl Med.* 2009;**1(11)**:11ps12.

151 Kantoff PW et al. Sipuleucel-T immunotherapy for castration-resistant prostate cancer. *N Engl J Med.* 2010;**363(5)**:411–422.

158 Hanley PJ et al. Functionally active virus-specific T cells that target CMV, adenovirus, and EBV can be expanded from naive T-cell populations in cord blood and will target a range of viral epitopes. *Blood.* 2009;**114(9)**:1958–1967.

161 Straathof KC et al. An inducible caspase 9 safety switch for T-cell therapy. *Blood.* 2005;**105(11)**:4247–4254.

163 Ciceri F et al. Infusion of suicide-gene-engineered donor lymphocytes after family haploidentical haemopoietic stem-cell transplantation for leukaemia (the TK007 trial): a non-randomised phase I-II study. *Lancet Oncol.* 2009;**10(5)**:489–500.

164 Couzin-Frankel J. Breakthrough of the year 2013. Cancer immunotherapy. *Science.* 2013;**342(6165)**:1432–1433.

165 Rosenberg SA, Restifo NP. Adoptive cell transfer as personalized immunotherapy for human cancer. *Science.* 2015;**348(6230)**:62–68.

67 Cancer immunotherapy

Padmanee Sharma, MD, PhD ▪ Sumit K. Subudhi, MD, PhD ▪ Karl Peggs, MD, MA, MRCP, FRCPath ▪
Sangeeta Goswami, MD, PhD ▪ Jianjun Gao, MD, PhD ▪ Sergio Quezada, PhD ▪ James P. Allison, PhD

Overview

The basic principles that guide cancer immunology are immune surveillance, immune editing, and immune tolerance. Rapid increase in the knowledge of the mechanistic details of these basic principles has led to clinical success in the treatment of cancer. In this chapter, we discuss the basic principles and recent advances in the field of basic and clinical immunotherapy that has given credence to the long-held belief that the immune system can be used to treat cancer. Further, we also focus on the role of combining different types of immunotherapies and other therapeutic modalities in the treatment of cancer.

Immunosurveillance

The idea that the immune system is capable of recognizing and responding to cancer is not novel. Paul Ehrlich (1854–1915) was perhaps first among the early visionaries to speculate that the immune system played a key role in suppressing tumors and that the incidence of cancer would be much greater were it not for the ability of the immune system to identify and eliminate nascent tumor cells, a concept that would later become known as the "immune surveillance" hypothesis when revisited over 50 years later by F. Macfarlane Burnet and Lewis Thomas.[1–3] However, proof of concept remained elusive. While it was established that chemically induced tumors were immunogenic in murine models, spontaneously arising tumors behaved differently and were not rejected in similar experimental systems.[4] These data informed a growing consensus that naturally arising tumors were nonimmunogenic and that the antigens targeted by the immune system in chemically induced tumors were perhaps unique to this setting. Moreover, profoundly immunosuppressed athymic mice did not have an increased frequency of tumors induced by a chemical carcinogen.[5] Even though a notable excess of a variety of cancers occurring in immunosuppressed organ transplant recipients was recognized as inferential that immune surveillance occurred in humans, it remained frustratingly apparent by the early 1980s that definitive support from murine models was still lacking.[3] Furthermore, while certain tumors were many hundred-fold more common in immune-suppressed individuals (e.g., some skin cancers, Kaposi's sarcoma, and lymphomas), the frequency of noncutaneous, non-virally induced cancers was generally not increased, suggesting a potentially unique role for immune surveillance in malignancies associated with oncogenic viruses.[6,7] It was at this time that further inferential evidence in humans was beginning to emerge from the demonstration of increased rates of malignancies in patients with the newly defined acquired immunodeficiency syndrome.[8,9] However, the marked association with virally induced cancers was similarly striking.

Multiple strands of evidence would need to coalesce to rekindle enthusiasm for the therapeutic potential of immune-based strategies. Aline van Pel, Thierry Boon, and Pierre van der Bruggen demonstrated that specific immunity to spontaneous tumors could be induced by vaccinating mice with mutagenized tumor cells[10] and that tumor-specific antigens could be recognized by human cytolytic T cells.[11] Their studies showed that spontaneous tumors were not inherently deficient in tumor antigens but rather failed to stimulate an effective immune response. Critically, this failure could be overcome by vaccination in mouse models. The molecular definition of tumor antigens revolutionized the field of tumor immunology by legitimizing the mechanism by which the adaptive immune system discriminates between normal and neoplastic cells. The detection of tumor-specific responses in humans fueled speculation that these responses could be similarly manipulated to induce tumor eradication.[12] Simultaneously, it engendered rapid development of a new field within tumor immunology searching for tumor-associated antigens. Many tumor antigens have since been cloned. They can be broadly segregated into five major categories: (1) differentiation antigens, for example, melanocyte differentiation antigens, tyrosinase, gp-100, and Melan-A/MART-1; (2) mutational antigens, for example, abnormal forms of the tumor suppressor p53; (3) over-expressed normal antigens, for example, HER-2/neu and galectin-9; (4) cancer–testis (CT) antigens, for example, MAGE, LAGE, and NY-ESO-1; and (5) viral antigens, for example, EBV and HERV.[13,14]

Immunoediting

The demonstration of tumor-specific antigens in spontaneously arising tumors that could be recognized by the immune system gave further credence to the theory of immune surveillance but fell short of providing definitive proof. Antigenicity is necessary but not sufficient for immunogenicity. In 2001, Robert Schreiber in collaboration with Lloyd Old demonstrated that T lymphocytes and the immune stimulator IFN-γ cooperated to inhibit the development of spontaneous and carcinogen-induced tumors in mice genetically engineered to lack a functional immune system (RAG-2$^{-/-}$),[15] but that some tumor cells escape detection and eventually cause cancer. They posited that driven by the selective pressure exerted by the immune system, the tumor cell population undergoes "immunoediting" becoming serially less immunogenic than the starting population, through a Darwinian environmental selection. Tumor cells from immunodeficient mice were more immunogenic than those from immunocompetent mice. Although sustaining the concept of immune surveillance, these data raised a potentially formidable obstacle to the delivery of clinically useful immunotherapies, suggesting that by the time a cancer becomes detectable it is already beyond the capabilities of the host immune system to eradicate it. Critically from the therapeutic standpoint,

2s

Holland-Frei Cancer Medicine, Ninth Edition. Edited by Robert C. Bast Jr., Carlo M. Croce, William N. Hait, Waun Ki Hong, Donald W. Kufe, Martine Piccart-Gebhart, Raphael E. Pollock, Ralph R. Weichselbaum, Hongyang Wang, and James F. Holland.
© 2017 John Wiley & Sons, Inc. ISBN: 978-1-118-93469-2

however, they showed that it was possible to make these cells visible to the immune system by increasing their antigen expression. Similar findings were obtained in RAG-1$^{-/-}$ mice,[16] and additional studies in mice specifically deficient in αβ or γδ T cells demonstrated that both cell types play critical and distinct roles in immune surveillance.[17-19] Natural killer (NK) and natural killer T (NKT) cells were also implicated as mediators of protection in experiments in which they were depleted with either anti-NK1.1 monoclonal antibody or anti-asialo-GM1 before challenge with a chemical carcinogen.[16] Further dissection of the critical effector mechanisms underlying host resistance to both chemically induced and spontaneous tumors has emerged from studies on IFN-γ and perforin demonstrating that deficiencies in either of these key immunologic molecules increases susceptibility to tumor growth.[15,20-26]

Immunoediting consists of three processes that occur either concurrently or sequentially.[27-30] First, "elimination" in which immunity functions as an extrinsic tumor suppressor (equivalent to the original concept of immunosurveillance); second, "equilibrium" in which cancer cells survive but are held in check by the immune system; and third "escape" in which variant cancer cells with either reduced immunogenicity or the capacity to attenuate or subvert immune responses grow into clinically apparent cancers. Data documenting the equilibrium process has remained relatively elusive and largely inferred from clinical observation. For example, the development of melanoma of donor origin in two recipients of renal allografts from the same donor who had been considered cured of melanoma treated 16 years previously.[31] More recently, Schreiber's group has shown clearer evidence to support the existence of equilibrium in a chemically induced primary murine cancer model.[32] Following exposure to the carcinogen, approximately 20% of animals developed fatal tumors but some survived with no overt evidence of tumor growth (apparent elimination). Immune suppression in these mice, however, resulted in the unmasking of dormant tumors, which then spread, ultimately killing the host. This effect was observed either following T cell depletion or following neutralization of IFNγ or IL-12 but not following depletion of NK cells suggesting a specific role for adaptive immunity in the maintenance of equilibrium. Furthermore, examination of stable dormant lesions revealed cancerous cells with similar morphological features to those in progressive lesions but with a lower proliferative index and increased apoptosis. The lesions were infiltrated with T cells suggesting a possible ongoing interaction with the host immune system. Engraftment of these cancerous cells into immunodeficient mice following a short period of *ex vivo* culture resulted in tumor growth. In contrast, transfer into immunocompetent recipients failed to induce tumor growth. Finally, tumor outgrowth occasionally occurred following a period of dormancy in immunocompetent animals, and in these cases, tumor cells were able to grow following transfer to immunocompetent mice, suggesting they had become less immunogenic. These data support the idea that tumor cells are unedited in equilibrium but become edited when they spontaneously escape immune control.

Immune tolerance

In 2005, Gerald Willimsky and Thomas Blankenstein suggested that sporadic tumors do not lose immunogenicity as would be predicted by models invoking immunoediting as the major reason for tumor escape but rather induce tolerance to evade immune detection.[33] The idea itself was not new and indeed had been part of the original immunoediting model. The message was simple and had major

implications for the successful application of immune-based therapies. Progression of cancer may not depend solely on intrinsic adaptions of the tumor cells to evade detection but rather on changes exerted on host immunity to permit tumor growth. These mechanisms are neither mutually exclusive nor entirely separable, as upregulation of the surface expression of immunoinhibitory ligands by tumor cells can potentially abrogate immune responses just as efficiently as downregulation of immunostimulatory elements. Their studies involved the use of mouse model in which a viral cancer-promoting gene (SV40 large T) was controlled to activate rarely in random tissues. Although immune responses to the SV40 large T protein were initially detected in the mice, they subsequently developed immune tolerance, while the tumors remained capable of eliciting vigorous immunity when transferred into identical but tumor-free mice (with no clear evidence for immunoediting).

The apparent contradictions between this study and those supporting a more central importance for tumor-intrinsic editing may reflect differences in inherent tumor immunogenicity. More immunogenic tumors will, by definition, generate a more robust immune response. This likely relates partly to the ability of dendritic cells (DCs) to present tumor debris in an "immunogenic" manner, which in itself may reflect activation by secondary signals. In this setting, evolutionary pressures may be higher and immunoediting may be critical to immune evasion. For less immunogenic tumors that do not efficiently activate cellular antigen-presenting machinery, arousal of the immune system is minimal and escape variants are therefore less likely to be sculpted by immunoediting. In these cases, tolerance or immunological ignorance may play variable roles.

Early failures—lessons learnt

The apparent confirmation of the validity of the immune surveillance hypothesis led to great enthusiasm for the development of immune-based anticancer therapies. However, attempts to target human cancers by immunotherapy have been significantly less successful than initially envisaged, leading to the marginalization of immunotherapies from the mainstream of oncologic practice. In patients presenting with cancer, endogenous antitumor immunity has been insufficient to eliminate the tumor. Immunological ignorance may contribute to tumor outgrowth, but antitumor responses are detectable in many of these patients. Indeed, it is clear from the detailed studies of immunoediting in mouse models that even when immunosurveillance fails, the relationship between the immune response and cancer continues to evolve. It is, therefore, likely that failure to eradicate tumors relates to limitations of effector function of the tumor-specific T cells. For maximal antitumor responses, it is necessary for appropriately targeted and activated effectors expressing T cell receptors (TCR) of sufficient avidity to migrate into tumor sites and maintain effector function within immunologically hostile tumor microenvironments. The presence of even large numbers of T cells capable of recognizing tumors is not singularly sufficient to mediate tumor regression, as evidenced by unrestricted tumor growth in TCR transgenic mice in which all of the T cells are capable of recognizing the tumor antigen.[34] Clinical studies of active immunization that have shown tumor growth can go unimpeded despite expansion of cancer cell-reactive T cells to 40% of the circulating CD8$^+$ T cell repertoire.[35] There is now ample experimental evidence that functional systemic antitumor activity may not translate into tumor rejection, either because of lack of infiltration of T cells into the tumor[36] or because of local suppression of function within the tumor microenvironment. Although tumor-specific immunity is compromised in tumor-bearing mice, there is often no generalized immune deficiency,[37] indicating that tumors can specifically suppress the induction of effective antitumor immunity. This concept is perhaps best highlighted by concomitant immunity, wherein a mouse injected with a tumor will reject a subsequent challenge with the same tumor at a distant site, despite continued growth at the site of initial challenge.[38–40] Intriguingly, however, it has been known for some time that the initial generation of concomitant immunity is eventually subverted during primary tumor progression by the establishment of CD4[+] T cell-mediated immune suppression.[41,42] Despite these findings, the majority of approaches to tumor immunotherapy have until recently remained grounded in infectious disease principles. It had been established in the 1980s that antigen-specific CD8[+] cytotoxic T cells (CTLs) were able to induce fully protective immunity against the influenza virus, leading to the development of effective vaccines.[43] The critical role of DCs in mediating these immune responses was recognized soon thereafter in the work of Ralph Steinman and others.[44] On the basis of growing evidence that tumors express antigens that can be presented by professional antigen-presenting cells (APCs) to induce the generation of tumor-specific CTLs, tumor immunotherapists aimed to parallel the successes achieved in developing vaccines for infectious diseases. Strategies have included vaccination with peptide, DNA, or antigen-pulsed DCs. Alternate approaches have been pursued based on directly enhancing effector number or function by adoptive transfer of T cells expanded from tumor-infiltrating lymphocytes (TILs), T cells activated *ex vivo* with cytokines, T cells together with cytokines, and more recently, T cells engineered to express receptors specific for tumor-associated antigens [either TCR or chimeric antigen receptors (CAR)].[45–49] While these approaches have resulted in some impressive responses (reviewed later), they all potentially remain limited by the locally immuno-suppressive microenvironment within the tumor, as evidenced by the evolution of such strategies to incorporate lymphodepleting or nonmyeloablative conditioning to enhance responses. As tumors can be viewed as taking advantage of immunological ignorance, anergy, and suppression, effectively subjugating host responses to create isolated nodes of immune privilege within an otherwise immunologically intact host, they share many similarities with chronic pathogens such as *Mycobacterium tuberculosis*, *Listeria monocytogenes*, and *Leishmania major*. In this context, the challenges of delivering effective vaccines or immunotherapies are much more closely aligned with those associated with therapy of these established chronic infections than with acute infectious pathogens, in which the majority of the successes have come with prophylactic vaccination strategies. Further consideration of the mechanisms underlying the tumor escape phase of the immunoediting model may enlighten strategies to enhance the effectiveness of immunotherapies.

Mediators of immune escape

As previously discussed, the significant changes occurring in the escape phase may be broadly considered as those intrinsic to the tumor cells themselves and those involving the local tumor microenvironment, although the two overlap. Classic examples of the former include downregulation of costimulatory molecules (e.g., B7 molecules) by the tumor leading to activation of tumor-reactive T cells in the absence of appropriate costimulation and induction of anergy[50] or tumor antigen loss or downregulation of major histocompatibility complex (MHC) molecules, which can render the tumor cells essentially invisible to

the immune system.[51] Further examples include mutations conferring increased resistance to apoptosis induction or cell-mediated cytotoxicity, such as overexpression of antiapoptotic molecules (e.g., FLIP and BCL-X$_L$),[52,53] and mutations in FAS or the TRAIL-R (TNF-related apoptosis-inducing ligand receptor) death receptor 5 (DR5).[54–56] Increased expression of T cell inhibitory molecules such as programmed cell death ligand 1 (PD-L1), B7-H3, B7x, HLA-G, and HLA-E by the tumor cells themselves or surrounding parenchyma (stromal or APCs) can directly inhibit effector T cell function, and in many cases, expression levels by the tumor or its microenvironment have been found to correlate inversely with tumor outcomes.[57–65] Further proposed mediators of local immune suppression include soluble suppressive factors elaborated by the tumor or parenchyma such as IL-10, TGF-β, VEGF, or gangliosides.[66–72] Indoleamine 2,3-dioxygenase (IDO) expression by tumor cells or IDO-competent APCs, such as some plasmacytoid dendritic cells (pDCs), can also contribute to acquired tolerance, both by direct suppression of T cells and by enhancement of local regulatory T cell-mediated suppression.[73,74] IDO catalyzes the rate-limiting step in tryptophan degradation, and the combination of local reduction in tryptophan levels (possibly via the intermediacy of causing cellular stress responses in effector T cells) and the production of immunomodulatory tryptophan metabolites appears to exert tolerogenic activity. Furthermore, IDO-expressing pDCs resident within tumor-draining lymph nodes appear to directly activate mature regulatory T cells, which can subsequently cause upregulation of PD-L1 by other DCs, which in turn inhibits effector T cell proliferation.[75] It has become clear that these regulatory networks are therefore extremely complex.[76] The presence of an array of other cell types capable of actively suppressing immune reactions such as CD4[+]CD25[+] regulatory T cells (T$_{reg}$), IL-10-secreting regulatory T cells, CD1d-restricted (NKT) T cells, immature and plasmacytoid DCs (iDCs and pDCs), and myeloid-derived suppressor cells (MDSCs) (noncell-autonomous suppression) within the tumor or tumor-draining lymph nodes is clearly critical to induction and/or maintenance of local immune privilege in a number of systems.[74,77] Such cells may be preferentially recruited to these sites or expanded or induced therein.

Noncell-autonomous suppression

A number of CD4[+] T cell subtypes with regulatory or suppressive activity are now recognized. They fall broadly into one of two categories: those which are produced by the thymus, express CD4, CD25, GITR, OX40 and CTLA-4, and appear crucially dependent on the expression of the X-linked forkhead/winged helix transcription factor, Foxp3, for their development (so-called "naturally occurring" regulatory T cells)[78–84] and those which arise from naïve CD4[+] T cells as a result of "tolerogenic" encounters in the periphery. The latter "inducible" or "adaptive" regulatory T cells include interleukin (IL)-10-producing, Foxp3-negative Tr1 cells,[85–87] transforming growth factor-β (TGFβ)-producing Th3 cells,[88,89] and extra-thymically generated CD4[+]CD25[+]Foxp3[+] iT$_{reg}$ cells.[90–95] In addition, CD4[+]CD25[-]Foxp3[+] T cells with regulatory capabilities have been recognized.[96] The acquisition of regulatory phenotype and suppressive functions by conventional nonregulatory CD4[+] T cells following exposure to antigens under certain conditions is now recognized as a major contributor to the maintenance of T cell homeostasis and control of inflammation. Of particular note, as thymic involution occurs relatively early in humans compared to mice and telomere length in human T$_{reg}$ is considerably shorter, it is conceivable that peripheral conversion plays a far more important role in the maintenance of tolerance (and perhaps in immune subversion by tumors) in humans than in mice.[97-99] Furthermore, if antigen encounter is required for conversion, it seems plausible that the regulatory pool expands at the expense of potential effector T cells, as precursors recognizing tumor antigens will be redirected into a suppressor rather than effector phenotype.[96,100,101] Characterization of the conditions that drive such peripheral conversion is ongoing, but factors such as suboptimal antigen stimulation in combination with TGF-β appear to be important, both of which are likely to be relevant within the tumor microenvironment.[93,102] IDO produced by either tumor cells or parenchyma (e.g., pDCs) also favors conversion,[75,103,104] and retinoic acid appears to be a key mediator in establishing intestinal tolerance.[105-108] Regulatory T cells require TCR triggering to become functional, and at least some tumor-associated T_{reg} are specific for tumor antigens,[109] but once activated, they suppress in an antigen-independent manner. While adaptive Tr1 and Th3 cells exert suppression mostly through soluble factors (IL-10 and/or TGF-β), their Foxp3$^+$ counterparts suppress via a variety of mechanisms, the relative importance of which remain to be fully elucidated in any given situation. Possible mechanisms include those involving CTLA-4, membrane-bound TGF-β, and pericellular generation of adenosine.[110-116] Their expansive capacity to suppress multiple immune effector populations, including CD4$^+$ and CD8$^+$ T cells, B cells, and NK cells,[117] makes them potentially attractive "nodal" targets for therapeutic intervention within immunosuppressive networks. To add further to this complexity, CD8$^+$ T cells with suppressor activity have also been described.[118-121] The dominant inhibitory potential of regulatory T cell populations in murine models of malignancy is well established,[122] and more recently, their potential role in human malignancies has been demonstrated.[123] The mechanisms driving regulatory T cell expansion and accumulation in patients with cancer are not fully understood, but both proliferation of pre-existing T_{reg} and conversion from naïve precursors are likely to be involved.[101,124,125] Their relative abundance predicts for tumor outcomes in murine models[126,127] and correlates inversely with outcomes in several epithelial carcinomas, including ovarian,[123,128] breast,[129] and hepatocellular carcinoma.[130] Intriguingly, in hematological malignancies, this association is reversed and high levels of regulatory T cells appear to confer improved prognoses (e.g., cutaneous T cell, follicular, and Hodgkin lymphoma.[131-133] The level of infiltration of a tumor by regulatory T cells alone may not be the best predictor of outcome. Hodgkin lymphoma tumors contain significant populations of both IL-10-secreting Tr1 and CD4$^+$CD25$^+$ regulatory T cells, which induce a profoundly immunosuppressive environment.[134] Combined assessment of cells expressing Foxp3$^+$ and of cells expressing TIA-1 (cytotoxic granule-associated RNA binding protein) offers a better predictor of response than either alone,[133] highlighting the potential importance of assessing the relative prevalence of multiple infiltrating cellular populations. Indeed, identification of specific immunological signatures (based on flow cytometry, PCR, or microarray analyses[135]) that predict outcomes or guide the institution or monitoring of therapies would be useful adjuncts to modern clinical practice. For example, it is plausible that tumors that contain few TILs, including T_{reg}, will respond well to treatments that aim to enhance CTL numbers, function, or migration, while those that contain significant numbers of T_{reg} would benefit from therapies aimed at reducing T_{reg} number or function. In addition, T_{reg} represent another regulatory mechanism that may be enhanced in response to, and hence limit the efficacy of, current immunotherapeutic interventions. For example, IL-2 has entered clinical trials for a number of human cancers

such as melanoma, renal cell carcinoma, rhabdomyosarcoma, and ovarian cancer. Its initial use was based on the idea that it may directly enhance effector function of both innate and adaptive immune systems. However, IL-2 is recognized as crucial for the homeostasis and function of CD4$^+$CD25$^+$ regulatory T cells *in vivo*,[136-138] and administration to patients with cancer results in increases in the numbers of peripheral T_{reg} cells and stimulation of expression of CXC-chemokine receptor 4 (CXCR4) and CCR4 on T_{reg} promoting their migration toward CXCL12 and CCL2 within the tumor microenvironment.[139-141] As the targets of many cancer vaccination strategies are self-antigens, it is perhaps no surprise that "therapeutic" cancer vaccines can induce amplification of tumor-specific regulatory T cells.[96,142,143] The "immunogenicity" or "tolerogenicity" of DCs thus becomes an increasingly important consideration in vaccination programs as even conventionally "mature" DCs can activate and expand autoantigen-specific T_{reg} cells.[144,145]

Multiple suppressive APC populations play a part in the generation of local immune privilege within tumors. Developing tumors may selectively recruit suppressive APCs or convert stimulatory APCs into suppressors, mirroring the situation with suppressive T cell populations. The molecular mechanisms underpinning active immune suppression by DC and myeloid populations have not been fully elucidated but include secretion of IL-10 and TGF-β, expression of FAS ligand, PDL1, and elaboration of intracellular IDO.[146-150] IDO-competent DCs can induce apoptosis of activated T cells or either T cell anergy or conversion of effectors into T_{reg} as previously outlined.[75,103,151,152] The local balance of stimulatory versus suppressive APCs is probably critical in determining the eventual outcome of T cell encounter with antigen in these sites. It has also become clear that the interaction between DCs and T_{reg} is likely a two-way process.[153-155] MDSCs are a heterogeneous group of cellular precursors of macrophages, granulocytes, DCs, and myeloid cells at earlier stages of differentiation, which express both the myeloid differentiation antigen Gr-1 (Ly6G and Ly6C) and CD11b in mice, and are generally defined as CD14$^-$CD11b$^+$ cells in humans (expressing CD33 but lacking expression of mature myeloid or lymphoid markers).[156-158] Specific phenotypic markers that are reflective of suppressor function remain relatively poorly defined.[159] They consist of two major subsets of Ly6G$^+$Ly6C^{low} granulocytic and Ly6G$^-$Ly6C^{high} monocytic cells in mice. Numbers may correlate with clinical outcomes in human cancer.[160] Several tumor-derived cytokines have been implicated in the expansion of MDSC, including VEGF, IL-1β, and GM-CSF.[161-163] The mechanism of MDSC-mediated suppression is complex, involving contributions from either iNOS or arginase 1,[147,164-167] which enable MDSCs to inhibit T cell responses in various ways, including induction of apoptosis, inhibition of proliferation, or induction of a regulatory phenotype. Nitration of tyrosines in the TCR-CD8 complex appears to render CD8-expressing T cells unable to bind peptide-MHC complexes and to respond to the specific peptide, although they retain their ability to respond to nonspecific stimulation.[168] Type 2 macrophages found at tumor sites have also been implicated in suppression of tumor immunity and seem to share some functional properties with immature myeloid cells.[169,170]

Even in those cancer immunotherapies that succeed in inducing systemic immunity, translation into clinically significant effects has been rare. It is likely that these mechanisms will need to be addressed in order to improve outcomes. What remains wholly unclear is how effectively this aim can be met and how many of the disparate targets will need to be tackled at any one time in order to generate locally curative immunity.

Moving toward clinically effective immunotherapies

In 1891, William Coley (1862–1936), a surgeon at New York Cancer Hospital which later became part of the Memorial Sloan-Kettering Cancer Center, found a patient who had been seen 7 years earlier with an inoperable malignant tumor in his neck, which had disappeared following cutaneous erysipelas caused by *Streptococcus pyogenes*.[171] Coley reasoned that somehow the infection had been the precipitant of the remarkable recovery and found more than 20 published accounts before 1890 linking infection with erysipelas and antitumor responses. On this background, he pursued his own clinical trial using live bacteria, evolving to the use of heat-killed bacteria following some infection-related deaths.[172,173] It is remarkable to consider that even a minority of these patients were cured. The first patient he infected with erysipelas was apparently cured, dying 10 years later of unknown causes, as was the first patient treated with his mixed Coley Toxins, dying 25 years later of a heart attack. Ultimately, the antitumor effects were probably attributable to the production of tumor necrosis factor (TNF) in response to bacterial endotoxins.[174,175] While TNF itself has proven too toxic for reliable clinical usage, it is perhaps fitting that members of the TNF superfamily and their receptors remain important targets for current approaches to immunotherapy.

Adoptive cell therapy and the development of personalized immunotherapies

The growing appreciation that tumor-bearing hosts often do mount antitumor responses and that the greatest concentration of accessible tumor-specific cells may reside within the tumor itself (albeit held in check by local immunosuppressive factors) has informed the development of the field of adoptive cellular therapy (ACT). Furthermore, the failure of active immunization to affect major clinical responses has clearly not always reflected a lack of systemic antitumor immunity, although it has been argued that at least part of this failure relates to stimulation mainly of low-avidity effector T cells, itself reflecting the impact of central deletional tolerance on the anti-self T cell repertoire. These cells may be detectable by conventional immune monitoring techniques but have little chance of rejecting established tumors, particularly as access to and function within the tumor microenvironment are also likely to be limiting factors. Adoptive immunotherapy allows the identification of rare cells with relatively high affinity for tumor antigen that can be selected *in vitro* and expanded before transfer to the host. These cells can be activated *ex vivo* and directly administered, in the hope of avoiding the tolerizing factors present at the tumor site. Initially based on the idea that significantly increasing the number of tumor-reactive T cells will bypass all peripheral and local regulatory mechanisms, flooding the tumor and leading to prompt tumor rejection, modern approaches now recognize the importance of further manipulation of the host to optimize the chances of therapeutic success. These approaches have been developed in parallel with, and in many cases informed, studies advancing our knowledge of the factors limiting antitumor immunity, establishing that the administration of large numbers of activated high-affinity "tumor-specific" T cells to a lymphodepleted host can overcome inhibitory factors and mediate effective cancer immunotherapy in some cases of human malignancy, particularly melanoma. Approaches to date have been largely based on the *in vitro* expansion of T cells obtained from tumor infiltrates and to a lesser degree from peripheral blood or lymph nodes biopsies. Transfers are often combined with administration of the T cell growth factor IL-2. It is likely that such strategies will continue to evolve, incorporating advances in immunostimulatory antibody research (see the following text).

Much of the pioneering work that laid the foundations for subsequent investigation of passive anticancer immunotherapy through ACT was performed by Nicholas Mitchison in the early 1950s,[176,177] and it is perhaps germane to reflect that the enhancing activity of host irradiation and the significance of antigen dose in determining immune response were already established in these seminal works.[178–180] The further development of ACT owes much to work of the groups of Alexander Fefer, Martin Cheever, and Philip Greenberg at University of Washington, as well as those of Steven Rosenberg and Nicholas Restifo at National Cancer Institute. Fefer advanced the concept of "chemoimmunotherapy" in the late 1960s, demonstrating that an established syngeneic lymphoma (FBL-3 or Friend virus-induced lymphoma) could be eradicated after therapeutic combination of high doses of the alkylating agent cyclophosphamide and the transfer of immune cells from a mouse previously sensitized (or challenged) with the same tumor.[181] Further studies helped to define some of the mechanisms underpinning this antitumor activity, demonstrating that it was either directed against tumor or virus antigens,[182,183] that T cells were the major mediators,[184] and that this activity could also be isolated from nonsensitized mice, although with a much diminished potency.[185] This last point is significant as it suggests that a population of tumor-reactive T cells may be present in naive animals. The work was extended to show that antitumor activity was enhanced in cells that had been resensitized and expanded with irradiated tumor *in vitro*,[186–192] or even with cells that had been only primarily sensitized *in vitro*.[189] An important advance during this work was the introduction of IL-2 in the *in vitro* system that allowed further expansion of tumor-reactive T cells.[189] Finally, it was demonstrated that tumor-reactive T cells could be cultured *in vitro* for long periods of time and that after adoptive transfer they would proliferate and mediate specific tumor rejection that could be significantly augmented by the *in vivo* administration of IL-2.[190–192] These studies were among the first to highlight the potential benefits of the use of IL-2 both *in vitro* and *in vivo* in mediating efficient expansion and enhancing tumor rejection.

Contemporaneously, Rosenberg also demonstrated the benefits of IL-2 in cancer immunotherapy. In what would become one of the cornerstones of ACT, a series of studies were published on the use of "T cell growth factor" (TCGF or IL-2) to clone and expand T cells,[45,193,194] including its use for the isolation and expansion of T cells infiltrating solid tumors.[195] Importantly, human lymphocytes grown in TCGF were capable of killing autologous tumor cells *in vitro*.[196] This initial observation led to a series of publications documenting the role of IL-2 in the "Lymphokine-Activated Killer" (LAK) cell phenomena[197] and the capacity of these cells to kill fresh tumor cells *in vitro* and to induce regression of established disseminated lymphoma after adoptive transfer in animal models.[198] These studies were not limited to lymphoma and follow-up studies rapidly transitioned to treatment of established murine melanoma.[199] One notable feature of Rosenberg's approach to immunotherapy was its fast translation into clinical trials. In early 1984, the first phase I study on the use of LAK cells in humans was published.[200] This trial demonstrated proof of concept, showing that large numbers of cells could be obtained by *in vitro* expansion of lymphocytes derived from peripheral blood, which could then be safely transferred back into patients with cancer. The study also documented evidence of migration of these cells into several organs and tissues including tumor. Two additional studies would be instrumental in the advancement of ACT into the clinical setting, both relating to the *in vivo* administration of IL-2 in murine models.[201,202] Following phase I assessment of the safety of systemic administration of IL-2 in humans,[203] a much larger study combining LAK and IL-2 administration was performed[204,205] in which more than 100 patients were treated with several courses of IL-2 and very high numbers of autologous LAK cells (up to 18.4×10^{10} cells). Complete or partial responses were seen in 21% of patients.[205] Despite the favorable results obtained in these early clinical trials, data from murine models would redirect research away from LAK cells and toward the transfer of highly specific tumor-reactive T cells. The new approach was based in the isolation and *in vitro* expansion of TILs with IL-2.[195] These expanded TILs were 50–100 times more efficient than LAK cells in the treatment of various types of tumors and their potency was significantly enhanced when their transfer was combined with *in vivo* administration of cyclophosphamide and IL-2.[45] Clinical trials mirroring the murine experience and combining cyclophosphamide, TILs, and IL-2 have yielded complete and partial responses in up to 31% of patients with metastatic melanoma.[206]

These early studies have helped to inform the evolution of ACT as a form of personalized immunotherapy.[207–209] The transition of ACT into the clinical setting has, however, not been without difficulties. These can be considered in two groups: factors relating to difficulties in generating appropriate products for adoptive transfer and factors relating to host or tumor resistance to transferred populations.

Generation of cellular therapy products

One major limitation has been the difficulty in accessing tumor samples containing sufficient numbers of viable TILs for successful isolation and expansion, which remains a limiting step in 60–70% of cases.[210] Alternative strategies for isolation of tumor-reactive lymphocytes (TRLs) would facilitate more widespread application. Such approaches include the use of T cells from peripheral blood or lymph node biopsies.[211–214] Stimulation with antibodies directed against CD3 and the costimulatory receptor CD28 expressed on T cells are now widely used for the *ex vivo* expansion of large numbers of TRLs, while 4-1BB (see below) has recently attracted more attention both for activation and selection protocols.[214–218] The identification and cloning of T cells with specificity to antigens that are either more abundant on or, less commonly, specific to tumor cells (NY-ESO-1, MART-1, tyrosinase, gp100, p53) have also contributed greatly to the development of alternatives to isolation of TILs. *In vitro* enrichment of such TRLs from peripheral blood by stimulation with their cognate antigen can be followed by expansion protocols as previously outlined. Much has been learnt about the optimal characteristics of the transferred cells, in terms of maximizing persistence and antitumor activity. Long-term *in vitro* culture has been demonstrated to be detrimental and the level of differentiation of T cells to be critical.[219] IL-2 drives differentiation of T cells to intermediate and late effector stages of differentiation. Furthermore, IL-2 may not be the optimal cytokine to use to enhance activity *in vivo* as it also expands T_{reg} and is associated with significant toxicity. The first issue may be addressed by the use of IL-7, IL-15, and IL-21, which seem to more specifically target effector T cells when applied either alone or in combination,[220] rescuing tolerant CD8$^+$ T cells,[221] and generating less differentiated cells that appear to mediate greater antitumor immunity.[222–224] IL-2 seems to be required not only for the expansion but also for the long-term persistence of the adoptively transferred T cells. More recent work in murine models suggests that cotransfer of CD4$^+$ T cells can supply IL-2 and sustain TRLs for long periods of time

therefore increasing the antitumor effect of ACT.[225–227] Numerous studies have demonstrated the requirement for CD4$^+$ T cell help in the generation and/or maintenance of CD8$^+$ T cell memory. In addition to provision of cytokine support, they have roles in DC conditioning and in recruitment and activation of macrophages and eosinophils, which can mediate antitumor effects.[224,228,229]

More recent efforts have focused on genetic modification of T cells to engineer improved antitumor effects. Such approaches include the transfer of CAR that have antibody-based external receptor structures and cytosolic domains that encode signal transduction modules of the TCR.[230] These allow redirection of T cell specificity in an MHC unrestricted manner, while delivering the equivalent intracellular signaling of TCR ligation. Furthermore, the impact of triggering can be enhanced by engineering the cytosolic domain for additional provision of counterfeit costimulatory signaling following ligation (mimicking CD28, 4-1BB, or OX40 ligation). Although incorporation of a CD28 component results in IL-2 release and limited proliferation (plus enhanced resistance to the suppressive effects of T_{reg}[231]), T cell activation remains incomplete and can be further enhanced by inclusion of the 4-1BB or OX40 signaling domains within the construct.[232,233] A number of early trials have suggested that persistence of transgene-expressing cells may be limited to periods of days to weeks following transfer.[49,234–237] This may relate in part to the potential immunogenicity of the CAR. However, lessons learnt from earlier ACT studies may also be pertinent, and current approaches are focusing on the use of central rather than effector memory populations[238,239] and on the use of T cells specific for herpes viruses that are maintained at relatively high levels in humans owing to persistent stimulation via their native TCR by the "latent" viral reservoir.[49] Central memory cells represent the least differentiated end of the spectrum of antigen-experienced T cells and retain the developmental options of naive T cells including the capacity for marked clonal expansion. An alternative strategy to redirect T cell specificity relies on transduction of TCR genes from tumor-reactive clones, although this has the relative disadvantage of conferring MHC-restricted targeting.[240–242] In the first clinical trial using this approach, a MART-1-reactive TCR was transduced into human lymphocytes, inducing the capacity to secrete effector cytokines and display lytic activity when coincubated with MART-1$^+$ tumor cells. Following recipient lymphodepletion, these cells were infused into patients with melanoma who subsequently received infusions of IL-2 with the suggestion that the T cells may have effected clinical responses in 2/17 patients.[48] Potential factors limiting efficacy in this study include variable persistence of gene-modified cells and relatively low levels of surface expression of the introduced TCR. The latter relates to competition of exogenous TCR chains with endogenous TCR chains for assembly with CD3 components and also to the formation of mixed dimers of exogenous and endogenous TCR chains, restricting avidity.[243] Indeed, gene optimization that elicits only modest increases in TCR expression may result in marked enhancement of antitumor activity.[244] An alternate and perhaps complementary approach is to engineer cells in ways to enhance survival, for example, by transducing cells with chimeric GM-CSF-IL-2 receptors (designed to deliver an IL-2 signal when binding GM-CSF in an autocrine loop[245]), CD28,[246] or the catalytic subunit of telomerase.[247] The ability to further modify these lymphocytes, to make them less subject to the suppressive influences present in the tumor microenvironment such as the introduction of genes encoding dominant-negative TGF-β or inhibitory RNAs to prevent the expression of inhibitory molecules such as CTLA-4 and PD-1, could potentially further enhance the activity of the transferred cells.[248] Alternatively, overexpression of selected costimulatory ligands may induce auto- and transcostimulation, resulting in potent antitumor activity.[249]

The role of lymphodepletion

Transfer of tumor-specific T cells into unmanipulated hosts is often accompanied by a failure to demonstrate engraftment or persistence of transferred cells, or only modest antitumor effects on bulky tumors,[250-252] and it is likely that further attention to both intrinsic and extrinsic inhibitory factors will be critical to successful clinical application. Profound lymphodepletion of the host substantially increases the effectiveness of cell transfer therapy, likely by a number of mechanisms including elimination of cytokine sinks (lymphocytes competing with transferred cells for homeostatic cytokines such as IL-7 and IL-15), elimination of T_{reg} and myeloid suppressor cells, and provision of an environment driving homeostatic proliferation.[225,238,253-255] The T_{reg} content of the adoptively transferred population may also be important.[225] In addition to effects on immune cells, host irradiation can sensitize the stromal cells surrounding the tumor[256] and induce upregulation of adhesion molecules on tumor vasculature.[257,258] Finally, host irradiation releases LPS from commensal gut micro-flora, which further matures DCs to activate tumor-reactive T cells,[259] and escalation to ablative conditioning with hematopoietic stem cell rescue may further promote the expansion and function of adoptively transferred CD8[+] T cells.[260]

Current position of adoptive T cell transfer

Experience with ACT is, therefore, generally encouraging, but it is important to recognize that use of TILs may favor inclusion of those with an immune system inherently more capable of mediating antitumor activity. As the level of tumor infiltration with TILs has been shown to correlate with outcome in a number of studies of human malignancy, the ability to generate a therapeutic product from TILs could be a predictive biomarker for outcome. The achievement of higher response rates in the significantly less selected groups receiving CAR- or TCR-transduced ACT will be an important step forward in this regard, but current results have demonstrated results more typical of other single-agent immunotherapeutic approaches. In the absence of large randomized studies, it is impossible to assess the relative contributions of lymphodepleting chemoradiotherapy, IL-2, and ACT to overall results. The number of randomized studies performed in the field remains limited (reviewed in[211]) and only one of these had a positive outcome. Intriguingly, this was in patients with hepatocellular carcinoma rather than the more commonly treated melanoma or renal cancer. Patients received peripheral blood T cells activated *in vitro* with anti-CD3 and IL-2 in the adjuvant setting following surgical resection of the primary tumor ($n = 150$). Tumor recurrence was reduced 41% in those receiving ACT with longer progression-free survival ($p = 0.01$), and a trend toward longer overall survival ($p = 0.09$).[261] There was no such benefit in a more recent trial of patients with stage III melanoma randomized to receive TIL plus IL-2 or IL-2 alone.[262,263] One further major problem with the application of ACT is that it is a highly personalized treatment and does not easily fit into current modes of oncological practice. Generation of appropriate cellular products is labor-intensive and requires significant laboratory expertise. Furthermore, each patient essentially requires the generation of new reagent limiting the opportunities for easy commercialization, and suggesting that delivery may be considered more service-oriented rather than product-related (as in the case

of most drugs). This aspect, combined with increasing awareness that minimizing *ex vivo* T cell manipulation may be advantageous in terms of clinical outcomes, is driving the current evolution of clinical strategies. The issue is also informed by topical debate concerning the nature of the best targets for immunotherapy in terms of public versus private antigens. While we have historically focused on "public" or shared tumor antigens such as MART-1 and gp100, accepting that antitumor efficacy may then be inextricably linked to tissue-specific toxicity, "private" or patient-specific antigens generated as a consequence of the evolution of the malignant phenotype and inherent genetic instability within these lesions have a number of attractive advantages,[264,265] an idea we shall return to later.[266] The acceptance of tissue-specific toxicity leads to the concept of "dispensable tissues,"[267] which may be acceptable in the case of vitiligo with therapies targeting melanoma or B cell deficiency following anti-CD20 therapy but will be more of an issue if the target is shared by a vital organ.[235] The parallel development of "off the shelf" reagents for enhancing immunity offers a number of interesting approaches to further enhance the efficacy of ACT. The recently reported clinical successes with genetically modified T cell therapies[268] and renewed interest by pharmaceutical companies to develop these strategies for eventual approval of ACT for the treatment of patients holds great promise for the future.

Promoting DC function

Detailed discussion of the newer approaches aimed at enhancing antigen presentation in efforts to improve antitumor immunity is beyond the scope of this chapter. However, a few deserve brief mention. DCs are uniquely specialized to present processed antigens to stimulate antigen-specific effector responses. Progress in our understanding of factors associated with DC-induced immunogenicity rather than tolerogenicity has informed the development of clinical therapeutics, yet it remains apparent that even conventionally "mature" DCs (with high levels of expression of costimulatory molecules) can mediate immune suppressive activity.[142,269-271] Cytokines known to enhance DC immunogenicity (e.g., IFNs, IL-15, TNF, and IL-1) are generally insufficient to induce robust adaptive immunity when given in isolation.[272]

Toll-like receptor (TLR) agonists are showing some early promise in clinical studies, particularly in combination with other therapeutic modalities. Unmethylated CpG oligodeoxynucleotides (ODNs) bind TLR9 on pDCs and B cells, inducing Th1 polarized immune responses and regression of established tumors in mice, as well as activity in phase I and II clinical trials.[273-280] TLR9-activated APCs activate NK cells, enhance expression of Fc receptors on polymorphonuclear leukocytes, and promote CTL activation. However, it is important to remain aware that in some settings TLR ligands provoke immunosuppressive or tolerogenic responses.[281,282] The context of TLR signaling may well be important and much remains to be learnt about how the immune system discriminates between pathogenic inflammatory insults and the "beneficial" inflammation associated with commensal organisms or wound healing in order to iterate either immune activation or suppression in the light of apparently similar inflammatory signaling. The imidazoquinolone Imiquimod ligates TLR7 (and to a lesser degree TLR8) and when applied topically stimulates recruitment of pDCs and myeloid-derived DCs into tumors, both of which are implicated in subsequent antitumor activity.[283] It may also directly induce upregulation of vascular E-selectin and inhibit regulatory T cell function (including both T_{reg} and novel γδ suppressor populations),[284-286] and has been demonstrated to exhibit exciting clinical activity in vulval intraepithelial neoplasias.[287,288] Activation of invariant NKT cells by the CD1d-reactive glycolipids α-galactosylceramide (a-GalCer) or its analog a-C-galactosylceramide (a-C-GalCer) provides an alternative route to DC maturation, enhancing antitumor activity in a number of murine models.[289-291] Both CpG and imiquimod also induced increased levels of tumor antigen-specific T cells in melanoma patients vaccinated with recombinant protein tumor antigen NY-ESO-1.[292,293]

Another attractive target for enhancing APC performance is CD40. This molecule belongs to the tumor necrosis factor receptor (TNFR) superfamily (see below), and ligation is crucial for development of competent cellular immune responses, at least in part through the induction of IL-12 secretion by DCs. It is also critical for affinity maturation and heavy chain class switching during humoral responses.[228,294] It is constitutively expressed by B cells and DCs and is also expressed by macrophages, T cells, and nonhematopoietic cells such as vascular endothelium.[295] Its ligand CD40L is principally expressed by activated CD4+ T helper cells, although it is also expressed by plasmacytoid DCs, activated NK cells, and platelets. CD40 ligation is critical for licensing of DCs, providing the temporal bridge between CD4+ T cell help and effective generation of CD8+ CTL responses by "conditioning" DCs (enhancing activation and costimulatory capacity). This activity may be reliant on CD27:CD70 interactions, as blocking CD70 during anti-CD40 treatment abrogates protection in a murine lymphoma model.[296] CD40 stimulation can potentially effect antitumor responses in a number of ways.[297,298] Firstly, the expression of CD40 by a number of lymphoma and carcinoma tumor cells suggests that monoclonal antibodies to CD40 could elicit complement-dependent cellular cytotoxicity (CDC) or antibody-dependent cellular cytotoxicity (ADCC). Secondly, CD40 signaling has been reported to directly induce apoptosis in some tumor cells, notably in high grade B cell non-Hodgkin lymphomas and epithelial carcinomas.[299-301] Finally, by enhancing antigen-presenting capacity CD40 ligation may directly, particularly in the case of B cell lymphomas, or indirectly enhance presentation of tumor antigens to the immune system, at least partially overcoming the requirement for CD4+ T cell help in the generation of effective and durable antitumor CTL responses.[302-304] CD40 ligation by either CD40L or stimulatory anti-CD40 monoclonal antibodies *in vitro* or *in vivo* enhances antitumor vaccine efficiency in a number of murine models of malignancy.[297,305] By extension, forced expression of CD40L by either DC vaccines or B cell tumors such as chronic lymphocytic leukemia using recombinant adenoviral vectors can enhance antitumor T cell responses and induce some level of clinical response.[306,307] Of note, however, these responses may be transient and associated with rapid engagement of host immune inhibitory circuits (e.g., T_reg), suggesting that combinatorial approaches might be more effective.[143] Clinical trials with recombinant CD40L trimer or anti-CD40 antibodies have suggested that *in vivo* triggering of CD40 on tumors and/or APCs can induce responses in a minority of patients, particularly in B cell lymphomas or melanoma, although toxicities including systemic inflammatory syndromes and venous thromboses have been documented.[308-310] A novel approach utilized electroporation to introduce mRNA encoding CD40 ligand, constitutively active TLR4, CD70, and multiple melanoma tumor antigens into autologous DCs (TriMix-DC). Tumor regressions were observed in 6 of 17 patients who had received interferon-α-2b in combination with TriMix-DC.[311] Further, combination of anti-CD40 antibody and chemotherapy agent, gemcitabine, showed tumor regression in both human and mice.[312] Antitumor responses were attributed to activated

macrophages that infiltrated tumor stroma. These agents may prove to be valuable components of future therapeutic combinatorial strategies.[313]

Directly promoting T cell function

Immune activation is critically regulated by two major families of coreceptors expressed by T cells: the immunoglobulin-like (Ig) superfamily and the TNFR superfamily.[314,315] Costimulatory members of the former include CD28 and inducible T-cell costimulator (ICOS), while OX40, CD27, 4-1BB, CD30, GITR (glucocorticoid-induced TNFR family related gene), and HVEM (herpes-virus entry mediator) are members of the latter. The most well-established inhibitory members of the immunoglobulin "costimulatory" family include cytotoxic T-lymphocyte-associated-antigen 4 (CTLA-4) and programmed cell death 1 (PD1). B- and T-lymphocyte attenuator (BTLA) is the most recently described member of the family and also appears to mediate inhibitory effects on T cell activation.[316] The identities of the receptors for the newer members of the B7 ligand family (B7-H3 and B7x/B7-H4) remain elusive, but these receptors may also mediate significant inhibitory activity, perhaps more so in the periphery given the tissue distribution of these more recently identified ligands. Stimulatory or blocking monoclonal antibodies (Figure 1) are being extensively investigated for their abilities to enhance T cell numbers, function, and maintenance of immunological memory.[317,318]

Stimulatory antibodies to 4-1BB (CD137), OX40 (CD134), and GITR—accentuating the positive?

A number of the members of the TNFR family are appealing candidates for the development of targeted therapeutics. To date, there has been relatively little data regarding agonistic anti-CD27 antibodies in murine tumor models, although it does appear to be a potentially interesting target for boosting antitumor immunity.[296] Greater attention has been focused on 4-1BB and OX40. 4-1BB is expressed on activated T cells (including T_reg and NKT cells), activated NK and DCs, eosinophils, mast cells, and endothelial cells in some metastatic tumors.[315,319-321] Its ligand 4-1BBL is expressed on activated DCs, B cells, and macrophages. Ligation on T cells results in upregulation of antiapoptotic genes and protection from activation-induced cell death (AICD),[322] enhancing establishment of durable memory CTLs.[323] The upregulation of 4-1BB on antigen-experienced T cells suggests that anti-4-1BB may differentially target these primed T cells, preferentially influencing those T cells with highest avidity receptors and partially explaining why 4-1BB costimulation may be superior to CD28 costimulation for the generation of antigen-specific cells for adoptive therapies.[217] While it is assumed that costimulation of CD8+ T cells is the principal mechanism of action of anti-4-1BB, various other immunomodulatory activities may contribute. In this respect, a common theme developing in our understanding of the function of immunostimulatory antibodies is their possible multiplicity of function, reflecting the cellular distribution of the receptors. Thus, (1) activation of APCs,[324] (2) reduction in T_reg suppressive capacity[325] or enhancement of effector resistance to suppression,[326] and (3) costimulation of CD4+ and CD8+ T cells are all supported by experimental data. Furthermore, activated NK cells (possibly equivalent to interferon-producing killer DCs), IKDC,[327-329] and NKT cells may be relevant targets for antitumor activity.[320,321,330,331]

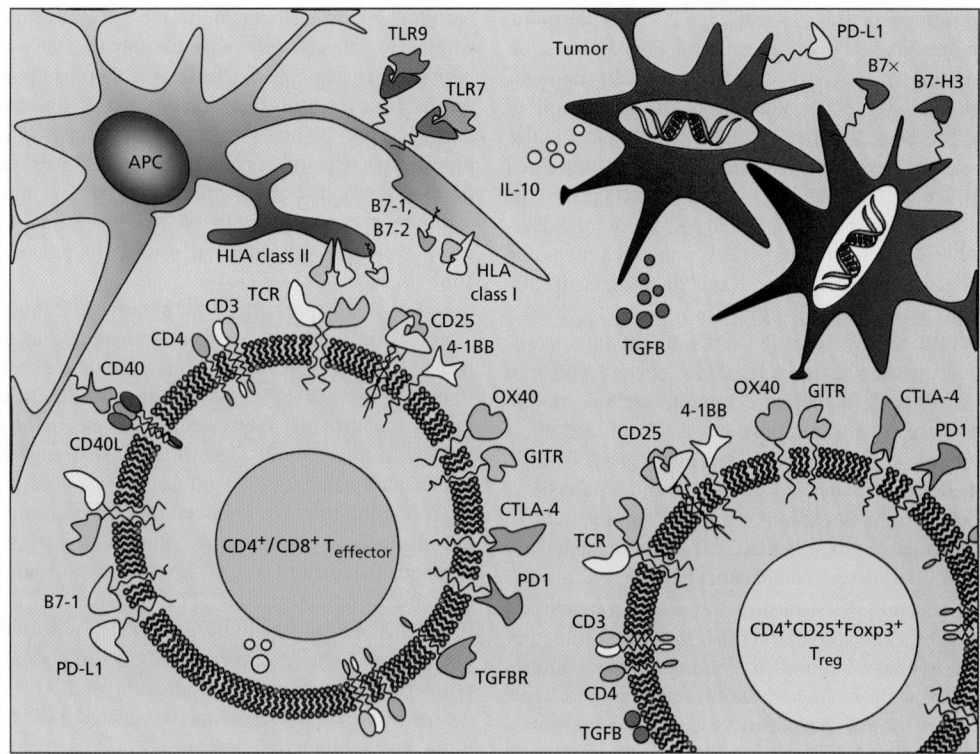

Figure 1 **Potential targets for immunostimulatory therapies**. The majority of T cell coreceptors that are upregulated upon activation of effector cells are also expressed by regulatory T cell populations and both cell types may be important targets for therapeutic interventions.

Reverse signaling into cells expressing the ligands for a number of Ig or TNFR superfamily members (see also GITR:GITRL, CTLA-4:B7, and PD-1:PD-L1 below) is another recurring theme of recent investigations into immune modulating functions of these molecules. In the case of 4-1BBL, this may result in enhanced production of inflammatory mediators or enhanced cell adhesion, facilitating egress of immune effectors into sites of inflammation.[332,333] There are conflicting data as to whether 4-1BB ligation on T_{reg} results in enhanced or reduced suppressive capacity,[325,334,335] and synergy of antitumor activity with approaches that are thought to target T_{reg} number or function has been taken as evidence that any 4-1BB-mediated inhibitory effects on T_{reg} function may be relatively modest.[336-338] Forced expression of 4-1BBL in murine tumors enhances immunogenicity, reducing engraftment rates in immune competent recipients, although growth of untransfected cells is only modestly affected in relatively poorly immunogenic tumors.[320] Agonistic anti-4-1BB monoclonal antibodies enhance antitumor CTL responses, enabling rejection of established syngeneic tumor cell lines.[339-341] Activity appears critically dependent on CD8+ T cells and (in most studies) NK cells, with the role of CD4+ T cells varying in different tumor models.[320,340-343] Just as with other immunostimulatory antibodies, combination with vaccination strategies enhances activity in poorly immunogenic tumor models.[344,345] Coadministration with transgenic tumor-specific CTL enhances antitumor activity, apparently via a reduction in AICD rather than enhanced proliferation.[346] These data demonstrate the activity of anti-4-1BB antibodies in the absence of CD4+ T cell help, albeit in immunodeficient hosts (RAG2−/−) lacking normal regulatory mechanisms. Early experience with a humanized clinical grade antibody (BMS-663513/Urelumab) has targeted mainly patients with melanoma and renal cell carcinoma.[347] The antibody initially appeared to be well tolerated with some evidence of activity (6% partial responses in melanoma patients), once again demonstrating

the probable need to evaluate combinatorial approaches (and also define the optimal dosing strategy).[336,348,349]

Two particularly intriguing and seemingly paradoxical features of anti-4-1BB monoclonal antibodies are their ability to ameliorate autoimmunity[350-352] and to suppress humoral immunity in mice.[353] Although the precise mechanism(s) remain obscure, possibilities include effects on T_{reg} function, interference with CD4+ T cell activation (possibly via the intermediacy of expansion of IFNγ-secreting CD11c+CD8+ T cells[354]), or IFNγ-dependent induction of IDO.[351,352] This highlights the potential importance of the timing of immunomodulatory interventions, as CD4 downregulation may be induced by AICD, which can also occur in CD8+ T cells if exposure to anti-4-1BB occurs immediately after antigen encounter.[355,356] While this suppressive activity has been proposed to be advantageous in terms of limiting possible antibody-mediated toxicities, it is recognized that it might also be deleterious to the development of optimal anticancer immunity. Preclinical studies with anti-CD137 in murine models showed promising activity in combination with antibodies directly targeting the tumor. Most recently, it was shown that anti-CD137 increases efficacy of cetuximab (anti-EGFR mAb) in murine xenograft models,[357] making it another suitable target for combination therapy. Clinical studies with PF-05082566 (Pfizer, anti-CD137) in combination with rituximab in B cell lymphoma and MK-3475 (anti-PD-1) in solid tumor is currently ongoing.

OX40 is expressed transiently on activated CD4+ and CD8+ T cells, functioning as a late costimulatory receptor.[315,358] It is also expressed by NKT cells, where triggering may be required for optimal activation by a-GalCer,[359] and T_{reg}. Its ligand OX40L is expressed in a similar distribution to 4-1BBL, on activated DCs, B cells, and macrophages, as well as activated T cells and endothelial cells.[315] OX40 ligation regulates CD4+ and CD8+ T cell survival and memory generation, preventing T cell tolerance.[360-363] It also impairs the suppressor functions of T_{reg}.[364,365] Furthermore, OX40 triggering appears to be antagonistic for Foxp3 induction in antigen-responding naïve CD4$^+$ T cells, effectively suppressing the generation of iT_{reg},[366,367] and blocks the generation of IL-10-producing Tr1 cells,[368] suggesting that OX40 may antagonize the generation of a number of different inducible regulatory T cell populations. 4-1BB and OX40 act independently to facilitate robust CD8 and CD4 recall responses, overlapping in their intracellular signaling pathways,[369] yet neither 4-1BB nor GITR signaling seem to block the generation of Tr1,[368] and there are currently no reports illustrating whether they influence Foxp3$^+$ iT_{reg} induction. As with 4-1BBL, forced expression of OX40L by tumor cells increases immunogenicity, with tumor rejection dependent on both CD4$^+$ and CD8$^+$ T cells.[370] Furthermore, intratumoral injection of DCs modified to have enhanced expression of OX40L can effect tumor rejection in murine models that is dependent on CD8$^+$ CTL responses, themselves dependent on CD4$^+$ T cells and NKT cells.[359] Agonistic anti-OX40 antibodies also increase antitumor activity in a number of transplantable tumor models.[371] Concomitant activity on both effector and regulatory compartments may be a prerequisite of effective rejection of established tumors.[81] In preclinical models, OX40 ligation enhances several other immunostimulatory approaches.[372–376] A phase I clinical trial using a mouse monoclonal antibody that agonizes human OX40 signaling in patients with advanced cancer showed that patients treated with one course of the anti-OX40 mAb (9B12) had an acceptable toxicity profile and regression of at least one metastatic lesion in 12 of 30 patients.[377]

In common with both 4-1BB and OX40, GITR is transiently expressed on activated T cells.[378,379] It is also constitutively expressed at high levels on T_{reg} with further induction following activation.[380,381] Its ligand GITRL is expressed at low levels on B cells, macrophages, and some DCs, transiently increasing following activation. GITR ligation stimulates both proliferation and function of CD4$^+$ and CD8$^+$ T cells.[382] Its activity on T_{reg} has remained more contentious.[383,384] Anti-GITR antibodies reduce suppression in cocultures of CD4$^+$CD25$^-$ effectors and CD4$^+$CD25$^+$ T_{reg}, but whether this relates to reduced T_{reg} suppressor function, increased resistance of effectors to the preserved suppressor function of T_{reg}, or a combination of both, has yet to be definitively demonstrated. Experiments using mixtures of GITR$^{+/+}$ and GITR$^{-/-}$ effector and regulatory cells suggest that ligation of GITR on the effector population rather than the regulatory population is critical for abrogating suppression,[384] suggesting that enhanced effector resistance to suppression may be key in *in vitro* assays. Injection of adenovirus expressing recombinant GITRL into B16 melanoma promotes T cell infiltration and reduced tumor volumes,[385] while agonistic anti-GITR antibodies have been shown to enhance both rejection of established methylcholanthrene-induced fibrosarcomas and to enhance systemic antitumor responses and concomitant immunity when given following B16 melanoma challenge.[386,387] Furthermore, the same antibody also enhances the impact of DNA vaccination in terms of generation of systemic immunity and enhancing resistance to challenge with murine melanoma.[388]

Stimulation through checkpoint blockade of CTLA-4 (CD152), PD-1 (CD279), PD-L1 (CD274)—eliminating the negative

In contrast to the TNFR superfamily, the existence of coinhibitory receptors mediating direct downregulation of lymphocyte activation and/or effector function has been a recognized feature of the Ig superfamily for some time. Indeed, the coinhibitory

receptor–ligand members outnumber the costimulatory members within this superfamily, engendering the idea of regulatory or inhibitory checkpoint blockade as a therapeutic anticancer strategy by James Allison two decades ago.[389] Blockade of inhibitory immune checkpoints for therapeutic benefit offers considerable promise, particularly as combination with other treatment modalities that promote cross-priming of antitumor immunity may yield additive or synergistic activity. The first strategy shown in both murine models and patients to elicit regression of tumors was antibody blockade of CTLA-4.[389,390]

CTLA-4 is expressed by activated CD4$^+$ and CD8$^+$ T cells, although its surface expression is tightly regulated with a short half-life. While expression is difficult to detect on resting T cells, it influences some of the earliest events in T cell activation,[391,392] being rapidly mobilized from intracellular vesicles in the proximity to the MTOC to the immune synapse after TCR engagement.[393] In the unphosphorylated state, an intracellular localization motif mediates rapid binding to AP-2, endocytosis, and lysosomal targeting.[394] It is constitutively expressed by natural and inducible Foxp3$^+$ T_{reg}, although the majority of CTLA-4 is again found intracellularly, even following activation. CTLA-4 shares the B7-1 (CD80) and B7-2 (CD86) ligands with CD28, a critical costimulatory molecule. Ligation of CD28 in concert with TCR stimulation enhances T cell proliferation by inducing production of IL-2 and antiapoptotic factors, decreasing the number of ligated TCR that are required for a given biological response.[395] CTLA-4 engagement selectively blocks augmentation of gene regulations by CD28-mediated costimulation but does not ablate gene regulation induced by TCR triggering alone.[396] The function of CTLA-4 as a negative regulator of CD28-dependent T cell responses is most strikingly demonstrated by the phenotype of CTLA-4 knock-out mice, which succumb to a rapidly lethal polyclonal CD4-dependent lymphoproliferation within 3–4 weeks of birth.[397,398] CTLA-4 has significantly higher affinities for both B7 ligands than does CD28 and has a higher affinity for B7-1 than B7-2, whereas that of CD28 for B7-2 appears greater than that for B7-1.[399] Although initial measurements suggested a 100- to 1000-fold increased affinity and avidity for CTLA-4:B7 interactions, more recent data using surface plasmon resonance experiments revealed that the interactions between these molecules are 10-fold weaker owing to rapid dissociation rates. Accumulation of both CD28 and CTLA-4 at the synapse is influenced by ligand binding. CD28 is recruited to the synapse in the absence of B7-1 and B7-2 binding but is not effectively stabilized there, and its localization can be disrupted by CTLA-4. The latter is more critically dependent on ligand binding for concentration at the synapse.[400] CTLA-4 may, therefore, both out-compete CD28 for ligand, particularly when ligand densities are limiting and be able to exclude CD28 from the immunological synapse by virtue of the generation of extended high-affinity lattices of alternating CTLA-4 and B7-1 homodimers.[401] For this reason, the tight spatial and temporal regulation of CTLA-4 expression is likely to be critical for determining the outcome of CD28-mediated signaling. Furthermore, CTLA-4 ligation induces decreased production of cytokines (particularly IL-2 and its receptor) and cell cycle arrest in G_1, suggesting that both ligation-dependent and ligation-independent mechanisms contribute to its negative regulatory function. Finally, CTLA-4 has an important role in T_{reg}-mediated suppression, as evidenced by the recent demonstration that T_{reg}-specific CTLA-4 deficiency in conditional knock-out (CKO) mice is associated with a profound reduction in their suppressive capacity.[112] CKO mice developed a lethal autoimmune lymphoproliferative syndrome with a slightly slower tempo than CTLA-4$^{-/-}$ mice. The mechanism(s) by which CTLA-4 mediates these T_{reg}-associated effects remain(s) unclear but may be dependent on reverse signaling into B7-expressing cells.[110,111] Certain subsets of DCs are induced to express IDO subsequent to CTLA-4 binding to DC-associated B7,[110,402] and induction of constitutive expression of inducible cAMP early repressor/cAMP response element modulator (ICER/CREM) attenuates IL-2 production in activated $CD25^+Foxp3^-$ T cell effectors following similar B7-mediated "signaling".[111] Furthermore, T_{reg}-mediated suppression during *in vitro* suppressor assays is associated with reduced activation of APCs (evidenced by reduced surface expression of B7 molecules[112]).

Antibody-mediated blockade of CTLA-4 is particularly effective at enhancing secondary immune responses, more markedly in $CD4^+$ T cells. While often having only modest effects as a monotherapy in preclinical tumor models of poorly immunogenic tumors, anti-CTLA-4 synergizes with a number of other antitumor immunotherapies (reviewed in Refs 314, 318). These promising preclinical results of CTLA-4 inhibitors led to the clinical development of two humanized monoclonal antibodies that block the function of CTLA-4: ipilimumab (IgG1) and tremelimumab (IgG2). Tremelimumab demonstrated durable responses in early clinical trials[403–405]; however, in a phase III randomized clinical trial, it failed to demonstrate an overall survival advantage when compared with chemotherapy (dacarbazine or temozolomide) in patients with advanced melanoma.[406] The failure to demonstrate a survival advantage by tremelimumab may be related to clinical trial design problems rather than lack of biological activity of the agent. Clinical development of ipilimumab is quite advanced, with objective responses observed in patients with melanoma, prostate, ovarian, renal, colorectal, and lung cancers. In two randomized controlled phase III clinical trials in patients with advanced melanoma, ipilimumab improved survival.[407,408] More remarkable is that the survival benefit persisted for approximately 20% patients for greater than 4 years, with the benefit extending up to 10 years in some patients.[409] The success of these trials led to the FDA approval of ipilimumab as a first- and second-line agent in advanced melanoma. It should be noted that the phase III results of ipilimumab in chemotherapy-refractory advanced prostate cancer was recently reported, and it improved median progression-free survival when compared to placebo; however, it barely failed to meet statistical significance ($P = 0.053$) in promoting a survival benefit.[410] A second trial compared the efficacy of ipilimumab and a placebo in chemotherapy-naïve metastatic prostate cancer patients. This phase III trial has completed accrual, and the results will be reported shortly.

A number of factors have been proposed to potentially serve as biomarkers for response to ipilimumab therapy. Recent studies suggest that an increase in TILs correlates with clinical response of anti-CTLA-4 therapy.[411] In addition, sustained ICOS expression on CD4 T cells has also been observed to correlate with survival of melanoma patients treated with anti-CTLA-4 therapy.[412,413] Consistent with this observation, increased frequency of ICOS+ CD4 T cells can also serve as a pharmacodynamic biomarker for anti-CTLA-4 therapy.[414] As described above, ICOS is one of the costimulatory receptors of T cells. Preclinical study shows that engagement of the ICOS pathway markedly enhances efficacy of CTLA-4 blockade in cancer immunotherapy.[415]

PD-1 is more broadly expressed than CD28 or CTLA-4. It can be detected on activated $CD4^+$ and $CD8^+$ T cells, as well as B cells, monocytes, and at lower levels on NKT cells. It binds to two separate ligands, PD-L1 and PD-L2, which exhibit distinct expression profiles (reviewed in Ref. 150). PD-L1 is broadly expressed and can be detected on resting and activated T cells (including $CD4^+CD25^+Foxp3^+$ regulatory T cells), B cells, macrophages, DCs,

and mast cells. In addition, its expression on nonhematopoietic cells (including cornea, lung, pancreatic islets, placental syncytiotrophoblast, keratinocytes, and vascular endothelium) may have relevance to the function of this receptor–ligand pair. This broad nonhematopoietic expression pattern suggests that inhibition through the PD-L1/PD-1 axis may not be restricted solely to the interaction of T cells and professional APCs but that it may also be relevant during the effector phase of the immune response in peripheral tissues, perhaps helping to prevent immune mediated tissue damage directly at the tissue interface. By comparison, PD-L2 has a much more limited expression profile. It is not expressed on naïve nor activated T cells but is instead restricted to activated macrophages, myeloid DCs, and mast cells, suggesting that it fulfills a role that differs from that of PD-L1. The phenotype of $PD-1^{-/-}$ mice provides perhaps the most direct evidence for an inhibitory role of this receptor.[416,417] These mice can develop an array of autoimmune pathologies characterized by high titers of autoantibodies, in keeping with a negative regulatory effect on T and/or B cells. PD-L1 and PD-L2 may also regulate T cell responses through reverse signaling. Cross-linking antibodies against PD-L2 directly induce DCs to produce immunomodulatory cytokines such as IL-6 and TNF-α,[418,419] at the same time as protecting them from cell death.[420] In addition, PD-1-Ig inhibits DC activation and increases IL-10 production independently of any influence on IDO.[421]

PD-L1 was shown to bind B7-1 with an affinity intermediate between those of CTLA-4 and CD28 for B7-1.[422] This interaction was specific and bidirectional, allowing suppression of T cell proliferation and cytokine production either through B7-1 or PD-L1. T cell activation signals delivered through the TCR and CD28 will thus be integrated with cell intrinsic coinhibitory signals delivered through CTLA-4 and PD-L1 (via B7-1 on the APC, and potentially also via B7-1 and PD-1 on other T cells), and PD-1 and B7-1 (via PD-L1 on the APC, and potentially via CTLA-4, PD-1, and PD-L1 on other T cells). Finally, inhibitory signaling through PD-1 and B7-1 (via PD-L1 on nonhematopoietic tissues) may influence the final outcome of antigen encounter in the periphery. This leads to an almost bewildering complexity of possible cell intrinsic inhibitory signals, that is, almost certainly further complicated by the influence of the temporal expression profiles of the various "receptors" and "ligands". The hierarchy of the relative importance of individual elements remains unclear and is likely to differ between T cell subsets. It is also likely that there is some redundancy within such complex and apparently overlapping systems. The physiological relevance of some of these findings also remains uncertain, but members of the PD-1:PD-L1/PD-L2 grouping clearly make attractive therapeutic targets for attempts to enhance antitumor immunity. Combinatorial blockade of CTLA-4 and PD-L1 might concomitantly eliminate cell intrinsic negative signaling through CTLA-4, B7-1, PD-L1, and PD-1 while favoring positive signaling through CD28. Recent data highlights the relevance of this pathway to chronic T cell responses to pathogens.[423–426] During chronic LCMV infection, antigen-specific $CD8^+$ T cells are impaired. These "exhausted" T cells demonstrate a selective upregulation of PD-1 and *in vivo* administration of anti-PD-L1 antibodies restores their activity as indicated by increased proliferation and cytokine production and by a significant reduction in viral load.[423] Similarly, upregulation of PD-1 on HIV-specific $CD8^+$ T cells has been associated with T cell exhaustion and disease progression in humans.[424] Finally, it was shown that in HIV patients with progressive disease both PD-1 and CTLA-4 are upregulated on virus-specific $CD4^+$ T cells and that their expression directly correlates with disease progression and inability to produce IL-2 upon restimulation.[427] Together these data suggest that blockade of PD-1 and/or PD-L1 can restore functionality of the T cell compartment and could be applied, not only to reinvigorate responses to chronic infections but also to enhance T cell activity toward other chronic pathologies such as cancer.

PD-L1 is expressed by a variety of human and murine tumors, and PD-1 expressed by TILs, leading to the hypothesis that they may be important in restricting intratumor effector T cell responses. In humans, myeloid DCs isolated from tumor or lymph nodes from ovarian carcinoma patients express high levels of PD-L1 and are capable of enhancing T cell activity only following PD-L1 blockade.[428] Likewise plasmacytoid DCs in tumor-draining lymph nodes produce high levels of IDO, which results in regulatory T cell activation, upregulation of PD-L1 on the DCs, and negative regulation of T cell responses.[75] PD-L1 is expressed on several human carcinomas (mammary, cervical, lung, ovarian, colonic, renal), as well as melanoma, glioblastoma, and some hematopoietic malignancies.[57,429-433] Its expression has been directly correlated with poor prognosis in bladder, breast, kidney, gastric, and pancreatic cancer.[59,431,434] Forced expression of PD-L1 on murine tumor lines diminished T cell activation and tumor killing *in vitro*, and markedly enhanced tumor growth *in vivo*, while anti-PD-L1 antibodies blocked these effects.[435,436] In the 4T1 mammary carcinoma model, PD-L1 is upregulated *in vivo* by the tumor, making it refractory to immunotherapy with the anti-4-1BB antibody. Coadministration with anti-PD-L1 resulted in dramatic tumor rejection.[437] Likewise, anti-PD-L1 antibody delayed *in vivo* growth of PD-L1-expressing murine myeloma cell lines. PD-L1 blockade has also been shown to synergize with ACT to induce rejection of squamous cell carcinoma.[436] Furthermore, adoptive transfer of PD1$^{-/-}$ tumor-reactive CD8$^+$ T cells caused rejection of B16 melanoma while neither wild type nor CTLA-4$^{-/-}$ tumor-reactive CD8$^+$ T cells were capable of inducing rejection.[429] In this study, blockade of PD-L1 in the effector phase but not during T cell priming also mimicked the results obtained with CD8$^+$ PD-1$^{-/-}$ T cells. This is in keeping with a model wherein CTLA-4 may play a more vital role in the control of CD4$^+$ T cell responses,[438] whereas PD-1 is essential in the regulation of CD8$^+$ effector T cell responses within the tumor.

While PD-L1 blockade has been proven effective at enhancing antitumor T cell responses, very few studies have examined the ability of PD-1 blockade to directly promote antitumor T cell responses *in vivo*. Among these, anti-PD-1 antibodies (as well as genetic ablation) were shown to reduce dissemination of B16 melanoma to the liver following injection into the spleen. In the same study, CT26 colon carcinoma injected intravenously was prevented from disseminating to the lungs by anti-PD-1 therapy.[439] A more recent study also demonstrated that PD-1 (as well as PD-L1) blockade resulted in a small but significant decrease in growth of murine pancreatic carcinoma.[440]

These preclinical successes have translated into the clinic. In a phase I clinical trial, a fully human IgG4 anti-PD-1 mAb (nivolumab) was evaluated in patients with relapsed or refractory Hodgkin's lymphoma and demonstrated objective responses in 20 patients (87%), including 17% with a complete response.[441] In a separate phase I clinical trial, nivolumab showed an 18%, 27%, and 28% objective response rates in patients with advanced NSCLC, RCC, and melanoma.[442] A randomized controlled phase III clinical study compared nivolumab versus chemotherapy (dacarbazine) in patients with previously untreated melanoma (without the BRAF mutation), and the overall response rate favored nivolumab (40% vs 14%).[443] Another phase III clinical trial compared nivolumab versus chemotherapy (dacarbazine or carboplatin plus paclitaxel) in ipilimumab-refractory advanced melanoma patients induced an

overall response rate of 32% versus 11%, respectively[444]; leading to the accelerated FDA approval of nivolumab for patients with unresectable or metastatic melanoma who no longer respond to other drugs.

Consistent with these findings, another drug targeting PD-1, pembrolizumab (humanized IgG4 mAb), demonstrated an overall response rate of 26% in ipilimumab-refractory advanced melanoma patients in a phase I clinical trial, which prompted its accelerated FDA approval.[445] Pembrolizumab also had an overall response rate of 53% in patients with Hodgkin's lymphoma who had failed brentuximab vedotin.[446] These studies show that nivolumab and pembrolizumab have significant clinical activity in a variety of heavily pretreated patients with solid tumor malignancies, but they also appear to be highly active in a greater proportion of patients with hematological malignancies.

Promising clinical results were also observed with drugs targeting the ligand to PD-1, PD-L1. A phase I trial with anti-PD-L1 (human IgG4 mAb; BMS-936559) demonstrated an objective response rate of 6–17% in patients with advanced NSCLC, melanoma, and RCC.[447] Another agent targeting PD-L1, MPDL3280A (human IgG1), was engineered with a modification in the Fc domain that eradicates ADCC. MPDL3280A showed objective responses rate 13–26% in multiple solid tumor malignancies, including NSCLC, melanoma, RCC, colorectal cancer, gastric cancer, and head and neck squamous cell carcinoma.[448] Remarkably, MPDL3280A also had a 26% objective response rate in bladder cancer, a malignancy in which there have been no successful therapeutic developments in the past three decades.[449] It should be noted that other drugs targeting PD-1, pidilizumab (humanized IgG1 mAb) and MEDI0680 (humanized IgG4 mAb), and PD-L1, MEDI4736 (human IgG1 mAb) and MSB0010718C (human IgG1 mAb), are currently being evaluated in a number of different malignancies. These results show that monotherapies drugs targeting the immune checkpoints, CTLA-4, PD-1, and PD-L1, are likely to become the standard of care in multiple malignancies other than just melanoma.

Other inhibitory members of the Ig superfamily offer further possible targets for coinhibitory blockade although the impact such interventions would have on antitumor activity remains more speculative at present. Thus, the as yet unidentified receptor for the B7x (B7-H4) ligand[450-452] offers one such possibility.[453,454] The current literature on B7-H3 and antitumor responses remains somewhat contradictory (reviewed in Ref. 314). BTLA (B- and T-lymphocyte attenuator, CD272) is also a potential target, offering the unique example of an Ig superfamily member whose ligand is a member of the TNF receptor family (HVEM),[455] establishing a previously unsuspected link between these two important families of costimulatory molecules (reviewed in Ref. 456).

Targeting T$_{reg}$ suppressive capacity

Approaches aimed at reducing suppressor function or T$_{reg}$ numbers are attractive therapeutic strategies given the apparent importance of T$_{reg}$ populations in mediating local immune privilege within tumor sites. Small molecule inhibitors of T$_{reg}$ function would be useful additions to our current therapeutic armamentarium. From the preceding discussions, it is apparent that therapies directed toward members of both the Ig and TNFR superfamilies potentially act on regulatory and effector compartments. This duality of function simultaneously enhancing effector function and reducing suppressor function (and/or increasing resistance to suppression) may be critical to the early successes these approaches have enjoyed in preclinical and clinical applications. TLR8 triggering also appears to reverse T$_{reg}$-mediated suppression and to have additional inhibitory effects on suppressive γδ populations.[285,286]

An alternative approach to reducing suppressive capacity of T_{reg} is that of depletion. The recognition that subversion of regulatory T cells may play a critical role in establishing and maintaining intratumoral tolerance is partly based on observations of tumor outcomes following CD25-directed depletion. Anti-CD25 monoclonal antibodies (e.g., PC61) have antitumor activity in a number of murine tumor models[122,457–460] While effective when given before tumor engraftment, they have only limited activity in the therapeutic setting once tumor growth is established. Rather than relating to depletion of activated effectors as initially surmised, it is now recognized that failure in the therapeutic setting may relate to lack of effector infiltration and accumulation within established tumors, further illustrating the principle that systemic generation of immune responses may be insufficient to effect antitumor activity.[36] Furthermore, depletion of T_{reg} may be relatively short-lived, both because of rapid proliferation of naturally occurring T_{reg} and peripheral conversion of $CD4^+Foxp3^-$ precursors.[97,100] The duration of depletion likely relates to the functional half-life of the depleting agent. Studies in humans have used either IL-2 or anti-CD25 as a delivery vehicle for a variety of toxins. Denileukin diftitox (Ontak) is a fusion protein consisting of the IL-2 and the diphtheria toxin that directs the cytocidal action of diphtheria toxin to cells that overexpress the IL-2 receptor. *Ex vivo* studies indicate that it interacts with the high- and intermediate-affinity IL-2 receptor on the cell surface and undergoes internalization. Subsequent cleavage in the endosome releases the diphtheria toxin into the cytosol, which then inhibits cellular protein synthesis, resulting in rapid cell death. It is characterized by a relatively short half-life (60 min) compared with monoclonal antibodies. Preliminary studies in ovarian and renal cell carcinoma demonstrate an early reduction in circulating T_{reg} cells following denileukin diftitox therapy with preservation of the $CD4^+CD25^{int}$ memory T cell pool,[461] but possible depletion of $CD25^+$ effector cells with prolonged/repeated administration.[462] Administration before tumor RNA-transfected DC vaccines enhanced tumor immunity as measured by subsequent *in vitro* analyses of cytokine production in recall responses to the DC vaccine.[461] The *in vivo* antitumor efficacy is still under preclinical evaluation. However, the data from murine models suggest that the demonstration of antitumor activity may be more difficult than enhancement of systemic immunity, and the issue of the duration of depletion that can be achieved remains perhaps critical.[463,464] The same issues may pertain to other depletion strategies, such as those using fusions of anti-CD25 monoclonal antibody to a truncated form of the bacterial Pseudomonas exotoxin A,[465] or conjugated to ricin.[466] For these reasons, approaches that target T_{reg} function rather than number have potential advantages. Furthermore, if such approaches could be targeted to the tumor microenvironment, systemic toxicities, and particularly the risk of harmful autoimmunity, might be restricted. Our knowledge of the pathways involved in T_{reg} generation and accumulation within the tumor now allows consideration of a number of novel therapeutic strategies. Thus, inhibition of the IDO pathway or TGF-β might reduce the rate of peripheral conversion and influence immune privilege status within the tumor.[125,467–470]

Cytokines—intercellular mediators of immunity

Some of the possible uses of cytokines have been described in the section on ACT. Few have shown evidence of a potent ability to enhance antitumor activity *in vivo*, partially because of their pleiotropic effects and adverse side effect profiles at high doses (e.g., IL-2 and type I IFN). IL-15 and IL-21, both members of the common γ-chain group, have attracted more attention recently. IL-15 is likely to have differing roles in mouse and human $CD4^+$ memory T cell homeostasis, as human $CD4^+$ memory cells constitutively produce and proliferate in response to it while it is not produced by mouse T cells.[471,472] Other sources of physiologically active IL-15 include monocytes, macrophages, DCs, and stromal cells. It is recognized to activate NK cells, be critically involved in the maintenance of durable high-avidity $CD8^+$ memory T cell responses, and to promote MHC class I expression by DCs.[473,474] IL-15 is capable of enhancing $CD8^+$ T cell responses to vaccines and to enhance antitumor activity when either supplied exogenously or engineered to be secreted by tumor vaccines.[220,223,475] IL-15-based superagonist ALT-803 promotes the antigen-independent conversion of memory $CD8^+$ T cells into innate-like effector cells with antitumor activity in murine models of cancer.[476] Currently, phase I studies are going on using ALT-803 in hematological and solid malignancies. IL-21 is produced by NKT and $CD4^+$ T cells and enhances the proliferation and function of $CD8^+$ T cells, NK, and NKT cells, as well as influencing B cell differentiation.[477] Furthermore, it appears to reduce the suppressive capacity of T_{reg}.[478] It has been demonstrated to enhance antitumor activity in a number of preclinical murine models either as a monotherapy or in combinatorial approaches with other cytokines (IL-15, IL-2), apoptosis-inducing antibodies (anti-DR5), CD1d reactive glycolipids (aGalCer), or costimulatory agonists.[479–482] Early phase clinical studies of recombinant human IL-21 suggest that it is relatively well tolerated and mediates biological activity in terms of activation of NK and $CD8^+$ T cells, although it is too early to assess possible antitumor efficacy.[483,484]

Not all cytokines are immunostimulatory. Tumor cells can produce immunosuppressive cytokines or induce their production by regulatory infiltrates or stromal cells. Both IL-10 and TGF-β provide possible targets for therapeutic intervention. Targeting TGF-β has shown efficacy in murine tumor models[67,69] and clinical grade antibodies (used in systemic sclerosis) are available, as are those for IL-10.

Combinatorial immunotherapeutics

It is clear from preclinical models and early clinical experience that multimodal approaches may be required to successfully eradicate poorly immunogenic tumors. The recent literature demonstrates the potential for many combinations to give synergistic or additive effects. Attempting to rationally choose which are likely to be the best approaches is very challenging, but considering approaches under a number of basic headings allows the identification of potentially attractive combinations. We can perhaps simplistically think of modern strategies as (1) improving antigen presentation or immunogenicity (e.g., vaccines, CpG), (2) improving T effector function, numbers, or persistence directly (e.g., agonistic anti-TNFR antibodies, cytokines), (3) removing or disabling immunological checkpoints, either cell intrinsic or cell extrinsic (e.g., CTLA-4 or PD-1 blockade, regulatory T cell depletion, and possibly agonistic anti-TNFR antibodies), (4) "resetting" the system and taking advantage of proliferative advantages in a lymphopenic environment (e.g., ACT), and (5) improving antigen specificity or TCR avidity for tumor antigens (e.g., CAR and TCR gene therapies). It has also become apparent that some agents bridge these categories, so the duality of enhancing effector function and reducing suppression afforded by, for example, CTLA-4 blockade, or OX40 stimulation, may be achieved with one agent. As recent data highlight the ability of regulatory checkpoints to limit the efficacy of any directly stimulatory strategy, the inclusion of at least one therapy aimed at disabling immune checkpoints is theoretically attractive. So, for example, combination of anti-CTLA-4 with vaccines,[466,485,486] regulatory T cell depletion,[487] or anti-4-1BB[488] markedly enhances activity. Similarly, diverse synergy is seen when combining anti-4-1BB antibodies with other modalities.[330,348,372] One example of combining three of these strategies is provided in a preclinical model using antibodies directed toward the death-inducing TRAIL-R, CD40, and 4-1BB, which has been shown to augment antitumor activity in TRAIL-sensitive murine tumor models.[313] Induction of tumor apoptosis and antigen release from tumor cells and recruitment of innate immune cells into the tumor site by anti-DR5 (anti-TRAIL-R), coupled with augmentation of DC function induced by anti-CD40, and improved induction, activation and survival of tumor-specific CTL facilitated by anti-4-1BB (possibly with further effects on T_{reg}), are all likely to be important contributors to the favorable antitumor activity.[489,490] Furthermore, anti-CD40 can be substituted by CpG, utilizing NKT activation to amplify DC function, with similar results.[331] One potential advantage of approaches relying on the synergy of multiple components is that they might reduce the toxicity induced by higher doses of each agent administered as monotherapy (e.g., immune responses may be constrained toward tumor-related antigens rather than ubiquitous self-antigens). Appropriate timing of sequential therapies is likely to become an important factor in such combinatorial approaches.

Preclinical studies have shown that concurrent targeting of CTLA-4 and PD-1 significantly improves therapeutic efficacy when compared to the monotherapies.[491] A phase I clinical trial evaluated the concurrent treatment of advanced melanoma with ipilimumab plus nivolumab using various doses of both drugs (four cohorts). The objective response rate was 40% when all four cohorts were included and 53% in the cohort representing the maximum dose that was associated with an acceptable level of toxicities.[492] This latter cohort was also associated with an unprecedented 1- and 2-year overall survival rate of 94% and 88%.

In patients with metastatic renal cell carcinoma, optimal combination of ipilimumab and nivolumab resulted in a response rate of about 40% at 6 months of treatment.[493] Combination strategies using anti-PD1 (nivolumab) with targeted agents tyrosine kinase inhibitors sunitinib and pazopanib have also led to 6-month response rate of 52% and 45%, respectively, in patients with metastatic renal cell carcinoma.[494] Phase III trials with anti-CTLA-4 and anti-PD-1 are now ongoing.

Immunotherapy agents elicit different toxicities

As is the case for clinical responses, adverse events associated with anti-CTLA-4 and anti-PD-1 therapies are different from those seen with conventional chemotherapeutic agents and appear to be related to the systemic activation of the immune system and development of inflammatory-like conditions such as colitis, uveitis, hypophysitis, and dermatitis.[495-500] These adverse events have been termed immune-related adverse events or irAEs. Most irAEs have been manageable and reverse either spontaneously or with corticosteroids. Unlike previously approved cytokine therapies such as high-dose IL-2, which requires a medical setting comparable to an intensive care unit for administration owing to its potential serious toxicities related to capillary leak syndrome,[501] anti-CTLA-4

therapy is administered in clinical trials as a single intravenous infusion per dose in an outpatient setting. Most irAEs that occur as a result of treatment can be managed in the outpatient setting. The use of corticosteroids to treat irAEs does not appear to affect the antitumor action of anti-CTLA-4 antibody.[502]

Paradigm shift—from immune adjuvants to immunosupportive therapies?

Recent attention has also focused on the potential for immunotherapies to augment conventional chemotherapy or radiotherapy[503] and trying to optimize the immunogenicity of cell death. Cytotoxic chemotherapies appear to be capable of inducing an appropriate milieu for presentation of tumor antigens.[504] Further beneficial effects likely include increased antigen cross-presentation,[505] partial activation of DCs,[506] and partial sensitization of tumor cells for cytotoxic T cell-mediated lysis.[507] While there is currently scant evidence from studies in humans to define the relative importance of these considerations to therapeutic outcomes, the attraction of enhancing the immunogenicity of cell death *in vivo*, and one shared by agents such as CpG, is that the tumor might be turned into its own polyvalent cellular vaccine, allowing presentation of private tumor epitopes and favoring tumor-specific immunity. This would obviate the requirement for an absolute knowledge of the relevant target antigens. We are beginning to appreciate the impact of genetic instability within tumors on the generation of potentially immunogenic neo-antigens,[508,509] and it is possible that we will shift to a position wherein conventional anticancer therapies become viewed as immunosupportive, rather than one in which cancer immunotherapies are viewed as adjuvants.

Major challenges will need to be faced in the coming years. Identification of the best combinatorial strategies will continue to be informed by careful mechanistic studies in mouse models. The identification of robust predictors of response will perhaps parallel attempts to tailor chemotherapeutics according to the genetic profile of the tumor or of tumor infiltrates. Finally, attempts to manipulate the host in order to achieve such favorable immunological profiles will be required to prove the therapeutic worth of cancer immunotherapies in comparative studies, confirming them to be much more than modern biomarkers for disease outcome.

Key references

The complete reference list can be found on the Wiley Companion Digital Edition of this title (see inside front cover for login instructions).

11 van der Bruggen P et al. A gene encoding an antigen recognized by cytolytic T lymphocytes on a human melanoma. *Science.* 1991;**254**(**5038**):1643–1647.

13 Boon T, van der Bruggen P. Human tumor antigens recognized by T lymphocytes. *J Exp Med.* 1996;**183**:725–729.

15 Shankaran V et al. IFN-gamma and lymphocytes prevent primary tumor development and shape tumor immunogenicity. *Nature.* 2001;**410**:1107–1111.

25 Smyth MJ et al. Perforin-mediated cytotoxicity is critical for surveillance of spontaneous lymphoma. *J Exp Med.* 2000;**192**(**5**):755–760.

27 Dunn GP et al. Cancer immunoediting: from immunosurveillance to tumor escape. *Nat Immunol.* 2002;**3**(**11**):991–998.

34 Overwijk WW et al. Tumor regression and autoimmunity after reversal of a functionally tolerant state of self-reactive CD8+ T cells. *J Exp Med.* 2003;**198**(**4**):569–580.

35 Rosenberg SA et al. Tumor progression can occur despite the induction of very high levels of self/tumor antigen-specific CD8+ T cells in patients with melanoma. *J Immunol.* 2005;**175**(**9**):6169–6176.

45 Rosenberg SA, Spiess P, Lafreniere R. A new approach to the adoptive immunotherapy of cancer with tumor-infiltrating lymphocytes. *Science.* 1986;**233**(**4770**):1318–1321.

48 Morgan RA et al. Cancer regression in patients after transfer of genetically engineered lymphocytes. *Science.* 2006;**314**(**5796**):126–129.

57 Dong H et al. Tumor-associated B7-H1 promotes T-cell apoptosis: A potential mechanism of immune evasion. *Nat Med.* 2002;**8**(**8**):793–800.

82 Fontenot JD, Gavin MA, Rudensky AY. Foxp3 programs the development and function of CD4+CD25+ regulatory T cells. *Nat Immunol.* 2003;**4**(**4**):330–336.

83 Gavin MA et al. Foxp3-dependent programme of regulatory T-cell differentiation. *Nature.* 2007;**445**(**7129**):771–775.

84 Zheng Y, Rudensky AY. Foxp3 in control of the regulatory T cell lineage. *Nat Immunol.* 2007;**8**(**5**):457–462.

126 Quezada SA et al. CTLA4 blockade and GM-CSF combination immunotherapy alters the intratumor balance of effector and regulatory T cells. *J Clin Invest.* 2006;**116**(**7**):1935–1945.

171 Hall SS. A commotion in the blood: Life, death and the immune system. New York: Henry Holt and Company; 1997.

172 Coley WB II. Contribution to the Knowledge of Sarcoma. *Ann Surg.* 1891;**14**(**3**):199–220.

173 Coley WB. End results in Hodgkin's disease and lymphosarcoma treated by the mixed toxins of erysipelas and Bacillus prodigiosus, alone or combined with radiation. *Ann Surg.* 1928;**88**(**4**):641–667.

174 Old LJ. Tumour necrosis factor. Another chapter in the long history of endotoxin. *Nature.* 1987;**330**(**6149**):602–603.

217 Zhang H et al. 4-1BB is superior to CD28 costimulation for generating CD8+ cytotoxic lymphocytes for adoptive immunotherapy. *J Immunol.* 2007;**179**(**7**):4910–4918.

265 Segal NH et al. Epitope landscape in breast and colorectal cancer. *Cancer Res.* 2008;**68**(**3**):889–892.

268 Maude SL et al. Chimeric antigen receptor T cells for sustained remissions in leukemia. *N Engl J Med.* 2014;**371**(**16**):1507–1517.

357 Kohrt HE et al. Targeting CD137 enhances the efficacy of cetuximab. *J Clin Invest.* 2014;**124**(**6**):2668–2682.

371 Weinberg AD et al. Engagement of the OX-40 receptor in vivo enhances antitumor immunity. *J Immunol.* 2000;**164**(**4**):2160–2169.

389 Leach DR, Krummel MF, Allison JP. Enhancement of antitumor immunity by CTLA-4 blockade. *Science.* 1996;**271**(**5256**):1734–1736.

397 Waterhouse P et al. Lymphoproliferative disorders with early lethality in mice deficient in Ctla-4. *Science.* 1995;**270**(**5238**):985–988.

407 Hodi FS et al. Improved survival with ipilimumab in patients with metastatic melanoma. *N Engl J Med.* 2010;**363**(**8**):711–723.

409 Schadendorf D, et al. Pooled analysis of long-term survival data from phase II and phase III trials of ipilimumab in metastatic or locally advanced, unresectable melanoma. Presented at the 38th Congress of the European Society for Medical Oncology (ESMO), Amsterdam, Netherlands, September 27-October 1, 2013.

415 Fan X et al. Engagement of the ICOS pathway markedly enhances efficacy of CTLA-4 blockade in cancer immunotherapy. *J Exp Med.* 2014;**211**(**4**):715–725.

441 Ansell SM et al. PD-1 blockade with nivolumab in relapsed or refractory Hodgkin's lymphoma. *N Engl J Med.* 2015;**372**(**4**):311–319.

443 Robert C et al. Nivolumab in previously untreated melanoma without BRAF mutation. *N Engl J Med.* 2015;**372**(**4**):320–330.

492 Wolchok JD et al. Nivolumab plus ipilimumab in advanced melanoma. *N Engl J Med.* 2013;**369**(**2**):122–133.

508 Gubin MM et al. Checkpoint blockade cancer immunotherapy targets tumour-specific mutant antigens. *Nature.* 2014;**515**(**7528**):577–581.

509 Linnemann C et al. High-throughput epitope discovery reveals frequent recognition of neo-antigens by CD4+ T cells in human melanoma. *Nat Med.* 2015;**21**(**1**):81–85.

68 Cancer gene therapy

Haruko Tashiro, MD, PhD ▪ Malcolm Brenner, MB, PhD

Overview

Gene therapy of cancer has shown increasingly encouraging results and now is ready to enter mainstream oncological practice. Gene transfer can modify the cellular phenotype and behavior of malignant cells or host immune cells in order to modulate tumor responses. In this chapter, we discuss both of the above approaches and describe the vector systems that are able to produce the intended genetic modifications. We describe current clinical successes of gene therapy and outline the challenges it has yet to overcome. The success of either approach depends on efficient, safe gene transfer with vectors that can either integrate (e.g., retroviral, lentiviral, or adeno-associated viral, or transposons) or not integrate (e.g., adenoviral, herpesviral, or nonviral) into the human genome. To date, reversing the phenotype of all stem cells within a cancer has not proven feasible, and infectious cytolytic viral therapy has not yet had a significant impact in the clinic. Enhancement of active cancer immunotherapy with forced expression of antigens and cytokines or the enhancement of adoptive immunotherapy by engineering T lymphocytes with specific T-cell receptors and chimeric antigen receptors shows greater immediate promise, although ultimately a combination of multiple approaches will prove optimal.

Introduction

A range of tumor-targeted and immunomodulatory antibodies have recently been added to the conventional therapeutic tools of cancer, which until recently consisted of surgery, chemotherapy, and radiotherapy. In this chapter, we describe gene transfer, another treatment approach that has been in development and is now showing remarkable results, though currently only in a limited range of disorders. The intent of gene transfer in cancer is to modify the cellular phenotype and behavior of normal or malignant cells and thereby control or eradicate the tumor. The new genetic material may be transferred to cells *ex vivo* followed by cell infusion, or directly to the cells *in vivo*; the modification may be intended to be permanent or temporary.

Delivery of genetic material to target cells

The ideal gene delivery system (vector) is safe, efficient, and suitable for use in a wide range of applications; such a vector does not yet exist. Instead, gene delivery vectors, which may be of viral or nonviral origin, each have their own strengths and limitations (Table 1) and should be chosen for any given application based on balancing their desirable properties with their limitations.

Viral vectors

Viruses reproduce by efficiently inserting their genetic information into target cells. Investigators have exploited this property by modifying viruses in such a way that they retain their ability to insert therapeutic genetic material but no longer cause disease in the host. Several different vectors have been used for this purpose.

Integrating vectors

Retrovirus vectors

Retroviruses are enveloped, single-stranded RNA viruses, and vectors have been derived from several different retroviral family members, including γ-retroviruses (e.g., murine leukemia virus or MLV—one of the first and still most widely used retroviral vectors)[1] and human immunodeficiency virus (HIV-1, also now widely used[2,3]). Other retroviruses including simian immunodeficiency virus (SIV), bovine immunodeficiency virus, feline immunodeficiency virus, equine infectious anemia virus (EIAV), foamy virus, bovine leukemia virus, Rous sarcoma virus (RSV), spleen necrosis virus, and mouse mammary tumor virus have also been developed as potential vectors. These vectors integrate in the host cell DNA and therefore can provide stable expression even in a dividing cell population.

γ-Retroviral vectors (e.g., MLV)

Wild-type MLV retrovirus contains 5′ and 3′ long-terminal repeats (LTRs) that are responsible for integration and act as promoters. Between the LTRs are three sequences necessary for viral replication and packaging: *gag*, which encodes three proteins that contribute to the virion structure; *pol*, which encodes reverse transcriptase, integrase, and ribonuclease H (RNaseH) necessary for replication; and *env*, which encodes the envelope glycoprotein. Recombinant retroviral vectors are made replication-defective by removing the *gag*, *pol*, and *env* gene sequences from the viral nucleic acid backbone and replacing them with a cargo consisting of the therapeutic sequences of interest. These "gutted" vectors are manufactured in a producer cell line, in which the missing viral genes have been stably integrated in trans and are therefore able to produce infectious but nonreplicative particles containing enough reverse transcriptase to initiate the formation of a double-stranded DNA molecule that is then integrated into the DNA of the cell targeted for gene transfer.

As mentioned above, stable integration of retroviral sequences into the host cell genome[4] means that any modification is stable and will be passed to all daughter cells. Although this property is a critical advantage when stable alteration is required in a rapidly dividing population, γ-retroviral vectors have several limitations. As stable transduction and integration occur in S-phase cells and the preintegration complex is unstable, γ-retroviruses only integrate efficiently in actively dividing cells and not in slowly dividing or quiescent cells. Moreover, retroviral vector integration is by definition a mutational event, and as integration may favor the control regions of active genes, insertional mutagenesis can result—and has resulted—in transformation of the transduced target cell.[5,6] In

Holland-Frei Cancer Medicine, Ninth Edition. Edited by Robert C. Bast Jr., Carlo M. Croce, William N. Hait, Waun Ki Hong, Donald W. Kufe, Martine Piccart-Gebhart, Raphael E. Pollock, Ralph R. Weichselbaum, Hongyang Wang, and James F. Holland.
© 2017 John Wiley & Sons, Inc. ISBN: 978-1-118-93469-2

Table 1 Advantages and disadvantages of cancer gene therapy vectors.

	Advantages	Disadvantages
Integration of vector sequence into the genome		
Retrovirus	Stable genome integration	Integration only in dividing cells
	Long-term gene expression	Potential insertional mutagenesis
	Low immunogenicity	Inefficient *in vivo* gene delivery
	Relatively large insert size: 7–8 kb	
Lentivirus	Transduces nondividing cells	Potential insertional mutagenesis
	Long-term gene expression	Inefficient *in vivo* gene delivery
	Low immunogenicity	
Adeno-associated virus	Long-term gene expression	Potential insertional mutagenesis
	Transduces nondividing cells	Limited insert size: 4 kb
Nonintegration of vector sequence into the genome		
Adenovirus	High titer	Transient expression
	High transduction efficacy	Immune-related toxicity with repeated administration
	Transduces nondividing cells	Limited insert size: 7–8 kb (first generation)
	Limited immunogenicity	
Herpes virus	Large insert size: 30 kb	Cytotoxic
	Neuronal tropism	Transient expression
Nonviral DNA delivery	Large insert size	Transient gene expression
	Low immunogenicity	Inefficient *in vivo* delivery
	Can be used repeatedly	

addition, insert size is limited. Replication-incompetent γ-retroviral vectors made by a producer cell contain only the retroviral LTRs and the packaging signal. In principle, therefore, these vectors should have room for 7–8 kb of sequences of interest. Unfortunately, packaging constraints of the substituted "alien" sequences substantially reduce this limit.[7] Finally, retroviruses are unstable in primate complement and cannot be used readily for *in vivo* transduction. Owing to these limitations, generally retroviruses have been used for *in vitro* transduction of specific target cells before their transfer to the patient.

Lentiviral vectors

HIV-derived lentivirus vectors were the first to be developed and have been widely used both experimentally and clinically. Lentiviral vectors are usually engineered from the HIV-1 genome that contains the *gag-pro-pol* and *env* genes and two regulatory genes, *rev* and *tat* that are required for viral replication. The HIV-1 genome also has four accessory genes, *vif*, *vrp*, *vpu*, and *nef* that encode critical virulence factors. These genes are flanked by two LTRs. Recombinant lentiviral vectors are engineered by removing the majority of the HIV genes leaving the LTRs, packaging signal, and other regulatory elements.[8] First-generation packaging plasmids provide all *gag* and *pol* sequences, the viral regulatory genes, and the accessory genes. In second-generation lentiviral vectors, the four accessory genes are removed. To further reduce the risk of recombination and production of genetically modified infectious lentiviruses, third-generation vectors consist of a split-genome packaging system in which the *rev* gene is expressed from a separate plasmid and the 5′ LTR from the transfer construct[9]; moreover, in the latest generation vector, *rev* and *tat* genes are provided by a fourth plasmid.[10] As opposed to the stable packaging cell lines used for γ-retroviruses, the requirement for a multiple plasmid system to produce lentiviral vectors for human use has made it difficult to scale up production or reduce costs of

manufacture for larger clinical trials. Efforts continue to be made to generate a stable producer line that is safe and produces high-titer vector. Despite difficulties in production, lentiviruses have several advantages over γ-retroviruses. They can more readily infect nondividing and dividing cells,[11] although integration of the stable preintegration complex occurs at a high rate only when the cell enters cycle. Substitution of different viral envelopes modifies and broadens the viral tropism for target cells.[12] Initial clinical studies with lentiviral vectors evaluated the safety of an antisense gene against the HIV envelope in patients with HIV, but more recent attention has focused on the use of lentiviral vectors to transduce T cells to express tumor-directed receptors.[13]

Adeno-associated virus vectors

Adeno-associated viruses (AAV) are small, nonenveloped, single-stranded DNA viruses that are not known to cause disease in human or other animals[14] and require a helper virus (adenovirus, herpes simplex, or vaccinia virus) for the replication and production of new viral particles.[15] The AAV genome is composed of *rep*, which is required for virus replication, and *cap*, which encodes the viral capsid. There are at least 11 serotypes of AAV that differ primarily in their external capsid proteins and that bind to different cellular receptors and hence infect different targets. Recombinant AAV vectors are engineered by the removal of *rep* and *cap* genes but retain the AAV inverted terminal repeats (ITRs) flanking a gene of interest. rAAV has limited cargo capacity, and although widely and successfully used for the treatment of monogenic disorders, production is difficult to scale. So far, the virus has been rarely used in clinical cancer gene therapy.[16,17]

Nonintegrating viral vectors

Adenovirus vectors

Adenoviruses are nonenveloped, linear double-stranded large DNA viruses. A set of early genes (E1A, E1B, E2A, E2B, E3, and E4) encode regulatory proteins that serve to initiate cell proliferation, DNA replication, and down modulation of host immune defenses. The late genes (L1–L5) encode structural proteins. Importantly, adenoviruses are assigned to a species (A–F) and serotype according to the composition of their capsid, the knob/fiber of which attaches to one or more cellular receptors; cellular receptor usage is influenced by both species and serotype.[18] These molecular interactions lead to receptor-mediated endocytosis,[19] internalization, and uncoating of the virus. Adenoviruses can infect many normal and malignant cell types, irrespective of whether they are dividing or nondividing, but they do not integrate in host cell DNA and so the genetic modification is gradually lost in succeeding generations of dividing cells.

Recombinant adenovirus vectors are engineered from adenoviruses by the removal of one or more early genes including E1, which regulates replication, and E3, which diminishes immune recognition. The missing E1 genes are provided in trans by a packaging (or helper) cell line to produce replication-incompetent adenoviruses with room for up to 7–8 kb of new genetic material.[20] Second-generation adenoviruses have been developed in which E2 and E4 along with E1 and E3 are deleted, providing up to a 14 kb insert. They are, however, usually produced at a lower titer.[21] As adenovirus vectors do not integrate into the host cell genome, insertional mutagenesis does not occur but gene expression is only transient in dividing cells. Adenoviral vectors are also highly proinflammatory and favor an immune response against transduced cells and the transgenes they express.[22,23] While both of these characteristics make adenoviral vectors unsuited for long-term treatment of monogenic disorders, they may be beneficial for applications in cancer therapies, such as tumor vaccines, in which transient, high-level expression of an immunogenic transgene may be highly desirable.

Two major variants of adenoviral vectors are currently in clinical development.[22,23] Removal of all viral genes, except those that are required for packaging and replication, produces helper-dependent (or "gutless") adenoviral vectors (HD-Ad) that have lower immunogenicity and greater cargo capacity. Conversely, limitation or modification of the gene deletions can produce conditionally replication-competent adenoviral vectors (CRAD), capable of replicating in—and hence destroying—malignant cells, while sparing normal tissues. These oncolytic CRADs are made selective for tumor cells either because of their requirement for transcriptional regulators present at higher level in malignant than in normal cells or because investigators substitute tumor-"specific" promoters for viral promoters of critical replicative genes.[24,25]

Other nonintegrating viral vectors
Herpes viruses (HSV) are large (~186 nm), enveloped, double-stranded DNA viruses. Their linear double-stranded DNA genome is composed of unique long (UL) and unique short (US) coding regions, both flanked by terminal repeat sequence.[26] Although HSV encodes ~90 genes, many of these genes can be removed without inhibiting genome replication or the packaging of the virus.[27] Therefore, HSV vectors are able to carry large DNA sequences (up to 30 kb). Replication-competent HSV have also been developed and are being studied as oncolytic viruses in several different tumor types.[28–30] Vaccinia viruses are large DNA viruses that replicate cytoplasmically. Modified vaccinia virus Ankara (MVA) has had 31 kb deleted from the parental vaccinia genome, including the K1L, N1L, and A52R genes that regulate innate immune responses,[31] while MVA and Copenhagen-derived vaccine strains are being investigated currently as oncolytic viruses in cancer.[32] High immunogenicity that terminates the oncolytic response is one of the problems for clinical use.[33]

Nonviral vectors

Although viral vectors deliver genes with reasonably high efficiency, they have several drawbacks including cost and complexity of manufacture and the scalability of the production of some of the agents (e.g., lentiviruses and rAAV). Moreover, recognition of viral proteins by antibodies or cell-mediated immunity may limit systemic and/or repeated delivery of the vector, or the durability of transgene expression. Other limitations of viral vectors include insertional mutagenesis produced by some viral vectors and the limited size of the encoded transgenes.

Therefore, much effort has been devoted to increasing the efficiency of nonviral delivery of plasmid DNA in a way that efficiently allows the DNA to escape nuclease-mediated degradation.[34] Plasmid delivery can be effected by physical methods that disrupt the cell membrane (e.g., by electroporation, ultrasound, and hydrodynamic injection) or by chemicals that induce endocytosis,[35] such as cationic polymers or lipids. Unlike conventional nonviral vectors, a plasmid that adds transposons/transposase elements to the genes of interest will integrate in host cell DNA, and is being used ex vivo to produce stable gene transfer and expression in T lymphocytes. Nonviral gene delivery methods are generally less immunogenic and toxic, but efficiency *in vivo* remains low and transgene expression is modest. As yet, these approaches have not been widely adopted for cancer therapy.

Targets of gene therapy

As cancer is an acquired genetic disorder, in principle, gene therapy could be used to correct the disorder by, for example, replacing an inactive gene with an active one or neutralizing hyperfunctional genes. Although in several reports gene therapy has proven successful for the treatment of *p53*-deficient tumors,[36] engineering gene therapies that directly target cancer cells is difficult for many reasons. Unlikely monogenic hereditary diseases, gene therapies targeting cancer cells require modification of the complete population of tumor cells, which is usually extremely large. As described above, highly efficient gene delivery systems have not yet been established. Even if they were available, correction of a single abnormality may be insufficient to repair the transformed phenotype. Therefore, alternative strategies have been explored that target normal host tissue for anticancer therapy.

Gene therapy strategies that directly attack tumors

Prodrug-metabolizing enzymes
Transfer of genes encoding prodrug-metabolizing enzymes may partially overcome inefficient gene transfer, as these genes encode enzymes that convert harmless small molecule prodrugs into lethal cytotoxins that are then released into the general area of the tumor. Herpes simplex virus-derived thymidine kinase (HSV-tk) gene has been widely investigated for this purpose. The HSV-tk, which is encoded by the transferred gene, phosphorylates nontoxic prodrugs, such as acyclovir, valacyclovir, and ganciclovir, into toxic metabolites that inhibit cellular DNA synthesis and replication. Aside from the direct cytotoxic effect to the transduced cancer cells, this approach also has an indirect bystander cytotoxic effect,[37] as the metabolites can be transported from the transgene-expressing cells to adjacent nontransduced cells through gap junction intercellular communication.[38,39] One randomized Phase 3 clinical trial of HSV-tk gene therapy for patients with glioma employed this concept by injecting adenoviral vectors peri-lesionally.[40] As perilesional injections are not always feasible, tumor cells can be targeted through other means, such as vectors that can only transduce dividing cells, the use of enzyme-prodrug systems whose products are pharmacologically active only in dividing cells, or the use of a vector that is targeted to a receptor of tumor-restricted distribution.[41]

Virotherapy or viral oncolysis
Several case reports have documented spontaneous tumor regressions after viral infections.[42,43] As more detailed knowledge of the molecular biology of viruses and cancers has developed, oncolytic viruses that enter or replicate only in tumor cells have been engineered. Several of these oncolytic viruses are natural viral species that selectively infect and kill cancer cells. For example, H1 autonomously replicating parvovirus, reovirus, Newcastle disease virus, Mumps virus, and Moloney leukemia virus are all cancer specific. Other viruses such as measles, adenovirus, vesicular stomatitis virus, vaccinia, and herpes simplex virus require genetic modification to become cancer specific.[44] For example, in ONYX-015, there is deletion of the E1B region that normally binds to and inactivates the *p53* gene to allow viral replication. As a result, ONYX-015 is unable to block *p53* function and can replicate only in malignant cells, most of which are functionally *p53* defective.[45]

Oncolytic virus can kill tumor cells not only by direct lysis (their cytopathic effect) but also by indirect mechanisms such as the destruction of tumor blood vessels or amplification of specific anticancer immune responses. Thus, oncolytic viruses can be further modified to deliver therapeutic genes that induce T-cell chemotaxis (e.g., Rantes) or immunomodulation [e.g., GM-CSF (granulocyte-macrophage colony-stimulating factor), IL-2, IL-12, or IL-15][46–50] or to deliver a prodrug-converting enzyme that turns an otherwise inert agent into a cytotoxic drug at high concentration in the tumor (see section titled "Prodrug-metabolizing enzymes").[51]

Although several oncolytic virus clinical trials have proven the safety of this approach, with few exceptions[52] the clinical efficacy has not met the high expectations raised by promising preclinical studies. There are a number of obstacles that hamper the spread of viruses into target cells. When viruses are injected systemically, they can be cleared from the bloodstream before they reach the tumor cells by neutralizing antibodies, complement proteins, or the reticuloendothelial system.[53–55] In addition, the initial tumor transduction rate may not be high enough for efficient subsequent viral replication. To overcome these obstacles, several strategies have been investigated, such as delivering OV using mesenchymal stem cells to shield them from the immune response[56] and prior administration of immunosuppressive drugs.[57]

Induce host immunity to cancer by vaccines

Unlike vaccines against infectious agents, cancer vaccines are not used for the prevention of disease, but for its treatment, by augmenting the patients' own immune systems to recognize and attack the cancer cells. Although vaccines against human tumors have been investigated for more than 100 years, effective agents have yet to be fully established, and less than 10% of cancer vaccine recipients benefit from the treatment.[41] There is nonetheless a strong rationale for the continued exploration of these agents. Many cancer cells express tumor-associated antigens (TAAs), but effective immunity against TAAs are lacking because cancer cells escape from host immune surveillance (Figure 1). Tumor escape mechanisms include the downregulation of costimulatory molecules, expression of immune-inhibitory receptors/ligands such as PDL-1, secretion of a multiplicity of soluble immune-inhibitory factors, such as transforming growth factor-β (TGF-β), IL-10 and enzyme inhibitory ligands such as FasL or TRAIL, and the induction of regulatory T cells (T reg) or myeloid-derived suppressor cells.[58] Vaccination is intended to elicit host immunity against tolerized TAAs by coadministering the antigen with potent immunostimulatory signals. Target antigens have included oncoproteins, oncofetal antigens, differentiation-associated proteins, and viral proteins. Efforts have also been made to capture immune responses against an individual's unique tumor-associated neoantigens (antigens arising from mutations specific to each tumor).[59] Thus, TAAs have been given as (1) injections of peptides or proteins in immune adjuvants,[60] (2) components of recombinant viruses or other recombinant microorganisms to capitalize on the proinflammatory innate and adaptive immune responses induced by these organisms,[61] (3) protein, peptide-activated dendritic cells (DCs),[62] or (4) mRNA from tumor cells or tumor cells themselves modified to express immunostimulatory genes, both of which are intended to capture immune responses against neoantigens.[63] For this last application, investigators often use combinations of immunomodulatory genes to elicit robust T-cell responses including IL-2[63] and GM-CSF[64] with costimulatory molecules such as CD40L.[63,65]

Despite many years of effort, only one cancer vaccine (Provenge) has been licensed by the FDA. This vaccine is used to treat advanced prostate cancer and expresses a fusion protein of prostatic acid phosphatase with GM-CSF.[62] Provenge is produced following the *ex vivo* transduction of the patients' own antigen-presenting cell population in peripheral blood. While vaccine therapy alone has rarely been powerful enough to elicit curative immune responses, the combination of vaccines and checkpoint antibodies for T cells, such as CTLA4 mAb or PD-1 mAb, may augment this therapy's efficacy and reanimate the field.

Modifying host immune effector cells

One of the limitations of cancer vaccines is that the immune responses they are supposed to induce *in vivo* may be blocked or subverted by the immune evasion strategies of malignant cells and the tumor microenvironment these cells produce (Figure 1). An alternative approach is to prepare effector cells *ex vivo* that are engineered to be specific for the tumor and are also engineered to counteract whatever immune evasion strategies the tumor uses. These modified effector cells can then be returned to the patient.

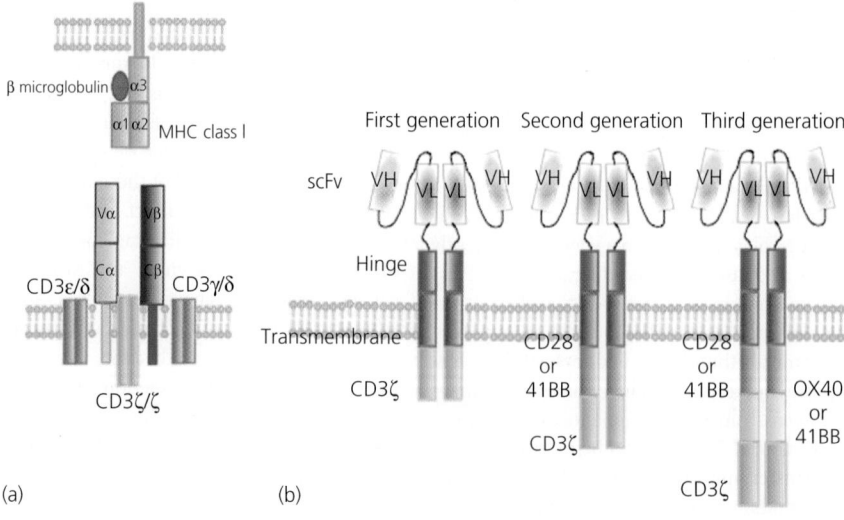

Figure 1 Transgenic T-cell receptors. (a) Transgenic α and β T-cell receptors, which need HLA to recognize the targeted antigen, and (b) chimeric antigen receptors, which recognize the antigen in HLA unrestricted manner. For endodomains, first-generation CAR has only CD3ζ and second- and third-generation CARs also have costimulatory molecules. scFV, single chain variable fragment.

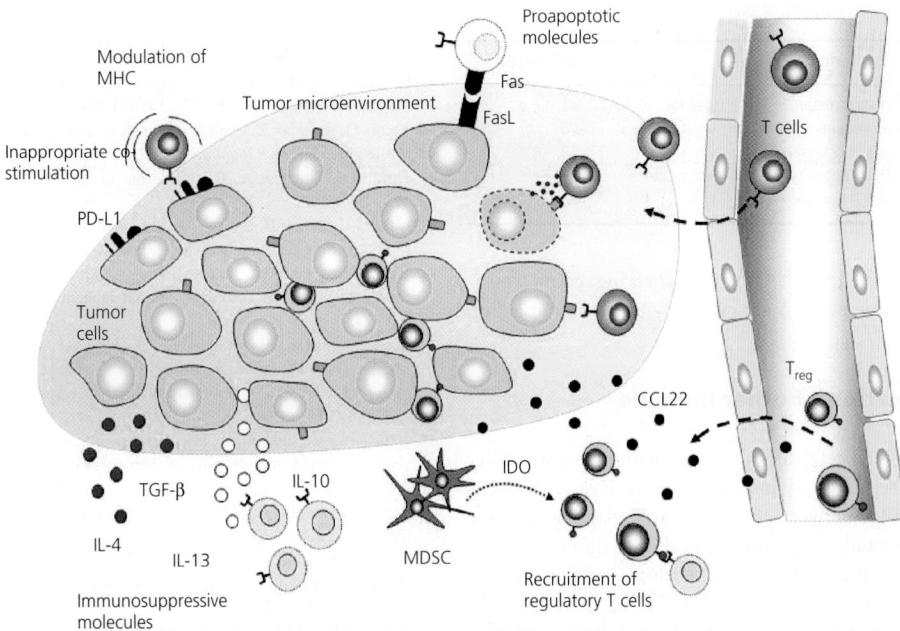

Figure 2 Tumor evasion mechanism. The tumor microenvironment consists of tumor cells and several kinds of immunosuppressive cells, such as T_reg and MDSCs. Tumor cells themselves express FasL to induce cytotoxic T lymphocytes (CTLs) apoptosis and PD-L1 to inhibit CTL functions. In addition, they secrete immunosuppressive molecules TGF-un IL-10, IL4, and IL-13.

Generating tumor specificity

T cells can be engineered to be tumor specific by transferring sequences encoding standardized TAA-specific receptors into bulk T-cell populations. Two types of receptors have been used: "natural" α and β T-cell receptors (TCRs) or artificial chimeric antigen receptors (CARs), so called because they are chimeras of a tumor–antigen-binding domain and a TCR-signaling domain. The TCR α and β chains are encoded by *TRA* and *TRB* genes and have been cloned for several different TAA epitopes.[66] These synthetic TCR can be modified to be of high affinity in an attempt to increase their effectiveness once transferred into T cells,[67] but sometimes at the cost of generating unwanted cross-reactivities.[68–71] Several clinical trials have been performed,[68–70] some of which have shown significant efficacy such as in melanoma, colorectal cancer, and myeloma, although off-target or "on-target antigen but off-tumor" toxicities remain a concern.

The major limitations of TCR-gene therapy are that each TCR recognizes only a small portion of a total tumor antigen (an epitope), which may be lost ("edited") by the tumor, and that the recognition of this epitope is moreover limited to a particular MHC polymorphism, restricting activity to those individuals who share that human leukocyte antigen (HLA) type. CAR-transduced T cells may allow engagement of a larger antigenic component than the 9–14 peptides recognized by the TCR. CAR T cells can also overcome the limitation of HLA restriction and recognize carbohydrate and other nonprotein antigens. CARs are composed of an extracellular domain that binds to the intended antigen, a transmembrane domain, and one or more intracellular signaling domains (Figure 2). Most commonly, the extracellular domain is derived from the antigen-binding portion of a monoclonal antibody targeting the intended antigen and the intracellular signaling domain (endodomain) comes from the CD3ζ component of the TCR.[41] Initial CAR T-cell efficacies were modest because CAR stimulation alone was insufficient to fully activate CAR T cells, producing limited expansion

and persistence *in vivo*. Second-generation CARs were created that added one or more of the costimulatory signals that T cells need to pass through sequential activation barriers, such as the signaling domains from CD27, CD28, 41BB, OX40, or ICOS. When these second-generation CARs are coupled with an exodomain that binds CD19, an antigen present on most normal and many B cell malignancies, CAR T cells produce striking results in the treatment of B cell malignancies. For example, CD19 CAR T cells have a 90% CR rate for relapsed/resistant B-ALL.[13,72]

Engineering T cells for efficacy against solid tumors

Extending CAR T cell successes from B cell malignancies to solid tumors will be challenging. One of the unwanted effects of CD19 CAR T cells is the destruction of normal B cells, which also express CD19, but this effect may be compensated for by infusion of immunoglobulin preparations. Solid tumors also share antigens with other organs, and few other normal cell types are as dispensable as B cells. There are a limited number of truly unique TAAs that can be recognized by antibodies or other antigen-recognition domains suitable for inclusion in CARs. Moreover, T cells traffic poorly to many tumor sites. In addition, once there, T cells encounter an immunosuppressive tumor microenvironment[73] (Figure 1) mediated by the recruitment of inhibitory cells (e.g., myeloid suppressor cells and regulatory T cells), the expression of inhibitory molecules (e.g., PDL1 and FasL), and the production of soluble inhibitory molecules/Th2-polarizing cytokines (e.g., adenosine, IDO, TGF-β, IL-6, IL-10, and PGE-2). Therefore, investigators are engineering T cells to improve the tumor migration of adoptively transferred T cells and their proliferation and survival *in vivo*. For example, to resist TGFβ, a dominant-negative TGF-β receptor type II has been expressed in tumor-directed T cells. TGF-β receptor type II expression induces resistance to tumor-secreted TGF-β and is showing

Table 2 Countermeasures to tumor immune evasion.

Targets	Gene modification	References
TGF-β	Dominant-negative TGF-β receptor	74
Fas L	Downregulation of Fas	76
IDO, arginase	GCN2 knockdown	77, 78
IL-10	IL-10 receptor 1/IgG1-Fc fusion proteins	79
IL-4	IL-4/IL-7 chimeric receptor	80

promising clinical benefits.[74,75] Other engineering countermeasures to tumor immune evasion are currently under investigation (Table 2).

Genetic modification of other immune system cells

Both natural killer (NK) cells and invariant chain or natural killer T (NKT) cells can be activated and expanded *ex vivo*. These cells form part of the bridge between the innate and adaptive immune responses, and once retargeted to tumors may have significant antitumor activity. All of the studies described for T cells are in the process of being replicated for NK and NKT cell populations; the next few years will reveal their potency, safety, and the durability of any antitumor activity.

Safety

Although immunotherapy with adoptively transferred T cells has produced striking results, like any potent therapy, the risk is considerable. Apart from fatal cross-reactivities with normal tissues, induction of cytokine release syndrome (or systemic inflammatory response syndrome) has been reported after the administration of some T-cell therapies, particularly CD19 CAR T cells. As these events may be lethal, investigators are developing and testing several safety or suicide systems that may allow rapid control of the treatment. They include cytotoxic antibodies, prodrug-metabolizing enzymes, and inducible apoptosis genes.[81–84]

Conclusion: How will cancer gene therapy enter clinical practice?

Now that the role of gene therapy for cancer is becoming clearer, the pharmaceutical industry and healthcare providers will have to begin to assess the high cost of developing, manufacturing, and delivering these individualized therapies. As optimal results may be obtained only when multiple biological therapies are combined (e.g., engineered T cells, oncolytic viruses, and checkpoint antibodies), the pharmacoeconomics will need to be carefully addressed by healthcare services experts and an adequate case made for their widespread substitution for conventional therapy. Although we believe that such a case will indeed be made, this remains one more in the long list of the challenges that cancer gene therapy will face before it truly becomes frontline treatment of cancer.

Key references

The complete reference list can be found on the Wiley Companion Digital Edition of this title (see inside front cover for login instructions).

1 Miller AD. Retroviral vectors. *Curr Top Microbiol Immunol.* 1992;**158**:1–24.

2 Reiser J, Harmison G, Kluepfel-Stahl S, Brady RO, Karlsson S, Schubert M. Transduction of nondividing cells using pseudotyped defective high-titer HIV type 1 particles. *Proc Natl Acad Sci U S A.* 1996;**93**(26):15266–15271.

3 Goyvaerts C, Kurt de G, Van Lint S, et al. Immunogenicity of targeted lentivectors. *Oncotarget.* 2014;**5**(3):704–715.

7 Mann R, Mulligan RC, Baltimore D. Construction of a retrovirus packaging mutant and its use to produce helper-free defective retrovirus. *Cell.* 1983;**33**(1):153–159.

8 Liechtenstein T, Perez-Janices N, Bricogne C, et al. Immune modulation by genetic modification of dendritic cells with lentiviral vectors. *Virus Res.* 2013;**176**(1–2):1–15.

10 Escors D, Breckpot K. Lentiviral vectors in gene therapy: their current status and future potential. *Arch Immunol Ther Exp (Warsz).* 2010;**58**(2):107–119.

11 Durand S, Cimarelli A. The inside out of lentiviral vectors. *Viruses.* 2011;**3**(2):132–159.

12 Naldini L, Blomer U, Gallay P, et al. In vivo gene delivery and stable transduction of nondividing cells by a lentiviral vector. *Science.* 1996;**272**(5259):263–267.

13 Porter DL, Levine BL, Kalos M, Bagg A, June CH. Chimeric antigen receptor-modified T cells in chronic lymphoid leukemia. *N Engl J Med.* 2011;**365**(8):725–733.

14 Basner-Tschakarjan E, Mingozzi F. Cell-mediated immunity to AAV vectors, evolving concepts and potential solutions. *Front Immunol.* 2014;**5**:350.

15 Flotte TR, Carter BJ. Adeno-associated virus vectors for gene therapy. *Gene Ther.* 1995;**2**(6):357–362.

16 Nathwani AC, Tuddenham EG, Rangarajan S, et al. Adenovirus-associated virus vector-mediated gene transfer in hemophilia B. *N Engl J Med.* 2011;**365**(25):2357–2365.

20 Berns KI, Giraud C. Adenovirus and adeno-associated virus as vectors for gene therapy. *Ann N Y Acad Sci.* 1995;**772**:95–104.

26 Wadsworth S, Jacob RJ, Roizman B. Anatomy of herpes simplex virus DNA. II. Size, composition, and arrangement of inverted terminal repetitions. *J Virol.* 1975;**15**(6):1487–1497.

27 Lentz TB, Gray SJ, Samulski RJ. Viral vectors for gene delivery to the central nervous system. *Neurobiol Dis.* 2012;**48**(2):179–188.

32 Gomez CE, Najera JL, Krupa M, Esteban M. The poxvirus vectors MVA and NYVAC as gene delivery systems for vaccination against infectious diseases and cancer. *Curr Gene Ther.* 2008;**8**(2):97–120.

33 Whitman ED, Tsung K, Paxson J, Norton JA. In vitro and in vivo kinetics of recombinant vaccinia virus cancer-gene therapy. *Surgery.* 1994;**116**(2):183–188.

34 Al-Dosari MS, Gao X. Nonviral gene delivery: principle, limitations, and recent progress. *AAPS J.* 2009;**11**(4):671–681.

35 Niidome T, Huang L. Gene therapy progress and prospects: nonviral vectors. *Gene Ther.* 2002;**9**(24):1647–1652.

36 Atencio IA, Grace M, Bordens R, et al. Biological activities of a recombinant adenovirus p53 (SCH 58500) administered by hepatic arterial infusion in a Phase 1 colorectal cancer trial. *Cancer Gene Ther.* 2006;**13**(2):169–181.

37 Freeman SM, Abboud CN, Whartenby KA, et al. The "bystander effect": tumor regression when a fraction of the tumor mass is genetically modified. *Cancer Res.* 1993;**53**(21):5274–5283.

40 Westphal M, Yla-Herttuala S, Martin J, et al. Adenovirus-mediated gene therapy with sitimagene ceradenovec followed by intravenous ganciclovir for patients with operable high-grade glioma (ASPECT): a randomised, open-label, phase 3 trial. *Lancet Oncol.* 2013;**14**(9):823–833.

41 Brenner MK, Gottschalk S, Leen AM, Vera JF. Is cancer gene therapy an empty suit? *Lancet Oncol.* 2013;**14**(11):e447–e456.

43 Taqi AM, Abdurrahman MB, Yakubu AM, Fleming AF. Regression of Hodgkin's disease after measles. *Lancet.* 1981;**1**(8229):1112.

44 Russell SJ, Peng KW, Bell JC. Oncolytic virotherapy. *Nat Biotechnol.* 2012;**30**(7):658–670.

45 Heise C, Sampson-Johannes A, Williams A, McCormick F, Von Hoff DD, Kirn DH. ONYX-015, an E1B gene-attenuated adenovirus, causes tumor-specific cytolysis and antitumoral efficacy that can be augmented by standard chemotherapeutic agents. *Nat Med.* 1997;**3**(6):639–645.

48 Senzer NN, Kaufman HL, Amatruda T, et al. Phase II clinical trial of a granulocyte-macrophage colony-stimulating factor-encoding, second-generation oncolytic herpesvirus in patients with unresectable metastatic melanoma. *J Clin Oncol.* 2009;**27**(34):5763–5771.

51 Agarwalla PK, Aghi MK. Oncolytic herpes simplex virus engineering and preparation. *Methods Mol Biol.* 2012;**797**:1–19.

54 Bessis N, GarciaCozar FJ, Boissier MC. Immune responses to gene therapy vectors: influence on vector function and effector mechanisms. *Gene Ther.* 2004;**11**(Suppl 1):S10–S17.

55 Muharemagic D, Zamay A, Ghobadloo SM, et al. Aptamer-facilitated protection of oncolytic virus from neutralizing antibodies. *Mol Ther Nucleic Acids.* 2014;**3**:e167.

58 Whiteside TL. Immune suppression in cancer: effects on immune cells, mechanisms and future therapeutic intervention. *Semin Cancer Biol.* 2006;**16**(1):3–15.

59 Schlom J. Therapeutic cancer vaccines: current status and moving forward. *J Natl Cancer Inst.* 2012;**104**(8):599–613.

61 Moss B. Genetically engineered poxviruses for recombinant gene expression, vaccination, and safety. *Proc Natl Acad Sci U S A.* 1996;**93**(21):11341–11348.

62 Kantoff PW, Higano CS, Shore ND, et al. Sipuleucel-T immunotherapy for castration-resistant prostate cancer. *N Engl J Med.* 2010;**363**(5):411–422.

65 Dessureault S, Noyes D, Lee D, et al. A phase-I trial using a universal GM-CSF-producing and CD40L-expressing bystander cell line (GM.CD40L) in the formulation of autologous tumor cell-based vaccines for cancer patients with stage IV disease. *Ann Surg Oncol*. 2007;**14**(**2**): 869–884.

67 Li LP, Lampert JC, Chen X, et al. Transgenic mice with a diverse human T cell antigen receptor repertoire. *Nat Med*. 2010;**16**(**9**):1029–1034.

72 Maude SL, Frey N, Shaw PA, et al. Chimeric antigen receptor T cells for sustained remissions in leukemia. *N Engl J Med*. 2014;**371**(**16**):1507–1517.

73 Han EQ, Li XL, Wang CR, Li TF, Han SY. Chimeric antigen receptor-engineered T cells for cancer immunotherapy: progress and challenges. *J Hematol Oncol*. 2013;**6**:47.

74 Bollard CM, Rossig C, Calonge MJ, et al. Adapting a transforming growth factor beta-related tumor protection strategy to enhance antitumor immunity. *Blood*. 2002;**99**(**9**):3179–3187.

81 Marin V, Cribioli E, Philip B, et al. Comparison of different suicide-gene strategies for the safety improvement of genetically manipulated T cells. *Hum Gene Ther Methods*. 2012;**23**(**6**):376–386.

69 Cancer nanotechnology

Yanlan Liu, PhD ▪ Danny Liu ▪ Jinjun Shi, PhD ▪ Robert S. Langer, ScD

Overview

The advances in state-of-the-art nanotechnologies have offered exciting opportunities to overcome many obstacles that contribute to the high mortality and recurrence of cancer, such as suboptimal pharmacokinetics and therapeutic efficacy of anticancer drugs, severe adverse effects, development of drug resistance, and cancer metastases. Here, we highlight the clinical stage nanoparticle technologies applied in conventional cancer therapies and for the development of novel classes of anticancer therapeutics. We also discuss recent cutting-edge research efforts in this exciting field, which could lead to more effective therapeutic nanoparticles for cancer treatment.

Introduction

Despite the exciting progress in cancer biology, diagnosis, and therapy, the global burden of cancer—one of the most devastating diseases worldwide—continues to grow at an alarming pace. According to the *World Cancer Report 2014*, it is expected that new cancer cases will rise from an estimated 14 million annually in 2012 to 22 million within the next 20 years, and cancer deaths from 8.2 million to 13 million per year over the same period.[1] Considering limitations in conventional cancer therapeutics, such as unfavorable pharmacokinetics, adverse effects, and development of drug resistance,[2] new strategies are therefore essential to improve therapy outcomes and address the rising cancer burden.

Over the past 20 years since the FDA approval of the first anticancer therapeutic nanoparticle Doxil (liposomal doxorubicin), nanotechnology has demonstrated tremendous potential for enhanced cancer treatment.[3–5] For example, nanoparticles can favorably modulate pharmacokinetic and biodistribution profiles of drug molecules to improve their therapeutic efficacy and/or reduce unintended adverse effects.[6] With unique physicochemical features, some nanomaterials themselves possess therapeutic action, such as iron oxide nanoparticles for hyperthermia cancer treatment.[7] To date, approximately 10 cancer nanotherapeutics have been approved for clinical use, and many are currently in clinical trials (Table 1).[8] This chapter overviews the clinical stage nanotechnologies in cancer therapies,and discusses recent cutting-edge research in the cancer nanotechnology field.

Clinical stage cancer nanotechnologies

What makes nanotechnology particularly impactful in cancer therapy is that it possesses a variety of distinctive features for drug delivery. With nanotechnology, it may be possible to (1) improve the delivery of therapeutic molecules (e.g., hydrophobic drugs) and protect them from premature degradation, clearance, or interaction with biological environments;[9,10] (2) deliver drugs more selectively to tumor cells by modifying the nanoparticles with targeting ligands;[11,12] (3) pack both imaging and therapeutic agents together for real-time feedback on drug delivery and for patient selection;[13] (4) cross-tight endothelial and epithelial barriers;[14,15] (5) codeliver multiple drugs to improve therapeutic efficacy through synergistic effects and/or to overcome drug resistance;[16,17] (6) control sustained drug release to reduce administration frequency; (7) protect nucleic acids from enzymatic degradation and facilitate their intracellular uptake and endosomal escape;[18] among others. Furthermore, some nanoparticles have inherent thermotherapy capabilities activated upon local stimulation, which make them invaluable in terms of surmounting the resistance of tumor cells to chemotherapeutic drugs and avoiding systemic adverse effects. Given these merits, nanotechnology has extraordinary potential to address obstacles existing in conventional cancer therapies and to develop novel classes of anticancer therapeutics. Here, we discuss the clinical stage nanotechnologies used in different cancer therapy modalities, such as chemotherapy, radiotherapy, hyperthermia therapy, gene therapy, and active immunotherapy (Table 1).

Chemotherapy

One major advantage of chemotherapy lies in its ability to systemically attack cancers. Unfortunately, owing to the suboptimal pharmacokinetic profiles, only a small fraction of the administered drugs can be delivered to tumor. Their nonspecific delivery to healthy cells also makes severe side effects inevitable. Nanoparticle technologies have thereby emerged as a promising way for efficient delivery of drugs to tumor tissue while reducing their side effects.[19,20] It has been recognized that the tumor surroundings are dense with leaky blood vessels. Together with the lack of functional lymphatic drainage, nanoparticles are allowed to extravasate out of circulation and accumulate in tumor tissue (Figure 1a), which is denoted as the enhanced permeability and retention (EPR) effect.[21] On the basis of the EPR effect, various nanoparticle platforms have been developed and approximately ten were introduced into the market, including Doxil, Abraxane, and Genexol-PM.[8]

To further improve specificity of nanoparticle delivery, active targeting has been proposed and advanced into clinical investigation by modifying the nanoparticle surface with targeting moieties, which can selectively recognize tumor cell-specific receptors. The targeting ligands can be antibodies, aptamers, peptides, carbohydrates, small molecules, or others.[22] Through receptor-mediated endocytosis, targeted delivery can increase nanoparticle retention and cellular uptake, thus significantly enhancing therapeutic efficacy (Figure 1b).[23] A recent representative example is BIND-014, a docetaxel-loaded polymer nanoparticles decorated with small molecules against prostate-specific membrane antigen (PSMA), which has been developed by BIND Therapeutics and is now in phase II clinical trials for the treatment of solid tumors. In xenograft animals treated with BIND-014, the docetaxel concentration in

Holland-Frei Cancer Medicine, Ninth Edition. Edited by Robert C. Bast Jr., Carlo M. Croce, William N. Hait, Waun Ki Hong, Donald W. Kufe, Martine Piccart-Gebhart, Raphael E. Pollock, Ralph R. Weichselbaum, Hongyang Wang, and James F. Holland.
© 2017 John Wiley & Sons, Inc. ISBN: 978-1-118-93469-2

Table 1 Representative clinical stage nanotechnologies in cancer therapies.

Category		Product	Description	Indications	Clinical state
Chemotherapy	Passive targeting	Doxil	PEGylated liposomal doxorubicin	Ovarian cancer, Kaposi sarcoma, multiple myeloma	FDA approval in 1995
		DaunoXome	Daunorubicin-loaded lipid vesicles	Advanced HIV-related Kaposi sarcoma	FDA approval in 1996
		Mepact	Liposomal muramyl tripeptide phosphatidyl-ethanolamine	Nonmetastatic, resectable osteosarcoma	Approved in Europe, Phase III in the United States
		Myocet	Liposomal doxorubicin	Metastatic breast cancer	Approved in Europe and Canada
		Abraxane	Nanoparticle albumin-bond (Nab)-paclitaxel	Metastatic pancreatic cancer, nonsmall-cell lung cancer, breast cancer	FDA approval in 2005
		Genexol-PM	Paclitaxel-loaded polymeric micelles	Breast cancer	Approved in South Korea, Phase IV in the United States
	Active targeting	BIND-014	Docetaxel-loaded polymer nanoparticle coated with a small molecule for targeting PSMA	Nonsmall-cell lung cancer, metastatic castration-resistant prostate cancer	Phase II
		MM-302	Doxorubicin-loaded liposome modified with antibody fragment for targeting tumor antigen	HER2 positive breast cancer	Phase III
		MBP-426	Oxaliplatin-loaded liposome coated with transferrin for targeting transferrin receptor	Gastric, esophageal, gastroesophageal adenocarcinoma	Phase Ib/II
	Stimuli-responsive targeting	MTC-DOX	Doxorubicin is bound to microscopic beads of activated carbon and iron as a magnetic-targeted carrier (MTC)	Adult primary hepatocellular carcinoma liver cancer	Phase III
		ThermoDox	Doxorubicin is encapsulated in thermally sensitive liposomes	Hepatocellular carcinoma	Phase III
Radiotherapy		NBTXR3	Hafnium oxide nanoparticles	Soft tissue sarcoma, locally advanced squamous cell carcinoma of the oral cavity or oropharynx	Phase I
Hyperthermia		NanoTherm	Aminosilane-coated iron oxide nanoparticles	Glioblastoma	European Union regulatory approval
		AuroLase	Silica core with a gold nanoshell	Refractory head and neck cancer, and primary and/or metastatic lung tumors	Phase I
Gene therapy		CALAA-01	Transferrin-decorated cyclodextrin polymer nanoparticle containing siRNA against the M2 subunit of ribonucleotide reductase	Solid tumors	Phase I
		ALN-VSP02	A lipid nanoparticle containing siRNAs against kinesin spindle protein and VEGF	Solid tumors	Phase I
		Atu027	Liposome containing a modified siRNA against protein kinase N3	Advanced or metastatic pancreatic cancer	Phase I/II
		SGT53-01	p53 gene-loaded liposome coated with antibody fragment for targeting transferrin receptor	Solid tumors	Phase Ib
Active immunotherapy		Lipovaxin-MM	Liposome-based vaccine loaded with melanoma antigens	Melanoma	Phase I
		dHER2 + AS15	Liposomal vaccine consisting of a HER2/neu peptide (dHER2) combined with the immunoadjuvant AS15	Metastatic breast cancer	Phase I/II
		DPX-0907	Multitumor-associated antigens-loaded liposome	HLA-A2 positive advanced stage ovarian, breast, and prostate cancer	Phase I
		Tecemotide	Liposome-encapsulated MUC1 antigen	Nonsmall-cell lung cancer	Phase III

tumor was sevenfold higher than that treated with conventional docetaxel (taxotere) 12 h after intravenous injection. Clinical data in patients with metastatic cholangiocarcinoma showed that tumor shrinkage was achieved at a dose of docetaxel that corresponds to only 20% of the typical dose for doctaxel.[24]

In addition to increasing specificity, avoiding the premature release of drugs before they reach the tumor may be equally important for maximizing therapeutic efficacy and minimizing adverse effects. Stimuli-responsive nanoparticles have shown promising potential for this purpose, as they only become active in the tumor microenvironment (TME) (Figure 1f).[25] Generally, these nanoparticles are designed to recognize subtle environmental changes associated with tumor pathological situations (e.g., pH, redox, and enzyme) or to be activated by external stimuli (e.g.,

heat, light, magnetic field, and ultrasound).[26] To some extent, external stimulation allows for tailored drug release profiles with excellent temporal, spatial, and dosage control.[27] In particular, noninvasive magnetic field- and ultrasound-responsive nanoparticle delivery systems have gained a lot attention as there are nominal limits in tissue penetration for these modalities.[25,26] At present, doxorubicin-loaded thermo-responsive liposomes are being investigated in phase II trials for the treatment of colorectal liver metastasis, bone metastases, and breast cancer and have even reached phase III trials for hepatocellular carcinoma therapy.[26]

Radiotherapy

In conventional radiotherapy, high-energy ionizing radiations such as gamma and X-rays are generally used to ionize cellular

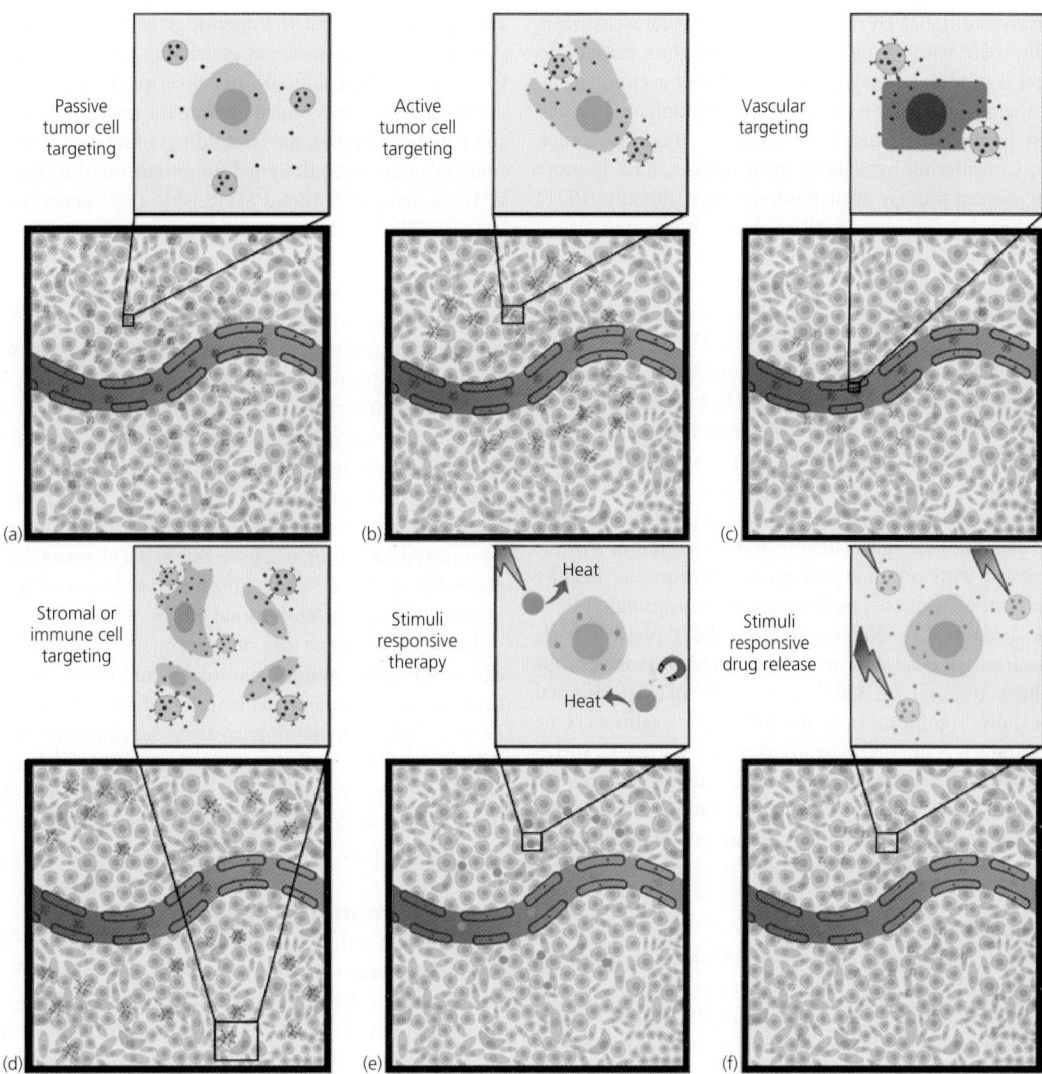

Figure 1 Schematic illustration of different nanotherapy strategies in cancer treatment. (a) Nontargeted nanoparticles passively extravasate out of the leaky vasculature for tumor accumulation through the EPR effect. The drug molecules may be released from the nanoparticles and diffuse throughout the tissue for bioactivity. (b) For active tumor cell targeting, the nanoparticles are modified with targeting ligands, which recognize receptors present on tumor cell surface. The receptor-mediated endocytosis leads to enhanced accumulation and cell uptake of nanoparticles. (c, d) By incorporating ligands that bind to the receptors on the surface of endothelial cells (c) or stromal/immune cells (d), nanoparticles can actively target tumor microenvironment for cancer therapy. (e) Some nanoparticles can generate heat under an alternating magnetic field or laser irradiation for cancer hyperthermia therapy. (f) Some nanoparticles become therapeutically active by releasing the payloads under either endogenous stimuli (e.g., pH, enzyme, and redox) or exogenous stimuli (e.g., light, heat, magnetic field, or ultrasound).

components and/or water to generate free radicals for DNA damage in tumor cells. However, the effectiveness of radiotherapy is limited by the tolerance of normal tissue to ionizing radiation dose and the development of radiation resistance of cancer cells.[28] Nowadays, several approaches have been proposed to address these issues. Introducing nanoscale radiosensitizers (e.g., gold, gadolinium, and iron oxide nanoparticles) into the X-ray pathway is considered an effective way to eradicate tumors at a lower dose of radiation.[29] These materials have higher electron density than water in tissues, enabling strong interaction with X-rays and allowing for more localized and consolidated damage to tumor. Currently, a new radiation NanoXray (developed by Nanobiotix) based on hafnium oxide nanoparticles is in clinical testing for patients with different soft tissue sarcoma.

An alternative way to enhance radiotherapeutic efficacy is to protect surrounding healthy tissues from damage or make them less radiation sensitive. Nanoparticles containing small molecules

with radioprotective effects (e.g., cysteine, citicoline, and amifostine) have been investigated. Oral administration of these particles has shown radioprotective effects in both mammalian cells and rats during radiation exposure.[30–32] Furthermore, nanoparticles loaded with therapeutics against radiation-resistant biological pathways (e.g., survivin and epidermal growth factor receptor) have shown the ability to overcome the resistance of tumor to radiation therapy.[33,34] All these nanoparticle strategies could lead to further improvement in clinical radiotherapy.

Hyperthermia therapy

Owing to low host toxicity, ease of control, and absent/low resistance, hyperthermia treatment methods such as photothermal therapy (PTT) and magnetothermal therapy may be considered for cancer therapy, especially for drug-resistant cancers. Distinct from traditional therapies, PTT relies on photosensitizers to absorb light and convert it into heat to kill cells in its vicinity.[35] Its key advantage over traditional chemotherapy is that photosensitizers are minimally toxic without light exposure and thus damage to healthy tissues is minimal even with photosensitizer accumulation. Unlike radiotherapy, the light used in PTT is nonionizing [usually near-infrared light (NIR)], hence its effect on tissues is much less invasive. Considering hypoxia in most tumors, PTT is more attractive for cancer therapy than photodynamic therapy (PDT) currently used in the clinic because PTT does not require oxygen, while PDT utilizes UV or visible light to activate photosensitizers to generate toxic reactive oxygen in the present of oxygen.[36] Moreover, NIR involved in PTT has much deeper penetration than UV or visible light typically used in PDT.[37] Nevertheless, low molecular weight PTT agents tend to aggregate in aqueous solution, nonspecifically bind to proteins and lack target specificity. A large number of nanoparticles have therefore been investigated as PTT agents including carbon-based nanomaterials, semiconductor nanocrystals, metallic nanoparticles, rare earth ion-doped nanocrystals, and organic nanoparticles. *In vivo* preclinical results of these PTT nanoparticle agents demonstrated that tumor shrinking was achieved with minimal damage to surrounding healthy tissues.[38] Currently, AuroLase (a gold nanoshell-encapsulated silica nanoparticle developed by Nanospectra) is under phase I trials for PTT of refractory head and neck cancer, and primary and/or metastatic lung tumors. In addition to PTT, magnetothermal therapy also shows significant potential for cancer treatment. One successful example is NanoTherm (iron oxide nanoparticles), which recently received EU Regulatory Approval as medical devices for glioblastoma treatment. Interestingly, these nanoparticles could also be used for X-ray CT or MRI imaging, thus enabling diagnosis, patient selection, and/or response tracking.

Gene therapy

Advances in cancer genetics and tumor-specific signaling pathways that are critical for tumor development/metastasis have given rise to the application of gene therapy in cancer treatment. The advantage of gene therapy over other anticancer strategies is that, in principle, we can rationally design nucleic acids (e.g., DNA, siRNA, antisense, and mRNA) to specifically regulate the expression of virtually any gene of interest. RNA interference (RNAi) technology, which can specifically silence the expression of target genes, represents a revolution in gene therapy and holds great promise for cancer research and therapy.[39–41] For instance, it provides a rapid approach to study the genetic alterations in human cancers, many of which are considered as "undruggable" targets and/or require complex and time-consuming development of effective inhibitors.[42,43] However, the ubiquitous application of RNAi in cancer treatment is hindered by the challenge of safe and effective delivery of RNAi agents such as small interfering RNA (siRNA) to tumors. As siRNA molecules are susceptible to degradation by endogenous enzymes and cannot readily cross cellular membrane owing to their polyanionic and macromolecular characteristics, a variety of nanoparticle vehicles have been extensively explored to protect siRNA and facilitate its delivery into the tumor cell cytosol where the RNAi machinery resides.[18,44] To date, several cationic lipid- or polymer-based siRNA nanoparticles, including CALAA-01, ALN-VSP02, Atu027, and others, have entered phase I or II clinical trials to treat different types of cancer.[18] RNAi nanotechnology has also shown potential in reversing drug resistance. By downregulating overexpressed antiapoptotic regulators (e.g., Bcl-2) and transporters (e.g., P-glycoprotein), or by suppressing of DNA repair pathways, drug resistant tumor cells can be resensitized.[45–47]

Distinct from gene silencing by siRNA or antisense, DNA-mediated gene therapy aims to replace a mutated gene in tumor cells with a functional, therapeutic gene. However, similar to siRNA delivery, the main problem restricting the *in vivo* applications of gene therapy is the difficulty of delivering the fragile, large, and negatively charged DNA molecules into the nucleus of tumor cells. Over the past few decades, an astounding amount of positively charged materials have been designed for enhancing the safety and efficacy of DNA delivery.[48] Today, SGT53-01, a p53 gene-loaded liposome coated with transferrin, is currently undergoing phase I clinical trials for treatment of solid tumors.[49] In addition to DNA, mRNA is also emerging as a promising therapeutic nucleic acid in recent years. Its therapeutic mechanism is similar to that of DNA-mediated gene therapy, but to some extent, mRNA would be more efficient as it does not require nuclear localization/transcription. Furthermore, mRNA has little chance of interacting with the host genome, thus excluding potentially detrimental genomic integration.[50] Naked and protamine-protected mRNAs are currently in active clinical trials for cancer treatment.[51,52] Although there is no clinical trial underway, a growing number of studies have shown that mRNA formulated in nanoparticles exhibited enhanced translation and generated a more robust immune response owing to improved intracellular uptake/endosomal escape.[53]

Taken together, the idea of using nucleic acids as therapeutics for cancer therapy is straightforward, but successful application of gene therapy faces the major challenge of safe and effective gene delivery *in vivo*. While remaining elusive, development of nanoparticle delivery vehicles with long blood circulation time, high tumor accumulation, uniform tissue penetration, and efficient cellular uptake and endosomal escape represents a great opportunity in the gene therapy field.

Active immunotherapy

In contrast to the therapy modalities mentioned above, active immunotherapy (or cancer vaccine) provides a unique strategy for cancer treatment by provoking the host's immune system to fight tumor cells. As immune systems are robust, have the capacity for memory, and possess exquisite specificity, active immunotherapy might achieve complete and long-lasting cancer cures with minimal detriment to health.[54] However, only a few vaccines have demonstrated sufficient efficacy for clinical use. The major reasons that contribute to these limited clinical responses may be the physical barriers imposed by the TME, host-derived immunosuppressive effects, or tumor escape from immune effector function.[55] Nanotechnology is gaining momentum in this field and becoming increasingly attractive as potent carriers for effective delivery of vaccine antigens and adjuvants. First, nanoparticles can be engineered for rapid phagocytosis by immune cells and can protect antigens (e.g., peptides, proteins and nucleic acids) from premature enzymatic and proteolytic degradation.[56] In particular, they allow for more effective antigen uptake in some immune cells such as dendritic cells (DCs), as compared to free antigens.[57] By surface coating with a proprietary DC-specific antibody fragment, a targeted liposomal vaccine, lipovaxin-MM (currently phase I study) can deliver multiple antigens to DCs effectively owing to the ligand-receptor interactions. Second, nanoparticles can package antigen and adjuvant for transport to the targeted site simultaneously, which could be crucial for ideal immunotherapy. For instance, by coloading tumor-associated antigen HER2/neu and adjuvant AS15 with potential immunostimulatory and antineoplastic activities into the liposome, this vaccine can stimulate the host immune response to mount a cytotoxic T-lymphocyte response, leading to tumor cell lysis, and is now in phase II clinical studies for metastatic breast cancer. Compared to liposomes, biodegradable polymer nanoparticles can not only regulate the pharmacokinetic and distribution profile of antigens/adjuvants but also exhibit additional unique features such as sustained release of antigens/adjuvants at the target site and eliminating the need for repeated doses.[58] A recent study by Selecta Biosciences further shows that adjuvant-carrying polymeric nanoparticles can augment the immune response to encapsulated antigen and exhibit strong local immune activation without inducing systemic cytokine release.[59]

Recent advances in cancer nanotechnologies

Despite the fascinating achievements mentioned earlier, the potential of cancer nanotechnologies may be far from being fully realized. In the following section, we briefly discuss some recent exciting advances in this field, which from our perspective may enable the development of more effective cancer nanotherapeutics.

One major challenge for effective systemic drug delivery to tumor tissues is to avoid the recognition of nanoparticles by mononuclear phagocyte system (MPS) in liver and spleen for long blood circulation. This can therefore facilitate time-dependent extravasation of nanoparticles through the leaky tumor microvasculature and lead to effective tumor accumulation. Nanoparticle physicochemical properties, such as size, shape, surface PEG charge, and surface modification (e.g., PEGylation), were previously shown to impact the circulation and tumor accumulation.[60–64] Recently, a new concept for effectively evading the MPS system by incorporating cellular membranes on NP surface has moved into the spotlight. By using natural erythrocyte membranes as coating shells, it was observed that the circulation half-life of cell membrane-coated nanoparticles in blood was 2.5-fold higher than PEG-coated nanoparticles.[65] Furthermore, the cellular membrane can also retain its inherent functions, leading to the active delivery of nanotherapeutics to tumor. For example, by coating with leukocyte membranes, a new generation of nanotherapeutics has demonstrated the ability to avoid opsonization, delay liver clearance, and recognize and bind tumor endothelium in an active manner.[66] Another thought-provoking concept to inhibit phagocytic clearance is to decorate nanoparticles with a "marker of self" ligand such as CD47 or its peptide variant.[67] Such ligands can impede phagocytosis of "self" cells or nanoparticles by signaling through the phagocyte receptor CD172a, thus delaying macrophage-mediated clearance of nanoparticles and promoting blood circulation for more effective drug delivery to tumors.

TME has been gradually recognized as a key contributor to tumor growth, progression, and metastasis and can therefore be considered as a potential target for effective cancer therapy.[68] Vascular endothelium performs critical functions such as transporting oxygen and nutrients from the bloodstream to tissues, controlling blood flow and trafficking blood cells. Its abnormalities are always implicated in the pathogenesis of tumor progression and metastasis.[69] Nanoparticles carrying drugs or siRNAs targeting dysfunctional tumor vascular endothelium have thus been a growing interest in cancer treatment (Figure 1c).[70] A specific polymeric nanoparticle platform has recently been developed for selective siRNA delivery to lung endothelial cells, leading to effective silencing of five endothelial genes (Tie1, Tie2, VEcad, VEGFR-2, and ICAM-2) without significant reduction of gene expression in pulmonary immune cells, hepatocytes, or peritoneal immune cells.[71] Another strategy is to target tumor-associated inflammation, such as inhibiting the infiltration of tumor-associated macrophages (Figure 1d).[72,73] Attention has also been given to targeting the communication between cancer cells and TME. One recent example is the active delivery of Bortezomib using biodegradable PLGA-PEG polymer to increase osteogenic differentiating and bond strength, which in turn significantly inhibited tumor growth in bone, the most common metastatic site for

many cancers.[74] In addition, some highly cytotoxic chemotherapeutic drugs can be administrated as "prodrugs" and then activated by TME (e.g., pH, enzyme, and hypoxia) into cytotoxic products.[75]

Although in an early state, the development of nanotherapeutics for noninvasive administration through oral, nasal, or ocular routes is constantly growing and showing many merits over systemic injection. Drug delivery through a nasal route is advantageous for treatment of lung cancer because it allows nanotherapeutics to bypass high liver uptake and avoid repeated administration. In a recent *in vivo* study using inhalable doxorubicin-encapsulated nanoparticles to treat lung cancer, highly significant improvement in survival was observed compared to intravenous injection groups.[76] On the other hand, cancer patients who require frequent administration of drugs would benefit from oral delivery because of the convenience and compliance, but this approach is limited by insufficient intestinal absorption of drugs owing to intestinal mucosal barrier. Very recently, IgG Fc fragments have been conjugated to polymer nanoparticles, which can effectively target neonatal Fc (FcRn) receptors and be transported across intestinal epithelium after oral administration and reach systemic circulation with mean absorption efficiency 10 times higher than nontargeted nanoparticles.[15] These targeted nanoparticles offer new hope for developing oral delivery nanotherapeutics for cancer treatment.

Summary

Clinical success in cancer nanomedicine has become a driving force behind the development of new nanoparticle technologies for safer and more effective treatment and the pursuit of personalized nanotherapeutics. Meanwhile, we have also realized how challenging the cancer nanotechnology field is due to the complexity and heterogeneity of cancer and the encumbrances in clinical translation. The convergence of nanotechnology with tumor biology and other biological/biomedical sciences will therefore be crucial for realizing the full potential of cancer nanotechnology. We expect that this chapter can encourage physicians, scientists, engineers, and others from different areas of expertise to become involved in this exciting field and promote the widespread application of nanotechnologies for cancer management.

Acknowledgments

This work was supported by NIH grants R00CA160350 (J.S.) and U54-CA151884 (R.L.); David Koch—Prostate Cancer Foundation Program in Nanotherapeutics (R.L.); Movember-PCF Challenge Award (J.S.); and PCF Young Investigator Award (J.S.).

Key references

The complete reference list can be found on the Wiley Companion Digital Edition of this title (see inside front cover for login instructions).

1 Stewart BW, Wild CP. *World Cancer Report 2014.* IARC: Lyon; 2014.

4 Hubbell JA, Langer R. Translating materials design to the clinic. *Nat Mater.* 2013;**12**:963–966.

9 Farokhzad OC, Langer R. Impact of nanotechnology on drug delivery. *ACS Nano.* 2009;**3**:16–20.

11 Langer R. Drug delivery and targeting. *Nature.* 1998;**392**:5–10.

15 Pridgen EM, Alexis F, Kuo TT, et al. Transepithelial transport of Fc-targeted nanoparticles by the neonatal fc receptor for oral delivery. *Sci Transl Med.* 2013;**5**:213ra167.

18 Kanasty R, Dorkin JR, Vegas A, et al. Delivery materials for siRNA therapeutics. *Nat Mater*. 2013;**12**:967–977.

21 Matsumura Y, Maeda H. A new concept for macromolecular therapeutics in cancer chemotherapy: Mechanism of tumoritropic accumulation of proteins and the antitumor agent SMANCS. *Cancer Res*. 1986;**46**:6387–6392.

22 Peer D, Karp JM, Hong S, et al. Nanocarriers as an emerging platform for cancer therapy. *Nat Nanotech*. 2007;**2**:751–760.

24 Hrkach J, Hoff DV, Ali MM, et al. Preclinical development and clinical translation of a PSMA-targeted docetaxel nanoparticle with a differentiated pharmacological profile. *Sci Transl Med*. 2012;**4**:128ra39.

26 Mura S, Nicolas J, Couvreur P. Stimuli-responsive drug-delivery systems in clinical trials. *Nat Mater*. 2013;**12**:991–1003.

29 Kwatra D, Venugopal A, Anant S. Nanoparticles in radiation therapy: a summary of various approaches to enhance radiosensitization in cancer. *Transl Cancer Res*. 2013;**2**:330–342.

38 Jaque D, Maestro ML, Rosal B, et al. Nanoparticles for photothermal therapies. *Nanoscale*. 2014;**6**:9494–9530.

41 Whitehead KA, Langer R, Anderson DG. Knocking down barriers: advances in siRNA delivery. *Nat Rev Drug Discov*. 2009;**8**:129–138.

56 Smith DM, Simon JK, Baker JR Jr. Applications of nanotechnology for immunology. *Nat Rev Immunol*. 2013;**13**:592–605.

65 Hu CMJ, Aryal S, Cheung C, et al. Erythrocyte membrane-camouflaged polymeric nanoparticles as a biomimetic delivery platform. *Proc Natl Acad Sci U S A*. 2011;**108**:10980–10985.

67 Rodriguez PL, Harada T, Christian DA, et al. Minimal "self" peptides that inhibit phagocytic clearance and enhance delivery of nanoparticles. *Science*. 2013;**339**:971–975.

68 Albini A, Sporn MB. The tumour microenvironment as a target for chemoprevention. *Nat Rev Cancer*. 2007;**7**:139–145.

71 Dahlman JE, Barnes C, et al. In vivo endothelial siRNA delivery using polymeric nanoparticles with low molecular weight. *Nat Nanotechnol*. 2014;**9**:648–655.

70 Hematopoietic cell transplantation

Roy Jones, MD, PhD ▪ *Elizabeth Shpall, MD* ▪ *Richard Champlin, MD*

Overview

Hematopoietic cell transplantation is an effective therapy for a variety of hematologic malignancies and selected other cancers, immunodeficiency states, and genetic disorders. Refinement of methods has allowed the application of this technique to older patients as well as the use of human leukocyte antigen mismatched donors and products. While toxic, the majority of these treatments have curative potential for otherwise fatal cancers. The immunotherapeutic activity of allotransplantation provides both therapeutic benefit and lessons for future immune treatments of cancer.

Hematopoietic cell transplantation involves engraftment of stem cells that can be collected from the bone marrow, peripheral blood, or umbilical cord blood (UCB). Allogeneic transplants are obtained from another individual. Autologous transplants involve use of a patient's own hematopoietic cells, usually after cryopreservation. Syngeneic transplants are between genetically identical twins.

Hematopoietic transplantation is an effective treatment for many life-threatening hematologic, immune, metabolic, and neoplastic diseases (Table 1).[1,2] The basis for autologous hematopoietic cell transplantation is to use patient-derived hematopoietic stem cells to prevent otherwise lethal myelosuppression from intensive treatment. More recently, autologous cells manipulated *in vitro* to produce augmented immune effects are being explored. The basis of allogeneic hematopoietic transplantation is the engraftment of donor-derived stem cells; in the recipient, these cells reconstitute hematopoiesis and immunity. Following successful transplantation, recipients are considered chimeras with hematopoietic and immune cells derived from the donor. Recently, it has been recognized that hematopoietic stem cells are capable of limited differentiation into nonhematopoietic tissues[4] including mesenchymal cells,[5,6] liver,[7,8] cardiovascular tissues,[9] and, possibly, neural tissue.[10] There is considerable interest in stem cell transplantation for restoration of damaged or diseased organs and tissues.[11,12]

Methods of transplantation

In most cases, transplanted hematopoietic cells are infused following intensive chemotherapy, irradiation, or other therapies such as antibodies. Over time, a variety of chemotherapeutic agents has been explored for use in transplantation, emphasizing the alkylating agents cyclophosphamide, busulfan, melphalan, thiotepa, and carmustine (BCNU). Total body radiation (TBI) is also employed. In allogeneic transplantation, these drugs are often combined with agents designed to produce additional tumor killing and immunosuppression, such as fludarabine.[13]

The existence of graft-versus-malignancy (GVM) effect is now well-established as an important component of therapeutic activity for allotransplantation.[14] This alloimmune effect is often associated with normal tissue toxicity and termed graft-versus-host disease (GVHD). A major focus of allotransplant research is the exploration of specific cell types and techniques that might produce GVM without GVHD.[15] Donor lymphocyte infusions (DLI) following transplantation can be used to augment the GVM effect.[16]

Hematopoietic transplantation as treatment for malignancies

Most hematopoietic transplants have been performed for treatment of hematologic malignancies.[17] Many chemotherapy drugs (predominantly alkylating agents[18]) and irradiation produce a dose-dependent antitumor response. Myelosuppression is the dose-limiting toxicity of many chemotherapeutic agents and whole-body irradiation. Doses of many agents can be escalated three- to fivefold above conventional maximally tolerated dose if followed by autologous or allogeneic transplantation to restore hematopoiesis (Figure 1).

Autologous transplantation

As a general rule, autologous hematopoietic transplantation is most effective in patients with malignancies shown to be responsive to conventional treatment immediately before the transplant regimen.[19] Factors known to predispose to treatment failure include higher volume residual tumor,[20,21] tumor types not known to exhibit a steep dose-killing relationship,[22] or treatment of patients at high risk for toxicities from the proposed treatment regimen.

Immune augmentation strategies used in the posttransplant setting are being actively explored to avoid the prolonged immunosuppression that follows transplantation and may increase the risk of relapse.[23] An additional factor that might predispose to relapse is contamination of the harvested cells with tumor. Although limited investigation using gene-marked tumor cells has shown that cryopreserved tumor cells can engraft and contribute to relapse, the clinical importance of this phenomenon is unclear.[24] Malignancies shown to be cured by autologous hematopoietic cell transplantation include intermediate grade and other selected lymphomas,[25] Hodgkin's disease,[26] acute lymphoblastic leukemia,[27,28] and acute myelogenous leukemia (AML).[29,30] Although not proven to be curative, major improvement in survival in myeloma patients receiving autologous transplantation has made the technique a standard treatment for appropriate patients with this condition.[31,32] Benefit is likely for patients with germ cell cancers,[33] low grade lymphomas,[34] and a variety of pediatric solid tumors.[35]

Holland-Frei Cancer Medicine, Ninth Edition. Edited by Robert C. Bast Jr., Carlo M. Croce, William N. Hait, Waun Ki Hong, Donald W. Kufe, Martine Piccart-Gebhart, Raphael E. Pollock, Ralph R. Weichselbaum, Hongyang Wang, and James F. Holland.
© 2017 John Wiley & Sons, Inc. ISBN: 978-1-118-93469-2

Table 1 Diseases treated with hematopoietic transplantation.

Malignant
- Acute myelogenous leukemia
- Myelodysplastic syndromes
- Acute lymphoblastic leukemia
- Chronic myelogenous leukemia and myeloproliferative disorders
- Chronic lymphocytic leukemia
- Non-Hodgkin lymphoma
- Hodgkin disease
- Multiple myeloma and amyloidosis
- Solid tumors: breast, testicular, ovarian, and small cell lung cancer
- Pediatric solid tumors: neuroblastoma, Ewing sarcoma, medulloblastoma, renal cell cancer, melanoma

Nonmalignant
- Aplastic anemia and related bone marrow failure states
- Hemoglobinopathies: thalassemia, sickle cell anemia
- Congenital disorders of hematopoiesis
- Fanconi anemia and related syndromes
- Congenital immune deficiencies: severe combined immune deficiency, Wiskott–Aldrich syndrome, chronic granulomatous disease, and related syndromes
- Inborn errors of metabolism
- Autoimmune disorders

Allogeneic transplantation

Allogeneic hematopoietic transplants combine cytotoxic treatments with the immune-mediated GVM effect. Donor-derived lymphoid cells may react against and eradicate malignant cells that survive high-dose cytotoxic therapy.[36,37] Patients with acute or chronic GVHD have reduced risk of relapse, suggesting a relationship between GVM and GVHD.[38,39] The most direct evidence for GVM comes from the observation that DLI can reinduce remission in patients who relapse posttransplant.[40,41]

There are major differences among malignancies in their susceptibility to GVM effects. Indolent myeloid and lymphoid malignancies

are highly sensitive to this process, as evidenced by durable remissions after modulation of immunosuppression or DLI in patients who have relapsed after an allogeneic transplant. GVM effects have been best documented in patients with chronic myelogenous leukemia (CML).

GVM effects also occur but with lesser intensity against other hematologic malignancies including AML, multiple myeloma (MM), Hodgkin's disease, and intermediate-grade lymphoma. In these diagnoses, allogeneic transplants produce a greater frequency of durable remissions than syngeneic or autologous transplants, but these disorders respond less frequently to DLI and responses are usually transient. Acute lymphoblastic leukemia and high-grade lymphoma appear relatively insensitive to graft-versus-leukemia (GVL) effects,[42] although patients with GVHD do have a reduced risk of relapse in some studies.[43]

GVM effects may be directed against a number of potential target antigens. Development of methods to separate GVM effects and GVHD and generate antigen-specific antitumor responses is a major goal of ongoing research. For example, natural killer (NK) cells may produce GVM with decreased risk of GVHD,[44] and regulatory T cells (Treg) may moderate GVHD with lesser effects on GVM.[45]

Donor selection

Autologous transplantation

Autologous transplants use the patient as their own donor. In the closely related special case, syngeneic transplants are donations from a genetically identical twin. Autologous transplants require no histocompatibility matching but often come from patients who have received extensive prior chemotherapy. This treatment often compromises marrow stem cell function making adequate stem cell collection more difficult. Stem cells can be

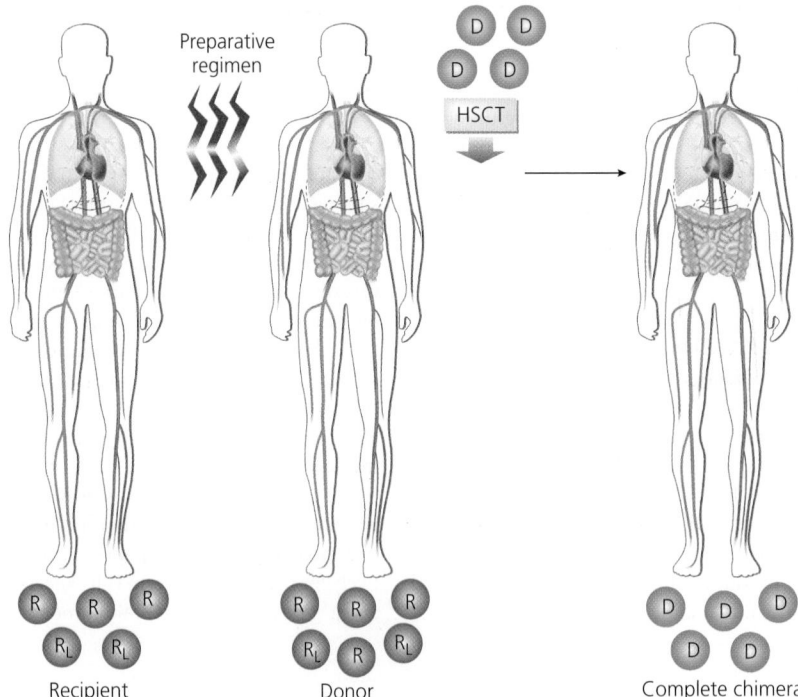

Preparative regimen

HSCT

Recipient   Donor   Complete chimera

Figure 1 Scheme of allogeneic hematopoietic transplantation. The recipient receives a myeloablative preparative regimen designed to eradicate malignant and normal cells. The recipient then receives donor hematopoietic cells that restore hematopoiesis. Abbreviations: D, donor hematopoietic cells; HSCT, hematopoietic stem cell transplant; R, recipient's normal bone marrow cells; RL, recipient's leukemia cells in bone marrow.

collected from the peripheral blood following mobilization with hematopoietic stimulants [G-CSF (granulocyte colony-stimulating factor), chemotherapy] or from bone marrow. A minimum of 2×10^6 CD34 cells/kg recipient body weight is required for satisfactory engraftment. Tumor contamination of collected cells represents a possible source of relapse and patients with significant tumor infiltration of marrow may be less desirable autotransplant candidates.[46,47] Various "purging" techniques to reduce or eliminate tumor cell contamination *in vitro* are being investigated.

Patients undergo collection of bone marrow or peripheral blood progenitor cells that are then cryopreserved in a viable state. Patients subsequently receive high-dose myelosuppressive therapy to eradicate the malignancy, followed by reinfusion of the stored cells to reconstitute hematopoiesis. Autologous hematopoietic cells can potentially be used as vehicles for gene therapy designed to correct deficiency states.

Allogeneic transplantation

Allogeneic transplants are collected from related or unrelated donors. The human leukocyte antigen (HLA) system is the major histocompatibility complex (MHC) in man, and the results of allogeneic transplantation depend on the histocompatibility between donor and recipient. The HLA system is encoded by several closely linked loci on the short arm of chromosome 6.[48,49] Class I loci include HLA-A, -B, and -C alleles. The class II region includes DR, DQ, and DP loci.

Historically, transplants have been from HLA-identical sibling donors. The HLA genes are inherited as a haplotype with one haplotype derived from each parent. There is approximately a one in four chance that any given sibling will be HLA matched with a potential recipient. Registries of potential unrelated donors have been established to provide hematopoietic transplants for patients lacking a histocompatible relative. HLA gene frequencies vary considerably among racial and ethnic groups, and patients are most likely to find transplants among potential donors of their own genetic background. Linkage disequilibrium occurs such that some haplotypes occur commonly, but approximately half of the population have rare haplotypes. There are now over 18 million potential unrelated bone marrow donors accessible in registries worldwide, and approximately half of patients can access an HLA-A, -B, -C, -DR-, and -DQ identical donor. Ten-antigen matched unrelated donor transplants now have outcomes that approximate those for histocompatible sibling donors.[50,51]

Transplant recipients who are mismatched at one or more loci are at higher risk of graft rejection, GVHD, and associated complications. One haplotype-identical related donors are readily available for most patients. The use of posttransplant high-dose cyclophosphamide has been shown to moderate GVHD risk and make haploidentical-related transplants increasingly possible.[52] In addition, UCB is now frequently used.[53,54] Constraints for HLA matching of UCB are much less than that for other cell sources, with mismatches at 2 of 6 HLA-A, -B, and DR loci being acceptable.[55] Owing to the size of the units, UCB transplants have been most successful in children but can also be accomplished in adults when large or multiple cord products are used. Delayed immune reconstitution and a high frequency of opportunistic infections remain major complications of both these techniques.

Like autotransplantation, allogeneic cells are usually administered after an intensive chemotherapy program. In addition to tumor killing, these programs are also designed to produce immunosuppression sufficient to facilitate engraftment of the allo cells. The intensity required is, in part, proportional to the immunocompetence of the recipient. After hematopoietic recovery, the degree of donor engraftment relative to host hematopoiesis (termed chimerism) is most commonly measured by PCR of DNA-restriction fragment length polymorphisms of the donor. In some circumstances, reduced-intensity chemotherapy is used to decrease regimen-related toxicity or to produce a mixed chimeric state. Delayed DLI can be used subsequently to produce full donor chimerism.[56] This technique is particularly useful when older patients are treated.[57,58]

Nonablative hematopoietic transplant

The recipient, a patient with normal and malignant leukemia cells in the bone marrow, receives a nonmyeloablative preparative regimen designed to prevent rejection of the transplant. The patient receives hematopoietic cells from the donor, which, after engraftment, produces a state of mixed chimerism in which both donor- and recipient-derived cells coexist (Figure 2). A subsequent graft-versus-hematopoietic effect may then occur, which eradicates residual normal and malignant cells of host origin, resulting in complete chimerism (presence of only donor derived hematopoietic and immune cells). A DLI may be administered to augment the GVM effect.

Selection of autologous or allogeneic transplantation

Selection of the type of transplantation for a patient, autologous or allogeneic, depends on the type of malignancy, age of the recipient, availability of a suitable donor, ability to collect a tumor-free autograft, stage and status of disease (bone marrow involvement, bulk of disease, chemosensitivity to conventional chemotherapy), and the malignancy's susceptibility to GVM effects.

Autologous transplantation is readily available, and there is no need to identify an HLA-matched donor. Autologous transplants have a lower risk of life-threatening complications; there are no risk of GVHD and no need for immunosuppressive therapy to prevent GVHD and graft rejection. Immune reconstitution is more rapid than after an allogeneic transplant and there is a lower risk of opportunistic infections. Graft failure occurs rarely. Treatment-related mortality is lower than 5% in most studies, and elderly patients can tolerate treatment relatively well.[59,60] However, autologous transplants have several drawbacks. Clonogenic tumor cells involving blood or bone marrow can contribute to relapse. Autologous transplantation relies solely on the effect of high-dose cytoreductive treatment for tumor eradication and lacks the immune-mediated GVM effect resulting after allogeneic transplantation. In most malignancies, relapse rates are higher after autologous transplants than after allogeneic transplantation, although this is often offset by a lower rate of treatment-related mortality. Patients with extensive prior therapy are at high risk for developing myelodysplasia and secondary acute leukemia after autologous hematopoietic transplantation.[61,62]

Allogeneic transplantation has the advantage that the graft is free of contaminating tumor cells and includes donor-derived immunocompetent cells that may produce an immune GVM effect. Allogeneic transplants may be associated with a number of potentially fatal complications such as regimen-related organ toxicity, graft failure, and GVHD. Immune reconstitution is slower after allogeneic transplantation and opportunistic infections are more frequent. Treatment-related mortality is significantly higher than with autologous transplantation.

In general, allogeneic transplants have been used in the treatment of leukemias and myelodysplastic syndromes (MDS). Autologous transplants have been used more often in solid tumors, lymphoma, and myeloma, although nonablative allogeneic transplants are under evaluation in these disorders as a means to induce GVM effects.

The outcome of transplantation relates to the selection of patients and timing of transplant during the natural history of the malignancy. The best results occur when the transplant is performed early in the disease course, when the malignancy is still sensitive to chemoradiotherapy treatment, and when the tumor burden is low. Conversely, transplants done as a last resort are associated with high rates of both relapse and treatment-related toxicity. Responsiveness to conventional-dose chemotherapy is a major predictive factor for the outcome of hematopoietic transplant. The best results have been achieved in patients with chemosensitive relapse or when transplant is performed in high-risk patients as consolidation of response, particularly in patients with minimal disease at the time of transplant. Primary resistance can sometimes be overcome by dose-intense treatment, such as in patients with acute leukemia, Hodgkin's disease, or MM who have failed to achieve an initial remission. However, patients with bulky disease, refractory relapse, or multiple relapses of their malignancy have a poor prognosis.

Pretransplant therapy

Autologous transplantation

Early autologous treatment regimens were copied from the allogeneic experience and utilized cyclophosphamide plus either TBI or busulfan. TBI has the advantage of being able to be delivered in precise dose and with protection of vulnerable organs such as lungs and kidneys. TBI is suboptimal for the treatment of bulk tumor masses where hypoxia and resistance may characterize deep-seated tumor cells. In contrast, chemotherapy agents such as busulfan

penetrate tumor vascularity and reach deep-seated tumors more effectively.

Alkylating agents are the most commonly used drugs in transplant regimens because they usually kill tumor cells in proportion to increasing dose. The most commonly used alkylating agents include cyclophosphamide, melphalan, busulfan, BCNU, and thiotepa. The platinum derivatives, carboplatin[63] and cisplatin,[64] are also used. Other commonly used nonalkylators are etoposide (VP-16), cytosine arabinoside, and fludarabine. The most frequently used chemotherapy regimen is BCNU, etoposide, Ara-C, and melphalan (BEAM), commonly used for Hodgkin disease and lymphomas.[65] The ifosfamide, carboplatin, and etoposide (ICE) regimen is also used for these diseases. In recent years, monoclonal antibodies have proven to be useful when added to standard treatments for leukemia and lymphoma. The anti-CD20 monoclonal antibody rituximab, shown to improve the survival of patients with intermediate grade lymphoma when combined with cyclophosphamide, doxorubicin, vincristine, and prednisone (CHOP) chemotherapy, appears to improve the effectiveness of BEAM.[66]

Allogeneic transplantation

The preparative regimen generally involves chemotherapy drugs alone or with TBI. The classical "myeloablative" regimens used in the treatment of leukemia are designed to ablate both hematopoiesis and immunity in the recipient and typically involve the combination of high-dose cyclophosphamide with either TBI[67,68] or high-dose busulfan.[69,70]

The toxicity of high-dose myeloablative therapy limits the use of this modality to relatively young patients in good medical condition. The discovery of the curative potential of the immune-mediated GVM effect has led to a novel approach using lower dose, reduced intensity preparative regimens as a means to reduce the toxicity of allogeneic hematopoietic transplantation. These reduced intensity conditioning regimens have been designed not to fully eradicate the malignancy, but rather to provide sufficient immunosuppression to achieve engraftment and to allow induction of GVM (Figure 2).[71,72]

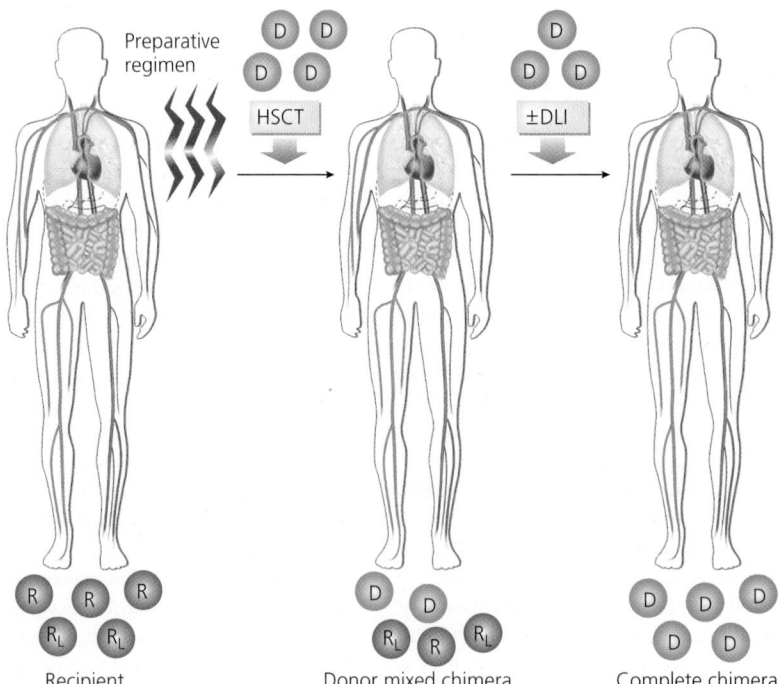

Figure 2 Scheme of nonablative allogeneic hematopoietic transplantation. Abbreviations: D, donor hematopoietic cells; DLI, donor lymphocyte infusion; HSCT, hematopoietic stem cell transplant; R, recipient's normal bone marrow cells; RL, recipient's leukemia cells in bone marrow.

These regimens can be tolerated by older patients and those with comorbidities who are not eligible to receive an ablative preparative regimen. Most reduced-intensity regimens include a purine analog, such as fludarabine, combined with an alkylating agent (cyclophosphamide, melphalan, or busulfan), or low-dose TBI. Engraftment has been achieved in most patients, and this approach is effective against a range of hematologic malignancies. Antithymocyte globulin is often added to produce additional immune suppression.

Complications of hematopoietic transplantation

Intensive chemoradiotherapy and hematopoietic transplantations may be associated with a number of serious complications as listed in Table 2. These include immune-mediated processes such as graft rejection and GVHD, toxicities resulting from the pretransplant conditioning regimen, infections owing to neutropenia, and posttransplant immune deficiency.

Graft rejection and graft failure

Graft failure is defined as the failure to establish hematopoietic engraftment (primary graft failure) or loss of an established graft (secondary graft failure). Graft failure after autologous transplant occurs rarely and is most often related to infusion of an inadequate number of viable stem cells.

Graft failure after allogeneic transplantation is also caused by immunologic graft rejection.[73,74] With current regimens, rejection occurs in fewer than 2% of transplants from an HLA-identical sibling. The risk is increased in recipients of HLA-mismatched grafts.[75,76] Donor CD8+ T lymphocytes provide a graft-facilitating effect, and T lymphocyte depletion from the allogeneic graft increases the risk of graft failure.[77,78] Cord blood transplants containing a lower number of CD34+ and CD8+ cells are more prone to engraftment failure.

Secondary graft failure or poor graft function may be caused by administration of myelosuppressive drugs, GVHD, and infections in the early posttransplant period. Ganciclovir or

Table 2 Complications after hematopoietic transplantation.

Immune complications
• Graft rejection
• Acute and chronic graft-versus-host disease
Regimen-related toxicity of the preparative regimen
• Mucositis and gastroenteritis
• Veno-occlusive disease of the liver
• Diffuse alveolar hemorrhage and interstitial pneumonitis
• Hemorrhagic cystitis
Hematologic complications
• Hemolytic anemia
• Thrombotic thrombocytopenic purpura and hemolytic disorders
Infections and immunodeficiency
• EBV-associated lymphoproliferative disease
Late complications
• Growth disturbances
• Hypothyroidism
• Sterility and hypogonadism
• Cataracts
• Avascular necrosis
• Secondary malignancies

Abbreviation: EBV, Epstein–Barr virus.

trimethoprim-sulfamethoxazole can produce pancytopenia, which is usually reversible after discontinuation of drug. Cytomegalovirus (CMV),[79] parvovirus,[80] human herpesvirus,[81,82] and mycobacterial and fungal infections may also compromise the graft. Poor engraftment may also result from microenvironment or marrow stroma dysfunction related to the patient's underlying disease or prior therapy.

Graft failure that is not due to rejection can often be successfully treated with G-CSF or second hematopoietic stem cell infusion from the same donor or an alternative donor.

Graft-versus-host disease

GVHD is a major, potentially life-threatening complication of allogeneic hematopoietic transplantation. Acute and chronic GVHD are distinct but interrelated syndromes. Acute GVHD typically occurs within the first 100 days posttransplant and results from reactivity of mature donor T lymphocytes present in the graft directed against disparate major or minor histocompatibility antigens of the recipient (the host).[83] Acute GVHD involves the skin, gastrointestinal (GI) tract, and liver as the primary target tissues. The hematopoietic and immune systems are also involved. A maculopapular rash is usually the first presentation and is typically pruritic and confluent. When severe, generalized erythroderma, bullae, and desquamation may occur. Acute GVHD of the liver targets the biliary epithelium and produces cholestatic hepatitis with marked elevation of bilirubin and alkaline phosphatase. GVHD can affect the entire GI tract, targeting epithelial cells. GI GVHD characteristically produces secretory diarrhea, abdominal pain, and on rare occasions, ileus. Upper GI GVHD produces nausea, vomiting, and anorexia, all which may occur without lower GI tract or other tissue involvement.[84] Conjunctivitis and other ocular manifestations, anemia, and thrombocytopenia often occur.

Severe GVHD is associated with a poor prognosis because of direct tissue damage, debilitation, and severe immunodeficiency caused by the GVHD process itself and by its treatment with immunosuppressive drugs.

The most important factor predicting the risk of GVHD is HLA disparity between the donor and recipient.[85–88] With current immunosuppressive prophylaxis, acute GVHD occurs in 25–50% of patients after transplants from an HLA identical sibling; this may be related to disparity between minor histocompatibility antigens. A higher incidence up to 61–90% has been reported following transplants from mismatched and unrelated donors. Results are improving for unrelated donor transplantation with the use of more precise molecular histocompatibility typing to identify donors. Older age is associated with an increased incidence of acute and chronic GVHD. Less intensive, nonmyeloablative conditioning regimens may also limit the severity of GVHD, presumably owing to reduction in tissue damage limiting the proinflammatory phase that facilitates development of GVHD.

Pharmacologic immunosuppression is generally administered for the first 6 months posttransplant to reduce the incidence and severity of GVHD. The current standard of care combines either cyclosporine or tacrolimus with a short course of methotrexate.[89,90] Corticosteroids are the first line of therapy in patients who develop acute GVHD. Approximately half of patients have a sustained response,[91] and the steroid dose can be gradually tapered off. Steroid-resistant GVHD has an unfavorable prognosis. The prognosis is best for GVHD limited to the skin. Acute GVHD involving the liver or multiple organs has a poorer prognosis than other sites. A number of other immunosuppressive agents are being studied. For mismatched grafts, recent studies have demonstrated that the use of post-transplant cyclophosphamide can decrease the risk of GVHD and permit related haploidentical transplants to be performed with acceptable risk.[92]

Chronic GVHD is a related syndrome affecting 25–60% of recipients of allogeneic transplantation who survive more than 6 months after transplant.[93] It most often occurs between 80 and 200 days after transplant, but onset may be delayed to the second year. Chronic GVHD is more common in older patients and in patients with prior acute GVHD although approximately one-third of affected patients have a *de novo* presentation without prior acute GVHD.[94] Chronic GVHD is more prevalent after transplants with peripheral blood stem cells than with marrow transplantation.[95]

Chronic GVHD has multiple clinical manifestations similar to those seen in several autoimmune disorders such as progressive systemic sclerosis, Sjögren syndrome, and primary biliary cirrhosis. Chronic GVHD is associated with profound immunosuppression and a major risk to the patients of opportunistic infections. Bronchiolitis obliterans without other major manifestations of chronic GVHD and intestinal involvement with anorexia, dysphagia, malabsorption, and wasting may occur. Polymyositis, serositis, and autoimmune manifestations occur rarely. Chronic GVHD may become a chronic debilitating disease affecting quality of life and remains the major determinant of late transplant-related morbidity. Progressive onset of extensive chronic GVHD from acute GVHD and the presence of thrombocytopenia are poor prognostic factors (Table 3).[96]

Corticosteroids are the first line of therapy for chronic GVHD.[97] The chronic nature of this syndrome requires long-term therapy for at least 6–9 months, using the lowest steroid doses, which control symptoms. Alternate day dosage may be preferable to minimize the complications resulting from chronic steroid therapy. Cyclosporine or tacrolimus may be used in combination with corticosteroids in high-risk patients.[98,99] Combinations of immunosuppressive agents may improve control of the direct manifestations of chronic GVHD, but they increase the risk of infectious morbidity and mortality. Photopheresis can be used as a steroid-sparing immune-modulatory treatment.[100]

Regimen-related toxicity

Myeloablative preparative regimens used to cytoreduce the malignancy approach the limit of tolerance for several tissues. The GI tract, kidneys, lungs, and liver are the most susceptible to toxic damage, but severe toxicity may also involve the heart, bladder, nervous system, and other tissues. The actual risk for toxicity varies among regimens and their relative dose intensity. Specific determinants include the toxicity profiles of the involved agents and their interactions that are affected by coexisting organ dysfunction, the effects of the diseases and prior therapy, and infections. Most toxicities are experienced during the first 30 days posttransplant, but regimen-related hepatic injury [hepatic veno-occlusive disease (VOD)], pulmonary toxicity, and neurologic effects may be delayed for several months.

VOD of the liver frequently occurs after TBI, busulfan, BCNU, thiotepa, carboplatin, and etoposide-containing regimens.[101] The clinical syndrome is characterized by painful hepatic enlargement, ascites, generalized fluid retention, and striking elevation of serum bilirubin. There is no proven treatment other than supportive care, and factors predicting the probability of a fatal outcome from VOD have been described.[102] Pulmonary toxicity directly related to drug injury is most commonly caused by BCNU, the frequency varying from 5% to 60% with increasing dose.[103] Virtually every alkylating agent used in transplantation has been associated with pulmonary toxicity, however, much less commonly than with BCNU. This injury typically occurs between 3 and 12 weeks following transplant and usually produces progressive shortness of breath, cough, and diffuse interstitial abnormalities on chest radiograph or CT scan. If infection is excluded, steroid treatment can

Table 3 Clinical staging and grading of graft-versus-host disease (GVHD).

Stage	Acute GVHD Skin[a]	Liver[b]	Gut[b]
1	Maculopapular rash <25%	Bilirubin 2–3 mg/dL	Diarrhea 500–1000 mL or persistent nausea[c]
2	Maculopapular rash 25–50%	Bilirubin 3–6 mg/dL	Diarrhea 1000–1500 mL
3	Generalized erythroderma	Bilirubin 6–15 mg/dL	Diarrhea >1500 mL
4	Desquamation and bulla	Bilirubin >15 mg/dL	Severe abdominal pain or ileus

Overall grade[d]	Severity	Skin		Liver		Gut
0	None	0	—	0	—	0
I	Mild	1–2	—	0	—	0
II	Moderate	3	or	1 or	or	1
III	Severe	—	—	2–3 or	—	2–3
IV[e]	Life threatening	4	or	4 or	or	—4

Chronic GVHD

Limited	Localized skin involvement *and/or* hepatic dysfunction
Extensive	1. Generalized skin involvement *or* 2. Localized skin involvement *and/or* hepatic dysfunction, *plus* any of the following: 　(a) liver histology showing chronic aggressive hepatitis, bridging necrosis, or cirrhosis 　(b) eye involvement (Schirmer test <5 mm wetting) 　(c) involvement of mucosalivary glands or oral mucosa 　(d) involvement of any other target organ

[a]Extents determined by rule of nines or burn chart.
[b]Downgrade one stage for additional causes of elevated bilirubin or diarrhea.
[c]Requires histologic evidence of GVHD in the stomach or duodenum.
[d]Minimal organ stage required to determine grade.
[e]Grade IV may also be determined with lower organ involvement with extreme decrease in performance status.
Sources: From Refs 117, 118, 137.

produce total reversal of this side effect.[104] Cardiac toxicity, usually manifests temporary myocardial injury and decline in cardiac ejection fraction, is also produced by a variety of alkylating agent regimens. Although most commonly asymptomatic and lasting only 1–3 months, it can occur in 20–40% of patients in selected regimens.[105] Irreversible cardiac failure can be seen but is much less common.

Hematologic complications

Hemolytic reactions may result from ABO blood group incompatibility between the donor and recipient.[106] ABO incompatibility is not a contraindication for allogeneic transplant. Red blood cells should be removed from the donor graft to prevent acute hemolytic reaction in cases with major ABO incompatibility and plasma should be removed in pairs with minor ABO incompatibility.

Atypical thrombotic thrombocytopenic purpura (TTP) may occur after hematopoietic transplantation.[107] Factors implicated in initiating endothelial injury include chemotherapeutic agents, irradiation, cyclosporine and tacrolimus, CMV and fungal infections, and cytokine-release syndromes.

Immunodeficiency and infections

Recipients of hematopoietic transplants have a severe immunodeficiency involving both T and B cells.[108] HLA-mismatched or unrelated and cord blood transplants have a more severe and prolonged immunodeficiency and risk for opportunistic infections. Recipients of autologous and syngeneic transplants also have a period of immunodeficiency but recovery is more rapid. Recipients of hematopoietic transplants may be susceptible to unusual opportunistic infections and to acute overwhelming infections. Prophylactic strategies against an array of potential infections and rapid recognition and treatment of infections are an essential part of successful management of transplant recipients.[109] Immunoglobulin replacement therapy should be considered in patients with documented immunoglobulin deficiency. Revaccinations should be performed upon immune recovery and are typically carried out 6 months posttransplant.

Posttransplant lymphoproliferative disease (PTLD) is a life-threatening complication of allogeneic transplantation.[110] It is more prevalent in recipients of mismatched or UCB grafts, and especially in those treated with aggressive immunosuppressive treatment including higher doses of ATG. PTLD in hematopoietic transplant recipients arises from the transformation of donor-derived B-lymphocytes by Epstein–Barr virus (EBV) infection. Treatment includes withdrawal of immunosuppression and administration of rituximab. Cellular therapy with donor or EBV-sensitized[111] lymphocyte infusions can have dramatic results in controlling PTLD.[112] Patients with increasing levels of EBV DNA are at highest risk for lymphoproliferative disease and are candidates for preemptive immunotherapy with rituximab.

Late effects

Late complications of hematopoietic transplantation include delayed effects of high-dose therapy, indolent infections, transfusion-related complications, and chronic GVHD. Late toxicity of high-dose therapy can produce cataracts, pulmonary fibrosis, dental abnormalities, hypothyroidism, hypogonadism, growth retardation, osteoporosis, and avascular necrosis of the hip or other bones. Permanent sterility occurs in most patients. There is an increased risk of solid and hematologic secondary tumors after hematopoietic transplantation. Solid tumors such as head and neck cancers, squamous cell carcinomas, melanomas, and brain, breast, and thyroid cancers may be more common in recipients of

TBI-containing regimens and the cumulative incidence is up to 7–10% at 15 years. Myelodysplasia and secondary leukemia occur more commonly after autologous transplant, occurring in 4–18% of patients within 2.5–8.5 years of transplant.[113,114]

Indications for hematopoietic transplantation

Acute myeloid leukemia (AML)

Hematopoietic cellular transplantation has been extensively evaluated for the treatment of patients with AML.[115,116] Myeloablative transplants have been used in younger patients. AML is more common with advanced age, however, so that reduced intensity transplantation, often based on a busulfan/fludarabine regimen, is now commonly used in fit patients up to 70 years of age. Most patients achieve complete remission after high dose therapy and hematopoietic transplantation. The major causes of treatment failure are GVHD, regimen-related toxicity, infections, and recurrent leukemia. More intensive regimens designed to have greater antileukemic activity by increasing the TBI dose or adding additional chemotherapeutic agents have produced additional toxicity, and overall survival has not improved.[117] The outcome after allogeneic transplantation is primarily dependent on the disease status (remission versus relapse), cytogenetic and mutational abnormality of the leukemia, patient age, and histocompatibility between donor and recipient.[118] For patients in remission, long-term disease-free survival is 40–65%.[119,120] An increasing number of patients with intermediate or high-risk prognostic features and fully matched donors are being transplanted in first complete remission. For patients with a favorable prognosis such as those with t8;21, t15;17, or inv 16 abnormalities, transplant is usually deferred until relapse and reinduction of remission.

The risks of allogeneic transplantation are increased in patients without an HLA-identical donor. Transplants from a related mismatched donor or using an UCB product should generally be considered in younger patients after relapse, those with poor-risk cytogenetic abnormalities, or patients with an antecedent hematologic disorder.[121]

Myelodysplastic syndromes (MDS)

MDS are a group of clonal hematologic disorders manifested by peripheral cytopenias and a high risk of transformation to AML. The International Prognostic Score (IPPS) defines low-, intermediate-, and high-risk groups based on marrow blast percentage, cytopenias, and karyotype.[122] The median survival of patients with low-risk IPPS scores is 5.7 years, but it is only 0.4 years for high-risk patients.

Allogeneic transplantation is a potentially curative treatment for MDS;[123,124] however, the timing of transplantation is controversial. Patients with high-risk disease, excess blasts, severe neutropenia, transfusion dependency, and high-risk cytogenetic abnormalities are considered candidates. Stable patients with low-risk disease may have extended survival with conservative therapy and should generally not be offered transplant until disease progression. The conditioning regimens used are similar to those used for AML, and prospect for long-term remission is equal to or perhaps slightly better than that for AML.

Acute lymphoblastic leukemia (ALL)

Intensive chemotherapy regimens have resulted in cure for 80–90% of children with ALL but only 30–35% of adults.[125] As with AML, poor prognosis adult patients such as those with the t9;22 Philadelphia chromosome and select other genetic markers are generally transplanted in first remission, others only following one or more relapses. The prognosis of patients with chemotherapy-resistant relapse is poor.

The most common preparative regimen used for transplants in ALL includes high-dose cyclophosphamide and TBI with or without other chemotherapeutic agents. TBI-containing regimens may be associated with improved disease-free survival, in comparison to non-TBI-containing regimens.[126] Chemotherapy-only regimens are being actively explored.

Chronic myeloid leukemia (CML)

The use of transplantation to treat CML has declined markedly in the past decade owing to the success of inhibitors of the BCR-ABL tyrosine kinase (TK), such as imatinib, to treat this condition. These oral medications produce multiyear remissions for most patients. Several next generation TK inhibitors can overcome common resistance mechanisms. As a result, transplant is reserved for patients with progressive leukemia after failure of two or more TK inhibitors, patients intolerant of these drugs, or those developing blast crisis, the late acute phase of CML.

Transplant regimens are those commonly used for AML and produce similar and often slightly superior outcomes. Early transplant failures can often be returned to complete remission through the administration of DLI.[127,128] While these infusions risk GVHD, CML is very sensitive to their use. CML was perhaps the earliest example of the use of PCR-based molecular detection (in this case, BCR-ABL) of minimal disease, which enhances the value of DLI immunotherapy administered at that time.

Hematopoietic transplantation has been used for the treatment of other myeloproliferative disorders.[129,130] The appropriate timing of transplantation is less well defined. Most researchers require the patient to be transfusion dependent to justify the risks inherent with hematopoietic transplantation.[131]

Chronic lymphocytic leukemia (CLL)

CLL is an indolent lymphoid malignancy; median survival exceeds 10 years.[132,133] The National Cancer Institute sponsored Working Group recommends use of the "3-risk group" modification of the original five-stage Rai staging system.[134] Median survival is >14, 8 and 4 years for the low-, intermediate-, and high-risk groups. Adverse prognostic factors are loss of immunoglobulin gene rearrangement, expression of CD38, and higher levels of beta2-microglobulin.[135]

Chemotherapy is generally recommended if the disease causes symptoms or impaired performance status.[136] Chemotherapy involving fludarabine, rituximab, cyclophosphamide, and more recently ibrutinib has produced major improvements in disease response and survival for symptomatic patients, but CLL is still considered incurable using standard treatment strategies. Allogeneic transplantation is being increasingly studied.[137,138] Patients with chemosensitive disease have better outcome following transplant. An International Bone Marrow Transplant Registry (IBMTR) analysis showed not only a 3-year survival of 46% but also a high risk for transplant-related mortality.[139] A GVL effect has been shown in this disease[140] and this has led to studies using nonmyeloablative conditioning to reduce toxicity and to extend the use of allogeneic transplantation options to the treatment of patients up to age 75. Encouraging preliminary results have been reported by many groups using this strategy.

The optimal timing of allogeneic transplantation is controversial. Given the risks of allogeneic transplantation and the indolent course of newly diagnosed patients, it is generally recommended that the procedure be considered only after failure of initial therapy. The prognosis is relatively poor if the procedure is delayed until after multiple relapses or after development of refractoriness to chemotherapy.

Non-Hodgkin lymphoma

The non-Hodgkin lymphomas are a heterogeneous group of malignancies with indolent to highly aggressive natural histories. Treatment with both standard and transplant-based therapies depends on the histologic subtype and prognostic factors operative in each patient. Lymphomas can be grouped into major categories: low-, intermediate-, and high grade. The low-grade lymphomas are often associated with t,[14,18] resulting in rearrangement of the BCL2 gene. Low-grade lymphoma patients have a median survival of 7–15 years.[141] The major factors influencing prognosis include stage, lactic dehydrogenase, and beta2-microglobin level.

High-dose chemotherapy with autologous hematopoietic transplantation has been extensively evaluated for low-grade lymphoma, producing rates of complete remission over 80%. Many studies have used marrow or blood stem cell autografts depleted of malignant cells using anti-B-cell monoclonal antibodies, a process which may achieve prolonged remissions.[142,143] Achievement of molecular complete remissions in which BCL2 rearrangement is undetectable by PCR analysis has been associated with prolonged disease-free survival. There is controversy, however, regarding the role of autologous transplantation in this disease. Long-term survival is similar after autologous hematopoietic transplantation and with conservative forms of standard-dose chemotherapy.[144] There is a risk of secondary myelodysplasia and acute leukemia after autotransplants in this disease, particularly in heavily pretreated patients.[145,146] Recent data suggests that a minority of patients treated after failure of initial systemic treatment can achieve multiyear relapse-free survival that may produce outcomes superior to conventional treatment.

Allogeneic bone marrow transplantation has also been evaluated in patients with low-grade lymphoma. High-dose cyclophosphamide and TBI or BEAM, both often combined with rituximab, are the most commonly used preparative regimens. Several groups have reported extended disease-free survival in patients with far advanced disease. Relapse rates after allogeneic transplants have been substantially lower than with transplantation of purged autologous transplants, most likely due to the GVL effect.[147,148] The recent encouraging results using nonmyeloablative preparative regimens reduce the risk of treatment-related mortality and the majority of patients achieve prolonged complete remissions. This option is increasingly being used for younger high-risk patients after failure of initial chemotherapy.[149] Mantle cell lymphoma is associated with a poor prognosis, particularly if the patients have intermediate or high-risk features using the MIPI scale.[150] Autologous hematopoietic transplants can be effective in chemoresponsive patients in first remission. Following relapse, however, most patients are currently treated with allogeneic transplants using reduced intensity conditioning regimens. Like CLL and low-grade lymphomas, a substantial GVL effect enhancing responses is seen.

Intermediate- and high-grade lymphomas are aggressive malignancies with a short natural history in the absence of effective therapy. These disorders are responsive to combination chemotherapy, and a fraction of patients achieve durable remissions. Standard chemotherapy for large cell lymphoma results in cure in approximately 40–60% for newly diagnosed patients with diffuse large cell lymphoma. High-, intermediate- and low-risk groups have been defined.

High-dose chemotherapy and autologous transplantation improve cure rates for patients with recurrent large cell lymphoma who respond to salvage chemotherapy.[151,152] The Parma study randomized patients younger than 60 years with chemosensitive relapse to further conventional chemotherapy or autologous transplantation and demonstrated substantial benefit for the latter.[153] Patients with chemotherapy-resistant disease and those with multiple relapses have poor results but can be considered for novel preparative regimens with autologous transplant or allogeneic transplantation using myeloablative regimens.

High-dose therapy with allogeneic transplantation has been examined in a number of studies in patients with intermediate or high-grade lymphoma. Several studies reported a decreased recurrence rate compared to autologous transplants, but the benefit is off-set by higher rates of treatment-related mortality.[154] Many physicians have reserved allotransplantation for patients having a poor prognosis with alternative modalities, such as a relatively poor response to chemotherapy or patients in which autologous transplants were not feasible.

Hodgkin's disease

Patients failing to achieve a complete remission with initial chemotherapy can be salvaged with autologous transplantation in approximately one-third of cases. For patients with recurrent Hodgkin's disease, particularly with shorter relapse-free intervals, high-dose chemotherapy and autologous hematopoietic transplantation results in a complete remission rate of 50–80% and a 40–60% disease-free survival at 3–5 years posttransplant.[155,156] The BEAM and cyclophosphamide, carmustine, etoposide preparative regimens have been most frequently used. Numerous phase 2 studies have suggested that high-dose chemotherapy improves disease-free survival and possibly overall survival compared to standard chemotherapy in this setting.

Allogeneic transplants using nonmyeloablative techniques have been primarily reserved for patients progressing after autotransplantation or patients with inadequate marrow reserve.[157]

Multiple myeloma

Standard chemotherapy for myeloma can control the disease for variable periods, but even with newer regimens containing lenalidomide and/or proteasome inhibitors, only 20–30% achieve complete remission. Increasing numbers of randomized and historically controlled trials suggest that the addition of autologous transplantation to standard chemotherapy improves disease-free and overall survival. High-dose chemotherapy with autologous hematopoietic transplantation is now considered a standard treatment for patients with intermediate or high-tumor-mass MM. High-dose therapy and autologous transplantation delays relapse but is not curative, and almost all patients ultimately develop recurrent disease.

Chemosensitivity of the tumor is a major determinant of transplant outcome. Patients with chemosensitive disease who received transplants within the first year had a more favorable outcome, and 40–50% may achieve CR. Encouraging results have also been achieved in patients with primary refractory disease if transplanted early in the course of disease,[158,159] but treatment is of only limited value in advanced resistant disease, and especially in patients with refractory relapse.[160] High beta2-microglobulin level and several cytogenetic abnormalities are the most prominent adverse prognostic factors.[161,162] Autologous transplants for myeloma commonly use single-agent melphalan and produce a toxic mortality risk of only 1–2% even in elderly patients. The use of two sequential (or tandem) transplants may produce superior overall and relapse-free survival and are frequently employed.[163] Most studies

have suggested a better outcome when autologous hematopoietic transplantation is performed early after achievement of a myeloma response. A randomized French study of early versus late transplant did not show any survival difference, but patients randomized to early transplant enjoyed longer periods of time without need for chemotherapy.[164]

Allogeneic transplants can cure myeloma in 30–40% of patients but are accompanied by high rates of regimen-related toxicity and infection. Reduced-intensity conditioning and exploitation of GVM effects have increased the effectiveness of allotransplant but its use after failure of autotransplant remains investigational. Other plasma cell dyscrasias have also been effectively treated with high-dose melphalan and autologous hematopoietic transplantation. Amyloidosis may benefit, as suggested by the majority of recent studies. Treatment-related fatality rates are considerably higher than for myeloma, however, often as high as 8–12%.

Solid tumors

High-dose chemotherapy with autologous hematopoietic transplantation has been studied in both breast and ovarian cancer, but results are conflicting and this technique is not currently a part of routine treatment of these diseases.

A similar approach with autologous transplantation has been used for the treatment of other chemotherapy-responsive solid tumors in adults, including testicular or mediastinal germ cell tumors. Recent data suggests improved relapse-free survival for relapsed and refractory patients.[165]

Autologous transplants have been studied in a range of pediatric solid tumors such as neuroblastoma and Ewing sarcoma; tumors that are highly sensitive to chemotherapy and irradiation yet have a poor prognosis in patients with advanced disease.[166,167]

Aplastic anemia

Severe aplastic anemia (AA) is defined as marrow cellularity of less than 25%, with either neutrophil count $<0.5 \times 10^9$/L, platelet count $<20 \times 10^9$/L, or total reticulocyte count $<40 \times 10^9$/L. Without effective therapy, more than 50% of patients with severe AA may die within 6 months of diagnosis. Effective treatments for AA include immunosuppressive therapy (such as cyclosporine and ATG)[168] and hematopoietic transplantation.

Allotransplant can provide effective treatment for patients unresponsive to immunosuppressive agents. Multiple blood transfusions may sensitize the recipient against the donor and increase the risk of rejection. With current regimens, early transplant, a judicious transfusion policy, and improved supportive care systems, less than 10% reject the grafts and long-term survival can be achieved in 80–90% of recipients of marrow from an HLA-matched sibling donor. Allotransplant from unrelated or mismatched donors is being actively studied but carries a higher risk of transplant complications.

Congenital metabolic and immune disorders

Allogeneic transplantation is a potentially curative treatment for several congenital disorders of the hematopoietic and immune systems. Thalassemia[169] and sickle cell anemia[170] are among the most common nonmalignant hematological disorders curable with transplant. Fanconi anemia has been treated similarly to AA but with very low-dose conditioning regimen owing to the known sensitivity of these patients to the effects of irradiation and alkylating agents.[171,172] Allogeneic transplantation has been the treatment of choice for infants with severe combined immunodeficiency.[173] Engraftment can be achieved in many patients even without conditioning in this disorder. Allogeneic transplantation has been able to reverse the bone sclerosis in osteopetrosis.[174] The results in lipid storage diseases have been inconsistent.[175] For patients without a matched sibling, both unrelated donor transplants or mismatched-related transplants have been successful.[176] In most disorders, outcome was better when transplants were given early. In the future, gene modification of autologous cells may be a curative approach for some of these disorders.[177]

There has been increasing interest over the last few years in autologous transplantation with or without T-cell depletion of the graft for the treatment of autoimmune disorders.[178] The goal is to ablate the abnormal immune response and reconstitute immunity from hematopoietic stem cells and progenitors. Encouraging results have been reported in a limited number of patients with rheumatoid arthritis, systemic lupus erythematosus, multiple sclerosis, myasthenia gravis, and other disorders.

Future directions

Over the last decade, hematopoietic transplantation has become a much safer procedure, applicable to a larger patient population in a variety of disease processes. The use of hematopoietic transplantation is likely to evolve with the development of molecularly directed anticancer therapies and with improved methods to selectively target and modulate immunity. Targeted radiation therapies, such as monoclonal antibody–radionuclide immunoconjugates and bone-seeking isotopes, are under active evaluation as a means to target radiotherapy to the tumor; this approach has little systemic toxicity other than myelosuppression. It may be possible to further improve results by using strategies to overcome drug resistance mechanisms such as administration of inhibitors of DNA repair processes, glutathione conjugation, or other mechanisms. Near-term improvements in autotransplantation will emphasize incorporation of newer therapeutics, particularly targeted agents, and supplementary immune augmentation techniques.

The GVM effect associated with allogeneic transplants illustrates the capability of the immune system in eradicating cancer. Strategies to enhance immune antitumor mechanisms with both allogeneic and autologous transplants are under active investigation. The major goal is to separate the beneficial GVM effect from GVHD. Tumor vaccines have been generated by *ex vivo* transfection of tumors with genes (to improve antigen presentation), costimulatory molecules, and various cytokines to enhance the immune response directed against the tumor. Selected lymphocyte subfractions (NK cells, regulatory T cells, and cells engineered to express chimeric antigen receptors to facilitate engagement of tumor cells by cytotoxic T cells) are being actively studied to improve antitumor effects while reducing the risk of GVHD. In the allogeneic transplant setting, efforts are being directed at expanding the donor pool and reducing the toxicity of the procedure. The majority of patients who are candidates for allogeneic transplant do not have an HLA-matched sibling donor. Further development of international unrelated donor registries for bone marrow, blood stem cells, and cord blood will increase the likelihood of finding a well-matched donor. Special attention is given to representation of ethnic minorities in these registries. New molecular methods to improve the precision of histocompatibility matching may decrease the risk of rejection and GVHD. Another approach is to use related partially matched donors. This technique, along with greater availability of banked UCB, will hopefully allow the substantial majority of patients requiring allotransplantation to have access to a suitable donor product. Considerable progress in supportive care has made allogeneic transplants increasingly safe by preventing infections and transplant-related complications. The finding that GVL is responsible for much of the therapeutic potential of allogeneic

transplants has opened the way for the use of nonmyeloablative regimens as a means to allow engraftment of donor cells with reduced toxicity. Providing GVL as the primary treatment requires carefully planned prospective clinical trials to define the role of this strategy, the diseases, and the patient population for which it will be useful.

Key references

The complete reference list can be found on the Wiley Companion Digital Edition of this title (see inside front cover for login instructions).

1 Thomas ED, Storb R, Clift RA, et al. Bone-marrow transplantation (second of two parts). *N Engl J Med.* 1975;**292**:895–902.
2 Thomas ED, Buckner CD, Banaji M, et al. One hundred patients with acute leukemia treated by chemotherapy, total body irradiation, and allogeneic marrow transplantation. *Blood.* 1977;**49**:511–533.
4 Anderson DJ, Gage FH, Weissman IL, et al. Can stem cells cross lineage boundaries? *Nat Med.* 2001;**7**:393–395.
11 Korbling M, Katz RL, Khanna A, et al. Hepatocytes and epithelial cells of donor origin in recipients of peripheral blood stem cells. *N Engl J Med.* 2002;**346**:738–746.
13 de Lima M, Couriel D, Thall PF, et al. Once-daily intravenous busulfan and fludarabine: clinical and pharmacokinetic results of a myeloablative, reduced-toxicity conditioning regimen for allogeneic stem cell transplantation in AML and MDS. *Blood.* 2004;**104**:857–864.
17 Thomas ED. Karnofsky Memorial Lecture. Marrow transplantation for malignant diseases. *J Clin Oncol.* 1983;**1**:517–531.
18 Frei E 3rd, Holden SA, Gonin R, et al. Antitumor alkylating agents: in vitro cross-resistance and collateral sensitivity studies. *Cancer Chemother Pharmacol.* 1993;**33**:113–122.
24 Brenner MK, Rill DR, Moen RC, et al. Gene marking to trace origin of relapse after autologous bone marrow transplantation. *Lancet.* 1993:34185–34186.
25 Ferrara JL, Deeg HJ. Graft-versus-host disease. *N Engl J Med.* 1991;**324**:667–674.
31 Attal M, Harousseau J-L, Stoppa A-M, et al. A prospective, randomized trial of autologous bone marrow transplantation and chemotherapy in multiple myeloma. *N Engl J Med.* 1996;**335**:91–97.
37 Champlin R, Khouri I, Shimoni A, et al. Harnessing graft-versus-malignancy: non-myeloablative preparative regimens for allogeneic hematopoietic transplantation, an evolving strategy for adoptive immunotherapy. *Br J Hematol.* 2000;**111**:18–29.
39 Sullivan KM, Weiden PL, Storb R, et al. Influence of acute and chronic graft-versus-host disease on relapse and survival after bone marrow transplantation from HLA-identical siblings as treatment of acute and chronic leukemia. *Blood.* 1989;**73**:1720–1728.
41 Kolb HJ, Schattenberg A, Goldman JM, et al. Graft-versus leukemia effect of donor lymphocyte transfusions in marrow grafted patients. European Group for Blood and Marrow Transplantation Working Party Chronic Leukemia. *Blood.* 1995;**86**:2041–2050.
48 Hansen JA, Choo SY, Geraghty DE, et al. The HLA system in clinical marrow transplantation. *Hematol Oncol Clin N Am.* 1990;**4**:507–515.
49 Kernan NA, Bartsch G, Ash RC, et al. Analysis of 462 transplantations from unrelated donors facilitated by the National Marrow Donor Program. *N Engl J Med.* 1993;**328**:593–602.
52 Bayraktar UD, Champlin RE, Ciurea SO, et al. Progress in haploidentical stem cell transplantation. *Biol Blood Marrow Transplant.* 2012;**18**:372–380.
54 Rocha V, Labopin M, Sanz G, Arcese W, et al. Transplants of umbilical cord blood or bone marrow from unrelated donors in adults with acute leukemia. *N Engl J Med.* 2004;**35**:2276–2285.
62 Armitage JO. Myelodysplasia and acute leukemia after autologous bone marrow transplantation. *J Clin Oncol.* 2000;**18**:945–946.
64 Martelli M, Vignetti M, Zinzani PL, et al. High-dose chemotherapy followed by autologous bone marrow transplantation versus dexamethasone, cisplatin, and cytarabine in aggressive non-Hodgkin's lymphoma with partial response to front-line chemotherapy: a prospective randomized italian multicenter study. *J Clin Oncol.* 1996;**14**:534–542.
67 Clift RA, Buckner CD. Marrow transplantation for acute myeloid leukemia. *Cancer Invest.* 1998;**16**:53–61.
71 Giralt S, Estey E, Albitar M, et al. Engraftment of allogeneic hematopoietic progenitor cells with purine analog-containing chemotherapy: harnessing graft-versus-leukemia without myeloablative therapy. *Blood.* 1997;**89**:4531–4536.
83 Ferrara JL, Deeg HJ. Graft-versus-host disease. *N Engl J Med.* 1991;**324**:667–674.
90 Przepiorka D, Ippoliti C, Khouri I, et al. Tacrolimus and minidose methotrexate for prevention of acute graft-versus-host disease after matched unrelated donor marrow transplantation. *Blood.* 1996;**88**:4383–4389.

92 Bolaños-Meade J, Fuchs EJ, Luznik L, et al. HLA-haploidentical bone marrow transplantation with post-transplant cyclophosphamide expands the donor pool for patients with sickle cell disease. *Blood* 2012;**120**:4285–4291.

93 Sullivan KM, Agura E, Anasetti C, et al. Chronic graft-versus-host disease and other late complications of bone marrow transplantation. *Semin Hematol.* 1991;**28**:250–259.

101 Shulman HM, Hinterberger W. Hepatic veno-occlusive disease—liver toxicity syndrome after bone marrow transplantation. *Bone Marrow Transplant.* 1992;**10**:197–214.

105 Gottdiener JS, Appelbaum FR, Ferrans VJ, et al. Cardiotoxicity associated with high-dose cyclophosphamide therapy. *Arch Intern Med.* 1981;**141**:758–763.

112 Heslop HE, Slobod KS, Pule MA, et al. Long-term outcome of EBV-specific T-cell infusions to prevent or treat EBV-related lymphoproliferative disease in transplant recipients. *Blood.* 2010;**115**:925–935.

117 Appelbaum FR, Fisher LD, Thomas ED. Chemotherapy v marrow transplantation for adults with acute nonlymphocytic leukemia: a five-year follow-up. *Blood.* 1988;**72**:179–184.

129 Anderson JE, Sale G, Appelbaum FR, et al. Allogeneic marrow transplantation for primary myelofibrosis and myelofibrosis secondary to polycythaemia vera or essential thrombocytosis. *Br J Haematol.* 1997;**98**:1010–1016.

138 Khouri IF, Keating MJ, Vriesendorp HM, et al. Autologous and allogeneic bone marrow transplantation for chronic lymphocytic leukemia: preliminary results. *J Clin Oncol.* 1994;**12**:748–758.

154 Chopra R, Goldstone AH, Pearce R, et al. Autologous versus allogeneic bone marrow transplantation for non-Hodgkin's lymphoma: a case-controlled analysis of the European Bone Marrow Transplant Group Registry data. *J Clin Oncol* 1992;**10**:1690–1695.

159 Alexanian R, Dimopoulos MA, Hester J, et al. Early myeloablative therapy for multiple myeloma. *Blood.* 1994;**84**:4278–4282.

163 Moreau P, Hullin C, Garban F, et al. Tandem autologous stem cell transplantation in high-risk de novo multiple myeloma: final results of the prospective and randomized IFM 99–04 protocol. *Blood.* 2006;**107**:397–403.

165 Nieto Y. Transplantation for refractory germ cell tumors: does it really make a difference? *Curr Oncol Rep.* 2013;**15**:232–238.

167 Fraser CJ, Weigel BJ, Perentesis JP, et al. Autologous stem cell transplantation for high-risk Ewing's sarcoma and other pediatric solid tumors. *Bone Marrow Transplant.* 2006;**37**:175–181.

168 Bacigalupo A, Bruno B, Saracco P, et al. Antilymphocyte globulin, cyclosporine, prednisolone, and granulocyte colony-stimulating factor for severe aplastic anemia: an update of the GITMO/EBMT study on 100 patients. European Group for Blood and Marrow Transplantation (EBMT) Working Party on Severe Aplastic Anemia and the Gruppo Italiano Trapianti di Midolio Osseo (GITMO). *Blood.* 2000;**95**:1931–1934.

170 Walters MC, Storb R, Patience M, et al. Impact of bone marrow transplantation for symptomatic sickle cell disease: an interim report. Multicenter investigation of bone marrow transplantation for sickle cell disease. *Blood.* 2000;**95**:1918–1924.

176 Filipovich AH, Shapiro RS, Ramsay NK, et al. Unrelated donor bone marrow transplantation for correction of lethal congenital immunodeficiencies. *Blood* 1992;**80**:270–276.

178 van Bekkum DW. Autologous stem cell therapy for treatment of severe inflammatory autoimmune diseases. *Neth J Med.* 1998;**53**:130–133.

Special Populations

PART 10

Special Populations

71 Principles of pediatric oncology

Teena Bhatla, MD ▪ William L. Carroll, MD

Overview

Pediatric malignancies differ from those that occur in adults in their relative incidence, pathological type, clinical presentation, and prognosis. The last several decades of the twentieth century have been a period of enormous accomplishment in the field of pediatric cancer research and outcomes have steadily improved largely due to results from large well-controlled clinical trials conducted by various cooperative groups at the national and international level. This chapter seeks to provide a broad overview of pediatric oncology, outlining the several common cancer types that are unique to the pediatric age group.

Introduction and epidemiology

Cancer is a relatively rare disease in childhood, yet cancer remains the second leading cause of death in children after accidents. The spectrum of cancer types in children is distinctly different compared to adults. Although epithelial tumors (carcinomas) dominate the adult cancer spectrum, childhood cancers tend to be of hematopoietic (e.g., leukemias, lymphomas), mesenchymal (sarcomas), and neuroectodermal (e.g., neuroblastomas (NBs), gliomas, medulloblastomas) origin. Acute lymphoblastic leukemia (ALL) and brain tumors are the most common childhood cancers accounting for 25% and 20%, respectively, of all cases. The incidence of the most common childhood tumors is illustrated in Figure 1 and Table 1, but it should be noted that incidence can vary according to ethnic and geographic factors. For example, Burkitt lymphoma accounts for 50% of all childhood cancer in equatorial Africa.

There is a suggestion that the incidence of cancer is rising particularly among certain subtypes of childhood tumors, but better reporting of cases and improved diagnostic imaging may account for some of this trend.[1] The etiologies of most childhood cancers remain uncertain. Environmental influences are less likely to play a role in children with radiation being the most well-established risk factor. Breakthroughs in next-generation sequencing technologies also indicate that childhood tumors have a much lower mutational burden compared to malignancies of adults, and this would also suggest that the environment plays a less important role in tumor initiation.[2]

Genetic predisposition causes about 5% of all cancers in the pediatric age group although this figure may increase with recent results from next-generation sequencing revealing unrecognized mutations in cancer predisposition genes. About a third of all cases of retinoblastoma (RB) are caused by a germline mutation in *RB*1 and children with Down syndrome (DS) have 20-fold increased incidence of leukemia (lymphoid and myeloid). Other hereditary syndromes, such as neurofibromatosis 1 (brain tumors),

Beckwith–Wiedemann [Wilm's tumor (WT), hepatoblastoma (HB), rhabdomyosarcoma (RMS)], Li–Fraumeni (sarcomas, carcinomas), Gorlin's (medulloblastoma, skin cancer), and ataxia telangiectasia (leukemia, lymphoma), account for a small, but important fraction of childhood cancers. Often these familial syndromes paved the way for identification of genes that play a role in the much more common sporadic forms of the disease.

In addition, more subtle "host" genetic variation (compared to the syndromes described above) has been suggested by the identification of genetic variations (single nucleotide polymorphisms or "SNPs") that account for an increased risk of cancer and may impact on outcome and side effects of therapy. For example, germline SNPs in *ARID5B, IKZF1, CEBPE, PIP4K2A,* and *CDKN2A-CDKN2B* influence susceptibility to ALL and *GATA3* variants are associated with a particular subtype of ALL called "Ph-like" ALL (see below).[3]

The dramatic improvement in outcome for childhood cancer represents one of the greatest success stories in the history of the "War on Cancer" that began in earnest in 1971. At that time, roughly 60% of all children less than 20 years of age survived 5 years from diagnosis, whereas today, the figure is more than 80% (Figure 2 and Table 2). There are many reasons for these advances including the commitment to multidisciplinary care and highly disciplined clinical trials directed by nation and worldwide consortiums such as the Children's Oncology Group (COG). Interestingly, many of the same chemotherapeutic agents developed decades ago are still used today, but augmentation of doses and schedules have been realized through advances in supportive care and treatment intensification has improved outcome for almost all tumors. Lastly, risk-adapted therapy, tailoring treatment based on prognostically relevant clinical and laboratory variables, has allowed intensification of treatment for those patients most likely to benefit while avoiding more toxic therapy for those patients predicted to have an excellent outcome with standard treatment. Survival rates have been most dramatic for ALL (10% in the 1960s to greater than 90% today), the most common malignancy, but survival rates remain low for patients with certain brain tumors, metastatic solid tumors, and relapsed disease. Moreover, while mortality has decreased by approximately 50%, close to 2000 children die each year in the United States.[4] Thus, more effective treatments are urgently needed, and the cost of cure is substantial with short and long side effects, so more targeted, less toxic treatments are a priority also.

Childhood acute lymphoblastic leukemia (ALL)

ALL is the most common malignancy in children in the United States. The peak incidence is between 2 and 6 years of age, and there is a slight male predominance. Stepwise gains in outcome in childhood ALL equal or surpass gains in other areas of childhood cancer have come through the results of large international cooperative

Holland-Frei Cancer Medicine, Ninth Edition. Edited by Robert C. Bast Jr., Carlo M. Croce, William N. Hait, Waun Ki Hong, Donald W. Kufe, Martine Piccart-Gebhart, Raphael E. Pollock, Ralph R. Weichselbaum, Hongyang Wang, and James F. Holland.
© 2017 John Wiley & Sons, Inc. ISBN: 978-1-118-93469-2

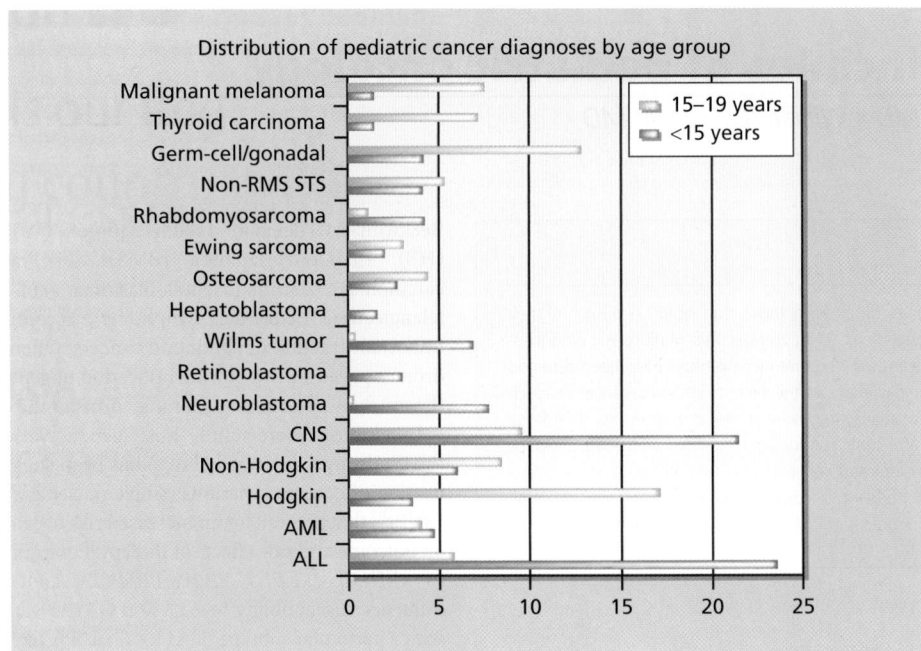

Figure 1 Distribution of pediatric cancer diagnoses by age group. *Abbreviations*: ALL, acute lymphoblastic leukemia; AML, acute myelogenous leukemia; CNS, central nervous system; RMS, rhabdomyosarcoma; STS, soft tissue sarcoma.

Table 1 Age-adjusted and age-specific SEER annual incidence rates per million population for childhood cancer, 2007–2011.

Cancer type (ICCC group)	Age at diagnosis						
	0–14	0–19	<1	1–4	5–9	10–14	15–19
All groups combined (including benign CNS tumors)	172.8	191.2	253.4	228.1	137.2	150.9	246.2
All leukemia	54.4	49.4	51.7	95.0	44.5	33.9	34.5
Acute lymphoblastic leukemia (ALL)	41.9	35.9	20.3	79.7	37.1	22.1	18.2
Acute myeloid leukemia (AML)	8.0	8.5	18.9	10.6	4.5	7.4	9.9
All CNS	44.3	45.1	48.8	49.4	43.1	40.6	47.8
Ependymoma and choroid plexus tumors	4.0	3.7	8.8	6.9	2.6	2.4	2.8
Astrocytoma	16.7	15.6	15.5	18.7	17.1	15.2	12.2
Embryonal tumors	7.6	6.4	12.5	11.3	7.4	4.1	2.7
Hodgkin lymphoma	5.9	12.4	—	1.1	5.0	11.6	31.8
NHL (excluding Burkitt lymphoma)	6.8	8.6	—	4.5	6.9	9.5	14.1
Burkitt lymphoma	2.6	2.6	—	1.7	3.4	3.0	2.4
Neuroblastoma and ganglioneuro blastoma	10.6	8.1	51.0	20.9	4.3	1.2	0.9
Retinoblastoma	4.2	3.1	27.7	8.7	—	—	—
Wilms' tumor and other nonepithelial renal tumor	8.4	6.8	15.3	19.8	5.8	1.1	1.9
Hepatoblastoma	2.9	2.5	10.1	6.4	0.8	0.9	1.5
Osteosarcoma	4.2	5.1	—	—	3.3	8.5	7.7
Ewing sarcoma	2.5	2.8	—	1.1	2.2	4.3	3.5
Soft tissue sarcomas	11.2	12.4	19.6	11.0	8.8	12.2	15.6
Rhabdomyosarcoma and embryonal sarcoma	5.4	4.9	5.8	7.7	4.9	4.1	3.5
Germ cell tumors	6.0	12.2	18.9	4.0	3.2	7.8	30.7
Carcinomas	6.8	17.6	—	1.8	4.0	14.3	49.7
Adrenocortical carcinoma	0.3	0.2	—	—	—	—	—
Thyroid carcinoma	2.8	8.3	—	—	1.3	6.8	24.6
Nasopharyngeal carcinoma	0.3	0.6	—	—	—	0.8	1.4
Malignant melanoma	1.8	4.3	—	0.9	1.3	3.1	11.7

groups. Refined risk-adapted approaches for therapy allocation and dose/schedule intensification of therapy have been primarily responsible for improving the overall survival rate to more than 90%.[6]

Although the exact etiology of childhood ALL is unclear, genetic factors play a significant role in the etiology of childhood ALL in selected cases. Various constitutional chromosomal abnormalities have been associated with pediatric ALL, such as DS, Bloom's syndrome, Fanconi anemia, and ataxia telangiectasia. Of these,

DS-ALL deserves special attention. Children with DS have 10–20 times higher risk of developing leukemia compared to children without DS. These children have unique clinical and biological characteristics that affect their treatment and outcome. Notably, T-cell and mature B-cell immunophenotype, and favorable cytogenetic features such as hyperdiploidy and the *ETV6-RUNX1* translocation are not as common in this group of patients. Novel somatic alterations such as JAK2-activating mutations are found in about 20% of DS-ALL, while CRLF2 alterations (*P2RY8-CRLF2* fusion) has been

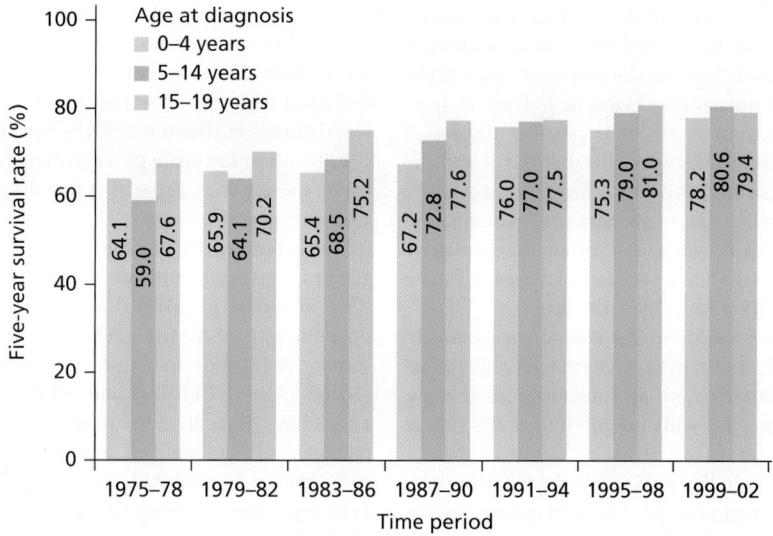

Figure 2 Five-year survival rates for all cancers by age group and period of diagnosis from 1975–2002. Source: Smith et al. 2010.[5] Reprinted with permission. © 2010 American Society of Clinical Oncology. All rights reserved.

Table 2 Five-year relative survival rates (percent) (SEER.cancer.gov/csr/1975_2011).

Site (ages 0–14)	1975–1977	1978–1980	1981–1983	1984–1986	1987–1989	1990–1992	1993–1995	1996–2002	2004–2010
All sites	58	62.6	66.7	68.2	71.4	75.4	77.0	79.4	83.1
Bone and joint	51.3	48.7	56.8	59.4	66.8	66.8	73.9	71.6	78.9
Brain and CNS	56.9	57.7	56.0	61.8	63.8	64.0	70.1	74.1	74.1
Hodgkin lymphoma	80.3	87.7	87.7	90.8	87.1	96.7	94.6	95.3	97.6
ALL	57.6	66.4	71.3	72.5	77.7	83.0	83.8	87.0	91.8
AML	18.8	25.8	26.7	30.0	36.2	41.0	41.0	53.1	66.3
Neuroblastoma	52.4	56.9	54.5	52.0	61.9	76.6	67.2	68.7	76.6
NHL	42.6	52.7	66.9	70.3	70.7	75.9	80.6	86.0	85.6
Soft tissue	61.0	74.3	69.2	73.4	65.4	79.2	76.4	71.7	81.3
Wilms tumor	73.1	78.6	86.4	90.7	92.2	91.9	91.4	92.1	91.7

Site (ages 0–19)	1975–1977	1978–1980	1981–1983	1984–1986	1987–1989	1990–1992	1993–1995	1996–2002	2004–2010
All sites	61.5	65.2	68.0	70.6	73.3	76.0	77.4	79.5	83.5
Bone and joint	51.1	48.4	51.2	57.2	63.5	68.2	68.6	68.0	75.5
Brain and CNS	58.7	58.1	57.6	64.0	65.9	66.1	71.0	75.1	74.0
Hodgkin lymphoma	86.0	88.7	85.4	90.8	88.9	94.2	93.9	95.1	97.3
ALL	54.1	62.4	67.1	70.1	75.0	79.7	81.3	83.5	90.0
AML	18.7	26.2	26.4	31.7	36.9	41.0	39.4	48.4	65.1
Neuroblastoma	52.7	57.0	53.4	52.0	60.5	76.3	67.0	69.0	76.3
NHL	43.4	53.9	63.5	68.1	70.3	72.1	77.8	81.9	83.9
Soft tissue	65.2	68.8	68.2	72.4	67.2	68.9	73.8	70.9	78.1
Wilms tumor	72.6	78.0	86.5	91.0	92.2	91.3	91.5	92.1	91.5

observed in about 50% of DS-ALL cases.[7,8] DS-ALL children are more prone to methotrexate-related toxicities, with more frequent mucositis and infectious complications. In general, prognosis of DS-ALL is worse than non-DS ALL, however, enhanced supportive measures have improved the outcome. More recently, genome-wide association studies (GWAS) have identified inherited genetic variation at the *GATA3* locus being associated with ALL in adolescents and young adults (AYAs) population.[9]

Children with ALL usually presents with signs and symptoms suggestive of bone marrow infiltration, manifesting as fever (60%), bleeding symptoms (50%), and bone pain (30%). Child may present with a limp or refusal to walk. Lymphadenopathy and hepatosplenomegaly are present in about half to two-thirds of cases and is usually asymptomatic. Rarely, patients may present with symptoms suggestive of extramedullary spread, such as CNS involvement, testicular enlargement, and ocular changes. The

diagnosis is typically made by bone marrow aspiration and/or biopsy. Multiple cell surface antigen markers, cytogenetic, and less commonly histochemical staining abnormalities in the leukemic cells are used to establish the diagnosis of ALL subtype and result in specific therapeutic decisions.[10] About 85% of cases of childhood ALL express membrane markers consistent with B-precursor lineage, and about 15% express T-lineage markers. Although age and initial white blood cell (WBC) count at the time of disease presentation remain important predictors of outcome, other factors such as blast immunophenotype and cytogenetics, CNS involvement, and early response to chemotherapy are currently being utilized for risk stratification. Cytological confirmation of leukemic cells in cerebrospinal fluid (CSF) is required for the diagnosis of CNS leukemia. Standard or average risk patients are defined as age between 1 and 9 years with an initial WBC count of less than 50,000/mm³, while age more than 10 years with a presenting WBC of more than 50,000/mm³ are classified into high-risk disease category. Risk assessment is further refined by presence or absence of favorable [e.g., hyperdiploidy (specifically trisomies 4 and 10) or *EVT6/RUNX1* fusion] and unfavorable cytogenetic features (e.g., hypodiploidy or iAMP21), overt CNS and testicular disease at diagnosis, and minimal residual disease (MRD) at day 8 and the end of induction chemotherapy. Philadelphia chromosome positive (ph+) ALL or t(9:22) occurs in 2–3% of pediatric ALL patients, and historically has been associated with a poor prognosis, now have much better outcome with the incorporation of tyrosine kinase inhibitors (TKI) in combination with chemotherapy.

Contemporary therapies include several components, namely, induction, presymptomatic, or prophylactic central nervous system therapy, postinduction intensification, and maintenance therapy. This design of current treatments will cure more than 80–90% of patients overall.[6]

Additional recent advances in therapy include the following:

- Current frontline therapy regimens are tailored to risk category as assessed by clinical features and biologic profile.[10]
- The substitution of dexamethasone for prednisone has improved the survival for standard risk patients, while no event-free survival (EFS) advantage has been noted for patients more than 10 years of age. In addition, there was significantly increased rate of osteonecrosis in patients more than 10 years of age.[11]
- Initial response to therapy determined by day 8 peripheral blood and/or bone marrow assessment of MRD at end induction (day 29) is an important predictor of outcome and is now utilized in risk-adjusted treatment approaches.[12]
- Postinduction intensification (or delayed intensification) improves outcome for both high and standard risk, B-precursor and T-lineage patients particularly when augmented regimens were utilized.[13] However, there was no additional benefit of second delayed intensification.[13]
- Improved outcome associated with specific cytogenetic aberrations including hyperdiploidy, trisomy 4, 10, and t(12;21) (ETV6-RUNX1) and these patients are now classified as having low-risk disease, and receive less intensive chemotherapy if MRD is negative at day 8 and at day 29.[14]
- High-dose methotrexate given during interim maintenance improves outcome in high-risk patients.[15]
- Current systemic therapy allows elimination of cranial irradiation for almost all patients except those who have overt CNS disease at diagnosis.[16]
- Review of comparative outcome results of AYAs treated with pediatric or adult protocol-based therapy has shown improved outcomes for those treated utilizing the pediatric approach. However, treatment mortality comprises a larger percentage of adverse events than in younger children.[17,18]
- Ph+ pediatric ALL can be treated with aggressive chemotherapy and concomitant targeted therapy with tyrosine kinase inhibitor—imatinib or dasatinib—leading to remarkable improvement in EFS without the need for stem cell transplantation.[19]
- Hematopoietic stem cell transplantation (HSCT) has a limited role in newly diagnosed ALL, except in refractory settings, those with hypodiploidy and possibly those patients with persistently high MRD at later time points. Early relapsed ALL (bone marrow relapse within 36 months from initial diagnosis or while in therapy) generally undergo HSCT, while late relapsed cases are treated with chemotherapy, and HSCT is considered on individual basis.

In addition to the disease- and treatment-related prognostic variables, recent studies have highlighted the importance of host factors in governing the disease outcome as well. Host factors refer to differences among patients with regard to drug absorption, metabolism, and sensitivity. Considerable heterogeneity has been described with respect to host pharmacology of thiopurines[20] and vincristine.[21] Furthermore, SNPs have been identified to be associated with unfavorable pharmacokinetics of various antileukemic chemotherapeutics, suggesting that drug disposition influences the risk of relapse.[22]

The heterogeneity of childhood ALL is reflected in emerging genomic and epigenomic studies. DNA copy number abnormalities were identified in genes that encode regulators of B-cell development, as *CDKN2A/B*, *PAX5*, *IKZF1*, and *EBF1*.[23] In addition, somatic mutations in *JAK2*, alterations in RAS pathway genes (*NRAS*, *KRAS*, *PTPN11*, and *NF1*) and *CRLF2* genomic alterations have been identified with increased frequency in high-risk patients.[24,25] *JAK1* and *JAK2* mutations have previously been shown to be mutated in DS-ALL and T-cell ALL as well.[8] Furthermore, gene expression profiling has identified a subset of patients whose blasts share a gene expression profile observed in patients with Ph+ ALL but who lack the BCR-ABL1 fusion protein. Such patients are called "Ph-like" ALL.[26] Ph-like ALL is associated with worse outcomes and deletions or mutations of IKZF1 are a characteristic feature of both Ph-positive and Ph-like ALL.[27] This subgroup harbors tyrosine kinase fusions other than BCR-ABL, including *ABL1*, *ABL2*, *CSF1R*, and *PDGFR* fusions, and are candidates for treatment with tyrosine kinase inhibitors,[28] while another subset of these patients harboring *JAK* mutations are candidates for JAK inhibitors.[29] This approach is currently under evaluation in the high-risk ALL trial through COG.

Although significant advances have been made in the outcomes of newly diagnosed ALL over the past four decades, infant ALL and early relapsed ALL are the two subgroups whose outcome remains dismal, and there is an urgent need of innovative strategies for these patients. Because of increased FLT3 (a tyrosine kinase) expression in infant ALL, the incorporation of the FLT3 inhibitor lestaurtinib on the standard intensive chemotherapy backbone in infant leukemia is currently being investigated. Also given the unique biology of infant ALL with the majority of patients having rearrangement of the *MLL* gene on 11q23, the protein DOT1L is recruited to MLL target genes resulting in aberrant expression of genes. DOT1L inhibitors are in clinical trials.

For relapsed ALL, various novel treatment strategies are emerging including molecularly targeted agents and cellular therapies. Recently, bispecific T-cell engager antibodies have gained considerable attention. These proteins have both T-cell specific and B-cell specific regions, thereby directing the patient's own cytotoxic T cells to the malignant tumor cells. Blinatumomab, a bispecific CD19-directed CD3 T-cell engager, has shown single agent activity and safety in children with multiple recurrent and refractory B-ALL, and is currently in clinical trial for children with B-ALL at first relapse through COG. Recent developments in cellular- and immune-based therapy have led to another major leap in the treatment of relapsed and refractory ALL. Chimeric antigen receptors (CARs)-modified T cells are genetically engineered to express antibodies directed against tumor antigens (CD19 for B-ALL) as well as T-cell activation molecules. They have shown great promise for long-term remission and possibly cure for this group of patients with extremely poor prognosis.[30]

Acute myeloid leukemia (AML) in children

AML comprises about 20% of pediatric leukemia and chronic myeloid leukemia is detected in about 1–2%. Similar to ALL, the development of AML has also been associated with various inherited and acquired predisposition syndromes, such as DS, bone marrow failure syndromes such as Fanconi anemia, dyskeratosis congenita, severe congenital neutropenia (Kostmann syndrome), Diamond–Blackfan anemia, as well as acquired aplastic anemia. Patients treated with chemotherapy (particularly alkylating agents and topoisomerase inhibitors) and radiation therapy are at risk of developing therapy-related AML (t-AML). The presentation of AML is similar to that of ALL; occasionally, child may present with violaceous, raised, plaque-like lesions on the skin or gums, called chloromas, which is an extramedullary manifestation of AML. Patients with acute promyelocytic leukemia (APL), a distinct AML subtype, characterized by t(15:17) or *PML-RARA* fusion, often present with severe coagulopathy and frequently have hyperleucocytosis.

Compared to ALL, pediatric AML is less responsive to available chemotherapy. AML survival has recently improved with cure rates approaching up to 60–70% in the pediatric population.[31] This has been achieved by dose intensification, improved supportive measures, results from large clinical trials, and better understanding of the biology and heterogeneity of this disease. Unlike ALL, age and WBC are not considered as independent prognostic variables for stratification. In fact, cytogenetic and molecular characteristics and response to induction chemotherapy are utilized in current treatment schema for risk-adapted therapy.[32,33] Presence of inversion 16, t(8;21) and t(15;17), biallelic *CEBPA* mutations, and *NPM1* mutations are considered as favorable, while monosomy 7, monosomy 5/del(5q), and FLT3-ITD with high allelic ratio are considered unfavorable characteristics. AML therapy consists of remission induction, prophylactic CNS-directed therapy, and postremission therapy. Chemotherapy regimens are intensive requiring prolonged hospitalizations and aggressive supportive measures. After initial 1–2 induction courses and upon achieving morphological remission (less than 5% blasts in marrow), postremission therapy is administered, which may comprise additional intensive chemotherapy or HSCT depending on the cytogenetic risk factors and the depth of response (MRD status) to induction chemotherapy. Prolonged maintenance courses have been shown to be inferior and are not incorporated in current regimens except in APL. APL treatment requires rapid initiation of all-trans retinoic acid (ATRA), a differentiation-inducing agent, with concomitant chemotherapy along with aggressive supportive measures, followed by prolonged maintenance phase consisting of ATRA, 6-mercaptopurine, and methotrexate. This regimen leads to the EFS of 70–80%, without the use of HSCT in first complete remission in APL.[34] Arsenic trioxide has been shown as active agent against APL, and early experience in children with APL has shown encouraging results.

As the more intensive induction regimens have been maximally intensified, new active agents and strategies are needed. Currently, COG is studying in randomized study design the effect incorporating bortezomib, a proteasome inhibitor in FLT3-ITD-negative patients or sorafenib, a multitarget tyrosine kinase inhibitor that targets *FLT3*, *c-KIT*, *PDGF*, *VEGF*, and *MEK/ERK/RAF* pathway, for patients with high allelic ratio FLT3-ITD-positive AML, to the standard chemotherapy backbone for AML. In addition, epigenetic modifiers, such as vorinostat and 5-azacytadine, monoclonal antibodies against myeloid cell surface antigens, and various transplantation conditioning regimen and graft sources are currently being explored to improve the outcomes of pediatric AML.

Non-Hodgkin lymphoma in children (NHL)

Approximately 15% of all childhood cancers diagnosed in the United States are lymphomas. Sixty percent of all childhood lymphomas are classified as NHLs, representing 3% of all childhood malignancies for children younger than 5 years, and 8–9% for children and adolescents 5–19 years of age. In contrast to adults where most NHLs are low or intermediate grade, almost all NHL in children are high grade. There are three major subtypes of childhood NHL: (1) mature B-cell lymphoma predominantly Burkitt's lymphoma (classic and atypical) or diffuse large B-cell lymphoma (DL-BCL), (2) precursor T-cell lymphoma or lymphoblastic lymphoma, and (3) mature T-cell or null cell lymphomas, anaplastic large-cell lymphoma (ALCL). The World Health Organization (WHO) classifies ALCL as a peripheral T-cell lymphoma. The distribution of these histologic subtypes includes approximately 40% Burkitt lymphoma, 30% lymphoblastic lymphoma, 20% diffuse large B cell, and 10% ALCL. Burkitt's lymphoma tumor cells are characterized by a chromosomal translocation juxtaposing the *c-myc* oncogene and immunoglobulin locus regulatory elements t(8;14), rarely t(8;22) or t(2;8). Similarly, more than 90% of pediatric ALCL have a characteristic chromosomal rearrangement involving the *ALK* gene t(2;5).

Presence of bulky disease poses two potentially life-threatening situations that are often the presenting feature in children with NHL. First is the tumor lysis syndrome resulting in major electrolyte imbalances, most notably, hyperuricemia, hyperkalemia, and hyperphosphatemia. Aggressive hydration, allopurinol, or rasburicase (urate oxidase) are used in such situations along with other supportive measures. Second is the presence of large mediastinal masses especially seen in lymphoblastic lymphoma, posing a risk of cardiac or respiratory arrest (superior vena cava syndrome).

The primary modality of treatment of all histologic types and stages of childhood NHL is multiagent chemotherapy. The exact regimen of chemotherapy with or without intrathecal therapy and the intensity and length of treatment are usually dictated by the extent of disease and the histologic subtype. Although Burkitt's lymphoma, DL-BCL, and ALCL are treated with short intensive courses of chemotherapy, lymphoblastic lymphoma is treated based on ALL regimens consisting of long maintenance phase. The role of surgery is critically important in the diagnosis and staging process, but it has a limited role in the overall treatment of childhood NHL. There is minimal to no role of radiation therapy in the overall treatment of childhood NHL.

The prognosis for children and adolescents with NHL, both with limited-stage and advanced-stage disease, has improved significantly over the past two decades. Except for rare subtypes, the chance of being alive and disease free at 5 years for limited-stage and advanced-stage disease B NHL is 95% and 80%, respectively.[35] The prognosis for advanced lymphoblastic NHL in children and adolescents has now increased to over 85% survival.[36] The prognosis, however, for the most advanced childhood and adolescent ALCL is still less than 70% at 7 years of follow-up.[37]

Recently, therapeutic strategies for childhood NHL are incorporating surface, intracellular, and molecular targets in order to not only improve the overall cure rates of advanced-stage disease but to minimize the collateral damage from the chemotherapy agents. Rituximab is a monoclonal antibody targeting the CD20 antigen, expressed by Burkitt's lymphoma and DLBCL in children. The COG has demonstrated safety and tolerability of adding rituximab to the standard chemotherapy backbone in children and adolescents, with a 3-year EFS of 90% in patients with advanced mature B-cell lymphoma (with bone marrow and CNS involvement).[38] Likewise, the promising activity of crizotinib (targeting *ALK*)[39] and brentuximab vedotin (monoclonal anti-CD30 antibody)[40] in relapsed ALCL has now led to a randomized phase 2 trial of adding these agents in combination with chemotherapy in newly diagnosed ALCL.

Hodgkin disease (HD)

HD accounts for approximately 5% of pediatric malignancies in developed countries. Reed–Strenberg (RS) cells (multinucleated giant cells) are the hallmark of HD, which are present in a background of inflammatory cells consisting of eosinophils, small lymphocytes, plasma cells, neutrophils, histiocytes, and fibroblasts. RS cells nearly always express CD30, while CD15 is expressed in approximately 70% of cases. Two broad pathologic categories of HD are classical Hodgkin's lymphoma and nodular lymphocyte predominant. Classical Hodgkin's lymphoma accounts for the majority of cases of childhood HD, while nodular lymphocyte predominant Hodgkin's lymphoma occurs only in 5–10% cases.

The cure rate for pediatric patients with HD is greater than 90%. Standard therapy for pediatric patients with HD includes combination chemotherapy and low-dose involved-field radiotherapy (RT). Clinical research in pediatric HD aims to delineate minimal treatment necessary for cure and eliminate or minimize late sequelae of treatment.

PET scans have been demonstrated to be useful biomarkers of early response and useful in response-based therapy approaches to determine which patients would be eligible for treatment with chemotherapy alone or those that require intensification of therapy. The recently completed COG HD trial demonstrated successful omission of involved field RT without comprising outcome in intermediate-risk patients who show rapid response (PET-CT-negative disease), to two cycles of ABVE-PC (doxorubicin, bleomycin, vincristine, etoposide, prednisone, cyclophosphamide) and a complete response after four cycles.[41] Management of relapsed/refractory HD remains challenging, and currently high-dose chemotherapy followed by autologous HSCT is considered standard of care for most patients. Recently, brentuximab vedotin (CD30-directed antibody drug conjugate) is being used in combination with chemotherapy for relapsed/refractory disease. Study of the biology of the RS cell in an effort to identify new therapeutic targets is also receiving significant attention.

Renal tumors

Wilms tumor

WT accounts for over 90% of renal tumors in children and 6% of childhood cancers in general. Today survival rates for all patients exceeds 90% and even patients presenting with metastatic disease have an event-free survival rate of 80% at 2 years.[42] The typical clinical presentation is that of a well-appearing child who has an abdominal mass noted as an incidental finding. Over 90% of patients have a unilateral tumor with multicentric or bilateral tumors accounting for the remainder of cases. Patients with unilateral tumors present on average at 36.5 months (males) to 42.5 months (girls), while those with bilateral disease present earlier in life (33–35 months) reflecting a genetic predisposition.[43]

Many congenital syndromes are associated with WT and analyses of such cases led to the discovery of tumor suppressor genes involved in the pathogenesis of both inherited and sporadic cases. Children with the WAGR (WT, aniridia, genitourinary abnormalities, and mental retardation) syndrome have a greatly increased risk of WT, and this syndrome is associated with constitutional

(germline) deletions at 11p13. Within the deleted region lies the WT1 gene responsible for the risk of WT (as well as PAX5 responsible for aniridia). Disease pathogenesis follows a classic two-hit model with the tumor having lost both WT1 alleles. Likewise, the Denys–Drash syndrome (pseudohermaphroditism, degenerative renal disease) is associated with constitutional mutations of WT1 and tumors contain mutations in both alleles. Somatic mutations of WT1 are seen in 10–20% of sporadic WT.[44]

A second tumor suppressor gene, WT2, has been mapped to 11p15.5. Abnormalities of this region are associated with another syndrome where the risk of WT is particularly high, the Beckwith–Wiedemann syndrome (macroglossia, omphalocele, visceromegaly, and hemihypertrophy). This region encodes a large number of imprinted genes including insulin-like growth factor 2 (*IGF2*) and *H19*, which encodes a noncoding RNA that acts as a tumor suppressor gene.[45] Somatic loss of heterozygosity (LOH) of WT2 is the most common defect in sporadic WT occurring in up to 80% of cases. Other mutations are seen in WT including *WTX* (32%), *CTNNB1* (encoding β-catenin, 15%), and *T53* (5%).[44]

WT presents typically as a well-circumscribed heterogeneously enhancing mass originating from kidney (Figure 3a). Pathologically, WT typically shows a triphasic pattern composed of blastemal, epithelial, and stromal cell types, although in some cases only one or two of these cell types may be visualized. Anaplasia is characterized by markedly enlarged nuclei, pleomorphism, and polyploidy mitotic features, and these are associated with a poor prognosis. Anaplasia may be focal or diffuse and is seen in 5% of tumors.[46] In the absence of anaplasia, WTs are classified as having "favorable histology." Nephrogenic rests are precursor lesions and represent persistent nephroblastic tissue that has not undergone full differentiation.[47] Patients with nephrogenic rests (30% sporadic and 100% bilateral WTs) may be at risk for the development of a subsequent WT. There are two types of nephrogenic rests based on location: perilobar and intralobar. Most nephrogenic rests undergo gradual resolution.

Therapy for WT involves surgical resection and chemotherapy with radiation reserved for more advanced stages. Worldwide there are two general approaches that lead to equivalent outcomes. In North America (based on practices established by the National Wilms Tumor Study Group (NWTSG) and now COG), most cases are treated by initial surgery (nephrectomy and lymph node sampling) followed by chemotherapy.[42] In Europe (Societe Internationale d'Oncologie Pediatrique or SIOP), neoadjuvant therapy is advocated with delayed surgery. The advantage of the North American approach is that it allows for full, unaltered evaluation of all tumor tissue and accurate staging, while the SIOP approach allows for preoperative tumor shrinkage thereby making resection easier and decreasing the risk of spillage.[48,49]

The usual definitive surgical approach to WT is a radical nephrectomy through a wide abdominal incision. The adrenal gland is removed and regional lymph nodes are sampled. More recently, a flank approach is being used and there is a question whether adrenalectomy is needed.[50] Given the risk of second WTs, a partial nephrectomy or "nephron sparing" surgery is used for patients with bilateral tumors but also this is increasingly being considered for unilateral favorable histology tumors, especially in the neoadjuvant setting where there is assurance of negative margins due to an excellent response to chemotherapy. Finally, laparoscopic-/robotic-assisted resections are being explored by some surgeons.

Treatment of WT includes nephrectomy and stage-dependent chemotherapy with or without radiation to the abdomen and/or lungs. There are subtle differences in staging between the COG and

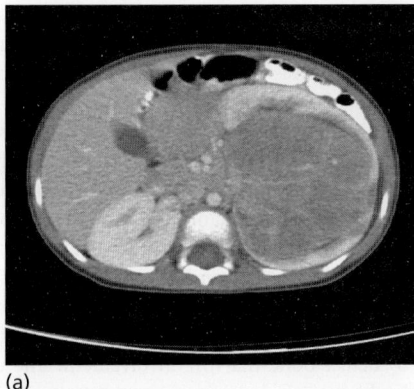
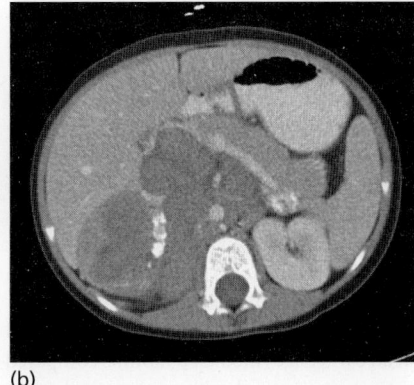

(a)   (b)

Figure 3 Computed tomographic (CT) imaging characteristics of common childhood abdominal tumors. (a) Wilm's tumor: axial contrast-enhanced CT images of the abdomen showing a large well circumscribed heterogeneous left renal mass that does not cross the midline. (b) Neuroblastoma: axial contrast-enhanced CT images of the abdomen demonstrating a large lobulated heterogeneous mass in the right upper quadrant that crosses the midline with characteristic encasement of aorta and displacement of superior mesenteric vein, splenic vein, and pancreas anteriorly. Dense calcifications are present within the mass.

SIOP approaches, but in general, complete resection of tumor with an intact capsule and no extension to the renal sinus is stage I. Stage II tumors are those completely resected, but the tumor extends beyond the capsule or into the renal sinus while incompletely resected tumors or those with lymph node involvement, tumor spillage, and/or positive surgical margins are declared stage III. Stage IV indicates metastatic hematogenous spread (usually lung but also liver, brain, or bone). Preoperative evaluation includes a CT of the abdomen and pelvis and Doppler ultrasound if there is concern about tumor thrombus in the inferior vena cava. Magnetic resonance imaging (MRI) may be useful for following nephrogenic rests and aid in surgical planning for patients with bilateral tumors.

Once removed, the tumors are evaluated pathologically to validate the diagnosis and examine sections for the presence of anaplasia. In addition, certain molecular markers may portend for a worse prognosis such as LOH at 1p and 16q, and these genetic lesions have been uniformly assessed on recent protocols.[42]

Patients less than 2 years with stage I favorable histology tumors weighing less than 550 g may be treated with nephrectomy only as the small minority who relapse can be salvaged with chemotherapy and RT. Patients with stage I and II tumors (without LOH at 1p and 16q) are treated with vincristine and dactinomycin (18 weeks), while stage III patients receive vincristine, dactinomycin, and doxorubicin with abdominal irradiation (24 weeks). Patients with LOH at 1p and 16q are upstaged and require additional therapy. Many different drug combinations have been assessed for favorable histology stage IV patients, but none have seemed to improve outcome over the three drug combination given with abdominal and chest irradiation. Those patients whose metastatic lesions regress early in therapy may not require chest XRT, whereas those patients whose lesions do not regress early require chest irradiation and may benefit from additional chemotherapy. The presence of anaplasia is associated with an inferior prognosis and therapy is modified based on whether the anaplasia is diffuse or focal as well as stage. For example, patients with stage II–IV tumors showing diffuse anaplasia are treated with combination therapy including vincristine, doxorubicin, cyclophosphamide, carboplatin, etoposide although the optimal regimen has yet to be established.

Patients with bilateral tumors and those with unilateral tumors and a congenital predisposition syndrome pose a special challenge as these patients are at risk for subsequent tumors. These patients can be treated with preoperative chemotherapy [vincristine,

dactinomycin (unilateral tumors with predisposition syndrome) ±doxorubicin (bilateral tumors)] and undergo nephron sparing surgery at weeks 6 or 12 depending on optimal response. Such patients usually do not require an initial biopsy given the typical clinical and radiographic presentation. Therapy after resection is guided by stage and histology of the resected specimen.

The outcomes for all stages of favorable histology WT is excellent with 10-year relapse-free survival rates of 91% (stage I), 85% (stage II), 84% (stage III), and 75% (stage IV) while historically patients with anaplastic tumors have a worse outcome (10-year relapse-free survival 43% (stages I–III), 18% (stage IV)). Patients with bilateral tumors have an intermediate 10-year relapse-free outcome of approximately 65% (overall survival 78%).[42]

Other renal tumors

Renal cell carcinomas, clear cell sarcomas of the kidney and malignant rhabdoid tumors constitute 5.9%, 3.5%, and 1.6% of all renal tumors in children. Children with renal cell carcinoma present with abdominal pain, hematuria, and an abdominal mass on examination. Many conditions are associated with renal cell carcinoma including von Hippel–Lindau disease, familial renal cell carcinoma and previous therapy for malignancy. Pediatric renal cell carcinomas differ from adults in that a higher proportion are papillary and not otherwise specified, and the clear cell and chromophobe variants are less common.[51,52] Most tumors in childhood are characterized by translocations involving *transcription factor E3* gene (*TFE3*) located on Xp11.2 with a variety of fusion partners. Children tend to present at a more advanced stage compared to adults. Radical nephrectomy with lymph node dissection remains the primary treatment. Survival rates at 4 years are 92%, 85%, and 73% for stages I, II, and II respectively while outcome for stage IV disease remains dismal (14%).[42,53] Optimal therapy for patients with unresectable or metastatic disease has not been defined but there is great interest in using tyrosine kinase inhibitors (sunitinib and others) in translocation positive renal cell carcinoma.[42]

Clear cell sarcomas are a distinct group of tumors with the histological appearance of nests of cells separated by organized fibrovascular septa. The molecular pathogenesis is unknown for most tumors although a t(10;17)(q22,p13) is noted in a small subgroup of these cases. Clear cell sarcomas can metastasize to bone and brain in addition to lung and liver but most patients present with localized disease. Historically these patients have been classified as unfavorable but incremental improvements have been achieved over successive NWTS trials. Patients treated on a regimen of vincristine, doxorubicin, cyclophosphamide, and etoposide with radiation therapy to the tumor bed had a 5 year EFS of 79%.[42,54]

Malignant rhabdoid tumors present at a younger age compared to WT and symptoms include fever and gross hematuria.[55] The majority of patients have advanced disease and up to 15% have associated CNS lesions. Histologically, the tumor is composed of large cells, prominent nucleoli, and eosinophilic cytoplasmic granules. These tumors are due to biallelic inactivation (mutation and/or deletion) of the *SMARCB1* gene on 22q (also known as *INI1*) which encodes a member of a chromatin remodeling complex.[56] About a third of patients harbor a germline mutation in *SMARCB1* and these children present at an earlier age (median 5 months compared to 18 months). Most patients are treated with surgery, radiation, and multiagent chemotherapy but optimal drug combinations have yet to be identified. Young age, advanced stage and the presence of CNS disease are adverse prognostic factor. Four year relapse-free survival is 50%, 33%, 33%, and 21% for stages I, II, II, and IV respectively.[42]

Congenital mesoblastic nephroma typically occurs in infancy and present as unilateral abdominal tumors. Two patterns exist, classic and cellular. The cellular form of mesoblastic nephroma is characterized by the *ETV6/NTRK3* fusion transcript (t(12;15)(p13;q25) identical to infantile fibrosarcoma.[57] These tumors are treated by complete resection without need for adjuvant therapy since metastasis is quite rare. Overall survival rates are approximately 95%.[58]

Neuroblastoma

NB is the most common extracranial solid tumor of children and accounts for 8–10% of all childhood cancers. This tumor represents transformation of precursor neural crest cells that were destined to form sympathetic ganglia and the adrenal medulla. It is the most common tumor of infancy and the median age of presentation is 18 months.[59] Curiously the disease has a wide clinical and biological spectrum ranging from spontaneous regression of widespread disease in infants to unrelenting, aggressive disease usually in older children. About 2% of cases are familial in nature and 50% of these patients carry germline mutations in the anaplastic lymphoma kinase gene, *ALK,* while a much smaller number of familial cases are due to mutations in *Phox2b* in association with other neurocristopathies like Hirschsprung's disease.[60-62] It is likely that additional steps are required for full transformation since only 50% of germline carriers of *ALK* mutations develop NB.[63] Indeed GWAS have identified a number of predisposition loci yet their contribution to most sporadic cases is likely to be quite modest.[64] *ALK* mutations and amplifications are seen in 8–12% and 2–3% respectively of sporadic cases and *Phox2b* mutations have been detected in 2% of sporadic tumors.[65]

The clinical presentation of NB is dependent on the location of the primary tumor but a majority of patients have symptoms due to widespread disease at initial diagnosis such as fever, weight loss, irritability, bone pain, and cytopenias. Two-thirds of cases are associated with an abdominal primary and the great majority of NBs are located in the adrenal gland (Figure 3b). Children may present with abdominal pain, constipation, and distention. A large abdominal mass that typically crosses the midline is detected on physical examination. Cervical and thoracic tumors (posterior mediastinum) can be associated with Horner syndrome. Presacral and paraspinal tumors may present with cord compression such as urinary retention, motor weakness, and clonus. Finally, NB may present with an unusual paraneoplastic syndrome characterized by opsoclonus myoclonus syndrome (OMS), where children typically manifest darting eye movements and myoclonic jerks with or without ataxia.[66] Interestingly, OMS is often associated with favorable prognosis tumors, but unfortunately, neurological symptoms persist after effective treatment of the NB.

Initial evaluation of NB includes cross-sectional imaging with CT or MRI of the chest, abdomen and pelvis to determine local, regional (including extradural extension), and distant sites of disease. Metaiobenzlguanidine (MIBG) is a norepinephrine analogue selectively taken up by sympathetic nervous tissue and is used to assess disease location not picked up by CT or MRI. Most tumors are MIBG avid but for those that are not avid, FDG-PET may be used. Bilateral bone marrow aspirates and biopsies are required to detect bone marrow involvement. The diagnosis is confirmed by biopsy of the primary or distant site involvement, or characteristic tumor cell in the bone marrow with elevated levels of vanillylmandelic acid (VMA) and homovanillic acid (HVA) in the urine.

Histologically, tumors can display a range of cellular differentiation from ganglioneuroma (differentiated) to ganglioneuroblastoma to typical NB. Typically, the tumor is composed of small round blue cells with rosettes. Histologically, tumors can be classified as favorable or unfavorable based on age, the degree of differentiation (differentiated associated with better prognosis), Schwannian stromal content, and the karyorrhexis index [MKI, the number of mitosis and karyorrhexis (fragmented nuclei) per 5000 cells, less than 100 or 200 MKI (depending on stroma, age, and degree of differentiation) is associated with a better prognosis].[67]

An International Neuroblastoma Staging System (INSS) was developed to harmonize approaches and analyses of outcome worldwide (Table 3).[68] It is noteworthy that children with 4S disease have a high degree of spontaneous regression in spite of widespread disease. More recently, this has been replaced by the International Neuroblastoma Risk Group (INRG) stratification system based on radiographic features that indicate resectability and the presence of widespread metastatic disease: L1 (localized tumors confined to one body compartment), L2 (locoregional tumor with involvement of adjacent structures), M (distant metastasis), and MS (metastatic disease in children <18 months confined to skin, liver, and/or bone marrow).[69]

Treatment stratification is based on a number of clinical and biological variables that allow classification into low-, intermediate-, and high-risk categories. Two of the most important risk factors are age and stage with children less than 18 months of age having a distinctly better prognosis than older children. The overall survival of children with INSS stages 1, 2, 3, and 4S is 91±1% compared to 42±1% for stage IV disease.[70] NB was one of the first human tumors where genetic stratification has had a significant impact. *MYCN* amplification (>4 fold increase of MYCN signals compared to the control) is observed in 20% of cases and portends aggressive disease. Ploidy is also predictive of survival especially in infants and patients with localized disease, where hyperdiploidy is associated with a good prognosis. The COG uses age, stage, histology, *MYCN* status, and ploidy to classify patients into low- (40% tumors, EFS >95%), intermediate- (20%, EFS 80–95%), and high-risk (40%, EFS 40–50%) categories.[65] Additional genetic risk factors impact prognosis including allelic gains at 17q and LOH at 1p36 and 11q, all of which are associated with a poor prognosis. In addition to the variables used for the COG risk classification, 11q aberrations are used in the INRG classification system.[70] Newer classification approaches include the integration of segmental chromosome gains or losses. Although gains of whole chromosomes have been associated with a good prognosis, segmental gains or losses are associated with a poor prognosis particularly segmental loss at 1p,

Table 3 International neuroblastoma staging system (INSS)[67].

Stage I	Localized tumor with complete gross excision ($\pm$ microscopic disease), ipsilateral lymph nodes negative.
Stage IIA	Localized tumor, incomplete resection, ipsilateral nonadherent lymph nodes negative.
Stage IIB	Localized tumor with or without gross excision, ipsilateral lymph nodes positive, contralateral nodes negative.
Stage III	Unresectable unilateral tumor that crosses the midline ($\pm$ lymph nodes), unilateral tumor with contralateral lymph node involvement, midline tumor with bilateral extension, or lymph node involvement.
Stage IV	Disseminated disease to distant lymph nodes, skin, liver, bone, bone marrow, and other organs.
Stage IVS	Localized primary tumor (e.g., defined as I, 2A, or 2B) in infants less than 1 year of age with disseminated disease to the skin, liver, and/or limited bone marrow involvement (tumor cells <10% nucleated cells).

3p, 4p, 11q or gains at 1q, 2p, or 17q. Future studies will factor these variables into classification of lower risk disease.[71]

Treatment for patients with low-risk disease (INSS 1, biologically favorable INSS 2A, 2B) is surgery alone with chemotherapy reserved for patients with life-threatening symptoms or for the minority of patients whose disease progresses or reoccurs.[71] There is a subset of patients less than 6 months of age with small adrenal primaries whose tumors may regress without surgery.[72] Most stage IV-S patients undergo spontaneous regression, but some infants present with massive hepatomegaly and associated respiratory distress necessitating immediate management with low-dose chemotherapy and/or irradiation. Intermediate-risk patients (e.g., INSS stage III and most stage IV <18 months, INRG L2 and M < 18 months if diploid) are treated with surgery and moderately intensive chemotherapy that includes carboplatin or cisplatin, etoposide, cyclophosphamide, and doxorubicin for 2–8 cycles depending on initial tumor response and other prognostic markers such as segmental chromosome abnormalities. In some cases, surgery may be avoided altogether as well as chemotherapy (L2 < 18 months).

Treatment of high-risk disease remains a challenge, but stepwise improvements have occurred through the use of myeloablative regimens, differentiation therapy, and most recently, immunotherapy.[73,74] Initial therapy consists of six cycles of dose-intensive chemotherapy with cyclophosphamide, topotecan, cisplatin, etoposide, doxorubicin, and vincristine, or similar agents. Surgery (before consolidation with myeloablative chemotherapy) and irradiation therapy (after consolidation) to minimize tumor burden is routinely used in the high-risk setting. Multiple studies have demonstrated that consolidation with myeloablative chemotherapy followed by autologous peripheral blood stem cell re-infusion improves outcome.[75] Studies have shown no benefit to purging the stem cell source, and stem cells are usually harvested after two cycles of chemotherapy.[76] Data exist to indicate that myeloablation with busulfan–melphalan is superior to other regimens and that "tandem" courses of high-dose chemotherapy with stem cell rescue may be beneficial over a single course.[77] An upcoming COG study will look at the benefit of targeted ^{131}I-MIBG prior to consolidation in the newly diagnosed setting.[71]

The use of biological approaches has also improved outcome for patients with high-risk disease. Cis-retinoic acid has long been noted to differentiate tumor cells in culture, but early use in the treatment of relapsed or refractory disease was disappointing. However, a randomized trial examining its impact when delivered after cytotoxic therapy in the setting of MRD for high-risk patients showed a substantial benefit and its use is currently being evaluated in patients with lower risk disease.[78] The additional use of the anti-GD2 monoclonal antibody (mab) ch 14.18 in conjunction with granulocyte–monocyte colony-stimulating factor and interleukin-2 increased the 2-year survival significantly (66% $\pm$ 5% with mab vs 46% $\pm$ 5% without mab).[74]

Therapy for refractory patients and those who relapse remain unsatisfactory. Whole genome copy number analysis and sequencing have discovered 12% of patients with ALK aberrations, and such patients may benefit from ALK inhibitors such as crizotinib that is the current focus of early phase investigations. Somatic alterations of other genes were much less frequent including *ATRX*, *ARID1A*, and *PTPN11* (regulates ras pathway), but as yet, targeted therapy is not available. The neurotropin receptor TrkB is expressed on high-risk NBs and targeting these pathways remains a potential therapeutic opportunity even though early experience with lestaurtinib was negative.[79] The nuclear transcription MYCN, like other transcription factors, has been difficult to target, but new approaches targeting bromodomain and extraterminal (BET) bromodomain proteins that regulate chromatin have shown striking efficacy in preclinical models of Myc-amplified tumors, and therapeutic compounds are in early phase investigation.[80]

Pediatric bone tumors

Malignant primary bone tumors that occur in both younger and older patients have important differences in pathogenesis, presentation, and treatment, and these differences will be highlighted. Although primary bone tumors are rare, they are the sixth most common malignant neoplasm in children and the third most frequent neoplasm in AYAs. Malignant bone tumors occur in the United States at an annual rate of approximately 8.7 cases per million children and adolescents younger than 20 years. Only half the bone tumors in childhood are malignant, and of these, osteosarcoma (OS) is the most frequent, accounting for approximately 35% of all primary sarcomas of bone. Ewing sarcoma (EWS), the second most frequent primary bone cancer, is more common than OS in children younger than 10 years.

Osteosarcoma

OS, the most common primary malignant bone tumor, is composed of spindle cells producing osteoid. It is a highly aggressive neoplasm for which dramatic progress has been made in treatment and outcome during the past several decades. OS is primarily a disease of AYAs, although it can also occur in older patients. OS has a bimodal age distribution, with the first peak in the second decade of life during the adolescent growth spurt, and the second among older adults. It is estimated that approximately 400 children and adolescents less than 20 years of age are diagnosed each year in the United States. It is extremely rare before the age of 5 years. The most common clinical presentation is pain with or without an associated soft tissue mass in the involved region of bone. Among young patients, the most common location is the metaphysis of a long bone. Approximately, half of all OSs originate around the knee joint.

The peak age coincides with a period of rapid bone growth in young people, suggesting a correlation between rapid bone growth and the evolution of OS. Radiation exposure is another well-documented etiologic factor. The incidence of OS is dramatically increased among survivors of RB. In the hereditary form of this disorder, germline mutations of the RB gene are common. This is the likely basis for the increased frequency of secondary cancers in this population, as the rate in survivors of unilateral sporadic RB is much less. Germline mutations in the P53 gene can lead to a high risk of developing malignancies, including OS, which has been described as the Li–Fraumeni syndrome. Most OSs, including those in children and adolescents, are of the osteoblastic subtype. The current WHO classification recognizes two additional subtypes of conventional OS: chondroblastic and fibroblastic based on the predominant pattern of differentiation. Telangiectatic OS is a rare subtype, which appears as a purely lytic lesion on plain radiographs and thus, may be confused with aneurysmal bone cyst or giant cell tumor.

Similar to other sarcomas in young patients (typically high grade), OS metastasizes very early in its evolution. Approximately 20% of patients present with radiographically detectable metastases, most frequently to the lung, while almost all newly diagnosed patients with OS have at least micrometastatic disease as evidenced by the fact that if treated by surgical resection alone, 80% will relapse in the lung within 2 years.[81] Death from OS is almost always the result of progressive pulmonary metastasis with respiratory failure, pulmonary hemorrhage, pneumothorax, or superior vena cava obstruction. The diagnosis of OS is typically suspected by the radiographic appearance of the affected lesion. OS can present as a lytic, sclerotic, or a mixed lytic–sclerotic lesion. The diagnosis of OS is dependent on a biopsy for histologic examination providing a pathological diagnosis. OS is a pleomorphic, spindle cell tumor that forms an extracellular matrix consisting mostly of osteoid. Immunohistochemistry and cytogenetics are not helpful in diagnosing OS. Patients with OS should undergo a staging work-up to determine the extent of disease at presentation, which includes plain radiographs and MRI of the involved bone and should capture the adjoining joints, noncontrast chest CT, a bone scan, and/or a PET scan.

Multiagent systemic chemotherapy, along with local and metastatic disease control with surgery, is the standard of care.[81] The standard chemotherapy of patients with nonmetastatic OS, although variable, includes the use of cisplatin and doxorubicin with the addition of high-dose methotrexate. Advances made in surgical techniques have significantly improved the clinical practice and functional limb salvage options available for patients. *Rosen* et al. introduced the concept of chemotherapy prior to surgical resection.[82] Although no differences in outcome are reported with the incorporation of neoadjuvant chemotherapy versus upfront surgery followed by adjuvant chemotherapy, neoadjuvant chemotherapy does provide several potential advantages, including better resectability if tumor shrinks, improved surgical planning and endoprosthetic customization, treatment of micrometastatic disease and above all, the ability to assess the response to chemotherapy. A strong correlation between the degree of necrosis and the probability of subsequent DFS was observed,[83] which has subsequently been confirmed in multiple clinical trials. Soon after the identification of the prognostic value of the degree of necrosis following induction chemotherapy, it was suggested that chemotherapy be modified for the patients with less necrosis. Despite an early report of benefit, intensified regimens including ifosfamide and etoposide have not improved outcome for poor responders.[84] Because complete surgical resection is imperative for the cure of OS, surgical resectability is an important prognostic factor, therefore patients presenting with axial skeleton tumors fare worse than those having tumors in appendicular skeleton.

The standard management for patients with metastatic disease at the time of initial diagnosis follows the same general principles as those who present with localized disease. The outcome of OS patients depends on several factors. The most consistent prognostic factor at diagnosis is the presence of clinically detectable metastases, which confers an unfavorable prognosis. In patients with metastatic disease at diagnosis, the number of pulmonary nodules, as well as, whether they are unilateral or bilateral is also of prognostic significance. With currently available regimens, approximately 60–70% of patients with nonmetastatic OS of the extremity will survive without evidence of recurrence. In most large reported studies, only 10–20% of patients who present with clinically detectable metastatic disease survive. OS is resistant to radiation therapy, thus it is not a part of standard OS treatment and is reserved for pain/symptoms relief in palliative care settings only.

The survival of patients with OS appears to have reached a plateau. At present, none of the agents in early phase clinical trials have shown promise to move them in the frontline therapy. Research is ongoing to elucidate novel molecular targets in OS, of which anti-GD2 antibody and RANKL antibody are of particular interest.[85]

Ewing sarcoma

EWS is the second most common primary malignant bone tumor in children and adolescents. EWS is a part of peripheral primitive neuroectodermal tumors (PPNETs). In the early 1980s, EWS and PPNET were both found to contain the same reciprocal translocation between chromosomes 11 and 22, t(11;22) (q24;q12).[86,87] Later that decade, similar patterns of oncogene expression (c-myc, N-myc, c-myb, and c-mil/raf-1) were seen among these tumors. The combination of the shared translocation, cellular physiology, and clinical response has led to categorizing these tumors into the Ewing sarcoma family of tumors (EWSFTs). The EWSFT includes EWS, PPNET, neuroepithelioma, atypical EWS, and Askin tumor (an EWSFT of the chest wall).

Most cases are thought to be sporadic, but family members of EWSFT patients have an increased incidence of neuroectodermal and stomach malignancies.[88] EWSFT are thought to derive from cells of neuroectodermal origin, possibly postganglionic cholinergic neurons, although the exact cell of origin has yet to be identified. The immunohistochemical hallmark of EWSFT is diffuse membranous staining for CD99 (MIC2), which is present in greater than 90% of EWSFT. Undifferentiated tumors are negative for other markers except vimentin and FLI-1, whereas more differentiated tumors variably express additional markers, including neuron-specific enolase, S-100, neurofilaments, CD57, and synaptophysin. Muscle and lymphoid markers are negative. The translocation t(11;22)(q24;q12), or another related translocation, occurs in greater than 95% of EWSFT. Some argue that such a translocation is pathognomonic and is both necessary and sufficient for a diagnosis of EWSFT. The classic t(11;22)(q24;q12) translocation joins the EWS gene located on chromosome 22 to an ets-family gene, *FLI1* (Friend Leukemia Insertion), located on chromosome 11. Other ets-family partners are *ERG* t(21;22), *ETV1* t(7;22), and *E1AF* t(17;22). Standard cytogenetics and fluorescence *in situ* hybridization (FISH) can reveal this anomaly and additional karyotypic abnormalities, including trisomies 8 and 12, and chromosomes 1 and 16 abnormalities. Some of the t(21;22) translocations remain cryptic by standard cytogenetic techniques and require reverse transcription polymerase chain reaction or FISH.

The incidence of EWSFT peaks in the latter half of the second decade of life. An enigma in EWSFT is its racial distribution. The incidence in whites is at least ninefold higher than in blacks. EWS arises most commonly in the bone, but it can also originate in extraosseous soft tissues. Frequent primary sites include the pelvis (25%), femur (16%), ribs (12%), and spine (8%). Approximately 25% of patients present with metastatic disease. Of these, 37% (or 9% of all patients) have metastases confined to the lung or pleura. The remaining patients have bone and/or bone marrow metastases, either alone or in addition to pulmonary/pleural disease. Rarely, patients with bone marrow metastases have extensive infiltration and present with systemic symptoms. Diagnosis is typically done by tumor biopsy. Staging work-up typically includes MRI/CT of the primary site, CT scan of the chest to evaluate for lung metastasis, bone scan and bone marrow aspiration, and biopsy. Recently, FDG-PET/CT is replacing bone scan for EWS metastatic work-up. The most consistent prognostic factor is the presence of metastatic disease at diagnosis. The presence of an axial tumor, older age at diagnosis, larger size of primary tumor, and poor histologic response after induction chemotherapy are other adverse prognostic indicators in EWS.

The successful management of patients with ESFT requires the use of both local and systemic therapy. Both surgery and radiation therapy are utilized for local control, while systemic control is achieved by chemotherapy. EWS, unlike OS, is quite radioresponsive, and RT is considered a standard option for definitive local control. Radiotherapy can be used as an alternative to disfiguring surgery such as amputation. Alkylating agents (cyclophosphamide, ifosfamide, melphalan, and busulfan) and doxorubicin are the most active single agents in EWS, while addition of ifosfamide plus etoposide has led to significant increase in EFS and OS, particularly for localized disease.[89] Recently, the COG has shown superior efficacy of dose-intensive therapy administered every 2 weeks with filgrastim support compared to the conventional every-3-week therapy for patients with initially localized disease.[90] Altogether, these measures have increased 5-year EFS of localized EWS to approximately 75%.

EWS patients with disease metastatic at initial diagnosis have a poor outcome. Patients with multiple sites of metastases have the lowest survival rates. Patients with metastases confined to the lungs may represent a group of patients with better prognosis than patients with bone or bone marrow metastases. Overall cure rates for metastatic EWS remains 20%, utilizing the standard interval-compressed chemotherapy including ifosfamide and etoposide as described above for localized disease along with local control of primary and metastatic sites utilizing surgery and radiation therapy. Myeloablative chemotherapy followed by autologous stem cell rescue has not shown significant improvement in overall survival.[91]

Moving forward, based on feasibility of adding topotecan/cyclophosphamide in a pilot study, COG is running a phase 3 randomized trial for patients with localized EWS. The insulin-like growth factor type I receptor (IGF-1R) is critical for transformation and growth of ESFT,[92] and incorporation of antibody against IGF-1R with intensified chemotherapy backbone is being investigated through the COG for newly diagnosed metastatic EWS patients. In addition, mTOR inhibitors are being tested in relapse and refractory EWS.[85]

Soft tissue sarcomas

Soft tissue sarcomas represent a widely heterogeneous group of malignancies that in aggregate account for 7.4% of cancers in children and adolescents up to 19 years of age. Approximately 800–900 cases are diagnosed per year in the United States.[1] The most common soft tissue sarcoma is RMS that is derived in large part from striated muscle, while others originate from fibrous connective tissue (fibrosarcoma), smooth muscle (leiomyosarcoma), and fat (liposarcoma). Synovial cell sarcoma is now thought to originate in precursor cells distinct from those that lead to synovium.

Rhabdomyosarcoma

RMS accounts for 50% of soft tissue tumors in children less than 14 years of age. By far, most cases of RMS are sporadic although cases have been described in association with NF-1, Costello syndrome, Beckwith–Wiedemann syndrome, and Li–Fraumeni syndrome. The histologic hallmark of RMS, a small round blue cell tumor, is evidence of skeletal muscle differentiation most often validated by immunohistochemistry (MyoD, myogenin, muscle specific actin, myoglobin, and desmin). RMS is composed of two histologic subtypes. Embryonal RMS (ERMS, 60–75% of cases) is characterized by spindle cells with myxoid areas, whereas alveolar RMS typically shows oval cells forming alveolar spaces surrounded by fibrous septae.[93] The majority of alveolar cases are characterized by translocations between the DNA-binding domains of PAX3 (55% of ARMS) or PAX7 (20%) and FOXO1. About 15% of ARMS are fusion negative. The outcome for ERMS is superior to that of ARMS, and patients with fusion-negative ARMS have a better outcome compared to fusion-positive cases.[94] Interestingly, ERMS is associated with a higher mutational burden and frequent alterations of RAS pathway genes.[95]

The clinical presentation of RMS depends on location. About 40% of RMS occur in the head, neck, and orbit. Symptoms can include a painless mass (superficial head and neck primary tumors), proptosis, and esotropia (orbital tumors), snoring, recurrent unilateral epistaxis, sinusitis, and cranial nerve palsies (nasopharyngeal and paranasal lesions). Genitourinary RMS accounts for 20% of cases, and bladder/prostate lesions can lead to urinary obstruction. Approximately, 20% occur in the extremities and usually present as a painless mass. Extremity tumors tend to be of the alveolar subtype, whereas the majority of tumors located in the head, neck, and GU sites are ERMS. The botryoid variant of ERMS arises under mucosal surfaces (e.g., vagina, nasopharynx) and can present as a protruding grape-like mass.

The clinical evaluation of patients includes cross-sectional imaging (CT or MRI) of the primary with evaluation of possible metastatic disease (chest CT, bilateral bone marrow aspirates and biopsies, and bone scan). Approximately, 15% of patients will have metastatic disease at diagnosis, most commonly lung followed by bone marrow, lymph node, and bone. RMS is classified according to well-documented determinants of prognosis such as age, location of the primary tumor, extent of disease (group), histologic subtype, and stage. The stage incorporates the site of the primary (favorable site vs unfavorable site) and a pretreatment assessment of tumor size (confined to organ, T1 vs extension, T2; size ≤ 5 cm or >5 cm), nodal status (N_0 uninvolved, N_1, involved, N_X unknown), and metastasis (M_0 or M_1). Favorable sites include the orbit, nonparameningeal head and neck, biliary, and non-bladder/prostate genitourinary sites. The group is dependent on the surgical resectability (Group 1—completely resected, Group II—gross total resection with evidence of regional spread, Group III—gross residual disease, Group IV—distant metastasis at diagnosis). Regional lymph nodes should be sampled in cases of RMS located in the extremities. Of note, initial response to chemotherapy has not been proven to be prognostic in COG studies. These variables have been used to develop a risk stratification used in COG trials (Table 4).[96]

Treatment for RMS requires a mulitdisciplinary approach. The chemotherapeutic agents most beneficial are vincristine, dactinomycin, and cyclophosphamide (VAC). Patients with low-risk

Risk group	Stage	Group	Histology	Percent of cases	EFS
Low, subset 1	I	I–II	ERMS	27%	85–95%
	I	III (orbit)	ERMS		
	II	I–II	ERMS		
Low, subset 2	I	III (non-orbit)	ERMS	5%	70–85%
	III	I–II	ERMS		
Intermediate	II–III	III	ERMS	27%	73%
	I–III	I–III	ARMS	25%	65%
High	IV	IV	ERMS	8%	35%
	IV	IV	ARMS	8%	15%

Source: Hawkins et al. 2013.[96] Reproduced with permission from John Wiley & Sons.

disease, subset 1, can be effectively managed with a short course of VAC treatment where the dose of cytoxan is minimized to avoid infertility, whereas a higher dose of the drug is required for subset 2 patients.[97] Patients with Group II and III tumors receive irradiation. There have been many attempts to improve outcome for intermediate-risk patients with the addition of agents such as etoposide, carboplatin, ifosfamide, and topotecan to VAC, but to date such efforts have been disappointing. A recently completed COG study looked at the addition of vincristine/irinotecan (V/I) to VAC, and while EFS was not improved, there was less hematologic toxicity and the total dose of cytoxan was lower. Thus, moving forward VAC/VI is likely the standard of care for intermediate-risk RMS.[98] There has been little improvement in outcome for high-risk disease, but the use of interval compressed ifosfamide/etoposide and vincristine/doxorubicin/cyclophosphamide may be associated with a substantial gains for high-risk ERMS. A number of drugs are being considered or are under investigation including some of which are aimed at molecular targets such as IGF-1R (autocrine activation), ALK (amplified), C- Met (overexpressed), and RAS (mutated in ERMS).[96,99]

Nonrhabdomyosarcoma soft tissue sarcomas

Nonrhabdomyosarcoma soft tissue sarcomas (NRSTS) represent a wide variety of tumors with distinct genetic, pathologic, and clinical profiles. They tend to occur in older patients and most are located in the extremities. Many are associated with distinct genetic lesions that are diagnostic such as synovial sarcoma (t(X;18)p11;q11) (SYT-SS1 and SYT-SSX2). The mainstay of treatment is surgery, and irradiation is used for patients with high-grade lesions and positive margins. The impact of chemotherapy is less certain, but neoadjuvant therapy may be indicated to improve chances of surgical excision. The use of adjuvant chemotherapy in addition to irradiation for larger grossly resected tumors is more controversial but was recommended in the recent COG protocol for these tumors.[100] Table 5 summarizes risk groups and outcomes.[96,101]

Table 5 Nonrhabdomyosarcoma prognostic groups.

Risk group	Gross resection	Grade	Size	Distant metastasis	Percent of NRSTS	5-Year survival
Low	Yes	Low	Any	No	60%	90%
	Yes	High	<5 cm	No		
Intermediate	Yes	High	>5 cm	No	30%	50%
	No	Any	Any	No		
High	Any	Any	Any	Yes	10%	15%

Source: Data from Refs 96, 100.

Central nervous system tumors

Significant differences in epidemiology, molecular genetics, and biology distinguish CNS tumors of the infant and child from those arising in adulthood. Because of these differences, important aspects of clinical presentation, treatment, and outcome are uniquely related to childhood CNS tumors.

Malignant CNS tumors are the most common solid tumor of childhood, with 2200 new cases per year in the United States. Pediatric brain tumors vary considerably in their histological, topographical, and gender distribution throughout childhood and adolescence. Boys are more commonly affected than girls in all age groups, but this increase is accounted for mostly by medulloblastoma, PNET, and ependymoma. Over 90% of CNS tumors in children are primary brain tumors. Survival has improved from 60% in 1975–1984 to 65% in 1985–1994 to 73.3% in 1995–2011, and survival is noted to improve with increasing age: 45% in those aged less than 1 year, 59% in those aged 1–4 years, 64% in 5–9 year olds, 70% in 10–14 year olds, and 77% in 15–19 year olds. The main histological entities in children are pilocytic astrocytomas (23.5%), followed by medulloblastomas (16.3%), ependymomas (10.1%), anaplastic astrocytomas and glioblastomas (7.2% each), and craniopharyngiomas (5.6%),[102] while high-grade glial tumors, anaplastic astrocytoma, and glioblastoma account for majority of adult brain tumors, followed by meningiomas and other mesenchymal tumors.

In the United States, CNS tumors are the most common cause of death due to cancer in childhood, accounting for 24% of cancer-related deaths. Morbidity as a result of increasingly successful treatment approaches remains high and includes cognitive, memory, and learning impairment, neuroendocrine deficiencies, hearing deficits, sterility, and secondary cancers.

The etiology of CNS tumors remains mostly unknown. The known risk factors include (1) gender (male), (2) therapeutic doses of ionizing radiation to the head (e.g., for leukemia or prior brain tumor), and (3) genetic syndromes such as neurofibromatosis, tuberous sclerosis, nevoid basal cell carcinoma syndrome (Gorlin syndrome), Turcot's syndrome, and Li–Fraumeni syndrome.

Embryonal tumors of the central nervous system comprise a group of tumors that share a histologically similar, undifferentiated morphology and represent the most common malignant brain tumor group in children (21%). The incidence is constant from infancy to 3 years of age and then a steady decline is observed thereafter. This group includes the primitive neuroectodermal tumors (PNETs), ependymoblastoma, and atypical teratoid rhabdoid tumor (AT/RT). PNETs are a group of highly malignant tumors composed of small round blue cells of neuroectodermal origin. PNETs are further subdivided by anatomic location into medulloblastoma (posterior fossa) and supratentorial PNET. Controversy has existed regarding the class division between supratentorial PNET and medulloblastoma, but the preponderance of molecular genetic, biologic, and clinical evidence validates this division.[103]

Medulloblastoma is the most common malignant brain tumor in children, with a bimodal peak age distribution first being between 3 and 4 years and again between 8 and 10 years of age. It has a typical radiographic presentation of a solid midline posterior fossa mass that arises from cerebellum and occupies the fourth ventricle (Figure 4a). Surgery (preferred gross total resection) and cranio-spinal irradiation have been essential elements of successful therapy for medulloblastoma. However, to reduce late effects, especially in very young children, the incorporation of chemotherapy has permitted a reduction in radiation dose. Recently, tandem high-dose chemotherapy with stem cell rescue has demonstrated even further benefit without compromising survival in high-risk medulloblastomas.

More recently, medulloblastomas have been categorized into four groups by transcriptional profiling: WNT, Sonic Hedgehog (SHH), group C, and group D.[104] Tumors displaying WNT pathway activation, comprises of 10% of tumors, while approximately 30% exhibit activation of SHH pathway as a result of mutation of *PTCH1* or the *SMO* gene, both associated with favorable prognosis. Group C constitutes tumors with a poor prognosis, irrespective of their metastatic status. Ongoing research is examining treatment stratification by subgroup and potentially new targets for more effective and less toxic therapies.

AT/RT is an aggressively malignant, primitive tumor most often arising in children younger than 2 years of age. These tumors have only recently been recognized as an entity distinct from PNET due to their histological similarity with two-thirds containing foci morphologically indistinct from PNET. Approximately half of AT/RTs arise in the infratentorial compartment with a propensity to invade the cerebello-pontine angle. Because of its association with chromosome 22 deletion and mutation of *SMARCB1/INI1* (tumor suppressor gene), analysis of these markers in infants and children with presumed medulloblastoma/PNET is being used as a molecular diagnostic tool for this tumor. This disease is often fatal despite aggressive treatment.

Ependymoma makes up approximately 10% of childhood CNS tumors with approximately two-thirds occurring infratentorially. Greater than half of these tumors occur in children less than 5 years of age with a peak during the second year of life. The addition of chemotherapy to surgery and RT for childhood ependymoma has not been proven to impact overall survival, although studies are ongoing to investigate this further.

Glial neoplasms range from benign low-grade gliomas, which can be resected and/or observed to aggressive high-grade gliomas, which have extremely poor outcome. Low-grade gliomas broadly encompass both pilocytic astrocytomas (WHO grade 1) and diffuse fibrillary and pilomyxoid astrocytomas (WHO grade 2), while high-grade gliomas comprises of anaplastic astrocytoma (WHO grade 3) and glioblastomas (WHO grade 4). The incidence of cortical astrocytomas increases with age, having a first peak at age 5 and again at age 13. In children, brain stem and cerebellar astrocytomas are as common as cortical tumors. Cerebellar astrocytoma is found almost exclusively in children, occurring most frequently between ages 4 and 9. Juvenile pilocytic astrocytoma (JPA) is the most common subtype, accounting for 85% of cerebellar astrocytomas

(Figure 4b). Diffuse astrocytoma is the next most common, whereas malignant astrocytoma is rare in this location. Total surgical resection is curative in 95–100%. JPAs may stabilize for long periods of time or even spontaneously regress; however, the behavior of cerebellar astrocytomas in children with neurofibromatosis type I (NF-1) may be more aggressive. Gliomas of the visual pathway, hypothalamus, and thalamus comprise a relatively common form of childhood astrocytoma. Tumors of the optic chiasm and hypothalamus are usually low grade, whereas thalamic tumors tend to be more variable. About 20% of children with NF-1 will develop visual pathway tumors, predominantly JPA, during childhood. These tumors present most frequently between 5 and 10 years of age. Recent studies have highlighted the role of MAPK/ERK pathway in the oncogenesis of these tumors. Although IDH1 mutations characterize the vast majority of low-grade and secondary high-grade gliomas in adults,[105] the majority of pediatric low-grade gliomas harbor BRAF alterations in the form of *BRAF* gene rearrangement and fusion and/or point mutation.[106,107] Efforts are underway to exploit these pathways for molecularly targeted therapy for the low-grade gliomas in children.

Brain stem gliomas (BSG) comprise 10–15% of all pediatric CNS tumors and are generally uncommon in the adult population. Peak incidence is between 5 and 9 years of age, but it may occur anytime during childhood. BSGs most commonly arise in the pons (diffuse intrinsic), in which location they typically resemble adult glioblastomas multiforme (GBM) and have an almost uniformly dismal prognosis (Figure 4c). In contrast, those arising from midbrain or medulla are likely to be low-grade lesions that have a more indolent course and better outcome. Surgery and postoperative radiation therapy are the mainstay of therapy in children with high-grade gliomas. Recently, sequencing studies have shown recurrent but mutually exclusive mutations in histone H3F3A and IDH1 in about 30–40% of pediatric glioblastomas,[108] suggesting disrupted epigenetic regulatory mechanisms, which can be further exploited for therapeutic targeting.

Intracranial germ cell tumors (IGCTs) account for less than 5% of pediatric CNS tumors but are primarily seen in children and adolescents, with 90% occurring in those less than 20 years. Incidence peaks at age 10–12 years. They account for nearly 50% of all pineal region tumors of childhood. Germinomas account for approximately two-thirds of IGCTs, while the remaining third are nongerminomatous germ cell tumors (GCTs), including yolk sac tumor, choriocarcinoma, mixed GCTs, and mature and immature teratomas. Elevation of serum and CSF tumor markers as AFP and

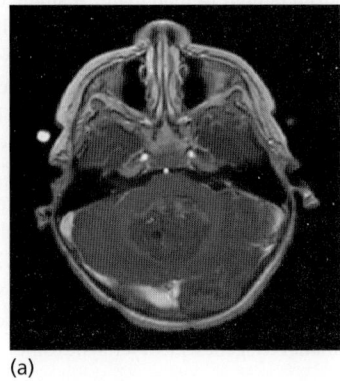 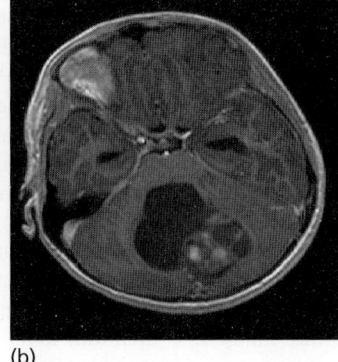 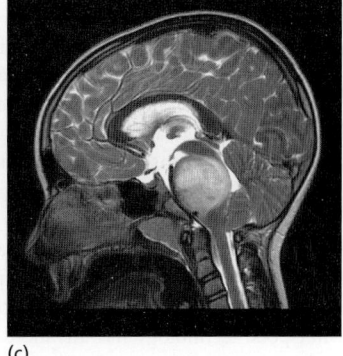

(a)   (b)   (c)

Figure 4 MRI imaging findings of common pediatric brain tumors. (a) Axial T1 image with contrast showing a midline tumor in the cerebellum, and pathology consistent with medulloblastoma. (b) T1-weighted axial MRI image with contrast of typical pilocytic astrocytoma in the cerebellum of a 5-year-old child showing heterogeneously enhancing mural nodule and intratumoral cysts, dilated temporal horns bilaterally suggestive of hydrocephalus. (c) T2-weighted sagittal view showing diffuse enlargement of pons in a patient with diffuse intrinsic pontine glioma.

β-HCG along with radiologic findings can be used as surrogate diagnostic markers, but when the results of tumor markers are equivocal, tumor biopsy is performed for definitive diagnosis. Germinomas are highly radiosensitive and 5-year overall survival is more than 90% with radiation alone. COG is currently investigating the effect of chemotherapy followed by response-based radiation therapy, in order to minimize the radiation dose and subsequent long-term side effects.

Less-frequently encountered tumors

Individually, RB, GCTs, liver tumors, and carcinomas are less frequently encountered tumors in pediatrics, but collectively, however, these neoplasms account for up to 18% of all cancers seen in children and adolescents. Moreover, the incidence of some of these tumors, such as germ cell (GCT) malignancies and certain carcinomas, is significantly higher in older patients, those aged between 15 and 19 years, a population that has been under-represented in prospective cooperative national trials.

Retinoblastoma

RB is the most frequent neoplasm of the eye in childhood and represents 3% of all pediatric cancers. An estimated 200–300 children develop RB each year. Most patients present in infancy during the first 2 years of life (two-thirds of cases, 95% <5 years) and the tumor originates in the retina with usual extension into the vitreous cavity.[109] Common symptoms are leukocoria and strabismus. RB presents in two distinct clinical forms: (1) bilateral or multifocal, hereditary (25% of cases), characterized by the presence of germline mutations of the RB1 gene either inherited from an affected parent (25%) or as a result of a new germline mutation, and (2) unilateral (75% of cases). About 90% of unilateral cases are nonhereditary. Patients with bilateral RB present at an earlier age (<1 year) compared to children with unilateral nonhereditary disease (2–3 years).

Based on clinical forms of the disease Knudsen proposed the classic "two-hit" hypothesis in 1971 where two mutational events were needed in a retinal cell for transformation.[110] Further analyses indicated that the two events were in fact disruption of both alleles of a single gene, a tumor suppressor gene. The RB1 gene, located in chromosome 13q14, was identified and cloned in 1986.[111] The product of RB1 (pRb) is a 110-kd nuclear phosphoprotein that acts by influencing the transcription of several genes involved in cell cycle progression. The level of pRb phosphorylation varies throughout the cell cycle and inactivation removes the pRb constraint on cell cycle control, with the consequence of deregulated cell proliferation.

Patients with hereditary RB are born with a germline defect in RB1 and inactivation of the other RB1 allele is a somatic event, whereas unilateral or nonhereditary tumors have somatic inactivation of both alleles. The RB1 gene is large containing 27 exons over about 200 kb of DNA, and mutations have been described in almost every exon. Nonsense and frameshift mutations are the most common germline and somatic events (>80%), although deletions are also seen (10–20%).[112] Although loss of RB1 is the critical step in tumor pathogenesis, it is clear that additional events are required for tumor development. All patients with RB require genetic counseling and genetic testing. Although there are no mutational hotspots, technology has advanced so that almost all cases of germline predisposition can be identified.

Suspected cases of RB are diagnosed by an experienced ophthalmologist by an exam under anesthesia with a dilated pupil. Imaging studies such as MRI, CT, and ultrasound are helpful in distinguishing RB from other causes of leukocoria (retrolental fibrodysplasia, Coats disease, toxocariasis, and toxoplasmosis) and to assess extraocular extension. CT may be used with caution given the increased risk of secondary tumors associated with radiation in patients with hereditary forms of the disease. Many staging systems are currently in use to predict outcome and guide therapy.[113]

The goals of therapy are to eradicate the tumor optimizing cure, preserve vision, and avoid long-term complications particularly second malignancies. Typically patients with unilateral tumors present with large tumors where there is little chance for preserving vision. Enucleation is curative in more than 90% of cases of unilateral tumors. Careful pathological examination of the resected specimen by an experienced ocular pathologist is needed to determine if any features associated with metastatic disease are present: vitreous seeding, massive choroidal involvement, tumor beyond lamina cribrosa, and scleral/extrascleral extension. These features would dictate the use of chemotherapy, usually with combinations of the effective drugs including vincristine, doxorubicin, cyclophosphamide, carboplatin, and etoposide. For small tumors where vision preservation is possible, chemotherapy and local control with photocoagulation, cryotherapy, and thermotherapy may be considered.[114] Direct ocular delivery of chemotherapy via the ophthalmic artery has been used with increasing frequency.[115] RB is particularly radiation sensitive, but given concerns about second malignancies, it is usually reserved for salvage. Chemotherapy (systemic ± periocular or subtenon administration) is given to patients with bilateral tumors to lower tumor burden followed by local control measures.[109,116,117] This has resulted in higher eye salvage rates and decreased and delayed use of radiation therapy.

The risk of secondary tumors is strikingly higher for patients with the hereditary form of RB and risk is further increased by irradiation therapy.[118] Bone (OS) and soft tissue sarcomas, tumors of the nasal cavity, and melanoma are the most common secondary cancers. Given the association with radiation, many tumors originate in the head and neck area, but as germline mutations predispose to subsequent cancers independent of irradiation (and chemotherapy), many tumors are outside of the original radiation field.

Germ cell tumors

GCTs account for about 3.5% of tumors in children and adolescents and 60% originate in extragonadal sites. This distribution is related in part to the aberrant migration of primordial germ cells in the developing embryo and persistence at sites outside their normal destination into the ovary or testes. GCTs display a wide spectrum of clinical presentations depending on primary site and pathological features that range from benign to malignant. A single tumor may show a variety of tissue types and both benign and malignant elements. The age distribution follows a bimodal pattern, with a peak during the first 3 years of life and a second peak in late adolescence. In general, females have a higher overall incidence of GCT, although males are more at risk of malignant GCT. Cryptorchidism is a risk factor for the subsequent development of testicular GCT, and interestingly, this increased risk extends to the normally descended contralateral testis.[119] Surgical or hormonal correction ameliorates but does not eliminate the risk. Klinefelter syndrome (47 XXY) is also associated with an increased risk of GCT, and all males with mediastinal GCT should be screened for this condition.[120] Likewise, children with 46 XY gonadal dysgenesis (Swyer syndrome) are predisposed to GCTs.

The pathological classification of GCTs is partly predicated on their histopathological origin (germinoma vs nongerminoma) and whether they are benign or malignant (mature teratomas, immature teratomas, and malignant GCTs).[121] Teratomas contain tissues from multiple embryonic germ layers (endoderm, mesoderm, and ecto-derm) with varying degrees of differentiation. They are classified into three categories: benign, immature, and malignant teratomas [malignant GCT of mixed histologies (discussed below)]. Benign teratomas contain well-differentiated tissues such as cartilage, squamous epithelium, smooth muscle, and some may contain more complex structures such as teeth, salivary glands, and so on. Mature teratomas are commonly observed in the sacrococcygeal region and ovary. Immature teratomas contain immature elements usually neuroepithelium, but can also be immature mesenchyma or renal blastema. Immature teratomas usually occur in the ovaries and rarely in extraovarian sites. They are graded into four categories according to the degree of maturation. Grades 0–2 usually have a benign behavior. Another benign GCT is gonadoblastoma that occurs exclusively in dysgenetic gonads.

Malignant GCTs include a spectrum of tumors that are summarized in Table 6. Symptoms are related to the site of the primary tumor. Cytogenetic and molecular studies have confirmed that childhood GCTs constitute a group of distinct entities. A distinct chromosomal aberration, i(12p), is often seen in adult GCT. In children, however, the i(12p) is found almost exclusively in gonadal and extragonadal (usually mediastinal) tumors of adolescent males.[122] Gains in chromosomes 1q, 2, 3, 7, 8, 12, and 14 have been described in tumors originating in prepubertal females, whereas tumors in prepubertal males have been found to have gains in chromosomes 1q, 7, and 21, and losses in chromosome 1p.[122] Finally, del 1p36 is a common finding in extragonadal and testicular tumors in young children with yolk sac tumor (YST).[123] Recently, LIN28 a key regulator of BLIMP1, which is essential for the development of embryonic germ cells has been shown to be overexpressed in GCTs.[124] The sacrococcyx is the most common location of GCTs in children.[125] Most occur in the first 2 years of life. Two-thirds of these tumors are mature or immature teratomas, and symptoms include a visible mass, urinary retention, constipation, and weakness of the lower extremities due to compression. The ovary is the second most common site and abdominal pain is the most common symptom. Torsion of the ovary may precipitate acute pain. Almost 70% of ovarian GCTs are benign teratomas. Dysgerminoma and malignant tumors of mixed histology account for 80% of malignant ovarian GCTs with most of the remainder being yolk sac tumors. About 10% occur in the testes and these cases present as slowly growing masses. Two-thirds of these cases are yolk sac tumors. Mediastinal GCTs account for 4% of cases, and patients present with wheezing, cough, and shortness of breath. There is a strong male bias and most cases occur in children over 10 years. About 3% of GCTs occur in the CNS.

The diagnostic evaluation includes cross-sectional imaging to assess the extent of primary disease and potential dissemination (lymph nodes, intracavitary seeding, lungs, liver, and possibly the CNS) and tumor markers. Many staging systems exist for GCTs, and there are current efforts to decide on a consensus staging system to be shared by pediatric, adult, and gynecologic oncologists.[126] Most of the current systems rely on age, extent of disease including resectability, lymph node involvement, and presence of metastasis.[126] Therapy is based on the biology of individual tumor subtypes and stage.[127] Mature teratomas are treated with surgery alone as are immature teratomas. The use of chemotherapy in incompletely resected immature teratomas is controversial. Stage I completely resected testicular and ovarian (dysgerminoma) tumors can be treated with surgery alone and observation (including regression of tumor markers) as most patients (>80%) are cured and salvage with chemotherapy is quite high for the minority who recur. In general, retroperitoneal lymph node dissections are not performed in children with testicular GCT. Note stage I nongerminoma ovarian tumors may also be treated with surgery followed by observation. The relapse rate is significantly higher than for ovarian dysgerminoma, but salvage is also high.[128] Surgery and chemotherapy are recommended for stage II–IV ovarian and testicular tumors. The standard chemotherapy used includes cis-platinum, etoposide, and bleomycin (PEB) for four to six cycles depending on stage and response to chemotherapy (including assessment after second look surgery). The cure rate for these tumors is more than 90%. Likewise, all patients with extragonadal GCT benefit from surgery and chemotherapy (four cycles stage I–II, six cycles stage III–IV) with overall survival of 90% and 70% (metastatic mediastinal)—80% respectively for stage I–II and II–IV disease.[129]

Liver tumors

Malignant tumors of the liver account for 1% of all childhood cancers with hepatoblastoma (HB) accounting for 43% of all hepatic tumors (benign and malignant) followed by hepatocellular

Table 6 Malignant germ cell tumors.

Tumor	Frequency	Clinical features	Histology	Common locations	Tumor markers
Unipotential variants					
Germinoma Seminoma (testes) Dysgerminoma (ovary) Germinoma (extragonadal)	12%	Older age	Large cells with clear cytoplasm	Ovary, anterior mediastinum, brain, testes (much older pts.)	Negative (mildly elevated HCG may be seen in selected cases)
Totipotential variants					
Embryonal carcinoma	8%		Similar to yolk sac tumors, but cells are larger, with a major epithelial pattern	Testes, many locations	Negative or mildly elevated
Yolk sac (endodermal sinus tumor)	55%		Pseudopapillary (Schiller–Duval bodies), reticular, polyvesicular and solid patterns	Ovary, testicle sacrococcygeal location	Elevated AFP, normal HCG
Choriocarcinoma	1% (nongestational)	High likelihood of disseminated disease	Cytotrophoblasts and syncytiotrophoblasts	Ovary, testicle, extragonadal	Elevated HCG
Malignant germ cell tumors of mixed histology	24%		Composed of immature and mature teratoma but also composed of one or more types of malignant GCT	Ovary, testicle, extragonadal	Elevated AFB and/or HCG

carcinoma (HCC). HB is a disease of young infants with cases infrequently observed after 4 years of age. The incidence of HB has been rising possibly due to its association with prematurity and low birth weight.[130] HB has been associated with constitutional syndromes including familial adenomatous polyposis and Beckwith–Wiedemann syndrome. Patients usually present with an asymptomatic abdominal mass noted by parents or pediatrician. HB is an embryonal tumor that histologically recapitulates liver development and there are four recognized subtypes: epithelial (embryonal and fetal patterns, 67%), mesenchymal (epithelial and mesenchymal, 21%), pure well-differentiated fetal (7%), and small cell undifferentiated (5%).[131] The fetal histology is associated with a particularly favorable outcome. The most prevalent somatic lesion in HB is deletion or mutation of exon 3 of CTNNB1 (β-catenin) that leads to activation of the Wnt pathway.[132,133]

The outcome for children with HB has improved due to enhanced surgical techniques and the introduction of platinum-based chemotherapy. Currently, the 5-year overall survival rate is approximately 70%. A pretreatment extent of disease (PRETEXT) is now used to stratify therapy for HB and therefore a detailed assessment of the primary hepatic lesion is mandatory to determine resectability.[134] As 20–30% of patients may present with lung metastasis, cross-sectional imaging of the lung is also part of staging. AFP is a very sensitive diagnostic marker and is essential for assessing response to therapy. PRETEXT is based on involvement of the four major liver sections and the presence of venous, portal, and extrahepatic involvement as well as metastatic disease. Surgical resection with clear margins is the primary goal of treatment. Although PRETEXT I and II tumors may be candidates for upfront resection, many centers favor neoadjuvant therapy for all PRETEXT stages. Tumors are usually sensitive to therapy (usually cisplatin, 5-flourouricil, and vincristine ± doxorubicin). The use of dose dense treatment and integration of new agents including irinotecan and temsirolimus are currently being evaluated for children with high-risk disease.[127] Patients with PRETEXT IV disease or venous and/or portal involvement following chemotherapy are referred for liver transplantation, although complete regression (by chemotherapy ± surgery) of all metastatic lesions is required before proceeding with organ transplantation.

Hepatocellular carcinoma (HCC) is a disease of older adolescents and adults. Although HCC in adults is associated with pre-existing liver disease [hepatitis B and C, inflammatory liver disease, cirrhosis (tyrosinemia, biliary)] less than a third of patients diagnosed in Western countries have a history of liver disease.[135] In contrast to patients with HB, patients with HCC usually have constitutional symptoms such as weight loss, anorexia, and vomiting. Microscopically, HCC differs from HB in that tumor cells are larger, have defined borders, distinct nucleoli, and tumors have a high degree of vascular invasion. Transitional liver tumors display pathologic and genetic features of both HB and HCC. HCCs show an increased overall mutational burden than HB, but far fewer mutations in CTNNB1 and have multiple copy number variations.[136] Mutations in TP53 and epigenetic modifiers are frequent. Outcomes for HCC have been disappointing with no improvement over the past two decades in sharp contrast to advances made for other childhood tumors.[137] Complete surgical excision is the most important prognostic variable, but most patients present with advanced disease. For early stage tumors, complete resection followed by adjuvant chemotherapy is recommended, while neoadjuvant chemotherapy (with the hope of improving resection) is recommended for more advance stages (e.g., PRETEXT III). Patients who present with metastatic disease have a dismal outcome.

Carcinomas and melanoma

Carcinomas and melanoma account for approximately 9% of all cases of cancer in children. In the SEER database, the distribution of these malignancies is as follows: thyroid carcinoma, 35%; melanomas, 31%; adrenocortical carcinomas, 1.3%; nasopharyngeal carcinoma, 4.5%; and other skin carcinomas, 0.5%. Most carcinomas (75%) occur in the 15- to 19-year-old age group. In patients aged 15–19 years, thyroid cancer and melanoma account for more than 14% of the malignancies seen in this age group.

About 90% of thyroid carcinomas are papillary carcinomas, and the BRAFV600E mutation seen in adults is rare in children.[138] These tumors are treated by surgical resection and radioactive iodine ablation with 10-year survival rates exceeding 90%.[139] Patients require lifelong thyroid hormone replacement. Medullary carcinoma is usually familial (multiple endocrine neoplasia II) and is particularly aggressive.[140] Patients may be candidates for inhibitors of RET kinase. Most patients (90%) with melanoma have localized disease at initial evaluation, the most common site being the trunk, although patients younger than 20 years are more likely than adults to have disease primarily in the head and neck.[141] Like their adult counterpart, the majority of pediatric melanomas contain the BRAFV600E mutation. Survival rates are similar for patients younger than 20 and older than 20 years of age, and the prognosis appears to be stage dependent.[142] In the 15- to 19-year-old age group, the incidence of cutaneous melanoma increased at a rate of 2% per year between 1973 and 2006, but more recent reports show a decreasing trend among children.[1]

Late effects and quality of survivorship

With the use of multimodal and risk-based treatment, the overall 5-year survival rate of more than 12,500 children and adolescents (age 0–19) diagnosed with cancer each year in the United States is approaching 80% (SEER). The improvement in survival has resulted in about 1 in 810 individuals under the age of 20 and 1 in 640 individuals between the ages 20 and 39 years representing childhood cancer survivors.

The late sequelae of cancer treatment can cause chronic medical problems and involve all organ systems. Overall mortality among childhood cancer survivors has been described to be 10-fold that of the general population. The Childhood Cancer Survivor Study (CCSS) assessed overall and cause-specific mortality in a retrospective cohort of 20,227 five-year survivors and demonstrated a 10.8-fold excess in overall mortality.[143] Risk of death was statistically significantly higher in females, individuals diagnosed with cancer before the age of 5 years, and those with an initial diagnosis of leukemia or brain tumor. The excess mortality was due to death from primary cancer, second cancer, cardiotoxicity, and noncancer death, and existing up to 25 years after the initial cancer diagnosis.

The more commonly reported second primary cancers are breast, bone, and thyroid cancers, therapy-related myelodysplasia, and acute myeloid leukemia. Female survivors who were treated with chest or mantle radiation for a pediatric malignancy face a significantly increased risk of breast cancer.

Genetic predisposition was first noted to have a substantial impact on the risk of secondary sarcomas among patients with the genetic form of RB. This risk is further increased by radiation treatment and increases with the total dose of radiation delivered. Patients with a family history of early onset cancers have also been shown to be at an increased risk of developing a second cancer. Members of families with Li–Fraumeni syndrome have been reported to be at increased risk of multiple subsequent cancers, with the highest risk observed among survivors of childhood cancer.[144] The subsequent cancers reported in this population were characteristic of Li–Fraumeni syndrome. It therefore appears that germline mutations in tumor suppressor genes, as occurring in Li–Fraumeni syndrome, might interact with therapeutic exposures to result in an increased risk of second cancers.

Several genetic polymorphisms of enzymes capable of metabolic activation or detoxification of anticancer drugs, such as NAD(P)H:quinone oxidoreductase (NQO1), glutathione S-transferase (GST)-M1 and -T1, and CYP3A4, have been examined for their role in the development of therapy-related leukemia or myelodysplasia. These studies indicate that NQO1 polymorphism is significantly associated with the genetic risk of therapy-related acute leukemia and myelodysplasia. In addition, individuals with CYP3A4-W genotype may be at increased risk of treatment-related leukemia, presumably by increasing the production of reactive intermediates that damage DNA.[145,146]

Because subsequent malignancies remain a significant threat to the health of survivors treated for cancer during childhood, vigilant screening is important for those at risk. Risk of secondary acute myeloid leukemia is associated with exposure to topoisomerase II inhibitors (i.e., epipodophyllotoxins and anthracyclines) for up to 10 years and with alkylating agents for up to 15 years. In addition, there is a significant risk of breast cancer (females) and other solid tumors for survivors of Hodgkin disease who were treated with radiation therapy.

Neurocognitive sequelae of treatment of childhood cancer occur because of radiation to the whole brain, systemic therapy with high-dose methotrexate or cytarabine, or with intrathecal methotrexate and other agents. Children with a history of brain tumors, ALL, or NHL are most likely to be affected. Risk factors include increasing radiation dose, young age at the time of treatment, treatment with both cranial radiation and systemic or intrathecal chemotherapy, and female gender.[147–149] Severe deficits are most frequently noted in children with brain tumors treated with radiation therapy and in children who were less than 5 years of age at the time of treatment.

Chronic cardiotoxicity usually manifests itself as cardiomyopathy, pericarditis, and congestive heart failure. Childhood cancer survivors in the CCSS who were treated with chest or spinal radiation had a more than twofold increased risk of death related to cardiac disease in comparison with the standard US population.[150] The anthracyclines, doxorubicin and daunomycin, are well-known causes of cardiomyopathy.[151,152] The incidence of cardiomyopathy is dose-dependent and may exceed 30% among patients who received cumulative doses of anthracyclines in excess of $300 \, mg/m^2$. A cumulative dose of anthracyclines greater than $300 \, mg/m^2$ was associated with an increased risk of clinical heart failure (relative risk 11.8) compared to a cumulative dose lower than $300 \, mg/m^2$. The estimated risk of clinical heart failure increased with time and approached 5% after 15 years. These studies and others emphasize that cardiomyopathy can occur many years after completion of therapy (15–20 years) and that the onset may be spontaneous or coincide with exertion or pregnancy.

Pulmonary fibrosis and pneumonitis can result from pulmonary radiation. Thus, these problems are seen most often in patients with thoracic malignancies, notably Hodgkin disease. In addition to radiation therapy, a growing list of chemotherapeutic agents appears to be responsible for pulmonary disease in long-term survivors. Bleomycin toxicity is the prototype for chemotherapy-related lung injury. Although interstitial pneumonitis and pulmonary fibrosis have been reported in children, clinically apparent bleomycin pneumonopathy is most frequent in older adults. The chronic lung toxicity usually follows persistence or progression of abnormalities developing within 3 months of therapy. Alkylating agents also are believed to cause chronic lung injury. Following HSCT, both restrictive and obstructive lung disease, including bronchiolitis obliterans are well described.[153]

Chronic fibrosis of the liver is associated with radiation. Chemotherapy, even in the absence of radiation therapy, may be a cause of chronic hepatopathy. Viral hepatitis, most often related to transfusion of blood products prior to 1992, is another cause of chronic liver disease in long-term survivors.[154]

Damage to the proximal renal tubule from chemotherapy can cause Fanconi renal syndrome (hypokalemia, hypophosphatemia, glucosuria, proteinuria, renal tubular acidosis, and rickets). Children at particular risk include those who received treatment with more than one nephrotoxic agent and those with concomitant renal damage related to surgery or radiation.[155] Electrolyte wasting associated with ifosfamide therapy and hypomagnesemia associated with cisplatin therapy appear to persist in some children. Cyclophosphamide and ifosfamide are both capable of inducing hemorrhagic cystitis as a result of accumulation of acrolein in the bladder. Radiation to the pelvis or bladder can result in fibrosis and scarring, with resultant decreased bladder capacity and predisposition to urinary tract infections. Bladder cancer has developed in some patients who received bladder-toxic agents during treatment of childhood cancer. Yearly urinalysis should be done in these patients to evaluate for the presence of microscopic hematuria.

Decreased linear growth is a common problem during therapy in children with cancer. Although catch-up growth may occur, such that the premorbid growth status is regained, in some instances, short stature is permanent or even progressive. Severe growth retardation, defined as a standing height below the fifth percentile, has been observed in as many as 30–35% of survivors of childhood brain tumors[156] and in 10–15% of patients treated with some antileukemia regimens.[157] Whole-brain irradiation is a major risk factor for short stature, especially in doses exceeding 18 Gy.

Observational studies indicate that obesity as measured by weight or body mass index (BMI) has been reported in children with ALL and brain tumors treated with conventional therapy or BMT.[158] This problem has its onset either during therapy or within the first year after discontinuation of therapy and may either progress or stabilize. In addition, hypothyroidism is a common late effect and usually is due to radiation to the neck for a nonthyroid malignancy, which contributes to obesity.

All therapeutic modalities (radiation, surgery, or chemotherapy) cause both germ cell depletion and abnormalities of gonadal endocrine function among male cancer survivors.[159] Radiation to the testes is known to result in germinal loss with decrease in testicular volume and sperm production, and increases in follicle-stimulating hormone (FSH). Effects are dose-dependent, following fractionated exposures of 0.1–6 Gy. All males treated with inverted-Y radiation for HD at a cumulative testicular dose of 1.4–3.0 Gy become azoospermic without recovery after 2–40 months of follow-up, despite lead shielding of the scrotum. At doses of 4–6 Gy, azoospermia may persist for at least 3–5 years, and at doses above 6 Gy, usually appears to be irreversible. Alkylating agents decrease spermatogenesis in long-term survivors of cancer, and the effects are dose-dependent. Gonadal damage following cumulative doses lower than $7.5 \, mg/m^2$ of mechlorethamine or $200 \, mg/kg$ of cyclophosphamide as used in HSCT has been shown to be reversible in up to 70% of patients after therapy-free intervals of several years.

The gonadal toxicities are of serious concern to patients and their families. This concern has popularized pretreatment sperm banking. Unlike the males, germ cell failure and loss of ovarian endocrine function usually occur concomitantly in females. Following radiation therapy, manifestations are both age-dependent and dose-dependent. Prepubertal ovaries are relatively radioresistant because of the higher number of primordial follicles. Ovarian failure has also been associated with chemotherapy, such as single alkylating agents (cyclophosphamide, busulfan, nitrogen mustard) or as combination therapy. A report from the CCSS of 4029 pregnancies in 1915 female 5-year survivors of childhood cancer did not identify excess adverse outcomes for chemotherapeutic agents.[160] A companion study of 2323 pregnancies in partners of 1427 male survivors reported 69% live births, 1% stillbirths, 13% miscarriages, and 13% abortions (5% of outcomes were not accounted for).[161] The probability of a pregnancy ending in a live birth was significantly less than that for partners of male sibling controls (RR 0.8, $p = 0.007$).

Patients who desire to have children after completion of therapy may require care in high-risk obstetrical clinics, especially those who have a discussion of sperm banking storage received abdominal or pelvic irradiation. Because much remains unknown about the problems of children born to survivors of childhood cancer, long-term general follow-up should be emphasized.

Several potentially ototoxic agents are commonly used in the treatment of children with malignancies, including platinum-based chemotherapy, aminoglycoside antibiotics, loop diuretics, and RT. These agents are all capable of causing sensorineural hearing loss. Very young children who received ototoxic agents during their cancer treatment and whose speech has not yet developed should undergo audiologic evaluations to determine whether they require intervention. Interventions to assist children experiencing hearing loss because of cancer treatment include the use of hearing aids and other assistive devices, along with preferential seating in the front of the classroom. Musculoskeletal problems after childhood cancer involve bony abnormalities, such as scoliosis, atrophy, or hypoplasia; avascular necrosis (AVN); and osteoporosis (bone density ≥2.5 SD below mean)/osteopenia (bone density 1–2.5 SD below mean), especially with the use of steroids in ALL treatment.

Providing appropriate health care for survivors of cancer is emerging as one of the major challenges in medicine. Childhood cancer survivors, an especially high-risk population, seek and receive care from a wide variety of health care professionals, including oncologists, medical and pediatric specialists, surgeons, primary care physicians, gynecologists, nurses, psychologists, and social workers. The challenge arises from the heterogeneity of this patient population treated with numerous therapeutic modalities in an era of rapidly advancing understanding of late effects. The COG has recently updated risk-based, exposure-related guidelines [Long-Term Follow-Up Guidelines for Survivors of Childhood, Adolescent, and Young-adult Cancers, (version 4.0, 2013)] specifically designed to direct follow-up care for patients who were diagnosed and treated for pediatric malignancies. These guidelines represent a set of comprehensive screening recommendations that are clinically relevant and can be used to standardize and direct the follow-up care for this group of cancer survivors with specialized health care needs. <www.survivorshipguidelines.org>.

Acknowledgments

The authors acknowledge the previous contributors to this chapter as their work enabled the summary present here and the bibliography. They are Maura O'Leary, MD; Gregory H. Reaman, MD; Les Robison, PhD; Smita Bhatia, MD, MPH; Paul Gaynon, MD; Anne Angiolillo, MD; Janet Franklin, MD; Richard Aplenc, MD, MSCE; Beverly Lange, MD; Tobey McDonald, MD; Brian Rood, MD; James Nachman, MD; Mitchell Cairo, MD; Elizabeth Raetz, MD; Sherrie Perkins, MD; Carlos Rodriguez-Galindo, MD; Alberto Pappo, MD; Paul Grundy, MD; Jeffrey Dome, MD; John Kalapurakal, MD; Elizabeth Perlman, MD; Michael Ritchey, MD; John Maris, MD Suzanne Shustermann, MD; William Meyer,; MD; Kadria Sayed, MD; David Parham, MD; Richard Gorlick, MD, FAAP; Mark Bernstein, MD, FRCP(C); Jeffrey Toretsky, MD; R. Lor Randall, MD,FACS; Mark Gebhardt, MD; Lisa Teot, MD; Suzzane Wolden, MD; and Neyssa Marina, MD.

Key references

The complete reference list can be found on the Wiley Companion Digital Edition of this title (see inside front cover for login instructions).

1 Siegel DA, King J, Tai E, Buchanan N, Ajani UA, Li J. Cancer incidence rates and trends among children and adolescents in the United States, 2001–2009. *Pediatrics.* 2014;**134**(4):e945–e955.

2 Vogelstein B, Papadopoulos N, Velculescu VE, Zhou S, Diaz LA Jr, Kinzler KW. Cancer genome landscapes. *Science.* 2013;**339**(6127):1546–1558.

4 Smith MA, Altekruse SF, Adamson PC, Reaman GH, Seibel NL. Declining childhood and adolescent cancer mortality. *Cancer.* 2014;**120**(16):2497–2506.

6 Hunger SP, Lu X, Devidas M, et al. Improved survival for children and adolescents with acute lymphoblastic leukemia between 1990 and 2005: a report from the children's oncology group. *J Clin Oncol.* 2012;**30**(14):1663–1669.

10 Schultz KR, Pullen DJ, Sather HN, et al. Risk- and response-based classification of childhood B-precursor acute lymphoblastic leukemia: a combined analysis of prognostic markers from the pediatric oncology group (POG) and children's cancer group (CCG). *Blood.* 2007;**109**(3):926–935.

12 Borowitz MJ, Devidas M, Hunger SP, et al. Clinical significance of minimal residual disease in childhood acute lymphoblastic leukemia and its relationship to other prognostic factors: a children's oncology group study. *Blood.* 2008;**111**(12):5477–5485.

16 Pui C-H, Campana D, Pei D, et al. Treating childhood acute lymphoblastic leukemia without cranial irradiation. *N Engl J Med.* 2009;**360**(26):2730–2741.

19 Schultz KR, Carroll A, Heerema NA, et al. Long-term follow-up of imatinib in pediatric Philadelphia chromosome-positive acute lymphoblastic leukemia: children's oncology group study AALL0031. *Leukemia.* 2014;**28**(7):1467–1471.

31 Gamis AS, Alonzo TA, Perentesis JP, Meshinchi S. Children's oncology group's 2013 blueprint for research: acute myeloid leukemia. *Pediatr Blood Cancer.* 2013;**60**(6):964–971.

35 Cairo MS, Gerrard M, Sposto R, et al. Results of a randomized international study of high-risk central nervous system B non-Hodgkin lymphoma and B acute lymphoblastic leukemia in children and adolescents. *Blood.* 2007;**109**(7):2736–2743.

38 Goldman S, Smith L, Galardy P, et al. Rituximab with chemotherapy in children and adolescents with central nervous system and/or bone marrow-positive Burkitt lymphoma/leukaemia: a children's oncology group Report. *Br J Haematol.* 2014;**167**(3):394–401.

39 Mosse YP, Lim MS, Voss SD, et al. Safety and activity of crizotinib for paediatric patients with refractory solid tumours or anaplastic large-cell lymphoma: a children's oncology group phase 1 consortium study. *Lancet Oncol.* 2013;**14**(6):472–480.

40 Gopal AK, Chen R, Smith SE, et al. Durable remissions in a pivotal phase 2 study of brentuximab vedotin in relapsed or refractory Hodgkin lymphoma. *Blood.* 2015;**125**(8):1236–1243.

41 Friedman DL, Chen L, Wolden S, et al. Dose-intensive response-based chemotherapy and radiation therapy for children and adolescents with newly diagnosed intermediate-risk hodgkin lymphoma: a report from the Children's Oncology Group Study AHOD0031. *J Clin Oncol.* 2014;**32**(32):3651–3658.

42 Dome JS, Fernandez CV, Mullen EA, et al. Children's oncology group's 2013 blueprint for research: renal tumors. *Pediatr Blood Cancer.* 2013;**60**(6):994–1000.

49 Lemerle J, Voute PA, Tournade MF, et al. Effectiveness of preoperative chemotherapy in Wilms' tumor: results of an International Society of Paediatric Oncology (SIOP) clinical trial. *J Clin Oncol.* 1983;**1**(10):604–609.

59 London WB, Castleberry RP, Matthay KK, et al. Evidence for an age cutoff greater than 365 days for neuroblastoma risk group stratification in the children's oncology group. *J Clin Oncol.* 2005;**23**(27):6459–6465.

64 Maris JM. Recent advances in neuroblastoma. *N Engl J Med.* 2010;**362**(23):2202–2211.

70 Cohn SL, Pearson AD, London WB, et al. The International Neuroblastoma Risk Group (INRG) classification system: an INRG Task Force report. *J Clin Oncol.* 2009;**27**(**2**):289–297.

71 Park JR, Bagatell R, London WB, et al. Children's oncology group's 2013 blueprint for research: neuroblastoma. *Pediatr Blood Cancer.* 2013;**60**(**6**):985–993.

74 Yu AL, Gilman AL, Ozkaynak MF, et al. Anti-GD2 antibody with GM-CSF, interleukin-2, and isotretinoin for neuroblastoma. *N Engl J Med.* 2010;**363**(**14**):1324–1334.

81 Link MP, Goorin AM, Miser AW, et al. The effect of adjuvant chemotherapy on relapse-free survival in patients with osteosarcoma of the extremity. *N Engl J Med.* 1986;**314**(**25**):1600–1606.

85 Gorlick R, Janeway K, Lessnick S, Randall RL, Marina N, on behalf of the COG-BTC. Children's oncology group's 2013 blueprint for research: bone tumors. *Pediatr Blood Cancer.* 2013;**60**(**6**):1009–1015.

89 Grier HE, Krailo MD, Tarbell NJ, et al. Addition of ifosfamide and etoposide to standard chemotherapy for Ewing's sarcoma and primitive neuroectodermal tumor of bone. *N Engl J Med.* 2003;**348**(**8**):694–701.

90 Womer RB, West DC, Krailo MD, et al. Randomized controlled trial of interval-compressed chemotherapy for the treatment of localized Ewing sarcoma: a report from the children's oncology group. *J Clin Oncol.* 2012;**30**(**33**):4148–4154.

93 Pappo AS, Shapiro DN, Crist WM, Maurer HM. Biology and therapy of pediatric rhabdomyosarcoma. *J Clin Oncol.* 1995;**13**(**8**):2123–2139.

96 Hawkins DS, Spunt SL, Skapek SX. Children's oncology group's 2013 blueprint for research: soft tissue sarcomas. *Pediatr Blood Cancer.* 2013;**60**(**6**):1001–1008.

97 Walterhouse DO, Pappo AS, Meza JL, et al. Shorter-duration therapy using vincristine, dactinomycin, and lower-dose cyclophosphamide with or without radiotherapy for patients with newly diagnosed low-risk rhabdomyosarcoma: a report from the Soft Tissue Sarcoma Committee of the Children's Oncology Group. *J Clin Oncol.* 2014;**32**(**31**):3547–3552.

98 Hawkins DSAJ, Mascarenhas L. Vincristine, dactinomycin, cyclophosphamide (VAC) versus VAC/V plus irinotecan (VI) for intermediate-risk rhabdomyosarcoma (IRRMS): a report from the Children's Oncology Group Soft Tissue Sarcoma Committee. American Soceity of Clinical Oncology ASCO annual meeting abstract. *J Clin Oncol.* 2014;**32**:5s(suppl; abstr 10004).

100 Spunt SLML, Anderson JR. Risk-based treatment for nonrhabdomyosarcoma soft tissue sarcomas (NRSTS) in patients under 30 years of age: children's oncology group study ARST0332. American Soceity of Clinical Oncology ASCO annual meeting abstract. *J Clin Oncol.* 2014;**32**:5s(suppl; abstr 10008).

102 Rickert C, Paulus W. Epidemiology of central nervous system tumors in childhood and adolescence based on the new WHO classification. *Childs Nerv Syst.* 2001;**17**(**9**):503–511.

104 Northcott PA, Korshunov A, Witt H, et al. Medulloblastoma comprises four distinct molecular variants. *J Clin Oncol.* 2011;**29**(**11**):1408–1414.

109 Rodriguez-Galindo C, Orbach DB, VanderVeen D. Retinoblastoma. *Pediatr Clin North Am.* 2015;**62**(**1**):201–223.

126 Frazier AL, Hale JP, Rodriguez-Galindo C, et al. Revised risk classification for pediatric extracranial germ cell tumors based on 25 years of clinical trial data from the United kingdom and United States. *J Clin Oncol.* 2015;**33**(**2**):195–201.

127 Rodriguez-Galindo C, Krailo M, Frazier L, et al. Children's Oncology Group's 2013 blueprint for research: rare tumors. *Pediatr Blood Cancer.* 2013;**60**(**6**):1016–1021.

128 Billmire DF, Cullen JW, Rescorla FJ, et al. Surveillance after initial surgery for pediatric and adolescent girls with stage I ovarian germ cell tumors: report from the children's oncology group. *J Clin Oncol.* 2014;**32**(**5**):465–470.

134 Brown J, Perilongo G, Shafford E, et al. Pretreatment prognostic factors for children with hepatoblastoma—results from the International Society of Paediatric Oncology (SIOP) study SIOPEL 1. *Eur J Cancer.* 2000;**36**(**11**):1418–1425.

147 Mulhern RK, Merchant TE, Gajjar A, Reddick WE, Kun LE. Late neurocognitive sequelae in survivors of brain tumours in childhood. *Lancet Oncol.* 2004;**5**(**7**):399–408.

149 Krull KR, Brinkman TM, Li C, et al. Neurocognitive outcomes decades after treatment for childhood acute lymphoblastic leukemia: a report from the St Jude lifetime cohort study. *J Clin Oncol.* 2013;**31**(**35**):4407–4415.

152 van der Pal HJ, van Dalen EC, van Delden E, et al. High risk of symptomatic cardiac events in childhood cancer survivors. *J Clin Oncol.* 2012;**30**(**13**):1429–1437.

72 Cancer and pregnancy

Jennifer K. Litton, MD

Overview

The diagnosis of cancer during pregnancy is a clinical and emotional challenge for both the patient and the caregivers. A multidisciplinary approach including medical oncologists, surgeons, radiation oncologists, and obstetrics is vital to coordinate the treatment of the mother and the monitoring of the fetus. The available data regarding the treatment of cancer during pregnancy, including staging, surgery, radiation, and systemic therapy as well as outcomes for the patients and the children exposed to chemotherapy *in utero* is reviewed.

The diagnosis of cancer during pregnancy presents a complex set of challenges for the patient, family members, and physicians. The welfare of the mother may be perceived to be threatened by the pregnancy owing to concerns regarding the disease, diagnostic and therapeutic procedures required for treatment, and a desire to avoid harm to the fetus during treatment for the mother's malignancy. Many have perceived that treatment may require compromise of the wellbeing of either the mother or the fetus. However, in some circumstances, fetal death may be an unavoidable consequence of cancer treatment. Frequently, however, judicious decision making not only can provide appropriate cancer care for the pregnant woman but also will preserve the pregnancy through successful labor and delivery.

Many issues arise in the realm of concurrent cancer and pregnancy (Table 1). The data for specific tumor types, diagnostic procedures, therapeutic interventions, and long-term cancer outcomes have been derived primarily from case reports, small case series, and retrospective reviews. Controlled studies are rare, and prospective data is even rarer. Data on labor and delivery outcomes for patients completing pregnancy remains scarce, as are long-term data on growth and development of children exposed to cancer treatment *in utero*. Over the past decade, the treatment for cancer during pregnancy has evolved and is now within guidelines of care for several tumor types as cohort descriptions and prospective case series have been reported.[1] With that, there is emerging data on outcomes of patients as well as small, but emerging data on the children exposed to chemotherapy *in utero*.

Cancer and pregnancy epidemiology

The diagnosis of cancer during pregnancy is rare and tracking the true incidence remains challenging. Much of the data includes pregnancy-associated breast cancers, defined as those cancers diagnosed both during pregnancy and within the 1-year period after delivery. With emerging data that biology and outcomes may be influenced by the timing of diagnosis, evaluating and reporting these incidences separately may be important. Smith et al.[2] used the California Cancer Registry, evaluating 4,846,505 women of whom 4539 had an identified invasive malignancy either during pregnancy or within 12 months after delivery. In this analysis, cancer occurred in approximately 1 in 1000 deliveries from 1991 through 1999. However, 64% of these cases occurred within the 12 months after delivery. Per 1000 live singleton births, the most common tumor types were breast (0.19), thyroid (0.14), cervix (0.12), melanoma (0.09), Hodgkin's disease (0.05), ovarian leukemia (0.05), and acute leukemia (0.04). In an Australian linkage study between 1994 and 2008, 1798 pregnancy-associated cancers, encompassing diagnoses both during and within 1 year from delivery, were identified in 1,309,501 deliveries.[3] Four hundred and ninety five of these cancers were identified during pregnancy. During pregnancy, the most common cancer identified in this cohort was melanoma (15.1/100,00), breast (7.3/100,000), thyroid (3.2/100,000), and gynecological (3.9/100,000). However, cancer from nearly any anatomic location can occur with pregnancy.

Interestingly, in this study from Australia, and others, the incidence of pregnancy-associated breast cancer has been increasing. This may be secondary to increasing maternal age as well as other changes in epidemiological risk factors. In the Australian cohort, from 1994 to 2007, the incidence of pregnancy-associated breast cancer increased from 112.3 to 191.5/100,000 deliveries. A Swedish registry also showed a trend to increasing incidence that may be partially explained by advancing maternal age, with an increase of 16.0 to 37.4 cases per 100,000 deliveries from the beginning to the end of cohorts collected from 1963 to 2002.[4] This may also be influenced as further advances in reproductive technologies are making pregnancies more accessible to older women.

Diagnosis and staging

A biopsy, with review of cytologic and histologic materials, is required for the diagnosis of any malignancy during pregnancy. The type of biopsy is determined by the accessibility of the disease site and the quantity of material required.

If a surgical biopsy if required, the anatomic location of the biopsy and the gestational age of the fetus are factors to be considered before proceeding. A surgical biopsy can be performed safely.[1,5,6] It is imperative that adequate material for pathologic diagnosis and required studies be obtained; for example, hormone receptors and HER-2/neu status are necessary for the proper evaluation of breast cancer, and morphologic and immuno-phenotyping of lymphomas and leukemias is essential to their optimal assessment and treatment.

Staging provides guidance for discussions regarding cancer prognosis, recommended loco-regional and/or systemic therapies, and potential risks of treatment in relation to benefit and outcome for the patient. Frequently, staging assessment in the non-pregnant patient involves exposure to ionizing radiation, which is to be avoided whenever possible during pregnancy. The impact of

Holland-Frei Cancer Medicine, Ninth Edition. Edited by Robert C. Bast Jr., Carlo M. Croce, William N. Hait, Waun Ki Hong, Donald W. Kufe, Martine Piccart-Gebhart, Raphael E. Pollock, Ralph R. Weichselbaum, Hongyang Wang, and James F. Holland.
© 2017 John Wiley & Sons, Inc. ISBN: 978-1-118-93469-2

Table 1 Issues related to cancer and pregnancy.

Impact of cancer on pregnancy
Impact of pregnancy on cancer
Termination of pregnancy/fetal death with cancer treatment
Diagnostic procedures and staging during pregnancy
Cancer treatment, maternal effects
Cancer treatment, fetal effects
Placental metastasis
Transplacental malignancy
Long-term outcome for children
Ethical, moral, and legal concerns
The UNKNOWN

radiation upon the fetus varies with respect to fetal gestational age. Pre-implantation and fetal organogenesis are most sensitive to the negative effects of radiation exposure.[7] Fetal exposures of < 5 cGy are not thought to be harmful.[8] With abdominal computerized tomography, exposure may be as high as 30 mSv. As a consequence of known fetal toxicity associated with exposure to ionizing radiation during pregnancy, abdominal shielding and non-ionizing techniques should be used whenever possible during these imaging procedures.[8] Ultrasonography (US) for breast, liver, and other abdominal organ imaging can also contribute to the staging evaluation without ionizing radiation. Magnetic resonance imaging (MRI) can be used to assess for bone and liver diseases, as well as fetal abnormalities, if required.[9,10] The use of gadolinium as a contrast agent for MRI during pregnancy remains controversial. Although multiple case reports have not demonstrated an increase in adverse effects to the fetus, gadolinium is often avoided if possible owing to lack of toxicity information.[11-13] Accurate determination of disease stage is essential in ensuring accurate cancer treatment decisions, and findings during the staging process also may influence the woman's decision regarding the maintenance of her pregnancy.

The use of PET/CT scanning has become standard in the treatment and evaluation of lymphomas and has had an increase in use in evaluation of metastatic disease in solid tumors as well. There is very limited data regarding the use of PET/CT in the pregnant breast cancer patient. Evidence that FDG crosses the placenta and can accumulate in fetal brain, bladder, and cardiac tissue has been demonstrated in animal studies.[14] Zanotti-Fregonara et al.[15] estimated that the FDG uptake by embryo tissues in early pregnancy is at least 3.3E-2mGy/MBq in a patient found to be pregnant at the time of scanning. Few other case reports exist. Hove et al.[16] describe an 18-year-old woman with Hodgkin's disease who underwent PET/CT. There was significant uptake in the fetal myocardium. The patient developed HELLP syndrome and the child was delivered at 31 weeks by caesarian section. Therefore, there is insufficient safety data to support the use of PET/CT scanning during pregnancy and should be delayed until after delivery whenever possible.

Cancer treatment during pregnancy

The optimal treatment of cancer during pregnancy requires a meticulously coordinated multidisciplinary approach. Careful and repeated consultations with the obstetrician and/or maternal fetal medicine specialist are essential during the course of the pregnancy. Accurate assessment of fetal age, maturation, and the expected delivery date must be performed before treatment planning. The therapeutic options for the pregnant patient do not differ from those of the non-pregnant patient with cancer, but the application of treatment may be more complex. When evaluating multiple tumor types during pregnancy, Stensheim et al.[17] described 516

women from Norwegian health registries with no difference identified in cause-specific death. However, it is interesting to note that when diagnosed instead during lactation, there was an increase in both breast and ovarian death rates. Outcomes in large cohorts are otherwise described with cancer-specific sites and the timing and treatment are important in relation to the outcomes of the patient.

Surgery

Surgery remains the mainstay for treatment of solid tumors, and pregnancy is not a contraindication for cancer surgery. Mazze and Kallen[6] have reported on a registry series of 5405 pregnant patients on whom emergency surgery was performed. They did not observe an increased incidence of congenital malformations or stillbirths in women who had surgical procedures while pregnant. An increased frequency of low- and very low birth-weight infants was noted and attributed to prematurity and intrauterine growth retardation and may have been influenced by the underlying reason behind the necessary surgery. No specific type of surgical procedure or anesthesia was associated with an increase in adverse reproductive outcomes. In a case-control study, Duncan et al.[18] did not observe an increase in congenital anomalies in 2565 pregnant women who had surgery while pregnant, when compared to control patients who did not have surgery. If warranted by tumor type and disease stage, surgery should proceed and should be coordinated with the obstetrician, anesthesiologist, and neonatal specialist.

Radiation

Pregnancy has been considered an absolute contraindication to radiation therapy for cancer. Radiation therapy for cervical cancer during pregnancy usually leads to fetal death and spontaneous abortion.[19] The fetus is most sensitive to malformation from radiation exposure 2 to 8 weeks after conception, whereas exposure from 8 to 25 weeks of gestation may have a greater risk of mental retardation.[7] Nevertheless, successful radiation therapy of pregnant women with Hodgkin's disease has been reported.[20] If radiation is warranted, appropriate fetal shielding, careful dosimetry calculations, and estimates of fetal dose exposure are necessary. However, owing to the very limited safety, data should be considered only in very select cases.[21-25] Radiation therapy for breast cancer, following mastectomy or breast conservation surgery, can usually be delayed until the postpartum period, especially if chemotherapy is administered.

Systemic therapy

Many different agents have been reported to have been used in pregnancy. Representative chemotherapeutic, hormone, and biologic agents are listed in Table 2.

Systemic therapy is of concern because of the potential deleterious effects on the fetus. Physiologic changes associated with pregnancy (elevated blood volume, increased cardiac output, amplified glomerular filtration rate, and changes in circulating protein levels) make predictions about drug pharmacokinetics uncertain at best.[26] In addition, systemic agents are designed to be anti-proliferative compounds, and their administration during pregnancy poses genuine risk to the developing fetus. Potential concerns include stillbirth, spontaneous abortion, fetal malformations/teratogenesis, organ-specific toxicities, intrauterine growth retardation with low birth weight, and premature delivery.[27]

Table 2 Drugs reported to have been used during pregnancy.

Regimens	Systemic therapies	
MACOP-B	Hydroxyurea	α-Interferon
MOPP-ABVD	All-trans retinoic acid	Rituximab
FAC	Methotrexate	Trastuzumab
CMF	Doxorubicin/epirubicin	Lapatinib
AC	Cyclophosphamide and nitrogen mustard	Imatinib
VACOP-B	Vincristine and triethylene melamine	Prednisone
CHOP	Bleomycin	Tamoxifen
BEP	Cisplatin	Erythropoietin
	Vinorelbine, vinblastine, and vincristine	Filgrastim
	Paclitaxel	Dasatinib
	Docetaxel	
	Etoposide	
	Idarubicin and daunorubicin	
	Cytosine-arabinosine	
	5-Fluororucil, busulfan	
	Teniposide	
	6-Mercaptopurine	
	Dacarbazine	
	Aminopterin	
	Actimomycin D	
	Procarbazine	
	Amsacrine	
	L-asparaginase	

ABVD, Adriamycin (doxorubicin), bleomycin, vinblastine, and dacarbazine; AC, Adriamycin (doxorubicin) and cyclophosphamide; CMF, cyclophosphamide, methotrexate, and 5-fluorouracil; FAC, 5-fluorouracil, Adriamycin (doxorubicin), and cyclophosphamide; MACOP-B, methotrexate, Adriamycin (doxorubicin), cyclophosphamide, Oncovin (vincristine), prednisone, and bleomycin; MOPP, mechlorethamine, Oncovin (vincristine) procarbazine, and prednisone; and VACOP-B, VePesid (etoposide), Adriamycin (doxorubicin), cyclophosphamide, Oncovin (vincristine), prednisone, and bleomycin.

In addition to cytotoxic therapy, there are also reports regarding supportive medications. Erythropoietin use during pregnancy was reported by Scott et al.[28] as well as others. No maternal or fetal toxicities have been noted. FDA Black Box warnings about the use of erythropoietin in breast cancer patients would apply to the pregnant patient as well, even in the absence of specific risk data in these patients. Dale et al.[29] found that the use of filgrastim during pregnancy was not associated with a change in neonatal outcome, when compared to untreated patients. There have been limited case reports of the safe use of pegfilgrastim during pregnancy after dose-dense chemotherapy for breast cancer.[30] Dexamethasone and lorazepam have also been reported as premedications without significant toxicity.[9]

Outcomes in the children exposed to chemotherapy *in utero*

The fetal risks related to chemotherapy appear to be greatest during the first trimester of pregnancy. Doll et al.[27] reviewed antineoplastic agents and fetal malformations in relation to the trimester of pregnancy. They reported that *in utero* exposure to systemic agents was associated fetal malformation risks of 14% and 19% for alkylating agents and antimetabolites, respectively. A similar review of second- and third-trimester exposure demonstrated a 1.3% incidence of fetal malformation. Thus, they concluded that single-agent or combination chemotherapy could be given during the second and third trimesters with low risk of fetal malformation, but these agents should be avoided during the first trimester of pregnancy. Similarly, in a review of cytotoxic agents used during pregnancy, Ebert et al.[26] collected 217 cases from the literature published between 1983 and 1995. They classified the use of the agents by disease category and analyzed outcome of pregnancy in

relation to agent, dose, and gestational age at exposure. There were 94 cases of leukemia, 57 cases of lymphoma, 26 cases of breast or ovarian cancer, 16 cases of cytotoxic therapy used for rheumatic diseases, and the remainder of the malignancies. Eighteen newborns were reported to have congenital developmental abnormalities. Of these 18 newborns, 15 neonates had been exposed to cytotoxic drugs during the first trimester. Chromosomal abnormalities were noted in two neonates who had experienced exposure to cytotoxic agents during the first trimester.[26] Antimetabolite use was found in 50% of the neonates with congenital abnormalities following first trimester exposure to chemotherapy. Of the reviewed cases, 82.3% of leukemia patients, 75.4% of lymphoma patients, and 75% of breast or ovary cancer patients with associated pregnancies were reported to have live births with normally developed neonates. Germann et al.[31] collected data involving 160 patients who received anthracyclines during pregnancy. In this group, five cases of fetal malformations (3%) were found, with three cases occurring with the use of chemotherapy in the first trimester. The remaining two cases of fetal malformation occurred after chemotherapy administration in the second trimester; one involved Down's syndrome unrelated to chemotherapy, and the other involved a congenital adherence of the iris to the cornea that demonstrated no clinical consequence. The combination chemotherapy regimens associated with fetal malformations included cytosine arabinoside or cyclophosphamide. As these initial reports that there have been multiple case studies showing safety of systemic therapy with anthracyclines and taxanes as well as limited information regarding platinums when treated in the second and third trimesters.[32–34] Systemic treatment, especially with antimetabolites such as methotrexate, should be avoided during the first trimester of pregnancy except in circumstances in which delay in cancer treatment would jeopardize the life of the patient, such as acute leukemia.

A long-term report on children exposed to chemotherapy *in utero* during treatment of mothers for a variety of hematologic malignancies has been presented by Aviles and Neri.[35] They described 84 children followed a median of 18.7 years. Thirty-eight had been exposed to chemotherapy *in utero* during the first trimester of pregnancy. Fertility was reported to be preserved, some of the chemotherapy-exposed children having become parents. No learning, neurologic, or psychological problems were reported for any of the *in utero* chemotherapy-exposed subjects. Van Calsteren et al.[36] report on ten children from nine pregnancies exposed to chemotherapy *in utero* for differing primary cancers. The children who were born prematurely had multiple abnormalities ranging from speech delay to mental and motor retardation. These were children born at less than 33 weeks gestation. Echocardiograms were also obtained demonstrating a tendency towards a thinner ventricular wall. Abdel-Hady et al.[37] describe 118 children born to mothers who received chemotherapy during pregnancy with no significant difference when compared to a control group of children.

Much of the data in the children exposed to chemotherapy has come from studies of breast cancer diagnosed and treated during pregnancy. Murthy et al.[38] have updated on the outcomes of the children exposed to chemotherapy *in utero*. Complications for the neonate included prematurity, neutropenia, tachypnea of the newborn, and respiratory distress syndrome. One case of spontaneous cryptogenic intracranial hemorrhage occurred which all resolved. There were three congenital abnormalities reported which included Down syndrome (1), congenital ureteral reflux (1), and clubfoot (1).[38] Cardonick et al.[39] also described a voluntary registry of outcomes in children exposed to chemotherapy demonstrating a 3.8% rate of congenital malformations which is similar to the national average of pregnant patients without cancer. Loibl et al.[40] reviewed a registry of patients diagnosed with breast cancer during pregnancy from multiple different European sites. Of the 447 patients followed, 197 received chemotherapy during pregnancy from 2003 to 2011. Of these, 22 babies had reported complications and were delivered before the 37th week with four congenital malformations (trisomy 18, rectal atresia, polydactylia, and craniosynostosis). Nine of these babies were delivered after the 37th week with three malformations (asymmetric head, polydactyly, and Moebius syndrome). When evaluating for longer term outcomes in children exposed to chemotherapy *in utero*, Amant et al.[41] described 70 children and evaluated that for neurocognitive and cardiac outcomes as well as general health, there was no significant finding except for those children who were born prematurely. Both of these studies highlight the need for to avoid iatrogenic preterm delivery whenever possible, with holding treatment past the 35th week of pregnancy in order to avoid blood nadirs and allowing the children to proceed full term.

Specific cancers

Breast cancer

The diagnosis of breast cancer during pregnancy is often delayed, presumably due to the anatomical and physiologic changes in the pregnant breast.[42] However, women with breast cancer during pregnancy have demonstrated the same survival rates, stage for stage, as non-pregnant patients with breast cancer.[34,43,44] Imaging, local, and systemic therapies have been well described in the successful treatment of breast cancer diagnosed during pregnancy.

Imaging of the breast in women with a palpable mass or thickening is warranted, especially if it persists for 2 weeks or longer. Mammography and US may confirm the presence of a malignant mass. Although Max and Klamer reported normal mammograms in six of eight women with breast cancer during pregnancy, others have reported abnormal mammograms in the majority of women with pregnancy and breast cancer (18 of 23 and 5 of 8).[45–47] There are limited data on US; Liberman reported positive findings in six of six patients, and Samuels found positive findings in two of four patients.[46,47] Yang et al.[48] diagnosed 100% of the masses as well as axillary metastases in 18 of 20 women. US was also shown to be effective for restaging to evaluate response to pre-operative chemotherapy in the pregnant breast.[48] US may be useful for guiding either fine needle aspiration (FNA) or core biopsy in order to confirm a diagnosis of malignancy.[49–51] Chest radiography, liver US, and MRI of the thoracic/lumbar spine can be used to assess for extant organ metastasis.[1,9]

Lymph node evaluations can be tailored to clinical findings. If clinically suspicious regional nodes are identified on physical examination or by imaging techniques, an FNA that is guided by palpation or US can be utilized to confirm metastases. The theoretical dosage of radiation that would be absorbed by the fetus following sentinel lymph node biopsy has been calculated to be less than 5 cGy.[52,53] Khera et al.[54] have reported their experience with sentinel node procedures in the pregnant patient. Ten patients had sentinel node procedures, six with blue dye and Tc99m, two with Tc99m alone, and two with blue dye alone. No adverse sequelae were reported for nine neonates. One woman chose elective termination of pregnancy. Gropper et al.[55] have published their series of 25 women who underwent sentinel lymph node dissections during pregnancy with no procedure complications. Gentilini et al. have performed the technique on 12 patients with one child born with a ventricular septal defect.[10]

Breast-conserving surgery is possible with postpartum breast irradiation. Pre- or postoperative chemotherapy is used with the same criteria for selection of therapy as in the non-pregnant patient. However, breast-conserving therapy should be considered only when radiation can be given in a timely manner after delivery. Often, given the timing of chemotherapy, this will allow for postpartum radiation. Dominici et al.[49] have described a single institution experience of mastectomy versus breast-conserving surgery as well as biopsy procedures with no significant difference in wound complications or complications from FNA or core biopsies.

Other agents have been described in the literature to treat breast cancer and include vinorelbine, paclitaxel, docetaxel, and cisplatin.[56,57] The use of taxanes, both paclitaxel and docetaxel, has been described also in the second and third trimesters[56,58–65] with all available follow-up data reported healthy children.[56] Vinorelbine has been reported to be used in both adjuvant and metastatic settings, with five of the six children reported healthy at 6–35 months of follow-up. Information on one of the children was not available in the literature. Neonatal complications included one episode of grade 4 neutropenia and transient cytopenia at day 6 of life.[63,66–68] Multiple case reports of trastuzumab administered during pregnancy have been identified. This has been associated with oligo- and anhydramnios with its use was described in case reports.[62,66,69–73] One case was of reversible heart failure in the mother with no anhydramnios in the fetus was reported.[71] One of the children born developed respiratory failure, capillary leak syndrome, infections, and necrotizing enterocolitis, dying from multiple organ failure 21 weeks after delivery.[73] In addition, Bader et al.[62] described a case of reversible renal failure in the fetus. One report of the use of lapatinib was recently described in a patient who conceived while on lapatinib. Despite approximately 11 weeks of exposure, the pregnancy was otherwise uncomplicated with the delivery of a healthy baby.[74] Routine administration of biologic agents is not recommended during pregnancy and trastuzumab now has an FDA Category D rating.

Tamoxifen is a standard treatment for hormone receptor positive tumors in pre-menopausal women. Although some case reports of tamoxifen fetal exposure demonstrated no effect on the newborn, there are other reports including Goldenhar syndrome (microtia, preauricular skin tags, and hemifacial microsomia),[75] ambiguous genitalia, and other birth defects. In addition, vaginal bleeding and spontaneous abortion have also been reported.[75–79] Braems et al.[80] described 11 babies with congenital malformations out of 44 live births and 3 stillbirths. Aromatase inhibitors are not indicated as a single agent in pre-menopausal women and should not be used in conjunction with ovarian suppression in a pregnant patient. Endocrine therapy should be delayed until after delivery.

Outcomes of pregnant breast cancer patients appear to be similar to non-pregnant cancer patients when treated with appropriate therapies in the second and third trimesters. Litton et al.[81] have described the outcomes of a single institution cohort treated at the University of Texas MD Anderson Cancer Center since 1989 where all women presented for early-stage breast cancer and received chemotherapy with 5-fluoruracil, doxorubicin, and cyclophosphamide (FAC) in the second and third trimesters of pregnancy. There were all live births. Rouzier et al.[82] reviewed 48 patients with pregnancy-associated breast cancer and have concluded that chemosensitivity and pathological response rates were modeled to be similar in pregnant and non-pregnant breast cancer patients. Amant et al. compared 311 women to 865 non-pregnant breast cancer patients with no statistically significant difference in OS.

Azim et al.[33] performed a meta-analysis of 30 studies of PABC which did show a higher risk of relapse and death. However, this did not hold true for the diagnosis during pregnancy which may further emphasize the importance of separating the situations of being diagnosed during versus after pregnancy. This analysis also included multiple older studies that either delayed or gave substandard therapy to pregnant patients that may also have affected survival outcomes.

Thyroid cancer

In pregnant women, thyroid cancer presents most often as an asymptomatic nodule in the neck. Ultrasound evaluation can confirm the size and solid character of the nodule. FNA biopsy is the most reliable diagnostic test and is safe and accurate during pregnancy.[83-85] Most often, pregnancy-associated thyroid cancers are differentiated thyroid cancers (DTC). Radioiodine scans and therapeutic radioiodine should not be given during pregnancy and can be safely delayed until after delivery.[86] Thyroid surgery can be delayed until after delivery for many patients, especially if the diagnosis is made during the third trimester of pregnancy.[86,87] If warranted, thyroid resection can be done under local anesthesia.[88] Moosa and Mazzaferi[89] reported on 61 pregnant patients with thyroid cancer and 528 age-matched non-pregnant controls. They reviewed diagnosis, treatment, and outcome for the two cohorts. Seventy-four percent of the pregnant patients had been discovered to possess an asymptomatic thyroid nodule during routine examinations. Twenty percent of the pregnant patients underwent thyroid surgery during the second trimester, while 77% of patients underwent surgery following delivery. Thirty percent of the patients received postoperative iodine-131 therapy; all of these treatments were administered postpartum. The presence of pregnancy or delayed surgery did not result in differences in cancer recurrence, distant recurrence, or death. On the basis of these findings, Moosa and Mazzaferi[89] concluded that treatment for thyroid cancer during pregnancy may be delayed until after delivery in most patients. In addition,, Yasmeen et al.[90] reviewed data from the California Cancer Registry of 595 women diagnosed with thyroid cancer within 9 months antepartum to 12 months postpartum, compared to matched non-pregnant counterparts, and no significant differences were found in overall survival, maternal, or fetal outcomes. Alves et al.[91] performed a systematic review of four studies in total, including the two mentioned earlier, and there was no change in long-term survival outcomes between pregnant and non-pregnant DTC patients.

Cervical cancer

Evaluation of extent of disease for diagnosed cervical cancer includes physical examination and assessment of pelvic anatomic structures by MRI. Laparoscopic lymph node surgery has been reported.[92] Treatment options vary with disease stage, gestational age at diagnosis, and the desires of the patient. For stage I disease, Sorosky et al.[93] have reported a favorable outcome with only planned follow-up observation until the third trimester. They followed eight women with stage I disease, <2.5 cm in dimension, for a mean interval of 109 days. All patients underwent delivery via caesarean delivery, followed by radical hysterectomy. Serial MRIs was used to follow the disease for two patients, and no clinical disease progression was noted. After treatment, all patients were alive and free of disease at a mean follow-up of 37 months.

In a review of 22 patients with cervical cancer diagnosed during pregnancy or within 12 months postpartum, Allen et al.[94] noted 20 live deliveries and only one disease recurrence. Nine of eleven patients with microinvasive disease were treated with core biopsy only. Ten patients with stage IB or IIA disease were treated with radical hysterectomy, and one patient with stage IIIB disease received

chemotherapy, radiation therapy, and simple hysterectomy as treatment. Allen recommended all pregnant women undergo cervical cytologic evaluation. Cone biopsy is safe in pregnancy and may be adequate treatment for microinvasive disease.[94]

Outcome and recurrence risk have been assessed in relation to method of delivery for women diagnosed with cervix cancer during pregnancy or within 6 months postpartum. Sood et al.[95] followed 83 pregnant women with cervical cancer; 56 of these patients were diagnosed with during pregnancy, and 27 patients were diagnosed postpartum. As the risk of recurrence was increased in those diagnosed postpartum who delivered vaginally, Sood et al. concluded that women with cervical cancer should be delivered by caesarean. However, van der Vange et al.,[96] in a case-control study, reported that mode of delivery had no effect on survival. Overall, they noted no difference in survival of pregnant patients with cervical cancer compared to the non-pregnant group. Systemic chemotherapy for cervical cancer can be effective when given during pregnancy. Most of the reported therapies have been platinum based and administered with several other agents such as vincristine and bleomycin.[97] However, neoadjuvant chemotherapy regimens have been described and include paclitaxel plus either cisplatin or carboplatin.[97-99] There are several case reports describing the use of neoadjuvant cisplatin-based regimens with either taxane or vinorelbine used in order to preserve the pregnancy until the fetus is viable with good maternal and fetal outcomes.[100-102]

Treatment of the pregnant patient with cervical cancer requires careful consideration of disease stage and gestational age. Early in pregnancy with early stage disease, pregnancy termination followed by cancer treatment may be appropriate. Alternatively, planned delay in cancer treatment with careful monitoring of disease may allow for successful completion of the pregnancy.[93] Radiation therapy will likely cause fetal death and usually results in spontaneous abortion.[19]

As a significant population of patients is diagnosed with cervical cancer while in childbearing age, the concern for preservation of fertility has led to the utilization of radical vaginal trachelectomy with pelvic lymphadenectomy, instead of radical hysterectomy, in select patients with Stage I cervical cancer. Burnett et al.[103] made this procedure available to 21 patients over a period of 6 years with 18 of 21 patients received radical trachelectomy in order to preserve fertility. Within this group, one patient gave birth to healthy twins, delivered at 24 weeks, following superovulation treatment. One patient delivered a singleton term infant via caesarean hysterectomy; no residual disease was found in the cervix. The last patient most likely became pregnant in the week before the radical vaginal trachelectomy. She had spontaneous rupture of membranes at 20 weeks gestation, requiring hysterotomy for evacuation of the uterus with subsequent neonatal demise. Multiple other groups have described success in this procedure for fertility preservation.[104,105] There are only a few case reports of this procedure done during pregnancy and therefore its use remains controversial.[98,106]

There remain limitations on survival outcome in women diagnosed with cervical cancer diagnosed during pregnancy. Nguyen et al.[107] concluded that tumor characteristics and maternal survival were not adversely affected by pregnancy, nor was pregnancy adversely affected by cervical cancer. Similar conclusions were reached by van der Vange and colleagues in a case-control study. They reported on 23 patients diagnosed during pregnancy and 24 patients diagnosed within 6 months postpartum. Thirty-nine patients had early stage disease. No difference in survival was noted for cases compared to controls. They noted that the delivery method had no effect on survival, thus concluding that prognosis for early stage cervical cancer is similar in pregnant and non-pregnant women.[96,108] Zemlickis et al.[109] reported on a long-term follow-up of cervical cancer outcome in a case-control study of pregnant women. No survival differences were observed. When compared to matched controls, patients with invasive cervical cancer were more likely to give birth to children who had lower birth weights. No adverse impact of pregnancy on cervix cancer outcome could be demonstrated.

Hodgkin's disease and non-Hodgkin's lymphoma

The presentation of Hodgkin's disease during pregnancy does not differ from that of the non-pregnant patient, with lymphadenopathy being the most common method of presentation.[110] The diagnosis is established by lymph node biopsy, with sufficient material to confirm specific type of disease.[111] Staging assessment, in addition to medical history and physical examination, can include an abdominal shielded chest radiograph, abdominal US, and MRI to document disease location and extent in order to assist treatment planning. For supradiaphragmatic disease, radiation therapy can be completed successfully while maintaining the pregnancy with uterine/fetal shielding.[20,22,111–113] Radiation therapy during pregnancy for stage IA and IIA Hodgkin's disease has been reported by Woo et al.[20] Sixteen patients received radiation to the neck (2), neck and mediastinum (3), or mantle.[114] Fetal radiation dose estimates were determined for nine patients. Reported doses ranged from 1.4 to 5.5 cGy for photon therapy and 10 to 13.6 cGy for cobalt therapy. There were 16 normal full-term infants, and the 10-year patient survival rate was 71%.[20] This outcome is similar to an earlier report by Jacobs et al.,[113] who reported on the use of radiation therapy involving the neck and mediastinum during the second and third trimesters of pregnancy. Supradiaphragmatic radiation therapy can be accomplished while maintaining a viable pregnancy. There are limited data regarding the impact of Hodgkin's disease on pregnancy and the effects of pregnancy upon disease prognosis. Anselmo et al.[115] concluded that the prognosis of Hodgkin's disease was not affected by pregnancy. Tawil et al.,[112] reporting on their experience with 12 patients with Hodgkin's disease and pregnancy, concluded that pregnancy did not significantly affect the course of the malignancy, and the presence of this malignancy did not affect pregnancy outcome. Examining pregnancy outcome, Zuazu et al.[116] found no increase in the complication rate of pregnancy in 56 patients with leukemia or lymphoma. In those patients treated with systemic chemotherapy, there was no increase in incidence of fetal malformations. In the Gelb series, patients were treated with a variety of systemic chemotherapy agent combinations, including MOPP (mechlorethamine, vincristine, procarbazine, prednisone), ABV (doxorubicin, bleomycin, vinblastine), COP (cyclophosphamide, vincristine, prednisone), and CHOP (cyclophosphamide, doxorubicin, vincristine, prednisone).[110] No fetal malformations were reported. Fifteen patients were alive and disease free. Gelb and colleagues concluded that otherwise indicated systemic therapy should not be delayed because of pregnancy.

Non-Hodgkin's lymphoma during pregnancy presents at more advanced stage and has more aggressive biologic behavior than Hodgkin's disease during pregnancy.[110,117,118] The clinical behavior of non-Hodgkin's lymphoma appears to be the same with or without pregnancy.[110] Because the majority of patients present with advanced stage disease, systemic chemotherapy is warranted. Combination chemotherapy has been reported to be used with some success. Agents used have included epirubicin, vincristine, prednisone, etoposide, cyclophosphamide, doxorubicin, and bleomycin in various combinations (VACOP-B and MACOP-B).[119–121] There have been several reports of the use of rituximab during pregnancy. Herold et al.[122] utilized a combination of rituximab, doxorubicin, vincristine, and prednisolone to treat a female with bulky stage IIA NHL. At the time of initiation of therapy, the patient was in her 21st week of pregnancy. She responded well to therapy and delivered a healthy infant at 35 weeks via caesarean section; the child demonstrated a normal B cell population. Kimby et al.[123] treated a patient with Stage IIB NHL with weekly rituximab for four cycles. The patient reported conception occurrence between the first and second infusions of rituximab. She delivered at healthy baby girl at 40 weeks. The infant demonstrated a low granulocyte count at birth, but her hematologic parameters had recovered by 18 months of age. Since that time, there have been multiple reports of rituximab, cyclophosphamide, doxorubicin, vincristine, and prednisone (R-CHOP) during pregnancy for diffuse large B cell lymphoma with reports of fetal leukopenia but with only preterm birth complicating the pregnancy.[124,125]

In one of the largest reported multicenter, retrospective analyses, Evens et al.[125] identified 90 patients diagnosed with either Hodgkin's or non-Hodgkin's lymphoma during pregnancy. Six of the women terminated their pregnancy. Fifty-six women received chemotherapy during pregnancy that included R-CHOP as well as other modified regimens that included etoposide, bleomycin, dacarbazine, cytarabine, and cisplatin. Pretreatment also included steroids and growth factor support. One child was born with a malformation with microcephaly. There was an increase in induction of labor and therefore also c-sections and NICU admissions. The authors reported that the survival was in line with expected outcomes of similar lymphoma patients. Aviles et al.[126] reported the outcome of 16 patients treated for non-Hodgkin's lymphoma during pregnancy, including eight during the first trimester. No congenital malformations were noted, and normal deliveries were reported. They concluded that pregnancy was not a contraindication to treating non-Hodgkin's lymphoma and that long-term remission was possible. Burkitt's lymphoma, anaplastic large cell lymphoma, and T-cell lymphoma have also all been reported in association with pregnancy.[127–131]

Ovarian cancer

In a review of adnexal masses during pregnancy, one ovarian cancer was found in 125 patients. There were 40 dermoids, 15 endometriomas, 14 cysts, 13 cystoadenomas, 9 tubal cysts, and 4 fibroids, a 0.8% malignancy rate.[132] In a retrospective review, Sayedur et al.[133] identified nine cases of ovarian cancer and pregnancy over 24 years, an incidence of 0.08/1000 pregnant women. For pregnant women, adnexal masses are more frequent, likely to be benign and management decisions are becoming more complex. US, percutaneous aspiration, and surgical intervention are possible.

In a study by Platek et al.,[134] 31 patients of 43,372 deliveries were found to have adnexal masses > 6 cm persistent beyond 16 weeks of gestation. No ovarian cancers were diagnosed. When malignancies have been found, germ cell tumors and epithelial cancers of low malignant potential were most common.[135] The pathology of ovarian cancer during pregnancy was reviewed by Dgani et al.[136] They recorded data on 23 patients over a 24-year period. Borderline carcinomas were most frequent (35%), followed by invasive epithelial tumors (30%), dysgerminomas (17%), and granulosa cell tumors (13%). Early stage disease was common; 74% of patients were stage I.

In the series of Sayedur et al.,[133] seven of the nine patients had stage I epithelial tumors. Five patients were treated with salpingo-oophorectomy, three with total abdominal hysterectomy and bilateral salpingo-oophorectomy with omentectomy. They reported 100% survival for stage I disease and 78% 5-year survival overall. Conservative surgery for early stage disease and low malignant potential tumors may preserve fertility. In the Dgani series, 14 of the 23 patients delivered live neonates.[136] Dgani concluded that the overall prognosis for ovarian cancer during pregnancy is better than ovarian tumors in general because of early stage at diagnosis and tumors of low malignant potential.

Chemotherapy for more advanced-stage disease has been reported primarily as case reports. Cisplatin, carboplatin, doxorubicin, bleomycin, cyclophosphamide, and, most recently, paclitaxel have all been given for treatment of ovarian cancer during pregnancy.[99,137-139]

Acute and chronic leukemia

Acute leukemia

Acute leukemia occurring during pregnancy presents unique circumstances because of bone marrow failure and the attendant cytopenias that may occur. Myeloid leukemias are more common than lymphoid. The presenting signs and symptoms are not different from those of the non-pregnant patient. The diagnosis is made by bone marrow aspiration, and standard classification is used for sub-typing. In a series from the Mayo Clinic, 17 pregnant patients with acute leukemia were seen in a 37-year period. Fifteen of the seventeen patients were diagnosed with acute myeloid disease. The majority of these individuals presented during the first or second trimester of pregnancy. Five of nine patients treated with chemotherapy during pregnancy had long-term complete remissions, whereas three of four patients who delayed treatment until after delivery died of disease. No fetal malformations were noted in those treated with chemotherapy during pregnancy.[140]

Cardonick and Iacobucci[141] performed an analysis of 152 patients who were treated for acute lymphoblastic leukemia (63 cases) or acute myelogenous leukemia (89 cases). They found that 6 neonates developed congenital abnormalities and 12 neonates demonstrated intrauterine growth retardation. There were 11 cases of intrauterine fetal death and two neonatal deaths. All cases of abnormalities occurred in association with first trimester usage of cytarabine or thioguanine, as monotherapy or in combination with an anthracycline. However, combinations of vincristine, mercaptopurine, doxorubicin or daunorubicin, cyclophosphamide, prednisone, and methotrexate were used in all trimesters.

Acute promyelocytic leukemia (APL) is of special interest because of the use of all-trans retinoic acid (ATRA) in the treatment program. Retinoids have known teratogenic effects.[142] However, a number of case reports have documented fetal safety and favorable patient outcome with the use of ATRA for APL.[143,144]

Chronic leukemia

Pregnancy and chronic lymphocytic leukemia (CLL) is extraordinarily rare.[145,146] Welsh et al.[146] reported a case of CLL with pregnancy and noted a substantial decrease in white blood cells after delivery. They noted that this apparent hematologic remission was not accompanied by clonal remission. Gurman described a case of a patient who became pregnant shortly after her diagnosis of CLL. She received no cytotoxic therapy, and she delivered a healthy infant at 39 weeks gestation.[31] Her third trimester was complicated by gestational diabetes and preeclampsia. Unlike the Welsh report, which demonstrated elevated numbers of lymphocytes in the intervillous space, the latter case demonstrated no lymphocytic infiltration of the placenta. Ali et al.[147] treated a patient who was diagnosed with CLL during her 17th week of gestation. She received three courses of leukapheresis at the 25th, 30th, and 38th week of gestation in order

Table 3 Placental metastases.

Tumor type
Small-cell lung cancer[166]
Melanoma[166]
Pancreas[168]
Breast[169]
Medulloblastoma[170]
Large cell lung cancer[171]
B-cell lymphoma[172]
T-cell lymphoma[173]
Non-Hodgkin's lymphoma[174]
Large cell lymphoma[129]

to maintain her WBC count below 100×10^9/L. She delivered a normal infant at 39 weeks of gestation.

Chronic myeloid leukemia has been treated during pregnancy with interferon α, hydroxyurea and leukapheresis, and leukapheresis alone.[148-151] No untoward effects of treatment on fetal growth, nor development or complications of labor and delivery have been reported.

Sustaining the pregnancy until delivery is feasible. Limited data suggest that pregnancy has no effect on CML long-term outcome; however, there are no case-control studies. Although limited data from animal studies suggest that imatinib may have teratogenic properties, there is increasing, but conflicting data on imatinib use during pregnancy. Yilmaz et al.[152] described three patients exposed to imatinib during pregnancy, all with healthy neonates at delivery. Prabhash et al.[153] described two cases of normal births after imatinib exposure and continuation of imatinib therapy throughout the pregnancy. Ault et al. described 19 pregnancies involving 18 patients who conceived while receiving imatinib. All female patients discontinued therapy at the time the pregnancy was discovered. Three pregnancies ended in spontaneous abortion and one with an elective abortion. Two of the 16 babies had abnormalities; one with hypospadias and another with rotation of the small intestine. The authors concluded that patients should use contraception as the discontinuation of imatinib may lead to loss of disease response. Another case report describes the development of a meningocele and death of the fetus exposed to imatinib.[154] Yadav et al.[155] described another woman who received hydroxyurea and imatinib during the third trimester with fetal complications of IUGR and oligohydramnios. However, the child developed normally after delivery. Alizadeh et al.[156] described 22 pregnancies in 14 patients or in the partner of a male patient exposed to tyrosine kinases for CML with only 1 with an atrial septal defect. Therefore, patients should be encouraged to continue with contraception while on imatinib given these scant and conflicting reports; however, some patients have maintained imatinib therapy during pregnancy. This may be an option for some women, only after detailed and deliberative discussion with the treating team regarding risks and the limits of available information.

Melanoma

Surgical management remains the mainstay of treatment for newly diagnosed melanoma during pregnancy. There have been multiple reports of melanoma diagnosed during pregnancy. Johansson et al.[157] described the Swedish registry of 1019 women with pregnancy-associated melanoma. Of these there was no difference in cause-specific mortality in pregnant versus non-pregnant patients. However, Bannister-Tyrell et al.[158] have described an Australian experience of 577 pregnancy-associated melanomas, of which 195 were diagnosed during pregnancy. However, in this

Table 4 Multidisciplinary approach to the pregnant patient with cancer.

Diagnosis and treatment planning	Considerations
Confirm diagnosis	Cytology and histology
Assess extent of disease	Staging, physical exam, organ function, and metastatic disease
Disease-related prognosis independent of pregnancy	
Assess pregnancy	Comorbidities—age, diabetes, and cardiac function
	Gestational age
	Expected delivery date
Review treatment options	*For Patient*:
	Anticipated benefits for the patient
	"Cure," prolongation of life, improve or delay symptoms
	For Fetus:
	Anticipated outcome
	Maintaining pregnancy
	Anticipated risks for fetus
Plan and implement treatment plan	
Reevaluate patient and fetus at frequent intervals	
Multidisciplinary treatment team members	Patient
	Obstetrician
	Oncologists-surgical, radiation, medical, gynecologist, and radiation physicist
	Nurses
	Ethicists
	Social service
	Pastoral care

group, there was an association with detection of the melanoma at more advanced stages.

Transplacental malignancy and placental metastasis

A number of case reports have noted transplacental passage of malignancy from mother to neonate.[159-167] Catlin et al.[159] reported a neonatal death related to the transplacental passage of maternal natural killer cell lymphoma. Successful treatment of maternal transplacental small-cell lung cancer has been noted.[166] Teksam presented a striking case of a 33-week neonate who was emergently delivered after her mother was diagnosed with lung cancer. Owing to the presence of placental metastases, the infant underwent initial screening with brain MRI and chest/abdomen CT, both of which were apparently normal. Unfortunately, serial examinations demonstrated development of a cerebellar tumor that significantly improved after chemotherapy, but the mass progressed a few months afterward. Biopsy and resection confirmed that the neoplasm was metastatic lung cancer. Additional metastatic lesions were identified in the frontal and temporal lobes on follow-up MRI.[167]

Leukemia cell identification in circulation in a neonate born to a mother with ALL has also been reported. However, leukemic cell engraftment and neonatal disease were not observed.[164] Acute monocytic leukemia transmission from mother to fetus has been documented.[162]

Alexander et al.[163] reviewed 87 cases of fetal or placental metastases; they found that malignant melanoma affected 31% of these patients, making melanoma the most common malignancy to involve both the fetus and placenta.

Dildy and colleagues reviewed placental metastases and reported 52 cases in 1989. Solid tumors and hematologic malignancies have

been noted to involve the placenta (Table 3).[129,168-176] Systematic evaluation of the placenta at the time of delivery of the pregnant woman with cancer has not been routine. However, new technologies are being evaluated for easier identification of possible transplacental transfer of malignancies.

Conclusion

Cancer and pregnancy presents a unique opportunity for multispecialty oncologic and prenatal care. The gathering and discussion of data to be utilized in treatment planning requires careful coordination with obstetrical, surgical, and anesthesiology colleagues. Given the concern for the well being of both the mother and the fetus, support for and reassurance of the patient during the decision process becomes a paramount duty for physicians. It is possible to have a favorable outcome for mother and child. An outline of a sequential approach to multispecialty management for cancer and pregnancy is presented in Table 4.

Key references

The complete reference list can be found on the Wiley Companion Digital Edition of this title (see inside front cover for login instructions).

1 Peccatori FA, Azim HA, Orecchia R, et al. Cancer, pregnancy and fertility: ESMO Clinical Practice Guidelines for diagnosis, treatment and follow-up. *Ann Oncol.* 2013;24:vi160–vi170.

5 Dominici LS, Kuerer HM, Babiera G, et al. Wound complications from surgery in pregnancy-associated breast cancer (PABC). *Breast Dis.* 2010;31:1–5.

6 Mazze R, Kallen B. Reproductive outcome after anesthesia and operation during pregnancy: a registry study of 5405 cases. *J Obstet Gynecol.* 1989;161:1178.

9 Hahn K, Johnson P, Gordon N, et al. Treatment of pregnant breast cancer patients and outcomes of children exposed to chemotherapy in utero. *Cancer.* 2006;107:1219–1226.

11 De Santis M, Straface G, Cavaliere AF, et al. Gadolinium periconceptional exposure: pregnancy and neonatal outcome. *Acta Obstet Gynecol Scand.* 2007;86:99–101.

17 Stensheim H, Moller B, van Dijk T, et al. Cause-specific survival for women diagnosed with cancer during pregnancy or lactation: a registry-based cohort study. *J Clin Oncol.* 2009;27:45–51.

20 Woo S, Fuller L, Cundiff J, et al. Radiotherapy during pregnancy for clinical stages IA-IIA Hodgkin's disease. *Int J Radiat Oncol Biol Phys.* 1992;23:407.

27 Doll D, Ringenberg Q, Yarbro J. Antineoplastic agents in pregnancy. *Semin Oncol.* 1989;16:337–346.

30 Cardonick E, Gilmandyar D, Somer RA. Maternal and neonatal outcomes of dose-dense chemotherapy for breast cancer in pregnancy. *Obstet Gynecol.* 2012;120:1267–1272.

31 Germann N, Goffinet F, Goldwasser F. Anthracyclines during pregnancy: embryo-fetal outcome in 160 patients. *Ann Oncol.* 2004;15:146–150.

32 Cardonick E, Bhat A, Gilmandyar D, et al. Maternal and fetal outcomes of taxane chemotherapy in breast and ovarian cancer during pregnancy: case series and review of the literature. *Ann Oncol.* 2012;23:3016–3023.

33 Azim HA Jr, Santoro L, Russell-Edu W, et al. Prognosis of pregnancy-associated breast cancer: a meta-analysis of 30 studies. *Cancer Treat Rev.* 2012;38:834–842.

34 Litton J, Warneke C, Hahn K, et al. Case control study of women treated with chemotherapy for breast cancer during pregnancy as compared with non-pregnant breast cancer patients. *Oncologist.* 2013;18(4):369–376.

35 Aviles A, Neri N. Hematologic malignancies and pregnancy: a final report of 84 children who received chemotherapy in utero. *Clin Lymphoma.* 2001;2:173–177.

36 Van Calsteren K, Berteloot P, Hanssens M, et al. In utero exposure to chemotherapy: effect on cardiac and neurologic outcome. *J Clin Oncol.* 2006;24:e16–e17.

37 Abdel-Hady el S, Hemida RA, Gamal A, et al. Cancer during pregnancy: perinatal outcome after in utero exposure to chemotherapy. *Arch Gynecol Obstet.* 2012;286:283–286.

38 Murthy R, Theriault R, Barnett C, et al. Outcomes of children exposed in utero to chemotherapy for breast cancer. *Breast Cancer Res.* 2014;16:3414.

39 Cardonick EMD, Dougherty RMD, Grana GMD, et al. Breast cancer during pregnancy: maternal and fetal outcomes. *Cancer J.* 2010;16(1):76–82.

40 Loibl S, Han SN, von Minckwitz G, et al. Treatment of breast cancer during pregnancy: an observational study. *Lancet Oncol.* 2012;13:887–896.

41 Amant F, Van Calsteren K, Halaska MJ, et al. Long-term cognitive and cardiac outcomes after prenatal exposure to chemotherapy in children aged 18 months or older: an observational study. *Lancet Oncol.* 2012;13:256–264.

48 Yang WT, Dryden MJ, Gwyn K, et al. Imaging of breast cancer diagnosed and treated with chemotherapy during pregnancy. *Radiology.* 2006;**239**:52–60.

54 Khera SY, Kiluk JV, Hasson DM, et al. Pregnancy-associated breast cancer patients can safely undergo lymphatic mapping. *Breast J.* 2008;**14**:250–254.

56 Mir O, Berveiller P, Ropert S, et al. Emerging therapeutic options for breast cancer chemotherapy during pregnancy. *Ann Oncol.* 2008;**19**:607–613.

58 Mir O, Berveiller P, Goffinet F, et al. Taxanes for breast cancer during pregnancy: a systematic review. *Ann Oncol.* 2009;**21**:425–433.

62 Bader AA, Schlembach D, Tamussino KF, et al. Anhydramnios associated with administration of trastuzumab and paclitaxel for metastatic breast cancer during pregnancy. *Lancet Oncol.* 2007;**8**:79–81.

70 Pant S, Landon MB, Blumenfeld M, et al. Treatment of breast cancer with trastuzumab during pregnancy. *J Clin Oncol.* 2008;**26**:1567–1569.

71 Shrim A, Garcia-Bournissen F, Maxwell C, et al. Favorable pregnancy outcome following Trastuzumab (Herceptin(R)) use during pregnancy – Case report and updated literature review. *Reprod Toxicol.* 2007;**23**:611–613.

72 Shrim A, Garcia-Bournissen F, Maxwell C, et al. Trastuzumab treatment for breast cancer during pregnancy. *Can Fam Physician.* 2008;**54**:31–32.

98 Amant F, Halaska MJ, Fumagalli M, et al. Gynecologic cancers in pregnancy: guidelines of a second international consensus meeting. *Int J Gynecol Cancer.* 2014;**24**:394–403. doi: 10.1097/IGC.0000000000000062.

126 Aviles A, Diaz-Maqueo JC, Torras V, et al. Non-Hodgkin's lymphomas and pregnancy: presentation of 16 cases. *Gynecol Oncol.* 1990;**37**:335–337.

171 Dildy GA 3rd, Moise KJ Jr, Carpenter RJ Jr, et al. Maternal malignancy metastatic to the products of conception: a review. *Obstet Gynecol Surv.* 1989;**44**:535–540.

73 Cancer and aging

Arti Hurria, MD ▪ Hyman B. Muss, MD ▪ Harvey J. Cohen, MD

Overview

Cancer is a disease of aging. Approximately sixty percent of all cancers and seventy percent of cancer mortality occurs in people >/= age 65. The number of older adults with cancer is on the rise as the US population is aging. However, there is great heterogeneity in the health status of older adults which may impact cancer treatment decisions and outcomes. This chapter will review the principles of geriatric assessment and frailty, the biology of cancer and aging, as well as the unique issues and considerations in caring for older patients with cancer during treatment and into the survivorship years.

Cancer is a disease that disproportionately affects older patients. Almost 60% of all cancers occur in people ≥age 65. People aged 65 and older have a ninefold increase in the incidence of cancer and an 18-fold increase in cancer mortality in comparison to people younger than age 65 (Table 1).[2] The number of older people with cancer is continuously growing as the population is aging. In the United States, in 1900, 3.1 million people were of age 65 and older. Over the century, this number increased approximately 10-fold, so that in the year 2000 there were 35 million people aged 65 and older. This number is expected to double yet again, thus in 2030, it is projected that there will be 71.5 million people over the age of 65, accounting for 20% of the population[3,4] (Table 2).

Among those over the age 65, there has been an age shift over time, leading to an increase in the older segment of the population. For example, during the 1990s the number aged 85 and older increased by 38%, the number aged 75 to 84 increased by 23%, and the number aged 65 to 74 increased by less than 2%. By 2030, the number ≥ age 85 is expected to double.[3] Those who live to age 100 and beyond, the "centenarians," are the fastest growing segment of the older population. On the basis of these statistics, oncologists inevitably care for a large number of older patients. There is no standard chronological age at which a person is considered "older." Historically, aged ≥ 65 was used for two reasons:

1. this was the traditional age for retirement and
2. people in the United States become eligible for entitlement programs (Social Security, Medicare).

As our population ages, we see much heterogeneity in the aged ≥ 65 population, with many individuals continuing to work and function similarly to younger counterparts. Therefore, this chapter focuses on defining characteristics to understand "functional age," rather than "chronological age" to distinguish the "older" patient. This chapter is also dedicated to discussing the unique issues and considerations in caring for an older patient with cancer.

Life expectancy and aging

Statistics regarding average life expectancy are useful to consider when caring for an older patient. The average life expectancy at birth is 76.5 years. As an individual ages, the average projected life expectancy increases. For example, a person who lives to 65 years of age has an average life expectancy of 19.1 years, placing their projected age of death at 84.1 years. A person who lives to 80 years of age has an average projected life expectancy of 9.1 years, placing the projected age of death at 89.1 years. Even the 100-year-old person has an average life expectancy of 2.3 years, placing their average projected age of death at 102.3 years. One may think of this as a "survival of the fittest" phenomenon, in which the absolute life expectancy increases as one ages (Table 3).[5]

The biology of cancer and aging

Aging can be defined as "the process that converts healthy adults into frail ones with diminished reserves in most physiologic systems and an exponentially increasing vulnerability to disease and death".[6] Despite the universality of this definition, aging is clearly a heterogeneous process. Each individual ages at a unique pace and demonstrates varying manifestations of vulnerability. Although much progress has been made, the mechanisms of both aging and neoplasia are incompletely understood and therefore theories about the association of these two processes are an area of active research.[7,8] It has been suggested that cancer and aging are two sides of the same coin with the control of tissue renewal and repair being a pivotal point with excess proliferation leading to neoplasia and decline in cell growth and function resulting in senescence.[9,10] P16INK expression may play a key role in this branch point as may metabolic stress resistance pathways and waste management controls via autophagy pathways.[11,12]

Other theories of the association with aging and neoplasia[13,14] include longer duration of exposure (time) and possibly increased susceptibility to oxidative stress and carcinogens; age-induced increase in DNA instability resulting in higher mutation potential that could result in both oncogene activation or amplification or tumor suppressor gene defects; a decrease in DNA repair with age, which might enhance the predisposition to the genetic defects; age-related telomere shortening, which might increase the above-mentioned DNA instability; immune dysregulation, which may decrease immune surveillance and allow the emergence of malignant clones but may also create a pro-inflammatory environment favoring the growth of malignant cells; and finally an altered microenvironment, including the presence of senescent cells that may secrete proinflammatory and carcinogenic cytokines.[14–16] These theories do not explain why there is a decrease in cancer incidence in the older segment of the population. In a autopsy study of 507 patients over 75 years of age, the prevalence of cancer at the time of autopsy decreased with increasing age (35% age

Holland-Frei Cancer Medicine, Ninth Edition. Edited by Robert C. Bast Jr., Carlo M. Croce, William N. Hait, Waun Ki Hong, Donald W. Kufe, Martine Piccart-Gebhart, Raphael E. Pollock, Ralph R. Weichselbaum, Hongyang Wang, and James F. Holland.
© 2017 John Wiley & Sons, Inc. ISBN: 978-1-118-93469-2

Table 1 Ninefold increase in cancer incidence and 18-fold increase in cancer mortality with age < 65.

Age	Incidence (per 100,000)	Mortality (per 100,000)
<age 65	223.8	56.1
≥age 65	2095.8	1008.4

Source: Data derived from SEER for 1975–2011 Incidence and 1975–2010 for Mortality.[1]

Table 2 The growing US population aged 65 and older 1.2.

Year	Million	Percentage of population
1900	3.1	4.1
2000	35.0	12.4
2030	71.5	19.7

Table 3 Average life expectancy.

Age now	Life expectancy	Age of death
65	19.1	84.1
70	15.5	85.5
75	12.1	87.1
80	9.1	89.1
85	6.6	91.6
90	4.7	94.7
95	3.3	98.3
100	2.3	102.3

Source: Data derived from the National Vital Statistics Report 5.

75 to 79, 20% age 95 to 99, and 16% in centenarians). This has been confirmed in a detailed demographic study and suggests that research into the cause of this phenomenon may be enlightening regarding the overall relationship of aging and cancer.[17]

Physiologic changes with aging

Physiologic changes occur in each organ system with aging, independent of disease. Most organ systems show a linear physiological decline beginning at 30 years of age. This decline occurs at variable rates between individuals and across organ systems. The consequence of these changes during normal activity is minimal; however, during times of stress the decreased reserve becomes more apparent.[18]

As the cardiovascular system ages, there is a decrease in cardiac output, decrease in maximal heart rate, and prolonged recovery following exertion. During times of stress, there is a decreased response to catecholamines. As the pulmonary system ages, there is a decreased response to hypoxemia or hypercapnia, decreased elasticity in the lung tissue, increased ventilation–perfusion mismatch, and decreased forced expiratory volume. Endocrine changes with aging include a decrease in certain hormone levels and an increase in others. For example, there is a decrease in insulin-like growth factor, growth hormone, renin, aldosterone, dehydroepiandrosterone, and sex steroids and increase in insulin, norepinephrine, parathyroid hormone, vasopressin, and atrial natriuretic peptide. Changes to the neurological system with aging include neuronal loss, decrease in brain weight, decreased vision, loss in high frequency and low frequency hearing, and alterations in both taste and smell. Changes in the immune system manifest as decrease in thymic mass, decreased production of thymic hormones, decrease in naive lymphocytes, and a decrease in antibody response.[18]

There is a decrease in hepatic and renal mass with aging. Autopsy studies demonstrate a decrease in liver volume with aging by approximately 25% to 50%. In addition, there is decreased hepatic blood flow, estimated at a 10% to 15% decrease in liver perfusion, even after taking into account the decrease in liver volume.[19–21] Renal mass decreases by 25% to 30% over the lifespan, leading to a decreased number of functional nephrons. Renal blood flow decreases by 1% per year after 50 years of age and glomerular filtration decreases by 1 mL/min/year after the age of 40.[19,21]

Hematopoietic changes with aging include a decrease in bone marrow mass and increase in bone marrow fat. Despite this, peripheral blood cell concentrations in healthy older patients are similar to those of younger patients.[22]

The frail older patient

The term "frail" is used to describe a subset of older patients with a critically reduced functional reserve that places them at risk for dependency, institutionalization, illness, hospitalization, and mortality.[23] A proposed definition of frailty is "a state of age-related physiologic vulnerability resulting from impaired homeostatic reserve and reduced capacity of the organism to withstand stress." Therefore, the clinical syndrome of frailty is proposed to be a dynamic consequence of a negative energy balance; for example, starting with undernutrition that leads to loss of muscle and bone mass and contributes to further decline in activity level and strength. This, in combination with decreased reserve, contributes to the increased vulnerability of the frail patient. The end result is failure to thrive, which is a syndrome of unexplained weight loss, decreased muscle mass, and metabolic abnormalities including a decrease in albumin, creatinine, cholesterol, and hemoglobin. Immune dysfunction and chronic inflammation may play a role in frailty. Markers of inflammation are associated with aging and frailty including the cytokine interleukin 6 (IL 6) and the acute phase reactant, C-reactive protein (CRP).[24–26] In addition, elevations in plasma D dimer have been associated with age. Both IL 6 and D dimer have been predictive of mortality and functional decline.[23,27,28]

A phenotype for frailty was developed in a prospective observational study of 5317 community-dwelling men and women age ≥ 65. The "frailty phenotype" was defined as a clinical syndrome in which three or more of the following criteria are present: (1) unintentional weight loss ≥ 10 lbs in past year, (2) self-reported exhaustion, (3) weakness defined as the lowest twentieth percentile in grip strength adjusted for gender and body mass index, (4) slow walking speed defined as the lowest twentieth percentile on a timed walk of 15 feet, and (5) low physical activity defined as the lowest quintile of kilocalories per week. Individuals with one or two of the criteria were categorized as an "intermediate or prefrail phenotype." Patients defined as frail or prefrail, compared with nonfrail, had a higher incidence of 3- and 7-year mortality, hospitalization, incident falls, progressive decline in ability to complete activities of daily living (ADL), and decreased mobility. On the basis of these criteria, 7% of community-dwelling individuals age 65 and older were frail and 47% were prefrail. The prevalence of frailty and prefrailty was greater in women than men and increased with age.[29] Frailty is also associated with an increased risk of recurrent falls, hip fracture, and any nonspine fractures.[30]

Another method of measuring frailty was developed by Rockwood and colleagues in which frailty is viewed as an accumulation of deficits.[31] This frailty index is based on the premise that while individual deficit may not have a discernible threat to mortality (or other outcomes), the accumulation of these individual deficits will add up to poorer outcomes in the geriatric population. For example, in general populations of older people, the accumulation of deficits has been demonstrated to predict hospitalization, institutionalization, and death.[32,33] In comparison to the phenotype model developed by Fried and colleagues, which requires the knowledge of specific parameters, the deficits accumulation method can be used for virtually any data set which captures geriatric assessment variables if enough variables are collected. Future research is needed to identify the utility of these different methods of measuring frailty in predicting outcomes in older adults with cancer.

Frail older patients with cancer represent a unique subset of patients that pose challenging therapeutic decisions. The aforementioned geriatric measures of frailty have not been widely studied in older adults with cancer, where there may be additional outcomes of interest. For example, a consensus statement on research recommendations for older adults with cancer proposed that an oncologic definition of frailty should assess the risk for toxicity to cancer treatment.[34] An important initial step in evaluation of the frail patient is to determine whether the cancer is likely to decrease the patient's life expectancy. In a model proposed by Balducci and Stanta,[35] one would consider treatment of the cancer if it was impacting the patient's life expectancy or if it was causing a compromise in quality of life. The goal of treatment must be determined: life prolonging versus palliation. Treatment decisions involve weighing the risks and benefits with the patient and caregiver. As the nation is aging, there will be a rise in the number of frail older patients with cancer. Clinical trials focusing on efficacy and tolerability of treatment within this patient population are needed.[36]

Evaluation of the older patient: geriatric assessment

The term "geriatric assessment" was defined at a consensus conference in 1989 as "a multi-dimensional inter-disciplinary patient evaluation that leads to the identification of patient's problems."[37] The assessment includes an evaluation of the older person's functional status (ability to live independently at home and in the community), comorbid medical conditions, cognition, psychological status, social functioning and support, medication review, and nutritional status (Table 4). This comprehensive assessment allows for identification of areas of vulnerability and a multidisciplinary plan to address these areas. In addition, geriatric assessment provides valuable information regarding prognostic factors for morbidity and mortality in the older patient.[38] Each domain of a geriatric assessment is reviewed in the following section.

Functional status

Assessment of functional status includes an evaluation of an individual's ability to live independently at home and in the community. Traditional assessment measures are "ADL" and "instrumental activities of daily living" (IADL) (Table 5). ADL are basic self-care skills, such as ability to bathe, dress, toilet, transfer, maintain continence, and feed oneself. These activities are essential in order for one to maintain independence in the home. The need for assistance with ADL has been predictive of cognitive impairment and greater resource requirement,[39] nursing home placement,[40] prolonged hospital stay, and worsening of function in the hospital.[41]

IADL include those self-care skills that allow one to live independently in the community. These include ability to telephone, shop, travel, prepare meals, do housework, take medications, and manage one's finances. In a study by Reuben and colleagues of 282 patients

Table 4 Key components of a comprehensive geriatric assessment.

Functional status
Comorbid (co-existing) medical conditions
Cognition
Psychological status
Social functioning and support
Socioeconomic issues
Medication review
Nutritional status

Table 5 Functional status assessment.

Activities of daily living	Instrumental activities of daily living
Bathing	Telephone
Dressing	Traveling
Toileting	Shopping
Transfer	Preparing meals
Continence	Housework
Eating	Medication management
	Money management

aged 64 and older, dependence in IADL (such as housework, shopping, and driving, scored as a continuous variables) was an independent predictor of mortality ($p < 0.0001$).[42] The need for assistance with IADL is predictive of risk of cognitive impairment.[43] Individuals who require assistance with IADL often need assistance to maintain independence in the community.

Cancer in an older patient is associated with an increased need for assistance in daily activities. In a large study of older patients, individuals with cancer had more limitations in ADL and IADL than individuals without cancer and required more healthcare use.[44,45] The need for assistance with IADLs has been associated with poorer overall survival[46,47] and increased risk of chemotherapy toxicity in older adults with cancer.[48–50] For example, the need for assistance with IADL and poorer quality of life are associated with poorer overall survival among older adults with lung cancer.[47] In a study of older adults with ovarian cancer, predictors of chemotherapy toxicity included a poor performance status (Eastern Cooperative Oncology Group performance status of <2) and functional dependence (defined as living at home with assistance or living with assistance in a specialized institution).[51]

Comorbid medical conditions

Comorbidity is defined as a concurrent medical problem that is a competing source of morbidity or mortality. In a study by Yancik and colleagues, summary data on comorbidity were collected on 7600 patients aged ≥ 55 years. The most common concurrent medical problems included hypertension (42.9%), heart-related conditions (39.1%), and arthritis (34.9%). The number of comorbid conditions increased with age. Patients aged 55 to 64 had an average of 2.9 comorbid conditions, patients aged 65 to 74 had 3.6 comorbid conditions, and those 75 and older had 4.2 medical conditions (Table 6).[3] The association between comorbidity and survival in patients with cancer is independent of a patient's functional status.[52] Therefore, each is an important domain to assess. The potential impact of a new disease as a competing cause of mortality decreases with increasing age secondary to the decrease in absolute projected life expectancy.[53] For example, consider the impact of a disease with a projected 50% mortality over 5 years in a 65-year-old person in comparison to an 85-year-old person.

Table 6 Rank order of major condition, >10% of study sample.

Condition	Percent
Hypertension	42.9
Heart-related conditions	39.1
Arthritis	34.9
Gastrointestinal problems	31.0
Anemia	22.6
Eye problems	19.0
Urinary tract	18.0
Previous cancers	15.4
Gallbladder problems	14.9
Chronic obstructive pulmonary disease	14.5
Diabetes	12.8
Fracture	10.8
Gland disorders	10.6

This disease will decrease the 65-year-old person's average life expectancy by approximately 10 years, whereas because the absolute projected life expectancy of an 85-year-old person is less than that of a 65-year-old person, it will decrease an 85-year-old person's average life expectancy by only about 2 years.[53] A study by Piccirillo et al.[54] with evaluative data of over 27,000 patients demonstrated that among individuals with cancer, the mean number of comorbid conditions and the severity of the comorbid conditions increase with age.

The level of comorbidity has been shown to affect functional recovery following surgical treatment for breast cancer. In a study of older women with breast cancer, women with >2 comorbid conditions were less likely following surgery to become independent in completing IADL and more likely to experience difficulty completing tasks requiring upper body strength.[55]

Comorbid medical conditions also impact the likelihood of receipt and tolerance of chemotherapy. Data from the Surveillance, Epidemiology, and End Results-Medicare database demonstrates that older patients with colon cancer who have a history of heart failure, diabetes, or chronic obstructive pulmonary disease are less likely to receive adjuvant chemotherapy.[56] In a clinical trial of older adults with lung cancer, patients with higher levels of comorbidity were more likely to discontinue chemotherapy.[57]

Nutrition

Poor nutritional status is an independent predictor of functional dependency and survival. In a prospective cohort study of 214 older community-dwelling adults, a low body mass index defined as a body mass index $< 22 \text{ kg/m}^2$ was associated with dependency in ADL [odds ratio 1.21; 95% confidence interval (CI) 1.01–1.45]. After adjusting for potential confounding factors including age, gender, mental status, comorbidity, and functional dependency, body mass index $< 22 \text{ kg/m}^2$ was associated with decreased 1-year survival [relative risk (RR) 0.85, 95% CI 0.74–0.97].[58] However, conflicting data has shown that among hospitalized old adults, a BMI ≥ 30 was associated with better 4-year all-cause mortality, while lower BMI was not associated with increased risk of mortality.[59]

Weight change over a 3-year period was recorded in a study of 4714 community-dwelling adults, aged 65 and older. Weight change, defined as a 5% or greater loss or gain in weight over a 3-year period, occurred in 34.6% of women and 27.3% of men. A higher proportion of participants lost weight than gained weight. Weight loss, and not weight gain, was associated with an increased risk of mortality (Hazard ratio = 1.67, 95% CI = 1.29–2.15).[60]

The prognostic effect of unintentional weight loss in patients with cancer was evaluated in a study of 3047 patients enrolled in Eastern Cooperative Oncology Group chemotherapy trials. Weight loss during the 6 months before chemotherapy was associated with poorer survival (statistically significant in 9 out of 12 tumor types). In addition, weight loss was associated with lower chemotherapy response rates (significant only in patients with breast cancer). Decreasing weight correlated with decreased performance status in all tumor types except pancreatic and gastric cancer.[61]

Cognition

The presence of dementia is an independent prognostic indicator of survival.[62,63] In a study by Wolfson and colleagues, 10,263 people aged 65 and older were screened for dementia. Of these, 821 people had a diagnosis of probable Alzheimer's disease, possible Alzheimer's disease, or vascular dementia. The median survival of these patients was 3.3 years (3.1 years if a diagnosis of probable Alzheimer's disease, 3.5 years if possible Alzheimer's disease, and 3.3 years if vascular dementia).[63]

A baseline assessment of cognition in an older patient with cancer is important for several reasons. First, if a person has a rapid change in memory or new cognitive deficits, metastatic disease to the brain should be excluded. Second, the degree of cognitive impairment will need to be considered when devising a treatment plan. For example, all oral medications and especially chemotherapy drugs should be used with caution in patients with cognitive impairment. Correct dosing for oral chemotherapy is as important as with intravenous chemotherapy, so that if the patient takes an incorrect dose, the side effects could be serious or even fatal. The role of the patient's family or caregiver is critical in maintaining safety. A patient with cognitive impairment will need assistance in remembering instructions regarding use of supportive medications such as antiemetics. A caregiver will need to be aware of potential side effects of treatment that would necessitate medical attention. The presence of cognitive impairment is associated with increased risk of hospitalization and poorer chemotherapy tolerance.[49,64]

Psychological state and social support

Older patients with cancer often demonstrate better psychological functioning in comparison to younger patients. Following a diagnosis of breast cancer, older women demonstrate better mental health and well-being in comparison to younger patients.[65] In women < age 65, a recent diagnosis of breast cancer produced a marked increase in anxiety and depression and decreased morale in comparison to people of the same age who had a diagnosis over 5 years prior. In comparison, for women ≥ 65 years of age, a more recent diagnosis did not affect their level of anxiety, depression, or morale in comparison to age counterparts with a diagnosis greater than 5 years ago.[66,67]

The presence of social support plays an important role in the psychological functioning of the older patient. Significant predictors of severe psychological distress in women of breast cancer of any age include being divorced or separated and having less social support.[68] Social support can serve as a buffer against the psychological impact of a stressful life event.

In addition, social isolation is an independent predictor of mortality. This was demonstrated in a study by Seeman and colleagues in which they examined the importance of four measures of social support: (1) marital status, (2) close contact with two or more close friends/relatives, (3) regular church attendance, and (4) membership in other types of groups. The presence of social ties was related to survival, independent of age. The relative hazard for increased 5-year mortality among men and women in three community-based cohorts ranged from 1.97 to 3.06 for participants with no social ties in comparison to those with all four social ties.[68] In another study of 282 patients aged 65 and older, living alone was independently predictive of risk of death.[42]

Medication review: evaluation for polypharmacy

A review of the patient's medication list is an important part of the geriatric assessment. In addition, one must consider whether newly prescribed medications may cause an adverse effect or drug interaction. Older patients are more vulnerable to adverse drug events than younger patients. Approximately one-fifth of hospital admissions in older patients are secondary to adverse drug events.[19] This is partly because older patients use more medications than younger patients. The average number of medications taken by an older patient with cancer is 5 ± 4 drugs.[69]

Contributing to the risk of adverse drug events are the changes in pharmacokinetics and pharmacodynamics that occur with aging. These changes should be considered with the dosing of any medication, including chemotherapy. There are age-related changes in the gastrointestinal tract such as decreased acid secretion and fewer villi in mucosal surfaces. There are significant changes in volume of distribution including increased body fat (leading to slower metabolism of lipid soluble drugs), decrease in total body water (leading to an increase in the plasma level of water-soluble drugs), decrease in lean body mass, decrease in serum albumin, and decrease in hemoglobin.[20] Hepatic metabolism changes with aging, secondary to decreased liver volume and decreased hepatic blood flow. Phase I hepatic reactions (oxidation, deamination, hydroxylation) decrease with aging. These include reactions mediated via cytochrome P-450, decreasing by approximately 30% in older patients. There is no significant change in phase II hepatic reactions (conjugation: acetylation, glucuronidation, sulfation) with aging.[19–21] Renal mass decreases by 25–30% over the lifespan, leading to a decreased number of functional nephrons. Consequently, there is a decrease in glomerular filtration, tubular secretion, and reabsorption with aging. Therefore, drugs dependent on renal clearance have a longer half-life in older patients and drug dosing may need to be adjusted based on creatinine clearance.

Comprehensive geriatric assessment

Geriatric assessment is a comprehensive approach to the evaluation of the older patient, with an evaluation of the domains described above: functional status, comorbidity, cognition, nutritional status, psychological state and social support, and medication review. Studies regarding the value of this assessment have been conflicting; however, a meta-analysis of the controlled trials by Stuck and colleagues suggests a benefit to geriatric assessment. This meta-analysis of 28 controlled trials comprising 4959 participants and 4912 controls randomized to one of five comprehensive geriatric assessment programs demonstrated that a geriatric evaluation and management unit (inpatient unit for geriatric assessment and rehabilitation) reduced mortality by 35% at 6 months and a home assessment service (in-home geriatric assessment) reduced mortality by 14% at 36 months via early identification and treatment of problems.[70] A more recently published multisite randomized, controlled trial of inpatient and outpatient geriatric evaluation and management demonstrated that geriatric evaluation and management reduced functional decline and improved mental health but had no effect on survival.[71]

The role of geriatric assessment in care of the older cancer patient is an area under active research. A systematic review of geriatric assessment studies in older adults with cancer confirmed that performing a geriatric assessment is feasible in oncology practice and can identify older adults at risk for adverse outcomes; however, additional studies are needed regarding the impact of geriatric assessment results on oncology decision-making and interventions to improve outcomes.[72,73] Balducci[74] studied geriatric assessment in the evaluation of the older patient with cancer and found that this assessment helped to characterize patients of the same chronological age by identifying impairment in the following areas: dependency in functional status (18% ADL, 72% IADL), serious comorbidity (36% by Charlson scale, 94% by Cumulative Illness Rating Scale—Geriatrics), memory impairment (22%), poor nutrition (19%), and polypharmacy (41%). Garman et al.[75] performed a retrospective chart review of older patients with cancer admitted to an inpatient Geriatric Evaluation and Management Unit, in which a comprehensive geriatric assessment was used to identify goals of care. These goals were accomplished in over 75% of cases: 73% in symptom management, 79% in functional improvement, and 100% in disposition and caregiver support. Other studies have demonstrated that domains of a geriatric assessment can predict survival and toxicity to chemotherapy in older adults with cancer.[47,51] Geriatric assessment and intervention can lead to improve pain control, mental health, and emotional well-being among older adults with cancer.[76]

The information derived from a geriatric assessment could be potentially valuable to oncologists for several reasons. First, it would help the clinician get a sense of the "functional age" of the patient. Second, it would identify patients at high risk for functional decline or toxicity to treatment, for whom targeted intervention may be beneficial. Third, it would provide valuable information regarding older patients in clinical trials, allowing us to standardize patient characteristics across studies and to control for possible confounding factors contributing to mortality.

A traditional comprehensive geriatric assessment is a multidisciplinary assessment that can take 2 h to perform. Because of the time-intensive nature, it is often not feasible in a busy oncology practice. Therefore, other means of performing geriatric assessment are under study. The Cancer and Leukemia Group B (CALGB) is developing a short geriatric assessment tool. Pilot data demonstrated that this brief but comprehensive, mainly self-administered geriatric assessment questionnaire is feasible in the setting of an outpatient oncology clinic[77] and cooperative group.[78] This geriatric assessment will be collected as baseline information in subsequent clinical trials. Other authors have reported on the feasibility of a geriatric assessment that is mailed to the patient to complete before the office visit.[79,80] There are several abbreviated geriatric assessment screening tools that are available; however, there is no consensus regarding the optimal screening tool to identify patients who would benefit from a more detailed geriatric assessment.[34]

A proposed framework depicting the factors to consider in decision-making for an older patient with cancer is described in the Comprehensive Geriatric Model, developed by Cohen and DeMaria.[81] This model summarizes the key aspects critical to the care of the older patient including social, psychological, and biological factors that may impact on the host, the disease, and the outcomes from treatment. In this model, chronological age plays a role by defining the decreased functional reserve that can occur with aging, but subsequent factors including biological, social, and psychological factors unique to the individual patient are factored into decision-making. This is a dynamic process in which alterations in one domain can subsequently impact upon the other domains within the model.

Knowledge about older cancer patients: underrepresentation on clinical trials

Despite the aging population and the association of cancer with aging, data regarding the benefits and risks of treatment of the older cancer patient are limited. This is secondary to limited involvement of older patients on clinical trials. The Southwest Oncology Group analyzed 164 clinical trials from 1993 to 1996 and comprised of 16,396 patients. They found that only 25% of the patients on clinical trial were aged 65 and older. This underrepresentation was across 15 cancer types, except lymphoma. Older patients with breast cancer were the least represented, with only 9% of patients over the age of 65.[82]

Similar data regarding the underrepresentation of the older patient are seen in Canadian trials. Enrollment on clinical trials by age was analyzed from 1993 to 1996. Fifty-eight percent of the Canadian population with cancer is ≥age of 65, whereas only 22% of patients enrolled on trial were ≥age of 65.[83]

The representation on clinical trials worsens with increasing age. The National Cancer Institute analyzed enrollment of patients ≥ age of 65 and patients ≥ age of 75. Data from 23,000 patients across 500 therapeutic trials were analyzed. They found an underrepresentation of patients over the age of 65 on clinical trial; however, this was even more pronounced for patients ≥ age of 75. Only 11% of men on clinical trial were over the age of 75 and only 5% of women were over the age of 75. There was a striking underrepresentation of older patients with breast cancer, with only 2.7% being over the age of 75. This study demonstrated that with increasing age, there is even less representation on clinical trial.[84] A review of enrollment on NCI adult cooperative group clinical trials from 2001 to 2011 shows continued underrepresentation of older adults.[36]

Understanding barriers to clinical trial enrollment

The CALGB Committee on Cancer in the Elderly developed a study to understand barriers to participation of older patients on cancer treatment trials. Women with breast cancer, <age of 65 and ≥age of 65, were paired by physician and stage. The trial sought to determine the frequency with which each group was offered enrollment on clinical trial and likelihood of accepting treatment on trial. The results demonstrated that older women were less likely to be offered enrollment onto clinical trial than younger women (51% < age 65 vs 35% ≥ age 65; $p = 0.06$): however, if offered, older women would be as likely to accept enrollment on trial as younger women (56% < age 65 vs 50% ≥ age 65; $p = 0.67$). Physicians did not offer a clinical trial to older patients because (1) physicians were concerned about the toxicity of treatment in older patients and (2) physicians were concerned regarding the impact of comorbid diseases.[85] The most common physician recommendations of ways to improve accrual of older patients to clinical trials include providing clinic personnel to explain trials to older patients and their families, providing educational materials about clinical trials for patients and families, and providing transportation to make it easier for older patients to participate in clinical trials.[86,87]

Cancer screening in the elderly

National organizations publish screening recommendations for the public as a whole; however, few provide guidelines for cancer screening in the elderly. Moreover, randomized trials of screening interventions have rarely included meaningful sample sizes of older persons. The American Geriatrics Society (AGS) recommends that cancer screening be individualized, rather than setting guidelines strictly by age, taking into account the patient's preferences, life expectancy, and the risks and benefits of the screening test. In their recent recommendations as part of the "Choosing Wisely" campaign, they recommend no routine screening for prostate, colon, or breast cancer in patients with an estimated life expectancy less than 10 years.[88] General guidelines to help steer these discussions with patients at average risk for developing these cancers are summarized in the following section.

Breast cancer

Breast cancer screening traditionally consists of mammography, clinical breast exam, and breast self-exam. The American Cancer Society (ACS) recommends continuing breast cancer screening as long as a woman is in good health and is a candidate for treatment.[89] The AGS suggests to not screen women with estimated life expectancies less than 10 years. In a recent review of mammographic screening in older women, it was recommended that screening mammography be stopped for women with a less than 10 year life expectancy.[90] We suggest annual or biennial screening only for older women with estimated survival of at least 10 years.

Cervical cancer

The ACS guidelines for cervical cancer screening recommend that women aged 65 and older may cease screening with the Papanicolaou (Pap) smear if there are three or more documented, consecutive, normal Pap smears or two or more consecutive Pap and HPV tests within the past 10 years (with the most recent test in last 5 years).[91] The US Preventative Service Task Force recommends discontinuing cytologic screening for women aged 65 and older who have had adequate screening with normal results.[89]

Prostate cancer

Screening for prostate cancer consists of a digital rectal exam and prostate specific antigen (PSA) test. The ACS recommends offering annual screening for prostate cancer, with digital rectal exam and PSA test, beginning at the age of 50 in patients at average risk and continued in men who have a life expectancy of at least 10 years. The benefits and limitations of testing should be discussed with the patient so that an informed decision regarding screening is made.[91] The US Preventative Service Task Force 2012 updated guidelines recommend against PSA screening for prostate cancer regardless of age.[92] We agree with the AGS and suggest that the risks and benefits of screening be discussed only in men with life expectancies greater that 10 years.[93]

Colon cancer

The ACS recommends that adults at average risk begin screening for colorectal cancer at 50 years of age. There are many options for colon cancer screening including annual fecal occult blood testing, flexible sigmoidoscopy every 5 years, annual fecal occult blood testing plus flexible sigmoidoscopy every 5 years, colonoscopy every 10 years, or double contrast barium enema every 5 years.[89] The US Preventative Services Task Force acknowledges the appropriate age at which to discontinue colorectal cancer screening is unknown, because screening studies have generally been restricted to patients younger than the age of 80.[94] They recommend discontinuing screening in patients whose age or comorbid conditions limit life expectancy.[95] We side with the AGS and do not recommend screening patients with life expectancies of less than 10 years.[93]

Lung cancer

The ACS recommends lung cancer screening in current and former smokers aged 55–74 in good health and with a 30 pack-year history.[91] The risks and benefits of screening need to be carefully explained in this population[96] and smoking cessation should be the highest priority. The American Association for Thoracic surgery and the USPSTF increased the upper age limit for screening to age 79 and age 80, respectively.[97,98] We concur with extending the upper age limit to 80 years of age.

Treatment tolerance of the older patient

Surgery

Surgery is the primary treatment for the majority of solid tumors. Failure to obtain definitive surgical treatment is associated with an increased mortality from disease regardless of age. For example, in a study performed by the Cancer Research UK Breast Cancer Trials Group, 455 women older than 70 years of age, with operable breast cancer, were randomized to treatment with tamoxifen alone versus tamoxifen plus surgery. At 12.7 years of follow-up, women who did not undergo surgery had an increase in breast cancer mortality (Hazard ratio 1.68; 95% CI 1.15–2.47).[99] Therefore, if possible, older women should undergo primary surgical removal of breast cancer in order to decrease their risk of breast cancer mortality.

Several studies have demonstrated that advanced age alone should not be a reason to deny surgical treatment for colorectal cancer.[100–103] Risk of surgical morbidity and mortality is increased with intra-abdominal surgery or those performed under an emergency situation; however, even in these high-risk situations, older patients benefit from surgical management. In a study of emergency colorectal surgery, older and younger patients had a similar primary resection rate (95% > age 70, 89% ≤ age 70; $p = 0.70$) and primary anastomosis rate (84% > age 70, 78% ≥ age 70; $p = 0.64$). Older patients had a higher incidence of postoperative cardiopulmonary complications but no statistically significant difference in mortality (9% > age 70, 5% ≥ age 70; $p = 0.48$).[100] The PACE tool utilizes geriatric assessment items to identify older adults with cancer at risk for surgical complications.[104,105]

Radiation therapy

Radiation therapy is commonly used for both curative and palliative intent in the older patient. Studies have demonstrated that treatment tolerance in younger and older patients is similar.[106,107] In a study of 1208 patients receiving thoracic irradiation, age had no impact on the acute or late radiation toxicities. Patients were divided into 6 age groups, ranging from <50 to >70. There was no significant difference in acute toxicities such as nausea, dyspnea, esophagitis, or weakness and there was no significant difference in survival between age groups ($p = 0.82$). Older patients were more likely to experience weight loss than younger patients ($p = 0.002$).[107] Therefore, close attention should be paid to nutritional status in older patients receiving radiation.

Treatment tolerance to radiation and efficacy of radiation therapy in the "oldest old" patient has also been demonstrated. In a retrospective review of 191 patients ≥ age of 80, 94% were able to complete treatment without complications. A response to treatment was seen in 77% of patients treated for curative intent and 81% of patients treated for palliative intent. Six percent of patients required treatment interruption, secondary to weight loss from diarrhea, dysphagia, or progressive disease. This occurred more commonly in patients who were treated with large treatment fields. Of patients receiving treatment for aero-digestive tract cancer, 20% of patients had grade 3 mucositis and 2% of patients had grade 4 mucositis, reinforcing the need for careful attention to nutritional status and weight loss in older patients.[108]

Other studies have sought to determine whether there is a subgroup of older patients with low risk disease in which radiation therapy can be eliminated. A study performed by the CALGB randomized 636 women aged 70 and older with clinical stage I, estrogen-receptor-positive breast cancer who underwent a lumpectomy to treatment with radiation to the affected breast and tamoxifen, or tamoxifen alone. The women treated with tamoxifen alone had more locoregional recurrences at 5 years of follow-up: 4% in the tamoxifen alone arm versus 1% in the tamoxifen and radiation arm ($p < 0.001$); however, there was no difference in breast cancer-specific mortality or 5-year rates of overall survival.[109]

Chemotherapy

Several studies have sought to determine whether treatment on chemotherapy trials is more toxic for older patients.[110] A study by the Piedmont Oncology Association was a case control study of women with metastatic breast cancer enrolled on clinical trials. The women were divided into three groups, by age: <50, 50 to 69, and >70. The study demonstrated that older women receiving treatment on clinical trial had no significant difference in the incidence of toxic effects, dose delivery, or dose delays in comparison to younger women. In addition, there was no difference in response, time to disease progression, or survival. Therefore, older women who received treatment on clinical trial not only tolerated the treatment but also equally benefited from this treatment.[111] An analysis of phase II trials at Illinois Cancer Center found similar results. Older and younger patients had no difference in toxic effects, need for dose reduction, or need for treatment interruption or delay. In addition, there was no difference in response to treatment.[112] In contrast, an analysis of three CALGB clinical trials for the adjuvant treatment of patient with node-positive breast cancer demonstrated that older adults were more likely to experience a grade 4 hematologic toxicity and were more likely to discontinue therapy because of toxicity. In addition, older adults were more likely to die of acute myelogenous leukemia or myelodysplastic syndrome.[113]

A limitation in interpreting these studies is that geriatric assessment information was not collected. Therefore, it is not clear whether the older patients who enrolled on these clinical trials are representative of the patients cared for in everyday practice. As so few older patients are offered entry on clinical trial, the older patients represented on clinical trials may have a younger "functional age." Therefore, incorporating geriatric assessment into clinical trials would be a valuable way of standardizing possible confounding factors across patients of the same chronological age, helping to determine the "functional age" of the patients represented. Clinical trials focusing on the older patient are needed in order to optimize care of this patient population. Developing a registry of older patients with selected diseases (breast cancer, colon cancer, intermediate grade lymphoma, etc.) and treated with chemotherapy with curative intent would provide a database with which to evaluate patterns of care and outcomes.

Survivorship

Accompanying the increasing number of older people with cancer and improvements in treatment, the number of older cancer survivors is also increasing. It is estimated that by 2020 two-thirds of cancer survivors will be over the age of 65. The aging cancer survivor is dealing with the simultaneous and often interacting impact of their aging physiology, the accumulation of multiple chronic conditions, geriatric syndromes, the after effects of cancer, and the late effects of cancer treatment.[114] The latter's impact on multiple organ systems may to an extent mimic the aging phenotype.[114] The management of this challenging situation requires a coordinated effort among oncologists and primary care providers with effective information exchange. A shared geriatrics-oriented survivorship care plan, fueled by a comprehensive geriatric assessment, may be the most effective way to accomplish this.[115,116] The patient has a role to play as well and using the cancer survivorship status as a teachable moment, improved outcomes can be obtained with lifestyle oriented interventions in addition to careful follow-up.[117]

Conclusions

Cancer is a disease that disproportionately affects older patients. Data regarding the care of these patients are limited secondary to the underrepresentation of older patients on clinical trials. In moving forward, an effort should be made to include older patients on clinical trial, in order to increase our understanding about the optimal way to care for this growing population. Incorporation of geriatric assessment in the care of the older patient will provide information regarding prognostic factors that distinguish two individuals of the same chronological age, thereby helping us understand "functional age" and risk of chemotherapy side effects. Brief, comprehensive geriatric assessment screening tools for older oncology patients have been developed.

Key references

The complete reference list can be found on the Wiley Companion Digital Edition of this title (see inside front cover for login instructions).

3 Yancik R. Cancer burden in the aged: an epidemiologic and demographic overview. *Cancer*. 1997;**80**:1273–1283.

11 Liu Y, Johnson SM, Fedoriw Y, et al. Expression of p16(INK4a) prevents cancer and promotes aging in lymphocytes. *Blood*. 2011;**117**:3257–3267.

12 Finkel T, Serrano M, Blasco MA. The common biology of cancer and ageing. *Nature*. 2007;**448**:767–774.

13 Irminger-Finger I. Science of cancer and aging. *J Clin Oncol*. 2007b;**25**:1844–1851.

16 Campisi J. Aging, cellular senescence, and cancer. *Annu Rev Physiol*. 2013;**75**: 685–705.

24 Leng SX, Xue QL, Tian J, Walston JD, Fried LP. Inflammation and frailty in older women. *J Am Geriatr Soc*. 2007;**55**:864–871.

25 Walston J, Mcburnie MA, Newman A, et al. Frailty and activation of the inflammation and coagulation systems with and without clinical comorbidities: results from the Cardiovascular Health Study. *Arch Intern Med*. 2002;**162**:2333–2341.

26 Cohen HJ, Pieper CF, Harris T, Rao KM, Currie MS. The association of plasma IL-6 levels with functional disability in community-dwelling elderly. *J Gerontol A Biol Sci Med Sci*. 1997;**52**:M201–M208.

27 Cohen HJ. In search of the underlying mechanisms of frailty. *J Gerontol A Biol Sci Med Sci*. 2000;**55**:706–708.

28 Cohen HJ, Harris T, Pieper CF. Coagulation and activation of inflammatory pathways in the development of functional decline and mortality in the elderly. *Am J Med*. 2003;**114**:180–187.

29 Fried LP, Tangen CM, Walston J, et al. Frailty in older adults: evidence for a phenotype. *J Gerontol A Biol Sci Med Sci*. 2001;**56**:M146–M156.

31 Rockwood K, Mitnitski A. Frailty in relation to the accumulation of deficits. *J Gerontol A Biol Sci Med Sci*. 2007;**62**:722–727.

33 Song X, Mitnitski A, Rockwood K. Prevalence and 10-year outcomes of frailty in older adults in relation to deficit accumulation. *J Am Geriatr Soc*. 2010;**58**:681–687.

34 Decoster L, Van Puyvelde K, Mohile S, et al. Screening tools for multidimensional health problems warranting a geriatric assessment in older cancer patients: an update on SIOG recommendationsdagger. *Ann Oncol*. 2014;**26**(2):288–300.

36 Hurria A, Dale W, Mooney M, et al. Designing therapeutic clinical trials for older and frail adults with cancer: U13 conference recommendations. *J Clin Oncol*. 2014;**32**(24):2587–2594.

38 Wildiers H, Heeren P, Puts M, et al. International Society of Geriatric Oncology Consensus on Geriatric Assessment in Older Patients With Cancer. *J Clin Oncol*. 2014;**32**:2595.

44 Mohile SG, Xian Y, Dale W, et al. Association of a cancer diagnosis with vulnerability and frailty in older Medicare beneficiaries. *J Natl Cancer Inst*. 2009;**101**:1206–1215.

47 Maione P, Perrone F, Gallo C, et al. Pretreatment quality of life and functional status assessment significantly predict survival of elderly patients with advanced non-small-cell lung cancer receiving chemotherapy: a prognostic analysis of the multicenter Italian lung cancer in the elderly study. *J Clin Oncol*. 2005;**23**:6865–6872.

48 Hurria A, Togawa K, Mohile SG, et al. Predicting chemotherapy toxicity in older adults with cancer: a prospective multicenter study. *J Clin Oncol*. 2011b;**29**:3457–3465.

50 Extermann M, Boler I, Reich RR, et al. Predicting the risk of chemotherapy toxicity in older patients: the Chemotherapy Risk Assessment Scale for High-Age Patients (CRASH) score. *Cancer*. 2012;**118**:3377–3386.

51 Freyer G, Geay JF, Touzet S, et al. Comprehensive geriatric assessment predicts tolerance to chemotherapy and survival in elderly patients with advanced ovarian carcinoma: a GINECO study. *Ann Oncol*. 2005;**16**:1795–1800.

53 Welch HG, Albertsen PC, Nease RF, Bubolz TA, Wasson JH. Estimating treatment benefits for the elderly: the effect of competing risks. *Ann Intern Med*. 1996;**124**:577–584.

56 Gross CP, Mcavay GJ, Guo Z, Tinetti ME. The impact of chronic illnesses on the use and effectiveness of adjuvant chemotherapy for colon cancer. *Cancer*. 2007;**109**:2410–2419.

57 Frasci G, Lorusso V, Panza N, et al. Gemcitabine plus vinorelbine versus vinorelbine alone in elderly patients with advanced non-small-cell lung cancer. *J Clin Oncol*. 2000;**18**:2529–2536.

67 Kornblith AB, Dowell JM, Herndon JE 2nd, et al. Telephone monitoring of distress in patients aged 65 years or older with advanced stage cancer: a cancer and leukemia group B study. *Cancer*. 2006;**107**:2706–2714.

70 Stuck AE, Siu AL, Wieland GD, Adams J, Rubenstein LZ. Comprehensive geriatric assessment: a meta-analysis of controlled trials. *Lancet*. 1993;**342**: 1032–1036.

71 Cohen HJ, Feussner JR, Weinberger M, et al. A controlled trial of inpatient and outpatient geriatric evaluation and management. *N Engl J Med*. 2002;**346**: 905–912.

73 Puts MT, Santos B, Hardt J, et al. An update on a systematic review of the use of geriatric assessment for older adults in oncology. *Ann Oncol*. 2014;**25**:307–315.

76 Rao AV, Hsieh F, Feussner JR, Cohen HJ. Geriatric evaluation and management units in the care of the frail elderly cancer patient. *J Gerontol A Biol Sci Med Sci*. 2005;**60**:798–803.

78 Hurria A, Cirrincione CT, Muss HB, et al. Implementing a geriatric assessment in cooperative group clinical cancer trials: CALGB 360401. *J Clin Oncol*. 2011a;**29**:1290–1296.

79 Ingram SS, Seo PH, Martell RE, et al. Comprehensive assessment of the elderly cancer patient: the feasibility of self-report methodology. *J Clin Oncol*. 2002;**20**:770–775.

82 Hutchins LF, Unger JM, Crowley JJ, Coltman CA Jr, Albain KS. Underrepresentation of patients 65 years of age or older in cancer- treatment trials. *N Engl J Med*. 1999;**341**:2061–2067.

85 Kemeny MM, Peterson BL, Kornblith AB, et al. Barriers to clinical trial participation by older women with breast cancer. *J Clin Oncol*. 2003;**21**:2268–2275.

86 Dale W, Mohile SG, Eldadah BA, et al. Biological, clinical, and psychosocial correlates at the interface of cancer and aging research. *J Natl Cancer Inst*. 2012;**104**:581–589.

87 Kornblith AB, Kemeny M, Peterson BL, et al. Survey of oncologists' perceptions of barriers to accrual of older patients with breast carcinoma to clinical trials. *Cancer*. 2002;**95**:989–996.

90 Walter LC, Schonberg MA. Screening mammography in older women: a review. *JAMA*. 2014;**311**:1336–1347.

95 U.S. Preventive Services Task Force. Screening for colorectal cancer: recommendation and rationale. *Ann Intern Med*. 2002;**137**:129–131.

104 Audisio RA, Participants P, Pope D, Ramesh HSJ, Gennari R, Van Leeuwen BL. Shall we operate? Preoperative assessment in elderly cancer patients (PACE) can help - A SIOG surgical task force prospective study. *Crit Rev Oncol Hematol*. 2008;**65**:156–163.

113 Muss HB, Berry DA, Cirrincione C, et al. Toxicity of older and younger patients treated with adjuvant chemotherapy for node-positive breast cancer: the Cancer and Leukemia Group B Experience. *J Clin Oncol*. 2007;**25**:3699–3704.

117 Demark-Wahnefried W, Morey MC, Sloane R, et al. Reach out to enhance wellness home-based diet-exercise intervention promotes reproducible and sustainable long-term improvements in health behaviors, body weight, and physical functioning in older, overweight/obese cancer survivors. *J Clin Oncol*. 2012;**30**: 2354–2361.

74 Disparities in cancer care

Otis W. Brawley, MD, MACP

Overview

Differences in healthcare outcome have become increasingly apparent over the past 50 years. It is especially apparent in cancer, a discipline that has had tremendous advancement. Ironically, the more progress that is made, the greater the disparities become. There are populations that do not enjoy the progress usually because of socioeconomic differences. The field of health disparities has grown into its own discipline within epidemiology. It involves population categorization by race, area of geographic origin, socioecomic status, and so on. The discipline looks at differences in risk of cancer, risk of death, survival, and the survival experience.

A number of well-designed studies show that equal treatment yields equal outcome among equal patients whether one categorizes population by race, socioeconomics, or other major factors. If people with the same genetic markers are compared, race for example is not a factor in outcome unless it is allowed to be. Numerous patterns of care studies demonstrate that there is not equal treatment by race in the United States. The discipline of health disparities has progressed to include assessment of interventions to reduce disparities.

The advent of precision medicine and tailored therapy will make categorization using genes and polymorphisms more important. The crude categories of race and ethnicity and even socioeconomic status will only be important in terms of social issues such as access to care and equality of treatment.

Social interventions to overcome disparities and bring about equity include efforts to (1) increase cultural competence and understanding of the patient among healthcare providers; (2) increase access to care; and (3) improve communications and educate those needing service.

Introduction

Over the past 50 years, there has been tremendous progress in healthcare and especially in the prevention and treatment of cancer. This progress has led to an increasing appreciation of the differences in outcomes among populations. The first studies to discuss the fact that some populations had higher rates of death from certain cancers were conducted in the late 1960s and published in the early 1970s.[1,2] These studies noted that Black-Americans have higher death rates than Whites. The area has grown to encompass other racial groups and the poor. As the issue became more broadly understood and the discipline matured, health disparities and health equity became a political issue. Indeed, the discipline was an influence on healthcare reform legislation, as well as legislation on the design and recruitment to US government funded clinical trials.

Reporting and understanding population differences in cancer incidence and outcome is important. The causes of cancer are both genetic and environmental. When the populations and the differences between them are truly understood, reasonable hypothesis can be generated about the factors that cause or prevent cancer, as well as the factors that make cancers more or less aggressive. With rigorous careful study of the well-defined populations, one can also increase knowledge about the efficacy and effectiveness of preventive and treatment interventions.

The birth of a discipline

The US National Cancer Institute established the Surveillance, Epidemiology, and End Results (SEER) program in the early 1970s as part of the implementation of the National Cancer Act. This program collects cancer incidence and mortality data from a number of population-based registries around the United States. Before SEER, there was extremely limited cancer incidence data. Even today SEER does not provide a fully representative sample of the country for calculation of incidence rates. SEER publishes cancer incidence and mortality data as well as 5-year survival rates by race and gender annually. This data is publically available at www.cancer.gov/statistics.

Through its "Black–White Studies" in the 1980s and 1990s, SEER clearly documented Black–White racial disparities in cancer incidence, mortality, and survival. The SEER studies also demonstrated differences in treatment patterns with a higher proportion of Blacks getting inappropriate cancer care.

Interest in other diseases also contributed to the birth of the academic discipline. As cancer disparities were studied, disparities in cardiovascular disease, especially hypertension was also being defined. Interest in the genetic blood disorder known as sickle cell anemia was also increasing.

The discipline was first called "minority health research" and later "special populations' research." It has now evolved into the field of "health disparities" and some are now even referring to it as "health equity." As the field has matured, the questions have become better defined and some of the solutions better elucidated. It has remained the study of the underserved, those who do not receive adequate preventive and treatment services. Today, the field of health disparities is far more than cultural competence among healthcare providers and developing specific interventions to overcome health disparities. It is transdisciplinary integrating basic science, clinical science, epidemiology, and social science.

Defining health disparities

The National Cancer Institute (NCI) defines "cancer health disparities" as adverse differences in cancer incidence, cancer prevalence, cancer mortality, cancer survivorship, and burden of cancer or related health conditions that exist among specific population groups in the United States. Translated, disparities in health are the concept that some populations do worse than others.

Holland-Frei Cancer Medicine, Ninth Edition. Edited by Robert C. Bast Jr., Carlo M. Croce, William N. Hait, Waun Ki Hong, Donald W. Kufe, Martine Piccart-Gebhart, Raphael E. Pollock, Ralph R. Weichselbaum, Hongyang Wang, and James F. Holland.
© 2017 John Wiley & Sons, Inc. ISBN: 978-1-118-93469-2

Factors measured

Health disparities are differences between populations. A number of outcomes can be measured and compared. Most common are as follows:

Incidence—usually expressed as the number diagnosed with the disease in a given year per 100,000 in the population. Incidence rates are the equivalent of the population's risk of developing a disease. Individuals from groups with a higher incidence of a disease have a higher risk of getting that disease.

Mortality—usually expressed as the number dying due to the disease in a given year per 100,000 in the population. Mortality rates are the equivalent of the population's risk of death from the disease. Individuals from groups with a higher mortality from a disease have a higher risk of dying from that disease.

Incidence and mortality are often "age adjusted" to a standard population to remove the effects of two populations having different age distributions. Age adjustment is also used to remove the effect of a population aging over time. Age is a risk factor for many cancers. A population having a higher age-adjusted incidence in 1990 compared to 1960 is not because there are more older people alive in that population in 1990 compared to 1960.

Survival rates—the median time from diagnosis to death for a cohort or the percent alive 5 years after diagnosis.

Prevalence—the proportion of a population that has a disease or risk factor for a disease.

Differences in patterns of care (screening and treatment) are also measured. This refers to the proportion of two or more groups getting a treatment standard to the condition. In more sophisticated analyses, it can be the proportion of a group getting high-quality treatment compared to another group.

Less commonly, and not in the NCI definition, disparities in morbidity, comorbid disease, and quality of life are measured outcomes.

Population categorization

While the field started by looking at Black and White race, it has evolved to the point that "populations" can be defined by race, ethnicity and culture, area of geographic origin, socioeconomic status (SES), and other factors. Clearly defining populations is extremely important in doing good health disparities research.

Race is a concept first put forth about 350 years ago. The initial categories were Caucasian, Negroid or African, and Mongoloid or Asian.[3] These categories had to do with skin color, facial traits, and presumed geographic area of origin. Distinct racial groups do not exist. Based purely on visible traits, racial groups are overlapping populations. The anthropology community has never accepted race as a biologic categorization.

The US Office of Management and Budget (OMB) defines race for use in government collection of data. The OMB definition is used most importantly in the decennial census, but, by legislation, is also used to describe the populations enrolled in federally funded clinical trials.

The OMB directive specifically states that its racial categories reflect a social definition of race as recognized in the United States and that the definition is not an attempt to define race biologically, anthropologically, or genetically. The OMB racial definition has changed over time. A person from the Indian subcontinent of Asia who migrated to the United States before the 1950 census has been considered three different races over the past 65 years. The current definition was published in 1997 (Table 1).

In collecting race data, the OMB has one "ethnicity" question. Ethnicity is defined by the OMB for government data as simply "Hispanic" or "non-Hispanic."

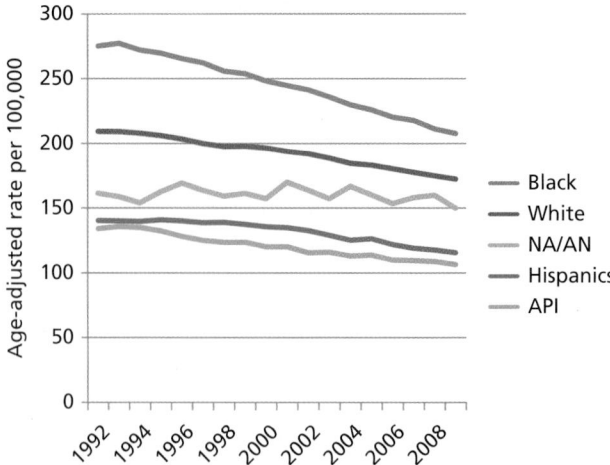

Figure 1 Age-Adjusted Cancer Mortality Rate 1990–2010 by 1990 OMB racial/ethnic category. Note: Age-adjusted mortality rates have declined significantly over the past 20 years for all but Native American/Alaskan Natives. The Native American/Alaskan Native (NA/AN), Hispanic and Asian-Islander (API) death rates are lower rates compared to Whites who have lower rates than Blacks. This graph uses the category Asian-Pacific Islander, which was the category used until 2000. Native Hawaiians are included in the Native American/Alaskan Native Category.

The National Cancer Institute SEER Program and the National Center for Health Statistics of the Centers for Disease Control and Prevention publish health data using OMB definitions. They are dependent on US Census data for the denominators to calculate incidence and mortality rates. Mortality trends by OMB Race/Ethnicity Criteria as published by the NCI SEER are plotted in Figure 1. This plot uses the definition used in the 1990 census.

Race is a useful category to collect data if viewed as a social definition. Some populations do bear an unequal burden. There are civil rights issues such as discrimination and differences in access to care that determine outcomes.

Ethnicity and culture as used in academic study is a very broad term that encompasses human identity. It is not static or mutually exclusive. It is fluid and without definite boundaries. In social research, ethnic groups are distinguished by specifying the nature and source of human variation (e.g., behavior, lifestyle habits, and other environmental influences) and their relationship to health. When used appropriately, populations of one nationality can have a number of ethnicities.

This is a more scientific categorization than race as it relates to environmental influences such as diet and other extrinsic influences that may increase or decrease the likelihood of an illness. Even such habits as how one smokes cigarettes or engages in sexual activity are influenced by ethnicity and culture.

While ethnicity and culture is related to factors that cause cancer, there are also ethnic and cultural influences on ones acceptance of a disease and in how one seeks and accepts therapy.

Area of geographic origin is more scientific than race. Many confuse race and area of geographic origin and there is some overlap. Many people have several areas of geographic origin because of the commingling of populations over the centuries.

A number of genetic traits correlate with area of geographic origin. For example, sickle cell disease is a genetic disease of people from the Mediterranean basin and sub-Saharan Africa. There are people from Spain, Italy, Greece, Syria, Turkey, and Lebanon with Sickle cell disease. Natives of southern Africa do not have sickle cell

Table 1 US Government definitions of race and ethnicity year 2000 census.

White	A person having origins in any of the original peoples of Europe, the Middle East, or North Africa. It includes people who indicate their race as "White" or report entries such as Irish, German, Italian, Lebanese, Arab, Moroccan, or Caucasian
Black or African American	A person having origins in any of the Black racial groups of Africa. It includes people who indicate their race as "Black, African Am., or Negro"; or report entries such as African American, Kenyan, Nigerian, or Haitian
American Indian and Alaska Native	A person having origins in any of the original peoples of North and South America (including Central America) and who maintains tribal affiliation or community attachment. This category includes people who indicate their race as "American Indian or Alaska Native" or report entries such as Navajo, Blackfeet, Inupiat, Yup'ik, or Central American Indian groups or South American Indian groups
Asian	A person having origins in any of the original peoples of the Far East, Southeast Asia, or the Indian subcontinent including, for example, Cambodia, China, India, Japan, Korea, Malaysia, Pakistan, the Philippine Islands, Thailand, and Vietnam. It includes people who indicate their race as "Asian Indian," "Chinese," "Filipino," "Korean," "Japanese," "Vietnamese," and "Other Asian" or provide other detailed Asian responses
Native Hawaiian and Other Pacific Islander	A person having origins in any of the original peoples of Hawaii, Guam, Samoa, or other Pacific Islands. It includes people who indicate their race as "Native Hawaiian," "Guamanian or Chamorro," "Samoan," and "Other Pacific Islander" or provide other detailed Pacific Islander responses

disease. There are people who we consider White who get sickle cell disease and people who we consider Black who do not.

While a genetic trait can have a higher prevalence among people from a specific geographic area, its important to realize while the prevalence can be higher, the people of that area likely do not monopolize that trait. For example, cystic fibrosis is more common among, but not exclusive to those originating in northern Europe and alcohol dehydrogenase deficiency is common, but not exclusive to those from Japan.

Ancestry is yet another way of categorizing populations. Ancestry is of course linked to race and area of geographic origin. Use of race can be especially problematic as people transcend racial boundaries. When one considers ancestry, it may be a bit easier to appreciate the effect of family and admixture. Genetic influences often parallel ancestry.

Some of the Black–White differences in breast and prostate cancer might be due to differences in genetics that better parallels ancestry or area of geographic origin more so than race.

SES is defined by education, income, and occupation. While the social determinants of health are extremely important, there is controversy over how well SES can be used to define the human condition. The European literature uses a concept called "deprivation." The "deprivation index," calculated during the decennial census in Scotland, takes a number of markers of wealth, education, and social status into account.[4]

SES or social deprivation determines where we live, birthing habits, diet, and even how or if we consume healthcare. Education is particularly important, Americans with the least education are more than twice as likely to die of cancer as compared to the most educated.[5–7]

There can also be population differences in stage at diagnosis and differences in the distribution of pathologies by SES. Differences in the uptake of screening by SES can lead to a higher proportion of the wealthy being diagnosed with early-stage disease when compared to lower SES cohorts. A group of people who participate in screening and indeed are more likely to get high quality screening are more likely to do well. In a disease with substantial overdiagnosis, the differences can be even more dramatic.

Relationships among population categories

Race is perhaps better seen as a characteristic and not a category or subtype. Much emphasis is placed on racial groups and differences in outcome among racial groups. The emphasis is partly due to the

American obsession with race and the fact that most American data on population differences is collected based on the US government definition of race. Outcomes data based on ethnicity, SES, or ancestry is not easily obtainable. While the racial categories are not based in biology, they do have some relevance for what they are, a sociopolitical construct that can be related to ethnicity, area of geographic origin and SES.

Unfortunately, the medical literature is filled with the "medicalization of race." There are a number papers to suggest that genetics defines differences among the races and these differences are the cause of a number of disparities.[8] Some of these papers should be discussing ancestry, which is different from race, and others often ignore the fact that there are clear correlations between race and SES. Low SES can be a cause of disparity. Race can also correlate with ethnicity and culture, which leads to behavior. Some behaviors increase risk of disease.

While there can be a correlation between race and cancer outcomes, it is important to remember that correlation does not necessarily mean causation. Racial differences are often due to social issues such as discrimination in education and in the provision of healthcare. Many in medicine falsely consider race a biologic categorization, thinking of race to be defined by genes. Sickle cell disease is a genetic, inherited condition. In the United States, it was and is still wrongly viewed as a "Black disease." This helped reinforce many of the views regarding race, genetics, and risk of disease. We often hear about race as a biologic category influencing disease in the discussion of prostate cancer incidence and mortality or in the discussion of the higher prevalence of triple negative breast cancer in Black women compared to Whites.

There is a lack of well-defined universal terminology in describing the above-mentioned categories making it difficult to assemble information on disparate/underserved populations. SES often includes education and income and even measures of wealth, but neglects to capture status in the social hierarchy. The European social science concept, deprivation and the deprivation index, takes social hierarchy and SES into account. It is a more precise tool than SES for measuring social situation.

Even using the crude measure of SES, there are clear correlations between race and SES. As a result, the effect of SES on risk of a bad health outcome is often and can easily be misattributed to race. Indeed, researchers often toss a SES measure into a model without considering the potential cause or contributory role or conclude that a racial/ethnic difference must be genetic or cultural after one or two SES measures are controlled for.

SES is often correlated with a higher risk of certain cancers because the poor have a higher prevalence of habits associated with disease risk. These habits are often due to poverty. For example:

- High caloric intake, lack of physical activity, and obesity are habits causally associated with more than a dozen cancers.[9] It is estimated that this triad is responsible for nearly a third of all cancers in the United States and it is a growing problem internationally. Those with lower SES in the United States have a higher prevalence of obesity.[10] The less educated and poor do tend to consume more calories per day. Processed calorie dense high-carbohydrate foods are less expensive than low calorie protein-rich foods.[11]
- Lung cancer and a number of smoking-related cancers are more common in the poor versus the middle class. Adults living below the poverty line are more likely to smoke compared to adults in America's middle class (30% prevalence vs 6% of Americans with a college degree).[12]
- The poor or those of lower SES are less likely to engage in medical preventive services. Surveys show that they are less likely to receive commonly accepted screening for breast or colon cancer.[13]

SES, ethnicity, and culture can come together to increase cancer risk. It can lead to a cancer causing infectious disease to be endemic within a group of people, however defined. This can lead to increased risk of a cancer in that group. This has been seen in cervical cancer owing to human papilloma virus, especially in people lacking access to preventive services. The increased risk of hepatoma among people from southeast Asia is another example. It is linked to hepatitis B that has a high prevalence in that population.[14] There are also studies to show that migration of cohorts from areas of low cancer risk in Asia to and acculturation in the United States increases risk of cancer within two generations.[15]

Disparities in treatment patterns

Many of the early health disparities studies focused on the fact that there are significant disparities in the quality of treatment received. In the initial studies, a higher proportion of Whites receive high-quality treatment compared to Blacks. Studies suggested that a number of factors lead to differences in treatment received.[16,17] Poverty, lack of insurance, or social disenfranchisement puts a patient at higher risk of receiving poor-quality healthcare or being underserved.[18]

Some patients:

- Decline therapy due to their culture discouraging acceptance or cultural differences with the healthcare provider.
- Do not adhere to prescribed regimens due to illiteracy or lack of medical sophistication.
- Do not adhere to prescribed therapy due to inconvenience of getting care.
- Cannot receive preferred more aggressive therapies due to comorbid diseases more common in disparate populations.
- Are not offered needed care due to racism or discrimination based on SES.

Awareness of these issues is extremely important and the biggest hurdle to overcoming them. Healthcare providers sensitive to these issues are often able to provide better service.[19] There has been a move toward training physicians to provide "culturally competent" care.[20] The American Society of Clinical Oncology and others offer courses on communicating to patients from backgrounds different from the provider www.university.asco.org/cultural-competence-oncology-practice.

The fact that some groups are more likely to receive poor quality of treatment has been most rigorously studied in breast cancer. Lund et al.[21] studied treatment patterns in metropolitan Atlanta over a 2-year period (2000 and 2001). Assessing women diagnosed with a localized breast cancer, they found that 7% of Black and 2% of White received no therapy within the first year after diagnosis.

Others have demonstrated that minority race, lack of education, lack of insurance, and lower SES are variables predicting for patients more likely to get inadequate care.[17,22] When these studies are assessed with logistic regression, regardless of race, less educated breast cancer patients are more likely to receive nonstandard breast cancer treatment regimens and less likely to receive adequate chemotherapy dosing.[10,23] Obese breast cancer patients are also less likely to receive adequate dosing of chemotherapy.

Disparities in quality of care lead to disparities in prognosis and treatment

While race does not appear to be the direct cause of these disparities in care given, race does translate into a higher proportion of Black or African-American Women receiving poor cancer treatment. This is because compared to Whites, a higher proportion of Black or African-American women have less than a high school education, and a higher proportion are obese. Approximately, 50% of Black women are obese compared to 34% of Whites. The disparate treatment of the less educated, the poor and the obese translates into a higher proportion of Blacks receiving less than optimal care compared to Whites. Again, the difference between correlation and causation is important.

Variable access to quality care by race can lead to differences in outcome in unsuspecting ways and lead to erroneous assumptions. For example, there is a Black–White disparity in American colorectal cancer death rates. Blacks have higher mortality rates and inferior 5-year survival rates when compared to Whites at each stage. This has led some to suggest that colorectal cancer is more aggressive in Blacks. It should be noted that Black–White colorectal mortality rates were very similar in the 1970s and the disparity in death rate has increased every year since 1981. The mortality disparity is greater in 2011 than at anytime despite the decline in mortality rates for both races.

Patterns of care studies suggest that Blacks with stage 3 disease are less likely to receive adjuvant chemotherapy and part of the disparity in stage 3 disease might be due to disparities in treatment. One might be tempted to stop here, but looking further, there are studies to show that Blacks tend to be treated in hospitals that are overcrowded and resource limited.[24] They are more likely to get fewer lymph nodes resected at surgery and they are less likely to have a thorough pathologic examination of those nodes. Translated, a proportion of the Blacks diagnosed with stage 1 and 2 cancer would have been diagnosed with stage 3 colorectal if they had received appropriate surgery and pathologic evaluation. These true stage 3 patients would improve the survival rates of Black stage 3 patients by their inclusion and improve the survival of Black stage 1 and 2 patients by their exclusion.

This is a classic Will Rogers' phenomenon.[25] Blacks of each stage have inferior 5-year survival because of disparities in treatment and staging. When assessed in an equal access system, racial differences in outcome decrease dramatically.[26]

Genetic expression—race, ancestry, ethnicity, and culture

Still within colorectal stage with good treatment, there are disparities in outcome. Black survival is slightly inferior to White survival.

EMAST, a marker of microsatellite instability, confers a poorer prognosis and is more common among Blacks or African-Americans. EMAST appears to be an acquired defect associated with inflammation.[27] The role of diet, microbiome, and accumulation of EMAST is an important issue when studying Black–White colon cancer disparities. This is an example of diet, an element of ethnicity and culture, paralleling race or ancestry and affecting the genetic expression and biologic behavior of a tumor.

Some extrinsic influences associated with race, ethnicity, and culture and even socioeconomics can affect genetic expression within a malignancy. A higher proportion of American White women are middle class and college educated. Middle class, college educated women often delay childbirth to establish a career. Having a first term pregnancy after the age of thirty is a risk factor, not just for breast cancer, but estrogen receptor positive breast cancer. Indeed, this is likely the reason that White American women have a higher incidence of breast cancer compared to Black American women. This is also the reason that White women have a higher incidence of estrogen receptor positive disease.[28]

Studies of White breast cancer patients in the United States and Scotland suggest that middle class social status in childhood is associated with a higher risk of estrogen receptor positive breast cancer in adulthood. Poverty in childhood is associated with estrogen receptor negative disease in later life.[29,30] Differences in diet and patterns of weight gain in childhood are thought to be causal. Duration of breast feeding, number of children breast-fed, and length of breast feeding have all been correlated with a lowered risk of basal-like breast cancer, but not a reduced risk of better prognosis luminal A disease.[31]

In the United States, the Black and Hispanic female population has disproportionately high number who are overweight and obese. This may be due to ethnicity and culture as well as SES. Obesity, or more specifically weight gain in adulthood, is thought a risk factor for postmenopausal breast cancer.[32] Differing pathologic trends seen in Black and White American women may be due to these influences.[31]

The understanding of the environmental influences associated with SES, ethnicity, and culture in the groups being compared can be especially useful. An understanding of the genetic polymorphisms and mutations (markers) that are associated with area of geographic origin and conserved because of ethnicity and culture is also helpful. As the field of epigenetics progresses, the affect of extrinsic influences will be even better appreciated.

Population and genetic differences

While evidence suggests that differences among broad ill-defined population categories have been overemphasized, there are intrinsic genetic differences between well-defined populations. Race is not the appropriate way to define those populations. Intrinsic genetics markers better correlate with ancestry, area of geographic origin, and sometimes with ethnicity and culture. Genetic differences correlated or associated with race should most often be considered familial or ancestral. A gene or series of genes can be conserved among families. Even then, the prevalence of a polymorphism or gene may be higher in a specific population, but that population is unlikely to monopolize that gene.[33]

A closed society will conserve genetic traits within that society. Segregation on the basis of race, ethnicity and culture, area of geographic origin, or other factors can lead to preservation of a specific gene or series of genes in the segregated population. This is demonstrated in several genetic diseases such as Tay Sachs disease, cystic fibrosis, and sickle cell disease.[34] Each of these diseases has a higher prevalence in, but is not exclusive to, a specific group.

Perhaps the best example is that of BRCA mutations. Women with certain mutations of the BRCA-1 and BRCA-2 genes are at higher risk than average risk for the development of breast and ovarian cancer. Mutations of BRCA-1 and BRCA-2 have been found in women of all races, but three specific mutations are common, but not exclusive, to people who identify themselves as being of Ashkenazi Jewish ancestry.[33,35] Population modeling suggests that these specific mutations are linked to a small number of individuals living about 1000–1200 years ago. These mutations are considered ancestral and are common among Jewish families owing to ethnic segregation among families.

Pharmacogenomics

There is clinically relevant variability in drug response due to differences in the enzymes that metabolize drugs. These differences can vary by populations as categorized by race, ethnicity, ancestry, and area of geographic origin or even at times SES. Extrinsic factors such as diet and use of some medicines can up or down regulate hepatic enzyme expression. The same pathways through which drugs are metabolized are often involved in the detoxification of environmental toxins and carcinogens, and thus variations in detoxification enzymes may lead to variations in cancer risk.

The physician is, of course, interested in how his or her individual patient metabolizes drugs to be prescribed. One can sometimes use a form of "population profiling" to assess an individual for certain common drug treatment issues. For example, approximately 10% of persons from certain areas of Asia develop severe cutaneous adverse reactions such as Stevens–Johnson Syndrome, when administered carbamazepine.[36] This might be a reasonable justification for avoiding use of carbamazepine in people whose ancestry includes an area of geographic origin in Malaysia, Singapore, Thailand, or India. If carbamazepine must be used, careful monitoring or testing for certain allele frequencies of HLA-B*1502 might be in order.

Tacrolimus has been well studied in renal transplant patients. This drug, which is structurally related to several anticancer drugs, is metabolized by CYP3A. In clinical use, some Black or African-American kidney transplant patients require higher tacrolimus doses to reach trough concentrations similar to those observed in White patients. This is due to differences in polymorphisms of CYP3A. Even within a specific group, there can be substantial variability in pharmacology. Within Blacks, there is a three to fivefold range in 12-h postdose tacrolimus concentrations.[37] Special attention to pharmacokinetics is needed in all patients treated with this drug.

Among cancer drugs, population differences of polymorphisms of UGT1A1 affect the dosing and efficacy of irinotecan.[38] Indeed, some suggest pharmacogenetic testing before use of this drug. Differences in ABCG2 affect the dosing and efficacy of topotecan, irinotecan, mitoxantrone, doxorubicin, and methotrexate.[36]

This is not a new concept, indeed in the genomic age, it is an old concept reapplied. For decades, we have appreciated that glucose-6-phosphate dehydrogenase (G6PD) deficiency is more common among people whose ancestry includes people of Mediterranean or Africa origin. Indeed, it is the most common human enzyme defect. Those with the deficiency are at risk of hemolysis when taking sulfa antibiotics, antimalarial, or certain other drugs.

US Government rules on minority inclusion in clinical trials

The US Government rules are the result of concerns that "racial minorities and women do not benefit from federally sponsored research because they do not participate in it."

The clinical trialist doing research with funding from the US National Institute of Health must report the race and gender of patients accrued to trials on an annual basis. While the NIH is legally obligated to require this information for all phase 3 clinical trials, NIH and other government agencies often require this information for all their trials involving human subjects.

The NIH revitalization of 1993, Public Law 103-43, mandates inclusion of women and minorities in clinical research. Specifically, it states, "the Director of the NIH shall ensure that trials are designed and carried out in a manner sufficient to provide valid analysis of whether the variables being studied in the trial effect women or members of minority groups as the case may be differently than other subjects in the trial." The stated goal of the legislation is to increase the opportunities for obtaining critically important information with which to enhance health and treat disease among all Americans and to detect and account for significant differences between genders or racial and ethnic groups where they exist and to identify more subtle differences that might warrant further exploration in targeted studies.[39]

The Revitalization Act is interpreted as demanding diverse representation on Federally sponsored trials, especially phase III trials. The funded researcher must make a good faith effort to accrue minorities and women proportionate to the US population.[39]

The legislation is controversial in that it is scientifically flawed. It calls for subset analysis to assess racial and ethnic differences. It uses race and ethnicity as if they define biological categories.[39] An additional issue is the legislation calls for subset analysis. A cardinal rule of clinical trialist is subset analyses are often wrong and should only be used to establish a hypothesis to be tested in a more rigorous study. A subset analysis is post hoc, retrospective, and underpowered. Power could be increased by oversampling minorities, but this creates ethical concerns in that a disproportionately greater number of minorities would be subjected to the risk of the study compared to majority Whites.

Interestingly, the law was written after a subset analysis of a study suggested that zidovudine was less effective among the Black or African population.[40,41] The result is many Blacks with HIV stopped taking or refused to start antiviral therapies. It was not widely appreciated that later studies showed that equal treatment yielded equal outcome among equal patients. A higher proportion of Black participants in the original study started therapy with more advanced HIV disease and were less likely to adhere to the prescribed regimen for social reasons.[42] Factors associated with SES again causing a difference in outcome which some interpreted as due to an inherent racial-biologic difference.

The lawmakers who wrote the NIH Revitalization assumed that disparities exist because the drugs and therapies used in the treatment of major diseases have not been tested in minorities and women. Some actually believed that disease like cancer are different in the different races. Other believed that drugs or therapies have different affects in Blacks versus Whites.[43] Ignored is an important fact; many of the racial differences are because minority and poor patients do not get the treatment that is known beneficial to them and treatments not administered certainly do not work.

If health disparities are to be overcome and we are to have equity, it is best to embed good disparities related research questions into cancer treatment, prevention, screening, and control trials.

This can provide more robust statistical power to address important questions.

Diverse enrollment in clinical trials is important. In the study of interventions and outcomes, there is the concept of efficacy and effectiveness. Efficacy is how well an intervention works in an ideal clinical environment. Effectiveness is how well that intervention works in a "real-world" situation. It is important that persons from all communities participate in clinical trials. An effort to do research in the community where the majority of cancer care is provided is an effort to make results more broadly pertinent. Study of accrual to NCI funded treatment studies has for some time shown relative racial/ethnic balance in clinical trial enrollment and refusal rates.[44,45] Indeed, there is interest in inclusion of the elderly, people with comorbid diseases in clinical trials to get more realistic findings.[46]

Summary

Health disparities or health equity research and programs are important. It is paramount that we carefully define our measures of outcome and the populations being compared. There are differences in disease incidence and outcome by population, however defined.

An important fact is a number of well-designed studies and meta-analysis of studies show that equal treatment yields equal outcome among equal patients.[26] If people with the same genetic markers are compared, race is not a factor in outcome unless it is allowed to be. Rarely discussed is the fact that numerous patterns of care studies demonstrate that there is not equal treatment. Often find the discussion focuses on is a particular breast cancer drug is as effective in Blacks as it is in Whites, but it is forgotten that a substantial proportion of Blacks do not get adequate treatment to include surgery as well as chemotherapy and radiation.

With scientific progress, our understanding of cancer improves. We better appreciate its causes, biologic behaviors, and treatments. We are quickly moving into an era of personalized medicine in which genetics and genomics become very relevant. The advent of precision medicine and tailored therapy will make categorization using genes and polymorphisms more important. The crude categories of race and ethnicity and even SES will only be important in terms of social issues such as access to care and equality of treatment.

Social interventions to overcome disparities and bring about equity include efforts to:
- Increase cultural competence and understanding of the patient among healthcare providers
- Increase access to care
  ◦ Provision of insurance
  ◦ Staffing community health centers
  ◦ Attention to the patients social situation
- Improve communications and educate those needing service
  ◦ Targeted messaging
  ◦ Patient navigation

References

1 Fontaine SA, Henschke UK, Leffall LD Jr, et al. Comparison of the cancer deaths in the black and white U.S.A. population from 1949 to 1967. *Med Ann Dist Columbia.* 1972;**41**:293–298.

2 Burbank F, Fraumeni JF Jr. U.S. cancer mortality: nonwhite predominance. *J Natl Cancer Inst.* 1972;**49**:649–659.

3 Witzig R. The medicalization of race: scientific legitimization of a flawed social construct. *Ann Intern Med.* 1996;**125**:675–679.

4 Brewster DH, Black RJ. Breast, lung and colorectal cancer incidence and survival in South Thames Region, 1987-1992: the effect of social deprivation. *J Public Health Med.* 1998;**20**:236–238.

5 Siegel R, Ward E, Brawley O, Jemal A. Cancer statistics, 2011: the impact of eliminating socioeconomic and racial disparities on premature cancer deaths. *CA Cancer J Clin*. 2011;**61**:212–236.

6 Jemal A, Siegel R, Xu J, Ward E. Cancer statistics, 2010. *CA Cancer J Clin*. 2010;**60**:277–300.

7 Jemal A, Simard EP, Xu J, Ma J, Anderson RN. Selected cancers with increasing mortality rates by educational attainment in 26 states in the United States, 1993-2007. *Cancer Causes Control*. 2013;**24**:559–565.

8 Goldson A, Henschke U, Leffall LD, Schneider RL. Is there a genetic basis for the differences in cancer incidence between Afro-Americans and Euro-Americans? *J Natl Med Assoc*. 1981;**73**:701–706.

9 Calle EE, Rodriguez C, Walker-Thurmond K, Thun MJ. Overweight, obesity, and mortality from cancer in a prospectively studied cohort of U.S. adults. *N Engl J Med*. 2003;**348**:1625–1638.

10 Griggs JJ, Culakova E, Sorbero ME, et al. Effect of patient socioeconomic status and body mass index on the quality of breast cancer adjuvant chemotherapy. *J Clin Oncol*. 2007;**25**:277–284.

11 Harrington J, Fitzgerald AP, Layte R, Lutomski J, Molcho M, Perry IJ. Sociodemographic, health and lifestyle predictors of poor diets. *Public Health Nutr*. 2011;**14**:2166–2175.

12 Jamal A, Agaku IT, O'Connor E, King BA, Kenemer JB, Neff L. Current cigarette smoking among adults—United States, 2005-2013. *MMWR Morb Mortal Wkly Rep*. 2014;**63**:1108–1112.

13 Cancer screening—United States, 2010. *MMWR Morb Mortal Wkly Rep*. 2012;**61**:41–45.

14 Characteristics of persons with chronic hepatitis B—San Francisco, California, 2006. *MMWR Morb Mortal Wkly Rep*. 2007;**56**:446–448.

15 Shimizu H, Ross RK, Bernstein L, Yatani R, Henderson BE, Mack TM. Cancers of the prostate and breast among Japanese and white immigrants in Los Angeles County. *Br J Cancer*. 1991;**63**:963–966.

16 Simon MS, Lamerato L, Krajenta R, et al. Racial differences in the use of adjuvant chemotherapy for breast cancer in a large urban integrated health system. *Int J Breast Cancer*. 2012;**2012**:453985.

17 Wu XC, Lund MJ, Kimmick GG, et al. Influence of race, insurance, socioeconomic status, and hospital type on receipt of guideline-concordant adjuvant systemic therapy for locoregional breast cancers. *J Clin Oncol*. 2012;**30**:142–150.

18 Shavers VL, Brown ML. Racial and ethnic disparities in the receipt of cancer treatment. *J Natl Cancer Inst*. 2002;**94**:334–357.

19 Moy B, Polite BN, Halpern MT, et al. American Society of Clinical Oncology policy statement: opportunities in the patient protection and affordable care act to reduce cancer care disparities. *J Clin Oncol*. 2011;**29**:3816–3824. doi: 10.1200/JCO.2011.35.8903. Epub 2011 Aug 1.

20 Betancourt JR, Green AR, Carrillo JE, Park ER. Cultural competence and health care disparities: key perspectives and trends. *Health Aff*. 2005;**24**:499–505.

21 Lund MJ, Brawley OP, Ward KC, Young JL, Gabram SS, Eley JW. Parity and disparity in first course treatment of invasive breast cancer. *Breast Cancer Res Treat*. 2008;**109**:545–557.

22 Short LJ, Fisher MD, Wahl PM, et al. Disparities in medical care among commercially insured patients with newly diagnosed breast cancer: opportunities for intervention. *Cancer*. 2010;**116**:193–202.

23 Griggs JJ, Hawley ST, Graff JJ, et al. Factors associated with receipt of breast cancer adjuvant chemotherapy in a diverse population-based sample. *J Clin Oncol*. 2012;**30**:3058–3064.

24 Breslin TM, Morris AM, Gu N, et al. Hospital factors and racial disparities in mortality after surgery for breast and colon cancer. *J Clin Oncol*. 2009;**27**:3945–3950.

25 Feinstein AR, Sosin DM, Wells CK. The Will Rogers phenomenon. Stage migration and new diagnostic techniques as a source of misleading statistics for survival in cancer. *N Engl J Med*. 1985;**312**:1604–1608.

26 Bach PB, Schrag D, Brawley OW, Galaznik A, Yakren S, Begg CB. Survival of blacks and whites after a cancer diagnosis. *JAMA*. 2002;**287**:2106–2113.

27 Grady WM, Carethers JM. Genomic and epigenetic instability in colorectal cancer pathogenesis. *Gastroenterology*. 2008;**135**:1079–1099.

28 Chu KC, Anderson WF, Fritz A, Ries LA, Brawley OW. Frequency distributions of breast cancer characteristics classified by estrogen receptor and progesterone receptor status for eight racial/ethnic groups. *Cancer*. 2001;**92**:37–45.

29 Gordon NH. Association of education and income with estrogen receptor status in primary breast cancer. *Am J Epidemiol*. 1995;**142**:796–803.

30 Thomson CS, Hole DJ, Twelves CJ, Brewster DH, Black RJ. Prognostic factors in women with breast cancer: distribution by socioeconomic status and effect on differences in survival. *J Epidemiol Community Health*. 2001;**55**:308–315.

31 Millikan RC, Newman B, Tse CK, et al. Epidemiology of basal-like breast cancer. *Breast Cancer Res Treat*. 2008;**109**:123–139.

32 Brawley OW. Health disparities in breast cancer. *Obstet Gynecol Clin North Am*. 2013;**40**:513–523. doi: 10.1016/j.ogc.2013.06.001.

33 Berman DB, Wagner-Costalas J, Schultz DC, Lynch HT, Daly M, Godwin AK. Two distinct origins of a common BRCA1 mutation in breast-ovarian cancer families: a genetic study of 15 185delAG-mutation kindreds. *Am J Hum Genet*. 1996;**58**:1166–1176.

34 Liu E. The uncoupling of race and cancer genetics. *Cancer*. 1998;**83**:1765–1769.

35 Offit K, Gilewski T, McGuire P, et al. Germline BRCA1 185delAG mutations in Jewish women with breast cancer. *Lancet*. 1996;**347**:1643–1645.

36 Yasuda SU, Zhang L, Huang SM. The role of ethnicity in variability in response to drugs: focus on clinical pharmacology studies. *Clin Pharmacol Ther*. 2008;**84**:417–423.

37 Vadivel N, Garg A, Holt DW, Chang RW, MacPhee IA. Tacrolimus dose in black renal transplant recipients. *Transplantation*. 2007;**83**:997–999.

38 McLeod HL, Sargent DJ, Marsh S, et al. Pharmacogenetic predictors of adverse events and response to chemotherapy in metastatic colorectal cancer: results from North American Gastrointestinal Intergroup Trial N9741. *J Clin Oncol*. 2010;**28**:3227–3233.

39 Freedman LS, Simon R, Foulkes MA, et al. Inclusion of women and minorities in clinical trials and the NIH Revitalization Act of 1993—the perspective of NIH clinical trialists. *Control Clin Trials*. 1995;**16**:277–285; discussion 86–89, 93–309.

40 Hamilton JD, Hartigan PM, Simberkoff MS. The effect of zidovudine on patient subgroups. *JAMA*. 1992;**267**:2472–2473.

41 Rothenberg R, Woelfel M, Stoneburner R, Milberg J, Parker R, Truman B. Survival with the acquired immunodeficiency syndrome. Experience with 5833 cases in New York City. *N Engl J Med*. 1987;**317**:1297–1302.

42 Easterbrook PJ, Keruly JC, Creagh-Kirk T, Richman DD, Chaisson RE, Moore RD. Racial and ethnic differences in outcome in zidovudine-treated patients with advanced HIV disease. Zidovudine Epidemiology Study Group. *JAMA*. 1991;**266**:2713–2718.

43 Brawley O. Response to "inclusion of women and minorities in clinical trials and the NIH Revitalization Act of 1993—the perspective of NIH clinical trialists". *Control Clin Trials*. 1995;**16**:293–295.

44 Wendler D, Kington R, Madans J, et al. Are racial and ethnic minorities less willing to participate in health research? *PLoS Med*. 2006;**3**:e19.

45 Langford AT, Resnicow K, Dimond EP, et al. Racial/ethnic differences in clinical trial enrollment, refusal rates, ineligibility, and reasons for decline among patients at sites in the National Cancer Institute's Community Cancer Centers Program. *Cancer*. 2014;**120**:877–884.

46 Unger JM, Coltman CA Jr, Crowley JJ, et al. Impact of the year 2000 Medicare policy change on older patient enrollment to cancer clinical trials. *J Clin Oncol*. 2006;**24**:141–144.

75 Neoplasms in acquired immunodeficiency syndrome

Jeremy S. Abramson, MD, MMSc ▪ *David T. Scadden, MD*

Overview

Immunodeficiency of multiple etiologies is associated with an increased risk of malignancy, particularly lymphoma. The risk is variable, depending on the severity and extent of the immunologic abnormality. In the setting of the acquired immunodeficiency syndrome (AIDS) secondary to human immunodeficiency virus type 1 (HIV-1) infection, the range of tumor types is more extensive. Yet, the tumors are generally associated with oncogenic viruses and may be considered secondary, opportunistic neoplasms. Etiologic factors contributing to them include poor control of oncogenic viruses, altered cytokine regulation owing to HIV effects on immune cells and tissue stimulation from other AIDS-associated events. The interplay of immunity, infection, and oncogenesis is central to AIDS-related malignancies.

The spectrum of the tumor types seen in the context of immunodeficiency extends beyond that of lymphoma, but is quite limited. There appears to be little interaction between the conditions that predispose to the emergence of epithelial malignancies seen in the general population and immunodeficiency. Rather, immunodeficiency tumors represent a narrow subset of neoplasms, some of which are seen with only very low incidence in the general population. For example, primary central nervous system (PCNS) lymphoma and Kaposi sarcoma (KS) are extremely rare entities in all but the immunodeficient population, where they compose a large proportion of tumors. In addition, the incidence of specific tumor types varies according to the immunodeficient state. Non-Hodgkin lymphoma (NHL) is a common theme among all of the immunodeficiencies, yet in AIDS there is a broader spectrum of histologic subtypes than are seen in other immunodeficient states. KS is increased in subgroups of patients with HIV-related and pharmacologically induced immunodeficiency. Cutaneous tumors are common in many immunodeficient states, but the increase in squamous cell tumors of the skin is higher in the post solid-organ-transplantation population than in those with HIV-related immunodeficiency. In the latter, papillomavirus-related squamous cell neoplasia of the anogenital region predominates (Table 1).

Shared among the tumors related to immunodeficient states is the frequent association with an infectious pathogen. The presence of Epstein–Barr virus (EBV) in immunodeficiency-related lymphomas is well known and likely a result of the direct stimulation that the virus provides to B-cell proliferation. In the absence of effective immunologic targeting of cells expressing EBV latency gene products, the overgrowth of cells may proceed unchecked, with the subsequent emergence of a transformed cell. This model for the direct ability of viruses to induce cell proliferation is a paradigm that may be applied to human papilloma virus (HPV)-related tumors as well. However, the model is less easily applied to the KS-associated herpesvirus/human herpesvirus-8 (KSHV/HHV8)-related tumors. The tumors associated with KSHV/HHV8 are more varied and are of less clear pathophysiologic relationship to viral gene products issues that are discussed in greater depth in sections that follow. In general, the tumors that do emerge in immunodeficiency are those in which a secondary pathogen can be implicated (Table 2). Immunodeficiency further leads to a failure of innate host tumor surveillance. In essence, the concept of inadequate immunologic control provides a unifying mechanism, and these tumors may be considered opportunistic malignancies, much the way in which specific infections are considered opportunistic infections. Indeed, the opportunistic malignancies of the immunocompromised patient represent the overlap between infectious diseases and oncology and provide unique insight into the intersection of immune function and tumor development.

Epidemiology

The spectrum of tumors in the context of HIV-1 infection varies on the basis of risk group and is substantially affected by the use of modern combination antiretroviral therapy (cART).

Pre-cART

cART did not become available until 1996, with the introduction of the protease-inhibitor class of anti-HIV medications. Widespread use of protease inhibitors occurred rapidly in the United States, Western Europe, and Australia, altering the death rate and complication rate of HIV disease. The spectrum of opportunistic diseases also changed,[1,2] with an impact on malignant disease, discussed in the section "Post-cART." Given the ongoing lack of access to cART in much of the developing world, and the number of patients unable to take or having failed cART, the profile of AIDS-related malignancies in the pre-cART era is still of considerable importance.

One of the first manifestations of the AIDS epidemic was the cluster of cases of a rare malignancy among men who have sex with men in the coastal cities of the United States. That tumor, KS, was identified as an AIDS-defining illness with the first attempt at classifying the immunodeficiency syndrome by the Centers for Disease Control and Prevention (CDC).[3] The prevalence of KS among HIV-infected patients was approximately 20% early in the AIDS epidemic, but clearly was noted to be highest among patients whose risk factor for HIV transmission was men having sex with men.[4] KS prevalence was substantially lower in the groups infected by blood products or through parenteral drug use.[5] Subsequent behavioral studies indicated that specific types of sexual practice, including promiscuity and oral–fecal contact,[6] had the highest risk and substantiated the impression that KS might be a manifestation of a secondary, transmissible pathogen. Indeed, it was strong epidemiologic data that galvanized efforts to identify a pathogen and that led to the molecular cloning of the KSHV, also known as HHV8.[7]

The second most common malignancy, which was recognized in 1984 to be increased among young men who have sex with men, was NHL. This disease was added to the list of AIDS-defining complications in the first revision of the CDC criteria for AIDS. It was noted that lymphomas that occurred in this population were generally of high-grade histology and followed extremely aggressive clinical courses. Unlike KS, this complication was much more

Holland-Frei Cancer Medicine, Ninth Edition. Edited by Robert C. Bast Jr., Carlo M. Croce, William N. Hait, Waun Ki Hong, Donald W. Kufe, Martine Piccart-Gebhart, Raphael E. Pollock, Ralph R. Weichselbaum, Hongyang Wang, and James F. Holland.
© 2017 John Wiley & Sons, Inc. ISBN: 978-1-118-93469-2

Table 1 Tumor types with increased incidence in HIV disease.

Kaposi sarcoma
Non-Hodgkin lymphoma
    Diffuse large B-cell lymphoma
    Burkitt lymphoma
    Plasmablastic lymphoma
    Primary effusion lymphoma
    Primary CNS lymphoma
Squamous cell neoplasia
Hodgkin lymphoma
Leiomyosarcoma (in children)
Plasmacytoma
Seminoma
Skin cancers
Lung cancer
Osopharyngeal cancer
Liver cancer
Prostate cancer

Table 2 Secondary virus infections associated with AIDS-related malignancies.

Virus	Tumor
EBV	NHL (PCNSL; most systemic DLBCL; PBL)
	HL
	Leiomyosarcoma (children)
KSHV/HHV8	KS
	NHL (PEL) Multicentric Castleman disease (premalignant)
HPV	Squamous cell neoplasia

Abbreviations: ARL, AIDS-related lymphoma; EBV, Epstein–Barr virus HL, Hodgkin lymphoma; HPV, human papillomavirus; KS, Kaposi sarcoma; KSHV, Kaposi sarcoma herpesvirus; NHL, non-Hodgkin lymphoma; PCNS, primary central nervous system; PBL, plasmablastic lymphoma; PEL, primary effusion lymphoma; DLBCL, diffuse large B-cell lymphoma.

broadly based in the risk groups for HIV infection. All groups had a high relative risk, estimated to be approximately 60-fold above that of the general population.[6,8–10] Subsets of infected individuals have been noted to have somewhat greater or lesser risk, such as the hemophiliac population, in which at least one study has noted an increased risk.[6,10] Similarly, it has been noted that risk among intravenous drug users or those from the Caribbean basin may be lower, but concern about confounding issues of care and surveillance complicate that analysis. However, the potential for important cofactors of lymphomagenesis within these subsets remains, and attention to this possibility may yield important information about the process of lymphocyte transformation.

The third most common malignancy occurring in the setting of HIV disease are anogenital squamous cell neoplasms, which are invariably associated with HPV infection of oncogenic serotypes. The majority, however, appear to be *in situ* carcinomas or high-grade intraepithelial neoplasia, while an increased incidence of invasive cancer remains controversial.[11,12] HPV-associated head and neck cancers may also be increasing in prevalence, related to the high seroprevalence of HPV, as well as additional concomitant risk factors for head and neck cancers including immunosuppression, tobacco, and alcohol use.

Post-cART

The introduction of cART has resulted in profound and dramatic changes in the nature of HIV disease. The inexorable decline in immune function and its attendant ravaging secondary infections and tumors in many cases is stopped, and indeed reversed, when combination therapy with protease inhibitors is introduced. The improvement in those patients with advanced disease has led to widespread use of the agents, including among those individuals who have recently acquired HIV-1 infection. The result has been a precipitous decline in the rate of death from AIDS in populations with access to the medications. Although death and debility from AIDS has decreased dramatically, there has not been a similar decline in new cases of HIV infection. Therefore, the total population with HIV infection in the West is rising, and those infected are living longer; globally, the epidemic goes unabated. Some changes in the epidemiology of malignancies in HIV infection have been immediately evident since cART was introduced, but the impact of longer periods of more modest immune dysfunction or even of the antiretroviral drugs themselves is only now becoming understood.

An observation immediately evident in the clinical care of patients with advanced HIV disease was the regression of KS following successful HIV suppression on cART. The impact on new cases of KS was also rapidly noticeable, and epidemiologic data have substantiated the magnitude of those clinically apparent effects. Multiple studies from sites in the United States, Europe, and Australia indicate the widespread decline in KS, with estimates of decline in incidence as high as 80-fold.[13–16] The risk for development of KS, both pre- and post-cART, correlates directly with the depth of CD4 count suppression,[17] though cases of KS in patients with increased CD4 counts are being increasingly reported in the post-cART era,[18,19] where the disease may be more localized to the skin of the lower extremities with less visceral dissemination, more akin to endemic KS seen in non-HIV-infected individuals in the Mediterranean basin.

As with KS, changes in the incidence of primary central nervous system lymphoma (PCNSL) are dramatic. Although this complication of advanced HIV disease was much less common than KS, and its decline was therefore less well documented, the impact in clinical terms has been comparable in magnitude. Cases are rarely seen except among those who have failed or have not been receiving antiretroviral therapy. This is a complication of severe immune suppression that, like the post-transplantation setting, is virtually uniformly associated with EBV detectable in tumor tissue. In general, the EBV latency genes expressed in these tumors are type III or those of lymphoproliferative disease (EBNA1-6, LMP1, and LMP2).[20] These and other features distinguish PCNS lymphoma from other AIDS-related lymphomas (ARL) and may be the basis for clear differences in the impact of cART.

The incidence of systemic AIDS-related NHL has also decreased in the cART era, and the pattern of lymphoma subtypes in this population has also evolved.[21–24] Early in the cART era, it became clear that there was significant variability in the impact of cART among lymphoma subtypes, with the greatest risk reduction seen in PCNSL and immunoblastic diffuse large B-cell lymphoma (DLBCL), while the incidence of Burkitt lymphoma (BL) and Hodgkin lymphoma (HL) did not decline.[22,25] One recent study of a cohort of 23,050 HIV-positive individuals in the United States found that 476 (2%) developed lymphoma between 1996 and 2010, among which 83% were NHLs and 17% were HL.[26] The most common subtype in the cART era is DLBCL, accounting for 42% of cases, and it is also the most common type of NHL in non-HIV-infected individuals. BL accounted for 12% of cases, which is a significantly greater proportion compared to the general population. PCNSL has declined the most dramatically in incidence compared to the pre-cART era, accounting for only 11% of NHLs in this cohort. The risk for most HIV-related lymphomas correlates directly with decline in CD4 count, though less so for BL and HL than other histologies.[17] Median CD4 counts in DLBCL and BL in this modern cohort were 68 and 118 cells/µL, respectively. Reflecting the HIV-infected patient population in the pre-cART era, the median CD4 count was lowest in PCNSL in this modern analysis with a median of 14 cells/µL.

The differential impact of cART within lymphoma subsets highlights biologic differences between these tumor types and suggests differential immune participation in tumor development.

Kaposi sarcoma (KS)

It was the announcement of clustered cases of KS in Los Angeles and New York that made headlines and first brought the AIDS epidemic to public awareness in 1981.[27] Having originally been described by the Hungarian dermatologist Moritz Kaposi in 1872,[28] KS was regarded as a tumor that generally had an indolent course in elderly men of Mediterranean extraction, but which could be problematic in the context of immunosuppressive medication for organ transplantation. It was this latter association that helped focus attention on an immune alteration spreading among subcommunities in urban centers. Recognized as a common entity among HIV-positive men who have sex with men, but not among groups with other risk factors for HIV infection (such as blood product exposure),[5,25] it was long suspected as being related to a second cofactor.[29] A number of potential culprits were examined; none proved tenable until the identification of KSHV/HHV8. This virus was first recognized through the use of a genetic comparison of tissues from individuals with and without KS. A deoxyribonucleic acid (DNA) fragment that had partial homology with other members of the gamma-herpesvirus family was consistently noted.[7] This subset of the herpesviruses includes several viruses with oncogenic potential, such as EBV, associated with a number of tumors and *herpesvirus saimiri* (HVS), associated with the ability to transform T cells. Because of the company KSHV/HHV8 kept and the high frequency of detectable signature DNA sequences in KS lesions, this virus rapidly and justifiably became the focus of investigation for a pathophysiologic basis of KS.

Viral epidemiology

KSHV/HHV8 is a 165-kilobase (kb) double-stranded DNA virus with features strongly supporting its causative role in clinical KS. There are data indicating that KSHV/HHV8 infection precedes tumor formation,[29,30] that populations with high seroprevalence for KSHV/HHV8 are also those with a high incidence of KS,[25] and that the virus infects cell types within tumors.[29]

The definition of prior exposure to KSHV/HHV8 depends on documentation of antibodies specifically reactive against the virus. There have been a number of assays that have been tested with variable results. Data indicate seropositivity estimated at 3.5% in North America, up to 25% in the peoples of the Mediterranean basin, and up to 89% in sub-Saharan African populations.[31–33]

The much-suspected role of sexual transmission has been convincingly demonstrated in a longitudinal study of men in San Francisco over a 10-year period. Among exclusively heterosexual men, no KSHV/HHV8 seropositivity was detected; however, among men who have sex with men, the incidence of seroconversion was linearly related to the number of male sexual-intercourse contacts.[34] Men who had more than 250 sexual partners in the preceding 2 years had a seropositivity rate of 65%. Yet, sexual transmission is not the exclusive basis of virus spread. KSHV/HHV8 can be identified in saliva, and it is thought that oral transmission can rarely occur.[35] The higher incidence of KSHV/HHV8 seropositivity among family members in areas of endemic KS and given that children are often infected in sub-Saharan Africa indicate that nonsexual means

of transmission do occur, but the specific basis is still to be fully defined.

Clinical manifestations

KS characteristically appears as pigmented macular-papular lesions on mucocutaneous surfaces (Figures 1 and 2). It is typically violaceous or erythematous in hue and may be associated with an ecchymotic halo. Typically, the lesions are multifocal and do not have a predictable order or pace of progression. Lesions may present as solitary nodules or plaques, but may also occur in clusters or simultaneously in multiple well-segregated sites. Although classic or endemic KS often favors the lower extremities, the pattern of involvement is much less predictable in the setting of HIV infection. Virtually any mucocutaneous site may be involved. On the face, the ears and nose are often affected, resulting in profound disfigurement. In addition to the disabling cosmetic effects of KS, lesions do occasionally become thick, uncomfortable plaques and can ulcerate with possible superinfection. Lesions are not generally

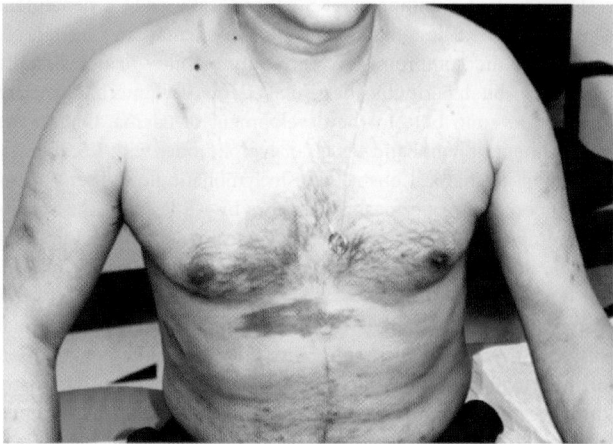

Figure 1 Cutaneous Kaposi sarcoma in a white patient with advanced HIV disease. The violaceous plaques on the chest are of characteristic appearance. These lesions entirely resolved on paclitaxel chemotherapy and antiretroviral medication.

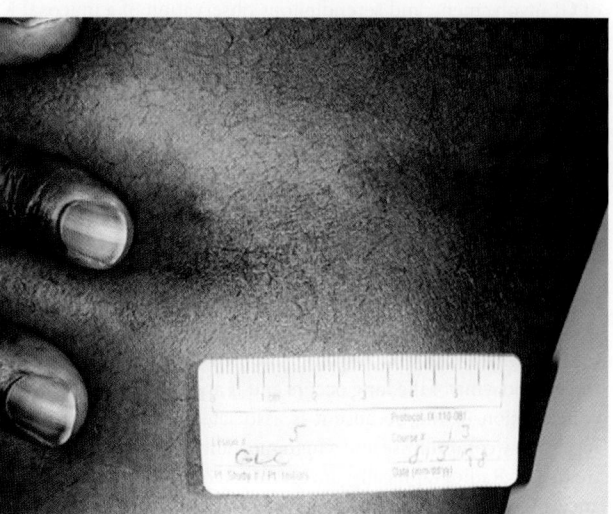

Figure 2 Kaposi sarcoma in an African American male with HIV-1 infection. Skin tone can make the lesions less readily distinguishable from other cutaneous processes and quite distinct from the appearance in lighter skinned individuals.

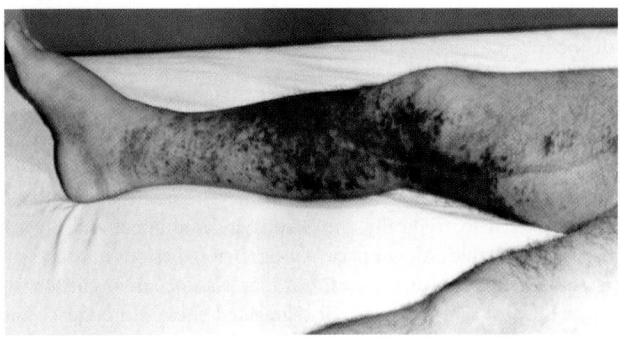

Figure 3 Lower extremity involvement by Kaposi sarcoma can result in marked edema and limited mobility. This patient had pedal edema that had limited response to chemotherapy despite marked improvement in the circumferential Kaposi sarcoma.

destructive, however. The integument or mucous membrane overlying a lesion is most often intact, and deep invasion into muscle or bone generally does not occur.

Edema often accompanies KS either locally or at a dependent site distal to KS lesions (Figure 3). The edema can be marked, with profound compromise of extremity mobility or occasionally with periorbital, peripubic, or genital edema. Two mechanisms are thought to contribute to the development of edema. One is the involvement of lymphatic vessels or lymph nodes with KS, thereby causing a mechanical obstruction to lymphatic flow. The other is the elaboration of permeability factors by KS lesions. The vessels that compose a KS lesion are themselves leaky, with extravasation of plasma proteins and cells into surrounding soft tissue. In addition, the vascular endothelial growth factor (VEGF) produced by KS lesions can alter the integrity of surrounding otherwise-normal vessels, increasing their permeability, and, thus, their contribution of fluid to interstitial fluid. The increased demand on lymphatic drainage and the compromised egress of lymph results in thickened skin locally and frank edema distally.

Involvement of organs other than lymph nodes and skin occurs frequently. The most common site is the gastrointestinal (GI) tract, where mucosal-based lesions are commonly observed in the course of endoscopic examination. The physiologic significance of these lesions is often minimal, however. Most patients will be unaware of GI involvement, and serendipitous observation of a mucosal KS lesion should not trigger a reflex to undertake aggressive therapy. However, there are some individuals for whom GI KS can be a symptomatic and even life-threatening complication. Massive bleeding has been observed, as has intussusception.

Pulmonary involvement may take several forms. Pleural-surface studding with KS lesions can result in pleural effusions, which are often bloody, but which do not have a characteristic set of diagnostic findings or cytologic abnormalities. Bronchial mucosa may be involved and, like GI mucosal surfaces, may be incidentally noted during bronchoscopic examination. The lesions are generally not destructive; but depending on location, they may be responsible for bronchial irritation, coughing, and hemoptysis. Involvement of the parenchyma of the lung occurs and is arguably the most serious complication of KS, because it is associated with life-threatening respiratory compromise and a high mortality rate if unsatisfactorily treated.[36] Radiographically, involvement often takes the appearance of peribronchiolar cuffing on computed tomography (CT). Pathologically, this infiltration may extend into fine interstitial tissue and affect airspace function. This results in either a patchy or diffuse reticulonodular appearance on X-rays. The diagnosis of KS involvement of the lung is often difficult to firmly establish

short of parenchymal thoracoscopic or open biopsy. Bronchoscopy is useful in assessing alternative infectious explanations for clinical findings and may identify mucosal lesions. However, mucosal lesions do not necessarily coincide with parenchymal infiltration, and transbronchial biopsy is often unrevealing. Notably, KS of the bronchial mucosa may coexist with opportunistic infections of the lung parenchyma, such as *Pneumocystis jiroveci* (*P. jiroveci*), cytomegalovirus (CMV) and others, so clinicians must maintain a broad differential diagnosis regarding lung findings in HIV patients, particularly with low CD4 counts. In some circumstances, the use of a therapeutic trial may also be helpful in establishing a presumptive diagnosis. If thorough microbiologic evaluation has been unrevealing, the chemotherapeutic agents discussed below have been well tolerated and associated with high rates of response, such that their use in select patients may be justified as a test for chemotherapy responsiveness of a parenchymal infiltrate. Such a strategy is generally reserved for those patients in whom (1) there is a diagnosis of KS already established from involvement of other sites, (2) there are no symptoms suggesting infection, or (3) aggressive assessment for infection is negative and there are no other contraindications to cytotoxic chemotherapy.

In addition to lung, GI tract, and lymph nodes, special sites of concern are areas of the upper airway. Involvement of the mucosa of the mouth, sinuses, pharynx, and larynx can result in distortion of soft tissues such that airway compromise or alteration of food ingestion can occur. These are lesions that generally respond rapidly to therapy and do not invade deeper structures. Therapeutic approaches are discussed in the section "Treatment."

Given the common involvement beyond the readily apparent skin or oral mucous membranes, extensive staging evaluations are often considered. Although the bulk of tumor does influence prognosis, other characteristics of the patient's immune and general health were incorporated into a KS staging system by the AIDS Clinical Trials Group (ACTG), based on pre-cART data on KS patients (Table 3).[38] In the cART era, tumor extent and concomitant systemic illness appear to the most powerful predictors of prognosis in this model, with limited tumor involvement and lack of opportunistic infections predicting a 3-year overall survival of approximately 90%, compared to only 50% with extensive or visceral disease and presence of other HIV-related complications.[39] An alternative prognostic model has been proposed in the cART era based on multivariate analysis in 326 AIDS-associated KS patients, which identified four favorable prognostic variables by multivariate analysis: (1) having KS as the AIDS-defining illness, (2) increasing CD4 count, (3) age <50 years, and (4) absence of another AIDS-associated illness.[40] These variables generated risk scores predicting for 5-year overall survival ranging from 98% in the most favorable cohort, to only 8% in the least.

The staging performed at diagnosis is often based on clinical presentation, with radiographic studies limited to a chest x-ray unless symptoms dictate otherwise. Testing of stool for fecal occult blood is a reasonable screening test for GI involvement, though specificity is poor. If localizing symptoms do suggest organ involvement, then more extensive radiographic and procedural interventions are appropriate, but they cannot be recommended routinely. Criteria for staging do include assessment of the underlying HIV infection, and all patients should have a careful history regarding medications, other complications of HIV infections, and documentation of the CD4 count in the blood.

Establishing the diagnosis of KS generally depends on simple punch biopsy of the skin or a snip biopsy of mucosal surfaces. The CDC criteria for an AIDS-defining diagnosis of KS do not require

Table 3 Staging classification for AIDS-related Kaposi sarcoma.

	Good risk[a]	Poor risk (1)[b]
Tumor (T)	Small tumor burden with limited involvement of one or more	Large tumor burden
		Oral
	Lymph nodes	Gastrointestinal
	Skin	Pulmonary
	Other[c]	Other visceral with involvement of tumor associated edema or ulceration
Immune system (I)	CD^{4+} cells >200 mm^3	CD^{4+} cells <200 mm^3
Systematic illness (S)	No opportunistic infection (including thrush), or B symptoms[d]	History of opportunistic infection or thrush B symptoms[d]
		Other HIV-related illness (e.g., NHL or other malig-nancy, neuro-logic disease, wasting syndrome)

[a]All the parameters listed.
[b]Any of the parameters listed.
[c]Limited oral disease is confined to the palate and is not nodular.
[d]B symptoms are unexplained fever, night sweats, weight loss of more than 10% of body weight, or diarrhea persisting for more than 2 weeks.
Abbreviations: HIV, human immunodeficiency virus; NHL, non-Hodgkin lymphoma.
Source: Krown 1989.[37]

histologic confirmation if assessment is by an experienced clinician. However, biopsy is strongly recommended, given the broad differential diagnosis for nonblanching lesions resembling KS,[38] including bacillary angiomatosis (usually caused by *Bartonella* infection, with increased frequency in advanced HIV-infection patients); hematoma; purpura; sarcoid plaques; lichen planus; pyogenic granuloma; mycosis fungoides; secondary syphilis; pityriasis rosea; drug-related erythema multiforme; prurigo nodularis; nevi; vascular lesions of the phakomatoses; epithelioid hemangioendothelioma; angiosarcoma; melanoma; and basal cell carcinoma.

Pathology and pathogenesis

The histologic appearance of KS belies its unclear association with the term "sarcoma." No monomorphic array of mesenchymally derived cells is seen. Rather, the lesions are composed of endothelial cells lining ectatic vascular spaces surrounded by spindle cells of variable extent admixed with mononuclear immune cells and extravasated red blood cells. It is the red blood cells that provide the pigment to KS lesions and their breakdown that leads to the ecchymotic halo seen in actively growing lesions. The hemosiderin deposited locally yields a pigmented lesion that may remain even after effective therapy reverses the proliferative spindle and endothelial cell components. Cutaneous lesions are generally within the dermis and deep invasion to muscle is generally not seen.

The origins of the endothelial and spindle cell components remain controversial. The endothelial cells of KS lesions express the VEGF-C receptor characteristic of lymphatic endothelium and do not have detectable nitric oxide synthase, generally present in vascular endothelium.[41,42] The finding that the spindle cell expresses the mannose-binding receptor and CD68 suggests that the origin may be a macrophage-like cell type, perhaps emanating from the sinuses of secondary lymphoid organs and circulating in the blood before ultimately assuming its role in a KS lesion.[43]

The difficulty in defining the cell of origin emanates from its complex histology and the limitations of the available *in vitro* or *in vivo* models. *In vitro* culture has been established for some cell types, and outgrowth of cell lines has been documented, although the relationship to the primary disease process is unclear. *In vivo* transplantation of KS tissue into immunodeficient mice has resulted in tumors, but these are of murine origin. The potential for cytokine elaboration driving lesion development was hypothesized, and studies have extensively characterized cytokine production by KS lesions.[44–46] The cytokines, particularly VEGF and basic fibroblast

growth factor (bFGF), may play a role in the paracrine or autocrine sustenance of KS. Antibodies to bFGF block the proliferation of KS cells and prevent them from entering the S-phase of the cell cycle, even in the presence of exogenous growth factors like the interleukin (IL)-6–IL-6R complex, IL-10, tumor necrosis factor (TNF)-α, and oncostatin M.[47] But exogenous growth factors do not completely explain the phenotype and growth potential of KS cells, which overexpress the antiapoptotic *bcl-2* gene independently of any factors contained in conditioned medium from these cells.[48]

KSHV/HHV8 appears necessary for the induction of KS and is found in KS lesions regardless of whether the underlying context is HIV disease, organ transplantation, or endemic KS. However, the specific mechanism by which the virus participates in the oncogenic process is unclear and does not readily fit into paradigms established by other virus-related neoplastic disease. The latent genes implicated in EBV-induced transformation do not have homologs in KSHV/HHV8. The genes of HVS, which are known to transform cells, have homology only in the genome of a KSHV/HHV8 gene, *K1*, that is capable of transforming an immortalized cell line.[49] However, this gene is not expressed in the latent phase of the KSHV/HHV8 life cycle. Similarly, a chemokine receptor-like KSHV/HHV8 gene product, open reading frame (ORF 74), is constitutively activated and is capable of transforming cells when transduced as a single gene; but it is also a lytic-phase gene.[50] The encoded viral G-protein-coupled receptor activates multiple signaling pathways including the phosphatidylinositol-3 kinase (PI3K)/AKT, mitogen-activated protein kinase (MAPK), and Janus kinase/signal transducer and activator of transcription (JAK/STAT) pathways.[51–53] These pathways exert protean antiapoptotic and proliferative effects that promote tumorigenesis. Two other gene products, K9 (a homolog of the interferon regulatory factor family) and K12 (with no clear gene family homology), are capable of transforming cell lines when transduced but are not expressed in latent phase.[54–57] The lack of clear association with the latent phase would suggest that these gene products are not transforming in cis, but whether they may transform in trans cannot be excluded. A number of other mechanisms, including those that may be capable of acting at a distance, have been raised as possibilities for KSHV/HHV8. These include the chemokine-related gene products, vMIP-I (K6) and vMIP-II (K4), or the IL-6 homolog, K2. Each is capable of interacting with cognate receptors on target cells, either acting as agonists (K2 and K6) or antagonists (K4).[58,59] Finally, there are KSHV/HHV8 gene products that have antiapoptotic effects and that may enhance tumorigenicity. ORF 16 encodes a bcl-2-related gene product,[60] and ORF 71 (K131) encodes a functional member of the Fas-associated death domain-like IL-10-converting enzyme-inhibitory protein (FLIP) family of antiapoptotic genes.[61] The vFLIP of KSHV/HHV8 protects cells from Fas-mediated cell death and can enhance tumor progression of cell lines transplanted *in vivo*. KSHV/HHV8 further induces transcription of hypoxia-induced factor 1 alpha (HIF1alpha) and HIF2alpha resulting in upregulation of the proangiogenic factor, VEGF, as well as other proangiogenic and antiapoptotic factors[62,63] VEGF and VEGF receptors are richly expressed within KS lesions and appear to play a critical role in pathogenesis.[64,65] KSHV/HHV8 has further been shown to encode a microRNA that downregulates thrombospondin 1, a negative regulator of angiogenesis and tumor suppressor.[66] Thus, KSHV/HHV8 encodes a range of gene products with potential for altering the growth, death, and immunologic characteristics of infected cells. It is not clear which of these mechanisms will be seen to play a dominant role in oncogenesis; further investigations into the process will certainly lead to new insights into viral-induced tumors and open new avenues for therapeutic attack.

The prevalence of KS in populations, (1) that are HIV infected, (2) that have undergone solid organ transplantation, (3) that are aged, and (4) that are of Mediterranean extraction, or live in economically disadvantaged parts of tropical Africa, suggests that expression of a KS disease phenotype requires a degree of immunosuppression. The advent of cART for HIV infection treatment offers dramatic support to a central role for immune suppression: Complete remissions of cutaneous and pulmonary KS are well recognized in the context of increases in CD4 count and declines in HIV load induced by cART.[67,68] Although HIV-induced immunodeficiency is only one type of immune abnormality that may predispose to KS, the relative risk among the population co-infected with HIV and KSHV/HHV8 is strikingly high, suggesting the potential for interaction between the two viruses in the pathogenesis of tumor. The HIV gene product, *tat*, affects KSHV/HHV8 replication itself,[69] alters cytokine and cytokine receptor expression in target cells, and leads to proangiogenic effects.[70,71] Expression of *tat* may induce the lytic phase of KSHV/HHV8, resulting in increased viral transcripts, IL6 production, and stimulation of the JAK/STAT proliferation pathway, which offers a pathophysiologic rationale for the preferential occurrence of KS in HIV-infected patients versus solid-organ transplant recipients and other immunosuppressed populations.[51] Retrospective analysis of the incidence of KS among HIV-infected patients receiving antiherpesvirus medications has suggested a direct role of replicating KSHV/HHV8 in the pathologic process. In several studies, there was a decreased incidence of KS in patients treated with ganciclovir or foscarnet.[72-75] Therefore, suppression of replicating virus appears to lower the risk of KS. A randomized controlled clinical trial of valganciclovir in HHV8 seropositive individuals has also been shown to significantly decrease HHV8 replication,[76] though benefits on clinically meaningful endpoints has yet to be established. Although transformation is generally associated with the latent phase of herpesvirus infection, control of the lytic phase (the only time at which the anti-herpesvirus medications have known activity) may limit the potential for transformation.

Control of virus by immunologic means also appears to be highly relevant to the risk of developing KS. It has long been known that there is an increased risk of KS in the context of multiple types of immunologic deficiency. The definition of epitopes of the virus that are recognized by cytotoxic T lymphocytes (CTLs) will allow for further definition of this important point and potentially lead to vaccine strategies.

Treatment

Treatment of KS should be guided by the impact of the tumor on the patient. The goals of treating this disease are to palliate symptoms, alleviate organ compromise, reduce edema, and improve quality of life and ultimately overall survival in affected patients. The variability in the course of HIV-infected patients with KS and the lack of clear association of tumor control with mortality suggests that aggressive therapy may not always be an appropriate response to the diagnosis of KS. This is particularly true among patients with advanced HIV disease or untreated HIV disease. In that setting, the toxicity of cytotoxic therapy may be daunting, and the potential therapeutic effect of anti-HIV medications is considerable. Suppressing HIV replication is associated with a rise in CD4 count, with attendant improvement in immunologic function, and also reduction in whatever the direct contribution of HIV to the pathophysiology of KS might be. The net result is a high frequency of clinical improvement among patients with established KS and, occasionally, complete eradication, simply by the introduction of cART. Therefore, for patients in whom the impact of KS is not organ threatening or profoundly symptomatic, a therapeutic trial of antiretroviral therapy alone is appropriate first-line therapy (Figure 4). This strategy was validated in a phase III placebo-controlled trial in sub-Saharan Africa, where 59 subjects were randomly assigned to cART alone or cART plus combination chemotherapy.[77] Subjects treated with chemotherapy had a higher overall response rate at 1 year (66% vs. 39%), but no difference in overall survival. CD4 count and quality of life improved in both arms, without a statistically significant difference.

In patients with highly symptomatic or organ-threatening disease, a more aggressive approach is warranted, concurrent with cART. Though anti-HIV therapy is an important component in the treatment of HIV-related KS, it should be recognized that not all patients will experience an improvement in their KS with antiretroviral therapy, and that improvement, when it occurs, may only be noted only after 4–8 weeks of therapy. If the patients do not show an improvement in KS by 12 weeks of initiation of anti-HIV therapy, it is unlikely that their disease will be controlled by that intervention alone; additional treatment options must then be considered. Another important phenomenon is that some patients will experience a flare of their KS shortly after beginning cART, evidenced by a rapid increase in size and number of KS lesions. Such flares may be self-limited and can regress with ongoing cART; however, this warrants close attention by treating physicians and consideration of additional KS-directed therapy if a flare becomes clinically significant. In contrast to antiretroviral drugs for HIV, anti-herpesvirus medications do not appear to have a therapeutic role in the management of active KS, where objective responses to ganciclovir and valganciclovir have not been observed. Anti-herpesvirus agents currently available, therefore, cannot be recommended as anti-KS therapy at this time.

Local antitumor chemotherapy

Therapies directed at KS tumors can be divided into either local or systemic therapies. Local therapies offer the benefit of deferring systemic chemotherapies and their attendant risks of increased immunosuppression in an already vulnerable patient population. The selection of a local therapy may be influenced by certain factors, such as the extent and location of the lesions (e.g., small, singular lesions on the trunk or on an extremity) and the rapidity of clinical change (e.g., indolent development of new lesions over months rather than weeks). Options for local therapy include intralesional injection of vinblastine, topical retinoid, radiotherapy and cryotherapy, among others.

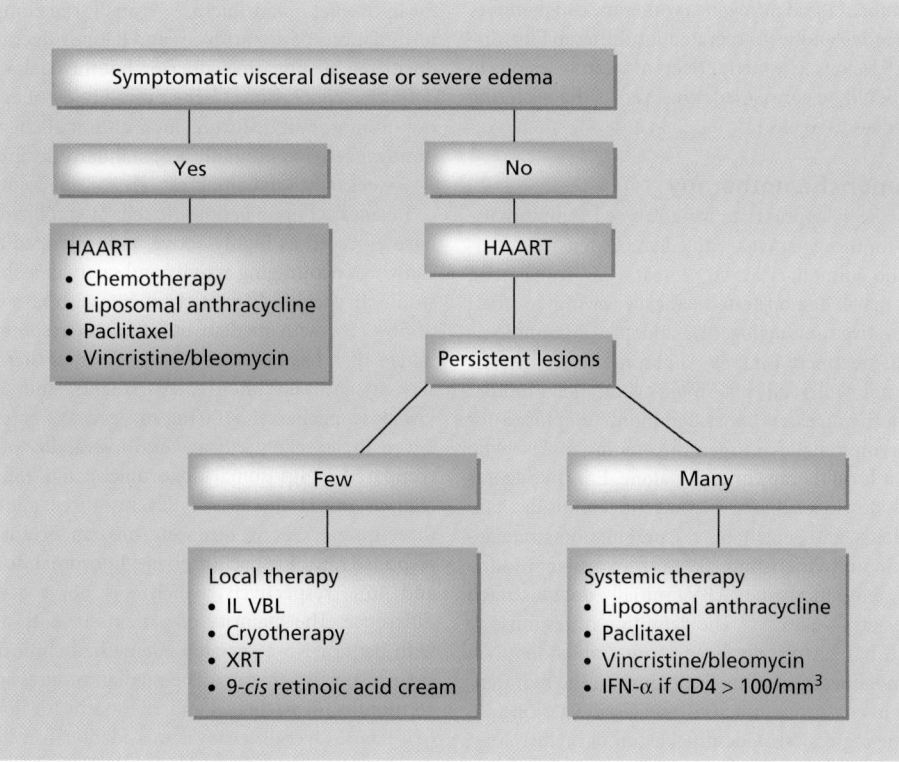

Figure 4 Treatment schema for patients with Kaposi sarcoma. *Abbreviations*: HAART, highly active antiretroviral therapy; IFN-α, interferon-α; IL, interleukin; VBL, vinblastine; XRT, radiation therapy.

For patients who have a small number of lesions that are unresponsive to anti-HIV medications, or who require more rapid improvement than the anti-HIV medications may offer, intralesional injection of vinblastine is a reasonable first-line approach. In particular, palatal or buccal mucosa lesions respond promptly to intralesional vinblastine.[78] Practitioners most commonly use vinblastine at 0.1–0.4 mg/mL, injecting approximately 0.1–0.2 mL into a 1 cm^2 lesion. Local discomfort may be considerable, and so the vinblastine may be admixed 1:1 with lidocaine to improve tolerability. Local reaction is generally modest, but skin breakdown can occur. Unfortunately, responses are usually short-lived, with most lesions progressing after a few months.

Topical 9-cis-retinoic acid (alitretinoin) gel has also been approved for treatment of cutaneous KS based on a randomized placebo-controlled trial in 139 patients, which demonstrated a sixfold higher response rate in the retinoic acid–treated group, as compared with the placebo-treated group.[79] The difficulty with this medication is its potential for inducing an irritating local reaction when applied to normal skin. Consequently, patients must be counseled to be fastidious in their application of the compound exclusively to affected skin. Even with such care, some patients develop local reactions that may be troubling. Responses are not immediate, and may not be observed for 1–2 months after initiation of treatment, so patience is required. Of note, the same compound appears to have activity when given systemically. In two open-label multicenter trials, the tumor response rate was nearly 40%.[80] Headache, dry skin, hyperlipidemia, and pancreatitis were notable toxicities.

Radiation therapy

Radiation therapy using either orthovoltage or electron beam may provide highly effective locoregional control of KS, even at relatively low doses. The great majority of treated patients will experience an objective response, many of which will be complete. A French study of 643 patients with AIDS-associated KS found a complete response rate of 92% when 20 Gy was delivered over 2 weeks, followed 2 weeks later with 10 Gy over 1 week.[81] Modifications in dose schedule may reduce the complexity for patients. A 36-person study administered a total of 21 Gy in thrice weekly fractions for 2 weeks, achieving an overall response rate of 91% with complete response rate of 80%.[82] Treatment with as little as one 8 Gy fraction has been reported to achieve a response in approximately three-quarters of patients.[83,84] Tolerance of therapy is generally good, though acute and late toxicities may occur including increased edema, ulceration, and chronic skin injury. Caution must be used when targeting mucous membranes, as the sensitivity of patients with AIDS to mucositis from radiation therapy appears to be heightened, and debilitating complications can occur.

Photodynamic therapy is an experimental modality employing light activation photosensitizing drugs to result in local tumor necrosis. A study of the photosensitizer photophrin in nearly 350 KS lesions yielded a 96% response rate, one-third of which were complete.[85]

Cryotherapy

Liquid nitrogen cryotherapy has been evaluated in a phase II clinical trial for local control of cutaneous KS.[86] Twenty patients had 2–4 lesions and could be treated every 3 weeks until achievement of maximal response. Complete responses were observed in 80% of lesions with an average of three treatments per lesion (range 1–8). A subsequent retrospective analysis of 30 patients reported a complete response rate in 63% of patients with a mean of 3 sessions required per patient, and many of the remissions were sustained.[87] Blistering occurs frequently with this technique, but bleeding, pain, and infection are uncommon. Liquid nitrogen cryotherapy can therefore be considered an effective and well-tolerated local therapy for discrete symptomatic KS lesions. Cosmetic effects of treating lesions in highly visible sites should be considered, however, as the blistering can be unsightly for days to weeks.

Systemic antitumor chemotherapy

Systemic therapy for KS is appropriate for advanced symptomatic disease, particularly for those patients with edema, extensive mucocutaneous disease, and pulmonary or symptomatic GI involvement. Type 1 interferons have demonstrated efficacy owing to their antiviral, antiproliferative, antiangiogenic, and pro-immunologic activities, though this treatment is rarely employed due to the slow onset of action and poor tolerability.[88] Single-agent and combination cytotoxic chemotherapies are most commonly employed for those patients with symptomatic or organ threatening disease who are not candidates for local therapy or cART alone. Effective agents in this disease include doxorubicin, bleomycin, etoposide, taxanes, the vinca alkaloids, and gemcitabine. Combination strategies with either bleomycin and vincristine (BV) or doxorubicin (adriamycin), bleomycin, and vincristine (ABV) initially demonstrated tumor response rates of 57–88%.[89,90] The definition of response to chemotherapy in KS has historically been more ambiguous than with most other tumors because of the limitations of the bidimensional measurement in cutaneous, mucosal, and visceral lesions. KS can undergo complete regression of identifiable tumor on histology, yet the region of hyperpigmentation may not change in size. What does change is the nodularity of the lesion, the color characteristics (from a violaceous or salmon color to a gray-brown hemosiderin stain), and, when present initially, associated edema. Responses in the early literature are difficult to assess due to lack of uniform response criteria, while more recent studies have benefited by the introduction of standard response criteria initially defined within the ACTG and refined by a joint effort of the AIDS Malignancy Consortium, the National Cancer Institute, and the US Food and Drug Administration (FDA).

Combination cytotoxic therapy with ABV has served as a standard for comparison with newer treatment regimens. Although this regimen produces a substantial response rate, side effects are common, most prominently nausea, alopecia, fatigue, peripheral neuropathy, acral cyanosis, Raynaud phenomenon, cytopenias, and infection.[91] These toxicities can be quite debilitating in a patient population on numerous other medications and often dealing with numerous other medical problems. The impetus for an active, but more easily tolerated, treatment program has therefore been particularly acute in KS. The liposomal encapsulated anthracyclines have provided that option and have emerged as a highly effective and tolerable treatment option. The leaky vasculature composing KS lesions predisposes to deposition of the drug, and lesion concentrations of drug have been shown to be almost an order of magnitude higher than in noninvolved tissue.[92] Furthermore, the side effect profiles of these agents are more favorable. Two phase III studies with approximately 250 HIV-related KS patients in each found liposomal doxorubicin monotherapy superior to traditional cytotoxic combinations of either ABV or BV. Liposomal doxorubicin achieved responses in 46–58% of patients, compared to 25% with the traditional two- and three-drug combinations.[93,94] Time to response and tolerability were both improved in the liposomal doxorubicin–treated patients, as was health-related quality of life,[95] though survival differences were observed. A large randomized study comparing the traditional ABV combination with liposomal daunorubicin found the liposomal drug to have less toxicity, but the tumor response rate was equivalent and not as high as that found

for liposomal doxorubicin.[96] A small trial compared the liposomal formulations of doxorubicin and daunorubicin, with the liposomal doxorubicin appearing superior, but the trial was too small to draw definitive conclusions.[97] The overall body of evidence supports the use of liposomal doxorubicin as an initial chemotherapy of choice in advanced symptomatic KS; standard dosing is 20 mg/m^2 every 2–3 weeks until maximal response or unacceptable toxicity.

Taxanes act upon neoplastic cells by stabilizing microtubules, and have emerged as highly active, well-tolerated agents for KS. After showing encouraging activity and safety in a phase I trial,[98] phase II studies in previously treated patients with KS showed response rates of 56–71% with median durations of response of 9–10 months, longer than has been seen with any other therapy.[99] Responses are seen in anthracycline-treated patients, and patients can tolerate low-dose paclitaxel (100 mg/m^2 every 2 weeks) extremely well. Given the excellent efficacy and tolerability of paclitaxel, this was compared to liposomal doxorubicin in a randomized controlled trial as initial therapy.[100] Seventy-three patients were enrolled, three-quarters of whom were on concurrent cART. The overall response rates for paclitaxel and liposomal doxorubicin were 56% and 46%, respectively, which was not a statistically significant difference. The majority of patients in both arms who presented with pain or KS-associated edema had clinical improvement with their respective therapy. The median progression-free survival was 18 months for paclitaxel and 12 months for liposomal doxorubicin ($p = 0.66$). Overall survival was identical in both arms, and both agents were well tolerated overall. Based on the aggregated data, either liposomal doxorubicin or paclitaxel can be considered an appropriate frontline systemic therapy for KS, with the alternate agent reserved for therapy at relapse if required. At our center, we typically employ liposomal doxorubicin as frontline therapy if there are not contraindications to anthracycline use, and reserve paclitaxel for relapsed disease. For patients who quickly progress off therapy, paclitaxel can be continued as ongoing maintenance therapy; and some patients have received this therapy for over 2 years at our center, with ongoing excellent tumor control. The newer taxane, docetaxel, also has demonstrated efficacy in advanced KS, including patients who have previously received anthracyclines or even paclitaxel, though neutropenia has been a problem.[101,102] We currently would not recommend docetaxel outside of a clinical trial.

Novel therapies

The highly vascular nature of KS lesions and their ready accessibility to study have made KS a candidate disease for assessment of anti-angiogenesis agents. A number of clinical trials involving a range of different agents have occurred or are under way. Bevacizumab is a monoclonal antibody against VEGF-A that was evaluated in a phase II clinical trial of HIV-associated KS patients who did not respond to cART alone.[103] This was an overall high-risk population and the majority of patients had previously been treated with chemotherapy (most commonly liposomal doxorubicin), with a median time since last chemotherapy of 3 months. Bevacizumab was administered intravenously at 15 mg/kg on a 21-day cycle to a total of 17 subjects. The overall response rate was 31%, with 3 patients achieving a complete response. The median number of cycles administered was 10 (range 1–37), and the median time to progression was 8 months. Given the high-risk and pretreated nature of the study population, these results suggest encouraging activity of bevacizumab in HIV-associated KS. Studies combining bevacizumab with other agents are ongoing. The agent thalidomide has a number of properties, including inhibiting angiogenesis, and has been assessed in early-phase studies in patients with KS.

A phase II study with 20 patients demonstrated partial responses in 8 patients and a median time to progression of 7 months.[104] Neutropenia, depression, somnolence, and neuropathy were notable toxicities. The next-generation agent lenalidomide has shown responses in case reports, and a prospective trial for lenalidomide in KS is ongoing.[105,106]

Membrane metalloproteinases (MMPs) are overexpressed in KS cells and may facilitate tumor invasion and metastasis.[107] The MMP inhibitor COL-3 demonstrated efficacy and safety in a 75-patient randomized phase II trial of low-dose and high-dose oral COL-3.[108] The overall response rate was 41% in the low-dose and 29% in the high-dose group, with responses correlating with decline in plasma MMP levels. Rashes and photosensitivity were the most frequent adverse events.

KSHV/HHV8 induces the PI3K/AKT/mTOR pathway, resulting in pro-proliferative and anti-apoptotic effects which contribute to KS pathogenesis.[53] Targeting of the mTOR pathway has therefore garnered attention as a rational therapeutic target in this disease. Enthusiasm for this strategy was generated by a report of 15 patients with KS post renal transplantation who had a striking 100% complete response rate when immunosuppression was changed from cyclosporine to sirolimus.[109] A small study by the AIDS Malignancy Consortium of seven subjects with HIV-associated KS on cART showed responses in three subjects, all of whom were on protease-inhibitor-containing therapy which resulted in higher sirolimus exposure.[110] The drug was well tolerated and did not result in significant changes in HIV viral load or a significant decrease in CD4 counts. Additional data will hopefully further inform the role of this agent in HIV-associated KS.

Tyrosine kinase inhibitors have attracted attention as a possible treatment strategy in KS due to the role of platelet-derived growth factor (PDGF) and c-KIT activation in KS biology.[111,112] The AIDS Malignancy Consortium conducted a 30-person phase II trial of imatinib mesylate in HIV-associated KS.[113] Seventy-seven percent of patients had prior cART, and 57% had prior chemotherapy for KS. The overall response rate was 33%, all partial responses, with a median time to response of 21 weeks. Among responders, the median duration of response was 9 months.

The viral process underlying KS and the relationship of the disease to immune function also suggests that immunologic approaches may ultimately have therapeutic value. KSHV/HHV8 can alter both macrophage and CTL function. Macrophage inhibitory chemokines are encoded by the virus and produced in KSHV/HHV8-infected cells. The cells also produce an OX-2 homolog termed K-14. OX-2 receptors are present on monocyte/macrophages and stimulation dampens the ability of macrophages to be activated by other stimuli. K14 is capable of reducing activated macrophage production of inflammatory cytokines, possibly restricting host response to KSHV/HHV8.[114] In addition, KSHV/HHV8 encodes genes that alter the ability of infected cells to be targeted by CTLs. The K3 and K5 viral gene products limit CTL engagement of MHC class I molecules, and K5 also inhibits interaction with the coreceptor (B7) complex necessary for CTL activation.[115] However, a number of reports have defined epitopes within KSHV/HHV8 gene products that are recognized by CTLs.[116,117] Definition of whether reactivity to certain epitopes associates with protection from disease and whether immune inhibitory pathways may be further considered if a vaccine or adoptive cell therapies become of interest in this disease.

Non-Hodgkin lymphoma (NHL)

Lymphoproliferation occurs in the context of immunodeficiency of many different types. It is a common complication in individuals born with congenital abnormalities of T-cell function, individuals receiving immunosuppressive medications for organ transplantation, and in individuals with HIV infection. The common theme among these is the role of EBV going unchecked in its ability to induce B-cell proliferation. However, only a minority of ARL resembles the lymphoproliferative disease of the congenital or post-transplantation setting. ARL comprises a complex set of tumors with challenging clinical scenarios. It has been, and remains, the most lethal complication of HIV infection, demanding new approaches and new understanding of the pathophysiology underlying it. The most common ARL is DLBCL, followed by BL, PCNSL, primary effusion lymphoma (PEL) plasmablastic lymphoma (PBL), and rarely peripheral T-cell lymphomas (PTCL). These entities show significant variation in incidence based on the depth of HIV-related immunosuppression.

Epidemiology

The association of NHL with HIV infection was evident within the first half-decade of the AIDS epidemic, when an unusual number of lymphomas among young men became evident in cancer registries in California. The first revision of the definition of AIDS by the CDC, in 1987, included NHL, and it has remained an important and devastating manifestation of HIV infection. Unlike KS, in which select subsets of HIV-infected individuals have a unique risk, NHL is more uniformly distributed among risk groups for HIV, with little variation. What variation is present may be attributable partly to issues of care.

The risk of NHL among HIV-infected individuals is in part determined by the level of immunosuppression, with higher risk noted among those with low CD4 cell counts; however, specific subsets of lymphoma have a stronger association with severe immunosuppression than others. The occurrence of PCNSL is restricted to those with very advanced immunodeficiency, as are the PEL and PBL subsets of systemic ARLs. These manifestations of profound immune dysfunction have significantly decreased in incidence since the advent of cART. Among the other ARLs, DLBCL has declined in incidence due to cART, but continues to be the most common ARL. Unlike other subtypes of ARL, BL occurs most commonly in the setting of preserved immune function, and constitutes an increasing proportion of ARLs over time as individuals enjoy longer lives with well-controlled HIV.[26,118] The median CD4 counts in most treatment reports of ARLs are in the range of 50–100 cells/mm³, with the BL group often having a CD4 count >200 cells/mm³. In contrast, reports of patients with PCNSL demonstrate profound CD4 count depression).[26,119] Thus, NHL may occur across a broad range of contexts in HIV disease, including those with virtually no other manifestations of immunosuppression, and may be the presenting illness of HIV infection. Possible unrecognized HIV infection should therefore be considered in any person presenting with an NHL histology that may occur in the context of HIV infection. The duration and severity of persistent immunosuppression is important in determining risk for developing an ARL, with a relative hazard of approximately 1.4 for each 50% decline in CD4 count. Reassuringly, as the CD4 count responds to cART, the risk of lymphoma reduces, but there is a lag time of approximately 1 year, somewhat longer than for other opportunistic diseases.[21] Interestingly, the reduction in risk appears to proceed with longer time on cART in parallel and likely reflects the gradual repair in immune function seen over long periods of time on cART. Immune function is accompanied by HIV ribonucleic acid (RNA) level as a predictor of ARL risk. In the EuroSIDA study, each log of HIV RNA was associated with a relative hazard of 1.51.[21] Therefore, controlling HIV is a critical determinant of ARL, presumably because of the immunologic alterations it engenders, though other pathophysiologic mechanisms may also participate.

Pathology and pathogenesis

The development of lymphoma among HIV-infected individuals is virtually always associated with transformation of a B cell, a cell type that HIV itself is unable to infect. Thus, HIV does not play a direct role in the development of most ARL; rather, it provides the background immunosuppression either for transforming viruses or for proliferative triggers for B cells to go unabated. The rare exception to this is a small subset of tumors of T-cell origin (PTCL).

HIV-associated PTCL is distinctly uncommon, but includes a spectrum of clinicopathologic entities.[24,120-122] In one subset, the HIV genome has been identified either in the T cells or in tumor-associated macrophages. Definition of the HIV chromosomal integration site revealed a preferential localization to a region upstream of the c-*fes* proto-oncogene, a finding that suggests a direct role for HIV in tumor pathogenesis.[123]

Although HIV may not be present in any but the rare PTCL, other viruses are often present and play a crucial pathogenetic role in lymphomagenesis. Most notably, EBV is common in certain systemic ARLs and virtually all cases of PCNSL. The biology by which this gamma-herpesvirus exerts its effects is being unraveled through molecular analyses and perhaps is most clearly defined for the PCNS lymphomas and post-transplantation lymphoproliferative diseases (PTLDs). In that context, specific expression of latent virus genes is characteristic of a so-called type III pattern. These genes include the *LMP1, LMP2,* and *EBNA1* through *EBNA6.* The *LMP1* gene has been extensively studied as a potentially direct mediator of B-cell proliferation and has been shown to interact with the tumor necrosis factor receptor (TNFR)-signaling pathway.[124,125] LMP1 is expressed in primary tumor tissue from patients with PTLD and ARL and is associated with activation of NFκB, a critical regulator of survival in normal and malignant B cells.[126] LMP1 is a six-transmembrane-spanning molecule with a cytoplasmic carboxy terminus capable of interacting with the TNFR II-associated factors (TRAFs) that mediate downstream transcription factor activation.[125,127,128] Aggregation of the cytoplasmic domains of *LMP1* mimic activated TNFR II, thereby providing a stimulus resembling constitutively activated receptor.[129] The activated pathways are similar to those of the TNFR family member CD30, involving the transcriptional regulators NFκB and cjun.[129,130] Potential downstream targets of these regulators are the pro-proliferative cytokines, IL-6 and IL-10.

A number of mutations within the carboxy terminus of LMP1 have been noted, and there are some data to support the possibility that these are associated with HIV-associated NHL and HL.[129,131-133] However, other studies have indicated that the frequency of such mutations is no greater among those with lymphoproliferative disease than it is among patients in an unaffected control group.[132] The concept that molecular evolution of persistent EBV infection may lead to alteration in the malignant potential of select latently infected B cells is an appealing hypothesis that remains speculative at this time.

The proportion of tumors associated with EBV varies by histologic subtype. EBV is present in virtually all cases of PCNSL and PBL, and in approximately 80% and 30% of HIV-related DLBCL and BL, respectively.[134-137] This finding leaves a large fraction of systemic ARLs without a clear association with an oncogenic

virus; among these, however, a small proportion is linked to KSHV/HHV8. PEL is a unique ARL subtype typically seen in patients with profound immunosuppression, and presents as a fluid collection without tumor mass in the involved body cavity, which may be the pleural space, peritoneum, or pericardium.[138] The tumor cells generally do not express most B-, T-, or even hematopoietic-cell surface markers (they are CD45, CD3, and CD19 negative). Molecular analysis of the cells demonstrates that they have undergone immunoglobulin gene rearrangement consistent with an origin in the B-cell lineage. All such tumors identified to date include the KSHV/HHV8 genome, and most have evidence of EBV co-infection. Notably, nearly all cases of PEL express the CD30 surface antigen. CD30 is the target of brentuximab vedotin, and anti-CD30 monoclonal antibody covalently bound to the microtubule toxin monomethyl auristatin E (MMAE). This drug is FDA approved for other relapsed CD30-expressing lymphomas, HL, and anaplastic large cell lymphoma. Based on the CD30 expression in PEL, brentuximab vedotin was evaluated in PEL cell lines where it resulted in decreased proliferation and apoptosis.[139] *In vivo* evaluation in mouse xenografts with PEL cell lines resulted in tumor progression and prolonged survival. These intriguing *in vivo* and xenograft data warrant clinical evaluation of brentuximab vedotin in this rare but currently unmet medical need.

The ability of KSHV/HHV8 to infect B cells *in vitro* has been shown, whereas the impact of that infection has been difficult to discern *in vitro.* No clear association of virus infection with altered B-cell growth kinetics, as with EBV, has been noted with KSHV/HHV8. However, the close clinical and pathologic relationship of KSHV/HHV8 to PEL is compelling evidence for a direct relationship between KSHV/HHV8 and B-cell oncogenesis. PEL cells are latently infected with KSHV/HHV8, and so latent gene products likely play a dominant role in disease pathogenesis. Specifically, LANA-1, LANA-2, v-cyclin, v-FLIP, and viral IL6 are all transcribed from a common promoter and are constitutively expressed in PEL cells, where they promote cellular proliferation and survival through various mechanisms.[140]

Among the possible contributions of viruses to malignant transformation is alteration in the immunologic reactivity to neoplastic cells. Mechanisms include the ability of EBV EBNA1 to alter antigen-processing pathways and thereby potentially mask EBV-infected cells from CTL reactivity.[141] Although the specific details of the mechanism remain to be elucidated, it appears that KSHV/HHV8 exerts a similar effect on infected transformed cells. In addition, viral gene products may be elaborated by infected cells and may impact immune effector cells. For example, EBV encodes a viral IL-10 homolog (BRCF-1) with biologic activity, mimicking that of endogenous IL-10.[142] Cell lines and tumors from AIDS patients and animal models of ARL indicate that IL-10 is produced,[142-145] and that it potentially exerts an inhibitory influence on the T-helper cell (TH1) response. IL-10 potently suppresses interferon-α and IL-2 production by effector cells of the TH1 response and is a B-cell mitogen.

Other cytokines potentially participating in altered reactivity to malignant cells include IL-6, which, in addition to serving as a proliferative stimulus to B cells, may act to alter cell sensitivity to immune killing. Specifically, IL-6 has been shown to reduce the ability of EBV-positive cells to be lysed by antigen-specific CTL from HIV-1–positive individuals.[146] IL-6 levels have been noted to be elevated in the serum of patients with AIDS and may be associated with the development of NHL.[147] The CD40 and CD40 ligand (CD40L) interaction has also been hypothesized to participate in the development of HIV-related lymphomas. Activation of this TNFR family pathway alters the proliferation, differentiation, and survival of B cells that serve as a key mechanism of interaction of the B- and T-cell-mediated immune mechanisms. The infection of microvascular endothelial cells from the bone marrow and CNS has been shown to result in altered CD40 signaling that upregulates adhesive interactions with B cells and possibly explains the potential for extranodal lymphoma in HIV-infected individuals.[148]

Chemokine pathways may also contribute to the unique susceptibility of HIV-infected patients for lymphomagenesis. Patients with a genetic variant in the CXC chemokine, stroma-derived growth factor-1 (SDF-1), have an excess risk of developing the BL subtype of ARL.[149] This chemokine is a known B-cell mitogen and by exerting chemokinetic effects, may contribute to a proliferative stimulus for patients with the genetic variant. The presence of this variant has been suggested to possibly provide a method of identifying those patients with increased risk of lymphoma, although the potential for this risk factor remains speculative at this time.

Genetic mutations in the tumor cells have been well characterized and are related to the specific histologic subtype. DLBCLs exhibit a Bcl-6 rearrangement in approximately 33% of cases, a c-*myc* rearrangement in as high as 40%, and a TP53 mutation in approximately 25%.[150,151] In contrast, BLs seen in AIDS have c-*myc* rearrangements but not *Bcl-6*, and rarely have TP53 mutations.[152–154] The presence of EBV is variably associated with either the c-*myc* or *Bcl-6* rearrangements in BL and DLBCL, respectively. The finding that rearranged c-*myc* gene juxtaposes with the immunoglobulin gene heavy chain switch region suggests that the malignant event is occurring proximate to the time of immunoglobulin class switching. This relatively late event in B-cell ontogeny is indicative of transformation in a relatively mature germinal center B cell.

Clinical manifestations

ARLs are generally extremely aggressive, high-grade lymphomas. The presenting clinical features of systemic ARLs are similar to those of aggressive NHLs in the immunocompetent host, though HIV-infected patients are likelier to present with advanced-stage disease and frequent involvement of extranodal sites. Extranodal involvement occurs in the majority of patients,[155] and lymphoma restricted to extranodal sites may be seen in approximately half of the patients. Particular sites of involvement are favored by specific histologic types. Among those patients with BL, bone marrow and leptomeningeal disease occur in approximately one-quarter, while DLBCL favors the GI tract and liver as well as brain parenchyma and leptomeninges, though no extranodal site is immune from lymphoma involvement.

Systemic "B" symptoms of significant weight loss, fevers, and drenching night sweats are common. Given the immunosuppressed nature of these patients, a thorough microbiologic evaluation is required to exclude concomitant bacterial, mycobacterial, viral, fungal, or parasitic disease. KSHV/HHV8-associated multicentric Castleman disease (MCD) should also be considered in the differential diagnosis, as discussed below.

PEL is usually an end-stage complication of HIV-induced immunosuppression occurring generally with a CD4 count of <50 cells/mm^3 and has occasionally been observed in other types of immunosuppression, including that associated with organ transplantation. The common sites of involvement with this tumor are the peritoneal cavity, pleural space, and pericardium.[156] Involvement of the bone marrow has been observed with progressive disease, and rare cases of extracavitary PEL do occur, usually involving other extranodal locations.[157–159] The approach to this patient population is similar to any other systemic ARL, including evaluation of the CNS.

Plasma cell disorders are increased in the setting of HIV infection and are also fairly heterogeneous. Rare cases of highly aggressive PBL of the jaw and oral cavity occurs most frequently in severely immunosuppressed patients, usually with CD4 counts below 50 cells/mm^3, but may occur in patients with less profound immune dysfunction.[136] Histopathology has indicated that these tumors mark as plasma cells with MUM1, CD138, and CD38 and are often negative for typical lymphoid markers, such as CD45 (leukocyte common antigen) and CD20. EBV is uniformly present with a lower frequency of KSHV/HHV8. PBL is a highly aggressive disease. The Ki67 proliferation fraction is usually >90%, and MYC translocations are detected in approximately half of the patients.[160] Extramedullary plasmacytomas and overt multiple myeloma with paraprotein specific for HIV antigens have also been reported. Treatment of plasmacytoma and multiple myeloma should be based on standard guidelines for these diseases outside the context of HIV infection. The optimal care for PBL remains undefined, but CHOP (cyclophosphamide, doxorubicin, vincristine, and prednisone), as would be used for DLBCL, has produced very poor results. Given the rapid disease kinetics and often MYC translocation, therapies typically directed at BL are often used in patients who can tolerate such therapy.

PCNSL represents 15–20% of all HIV-related lymphomas, and is generally a manifestation of severe immunosuppression. Mean CD4 counts are <30 cells/mm^3, there is commonly a previous history of an AIDS-defining complication, and the EBV genome is invariably present in the tumor.[161] Histologically, these tumors have an immunoblastic diffuse large B-cell appearance and express a type III pattern of EBV latent gene products.[162] The clinical approach to these patients is detailed in a later section.

MCD, or angiofollicular lymph node hyperplasia, may occur in patients with advanced HIV disease and mimic the presentation of an ARL or infectious disease.[163] MCD is a polyclonal disease that is uniformly associated with KSHV/HHV8 in the HIV-infected patient and may exhibit a rapidly progressive, lethal course. Both the hyaline-vascular and plasma cell subtypes of MCD have been reported in AIDS, but the plasma cell histology type is far more common. KSHV/HHV8 is found in the involved nodes, and there is a high prevalence of co-incident or subsequent KS.[163] Fever, lymphadenoapthy, hepatosplenomegaly, and anemia are present in virtually all patients; and IL-6 is abundantly produced in MCD and plays a critical role in the pathophysiology, via activation of the JAK/STAT pathway, and promotion of angiogenesis and proliferation.[164–166] A monoclonal antibody against IL-6 has shown clinical efficacy in the treatment of HIV-negative HHV8-negative MCD,[167] but clinical efficacy in HIV-associated MCD has yet to be established. Patients with MCD may present with a synchronous ARL, and an ARL may occur subsequent to the diagnosis of MCD; so diagnostic vigilance is required with a low threshold for repeat biopsy in the setting of progression or relapse, or based on a change in clinical behavior.

Clinical approach

Evaluation of patients with ARL follows staging procedures for other types of NHL, with several caveats specific to the HIV-infected population. First, the frequent involvement of the CNS mandates a more thorough assessment of the CNS than in HIV-negative counterparts, including sampling of the cerebrospinal fluid (CSF) in the majority of patients at diagnosis, and consideration of neuroimaging, particularly in the presence of neurologic signs or symptoms. CSF sampling can be omitted in selected patients with no neurologic symptoms and low-risk features including limited stage disease, absence of extranodal disease, and normal LDH. Second, the potential for co-incident opportunistic infection must be kept in mind when evaluating a patient with "B" symptoms or suspicious radiographic findings. Microbiologic evaluation is particularly important for that population with CD4 counts <200 cells/mm³ in whom the risk of opportunistic disease is increased, and is a necessity for those with <50 cells/mm³. Depending on the clinical scenario, particular concern should be paid to the possible presence of active *P. jiroveci* (formerly *Pneumocystis carinii*), CMV, *Toxoplasma gondii*, *Mycobacterium avium complex*, *Mycobacterium tuberculosis*, and *Cryptococcus*. Hepatitis B and C serologies should be evaluated in all patients since co-infection may occur. Third, assessment of the status of the HIV disease is critical in defining the therapeutic approach. CD4 cells should be measured as well as plasma HIV RNA, and a detailed history of previous antiretroviral therapy and opportunistic disease should be obtained. Those patients for whom NHL represents a manifestation of end-stage, treatment-refractory HIV disease should be considered for palliative intent. For the majority of patients, however, viral suppression on cART offers an open-ended prognosis from HIV-1 infection, and the emphasis should be on curing the lymphoma—a concept not realistically considered in the pre-cART era, but of substantial importance since the availability of cART in 1996. Selecting a cART regimen appropriate for the patient involves weighing where the patient may lie in the continuum of HIV disease as well as consideration of drug–drug interactions, and should be performed collaboratively with an infectious disease specialist.

Prognostic factors

Prognosis in patients with ARL has generally been poor; but with the advent of cART, the improved prognosis from HIV-1 itself, as well as the improved tolerance of chemotherapy, long-term outcome in patients with ARL has substantially improved. Prior to the advent of cART, the median survival for patients with HIV-associated DLBCL was 8 months compared to 43 months in the setting of cART.[168] Poor prognostic factors in ARL prior to the introduction of cART included age >35 years, intravenous drug use, and stages III/IV disease, which predicted overall survival ranging from 46 weeks in the most favorable subgroup to 18 weeks in the least.[169] The International Prognostic Index (IPI) is the most commonly used risk stratification tool in the setting of non-HIV-related aggressive lymphoma,[170] and has been evaluated in ARL. In the pre-cART era, outcome was poor in all IPI subgroups; however, since the advent of cART, the IPI separates three risk groups with risk scores of 0–2, 3, and 4–5 predicting 3-year overall survivals of 64%, 50%, and 13%, respectively.[171] None of these patients, however, received rituximab, which is now included in the therapy for the majority of patients with CD20+ lymphomas, as discussed below. A prognostic score has been developed in the cART and rituximab era based on an analysis of 487 ARL patients treated on prospective clinical trials with rituximab-containing chemotherapy.[172] The majority of patients had DLBCL (70%), with most remaining patients having BL. The median CD4 was 174 cells/µL and 40% had a prior diagnosis of AIDS. The most common chemotherapy regimen administered was R-CHOP (49%), followed by EPOCH-R (19%), the GMALL regimen (16%), and CDE (cyclophosphamide, doxorubicin, etoposide, 15%). Based on significant prognostic factors on multivariable analysis, a prognostic model was developed incorporating the traditional age-adjusted IPI risk factors (advanced stage, poor performance status, and elevated LDH), with the addition of CD4 count, HIV viral load, history of AIDS, and number of extranodal sites. These prognostic factors generated three risk groups with 5-year overall survival in the low, intermediate, and high-risk groups of 78%, 60%, and

50%, respectively, which appeared to be a superior predictor than the traditional IPI. These data demonstrate the high curability of ARLs using modern therapies and concurrent cART. Additional studies have also non-center marker expression (BCL-6 and CD10 negative, MUM1/IRF4, or CD138 positive) to be associated with a shorter disease-free survival, analogous to HIV-negative DLBCL.[173] BL demonstrates an extremely poor outcome when treated with traditional DLBCL-type regimens like CHOP, but modern data demonstrate that HIV-related BL patients fare just as well as their HIV-negative counterparts when treated with combination regimens typically used in adults with non-HIV-associated BL.[171,174–176] In considering prognosis of ARL patients, the status of HIV disease itself must always be carefully considered given that tolerance of therapy is significantly poorer in patients with advanced AIDS failing antiretroviral therapy.

Treatment

Early in the AIDS epidemic, the aggressive nature of the lymphomas observed was met with an aggressive clinical approach to therapy. The result was severe toxicity and frequent treatment-related death. Since that time, however, prophylactic therapy for opportunistic infections has improved, as has supportive care with hematopoietic growth factors, thus easing the tolerability of chemotherapy. Low-dose chemotherapy regimens were developed with the goal of minimizing treatment-associated toxicity in the setting of AIDS, but demonstrated uniformly poor results in the pre-cART era. With cART and supportive care, however, it became clear that patients with ARL could then be treated with the same standard dose chemotherapy regimens administered to their HIV-negative counterparts, with much improved outcomes compared to the pre-cART era. Accordingly, reduced dose regimens rarely have a role in modern ARL therapy.

The most commonly employed regimens for ARL in the modern era are CHOP and EPOCH, with the addition of rituximab for CD20+ cases (see further discussion below) (Table 4).

Standard cytotoxic chemotherapy plus antiretroviral therapy

Early in the ART era, combination of antiviral therapy with chemotherapy proved difficult due to drug–drug interactions and overlapping toxicities including bone marrow suppression and peripheral neuropathy, among others. This led to some early debate on whether ART should be administered concurrently with chemotherapy or be held during cancer therapy. Given the advances in modern cART, however, the toxicities and drug–drug interactions are reduced and highly manageable. It has also become clear that concurrent cART decreases complications of AIDS during therapy and improves the ability to administer full-dose chemotherapy with curative intent. Accordingly, concurrent administration of cART with chemotherapy in ARL is the modern standard of care.

This approach was validated by a trial of CHOP plus indinavir, d4T, and 3TC conducted by the AIDS Malignancy Consortium and involved a cohort of patients receiving low-dose CHOP and a subsequent cohort receiving full-dose CHOP plus the same antiretroviral regimen.[177] This study indicated that the combination did not result in unexpected severe or more frequent toxicities. Pharmacologic analysis tested the possibility both of antineoplastic drugs affecting protease inhibitor levels and of antiviral therapies altering cytotoxic drug metabolism. No alterations in levels of indinavir or doxorubicin were noted, although a reduction in cyclophosphamide clearance of approximately 50% was observed.

The United States National Cancer Institute tested infusional dose-adjusted EPOCH without concomitant cART.[178] The etoposide, vincristine, and doxorubicin were given as a 96-h continuous

Table 4 Commonly used therapy regimens for AIDS-related lymphoma.

Therapy regimen	Dose and schedule
CHOP (+/– Rituximab based on CD20 expression)[a]	
Cyclophosphamide	750 mg/m^2, IVPB, day 1
Doxorubicin	50 mg/m^2, IVPB day 1
Vincristine	1.4 mg/m^2 (not to exceed 2 mg), IVPB, day 1
Prednisone (each cycle q 21–28 d)	100 mg, po, days 1–5
Rituximab (if included)	375 mg/m^2, day 1
Supportive care includes concurrent cART and prophylaxis against *P. jiroveci* and herpesviruses	
EPOCH regimen (+/– Rituximab based on CD20 expression)[a]	
Etoposide	50/m^2, CI, days 1–4
Vincristine	0.4 mg/m^2, CI, days 1–4
Doxorubicin	10 mg/m^2, CI, days 1–4
Prednisone	60 mg/m^2, po, days 1–5
Cyclophosphamide	375 mg/m^2, IV, day 5
Rituximab (if included)	375 mg/m^2, day 1 (or on day 1 and day 5 if administering as SC-EPOCH-RR)
Supportive care includes concurrent cART in most patients and prophylaxis against *P. jiroveci* and herpesviruses, and a proton-pump inhibitor	

Abbreviations: CHOP, cyclophosphamide, hydroxydaunomycin (doxorubicin, adriamycin), Oncovin (vincristine), prednisone; CNS, central nervous system; EPOCH, etoposide, prednisone, Oncovin (vincristine), cyclophosphamide, hydroxyldaunomycin (doxorubicin, adriamycin); G-CSF, granulocyte stimulating factor; IV, intravenously; po, per os (orally); SC-EPOCH-RR, short-course-EPOCH with 2 doses of rituximab per cycle.
[a]CNS prophylaxis with intrathecal methotrexate should be included for the majority of patients, but may be omitted in selected low-risk patients with limited-stage disease, normal LDH, and absence of extranodal disease.

infusion, followed by bolus cyclophosphamide on day 5; the cyclophosphamide dose was modified based on baseline CD4 count and neutropenia during the prior cycle. Intrathecal methotrexate was administered with each cycle for CNS prophylaxis. Holding antiviral therapy resulted in a rise in HIV RNA during cancer chemotherapy that reverted to entry levels when antivirals were resumed following completion of chemotherapy. Clinical outcome was the best reported to date in ARL patients with 74% of patients achieving a complete response and 5-year disease-free and overall survivals of 92% and 60%, respectively. Continuous-infusion regimens have also been combined with antiviral therapy as initial treatment of ARL. The CDE regimen (cyclophosphamide 800 mg/m^2, doxorubicin 50 mg/m^2, etoposide 240 mg/m^2, by continuous 96-h infusion) was tested in 98 patients with concomitant cART (dideoxyinosine [ddi] monotherapy was used in the first 43 patients) resulted in a complete response rate of 45%, with 43% of patients alive after 2 years.[179] Patients treated with concomitant cART versus ddi had an improved overall survival owing to decreased hematologic toxicity and treatment-associated death. These trials support that combining antivirals and antitumor therapy appears safe and effective. The short-term consequences of holding antiretroviral therapy appear to be acceptable in selected low-risk patients with reasonable immune function; but this should be done cautiously, with initiation of cART once feasible.

BL patients have traditionally been included in trials with other ARLs and have not clearly had a worse outcome from HIV-related DLBCL, though the majority of these trials were conducted prior to cART when outcomes were uniformly poor. Modern evidence suggests that patients with HIV-related BL experience similarly encouraging outcomes to non-HIV-infected patients when treated with intensive multiagent chemotherapy.[174,175]

Monoclonal antibody therapy
Efforts to improve the outcome for patients with ARL have included the addition of the humanized anti-CD20 antibody rituximab, which has shown a survival benefit when combined with CHOP chemotherapy in HIV-negative DLBCL.[180] A multicenter randomized phase III trial testing CHOP versus CHOP plus rituximab (R-CHOP), however, demonstrated that in the setting of AIDS,

patients did not have an improvement in overall outcome with the addition of rituximab.[181] There was a trend toward improved response (58% vs. 47%) with rituximab that did not reach statistical significance; however, this was outweighed by an increased rate of infection-related death (14% vs. 2%). Most deaths in the rituximab arm were in patients with CD4 counts <100 cells/mm^3, with 60% of deaths occurring at a CD4 count <50 cells/mm^3. Further complicating analysis of this trial is a 3-month maintenance rituximab period following initial R-CHOP, during which time 40% of infection-related deaths occurred. Subsequent phase II studies, however, showed that rituximab could be added to standard chemotherapy for ARL with the suggestion of improved clinical outcomes,[175,182–185] and a meta-analysis of 1060 ARL patients treated on prospective clinical trials with rituximab plus chemotherapy or chemotherapy alone demonstrated an improved survival in rituximab-treated patients.[186] Accordingly, inclusion of rituximab is considered standard for patients with ARL in the modern era, but patients with low CD4 counts continue to be at increased risk for treatment-associated complications and must be followed up closely and receive maximal supportive care including prophylactic antibiotics and growth factor support.

The optimal chemoimmunotherapy strategy remains a subject of debate. R-CHOP and EPOCH-R are both considered standard regimens for HIV-associated DLBCL. A pooled analysis of 150 patients with HIV-associated CD20+ NHL treated on AIDS Malignancy Consortium studies found EPOCH-R to be associated with an improved event-free survival (hazard ratio [HR] 0.40; 95% confidence intervals [CI], 0.23, 0.69; $P < 0.001$) and overall survival (HR, 0.38; 95% CI, 0.21, 0.69; $P < 0.01$),[187] making this a preferred regimen for most patients. Studies of EPOCH-R have also shown that concurrent administration of rituximab on day 1 of each chemotherapy cycle appears to offer improved disease control compared to sequential treatment of EPOCH followed by rituximab, and that ARL patients may be treated with fewer chemotherapy cycles if rituximab is administered twice per cycle (short-course EPOCH-RR).[184,185] Both standard EPOCH-R and short-course EPOCH-RR can be considered appropriate regimens for CD20+ ARL patients. Though primarily studied without concurrent cART, EPOCH-R can be safely combined with cART and this is recommended as standard practice. Routine prophylaxis on EPOCH-R also includes routine white cell growth factor support, and prophylaxis against *P. jiroveci*, herpesvirus infections, and gastric ulcers with a proton pump inhibitor.

BL patients may be treated with the same intensive chemotherapy regimens plus rituximab, as have been used for non-HIV-infected BL patients.[174] The safety of high-intensity regimens in HIV infection may reflect the generally improved HIV control and CD4 count relative to other ARL subsets. More recently, the short-course EPOCH-RR regimen (rituximab is given twice per cycle) has been evaluated in 11 HIV-associated BL with a 6-year overall survival of 90%.[175] These encouraging data warrant further evaluation in a larger cohort of HIV-associated BL patients. PBL is a highly aggressive lymphoma, often also including an MYC translocation, that is usually treated similarly to BL. Our practice is to use EPOCH in the majority of PBL patients. Rituximab usually has no role as these cases are typically CD20 negative, but rituximab should be included for rare CD20 positive cases. Multiple case reports have demonstrated responses to the proteasome inhibitor bortezomib, so this can be considered an option for relapsed disease.[188-192] As with other ARLs, concurrent cART is recommended for all patients.

CNS prophylaxis
The role of CNS prophylaxis has been much debated. Although early studies indicated a very high incidence of CNS involvement or relapse, the usefulness of routine CNS prophylaxis has never been rigorously studied in this patient population. The approach to this issue is center dependent, and many centers treat all patients with an intrathecal chemotherapy injection (most commonly methotrexate) with every cycle of systemic chemotherapy. The practice at other centers has been to reserve this treatment for patients with Burkitt histology or bone marrow, testicular, or Waldeyer ring involvement, or for patients with multiple extranodal sites of disease and an elevated LDH. It is our practice to include intrathecal methotrexate as a CNS prophylaxis in the treatment program for the majority of patients with DLBCL, but to omit it in patients with very low-risk features including limited-stage disease, absence of extranodal involvement, and normal LDH. All patients with the highly aggressive BL and PBL histologies require CNS prophylaxis.

Treatment of relapsed or refractory disease
Treatment of relapsed aggressive lymphoma in non-HIV-infected individuals incorporates the use of high-dose chemotherapy with autologous stem cell rescue (ASCT), an approach which has been proved to cure more patients than standard dose chemotherapy alone.[193] Myeloablative chemotherapy in the setting of HIV infection carries substantially increased risks of morbidity and mortality, though evidence suggests it can be performed effectively in the cART era. In one study including 50 patients with relapsed ARL, 27 actually proceeded to peripheral blood stem cell transplant with a 4-year progression-free and overall survival of 76% and 75%, respectively. The overall survival for all 50 patients was 50%, reflecting the poor outcomes in patients who did not proceed to transplant.[194] The reasons for not being transplanted were primarily chemotherapy-resistant disease (14), failure of stem cell mobilization (6), and early toxic death (2). Multiple other reported experiences for ASCT in relapsed ARL have similarly reported encouraging rates of cure.[195,196] Of note, the modern availability of the CXCR4 antagonist plerixafor to improve stem cell mobilization will likely decrease the risk of mobilization failures, as it has on the non-HIV population.[197] ASCT should therefore be considered the treatment of choice for relapsed ARL patients considered fit enough to undergo high-dose therapy. Such transplants should only be

performed at centers experienced in stem cell transplantation for this uniquely high-risk population of patients.

Allogeneic stem cell transplantation (alloSCT) in HIV-infected patients using fully myeloablative conditioning has been reported and carries marked infection-related toxicity in addition to graft versus host disease and progressive lymphoma.[198-200] Non-myeloablative alloSCT using a reduced intensity conditioning regimen, however, appears feasible in a small series of patients with HIV and relapsed hematologic malignancy, with reduced toxicity.[201,202] AlloSCT has also resulted in the only known cure of HIV. This is the remarkable case of Timothy Ray Brown, also known as the Berlin patient, who had HIV and developed acute myelogenous leukemia (AML).[203] He was given an alloSCT with donor stem cells harboring the 32 base pair deletion in CCR5, which confers resistance against HIV infection by preventing viral entry. Mr. Brown remains free of AML as well as without detectable HIV in the blood or tissues, and is off all antiretroviral therapy. Two additional cases of HIV patients treated with alloSCT and concurrent cART for relapsed hematologic malignancies using stem cells from a CCR wild type donor initially found no evidence of persisting HIV infection post transplant, but subsequently identified viral relapse in the two patients at 12 and 32 weeks, respectively.[204] These patients demonstrate that alloSCT and cART may significantly reduce the HIV reservoir, but does not eradicate it when using CCR wild-type stem cells, perhaps due to persistence of the virus in tissue reservoirs post transplant. Genetic engineering methods that produce mutant CCR5 in donor stem cells that prevent HIV viral entry in transplanted patients, as was seen in the Berlin patient, warrant investigation.

Supportive care
All patients should be considered for prophylaxis for opportunistic infections. Reduction in CD4 count by approximately half can be expected during chemotherapy, and *P. jiroveci* prophylaxis is recommended even if entry CD4 count exceed 200 cells/mm^3. The other prophylactic therapies standardly used in advanced HIV disease are also applied to this population.

Growth factor use is often required, given the noted increased sensitivity to myelotoxic injury in patients with HIV disease. A single randomized trial of CHOP versus CHOP plus GM-CSF found a significant decrease in the incidence of fever and neutropenia and days of hospitalization in the cohort receiving prophylactic growth factor,[205] though this trial antedated the use of protease inhibitors, which has generally improved patients' tolerance of chemotherapy. Given the increased incidence of neutropenia and infections on chemotherapy in HIV patients, we recommend routine use of G-CSF support in the majority of patients receiving combination chemotherapy regimens for ARL.

Treatment of malignancy concurrent with HIV also warrants careful attention to possible drug–drug interactions. Many protease inhibitors such as darunavir, indinavir, ritonavir, and saquinavir inhibit CYP3A4, which is responsible for metabolizing vinca alkaloids as well as taxanes. Accordingly, patients on these antiretroviral drugs will have higher chemotherapy levels and must be monitored for higher risks of marrow toxicity and neuropathy, and the dose reduced accordingly. Similarly, non-nucleoside reverse transcriptase inhibitors like efavirenz and nevirapine will induce CYP3A4 and thus theoretically lead to subtherapeutic levels of substrate chemotherapies. Empiric dose escalation of chemotherapy in this setting, however, is not recommended. In general, zidovudine should be avoided with cART due to myelotoxicity, and caution should also be used with stavudine and didanosine due to peripheral neuropathy.

Primary CNS lymphoma

A brain mass in the context of HIV infection can be caused by a number of infections and neoplastic processes, and thereby poses a substantial diagnostic challenge. Most commonly seen in AIDS patients are *T. gondii* abscess, PCNS lymphoma, mycobacterial or bacterial abscess, and progressive multifocal leukoencephalopathy (PML). Criteria for distinguishing among these entities remain imperfect without tissue sampling, but for those patients in whom biopsy is not possible or is refused, certain parameters can raise or lower the likelihood of a lymphoma diagnosis, and the use of PCR analysis for EBV DNA in the CSF has greatly improved the reliability of a diagnosis without histologic confirmation.

In general, PCNSL, PML, and toxoplasmosis are complications of far advanced immunosuppression with CD4 counts of <50 cells/mm^3. This patient population is often on trimethoprim-sulfamethoxazole prophylaxis for *P. jiroveci*, which provides excellent protection against *Toxoplasma*. For those patients in whom a *Toxoplasma* antibody titer is negative and who have been on such prophylaxis, the likelihood of a lymphoma diagnosis in the setting of a CNS mass lesion has been documented to be 74%.[206] Additional information can be gained from PCR analysis for the EBV genome in CSF samples. Detection of EBV in the CSF has been reported to have specificity for lymphoma approximating 100%.[206,207] Sensitivity may be only 80% and there are rare cases of EBV+ CSF where no lymphoma is diagnosed, but this test has become extremely useful in assessing the patient who is unable or unwilling to undergo a definitive histologically defining procedure.

Radiographic features more suggestive of lymphoma include central location, lack of multifocality, and size >2 cm.[208] In addition, a lesion that crosses the midline is highly likely to be a neoplastic process. Single-photon emission computed tomography (SPECT) or positron emission tomography (PET) can also help distinguish lymphoma from abscess. The combination of one of these imaging techniques with a positive DNA PCR for EBV is now often considered sufficient evidence for initiation of therapy. If these tests do not clearly delineate the process and a biopsy is not feasible, empiric anti-Toxoplasma therapy may be used as a diagnostic as well as therapeutic tool. Initiation of sulfadiazine or clindamycin with pyrimethamine generally halts the progression by 5 days and results in clinical or radiographic improvement by 14 days.[209,210] For those in whom these milestones are not met, the likelihood of toxoplasmosis is low.

Therapy for PCNSL remains very limited, and with poor outcome. Radiation with or without chemotherapy, has been the mainstay of care, with response rates ranging from 60% to 79%, but durable remissions are uncommon. Outcomes do appear improved in the cART era.[161,211–213] High-dose methotrexate-based therapy has been the mainstay of therapy in PCNSL in non-HIV-infected patients, where response rates are high and may result in sustained remissions. Such chemotherapy has been limited in HIV patients based on data from the pre-cART era when outcomes were extremely poor due to high rates of toxicity and infectious complications.[213] Even in the cART era, however, PCNSL patients often have advanced HIV and very low CD4 counts, and thus remain at high risk. Among HIV-associated PCNSL with CD4 counts >100 cells/mm^3 and in otherwise good health, methotrexate-based therapy including rituximab should be considered. Combination of cytotoxic chemotherapy and radiation therapy has been tested, with disappointing effect on the tumors and unacceptable toxicity. In spite of the fact that EBV genome is associated with PCNSL, it is generally in the latent phase and therefore unlikely to be sensitive to lytic-phase-specific antiviral agents. Nonetheless, limited experience with the use of ganciclovir in combination with zidovudine

and IL-2 has suggested antitumor activity.[214] The ultimate use of these agents or other EBV-directed genetic or chemical manipulations awaits careful assessment in clinical trial. The relationship of the disease to poor immunologic function does provide the rationale, however, for emphasizing optimization of anti-HIV therapy as a component of antitumor therapy. The overall poor outcome for these patients also strongly advocates the encouragement of patients to participate in clinical protocols testing novel approaches.

The use of steroids in this patient population has engendered concern because of the potential worsening of immunosuppression. There is an absence of data regarding this point, but the opportunity to reduce edema and mass effect should not be avoided out of concern for immunosuppression. Rather, the tapering of steroids should be as rapid as is tolerated, and vigilance regarding the development of concurrent infection should be maintained. In the era preceding cART, death was as commonly caused by secondary events as by tumor.[215] For those patients who present with PCNSL who have not been receiving cART, initiating antiretroviral therapy should be considered a priority, as anecdotal reports have emerged of long-term survivors among the group gaining control of HIV-1.[216,217]

Multicentric Castleman disease

MCD is a lymphoproliferative disorder associated with KSHV/HHV, usually seen in the setting of advanced HIV infection. Patients typically present with a systemic syndrome of fevers, malaise, diffuse lymphadenopathy, hepatosplenomegaly, edema, effusions, and anemia. Though not a clonal process, MCD can transform into DLBCL, so attention to the possibility of a high-grade transformation should be paid both at the time of initial diagnosis and subsequent recurrence. Patients may also present with other concomitant HHV8-associated malignancies, KS or PEL, or with opportunistic infections given the usually low CD4 count at diagnosis. All patients should be treated with cART, though antiretrovirals alone are unlikely to produce remissions. While antiviral therapy against HIV has not been shown to successfully treat MCD, antiviral therapy against HHV8 may be effective given that HHV8 lytic replication is common in MCL and thus may be medically targeted. A prospective trial of high-dose zidovudine plus valganciclovir in 14 patients with symptomatic HIV- and HHV-8 associated MCD found an overall clinical and complete response rate of 86% and 50%, respectively.[218] Traditional chemotherapy agents alone have proved disappointing historically, though small, have reported efficacy with single-agent alkylators, vinblastine, oral etoposide, thalidomide, or liposomal doxorubicin.[163,219–223] Rituximab has been tested in MCD given the robust presence of CD20+ B cells. A prospective trial of rituximab monotherapy in 24 patients with chemotherapy-dependent HIV-associated MCD reported sustained remissions in 71% of patients after 1 year; responses to rituximab in patients previously treated with rituximab have been reported as well.[224,225] Of note, patients with MCD and concomitant KS may experience a flare of KS while on rituximab, so this warrants careful attention by the treating clinician. For patients with highly aggressive disease, or disease progressing on rituximab monotherapy, rituximab has been combined with either etoposide or liposomal doxorubicin with encouraging results.[226,227] The combination of rituximab and liposomal doxorubicin may be a particularly appealing combination for patients with concurrent KS and MCD. More recently, the anti-IL-6R monoclonal antibody siltuximab has been FDA approved in HIV-negative HHV8-negative MCD based on a randomized trial showing that 34% of patients treated with siltuximab achieved a durable clinical and radiological response, compared to 0% in the placebo arm.[167] This data cannot easily be extrapolated to HIV-associated MCD, however, where viral IL-6 is produced by HHV8, and is not targeted by the siltuximab antibody. IL-6 targeted agents warrant evaluation in HIV patients in the context of a clinical trial.

For initial therapy of MCD, we recommend rituximab along with concurrent cART in the majority of patients. Liposomal doxorubicin or etoposide can be added for rapidly progressive or resistant disease, with more intensive therapy like CHOP[228] reserved for rare fulminantly progressing cases, or those with high-grade transformation. High-dose zidovudine with valganciclovir may also be considered.

Hodgkin lymphoma (HL)

Although not officially an AIDS-defining tumor, HL is increased in frequency in HIV-infected patients and has a number of unique characteristics distinguishing it from HL outside the context of AIDS.

Epidemiology

The risk of HL in patients infected with HIV-1 is estimated to be 2.5- to 8.5-fold above that of the uninfected population.[9,229–231] This risk appears to be uniformly increased across the risk groups for HIV infection, independent of age or gender.[232] Notwithstanding the increase in relative risk in the HIV-infected population, the overall magnitude of the problem is still relatively small compared with that of NHL. Unlike most AIDS-associated NHL, the incidence of HL in HIV infection has not decreased in the cART era, and may even be increased.[123,233,234] The cause of this surprising increase is speculative, but it may be due to the critical role host CD4-positive T-cell signaling plays in the microenvironment of HL. Indeed, HL is more likely to occur at moderately decreased CD4 counts than in the setting of severe immunodeficiency.

Pathology and pathogenesis

HL in the context of HIV infection has pathologic features that distinguish it from the seronegative population. In particular, there is a much higher frequency of the mixed-cellularity subtype, with a corresponding reduction in the relative proportion of patients with nodular sclerosis histology. The overall frequency of mixed-cellularity or lymphocyte-depleted histology was found to be two-thirds of the cases in the HIV-1-positive context compared with only 29% in uninfected patients.[235] In addition, the presence of EBV in HL tissue is markedly increased in HIV-infected individuals. Estimates ranged from 80% to 100% in contrast to the HIV-negative population.[234,236] Of note, expression of the EBV LMP1, but not EBNA2, latency genes is in a type 2 pattern. Thus, the EBV genome is identified with high-frequency in HIV-infected HL and is considered likely to play an etiologic role.

In addition to the presence of EBV, there are other molecular characteristics of HL unique to the HIV-infected population. The transcription factor Bcl-6 expressed in germinal-center B cells, is present on Reed–Sternberg cells from both HIV-1-infected and uninfected individuals whereas, syndecan-1 (a proteoglycan associated with the post-terminal center) is restricted to the HIV-1-positive population.[237,238] Therefore, the postgerminal-center B cell may be the cell of origin in HIV-1-related HL, as opposed to the germinal-center cell of origin presumed to be the source of Reed–Sternberg cells in the uninfected population.

Clinical features

HL in patients with HIV is typically of advanced stage and associated with B symptoms.[239,240] Stage III or IV disease has been documented in approximately 80% of patients with HIV-associated HL at the time of diagnosis, as compared with just under half in HL patients without HIV. Like ARL, the location of HL in the setting of HIV-1 infection is often extranodal, involving the bone marrow in up to 50% of patients. Other sites include the tongue, rectum, skin, and lung, and extranodal disease may be the site of presentation. Staging strategies should be the same as those in HL patients outside the context of HIV-1, with particular attention to possible microbiologic explanations for B symptoms.

Treatment

The clinical treatment approach to patients with HL in the setting of HIV infection is similar to that in other contexts; and radiation therapy, chemotherapy, or combined radiation and chemotherapy should be applied as appropriate for stage, similar to guidelines for treatment outside the setting of HIV infection.

Though pre-cART outcomes of AIDS-associated HL were quite poor, with a median survival of <2 years,[241] modern treatment in the setting of antiretroviral therapy has shown encouraging rates of cure.[240] Patients with advanced-stage disease treated with standard Adriamycin (doxorubicin), bleomycin, vinblastine, and dacarbazine (ABVD), and concomitant cART were reported to achieve complete responses in 87% of cases with 5-year event-free and overall survivals of 71% and 76%, respectively.[242] Favorable outcomes have also been observed with the bleomycin, etoposide, Adriamycin (doxorubicin), cyclophosphamide, Oncovin (vincristine), procarbazine, and prednisone (BEACOPP), and Stanford V (doxorubicin, vinblastine, mechlorethamine, etoposide, vincristine, bleomycin, prednisone, and radiotherapy) regimens, when given with concomitant cART.[243,244]

The underlying level of immunosuppression and overall performance status of the patient must be considered before embarking on these therapies, and, in general, prophylaxis for *P. jiroveci* is recommended for all patients regardless of CD4 count. Treatment complications, including myelosuppression and opportunistic infections, may be expected to be more severe among patients with advanced AIDS; however, cure of HL is a realistic aim in the setting of HIV infection, and antitumor therapy dose reduction should be contemplated only in patients with advanced AIDS who have demonstrated intolerance to the standard-dose regimens. As with the treatment of NHL, treating clinicians must be vigilant for drug–drug interactions between chemotherapy and cART.

Squamous cell neoplasia

The issue of HPV-related disease is an increasing concern in the HIV epidemic for several reasons, including (1) the increasing frequency of women infected by HIV, (2) the rampant progression of HIV disease in parts of the world where there is already a high incidence of cervical cancer and limited screening for cervical disease, and (3) the extension in overall survival of HIV-infected individuals. The nature of the abnormalities is fairly broad in scope and includes anogenital, conjunctival, oropharyngeal, and cutaneous neoplasia.

Epidemiology

The increased frequency of squamous cell neoplasia in HIV-infected individuals has been well documented, and has not decreased since the introduction of cART, may be increasing.[12,245,246] The single AIDS-defining disease among the HPV-related tumors is that of invasive cervical carcinoma, though there is controversy as to whether this malignancy is increased in frequency in the setting of HIV infection. However, it is very clear that intraepithelial neoplasia of both the uterine cervix and the anus is increased. HIV-infected men who have sex with men have a particularly high incidence of squamous cell abnormalities and a markedly increased risk of high-grade anal intraepithelial neoplasia and anal cancer, which has the most rapidly rising incidence of all malignancies in the cART era.[12] Indirect evidence that immune suppression augments this cancer risk comes from an analysis of AIDS and cancer registries. In a retrospective study of more than 300,000 HIV patients, the incidence of *in situ* and invasive cancers was significantly higher in the 5 years following an AIDS-defining illness than in the 5 years preceding it.[245] Among women, cervical, vulvar/vaginal, and anal cancers were increased, while among men, anal, penile, tonsillar, and conjunctival cancers were increased.

Pathology and pathogenesis

The association of specific subtypes of HPV with a potential for epidermal cell transformation has been long established, and the frequency of HPV-16, -18, and -19, is reported to be increased in HIV-infected individuals.[247] The frequency of multiple subtypes of HPV has also been assessed and found to be markedly increased in the HIV-infected population (73% of HIV-1-infected men who have sex with men, as compared with 23% of uninfected men).[247,248] The incidence of high-grade intraepithelial neoplasia of the anus has been estimated to be as high as 48% among HIV-1-positive men who have sex with men over a 4-year interval and was associated with the presence of multiple HPV subtypes, persistent anal infection, and high-level infection with oncogenic HPV subtypes.[249] Screening for intraepithelial neoplasia among HIV-1–infected men who have sex with men has demonstrated a prevalence of high-grade anal intraepithelial neoplasia (or carcinoma *in situ* [CIS]) of 36% compared with 7% of HIV-1-negative men who have sex with men.[250] Most often, these lesions on the anus and uterine cervix are not solitary sites but rather represent one of multiple areas of dysplasia and are therefore difficult to satisfactorily treat, particularly on the anus. Patients with a history of high-grade intraepithelial neoplasia may often have recurrence following attempts at excision, cryotherapy, or topical treatment because of the ubiquitous nature of the HPV infection locally and the tendency of that virus to continue to have effects on local tissue.

A critical issue in evaluating the magnitude of this problem is the risk of progression of intraepithelial neoplasia to frank invasive cancer. This issue remains ill defined and highly controversial. If the risk is estimated at 1% or above, cost–benefit analyses have indicated that ongoing screening is justified.[251] The lack of large increases in the frequency of invasive anogenital cancer among HIV risk groups suggests that the risk is relatively small. However, the potential for frank invasion is not zero, and, therefore, vigilance among patients with HIV disease is warranted.

The risk of some opportunistic neoplasms is clearly diminished in the context of aggressive therapy for HIV and suppression of HIV replication. There have been conflicting reports of whether HPV-related tumors are among those responsive to improved anti-HIV therapy. Some reports have indicated that some individuals may experience improvement in HPV-related neoplasia;[252] however, the bulk of data suggests that antiretroviral therapy has little impact on the incidence of dysplasia or invasive anal cancer.[253] At present, the complete suppression of HIV should not be regarded as a fail-safe defense against the development of HPV-related tumors.

Clinical presentation

HPV disease may present anywhere along the continuum of condyloma acuminatum to invasive anal cancer. Patients who have anal dysplasia may or may not have symptoms associated with it. Common practice with patients with a history of high-grade anal dysplasia is to perform an anoscopic examination and possible biopsy, even if the diagnostic lesion is on the anal verge, to assess for possible invasive disease out of the external examination field. Some centers perform anal Papanicolaou (Pap) evaluation for HIV-infected individuals, where it has been shown to be effective at identifying premalignant lesions. One study in 245 men found that 96% of anal Pap smears were interpretable with two-thirds of men screened having an abnormal cytology.[254] High-resolution anoscopy and biopsy demonstrated a positive predictive value of 96% for detection of anal dysplasia by cytologic screening. The clinical relevance of early cytologic detection remains unclear, though early lesions may benefit from local therapy. Given the rising incidence of HPV-associated anal cancer in HIV-infected individuals, anal Pap smears may be considered in high-risk individuals, such as men who have sex with men.

For women with HIV infection, the standard practices and recommendations for cervical screening are to be followed, with increased vigilance for those with severe immunosuppression. For HIV-infected women with CD4 counts of <200 cells/mm^3, the recommendation is for Pap smears to be performed semiannually.

HPV vaccination is a vital tool in the prevention of cervical cancer where it has been proved to decrease the incidence of high-grade cervical intraepithelial neoplasia related to HPV,[255] and is now considered a standard vaccine in young girls. HPV vaccination of boys has been more controversial, though it may reduce their incidence of HPV-associated neoplasia as well as prevent transmission of HPV to women, thus contributing to a reduced incidence of cervical cancer. A quadrivalent HPV vaccine was administered to 4065 males aged 16–26 in a randomized placebo-controlled trial, and found a reduction in HPV infection as well as in HPV-associated external genital lesions.[256] A substudy of MSM also found the vaccine to be effective in this population, and to reduce the incidence of high-grade anal intraepithelial neoplasia. Based on these data, HPV vaccination is now recommended for all males up to age 21 and MSM up until age 26.

Treatment

Treatment guidelines for dysplasia and carcinoma of the uterine cervix are well defined and should be followed in the setting of HIV infection. Management of anal disease is less clear.

High-grade intraepithelial neoplasia or CIS at the anal verge may be treated with topical imiquimod or 5-fluorouracil, while lesions in the anal canal may be treated with surgical excision, cryotherapy, or laser ablation. Given the ambiguity of risk for progression to frank invasive cancer, these lesions may be followed with vigilant monitoring alone, and spontaneous regression of anal intraepithelial neoplasia may occur.[257] For patients with invasive carcinoma of the anus, treatment guidelines recommending a combination of chemotherapy and radiation therapy should be followed as in non-HIV-infected individuals; this treatment has been reasonably well tolerated in the HIV-infected population.[258,259] There is a distinct increased sensitivity to mucosal injury with radiation in HIV disease, and, therefore, close interaction between the medical and radiation oncologists is essential. If patients have very advanced HIV disease failing antiretrovirals, a conservative approach to management of the malignancy may be warranted, but this requires case-by-case assessment.

Other non-AIDS defining cancers

A number of other non-AIDS defining malignancies occur at a relatively increased risk in HIV-infected individuals, even in the cART era; these include cancers of the lung, oropharynx, liver, prostate, testes, and skin.[231,260–263] Among skin cancers, melanoma, basal cell, and squamous cell cancers all occur at increased rates. Merkel cell carcinoma (MCC) is a very rare neural-crest-derived skin cancer that has also been shown to be increased in the setting of AIDS, as well as in solid organ transplant recipients.[264,265] Though generally a disease of the aged, MCC in immunosuppressed patients tends to occur at a significantly younger age and carries an aggressive natural history. The association of this rare skin cancer with immunosuppressed patients prompted a search for an underlying infectious pathogen, which recently resulted in the identification of a previously unknown polyomavirus, now called Merkel cell polyomavirus (MCV).[266] MCV DNA was found to be integrated into the tumor cell genome in the majority of MCCs but not in control tissues, and the pattern of integration suggested that infection preceded clonal expansion of the tumor cells. These data suggest a pivotal role for this novel polyomavirus in the pathogenesis of MCC, though the exact nature of this role has yet to be determined. Identification of the MCV highlights the potential role of other undiscovered viruses in immunosuppression-related malignancies where a pathogen has not yet been identified, and remains an area of ongoing investigation.

Key references

The complete reference list can be found on the Wiley Companion Digital Edition of this title (see inside front cover for login instructions).

1 Palella FJ Jr, Delaney KM, Moorman AC, et al. Declining morbidity and mortality among patients with advanced human immunodeficiency virus infection. HIV Outpatient study investigators. *N Engl J Med.* 1998;**338**:853–860.

7 Chang Y, Cesarman E, Pessin MS, et al. Identification of herpesvirus-like DNA sequences in AIDS-associated Kaposi's sarcoma. *Science.* 1994;**266**:1865–1869.

12 Simard EP, Pfeiffer RM, Engels EA. Spectrum of cancer risk late after AIDS onset in the United States. *Arch Intern Med.* 2010;**170**:1337–1345.

14 Buchbinder SP, Holmberg SD, Scheer S, et al. Combination antiretroviral therapy and incidence of AIDS-related malignancies. *J Acquir Immune Defic Syndr.* 1999;**21(Suppl 1)**:S23–S26.

17 Biggar RJ, Chaturvedi AK, Goedert JJ, Engels EA. AIDS-related cancer and severity of immunosuppression in persons with AIDS. *J Natl Cancer Inst.* 2007;**99**:962–972.

20 Young L, Alfieri C, Hennessy K, et al. Expression of Epstein-Barr virus transformation-associated genes in tissues of patients with EBV lymphoproliferative disease. *N Engl J Med.* 1989;**321**:1080–1085.

24 Gibson TM, Morton LM, Shiels MS, et al. Risk of non-Hodgkin lymphoma subtypes in HIV-infected people during the HAART era: a population-based study. *AIDS.* 2014;**28**:2313–2318.

25 Kedes DH, Operskalski E, Busch M, et al. The seroepidemiology of human herpesvirus 8 (Kaposi's sarcoma-associated herpesvirus): distribution of infection in KS risk groups and evidence for sexual transmission. *Nat Med.* 1996;**2**:918–924.

38 Krown SE, Testa MA, Huang J. AIDS-related Kaposi's sarcoma: prospective validation of the AIDS Clinical Trials Group staging classification. AIDS Clinical Trials Group Oncology Committee. *J Clin Oncol.* 1997;**15**:3085–3092.

40 Stebbing J, Sanitt A, Nelson M, et al. A prognostic index for AIDS-associated Kaposi's sarcoma in the era of highly active antiretroviral therapy. *Lancet.* 2006;**367**:1495–1502.

50 Bais C, Santomasso B, Coso O, et al. G-protein-coupled receptor of Kaposi's sarcoma-associated herpesvirus is a viral oncogene and angiogenesis activator. *Nature.* 1998;**391**:86–89.

69 Harrington W Jr, Sieczkowski L, Sosa C, et al. Activation of HHV-8 by HIV-1 tat. *Lancet.* 1997;**349**:774–775.

77 Mosam A, Shaik F, Uldrick TS, et al. A randomized controlled trial of highly active antiretroviral therapy versus highly active antiretroviral therapy and chemotherapy in therapy-naive patients with HIV-associated Kaposi sarcoma in South Africa. *J Acquir Immune Defic Syndr.* 2012;**60**:150–157.

93 Northfelt DW, Dezube BJ, Thommes JA, et al. Pegylated-liposomal doxorubicin versus doxorubicin, bleomycin, and vincristine in the treatment of AIDS-related Kaposi's sarcoma: results of a randomized phase III clinical trial. *J Clin Oncol.* 1998;**16**:2445–2451.

100 Cianfrocca M, Lee S, Von Roenn J, et al. Randomized trial of paclitaxel versus pegylated liposomal doxorubicin for advanced human immunodeficiency virus-associated Kaposi sarcoma: evidence of symptom palliation from chemotherapy. *Cancer.* 2010;**116**:3969–3977.

125 Mosialos G, Birkenbach M, Yalamanchili R, et al. The Epstein-Barr virus transforming protein LMP1 engages signaling proteins for the tumor necrosis factor receptor family. *Cell.* 1995;**80**:389–399.

126 Liebowitz D. Epstein-Barr virus and a cellular signaling pathway in lymphomas from immunosuppressed patients. *N Engl J Med.* 1998;**338**:1413–1421.

136 Delecluse HJ, Anagnostopoulos I, Dallenbach F, et al. Plasmablastic lymphomas of the oral cavity: a new entity associated with the human immunodeficiency virus infection. *Blood.* 1997;**89**:1413–1420.

156 Nador RG, Cesarman E, Chadburn A, et al. Primary effusion lymphoma: a distinct clinicopathologic entity associated with the Kaposi's sarcoma-associated herpes virus. *Blood.* 1996;**88**:645–656.

161 Uldrick TS, Pipkin S, Scheer S, Hessol NA. Factors associated with survival among patients with AIDS-related primary central nervous system lymphoma. *AIDS.* 2014;**28**:397–405.

163 Oksenhendler E, Duarte M, Soulier J, et al. Multicentric Castleman's disease in HIV infection: a clinical and pathological study of 20 patients. *AIDS.* 1996;**10**:61–67.

172 Barta SK, Xue X, Wang D, et al. A new prognostic score for AIDS-related lymphomas in the Rituximab-era. *Haematologica.* 2014;**99**:1731–1737.

174 Barnes JA, Lacasce AS, Feng Y, et al. Evaluation of the addition of rituximab to CODOX-M/IVAC for Burkitt's lymphoma: a retrospective analysis. *Ann Oncol.* 2011;**22**:1859–1864.

175 Dunleavy K, Pittaluga S, Shovlin M, et al. Low-intensity therapy in adults with Burkitt's lymphoma. *N Engl J Med.* 2013;**369**:1915–1925.

181 Kaplan LD, Lee JY, Ambinder RF, et al. Rituximab does not improve clinical outcome in a randomized phase 3 trial of CHOP with or without rituximab in patients with HIV-associated non-Hodgkin lymphoma: AIDS-malignancies consortium trial 010. *Blood.* 2005;**106**:1538–1543.

185 Dunleavy K, Little RF, Pittaluga S, et al. The role of tumor histogenesis, FDG-PET, and short-course EPOCH with dose-dense rituximab (SC-EPOCH-RR) in HIV-associated diffuse large B-cell lymphoma. *Blood.* 2010;**115**:3017–3024.

187 Barta SK, Lee JY, Kaplan LD, et al. Pooled analysis of AIDS malignancy consortium trials evaluating rituximab plus CHOP or infusional EPOCH chemotherapy in HIV-associated non-Hodgkin lymphoma. *Cancer.* 2012;**118**:3977–3983.

194 Re A, Michieli M, Casari S, et al. High-dose therapy and autologous peripheral blood stem cell transplantation as salvage treatment for AIDS-related lymphoma: long-term results of the Italian Cooperative Group on AIDS and Tumors (GICAT) study with analysis of prognostic factors. *Blood.* 2009;**114**:1306–1313.

203 Hutter G, Nowak D, Mossner M, et al. Long-term control of HIV by CCR5 Delta32/Delta32 stem-cell transplantation. *N Engl J Med.* 2009;**360**:692–698.

212 Hoffmann C, Tabrizian S, Wolf E, et al. Survival of AIDS patients with primary central nervous system lymphoma is dramatically improved by HAART-induced immune recovery. *AIDS.* 2001;**15**:2119–2127.

224 Gerard L, Berezne A, Galicier L, et al. Prospective study of rituximab in chemotherapy-dependent human immunodeficiency virus associated multicentric Castleman's disease: ANRS 117 CastlemaB Trial. *J Clin Oncol.* 2007;**25**:3350–3356.

227 Uldrick TS, Polizzotto MN, Aleman K, et al. Rituximab plus liposomal doxorubicin in HIV-infected patients with KSHV-associated multicentric Castleman disease. *Blood.* 2014;**124**:3544–3552.

234 Biggar RJ, Jaffe ES, Goedert JJ, et al. Hodgkin lymphoma and immunodeficiency in persons with HIV/AIDS. *Blood.* 2006;**108**:3786–3791.

242 Xicoy B, Ribera JM, Miralles P, et al. Results of treatment with doxorubicin, bleomycin, vinblastine and dacarbazine and highly active antiretroviral therapy in advanced stage, human immunodeficiency virus-related Hodgkin's lymphoma. *Haematologica.* 2007;**92**:191–198.

245 Frisch M, Biggar RJ, Goedert JJ. Human papillomavirus-associated cancers in patients with human immunodeficiency virus infection and acquired immunodeficiency syndrome. *J Natl Cancer Inst.* 2000;**92**:1500–1510.

246 Palefsky JM, Holly EA, Efirdc JT, et al. Anal intraepithelial neoplasia in the highly active antiretroviral therapy era among HIV-positive men who have sex with men. *AIDS.* 2005;**19**:1407–1414.

255 The FUTURE II Study Group. Quadrivalent vaccine against human papillomavirus to prevent high-grade cervical lesions. *N Engl J Med.* 2007;**356**:1915–1927.

256 Giuliano AR, Palefsky JM, Goldstone S, et al. Efficacy of quadrivalent HPV vaccine against HPV Infection and disease in males. *N Engl J Med.* 2011;**364**:401–411.

257 Tong WW, Jin F, McHugh LC, et al. Progression to and spontaneous regression of high-grade anal squamous intraepithelial lesions in HIV-infected and uninfected men. *AIDS.* 2013;**27**:2233–2243.

261 Clifford GM, Polesel J, Rickenbach M, et al. Cancer risk in the Swiss HIV Cohort Study: associations with immunodeficiency, smoking, and highly active antiretroviral therapy. *J Natl Cancer Inst.* 2005;**97**:425–432.

76 Cancer survivorship: new challenge in cancer medicine

Julia H. Rowland, PhD

Overview

As the population of cancer survivors continues to increase, so too has attention to the long-term care needs of these individuals after treatment ends. While most survivors adapt well post-treatment, many experience lingering effects of their illness. In some cases, these effects become permanent and raise challenges to recovery and adaptation. In this chapter, we outline some of the common persistent sequelae of cancer and their management and review the emerging guidelines for survivorship care planning. Models of follow-up care after cancer are discussed, along with the needs and support of informal cancer caregivers in this process. Recommendations for future directions in survivorship research and care are provided.

Introduction

A quick glance through the chapters of the ninth edition of this classic volume reveals how very far we have come in advancing the science and art of cancer medicine. Arguably, the greatest measure of the progress made is the growing population of cancer survivors. While a testament to the many successes achieved, this population is at the same time a reminder that a focus on cure is not enough; we must attend equally to the life to which we return each patient treated. How best to care for patients after primary treatment ends and there is no evidence of disease, is one of the emerging challenges for healthcare providers.

In this chapter, we will review the magnitude of the challenge clinicians—along with cancer survivors themselves and their loved ones—face after cancer. Survivors of childhood cancer have been at the vanguard of the survivorship movement in the United States, in part because of the truly dramatic progress made in curing cancers in this youngest population. The special challenges to and guidelines for their long-term care are well detailed elsewhere.[1-8] In this chapter, we will restrict our review to the post-treatment recovery and care of individuals diagnosed as adults.

Cancer survivorship: a brief history

Before the 1970s, the picture for most patients diagnosed with cancer was bleak. There were few effective treatment options, and most entailed serious adverse effects that were often poorly controlled.[9,10] In this earlier period, a major focus was on helping people die of their disease, not live with it. The "survivors" in this earlier period were more often grieving family members than patients themselves. As our ability expanded to both cure and control the many diseases we call cancer, this picture changed dramatically.

The origins of the survivorship movement are often attributed to two events. The first was the publication in 1985 in the *New England Journal of Medicine* of a piece by a young physician, Dr. Fitzhugh Mullan, entitled "Seasons of Survival."[11] In this commentary, Mullan describes his personal experience with cancer and provided, for the first time, language for thinking about an expanded cancer trajectory. The following year, a group of 23 individuals, including Mullan, gathered in Albuquerque, New Mexico, and founded what is now known as the National Coalition for Cancer Survivorship (NCCS). This group proposed a new definition of the term "cancer survivor." Until then, the term "cancer survivor" referred to someone who had remained disease-free for a minimum of 5 years. The coalition members argued that a "cancer survivor" should refer to anyone with cancer, from the moment of diagnosis and for the balance of his or her life. The intent of the NCCS founders was not to label individuals. Rather, they wanted first to convey a message of hope to those newly diagnosed with cancer that life was not over, and second, to promote a dialogue between patients and their physicians about the impact that different treatment options might have on survivors' future health and functioning (i.e., to foster informed, patient-centered decision making). Although some persons with a cancer history do not consider themselves to be survivors,[12,13] the language helped launch a survivorship movement globally.

Since 1986, the field of cancer survivorship has come into its own. The past dozen years in particular have seen national attention paid to the topic of cancer survivorship. This is reflected in the publication of five major reports addressing the status of the research and care of those living with cancer, including two volumes produced by the Institute of Medicine (IOM) on childhood[1] and adult cancer survivorship,[14] a report by the Centers for Disease Control and Prevention (CDC) and the Lance Armstrong Foundation calling for a national action plan around cancer survivorship,[15] and two reports from the President's Cancer Panel.[16,17] Major noncancer and cancer scientific journals have devoted special issues to this aspect of the cancer control continuum,[18-21] texts have appeared summarizing our accomplishments in the field of survivorship research and promoting evidence-based care,[22,23] and the field now has a scientific journal dedicated to this burgeoning area of science.[24] Importantly, cancer survivorship is recognized to represent a discrete place on the cancer control continuum, bringing its own unique set of concerns and challenges. The key driver behind attention to this field has been the sheer numbers (Figure 1).

Magnitude of the problem

Cancer prevalence

As of January 1, 2014, there were an estimated 14.5 million cancer survivors in the United States alone.[25] Globally, figures suggest that

Holland-Frei Cancer Medicine, Ninth Edition. Edited by Robert C. Bast Jr., Carlo M. Croce, William N. Hait, Waun Ki Hong, Donald W. Kufe, Martine Piccart-Gebhart, Raphael E. Pollock, Ralph R. Weichselbaum, Hongyang Wang, and James F. Holland.
© 2017 John Wiley & Sons, Inc. ISBN: 978-1-118-93469-2

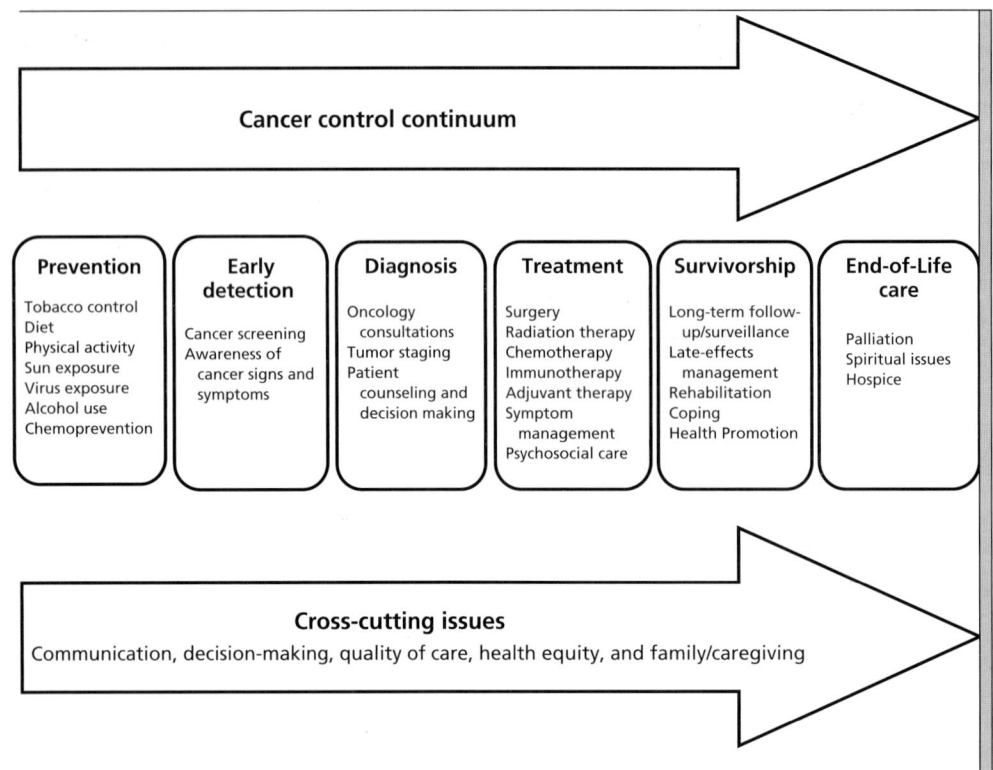

Figure 1 Cancer control continuum—elaborated. Source: Adapted from http://cancercontrol.cancer.gov/od/continuum.html.

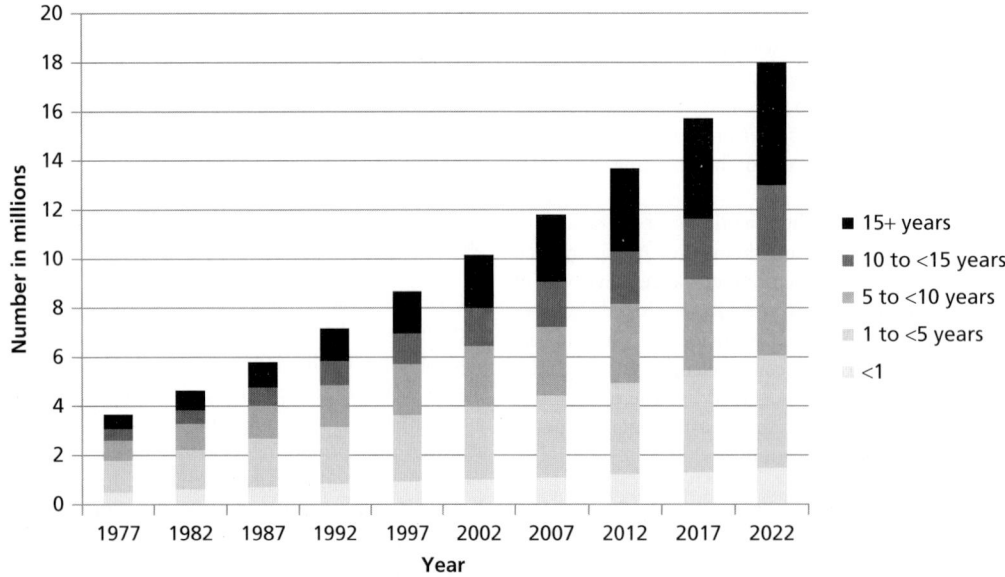

Figure 2 Estimated and projected number of cancer survivors in the United States from 1977 to 2022 by years since diagnosis. Source: de Moor 2013.[27]

there are over 32.6 million cancer survivors worldwide, although this represents a minimum count as most countries can only project prevalence up to 5 years post diagnosis.[26] As reflected in Figure 2, the number of cancer survivors has increased steadily over the past 45 years. In 1971, when President Nixon signed the National Cancer Act and declared the "war on cancer," there were an estimated three million survivors. By 2024, this number will climb to 19 million. The increase in numbers is due in part to advances in early detection, treatment efficacy, and supportive care. Breakthrough discoveries notwithstanding, however, the biggest contributor to growth

in cancer prevalence in the decade to come will be the aging of the population.[28]

Today, over 60% of those diagnosed are aged 65 and older. With the Baby Boomer generation turning 65 at a rate of approximately 11,000 a day (since January 2011), it is estimated that 11 million cancer survivors will be older adults by 2020, representing a 42% increase in their numbers in just one decade (2010–2020).[29]

In addition to their growing numbers, today's cancer survivors are also living longer. In 2014, 41% of survivors were diagnosed 10 or more years ago, and an impressive 15% were diagnosed 20 or more years earlier (Figure 2).[27] *Healthy People 2020* has a target goal to increase the proportion of cancer survivors who are living 5 years or longer after cancer to 72.8%.[30] While we have surpassed this figure for those diagnosed as children (age <15), where 10-year survival is now >77%, this is definitely a challenge goal in adult onset cancers. Approximately 68% of adults diagnosed today can expect to be alive in 5 years. Unknown in all of these figures is the well-being or disease status of this burgeoning population. Beyond estimates for the number of individuals within 1 year of diagnosis, and 1-year from death, our Surveillance Epidemiology and End Results (SEER) registry data provide limited information about the health status of the cancer survivor population. This constitutes an important gap in our knowledge base. Of note, *Healthy People 2020* also has a goal to increase the mental and physical health-related quality of life (HRQOL) of cancer survivors.[30] How we are to measure this effect remains unclear.

Cancer's long-term and late effects

Research among long-term cancer survivors has grown in parallel to their growing numbers. Clear from this science and the testimony of survivors themselves is that being told you are cancer-free does not mean you are free of the cancer experience. As one survivor put it, "It's not over when it is over."

Cancer has the capacity to affect virtually every aspect of an individual's life and function: physical, psychological, social, economic, and existential (Table 1). Some of these effects are acute and resolve quickly once treatment ends (e.g., nausea and vomiting, and hair loss). Others become more chronic, arising during active treatment and persisting over time (e.g., fatigue, sexual dysfunction, memory problems, bladder, and bowel problems). While some of these latter symptoms may resolve in the longer term, other sequelae of cancer and its treatment can be permanent (e.g., infertility and amputation). Further, as survivors are living longer, they are surviving long enough to experience effects once considered only as "putative" risks secondary to some treatments (e.g., radiation therapy and certain chemotherapeutic agents). A third category of effects are those that are late-occurring, defined as manifesting 6 months or more after treatment. In addition to recurrence or second cancer,[31,32] risks for other chronic health conditions (e.g., cardiovascular disease, diabetes, and osteoporosis) is also increased.[33,34] Depending on the age of the survivor, these conditions may be of more concern than the cancer itself.[35]

Overall, most survivors are remarkably resilient, coping well with what at times can be lengthy as well as physically rigorous treatments. Although a significant subset continues to struggle with emotional distress, by a year or more after treatment, most cancer survivors report levels of emotional well-being equivalent to or better than their peers without a cancer history.[36] When

Table 1 Potential long term and late effects of cancer and its treatment.

Physical/Medical (e.g., second cancers/recurrence, cardiac dysfunction, pain, fatigue, memory problems, sleep disturbance, sexual impairment, infertility, and loss of bowel/bladder control)
Psychological (e.g., fear of recurrence, depression, anxiety, lowered self-esteem, and altered body image)
Social (e.g., changes in interpersonal relationships, altered family functioning/dynamics, social isolation, altered intimacy, problems advancing at work/returning to school)
Financial (e.g., concerns regarding health or life insurance access/coverage, financial strain due to cost of care/job loss)
Existential/spiritual issues (e.g., disillusionment, loss of faith, altered sense of purpose or meaning, appreciation of life, benefit finding, and post-traumatic growth)

it comes to physical health, the picture is different. Compared with those without a cancer history, survivors demonstrate worse physical functioning, higher rates of disability, and more unemployment.[37–39] Further, research suggests that lingering physical symptoms commonly occur in clusters (e.g., pain, sleep problems, and fatigue) and greater symptom burden is associated with increased risk of poor quality of life.[40]

The provision of detail about each of the lingering effects of cancer is beyond the scope of this chapter (for reviews, see Refs 41–43). However, four persistent effects are worth discussing here because they are common across a number of cancers and troubling: fear of recurrence, fatigue, depression, and memory problems. Perhaps the most universal effect of surviving cancer is worry that the disease will return.[44] Fear of recurrence can be exacerbated by a variety of triggers (e.g., coming for routine follow-up visits, anniversary dates of diagnosis or treatment, death of a fellow or publicly visible cancer survivor, and any unexplained ache or pain),[45] and healthcare professionals see this response as challenging to manage.[46] Reassurance that such anxiety is normal and often diminishes over time, along with counsel about what is or, more important, is not a worrisome sign or symptom generally helps to allay concerns. In cases where fear persists and is interfering with daily function and/or recommended follow-up care, referral for brief counseling to see what may be contributing to the anxiety, to learn some relaxation techniques, and to obtain social support can be helpful. Of note, survivors who continue on long-term therapies (e.g., use of adjuvant hormonal therapy among breast cancer survivors) may feel less anxious about the disease coming back. These individuals often report being reassured by the sense that they are doing something active to reduce risk of recurrence.

Fatigue, common during treatment, persists in approximately a quarter to a third of long-term survivors.[47,48] The mechanisms of risk for long-term fatigue are not well understood.[49] The importance of addressing this troubling effect of cancer and its therapy is reflected in the American Society of Clinical Oncology (ASCO) guideline for assessment of this symptom post-treatment.[50] To date, few interventions appear to mitigate cancer-related fatigue, with the exception of exercise. While seemingly counterintuitive, patients who remain physically active during and after treatment report lower, not higher levels of fatigue.[51] After ruling out possible physiologic causes of fatigue (e.g., anemia, infection), reassurance that fatigue generally abates over time, albeit far more slowly than once thought, can be helpful in reducing distress about this lingering effect.

Prevalence rates of depression or depressive symptoms among cancer survivors are higher than that observed in the general public, particularly in the early 1–2 years post-treatment.[52] Depression is not only painful, but is also associated with delay in return to work and lower adherence to medical regimens in survivors.[53] Younger age, being female, and prior history of depression are all associated with increased risk for depression among cancer survivors, yet many survivors experience depression for the first time after a cancer diagnosis.[54–56] Survivors and their clinicians need to be aware that cancer treatments can induce depression especially as many people believe that their symptoms are a sign of poor coping or mistakenly assume that depressed mood is expected in the face of cancer.[55] Because of the risk for higher all-cause mortality associated with depression, routinely screening for symptoms of depression and referring for treatment is important. Excellent algorithms exist for caring for individuals who are found to be depressed; many can benefit from psychotherapy alone without the need for added medications that many cancer survivors report they are reluctant to take.[57,58]

Although long dismissed in the clinical setting, growing attention is now being paid to survivors' complaints of chronic difficulties post-treatment with memory and concentration. Neurocognitive dysfunction (i.e., difficulty remembering things, thinking clearly and focusing attention, also referred to as "chemo-brain" or "chemo-fog") is a real and persistent effect of cancer that, more recent studies suggest, may affect between 15% and 25% of survivors in the early re-entry period, with a range as high as 61%.[59] The etiology of cancer-related cognitive impairment is multifactorial and may involve systemic proinflammatory cytokines that cross the blood–brain barrier, exposure to chemotherapy, hormonal and biotherapies, and direct treatment toxicities (e.g., surgery, radiation to the brain).[60,61] Both older age and lower cognitive reserve increase risk for cognitive problems after chemotherapy, findings that contribute to the emerging hypothesis that cancer treatments accelerate the aging process.[61] A number of promising interventions have been developed to help childhood cancer survivors manage cognitive problems resulting from cancer,[62] and more recently, cognitive behavioral therapy interventions are being explored among adult survivors.[63]

Providing survivorship care

Transitioning to recovery

For many survivors, the relief of completing treatment may be tempered by concerns about what the future holds. The stress associated with transitioning to recovery and life *after* (instead of with) cancer has multiple sources. First and foremost among these is worry that the cancer will return now that therapy has stopped. General levels of anxiety may increase as patients transition off treatment. Fear in the survivor can have an adverse effect on family quality of life; the reverse also is true, with family members' fears negatively influencing the quality of life of the survivor.[64] When activated, fear may also lead to disruptive behavior such as heightened body monitoring and anxiety well in advance of a doctor visit, and worry about the future. In some instances, severely disabling reactions can occur including hypochondriac-like preoccupation with health at one extreme, or avoidance and denial at the other, along with inability to plan for the future, and despair. Interventions are being developed to help survivors cope successfully with uncertainty.[65]

Survivors can be taken by surprise by what feels like a paradoxical response to ending treatment, a combination of joy and anxiety. Persistent symptoms (e.g., fatigue, memory problems, and pain syndromes) contribute to a sense of diminished well-being and can lead a survivor to feel she is less well than when treatment was initiated. Loss of the supportive therapy environment (including relationships with staff and fellow patients) must be negotiated. All of this generally occurs in a setting in which family and friends, and even survivors themselves, are ready for everything to be back to "normal."

Key to navigating this transition is acknowledging that it can be stressful. Having a plan of action for the future is also helpful. In this context, the current demand for the development and delivery of survivorship care plans (SCPs) may provide a ready solution to aid smooth coordination of post-treatment care.

Standards for survivorship care

One of the key recommendations in both the President's Cancer Panel report on cancer survivorship[16] and the IOM report, *From Cancer Patient to Cancer Survivor: Lost in Transition* (whose title aptly describes the survivor's dilemma when treatment ends[14]), is

that clinicians should provide patients with a comprehensive treatment summary and a tailored plan for follow-up care. Together, these documents comprise what is known as a survivorship care plan or SCP. Although there is not yet consensus on a standard SCP format or content, several common elements are recommended for inclusion. The treatment summary should provide details about the specific cancer (e.g., diagnosis, stage, pathology, and genetic markers if relevant), type of treatments received (e.g., chemotherapy, radiotherapy with dosing and target area as appropriate, hormonal therapy, and biologic agent use), toxicities experienced, treatment response, and risk for late effects, along with the name and contact information for treating physicians. This information is then used to generate a unique plan of post-treatment care. The IOM[14] identified 11 elements as part of this document that can be summarized in four broad categories: (1) surveillance for recurrence or new cancers including the nature and timing of these tests; (2) assessment and treatment of or referral to community resources for help with persistent effects of cancer, encompassing psychosocial as well as physical sequelae, acknowledging that psychosocial effects of survival are often overlooked[66]; (3) recommendations for prevention of future cancer or adverse health conditions, including lifestyle recommendations and potential referral for genetic testing; and (4) specification regarding the components of follow-up care, as well as the contact information for the clinician(s) responsible for delivering follow-up care (Table 2).

Despite being strongly recommended in two national reports, use of SCPs has been slow to catch on. In their review of the literature on use of SCPs, Mayer et al.[67] arrive at several overarching conclusions: SCPs are broadly endorsed by both patients and providers, but in practice remain underutilized, with large numbers of clinicians reporting failure to deliver these or patients to receive same; while agreement exists among both providers and patients on preferred SCP content, the timing of delivery and who should deliver these is unclear; and finally, limited data exist on the impact of SCP implementation, raising concern about what, if any, difference these documents will make in care delivery or outcomes. These challenges notwithstanding, pressure to embrace SCP use is growing.

In an important step toward making treatment summaries and care plans a part of quality care, ASCO decided to incorporate relevant measures as part of its Quality Oncology Practice Initiative (QOPI). A voluntary program opened to ASCO members in 2006, QOPI was created to promote excellence in cancer care by helping oncologists create a culture of self-examination and improvement. In 2008, ASCO added three items to its core set of questions inquiring whether a chemotherapy treatment summary

Table 2 Essential elements of survivorship care.

Surveillance for recurrence or new cancer (e.g., tests to be performed and their periodicity and changes to be monitored)

Assessment and treatment or referral for persistent effects including medical problems (e.g., depression, lymphedema, sexual dysfunction, and functional impairment), symptoms (e.g., pain and fatigue), psychological distress experienced by cancer survivors and their caregivers; and concerns related to employment, insurance, and disability; use of rehabilitation as indicated

Prevention of late effects (e.g., second cancers, cardiac problems, and osteoporosis) accompanied by use of genetic testing as indicated; including a focus on health promotion (e.g., diet, weight, physical activity, and sun block use), and management of comorbid conditions

Coordination of care (e.g., including frequency of visits, tests and who is performing these) between specialists and primary care providers to ensure that all of the survivor's health needs are met

Source: Adapted from Hewitt 2006.[14]

was completed, a copy was provided to the patient, and a copy was also sent or communicated to another practitioner, all within 3 months of chemotherapy end. Somewhat complex templates for cancer surveillance for breast, colorectal, and prostate cancer were a regular feature on the ASCO web site. More recently, ASCO released a short SCP template.[68] An online tool for building SCPs, *Journey Forward*, is also readily available, the result of a collaboration of oncology experts, industry, a health insurer, and advocacy groups (http://journeyforward.org/). A number of the key oncology electronic software vendors have begun to develop tools for this purpose as well although lack of interoperability among platforms creates a barrier to their intent, namely, to share information and maximize coordination of care. Key hurdles to optimal SCP use are the personnel time it takes to generate them, lack of easy IT integration to facilitate data capture and exchange, and limited evidence-based guidelines with which to inform recommended care.[69] Busy clinicians are hardpressed to use these documents and provide high-quality care because of limited time and budgets. At the same time, SCPs are of limited utility without the intended conversation between patient and provider on their content and use; without these informing dialogues, they are just another piece of paper.

Despite the legitimate concerns about their use, starting in 2015, the American College of Surgeon's Commission on Cancer is including development and delivery of SCPs as an accreditation criterion.[70] Ideally, this action will stimulate thoughtful research regarding who should create and deliver these documents, what is the best approach to doing this, when in the course of care this process should be initiated, and who will pay for this activity. Importantly, understanding whether or not use of SCPs improves patient, provider and system function will be critical.

Models of survivorship care

While it is increasingly recognized that cancer survivors need to be followed for life after treatment, little consensus exists about how this should be done. Anticipated shortages of oncology providers,[71] coupled with growing pressure for these professionals to see new patients, makes solving the question of who should provide cancer-related follow-up care a paramount concern.

A number of papers have called for consideration of a shared-care model in which primary care physicians (PCPs) have primary responsibility for follow-up with referral back to oncology or other specialists as needed.[72–74] In this model, it is essential that the oncologist provide the PCP with an SCP to communicate key information about the survivor's illness history, surveillance recommendations, and potential late complications for which to monitor. One large survey suggests that many US PCPs prefer a shared-care model; fewer prefer an oncologist-led model, a PCP-led model, or other specialty survivorship clinics.[75,76] This same study reported PCPs' confidence regarding their knowledge of survivorship care may be less than optimal.[77] However, international studies have found comparable time to recurrence, quality of life, and psychological functioning among survivors followed up by oncology and those followed up in primary care with some element of guidance (e.g., one page of follow-up instructions).[78,79]

Other models of follow-up care have also been launched, the most common of these developed at large comprehensive cancer centers, being multidisciplinary, specialized survivorship clinics.[80] These tend to offer one of two models: (1) a consultative program in which patients can come at any point post-treatment for review of their history, current function and risk for future problems, and leave with recommendations for care of current problems and an outline of proposed future care to share with their providers; or (2) a full-service program in which survivors can come for regular visits for some specified period of time (e.g., 2–5 years) after cancer treatment. A third model involves nurse-led care in which the nurse serves as a conduit between the care team and the survivor.[81–83] Evolution of a given program often reflects the resources of the clinic or facility, the patient population being served, and more generally, the passion of a key leader or leaders to bring the program together and champion funding support for the enterprise. Sustainability for survivorship care programs is a central concern as there is as yet no clear system for reimbursing this care. Models for financing include fee-for-service, insurance reimbursement, research grants, philanthropy, and dedicated program-specific fund raising. Some larger centers see inclusion of a survivorship clinic as "value added" to their operation and will put resources toward support of these programs in the expectation that they will bring more new patients (as well as survivors) to their high-quality facility.

Because of the complexity of cancer and its treatment and the wide variation in what patients bring to their cancer experience (e.g., with respect to pre-existing medical history, function and psychosocial resources), it is clear that one size does not fit all when it comes to models of survivorship care. Additional calls have been made to develop risk-stratified approaches to post-treatment care. In this approach, clinician specialty and visit frequency depend on survivor needs and risk for recurrence and late effects.[84,85] Low-risk survivors (e.g., early-stage breast or colorectal cancer receiving surgery only) may be transferred right back to primary care shortly after conclusion of treatment. High-risk survivors (e.g., those undergoing stem-cell transplant or with more complex care needs) would be seen regularly by oncology with routine care addressed by the PCP.[72,73] A risk-stratified model of care is currently being tested in Great Britain (http://www.ncsi.org.uk/what-we-are-doing/risk-stratified-pathways-of-care/risk-stratification/). For this type of care to become more common, evidence-based predictive models are needed for survivors most likely to experience negative sequelae after cancer.

Regardless of the model used, two central tenets of survivorship care remain constant: coordination of care is critical if survivors are to receive optimal post-treatment follow-up, and survivors themselves necessarily play an important role in their healthcare and outcomes. While current survivorship care in the United States involves multiple providers from a variety of specialties,[86] no system for communication and coordination among these individuals or teams has been established.[87] Furthermore, until such time as there is consensus about which providers are responsible for, or appropriately skilled in, the essential components of survivorship care,[77,88,89] survivors are at risk of care that is potentially duplicative, inappropriate (e.g., over testing in the absence of proven utility of special scans or tumor markers), or ineffective in reducing cancer-related morbidity. Even some oncologists report incomplete knowledge of the late effects of cancer treatment.[90] To maximize the efficiency and effectiveness of survivorship care, clear communication is crucial at the end of cancer treatment between patients and their providers, as well as cancer providers and their patients' PCP and other specialists, about who is going to provide what kind of care, and when and where this will be delivered. Increased efforts are needed in training diverse healthcare providers about the long-term and late effects of cancer and developing guidelines for delivery of optimal survivorship care. Toward this latter goal, guidelines released by the National Comprehensive Cancer Network (NCCN),[91,92] ASCO,[68,93] and the American Cancer Society (ACS)[94] are already available for advancing survivorship care. Similar efforts are occurring globally.[95]

For their part, survivors may expect that if they continue to see their oncologist years after treatment, he or she is providing primary care.[96] In addition to serving as a communication vehicle between clinicians, SCPs can facilitate survivors' education about their role in managing post-treatment health. Self-management interventions have been shown to improve survivors' quality of life, psychological functioning, and health behaviors. The care received is also more likely to be consonant with survivors' needs and goals when survivors actively participate in treatment-related decision making.[97]

Rehabilitation and health promotion

As the goal of cancer therapy expands beyond merely curing or controlling disease to optimizing function and quality of life after cancer, two additional aspects of care have emerged as central to these aims: rehabilitation and health promotion. Use of cancer-related rehabilitation in the United States has diminished over time, in part reflecting earlier diagnosis (hence less need for more aggressive treatments) and broader use of more limb- and tissue-sparing approaches to surgery. Concern about the persistent effects of cancer and its treatment, however, are causing clinicians to rethink use of these services, access to which remain a standard of care in many countries outside the United States.[98,99] Survivors report multiple rehabilitative needs after cancer,[100] and research suggests that attending to these, both preventively and after the fact,[101] can reduce cancer-related morbidity and mortality. A licensed program designed to meet the rehabilitative needs of cancer survivors has been adopted by several sites across the United States.[102] In 2013, the Commission on Accreditation of Rehabilitative Facilities (CARF) developed certification standards for cancer rehabilitation.[103] How quickly incorporation of these types of services occurs in large cancer centers remains to be seen.

Interest in health promotion after cancer has grown in the past decade driven by multiple factors, including demand by survivors themselves. Most cancer survivors are older, often present with comorbid conditions that are exacerbated by cancer treatment or are at increased risk for comorbid health problems (e.g., cardiac problems, obesity, and osteoporosis) as a function of treatment, develop poor health habits while in active treatment (sedentary and poor diet), are aging, and could benefit from lifestyle interventions. Importantly, survivors often ask their care team what they can do to reduce the risk of a recurrence and regain health after cancer. Because of these factors, researchers see cancer as a "teachable moment."[104]

The benefits of healthy lifestyle are well known in association with prevention of cancer, covered elsewhere in this volume. Among cancer survivors, observational studies suggest that smoking cessation, increased physical activity, and weight control may reduce the risk of cancer recurrence, cancer specific mortality, and overall mortality,[105–107] although randomized clinical trials are still needed to support causal statements about the effects of behavior change. The consistency of the data behind the benefits of remaining or becoming more physically active during and after cancer is sufficient for clinicians to recommend their patients strive to be up and about right from the start of treatment. The ACS provides and regularly updates guidelines for cancer survivors about nutrition and physical activity after cancer.[108] While some survivors change their behavior spontaneously,[109] many do not.[110] Survivorship care provides an important opportunity for clinicians to support cancer survivors' efforts to make changes in dietary behaviors, levels of physical activity, smoking, and stress management that have the potential to reduce risk of recurrence, second malignancies, and comorbid health conditions, an opportunity currently being missed by many practitioners.[111,112] More research is urgently needed on how providers can effectively deliver health promotion assistance and how survivors can successfully implement and sustain beneficial changes.

Families and informal caregivers

Because the advocacy community considers informal caregivers to be cosurvivors, no discussion of survivorship care is complete without consideration of the family caregiver. With the majority of cancer care now delivered in the outpatient setting and many more individuals living long-term after cancer, large numbers of whom will live with cancer as a chronic illness, the burden of cancer on families is rising rapidly. Research suggests that family caregivers frequently feel ill-prepared for the demands of care for their loved one, receive little or no guidance on what to do, and often strain under the demands of competing roles, including holding jobs, managing children, and caring for their own health.[113] One study found that two out of five caregivers experience moderate psychological distress and one out of five desires formal support.[114] Caregivers may worry more about recurrence than the survivor.[64] Unrealistic expectations for a speedy return to life as usual can contribute to anxiety that lingering symptoms may reflect return of the disease and resentment that recovery is taking too long and lead to disruptions in family functioning.

Providing both cancer survivors and their caregivers with information about what to expect in the first 6 months after treatment ends is vital to reduce distress in both parties. Dyadic studies indicate that health outcomes in both patients and their caregiver partners are mutually dependent.[115–117] Because family caregivers, like their care recipients, tend to be older adults and at risk of their own comorbid health conditions (including cancer), it is possible that healthy lifestyle education efforts with the survivor may also benefit the caregiver, although this effect remains to be tested. Moreover, involvement of family caregivers can be critical to ensuring survivors' adherence to recommended adjuvant therapies, follow-up visits, and symptom control and reporting. Thus, ensuring that this vital support system is functioning well can provide an enormous asset to providers in effectively managing their patients' care. Already a number of cancer centers are striving to include services for caregivers as part of their comprehensive care.[118]

Conclusion

The growing population of cancer survivors has taught us several lessons. First, that cancer survivorship—defined as the period that extends from completion of curative therapy until recurrence or death from cancer or another event—represents a distinct phase along the cancer control continuum. It brings its own unique set of challenges and opportunities for recovery and growth. Second, the majority of survivors will live years beyond their initial diagnosis. Those treated as children, adolescents, or young adults have the potential to live a lifetime with a cancer history. However, few of our current therapies are entirely benign; most have some degree of associated toxicity and a number produce considerable adverse physical as well as psychosocial sequelae. Consequently, third, all of these chronic and late effects must be tracked and actively addressed. Fourth, while a subset of survivors continues to struggle after cancer treatment ends, most are remarkably resilient. Nevertheless, the capacity of survivors and their healthcare providers to realize the shared goal of good quality of life and function requires collaboration and communication between both groups. Defining and delivering high-quality survivorship care, albeit a high-end problem, constitutes a significant challenge for cancer medicine. Success, in our efforts to reduce undue suffering and premature death due to cancer, will require continued investment in survivorship research. It will also require enhanced commitment to the training and support of current and future generations of multidisciplinary providers who care long term for those treated for cancer. While a number of questions remain about how to achieve these lofty goals, the resources to do so are evolving rapidly. Further, a number of evidence-based programs have evolved to address survivors' post-treatment needs. Though far from perfect, these are good enough to begin disseminating.[119] Increased attention will be needed, nevertheless, to promote tailoring of care to older adult cancer survivors, a surprisingly neglected population.[120] Along with interest in the field of cancer survivorship more generally, the number of survivorship scientists and practitioners is expanding steadily both in the United States and abroad.[121,122] There is broadening public awareness of the importance of managing the care of those with chronic illnesses like cancer, and the advocacy community championing cancer survivorship needs remains strong. The next decade will permit us to promote and measure the impact of collective efforts to enable more survivors and their families to thrive after cancer.

Summary

- The number of individuals in the United States with a cancer history will continue to grow over the next two decades, driven largely by the aging of the population. By 2022, there will be 18 million cancer survivors, approximately two-thirds of whom will be age 65 or older.

- Cancer survivorship—defined as the period that extends from completion of curative therapy until recurrence or death from cancer or another event—represents a unique place on the cancer control continuum and is accompanied by its own set of health care challenges.

- Cancer and its treatment can cause a variety of persistent (e.g., pain, fatigue, memory problems, and sexual dysfunction) as well as late-occurring (e.g., second cancers, cardiac problems, diabetes, osteoporosis, and depression) adverse sequelae. Often occurring in clusters, these effects can have a negative impact on every aspect of a survivor's life: physical, psychological, social, economic, and existential.

- Most cancer survivors are remarkably resilient and adapt well after cancer. However, a significant subset struggle with the aftermath of their illness. Use of systematic assessment at the end of treatment with early identification and referral of those in need of additional support is important.

- Use of SCPs to improve quality of and communication around post-treatment care is growing. In addition to a treatment summary, essential elements of an SCP include plans for (1) surveillance for recurrent or new cancers; (2) assessment and treatment of persistent effects of cancer; (3) prevention of late consequences, including use of genetic testing and health promotion; and (4) coordination of care.

- No consensus exists on the best model for follow-up care delivery. Currently, multiple models are being examined. Interest is growing in the development of models that (1) involve shared care between oncology and primary care providers and (2) are structured around risk-based algorithms (e.g., survivors with early-stage disease and minimal treatment would return quickly to their PCP, whereas those at high risk of recurrence would remain more closely connected with oncology care teams and centers).

- Survivorship may provide a "teachable moment" for clinicians to help cancer survivors pursue healthy lifestyles and behaviors.

- Attention must be given to the psychological and physical well-being of family caregivers in the recovery process. Viewed as "secondary survivors," informal caregivers play an important role in survivors' recovery and yet may struggle themselves with this transition to a "new normal."

Key references

The complete reference list can be found on the Wiley Companion Digital Edition of this title (see inside front cover for login instructions).

1 Hewitt M, Weiner SL, Simone JV (eds.). *Childhood Cancer Survivorship: Improving Care and Quality of Life.* Washington, DC: The National Academies Press, 2003.

4 Phillips SM, Padgett L, Leisenring W, et al. Survivors of childhood cancer in the United States: prevalence and burden of morbidity. *Cancer Epidemiol Biomarkers Prev.* 2015;**24**:653–663.

7 Children's Oncology Group Guidelines (2015) *Long-Term Follow-up Guidelines,* http://www.childrensoncologygroup.org/index.php/survivorshipguidelines (accessed 12 January 2015).

11 Mullan F. Seasons of survival: reflections of a physician with cancer. *N Engl J Med.* 1985;**313**:270–273.

14 Hewitt M, Greenfield S, Stovall E (eds.). *From Cancer Patient to Cancer Survivor: Lost in Transition.* Institute of Medicine, National Academies Press: Washington, DC, 2006.

16 National Cancer Institute. *President's Cancer Panel, 2003–2004 Annual Report: Living Beyond Cancer: Finding a New Balance* (NIH publication No. P986). Washington, DC: National Institutes of Health; 2004.

25 *American Cancer Society.* Cancer Treatment & Survivorship. Facts & Figures 2014-2015. Atlanta, GA: American Cancer Society, 2014.

29 Parry C, Kent EE, Mariotto AB, Alfano CM, Rowland JH. Cancer survivors: a booming population. *Cancer Epidemiol Biomarkers Prev.* 2011;**20**:1996–2005.

36 Reeve BB, Potosky AL, Smith AW, et al. Impact of cancer on health-related quality of life of older Americans. *J Natl Cancer Inst.* 2009;**101**:860–868.

37 Smith AW, Reeve BB, Bellizzi KM, et al. Cancer, comorbidities, and health-related quality of life of older adults. *Health Care Financ Rev.* 2008;**29**:41–56.

39 Farley Short P, Vasey JJ, Moran JR. Long-term effects of cancer survivorship on the employment of older workers. *Health Serv Res.* 2008;**43**(1 Pt 1):193–210.

44 Koch L, Jansen L, Brenner H, Arndt V. Fear of recurrence and disease progression in long-term (≥5 years) cancer survivors – a systematic review of quantitative studies. *Psychooncology.* 2013;**22**:1–11.

47 Bower JE, Ganz PA, Desmond KA, et al. Fatigue in long-term breast carcinoma survivors: a longitudinal investigation. *Cancer* 2006 ;**106**:751-758.

53 Mitchell AJ, Ferguson DW, Gill J, et al. Depression and anxiety in long-term cancer survivors compared with spouses and healthy controls: a systematic review and meta-analysis. *Lancet Oncol.* 2013;**14**:721–732.

57 Andersen B, DeRubeis RJ, Berman BS, et al. Screening, assessment and care of anxiety and depressive symptoms in adults with cancer: an American Society of Clinical Oncology guideline adaptation. *J Clin Oncol.* 2014;**32**:1605–1619.

58 Faller H, Schuler M, Richard M, et al. Effects of psycho-oncologic interventions on emotional distress and quality of life in adult patients with cancer: systematic review and meta-analysis. *J Clin Oncol.* 2013;**31**:782–793.

59 Ahles TA, Root JC, Ryan EL. Cancer- and cancer treatment-associated cognitive change: an update on the state of the science. *J Clin Oncol.* 2012;**20**:2675–3686.

66 Adler NE, Page AEK (eds.). *Cancer Care for the Whole Patient: Meeting Psychosocial Health Needs.* Institute of Medicine, Committee on Psychosocial Services to Cancer Patients/Families in a Community Setting, Academies Press: Washington, DC, 2008.

67 Mayer DK, Birken SA, Check DK, Chen RC. Summing it up: an integrative review of studies of cancer survivorship care plans (2006-2013). *Cancer.* 2014;**121**:978–996 [Epub ahead of print].

68 Mayer DK, Nekhlyudov L, Snyder CF, et al. American Society of Clinical Oncology clinical expert statement on cancer survivorship care planning. *J Oncol Pract.* 2014;**10**:345–351.

72 Howell D, Hack TF, Oliver TK, et al. Models of care for post-treatment follow-up of adult cancer survivors: a systematic review and quality appraisal of the evidence. *J Cancer Surviv.* 2012;**6**:359–371.

73 Oeffinger KC, McCabe MS. Models for delivering survivorship care. *J Clin Oncol.* 2006;**24**:5117–5124.

75 Potosky AL, Han PKJ, Rowland J, et al. Differences between primary care physicians' and oncologists' knowledge, attitudes and practices regarding the care of cancer survivors. *J Gen Intern Med.* 2011;**26**:1403–1410.

78 Grunfeld E, Levine MN, Julian JA, et al. Randomized trial of long-term follow-up for early-stage breast cancer: a comparison of family physician versus specialist care. *J Clin Oncol.* 2006;**24**:848–855.

90 Nekhlyudov L, Aziz NM, Lerro C, Virgo KS. Oncologists' and primary care physicians' awareness of late and long-term effects of chemotherapy: implications for care of the growing population of survivors. *J Oncol Pract.* 2014;**10**:e29–e36.

91 Denlinger CS, Carlson RW, Are M, et al. Survivorship: introduction and definition. *J Natl Compr Canc Netw.* 2014;**12**:34–45.

92 Denlinger CS, Ligibel JA, Are M, et al. Survivorship: screening for cancer and treatment effects Version 2.2014. *J Natl Compr Canc Netw.* 2014;**12**:1526–1531.

93 McCabe MS, Bhatia S, Oeffinger KC, et al. American Society of Clinical Oncology statement: achieving high-quality cancer survivorship care. *J Clin Oncol.* 2013;**31**:631–640.

94 Skolarus TA, Wolf AM, Erb NL, et al. American Cancer Society prostate cancer survivorship care guidelines. *CA Cancer J Clin*. 2014;**64**:225–249.

95 Cancer Journey Survivorship Expert Panel, Howell D, Hack TF, Oliver TK, et al. Survivorship services for adult cancer populations: a pan-Canadian guideline. *Curr Oncol*. 2011;**18**:e265–e281.

98 Stubblefield MD, Hubbard G, Cheville A, et al. Current perspectives and emerging issues on cancer rehabilitation. *Cancer*. 2013;**119**:2170–2178.

99 Alfano CM, Ganz PA, Rowland JH, Hahn EE. Cancer survivorship and cancer rehabilitation: revitalizing the link. *J Clin Oncol*. 2012;**30**:904–906.

104 Demark-Wahnefried W, Aziz NM, Rowland JH, Pinto BM. Riding the crest of the teachable moment: promoting long-term health after the diagnosis of cancer. *J Clin Oncol*. 2005;**23**:5814–5830.

108 Rock CL, Doyle C, Demark-Wahnefried W, et al. Nutrition and physical activity guidelines for cancer survivors. *CA Cancer J Clin*. 2012;**62**:243–274.

110 Underwood JM, Townsend JS, Stewart SL, et al. Surveillance of demographic characteristics and health behaviors among adult cancer survivors—behavioral Risk Factor Surveillance System, United States, 2009. *MMWR Surveill Summ*. 2012;**61**:1–23.

113 Van Ryn M, Sanders S, Kahn K, et al. Objective burden, resources, and other stressors among informal cancer caregivers: a hidden quality issue? *Psychooncology*. 2011;**20**:44–52.

117 Waldron EA, Janke EA, Bechtel CE, et al. A systematic review of psychosocial interventions to improve cancer caregiver quality of life. *Psychooncology*. 2013;**22**:1200–1207.

118 Matson M, Song L, Mayer DK. Putting together the pieces of the puzzle: identifying existing evidence-based resources to support the cancer caregiver. *Clin J Oncol Nurs*. 2014;**18**:619–621.

119 Earle CC, Ganz PA. Cancer survivorship care: don't let the perfect be the enemy of the good. *J Clin Oncol*. 2012;**30**:3764–3768.

122 Stein K, Mattioli V. Dialogues on cancer survivorship: a new model of international cooperation. *Cancer*. 2013;**119**(**Suppl 11**):2083–2085.

Disease Sites

PART 11

Disease Sites

77 Primary and metastatic neoplasms of the brain in adults

Lisa M. DeAngelis, MD, FAAN

Overview

Primary brain tumors are uncommon but aggressive neoplasms even when histology is low grade. Secondary, or metastatic, tumors are at least 3 times more common than all primary tumors combined. Diagnosis is easily established by magnetic resonance imaging (MRI), and surgical resection provides histologic confirmation and decompression; surgery alone may suffice for low-grade tumors and most extra-axial tumors such as meningiomas. Treatment of parenchymal brain tumors, primary or metastatic, often requires a combination of radiotherapy and chemotherapy, which may improve patient function and control disease but rarely achieves cure.

Introduction

Tumors of the central nervous system (CNS) are a heterogeneous group of both benign and malignant intracranial neoplasms. CNS tumors are classified into two groups: those that grow within the brain (intracerebral) and those that grow outside the brain (extra-cerebral). Historically, CNS tumors have been intractable to standard therapies of surgical resection, radiotherapy (RT), and chemotherapy. However, over the past several decades, advances in diagnostic imaging, surgical techniques, radiation oncology, and chemotherapy have improved survival and quality of life. Most important, we are acquiring a better understanding of the molecular events associated with the malignant phenotype of a brain tumor, which has led to several novel chemotherapeutic approaches to their treatment.

Epidemiology

Primary intracranial tumors are uncommon. The overall annual incidence of brain tumors, both benign and malignant, in the United States is estimated at 21.03 cases per 100,000 person-years leading to an estimated 63,000 new cases diagnosed each year (Central Brain Tumor Registry of the United States Statistical Report [CBTRUS] 2006–2010).[1] More than 26% are gliomas, and almost three-quarters of these are high grade with a higher incidence in men (7.76 per 100,000 person-years) than in women (5.60 per 100,000 person-years).[1]

The incidence and histologic type of intracranial tumor differs by race, gender, and age.[1] The overall incidence of brain tumors (especially gliomas) is greater in Whites than Blacks. However, meningiomas are more frequent in Blacks than Whites. Pituitary adenomas are also more common in Blacks than Whites. Gender differences are apparent. The male to female ratio is 1.3 for oligodendrogliomas, 1.38 for astrocytomas, and 0.77 for malignant meningiomas, and for benign meningiomas, the male to female ratio is 0.44. Lymphomas and germ cell tumors are more common in males, 1.31 and 2.33, respectively.

CNS tumors can occur at any age, but the incidence and histologic type vary by age. There is a small peak before age 10 and a steady rise from age 15. The average age of onset for all primary brain tumors is 54 years. The average age of onset of glioblastoma (GBM) and meningioma is 62 years, whereas for oligodendroglioma the mean age of onset is 16 years. The CBTRUS data show that the highest incidence for all brain tumors occurs in the 75- to 84-year-old age group, with GBMs occurring most frequently in patients older than 65 years. Survival is directly related to patient age and tumor histology. For instance, the 5-year relative survival rate for patients with pilocytic astrocytomas (a common childhood tumor) is 94.4%, compared to 4.7% in patients with GBMs. Other important prognostic factors include extent of disease, extent of resection, and tumor location.

Risk factors

There have been a large number of studies examining the relationship between the environment and the occurrence of brain tumors, but only two unequivocal risk factors have been identified: ionizing radiation and immune suppression (Table 1). The role of low- and high-dose therapeutic ionizing radiation as a significant risk factor for brain tumors has been confirmed in many studies. Irradiation for intracranial tumors, e.g., medulloblastoma or extracranial head and neck cancers, including prophylactic irradiation for leukemia, increase the incidence of both gliomas and sarcomas sevenfold in those who survive more than 3 years. The cumulative relative risk of secondary brain tumors in patients treated with cranial irradiation ranges from 5.65 to 10.9; approximately two-thirds of the tumors are gliomas and one-third are meningiomas.[2] High-grade gliomas have a median latency of 9.1 years from cranial RT compared to 19 years for meningiomas. Low-dose radiation such as that used to treat tinea capitis, a fungal infection of the scalp, and skin hemangiomas in children is associated with an increased risk of brain tumors. A relative risk of 18, 10, and 3 have been observed for nerve sheath tumor, malignant meningioma, and glioma, respectively.

Congenital or acquired immune suppression, such as human immunodeficiency virus (HIV) infection, or the use of immunosuppressive drugs after organ transplantation, increases the incidence of primary central nervous system lymphoma (PCNSL).[3] HIV infection may also increase the frequency of glioma and intracranial leiomyosarcomas. PCNSL in immunosuppressed patients is driven by a pre-existing latent Epstein–Barr viral infection of B-lymphocytes. When a lymphoma occurs in an immunosuppressed patient, it is twice as likely to occur in the brain as elsewhere in the body.

Other studies of environmental risk factors are less convincing than those of ionizing radiation and immunosuppression,

Holland-Frei Cancer Medicine, Ninth Edition. Edited by Robert C. Bast Jr., Carlo M. Croce, William N. Hait, Waun Ki Hong, Donald W. Kufe, Martine Piccart-Gebhart, Raphael E. Pollock, Ralph R. Weichselbaum, Hongyang Wang, and James F. Holland.
© 2017 John Wiley & Sons, Inc. ISBN: 978-1-118-93469-2

Definite risk factors
Ionizing radiation
Hereditary syndromes
Family history of brain tumors
Immunosuppression

including dietary exposure to N-nitrosourea compounds, occupational exposure to pesticide and fertilizer manufacturing, formaldehyde, synthetic rubber production, vinyl chloride synthesis, and petrochemical industries. Additional research evaluating the association of brain tumors with head trauma, cigarette smoking, seizure history, maternal alcohol use, and infection has been inconclusive.

Exposure to electromagnetic fields (EMF), especially through the use of cellular phones, has been of interest. Most studies have demonstrated no association between cellular phone use and brain tumors, but there may be a dose relationship to brain tumor risk.[4,5] Recent data suggest a history of allergies or atopic disease may be protective against glioma development. In addition, large genome-wide association studies point to eight germline DNA single nucleotide polymorphisms in seven genes that predispose to glioma formation or specific glioma grade or subtypes; the mechanism of this predisposition is unknown.[6]

Molecular genetics

There is evidence that somatic mutations in different molecular pathways may lead to the development of an identically appearing GBM. There appear to be at least four different molecular subclasses of GMB that include (1) *classical* characterized by EGFR amplification/mutation and p53 mutation, (2) *proneural* characterized by alterations in PDGFRA and isocitrate dehydrogenase (*IDH*) mutations, (3) *mesenchymal* characterized by NF1 dysfunction, and (4) *neural* with EGFR overactivity and displaying neural markers.[7] At the present time, this molecular classification scheme does not drive treatment selection or prognosis. Lower grade gliomas with either astrocytic or oligodendroglial features are characterized by IDH mutations, primarily the *IDHR132H* mutation in 70%.[8] This mutation leads to the formation of the oncometabolite, 2 hydroxyglutarate (2HG), which has become both a diagnostic and therapeutic target using magnetic resonance (MR) spectroscopy and novel IDH1 inhibitors. *IDH1* mutations are thought to arise early in gliomagenesis, but they are noticeably lacking in primary GBMs, or those that present in older age as *de novo* GBMs.

In addition to oncogene amplification and tumor suppressor gene inactivation, malignant tumors acquire the ability to invade adjacent neural structures and form a new blood supply via angiogenesis. Glial tumors are extremely invasive neoplasms and typically extend well beyond their macroscopic or imaging borders. Angiogenesis leads to vascular hyperplasia, which is the pathologic hallmark of a GBM. Vascular endothelial growth factor (VEGF) is one of the key stimulants to angiogenesis in gliomas. VEGF is not expressed in normal brain endothelium but is upregulated in gliomas by local hypoxia. VEGF also increases vascular permeability and plays a role in the peritumoral edema seen in malignant gliomas.

Familial tumor syndromes of the CNS

Familial brain tumor syndromes are a heterogeneous group of disorders characterized by an association of brain tumors with systemic features, primarily dermatologic (Table 2).

Neurofibromatosis 1

Neurofibromatosis 1 (NF-1), also known as von Recklinghausen disease, is the most common hereditary disease predisposing to CNS cancer, with a prevalence of 1 in 4000. The incidence is equal in men and women. It is an autosomal dominant disorder with 100% penetrance but is highly variable in its expressivity with both minimally and severely affected individuals within the same family. The NF-1 gene has been mapped to chromosome 17q11.2 and encodes a tumor suppressor, neurofibromin.

The predominant CNS tumors in NF-1 are optic pathway and brainstem gliomas. Optic pathway gliomas are usually pilocytic astrocytomas and brainstem gliomas are astrocytomas. The typical peripheral nerve tumor is the plexiform neurofibroma, which often involves the paraspinal and cranial nerves. Other NF-1 related tumors include malignant schwannomas, rhabdomyosarcomas, and GBMs.

Neurofibromatosis 2

Neurofibromatosis 2 (NF-2), known as central neurofibromatosis, is an autosomal dominant disorder that accounts for only 10% of all neurofibromatosis cases. The NF-2 gene is a tumor suppressor gene located on chromosome 22q12.2, which encodes a tumor suppressor, merlin. The predominant CNS tumors in NF-2 are vestibular schwannomas, often bilateral, and meningiomas.

Tuberous sclerosis

Tuberous sclerosis (TS) is an autosomal dominant disorder. It has been mapped to two different loci: TS complex 1 located on chromosome 9q34.14 encodes the protein hamartin and TS complex 2 located on chromosome 16p13.3 encodes the protein tuberin. The classic clinical triad of mental retardation, seizures, and facial angiofibromas occurs only in the most severe cases. Skin lesions are seen in 96% of patients, including angiofibromas, uncal fibromas, hypomelanotic skin patches known as "ash leaf spots," and dental pits. The hallmark CNS tumor is the subependymal giant cell astrocytoma (SEGA). Although pathologically benign, SEGAs are driven by mTOR overactivity and recent work has demonstrated the value of mTOR inhibition with drugs such as everolimus causing tumor regression and improved seizure control.[9]

von Hippel–Lindau disease

von Hippel–Lindau (VHL) disease is a tumor syndrome involving multiple organ systems leading to hemangioblastomas in the cerebellum, spinal cord, and retina and pheochromocytomas and renal cell carcinoma. Other less common lesions include pancreatic and renal cysts and endolymphatic sac tumors. The hemangioblastomas are associated with overexpression of VEGF. VHL is an autosomal dominant disorder mapped to chromosome 3p25-p26. It has a high penetrance but variable expressivity.

Li–Fraumeni syndrome

Li–Fraumeni syndrome is a rare autosomal dominant disorder seen in children and young adults leading to multiple different tumors. It is caused by germ line mutations of p53. However, some families do not have the p53 mutation and their genetic defect is unknown. Overall penetrance of the gene is about 50%

Table 2 CNS tumor syndromes.

Disorders	CNS tumors	Tumors of other organs and tissues	Skin lesions	Genes	Chromosomes
Neurofibromatosis-1	Glioma, neurofibroma	Iris hamartoma, osseous lesions, pheochromocytoma, leukemia	Café au-lait spots, cutaneous axillary freckling, neurofibromas	NF1	17q11.2
Neurofibromatosis-2	Vestibular Schwannoma, Meningioma	Posterior lens opacities, retinal hamartoma	None	NF2	22q12.2
von Hippel–Lindau disease	Hemangioblastoma	Retinal hemangioblastoma, renal cell carcinoma, pheochromocytoma, visceral cysts, endolymphatic sac tumor	None	VHL	3p25-p26
Tuberous sclerosis	Subependymal giant cell astrocytoma (SEGA)	Cardiac rhabdomyoma, adenomatous polyps of the duodenum and small intestine, cysts of the lung and kidney, lymphangioleiomyomatosis, renal angiomyolipoma	Cutaneous Angiofibroma ("adenoma sebaceum"), peau de chagrin, subungual fibromas	TSC1, TSC2	9q34.14, 16p13.3
Li–Fraumeni syndrome	Gliomas (10%)	Breast carcinoma; bone and soft tissue sarcoma; adrenocortical, lung, and GI carcinoma; leukemia	None	P53	17p13.1
Cowden disease	Cerebellar mass (Lhermitte Duclos disease)	Hamartomatous polyps of the eye, colon, and thyroid; breast carcinoma, thyroid cancer	Multiple trichilemmomas, fibromas	PTEN	10q22.3
Brain tumor-polyposis syndrome type 1	Malignant glioma	Colorectal adenomas, colon carcinoma, No polyps		MLH1 MSH2 MSH6 PMS2	3p21.3 2p21-22 2p16 7p22.1
Brain tumor-polyposis syndrome type 2	Medulloblastoma	Colon cancer, colonic polyps		APC	5q21
Nevoid basal cell carcinoma syndrome (Gorlin syndrome)	Medulloblastoma (anaplastic)	Jaw cysts, ovarian fibromas, skeletal abnormalities	Multiple basal cell carcinomas, palmar and plantar pits	PTCH	9q22.3-31
Retinoblastoma	Pineal tumor	Retinal tumor, osteosarcomas and other tumors	None	RBI	13q14
Bloom syndrome	Medulloblastoma meningioma	Characteristic face and voice, gonadal failure, diabetes, immunodeficiency	Sun sensitivity, patches of hyper-and hypopigmentation	BLM	15q26.1
Fanconi anemia	Astrocytoma, medulloblastoma	Anemia, skeletal malformations, enlarged cerebral ventricles, gastrointestinal malformations, AML	Café au-lait spots, hyper- and hypopigmentation	FANCA	16q24.3
Familial melanoma	Astrocytoma	Melanoma, pancreas, breast	Nevi	CDKN2A p16(1NK4)	9p21.3
Rhabdoid predisposition syndrome	PNET, choroid plexus carcinoma	Renal tumors, extrarenal malignant rhabdoid tumors	None	HSNFA/INH1	22q11
Multiple endocrine neoplasia (MEN-1 Carney complex)	Pituitary adenomas	Hyperparathyroidism, gastrinoma, insulinoma, thyroid/bronchial carcinoid	Facial angiofibroma, lipoma, collagenoma	MEN1	11q13
Ataxia-telangiectasia	Astrocytoma, medulloblastoma, cerebellar ataxia	Lymphomas, hypogonadism, radiationsensitivity, insulin resistance, premature aging, small stature	Telangiectasias	ATM	11q22-q23

PNET, primitive neuroectodermal tumor; AML, acute myelogenous leukemia.

by age 30 and 90% by age 60. Common tumors include breast, osteosarcoma, and brain tumors, primarily high-grade gliomas. Some develop medulloblastomas and supratentorial primitive neuroectodermal tumors (PNET). Other less common tumors include soft tissue sarcomas, leukemia, and lung, adrenal, gastric, and colon cancers.

Brain tumor-polyposis/GI cancer syndromes
These hereditary syndromes are characterized by colon carcinoma with or without associated polyposis and malignant brain tumors. The two broad variants of brain tumor-polyposis syndrome vary in their association with malignant brain tumors: type 1 is associated with malignant gliomas and type 2 is associated with medulloblastoma. These syndromes incorporate autosomal dominant and autosomal recessive syndromes. The type 1 brain tumor-polyposis syndrome may not have polyposis and is due to mutations in one

of the mismatch repair genes; these syndromes have also been called Turcot, Lynch, Muir-Torres, or Gardner syndrome. The type 2 brain tumor-polyposis syndrome is usually due to a germline mutation in the *APC* gene which has also been described as Turcot syndrome.

Histological classification of CNS tumors
WHO classifies tumors by their patterns of differentiation and presumed cell of origin. The majority of primary CNS tumors are neuroepithelial and the cell of origin is the glial cell (usually astrocyte) (Table 3).[10] The remainder arise from meningeal, pituitary, lymphocytic, or germ cells. Neurons constitute less than 10% of brain cells and are an uncommon source of CNS neoplasms.

In general, children most frequently develop PNETs, low-grade astrocytomas, and ependymomas; 70% are infratentorial and occur

Table 3 Partial WHO list of common tumors of neuroepithelial tissue.

I.   Astrocytic tumors
1. Diffuse astrocytoma, grade 2
2. Anaplastic astrocytoma, grade 3
3. Glioblastoma (giant cell, gliosarcoma variants), grade 4
4. Pilocytic astrocytoma, grade 1
5. Pleomorphic xanthoastrocytoma, grade 2
6. Subependymal giant cell astrocytoma, grade 1

II. Oligodendroglial tumors
1. Oligodendroglioma, grade 2
2. Anaplastic oligodendroglioma, grade 3
3. Oligoastrocytoma, grade 2
4. Anaplastic oligoastrocytoma, grade 3

III. Ependymal tumors
1. Ependymoma, grade 2
2. Anaplastic ependymoma, grade 3
3. Myxopapillary ependymoma, grade 1
4. Subependymoma, grade 1

IV. Choroid plexus tumors
1. Choroid plexus papilloma, grade 1
2. Choroid plexus carcinoma, grade 3

V.   Neuronal and mixed neuronal-glial tumors
1. Gangliocytoma, grade 2
2. Ganglioglioma, grade 2
3. Anaplastic ganglioglioma, grade 3
4. Dysembryoplastic neuroepithelial tumor (DNET), grade 1
5. Central neurocytoma, grade 2

VI. Pineal tumors
1. Pineocytoma, grade 1
2. Pineal parenchymal tumor of intermediate differentiation, grade 2
3. Pineoblastoma, grade 3

VII. Embryonal tumors
1. Medulloblastoma (desmoplastic, large cell, melanotic, medullomyoblastoma)
2. CNS primitive neuroectodermal tumors (PNETs)
   (a) Neuroblastoma
   (b) Ganglioneuroblastoma
   (c) Ependymoblastoma
   (d) Medulloepithelioma

near the midline. In contrast, adults usually present with supratentorial tumors that are off the midline and are higher grade astrocytic tumors. GBM, a WHO grade 4 tumor, is hypercellular with nuclear pleomorphism, mitotic figures, endothelial proliferation, and necrosis. Gliosarcomas display the typical pathologic features of GBM in combination with densely packed spindle-shaped cells in herring bone patterns. Gliosarcomas have the same prognosis as GBM and are treated identically. Anaplastic astrocytomas (AA), WHO grade 3 tumors, also have increased cellularity, nuclear atypia, and mitoses, but necrosis and microvascular proliferation are absent. WHO grade 2 astrocytomas typically comprise a fairly uniform group of astrocytes in a background of fibrillary matrix. There is less cellular pleomorphism, and mitoses are rare; there is an absence of vascular proliferation and necrosis. Grade 2 and 3 tumors with an *IDH* mutation have a better prognosis than tumors matched for type and grade without an *IDH* mutation.

Glial tumors can be very heterogeneous; there can be different grades and even different histologic features with astrocytic and oligodendroglial appearing regions within the same tumor. This can be challenging diagnostically and highlights the need to get an adequate pathologic sample for examination. The highest grade found within the lesion determines the diagnosis and dictates

treatment. Grade 1 tumors, juvenile pilocytic astrocytomas (JPA), occur almost exclusively in children. They are characterized by low cellularity, Rosenthal fibers, and cysts, and they do not infiltrate surrounding tissue extensively. They may contain rare mitoses and hyperchromatic nuclei, although these are not features of malignancy in these tumors. In young children, they occur most commonly in the cerebellar hemispheres where they have a 95% 5-year progression-free survival (PFS) rate after complete resection. The other low-grade glial tumors also tend to be discreet and less infiltrative. These include pleomorphic xanthoastrocytoma (PXA), ganglioglioma, neurocytoma, and dysembryoplastic neuroepithelial tumor (DNET). These tumors usually require an experienced neuropathologist to diagnose.

Oligodendrogliomas are characterized by a relatively uniform array of small round cells with artifactual perinuclear halos in a background of fine capillary ("chicken-wire") vasculature. They are typically described as having a "fried-egg" appearance. Occasionally, oligodendrogliomas have features of anaplasia, pleomorphism, and necrosis and are classified as grade 3 anaplastic oligodendrogliomas (AO). They have a better clinical prognosis than their astrocytic counterparts. Some oligodendrogliomas have loss of heterozygosity on chromosomes 1p and 19q due to a translocation. Tumors with 1p19q codeletion have a better prognosis and are more responsive to therapy. Tumors containing a mutation in *IDH* and have 1p19q codeletion have the best prognosis.

PNETs are a group of neoplasms characterized by undifferentiated small blue cells with Homer–Wright rosettes (cells arranged around a true lumen). They are usually fast growing and often disseminate along CSF pathways. They are most common in children and are often found in the cerebellum (medulloblastoma) and in the pineal gland (pinealoblastoma). Although these lesions are histologically identical, the medulloblastoma is more amenable to treatment and has a better outcome.

Ependymomas arise from ependymal cells that line the ventricles and spinal canal. They arise wherever ependymal cells are present and have a predilection for the fourth ventricle. They are the most frequent neuroepithelial tumor of the spinal cord, accounting for more than 50% of spinal gliomas in both children and adults. They are histologically characterized by perivascular pseudorosettes (tumor cells arranged radially around blood vessels) and Homer–Wright rosettes. These tumors are usually low grade but can be aggressive and spread along CSF pathways.

Clinical presentation

Patients with brain tumors may present with generalized, nonfocal symptoms and signs or with focal manifestations related to the specific location of the tumor in the brain.[10] Factors that contribute to the presenting symptoms and signs include tumor location, size, and growth rate. Supratentorial tumors are more likely to present with seizure, whereas infratentorial tumors more commonly present with headache, nausea, and vomiting. Superficial cortical tumors are more likely to cause seizure, whereas deeper tumors are more likely to cause personality and cognitive changes. Seizure is the presenting symptom in about 20% of patients with malignant brain tumors, but is the initial manifestation in approximately 90% of those with low-grade tumors. Tumors in eloquent areas of the brain will cause focal symptoms such as aphasia, hemiparesis, or sensory loss. Tumors in the brainstem typically present with cranial nerve deficits such as diplopia or facial weakness. Tumors of the cerebellum may cause ipsilateral ataxia, unsteady gait, and nystagmus.

Symptoms usually evolve over several weeks; sometimes the symptoms begin acutely, corresponding to a hemorrhage into a metastasis or glial tumor, or a seizure with a prolonged postictal state. GBM and oligodendrogliomas of any grade have a 5–10% risk of hemorrhage. Any intracranial metastatic tumor can hemorrhage, but certain tumors, such as melanoma, thyroid, renal, and choriocarcinoma, have a propensity to bleed; however, lung cancer is the most common source of a hemorrhagic brain metastasis because of its high frequency of CNS metastases. On occasion, focal seizures can cause neurologic signs that do not resolve completely.

Diagnostic neuroimaging

Patients with symptoms and signs suggestive of an intracranial lesion should have a magnetic resonance imaging (MRI) study; it is the modality of choice for CNS tumors and CT should be used only in those patients unable to get an MRI.

High-grade tumors such as GBM disrupt the blood–brain barrier and have the characteristic appearance of a hypointense center surrounded by a hyperintense irregular rim of contrast enhancement (Figure 1). Almost 95% of GBMs will enhance with gadolinium. Anaplastic gliomas enhance less frequently, particularly in younger adults, and they may be confused with lower grade gliomas radiographically (Figure 2). GBMs also have a greater tendency to spread along white matter tracts, particularly the corpus callosum, and to cross to the contralateral cerebral hemisphere. In comparison, low-grade tumors have an intact blood–brain barrier and usually do not contrast enhance. An exception is the JPA, a grade 1 tumor that has areas of dense enhancement. Fluid-attenuated inversion recovery (FLAIR) sequences provide rapid distinction between normal brain and brain tumor or edema and provide the best images to delineate the radiographic extent of the lesion (Figure 3). On FLAIR imaging, however, infiltrative tumor cannot be differentiated from edema. Diffusion-weighted imaging (DWI) assesses the mobility of water molecules and may differentiate between ischemia and tumor. Perfusion images measure blood volume and vascularity and correlate with tumor grade and with ^{18}fluorodeoxyglucose (FDG) positron emission tomography (PET) studies.

On MRI, metastases are usually spherical and have more regular margins than primary tumors. They are usually found at gray–white matter junctions in watershed areas of the brain. When small, they uniformly contrast enhance, and when larger, they may ring enhance. The tumor is usually surrounded by substantial edema. Very small metastases may appear as small dots of contrast enhancement with or without hyperintensity on the FLAIR image; they usually lack surrounding edema. Fifty percent of patients have a single identifiable brain metastasis, 20% have two metastases, 13% have three and the remainder have more than three. There are some limitations to MRI, and the differential diagnosis of a brain tumor includes radiation necrosis, ischemic stroke, infection, inflammatory process, and demyelination.

Other imaging techniques

PET has several uses in the diagnosis of brain tumors. PET can help distinguish between recurrent tumor and radiation necrosis, may differentiate low-grade from high-grade lesions, and may guide stereotactic biopsy to the site of high-grade tumor within an apparently low-grade lesion seen on MRI (Figure 4). PET is performed by injecting substances such as glucose, an amino acid such as methionine, or even a nucleotide labeled with a positron-emitting isotope such as O15, C11, N13, and F18. FDG is the most commonly used isotope for evaluating brain tumors, and defines the metabolic rate

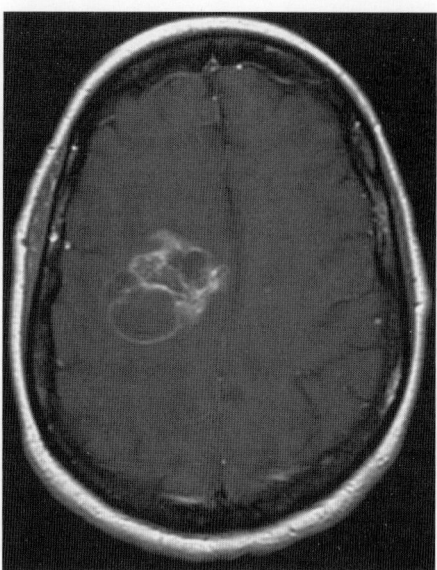

Figure 1 Glioblastoma. This is a postgadolinium T1-weighted MRI of a right posterior frontal glioblastoma. There is irregular contrast enhancement with focal areas of necrosis.

of the lesion being examined. Hypermetabolism (increased FDG uptake) is common in high-grade tumors and hypometabolism (low FDG uptake) is common in low-grade tumors. FDG PET may help distinguish radiation necrosis from recurrent tumor. Whereas both may appear similar on MRI, radiation necrosis is typically, but not always, hypometabolic on PET in comparison to recurrent high-grade tumor, which is either isometabolic with normal brain or hypermetabolic on PET.

Functional magnetic resonance imaging (fMRI) maps the functional organization of the brain, particularly the primary motor, sensory, and language cortices. fMRI is based on the concept that increased neuronal activity results in increased cerebral blood flow (CBF), causing a focal change in the oxyhemoglobin to deoxyhemoglobin ratio leading to increased signal on MRI. The fMRI is useful in presurgical planning and allows a surgeon to map eloquent cortex and then plan resection while preserving neurologic function; this facilitates maximal resection without neurologic deficit.

Principles of therapy

Treatment of a brain tumor includes both definitive and supportive therapy. Definitive therapy encompasses surgery, radiation therapy, and chemotherapy. Supportive therapy considers management of tumor symptoms such as treatment of focal and general symptoms with corticosteroids, seizure control with antiepileptic medication, treatment of deep venous thrombosis (DVT) with anticoagulants, and the provision of psychosocial support when needed.

Supportive therapy
In addition to surgery, RT, and chemotherapy, where the goal of treatment is to extend survival, various types of supportive therapy are also required to treat a patient's neurologic symptoms and improve their quality of life.

All seizures from a brain tumor begin as a focal seizure even if the focality is not observed clinically. Patients with brain tumors who have had a seizure either at presentation or during the course of their treatment should be treated with an antiepileptic drug (AED). The optimal AED does not affect the hepatic microsomal system, which can alter the metabolism of chemotherapeutic

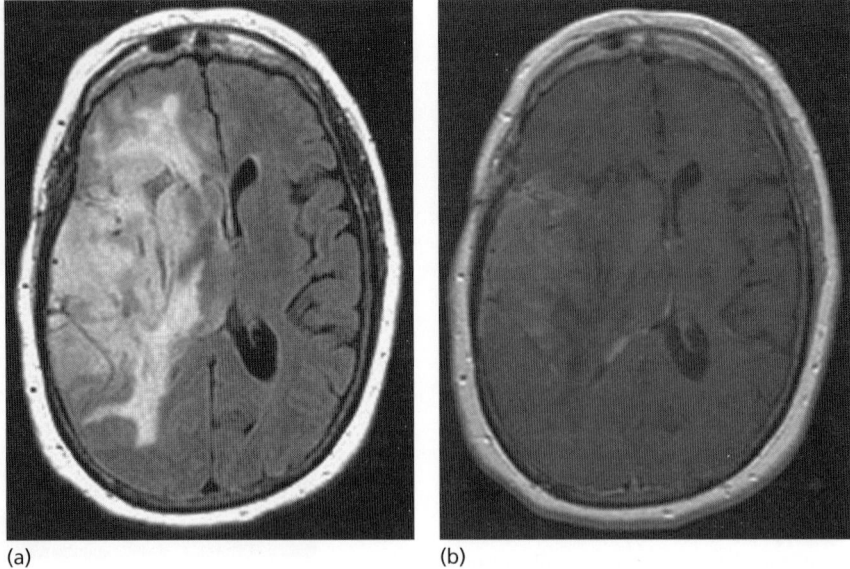

(a)   (b)

Figure 2 Anaplastic oligodendroglioma. (a) FLAIR image showing extensive tumor infiltrating the right hemisphere. (b) Patchy enhancement is seen throughout the tumor.

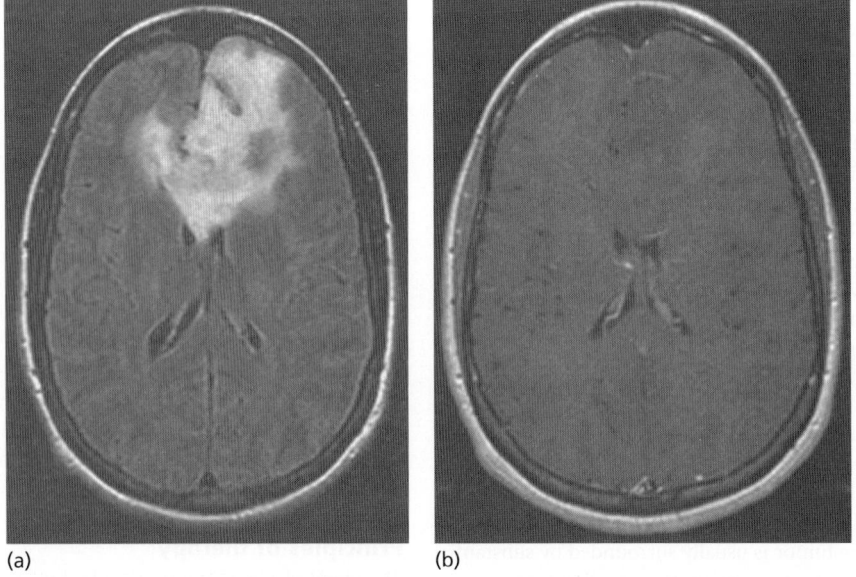

(a)   (b)

Figure 3 Low-grade glioma. (a) FLAIR image demonstrating extensive infiltrative disease predominantly of the left frontal lobe extending across the anterior corpus callosum and involving the deep right frontal white matter. (b) Postcontrast images show no evidence of enhancement of this large lesion.

agents; common choices include levetiracetam, topiramate, or zonisamide. AEDs do not prevent seizures in patients with brain tumors who have never had a seizure, and they should be avoided in this situation.[10]

Corticosteroids dramatically relieve the symptoms from edema caused by brain tumors, thus reducing intracranial pressure. Symptomatic improvement usually takes hours and patients may be symptom free within 24–48 h. Corticosteroids are indicated in all symptomatic patients with brain tumors, except those with presumed PCNSL where corticosteroids may cause tumor necrosis owing to their lympholytic effect, compromising a histologic diagnosis if the steroids are administered before biopsy.

The optimal dose of corticosteroid is unclear. A common starting dose is 16 mg of dexamethasone per day divided in two doses as the drug is long-acting. The dose should be titrated to the lowest dose commensurate with good neurologic function. For patients on steroids longer than 6 weeks, prophylactic treatment for *Pneumocystis jirovecii* infection is indicated.

DVT is a common complication of brain tumors. Factors that contribute to its development include immobility, neurosurgery, the release of thromboplastins from the brain, and hypercoagulability related to cancer and chemotherapy. The use of prophylactic and therapeutic anticoagulation is safe and effective and does not increase the risk of intratumoral hemorrhage.[11] Anticoagulants, including low molecular weight heparin and the newer inhibitors of thrombin or factor Xa, are the agents of choice. Vena cava filters should be reserved for those with absolute contraindications to anticoagulation.

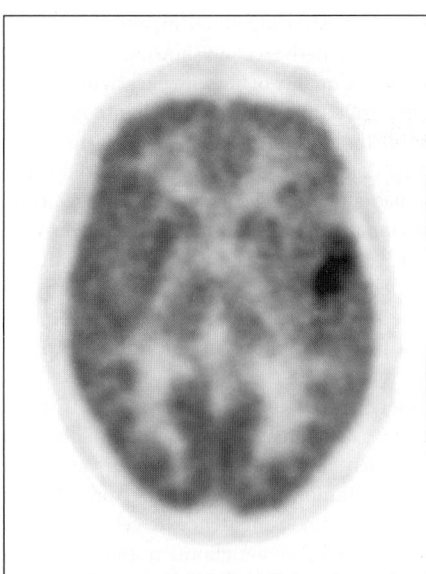

Figure 4 Low-grade glioma. This is an FDG PET image of a left temporal low-grade glioma showing an area of focal hypermetabolism that corresponded to a focal area of anaplasia.

Surgery

Surgery is the most important single modality in the treatment of brain tumors. The goals of surgery are multifactorial: establish a tissue diagnosis, decompress the tumor mass, alleviate symptoms, and reduce steroid dose. The ultimate goal of surgery is gross total resection. Biopsy, in particular stereotactic needle biopsy, is indicated for (1) a surgically inaccessible tumor such as those in the brainstem, basal ganglia, or thalamus, (2) multifocal tumors or gliomatosis cerebri, (3) a patient with medical comorbidity resulting in a high surgical/anesthetic risk. Needle biopsies have several limitations. There is a limited tissue sample that can often compromise accurate diagnosis, both with respect to tumor type and grade. Benign tumors or grade 1 gliomas may be cured by complete removal. For tumors that cannot be cured, such as all infiltrative gliomas, extent of resection is a significant prognostic factor, and biopsy alone confers inferior survival compared with more extensive resection. A retrospective analysis of three prospective RTOG randomized trials of 645 GBM patients revealed a statistically significant improvement in survival between GBM patients who had gross total resection (median 11.3 months) vs. those who had biopsy only (median 6.6 months)[12]; comparable data are available for low-grade gliomas (LGGs). Furthermore, resection usually improves neurologic function, not worsen it. In a prospective multi-institutional series, the morbidity among 408 patients undergoing craniotomy for newly diagnosed malignant glioma was 24%; mortality was 1.5%. Fifty-three percent of patients improved neurologically after craniotomy, and only 8% were neurologically worse.[13] Preoperative fMRI (see earlier text) and awake intraoperative cortical mapping are techniques that facilitate tumor removal without neurologic injury.

Radiation therapy

RT is an effective adjuvant treatment for malignant glioma. For some tumors, such as germinomas, RT is curative. In prospective trials, RT gives better survival than surgery alone, or surgery plus chemotherapy. In the original 1978 Brain Tumor Study Group report of high-grade glioma, the median survival of patients treated

by surgery alone was 14 weeks, whereas those receiving postoperative whole-brain radiotherapy (WBRT) of 50–60 Gy was 36 weeks. Improved RT techniques now allow for higher doses to the tumor while sparing normal brain. Focal RT is delivered to the area of abnormal FLAIR signal on MRI scan with a margin of 2–3 cm, followed by a cone down to the enhancing area. Standard fractionated external beam RT involves delivering the optimum dose of 60 Gy in daily fractions of 1.8–2.0 Gy/day over 6 weeks. Modern techniques involve intensity-modulated radiation therapy (IMRT), which conforms the dose to the shape of the target volume, sparing adjacent critical structures.

Stereotactic radiosurgery (SRS) is another technique used to treat some brain tumors, particularly metastases. SRS delivers highly focal RT to a clearly defined small target, typically in a single dose. SRS can be delivered by a gamma knife (cobalt 60 sources), linear accelerator, or Cyberknife with equivalent results. To maintain a steep dose gradient, the target volume must be small—less than 4 cm. Radiosurgery is primarily used to treat small lesions such as metastatic tumors, meningiomas, acoustic neuromas, and pituitary adenomas. It is rarely used in the treatment of malignant glioma because this infiltrative disease does not lend itself to focused RT.

Protons, neutrons, and heavy charged particles have also been used to treat CNS tumors. Proton beams interact with nuclei of atoms rather than their electrons. Large doses of radiation are deposited in a targeted area sparing adjacent tissue. Charged particles can have an abrupt fall off sparing sensitive structures that could not withstand therapeutic irradiation. This technique is ideal for skull base tumors such as chordomas, meningiomas, and chondrosarcomas, lesions adjacent to the optic nerves, chiasm, and brainstem. Proton therapy is also used to a greater extent in pediatrics to limit RT exposure to developing organs, but its superiority to standard RT has not yet been established.[14]

Chemotherapy

Chemotherapeutic drugs have traditionally been unsuccessful in the treatment of most brain tumors. Some exceptions include PCNSL, germinomas, and some oligodendrogliomas. The role of chemotherapy in the treatment of astrocytomas is limited with respect to extending survival compared with surgery and radiation alone. There are no adequate chemotherapeutic agents for acoustic neuromas and meningiomas.

There are several problems specific to the chemotherapy of brain tumors. These include the role of the blood–brain barrier, the paucity of lymphatics in the brain, the heterogeneity of gliomas, the intrinsic resistance of gliomas, and a low therapeutic/toxic ratio. Many chemotherapy agents cannot penetrate a tumor in the brain owing to an intact blood–brain barrier. In tumors such as metastases and high-grade gliomas, there is disruption of the blood–brain barrier allowing variable penetration of water-soluble chemotherapeutic agents to the tumor. However, in certain tumors such as LGGs, the blood–brain barrier is intact and water-soluble chemotherapeutic agents cannot reach the disease. In high-grade gliomas, the blood–brain barrier is intact at the infiltrative margin of the tumor, where the cells are most viable. Many attempts have been made to disrupt the blood–brain barrier in the treatment of brain tumors, such as opening the blood–brain barrier with a hyperosmolar agent such as intraarterial mannitol. Other attempts include intraarterial infusions, intratumoral injections via catheters, implanting drug-impregnated wafers, and drugs altered to cross the blood–brain barrier. None has yet proved to be more effective, and many are more toxic than conventional routes.

In addition to the blood–brain barrier, most brain tumors have intrinsic resistance to conventional chemotherapeutic agents, and therefore, most are ineffective even if they achieve adequate concentrations in tumor tissue. The exception to this is the growing role of systemic chemotherapy to treat brain metastases. When RT or chemotherapy does succeed in killing tumor cells, the deficiency of a lymphatic system in the brain prevents the easy removal of detritus caused by treatment. Thus, necrotic tissue may serve as a nidus for edema and worsening neurologic function. Specific drugs will be discussed by tumor type.

Glioblastoma and anaplastic astrocytoma

GBM is a disease of advancing age where the mean age is 54 years, compared with a mean age of 45 years for AA. The median survival for AA ranges between 3 and 5 years and for GBM is about 18 months. Favorable prognostic factors include younger age, a high Karnofsky performance score (KPS), AA vs. GBM histology, and surgical resection vs. biopsy alone.[10]

For newly diagnosed GBM, the standard treatment following surgical resection is RT (60 Gy in 1.8–2.0 fractions) with concurrent daily temozolomide followed by at least six cycles of adjuvant temozolomide. A prospective randomized trial of 573 patients aged ≤70 years with newly diagnosed GBM showed that patients treated with RT plus continuous daily temozolomide (75 mg/m^2/day) followed by 6 months of adjuvant temozolomide (150–200 mg/m^2/day for 5 days of a 28-day cycle) had a median survival of 14.6 months compared with 12.1 months in patients treated with RT alone. More importantly, the 2-year survival rate was 26.5% compared with 10.4%.[15] There was minimal toxicity in the combined RT/chemotherapy group. The significance of the DNA repair enzyme, MGMT, was also demonstrated. Hegi et al.[16] analyzed the methylation status of the *MGMT* promotor in approximately one-half of the subjects from the phase III study. There was a distinct survival advantage for any patient whose promotor was methylated and therefore less active. Median survival of patients treated with RT plus temozolomide was 21.7 months for those with a methylated *MGMT* promotor and 15.3 months for those without ($p = 0.007$). Although patients whose tumors have a methylated promotor benefitted the most from the addition of temozolomide, there was some benefit with the addition of temozolomide even in patients whose tumor had an unmethylated *MGMT* promoter.

Elderly patients (>70 years of age) treated with surgery and RT survive longer than those treated with surgery alone, but the prognosis still remains poor.[17] Reducing the dose and duration of RT for patients over 70 years (45 Gy/25 fractions) has comparable efficacy to the more protracted regimens. Alternatively, temozolomide alone may be equally efficacious. There are no definitive data for chemoradiation in the elderly.

Despite standard therapy, almost all patients will recur, usually at the original location. Treatment options at relapse include re-resection, rarely re-irradiation with highly focused RT such as SRS with or without bevacizumab, and a change in systemic chemotherapy. Bevacizumab is FDA approved for recurrent GMB as a single agent based on a randomized phase II trial demonstrating a 6-month PFS rate of 30% and a median survival of 9 months, which was identical to the combination of bevacizumab and irinotecan.[18] These preliminary data led to two large randomized phase III trials of standard chemoradiation with or without bevacizumab for newly diagnosed GBM.[19,20,] Both studies demonstrated a statistically significant prolongation of PFS (median 6–7 months to 10.7 months), but no effect on overall survival (median 15–16 months). However, the two studies differed in their quality of life

data with one study showing better maintenance of quality of life with bevacizumab, and the second showing an increase in symptom burden and a worse quality of life with bevacizumab. On the basis of these data, incorporation of bevacizumab into initial therapy is not recommended. In addition, preliminary data from a randomized European trial suggest that bevacizumab plus lomustine is superior to bevacizumab alone for recurrent GBM, suggesting that single agent bevacizumab is inadequate at progression; final results of this study are not yet available. The molecular profiling of malignant gliomas has led to the targeting of specific pathways in tumor growth. There are several ongoing trials for recurrent GBM looking at the role of EGFR inhibitors, mTOR inhibitors, PKC inhibitors, and interruptions in RAS signaling.[21]

Immunotherapy has emerged as a novel treatment strategy for gliomas given its recent success in other solid tumors.[22] This has taken a variety of approaches including vaccine development using processed tumor antigens, often from the patient's own tumor. Immunotherapy using dendritic cells or a peptide vaccine is capable of producing an antiglioma response. Early results from a randomized phase III trial of a vaccine targeting EGFRvIII suggest a survival benefit when added to the standard treatment at diagnosis; unfortunately, this is applicable to only approximately 20% of patients. Dendritic cell vaccinations may increase the sensitivity of tumor cells to chemotherapy and improve survival. Other immunotherapeutic approaches, such as immune checkpoint inhibitors, including anti-CTLA4, anti-PD1, and anti-PDL1 agents, are also being explored in ongoing trials.

While tumor progression is inevitable and median survival for GBM remains at 18 months, there is a growing minority of patients surviving several years with excellent functional status who are benefitting from many of these new approaches.

Anaplastic gliomas

AA is much rarer than GBM and consequently there have been few trials studying grade III tumors exclusively. An ongoing randomized trial evaluating the role of adding temozolomide to RT will provide guidance in the future, but off-study most have adopted a treatment approach identical to GBM for newly diagnosed patients. A phase III trial of all types of grade III gliomas demonstrated that outcome was unaffected by whether a patient started with RT alone or even chemotherapy alone when the other modality is employed at progression.[23] However, most use RT plus temozolomide at diagnosis.

Low-grade gliomas and oligodendrogliomas

LGGs include astrocytomas, oligodendrogliomas, and mixed oligoastrocytomas.[1] There is great histologic diversity to LGGs that makes generalizations about their treatment and prognosis difficult. In general, they are slow-growing tumors that may not require immediate therapeutic intervention. However, their major risk lies in their tendency to transform to a higher grade glioma at which time their prognosis is dictated by the new histology.

LGGs constitute approximately 10% of all primary brain tumors.[1] The median age at diagnosis is 37 years, and young age is an important positive prognostic factor. Oligodendrogliomas have a tendency to arise in the white matter of the frontal (40%), parietal (30%), and temporal (20%) lobes of young adults. They represent 10% of all LGGs in adults and 5% of LGGs in children.

Seizure is the initial symptom in 60–80% of patients, and the majority of seizures are focal. Most patients are neurologically well at presentation with 90% having a KPS of 90–100 at diagnosis.

Patients with LGGs have a better prognosis than those with malignant gliomas, but almost all will die from their disease. The median survival for a low-grade oligodendroglioma is 9.8 years compared with 4.7 years for a low-grade astrocytoma.

At present, the only agreed upon intervention in the management of LGGs is obtaining tissue for histologic diagnosis. There is growing evidence to suggest that a complete resection at diagnosis is a favorable prognostic factor. A recent review of 216 patients with LGG who underwent surgical resection demonstrated that after adjusting for age, KPS, tumor location, and histology, the extent of resection remained a significant factor in overall survival and PFS.[24] In addition, there was no association between extent of resection and postoperative neurologic deficit. Most series report 80% or greater 5-year survival rates in patients who undergo gross total resection based on review of immediate postoperative MRIs. These data strongly argue for achieving a maximal resection in LGGs.

The timing of RT in the treatment of LGG is also controversial. The European Organization for Research and Treatment of Cancer (EORTC) conducted a prospective phase III trial in adults with supratentorial LGGs, randomizing them to observation only or to initial treatment with radiation alone.[25] The median PFS was 5.3 years in the treated group compared with 3.4 years in the observation arm ($p < 0.0001$). However, the overall survival rate was similar (median 7.4 and 7.2 years, respectively). Two-thirds of patients in the observation arm eventually received RT. Therefore, observation and deferral of RT may be justified without compromising overall survival depending upon the clinical situation. However, there is growing consensus that high-risk patients, variably defined as those with poorly controlled seizures or serious neurologic deficits, residual tumor volume >4–6 cm and older age, need immediate treatment.

The dose of RT was examined in two prospective randomized trials comparing low-dose radiation (45–50 Gy) to a higher dose (59.4–64 Gy).[26,27] There was no difference in PFS or overall survival between low- and high-dose groups, but higher RT doses were associated with greater toxicity, so lower doses are standard. Importantly, the role of adjuvant chemotherapy has been clarified recently. In a large prospective trial (RTOG 9802), patients were stratified based on risk factors (age and extent of resection) into favorable and unfavorable patients. Favorable patients were observed (group 1) and unfavorable patients were randomized to RT+/− procarbazine, CCNU, and vincristine (PCV) (groups 2 and 3). The addition of PCV to RT significantly prolonged median survival from 7.8 years to 13.3 years in high-risk patients.[28]

Several series have shown that temozolomide has activity in patients with LGGs who have had progression after radiation.[29] Among these patients, 47–67% had tumor shrinkage (>25%) with a median PFS of 10–22 months. Several small studies have explored the use of temozolomide as the initial postsurgical therapy for LGGs.[30] Response rates, when minor responses are included, range from 31 to 61%, and median time to progression was 31–36 months. Many have used these data to suggest that temozolomide can replace PCV when used together with RT for the initial treatment of LGGs because of its markedly lower toxicity profile.

LGGs with 1p and 19q chromosomal deletions respond better to chemotherapy and those with both an *IDH* mutation and 1p19q codeletion respond best and have the longest survival. Increasingly, diagnostic classification of the grade II and III tumors is relying upon their molecular profile and not their histologic appearance, which is subject to variable interpretation. Codeletion of 1p19q was first recognized in oligodendrogliomas and was appreciated as both a prognostic and predictive factor in the uncommon AO.

The median overall survival in AO without 1p19q loss is 2 to 3 years, but greater than 6 to 7 years in patients with tumors with combined 1p19q loss. One study showed that 100% of AO patients with 1p or combined 1p19q loss had an objective response to PCV chemotherapy in contrast to a 25–31% response rate when these alleles were retained.[31] The 5-year survival rate for patients with tumors with 1p19q loss is 95% as opposed to 25% for those whose tumor retained these alleles. No formal comparison between PCV and temozolomide is available, although some retrospective data suggest PCV may be superior.[32]

There have been two large randomized trials of patients with AO at initial diagnosis.[33,34] Both examined the administration of RT +/− PCV chemotherapy; one trial used PCV in the neoadjuvant setting and the second used it following RT. Both trials demonstrated that chemotherapy significantly prolonged PFS and overall survival was prolonged for the entire group in one study. However, both studies demonstrated dramatic prolongation of median overall survival with RT and PCV in the 1p19q codeleted group (e.g., median 14.7 vs. 7.3 years). Therefore, the standard of care is to treat such patients with RT and chemotherapy. Whether PCV must be the regimen of choice is unknown as temozolomide is clearly effective and better tolerated. The chemosensitivity of AO has made upfront chemotherapy attractive in an effort to defer radiation and its potential toxicity in long-term survivors. A few small studies using temozolomide exist. One trial of upfront temozolomide alone shows a short time to progression (8 months) in patients who did not have 1p loss, in contrast to patients with 1p loss who were free from progression at 24 months.[35] In a phase II trial of 69 patients with newly diagnosed AO, an intensive PCV regimen was followed by high-dose thiotepa with autologous stem cell rescue, without RT.[36] The median PFS in the 39 patients who received the stem cell procedure was 78 months and the overall survival has not been reached. These data provide conflicting information regarding the optimal approach to patients with AO, but a clear standard is RT plus chemotherapy.

Ependymoma

Ependymomas account for approximately 2% of all intracranial tumors in adults and 5% in children. Ependymomas are derived from ependymal cells that tend to occur along the surfaces of the ventricles. They may also occur in the brain parenchyma adjacent to the ventricles or anywhere along the spinal canal. More than 60% of ependymomas occur in the posterior fossa and arise from the caudal floor of the fourth ventricle. Supratentorial ependymomas are typically parenchymal rather than intraventricular in location and most common in the frontal and parietal lobes. They can extend along the subarachnoid space and seed the CSF.

The WHO divides ependymomas into ependymomas (WHO grade II), anaplastic ependymomas (WHO grade III), subependymomas, and myxopapillary ependymomas (both WHO grade I). Although histologically identical, the molecular profile of ependymomas varies with location: supratentorial, posterior, and spinal. Supratentorial ependymomas are characterized by an oncogenic fusion of RELA and an unknown gene, C11orf95, which spontaneously drives NF-kB signaling.[37] Good molecular prognostic factors in intracranial ependymomas, which include both supra- and infratentorial lesions, include gains in chromosomes 9, 15q, and 18 and loss of 6, whereas gain of 1q or homozygous deletion of *CDKN2A* is associated with significantly shorter PFS and overall survival.[38]

Clinical findings depend on the tumor location. Infratentorial ependymomas most commonly cause brainstem compression or CSF obstruction leading to headache, nausea, and vomiting. Supratentorial tumors may present with seizure or focal deficits. MR scan demonstrates a tumor that is heterogeneously hypo- and isointense on T1 and hyperintense on T2 and may or may not enhance. Calcification is present in 60% of infratentorial tumors and areas of necrosis and cysts are seen in 80% of tumors.

The initial treatment of ependymomas is surgical. A gross total resection will prolong survival but may not always be possible depending upon the tumor location. A complete resection of a grade II tumor does not require additional treatment. However, subtotal resection of a grade II lesion or identification of an anaplastic ependymoma (grade III), regardless of extent of resection, should be followed by focal RT.

Radiotherapy is delivered to the tumor bed and not to the entire neuraxis unless CSF spread is documented at diagnosis on spine MRI or CSF cytology, which should be done in all patients for staging. Ependymomas are primarily chemoresistant tumors, and there is no role for routine adjuvant chemotherapy. At recurrence, some investigators have reported response rates of up to 65% with platinum drugs; others have reported responses with nitrosoureas, etoposide, or even bevacizumab, but temozolomide is not the agent of choice.[39]

Primary central nervous system lymphoma

PCNSL is a non-Hodgkin lymphoma typically of the diffuse large B-cell subtype, restricted to the brain, CSF, spinal cord, or eyes. It accounts for 2% of all brain tumors.[1] It is more common in the immunosuppressed patient where it is usually associated with the Epstein–Barr virus.

The median age at PCNSL diagnosis is 60 although immunocompromised patients are younger. Older age and poor performance status are associated with shorter survival. Multiple lesions occur in 30–40% of sporadic cases. PCNSL grows rapidly, so symptoms are usually present for only a few weeks before diagnosis. The most common presenting symptoms are cognitive deficits or personality changes that can be attributed to the tumor's predilection for the frontal lobe and its tendency for multifocality (Figure 5). Ocular involvement of PCNSL is common. It may be the initial manifestation of the disease, or occur at relapse. Patients who develop ocular lymphoma first have a 50–80% chance of developing cerebral lymphoma. The diagnosis of isolated ocular lymphoma can be difficult because symptoms often mimic benign inflammatory conditions such as uveitis. Diagnosis is made from slit lamp exam, ocular ultrasound, and often vitreal biopsy. Staging evaluation should include an ocular exam and lumbar puncture for cytologic evaluation in every patient with cerebral PCNSL as well as a systemic evaluation.

PCNSL is a highly treatable disease. It is very chemo- and radiosensitive, similar to systemic non-Hodgkin lymphoma. Despite this sensitivity to treatment, PCNSL has a high recurrence rate with a 5-year survival of 25–50%. There are differing reports on the therapeutic value of surgical resection, but most patients are diagnosed by biopsy alone as resection is usually not feasible. Owing to their oncolytic effect on malignant lymphocytes, steroids should be held before surgical biopsy so as not to interfere with the pathologic diagnosis.

Modern treatment of PCNSL is based on high-dose methotrexate regimens. Standard chemotherapy regimens for systemic lymphoma such as CHOP (cyclophosphamide, doxorubicin, vincristine, and prednisone) are not beneficial and should be avoided. Methotrexate is the most effective and commonly used drug for the treatment of PCNSL. High-dose methotrexate (doses of 3–8 gm/M^2) with leucovorin rescue produces response rates of 60–90% when used as a single agent or in combination with other drugs. A wide range of high-dose methotrexate regimens are reported in the literature, and they can achieve a median overall survival of 30–60 months. Other drugs commonly employed with methotrexate include cytarabine, procarbazine, and temozolomide. Methotrexate-based regimens have been consolidated using various approaches including autologous stem cell transplantation (highly selected patients), low-dose WBRT of 2340 cGy (theoretic potential for neurotoxicity), and continuous infusion of etoposide and high-dose cytarabine (severe systemic toxicity).[40–42] Rituximab has been added to most regimens despite its poor penetration into the CNS; efficacy has been observed. The optimal approach will be clarified by the completion of multiple ongoing randomized studies. A large phase III trial failed to demonstrate a survival benefit when full dose WBRT radiotherapy of 4500 cGy was added to methotrexate and this approach has largely been abandoned owing to the enhanced

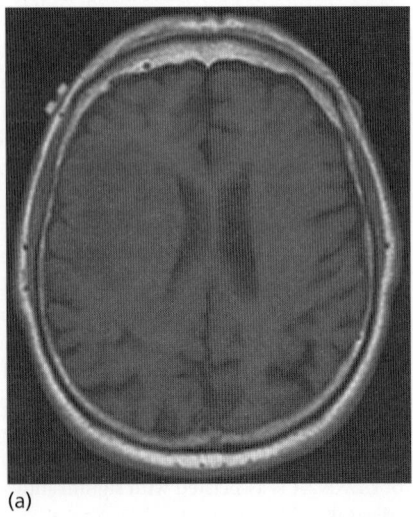
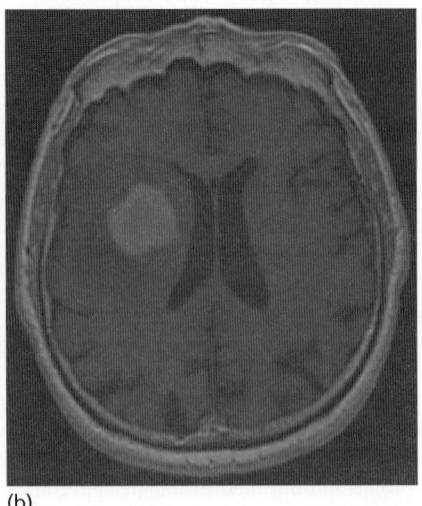

(a) (b)

Figure 5 PCNSL. Pre-gadolinium (a) and postgadolinium (b) images of a right frontal diffusely enhancing PCNSL. Note the edema that surrounds the enhancing mass.

neurotoxicity seen in long-term survivors, especially among older patients.[43]

Meningioma

Meningiomas account for approximately 25% of intracranial tumors. They are extra-axial and arise from arachnoidal cap cells rather than the dura itself. They are more common in women than in men.[1] Approximately 85% of meningiomas are supratentorial, and multiple meningiomas occur in 10% of sporadic cases. Ionizing radiation is the only established risk factor for meningioma. Both low- and high-dose radiation have been associated with the development of meningiomas. These meningiomas are more often atypical or malignant and are often multifocal.

Recent molecular profiling work demonstrates that the tumor suppressor NF2 is inactivated in about one-half of patients. Approximately 25% have *TRAF7* mutations with co-occurrence of the K409Q mutation in KLF4, a transcription factor. Approximately 20% had an E17K mutation in AKT1, which often co-occurred with *TRAF7* mutations. Finally, about 5% had mutations in SMO, which activated the Hedgehog signaling pathway. Each of the mutations conferred geographic localization of the tumor at the skull base, usually anterior, and distinct from the NF2 mutations, which had no genetic overlap and occurred in the posterior skull base.[44,45] These interesting biologic insights do not yet provide a therapeutic pathway but they may in the future.

The prognosis after treatment of meningiomas depends on the histology of the tumor and the extent of resection. Age at diagnosis and tumor size may also play a role. Younger patients fare better than the elderly. The recurrence rate for a completely resected typical meningioma is 20% at 5 years and 25% at 10 years. Tumors that are incompletely resected have about a 60% chance of recurrence without RT. McCarthy et al.[46] published a survey of more than 9000 patients with meningiomas treated in the United States and included in the National Cancer Data Base. The 5-year overall survival was 60%, 81% for patients < 65 years, and 56% for patients > 65 years. The estimated 5-year survival for benign tumors was 75% and 55% for malignant tumors. Population-based studies reported a 5-year survival rate near 90%.

Typically, meningiomas compress rather than invade adjacent brain. However, they may invade venous structures such as the superior sagittal sinus. The histologic appearance of meningiomas may vary, but only those with rhabdoid or clear cell features are more aggressive and carry a worse prognosis. Atypical meningiomas have a higher mitotic index as well as increased cellularity, a high nucleus/cytoplasm ratio, prominent nucleoli, necrosis, and patternless growth. A malignant meningioma must have at least 20 mitoses per 10 high-power fields or histology resembling carcinoma or sarcoma. Whereas only 1% of meningiomas metastasize, about one-half of malignant meningiomas metastasize, usually to liver, bone, and lung.

Most meningiomas are very slow growing and may be asymptomatic; many are found incidentally on imaging done for other reasons. Meningiomas produce symptoms and signs by compressing brain structures and causing edema or hydrocephalus. Although most meningiomas do not cause significant brain edema, secretory meningiomas may cause edema resulting in significant neurologic symptoms. Convexity meningiomas may cause seizure. Meningiomas in particular locations may have typical clinical syndromes, such as cavernous sinus meningiomas that cause diplopia, proptosis, and other oculomotor abnormalities.

CT and MRI readily diagnose meningiomas. On CT, meningiomas are hyperdense extra-axial masses. Calcification is present in

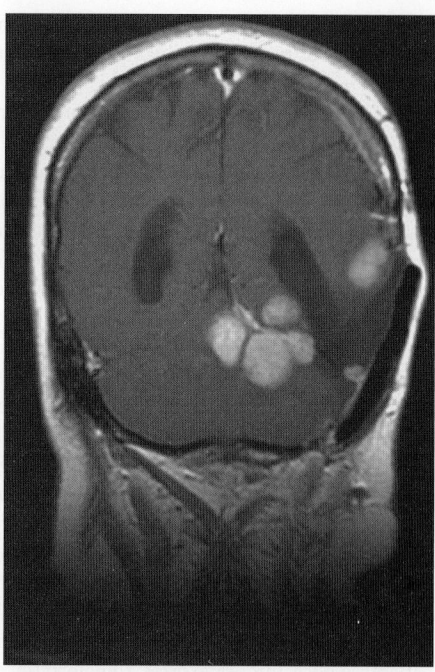

Figure 6 Meningioma. A coronal postgadolinium MRI of a multilobulated meningioma extending below and above the tentorium. There is a second lesion in the left occipito-parietal cortex.

25%. Meningiomas demonstrate dense uniform contrast enhancement. Atypical, malignant, and large meningiomas more commonly cause surrounding brain edema. On T1- and T2-weighted MRI images, most meningiomas have signal intensity similar to surrounding grey matter. They enhance diffusely and a dural tail seen on contrast-enhanced images is characteristic (Figure 6). Some tumors may have flow voids indicating marked vascularity. The first step in the management of a patient with a meningioma is to decide whether treatment is necessary. Many meningiomas may be followed for years if they do not exhibit growth or cause neurologic symptoms. If seizures are the only symptom and are well controlled with medication, surgical resection may not be necessary. Some meningiomas are not resected because tumor removal may be dangerous. This is usually the case for lesions located at the skull base and cavernous sinus. These meningiomas may encase portions of the intracavernous carotid artery as well as multiple cranial nerves.

Surgery is definitive and if the tumor can be removed completely, a cure may be achieved. Meningiomas with the best potential for complete removal are those located along the convexity. Preoperative embolization may be done to reduce the size and vascularity of the tumor, making resection easier. Even in those patients in whom a complete removal has been accomplished, approximately 15–20% of these tumors will recur and may require additional surgery or RT.

RT is used in the treatment of inoperable meningiomas in partially resected tumors in some patients at recurrence, and in all malignant tumors regardless of resection.[47] The role of RT in atypical meningiomas is unclear. Recent data suggest that RT can be effective, particularly in prolonging PFS for patients with atypical tumors, but this is true for a minority of patients and the effect on overall survival is less clear. In addition, new 3D planning techniques and stereotactically guided conformational RT allow for reductions in the volume of normal tissue irradiated and less neurotoxicity. The use of protons in the treatment of some meningiomas has also been of benefit in reducing toxicity and delaying recurrence.

Stereotactic RT is an important treatment option for atypical, malignant, and recurrent meningioma. Radiosurgery has also become an option for small typical meningiomas less than 3 cm. In a retrospective comparison of 198 adult patients who underwent either surgical resection or radiosurgery as initial treatment of their meningioma, both modalities had equivalent tumor control. Tumor control rates with SRS are higher than 90% in most series with complication rates less than 5%.

There is a small group of patients in whom, despite multiple surgical resections and RT, the meningioma recurs. In these patients, medical therapy may be considered but is generally ineffective.[48] The progesterone antagonist, mifepristone, initially appeared effective, but this was not sustained with further testing. To date, no effective chemotherapy has been found to treat meningioma. There have been some attempts with anthracyclines, cisplatin, and irinotecan but without definite success. There are several small series of patients with recurrent meningioma that report a response to hydroxyurea, but most patients do not appear to benefit. Sunitinib has been reported effective.[49] Pasireotide may be helpful in those patients whose tumors express somatostatin receptor.[50] Bevacizumab has been helpful in reducing edema or in treating radionecrosis of underlying brain if present, but does not shrink the tumor, regardless of grade.

Brain metastasis

Metastasis is the most common tumor affecting the brain with approximately 70,000 patients diagnosed with symptomatic intracranial metastases annually. Most brain metastases present late during the course of a widely metastatic cancer, but in a smaller percentage of patients, a brain metastasis may be the first evidence that the patient has cancer; alternatively, a patient with cancer believed to be localized may have an asymptomatic brain metastasis found on screening neuroimaging. With more effective systemic therapy, brain metastases are increasingly emerging as the sole site of relapse in patients with otherwise controlled cancer.[51,52]

The most common sources of brain metastases are lung and breast carcinoma and melanoma (Table 4). However, any malignant neoplasm can metastasize to the brain and it is likely that there will be an increasing number of metastases from what are believed to be uncommon sites, e.g., ovary or prostate.[51,52] In as many as 10% of patients with brain metastases, no primary tumor is found on initial search although immunocytochemical analysis of the brain metastasis may help identify the primary site. On rare occasions, the primary tumor is not identifiable even at autopsy.

Pathophysiology of the metastatic process

To reach the brain, a systemic cancer must develop its own blood supply, invade local tissues, and enter the circulation either by invading venules or lymph channels that eventually reach the venous circulation (Figure 7).[52,54] Because systemic tumors enter the venous circulation and, ultimately, the right side of the heart, the first capillary bed they encounter is in the lung. Accordingly, the majority of patients with brain metastases have either primary lung tumors or lung metastases at the time the brain lesions become symptomatic. To reach the arterial circulation, the tumor must (1) grow in the lung and seed the pulmonary venous circulation,[14] (2) traverse the lung capillary bed to enter the left side of the heart, or (3) cross a patent

Table 4 Source of brain metastases in 729 patients.

Primary tumor	Total (%)	Single	Multiple
Lung cancer	288 (39)	137	151
nonsmall cell	178	89	89
small cell	110	48	62
Breast	121 (17)	59	62
Melanoma	80 (11)	39	41
Genitourinary	81 (11)	49	32
Renal cell	45	25	20
Bladder	14	9	5
Prostate	11	9	2
Testicular	11	6	5
Gynecologic	52 (7)	28	24
Uterine/vulvar	38	20	18
Ovarian	14	8	6
Gastrointestinal	45 (6)	30	15
Unknown	33 (5)	23	10
Miscellaneous	29 (4)	19	10
Total	729	384	345

Data from Ref. 53.

foramen ovale to enter the left heart directly. Some have proposed that tumor reaches the brain via the vertebral venous system (Batson's plexus) to explain the absence of lung metastases.

Two factors promote intracranial metastases: (1) In the resting state, the brain receives 15–20% of the body's blood flow, enhancing the probability that circulating tumor cells will reach the brain. (2) Certain tumor cells find the brain a propitious place for arrest and growth, such as small-cell lung carcinoma. Once in the intracranial cavity, the tumor must arrest within the capillary bed, cross the endothelium and vessel wall, grow within the organ, vascularize itself through the process of angiogenesis, and then grow large enough to cause symptoms. At each step in the metastatic process, the tumor cells may fail, so that only a fraction of cells that reach the circulation ever become metastases.

Tumors may metastasize to virtually any portion of the intracranial cavity, but the overall distribution of brain metastasis is also determined by the size of the region and its vasculature. Thus, about 85% of brain metastases are found in the cerebral hemispheres, 10–15% in the cerebellum, and only approximately 3% are found in the brainstem, comparable to the distribution of blood flow to these areas.

In patients whose systemic tumor is otherwise controlled, the brain is often a site for isolated metastatic disease. Neither blood flow nor the nature of the CNS microenvironment fully explains this phenomenon, but the blood–brain barrier may. The CNS as a sanctuary site of microscopic disease may apply to breast, small-cell lung, and perhaps other cancers with effective systemic treatment using water-soluble agents unable to penetrate an intact blood–brain barrier. When a chemosensitive tumor has relapsed in the CNS, it does not necessarily mean that the CNS disease is resistant to the chemotherapeutic agents that controlled the systemic tumor. The blood–brain barrier may have prevented those tumor cells from ever seeing a significant concentration of the drug, thus preserving the tumor cells' intrinsic chemosensitivity to that agent, which may then be demonstrated by changing the dose or schedule to achieve higher drug concentration in the brain.

Treatment

The therapeutic approach to patients with brain metastases depends on the number and location of metastases, on the biology of the primary tumor, and on the extent of systemic disease.

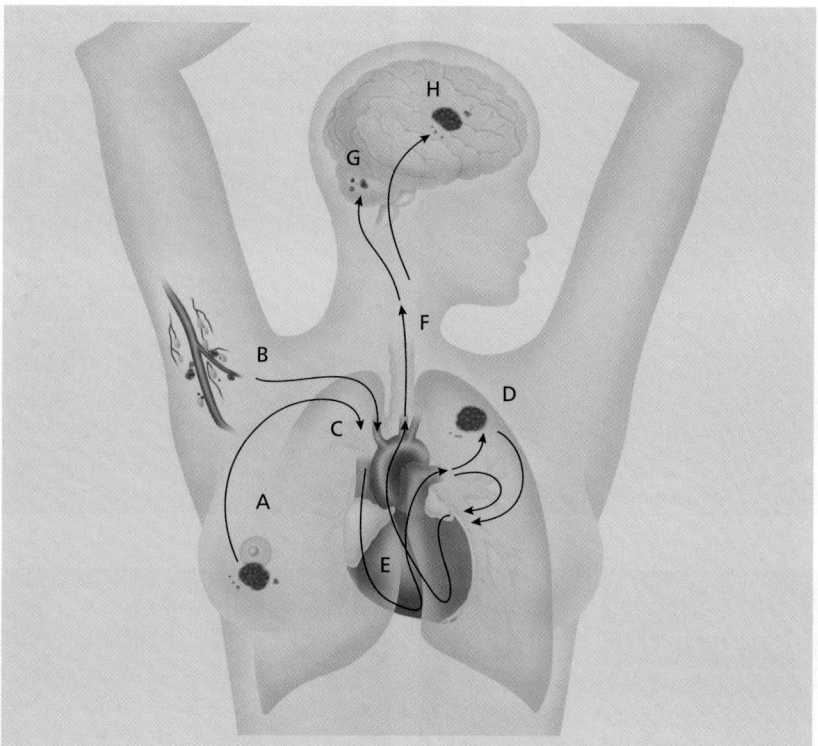

Figure 7 Pathophysiology of the metastatic process. Metastasis is a multistep process. In this illustration: (A) malignant neoplasm arises in an organ distant from the central nervous system and, as it grows, it develops its own vascular supply. (B) Clone(s) of malignant cells with metastatic potential enter blood or lymph channels and eventually reach the venous circulation. (C) The malignant cells enter the right heart with the venous circulation and either exit through the pulmonary artery to the lung (D), or cross a patent foramen ovale (D), to enter the systemic circulation. Most tumors that enter the lung either arrest in the pulmonary capillary bed, grow as pulmonary metastases and subsequently seed the pulmonary venous circulation, or, alternately, (E), transverse the pulmonary vascular bed without arresting (E), to enter the pulmonary venous circulation. Malignant clones in the pulmonary venous circulation then enter the left heart and exit into the systemic circulation (F), along with those cells that may have crossed a patent foramen ovale (F). Once in the systemic circulation, the likelihood of entering the cerebral circulation is high because, in the resting state, 15–20% of cardiac output supplies the central nervous system. Tumor cells entering the cerebral circulation must then arrest in brain capillaries or venules, cross the vessel wall, and grow within the brain (G, H). Source: DeAngelis and Posner, 2008.[52] Reproduced with permission from Oxford University Press.

Surgery

Two controlled trials clearly indicate that for patients with a single brain metastasis, surgical removal followed by WBRT is superior to WBRT alone, both in preventing brain relapse and in improving quality of life.[55,56] A third trial found no benefit, but many of the patients randomized to radiotherapy alone underwent resection at relapse.[57] In patients whose systemic disease is quiescent or controllable, surgical removal of a single brain metastasis substantially improves survival; 2-year survivals are 15–20%, depending on the primary tumor, and 5-year survival rates are approximately 10%. Retrospective analysis supports the resection of two or even three metastases, with an outcome comparable to a surgically treated single brain metastasis.

A randomized controlled trial indicates that patients with a single resected metastasis who receive postoperative WBRT have fewer recurrences in the brain and are less likely to die of neurologic causes than are similar patients treated with surgery alone.[58] However, overall survival was comparable between the two groups because patients with controlled cerebral disease died of progressive systemic tumor. These data suggest that an appropriate patient with a single, surgically accessible brain metastasis should have that metastasis removed and receive postoperative WBRT. However, because of the toxicity of WBRT, particularly in the over 60 age group, many physicians do not use it in the immediate postoperative period, but reserve radiation until relapse, even though RT may be less effective once a tumor has recurred.

Radiation therapy

The time-honored treatment of brain metastases has been WBRT, delivering 3000 cGy in 10 fractions. For patients with extensive systemic disease or multiple brain metastases, this remains the best option. Most patients improve with steroids and RT (Figure 8) and are less likely to die of their neurologic disease than are patients who do not receive this treatment. However, survival is short, with a median of 4–6 months, because most patients die of uncontrolled systemic tumor. In occasional patients, RT actually sterilizes the brain metastases and they do not recur. Because of late-delayed radiation toxicity in those patients whose systemic prognosis is more than a year, we recommend a dose of 4000–5000 cGy given in 180–200 cGy fractions. The lower dose per fraction reduces the risk of radiation toxicity but cognitive dysfunction may occur even with small fractions, especially if the patient is elderly. Cognitive deficits from RT are more severe in adults over 60 years of age, and in those who receive extensive chemotherapy. Nevertheless, even young adults often complain of memory loss after WBRT.

Radiosurgery

Radiosurgery is increasingly employed instead of surgery for the treatment of single or even multiple brain metastases that are <3–4 cm in diameter.[52,59–61] SRS can be delivered either using the gamma knife, linear accelerator, or Cyberknife, all with equal efficacy. It is usually given as a single dose but it can be fractionated.

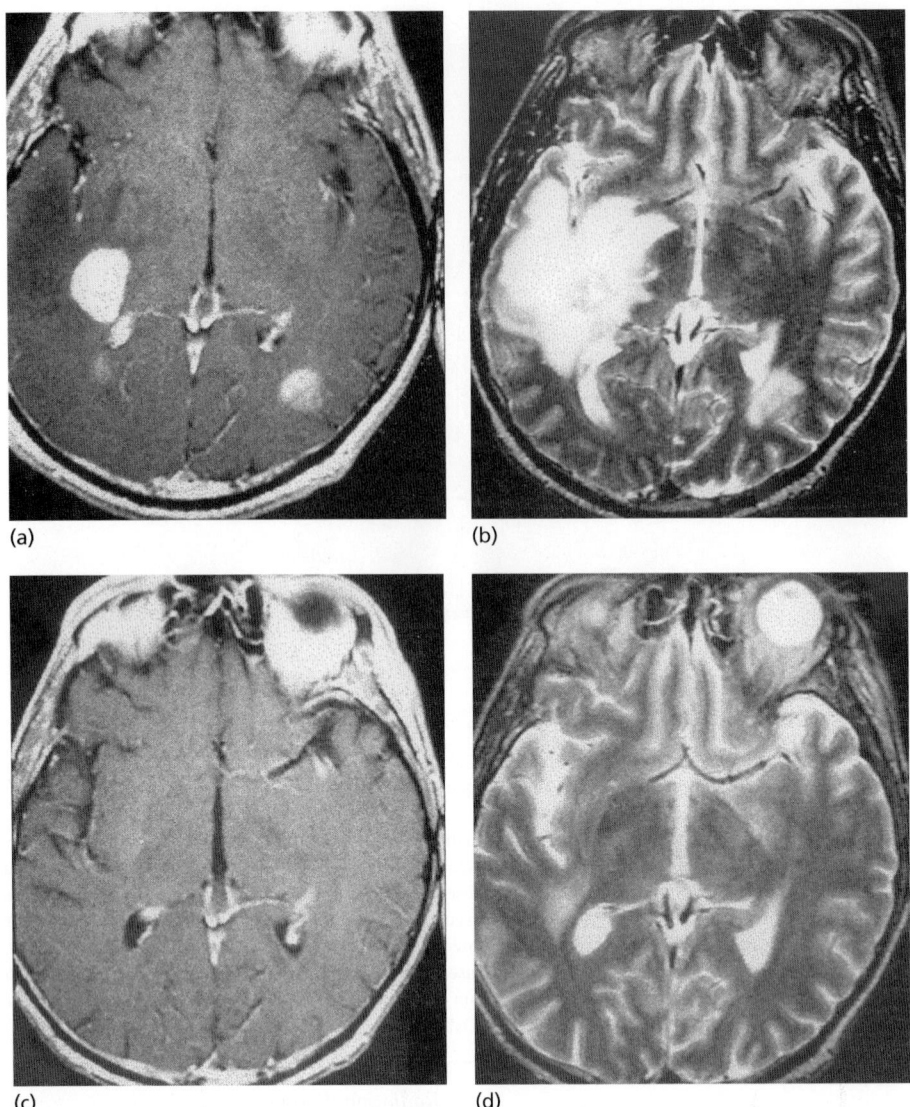

Figure 8 Metastatic small-cell lung cancer before and after radiation therapy. (a) The T1-weighted image before radiation shows two of the multiple contrast enhancing metastases; the larger is surrounded by hypointense brain edema. (b) The T2-weighted image before radiation shows hyperintense edema surrounding the relatively hypointense tumor. (c, d) MRI scans after radiation show an excellent response to radiation therapy.

The treatment appears to be most effective against those tumors that are relatively resistant to conventional external beam RT, such as melanoma and renal cell carcinoma. Most report approximately 80% tumor control defined as disappearance, decrease in size, or stability of the treated lesion. Postradiosurgery MRI may show a transient increase in tumor size because of radiation injury or tumor necrosis. This can resolve over a few months and, therefore, an increase in lesion size a few weeks to months after SRS does not necessarily indicate tumor progression. Local control may be maintained over 2 years in 60% of patients, but with increasing survival, symptomatic recurrence becomes increasingly likely. Radiosurgery has advantages over surgery in that it is relatively noninvasive, does not require hospitalization, and can often reach areas that are surgically inaccessible. SRS has the disadvantage that it is not useful for tumors larger than 3–4 cm and should be avoided for lesions with extensive uncontrolled edema.

A randomized, prospective trial comparing WBRT and WBRT followed by a SRS boost in 331 patients with one to three newly diagnosed brain metastases showed no survival advantage with the addition of radiosurgery to WBRT.[62] A separate randomized controlled trial examined SRS with and without WBRT in patients with 1–4 brain metastases. Similar to the findings in the postoperative WBRT study, WBRT significantly reduced brain recurrence but had no effect on survival.[63] Furthermore, these authors demonstrated that cognitive function was better when CNS disease was controlled even when WBRT was necessary to achieve that control; they did observe that WBRT could contribute to impaired neurocognitive function in some long-term survivors.[64] Thus, the decision to use postoperative or post-SRS WBRT should be individualized.

There have been no randomized, prospective studies comparing neurosurgery and radiosurgery as treatment of solitary brain metastasis, and retrospective studies have shown conflicting results. However, most agree that they achieve comparable degrees of local control. At this time, we use surgery to resect lesions from accessible locations if they are >3–4 cm, are associated with significant vasogenic edema or hemorrhage, arise from a radioresistant primary, or cause obstruction of CSF flow. SRS is an excellent option for smaller lesions or those in a surgically inaccessible location; we rarely treat more than three lesions in a patient and usually do not administer WBRT concurrently.

Chemotherapy

Chemotherapy is increasingly recognized as efficacious for brain metastases from chemosensitive systemic cancers. These include germ cell tumors, breast cancer, small-cell lung cancer, and others.[52,59,65,66] Chemotherapy is often reserved for patients whose brain metastases have recurred after surgery or WBRT, but chemotherapy may also be considered in asymptomatic patients with brain metastases discovered on a screening MRI who are scheduled to receive chemotherapy for their systemic disease.

There are several reasons for administering chemotherapy before radiation: (1) It is useful to judge tumor response to chemotherapy before initiating RT. If the tumor is responsive, the chemotherapy can be continued. (2) RT decreases the blood supply to the tumor, but may increase it to the brain, and thus may decrease the amount of chemotherapeutic agent that reaches the metastases but enhance exposure of normal brain to chemotherapy toxicity. (3) Some evidence suggests that chemotherapy delivered before radiation is less neurotoxic than the converse because RT may open the blood–brain barrier and allow entry of potentially toxic agents that are given post-RT. The evidence is best for methotrexate but may apply to other drugs as well.

In addition to standard chemotherapeutic agents, small-molecule inhibitors may be effective against brain metastases. This has been best observed with erlotinib in non-small cell lung cancer, sunitinib for renal cancer, and vemurafenib for melanoma.[67,68] Furthermore, changing the dosing schedule to a weekly high-dose regimen that enhances CNS drug penetration improves CNS tumor response. Initial reports of lapatinib's efficacy against brain metastases from breast cancer failed to meet the expected response rate in a phase II trial.[69]

Prognosis

Patients treated with WBRT have a median survival of 4–6 months, and those treated by surgery followed by WBRT have a median survival of about 9 months. Patients with controlled systemic disease treated by surgery and radiation have a 10–15% 5-year survival. Prolonged survival can also be seen after SRS.[52]

Prognostic factors include mental status, response to steroids, activity of the systemic tumor, and treatment modality. In one series, site of the primary tumor, age, and the number of brain metastases were prognostic factors, although with lesser importance than those indicated above. In patients with lung primaries, male sex was a significant adverse factor. In patients with breast primaries, the interval between the primary tumor and the development of brain metastases was also significant, with a longer interval correlating with better survival. The RTOG performed a recursive partitioning analysis of prognostic factors in 1200 patients with brain metastases treated with WBRT in three RTOG trials.[70] They segregated patients into three classes based only on KPS, age, and the presence of extracranial metastases. Class 1 patients had a KPS $\geq$ 70, were <65 years of age, and had a controlled primary and no extracranial metastasis; median survival was 7.1 months. Class 3 patients had a KPS < 70 and a median survival of 2.3 months. Class 2 included all other patients and had a median survival of 4.2 months. This classification scheme may apply to patients treated with surgery and radiosurgery.[71]

Key references

The complete reference list can be found on the Wiley Companion Digital Edition of this title (see inside front cover for login instructions).

1 Ostrom QT, Gittleman H, Farah P, et al. CBTRUS statistical report: primary brain and central nervous system tumors diagnosed in the United States 2006–2010. *Neuro Oncol.* 2013;**15**:ii1–ii56.

4 Coureau G, Bouvier G, Lebailly P, et al. Mobile phone use and brain tumours in the CERENAT case–control study. *Occup Environ Med.* 2014;**71**:514–522.

6 Ostrom QT, Bauchet L, Davis FG, et al. The epidemiology of glioma in adults: a "state of the science" review. *Neuro Oncol.* 2014;**16**:896–913.

7 Huse JT, Holland E, DeAngelis LM. Glioblastoma: molecular analysis and clinical implications. *Annu Rev Med.* 2013;**64**:59–70.

8 Cohen AL, Colman H. Glioma biology and molecular markers. *Cancer Treat Res.* 2015;**163**:15–30.

10 Omuro A, DeAngelis LM. Glioblastoma and other malignant gliomas: a clinical review. *JAMA.* 2013;**310**:1842–1850.

13 Chang SM, Parney IF, McDermott M, et al. Perioperative complications and neurological outcomes of first and second craniotomies among patients enrolled in the Glioma Outcome Project. *J Neurosurg.* 2003;**98**:1175–1181.

14 Merchant TE, Farr JB. Proton beam therapy: a fad or a new standard of care. *Curr Opin Pediatr.* 2014;**26**:3–8.

15 Stupp R, Hegi ME, Mason WP, et al. Effects of radiotherapy with concomitant and adjuvant temozolomide versus radiotherapy alone on survival in glioblastoma in a randomised phase III study: 5-year analysis of the EORTC-NCIC trial. *Lancet Oncol.* 2009;**10**:459–466.

18 Friedman HS, Prados MD, Wen PY, et al. Bevacizumab alone and in combination with irinotecan in recurrent glioblastoma. *J Clin Oncol.* 2009;**27**:4733–4740.

19 Chinot OL, Wick W, Mason W, et al. Bevacizumab plus radiotherapy-temozolomide for newly diagnosed glioblastoma. *N Engl J Med.* 2014;**370**:709–722.

20 Gilbert MR, Dignam JJ, Armstrong TS, et al. A randomized trial of bevacizumab for newly diagnosed glioblastoma. *N Engl J Med.* 2014;**370**:699–708.

21 Thomas AA, Brennan CW, DeAngelis LM, Omuro AM. Emerging therapies for glioblastoma. *JAMA Neurol.* 2014;**71**:1437–1444.

22 Reardon DA, Freeman G, Wu C, et al. Immunotherapy advances for glioblastoma. *Neuro Oncol.* 2014;**16**:1441–1458.

23 Wick W, Hartmann C, Engel C, et al. NOA-04 randomized phase III trial of sequential radiochemotherapy of anaplastic glioma with procarbazine, lomustine, and vincristine or temozolomide. *J Clin Oncol.* 2009;**27**:5874–5880.

25 van den Bent MJ, Afra D, de Witte O, et al. Long-term efficacy of early versus delayed radiotherapy for low-grade astrocytoma and oligodendroglioma in adults: the EORTC 22845 randomised trial. *Lancet.* 2005;**366**:985–990.

28 van den Bent MJ. Practice changing mature results of RTOG study 9802: another positive PCV trial makes adjuvant chemotherapy part of standard of care in low-grade glioma. *Neuro Oncol.* 2014;**16**:1570–1574.

31 Jenkins RB, Blair H, Ballman KV, et al. A t(1;19)(q10;p10) mediates the combined deletions of 1p and 19q and predicts a better prognosis of patients with oligodendroglioma. *Cancer Res.* 2006;**66**:9852–9861.

32 Lassman AB, Iwamoto FM, Cloughesy TF, et al. International retrospective study of over 1000 adults with anaplastic oligodendroglial tumors. *Neuro Oncol.* 2011;**13**:649–659.

33 Cairncross G, Wang M, Shaw E, et al. Phase III trial of chemoradiotherapy for anaplastic oligodendroglioma: long-term results of RTOG 9402. *J Clin Oncol.* 2013;**31**:337–343.

34 van den Bent MJ, Brandes AA, Taphoorn MJ, et al. Adjuvant procarbazine, lomustine, and vincristine chemotherapy in newly diagnosed anaplastic oligodendroglioma: long-term follow-up of EORTC brain tumor group study 26951. *J Clin Oncol.* 2013;**31**:344–350.

37 Parker M, Mohankumar KM, Punchihewa C, et al. C11orf95-RELA fusions drive oncogenic NF-κB signalling in ependymoma. *Nature.* 2014;**506**:451–455.

39 Green RM, Cloughesy TF, Stupp R, et al. Bevacizumab for recurrent ependymoma. *Neurology.* 2009;**73**:1677–1680.

40 Morris PG, Correa DD, Yahalom J, et al. Rituximab, methotrexate, procarbazine, and vincristine followed by consolidation reduced-dose whole-brain radiotherapy and cytarabine in newly diagnosed primary CNS lymphoma: final results and long-term outcome. *J Clin Oncol.* 2013;**31**:3971–3979.

41 Rubenstein JL, Hsi ED, Johnson JL, et al. Intensive chemotherapy and immunotherapy in patients with newly diagnosed primary CNS lymphoma: CALGB 50202 (Alliance 50202). *J Clin Oncol.* 2013;**31**:3061–3068.

42 Omuro A, Correa DD, DeAngelis LM, et al. R-MPV followed by high-dose chemotherapy with TBC and autologous stem-cell transplant for newly diagnosed primary CNS lymphoma. *Blood.* 2015;**125**(**9**):1403–10.

43 Thiel E, Korfel A, Martus P, et al. High-dose methotrexate with or without whole brain radiotherapy for primary CNS lymphoma (G-PCNSL-SG-1): a phase 3, randomised, non-inferiority trial. *Lancet Oncol.* 2010;**11**:1036–1047.

44 Clark VE, Erson-Omay EZ, Serin A, et al. Genomic analysis of non-NF2 meningiomas reveals mutations in TRAF7, KLF4, AKT1, and SMO. *Science.* 2013;**339**:1077–1080.

48 Kaley T, Barani I, Chamberlain M, et al. Historical benchmarks for medical therapy trials in surgery- and radiation-refractory meningioma: a RANO review. *Neuro Oncol.* 2014;**16**:829–840.

51 Kastritis E, Efstathiou E, Gika D, et al. Brain metastases as isolated site of relapse in patients with epithelial ovarian cancer previously treated with platinum and paclitaxel-based chemotherapy. *Int J Gynecol Cancer.* 2006;**16**:994–999.

52 DeAngelis LM, Posner JB. *Neurologic Complications of Cancer*, 2nd edition. New York: Oxford University Press; 2008.

53 Kleihues P, Cavenee WK (eds). *Pathology and genetics. Tumors of the nervous system. World Health Organization Classification of Tumors.* Lyon: International Agency for Research on Cancer (IARC) Press; 2000:6–7.

55 Patchell RA, Tibbs PA, Walsh JW, et al. A randomized trial of surgery in the treatment of single metastases to the brain. *N Engl J Med.* 1990;**322**:494–500.

56 Vecht CJ, Haaxma-Reiche H, Noordijk EM, et al. Treatment of single brain metastasis: radiotherapy alone or combined with neurosurgery? *Ann Neurol.* 1993;**33**:583–590.

58 Patchell RA, Tibbs PA, Regine WF, et al. Postoperative radiotherapy in the treatment of single metastases to the brain: a randomized trial. *JAMA.* 1998;**280**:1485–1489.

59 Bertolini F, Spallanzani A, Fontana A, Depenni R, Luppi G. Brain metastases: an overview. *CNS Oncol.* 2015;**4**:37–46.

62 Andrews DW, Scott CB, Sperduto PW, et al. Whole brain radiation therapy with or without stereotactic radiosurgery boost for patients with one to three brain metastases: phase III results of the RTOG 9508 randomised trial. *Lancet.* 2004;**363**:1665–1672.

63 Aoyama H, Shirato H, Tago M, et al. Stereotactic radiosurgery plus whole-brain radiation therapy vs stereotactic radiosurgery alone for treatment of brain metastases: a randomized controlled trial. *JAMA.* 2006;**295**:2483–2491.

65 Brastianos HC, Cahill DP, Brastianos PK. Systemic therapy of brain metastases. *Curr Neurol Neurosci Rep.* 2015;**15**:518.

68 Grommes C, Oxnard GR, Kris MG, et al. "Pulsatile" high-dose weekly erlotinib for CNS metastases from EGFR mutant non-small cell lung cancer. *Neuro Oncol.* 2011;**13**:1364–1369.

71 Regine WF, Rogozinska A, Kryscio RJ, et al. Recursive partitioning analysis classifications I and II: applicability evaluated in a randomized trial for resected single brain metastases. *Am J Clin Oncol.* 2004;**27**:505–509.

78 Neoplasms of the eye

Jasmine H. Francis, MD ▪ Amy C. Schefler, MD, FACS ▪ David H. Abramson, MD

Overview

Cancers involving the eye are less common compared to lung, prostate and breast cancer. However, they pose a special challenge because they can influence both life and vision. The field of ophthalmic oncology focuses on these two elements: improving efficacy to treat the disease and save life, and limiting the consequence of treatment to maintain vision. The eye itself is composed of a variety of distinct tissues and ophthalmic malignancies can affect a number of these anatomical areas. This makes the topic of neoplasms of the eye heterogeneous in origin, pathogenesis, prognosis, and treatment.

Introduction

This chapter reviews benign and malignant ocular, orbital, and lid tumors in both children and adults. The most common of these are listed in Table 1.

Pediatric ophthalmic oncology: ocular diseases

Benign disease

Benign pediatric ocular lesions are very rare. Choroidal nevi, which are present in more than 10% of the adult population, are rare before puberty and are never seen in the infant. Conjunctival and iris nevi are also extremely rare in prepubertal children. Iris nevi detected in children often represent Lisch nodules, a manifestation of neurofibromatosis type 1.

Benign retinal tumors are also rare. When found they are usually astrocytic hamartomas and are frequently part of the tuberous sclerosis syndrome. When viewed with indirect ophthalmoscopy, astrocytic hamartomas usually have a thin, transparent membrane overlying the retina and typically obscure retinal blood vessels. They may enlarge and calcify with time. They may be confused with myelinated nerve fibers, which are white, follow the distribution of the nerve fiber layer, and obscure retinal vessels.

Hamartomas of the retinal pigment epithelium are rare in children. They are frequently near the optic disc and are pigmented, with distortion of retinal vessels and a slightly opaque appearance. They have no malignant potential.

Primary malignant disease (retinoblastoma)

Introduction to retinoblastoma

The most common primary ocular malignancy of childhood is retinoblastoma.[1] Retinoblastoma arises from a cone precursor cell.[2] Although retinoblastoma is relatively rare, it has been the subject of great interest because of its well-studied genetic inheritance pattern and molecular biology.

Retinoblastoma has an incidence rate of 1 in 18,000–30,000 live births worldwide. Surveys suggest a relatively constant occurrence in this century. The incidence in the United States is relatively low, at 3.58 cases for each million children under the age of 15 years, and decreases with advancing age. The overall median age at diagnosis in the United States is 18 months, with the median age of diagnosis of bilateral cases occurring at 12 months and of unilateral cases at 24 months. In rare instances, retinoblastoma is detected prenatally via ultrasound or during adulthood.

Survival rates for retinoblastoma patients in the developed world have increased dramatically over the past century. The mortality of retinoblastoma was reported as 83% in 1897 in children who were treated with enucleation, and as 43% in all children in 1916.[3] In contrast, cancer registry reports in Europe and the United States have demonstrated 5-year survival rates of 90% and 98%, respectively. The improved survival rate is due to earlier detection of the tumor and improved techniques for local tumor control. In contrast to developed countries, however, developing nations report dramatically low survival rates, as patients in these countries typically present with widespread metastatic disease. Worldwide approximately 50% of patients still die of metastatic retinoblastoma.

There are no differences in incidence by sex, race, or right versus left eye. Some data suggest geographic clustering, but convincing evidence is lacking. Retinoblastoma does appear to occur more commonly in poor patients worldwide.

Molecular biology of retinoblastoma

The traditional view of retinoblastoma genetics, widely held until recently, was that the disease occurs in two forms, germinal and nongerminal. Both forms occur as a result of loss or mutation of both alleles of the retinoblastoma gene (*rb1*). In nongerminal cases, both *rb1* alleles are inactivated somatically in a single developing retinal progenitor cell, whereas in germinal cases, the first mutation occurs in the germline and only the second mutation is somatic. Nongerminal retinoblastoma is always unilateral and unifocal, although the tumor may break apart resulting in hundreds of tiny intraocular seeds. Recent evidence has indicated

Holland-Frei Cancer Medicine, Ninth Edition. Edited by Robert C. Bast Jr., Carlo M. Croce, William N. Hait, Waun Ki Hong, Donald W. Kufe, Martine Piccart-Gebhart, Raphael E. Pollock, Ralph R. Weichselbaum, Hongyang Wang, and James F. Holland.
© 2017 John Wiley & Sons, Inc. ISBN: 978-1-118-93469-2

Disease sites

Table 1 Most common ophthalmic neoplasms, benign and malignant.

	Benign	Malignant	
		Primary	Secondary
Children			
Ocular	—	Retinoblastoma	Leukemia
Orbital	Capillary hemangioma	Rhabdomyosarcoma	Leukemia
Adult			
Ocular	Choroid nevus	Uveal melanoma	Metastasis (lung, breast)
Orbital	Cavernous hemangioma	Lymphoma	Sinus cancer
Lids	Chalazion	Basal cell carcinoma	Lymphoma

that nearly all retinoblastoma patients probably demonstrate a degree of mosaicism for the *rb1* mutation. Furthermore, evidence suggests that genomic instability, microsatellite instability, defects of the DNA mismatch repair system, and alterations in DNA methylation and acetylation/deacetylation may also be necessary for the malignant transformation of retinoblastoma after the loss of pRB.[4]

The proposed retinoblastoma gene was localized to chromosome 13ql4 through deletion studies and linkage analysis. The protein is a regulator at the cell cycle checkpoint between G1 and entry into the S-phase (Figure 1). Loss of normal *rb1* function, as in the case of the tumors, allows for uncontrolled entry into the S-phase and more rapid cell division. Recently, it was discovered that *Rb1* wild-type tumors may occur in the context of MYCN oncogene amplification.[5]

Rb1 was the first tumor suppressor gene to be identified. The tumor-suppressive function of the *rb1* gene was confirmed in studies that demonstrated the loss of both alleles of the gene in tumor tissue specimens. Later studies showed that a germinal *rb1* mutation was present in virtually all retinoblastoma kindreds and that inheritance of the mutant *rb1* allele predicted disease.[6] The tumor-suppressive function of the gene has furthermore been demonstrated in transfection studies showing that the introduction of wild-type expression in pRB-defective cell lines partially reverses the malignant phenotype.

Genetic testing

Both population data gathered from families and our current understanding of the molecular mechanisms of inheritance of the disease have enabled us to predict the likelihood that new offspring in families affected by retinoblastoma will develop the disease (Table 2). Karyotypic studies, which analyze the morphology of entire chromosomes, are generally not useful for the clinical diagnosis of retinoblastoma because they can only identify deletions spanning 2–5 million base pairs and only 3–5% of retinoblastoma patients carry deletions this large.[7] Instead, more sophisticated indirect and direct techniques that detect smaller mutations are used. At the present time, a single genetic test is unlikely to detect all germline RB gene mutations in patients with retinoblastoma because of the variety of types and locations of mutations that occur. However, adaptation of a routine clinical protocol including a series of complementary tests based on the observation that most mutations alter the protein size and disrupt the large pocket domain may be able to rapidly detect the majority of mutations.[8]

Presenting signs and symptoms of retinoblastoma

The most common presenting signs and symptoms of retinoblastoma vary depending on the socioeconomic conditions in which the patient presents. In developing countries, children have often developed extraocular disease before they are diagnosed and frequently present with proptosis and an orbital mass (Figure 2). These children are older at diagnosis (age 4–6 years) compared patients in the United States and few survive. Many large retrospective studies over the past quarter-century have examined the most common presentations of retinoblastoma in large developed nations.[8] In the United States, the most common presenting sign (60% of cases) is leukocoria, a white pupillary reflex (Figure 3). The reflex is caused either by the reflection of incoming light off the tumor or by the retinal detachment caused by the underlying tumor.

Presenting signs in the United States that occur less commonly include strabismus (misalignment of the eyes), inflammatory signs (mimicking orbital cellulitis), anisocoria (different sized pupils), heterochromia (different colored irides), hyphema (blood in the anterior chamber), tumor hypopyon (tumor in the anterior chamber), and nystagmus. Two large retrospective studies on large populations of retinoblastoma patients have recently examined the patterns of detection of retinoblastoma in the United States. The vast majority of patients' disease was discovered by a family member

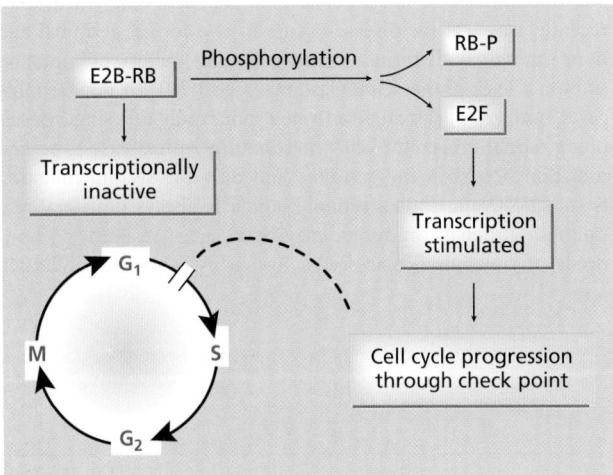

Figure 1 Artistic rendition of molecular mechanism of retinoblastoma gene action.

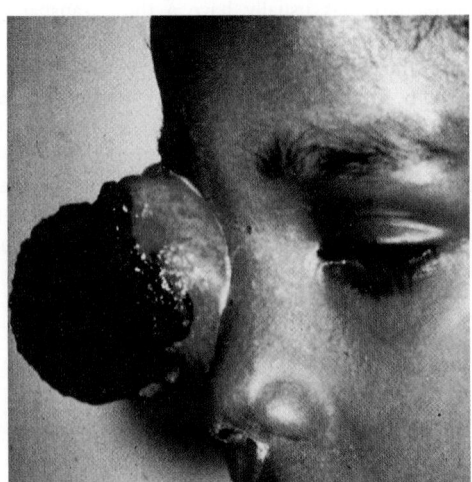

Figure 2 Advanced orbital presentation of retinoblastoma. Source: Courtesy of A. Wachtel, M.D., Lima, Peru.

Table 2 Genetic counseling for retinoblastoma.

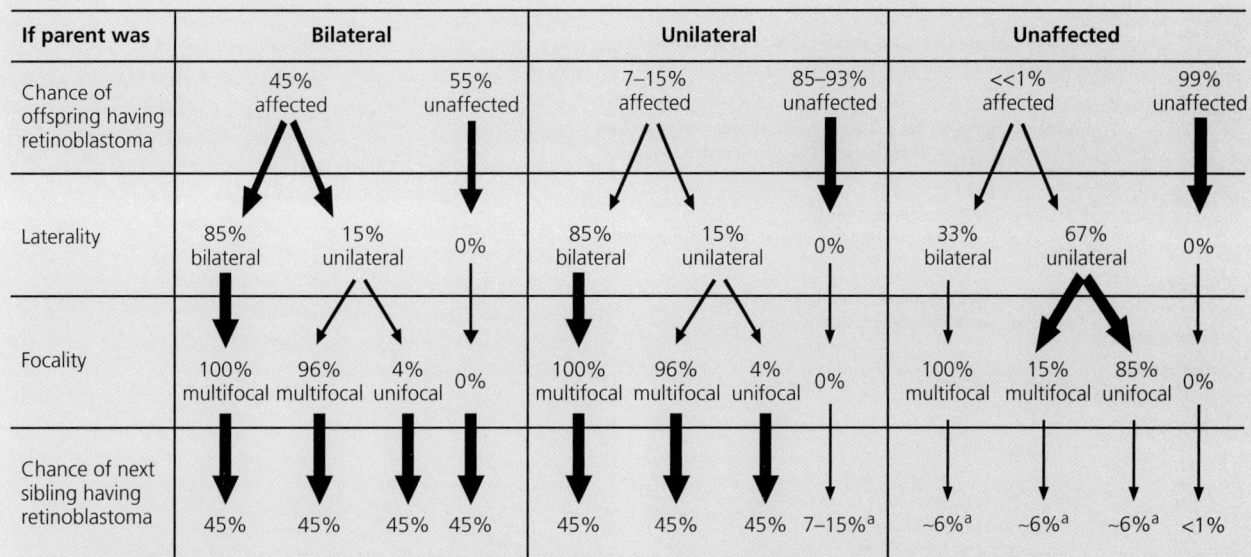

If parent was	Bilateral				Unilateral				Unaffected			
Chance of offspring having retinoblastoma	45% affected		55% unaffected		7–15% affected		85–93% unaffected		<<1% affected		99% unaffected	
Laterality	85% bilateral	15% unilateral	0%		85% bilateral	15% unilateral	0%		33% bilateral	67% unilateral	0%	
Focality	100% multifocal	96% multifocal	4% unifocal	0%	100% multifocal	96% multifocal	4% unifocal	0%	100% multifocal	15% multifocal	85% unifocal	0%
Chance of next sibling having retinoblastoma	45%	45%	45%	45%	45%	45%	45%	7–15%[a]	~6%[a]	~6%[a]	~6%[a]	<1%

[a]If parent is a carrier, then the chance of next sibling having retinoblastoma is 45%.

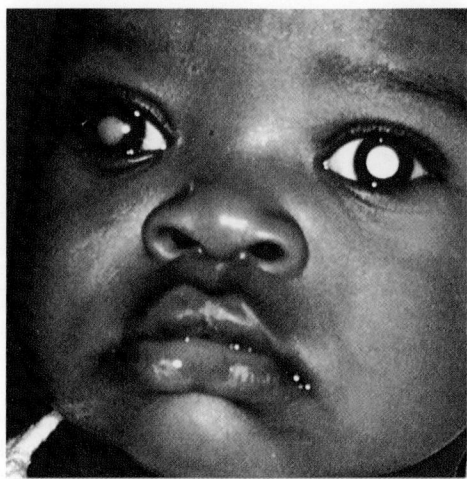

Figure 3 Leukocoria (white pupillary reflex) caused by retinoblastoma. The tumor can be seen in the vitreous. There are seeds in the anterior chamber, anterior to the iris.

(80%) rather than by a pediatrician (8%) or an ophthalmologist (10%).[8]

Diagnostic testing

The differential diagnosis of retinoblastoma includes lesions that can simulate a solitary ocular tumor such as astrocytic hamartomas and toxocara canis and lesions that can cause a total retinal detachment such as Coats' disease, retinopathy of prematurity, and persistent hyperplastic primary vitreous [persistent fetal vasculature (PFV) syndrome] (Table 3). Patients suspected of having retinoblastoma should undergo indirect ophthalmoscopy and fundus photography as well as ophthalmic ultrasonography. Ultrasonography is useful as it demonstrates masses with high reflectivity that block sound, causing characteristic shadowing behind the tumor. Needle biopsies are rarely performed for suspected retinoblastoma, as puncturing the eye and aspiration can lead to tumor seeding with orbital invasion and even death from metastatic disease.

Table 3 Lesions simulating retinoblastoma.

Solitary ocular tumor
    Astrocytic hamartoma
    Toxocara canis
Total retinal detachment
    Coats' disease
    Retinopathy of prematurity
    Persistent fetal vasculature (PFV)

Staging of intraocular retinoblastoma

The Reese–Ellsworth classification scheme was the worldwide gold standard for describing intraocular tumors (Table 4a).[9] It is not a true staging scheme (for untreated patients do not progress from group I to higher groups), but it has served as an excellent ocular reference for comparison of different series and treatment schemes. A higher numeric classification signified that a tumor was more anterior and that there was a decreased success rate in treating the lesion with lateral port external-beam radiation. Its usefulness has been questioned by many ophthalmic oncologists, who feel that it is no longer appropriate given the current trend away from the use of external-beam radiation. An alternate classification system was developed and has been used clinically by several centers in a collaborative study (Table 4b).[10] It has been shown to correlate with the response to treatment of intraocular disease with systemic chemotherapy combined with focal therapy. As with the Reese–Ellsworth classification, this system may also become antiquated as treatment trends inevitably change in the future.

Treatment of intraocular retinoblastoma

Survival rates in excess of 95% are currently achieved for most patients treated at major centers in developed countries with a multimodal treatment approach that may include enucleation, external-beam radiation, brachytherapy, transpupillary thermotherapy (TTT), cryotherapy, and chemotherapy (systemic, intra-arterial, periocular, and intravitreal). The treatment strategy

Table 4 (a) Reese–Ellsworth scheme for intraocular retinoblastoma. (b) New international classification for retinoblastoma.

(a)

Group I
- Solitary tumor, <4 disc diameters in size, at or behind the equator
- Multiple tumors, none over 4 disc diameters in size, all at or behind the equator

Group II
- Solitary tumor, 4–10 disc diameters in size, at or behind the equator
- Multiple tumors, 4–10 disc diameters in size, behind the equator

Group III
- Any lesion anterior to the equator
- Solitary tumors larger than 10 disc diameters behind the equator

Group IV
- Multiple tumors, some larger than 10 disc diameters
- Any lesion extending anteriorly to the ora serrata

Group V
- Massive tumors involving over half the retina
- Vitreous seeding

(b)

Group A Rb ≤ 3 mm in basal dimension or thickness

Group B Rb > 3 mm or with one or more of the following:
- Macular location (≤3 mm to foveola)
- Juxtapapillary location (≤1.5 mm to optic nerve)
- Additional subretinal fluid (≤3 mm from margin)

Group C Retinoblastoma tumor with one of the following:
- Subretinal seeds ≤ 3 mm
- Vitreous seeds ≤ 3 mm
- Both subretinal and vitreous seeds ≤ 3 mm

Group D Retinoblastoma tumor with one of the following:
- Subretinal seeds > 3 mm
- Vitreous seeds > 3 mm
- Both subretinal and vitreous seeds > 3 mm

Group E Extensive retinoblastoma occupying >50% of globe or any of the following:
- Neovascular glaucoma
- Opaque media from vitreous hemorrhage in anterior chamber, vitreous, or subretinal space
- Invasion of postlaminar optic nerve, choroid (>2 mm), sclera, orbit, or anterior chamber

for each patient depends on several factors: involvement of one or both eyes, heredity of the disease, age of the patient, tumor volume and localization, stage of disease (including Reese–Ellsworth classification), and presence of extraocular disease.[1]

Enucleation

Enucleation is surgical removal of the eye without resecting the lids or extraocular muscles.[1] Patients considered for enucleation include those with advanced retinoblastoma in one or both eyes, active tumor in a blind eye, and painful glaucoma from tumor invasion.

External-beam radiation

External-beam radiation, once employed in many patients with intraocular retinoblastoma, has fallen out of favor due to its contribution to the development of second nonocular cancers in germinal retinoblastoma patients.[1] When radiation is given, it is often used as a last resort salvage therapy after other therapies have failed.

Transpupillary thermotherapy (TTT)

TTT is a treatment modality for retinoblastoma that is delivered using modifications to the hardware and software of the infrared diode laser.[1] TTT is used to treat selected small retinoblastomas, typically those located in the posterior aspect of the globe. A study examining the use of TTT as single modality therapy for small tumors found that 92% of tumors 1.5 disc diameters or less in base diameter were successfully cured with TTT alone.

Cryotherapy

Cryotherapy is used as a primary treatment for small peripheral retinoblastomas or as adjuvant or secondary treatment for tumors treated by other modalities.[1] Rapid freezing (−90°C per minute) results in intracellular ice crystal formation, protein denaturation, pH changes, and finally cell membrane rupture. All studies examining the use of cryotherapy alone have demonstrated 90–100% cure rates in tumors that are <3 mm in diameter and <1 mm in thickness with minimal complications.

Brachytherapy

Episcleral brachytherapy was pioneered in 1933 by the British ophthalmologist Henry Stallard. Radioactive plaques can be used as primary therapy and their relative indications include tumors that are classified as Reese–Ellsworth stage IVa or less and tumors that are between 4 and 10 disc diameters in size. Brachytherapy can also be used as a salvage technique in eyes that have failed other types of therapy including intra-arterial chemotherapy, external-beam radiation, photocoagulation, or cryotherapy. [125]Iodine is currently the most commonly used isotope in brachytherapy for retinoblastoma. This isotope is advantageous because the radioactive seeds can be placed into a custom-built plaque designed to match the size of the lesion.

Systemic chemotherapy

Chemoreduction can be used to shrink these tumors so that focal treatments such as cryotherapy, thermotherapy, or radioactive plaques can be administered afterword.[1] Most studies of chemoreduction for retinoblastoma since 1996 have utilized vincristine, carboplatin, and an epipodophyllotoxin, either etoposide or teniposide. The addition of cyclosporine as a P-glycoprotein inhibitor has also been suggested to decrease multidrug resistance.[11] Choice of agents and number and frequency of cycles vary currently at different institutions.

For patients with Reese–Ellsworth groups I–III eyes patients, many authors have demonstrated that enucleation can be successfully avoided almost 100% of the time. Results for patients with Reese–Ellsworth groups IV and V eyes have been more discouraging. In a meta-analysis of patients treated with chemoreduction, 37% of eyes avoided *both* external-beam radiation and enucleation. Forty-one percent of eyes required radiation but avoided enucleation, and 40% of eyes required enucleation (with or without prior radiation).[12] Owing to concerns of short- and long-term toxicity, many centers have abandoned systemic chemotherapy as primary treatment of retinoblastoma in favor of more focal chemotherapy techniques.

Intra-arterial chemotherapy

Clinicians in Japan were the first to postulate that another method of local drug delivery, intra-arterial infusions of chemotherapy, may increase penetration of the drug into small intraocular tumors and decrease systemic side effects.[13] Our group introduced a technique in which the ophthalmic artery is selectively cannulated and a combination of up to three drugs (melphalan, topotecan, and carboplatin) are injected at the ostium.[1] Other techniques to access the ophthalmic artery include catheterization of the middle meningeal artery or the use of a balloon. Treatment typically consists of monthly infusions given an average of three times. This technique has been adopted by many centers worldwide and is our primary method of treatment for both unilateral and bilateral retinoblastoma. It can be used to treat eyes of all classifications, whether naïve or prior treated, and bilateral cases can be infused in the same session with tandem therapy. In children <3 months of age or 6 kg, bridge therapy is employed: single-agent carboplatin is given until the child reaches an adequate age and weight for intra-arterial chemotherapy. Two-year Kaplan–Meier estimates of ocular event-free survival are estimated at 82% for naïve eyes and 60% for prior treated eyes,[14] although with the recent adoption of intravitreal chemotherapy, these numbers are likely higher (Figure 4).

Ocular side effects are minimal and may include periocular inflammation, medial forehead erythema, and chorioretinal changes.[14] Electroretinogram monitoring of retinal function demonstrates that carboplatin and topotecan have no impact on retinal function; and while melphalan may have an effect, these changes are minimal and likely clinically irrelevant. Approximately 30% of children have at least one episode of grade 3 or 4 hematotoxicity during their treatment course (particularly when melphalan dose exceeds 0.4 mg/kg) and therefore monitoring of blood counts

is advised. Vascular complication is a rare complication and no death has been reported from this procedure.

Periocular chemotherapy

Periocular injections of carboplatin or topotecan have been used, particularly as salvage or adjuvant treatment. However, side effects, particularly with carboplatin, include scarring and loss of vision. Furthermore, its long-term efficacy of this delivery method has been questioned.

Intravitreal chemotherapy

Injections through the wall of the eye and into the vitreous were historically avoided owing to concerns of extraocular extension of tumor through the needle tract. However, the adoption of safety-enhanced techniques and an exceedingly low calculated risk of extraocular extension have lessened these fears. Intravitreal injections of chemotherapy typically consist of melphalan, but have included carboplatin and topotecan, given weekly up to eight times. This modality is rapidly becoming the optimal method for treating vitreous seeding with ocular survival rates reportedly as high as 83–100%. However, electroretinogram recordings have revealed that for every 30 μg injection of melphalan, the retina function decreases by 5% and future work may mitigate this toxicity either with other drugs or alterations to the delivery method.[15]

Treatment of extraocular retinoblastoma

In the most developed nations, extraocular disease occurs only in a small minority of patients. For more complete information on the treatment of extraocular retinoblastoma, the reader is encouraged to consult more extensive sources.[16,17]

Second malignancies

In 1949, it was first recognized that some retinoblastoma patients develop second nonocular neoplasms years after the successful treatment of the eye cancer. Since then, the incidence of additional nonocular cancers in survivors of retinoblastoma who carry the *rb1* mutation has been reviewed extensively.[18] Previous analyses have also shown that additional nonocular cancers are the leading cause of death in survivors of germinal retinoblastoma in the United States. Of the survivors of germinal retinoblastoma, cumulative incidence reports of second malignancies vary, but most large studies with adequate long-term follow-up have reported yearly incidence rates of approximately 0.5–1% per year.[18,19]

Several clinical risk factors and treatment-related exposures have been shown to have an association with the development of second nonocular cancers in retinoblastoma survivors (Table 5). For instance, external-beam radiation increases the risk of development of second cancers in a dose-dependent manner. Secondary acute myeloblastic leukemia (AML) has been linked to the use of etoposide (an epipodophyllotoxin) in systemic chemotherapy regimens for retinoblastoma.

Second malignancies observed in retinoblastoma survivors in the United States include, in order from most common to least, osteogenic sarcomas of the skull and long bones, soft tissue sarcomas, pineoblastomas, cutaneous melanomas, brain tumors, Hodgkin's disease, lung cancer, breast cancer, salivary gland, and oral cancers. This reflects a cohort who historically received large doses of external-beam radiation. In the United Kingdom, a study published several years ago offers unique insight into the types of malignancies that develop in patients not treated with external-beam radiation.[20] Patients in the study, who were all over 25 years of age at follow-up, had a much higher risk of

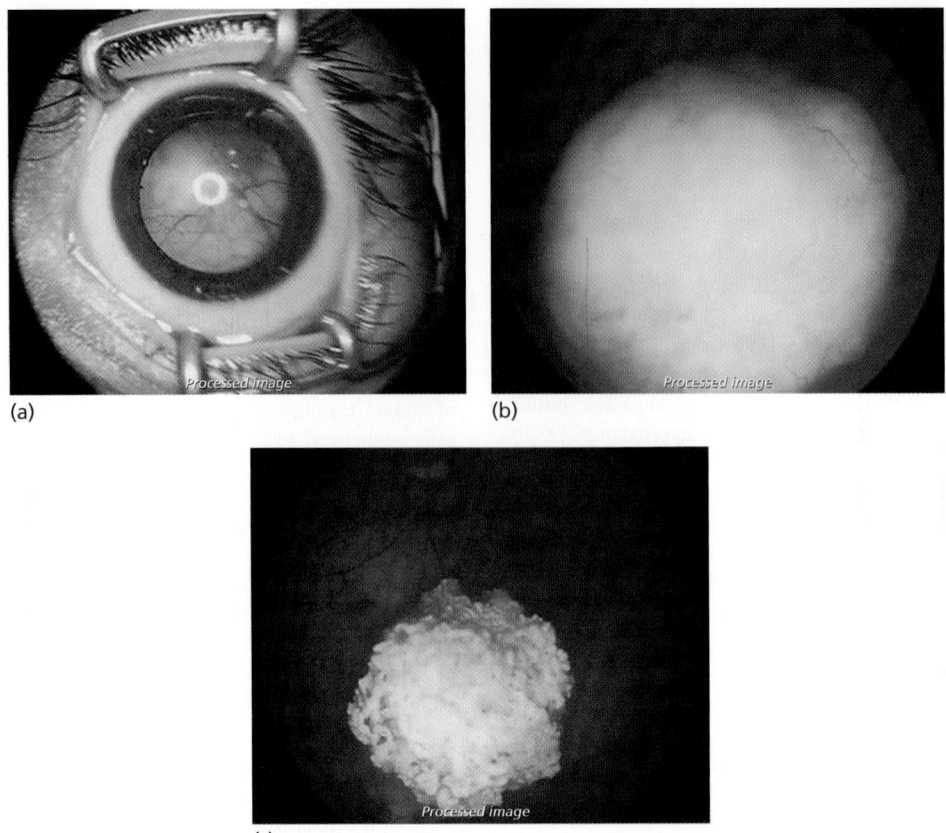

(a)

(b)

(c)

Figure 4 (a) An example of the typical patient undergoing intra-arterial chemotherapy. The globe is full of retinoblastoma with a total retinal detachment visible behind the lens. (b) Fundus photograph before intra-arterial chemotherapy. Note that the large tumor is obscuring the optic nerve head. (c) Fundus photograph after intra-arterial chemotherapy. The tumor has become calcified and there are no vitreous seeds visible. The optic nerve head can now be visualized above the tumor. The retina is flat.

Table 5 Risk factors for second nonocular cancer development in retinoblastoma survivors.

Factor	Strength of association with incidence of second cancers
Presence of germinal mutation in *rb1* gene	Definite causation (necessary risk factor)
Dose of external-beam radiation	Dose-dependent causation
External-beam radiation given at <1 year of age	Very likely association
Presence of lipomas	Definite association (noncausative)
Smoking	Definite causation
Chemotherapy	Possible association
Sun exposure	Possible association
Growth hormone	Possible association

developing epithelial cancers (notably lung, bladder, and probably breast) than of developing sarcomas and other early onset cancers compared to patients in the United States who received radiation.

Secondary malignant disease (leukemia)

Childhood acute lymphocytic leukemia (ALL) is the most common malignant tumor that involves the eyes of children. Leukemia primarily involves the uveal tract: the iris, ciliary body, and/or choroid. It can also involve the retina, optic nerve, and orbit.

Leukemic iris infiltrates can appear as creamy clusters of cells floating on the surface of the iris. When iris infiltrates are present, they can manifest as heterochromia (different color irides), cells in the anterior chamber (tumor hypopyon mimicking idiopathic iritis), or bleeding in the anterior chamber (hyphema). Hyphema can be associated with glaucoma and a painful, photophobic, red, sensitive eye. In contrast to iris involvement, leukemic infiltration is virtually impossible to detect ophthalmoscopically in the ciliary body or choroid because ALL diffusely invades the choroidal blood vessels. This subtle thickening is often detectable only by B-scan ultrasound.[21] Leukemic infiltration in the choroid has been identified in 90% of eyes at autopsy after death from leukemia. Retinal involvement is rare.

Leukemic infiltration of the eye can present in different time sequences in relation to the overall presentation of the disease. Most commonly, the infiltration presents simultaneously with the initial presentation of the leukemia. The majority of patients with ALL demonstrate ultrasonic ocular findings at presentation. When the leukemia is treated, the choroidal involvement usually disappears within days. Leukemic infiltration of the eye can also present as an isolated site of relapse following induction treatment and CNS (central nervous system) radiation prophylaxis. In these children, the CNS has often been treated with radiation but the eye has escaped treatment, functioning as a sanctuary site. Treatment of the eye alone in such cases may be justified. Finally, leukemic infiltration can present as a sign of CNS recurrence with or without evidence of a gross mass in the CNS. These patients frequently have leukemic cells near the posterior pole and in the vitreous. In these cases, the tumor cells enter the eye via the optic nerve, which has been seeded directly from the CNS. In these cases, treatment to the brain with chemotherapy or external-beam radiation is generally considered.

Pediatric ophthalmic oncology: orbital diseases

Benign disease

Capillary hemangiomas

Benign tumors of the orbit in children are frequently incidental problems detected on CT (computed tomography) scan or observed because of lid or orbital asymmetry. Many require no treatment. The most common benign orbital tumor of childhood is the capillary hemangioma.[22] On CT, capillary hemangiomas are usually associated with congenitally enlarged orbits while rhabdomyosarcomas are not.

Treatment of these hemangiomas is frustrating. The tumors respond to low-dose radiation and we have used fractionated doses up to 800 cGy with success. There have also been several reports of treatment with recombinant interferon alpha.[23] Local injections of short- and long-acting steroids are probably the treatment of choice when mandated by visual or overwhelming cosmetic reasons. When capillary hemangiomas occur on the skin, they can be treated with a topical β-blocker.

Dermoid cysts

Dermoid cysts are benign and represent congenital ectodermal rests. Treatment is surgical, but utmost care must be taken because some have bilobed posterior orbital extensions that can extend intracranially.

Lymphangioma

Despite the fact that lymphatics do not exist in the orbit, benign lymphangiomas do.[24] These tumors are thought to be congenital and have no malignant potential, but in contrast to hemangiomas are rarely present at birth. They are most commonly seen at around age 6 with explosive proptosis caused by bleeding of the tumor into the cystic spaces referred to as *chocolate cysts*. Treatment is difficult. They do not respond to steroids or radiation. Surgery with electrocautery laser is the treatment of choice. Satisfactory cosmetic results are difficult to attain.

Malignant disease

Rhabdomyosarcoma

The most common primary malignant orbital tumor of childhood is rhabdomyosarcoma. The average age at diagnosis is 6–10 years with equal incidence in both sexes and both orbits. Although the hallmark presentation of an orbital rhabdomyosarcoma is rapid, progressive, painless proptosis, patients can present with a less dramatic course with slow, progressive proptosis or with ptosis, strabismus, or a subconjunctival fleshy mass. The diagnosis of rhabdomyosarcoma should be considered whenever rapid progressive proptosis occurs in the first 20 years of life. The most common location in the orbit is superonasal. CT or MRI (magnetic resonance imaging) scans can help define the extent of the tumor.

Urgent biopsy is mandatory. All attempts should be made to biopsy the lesion directly without going through the sinuses or skull because of the possibility of causing metastatic disease by tracking tumor cells along the biopsy path. The most common histologic type is an embryonal rhabdomyosarcoma. When rhabdomyosarcomas present in the inferior orbit they are usually histologically alveolar type. These malignancies do not originate from extraocular muscles but from undifferentiated pluripotential mesenchymal elements in the orbital soft issues.

External-beam radiation was first utilized in the mid-1960s and later combined with chemotherapy producing excellent local cures and better than 90% long-term survival. The Intergroup Rhabdomyosarcoma studies in the 1980s demonstrated that the most effective combination for disease localized to the orbit was vincristine, actinomycin-D and radiation. In giving radiation, the eye was not spared or shielded. Long-term follow-up demonstrated that after a median of 7 years, only 14% of such eyes were enucleated, but vision was impaired in 70% of them.[25] A meta-analysis completed by four international collaborative groups found no significant difference in survival for those patients treated with chemotherapy alone versus chemotherapy plus radiation.[26]

Adult ophthalmic oncology: ocular diseases

Benign disease

Benign tumors of the lid, conjunctiva, iris, and choroid are common while those of the retina and cornea are rare. Benign tumors of the lens and vitreous do not occur. The most important benign tumors of the eye in adults are the choroidal nevi.

Choroidal nevi

Choroidal nevi are never present at birth, but generally present around puberty. In the United States, 10–13% of the adult population have choroidal nevi. They are racially related; choroidal nevi in blacks are very rare.

Choroidal nevi are flat, pigmented benign lesions with edges that can be feathered and irregular or rounded (Figure 5). They are usually slate-gray to light chocolate in color. Over time (months to years), there can be associated changes visible by ophthalmoscopy. Many demonstrate changes on their surface such as drusen or have associated findings such as subretinal fluid or neovascular membranes. They may also cause visual field defects. As 10% of the adult population has choroidal nevi and there are only 1500 choroidal melanomas in the United States yearly, it is assumed that

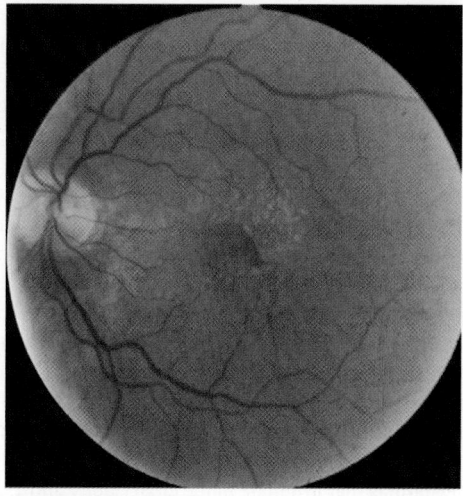

Figure 5 Choroidal nevus located inferior to the macula. Note the yellow drusen indicating benign status.

Table 6 Predictive factors: nevus to melanoma transformation.

- *Size*: The greater the thickness of a choroidal nevus, the greater the chance of it becoming a melanoma. Of nevi 2.5 mm in thickness, approximately 1% per month become melanomas.
- *Location*: Nevi at the posterior portion of the eye more commonly become melanomas than those situated anteriorly.
- *Orange Pigment*: When choroidal nevi develop orange pigment on their surface, the chance of a melanoma developing greatly increases.
- *Serous Fluid*: Serous fluid in the form of an overlying retinal detachment can be seen with nevi, but such nevi more likely become melanomas.
- *Absence of Drusen*: Drusen are a strong indicator of chronicity and benignity and lesions with drusen rarely transform.
- *Hot Spots* on fluorescein angiography
- *Symptoms* (decreased vision or visual field defect)

the chance of a choroidal nevus becoming a melanoma is <1 in 6000. A number of studies have now demonstrated which nevi are more likely to undergo malignant transformation. The predictive factors are shown in Table 6.

A melanocytoma is a special type of choroidal nevus often observed in darker-skinned Caucasians of Mediterranean origin. Melanocytomas are brown-black lesions that most commonly originate from the optic nerve head, but can evolve from the choroid, ciliary body, or iris. The lesions may be several millimeters high, can grow slowly, and can affect the visual field or visual acuity. Pathologically, the lesion is a magnocellular nevus with jet black pigmentation. While the lesions are benign, rare cases of transformation to malignancy have been recorded although no deaths have been documented.

The differential diagnosis of a choroidal nevus includes congenital hyperplasia of the retinal pigment epithelium (CHRPE), hamartomas of the retinal pigment epithelium, and hemorrhages within the retina, especially hemorrhages beneath the retinal pigment epithelium (most commonly associated with age-related macular degeneration). Ophthalmoscopic appearance and results of a fluorescein angiogram and ultrasonography are used to distinguish these lesions from each other.

Iris nevi and melanomas

Iris nevi are benign lesions of the iris that appear on slit lamp examination as pigmented flat areas. They are common, may be multiple, and occur more often in blue-eyed patients. Like choroidal nevi, iris nevi are rarely present at birth and present around puberty. Rarely, they can appear elevated and can grow and shed pigmented cells into the anterior chamber angle, clogging the trabecular meshwork and causing a severe secondary glaucoma that can blind the eye. These lesions have often been referred to as iris melanomas. Widespread metastases, however, are seen rarely if ever. Many clinicians have theorized that the reason for the less aggressive behavior observed in iris melanomas versus choroidal melanomas is simply the smaller size of these lesions. However, studies suggest that they are distinctly different from choroidal lesions in that a significant percentage demonstrate an activating mutation in exon 15 of the BRAF gene, which is common in cutaneous melanoma, but almost never seen in choroidal lesions. Management of iris melanoma is based on the presence or absence of glaucoma and should not be guided by a need to prevent metastases. Melanomas that originate in the ciliary body and extend into the iris, however, often demonstrate very aggressive behavior and can metastasize.

Malignant disease

Introduction to choroidal melanoma

Choroidal melanoma is the most common primary ocular malignant tumor in adults in the United States but the second most common worldwide (after retinoblastoma). There are about 1500 new cases per year of choroidal malignant melanoma in the United States. The average age at diagnosis is 55–65 years with men and women equally affected and no predilection for right versus left eye. In the United States, 99% of choroidal melanomas occur in Caucasians. The most common way in which the tumor is detected is on routine exam (41%). Men more often present with symptoms and when there are symptoms, the right eye is more often found to have the tumor. The most common symptom is a perceived deficit in the peripheral visual field followed by decreased vision. The lesion is not painful, unlike metastatic tumors to the eye in which pain is not unusual.

Melanomas of the choroid originate in melanocytes that normally lie within the choroid. The choroid, the layer between the sclera and retina is a rich, high-flow syncytium of vascular lobules that not only supply blood to the photoreceptors (rods and cones) of the retina but also serve as a heat sink to dissipate heat energy liberated by absorbed visible light.

Whether all melanomas of the choroid originate from choroidal nevi is not known, but patients with flat, pigmented, untreated nevi followed for more than 20 years have developed melanomas arising from the previously dormant lesion. The cause of choroidal melanomas is unknown but predisposing medical conditions include melanosis oculi (nevus of Ota) and dysplastic nevus syndrome. Medications that have been shown to cause increased growth of the tumors include estrogen replacement therapy and levodopa. Occupational associations include agriculture and farming work and several industrial operations, including welding. Mutually exclusive mutations in GNAQ/GNA11 occur in almost all choroidal nevi and melanomas, and the addition of a BAP1 mutation is believed to be a genetic event that is associated with malignant transformation of these lesions.[27]

Diagnosis of choroidal melanoma

The diagnosis of choroidal melanoma can usually be made on the basis of ophthalmoscopic examination alone. The lesions most often appear as elevated, dome-shaped masses that can rupture Bruch's membrane (Figure 6). When Bruch's membrane is ruptured, the tumors are referred to as mushroom shaped or collar button because of their characteristic shape. The lesions can also be multilobed or flat and diffuse. Lesion color varies from patient to patient and from area to area within the tumor. As many as 40% of the tumors have no pigment clinically. When pigmented, the tumors are frequently a dusky gray to charcoal in color but occasionally they are deep brown.

Ocular ultrasonography and sometimes fluorescein angiography can also aid in diagnosis. All choroidal melanomas have associated retinal detachments. In some cases, it may be difficult to detect the detachments ophthalmoscopically, while in others the retinal detachment may be so extensive that the melanoma is not seen clinically. Typically, the B-scan ultrasound demonstrates an elevated solid tumor and the A-scan demonstrates medium to low reflectivity. With the use of rigorous and standardized ophthalmic and systemic examinations, a diagnostic accuracy of 99.7% was reached in the Collaborative Ocular Melanoma Study (COMS).[28] As clinical accuracy is so high, needle biopsy for diagnosis is rarely needed.

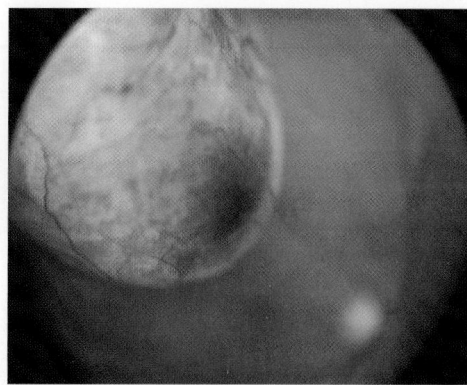

Figure 6 Malignant melanoma of the choroid.

As there are no lymphatics in the eye or within the orbit, melanomas of the choroid metastasize through vascular channels. Approximately 68% of single-site metastases occur within the liver. The median survival has been reported as 6 months to 1 year.[29]

Clinical and pathologic risk factors

A number of clinical and pathological features have been shown to correlate with patient survival.[30] First, larger tumors, measured clinically using the height and/or greatest base diameter to volume, are more likely to metastasize. Second, location of the melanoma affects prognosis. Patients with melanomas originating in the iris have the best outcome. Ciliary body melanomas have a threefold mortality compared with choroidal melanomas. Third, patients younger than 60 have better survival than those older than 60. Fourth, patients with extraocular extension have higher mortality rates than those who do not. Finally, many pathologic features (only available in cases where the eye has been removed) correlate with survival and are covered extensively elsewhere. The best known of these is cell type. Epithelioid cells, which are larger and more pleomorphic, are more likely to be contained in large tumors and carry a worse prognosis.

The COMS group, which included 44 institutions across the United States, was a series of prospective, randomized clinical trials and other reports on the prognosis and treatment of small, medium, and large choroidal melanomas. The COMS size classification scheme is shown in Table 7 and the results of the studies are detailed in Table 8.

Genetic analysis

In recent years, interest in analysis of chromosomal changes and gene expression patterns in choroidal melanoma has greatly increased. Several chromosomal abnormalities, including gain or loss of chromosomal material in chromosomes 3, 6, and 8, have been detected in primary uveal melanoma tissue and have been associated with metastasis. Monosomy 3 in uveal melanoma is a

statistically significant predictor of both relapse-free and overall survival.[31]

Gene expression microarray analysis is used to distinguish 2 groups: class 1 (low-grade tumors) and class 2 (high-grade tumors).[32] These classifications strongly predicted metastatic death with a 95% Kaplan–Meier-based survival prediction at 92 months of 95% in class 1 and 31% in class 2. In one study, the classifications outperformed other clinical and pathologic prognostic indicators. Specific gene mutations have been identified to correlate with survival: for instance, somatic BAP1 mutations are found is 84% of high-risk class 2 tumors.[32] Furthermore, germline BAP1 mutations may occur in 3–5% of patients with choroidal nevi or melanomas and have been associated with a hereditary cancer syndrome consisting of malignancies such as mesothelioma and cancers of the kidney and stomach. Recently two other mutations (SF3B1 and EIF1AX) have reportedly been associated with a more favorable prognosis and are more commonly found in male patients.[33]

The number of clinical centers performing karyotyping, single nucleotide polymorphism (SNP) analysis, fluorescent *in situ* hybridization (FISH) analysis, and/or comparative genomic hybridization (CGH) on fine-needle aspiration and enucleation specimens has dramatically increased in the last few years. Some groups have also begun to perform FISH or microsatellite array on fine-needle aspiration biopsy specimens. Biopsies have been attempted via pars plana and transscleral approaches. Because few effective treatments are available for metastatic uveal melanoma at this time, it is unclear what, if any, interventions or screening programs for metastases should be offered to patients whose lesions are shown to be high risk for metastasis on biopsy. Nonetheless, as new treatments (such as selumetinib[34]) or prophylactic drugs for metastatic melanoma are developed and available for clinical trials, it will be important to identify which patients are appropriate for entry into such studies.

Treatment and prognosis of small melanomas

In the COMS, the definition of a small melanoma was a lesion that was 1–2.5 mm in thickness and 5–16 mm in largest basal diameter. This observational study demonstrated that, of choroidal melanomas initially managed by observation, 21% demonstrated growth to medium or large tumors by 2 years and 31% by 5 years. However, there were no defined criteria or threshold for treatment and this group may have included patients whose lesions demonstrated no growth or high-risk features. Factors significantly associated with growth by statistical analysis in the study were greater initial tumor thickness and diameter, presence of orange pigment, absence of drusen, and absence of areas of retinal pigment epithelial changes adjacent to the tumor (Table 6).

As the COMS brachytherapy trials were published, most ophthalmologists in the United States have continued to use the COMS tumor size guidelines in order to designate a tumor as medium and institute brachytherapy. Nonetheless, some investigators have raised the question of whether small melanomas should also be treated with brachytherapy and/or biopsied for gene profiles. Although the COMS indicated that the long-term mortality rate for these patients is low (8-year all-cause mortality of 14.9%),[35] it may be significant enough to justify the consideration of brachytherapy in these patients. There has been only one study examining the outcomes of patients with small melanomas initially observed, then treated with a standardized brachytherapy protocol after growth or new orange pigment was observed. The melanoma-specific 5-year mortality rate for the tumors in the COMS small tumor study was 1%[35]; however, the calculation of this rate included a substantial number of patients whose suspected tumors did not grow and were

Table 7 Final size classifications of choroidal melanomas in the collaborative ocular melanoma studies (COMS).

	Small melanomas (mm)	Medium melanomas	Large melanomas
Apical height	1–2.5	2.5–10 mm AND	>10 mm OR
Largest basal diameter	5–16	<16 mm	Greater than 16 mm (when 2 mm or greater in height)

Table 8 Results of the collaborative ocular melanoma study (COMS).

	Small	Medium	Large
Reference	*Arch Ophthalmol*. December 1997; 115(12):1537–1544	*Arch Ophthalmol*. July 2001; 119(7):969–982	*Am J Ophthalmol*. June 1998; 125(6):779–796
Type of study	Nonrandomized, prospective follow-up	Prospective randomized clinical trial	Prospective randomized clinical trial
Number of patients in study	204	1317	1003
Size of melanomas included in study	Apical height: 1.0–2.5 mm	Apical height: 2.5–10.0 mm	Apical height: 10.0 mm or larger
	Largest basal diameter: 5 mm	Largest basal diameter: 5–16 mm	Largest basal diameter: 16 mm or larger
Objective of study	To describe time to tumor growth and determine baseline characteristics associated with growth of small tumors	^{125}I brachytherapy versus enucleation for treatment of medium tumors	Pre-enucleation radiation versus enucleation alone for treatment of large tumors
Findings of study	21% grew by 2 years	No clinically or statistically significant difference in survival rates between the two treatments for up to 12 years after treatment	No significant difference in survival rates between the two treatments
	31% grew by 5 years		Age and largest basal diameter of the tumor are the only factors that affect prognosis
	Characteristics associated with growth: initial tumor thickness and diameter, presence of orange pigment, absence of drusen, absence of retinal pigment epithelial changes		

never treated. A randomized, prospective trial of visual and survival outcomes in patients managed by observation versus prompt treatment is needed to answer this critical question.

Treatment and prognosis of medium melanomas

The COMS completed a prospective, randomized clinical trial enrolling 1317 patients with medium-sized melanomas in which patients were randomly assigned to enucleation or brachytherapy with ^{125}I plaques at a tumor dose of 10,000 cGy.[36] The study concluded mortality rates following brachytherapy (81% 5-year survival) did not differ from mortality rates following enucleation (82% 5-year survival) for up to 12 years after treatment. Given the findings of this study, patients with medium-sized melanomas are offered both enucleation and brachytherapy as potential treatment options. Brachytherapy with ^{125}I plaques is usually administered at doses of 7500–10,000 cGy to the tumor apex. The fractionation schemes vary markedly without an apparent effect on local control, metastasis, or complications. Complications include radiation retinopathy and optic neuropathy. As a result of these complications, 43% of patients have 20/200 vision or worse by 3 years of follow-up.

Treatment and prognosis of large melanomas

In the past, patients with large tumors were generally treated with enucleation, with or without preoperative radiation. The COMS prospective, randomized clinical trial for patients with large tumors found that there was no survival difference between patients treated with enucleation alone (5-year survival 57%) and patients treated with pre-enucleation radiation (5-year survival 62%).[37] The patients assigned to the pre-enucleation radiation group in this study were treated with five fractions of 200 cGy external-beam radiation and enucleation within 72 h. Patients with large melanomas are now generally treated with enucleation alone.

Ocular surface squamous neoplasia (OSSN)

Ocular surface squamous neoplasia (OSSN) is the term that refers to both intraepithelial neoplasia and squamous cell carcinoma of the conjunctiva/cornea. The incidence of this disease has geographic variability, with some of the highest rates in Africa. Ultraviolet radiation is an important risk factor, but viral, particularly human papilloma virus, and genetic etiologies are also believed to be implicated. Squamous cell carcinoma is more aggressive in patients with human immunodeficiency virus.

OSSN has variability in its appearance, but typically presents as a slowly progressive redness or irritation of the eye often with leukoplakia. Lesions can be isolated, but as they progress, they can invade into the adjacent skin, orbit, sclera, and interior of the eye. Well-circumscribed lesions can be removed with excisional biopsy and an adequate tissue margin with adjuvant cryotherapy and/or topical chemotherapy. In more extensive and advanced cases, radiation or even exenteration (removal of orbital contents) may be indicated. The risk of metastases from squamous cell carcinoma ranges from <1% to 8% and is more common in mucoepidermoid/spindle cell subtypes, tumors with a high mitotic index, or those that recur or invade the eyelid and orbit. Metastases are typically first found in the adjacent lymph nodes.

Metastatic disease

The most common malignant neoplasm in the eye or orbit, in children or adults, is metastatic carcinoma to the choroid. While there are only 350 cases of retinoblastoma and 1500 cases of choroidal melanoma yearly in the United States, it is estimated that 30,000–100,000 patients with cancer develop metastases to the eye each year.

Most cancers metastasize to the uveal tract (iris, ciliary body, and choroid), with choroidal metastases occurring most frequently. Metastases to the lids, conjunctiva, optic nerve, orbit, extraocular muscles, and orbital bones are also reported. Metastases to the retina are rare.

Choroidal metastases are usually amelanotic, multiple, bilateral, minimally elevated, and painful when situated around the optic nerve or invading the sclera. In contrast, ocular melanomas are typically pigmented, solitary, unilateral, significantly elevated, and painless. Metastatic tumors, such as ocular melanomas, always have an associated serous detachment but the amount of detachment is proportionally greater with metastases. Ultrasonographically, most metastases have high reflectivity on ultrasound. Most ocular melanomas are detected on routine examinations, whereas ocular metastases are typically identified because of symptoms of decreased visual field and diminished visual acuity owing to serous retinal detachments.

Metastasis to the eye most commonly occurs in adults aged 55–65, the same age distribution as that for ocular melanomas. Metastases originate most commonly from a primary lung cancer and second most commonly from a primary breast cancer. As many as 34% of patients who present with metastases to the choroid have no previously known history of a primary cancer.[38] Many other cancers metastasize to the eye, including G.I., prostate (though more commonly to orbital bones), thyroid, ovarian, and cutaneous melanoma. Virtually all cancers have been found to be capable of metastasizing to the eye.

The most striking feature of metastatic ocular lesions is their association with concurrent CNS metastases. While the true concordance of these two lesions is unknown, it has been our experience that more than 75% of cases of ocular metastasis have concurrent CNS disease, although frequently the CNS disease is initially undetectable with imaging. It has therefore been speculated that some ocular metastases do not arrive through blood-borne routes but that CNS metastases may actually seed the choroid via the subarachnoid space as they do in childhood leukemia.

Treatment for ocular metastasis is considered when symptoms of diminished vision, pain, or diplopia are present. Treating the ocular lesion rarely has an impact on survival, except in carcinoid metastases, but may significantly alter the quality of life. Many ocular metastases respond to chemotherapy, targeted molecules, and biologics the way other systemic metastases respond. Chemotherapy and/or hormonal manipulation with the additional of intravitreal injections of anti-VEGF (vascular endothelial growth factor) may cause rapid regression of the tumor and of subretinal fluid. External-beam radiation and photodynamic therapy are used to palliate symptoms from ocular metastases. Except for carcinoid and breast cancer, however, median survival in patients with metastatic choroidal lesions is just over 6 months.

Cancer-associated retinopathy (CAR)

Cancer-associated retinopathy (CAR) is a paraneoplastic disorder characterized by visual loss in patients with cancer. Patients report photopsias or entopic phenomenon as well as light sensitivity and night blindness. Examination reveals decreased visual acuity, decreased color vision, and scotomas. A CAR antibody, a 23 kDa protein commonly found on blood testing, is known to be specific for a photoreceptor and bipolar cell-specific calcium binding protein. The underlying tumor is thought to express recoverin and stimulate this antibody response. The circulating antibodies then react with the retina resulting in photoreceptor degeneration. Although antibodies to recoverin account for the majority of cases, additional antibodies to 46, 45, 60, and 65 kDa proteins have been described. Lung cancer, endometrial sarcoma, lymphoma, and prostate cancer have been associated with the syndrome. Treatment is difficult. Steroids, plasmapheresis, intravenous immunoglobulin (IVIG), and treatment of the underlying tumor have been attempted. Although individual successes have been reported, most patients have little improvement and there is no clear consensus as to the best treatment.[39]

Ocular lymphoid tumors

Non-Hodgkin lymphomas can occasionally infiltrate the intraocular tissues and become clinically apparent even before identification of the systemic disease. Immunocompromised patients, especially those with viral illness such as those with HIV/AIDS (human immunodeficiency virus infection and acquired immune deficiency syndrome), show an increased incidence of this disease.

Primary malignant lymphomas of the eye have historically been called *reticulum cell sarcoma* or *microgliomatosis* and usually present with cells in the vitreous with associated retinal and optic nerve involvement. Diagnosis is made by vitrectomy or lumbar puncture. Treatment is accomplished with systemic steroids

and external-beam radiation therapy of 2400 cGy to the affected eye and/or chemotherapy. Intravitreal injections of rituximab or methotrexate have been used, particularly in cases of visual decline from intraocular disease. These patients frequently have CNS disease but rarely have systemic disease. There is controversy about whether to treat the brain in those cases in which diagnostic lumbar puncture and MRI demonstrate no disease. Median survival is 3.5 years and is usually determined by the extent of brain involvement. Treatment of ocular lesions does not seem to affect the appearance or extraocular sites in the future.

Uveal lymphoid infiltration is a rare disorder characterized by localized or diffuse infiltration of the uveal tract by lymphoid cells. Patients typically present with painless, progressive visual loss. Nodular amelanotic thickening of the choroid or exudative retinal detachment with secondary glaucoma can be present. Biopsy confirmation should be targeted to the most accessible tissue. Management emphasizes globe conservation aimed at visual presentation and generally involves oral steroids and/or external-beam radiation. Prognosis for survival is excellent and generally based on the degree of systemic involvement. Associated CNS involvement is rare.

Adult ophthalmic oncology: orbital diseases

Introduction to orbital tumors

Fortunately, malignant tumors of the orbit are unusual. Neoplasms account for approximately 20–25% of orbital disease and are most common in patients in their sixties or older. Malignant primary cancers of the orbit that do require biopsy and surgical management include lacrimal gland tumors and orbital lymphoma.

All cases of suspected orbital tumor should undergo imaging, including ophthalmic ultrasound, CT scans with or without contrast, and/or MRI with or without contrast in order to define more clearly the location and characteristics of the tumor.

Benign and malignant disease

Well-delineated orbital masses

The most common benign orbital tumor of adults is the cavernous hemangioma. Patients have slowly progressive painless proptosis with a mass indenting the globe, showing striae in the retina and a flattened globe on imaging studies. Treatment is surgical, and complete removal is possible. Other well-circumscribed lesions include neurofibromas, schwannomas, hemangiopericytomas, meningioma, and gliomas.

A mucocele or mucopyocele is a cystic, encapsulated mass originating in a paranasal sinus (usually the frontal sinus) that follows repeated bouts of sinusitis often leading to recurrent orbital cellulitis. It is the most common cause of proptosis in children. The bony wall is not intact on imaging studies. Treatment involves antibiotics. Surgical drainage is necessary if antibiotics fail to achieve resolution of the pyomucocele or if optic nerve compression is present.

Diffuse orbital masses

Diffuse orbital masses usually require a biopsy and include orbital lymphoma, orbital cellulitis, fibrous histiocytoma (benign and malignant), neurofibromas, and sarcomas. Lymphoproliferative neoplasms account for >20% of all orbital mass lesions. The incidence of non-Hodgkins lymphoma of all anatomic sites has been increasing at a rate of 3–4% per year and orbital lymphomas have been increasing at an even greater rate, although the factors responsible for this rise are poorly understood. Historically, lymphoid tumors were classified as either active lymphoid hyperplasia or malignant lymphoma. More recently, it has been recognized that lymphoproliferative lesions represent a continuum and that ultimate behavior is difficult to predict. Currently, 70–90% of orbital lymphoproliferative lesions are designated as malignant lymphomas on the basis of molecular genetic studies and monoclonal cell surface markers.

The typical lymphoproliferative lesion presents as a gradually progressive painless mass. It can be located anteriorly in the orbit or beneath the conjunctiva. Orbital imaging reveals the characteristic molding of the tumor around normal structures, and bony erosion is rare except in high-grade lesions. Up to 50% of all lesions arise in the lacrimal fossa, and up to 17% of lesions occur bilaterally. For all lesions, early biopsy is recommended to establish a diagnosis and characterize the lesions to reflect distinct morphologic, immunologic, cytogenetic, and molecular properties under the Revised European American Lymphoma (REAL) classification.[40] This classification has been shown to predict differences in the clinical behavior of these lesions. The classification allocates adnexal lymphomas to one of five categories: marginal zone lymphoma (MALT), diffuse lymphoplasmacytoid/lymphoplasmacytic lymphoma, follicle center lymphoma, diffuse large B-cell lymphoma, and other rare lymphomas.

Management of adnexal lymphoma involves a metastatic work-up by an oncologist. Ocular disease is generally treated with 2000–3000 cGy of external-beam radiation therapy, which results in local control in virtually all cases and may prevent systemic spread. However, at least 50% of patients eventually have systemic lymphoma detected and treatment of systemic dissemination is based on the pathologic grade of the lesion and its characteristic degree of aggressiveness. Some indolent lymphomas are refractory to chemotherapy and are associated with long-term survival, whereas more aggressive lymphomas may be cured with aggressive chemotherapy and/or radiation.

Some studies suggest that patients with bilateral orbital involvement have a poorer prognosis. Conjunctival lesions have the lowest likelihood (20%) of developing systemic disease. Eyelid lymphomas have the highest likelihood (67%), with orbital lesions in between (35%).

Lacrimal gland tumors

Lacrimal gland tumors can be easily identified with ophthalmic ultrasonography, but a more clear definition of tumor location, especially bony involvement, is best demonstrated with CT scans. When lacrimal gland masses are bilateral on orbital imaging, they generally represent lesions such as sarcoid, orbital pseudotumor, or lymphoma. Of those lacrimal gland masses not presenting with inflammatory signs, the majority represent lymphoproliferative disorders, as fully 50% of orbital lymphomas develop in the lacrimal fossa. Only a minority of lacrimal fossa lesions are primary epithelial neoplasms of the lacrimal gland. Biopsy is necessary in suspected cases to establish a pathologic diagnosis.

Approximately 50% of primary epithelial neoplasms of the lacrimal gland are benign mixed tumors (pleomorphic adenomas) and about 50% are carcinomas. Approximately half of the carcinomas are adenoid cystic tumors (Figure 7), and the remainder include malignant mixed tumors, primary adenocarcinomas,

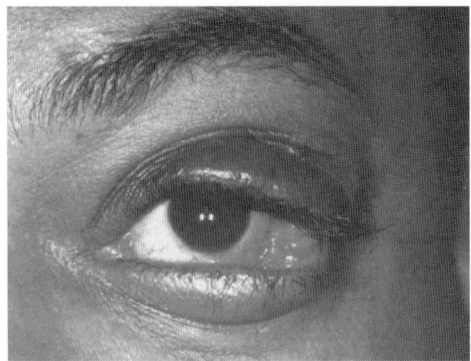

Figure 7 Adenoid cystic carcinoma of the lacrimal gland in a patient who underwent 2 biopsies of the mass, both of which were equivocal. The patient developed metastases to the parotid gland and later died.

mucoepidermoid carcinomas, and squamous carcinomas. Treatment for primary malignant lacrimal gland tumors includes excisional surgery and radiation therapy. Except for pleomorphic adenomas that undergo successful surgical removal without a preliminary biopsy (with resultant tumor capsule rupture, increasing risk of recurrence), the clinical course for most of these tumors is that of multiple painful recurrences with ultimate mortality from intracranial extension or systemic metastases, often occurring a decade or more after initial presentation.

References

1 Abramson DH. Retinoblastoma: saving life with vision. *Annu Rev Med*. 2014;**65**:171–184.

2 Xu XL, Singh HP, Wang L, et al. Rb suppresses human cone-precursor-derived retinoblastoma tumours. *Nature*. 2014;**514**:385–388.

3 Albert DM. Historic review of retinoblastoma. *Ophthalmology*. 1987;**94**:654–662.

4 Dimaras H, Khetan V, Halliday W, et al. Loss of RB1 induces non-proliferative retinoma: increasing genomic instability correlates with progression to retinoblastoma. *Hum Mol Genet*. 2008;**17**:1363–1372.

5 Rushlow DE, Mol BM, Kennett JY, et al. Characterisation of retinoblastomas without RB1 mutations: genomic, gene expression, and clinical studies. *Lancet Oncol*. 2013;**14**:327–334.

6 Dunn JM, Phillips RA, Becker AJ, Gallie BL. Identification of germline and somatic mutations affecting the retinoblastoma gene. *Science*. 1988;**241**: 1797–1800.

7 Harbour JW. Overview of RB gene mutations in patients with retinoblastoma. Implications for clinical genetic screening. *Ophthalmology*. 1998;**105**:1442–1447.

8 Abramson DH, Beaverson K, Sangani P, et al. Screening for retinoblastoma: presenting signs as prognosticators of patient and ocular survival. *Pediatrics*. 2003;**112**:1248–1255.

9 Reese AB. *Tumors of the Eye*, 3rd ed. New York: Harper and Row; 1976.

10 Murphree AL. The case for a new evidence-based group classification of intraocular retinoblastoma: linking natural history with clinical outcomes. In: *International Conference of Ocular Oncology*, September 3, 2005; Whistler, Canada.

11 Chan HS, DeBoer G, Thiessen JJ, et al. Combining cyclosporin with chemotherapy controls intraocular retinoblastoma without requiring radiation. *Clin Cancer Res*. 1996;**2**:1499–1508.

12 Abramson DH, Schefler AC. Update on retinoblastoma. *Retina*. 2004;**24**:828–848.

13 Yamane T, Kaneko A, Mohri M. The technique of ophthalmic arterial infusion therapy for patients with intraocular retinoblastoma. *Int J Clin Oncol*. 2004;**9**:69–73.

14 Gobin YP, Dunkel IJ, Marr BP, Brodie SE, Abramson DH. Intra-arterial chemotherapy for the management of retinoblastoma: four-year experience. *Arch Ophthalmol*. 2011 Jun;**129**(**6**):732–737.

15 Francis JH, Schaiquevich P, Buitrago E, et al. Local and systemic toxicity of intravitreal melphalan for vitreous seeding in retinoblastoma: a preclinical and clinical study. *Ophthalmology*. 2014;**121**(**9**):1810–1817.

16 Chantada G, Fandino A, Davila MT, et al. Results of a prospective study for the treatment of retinoblastoma. *Cancer*. 2004;**100**:834–842.

17 Dunkel IJ, Aledo A, Kernan NA, et al. Successful treatment of metastatic retinoblastoma. *Cancer*. 2000;**89**:2117–2121.

18 Abramson DH. Second nonocular cancers in retinoblastoma: a unified hypothesis. *The Franceschetti Lecture Ophthalmic Genet*. 1999;**20**:193–204.

19 Moll AC, Imhof SM, Schouten-Van Meeteren AY, Kuik DJ, Hofman P, Boers M. Second primary tumors in hereditary retinoblastoma: a register-based study, 1945–1997: is there an age effect on radiation-related risk? *Ophthalmology*. 2001;**108**:1109–1114.

20 Fletcher O, Easton D, Anderson K, Gilham C, Jay M, Peto J. Lifetime risks of common cancers among retinoblastoma survivors. *J Natl Cancer Inst*. 2004;**96**:357–363.

21 Abramson DH, Jereb B, Wollner N, Murphy L, Ellsworth RM. Leukemic ophthalmopathy detected by ultrasound. *J Pediatr Ophthalmol Strabismus*. 1983;**20**:92–97.

22 Haik BG. Vascular tumors of the orbit. In: Hornblass A, ed. *Ophthalmic and Orbital Plastic Reconstructive Surgery*. Baltimore: Williams and Wilkins; 1989:509–517.

23 Teske S, Ohlrich SJ, Gole G, Spiro P, Miller M, Sullivan TJ. Treatment of orbital capillary haemangioma with interferon. *Aust N Z J Ophthalmol*. 1994;**22**:13–17.

24 Jones IS. Lymphangiomas of the ocular adnexae: an analysis of 62 cases. *Am J Ophthalmol*. 1961;**51**:481–509.

25 Raney RB, Anderson JR, Kollath J, et al. Late effects of therapy in 94 patients with localized rhabdomyosarcoma of the orbit: report from the Intergroup Rhabdomyosarcoma Study (IRS)-III, 1984–1991. *Med Pediatr Oncol*. 2000;**34**:413–420.

26 Oberlin O, Rey A, Anderson J, et al. Treatment of orbital rhabdomyosarcoma: survival and late effects of treatment–results of an international workshop. *J Clin Oncol*. 2001;**19**:197–204.

27 Harbour JW, Onken MD, Roberson EDO, et al. Frequent mutation of BAP1 in metastasizing uveal melanomas. *Science*. 2010;**330**:1410–1413.

28 Collaborative Ocular Melanoma Study Group. Accuracy of diagnosis of choroidal melanomas in the Collaborative Ocular Melanoma Study. COMS report no. 1. *Arch Ophthalmol*. 1990;**108**:1268–1273.

29 Collaborative Ocular Melanoma Study Group. Assessment of metastatic disease status at death in 435 patients with large choroidal melanoma in the Collaborative Ocular Melanoma Study (COMS): COMS report no. 15. *Arch Ophthalmol*. 2001;**119**:670–676.

30 Shields JA, Shields CL, Donoso LA. Management of posterior uveal melanoma. *Surv Ophthalmol*. 1991;**36**:161–195.

31 Prescher G, Bornfeld N, Hirche H, Horsthemke B, Jockel KH, Becher R. Prognostic implications of monosomy 3 in uveal melanoma. *Lancet*. 1996;**347**:1222–1225.

32 Onken MD, Worley LA, Ehlers JP, Harbour JW. Gene expression profiling in uveal melanoma reveals two molecular classes and predicts metastatic death. *Cancer Res*. 2004;**64**:7205–7209.

33 Martin M, Maßhöfer L, Temming P, et al. Exome sequencing identifies recurrent somatic mutations in EIF1AX and SF3B1 in uveal melanoma with disomy 3. *Nat Genet*. 2013;**45**:933–936.

34 Carvajal RD, Sosman JA, Quevedo JF, et al. Effect of selumetinib vs chemotherapy on progression-free survival in uveal melanoma: a randomized clinical trial. *JAMA*. 2014;**311**:2397–2405.

35 Collaborative Ocular Melanoma Study Group. Mortality in patients with small choroidal melanoma. COMS report no. 4. The Collaborative Ocular Melanoma Study Group. *Arch Ophthalmol*. 1997;**115**:886–893.

36 Diener-West M, Earle JD, Fine SL, et al. The COMS randomized trial of iodine 125 brachytherapy for choroidal melanoma, III: initial mortality findings. COMS Report No. 18. *Arch Ophthalmol*. 2001;**119**:969–982.

37 Collaborative Ocular Melanoma Study Group. The Collaborative Ocular Melanoma Study (COMS) randomized trial of pre-enucleation radiation of large choroidal melanoma II: initial mortality findings. COMS report no. 10. *Am J Ophthalmol*. 1998;**125**:779–796.

38 Shields CL, Shields JA, Gross NE, Schwartz GP, Lally SE. Survey of 520 eyes with uveal metastases. *Ophthalmology*. 1997;**104**:1265–1276.

39 Keltner JL, Thirkill CE, Tyler NK, Roth AM. Management and monitoring of cancer-associated retinopathy. *Arch Ophthalmol*. 1992;**110**:48–53.

40 Coupland SE, Krause L, Delecluse HJ, et al. Lymphoproliferative lesions of the ocular adnexa. Analysis of 112 cases. *Ophthalmology*. 1998;**105**:1430–1441.

79 Neoplasms of the endocrine glands: pituitary neoplasms

Chirag D. Gandhi, MD, FACS, FAANS ▪ Margaret Pain, MD ▪ Kalmon D. Post, MD, FACS, FAANS

Overview

Pituitary neoplasms represent a phenotypically and pathologically diverse family of tumors. Treatment and classification are both patient and tumor specific as symptoms may derive from abnormal hormone production, compression of adjacent nervous system structures, and, in rare cases, metastases. Transsphenoidal surgery represents a common and well-tolerated treatment for most pituitary adenomas; however, advances in radiation and chemotherapy have increased treatment options, enhancing treatment efficacy, and eligibility.

Pituitary adenomas are epithelial tumors arising from the adeno-hypophysis that can manifest with neurological symptoms from local mass effect such as headaches, visual disturbances, increased intracranial pressure, and cranial nerve palsies or as a variety of clinical entities depending on the hormones they secrete. In rare cases (<1%), patients can also present with diabetes insipidus. Pituitary adenomas constitute 10–15% of intracranial tumors, although the incidence is as high as 24% in autopsy series. They are most common in the third and fourth decades of life and overall affect both sexes equally. However, there are differences in frequency of certain subtypes between the sexes. Cushing's disease, for example, is more common in women; Prolactin (PRL)-secreting adenomas are more common in young women; and null-cell adenomas, onco-cytomas, and gonadotropin-secreting adenomas are more common in men.

Distinction between pituitary neoplasm subtypes has been refined progressively as we have come to understand more about the pathology and biochemistry of the pituitary gland. Early on, tumors were classified based on the light microscopy characteristics of the predominant cell cytoplasm and were therefore divided into categories as acidophilic, basophilic, or chromophobic tumors. Acidophils were thought to produce excess amounts of growth hormone (GH) and were linked to acromegaly and gigantism; basophils were thought to secrete adrenocorticotrophic hormone (ACTH) and to cause Cushing's disease; and chromophobes were regarded as hormonally inactive. This system has become too simplistic for modern treatment algorithms as hormone secretion is only loosely associated with hematoxylin and eosin staining. It has been well established that both acidophilic and basophilic adenomas may secrete other hormones and that chromophobes can be hormonally active capable of secreting GH, PRL, ACTH, thyroid-secreting hormone (TSH), follicle-stimulating hormone (FSH), luteinizing hormone (LH), or α-subunit.[1]

From a medical perspective, tumors are frequently categorized based on the predominant hormone that they secrete.[2,3] Tumors are further categorized as hormonally active or inactive and are considered active only if the amount of hormone they secrete exceeds normal levels in the blood and is clinically evident. Inactive adenomas contain secretory and cellular components necessary for hormone production, but they are not associated with clinical or biochemical evidence of hormone excess. There are several theories about the etiology of inactive adenomas. One theory is that the gland cells become neoplastic but inherently have low hormone production. Another proposed theory is that the cells produce abnormal hormone that is not recognized by antibodies in the standard radioimmunoassays, and finally that the cells have lost the ability to produce hormone through some acquired genetic defect.[4] This functional classification is now being further modified to incorporate recent advances in molecular and immunohistochemical advances in pituitary research.

Anatomically and radiologically, tumors can also be classified based on their relationship to and involvement within the cavernous sinus. Magnetic resonance imaging (MRI) is the modality of choice and should be requested with a special consideration given toward imaging the pituitary. This can usually be achieved by obtaining thin slices through the pituitary in the coronal and sagittal planes (Figure 1). With high sensitivity for intracranial pathology, coronal T_2-weighted images give greater clarity to possible optic chiasm displacement as well as hemorrhagic and cystic changes within the tumor. Gadolinium contrast enhancement is essential for increasing the diagnostic yield for microadenomas (<10 mm) and is also useful in delineating normal from abnormal tissue in macroadenomas (T_1-weighted images pre- and postgadolinium).[5] In general, pituitary adenomas appear as a hypointense lesion on a T_1 precontrast image and will enhance less than normal pituitary tissue on T1 postcontrast series. Radiographic appearance has been used to further categorize parasellar invasive tumors according to the schema derived by Jules Hardy and/or Engelbert Knosp (Figure 2). The Knosp classification scheme has emerged as a relevant strategy for preoperative prediction of cavernous sinus invasion. Briefly, the MRI appearance of the tumor and its influence on the medial wall of the sinus relative to the position of the intracavernous internal carotid artery are used to estimate the likelihood of invasion. Increasing mass effect of the tumor on the medial wall correlates with increased likelihood of invasiveness. When compared with noninvasive tumors, invasive tumors are more likely to demonstrate aggressive behavior.[7]

Molecular biological investigation into pituitary tumorigenesis has demonstrated that adenomas are a result of monoclonal proliferation[8–10] and that neoplastic progression is related to both oncogenes and dysfunctional tumor suppression. Although several mutations have been implicated in pituitary tumorigenesis, only one mutation has been identified with significant prevalence in affected patients. Approximately 10–40% of GH-secreting adenomas result from a point mutation affecting the α-chain of the GTP-binding

Holland-Frei Cancer Medicine, Ninth Edition. Edited by Robert C. Bast Jr., Carlo M. Croce, William N. Hait, Waun Ki Hong, Donald W. Kufe, Martine Piccart-Gebhart, Raphael E. Pollock, Ralph R. Weichselbaum, Hongyang Wang, and James F. Holland.
© 2017 John Wiley & Sons, Inc. ISBN: 978-1-118-93469-2

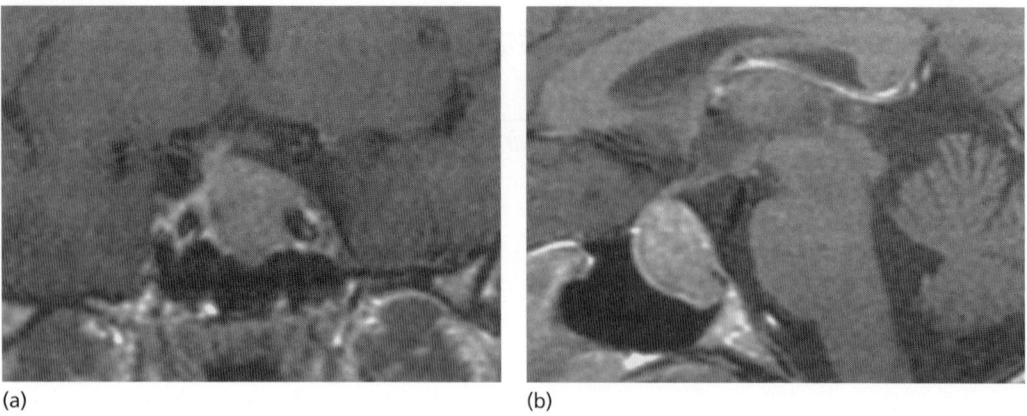

(a)   (b)

Figure 1 A 38-year-old woman with an ACTH-secreting adenoma. (a) Coronal T1-weighted magnetic resonance with contrast demonstrates a hypointense macroadenoma within the sella that extends into the left cavernous sinus and encases part of the carotid artery. (b) Sagittal T1-weighted magnetic resonance with contrast demonstrates a hyperintense macroadenoma within the sella.

Sella turcica radiological classification	Extrasellar extensions				
	Suprasellar			Parasellar	
Grade 0 (normal)	A	B	C	D	E
Grade I					
Grade II					
Grade III					
Grade IV	Symmetrical			Asymmetrical	

(a)   (b)

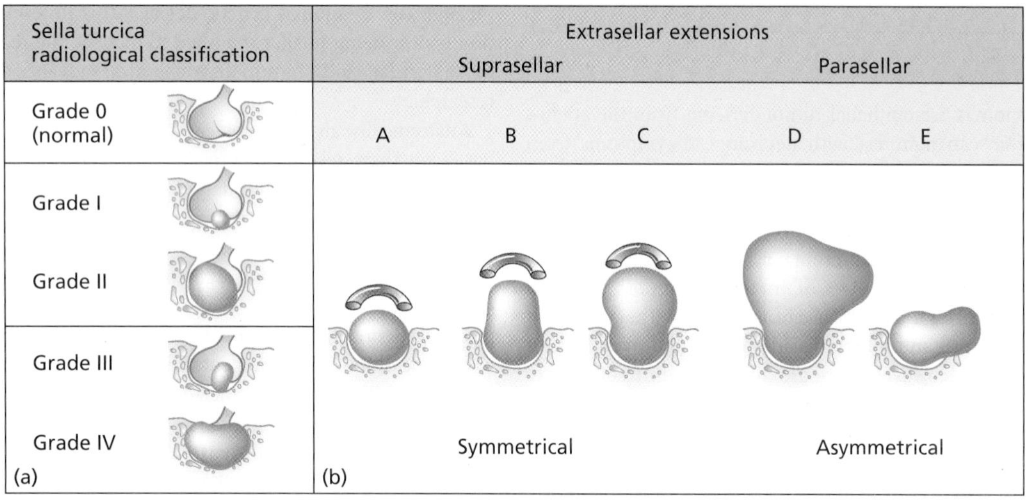

Figure 2 (a) Hardy's classification of pituitary adenomas. Grade I and II are enclosed within the sella. Grades III and IV are invasive. Extrasellar classifications A, B, and C are increasing amounts of direct suprasellar adenomas. D is asymmetric extension, and E is lateral extension into the cavernous sinus. Source: Adapted from Hardy J and Somma M.[6] (b) Knosp classification of cavernous sinus invasion. Source: Woodworth, GF et al. J. Neurosurgery 120:1086–1094, 2014.

protein, leading to constitutive cAMP activation. It is postulated that the elevated cAMP formation leads to GH hypersecretion and adenoma proliferation.[11] Although it has been theorized that adenomas with this gsp oncogene mutation are smaller and more sensitive to medical therapy, recent studies have failed to demonstrate any phenotypic differences between patient with the mutation and those without it.[12] Many other additional factors have been identified to influence tumor progression. Oncogenes linked to adenoma progression include cAMP-responsive nuclear transcription factor, CREB, which is thought to be promoted by the overexpression of Gsα[12]; ras oncogene mutations that have been detected in aggressive prolactinomas[13]; and the pituitary tumor transforming gene (PTTG) thought to be a marker for invasiveness in secretory adenomas.[14,15] Tumor suppressor genes such as Rb, menin, TP53, p27, p16,[16,17] hormone-promoting factors such as hypothalamic neurohormones, and locally produced growth factors and cytokines are also being studied for their contribution to adenoma growth.[18] With research into galectin-3 (Gal-3), a therapeutic drug target found only in PRL- and ACTH-secreting tumors, as well as nuclear receptor, peroxisome proliferator-activated receptor gamma (PPAR-γ), isolated from a number of studied adenomas, there is promise for novel drug development.[19–21]

Evaluation of a patient with suspected or known pituitary adenoma requires both complete radiographic and endocrinological and potentially genetic assessment before initiation of therapy.[22] Endocrine assessment should include a complete metabolic panel, pregnancy test, serum GH, insulin-like growth factor (IGF-1), TSH, free T4, T3, PRL, ACTH, cortisol, LH, FSH, and testosterone. Following these tests, the determination of further medical or surgical treatments can be made.

Surgery is the preferred and definitive treatment of all pituitary adenomas with the exception of prolactinomas and asymptomatic, hormonally inactive tumors (incidentalomas). On the basis of the innovative work of Cushing, Guiot, and Hardy, the transsphenoidal approach is the preferred surgical technique for most adenomas and is associated with minimal morbidity and rapid recovery.[23,24] The goals of surgery include the reduction of tumor-related mass effect on adjacent structures, the cessation of endocrine hyperactivity, and the preservation or restoration of normal pituitary function. Adjuvant treatment can then be initiated based on the histopathology and immunochemistry, postoperative hormone secretory status, and the degree of extrasellar extension. In contrast, prolactinomas frequently respond well to medical therapy and incidental tumors require only observation until they are associated with symptoms.

Finally, a small percentage of pituitary neoplasms demonstrate aggressive behavior or carcinomatous change. Hormonally active tumors usually require hormone-specific therapy but this may not be sufficient for disease control. Temozolomide, an oral alkylating agent, has emerged as an effective adjunctive therapy for these patients.[25] Its efficacy is explained by the phenotype of low O[6]-methylguanine-DNA methyltransferase (MGMT) expression frequently found in aggressive pituitary neoplasms.[26]

Prolactin-secreting pituitary adenomas

Prolactinomas are the most commonly diagnosed pituitary adenoma, representing approximately 30% of cases.[27] Although rarely life threatening, when symptomatic, they can present with clinical findings relating to hyperprolactinemia (abnormal reproductive or sexual function) or mass effect on adjacent structures owing to size. Because of their reliable responsiveness to medical management, chemotherapeutics are often the first-line treatment for these tumors (Figure 3). However, surgical treatment has been shown to be equally effective and may be indicated at a primary intervention for certain cases.

Clinical presentation

Although autopsy studies have demonstrated that prolactinomas have similar prevalence between the genders, women are four times more likely than men to become symptomatic. In women of reproductive age, hyperprolactinemia may cause oligomenorrhea, secondary amenorrhea, galactorrhea, and sterility. Less common symptoms in this population are decreased libido, dry vaginal mucosa caused by estrogen deficiency, weight gain, and psychological symptoms such as depression and anxiety. Prolactinomas account for approximately 5% of women with primary amenorrhea and 25% of women with secondary amenorrhea (excluding pregnancy).[28] When the presentations of amenorrhea are accompanied by concomitant galactorrhea, the incidence of prolactinoma increases to 70–80%.[29]

In men and postmenopausal women, where symptomatic hyperprolactinemia is much more subtle, the tumors may grow to much larger sizes and are detected only when they begin to produce symptoms related to mass effect. Macroadenoma-related mass effect may result in headaches, visual disturbances (typically bitemporal hemianopsia as a result of chiasmatic compression), hypopituitarism, ophthalmoplegia, and, rarely, noncommunicating

hydrocephalus from obstruction of the foramen of Monro. Men may also experience a diminished libido, impotence, gynecomastia, and infertility from decreased androgen production. The mechanism of hypogonadism caused by hyperprolactinemia is still controversial. One possibility is that PRL alters the hypothalamic release of gonadotropin-releasing hormone (GnRH) through dopamine inhibition, which in turn causes disruptions in the normal pulsatile secretion of LH.[30] Prolonged periods of hyperprolactinemia have also been linked to bone demineralization by way of hypogonadism as bone density is normal in eumenorrheic hyperprolactinemic women.[31]

Diagnosis

Beside prolactinomas, hyperprolactinemia can be associated with a variety of causes such as pregnancy, hypothyroidism, PRL-stimulating drugs (e.g., phenothiazines, butyrophenones, and metoclopramide), and renal failure that need to be considered in the differential diagnosis. In addition, physiological hyperprolactinemia can occur from psychological and physical stresses, such as exercise, surgery, and hypoglycemia, but the PRL level rarely excessed 40 ng/mL in these cases.[32] A definitive diagnosis of prolactinoma is difficult and in most cases requires radiographic evidence in addition to elevated PRL levels. In men, a basal PRL value greater than 100 ng/mL is almost always indicative of a prolactinoma. In women, PRL levels of 100–200 ng/mL should raise suspicion for prolactinoma, while a level of over 200 ng/mL is highly suggestive of prolactinoma.[33,34] The greatest diagnostic uncertainty lies in patients with PRL levels between 50 and 100 ng/mL. Within this range, hyperprolactinemia may also be related to "stalk effect," where mass of a tumor interferes with the flow of prolactin-inhibitory factor (PRIF) from the hypothalamus. Although various endocrine stimulation tests to differentiate these two possibilities have been suggested, they have not been proven reliable.[35]

Serum PRL levels are an index of secretory activity and have been found to be associated with the size of the prolactinoma (excluding cystic or necrotic components). Eighty percent of tumors producing less than 200 ng/mL are microadenomas, while at levels above 200 ng/mL only 20% are microadenomas. This relationship becomes unreliable for very large tumors (>4 cm). While the total PRL level may usually correlate with size and may even be greater than 1000 ng/mL, the laboratory value may be falsely low (25–150 ng/mL) and not reflect the actual serum concentration because of a phenomenon known as the "Hook effect."[36,37] Briefly,

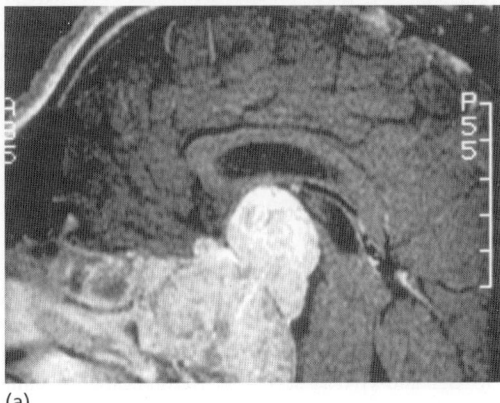
(a)

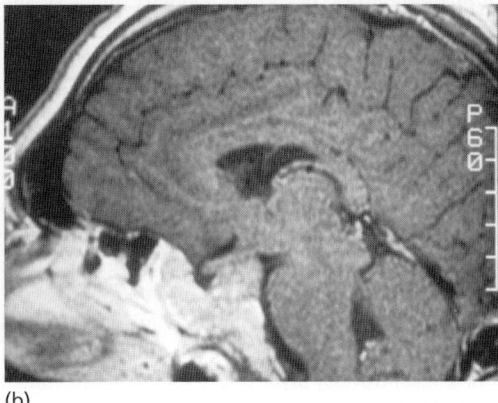
(b)

Figure 3 A 52-year-old male with diminished libido and a macroprolactinoma. (a) Sagittal T1-weighted magnetic resonance with contrast demonstrates a large sellar/suprasellar adenoma with compression of the optic chiasm. (b) Sagittal T1-weighted with contrast demonstrates a significant reduction in tumor volume after being treated medically with bromocriptine.

the Hook effect results from saturation of the antibody binding sites during the radioimmunoassay and therefore distorting the binding curve. This can be resolved by performing serial dilutions and should be considered for all giant pituitary adenomas.

Treatment

The treatment options available to a patient with a prolactinoma include observation, medical therapy, surgery, and radiotherapy. Treatment decisions should take into consideration the tumor size, PRL level, clinical manifestations, tolerance of medical therapy, and the desire for fertility. The vast majority of microprolactinomas (<10 mm) do not increase in size.[34] Together with autopsy studies suggesting higher prevalence of undiagnosed tumors within the population, many clinicians and patient opt for observation and against treatment for microadenomas in the absence of clinical hyperprolactinemia, normal pituitary function, and no desire for pregnancy.

Dopamine agonists have been shown to be highly effective in suppressing tumor growth and PRL production because dopamine, when secreted by the hypothalamus, is an endogenous inhibitor of PRL production. Bromocriptine was the first dopamine agonist to be used for treatment of prolactinomas, but newer agents such as cabergoline, quinagolide, lisuride, and terguride have also gained widespread acceptance. On a molecular level, dopamine agonists selectively activate type D2 dopamine receptors, thereby blocking transcription of the PRL gene.[38] The shrinkage of PRL cells results in amyloid deposition and fibrosis of the tumor.[39] Dopamine agonists have been shown to have a high response rate with normalization of PRL levels in 70–80% of patients, tumor shrinkage in 80–90%, and restoration of ovulation in 80–90%.[40] On the basis of these results, some argue that medical treatment should be used in all patients except the 10% who experience significant side effects.[41] In addition, there is evidence to suggest that a significant percentage of patients who respond to cabergoline with normalization of PRL levels and tumor shrinkage will remain in remission following discontinuation of the drug after 2 years.[42,43] However, even in patients who have optimal response to cabergoline (normalization of PRL, tumor volume reduction, no invasion of critical structures, or optic chiasm compression), the majority do experience recurrence and so close follow-up after treatment discontinuation is critical.[43]

Dopamine agonists do have some significant disadvantages that may temper their use. For many patients, the effects are reversible and therefore lifelong compliance is needed to control the disease. In addition, significant side effects such as nausea, vomiting, postural hypotension, headaches, XX depression, and anxiety have been reported with medication use. In cases of pituitary apoplexy and in tumors with large cystic components, dopamine agonists are not effective in shrinkage as tumor size is not correlated with tumor cellularity. More harmful side effects of dopamine agonists have also been reported. At much higher doses of cabergoline than the maximum dose used for prolactinomas, cardiac toxicity has occurred. Although subclinical valvular fibrosis and trace mitral regurgitation with cabergoline therapy of prolactinomas has been reported, no patients experienced clinically significant change in cardiac function as a result.[44,45,136] Finally, dopamine agonists are not always effective for the treatment of prolactinomas. Bromocriptine resistance may be an indicator of increased tumor aggressiveness, and there may be an association between gand medication resistance.[46]

Currently, there is controversy in the role of surgery for treatment of prolactinomas. With requirement for strict long-term compliance and frequent medical follow-up, some argue that surgery should be the initial treatment with medical therapy as an adjunct only in cases without remission.[47] The rate of long-term remission after surgery varies significantly with preoperative PRL levels and tumor size. Remission rates are best, 50–80%, for microadenomas with preoperative PRL levels of less than 200 ng/mL.[40,47–49] Rates drop significantly for macroadenomas and in patients with PRL levels of 200–500 ng/mL. Surgery has not been shown to be useful in giant adenomas and tumors with PRL levels greater than 500 ng/mL, as a complete resection is rarely possible. Even in these patients, however, dopamine agonists appear to be beneficial. Meta-analysis has found that three-fourths of patients experienced significant reduction in tumor volume and normalization of PRL level in 60–70%.[50] There is evidence to suggest that surgery is more effective when dopamine agonists are used as neo-adjuvant therapy.[51] In addition, some have demonstrated that surgery to be beneficial in cases of dopamine resistance as partial tumor resection was associated with better hormonal control and lower doses of dopamine agonists.[52,53] Overall, there is an inverse correlation between PRL levels and remission rates.

Conventional radiotherapy is generally not considered a primary mode of treatment.[54] The use of stereotactic radiosurgery as either a primary[55] or adjuvant[56] therapy is becoming increasingly common. Radiosurgery has been shown to be successful in decreasing PRL levels (and in one study, 30% of patients achieved an endocrinological cure.[57] As radiotherapy is rarely used alone, these data may be skewed by confounding factors.

Medical therapy by means of dopamine agonists remains the first-line treatment for most prolactinomas[58] This treatment should be considered for all patients, including those desiring pregnancy and those with primary amenorrhea.

For tumors larger than 2 cm or with PRL levels between 200 and 500 ng/mL, neo-adjuvant treatment with dopamine agonists appears to reduce tumor volume, followed by surgery. Any residual tumor can then be treated medically. For very large, invasive, or tumors associated with PRL levels of greater than 500 ng/mL, medical therapy should be the primary treatment modality.[50]

Special consideration should be given to patients with prolactinomas during pregnancy. There is a small but serious risk of rapid expansion of the tumor off medication. Complications related to this growth occur primarily from macroadenomas with suprasellar extension; they are much less frequent for microadenomas.[59] If these patients become symptomatic, a dopamine agonist can be administered. Both bromocriptine and cabergolide are US FDA pregnancy category B, indicating that animal studies have not shown risk to the fetus but that randomized, controlled trials in humans are inadequate to assess the risk comprehensively.[60,61] During pregnancy, surgery should be undertaken only if the tumor does not respond to medical treatment or if there are progressive neurological symptoms. To reduce the risk of pregnancy-related complications, patients with macroadenomas who desire pregnancy should undergo transsphenoidal resection before conception or remain on bromocriptine throughout the pregnancy.

Growth hormone-secreting pituitary adenomas

GH secretion is under hypothalamic control through somatostatin and growth hormone-releasing hormone (GHRH). Upon release, GH causes the production of IGF-1 from the liver, which affects bone and tissue growth and provides negative-feedback inhibition to GH and GHRH secretion. Acromegaly, the clinical condition associated with GH-producing adenomas, results in autonomous GH secretion and loss of this negative-feedback inhibition. However, the clinical manifestations of GH-secreting tumors have been found to correlate better with IGF-1 levels than with GH levels.

Clinical presentation

GH-secreting pituitary adenomas account for about 30% of all endocrine-active pituitary tumors. Most patients present in their third to fifth decade with macroadenomas and a long history of subclinical symptoms that usually ranges between 4 and 10 years.[62] GH excess classically presents as acromegaly or gigantism, both marked by an insidious coarsening of features with frontal bossing and prognathism, macroglossia, and exaggerated acral growth. Patients are also found to develop organomegaly, hypertension, cardiomyopathy, congestive heart failure, restrictive lung disease, sleep apnea, and arthropathies. In addition, a very high percentage of these patients develop impaired glucose metabolism and diabetes mellitus. Common presenting symptoms include fatigue, headaches, arthralgias, oily skin, and hyperhidrosis. For patients with variant tumors that also cosecrete PRL, amenorrhea, galactorrhea, and loss of libido may also be present. With an insidious onset and high rate of medical comorbidities at time of presentation, untreated patients have a high rate of early mortality- as high as 50% at 50 years old and 2–3 times that of the general population.[63]

Diagnosis

Acromegaly is frequently suspected based on change of appearance and sub-clinical history. Hormone hypersecretion can be assessed through analysis of basal fasting GH levels or age- and gender-adjusted IGF-1. Elevated basal fasting GH levels greater than 2.5 ng/mL suggest acromegaly. However, because GH has both a short half-life and is secreted in a pulsatile manner, assessment of IGF-1 often generates a more accurate assessment of GH excess.[64] Dynamic testing is typically reserved for monitoring therapeutic efficacy. The oral glucose tolerance test (OGTT) tracks GH response to a large oral glucose load (75–100g). Normal patients respond to the glucose load with GH suppression and levels fall below 1 ng/mL. Loss of glucose-induced suppression is diagnostic for a GH—secreting tumor. A study of 92 patients with acromegaly suggests that nadir levels of GH did not vary significantly based on either age or gender.[65]

Although rare, ectopic GHRH has been reported to account for approximately 1% of acromegaly cases. When responsible for GH excess, the ectopic GHRH production can usually be attributed to tumors in the chest or abdomen. To avoid unnecessary surgery, image confirmation of a pituitary tumor should be obtained after making a clinical and biochemical diagnosis.

Treatment

The clinical definition for cure of acromegaly has been refined several times since the introduction of the GH assay in the 1960s. Currently, the biochemical goals of therapy are to reduce basal GH levels to less than 2.5 ng/mL, normalize IGF-1 levels, and achieve a nadir GH level of less than 1 ng/mL during an OGTT.[66] A complete cure should lead to recovery of normal pituitary function and, in most cases, a slow reversal of both cosmetic and physiological abnormalities.

Transsphenoidal surgery remains the first-line therapy for GH-secreting tumors.[63] The advantages of surgery include a prompt decrease in GH levels and a tissue diagnosis. At our institution, a 14-year review of 115 patients demonstrated that surgery alone produced biochemical remission in 61% of cases.[67] The rate was 88% for microadenomas and 53% for macroadenomas. There was a negative correlation of surgical outcome with tumor size and preoperative GH levels. Immediate postoperative GH levels were found to correlate with long-term outcome. In cases where the postoperative GH level was less than 3 ng/mL, the chance of a favorable long-term outcome was 89%. Postoperative radiotherapy was given

to 32 patients and led to remission in 31% of these patients. An additional three patients achieved remission with a combination of surgery, radiotherapy, and medical treatment. The overall complication rate was 6.9% with no CSF leaks, meningitis, permanent diabetes insipidus, or new hypopituitarism. The recurrence rate was 5.4%. Other published studies reflect similar results.[68,69]

Both radiotherapy and radiosurgery have been used for treatment of acromegaly. The use of conventional external beam radiation has been found to reduce GH levels to less than 5 ng/mL in 50–70% of cases, but the effects can take as long as a decade to occur.[70] Hypopituitarism has been found in 50% of patients 10 years after irradiation, with an increasing incidence annually thereafter.[71] Radiosurgery has demonstrated normalization of GH levels within 3–5 years.[72] The likelihood of hypopituitarism is similar. In addition, radiation to sensitive adjacent structures such as the optic chiasm remains a concern and a 4-mm safety boundary is recommended for radiotherapy for all pituitary adenomas. In general, radiosurgery continues to be an adjunctive therapy after failed transsphenoidal surgery.[68,73,74] These results are somewhat difficult to interpret as the definition of "normal" was inconsistent.[57] Endocrine cure rates in a variety of small studies were found to range from 0% to 96% and improvement in 0–67%. Out of the 20 studies reviewed, 6 did not cite their criteria for cure, and 11 of 14 used different criteria to define cure. Unfortunately, the studies are further confounded by the inconsistent use of somatostatin analogs in patients undergoing radiosurgery. Current studies on the efficacy of radiosurgery also have limited long-term follow-up. Additional randomized studies are needed. A more recent retrospective study assessed endocrine cure rates by normal OGTT for patients with adjuvant radiosurgery and found that 65% of patients achieved remission at 61.5 months with a trend toward increased remission at later time points.[75] In spite of normalization of the oral glucose tolerance, a subset of patients experience persistent elevation of IGF-1 after radiotherapy, demonstrating persistent pituitary axis dysfunction and subtle clinical symptoms of acromegaly.[76]

Medical management as the primary or adjuvant treatment of acromegaly remains a controversial topic. In patients with no visual loss, some endocrinologists have advocated treatment with somatostatin analogs as the first-line therapy.[77] However, in the context of the significant long-term morbidity associated with acromegaly, most practitioners recommend surgery as the first-line treatment with adjuvant medical or radiotherapy, if needed. Three classes of drugs are used to treat acromegaly: dopamine agonists, somatostatin analogs, and GH-receptor blockers. Dopamine agonists such as bromocriptine and cabergoline have been shown to provide symptomatic relief in some acromegalic patients.[78] Although they have limited efficacy, these medications remain popular treatments for acromegaly because of their low cost and oral administration. In comparison, somatostatin analogs have been shown to be more effective. Octreotide was found to normalize IGF-1 and reduce GH levels to less than 5 ng/mL in approximately 50% of patients.[79] The long-acting analogs such as lanreotide and octreotide LAR are slightly more effective and reduce GH to less than 2.5 ng/mL for 70% of patients and normalize IGF-1 in 88% of patients.[80–82] Another class of medication for treatment of acromegaly are GH-receptor antagonists. At this time, pegvisomant is the only medication in this class with FDA approval. This class of medications is unique in that the site of action is not within the pituitary gland but rather on the receptors for GH. By preventing dimerization of the GH receptor, pegvisomant inhibits production of IGF-1, the hormone responsible for most of the clinical sequelae of acromegaly. Because it does not affect tumor size or GH production, this medication is typically reserved for cases of acromegaly that are refractory to other treatments. The medication has notable side effects including hepatic transaminitis and an association with rare tumor growth.[83] Because of this, it is recommended that patients prescribed pegvisomant be monitored with regular MRI exams and liver function tests.

Medical treatment demonstrates good results with regard to management of the clinical effects of GH excess. It has been found to provide symptomatic relief of headaches and hyperhidrosis as well as to improve arthropathy and cardiac function. If the medication is able to normalize IGF-1 levels and GH levels in the OGTT, patients experience significant improvement in left ventricular ejection fraction. This is especially notable as patients with uncontrolled acromegaly tend to also have deterioration of LVEF.[84,85] Unlike prolactinomas, medication does not cure acromegaly. Although current medical therapies are well tolerated and demonstrate good efficacy, lifelong treatment is required in order to avoid recurrence. This presents a serious downside to medical therapy as its success is both expensive and dependent on long-term compliance. Because of this, many practitioners and patients use chemotherapy as an adjuvant to either surgery or radiotherapy. There has not been statistically significant benefit demonstrated for the use of neo-adjuvant somatostatin analog treatment.[86]

A minority (20–30%) of GH-secreting adenomas also secrete PRL. If symptomatic, patients may experience amenorrhea, galactorrhea, impotence, or loss of libido. Dopamine agonists are particularly effective in the treatment of mixed GH- and PRL-secreting tumors, but transsphenoidal surgery still remains the first-line treatment.[87]

Adrenocorticotrophic hormone-secreting adenomas

Cushing's disease represents the most frequent cause of clinical hypercortisolism, or "Cushing's syndrome." ACTH-producing tumors stimulate adrenal hyperplasia and ultimately result in hypercortisolism. Many consider Cushing's disease the most challenging pituitary endocrinopathy both to diagnose and to treat. Tumors are often small and evade detection by radiological imaging. Macroadenomas are often aggressive and have a high rate of recurrence. Demographically, Cushing's disease is nine times more common in women with a peak incidence in the third and fourth decades of life.

Clinical presentation

Only about 10–20% of ACTH-secreting adenomas are large enough to produce mass effect with resultant visual field deficits, cranial neuropathies, or hypopituitarism. The majority of tumors are less than 5 mm and present with clinical hypercortisolism. Common presenting features of Cushing's disease include central obesity, moon facies, buffalo hump, hirsuitism, purple abdominal striae, and acne. Other clinical findings include hypertension, osteopenia, proximal myopathy, diabetes mellitus, and, very frequently, psychiatric disorders. Affected patients experience significant morbidity from the condition with a 5-year mortality rate of 50% in those left untreated.[88] The increased morbidity and mortality are unique to secretory Cushing's disease patients, thought to be sequelae of increased cortisol exposure. Among the predictors of increased mortality in Cushing's patients, duration of clinical hypercortisolism, preoperative ACTH concentration, and depression have been shown to be significant.[89]

Diagnosis

Accurate diagnosis of Cushing's disease depends on identifying evidence of hypercortisolism and localizing the pathology to the pituitary gland. Accuracy in diagnosis approaches 100% with a complete workup;[90] however, each individual test has a failure rate of 10–30% (Table 1).[91]

Hypercortisolism can be demonstrated through elevation in 24-h urinary free cortisol and 17-OH corticosteroids. Assays for midnight salivary cortisol have also been shown to be both sensitive and specific for hypercortisolism.[92] The etiology of hypercortisolism should be assessed first with a low-dose dexamethasone suppression test. This test assesses functioning of the hypothalamic–pituitary–adrenal negative-feedback loop for cortisol secretion. Patients with Cushing's disease will have hypercortisolism that persists in spite of a low-dose bolus of dexamethasone. However, 95% of Cushing's disease patients demonstrate a 50% decrease in plasma cortisol when a high dose of

Table 1 Biochemical evaluation for Cushing syndrome.

A. Screening for Cushing syndrome
  1 Measurement of 24 h UFC in two or three collections. Test is unequivocal for hypercortisolism if the cortisol level is fourfold that of normal in two of three screens. If equivocal, proceed to the low-dose DST. Salivary cortisol levels are also highly sensitive and specific
  2 Low-dose DST. 1 mg dexamethasone is administered at 11 p.m. and serum cortisol is drawn the following day at 8 a.m. A 2-day test is also commonly performed
       If < 5 µg/dL: Cushing syndrome is excluded
       If 5–10 µg/dL: Indeterminate and retesting is necessary
       If > 10 µg/dL: Cushing syndrome is probably present

B. Tests to distinguish primary Cushing disease from ectopic or adrenal tumors
  1 Serum ACTH is low in adrenal tumors. Plasma ACTH (values > 10 pg/mL are suggestive of ACTH-dependent disease; values < 5 pg/mL are suggestive of ACTH-independent disease)
       Abdominal CT can help identify a unilateral adrenal mass or bilateral adrenal enlargement in ACTH-dependent cases
  2 High-dose DST. 8 mg of dexamethasone is administered at 11 p.m. and serum cortisol is drawn the following day at 8 a.m. A 2-day test is also commonly performed
       In 95% of cases of Cushing disease, plasma cortisol is suppressed by 50%
       No suppression is seen with ectopic or adrenal sources
  3 CRH stimulation test. Can be used after an equivocal high-dose DST
       Cushing disease responds to CRH with further increases in plasma cortisol levels
       Ectopic and adrenal tumors do not respond to CRH
  4 IPSS is reserved for persistent equivocal testing or in re-operations in which IPSS was not initially performed
       After CRH administration, an inferior petrosal sinus/plasma ACTH gradient > 3 : 1 is suggestive of Cushing disease and aids with lateralization

Abbreviations: DST, dexamethasone suppression test; UFC, urinary free cortisol; CRH, corticotrophin releasing hormone; IPSS, inferior petrosal sinus sampling.

dexamethasone is used. Plasma ACTH levels should be assessed to differentiate a diagnosis of Cushing's disease from adrenal causes of hypercortisolism.[93] Diagnostic sensitivity for Cushing's disease can be further increased if a corticotrophin-releasing hormone (CRH) stimulation test is added to the workup.[94] Finally, inferior petrosal sinus sampling (IPSS) can be performed to improve tumor localization and diagnostic specificity if the previous workup is not definitive. While MRI is a sensitive study for tumor localization for tumors larger than 3 mm in diameter, conventional sequences fail to detect a high percentage of tumors.[95] However, with optimization of T1 postcontrast sequences or utilizing spoiled gradient recalled acquisition (SPGR), significantly more tumors can be visualized.[95,96] IPSS and cavernous sinus sampling can be helpful in these situations as they can confirm a pituitary pathology but laterality is incorrect in 25–30% of exams.[97]

Treatment

Transsphenoidal surgery is the first-line treatment for Cushing's disease. The overall remission rate following surgery ranges from 76% to 91%.[98] Microadenomas tended to have slightly better outcomes with remission rates between 84% and 94%[98] The major determining factor for success was the ability to localize the tumor on MRI.[99] In contrast, remission rates for macroadenomas appear to depend chiefly on the degree of invasiveness. Surgery alone achieves remission for 64% of patients, and when combined with adjuvant radiotherapy or radiosurgery, this number improves to 83% and 70%, respectively.[98,100]

While the postoperative course is unique for every patient, many patients with a successful tumor resection experience a rapid decline in their serum cortisol and ACTH levels. In some patients, this leads to life-threatening hypocortisolism (Addisonian crisis). Most patients require replacement therapy for up to 1 year as their hypothalamic–pituitary–adrenal axis recovers from the chronic ACTH overstimulation. Good prognostic factors for full postoperative remission include lower than normal serums levels of cortisol and ACTH. However, even with immediate improvement in serum cortisol, 15–25% of patients experience a recurrence.[21,101] In our experience, even normal cortisol and restoration of a normal response to dexamethasone suppression do not guarantee lasting remission. Because of this, long-term follow-up is essential in these patients.

Radiotherapy and radiosurgery are frequently used as adjuvant treatment when surgical results are inadequate. Conventional radiotherapy cure rates are as high as 90% at 5 years post-treatment.[102] However, a large proportion of these patients began to experience hypopituitarism in later years and 5% developed Nelson's syndrome.[102] Conventional radiation is not used as a primary modality because the effects of treatment take several years to develop while the symptoms and morbidities of Cushing's disease persist. In contrast, radiosurgery for Cushing's disease produces results much sooner. Remission is achieved in 35–90% of patients with much lower rates of hypopituitarism.[103,104] Full interpretation of these data is complicated by the fact that there was discrepancy in what constituted a "cure" and long-term follow-up was limited.

While medical therapy is not recommended as a primary treatment of Cushing's disease, it may be suitable for patients who do not experience improvement after surgery or who are otherwise not good candidates for surgery. Pasireotide was approved by the US FDA for these indications in 2012. A somatostatin analog with high specificity for the somatostatin receptor 5, it has been shown to be clinically effective in reduction of cortisol levels and should be considered the preferred medication to treat Cushing's disease.[105] In addition, chemotherapy can temporize patients with

severe hypercortisolism as they await surgery. In these cases, ketoconazole is often the drug of choice as it works to block adrenal steroid synthesis. Up to 90% of patients experience normalization of serum cortisol and ACTH while taking ketoconazole. However, the effects of this medication end immediately after cessation and patients on this medication must be closely monitored for hepatotoxicity.[106] Other medical treatments for Cushing's disease include aminoglutethimide, metyrapone, mitotane, and cyproheptadine. Dopamine agonists such as cabergoline have also been shown to be successful in the treatment of ACTH-secreting tumors. After 3 months of cabergoline treatment, 60% of patients demonstrated cortisol inhibition and 40% had normalization of cortisol secretion.[107] This finding could be explained by the observation that the majority of ACTH-secreting adenomas demonstrate positive dopamine receptor (D2) immunostaining.[107]

There are more radical surgical options for patients who do not respond to the above measures. Total adrenalectomy offers absolute control of cortisol secretion but requires lifelong dependence on exogenous glucocorticoid and mineralocorticoid replacement. Nelson's syndrome, a rapid enlargement of the pituitary adenoma from loss of cortisol negative-feedback inhibition, results in 10–30% of patients.[108] Nelson's syndrome typically presents with hyperpigmentation caused by stimulation of melanocytes by elevated ACTH. Most patients with Nelson's syndrome harbor large, invasive pituitary adenomas. Studies examining the effectiveness of neurosurgery for treatment of Nelson's syndrome have demonstrated variable rates of success.[109–111] There appears to be some prophylactic value in hypophyseal radiosurgery before adrenalectomy.[112]

In the event that ACTH and cortisol levels remain elevated after surgery, additional exploration of the pituitary is usually effective.[113] To increase the likelihood of success during the second surgery, IPSS should be performed before the operation. A complete hypophysectomy can be considered if previous treatments were unsuccessful but it is rarely indicated.

Silent ACTH-secreting adenomas

There is a subset of pituitary adenomas where immunohistochemical staining suggests ACTH production but the patient does not have clinical evidence of hypercortisolism. The exact incidence of this phenomenon is unclear but has been reported to be between 6% and 43%.[114] There is evidence that these tumors behave more aggressively than other ACTH-producing tumors and have a 37% rate of recurrence.[115,116] However, when compared to ACTH-negative nonfunctioning pituitary adenomas, these tumors demonstrated similar regrowth rates.[117] A subset of patients with these tumors also goes on to develop HPA axis dysfunction postoperatively and require postoperative steroid replacement.[114]

Gonadotropin-secreting and nonsecretory pituitary adenomas

Approximately one-third of pituitary tumors are considered nonsecretory adenomas. The peak incidence is in the fifth decade and patients typically present with symptomatic hypopituitarism, visual field defects, and visual concerns. Despite their similar clinical presentation, these tumors comprise a heterogeneous group of pathologies. Ultrastructural examination frequently demonstrates secretory granules and staining to suggest production of FH, LSH, and the α-subunit. A smaller subset produces other anterior pituitary hormones without clinical manifestation.[118] With such a heterogeneous group of tumors, there is no clear or consistent treatment algorithm or prognosis.

Clinical presentation

Because they are not associated with hypersecretion syndromes, patients with these tumors usually present with symptoms of mass effect. This can range from hypopituitarism to vision changes or headaches. The majority of cases are associated with a macroadenoma.

Treatment

Surgery remains the primary treatment of patients with inactive adenomas. The goals are to relieve the mass effect, restore pituitary function, and obtain a tissue diagnosis. As with other pituitary adenomas, a transsphenoidal approach is often preferred unless there is significant extrasellar extension. With no clear criteria for what is considered a cure, surgical efficacy is not as well described as with other tumors. Many patients do experience improvement in preoperative symptoms, and 70–80% experience significant improvement in visual function.[119] Nearly 100% experience improvement in headaches[120] and 15–57% with improvement in pituitary function.[119] However, this improvement is largely due to decompression of mass effect and should not be taken to be indicative of complete remission. The extent of resection should be assessed routinely with an MRI 3–4 months postoperatively. Imaging acquired earlier than this is often confounded by edema and otherwise normal postoperative changes. Residual tumor is identified in 66–86% of patients but the rate of recurrence is highly variable.[121,122]

Radiotherapy or radiosurgery is increasingly utilized either for primary or adjuvant treatment of nonsecretory adenomas. A recent multicenter study analyzing the safety and efficacy of radiosurgery for residual lesions found that overall tumor control was achieved in greater than 90% of patients at follow-up with low incidence of side effects.[123] The same group later went on to study radiosurgery as a primary treatment modality in patients not well suited for surgery. They found tumor control in 85% of patients at 10 years with a 24% rate of new or worsened hypopituitarism.[124] Because of the risks of radiation to the pituitary, many clinicians advocate reserving radiotherapy only for tumors that demonstrate growth in serial postoperative imaging.[125,126] Studies of the natural history of these tumors have demonstrated a difference in growth patterns and proliferation index (MIB-1) between patients younger patients and those 61 years of age or older.[127] Time to tumor doubling was significantly longer for older patients, suggesting that adjuvant treatment may not always be necessary in this age group.

In addition, medical therapy has only limited efficacy for this class of tumors. In a study of nine patients with nonsecretory adenomas treated for 1 year with cabergoline, tumor dopamine reception expression was demonstrated in 67%, but only 56% demonstrated response to cabergoline.[128] This response was clinically significant in only two patients. Other medical treatments such as bromocriptine, other dopamine agonists, octreotide, and GnRH agonists or antagonists have been used but their results have been inconsistent.

TSH-secreting pituitary adenomas

TSH-secreting adenomas are the least common variant of pituitary tumors, representing only 1–2% of cases.[129]

Clinical presentation

Patients present with signs and symptoms suggestive of hyperthyroidism, such as heat intolerance, diarrhea, visual changes, weight loss, tremulousness, fatigue, and exophthalmos. This frequently leads to a work up and presumptive diagnosis of Graves' disease.

As a result, patients with TSH-secreting pituitary adenomas are often diagnosed later in their course of illness, when their tumors are large and locally invasive. Thus, they may also suffer from symptoms related to tumor mass effect, such as headaches, vision changes, and hypopituitarism.[130]

Diagnosis

The majority of TSH-secreting adenomas is associated with elevated levels of TSH, in spite of elevated T3 and free T4. There is increased diagnostic sensitivity with an increased α-subunit/TSH ratio. Finally, ultrasensitive immunometric TSH assays allow for distinction between patients with primary hyperthyroidism from those with central hypothyroidism or resistance to thyroid hormone.

Treatment

Hyperthyroidism presents significant anesthesia and surgical risk owing to its effects on heart rate and cardiac function. Therefore, treatment of hyperthyroidism before surgery is essential. This is frequently accomplished through beta blockade. If surgery is nonemergent, an antithyroid drug (propylthiouracil or methimazole) may also be added. Transsphenoidal surgery is the primary treatment for this type of tumor but is associated with low rates of remission (35–62%). When adjuvant medical therapy or radiotherapy is added, the rate of remission increases to 55–81%.[131-134] Remission is frequently characterized by resolution of clinical symptoms of hyperthyroidism. The criteria for remission are not well established. External radiation is used if clinical remission is not attained with surgery alone but is not used as first-line treatment.

Octreotide has demonstrated clinical efficacy in 92% of cases and is associated with a normalization of TSH and tumor shrinkage for the vast majority.[135] While useful as an adjuvant therapy, significant long-term costs and continued compliance make octreotide unpopular for the primary treatment modality. Recent reports suggest that lanreotide, a long-acting octreotide analog, may have similar efficacy while avoiding some of the downsides of octreotide.

Conclusion

Pituitary adenomas are a heterogeneous group of tumors requiring treatments specific to their underlying pathology. Transsphenoidal surgery remains the most common intervention while medical and radiation therapies play important roles in long-term control. As our understanding of molecular biology, drug development, and radiosurgery evolves, there will no doubt be further improvements to clinical outcomes and patient satisfaction.

Summary

Pituitary neoplasms arise from the adenohypophysis and can be classified based on their cell type as well as their radiographic appearance. Transsphenoidal surgery is the treatment of choice for all adenomas except prolactinomas, for which medical therapy is the primary therapy. Hormone-specific chemotherapy and radiotherapy have demonstrated clinical benefit for many tumor subtypes. Prognosis depends heavily on hormonal control as the systemic effects from hormone overproduction are often more severe than mass effect from the neoplasm. Research developments into the genetics of these tumors as well as their tumor biology have led to a number of promising targets for future therapies.

Key references

The complete reference list can be found on the Wiley Companion Digital Edition of this title (see inside front cover for login instructions).

4 Kovacs K, Horvath E, Vidal S. Classification of pituitary adenomas. *J Neurooncol.* 2001;**54**:121.

7 Knosp E, Steiner E, Klaus K, Matula C. Pituitary adenomas with invasion of the cavernous sinus space: imaging classification compared with surgical findings. *Neurosurgery.* 1993;**33(4)**:610.

10 Yu R, Melmed S. Oncogene activation in pituitary tumors. *Brain Pathol.* 2001;**11**:328.

15 Mete O, Ezzat S, Asa SL. Biomarkers of aggressive pituitary adenomas. *J Mol Endocrinol.* 2012;**49**:R69.

18 Salehi F, Agur A, Scheithauer BW, Kovacs K, Lloyd RV, Cusimano M. Biomarkers of pituitary neoplasms: a review. *Neurosurgery.* 2010;**67**:1790.

22 Syro LV, Builes CE, Di Leva A, Sav A, Rotondo F, Kovacs K. Improving differential diagnosis of pituitary adenomas. *Expert Rev Endocrinol Metab.* 2014;**9(4)**:377.

25 Syro LV, Ortiz LD, Scheithauer BW, et al. Treatment of pituitary neoplasms with temozolomide: a review. *Cancer.* 2011;**117**:454.

26 McCormack A, Kaplan W, Gill AJ, et al. MGMT expression and pituitary tumors: relationship to tumor biology. *Pituitary.* 2013;**16**:208.

43 Kharlip J, Salvatori R, Yenokyan G, Wand GS. Recurrence of hyperprolactine-mia after withdrawal of long-term cabergoline therapy. *J Clin Endocrinol Metab.* 2009;**94(7)**:2428.

44 Boguszewski CL, dos Santos CM, Sakamoto KS, Marini LC, de Souza AM, Azevedo M. A comparison of cabergoline and bromocriptine on the risk of valvular heart disease in patients with prolactinomas. *Pituitary.* 2012;**15**:44.

50 Maiter D, Delgrange E. The challenges in managing giant prolactinomas. *Eur J Endocrinol.* 2014;**170**:R213.

53 Vrooanen L, Jaffrain-Rea ML, Petrossians P, et al. Prolactinomas resistant to stan-dard doses of cabergoline: a multicenter study of 92 patients. *Eur J Endocrinol.* 2012;**167**:651.

58 Bloomgarden E, Molitch ME. Surgical treatment of prolactinomas: cons. *Endocrine.* 2014. PMID: 25112227.

59 Molitch ME. Pregnancy and the hyperprolactinemic woman. *N Engl J Med.* 1985;**312**:1364.

63 Melmed S, Casanueva FF, Cavagnini F, et al. Guidelines for acromegaly manage-ment. *J Clin Endocrinol Metab.* 2002;**87**:4054.

67 Freda PU, Wardlaw SL, Post KD. Long-term endocrinological follow-up evalu-ation in 115 patients who underwent transsphenoidal surgery for acromegaly. *J Neurosurg.* 1998;**89**:353.

76 Elias PCL, Lugao HB, Pereira MC, Machado HR, de Castro M, Moreira AC. Discordant nadir GH after oral glucose and IGF-1 levels on treated acromegaly: refining the biochemical markers of mild disease activity. *Horm Metab Res.* 2010;**42**:50.

82 Ayuk J, Stewart SE, Stewart PM, Sheppard MC. Long-term safety and efficacy of depot long-acting somatostatin analogs for the treatment of acromegaly. *J Clin Endocrinol Metab.* 2002;**87**:4142.

83 Van der Lely AJ, Hutson RK, Trainer PJ, et al. Long-term treatment of acromegaly with pegvisomant, a growth hormone receptor antagonist. *Lancet.* 2001;**358**:1754.

85 Colao A, Cuocolo A, Marzullo P, et al. Is the acromegalic cardiomyopathy reversible? Effect fo 5-year normalization of growth hormone and insulin-like growth factor I levels on cardiac performance. *J Clin Endocrinol Metab.* 2001;**86**:1551.

86 Fougner SL, Bollerslev J, Svartberg J, Oksnes M, Cooper J, Carlsen SM. Pre-operative octreotide treatment of acromegaly: long-term results of a randomized controlled trial. *Eur J Endocrinol.* 2014;**171**:229.

87 Freda PU, Reyes CM, Nuruzzaman AT, Sundeen RE, Khandji AG, Post KD. Caber-goline therapy of growth hormone & growth hormone/prolactin secreting tumors. *Pituitary.* 2004;**7**:21.

89 Lambert JK, Goldberg L, Fayngold S, Kostadinov J, Post KD, Geer EB. Predictors of mortality and long-term outcomes in treated Cushing's disease: a study of 346 patients. *J Clin Endocrinol Metab.* 2013;**98**:1022.

96 Chowdhury IF, Sinaii N, Oldfield EH, Patronas N, Nieman LK. A change in pitu-itary magnetic resonance imaging protocols detects ACTH-secreting tumours in patients with previously negative results. *Clin Endocrinol.* 2010;**72**:502.

100 Sheehan JP, Xu Z, Salvetti DJ, Schmitt PJ, Vance ML. Results of gamma knife surgery for Cushing's disease. *J Neurosurg.* 2013;**119**:1486.

101 Bochicchio D, Losa M, Buchfelder M. Factors influencing the immediate and late outcome of Cushi'g's disease treated by transsphenoidal surgery: a retrospective study by the European Cushing's Disease Survey Group. *J Clin Endocrinol Metab.* 1995;**80**:3114.

104 Sheehan JM, Vance ML, Sheehan JP, Ellegala DB, Laws ER Jr. Radiosurgery for Cushing's disease after failed transsphenoidal surgery. *J Neurosurg.* 2000;**93**:738.

105 Colao A, Petersenn S, Newell-Price J, et al. A 12-month phase 3 study of pasireotide in Cushing's disease. *N Eng J Med.* 2012;**366(10)**:914.

107 Pivonello R, Ferone D, de Herder WW, et al. Dopamine receptor expression and function in corticotroph pituitary tumors. *J Clin Endocrinol Metab.* 2004;**89**:2452.

112 Mehta GU, Sheehan JP, Vance ML. Effect of stereotactic radiosurgery before bilat-eral adrenalectomy for Cushing's disease on the incidence of Nelson's syndrome. *J Neurosurg.* 2013;**119**:1493.

117 Ioachimescu AG, Eiland L, Chhabra VS, et al. Silent corticotroph adenomas: Emory University cohort and comparison with ACTH-negative nonfunctioning pituitary adenomas. *Neurosurgery.* 2012;**71**:296.

118 Black PM, Hsu DW, Klibanski A, et al. Hormone production in clinically nonfunc-tioning pituitary adenomas. *J Neurosurg.* 1987;**66**:244.

122 Colao A, Cerbone G, Cappabianca P, et al. Effect of surgery and radiotherapy on visual and endocrine function in nonfunctioning pituitary adenomas. *J Endocrinol Invest.* 1998;**21**:284.

123 Sheehan JP, Starke RM, Mathieu D, et al. Gamma knife radiosurgery for the man-agement of nonfunctioning pituitary adenomas: a multicenter study. *J Neurosurg.* 2013;**119**:446.

124 Lee C, Kano H, Yang H, et al. Initial gamma knife radiosurgery for nonfunctioning pituitary adenomas. *J Neurosurg.* 2014;**120**:647.

128 Pivonello R, Matrone C, Filippella M, et al. Dopamine receptor expression and function in clinically nonfunctioning pituitary tumors: comparison with the effec-tiveness of cabergoline treatment. *J Clin Endocrinol Metab.* 2004;**89**:1674.

134 Malchiodi E, Profka E, Ferrante E, et al. Thyrotropin-secreting pituitary ade-nomas: outcome of pituitary surgery and irradiation. *J Clin Endocrinol Metab.* 2014;**99**:2069.

136 Schade R, Andersohn F, Suizza S, Haverkamp W, Garbe E. Dopamine agonists and the risk of cardiac-valve regurgitation. *N Eng J Med.* 2007;**356**:29.

80 Neoplasms of the thyroid

Steven I. Sherman, MD ▪ Maria E. Cabanillas, MD ▪ Stephen Y. Lai, MD, PhD

Overview

Thyroid carcinomas, particularly, papillary cancers, exhibit increasing incidence but, generally, low risk for mortality. An optimal approach to an undiagnosed thyroid mass relies upon ultrasound characterization and guided fine needle aspiration of lesions at risk for clinically significant malignancy. Given the absence of prospective trials, controversy continues over the most appropriate initial treatment strategy for differentiated carcinoma, including extent of thyroidectomy and neck dissection and use of adjuvant radioiodine. Medullary carcinoma is treated initially with thyroidectomy, central and possible lateral neck dissections, and early evaluation to distinguish sporadic from hereditary disease. Recent developments in systemic, targeted therapies have led to multiple anti-angiogenic drugs available to treat progressive metastatic differentiated or medullary carcinoma with significant improvement in progression-free survival, though improvements in overall survival are lacking. In distinct contrast, anaplastic carcinoma remains one of the most fulminantly aggressive malignancies, with limited and generally palliative benefit only from selected use of multimodality therapy with surgery, radiation, and chemotherapy.

Historical perspective

Thyroid carcinoma, historically an uncommon disease, has transformed into one of the most commonly diagnosed malignancies, with escalating worldwide incidence. Although most patients require localized therapy only, treatment of advanced disease has changed with advent of targeted therapies. Even initial treatment has undergone revision, with recognition that more conservative approaches are sufficient.

Incidence and epidemiology—local and worldwide

About 62,450 persons were diagnosed in 2015 with carcinoma of the thyroid gland in the United States, with disease-related mortality of nearly 2000.[1] Globally, the incidence is six times higher, whereas disease-related mortality is >20 times higher.[2] Female incidence is about twice that of males, peaking in South Korea, where thyroid cancer is the leading malignancy diagnosed in women. The escalating incidence is seen primarily in small tumors confined to the gland and has been associated with increased thyroid imaging, higher socioeconomic status, and "overdiagnosis."[3]

Differentiated thyroid carcinomas (DTC), derived from the hormone-producing follicular epithelial cells, account for 96% of thyroid cancers, including papillary thyroid cancer (PTC), follicular thyroid cancer (FTC), and oxyphilic carcinomas (88%, 6%, and 2%, respectively).[4] Another 2% are medullary thyroid cancer (MTC) carcinomas, derived from neuroendocrine "C" cells, and

the remaining 1% are poorly differentiated thyroid cancer (PDTC) carcinoma or highly aggressive, undifferentiated, anaplastic thyroid cancer (ATC) carcinomas.

Risk factors—genetic, behavioral, environmental

Although most lack an obvious cause for DTC, the best established risk factor is radiation exposure, especially during childhood and adolescence. Between 0.1 and 10 Gy of exposure, the excess relative risk is 7.7 per Gy, with risk leveling above 10 Gy and after age 20 at time of exposure.[5] Obesity has also been associated with higher risk of DTC (relative risk about 1.3).[6] Iodine deficiency has been associated with a higher frequency of FTC, and possibly contributes to risk for ATC.[7] DTC is a component of certain genetic syndromes, including familial adenomatous polyposis, Cowden syndrome, and Carney complex.[8,9] Familial nonmedullary carcinoma, occurring in at least two first-degree relatives, has been reported in 5% of all PTC patients, although genetic loci and mechanisms are unclear.[10] Hereditary MTC syndromes, including subtypes of multiple endocrine neoplasia (MEN) type 2A and MEN2B, account for 25% of all cases of MTC; environmental factors are not known to influence development of MTC.[11]

Prevention

Other than use of potassium iodide prophylaxis in the setting of a nuclear accident or mechanical shielding of the thyroid from external radiation,[12] there is no known strategy to prevent development of DTC. Thyroidectomy following prospective screening of children at high risk for hereditary MTC may prevent development of aggressive malignancy.[13]

Pathology

Conventional PTCs are characterized by papillae with a fibrovascular core surrounded by tumor cells with large, oval, often overlapping nuclei containing hypodense powdery chromatin, cytoplasmic pseudoinclusions, and grooves (Figure 1). The follicular variant accounts for about 10% of PTCs, with cells displaying nuclear features of PTC but organized into follicles rather than papillae. In contrast, the uncommon tall cell variant of PTC is a more aggressive tumor, characterized by eosinophilic tumor cells that are twice as tall as they are wide. The primary tumors are larger, invasive, and frequently metastatic.

FTCs are distinguished from follicular adenomas by demonstrating invasiveness in one or more foci along the capsule or across vascular endothelial walls. The extent of invasion separates FTC into minimally invasive and widely invasive lesions, the former demonstrating only scattered foci of capsular or vascular invasion.

Holland-Frei Cancer Medicine, Ninth Edition. Edited by Robert C. Bast Jr., Carlo M. Croce, William N. Hait, Waun Ki Hong, Donald W. Kufe, Martine Piccart-Gebhart, Raphael E. Pollock, Ralph R. Weichselbaum, Hongyang Wang, and James F. Holland.
© 2017 John Wiley & Sons, Inc. ISBN: 978-1-118-93469-2

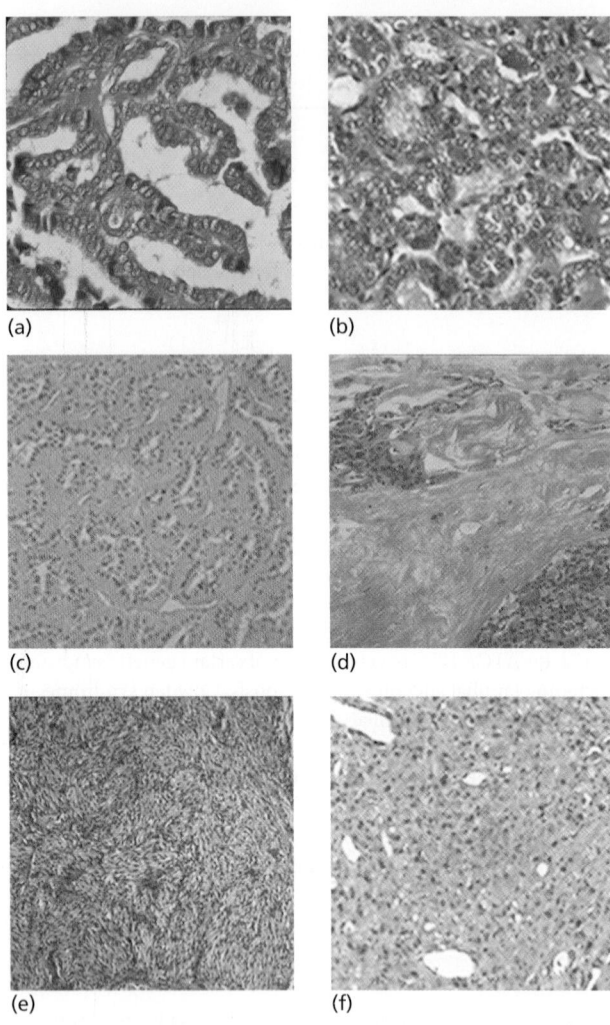

(a)

(b)

(c)

(d)

(e)

(f)

Figure 1 Pathologic features of thyroid carcinoma. (a) Papillary carcinoma, with characteristic fibrovascular papillary formation, crowded nuclei, and nuclear clearing. (b) Follicular variant of papillary carcinoma, with typical cells of papillary carcinoma in follicular formations. (c) Tall cell variant of papillary carcinoma, with cells at least twice as tall as they are wide and eosinophilic cytoplasm. (d) Follicular carcinoma, demonstrating invasion across a thick capsule into neighboring thyroid. (e) Medullary thyroid carcinoma, with nests of spindle-shaped cells. Such nests are often interspersed with clusters of round-to-oval cells. (f) Anaplastic carcinoma, showing large, discohesive, pleomorphic tumor cells. Source: Courtesy of Michelle D. Williams M.D.

Cytologic features do not reliably distinguish benign from malignant follicular lesions. Oxyphilic (or Hürthle cell) neoplasms are formed by cells containing numerous mitochondria, imparting a granular, eosinophilic cytoplasmic appearance.[14] Most have a follicular architecture and are diagnosed as carcinomas by the presence of invasion.

PDTC is often considered intermediate between DTC and ATC and may represent a partial dedifferentiated state. Cells tend to be nested with solid or insular architectural patterns, without the nuclear features of PTC. Diagnostic criteria also require one of (1) convoluted nuclei, (2) tumor necrosis, or (3) at least three mitoses per high power field.[15] ATC is usually macroscopically infiltrative; microscopically, the tumor is heterogeneous, with pleomorphic nuclei, sheets of spindle, epithelioid, or giant cells, areas of necrosis, and extensive inflammatory infiltrate. While PTC, FTC, and even PDTC generally stain positive for thyroglobulin (Tg) and other

follicular cell-specific antigens, ATC may stain only for cytokeratin and PAX8.[16]

MTCs commonly contain nests and sheets of rounded or spindle-shaped neuroendocrine cells, surrounded by a fibrovascular stroma. Nuclei tend to have speckled chromatin, and the cytoplasm is usually granular and eosinophilic. Amyloid deposition within the stroma is pathognomonic. Calcitonin and neuroendocrine immunohistochemical markers are usually detected. MTC in hereditary syndromes arises from a background of C cell hyperplasia.

Pathogenesis and natural history

Molecular alterations

Oncogenes associated with PTC include mutually exclusive activating mutations in *BRAF* (62%), *RAS* (13%), and *RET/PTC* chromosomal rearrangements (7%), all upstream of the mitogen-activated protein (MAP) kinase.[17] *BRAF* mutations are most common in conventional PTC and tall cell variants, whereas *RAS* mutations are seen in the follicular variant of PTC and FTC. Comprehensive analysis of genomic, transcriptional, epigenetic, and microRNA changes identifies clear signaling differences between *BRAF* and *RAS*-type tumors.[17] In FTC, chromosomal rearrangements fusing a thyroid-specific transcription factor to peroxisome proliferator-activated receptor gamma-1 to form the PAX8-PPARγ oncogene may also be seen.[18] In PDTC and ATC (which may arise from pre-existing DTC), coexisting mutations are more common, including *RAS*, *BRAF*, *TP53*, *CTNNB1*, *PIK3CA*, and *PTEN* mutations and loss of heterozygosity. Other factors contributing to progression of DTC include overexpression of other intracellular kinases, deoxyribonucleic acid hypermethylation and histone deacetylation leading to silencing of tumor-suppressor genes, and cell-cycle dysregulation.[17,19]

Mutations in exons 8, 10, 11, and 13–16 of the tyrosine kinase receptor *RET* occur in nearly all families with hereditary MTC.[10,11] Somatic mutations are also found in 40–50% of sporadic MTC tumors, particularly the highly activating codon 918 mutation associated with poorer patient prognosis.[20] Strong genotype–phenotype correlations allow stratification of mutations to predict disease aggressiveness.[21] *RAS* mutations are reported in 20–70% of sporadic MTC lacking *RET* changes.

Screening

RET mutations in hereditary MTC are inherited in an autosomal dominant manner with generally high penetrance. In addition to known kindreds, about 6% of patients with clinically sporadic MTC carry a germ line mutation in *RET*, leading to identification of new families.[22] Genetic counseling and testing for *RET* proto-oncogene mutations should be offered to all patients newly diagnosed with clinically apparent sporadic MTC, as well as for screening children and adults in known families with inherited forms of MTC.[21,23] In the patient with clinically sporadic MTC, the likelihood of a false negative *RET* germ line test for familial disease is <1%; however, if the family history is suggestive for an autosomal inherited disorder, complete sequencing of *RET* can be considered, and the family should be screened clinically and biochemically for possible MTC. For patients with familial adenomatous polyposis or Cowden syndrome, at higher risk for DTC, annual examination and possible ultrasound of the thyroid have been suggested.[24]

Diagnosis

While about 5% of individuals have a palpable thyroid nodule, and ultrasonography reveals nodules in up to half of individuals without palpable lesions, only 5% of nodules are malignant.[25,26] Most are asymptomatic, and few clinical features are specific for malignancy. Sonographic criteria that increase malignancy likelihood include microcalcifications, irregular margins, and shape taller than wide.[27] Incidentally detected thyroid nodules are also seen in 1–2% of fluorodeoxyglucose-positron emission tomography (FDG-PET) scans, for which the risk of malignancy is 40%.[28] Thyroid ultrasound with cytologic examination of a fine needle aspirate (FNA) of solitary nodules at least 1 cm in size is the most appropriate diagnostic procedure; in the setting of multiple nodules, those with suspicious sonographic appearances (and if none are present, the largest) should be preferentially aspirated.[29] PTC, MTC, and ATC can be readily diagnosed on the basis of cytologic criteria.[30] The false-positive and false-negative rates for nodules characterized as "malignant" and "benign," respectively, are <5%. However, as FTC is distinguished from benign follicular adenoma by invasion through the tumor capsule or vascular wall, these nodules are usually reported cytologically (along with follicular variants of PTC) as indeterminate follicular lesions or neoplasms, with an overall 20% risk of malignancy.[30,31] Molecular testing with a gene expression classifier can reduce the risk of malignancy in indeterminate nodules to as low as 5%; detection of *BRAF* mutations, although uncommon in indeterminate nodules, carries a very high positive predictive value for malignancy.[32–35] Although not routinely recommended for initial nodule evaluation, a random serum calcitonin level >100 pg/mL has high predictive value for MTC. Once malignancy is suspected, ultrasonography of the nodal chains in the neck is recommended before surgery; computed tomography (CT) or magnetic resonance imaging (MRI) may also provide occasional benefit in surgical planning for invasive or bulky disease.

Patients with aggressive disease, especially PDTC and ATC, commonly present with extensive local invasion and distant metastases.[36] The lungs and pleura are the most common sites of distant metastases, being seen in up to 90% of patients with distant disease, followed by bones, brain, skin, liver, and kidneys. CT of the neck and mediastinum can accurately determine the extent of the thyroid tumor and identify tumor invasion of the great vessels and upper aerodigestive tract structures. Metastatic work-up to detect distant disease is necessary but should not delay therapy.[37]

In half of MTC patients, metastatic cervical adenopathy is noted at initial presentation, and symptoms of upper aerodigestive tract compression or invasion are reported in up to 15% of patients with sporadic disease. Distant metastases are most commonly found in the liver. The ability of the tumor to over-secrete measurable quantities of Ct, occasionally along with other peptides and biogenic amines such as adrenocorticotrophic hormone or calcitonin gene-related peptide, leads to unexplained diarrhea or symptoms of Cushing syndrome in many patients.

TNM staging, classification

The seventh edition of the American Joint Committee on Cancer (AJCC)/UICC (Union for International Cancer Control) staging system is recommended for standard clinicopathologic staging and assessment of risk for mortality for all thyroid cancers (Table 1).[21,37,38,40] However, there are significant concerns that it may overestimate risk for small tumors and underestimate risk for young patients with DTC.[41,42] The important prognostic value of

histologic subtypes of DTC is also excluded. Risk for DTC recurrence may be better predicted by other proposed schemes following completion of initial therapy.[40,43,44]

Prognostic factors

In the Surveillance, Epidemiology, and End Results (SEER) report of 15,700 patients, the overall 10-year age- and gender-corrected survival rates were 98% for PTC, 92% for FTC, 80% for MTC, and 13% for ATC.[45] Older age at diagnosis and greater extent of disease including increasing tumor size, extrathyroidal invasion and distant metastases, are associated with a worse prognosis, independent of the type of cancer. In PTC, *BRAF* mutations may be prognostic for

Table 1 Tumor, node, metastases (TNM): The American Joint Committee on Cancer (AJCC) Staging Scheme for Thyroid Carcinomas (Seventh Edition).[38]

T: Tumor status	
T0	No evidence of primary tumor
T1a	Tumor ≤1 cm, without extrathyroidal extension
T1b	Tumor >1 cm but ≤2 cm in greatest dimension, without extrathyroidal extension
T2	Tumor >2 cm but ≤4 cm in greatest dimension, without extrathyroidal extension
T3	Tumor >4 cm in greatest dimension limited to the thyroid -or- Any size tumor with minimal extrathyroid extension (e.g., extension into sternothyroid muscle or perithyroidal soft tissues)
T4a	Tumor of any size extending beyond the thyroid capsule to invade subcutaneous soft tissues, larynx, trachea, esophagus, or recurrent laryngeal nerve
T4b	Tumor of any size invading prevertebral fascia or encasing carotid artery or mediastinal vessels
Tx	Tumor status unknown

N: Regional node status	
N0	No metastatic nodes
N1a	Metastases to level VI (pretracheal, paratracheal, and prelaryngeal/Delphian lymph nodes)
N1b	Metastases to unilateral, bilateral, or contralateral cervical (level I, II, III, IV, or V) or retropharyngeal or superior mediastinal lymph nodes (level VII)
Nx	Nodes status unknown

M: Distant metastases	
M0	No distant metastases
M1	Distant metastases
Mx	Metastases status unknown

	<45 years	≥45 years
Stage assignments: differentiated thyroid carcinoma		
Stage I	Any T, any N, M0	T1, N0 M0
Stage II	Any T, any N, M1	T2, N0, M0
Stage III		T3, N0, M0
		T1–3, N1a, M0
Stage IV		A: T4a, any N, M0
		Any T, N1b, M0
		B: T4b, any N, M0
		C: Any T, any N, M1
Stage assignments: medullary thyroid carcinoma		
Stage I	T1, N0, M0	
Stage II	T2–3, N0, M0	
Stage III	T1–3, N1a, M0	
Stage IVA	T4a, N0, M0	
Stage IVB	T4a, N1a, M0	
	Any T, N1b, M0	
Stage IVC	Any T, any N, M1	
Anaplastic thyroid carcinoma		
All are classified as stage IV		

Source: Edge 2010. Reproduced with permission of Springer.

locoregional recurrence and perhaps mortality, whereas in MTC, *RET* M918T mutations are associated with worse outcomes.[20,46-48]

Multidisciplinary care

Surgery—standard operations, complications, outcomes

Total thyroidectomy has been the initial surgical procedure advocated for most patients with DTC, given that (1) foci of PTC are commonly bilateral[49,50]; (2) contralateral recurrence occurs in 5–10% of patients who undergo unilateral surgery; and (3) efficacy of therapy with radioiodine is maximized by total resection. Earlier cohort studies support the contention that recurrence rates are 2–3 times higher following lobectomy compared with total thyroidectomy for primary PTC >1 cm, with possible improvements in survival in multivariate analyses.[51-53] More recently, larger studies have challenged these conclusions, suggesting no improvement in survival following total thyroidectomy.[54,55] Active surveillance has even been advocated for selected patients with small PTC confined to the gland, given infrequent progression on serial imaging.[56] In the absence of randomized prospective trials, total thyroidectomy is recommended for DTC patients with primary tumors >4 cm or clinical evidence preoperatively of extrathyroidal invasion or nodal or distant metastases. Either total thyroidectomy or ipsilateral lobectomy may be appropriate for smaller primary tumors without metastatic or invasive disease and lobectomy or active surveillance optimal for subcentimeter primary tumors.

Although microscopic regional nodes with PTC occur in up to 80% of patients, only about 35% have clinical cervical or mediastinal node metastasis, typically in lateral cervical compartments.[57] With clinically involved lateral neck disease, a comprehensive neck dissection (levels II–V) should be performed.[58,59] While resection of clinically involved central compartment (level VI and superior mediastinal nodes) nodes has been associated with improved survival and is commonly recommended, the potential benefit of prophylactic central neck dissection may outweigh the potential surgical morbidity only when performed by experienced thyroid surgeons.[60] In the presence of invasion of aerodigestive tract structures, similar survival rates are achieved from either complete surgical resection or shave excision leaving only microscopic residual disease.[61] However, half of patients die within 4 years following shave excision for frank cartilage destruction or intraluminal involvement. Surgery in patients with extensively invasive thyroid carcinoma should aim, therefore, to remove all gross tumors, maximizing functionality, unless the disease is unresectable or patient refuses the proposed surgery.[62]

For newly diagnosed MTC, serum calcium and plasma-free metanephrines should be measured to exclude coexistent hyperparathyroidism and pheochromocytoma, unless MEN2 has been ruled out by germ line *RET* testing. Total thyroidectomy is indicated in all patients with MTC, especially given the high frequency of bilateral disease in both sporadic and familial disease, and has been associated with improved survival.[21,63] Even in the absence of clinically detectable nodal metastases, central neck compartment dissection should be performed in all patients, and ipsilateral lateral neck and/or mediastinal dissections should be strongly considered when the primary tumor is >1 cm or when central compartment disease is present. Disfiguring radical neck dissections do not improve prognosis and are not indicated. In the presence of grossly invasive disease, more extended procedures with resection of involved neck structures may be appropriate, but function-preserving approaches are preferred.

Given the identification of patients with malignant disease as early as age 6 years, prophylactic thyroidectomy by age 5 is recommended for carriers of a familial *RET* mutation; given potential for earlier metastatic disease, surgery should be performed by age 1 year in children with MEN2B. Of 50 *RET* mutation carriers, 88% had normal levels of plasma calcitonin when evaluated 5–10 years after prophylactic thyroidectomy.[13] Surveillance with calcitonin measurements, thyroid ultrasound and delayed surgery may be appropriate for children with the least virulent *RET* mutations in codons 768, 790, 791, 804, and 891, particularly if the family history is of less aggressive disease.[23]

Minimally invasive surgical approaches, including approach to the thyroid from remote incisions in the axilla, may improve cosmesis and decrease postoperative discomfort.[64,65] These approaches afford surgeons superior visualization of critical structures through the use of endoscopic instruments. Robotic technology provides novel surgical approaches to the thyroid gland, including true three-dimensional visualization, highly articulated endo-wrist capability, and motion scaling. Natural orifice techniques are being developed, including transoral endoscopic thyroidectomy adopted for robotic instrumentation.[66,67] Implementing these approaches requires documenting improved operative outcomes relative to traditional open surgeries.[68,69]

Except for patients whose tumors are small and confined entirely to the thyroid, total thyroidectomy with complete tumor resection does not prolong survival in ATC.[70,71] Grossly incomplete resection is often of little palliative benefit given the rapid rate of tumor growth and high rate of distant metastases.

Radiation oncology—standard approaches, modalities, complications, and outcomes

Radioiodine

Adjuvant radioiodine therapy following primary surgery for DTC aims to destroy any residual microscopic foci of disease within a thyroid bed remnant or in regional nodal metastases, and should increase the predictive value of subsequent serum Tg measurements for detection of recurrent or metastatic disease by eliminating residual normal thyroid cells (referred to as "ablation"). Conflicting data have been reported from multiple retrospective studies of the efficacy of radioiodine.[72] In a recent multicenter thyroid cancer registry, improved survival was associated with postoperative radioiodine use in stages II–IV disease patients after adjustment for extent of thyroidectomy, and in stage III–IV patients when also adjusted for thyroid hormone suppression therapy.[52] For patients with residual disease or metastases, radioiodine therapy is recommended. In contrast, ablation may be withheld for patients with small solitary primary tumors without evidence of extrathyroidal invasion or metastasis. As MTC and ATC lack the capacity to concentrate iodine, radioiodine has no role in their management.

The efficacy of radioiodine depends on patient preparation, tumor-specific characteristics, sites of disease, and administered radioiodine activity. Iodide uptake by thyroid tissue is stimulated by thyrotropin (thyroid stimulating hormone, TSH) and is suppressed by increased endogenous iodide stores. Sufficiently elevated TSH levels can result from either endogenous production following thyroid hormone withdrawal or exogenously administered recombinant human TSH.[73] Diagnostic whole body radioiodine scans for localization of uptake before ablation or therapy are frequently performed 24–72 h after administration of 2–5 mCi of either ^{123}I or ^{131}I.[74,75] Most patients demonstrate significant uptake of radioiodine within the thyroid bed following thyroidectomy, presumably from normal residual thyroid. However, scanning before ablation may be considered optional for patients who are apparently free from gross metastases.[40,76]

[131]I, 30–100 mCi, is routinely administered if thyroid bed uptake is visualized on diagnostic scanning, or empirically if no pretherapy scanning has been performed in a patient selected for adjuvant treatment. Higher amounts, 150–200 mCi, are given if scanning demonstrates uptake in locoregional or distant metastatic disease. [131]I treatment of regional nodal metastases yields a complete response in 80% of patients but can be suboptimal in those with residual bulky disease.[77] Patients treated for iodine-concentrating pulmonary metastases, which occur in 5% of DTC patients, have a 5-year survival rate of 60–80%, as compared with 30% for those whose tumors do not concentrate iodine.[78,79] Long-term survival is highest in those patients with micronodular pulmonary metastases identified only by ^{131}I scanning.[78] [131]I treatment, 200 mCi, of skeletal metastases may yield complete resolution of disease in fewer than 10% of treated patients and partial remission in only 35%.[80] Following surgical debulking, radioiodine therapy can also be administered to patients with iodine-concentrating intracerebral metastases.[81]

Transient complications of radioiodine include sialoadenitis, oligospermia, leukopenia, and ovarian failure.[82,83] Chronically, radioiodine is associated with dose-related development of secondary neoplasms, including colorectal carcinoma, salivary tumors, and acute leukemias (excess absolute risks: 14.4 solid cancers and 0.8 leukemias per GBq of ^{131}I at 10,000 person-years of follow-up).[84] Patients who receive repeated doses of radioiodine treatment for diffuse pulmonary metastases, rarely, can develop pulmonary fibrosis.

External beam radiation therapy (EBRT)

EBRT (external beam radiation therapy) may be effective adjuvant therapy to prevent locoregional recurrence in older patients with grossly invasive PTC.[85,86] In a review of 282 patients treated with EBRT, a subgroup of 155 PTC patients with presumed microscopic residual disease experienced significant reduction in 10-year rates of locoregional control (93% vs 78%) and disease-specific survival (100% vs 95%).[87] Adjuvant EBRT is likely of little benefit to those younger than age 45 years, and esophageal and tracheal side effects may be poorly tolerated by the more elderly patient. Intensity-modulated radiotherapy (IMRT) may be associated with reduced short-term toxicity.[88] EBRT, 40–50 Gy to the thyroid bed, is recommended in the setting of gross extrathyroidal invasion with presumed microscopic residual disease, as well as following incomplete resection near aerodigestive structures.

For MTC, EBRT should be considered after maximal surgical therapy for those at high risk for regional recurrence, owing to gross extraglandular invasion or extensive bulky nodal metastases. In one study, the 10 years locoregional relapse-free rate was 86% after adjuvant EBRT, as compared with 52% for those patients who did not receive such therapy.[89] With conformal or IMRT, 60 Gy administered in 30 fractions, local control is readily achieved with acceptable toxicity even in the setting of distant metastases.[90]

For ATC, primary treatment with EBRT, administered in conventional doses, does not prolong survival, despite initial response in up to 40% of patients.[91,92] Hyperfractionated radiotherapy, combined with radiosensitizing chemotherapy, may increase the local response rate to about 80%, with subsequent median survival of 1 year with eventual mortality from distant metastases.

Thyroid hormone treatment

DTC patients require life-long thyroid hormone administration to treat postsurgical hypothyroidism and minimize TSH stimulation to tumor growth. With TSH-suppressive thyroid hormone therapy, both overall survival and disease-free survival may be improved two- to threefold, particularly in stage III and IV patients.[52] Lesser degrees of suppression may also improve overall survival in stage I and II patients.[52,93] However, potential morbidity from overly aggressive thyroid hormone therapy includes acceleration of osteoporosis,[94] provocation of atrial fibrillation,[95] and possibly, cardiac hypertrophy and dysfunction and impaired quality of life.[96] During initial follow-up, patients at lower risk for thyroid cancer recurrence and mortality should have their TSH levels maintained between 0.1 and 0.5 mU/L, whereas patients at higher risk should have TSH levels suppressed to <0.1 mU/L.[40] Patients who remain disease free for 5–10 years may potentially have their degree of TSH suppression reduced by lowering their doses of thyroid hormone. However, those with metastatic disease should have TSH levels maintained below 0.1 mU/L as tolerated.[97] Following surgery for MTC, thyroid hormone therapy is indicated, but TSH suppression is not appropriate as C cells lack TSH receptors.

Monitoring for recurrence

Serum biomarker monitoring

Measurement of serum Tg, a characteristic product of follicular cells, aids detection of residual, recurrent, or metastatic DTC, given the correlation between tumor size and Tg level. After thyroidectomy and remnant ablation, serum Tg concentration should approach undetectability but may take several years to decline to nadir following primary therapy.[98] Detection of residual cancer is enhanced by elevation of serum TSH, which stimulates Tg production; sensitivity of Tg following TSH stimulation is 85–95% but as low as 50% during TSH suppression or with dedifferentiated tumors.[99] Tg assays with functional sensitivities as low as 0.1 ng/mL may obviate need for TSH stimulation.[100] Tg levels that double in <1 year are associated with worse recurrence rates and mortality.[101,102]

Ct and CEA levels are similarly valuable biomarkers for MTC. Most patients with detectable serum calcitonin values postoperatively have residual disease. Values <150 pg/mL can be followed conservatively, but values >150 pg/mL should be re-evaluated for either residual resectable disease in the neck or the presence of distant metastases. Five-year survival rates of 100%, 92%, and 25% are reported in patients with postoperative calcitonin levels that double in >24, 6–24, and <6 months, respectively.[103,104]

Diagnostic imaging

Follow-up imaging for most DTC and MTC patients is based on cervical ultrasound, which accurately identifies locoregional metastases and recurrence measuring several millimeters in diameter. Ultrasound facilitates confirmatory FNA of suspicious lesions, sensitivity of which can be enhanced by measurement of either Tg or calcitonin in the needle washout.[105–108] Further imaging should be performed to identify foci of disease that could be surgically resected or treated by other means. For DTC patients, radioiodine scans may detect residual or metastatic disease that could respond to further therapy. Contrast-enhanced CT of the neck and chest is appropriate when Tg levels are elevated during follow-up, and FDG-PET imaging can be useful when Tg levels are >10 ng/mL and radioiodine imaging is negative and in mitochondria-rich oxyphilic tumors.[109,110] For MTC, contrast-enhanced CT of neck, chest, and liver (with three-phase enhancement) and MRI of the axial skeleton are appropriate when calcitonin levels exceed 150 pg/mL.[21,111]

Management of recurrent or metastatic disease

Surgery

Comprehensive neck dissection (levels II–V) should be performed for DTC patients with metastatic nodes >1 cm in diameter, though undetectable thyroglobulin levels result in fewer than half of patients.[112,113] Recurrence of disease may require re-exploration of the thyroid bed or dissection of the central and/or lateral nodes, although there may be higher risk for complications given fibrosis from prior surgery.[114] With aerodigestive tract invasion, complete surgical excision of gross disease can improve survival, but may require more extensive procedures such as tracheal resection and anastomosis or pharyngectomy. Tracheal stents, tracheotomy, and laser ablation or partial excision can be of palliative value. Among patients with brain metastases, resection or radiosurgery may improve survival.[81,115] In MTC, reoperative lymphadenectomy or excision of palpable disease rarely normalizes serum calcitonin levels, and thus, only patients with gross disease in the neck should undergo reoperative neck surgery.

Radioiodine

Repeat treatment with ^{131}I can be beneficial for patients with metastatic DTC identified by radioiodine imaging, though cumulative ^{131}I activities >600 mCi are rarely effective.[78] Radioiodine-refractory disease is characterized by tumors detectable on CT or MRI but lacking uptake on radioiodine imaging, or disease that progresses radiographically despite uptake of prior radioiodine therapy.

External-beam radiation

Patients with unresectable invasive disease in the neck may benefit from EBRT, with 5-year local control and disease-specific survival rates of about 65%.[87] EBRT can also palliate patients with painful skeletal metastases. Radiation doses of 50 Gy in 25 fractions may be given for solitary lesions, but reduced doses should be administered for vertebral foci.

Chemotherapy

Multitargeted kinase inhibitors are indicated treatment for DTC and MTC patients with multiple measurable, progressive metastases in one or more organs.[116] Targets contributing to efficacy of these agents include pro-angiogenic receptors, such as the vascular endothelial growth factor receptor (VEGFR) and fibroblast growth factor receptor (FGFR). In addition to being pro-angiogenic, these receptor kinases also have been identified on tumor cells themselves, likely contributing to tumor proliferation. Activated signaling in BRAF-mutated PTC and RET-mutated MTC suggests additional targets for more selective kinase inhibitors.

Lenvatinib and sorafenib both prolong progression-free survival (PFS) in DTC patients with progressive radioiodine-refractory disease.[117,118] In the SELECT phase III trial of lenvatinib, median PFS was markedly prolonged compared with placebo, 18.3 months versus 3.6 months [hazard ratio (HR) 0.21, 99% confidence interval (CI) 0.14–0.31; $p < 0.0001$].[117] Response rate with lenvatinib was 65%, including four patients with prolonged complete responses. Common lenvatinib-related adverse events included hypertension, diarrhea, fatigue, decreased appetite, nausea, vomiting, decreased weight, and stomatitis. In the DECISION phase III trial of sorafenib,

median PFS was prolonged compared with placebo, 10.8 versus 5.8 months (HR 0.59, 95% CI 0.45–0.76; $p < 0.0001$).[118] Response rate with sorafenib was 12%, all partial responses. Common sorafenib-related adverse events included palmar-plantar erythrodysesthesia, diarrhea, alopecia, rash, fatigue, weight loss, and hypertension. Other kinase inhibitors with evidence of efficacy in advanced DTC include the multitargeted agents vandetanib[119] and pazopanib,[120] and the BRAF inhibitors vemurafenib[121] and dabrafenib.[122]

In patients with progressive MTC, cabozantinib and vandetanib both prolong PFS.[123,124] In the EXAM phase III trial of cabozantinib in patients with progressive MTC, median PFS was prolonged compared with placebo, 11.2 months versus 4.0 months (HR, 0.28, 95% CI 0.19–0.40; $p < 0.001$). Response rate was 28%, all partial responses. In subgroup analysis, patients whose tumors contained either RET or RAS mutations were more likely to benefit, whereas no improvement in PFS was seen in those lacking either of these mutations.[125] Common cabozantinib-related adverse events included diarrhea, palmar-plantar erythrodysesthesia, decreased weight, nausea, and fatigue. In the ZETA phase III trial of vandetanib in patients with MTC, median PFS was prolonged compared with placebo, 30.5 months versus 19.3 months (HR 0.46, 95% CI, 0.31–0.69, $p < 0.001$). Subgroup analysis suggested PFS improvements in patients with progressive disease as well as those with RET M918T mutations. Common vandetanib-related adverse events included diarrhea, rash, nausea, hypertension, and headache; prolongation of cardiac QT intervals warrants careful observation of electrolytes and electrocardiography (ECG) monitoring during therapy.

Cytotoxic chemotherapy is of limited value in both DTC and MTC.[126] Combination doxorubicin and cisplatin was compared with doxorubicin alone in a randomized trial for metastatic DTC; objective responses were seen in only 16% with combination therapy including two durable complete responses, whereas 31% had partial responses with doxorubicin monotherapy.[127] In MTC, responses in up to 30% of patients may be seen with dacarbazine combined with other agents including vincristine, 5-fluorouracil, cyclophosphamide, or doxorubicin.[128]

In ATC, paclitaxel may yield short-term stabilization and palliative benefit in a minority of patients.[129] Although formal trials documenting benefit are lacking, consensus guidelines recommend combination regimens including taxanes, anthracyclines, and platinum-containing compounds.[37] A randomized phase III trial of fosbretabulin, paclitaxel and carboplatin versus paclitaxel and carboplatin demonstrated no improvement in survival although enrollment was incomplete.[130] Despite preclinical suggestions of efficacy, neither sorafenib nor pazopanib demonstrated single agent activity.[131,132]

Key references

The complete reference list can be found on the Wiley Companion Digital Edition of this title (see inside front cover for login instructions).

3 Davies L, Welch HG. Current thyroid cancer trends in the United States. *JAMA Otolaryngol Head Neck Surg.* 2014;**140**:317–322.

11 Wells SA Jr, Pacini F, Robinson BG, et al. Multiple endocrine neoplasia type 2 and familial medullary thyroid carcinoma: an update. *J Clin Endocrinol Metab.* 2013;**98**:3149–3164.

13 Skinner MA, Moley JA, Dilley WG, et al. Prophylactic thyroidectomy in multiple endocrine neoplasia type 2A. *N Engl J Med.* 2005;**353**:1105–1113.

15 Volante M, Collini P, Nikiforov YE, et al. Poorly differentiated thyroid carcinoma: the Turin proposal for the use of uniform diagnostic criteria and an algorithmic diagnostic approach. *Am J Surg Pathol.* 2007;**31**:1256–1264.

17 Cancer Genome Atlas Research Network. Integrated genomic characterization of papillary thyroid carcinoma. *Cell.* 2014;**159**:676–690.

20 Elisei R, Cosci B, Romei C, et al. Prognostic significance of somatic RET oncogene mutations in sporadic medullary thyroid cancer: a 10-year follow-up study. *J Clin Endocrinol Metab.* 2008;**93**:682–687.

21 Wells SA Jr, Asa SL, Dralle H, et al. Revised American Thyroid Association guidelines for the management of medullary thyroid carcinoma. *Thyroid.* 2015;**25**(**6**):567–610. Epub Mar 26 2015.

28 Cibas ES, Alexander EK, Benson CB, et al. Indications for thyroid FNA and pre-FNA requirements: a synopsis of the National Cancer Institute Thyroid Fine-Needle Aspiration State of the Science Conference. *Diagn Cytopathol.* 2008;**36**:390–399.

30 Baloch ZW, LiVolsi VA, Asa SL, et al. Diagnostic terminology and morphologic criteria for cytologic diagnosis of thyroid lesions: a synopsis of the National Cancer Institute Thyroid Fine-Needle Aspiration State of the Science Conference. *Diagn Cytopathol.* 2008;**36**:425–437.

32 Alexander EK, Kennedy GC, Baloch ZW, et al. Preoperative diagnosis of benign thyroid nodules with indeterminate cytology. *N Engl J Med.* 2012;**367**:705–715.

33 Nikiforova MN, Wald AI, Roy S, et al. Targeted next-generation sequencing panel (ThyroSeq) for detection of mutations in thyroid cancer. *J Clin Endocrinol Metab.* 2013;**98**:E1852–E1860.

34 Nikiforov YE, Carty SE, Chiosea SI, et al. Highly accurate diagnosis of cancer in thyroid nodules with follicular neoplasm/suspicious for a follicular neoplasm cytology by ThyroSeq v2 next-generation sequencing assay. *Cancer.* 2014;**120**:3627–3634.

37 Smallridge RC, Ain KB, Asa SL, et al. American Thyroid Association guidelines for management of patients with anaplastic thyroid cancer. *Thyroid.* 2012;**22**:1104–1139.

43 Tuttle RM, Tala H, Shah J, et al. Estimating risk of recurrence in differentiated thyroid cancer after total thyroidectomy and radioactive iodine remnant ablation: using response to therapy variables to modify the initial risk estimates predicted by the new American Thyroid Association staging system. *Thyroid.* 2010;**20**:1341–1349.

45 Gilliland FD, Hunt WC, Morris DM, et al. Prognostic factors for thyroid carcinoma: a population-based study of 15,698 cases from the Surveillance, Epidemiology and End Results (SEER) program 1973–1991. *Cancer.* 1997;**79**:564–573.

47 Xing M, Alzahrani AS, Carson KA, et al. Association between BRAF V600E mutation and mortality in patients with papillary thyroid cancer. *JAMA.* 2013;**309**:1493–1501.

52 Jonklaas J, Sarlis NJ, Litofsky D, et al. Outcomes of patients with differentiated thyroid carcinoma following initial therapy. *Thyroid.* 2006;**16**:1229–1242.

53 Bilimoria KY, Bentrem DJ, Ko CY, et al. Extent of surgery affects survival for papillary thyroid cancer. *Ann Surg.* 2007;**246**:375–381; discussion 381–374.

54 Adam MA, Pura J, Gu L, et al. Extent of surgery for papillary thyroid cancer is not associated with survival: an analysis of 61,775 patients. *Ann Surg.* 2014;**260**:601–605; discussion 605–607.

56 Ito Y, Miyauchi A, Inoue H, et al. An observational trial for papillary thyroid microcarcinoma in Japanese patients. *World J Surg.* 2010;**34**:28–35.

61 Gillenwater AM, Goepfert H. Surgical management of laryngotracheal and esophageal involvement by locally advanced thyroid cancer. *Semin Surg Oncol.* 1999;**16**:19–29.

71 Haigh PI, Ituarte PHG, Wu HS, et al. Completely resected anaplastic thyroid carcinoma combined with adjuvant chemotherapy and irradiation is associated with prolonged survival. *Cancer.* 2001;**91**:2335–2342.

73 Pacini F, Ladenson PW, Schlumberger M, et al. Radioiodine ablation of thyroid remnants after preparation with recombinant human thyrotropin in differentiated thyroid carcinoma: results of an international, randomized, controlled study. *J Clin Endocrinol Metab.* 2006;**91**:926–932.

76 Cailleux AF, Baudin E, Travagli JP, et al. Is diagnostic iodine-131 scanning useful after total thyroid ablation for differentiated thyroid cancer? *J Clin Endocrinol Metab.* 2000;**85**:175–178.

77 Maxon HR, Englaro EE, Thomas SR, et al. Radioiodine-131 therapy for well-differentiated thyroid cancer – a quantitative radiation dosimetric approach: outcome and validation in 85 patients. *J Nucl Med.* 1992;**33**:1132–1136.

78 Durante C, Haddy N, Baudin E, et al. Long-term outcome of 444 patients with distant metastases from papillary and follicular thyroid carcinoma: benefits and limits of radioiodine therapy. *J Clin Endocrinol Metab.* 2006;**91**:2892–2899.

84 Rubino C, de Vathaire F, Dottorini ME, et al. Second primary malignancies in thyroid cancer patients. *Br J Cancer.* 2003;**89**:1638–1644.

96 Biondi B, Cooper DS. Benefits of thyrotropin suppression versus the risks of adverse effects in differentiated thyroid cancer. *Thyroid.* 2010;**20**:135–146.

97 Carhill A, Litofsky D, Ain K, et al. Long-term moderate thyroid hormone suppression therapy is associated with improved outcomes in differentiated thyroid carcinoma: National Thyroid Cancer Treatment Cooperative Study Group Registry analysis 1987–2012. *Thyroid.* 2014;**24**(**S1**):A6.

98 Pacini F, Agate L, Elisei R, et al. Outcome of differentiated thyroid cancer with detectable serum Tg and negative diagnostic 131I whole body scan: comparison of patients treated with high 131I activities versus untreated patients. *J Clin Endocrinol Metab.* 2001;**86**:4092–4097.

99 Haugen BR, Pacini F, Reiners C, et al. A comparison of recombinant human thyrotropin and thyroid hormone withdrawal for the detection of thyroid remnant or cancer. *J Clin Endocrinol Metab.* 1999;**84**:3877–3885.

100 Castagna MG, Tala Jury HP, Cipri C, et al. The use of ultrasensitive thyroglobulin assays reduces but does not abolish the need for TSH stimulation in patients with differentiated thyroid carcinoma. *J Endocrinol Invest.* 2011;**34**:e219–e223.

102 Pacini F, Sabra MM, Tuttle RM. Clinical relevance of thyroglobulin doubling time in the management of patients with differentiated thyroid cancer. *Thyroid.* 2011;**21**:691–692.

103 Giraudet AL, Al Ghulzan A, Auperin A, et al. Progression of medullary thyroid carcinoma: assessment with calcitonin and carcinoembryonic antigen doubling times. *Eur J Endocrinol.* 2008;**158**:239–246.

109 Leboulleux S, Schroeder PR, Schlumberger M, et al. The role of PET in follow-up of patients treated for differentiated epithelial thyroid cancers. *Nat Clin Pract Endocrinol Metab.* 2007;**3**:112–121.

117 Schlumberger M, Tahara M, Wirth LJ, et al. Lenvatinib versus placebo in radioiodine-refractory thyroid cancer. *N Engl J Med.* 2015;**372**:621–630.

118 Brose MS, Nutting CM, Jarzab B, et al. Sorafenib in radioactive iodine-refractory, locally advanced or metastatic differentiated thyroid cancer: a randomised, double-blind, phase 3 trial. *Lancet.* 2014;**384**:319–328.

123 Elisei R, Schlumberger MJ, Muller SP, et al. Cabozantinib in progressive medullary thyroid cancer. *J Clin Oncol.* 2013;**31**:3639–3646.

124 Wells SA Jr, Robinson BG, Gagel RF, et al. Vandetanib in patients with locally advanced or metastatic medullary thyroid cancer: a randomized, double-blind phase III trial. *J Clin Oncol.* 2012;**30**:134–141.

129 Ain KB, Egorin MJ, DeSimone PA. Treatment of anaplastic thyroid carcinoma with paclitaxel: phase 2 trial using ninety-six-hour infusion. *Thyroid.* 2000;**10**:587–594.

81 Neoplasms of the adrenal cortex

Tito Fojo, MD, PhD

Overview

Adrenocortical cancer (ACC) is a rare malignancy, with varied presentations and a poor prognosis. Imaging studies have emerged as central to a work up, and in most cases a biopsy is not needed and should not be performed. Pathologic examination is very valuable with the Weiss criteria used to discriminate a small adenomas from carcinomas. Management is multidisciplinary and includes surgical resection or ablation, oral mitotane, intravenous chemotherapy, and palliative radiation. Surgery remains the only proven curative option, must be considered at presentation, and relapse with laparoscopic resection avoided. Mitotane is approved for the treatment of inoperable functional and nonfunctional ACC and its clinical value is primarily as an anti-hormonal agent. In a patient whose tumor is producing an excess of hormones mitotane is indispensable, however, its use in the adjuvant setting is uncertain. Replacement steroids are needed. Systemic chemotherapy using mitotane in combination with etoposide, doxorubicin, and cisplatin (EDP-M) or with streptozotocin (S-M) are the preferred options. These should not be discarded in favor of a "novel targeted therapy", none of which have shown any proven efficacy. Increasing evidence suggests that palliative radiation therapy is beneficial for patients with metastatic disease. Radiofrequency ablation (RFA) or cryoablation have emerged as surgical adjuncts or stand-alone modalities for recurrences. As with most rare diseases, enrollment in clinical trials is strongly encouraged.

Introduction

Adrenocortical cancer (ACC) is a rare malignancy, with an estimated incidence of 1.5–2 per million per year. Patients can present without symptoms, with local symptoms from a large, locally invasive primary tumor, or with the systemic manifestations of endocrine hypersecretion. A multidisciplinary approach to treatment is essential as the disease presents many management challenges.

General

The 5-year survival is ≈10–25% with average survival from diagnosis of ≈14.5 months. Biochemical evidence of hormone excess can be found in ≈50% with ≈10–20% presenting with Cushing's syndrome. Other symptoms include hirsutism in females and gynecomastia in males. Several reviews provide in-depth summaries.[1–5]

Evaluation and work-up

Initial evaluation should include a history, physical examination, with blood and urine studies to determine if tumor is functional. Computed tomography (CT) or magnetic resonance imaging (MRI) is often diagnostic. Both can help differentiate benign adenomas from malignant lesions.[6–9] MRI is superior in identifying liver metastases and extent of vascular invasion, especially the inferior vena cava. ^{18}F-fluorodeoxyglucose positron emission tomography (FDG-PET) can help assess extent of disease and may be valuable before a major surgery. However, FDG-PET is not of value for monitoring progress and should not be used as the primary modality.[10–13]

The role of a biopsy

Most patients presenting with an adrenal mass suspicious for malignancy should have surgery and not a diagnostic biopsy given risk of seeding tumor, and difficulty differentiating benign from malignant in a small biopsy.[14–16] Surgery can be performed without a biopsy in a patient (1) with evidence of hormone excess, where diagnosis of ACC is not in doubt or (2) without evidence of hormone production but with an isolated adrenal mass found during evaluation or incidentally on an imaging scan. Only with widespread metastases that make surgical resection unlikely to provide benefit or if disease elsewhere suggests a primary location other than adrenal, should a biopsy be performed.

Pathology

To distinguish a small ACC without local spread or distant metastases from a benign adenoma, the "Weiss criteria," first proposed in 1984, are used.[17–22] Weiss, noted nine criteria most useful in distinguishing malignant from benign: (1) nuclear grade III/IV, (2) mitotic rate >5 per 50 high-power fields, (3) atypical mitoses, (4) tumors with ≤25% clear cells, (5) diffuse architecture, (6) microscopic necrosis, (7) venous invasion, (8) sinusoidal invasion, and (9) capsular invasion. The presence of ≥3 criteria is the threshold for malignancy.

The Weiss criteria were developed to discriminate a small adenomas from carcinomas, but their prognostic value in larger tumors is not established. In 42 patients with a diagnosis of ACC, only mitotic rate had a *strong* statistical association with outcome.[18] Tumor weight >250 g, size >10 cm, atypical mitoses, and capsular invasion showed a marginal association with poor survival ($P < 0.06$). However, other criteria were not associated with survival. A recent study confirmed the importance of mitotic rate.[22]

Management of ACC

Options include surgical resection or ablation, oral mitotane, intravenous chemotherapy, and palliative radiation. Although controlled trials are generally lacking, this does not mean evidence is lacking nor does it mean anything is an option.

Holland-Frei Cancer Medicine, Ninth Edition. Edited by Robert C. Bast Jr., Carlo M. Croce, William N. Hait, Waun Ki Hong, Donald W. Kufe, Martine Piccart-Gebhart, Raphael E. Pollock, Ralph R. Weichselbaum, Hongyang Wang, and James F. Holland.
© 2017 John Wiley & Sons, Inc. ISBN: 978-1-118-93469-2

Surgical resection

Surgery remains the only proven curative option and must be considered at presentation and relapse. At presentation consider only complete resection of local disease given survival <1 year in patients with incomplete resection.[2,23,24] The key at presentation is an open procedure by an experienced oncologic surgeon. While some argue laparoscopic surgery can be used in selected patients, the occurrence of peritoneal dissemination—a lethal complication—should discourage any approach other than open resection. Laparoscopic surgery for adrenal incidentalomas that do not seed the abdomen is appropriate. However, intraoperative tumor spill rates as high as 50%—even by experienced surgeons—have been reported.[25,26] A study summarizing outcomes in 152 ACC patients[27] concluded that for ACCs ≤ 10 cm in diameter, laparoscopic was not inferior to open adrenalectomy. However, after extensive preselection only 23% underwent laparoscopy with one-third converted to open. These results in specialized referral centers have very limited to no applicability in the general community. In addition, laparoscopic resections have a higher incidence of positive margins and more rapid recurrence. A systematic review of laparoscopic surgery concluded, "There is no prospective randomized series to guide or endorse the use of laparoscopic resection for adrenocortical carcinoma."[28]

At the time of relapse, aggressive surgery may emerge as the preferred option especially in patients with less aggressive clinical presentations and a slower pace of tumor growth.[29,30] It must be recognized that studies addressing this approach have an inherent bias: those undergoing surgery likely have more limited disease, a better performance status, and possibly tumors with "more indolent biology."

Mitotane

Initially identified as an adrenolytic agent, mitotane is approved for the treatment of inoperable functional and nonfunctional ACC. However, its tumoricidal activity is limited and its clinical value is primarily an antihormonal agent, with data suggesting that mitotane modifies peripheral metabolism of steroids. *In a patient whose tumor is producing an excess of hormones,* mitotane is indispensable, must be started as soon as possible, and continues indefinitely, even if disease progression occurs.

Mitotane's use in the adjuvant setting is uncertain. Several small and one large study encumbered by the biases all retrospective studies must bear suggest adjuvant mitotane continued indefinitely, can delay and possibly prevent a recurrence of disease.[31,32] Identifying those who will benefit is important as only a fraction of patients tolerate mitotane well. Mitotane therapy should be viewed as a marathon not a sprint and its administration adjusted accordingly. Starting at 1–2 g/day it should be gradually advanced until a maximum dose of 4–6 g/day is reached 2–3 months later. Serum levels guide adjustments beyond that and eventually as little as 0.5–1 g/day is needed. Replacement steroids can start with mitotane or when clinical or laboratory parameters indicate incipient adrenal insufficiency. Give hydrocortisone and fludrocortisone and instruct the patient to wear a bracelet labeled adrenal insufficiency. When discontinued, mitotane elimination takes months and supplementation is required 6–12 additional months.

Systemic chemotherapy

Two therapeutic regimens have emerged as the preferred options for ACC both using mitotane in combination with etoposide, doxorubicin, and cisplatin (EDP-M) or with streptozotocin (S-M). These should not be discarded in favor of a "novel targeted therapy," none of which have any proven efficacy. Both regimens were evaluated in the FIRM-ACT trial,[33] which found significantly better response rate (23.2% vs 9.2%, P < 0.001) and progression-free survival (PFS) (5.0 vs 2.1 months, HR 0.55 and P < 0.001) with EDP-M than with S-M as first-line therapy, with similar rates of toxic events. There was no significant difference in overall survival, possibly owing to crossover. Importantly, as the 185 patients who received EDP-M as second line had a similar median PFS, there exists a window to enroll in an experimental regimen. The FIRM-ACT results also suggest that the therapies are not cross-resistant and thus may be administered in succession.

Finally, ≥50% of patients with ACC have undergone a nephrectomy often prompting the use of carboplatin instead of cisplatin. However, given that in other cancers the activity profiles have been dissimilar, the drug of choice should remain cisplatin.

Radiation therapy

Increasing evidence suggests palliative radiation therapy is beneficial for patients with metastatic disease. Its use for other than palliation is not supported by data nor its use following primary surgery. Initial studies found no benefit from adjuvant radiation, and although later studies using better techniques claim benefit with little toxicity, this should not be routinely adapted.[34,35] Benefit is uncertain but harm is guaranteed—including acute complications of radiation and the likelihood, a subsequent surgery that may be the only curative option will be made more difficult. Only in a patient with known positive margins after surgery performed by a highly qualified surgical oncologist would one consider post-surgical radiation and then only if reoperation is deemed not possible owing to associated comorbidities.

Interventional radiology as a treatment modality

Given the value of surgery in the management of ACC, radiofrequency ablation (RFA) or cryoablation has emerged as surgical adjuncts or stand-alone modalities for recurrences.[36] In the decision paradigm, ablation should be viewed as surgical interventions, albeit less invasive. The value of embolization to reduce tumor size and reduce vascular supply making a subsequent surgical intervention is established, albeit not with randomized data.

Management of hormonal excess and deficiency

In the preoperative setting assesses a patient's hormonal status, as any functioning tumor can suppress corticotropin with involution of the contralateral adrenal. In this way, determine the need for steroid replacement in the postoperative period.

The severe consequences of uncontrolled hormone production and the need for aggressive and sustained attention must be recognized.[37] Using chemotherapy to solve the problem of hormonal excess is a flawed strategy. In addition to mitotane, the cornerstone for managing hormonal excess, ketoconazole, metyrapone, and etomidate should be added singly or in combination. The management must be proactive and forward thinking.

Conclusion

Surgery remains the cornerstone for managing ACC, with RFA and cryoablation of value. Chemotherapy has a role in many patients but new paradigms are needed and referral to clinical trials is essential. Radiation therapy should be reserved for palliative indications. Attention must be given to hormonal excess as in patients with this complication, it is the major factor affecting the quality of their life. A multidisciplinary effort is mandatory.

References

1 Fassnacht M, Kroiss M, Allolio B. Update in adrenocortical carcinoma. *J Clin Endocrinol Metab*. 2013;**98**:4551–4564.

2 Ayala-Ramirez M, Jasim S, Feng L, et al. Adrenocortical carcinoma: clinical outcomes and prognosis of 330 patients at a tertiary care center. *Eur J Endocrinol*. 2013;**169**:891–899.

3 Else T, Kim AC, Sabolch A, et al. Adrenocortical carcinoma. *Endocr Rev*. 2014;**35**:282–326.

4 Terzolo M, Daffara F, Ardito A, et al. Management of adrenal cancer: a 2013 update. *J Endocrinol Invest*. 2014;**37**:207–217.

5 Ronchi CL, Kroiss M, Sbiera S, et al. EJE prize 2014: current and evolving treatment options in adrenocortical carcinoma: where do we stand and where do we want to go? *Eur J Endocrinol*. 2014;**171**:R1–R11.

6 Korobkin M, Brodeur FJ, Yutzy GG, et al. Differentiation of adrenal adenomas from nonadenomas using CT attenuation values. *AJR Am J Roentgenol*. 1966;**166**:531–536.

7 Mitchell DG, Crovello M, Matteucci T, et al. Benign adrenocortical masses: diagnosis with chemical shift MR imaging. *Radiology*. 1992;**185**:345–351.

8 Outwater EK, Siegelman ES, Huang AB, et al. Adrenal masses: correlation between CT attenuation value and chemical shift ratio at MR imaging with in-phase and opposed-phase sequences. *Radiology*. 1996;**200**:749–752.

9 Goldfarb DA, Novick AC, Lorig R, et al. Magnetic resonance imaging for assessment of vena caval tumor thrombi: a comparative study with venacavography and computerized tomography scanning. *J Urol*. 1990;**144**:1100–1103.

10 Groussin L, Bonardel G, Silvéra S, et al. 18F-fluorodeoxyglucose positron emission tomography for the diagnosis of adrenocortical tumors: a prospective study in 77 operated patients. *J Clin Endocrinol Metab*. 2009;**94**:1713–1722.

11 Nunes ML, Rault A, Teynie J, et al. 18F-FDG-PET for the identification of adrenocortical carcinomas among indeterminate adrenal tumors at computed tomography scanning. *World J Surg*. 2010;**34**:1506–1510.

12 Ansquer C, Scigliano S, Mirallié E, et al. 18F-FDG PET/CT in the characterization and surgical decision concerning adrenal masses: a prospective multicentre evaluation. *Eur J Nucl Med Mol Imaging*. 2010;**37**:1669–1678.

13 Takeuchi S, Balachandran A, Habra MA, et al. Impact of 18F-FDG PET/CT on the management of adrenocortical carcinoma: analysis of 106 patients. *Eur J Nucl Med Mol Imaging*. 2014;**41**:2066–2073.

14 Mazzaglia PJ, Monchik JM. Limited value of adrenal biopsy in the evaluation of adrenal neoplasm: a decade of experience. *Arch Surg*. 2009;**144**:465–470.

15 Osman Y, El-Mekresh M, Gomha AM, et al. Percutaneous adrenal biopsy for indeterminate adrenal lesion: complications and diagnostic accuracy. *Urol Int*. 2010;**84**:315–318.

16 Williams AR, Hammer GD, Else T. Transcutaneous biopsy of adrenocortical carcinoma is rarely helpful in diagnosis, potentially harmful, but does not affect patient outcome. *Eur J Endocrinol*. 2014;**170**:829–835.

17 Weiss LM. Comparative histologic study of 43 metastasizing and nonmetastasizing adrenocortical tumors. *Am J Surg Pathol*. 1984;**8**:163–169.

18 Weiss LM, Medeiros LJ, Vickery AL Jr. Pathologic features of prognostic significance in adrenocortical carcinoma. *Am J Surg Pathol*. 1989;**13**:202–206.

19 Gicquel C, Bertagna X, Gaston V, et al. Molecular markers and long-term recurrences in a large cohort of patients with sporadic adrenocortical tumors. *Cancer Res*. 2001;**61**:6762–6767.

20 Lau SK, Weiss LM. The Weiss system for evaluating adrenocortical neoplasms: 25 years later. *Hum Pathol*. 2009;**40**:757–768.

21 Jain M, Kapoor S, Mishra A, et al. Weiss criteria in large adrenocortical tumors: a validation study. *Indian J Pathol Microbiol*. 2010;**53**:222–226.

22 Volante M, Bollito E, Sperone P, et al. Clinicopathological study of a series of 92 adrenocortical carcinomas: from a proposal of simplified diagnostic algorithm to prognostic stratification. *Histopathology*. 2009;**55**:535–543.

23 Henley DJ, van Heerden JA, Grant CS, et al. Adrenal cortical carcinoma—a continuing challenge. *Surgery*. 1983;**94**:926–931.

24 Pommier RF, Brennan MF. An eleven-year experience with adrenocortical carcinoma. *Surgery*. 1992;**112**:963–970.

25 Leboulleux S, Deandreis D, Al Ghuzlan A, et al. Adrenocortical carcinoma: is the surgical approach a risk factor of peritoneal carcinomatosis? *Eur J Endocrinol*. 2010;**162**:1147–1153.

26 Miller BS, Ammori JB, Gauger PG, et al. Laparoscopic resection is inappropriate in patients with known or suspected adrenocortical carcinoma. *World J Surg*. 2010;**34**:1380–1385.

27 Brix D, Allolio B, Fenske W, et al. Laparoscopic versus open adrenalectomy for adrenocortical carcinoma: surgical and oncologic outcome in 152 patients. *Eur Urol*. 2010;**58**:609–615.

28 Angst E, Hiatt JR, Gloor B, et al. Laparoscopic surgery for cancer: a systematic review and a way forward. *J Am Coll Surg*. 2010;**211**:412–423.

29 Wängberg B, Khorram-Manesh A, Jansson S, et al. The long-term survival in adrenocortical carcinoma with active surgical management and use of monitored mitotane. *Endocr Relat Cancer*. 2010;**17**:265–272.

30 Bellantone R, Ferrante A, Boscherini M, et al. Role of reoperation in recurrence of adrenal cortical carcinoma: results from 188 cases collected in the Italian National Registry for Adrenal Cortical Carcinoma. *Surgery*. 1997;**122**:1212–1218.

31 Terzolo M, Angeli A, Fassnacht M, et al. Adjuvant mitotane treatment for adrenocortical carcinoma. *N Engl J Med*. 2007;**356**:2372–2380.

32 Huang H, Fojo T. Adjuvant mitotane for adrenocortical cancer—a recurring controversy. *J Clin Endocrinol Metab*. 2008;**93**:3730–3732.

33 Fassnacht M, Terzolo M, Allolio B, et al. Combination chemotherapy in advanced adrenocortical carcinoma. FIRM-ACT Study Group. *N Engl J Med*. 2012;**366**:2189–2197.

34 Markoe AM, Serber W, Micaily B, et al. Radiation therapy for adjunctive treatment of adrenal cortical carcinoma. *Am J Clin Oncol*. 1991;**14**:170–174.

35 Fassnacht M, Hahner S, Polat B, et al. Efficacy of adjuvant radiotherapy of the tumor bed on local recurrence of adrenocortical carcinoma. *J Clin Endocrinol Metab*. 2006;**91**:4501–4504.

36 Wood BJ, Abraham J, Hvizda JL, et al. Radiofrequency ablation of adrenal tumors and adrenocortical carcinoma metastases. *Cancer*. 2003;**97**:554–560.

37 Veytsman I, Nieman L, Fojo T. Management of endocrine manifestations and the use of mitotane as a chemotherapeutic agent for adrenocortical carcinoma. *J Clin Oncol*. 2009;**27**:4619–4629.

82 Tumors of the diffuse neuroendocrine and gastroenteropancreatic system

Evan Vosburgh, MD

Overview

The diffuse neuroendocrine system (DES) is represented by a small number of cells spread through the body, and the tumors that derive from these cells present a wide spectrum of epidemiologic, pathologic, biologic, genetic, and clinical features. Clinical and scientific investigation of the inherited multiple endocrine neoplasia (e.g., MEN-1, MEN-2) syndromes, and the various unique clinical syndromes secondary to secretion of specific peptides (e.g., insulinomas, glucagonomas, VIPomas) are challenging. Clinical presentation can be dramatic, nonspecific, or incidentally noted in absence of symptoms. Tumors might be small, difficult to detect tumors (<1 cm in size) or bulky hepatic metastases in a well patient. Cancer registry data show five-year survivals for tumors of the neuroendocrine system that have not improved in the past several decades, and that remain about 30–60%. The same registry data documents a rising and unexplained incidence of these tumors, particularly the neuroendocrine tumors of the gastroenteropancreatic system (GEP-NETs), that when coupled with the long average survival results in prevalence figures similar to cancers such as testicular, ovarian, and multiple myeloma.

Recent advances in understanding of the genetics, biology, clinical features, and response to therapy are better defining subtypes of neuroendocrine tumors once clustered and studied as "carcinoids." Revised histologic grouping and staging are informing ongoing clinical trials and are providing more informed clinical care of these diverse tumors. Recent approvals of several targeted therapies with progression-free survival benefit suggest that the status quo is changing for tumors of the DES.

Recent advances in understanding of the genetics, biology, clinical features, and response to therapy are better defining subtypes of neuroendocrine tumors once clustered and studied as "carcinoids." Revised histologic grouping and staging are informing ongoing clinical trials and are providing more informed clinical care of these diverse tumors. Recent approvals of several targeted therapies with progression-free survival benefit suggest that the status quo is changing for tumors of the DES.

This chapter will focus on the gastroenteropancreatic neuroendocrine tumors (GEP-NETs), representing the majority of all NETs:

- GI-NET (gastrointestinal neuroendocrine tumors)—often referred to by the term "carcinoid."
- PNET (pancreatic neuroendocrine tumors)—both nonsecretory and those defined by secretion of specific peptides (i.e., insulinomas).
- MEN-1 & MEN-2 (multiple endocrine neoplasia syndromes) and MTC (medullary thyroid carcinoma). Cancer syndromes with defined gene mutations.
- Pheochromocytoma and parathyroid tumors—both as sporadic cases and in association with MEN syndromes.

Epidemiology

One of the challenges facing the classification systems over the past century for *carcinoid* and related neuroendocrine tumors is that the histology is not particularly informative and tends to be similar for benign and malignant biologic phenotypes. One distinction that has been maintained with some consistency over time has been the separation of classic *carcinoid* tumors of the GI tract from the pancreatic islet cell tumors or PNETs.

In comprehensive epidemiologic reviews of *carcinoid* tumors, Modlin et al.[1] and Yao et al.[2] report SEER (Surveillance, Epidemiology, and End Results) cancer registry data of incidence and prevalence spanning over a half century. The multidecade analysis of over 13,000 and 35,000 cases respectively show an increase in overall incidence for the past 30 years. Over 65% of NET are in the two broad groups of tumors, *carcinoid* (renamed GI-NET), and islet cell tumors (renamed PNET), together referred to as GEP-NET (Figure 1). Within the GI-NET, the small bowel remains the most common site with a stable incidence over time, as opposed to the gastric and rectal carcinoids that have increased in recent decades. The PNET are divided roughly into nonfunctional PNET and functional PNET. Functional PNET in order of decreasing incidence are gastrinoma, insulinoma, VIPoma, glucagonoma, and the very rare neurotensinoma, somatostatinoma, and other ectopic hormone-secreting tumors. The changes in gastric and rectal incidence are thought to represent an increased detection rate with the increasing use of upper and lower endoscopies. Over the same period, the incidence of carcinoids of the appendix decreased, perhaps reflecting the decrease in open abdominal procedures and

Holland-Frei Cancer Medicine, Ninth Edition. Edited by Robert C. Bast Jr., Carlo M. Croce, William N. Hait, Waun Ki Hong, Donald W. Kufe, Martine Piccart-Gebhart, Raphael E. Pollock, Ralph R. Weichselbaum, Hongyang Wang, and James F. Holland.
© 2017 John Wiley & Sons, Inc. ISBN: 978-1-118-93469-2

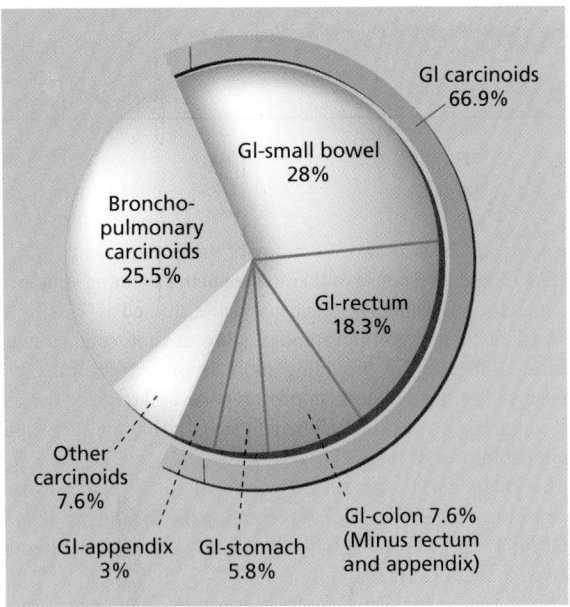

Figure 1 Estimated relative incidence of neuroendocrine tumors (NET) by anatomical site. Compiled for illustrative purpose from numerous publications, and estimated by combining classification systems that have varied over time and by source. Data from[1]

bystander appendectomies.[1] The gastric, rectal and appendiceal NET are often diagnosed incidentally and as superficial lesions whose management is not discussed in this chapter.

The over 50 years of data documents little change in overall survival, survival by site and extent of disease, including documentation of metastatic disease at diagnosis in a relatively constant 10-12%. It should be noted that the low incidence of GEP-NET tumors is somewhat deceptive, as Yao et al.[2] demonstrated that the overall survival that exceeds many other tumors types translates to *prevalence* figures of GEP-NET that exceed other gastrointestinal tumors including esophageal, gastric, pancreatic, and hepatobiliary.

The diffuse endocrine system

The diffuse endocrine system (DES) had its descriptive origins in early histology and cell biology that defined a population of normal chromium-avid epithelial cells widely scattered through the intestinal tract (enterochromaffin cells) and organs including brain, parathyroid, pituitary, thyroid, lungs, adrenal glands (chromaffin or clear cells).[3] In the gastrointestinal (GI) tract, cells of the DES are found from the stomach to rectum and represent less than 1% of the surrounding cell population. The cells of the gut DES share phenotypic and biochemical features with neural cells. Along with the large core dense vesicles (LCDV) of endocrine cells, the DES cells also contain synaptic-like microvesicles (SLMV) characteristic of the synaptic regions of neural cells. The complex and diverse biochemistry and control of secretion of over 100 amines, peptides, and eicosanoids from the LCDV and SLMV of the DES cells is discussed in detail by Weidenmann et al.[4] Cells of the DES may or may not share a single embryologic origin. However, it is known that gut enteroendocrine cells arise from gut endoderm,[5] and the four epithelial cell types of the gut, including neuroendocrine cells, are derived from a common pluripotential stem cell found in the intestinal crypts,[6] a stem cell characterized by expression of leucine-rich repeat-containing G-protein coupled receptor 5 (LGR5).[7] The pancreatic neuroendocrine cells are derived from

pluripotent cell of the islets of Langerhans. The genetic, epigenetic, and biological characterization of the cells of origin and determinates of the numerous phenotypes of NET tumors are only just beginning to be defined.

Neuroendocrine markers

Neuroendocrine markers are utilized in the histologic and immunohistochemical categorization of NETs, and to some degree as clinical markers for diagnosis and assessment of response and relapse. Markers include:

Serotonin and Metabolites—The rate-limiting step in NETs that synthesize and secrete serotonin is the conversion of tryptophan into 5-hydroxytryptophan (5-HTP). 5-HTP is rapidly converted to 5-hydroxytryptamine that is either stored in the neurosecretory granules or may be secreted directly into the vascular compartment where it is converted into the urinary metabolite 5-hydroxyindoleacetic acid (5-HIAA).[8] The quantification of 5-HIAA in a 24-h urine collection is the best characterized and most frequently used clinical assay for diagnosis and follow-up for those NETs that synthesize and secrete serotonin.[9]

Chromogranin A (CgA) is a member of the chromogranin family of glycoproteins that are stored along with numerous peptide hormones in the large dense core vesicles (LDCV) of endocrine and neuroendocrine cells.[10] It therefore can serve as an immunohistochemical marker for tissue staining and a plasma marker. CgA has been generally accepted as the most useful diagnostic marker for GEP-NET patients with sensitivity above 90%.[11] The CgA level correlates with metastatic versus nonmetastatic disease at presentation and can be used to follow patients for relapse following surgery.[12]

Synaptophysin (p38) is a major neuronal protein concentrated in the membrane of small synaptic vesicles of nerve cells.[13] Weidenmann et al.[14] demonstrated the presence of synaptophysin in a wide range of normal neuroendocrine cells and neuroendocrine tumors.

Neuron-Specific Enolase (NSE) was demonstrated by Bishop and colleagues[15] to be found in all identifiable endocrine and nerve cells of the GI tract and pancreas. NSE has replaced earlier histologic argentaffin stains as a general cytosolic marker of normal neuroendocrine cells and tumors.

Somatostatin and somatostatin receptors

The biology of somatostatin and the somatostatin receptors (SSTRs) and their expression on GEP-NET have yielded information that remains central to the diagnosis and therapy of this group of tumors. Somatostatin analogues are early examples of *targeted* cancer therapy and have broad symptomatic benefit and limited antiproliferative activity that have contributed greatly to the medical and surgical management of NET. The development of radioconjugated somatostatin analogues as imaging agents provide valuable clinical data, and the further extension of these agents as peptide receptor radiotherapy (PRRT) resulted in measurable responses in refractory patients.

Somatostatin is a peptide that inhibits a wide variety of physiologic activities, the most relevant for the treatment of NET being the inhibition of hormone secretion. Somatostatin is found in the central nervous system, hypothalamic pituitary system, GI tract, exocrine and endocrine pancreas, and immune effector cells. It exists as somatostatin-28 and somatostatin-14.[16]

Somatostatin and analogues bind at the plasma membrane with varying affinities to a family of G-protein–coupled receptors (GPCR) subtypes, referred to as SSTR isoforms 1–5, resulting in a decrease in cellular proliferation and induction of apoptosis.[17,18]

The GEP-NET, particularly tumors of the small bowel and pancreatic islets, express multiple SSTR subtypes, the most common and highest density being SSTR2 in over 80% of cases, followed by SSTR5.[19–21] The expression of SSTR2 has been central to the development of somatostatin analogues as therapy to control secretory symptoms, for diagnostic and follow-up nuclear imaging, and for the emerging therapeutic option of PRRT.

Histology and staging of neuroendocrine tumors

Modlin[22] detailed the rich history of NET dating from Siegfried Oberndorfer's 1907 description of a group of monotonous-appearing GI tumors labeled "karzinoide" (carcinoid = carcinoma-like), as distinct from the more aggressive adenocarcinomas. The term *carcinoid* has, for almost 100 years, been generally applied to all tumors of the DES that share a similar histological appearance described as monotonous small cells with regular, well-rounded nuclei with insular, trabecular, glandular, undifferentiated, and mixed growth patterns.[23] With an increased understanding of the DES, more specifically the GEP cells, and the parallels between normal cell types and specific tumor types, the description and classification of "carcinoids" has evolved, and a series of revised classifications systems have been made to further classify tumors into more biologically and clinically relevant groups.

Histology and staging

Recognizing the importance of site of origin, differentiation, the revised WHO classification published in 2000 by Solcia et al.[24] adapted the term (*neuro*) *endocrine* to avoid the inconsistent historical definitions of *carcinoid*. The 2000 WHO classification introduced the term GEP-NET, and defined three broad groups based on differentiation, leaving site of origin as the lead descriptor to accommodate the breadth of NET subtypes. More recent refinements by UICC/AJCC/WHO[25] and modifications by the European Neuroendocrine Society (ENETS)[26] and North American Neuroendocrine Tumor Society (NANETS)[27] recognize the common and shared importance of histologic *differentiation*, and placed further emphasis on *grade* as determined by mitotic rate and/or Ki67 percentage (Table 1). TMN staging was incorporated for the first time in 2010,[28] and prospective and retrospective validation of its prognostic use are ongoing.

Clinical features of tumors of the DES

Generally speaking, tumors of the DES are difficult to recognize at initial presentation. Pulmonary nodules, pancreatic masses, hepatic metastases, and gastric and rectal lesions at endoscopy often are thought to be more common malignancies prior to pathology reports being issued. The early symptoms are often

Table 1 Classification of GEP-NET.

WHO 2010 Nomenclature	AJCC/ENETs Nomenclature
Neuroendocrine neoplasm, grade 1	Neuroendocrine tumor, grade 1
Neuroendocrine neoplasm, grade 2	Neuroendocrine tumor, grade 2
Neuroendocrine carcinoma, grade 3	Neuroendocrine carcinoma, grade 3
• Small cell carcinoma	• Small cell carcinoma
• Large cell neuroendocrine carcinoma	• Large cell neuroendocrine carcinoma

Both systems emphasize the importance of grade, as determined by mitoses/hpf or Ki-67 percentage. Data from[25–27]

nonspecific (i.e., abdominal pain and diarrhea), and even when more dramatic or classic secretory symptoms occur, the primary tumors are often small and difficult to localize. Patients often have long-standing symptoms and are diagnosed following the development of symptoms related to more advanced local or distant metastatic disease. However, once the diagnosis is considered, advancements in nonspecific (i.e., CgA) and specific tumor markers (i.e., 5-HIAA, gastrin) along with the imaging capabilities with radio-labeled somatostatin analogues, complemented by ultrasound, computed tomography (CT), magnetic resonance imaging (MRI), and positron emission tomography (PET) scanning, permit a strong presumptive or confirmed diagnosis to guide medical and surgical management. The variability in the location, secretory status, and biological behavior of these rare tumors has made clinical investigation difficult. Despite the lack of comparative trials, consensus based on clinical evidence is available for guiding management of NET.[29]

Imaging

Somatostatin receptor scintigraphy (SRS) is central to the diagnosis and localization of most cases of GEP-NET. The OctreoScan™, ([[111]Indium-DPTA-pentreotide]), has for decades been the scan of choice, now just recently being replaced in some institutions by the increased specificity and sensitivity of ^{68}Ga-PET/CT.[30] The low proliferative capacity of neuroendocrine tumors is thought to account for the low sensitivity of standard [18]FDG-PET.[31] CT and MRI generally provide further anatomical definition of SRS-documented disease and are more useful than SRS in following tumor growth or response.[32] Most reports support SRS as the initial imaging modality for locating both primary and metastatic lesions (including bone) in patients with confirmed and suspected GEP-NET, except those with insulinoma.[33,34] A European multicenter trial in 350 patients with a histologically or biochemically proven neuroendocrine gastroenteropancreatic (GEP-NET) tumors compared conventional imaging methods (positive in 88% of cases) to SRS (positive in 80% of cases). The SRS detection rates varied with tumor type: glucagonomas (100%), VIPomas (88%), GI-NET (87%), and nonfunctioning PNET (82%). The low detection rate (46%) noted for insulinomas is related to the lower density of SSTR2 on insulinoma cells. Fasting insulin levels coupled with endoscopic ultrasound (EUS) is the most sensitive method of preoperative localization for insulinomas.[35]

Gastrointestinal neuroendocrine tumors (GI-NETs)

Well-differentiated neuroendocrine tumors of the small bowel (GI-NETs) are the most common neuroendocrine tumors. In the small bowel, where tumors in general are rare, they account for 13–34% of all tumors and 17–46% of all malignant tumors.[36]

GI-NETs have been reported from the first to the tenth decade. Modlin et al.[1] reported the average age at diagnosis has increased from 59.9 to 61.4 years over several decades. Except for the small percentage of patients who present with undifferentiated neuroendocrine carcinomas,[37] GI-NETs are generally slow growing, often remain undiagnosed for many years, and sometimes are recognized only by symptoms related to metastatic spread to lymph nodes, liver, and, less often, bone.

Small bowel GI-NET can present with small bowel obstruction, abdominal pain, diarrhea, or GI bleeding. Because tumors located in the distal small bowel in most cases have a low intramural profile (Figure 2), it is not surprising that many of these tumors can grow to larger than 2 cm and remain undiagnosed. The ability of small

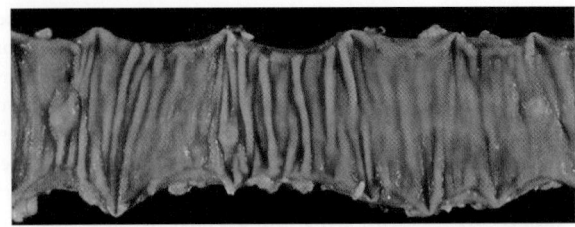

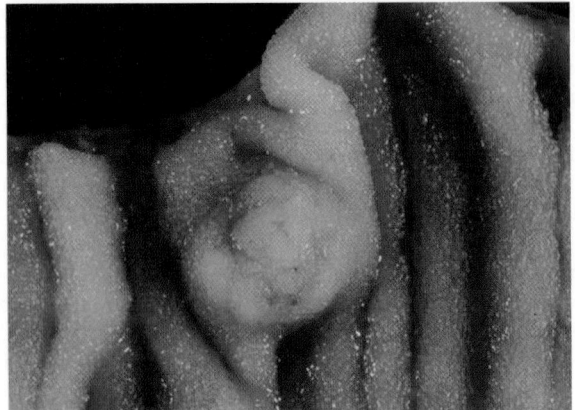

Figure 2 Multiple carcinoids of the small bowel. Three small (<1 cm) intestinal carcinoids found in a young male on inspection of the terminal ileum at colonoscopy. Source: Courtesy of Ed Uthman, MD.

tumors to cause significant local symptoms is in part related to the development of events such as ischemia, strangulation, and intussusception from the marked fibrotic reaction they produce. The likelihood of metastases relates to tumor size. The incidence of metastases associated with ileal GI-NET is less than 15% with a tumor smaller than 1 cm, but increases to 95% with tumors larger than 2 cm. When not diagnosed incidentally during a surgical or endoscopic procedure, the confirmation of GI-NET tumors might be made only after lengthy evaluation of abdominal complaints or iron-deficiency anemia, or astute recognition of the *carcinoid syndrome*.

Carcinoid syndrome

Carcinoid syndrome occurs at diagnosis in less than 10% of patients with small bowel GI-NET tumors, but small bowel GI-NET account for upwards of 90% of patients with the carcinoid syndrome.[38] Over 90% of cases of carcinoid syndrome only occur after metastatic spread to the liver, with principal features of diarrhea (83%), flushing (49%), wheezing (6%), abdominal pain, and very rarely, pellagra.[37,39] Serotonin and its metabolites are thought to account for the majority of carcinoid syndrome symptoms, but other mediators, such as prostaglandins, substance P, kallikrein, dopamine, and neuropeptide K, may also be involved.[9] No single measurement detects all cases of carcinoid syndrome, although the urine 5-HIAA appears to be the best screening procedure, detecting about 84% of patients with NET-related carcinoid syndrome.[40] False positives can occur with ingestion of serotonin rich foods, such as nuts, avocados, kiwi, pineapple, and bananas.[41] CgA has been found to be elevated in 100% of carcinoid syndrome patients, but is lacking in specificity of tumor location because it is elevated in PNET and other neuroendocrine tumors.[42]

Carcinoid heart disease

Carcinoid heart disease develops in half to two-thirds of patients with the *carcinoid syndrome*[43,44] and is characterized by predominantly right-sided valvular lesions described as plaques with proliferation of myofibroblasts and dense extracellular collagen and myxoid deposits.[45] The cardiac disease is a structural disease with thickening and retraction of the valves causing regurgitation (followed later by fusion of fibrous changes to cause stenosis) resulting most often in right-sided congestive heart failure.[46] Moller et al.[47] reported on over 100 patients followed with serial echocardiograms or referred for surgery based on initial echocardiograms and found median survival of 1.6 years for those with documented carcinoid heart disease versus 4.6 years for those without carcinoid heart disease. Peak 5-HIAA levels and prior chemotherapy were independent predictors of progression of carcinoid heart disease. Indirect evidence of the role of serotonin and metabolites includes the histologic similarities to the valvular lesions seen with the diet drugs fenfluramine-phentermine.[48] Studies to date suggest that control of serotonin (5-HIAA) levels *after* carcinoid heart disease that has been established does not prevent progression of valvular disease.[47,49] It is generally accepted, but not proven, that early and improved control of serotonin secretion at diagnosis with somatostatin analogues has reduced the incidence of symptomatic carcinoid heart disease.

Pancreatic net (PNET) (islet-cell tumors)

The second most common GEP-NET occurs in the pancreas. As a group, they have histologic features that are similar to other GEP-NET.[50] The PNET represent about 15% of all GEP-NET, but represent only a small fraction, 1–2%, of all pancreatic tumors. Nonfunctioning PNET and gastrinoma are the most common PNETs, followed by insulinoma and a list of increasingly rare tumors defined by the clinical syndromes associated with their specific secretory products (Table 2).

Nonfunctioning PNET

Nonfunctioning PNET have no specific clinical syndrome, despite staining for one or more peptides and amines or even having quantifiable serum levels of certain neuroendocrine markers. Nonfunctional PNETs account for about 15–30% of the PNET, often diagnosed in the fourth or fifth decade of life, presenting with bulky disease causing abdominal pain in 36%, jaundice in 28%, and or as an incidental finding at surgery in 16%.[51] There is a high reported incidence of local or distant metastases at diagnosis that ranges from 60% to 90%. Serum CgA is elevated in close to 100% of nonfunctioning PNETs.[42] SRS, CT and MRI are used to stage and follow for recurrence and development of metastatic disease.

As for most GEP-NET, the treatment of choice and the only therapy that can achieve a cure is surgery. Given the late presentation and high percentage of patients with metastatic disease at presentation, surgical cure is not often possible for a nonfunctional PNET. However, procedures such as surgical debunking and relief of biliary obstruction can provide significant palliation. The impact of earlier detection due to increased use of imaging has yet to be documented.

Gastrinoma

The gastrinoma syndrome, also named the Zollinger–Ellison Syndrome (ZES), originated with a report of two patients with severe peptic ulcer disease and non β islet-cell tumors of the pancreas,[52] with later identification of gastrin as the secreted hormone.[53] Gastrinoma patients have a severe ulcer diathesis and persistently elevated basal gastric acid hypersecretion. The acid hypersecretion is also responsible for the frequent symptom of diarrhea, the only symptom in upwards of 20% of patients.[54] Gastrinomas account for about 25%

Table 2 The Clinical Syndromes.

Clinical Syndrome	Tumor Type	Site	Hormone(s)
Flushing/diarrhea/wheezing	Carcinoid	Mid foregut	Serotonin, substance P
		Pancreas/foregut Adrenal medulla	NKA, TCT, PP, CGRP, VIP
Ulcer disease	Gastrinoma	Pancreas (85%), duodenum (15%)	Gastrin
Hypoglycemia	Insulinoma sarcomas	Pancreas/uterus	Insulin/TNF
	Hepatoma	Retroperitoneal liver	IGF/BP
Dermatitis/dementia	Glucagonoma	Pancreas	Glucagon
Diabetes/DVT			
Diabetes/steatorrhea	Somatostatinoma	Pancreas	Somatostatin
Cholelithiasis/neurofibromatosis	Somatostatinoma	Duodenum	Somatostatin
Silent/liver mets	PPoma	Pancreas	PP
Acromegaly	GEP	Pancreas	GH (GHRH)
Cushing	GEP	Pancreas	ACTH/CRF
Hypercalcemia	VIPoma	Pancreas	VIP
	GEP	Pancreas	PTHrP
Pigmentation	GEP	Pancreas	MSH

Abbreviations: ACTH, adrenocorticotropic hormone (corticotrophin); BP, binding protein; CGRP, calcitonin gene, related peptide; CRF, corticotropin releasing factor; DVT, deep venous thrombosis; GEP, gastroenteropancreatic; GH, growth hormone, somatotropin; GHRH, growth hormone-releasing hormone; IGF, insulin-like growth factor; MSH, melanocyte stimulating hormone; NKA, neurokinin A; PP, pancreatic polypeptide; PTHrP, parathyroid hormone related peptide; TCT, thyrocalcitonin; TNF, tumor necrosis factor; VIP, vasoactive intestinal peptide; WDHHA, watery diarrhea, hypokalemia, hypochlorhydria, and acidosis.

of all PNET, are found primarily in the duodenum (70%) and pancreas (25%), and demonstrate malignant behavior in approximately 50% of cases.[55,56] About 20% of gastrinoma patients are eventually found to have germline mutations in *MEN-1*,[54] and their presentation and course differ from sporadic cases (see MEN-1 Syndrome).

The diagnosis requires the demonstration of an elevated fasting serum gastrin and elevated basal acid output, both also seen in *Helicobacter pylori* infection, antisecretory therapy (i.e., omeprazole), chronic gastritis, pernicious anemia, atrophic gastritis, and postvagotomy states.[57] The most sensitive and accurate test remains the secretin stimulation test.[58]

Treatment of the gastrinoma syndrome with medical therapy (i.e., omeprazole) is successful in about 95% of patients,[59] such that the long-term survival of patients with very slow growing gastrinomas is now determined largely by the eventual malignant behavior of the tumor rather than ulcer diathesis and diarrhea.[60] Surgery has evolved from gastric resections to control ulcer disease to complex surgery using pre- and intraoperative imaging to localize and resect often small local and regional metastatic disease. The overall survival rate for gastrinomas at 5 years, excluding patients with MEN-1, is between 60% and 80%, and at 10 years is between 45% and 75%.[56,61,62]

Insulinoma

Insulinomas were first described by Whipple in a 1938 report of 30 patients with pancreatic adenomas and hypoglycemia.[63] Insulinomas are the second most common functioning PNET, with an incidence of 0.8–0.9 cases per million. Overall, the incidence of metastatic disease, about 5–15%, is low compared with other PNET. The tumors are often well encapsulated as a single solitary nodule, or multiple nodules evenly distributed throughout the pancreas.[64] The finding of multiple insulinomas should prompt testing for MEN-1.[65] In a prospective database of patients operated for insulinomas, 88% of MEN-1 patients had multifocal lesions versus only 4% of nonMEN-1 patients.[66]

Almost all cases of insulinoma present with symptoms of hypoglycemia, with neuroglycopenic symptoms (visual complaints, altered consciousness, weakness) more common than adrenergic symptoms alone (sweating, tremulousness).[64] Diagnosis of suspected cases is made by a supervised fast, where over 90% of patients will develop a serum glucose of <50 mg/dL during a 48-h

fast, and the corresponding serum insulin level at the time of hypoglycemia will equal or exceed 5 U/mL.[67]

With surgery, 80–90% of all insulinoma patients will be cured.[64] EUS, which has a reported sensitivity of 80%, can localize tumors < 1 cm,[68] and intraoperative ultrasound (IOUS) can be used to avoid blind pancreatic resections when EUS cannot localize a lesion. A diet of small, frequent meals coupled with medical therapy with diazoxide to directly block release of insulin from the β-cell along with octreotide can control symptoms in as many as 60% of patients preoperatively or with unresectable lesions.[69]

VIPoma

The VIPoma (vasoactive intestinal polypeptide) was first described by Verner and Morrison[70] followed by a review of 55 patients with the WDHA syndrome (watery diarrhea, hypokalemia, and achlorhydria).[71] The VIPomas are quite rare, accounting for only about 5% of PNET, and unlike other PNETs, have distinct adult and pediatric subsets of patients. In adults, 90% of the tumors are found in the pancreas, most often as solitary nodules and upwards of 60% of cases present with or develop metastatic disease. In children, most VIP-secreting tumors are extrapancreatic and are neurogenic in origin, with the most common histology being ganglioneuroblastomas and ganglioneuromas.[72] The diagnosis requires the documentation of elevated plasma VIP concentrations and documentation of large volume secretory diarrhea.[73]

Octreotide controls symptoms in over 80% of patients, corresponding with a drop in the VIP plasma level.[69] Long et al.[72] reported that in 52 patients with pancreatic VIPomas, the average lesion was 9 cm in diameter, and thus readily visible by CT or ultrasound. Some VIPomas require angiography with or without selective venous sampling for VIP levels.[73] Complete resections have resulted in long-term control of symptoms in 30–50% of adult patients.[74]

Glucagonoma

Glucagonoma was first reported in 1966 by McGavran et al.,[75] who called attention to a syndrome that included acquired diabetes and glucagon-producing tumors. This rare tumor, estimated to account for 1% of GEP-NET, was later recognized to include a characteristic skin rash labeled *necrolytic migratory erythema* (NME).[76,77] The tumor occurs almost exclusively in adults over 40 years of age and has been associated with MEN-1 in a few cases.[78]

The largest single-institution experience by the Mayo Clinic reported on 21 patients seen between 1975 and 1991.[79] The main presenting features of the glucagonoma syndrome included weight loss (71%), NME rash (67%), mild diabetes mellitus (38%), diarrhea (29%), and painful glossitis and angular stomatitis (29%).

Glucagonomas are almost all found as single lesions in the pancreas (tail > body), averaging 5–10 cm in size, and metastatic disease is already present in over 60% of patients, most often to the liver.[80] If the diagnosis is made while the tumor is still localized, surgical resection can be curative.[81] Due to the slow growth of tumors and available therapies, the 10 years survival is 51.6% for patients with metastases and 64.3% for patients without metastases at diagnosis.[82] Both the NME rash and diarrhea, but generally not the glucose intolerance/diabetes, respond to octreotide in over 50% of the patients, with complete disappearance of symptoms in about 30% of patients.[69]

Somatostatinoma

Somatostatinomas are rare PNET, with about 50 cases reported to date. The first cases were reported in 1977 by Ganda et al.[83] and Larsson et al.[84] Krejs et al.[85] reported a series of 8 cases in 1979, and Vinik et al.[86] reported the largest review on 48 cases in 1986. Somatostatinomas are rarely seen in association with MEN-1.[78]

Despite a defined clinical syndrome of diabetes, diarrhea, steatorrhea, gallbladder disease, hypochlorhydria, and weight loss,[87] most cases are diagnosed at laparotomy or laparoscopy, or identified on imaging studies for abdominal complaints or jaundice. A markedly elevated plasma level of somatostatin is thought to be responsible for the majority of symptoms. The tumors tend to present as large masses, reflecting the high levels of somatostatin thought necessary to create symptoms. At diagnosis, 85% of the pancreatic and 50% of the intestinal primaries had evidence of metastatic spread.[88] Though the data are minimal; the outlook for those with somatostatinomas is poor, given the high incidence of malignant spread. Close to half of reported patients died within a year and others survived up to as long as 5 years.[87]

Therapy for GEP-NET

In general, GEP-NET are slow growing and symptoms are most often attributable to secretory products or pain from bulky disease. For those patients whose tumors are not resectable at diagnosis or who later develop metastatic disease, the focus is on control of symptoms. The use of the long-acting somatostatin analogues to decrease secretion of vasoactive and other hormones, combined with bulk-reducing procedures primarily directed at hepatic lesions, the quality of life of GEP-NET patients can be maintained for extended periods of time. Recent data demonstrates for selected patients, somatostatin analogues, sunitinib, and everolimus can prolong progression-free survival in patients with metastatic disease.

Surgery primary

Prophylactic treatment with a somatostatin analogue should be considered before all surgical procedures in GEP-NET patients to avoid precipitation of the *carcinoid syndrome* or other secretory crises.[89] Gastric and duodenal GEP-NET can, in selected cases with tumors <1 cm, be excised endoscopically.[90] GI-NETs of the small bowel that appear localized should be resected en bloc with lymphadenectomy and removal of the mesentery.[91] GI-NETs of the appendix are generally treated by appendectomy if <2 cm, and resection if >2 cm.[92]

Liver-directed therapies

Given the high frequency of metastatic spread to the liver, a number of liver-directed therapies have been used in the management of GEP-NETs. It is estimated that >90% of patients with hepatic metastases have lesions that are too large, too numerous, or too diffuse to permit resection. Hepatic Resections: Que et al.[93] recently performed a meta-analysis summarizing reports of involving hemihepatectomy, trisegmentectomy, or wedge resection for GEP-NET. The operative mortality after partial hepatectomy for GEP-NETs in this series was 2.3%. More than 80% had improvement in symptoms related to hormone excess (i.e., carcinoid syndrome), and the duration of response ranged from 4 to 120 months.

Radiofrequency ablation

Radiofrequency ablation (RFA) has been used in these patients to reduce bulk of disease and control symptoms. The largest series to date of RFA in metastatic neuroendocrine tumors involving patients treated over a 10-year period at a single institution demonstrated perioperative morbidity of <5%, a 90% partial and 72% complete relief of symptoms, and median duration of symptom control of approximately one year.[94]

Hepatic artery vaso-occlusive therapy

Overall, vascular-occlusion therapies have led to biochemical responses as high as 50%, and tumor reduction as high as 40%, all generally of short duration.[95] Hepatic arterial occlusion combined with sequential chemotherapy has resulted in biochemical responses as high as 80%, with a median duration of response of 18 months or more.[96–98]

Hepatic transplantation

A recent review of the first 103 liver transplants in Europe for NET tumors showed 5-year overall and disease-free survival of 46% and 24% respectively.[99] However, the restrictive transplant criteria, significant morbidity and mortality of the procedure, and the general lack of transplantable organs make transplant a limited therapeutic option.

Somatostatin analogues

Somatostatin analogues have had a major impact on the flushing, diarrhea, and wheezing in patients with metastatic carcinoid and the carcinoid syndrome and can control many of the other secretory symptoms associated with various NET. Yao's analysis of SEER data has shown an increase in survival in GEP-NET following the introduction of octreotide in the United States in 1998,[2] perhaps reflecting an antiproliferative effect combined with reduced risks of surgery, allowing patients to benefit from more aggressive approach to metastatic disease. Janson et al.[100] and Kvols et al.[101] have shown that a positive SRS (OctreoScan™) predicts for patient symptomatic response to somatostatin analogues. Octreotide, a long-acting formulation (somatostatin-LAR)[102] and recently approved lanreotide are available in the United States.[103] SOM 230 (pasreotide), a somatostatin analogue with broad binding affinity to SSTR1-5, is currently in phase III development for GEP-NET, and recently approved in the United States for Cushing's disease.[103]

Use of somatostatin analogues over many decades, both short and long acting formulations,[104,105] are associated with biochemical responses in 70–80% of patients, symptomatic control of diarrhea and flushing in over 80% of patients, and a decrease in 5-HIAA levels (if elevated at baseline) in over 70% of patients.[106,107] Recent studies of somatostatin analogues in *asymptomatic* GEP-NET patients with significant tumor burden have shown clinical benefit beyond symptom control. The PROMID trial was a phase III, randomized, placebo-controlled, double-blind study of small bowel GI-NET patients with minimally or asymptomatic metastatic disease that compared long-acting octreotide to placebo. The median time to progression for octreotide was 14.3 months and placebo was 6.0 months, with stable disease at 6 months for octreotide of 67% and placebo of 37%. Median overall survival was not assessed owing to a crossover design.[108] The CLARINET trial was a phase III, randomized, placebo-controlled, double-blind study of both well-differentiated GI-NET and PNET patients with asymptomatic but progressive metastatic disease. The trial compared long-acting lanreotide to placebo. The primary end point of progression-free survival was significantly greater for lanreotide (not reached) versus 18 months for placebo, with no significant difference in overall survival.[109]

Biologic agents

Oberg pioneered the use of leukocyte interferon in GEP-NET[110] and reviewed the early trials in 2000[112] demonstrating a biochemical response in 63–77% of patients, with stable disease reported in over 50%, and a rare complete or partial tumor response. One of the few multicenter, randomized, comparative trials done in the field of GEP-NET to date, however, showed that the objective responses were no higher with the combination as compared with either agent alone.[111] Though a higher symptomatic and biochemical response rate was seen in the combination therapy group, it was at the expense of increased toxicity.

Peptide receptor radiotherapy (PRRT)

Targeting the SSTR provided by somatostatin analogues has led to the development of PRRT reagents for GEP-NET whereby the localization with the Octreoscan documents the opportunity for selective delivery of a radiopharmaceutical at the site of SSTR2, 5 expressing tumors.[112] Trials of several different radionuclide-somatostatin analogue combinations have been studied in phase I, II clinical trials, but no phase III trials have been completed. Response rates (CR + PR) ranging from about 10–30%, with 40–60% of patients developing stable disease have been reported.[113,114] Currently no PRRT are approved for therapeutic indications, and they remain available only through clinical trials or for compassionate use in selected centers in Europe.

Cytotoxic chemotherapy for GEP-NET

Several authors have reviewed the history of treatment of GEP-NET, with single-agent and multiagent chemotherapy.[9,115] In the absence of randomized trials that contain a no-treatment arm, there is no persuasive evidence that single-agent or combination chemotherapy provides any significant impact on disease progression or on survival in patients with metastatic NET. The approved agents, DTIC and Streptozocin, have significant toxicities and questionable benefit. Recent studies of temozolomide, in combination with thalidomide,[116] or in a retrospective study with capecitabine[117] are encouraging. Chemotherapy is generally reserved to provide palliation of hormone excess and symptoms related to tumor bulk.

Targeted therapies

Early phase trials have been completed for several targeted therapies. Minimal or no response was seen in phase II studies of the tyrosine kinases inhibitors imatinib[118] and gefitinib.[119] More encouraging are the responses seen in phase II trials of the VEGF inhibitor bevacizumab.[120] A series of clinical trials has led to FDA approval in 2011 for both everolimus and sunitinib for PNET. GI-NET patients were included in the trials and responded, but below the level required for approval.

Everolimus, an oral inhibitor of m-TOR, studied in the RADIANT-3 phase III, randomized, placebo-controlled study of well differentiated PNET patients with advanced and progressive disease demonstrated a median PFS of 11.0 months for everolimus versus 4.6 months for placebo.[121] The earlier RADIANT-2 phase III, randomized, placebo-controlled study of well differentiated GI-NET patients with advanced and progressive disease and carcinoid syndrome, demonstrated a non-significant difference in median PFS of 16.4 months for everolimus versus 11.3 months for placebo.[122]

Sunitinib, and oral multi-tyrosine kinase inhibitor, was shown in a phase III, randomized, placebo-controlled study of well differentiated PNET that were locally advanced or metastatic and with recent progression, to have a PFS of 11.4 months versus 5.5 months for placebo. Though assessments were confounded by early closure by a data safety committee, and possible bias from investigator response assessment, the FDA approved sunitinib for this indication after an independent data review.[123]

MEN syndromes

The MEN-1 and MEN-2 syndromes, first referred to as Werner syndrome, were based on the author's observation of groups of individuals with multiple adenomas that appeared to be inherited in an autosomal dominant pattern.[124] The MEN-1 and MEN-2 syndromes differ in genetics, clinical presentation, the type and frequency of involvement of certain endocrine tissues, preventive and therapeutic surgery, and follow-up of affected individuals and family members. The neuroendocrine tumors that occur within the MEN syndromes have both similarities and differences to the same tumors when they occur sporadically.

MEN-1 syndrome

A somewhat unpredictable cluster of neuroendocrine and nonendocrine tumors from a total of about 20 different histologic types characterizes MEN-1 syndrome cases and families (Table 3). Though there is no "typical" grouping of neuroendocrine tumors, data from many families show that the most common tumors are parathyroid (including hyperplasia) (90%), enteropancreatic (70%), and anterior pituitary (25%).[126] A practical clinical guideline for diagnosis of an MEN-1 individual is to have two of the three

Table 3 MEN-1 Tumor Type Distribution and Estimated Penetrance (%) by Age 40 Years.

Endocrine Tumors (Common)	Endocrine Tumors (Less Common)	Nonendocrine Features
Parathyroid adenoma (90%)	Thymic carcinoid (2%)	Collagenomas (70%)
Gastrinoma (40%) PP (nonfunctioning) oma (20%)	Bronchial carcinoid (2%) PNET (VIPoma, glucagonoma, etc) (2%)	Facial angiofibromas (85%)
Prolactinoma (20%)	ACTH, GH (2%)	Lipomas (30%)
Insulinoma (10%)	Pheochromocytoma (<1%)	
ECL tumor (10%)	TSH (rare)	

[a]Nonfunctioning adrenal tumors are found in as high as 25% of MEN-1 patients on full evaluation.

Source: Data taken in part from Giusti et al.[125]

principal tumors diagnosed, and a MEN-1 family would involve at least one case as defined above and at least one first-degree relative with at least one of the principal tumor types.

About 80% of familial MEN-1 individuals and about 50% of sporadic MEN-1 individuals have a heterozygous germline mutation in the *MEN-1* gene.[127,128] A recent update described 1336 mutations spread across the coding region of the *MEN-1* gene.[129] MENIN, the product of the *MEN-1* gene, acts as a tumor suppressor with the various mutations resulting in loss-of-function. Despite the varied genotypes, no correlation of genotype to clinical phenotype has been determined that could allow a more focused algorithm to justify preventive surgery and a more focused screening of affected family members with specific mutations.[129]

MEN-1 and parathyroid lesions

Most patients first present with symptoms of hyperparathyroidism (HPT), asymptomatic hypercalcemia, or if in a known MEN-1 family undergoing screening, with biochemical or imaging evidence of parathyroid tumor(s). The average age of onset is 25–30 years old, and by age 50, nearly 100% of the MEN-1 patients will have evidence of HPT. In contrast, only 2–4% of cases of sporadic HPT investigated will be found to have mutations in the *MEN-1* gene,[130] and the average age of onset is 55–60 years old.

MEN-1 and gastrinoma

Gastrinomas are the next most common "tumor" to follow HPT in MEN-1 patients.

Approximately 20% of gastrinomas are associated with the MEN-1 syndrome,[54] present at an earlier age, often are multiple small or undetectable primaries, and are less frequently (7–12%) malignant than sporadic gastrinomas. When there is no evidence of metastatic disease and venous sampling demonstrates an anatomically localized source of gastrin, enucleation (pancreatic head), or resection (body or tail) may offer excellent palliation, but rarely a cure.[9] It is generally recommended to avoid surgery and manage medically with periodic evaluations for radiological progression of tumors.

MEN-1 medical and surgical management

The clinical features of patients with MEN-1 depend entirely upon the natural history of the individual tumors and endocrine hyperfunction. Treatment of the MEN-1 syndrome is dependent on the phenotypic expression in the individual patient. Most patients with MEN-1 pancreatic disease requiring surgical intervention present with a syndrome caused by hypersecretion of a specific hormone such as gastrin, insulin, VIP, or glucagon. Overall, patients with familial MEN-1 neoplasms have longer survival than patients with sporadic endocrine pancreatic tumors.[9] Regardless of initial findings; MEN-1 patients must be followed for life for involvement of the pituitary gland, parathyroid glands, endocrine pancreas or duodenum, adrenal glands, thymus, and lungs (bronchial carcinoids). Family members who are screened with *MEN-1* gene sequencing and are found to be positive should undergo similar lifelong surveillance.[131]

MEN-2 syndromes

The MEN-2 syndromes represent several distinct clusters of neuroendocrine tumors with an association between specific gene mutations of the *RET* proto-oncogene and phenotype. MEN-2A patients are characterized by MTC (95%), pheochromocytoma (50%), and hyperplasia/adenoma of the parathyroid

Table 4 Classification of MEN-2 Syndromes.

	MEN-2 Cases	MTC	Pheo	Parathyroid Hyperplasia/Adenoma
MEN-2A	60–90%	95%	50%	20–30%
MEN-2B	5%	100%	50%	Uncommon
FMTC	5–35%	100%	0%	0%

Abbreviations: FMTC, familial medullary thyroid carcinoma; MTC, medullary thyroid carcinoma; Pheo, pheochromocytoma.
Source: Data from Moline et al.[133]

glands (15–30%) of cases.[132] MEN-2B patients have MTC (100%), pheochromocytoma (50%), and varied reported incidences of mucosal neuromas and marfanoid body habitus (Table 4).[132,134] There have been almost 1000 MEN-2 families reported worldwide, with the subtype MEN-2B representing about 80% of families.[135] Over 70 distinct *RET* mutations have been identified, and with increasing data on large kindreds, the genotype–phenotype relationships with each mutation have become *less* distinct than originally reported.[136]

Medullary thyroid carcinoma

MTC represents about 5–10% of new cases of thyroid cancers, or about 1000 cases per year in the United States. Of these, about 75% have no family history of MTC (sporadic MTC) and are generally diagnosed around the age of 50–60 years.[137] Both MEN-2A and 2B patients are at high risk of MTC (Table 4). MEN-2A patients often present with MTC before pheochromocytoma or parathyroid disease. In known MEN-2A families, biochemical evidence of MTC usually occurs between the ages of 5 and 25 years.[138] The MEN-2B patients have an earlier age of onset of cancers and a more aggressive phenotype of MTC leading to a worse prognosis compared with MEN-2A patients.[139,140] Fortunately, some of these children are recognized prior to the diagnosis of MTC based on genetic screening or clinical recognition of marfanoid body habitus and mucosal neuromas.[141] MTC is suspected in the presence of elevated serum calcitonin levels, a sensitive and specific marker. Patients not identified by genetic testing or biochemical screening, about 30% of MTC patients, will present with a (painful) neck mass, and/or diarrhea associated with high calcitonin levels. Unfortunately most of these patients already have local or distant spread of their tumors.[137]

Familial medullary thyroid carcinoma

The designation of familial medullary thyroid carcinoma (FMTC), as opposed to MEN-2A, MEN-2B, and sporadic MTC, is defined as families with four or more cases of MTC in the absence of a diagnosis of pheochromocytoma or parathyroid hyperplasia/adenoma. Of these cases, almost 90% will be found to have an identifiable *RET* mutation.[142] It is recommended that all FMTC cases undergo regular screening tests for pheochromocytoma and parathyroid disease given that some families are later classified as MEN-2A or 2B.[143] The therapy for FMTC is the same as for MTC in association with MEN-2A, MEN-2B, though the clinical course and prognosis is more favorable for FMTC.[142]

Treatment of medullary thyroid carcinoma

Prophylactic thyroidectomy (and autotransplant of parathyroid tissue) is accepted therapy for MEN-2B patients with documented *RET* germline mutations. The timing of the surgery, still controversial, can in fact be guided by the specific *RET* codon affected.[126] Treatment of established MTC involves total thyroidectomy and lymph node dissection in almost all cases, followed by lifelong thyroid replacement. Of these patients, approximately 50% will develop recurrent disease,[144] necessitating yearly screening with a calcitonin stimulation test. Clinical studies of chemotherapy and radiotherapy have not demonstrated any durable responses.[145] However, clinical investigation of various targeted multikinase inhibitors have shown promising results, and led to the recent FDA approval of two new agents for MTC.

Vandetanib is an oral inhibitor of VEGF2-3, RET, EGFR that in a phase III randomized, placebo-controlled trial against placebo achieved the primary endpoint of an increase in progression-free survival of 30.5 months versus 19.3 months for placebo.[146] Partial response of 45% was seen, with even higher biochemical responses in calcitonin and CEA. No overall survival benefit has been demonstrated as yet, and significant toxicity including QTc prolongation requiring a *black box warning* was required at FDA approval in 2011.[147]

Cabozantinib is an oral inhibitor VEGF2-3, RET, MET that in a phase III randomized, placebo-controlled trial of patients (with documented recent progression) against placebo achieved the primary endpoint of an increase in progression-free survival of 11.2 months versus 4.0 months for placebo. Partial response was 28%, with no overall survival benefit yet demonstrated. Toxicities were similar to vandetanib, excluding effects on QTc.[148]

Clinical trials of vandetanib, cabozantinib, and several other multikinase inhibitors alone and in combination are ongoing.[149]

Pheochromocytoma

Pheochromocytomas arise in the chromaffin cells of the adrenal medulla. Paragangliomas of the sympathetic nervous system, often called extra-adrenal pheochromocytomas, are most often located in the retroperitoneum. Paragangliomas of the parasympathetic nervous system are often located in the region of the aortic arch, neck, and base of skull (i.e., carotid body paragangliomas).[150] Mayo Clinic data estimates that approximately 800 cases of pheochromocytoma are diagnosed in the United States each year.[151] They are found in approximately 0.05–0.1% of hypertensive patients.[152]

Clinical features and diagnosis

Discussions of the diagnosis and management of pheochromocytoma often consider the "rough rule of tens": 10% of neoplasms occur in children, 10% of sporadic cases are bilateral, 10% are extra-adrenal, and 10% are malignant. Previously, this rule included that 10% of pheochromocytomas were familial, but recent updates document that over 40% of pheochromocytoma patients without personal or family history of associated endocrine neoplasia have a germ-line mutation in one of the following genes: *VHL, RET, NF-1, MEN-1*, succinate dehydrogenase subunits D,B,C (*SDHD, SDHB, SDHC, SDHAF2), SMAD4, ENG, ALK1, TMEM127, MAX, HIF2A*.[153,154] It is now recommended that genetic counseling and possible genetic testing, be considered for all patients diagnosed with pheochromocytoma, particularly those diagnosed under age 50 years with a family history or multifocal disease.[155]

Patients may present anywhere in the spectrum from normotensive and asymptomatic to a severe, life-threatening hypertensive crisis. The fundamental basis for the diagnosis of pheochromocytoma is a high index of clinical suspicion with confirmation by biochemical determinations for catecholamines or catecholamine metabolites by assays for plasma metanephrines or the more widely available measurements of 24-hour urinary excretion for catecholamines, metanephrines, or vanillylmandelic acid (VMA).[156] CT scanning, as well as MRI, can visualize over 90% of adrenal pheochromocytomas in patients with biochemical evidence of a pheochromocytoma.[157]

Surgical management of benign or recurrent resectable disease

Nearly all benign pheochromocytomas can be cured by surgical resection. Because of its slow growth rate and accompanying significant morbidity, complete resection of local recurrence or limited metastases of malignant pheochromocytoma should be attempted. The value of debulking surgery for patients whose tumor cannot be completely resected is not established, but reports of successful control of symptoms following surgery have been reported.[158] An international consensus on preoperative management summarizes the critical need to control blood pressure, manage cardiac rate and rhythm, normalize fluid status and prevent a "catecholamine storm" at the time of invasive procedures and surgery.[159]

Medical treatment of recurrent or metastatic disease

It is estimated that only about 5–25% of all pheochromocytomas are malignant.[151] The CVD (cyclophosphamide, vincristine, and dacarbazine) regimen that is effective in children with advanced neuroblastoma is considered the preferred treatment of symptomatic, disseminated pheochromocytoma.[160]

MEN-2 and pheochromocytoma

Pheochromocytomas in MEN-2 patients are diagnosed between the ages of 20–30 years, earlier than the sporadic pheochromocytomas diagnosed between 35–45 years old,[161] in part owing to MEN-2 patients being actively screened. About 25% of MEN-2A patients present with pheochromocytoma as their first tumor.[162,163] Up to 75% of patients are diagnosed concurrently with MTC.[161] MEN-2 patients with pheochromocytomas develop bilateral tumors and appear to have a lower incidence of malignant transformation than patients with sporadic tumors.[164] Given the low incidence of malignancy in MEN-2 patients, unilateral or bilateral subtotal resection with preservation of adrenocortical function can be considered in this population to avoid lifelong replacement therapy. The MEN-2A patients are often asymptomatic, but can develop hypertensive crises during surgery undertaken for HPT or MTC. Therefore, all patients with MEN-2 should be carefully screened for the presence of pheochromocytoma before any surgery or invasive procedure and, if present, treated with α-adrenergic blockade to control blood pressure.[159]

Within MEN-2 families, the specific *RET* mutation at codon 634 is highly associated with the presence or eventual development of pheochromocytoma and should be considered in following these patients. Overall, the general recommendation is to screen all MEN-2 patients for pheochromocytoma on a yearly basis.[155]

Key references

The complete reference list can be found on the Wiley Companion Digital Edition of this title (see inside front cover for login instructions).

2   Yao JC, Hassan M, Phan A, et al. One hundred years after "carcinoid": epidemiology of and prognostic factors for neuroendocrine tumors in 35,825 cases in the United States. *J Clin Oncol.* 2008;**26**:3063–3072.

7   Clevers H. The intestinal crypt, a prototype stem cell compartment. *Cell.* 2013;**154**:274–284.

11 Oberg K. Biochemical diagnosis of neuroendocrine GEP tumor. *Yale J Biol Med.* 1997;**70**:501–508.

12 Nehar D, Lombard-Bohas C, Olivieri S, et al. Interest of Chromogranin A for the diagnosis and follow-up of endocrine tumors. *Clin Endocrinol* (Oxford). 2004;**60**:644–652.

16 Lamberts SW, van der Lely AJ, de Herder WW, et al. Octreotide. *N Engl J Med.* 1996;**334**:246–254.

22 For a definitive historical discussion on carcinoid tumors, the reader is encouraged to read:Modlin IM, Shapiro MD, Kidd M. Siegfried Oberndorfer: origins and perspectives of carcinoid tumors. *Hum Pathol.* 2004;**35**:1440–1451.

27 Klimstra DS, Modlin IR, Coppola D, et al. The pathologic classification of neuroendocrine tumors. A review of nomenclature, grading, and staging systems. *Pancreas.* 2010;**39**:707–712.

36 Moertel CG, Sauer WG, Docherty MB, Baggenstoss AH. Life history of the carcinoid tumor of the small intestine. *Cancer.* 1961;**14**:291–293.

37 Kulke MH, Mayer RJ. Carcinoid tumors. *N Engl J Med.* 1999;**340**:858–868.

45 Simula DV, Edwards WD, Tazelaar HD, et al. Surgical pathology of carcinoid heart disease: a study of 139 values from 75 patients spanning over 20 years. *Mayo Clin Proc.* 2002;**77**:139–147.

52 Zollinger RM, Ellison EH. Primary peptic ulceration of the jejunum associated with islet cell tumors of the pancreas. *Ann Surg.* 1955;**142**:709–723.

59 Metz DC, Strader DB, Orbuch M, et al. Use of omeprazole in Zollinger-Ellison: a prospective nine-year study of efficacy and safety. *Aliment Pharmacol Ther.* 1993;**7**:597–610.

60 Norton JA, Fraker DL, Alexander HR, et al. Surgery increases survival in patients with gastrinoma. *Ann Surg.* 2006;**244**:410–419.

65 Marx S, Spiegel AM, Skarulis MC, et al. Multiple endocrine neoplasia type 1: clinical and genetic topics. *Ann Intern Med.* 1998;**129**:484–494.

71 Verner JV, Morrison AB. Endocrine pancreatic disease with diarrhea: report of a case due to diffuse hyperplasia of non-beta islet tissue with a review of 54 additional cases. *Arch Intern Med.* 1974;**133**:492–499.

75 McGavran MH, Unger RH, Recant L, et al. A glucagon secreting alpha-cell carcinoma of the pancreas. *N Engl J Med.* 1966;**274**:1408–1413.

84 Larsson LI, Hirsch MA, Holst J, et al. Pancreatic somatostatinoma clinical features and physiologic implications. *Lancet.* 1977;**1**:666–668.

86 Vinik AI, Strodel WE, Eckhauser FE, et al. Somatostatinomas, PPomas, neurotensinomas. *Semin Oncol.* 1987;**14**:263–281.

93 Que FG, Nagorney DM, Batts KP, et al. Hepatic resection for metastatic neuroendocrine carcinomas. *Am J Surg.* 1995;**169**:36–43.

94 Mazzaglai PJ, Berber E, Milas M, Siperstein AE. Laparoscopic radiofrequency ablation of neuroendocrine liver metastases: a 10-year experience evaluating predictors of survival. *Surgery.* 2007;**142**:10–19.

98 Del Prete M, Fiore F, Modica R, et al. Hepatic arterial embolization in patients with neuroendocrine tumors. *J Exp Clin Canc Res.* 2014;**33**:43–51.

101 Kvols LK, Reubi JC, Horisberger U, et al. The presence of somatostatin receptors in malignant neuroendocrine tumor tissue predicts responsiveness to octreotide. *Yale J Biol Med.* 1992;**65**:505–18.

111 Faiss S, Pape UF, Bohmig M, et al. Prospective, randomized, multicenter trial on the antiproliferative effect of lanreotide, interferon alfa, and their combination for therapy of metastatic neuroendocrine gastroenteropancreatic tumors—the International Lanreotide and Interferon Alfa Study Group. *J Clin Oncol.* 2003;**21**:2689–96.

114 Kwekkeboom DJ, Bakker WH, Kam BL, et al. Treatment with Lu-177 DOTA-Tyr3-octreotate in patients with neuroendocrine tumors: interim results. *Eur J Nucl Med Mol Imaging.* 2003;**30**:S231.

117 Strosberg JR, Fine RL, Choi J, et al. First-line chemotherapy with capecitabine and temozolomide in patients with metastatic pancreatic endocrine carcinomas. *Cancer.* 2011;**117**:268–275.

121 Yao JC, Shah MH, Ito T, et al. Everolimus for advanced pancreatic neuroendocrine tumors. *N Engl J Med.* 2011;**364**:514–523.

123 Raymond E, Dahan L, Raoul J-L, et al. Sunitinib maleate for the treatment of pancreatic neuroendocrine tumors. *N Engl J Med.* 2011;**364**:501–513.

126 Brandi ML, Gagel RF, Andeli A, et al. CONSENSUS: Guidelines for diagnosis and therapy of MEN type I and type 2. *J Clin Endo Metab.* 2001;**86**:5658–5671.

129 Lemos MC, Thakker RV. Multiple endocrine neoplasia type I (MEN1): analysis of 1336 mutations reported in the first decade following identification of the gene. *Hum Mutat.* 2008;**29**:22–32.

131 Thakur RV. Multiple Endocrine neoplasia, type I (MEN1). *Best Practice & Res Clin Endocrinol & Metab 2010.* 2013;**24**:355–370.

138 Lips CJ, Landsvater RM, Hoppener JW, et al. Clinical screening as compared with DNA analysis in families with multiple endocrine neoplasia type 2A. *N Engl J Med.* 1994;**331**:828–835.

146 Wells SA, Robinson BG, Gagel RF, et al. Vandetinib in patients with locally advanced or metastatic meduallry thyroid cancer: A randomized, double-blind phase III trial. *J Clin Oncol.* 2013;**30**:134–141.

148 Eisei R, Schulmberger MJ, Muller SP, et al. Cabozantinib in progressive medullary thyroid cancer. *J Clin Oncol.* 2013;**31**:3639–3646.

152 Pacak K, Linehan WM, Eisenhofer G, et al. Recent advances in genetics, diagnosis, localization, and treatment of pheochromocytoma. *Ann Intern Med.* 2001;**134**:315–329.

83 Neoplasms of the head and neck

Renata Ferrarotto, MD ▪ *Merrill S. Kies, MD* ▪ *Adam S. Garden, MD* ▪ *Michael E. Kupferman, MD*

Overview

Head and neck cancers (HNCs) comprise a diverse group of malignancies affecting the upper aerodigestive tract. The most common tumor type is squamous cell carcinoma. While the main risk factors for HNC remain tobacco and alcohol abuse, oncogenic viruses such as human papilloma virus and Epstein–Barr virus play a major carcinogenic role in tumors of the oropharynx and nasopharynx, respectively. The management of head and neck malignancies is site and histology specific, and requires a multidisciplinary team approach. In this chapter, we review the current knowledge of HNC, with focus on squamous and salivary cancers, and discuss ongoing and future research aiming to improve the management and outcomes of patients with these malignancies.

Introduction

Approximately 62,000 new cases of head and neck cancer (HNC) will be diagnosed in the United States and over 13,000 Americans will die from these malignancies in 2016, accounting for 4% of all new cancer cases and 2% of cancer deaths annually.[1,2] Tobacco and alcohol are the primary etiologic agents for squamous cell carcinomas (SCCs).[3] However, a rising proportion of these cancers (particularly those found in the oropharynx) are attributable to oncogenic human papilloma virus (HPV)[4] and the preventive efficacy of population-wide HPV vaccination on incidence rates has yet to be determined. HNCs have a much greater impact in certain parts of the world, especially where cigarette smoking and/or chewing of carcinogenic stimulants is more prevalent.[1,5,6] The more widespread adoption of multidisciplinary care likely underlies improvements in survival rates for some sites (nasopharynx and oropharynx);[7] however, long-term survival rates are stagnant for other sites.[8]

Despite marked advances in reconstructive surgery, rehabilitation, and intensity-modulated radiotherapy (IMRT), head and neck squamous cell carcinoma (HNSCC) patients continue to have significant functional deficits which affect quality of life. Combined-modality approaches involving chemotherapy and radiation are now standards of care for "nonsurgical" locally advanced disease with objectives of disease eradication and organ preservation. Understanding the biology of HNC and developing molecularly targeted therapeutic agents and chemoprevention strategies have advanced substantially. These new therapeutic and preventive approaches appear to hold great promise for improving the control of HNC and its sequelae. This chapter reviews the current status of and future investigative directions for the epidemiology, biology, diagnosis, and therapy of HNC.

Descriptive epidemiology

Incidence

In the United States, estimates for 2015 are for approximately 45,780 new cases of oral cavity and oropharynx cancer, 13,560 new cases of laryngeal cancer, 3200 nasopharyngeal carcinoma (NPC), 3100 malignant salivary gland tumors, and 2000 nasal cavity and paranasal sinus neoplasias.[2] The United States has benefited from tobacco control efforts with declining smoking prevalence beginning in the 1960s and subsequent declines in incidence rates for most HNC beginning in the 1980s.[9] Approximately one in two oral cavity cancers occur in women, while only one in four pharyngeal and laryngeal cancers occur in women. Death rates from oral cavity and pharyngeal cancers have declined among whites and blacks over the years from 1993 to 2007, the largest changes in black men and women with 12 years of education. Although blacks and whites have similar rates of oral cavity/pharyngeal cancer, black men have double the rate of laryngeal cancer of white men; and black women have a 40% higher rate of laryngeal cancer than that of white women. Hispanics have the lowest incidence of oral cavity/pharyngeal cancer, and Asians have the lowest rates of laryngeal cancer.[10] The median age at diagnosis for HNSCC is approximately 60 years, but the incidence of these cancers in young adults (age <45 years) appears to be increasing, related to increasing numbers of oropharyngeal cancers associated with oncogenic HPV.[4] HPV-positive oropharyngeal cancers are more common in white men, presumably related to the prevalence of oral sexual practices.[9]

Worldwide, HNC incidence was approximately 550,000 cases in 2011. Melanesia has the highest incidence of oral cavity cancer (36 : 100,000), followed by South-Central Asia, and Central and Eastern Europe.[10] While mortality rates attributed to oral cavity cancer have been decreasing in most countries in Europe and Asia, rates continue to increase in Eastern European countries, particularly in females, reflecting the tobacco epidemic in that region. Although 80% of HNC cases in South-Central Asia are oral cavity and pharyngeal (excluding nasopharyngeal), in other regions of the world, laryngeal and nasopharyngeal cancers are more common. Laryngeal cancer accounts for approximately one-third of HNC in the developed world, and approximately 40% of cases in Southern and Eastern Europe. In South-Eastern Asia, nasopharynx carcinoma is the sixth most common malignancy overall in males, accounting for ~70% of all HNC in countries like Malaysia, Indonesia and Singapore.[10]

Prevalence

Highlighting the impact of cancer survivorship, approximately 350,000 individuals were living in the United States with a history of HNC in November, 2007. As expected, the sex distribution of these prevalent cases reflects the sex of the incident cases. However,

Holland-Frei Cancer Medicine, Ninth Edition. Edited by Robert C. Bast Jr., Carlo M. Croce, William N. Hait, Waun Ki Hong, Donald W. Kufe, Martine Piccart-Gebhart, Raphael E. Pollock, Ralph R. Weichselbaum, Hongyang Wang, and James F. Holland.
© 2017 John Wiley & Sons, Inc. ISBN: 978-1-118-93469-2

African Americans accounted for only 11.5% and 7.3% of the prevalent population of individuals with a history of laryngeal and oral cavity/pharyngeal cancer, respectively. These small percentages likely reflect the poorer overall survival (OS) of African Americans diagnosed with HNSCC. Over the past decade, African Americans have demonstrated survival rates approximately 20% and 15% worse than whites for oral cavity/pharyngeal and for laryngeal cancer, respectively.[11]

Mortality

In 2015 in the United States, 8650 deaths will be attributed to oral cavity and oropharyngeal cancer, and 3640 to laryngeal cancer.[2] Broader use of and improvements in multidisciplinary care, and the declining incidence attributable to tobacco control, likely underlie the significantly improved survival rates for nasopharyngeal, oropharyngeal, and hypopharyngeal cancer patients, and trends toward improved oral cavity cancer survival rates; however, laryngeal cancer survival rates appear to be worsening.[7,8] As with other cancer sites, mortality/incidence ratios for HNC are much higher in developing countries as compared with the United States.[1,10]

Risk factors

Tobacco

In the late 1950s, a landmark case-control study by Dr. Ernst Wynder established the link between tobacco use and oral cavity cancer. A year later, a cohort study of over 180,000 men demonstrated an increased risk of death from HNSCC in cigarette smokers as compared with men who never smoked.[12] In 1964, the Advisory Committee to the Surgeon General on Smoking and Health published its report linking smoking to cancer.[13] The strength and consistency of the association between smoking and HNSCC have been demonstrated in numerous case-control and cohort studies with significant relative risks or odds ratios in the 5- to 25-fold range.[14,15] Furthermore, a dose–response effect is consistently shown between the duration and dose of smoking with increasing risk of HNSCC and between the time since quitting and the decreasing risk of HNSCC. Other mucosal malignancies of the head and neck such as NPC and sinonasal malignancies have a weaker association with tobacco smoking.[16]

Although the risk of bronchogenic carcinoma appears to be less significant for cigar and pipe smokers than for cigarette smokers, these forms of tobacco use are also clearly associated with an increased risk of HNSCC.[17] The pooling of saliva containing carcinogens in gravity-dependent regions may account for the site distribution of HNSCC based on consumption patterns; in the United States, floor of mouth (FOM), laryngeal, and hypopharyngeal cancers are almost exclusively found in smokers. Smokeless tobacco and related product users and pipe smokers often have a habitual position for the quid or pipe stem, and these products are also associated with cancer of the oral cavity. In South-Central Asia where the use of such products is common, the gingivobuccal region is the most common site for HNSCC.[6,18]

Although smoking rates are declining in the developed world, they are rising in developing countries. In 1965, 42.4% of the U.S. adult population was actively smoking, while in 2013 only 17.8% were current smokers.[19] Although the reduction in cigarette smoking has been much greater in men over the past three decades, the rate of current cigarette use remains higher in men (20.5%) than in women (15.3%), and 26.1% of Native Americans continue to smoke.[20] Worldwide, striking variations in HNC sites and incidence are seen among different regions, cultures, and demographic groups and are due, in large part, to differing patterns of tobacco and other

substance abuse. For instance, in South-Central Asia, "pano" (betel leaf, lime, catechu, and areca nut) is commonly chewed and is a strong risk factor independent of tobacco use for carcinoma of the oral cavity, one of the most common cancers in men and women in this region.[10,21]

Alcohol

Alcohol, too, is an important promoter of carcinogenesis in at least 30% of HNSCCs.[10,22] Furthermore, alcohol appears to have an effect on HNSCC risk independent of tobacco smoking, but these effects are consistently significant only at the highest level of alcohol consumption.[23] Although studies attempting to correlate the type of alcoholic beverage with specific cancer risks have been conflicting, most investigators believe that ethanol itself is the main causative factor. Nevertheless, it appears that the major clinical significance of alcohol consumption is that it potentiates the carcinogenic effect of tobacco. The synergistic relationship between smoking and alcohol results in a 30-fold increased risk of HNC.[22,24]

Infectious agents

Although various infectious agents have been suggested to play a role in head and neck carcinogenesis, current scientific evidence implicates only Epstein–Barr virus (EBV) and HPV as etiologic agents. Although herpes simplex viruses have been suggested as a risk factor for oral cavity cancer,[25] and *Helicobacter pylori* for laryngeal cancer,[26] confirmation is lacking.

Human papilloma virus

In contrast to non-oropharyngeal cancers, the incidence of oropharyngeal squamous cell carcinoma (OPSCC) has increased in recent decades, specifically among younger age groups,[27–31] given the rising incidence of oropharyngeal cancers associated with HPV infection.[32,33] HPV is associated with approximately 70% of OPSCC in the United States.[34] HPV may also play a role in the etiology of SCCs arising in the sinonasal tract.[35]

HPVs are deoxyribonucleic acid (DNA) viruses with a unique affinity for human epithelia, and HPV-associated cancers arise from the tonsillar crypts without an overlying epithelial dysplasia. HPV has been well established as an etiologic agent in cervical and anal cancer,[36] and over the past decade, several investigators have indicated that infection with HPV is a significant risk factor for oropharyngeal carcinoma.[37–44] Over 120 different HPV types have been isolated, with low-risk types (e.g., HPV 6, 11) inducing benign hyperproliferation of the epithelium, leading to lesions such as papillomas and warts, and high-risk types (e.g., HPV 16, 18, 31, 33, 35) associated with carcinogenesis.[45] The prototypical oncogenic types 16 and 18 account for over 90% of HPV-related OPSCC, and are capable of malignant transformation of primary human keratinocytes from genital or upper respiratory tract epithelia.[46] This transforming potential is attributed to the two HPV oncoproteins, E6 and E7, that inactivate two human tumor-suppressor proteins, p53 and pRb, respectively.[47,48] These viral oncoproteins are not only necessary for transformation but also stimulate cellular proliferation, delay cellular differentiation, increase the frequency of spontaneous and mutagen-induced mutations, and promote focal and broad chromosomal instability in transfected cell lines.[49] Furthermore, in order to maintain a malignant phenotype, a transcriptionally active viral genome appears to be necessary.[50–53]

The risk factors associated with HPV-associated OPSCC are distinct from HPV-negative tumors, and include oral sexual behaviors and marijuana use. Furthermore, a dose–response relationship has been identified between the risk of developing

HPV-positive OPSCC with number of oral sex partners and joint years of marijuana use.[54] Although oropharyngeal cancer patients presenting without the classic tobacco exposures more commonly have HPV-16-associated tumors,[37] it is also possible that there may be synergistic interactions between the traditional oropharyngeal risk factors of tobacco and alcohol with HPV.[41] The potential effect of HPV-16 immunizations in the prevention of cervical carcinomas may help prevent oropharyngeal cancers as well.[4]

EBV
The epidemiologic link between EBV and NPC is quite strong,[42,43] and is further supported by the identification of EBV DNA in premalignant nasopharyngeal lesions. Although World Health Organization (WHO) types II and III are overwhelmingly positive for EBV, the virus is also associated with well-differentiated (WHO type I) NPC.[46] Both serologic and mucosal swab evidence of EBV infection has been used to enhance screening for NPC in endemic areas.[42] Evidence of EBV DNA in cervical lymph node metastases of unknown primary origin has been used to identify nasopharyngeal primaries. More recently, the detection of EBV DNA in peripheral blood (both cellular and cell-free component) has demonstrated prognostic significance for predicting survival and distant metastases and may become a biomarker to follow up on these patients.[51]

Genetic susceptibility
Since only a fraction of smokers develop cancer, variations in genetic susceptibility may be equally important in disease etiology. A genetic component to this disease is also supported by large family studies demonstrating a three- to eightfold increased risk of HNSCC in first-degree relatives of patients with HNSCC.[53,55] According to this hypothesis, inherited differences in the efficiencies of carcinogen metabolizing systems, DNA repair systems, and/or cell-cycle control/apoptosis systems influence risk of tobacco-induced cancers.[56,57] Identifying such at-risk individuals in the general population by use of biomarker assays would have a profound impact on primary prevention, early detection, and secondary prevention strategies. Three recent high-impact publications of genome-wide association studies have identified the same lung cancer susceptibility locus in separate populations.[54,58,59] These studies will likely be followed in the near future by similar explorations of genome-wide HNSCC association studies and suggest that tailored prevention of tobacco-associated cancers may be a realistic goal.

Environmental tobacco smoke
In a study of 173 cases of HNSCC and 176 cancer-free controls, environmental tobacco smoke was associated with a more than twofold increased risk of HNSCC, and a dose–response relationship was also observed.[60] In a separate study of 44 nonsmokers with HNSCC and 132 cancer-free nonsmoker controls, environmental tobacco smoke was associated with a significantly increased risk of HNSCC, and this was particularly true for females and for those reporting exposure at work.[61]

Laryngopharyngeal reflux
Observational and anecdotal studies have long suggested that gastroesophageal reflux (GERD) may be associated with laryngeal cancer.[62,63] Furthermore, multiple studies have documented a high prevalence of gastric reflux into the laryngopharynx in patients with laryngeal cancer via 24-h pH probe monitoring.[64] A case-control study of 10,140 hospitalized patients and 12,061 outpatients with

laryngeal and pharyngeal cancer and 40,561 hospitalized and 48,244 outpatient controls has been performed using U.S. Department of Veterans Affairs databases.[65] The diagnosis of GERD was associated with a significantly elevated risk of laryngeal cancer (OR, odds ratio = 2.4 and OR = 2.3 for hospitalized and outpatient groups, respectively) and of pharyngeal cancer (OR = 2.4 and OR = 1.9 for hospitalized and outpatient groups, respectively). However, a large Swedish cohort study of 66,965 patients with discharge diagnoses of heartburn, hiatal hernia, or esophagitis with a follow-up of 376,622 person-years concluded that there was no evidence of a causal association between GERD and either laryngeal or pharyngeal cancer.[66]

Marijuana
Marijuana smoke has a four times higher tar burden and a 50% higher concentration of benzopyrene and aromatic hydrocarbons than does tobacco smoke. Although anecdotal evidence has long suggested that marijuana is a risk factor for HNSCC, few reports have found direct evidence of marijuana as an etiologic factor for HNSCC because most users of marijuana are also exposed to tobacco and alcohol.[67,68] A recent case-control study including 240 HNSCC patients and 322 cancer-free controls demonstrated a positive association of fivefold between marijuana use and HPV-related HNSCC, with a dose–response relationship.[69] However, a large retrospective cohort of 64,855 health maintenance organization (HMO) members found no association of marijuana use with tobacco-related cancers.[70] Problems of underreporting of marijuana use and limited sample size of heavy users limit conclusions regarding marijuana use and HNSCC risk.[71]

Diet
Epidemiologic evidence from case-control studies suggests that diets high in animal fats and low in fruits and vegetables may be risk factors for HNSCC.[72,73] Case-control studies have correlated salted fish consumption with NPC risk, which may be due to the high content of nitrosamine compounds in preserved foods.[74,75] Some evidence suggests vitamin A and beta-carotene may be responsible for the protective effect of diets high in fruits and vegetables, and carotenoid deficiency has been considered to be a risk factor for HNSCC and lung cancers.[76] It is not known, however, which of the more than 500 carotenoids are protective, what chemical interactions may occur, or what protective role other micronutrients in carotenoid-rich foods may play. Others have found that total intake of vitamins C and E are also protective.[73] Moreover, diets are complex and difficult to assess and validate; in particular, there are often inaccuracies in translating foods into constituent nutrients. It may be impossible to determine which of the vast array of compounds is most beneficial, and controlling for other dietary variables and confounding risk factors has remained a difficult methodological problem.

Occupation/air pollution
Although occupational exposures probably play a minor role overall in the development of HNSCC, they are major risk factors for malignancies of the sinonasal region.[77-79] The most important exposures occur in the metalworking, refining, woodworking, and leather/textile industries.[77,78] Indoor air pollution is a significant problem in much of the developing world where indoor stoves using biomass or fossil fuels are the primary method of cooking and heating. Although controversial, an expert committee of the National Academy of Sciences has concluded that there is sufficient

evidence to consider asbestos as a significant independent risk factor for laryngeal cancer.[80]

Radiation

No significant association has been demonstrated between ionizing radiation and the development of HNSCC. However, SCCs of the lip, like skin cancers, are associated with ultraviolet radiation exposure. Furthermore, exposure to gamma radiation is associated with thyroid cancers, sarcomas of the head and neck, salivary gland malignancies, and paranasal sinus cancers. Although therapeutic irradiation of HNC does not appear to induce second primary SCCs of the aerodigestive tract, it is associated with an increased risk of sarcomas of the head and neck.[81] This is a particular concern for children requiring radiotherapy. Furthermore, environmental, medical diagnostic, and therapeutic radiation exposure to the head and neck are all significantly associated with salivary gland malignancies, with a dose–response relationship.[82,83] Mucoepidermoid carcinomas (MECs) appear to be the most common radiation-induced salivary malignancy.[82,83] Occupational studies have suggested that indoor exposure to radon gas or volatile chemicals may also increase the risk for HNSCC.[79]

Ultimately, the public health goal is better prevention and early detection of these malignancies by reducing the use of tobacco and alcohol, preventive vaccination against high-risk oncogenic HPV, discovering and avoiding other causative agents, and identifying the genetically susceptible. Unfortunately, HNSCC screening has not been effective, likely due to the rarity of the disease and expertise required for examination.[84] However, in parts of the world where HNSCC accounts for a major portion of the cancer burden, prevention and screening programs have had some measure of efficacy where implemented.[6]

Pathologic assessment and biology

Aside from stating that a particular tumor is SCC, additional information reported by the pathologist usually includes tumor grade or differentiation. Unfortunately, differentiation factors have not been consistently accurate in reflecting the biologic aggressiveness of HNSCC.[85] Prognosis is influenced by many factors other than grade.[86,87] These include tumor size, nodal status, site, surface expression of epidermal growth factor receptor (EGFR), host immune response, age, and performance status. P16 expression/HPV status is the strongest independent prognostic factor for survival among patients with OPSCC.[88]

Features reflecting aggressive disease include lymphatic invasion, perineural invasion, lymph node metastases, and penetration of the tumor through the capsule of involved lymph nodes (extracapsular spread [ECS]). A complete discussion of the molecular pathology underpinning HNSCC is beyond the scope of this chapter, and the reader is referred to some of the many reviews in this area.[89,90] Intense investigation is ongoing regarding the complex interplay of cellular and genetic alterations that contribute to carcinogenesis and the metastatic phenotype in HNSCC. The fundamental roles of p53, dysregulated receptor tyrosine kinase signaling, apoptotic resistance, angiogenesis, and chemotherapeutic resistance are under active study.

Anatomy

The term "cancer of the head and neck" refers to a diverse collection of neoplasms arising from the anatomic sites that make up the upper aerodigestive tract (UADT). This chapter, however, deals predominantly with SCC, as it accounts for approximately 90% of malignancies in this region. The UADT consists of a complex mucosa-covered conduit for food and air that extends from the vermilion surface of the lips to the cervical esophagus. In common usage, this terminology has been applied primarily to those cancers arising from the mucosal surfaces of the lips, oral cavity, pharynx, larynx, and cervical esophagus. Included in this designation, however, are other important sites, such as the nose and paranasal sinuses, salivary glands (major and minor), thyroid and parathyroid, and skin (both melanoma and nonmelanoma skin cancers). Some cancers arising in this region are typically excluded from the generic designation of HNC. Examples are tumors of the central nervous system, ocular neoplasms, and primary tumors of lymphatic origin.

Because of the diversity of sites and tissues of origin, the biology of tumor growth, patterns of metastases, and natural boundaries for tumor extension, signs and symptoms of disease are quite varied. The anatomy of the region has also dictated that optimal evaluation, diagnosis, and treatment require specific multidisciplinary expertise, including neurosurgery, otolaryngology, head and neck surgery, oral and maxillofacial surgery, cosmetic and reconstructive disciplines, and specialists in radiology, pathology, radiation therapy, and medical oncology. Although the anatomic structures are only millimeters apart, the low metastatic potential and high curability of vocal cord cancers stand in contrast to the early dissemination and poor prognosis of stage-matched pyriform sinus cancers.[91] Clinical differences between cancers in different sites are explained by anatomic factors and major biologic differences. Regrettably, the relatively small number of HNC patients often requires grouping patients for trials. Associated morbidities of disease and treatment involve the special senses to varying degrees, notably speech, mastication and swallowing, smell, and respiratory function, all critically important for social interaction, a good quality of life, and ultimately, survival.

Oral cavity

The oral cavity is defined as starting at the vermilion border of the lips and extending posteriorly to include the lips, buccal mucosa, anterior tongue, floor of the mouth (FOM), hard palate, upper and lower gingiva, and retromolar trigone. The tongue occupies a major portion of the oral cavity and is contiguous with the FOM. The gingival mucosa overlying the mandibular and maxillary alveolar ridges adheres to the underlying periosteum. The hard palate forms the roof of the oral cavity and consists of mucosa overlying the palatine portion of the maxilla extending from the superior alveolar ridge to the junction with the soft palate, which is the anterior border of the oropharynx. Although the delineation between the oral cavity and oropharynx might seem artificial, the distinction is important because of varying natural history and sensitivity to nonsurgical therapy and numerous functional considerations after surgical resection, which is the mainstay of treatment for this subgroup of diseases.

Pharynx

The pharynx is a musculomembranous tube suspended from the skull base to the level of the sixth cervical vertebra, supported by overlapping constrictor muscles and other muscles arising from the styloid process and skull base. This conduit communicates with the oral cavity anteriorly, the nasopharynx superiorly, and the hypopharynx and larynx inferiorly. It is divided into four sites of clinical importance: the tonsillar area, which makes up the major portion of the lateral pharyngeal wall and blends with the tongue base, soft palate and retromolar trigone, the tongue base, and the posterior pharyngeal wall. Innervation of the pharynx is via the pharyngeal plexus, with contributions from the glossopharyngeal (sensory) and vagus nerves (motor and sensory).

The hypopharynx is divided into three distinct regions: the pyriform sinuses; the posterior surface of the larynx (postcricoid area); and the inferior, posterior, and lateral pharyngeal walls. The pyriform sinuses are paired mucosal pouches wrapped around the larynx, which funnel food around the larynx and into the esophagus. They are bounded superiorly by the pharyngoepiglottic folds and inferiorly by the cricoid cartilage. The sinuses come together at the esophageal introitus and cervical esophagus at the level of C6.

Larynx

The larynx consists of a mucosa-covered cartilaginous framework (thyroid and cricoid cartilages) suspended from the hyoid bone above by the thyrohyoid membrane and attached below to the trachea. The opening to the larynx is continuous with the pharyngeal airway. Unlike the rest of the pharynx, the mucosa of the larynx consists largely of columnar, ciliated, respiratory-type epithelium. Stratified squamous epithelium is found on the upper posterior epiglottis, aryepiglottic folds, and true vocal folds. Notably, lymphatics in the upper larynx are sparse in the true vocal folds, or glottis.

The larynx is divided into three anatomic regions: the supraglottic, glottic, and subglottic larynx. The supraglottic larynx includes the epiglottis, aryepiglottic folds, laryngeal surface of the arytenoids, false vocal cords, and ventricles. The glottic larynx consists of both true vocal cords and the mucosa of the anterior and posterior commissures. It extends from the lateral-most apex of the laryngeal ventricle to 1 cm below the free edge of the vocal folds toward the cricoid. It has few, if any, lymphatics. The subglottic larynx consists of the region bounded by the glottis above and the inferior border of the cricoid cartilage. Lymphatic supply to the subglottic larynx is extensive and bilateral. The infraglottic lymphatics drain to the cervical nodes through the cricothyroid membrane, while supraglottic lymphatics drain through the thyrohyoid membrane.

Nose and paranasal sinuses

The term "nose and paranasal sinuses" refers to the region of the UADT that starts at the vestibule of the nose anteriorly, is covered by squamous epithelium, and extends posteriorly to the choana, where the nasopharynx begins. By definition, paranasal sinus malignancy does not include the nasopharynx unless by extension. It does include the paranasal sinuses, specifically, the maxillary, ethmoid, frontal, and sphenoid sinuses. Although the most common malignancy of the nose and paranasal sinuses is SCC, the nose and paranasal sinuses pose a particular set of problems that deserve separate consideration. Moreover, nonsquamous cancers may also occur with distinctive patterns of tumor progression and requirements for effective therapy.

Neck

Anatomic considerations in the treatment of cancers of the head and neck must include a thorough understanding of the neural, vascular, and, especially, the lymphatic structures of the neck. Detailed anatomic studies have described the organization of the lymphatic drainage of the UADT. Specific regions of the head and neck and the tumors that arise therein have lymphatic drainage that is consistent and predictable. There are 12 major groups of lymph nodes (six each bilaterally) in the head and neck (Figure 1),[92] although only levels I to V play a major role in HNSCC. Primary and secondary echelons of lymph node drainage have been defined for each major region of the head and neck mucosa. A standard rule

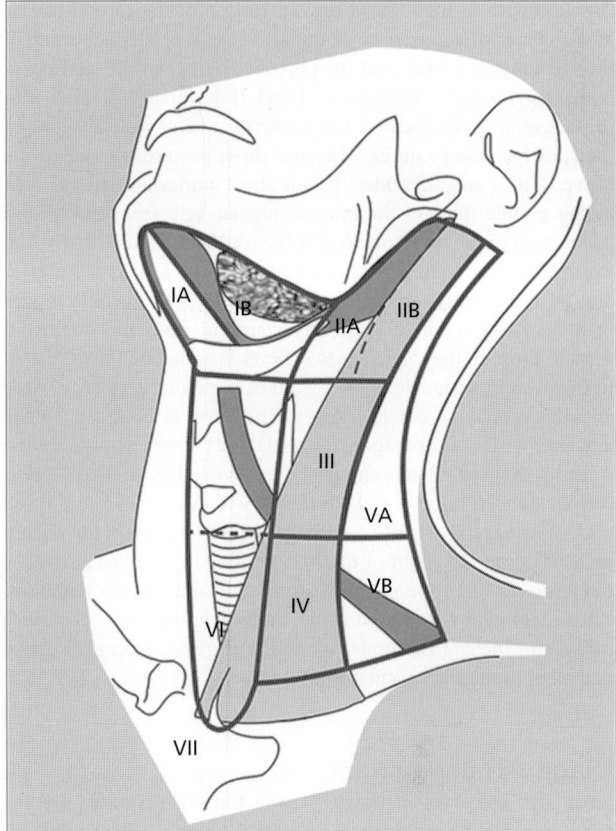

Figure 1 Nodal levels in the head and neck.

of thumb is that the lymphatic drainage for any particular region is predicted by the arterial supply of that region. The lip, cheek, and anterior gingiva drain into the submandibular and submental lymph node groups. In addition, the cheek and upper lip also drain into the inferior parotid and facial nodes, while the posterior gingiva and palate drain into the internal jugular chain and lateral retropharyngeal groups. Lymphatic drainage for the mobile tongue is into the internal jugular, subdigastric, omohyoid, submandibular, and submental nodal groups. Midline lesions often drain bilaterally. Although metastases to the lower neck nodes are infrequent from the oral cavity, generally the more anterior the tumor location in the tongue, the more likely it is that metastases also will spread to lower jugular nodes. FOM drainage is similar to that of the tongue. The upper portion of the pharynx drains directly into the upper cervical lymph nodes along the internal jugular chain. The oropharynx and tonsil drain through the parapharyngeal space into the midjugular region, particularly into the jugulodigastric nodes. Retro and lateral pharyngeal nodes can also be involved. The regions of the hypopharynx and larynx drain primarily along the routes of their vascular supply to either the deep cervical nodes along the midjugular (upper pharynx, larynx) or the deep nodes along the lower jugular and paratracheal region (lower pharynx, larynx).

For the purposes of local treatment, the various lymph node groups of the neck have been divided into levels. Level I includes the submental group of nodes (IA), located within the triangle bounded by the anterior belly of the digastric muscles and the hyoid bone, and the submandibular group (IB), bounded by both bellies of the digastric muscle and the body of the mandible. Level II nodes consist of the upper jugular lymph nodes located in proximity to the upper third of the internal jugular vein and extending from the skull base to the level of the bifurcation of the carotid artery. The anterior and posterior boundaries are the lateral border of the sternohyoid muscle and the posterior border of the sternocleidomastoid muscle, respectively. Level II is further divided into those lymph nodes located anteroinferior to the vertical plane of the spinal accessory nerve (IIA) and those posterosuperior to the nerve (IIB). Level III nodes include those nodes located adjacent to the middle third of the internal jugular vein from the carotid bifurcation to the plane marked by the omohyoid muscle's crossing over the jugular vein (the level of the cricoid cartilage). Anterior and posterior boundaries are the same as level II. Level IV nodes include the lower jugular group extending from the omohyoid muscle above to the clavicle below. Level V nodes are those located in the posterior triangle in the region of the spinal accessory nerve and the transverse cervical artery. This level is bounded by the anterior border of the trapezius muscle, the posterior border of the sternocleidomastoid muscle, and the clavicle below. This level is further divided into Va and Vb nodes, with Va nodes being those nodes located above the plane along the inferior edge of the cricoid and including the chain of nodes superior to the spinal accessory nerve posterior to the sternocleidomastoid muscle. Vb nodes are the nodes below the cricoid plane, inferior to the spinal accessory nerve and include the nodes along the transverse cervical artery and all of the supraclavicular fossa.

Diagnosis and staging

Since site and stage of disease at the time of diagnosis are the most important prognostic factors in the treatment of HNSCC, the identification and treatment of early-stage cancers generally correlates with excellent survival. Most dysplastic lesions or *in situ* carcinomas of the oral mucosa occur as red (erythroplasia) or white (leukoplakia) patches that may be readily apparent on visual examination. In areas less easily visualized directly, such as the larynx and hypopharynx, early lesions cause such symptoms as chronic hoarseness and sore throat and, with progression, referred otalgia or dysphagia. Such symptoms demand visualization of the larynx and hypopharynx usually by fiberoptic approaches.

Dysphagia, odynophagia, otalgia, hoarseness, mucosal irregularities and ulceration, oral or oropharyngeal pain, weight loss, and the presence of an unexplained neck mass are the most common presenting symptoms of invasive HNSCC. The predominant symptoms vary with the site: chronic dysphagia or odynophagia demands thorough visualization of the oropharynx, hypopharynx, and esophagus; chronic hoarseness demands visualization of the larynx; chronic unilateral serous otitis media in an adult may be a result of cancer of the nasopharynx blocking the eustachian tube; and unilateral nasal polyps, nasal obstruction, or epistaxis is a common presenting sign of nasal cavity or paranasal sinus neoplasms. A firm or hard unilateral cervical mass represents malignancy until proved otherwise. In persons older than 20 years, such a mass represents neoplasm more than 80% of the time, and 60% of these neoplasms are due to metastatic spread from an UADT primary.

In patients presenting with a suspicious neck mass, a complete head and neck examination usually reveals the primary malignant tumor (Figure 2). If it does not, a thorough search for occult primary cancers both above and below the clavicles is warranted. Technologic advances in fiberoptics and in flexible and rigid endoscopes now provide excellent upper airway visualization and biopsy capabilities that can be performed routinely in the clinic setting.[93] Endoscopic evaluation should include the nasopharynx, oropharynx, hypopharynx, larynx, and upper esophagus. Endoscopic evaluation should be accompanied by chest radiography

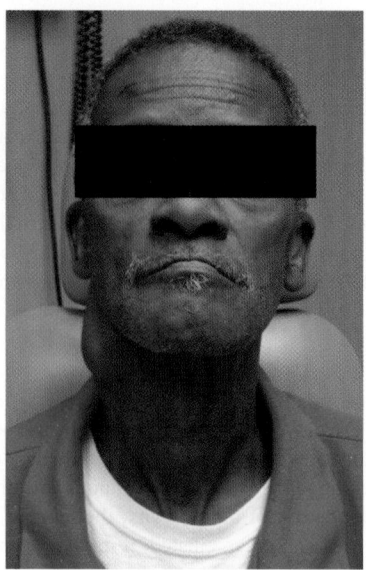

Figure 2 Untreated N3 disease in a patient with HNSCC.

and axial imaging of the head and neck. If these fail to reveal a primary, then consideration should be given for esophagoscopy as well, since it is more sensitive for mucosal lesions of the esophagus than is computed tomography (CT). Most commonly, occult primaries responsible for neck metastases occur in the nasopharynx, tongue base, tonsil, or hypopharynx. In the absence of an identifiable mass, directed biopsies of these sites are indicated during endoscopic evaluation, and, if present, bilateral tonsillectomies should be performed if a primary is not identified. Metastasis to a solitary left supraclavicular lymph node (Virchow's node) is occasionally seen with infraclavicular cancer, especially colon cancer. Generally, isolated metastatic supraclavicular masses (level IV) derive from breast, lung, or infradiaphragmatic neoplasms. Thyroid malignancies may also metastasize to this area.

Imaging with CT and magnetic resonance imaging (MRI) is frequently used to supplement the clinical evaluation and staging of the primary tumor and regional lymph nodes. Ultrasonography, when combined with fine-needle aspiration (FNA) technique, is an effective means for staging the neck, thyroid, and salivary glands. Open biopsies should be performed only after attempts by FNA of suspicious nodes are nondiagnostic. If an excisional biopsy is required because FNA is inconclusive or not feasible, then the surgeon and patient should discuss the advisability of neck dissection if the mass should prove to be metastatic SCC. The potential ramifications of false-negative results on FNA are inherently obvious. Accuracy of the cytological interpretation of the aspirate is directly dependent on the skill and experience of the ultrasonographer and pathologist.

Positron emission tomography (PET) imaging has a demonstrated role in management of HNC. Highly elevated primary tumor fluorodeoxyglucose standardized uptake values (FDG SUVs) may predict for more aggressive disease and inferior treatment outcomes.[94–96] FDG-PET can provide over 90% sensitivity and specificity for upfront staging of both primary and cervical neck nodal disease,[97] can localize occult local primary disease,[98,99] or distant metastases[100] not elicited by anatomic imaging or physical examination. Combined FDG-PET/CT imaging may further improve neck staging accuracy results.[101,102] Incremental superiority of FDG-PET for regional staging of the neck relative to CT or MRI alone was confirmed by a meta-analysis of retrospective and prospective studies encompassing over 1200 FDG-PET imaging cases with confirmatory neck dissection pathology.[103]

Analysis of this dataset revealed FDG-PET to be sensitive (79%) and specific (86%) for this indication. Recent prospective series in early-intermediate T-stage oral cavity and oropharyngeal cancer patients suggest that FDG-PET can potentially guide more appropriate management of clinically N0 patients when directly correlated with CT and sentinel node biopsy[104] or with CT/MRI findings.[105]

Considerable interest has recently focused on FDG-PET monitoring of disease response to radiotherapy or chemoradiotherapy. A number of groups have found that FDG-PET posttreatment restaging provides high negative predictive power;[106–108] accordingly, there is now growing acceptance of withholding consolidative neck dissection following radiotherapy in the absence of residual FDG-avid adenopathy,[109] although others argue that expert clinical interpretation of serial CT imaging could achieve similar results.[61,110] FDG-PET/CT may eventually prove useful for improving delineation of disease targets for advanced radiotherapy planning.[111] However, challenges for this remain, particularly for identification of validated thresholding techniques to precisely distinguish FDG-avid disease from bystander tissues.[112,113] At MD Anderson Cancer Center, we routinely use FDG-PET/CT to supplement anatomic imaging and clinical examination for radiotherapy planning; however, we do not use negative FDG-PET results to defer treatment of suspicious findings identified by examination or conventional restaging techniques after chemotherapy.

Staging criteria for cancers arising in the UADT, paranasal sinuses, and salivary glands have been developed by the American Joint Committee on Cancer (AJCC) (Table 1). The criteria undergo regular reevaluation and modification. The most current version referred to in this chapter is the 7th edition.[114] The stage groupings are based on T (primary tumor), N (regional node), and M (distant metastasis) designations. Because of variations in the growth, behavior, and prognosis of HNCs according to site of origin and extent, differences exist in the staging criteria for each anatomic site. However, except for tumors arising in the nasopharynx and those of the thyroid, there is uniformity in the nodal staging criteria and stage grouping (Table 2).

Careful documentation of tumor extent and accurate staging classification are crucial for discussions of the results of different treatment approaches. Restaging after treatment or for recurrent cancers must be clearly designated and separate from the primary staging of previously untreated cancers. Postsurgical, or pathologic, staging is important in the primary treatment of HNC because of the increasing use of postoperative radiation therapy (PORT) and/or adjuvant chemotherapy for patients with locally aggressive tumors, ECS into the soft tissues of the neck, close or positive margins, and perineural invasion.

Table 1 AJCC clinical tumor stage and groupings for head and neck cancer.

Stage 0	Tis	N0	M0
Stage I	T1	N0	M0
Stage II	T2	N0	M0
Stage III	T3	N0	M0
	T1	N1	M0
	T2	N1	M0
	T3	N1	M0
Stage IVA	T4a	N0, N1, or N2	M0
	Any T	N2	M0
Stage IVB	Any T	N3	M0
	T4b	Any N	M0
Stage IVC	Any T	Any N	M1

Source: Edge 2010.[114] Reproduced with permission of Springer.

Table 2 AJCC clinical tumor staging characteristics for regional lymph nodes and distant metastases.

Regional lymph nodes	
Nx	Regional lymph nodes cannot be assessed
N0	No evidence of regional lymph node metastases
N1	Metastasis in single, ipsilateral regional lymph node <3 cm in greatest dimension
N2a	Metastasis in single, ipsilateral regional lymph node between 3 and 6 cm in greatest dimension
N2b	Metastasis in multiple ipsilateral regional lymph nodes, none >6 cm in greatest dimension
N2c	Metastasis in bilateral or contralateral regional lymph nodes, none >6 cm in greatest dimension
N3	Metastasis to regional lymph node >6 cm in greatest dimension
Distant metastases	
Mx	Presence of distant metastasis cannot be assessed
M0	No evidence of distant metastasis
M1	Distant metastases are present in one or more locations

Source: Edge 2010.[114] Reproduced with permission of Springer.

It should be noted, however, that as good as the widely accepted AJCC staging system is for HNC, it still falls short in that it too often fails to distinguish between deeply infiltrative tumors and those that are superficial or exophytic. Experience shows that this distinction is an important one and can have a significant impact on survival. Moreover, the recent emergence of HPV-positive cancers presents an essentially distinctive group of patients for whom some of the older baseline staging data may not be fully applicable.[115] Future revisions to the AJCC for HPV status, particularly for oropharyngeal cancers, are anticipated.

General principles of treatment

After a histological diagnosis has been established and tumor extent determined, the selection of appropriate treatment of a specific cancer depends on a complex array of variables, including tumor site and stage, HPV status, prognosis, relative morbidity of various treatment options, patient performance and nutritional status, concurrent health problems, social and logistic factors, therapeutic options for potential recurrences or second primaries, and patient preference. These variables are each considered with respect to the established effectiveness of various treatment regimens available.

The overall management goals in treating patients with HNC are to achieve the highest cure rates at the lowest cost in terms of functional and cosmetic morbidity. The achievement of these goals requires the close cooperation of an interdisciplinary team of practitioners representing surgery, radiation and medical oncology, prosthodontics, dentistry, speech language pathology, social services, dietetics, physical and rehabilitative medicine, pathology, nursing, and often psychiatry.

Effective rehabilitation is an important part of the overall treatment of HNC. Modern advances in surgical reconstruction, microvascular free-tissue transfer, and prosthodontics have significantly improved posttreatment function.[116] Rehabilitation concerns must be addressed at initial treatment planning and carefully integrated with the various treatment modalities used. Pretreatment dental evaluations, and speech and swallowing assessments should be routinely performed. Needed dental care and/or extractions should be performed prior to radiation to reduce the risks of dental-associated mucositis and osteoradionecrosis. The overall impact of treatment and rehabilitation on patient quality of life is an important issue that may require specialized social or psychiatric support systems for the patient and family. Furthermore, attention must be paid to nutritional support, and early intervention with the placement of enteral access for gastrostomy feeding should be entertained in selected patients. Contemporary combined approaches of chemotherapy and radiotherapy are often associated with severe mucocutaneous treatment effects that must be addressed. Finally, the prolonged nature of treatment for advanced disease, which may extend over many months, requires consideration of the social and financial impact of treatment decisions on the patient, the family, and the patient's career.

Biopsies of primary tumors need not be excisional unless the biopsy procedure is sufficient for local control. Oncologic principles of surgical resection must not be compromised by ill-conceived reconstructive efforts or attempts at modifying the necessary resection in order to minimize functional or cosmetic morbidity. Gross residual cancer or positive surgical margins after tumor resection portend high risk for treatment failure. Appropriate management must also include the use of precise modern techniques of conservative surgical resection (e.g., partial laryngectomy and functional neck dissection) that, in selected patients, have cure rates similar to those of more radical techniques.

Oral premalignancy

Appropriate management of leukoplakia and erythroplakia lesions includes a high index of suspicion, particularly in high-risk individuals. Although both lesions are considered premalignant, erythroplasia lesions are of greater clinical concern, since approximately half of these lesions contain carcinoma *in situ* (CIS) or invasive cancer. Erythroplakia mandates biopsy to rule out invasive cancer. The management of erythroplakia and leukoplakia depends on the location, extent, and histology. The diffuse field effect and multifocal nature of the epithelial carcinogenic process support the need for effective prevention. Various molecular markers, including aneuploidy, loss of heterozygosity (LOH) and podoplanin expression portend a high risk of transformation in dysplastic oral intraepithelial neoplasia (IEN).[117–119] White lesions can be confused with mucositis; lichen planus; local tissue irritation from mechanical, thermal, or chemical trauma; histoplasmosis; candidiasis; and other infectious processes.

Topical supravital staining with toluidine blue of suspicious lesions can be helpful in identifying areas for biopsy and in screening high-risk populations. Toluidine blue staining was found to be associated with LOH in dysplastic, minimally dysplastic, or nondysplastic oral IEN, which suggests the potential of toluidine blue for identifying oral IEN with a high risk of cancer and perhaps for helping guide surgical margin widths.[120,121] Lesions that persist despite the removal of local irritating factors, or those that are associated with ulceration, vertical growth, induration, a recent change in size, or pain, should be sampled by biopsy and/or excised. Despite aggressive local therapy, complete surgical resection (as defined by the absence of dysplasia at the margins) does not prevent oral carcinoma development in cases of aneuploid dysplastic leukoplakia.[118] In this context, a targeted therapy prevention approach has been tested in a phase II randomized trial (EPOC). This study compared erlotinib, an EGFR inhibitor, versus placebo in patients with high-risk oral premalignant lesions harboring LOH. Despite the negative results for the overall population, there was a trend toward improved oral cancer-free survival in patients who did not have a prior oral cancer.[122] Future research in this area should evaluate the roles of optimal surgical margin width and complete

resection as confirmed by molecular analyses in reducing the cancer risk associated with molecularly defined high-risk oral IEN.

Overview of natural history and treatment by site

Oral cavity

Both tumor and treatment may significantly compromise speech and deglutition, particularly for those patients in whom cancer involves the tongue, FOM, or mandible. Despite the fact that this region is readily amenable to visual examination and bimanual palpation, more than 50% of patients are diagnosed in advanced stages. The current T staging of oral cavity primaries is presented in Table 3.

Lips

SCCs of the mucosal surface of the lips are the most common oral cavity cancers. An important distinction must be made with cancers of the skin surrounding the lips, which are considered cutaneous malignancies. Over 90% occur on the lower lip, usually on the exposed vermilion border, midway between the midline and the oral commissure.[123] Well-differentiated and verrucous cancers rarely metastasize. Poorly differentiated and spindle cell varieties tend to grow aggressively and metastasize commonly. Perineural infiltration of large nerves is indicative of aggressive disease and often requires combined therapies.

Considerations in the treatment of lip cancers include (1) oncological control of the disease, (2) a functional oral sphincter with oral competence, and (3) acceptable cosmetic outcome. These goals may be achieved with either primary radiation or surgery when the tumors are less than 2 cm in size or very superficial. Larger or deeply invasive lesions, however, are best treated with surgical resection and reconstruction, which allow for greater accuracy in evaluating the extent of tumor and nerve or lymphatic involvement. Frequently, adjacent precancerous changes are present, which can also be treated with surgery (lip shaving and advancement) to prevent recurrences or the development of second primary tumors.[124,125] For larger lesions, primary reconstruction with local, regional, and sometimes free-tissue flaps avoids defects that result from tissue loss with radiotherapy, provides for future reconstructive and treatment options, and decreases the risk of osteoradionecrosis of

Table 3 Primary tumor staging characteristics for oral cavity and oropharynx carcinoma.

Tx	Primary tumor cannot be assessed (as occurs after excisional biopsy)
T0	No evidence of primary (as in unknown primary tumors)
Tis	Carcinoma *in situ*
T1	Tumor is 2 cm or less in greatest dimension
T2	Tumor is between 2 and 4 cm in greatest dimension
T3	Tumor is >4 cm in greatest dimension
T4	A: Moderately advanced local disease: Tumor invades adjacent structures (through cortical bone, maxillary sinus, skin, tongue musculature, deep tissue, nerves) B: Very advanced local disease: Oral cavity: tumor invades masticator space, pterygoid plates, skull base, encases carotid artery Oropharynx: tumor invades prevertebral fascia, encases carotid artery, or involves mediastinal structures

the mandible. Lesions demonstrating extensive infiltration, bone involvement, or lymphatic metastases should be managed with combined surgery and PORT.

Radiation therapy techniques for management of lip cancers include external irradiation, interstitial implants, and combinations of both. Local tumor control rates with irradiation exceed 80%,[126,127] with determinant survival at 5 years (including surgical salvage) in excess of 95%. Similar tumor control and survival rates are reported with primary surgical excision.[128] Regional metastasis decreases the survival rates to approximately 55%.[129,130] The 5-year survival rates for patients with carcinomas of the upper lip are lower than for those with similar lower lip lesions and range from 40% to 60%.[131] Involvement of both lips and the lateral commissure is uncommon. The prognosis for commissure lesions is not as good as for cancers of other areas of the lip.

Tongue

Tongue cancers account for approximately 25% of oral cavity SCCs and most commonly arise in the anterior two-thirds of the tongue on the lateral or ventral surface. Infiltration of the underlying tongue musculature occurs early. The biologic aggressiveness of T1 and T2 (<4 cm) tongue cancers is noteworthy and is reflected in higher rates of occult regional metastases than those of similarly staged lesions arising from other oral sites. Occult nodal metastases are present in 30–40% of early lesions.[132] Bilateral nodal involvement can occur with cancers of the tip or the midline of the tongue. Locoregional recurrence in patients with tongue cancer accounts for 60–70% of cancer deaths. Distant metastases account for 10–15% of deaths, and second primaries in the UADT account for approximately 20–40%.[132,133] The management of carcinomas of the tongue has been significantly influenced by an increased appreciation of the aggressiveness of seemingly small but deeply infiltrative lesions, the high rate of occult lymph node metastases, and improvements in soft tissue and bony reconstruction. Although surgical excision alone has been the mainstay of treatment, combined surgery and adjuvant radiation therapy to include the primary site and regional nodes is commonly used for advanced cancers (stages III and IV) and is being used increasingly for small stage II cancers that exhibit pathologic indicators of lymph node metastasis or perineural invasion (Figure 3). Postoperative chemoradiotherapy is indicated for adverse pathologic findings of perineural invasion, nodal ECS, or close surgical margins.[134]

For stage I cancers, surgical excision is effective and expeditious, with excellent preservation of function. For stage II lesions that are infiltrative, hemiglossectomy or partial glossectomy achieves excellent tumor control rates and should be combined with dissection of neck nodes at risk (supraomohyoid dissection) to provide accurate information about staging and determine the need for PORT. Free-tissue transfer reconstruction can significantly offset the morbidity of hemiglossectomy.

Extension of cancer to the FOM or the mandible may necessitate partial mandibulectomy or segmental mandibular resection. Modern reconstructive techniques with vascularized composite bone and soft tissue free flaps, titanium metal prostheses, and dental implants have improved the functional and cosmetic results of major mandibular resections. An elective neck dissection is recommended for lesions with >4 mm of invasion owing to the risk of occult nodal disease.

For more advanced primary lesions (stages III and IV), surgery and postoperative external beam radiation are generally used. No prospective controlled trials have proved the superiority of combined therapy over surgery alone for disease without nodal

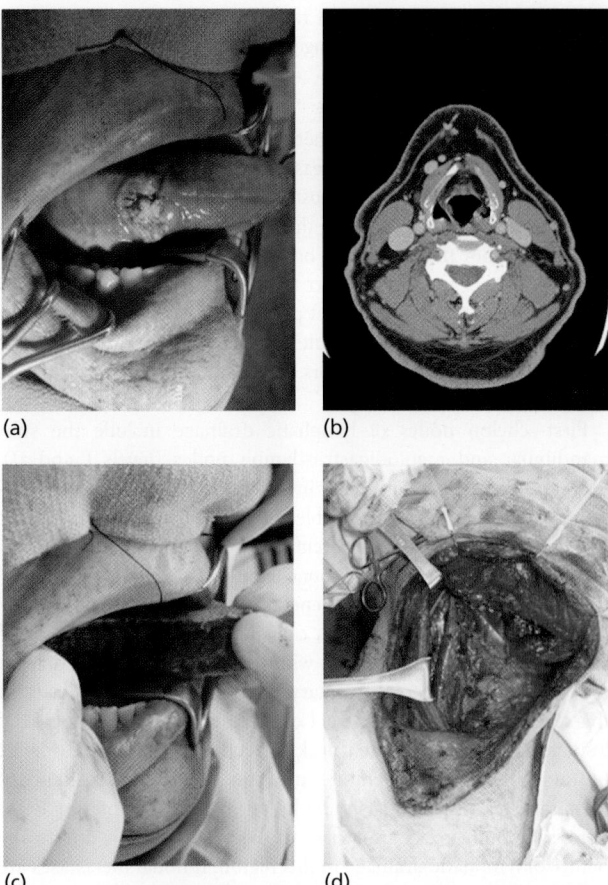

(a)   (b)

(c)   (d)

Figure 3 (a) T1 N0 SCCA of the oral cavity. (b) CT scan revealing no lymphatic metastasis. (c) Hemiglossectomy resection. (d) Staging supraomohyoid neck dissection.

metastases, but retrospective studies indicate improved locoregional control rates.[135–138] These improvements have generally been offset, in part, by an increased frequency of distant metastases and second primaries. Surgical management generally consists of partial glossectomy and neck dissection, with the mandible being spared unless directly involved. In instances with limited periosteal invasion, partial mandibular resections that spare mandibular continuity and maintain function can be performed. When tumors extend to the midline or involve the tongue base, subtotal or total glossectomy may be necessary. Continued advances in reconstructive techniques have improved the functional results of these aggressive resections. Provision for temporary tracheostomy and prolonged enteral nutrition should be made. Total glossectomy or sacrifice of both hypoglossal nerves frequently necessitates permanent feeding gastrostomy. Current experience indicates that total glossectomy can, in highly select patients, be accomplished without the need for laryngectomy, although prolonged or even permanent parenteral feeding will likely be required.[139] PORT is generally administered within 4–6 weeks of surgery. High-risk surgical margins or ECS can be treated to a high-dose or with concomitant chemoradiotherapy. For advanced oral cavity cancers, both ipsilateral and contralateral necks are irradiated, with the dosage determined by the extent of disease. Close surgical margins are often treated to high doses (66–70 Gy) because of the difficulty in eradicating even small amounts of tumor in the tongue after glossectomy. Even with combined therapy, estimated 2-year disease-free survival (DFS) and OS rates for advanced disease are about 50%. The 5-year survival rates range from 50% to 70% for stages I and II to 15–30% for stages III and IV.[140–144]

Floor of mouth (FOM)

FOM cancers occur with a frequency similar to that of tongue cancer. Early spread to adjacent areas (gingiva and periosteum of the mandible) is common. The periosteum of the mandible is a natural barrier to invasion. Fixation of the tongue is a sign of deep invasion. The tumor may extend to or through the mylohyoid muscle, which serves as a natural barrier to direct spread below the hyoid bone. Lymph node metastases at presentation are seen in approximately 40% of patients. The occult metastatic rate increases with the T stage of the primary: T2 tumors have a 40% and T3 tumors a 70% occult metastasis rate.[145,146]

First-echelon nodes of lymphatic drainage include the submandibular and jugulodigastric lymph nodes (levels I and II). Evaluation for early mandibular involvement is facilitated by palpation. since fixation to the mandible indicates periosteal involvement and direct bone invasion is present in 50–60% of such tumors. This distinction is often aided with bone windows on CT.

Small cancers (T1, T2) are generally treated effectively by wide resection. Lateral FOM tumors can often be resected transorally and the resection defect closed with the advancement of adjacent mucosa, skin grafts, or secondary intention. Sialodochoplasty of the severed submandibular duct can be performed for superficial lesions. An elective selected neck dissection is performed for T1 tumors with more than 4 mm of invasion and for all T2-4 cancers. Bilateral neck dissections should be performed for anterior FOM lesions, as both necks are at risk for occult metastasis due to the nature of lymphatic drainage in this region. If nodal metastases are present, therapeutic neck dissection is indicated. Surgery remains the mainstay of treatment of early FOM malignancies, achieving excellent functional and curative results.

More advanced FOM cancers (T3, T4) are generally treated with resection combined with similar approaches to that described for oral tongue cancers in the prior section (Figure 4). Again, mandibular continuity-sparing procedures with cortical resections can often be employed. In these instances, we have found fasciocutaneous flaps to offer excellent FOM and tongue reconstructive potential. Large mucosal and soft tissue surgical defects are typically reconstructed with free-tissue transfers, and contemporary management of mandibular defects entails bony reconstruction with either a fibula or scapula free flap.

Treatment results are influenced by the size of the primary tumor, presence of lymph node metastases, degree of mandibular involvement, and adequacy of resection. The 5-year survival rates for stage I and II FOM carcinomas range around 80%.[146] Cancers that cross the

midline or involve the tongue or the mandible are associated with 5-year survival rates of 50–60%.[147] Survival rates for more advanced lesions (stages III and IV) are less than 50%. The major advantage of combined treatment (radiation and surgery) in these patients is improved control of neck disease. Recurrence in the untreated, clinically negative neck is the most frequent site of failure in patients treated only with surgery.[148] For patients with multiple nodal metastases, induction chemotherapy (IC) is under study[149] as there is high risk for later development of distant metastases. Continuing surveillance for metachronous second primary cancers in the head and neck, esophagus, or lungs is advised.[150,151]

Gingival and buccal mucosa

Gingival cancers occur most commonly (80%) in the lower gingiva, posterior to the bicuspids. For both sites, trismus is an ominous sign indicating extension to the masseter or pterygoid muscles. Occult nodal metastases have been documented in as high as 30% of buccal cancers and elective neck dissection recommended in all but the earliest of cancers.[152] Exophytic tumors tend to be papillary or verrucous in appearance and can be confused with benign hyperkeratosis.

Small, superficial gingival cancers can be effectively treated with surgical resection transorally with excellent preservation of function. Even larger lesions requiring partial maxillectomy or alveolectomy can be resected without external incision. For larger lesions (T3 and T4), segmental mandibulectomy and/or maxillectomy is required, and adjuvant radiation is frequently recommended (Figure 5). Elective neck dissection should be performed for advanced lesions of the mandibular gingival, as these lesions tend to have occult metastases. Limited data are available on the behavior of maxillary ridge and hard palate cancers, but these lesions can metastasize to the lateral neck nodes, and thus elective management of the neck is strongly encouraged, whether with neck dissection or neck irradiation.[153] Clinically positive neck nodes warrant neck dissection at the time of the resection of the primary tumor.

OS rates for gingival and buccal cancers depend on tumor size, bone involvement, and node metastases. Surgical results are clearly superior to those of radiation when bone involvement is present.[152,154]

Retromolar trigone

Cancers arising in the retromolar trigone are rarely confined to that gingiva, but often involve adjacent buccal mucosa, anterior tonsillar pillar, the FOM, and/or posterior gingiva. The risk of clinically positive and occult lymph node metastases is higher than with other gingival cancers. Frequent involvement of periosteum mandates partial

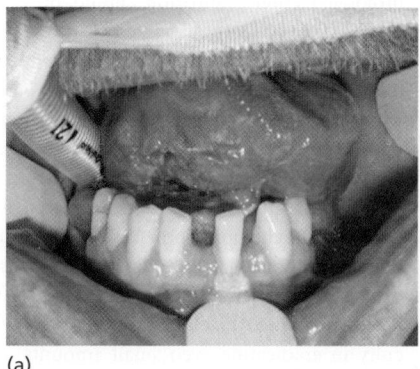
(a)

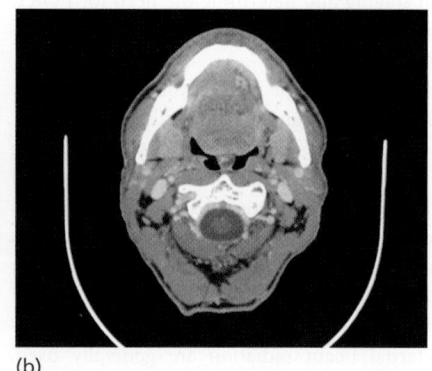
(b)

Figure 4 (a) T3 N0 floor of mouth SCCA. (b) Deep infiltration of the intrinsic tongue musculature on axial imaging.

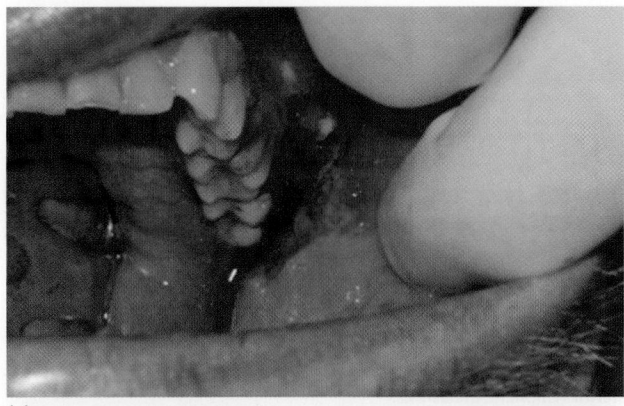

(a)

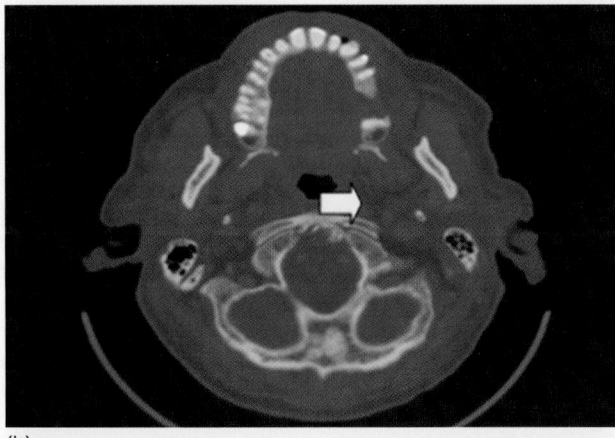

(b)

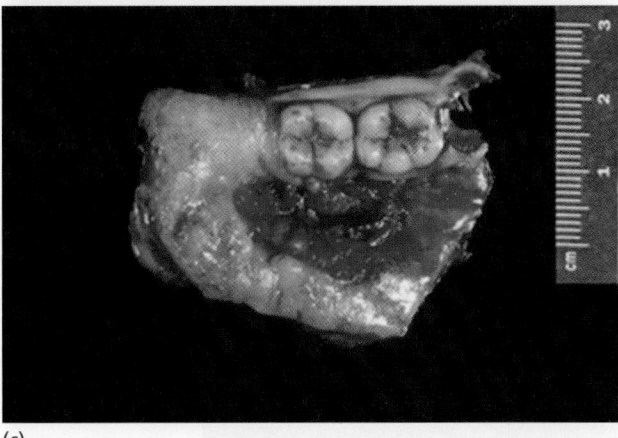

(c)

Figure 5 (a) T4 N0 SCCA of the oral cavity (buccal mucosa). (b) CT scan demonstrating bony destruction of the hard palate. (c) Specimen resected during infrastructure maxillectomy.

(rim or marginal) mandibulectomy as part of the surgical management, even for small lesions. Primary radiation therapy is reserved for superficial lesions that cover a large surface area, such as extension to the soft palate or buccal mucosa, and remain mobile. Moderately advanced or deeply invasive lesions are best treated with surgical resection (mandibulectomy and neck dissection), followed by postoperative adjuvant therapy, as indicated.

Oropharynx

The clinical staging of oropharyngeal cancers is similar to the staging of oral cavity cancers (Table 3). Tumors arise most commonly from the palatine arch, which includes the tonsillar fossa and base of the tongue. The recent identification of HPV as the major etiological factor in the development of OPSCC has led to a recognition of a distinct disease phenotype. Many of these patients are younger and without any history of smoking, and molecular analysis of these tumors reveals the presence of HPV DNA. Clinically, HPV-associated tumors are small, but the nodal burden is more robust.[37] Aside from a cervical mass of unknown etiology, the most common presenting symptom is chronic odynophagia (often unilateral) and referred otalgia. Change in voice, dysphagia, and trismus are late signs. Regional lymphatic metastases occur frequently and are related to the depth of tumor invasion and tumor size. Upper cervical nodes are generally first involved, but lower nodes can become clinically involved with skipping of the upper first-echelon nodes. Bilateral lymphatic metastases can occur, particularly with cancers of the soft palate, tongue base, and midline pharyngeal wall. The retropharyngeal lymph nodes are also common sites of metastasis and warrant evaluation when planning treatment.

Management of oropharyngeal cancers is very challenging, given the essential role this anatomic site plays in breathing, speech, and swallowing. Therefore, the goal of treatment is to not only achieve oncologic cure but also to preserve the multimodal function of the oropharynx. Traditional surgical approaches to the oropharynx are associated with significant morbidity, which prompted a shift toward nonsurgical modalities in the 1990s, specifically utilizing radiation or chemoradiation, which have been the mainstay therapeutic approaches for the past 15–20 years.[155,156] However, recent technological innovations have led to a resurrection of surgical options through a transoral robotic approach (TORS), which allows for adjuvant therapy to be modified on the basis of pathological findings of disease. This novel paradigm can reduce radiation doses and may theoretically decrease long-term side effects. These advantages become imperative considering the emerging population of young patients with HPV-related cancer.

Tumor-related contraindications for TORS include unresectable cervical lymphadenopathy, mandibular invasion, pharyngeal wall or tongue base involvement requiring resection of greater than 50% of these sites, radiologic evidence of carotid involvement, and fixation to the prevertebral fascia. The other limitation of TORS is access, and therefore a thorough preoperative assessment of the patient and tumor characteristics is essential. This should include an evaluation of the dentition, presence of trismus or tori, tongue size, degree of neck extension, sequelae of previous treatment, and the tumor extent. The oncologic outcomes for robotic surgery have been favorable thus far, with OS and DFS rates ranging 82–100% and 86–96%, respectively. Although the role of TORS is still being determined, early oncologic results from several case series are comparable to the outcomes observed with radiation or concurrent chemoradiation.[157]

Tonsil

The traditional treatment of stage I and II tonsillar neoplasms is radiation therapy as a single modality. Transoral wide local excision of small, superficial lesions may be locally effective, but does not address the high potential of occult lymph node metastasis. While surgery and primary radiation offer comparable locoregional control for small tumors, patients with HPV-negative tumors may more often require PORT.[158] For patients with early-stage HPV-positive tumors, TORS with neck dissection offers excellent local-regional control, without the need for adjuvant radiotherapy.[157] Surgical management of advanced cancers results in poor patient function and, therefore, combined chemotherapy and radiotherapy approaches are utilized (Figure 6). For patients with nodal disease

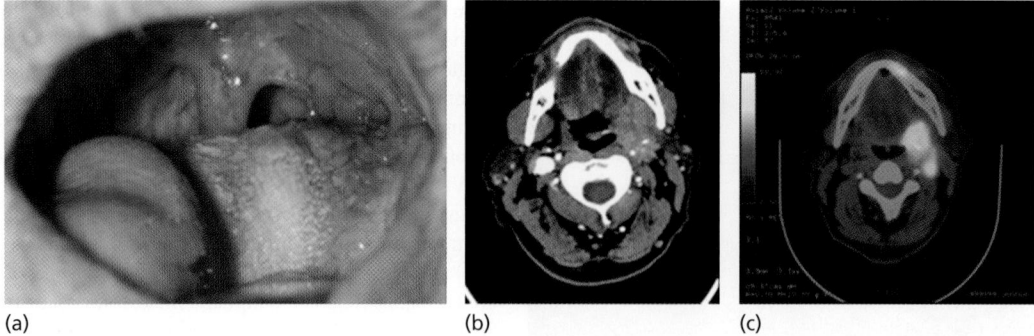

(a)　　　　　　　　　　　(b)　　　　　　　　　　　(c)

Figure 6 (a) T2 N2b SCCA of the oropharynx, clinically small lesion. (b) Deep infiltration into the parapharyngeal space is evident on CT scanning. (c) On PET-CT imaging, two distinct lesions are evident, the primary tumor and a posterior lymphatic metastasis.

(N1-2), the addition of PORT to TORS is associated with excellent oncological and functional outcomes, and spares the need for concurrent chemoradiotherapy. There is a growing rationale for avoiding XRT, particularly among patients with p16-positive (HPV-related) small tumors (T1–2) and small volume neck disease (N1), and this approach is currently under investigation in a multi-institutional clinical trial (ECOG 3311).

Alternatively, radiation for early tonsillar cancers offers the advantage of treating upper echelon lymph nodes along with the primary tumor. Treatment is usually unilateral unless extension to the tongue base or midline soft palate is present.[159] Ipsilateral treatment portals allow sparing of the contralateral mucosa and salivary glands. Modern treatment techniques, such as IMRT, permit conformal dose delivery which can reduce the potential morbidity of radiation treatment, particularly by reducing radiation-related xerostomia. Initial institutional reports have indicated encouraging treatment outcomes with the use of IMRT in oropharyngeal cancer patients;[160–164] this is discussed in greater detail in the section titled "Radiotherapy."

Survival rates for patients with advanced (stage III/IV) tumors vary according to HPV/p16 expression status and smoking history. Patients with HPV-positive tumors and less than 10 pack-year smoking history (low-risk) treated with the combination of chemotherapy and radiotherapy have a 3-year survival rate of 93%; while a smoking history of more than 10 pack-years and HPV-/p16-negative tumor undergoing chemoradiation have a 3-year survival rate of 46.2%.[88] In general, surgery is rarely recommended for advanced tonsillar tumors unless the mandible is grossly invaded. When surgery is planned, postoperative concurrent therapy should be anticipated in the properly selected patient.

Tongue base

Cancers of the base of the tongue pose a more difficult therapeutic problem than do tonsillar carcinomas, particularly for HPV-negative malignancies. Most patients with HPV-negative tumors present with advanced primary site disease due to the silent nature of these tumors, resulting in frequent regional metastases, greater treatment morbidity, and poor patient survival. Due to the aggressive nature of HPV-negative tumors, most are treated with definitive radiation with or without chemotherapy, although a role for TORS is currently under clinical investigation. Owing to the rich network of lymphatics present in the base of the tongue, 75% of patients will present with stage III or IV disease (Figure 7). Understaging of the primary tumor is common because these cancers tend to be diffusely infiltrative beyond their clinical appearance.[165]

The results of radiation therapy alone as definitive treatment of small primary tumors (T1, T2) are better for exophytic than for deeply invasive tumors.[166] Radiation alone is generally reserved for those patients without clinical nodal metastases, but can be combined with planned neck dissection for patients with clinically positive nodes that persist after the completion of radiation-based approaches.

Surgical management of early primary tongue-base tumors (T1–2) achieves results similar to those from radiation alone. Advances in robotic surgery have prompted the application of this

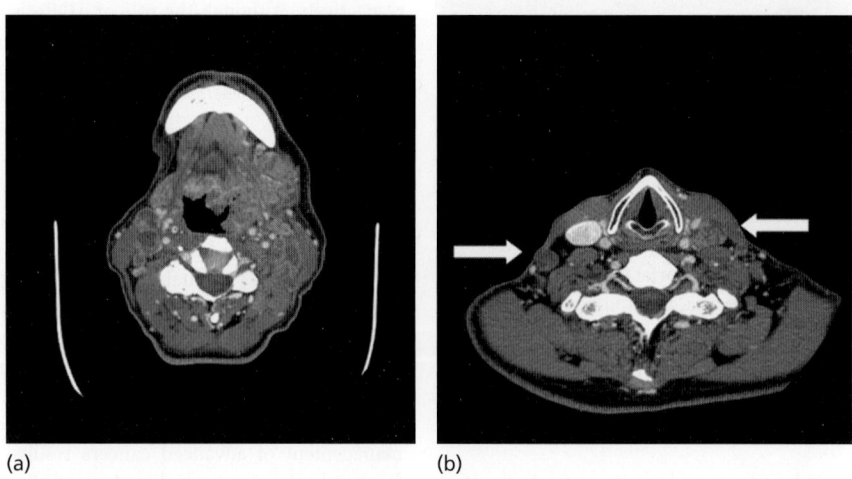

(a)　　　　　　　　　　　(b)

Figure 7 (a) Massive T4 N2c SCCA of the oropharynx (left base of tongue). (b) Multilevel bilateral nodal metastases present.

technology in the management of tongue-base cancers, and is now a well-established approach in the HPV-positive population.[167] Elective neck dissection can serve as a staging procedure, thereby providing a rationale for adjuvant radiation therapy. To date, no prospective randomized trial data that compare surgery alone with combined surgery with either preoperative or postoperative radiation are available.

Radiation therapy is a standard approach for definitive treatment for the oropharynx which combines the goal of an oncological cure with organ preservation. The current XRT regimens are the results of several large randomized trials that have demonstrated favorable OS and DFS,[168] although permanent dysphagia and gastrostomy tube usage rates remain substantial.[156] Total radiation dosages and overall treatment times are regarded as important variables for oncologic response and for tissue toxicity. Several studies have shown that altered fractionation improved the locoregional rate, and a meta-analysis of 15 trials demonstrated a survival advantage with altered fractionation regimens.[169] Since cancers of the oropharynx are adjacent to several critical structures, the ideal dose distributions would tightly conform to the target area and spare the nonaffected surrounding tissue, which has led to the use of IMRT as a standard of care for HNSCC.[170]

The classic pattern of relapse after RT in OPSCC has been locoregional recurrence, attributed to the development of radioresistant tumor cells that persist after treatment. To overcome this resistance, chemotherapy has been added to sensitize the tumor cells to the damaging effects of ionizing radiation. For patients with locally advanced oropharyngeal cancer, a pivotal randomized phase III trial by the French GORTEC group revealed an improvement in both progression-free survival (PFS) and 5-year OS for patients receiving combined modality therapy (42% and 51%) versus radiation therapy alone (22.4% and 15.8%) and improvement in locoregional control rates in the chemoradiation arm (66%) versus radiation therapy alone (42%). Despite these benefits, similar rates of distant metastases were observed in both arms (11%) and more significant side effects, including hematologic toxicities and grades 3 and 4 mucositis were observed in the chemotherapy arm.[171,172] These toxicities led to a higher rate of temporary gastrostomy tube usage in the combination arm compared to the radiation therapy alone arm. Taken together, these results suggest that the addition of chemotherapy concurrently to radiation therapy improves locoregional control, which translates into both a PFS and OS benefit for these patients, at the expense of more acute toxicities.

The risk of recurrence for locally advanced OPSCC following surgical resection has traditionally been high. For patients with high-risk features, including perineural invasion, multiple positive nodes, and advanced T stage, PORT has been shown to decrease locoregional recurrences. Furthermore, it has been shown that the addition of chemotherapy given concurrently with radiation can improve locoregional control rates in patients with high-risk features, particularly when surgical margins are positive or ECS is present.[134,173] Thus, patients who undergo surgical resection for OPSCC should be considered for adjuvant chemoradiotherapy when adverse pathological features are present. Whether this treatment paradigm is necessary for HPV-positive patients is currently under investigation.

Soft palate and pharyngeal wall

Cancers of the soft palate and pharyngeal wall are less common than other oropharyngeal neoplasms. Many soft palate and posterior wall cancers tend to be superficial. Advanced lesions with deep invasion have ready access to the prevertebral fascia, infratemporal fossa, and skull base and can be associated with extensive submucosal spread with clinical skip areas.

Radiation-based approaches as curative treatment are preferred in most cases, even for T3 primary tumors. Resection of most soft palate lesions is associated with severe functional disability. The rates of occult regional metastases are difficult to determine because elective irradiation of bilateral nodal groups is included as part of primary treatment and must include the retropharyngeal lymphatics. Clinically positive lymph nodes at presentation occur in 30% of patients.[174] Small primary tumors with positive nodes can be effectively treated with definitive radiation to the primary tumor and neck. Neck dissections should be performed if disease in the neck persists at 6 to 8 weeks following the completion of XRT. Pharyngeal wall cancers or palate cancers with extension to the tonsil and those cases with advanced regional metastases are usually treated with combined chemoradiotherapy approaches unless gross mandibular involvement is noted. Overall 5-year survival rates for soft palate and faucial pillar cancers are 60–70% and range from 80% to 90% for T1 and T2 lesions to 30–60% for stages III and IV lesions.[175]

Hypopharynx

The hypopharynx represents one of the most lethal sites for HNSCC. Lymph node metastases are clinically evident at time of diagnosis in 70–80% of patients.[176] Primary tumor extension beyond the hypopharynx is common.[177] Hypopharyngeal cancers are characterized by a propensity to spread submucosally to involve the oropharynx or esophagus. Ulcerated deep infiltration and skip areas are anticipated. This leads to difficulties in adequately assessing the margins of the tumor and contributes to poor local tumor control, even with the addition of adjuvant radiation. More than 75% of hypopharyngeal cancers arise in the pyriform sinus, while 20% occur in the posterior pharyngeal wall (Figure 8). Postcricoid cancers are rare (<5%). Because of the locale of hypopharyngeal cancers, their growth patterns and proximity to the larynx, surgical management often entails total laryngopharyngectomy. Extension to the esophagus will necessitate a cervical esophagectomy.

The staging of hypopharyngeal cancer is based on the subsite involved, the size of the tumor, the presence of vocal cord fixation, and the extent of lymph node metastases.[114] Staging is critical for treatment planning and must include endoscopic evaluation.[178]

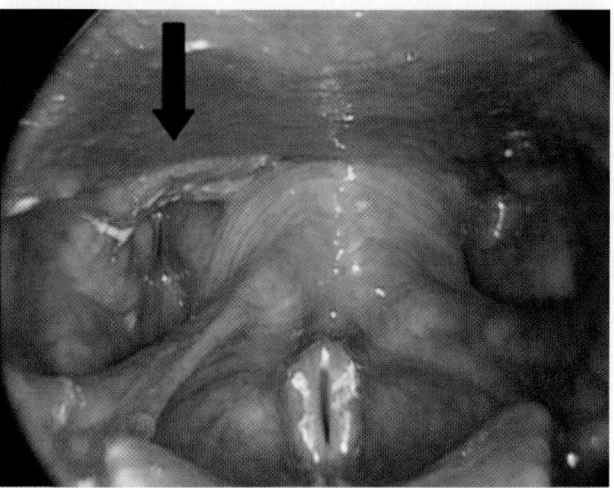

Figure 8 T1 SCCA of the hypopharynx, involving the posterior pharyngeal wall and extending into the esophageal inlet.

Because of the necessity to remove the larynx as part of the surgical treatment of most hypopharyngeal cancers, radiation therapy for early T1 and T2 and in combination with chemotherapy for T3 disease has been investigated.[179] Retrospective analyses have consistently demonstrated that survival rates are lower and locoregional failure rates higher with radiation alone as compared with surgery or surgery and radiotherapy.[180,181]

Nevertheless, the functional implications of primary surgery for even the earliest of hypopharyngeal cancers have brought about the primary role of radiation-based approaches. For small (T1) cancers of the hypopharynx, and particularly for superficial posterior pharyngeal wall lesions, radiation therapy alone has been used effectively, with surgery reserved for salvage.[182] Radiation therapy offers the advantage of treating bilateral occult lymph node disease, including that of retropharyngeal nodes, which are frequently involved when cancer arises from the posterior pharyngeal wall. Most patients, however, present with advanced primary tumors (T3–4) and positive lymph nodes. In such patients, local control rates with radiation alone decrease to 50% and salvage surgery is rarely successful. Thus, surgical management remains the mainstay of treatment of most advanced hypopharyngeal cancers. This is especially true when function is poor at diagnosis.

Tumors arising in the lower hypopharynx or postcricoid mucosa often spread to involve the esophagus. Distal submucosal spread into the esophagus can be extensive and requires partial or total esophagectomy. Reconstruction with transposition of the stomach (gastric pull-up), jejunal free graft, or tubed fasciocutaneous free flap is currently recommended.[183–185] With improved locoregional control following the advent of total laryngopharyngectomy and PORT, disease recurrence more commonly occurs in distant sites (i.e., the lung). Treatment approaches with combined preoperative or postoperative radiation have dramatically improved the control of locoregional disease, but survival rates have not improved as substantially over those with surgery alone because of the increased rates of distant metastases. Postoperative radiation is currently preferred to preoperative radiation because of its lower local recurrence rates, fewer complications, and less difficulty in accurately assessing tumor margins.[180,186] The presence of lymph node metastases, extracapsular lymph node involvement, and direct extension of the primary tumor into the soft tissues of the neck are adverse prognostic factors and are indications for postoperative chemoradiotherapy.[187,188]

Overall 5-year survival rates range from 10% to 30% for posterior pharyngeal wall cancers and from 20% to 40% for pyriform sinus cancers. The rates of distant metastases range from 20% to 50%[123,127] and increase with the extent of lymph node disease.[176,189–191]

Larynx

Because of the prominent role the larynx plays in communication, swallowing, respiration, and protection of the lower airway, the treatment of cancer of the larynx presents formidable dilemmas regarding functional consequences in addition to the intrinsic threat to life posed by these cancers. More so than with any other site of HNC, quality-of-life issues have been incorporated into treatment decisions and have echoed throughout the management strategy of the other head and neck sites.

The larynx is divided into three subsites: supraglottic, glottic, and subglottic. Each site is associated with differences in patterns of local spread, risks of lymphatic metastasis, and control rates. Anatomic studies of the vascular and lymphatic compartments of the larynx have defined natural anatomic barriers to cancer spread within the larynx and have contributed to the development of select surgical procedures for partial laryngeal resections of certain cancers.[192,193]

The true vocal cords present an effective boundary between supraglottic and subglottic lymphatic spread within the larynx. This anatomic barrier can be compromised by tumors involving the anterior or posterior commissures and with deeply invasive tumors that extend vertically across the true and false vocal cords (transglottic cancers). Normally, the inner perichondrium of the thyroid cartilage also presents an effective barrier to cancer spread. However, cancer involvement of the anterior commissure or transglottic extension is associated with invasion of the thyroid cartilage in 40–60% of cases.[194]

Early diagnosis is critical for achieving high survival rates and larynx preservation. Most cancers that are diagnosed at an early stage arise in the glottic larynx. This is because minimal changes of the vibrating vocal cord from tumor growth result in dysphonia or hoarseness. Supraglottic cancers are usually more advanced than glottic cancers at the time of diagnosis because they do not generally produce early symptoms of hoarseness. Rather, the earliest symptoms of a supraglottic cancer are usually sore throat, dysphagia, referred otalgia, or the development of a neck mass representing regional metastasis. Airway compromise may be an early symptom with subglottic cancer.

Modern clinical evaluation of laryngeal cancers includes fiberoptic laryngoscopy, direct laryngoscopy, CT, or MRI of the larynx and neck, as well as videostroboscopic analysis (Figure 9). Radiological imaging is of value in assessing direct extension to the preepiglottic and paraglottic spaces, detecting cartilage invasion, and evaluating the soft tissues and lymph nodes of the neck. However, the precise evaluation of tumor extent still requires direct laryngoscopy under anesthesia. With large, obstructive tumors, tracheostomy may be required. In some patients, debulking the tumor mass at the

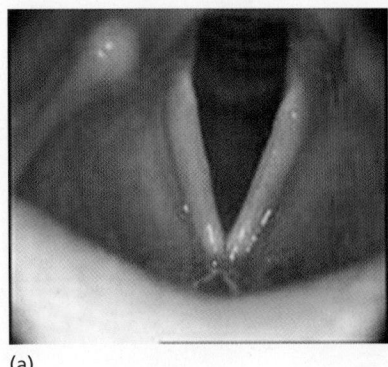
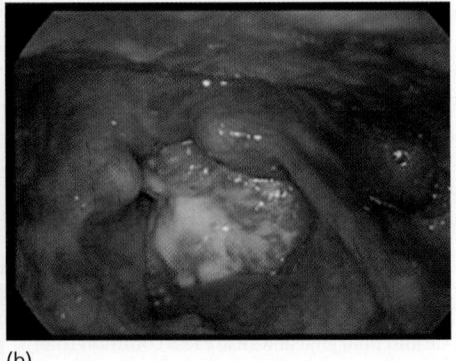

(a)   (b)

Figure 9 (a) Normal larynx. (b) T3 left glottic SCCA, with obliteration of the normal vocal cord anatomy. Extension onto the supraglottis and onto the arytenoid is evident.

time of direct laryngoscopy can obviate the need for tracheostomy and thereby reduce the potential risk of tumor seeding of the tracheostomy site. Even with precise clinical evaluation, inaccurate estimation of tumor extent (usually underestimation) occurs in 30–40% of cases.[195,196]

Supraglottic primary tumors account for approximately 35% of all laryngeal cancers.[8] The staging of supraglottic cancers is based on the subsite or region of the supraglottis involved. Subsites include the false vocal cords, arytenoids, lingual and laryngeal surfaces of the epiglottis, and aryepiglottic folds. The epiglottis itself is also subdivided into the region extending above the plane of the hyoid and that below the hyoid. Suprahyoid tumors tend to have a better prognosis than infrahyoid, with the exception of those invading the aryepiglottic fold to involve the pyriform sinus. This, again, is due to the richer network of lymphatics in the infrahyoid portion of the epiglottis. Early cancers (T1 and T2) can involve one or more subsites but have normal vocal cord motion. Those cancers that cause fixation of the arytenoid or involve the postcricoid region, medial wall of the pyriform sinus, or preepiglottic space are staged T3. Those that extend beyond the larynx or invade thyroid cartilage are staged T4.

Functional and anatomic features also determine the staging of glottic carcinomas. Cancers limited to the true vocal cords are T1, those with extension to an adjacent site or with impaired cord mobility are T2, arytenoid fixation and vocal cord immobility upstages a lesion to a T3. Those tumors with cartilage involvement or extension outside the larynx are T4.

True subglottic cancers that are limited to the subglottic region (T1) or to the subglottis and true vocal cords (T2) are early cancers. Fixation of the vocal cord (T3) and cartilage invasion or extension outside the larynx (T4) is associated with a worse prognosis. The nodal classification for staging is the same as for other HNSCC sites.

Although controversy exists regarding the optimal treatment for larynx cancer, at the University of Texas MD Anderson Cancer Center, curative radiotherapy is generally the treatment of choice for early-stage laryngeal lesions. For moderately advanced lesions, one must consider the trade-offs between definitive radiotherapy with salvage surgery held in reserve versus definitive surgery or combined chemotherapy and radiation therapy approaches. A number of factors, aside from stage, warrant consideration in determining the optimal treatment strategy, including patient's age, medical comorbidities, laryngeal function, and rehabilitative potential. Advanced T4 lesions are treated with surgery and PORT.

Radiation therapy remains the management of choice for early glottic cancers. Nevertheless, in some instances, patients may choose conservation laryngeal surgery, including endoscopic laser excision of localized lesions, or partial laryngeal surgery. Both require frozen-section analysis of margins if the patient and tumor factors support such an approach. In addition, conservation laryngeal surgical salvage is effective in those 10–20% of cases in which external beam therapy has been unsuccessful for stages I and II cancers.

The treatment of more advanced laryngeal cancers (T3 and T4) has historically included surgery with or without radiation therapy. Prospective randomized studies have shown convincingly that chemotherapy and radiation therapy (including surgical salvage) are equally effective in the long-term survival of patients with T3 laryngeal cancers as compared with surgery with or without radiation therapy. It is important to note that approximately 60% of patients may preserve their larynx, and thus quality of life has significantly improved.[197–199] Speech communication profiles are clearly better in the group of patients randomized to the larynx preservation arm, but there was no determination of swallowing

function.[200] However, local control was poorer for patients with T4 lesions. Current standard of care argues that laryngeal preservation approaches or protocols be considered in treating such patients, with the corollary that patients with poor function at diagnosis will likely have poor laryngeal function after conservation treatment. Thus, a primary surgical approach should be strongly considered for patients with significant aspiration based on pretreatment swallowing studies. In addition, due to the toxicity of combined chemoradiotherapy regimens, those with pulmonary and cardiac comorbidities that may limit treatment intensity may be best managed with surgery and radiotherapy.

Many surgical procedures for laryngeal carcinoma involve the creation of a tracheal stoma. This area is at significant risk of tumor recurrence, which is most likely associated with paratracheal nodal metastases. For this reason, bilateral paratracheal dissections should be performed in T4 glottic cancers and radiation therapy provided postoperatively if metastases to this echelon of nodes are found pathologically. Once a stomal recurrence has developed, the prognosis is grave regardless of salvage treatment, with a reported 5-year survival of 17%.[201] If risk factors for stomal recurrence are present, then the tracheal stoma should be irradiated as part of the initial management.

Supraglottic cancers

Important factors in selecting therapy for supraglottic cancers are tumor location, cord fixation, and pre-epiglottic extension. Tumors limited to the suprahyoid epiglottis are amenable to radiation with fields that encompass neck regions at risk of lymphatic metastases. In addition, some proponents of limited surgical interventions recommend endoscopic laser excision separate from management of the neck. Tumors involving the aryepiglottic folds, pyriform sinuses, or infrahyoid epiglottis tend to be more aggressive, are deeply infiltrative, and frequently involve the pre-epiglottic space. Radiation alone is less effective than surgery, resulting in more frequent local recurrences that require surgical salvage. The addition of systemic concurrent chemotherapy will positively impact the outcomes of patients with these tumors. Persistent postradiation edema of the supraglottic larynx is not uncommon and contributes to difficulty in detecting recurrence, which occurs in 40–50% of cases.[202,203] Most patients who have recurrence will ultimately require a salvage total laryngectomy.

In any patient undergoing partial laryngectomy, preoperative consent should be obtained for total laryngectomy in case the surgical findings dictate that more extensive surgery is needed. Approximately 20% of patients require prolonged tracheostomy, and this is usually related to edema secondary to PORT. The rates of persistent swallowing difficulties are low, however, and the need for completion laryngectomy for persistent aspiration ranges only from 0% to 5%.[204,205]

The frequency of neck node metastases is at least 20% with T2 or greater tumors. Treatment of the clinically negative neck may be accomplished with surgery or radiation.[206] Cure rates range from 73% to 75% for radiotherapy and increase to 80–85% with the addition of surgical salvage.[207–209] Most recurrences are local, and preservation of voice is successful in 65–70% of patients when salvage surgery is included.[207]

The treatment of more advanced supraglottic cancers (T3, T4) remains controversial, with laryngeal preservation remaining a focus of treatment (Figure 10). Combined chemoradiotherapy is often curative, but toxicities remain significant. As described, patients with T4 lesions are best managed with laryngectomy and radiotherapy, as cartilage and bone invasion are difficult to control with radiation. However, some experienced centers have

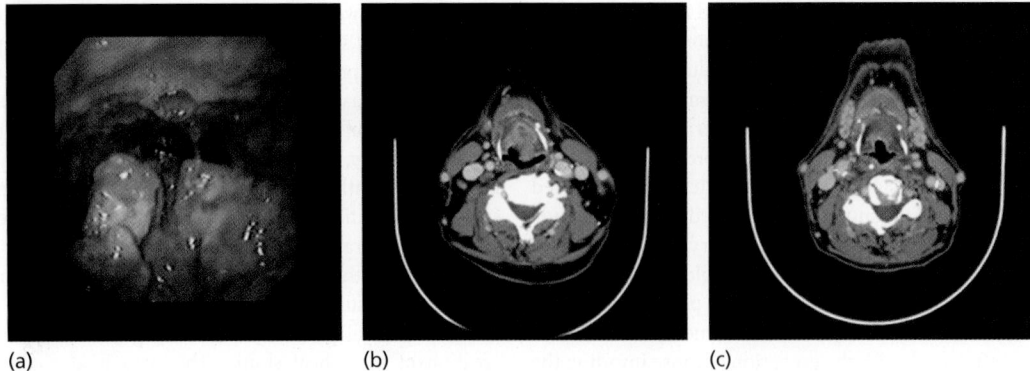
(a) (b) (c)

Figure 10 (a) T3 N0 SCCA of the supraglottis. Destruction of the epiglottis is evident. (b) Invasion of the pre-epiglottic space is seen on CT scan, prior to concurrent chemoradiotherapy. (c) Posttreatment imaging, demonstrating a complete response at the primary site.

treated patients having minimal laryngeal framework invasion with combined chemoradiotherapy with high success. One area of controversy surrounds the management of patients with bulky T3 lesions and poor pretreatment function. These patients may require long-term or permanent enteral nutrition and tracheostomy for significant aspiration, and may ultimately require a laryngectomy for pulmonary toilet. One novel approach that has been advocated is to utilize IC to assess both tumor and functional responses. Those with improvement of their function after one cycle of chemotherapy may tolerate concurrent chemoradiotherapy and avoid laryngectomy. Alternatively, those with minimal or no response would be best managed with surgery and PORT.

Although the stigma of laryngectomy remains, contemporary postoperative laryngeal rehabilitation offers quite acceptable functional outcomes. The advent of tracheo-esophageal punctures (TEP), in conjunction with intense rehabilitation, has markedly improved the functional outcomes of laryngectomized patients. A laryngeal speech can be realized within 2 weeks of surgery. In the salvage surgical setting, TEP placement should be deferred for at least 3 months while the surgical site matures. Early TEP placement resulted in fistula formation and poor wound healing.

Planned neck dissection at the conclusion of treatment for N2 disease or greater is often performed. In the clinically negative neck, elective neck dissection revealed metastases in 15–30% of patients, and thus bilateral elective neck irradiation is warranted. Failure to control disease in the neck is a major cause of mortality in supraglottic cancers. In most reports, radiation alone for the control of supraglottic cancers with N2 or N3 nodes is inferior to combined therapy. Overall 5-year survival rates for supraglottic cancers range from 40% to 50%. Local failures occur in approximately 10% of patients and regional failures in 15–20%. Rates of distant metastases range from 11% to 18%, with rates approaching 30% in patients with stage IV disease. Second primaries (20–25% of failures) are a major cause of death and intercurrent illness accounts for up to 20% of deaths.[209-211]

Glottic and subglottic cancers

The treatment of glottic cancer is greatly influenced by the secondary goal of voice preservation. For small cancers (T1, T2) with mobile vocal cords, radiation therapy alone achieves excellent local control rates of 80–95% and OS rates similar to those for surgical resection.[212,213] Voice quality, although often impaired by radiation, is generally better than that following surgical resection.[214] Local recurrences after definitive radiation can often be salvaged by subsequent surgery. Tumor involvement of the anterior commissure or arytenoids has been associated with higher local recurrence rates

for radiation alone, but this may have been related to understaging. The "irradiate-and-watch" treatment strategy is predicated on close follow-up in order to detect recurrences when they are still salvageable by surgery. Delay in the diagnosis of recurrent glottic cancers after radiation is more frequent than with supraglottic cancers and may require total laryngectomy for cure. Partial laser resection is another primary or salvage treatment option of glottic carcinomas.

Lesions with impaired mobility owing to muscle invasion behave more like T3 cancers and have a poorer prognosis with radiotherapy alone.[215-218] Transglottic cancers and those with subglottic extension have higher rates of regional metastases and more often require total laryngectomy for cure (Figure 11). In selected patients with these more advanced lesions, extended supraglottic laryngectomy or supracricoid partial laryngectomy may effectively salvage the patient and avoid a permanent stoma.[219] Voice quality is typically poor with these procedures, and permanent tracheostomy may be needed. In addition, these procedures are technically challenging and require a high level of training and experience.

The design of radiation treatment must be tailored to the individual patient, but some general comments can be made. Early-stage (T1–2, N0) glottic lesions are treated with conventional fields localized to the larynx only; for T2 tumors with significant subglottic spread, the upper trachea is also included. T1 tumors are typically treated once-daily to doses of approximately 6300–6600 cGy, while T2 tumors are treated more aggressively with twice-daily or concurrent-boost fractionation.[220] T2 tumors with bulky subglottic extension or with anterior involvement with potential extralaryngeal spread outside the thyroid cartilage are at higher risk for treatment failure, and can be considered for concurrent chemoradiotherapy. There has been recent interest in using IMRT to minimize dose to the adjacent carotid vessels; and for very early lesions, there have also been reports of single vocal cord irradiation[221] to further reduce the volume of irradiated tissue. Management of advanced T3 glottic cancers has historically consisted of total laryngectomy with or without PORT. Although older series show suboptimal control rates (20–35%) and survival rates (10–50%) for unselected sets of T3 and T4 tumors treated with radiation alone, it is now recognized that with proper selection, radiotherapy control rates for T3 lesions can approach 70–80%,[222,223] which is enhanced by the addition of platinum-based chemotherapy. In patients without regional metastases, local tumor control rates with surgery alone are excellent. Significant increases in local control with the addition of radiation therapy have not been clearly demonstrated. However, in patients with regional metastases, overall prognosis is poor and recurrence in the neck is a major problem when surgery alone is used. Improved regional

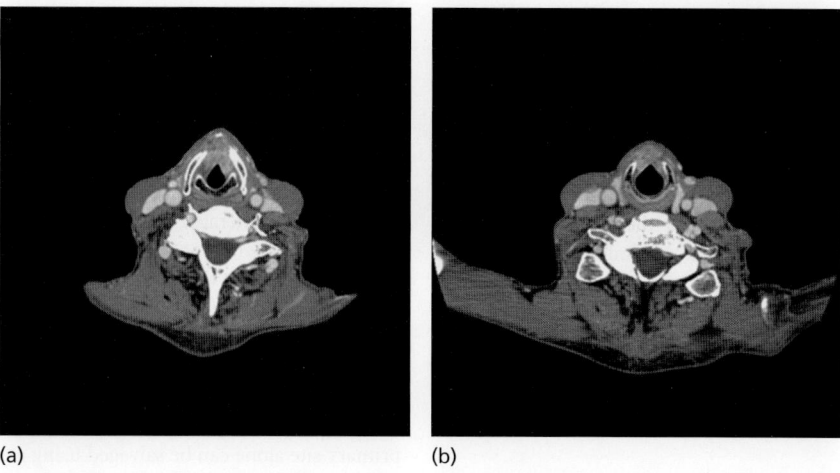

(a)   (b)

Figure 11 Small volume laryngeal SCCA with both glottic (a) and subglottic (b) involvement. The lesion is staged T4 due to the extensive cartilagenous invasion, with extension into the soft tissue of the neck.

tumor control rates are achieved with the addition of adjuvant radiation therapy.[224] Because rates of occult regional metastases approach 30% in patients with advanced glottic (T3, T4) cancers, elective modified or selective node dissections for staging purposes are recommended when surgery is performed for primary disease. Demonstration of histologically positive nodal metastases has been used as an indication for PORT. Surgery alone is curative in 50–80% of patients without nodal metastases,[216,225–228] but this decreases to less than 40% if metastases are present.[216,229,230]

As T3–4 tumors have a greater propensity for nodal metastases, larger radiation fields that encompass levels 2–4 are recommended. In the postoperative setting, radiation targets include the tumor bed and draining lymphatics including the upper paratracheal nodes. The stoma is included in the treatment fields, particularly when there is subglottic or nodal disease (especially with ECS) or when a tracheostomy was done emergently prior to oncologic therapy.

Subsets of laryngeal cancers that warrant special consideration are those that involve both the glottic and supraglottic regions (transglottic). These cancers are usually advanced and are associated with a high incidence (30–50%) of regional metastases.[231,232] These tumors can be difficult to control with radiation alone, and may warrant the addition of chemotherapy in the treatment plan.

Distant spread is approximately four times more common with supraglottic than with glottic cancers.[233] Rates of distant metastases associated with glottic cancer have increased, however, with the use of combined therapy and have been reported in approximately 20% of patients with advanced disease. Rates appear to be directly related to the extent of nodal disease, with reported rates as high as 40–50% in patients with N2 or N3 disease.[234]

Subglottic carcinomas are a rare variant of squamous carcinomas of the larynx possessing a high risk for paratracheal metastases, local recurrence, and death from disease. Surgery is the preferred therapy except in early superficial diseases of this site.[235,236] Tumors originating from or involving the subglottic larynx can spread to the upper paratracheal nodes as well as to the nodes in the cervical chain; therefore, radiation fields for this disease must include the upper mediastinum.[237]

Carcinoma in situ (CIS)

A special issue relates to the treatment of CIS of the vocal cords. This disease often can be managed with vocal cord stripping, but if enough serial sections are examined, foci of invasive carcinoma are often found. For diffuse CIS of the glottis, radiation therapy has been advocated, due to significant risk of malignant transformation and the inability to clear this disease surgically. Very superficial cancers limited to the free edge of the vocal cord or CIS can be effectively treated by limited excision by conventional means or with laser excision, with excellent voice preservation.[238] More extensive disease requires cordectomy, vertical hemilaryngectomy, or supracricoid laryngectomy.

Nonsurgical treatment

There has been an increasing focus on the use of chemotherapy in the management of laryngeal cancers of all stages. Randomized trials have demonstrated that the concurrent administration of chemotherapy and radiotherapy improves local-regional disease control and OS in patients with locally advanced HNSCC. IC has long been recognized as highly active, with clinical partial and complete responses observed in 80–90% of patients.[239–241] It was postulated that a substantial response to initial treatment with chemotherapy would lead to an improvement of therapeutic efficacy for surgery or radiotherapy. This led to the Department of Veterans Affairs Laryngeal Cancer Study,[155] in which 332 patients with stage III or IV SCC of the larynx were randomized to receive either IC consisting of cisplatin and fluorouracil followed by radiotherapy or surgery and PORT. Patients who experienced no tumor response to chemotherapy or those who had locally persistent or recurrent cancer underwent salvage laryngectomy. Two-year survival for both treatment groups was 68%, and 41% of patients randomly assigned to the experimental arm were alive with a functional larynx at 2 years. Thus, the efficacy of chemotherapy followed by radiotherapy (with surgical salvage) was similar to that of surgery followed by radiotherapy and established organ preservation as a realistic goal of nonsurgical treatment administered with curative intent. Lefebvre et al.[179] later reported the potential for effective sequential IC followed by radiotherapy in a European trial involving patients with cancers of the hypopharynx.

In the Veterans Affairs study, there were observed trends in patterns of tumor relapse, with 20% of patients in the chemotherapy arm having locoregional recurrence versus 7% in the surgery arm. Distant disease recurrence was more likely in the surgical arm, affecting 17% of patients versus 11% in the chemotherapy/radiotherapy group. Salvage laryngectomy was required more often in patients with glottic cancer than in those with supraglottic primary sites (43% vs 31%), in patients with fixed vocal cords than in those with mobile vocal cords (41% vs 29%), and in patients with gross invasion of thyroid cartilage compared with patients without (41% vs 35%). Salvage laryngectomy was required in 56% of patients with T4 cancers compared with 29% of patients with smaller primary tumors ($p = 0.001$).

The Veterans Affairs Larynx study prompted further investigations of sequential chemotherapy and radiotherapy in the treatment of intermediate-stage larynx cancer. These trials indicate that for patients with intermediate-stage SCC of the larynx, a combined treatment program with the objectives of tumor eradication and laryngeal preservation is appropriate. It is also important to recognize that patients with locally advanced destructive primary laryngeal cancers were not included in the multi-institutional trial. These patients may require total laryngectomy for optimal tumor control and to preserve swallowing function.

Nasopharynx

Presentation and staging
In the United States, NPC accounts for 2% of all HNSCC. Its unusual epidemiologic and natural history features include a remarkable tendency toward early regional and distant dissemination. NPC also is extremely sensitive to radiotherapy and cytotoxic chemotherapy.

The nasopharynx is a chamber bounded anteriorly by the choana of the nasal cavity, superiorly by the clivus, and inferiorly by the soft palate. Its posterior wall is the mucosa that overlies the superior constrictor muscles of the pharynx and the C1 and C2 vertebral bodies. The lateral walls contain the eustachian tube orifices. The region is richly endowed with lymphatics that drain to the retropharyngeal and deep cervical nodes.

Malignant neoplasms of the nasopharynx are primarily epithelial, with the presence of keratin associated with a poorer prognosis. The WHO recognizes three histopathologic types of NPC: type 1, differentiated SCC (of varying degrees); type 2, nonkeratinizing carcinoma; and type 3, undifferentiated lymphoepithelial carcinoma. Mixed patterns are common.

About one-third of patients present with a neck mass without other complaints, and about 70–75% of patients have enlarged neck nodes at presentation. Other common symptoms are epistaxis, nasal stuffiness, headache, and hearing loss (generally unilateral). The tumor can spread laterally and superiorly to cause bony destruction of the base of the skull. Frequently, there are cranial nerve findings, with the sixth nerve being most commonly involved. There are two principal cranial nerve syndromes associated with NPC: (1) the retroparotidian syndrome, involving cranial nerves IX, X, XI, and XII and (2) the petrosphenoidal syndrome, involving cranial nerves III, IV, V, and VI (and occasionally cranial nerve II via extension through the foramen lacerum into the middle cranial fossa). Evaluation of the nasopharynx should consist of direct visualization with a fiberoptic scope. An MRI scan is important in evaluating base-of-skull involvement and the possible presence of occult-involved lymph nodes.

The most recent revision of the AJCC/Union Internationale Contre le Cancer (UICC) staging system recognizes the uniqueness of NPC among other head and neck tumors.[114]

Treatment
Standard treatment of NPC is radiation therapy or concurrent chemoradiotherapy for early and locally advanced disease, respectively. Surgical resection even for early-stage disease is technically difficult because of the anatomic location of the primary tumor and frequent bilateral cervical and retropharyngeal node involvement. The role of the surgeon is limited to obtaining tissue for diagnosis,

resecting residual adenopathy after definitive radiotherapy, and surgery for rare non-WHO histologies such as adenoid cystic carcinoma.[242] Prior to initiating therapy, dental consultation is advised since it is necessary to irradiate the parotid glands bilaterally, and the resulting xerostomia predisposes to serious oral problems.

The nasopharynx is a disease site for which IMRT has been utilized in an attempt to improve the therapeutic index of external beam radiotherapy. Increasing the conformality of radiation delivery is desired, given the many critical neural, vascular, and soft tissues surrounding this anatomic site.

A clear correlation exists between the degree of cervical adenopathy and the subsequent development of distant metastases, with patients with bilateral adenopathy having an 80% 5-year actuarial risk of distant metastases. Common sites of distant metastases are the lung, bone, and liver. In selected cases, a failure at the primary site alone can be salvaged using a combination of external beam radiotherapy and an intracavitary implant.[243,244] Five-year local control rates were the best for patients with persistent disease (87.2%) versus those with a first recurrence (62.7%) or a second recurrence (23.4%, $p = 0.0004$). Overall 5-year survival rates for these three patient groups were 79.1%, 53.6%, and 42.9%, respectively.

The efficacy and toxicity of systemic therapy is presently evaluated in trials that include NPC as a distinct entity, and efforts are made to define patient cohorts according to the WHO classification. Including NPC with squamous cancers in studies of other head and neck sites will confound study outcomes in part because of the exquisite sensitivity of NPC to chemotherapy and radiation, but also because of the distinctive patient demographics and patterns of tumor recurrence in NPC.

Reports of phase II trials demonstrate single-agent activity for cisplatin, carboplatin, fluorouracil, bleomycin, methotrexate, anthracycline, vinca alkaloids, and taxanes.[245,246] Response rates range from 20% to 60%. More recent reports of cisplatin-based drug combinations describe tumor responses in 50–80% of patients, clinically complete in 20–25% of these.[247–250] Moreover, Fandi et al.[251] have reported durable disease remissions in a cohort of patients followed up over a period of years. Chan et al.[252] have reported that the combination of carboplatin and cetuximab, a chimeric monoclonal antibody directed against EGFR, has activity (overall disease-control rate 60%) even in heavily previously treated NPC patients.

For patients with stage III or IV at diagnosis, chemoradiotherapy has become the standard of care. In the United States, an Intergroup Cooperative Study (IG0099) tested radiotherapy-alone arm versus an experimental arm consisting of concurrent cisplatin given on days 1, 22, and 43 during radiotherapy followed by three courses of adjuvant cisplatin and 5-FU chemotherapy.[253] A total of 147 evaluable patients with stages III and IV tumors were enrolled. Notably, approximately one-third of patients were classified WHO 1, unlike most reports from the Pacific Rim in which >95% of patients are WHO 2/3. At 3 years, there was improved PFS (69% vs 24%, $p = 0.001$), improved OS (76% vs 46%, $p = 0.005$), and reduced distant metastases (13% vs 35%, $p = 0.002$) for the experimental arm. The results of this trial established the standard of care in the United States. These data were corroborated by another randomized phase III trial, which compared concurrent cisplatin (40 mg/m^2 weekly) and radiotherapy with radiotherapy alone in 350 patients with local and regionally advanced (N2 and N3, or N1 with nodal disease ≥4 cm) NPC.[254] This study found that treatment with combined chemotherapy plus radiotherapy prolonged PFS. The treatment effect had a notable covariate interaction with tumor stage, and subgroup analysis showed a significant difference in

Table 4 Selected concurrent chemoradiotherapy trials in locally advanced NPC.

Study	n	Treatment arms	Outcomes
Al-Sarraf et al.[253]	78	cddp 100 mg/m^2 weeks 1,4,7-RT + adj cddp/fu	5-Year PFS 58% and OS 67% CM vs 29% 29% and 37% RT
	69	RT	($p < 0.001$)
Lin et al.[256]	141	cddp 20 mg/m^2/day + fu 400 mg/m^2/day 96 h infusion weeks 1 + 5-RT	5-Year PFS 72% and OS 72% CM vs 53% and 54% RT
	143	RT	($p = 0.001 + 0.002$)
Chan et al.[254,255]	174	cddp 40 mg/m^2 weekly RT	5-Year PFS 60% and OS 70% CM vs 52% and 59% RT
	176	RT	($p = 0.06 + 0.05$)
Hui et al.[257]	34	Doc 75 mg/m^2 + cddp 75 mg/m^2 × 2	3-Year PFS 88% and OS 94% vs 60% ($p = 0.12$) and 68% ($p = 0.01$)
	31	→ CRT CRT	

Abbreviations: cddp, cisplatin; CM, combined modality; doc, docetaxel; fu, fluorouracil; OS, overall survival; PFS, progression-free survival; RT, radiotherapy.

patients with T3 disease in favor of the concurrent-therapy arm ($p = 0.0075$). The time to first distant failure also was statistically prolonged in patients with T3 tumors in the concurrent-treatment arm ($p = 0.016$). An updated report[255] concludes that OS benefit after chemoradiotherapy was most clearly obtained in patients with T3/4 staging ($p = 0.013$). Lin et al.[256] conducted a prospective phase III trial with randomization to radiation therapy alone or XRT with two cycles of concurrent cisplatin and fluorouracil administered during weeks 1 and 5 of XRT. OS again favored the combined treatment arm (Table 4).

Alternatively, strategies with IC have much appeal because of the high risk of systemic tumor dissemination in patients with NPC. However, a survival advantage for this approach has not been conclusively demonstrated. Chua et al.[258] have analyzed pooled data from two large phase III trials investigating the role of IC in NPC. In these trials, a total of 784 patients were randomized to receive 2–3 cycles of cisplatin-based combination drug therapy followed by XRT or radiotherapy alone. The 5-year relapse-free survival was 50.9% and 42.7%, respectively ($p = 0.014$), and disease-specific survival was 63.5% and 58.1% ($p = 0.029$). OS was not found to be significantly different between the arms ($p = 0.092$). Hui et al.[257] have recently reported favorable PFS and OS results in a phase II study of induction cisplatin and docetaxel followed by chemoradiotherapy. Phase III trials investigating the value of IC are under way. NRG-HN001 is an ongoing phase II/III study investigating the value of measuring plasma EBV DNA as a marker of efficacy of concurrent chemoradiotherapy. With undetectable DNA, patients are randomized to observation or adjuvant chemotherapy. Patients with detectable DNA after chemoradiotherapy receive additional treatment, testing an alternative regimen consisting of paclitaxel and gemcitabine versus cisplatin and fluorouracil.

Nose and paranasal sinuses

The nose and the paranasal sinuses pose a unique set of problems that deserve separate consideration from SCC of the UADT. The three most common malignant histologies of the paranasal sinuses are SCC, adenocarcinoma, and adenoid cystic carcinoma, but a number of other histologies are prevalent in this region, including sinonasal undifferentiated carcinoma (SNUC), neuroendocrine carcinoma, and esthesioneuroblastoma (often referred to as olfactory neuroblastoma).

Cancer of the nose and paranasal sinuses is relatively rare. It accounts for approximately 3% of cancers of the UADT and tends to occur in the fifth decade of life.[259] These tumors tend to be asymptomatic and usually contained within either a sinus or the nasal cavity. Early symptoms usually include nasal airway obstruction, rhinorrhea, sinusitis, epistaxis, and, occasionally, dental problems such as dental pain, numbness, and loose teeth. Late symptoms include cranial nerve deficits, proptosis, facial pain and swelling, ulceration through the palate, and trismus, all of which are ominous signs (Figure 12).

The diagnosis of nose and paranasal sinus cancers is made by having a high index of suspicion in a patient who presents with nasal airway obstruction and a nasal mass. A thorough endoscopic or fiberoptic examination of the entire nasal cavity is critical to rule out benign disease such as nasal polyposis or sinusitis. Biopsy is indicated when a mass is found. Great care should be taken as these lesions can hemorrhage, especially neuroendocrine carcinoma and

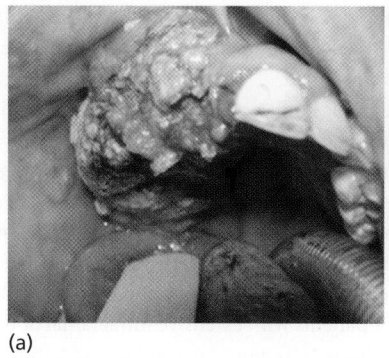
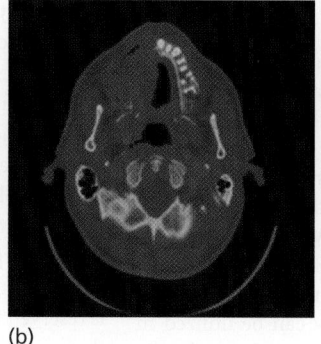
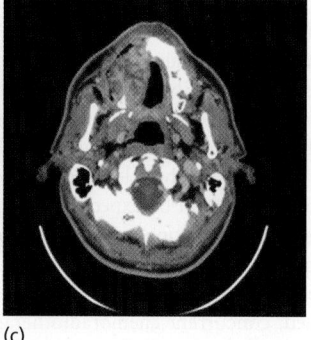

(a)   (b)   (c)

Figure 12 (a) T4 SCCA of the maxillary sinus, with extension into the oral cavity. (b) Bone windows on CT scan reveals complete replacement of the maxillary sinus with tumor and destruction of the pterygoid plates. (c) Soft tissue windows reveal extraosseous extension into the midface.

esthesioneuroblastoma. When taking a patient to the operating room for an endoscopic examination and biopsy, a frozen section should be obtained. It is critical to consider minimizing exposure of uninvolved structures; therefore, biopsy only should be performed without Caldwell Luc procedures, septoplasty, or entry into uninvolved sinuses. Imaging plays an important part in not only the diagnosis and staging of these lesions but also the surgical planning. The combination of CT and MRI provides useful information, especially with regard to skull-base involvement.

Because these malignancies rarely present as early stage, the accepted staging systems are not commonly used in clinical practice. Special note is made of "Ohngren's line," or the malignant plane. The plane is defined by an imaginary line drawn from the medial canthus to the ipsilateral angle of mandible and passes through the infraorbital foramen. Tumors above this line (suprastructure) are unfavorable, while those below (infrastructure) are considered favorable.

Treatment

Treatment of neoplasms of the sinonasal cavity is primarily determined by the histology. Traditionally, surgery with PORT has been advocated for many of these tumors. Although very effective for smaller tumors of selected histologies, this approach provides poor control for advanced disease involving the orbit, skull base and soft tissues of the face. An IC-based approach, with patients triaged to either concurrent chemoradiotherapy or surgery with PORT based on the response to chemotherapy is currently under investigation among patients with advanced tumors (clinical trial registration number NCT00707473).[260]

A complete discussion of the surgical management of paranasal sinus malignancies is beyond the scope of this chapter, but highlights of surgical considerations are briefly presented. Surgical approaches include (1) open transfacial, (2) midface degloving/sublabial, and (3) endoscopic. Surgical resections include (1) medial maxillectomy, (2) infrastructure maxillectomy, (3) total maxillectomy with or without orbital exenteration, and (4) craniofacial resection. The approach and resection utilized should be personalized, based on tumor location, extent, histology, cosmesis, and patient preference.

The endoscopic approach is being increasingly used in the management of paranasal sinus cancers. It provides excellent visualization with angled telescopes, the ability to remove bone with high-speed drills and soft tissue with microdebriders and can also be complemented by intraoperative surgical navigation. However, this approach requires a high degree of comfort with the technology and experience with endoscopic techniques, as well as the ability to convert to an open approach when necessary. Some of the limitations include inability to repair large defects, access to the orbit, and the need for an experienced surgical assistant for a two-handed technique.

Radiotherapy plays a major role in the management of sinonasal malignancies. It is used both preoperatively and postoperatively and, in select cases, as definitive therapy for small T1 and T2 lesions, especially those limited to the nasal vestibule and anterior nasal cavity.[261] In this situation, high locoregional control rates and good cosmetic outcome should be expected. With the increased use of radiotherapy in combination with surgery, ever-improving rates of locoregional control have been achieved. Surgery with PORT remains the standard of care for advanced sinonasal cavity tumors. As mentioned, concurrent chemoradiotherapy can be utilized in selected patients. Patients with inoperable tumors or those who are not considered good surgical candidates may be best treated with radiation therapy alone for local control and palliation.

Treatment-related sequelae from radiation to the paranasal sinuses and skull base are common. Acute complications include skin desquamation, nasal dryness, mucositis, xerophthalmia, and fistula formation. Chronic side effects include nasal dryness, xerophthalmia, visual impairment, atrophic rhinitis, osteoradionecrosis, and pituitary dysfunction. Dry eye can range from mild dryness to corneal ulceration, and even blindness. Enucleation may be necessary for debilitating ophthalmoplegia. Although the retina, like most neural structures, is radioresistant, visual impairment can occur as a result of damage to the lens and/or microvasculature that support both the retina and optic nerve. Frontal lobe necrosis is a devastating complication that may require neurosurgical intervention.

Although chemotherapy as a component of concurrent treatment with radiation is covered more extensively in a separate section, some aspects of chemotherapy are mentioned briefly here. The use of IC in selected patients with involvement of the eye has shown promising results in preserving the orbit.[262] Choi and colleagues reported results of concurrent chemoradiotherapy and investigators at the University of Chicago have used IC with cisplatin and infusional 5-FU to achieve improved rates of locoregional control and preserve the eye.[262,263] Studies at various centers are currently ongoing to validate the use of this approach for advanced sinonasal malignancies. Some investigators have utilized intra-arterial chemotherapy followed by surgery and/or radiation therapy for advanced sinonasal malignancies.[264–266] Although these studies have shown some benefit with regard to locoregional control, the morbidity associated with intra-arterial therapy does not appear to justify this approach. For patients with unresectable skull-base neoplasms, concurrent chemoradiotherapy is a reasonable approach that may offer locoregional control in up to 50% of patients.[262] SNUC, neuroendocrine carcinoma, and esthesioneuroblastoma represent a spectrum of tumors with neuroendocrine differentiation that can be difficult to distinguish histologically. Immunohistochemistry is often necessary to accurately diagnose these lesions, which may also be confused with sinonasal melanoma, rhabdomyosarcoma, PNET, or lymphoma. An experienced head and neck pathologist should be consulted prior to determining a treatment plan.

SNUC is a rare but lethal cancer typically presenting as advanced disease in elderly patients. Traditional treatment has been surgery followed by PORT, but this has provided poor long-term control. These tumors may be chemosensitive and a response to IC may identity patients for concurrent chemoradiotherapy as definitive treatment.[267–269] Surgical salvage has a uniformly dismal prognosis, but in light of the poor locoregional control achieved with traditional surgery and PORT, most agree that study of concurrent chemoradiotherapy is warranted.

Esthesioneuroblastoma is a rare neoplasm emanating from the olfactory neurofilaments at the cribriform plate. Invasion of the anterior cranial fossa occurs early in the disease process, and eventually involves the brain parenchyma (Figure 13). Patients often present with nasal obstruction and epistaxis. Treatment centers around surgical resection and PORT, which offers effective locoregional control and favorable survival outcomes.[270] Chemotherapy is reserved for patients with extensive intracranial or orbital disease that would otherwise require an extensive resection. It may also be used in the neoadjuvant setting as a cytoreductive approach to allow complete surgical resection.[271]

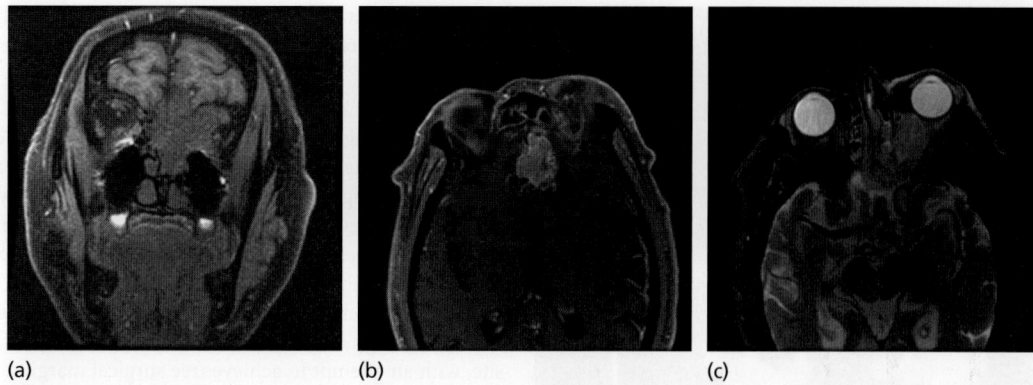

Figure 13 (a) Esthesioneuroblastoma involving the central skull base, with intracranial extension. (b) Involvement of the left frontal lobe on MRI. (c) Invasion of the left orbital apex.

Salivary glands

Anatomy

Salivary gland tissue is ubiquitous in the submucosa of the upper gastrointestinal tract and with three major salivary glands: parotid, submaxillary (or submandibular), and sublingual glands. The most common sites of tumors of minor salivary glands are the palate, the base of the tongue, and the buccal mucosa.[272]

The majority of salivary gland tumors arise in the parotid glands, and although nearly 80% of these are benign, these glands are the origin of the majority of malignant tumors. Tumors arising in the submandibular, sublingual, or minor salivary glands are more likely to be malignant.

The largest salivary glands are the parotids, which are located on the cheeks anterior to the external auditory canal and pinna. The gland wraps around the mandible, and as the facial nerve passes through the parotid, it divides it into superficial, or lateral, and deep lobes. About 80% of the gland lies lateral to the facial nerve, and 20% lies deep to this nerve, behind and medial to the mandible. The internal carotid artery, the internal jugular vein, the cervical sympathetic chain, and cranial nerves IX, X, and XI are in close proximity to the deep lobe of the parotid. The lymphatic drainage of parotid tumors is into intraparotid lymph nodes, external jugular chain, and the upper jugular lymph nodes (levels II and III). Additional lymphatic drainage is into adjacent levels, including the posterior triangle or level V. The presence of nerves within the parotid gland, especially the facial nerve and the auriculotemporal branch of the trigeminal, can be involved by tumors, especially adenoid cystic carcinoma and SCC. Any parotid mass warrants evaluation, and surgical excision is often the only solution since progression of even benign neoplasms may not only cause facial asymmetry but also place the facial nerve at risk. Further, benign lesions may transform into high-grade malignancies over time, as in the case of carcinoma ex-pleomorphica.

The second largest glands are the submandibular glands, located in the triangle formed by the two bellies of the digastric muscle and the mandible. Malignant tumors in this location can spread to the lymph nodes in levels II, III, and IV, as well as grow along the nerves, preferentially the branches of the lingual nerve, and occasionally the mandibular branch of the facial nerve.

The sublingual glands are the smallest of the major salivary glands and are formed of a conglomeration of glands located underneath the mucosa of the FOM and surrounding the excretory duct of the submandibular gland, Wharton's duct.

Diagnosis

The clinical presentation of malignant salivary gland tumors is variable, depending on the site and histology. The presence of a facial nerve paralysis is uncommon but generally indicates a malignant lesion. Tumors of the deep lobe of the parotid are notorious for producing dysphagia and submucosal deformity of the soft palate. When major invasion of the parapharyngeal space occurs, involvement of cranial nerves IX, X, XI, and even XII can occur. The usual presentation of submandibular gland tumors is a painless swelling below the mandible, and such tumors need to be distinguished from the much more frequent bacterial sialoadenitis of this gland.

On physical examination, a palpable mass without superficial ulceration of either skin or mucosa is the most frequent finding. An important cytological diagnostic procedure to be considered is FNA, which can exclude or confirm neoplasia. This procedure, especially in the parotid and submandibular gland, has gained increasing acceptance and should be considered whenever the information that can be obtained will have an impact on treatment or prognosis. The accurate typing of tumor is often less important and may be deferred to the definitive histological examination. This has to be applied judiciously in spite of the high accuracy reported by experts (i.e., sensitivity, 94%; specificity, 97%; accuracy, 95%).[273]

Histopathology

Benign lesions are the most frequent tumor of the parotid gland. The histological classification of malignant salivary tumors has been reviewed and expanded over the years and the present WHO classification is the most often quoted (Table 5).[274] MEC is the most frequent cancer of the parotid gland and is classified into high-grade, intermediate, and low-grade tumors (Figure 14).[275,276] Low-grade MEC is characterized by a slow growth rate, a low recurrence rate after complete surgical excision (about 15%), and rare incidence of metastasis. High-grade tumors are more aggressive, and the local recurrence rate after surgery alone approaches 60%.[277] Local recurrences and distant metastases may occur many years after treatment. About 50% of patients with high-grade MEC

Table 5 Most common malignant tumors of salivary glands.

Mucoepidermoid carcinoma (low, intermediate, or high grade)
Acinic cell carcinoma
Adenoid cystic carcinoma
Adenocarcinoma
Malignant mixed tumor (carcinoma-expleomorphic adenoma)
Squamous cell carcinoma

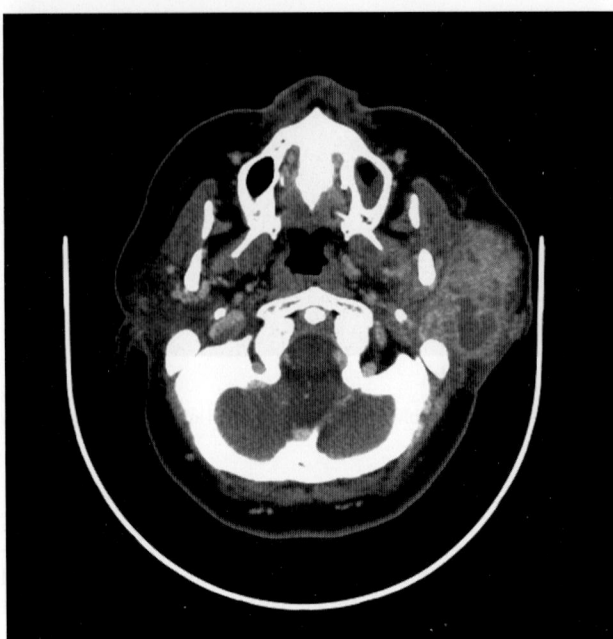

Figure 14 Mucoepidermoid carcinoma of the left parotid gland.

present with regional metastases, and 30% develop metastases at distant sites.[275,278] Acinic cell carcinomas are usually well differentiated and account for approximately 13% of the cancers arising from the parotid glands. Lymph node metastases occur in about 15% of cases. Local recurrence and distant metastases may occur many years after treatment.[279] Adenoid cystic carcinoma accounts for approximately 10% of parotid gland malignancies but it accounts for 60% of malignant neoplasms of the submandibular or minor salivary glands.[272,280] Three subtypes that correlate to biological behavior—cribiriform, tubular, and solid (most aggressive)—have been identified. A remarkable feature of this neoplasm is its propensity to invade major nerves and spread along the endoneural and perineural sheaths. This has significant prognostic importance and must be taken into account when deciding treatment and, specifically, when considering PORT. Although these tumors often follow an indolent course, as many as 40% of patients ultimately develop regional and distant metastases.[280]

Adenocarcinomas are more common in the minor salivary glands. The majority of them are high-grade tumors. About 36% of patients either present with or subsequently develop regional lymph node metastases; therefore, the regional lymph nodes need to be addressed in treatment strategies for high-grade adenocarcinomas.[281] Lung and bone are frequent sites of distant metastases.

Carcinoma ex-pleomorphic arises from preexisting benign pleomorphic adenoma. The risk of malignant transformation increases with time and age of the patient. Of adenomas of less than 5 years' duration, 1.6% can dedifferentiate; when present for more than 15 years, the dedifferentiation rate increases to 9.4%.[282] True malignant mixed tumors are rare, constituting only 2–5% of all malignant salivary gland tumors. These are typically aggressive tumors. A histology that deserves mention is salivary ductal carcinoma, which appears microscopically similar to breast carcinoma. Primary SCC of the salivary gland is rare, accounting for less than 3% of parotid neoplasms. This lesion must be distinguished from metastatic SCC to the parotid lymph nodes from cutaneous malignancies or from other sites. Primary SCCs of the parotid gland may develop regional

lymph node metastases in 50% of patients, a clinical feature that must be considered when patients are treated by surgery and PORT.

Treatment

The accepted staging system for salivary gland tumors can be found in the monographs of the AJCC and UICC.[114] The treatment of benign and malignant salivary gland tumors is surgery. Early-stage (T1 or T2) and especially low-grade tumors should be treated with comprehensive excision with free surgical margins. Such tumors arising in the parotid gland are generally treated by parotidectomy with preservation of the facial nerve. Early-stage high-grade tumors of any histology are treated with surgical resection of the primary site, with an attempt to achieve free surgical margins. This often is not possible, and microscopic spread, especially of adenoid cystic carcinoma, may occur along tissue planes, submucosal spaces, and perineural pathways. The dissection of regional lymph nodes should be done judiciously; elective nodal dissection is seldom indicated except in high-grade malignancies, especially salivary duct carcinoma, MEC, and SCC.[283] Salivary gland malignancies were thought to be resistant to conventional photon radiation, but over the years it has become established that postoperative irradiation is highly effective for eradicating subclinical disease.[280,284,285]

PORT is also indicated for major and minor salivary gland cancers when (1) the tumor is high grade or is metastatic SCC, regardless of surgical margins; (2) the surgical margins are close or microscopically positive, regardless of grade; (3) a resection has been performed for a recurrent cancer, regardless of the histology or margin status; (4) the tumor has invaded beyond the capsule of the gland into skin, bone, nerve, or glandular tissue; (5) regional lymph nodes contain metastatic cancer; or (6) if there is gross residual or unresectable disease. In addition, preoperative radiotherapy prior to planned surgery may facilitate parotidectomy in advanced cases and allow preservation of the facial nerve.[284,286] If the facial nerve is involved at presentation, surgery and PORT are favored.

For T3 and T4 parotid cancer, unless the facial nerve is circumferentially encompassed by tumor or grossly enlarged by cancer, nerve-sparing surgery may be used followed by radiotherapy. Radiation therapy doses to the primary site and involved structures are in the range of 55–65 Gy. Generally, for low-grade MEC and acinic cell carcinomas, it is not necessary to treat the clinically uninvolved neck. For all other high-grade histologies, the neck nodal drainage is generally treated to doses in the range of 50 Gy. In the case of adenoid cystic carcinomas, the radiation fields should include the anatomic course of named nerve trunks to the base of the skull.[280] Management of the facial nerve is one of the more controversial and complex issues surrounding the treatment of salivary gland cancers. Resection of the nerve results in profound cosmetic and functional deficits. Even resection of a single branch, particularly the frontal branch, can lead to significant morbidity. Thus, patients must be extensively counseled preoperatively regarding the intraoperative management of the nerve. Compromised function preoperatively portends poor functional outcome, even with nerve grafting. When the normally functioning facial nerve is found intraoperatively to be involved by cancer and cannot be preserved, resection and primary nerve grafting should be performed. PORT can be administered to nerve grafts, although the long-term functional outcomes remain suboptimal.

The results of treatment depend on histological type and tumor site. In a series from the University of Texas MD Anderson Cancer Center, 5-year survival rates were 100% for patients with acinic cell carcinoma, 95% for patients with adenoid cystic carcinoma, 90% for patients with low-grade MEC, 80% for patients with high-grade MEC, 70% for patients with adenocarcinoma, and 59% for patients with malignant mixed tumors.[281,284] At the Princess Margaret Hospital, primary parotid disease was controlled by surgery alone in 24% of cases and by surgery and radiotherapy in 74% of cases.[287]

Minor salivary gland tumors, especially tumors in the paranasal sinuses, often present with advanced-stage disease. In the MD Anderson series, the 2-year local control rate was 47% in patients treated with surgery alone and 76% in patients treated with surgery and PORT.[284,288,289]

For patients with large inoperable salivary gland tumors or for patients who are at high risk of local recurrence after an incomplete resection, fast-neutron radiotherapy is an alternative to standard XRT. Fast neutrons have different radiobiological properties when compared with standard radiation, and *in vivo* data from Battermann et al.[290] on the response of pulmonary metastases to fractionated radiotherapy show a relative biologic effectiveness (RBE) factor in the range of 8.0 for salivary gland tumors, compared with RBEs in the range of 3.0 to 3.5 for late effects in most normal tissues. To put this in perspective, if one were to give a dose of 20 neutron-Gy to a parotid tumor, the biologic effect in terms of the mucosa and temporomandibular joint would be equivalent to 60–70 photon-Gy, but the biologic effect on the tumor would be equivalent to 160 photon-Gy—a theoretical therapeutic gain of a factor of 2.3 to 2.6.

The Radiation Therapy Oncology Group (RTOG) in the United States and the Medical Research Council (MRC) in the United Kingdom performed a phase III randomized clinical trial to compare fast-neutron radiotherapy versus conventional photon irradiation for inoperable salivary gland tumors. The fast-neutron group achieved significantly improved tumor clearance at both the primary site and in the regional lymph nodes. At the 2-year endpoint, the local/regional control rates were 67% for the neutron group compared with 17% for the photon group ($p < 0.005$), and survivals were 62% for the neutron group compared with 25% for the photon group ($p = 0.1$). Because of the significantly greater locoregional control rate achieved in the fast-neutron group, the study was closed early for ethical reasons. Ten-year data continued to show improved locoregional control on the neutron arm (56% vs 17%, $p = 0.009$) but no difference in OS because of deaths from distant metastases.[291]

As neutron therapy is only available in very few centers, and results of neutrons are mixed and dependent on the site of disease, other alternatives for inoperable salivary gland cancers have been studied, albeit the reports are very small retrospective series. Samant et al.[292] describe encouraging results in patients with unresectable adenoid cystic carcinoma treated with concurrent chemoradiation. A team from Massachusetts General Hospital[293] has described encouraging outcomes of patients with adenoid cystic carcinoma involving the skull base treated with proton therapy. Intrigued with the role of high-energy particle therapy, German investigators have performed a small phase II trial (COSMIC) combining IMRT with a carbon ion boost. Results are very preliminary, but the response rate in 16 patients with unresected malignant salivary gland tumors was 69%.[294]

Systemic therapy

Systemic therapy for salivary cancer remains an investigational endeavor, with no standard regimen universally accepted. Chemotherapy may be used in the primary management of patients with locally advanced and unresectable disease concurrently with radiation therapy. More often, chemotherapy becomes a treatment option for patients with distant disease recurrence. Previous studies have demonstrated single-agent activity for methotrexate, doxorubicin, cisplatin, 5-FU, vinca alkaloids, and taxanes. Response

rates are in the range of 15–20%. Combination therapy provides some increase in response but with no clear survival advantages. A regimen with cyclophosphamide, doxorubicin, and cisplatin (CAP) has produced responses in 40–50% of patients treated, with duration 4–6 months.[295] Cisplatin and vinorelbine render responses in 44–54% of patients.[296,297] Responses are more often observed in patients with adenocarcinomas, and less likely in adenoid cystic carcinoma. Anti-VEGF inhibitors such as sunitinib and axitinib have demonstrated minimum activity with mostly disease stabilization in metastatic adenoid cystic carcinomas.[298,299]

A decision to proceed with systemic therapy should be considered with attention given to tumor histology, stage, time to disease progression after primary therapy, patient performance status, and the pace of disease progression. Efforts are also under way to identify molecular markers, which may enhance our ability to individualize therapy. Most head and neck oncologists tend to separate patients with adenoid cystic carcinoma from others in developing a treatment strategy. As metastatic adenoid cystic carcinoma will often be indolent in its growth pattern, a short period of observation is typically indicated. At times, there may be only slow growth over a period of years. However, if serial evaluations show more aggressive cancer, then it would be appropriate to consider an investigational trial or chemotherapy.[295,300–303] In patients with high-grade MEC or salivary duct adenocarcinoma, traditional cisplatin-based chemotherapy combinations may be more routinely active. Taxanes are active as single agents and are being tested in combination chemotherapy regimens.[304]

Approximately 70% of salivary gland malignancies overexpress EGFR. Our group conducted a clinical trial with gefitinib, a small-molecule EGFR tyrosine kinase inhibitor, in patients with advanced salivary tumors; however, no tumor responses were seen.[305] A high level of c-KIT expression has been identified in adenoid cystic carcinoma, but preliminary trials with imatinib mesylate, a tyrosine kinase inhibitor against KIT, have not demonstrated clinical benefit.[306] Salivary duct carcinomas overexpress HER2 in up to 50% of cases, and approximately 20% are HER2 amplified.[307] Androgen receptor overexpression is seen in 80% of salivary duct carcinomas. Responses to trastuzumab, a monoclonal antibody that targets HER2, and to androgen blockage have been reported.[308–311] A clinical trial investigating the role of hormone manipulation in androgen-receptor-positive salivary duct carcinoma is planned (clinical trial identification NCT 01969578). Given the relative rarity of salivary cancers in general, formal trials require collaboration among multiple, large tertiary centers or implementation through the cooperative oncology group mechanism.

Radiation therapy

Radiotherapy plays an integral role in the treatment of most HNCs. Used as the sole modality for the treatment of selected early-stage disease, radiation gives comparable results to a surgical resection, often with less morbidity. Radiation therapy is the treatment of choice for early-stage NPC. It is also a very effective therapy for early-stage oropharynx cancers, though the advent of minimally invasive intraoral approaches has raised the question of whether surgery or radiation is preferred for these cancers. Radiation (combined external beam and brachytherapy) is also an alternative to surgery for early cancers of the oral cavity, particularly the mobile tongue, and while not commonly used in the United States, it is common practice in some international centers. For tumors arising in the larynx, radiation may be preferred to surgery because it can offer retention of function and good vocal quality.

For advanced-sized lesions, radiation is used as a component of multimodality therapy. For patients planned for surgery, radiation is often used as an adjuvant in order to improve locoregional control. The sequencing for radiation when combined with surgery has been a topic of debate, as preoperative and postoperative radiation has advantages and disadvantages. The RTOG conducted a randomized trial comparing preoperative and postoperative radiation, and concluded that postoperative radiation resulted in improved local-regional control with a suggestion of an improvement in survival.[312] The results of this study combined with general practice patterns have led to performing radiation postoperatively. A principle advantage of performing surgery first is that pathology can be assessed. Currently, a trichotomous risk assessment system is used, assigning patients into "low", "intermediate" and "high"-risk categories. For low-risk patients, recurrence is uncommon; therefore, the benefits of adjuvant treatment may not be warranted. High-risk patients, typically those with inadequate surgical margins or extracapsular nodal disease, have a very high rate of recurrence such that prior and current studies are assessing methods to enhance adjuvant radiation by altered radiation fractionation or chemosensitization.[313]

When used as an adjuvant, it is important that there be good communication between the surgeon and the radiation oncologist in order to avoid inadvertent delays that can compromise outcome. Several groups have highlighted the importance of minimizing the treatment "package" time, the time from surgery to the completion of PORT, to maximize local and regional control.[314,315]

For advanced tumors arising in certain sites, such as the pharynx and larynx, nonoperative therapy, consisting of combined radiation and chemotherapy, may be preferred. Combination chemotherapy and radiation is the preferred treatment for advanced NPC and locally advanced oropharyngeal cancer. In particular, HPV-associated cancers of the oropharynx have been demonstrated to be very responsive to chemotherapy and radiation, with high survival rates seen in patients treated with concurrent chemoradiation.[88] The optimal therapy (see above) for advanced laryngeal and hypopharyngeal cancer remains a topic of controversy. The concept of laryngeal preservation remains an exciting idea; however, several decades of study have led investigators to be more cautious with the realization that larynx preservation may come with a trade-off of increased dysphagia and risk of aspiration. Further, some have questioned whether the zeal for laryngeal preservation has led to a decrease in the survival rate of patients with locally advanced laryngeal cancer.[8]

Ionizing radiation (high-energy photons, electrons, neutrons, protons, and other charged particles) interacts with matter in subtle ways and should not be thought of as simply a form of cautery.[316] Tumors and normal tissues can vary dramatically in their ability to repair the cellular damage caused by ionizing radiation. This makes it possible to use treatments such as chemotherapy and hyperthermia to reduce the repair capability of tumors and to design fractionation schemes that effectively widen the therapeutic window between tumor control and normal tissue damage. HNSCCs are generally characterized as being "moderately radiosensitive," meaning that fairly large amounts of radiation must be delivered in order to achieve a high probability of tumor control. Fortunately, the required doses are within the tolerance range of most tissues in the head and neck.

The effectiveness of a given dose of radiation depends on how it is given.[317] In the United States, the traditional "curative" treatment regimen consists of giving 180–200 cGy once a day for 5 days a week to a total dose of 6500–7400 cGy; in the United Kingdom and Canada, higher daily doses of 220–250 cGy are given once a day for

5 days a week to a total dose of 5000–5500 cGy. These two schemas have evolved empirically; and a review of the literature indicates that they provide comparable tumor control, with the main debate relating to differences in complications. Various altered fractionation regimens have been compared with the standard regimens in clinical trials and some of these appear to be evolving into new "standards".

Radiation kills the stem cells in the basal layer of the skin and mucosa; and several weeks later, the cells in the more superficial protective layers are not adequately replaced when they are lost through normal physiologic processes. This denudes the epithelium, giving rise to a mucosal reaction that can greatly inhibit a patient's ability to swallow solids and liquids. This does not occur immediately but is progressive after several weeks of radiotherapy. The use of concurrent chemotherapy and/or altered fractionation treatment regimens can make this reaction occur sooner and be more severe. Patients must be monitored closely to ensure that they maintain adequate nutrition during therapy, and often a feeding tube is required. Placement of such a tube is preferable to giving the patient a break in therapy, which can lower the tumor control probability due to repopulation.[318–320] A similar reaction can occur in the skin in the treatment portals, giving rise to a severe sunburn-like reaction. Radiation to the head and neck area can cause significant changes in salivary gland function and taste perception.[321–323] Radioprotectors and salivary stimulants have been extensively studied and have limited success in minimizing xerostomia. The more significant advances in xerostomia reduction have been in using the newer conformal techniques to lower the dose to the salivary glands.[324] The severity and duration of these changes are dose dependent. There is transient loss of saliva and taste after doses of 1000–1500 cGy; however, these lower doses often do not cause permanent late effects. Doses of 7000 cGy almost always cause permanent changes. Studies by the Universities of Michigan and Utrecht[325] have demonstrated the absence of a threshold dose for gland damage, and the TD (50), or dose leading to 50% complication probability in the parotid gland, is 40 Gy.

Both the decrease in the amount of saliva and the changes in its chemical composition allow changes in the distribution of microorganisms inhabiting the mouth, which in turn can markedly increase the risk of dental caries. Aggressive dental prophylaxis prior to beginning radiotherapy is mandatory in the dentulous patient because the incidence of osteoradionecrosis can be considerably reduced if the necessary repairs and/or extractions are done prior to treatment rather than in heavily irradiated tissues.[326] If extractions are necessary, a delay of 2–3 weeks between the extractions and the initiation of radiotherapy is necessary in order to allow for adequate healing. If extractions or other invasive procedures are required after high-dose XRT, hyperbaric oxygen treatments are helpful in reducing the risk of osteoradionecrosis, particularly if the mandible is involved.[327,328]

Technologic advances

Modern radiotherapy centers use sophisticated linear accelerators producing photon beams of different energies and megavoltage electron beams that can easily treat posterior neck lymph nodes without risk of spinal cord damage. Computer-controlled multileaf collimators facilitate custom blocking techniques to spare uninvolved normal tissues. CT and MRI are used to locate tumors, with many radiation oncology centers having dedicated scanners used exclusively for simulation and treatment planning. CT, MRI, and PET scans are fused to give the clinician a broader perspective in locating regions at risk of tumor.

Intensity-modulated radiotherapy (IMRT)

The principal goal of radiation is to deliver the appropriate dose to areas harboring cancer, while avoiding radiation to adjacent normal tissues. This concept is referred to as conformal therapy. IMRT was developed during the last decade of the twentieth century and is currently an accepted standard for achieving conformal therapy in HNC. In this approach, many different treatment fields are used, with each field being divided into multiple segments, and each segment delivering a prescribed amount of radiation.[329] Recently, these techniques have further evolved in that the treatment can be delivered dynamically, with either treatment accelerators built with computed tomographic units, or with arc-rotational techniques (volumetric-modulated arc therapy). These techniques allow for a continued rotation of the therapy machine as well as a fluid change in the field collimation, ideally achieving even more conformality.

These IMRT systems are further enhanced by software innovations that allow for inverse treatment planning. This form of planning enables the clinician to specify normal tissue dose constraints in combination with specific dose goals to be delivered to the treatment target. In HNCs, there often are critical normal structures in close proximity to the tumor, and achieving a sharp dose gradient around the target while limiting the normal tissue dose offers the potential for significant therapeutic gain. The ability to reduce the dose to the parotid glands and to reduce the subsequent xerostomia experienced by the patient is an important advantage of this technique, and has been demonstrated in several trials including the randomized phase III PARSPORT trial.[324] Likewise, additional anatomic regions important for functional swallowing, such as larynx and pharyngeal constrictor muscles, are being identified for future IMRT dose-sparing strategies to improve functional recovery following treatment.[330]

The advantages of improved tumor imaging are obvious as there should be fewer "marginal misses" than in the past. Another advantage relates to being able to give higher radiation doses to the tumor in a safe manner. In the case of HNSCC, dose–response curves generally exhibit a steep region, wherein modest increases in radiation dose will give rise to significant improvement in outcome.[331–333] Taking oropharyngeal cancer as an example, Setton et al.[334] from the Memorial Sloan-Kettering Cancer Center reported results for 442 patients with oropharyngeal primaries (73% of whom had stage IV disease) treated with IMRT and a median follow-up for survivors of 37 months. Three-year estimates of local progression-free, regional progression-free, distant metastases-free, and OS were 95%, 94%, 87%, and 85%, respectively. Reported grade 2 or greater late xerostomia severity was 29%. Garden et al.[163] reported our results from the MD Anderson Cancer Center for 776 patients with oropharyngeal cancer treated with IMRT from 2000 to 2007. Median follow-up was 54 months. The 5-year actuarial locoregional control, recurrence-free, and OS rates were 84%, 90%, and 82%, respectively. Additional series echo these encouraging locoregional disease-control rates for oropharyngeal disease.[160,162,164] Similar excellent results are seen for NPC, a disease that often approximates critical neural structures adding to the complexity of treatment. The RTOG phase II study 0225 tested the feasibility of transporting IMRT for NPC to a multi-institutional setting. The estimated 2-year PFS was nearly 93%.[335] More recently, large series, particularly from China where NPC is endemic, report similar high rates of disease control.[336]

Given the complexity of IMRT treatment planning and delivery, rigorous quality assurance and technical support, as well as adequate clinician experience are critical to its ultimate effectiveness.[337]

Combined surgery and radiotherapy

Radiotherapy is often given as an adjuvant to surgery for moderately advanced but resectable tumors. For most head and neck sites, giving adjuvant radiotherapy improves local control for T3 or T4 primaries or in situations where there is pathologic involvement of cervical lymph nodes.

Radiotherapy can be given either preoperatively or postoperatively. The aims of preoperative radiotherapy are to sterilize microscopic disease outside the resection field and to shrink the tumor bulk. Theoretically, preoperative radiotherapy should also reduce the risk of disseminating viable tumor cells at the time of surgery. Dosages of 5000 cGy over 5 to 5.5 weeks are generally given, with no significant wound healing problems occurring at this dosage. Preoperative radiotherapy is rarely indicated today.

In the postoperative setting, the surgical procedure has disrupted the regional blood supply. Conventional wisdom suggests that higher doses of radiation are needed because of the increased likelihood of hypoxic tumor cells, which would be more radioresistant than their well-oxygenated counterparts. Generally, 5500–6000 cGy in 180–200 cGy fractions are given for microscopic residual disease. If the surgical margins are grossly positive or if there is a high likelihood of macroscopic residual disease, higher doses are used. Peters et al.[338] have shown that at least 6300 cGy should be given if extracapsular nodal extension is found in the operative specimen. PORT has the advantage of being given only to those patients thought to be at significant risk of locoregional recurrence based on a review of the pathologic data. It has the additional advantage of not delaying the surgical procedure, which is the most important treatment modality for patients with advanced, operable tumors.

Although it is generally felt that there is little use for a debulking surgical procedure, there may be situations where a gross total resection followed by high-dose radiotherapy is preferable to treatment with radiotherapy alone. An analysis by the Head and Neck Intergroup (IG0034) showed that excluded patients with positive surgical margins had improved locoregional tumor control compared with matched cohorts from the RTOG databases of patients treated with radiotherapy alone.[339] At 4 years, respective locoregional control rates were 44% versus 24% ($p = 0.007$). Since this was not a randomized study, the authors do not argue for changing traditional resectability criteria, but, rather, testing this concept in the context of a controlled clinical trial.

Locoregional disease relapse following surgery is particularly common in patients with positive surgical margins, extracapsular nodal disease, or multiple positive nodes. Based on retrospective analyses,[340,341] adjuvant radiation reduces the relative risk of relapse by approximately 50%; however, locoregional recurrence rates remain as high as 35–60% in this population.[342] Two landmark multi-institutional phase III trials demonstrated improved outcomes with concurrent chemoradiation in patients with high risk of recurrence following surgery. In the first trial,[173] the EORTC randomized 334 subjects to 66 Gy with or without cisplatin 100 mg/m^2 × 3 cycles. Estimated 3-year local control (85% vs 70%), DFS (60% vs 40%), and OS (65% vs 50%) were improved by the addition of cisplatin. Acute toxicity was exacerbated by chemotherapy, but severity of late effects purportedly remained equivalent. The RTOG conducted a complementary trial,[134] randomizing 459 patients to nearly identical treatment arms as the EORTC trial: 60–66 Gy with or without cisplatin 100 mg/m^2 × 3 cycles. Chemotherapy improved estimated 2-year local control (82% vs 72%, $p = 0.01$) and DFS (70% vs 60%, $p = 0.05$). As with the EORTC trial, this was at the cost of higher acute grade 3 or greater toxicity. The trials had different inclusion criteria, study populations, and follow-up intervals. However, joint reanalysis of both trials strongly suggested significant clinical benefit to combined adjuvant therapy for patients with either positive surgical margins or extracapsular nodal disease.[173]

Systemic therapy

Chemotherapy and radiation for locally advanced disease

Induction chemotherapy

Treatment with chemotherapy used in sequence before surgery or radiotherapy—known as induction or neoadjuvant chemotherapy—has potential advantages. It is feasible. Drug activity may be optimal because there has been no disruption of normal vascularity. Effective systemic therapy in this setting is likely to induce a favorable tumor response and there is a reduction in the risk of distant disease recurrence.[155,199,343,344] The potential for IC to affect local disease control following surgery or radiotherapy continues to be under study. Early trials demonstrated that PF is a highly active regimen;[345] a substantial response to chemotherapy predicts tumor sensitivity to radiotherapy; and that there appeared not to be a major adverse effect on surgical or radiotherapy morbidity.[344]

Discussed in part above, the VA Laryngeal Cancer Study Group[155] demonstrated the feasibility of induction PF followed by radiotherapy for patients with stage III/IV SCC of the larynx. Patients were randomly assigned to receive standard laryngectomy and PORT or 2–3 cycles of PF followed by radiotherapy. Surgery was reserved for salvage of patients with persistent or progressive disease. After 3 years' follow-up, 66% of surviving patients in the induction therapy group had a preserved and functional larynx. Moreover, there were no OS differences between the treatment arms. A subsequent study conducted by the EORTC in patients with squamous cancer of the hypopharyx compared induction PF followed by radiotherapy in responding patients to laryngopharyngectomy and radiation.[179] No survival differences were observed and 28% of the chemotherapy group survived with a functional larynx. The larynx preservation rate at 3 years was 42%. These studies demonstrated the potential for sequential chemotherapy and radiotherapy to be effective treatment strategies and that anatomic organ preservation is a reasonable therapeutic objective for many patients.

In follow-up to the VA study,[199] the Head and Neck Intergroup conducted a prospective three-arm study with sequential PF and radiotherapy as the control arm compared to concurrent cisplatin and radiotherapy, and radiotherapy administered as a single modality. Surgical salvage was implemented for patients with persistent or progressive tumor. For entry, patients had stage III/VI disease, but T1 and advanced T4 lesions were not eligible. The concurrent arm produced superior local disease control resulting in larynx preservation at 10 years in 82% versus 68% in patients receiving sequential chemotherapy and radiation and 64% in patients treated with radiation alone. However, gains in disease control seemed to have been negated by an increase in the number of non-cancer-related deaths in the concurrent arm; thus, there were no significant survival differences observed between the concurrent and sequential treatment arms.[346] A sequence of studies has focused on the addition of taxanes to the PF regimen to advance the antitumor activity. The EORTC studied 358 patients in a prospective trial (TAX323)[347] comparing induction PF versus docetaxel, cisplatin and fluorouracil (TPF). After IC for four cycles, all patients received radiotherapy as a single modality. With a median follow-up of 32 months, TPF produced superior tumor responses, a PFS advantage

with HR 0.72, and increased survival, HR 0.73. In the TAX 324 phase III trial[348] 501 patients were randomized to receive IC with docetaxel (75 mg/m^2), cisplatin (100 mg/m^2), and fluorouracil (1000 mg/m^2/day continuous infusion × 4 days) or the standard PF regimen. After three cycles, chemoradiotherapy with weekly carboplatin was administered. A fraction of patients underwent surgery for advanced nodal disease. A significant difference in DFS and OS was obtained, with 62% of patients receiving TPF alive at 36 months compared to 48% of the control group.

To build on the more modern IC platform of incorporating a taxane, GORTEC conducted the TREMPLIN phase II randomized trial comparing concurrent cisplatin versus concurrent cetuximab following a partial response to induction TPF.[349] OS was equivalent in both arms, and the authors concluded they could not determine the optimal regimen to test against a control of IC followed by radiation alone.

While the addition of docetaxel to the PF backbone chemotherapy regimen improved outcomes in TAX323 and 324, it remained undetermined if the three-drug IC regimen was superior to concurrent chemoradiation. At least four clinical trials attempted to answer this question. The PARADIGM study randomized 145 unresectable stage III or IV HNSCC patients to receive TPF followed by concurrent chemoradiation with carboplatin (for patients who responded to IC) or docetaxel (for nonresponders to IC), versus concurrent radiation therapy with cisplatin (100 mg/m^2 every 3 weeks × 2 doses). The 3 year OS was not statistically different between the two groups (73% in the IC arm vs 78% in the concurrent chemoradiation arm). Higher hematological toxicity and one treatment-related death was seen in the IC arm. Given slow accrual, the study did not meet its patient target number, limiting its power and interpretation.[350] The DeCIDE trial included 285 patients with N2 or N3 nodal status (therefore, with a higher risk of distant recurrence). Patients were randomized to receive two cycles of TPF followed by concurrent chemoradiation with DFHX (docetaxel, 5-fluorouracil, and hydroxyurea) versus the same concurrent definitive chemoradiation regimen. Once again, due to slow accrual, sample size was adjusted and the study was closed early. The 3-year OS rates were similar between the two groups, with 75% in the IC arm and 73% in the concurrent chemoradiation arm. Significantly lower distant metastasis was seen in the group that received IC (10% vs 19%, $p = 0.025$) and there was a trend to survival benefit for the patients with N2c and N3 disease who received IC ($p = 0.19$).[351] Both PARADIGM and DeCIDE were underpowered studies. Patient outcomes were better than historical control, most likely because the majority of the population had oropharynx carcinoma primaries, possibly HPV related. Hitt et al.[352] evaluated in a randomized phase III trial IC with either PF or TPF followed by concurrent chemoradiation with high-dose cisplatin versus the same concurrent chemoradiation schema. There was no difference in median PFS, time to treatment failure, or OS between the two arms. Preliminary results of a phase II/III European trial presented at the 2014 ASCO meeting, evaluated induction TPF versus no IC followed by chemoradiation with either cetuximab or PF in 415 patients. The median survival was of 53.7 months in the induction arm versus 30.3 months in the upfront chemoradiation arm (HR 0.72, $p = 0.025$), with a reduced risk of distant metastases in patients who received IC. The difference in outcomes observed in this trial versus DeCIDE and PARADIGM is likely due to different patient populations and inclusion criteria.[353]

Based on the results of these trials, together with the MACH-NC meta-analysis,[168] concurrent chemoradiation with cisplatin remains as standard of care treatment for locally advanced HNSCC. Given the reduction in distant metastasis rates, further studies with IC in a risk-stratified population based on HPV status, smoking history, N stage, and molecular markers correlates might identify the population that will benefit the most from this treatment strategy. In our institution, IC is used for a larynx preservation approach and in selected oropharynx cases, in patients with bulk N2c/N3 disease, low neck adenopathy, and with good performance status.

Concurrent chemotherapy and radiation

A sequence of randomized trials[171,199,354–361] and meta-analysis[362] demonstrate that the concurrent administration of chemotherapy and radiation leads to improved local control and OS in patients with locally advanced SCC, particularly of the oropharynx. However, most reported trials include patients with invasive SCC from a mix of primary sites. Scrutiny of these manuscripts is advised as the percentage of patients with oral cavity, pharyngeal, and laryngeal primary sites may vary in reports from different centers, and this may markedly affect study outcomes. It should be emphasized that concurrent chemoradiotherapy is associated with marked, acute mucocutaneous toxicity requiring expert supportive medical care. Speech and swallow rehabilitation consultation is routinely needed. Gastrostomy feeding tubes are placed in a high percentage of patients. The risk of long-term complications such as osteonecrosis and oropharyngeal fibrosis are under study.

Oral cavity primary tumors are most often approached surgically if there are no medical contraindications. Depending upon tumor histology, size, pathologic margins, and the extent of nodal involvement, PORT is administered. Patients with positive surgical margins or nodal ECS are more likely to benefit from adjuvant concurrent chemoradiation rather than radiotherapy administered as a single modality, as previously discussed.[134,173,313]

With regard to toxicity, usually a brisk mucocutaneous reaction occurs with chemoradiation, necessitating the use of oral rinses for hygiene, analgesics, attention to fluid and calorie intake, and involvement of speech and swallowing rehabilitation specialists. Moreover, there is concern that long-term xerostomia, fibrosis, and related swallowing dysfunction may be more likely after concurrent chemoradiotherapy than radiation therapy alone. Long-term functional data for most patients have not been routinely reported. In the Intergroup larynx trial[199] and the postoperative chemoradiotherapy trials,[134,173,313] there appeared not to be a high risk of chronic deleterious effects of combined therapy relative to control groups treated with radiotherapy alone. Setton et al.[363] reported on nearly 1500 oropharyngeal cancer patients treated with concurrent chemotherapy and radiation. The 2-year gastrostomy tube dependence rate was 4.4%. A prospective study conducted at the MD Anderson Cancer Center evaluating the long-term outcomes of 47 patients who underwent IC followed by a risk-adjusted local treatment, including radiation therapy, concurrent chemoradiation, or surgery for oral cavity primary, demonstrated at 2 years a nonsignificant 13% average reduction in swallowing efficiency relative to baseline ($p = 0.191$), a rate of chronic dysphagia of 7.1%, and gastrostomy dependency in 4.8% of the patients.[364]

In a landmark study, Bonner et al.[365] conducted a prospectively randomized trial in which previously untreated patients with locally advanced SCC of the oropharynx, hypopharynx, or larynx received definitive radiotherapy with or without cetuximab. Cetuximab is a chimeric human and murine monoclonal antibody directed against the EGFR. In this phase III trial, 424 patients were entered and median duration of follow-up was 38 months. Notably, there was no increase in severe-grade radiation-related mucocutaneous toxicity. Moreover, median survival (28 months vs 54 months) and 3-year survival (44% vs 57%) favored the combined therapy arm with a significant advantage in locoregional tumor control. This study led

Table 6 EGFR-based bioradiotherapy with Panitumumab (P).

	N	2-Year LRC (%)
Concert 1		
CT – RT	63	68
CT – RT + P	87	61
Concert 2		
CT – RT	61	61
P – RT	90	51

LRC, locoregional control.

to the approval of cetuximab to be administered concurrently with radiation therapy for locally advanced HNSCC.

A follow-up phase III study, RTOG 0522, evaluated the addition of cetuximab to the standard concurrent cisplatin and radiotherapy treatment in 891 patients with stage III or IV HNSCC. Patients were randomized to receive radiation and cisplatin with or without cetuximab. The addition of cetuximab to cisplatin-radiation led to significantly more interruptions in treatment, an increased rate of acute grades 3 and 4 toxicity, and was not associated with improved patient outcomes.[366] Concert 1 and 2 trials have further explored bioradiotherapy with panitumumab (Table 6),[367,368] showing no OS or local disease control advantage after matching chemoradiotherapy with the addition or substitution of the antibody.

Thus, the current standard of care for patients with stage III and IV HNSCC, who are not candidates for surgery, is to be treated with definitive concurrent chemoradiotherapy. Cisplatin $100 \, mg/m^2$ administered on weeks 1, 4, and 7 with once-daily radiotherapy, or cisplatin $40 \, mg/m^2$ weekly, are widely accepted. Concurrent radiation therapy with cetuximab is an alternative for patients not eligible to receive cisplatin (e.g., renal insufficiency, hearing loss, advanced age, or poor performance status).

Given that patients with HPV-related OPSCC have a better prognosis and treatment outcomes, de-escalation therapy is being extensively studied in this patient population. The ongoing RTOG 1016 trial is randomizing patients with HPV-related OPSCC to receive definitive radiation therapy with cisplatin versus cetuximab. Accrual has been completed and results are awaited.

Recurrent and metastatic disease: cytotoxics

Activity of cytotoxic chemotherapy with single agents has been demonstrated in phase II trials, and expected response rates for multiple drugs are presented in Table 7. Benefit is more likely to be obtained in patients with ECOG performance status 0 or 1; in patients presenting with recurrence greater than 6 months from primary therapy; and in patients with sites of involvement not previously radiated.

Phase III studies have directly compared cisplatin and methotrexate (randomized, two-arm design). In one of these studies, Hong

Table 7 Single-agent activity in recurrent head and neck cancer.

Agent	Approximate response (%)
Methotrexate	25
Bleomycin	15
Cisplatin	25
Carboplatin	20
5-Fluorouracil	15
Paclitaxel	30
Docetaxel	30
Ifosfamide	20
Cetuximab	13

Table 8 Selected randomized phase III trials of chemotherapy in recurrent or metastatic squamous cell carcinoma of the head and neck.

Trial	No. of patients	Regimen	Response rate (%)	Survival (*p* value)
Jacobs et al.[373]	79	cddp/fu	32	NS
	83	Cddp	17	
	83	Fu	13	
Forastiere et al.[374]	87	cddp/fu	32	NS
	86	cbdca/fu	21	
	88	Mtx	10	
Clavel et al.[375]	127	cddp/mtx/bleo/vcr	34	NS
	116	cddp/fu	31	
	122	Cddp	15	
Schrijvers et al.[376]	122	cddp/fu/ifnα-2b	47	NS
	122	cddp/fu	38	
Forastiere et al.[377]	101	cddp/pac (high dose)	35	NS
	98	cddp/pac (low dose)	36	
Gibson et al.[378]	104	cddp/fu	22	NS
	100	cddp/pac	28	
Vermorken et al.[347]	215	platin/fu	20	7.4 mos median
	219	platin/fu—cet	36	10.1 mos median *p* = 0.04

Abbreviations: bleo, bleomycin; cbdca, carboplatin; cddp, cisplatin; fu, fluorouracil; ifnα-2b, interferon alfa-2b; mtx, methotrexate; NS, not statistically significant; pac, paclitaxel; vcr, vincristine.

et al.[369] gave cisplatin at 50 mg/m^2 on days 1 and 8 every month versus methotrexate at 40–60 mg/m^2/week. Response rates were 28.6% and 23.5%, respectively. The taxanes constitute a distinctive class of established active agents in HNSCC.[370–372] Use of docetaxel has produced response rates ranging from 21% to 42% in phase II studies in patients who had not previously received palliative chemotherapy.[370,372]

Combination chemotherapy may produce responses in 30–40% of patients, but without significant survival advantages over single-agent therapy, which is usually in the range of 6–9 months (Table 8). Gibson et al.[378] conducted a prospective phase III trial comparing cisplatin and infusional fluorouracil with cisplatin and paclitaxel in 218 patients. There was no difference in response rate (27% and 26%, respectively) or median survival (8.7 months vs 8.1 months). Toxicity was similar.

In a randomized phase III prospective trial, Vermorken et al.[379] evaluated the addition of cetuximab to the platin-fluorouracil combination in 442 patients with recurrent or metastatic HNSCC. A response advantage and improved median survival from 7.4 to 10.1 months was observed. There was no unusual toxicity. This regimen has become the standard-of-care first-line therapy for suitable patients.

OS for patients with recurrent or metastatic HNSCC remains poor. Only approximately 30% of patients survive 1 year, highlighting the pressing need for new drug development and more efficacious systemic therapy strategies.

Novel therapeutics

Invasive SCCs emerge after the accumulation of multiple genomic events in a multistep process. There appear to be essential molecular alterations that are biologically significant, which confer a survival advantage for cancer cells and which constitute the process of carcinogenesis.[380] As we understand better the underlying cancer biology, potential therapeutic targets have been identified and are leading to innovative treatment strategies.

Epidermal growth factor receptor

EGFR is a transmembrane glycoprotein, activation of which triggers a cascade of downstream intracellular signaling events important for regulation of epithelial cell growth.[381–385] EGF and transforming growth factor-alpha (TGF-α) are ligands for the receptor. Overexpression of EGFR or TGF-α has been observed in approximately 90% of HNSCC.[384]

Gefitinib and erlotinib are small-molecule inhibitors of EGFR. Both agents have been tested as single agents in recurrent or metastatic HNSCC, showing minimum clinical activity.[386,387] Afatinib and dacomitinib, second-generation EGFR inhibitors, are under investigation in platinum refractory metastatic HNSCC. Preliminary results demonstrate some activity with responses rates around 10%.[388]

Cetuximab is a monoclonal antibody directed against the extracellular portion of EGFR. Binding of the monoclonal antibody competes with ligand activation and prevents receptor dimerization, with consequent abrogation of multiple downstream signals. Vermorken et al.[389] have reported responses in 13% of platin-refractory patients treated with cetuximab single agent. As previously mentioned, Vermorken et al.[379] have demonstrated in a phase III trial that the addition of cetuximab to cisplatin or carboplatin and fluorouracil favorably affects tumor response and improved overall median survival by 2.7 months (from 7.4 to 10.1 months in the cetuximab group). Bonner et al.[365] have also reported, as discussed earlier, an increase in local tumor control and OS in the radiotherapy plus cetuximab combination arm versus radiotherapy alone.

An association between skin rash and tumor response has been repeatedly observed[343,390] and needs further exploration, possibly by escalating cetuximab dose until rash or dose-limiting toxicities develop. To date, cetuximab is the only Food and Drug Administration—approved targeted therapy for the treatment of HNSCC.

Angiogenesis

New blood vessel formation is a necessary process for tumor growth. Vascular endothelial growth factor (VEGF) is a multifunctional cytokine and a potent stimulator of the growth of endothelial cells. Increased VEGF protein expression is seen in many cancers, including HNSCC.[391,392]

Bevacizumab prevents VEGF binding to receptor tyrosine kinases (VEGFR1 and VEGFR2) with resultant inhibition of tumor cell growth. Argiris et al.[393] evaluated in a single-arm phase II trial the activity of cetuximab and bevacizumab in 46 patients with recurrent or metastatic HNSCC that received up to one line of systemic therapy. The overall response rate was 16% and median PFS and OS were 2.8 and 7.5 months, respectively. A large phase III trial (E1305) with platin and docetaxel or platin and 5-fluorouracil plus or minus bevacizumab for patients with recurrent or metastatic HNSCC has been conducted and results are awaited (Clinical trial reference number NCT00588770). Newer generation small-molecule VEGFR inhibitors axitinib and pazopanib are currently being investigated clinically. Sorafenib and sunitinib are small-molecule pan-receptor tyrosine kinase inhibitors, with multiple targets including VEGFR. They have been tested in metastatic HNSCC with modest activity.[394,395]

Phosphatidylinositol-3 kinase (PI3K)

Advances in next-generation sequencing have revealed recurrent genetic alterations in HNSCC. The most frequent potentially targetable alterations consist of activation of the PI3K (phosphatidylinositol-3 kinase) pathway, either by PIK3CA mutations or amplification (~35%) or PTEN loss (~5%).[396,397] The PI3K/AKT/mTOR pathway is important in regulating the cell cycle and its deregulation is involved in cancer cell proliferation. Various clinical trials with PI3K inhibitors as single agent or combined with other targeted therapy (e.g., EGFR inhibitors or MEK inhibitors) are being conducted in HNSCC.

Gene therapy

Approaches utilizing adenovirus-mediated wild-type *TP53* gene transfer have generated excitement following the demonstration of tumor responses in some patients.[398] Khuri et al.[399] conducted a multicenter phase II trial combining ONYX-015, which is a selective replicating adenovirus, with cisplatin and 5-FU in treating patients with advanced HNSCC. A response rate of 52% was observed in 30 patients with fully evaluable tumors. In a subset analysis of patients with tumors injectable and not accessible for injection, there was a substantial difference with tumor responses observed more often after chemotherapy and ONYX-015 administration ($p = 0.006$). Ongoing trials with TP53 replacement strategies continue for patients with recurrent HNSCC accessible to injection and as a chemoprevention strategy.

Immunotherapy

Recently, a new class of drugs that enhances antitumor immunity has emerged and is transforming the medical oncology field. One of the most promising pathways for manipulation involves programmed death ligand 1 (PD-L1). PD-L1 can be overexpressed in solid tumors, and upon binding to PD-1 expressing tumor-infiltrating T cells, it inhibits its activity and promotes immune tolerance, protecting the tumor cells from apoptosis. Blockage of PD-1-PD-L1 interaction enhances immune function and has shown meaningful clinical activity.[400–402] Pembrolizumab and nivolumab, humanized monoclonal antibodies that target PD-1, have been approved for the treatment of metastatic refractory melanoma; and, more recently, nivolumab was approved as second-line therapy for lung SCC. The activity of these antibodies seems to correlate with PD-L1 expression in the tumor and/or stroma cells.

Preliminary results of the head and neck cohort of the KEYNOTE-012 phase I trial showed that 78% of the 104 patients with refractory metastatic/recurrent HNSCC screened expressed PD-L1 in at least 1% of the cells in the tumor microenvironment. Out of the 51 patients evaluable for response, 51% experienced decreased tumor burden, with an overall response rate by RECIST of 20%, irrespective of HPV status.[403] Eight patients had disease

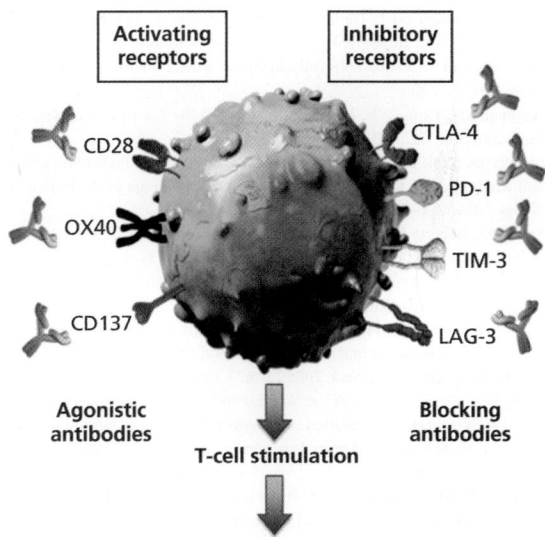

Figure 15 Activating and inhibitory receptor in T-cells. Source: Mellman 2011.[404] Reproduced with permission of Nature Publishing Group.

stability over 6 months, and seven remained on treatment when the preliminary data of the study were presented. Treatment was well tolerated overall, with the main side effects being fatigue, pruritus, and rash.

Given these encouraging early results, numerous immunotherapy clinical trials with checkpoint inhibitors, costimulatory agonists, vaccines, and adoptive T-cell transfer are being conducted in HNSCC and hold great promise for the near future (Figure 15).

Current directions

Systemic therapy is an integral part of HNC treatment. Many patients with locally advanced disease are treated with chemotherapy and radiation. The increasing appreciation of HPV as an etiologic and favorable prognostic factor can be expected to affect patient management and de-escalation clinical studies are currently ongoing. Options for the treatment of recurrent disease now include reirradiation, cytotoxic chemotherapy, and molecularly targeted therapy. Insights into the genomics of HNC are leading to multiple targeted therapy trials in specific subgroups. The preliminary results of checkpoint inhibitors in metastatic HNSCC hold promise and might add to the systemic therapy armamentarium in the near future.

Key references

The complete reference list can be found on the Wiley Companion Digital Edition of this title (see inside front cover for login instructions).

4 Sturgis EM, Cinciripini PM. Trends in head and neck cancer incidence in relation to smoking prevalence: an emerging epidemic of human papillomavirus-associated cancers? *Cancer*. 2007;**110**:1429–1435.

29 D'Souza G, Kreimer AR, Viscidi R, et al. Case-control study of human papillomavirus and oropharyngeal cancer. *N Engl J Med*. 2007;**356**:1944–1956.

42 Chien YC, Chen JY, Liu MY, et al. Serologic markers of Epstein-Barr virus infection and nasopharyngeal carcinoma in Taiwanese men. *N Engl J Med*. 2001;**345**:1877–1882.

88 Ang KK, Harris J, Wheeler R, et al. Human papillomavirus and survival of patients with oropharyngeal cancer. *N Engl J Med*. 2010;**363**:24–35.

94 Allal AS, Dulguerov P, Allaoua M, et al. Standardized uptake value of 2-[(18)F] fluoro-2-deoxy-D-glucose in predicting outcome in head and neck carcinomas treated by radiotherapy with or without chemotherapy. *J Clin Oncol*. 2002;**20**:1398–1404.

103 Kyzas PA, Evangelou E, Denaxa-Kyza D, Ioannidis JP. 18 F-fluorodeoxyglucose positron emission tomography to evaluate cervical node metastases in patients with head and neck squamous cell carcinoma: a meta-analysis. *J Natl Cancer Inst.* 2008;**100**:712–720.

119 Lippman SM, Hong WK. Molecular markers of the risk of oral cancer. *N Engl J Med.* 2001;**344**:1323–1326.

134 Cooper JS, Pajak TF, Forastiere AA, et al. Postoperative concurrent radiotherapy and chemotherapy for high-risk squamous-cell carcinoma of the head and neck. *N Engl J Med.* 2004;**350**:1937–1944.

144 Schiff BA, Roberts DB, El-Naggar A, Garden AS, Myers JN. Selective vs modified radical neck dissection and postoperative radiotherapy vs observation in the treatment of squamous cell carcinoma of the oral tongue. *Arch Otolaryngol Head Neck Surg.* 2005;**131**:874–878.

152 Diaz EM Jr, Holsinger FC, Zuniga ER, Roberts DB, Sorensen DM. Squamous cell carcinoma of the buccal mucosa: one institution's experience with 119 previously untreated patients. *Head Neck.* 2003;**25**:267–273.

155 Hong WK, Wolf GT, Fisher SG, et al. Induction chemotherapy plus radiation compared with surgery plus radiation in patients with advanced laryngeal cancer. The Department of Veterans Affairs Laryngeal Cancer Study Group. *N Engl J Med.* 1991;**324**:1685–1690.

156 Machtay M, Moughan J, Trotti A, et al. Factors associated with severe late toxicity after concurrent chemoradiation for locally advanced head and neck cancer: an RTOG analysis. *J Clin Oncol.* 2008;**26**:3582–3589.

157 Hinni ML, Nagel T, Howard B. Oropharyngeal cancer treatment: the role of transoral surgery. *Curr Opin Otolaryngol Head Neck Surg.* 2015;**23**:132–138.

166 Weber RS, Gidley P, Morrison WH, et al. Treatment selection for carcinoma of the base of the tongue. *Am J Surg.* 1990;**160**:415–419.

168 Pignon JP, le Maitre A, Maillard E, Bourhis J, Group M-NC. Meta-analysis of chemotherapy in head and neck cancer (MACH-NC): an update on 93 randomised trials and 17,346 patients. *Radiother Oncol.* 2009;**92**:4–14.

169 Bourhis J, Overgaard J, Audry H, et al. Hyperfractionated or accelerated radiotherapy in head and neck cancer: a meta-analysis. *Lancet.* 2006;**368**:843–854.

170 Marta GN, Silva V, de Andrade CH, et al. Intensity-modulated radiation therapy for head and neck cancer: systematic review and meta-analysis. *Radiother Oncol.* 2014;**110**:9–15.

171 Calais G, Alfonsi M, Bardet E, et al. Randomized trial of radiation therapy versus concomitant chemotherapy and radiation therapy for advanced-stage oropharynx carcinoma. *J Natl Cancer Inst.* 1999;**91**:2081–2086.

172 Denis F, Garaud P, Bardet E, et al. Final results of the 94-01 French Head and Neck Oncology and Radiotherapy Group randomized trial comparing radiotherapy alone with concomitant radiochemotherapy in advanced-stage oropharynx carcinoma. *J Clin Oncol.* 2004;**22**:69–76.

173 Bernier J, Domenge C, Ozsahin M, et al. Postoperative irradiation with or without concomitant chemotherapy for locally advanced head and neck cancer. *N Engl J Med.* 2004;**350**:1945–1952.

197 Hong WK, Lippman SM, Wolf GT. Recent advances in head and neck cancer—larynx preservation and cancer chemoprevention: the Seventeenth Annual Richard and Hinda Rosenthal Foundation Award Lecture. *Cancer Res.* 1993;**53**:5113–5120.

199 Forastiere AA, Goepfert H, Maor M, et al. Concurrent chemotherapy and radiotherapy for organ preservation in advanced laryngeal cancer. *N Engl J Med.* 2003;**349**:2091–2098.

251 Fandi A, Bachouchi M, Azli N, et al. Long-term disease-free survivors in metastatic undifferentiated carcinoma of nasopharyngeal type. *J Clin Oncol.* 2000;**18**:1324–1330.

253 Al-Sarraf M, LeBlanc M, Giri PG, et al. Chemoradiotherapy versus radiotherapy in patients with advanced nasopharyngeal cancer: phase III randomized Intergroup study 0099. *J Clin Oncol.* 1998;**16**:1310–1317.

255 Chan AT, Leung SF, Ngan RK, et al. Overall survival after concurrent cisplatin-radiotherapy compared with radiotherapy alone in locoregionally advanced nasopharyngeal carcinoma. *J Natl Cancer Inst.* 2005;**97**:536–539.

256 Lin JC, Jan JS, Hsu CY, Liang WM, Jiang RS, Wang WY. Phase III study of concurrent chemoradiotherapy versus radiotherapy alone for advanced nasopharyngeal carcinoma: positive effect on overall and progression-free survival. *J Clin Oncol.* 2003;**21**:631–637.

297 Airoldi M, Pedani F, Succo G, et al. Phase II randomized trial comparing vinorelbine versus vinorelbine plus cisplatin in patients with recurrent salivary gland malignancies. *Cancer.* 2001;**91**:541–547.

314 Ang KK, Trotti A, Brown BW, et al. Randomized trial addressing risk features and time factors of surgery plus radiotherapy in advanced head-and-neck cancer. *Int J Radiat Oncol Biol Phys.* 2001;**51**:571–578.

329 Leibel SA, Fuks Z, Zelefsky MJ, et al. Intensity-modulated radiotherapy. *Cancer J.* 2002;**8**:164–176.

346 Forastiere AA, Zhang Q, Weber RS, et al. Long-term results of RTOG 91-11: a comparison of three nonsurgical treatment strategies to preserve the larynx in patients with locally advanced larynx cancer. *J Clin Oncol.* 2013;**31**:845–852.

347 Vermorken JB, Remenar E, van Herpen C, et al. Cisplatin, fluorouracil, and docetaxel in unresectable head and neck cancer. *N Engl J Med.* 2007;**357**:1695–1704.

348 Posner MR, Hershock DM, Blajman CR, et al. Cisplatin and fluorouracil alone or with docetaxel in head and neck cancer. *N Engl J Med.* 2007;**357**:1705–1715.

350 Haddad R, O'Neill A, Rabinowits G, et al. Induction chemotherapy followed by concurrent chemoradiotherapy (sequential chemoradiotherapy) versus concurrent chemoradiotherapy alone in locally advanced head and neck cancer (PARADIGM): a randomised phase 3 trial. *Lancet Oncol.* 2013;**14**:257–264.

351 Cohen EE, Karrison TG, Kocherginsky M, et al. Phase III randomized trial of induction chemotherapy in patients with N2 or N3 locally advanced head and neck cancer. *J Clin Oncol.* 2014;**32**:2735–2743.

360 Staar S, Rudat V, Stuetzer H, et al. Intensified hyperfractionated accelerated radiotherapy limits the additional benefit of simultaneous chemotherapy—results of a multicentric randomized German trial in advanced head-and-neck cancer. *Int J Radiat Oncol Biol Phys.* 2001;**50**:1161–1171.

361 Wendt TG, Grabenbauer GG, Rodel CM, et al. Simultaneous radiochemotherapy versus radiotherapy alone in advanced head and neck cancer: a randomized multicenter study. *J Clin Oncol.* 1998;**16**:1318–1324.

362 Pignon JP, Bourhis J, Domenge C, Designe L. Chemotherapy added to locoregional treatment for head and neck squamous-cell carcinoma: three meta-analyses of updated individual data. MACH-NC Collaborative Group. Meta-Analysis of Chemotherapy on Head and Neck Cancer. *Lancet.* 2000;**355**:949–955.

365 Bonner JA, Harari PM, Giralt J, et al. Radiotherapy plus cetuximab for squamous-cell carcinoma of the head and neck. *N Engl J Med.* 2006;**354**:567–578.

366 Ang KK, Zhang Q, Rosenthal DI, et al. Randomized phase III trial of concurrent accelerated radiation plus cisplatin with or without cetuximab for stage III to IV head and neck carcinoma: RTOG 0522. *J Clin Oncol.* 2014;**32**:2940–2950.

379 Vermorken JB, Mesia R, Rivera F, et al. Platinum-based chemotherapy plus cetuximab in head and neck cancer. *N Engl J Med.* 2008;**359**:1116–1127.

389 Vermorken JB, Trigo J, Hitt R, et al. Open-label, uncontrolled, multicenter phase II study to evaluate the efficacy and toxicity of cetuximab as a single agent in patients with recurrent and/or metastatic squamous cell carcinoma of the head and neck who failed to respond to platinum-based therapy. *J Clin Oncol.* 2007;**25**:2171–2177.

403 Seiwert TY, Burtness B, Weiss J, et al. A phase Ib study of MK-3475 in patients with human papillomavirus (HPV)-associated and non-HPV-associated head and neck (H/N) cancer. *ASCO Meeting Abstracts.* 2014;**32**:6011.

84 Cancer of the lung

Charles Lu, MD, SM ▪ Daniel Morgensztern, MD ▪ Anne Chiang, MD, PhD ▪ Amir Onn, MD
▪ Boris Sepesi, MD ▪ Ara A. Vaporciyan, MD ▪ Joe Y. Chang, MD, PhD ▪ Ritsuko K. Komaki, MD
▪ Ignacio I. Wistuba, MD ▪ Roy S. Herbst, MD, PhD

Overview

Worldwide, lung cancer is responsible for the largest number of cancer-related deaths, and reducing tobacco consumption is the most effective way to reduce lung cancer mortality. Standard therapy options continue to include surgery, radiotherapy, and/or chemotherapy. As lung cancer is a heterogeneous disease, it is hoped that translational proteomic and genomic research will advance our understanding of driver molecular pathways and allow development of more effective, less toxic, targeted therapies. Recent developments in immunotherapy have generated significant excitement and represent a novel therapeutic strategy, which has already impacted current standard of care.

Etiology and epidemiology

Worldwide, lung cancer is the most common (1.61 million of 12.7 million new cases) and the deadliest (1.38 million of 7.6 million cancer-related deaths) form of cancer.[1] The US 2015 cancer statistics indicate that lung cancer is the second most common cancer for both men and women (14% and 13% of all cases, respectively), but, as in previous years for both sexes, it is the number one cause of cancer death (86,380 men, 28% of all cancer-related deaths, and 71,660 women, 26% of all cancer-related deaths). In fact, more people in the United States die of lung cancer than of the next three causes of cancer-related deaths combined, which are prostate, breast, and colorectal cancer.[2] In 1920, fewer than 1000 cases of lung cancer were reported, and it was regarded as a rare malignancy. Since the 1950s, however, lung cancer has been recognized as a major public health problem. The incidence of new cases rose first in men and reached a peak in the mid 1980s; a steady decline has been noted since then. The incidence in women increased until the late 1990s and has recently stabilized. These changes occurred in parallel to the widespread adoption of cigarette smoking by both sexes. The decline in lung cancer incidence and mortality among men has been explained by reduction in smoking rates.[3]

Smoking and lung cancer

Tobacco is the world's single most avoidable cause of death. Lung cancer is the most common tobacco-related cause of cancer mortality: one case occurs for every 3 million cigarettes smoked. As described by Proctor,[4] cancers caused by tobacco were among the earliest discovered environmental cancers. First reports on the association between tobacco use and cancer of the oral cavity and lip were published in Europe in the eighteenth and nineteenth centuries. More than 60 years ago, Muller in Germany was the first to recognize the positive association between cigarette smoking

and lung cancer. Since then, multiple epidemiological studies have confirmed these observations and elaborated on the molecular mechanisms of smoking carcinogenesis, providing sufficient evidence to establish a strong causal association between cigarette smoking and cancer of the aerodigestive tract, urinary bladder, kidney and uterine cervix, as well as myeloid leukemia. A meta-analysis of over 50 studies on never smokers showed a consistent and statistically significant association between exposure to environmental tobacco smoke and lung cancer risk.[4]

To date, smoking accounts for about 85–90% of lung cancer deaths in both sexes. The rate at which lung cancer develops is strongly correlated with the duration of tobacco exposure. After 45, 30, and 15 years of cigarette smoking, the annual incidence rates of lung cancer are 0.5%, 0.1%, and under 0.01%, respectively. Thus, a threefold increase in the duration of tobacco use can increase the annual incidence of lung cancer by 50-fold. As smoking ceases, the annual risk remains roughly constant thereafter. For instance, after 30 years of smoking, the risk is approximately 0.1%, and if a smoker stops after 30 years, this annual rate will persist indefinitely. Thus, 15 years later, the annual risk is 0.1% instead of 0.5%, which it would have been if smoking had continued. About 80% of the risk is, therefore, avoided by stopping smoking.[5]

Passive smoking

Smokers are not the only people at increased risk from exposure to tobacco smoke. "Passive smoking" from environmental tobacco smoke also increases the risk of lung cancer death. According to the Environmental Protection Agency, each year about 3000 nonsmoking adults die of lung cancer as a result of breathing the smoke of others' cigarettes. Analysis has shown that the sidestream smoke emitted from a smoldering cigarette between puffs contains virtually all carcinogenic compounds that have been identified in the mainstream smoke inhaled by smokers.

Familial predisposition

It is interesting that the vast majority of cigarette smokers, including heavy smokers, do not develop lung cancer. This suggests that cancer formation is dependent on an inherited predisposition or cofactors such as additional carcinogens. Studies that have compared risk factors of individuals with histologically confirmed lung cancer and of individuals with other smoking-related cancers found that having relatives with lung cancer did not increase the risk of developing lung cancer, but it did increase the risk of having cancer at some site.[6] This suggests a heritable variation in response to carcinogens. Respiratory diseases also predispose to development of lung cancer. Studies of families predisposed to lung cancer showed that the development of lung cancer in young individuals (aged 50 years or younger) was compatible with Mendelian codominant inheritance or a rare autosomal gene.[7]

Holland-Frei Cancer Medicine, Ninth Edition. Edited by Robert C. Bast Jr., Carlo M. Croce, William N. Hait, Waun Ki Hong, Donald W. Kufe, Martine Piccart-Gebhart, Raphael E. Pollock, Ralph R. Weichselbaum, Hongyang Wang, and James F. Holland.
© 2017 John Wiley & Sons, Inc. ISBN: 978-1-118-93469-2

Table 1 Documented occupational lung carcinogens.

Substance	Occupational exposures
Arsenic	Smelters, pesticide manufacturers
Asbestos	Miners, millers, insulators, railroad, and shipyard workers
Chloromethyl ethers	Ion-exchange resin manufacturers
Chromium	Chromate and pigment manufacturers
Hydrocarbons	Coal-gas workers, roofers
Mustard gas	Poison-gas manufacturers
Nickel	Refiners
Radiation	Miners of uranium and other ores

Source: Adapted from Roth 1989.[8]

Other environmental causes

Lung cancer occurs in association with occupational and environmental exposures to carcinogenic agents other than tobacco smoke. Occupational agents classified as group 1 carcinogens by the International Agency for Research on Cancer include inorganic arsenic, asbestos, bis(chloromethyl)ether, chromium (hexavalent), nickel and nickel compounds, polycyclic aromatic compounds, radon, and vinyl chloride. Group 2A of probable carcinogens includes acrylonitrile, beryllium, cadmium, formaldehyde, acetaldehyde, synthetic fibers, silica, and welding fumes. Currently, occupational exposures have been estimated to account for 5–15% of all lung cancer cases worldwide (Table 1).

Molecular pathogenesis

The rapidly developing technology of molecular biology has allowed the identification of multiple genes responsible for lung carcinogenesis. Interestingly, these genes are altered forms of genes normally present in eukaryotic cells. The plethora of genetic abnormalities and redundancy of altered pathways induced by tobacco and other carcinogens determines lung cancer heterogeneity, which is remarkable in comparison to that of other solid tumors. In this regard, it has to be remembered that individual tumors are characterized by specific genetic alternation(s) and that there is a gradual accumulation of abnormalities in a given tumor, from normal epithelium to invasive carcinoma. Table 2 lists genes that have been implicated in lung carcinogenesis. A detailed review of cancer biology may be found in other sections of this textbook.

Molecular abnormalities in premalignancy

Structural and genetic epithelial changes occur gradually, and invasive carcinoma develops 5–20 years after initial insult to the airways (Figure 1). Loss of specific chromosomal regions on a single allele [loss of heterozygosity (LOH)] has been detected frequently in lung cancers and bronchial epithelia exposed to tobacco carcinogens. The regions of the earliest and most frequent allelic loss are 3p21, 3p22–24, 3p25, and 9p21.[9] It is noteworthy that many of these changes are seen in histologically normal bronchial epithelium from smokers, but not nonsmokers.[10,11] However, these changes appear to become more frequent and extensive in terms of chromosome loss with advancing abnormality of premalignancy. In some cases, these molecular changes appear to be clonally independent. Methylated sequences of tumor suppressor gene promoters can be detected in tumors, smoking-damaged normal lung (preneoplastic changes), sputum, and blood. These represent attractive surrogate biomarkers for early detection and monitoring of chemoprevention, smoking cessation, and response to therapy. Recent advances in the characterization of molecular abnormalities

Table 2 Summary of molecular abnormalities associated with the NSCLC adenocarcinoma and squamous-cell carcinoma histologies.

Gene	Molecular change	Adenocarcinoma	Squamous-cell carcinoma
EGFR	Mutation	10–40%	Very rare
	Amplification/CNG[a]	15%	40%
	IHC[b] overexpression	15–39%	~58%
KRAS	Mutation	10–30%	Very rare
BRAF	Mutation	2%	3%
EML4-ALK	Translocation	13%	Very rare
ROS1	Translocation	1%	Very rare
RET	Translocation	1%	Very rare
LKB1	Mutation	8–30%	0–5%
HER2	Mutation	2–4%	Very rare
	Amplification	8%	2%
	IHC[b] overexpression	35%	1%
DDR2	Mutation	Very rare	4%
TP53	LOH[c] and mutations	50–70%	60–70%
FGFR1	Amplification	1–3%	8–22%
PIK3CA	Amplification/CNG[a]	2–6%	33–35%
	Mutation	2%	2%

[a]CNG, copy number gain.
[b]IHC, immunohistochemistry.
[c]LOH, loss of heterozygosity.

of lung cancer, including the reports of several novel molecular pathways involved in the pathogenesis of invasive squamous cell carcinoma (SCC) and adenocarcinoma of the lung identified using high-throughput technologies such as next-generation sequencing of tumoral DNA and RNA,[12,13] have been extended to the analysis of molecular changes involved in the development of preneoplastic lesions of the lung airway.[14] It has been shown that in lung adenocarcinoma harboring epidermal growth factor receptor (EGFR) mutations, those changes can be detected in bronchial normal epithelium adjacent to tumors.[15] In SCC, gene amplification and protein overexpression of the cell lineage gene SOX-2 have been detected in a subset of bronchial dysplasia in patients with invasive squamous tumors.[16,17] High-throughput microarray profiling studies of the lung airway has shown that global alterations in the gene expression of normal epithelial cells can (1) predict cancer development in smokers,[18] (2) identify the activation of pathways (e.g., PI3K) that can be potentially targeted using chemoprevention strategies,[19] and (3) better define the localized molecular field of cancerization that can explain the development of different histologies of lung cancer.[14,20,21]

Pathology of lung cancer

From histopathologic and biologic perspectives, lung cancer is a complex neoplasm. The 2004 WHO (World Health Organization) histologic classification of lung cancer has been recently revised with support from the pathology panel of the International Association for the Study of Lung Cancer (IASLC).[22] The new classification is based on the analysis of lung tumors by light microscopy with standard histology techniques and immunohistochemical analysis of proteins representing differentiation markers (Table 3).[22,23] The most common histologic types of lung cancer are non-small-cell lung carcinomas (NSCLC), which include SCC, adenocarcinoma [including minimally invasive adenocarcinoma (MIA) and large-cell carcinoma, and small-cell lung carcinomas (SCLC).[24] Lung neoplasms are generally classified by the best-differentiated region of the tumor and graded by its most poorly differentiated portion.

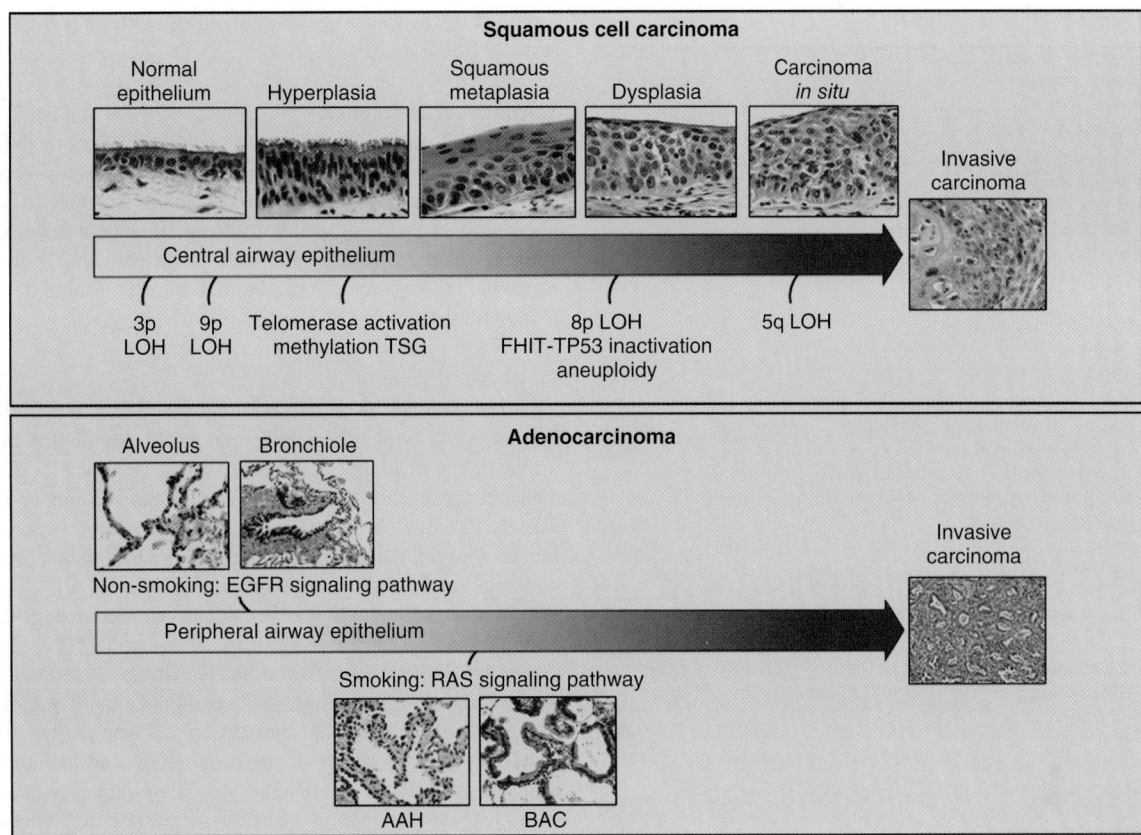

Figure 1 Summary of histopathologic and molecular changes involved in the pathogenesis of squamous-cell carcinoma and adenocarcinomas of the lung.

Precursor lesions

Lung cancers are believed to arise after the development of a series of progressive pathological changes (preneoplastic or precursor lesions) in the respiratory mucosa. The new WHO histological classification of preinvasive lesions of the lung lists three main morphologic forms: (1) squamous dysplasia and carcinoma *in situ* (CIS); (2) atypical adenomatous hyperplasia (AHH) and adenocarcinoma *in situ* (AIS); and (3) diffuse idiopathic pulmonary neuroendocrine cell hyperplasia (DIPNECH), which has been associated with the development of carcinoid tumors of the lung.[22,23] While the sequential preneoplastic changes have been defined for centrally arising squamous carcinomas, they have been poorly documented for large-cell carcinomas, adenocarcinomas, and SCLCs.[25,26]

Invasive tumors

Minimally invasive adenocarcinoma (MIA)

This lesion is defined as a small (≤3 cm), solitary adenocarcinoma with a predominantly lepidic pattern and with ≤5 mm invasion area in greatest dimension.[22,27] MIA is usually composed of nonmucinous cells, but infrequently, it may be mucinous. The measurement of the invasive area should include the presence of histological subtypes other than a lepidic pattern (i.e., acinar, papillary, micropapillary, and/or solid), or the identification of malignant cells clearly infiltrating stroma.[22] If a tumor invades lymphatics, blood vessels, or pleura or contains tumor necrosis, it should be diagnosed as invasive adenocarcinoma.

Adenocarcinoma

This tumor type accounts for nearly 40% of all lung cancers (Figure 2a, b). Most adenocarcinomas are histologically heterogeneous, and according to the new WHO classification, adenocarcinoma can be subclassified based on the predominant histological pattern present (i.e., acinar, papillary, solid with mucin production, micropapillary, and lepidic).[22] When tumor cells grow in a purely lepidic manner without evidence of invasion, they are regarded as AIS.[22] The solid adenocarcinoma pattern is, by definition, poorly differentiated, and these poorly differentiated tumors usually demonstrate mucus production as shown by mucicarmine or periodic acid-Schiff staining. Lung adenocarcinomas typically immunostain for thyroid transcription factor-1, Napsin A, and cytokeratin 7. There are four variants of adenocarcinoma tumors, including mucinous, colloid, fetal (low and high grade), and enteric. While adenocarcinomas of the lung spread primarily by lymphatic and hematogenous routes, aerogeneous dissemination often occurs in mucinous tumors and is characterized by spread of tumor cells through the airways forming lesions separate from the main mass.[28]

Squamous-cell carcinoma (SCC)

SCC accounts for approximately 30% of all lung cancers. Intercellular bridges, squamous pearl formation, and individual cell keratinization characterize squamous differentiation in this tumor type (Figure 2c). While all these features are very apparent in well-differentiated SCCs, they are difficult to find in poorly differentiated tumors. The histologic subtypes included in the new WHO classification include keratinizing, nonkeratinizing, and basaloid.[29] In tumors with keratinizing features, there is no need for immunohistochemistry analysis. The nonkeratinizing tumors necessitate immunohistochemistry examination to distinguish theses tumors from large-cell carcinoma with a null immunophenotype in surgical resections or other types of poorly differentiated NSCLCs. For such tumors, diffuse positive staining with p40, p63, and/or CK5 or

Table 3 Histological classification of lung cancer.

(I) Epithelial Tumors
(a) Benign
    (i) Papillomas
        (a) Squamous-cell papilloma
        (b) Glandular papilloma
        (c) Mixed squamous-cell and glandular papilloma
    (ii) Adenomas
        (a) Sclerosing pneumocytoma
        (b) Alveolar adenoma
        (c) Papillary adenoma
        (d) Mucinous cystadenoma
        (e) Pneumocytic adenomyoepithelioma
        (f) Mucous gland adenoma
(b) Preinvasive lesions
    1 Atypical alveolar hyperplasia (AAH)
    2 Adenocarcinoma in situ (AIS)
    3 Squamous dysplasia and carcinoma in situ
    4 Diffuse idiopathic pulmonary neuroendocrine cell hyperplasia
(c) Malignant
    (i) Adenocarcinoma
        (a) Minimally invasive adenocarcinoma (MIA)
        (b) Invasive adenocarcinoma
        (c) Variants of invasive adenocarcinoma: mucinous, colloid, fetal and enteric
    (ii) Squamous-cell carcinoma
        (a) Keratinizing
        (b) Nonkeratinizing
        (c) Basaloid carcinoma
    (iii) Adenosquamous carcinoma
    (iv) Sarcomatoid carcinoma
        (a) Pleomorphic
        (b) Spindle cell
        (c) Giant-cell carcinoma
        (d) Carcinosarcoma
        (e) Pulmonary blastoma
    (v) Large-cell carcinoma
    (vi) Neuroendocrine tumors
        (a) Typical carcinoid
        (b) Atypical carcinoid
        (c) Large-cell neuroendocrine carcinoma (LCNEC)
        (d) Small-cell carcinoma (SCLC)
    (vii) Other and unclassified carcinomas
        (a) Lymphoepithelioma-like carcinoma
        (b) NUT-carcinoma
    (viii) Salivary gland tumors
        • Mucoepidermoid carcinoma
        • Adenoid cystic carcinoma
        • Epithelial–myoepithelial carcinoma
        • Pleomorphic adenoma
(II) Mesenchymal tumors
(III) Lymphohistiocytic tumors
(IV) Tumors of ectopic origin
(V) Metastatic tumors

CK5/6 confirms their squamous phenotype and classification as a nonkeratinizing SCC. Both TTF-1 and mucin stains should be negative or only focally positive (<10% of cells with faint staining).

Approximately, 70% of SCCs of the lung present as central lung tumors.[30] The tumor may grow to a large size and central cavitation secondary to necrosis is a common gross finding.[31]

Adenosquamous carcinoma

Adenosquamous carcinoma of the lung is characterized by the presence of SCC and adenocarcinoma with each comprising at least 10% of the tumor.[32] They account for 0.4–4% of lung cancers and are usually located in the periphery of the lung and may contain a central scar. The routes of dissemination and metastasis are similar to other NSCLCs.

Sarcomatoid carcinomas

Sarcomatoid carcinomas of the lung are a group of poorly differentiated NSCLCs that contain a component of sarcoma or sarcoma-like (spindle and/or giant cell) differentiation.[33] Currently, there are five variants identified: pleomorphic carcinoma, spindle-cell carcinoma, giant-cell carcinoma, carcinosarcoma, and pulmonary blastoma.[33,34] Sarcomatoid carcinomas are rare tumors (0.3–1.3% of lung tumors).[33,35]

Large-cell carcinoma

Large-cell carcinoma is defined as an undifferentiated NSCLC that lacks the cytologic, architectural, and immunohistochemical features of SCC, adenocarcinoma, or SCLC (Figure 2d). Thus, it is a diagnosis of exclusion. Large-cell carcinomas account for approximately 10% of all lung cancers, and they represent a spectrum of morphology, most consisting of large cells with abundant cytoplasm and large nuclei with prominent nucleoli (Figure 2d).[31] The 2004 WHO classification listed four histological variants of large-cell carcinoma: large-cell neuroendocrine carcinoma (LCNEC), basaloid carcinoma, lymphoepithelioma-like carcinoma, clear-cell carcinoma, and large-cell carcinoma with rhabdoid phenotype. However, in the revised WHO classification, LCNEC is being reclassified into a new category (neuroendocrine carcinoma), and basaloid carcinoma is included as a variant of SCC. Pure large-cell carcinoma with clear cells or rhabdoid phenotype is extremely uncommon. If these components are detected in a large-cell carcinoma, their presence should be added in the description of the tumor.

Neuroendocrine tumors

Lung neuroendocrine tumors account for approximately 15% of lung cancers. They are composed of malignant cells showing neuroendocrine differentiation and representing a wide spectrum of tumors: typical and atypical carcinoids, considered low- and intermediate-grade malignancies, respectively, and LCNEC and SCLC, considered high-grade tumors (Figure 3a–c).

Carcinoid tumors

Carcinoid tumors are characterized by organoid growth pattern, uniform cytologic features, and immunohistochemical expression of neuroendocrine markers, such as chromogranin and synaptophysin (Figure 3c).[36] Carcinoid tumors have been divided into two categories, typical and atypical types, based on their clinical behavior and pathologic features, with atypical crinoids having more malignant histologic and clinical features.[37] Typical and atypical crinoids are also referred to as low- and intermediate-grade neuroendocrine carcinomas, respectively. Histologically, typical carcinoids show fewer than 2 mitoses per 2 mm^2 field and lack necrosis, while atypical carcinoids show 2–10 mitoses per 2 mm^2 field and/or foci of necrosis.[36] Typical carcinoids are uniformly distributed throughout the lungs, whereas atypical carcinoids are more commonly peripheral tumors.[38] Compared to typical carcinoids, atypical carcinoids have a larger tumor size and a higher rate of metastases, and their survival is significantly reduced.[38] At presentation, approximately 10–15% of typical and 40–50% of atypical carcinoids demonstrate regional lymph node metastases.[36]

Large-cell neuroendocrine carcinoma (LCNEC)

This tumor type is defined by the presence of large undifferentiated cells with prominent nucleoli, neuroendocrine pattern of growth,

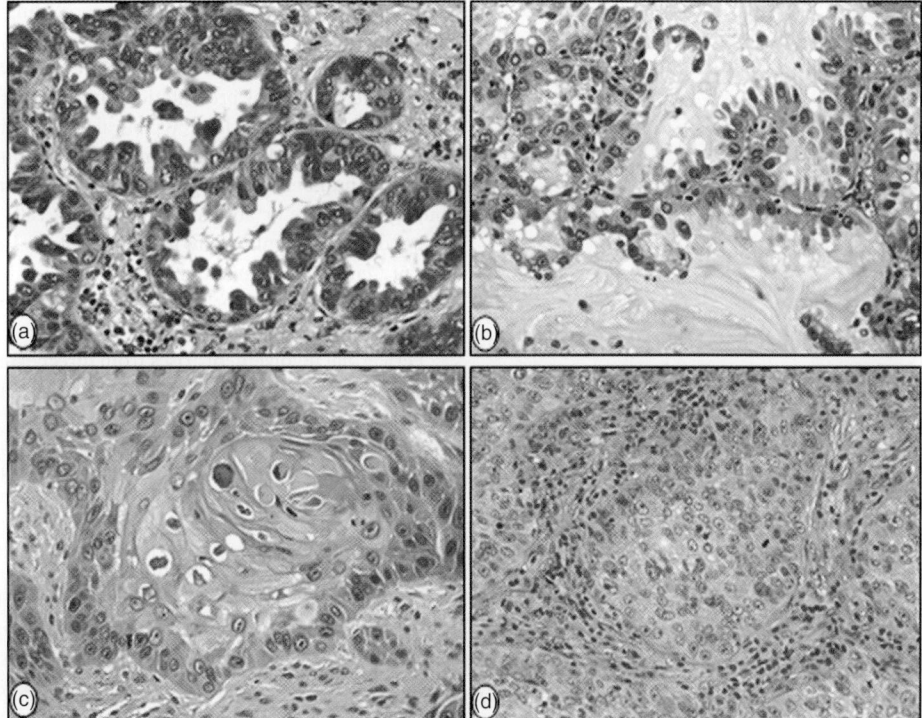

Figure 2 Histopathological characteristics of major forms of NSCLC: (a) invasive adenocarcinoma with acinar pattern, (b) adenocarcinoma with lepidic (noninvasive) pattern, (c) keratinizing squamous-cell carcinoma, and (d) large-cell carcinoma.

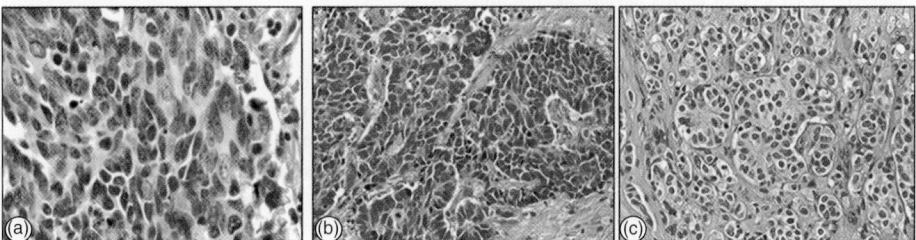

Figure 3 Neuroendocrine tumors of the lung: (a) SCLC, (b) LNEC, and (c) typical carcinoid.

high mitotic rate, and neuroendocrine differentiation demonstrated by immunohistochemistry (Figure 3b).[39] They are usually peripheral, nodular masses, with necrosis. LCNEC is considered an aggressive malignancy with a prognosis similar to SCLC.[39] The term combined LCNEC is used for tumors associated with other better differentiated types of NSCLC, mostly adenocarcinomas.

Small-cell lung carcinoma (SCLC)

This tumor type accounts for approximately 15% of all lung cancers.[29] They characteristically consist of small epithelial tumor cells with finely granular chromatin and absent or inconspicuous nucleoli (Figure 3a). Necrosis is frequent and extensive and the mitotic count is high. Although there is not a precise upper limit for cell size to be defined as small cell, it has been suggested that the cells should measure approximately the diameter of two or three small mature lymphocytes.[40] While SCLC represents a light microscopic diagnosis, electron microscopy shows neuroendocrine granules in at least two-thirds of cases and immunohistochemistry for neuroendocrine markers (chromogranin and synaptophysin) is positive in most (~90%) cases.[40,41] Less than 10% of SCLCs demonstrate a mixture with NSCLC histologic types, usually adenocarcinoma, SCC, or large-cell carcinoma, and they are termed combined SCLCs.

NSCLC histological classification applied to small biopsies and cytology specimens

In these tumor samples, the NSCLC diagnosis has been lumped together without attention to more specific histologic typing. One of the major recent changes in lung cancer pathology has been the development of standardized criteria and terminology for pathologic diagnosis of lung cancer in small biopsies and cytology.[42] In addition to the criteria and terminology, there is a paradigm shift for pathologists in tumor classification and management of specimens, which indicates the need to perform immunohistochemistry to further classify tumors formerly diagnosed as NSCLC not otherwise specified (NOS). Currently, if a NSCLC does not show clear glandular or squamous morphology in a small biopsy or cytology specimen, it is classified as NSCLC-NOS. Tumors with this morphology should be studied with limited special immunohistochemical markers to classify them further. It is recommended to use a single adenocarcinoma maker (i.e., TTF-1), a single squamous marker (i.e., p40 or p63), and/or mucin stains.[42] Tumors that are positive for an adenocarcinoma marker or mucin are classified as NSCLC, favor adenocarcinoma. Tumors that are positive for an SCC marker with negative adenocarcinoma marker are classified as NSCLC, favor SCC. Cytology is also a powerful diagnostic tool that can accurately subtype NSCLC in most cases, and immunohistochemistry is readily available if cell blocks are prepared for the cytology samples.

Clinical manifestations

Clinical presentation

Some patients present with an asymptomatic lesion were discovered incidentally on chest radiograph. The majority of lung cancers, however, are discovered because of the development of a new or worsening clinical symptom or sign. Although no set of signs or symptoms is pathognomonic for lung cancer, they may be divided into four categories: (1) those due to local tumor growth and intrathoracic spread, (2) those due to distant metastases, (3) nonspecific systemic symptoms, and (4) paraneoplastic syndromes.

Manifestations of local tumor growth and intrathoracic spread
Signs and symptoms referable to the primary tumor vary depending on location and size of the tumor. Centrally located tumors produce cough, a localized wheeze, hemoptysis, and symptoms and signs of airway obstruction and postobstructive pneumonitis such as dyspnea, fever, and productive cough. Peripheral tumors are more likely to be asymptomatic when they are small and confined within the lung; occasionally, cough and pleuritic chest pain may be evident.

Intrathoracic spread of lung cancer, either by direct extension or by lymphatic metastasis, is associated with a variety of sign and symptom complexes. Mediastinal invasion may be manifested as vague, poorly localized chest pain in association with other findings of nerve entrapment, vascular obstruction, and/or compression or invasion of the esophagus. One of the most common neurologic disorders arising from mediastinal involvement is hoarseness owing to entrapment of the recurrent laryngeal nerve. Because of its longer intrathoracic course, the left recurrent laryngeal nerve is more likely to be the source of hoarseness than the right recurrent laryngeal nerve.[43] Compression of the esophagus by the tumor also may lead to dysphagia. The formation of a tracheoesophageal or bronchoesophageal fistula, which occurs with a frequency of 0.16%, can be manifested by vigorous cough, especially on swallowing, and recurrent aspiration pneumonia.[44] Involvement of the phrenic nerve is associated with hiccups early, and later leads to paralysis and elevation of the hemidiaphragm with resulting dyspnea.

The principal vascular syndrome associated with the extension of lung cancer into the mediastinum is superior vena cava (SVC) syndrome, most commonly caused by invasion of the vein and extrinsic compression by the tumor, but also by intraluminal thrombosis.[45] Lung cancer accounts for 65–90% of all cases of SVC syndrome, and in approximately 85% of these cases, the primary lung tumor is on the right, primarily in the right upper lobe or right mainstem bronchus. Establishment of a histologic diagnosis is important before initiating treatment, because the SVC syndrome is no longer considered a radiotherapeutic emergency.

With apical tumors, the classic Pancoast's syndrome (lower brachial plexopathy, Horner's syndrome, and shoulder pain) is due to local invasion of the lower brachial plexus (C8 and T1 nerve roots), satellite ganglion, and chest wall.[46] The tumor may cause symptoms through involvement of the first or second rib or vertebrae and other nerve roots. The radiographic signs are those of an asymmetric apical cap or an apical mass. Most superior sulcus tumors are SCCs, although they may be adenocarcinomas,

or even in 1–2% of cases, SCLC, underscoring the importance of establishing a histologic diagnosis.

Approximately 15% of patients with lung cancer have pleural involvement at initial presentation, and 50% of patients with disseminated lung cancer develop pleural effusion during the course of their illness. A pleural effusion may cause dyspnea, cough, or chest pain.[47] A number of pathogenic mechanisms have been suggested, but the presence or absence of malignant cells in cytology specimens does not significantly influence survival outcome, although the presence of malignant cells in pleural washings at the time of pulmonary resection for lung cancer has been shown to have a negative impact survival.[48]

Pericardial involvement arises from direct extension of the tumor or as a result of retrograde spread through mediastinal and epicardial lymphatics. Lung cancer is the single most frequent source of pericardial metastases.[49] Clinical findings include cardiac dysrhythmias, enlargement of the cardiac silhouette, and, infrequently, cardiac tamponade (Table 4).

Manifestations of distant metastases
Approximately 60% of SCLC and 30–40% of NSCLC patients present with stage IV metastatic disease. Although lung cancer can metastasize to virtually any organ site, the most common sites of hematogenous spread that are clinically apparent are the central nervous system (CNS), bones, liver, and adrenal glands. Many of these patients do not have symptoms that can be attributed to a specific distant site.

Systemic, nonspecific signs, and symptoms
As shown in Table 5, systemic, nonspecific signs and symptoms are common in both SCLC and NSCLC. The 30% rate of anorexia is probably underreported. Weight loss, which is usually but not always accompanied by anorexia, occurs in approximately one-half of the patients and generalized weakness in one-third. Fever and anemia occur in fewer than 20% of the patients. Fever is generally not considered paraneoplastic in lung cancer patients; if present, it is usually associated with a documented infection (e.g., postobstructive pneumonia) or with liver metastases.

Paraneoplastic syndromes
Table 6 lists 21 paraneoplastic syndromes, which induce signs and symptoms away from the primary tumor or its metastasis. The major categories of paraneoplastic syndromes include endocrine, neurologic, cutaneous and musculoskeletal, and cardiovascular and hematological manifestations.[50]

Table 4 Clinical manifestations of lung cancer caused by local tumor growth and intrathoracic spread at presentation.

Clinical manifestation	Frequency (%)	
	SCLC	NSCLC
Cough	50–76	40
Dyspnea	34–40	30–40
Chest pain	35–36	25–40
Hemoptysis	15–23	15–35
Pneumonitis	21–25	13–24
SVC syndrome	12	<10
Pleural effusion	10–15	15
Pancoast syndrome	Rare	3
Pericardial effusion	Uncommon	Rare

NSCLC, nonsmall-cell lung cancer; SCLC, small-cell lung cancer; SVC, superior vena cava.

Table 5 Clinical manifestation caused by systemic effect at presentation.

Clinical manifestation	Frequency (%)	
	SCLC	NSCLC
Anorexia	30	30
Weight loss (≥10 lb)	35–52	45–52
Fatigue	23–42	35
Fever	11–15	7–16
Anemia	11–15	16–20

NSCLC, nonsmall-cell lung cancer; SCLC, small-cell lung cancer.

Table 6 Major paraneoplastic manifestations of lung cancer.

Syndrome	Clinical frequency (%)	Comments
Endocrine		
Inappropriate ADH	5–10	Mainly SCLC
Atrial natriuretic factor	?	—
Ectopic ACTH	3–7	Most commonly with SCLC
Hypercalcemia of malignancy	10	Most commonly with squamous-cell types
Gynecomastia	6	More with large-cell type
Other hormones	—	No significant clinical manifestations
Neurologic		
Eaton–Lambert	6	Mainly SCLC
Subacute sensory neuropathy	Rare	Mainly SCLC
Subacute cerebellar degeneration	Rare	Mainly SCLC
Limbic encephalopathy	Rare	Mainly SCLC
Visual paraneoplastic syndrome	Rare	Mainly SCLC
Subacute necrotic myelopathy	Rare	Mainly SCLC
Cutaneous/musculoskeletal		
Hypertrophic pulmonary osteoarthropathy	<10	More with adenocarcinoma
Acanthosis nigricans	Rare	—
Tylosis	Rare	—
Tylosis	Rare	—
Cardiovascular/hematologic		
Nonbacterial thrombotic endocarditis	Uncommon	More with adenocarcinoma
Migratory thrombophlebitis	Uncommon	More with adenocarcinoma
Hypercoagulable status	10–15%	Renal
Glomerulonephritis	Rare	—
Nephrotic syndrome	Rare	—

ADH, antidiuretic hormone; SCLC, small-cell lung cancer; ACTH, adrenocorticotropic hormone.

Endocrine syndromes

Syndrome of inappropriate secretion of antidiuretic hormone (SIADH)

Excess secretion of arginine-vasopressin associated with hyponatremia is the hallmark of SIADH (syndrome of inappropriate secretion of antidiuretic hormone). The cardinal findings are hyponatremia with corresponding serum hypo-osmolality; continued renal excretion of sodium; absence of fluid volume depletion; inappropriately high urine osmolality; and normal kidney, adrenal, and thyroid function. SIADH may be caused by a variety of malignant tumors, and SCLC is the most common (up to 15%, though only one-third are symptomatic). Water restriction is usually sufficient to control symptoms until systemic anticancer treatment is initiated, which typically leads to improvement or resolution of the

hyponatremia. Saline infusion, furosemide, or demeclocycline is infrequently required.

Syndrome of ectopic adrenocorticotropic hormone

Hyperadrenocorticism in association with ectopic adrenocorticotropic hormone (ACTH) production (>200 pg/mL) is a frequently observed hormonal syndrome in lung cancer, particularly in SCLC. Serum ACTH levels are elevated in 30–72% of SCLC patients, and cortisol secretion is abnormally regulated in 51%, but only 3–7% of SCLC patients become symptomatic. Patients with ectopic ACTH syndrome generally fit the demographic characteristics of lung cancer patients and rarely exhibit the classic cushingoid features of centripetal obesity or moon facies. Ectopic ACTH syndrome was found to be associated with frequent complications from chemotherapy and shortened survival in patients with SCLC.[51]

Other hormone production

Other hormones elevated in lung cancer, particularly in patients with SCLC, include calcitonin, growth hormone, prolactin, serotonin, insulin, gastrin, and melanocyte stimulating factors. In most cases, however, these laboratory abnormalities bear minimal clinical significance.

Hypercalcemia of malignancy

It has long been known that cancer patients may have hypercalcemia even without demonstrable bone metastases. Hypercalcemia has been reported to occur in up to 30% of patients with cancer at some time during the course of their disease. This incidence may be falling owing to the wide use of bisphosphonates in patients with multiple myeloma or breast cancer, although data are lacking. Hypercalcemia leads to progressive mental impairment, including coma, as well as renal failure. These complications are particularly common terminal events among patients with cancer. The detection of hypercalcemia in a patient with cancer signifies a very poor prognosis; approximately 50% of such patients die within 30 days. A parathyroid hormone-related protein has been shown to be responsible for the majority of cases of hypercalcemia of malignancy. SCC is the lung cancer mostly associated with hypercalcemia, and SCLC is rarely involved. Hypercalcemia may be completely reversible with effective treatment of the underlying cancer, and bisphosphonates may be used as a specific therapeutic modality.[52] Denosumab, a monoclonal antibody, which binds the bone resorption mediator RANKL, has recently been approved for hypercalcemia of malignancy refractory to bisphosphonate therapy.[53]

Neurologic syndromes

Neurologic syndromes associated with lung cancer may occur through autoimmune mechanisms, mainly in patients with SCLC. Symptoms may precede diagnosis of the cancer by many months or may be the first sign of tumor recurrence. The severity of neurologic symptoms is unrelated to tumor bulk, and a primary malignant lesion may be undetected before death, despite disabling symptoms. Most of these conditions are not specific for malignancy.

Eaton–Lambert syndrome

A myasthenia gravis-like disorder that was originally linked to SCLC but was found in other cancers, this syndrome, characterized by proximal limb muscle weakness and fatigue, is caused by the formation of IgG antibodies directed at calcium channels present in both the tumor and the neuromuscular junction. A type-1 antineuronal nuclear autoantibody (ANNA-1, also known as "anti-Hu") has been identified as a marker of neurological autoimmunity that is highly associated with SCLC (97%) and other paraneoplastic neurologic disorders.[54]

Subacute sensory neuropathy

This is the most characteristic peripheral neuropathy associated with SCLC. Clinical symptoms characterized by progressive impairment of all sensory modalities, with areflexia and marked sensory ataxia followed by stabilization after a period of weeks, may precede the diagnosis of SCLC by several months. It may be accompanied by more widespread evidence of paraneoplastic encephalitis, with cerebellar brainstem dysfunction and dementia.

Cutaneous and musculoskeletal syndromes

Digital clubbing and hypertrophic pulmonary osteoarthropathy (HPO) are the other major paraneoplastic syndromes associated with lung cancer, most commonly with NSCLC. Digital clubbing is more common than HPO, which often resembles rheumatoid arthritis. It is characterized by a symmetric polyarthritis (usually involving the ankles, wrists, and knees), proliferative periostitis of the long bones, and neurovascular changes of the hands and feet. Lung cancer accounts for more than 80% of cases of HPO in adults.[55] Radionuclide bone scans typically demonstrate increased uptake at the distal ends of the affected long bones, and the results may be confirmed by evidence of new bone formation on plain films; the spine is spared. The onset of HPO is often acute and may precede the diagnosis of cancer. A variety of underlying mechanisms have been suggested, including the release of platelet-derived growth factor by megakaryocytes or platelet clumps that bypass the pulmonary capillary network. The syndrome may resolve with response of the cancer to therapy. No effective form of treatment is recognized, including aspirin and nonsteroidal anti-inflammatory agents.

Cardiovascular and hematological manifestations

Arterial and, more commonly, venous thrombosis is a frequent complication of cancer and sometimes a harbinger of occult cancer. Moreover, the use of new and aggressive therapy for cancer increases the risk of thrombosis. The two most notable manifestations in lung cancer are nonbacterial thrombotic endocarditis (NBTE) and venous thromboembolism (VTE).

Diagnostic and staging techniques

Accurate clinical staging includes a combination of noninvasive and invasive procedures. Noninvasive studies include sputum cytology and imaging studies; most commonly used are chest radiography, computed tomography (CT) scanning, and positron emission tomography (PET) (usually PET–CT) scanning. For mediastinal or spinal lesions, magnetic resonance imaging (MRI) is considered. Invasive procedures include bronchoscopy, CT or ultrasound (US)-guided fine-needle aspiration (FNA) or biopsy, lymph node biopsy, and surgical (open) biopsy using mediastinoscopy or thoracoscopy. Patients who present with clinical or radiographic evidence of extensive disease (ED) usually require the least invasive procedure to establish both the diagnosis and disease stage. Cytologic or histologic confirmation through FNA or biopsy usually is sufficient to confirm suspicion of N3 or M1 disease. Thoracentesis or pericardiocentesis should be performed on associated effusions to assess malignant cytology. Tissue may be required for molecular assessment of the tumor to better select medical therapy. Therefore, in some cases repeated biopsy is needed.

Noninvasive studies

Sputum cytology

Cytologic evaluation of sputum, bronchial washings, bronchial brushings, and FNA specimens have high diagnostic yield, but the positive and negative predictive values of each and their accuracy of diagnosis certainly are dependent on sampling error, tissue preservation, processing quality, and observer experience. Sputum cytology is a simple test with a specificity rate of 99%. However, the sensitivity rate is approximately 70% for central tumors, and <50% for peripheral lesions. To increase the yield, three specimens are usually collected. In practice, more invasive measures to obtain a diagnosis are used in most cases.

Imaging

Lung cancer is generally first imaged by chest radiography. CT scan, PET/CT scan, and occasionally MRI are used to stage a known or suspected lung cancer and monitor response to therapy.

Chest radiography

Posterior–anterior and lateral chest radiographs remain the simplest method for identifying patients with lung cancer. It is widely available, has low cost and low radiation dose, but most cases are identified at an advanced stage. A standard chest radiograph can detect a lesion as small as 3 mm in diameter; however, unsuspected nodules generally are not seen unless larger than 5 mm in diameter. Associated atelectasis, postobstructive pneumonitis, abscess, bronchiolitis, pleural reaction, rib erosion, pleural effusion, or bulky mediastinal lymphadenopathy may be identified on radiographs, raising suspicions of a primary lung malignancy.

Plain chest radiography may identify abnormal pulmonary nodules. There are no absolute criteria to confirm a benign lesion on the basis of its radiographic appearance, but stability of size for 2 years and the presence of specific patterns of calcification (multipunctate foci, a dense central nidus, a popcorn ball, or laminated "bull's eye" appearance) are considered indicators of benignancy. However, some tumors such as AIS and typical carcinoids occasionally appear to be stable for 2 or more years.[56]

Computed tomography

As a single comprehensive study, CT scan remains the most effective noninvasive technique for evaluating suspected or known lung cancer and the mediastinum, which may contain associated metastatic disease. However, the accuracy of CT scanning in identifying metastatic disease in mediastinal lymph nodes is highly variable and its sensitivity ranges from 51% to 95%. Such a wide range in accuracy is secondary to variations in the criteria for nodal abnormality, which are based on size and shape of a lymph node, CT scanner differences, and nonuniformity in nodal mapping. A lymph node size ≥1 cm in shortest diameter has been generally accepted as the criterion of abnormal nodal enlargement. Approximately 8–15% of patients considered to have a negative CT scan for mediastinal nodal enlargement, with lymph nodes ≤1 cm, will ultimately be found to have mediastinal nodal involvement at the time of operation. Mediastinal lymph nodes that are ≥2 cm in diameter contain metastatic disease in over 90% of cases. Lymph nodes that are 1.5–2 cm in size contain disease in over 50% of cases. Lymph nodes that are 1–1.5 cm in size harbor metastatic disease in 15–30% of cases. The negative predictive accuracy of CT scan is 85–92% for mediastinal lymph node metastases. For these reasons, many centers are now using PET–CT imaging.

Magnetic resonance imaging

MRI is not used for the routine evaluation of patients with lung cancer, but it does have specific advantages over CT scan. Because of its heightened ability to discern neurologic and vascular structures, tumors that reside in close proximity to neurovascular structures may be more accurately assessed by MRI than by CT scan. MRI is most useful in evaluating patients with superior sulcus tumors.

Positron emission tomography

Over the past several years, PET scanning with 2-[18F]fluoro-2-deoxy-D-glucose (FDG-PET) has been increasingly used in the diagnosis, staging, and therapeutic monitoring of lung cancer. This test identifies areas of increased glucose metabolism, which is a common trait in pulmonary tumors. As commercial PET scanners provide nominal spatial resolution of 4.5–6.0 mm in the center of the axial field of view, even lesions that are ≤1 cm in diameter can be detected on the basis of an increased uptake of FDG. Although initially heralded as a reliable noninvasive method of identifying and staging pulmonary neoplasms, a number of limitations have become apparent. Many inflammatory processes such as abscesses and active granulomatous diseases, as well as hypoxic conditions such as those that exist after radiotherapy, may cause high FDG uptake and lead to false-positive results. Treatment-induced hypermetabolic inflammatory changes also may lead to difficulty differentiating between treatment effects and those of the residual tumor. False-negative results have occurred primarily in tumors with low glucose metabolism (carcinoid and AIS) and in small tumors, owing to the limited spatial resolution of current PET scanners.[57]

Integrated PET–CT

PET provides imprecise information on the exact location of focal abnormalities. Thus, even if the results of PET and CT scan are visually correlated, the precise location of lesions is sometimes difficult to determine. To overcome this limitation, integrated PET–CT was introduced.[58] Recent studies suggested that integrated PET–CT improved the diagnostic accuracy of NSCLC. Tumor staging was significantly more accurate with integrated PET–CT than with CT scan alone ($p = .001$), PET alone ($p < .001$), or visual correlation of PET and CT scan ($p = .013$); node staging was also significantly more accurate with integrated PET–CT than with PET alone ($p = .013$).[58] In patients with potentially resectable NSCLC, the accuracy of PET–CT is insufficient for mediastinal staging, and pathologic assessment of mediastinal lymph nodes remains the standard of care.[59] Randomized clinical trials (RCTs) suggest that PET–CT may help in the preoperative assessment of metastatic disease, potentially leading to the avoidance of unnecessary surgery.[60]

Invasive studies

Tissue is collected for histopathological diagnosis, molecular studies, and genetic testing. In most cases, FNA for cytological assessment does not suffice and core biopsies are recommended. Endobronchial and centrally located tumors are usually diagnosed with bronchoscopy, whereas peripheral lesions with CT- (or US-) guided biopsies. In many cases, the biopsy is targeted to a lesion that would determine the diagnosis and the stage of the disease. For example, biopsy of a contralateral lymph node should be considered in cases where it would alter the disease stage (N stage) and a biopsy of a liver lesion would confirm the diagnosis of the primary tumor and the presence of a metastasis (M stage). In this regard, one has to consider the potential differences in the genetic expression between the primary tumor and its metastatic lesions and to avoid a biopsy of a lesion in a bone because decalcification processes could alter the genetic expression of the tumor.

FNA biopsy

Transthoracic percutaneous needle biopsy (TPNB) has significantly heightened the ability to diagnose intrathoracic pathologic processes. With CT or US guidance, tissue samples can be obtained from poorly accessible sites in the lung, mediastinum, abdomen, and retroperitoneum. The procedure is performed under local anesthesia using a small-gauge needle to either aspirate or biopsy lesions. Aspirated material is immediately processed with optimal procedural coordination. Many centers use an on-site cytopathologist for interpretation. Should the material be inadequate, a repeat aspiration can be performed. TPNB has been shown to be over 90% effective in establishing a final diagnosis. The false-positive rate is low (1%) and the false-negative rate ranges from 23% to 29%.[61]

Fiberoptic bronchoscopy (FOB)

Fiberoptic bronchoscopy (FOB) is an essential and standard technique for the evaluation of patients with pulmonary neoplasms; it remains the most important procedure for determining the endobronchial extent of disease. FOB permits careful survey of the supraglottic, glottic, tracheal, and bronchial regions to the level of most subsegments. Tumor (T) status can be defined by measuring tumor proximity to the carina and various bronchi and by identifying unsuspected occult lesions that indicate multiplicity of disease. For lesions that are visible by endoscopy, an accurate histologic diagnosis can be achieved in over 90% of cases. For central lesions, cytologic studies via needle aspiration, washings, and brushings, coupled with biopsy, heighten the diagnostic yield to over 95%. Peripheral lesions not visible endoscopically may be approached by cytologic studies of brushings and bronchioloalveolar lavage (BAL), which yield a diagnosis in 50–60% of patients. Cytologic studies, coupled with transbronchial fine-needle aspiration (TBNA), greatly enhance diagnostic yield.

TBNA biopsy

TBNA biopsy was introduced by Wang and Terry[62] using FOB. It has been used most widely to sample endobronchial and peripheral lesions and significantly improves the diagnostic yield when coupled with standard diagnostic measures (washings, brushings, and biopsies). TBNA is best performed in a suite that is equipped with fluoroscopy to enhance localization of the lesion. One of the most important applications of TBNA is the evaluation of mediastinal lymphadenopathy. The true sensitivity and specificity of TBNA appear to range from 14% to 50% and 96% to 100%, respectively. Thus, negative results require definitive operative confirmation, but the risk of a false-positive finding appears to be quite low.[63]

Advances in bronchoscopy

The development of linear echo-endoscopes has opened up new diagnostic possibilities for patients with lung cancer. Transesophageal US-guided fine-needle aspiration (EUS-FNA) and transbronchial US-guided needle aspiration (EBUS-TBNA, endobronchial ultrasound transbronchial needle aspiration) are both minimally invasive diagnostic techniques that enable real-time controlled aspirations of mediastinal lymph nodes and centrally located lung tumors. Evolving reports using these technologies suggest that EBUS-FNA has higher sensitivity than TBNA and that EUS plus EBUS may allow near-complete minimally invasive mediastinal staging in patients with suspected lung cancer. These newer diagnostic technologies may serve as an alternative approach for mediastinal staging in patients with suspected lung cancer.[64] Electromagnetic registration and guidance combine virtual bronchoscopy, three-dimensional (3D) CT images, and a steerable probe to aid in the biopsy of lung lesions. The yield and safety of this technology are being tested in several centers.[65]

Mediastinoscopy

Transcervical mediastinoscopy is the best method for invasive evaluation of the middle mediastinum to include the peritracheal and subcarinal lymph nodes. The indication remains preoperative mediastinal nodal assessment in patients with CT scan evidence of cross-sectional lymph node enlargement of ≥1 cm. In such patients who are proven to have lung cancer, the chance that these nodes contain metastasis is over 7%. If the nodes are enlarged to 1.5–2 cm or more, the risk of having metastatic involvement is over 30%. The accuracy of cervical mediastinoscopy ranges from 80% to 90%, and the false-negative rate ranges from 10% to 12%. The lymph node station most commonly missampled is the subcarinal region, which is difficult to access in some patients. The subaortic and aortopulmonary window regions are inaccessible by standard cervical mediastinoscopy.[66] Extended cervical mediastinoscopy, a variation of standard mediastinoscopy, has been useful for staging lesions in the left upper lobe. The standard mediastinoscopy incision is used, with the plane of dissection extending anterior to the innominate artery and aorta, anterolaterally to the level of the aortopulmonary window. "Anterior mediastinotomy," originally described by McNeil and Chamberlain, permits direct visual access to the anterior mediastinum through the second, third, or fourth anterior interspace, with or without removal of a short portion of the adjacent cartilage. For right-sided lesions, the procedure provides access to the proximal pulmonary artery and SVC. The procedure is used on the left side to evaluate disease in the subaortic and lateral aortic regions.

Thoracoscopy

Thoracoscopy and video-assisted thoracoscopic surgery (VATS) are used in a broader range of applications, including resectional techniques. The VATS approach is used in many thoracic conditions, and its role continues to evolve regarding the evaluation and management of lung cancer. It is currently considered for the evaluation and treatment of pleural tumors and effusions and in the diagnosis of indeterminate pulmonary nodules, and has a complementary role to standard mediastinoscopy in the staging of mediastinal lymph nodes. It has also become an accepted approach for resection of peripheral early-stage lung cancer in many centers.[67]

Operative staging

Operative staging provides the opportunity to verify histologically the extent of gross and microscopic diseases. The surgeon is responsible for performing a complete nodal dissection or nodal sampling as an integral part of the thoracotomy. Lymph nodes are removed and labeled according to the location of the station on the regional station map (Figure 4).

Cancer screening and early detection

Because symptoms of early-stage localized disease are insidious and nonspecific, they are frequently attributed to the effects of smoking. By the time the patient seeks medical attention, the disease is usually advanced so that complete surgical resection is possible in fewer than 30% of cases, and the overall 5-year survival rate is <17%. Clearly, screening and early detection of cancer at a more treatable stage is a desirable goal.

In the 1970s, the National Cancer Institute (NCI) sponsored three separate RCTs to assess the efficacy of lung cancer screening in male smokers (aged 45 years or older who smoked at least one pack per day).[69] By 1978, a total of 31,360 patients had been enrolled, and the final results of all three studies were unable to demonstrate a disease-specific mortality reduction.[70]

The introduction of low-radiation-dose spiral computed tomography (LDCT) renewed interest in screening high-risk individuals for early lung cancer.[71] The NCI subsequently funded the National Lung Screening Trial (NLST), which enrolled 53,454 persons at high risk for lung cancer at 33 medical centers between 2002 and 2004. Eligible participants were between 55 and 74 years old, had a smoking history of at least 30 pack-years, and, if former smokers, had quit within the past 15 years and were randomly assigned to undergo three annual screenings with either LDCT or chest radiography. Subjects in the LDCT screening arm demonstrated a 20% reduction in lung cancer-specific mortality (95% CI, 6.8–26.7; $P = 0.004$).[72] The current US Preventive Services Task Force (USPSTF) recommends lung cancer screening with annual LDCT for asymptomatic adults between 55 and 80 years old with at least a 30 pack-year smoking history.[73]

Staging systems

Staging is the determination of the extent of disease, with the intent of grouping patients with similar levels of disease for analytical, therapeutic, and prognostic purposes. The staging of lung cancer provides a scale of relative disease, which can be assigned to all patients with primary lung malignancies. Accurate staging of lung cancer is essential for defining operability, for selecting treatment regimens, for predicting survival, and for reporting comparable end results.

The accuracy of staging depends on available clinical information and relies on preoperative and subsequent evaluations at different times during the course of the disease: clinical-diagnostic staging (c), surgical-evaluative staging (s), postsurgical resection-pathologic staging (p), retreatment staging (r), and autopsy staging (a).

Staging of NSCLC

The current seventh edition of the AJCC and UICC lung cancer staging system was updated in 2009 and is based on 67,725 cases treated from 1990 to 2000, derived from 46 sources in more than 19 countries.[74] This revision further improves the alignment of TNM (tumor, node, and metastasis) stage with prognosis and treatment (Tables 7–9).

Staging of SCLC

When the TNM system was first developed for NSCLC in the 1960s, it was not prognostic when applied to SCLC. This was most likely explained by the very low incidence of stage I or II SCLC and the fact that without chemotherapy, all patients with SCLC had very short survival. In a placebo-controlled trial of cyclophosphamide, the Veterans Administration Lung Group (VALG) developed a two-stage system for SCLC.[76] They separated patients into two groups, termed limited or extensive, based on whether or not their disease could be encompassed by a radiation port. The former group included those with malignant pleural effusion; the latter included all those with metastatic disease to distant sites. This classification was prognostic in patients on both arms of the trial, with median survival rates twice as long in limited stage patients. Through the past 20 years, the "limited" classification has been refined to identify those who are candidates for curative-intent chemoradiation.

As in NSCLC, the process of staging SCLC is key to determining therapy and prognosis. The main goal of thorough staging is to

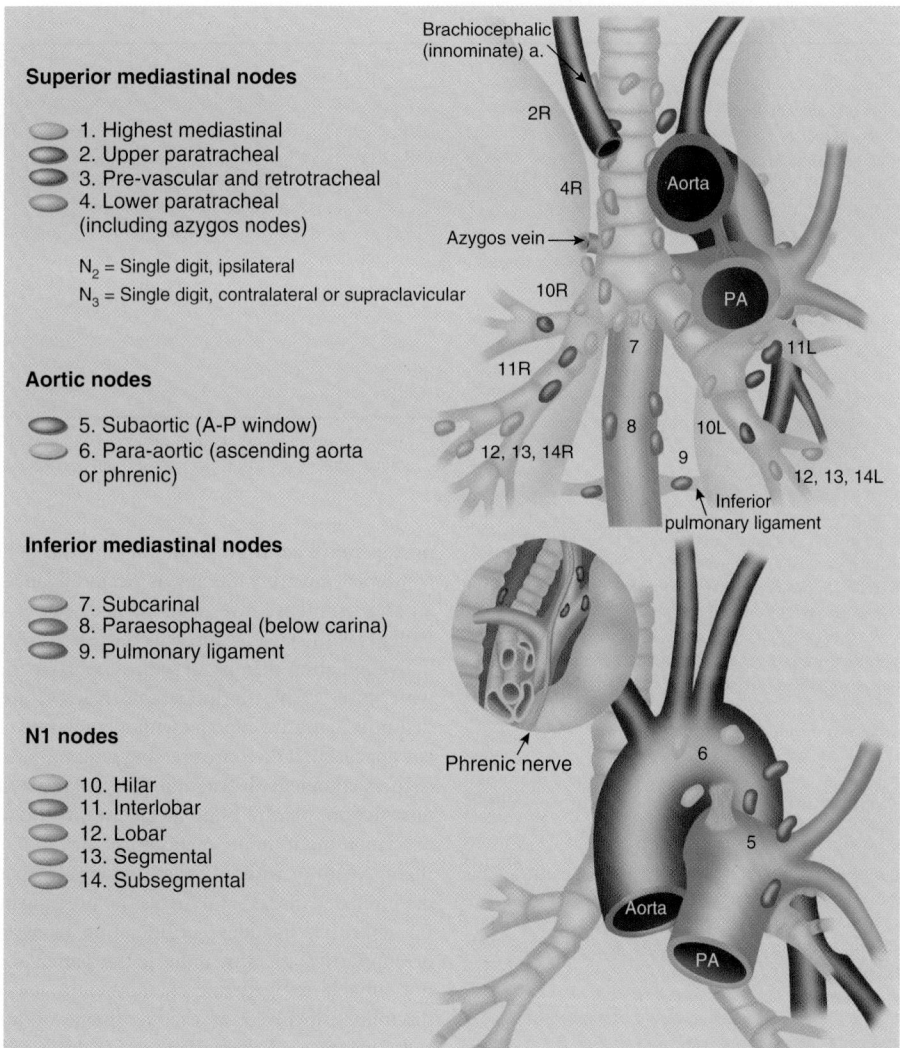

Superior mediastinal nodes

<ovals> 1. Highest mediastinal
2. Upper paratracheal
3. Pre-vascular and retrotracheal
4. Lower paratracheal
(including azygos nodes)

N_2 = Single digit, ipsilateral
N_3 = Single digit, contralateral or supraclavicular

Aortic nodes

5. Subaortic (A-P window)
6. Para-aortic (ascending aorta
or phrenic)

Inferior mediastinal nodes

7. Subcarinal
8. Paraesophageal (below carina)
9. Pulmonary ligament

N1 nodes

10. Hilar
11. Interlobar
12. Lobar
13. Segmental
14. Subsegmental

Brachiocephalic
(innominate) a.
2R
Aorta
4R
Azygos vein
10R
PA
11L
11R
7
8   10L
12, 13, 14R   9   12, 13, 14L
Inferior
pulmonary ligament
Phrenic nerve
6
5
Aorta
PA

Figure 4 Regional lymph node stations for the staging of lung cancer. The location of the lymph nodes and assigned numbers are determined by the surgeon at the time of operation. Source: Adapted from Onishi et al. 2004.[68]

identify patients who are candidates for curative-intent chemoradiation. Patients who have clinically evident metastatic disease (extensive stage) do not require thorough staging for all potential sites of spread. Because the major intent of staging is to determine therapy, the case can be made to image the brain in all patients as positive findings are an indication for eventual brain radiation.

General guidelines for lung cancer staging

Patients who present with a new lung lesion and no evidence of metastatic disease by history, physical examination, or chest radiography should undergo CT scanning of the chest, including the liver and adrenal glands. In some circumstances, when a clinical stage I malignancy is suspected, invasive diagnostic studies can be waived, and the patient can undergo resection for diagnosis and treatment. If a resection beyond a lobectomy is required or if the patient is a high surgical risk, it is best to attempt preoperative diagnosis of the lesion. If the patient requires pneumonectomy, a cancer diagnosis should be made before proceeding with the resection.

Asymptomatic patients who have no abnormal results on physical examination and who are potential surgical candidates with clinical stage I, stage II, or stage IIIAN1 disease can undergo resection. Patients with chest CT scan evidence of metastatic disease, particularly N2 or N3 disease, should undergo invasive studies, which may

include cervical mediastinoscopy. In some instances, FNA can be performed. For patients with potentially resectable stage III disease, the status of the mediastinal lymph nodes is the most important factor in determining therapy. If the lymph nodes are radiographically enlarged (>1 cm in cross-sectional diameter), histologic or cytologic evaluation is necessary before proceeding to thoracotomy.

If a diagnosis of SCLC is made, a thorough search for metastatic disease should be undertaken, followed by appropriate treatment with chemotherapy or chemoradiotherapy. In only 5% of cases can a patient with SCLC be considered for surgical intervention; these are cases of very early-stage disease, without evidence of nodal or metastatic disease.

If the history and physical examination are suggestive of metastatic disease, other noninvasive staging studies directed to the area of concern should be performed. In addition to a chest CT scan, these studies may include a PET/CT scan, a CT scan or MRI of the brain, bone scan, and a CT scan of the abdomen if the CT scan of the chest did not include the liver and adrenal glands.

Approximately 10% of all lung cancer patients have CNS metastases at the time of diagnosis. CNS metastases are more common in patients with SCLC. Occult brain metastases are present in approximately 3–6% of patients with NSCLC. CT scanning of the brain identified a 13% incidence of metastases in patients being evaluated

Table 7 TNM descriptors.

Primary tumor (T)

TX	Primary tumor cannot be assessed, or tumor proven by the presence of malignant cells in sputum or bronchial washings but not visualized by imaging or bronchoscopy
T0	No evidence of primary tumor
Tis	Carcinoma *in situ*
T1	Tumor ≤3 cm in greatest dimension, surrounded by lung or visceral pleura, without bronchoscopic evidence of invasion more proximal than the lobar bronchus[a] (i.e., not in the main bronchus)
	T1a tumor ≤2 cm[a]
	T1b tumor >2 cm but ≤ 3 cm
T2	Tumor >3 cm but ≤7 cm; or tumor with any of the following features:
	• Involves main bronchus, ≥2 cm distal to the carina
	• Invades the visceral pleura
	• Associated with atelectasis or obstructive pneumonitis that extends to the hilar region but does not involve the entire lung
	T2a tumor >3 cm but ≤5 cm
	T2b tumor >5 cm but ≤7 cm
T3	Tumor >7 cm or one that directly invades any of the following: chest wall (including superior sulcus tumors), diaphragm, mediastinal pleura, parietal pericardium; or tumor in the main bronchus, ≤2 cm distal to the carina but without involvement of the carina; or associated atelectasis or obstructive pneumonitis of the entire lung
T4	Tumor of any size that invades any of the following: mediastinum, heart, great vessels, trachea, esophagus, vertebral body, carina; or tumor nodules in a different ipsilateral lobe to that of the primary

Regional lymph nodes (N)

NX	Regional lymph nodes cannot be assessed
N0	No regional lymph node metastasis
N1	Metastasis to ipsilateral peribronchial and/or ipsilateral hilar lymph nodes, and intrapulmonary nodes involved by direct extension of the primary tumor
N2	Metastasis to ipsilateral mediastinal and/or subcarinal lymph node(s)
N3	Metastasis to contralateral mediastinal, contralateral hilar, ipsilateral, or contralateral scalene, or supraclavicular lymph node(s)

Distant metastasis (M)

MX	Presence of distant metastasis cannot be assessed
M0	No distant metastasis
M1	Distant metastasis present
	M1a separate tumor nodule(s) in a contralateral lobe; pleural nodules, or malignant pleural or pericardial effusion[b]
	M1b distant mets

[a]The uncommon superficial tumor of any size with its invasive component limited to the bronchial wall, which may extend proximal to the main bronchus, is also classified T1a.

[b]Most pleural effusions associated with lung cancer are due to tumor. However, there are a few patients in whom multiple cytopathologic examinations of pleural fluid show no tumor. In these cases, the fluid is nonbloody and is not an exudate. When these elements and clinical judgment dictate that the effusion is not related to the tumor, the effusion should be excluded as a staging element, and the patient's disease should be staged M0.

Source: Edge et al. 2010.[75] Reproduced with permission of Springer.

Table 8 Stage grouping in lung cancer: TNM subsets.[a]

Stage	TNM subset
0	Carcinoma *in situ*
IA	T1a–T1b N0 M0
IB	T2a N0 M0
IIA	T1a–T2a N1 M0
	T2b N0 M0
IIB	T2b N1 M0
	T3 N0 M0
IIIA	T1a–T3 N2 M0
	T3 N1 M0
	T4 N0–N1 M0
IIIB	T1a–T4 N3 M0
	T4 N2 M0
IV	Any T, Any N, M1a–M1b

[a]Staging is not relevant for occult carcinoma, designated TX N0 M0.

Source: Edge et al. 2010.[75] Reproduced with permission of Springer.

postoperative adjuvant chemotherapy and radiotherapy. The use of combined-modality therapy in locally advanced stage III NSCLC is an area of intense investigation, as discussed later in this chapter. Patients with stage IV disease are treated with chemotherapy, palliative radiation therapy, or with supportive therapy alone. Patients with unresectable or inoperable NSCLC are evaluated first for definitive, curative therapy with a combined chemoradiation therapy approach. If there are pressing symptomatic needs for palliation, such as complete obstruction of a major airway, hemoptysis, SVC obstruction, painful bony metastases in the weight-bearing areas, or symptomatic brain metastases, the initial treatment is radiotherapy with or without chemotherapy. If a patient has evidence of disseminated disease and there is no pressing need for radiotherapy, the approach includes consideration of systemic chemotherapy, or supportive therapy alone if the patient's general condition is not suitable for systemic chemotherapy. Each of the three main disciplines involved in the treatment of lung cancer—surgery, radiotherapy, and chemotherapy—is discussed individually. SCLC, whose treatment differs from that of NSCLC, is discussed as a separate section, albeit with similar organization.

Surgical treatment

Preoperative assessment

A patient who is considered for pulmonary resection should undergo preoperative evaluation by a thoracic surgeon. Lung cancer treatment outcomes are improved under the care of specialized thoracic surgeons.[80] There are many factors that influence patient selection for pulmonary resection, surgical approach, and the extent of surgical procedure. Known factors associated with increased perioperative morbidity and mortality include age, cigarette use, cardiac disease, restricted pulmonary function, and pneumonectomy. General PS graded by the Eastern Cooperative Oncology Group (ECOG) scale is another commonly quoted indicator of not only perioperative outcomes but also of the ability to tolerate any type of aggressive therapy.[81]

for resection, although only 21% of these were unsuspected by virtue of unremarkable neurologic examination findings. Because of this low incidence of occult brain metastases, particularly in patients with early clinical stages of disease, routine MRI or CT scanning of the brain is not required. MRI is more sensitive than CT scans for identifying and diagnosing asymptomatic metastatic disease to the brain.[77,78]

Therapy for NSCLC

In patients with NSCLC, the most important prognostic factor is tumor stage.[79] Surgery is the standard mode of treatment for patients with stage I and II tumors. Selected patients with stage III tumors may be candidates for surgical resection and may receive either preoperative chemotherapy (or chemoradiotherapy) or

Surgical technique

Conduct of anesthesia

Pulmonary resections are conducted under general anesthesia with selective single-lung ventilation. FOB is generally performed first to ensure the correct placement of an endotracheal tube and to

Table 9 Lymph node map definitions.

Nodal station	Anatomic landmarks
N2 nodes: all N2 nodes lie within the mediastinal pleural envelope	
1. Highest mediastinal nodes	Nodes lying above a horizontal line at the upper rim of the brachiocephalic (left innominate) vein where it ascends to the left, crossing in front of the trachea at its midline
2. Upper paratracheal nodes	Nodes lying above a horizontal line drawn tangential to the upper margin of the aortic arch and below the inferior boundary of No. 1 nodes
3. Prevascular and retrotracheal nodes	Prevascular and retrotracheal nodes may be designated 3A and 3P; midline nodes are considered to be ipsilateral
4. Lower paratracheal nodes	The lower paratracheal nodes on the right lie to the right of the midline of the trachea between a horizontal line drawn tangential to the upper margin of the aortic arch and a line extending across the right main bronchus at the upper margin of the upper lobe bronchus, and contained within the mediastinal pleural envelope; the lower paratracheal nodes on the left lie to the left of the midline of the trachea between a horizontal line drawn tangential to the upper margin of the aortic arch and a line extending across the left main bronchus at the level of the upper margin of the left upper lobe bronchus, medial to the ligamentum arteriosum and contained within the mediastinal pleural envelope. Researchers may wish to designate the lower paratracheal nodes as No. 4s (superior) and No. 4i (inferior) subsets for study purposes; the No. 4s nodes may be defined by a horizontal line extending across the trachea and drawn tangential to the cephalic border of the azygos vein; the No. 4i nodes may be defined by the lower boundary of No. 4s
5. Subaortic (aortopulmonary window)	Subaortic nodes are lateral to the ligamentum arteriosum or the aorta or left pulmonary artery and proximal to the first branch of the left pulmonary artery and lie within the mediastinal pleural envelope
6. Para-aortic nodes (ascending aorta or phrenic)	Nodes lying anterior and lateral to the ascending aorta and the aortic arch or the innominate artery, beneath a line tangential to the upper margin of the aortic arch
7. Subcarinal nodes	Nodes lying caudal to the carina of the trachea, but not associated with the lower lobe bronchi or arteries within the lung
8. Paraesophageal nodes (below carina)	Nodes lying adjacent to the wall of the esophagus and to the right or left of the midline, excluding subcarinal nodes
9. Pulmonary ligament nodes	Nodes lying within the pulmonary ligament, including those in the posterior wall and lower part of the inferior pulmonary vein
N1 nodes: all N1 nodes lie distal to the mediastinal pleural reflection and within the visceral pleura	
10. Hilar nodes	The proximal lobar nodes, distal to the mediastinal pleural reflection and the nodes adjacent to the bronchus intermedius on the right; radiographically, the hilar shadow may be created by enlargement of both hilar and interlobar nodes
11. Interlobar nodes	Nodes lying between the lobar bronchi
12. Lobar nodes	Nodes adjacent to the distal lobar bronchi
13. Segmental nodes	Nodes adjacent to the segmental bronchi
14. Subsegmental nodes	Nodes around the subsegmental bronchi

examine airways for the presence and extent of endobronchial disease or unexpected lesions.

Incisions

Several approaches and surgical techniques are used for the resection of pulmonary tumors. The decision about the approach and technique is based on the tumor size, location, and the relationship to other intrathoracic structures; patient's comorbidities and surgeon's experience are also taken into account. Options for surgical techniques include traditional open thoracotomy approach, video-assisted thoracic surgery (VATS), or robotic-assisted thoracic surgery (RATS).

Posterolateral thoracotomy with or without division of the latissimus dorsi muscle generally permits the best overall exposure to the pleural cavity and allows direct palpation of all structures within the hemithorax. Median sternotomy or clamshell incision can be used for resections of tumors located in the upper lobes or in cases of bilateral disease when exploration of both thoracic cavities is desired.

VATS has become a well-established tool in the armamentarium of thoracic surgeons.[82] Multiple investigators have shown the ability to perform anatomic lobectomies and even pneumonectomies using a VATS approach. There are sufficient data that the postoperative recovery is greatly shortened compared to standard rib spreading techniques. Other advantages include decreased postoperative air leaks, pneumonia, atrial fibrillation, length of stay, and mortality. These advantages have led some investigators to hypothesize that better tolerance of adjuvant chemotherapy will be seen following thoracoscopic lobectomy compared to open thoracotomy thus resulting in improved overall survival (OS). These claims have not been substantiated in an RCT.

The advent of robotic technology and RATS has further amplified the argument for performance of pulmonary resections without thoracotomy and rib spreading, and early outcomes of RATS lobectomy appear promising.[83] The cost of robotic technology is presently relatively high and it remains to be seen whether there is a demonstrable benefit of this technique over traditional VAT surgery.

Standard surgical procedures

Pneumonectomy, removal of the entire lung, is indicated for tumors that cannot be completely resected with a lesser procedure due to their central location and involvement of mainstem bronchus of main pulmonary artery, or due to transfissure involvement of multiple lobes. Adequate exposure for this procedure is generally obtained via posterolateral thoracotomy. Perioperative mortality after pneumonectomy is approximately 5%, with a range between 2% and 26% in some studies after neoadjuvant chemoradiation for locoregionally advanced disease. Right-sided pneumonectomy is regarded as the highest risk pulmonary procedure. Cardiopulmonary complications (pneumonia, acute respiratory distress syndrome, atelectasis, aspiration, atrial fibrillation, and myocardial infarction) are the most frequent morbidities associated with pulmonary resection and occur in approximately 20–30% of patients.[84–87]

Lobectomy is the most common type of resection performed for lung cancer. It is regarded as an oncologic standard for the

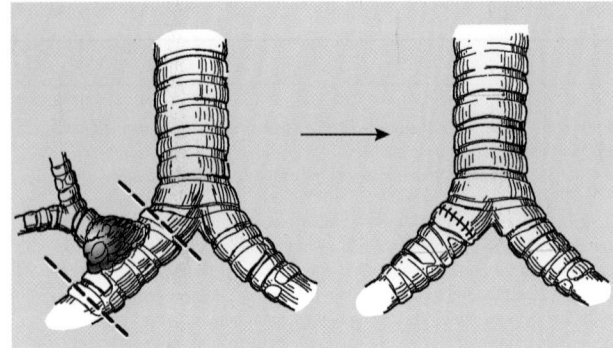

Figure 5 A standard right upper lobectomy cannot be performed in this circumstance because residual tumor will remain in the bronchial stump. Rather than performing a pneumonectomy, a sleeve lobectomy is performed to ensure negative margins while still preserving the right middle and lower lobes.

removal of lung cancer, as it extirpates the primary tumor with its lymphatic basins while sparing remaining functional lung parenchyma. Importantly, cancer survival is equivalent for patients undergoing lobectomy or pneumonectomy for all stages of disease when a complete resection is performed. Lobectomy requires isolation, ligation, and division of the individual arterial, venous, and bronchial branches supplying the lobe, along with the division of the interlobar fissure. Tumors that are close to the origin of a lobar bronchus require bronchial sleeve resection to obtain negative margin; this procedure spares functional lung parenchyma without compromising oncologic outcome (Figure 5). In selected patients, bronchial sleeve resection has proven to be a safe and effective method for pulmonary preservation, with cancer survival rates comparable to those following pneumonectomy.[88]

Sublobar resections refer to segmentectomy, wedge resection, and lumpectomy. Lung segments are distinct anatomic regions supplied by a named artery, vein, and bronchus; although parenchymal boarders of lung segments are not clearly visible. Each segment contributes approximately 5–6% of lung function so the loss of functional parenchyma is much less than with lobectomy. After isolation of bronchovascular structures, lung parenchyma of a given segment or segments is divided with a stapler. Segmentectomy is indicated in patients whose pulmonary function precludes lobar resection or in patients with tumors <2 cm in size. Whether segmentectomy is equivalent to lobectomy for T1A tumors is unclear, and this question is being addressed in two ongoing RCTs.

Wedge excision, in contrast, is performed without identifying bronchovascular anatomic landmarks. It is a simple and quick procedure for peripheral lesions. A stapling device is used to remove the lesion. The aim is to achieve a margin of normal tissue at least the same size as the tumor. Lesions that reside more deeply within the pulmonary tissue may be removed by precise local excision with laser or electrocautery assistance (lumpectomy). The pulmonary tissue is directly incised and the lesion is removed, with preservation of the surrounding lung. This technique is more applicable for benign lesions, or selected resection of metastases rather than lung cancer.

Positive margins (bronchial and parenchymal)

At the time of resection, the bronchial margin should be assessed by frozen section to ensure a complete resection. If the margin contains evidence of disease, all reasonable attempts to achieve a negative margin should be undertaken to minimize the risk of local recurrence. Several studies have shown that reasonable survival rates

can be achieved in the face of a positive bronchial margin. When microscopic disease or CIS exists within the mucosa, 5-year survival rate can approach 24%.[89] Shields and colleagues[90] also showed a reasonable survival rate in patients with carcinoma in the bronchial mucosa. In this cohort of patients, however, survival was poor when disease was present outside of the bronchial mucosa or within the peribronchial lymphatics, a finding similar to those of other studies.[89,91]

Radiotherapy

Radiation therapy for lung cancer has changed rapidly in the past decade. Our ability to define target volumes and avoid normal structures has been aided by advancements in four-dimensional (4D) CT technology and in FDG-PET scanning. It is now possible, moreover, to measure and account for individual variations in respiratory tumor motion. Treatment-planning algorithms can account for tissue heterogeneity and motion, which can improve dose distributions to target volumes. Three-dimensional conformal radiotherapy (3D CRT) is routinely achieved by using International Commission on Radiation Units and Measurements (ICRU) definitions of volumes and doses. Intensity-modulated radiotherapy (IMRT), including volumetric intensity-modulated arc therapy (VMAT) and stereotactic ablative radiotherapy (SABR), has been implemented clinically, and proton therapy has become a reality. We also look forward to the rational integration of new biologic therapies, including biomarker and pathway-targeted therapy and immunotherapy, into standard treatment.

More than 60% of lung cancer patients will receive radiotherapy at some point in their disease, 45% for initial treatment, and 17% for palliation.[92] This means that over 100,000 US patients with lung cancer are irradiated yearly. Experienced teams are required to manage the care of these patients optimally, particularly when combined-modality therapy is used; outcomes are demonstrably better when patients are treated by experienced personnel.[93,94]

Radiation treatment techniques and volumes for lung cancer

The ICRU has defined several important volumes for the modern treatment of lung cancer: gross tumor volume (GTV), clinical target volume (CTV), planning target volume (PTV), and internal target volume (ITV).

Gross tumor volume

GTV is defined as visible tumor by any imaging modality. FDG-PET scanning is important for radiation treatment planning.[95] It reduces interobserver differences in GTV contouring[96] and helps to categorize suspect mediastinal/hilar lymphadenopathy as either benign or malignant; higher standardized uptake values (SUVs) are predictive of metastatic disease and local failure. It also helps to identify tumors within an atelectatic lobe and thereby decrease the amount of normal lung irradiated. Finally, because FDG-PET scans detect distant metastases in about 30% of patients with NSCLC (particularly those with otherwise advanced disease), it can help significantly with patient triage.[97]

Clinical target volume

CTV is defined as the volume that is likely to contain gross and microscopic disease. To include the tumor within the CTV with 95% accuracy requires GTV to CTV expansions of 6 mm for squamous cancers and 8 mm for adenocarcinomas.[98] Expansions for other histologic types have not been determined, but a conservative approach would be to use 8 mm. Appropriate CTV for the mediastinum has not been rigorously determined. We empirically use

8-mm expansions around involved nodes (either gross involvement or FDG-PET positivity). Clinical editing of the CTV margin is needed to take anatomical boundaries and pattern of failure into consideration.

Planning target volume

PTV is defined as CTV with a margin to account for daily setup error and target motion. PTV takes setup uncertainty and motion into account. Setup uncertainty is likely both technique dependent and institution dependent and should be measured individually for each technique.

Accounting for respiratory-dependent tumor motion is similarly challenging and can be approached in several ways. It is clear, however, that two-dimensional (2D) measurement of tumor motion (e.g., fluoroscopy) is inadequate. Such motion is unpredictable and is independent of tumor size, location, and PFT (pulmonary function test) results.[99] Tumor motion should be assessed individually based on each patient's disease status, breath pattern, and other clinical conditions. 4D CT imaging showed that approximately 40% of lung cancers move more than 5 mm and 10% of lung cancers move more than 10 mm during the respiration. For patients with tumors moving <5 mm, simple expansion along the axis of motion is adequate. For patients with tumors moving more than 5 mm, particularly more than 10 mm, the treatment machine can be gated with respiration, the patient can use an assisted breath-hold technique, or an ITV-based approach can be used.

Internal target volume

ITV is an expansion of CTV in which target motion is explicitly measured and taken into account as defined by ICRU62. By using technologies such as multislice detectors and faster imaging reconstruction, we can image patients during real-time breathing and assess organ motion using 4D CT.[100] To determine the ITV from the 4D CT images, the tumor volume outlined on expiratory phase of the 4D images is registered on other phases of the images to create a union of target contours enclosing all possible positions of the target. The same principle can be applied to the images acquired with inspiration and expiration breath holds. Attention should be paid to irregular breathing and variation of breathing patterns over the course of the treatment and the effects of such on the ITV margin. Even with 4D CT, the free-breathing ITV is only a snapshot and a single stochastic sampling of the patient breathing during the 4D CT acquisitions. Thus, the true ITV margin should be enlarged on the basis of the uncertainty of patient's breathing during the treatment course.

Intensity-modulated radiation therapy (IMRT)

IMRT, including VMAT, can improve dose conformality and allow integrated dose escalation and dose "painting" within the PTV. Collectively, this leads to the delivery of higher radiation doses to high-risk areas of the tumor such as gross tumor, hypoxic areas, or areas showing high SUVs on PET–CT without increasing the number of treatment fractions and while minimizing exposure to normal tissues.[101,102] However, the application of IMRT to lung cancer has been delayed because of concerns that IMRT may deliver low yet damaging doses to larger volumes of normal lung tissue. Moreover, the possible movement of a tumor due to respiration introduces another level of complexity to both the IMRT dosimetry and the technique used.

Although IMRT may be effective in reducing normal tissue toxicity and improving tumor coverage, its high-dose gradient and conformity require a high level of precision in dose delivery and tumor localization. In the meantime, the complexity introduced by

tumor motion must be recognized when using IMRT. Unlike 3D CRT, IMRT treats only a portion of the target volume at a particular time. Concern has been expressed as to whether target motion and collimator motion during IMRT delivery have a significant interplay effect, thus degrading the planned dose distributions. For IMRT to be feasible and more effective in treating NSCLC, motion reduction techniques should be explored further, such as breath holding and tumor tracking. Our clinical data indicate that IMRT may reduce toxic effects in normal tissue in selected cases and allow further dose escalation.[103] When used appropriately, IMRT is the preferred radiotherapy modality for dose-escalated radiotherapy in lung cancer.[104]

Stereotactic ablative radiotherapy (SABR)

SABR, also called stereotactic body radiation therapy (SBRT), allows precise targeting and delivery of high doses of radiation therapy in <2 weeks. SABR for lung cancer uses elements of 3D CRT or IMRT/VMAT, incorporates a variety of systems for taking tumor motion into consideration, and decreases setup uncertainty by using image-guided radiotherapy techniques. Use of SABR reduces treatment volumes, facilitating hypofractionation with markedly increased daily doses (>10 Gy) and significant reduction in overall treatment times. The combination of multiple beam angles or arc therapy to achieve sharp dose gradients, high-precision localization, and a high dose per fraction in extracranial locations is referred to as SABR. This approach delivers a high biological effective dose (BED) to the target while minimizing toxic effects to normal tissues, which may improve local control and survival rates.

Onishi et al.[68] reported on the use of SABR for stage I NSCLC in their retrospective evaluation of results from a Japanese multi-institutional study. Patients with stage I NSCLC ($n = 245$; median age, 76 years; T1 N0 M0, $n = 155$; T2 N0 M0, $n = 90$) were treated with hypofractionated high-dose SABR. Stereotactic 3D treatment was delivered with noncoplanar dynamic arcs or multiple static ports. A total dose of 18–75 Gy at the isocenter was administered in 1–22 fractions. The median calculated BED was 108 Gy (range, 57–180 Gy). During follow-up (median, 24 months; range, 7–78 months), pulmonary complications of grade 2 or higher (according to the NCI's common terminology criteria) were observed in only six patients (2.4%). Local progression occurred in 33 patients (14.5%), and the local recurrence rates were 8.1% for patients with a BED = 100 Gy and 26.4% for those with a BED < 100 Gy ($p < .05$). The 3-year OS rates for medically operable patients were 88.4% for those with BED = 100 Gy and 69.4% for those with <100 Gy ($p < .05$). This analysis showed that hypofractionated high-dose SABR with BED < 150 Gy was feasible and beneficial for curative treatment of patients with stage I NSCLC. For all treatment methods and schedules, local control and survival rates were better when the BED was 100 Gy than when it was less. Survival rates in selected patients (medically operable, BED = 100 Gy) were excellent and were potentially comparable to those of surgery.

The treatment of more than 2000 patients with imaging-guided SABR (4D CT simulation and daily CT-on-rails for tumor localization and setup accuracy) at doses of 50 Gy delivered in four fractions (daily treatment for 4 days) or 70 Gy in 10 fractions was associated with local control rates at the primary site of higher than 95% with minimal toxicity, even for centrally located lesions when normal tissue dose constraints were respected.[105]

Proton therapy

The proton is a charged particle that, compared with the photon, possesses a well-defined range of penetration determined by both the beam's energy and the density of the tissue through which it passes. As the proton beam penetrates the body, the particles slow down and deposit the dose sharply near the end of its range, a phenomenon known as the Bragg peak. By modulating the Bragg peak across the target volume, proton beams can deliver a full, localized, uniform dose of energy to the treatment site while sparing the surrounding normal tissues. This therapy is ideal when organ preservation is paramount, such as in lung cancer. Clinical data using escalated/accelerated proton radiotherapy showed promising results comparable to those of surgical resection in stage IA cases.[106,107] The accuracy of target delineation and tumor motion consideration is critical for both proton and photon treatments. Proton treatment is more sensitive than photon therapy to anatomical motion, position uncertainties, and tissue inhomogeneity.[108]

Primary radiation therapy for stage I and II NSCLC

Patients who have surgically resectable NSCLC but are medically inoperable or who decline surgery should be considered for curative radiotherapy. Primary radiotherapy for early-stage NSCLC is considered standard treatment, and several studies have reported a benefit from dose escalation with regard to survival and local control in early-stage NSCLC.[109-112] Because early-stage NSCLC is not inherently a systemic disease at diagnosis, and as local control is poor after conventional radiotherapy, research measures aimed at improving survival should put significant emphasis on improving local tumor obliteration.

It should be kept in mind that lung cancer in such patients is always staged clinically, which makes comparison with surgically treated patients difficult. Several surgical series demonstrate a 24–37% upstaging of cT1–T2 N0 disease, which partially explains the poorer results seen in clinically staged irradiated patients.[113] As better screening tools for early-stage NSCLC are developed, however, the number of patients with small but medically inoperable tumors will increase.[71]

Postoperative radiotherapy (PORT)

PORT (postoperative radiotherapy) is currently contraindicated for patients with stage I completely resected disease on the basis of the PORT meta-analysis.[114] Data for stage II and higher disease neither support nor refute the use of PORT (because the hazard ratio error bars include 1.0), although it clearly improves regional control.

The use of PORT for stage II and III NSCLC was first tested in a controlled trial by the Lung Cancer Study Group, which randomized 210 patients to receive either 50 Gy in 25 fractions or no treatment.[115] Local recurrence rate was significantly reduced (3% vs 41%), but there was no effect on OS or disease-free survival (DFS) because of the high rate of distant failure. However, recent data from subgroup analyses of a phase III RCT examining surgical resection with/without adjuvant chemotherapy [ANITA (Adjuvant Navelbine International Trialist Association) trial] indicated that PORT may improve OS in patients with N2 disease.

In patients with resectable or marginally resectable NSCLC, 5-year survival rates and collective results of surgery alone for stage III (N2) ranged from 14% to 30%. Many patients who have clinical N0 disease are found to have occult mediastinal lymph node metastases. Approximately 15% of patients with resected T1 tumors have N2 disease, and 40–45% of patients with T2–T3 tumors will have N2 disease. Patients with incomplete resection, including positive margins, multiple levels of lymph node involvement, extracapsular extension, and N2 disease usually have poor local control, and PORT is usually indicated.

Preoperative chemotherapy and chemoradiotherapy

If N2 disease is bulky and the potential for complete resection is questionable, patients can be treated by neoadjuvant chemotherapy followed by surgery. Increasing numbers of patients with stage III disease undergo induction chemotherapy followed by surgery, based on the work of Rosell et al.[116] and Roth et al.[117] Findings from a phase II trial conducted by the Southwest Oncology Group (SWOG) found that concurrent induction chemoradiotherapy with etoposide and cisplatin (EP) in 74 patients with biopsy proven stage IIIA (N2) NSCLC may improve patient survival with reasonable toxicity.[118] Following this, the NCI launched a phase III multicenter for patients with biopsy-proven N2 disease and potentially resectable NSCLC (NCI Protocol INT 139). Patients were stratified by PS and T status and were randomized to receive induction chemoradiotherapy followed by surgery or chemotherapy with definitive radiotherapy. Results showed no differences in OS but better progression-free survival (PFS) in the group treated with surgery. Subgroup analysis revealed better survival for patients who underwent a lobectomy ($p = .002$). However, trimodality therapy was not optimal when a pneumonectomy was required owing to the high mortality risk. Finally, N0 status at surgery significantly predicted a higher 5-year survival rate. The study concluded that chemotherapy plus radiotherapy with or without resection (preferably lobectomy) are options for patients with stage IIIA (N2) NSCLC. Surgical resection after chemoradiation can be considered for fit patients if lobectomy is feasible.[119]

Radiation therapy for unresectable stage III NSCLC

For patients with unresectable stage III NSCLC, conventional radiotherapy alone resulted in a median survival time of 10 months and a 5-year survival rate of 5%. To improve outcomes, chemotherapy was added to radiotherapy. Chemotherapy and radiotherapy can be delivered sequentially or concurrently. The most well-known trial, reported by the Cancer and Leukemia Group B (CALGB), compared standard radiotherapy to 60 Gy to sequential cisplatin and vinblastine chemotherapy for two cycles followed by radiotherapy to 60 Gy. Median survival times and 5-year survival rates were superior for the chemoradiotherapy arm (13.8 months vs 9.7 months, 19% vs 7%, respectively).[120]

The RTOG subsequently conducted a three-arm trial (RTOG 88-08) comparing standard radiotherapy, sequential chemoradiotherapy (CALGB regimen), and 69.6-Gy hyperfractionated radiotherapy. Sequential chemoradiotherapy was statistically superior to standard and hyperfractionated radiotherapy.[121]

Schaake-Koning et al.[122] compared radiotherapy alone with radiotherapy plus daily cisplatin or weekly cisplatin. There was no difference in distant failure rates between the groups with or without cisplatin. However, the survival rate in the radiotherapy-plus-cisplatin group was 54% at 1 year, 26% at 2 years, and 16% at 3 years, compared with 46%, 13%, and 2% in the radiotherapy-alone group ($p = .009$). Therefore, this study showed that a gain in local tumor control seems to have translated into increased survival time.

Furuse and colleagues compared patients receiving two cycles of mitomycin, vindesine, and cisplatin given every 28 days concurrent with split-course radiotherapy (total dose of 56 Gy) with patients receiving two cycles of mitomycin, vindesine, and cisplatin followed by continuous radiotherapy (total dose of 56 Gy). The concurrent treatment yielded an improved 5-year survival rate compared with the sequential treatment.[123]

The RTOG conducted a three-arm RCT (RTOG 9410) to analyze whether the concurrent delivery of cisplatin-based chemotherapy with thoracic radiotherapy (TRT) improves survival compared with the sequential delivery of these therapies for patients with locally advanced, unresected stage II–III NSCLC. The sequential therapy consisted of cisplatin and vinblastine followed by 60 Gy of radiation. The concurrent treatment used the same chemotherapy with 60 Gy of radiation beginning on day 1 of chemotherapy. The third treatment was concurrent cisplatin and oral etoposide with 69.6 Gy of radiation in 1.2-Gy BID fractions beginning on day 1. RTOG 9410 demonstrated that the concurrent delivery of cisplatin-based chemotherapy with TRT conferred a greater long-term survival benefit than did the sequential delivery of these therapies.[124]

A third RCT comparing concurrent with sequential chemoradiotherapy also explored the use of consolidation chemotherapy.[125] In this phase III trial, patients were assigned to receive two cycles of cisplatin plus vinorelbine followed by 66 Gy of radiation or cisplatin/etoposide and concurrent radiation to 66 Gy followed by two cycles of consolidation chemotherapy with cisplatin and vinorelbine. Local control rates were improved with the concurrent regimen (40% vs 24%), and the median survival times and 4-year survival rates were numerically superior (but not statistically superior) in the concurrent arm of the trial (16.3 months vs 14.5 months and 21% vs 14%, respectively). However, the incidence of grade 3 esophagitis was significantly higher in the concurrent arm (32% vs 3%), and the toxic effects-related death rates were high in both arms (9.5% in the concurrent arm and 5.6% in the sequential arm).

These three phase III trials consistently demonstrated longer survival times for patients receiving concurrent chemoradiotherapy, and this difference was significant in two of the three trials. On the basis of these results, concurrent chemoradiotherapy has been the standard of care since 2001. It is important to note that toxic effects are significantly more common with concurrent chemoradiotherapy than with sequential chemoradiotherapy.

In RTOG 9410, the locoregional failure rate after concurrent chemoradiotherapy was still 34–43%. To improve the local control rate, three groups [RTOG, North Central Cancer Treatment Group (NCCTG), and the University of North Carolina (UNC)] have separately performed radiation dose-escalation trials for patients with inoperable stage III NSCLC and reported results supporting the safety of 74 Gy. UNC conducted a phase I/II dose-escalation clinical trial using high-dose 3D CRT (60–74 Gy) for inoperable stage IIIA/IIIB NSCLC with induction chemotherapy followed by concurrent chemoradiotherapy.[126] They reported a 3-year survival rate of 36% and a 13% locoregional relapse rate as the only site of failure. For patients who finished radiotherapy, the 3-year survival rate was 45%.

RTOG conducted a phase III study to compare conventional-dose (60 Gy) with escalated-dose (74 Gy) radiotherapy concurrently with weekly paclitaxel and carboplatin, with or without cetuximab, an antibody against EGFR, for patients with stage IIIA or IIIB NSCLC. Surprisingly, early analyses showed no improvement in OS with the higher radiation dose.[127] In fact, the high-dose arm had worse survival rates and greater toxicity. It is possible that 74 Gy is too toxic when delivered by the photon-based radiation technologies used in this trial. Further, the addition of cetuximab did not improve survival either.

Randomized trials have failed to identify an optimal concurrent chemotherapy doublet regimen. Several commonly used options include platinum (cisplatin or carboplatin) in combination with etoposide, paclitaxel, and pemetrexed.[128–130]

Systemic therapy for incurable, advanced-stage NSCLC

For patients with stage IV NSCLC, or those with recurrent disease, which is not amenable to curative surgery or radiotherapy, the goals of systemic therapy are to palliate symptoms and prolong survival. In a meta-analysis of 2714 patients enrolled into 16 RCTs comparing chemotherapy to best supportive care (BSC), there was a significant benefit from chemotherapy with increased median OS from 4.5 to 6 months and 1-year OS from 20% to 29% (HR 0.77; 95% CI 0.71–0.83, $P < 0.0001$).[131] Most trials included platinum-based doublets, which were the only chemotherapy regimens associated with a statistically significant improvement in OS.

First-line chemotherapy

Three large RCTs compared platinum-doublet to single-agent non-platinum chemotherapy. The Swedish Lung Cancer Study Group randomized 334 patients with advanced NSCLC to gemcitabine plus cisplatin or as single agent.[132] The platinum-doublet arm was associated with a significant improvement in overall response rate (30% vs 11%), median OS (10 months vs 8.6 months), and 1-year OS (40% vs 32%). Georgoulias et al.[133] compared docetaxel with cisplatin as single agent in 324 patients. Although the response rates were significantly higher in the combination arm (36% vs 22%), there were no significant differences in median OS (10.5 months vs 8 months) or 1-year OS (44% vs 43%). Similar results were observed in the CALGB 9730 study with 561 patients, where the combination of carboplatin plus paclitaxel was associated with increased response rates (30% vs 17%) but the median OS (8.8 months vs 6.7 months) and 1-year OS (37% vs 32%) did not reach statistical significance.[134] In contrast, two large studies showed a significant improvement in overall response rates, median OS, and 1-year OS for cisplatin doublets, using either gemcitabine or vinorelbine, compared to cisplatin alone.[135,136] Three large meta-analyses comparing platinum doublets to single-agent chemotherapy showed increased response rates and OS for doublets.[137–139] The addition of a third drug to the platinum regimen was associated with increased response rates but no improvement in OS.[137] With these data, the American Society of Clinical Oncology guidelines from 2009 recommended a platinum-based doublet as the initial treatment for patients with advanced NSCLC and ECOG PS of 0 or 1.[140]

Multiple studies showed either no significant differences or a small improvement for a particular chemotherapy combination.[141–143] In a large RCT, 1725 patients with previously untreated advanced-stage NSCLC were randomized to cisplatin plus gemcitabine or pemetrexed.[144] Similar to most previous studies comparing platinum-based doublets, there were no significant differences in median PFS or median OS. Nevertheless, this was the first study to show differences in outcomes for chemotherapy according to histology, with cisplatin plus pemetrexed associated with increased median OS in nonsquamous tumors (11.8 months vs 10.4 months, HR 0.84, $P = 0.005$) but not in squamous tumors (9.4 months vs 10.8 months, HR 1.23, P 0.05). Histology also played a role in a phase III trial comparing carboplatin plus paclitaxel or nab-paclitaxel in 1052 patients.[145] This study showed increased response rates (33% vs 25%, $P = 0.05$) but similar median PFS and OS. The improvement in response rates was observed only in patients with squamous-cell histology (41% vs 24%, $P < 0.001$), with nearly identical responses in adenocarcinoma (26% vs 27%).

As carboplatin has a similar mechanism of action compared to cisplatin, two meta-analyses examined whether it would have equivalent efficacy in NSCLC. One meta-analysis included 2948 patients from eight RCTs, while the other included 2968 patients from nine RCTs. Although treatment with cisplatin-based doublets demonstrated longer OS, the results did not reach statistical significance.[146,147] In subset analyses, cisplatin doublets were associated with improved OS in patients with stage IIIB, nonsquamous histology and in those treated with third-generation chemotherapy including paclitaxel, docetaxel, and gemcitabine. Carboplatin was associated with increased incidence of thrombocytopenia whereas cisplatin was associated with increased risk of nausea, vomiting, and nephrotoxicity. Therefore, despite the superiority of cisplatin-based doublets, the small improvement in OS and increased toxicity compared to carboplatin led to the acceptance of both platinum drugs in a population of incurable patients treated with palliative intent.

Monoclonal antibodies

Bevacizumab
Bevacizumab is a recombinant humanized antibody against circulating vascular endothelial growth factor (VEGF). In a phase II study comparing first-line carboplatin plus paclitaxel with or without bevacizumab in patients with advanced NSCLC, treatment with bevacizumab was associated with increased response rates and median OS.[148] Six patients experienced life-threatening bleeding of which four were fatal. All six patients had centrally located tumors, five had cavitation in the tumor either at baseline or after treatment with bevacizumab, and four patients had squamous-cell histology. The ECOG 4599 trial randomized 878 patients with recurrent or advanced NSCLC with predominantly nonsquamous histology, hemoptysis of less than half teaspoon per event, and no brain metastases, to carboplatin plus paclitaxel with or without bevacizumab.[149] The bevacizumab arm was associated with increased response rates (35% vs 15%, $P < 0.001$), PFS (6.2 months vs 4.5 months, HR 0.66, $P < 0.001$), and median OS (12.3 months vs 10.3 months, HR 0.79, $P = 0.003$). The addition of bevacizumab increased the incidence of neutropenia, neutropenic fever, thrombocytopenia, hypertension, proteinuria, and bleeding. The avastin in lung cancer (AVAiL) trial randomized 1043 patients to cisplatin plus gemcitabine alone or in combination with either low-dose (7.5 mg/kg) or high-dose bevacizumab (15 mg/kg).[150] The low-dose and high-dose bevacizumab arms demonstrated higher response rates (34.1% vs 30.4% vs 20.1%, $P = 0.003$), but there were no significant differences in median OS.[151]

Ramucirumab
Ramucirumab is a human monoclonal antibody against VEGF receptor 2. In a randomized trial comparing platinum plus pemetrexed with or without ramucirumab in 130 patients with previously untreated advanced-stage NSCLC, the addition of ramucirumab was associated with a nonsignificant increase in response rates (49.3% vs 38%, $P = 0.18$) and median PFS (7.2 months vs 5.6 months, HR 0.75, $P = 0.13$).[152]

Cetuximab
Cetuximab is a chimeric monoclonal antibody against EGFR. The addition of cetuximab to chemotherapy was evaluated in two large RCTs. In BMS099, 676 previously untreated patients with advanced-stage NSCLC were randomized to chemotherapy (platinum combined with paclitaxel or docetaxel) with or without cetuximab.[153] Although the cetuximab arm was associated with increased response rates (25.7% vs 17.2%, $P = 0.007$), PFS and OS were not significantly improved. In the first-line erbitux (FLEX) trial, 1125 patients were randomized to cisplatin plus vinorelbine alone or in combination with cetuximab.[154] The cetuximab arm was

associated with improved response rates (36% vs 19%, $P = 0.01$) but not median PFS (4.8 months for both arms). Nevertheless, the median OS was significantly increased in patients treated with cetuximab (11.3 months vs 10.1 months, HR 0.87, 95% CI 0.76–0.99, $P = 0.04$). Further analyses of the FLEX study showed that the benefit from the addition of cetuximab was seen only in patients with IHC H-score (calculated as the percentage of cells scoring weekly for EGFR X 1, plus percentage of cell scoring moderately X 2, plus percentage of cells scored strongly X 3, with the total ranging from 0 to 300) above 200 with a median OS of 12.2 months compared to 9.6 months in patients treated with chemotherapy alone.[155]

Duration of chemotherapy
Patients with advanced NSCLC who achieve clinical benefit, defined as the absence of progressive disease (PD), and tolerate treatment without major toxicities, should receive no more than four to six cycles of platinum-based therapy. Clinical trials comparing three to four cycles of chemotherapy to six cycles of continuation of therapy until tumor progression showed no benefit from more prolonged therapy.[156–158]

Maintenance therapy
Additional treatment after four to six cycles of platinum-based chemotherapy in patients without tumor progression is termed maintenance therapy. The main types of maintenance therapy include continuation of the nonplatinum drug alone, continuation of the monoclonal antibody alone, and switch therapy where a different nonplatinum drug is used. Several trials have evaluated the role of maintenance therapy in patients without tumor progression after four to six cycles of chemotherapy (Table 10).[164–168] These trials were restricted to patients with nonsquamous histology where the two main drugs used during the maintenance phase, pemetrexed and bevacizumab, are more effective and safer, respectively. The median OS was improved for maintenance pemetrexed compared to observation and the role of bevacizumab, either alone or in combination with pemetrexed, remains unclear.

Second-line chemotherapy
The benefit from second-line chemotherapy has been established by two randomized trials using docetaxel. In the TAX 320 study, 373 previously treated patients were randomized to docetaxel or a control regimen of ifosfamide or vinorelbine.[169] Docetaxel was administered as either 100 mg/m^2 (D100) or 75 mg/m^2 (D75) every 3 weeks. Response rates for D100, D75, and control arms were 10.8%, 6.7%, and 0.8%, respectively. The 1-year OS was significantly higher in the D75 arm compared to the control therapy (32% vs 19%, $P = 0.025$) but not in the D100 arm. Prior use of paclitaxel did not have an impact on the response or survival. The second trial had a similar design and randomized 203 previously treated patients with advanced NSCLC not previously exposed to paclitaxel, to docetaxel (D75 or D100) or BSC.[170] Similar to the TAX 320 study, D75 was associated with improved 1-year OS compared to D100 and BSC (37% vs 19% vs 19%) and less toxicity compared to D100. The second approved chemotherapy drug in the second-line setting was pemetrexed. A large RCT compared docetaxel 75 mg/m^2 to pemetrexed 500 mg/m^2, both administered every 3 weeks. Response rates and median PFS were similar, and there were no significant differences in median OS (8.3 months for pemetrexed vs 7.9 months for docetaxel) or 1-year OS.[171] Patients treated with docetaxel were more likely to have grade 3 or 4 neutropenia, febrile neutropenia, and alopecia compared to

Table 10 Maintenance chemotherapy.

Trial	Induction	Maintenance	PFS (months)	OS (months)
JMEN[159]	Platinum doublet	Pem versus Obs	4 versus 2 ($P < 0.001$)	13.4 versus 10.6 ($P = 0.01$)
PARAMOUNT[160]	CisPem	Pem versus Obs	4.4 versus 2.8 ($P < 0.01$)	16.9 versus 14 ($P = 0.01$)
AVAPERL[161]	CisPemBev	PemBev versus Bev	7.4 versus 3.7 ($P < 0.001$)	17.1 versus 13.1 ($P = 0.29$)
PRONOUNCE[162]	CarbPem	Pem	4.4 versus 5.5 ($P = 0.6$)	10.5 versus 11.7 ($P = 0.06$)
	CarbPacBev	Bev		
PointBreak[163]	CarbPemBev	PemBev	6 versus 5.6 ($P = 0.01$)	12.6 versus 13.4 ($P = 0.9$)
	CarbPacBev	Bev		
ECOG 5508	CarbPemBev	PemBev	Pending	Pending
		Pem		
		Bev		

Bev, bevacizumab; Carb, carboplatin; Cis, cisplatin; Pem, pemetrexed; Pac, paclitaxel; NR, not reached; Obs, observation.

pemetrexed. In the REVEL study, 1825 patients with advanced NSCLC progressing on first-line platinum-based chemotherapy were randomized to docetaxel alone or in combination with ramucirumab.[172] The addition of ramucirumab was associated with increased median PFS and OS (10.5 months vs 9.1 months, HR 0.86, 95% CI 0.75–0.98, $P = 002$). Two EGFR tyrosine kinase inhibitors (TKIs) were compared to BSC in patients with previously treated NSCLC. In the Iressa survival evaluation in lung cancer (ISEL) trial, 1692 patients were randomized to gefitinib (Iressa) or placebo.[173] Gefitinib was not associated with a significant improvement in median OS (5.6 months vs 5.1 months, HR 0.89, 95% CI 0.77–1.02, $P = 0.08$). In contrast, the NCIC-BR21, which randomized 731 patients to erlotinib or placebo, showed a significant improvement in median duration median OS (6.7 months vs 4.7 months, HR 0.70, 95% CI 0.58–0.85, $P < 0.0001$) in patients treated with erlotinib.[174] The currently approved regimens for previously treated advanced NSCLC currently include docetaxel, pemetrexed, erlotinib, and the combination of docetaxel plus ramucirumab.

Chemotherapy in the elderly

Approximately one-third of all patients with NSCLC are aged 70 years or older, and, although these patients are likely to have an increased risk of co-morbid conditions and impaired organ function, most studies have suggested that age alone should not be a factor in the decision to treat patients with chemotherapy. Retrospective studies of patients treated for advanced NSCLC found no major differences between patients older than and younger than 65 years of age,[175] and an analysis of age as a risk factor in chemotherapy trials found that the response, toxicity, and survival rates of elderly patients were similar to those of younger patients.[176] An international expert panel has published recommendations for elderly NSCLC patients. These include comprehensive geriatric assessment to better define prognosis and predict tolerance to treatment. The panel concluded that single-agent chemotherapy with a third-generation drug (vinorelbine, gemcitabine, or a taxane) is a reasonable option for nonselected elderly patients with advanced NSCLC and that platinum-based chemotherapy is a viable option for fit patients with adequate organ function.[177]

Targeted therapy

Epidermal growth factor receptor

Gefitinib was the first EGFR TKI tested in patients with advanced NSCLC. In the Iressa dose evaluation in advanced lung cancer (IDEAL) trials, patients with advanced NSCLC progressing after previous chemotherapy were randomized to gefitinib 250 or 500 mg.[178,179] The studies showed a response rate of approximately 10–18%, without significant differences between the two doses of gefitinib and increased rash with the higher dose. Clinical predictors for response included good PS, adenocarcinoma histology, female gender, and Japanese ethnicity. The discovery of EGFR mutations, mostly deletions in exon 19 and the substitution of arginine for leucine at position 858 (L858R), provided the biological explanation for the clinical predictors of response to EGFR TKIs.[180,181] In one of the studies, eight of the nine patients responding to gefitinib had EGFR mutations, which were more common in never smokers with adenocarcinoma histology.[180] In a Spanish study evaluating 2105 patients with nonsquamous NSCLC, 350 patients (16.6%) had EGFR mutation.[182] These mutations were most common in never smokers (37.7%). In the Memorial Sloan-Kettering Cancer Center experience, the presence of EGFR mutations in never smokers, former smokers, and current smokers with adenocarcinoma was 52%, 15%, and 6%, with the incidence of EGFR mutations inversely related to smoking burden.[183]

In a pooled analysis of outcomes for patients treated with EGFR TKIs, 78% with an EGFR mutation responded to therapy compared to only 10% with wild-type EGFR.[184] In order to compare the two approaches in a large RCT, the Iressa Pan Asia Study (IPASS) was designed to compare gefitinib to carboplatin plus paclitaxel in chemo-naive patients with advanced-stage NSCLC.[185] In patients with EGFR wild type, gefitinib was associated with decreased response rates (23.5% vs 1.1%) and median PFS (HR 2.85, 95% CI 2.05–3.98, $P < 0.001$). In contrast, in patients harboring EGFR mutations, response rates (71.2% vs 47.3%) and median PFS were higher for those treated with gefitinib (HR 0.48, 95% CI 0.36–0.64, $P < 0.001$). Several similar trials including only patients with EGFR mutant tumors have been conducted with similar results for patients treated with gefitinib[186,187] or erlotinib.[188,189]

More recent studies compared the second-generation EGFR TKI afatinib to chemotherapy. Second-generation EGFR TKIs are characterized by irreversible binding to the HER family including HER-2 and HER-4. In the Lux-Lung 3 and 6 studies of patients with previously untreated advanced-stage lung adenocarcinoma, afatinib was associated with improved PFS versus cisplatin plus pemetrexed or cisplatin plus gemcitabine, respectively.[190,191] Although combined analysis of the two trials showed no difference in OS between afatanib and chemo, a subset analysis showed that median OS was significantly higher in patients harboring the EGFR deletion 19 mutation, but not those with the L858R mutation.[192]

Despite the initial responses to EGFR-TKI therapy and prolonged median PFS compared to standard chemotherapy, virtually all EGFR mutant patients eventually developed acquired resistance to therapy.[193] The most common cause of acquired resistance to EGFR TKIs is the development of a secondary mutation in exon 20 (T790M).[194] Other potential causes include Met amplification,

PIK3CA mutations, HER-2 amplification, BRAF mutations, and SCLC transformation.[195,196] Third-generation EGFR TKIs are potent inhibitors of T790M tumors. Two drugs are in advanced stage of development. Early results from trials with CO-1686 in patients with T790M mutation showed 58% response rate and an estimated median PFS >12 months.[197] Similarly, impressive results were observed with AZD-9291 in such patients, where response rates and overall disease control were 64% and 94%, respectively.[198] Another approach in patients with acquired resistance to EGFR TKIs is the combination of afatinib and cetuximab. In a phase IB study, this combination was tested in 126 patients with acquired resistance to erlotinib or gefitinib.[199] The overall response rate was 29% with no significant differences between T790M positive and negative patients (32% and 25% respectively, $P = 0.34$).

Anaplastic lymphoma kinase

Anaplastic lymphoma kinase (ALK) fusions with EML4, KIF5B, TFG, and KLC1, among others, result in constitutive activation of ALK and its downstream signaling pathways.[200] Crizotinib is an oral ATP-competitive inhibitor of ALK, MET, and ROS1 tyrosine kinases. In an expanded cohort from a phase 1 trial including 82 patients with ALK fusion, response rate was 57% with an additional 33% of patients achieving stable disease (SD).[201] At the time of cutoff, the median PFS was not reached and the estimated probability of PFS at 6 months was 72%. In patients with ALK fusion, first-line crizotinib was associated with improved median PFS compared to platinum plus pemetrexed (10.7 months vs 7 months; HR 0.45, 95% CI 0.35–0.60, $P < 0.001$) without significant changes in median OS.[202] Similar findings were observed in the second-line setting where crizotinib was associated with increased median PFS compared to docetaxel or pemetrexed but no changes in median OS.[203] One option for patients who develop acquired resistance to crizotinib is the use of second-generation ALK inhibitors. In the dose escalation part of a phase 1 study, ceritinib was associated with a 58% response rate and a median PFS of 7 months, ranging from 6.9 months in patients previously treated with crizotinib to 10.4 months in those who had not received previous ALK directed therapy.[204]

Other targets

Several potentially targetable gene abnormalities have been described in NSCLC and are currently being investigated in clinical trials.[205] Among them, there has been recent data suggesting benefit from crizotinib in patients with ROS1 fusions.[206] In a phase II trial enrolling 50 patients with ROS1 fusions, the response rate was 72% with a median PFS of 19.2 months.[207] Although there are no direct inhibitors for KRAS mutations, downstream blockage with MEK inhibitors may play a role in the treatment of this patient population. In a phase 2 study randomizing 87 previously treated patients with advanced KRAS mutant NSCLC to docetaxel alone or in combination with selumetinib, the latter was associated with increased median PFS (5.3 months vs 2.1 months, $P = 0.01$) and a numerically superior median OS (9.4 months vs 5.2 months, $P = 0.21$).[208]

Immunotherapy

Immune check point pathways play a key role in regulating T-cell responses. Programmed cell death (PD1) is an inhibitory T-cell receptor that binds to its ligand PD-L1 in tumors. Preclinical studies have shown that inhibition of the PD-1/PD-L1 interaction may increase T-cell responses and induce an anti-tumor effect. Several drugs designed to block this pathway are under development including the anti-PD1 antibodies BMS-936558 (nivolumab) and MK-3475 (pembrolizumab) and the anti-PDL1 antibodies

MPDL-3280A and MEDI-4736.[209] In a phase 1 study evaluating the role of nivolumab in patients with NSCLC, renal cell carcinoma, and melanoma, there were 14 responses among the 122 patients with NSCLC.[210] All the responses occurred in patients treated with 3 or 10 mg/kg, including 6 out of 13 patients with squamous histology and 7 out of 44 patients with nonsquamous histology. In a study evaluating MPDL-3280A in multiple malignancies, the response rate in 53 patients with NSCLC was 34% with SD lasting 24 weeks or more in 17% of patients.[211] Treatment with PD-1/PD-L1 checkpoint inhibitors was well tolerated in both studies and the presence of PD-L1 expression in tumors was associated with responses.

Systemic therapy for potentially curable NSCLC

Adjuvant chemotherapy

The administration of chemotherapy after curative NSCLC surgical resection in order to improve OS is termed adjuvant chemotherapy. Despite undergoing resection, the majority of lung cancer patients experience recurrent and/or metastatic disease; two-thirds of these recurrences and metastases occur systemically. Therefore, supplementing surgery with chemotherapy is a rational treatment strategy.[212] A meta-analysis in 1995 compared surgery alone with surgery followed by cisplatin-based chemotherapy. This study included eight trials and 1394 patients and showed a 13% reduction in the risk of death, suggesting that adjuvant chemotherapy afforded an absolute benefit of 5% at 5 years ($p = .08$).[213] Subsequent randomized trials have demonstrated a modest benefit with adjuvant chemotherapy.[214-217] A pooled analysis of the five largest randomized trials conducted after the 1995 meta-analysis included 4584 patients. Improved survival was observed in stage II and III disease.[218] Current ASCO guidelines indicate that adjuvant cisplatin-based chemotherapy is recommended for routine use in patients with stage IIA, IIB, and IIIA disease, including selected patients older than 65 years. Although there has been a statistically significant OS benefit seen in several RCTs enrolling a range of people with completely resected NSCLC, results of subset analyses for patient populations with stage IB disease were not significant, and adjuvant chemotherapy in stage IB disease is not currently recommended for routine use. To date, very few patients with stage IA NSCLC have been enrolled onto RCTs of adjuvant therapy, and adjuvant chemotherapy is not recommended for this stage group.[219]

Neoadjuvant chemotherapy

The delivery of chemotherapy before surgical resection is termed neoadjuvant or induction chemotherapy. Potential advantages to neoadjuvant chemotherapy compared with adjuvant chemotherapy include improved chemotherapy compliance, lower pneumonectomy rates, and the ability to assess tumor responsiveness to chemotherapy. Although adjuvant chemotherapy remains the current standard of care for resectable NSCLC, clinical trial data indicate that neoadjuvant chemotherapy may confer a similar level of benefit.[220-223] A meta-analysis of 13 trials that randomized a total of 3224 patients demonstrated improved survival with neoadjuvant chemotherapy (HR 0.84, $P = 0.0001$).[224] Although these data indicate that neoadjuvant chemotherapy may be a reasonable approach for resectable NSCLC patients, few studies provide guidance regarding how to select patients for adjuvant versus neoadjuvant therapy.

Therapy for SCLC

SCLC differs from NSCLC in its rapid growth rate, propensity for early systemic spread, and short natural history. With the general acceptance of SCLC as a systemic disorder and recognition of the superiority of multimodal regimens over local therapy alone, chemotherapy became the cornerstone of SCLC management.[225]

Surgical treatment
Although it has been established that surgical resection does not customarily play a role in the treatment of SCLC, there are some clinical settings in which surgery may be of potential benefit, such as in the case of peripheral SCLC. Although two-thirds of patients have ED at the time of presentation, fewer than 5% present with the tumor confined to the lung, with or without N1 lymph node metastases. These patients commonly present with a solitary pulmonary nodule on an incidental chest radiograph. Overall 5-year survival rate for patients who have undergone surgery followed by adjuvant chemotherapy has been shown to range from 28% to 60% for patients with stage I disease and 20 to 35% for patients with T1 N1 disease.[226] A recent retrospective study showed a 5-year OS of 52.6% for all patients undergoing surgery and 45–51% for T1 N1 disease.[227] Isolated reports have described 5-year survival rates as high as 70–80% for some patients with very limited stage disease. The great disparity between the survival rates of these patients and those of the more common central SCLC has led to several hypotheses. Some investigators believe that these tumors represent a variant of SCLC with altered biology; however, others believe that these tumors are inaccurately diagnosed and may in fact be well or moderately differentiated neuroendocrine carcinomas (typical or atypical carcinoids).[228]

Although most patients with peripheral SCLC have the diagnosis made at the time of thoracotomy, a minority are diagnosed preoperatively with FNA. The rare but established presentation of SCLC as a peripheral lesion, along with the fact that NSCLC and carcinoids can be misdiagnosed as SCLC on FNA, should prompt the clinician to continue to consider the patient for surgical treatment rather than refer immediately for chemotherapy. In light of this preoperative diagnosis, staging should be even more thorough than usual to reflect the high incidence of occult mediastinal and systemic metastasis associated with SCLC. Thorough radiographic staging and mediastinoscopy are employed before consideration of surgery. The presence of mediastinal involvement would obviate the role of surgery, but the presence of hilar adenopathy on radiographic staging is not an absolute contraindication to surgery. These patients may still undergo exploration as a means of establishing the presence of disease within the hilar nodes and, in good candidates, resection can still be offered if a complete resection is possible. All patients with surgically treated SCLC should receive postoperative chemotherapy. In trials reported by the Veterans Administration Surgical Adjuvant Group, patients who received postoperative chemotherapy did better than those who did not. When the timing of chemotherapy was examined, there appeared to be no advantage to giving chemotherapy preoperatively.[225]

Radiotherapy
Surgical local control is applicable to a very small subset of patients with SCLC. The remainder requires some form of local control as part of their treatment, and radiotherapy fulfills this role. Two meta-analyses employing different methods confirmed the value of thoracic irradiation to decrease local recurrence and prolong survival. The first study, based on results from 11 trials, showed an absolute increase in OS rate of 5.4% at 2 years.[229] The second study collected data on 2140 patients from 13 RCTs comparing chemotherapy alone with chemotherapy plus thoracic irradiation and found an improvement in absolute survival rate of 5.4%, from 15% to 20.4%, at 3 years.[230] Of note, the trials included in these

meta-analyses were not recent studies, and none of them employed EP, the current standard chemotherapy regimen. In addition, these trials included both sequential and concurrent chemoradiotherapy.

Timing of thoracic radiotherapy relative to chemotherapy
The optimal schedule of chemoradiotherapy for limited disease (LD) SCLC continues to evolve. Earlier data from randomized trials, including meta-analyses, favored concurrent chemoradiotherapy and the administration of radiotherapy earlier in the course of treatment (i.e., during cycles 1–3 of chemotherapy).[231–237]

Fractionation of thoracic radiotherapy with concurrent chemotherapy
Because SCLC is radiosensitive, without a shoulder in the radiation dose–response curve, and has a rapid doubling time, the use of multiple reduced-dose fractions in theory may increase efficacy. This approach is also hypothesized to protect normal tissues from late effects, especially those with a shoulder in their dose response.[238] Several phase II trials of hyperfractionated and accelerated chemoradiation in LD SCLC patients yielded encouraging 2-year survival outcomes compared to historical controls with conventionally fractionated radiation.[239,240] Standard daily fractionation (1.8 Gy per fraction × 25 fractions in 5 weeks) and accelerated fractionation (1.5 Gy twice-daily × 30 fractions in 3 weeks) were compared in a pivotal intergroup phase III trial (INT-0096) of 417 patients with LD SCLC.[241] Concurrent chemotherapy consisted of cisplatin 60 mg/m^2 IV on day 1 and etoposide 120 mg/m^2 IV on days 1–3 for four cycles. The accelerated radiation was associated with prolonged median (23 months vs 19 months) and 5-year (26% vs 16%) survival compared with concurrent once-daily radiotherapy ($p = .04$). The only significant difference in toxicity between the arms was in grade 3 esophagitis, which was more frequent with twice-daily TRT (27% vs 11%, $p < .001$). Despite these favorable results, this approach has not been widely adopted in the community, possibly because of the difficulty of scheduling and the increased rate of esophagitis.[242]

Total tolerable dose
Radiation dose to the thorax is another controversial area.[243] A study by the National Cancer institute of Canada (NCIC) clearly demonstrated a dose response in the thorax: thoracic PFS was prolonged by giving 37.5 Gy in 15 fractions over 3 weeks rather than 25 Gy in 10 fractions over 2 weeks as consolidation after completion of induction chemotherapy.[244] Arriagada and colleagues published a report of 173 patients with LD SCLC treated in three consecutive trials. The total dose of TRT ranged from 45 to 65 Gy, administered by split courses interdigitating with chemotherapy. Dose of radiotherapy did not significantly impact local control or survival.[245] Strategies were considered that might increase the local control rate for concurrent chemotherapy and radiation therapy without increasing the esophageal toxicity rate to unacceptable levels. One strategy was to increase the total dose by administering daily thoracic radiation therapy at higher levels. Considering the value demonstrated by accelerated fractionation even to a total dose of just 45 Gy in 3 weeks, there was concern that a greater overall duration of thoracic radiation therapy might be disadvantageous.

Accelerated fractionation via concomitant boost is associated with improved locoregional control in patients with head and neck cancer compared to conventional daily fractionation.[246] This strategy uses once-daily irradiation through approximately 4–5 weeks of treatment and then twice-daily irradiation in approximately the last 2 weeks of treatment, delivering one daily fraction to the large field and one fraction to boost the dose to the small field. Thus, it is termed concomitant boost. Taking a lead from its success in head and neck cancer, the RTOG evaluated a similar strategy in phase I and II trials (RTOG 9712 and RTOG 0239, respectively) of concomitant boost radiation with concurrent EP in SCLC. The results showed an 18% rate of severe acute esophagitis (lower than the 27% previously noted in INT 0096) and a 2-year survival rate of 36.6% (lower than the 47% seen in INT 0096).[247,248]

Theorizing that daily radiation to a dose >45 Gy might be as efficacious as 45 Gy given twice-daily in 3 weeks, the CALGB compared the MTDs (maximum tolerated doses) of once-daily and twice-daily radiotherapy in LD SCLC patients.[249] Radiotherapy was started with the fourth cycle of chemotherapy, and the recommended phase II dose in the once-daily arm was 70 Gy. Not surprisingly, the MTD of the accelerated therapy was 45 Gy. A subsequent phase II trial (CALGB 39808) demonstrated that 70 Gy in daily fractions was feasible with carboplatin and etoposide after induction chemotherapy with paclitaxel and topotecan.[250] The median survival of 22.4 months reflects the best outcome reported for conventional daily fractionation in LD SCLC. The rate of grade 3–4 esophagitis was 21%, compared to 17% in RTOG 0239, and estimated in a much larger number of patients, 32% in INT-0096. A pooled analysis of patients treated on 3 CALGB trials (39808, 30002, 30206) using high-dose (70Gy) daily radiotherapy with concurrent chemotherapy following two cycles of induction chemotherapy showed a median survival of 19.9 months, with 2- and 5-year OS rates of 37% (95% CI: 31–44%) and 21% (95% CI: 16–27%), respectively.[251]

Given the reduced esophageal toxicity and predicted maintained efficacy of the radiation regimens in CALGB 39808 and RTOG 0239, a pivotal phase III trial is ongoing, comparing two experimental arms with a control arm of 45 Gy administered twice-daily, all with early concurrent EP (cycle 1).

Prophylactic cranial irradiation in SCLC
Symptomatic brain metastases are detected in approximately 10% of SCLC patients at initial presentation, and an additional 10% may have occult metastases on MRI or CT imaging, with the likelihood of new brain metastases developing increasingly with lengthening survival.[252] In the absence of specific therapy to the CNS, the actuarial cumulative probability reached 80% at 28 months of follow-up when the cases of CNS metastasis found at autopsy were included and 58% at 24 months when only clinical brain metastases were counted. At postmortem examination, much higher incidences were reported, ranging up to 65%. With the hope that the CNS would be the only site of residual disease, prophylactic cranial irradiation (PCI) was incorporated as an initial part of treatment of SCLC in the early 1970s.[225] A meta-analysis concluded that PCI prolongs both OS and DFS among SCLC patients in complete remission.[253] When patients with LD SCLC were evaluated before and after PCI, 83% (25/30 patients) were found to have minor cognitive dysfunction before PCI, and no significant differences were found in the comparison of pretreatment and post-treatment neuropsychological results.[254] An RCT comparing PCI at 25 or 35 Gy in 720 patients evaluated neurocognitive function and quality of life and found no significant differences between the two groups.[255] These data indicate that concerns over PCI-associated neurotoxicity should not deter patients from receiving PCI.

PCI may improve outcomes for patients with extensive stage disease (ED) that have responded to therapy. An RCT for patients with extensive SCLC who achieved a response to chemotherapy has shown that PCI reduced the incidence of symptomatic brain metastases and prolonged DFS and OS. PCI increased median survival from 5.4 to 6.7 months ($p = .003$), and 1-year survival rates were 27.1% in the PCI group compared to 13.3% in the control group ($p = .003$). This difference in survival in the PCI patients may be attributed in part to increased treatment for extra-CNS progression in that group (68% vs 45%) and a low rate of brain radiation for patients with brain recurrence on the control arm (59%). Effects of PCI on health-related quality of life were collected, with short-term results at 3 months showing a negative impact of PCI, especially on hair loss and fatigue, but similar cognitive and emotional functioning. Long-term results were unable to be assessed due to noncompletion of forms and small numbers.[256]

Chemotherapy
In its initial presentation, SCLC is sensitive to a variety of cytotoxins in the following drug classes: alkylators, anthracyclines, camptothecin derivatives, epipodophyllotoxins, platinating agents, vinca alkaloids, and taxanes. While the nitrogen mustard derivatives, methotrexate, vinorelbine, and gemcitabine, do have activity, they are less active than other drugs and not commonly utilized. Drugs considered active are associated with single-agent response rates generally >30%.

The combination of EP, first studied as a salvage regimen in the 1980s, has over the past 25 years become the standard of care for initial therapy of both LD and ED patients. RCTs have generally shown equivalent efficacy for EP and other more toxic regimens in patients with ED; thus, it is the standard based on higher therapeutic index.[257] In patients with LD, in combination with concurrent thoracic radiation, it was associated with survival impact when compared to cyclophosphamide, epirubicin, and vincristine.[258] This may relate to the ability to deliver full doses of EP in this setting without prohibitive midline, lung parenchymal, and bone marrow toxicity, that is observed with anthracycline-alkylator regimens.

Combination chemotherapy
The standard regimen for initial therapy in North America is the combination of EP. A minimum of four courses of EP is recommended based on a Southeastern Cancer Study Group phase III trial, which randomized patients to receive four courses of EP, six courses of cyclophosphamide, doxorubicin, and vincristine (CAV), or alternating EP and CAV.[257]

The Japanese Clinical Oncology Group (JCOG) trial 9511 randomized patients with ED to either EP or irinotecan and cisplatin (IP).[259] Patients in the IP arm had improved median and long-term survival, compared to patients on etoposide (median survival: 12.8 months vs 9.4 months, $p = .002$, 2-year survival: 20% vs 5%). The experimental arm in this study consisted of IP given at 4-week cycles. A slight modification of this schedule was used in a subsequent trial in North America, which attempted to confirm these findings.[260] However, this trial, in a predominantly Caucasian population, demonstrated no benefit for patients in the IP arm. Toxicities were different with more diarrhea due to irinotecan, and more myelosuppression in the EP arm. The results of SWOG 0124, replicating the dose and schedule of IP from JCOG 9511, also failed to confirm the benefit for IP over EP for patients with ED.[261] Interestingly, subsequent pooled analyses of JCOG 9511 and SWOG 0124 patients showed significant differences in response rates and survival for the IP arms across trials, but not for the EP arms. These data suggest that polymorphisms in genes involved in irinotecan metabolism may explain differences in toxicity and possibly efficacy between the Japanese and American patients.[262]

Carboplatin substitution for cisplatin in combination with etoposide has been studied in multiple RCTs and several meta-analyses.[263] The most recent meta-analysis analyzed 4 RCTs, including 663 LD and ED SCLC patients, and showed no difference between cisplatin and carboplatin with respect to OS, PFS, and response rate.[264] The median OS was 9.6 and 9.4 months for cisplatin and carboplatin, respectively (HR 1.08; $p = .37$). Further, carboplatin was substantially less toxic as regards emesis, nephrotoxicity, and neurotoxicity, while hematologic toxicity was higher. Current practice standards hold that carboplatin with etoposide is reasonable therapy for patients with ED and, based on favorable toxicity profile, is preferred in those with poor PS and/or significant comorbidities.

Carboplatin and irinotecan are other first-line options for ED SCLC patients. A randomized phase II trial found improvement in PFS with carboplatin and irinotecan versus carboplatin and etoposide.[265] A subsequent phase III trial comparing carboplatin and oral etoposide with carboplatin and irinotecan showed improvement in OS from 7.1 to 8.5 months ($p = .04$).[266] Other regimens including carboplatin with pemetrexed have been found to be inferior to carboplatin and etoposide.[267]

Management of the elderly

Currently representing more than one-third of patients with SCLC, the proportion of those aged >70 years will continue to increase in the future as our population ages. Although the heterogeneity in this group is substantial, there is general agreement that they represent a population at higher risk for treatment-related morbidity and mortality. Although RCTs are few in number, reducing the intensity of therapy in this group by using single agents or low-dose chemotherapy has been associated with inferior efficacy and shortened survival and is not recommended.[268,269] Multiple phase II trials of etoposide and carboplatin in this population have revealed good tolerance and reasonable efficacy.[270,271] In a phase II randomized trial, EP was safely given to elderly patients with granulocyte-colony stimulating factor (G-CSF) support and resulted in efficacy similar to outcomes in younger patients.[272]

Regarding management of the elderly patient with LD, an analysis of patients >70 years in INT-0096 reported an increased death rate in the first 6 months after randomization, with a 10% treatment-related death rate compared to the 1% rate in those <70 years.[273] Severe myelosuppressive toxicity was greater in the elderly compared to younger patients. Other toxicities were similar. Median (21.6 months vs 14.4 months) and 5-year (22% vs 16%) survival rates were worse in the elderly, reflecting, at least in part, the increased death rate during treatment and early in follow-up. These data suggest that the elderly with LD and retained performance status benefit from standard chemoradiation. However, this group should be carefully selected with respect to PS and deserve greater use of supportive care measures. Chemoradiation is recommended.

Special clinical situations

Brain metastases

Formerly, systemic chemotherapy was believed to play a limited role in the treatment of brain metastases because of the widely held view of the brain as a pharmacologic sanctuary. In the 1980s, several groups observed in prospective trials that systemic chemotherapy alone, without brain irradiation, could induce objective regression of brain lesions. These results indicate that once contrast-enhancing metastases are evident with MRI or CT, the blood–brain barrier is not intact and response rates to chemotherapy are similar in the brain and in extra-CNS sites.[274,275] First-line therapy with cranial irradiation may not be necessary, even though this has not been addressed in an RCT setting. Ultimate irradiation of the brain is indicated, however, given an increase in complete response rates

with its addition. A meta-analysis of three trials involving 192 patients noted no significant differences in OS for patients receiving whole-brain radiotherapy (WBRT) and topotecan versus no topotecan, teniposide with or without WBRT, and sequential versus concurrent chemoradiotherapy with teniposide and cisplatin.[276] For patients with intracranial relapse, the available data indicate that the efficacy of second-line chemotherapy is generally much less than in previously untreated patients, and initial WBRT is standard. Conversely, patients with recurrent brain metastases after previous cranial irradiation should not be denied a trial of systemic chemotherapy. Small studies investigating gamma knife radiosurgery in both the upfront and recurrent setting are ongoing.

Second-line therapy for SCLC

The prognosis is poor for patients who receive second-line therapy after relapse, with median survival generally in the range of 4–6 months. Response to additional therapy and survival from the time of relapse is influenced by response to initial chemotherapy and the progression-free interval following its completion. Giaccone et al.[277] were the first to observe this in a trial with teniposide reported in 1988. In this study, none of seven patients who had not responded to initial treatment responded to teniposide. Of 16 whose progression-free interval was ≤2.6 months, only two (12%) responded to teniposide. This contrasted with the 42% response rate (10/24) in those with response to initial chemotherapy and 53% response rate (9/17) with more prolonged progression-free interval. Although the numbers are small in each subgroup, these observations were confirmed in multiple trials that followed in the 1990s. Disease that relapses <2–3 months after first-line therapy is commonly termed refractory, and rates of response in this setting are lower than disease that relapses later, which is usually termed sensitive.

Although there is no generally accepted standard regimen for relapse, topotecan is the most extensively studied agent, and it is the only drug with an FDA (Food and Drug Administration) indication for treatment of sensitive relapse SCLC. This indication is derived from a trial that compared topotecan to CAV in patients who had responded to initial chemotherapy and relapsed ≥60 days after its completion.[161] The response rates were 24.3% in 107 topotecan-treated patients and 18.3% in 104 patients treated with CAV ($p = .285$). There was no difference in median time to progression or median survival duration between the two groups. Symptoms improved to a greater degree in the topotecan group than in the CAV group for four of eight categories evaluated, including dyspnea, anorexia, hoarseness, fatigue, and interference with daily activity ($p = .043$). Grade 4 neutropenia occurred in 38% of topotecan courses and 51% of CAV courses ($p < .001$). Grade 4 thrombocytopenia and grade 3 or 4 anemia occurred more frequently with topotecan, occurring in 10% and 18% of topotecan courses and 1% and 7% of CAV courses, respectively ($p < .001$ for both). Subsequent phase II and III RCTs compared oral versus intravenous topotecan and identified similar efficacy outcomes with the more convenient oral form. Toxicity is altered somewhat with the oral form producing less neutropenia but more diarrhea than the intravenous drug.[159,160,162] The use of weekly topotecan is controversial and is still under investigation.

Oral topotecan has been compared to BSC in a recent trial that documented the survival impact of second-line chemotherapy on SCLC. Patients with both refractory and sensitive relapse who were not candidates for standard intravenous therapy were randomized to BSC versus oral topotecan ($N = 141$).[163] Although response rates to topotecan were low at 7%, 44% of treated patients attained SD and had improved symptom control and maintenance of quality of life. The impact of topotecan on progression and survival was seen equally in patients with refractory or sensitive relapse. Median survival was 26 weeks versus 14 weeks for topotecan and control patients, respectively ($p = .0104$). Survival at 6 months was also favorably impacted by treatment, 49% versus 26%. The evidence for impact of chemotherapy in this setting was persuasive and should influence our use of chemotherapy in this setting both within and outside of clinical investigation.

Other choices for management of recurrent SCLC include use of the initial induction regimen, especially if PFS after discontinuation of induction is prolonged, typically 6 months or longer. Irinotecan, while not studied as extensively as topotecan in recurrent patients, appears to have similar benefits, alone or in combination with carboplatin.[278,279] Limited evaluation of taxanes and anthracyclines also suggests low-level activity in recurrent disease.[280] Amrubicin, an anthracycline, showed promising activity in the second-line setting, but preliminary results of a phase III RCT comparing amrubicin to topotecan did not meet its primary endpoint of OS or PFS, although response rate was improved (31% vs 17%, $P = 0.002$).[281–284] Palliative radiation to chest, brain, and bone is also effective and used commonly in drug-resistant and recurrent SCLC.

Targeted therapy

Efforts in genomic characterization of SCLC have employed multiple approaches, including whole-exome sequencing, transcriptome profiling, copy number and rearrangement analyses of tissue from both human and murine tumors, and circulating tumor cells (CTCs).[285–288] SCLC has a very high density of mutations per tumor, although many of these may be passenger, not driver, mutations. The most frequent mutations include those that inactivate the tumor suppressor genes TP53 and RB-1; other interesting observations include PTEN loss, MYC amplification, and alterations in genes involved in PI3K/AKT and stem cell signaling. Despite these research efforts, patients with SCLC have yet to benefit from

enhanced knowledge of the abnormal biology that is associated with its development and progression.

Conclusions and future prospects

Elimination of tobacco consumption is the most effective way to reduce lung cancer incidence. However, this goal remains elusive because of continuing social and economic pressures. Lung cancer also occurs in people who have never smoked. Lung cancer will continue to be a significant public health burden well into the twenty-first century. Thus, early detection and new therapeutic options are needed to improve the dismal rate of survival for lung cancer patients. The recent demonstration that low-dose chest CT scans can improve lung cancer mortality in high-risk populations is encouraging. Progress in defining the molecular events involved in lung cancer carcinogenesis and therapeutic resistance has been rapid over the last 15 years, and the potential benefits from this progress for patients may be substantial.

The mainstay of cancer therapy remains surgery, radiotherapy, and chemotherapy, and recent years have shown improvement in patient outcome by their combination and optimization (Figure 6). A large effort has been dedicated to further impact lung cancer outcome by adding biological therapy. Such an approach utilizes alteration of oncogene expression with recombinant gene constructs to allow reversal of the transformed phenotype. In addition, a wealth of biologically active agents that interfere with signal transduction events in the development and progression of lung cancer is now being explored. Rather than targeting the actual genetic errors, these treatments correct or interfere with the sequelae of those genetic changes. For example, genetic mutations that lead to increased expression or activity of a growth factor receptor could be targeted, either by blocking the receptor itself or by interfering with its downstream signal transduction pathways. The first drugs of this kind are the EGFR TKIs approved for the management of lung cancer. In parallel, monoclonal antibodies to VEGF are combined with conventional chemotherapy to improve survival of patients with lung cancer, colorectal cancer, breast cancer, and renal cell

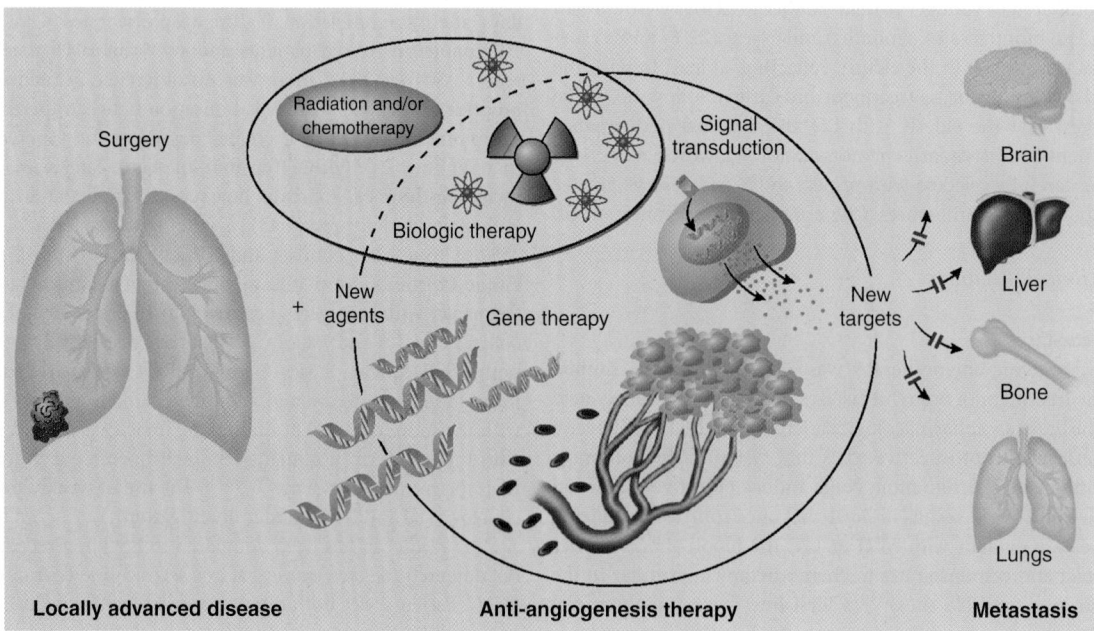

Figure 6 Most patients with nonsmall-cell lung cancer die from metastatic disease. Treatment in the locally advanced setting will likely require chemotherapy or radiation therapy in combination with biologic therapy to enhance its effectiveness and prevent metastatic spread of tumor.

carcinoma, among others. Immunotherapy has recently emerged as a promising therapeutic strategy, exemplified by the approval of nivolumab as a standard of care for the treatment of squamous-cell NSCLC, and the horizon looks bright with many clinical trials investigating new combination approaches.

In summary, lung cancer therapy efforts in recent years have focused on cancer prevention, early detection, and multimodality therapy. Improvements in systemic therapy (chemotherapy, molecular targeted therapy, and immunotherapy) will impact all stages of disease. As lung cancer is a heterogeneous disease, it will also be essential to identify and better understand specific molecular targets and select patients for therapy according to their tumor's biological profile. It is hoped that advances in translational proteomic and genomic research will be the key to identifying reliable, validated predictive biomarkers for these new targeted agents. Progress in these areas will hopefully lead to better control of this disease while minimizing treatment-related side effects.

Key references

The complete reference list can be found on the Wiley Companion Digital Edition of this title (see inside front cover for login instructions).

10 Mao L, Lee JS, Kurie JM, et al. Clonal genetic alterations in the lungs of current and former smokers. *J Natl Cancer Inst.* 1997;**89**:857–862.

11 Wistuba II, Lam S, Behrens C, et al. Molecular damage in the bronchial epithelium of current and former smokers. *J Natl Cancer Inst.* 1997;**89**:1366–1373.

13 Hammerman PS, Hayes DN, Wilkerson MD, et al. Comprehensive genomic characterization of squamous cell lung cancers. *Nature.* 2012;**489**:519–525.

14 Kadara H, Fujimoto J, Yoo SY, et al. Transcriptomic architecture of the adjacent airway field cancerization in non-small cell lung cancer. *J Natl Cancer Inst.* 2014;**106**:dju004.

46 Rusch VW. Management of Pancoast tumours. *Lancet Oncol.* 2006;**7**:997–1005.

64 Wallace MB, Pascual JMS, Raimondo M, et al. Minimally invasive endoscopic staging of suspected lung cancer. *JAMA.* 2008;**299**:540–546.

72 National Lung Screening Trial Research Team, Aberle DR, Adams AM, et al. Reduced lung-cancer mortality with low-dose computed tomographic screening. *N Engl J Med.* 2011;**365**:395–409.

73 Moyer VA. Screening for lung cancer: U.S. preventive services task force recommendation statement. *Ann Intern Med.* 2014;**160**:330–338.

74 Goldstraw P, Crowley J, Chansky K, et al. The IASLC lung cancer staging project: proposals for the revision of the TNM stage groupings in the forthcoming (seventh) edition of the TNM classification of malignant tumours. *J Thorac Oncol.* 2007;**2**:706–714.

104 Chang JY. Intensity-modulated radiotherapy, not 3 dimensional conformal, is the preferred technique for treating locally advanced lung cancer. *Semin Radiat Oncol.* 2015;**25**:110–116.

105 Chang JY, Li QQ, Xu QY, et al. Stereotactic ablative radiation therapy for centrally located early stage or isolated parenchymal recurrences of non-small cell lung cancer: how to fly in a "no fly zone". *Int J Radiat Oncol Biol Phys.* 2014;**88**:1120–1128.

119 Albain KS, Swann RS, Rusch VW, et al. Radiotherapy plus chemotherapy with or without surgical resection for stage III non-small cell lung cancer: a phase III randomised controlled trial. *Lancet.* 2009;**374**:379–386.

124 Curran WJ, Paulus R, Langer CJ, et al. Sequential vs concurrent chemoradiation for stage III non-small cell lung cancer: randomized phase III trial RTOG 9410. *J Natl Cancer Inst.* 2011;**103**:1452–1460.

144 Scagliotti GV, Parikh P, von Pawel J, et al. Phase III study comparing cisplatin plus gemcitabine with cisplatin plus pemetrexed in chemotherapy-naive patients with advanced-stage non-small-cell lung cancer. *J Clin Oncol.* 2008;**26**:3543–3551.

147 Ardizzoni A, Boni L, Tiseo M, et al. Cisplatin- versus carboplatin-based chemotherapy in first-line treatment of advanced non-small-cell lung cancer: an individual patient data meta-analysis. *J Natl Cancer Inst.* 2007;**99**:847–857.

149 Sandler A, Gray R, Perry MC, et al. Paclitaxel-carboplatin alone or with bevacizumab for non-small-cell lung cancer. *N Engl J Med.* 2006;**355**:2542–2550.

155 Pirker R, Pereira JR, von Pawel J, et al. EGFR expression as a predictor of survival for first-line chemotherapy plus cetuximab in patients with advanced non-small-cell lung cancer: analysis of data from the phase 3 FLEX study. *Lancet Oncol.* 2012;**13**:33–42.

165 Ciuleanu T, Brodowicz T, Zielinski C, et al. Maintenance pemetrexed plus best supportive care versus placebo plus best supportive care for non-small-cell lung cancer: a randomised, double-blind, phase 3 study. *Lancet.* 2009;**374**:1432–1440.

166 Paz-Ares L, de Marinis F, Dediu M, et al. Maintenance therapy with pemetrexed plus best supportive care versus placebo plus best supportive care after induction therapy with pemetrexed plus cisplatin for advanced non-squamous non-small-cell lung cancer (PARAMOUNT): a double-blind, phase 3, randomised controlled trial. *Lancet Oncol.* 2012;**13**:247–255.

168 Patel JD, Socinski MA, Garon EB, et al. PointBreak: a randomized phase iii study of pemetrexed plus carboplatin and bevacizumab followed by maintenance pemetrexed and bevacizumab versus paclitaxel plus carboplatin and bevacizumab followed by maintenance bevacizumab in patients with stage IIIB or IV nonsquamous non-small-cell lung cancer. *J Clin Oncol.* 2013;**31**:4349–4357.

172 Garon EB, Ciuleanu TE, Arrieta O, et al. Ramucirumab plus docetaxel versus placebo plus docetaxel for second-line treatment of stage IV non-small-cell lung cancer after disease progression on platinum-based therapy (REVEL): a multicentre, double-blind, randomised phase 3 trial. *Lancet.* 2014;**384**:665–673.

180 Lynch TJ, Bell DW, Sordella R, et al. Activating mutations in the epidermal growth factor receptor underlying responsiveness of non-small-cell lung cancer to gefitinib. *N Engl J Med.* 2004;**350**:2129–2139.

186 Maemondo M, Inoue A, Kobayashi K, et al. Gefitinib or chemotherapy for non-small-cell lung cancer with mutated EGFR. *N Engl J Med.* 2010;**362**:2380–2388.

188 Rosell R, Carcereny E, Gervais R, et al. Erlotinib versus standard chemotherapy as first-line treatment for European patients with advanced EGFR mutation-positive non-small-cell lung cancer (EURTAC): a multicentre, open-label, randomised phase 3 trial. *Lancet Oncol.* 2012;**13**:239–246.

190 Sequist LV, Yang JC, Yamamoto N, et al. Phase III study of afatinib or cisplatin plus pemetrexed in patients with metastatic lung adenocarcinoma with EGFR mutations. *J Clin Oncol.* 2013;**31**:3327–3334.

196 Camidge DR, Pao W, Sequist LV. Acquired resistance to TKIs in solid tumours: learning from lung cancer. *Nat Rev Clin Oncol.* 2014;**11**:473–481.

202 Solomon BJ, Mok T, Kim DW, et al. First-line crizotinib versus chemotherapy in ALK-positive lung cancer. *N Engl J Med.* 2014;**371**:2167–2177.

204 Shaw AT, Engelman JA. Ceritinib in ALK-rearranged non-small-cell lung cancer. *N Engl J Med.* 2014;**370**:2537–2539.

207 Shaw AT, Ou SH, Bang YJ, et al. Crizotinib in ROS1-rearranged non-small-cell lung cancer. *N Engl J Med.* 2014;**371**:1963–1971.

208 Janne PA, Shaw AT, Pereira JR, et al. Selumetinib plus docetaxel for KRAS-mutant advanced non-small-cell lung cancer: a randomised, multicentre, placebo-controlled, phase 2 study. *Lancet Oncol.* 2013;**14**:38–47.

210 Topalian SL, Hodi FS, Brahmer JR, et al. Safety, activity, and immune correlates of anti-PD-1 antibody in cancer. *N Engl J Med.* 2012;**366**:2443–2454.

211 Herbst RS, Soria JC, Kowanetz M, et al. Predictive correlates of response to the anti-PD-L1 antibody MPDL3280A in cancer patients. *Nature.* 2014;**515**:563–567.

214 Arriagada R, Bergman B, Dunant A, Le Chevalier T, Pignon JP, Vansteenkiste J. Cisplatin-based adjuvant chemotherapy in patients with completely resected non-small-cell lung cancer. *N Engl J Med.* 2004;**350**:351–360.

222 Pisters KM, Vallieres E, Crowley JJ, et al. Surgery with or without preoperative paclitaxel and carboplatin in early-stage non-small-cell lung cancer: Southwest Oncology Group Trial S9900, an intergroup, randomized, phase III trial. *J Clin Oncol.* 2010;**28**:1843–1849.

256 Slotman B, Faivre-Finn C, Kramer G, et al. Prophylactic cranial irradiation in extensive small-cell lung cancer. *N Engl J Med.* 2007;**357**:664–672.

261 Lara PN Jr, Natale R, Crowley J, et al. Phase III trial of irinotecan/cisplatin compared with etoposide/cisplatin in extensive-stage small-cell lung cancer: clinical and pharmacogenomic results from SWOG S0124. *J Clin Oncol.* 2009;**27**:2530–2535.

267 Socinski MA, Smit EF, Lorigan P, et al. Phase III study of pemetrexed plus carboplatin compared with etoposide plus carboplatin in chemotherapy-naive patients with extensive-stage small-cell lung cancer. *J Clin Oncol.* 2009;**27**:4787–4792.

283 Jotte R, Conkling P, Reynolds C, et al. Randomized phase II trial of single-agent amrubicin or topotecan as second-line treatment in patients with small-cell lung cancer sensitive to first-line platinum-based chemotherapy. *J Clin Oncol.* 2011;**29**:287–293.

285 Peifer M, Fernandez-Cuesta L, Sos ML, et al. Integrative genome analyses identify key somatic driver mutations of small-cell lung cancer. *Nat Genet.* 2012;**44**:1104–1110.

286 Rudin CM, Durinck S, Stawiski EW, et al. Comprehensive genomic analysis identifies SOX2 as a frequently amplified gene in small-cell lung cancer. *Nat Genet.* 2012;**44**:1111–1116.

85 Malignant pleural mesothelioma

Daniel R. Gomez, MD ▪ Anne S. Tsao, MD ▪ Haining Yang, PhD ▪ Harvey I. Pass, MD

Overview

Malignant pleural mesothelioma is an aggressive malignancy with an incidence that may be peaking worldwide in the next 5–10 years. While the majority of patients do ultimately die of this disease, there have been substantial treatment and diagnostic shifts over the past decade that may improve long-term outcomes. These changes include worldwide interest in defining early detection biomarkers for the disease, a debate as to the optimal surgical approach (extrapleural pneumonectomy vs lung-sparing methods such as pleurectomy/decortication), further refinement of radiation techniques that allow for conformal treatment fields and the delivery of radiation with the involved lung intact, and the emergence of systemic therapies that are targeted in nature and allow for the increased individualization of care. Indeed, prospective clinical trials assessing the safety and efficacy of novel treatment approaches will be essential to the standardization of paradigms that improve the outcomes. It is hoped that the maturation of these efforts will lead to an optimal approach in which earlier-stage patients will benefit from multiple modalities that will provide synergistic control while limiting toxicity, thereby increasing the number of long-term survivors over the next one to two decades.

Incidence and epidemiology

The incidence of mesothelioma has been underestimated in mortality statistics.[1] Presently, pleural mesotheliomas are responsible for approximately 15,000–20,000 deaths annually worldwide. Cases are clustered in areas of asbestos product plants and shipbuilding facilities, not only in the United States, but also in other industrialized countries, such as England.[2,3] Approximately, 3000 cases per year are diagnosed in the United States, and based on a latency period of approximately 20–40 years and estimated asbestos exposure rates, it has been projected that the incidence will peak in 2010–2015.[4] This timeframe is similar to what has been predicted in other countries, such as the United Kingdom, Australia, and the Netherlands.[5,6] The male to female ratio is approximately 4 : 1, and 80% arise from the pleura.[7] In autopsy studies, the frequency of malignant mesothelioma varies from 0.02% to 0.7%, with a rate of 0.2% in the largest series.[8] In most hospital series, the pleura is more often involved than the peritoneum, with a predominance of the right side over the left (60 : 40).[8] In some epidemiologic studies monitoring cohorts of asbestos workers, however, the peritoneal form is more common than the pleural. The mean age of patients is approximately 60 years, but the disease can occur at any age, including in childhood.[9,10]

Etiology

It has been well established that one of the primary causes of mesothelioma is *asbestos exposure*. It has been estimated that beginning at 15 years after onset of exposure, approximately 6–10% of asbestos workers older than age 35 years will die of mesothelioma.[11] Furthermore, from 1940 to 1979, approximately 27.5 million workers were occupationally exposed to asbestos in the United States, with a calculated annual death rate from mesothelioma of approximately 2000 in 1980 up to 3000 in the late 1990s.[12] Insulation, construction, shipyard industries, and automobile brakes are among the many sources of occupational exposure.[13] Although asbestos exposure and cigarette smoking act synergistically to produce lung cancer, smoking is not an established risk factor for mesothelioma, although an association between cigarettes using "micronite" filters has been postulated.[14] Exposure can also occur by household contamination of women and children, usually through the work clothes of an asbestos' worker. Other less-common causative agents include radiation therapy (RT), as has been observed in young adults who have received RT for Wilms tumor (WT) or for mediastinal lymphoma.[15]

The role of pleural plaques and their association with mesothelioma has been debated for several years. One recent study addressed this issue through a screening program in France for patients that had previous asbestos exposure. Specifically, 5287 males were followed for 7 years with CT (computed tomography) scans, and both the incidence of mesothelioma and subsequent survival were assessed. Overall, 17 patients were diagnosed with malignant pleural mesothelioma (MPM), and there was a significant association between pleural plaques, with a hazard ratio of 8.9. The authors concluded that the presence of pleural plaques appeared to be an "independent risk factor for mesothelioma.[16]"

Molecular biology of mesothelioma

Multiple cytogenetic and molecular abnormalities contribute to the development of MPM. Asbestos inhalation leads to deposition of fibers in the lung parenchyma with eventual migration and implantation of fibers in the pleural lining. Repeated episodes of inflammation and healing, oxygen free radical production from inflammatory cells and the iron moiety within asbestos, and direct damage to DNA by the fibers are generally accepted pathogenic features of asbestos exposure.[17] Karyotype and comparative genomic hybridization (CGH) analyses of primary MPM tumors and cell lines detected frequent deletions, duplications, and translocations with genomic losses more common than gains.[18] Deletions within chromosomes 1p, 3p, 4p, 4q, 6q, 9p, 13q, 14q, and 22q are common and notable for the loss of the tumor-suppressor genes *p16/CDKN2A*, p53, and NF2 located within these loci.[19]

HMGB1, tumor necrosis factor alpha (TNF-α) and NF-κ signaling play an important role in the survival of genetically damaged mesothelial cells.[20] HMGB1 is a typical DAMP (damage-associated molecular pattern)[21,22] and a key mediator of inflammation.[23] Moreover, it is a critical regulator in the initiation of asbestos-mediated

Holland-Frei Cancer Medicine, Ninth Edition. Edited by Robert C. Bast Jr., Carlo M. Croce, William N. Hait, Waun Ki Hong, Donald W. Kufe, Martine Piccart-Gebhart, Raphael E. Pollock, Ralph R. Weichselbaum, Hongyang Wang, and James F. Holland.
© 2017 John Wiley & Sons, Inc. ISBN: 978-1-118-93469-2

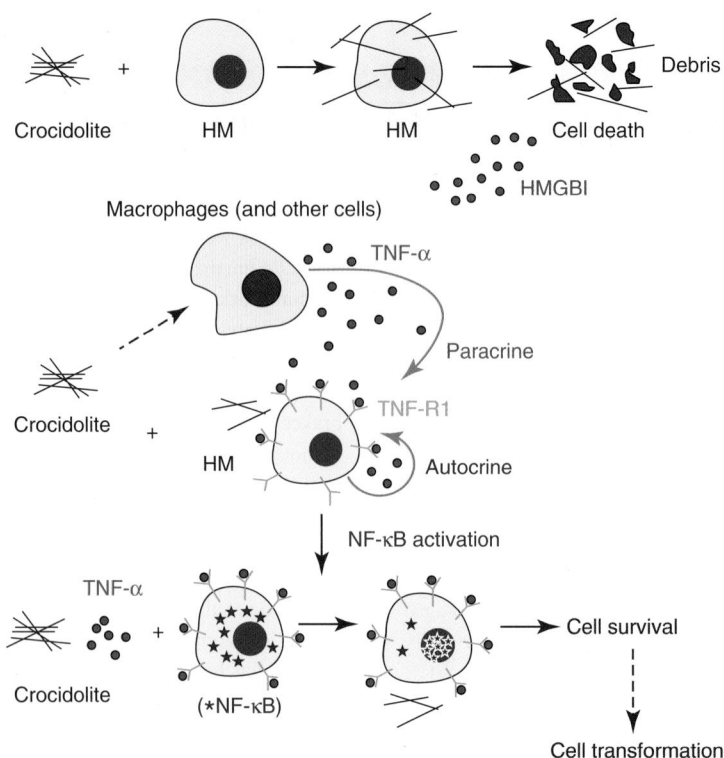

Figure 1 Mineral fiber carcinogenesis. Asbestos and erionite cause necrotic cell death in HM, which leads to the release of HMGB1 into the extracellular space. HMGB1 release causes macrophage accumulation, inflammatory response, and TNF-α secretion. TNF-α activates the NF-κB pathway, which increases HM survival after asbestos/erionite exposure. This allows HM with mineral fiber-induced DNA damage to survive and, if key genetic alterations accumulate, to eventually develop into MM. Source: Reproduced with permission of Haining Yang PhD, and Michele Carbone MD, PhD.

inflammation leading to the release of TNF-α and subsequent NF-κB signaling.[24] Phagocytic macrophages at sites of inflammation internalize asbestos and release mutagenic reactive oxygen species and numerous cytokines including TNF-α and interleukin-1 (IL)-1, which have been linked to asbestos-related carcinogenesis.[20,25] HMGB1 is also released by reactive macrophages, other inflammatory cells, and human mesothelial cells (HMC) upon exposure to asbestos.[24] During programmed necrosis, HMGB1 binds several proinflammatory molecules and triggers the inflammatory responses that distinguish this type of cell death from apoptosis. Secreted HMGB1 stimulates RAGE, TLR2, and TLR4 (the three main HMGB1 receptors) expressed on neighboring inflammatory cells such as macrophages and induces the release of TNF-α and IL-1β. Asbestos-mediated TNF-α signaling then induces the activation of NF-κB-dependent mechanisms, promoting the survival of HMCs after asbestos exposure,[24] and thus allowing HMCs with accumulated asbestos-induced genetic damage to survive, divide, and propagate genetic aberrations in premalignant cells that can give rise to a malignant clone. In addition, HMGB1 enhances the activity of NF-κB, which promotes tumor formation, progression, and metastasis.[26] HMGB1 has been found to be elevated in the serum of asbestos-exposed individuals and MM (multiple myeloma) patients, and investigations are underway to confirm the molecule as a biomarker for asbestos exposure (Figure 1).

Genetic predisposition to mesothelioma: the role of BAP1

Families have recently been identified in the United States, which appear to have unusual susceptibility to asbestos carcinogenesis, and these families have mutations of the BAP1 gene in their germline.[27] The familial susceptibility is associated with the presence of uveal

melanomas and other rare malignancies. BAP1 (BRCA-associated protein 1) has been identified as a novel MPM tumor-suppressor gene. BAP1 is located at the 3p21, a region frequently deleted in MM, and encodes for a deubiquitinase enzyme known to target histones and other proteins. Bott et al.[28] originally described the association of somatic mutations of BAP1 in 23% of mesothelioma samples. In a larger series of patients, the same group confirmed that somatic BAP1 mutations occur in about 20% of pleural MM and reported that the only clinical variable significantly different among those with and without BAP1 mutations was smoking (former or current), with BAP1 mutations more prevalent among smokers (75% vs 42%).[29] More recent studies have reported BAP1 gene alterations (either deletions or sequence-level mutations) in upward of 61% of MM samples,[30] and Arzt et al.,[31] with a separate cohort of 52 pleural MM, reported absence of BAP1 IHC staining in 60% of pleural MM, confirming previous results. In that study, there was no correlation between BAP1 expression and asbestos exposure, and these investigators suggested that expression of BAP1 in tumor samples is inversely correlated to survival.

BAP1 appears to exert its antitumor activities mainly in a BRCA-independent manner[27] with regulation of the cell epigenome, via modulation of histone H2A ubiquitination and chromatin accessibility[32]; however, the relevance of BAP1 to the biology of normal and cancer cells remains largely unexplained. In fact, manipulation of BAP1 in cancer cells has often yielded unexpected or even contradictory results. For example, silencing of BAP1 in MM and uveal melanoma cell lines resulted in reduced cell growth.[28,33]

Germline BAP1 mutations were first reported by Testa et al.[34] in two US families having a high frequency of MPMs. In the same study, 22% sporadic MM tumors harbored somatic BAP1 mutations. These findings have promoted speculation that BAP1 germline mutations can cause a novel cancer syndrome characterized by a significant excess of both pleural and peritoneal MM, uveal and cutaneous melanoma, and possibly other tumors.

Diagnosing and staging the patient with possible mesothelioma

Symptoms and signs

The onset of mesothelioma is associated with chest pain, dyspnea, or cough (Figure 2). Progressive invasion of the chest wall often leads to intractable pain. Pleural effusion is present initially in up to 95% of cases. Often the fluid is viscous owing to high content of hyaluronic acid. Later, tumor growth usually results in complete obliteration of the pleural space and encasement of the lung. Late symptoms of bulky mesotheliomas include mediastinal invasion with dysphagia, phrenic nerve paralysis, pericardial effusion, and superior vena cava syndrome.[35] Peritoneal involvement by mesothelioma is characterized by ascites and intestinal compromise leading to cachexia.

Laboratory evaluation

There are several laboratory abnormalities associated with mesothelioma. Of these, the presence of thrombocytosis with platelet counts >400,000 is probably the most common. Others include hypergammaglobulinemia, eosinophilia, anemia of chronic disease, elevated homocysteine levels, folic acid deficiency, and Vitamin B12 and Vitamin B6 deficiency.[35]

Histologic subtypes

There are three primary types of mesothelioma. The *epithelial type*, the *fibrous morphology type*, also called the *sarcomatoid* type, and a combination called *biphasic or mixed type*. The majority of mesotheliomas (50–70%) are of the epithelial type, 10% are sarcomatoid, and the remaining mesotheliomas are mixed. Immunohistochemical (IHC) markers are necessary to help distinguish between metastatic carcinomas and mesothelioma. These markers include positive pankeratin, keratin 5/6, calretinin, and WT-1. Negative markers include CEA, CD15, Ber-EP4, Moc-31, TTF-1, and B72.3. Such markers are important as mesothelioma may be difficult to distinguish from other malignancies, that is, biphasic mesotheliomas from carcinosarcomas or fibrous mesothelioma from metastatic pleural sarcomas.[36]

Several studies have examined the role of histologic subtype on prognosis. It has consistently been shown that epithelioid type has a better prognosis than the biphasic or sarcomatoid subtypes.[37] In addition to these histologies, several other, lower grade mesothelial tumors exist, such as *papillary mesothelioma*, which often occurs in the abdominal cavity, multicystic mesothelioma, which often presents in "clusters" and which can also present in the peritoneum, and adenomatoid mesothelioma, which is a benign mesothelial lesion in the genitourinary system. These subtypes typically have a more indolent course than the epithelioid, biphasic, or sarcomatoid histologies, though the clinical course can vary.[38]

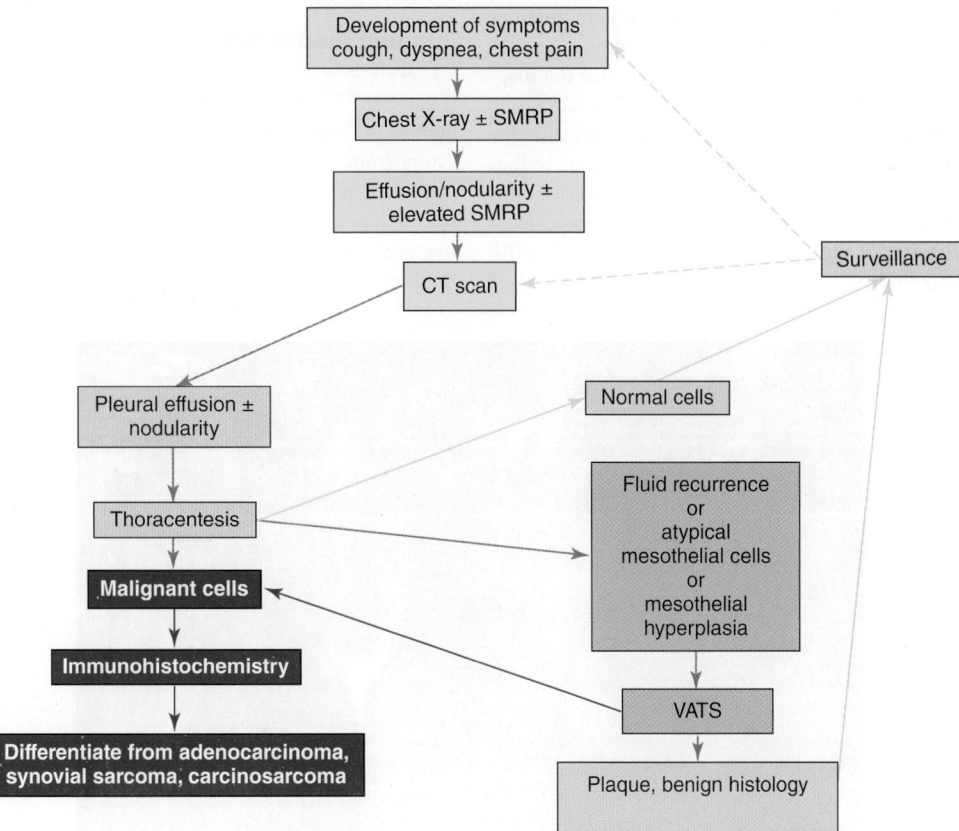

Figure 2 Algorithm for the work up of the asbestos-exposed individual who presents with new symptoms. Any new pleural effusion must have thoracentesis and immunohistochemical analyses. If atypical mesothelial cells are seen, thoracoscopy should be performed for histologic confirmation of malignancy or inflammatory disease.

Tumor markers

Two highly studied tumor markers for mesothelioma are osteopontin (OPN) and mesothelin (SMRP). OPN is a glycoprotein biomarker that is expressed by certain cancers, including lung, breast, colorectal, gastric, ovarian, and melanoma. OPN is also involved in cell-signaling pathways that are associated with asbestos-induced carcinogenesis. A recent study compared OPN levels in patients with mesothelioma with OPN levels in patients with asbestos-related diseases that were not malignant. This study revealed that OPN can be used to separate those patients that had asbestos exposure with mesothelioma from those who had asbestos exposure without malignancy.[39] A recent meta-analysis examined the utility of ostepontin in the diagnosis of mesothelioma over seven studies, and found a pooled sensitivity of 0.57 (95% CI 0.52–0.61), specificity of 0.81 (95% CI 0.79–0.84), positive likelihood ratio (PLR) of 3.78 (95% CI 2.23–6.41), and a negative likelihood ratio (NLR) of 0.51 (0.38–0.67). These results support the above correlation between OPN and mesothelioma.[40] OPN is limited by its lack of specificity and its performance is superior in plasma compared to serum.

SMRP originally described by Pastan,[41,42] is also a glycoprotein and is found in mesothelioma, ovarian cancer, and pancreatic cancer. Robinson et al.[43] demonstrated in 48 patients that SMRP is a serum biomarker with 83% sensitivity and 95% specificity and was confirmed to be a promising marker for MPM in blood and pleural fluid.[44] Serum SMRP levels were higher in MPM patients when compared to lung cancer patients, as were the SMRP levels in pleural fluid when compared to benign pleural fluid or other non-MPM pleural effusions.[44] Indeed, prior studies have suggested that the accuracy of detection is superior in pleural fluid than in serum,[45] though serum analysis is a more convenient measure of this factor. One recent study examined several combinations of serum markers as diagnostic tools for mesothelioma, and in particular to determine if other markers could enhance the diagnostic yield of using SMRP alone. The study found that combining SMRP and carcinoembryonic antigen (CEA) could improve the differentiation between mesothelioma and lung cancer, as well as the difference between mesothelioma and patients with asbestos exposure that do not have this disease.[46] A large meta-analysis has confirmed the report that the sensitivity and specificity of SMRP are similar in many studies.[47]

In addition to being used as a diagnostic tool, several studies have focused on these markers in tracking the course of disease. In one prospective study, 41 patients had 165 samples collected and disease status temporally assessed using response evaluation criteria in solid tumors (RECIST) criteria. The authors found that while SMRP was significantly correlated with a response, as measured by absolute change, RECIST criteria, or modified RECIST criteria, no such associations were found with OPN.[46] Another prospective study of 97 patients found that changes in soluble SMRP were associated with radiologic response, metabolically active tumor volume, and median survival.[48] Further validation of SMRP as a prognostic marker and a measure of tumor response is ongoing.

Several other potential tumor markers have been explored as having utility in this clinical scenario. One high-profile tumor marker that has been explored recently is fibulin-3, an extracellular protein located in the basement membrane of the vasculature. When assessing plasma fibulin-3 levels, the investigators found that this marker could distinguish between healthy patients with exposure to asbestos from those patients with malignancy in a cohort of over 200 patients, and this was confirmed by blinded validation studies.[49] Furthermore, when plasma fibulin-3 is analyzed in conjunction with that measured in the pleural effusion, it was found that the marker is effective in differentiating benign from both benign and other types of malignant effusions. The diagnostic ability of fibulin-3 has been confirmed in other studies.[50] In one study that compared soluble SMRP and fibulin-3 as a tumor markers, the investigators found that while SMRP was superior in diagnosis, fibulin-3 was better in assessing prognosis, thus implying utility of both markers in a complementary manner.[51]

Imaging modalities

CT scan is very useful for diagnosis and disease assessment (Figure 3).[52] Findings on CT scan include a pleural effusion, pleural nodularity, and concentric pleural thickening. However, investigators from Oxford recently estimated the positive and negative predictive values of approximately 400 patients undergoing a CT scan before thoracoscopy for diagnosis. They found that the positive predictive value of a CT scan that demonstrated "malignant" findings was 80%, while the negative predictive value was 65%.

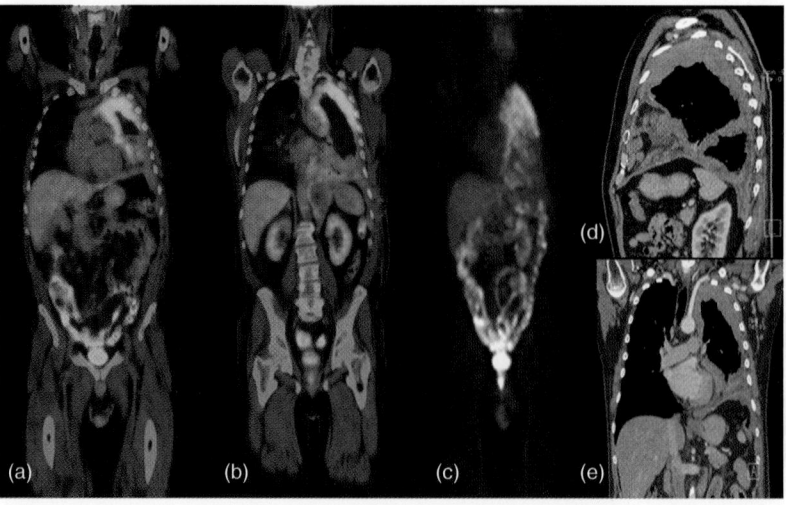

Figure 3 PET-CT and pleural mesothelioma. (a,b) Posterior and anterior views of the left chest reveals a bulky hypermetabolic tumor (c) maximum intensity projection (MIP) view confirming no disease outside the chest. (d) Sagittal view of CT image reveals bulky disease in the fissures. (e) Coronal view reveals abutment of the subclavian artery and possible diaphragmatic involvement.

Thus, CT scan alone appears to be insufficient in determining which patients undergo invasive pleural biopsies.[53]

Additional imaging modalities that can be used to stage mesothelioma include magnetic resonance imaging (MRI) and positron emission tomography (PET) scanning. MRI is not frequently used, but may be of additional benefit to detect diaphragm invasion, involvement of the endothoracic fascia, or an isolated area of chest wall involvement in patients that may be candidates for surgical resection. In addition, the role of PET/CT scanning has not been conclusively elucidated, and PET imaging is not recommended for diagnosis or staging in the 2014 National Comprehensive Cancer Network guidelines. However, many prior and ongoing studies are assessing this technique because of its utility in other thoracic malignancies such as lung cancer. In one study, PET was found to have a sensitivity of only 11% in detecting metastatic lymph-node disease[54]; however, the same study found that a high standardized uptake values (SUV) correlated with N2 disease at the time of resection. More recently, research from the same institution showed that an SUV value 10 greater correlated with a significantly shorter survival time and a 3.3 times greater risk of dying compared to SUV levels below 10.[55] This suggests that PET results may help to stratify patients for different treatments according to their metabolic activity. Integrated CT-PET is more informative than PET alone. In a study of 29 MPM patients, integrated CT-PET correctly assigned the overall stage in 72% of cases, showed increased sensitivity for T4 disease, 67% versus 19% for PET alone, identified 7 patients with extrathoracic disease missed by conventional radiographic studies, and identified 12 patients that would have been precluded from surgical resection based on conventional studies.[56] In addition, investigators from Memorial Sloan-Kettering Cancer Center examined the accuracy of PET scan in detecting histologic subtype. In 100 patients with MPM who underwent preoperative PET scans, they found that the mixed subtype of epithelioid mesothelioma had higher SUVs than patients with the nonpleomorphic subtype, thus supporting the conclusion that higher SUVs are correlated with aggressive disease.[57] Another recent study examined the prognostic significance of PET scan after neoadjuvant chemotherapy for resectable MPM in 50 patients, all of whom underwent EPP (extrapleural pneumonectomy) and postoperative hemithoracic radiotherapy. Metabolic response after neoadjuvant chemotherapy was significantly correlated with the overall survival, and the authors concluded that response to therapy may be integrated into the decision-making process for surgical resection after neoadjuvant chemotherapy.[58]

Surgical diagnosis and staging in mesothelioma

The interventions that can be used for diagnostic purposes in mesothelioma include thoracentesis with closed pleural biopsy, VATS (video-assisted thoracoscopy surgery) with pleural biopsy, and open pleural biopsy. It is important to have adequate tissue to classify not only whether the biopsy reveals mesothelioma, but also possibly the subtype of mesothelioma. Although cytologic diagnosis can be difficult, electron microscopy and IHC staining on a cell block of the pleural fluid can be performed to increase diagnostic yield up to 84% in suspected cases. Video-assisted thoracoscopy with direct biopsy and assessment of the involvement of the lung and pleura remains the gold standard for diagnosis. Studies have confirmed the utility of this technique among patients undergoing surgery for mesothelioma, but have also pointed out the difficulty in obtaining correct histologic diagnosis.[59] Information about parietal, visceral, and diaphragmatic pleural involvement can be

obtained, and this might have prognostic value for survival.[60] Open pleural biopsy is rarely performed, but may be required when there is no free pleural space.

Staging and prognostic indicators

The American Joint Committee on Cancer (AJCC) staging system for mesothelioma has been validated in a number of surgically based trials[61] and has been used since the 1990s. In order to improve the current staging system, an international database of over 2000 staged patients with MPM was analyzed by the International Association for the Study of Lung Cancer, and covariates predictive of survival included best staging information, age, sex, histology (epithelioid or not), and type of surgical procedure (palliative vs EPP or pleurectomy decortication).[62] Supplementary prognostic indicators complementing the international database include platelet count, white blood cell count, and the addition of adjuvant therapy.[63] Gill,[64] in a study of 88 epithelial MPMs having EPP, has expanded on the influence of tumor volume and survival in MPM stage-independent model of risk for death in patients having surgical cytoreduction as originally described by Pass et al.[65] In Gill's report, tumor volume, hemoglobin concentration, platelet count, pathologic TNM (tumour, node, and metastasis) category, and administration of adjuvant chemotherapy or RT were associated with survival.[64] Richards, using the same MPM cohorts as Gill from the Brigham and Women's Hospital series, has recently described a validated model for survival and time to recurrence in cytoreduced MPM using hemoglobin, CT volume, thickness of the fissures, and histological subtype (Table 1).[66]

Treatment

The treatment options for mesothelioma depend on several parameters, including performance status, medical comorbidities, pulmonary function, stage, and age of the patient as well other factors. Surgical options are considered as long as the bulk of the disease can be removed without leaving gross disease behind. If this cannot be accomplished, then supportive measures for palliation can be used (Table 2).

Supportive care

The median survival of MPM patients who select supportive care ranges only from 4[67] to 13 months,[68] and is influenced by multiple factors including the biology of the tumor as well as whether survival time is recorded from the time of symptom initiation or from the time of definitive diagnosis. There are a number of options for the control of pleural effusion, including repeated thoracenteses, talc pleurodesis, or placement of a Pleur X (Denver Biomedical, Denver, CO) catheter.[69] Failure of these techniques is usually associated with lung trapped by the tumor, a large solid tumor mass, a long history of effusion with multiple thoracenteses leading to loculations, age older than 70 years, or poor performance status. In such cases, the PleurX catheter with its one-way valve can be implanted under local anesthesia into pleural effusion, and patients can drain themselves at home using the available disposable drainage kits.[70] Recently, a randomized trial examined the influence of pleural fluid palliation in mesothelioma. The MesoVats trial was a randomization between 2003 and 2012 of 87 VAT pleurectomy or 88 talc pleurodesis for patients who were not considered for maximal cytoreductive techniques. There was no survival difference, but pleural effusion was better controlled with pleurectomy patients, and a significant

Table 1 The International Mesothelioma Interest Group (IMIG) staging system for pleural mesothelioma.

T1	
T1a	Tumor limited to the ipsilateral parietal ± mediastinal ± diaphragmatic pleura, no involvement of the visceral pleura
T1b	Tumor involving the ipsilateral parietal ± mediastinal ± diaphragmatic pleura, tumor also involving the visceral pleura
T2	Tumor involving each of the ipsilateral pleural surfaces (parietal, mediastinal, diaphragmatic, and visceral pleura) with at least one of the following features: • Involvement of diaphragmatic muscle • Extension of tumor from visceral pleura into the underlying pulmonary parenchyma
T3	Describes locally advanced but potentially resectable tumor Tumor involving all of the ipsilateral pleural surfaces (parietal, mediastinal, diaphragmatic, and visceral pleura) with at least one of the following features: • Involvement of the endothoracic fascia • Extension into the mediastinal fat • Solitary, completely resectable focus of tumor extending into the soft tissues of the chest wall • Nontransmural involvement of the pericardium
T4	Describes locally advanced technically unresectable tumor Tumor involving all the ipsilateral pleural surfaces (parietal, mediastinal, diaphragmatic, and visceral pleura) with at least one of the following features: • Diffuse extension or multifocal masses of tumor in the chest wall, with or without associated rib destruction • Direct transdiaphragmatic extension of tumor to the peritoneum • Direct extension of tumor to the contralateral pleura • Direct extension of tumor to mediastinal organs • Direct extension of tumor into the spine • Tumor extending through to the internal surface of the pericardium with or without a pericardial effusion; or tumor involving the myocardium
N-Lymph nodes	
NX	Regional lymph nodes cannot be assessed
N0	No regional lymph node metastases
N1	Metastases in the ipsilateral bronchopulmonar or hilar lymph nodes
N2	Metastases in the subcarinal or the ipsilateral mediastinal lymph nodes including the ipsilateral internal mammary nodes
N3	Metastases in the contralateral mediastinal, contralateral internal mammary, ipsilateral, or contralateral supraclavicular lymph nodes
M-Metastases	
MX	Presence of distant metastases cannot be assessed
M0	No distant metastasis
M1	Distant metastasis present
Stage I	
Ia	T1a N0 M0
Ib	T1b N0 M0
Stage II	T2 N0 M0
Stage III	Any T3 M0
	Any N1 M0
	Any N2 M0
Stage IV	Any T4
	Any N3
	Any M1

Abbreviations: T, primary tumor; T1, limited to ipsilateral pleura only (parietal pleura, visceral pleura); T2, superficial local invasion (diaphragm, endothoracic fascia, ipsilateral lung, and fissures); T3, deep local invasion (chest wall beyond endothoracic fascia); T4, extensive direct invasion (opposite pleura, peritoneum, and retroperitoneum); N, lymph nodes; N0, no positive lymph node; N1, positive ipsilateral hilar nodes; N2, positive mediastinal nodes; N3, positive contralateral hilar nodes; M, metastases; M0, no metastases; M1, metastases; blood-borne or lymphatic.
Source: Adapted from Rusch 1996.[61]

benefit in quality of life was recorded in favor of the pleurectomy group.[71]

Patients with chest-wall pain due to mesothelioma should be seen in consultation by a dedicated pain management team to consider narcotic control as well as novel pain-control techniques including outpatient epidural catheter use. Palliative radiotherapy is associated with a median survival of 4–5 months.[72,73]

Surgery for pleural mesothelioma

Maximal cytoreductive procedures
The goal of cytoreductive surgery in MPM should be the removal of all visible or palpable tumor (R0 or R1) or a "macroscopic complete resection" (MCR), regardless of whether that involves EPP or a lung-preserving operation. The Mesothelioma Domain of the International Association for the Study of Lung Cancer has defined uniform nomenclature for pleural mesothelioma resections[74] and includes EPP, extended pleurectomy and decortication (ePD)

(resection of the diaphragm and/or pericardium), and pleurectomy decortication as potential MCRs. Suspicion and documentation of disease outside the involved hemithorax eliminates the use of an MCR. Patients who present with ECOG performance status 2 or greater, or who have limiting cardiac reserve either with nonreversible myocardial ischemia or compromised ventricular function (ejection fraction <50%) are usually not candidates for cytoreductive procedures. Moreover, patients with compromised pulmonary-function testing who are not felt to be candidates for pneumonectomy must be carefully evaluated for either extended P/D in that the cytoreduction should not compromise the existing lung function but may recruit trapped lung and possibly improve dyspnea.

Extrapleural pneumonectomy (EPP)
As detailed in a recent systematic review of the use of EPP for MPM,[75] the median overall survival varies from 9.4 to 27.5 months, and 1-, 2-, and 5-year survival rates ranges from 36% to 83%, 5% to

Table 2 Treatment options for mesothelioma.

Supportive care	
Effusion control	Talc pleurodesis
	Vats assisted
	Slurry
	Pleurex catheter
	Repeated thoracenteses
Pain control	Narcotics
	Permanent epidural catheter
	Localized radiation
Surgery	Pleurectomy with decortication
	Extrapleural pneumonectomy
Chemotherapy[a]	Pemetrexed (Alimta) and cisplatin[a]
	Gemcitabine and cisplatin[a]
	Vinorelbine (Navelbine)
	Phase I/II trials with targeted agents
Multimodality therapy	Induction chemotherapy, surgery, and postoperative radiotherapy[b]
	Surgery and postoperative radiotherapy
	Surgery and postoperative chemotherapy
	Surgery and novel cytotoxic/targeted agents[b]
	Induction Radiation followed by surgery[b]
Novel intrapleural therapies	Hyperthermic chemoperfusion,[b] chemotherapy, povidone-iodine[b]
	Photodynamic therapy[b]
	Gene therapy[b]
Novel radiation techniques at selected centers	Intensity-modulated radiation therapy

[a]Most commonly used in recent phase II/III trials.
[b]Under investigation.

59%, and 0% to 24%, respectively (Figure 4). Overall perioperative mortality rates ranged from 0% to 11.8%, and centers routinely performing the operation have mortality rates close to 3% through improvements in preoperative staging, anesthesia, resection, reconstruction, and perioperative management of procedure-related complications.[76] The chief perioperative morbidities include atrial fibrillation, myocardial infarction, and pulmonary complications.[77] EPP *alone* does not appear to prolong survival. In most EPP series, median survival is <2 years, but 10–20% of patients are 5-year survivors. Patients with sarcomatoid histology and/or lymph-node involvement have an even poorer prognosis and should not be considered as candidates for EPP.[78]

Trimodality therapy and the move to lung-sparing techniques

Trimodality therapy consists of induction chemotherapy, followed by EPP, and RT either as hemithorax radiation to the pneumonectomy cavity or as intensity-modulated RT.[79] Overall, the studies of MPM trimodality therapy demonstrate a 3.1% mortality for EPP, along with a 27.7 month median survival in the 60% of presenting patients who complete the full package. The Mesothelioma and Radical Surgery (MARS) was an attempt to validate the use of EPP as part of this radical treatment package. MARS was originally designed as a randomized trial with 670 patients needed comparing induction chemotherapy, EPP, and postoperative RT to induction therapy but no EPP.[80] When difficulty arose in recruiting patients, an initial feasibility study was performed in 50 patients for EPP or no EPP. The study revealed nonsignificant differences in the 6, 12, 18, and median survivals comparing the surgery arm to the nonsurgical arm, with a median survival of 14.4 versus 19.5 months, respectively. The 18% operative mortality from EPP in MARS must be contrasted to the 3.1% operative mortality from other phase II trimodality trials (3.1%). Moreover, the lack of power of the study, the nonstandardization of the preoperative chemotherapy, and the

fact that only a third of the individuals received the full trimodality have diminished the impact of MARS.[81]

Nevertheless, the movement away from the idea that the only surgical MCR for MPM was EPP was already gaining momentum (Figure 5). A retrospective review of 663 consecutive patients (538 men and 125 women with MPM who underwent EPP or P/D at three US mesothelioma centers reported an operative mortality of 7% for EPP ($n = 27/385$) and 4% for P/D ($n = 13/278$).[82] Multivariate analysis demonstrated a 1.4-fold greater chance for death with EPP ($P < 0.001$) controlling for stage, histology, gender, and multimodality therapy. This study was the first to postulate that patients who underwent P/D could have comparable survival to those who underwent EPP; however, the reasons for such a conclusion were multifactorial and subject to selection bias. Other studies revealed a doubling of overall survival if the P/D is performed to remove all macroscopic disease in a compulsive manner.[83–90] In studies where a direct comparison of EPP and P/D performed by the same surgeon have been reported, P/D has less mortality, less morbidity, and a comparable overall survival to EPP. These findings are particularly striking for early-stage mesothelioma. As ePD is a less-extensive operation with lower morbidity and mortality than EPP, a newly designed MARS-2 trial will attempt to demonstrate whether this type of operation can offer survival and/or quality-of-life benefits to patients with MPM.[91] Patients with MPM registered on MARS-2 will receive two cycles of pemetrexed-platinum chemotherapy. Patients who do not progress on CT scan will then be randomized to up to four further cycles of pemetrexed-platinum chemotherapy or ePD followed by up to four further cycles of postoperative pemetrexed-platinum chemotherapy. An EORTC (European Organization for Research and Treatment of Cancer) trial will investigate the timing of the chemotherapy in combination with ePD.[92] Patients with MPM will be randomly allocated to ePD preceded or followed by four cycles of cisplatin/pemetrexed at standard doses. It is hoped that this randomized trial will address the feasibility of the operation in combination with standard (neo)-adjuvant chemotherapy and set the experimental arm of an ensuing phase III trial exploring the role of surgery in MPM or could be a standard arm for future trials of surgery in MPM.

Novel surgical strategies

An innovative phase I/II approach (surgery for mesothelioma after radiation therapy, SMART) using a short-accelerated course of high-dose hemithoracic intensity-modulated radiation therapy (IMRT) followed by EPP has been investigated by Cho et al.[93] Patients received 25 Gy in five daily fractions during 1 week to the entire ipsilateral hemithorax with concomitant 5 Gy boost to areas at risk followed by EPP within 1 week of completing neoadjuvant IMRT. Of the 25 patients accrued, IMRT was well tolerated with no grade 3+ toxicities, and EPP was performed 6 ± 2 days after completing IMRT without any perioperative mortality. After a median follow-up of 23 months, the cumulative 3-year survival reached 84% in epithelial subtypes compared with 13% in biphasic subtypes ($p = 0.0002$). A multicenter approach is planned for validation of these results.

At the University of Pennsylvania, a phase III trial of MCR with and without photodynamic therapy (PDT) is planned. Results with PDT have been associated with increased survival times with the conversion of MCR to lung sparing techniques such as standard or ePD.[94,95] Intrapleural hyperthermic perfusions are now more popular especially in Europe but differ from the studies in the United States in that these have not used cisplatinum/gemcitabine

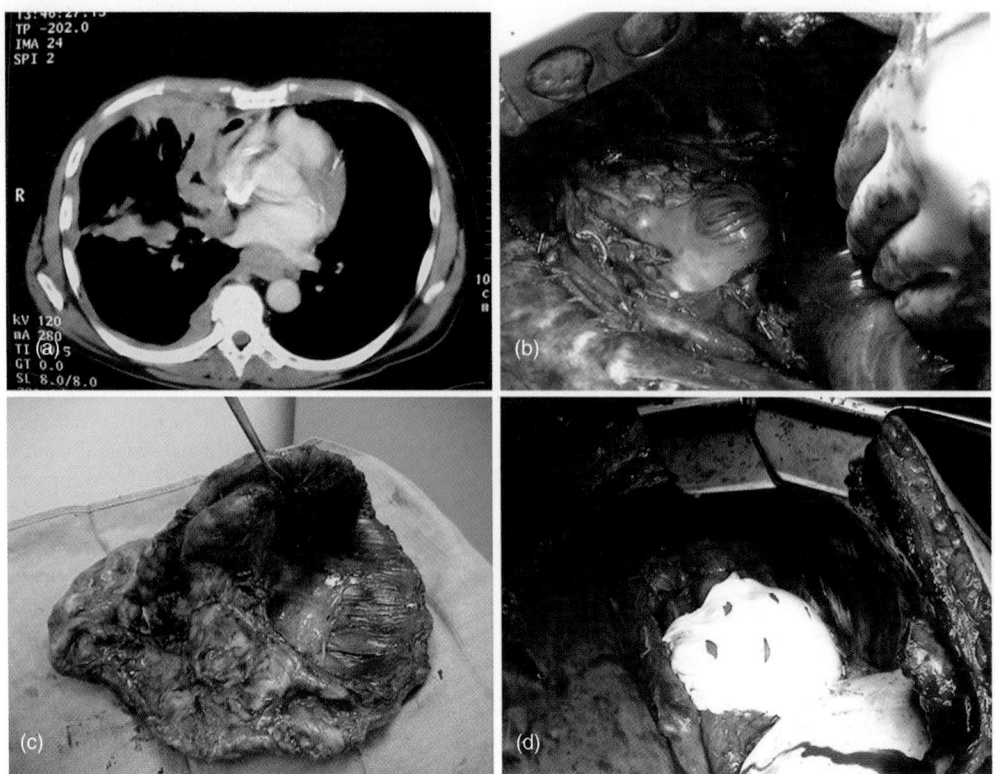

Figure 4 Extrapleural pneumonectomy for mesothelioma: (a) Computer tomography reveals thickened pleura, pericardium, and disease in the fissures. (b) Intraoperative view after the resection with hand on the liver. Stapled bronchial stump, right atrium, and extent of pericardiotomy are seen. (c) Operative specimen reveals diaphragmatic resection to the right and thickened pleura encasing the lung. (d) Reconstruction of the diaphragm and pericardium with Gore-Tex patches.

during the perfusion, electing to study warm povidone-iodine instead. Moreover, the perfusions are being performed chiefly in patients having pleurectomy-decortications.[96]

Radiation therapy for mesothelioma

RT is typically delivered in the adjuvant setting for MPM. The RT approach and risks are primarily determinant on the type of surgical resection involved, and can be divided into two categories: RT after EPP and RT after P/D or no surgery.

Adjuvant radiation therapy after extrapleural pneumonectomy

As mesothelioma is a malignancy that involves the pleura, it is generally accepted that even when specific regions are found to be involved with malignancy, the entire pleural cavity is at risk for disease. Therefore, attempts to control microscopic disease with RT have typically included treating the entire hemithorax, specifically the entire pleura +/− the ipsilateral lung and pericardium. Historically, hemithoracic radiation has been given using two-dimensional, or "conventional" techniques. These approaches utilize a limited number of fields and nonconformal methods. As a result, a great deal of dose heterogeneity typically occurs, with the target volume being underdosed and surrounding normal tissue, such as the esophagus, lung, heart, and spinal cord, receiving increased dose, or "hot spots." Rusch et al. performed a prospective phase II trial of surgical resection followed by hemithoracic radiation using conventional methods. From 1995 to 1998, approximately 90 patients at MSKCC (Memorial Sloan Kettering Cancer Center) underwent surgical resection (70% with EPP) and 57 then underwent hemithoracic RT to doses of 41.4–54 Gy.

The median survival was 17 months, with approximately 20% of these patients experiencing recurrence at the radiation treatment margins. Most patients that recurred experienced distant metastases.[97,98]

In the past decade, the conformal technique of IMRT has been advanced and applied to this clinical context. As a result, conformality has increased with this approach (Figure 6). Several institutions have reported their outcomes with this approach. In an early study from MD Anderson Cancer Center, 28 patients were treated with hemithoracic IMRT after EPP to doses of 45–50 Gy. One year OS and DFS were 65% and 88%, respectively, and 65% of patients had grade 2 or 3 nausea/vomiting.[99] These results have since been updated twice, in 2007[100,101] and 2013,[102] with the most recent study demonstrating 90% OS at 1 year and 71% at 2 years in this selected group of patients. Grade 3 toxicity was generally <20%, with 15–20% rates of grade 3 dermatitis and gastrointestinal side effects. It should be emphasized, however, that adhering to dose constraints is essential to minimize the risk of high-grade and potentially fatal toxicity. One early report by investigators at the Dana-Farber Cancer Institute demonstrated that 6 of 13 patients treated with IMRT after EPP experienced fatal radiation pneumonitis. While 11 of these patients also received heated intraoperative cisplatin, which may have contributed to this observation, the low-dose region to the remaining lung (particularly the percentage of lung receiving 20 Gy, or V20) was higher than our current acceptable levels.[103] Thus, conformality with IMRT comes with the tradeoff of a "low-dose radiation bath" to the remaining lung that needs to be closely monitored when performing RT planning.

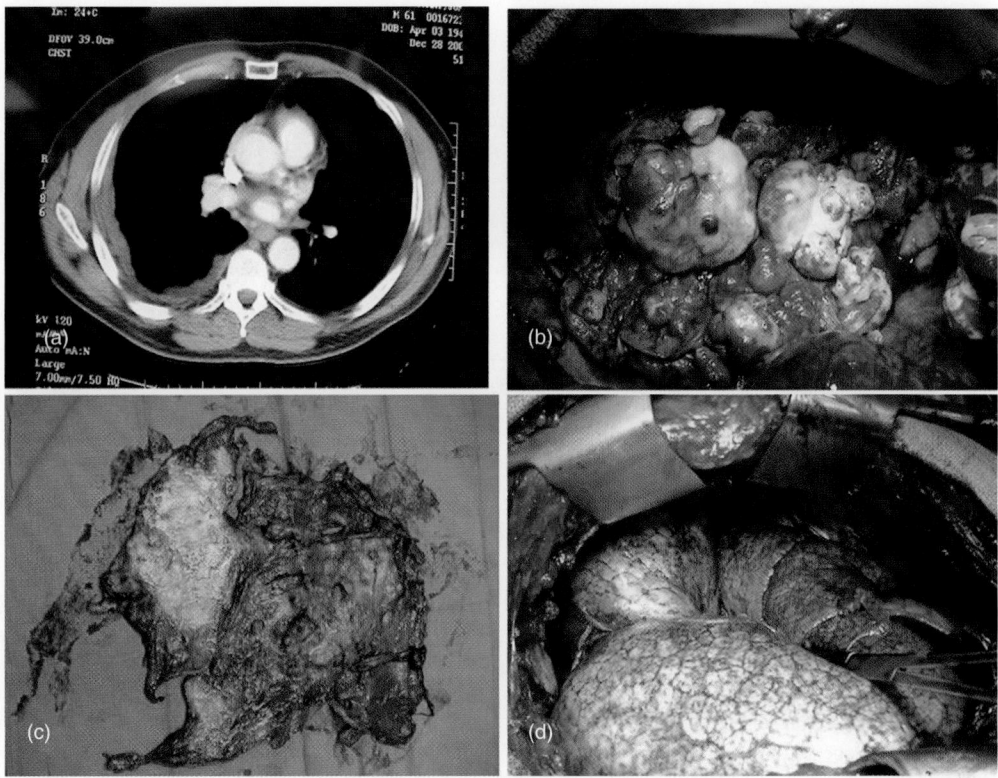

Figure 5 Pleurectomy for mesothelioma: (a) typical computer tomogram reveals thickened pleura; (b) operative view reveals disease primarily on the parietal pleura; (c) operative specimen; (d) completion of satisfactory cytoreduction with sparing and decortication of the lung.

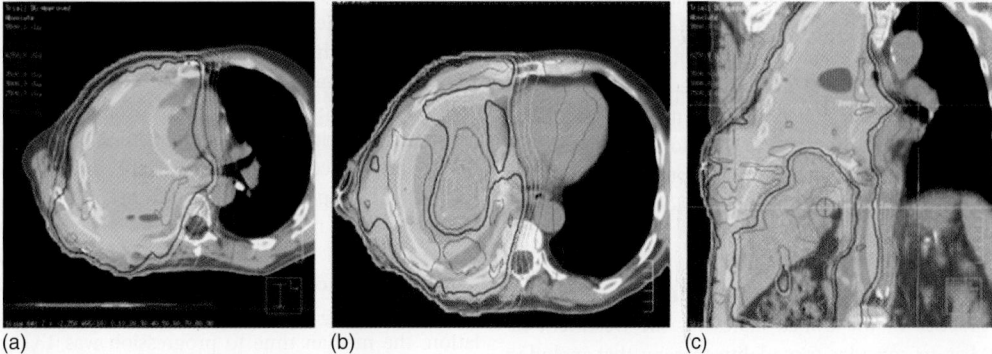

Figure 6 (a–c) Two axial slices and a coronal view of IMRT after extrapleural pneumonectomy. IMRT offers improved conformality and better dose homogeneity to both the target volume and critical normal structures.

Radiation therapy after pleurectomy/decortication (P/D) or unresectable disease

The role of RT after P/D is not yet established. Indeed, there are several reasons why hemithoracic radiation is more challenging when patients do not undergo an EPP. First, functional lung remains that exposes the patient to the risk of high-grade acute lung toxicity bilaterally. Second, presuming that the ipsilateral lung is contributing to the total lung function, because much of that lung will receive radiation dose, patients are at a higher risk for a substantial reduction in lung function after RT (compared to immediately postoperatively). Finally, by treating much of the ipsilateral lung and therefore deeming it to be nonfunctional, a "shunting" effect can be produced whereby perfusion continues in the ipsilateral lung, yet very little air exchange occurs. As a result, initial studies examining this approach demonstrated suboptimal outcomes. In one analysis from Memorial Sloan Kettering, 123 patients were treated with lung-sparing surgery

and underwent hemithoracic radiation using conventional techniques to a median total dose of 42.5 Gy, with approximately half of the patients also receiving brachytherapy. Local control was approximately 40%, with 38 cases of grade 3 toxicity and 7 cases of grade 4–5 toxicity. Thus, this technique was associated with low levels of local control and relatively high rates of toxicity.[104]

More recent studies have incorporated modern techniques into this paradigm, and several institutions have reported outcomes. Figure 7 demonstrates a patient that has received this treatment, with attempted sparing of the ipsilateral lung through the creation of a "rind" in treatment volume delineation. A study from Memorial Sloan Kettering reported results with 67 patients treated with either lung-sparing surgery or biopsy alone, and found a 1- and 2-year actuarial failure rate of 56% and 74%, respectively. Local recurrence was the dominant failure pattern, and patients undergoing a P/D increased the time to local recurrence (vs biopsy alone).[105] MD

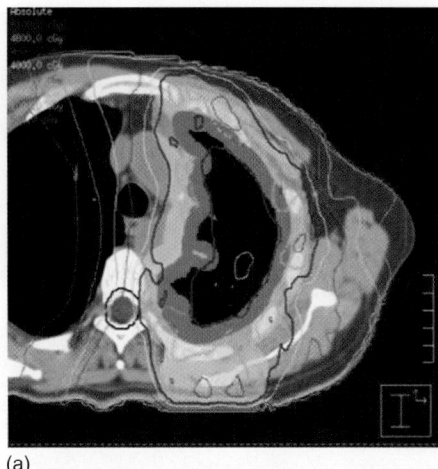 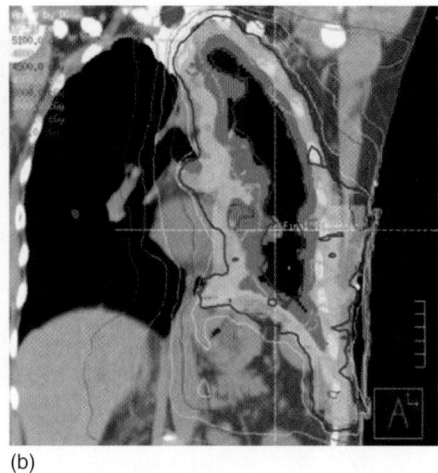

(a)   (b)

Figure 7 (a, b) An axial and a coronal view of a patient treated with IMRT after pleurectomy/decortication. A "rind" is created to attempt to spare the inner portion of the lung, though full sparing of the ipsilateral lung is typically not feasible.

Anderson Cancer Center also recently analyzed their data of 24 patients treated with IMRT after P/D, and found OS and PFS rates of 76% and 67% at 1 year, respectively, and 56% and 34% at 2 years, respectively. Measurable changes in pulmonary function were observed after surgery [21% forced vital capacity (FVC), 16% forced expiratory volume in one second (FEV1)], and again after hemithoracic IMRT (31% FVCand 25% FEV1). When comparing this group of patients to historical controls treated with EPP and adjuvant IMRT, no differences were found in high-grade toxicity, and both median OS (28.4 months vs 14.2 months, $p = 0.04$) and PFS (16.4 months vs 8.2 months) favored P/D.[106] Overall, prospective trials are needed to evaluate this approach and incorporate RT after P/D or in the setting of unresectable disease, and one such phase II trial is currently ongoing at Memorial Sloan Kettering and MD Anderson Cancer Center. In addition, the further advancement of radiation techniques such as proton-beam therapy may improve the extent of sparing that can be achieved when the lung is intact.

Systemic chemotherapy for mesothelioma

The standard practice in the United States for the treatment of resectable MPM is to consider trimodality therapy that includes four cycles of either neoadjuvant or adjuvant cisplatin-pemetrexed. However, several issues regarding the optimal sequence of trimodality therapy and the choice of systemic regimen remain unclear.

Neoadjuvant or adjuvant systemic therapy choices

The decision to administer neoadjuvant or adjuvant systemic therapy is made in a multidisciplinary setting. Neoadjuvant chemotherapy has the potential to adversely delay surgical resection or induce complications before resection. In addition, significant response rates with tumor shrinkage range between 29% and 44% with cisplatin-pemetrexed.[107,108] It is estimated from clinical trials that between 42% and 84% of the time, an EPP after neoadjuvant chemotherapy will be able to be completed.[107–113] Adjuvant chemotherapy does not compromise surgical resection, but does carry the risk of being unable to be administered after surgery and radiation because of diminished patient performance status. To date, there are no randomized trials comparing neoadjuvant or adjuvant therapy and both approaches are acceptable standard practice. A review of several prospective neoadjuvant clinical trials

reveals a median overall survival range of 16.6–25.5 months.[29–35] One adjuvant trial ($n = 20$) using platinum-gemcitabine or platinum-pemetrexed after EPP reported a comparable median overall survival of 17 months.[36,114]

The optimal systemic platinum-doublet is unknown for resectable MPM. Cisplatin-pemetrexed is commonly accepted as the standard of care in the United States; however, other countries prefer alternate regimens. De Perrot et al.[115] conducted a retrospective analysis ($n = 60$) on their centers' use of neoadjuvant chemotherapy and reported that there was no significant difference in survival outcomes. The neoadjuvant regimens assessed included cisplatin-vinorelbine, platinum-pemetrexed, cisplatin-raltitrexed, and cisplatin-gemcitabine.

With the risks in mind, neoadjuvant chemotherapy has the capability to yield prognostic information for surgical resection. In the largest neoadjuvant EPP trial ($n = 75$) completed to date, Krug et al.[107] reported that responding patients (defined as complete or partial response to neoadjuvant chemotherapy) had an improvement in the median overall survival (29.1 months compared to 13.9 months, $P = 0.076$) compared to patients who did not have a response.[107] In this trial, for the intent to treat population, the median time to progression was 13.1 months and the overall survival was 16.6 months. Taken together, the neoadjuvant platinum-doublet systemic therapy trials indicate that a need exists for better systemic agents with higher response rates, low toxicity, and capability to be given as maintenance therapy.

Several investigational approaches to neoadjuvant therapy with novel agents are being attempted in the resectable MPM population. An exploratory window of opportunity trial with neoadjuvant dasatinib was performed at the University of Texas M.D. Anderson Cancer Center. MPM cell lines and tumor cells have overexpression of activated Src kinase, and preclinical studies demonstrated antitumor efficacy of dasatinib.[116] This study has completed accrual and demonstrated that the biomarker Src kinase[Tyr419] was a pharmacodynamics marker and higher baseline levels were predictive of a metabolic response by PETCT to neoadjuvant dasatinib therapy. In addition, distinct patterns of PDGFRα and β expression by immunohistochemistry were predictive of sensitivity or resistance to dasatinib treatment. In addition, the Southwest Oncology Group (SWOG) is developing a neoadjuvant immunotherapy study in resectable MPM using an anti-PDL1 inhibitor. This study will utilize the immunotherapy agent as maintenance therapy after completion of trimodality treatment.

Memorial Sloan Kettering has been pioneering the use of an adjuvant WT-1 (Wilm's Tumor-1) vaccine in a Department of Defense-sponsored clinical trial.[117] The peptide vaccine delivered in the trial stimulates host T cells to identify and eliminate WT-1-expressing cells. Eligible patients must express WT-1 by immunohistochemistry on their mesothelioma tumor cells. In normal cells, WT-1 is a transcription factor that is present in young children but is lost once adulthood is reached.

Intrapleural and immunotherapy strategies

There has been significant research on intrapleural administration of chemotherapies for MPM. However, it is not standard of care and is recommended to only perform intrapleural therapy on a well-designed clinical trial. The premise behind the use of intrapleural treatment is to bring the agent into direct tumor cell contact and deliver high concentrations of the drug. In the past, intracavitary platinum-based regimens have been used with median PFS ranging between 7.5 and 13.6 months and median OS between 11.5 and 18.3 months.[118–123] The most significant adverse event identified in these studies was renal failure from systemic absorption of cisplatin. Hyperthermic intrapleural therapy administered after P/D yields median overall survival ranges between 9 and 13 months.[122,124–126]

Intrapleural gene therapy using adenovirus vectors containing the herpesvirus thymidine kinase (Ad-HSVtk) suicide gene[127–129] and an adenoviral vector containing an immune stimulant, interferon-β (Ad.hu.IFN-β)[130] has also been explored with some preliminary positive results for successful gene transfer into patient tumor cells. However, this strategy appears to primarily benefit patients with less bulky disease. Intrapleural cytokine administration has been reported in small studies to have a potential antitumor effect.[131–134] Gamma-interferon and interleukin-2 (IL-2) are the most common agents evaluated, with fever, flu-like symptoms, and catheter infections comprising the main toxic effects. Astoul et al.[132] reported that responders to IL-2 had significant overall survival benefit (28 months vs 8 months, $P = 0.01$). Lucchi et al.[131] reported the median overall survival of 26 months with a trial administering neoadjuvant intrapleural IL-2, P/D, adjuvant radiation, systemic IL-2 and cisplatin-gemcitabine chemotherapy, and then maintenance subcutaneous IL-2. Although the majority of the patients developed local recurrence, the use of immune modulatory agents is a worthwhile strategy in resectable MPM.

The role of immunotherapy in resectable mesothelioma is also being explored. Mesothelioma is considered an immunogenic disease and it is surmised that the addition of an anti-PDL1 inhibitor to cisplatin-pemetrexed in the neoadjuvant setting would be clinically beneficial. After surgical resection and adjuvant radiation treatment, maintenance immunotherapy to enhance t-cell activation against microscopic disease would potentially increase the overall survival outcomes. At ESMO 2014, Mansfield et al.[135] reported a 40% PD-L1 IHC expression in pleural mesotheliomas ($n = 224$) using a mouse monoclonal antihuman B7-H1 (clone 5H1-A3). A score of <5% IHC expression was considered negative. PD-L1 IHC expression was associated with more disease burden and less offers of surgery to the patient. In addition, PD-L1 IHC expression was associated with a worse survival (6 months vs 14 months, $p < 0.0001$).[135] SWOG is therefore initiating a neoadjuvant trial with cisplatin-pemetrexed with and without MPDL3280A, a PD-L1 inhibitor, in resectable MPM patients.

Systemic therapies for unresectable mesothelioma

In the front-line metastatic setting, cisplatin-pemetrexed is the Food and Drug Administration (FDA) approved regimen in the United States.[136] Vogelzang et al. conducted a randomized study of 456 patients and randomized them to cisplatin (75 mg/m^2 intravenous every 3 weeks) monotherapy or cisplatin (75 mg/m^2) and pemetrexed (500 mg/m^2) given intravenously every 3 weeks for a maximum of six cycles. The cisplatin-pemetrexed regimen improved the response rate (41.3% vs 16.7%, $p < 0.001$), time to progression (5.7 months vs 3.9 months, $p < 0.001$), and median overall survival (12.1 months vs 9.3 months, $p = 0.02$). The main grade 3/4 side effects experienced with the combination regimen in over 10% of patients were neutropenia, nausea/vomiting, and fatigue. Pemetrexed usage must be accompanied by vitamin B12 and folic acid supplementation. In addition, use of corticosteroids during pemetrexed administration is necessary.

Although there is no randomized clinical trial data on maintenance therapy, patients can be given platinum-pemetrexed for 4–6 cycles of therapy followed by pemetrexed maintenance therapy. In the treatment of nonsquamous nonsmall cell lung cancer, continuation maintenance therapy is a standard practice[137] and appears to work well for unresectable mesothelioma as well. A randomized trial was underway to evaluate this issue in mesothelioma, but accrual was problematic owing to the frequent use of maintenance pemetrexed. In patients who cannot tolerate platinum, single-agent pemetrexed can be given.[138]

In the unresectable setting, carboplatin is a very reasonable alternative to cisplatin and has demonstrated equivalent survival.[139,140] Other platinum-antifolate regimens (raltitrexed)[141] or platinum-gemcitabine[142,143] have been investigated and would be reasonable alternatives if a patient is unable to receive pemetrexed.

There are currently no FDA approved agents in the salvage setting for mesothelioma. Patients are encouraged to enroll in clinical trials with novel agents and immunotherapy. However, off-protocol, the agents that are most commonly prescribed include gemcitabine, vinorelbine, or the combination of gemcitabine–vinorelbine. Gemcitabine (1250 mg/m^2 intravenous on days 1, 8, and 15 of a 28-day cycle) has been reported to have response rate 7% and median OS of 8 months in the chemo-naïve setting.[144] Gemcitabine–vinorelbine (1000 mg/m^2 gemcitabine and 25 mg/m^2 vinorelbine on days 1 and 8 every 3 weeks for up to six cycles) has reported to have minor efficacy with a response rate of 7.4% and median time to progression of 2.8 months.[145] A phase II trial of single-agent vinorelbine ($n = 63$) reported a response rate of 16% and overall survival of 9.6 months.[146] A retrospective analysis[147] of 60 salvage mesothelioma patients conducted at Memorial Sloan Kettering treated in the second and third-line setting reported minimal response rates to either gemcitabine or vinorelbine but significant stabilization of disease. There was no significant gain in the overall survival benefit. Gemcitabine ($n = 27$) had a median PFS of 1.6 months and median OS of 4.9 months, while vinorelbine ($n = 45$) had a median PFS of 1.7 months and median OS of 5.4 months.

Biologic and novel-targeted agents

The use of novel biologic therapies has been an area of active research in MPM. The earliest biologic monotherapy studies, which were based on preclinical data demonstrating overexpression of the epidermal growth factor receptor (EGFR) and platelet-derived growth factor receptor (PDGFR) on MPM tumor cells, did not demonstrate significant response rates from either EGFR tyrosine kinase inhibitors (gefitinib or erlotinib)[69,70,148,149] or imatinib mesylate, a PDGFR inhibitor.[150] However, disease stabilization was noted in the imatinib mesylate monotherapy trials. The field has broadened significantly with several new targets and biologic agents.

Agents targeting angiogenesis

Mesothelioma tumor cells typically have high levels of vascular endothelial growth factor (VEGF) secretion, and high serum VEGF levels in patients are correlated to worse outcomes.[151] Bevacizumab, a monoclonal antibody to the ligand VEGF, has been the most studied agent so far in mesothelioma. A randomized frontline phase II trial compared cisplatin-gemcitabine with and without bevacizumab in 115 patients and showed that bevacizumab did not benefit survival nor response rates.[152] However, the subgroup analysis of patients with below the median VEGF levels who were treated with bevacizumab had improved progression-free ($p = 0.043$) and overall survival ($p = 0.028$). Two additional single-arm phase II trials utilizing platinum-pemetrexed with bevacizumab followed by maintenance bevacizumab have been conducted but have not demonstrated significant benefit in the unselected population and were not informative for biomarkers.[153,154] Dowell et al.[154] treated 53 mesothelioma patients with cisplatin-pemetrexed–bevacizumab and demonstrated a response rate of 34%, 6-month median progression-free survival of 6.9 months, and median overall survival of 14.8 months. Ceresoli et al.[153] evaluated 76 Italian patients with carboplatin-pemetrexed–bevacizumab and reported a 34% response rate, median progression-free survival of 6.9 months, and median overall survival 15.3 months. Of note, both trials had grade 3–4 small bowel perforation events (one case in the Dowell et al. trial and three cases in Ceresoli et al.). A phase III trial (IFCT-GFPC-0701 MAPS) comparing cisplatin-pemetrexed with and without bevacizumb is ongoing in France.[155] Taken together, these data indicate that antiangiogenic therapy may be beneficial for some MPM patients and that targeting the ligand VEGF may not be sufficient.

The SWOG is in the midst of conducting a phase I/II trial of cisplatin-pemetrexed with and without cediranib in chemo-naïve MPM patients (SWOG 0905). Cediranib is a VEGFR and PDGFR tyrosine kinase inhibitor. The results from the phase I portion of the trial were presented at ASCO 2013 and demonstrated a median PFS of 13–14 months and median OS of 14–16 months.[156] A small phase I trial of cisplatin-pemetrexed–imatinib mesylate ($n = 17$) with no maintenance therapy reported median PFS of 7.9 months and median OS of 8.8 months.[157] However, in the six patients who completed six cycles of the triplet regimen, median PFS was 9.6 months and median OS 22.4 months. Patients in the trial with higher-than-the-median p-PDGFRα IHC expression in baseline tumor biopsies had the best survival results.

In the salvage setting, several oral multikinase inhibitors that include VEGF/VEGFR pathway inhibition have been evaluated. Most of these trials to date have been in heavily pretreated patients and have utilized the novel agents as monotherapy drugs. It is surmised that antiangiogenic agents may need to be combined concurrently with other therapies (novel agents or chemotherapy) to have the greatest benefit. As an example, thalidomide as a single agent was reported to achieve disease stability,[158] but when investigated in an international trial with MPM patients receiving four cycles of platinum-pemetrexed followed by thalidomide or best supportive care, the trial was negative.[159]

In other salvage trials, monotherapy vatalanib (VEGFR-1, -2, and -3; PDGFR; and c-Kit) had an 11% response rate, a 66% stable-disease rate, median progression-free survival of 4.1 months, and median overall survival of 10 months.[160] CALGB 30307 administered sorafenib (VEGFR-2, PDGFR, and Raf) at 400 mg twice daily for MPM that was chemonaïve or previously treated with pemetrexed reported response rates of 4.4% and 38.8% disease stabilization, median failure-free survival of 4.1 months, and median overall survival of 10.4 months.[161–163] Interestingly, the chemonaïve patients had poorer survival outcomes than previously treated patients. Ceritinib monotherapy in SWOG 0509, a phase II trial of 54 previously treated MPM patients, had a 9% response rate with 34% stabilization of disease.[164] The median progression-free survival was 2.6 months, and the overall survival was 9.5 months. Sunitinib (VEGFR-2, PDGFR-β, c-Kit, and Flt-3) in both frontline and salvage therapy settings (National Cancer Institute of Canada, NCIC) has had limited activity.[165] Pazopanib (VEGFR-1, -2, and -3, and PDGFR) is under evaluation by the North Central Cancer Treatment Group.[166]

Ribonuclease inhibitors

Ranpirnase (Onconase, Alfacell Corporation) has target specificity to tumor cell tRNA and inhibits protein synthesis. This enables cell cycle arrest at the G_1 phase. A phase II MPM trial with ranpirnase resulted in a 5% response rate, a 43% stable disease rate, and a median overall survival of 6 months.[167] A phase III trial ($n = 105$) compared ranpirnase ($480 \, \mu g/m^2$ weekly) to doxorubicin ($60 \, mg/m^2$ every 3 weeks) and showed no difference in the overall survival in the intent-to-treat analysis. However, patients with CALGB prognostic groups 1–4 and EORTC risk criteria had a 2-month survival benefit when treated with ranpirnase over doxorubicin.[168] A large international phase III trial (P30-302) comparing doxorubicin to the combination of doxorubicin and ranpirnase did not reveal a survival effect for the ranpirnase arm.

Histone deacetylase inhibitors

Histone deacetylase inhibitors (HDACIs) are agents that prevent deacetylation and reinstate control over the cell cycle. Although preclinical studies have shown that HDACIs inhibit cell cycle progression and/or induce tumor apoptosis, the exact antitumor mechanism is unknown.[169] Suberoylanilide hydroxamic acid (SAHA), or vorinostat, an oral HDACI, was evaluated in an early phase I trial that included 13 mesothelioma patients (12 previously treated) and demonstrated two clinical partial responses.[170] An international randomized placebo-controlled phase III trial (VANTAGE 14) accrued 660 previously treated MPM patients and compared vorinostat to placebo. Unfortunately, the trial was negative for any overall survival benefit and the drug will not be developed further in mesothelioma (unpublished data).

Proteasome inhibitors

Proteasome complexes process ubiquinated proteins and regulate protein degradation. Blockade of proteasome activity leads to inhibition of nuclear factor-κB production and enables tumor cells apoptosis. Preclinical studies in cell lines and murine xenograft models treated with proteasome inhibition have shown antitumor activity.[171–173] Bortezomib is under evaluation in two European trials using single-agent bortezomib (ICORG/GIME) and the combination of cisplatin and bortezomib (EORTC).

Antimesothelin agents

SMRP is a cell-surface glycoprotein expressed on mesothelioma tumor cells. Anti-SMRP agents have been labeled with toxic molecules and have shown some significant antitumor activity against MPM.[174,175] SS1P, a recombinant anti-SMRP immunotoxin, was evaluated in a phase 1 trial in combination with cyclophosphamide and pentostatin, and reported 3 out of 10 patients having a major antitumor response.[176] In addition to SS1P, there are additional anti-SMRP therapies, Morab009 and an anti-SMRP vaccine.[175,177,178] In addition, CRS-207, a *Listeria monocytogene*-SMRP vaccine, is under evaluation in a phase I trial.[179]

Conclusion

Mesothelioma remains a very difficult malignancy to treat with poor survival overall. Several new approaches with regard to better staging may help select out the patients who are more appropriately treated with surgery. Multimodality therapy appears to be the most acceptable current approach for treatment. Several new drugs and immune therapies might alter the course of this disease, but overall it remains a challenge to all of those who continue to treat this entity.

Key references

The complete reference list can be found on the Wiley Companion Digital Edition of this title (see inside front cover for login instructions).

8 Hillerdal G. Malignant mesothelioma 1982: review of 4710 published cases. *Br J Dis Chest*. 1983;**77**(4):321–343.

17 Carbone M, Yang H. Molecular pathways: targeting mechanisms of asbestos and erionite carcinogenesis in mesothelioma. *Clin Cancer Res*. 2012;**18**(3):598–604.

20 Yang H, Bocchetta M, Kroczynska B, et al. TNF-alpha inhibits asbestos-induced cytotoxicity via a NF-kappaB-dependent pathway, a possible mechanism for asbestos-induced oncogenesis. *Proc Natl Acad Sci U S A*. 2006;**103**(27):10397–10402.

24 Yang H, Rivera Z, Jube S, et al. Programmed necrosis induced by asbestos in human mesothelial cells causes high-mobility group box 1 protein release and resultant inflammation. *Proc Natl Acad Sci U S A*. 2010;**107**(28):12611–12616.

27 Carbone M, Ferris LK, Baumann F, et al. BAP1 cancer syndrome: malignant mesothelioma, uveal and cutaneous melanoma, and MBAITs. *J Transl Med*. 2012;**10**:179.

28 Bott M, Brevet M, Taylor BS, et al. The nuclear deubiquitinase BAP1 is commonly inactivated by somatic mutations and 3p21.1 losses in malignant pleural mesothelioma. *Nat Genet*. 2011;**43**(7):668–672.

34 Testa JR, Cheung M, Pei J, et al. Germline BAP1 mutations predispose to malignant mesothelioma. *Nat Genet*. 2011;**43**(10):1022–1025.

39 Pass HI, Lott D, Lonardo F, et al. Asbestos exposure, pleural mesothelioma, and serum osteopontin levels. *N Engl J Med*. 2005;**353**(15):1564–1573.

43 Robinson BW, Creaney J, Lake R, et al. Mesothelin-family proteins and diagnosis of mesothelioma. *Lancet*. 2003;**362**(9396):1612–1616.

49 Pass HI, Levin SM, Harbut MR, et al. Fibulin-3 as a blood and effusion biomarker for pleural mesothelioma. *N Engl J Med*. 2012;**367**(15):1417–1427.

54 Flores RM, Akhurst T, Gonen M, Larson SM, Rusch VW. Positron emission tomography defines metastatic disease but not locoregional disease in patients with malignant pleural mesothelioma. *J Thorac Cardiovasc Surg*. 2003;**126**(1):11–16.

61 Rusch VW. A proposed new international TNM staging system for malignant pleural mesothelioma from the International Mesothelioma Interest Group. *Lung Cancer*. 1996;**14**(1):1–12.

62 Rusch VW, Giroux D, Kennedy C, et al. Initial analysis of the international association for the study of lung cancer mesothelioma database. *J Thorac Oncol*. 2012;**7**(11):1631–1639.

63 Pass HI, Giroux D, Kennedy C, et al. Supplementary prognostic variables for pleural mesothelioma: a report from the IASLC staging committee. *J Thorac Oncol*. 2014;**9**(6):856–864.

64 Gill RR, Richards WG, Yeap BY, et al. Epithelial malignant pleural mesothelioma after extrapleural pneumonectomy: stratification of survival with CT-derived tumor volume. *AJR Am J Roentgenol*. 2012;**198**(2):359–363.

65 Pass HI, Temeck BK, Kranda K, Steinberg SM, Feuerstein IR. Preoperative tumor volume is associated with outcome in malignant pleural mesothelioma. *J Thorac Cardiovasc Surg*. 1998;**115**(2):310–317.

71 Rintoul RC, Ritchie AJ, Edwards JG, et al. Efficacy and cost of video-assisted thoracoscopic partial pleurectomy versus talc pleurodesis in patients with malignant pleural mesothelioma (MesoVATS): an open-label, randomised, controlled trial.. *Lancet*. 2014;**84**(9948):1118–1127. doi: 10.1016/S0140-6736(14)60418-9. Epub 16 Jun 2014.

74 Rice D, Rusch V, Pass H, et al. Recommendations for uniform definitions of surgical techniques for malignant pleural mesothelioma: a consensus report of the international association for the study of lung cancer international staging committee and the international mesothelioma interest group. *J Thorac Oncol*. 2011;**6**(8):1304–1312.

75 Cao CQ, Yan TD, Bannon PG, McCaughan BC. A systematic review of extrapleural pneumonectomy for malignant pleural mesothelioma. *J Thorac Oncol*. 2010;**5**(10):1692–1703.

80 Treasure T, Lang-Lazdunski L, Waller D, et al. Extra-pleural pneumonectomy versus no extra-pleural pneumonectomy for patients with malignant pleural mesothelioma: clinical outcomes of the Mesothelioma and Radical Surgery (MARS) randomised feasibility study. *Lancet Oncol*. 2011;**12**(8):763–772.

81 Weder W, Stahel RA, Baas P, et al. The MARS feasibility trial: conclusions not supported by data. *Lancet Oncol*. 2011;**12**(12):1093–1094.

82 Flores RM, Pass HI, Seshan VE, et al. Extrapleural pneumonectomy versus pleurectomy/decortication in the surgical management of malignant pleural mesothelioma: results in 663 patients. *J Thorac Cardiovasc Surg*. 2008;**135**(3):620–626.

83 Cao C, Tian DH, Pataky KA, Yan TD. Systematic review of pleurectomy in the treatment of malignant pleural mesothelioma. *Lung Cancer*. 2013;**81**(3):319–327.

97 Rusch VW, Rosenzweig K, Venkatraman E, et al. A phase II trial of surgical resection and adjuvant high-dose hemithoracic radiation for malignant pleural mesothelioma. *J Thorac Cardiovasc Surg*. 2001;**122**(4):788–795.

98 Yajnik S, Rosenzweig KE, Mychalczak B, et al. Hemithoracic radiation after extrapleural pneumonectomy for malignant pleural mesothelioma. *Int J Radiat Oncol Biol Phys*. 2003;**56**(5):1319–1326.

99 Ahamad A, Stevens CW, Smythe WR, et al. Promising early local control of malignant pleural mesothelioma following postoperative intensity modulated radiotherapy (IMRT) to the chest. *Cancer J*. 2003;**9**(6):476–484.

105 Rimner A, Spratt DE, Zauderer MG, et al. Failure patterns after hemithoracic pleural intensity modulated radiation therapy for malignant pleural mesothelioma. *Int J Radiat Oncol Biol Phys*. 2014;**90**(2):394–401.

107 Krug LM, Pass HI, Rusch VW, et al. Multicenter phase II trial of neoadjuvant pemetrexed plus cisplatin followed by extrapleural pneumonectomy and radiation for malignant pleural mesothelioma. *J Clin Oncol*. 2009;**27**(18):3007–3013.

108 Van Schil PE, Baas P, Gaafar R, et al. Trimodality therapy for malignant pleural mesothelioma: results from an EORTC phase II multicentre trial. *Eur Respir J*. 2010;**36**(6):1362–1369.

110 Weder W, Stahel RA, Bernhard J, et al. Multicenter trial of neo-adjuvant chemotherapy followed by extrapleural pneumonectomy in malignant pleural mesothelioma. *Ann Oncol*. 2007;**18**(7):1196–1202.

117 Krug LM, Dao T, Brown AB, et al. WT1 peptide vaccinations induce CD4 and CD8 T cell immune responses in patients with mesothelioma and non-small cell lung cancer. *Cancer Immunol Immunother*. 2010;**59**(10):1467–1479.

119 Rusch VW, Figlin R, Godwin D, Piantadosi S. Intrapleural cisplatin and cytarabine in the management of malignant pleural effusions: a Lung Cancer Study Group trial. *J Clin Oncol*. 1991;**9**(2):313–319.

128 Sterman DH, Recio A, Vachani A, et al. Long-term follow-up of patients with malignant pleural mesothelioma receiving high-dose adenovirus herpes simplex thymidine kinase/ganciclovir suicide gene therapy. *Clin Cancer Res*. 2005;**11**(20):7444–7453.

132 Astoul P, Picat-Joossen D, Viallat JR, Boutin C. Intrapleural administration of interleukin-2 for the treatment of patients with malignant pleural mesothelioma: a Phase II study. *Cancer*. 1998;**83**(10):2099–2104.

136 Vogelzang NJ, Rusthoven JJ, Symanowski J, et al. Phase III study of pemetrexed in combination with cisplatin versus cisplatin alone in patients with malignant pleural mesothelioma. *J Clin Oncol*. 2003;**21**(14):2636–2644.

140 Castagneto B, Botta M, Aitini E, et al. Phase II study of pemetrexed in combination with carboplatin in patients with malignant pleural mesothelioma (MPM). *Ann Oncol*. 2008;**19**(2):370–373.

141 Van Meerbeeck JP, Gaafar R, Manegold C, et al. Randomized phase III study of cisplatin with or without raltitrexed in patients with malignant pleural mesothelioma: an intergroup study of the European Organisation for Research and Treatment of Cancer Lung Cancer Group and the National Cancer Institute of Canada. *J Clin Oncol*. 2005;**23**(28):6881–6889.

143 Nowak AK, Byrne MJ, Williamson R, et al. A multicentre phase II study of cisplatin and gemcitabine for malignant mesothelioma. *Br J Cancer*. 2002;**87**(5):491–496.

152 Kindler HL, Karrison TG, Gandara DR, et al. Multicenter, double-blind, placebo-controlled, randomized phase II trial of gemcitabine/cisplatin plus bevacizumab or placebo in patients with malignant mesothelioma. *J Clin Oncol*. 2012;**30**(20):2509–2515.

156 Tsao A, Moon J, Wistuba I, et al. A phase I study of cediranib (NSC #732208) in combination with cisplatinum and pemetrexed in chemonaive patients with malignant pleural mesothelioma (SWOG S0905). *J Clin Oncol*. 2013. Ref Type: Abstract;**31**.

157 Tsao AS, Harun N, Lee JJ, et al. Phase I trial of cisplatin, pemetrexed, and imatinib mesylate in chemonaive patients with unresectable malignant pleural mesothelioma. *Clin Lung Cancer*. 2014;**15**(3):197–201.

158 Baas P, Boogerd W, Dalesio O, Haringhuizen A, Custers F, van Zandwijk N. Thalidomide in patients with malignant pleural mesothelioma. *Lung Cancer*. 2005;**48**(2):291–296.

170 Krug LM, Curley T, Schwartz L, et al. Potential role of histone deacetylase inhibitors in mesothelioma: clinical experience with suberoylanilide hydroxamic acid. *Clin Lung Cancer*. 2006;7(**4**):257–261.

173 Fennell DA, McDowell C, Busacca S, et al. Phase II clinical trial of first or second-line treatment with bortezomib in patients with malignant pleural mesothelioma. *J Thorac Oncol*. 2012;7(**9**):1466–1470.

176 Hassan R, Miller AC, Sharon E, et al. Major cancer regressions in mesothelioma after treatment with an anti-mesothelin immunotoxin and immune suppression. *Sci Transl Med*. 2013;5(**208**):208ra147.

86 Thymomas and thymic tumors

Ronan J. Kelly, MD ▪ Alberto M. Marchevsky, MD

Overview

Thymomas, carcinomas, and other thymic neoplasms are rare and comprise fewer than 1.5% of all solid tumors. They are currently classified according to the recently updated (2015) histologic classification of the World Health Organization (WHO). The histologic features and classification criteria for thymomas and thymic carcinomas are reviewed in this chapter, with an emphasis on various diagnostic problems. Thymomas are staged according to the Masaoka–Koga system, although the American Joint Commission on Cancer (AJCC) is currently developing staging guidelines. There is some current uncertainty regarding how to stage thymic carcinomas. Thymoma patients with stages I and II are treated with radical thymectomy, whereas radiation therapy and chemotherapy are used in patients with more advanced stages. This chapter discusses in detail the current state of the art for the treatment of thymomas and other thymic neoplasms. The results of various therapeutic options are difficult to evaluate with certainty in the absence of a significant number of randomized clinical trials. Indeed, level I and II evidence is difficult to gather for patients with neoplasms that are rare, have a long natural history, and require follow-up for many years. The efforts of the International Thymic Malignancies Interest Group (ITMIG) to develop evidence-based guidelines for the diagnosis, staging, and treatment of thymic neoplasms are described.

Introduction

Thymic tumors are rare and comprise only 0.2–1.5% of all solid tumors or 0.13 per 100,000 person years in the United States.[1] As a result, traditional clinical research has been challenging in these tumors. A number of obstacles have also hindered our progress over the past few decades. One of the most compelling has been the lack of an International consensus surrounding appropriate histopathological and staging criteria. At least 15 different stage classifications have been proposed and used.[2] This has undoubtedly led to confusion among investigators and made it difficult to compare one clinical trial to another. To date, the most widely used staging classification systems have been the Masaoka and the subsequent Koga modification.[3,4] The vague wording and difficulty of interpretation in using these systems have hampered clinical research and made it difficult to collaborate on an International level. An ongoing effort by the International Thymic Malignancies Interest Group (ITMIG) and the International Association for the Study of Lung Cancer (IASLC) to develop a tumor, node, metastasis (TNM)-based staging system for thymic malignancies should lead to an official, stage classification system as proposed by the American Joint Committee on Cancer (AJCC) and the Union for International Cancer Control (UICC).

The World Health Organization (WHO) histological classification distinguishes thymomas (types A, AB, B1, B2, and B3) from thymic carcinomas (previously designated by WHO as type C) based on the morphology of epithelial tumor cells (with increasing degree of atypia along the spectrum from type A thymomas to thymic carcinomas), the proportion of lymphocytic involvement and resemblance to normal thymic tissue. Incremental improvements in our understanding of the molecular biology of both thymomas and thymic carcinomas have occurred in recent years, thanks to advanced technologies such as comparative genomic hybridization (CGH), expression array analysis, and next generation sequencing. It is becoming more apparent that the subclassifications of types A, AB, B1, B2, B3, and thymic carcinoma have different molecular features that may be clinically relevant. Genomic profiling distinguishes type B3 thymoma and thymic carcinoma as distinct entities from type A and type B2 thymoma. Furthermore, type B2 thymomas can be separated from other subgroups in that it has a more distinctly lymphocytic component than the other groups where epithelial cells predominate.[5] Next generation RNA sequencing has recently identified a large microRNA cluster on chromosome 19q13.42 in type A and type AB thymomas, while it is absent in type B thymomas and thymic carcinomas. This cluster has been shown to result in activation of the PI3K/AKT pathway, which suggests a possible role for PI3K inhibitors in these subtypes.[6] The presence of KIT mutations in thymic carcinomas is also well described, and although relatively rare, they can be successfully targeted with small molecules.

Surgical resection continues to be the cornerstone of therapy for early-stage disease while a multidisciplinary approach incorporating surgery, radiation, and chemotherapy is recommended in advanced or recurrent disease. In addition, intense interest is now focused on targeting the immune system in these most intriguing of tumors. Thymomas have been known to be associated with a variety of autoimmune disorders such as myasthenia gravis (MG), which have been linked to T-cell-mediated autoimmunity. Processes such as failure of positive and negative selection of T lymphocytes and defects in the autoimmune regulator gene (AIRE) have been proposed as theories underlying autoimmunity but additional research is required. Studies utilizing checkpoint inhibitors, for example, PD-1 inhibitors, are planned in the near future and immunotherapeutic strategies may hold promise for those patients with chemoresistant disease.

This chapter discusses the new histological and staging systems that are being developed and highlights some of the molecular biology breakthroughs that are improving our understanding of these rare tumors. In addition, we discuss the treatment of thymic malignancies focusing on surgery, radiotherapy (RT), and systemic therapy. Recent clinical trials involving chemotherapy and targeted therapeutics are emphasized and future targets are explored.

Incidence and epidemiology

Although thymic malignancies are relatively rare, they are among the most common mediastinal primary tumors with up to 50% of

Holland-Frei Cancer Medicine, Ninth Edition. Edited by Robert C. Bast Jr., Carlo M. Croce, William N. Hait, Waun Ki Hong, Donald W. Kufe, Martine Piccart-Gebhart, Raphael E. Pollock, Ralph R. Weichselbaum, Hongyang Wang, and James F. Holland.
© 2017 John Wiley & Sons, Inc. ISBN: 978-1-118-93469-2

anterior mediastinal masses proving to be of thymic descent.[7] Males have a slightly higher risk of developing thymomas than females, and the risk rises with age, reaching a peak in the seventh decade of life, which is in direct contrast to the progressive involution of the thymus with age.[8] Data from the National Cancer Institute's Surveillance, Epidemiology, and End Results (SEER) program collected for Hispanic and Asian/Pacific Islander subgroups has been available only since 1992 and 1998, respectively. Thymoma incidence in the United States is higher in African-Americans and especially Asian/Pacific Islanders than among whites or Hispanics. Furthermore, thymoma arises at a younger age among African-Americans than among whites (median age at diagnosis, 48 years vs 58 years; SEER data). Similarly, MG may be more common in African Americans than in whites.[9] Compared with controls, patients with thymoma are more likely to have an autoimmune disease at some point during their lives (32.7% vs 2.4%; $P <$ 0.001), most frequently MG (24.5%), systemic lupus erythematosus (2.4%), or red cell aplasia (1.2%).[10] Ethnic variations in terms of higher incidence rates and younger age at diagnosis suggest a role for genetic factors. The distribution of alleles at the HLA locus on chromosome 6 varies markedly across racial groups.[8] Both class I and class II HLA proteins are highly expressed on thymic epithelial cells.[11] Further research is needed to understand whether particular genetic variants (at HLA or other loci) predispose to thymoma. There are no known etiologic factors for thymic malignancies, although a few cases have developed following radiation therapy to the chest. Epstein–Barr virus (EBV) has been associated with thymic lymphoepithelioma, a rare variant of thymic carcinoma that is usually more frequent in young patients.[12] A few patients with the multiple endocrine neoplasm type I syndrome (MEN I) have had associated thymomas or neuroendocrine carcinomas of thymic origin.

Anatomic pathogenesis

Embryology and anatomy

The thymus is embryologically derived from the endodermal epithelium of the third pharyngeal pouches (which also give rise to the lower pair of parathyroid glands) and, less constantly, the fourth ones as well.[13,14] The right and left thymic anlagen migrate downward into the anterosuperior mediastinum, joining together without complete fusion to form a bilobate organ. Although most thymic tumors are located in the anterosuperior mediastinum, variations in migration account for the findings of gross or microscopic thymic tissue anywhere between the hyoid bone superiorly and the diaphragm inferiorly. Wide exposure of the mediastinum and even the neck is therefore necessary if surgical removal of the entire thymus is indicated, as in patients with thymoma or those with MG (with or without associated thymoma). The absolute weight of the thymus reaches its peak in the pubertal years (mean 34 ± 15 g between age 10 and 15 years) and then gradually decreases, although this age-related involution normally is never complete. Histologically, the normal thymus shows distinctive lobules with a sharp demarcation between the cortex, rich in lymphocytes, and the medulla, rich in epithelial cells and characteristic Hassall's corpuscles, formed by concentric layers of mature epithelial cells. The thymus plays a critical role in the maturation of bone marrow-derived lymphocytes into T cells and, as such, in cell-mediated immunity. It has a rich blood supply but no afferent lymphatics. Efferent lymphatics apparently originate from perivascular spaces and drain into the mediastinal and lower cervical nodes.

Table 1 Primary thymic neoplasms.

Thymic epithelial tumors
    Thymomas
    Thymic carcinoma

Germ cell tumors
    Seminoma
    Embryonal carcinoma
    Yolk sac tumor
    Choriocarcinoma
    Teratoma
    Mixed germ cell tumor
    Germ cell tumor with somatic-type malignancy
    Germ cell tumor with associated hematologic malignancy

Mediastinal lymphomas
    Primary mediastinal B-cell lymphoma
    Thymic extranodal marginal zone B-cell lymphoma of mucosa associated lymphoid tissue (MALT)
    T-cell lymphoma
    Hodgkin lymphoma
    Other

Histiocytic and dendritic cell tumors
Myeloid sarcoma
Mesenchymal tumors
    Thymolipoma
    Solitary fibrous tumor
    Sarcoma
    Other

Thymic neoplasms

The thymus can develop a variety of epithelial, germ cell, lymphoid, mesenchymal, and other neoplasms listed in Table 1.[13]

Pathology of thymic epithelial neoplasms

Thymic epithelial neoplasms include low-grade malignant lesions, designated as thymomas and malignant lesions of moderate to high-grade malignant potential classified as thymic carcinomas.[13,15,16]

Pathology of thymomas

Thymomas appear grossly as single or multiple, usually encapsulated neoplasms that range in size from microscopic lesions to large tumors replacing the entire anterior mediastinum and compressing the adjacent intrathoracic structures.[13,17–21] Grossly, most thymomas are well encapsulated and limited to the thymic gland (Figure 1) but some lesions are locally invasive extending into mediastinal soft tissues, superior vena cava and other vascular structures, lymph nodes, pleura, pericardium, trachea, and/or other intrathoracic structures adjacent to the thymus (Figure 2). On section, thymomas exhibit a distinctive fibrous capsule and multiple fibrous septa that divide the lesion into a characteristic lobulated appearance (Figure 3). They are usually solid tumors but can undergo cystic degeneration. Predominantly, cystic thymomas are distinguished from benign thymic cysts by the presence of focal solid areas.

Microscopically, thymomas are composed of epithelial cells with spindle-, oval-, or polygonal-shaped nuclei admixed with a variable number of mature lymphocytes. The epithelial and lymphoid cells of thymomas are arranged in solid sheets usually divided by fibrous septa in a somewhat lobulated appearance that can be observed at low-power microscopy in most thymomas (Figure 3).

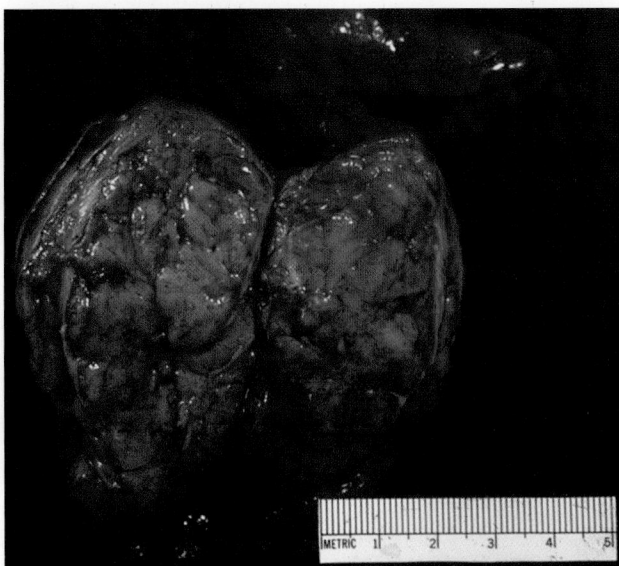

Figure 1 Gross photograph of thymoma showing an encapsulated tumor with a gray, soft surface exhibiting characteristic fibrous septa.

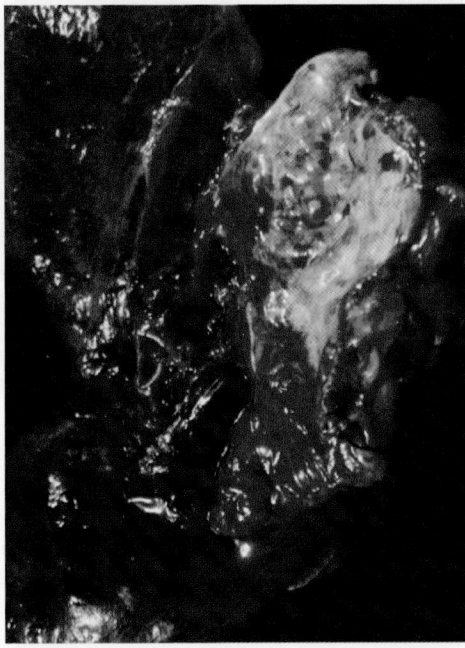

Figure 2 Gross photograph of invasive thymoma showing invasion of mediastinal soft tissues and bronchial wall.

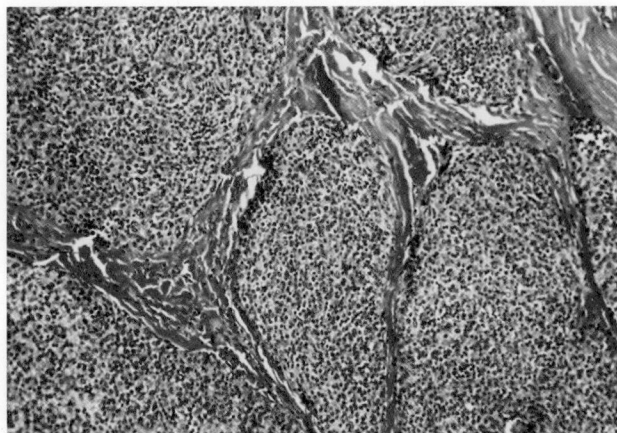

Figure 3 Photomicrograph of thymoma showing the characteristic lobulations of the lesion. The epithelial and lymphoid cells are separated by thin fibrous septa (H&E; ×40).

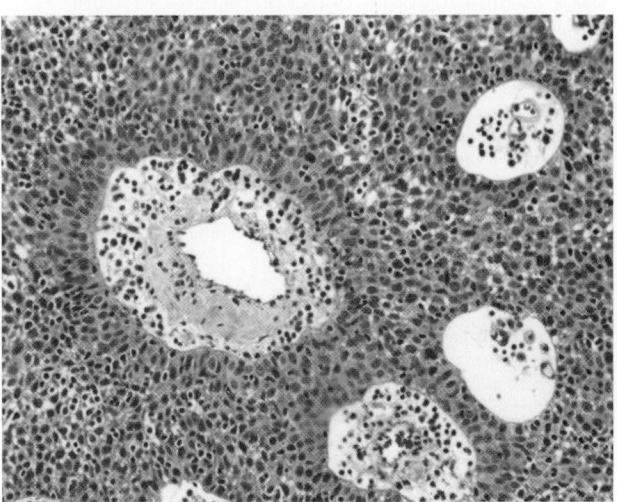

Figure 4 Photomicrograph of thymoma at higher power showing the tumor cells arranged around blood vessels, in a characteristic perivascular growth pattern. The tumor cells are polygonal, with minimal cytologic atypia. They are admixed with small mature lymphocytes (H&E; ×100).

Other histologic features of thymomas include perivascular spaces (Figure 4), medullary areas, pseudorosettes, gland-like structures, Hassall's corpuscles, areas of cystic degeneration, and less frequently hemorrhagic and/or calcified areas. Thymomas are often encapsulated, but can invade the capsule into adjacent tissues (Figure 5). Mitoses, cellular atypia, and necrosis are unusual in thymomas and should raise the suspicion of a thymic carcinoma.

World Health Organization classification of thymomas

Different classification schema have been proposed for the categorization of thymic epithelial neoplasms, but the most widely used classification scheme of these tumors has been proposed by the WHO in 1999 and has been modified in 2004 and 2015 (Table 2).

Thymomas A are composed predominantly of spindle epithelial cells with minimal numbers of lymphocytes (Figures 6 and 7).[19,20,22,23] Patients with thymoma A have a lower incidence of MG than those with other thymoma histologic types and a greater incidence of aplastic anemia. Thymomas B1–B3 are composed of polygonal epithelial cells that are designated as thymoma B and further subclassified into B1, B2, and B3 lesions. B1 thymomas are composed of inconspicuous polygonal epithelial cells admixed with a large number of mature lymphocytes. These lesions characteristically have scattered round, hypochromatic areas designated as medullary areas and have been described in the past as lymphocyte-predominant thymomas because of the sparsity of visible epithelial cells in histologic sections stained with hematoxylin and eosin (H&E). B2 thymomas are composed of polygonal cells that are more conspicuous than those seen in B1 lesions and frequently exhibit slight nuclear variability and focally prominent nucleoli (Figure 8). B3 thymomas, classified in other schema as "atypical thymoma," are composed of polygonal or spindled epithelial cells that exhibit moderate variability in

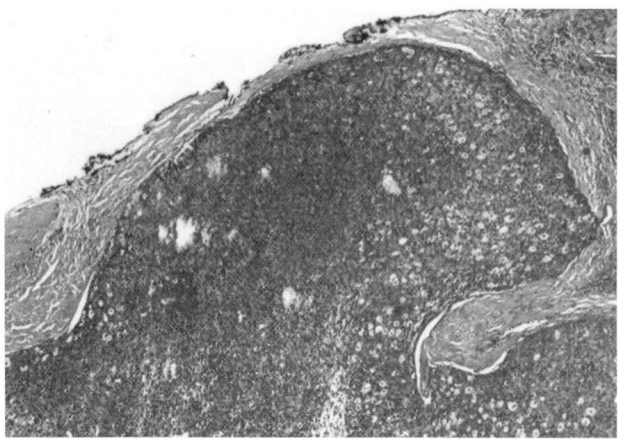

Figure 5 Photomicrograph of a thymoma showing invasion of the capsule (H&E; ×40).

Table 2 World Health Organization classification of thymomas and selected morphological features of the neoplasms.

Type A (spindle cell)
    Atypical type A (spindle cells with focal atypia)
Type AB (mixed spindle and polygonal cells)
Type B1 (lymphocyte-rich, scattered polygonal cells)
Type B2 (lymphocyte-rich with higher density of polygonal epithelial cells and
    focal, minimal atypia)
Type B3 (lymphocyte poor, polygonal cells with mild atypia)

Rare thymomas
- Micronodular thymoma
- Metaplastic thymoma
- Microscopic thymoma
- Sclerosing thymoma
- Lipofibroadenoma

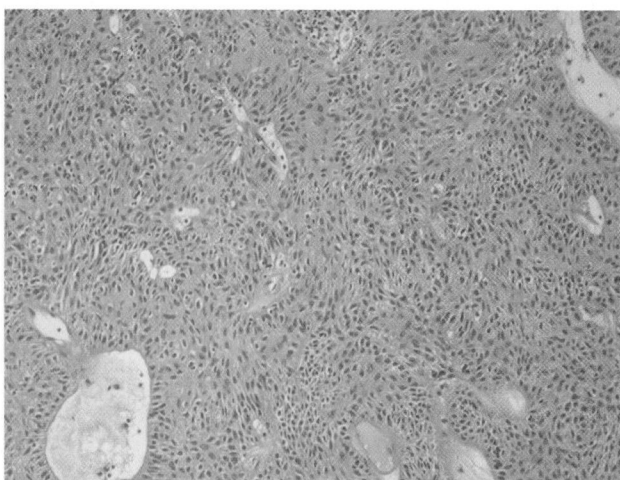

Figure 6 Photomicrograph of spindle cell thymoma (thymoma A). The tumor cells have elongated nuclei. Note the paucity of mature lymphocytes (H&E; ×100).

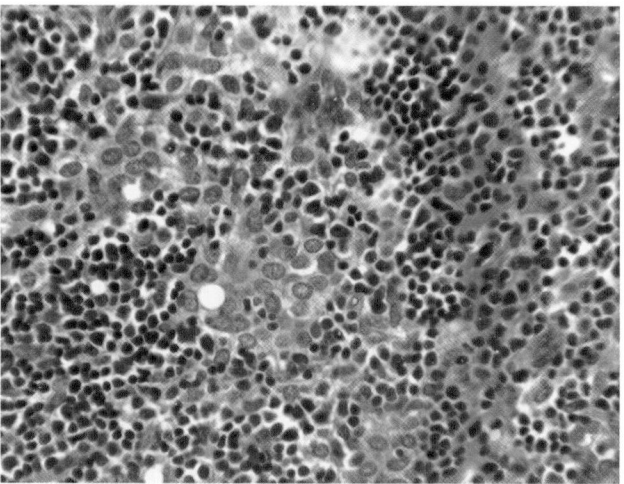

Figure 7 Photomicrograph of thymoma A showing small polygonal epithelial cells with round nuclei, lack of visible nucleoli and scanty cytoplasm. They are admixed with numerous lymphocytes (H&E; ×200).

cell size and shape (anisocytosis), focal nuclear hyperchromasia, and cytologic atypia. B3 thymomas characteristically have fewer lymphocytes than seen in B1 and B2 lesions and can be difficult to distinguish from low-grade thymic carcinomas. Thymomas AB have >5% lymphocytes and are composed of both spindle epithelial cells and polygonal cells. Thymomas are frequently heterogeneous neoplasms and can exhibit different WHO "types" on different sections taken from the same lesion.[24]

Immunohistochemistry and other ancillary techniques

The epithelial cells of thymomas exhibit cytoplasmic immunoreactivity to keratin AE1/AE3, a feature that is generally very helpful to confirm the diagnosis of thymoma on needle biopsies and other pathologic materials (Figure 9). A variety of other epitopes have been shown in the different WHO histologic types of thymomas, such as CD5, laminin, collagen IV, metallothionein, PE-53, cytokeratins such as CAM 5.2, CK7, CK14 and CK18, CD57, and others. However, they have limited diagnostic or prognostic value. CD5 is usually negative in thymomas other than thymoma C. Foxnl, CD205, and desmoglein-3 are novel markers of thymic epithelial cells that may be useful to distinguish different thymomas and thymic carcinoma.

Electron microscopy is seldom used for the routine diagnosis of thymomas.[13] The tumor cells reveal ultrastructural features that are characteristic for epithelial differentiation such as desmosomes, tonofilaments, elongated cell processes, and a lack of dense core granules. The malignant epithelial cells form an irregular mesh with multiple communicating spaces and channels containing mature lymphomas and resembling the normal ultrastructural features and microenvironment of the thymus gland.

Histologic prognostic features in thymomas

All thymomas are low-grade malignant neoplasms.[24-27] Thymomas A (spindle cell thymomas) have been considered as benign lesions in the past, but these lesions can recur or metastasize in a small number of patients. Patients with thymomas A, AB, and B1 appear to have the best prognosis, while those with thymomas B3 generally have more frequent recurrences and metastases and shorter survival.

Staging systems for thymomas

As it has been controversial whether thymomas are benign or malignant neoplasms, there is no current American Joint Commission on Cancer TNM system for thymomas. The most widely used system for staging these tumors is the Masaoka–Koga staging system given in Table 3.[28-32]

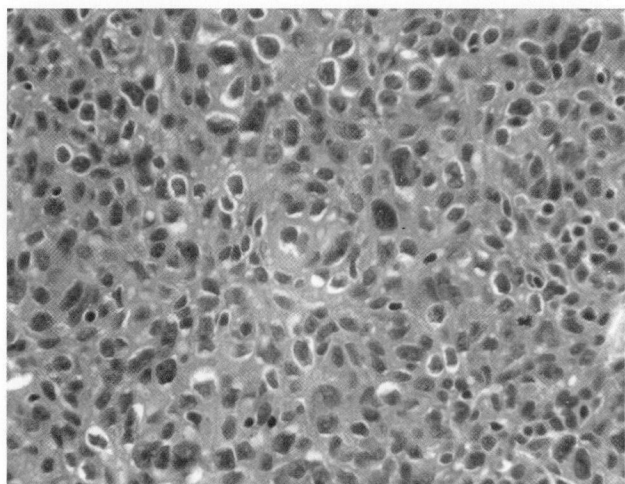

Figure 8 Photomicrograph of thymoma B3 (the so-called atypical thymoma). The tumor cells exhibit considerable variation in size and shape, hyperchromasia and somewhat irregular nuclear membranes. There are relatively few lymphocytes in the background (H&E; ×200).

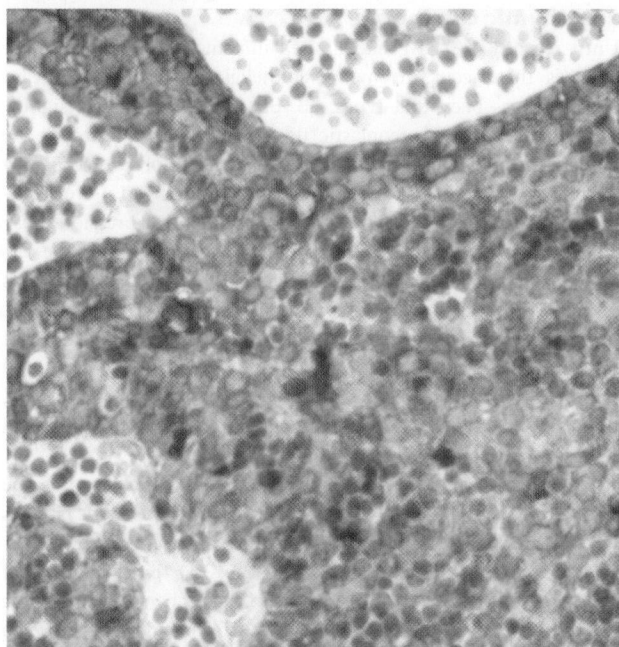

Figure 9 The epithelial cells of thymomas exhibit cytoplasmic immunoreactivity when stained for keratin AE1/AE2 (Immunostain; ×200).

Thymic carcinomas

Thymic carcinomas are unusual epithelial tumors comprising approximately 0.06% of thymic neoplasms and composed of epithelial cells that exhibit cytological features characteristic of malignancy, such as considerable pleomorphism, hyperchromasia, prominent nucleoli, increased mitotic activity, and/or necrosis.[22,28,31,33–38] A variety of histologic variants, described in Table 4, have been described. Squamous cell carcinomas are probably the most frequent variant of these neoplasms. Lymphoepithelioma of the thymus is a particularly interesting variant of thymic carcinoma frequently associated with the EBV expression and exhibits similar histopathologic features to those seen in the head and neck area.[16] Carcinoma with NUT, t(15;19) translocation is a recently described

Table 3 Masaoka–Koga staging of thymomas.

Stage	Extent of disease
I	Totally encapsulated
II	Microscopic (IIa) or macroscopic (IIb) transcapsular invasion into surrounding fat or mediastinal pleura
III	Invasion of surrounding organs (pericardium, lung, and great vessels)
IV	(A) Pleural or pericardial implants
	(B) Embolic metastasis

Table 4 World Health Organization classification of thymic carcinomas.

Squamous cell carcinoma
Basaloid carcinoma
Mucoepidermoid carcinoma
Lymphoepithelioma-like carcinoma
Clear cell carcinoma
Sarcomatoid carcinoma
Adenocarcinoma
NUT carcinoma
Undifferentiated carcinoma
Other rare thymic carcinomas

aggressive variant of thymic carcinomas that affects children and young adults.[34]

Thymic carcinoid and neuroendocrine tumors

Carcinoid tumors and other neuroendocrine neoplasms given in Table 5 can arise in the thymus.[23,39–43] They are more aggressive than their counterparts in the lung and other organs and with metastases at diagnosis in 30–40% of cases.[15] The association with Cushing syndrome with ectopic ACTH production in a patient with a thymic tumor should raise this possibility because it occurs in 30% of patients with thymic carcinoid tumor but not in patients with thymoma. Other paraneoplastic syndromes, such as osteoarthropathy and Eaton–Lambert syndrome, and an association with multiple endocrine neoplasia (type I or II) have been described.[39,43] Carcinoid syndrome has not been reported. Neuroendocrine tumors exhibit histopathologic features at low-power microscopy characteristic of neuroendocrine differentiation, including the formation of cellular nests, trabeculae, and pseudorosettes.[13] The tumor cells vary according to the cell type. Carcinoid tumors are composed of round to elongated nuclei with "salt-and-pepper" nuclear chromatin, variable hyperchromasia, and minimal pleomorphism. Typical carcinoid tumors usually lack mitosis and necrosis, while atypical carcinoid tumors exhibit low mitotic activity and focal areas of necrosis. Large cell neuroendocrine carcinoma of the thymus are composed of large, pleomorphic, hyperchromatic cells that can exhibit focally prominent nucleoli. Small cell carcinomas of the thymus are composed of small hyperchromatic cells with nuclear molding and inconspicuous nucleoli. Both variants of high-grade thymic neuroendocrine carcinomas exhibit frequent mitosis, usually higher than 10 mitosis in 10 high-power fields and extensive areas of necrosis. The tumor cells of all variants of thymic neuroendocrine carcinoma exhibit cytoplasmic immunoreactivity to chromogranin and synaptophysin and dense core neuroendocrine granules under electron microscopy. Immunostains for Ki-67 can be used to estimate the proliferative fraction of these lesions.

Table 5 Thymic neuroendocrine tumors.

Typical carcinoid
Atypical carcinoid
Large cell neuroendocrine carcinoma
Small cell carcinoma

Thymic lymphomas

Lymphomas are, with thymomas, the most common tumors of the thymus.[13,33,44–46] Although the thymus is a T-cell organ, the most frequent lymphomas of the thymus in adult patients are Hodgkin lymphoma and B-cell lymphomas (Table 3). Primary Hodgkin lymphoma of the thymus tends to be limited to the gland and is, as a rule, of the nodular sclerosis type. It is frequently associated with cystic change in the adjacent thymic tissue. B-cell lymphomas of the mediastinum frequently involve the thymus and lymph nodes and frequently exhibit histologic features that are unusual for B-cell lesions in other locations, such as sclerosis with compartmentalization of the tumor cells, clear cell features, and focal formation of cellular nests simulating an epithelial malignancy. They tend to follow an aggressive clinical course. Lymphomas involving the thymus and mediastinal lymph nodes in children include Burkitt's lymphoma, lymphoblastic lymphoma, and a lesion of T-cell origin. It is of prime importance to differentiate a lymphoma from a thymoma in view of the different therapeutic approaches. Special stains and electron microscopy may be necessary in difficult cases.

Germ cell tumors of the thymus

The thymus is a classic site of extragonadal primary germ cell tumors (Table 1). The most common ones are seminomas (sometimes difficult to differentiate from thymoma) and teratomas (mature or immature). Embryonal carcinomas, yolk sac tumors, teratocarcinomas, and choriocarcinomas have also been described.

Other thymic tumors

Other thymic tumors include thymolipomas, which may become quite large, thymic cysts, metastases to the thymus, and other neoplasms listed in Table 1.

TNM staging project—ITMIG/IASLC

As previously outlined, in the past 4 decades, at least 15 different stage classifications have been proposed for thymic malignancies.[47] The Masaoka staging system was originally proposed in 1981 and focuses on the integrity of the thymic capsule, the presence of micro or macroscopic invasion into adjacent structures, and metastatic spread.[3] An updated version from 1994 that is commonly used is the Masoka–Koga system.[4] It has long been recognized however that there is a significant need for an American Joint Committee on Cancer/Union for International Cancer Control (AJCC/UICC) validated stage classification system for thymic tumors. This will allow for consistent universal nomenclature facilitating multinational collaborative clinical research. A combined effort by ITMIG and the IASLC is now underway, and a database of more than 10,000 retrospective and prospective cases worldwide has been assembled.[47] The requirements for this staging system are that it has to contain nomenclature that describes the anatomic extent of the disease only, which is applicable to all types of thymic tumors and that it conforms to the TNM (tumor, node, metastases) structure. The T component of the proposed stage classification is divided into four categories or levels of involvement. A tumor is classified in

a particular level if one or more structures in that level is involved regardless of whether other structures of a lower level are involved or not. Encapsulation is of a tumor is not included as this does not have a clinically significant impact on outcomes as demonstrated in a retrospective database. T1a involves a tumor that is encapsulated or not with or without extension into mediastinal fat. Pathologically proven involvement of the pericardium is designated as T2 and several different structures are included in the T3 category including lung, brachiocephalic vein, SVC, chest wall, phrenic nerve, hilar, and pulmonary vessels. T4 lesions include several structures that indicate more extensive local involvement, for example, aorta, pulmonary artery, myocardium, trachea, and esophagus. Lymph node status "N" will be assigned into two groups according to their proximity to the thymus with N1 indicating anterior (perithymic) involvement and N2 disease indicating deep cervical or thoracic nodes. Finally, metastatic disease will be categorized as M1a indicating separate pleural or pericardial nodule(s) and M1b indicating a pulmonary intraparenchymal nodule or distant organ metastasis.[48] This proposed classification system will be applicable to both thymoma and thymic carcinoma, and it is hoped that it will allow for International stage classification consistency.

Molecular differences between thymoma and thymic carcinoma

Until recently, we have had limited information of the genomic changes that occur in thymic epithelial tumors. A significant challenge has been that types AB, B1, and B2 contain a significant number of non-neoplastic thymocytes that outnumber the malignant epithelial cells making CGH and fluorescence in situ hybridization (FISH) analyses challenging. Thanks to newer techniques such as next generation sequencing and expression array analysis, our knowledge of the tumor biology underlying the different phenotypes between thymomas and thymic carcinomas has improved in recent years. These studies have shown that thymic tumors as classified by the 2004 WHO system do have different molecular features. Genomic profiling distinguishes type B3 and thymic carcinoma from type A and type B2 thymomas. In addition, type B3 tends to have a more distinct lymphocytic component and thymic carcinomas are C-Kit positive.

The most frequent genetic alterations occur on chromosome 6p21.3 (MHC locus) and 6q25.2–25.3[5,49,50] Cytogenetic studies have demonstrated chromosomal abnormalities in all histological subtypes including the t(15;19)(q13:p13.1) translocation that generates the BRD4-NUT fusion gene that can occur in thymic carcinoma.[51] Molecular similarities do occur most notably between thymic carcinomas and type B3 thymomas where gain of 1q and loss of chromosome 6 is identified in both.[5] This may have implications for clinical trial design in future years with type B3 and thymic carcinoma being treated together. Additional data from CGH analysis performed on thymic carcinomas has demonstrated frequent copy number gains of 17q and 18 and loss of 3p, 16q, and 17p.[5,52] Further aberrations that have been described include multiple losses of genetic material and microsatellite instability (MSI) in different chromosomes (3p22–24.3, 3p14.2 (FHIT gene locus), 5q21 (APC gene), 6p21, 6p21–22.1, 7p21–22, 8q11.21–23, 13q14 (RB gene), and 17p13.1 (p53 gene).[52,53] In addition to the losses in the long arm of chromosome 6 the loss of heterozygosity (LOH) on chromosome 5 (5q21) (APC gene) may be the most significant. It has been demonstrated that alterations in chromosome 6 varies according to the WHO subtype (type A 10%, type AB 12%, type B 20–26%, and in thymic carcinoma 35%) and with clinical stage at diagnosis (stage I 7%, stage II 27%, stage III 21%, and stage IV 24%).[50] The most frequent LOHs (48.6%) occurred in region

6q25.2. Another hot spot showing LOH in 32.4% of tumors was located on 6q25.2–25.3. The third hot spot (30%) showing LOH appeared in region 6p21.31 including the MHC locus and the fourth (26.3%) was detected on 6q14.1–14.3. MSI has also been described on chromosome 6 in 10% of thymomas, more commonly in type B thymoma. Although the biological significance of many of these changes has yet to be determined, incremental benefits are being realized. The 6p23 region encompasses the *FOXC1* tumor suppressor gene, and chromosomal loss is correlated with lower protein expression. Patients with FOXC1 negative tumors have a shorter time to tumor progression and shorter disease-related survival.[54] Next generation RNA sequencing has shown that type A and type AB thymomas are significantly different from other subgroups. A large microRNA cluster on chromosome 19q13.42 has been shown to be significantly over-expressed in these groups, while it is absent in type B thymomas and thymic carcinoma.[6] This cluster has been shown to result in activation of the PI3K/AKT pathway by downregulating PTEN, which suggests a possible role for PI3K inhibitors in these subtypes.

Utilizing gene signatures to determine prognosis in thymic tumors

The main prognostic indicators in thymic malignancies are tumor stage, histologic subtype, and the extent of surgical resection. As our understanding of the underlying molecular biology improves gene signatures is seen as a next step in helping the oncologist move beyond clinical and morphological features to determine prognosis, aggressiveness of treatment, and extent of surveillance imaging. In an elegant study, whole genome expression was performed and the authors correlated their findings with outcomes in 34 patients with thymoma.[55] Unsupervised clustering of gene expression data identified four clusters of thymic tumors, which showed significant correlation with histological classification ($P = 0.002$). In addition, the authors identified a number of genes associated with clinical behavior of thymic tumors including stage, relapse, and metastasis and some were confirmed using qRT-PCR. Among the top genes chosen, Aldo-keto reductase family 1 B10 (*AKR1B10*) and junctophilin-1 (*JPH1*) were upregulated in both stage III and stage IV diseases. A hedgehog target gene, *COL11A1*, was downregulated in advanced stage disease. *AKR1B10* and *JPH1* showed a 5.96-fold ($P = 0.05$) and 3.01 ($P = 0.18$)-fold increase in metastasis positive tumors compared to nonmetastatic disease and *COL11A1* was decreased 12.5-fold ($P = 0.11$) in stage IV tumors. As a result of the differential expression levels of these genes, they were selected for validation by qRT-PCR, which confirmed the differential expression in the different phenotypes. The authors have developed a 9-gene signature that can be used to identify patients at high or low risk for developing metastases from thymomas. Additional validation studies are planned as is prospective evaluation in a clinical trial setting. In an effort to distinguish thymic carcinoma from thymoma, the same group has developed a 12-gene signature that may assist pathologists in difficult cases. Although gene signatures are not used clinically at present a validated signature would be of tremendous benefit in patients with Thymomas. These tumors can differ considerably with many being considered indolent requiring less surveillance than perhaps the more aggressive type B3 thymoma. In rare tumors with limited scope for randomized studies an improved understanding of poor prognostic indicators would be of tremendous benefit in the clinic.

Clinical features of thymomas

Most tumor-related symptoms are vague (cough, dyspnea, and chest pain) or secondary to local and regional mediastinal spread (pleural effusion, superior vena cava syndrome, or pericardial effusion) and, therefore, often indicate invasiveness. Occasionally, thymomas may present as diffuse pleural tumors and simulate malignant mesothelioma.[56] About half of thymomas occur in asymptomatic persons and are discovered fortuitously on a chest radiograph, which shows a retrosternal mass in the anterosuperior mediastinum forming a bulge in the cardiovascular silhouette. The tumor may be best seen on oblique and lateral views. Computed tomography (CT) is invaluable for detecting small thymomas and assessing possible invasion of surrounding structures, such as the mediastinum, pleura, and pericardium. It can show calcifications in or at the periphery of the tumor in approximately 20% of cases,[57] although they bear no relation to invasiveness. The presence of a fat plane all around the tumor is a good sign of noninvasiveness, but, conversely, fibrous adherence to surrounding structures may simulate invasion.[58] CT can also help differentiate thymomas from vascular structures and tumors, such as aneurysms, particularly when intravenous contrast is used.[58] Thymomas show increased T_1- and T_2-weighted image signal intensity by magnetic resonance imaging, but the role of that technique in detecting possible capsular and vascular invasion, compared with CT, needs to be further defined.[58] The use of positron emission tomography with 18-fluorodeoxyglucose to distinguish malignant from benign mediastinal tumors has been evaluated.[59] Thymic carcinomas and invasive thymomas show high uptake, whereas noninvasive thymomas show low uptake. It should be emphasized, however, that surgical exploration and pathologic evaluation remain the most reliable means to assess the invasiveness of thymomas.

Associated paraneoplastic syndromes

A remarkable number of paraneoplastic syndromes are associated with thymomas. They are mostly related to autoimmune mechanisms and are dominated by three characteristic entities (Table 3).

Myasthenia gravis

MG occurs in approximately 33–50% of patients with thymoma, and approximately 10% of patients who have MG have a thymoma.[60] Such patients are usually older than those with MG without thymoma, although the clinical signs of MG are similar in both groups. Few features distinguish the histologic appearance of thymomas in patients with MG; predominantly, spindle cell thymomas are rare in this group, and the surrounding thymic tissue reveals the presence of lymphoid follicles with germinal centers in approximately 50% of the cases (vs only 5–8% of cases involving thymomas without MG).[61] MG is an autoimmune disorder that is characterized by the presence of antibodies to the acetylcholine receptors of the neuromuscular junction. Such serum antibodies are found in 90% of patients with generalized MG.[58] The triggering mechanisms are unknown. Myoid cells in the normal thymus raise the possibility of *in situ* sensitization.[62] Serum striational antibodies directed against elements of the sarcomere, such as titin, are found in 80% of patients with MG and thymoma and in 25% of patients with thymoma but without MG.[58] Total thymectomy rather than thymomectomy is indicated in patients with MG, even in the absence of a thymoma (see the section titled "Surgery").

Red cell hypoplasia

Also called pure red cell aplasia (PRCA), red cell hypoplasia is an autoimmune disorder that is characterized by an acquired anemia with markedly decreased blood reticulocytes and a virtual absence of erythroblasts in the bone marrow.[61,63] There are often changes (an increase or a decrease) in white blood cell and/or platelet counts. PRCA is seen in approximately 5% of patients with thymoma, but 50% of patients with PRCA have a thymoma, which is of the spindle cell type in two-thirds of these patients.[61] PRCA generally occurs in patients older than 40 years of age who have thymoma, and the incidence of local invasion is not different from other thymomas. The bone marrow is usually quite cellular, and erythropoietin levels are typically high.[63] An immunoglobulin (Ig)G inhibitor of erythroblastic growth has been described in the serum of some patients.[63] Thymectomy produces remission of the anemia in approximately 30% of cases.[63] Corticosteroids and immunosuppressive agents are also effective. A prolonged complete remission (with tumor regression) was described in one case with the combination of octreotide and prednisone.[64]

Hypogammaglobulinomia

First reported by Good in 1954,[65] this acquired syndrome results in extreme susceptibility to recurrent, and often serious, infections. It occurs in approximately 5–10% of patients with thymoma, and a thymoma is found in 10% of patients with acquired hypogammaglobulinemia.[57,61] There is a decrease in all major Igs, particularly IgG and IgA, and decreased eosinophils in the blood and bone marrow. A combined deficit in cell-mediated immunity can also be seen. Almost a third of patients also have PRCA. Similar to those with PRCA, the age group is somewhat older (>40 years), and the thymoma is of the spindle cell type in 75% of cases.[61] The pathogenesis is obscure. There is a lack of pre-B cells, B cells, and plasma cells in the bone marrow, with decreased peripheral B cells.[66] Thymectomy does not result in any improvement; palliative treatment with Igs is indicated.[66]

A large number of other paraneoplastic syndromes or associated disorders have been described in patients with thymoma (Table 3). It is noteworthy that Cushing syndrome with ectopic adrenocorticotropin (ACTH) production is a typical feature of thymic carcinoids, not thymomas.[61]

Diagnosing an anterior mediastinal mass

The diagnosis of an anterior mediastinal mass is guided by the clinical suspicion of its etiology. A structured, clinically orientated approach increases efficacy and eliminates unnecessary investigations. Age and gender are the two most important features to consider from the outset as specific lesions tend to occur more commonly in certain demographic groups. Laboratory investigations include α-fetoprotein, β-human chorionic gonadotrophin, and lactate dehydrogenase. The causes include a wide variety of entities the most common of which include the following: thymic malignancy in approximately 35%, lymphoma in approximately 25% (Hodgkins lymphoma 13% and non-Hodgkins 12%), thyroid and other endocrine tumors in approximately 15%, benign teratoma in approximately 10%, malignant germ cell tumors in approximately 10% (seminoma 4%, nonseminoma 6%), and benign thymic lesions in approximately 5%. Invasive incisional biopsy techniques, with mediastinoscopy or mediastinotomy for thymoma, carry the risk of violating the tumor capsule and disseminating tumor cells.[67] Otherwise, percutaneous fine-needle aspiration or core biopsy under fluoroscopic or CT guidance is generally considered safe and effective. Combined with special stains and electron microscopy, if necessary, it has a sensitivity of 80% and specificity >90%.[57] It is of prime importance, however, to establish a firm pathologic diagnosis in view of the many other tumor types that may require specific therapies. The treatment of thymic malignancies is discussed in the following sections.

Therapy

Surgery

Because there are no reliable histologic criteria for the malignant nature of thymomas, all such tumors should be considered potentially malignant. Total thymectomy (rather than thymomectomy) is the procedure of choice, even for stage I-encapsulated tumors.[57] It is also the procedure indicated for patients with MG, with or without thymoma. The usual approach is by median sternotomy, although additional thoracic or cervical incisions may be necessary, and some surgeons advocate maximal thymectomy with exploration of all of the possible areas in which ectopic thymic tissue might be found.[68] There is a need for the surgeon to carefully explore the mediastinum for evidence of local invasion, which is the most reliable indication of malignancy and the most important prognostic factor. The tumor capsule should not be breached. Systematic microscopic examination is necessary to search for capsular invasion and to distinguish it from simple adhesions. Following total thymectomy, the recurrence rate is usually low (about 2%) for stage I-encapsulated thymomas.[61] Recently, video thoracoscopic approaches were performed for well-encapsulated small thymomas but the long-term results are unknown.[67]

In patients with thymoma and MG, remission of MG occurs in approximately 10–30% following thymectomy, often after a delay of up to 2 years or more, compared with a remission rate of approximately 40–80% after thymectomy for MG without a thymoma.[57,61,68,69] An additional fraction of patients shows improvement of MG. Early thymectomy (within 1 year) after onset of MG is associated with a higher percentage of less invasive thymomas.[70] Recurrence, and even first occurrence, of MG after apparent total thymectomy has been observed and could be related to tumor regrowth or persistent ectopic thymic tissue.[57] In the past, MG was a poor prognostic sign in patients with thymoma. Most recent surgical series, however, do not show a significant difference in survival for patients with thymoma, with or without MG.[3,71,72] Such a change is attributed to better surgical and anesthesia techniques, which have largely prevented postoperative deaths from MG.

Local invasion is seen in approximately 30–40% of thymomas at surgery,[3,71,72] but the slow-growing nature of the tumor and the rarity of distant metastases justify attempts at radical surgery. Identification of the phrenic, recurrent laryngeal, and vagus nerves is of major importance.[68] Extended resections—including one lung, one phrenic nerve, pericardium, or even resection and repair of great vessels, such as the innominate vein or superior vena cava—have been performed. They should be undertaken only if they lead to complete tumor resection. With modern techniques of peri- and postsurgical care, surgical mortality is low (0–5%), even in patients with MG.[3,68,72]

In four large series with a total of 744 patients, the 5- and 10-year survival rates were 75–85% and 63–80%, respectively, for patients with noninvasive encapsulated thymomas.[3,71,72] Survival figures for patients with invasive thymomas were 50–67% at 5 years and 30–53% at 10 years. While invasiveness is the major prognostic factor in patients with thymoma, most series also report a better prognosis for spindle cell thymomas and those with a higher ratio of lymphocytes to epithelial cells.[3,71,72] Local recurrences and/or metastases (often intrathoracic) may also be amenable to surgical resection.

Radiotherapy

Thymomas are radiosensitive, and the efficacy of RT has been emphasized in many reports. Following surgical biopsy, or partial excision, survival of more than 10 years after RT has been seen.[73] Most authors do not believe that it is only the lymphocytic component rather than the epithelial one that is sensitive to RT.[73]

The role of RT is best discussed according to stage. For stage I disease following total surgical resection, postoperative RT is not indicated in view of the very low relapse rates. For stage II and stage III diseases, the use of postoperative RT is recommended even after total surgical resection.[3,57,71,74] In a review of the literature, as well as their own experience, Curran and colleagues reported a 28% intrathoracic relapse rate after complete surgical resection without RT, as opposed to 5% when postoperative RT was given.[75] The latter figure may be unusual, however, because others have reported no such differences in favor of RT after complete surgical resection.[76] The systematic use of RT after complete resection has been recently questioned particularly for stage II patients, but the small number of cases and the retrospective nature of the collected data as well selection of patients do not allow a definitive conclusion in the absence of prospective randomized trials. The irradiated volume should include the mediastinum with adjacent areas and probably the supraclavicular areas, which are possible sites of relapse.[73] The total dose is usually about 45 Gy, with appropriate protection of the spinal cord, although doses of 50 Gy and higher have been given.[73,75] Radiation pneumonitis, mediastinitis, pericarditis, coronary artery fibrosis, hypothyroidism, and secondary cancers are potential complications.

RT is also given to patients with residual disease, following biopsy only or incomplete surgical resection for stage III disease. In 20 such cases, Curran and colleagues observed 4 mediastinal recurrences and 5 others outside the mediastinum, whereas no local relapse was seen when RT was given after total surgical resection for stage II or stage III disease.[75] Partial tumor debulking by surgery before RT in patients with stage III or stage IV disease does not appear to be beneficial.[77] The 5-year survival rate for such patients was 45% overall, including 61% for stage III and 23% for stage IV disease after RT. Collaboration between the surgeon and the radiotherapist is essential to delineate areas of tumor involvement by radiopaque clips and to plan the treatment.

Chemotherapy

Chemotherapy has activity in both the operable and the metastatic setting (Table 6). Cisplatin-based chemotherapy remains the standard of care in advanced stage disease. Combination chemotherapy regimens have shown higher response rates than single agent treatments. A four drug regimen of doxorubicin, cisplatin, vincristine, and cyclophosphamide (ADOC) was considered the standard of care for many years with reported overall response rate of 92% and a median survival of 15 months.[79] An intergroup trial however demonstrated the benefits of the 3 drug combination, cisplatin, doxorubicin, and cyclophosphamide (PAC) with an ORR of 50% and an MS of 38 months.[78] Various regimens include corticosteroids that have been shown to decrease tumor bulk in all histologic subtypes. The actual impact lies probably with a steroid-induced response in the lymphocytic component of the tumor rather than any anti-neoplastic effect on the malignant epithelial cells. A second three drug regimen that is commonly used is consists of cisplatin, doxorubicin, and methylprednisone (CAMP). This regimen was administered in the neoadjuvant setting and demonstrated an ORR of 93% with a 5-year OS of 81% in a small phase II trial consisting of 17 patients.[84] The EORTC investigated the doublet of cisplatin and etoposide in 16 patients and demonstrated a response rate of 56% and a median survival of 4.3 years.[80] The addition of ifosfamide to this doublet (VIP) demonstrated a partial response rate of 32% and an OS of 32 months albeit with higher toxicities.[81] A recently published phase II trial investigated carboplatin AUC5 and

Table 6 Selected studies of chemotherapy regimens used in thymic malignancies.

Regimen	Stage	CR + PR (%)
PAC[78]	IV	50
ADOC[79]	III/IV	90
PE[80]	IV	56
VIP[81]	III/IV	32
Carbo-Px[82]	IV	35
Pemetrexed[83]	IV	17

PAC, cisplatin, doxorubicin, cyclophosphamide; ADOC, doxorubicin, cisplatin, vincristine, cyclophosphamide; PE, cisplatin, etoposide; VIP, etoposide, ifosfamide, cisplatin; Carbo-Px, carboplatin, paclitaxel.

paclitaxel 225 mg/m^2 every 3 weeks up to a maximum of 6 cycles. An overall response rate of 33% and a progression free survival (PFS) of 19.8 months for thymomas and 6.2 months for thymic carcinomas in 34 treatment naïve patients was reported and this was very well tolerated.[82] A second multicenter trial investigated the efficacy of carboplatin/paclitaxel in 40 Japanese patients with newly diagnosed thymic carcinoma. An overall RR of 36% (95% CI, 21–53%; $P = 0.031$) and a median PFS of 8.1 months was seen with 1- and 2-year survival rates of 85% and 71%, respectively. The combination of carboplatin/paclitaxel is an effective regimen and if an anthracycline cannot be used then this doublet is a good choice in the first-line setting for thymic carcinoma.[85]

Second-line chemotherapy does have activity in thymic malignancies. A phase II study evaluated single agent pemetrexed at a dosage of 500 mg/m^2 every 3 weeks in 27 patients with previously treated unresectable stage IVA ($n = 16$) or stage IVB ($n = 11$) recurrent thymic malignancies.[83] The median number of cycles administered was 5 (range 1–6). In 23 fully evaluable patients, two complete and two partial responses (RECIST) were noted. All four responding patients had stage IVA thymoma.[83] Oral etoposide similarly may have some activity in pretreated patients with a response rate of 15% being reported.[86] Amrubicin in previously treated patients at a dosage of 35 mg/m^2 days 1–3 q3 weeks is currently being evaluated.[87]

In recent years that have been a number of small studies and case reports that have evaluated targeted therapies in thymic malignancies after progression on first-line therapy. Unfortunately, the results have been somewhat disappointing but given the rarity of these tumors and the fact that it is extremely challenging to preselect patients based on a certain molecular phenotype they are perhaps not unexpected. It is hoped that future molecular profiling "basket studies" enrolling multiple tumor types with selected oncogenic driver mutations will identify patients with thymic malignancies that have significant sensitivities to targeted therapy.

Targeted therapy—KIT, EGFR/HER2, VEGF

Although large randomized phase III trials are not possible in thymic malignancies, a number of small phase II studies and case reports (Table 7) have highlighted that a subset of patients do derive benefit from personalized medicine. KIT is frequently overexpressed in thymic carcinomas with IHC positivity occurring in up to 73–86% of tumors, but there is limited overexpression in thymomas with only 2% demonstrating positivity.[95,96] Unfortunately, despite the high frequency of KIT expression in thymic carcinomas, the rate of KIT mutations remains low at <10%. Case reports have identified that the type of KIT mutation determines the sensitivity to tyrosine kinase inhibitors. A number of mutations have been described, for example, V560 deletion[97] and L576P substitution[98] both found in exon 11, D820E mutation in exon 17,[99] and the

Table 7 Targeted therapies in thymic malignancies.

Drug	Number of patients	Thymoma	Thymic Ca	RR (%)
Gefitinib[88]	26	19	7	4
Erlotinib + Bev[89]	18	11	7	0
Imatinib[90]	15	12	3	0
Belinostat[91]	40	24	16	5
Cixutumumab[92]	49	37	12	10
Everolimus[93]	35	23	12	11
Sunitinib[94]	39	16	23	18

H697Y mutation found in exon 14.[52] V560 is highly sensitive to both sunitinib and imatinib, L576P has moderate sensitivity to sunitinib and low sensitivity to imatinib, whereas D820E is resistant to both TKIs indicating that "one size does not fit all" when it comes to mutation testing in thymic tumors. The rarity and the sensitivity of mutations explains the disappointing results of a small phase II trial that evaluated imatinib in patients with either type B3 thymoma or thymic carcinoma were no responses were seen.[100]

Epidermal growth factor receptor (EGFR) is similarly overexpressed (70% of thymomas and 50% of thymic carcinomas[96,101]) in thymic malignancies, but unfortunately somatic activating EGFR mutations are extremely rare.[98,102] There is no correlation between EGFR staining and histological subtype. EGFR gene amplification by FISH occurs in approximately 20% of thymic malignancies, most notably in type B3 thymomas and thymic carcinomas and is associated with more advanced stage and capsule invasion.[103] Not unexpectedly, there was no activity seen in a study that evaluated the efficacy of gefitinib 250 mg[88] or the combination of erlotinib and bevacizumab patients with progressive malignant thymic tumors.[89] Similarly, the EGFR monoclonal antibody cetuximab has limited efficacy although studies are ongoing.[90,104] At the present time, the evidence from the literature suggests that both EGFR tyrosine kinase inhibitors and monoclonal antibodies cannot be recommended to treat patients with thymic malignancies. Similarly, no cases of HER2 gene amplification by FISH have been detected[105] and there is no data to recommend HER2-targeted therapies in this disease setting.

Targeting angiogenesis, which is thought to play an important role in thymomagenesis, may be a more successful strategy. Vascular endothelial growth factor (VEGF)-A and VEGFR-1 and -2 are over-expressed in both thymomas and thymic carcinomas.[106,107] Although low response rates have been seen with bevacizumab, case reports involving sorafenib and sunitinib have highlighted the activity of these multikinase inhibitors predominantly in thymic carcinomas. Activity has been reported in a patient receiving sorafenib who had a missense mutation in exon 17 (D820E) of the c-KIT gene[99] and a second patient had prolonged stable disease (>9 months) in a nonmutated but high IHC expressing tumor for KIT, p53, and VEGF.[108] The multikinase inhibitor sunitinib has been evaluated in a phase II clinical trial involving 23 patients with thymic carcinoma. An impressive response rate compared to historical data of 26% and a disease control rate of 91% was reported.[109]

Other targets that have been evaluated include the insulin-like growth factor-1 (IGF-1)/IGF-1 receptor (IGF-1R), which has been identified as a poor prognostic indicator in thymic malignancies.[94,110] Expression of IGF-1R does differ between thymomas (4%) and thymic carcinomas (37%) indicating a possible difference in tumor biology that may be targetable.[94] A phase II study of cixutumumab, an IGF-1R monoclonal antibody in 49 patients with previously treated advanced thymic tumors, demonstrated a modest 14% response rate in thymomas but no activity in thymic

carcinoma.[92] Similarly histone deacetylase (HDAC) inhibitors have been evaluated in thymic tumors most notably the pan-HDAC inhibitor belinostat that demonstrated modest antitumor activity. In a phase I study of belinostat, a patient with thymoma had a minor response that lasted for 17 months on treatment;[111] therefore, a phase II trial in 41 patients (25 thymoma and 16 thymic carcinoma) in previously treated thymic malignancies was performed.[91] There were two partial responses in thymomas (response rate 8%) and no responses in thymic carcinomas. Ongoing studies targeting the mTOR pathway inhibitors are ongoing.[93] Future strategies targeting the PD-1/PD-L1 axis are planned. High PD-L1 expression ranging from 60% to 90% across the spectrum of thymic malignancies indicates that the use of checkpoint inhibitors may prove more successful than targeting individual genetic alterations although the concern about exacerbating autoimmune phenomenon mandates investigation in type B3/thymic carcinomas in the first instance.

Conclusion

Incremental improvements in our understanding of molecular biology allied with improvements in stage classification systems will it is hoped provide a uniform nomenclature and pathway toward larger collaborative efforts by providing consistency of communication across International boundaries. The ongoing TNM stage groupings that are being developed will provide a basis for the 8th edition of the AJCC/UICC stage classification due to be published in 2016. Surgical resection continues to be the cornerstone of therapy for early-stage disease while a multidisciplinary approach incorporating surgery, radiation, and chemotherapy is recommended in advanced or recurrent disease. Gene expression profiling and genomic clustering data indicating that the subclassifications of types A, AB, B1, B2, B3, and thymic carcinoma have different molecular features may allow for subset specific therapeutics. Clear differences have emerged between thymic carcinomas and type B3 thymomas when compared to type A and type B2 thymomas. It is hoped that molecular classification may be more useful to clinicians in the future than the current classification systems. Future strategies using prognostic and predictive biomarker or gene signatures may allow us to preselect patients for the most appropriate treatment. In addition, intense interest is now focused on targeting the immune system in these most intriguing of tumors. The association of thymic tumors with a wide variety of disorders secondary to T-cell-mediated autoimmunity allied to high PD-L1 expression indicates that checkpoint inhibitors such as PD-1 inhibitors may hold promise for patients with chemoresistant disease.

Key references

The complete reference list can be found on the Wiley Companion Digital Edition of this title (see inside front cover for login instructions).

1 Engels EA. Epidemiology of thymoma and associated malignancies. *J Thorac Oncol.* 2010;5:S260–S265.

3 Masaoka A, Monden Y, Nakahara K, et al. Follow-up study of thymomas with special reference to their clinical stages. *Cancer.* 1981;48:2485–2492.

4 Koga K, Matsuno Y, Noguchi M, et al. A review of 79 thymomas: modification of staging system and reappraisal of conventional division into invasive and non-invasive thymoma. *Pathol Int.* 1994;44:359–367.

13 Marchevsky AM, Wick MR. *Pathology of the Mediastinum.* Cambridge, UK: Cambridge Univ Press; 2014.

15 Travis WD, Brambilla E, Muller-Hermelink HK. *Pathology and Genetics of Tumours of the Lung, Pleura, Thymus and Heart (IARC WHO Classifications of Tumours.* Lyon, France: IARC Press; 2004.

16 Marx A, Strobel P, Badve SS, et al. ITMIG consensus statement on the use of the WHO histological classification of thymoma and thymic carcinoma: refined definitions, histological criteria, and reporting. *J Thorac Oncol.* 2014;9:596–611.

17 Suster S, Moran CA. Histologic classification of thymoma: the World Health Organization and beyond. *Hematol Oncol Clin North Am*. 2008;**22**:381–392.

22 Moser B, Scharitzer M, Hacker S, et al. Thymomas and thymic carcinomas: prognostic factors and multimodal management. *Thorac Cardiovasc Surg*. 2014;**62**:153–160.

24 Marchevsky AM, McKenna RJ Jr, Gupta R. Thymic epithelial neoplasms: a review of current concepts using an evidence-based pathology approach. *Hematol Oncol Clin North Am*. 2008;**22**:543–562.

25 Gupta R, Marchevsky AM, McKenna RJ, et al. Evidence-based pathology and the pathologic evaluation of thymomas: transcapsular invasion is not a significant prognostic feature. *Arch Pathol Lab Med*. 2008;**132**:926–930.

26 Marchevsky AM, Gupta R, Casadio C, et al. World Health Organization classification of thymomas provides significant prognostic information for selected stage III patients: evidence from an international thymoma study group. *Hum Pathol*. 2010;**41**:1413–1421.

27 Marchevsky AM, Gupta R, McKenna RJ, et al. Evidence-based pathology and the pathologic evaluation of thymomas: the World Health Organization classification can be simplified into only 3 categories other than thymic carcinoma. *Cancer*. 2008;**112**:2780–2788.

30 Detterbeck FC, Nicholson AG, Kondo K, et al. The Masaoka-Koga stage classification for thymic malignancies: clarification and definition of terms. *J Thorac Oncol*. 2011;**6**:S1710–S1716.

31 Ruffini E, Detterbeck F, Van Raemdonck D, et al. Tumours of the thymus: a cohort study of prognostic factors from the European Society of thoracic surgeons database. *Eur J Cardiothorac Surg*. 2014;**46**:361–368.

32 Detterbeck FC. Clinical value of the WHO classification system of thymoma. *Ann Thorac Surg*. 2006;**81**:2328–2334.

34 Gokmen-Polar Y, Cano OD, Kesler KA, et al. *NUT midline carcinomas in the thymic region*. Vol. **27**. Mod Pathol: ; 2014:1649–1656.

36 Kelly RJ. Thymoma versus thymic carcinoma: differences in biology impacting treatment. *J Natl Compr Canc Netw*. 2013;**11**:577–583.

37 Okuma Y, Hosomi Y, Watanabe K, et al. Clinicopathological analysis of thymic malignancies with a consistent retrospective database in a single institution: from Tokyo Metropolitan Cancer Center. *BMC Cancer*. 2014;**14**:349.

38 Ruffini E, Detterbeck F, Van Raemdonck D, et al. Thymic carcinoma: a cohort study of patients from the European society of thoracic surgeons database. *J Thorac Oncol*. 2014;**9**:541–548.

42 Moran CA, Suster S. Thymic neuroendocrine carcinomas with combined features ranging from well-differentiated (carcinoid) to small cell carcinoma. A clinicopathologic and immunohistochemical study of 11 cases. *Am J Clin Pathol*. 2000;**113**:345–350.

53 Kelly RJ, Petrini I, Rajan A, et al. Thymic malignancies: from clinical management to targeted therapies. *J Clin Oncol*. 2011;**29**:4820–4827.

81 Loehrer PJ Sr, Jiroutek M, Aisner S, et al. Combined etoposide, ifosfamide, and cisplatin in the treatment of patients with advanced thymoma and thymic carcinoma: an intergroup trial. *Cancer*. 2001;**91**:2010–2015.

82 Lemma GL, Lee JW, Aisner SC, et al. Phase II study of carboplatin and paclitaxel in advanced thymoma and thymic carcinoma. *J Clin Oncol*. 2011;**29**:2060–2065.

83 Loehrer PJ Sr, Yiannoutsos CT, Dropcho S, et al. A phase II trial of pemetrexed in patients with recurrent thymoma or thymic carcinoma. *J Clin Oncol* (Meeting Abstracts). 2006;**24**:7079.

85 Yoshihito Kogure FH, Yamanaka T. A multicenter prospective study of carboplatin and paclitaxel for advanced thymic carcinoma: West Japan Oncology Group 4207L. O3.1. *J Thorac Oncol*. 2013;**8**(**Supplement 1**).

86 Celine Boutros FF, Besse B. P2.03: oral etoposide in pretreated advanced thymoma and thymic carcinoma: a French experience. *J Thorac Oncol*. 2013;**8**(**Supplement 1**).

87 Heather Wakelee JR, Pedro-Salcedo MS. Stage 1 results of a 2-stage phase II trial of single agent Amrubicin in patients with previously treated thymic malignancies. O3.2. *J Thorac Oncol*. 2013;**8**(**Supplement 1**).

91 Giaccone G, Rajan A, Berman A, et al. Phase II study of belinostat in patients with recurrent or refractory advanced thymic epithelial tumors. *J Clin Oncol*. 2011;**29**:2052–2059.

92 Rajan A, Carter CA, Berman A, et al. Cixutumumab for patients with recurrent or refractory advanced thymic epithelial tumours: a multicentre, open-label, phase 2 trial. *Lancet Oncol*. 2014;**15**:191–200.

93 Wheler J, Hong D, Swisher SG, et al. Thymoma patients treated in a phase I clinic at MD Anderson Cancer Center: responses to mTOR inhibitors and molecular analyses. *Oncotarget*. 2013;**4**:890–898.

95 Pan CC, Chen PC, Chiang H. KIT (CD117) is frequently overexpressed in thymic carcinomas but is absent in thymomas. *J Pathol*. 2004;**202**:375–381.

96 Henley JD, Cummings OW, Loehrer PJ Sr. Tyrosine kinase receptor expression in thymomas. *J Cancer Res Clin Oncol*. 2004;**130**:222–224.

97 Strobel P, Hartmann M, Jakob A, et al. Thymic carcinoma with overexpression of mutated KIT and the response to imatinib. *N Engl J Med*. 2004;**350**:2625–2626.

98 Yoh K, Nishiwaki Y, Ishii G, et al. Mutational status of EGFR and KIT in thymoma and thymic carcinoma. *Lung Cancer*. 2008;**62**:316–320.

99 Bisagni G, Rossi G, Cavazza A, et al. Long lasting response to the multikinase inhibitor bay 43-9006 (Sorafenib) in a heavily pretreated metastatic thymic carcinoma. *J Thorac Oncol*. 2009;**4**:773–775.

100 Giaccone G, Rajan A, Ruijter R, et al. Imatinib mesylate in patients with WHO B3 thymomas and thymic carcinomas. *J Thorac Oncol*. 2009;**4**:1270–1273.

111 Steele NL, Plumb JA, Vidal L, et al. A phase 1 pharmacokinetic and pharmacodynamic study of the histone deacetylase inhibitor belinostat in patients with advanced solid tumors. *Clin Cancer Res*. 2008;**14**:804–810.

87 Tumors of the heart and great vessels

Anthony F. Yu, MD ▪ Sai-Ching Jim Yeung, MD, PhD, FACP ▪ Carmen P. Escalante, MD ▪ Sarina van der Zee, MD ▪ A. P. Chahinian, MD ▪ Valentin Fuster, MD, PhD

Overview

Primary tumors of the heart and great vessels are rare, but secondary tumors are significantly more common. Clinical manifestations of cardiac tumors depend on the location and size of the mass, not on the histopathology of the tumor. Several noninvasive imaging modalities including echocardiography, cardiac MRI, cardiac CT, and PET are currently available to provide complementary information on the location, extent, and tissue characteristics of a cardiac tumor. The clinical management of patients with cardiac tumors varies based on the type of tumor, clinical symptoms, and overall prognosis.

Introduction

Primary cardiac tumors are extremely rare, with a prevalence of <0.1% to 0.3% based on autopsy series.[1-4] More than 75% of primary cardiac tumors are benign (Table 1).[5,6] The majority of malignant primary cardiac tumors are sarcomas and lymphomas, which carry a poor prognosis despite treatment.[7,8] In contrast to primary cardiac tumors, metastases to the heart are relatively common.[2,9-11] While most primary tumors arise from the endocardium, followed by the myocardium and then the pericardium,[2] the latter is the most common site for metastases.[12]

Clinical features

The clinical manifestations of cardiac tumors frequently reflect the cardiac structure involved, tumor size, and the friability of the tumor rather than its histology.[12] The underlying mechanism responsible for clinical symptoms is varied and may include embolization, intracardiac or valvular obstruction, or direct invasion of myocardium or adjacent organs. The predominant site of common cardiac tumors is shown in Figure 1.

Tumors of the endocardial surface may present with valvular dysfunction or intracavitary obstruction. Right atrial tumors can lead to tricuspid valve obstruction and symptoms of right heart failure (i.e., fatigue, peripheral edema, ascites, hepatomegaly, jugular vein distention). Left atrial tumors tend to cause symptoms by obstructing blood flow and typically present with left heart failure symptoms (i.e., dyspnea, orthopnea, pulmonary edema, or hemoptysis). Myocardial invasion may present as arrhythmia, conduction abnormalities, systolic dysfunction, or diastolic dysfunction. Rarely, complete cavitary obstruction may lead to sudden death. Pericardial involvement can present as pleuritic chest pain or cardiac tamponade. Friable tumors, such as some myxomas and papillary fibroelastomas, may present with evidence of cerebral,

pulmonary, visceral, or peripheral emboli. Systemic manifestations, frequently seen in myxomas as well as malignant cardiac tumors, include fever, weight loss, myalgias, arthralgias, fatigue, and weakness.

Patients with cardiac tumors may present with the symptoms described above, or masses may be discovered incidentally on imaging studies, particularly when small in size. Physical examination may disclose a murmur, either systolic or diastolic, that varies with body position if the tumor is mobile. The characteristic "tumor plop" of a mobile tumor such as a myxoma is heard in diastole following the second heart sound and is thought to be due to the tension on the tumor stalk as the mass prolapses from atrium to ventricle or to the tumor striking the myocardium.[10] The tumor plop may be mistaken for a third heart sound or mitral opening snap. The electrocardiogram may show nonspecific ST-T abnormalities, atrial or ventricular arrhythmias, bundle branch block, or low voltage QRS complexes in the case of pericardial effusion. Chest X-ray findings include cardiomegaly and tumor calcification. Laboratory abnormalities include anemia (possibly hemolytic) or erythrocytosis, leukocytosis, thrombocytopenia, increased serum immunoglobulin levels, and elevated acute-phase reactants such as erythrocyte sedimentation rate and C-reactive protein.[10]

Diagnostic evaluation

Several cardiac imaging techniques are available for evaluation of patients with suspected cardiac masses. Two-dimensional transthoracic echocardiography (TTE) provides excellent spatial and temporal resolution of cardiac masses and is often the initial imaging modality of choice.[13] However, TTE can be limited by poor acoustic windows and lack of tissue characterization. Transesophageal echocardiography (TEE) allows for better tumor localization and characterization as well as assessment of intra- and extracardiac invasion. The use of contrast echocardiography may help to improve echocardiographic resolution and provide information on tumor vascularity.[14] Real-time three-dimensional echocardiography can offer incremental value over two-dimensional echocardiography by providing an accurate assessment of size and shape of the mass and enabling better localization of attachment point.[15]

Cardiac computed tomography (CT) and magnetic resonance imaging (MRI) provide cross-sectional images of the heart with high temporal and spatial resolution. Both modalities are able to depict intra- and extracardiac masses, as well as degree of myocardial or pericardial involvement, without limitations owing to body habitus or poor acoustic windows. Cardiac CT provides limited information regarding tissue characterization, but disadvantages of cardiac CT include radiation exposure and potential nephrotoxicity of contrast agents.[16] Cardiac MRI provides the highest degree of soft tissue contrast of any imaging modality and combines

Holland-Frei Cancer Medicine, Ninth Edition. Edited by Robert C. Bast Jr., Carlo M. Croce, William N. Hait, Waun Ki Hong, Donald W. Kufe, Martine Piccart-Gebhart, Raphael E. Pollock, Ralph R. Weichselbaum, Hongyang Wang, and James F. Holland.
© 2017 John Wiley & Sons, Inc. ISBN: 978-1-118-93469-2

Table 1 Type and frequency of primary tumors of the heart and pericardium in two series from the armed forces institute of pathology.

Type	1976–1993 series n	1976–1993 series %	Pre-1977 series n	Pre-1977 series %
Benign tumors				
Myxoma	114	27.9	130	29.3
Papillary fibroelastoma	31	7.6	42	9.5
Rhabdomyoma	20	4.9	36	8.1
Lipoma	2	0.5	45	10.1
Fibroma	20	4.9	17	3.8
Hemangioma	17	4.2	15	3.4
Atrioventricular nodal tumor	10	2.4	12	2.7
Teratoma	4	1.0	14	3.2
Lipomatous hypertrophy, atrial septum	12	2.9	0	0.0
Granular cell tumor	4	1.0	3	0.7
Lymphangioma	2	0.5	2	0.5
Benign fibrous tumor	3	0.7	0	0.0
Neurofibroma	0	0.0	3	0.7
Histiocytoid cardiomyopathy	2	0.5	0	0.0
Inflammatory pseudotumor	2	0.5	0	0.0
Myocytic hamartoma	2	0.5	0	0.0
Paraganglioma	2	0.5	0	0.0
Epithelioid hemangioendothelioma	1	0.2	0	0.0
Total	248	60.6	319	71.8
Malignant tumors				
Angiosarcoma	37	9.0	39	8.8
Unclassified sarcoma	35	8.6	0	0.0
Rhabdomyosarcoma	6	1.5	26	5.9
Mesothelioma	8	2.0	19	4.3
Fibrosarcoma	9	2.2	14	3.2
Osteosarcoma	13	3.2	5	1.1
Malignant fibrous histiocytoma	16	3.9	0	0.0
Lymphoma	7	1.7	7	1.6
Leiomyosarcoma	12	2.9	1	0.2
Myxosarcoma	8	2.0	0	0.0
Synovial sarcoma	5	1.2	1	0.2
Malignant teratoma	0	0.0	4	0.9
Neurogenic sarcoma	0	0.0	4	0.9
Thymoma[a]	0	0.0	4	0.9
Liposarcoma	2	0.5	1	0.2
Malignant schwannoma	2	0.5	0	0.0
Yolk sac tumor	1	0.2	0	0.0
Total	161	39.4	125	28.2
Total tumors	409		444	

[a]From thymic rests in the parietal pericardium.
Source: Adapted from Refs. 4 and 5. Cysts are excluded.

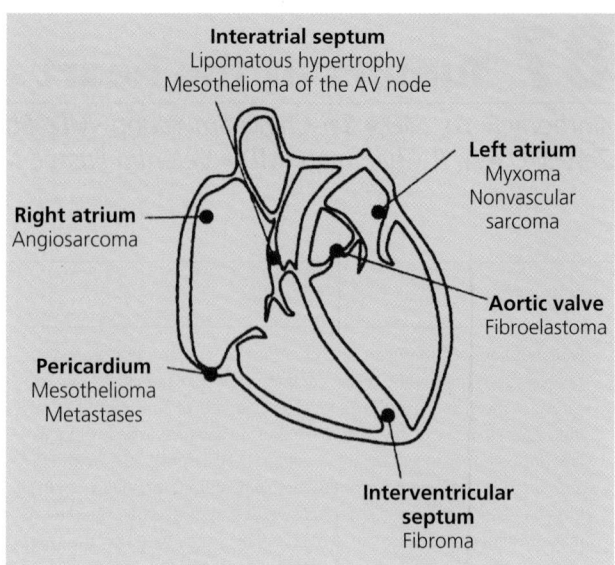

Figure 1 Predominant sites of common cardiac tumors.

Cardiac tumors

Benign primary cardiac tumors

Myxomas

Myxomas represent the most common primary cardiac tumor in the adult population. Histologically, these soft gelatinous tumors are thought to arise from the subendocardial mesenchyme and contain polygonal to stellate myxoma cells ("lepidic cells"), often around vascular channels in an eosinophilic matrix, with various areas of hemorrhage.[5] The cells are positive for factor VIII and can also express neuron-specific enolase and S-100 protein.[25] Most myxomas arise in the left atrium and are usually attached to the fossa ovalis. In a meta-analysis of 32 reports encompassing 1029 patients, 83% of myxomas were found to occur in the left atrium.[26] The remainder are found in the right atrium, or uncommonly, in the right or left ventricles. They often present as mobile masses attached by a stalk to the endocardial surface.[27] The mean age is 50 years at presentation, and more women are affected than men.[26] The classic clinical presentation includes a triad of constitutional symptoms, valvular obstruction, and embolization. Embolic phenomena, seen in 30–40% of patients, are more likely when the tumor surface is irregular (polypoid or myxoid) rather than smooth.[12] Surgery is generally recommended at the time of diagnosis owing to the risk of embolization or other cardiac complications, and involves en bloc resection along with margins of normal tissue and the fossa ovalis. Recurrence is rare but can occur in 2–5% of patients but long-term follow-up is necessary.[28–30]

Although most myxomas are sporadic, familial syndromes have been described. The Carney complex is an autosomal dominant multiple endocrine neoplasia syndrome that includes atrial myxomas and endocrine, neural and cutaneous tumors in addition to skin and mucosal pigmentation.[31–33] Mutations in *PRKAR1A*, a gene located on chromosome 17q22-24, which encodes a regulatory subunit of cyclic-AMP-dependent protein kinase A, have been identified in approximately one-half of affected patients.[34–37] A variant associated with distal arthrogryposis has been linked to a missense mutation in the myosin heavy-chain gene on 17p12-p13.1.[38] Familial myxomas present at a younger age, are more likely to be multiple, and are more likely to recur after

outstanding tumor localization, visualization of adjacent structures, and myocardial motion and perfusion assessment (Figure 2).[17–19] In addition, tailored imaging sequences allow more specific characterization of particular tumors.[18] Tissue characteristics of the cardiac mass can be evaluated using T1- and T2-weighted images, as well as enhancement with gadolinium contrast.[20] Although the spatial resolution of CT is greater than MRI, the soft tissue characterization of CT is inferior to MRI and thus, CT can be considered an intermediate modality appropriate in select patients.[16] Positron emission tomography (PET) can also help to identify cardiac involvement in patients with malignant tumors.[21] Cardiac angiography, once a mainstay in the diagnosis of cardiac tumors, has fallen out of use given the risk of embolization during the procedure.

When a cardiac mass is discovered on an imaging study, the differential diagnosis includes thrombus and vegetation, in addition to primary or secondary tumors.[22,23] Thrombi are usually seen in the context of underlying heart disease including arrhythmia (e.g., atrial fibrillation or atrial flutter), cardiomyopathy, or myocardial infarction. Normal anatomic variants, such as a prominent Eustachian valve or Chiari network, may also mimic cardiac tumors.[24]

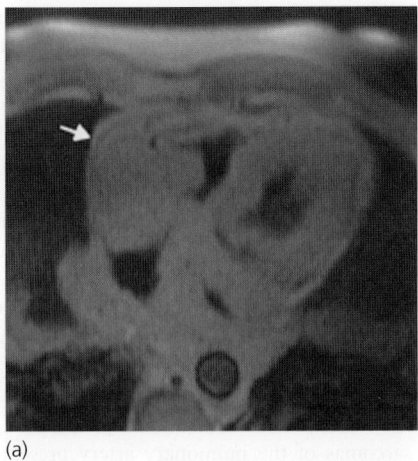 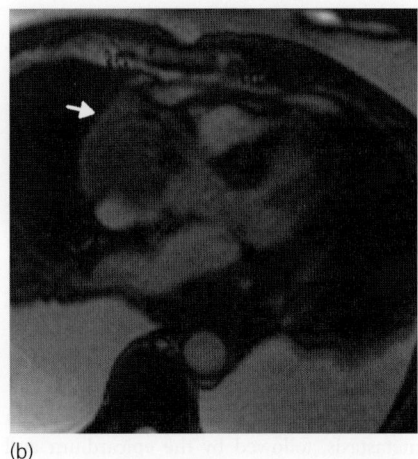

(a)   (b)

Figure 2 Cardiac MRI of a 69-year-old man with lymphoma demonstrating a large homogeneous mass (*arrows*) occupying most of the right atrium and extending into the right ventricle and posterior mediastinum. (a) Dark-blood image in the four-chamber view obtained using T2-weighted half-Fourier acquisition single-shot turbo spin echo. (b) Bright-blood image in the four-chamber view obtained using steady-state free precession; note the large bilateral pleural effusions.

resection than sporadic myxomas.[39] Identification of first-degree relatives facilitates the identification of myxomas at risk for embolization.

Papillary fibroelastomas
Papillary fibroelastomas are the most common primary tumor of the cardiac valves and are composed of papillary fronds similar to normal chordae tendineae. They usually arise from the valvular endocardium, most commonly the aortic valve, and occur over a wide range of ages.[40,41] Fibroelastomas may be asymptomatic (in ~30% of patients) or may present with transient ischemic attack, stroke, heart failure, angina, myocardial infarction, or sudden death. Surgical resection is recommended for patients with prior embolic events, as well as patients with large (≥1 cm) and mobile masses at high risk for embolization.[40,42,43]

Other benign tumors
Rhabdomyomas occur almost exclusively in children and are described below. Lipomatous septal hypertrophy is an exaggeration of the normal accumulation of fat within the atrial septum.[44] There is usually no role for surgical resection of lipomatous septal hypertrophy in the absence of symptoms such as vena cava obstruction, atrial arrhythmia, or congestive heart failure.[45,46] Lipomas and hemangiomas may be found anywhere in the heart. Fibromas primarily arise in the interventricular septum and more commonly affect the left ventricle.[47] Pericardial cysts are most common in the right costophrenic angle, and bronchogenic cysts can be found in the myocardium.[5] Paragangliomas and mesotheliomas may be benign or malignant. Mesotheliomas may be primary or metastatic to the pericardium or may occur in the AV node, presenting with AV block, arrhythmia, or sudden death.[48]

Malignant primary cardiac tumors

Sarcomas
Soft tissue sarcomas are the most common primary malignant neoplasm of the heart.[49] Angiosarcomas usually arise in the right atrium near the atrioventricular groove, although other chambers may be involved, and are associated with areas of hemorrhage, pericardial invasion, and effusion.[50] Angiosarcomas most commonly present between 20 and 50 years of

age, with a two- to threefold male predominance.[5] The clinical presentation may include palpitations, dyspnea, and chest pain (pleuritic and/or pericardial), or signs and symptoms related to congestive heart failure or thromboembolism. The relationship between cardiac angiosarcoma and Kaposi's sarcoma, in which cardiac involvement has been described, requires further investigation.[51,52] Rhabdomyosarcomas are the second most common malignant neoplasm of the heart and equally affect the right and left sided heart chambers.[53] Endomyocardial-based sarcomas, often with smooth muscle or myofibroblastic differentiation, are rare tumors usually located in the left atrium and consist of multiple subtypes, including undifferentiated pleomorphic sarcoma, osteosarcoma, leiomyosarcoma, fibrosarcoma, and myxofibrosarcoma.

The overall prognosis of cardiac sarcomas is poor, and aggressive local growth and metastatic spread are common. The median survival ranges from 6 to 12 months.[54,55] Complete surgical resection of cardiac sarcomas is the treatment of choice, although many patients develop recurrent disease. Orthotopic heart transplantation, at times combined with bilateral lung transplantation, has been described in a few small series and case reports. In most cases, heart transplantation followed by chemotherapy does not affect long-term outcome;[56] however, selected patients may have good outcomes with transplantation.[57,58]

Lymphomas
Primary cardiac lymphomas are rare and should be distinguished from systemic lymphoma with secondary cardiac involvement.[8] The typical sites are the atria, where infiltration of the wall is frequent, as well as the pericardium. Cardiac lymphoma may be seen in immunocompetent patients but is also associated with acquired immune deficiency syndrome and organ transplant-related immunosuppression. Unlike other cardiac tumors, the mainstay of treatment is chemotherapy, alone or in combination with radiation therapy, and occasionally autologous stem cell transplantation.[59,60]

Metastatic cardiac tumors
Secondary tumors of the heart are significantly more common than primary cardiac tumors.[61] Mechanisms of metastasis include direct extension, hematogenous spread, lymphatic spread, and cavoatrial

Table 2 Tumors likely to metastasize to the heart.

Melanoma
Malignant germ cell tumor
Leukemia and lymphoma
Breast carcinoma
Lung carcinoma
Hepatocellular carcinoma
Renal cell carcinoma
Sarcoma
Esophageal and gastric carcinoma
Mesothelioma (may be primary to pericardium or metastatic)

or pulmonary vein extension. The pericardium is the most common location for cardiac metastasis, followed by the epicardium and myocardium. Malignancies likely to metastasize to the heart are shown in Table 2.[27] In a recent postmortem review of 7289 cases with malignant neoplasms, the incidence of cardiac metastasis was 9.1%.[11] The frequency of heart metastases was, in decreasing order, mesothelioma (48.4%), melanoma (27.8%), lung adenocarcinoma (21%), poorly differentiated lung carcinoma (19.5%), squamous cell lung carcinoma (18.2%), and breast carcinoma (15.5%). Almost any cancer, however, can metastasize to the heart. A high frequency of cardiac metastasis and/or invasion can be seen in patients with malignant pleural mesothelioma.[62] In 19 autopsies, cardiac invasion was found in 14 (74%), with more than half involving the pericardium and more than one-quarter the myocardium.[63] Treatment is generally palliative.

Pediatric tumors

In contrast to adults, metastases to the heart are rarely observed in the pediatric population. Many cardiac neoplasms in children occur in the context of familial syndromes (see section on the Carney Complex, above). The majority are hamartomas. Rhabdomyomas account for the majority of pediatric cardiac tumors[64] and are associated with tuberous sclerosis, an autosomal dominant disorder characterized by benign neoplasms of the heart, kidneys, brain, lungs, and skin.[65] They occur most commonly in the ventricles and, in the context of familial syndromes, often regress spontaneously; surgical resection is usually necessary only if outflow tract obstruction is present.[66-68] Cardiac fibromas are mainly found in the ventricular septum and can grow to be quite large, often with areas of central calcification. Fibromas occur in a minority of patients with Gorlin syndrome, which is an autosomal dominant disorder presenting with multiple neoplasms, including basal cell carcinomas and medulloblastomas as well as odontogenic keratocysts and skeletal abnormalities.[69,70] Neurofibromas are found in patients with von Recklinghausen's disease.[27]

Tumors of the great vessels

Primary tumors involving the aorta, pulmonary artery, and vena cavae are rare, appearing in the literature mainly as case reports or in small retrospective case series.[71-73] Risk factors for the development of tumors of the great vessels remain poorly defined. Prior radiation exposure has been postulated as a possible causative factor.[74] Plastic polymers, such as Dacron, have been linked to aortic tumors in animal studies; nonetheless, aortic tumors arising around a Dacron graft in humans, although reported, are extremely rare.[75] Tumors of the great vessels typically present with thromboembolic events or an obstructive syndrome.[71] TEE and MRI are useful in differentiating tumors of the great vessels from intraluminal thrombus, mediastinal lymphadenopathy, or adjacent lung tumors.

Benign tumors of the aorta include endothelial papillary fibroelastomas arising in the aortic sinuses, which may present with intermittent prolapse into a coronary artery or with emboli to the heart or brain.[76] Intra-aortic myxomas have also been described, presenting with recurrent arterial emboli.[72]

Malignant tumors of the aorta and pulmonary artery are often aggressive, poorly differentiated sarcomas arising from intimal cells and showing myofibroblastic differentiation ("intimal type"). Rarely, malignant tumors of the great vessels are identified as angiosarcomas, leiomyosarcomas, hemangioendotheliomas, schwannomas, and fibrous histiocytomas.[71,77-79] Sarcomas of the inferior vena cava tend to be well-differentiated leiomyosarcomas.[80] Whereas sarcomas of the aorta present at a mean age of 62 years, sarcomas of the pulmonary artery present at a younger age. In a review of 60 cases of sarcoma involving the pulmonary trunk, the median age was 52 years, with a male-to-female ratio of 1:2 and a median duration of symptoms of 10 months.[81] The clinical picture was suggestive of pulmonary embolism, with dyspnea (70%), chest pain (48%), cough (34%), hemoptysis (30%), and syncope (25%). Metastases to lung (67%) and lymph node (20%) were common.

Although patients with tumors of the great vessels tend to present with advanced disease and prognosis is poor, a minority respond to resection and chemotherapy.[82] The cornerstone of therapy is complete surgical excision.[83] The use of various grafts has been advocated,[84] along with postoperative radiation and chemotherapy, often with an anthracycline-based regimen.[71,77] Although mean survival for patients with tumors of the great vessels is only 10 months, patients with sarcoma of the pulmonary artery may have a better prognosis compared with sarcoma of the aorta (23 vs 5 months).[71,84,85] Prolonged survival is extremely rare but has been reported.[86] For patients with unresectable disease, endovascular stent grafting may improve quality of life.[87]

Key references

The complete reference list can be found on the Wiley Companion Digital Edition of this title (see inside front cover for login instructions).

1 Bruce CJ. Cardiac tumours: diagnosis and management. *Heart.* 2011;**97**:151–160.
2 Lam KY, Dickens P, Chan AC. Tumors of the heart. A 20-year experience with a review of 12,485 consecutive autopsies. *Arch Pathol Lab Med.* 1993;**117**:1027–1031.
5 McAllister HA, Fenoglio JJ. *Tumors of the Cardiovascular System.* Washington: Armed Forces Institute of Pathology; 1978.
7 Shanmugam G Primary cardiac sarcoma. *Eur J Cardiothorac Surg.* 2006;**29**:925–932.
8 Simpson L, Kumar SK, Okuno SH, et al. Malignant primary cardiac tumors: review of a single institution experience.. *Cancer.* 2008;**112(11)**:2440.
11 Bussani R, De-Giorgio F, Abbate A, et al. Cardiac metastases. *J Clin Pathol.* 2007;**60**:27–34.
12 Burke A, Jeudy J Jr, Virmani R. Cardiac tumours: an update: Cardiac tumours. *Heart.* 2008;**94**:117–123.
13 Auger D, Pressacco J, Marcotte F, et al. Cardiac masses: an integrative approach using echocardiography and other imaging modalities. *Heart.* 2011;**97**:1101–1109.
14 Mulvagh SL, Rakowski H, Vannan MA, et al. American society of echocardiography consensus statement on the clinical applications of ultrasonic contrast agents in echocardiography. *J Am Soc Echocardiogr.* 2008;**21**:1179–1201; quiz 1281.
15 Zaragoza-Macias E, Chen MA, Gill EA. Real time three-dimensional echocardiography evaluation of intracardiac masses. *Echocardiography.* 2012;**29**:207–219.
16 Kassop D, Donovan MS, Cheezum MK, et al. Cardiac masses on cardiac CT: A review. *Curr Cardiovasc Imaging Rep.* 2014;**7**:9281.
19 Fussen S, De Boeck BW, Zellweger MJ, et al. Cardiovascular magnetic resonance imaging for diagnosis and clinical management of suspected cardiac masses and tumours. *Eur Heart J.* 2011;**32**:1551–1560.
20 Hoey ET, Mankad K, Puppala S, et al. MRI and CT appearances of cardiac tumours in adults. *Clin Radiol.* 2009;**64**:1214–1230.
21 Rahbar K, Seifarth H, Schafers M, et al. Differentiation of malignant and benign cardiac tumors using 18 F-FDG PET/CT. *J Nucl Med.* 2012;**53**:856–863.

24 Kim MJ, Jung HO. Anatomic variants mimicking pathology on echocardiography: differential diagnosis. *J Cardiovasc Ultrasound*. 2013;**21**:103–112.

27 Burke A, Virmani R. *Tumors of the Heart and Great Vessels, Atlas of Tumor Pathology*. Washington, DC: Armed Forces Institute of Pathology; 1996.

30 D'Alfonso A, Catania S, Pierri MD, et al. Atrial myxoma: a 25-year single-institutional follow-up study. *J Cardiovasc Med (Hagerstown)*. 2008;**9**:178–181.

31 Carney JA, Gordon H, Carpenter PC, et al. The complex of myxomas, spotty pigmentation, and endocrine overactivity. *Medicine (Baltimore)*. 1985;**64**:270–283.

33 Stratakis CA, Kirschner LS, Carney JA. Clinical and molecular features of the Carney complex: diagnostic criteria and recommendations for patient evaluation. *J Clin Endocrinol Metab*. 2001;**86**:4041–4046.

37 Carney JA. The complex of myxomas, spotty pigmentation, and endocrine overactivity. *Arch Intern Med*. 1987;**147**:418–419.

39 Carney JA. Differences between nonfamilial and familial cardiac myxoma. *Am J Surg Pathol*. 1985;**9**:53–55.

40 Sun JP, Asher CR, Yang XS, et al. Clinical and echocardiographic characteristics of papillary fibroelastomas: a retrospective and prospective study in 162 patients. *Circulation*. 2001;**103**:2687–2693.

41 Gowda RM, Khan IA, Nair CK, et al. Cardiac papillary fibroelastoma: a comprehensive analysis of 725 cases. *Am Heart J*. 2003;**146**:404–410.

46 Cale R, Andrade MJ, Canada M, et al. Lipomatous hypertrophy of the interatrial septum: report of two cases where histological examination and surgical intervention were unavoidable. *Eur J Echocardiogr*. 2009;**10**:876–879.

49 Yusuf SW, Bathina JD, Qureshi S, et al. Cardiac tumors in a tertiary care cancer hospital: clinical features, echocardiographic findings, treatment and outcomes. *Heart Int*. 2012;**7**:e4.

53 Castorino F, Masiello P, Quattrocchi E, et al. Primary cardiac rhabdomyosarcoma of the left atrium: an unusual presentation. *Tex Heart Inst J*. 2000;**27**:206–208.

54 Truong PT, Jones SO, Martens B, et al. Treatment and outcomes in adult patients with primary cardiac sarcoma: the British Columbia Cancer Agency experience. *Ann Surg Oncol*. 2009;**16**:3358–3365.

55 Hudzik B, Miszalski-Jamka K, Glowacki J, et al. Malignant tumors of the heart. *Cancer Epidemiology*. 2015;**39**:665–672.

57 Grandmougin D, Fayad G, Decoene C, et al. Total orthotopic heart transplantation for primary cardiac rhabdomyosarcoma: factors influencing long-term survival. *Ann Thorac Surg*. 2001;**71**:1438–1441.

61 Goldberg AD, Blankstein R, Padera RF. Tumors metastatic to the heart. *Circulation*. 2013;**128**:1790–1794.

64 Careddu L, Oppido G, Petridis FD, et al. Primary cardiac tumours in the paediatric population. *Multimed Man Cardiothorac Surg*. 2013;**2013**:mmt013.

65 Hinton RB, Prakash A, Romp RL, et al. Cardiovascular manifestations of tuberous sclerosis complex and summary of the revised diagnostic criteria and surveillance and management recommendations from the international tuberous sclerosis consensus group. *J Am Heart Assoc*. 2014;**3**.

66 Tao TY, Yahyavi-Firouz-Abadi N, Singh GK, and Bhalla S. Pediatric cardiac tumors: clinical and imaging features. *Radiographics*. 2014;**34**:1031–1046.

67 Sciacca P, Giacchi M, Mattia C, et al. Rhabdomyomas and tuberous sclerosis complex: our experience in 33 cases. *BMC Cardiovasc Disord*. 2014;**14**:66.

77 Blackmon SH, Rice DC, Correa AM, et al. Management of primary pulmonary artery sarcomas. *Ann Thorac Surg*. 2009;**87**:977–984.

80 Hollenbeck ST, Grobmyer SR, Kent KC, and Brenan MF. Surgical treatment and outcomes of patients with primary inferior vena cava leiomyosarcoma. *J Am Coll Surg*. 2003;**197**:575–579.

82 Mayer F, Aebert H, Rudert M, et al. Primary malignant sarcomas of the heart and great vessels in adult patients—a single-center experience. *Oncologist*. 2007;**12**:1134–1142.

83 Park BJ, Bacchetta M, Bains MS, et al. Surgical management of thoracic malignancies invading the heart or great vessels. *Ann Thorac Surg*. 2004;**78**:1024–1030.

86 Mattoo A, Fedullo PF, Kapelanski D, et al. Pulmonary artery sarcoma: a case report of surgical cure and 5-year follow-up. *Chest*. 2002;**122**:745–747.

87 Totaro M, Miraldi F, Ghiribelli C, et al. Cardiac angiosarcoma arising from pulmonary artery: endovascular treatment. *Ann Thorac Surg*. 2004;**78**:1468–1470.

88 Primary germ cell tumors of the thorax

John D. Hainsworth, MD ▪ *F. Anthony Greco, MD*

Overview

Primary germ cell tumors (GCT) of the thorax are rare but potentially curable. Benign teratomas account for approximately 60–70% and usually appear in young adults. The large majority of these tumors are curable with surgical excision. Malignant mediastinal GCT usually occur in young men and can be divided histologically into pure seminoma (~52% of cases) and various nonseminoma histologies. Pure seminomas are highly sensitive to chemotherapy; treatment with three cycles of bleomycin, etoposide, and cisplatin (BEP) as used in testicular cancer is curative in more than 80%. Selected patients with small (<6 cm) localized seminomas have high cure rates with radiation therapy alone. Nonseminomatous mediastinal GCT are associated with Klinefelter's syndrome (5–10% of cases) and are also associated with various acute leukemias. Optimal treatment includes four cycles of BEP chemotherapy (or an equivalent regimen), followed by resection of residual mediastinal masses. The cure rate for these relatively poor prognosis GCT is approximately 45%.

Mediastinal germ cell tumors (GCT), although rare, are of particular interest because they usually affect young males and because curative therapy is now available for many patients.

Benign teratomas of the mediastinum

Although benign teratomas of the mediastinum (mature cystic teratomas or dermoid tumors) account for only 3–12% of mediastinal tumors, they comprise 60–70% of all mediastinal GCT.[1,2] These tumors have been described in patients with ages ranging from 7 months to 65 years; however, most occur in young adults, with an approximately equal incidence in males and females.[2,3]

Benign mediastinal teratomas have a histologic appearance identical to that of benign teratomas arising in the more common ovarian location. On histologic examination, mature tissue from ectodermal, mesodermal, and endodermal germ cell layers is typically present. Mature tissue that recapitulates the histology of any human organ can be found in these tumors. However, the ectodermal component (i.e., skin, sebaceous tissue, neural tissue) usually predominates.[3]

Approximately 95% of benign teratomas arise in the anterior mediastinum; the remainder arise in the posterior mediastinum.[2,3] These tumors are slow growing, and 50–60% of patients are asymptomatic at the time of diagnosis by routine chest radiography.[3] When symptoms are present, dyspnea and substernal chest pain are the most common. Spontaneous rupture of the teratoma into the lung, tracheobronchial tree, pleura, or pericardium can cause an acute onset of symptoms, but these events occur late in the disease course. Cough productive of hair or sebum, caused by rupture into the tracheobronchial tree, is pathognomonic of a

benign mediastinal teratoma but occurs rarely. Superior vena cava syndrome is also rare and is a late manifestation. Serum levels of human chorionic gonadotropin (HCG) and alpha-fetoprotein are always normal in patients with benign teratoma.

Surgical excision is the treatment of choice for benign teratoma of the mediastinum. Surgical removal is sometimes difficult because of the large size and involvement of adjacent structures. Approximately 10–15% of patients require additional procedures (e.g., lobectomy, pericardiectomy) for complete tumor resection. Benign teratomas are resistant to radiation and cytotoxic drugs, and these modalities have no role in their treatment.

Tumor recurrence is rare following complete surgical resection.[2–4] Prolonged survival has been reported following subtotal resection of tumors involving vital mediastinal structures.

Malignant GCT

Etiology

Mediastinal GCT were initially thought to represent isolated metastases from an inapparent gonadal primary site. However, there is now abundant clinical evidence to substantiate the extragonadal origin of these tumors.[1,5]

Epidemiology

Malignant mediastinal GCT represent only 3–10% of tumors originating in the mediastinum, and only 1–5% of all germ cell neoplasms.[6] The great majority of mediastinal malignant GCT occur in males between 20 and 35 years of age. In the rare occurrences reported in females, mediastinal malignant GCT appear histologically and biologically identical to those occurring in males.

Patients with nonseminomatous extragonadal GCT have a subsequent increased risk of developing testicular cancer (approximately 10% at 10 years), strengthening the concept of a precursor abnormality in the germ cells of these patients.[7]

Histopathology

Mediastinal GCT appear to be histologically identical to GCT arising in the testis and contain the same range of histologic subtypes. However, the frequency of yolk sac tumor and teratocarcinoma is higher in mediastinal GCT, while embryonal carcinoma is less common. In a review of 229 malignant mediastinal GCT, pure seminoma was the most common histology, accounting for 52% of cases.[8] Nonseminomatous histologies included teratocarcinoma (20%), yolk sac tumor (17%), choriocarcinoma (3.4%), embryonal carcinoma (2.6%), and mixed nonseminomatous tumors (5.2%).

Clinical characteristics

Malignant mediastinal GCT are usually symptomatic at the time of diagnosis. Most mediastinal GCT are large and cause symptoms by

Holland-Frei Cancer Medicine, Ninth Edition. Edited by Robert C. Bast Jr., Carlo M. Croce, William N. Hait, Waun Ki Hong, Donald W. Kufe, Martine Piccart-Gebhart, Raphael E. Pollock, Ralph R. Weichselbaum, Hongyang Wang, and James F. Holland.
© 2017 John Wiley & Sons, Inc. ISBN: 978-1-118-93469-2

compressing or invading adjacent structures, including the lungs, pleura, pericardium, and chest wall. Pure seminomas are somewhat slower growing and have less potential for early metastasis than do tumors with nonseminomatous elements. Pure seminomas and tumors with nonseminomatous elements are therefore discussed separately, although substantial overlap exists in their clinical characteristics.

Seminoma

Seminomas grow relatively slowly and often become very large before causing symptoms. Tumors 20–30 cm in diameter can exist with minimal symptomatology. Approximately 20–30% of seminomas are detected by routine chest radiography while still asymptomatic.[9] The most common initial symptom is a sensation of pressure or dull retrosternal chest pain. Additional symptoms include exertional dyspnea, cough, dysphagia, and hoarseness. Superior vena cava syndrome develops in approximately 10% of patients. Systemic symptoms related to metastatic lesions are uncommon.

In order to be classified as a seminoma (or dysgerminoma in women), a mediastinal GCT must have no other histologic elements present. Tumors consisting of a mixture of seminoma and nonseminoma elements should be approached as nonseminomatous GCT.

At the time of diagnosis, only 30–40% of patients with mediastinal seminoma have localized disease; ramaining patients have one or more sites of distant metastases.[10] The regional lymph nodes (cervical, upper abdominal) are the most common metastatic sites; lung and bone are the most common visceral sites.[11]

Elevated serum levels of HCG are detected in up to 40% of mediastinal seminomas.[11] However, most of these are low-level elevations (2–10 ng/mL); levels of HCG exceeding 100 ng/mL are unusual and suggest the presence of nonseminomatous elements. The serum alpha-fetoprotein level is always normal in pure mediastinal seminoma, and any elevation of this tumor marker indicates the presence of nonseminomatous elements.

Nonseminomatous GCT

These rapidly growing neoplasms cause symptoms by compressing or invading local mediastinal structures, as seen in patients with mediastinal seminoma. Symptoms caused by metastases are much more common, as 85–95% of these patients have at least one metastatic site at the time of diagnosis.[12–14] Common metastatic sites include the lungs, pleura, lymph nodes (particularly supraclavicular and retroperitoneal), and liver. High levels of HCG are sometimes associated with gynecomastia. Constitutional symptoms are more common in these patients than in those with pure seminoma.

The serum tumor markers HCG and alpha-fetoprotein are usually abnormal in patients with mediastinal nonseminomatous GCT. Alpha-fetoprotein is elevated in 74–90% of patients, and elevation of HCG occurs in 30–38%.[15–17]

Approximately 5–10% of patients with mediastinal nonseminomatous GCT have Klinefelter syndrome.[18–20] The explanation for this association is unknown, but underlying germ cell defects related to the XXY chromosomal abnormality are likely to play a role.[21] The association of Klinefelter syndrome and mediastinal nonseminomatous GCT is specific; gonadal GCT show no association.[18,19]

Mediastinal nonseminomatous GCT are also associated with a variety of hematologic neoplasms including acute myeloid leukemia, acute nonlymphocytic leukemia, acute lymphocytic leukemia, erythroleukemia, acute megakaryocytic leukemia, myelodysplastic syndrome, and malignant histiocytosis.[22–28]

Hematologic neoplasms in this setting are not treatment-related but rather arise from clones of malignant lymphoblasts, myeloblasts, or progenitor cells contained within the GCT.[25–27]

Pretreatment evaluation and staging

The diagnosis of a mediastinal GCT should be considered in all young males with a mediastinal mass. In addition to physical examination and routine laboratory studies, initial evaluation should include CT of the chest and abdomen and determination of serum levels of HCG and alpha-fetoprotein. Any symptoms suggestive of distant metastases should be appropriately evaluated with radiologic studies.

In patients with suspected mediastinal GCT, a histologic diagnosis should be made using the least invasive approach because rapid initiation of definitive systemic therapy is important. Because these neoplasms are poorly differentiated, specimens obtained by fine-needle aspiration biopsy are sometimes insufficient for a definitive diagnosis. In such patients, surgical biopsy via median sternotomy or limited thoracotomy is indicated. Attempts at complete surgical resection of these mediastinal neoplasms are not indicated because curative results with other treatment modalities are superior.

Treatment of seminoma

Pure mediastinal seminomas are curable in the large majority of patients, even when metastatic at the time of diagnosis. These tumors are highly sensitive to radiation therapy and to combination chemotherapy, and the selection of treatment therefore depends on tumor stage and size, as well as the anticipated short- and long-term toxicity of treatment.

Chemotherapy

Cisplatin-based combination chemotherapy, as used in patients with advanced testicular cancer, is highly effective treatment for mediastinal seminoma. Patients who have no extrapulmonary 1 visceral metastases are classified as good risk GCT by the International Germ Cell Consensus Classification[29] and require first-line treatment with three cycles of combination chemotherapy. The most widely used combination regimen is bleomycin, etoposide, and cisplatin (BEP).[30] For patients with underlying pulmonary disease, or those who have had previous radiation therapy, bleomycin should be avoided; four cycles of etoposide/cisplatin are preferred. Patients with mediastinal seminoma and metastases to extrapulmonary sites have intermediate risk and therefore require four cycles of BEP. In this category, patients at risk for bleomycin toxicity should receive four courses of the VIP regimen (etoposide, ifosfamide, cisplatin).[31]

Cure rates higher than 80% have been reported in all series of patients treated with modern cisplatin-based regimens.[10–12,14,30,32–36] In the largest retrospective analysis, 47 of 51 patients achieved complete remission, with subsequent relapses in only 14%.[11]

Radiation therapy

Radiation therapy is also potentially curative for patients with mediastinal seminoma.[4,10,37,38] When localized tumors are <6 cm in diameter, the cure rate is high with radiation therapy or chemotherapy, and the choice of treatment should be individualized. For young patients without contraindications, curative treatment with chemotherapy avoids potential long-term consequences of mediastinal irradiation (e.g., coronary artery disease, valvular disease, constrictive pericarditis, second cancers), and is therefore the treatment of choice.[39,40] Patients with tumors <6 cm in diameter who are poor candidates for chemotherapy should have radiation therapy (35–50 Gy) using a field that includes the mediastinum and bilateral supraclavicular fossae. Patients who relapse after radiation therapy have a high salvage rate with chemotherapy.[12,30]

Residual mass

Following completion of chemotherapy, CT scans frequently show a residual mediastinal mass. In most published experience, residual masses <3 cm contain only fibrosis and necrotic tumor, whereas residual masses >3 cm have up to a 30% chance of containing residual viable cancer.[41,42] Therefore, careful follow-up without resection is recommended for patients with residual masses < 3 cm. Larger residual masses that are negative on PET scan can also be followed.[43,44] Follow-up includes CT scans every 3 months during the first year and every 6 months during the second year or until normal. This approach avoids a potentially difficult surgical procedure in most patients; intervention is necessary only if enlargement of masses is evident on serial scans.[41] Resection is recommended for residual masses > 3 cm. Patients with residual seminoma in the resected mass should have additional salvage chemotherapy or, in selected instances, radiation therapy to the mediastinum.

Treatment of nonseminomatous GCT

Most patients with mediastinal nonseminomatous GCT currently receive multimodality therapy, utilizing combination chemotherapy followed by surgical resection of residual mediastinal masses.

Chemotherapy

The use of cisplatin-based chemotherapy developed for the treatment of advanced nonseminomatous testicular neoplasms has improved the previously dismal outlook in patients with mediastinal nonseminomatous GCT. However, cure rates remain lower than those achieved in the treatment of testicular cancer.[12–17,32,33,36,45–48] Comparable long-term survival rates of 40–50% have been reported when testicular GCT with far advanced, bulky metastases are treated with similar cisplatin-based regimens.[29] Inherent biologic differences between mediastinal and testicular GCT also play a role in determining the relatively low cure rate.[49]

All patients with mediastinal nonseminomatous GCT have poor risk tumors; therefore, first-line treatment should include four courses of BEP or an equivalent regimen.[50] Following the completion of therapy, patients should be restaged with serum tumor markers and CT scans of the chest and abdomen.

Residual mass

Subsequent management is determined by the response to initial chemotherapy (Figure 1). Patients with normal CT scans and tumor marker levels require no further therapy. Approximately 20% of these patients subsequently relapse, with almost all relapses occurring during the first 2 years after completion of therapy. Standard follow-up of these patients includes monthly physical examination, chest radiography, and serum tumor marker determinations during the first year and similar evaluations every 2 months during the second year following therapy.

Most patients have residual radiographic abnormalities in the mediastinum after completion of chemotherapy.[16] In these patients, surgical resection of residual masses should be performed if technically feasible. Persistent elevation of serum tumor markers is not a contraindication to surgical resection in this setting.[51,52]

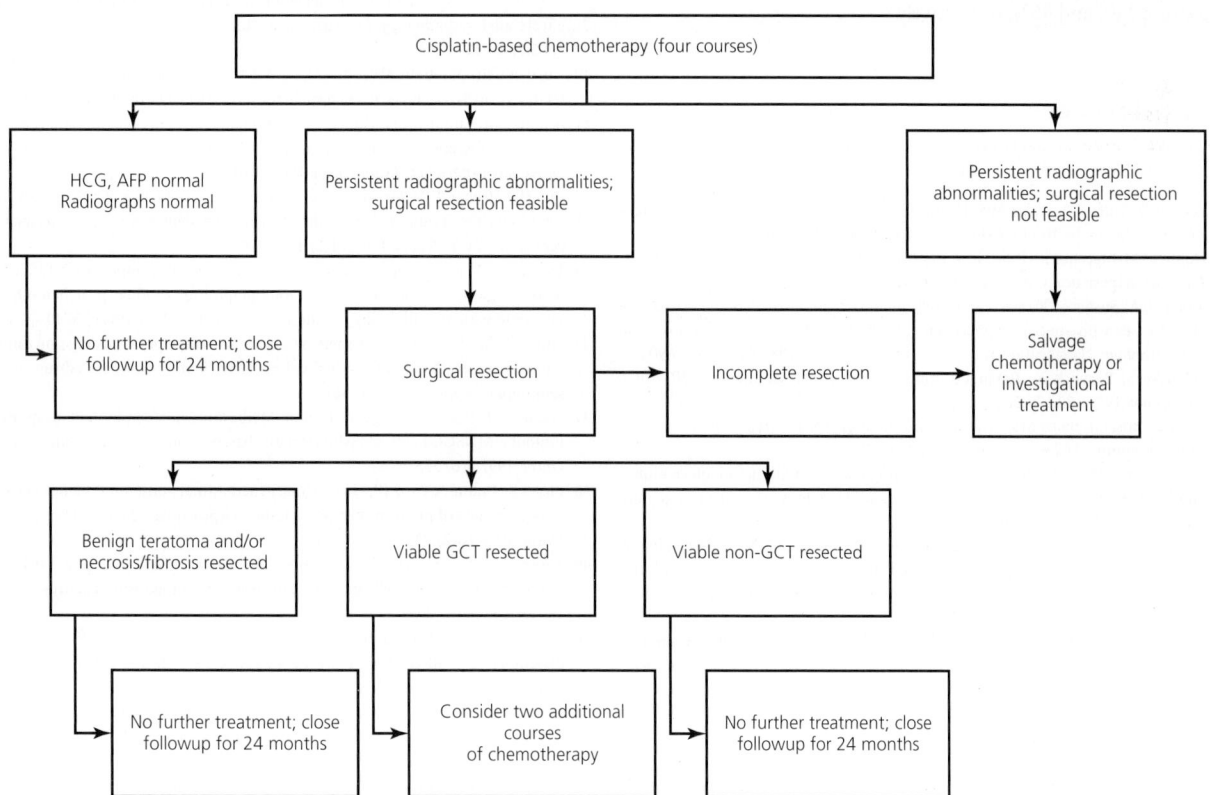

Figure 1 Management of mediastinal nonseminomatous germ cell tumors after completion of first-line chemotherapy.

Residual GCT is found in the resected specimen in a substantial proportion of patients (25–66%).[53–56] A few patients have residual cancer of various nongerm cell histologies (e.g., sarcoma, adenocarcinoma, neuroendocrine carcinoma).[55] The remainder of patients have benign teratoma, necrosis, or fibrosis without active carcinoma.

Complete surgical resection is curative for a substantial proportion of patients. Patients with no tumor remaining (i.e., necrotic tumor, fibrosis, and/or benign teratoma only) have a low risk of subsequent relapse (~20%).[53,55] Patients with resection of residual GCT have a high risk of future relapse; however, surgical resection is curative in 20–30%.[54,55] In these patients, two additional courses of chemotherapy postoperatively may reduce the recurrence rate. Most patients with residual nongerm cell histologies do poorly even with complete resection, although occasional long-term survivors have been reported.[55] Further systemic treatment after resection in these patients has been ineffective.

Recurrent/progressive disease

The prognosis is poor for patients in whom complete surgical resection is not feasible and in those who relapse after surgical resection. Standard second-line cisplatin-based regimens and high-dose chemotherapy regimens are curative in 20–50% of patients with recurrent testicular cancer but are effective in only 11% of patients with mediastinal nonseminomatous GCT.[51,52,57]

Prognosis

In a large retrospective multicenter study, 287 patients treated with current multimodality therapy were reviewed.[17] The complete response rate to chemotherapy was 19%; an additional 45% had normalization of tumor markers with a persistent mediastinal mass. Surgical resection of a residual mediastinal mass was required in 143 patients (50%). The 5-year progression-free and overall survival rates were 44% and 45%, respectively.

Key references

The complete reference list can be found on the Wiley Companion Digital Edition of this title (see inside front cover for login instructions).

3 Lewis BD, Hurt RD, Payne WS, Farrow GM, Knapp RH, Muhm JR. Benign teratomas of the mediastinum. *J Thorac Cardiovasc Surg*. 1983;**86**(5):727–731.

4 Dulmet EM, Macchiarini P, Suc B, Verley JM. Germ cell tumors of the mediastinum. A 30-year experience. *Cancer*. 1993;**72**(6):1894–1901.

8 Moran CA, Suster S. Primary germ cell tumors of the mediastinum: I. Analysis of 322 cases with special emphasis on teratomatous lesions and a proposal for histopathologic classification and clinical staging. *Cancer*. 1997;**80**(4):681–690.

9 Polansky S, Barwick K, Ravin C. Primary mediastinal seminoma. *AJR Am J Roentgenol*. 1979;**132**:17–21.

10 Jain KK, Bosl GJ, Bains MS, Whitmore WF, Golbey RB. The treatment of extragonadal seminoma. *J Clin Oncol*. 1984;**2**(7):820–827.

11 Bokemeyer C, Droz JP, Horwich A, et al. Extragonadal seminoma: an international multicenter analysis of prognostic factors and long term treatment outcome. *Cancer*. 2001;**91**(7):1394–1401.

13 Israel A, Bosl GJ, Golbey RB, Whitmore W Jr, Martini N. The results of chemotherapy for extragonadal germ-cell tumors in the cisplatin era: the Memorial Sloan-Kettering Cancer Center experience (1975 to 1982). *J Clin Oncol*. 1985;**3**(8):1073–1078.

15 Nichols CR, Saxman S, Williams SD, et al. Primary mediastinal nonseminomatous germ cell tumors. A modern single institution experience. *Cancer*. 1990;**65**(7):1641–1646.

16 Ganjoo KN, Rieger KM, Kesler KA, Sharma M, Heilman DK, Einhorn LH. Results of modern therapy for patients with mediastinal nonseminomatous germ cell tumors. *Cancer*. 2000;**88**(5):1051–1056.

17 Bokemeyer C, Nichols CR, Droz JP, et al. Extragonadal germ cell tumors of the mediastinum and retroperitoneum: results from an international analysis. *J Clin Oncol*. 2002;**20**(7):1864–1873.

20 Nichols CR, Heerema NA, Palmer C, Loehrer PJ Sr, Williams SD, Einhorn LH. Klinefelter's syndrome associated with mediastinal germ cell neoplasms. *J Clin Oncol*. 1987;**5**(8):1290–1294.

21 Carroll PR, Whitmore WF Jr, Richardson M, et al. Testicular failure in patients with extragonadal germ cell tumors. *Cancer*. 1987;**60**(1):108–113.

22 Nichols CR, Hoffman R, Einhorn LH, Williams SD, Wheeler LA, Garnick MB. Hematologic malignancies associated with primary mediastinal germ-cell tumors. *Ann Intern Med*. 1985;**102**(5):603–609.

23 Nichols CR, Roth BJ, Heerema N, Griep J, Tricot G. Hematologic neoplasia associated with primary mediastinal germ-cell tumors. *N Engl J Med*. 1990;**322**(20):1425–1429.

25 Orazi A, Neiman RS, Ulbright TM, Heerema NA, John K, Nichols CR. Hematopoietic precursor cells within the yolk sac tumor component are the source of secondary hematopoietic malignancies in patients with mediastinal germ cell tumors. *Cancer*. 1993;**71**(12):3873–3881.

27 Ladanyi M, Samaniego F, Reuter VE, et al. Cytogenetic and immunohistochemical evidence for the germ cell origin of a subset of acute leukemias associated with mediastinal germ cell tumors. *J Natl Cancer Inst*. 1990;**82**(3):221–227.

28 Hartmann JT, Nichols CR, Droz JP, et al. Hematologic disorders associated with primary mediastinal nonseminomatous germ cell tumors. *J Natl Cancer Inst*. 2000;**92**(1):54–61.

29 International Germ Cell Cancer Collaborative Group. International germ Cell Consensus Classification: a prognostic factor-based staging system for metastatic germ cell cancers. *J Clin Oncol*. 1997;**15**(2):594–603.

30 Loehrer PJ Sr, Birch R, Williams SD, Greco FA, Einhorn LH. Chemotherapy of metastatic seminoma: the Southeastern Cancer Study Group experience. *J Clin Oncol*. 1987;**5**(8):1212–1220.

31 Nichols CR, Catalano PJ, Crawford ED, Vogelzang NJ, Einhorn LH, Loehrer PJ. Randomized comparison of cisplatin and etoposide and either bleomycin or ifosfamide in treatment of advanced disseminated germ cell tumors: an Eastern Cooperative Oncology Group, Southwest Oncology Group, and Cancer and Leukemia Group B Study. *J Clin Oncol*. 1998;**16**(4):1287–1293.

35 Mencel PJ, Motzer RJ, Mazumdar M, Vlamis V, Bajorin DF, Bosl GJ. Advanced seminoma: treatment results, survival, and prognostic factors in 142 patients. *J Clin Oncol*. 1994;**12**(1):120–126.

36 Gerl A, Clemm C, Lamerz R, Wilmanns W. Cisplatin-based chemotherapy of primary extragonadal germ cell tumors. A single institution experience. *Cancer*. 1996;**77**(3):526–532.

38 Bush SE, Martinez A, Bagshaw MA. Primary mediastinal seminoma. *Cancer*. 1981;**48**(8):1877–1882.

39 Majewski W, Majewski S, Maciejewski A, Kolosza Z, Tarnawski R. Adverse effects after radiotherapy for early stage (I,IIa,IIb) seminoma. *Radiother Oncol*. 2005;**76**(3):257–263.

40 van den Belt-Dusebout AW, Nuver J, de Wit R, et al. Long-term risk of cardiovascular disease in 5-year survivors of testicular cancer. *J Clin Oncol*. 2006;**24**(3):467–475.

41 Schultz SM, Einhorn LH, Conces DJ Jr, Williams SD, Loehrer PJ. Management of postchemotherapy residual mass in patients with advanced seminoma: Indiana University experience. *J Clin Oncol*. 1989;**7**(10):1497–1503.

42 Puc HS, Heelan R, Mazumdar M, et al. Management of residual mass in advanced seminoma: results and recommendations from the Memorial Sloan-Kettering Cancer Center. *J Clin Oncol*. 1996;**14**(2):454–460.

43 De Santis M, Bokemeyer C, Becherer A, et al. Predictive impact of 2-18fluoro-2-deoxy-D-glucose positron emission tomography for residual postchemotherapy masses in patients with bulky seminoma. *J Clin Oncol*. 2001;**19**(17):3740–3744.

44 Hinz S, Schrader M, Kempkensteffen C, et al. The role of positron emission tomorgraphy in the evaluation of residual masses after chemotherapy for advanced stage seminoma. *J Urol*. 2008;**179**(936).

47 Hidalgo M, Paz-Ares L, Rivera F, et al. Mediastinal non-seminomatous germ cell tumours (MNSGCT) treated with cisplatin-based combination chemotherapy. *Ann Oncol*. 1997;**8**(6):555–559.

48 Fizazi K, Culine S, Droz JP, et al. Primary mediastinal nonseminomatous germ cell tumors: results of modern therapy including cisplatin-based chemotherapy. *J Clin Oncol*. 1998;**16**(2):725–732.

49 Toner GC, Geller NL, Lin SY, Bosl GJ. Extragonadal and poor risk nonseminomatous germ cell tumors. Survival and prognostic features. *Cancer*. 1991;**67**(8):2049–2057.

50 Williams SD, Birch R, Einhorn LH, Irwin L, Greco FA, Loehrer PJ. Treatment of disseminated germ-cell tumors with cisplatin, bleomycin, and either vinblastine or etoposide. *N Engl J Med*. 1987;**316**(23):1435–1440.

51 Saxman SB, Nichols CR, Einhorn LH. Salvage chemotherapy in patients with extragonadal germ cell tumors: the Indiana University experience. *J Clin Oncol*. 1994;**12**(7):1390–1393.

52 Hartmann JT, Einhorn L, Nichols CR, et al. Second-line chemotherapy in patients with relapsed extragonadal nonseminomatous germ cell tumors: results of an international multicenter analysis. *J Clin Oncol*. 2001;**19**(6):1641–1648.

53 Kesler KA, Rieger KM, Ganjoo KN, et al. Primary mediastinal nonseminomatous germ cell tumors: the influence of postchemotherapy pathology on long-term survival after surgery. *J Thorac Cardiovasc Surg*. 1999;**118**(**4**):692–700.

54 Vuky J, Bains M, Bacik J, et al. Role of postchemotherapy adjunctive surgery in the management of patients with nonseminoma arising from the mediastinum. *J Clin Oncol*. 2001;**19**(**3**):682–688.

55 Schneider BP, Kesler KA, Brooks JA, Yiannoutsos C, Einhorn LH. Outcome of patients with residual germ cell or non-germ cell malignancy after resection of primary mediastinal nonseminomatous germ cell cancer. *J Clin Oncol*. 2004;**22**(**7**):1195–1200.

56 Radaideh SM, Cook VC, Kesler KA, Einhorn LH. Outcome following resection for patients with primary mediastinal nonseminomatous germ-cell tumors and rising serum tumor markers post-chemotherapy. *Ann Oncol*. 2010;**21**(**4**): 804–807.

57 Broun ER, Nichols CR, Einhorn LH, Tricot GJ. Salvage therapy with high-dose chemotherapy and autologous bone marrow support in the treatment of primary nonseminomatous mediastinal germ cell tumors. *Cancer*. 1991;**68**(**7**): 1513–1515.

89 Neoplasms of the esophagus

Max W. Sung, MD ▪ *Virginia R. Litle, MD* ▪ *Steven J. Chmura, MD, PhD* ▪ *Stephen G. Swisher, MD, FACS* ▪ *David C. Rice, MB, BCh, BAO, FRCSI* ▪ *Jaffer A. Ajani, MD* ▪ *Ritsuko K. Komaki, MD* ▪ *Mark K. Ferguson, MD*

Overview

Esophageal cancer remains a leading cause of cancer deaths worldwide, sixth in men and ninth in women. In the past quarter century, esophageal cancer has changed from predominantly squamous-cell carcinoma to adenocarcinoma, but only in North America and Europe. The concurrent increase in cancers of the gastroesophageal junction has led to its currently inclusion in the AJCC TNM (tumor, node, metastasis) staging of esophageal cancer. Treatment options have expanded to include endoscopic mucosal resection for early-stage disease and neoadjuvant chemoradiation followed by surgery for intermediate stage disease. Surgical techniques have also evolved to include less invasive approaches using thoracoscopy and laparoscopy. Advances in systemic chemotherapy have also been reported, with the inclusion of hormonal and targeted therapies, for esophageal adenocarcinomas. A lethal disease when diagnosed in advanced stage, continued progress in therapeutic interventions can be anticipated with early-stage detection in high-risk patients, and the incorporation of molecular strategies in the treatment of advanced stage disease.

Historical perspectives

Esophageal cancer was recognized as early as the twelfth century, and pathologic descriptions were produced in the sixteenth and seventeenth centuries.[1] Initial attempts to treat the tumor included resection of a cervical esophageal cancer in 1877 and an intrathoracic cancer in 1913.[2,3] Surgical resection became the mainstay of therapy beginning in the 1940s. Radiotherapy was initially used in the 1920s, but it was not until the development of megavoltage techniques in the 1950s that this modality was used with any frequency. Active chemotherapeutic agents were first identified in the 1960s and have been increasingly incorporated into the treatment of advanced tumors.

Anatomy and histology

The esophagus is a muscular organ that extends from the cricopharyngeus muscle at its cephalad margin to the esophagogastric junction (EGJ). It is divided into regions on the basis of both anatomy and the proclivity for certain neoplasms to develop in specific regions (Figure 1). The cervical esophagus extends from the cricopharyngeus muscle to the thoracic inlet (15–18 cm from incisors). The upper third of the thoracic esophagus extends from the thoracic inlet to the tracheal bifurcation, just below the level of the aortic arch (18–24 cm). The middle thoracic esophagus extends from the tracheal bifurcation to a point midway between the carina and the EGJ (24–32 cm). The lower thoracic esophagus extends from this midway point to the EGJ (32–40 cm). Tumors of the EGJ and gastric cardia are often included in discussions of esophageal cancer because of their pathophysiologic similarities to adenocarcinomas of the distal esophagus.[4] Classifications of EGJ tumors have developed that define the different types of tumors according to the epicenter of the mass (i.e., type I, >1 cm above EGJ; type II, 1 cm above to 2 cm below EGJ; type III, >2–5 cm below EGJ).[5]

The muscle tissues of the esophagus are arranged in an outer longitudinal layer and an inner circular layer. The proximal one-third to one-half of the muscularis propria is derived from the bronchial arches, making it principally skeletal (striated) muscle and giving it the potential to develop rhabdomyosarcomas (Table 1). The remainder of the esophageal musculature comprises smooth muscle, as does the rest of the foregut, in which leiomyomas or leiomyosarcomas may occur. Fibrous, fatty, and connective tissues interspersed in the wall of the esophagus may also give rise to sarcomas.

The esophagus is lined over most of its length with squamous epithelium, which can give rise to squamous-cell carcinoma (SCC) and is the most common neoplasm of the esophagus in most of the world. These cancers occur most often in the cervical esophagus and in the upper and middle thoracic esophagus. Carcinosarcomas and spindle cell carcinomas, which are subtypes of squamous-cell cancer, infrequently occur in these regions. The distal 2–3 cm of the esophagus and the cardia is lined by columnar epithelium, in which adenocarcinomas may occur.[5] The development of intestinal metaplasia, known as Barrett esophagus, more proximally because of gastroesophageal reflux and other factors allows the development of adenocarcinomas in the middle and upper thoracic esophagus in isolated instances. Other cellular elements in the mucosa, submucosal glands, and muscularis propria may give rise to unusual neoplasms, such as small cell cancer, malignant melanoma, granular cell tumors, mucoepidermoid carcinoma, and adenoid cystic carcinoma.[6,7] The histologic types of benign and malignant tumors of the esophagus are given in Table 1.

Etiology

In most of the world, dietary and nutritional factors are the most common etiologic agents and are associated with the development of predominantly SCCs. Among the most frequently cited carcinogens are nitrosamines, which have been found to be in high concentrations in foods in endemic areas of esophageal cancer in northern China.[8] Contamination of food by fungi that reduce nitrate to nitrite may further aggravate this situation. Mechanical factors that have been cited include drinking beverages at excessively high temperatures and consumption of foods containing silica or other substances, such as crushed seeds, that directly

Holland-Frei Cancer Medicine, Ninth Edition. Edited by Robert C. Bast Jr., Carlo M. Croce, William N. Hait, Waun Ki Hong, Donald W. Kufe, Martine Piccart-Gebhart, Raphael E. Pollock, Ralph R. Weichselbaum, Hongyang Wang, and James F. Holland.
© 2017 John Wiley & Sons, Inc. ISBN: 978-1-118-93469-2

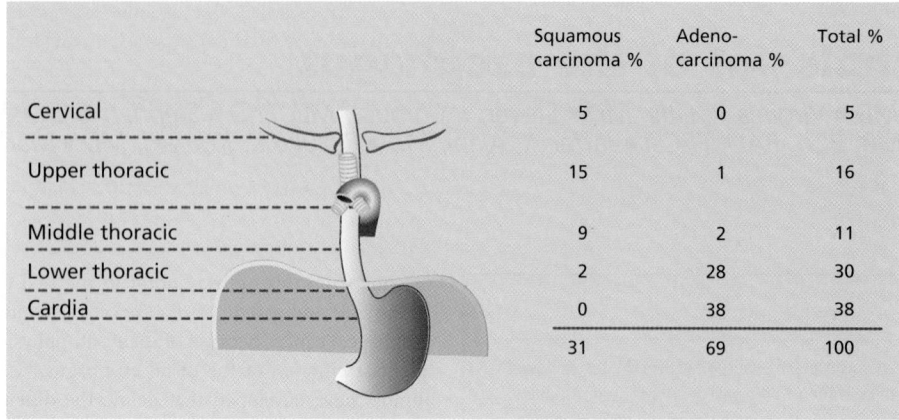

	Squamous carcinoma %	Adeno- carcinoma %	Total %
Cervical	5	0	5
Upper thoracic	15	1	16
Middle thoracic	9	2	11
Lower thoracic	2	28	30
Cardia	0	38	38
	31	69	100

Figure 1 The distribution of malignant neoplasms of the esophagus according to cell type and site of occurrence.

Table 1 Neoplasms of the esophagus.

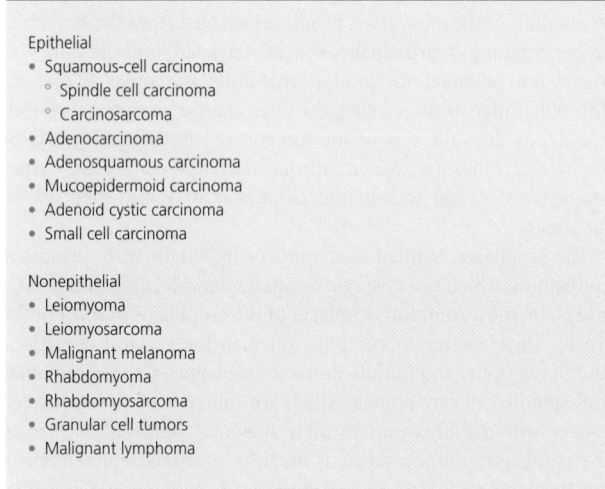

Epithelial
- Squamous-cell carcinoma
  - Spindle cell carcinoma
  - Carcinosarcoma
- Adenocarcinoma
- Adenosquamous carcinoma
- Mucoepidermoid carcinoma
- Adenoid cystic carcinoma
- Small cell carcinoma

Nonepithelial
- Leiomyoma
- Leiomyosarcoma
- Malignant melanoma
- Rhabdomyoma
- Rhabdomyosarcoma
- Granular cell tumors
- Malignant lymphoma

irritate the esophagus.[8,9] Deficiencies of folic acid, vitamins A and C, and riboflavin, molybdenum, and selenium also have been implicated in the development of esophageal neoplasms.[10,11,12a] Higher intake of fruits and vegetables, on the other hand, has been reported in a meta analysis of observational studies to be associated with a reduced risk of esophageal SCC.[12b]

In the western hemisphere, social factors figure more prominently in the development of esophageal cancer. Heavy alcohol consumption increases the risk of cancer 10–25 times, depending on the concentration of alcohol in the beverage.[13] Cigarette smoking has been linked to the development of both squamous-cell cancers and adenocarcinomas.[14] The combined exposure to low levels of tobacco and alcohol increases the risk of esophageal cancer by a factor of 10–20, whereas the synergistic effect of exposure to high levels of both alcohol and tobacco increases the risk by a factor of over 100.[15] Chronic esophageal injury due to gastroesophageal reflux has also been shown to be a risk factor for the development of adenocarcinoma, with severe, longstanding reflux symptoms increasing the risk of cancer by a factor of 40.[16] Chronic gastroesophageal reflux is believed to be etiologically related to the development of Barrett esophagus, which occurs primarily in white males and is associated with a 40-fold increase in the risk of adenocarcinoma of the esophagus.[17] A relationship between reflux and the development of squamous-cell cancers has also been suggested

in patients who consume a diet high in linoleic acid.[18] The lifetime risk of squamous-cell cancer of the esophagus is 5–10% in patients with esophageal achalasia, a 15-fold increase in incidence that is likely due to chronic irritation from retained food.[19–21]

Race and gender are associated with varying incidences of cancer of the esophagus in the western hemisphere. Men are more commonly affected than are women, blacks develop squamous-cell cancers more often than do whites, and white males develop adenocarcinomas more often than do females or individuals of other race groups.[22] However, none of these increased frequencies have yet been linked to genetic factors, and most have been explained by variations in socioeconomic status and the attendant social habits described earlier. The single proven genetic abnormality that is associated with a 25% lifetime incidence of squamous-cell cancer of the esophagus is tylosis A, the late-onset, familial form of palmar, and plantar hyperkeratosis.[23] A number of genetic alterations are associated with neoplasms of the esophagus, including allelic losses at chromosomes 3p, 5q, 9p, 9q, 13q, 17p, 17q, and 18q. Abnormalities of TP53, Rb, cyclin D1, and c-myc have also been associated with esophageal cancer development.[24]

Infectious agents, including human papillomavirus (HPV), have been implicated in the development of neoplasms of the esophagus. Transforming proteins from high-risk HPV subtypes 16, 18 cause loss of function of the tumor suppressor genes TP53 and Rb, resulting in abnormal proliferative states.[25] HPV has been documented in up to 50% of patients with squamous-cell cancers of the esophagus and appears to be more common in areas in which esophageal cancer is endemic.[26] These findings have not been universally reproducible, however.[27a] A systematic review and meta-analysis of 66 case–control studies suggests an association between HPV infection and esophageal SCC.[27b] There are significant variation and lack of consistency between studies; the International Agency for Research on Cancer (IARC) has concluded that the epidemiologic evidence of the association is inadequate.[27c]

Epidemiology

The most common esophageal neoplasm worldwide is SCC (90%); in the United States and Europe, the incidence of adenocarcinoma has been rising and has surpassed SCC (Figure 2). The incidence of esophageal cancer varies more worldwide than any other cancer. In the United States, the incidence of esophageal cancer is approximately seven cases per 100,000 people, whereas in high-risk areas in China, Iran, and Russia, it can be more than 100 per 100,000 people.[27d] In rural Linxian, China, esophageal cancer is the leading

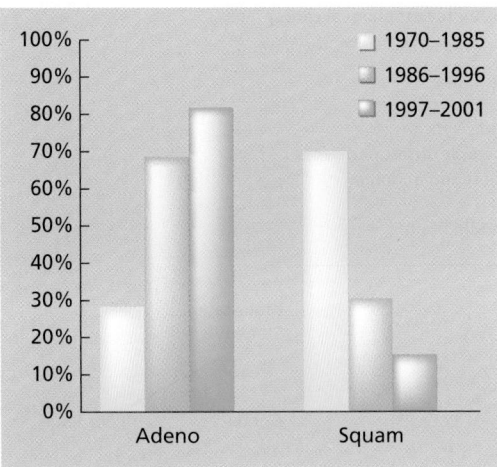

Figure 2 The proportion of adenocarcinoma and distal esophageal tumors has increased over time. *Abbreviations*: Adeno, adenocarcinoma and squam, squamous-cell carcinoma. Source: Hofsetter 2002.[28a] Reproduced with permission of Wolters Kluwer.

cause of death.[29,30a] These geographical variations imply a strong role for local environmental carcinogens in esophageal carcinogenesis. The long-term survival rate for patients with esophageal cancer, regardless of histology, is less than 10%, which is due, in large part, to the advanced stage at which these cancers are detected. Worldwide, the incidence and mortality for esophageal cancer are estimated to be 455,800 and 400.200, respectively, for 2012.[30b] For the United states, incidence and mortality for 2015 (excluding EGJ tumors) were estimated at 16,890 and 15,590, respectively.[31] The age-adjusted mortality rate from esophageal cancer in the United States has increased by 11% between 1975 and 2012.[32]

Besides geographical differences, there are other important differences that have been described in the Western hemisphere. Esophageal carcinoma is more common in men than in women regardless of the histologic subtype, and squamous-cell cancers tend to occur more frequently in blacks than in whites. In addition, there has been a striking increase in the incidence of adenocarcinoma in the United States and Europe, whereas SCC has remained stable.[33] Adenocarcinoma of the distal esophagus and cardia has risen by more than 350% among white males since the mid-1970s, increasing at a more rapid rate than any other solid tumor (Figure 2).[22,34-38] The reasons for these dramatic changes in the Western hemisphere are not clear but may include increased Barrett esophagus, gastroesophageal reflux, obesity, and over-the-counter medications as well as changing smoking and alcohol use.[16] In other areas of the world (outside Europe and North America), SCC of the esophagus predominates and adenocarcinoma has not increased.

Patients usually present because of complaints of dysphagia, which requires either the involvement of the entire circumference of the esophagus by the neoplasm or the growth of a large, polypoid obstructing mass. Dysphagia first develops in response to dense solid foods and progresses to result in difficulties with soft foods and then liquids. Accompanying vomiting and regurgitation are common. Symptoms of heartburn or gastroesophageal reflux (40%) are often associated and occur more frequently in patients with adenocarcinoma.[39] The most common symptom in the absence of dysphagia is pain (25% of cases).[39] It may be related to swallowing (odynophagia) or local extension of the tumor into adjacent structures such as the vertebral bodies, pleura, or mediastinum. In some instances, it may be due to bony metastases from systemic spread. Weight loss is noted in more than 70% of patients and is due to

the inability to swallow or systemic manifestations of the disease.[39] Patients with weight loss have a significantly worse prognosis in many series.[40,41]

The histology of the tumor depends in large part on its location. Adenocarcinoma is located predominantly in the lower esophagus, whereas SCC predominates in the cervical, upper, and middle esophagus (Figures 1 and 2). Unfortunately, because of the distensible nature of the esophagus, these symptoms often do not occur until the tumors are quite large and no longer localized to the esophagus.

In contrast to patients who present because of symptoms of dysphagia, a smaller subset of earlier stage adenocarcinoma patients are increasingly being identified in North America and Europe with endoscopic abnormalities noted during endoscopic surveillance for gastroesophageal reflux symptoms or Barrett's esophagus. These patients tend to present with smaller, earlier stage tumors that are more likely to be localized and amenable to treatment. In addition, in some areas of China where squamous-cell cancer is endemic, routine cytologic screening is performed, and if results are diagnostic or suspicious, follow-up endoscopy is performed. These mass screening efforts have led to early diagnosis in many areas of China, with 5-year survivals of more than 90%.[30a] The low incidence of esophageal cancer in most areas of the world, however, makes this type of mass screening impractical and cost ineffective from a public health standpoint.

Treatment overview

Patients who present with suspected esophageal cancer, because of either the above-mentioned symptoms or mass screening efforts, initially require pathologic confirmation of malignancy (see section titled "Diagnosis"). Once the pathologic diagnosis has been obtained, patients are assessed for therapy by determining the clinical stage (see the section titled "Staging Evaluation") of the tumor and the physiologic status of the patient (see section titled "Pretreatment Assessment"). With this information, an informed decision about treatment can be made that optimizes the chance to cure or palliate the disease while minimizing the treatment-related morbidity (see section titled "Therapy") (Figure 3).

Diagnosis

Symptomatic patients or patients in whom an esophageal mass is diagnosed by screening require endoscopy to enable biopsy for histologic examination and/or brushing for cytologic examination. The overall accuracy of histologic diagnosis of esophageal cancer using flexible endoscopy with biopsy is about 80%.[42,43] Endoscopically directed cytologic brushings have a diagnostic accuracy in excess of 90%. Combining these techniques yields an overall diagnostic accuracy of 98%.[42] If flexible endoscopic diagnostic techniques fail, rigid endoscopy with biopsy, which has a diagnostic accuracy close to 100%, should be considered.[43] In selected patients who have symptoms or findings on physical examination suggestive of metastatic disease, biopsy of the suspected metastatic site provides both a tissue diagnosis and a confirmation of stage.

Pretreatment assessment

In addition to a careful history and physical examination, the overall assessment of a patient with esophageal cancer focuses on specific concerns. Factors that are associated with treatment-related morbidity and mortality include patient age, a recent history of

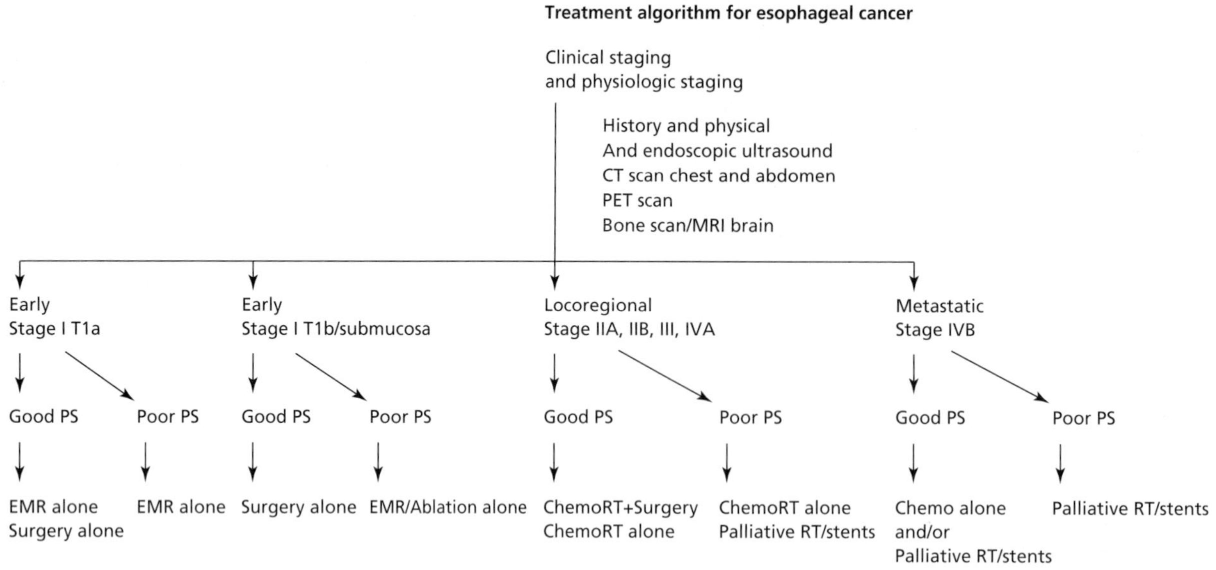

Treatment algorithm for esophageal cancer

Clinical staging
and physiologic staging

History and physical
And endoscopic ultrasound
CT scan chest and abdomen
PET scan
Bone scan/MRI brain

Early Stage I T1a	Early Stage I T1b/submucosa	Locoregional Stage IIA, IIB, III, IVA	Metastatic Stage IVB
Good PS / Poor PS	Good PS / Poor PS	Good PS / Poor PS	Good PS / Poor PS
EMR alone Surgery alone / EMR alone	Surgery alone / EMR/Ablation alone	ChemoRT+Surgery ChemoRT alone / ChemoRT alone Palliative RT/stents	Chemo alone and/or Palliative RT/stents / Palliative RT/stents

Figure 3 Current treatment recommendations for esophageal cancer based on performance status and clinical stage. *Abbreviations*: Chemo, chemotherapy; CT, computed tomography; MRI, magnetic resonance imaging; PET, positron emission tomography; PS, performance status; and RT, radiotherapy.

alcohol or tobacco abuse, body weight, recent weight loss, nutritional status, performance status, hepatic dysfunction, and renal dysfunction. Specific preoperative risk factors have been identified for esophageal resection and are therefore included in the physiologic assessment. Pulmonary complications are predicted by age, preoperative arterial oxygen tension, abnormal chest radiograph, and forced expiratory volume in one second (FEV_1).[44] Operative mortality is predicted by age, mid-arm circumference, history of smoking, incentive spirometry, performance status, and the frequency with which the operation is performed in an institution.[44,45] Any symptoms of cardiac disease necessitate careful evaluation with electrocardiography (ECG), echocardiography, stress tests, and coronary arteriography as indicated. Patients with significant coronary artery disease are at increased risk of morbidity and mortality. Cardiac intervention may be warranted before surgical treatment. These physiologic assessments allow patients to be classified as good or poor performance status, which then allows the aggressiveness of treatment to be tailored to their specific risks (Figure 3).

Staging evaluation

Assessment of stage permits medical practitioners to discuss the status of individual patients with accuracy, allows informed recommendations about therapy, and gives patients and their families necessary information about prognosis. The typical assessment for most patients often includes upper gastrointestinal endoscopy, contrast radiography of the esophagus, computed tomography (CT) of the chest and abdomen, endoscopic ultrasonography (EUS), and positron emission tomography (PET). Other examinations are selected on the basis of specific findings in individual patients, such as neurologic symptoms (magnetic resonance imaging [MRI] of brain), musculoskeletal symptoms (bone scan), or supraclavicular nodes (neck ultrasonography and biopsy). Staging techniques allow patients to be accurately placed into groups in which risk can be assessed as well as the optimum type of therapy selected.

Presentation

Contrast radiography of the esophagus

A contrast study of the esophagus is often the initial diagnostic examination obtained in patients with dysphagia. It allows confirmation of mucosal irregularity and serves as guide for subsequent endoscopy. It also allows evaluation of the esophagus and stomach distal to an area of stenosis, which cannot also be assessed by endoscopy if tight strictures exist.

Endoscopy

Upper gastrointestinal endoscopy allows a pathologic diagnosis to be obtained in the majority of patients. The gross appearance of the tumor can be categorized as advanced or superficial, and the extent of the tumor can be accurately determined. Additional unsuspected malignancies that may be present in up to 20% of patients with squamous-cell cancer may also be identified. Endoscopy also permits assessment of the mobility of a tumor, indicating whether it is fixed within the mediastinum.

Endoscopic ultrasonography

EUS improves the staging accuracy of primary tumors and regional and some nonregional lymph nodes. It has become an essential tool to help identify patients with early-stage carcinoma who may not need multimodality treatment (Figure 3). EUS depicts the normal esophagus as five alternating hyperechoic and hypoechoic layers representing the mucosa and lamina propria, muscularis mucosa, submucosa, muscularis propria, and adventitia. Depth of tumor invasion is determined by assessing the level to which the tumor extends. EUS is also useful for assessing whether there is involvement of the aorta, but airway invasion is not accurately determined because of interference of the ultrasound signal with the intratracheal air column. The accuracy of EUS determination of primary tumor stage is related to the pathologic tumor stage, being more accurate for more advanced stages of disease, with an overall accuracy of about 80%.[46–48] EUS is substantially less accurate in staging primary tumors after chemoradiotherapy is administered, primarily because of overstaging. The technique is not able to distinguish between treatment-induced fibrosis and residual tumor, leading to a mean overall accuracy in this setting of 45%.[49a,b]

In assessing lymph nodes with EUS, three criteria are used: size, border characteristics, and internal architecture. Lymph nodes that are enlarged, have a well-defined external border, and are characterized by relatively uniform, hypoechoic internal architecture are more likely to be malignant. Using these criteria, the overall accuracy of lymph node staging by EUS is about 75%.[47,50] After chemoradiotherapy, the accuracy of EUS for staging lymph nodes decreases to just over 50%.[49a] Development of fine needle aspiration techniques has allowed pathologic confirmation of enlarged lymph nodes in both regional and nonregional sites.[48–51]

CT of the chest and abdomen
CT has become a standard technique for esophageal cancer staging since its inception in the late 1970s because it has allowed better identification of patients with metastatic (M1b) and locally invasive tumors (T4). CT is not very accurate for determining the depth of the primary tumor (T) status, but it is helpful in identifying patients who might have direct invasion of local structures, such as the aorta or major airways, either of which precludes surgical intervention.[46] Aortic invasion is suspected when more than 25% of the aortic circumference is effaced by an esophageal cancer.

CT does not accurately determine lymph node (N) status as normal lymph nodes often vary in size according to their location in the mediastinum and abdomen, and a single size limit for nodes is not possible to establish. In addition, lymph nodes involved by metastatic spread are often not enlarged.[52–55] The sensitivity for CT detection of involved lymph nodes is therefore poor (30–60%), and the overall accuracy of nodal detection by CT is <60%.[56–58]

CT is most useful for detecting distant often unsuspected metastatic (M) disease. The most common sites for metastatic spread, aside from nonregional lymph nodes, are (in decreasing order of frequency) the liver, lung, peritoneum, adrenal gland, bone, and kidney. CT of the thorax and abdomen evaluates almost all these regions. Accuracy of the CT detection of liver metastases is in excess of 90%.[52,57,59,60]

Bronchoscopy
Bronchoscopy should be performed for all patients who are candidates for surgical therapy and whose tumors are adjacent to the trachea or mainstem bronchi, which typically are the mid-esophageal SCCs. This permits direct assessment of tumor invasion into the airway lumen or submucosa, which would be a contra-indication to surgical resection.

Magnetic resonance imaging
As a method for routine staging of esophageal neoplasms, MRI offers no advantages compared with CT and is therefore seldom used as it is a more difficult and expensive test to obtain. Both techniques have similar specificities, sensitivities, and overall accuracy for determining resectability with regard to direct invasion of the aorta and airway.[53,54,57] Neither test provides much useful information about regional or metastatic lymph nodes, and MRI offers no improvements over CT in evaluating the liver for metastatic disease. Whether advances in MRI technology will offer improved staging capabilities remains to be seen.

Positron emission tomography
PET scanning to detect involved lymph nodes and sites of metastatic disease through increased metabolism with 18F-fluorodeoxyglucose was introduced as an investigational staging technique for esophageal cancer in the mid-1990s. PET is most useful in helping identify patients with unsuspected metastatic disease. Given the possibility of false positive results from inflammation, biopsies are still required to definitively confirm metastatic disease in PET positive patients. The PET scan often serves as a guide to help identify suspected areas of metastatic disease for confirmatory biopsy. Another potential role for PET may be in determining response to chemotherapy and radiation therapy although false positives induced by chemotherapy and radiation-induced inflammation remain a problem.[61–63] PET may also have a role in identifying recurrent esophageal cancer by allowing targeting of unsuspected areas of increased metabolic activity.[64]

Bone scintigraphy
Bone scans have been used for decades for staging patients with esophageal neoplasms; however, PET-CT scan has essentially replaced bone scans in the work-up of esophageal cancer. In patients without bone pain or other evidence for metastatic disease, the overall likelihood of identifying skeletal metastases is <5%.[65]

Neck ultrasonography
Cervical and supraclavicular lymph nodes are affected by metastatic spread in up to 30% of patients with neoplasms of the thoracic esophagus, and most are not detectable on physical examination. The use of routine ultrasound examination of the neck in patients without palpable lymph nodes yields unsuspected nodal metastases in over 10% of patients.[66] The overall accuracy of cervical and supraclavicular nodal assessment with ultrasonography is about 90%.[67,68a] The addition of routine needle aspiration under ultrasound guidance for cytology may improve the yield of this potentially valuable technique.[68a] At the present time, however, this is not a commonly used screening technique and is reserved for cases where nodes are palpable to confirm metastatic disease

Minimally invasive surgical staging
Laparoscopy has been used since the early 1980s, and thoracoscopy has been used since the early 1990s in an effort to improve staging of esophageal neoplasms. Video-assisted thoracoscopic surgery (VATS) staging was studied in a CALGB study in 1995 and was found to be feasible and 88% accurate.[68b,c] With the current standard and accurate staging modalities of PET-CT and EUS, surgical staging is not routinely done except in conjunction with placement of a laparoscopic jejunostomy tube for nutritional support before chemoradiation therapy.

Biologic staging
A variety of biologic markers have been investigated for their utility in estimating prognosis in patients with esophageal neoplasms. These include growth factors (epidermal growth factor [EGF], transforming growth factor [TGF]-β, platelet-derived growth factor [PDGF]), oncogenes (*c-myc, int-2, hst-1, cyclin D, EGFR, HER-2/neu, h-ras*), tumor suppressor genes (*Rb, TP53, p73, APC, MCC, p27*), the cell adhesion molecule E-cadherin, the oncodevelopmental marker CEA, and deoxyribonucleic acid (DNA) content and ploidy.[69–71] To date, none of these techniques have become generally accepted staging techniques except in isolated referral centers.

TNM (tumor, node, metastasis) staging system
These pretreatment staging evaluations allow patients to be clinically staged by a cTNM (tumor, node, metastasis) staging system that can help determine the optimum therapy (Figure 3). The

Table 2 TNM staging system for esophageal neoplasms.

Primary tumor (T)	
TX	Primary tumor cannot be assessed
T0	No evidence of primary tumor
Tis	High-grade dysplasia
T1	Tumor invades lamina propria or submucosa
T2	Tumor invades muscularis propria
T3	Tumor invades adventitia
T4a	Resectable cancer invades adjacent structures such as pleura, pericardium, and diaphragm
T4b	Unresectable cancer invades adjacent structures such as aorta, vertebral body, and trachea
Regional lymph nodes (N)	
Any periesophageal lymph node from cervical nodes to celiac nodes	
NX	Regional lymph nodes cannot be assessed
N0	No regional lymph node metastases
N1	1–2 positive regional lymph nodes
N2	3–6 positive regional lymph nodes
N3	≥7 positive regional lymph nodes
Distant metastasis (M)	
MX	Distant metastasis cannot be assessed
M0	No distant metastasis
M1	Distant metastasis
Additions of nonanatomic cancer characteristics	
Histopathologic cell type	
Adenocarcinoma	
Squamous-cell carcinoma	
Histologic grade	
G1	Well differentiated
G2	Moderately differentiated
G3	Poorly differentiated
G4	Undifferentiated
Cancer location	
Upper thoracic	20–25 cm from incisors
Middle thoracic	>25–30 cm from incisors
Lower thoracic	>30–40 cm from incisors
Esophagogastric junction	Includes cancers whose epicenter is in the distal thoracic esophagus, esophagogastric junction, or within the proximal 5 cm of the stomach (cardia) that extend into the esophagogastric junction or distal thoracic esophagus (Siewert III). These stomach cancers are stage grouped similarly to adenocarcinoma of the esophagus

Adenocarcinoma stage groupings

Stage	T	N	M	G
Stage 0	Tis	N0	M0	G1
Stage IA	T1	N0	M0	G1–2
Stage IB	T1	N0	M0	G3
Stage IIA	T2	N0	M0	G1–2
	T2	N0	M0	G3
Stage IIB	T3	N0	M0	GAny
	T1–2	N1	M0	GAny
Stage IIIA	T1–2	N2	M0	GAny
	T3	N1	M0	GAny
	T4a	N0	M0	GAny
Stage IIIB	T3	N2	M0	GAny
Stage IIIC	T4a	N1–2	M0	GAny
	T4b	NAny	M0	GAny
	TAny	N3	M0	GAny
Stage IV	TAny	NAny	M1	GAny

Squamous-cell carcinoma stage groupings

Stage	T	N	M	G	Location
Stage 0	Tis	N0	M0	G1	Any
Stage IA	T1	N0	M0	G1	Any
Stage IB	T1	N0	M0	G2–3	Any
Stage IIA	T2–3	N0	M0	G1	Lower
	T2–3	N0	M0	G1	Upper, middle
Stage IIB	T2–3	N0	M0	G2–3	Lower
	T2–3	N0	M0	G2–3	Upper, middle
	T1–2	N1	M0	GAny	Any
Stage IIIA	T1–2	N2	M0	GAny	Any
	T3	N1	M0	GAny	Any
	T4a	N0	M0	GAny	Any
Stage IIIB	T3	N2	M0	GAny	Any
Stage IIIC	T4a	N1–2	M0	GAny	Any
	T4b	NAny	M0	GAny	Any
	TAny	N3	M0	GAny	Any
Stage IV	TAny	NAny	M1	GAny	Any

current staging system for esophageal cancer includes epithelial tumors of the cervical, thoracic, and intra-abdominal esophagus, as well as the EGJ (Table 2).[72a,b] Tumors are staged according to clinical findings from noninvasive tests and pathologic findings resulting from any invasive staging procedures. It is useful to specify lymph node locations during biopsy and resection because their location determines whether they are considered regional nodes or nonregional metastatic nodal disease (Figure 4). The prognosis of patients with esophageal cancer is determined by the depth of penetration of the primary tumor (transmural vs nontransmural), whether there is lymph node involvement, the relative number of lymph nodes involved, and whether distant metastases are present.[28,72,74–81,82–87] Nonanatomic classifications have been added, including histopathologic cell type (adenocarcinoma, SCC), histology grade (G1-4), and cancer location. The long-term survival in patients with esophageal neoplasms correlates well with the pathologic stage and histopathologic cell type (Figure 5).[74,80] The ability of the clinical cTNM staging system to accurately predict the pTNM status has improved with time as the use of endoscopic ultrasound, CT of the chest and abdomen, and PET scan has increased.[28a]

Therapy

Standard curative treatment options for esophageal cancer include surgical resection, external beam radiotherapy, chemotherapy, or combinations of two or three of these options. The selection of appropriate therapy is often challenging because few comparisons of these options have been performed in prospective, randomized manner. In addition, these trials have often been performed over a long time period with an inadequate number of patients during which significant changes in histology and types of treatment have occurred (i.e., different radiation equipment, dosages and fields, and different surgical techniques and chemotherapy agents). Clinical staging techniques have also evolved over time, leading to stage migration and poor correlation with pathologic stage, especially from studies before CT scan, endoscopic ultrasound, and PET.[28a] These problems make comparisons between different trials

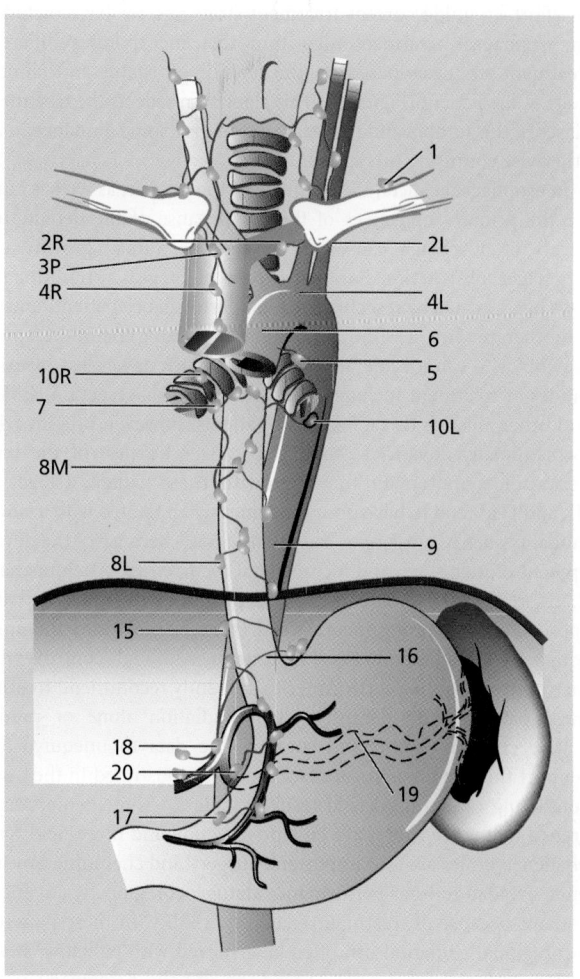

Figure 4 Lymph node staging map for neoplasms of the esophagus. Source: Ferguson 2010.[73] Reproduced with permission of Elsevier.

or treatment arms difficult. Treatment strategies have therefore evolved over time based on regional experiences and biases. In

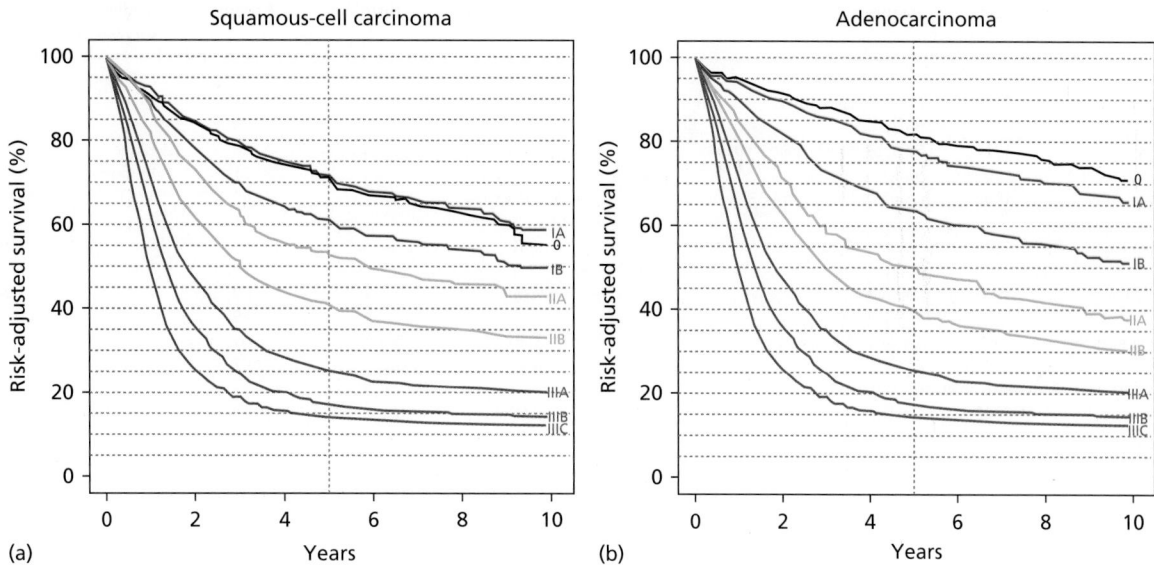

Figure 5 (a) Risk adjusted survival for squamous-cell carcinoma according to the ANCC Cancer Staging Manual, seventh edition. Source: Rice 2010.[72a] Reproduced with permission of Springer. (b) Risk-adjusted survival for adenocarcinoma according to the ANCC Cancer Staging Manual, seventh edition. Source: Rice 2010.[72b] Reproduced with permission of Springer.

an effort, to guide current treatment strategies, we have included an esophageal treatment algorithm that incorporates different treatment strategies based on the physiologic status and clinical stage of the patient (Figure 3). This algorithm reflects the treatment biases of the authors and is meant only to give some guidance in an otherwise confusing therapeutic arena.

In esophageal cancer, local control of the disease, as well as cure, are the primary objectives of therapy because of the debilitating effects of dysphagia caused by progressive tumor growth and esophageal obstruction. Early-stage cancers (stage 0, I) traditionally have been treated by resection in good performance patients and by radiotherapy with or without radiation-sensitizing chemotherapy in patients who cannot tolerate surgery. Recently, newer less invasive modes of treatment include endoscopic mucosal resection (EMR) and other ablative therapies. Most patients, however, present with locoregionally advanced esophageal cancer because of the long period of asymptomatic tumor growth. These patients (stages II, III, and IVa) tend to have poor outcomes when treated with a single modality such as surgery or radiation therapy because of the development of metastatic and locoregional recurrences. Attempts have therefore focused on treating these patients with multimodality approaches combining locoregional (surgery/radiation) therapies with systemic (chemotherapy) treatments. Although controversial, many oncologists in North America currently recommend treating these patients with definitive chemoradiation alone or preoperative chemoradiation and surgery. The data to unequivocally support these approaches are lacking as demonstrated in the often conflicting randomized trial results (Table 3). Some centers have argued that more aggressive en bloc resection and three-field lymphadenectomies are also important. Surgery and chemotherapy are often avoided in poor performance status locoregionally advanced patients because of treatment-related morbidity. In these patients, locoregional palliation can often be achieved with palliative stents and/or radiation. For patients who are initially recognized to be in advanced (metastatic) stages of disease, chemotherapy with or without palliative radiotherapy has been the mainstay of treatment.

The development of endoesophageal stents has provided additional locoregional palliation and has limited the need for palliative surgical bypass even in patients with tracheoesophageal fistulas (Figure 3).

Surgery

Esophagectomy remains the mainstay of treatment for locally or regionally advanced neoplasms of the esophagus. The major paradigm shift in the past 10–15 years has been management of superficial (clinical T1aN0) esophageal carcinomas in which EMR is used to stage and treat these intramucosal lesions. Even in more contemporary series mortality rates after esophagectomy can reach as high as 7% for early cancers , thus, a movement toward a less invasive approach for treatment of high-grade dysplasia and early esophageal cancer began almost 20 years ago.[28b] In the largest early series, Christian Ell and colleagues published their results of 61 patients with early carcinoma treated with EMR and after a mean 12-month follow-up. Eighty-six percentage of patients were still free of disease.[28c] Since then, numerous groups have concluded that EMR and ablation of the preneoplastic field of Barrett's esophagus are the standard of care for treatment of early cancers with eradication and 5-year survival rates reaching 80–90%.[28d,e]

Surgery however remains an integral element in multimodality therapy for regionally advanced cancers because patients who undergo preoperative (neoadjuvant) therapy have a 75% incidence of residual local disease amenable to resection, although this remains controversial as some oncologists argue that surgery should be reserved only for patients who relapse with locoregional disease. This idea of a salvage esophagectomy reserving resection only for those with recurrent disease after definitive chemoradiation therapy has been gaining traction but is associated with higher leak rates, conduit failures, lengths of stay, and 30-day mortality as compared with resection after neoadjuvant therapy. Indications for salvage esophagectomy continue to evolve as nonoperative therapies are refined.[28f]

Table 3 Results of randomized trials of definitive chemoradiotherapy for locoregionally advanced esophageal cancer.

Author	Year	Treatment	Technique	Histology	Patients	Median survival	p Value
Chemo/RT versus RT alone							
Roussel et al.[88]	1989	Methotrexate + 56 Gy	C ~ RT	S	77	9 mo	NS
		56 Gy			73	8 mo	
Araujo et al.[89]	1991	5-FU, bleomycin, mito + 50 Gy	C/RT	S	28	18 mo	NS
		50 Gy			31	16 mo	
Hatlevoll et al.[90]	1992	Cisplatin, bleomycin + 53 Gy	C ~ RT	S	46	6 mo	NS
		53 Gy			51	6 mo	
Slabber et al.[91]	1998	Cisplatin, 5-FU + 40 Gy	C/RT	S	34	6 mo	NS
		40 Gy			36	5 mo	
Smith et al.[92]	1998	Mitomycin, 5-FU + 40 Gy	C/RT	S > A	60	15 mo	.04
		40 Gy			59	9 mo	
Cooper et al.[93]	1999	Cisplatin, 5-FU + 50 Gy	C/RT	S > A	61	13 mo	.01
		64 Gy			62	9 mo	
Chemo/RT (high dose) versus chemo/RT (low dose)							
Minsky et al.[94]	2002	Cisplatin, 5-FU + 50 Gy	C/RT	S > A	10	18 mo	NS
		Cisplatin, 5-FU + 64y	C/RT		9	13 mo	
Chemo/RT/surgery versus chemo/RT alone							
Stahl et al.[95]	2005	Cis, 5-FU, Etop. ~ Cis, Etop. + 40 Gy ~ Surgery	C ~ C/RT ~ S	S	86	16.4 mo	NS
		Cis, 5-FU, Etop. ~ Cis, Etop. + 65 Gy	C ~ C/RT		86	14.9 mo	
Bedenne et al.[96a]	2007	Cis, 5-FU, + 46 Gy ~ Surgery	C/RT ~ S	S > A	129	17.7 mo	NS
		Cis, 5-FU, 66 Gy	CRT		130	19.3 mo	
Chemo/RT (5-FU) versus chemo/RT (no 5-FU)							
Ajani et al.[97]	2008	Cis, 5-FU, Paclitaxel ~ 5-FU, Paclitaxel + 50.4 Gy	C ~ RT	S > A	41	28.2 mo	NS
		Cis + Paclitaxel ~ Cis + Paclitaxel + 50.4 Gy	C ~ RT		43	14.9 mo	

Table 4 Operative approaches to resection for esophageal cancer.

Transthoracic
- Ivor Lewis (laparotomy, right thoracotomy, high intrathoracic anastomosis)
- McKeown modification of Ivor Lewis (cervical anastomosis)
- Left thoracotomy with intrathoracic anastomosis
- Left thoracotomy with cervical anastomosis
- Thoracoabdominal incision

Transhiatal
Minimally invasive
- Thoracoscopically assisted
- Laparoscopically assisted
- Thoracoscopic/laparoscopic

Approaches to resection

Surgical approaches to resection include a transthoracic operation, mobilization of the esophagus via a transhiatal route, and thoracoscopic/laparoscopic resection (Table 4; Figure 6).

Transthoracic approaches provide the ability to perform a more complete dissection of the primary tumor and lymph nodes than is possible using a transhiatal approach. The transhiatal approach

allows the operation to be done more quickly with fewer incisions and avoidance of a thoracic component thus minimizing postoperative pulmonary complications. In the mid-1990s, as laparoscopic approaches were advancing for benign disease, a minimally invasive approach was introduced for oncologic procedures as well. The laparoscopic transhiatal approach was reported as a technically feasible procedure for nine patients in the late 1990s.[28g] This was followed by advances in total thoracoscopic and laparoscopic approaches first as being feasible, then as associated with shorter length of stay and mortality rates less than 2%.[28h] Additional studies demonstrated morbidity rates dropping from 60% to 44% with a significant reduction in pulmonary complications as compared with the open approaches.[28i] The minimally invasive esophagectomy (MIE) has evolved from a three-hole-modified McKeown to the Ivor Lewis approach with an intrathoracic component. The benefit of this evolution was avoidance of recurrent laryngeal nerve injury and reduction in anastomotic leak rates.

The question of oncologic soundness with an MIE has been substantiated with longer follow-up. With the goal of retrieving more than 20 lymph nodes to adequately stage a patient with the current AJCC staging system, the median number of nodes is not diminished by a minimally invasive approach.[28i,j] Three-year

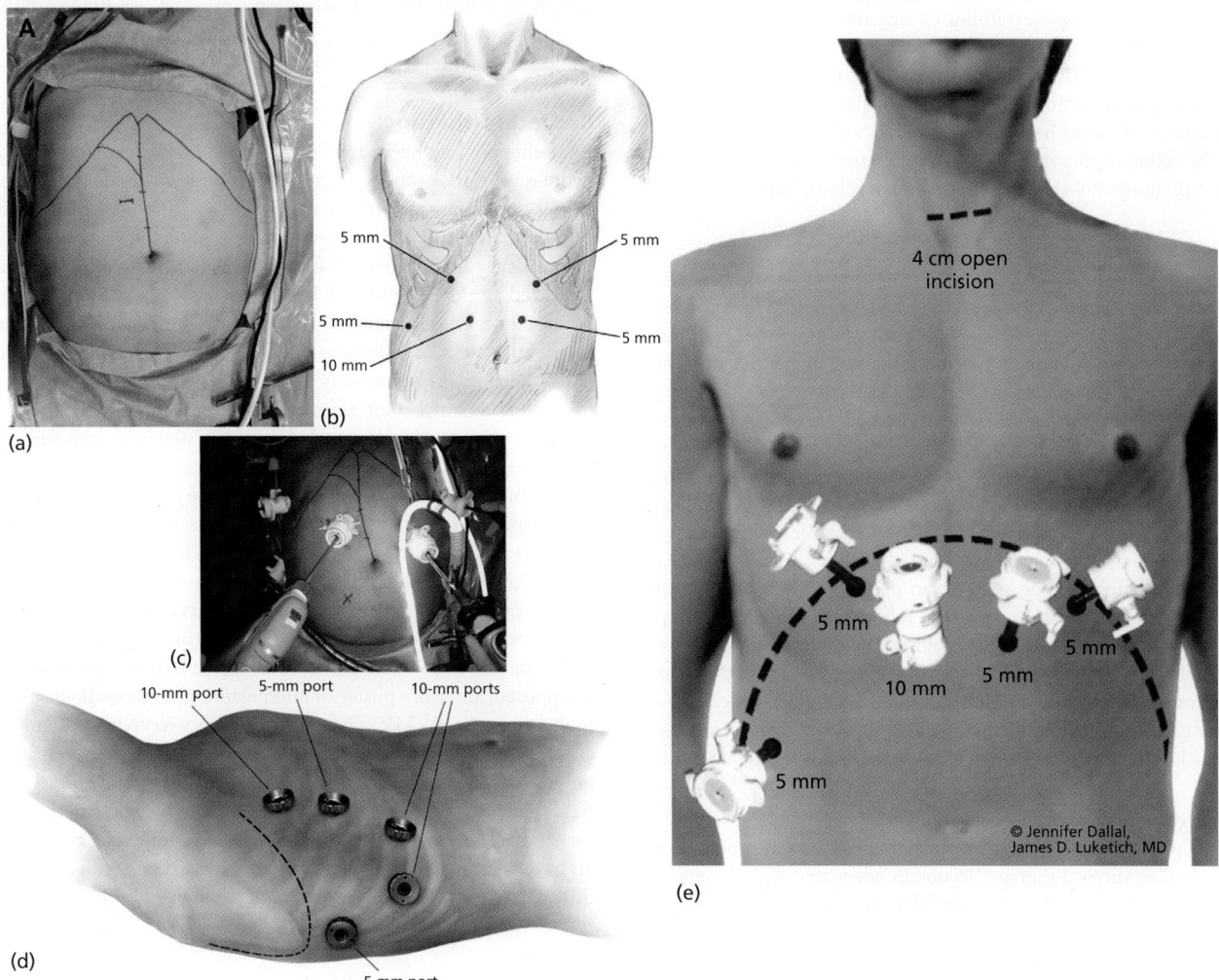

Figure 6 Approaches for esophagectomy. (a) Right thoracotomy and laparotomy with intrathoracic (Ivor Lewis operation) or cervical anastomosis (McKeown modification of Ivor Lewis esophagectomy). (b) Left thoracotomy, accessing the abdomen through a peripheral incision in the diaphragm, with intrathoracic or cervical anastomosis. (c) Transhiatal esophagectomy with cervical anastomosis. (d) Thoracoscopic esophagectomy: Port placement (MIE Ivor Lewis). (e) Laparoscopic esophagectomy: Port placement.

survival rates after MIE now approach 60% in experienced hands as reported in the intergroup study of 95 patients with locoregional recurrence rates as low as 7%.[28k]

The selection of an operative approach is dependent, in part, on tumor location and surgeon preference. Squamous-cell cancers are most often located in the middle and upper thoracic esophagus and are approached with open or minimally invasive transthoracic approaches with cervical anastomosis. In contrast, adenocarcinomas, which most often arise in the distal esophagus or cardia, are easily amenable to transthoracic and transhiatal approaches. Squamous-cell cancers are multifocal in nearly 20% of patients, and near-total esophagectomy is recommended to minimize the risk of performing an incomplete resection.[81] This usually necessitates a cervical anastomosis for reconstruction. In contrast, adenocarcinomas usually are not multifocal but tend to spread submucosally. When negative proximal and distal margins are obtained on frozen section at the time of operation, the extent of the esophageal resection is theoretically satisfactory.

Results from 44 published reports of transthoracic or transhiatal esophagectomy for cancer demonstrate a higher incidence of anastomotic complications in the latter group, but otherwise no important differences in operative morbidity or mortality and similar 5-year survival rates.[83-87,98a] Currently, the choice of the open versus minimally invasive approach to esophageal resection depends largely on the training, experience, and personal preference of the surgeon. The robot-assisted thoracoscopic esophagectomy (RATE or RAMIE) is also performed by a few surgical groups with varying reports of improved length of stay, overall morbidity, and number of nodes harvested compared with other approaches.[98b,c] The future of this approach may well remain within the realm of a small number of centers with dedicated robotic teams.

Effects of preoperative therapy

The use of preoperative therapy before surgery has the potential of increasing perioperative morbidity and mortality. One prospective randomized study reported that septic complications, respiratory complications, and operative mortality were higher in patients who underwent preoperative chemotherapy compared with surgery alone.[99] However, several other studies assessing neoadjuvant chemotherapy or chemoradiotherapy have shown no important differences in postoperative complications or operative mortality.[40,100-104] The complexity of esophageal surgery mandates that the procedure be performed at a high-volume referral center to minimize operative morbidity and mortality.[45] Medicare data suggest that high-volume centers can perform esophageal resections with a mortality of 3%, whereas less experienced centers have a mortality of 19%.[45] This morbidity and mortality may be even further increased when preoperative therapy is used. At less experienced centers, the morbidity and mortality of the procedure may be greater than the potential benefit, especially when considering the low likelihood of cure in locoregionally advanced patients.

Surgery for cervical esophageal cancer

Neoplasms of the cervical esophagus pose special problems with regard to surgical therapy. To obtain adequate surgical margins in tumors that extend to the cricopharyngeus muscle or invade the proximal trachea, it is necessary to include a laryngectomy as part of the resection, which adds substantial long-term morbidity to what is often a palliative not curative procedure. As a result, a higher percentage of patients with cervical esophageal cancer are treated nonsurgically than is the case for patients with cancers in other locations. Resection could provide good palliation for dysphagia but does not substantially influence long-term survival, and the

morbidity has led most people to recommend chemoradiation in this subset of patients.[105-108]

Reconstruction after esophagectomy

Reestablishing alimentary tract continuity after esophageal resection in a manner that permits ingestion of a normal diet is an important component of surgery for esophageal cancer. Options for reconstruction include using the stomach as a substitute or interposing a segment of colon or jejunum between the proximal esophageal remnant and the stomach (or duodenum after total gastrectomy). The use of the stomach for reconstruction is by far the most common technique because the stomach has the most reliable blood supply among any of the reconstructive options and because only a single anastomosis is required, compared with the three anastomoses necessary for bowel interposition. Cervical anastomoses are favored by some surgeons because they decrease the incidence of acid reflux into the esophageal remnant and because anastomotic leaks are usually easily managed by simple cervical drainage. The disadvantages of cervical anastomoses are a higher incidence of recurrent laryngeal nerve injury and more frequent anastomotic leaks. Whether the additional tumor-free proximal margin provided by a cervical anastomosis offers a survival advantage has not been proven.[109] Use of the posterior mediastinum (esophageal bed) for reconstruction optimizes emptying of the reconstructive organ but may predispose to tumor infiltration if a complete resection is not performed.[110]

Radiation therapy

Radiotherapy has been used for decades in the management of neoplasms of the esophagus and as with surgery targets the locoregional tumor rather than the systemic disease. The primary roles of radiotherapy, as with surgery, are as a potentially curative single modality for localized disease and as a palliative therapy for advanced tumors. Results of both uses have been disappointing because of a lack of complete response of the primary tumor and the development of radiation-induced strictures that limit its palliative benefits. More recently, the use of radiation has expanded to include an important adjuvant role in multimodality therapy to further improve the locoregional control obtained with surgery alone.

Treatment is planned to uniformly irradiate gross tumor and margins suspected of harboring microscopic disease, while minimizing injury to adjacent normal tissues, such as the lung, heart, and spinal cord. Regional nodal basins are usually included, typically cervical and supraclavicular nodes for cervical cancers, supraclavicular, and subcarinal lymph nodes for upper thoracic cancers, and celiac axis nodes for lower thoracic and cardiac cancers. Initial treatment is to opposed, anterior–posterior and posterior–anterior fields using high-energy (6–24 MV) photons. In patients receiving potentially curative high-dose therapy, the final treatments are delivered at an oblique angle to minimize the total dose to the spinal cord. Daily treatments of 1.8–2 Gy to a total of 60–70 Gy were formerly used for curative intent, although this has been modified as recent trials have demonstrated equal efficacy and less toxicity with the lower dose (50.4 Gy).[94] Palliative doses tend to be even lower to further reduce this morbidity (30–40 Gy).

Radiation as single modality therapy

The use of radiation therapy as a single modality for esophageal cancer is sometimes indicated as a potentially curative therapy in patients who are unable to tolerate (or who refuse) resection or combined definitive chemoradiotherapy. Radiation therapy alone achieves 5-year survival rates of 0–20% in patients without distant metastatic disease, with the majority of survival rates being less than 10%. Although low, these survival rates may be biased by patient selection as good performance status patients are usually treated with surgery while radiation is often reserved for the poor performance status group. Treatment of unresectable but localized esophageal cancer with radiotherapy yields results similar to those reported for potentially resectable cancers, with survival rates at 5 years of less than 10%.[88–93,111,112] One small randomized study has demonstrated increased survival with surgery alone versus radiation therapy alone, although the authors focused more on endpoints of quality of life.[113]

Radiotherapy as an adjuvant to resection

In an effort to obtain better local control of disease, radiotherapy has been used both preoperatively and postoperatively as an adjunct to resection (Table 5).[114–116,118,122] The interval between completion of radiotherapy and resection is typically 3–5 weeks (1 week/10 Gy), which is felt to minimize perioperative complications from bleeding and radiation-induced fibrosis. In the proper setting, postoperative complication and mortality rates are not increased by the administration of preoperative radiotherapy, although this may be contingent on performing the surgical procedure in a high-volume center.[45] Most randomized, controlled studies have not demonstrated a survival advantage compared with surgery alone although these studies were often performed with outdated radiation therapy techniques.[114–116,118,122] Meta-analysis of the combined data from all randomized studies that have been published do not demonstrate improved survival with preoperative radiotherapy.[123]

The use of radiotherapy postoperatively enables the administration of higher radiation doses than are feasible with preoperative radiotherapy although this treatment has been associated with increases in the incidence of anastomotic strictures and prolonged recovery from surgery, adversely affecting the quality of life.[117,120,121] There is also some evidence that median survival is worse in patients who undergo postoperative radiotherapy, compared with resection only, as a result of an earlier appearance of distant metastatic disease and because of irradiation-induced deaths, although selection bias may also play a role.[120] Postoperative irradiation appears to decrease the local recurrence rate but overall has no proven influence on long-term survival.

Intraluminal brachytherapy has been added in some centers to curative or palliative external beam radiotherapy in an effort to improve local control of disease. Doses of 10–20 Gy are administered after completion of external beam treatment in one or more fractions using Iridium-192. In patients with potentially curable disease, the addition of intraluminal brachytherapy appears to enhance locoregional control, compared with external beam radiotherapy alone, but is associated with a higher incidence of radiation-induced esophageal strictures.[119,124,125] Reducing the dose per fraction of intraluminal brachytherapy may in the future limit the incidence and severity of these local complications.[126] The use of brachytherapy in patients with unresectable or recurrent esophageal cancer is still under investigation but may provide better symptomatic relief than other modalities, such as gastric bypass surgery, chemotherapy, laser therapy, and stenting.[127–129]

Systemic therapy

A discussion of systemic chemotherapy for esophageal cancer must take into account the changing epidemiology of esophageal cancer in the past 50 years.

In the 1970s, when chemotherapy drugs were beginning to be tested in clinical trials, esophageal cancer was predominantly SCC histology and localized mostly in the upper two-thirds of the esophagus. Chemotherapy agents found to be effective were therefore not surprisingly ones that were also active for head and neck SCC.

In the past two decades, in the United States and other developed countries in the West, esophageal cancer has shifted to primarily adenocarcinoma histology and localized mainly in the distal third of the esophagus, the EGJ extending into the gastric cardia. Chemotherapy regimens tested to be effective are also active against gastric adenocarcinoma, which also led to the development of targeted therapy against the Her-2-neu receptor (trastuzumab) and the vascular endothelial growth receptor (bevacizumab, ramucirumab). SCC still remains the predominant histology for esophageal cancer in non-Western countries, including those in the esophageal cancer belt in central Asia, and in Africa and Southeast Asia.

Single-agent chemotherapy

Previous phase II trials have identified a number of chemotherapy drugs with 15–30% response rates when administered as single agent for esophageal cancer. These drugs included cisplatin, mitomycin, 5-FU, paclitaxel and vindesine.[130a] The responses were

Table 5 Results of randomized trials of pre- and postoperative radiotherapy for locoregionally advanced esophageal cancer

Authors	Year	Treatment	Histology	Patients (no.)	Five-year survival (%)	p Value
Preoperative RT versus surgery alone						
Launois et al.[114]	1981	Surgery alone	S	57	11.5	NS
		Surgery + 40 Gy		67	7.5	
Gignoux et al.[115]	1988	Surgery alone	S	106	10	NS
		Surgery + 33 Gy		102	9	
Wang et al.[116]	1989	Surgery alone	S	102	30	NS
		Surgery + 40 Gy		104	35	
Arnott et al.[117]	1992	Surgery alone	S	86	17	NS
		Surgery + 20 Gy		90	9	
Nygaard et al.[118]	1992	Surgery alone	S	41	4	.08
		Surgery + 35 Gy		48	18	
Postoperative RT versus surgery alone						
FUASR[119]	1991	Surgery alone	S	119	18	NS
		Surgery + 45–55 Gy		102	20	
Fok et al.[120]	1993	Surgery alone	S	65	11 (4 years)	NS
		Surgery + 49–52.5 Gy		65	11 (4 years)	
Ziernan[121]	1995	Surgery alone	S	35	20 (3 years)	NS
		Surgery + 56 Gy		33	23 (3 years)	

unfortunately short lived and did not lead to any meaningful prolongation of survival.

Multiagent chemotherapy

Combination of agents, which has been shown to have activity against esophageal cancer as single agents, has yielded response rates of up to 50% (Figure 3). The combination of bleomycin–vindesine–cisplatin has been reported with response rates of 53% and a median duration of response of 7 months.

A more commonly used and better-tolerated combination regimen is 5FU-cisplatin, which in a randomized phase II study versus cisplatin alone was shown to have superior response rates (35% vs 19%) but median survival remained similar (33 weeks vs 28 weeks).

The addition of paclitaxel to the 5FU-cisplatin backbone in a phase II trial has been reported with response rates of 48% with a median duration of response of 5.7 months and median survival of 10.8 months. It was further noted that response rates were comparable for SCC (50%) and adenocarcinoma (46%).[130b]

The paclitaxel–cisplatin combination without 5FU has also been found to be active for both SCC and adenocarcinoma in a phase II trial with response rates of 40% with clinical benefit (relief of dysphagia, weight gain) achieved in 70% of patients.[130c] The combination of paclitaxel-carboplatin in a phase II trial showed response rates of 43%, median duration of response 2.8 months, and median survival 9 months. One-year survival was 43%. The combination was well tolerated with no treatment-related deaths.[130d]

Epirubicin-cisplatin-5FU (ECF) has been previously shown to be an active regimen for gastric adenocarcinoma. Its activity in esophagogastric cancer (SCC/adenocarcinoma) was demonstrated in a phase III trial versus mitomycin–cisplatin-5FU with reported similar efficacy (response rates of 44.1% vs 42.4%, median survival of 9.4 months vs 8.7 months).[130e] The substitution of cisplatin and 5FU with oxaliplatin and oral capecitabine (EOX) was evaluated in a phase III trial (REAL-2) in 964 evaluable patients in a two-by-two design showed improved overall survival in the EOX group as compared to the ECF group, while progression-free survival and response rates were similar between the two groups.[130f]

The combination of irinotecan–cisplatin in a weekly regimen has been reported in a phase II trial to be active in esophageal cancer with response rates of 57%, median duration of response 4.2 months, and median actuarial survival 14.6 months. Similar response rates were observed for adenocarcinoma (52%) and SCC (66%).[130g]

Targeted Therapy

Trastuzumab, a monoclonal antibody directed against the Her-2-neu receptor, has been tested in the phase III ToGA trial of 5FU/capecitabine–cisplatin with and without trastuzumab.[130h] Patients with gastric or esophagogastric adenocarcinoma were eligible if their tumors were positive for positive Her-2-neu expression by IHC (1 to 3+) or FISH. Response rates were higher with trastuzumab (47% vs 35%) as was median survival (13.8 months vs 11.1 months). Further studies showed that trastuzumab was most effective for IHC 3+ tumors.

Ramucirumab, a monoclonal antibody that inhibits the VEGF-2 receptor, has been tested in the phase III REGARD trial versus placebo in previously treated gastric or esophagogastric adenocarcinoma.[130i] The study showed in favor of ramucirumab with median progression-free survival was 2.1 month versus 1.3 month, overall survival 5.2 month versus 3.8 months, response rates 8% versus 3%. Disease control rates (responses plus stable disease) were 49% for ramucirumab versus 23% for the placebo group. A survival benefit was seen for the combination of ramucirumab in combination with

paclitaxel in the phase III RAINBOW trial versus paclitaxel plus placebo in previously treated metastatic gastric or esophagogastric adenocarcinoma.[130j] The ramucirumab–paclitaxel combination was superior in median overall survival (9.6 months vs 7.4 months), progression-free survival (4.4 months vs 2.9 months), and response rates (28% vs 16%).

Bevacizumab, a monoclonal antibody directed against soluble VEGF, has been tested in combination with capecitabine–cisplatin in the phase III AVAGAST trial versus placebo plus capecitabine–cisplatin in patients with previously untreated gastric or esophagogastric adenocarcinoma. Although response rates and median progression-free survival were higher in the bevacizumab group (46% vs 37%, 6.7 months vs 5.3 months), no significant survival benefit was demonstrated (12.1 months vs 10.1 months).[130k]

Similarly, no survival benefit could be demonstrated in phase III trials of adding an anti-EGFR agent to chemotherapy in patients with gastric or esophagogastric adenocarcinoma. The phase III EXPAND trial of capecitabine–cisplatin with and without cetuximab showed median progression-free survival of 4.4 months versus 5.6 months for the control arm.[130l] In the phase III REAL3 trial, patients with esophagogastric adenocarcinoma were randomized to epirubicin–oxaliplatin–capecitabine with or without panitumumab.[130m] Median overall survival in an interim analysis was 8.8 months versus 11.3 months in favor of the control arm, and the study was halted.

Combined modality therapy

In locoregionally advanced esophageal cancer, combination chemotherapy has been investigated in combination with radiation or surgery to try to reduce the high rate of systemic relapse noted when surgery or radiation therapy alone is used. Attempts to use chemotherapy with surgery have included preoperative and postoperative strategies usually with cisplatin-based multiagent regimens. The randomized trials with preoperative chemotherapy usually consist of two or three chemotherapy cycles followed by resection. Some studies have also added postoperative chemotherapy to the regimen. There is no apparent difference in response to chemotherapy based on histology. There is no clear increase in perioperative complications noted with preoperative chemotherapy when the surgery is performed at an experienced center. As Table 6 demonstrates, recent randomized trials have demonstrated a survival benefit with preoperative chemotherapy especially when larger number of patients are randomized.[41,101,104,105,123,131–133,135] The reasons for the failure of the majority of trials may be due in part to the small numbers of patient in each study. Meta-analyses have suggested with larger number of patients that there is a significant benefit to preoperative chemotherapy especially in patients with adenocarcinoma.[136]

Postoperative chemotherapy (cisplatin, 5-FU) for patients after esophagectomy has not demonstrated to date a survival advantage compared with surgery alone and has been associated with increased treatment-related complications (Table 7).[137] Even in meta-analyses, there has not been a clear benefit demonstrated with postoperative chemotherapy.[143]

Definitive chemoradiotherapy with selective surgery has also been evaluated as a strategy to improve survival in locoregionally advanced esophageal cancer. These studies have used both sequential and concurrent treatment strategies. The concurrent use of chemotherapy and radiotherapy is theoretically appealing because, in addition to the systemic effects of chemotherapy, certain agents behave as radiosensitizers. Randomized studies with a concurrent strategy demonstrate an advantage to combined

Table 6 Results of randomized trials of pre- or postoperative chemotherapy for locoregionally advanced esophageal cancer.

Author (reference)	Year	Treatment	Histology	Patients (no.)	Resectability (%)	Operative mortality (%)	Median survival (mo)	p Value
Preoperative chemotherapy								
Roth et al.[41]	1988	Cisplatin, bleomycin, vindesine + surgery	S > A	19	—	10	9	NS
		Surgery alone		20	—	0	9	
Nygaard et al.[118]	1992	Cisplatin, bleomycin + surgery	S	50	58	10	*NS*	
		Surgery alone		41	69	13	7	
Schlag et al.[100]	1992	Cisplatin, 5-FU + surgery	S	21	69	—	6	NS
		Surgery alone		24	79	—	8	
Maipang et al.[131]	1994	Cisplatin, bleomycin, vinblastine + surgery	S	24	—	—	17	NS
		Surgery alone		22	—	—	17	
Ancona et al.[132]	1995	Cisplatin, 5-FU + surgery	S	35	78	7	—	NS
		Surgery alone		43	86	5	—	
Law et al.[103]	1997	Cisplatin, 5-FU + surgery	S	73	95	9	13	NS
		Surgery alone		74	89	8	17	
Kelsen et al.[104]	1998	Cisplatin, 5-FU + surgery	A > S	213	76	7	15	NS
		Surgery alone		227	89	6	16	
Clarke et al.[133]	2002	Cisplatin, 5-FU + surgery	A > S	400	78	10	17	<0.05
		Surgery alone		402	70	10	13	
Cunningham et al.[134]	2006	Epirubicin, cisplatin, 5-FU + surgery	A	250	69	6	23	<0.01
		Surgery alone	25% GEJ					
			75% Gastric	253	66	6	20	
Postoperative chemotherapy								
Ando et al.[123]	1997	Cisplatin, vindesine + surgery	S	105	—	—	58	NS
		Surgery alone		100	—	—	47	

Abbreviations: A, adenocarcinoma; NS, not significant; S, squamous cell; and 5-FU, 5-fluorouracil.

Table 7 Results of randomized trials of preoperative chemoradiotherapy for locoregionally advanced esophageal cancer.

Author (reference)	Year	Treatment	Histology	Patients (no.)	Technique	Operative mortality (%)	Median survival (mo)	p Value
LePrise et al.[137]	1994	Cisplatin, 5-FU + 20 Gy + surgery	S	41	Sequential	9	10	NS
		Surgery alone		45		7	10	
Walsh et al.[138]	1996	Cisplatin, 5-FU + 40 Gy + surgery	A	58	Concurrent	12	17	0.01
		Surgery alone		55		3	12	
Bosset et al.[139]	1997	Cisplatin + 37 Gy + surgery	S	143	Concurrent	12	19	NS
		Surgery alone		139		4	19	
Urba et al.[140]	2001	Cisplatin, 5-FU + 45 Gy + surgery	A	50	Concurrent	4	18	0.15
		Surgery alone		50		2	17	
Burmeister et al.[141]	2005	Cisplatin, 5-FU + 35 Gy + surgery	A,S	128	Concurrent	5	22	NS
		Surgery alone		128		5	19	
Tepper et al.[142]	2008	Cisplatin, 5-FU + 50.4 Gy + surgery	A > S	30	Concurrent	0	54	0.002
		Surgery alone		26		4	22	
Van Hagen et al.[96c]	2012	Paclitaxel, carboplatin + 41.4 Gy + surgery	A,S	178	Concurrent	4	49	0.003
		Surgery alone		188		4	24	
Mariette et al.[96d]	2014	Cisplatin, 5FU + 45 Gy + surgery	A,S	98	Concurrent	11	32	0.99
		Surgery alone		97		3	41	

Abbreviations: A, adenocarcinoma; NS, not significant; S, squamous cell; 5-FU, 5-fluorouracil.

treatment versus radiation therapy alone (Table 4).[88,90–92,95,111–113] Definitive chemoradiotherapy strategies with surgery used only as salvage appear most effective in SCC and less effective in adenocarcinoma where long-term survival is lower.[105] Two trials have been performed in Europe randomizing SCC patients to definitive chemoradiation or preoperative chemoradiotherapy and surgery.[95,96a] These studies demonstrated similar survivals between groups and suggest that definitive chemoradiation may be an acceptable strategy for SCC of the upper and middle esophagus. The optimum dose for definitive chemoradiotherapy is currently 50.4 Gy as suggested by a randomized trial in which increased doses of radiation were associated with increased treatment-related mortality without a survival advantage.[94] Interestingly, the higher dose had no impact on local failure or continued persistent disease. Both arms of the trial report roughly 50% local failure after 24 months of cumulative follow-up.

Preoperative chemoradiotherapy has also been investigated in locoregionally advanced esophageal cancer as a strategy in an attempt to reduce both the high locoregional and systemic relapse rate noted with surgery alone or preoperative chemotherapy and surgery. The theoretical advantages to preoperative as opposed to postoperative chemoradiation therapy include (1) the ability to control subclinical systemic metastases before the immune suppression that results from surgery; (2) downstaging locoregional disease to increase the likelihood of a complete resection at surgery; and (3) the ability to administer full doses of chemoradiation that would not be possible to administer postoperatively because of perioperative debility. As Table 7 demonstrates, the results are not consistent, although sequential chemoradiation does not appear to be beneficial.[95,137–141] There have been several trials that have been encouraging for concurrent preoperative chemoradiation in locoregionally advanced esophageal cancer especially in adenocarcinoma, but statistical significance has not been achieved in all trials. Meta analyses with larger numbers of patients have suggested that preoperative chemoradiation and preoperative chemotherapy have survival advantages compared with other strategies, although these studies are limited by different preclinical staging techniques and heterogenous patient populations (Figure 7).[136] A survival benefit for combined therapy is evident in most studies in patients who are found to have a complete pathologic response in the surgical specimen and have provided strong incentives to continue the investigations of this strategy. In addition, as surgery alone or radiation therapy alone has such poor outcomes, many oncologists currently use definitive chemoradiotherapy alone or preoperative chemoradiation and surgery for nonmetastatic, locoregionally advanced esophageal cancer (Figure 3). Two randomized trials from Europe have been reported comparing definitive chemoradiation versus preoperative chemoradiation and surgery in SCC.[95,96a] Preliminary results demonstrated improved locoregional control with surgery but no survival advantages. Although operative mortality was higher than expected, these trials suggest that definitive chemoradiation may be an acceptable strategy in SCC of the upper and middle esophagus especially in institutions where trimodality treatment-related mortality is high.[95,96a] The impact of neoadjuvant chemoradiotherapy on pathologic complete response and overall survival has been debated owing to lack of a survival benefit in most randomized trials. Most of these trials have been criticized for the poor design and lack of power to detect an overall survival benefit. A recent and updated meta-analysis of 12 surgery ± neoadjuvant chemoradiotherapy encompassing 1854 patients demonstrated that the hazard ratio for all-cause mortality was improved for neoadjuvant chemoradiotherapy (0.78, 95% CI 0.70–0.88; $p < 0.0001$). The benefit was seen for both the squamous (0.80, CI 0.68–0.93; $p = 0.004$) and adenocarcinoma (0.75, CI 0.59–0.95; $p = 0.02$) histologies. While increased postoperative morbidity and mortality were seen in this analysis, the impact on survival remained.

In an effort to decrease the operative mortality and maintain high rates of R0 resections, a phase II trial using paclitaxel and carboplatin with radiotherapy demonstrated low morbidity and 100% complete resection rates.[96b] The definitive phase III trial randomizing this regimen against surgery alone in patients with clinical stage T1N1, M0 or T2-3N0-1, M0 was recently reported.[96c] Of the 366 patients randomized, 75% were adenocarcinoma. Complete (R0) resection was obtained in 92% of the chemoradiotherapy arm versus 69% in the surgery alone arm ($p < 0.001$). Postoperative complications did not significantly differ between the arms. However, the primary endpoint of overall survival was significantly better in the chemoradiotherapy arm. With a median follow-up of 45 months, median overall survival was 49.4 months in the chemoradiotherapy arm versus 24 months in the surgery alone arm ($p = 0.003$). Overall 5-year survival was 47% versus 34%. Interestingly, the benefit in OS was maintained in both the squamous and the adenocarcinoma histologies.

On the basis of these randomized data and meta analysis, NCCN guidelines 3.2015 now recommended preoperative chemoradiation as a treatment choice for medically fit patients.

For patients with early-stage esophageal carcinoma (stage I or II), a randomized trial from Europe comparing neoadjuvant chemoradiotherapy (4500 cGY plus 5FU-cisplatin) following by surgery versus surgery alone reported interim analysis, which showed that 3-year overall survival was similar between the two groups: 47.5% versus 53.0% (HR 0.99). R0 resection rates were similar 93.8% versus 92.1% ($p = 0.749$), but postoperative mortality was higher in the neoadjuvant chemoradiotherapy group, 11.1% versus 3.4% ($p = 0.049$).[96d]

Recommendations for therapy

As our treatment algorithm suggests (Figure 3), good performance patients with localized, early-stage disease should undergo endoscopic resection or esophagectomy depending on tumor depth, whereas poor performance patients or patients refusing surgery can be treated with definitive chemoradiation or radiation alone. Locoregionally advanced esophageal cancer patients with good

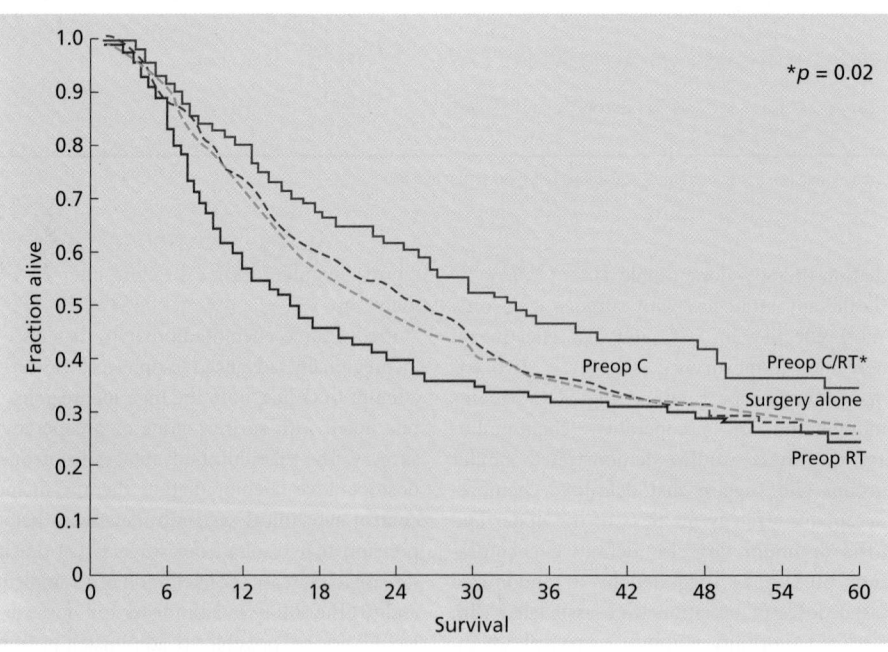

Figure 7 Improved long-term survival noted in patients undergoing preoperative chemoradiation (Preop C/RT) before surgery (surg) at the University of Texas M.D. Anderson Cancer Center ($n = 879$). Source: Hofsetter 2002.[28a] Reproduced with permission of Wolters Kluwer.

performance status are seldom cured with surgery or radiation therapy alone and may therefore be candidates for investigational trials, definitive chemoradiation, or preoperative chemoradiation and surgery. Poor performance patients with locoregionally advanced esophageal cancer should be treated with chemoradiation or palliative radiation therapy and/or stents. Metastatic esophageal cancer patients who are good performance status may be offered chemotherapy alone with the addition of palliative radiation and/or stents for locoregional control. Chemotherapy should not be used if the patients have a poor performance status as the focus should be on palliation.

Palliative therapy of esophageal obstruction

In patients with advanced esophageal cancer not amenable to potentially curative therapy, a primary goal of treatment is relief of dysphagia.[144] This can be accomplished with palliative resection, but high operative morbidity and mortality rates as well as the prolonged period of recovery that is necessary preclude meaningful palliation and most oncologists currently recommend nonsurgical means for palliation. External beam radiotherapy, as an isolated modality or in combination with chemotherapy, is noninvasive but requires considerable time to complete and results in strictures in up to 30% of patients. Intraluminal brachytherapy is another option that is considered in some centers.[145,146] Photocoagulative laser therapy is another option that is usually performed with an Nd:YAG laser, with an initial improvement in dysphagia in 85% of patients and a mean duration of response of less than 1 month. PDT offers a similar initial efficacy but provides a more enduring response, although skin photosensitivity is an undesirable side effect.[147]

The development of endoesophageal stents has offered another therapeutic option in these difficult patients. Endoesophageal stent placement has led to rapid and enduring improvement in swallowing for many patients with advanced disease who are obstructed locoregionally. The introduction of self-expanding wire mesh stents has greatly simplified stent placement and associated complications and has improved palliation of dysphagia, compared with plastic prostheses.[148,149] This method of palliation has provided a much less invasive mechanism to palliate these patients and has replaced surgical bypass as the primary modality to relieve dysphagia.

Malignant esophagorespiratory (tracheoesophageal) fistulas pose a special problem in patients with esophageal cancer. These patients were previously treated with surgical bypass although the high morbidity and short life expectancy of these patients were significant problems.[150] The introduction of coated wire mesh stents offers a better option for the treatment of such fistulas because they palliate dysphagia while occluding the fistula without requiring an extensive surgical procedure in an often debilitated and poor performance status patient.[151,152]

Key references

The complete reference list can be found on the Wiley Companion Digital Edition of this title (see inside front cover for login instructions).

4 Dolan K, Sutton R, Walker SJ, et al. New classification of oesophageal and gastric carcinomas derived from changing patterns in epidemiology. *Br J Cancer.* 1999;**80**:834–842.

13 Kjaerheim K, Gaard M, Andersen A. The role of alcohol, tobacco, and dietary factors in upper aerodigestive tract cancers: a prospective study of 10,900 Norwegian men. *Cancer Causes Control.* 1998;**9**:99–108.

24 Montesano R, Hollstein M, Hainaut P. Genetic alterations in esophageal cancer and their relevance to etiology and pathogenesis: a review. *Int J Cancer.* 1996;**69**:225–235.

31 Siegel RL, Miller KD, Jemal A. Cancer Statistics, 2015. *CA Cancer J Clin.* 2015;**65**:5–29.

35 Hesketh PJ, Clapp RW, Doos WG, et al. The increasing frequency of adenocarcinoma of the esophagus. *Cancer.* 1989;**64**:526–530.

39 Swisher SG, Hunt KK, Holmes EC, et al. Changes in the surgical management of esophageal cancer from 1970–1993. *Am J Surg.* 1995;**169**:609–614.

45 Swisher SG, DeFord L, Merriman KW, et al. Effect of operative volume on morbidity, mortality and hospital use after esophagectomy for cancer. *J Thorac Cardiovasc Surg.* 2000;**119**:1126–1134.

46 Tio TL, Coene PPLO, Luiken GJHM, et al. Endosonography in the clinical staging of esophageal carcinoma [abstract]. *Gastrointest Endosc.* 1990;**36**:S2–S10.

64 Flamen P, Lerut A, Van Cutsem E, et al. The utility of positron emission tomography for the diagnosis and staging of recurrent esophageal cancer. *J Thorac Cardiovasc Surg.* 2000;**120**:1085–1092.

70 Shimada Y, Imamura M, Shibagaki I, et al. Genetic alterations in patients with esophageal cancer with short-and long-term survival rates after curative esophagectomy. *Ann Surg.* 1997;**226**:162–168.

79 Tabira Y, Okuma T, Kondo K, et al. Indications for three-field dissection followed by esophagectomy for advanced carcinoma of the thoracic esophagus. *J Thorac Cardiovasc Surg.* 1999;**117**:239–245.

82 Jacobi CA, Zieren HU, Muller JM, et al. Surgical therapy of esophageal carcinoma: the influence of surgical approach and esophageal resection on cardiopulmonary function. *Eur J Cardio-Thorac Surg.* 1997;**11**:32–37.

83 Hulscher JBF, van Sandik JW, De Boer AGEM, et al. Extended transthoracic resection compared with limited transhiatal resection for adenocarcinoma of the esophagus. *New Engl J Med.* 2002;**347**:1662–1669.

94 Minsky BD, Pajak TF, Ginsberg RJ, et al. INT 0123 (Radiation Therapy Oncology Group 94–05) phase III trial of combined-modality therapy for esophageal cancer: high-dose versus standard-dose radiation therapy. *J Clin Oncol.* 2002;**20**:1167–1174.

101 Walsh TN, Noonan N, Hollywood D, et al. A comparison of multimodal therapy and surgery for esophageal adenocarcinoma. *N Engl J Med.* 1996;**335**:462–467.

117 Arnott SJ, Duncan W, Gignoux M, et al. Preoperative radiotherapy in esophageal carcinoma: a meta-analysis using individual patients data (Oesophageal Cancer Collaborative Group). *Int J Radiat Oncol Biol Phys.* 1998;**41**:579–583.

123 Ando N, Iizuka T, Kakegawa T, et al. A randomized trial of surgery with and without chemotherapy for localized squamous carcinoma of the thoracic esophagus: the Japan Clinical Oncology Group study. *J Thorac Cardiovasc Surg.* 1997;**114**:205–209.

141 Burmeister BH, Smithers BM, Fitzgerald L, et al. Surgery alone versus chemoradiotherapy followed by surgery for resectable cancer of the esophagus: a randomized controlled phase III trial. *Lancet Oncol.* 2005;**6**:659–668.

142 Tepper J, Krasna MJ, Niedzwiecki D, et al. Phase III trial of trimodality therapy with cisplatin fluorouracil, radiotherapy, and surgery compared with surgery alone for esophageal cancer; CALGB 9781. *J Clin Oncol.* 2008;**26**:1086–1092.

90 Carcinoma of the stomach

Carl Schmidt, MD ▪ Mariela Blum Murphy, MD ▪ James C. Yao, MD ▪ Christopher H. Crane, MD

Overview

Gastric cancer is the second most common cause of cancer-related death worldwide and risk factors include autoimmune gastritis, chronic *Helicobacter pylori* infection, obesity, and other causes. Some countries with higher incidence have established screening programs but methodology and eligibility remain controversial. Despite knowledge of risk factors and screening for high-risk populations, identification of earlier stage potentially curable disease remains a challenge.

Multiple genetic mutations are involved in gastric cancer pathogenesis, and mutations in the cellular adhesion protein CDH1 result in familial diffuse gastric cancer. Certain patterns of metastatic disease have been associated with particular molecular alterations. Increasing understanding of molecular pathways involved in gastric cancer has led to efficacious use of targeted biologic therapies with cytotoxic chemotherapy in the advanced setting, such as use of trastuzumab in patients with gastric cancer and *HER2/neu* overexpression.

Surgical resection is the primary potentially curative therapy in those without metastatic disease. Type of resection and extent of lymphadenectomy are not consistent, and standards for best practice are needed. Chemotherapy and radiation play an important role in the adjuvant setting and, therefore, decisions regarding choice and timing of these therapies require accurate staging by thorough evaluation with endoscopy, cross-sectional imaging and, in some cases, endoscopic ultrasound or positron emission tomography.

Palliative interventions and therapy are often important, both for patients with symptoms in the metastatic setting and after recurrence as cure is not achieved in either situation. Results of recent clinical trials are encouraging, and there have been multiple positive phase III trials in the adjuvant and metastatic setting during the past 10 years. Despite this, most people diagnosed with gastric cancer will die from it eventually, so much more research is needed.

Incidence and epidemiology

Despite a worldwide decline in gastric cancer incidence, gastric cancer remains the second most common cause of cancer-related death. Gastric cancer is particularly common in China (accounting for 42% of cases worldwide), South America, Eastern Europe, Japan, and Korea, where it is the most common malignancy.[1] The age-adjusted death rate has been on the decline in the United States over the past 30 years and was 3.8 per 100,000 in 2005.[2] However, this is mostly due to declining incidence; survival in patients with diagnosed gastric cancer remains poor with only modest improvements during recent years. According to the Surveillance, Epidemiology, and End Results (SEER) registry, the 5-year survival rate for gastric cancer (all stages) increased from 16.3% between 1975 and 1979 to 23% in 2000.[2] It should be noted these data predate the publication of major trials of multimodality therapy with positive results and widespread acceptance.

Risk factors

Environmental insults to the gastric mucosa may eventually lead to atrophic gastritis resulting in metaplasia, a precursor condition for some gastric cancers.[3] Other factors associated with increased risk include low serum ferritin levels, pernicious anemia, history of distal gastrectomy for peptic ulcer disease, and endemic *H. pylori* infection.[4-6] While some evidence is suggestive, it remains unknown whether eradicating *H. pylori* infection reduces the incidence of gastric cancer.[7] Behavioral associations with gastric cancer have long been thought to include dietary exposure to nitrates, nitrites, and bacterial or fungal contamination of food given decreasing incidence with the advent of refrigeration.[8] Studies have also documented increased incidence of proximal gastric cancers with obesity and a protective effect of physical activity on overall rates of gastric cancer.[9,10] Red meat consumption has been examined by multiple observational studies and found to be associated with increased risk of gastric cancer.[11,12] Some studies suggest a dose–response relationship between amount of red meat consumption and risk lending further support to this possibility. Consumption of fruit conversely may reduce the risk of gastric cancer.[13]

Familial clustering has been noted to occur in approximately 1% of gastric cancer cases. Germ line mutations account for only a small portion of these cases. Hereditary Diffuse Gastric Cancer (HDGC) syndrome results from germ line mutations of the CDH1 gene; however, CDH1 mutation accounts for only a small percentage of families with a history of diffuse gastric cancer. The CDH1 gene is involved in cellular adhesion, and defects in this gene are also associated with lobular breast cancer.[14] Affected individuals with gastric cancer inherit one copy of the defective CDH1 gene. Somatic mutation, deletion, or promoter methylation inactivates the other copy. Gastric cancers follow an autosomal dominant inheritance pattern with high penetrance.

Prophylactic gastrectomy is a consideration for members of families affected by HDGC syndrome. When prophylactic gastrectomy is performed, multifocal early gastric cancers are nearly always found in the resected specimen.[15] Genetic counseling is recommended in suspected cases, considering the degree of penetrance and age of onset of known cases of gastric cancer in the family and the paucity of long-term outcomes data for prophylactic gastrectomy. Worster et al.[16] studied the impact of prophylactic total gastrectomy on health-related quality of life (HRQOL). In 32 patients who underwent total gastrectomy, HRQOL was compared to 28 patients at risk for HDGC who did not undergo total gastrectomy. While physical and mental function returned to baseline by 12 months after operation, some symptoms persist, specifically, loose stools (70%), fatigue (63%), discomfort when eating (81%), reflux (63%), eating restrictions (45%), and body image (44%).

Holland-Frei Cancer Medicine, Ninth Edition. Edited by Robert C. Bast Jr., Carlo M. Croce, William N. Hait, Waun Ki Hong, Donald W. Kufe, Martine Piccart-Gebhart, Raphael E. Pollock, Ralph R. Weichselbaum, Hongyang Wang, and James F. Holland.
© 2017 John Wiley & Sons, Inc. ISBN: 978-1-118-93469-2

Gastric polyps occur in 27–70% of individuals with FAP (familial adenomatous polyposis).[17,18] While fundic gastric polyps are usually thought to be hamartomas, foveolar dysplasia and invasive adenocarcinoma have been described. Hereditary non-polyposis colorectal cancer (HNPCC) is a genetic disorder characterized by germ line mutations in a group of mismatch repair genes, including *hMSH2*, *hMLH1*, *hMSH6*, *hPMS1*, and *hPMS2*. Defects in these genes result in genomic instability characterized by microsatellite instability (MSI). Although colorectal and endometrial cancers are the most common manifestations of HNPCC, gastric carcinoma has also been observed. An analysis of the Korean Hereditary Tumor Registry showed a 3.2-fold increase in the relative risk of gastric cancer in families carrying the HNPCC mutation.[19] However, germ line mutation of one of the mismatch repair genes accounts for only a small percentage of gastric cancers with MSI.

- Gastric cancer is the second leading cause of cancer-related death worldwide
- Risk factors include autoimmune gastritis, *H. pylori* infection and obesity
- Germ line mutations in the CDH1 gene are associated with hereditary gastric cancer

---

Pathology

Adenocarcinoma is the dominant histology in gastric cancer. The Lauren and World Health Organization (WHO) classifications are the two major systems used. The Lauren's system classifies cancer as intestinal, diffuse, or mixed.[20] The simplicity of this system has resulted in widespread use. Intestinal-type gastric cancer is also called epidemic-type gastric cancer. It features a retained glandular structure and cellular polarity. Grossly, it usually has a sharp margin. It arises from the gastric mucosa and is associated with chronic gastritis, gastric atrophy, and intestinal metaplasia. The diffuse-type histology is associated with an invasive growth pattern. Scattered clusters of uniform-sized malignant cells frequently infiltrate the submucosa with little glandular formation and mucin production is common (Figure 1).

Studies of gastrectomy specimens obtained from patients without clinical disease have shown early diffuse-type gastric cancer arising below normal-appearing epithelium.[15] Tumor cells in this type appear to arise from the superficial layer of the lamina propria. An infiltrative growth pattern in diffuse-type gastric cancer often

results in the absence of a mass. The cancer may be difficult to identify using endoscopy, but thickened gastric folds and a difficult to distend stomach are hallmarks of diffuse gastric cancer. Malignant cells can infiltrate well beyond the apparent tumor margin. In advanced cases, this leads to the condition known as linitis plastic (leather-bottle-like stomach) characterized by involvement of the entire stomach, rapid progression, resistance to therapy, and poor prognosis.

Pathogenesis and natural history

Molecular alterations

Multiple molecular alterations are important in the pathogenesis of gastric cancer (Table 1). Epigenetic phenomena include hypermethylation of promoter regions for many genes including *CDH1*, *hMLH1*, and *p16*, which may be involved in early carcinogenesis.[21–27] Further, MSI caused by mutations in DNA repair genes has been reported in up to 39% of gastric cancers.[28] Tumor suppressor genes such as *p53*, *APC*, *MCC*, and *DCC* are also mutated in gastric cancer, and the incidence often varies with histology and stage.[29–31]

Loss of normal cellular adhesion is an important feature of human cancer development and prevalent in genetic alterations of gastric cancer. Diffuse-type gastric cancer is characterized by aberrant cellular adhesion with a pattern of infiltrative growth by a small cluster of or sometimes single tumor cells. The cadherin–catenin complex at the cell surface plays a critical role in cell adhesion and polarity, and up to 90% of gastric cancer cases have an abnormality in at least one component of the complex including CDH1 and α- and γ-catenin.[32,33] The *CD44* transmembrane glycoprotein, expressed in 31–72% of gastric cancers, may modulate invasion and metastasis.[34]

Similar to other adenocarcinomas, alterations in cellular signaling pathways occur in gastric cancer and provide potential targets for biologic therapies. *HER2/neu*, an oncogene in the *erbB* family of membrane receptor tyrosine kinases, is overexpressed in 10–38% of gastric cancer cases and is associated with intestinal-type distal cancer and worse prognosis.[30,35] Expression of other cellular receptors in gastric cancer correlates with oncogenic behavior, such as associations between the transmembrane receptor *EGFR* (epidermal growth factor receptor) with invasion and c-*Met* with peritoneal metastasis.[36] Angiogenesis appears essential for growth of gastric cancer and other solid tumors, and increased angiogenesis in gastric tumor specimens portends an unfavorable prognosis.[37] Vascular endothelial growth factor (*VEGF*) and basic fibroblast growth factor (*bFGF*) are major regulators of

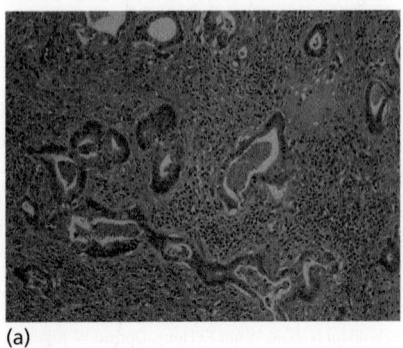 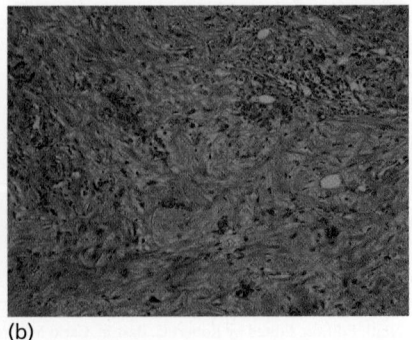

(a)   (b)

Figure 1 Photograph of histologic sections from intestinal (a) and diffuse (b) type gastric cancers.

Table 1 Molecular markers with clinicopathological correlations.

Marker	Involvement	Dominant histology	Clinical correlation
Epigenetic			
Hypermethylation	Common	Both	—
MSI	31–39%	Intestinal	Conflicting for survival, favorable or no difference
Tumor suppressor			
p53	47–74%	Both (intestinal early event and diffuse late event)	Correlates with stage in diffuse-type cancer
APC	8–34%	Intestinal	—
MCC	24–33%	Diffuse	—
DCC	12–49%	Intestinal	—
FHIT	49–67%	—	Correlates with stage, conflicting for survival
Adhesion			
CDH1	54–83%	Diffuse	—
α-Catenin	83–92%	Diffuse	—
γ-Catenin	91–100%	Diffuse	—
β-Catenin	—	Intestinal (GSK3β region)	Poor survival
CD44	31–72%	CD44v6-intestinal	CD44v6 in intestinal-type cancer correlates with inferior survival
Tyrosine kinases			
EGFR	35–81%	Both	Correlates with stage, conflicting for survival
HER2/neu	10–38%	Intestinal	Poor survival
PDGF α	42–45%	Both	Correlates with stage and poor survival
c-Met	34–71%	Diffuse	Correlates with stage and peritoneal metastasis
Angiogenesis			
VEGF	—	Intestinal	Correlates with hepatic metastasis
bFGF	—	Intestinal	Increased recurrence

angiogenesis, have prognostic value, and are potential targets for antiangiogenic therapy in patients with gastric cancer.[38,39] Expression of multiple transcription factors by gastric cancer cells, such as *Sp1* and *mTOR*, promotes abnormal cell growth, survival, and angiogenesis.[40,41]

Progression and patterns of metastasis

Gastric cancers metastasize in several ways. Adjacent organs such as the liver, diaphragm, pancreas, spleen, and colon (or its mesentery) may become involved by direct extension. Gastric cancers have a high tendency to spread through the lymphatic system to regional and distant nodes. Hematogenous metastatic disease is often found in the liver. Peritoneal metastatic disease is also common in the metastatic setting and may result in abdominal pain, bowel obstruction, cachexia, or all three. Japanese investigators have noted that histology and patient age may affect the pattern of spread of gastric cancer. In an autopsy study of 173 cases of gastric cancer, they found diffuse histology to be associated with peritoneal metastasis and intestinal histology to be associated with hepatic metastasis.[42] They also found peritoneal metastasis to be more common in younger patients. In another study, case records of 216 patients with synchronous peritoneal or hepatic metastasis found at surgical exploration more commonly had poorly differentiated histology associated with peritoneal metastases and well to moderately differentiated histology associated with hepatic metastases.[43]

On a molecular level, expression of *VEGF* and its receptor *KDR* has been associated with liver metastasis.[37,44] Expression of *VEGF-C*, which can cause neogenesis of lymphatic vessels, is associated with lymph node metastasis.[45,46] In addition, dysregulation of cellular adhesion is likely central to the development of peritoneal metastasis. *CD44H* has been linked with increased gastric cancer cell adhesion to mesothelial cells and increased peritoneal metastasis in animal models.[47] *C-met* amplification has also been linked with peritoneal metastasis.[36,48] Further translational research of the

molecular biology of metastasis may improve our ability to predict sites of failure and refine therapeutic strategies.

- Molecular alterations of many genes and cellular pathways are involved in the pathogenesis of gastric cancer including modifications in methylation of promoters, MSI, cellular adhesion, growth factors, and angiogenesis
- Metastatic involvement of regional lymph nodes is very common
- Peritoneal surfaces and liver are other common sites of metastasis

Screening

Large-scale screening programs have been established in several countries with a high incidence of gastric cancer, including Japan, Korea, Venezuela, and Chile. Available screening tests include, among others, upper gastrointestinal endoscopy and radiologic studies using oral contrast agents such as barium. The method for most efficacious screening remains controversial, and there is no uniformity in terms of recommended age, interval, or type of screening exam. Comparisons between screening methods by large controlled trials are lacking. Screening of asymptomatic people in countries with lower risk of gastric cancer, such as the United States, is not feasible or cost-effective.

Importantly, symptoms of gastric cancer are often nonspecific, leading to diagnosis at an advanced stage. This is caused in large part because both the stomach and abdominal cavity are large and distensible. Early symptoms, such as vague discomfort, episodic nausea/vomiting, or anorexia are common in patients without cancer. Thus, physicians may not attribute such symptoms to gastric cancer for many months. In fact, patients may undergo several months of therapy for presumptive peptic ulcer disease before a diagnosis of gastric cancer. As such, more research is needed to develop better methods of early detection even in countries with lower incidence.

Diagnosis

Common symptoms of gastric cancer at diagnosis include abdominal pain and weight loss. Although anemia is also a frequent finding, overt upper gastrointestinal bleeding is much less common. Dysphagia may occur predominantly in patients with proximal cancer, whereas nausea and vomiting are more common in patients with nonproximal cancer. Early satiety can be especially prominent in patients with linitis plastica. Abnormal physical examination findings often indicate advanced disease, such as a palpable epigastric mass that may indicate a large locally advanced tumor. Jaundice usually indicates hepatic metastasis or metastatic lymphadenopathy in the portal region.

There are several aspects of appropriate clinical staging of gastric cancer that should be performed in a stepwise manner. Potentially helpful laboratory studies include a complete blood count, electrolytes, blood urea nitrogen, creatinine, alkaline phosphatase, transaminases, and bilirubin. Evaluation of tumor markers CEA, CA19-9, and CA125 may be considered. At the time of referral to surgeon or oncologist, upper endoscopy has typically been performed and made the diagnosis. Endoscopic findings should be reviewed by the primary treating surgeon with regard to tumor size and location, especially for gastroesophageal junction (GEJ) tumors as some may be more appropriately treated like distal esophageal cancers. Computed tomography (CT) scan of the chest, abdomen, and pelvis is performed to provide further information about the primary tumor and detect evidence for malignant lymphadenopathy or metastatic disease including carcinomatosis. The finding of even a small amount of ascites may indicate peritoneal disease.

Endoscopic ultrasound (EUS) is accurate for assessing T stage and enables needle biopsy of suspicious perigastric nodes and even some left liver masses. EUS may not always be needed when CT scan findings are suggestive of advanced cancer. EUS should be considered for patients entering neoadjuvant therapy trials and for assessment of small masses amenable to endoscopic mucosal resection (EMR) or early-stage cancers for which operation without neoadjuvant therapy is considered. The role of positron emission tomography (PET) for gastric cancer is evolving; there is some evidence PET can be used to evaluate response to therapy.[49] Laparoscopy is controversial but considered essential by many for complete staging of gastric cancers. Laparoscopy results in upstaging in one-fifth to one-fourth of patients, primarily through detection of peritoneal metastases not seen on CT scans.[50-52]

TNM stage classification

Table 2 displays a portion of the current staging system for gastric cancer from the American Joint Committee on Cancer Staging Manual, seventh edition (Springer, New York 2010). This table applies to patients without metastatic disease (M1). In the current staging system, stages I to III are defined by various combinations of T (tumor) and N (nodal) stage without metastatic disease; prior versions of the system classified some patients with extensive nodal disease as stage IV. In the current system, stage IV disease is defined only by the presence of distant metastatic disease.

The following definitions are used to classify T and N stage:

- Tis—intraepithelial tumor with no invasion into lamina propria
- T1a—tumor invades lamina propria or muscularis mucosae
- T1b—tumor invades submucosa
- T2—tumor invades muscularis propria
- T3—tumor penetrates subserosal connective tissue without serosal invasion
- T4a—tumor invades serosa
- T4b—tumor invades adjacent organ or structure

Table 2 AJCC stage grouping for gastric cancer without distant metastatic disease.

T stage	Nodal stage			
	N0	**N1**	**N2**	**N3**
Tis	0			
T1a/b	IA	IB	IIA	IIB
T2	IB	IIA	IIB	IIIA
T3	IIA	IIB	IIIA	IIIB
T4a	IIB	IIIA	IIIB	IIIC
T4b	IIIB	IIIB	IIIC	IIIC

- N1—regional nodal metastases, 1–2 nodes
- N2—regional nodal metastases, 3–6 nodes
- N3a—regional nodal metastases, 7–15 nodes
- N3b—regional nodal metastases, 16 or more nodes

- Early gastric cancer may be detected by screening in countries with such programs
- Possible symptoms of gastric cancer include abdominal pain, bleeding, dysphagia, nausea, anorexia, weight loss, and early satiety
- Clinical staging is based on upper endoscopy and cross-sectional imaging of the chest, abdomen, and pelvis (typically CT scan)
- Other potentially useful staging studies include laparoscopy, EUS and PET

Multidisciplinary care

For patients with small tumors and low histologic grade, EMR is gaining acceptance as the primary method for local therapy. Such therapy is predicated on these tumors having a very low incidence of node-positive disease.[53] The incidence of nodal positivity with T1 tumors is approximately 10%, and other features of the primary tumor delineate patients with even lower risk. Tumors confined to the mucosa have a 1–3% incidence of nodal positivity versus a tumor with submucosal invasion with an incidence of up to 15%.[54] Other factors that increase the incidence of nodal disease include poor differentiation, signet-ring cells, lymphatic invasion, and tumor size >2 cm.[55] It is reasonable, therefore, to consider EMR for patients with small, well-differentiated T1 tumors confined to the mucosa. However, specialists at some high-volume centers have proposed expanded criteria for use of newer techniques using endoscopic submucosal dissection.[56] Removal of larger even ulcerated masses has been done. In our opinion, this more aggressive approach requires careful histological evaluation of the resected specimen and confirmation of T1a (mucosal) disease.

Surgery

The choice of operation for gastric cancer depends on tumor location, histological type, and disease stage. Gastrectomy is the most widely used approach for invasive gastric cancer, and the most common techniques are total gastrectomy, distal subtotal, and proximal subtotal gastrectomy. Segmental resection is less commonly used for invasive gastric cancer but is very common and appropriate for other gastric malignancies such as gastrointestinal stromal tumors. Prospective and randomized studies reveal no survival advantage of total gastrectomy for tumors of the distal stomach compared to distal subtotal gastrectomy when all disease is removed with adequate margins. Both techniques are associated with similar rates of mortality (1–3%), complications, and 5-year survival (around 60%).[57,58] In most series, the quality of life after subtotal gastrectomy is superior to that after total gastrectomy.[59,60]

Tumors of the proximal stomach and GEJ generally require more complex considerations for resection and reconstruction. Siewert's classification is very useful and commonly used to describe GEJ tumors.[61,62]:

- Type I: adenocarcinoma of the distal esophagus, which usually arises in Barrett's esophagus and may infiltrate the GE junction from above
- Type II: true carcinoma of the cardia arising immediately at the GEJ within 1 cm above and 2 cm below the junction
- Type III: subcardial gastric carcinoma infiltrating the junction and distal esophagus from below

In patients with an advanced tumor involving the GEJ, the site of origin (esophagus or stomach) may be unclear. Patients with type I tumors are often treated as distal esophagus cancers with consideration of preoperative chemoradiation for more advanced tumors and surgical resection using a gastric conduit with anastomosis in the neck or chest. In some cases, the jejunum or colon is used instead of the stomach for the conduit. Type II and III tumors may be removed with either total gastrectomy or proximal subtotal gastrectomy often through a transabdominal approach depending on the local extent of the tumor.[63,64] Total gastrectomy is generally favored in the United States over proximal gastrectomy because reflux esophagitis is rare after Roux-en-Y esophagojejunostomy reconstruction compared to roughly one-third of patients who will have significant reflux after proximal subtotal resection.[59,65,66] Further, proximal subtotal gastrectomy may fail to remove enough nodal tissue from the lesser curvature, a common site of nodal metastasis. However, some surgeons continue to advocate for proximal subtotal gastrectomy.[64]

The extent of lymph node dissection is one of the most controversial surgical topics in the management of gastric cancer. Radical lymph node dissection involves removal of lymph nodes beyond the usual field of gastrectomy. The Japanese Gastric Cancer Association defines extent of lymph node dissection using the designation "D."[67] Generally, D1 dissection includes perigastric lymph nodes. D2 dissection extends the lymphadenectomy to include nodes along the hepatic, left gastric, celiac, and splenic arteries (Figure 2). D3 dissection includes nodes along the porta hepatis and in the retropancreatic and periaortic regions.

The largest prospective study examining the potential benefit of extended lymphadenectomy is the Dutch D1D2 lymphadenectomy trial which randomized more than 1000 patients (711 treated with curative intent) to D1 or D2 lymphadenectomy in the setting of gastrectomy for cancer, with surgical quality carefully controlled.[68,69] Operative morbidity and mortality rates were significantly greater in the D2 group than in the D1 group (43% and 10%, respectively, vs 25% and 4%, $p < 0.01$). However, the increase in mortality rate was associated with either male patients undergoing D2 dissection or patients undergoing splenectomy and distal pancreatectomy for complete nodal dissection. Patients who underwent D2 dissection with preservation of the spleen/tail of the pancreas had operative mortality similar to that of patients who underwent D1 dissection. After median follow-up of 15.2 years, the D2 lymphadenectomy group had a higher disease-specific survival (DSS) rate compared to the D1 group and lower rates of local (12% vs 22%, $p = 0.02$) and regional (13% vs 19%, $p = 0.02$) recurrence.[70]

A recent trial from the Italian Gastric Cancer Study Group evaluated the role of modified organ-preserving D2 lymphadenectomy.[71] Patients with potentially curable gastric cancer were randomized

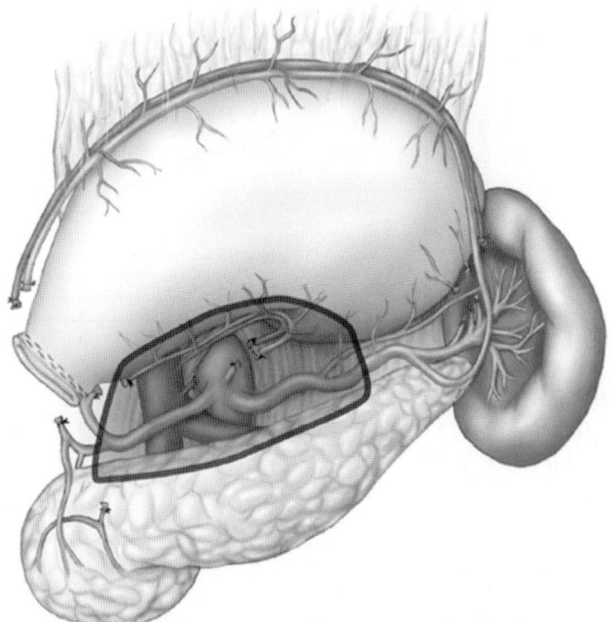

Figure 2 Area of critical modified D2 lymphadenectomy including celiac, hepatic, left gastric, and splenic artery lymph nodes (shaded area).

(intraoperative) to D1 or D2 dissection. Partial pancreatectomy or splenectomy was done only when local invasion was suspected. A total of 267 patients were randomized, and morbidity and mortality were 12% and 3%, respectively, for the D1 group and 18% and 2% for the D2 group. Five-year DSS rates were 71% and 73% for the D1 and D2 groups; subgroup analysis revealed that in patients with node-positive disease the 5-year DSS rate was 61% in the D2 group versus 46% in the D1 group. Further, in patients with T-stage 2–4 and positive lymph nodes, the 5-year DSS was 59% in the D2 arm versus 38% in the D1 arm (Figure 3). The National Comprehensive Cancer Network (NCCN) gastric cancer panel has recommended consideration of modified D2 lymphadenectomy sparing distal pancreas and spleen in the setting of gastrectomy for cancer if available from an experienced surgeon at a high-volume center.[72]

Linitis plastica is an extremely virulent form of gastric cancer and is considered incurable by many clinicians. Some feel that patients with linitis plastica should never undergo gastrectomy since at best the 5-year survival is <10%.[73] One approach to patients with linitis plastica is to evaluate with staging laparoscopy and, in the absence of metastatic disease, treat first with neoadjuvant therapy in the hope of selecting patients who do not develop metastatic disease for eventual gastrectomy. If a patient with linitis plastica has a positive margin of resection after operation, one should be cautious as to whether this deserves consideration or specific therapy given that isolated local recurrences are uncommon and rarely impact survival compared to the risk of metastatic disease. Recent evidence from the U.S. Gastric Cancer Collaborative suggests the traditional teaching that wide > 5 cm proximal margins are best for resection of distal cancers may not be necessary.[74] In their retrospective cohort study combining data from seven academic medical centers, the proximal margin distance was not an independent factor associated with overall survival (OS). Rather, T and N-stage were the primary associated factors, and a 3 cm margin was adequate in most patients.

While studies mentioned earlier indicate multivisceral resection should not be done routinely during lymphadenectomy, resection of other organs is sometimes needed when involved by the primary

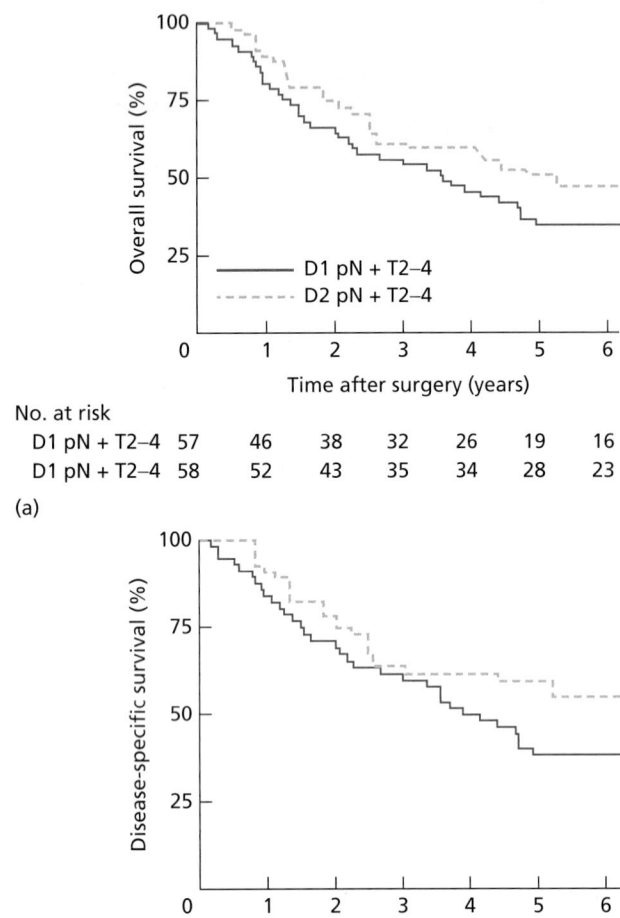

No. at risk
D1 pN + T2–4	57	46	38	32	26	19	16
D1 pN + T2–4	58	52	43	35	34	28	23

(a)

No. at risk
D1 pN + T2–4	56	46	38	32	26	19	16
D1 pN + T2–4	56	51	42	34	33	28	23

(b)

Figure 3 Kaplan–Meier curves of overall survival (a) and disease-specific survival (b) for patients with pathologic T2-4 and node-positive disease from the Italian Gastric Cancer Study Group D1D2 lymphadenectomy trial.[71]

tumor or grossly involved nodes. Investigators from Memorial Sloan-Kettering Cancer Center found that roughly one-third of 800 patients who underwent R0 resection of gastric cancer over 15 years required removal of at least one additional organ.[75,76] The operative mortality rate was 4% in these patients, similar to that reported in the Dutch trial for limited dissection and far lower than that for D2 dissection with adjacent organ resection. Interestingly, the likelihood of actual adjacent organ invasion was low (14%) after final pathological examination. The 5-year survival rate in these patients was 32% compared to 50% in patients who did not require multivisceral resection. These data support application of multivisceral resection when required to achieve R0 resection at centers where the operative mortality rate is low.

Minimally invasive approaches to the conduct of subtotal or total gastrectomy have increased in recent years using laparoscopy, computer-aided (robotic) surgery, or hybrid procedures. Prospective high-quality comparisons of these techniques to open surgery have not been done. There are multiple retrospective studies comparing them, which suggest that short- and long-term patient outcomes are improved or not adversely affected by minimally invasive techniques.[77,78] While operating time and cost may increase

with these approaches, especially early in the surgeon's learning curve, such costs may be balanced by other possible cost savings with shorter length of stay and more rapid overall recovery. However, all studies so far without randomization are subject to patient selection bias and, therefore, require caution when interpreting any possible benefits.

- EMR is considered with small T1a gastric cancers without adverse pathologic features
- Surgical resection is typically partial or total gastrectomy with upper abdominal (D1 or modified D2) lymphadenectomy
- Removal of other organs when needed due to local invasion is appropriate
- Use of laparoscopic and robotic techniques deserves further study

Radiation oncology

Use of postoperative chemoradiation for gastric cancer is supported by the results of the Intergroup trial (INT 0116).[79] Patients with gastric cancer after potentially curative resection were randomized to undergo postoperative chemoradiation with 45 Gray (Gy) external beam radiation with bolus fluorouracil (5-FU) or observation. The majority of the 556 evaluable patients had positive lymph nodes (85%) or T3/T4 tumors (68%). At 3 years, patients in the adjuvant chemoradiation arm had a 50% survival compared to 41% in the control arm ($p < 0.01$). There were increased gastrointestinal (33% grade 3/4) and hematological (54% grade 3/4) side effects in the therapy group. This trial established postoperative adjuvant chemoradiation as the standard of care for resected gastric cancer in the United States. There is no uniform agreement about which lymph node groups should be treated in the setting of gastric cancer, but treatment volumes should be tailored to the location of each individual tumor. There are detailed data regarding the risk of nodal involvement from lymphadenectomy series that can guide physicians.[80] Depending on the location of the primary tumor in the stomach, perigastric, gastroepiploic, celiac, porta hepatis, subpyloric, gastroduodenal, splenic-suprapancreatic, and retropancreaticoduodenal nodes can be at risk for metastatic spread. The gastric remnant, the perigastric nodes, and the branches of the celiac axis should be treated in all cases.

Primary systemic treatment

Preoperative chemotherapy

The Medical Research Council Adjuvant Gastric Infusional Chemotherapy (MAGIC) trial changed the landscape of treatment options for patients with locally advanced gastric cancer.[81] This randomized phase III trial compared surgery alone to surgery with three cycles of both preoperative and postoperative epirubicin, cisplatin, and 5-FU (ECF) chemotherapy. Among 503 patients accrued, ECF toxicity was manageable and the rates of postoperative morbidity and mortality were similar in the surgery alone and ECF groups. The resected tumors were smaller (3 cm vs 5 cm) with less advanced T and N stages than the ECF group. With a median follow-up of 4 years, patients in the ECF group had significantly better 5-year OS (36% vs 23%, $p < 0.01$) and disease-free survival (DFS) rates. This trial clearly establishes the perioperative ECF treatment regimen as a viable option for patients. It is important to realize only 42% of patients completed the prescribed protocol.

The French Action Clinique Coordonnées en Cancérologie Digestive (ACCORD-07) study confirmed the use of preoperative chemotherapy to be beneficial in patients with GEJ cancers despite closing prematurely due to low enrollment.[82] A total of 224 patients with adenocarcinoma of the lower esophagus, GEJ, or stomach (25%) were randomized to receive 2–3 cycles of 5-FU/cisplatin followed by surgery followed by 3–4 cycles of the same chemotherapy versus surgery alone. The median follow-up was 5.7 years. Only 50% of the patients received postoperative chemotherapy. Five-year survival rates were 38% in the chemotherapy/surgery group versus 24% in the surgery alone group. In contrast, a study by the European Organization for Research and Treatment of Cancer (EORTC) randomized patients with locally advanced adenocarcinoma of the stomach or GEJ to preoperative chemotherapy with cisplatin, leucovorin, and 5-FU followed by surgery or surgery alone. This trial did not find a survival difference between these two strategies but was possibly underpowered due to poor accrual.[83]

Postoperative adjuvant chemotherapy

Numerous trials of systemic chemotherapy for gastric cancer have been performed in the adjuvant setting. Many of the early trials were underpowered, included improper control groups or used suboptimal methodology. These limitations along with heterogeneous inclusion criteria rendered much of their results unreproducible.[84] Meta-analyses of these trials were fraught with difficulties and could not recommend a particular regimen. Nevertheless, two large analyses were performed with conflicting results.[85,86] Each analysis recommended treatment for subgroups such as patients with node-positive disease and Asian patients. Win and coauthors pooled data from several prospective studies to compare chemoradiation after R0 resection for gastric cancer to adjuvant chemotherapy.[87] The basic finding was that chemoradiation was associated with improved DFS without a difference in OS.

Most of the chemotherapy agents considered to be active against gastric cancer have reported response rates of 15–20% when administered alone which makes it uncertain whether any single-agent adjuvant therapy will have a strong benefit. Despite this, prolonged continuous administration of an oral 5-FU prodrug (S-1) has been attractive to a number of investigators with some promising results. Investigators in one study randomly assigned 1059 patients with stage II or III gastric cancer after R0 gastrectomy and D2 or higher lymphadenectomy to surgery alone or surgery and postoperative S-1.[88] Improved DFS and OS were observed in the S-1-treated group. The 3-year OS rates were 80.1% in the S-1-treated group and 70.1% in the surgery-alone group ($p < 0.01$). The update analysis after 5 years demonstrated 5-year OS was 71.7% in the S-1-treated group and 61.1% in the surgery-alone group.

It should be noted that the safety profile of S-1 differs between Western and Asian patients and that S-1 is currently not available in the United States. A Korean study, the capecitabine and oxaliplatin adjuvant study in stomach cancer (CLASSIC), examined the use of adjuvant chemotherapy with capecitabine and oxaliplatin for 6 months after gastrectomy with D2 lymphadenectomy versus surgery alone.[89] The study demonstrated a benefit in DFS and OS, specifically, 3 year-OS of 83% in the treatment group compared to 78% in the observation group. In a subgroup analysis, the survival benefit was lacking in patients with N0 disease. A published meta-analysis of 17 randomized controlled trials of adjuvant chemotherapy in gastric cancer demonstrated a statistically significantly benefit in OS and DFS for patients treated with fluorouracil-based adjuvant chemotherapy versus surgery alone.[90]

Integration of multimodal care

Surgery is the cornerstone of potentially curative therapy for localized gastric cancer, but the importance of adjuvant therapies cannot be overemphasized. Long-term survival rates with surgery alone remain suboptimal for all but the earliest gastric cancers (T1N0M0). As mentioned earlier, multicenter randomized studies demonstrate significant survival benefits for adjuvant therapy compared to surgery alone with two basic approaches (Table 3). Regardless of patient population, tumor location or extent of lymph node dissection, surgery alone is no longer adequate for patients with more than early gastric cancer who are fit for adjuvant therapy. A direct comparison across studies is not advisable due to differences in study design, patient population, proportion of patients with node positive disease, and extent of node dissection. It is perhaps interesting that many adjuvant therapy strategies and extended lymph node dissection are generally associated with a survival benefit around 10%.

We advise the following approach for consideration of adjuvant therapy. Patients with apparent early disease (stage IA) or patients with an indication for surgical resection first (acute bleeding or obstruction) should first undergo gastrectomy including modified D2 lymphadenectomy. Following this, postoperative chemoradiation as in the INT0116 study should be given to those with stage IB to IIIC on final pathology. Patients with more advanced disease should be considered for perioperative chemotherapy as in the MAGIC study. In either group, diagnostic laparoscopy with cytologic washings should be considered before choice of initial therapy. For institutions where this is not routine, laparoscopy or PET should be considered if any other studies

Table 3 Selected adjuvant therapy options.

Postoperative chemotherapy and chemoradiation (INT0116 study—MacDonald regimen)
Chemotherapy (one 28-day cycle)
- 5-FU 425 mg/m²/day IV on days 1–5
- Folinic acid 20 mg/m²/day IV on days 1–5

Chemoradiation (5 weeks)
- 5-FU 400 mg/m²/day IV on days 1–4 and on the last 3 days of radiotherapy
- Folinic acid 20 mg/m²/day IV on days 1–4 and on the last 3 days of radiotherapy
- External-beam radiation, 45 Gy at 1.8 Gy/day 5 days per week

1-month recovery period
Chemotherapy (two 28-day cycles)
- 5-FU 425 mg/m²/day IV on days 1–5
- Folinic acid 20 mg/m²/day IV on days 1–5

Perioperative chemotherapy (MAGIC trial regimen)
Chemotherapy ECF (three 21-day cycle)
- Epirubicin 50 mg/m² IV on day 1
- Cisplatin 60 mg/m² IV on day 1
- 5-FU 200 mg/m²/day CIV infusion on days 1–21

3–6 weeks recovery period
Surgical resection (gastrectomy/lymphadenectomy)
6–12 weeks recovery period
Chemotherapy ECF (three 21-day cycle)
- Epirubicin 50 mg/m² IV on day 1
- Cisplatin 60 mg/m² IV on day 1
- 5-FU 200 mg/m-/day CIV infusion on days 1–21

IV, intravenous and CIV, continuous intravenous infusion.

suggest possible metastatic disease. For Asian patients, postoperative chemotherapy with S-1 should be considered if available and when appropriate. Any patient eligible for clinical trials should be encouraged to enroll including nontherapeutic biomarker and other studies.

- It is proven that adjuvant therapy for most patients with gastric cancer is associated with higher cure rate than with surgical resection alone
- Randomized phase III trials support use of either perioperative chemotherapy or adjuvant postoperative chemotherapy combined with chemoradiation

---

Monitoring for recurrence

Surveillance for all patients after potentially curative therapy for gastric cancer is recommended by the NCCN gastric cancer panel.[91] Suggested follow-up studies include only history and physical examination routinely with laboratory studies, endoscopy, and imaging limited to the evaluation of specific symptoms or concerns. This approach is presumably influenced by the relatively limited benefit of any therapy in the recurrent or metastatic setting. It is important to evaluate patients after gastrectomy for nutritional deficiencies, particularly vitamin B_{12}, iron, and calcium.

Management of metastatic disease

Systemic therapy for advanced disease

For patients with advanced, recurrent or metastatic gastric cancer, therapy is mainly palliative. Despite numerous randomized trials, the survival rates in such patients remain poor. Poor performance status or multiple sites of metastases are associated with significantly worse outcomes. An analysis of the SEER registry showed only modest improvements in OS for patients with metastatic disease over the past three decades.[92] The median survival duration in unselected patients diagnosed with metastatic gastric cancer in 2004 was <5 months.[93] The median survival durations reported in clinical trials have ranged from 7 to 10 months. Considering this dismal prognosis, several investigators have examined systemic chemotherapy to evaluate its role for advanced gastric cancer.

Four small random assignment trials assessed the impact of palliative chemotherapy on survival duration and quality of life.[94-97] All four trials reported superior survival in patients receiving treatment when compared with those who received best supportive care (BSC). Those who received BSC had median survival ranging from 3 to 5 months, whereas those who received chemotherapy had median survival ranging from 8 to 12 months. Improvements in symptoms and quality of life were also apparent in the chemotherapy group. These findings are consistent with the fact that gastric cancer is a somewhat chemosensitive disease. Side effects of chemotherapy must be balanced against the potential benefits of it and symptoms associated with unchecked cancer growth. Palliative chemotherapy should be considered for most patients with an adequate performance status and nutritional support.

One difficult and controversial area is therapy for nonevaluable disease in asymptomatic patients (such as those with low-volume abdominal carcinomatosis). Although some advocate the immediate use of chemotherapy, others advise observation. The rationale for observation lies in the fact that only 30–40% of patients will

have an objective response to any particular chemotherapeutic regimen. Delaying treatment until the appearance of early symptoms or evaluable disease may spare patients from experiencing unnecessary toxic effects and preserve their quality of life. These patients should be closely observed with a medical history, physical examination, and CT scans if necessary. Treatment may be initiated when evaluable disease is established or symptoms appear, although if obstructive symptoms occur (due to peritoneal disease) systemic therapy may not be feasible.

A number of combination chemotherapy programs have been developed based on agents with known single agent activity in gastric cancer. One of the pivotal trials compared ECF with FAMTX (5-FU, doxorubicin, and methotrexate).[98] In this phase III trial, 274 patients received treatment. The response rate in the ECF group was 46%, whereas that in the FAMTX group was 21%. Moreover, the median survival duration was longer in the ECF arm (9 months vs 6 months; $p < 0.01$).[99] ECF has also been compared to the combination of mitomycin, cisplatin, and protracted venous infusion 5-FU (MCF) in previously untreated patients with advanced esophagogastric cancer.[100] In that trial, 580 patients received either ECF or MCF. The overall response rate was 42% with ECF and 44% with MCF ($p = 0.69$). There were only two deaths due to toxicity. Median survival was 9.4 months with ECF and 8.7 months with MCF ($p = 0.32$). This study confirmed the response and survival benefits of ECF.

Built on earlier success with the ECF regimen, the phase III study REAL-2 investigated the role of capecitabine and oxaliplatin in gastric and gastroesophageal cancer using a two-by-two design.[101] The study randomly assigned 1002 patients to treatment with either ECF or epirubicin and cisplatin plus capecitabine (ECX) or treatment with either epirubicin and oxaliplatin plus fluorouracil (EOF) or epirubicin and oxaliplatin plus capecitabine (EOX). Approximately 65% of patients had carcinoma of stomach or GEJ, and 88% had adenocarcinoma histology. Response rates and median OS were 41% and 9.9 months for ECF, 46% and 9.9 months for ECX, 42% and 9.3 months for EOF, and 48% and 11.2 months for EOX. Investigators concluded noninferiority of capecitabine compared to 5-FU and oxaliplatin compared to cisplatin. These findings were further confirmed in two phase III studies investigating the role of capecitabine or oxaliplatin in gastric cancer. In one study, 220 patients were randomly assigned to treatment with infusional 5-FU and leucovorin plus cisplatin (FLP) or 5-FU and leucovorin plus oxaliplatin (FLO).[102] While the response rates were higher in the FLO arm (34% vs 25%; $p < 0.01$), differences in time to progression were not statistically significant. A second contemporaneous phase III study compared cisplatin plus capecitabine (XP) and cisplatin plus 5-FU (FP).[103] Three-hundred-sixteen patients were randomly assigned to XP or FP. The response rate was higher in the XP group (41% vs 29%; $p = 0.03$). There were, however, no significant differences in progression-free survival (PFS) or OS.

Docetaxel-based chemotherapy regimens have also been extensively studied in patients with gastric cancer. A randomized phase III trial compared the combination of docetaxel, cisplatin, and 5-FU (DCF) with 5-FU plus cisplatin in a study that involved 445 patients.[104] Use of DCF resulted in a superior response rate (37% vs 25%; $p = 0.01$), PFS (median 5.6 months vs 3.4 months; $p < 0.01$) and OS (median 9.2 months vs 8.6 months; $p = 0.02$). However, the DCF regimen resulted in substantial treatment-related toxic effects. Specifically, 82% of the patients had grade 3/4 neutropenia, and 69% of the patients had at least one grade 3/4 treatment-related adverse event.

S-1 has been tested for efficacy in the advanced gastric cancer setting in several trials using differing combinations. Japanese investigators tested the combination of S-1 and cisplatin in a phase III trial (SPIRITS).[105] In this study, 305 patients were randomly assigned to treatment with S-1 or S-1 plus cisplatin. Response rate (54% vs 31%), PFS (median, 6 months vs 4 months; $p < 0.01$), and OS (median, 13 months vs 11 months; $p = 0.04$) were superior in the combination arm. Again, the toxicity profile of S-1 differs between Asian and Western patients due to differences in pharmacokinetics. A global phase III study which enrolled over 1000 patients compared S-1 or 5-FU plus cisplatin using a lower dose of S-1 and different schedule. Unfortunately, the study failed to achieve its primary endpoint of superior OS.[106]

Irinotecan in combination with 5-FU (IF) was compared to cisplatin and 5-FU (CF) in chemonaive patients with adenocarcinoma of the stomach or GEJ.[107] In this study, IF did not prolong OS over CF and the results of noninferiority of IF were borderline. Irinotecan plus S1 also failed to prolong OS compared with S-1 alone in a Japanese study.[108] However, a recent phase III trial of 416 patients reported the median time to treatment failure (TTF) was significantly longer with FOLFIRI than with ECX (5.1 months vs 4.2 months; $p < 0.01$).[109] There were no differences in PFS, median OS (9.5 months vs 9.7 months), or response rates. The irinotecan and 5-FU combination is an acceptable first-line regimen.

In the second-line setting, three agents have been shown to improve survival over BSC. The Arbeitgemeinschaft Internistische Onkologie (AIO) study compared irinotecan with BSC to BSC alone in patients with advanced gastric or GEJ adenocarcinoma.[110] Irinotecan showed an OS advantage over BSC. In the COUGAR-02 study, 186 patients were randomized to docetaxel with BSC versus BSC alone. The chemotherapy group had a median OS of 5.2 months compared to 3.6 months in the BSC group ($p = 0.01$).[111]

Molecularly targeted agents

Despite the incorporation of newer agents, the median survival of patients with advanced gastric cancer remains <1 year using cytotoxic chemotherapy. The addition of targeted agents has resulted in modest improvements in OS, PFS, and response rate. Molecular targeted agents are also being explored in the second-line setting. One of the most extensively studied receptors is the *EGFR* family. Several studies have investigated the addition of *EGFR* inhibitors to cytotoxic chemotherapy. Initial phase II trials had produced promising results. However, phase III trials rendered disappointing results. In the EXPAND trial, the addition of cetuximab (a chimeric monoclonal antibody (mAb) against *EGFR* to capecitabine and cisplatin (XP) provided no additional benefit over XP alone.[112] Furthermore, panitumumab (a fully humanized mAb against *EGFR*) resulted in worse OS of 8.8 months versus 11.3 months when added to epirubicin, oxaliplatin, and capecitabine (EOC) versus EOC alone.[113] The use of these two agents in gastric cancer is not recommended.

More promising results have been reported for other agents. *HER2/neu* (also a member of the *EGFR* family) is overexpressed in 20% of gastric and 30% of GEJ cancers. This receptor has been shown to be a key target for the treatment of these tumors. Trastuzumab (a humanized mAb) has been shown to prolong survival when added to chemotherapy with increase in OS from 11.1 to 13.8 months ($p < 0.01$).[114] As in other solid tumors, angiogenesis has been shown to be an important part of gastric cancer progression. Bevacizumab, a *VEGF* inhibitor, was studied in a phase III trial.[115] A total of 774 patients with advanced gastric or gastroesophageal cancer were randomized to receive bevacizumab or placebo plus cisplatin and capecitabine. The median OS was 12.1 months in the triple therapy group versus 10.1 months in the placebo group ($p < 0.01$). The PFS (6.7 months vs 5.3 months) and

response rate (46% vs 37%) were also improved in the bevacizumab group. However, the study did not reach its primary endpoint. Further subgroup analysis revealed that North and Latin American patients appeared to have a survival benefit with the addition of bevacizumab (median 11.5 months vs 6.8 months compared to placebo), whereas patients enrolled in Asia (90% from Japan and Korea) appeared to have no benefit. European patients had intermediate results.

The REGARD trial, a randomized phase III trial comparing ramucirumab versus placebo for patients with advanced, pretreated gastric cancer, was recently published.[116] Ramucirumab, a mAb that binds *VEGF-R2* and prevents its activation, improved OS over placebo (5.2 months vs 3.8 months, $p = 0.05$). The addition of paclitaxel to ramucirumab versus paclitaxel alone in a subsequent trial, the RAINBOW trial, has also shown a survival advantage of ramucirumab in advanced gastric cancer.[117] In that study, 665 patients were assigned to receive paclitaxel plus placebo or paclitaxel plus ramucirumab. The median OS was significantly longer in the ramucirumab plus paclitaxel group (9.6 months vs 7.4 months, $p = 0.02$). This combination has been proposed as the new standard second-line treatment for patients with advanced gastric cancer.

Other studies with targeted agents in pretreated patients with metastatic gastric cancer have been disappointing. The GRANITE-1 study randomized 656 patients to everolimus with BSC versus placebo with BSC.[118] Everolimus did not improve OS (median 5.4 months with everolimus and 4.3 months with placebo). Similarly, lapatinib was added to paclitaxel versus paclitaxel alone in 420 patients with *HER2/neu* positive gastric cancer.[119] Median OS was 11.0 months in the lapatinib and paclitaxel group versus 8.9 months in the paclitaxel alone group ($p = 0.21$). Despite different treatment strategies and incorporation of new targeted agents with standard chemotherapy, the outcome of patients with advanced gastric cancer remains poor; further research is certainly needed.

Supportive care

Patients with gastric cancer may present with symptoms including bleeding, obstruction, pain, early satiety, and weight loss. The indications for surgical resection of gastric cancer must be carefully considered in terms of intent of operation, whether for potential cure or palliation of symptoms or other cancer-related problems. Severe symptoms in patients without metastatic disease may prompt the decision to proceed with gastrectomy first followed by adjuvant therapy. For 307 patients with gastric cancer who underwent noncurative resection at Memorial Sloan-Kettering Cancer Center, roughly half of the patients had a truly palliative resection, most commonly for bleeding (20%), obstruction (43%), or pain (29%)..[120] In patients with metastatic disease, palliative gastrectomy is associated with high postoperative mortality (14%) and complications (27%).[121] In recent series, mortality has decreased to <5%, but caution remains important. Surgical bypass is also associated with high mortality in the palliative setting and frequently fails to achieve the desired benefit.[122,123]

When considering palliative resection, the surgeon should explicitly determine the degree of patient symptoms. For instance, while a patient with complete obstruction may only benefit from intervention such as resection, bypass, or endoscopic stenting, symptoms of incomplete obstruction may improve in up to 80% of patients with the use of chemotherapy.[124] Therefore, obstruction may be a relative indication for procedure rather than absolute. Pain in patients with gastric cancer may be caused by invasion of the celiac plexus, intestinal obstruction, or bone metastases. Obstruction can further confound the problem of pain management. In the absence of obstruction, short and long-acting oral narcotics are appropriate for pain. However, if obstruction is present, other methods must be employed.

Massive life-threatening bleeding may be treated with arterial embolization or endoscopy; however, resection may be required to control hemorrhage in some cases. Patients with significant bleeding from gastric cancer should be considered for resection, but without complete staging evaluation, one must be prepared that intraoperative findings of metastatic disease may change the intent of operation. In the metastatic setting, physicians must decide whether patients who are bleeding massively are surgical candidates and, if not, focus on BSC. Occasionally, endoscopic and embolization maneuvers can provide the necessary time to have these often difficult discussions. For patients who are experiencing slow oozing and need a transfusion every 1–2 weeks, endoscopy may be successful. Several series have indicated that 50–75% of patients experience improvement of bleeding, gastric outlet obstruction, and pain with chemoradiation.[125,126]

Treatment options for obstruction include laser recanalization, stenting, radiotherapy, bypass, drainage tubes, and resection. The technology of expandable stents has grown dramatically over the past two decades. Dormann reviewed 136 publications reporting the use of self-expanding metal stents for gastroduodenal malignancies in 32 case series and reported stent placement to be technically successful in over 90% of patients with no procedure-related mortality and a relatively low number of complications.[127] Relief of symptoms may be temporary; in 18% of cases, the stent became occluded secondary to tumor ingrowth. Generally, patients with malignant gastric outlet obstruction due to unresectable primary or metastatic cancers have poor survival (median around 2 months), but interventions such as endoscopic stenting or surgical bypass are associated with acceptable postprocedure quality of life.[128] In our opinion, surgical bypass should be considered for patients with high performance status and longer life expectancy. Patients with short length, single sites of obstruction located in the pylorus or early duodenum are excellent candidates for endoscopic stenting. Patients with poor performance status, rapidly progressive cancer, carcinomatosis, malignant ascites, multiple sites of obstruction, and very short life expectancy may be best served by percutaneous gastrostomy or no intervention.

Unmet needs and future directions

There are many opportunities for clinicians and researchers to develop improvements for the care of patients with gastric cancer. Many exciting studies have been published in recent years examining novel ways to improve outcomes, such as intravenous lidocaine infusion to improve postoperative pain control,[129] sentinel node mapping,[130,131] early postoperative enteral immunonutrition,[132] and improved pathologic staging through use of surgical *ex vivo* dissection.[133] Further advancements must continue to build upon the foundation of our collective understanding of the molecular pathogenesis of gastric cancers and robust high-quality clinical outcomes and comparative effectiveness research.

In the area of prevention and screening, several questions remain. Should we promote widespread efforts at *H. pylori* eradication? Should screening programs with upper endoscopy be developed for higher risk patients in the West? In terms of proper staging of gastric cancers, we have not yet defined which patients most benefit from pretreatment EUS or PET. With many methods available for surgical removal of gastric cancers including EMR and minimally invasive operations, developing widely accepted standards for the conduct of procedures, large registries, and public reporting of preoperative quality and long-term oncologic

outcomes is imperative. While some decisions such as palliative gastrectomy will always require an individualized approach, other considerations such as extent of lymphadenectomy may be best defined by evidence and best practice rather than individual surgeon bias.

Which patients should be chosen for the two basic adjuvant therapy strategies of preoperative chemotherapy or postoperative chemoradiation is not clear. Also, for patients who do not respond or progress after preoperative chemotherapy, what therapy should be given postoperatively, an alternate chemotherapy regimen or chemoradiation? Such questions regarding best therapy are only part of the puzzle. Management of challenging postoperative symptoms such as delayed gastric emptying or poor stomach function is ripe for novel research. There are many unmet needs in gastric cancer but, fortunately, there is high interest in ongoing research.

Conclusions

Fortunately, the incidence of gastric cancer is decreasing around the world. However, outcomes for many remain poor and overall cure rates low. Despite encouraging progress in all areas of gastric cancer treatment (surgery, chemotherapy, and radiation), many patients with gastric cancer still suffer symptoms, decreased HRQOL and will die eventually of disease despite best therapy. For the future, we must hope the ability to define at-risk populations will facilitate development of cost-effective screening programs and preventive measures. As we enter the age of molecular targeted therapy and personalized medicine, improvements in our understanding of molecular biology and molecular classification of gastric cancer may lead to the rational development of novel therapeutic strategies. The authors have a realistic hope that in our lifetime the landscape of gastric cancer will change such that most people are cured after therapy.

Key references

The complete reference list can be found on the Wiley Companion Digital Edition of this title (see inside front cover for login instructions).

7 Ford AC, Forman D, Hunt RH, Yuan Y, Moayyedi P. *Helicobacter pylori* eradication therapy to prevent gastric cancer in healthy asymptomatic infected individuals: systematic review and meta-analysis of randomised controlled trials. *BMJ* (Clinical research ed.). 2014;**348**:g3174.

14 Caldas C, Carneiro F, Lynch HT, et al. Familial gastric cancer: overview and guidelines for management. *J Med Genet*. 1999;**36**(**12**):873–880.

15 Huntsman DG, Carneiro F, Lewis FR, et al. Early gastric cancer in young, asymptomatic carriers of germ-line E-cadherin mutation. *N Engl J Med*. 2001;**344**(**25**):1904–1909.

20 Lauren P. The two histological main types of gastric carcinoma: diffuse and so-called intestinal-type carcinoma. An attempt at a histoclinical classification. *Acta Pathol Microbiol Scand*. 1965;**64**:31–49.

35 Lee EY, Cibull ML, Strodel WE, Haley JV. Expression of HER-2/neu oncoprotein and epidermal growth factor receptor and prognosis in gastric carcinoma. *Arch Pathol Lab Med*. 1994;**118**(**3**):235–239.

45 Yonemura Y, Endo Y, Fujita H, et al. Role of vascular endothelial growth factor C expression in the development of lymph node metastasis in gastric cancer. *Clin Cancer Res*. 1999;**5**(**7**):1823–1829.

49 Lordick F, Ott K, Krause BJ, et al. PET to assess early metabolic response and to guide treatment of adenocarcinoma of the oesophagogastric junction: the MUNICON phase II trial. *Lancet Oncology*. 2007;**8**(**9**):797–805.

52 Burke EC, Karpeh MS, Conlon KC, Brennan MF. Laparoscopy in the management of gastric adenocarcinoma. *Ann Surg*. 1997;**225**:262–267.

56 Gotoda T. Endoscopic resection of early gastric cancer. *Gastric Cancer*. 2007;**10**(**1**):1–11.

57 Bozzetti F, Marubini E, Bonfanti G, Miceli R, Piano C, Gennari L. Subtotal versus total gastrectomy for gastric cancer. Five year survival rates in a multicenter randomized Italian trial. *Ann Surg*. 1999;**230**:170–178.

62 Siewert J, Bottcher K, Stein H, Roder J, Busch R. Problem of proximal third gastric carcinoma. *World J Surg*. 1995;**19**:523–531.

66 Spector NM, Hicks FD, Pickleman J. Quality of life and symptoms after surgery for gastroesophageal cancer: a pilot study. *Gastroenterol Nurs.* 2002;**25**(3):120–125.

68 Bonenkamp JJ, Hermans J, Sasako M, van de Velde CJ. Extended lymph-node dissection for gastric cancer. Dutch Gastric Cancer Group. *N Engl J Med.* 1999;**340**(12):908–914.

69 Hartgrink HH, van de Velde CJ, Putter H, et al. Extended lymph node dissection for gastric cancer: who may benefit? Final results of the randomized Dutch gastric cancer group trial. *J Clin Oncol.* 2004;**22**(11):2069–2077.

70 Songun I, Putter H, Kranenbarg EM, Sasako M, van de Velde CJ. Surgical treatment of gastric cancer: 15-year follow-up results of the randomised nationwide Dutch D1D2 trial. *Lancet Oncol.* 2010;**11**(5):439–449.

74 Squires MH 3rd, Kooby DA, Pawlik TM, et al. Utility of the proximal margin frozen section for resection of gastric adenocarcinoma: a 7-Institution Study of the US Gastric Cancer Collaborative. *Ann Surg Oncol.* 2014;**21**(13):4202–4210.

78 Lee JH, Lee CM, Son SY, Ahn SH, Park do J, Kim HH. Laparoscopic versus open gastrectomy for gastric cancer: long-term oncologic results. *Surgery.* 2014;**155**(1):154–164.

79 Macdonald JS, Smalley SR, Benedetti J, et al. Chemoradiotherapy after surgery compared with surgery alone for adenocarcinoma of the stomach or gastroesophageal junction. *N Engl J Med.* 2001;**345**(10):725–730.

81 Cunningham D, Allum WH, Stenning SP, et al. Perioperative chemotherapy versus surgery alone for resectable gastroesophageal cancer. *N Engl J Med.* 2006;**355**(1):11–20.

82 Ychou M, Boige V, Pignon JP, et al. Perioperative chemotherapy compared with surgery alone for resectable gastroesophageal adenocarcinoma: an FNCLCC and FFCD multicenter phase III trial. *J Clin Oncol.* 2011;**29**(13):1715–1721.

83 Schuhmacher C, Gretschel S, Lordick F, et al. Neoadjuvant chemotherapy compared with surgery alone for locally advanced cancer of the stomach and cardia: European Organisation for Research and Treatment of Cancer randomized trial 40954. *J Clin Oncol.* 2010;**28**(35):5210–5218.

87 Min C, Bangalore S, Jhawar S, et al. Chemoradiation therapy versus chemotherapy alone for gastric cancer after R0 surgical resection: a meta-analysis of randomized trials. *Oncology.* 2014;**86**(2):79–85.

88 Sakuramoto S, Sasako M, Yamaguchi T, et al. Adjuvant chemotherapy for gastric cancer with S-1, an oral fluoropyrimidine. *N Engl J Med.* 2007;**357**(18):1810–1820.

89 Bang YJ, Kim YW, Yang HK, et al. Adjuvant capecitabine and oxaliplatin for gastric cancer after D2 gastrectomy (CLASSIC): a phase 3 open-label, randomised controlled trial. *Lancet.* 2012;**379**(9813):315–321.

94 Glimelius B, Ekstrom K, Hoffman K, et al. Randomized comparison between chemotherapy plus best supportive care with best supportive care in advanced gastric cancer. *Ann Oncol.* 1997;**8**(2):163–168.

98 Waters JS, Norman A, Cunningham D, et al. Long-term survival after epirubicin, cisplatin and fluorouracil for gastric cancer: results of a randomized trial. *Br J Cancer.* 1999;**80**(1–2):269–272.

101 Cunningham D, Starling N, Rao S, et al. Capecitabine and oxaliplatin for advanced esophagogastric cancer. *N Engl J Med.* 2008;**358**(1):36–46.

104 Van Cutsem E, Moiseyenko VM, Tjulandin S, et al. Phase III study of docetaxel and cisplatin plus fluorouracil compared with cisplatin and fluorouracil as first-line therapy for advanced gastric cancer: a report of the V325 Study Group. *J Clin Oncol.* 2006;**24**(31):4991–4997.

105 Koizumi W, Narahara H, Hara T, et al. S-1 plus cisplatin versus S-1 alone for first-line treatment of advanced gastric cancer (SPIRITS trial): a phase III trial. *Lancet Oncol.* 2008;**9**(3):215–221.

110 Thuss-Patience PC, Kretzschmar A, Bichev D, et al. Survival advantage for irinotecan versus best supportive care as second-line chemotherapy in gastric cancer – a randomised phase III study of the Arbeitsgemeinschaft Internistische Onkologie (AIO). *Eur J Cancer* (Oxford, England : 1990). 2011;**47**(15):2306–2314.

111 Ford HE, Marshall A, Bridgewater JA, et al. Docetaxel versus active symptom control for refractory oesophagogastric adenocarcinoma (COUGAR-02): an open-label, phase 3 randomised controlled trial. *Lancet Oncol.* 2014;**15**(1):78–86.

112 Lordick F, Kang YK, Chung HC, et al. Capecitabine and cisplatin with or without cetuximab for patients with previously untreated advanced gastric cancer (EXPAND): a randomised, open-label phase 3 trial. *Lancet Oncol.* 2013;**14**(6):490–499.

113 Waddell T, Chau I, Cunningham D, et al. Epirubicin, oxaliplatin, and capecitabine with or without panitumumab for patients with previously untreated advanced oesophagogastric cancer (REAL3): a randomised, open-label phase 3 trial. *Lancet Oncol.* 2013;**14**(6):481–489.

114 Bang YJ, Van Cutsem E, Feyereislova A, et al. Trastuzumab in combination with chemotherapy versus chemotherapy alone for treatment of HER2-positive advanced gastric or gastro-oesophageal junction cancer (ToGA): a phase 3, open-label, randomised controlled trial. *Lancet.* 2010;**376**(9742):687–697.

117 Wilke H, Muro K, Van Cutsem E, et al. Ramucirumab plus paclitaxel versus placebo plus paclitaxel in patients with previously treated advanced gastric or gastro-oesophageal junction adenocarcinoma (RAINBOW): a double-blind, randomised phase 3 trial. *Lancet Oncol.* 2014;**15**(11):1224–1235.

118 Ohtsu A, Ajani JA, Bai YX, et al. Everolimus for previously treated advanced gastric cancer: results of the randomized, double-blind, phase III GRANITE-1 study. *J Clin Oncol.* 2013;**31**(31):3935–3943.

119 Satoh T, Xu RH, Chung HC, et al. Lapatinib plus paclitaxel versus paclitaxel alone in the second-line treatment of HER2-amplified advanced gastric cancer in Asian populations: TyTAN – a randomized, phase III study. *J Clin Oncol.* 2014;**32**(19):2039–2049.

120 Miner TJ, Jaques DP, Karpeh MS, Brennan MF. Defining palliative surgery in patients receiving noncurative resections for gastric cancer. *J Am Coll Surg.* 2004;**198**(6):1013–1021.

121 Lasithiotakis K, Antoniou SA, Antoniou GA, Kaklamanos I, Zoras O. Gastrectomy for stage IV gastric cancer. a systematic review and meta-analysis. *Anticancer Res.* 2014;**34**(5):2079–2085.

127 Dormann A, Meisner S, Verin N, Wenk LA. Self-expanding metal stents for gastroduodenal malignancies: systematic review of their clinical effectiveness. *Endoscopy.* 2004;**36**(6):543–550.

91 Primary neoplasms of the liver

Junichi Shindoh, MD, PhD ▪ *Kristoffer W. Brudvik, MD, PhD* ▪ *Jean-Nicolas Vauthey, MD*

Overview

Primary liver cancer is the second leading cause of cancer death in men and the sixth leading cause among women. Hepatocellular carcinoma (HCC) constitutes 70–85% of primary hepatic neoplasms, followed by intrahepatic cholangiocarcinoma (ICC) (10–15%) and other less common hepatic malignancies (5%) such as hepatic angiosarcoma, epithelioid hemangioendothelioma, or hepatic lymphoma. Primary hepatic malignancies are generally associated with poor survival, and only a limited evidence of systemic therapy have been available, prevention, surveillance, early diagnosis, and multidisciplinary treatment approach are important factors to maximize treatment outcomes. In addition, most of the primary hepatic neoplasms are associated with chronic liver disease or cirrhosis, and the decreased hepatic functional reserve often precludes aggressive treatment for tumors. Therefore, for treatment selection, one should consider two intrinsic conflicting factors, curability and safety of treatment. Currently, several clinical staging systems and treatment algorithms are available to adequately select therapeutic options for HCC. The choice of therapy is individualized based on the tumor burden, degree of underlying liver disease, patient performance status, and the overall possibility of side effects or complications balanced with acceptable results. Selection of treatment should be determined in a multidisciplinary approach with the local expertise. The most curative treatment options including surgical resection, radiofrequency ablation, and orthotopic liver transplantation (OLT) should be the first priority as long as such treatments are approved. For the other hepatic malignancies, only limited clinical evidence is available and surgical resection or OLT is considered as the first-line treatment.

The liver is a specific site where all the visceral venous flow passes through before it reaches the heart. Therefore, the liver is the most common site of metastases from gastrointestinal malignancies which is termed secondary hepatic neoplasms. However, tumors can also arise from the cells within the liver and are termed primary hepatic neoplasms. Of the primary hepatic neoplasms, hepatocellular carcinoma (HCC) is the most common malignancy constituting 70–85% of the primary liver cancer, followed by intrahepatic cholangiocarcinoma (ICC) (10–15%) and other less common hepatic malignancies (5%) such as hepatic angiosarcoma, epithelioid hemangioendothelioma (EHE) or hemangiopericytoma, or hepatic lymphoma. Because primary hepatic malignancies are generally associated with poor survival and only a limited evidence of systemic therapy have been available, early diagnosis and multidisciplinary treatment approach are of most importance to expect favorable long-term outcomes. This chapter will review and discuss the clinical features and current treatment approaches for HCC, ICC, and the other less common primary liver cancers.

Hepatocellular carcinoma

Incidence and epidemiology

Primary liver cancer is the fifth most common cancer in men and the seventh in women, and the second leading cause of cancer death in men and the sixth leading cause among women, with about 695,500 deaths annually worldwide.[1] Nearly 85% of the cases occur in developing countries especially in sub-Saharan Africa and in East and Southeast Asia, with typical incidence rates of >20 per 100,000 individuals. The incidence rates are generally lowest in developed countries, with the exception of Japan where hepatitis C virus (HCV) infection is the most common cause for HCC.

Globally, the incidence of HCC is increasing in areas with historically low rates, including parts of Oceania, Central Europe, and North America.[2,3] A study reported in 2009 indicated that age-adjusted incidence rates of HCC tripled between 1975 and 2005 in the United States from 1.6 to 4.9 per 100,000 people.[2] In contrast, the incidences of liver cancer are decreasing in historically high-risk areas, such as China and Singapore, most likely due to reduction in hepatitis B virus (HBV) infection through improved public health.

The rates of HCC are more than twice as high in men as in women across geographic regions.[4] The incidence of HCC increases with age, although the age threshold varies among countries because of differences in predominant etiologies for HCC. The age threshold for HCC is generally younger when the predominant risk factor is vertical transmission of HBV (e.g., Southeast Asia and Africa), and older where acquired HCV infection during adulthood is the most common cause of HCC (e.g., Japan and United States).

Risk factors

Cirrhosis is the main risk factor and present in 80–90% of patients with HCC. It is hypothesized that chronic hepatocellular injury and inflammation from a variety of causes lead to cirrhosis and HCC as a result of hepatocyte regeneration and hyperplasia predisposing to mutations and malignant transformation.

Viral hepatitis (HBV and HCV)

It has been estimated that 75–80% of HCC are associated with chronic infections with HBV (50–55%) or HCV (25–30%).[5] Transmission of HBV occurs during delivery (vertical transmission), blood transfusions, sexual intercourse, or intravenous drug abuse. Transmission of HCV can also occur via parenteral exposure, however, primarily through blood transfusions and intravenous drug abuse.

HBV is a double-stranded DNA virus and chronic infection to HBV is the most common etiology for HCC, especially in China and Korea. Patients with positive hepatitis B surface antigen (HBsAg)

Holland-Frei Cancer Medicine, Ninth Edition. Edited by Robert C. Bast Jr., Carlo M. Croce, William N. Hait, Waun Ki Hong, Donald W. Kufe, Martine Piccart-Gebhart, Raphael E. Pollock, Ralph R. Weichselbaum, Hongyang Wang, and James F. Holland.
© 2017 John Wiley & Sons, Inc. ISBN: 978-1-118-93469-2

are at high risk of developing cirrhosis and HCC. However, it has been reported that those who are positive for anti-hepatitis B core antibodies (HBcAb) are also at high risk for HCC even when HBs-Ag is serologically negative.[6] In contrast to HCV-related HCC which usually arises in the liver with severe fibrosis or cirrhosis, approximately 20% of HBV-related HCC occurs in the absence of cirrhotic changes. A direct mutagenic effect that causes carcinogenesis has been postulated for HBV. Integration of HBV DNA in the host genome adjacent to cellular oncogenes or transactivating effect of the HBx protein on cellular gene expression may be attributable to the development of HCC without cirrhosis.[7–9] In fact, HBV-DNA integration has been detected in hepatocytes before tumor development among patients positive for HBsAg, which may enhance chromosomal instability and facilitate HCC development.[10,11]

HCV is a small, single-stranded RNA virus. The prevalence of HCV infection varies widely according to geographical areas. A meta-analysis of 21 case–control studies reported that HCC risk was 17 times higher among HCV-positive individuals as compared to HCV-negative individuals.[12] It has been suggested that oxidative stress is one of the mechanisms involved in inflammation-related carcinogenesis in patients infected with HCV.[13] In response to viral antigens, the activated macrophages and other recruited leukocytes release reactive oxygen species, causing areas of focal necrosis and compensatory cell division.[14] When these oxidants overwhelm the antioxidant defenses of neighboring cells, damages to biomolecules, particularly to oncogenes or tumor suppressor genes, may increase the carcinogenic potential of the underlying liver. HCV displays a high genetic variability. On the basis of nucleotide sequence homology, whole-sequenced HCV isolates are classified as genotype 1a, 1b, 2a, and 2b. The geographic distribution of these genotypes demonstrated that genotypes 1a, 1b, and 2a are predominant in Western countries and East Asia, whereas genotype 2b is predominant in the Middle East.[15] The HCV genotype 1b is reportedly more aggressive and more closely associated with advanced chronic liver diseases such as liver cirrhosis and HCC. However, these observations can be partially explained by the refractoriness to antiviral therapy, and recent studies have reported that lower HCV viral load is correlated with improved survival outcomes after surgical resection of HCC irrespective of the genotypes of HCV.[16,17]

Alcohol

Excessive alcohol consumption is a major risk factor for chronic liver disease and HCC, causing various degrees of liver damage from simple fat accumulation to cirrhosis. Various studies have concluded that excessive alcohol intake is an important risk factor for HCC development. A US case–control study demonstrated approximately threefold increase in HCC risk among individuals with heavy alcohol consumption defined as more than 60 ml ethanol per day.[18] HCC rarely develops in the absence of cirrhosis; however, the risk is increased with concurrent HBV or HCV infection.[19,20] A meta-analysis of 20 studies published between 1995 and 2004 that involved more than 15,000 patients with chronic HCV infection reported that the pooled relative risk of cirrhosis associated with heavy alcohol intake was 2.33, compared with no or low-quantity alcohol intake.[19] Therefore, alcohol consumption should be avoided among patients with viral hepatitis.

Aflatoxins

Aflatoxins (AFs) are potent hepatocarcinogens produced by *Aspergillus flavus* and *Aspergillus parasiticus* that grow readily on foods such as corn and peanuts stored in warm, damp conditions. There are four AF compounds: B_1, B_2, G_1, and G_2, and the most common and most toxic AF compound is AFB_1. When ingested, AFB_1 is metabolized to a highly active 8,9-epoxide metabolite, which can bind to and damage DNA. A consistent genetic mutation in codon 249 in the tumor suppressor p53 gene has been identified and positively correlated with AF exposure.[21,22] Although AFB_1 contributes to hepatocarcinogenesis, its role in pathogenesis of HCC is primarily mediated by its synergic effects on chronic hepatitis B because the areas where AFB_1 exposure is an environmental problem also have a high prevalence of chronic HBV infection. A prospective study from China showed that urinary excretion of AF metabolites was associated with increased risk for HCC up to fourfold, and HBV infection independently increased the risk sevenfold. However, the patients who excreted AFB_1 metabolites and had concomitant infection of HBV showed a 60-fold increase in risk of development of HCC.[23] These results suggest that prevention of HBV-related HCC would reduce the effects of AF on HCC risk.

Obesity

It is well established that obesity is significantly associated with a wide spectrum of hepatobiliary diseases, including fatty liver diseases, steatosis, steatohepatitis, and cryptogenic cirrhosis.[24,25] In a large prospective cohort study of more than 900,000 individuals in the United States followed up for a 16-year period, liver cancer mortality rates were five times greater among men with the greatest baseline body mass index (range, 35–40) compared with those with a normal body mass index, whereas the risk of liver cancer was not as increased in women, with a relative risk of 1.68.[26] Two other population-based studies from Northern Europe have also shown that obesity is correlated with increased HCC risk.[27,28]

Diabetes mellitus

Recently, diabetes has been recognized as a risk factor for chronic liver disease and HCC. Although adjustment of potential biases in cross-sectional and case–control studies is difficult, several studies have clearly demonstrated positive correlation between diabetes and HCC.[29–33] The postulated mechanisms for liver cell damage induced by type 2 diabetes mellitus involve insulin resistance and hyperinsulinemia.[34,35] Hyperinsulinemia reportedly reduces liver synthesis and blood levels of insulin growth factor-binding protein-1 (IGFBP-1), which increases (1) bioavailability of insulin-like growth factor-1 (IGF-1), (2) promotion of cellular proliferation, and (3) inhibition of apoptosis.[36] Excessive insulin binds to insulin receptor and activates its intrinsic tyrosine kinase, leading to phosphorylation of insulin receptor substrate-1 (IRS-1),[37] and hyperinsulinemia is also associated with production of reactive oxygen species, which may cause damage to DNA. Overexpression of IRS-1 is associated with decreased apoptosis, which is mediated by transforming growth factor β.[38] Given these evidences in basic researches and pathologic observation that HCC tumor cells overexpress both IGF-1 and IRS-1,[39] diabetes mellitus seems to contribute to liver cell damage and development of HCC.

Hemochromatosis

Hemochromatosis is an autosomal recessive genetic disorder of iron metabolism, with a prevalence rate of 2–5 per 1000 in the Caucasian population. In this inherited disorder, mutations have been documented in the *HFE* gene on chromosome 6 (Cys282Tyr [*C282Y*] and His63Asp [*H63D*]), the *HFR-2* gene on chromosome 1, and the *HFE-3* gene on chromosome 7. The *C282Y* mutation is the most commonly detected mutation and *C282Y* homozygotes or *C282Y/H63D* compound heterozygotes[40–42] is associated with increased absorption of dietary iron and accumulation in tissues such as the skin, heart, and liver, resulting in heart failure or liver cirrhosis.

There is growing evidence that even mild accumulation of iron is harmful to the liver, especially when other hepatotoxic factors such as chronic viral hepatitis or heavy alcohol intake are present. Iron enhances the pathogenicity of microorganisms, adversely affects the function of macrophages and lymphocytes, and enhances fibrogenic pathways.[43] A synergistic relationship between HCV infection and iron overload has been suggested,[44] and iron depletion has been reported to improve liver function tests in patients with chronic hepatitis C.[45] Although diagnosis of hemochromatosis is relatively difficult, treatment with therapeutic phlebotomy or iron chelation therapy before onset of cirrhosis may be effective in preventing the development of cirrhosis and HCC in these patients.

α_1-Antitrypsin deficiency

α_1-Antitrypsin deficiency (AATD) is an autosomal dominant disorder with mutations in the serine protease inhibitor (Pi) gene. Over 75 different Pi alleles have been identified, most of which are not associated with the disease,[46] and a relationship exists between Pi phenotypes and serum concentrations of α_1-antitrypsin. Typical clinical presentation of patients with AATD includes emphysema, hepatic necroinflammation, cirrhosis, and HCC. Because no effective medical treatment is available, liver transplantation is indicated for patients with decompensated cirrhosis in correcting the underlying metabolic disorder.

Other potential risk factors

The higher incidence of HCC reported in men compared to women suggest the influence of hormonal factors on hepatocarcinogenesis. Long-term use of oral contraceptives has been thought to be a potential risk factors for HCC; however, a review of 12 case–control studies have yielded an overall adjusted odds ratio of 1.6 (95% CI, 0.9–2.5),[47] and the correlation between the oral contraceptives and risk for HCC remains inconclusive.

Hypothyroidism has also been reported to be a potential risk factor for HCC especially in women.[48,49] Patients with hypothyroidism may experience weight gain[50] and insulin resistance,[51,52] both of which are significant factors for nonalcoholic steatohepatitis. Although the actual mechanism is unclear and only limited clinical evidence is available, development of chronic liver disease and hepatocarcinogenesis might be influenced by these hormonal factors to some extent.

Prevention

Prevention of HCC is highly dependent on avoiding the risk factors, adequate treatment for the underlying chronic liver disease, and early diagnosis of precursor lesions. Because the most common cause of HCC is cirrhosis associated with viral hepatitis, prevention of infection to HBV/HCV and treatment of chronic hepatitis with antiviral therapy are of most importance in cancer prevention.

For hepatitis B, parenteral exposure is the most common cause of transmission in developing countries and improvements in hygiene conditions and public education are essential to avoid viral transmission. In addition, vaccination and effective antiviral therapy are currently available for HBV. After the initiation of HBV vaccination, significant declines in the incidence of HCC have been documented in high-risk countries such as Taiwan.[53] When HBV infection has been established, various effective antiviral agents are currently available and reduction of viral load has reportedly correlated with reduced risk of HCC and improved survival outcomes in patients with chronic hepatitis B.[54–56]

For hepatitis C, interferon (IFN)-based combination treatment has been the standard of care and reduction of HCC risk has been shown especially in patients who achieved sustained viral response (SVR).[57–60] However, genetic variability of HCV highly affects the effectiveness of antiviral therapies. Although only a few clinical evidences are available, recently introduced new direct-acting antiviral agents (DAAs) have dramatically improved virologic response rate and will likely contribute to prevent HCC among patients with chronic hepatitis C in the near future.[61–63]

Pathology

The malignant transformation of hepatocytes to HCC is considered as a multistep process associated with genetic mutations, allelic losses, epigenetic alterations, and perturbation of molecular cellular pathways. However, the molecular process of carcinogenesis in HCC is poorly understood. The phenotypic expression of these potential multistep changes can be manifested by precursor lesions that can be distinguishable from surrounding regenerative nodules associated with cirrhosis with regard to size, color, texture, and degree of bulging of the cut surface. Changes in the tumor blood supply correspond to each step of the multistep process, from precursor lesions to classical HCC, and helps differential diagnosis on dynamic studies in CT or MRI (Figure 1).

Dysplastic nodules

It is commonly accepted that there is a stepwise progression from cirrhotic nodule to HCC. A unified nomenclature of such liver nodules has recently been reviewed by the International Working Party of the World Congress of Gastroenterology.[64] Dysplastic nodule (DN) is a distinct nodular lesion >5 mm in diameter and subclassified into low-grade dysplastic nodule (LGDN) and high-grade dysplastic nodule (HGDN). LGDNs show only mild dysplasia without architectural atypia, whereas HGDNs are characterized by architectural and/or cytologic atypia, which is insufficient for a diagnosis of HCC. HGDNs often show increased cell density with an irregular trabecular pattern. Small cell change (small cell dysplasia) is the most frequently seen form of cytologic atypia in HGDNs.

Early HCC

Early HCCs are vaguely nodular up to around 2 cm in diameter and are characterized by various combinations of the following major histologic features.[64]

1. Increased cell density more than two times that of the surrounding tissue, with an increased nuclear/cytoplasm ratio and irregular thin-trabecular pattern.
2. Varying numbers of portal tracts within the nodule (intratumoral portal tracts).
3. Pseudoglandular pattern.
4. Diffuse fatty change.
5. Varying numbers of unpaired arteries.

Distinguishing early HCCs from HGDNs is an unresolved challenge. Stromal invasion, defined as the presence of tumor cells invading into the portal tracts or fibrous septa, has been proposed as the most relevant feature discerning early HCC from HGDN. However, such feature may be difficult to identify, especially on biopsy specimens. In that context, a panel of three immunohistochemical markers of malignant transformation, heat shock protein 70, glutamine synthetase, and glypican 3, has been used to distinguish HCCs from HGDNs as well as CK 7 immunostaining for recognition of stromal invasion in early HCC.[65,66]

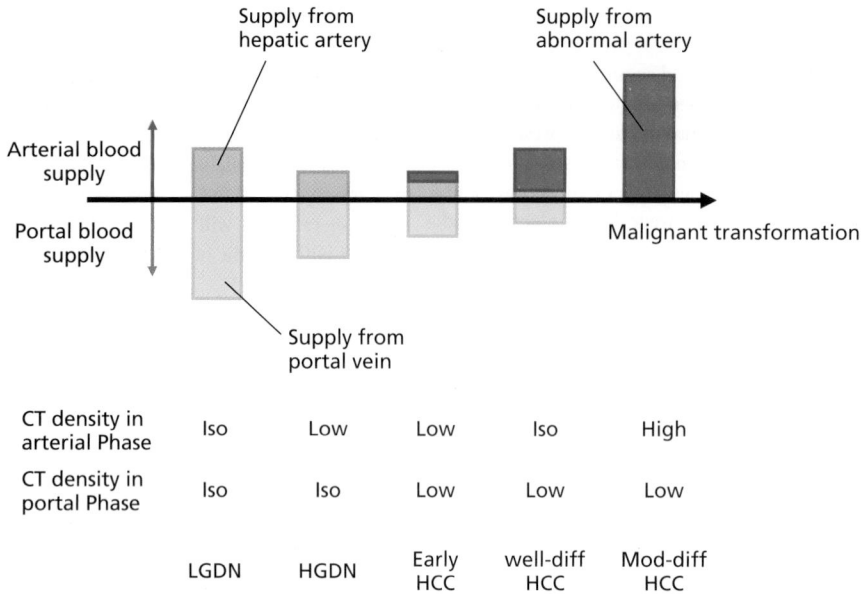

Figure 1 **A model of dynamic changes in blood supply from precursor lesions to classical hepatocellular carcinoma**. Dynamic changes in arterial and portal supply and exponential increase in abnormal arterial supply correlate with the typical patterns of enhancement in dynamic CT or MRI. *Abbreviations*: LGDN, low-grade dysplastic nodule; HGDN, high-grade dysplastic nodule; HCC, hepatocellular carcinoma; well-diff, well differentiated; mod-diff, moderately differentiated.

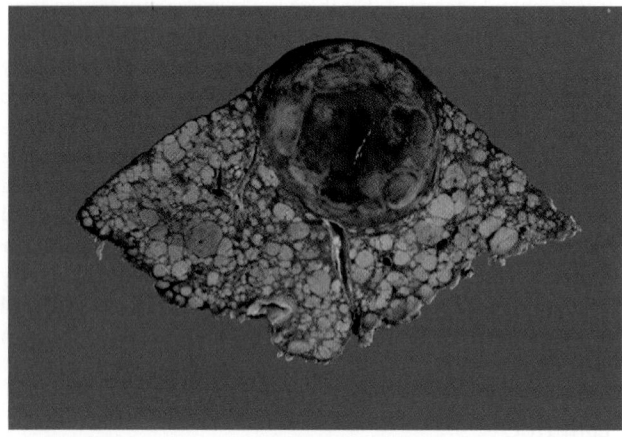

Figure 2 Gross appearance of hepatocellular carcinoma.

Macroscopic presentation of HCC

HCC forms a soft mass with a heterogeneous macroscopic appearance, polychrome with foci of hemorrhage or necrosis (Figure 2). Grossly, three main growth patterns that were described by Eggel in 1901 remain widely used.[67] The *nodular* type consists of well-circumscribed tumor nodules. *Massive* HCCs are circumscribed, huge tumor masses occupying most or all of a hepatic lobe. This type is commonly observed in patients without cirrhosis. The *diffuse* type is rare and characterized by innumerable indistinct small nodules studding the entire liver. The different patterns of growth are associated with various risks of spread, both intrahepatic and extrahepatic.[68] The Liver Cancer Study Group of Japan (LCSGJ) has proposed a modification, with the nodular category being divided into three subtypes: single nodular subtype, single nodular subtype with perinodular tumor growth, and confluent multinodular subtype.[69]

Multicentricity of tumor is noted in 16–74% of HCCs resected in cirrhotic livers.[68–72] Although it is sometimes difficult to distinguish intrahepatic metastases from HCCs generated by multicentric

neocarcinogenesis, tumor nodules are considered as intrahepatic metastases when (1) they show a portal vein tumor thrombus or grow contiguously with a thrombus, (2) multiple small satellite nodules surrounding a larger main tumor, or (3) a single lesion is adjacent to the main tumor but is significantly smaller in size and presents the same histology.[73]

Vascular invasion and formation of tumor thrombus are frequently observed especially in poorly differentiated HCC or large tumor. The portal vein is the most common site of vascular invasion, followed by hepatic veins, biliary tract, and hepatic arteries. The degree of tumor extension through the vascular structure is closely associated with prognosis. When a portal vein tumor thrombus extends up to the left or right portal pedicle (Vp3) or main portal trunk (Vp4), most patients develop recurrence and die within 2 years after surgery.[74]

Microscopic presentation of HCC

Grading of HCC has relied on Edmondson and Steiner classification for many years, which divided HCC into four grades from I to IV on the basis of histological differentiation.[75] Tumors with well-differentiated neoplastic hepatocytes arranged in thin trabeculae correspond to grade I. The larger and more atypical neoplastic cells are sometimes organized in an acinar pattern in grade II. Architectural and cytologic anaplasia are prominent in grade III, but the neoplastic cells are readily identified as hepatocytic in origin. When composed of markedly anaplastic neoplastic cells not readily identified as hepatocytic origin, the tumor is classified as grade IV.

Histologic variants of HCC

Fibrolamellar HCC

Fibrolamellar variant is a rare entity accounting for <1% of all cases of primary liver cancer, which is commonly encountered in young population without chronic liver disease. Fibrolamellar carcinomas are firm, sharply demarcated, and usually single tumors, ranging from 5 cm to over 20 cm. Histologically, it is characterized by the presence of lamellar stromal bands surrounding nests of large polygonal eosinophilic tumor cells with prominent nucleoli. Intensive surgical approaches have been reported to offer a chance of long-term survival despite occurrence of extrahepatic recurrences for patients with fibrolamellar HCC.[76]

Combined HCC and cholangiocarcinoma

Combined HCC and cholangiocarcinoma (HCC-CC) contain unequivocal elements of both HCC and ICC. These tumors show variable combinations of characteristic features of HCC (e.g., bile production, intercellular bile canaliculi, or a trabecular growth) as well as ICC (e.g., glandular structures, intracellular mucin production, or immunoreactivity for MUC-1, CK7, and CK19).[77–79] Although the surgical outcomes of combined HCC-CC remain indeterminate, intermediate postoperative long-term survival between HCC and ICC has been reported in several studies.[80,81]

Pathogenesis and natural history

The pathogenesis of HCC in cirrhosis is a multistep dedifferentiation process that progresses from regenerative nodule to dysplastic borderline nodule to frank HCC. DNs and early HCC are generally asymptomatic and are usually incidental findings on radiographic studies or detected as a result of screening procedures. Early HCC is a usually slow-growing lesion and remains indolent before acquiring oncological features of classical HCC. With stepwise sequence, small HCC acquires progression ability with angiogenesis, increases in tumor size, invades into the vascular structures, and metastasizes within the liver. These microscopic cancer spread process can evolve toward macroscopic formation of vascular tumor thrombi or multiple tumor presentation. HCC is characterized by early development of such intrahepatic metastasis, whereas distant organs are usually involved late in this disease. HCC usually remains asymptomatic until stretching liver capsule, compressing biliary structures, or tumor rupture with increase in size. In some cases, however, hyperbilirubinemia or hypercalcemia is observed without evidence of biliary obstruction or bone metastases as a paraneoplastic syndrome.

Dissemination or extrahepatic metastases occurs in later stages, primarily via the blood stream to the lungs, bones, and brain. The prognosis for patients with extrahepatic disease is dismal with overall survival up to 1 year depending on the extent of tumor involvement and other prognostic factors.

Screening and diagnosis

The primary objective of screening and surveillance for HCC should be to reduce mortality as much as possible in patients who actually develop the cancer and in an acceptably cost-effective manner. Surveillance is not recommended for the general population, given the low incidence of HCC among individuals with no risk factors. Therefore, the first step in HCC screening should be the identification of patients at risk of HCC development. Traditionally, two methodologies have been employed in HCC surveillance for high-risk patients: tumor marker determination, specifically serum alpha-fetoprotein (AFP) concentration, and diagnostic imaging studies.

The American Association for the Study of Liver Disease (AASLD) has established guidelines regarding the use of these screening techniques based on the best existing evidence.[82] The AASLD currently recommends serial hepatic ultrasound and serum AFP measurement every 6 to 12 months in at-risk populations (e.g., any patient with cirrhosis). Similarly, the Japanese Society of Hepatology has recommended hepatic ultrasound and serum

AFP/plasma des-gamma carboxyprothrombin (DCP) every 3 to 4 months and dynamic CT or MRI every 6–12 months for very high risk population (HBV-related cirrhosis or HCV-related cirrhosis) and hepatic ultrasound and tumor markers every 6 months for high-risk population (HBV-related chronic hepatitis, HCV-related chronic hepatitis, or cirrhosis with other etiologies) with or without dynamic CT or MRI every 6–12 months, as appropriate.[83] A randomized-controlled trial from China reported that the use of ultrasound and AFP enable early detection of HCC and lower HCC-related mortality by 37% in hepatitis B patients.[84] Various nonrandomized studies also confirmed prognostic improvement through regular surveillance programs among patients at high risk of HCC.[85–87] Regarding the interval of screening, recent meta-analysis revealed that every 6 months of surveillance is significantly better than every 12 months of screening in early detection of HCC. Sant et al.[88] reported that 70% of newly diagnosed HCC was within Milan criteria (solitary tumor ≤5 cm or ≤3 tumors with each tumor ≤3 cm)[89] when screened every 6 months or less, whereas the proportion of HCC within Milan criteria was 57% and the overall survival rate was inferior with surveillance every 6–12 months. When a suspected nodule was detected in the regular screening, a contrast-enhanced dynamic CT or MRI is needed. Because HCC is mainly fed by arterial flow, early enhancement and washout of contrast on the delayed phase of the scan are typical findings suggestive of HCC (Figure 3). These enhancement characteristics increase the specificity of the scan to >95%.[90]

An update of AASLD recommendations for diagnosis of HCC has been recently published (Figure 4).[91] These guidelines suggested that, for patients with cirrhosis, a liver mass detected on a radiographic study does not need biopsy confirmation for the diagnosis of HCC as long as the liver lesion exhibits typical vascular enhancement patterns on dynamic imaging studies with CT scan or MRI for lesions >1 cm in diameter. Lesions <1 cm in diameter should be followed with ultrasound every 3 months. If there is tumor growth or changes in character, further investigation is recommended according to size of tumor.

Staging

Because of close association of HCC with underlying chronic liver disease, the prognosis of patients with HCC depends on both the extent of malignant involvement and the severity of chronic liver disease. Thus, currently available staging systems for HCC are broadly divided into clinical and pathological staging systems. The clinical staging systems are particularly useful in guiding treatment selection, including Okuda staging system,[92] Cancer of the Liver Italian Program (CLIP) score,[93] and Barcelona Clinic Liver Cancer (BCLC) staging system.[94] The pathologic staging systems are established based on the surgical outcomes and include the LCSGJ staging system,[95] Japanese Integrated Staging (JIS) score,[96] Chinese University Prognostic Index (CUPI),[97] and American Joint Committee on Cancer/International Union Against Cancer (AJCC/UICC) staging system.[97] Each staging system has strengths and weaknesses. However, combining cancer staging with treatment algorithm is usually difficult, resulting in being too conservative in some cases for one therapy while being too aggressive regarding other therapy in other cases. Therefore, hepatic functional reserve and oncologic status of tumor should be classified separately.

Overall status of the hepatic functional reserve and risk of treatment are stratified by Child-Turcotte-Pugh (CTP) score, which is calculated by the presence of encephalopathy, the presence of ascites, serum bilirubin concentration, serum albumin concentration, and prothrombin time (Table 1). CTP score is nowadays included in various treatment algorithms for hepatic

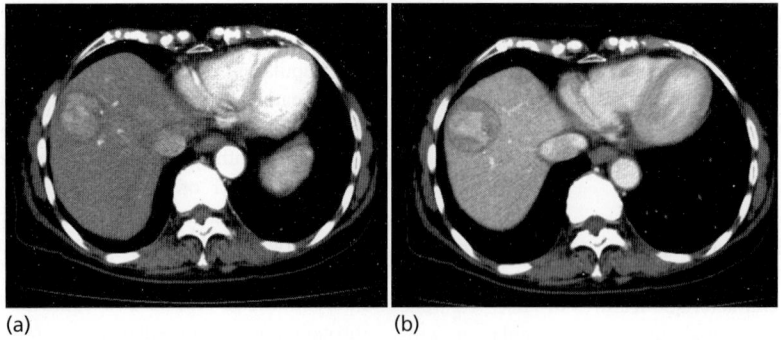

Figure 3 **Typical enhancement pattern of hepatocellular carcinoma in dynamic CT scan**. Early enhancement in the arterial phase (a) and washout in the late phase (b) are typically observed in moderately differentiated hepatocellular carcinoma.

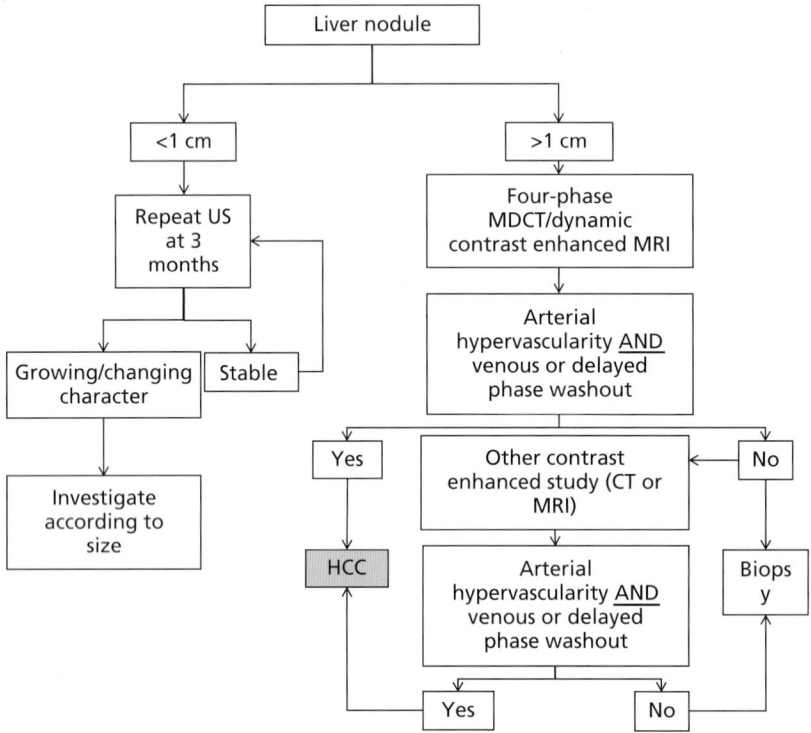

Figure 4 The American Association for the Study of Liver Disease (AASLD) diagnostic algorithm for suspected HCC. Source: Bruix 2005.[82] Reproduced with permission of Wiley.

neoplasms,[82,98,99] and liver resection is usually indicated for CTP class A patients or highly selected patients classified as CTP class B. Consensus exists that CTP class C patients should not undergo surgical resection owing to high perioperative mortality rate.[98]

The AJCC/UICC seventh edition TNM staging system (Table 2) is a modification of sixth edition, which was based on a study from the International Cooperative Study Group on Hepatocellular Carcinoma that included data from the United States, Japan, and France who all underwent surgical resection.[100] A major strength of the AJCC/UICC staging system was the use of centralized pathological review. Although the AJCC/UICC staging system was developed using a cohort dominated by hepatitis C-related HCC, it has also been independently validated in a Chinese cohort with a high prevalence of hepatitis B.[101] Recently, a new international multicenter study reported that microvascular invasion or tumor differentiation does not affect the surgical outcomes in small HCC measuring up to 2 cm, and this specific group of patients can be classified as a new subset of patients associated with good prognosis.[102]

Treatment

The choice of therapy for HCC is individualized based on the tumor burden, degree of underlying liver disease, patient performance status, and the overall possibility of side effects or complications balanced with acceptable results. BCLC staging system[94] is widely used to adequately stratify patients for specific therapies (Figure 5). However, the limitation of BCLC algorithm is that it is fairly conservative with regard to the application of surgical therapy (Figure 5, red color). Patients with larger solitary tumors are not considered as surgical candidates despite a growing experience with resection with acceptable outcomes (Figure 6) in this group.[102–104] Investigators have acknowledged that the BCLC algorithm limits resection criteria, and a modified BCLC algorithm has been proposed as a response to extend the indications for resection of HCC (Figure 7).[105] Resection guidelines currently used at MD Anderson Cancer center are summarized in Table 3. In the guidelines on liver cancer treatment proposed by the Japan Society of Hepatology,[99] surgical resection is currently indicated for CTP class A or class B patients with HCC ≤ 3 nodules irrespective of the size of each

Table 1 Child-Turcotte-Pugh (CTP) classification.

	Points		
	1	2	3
Albumin (g/dL)	>3.5	2.8–3.5	<2.8
Bilirubin (mg/dL)	<2.0	2.0–3.0	>3.0
Prothrombin time	—	—	—
Seconds	<4	4–6	>6
International normalized ratio (INR)	<1.7	1.7–2.3	>2.3
Ascites	None	Moderate	Severe
Encephalopathy	None	Grade I–II	Grade III–VI
CTP class A	5–6 Points	—	—
CTP class B	7–9 Points	—	—
CTP class C	10–15 Points	—	—

Table 2 American Joint Committee on Cancer/International Union Against Cancer (AJCC/UICC) seventh edition staging system for hepatocellular carcinoma.[97]

T classification	
T1	Solitary with no vascular invasion
T2	Solitary with vascular invasion or multifocal ≤5 cm
T3a	Multiple tumors >5 cm
T3b	Single tumor or multiple tumor of any size involving a major branch of the portal or hepatic vein
T4	Invasion of adjacent organs or perforation of visceral peritoneum
Stage grouping	
Stage I	T1N0M0
Stage II	T2N0M0
Stage IIIA	T3aN0M0
Stage IIIB	T3bN0M0
Stage IIIC	T4N0M0
Stage IVA	Any T N1M0
Stage IVB	AnyT Any N M1

Source: Edge 2010.[97] Reproduced with permission of Springer.

Table 3 MD Anderson Cancer Center liver resection criteria in patients with hepatocellular carcinoma.

Minor resection	
Child Pugh	A
Bilirubin	≤1.0 mg
Ascites	Absence
Platelets counts	>100,000/mm
Major resection	
Child Pugh	A
Bilirubin	≤1.0 mg
Ascites	Absence
Platelets counts	>100,000/mm
Portal hypertension	Absence
Future liver remnant	>40% or indication for portal vein embolization
Hypertrophy	>5% after portal vein embolization

tumor, whereas liver transplantation is limited only for CTP class C patients meeting with the Milan criteria. Selection of treatment should be determined in a multidisciplinary approach considering the local expertise. However, the most effective treatment including surgical resection, radiofrequency ablation (RFA), and orthotopic liver transplantation (OLT) should be the first priority as long as such treatments are permitted.

Surgical resection

For liver resection, strict assessment of hepatic functional reserve is needed for patients with HCC because HCC usually develops in an injured liver, and accordingly, maximum extent of resection is needed to be estimated carefully. Functional investigations have been proposed to better evaluate the severity of chronic liver disease. The measurement of indocyanine green retention rate at 15 min (ICG-R15) is the most frequently used test. For patients with obstructive jaundice or congenital intolerance to indocyanine green, ^{99m}Tc-galactosyl human serum albumin (GSA) scintigraphy sensitively estimates the hepatic functional reserve.

Liver resection is indicated only for CTP class A or B patients with controllable ascites and serum total bilirubin level of <2.0 mg/dL, and the maximum extent of resection can be determined based on the measurement of ICG-R15.[106] At the University of Tokyo, the maximum extent of resection is set up to 60% (right hepatectomy or trisectionectomy) for patients with ICG-R15 < 10%, up to 50% (left hepatectomy or sectorectomy) for those with ICG-R15 < 20%, segmentectomy for those with ICG-R15 < 30%, and only limited resection is indicated for patients with ICG-R15 > 30%. Following strictly this algorithm, no mortality due to hepatic insufficiency was reported in 1056 consecutive patients.[107] At MD Anderson Cancer Center, portal vein embolization (PVE) has been used to increase the candidacy of HCC patients for major hepatectomy and improve postoperative outcomes and safety.[108] The procedure has shown to be safe and well tolerated with increased survival rates.[109] In fact, PVE has another major benefit in HCC. Most patients with HCC have underlying cirrhosis and it is clinically challenging to assess liver function and make validated treatment decisions, especially when a major liver resection is required. The degree of hypertrophy after PVE is inversely associated with the regenerative potential of the liver. Subsequently, the degree of hypertrophy provides valuable information of potentially missed liver injury: <5% hypertrophy after PVE is associated with increased mortality after liver resection.[110]

Orthotopic liver transplantation (OLT)

Liver transplantation is another surgical approach with theoretically higher chance of eradication of tumor burden especially for patients with severe hepatic dysfunction. Clinical outcomes of liver transplantation for HCC were poor in the early era. However, after the landmark study by Mazzaferro et al.,[89] it has been widely recognized that preferable survival outcomes can be expected in a selected population with limited size and number of HCC (Milan criteria). The selection criteria for transplantation used by Mazzaferro et al.[89] was tumor diameter of 5 cm or less in patients with single HCC or 3 cm or less if the patient had two or three lesions. Nowadays, this criterion is extended with or without tumor markers or biopsy findings in several high-volume transplant centers.[111–122]

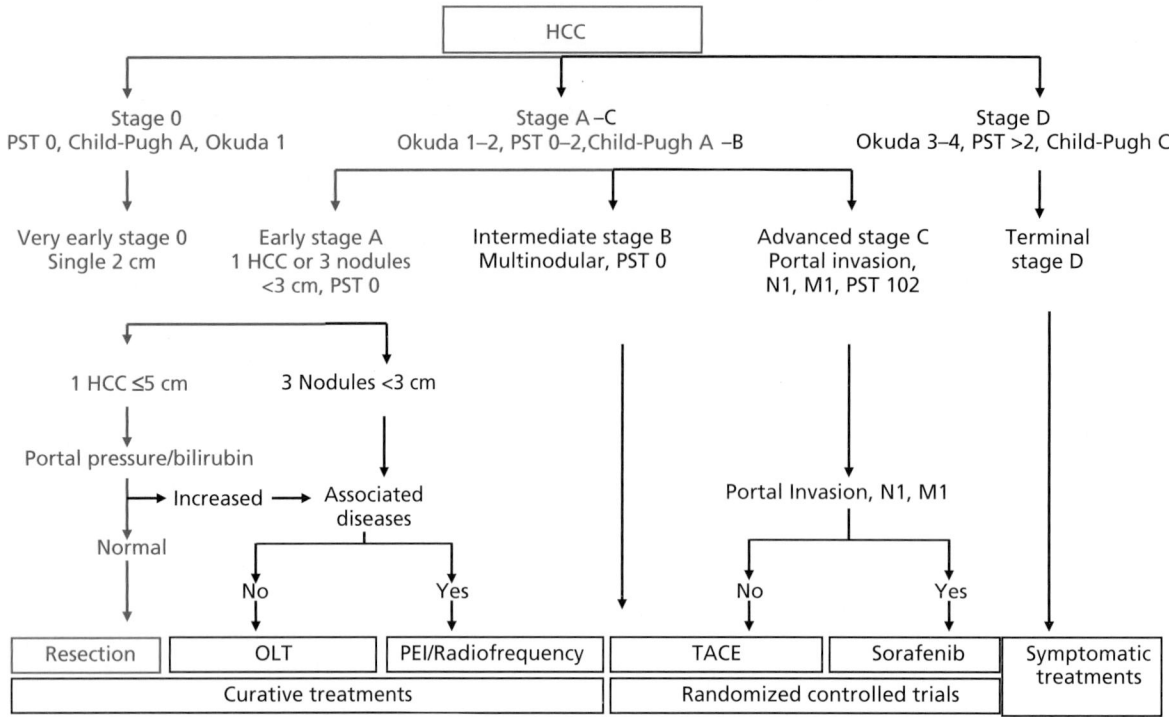

Figure 5 **BCLC algorithm for treatment selection in patients with HCC.** Red color indicates patients potentially candidates for resection according to the BCLC algorithm. Source: Llovet (2003). Reproduced with permission of Elsevier.

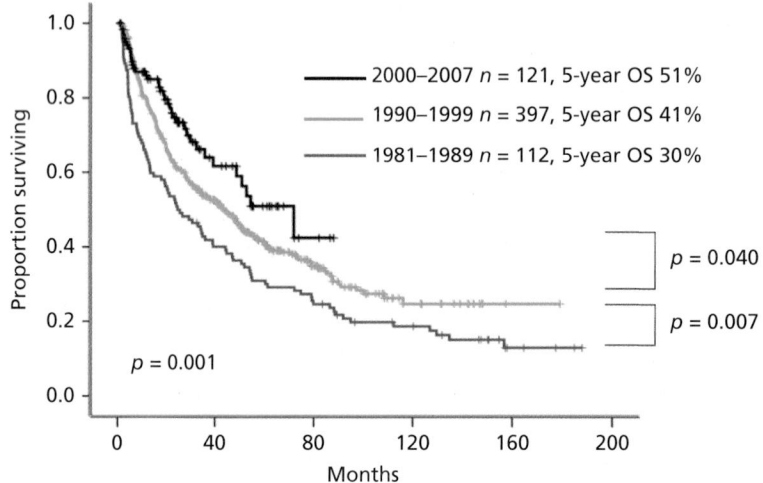

Figure 6 Kaplan–Meier plots of survival after resection of ≥4 segments in patients with HCC (*n* = 630) stratified by three different time periods. Source: Andreou 2013. Reproduced with permission of Springer.

Locoregional ablation therapies

Image-guided ablation is accepted as the best therapeutic choice for patients with early-stage HCC when surgical options are precluded. Several methods for local tumor destruction have been developed and clinically used over the two decades. RFA has shown superior ablative effect and greater survival benefit compared to conventional percutaneous technique, ethanol injection, in meta-analyses of randomized controlled trials,[123–127] and is now established as the standard ablative modality. Currently, thermal or nonthermal ablation methods including microwave ablation and irreversible electroporation are under investigation as potential alternatives to RFA.

Transarterial chemoembolization (TACE)

The normal liver receives dual blood supply from the hepatic artery (25%) and the portal vein (75%). HCC exhibits intense neo-angiogenic activity during its progression and is mostly dependent on the hepatic arterial supply. This provides the rationale of using arterial obstruction with or without regional chemotherapy as an effective therapeutic option for HCC. Transarterial therapies are usually considered palliative and should be offered to patients with intermediate stage disease without extra-hepatic metastases and sufficient hepatic functional reserve. The most commonly used agents for transarterial chemoembolization (TACE) are doxorubicin and cisplatin, followed by epirubicin, and none was found

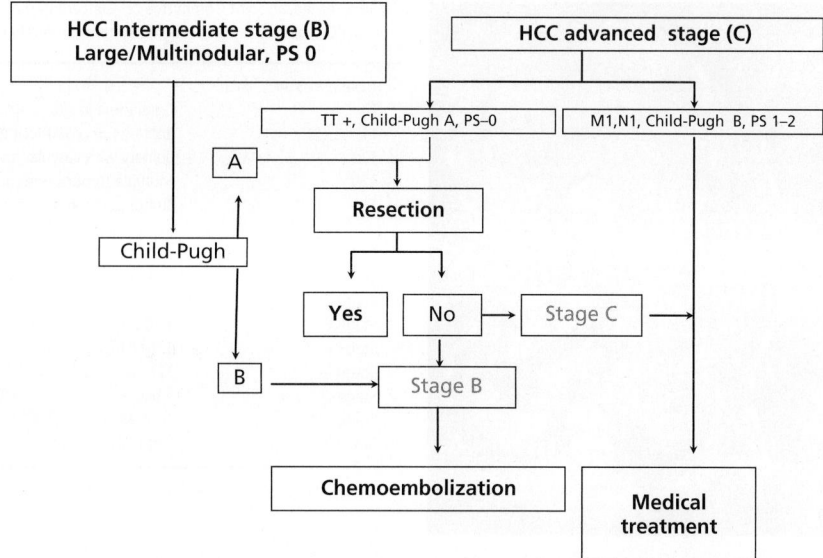

Figure 7 Modified BCLC algorithm extending resection indications in HCC. Source: Torzilli 2013.[109] Reproduced with permission of Wolters Kluwer Health.

superior to the others in RCTs.[128,129] Regarding the embolizing material, gelatin sponge (gelfoam) has conventionally been used. However, it could provide only short-term arterial occlusion up to 2 weeks. Currently, polyvinyl alcohol (PVA) particles are used in many centers, which offer permanent arterial occlusion and also achieves more distal embolization with its small particle size.[130] Drug-eluting beads have been recently developed to provide a combined local ischemic and cytotoxic effect. Although its superiority to conventional TACE remains controversial, at least equal efficacy and safety compared to conventional TACE have been shown in several studies.[131,132]

Systemic treatment

Systemic chemotherapy is commonly the only option for patients with advanced and/or disseminated disease in patients with HCC. For decades, various systemic therapies have been explored for the treatment of advanced HCC. Nevertheless, no satisfactory results have been obtained in cytotoxic chemotherapy so far. Sorafenib is a polyvalent molecule that has been shown in HCC cell line to inhibit the serine-threonine kinase Raf-1 and several receptor tyrosine kinases such as vascular endothelial growth factor receptor (VEGFR2), platelet-derived growth factor receptor (PDGFR), FLT3, Ret, and c-Kit. Two phase III studies: the SHARP trial[133] and the Asia-Pacific trial,[134] respectively, demonstrated survival benefit of sorafenib in patients with HCC, and this is only the biologic agent approved for clinical use in systemic therapy for HCC at present. However, the overall response rate was only 3% and there is no established treatment with sufficient tumor response rate.

Recently, our group has shown that cisplatin/interferon α-2b/doxorubicin/5-flurouracil (PIAF) combination therapy improves response, resectability, and patient survival in patients with initially unresectable HCC when limiting the indication only for patients with no hepatitis or cirrhosis.[135] As such, this traditional chemotherapy regimen might provide an option for unresectable HCC developed in noncirrhotic patients (Figures 8 and 9).

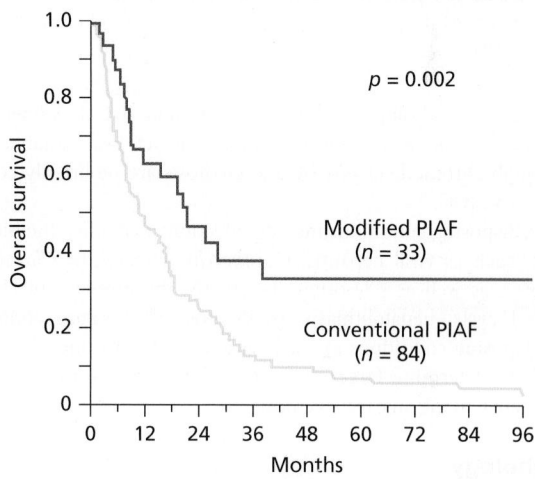

Figure 8 Kaplan–Meier plots of survival with initially unresectable HCC (*n* = 117) stratified on treatment with PIAF (cisplatin/interferon α2b/doxorubicin/5-flourouracil regimen). Source: Kaseb 2013.[135] Reproduced with permission of Wiley.

Intrahepatic cholangiocarcinoma

Incidence and epidemiology

ICC is the second most common primary hepatic malignancy after HCC. There is considerable geographic variation in the incidence of ICC, with a greater incidence in East Asia.[136] In the United States, the age-adjusted incidence of ICC increased from 0.32 in 1975 to 0.85 per 100,000 population in 2000 and has yet to plateau.[137] The overall survival rate in unresectable tumor is dismal, with 5-year survival rate of 5% to 10%. Because systemic therapy for ICC has not yet been established, surgical resection offers the only chance for cure. However, the overall survival after curative-intent surgery is disappointing, with a 5-year survival rate of 20% to 35%.[138]

Risk factors

ICC is thought to derive from a common hepatic progenitor cell that may also give rise to HCC,[139] and combined hepatocellular-CC

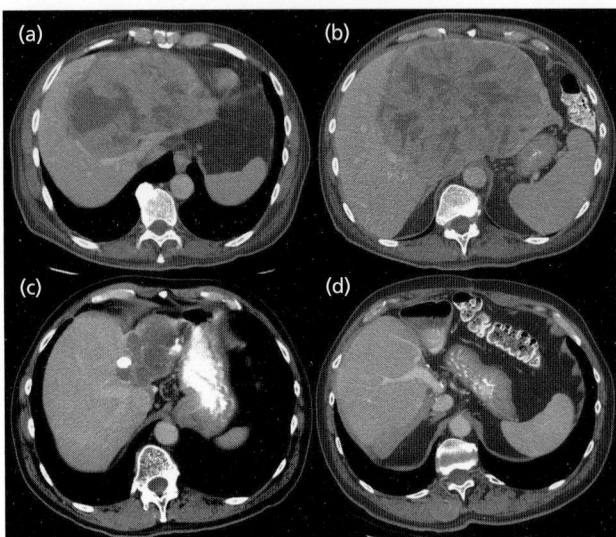

Table 4 American Joint Committee on Cancer/International Union Against Cancer (AJCC/UICC) seventh edition staging system for intrahepatic cholangiocarcinoma.[97]

T classification	
Tis	Carcinoma *in situ*
T1	Solitary tumor without vascular invasion
T2a	Solitary with vascular invasion
T2b	Multiple tumors, with or without vascular invasion
T3	Tumor perforating the visceral peritoneum or involving the local extrahepatic structures by direct invasion
T4	Tumor with periductal invasion
Stage grouping	
Stage 0	TisN0M0
Stage I	T1N0M0
Stage II	T2N0M0
Stage III	T3N0M0
Stage IVA	T4N0M0 or Any T N1 M0
Stage IVB	AnyT Any N M1

Source: Edge 2010.[97] Reproduced with permission of Springer.

Figure 9 Computed tomography of a 60-year-old male with large HCC. (a, b) A 15 cm in diameter HCC involving left lobe, right anterior sector and abutting the right hepatic vein. (c) After treatment with Platinum Interferon, Adriamycin, 5-flourouracil, and transarterial chemoembolization. (d) After extended left hepatectomy including resection of the caudate lobe and the inferior vena cava. The patient is alive without evidence of disease 8 years after surgery.

having histopathologic features of HCC and ICC is sometimes observed. Risk factors for ICC have not yet been established, although chronic liver disease and cirrhosis are reportedly correlated with ICC.

Predisposing conditions include infections that affect the biliary tract, such as viral hepatitis, *Opisthorchis viverini*, or *Clonorchis sinensis*, as well as sclerosing cholangitis, the presence of choledochal cysts, hepatolithiasis, or cirrhosis.[140] Because common predisposing conditions are lacking and rarity of tumor, it is difficult to determine target population for routine surveillance to facilitate making an early diagnosis.

Pathology

There are three morphologic subtypes of ICC that can be characterized on cross-sectional appearance: mass forming, periductal infiltrating, and intraductal growth (Figure 10). Mass-forming type is the most common subtype of ICC. Unlike with HCC, ICC shows invasive tumor growth without tumor capsule. Therefore, when a tumor is attaching to a major vascular structure, microscopic invasion to the vascular wall should be suspected and en-bloc resection is usually needed.

Diagnosis

On dynamic imaging studies, ICC is not enhanced owing to its hypovascular nature. However, various degrees of ring enhancement are observed surrounding the lesion, reflecting the fibrous connective tissue frequently observed around the tumor (Figure 11). In laboratory test, elevation of CEA or CA19-9 in primary solid liver lesion is suggestive of ICC.

Staging

Until the sixth edition, AJCC classification system for ICC was the same with that for HCC. In the 7th edition, however, an original staging system was adopted (Table 4) based on the survival outcomes of 598 patients who underwent liver resection of ICC from the SEER database.[141] This revised staging system has been validated externally and independently by the French Surgical Association (AFC)-IHCC 2009 study group.[142]

Treatment

For ICC, only surgical resection offers a chance of cure because there are no established other curative treatment options. Surgical treatment for ICC involves hepatectomy, extrahepatic bile duct resection, and systematic nodal dissection according to the extent of tumor. Significance of systematic nodal dissection remains controversial. However, nodal involvement is a significant prognostic factor for ICC,[141] and it has been reported that up to 30% of patient will have lymph node metastases.[143]

OLT for the treatment of CC has been reported with 5-year survival rates of 23%, with a median time to recurrence of 9 months,[144] both of which are significantly poor and insufficient compared to HCC. However, it has been reported that OLT in combination with neoadjuvant chemoradiation has 1-, 3-, 5-year survival rates of 92%, 82%, 82% compared to 82%, 48%, 21% with resection alone,[145] and OLT might be advantageous in selected patients.

For patients with advanced ICC, systemic chemotherapy has made some progress in the past decade. The response rate to single-agent 5-fluorouracil-based or gemcitabine-based systemic therapy is only about 10% to 30%.[146,147] The ABC-02 phase 3 randomized controlled trial, which studied 510 patients who had locally advanced or metastatic biliary tract cancer, has shown that the combination of gemcitabine plus cisplatin demonstrated improved progression-free survival and overall survival (11.7 vs 8.1 months) compared with gemcitabine alone,[148] and nowadays, doublet therapy with gemcitabine and cisplatin is considered the standard-of-care, first-line treatment for patients who have advanced cancer of the bile ducts and gallbladder. Recently, there has been growing interest in examining novel, targeted anticancer agents based on an existing understanding of the molecular carcinogenesis of biliary tract cancers.[140]

Hepatic angiosarcoma

Hepatic angiosarcoma is a rare tumor derived from the malignant transformation of hepatic endothelial cells, and close association with environmental carcinogens such as thorotrast (contrast agent used in 1940s and 1950s), vinyl chloride, arsenicals, and androgenic-anabolic steroids has been reported. Because no clear

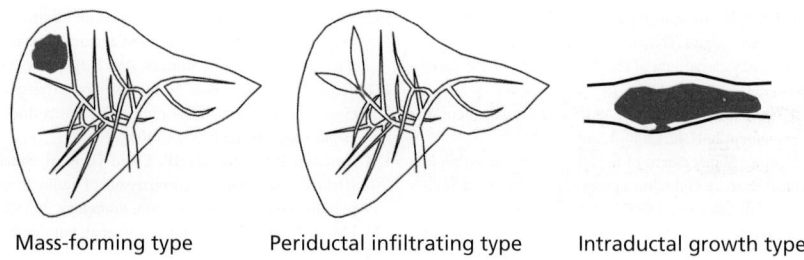

Mass-forming type   Periductal infiltrating type   Intraductal growth type

Figure 10 Gross classification of intrahepatic cholangiocarcinoma. Source: Adapted from Liver Cancer Study Group of Japan 2008.

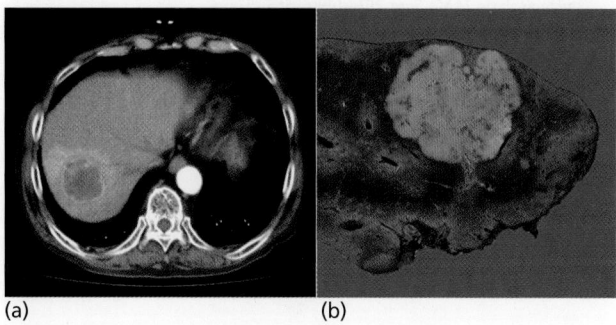

(a)   (b)

Figure 11 (a) Typical ring enhancement in enhanced CT scan and (b) gross appearance of intrahepatic cholangiocarcinoma.

etiology or association with chronic liver disease has been identified, hepatic angiosarcoma is usually advanced at the time of diagnosis. Although complete surgical resection or OLT may provide a chance of prolonged survival, prognosis is generally poor even after liver transplantation.[149] The efficacy of chemotherapy has not been well documented for this tumor.

Epithelioid hemangioendothelioma

EHE is a very rare, low-grade malignant neoplasm of endothelial origin with a reported incidence of <0.1 per 100,000 people.[150] EHE presents heterogeneous clinical features, nonspecific radiological characteristics, and a variable natural history.[151] The management options for EHE include liver resection, OLT, chemotherapy, and radiotherapy. However, it is difficult to compare the clinical outcomes among these therapeutic options because of the rarity of the disease. Favorable outcomes have been reported after liver resection for EHE, with 1- and 5-year survival rates of 100% and 75%, respectively.[152] However, owing to frequent diffuse presentation of the disease, liver resection is unsuitable in majority of the cases. The result of OLT is also encouraging with 1- and 5-year survival rates of 96% and 54.5%, respectively. A recent study has also shown favorable long-term outcomes after OLT with 5- and 10-year survival rates of 83% and 74%, irrespective of the presence of nodal involvement or extrahepatic disease.[153] Owing to the indolent nature of the disease, a recent study concluded that initial observation followed by resection or OLT in the patients who remained candidates for surgery could be beneficial to stratify treatment options.[154] However, because of the rarity of the disease, strong evidence-based management strategies are difficult to establish and large multicenter prospective trials maybe necessary for improved understanding of EHE.

Key references

The complete reference list can be found on the Wiley Companion Digital Edition of this title (see inside front cover for login instructions).

1 American Cancer Society. *Global Cancer Facts & Figures*. Atlanta, GA: American Cancer Society; 2007.

8 Moroy T, Marchio A, Etiemble J, et al. Rearrangement and enhanced expression of c-myc in hepatocellular carcinoma of hepatitis virus infected woodchucks. *Nature*. 1986;**324**:276–279.

9 Wang J, Chenivesse X, Henglein B, Brechot C. Hepatitis B virus integration in a cyclin A gene in a hepatocellular carcinoma. *Nature*. 1990;**343**:555–557.

10 Brechot C. Hepatitis B virus (HBV) and hepatocellular carcinoma. HBV DNA status and its implications. *J Hepatol*. 1987;**4**:269–279.

11 Brechot C, Pourcel C, Louise A, et al. Presence of integrated hepatitis B virus DNA sequences in cellular DNA of human hepatocellular carcinoma. *Nature*. 1980;**286**:533–535.

12 Donato F, Boffetta P, Puoti M. A meta-analysis of epidemiological studies on the combined effect of hepatitis B and C virus infections in causing hepatocellular carcinoma. *Int J Cancer*. 1998;**75**:347–354.

15 Dusheiko G, Schmilovitz-Weiss H, Brown D, et al. Hepatitis C virus genotypes: an investigation of type-specific differences in geographic origin and disease. *Hepatology*. 1994;**19**:13–18.

16 Shindoh J, Hasegawa K, Matsuyama Y, et al. Low hepatitis C viral load predicts better long-term outcomes in patients undergoing resection of hepatocellular carcinoma irrespective of serologic eradication of hepatitis C virus. *J Clin Oncol*. 2013;**31**:766–773.

18 Hassan MM, Spitz MR, Thomas MB, et al. Effect of different types of smoking and synergism with hepatitis C virus on risk of hepatocellular carcinoma in American men and women: case–control study. *Int J Cancer*. 2008;**123**:1883–1891.

19 Hutchinson SJ, Bird SM, Goldberg DJ. Influence of alcohol on the progression of hepatitis C virus infection: a meta-analysis. *Clin Gastroenterol Hepatol*. 2005;**3**:1150–1159.

20 Ikeda K, Saitoh S, Suzuki Y, et al. Disease progression and hepatocellular carcinogenesis in patients with chronic viral hepatitis: a prospective observation of 2215 patients. *J Hepatol*. 1998;**28**:930–938.

25 Tolman KG, Fonseca V, Tan MH, Dalpiaz A. Narrative review: hepatobiliary disease in type 2 diabetes mellitus. *Ann Intern Med*. 2004;**141**:946–956.

26 Calle EE, Rodriguez C, Walker-Thurmond K, Thun MJ. Overweight, obesity, and mortality from cancer in a prospectively studied cohort of U.S. adults. *N Engl J Med*. 2003;**348**:1625–1638.

30 El-Serag HB, Tran T, Everhart JE. Diabetes increases the risk of chronic liver disease and hepatocellular carcinoma. *Gastroenterology*. 2004;**126**:460–468.

40 Edwards CQ, Griffen LM, Goldgar D, et al. Prevalence of hemochromatosis among 11,065 presumably healthy blood donors. *N Engl J Med*. 1988;**318**:1355–1362.

61 Kumada H, Suzuki Y, Ikeda K, et al. Daclatasvir plus asunaprevir for chronic HCV genotype 1b infection. *Hepatology*. 2014;**59**:2083–2091.

62 Lawitz E, Poordad FF, Pang PS, et al. Sofosbuvir and ledipasvir fixed-dose combination with and without ribavirin in treatment-naive and previously treated patients with genotype 1 hepatitis C virus infection (LONESTAR): an open-label, randomised, phase 2 trial. *Lancet*. 2014;**383**:515–523.

63 Lawitz E, Sulkowski MS, Ghalib R, et al. Simeprevir plus sofosbuvir, with or without ribavirin, to treat chronic infection with hepatitis C virus genotype 1 in non-responders to pegylated interferon and ribavirin and treatment-naive patients: the COSMOS randomised study. *Lancet*. 2014;**384**(**9956**):1756–1765.

64 International Consensus Group for Hepatocellular Neoplasia. The International Consensus Group for Hepatocellular N Pathologic diagnosis of early hepatocellular carcinoma: a report of the international consensus group for hepatocellular neoplasia. *Hepatology*. 2009;**49**:658–664.

69 Liver Cancer Study Group of Japan. *The General Rules for the Clinical and Pathological Study of Primary Liver Cancer*, 5th ed. Tokyo: Kanehara; 2008.

75 Edmondson HA, Steiner PE. Primary carcinoma of the liver: a study of 100 cases among 48,900 necropsies. *Cancer*. 1954;**7**:462–503.

82 Bruix J, Sherman M. Practice Guidelines Committee AAftSoLD Management of hepatocellular carcinoma. *Hepatology*. 2005;**42**:1208–1236.

83 Kudo M, Izumi N, Kokudo N, et al. Management of hepatocellular carcinoma in Japan: Consensus-Based Clinical Practice Guidelines proposed by the Japan Society of Hepatology (JSH) 2010 updated version. *Dig Dis*. 2011;**29**:339–364.

91 Bruix J, Sherman M. American Association for the Study of Liver D Management of hepatocellular carcinoma: an update. *Hepatology*. 2011;**53**:1020–1022.

93 The Cancer of the Liver Italian Program (CLIP) Investigators. A new prognostic system for hepatocellular carcinoma: a retrospective study of 435 patients: the Cancer of the Liver Italian Program (CLIP) investigators. *Hepatology*. 1998;**28**:751–755.

94 Llovet JM, Bru C, Bruix J. Prognosis of hepatocellular carcinoma: the BCLC staging classification. *Semin Liver Dis*. 1999;**19**:329–338.

95 Makuuchi M, Belghiti J, Belli G, et al. IHPBA concordant classification of primary liver cancer: working group report. *J Hepatobiliary Pancreat Surg*. 2003;**10**:26–30.

97 Edge S, Byrd D, Compton C, et al. *AJCC Cancer Staging Manual*, 7th ed. New York: Springer; 2010.

100 Vauthey JN, Lauwers GY, Esnaola NF, et al. Simplified staging for hepatocellular carcinoma. *J Clin Oncol*. 2002;**20**:1527–1536.

102 Shindoh J, Andreou A, Aloia TA, et al. Microvascular invasion does not predict long-term survival in hepatocellular carcinoma up to 2 cm: reappraisal of the staging system for solitary tumors. *Ann Surg Oncol*. 2013;**20**:1223–1229.

121 Yao FY, Ferrell L, Bass NM, et al. Liver transplantation for hepatocellular carcinoma: expansion of the tumor size limits does not adversely impact survival. *Hepatology*. 2001;**33**:1394–1403.

124 Lencioni RA, Allgaier HP, Cioni D, et al. Small hepatocellular carcinoma in cirrhosis: randomized comparison of radio-frequency thermal ablation versus percutaneous ethanol injection. *Radiology*. 2003;**228**:235–240.

133 Llovet JM, Ricci S, Mazzaferro V, et al. Sorafenib in advanced hepatocellular carcinoma. *N Engl J Med*. 2008;**359**:378–390.

134 Cheng AL, Kang YK, Chen Z, et al. Efficacy and safety of sorafenib in patients in the Asia-Pacific region with advanced hepatocellular carcinoma: a phase III randomised, double-blind, placebo-controlled trial. *Lancet Oncol*. 2009;**10**:25–34.

138 Mavros MN, Economopoulos KP, Alexiou VG, Pawlik TM. Treatment and prognosis for patients with intrahepatic cholangiocarcinoma: systematic review and meta-analysis. *JAMA Surg*. 2014;**149**(**6**):565–574.

141 Nathan H, Aloia TA, Vauthey JN, et al. A proposed staging system for intrahepatic cholangiocarcinoma. *Ann Surg Oncol*. 2009;**16**:14–22.

151 Makhlouf HR, Ishak KG, Goodman ZD. Epithelioid hemangioendothelioma of the liver: a clinicopathologic study of 137 cases. *Cancer*. 1999;**85**:562–582.

92 Gallbladder and bile duct cancer

Ahmed O. Kaseb, MD ▪ Marc Uemura, MD ▪ Melanie B. Thomas, MD, MS ▪ Steven A. Curley, MD, FACS

Overview

Primary gallbladder and bile duct cancers are relatively rare tumors of the gastrointestinal tract. Both are mainly adenocarcinomas that start as abnormal growths within the mucous lining of the gallbladder and bile ducts. Bile duct tumors, or cholangiocarcinomas, are further differentiated by their location within the liver (intrahepatic) or outside the liver (extrahepatic). Both tumor types have distinct pathophysiologies and modes of hepatocarcinogenesis. Gallbladder cancers, for example, are associated with gallstones, chronic choleycystitis, and the porcelain gallbladder. They are commonly found incidentally on cholecystectomy specimens. On the other hand, cholangiocarcinomas have frequent associations with parasitic infections and other diseases causing chronic inflammation in the bile ducts (primary sclerosing cholangitis). While both gallbladder and cholangiocarcinomas can be cured if surgically resected, unresectable or advanced tumors have a poor prognosis and usually require systemic chemotherapy.

Gallbladder cancer

Adenocarcinoma of the gallbladder is the sixth most common digestive system malignancy in the United States. In Western countries such as the United States, where there is a lower incidence of hepatocellular carcinoma (HCC), gallbladder cancer is relatively more common. The American Cancer Society estimates that about 10,910 new cases of gallbladder cancer and bile duct cancer (excluding bile ducts within the liver) would be diagnosed in 2016 in the United States. About 3700 people died of these cancers in 2015. Of these new cases and deaths, about half are due to gallbladder cancer.[1] Between 1980 and 1995, mortality rates from gallbladder cancer decreased in the United States, Canada, Australia, and the United Kingdom, while increasing in Japan, Italy, Spain, and Chile.[2] Unlike HCC and cholangiocarcinoma, gallbladder carcinoma has a higher incidence in females than in males.[2] The preponderance of this cancer in females is even greater in patients <40 years old, with a female-to-male ratio of 20 : 1.[3]

Gallbladder carcinoma is more common in Southwest Native Americans than in the general American population. Incidence rates for U.S. white males, black males, and Native American males in New Mexico are 0.4, 0.6, and 3.8 cases per 100,000 per year, respectively. The corresponding rates for females are 1.0, 0.8, and 10.3.[2] Gallbladder carcinoma has been found in 6% of Southwest Native Americans undergoing biliary tract surgery.[4] Gallbladder carcinoma is the second most common gastrointestinal malignancy in this population, and the youngest reported case of gallbladder carcinoma occurred in an 11-year-old Navajo girl.[5]

Other human populations also have an increased incidence of gallbladder cancer. In Chile, the incidence of gallbladder cancer is rising, and gallbladder cancer is the number one cause of cancer mortality in Chilean women.[6] The geographic and population-based variations in the incidence of gallbladder cancer suggest that environmental risk factors, including carcinogens, infectious agents like *Salmonella typhi* and *Helicobacter pylori*, and diet have a role in gallbladder tumorigenesis.

Causative factors

There are no apparent associations between gallbladder carcinoma and hepatitis B or C virus infection, cirrhosis, or mycotoxin exposure. Similarly, chemical hepatocarcinogens have not been clearly demonstrated to increase the risk of developing gallbladder carcinoma. However, there are suggestions that workers exposed to carcinogenic substances, such as methylcholanthrene and nitrosamines, have a higher incidence and earlier onset of gallbladder carcinoma when compared with control populations.[7] There is a significant association between gallstones and gallbladder carcinoma, with gallstones present in 74–92% of patients with gallbladder carcinoma.[8,9] The risk of developing gallbladder carcinoma increases directly with increasing gallstone size.[10] Patients with gallstones 2.0–2.9 cm in diameter have a 2.4 times higher relative risk of developing gallbladder carcinoma, whereas patients with gallstones greater than 3.0 cm in diameter have a 10.1 times higher risk. Patients with long-standing chronic cholecystitis can develop calcification of the gallbladder wall, also known as porcelain gallbladder. It is possible that chronic inflammation and/or infection of the gallbladder increases the risk of developing gallbladder carcinoma because 22% of patients with calcified gallbladders have gallbladder carcinoma.[11] Furthermore, pathogenic bacteria are cultured from the gallbladders of patients with gallbladder cancer at a significantly greater frequency than from patients with simple cholelithiasis.[12] Cholelithiasis and cholecystitis are more common in females, which may in part explain the higher incidence of gallbladder carcinoma in females.[13]

Patients with these premalignant lesions may progress to invasive gallbladder carcinoma. Epithelial dysplasia, atypical hyperplasia, and carcinoma *in situ* have been identified in the gallbladder mucosa of 83%, 13.5%, and 3.5%, respectively, of patients undergoing cholecystectomy for cholelithiasis or cholecystitis.[14] Areas of mucosal dysplasia can be observed in >90% of patients with invasive gallbladder carcinoma.[15] There is also evidence that adenomatous polyps arising from the gallbladder mucosa are premalignant lesions. A review of 1605 cholecystectomies reported 11 benign adenomas, 7 adenomas with areas of malignant transformation, and 79 invasive gallbladder carcinomas.[16] There appears to be an increased expression of epithelial growth factors and proto-oncogene, particularly *ras*, in the progression from chronic cholecystitis to dysplasia and then to invasive carcinoma.[17] In patients with anomalous pancreaticobiliary ductal union, a condition known to be associated with an increased risk of developing gallbladder cancer, chronic inflammation results in hyperplasia of the gallbladder epithelium.[18] K-*ras* mutations were noted in some

Holland-Frei Cancer Medicine, Ninth Edition. Edited by Robert C. Bast Jr., Carlo M. Croce, William N. Hait, Waun Ki Hong, Donald W. Kufe, Martine Piccart-Gebhart, Raphael E. Pollock, Ralph R. Weichselbaum, Hongyang Wang, and James F. Holland.
© 2017 John Wiley & Sons, Inc. ISBN: 978-1-118-93469-2

of these patients with high-grade dysplasia, suggesting that mutations in this proto-oncogene may be an early event in gallbladder mucosal proliferation leading to carcinogenesis. Previous studies performed in patients with invasive gallbladder carcinoma have demonstrated that the majority have abnormal or mutated tumor suppressor (*p53* and *p16*), cell cycle regulation (cyclin E), and apoptosis regulation (Bc1-2) genes, as well as increased expression of angiogenesis factors (VEGF).[19,20] More recently, comprehensive genomic profiling has shown that invasive gallbladder carcinomas have alternations in other proteins necessary for cell cycle regulation (CDKN2B), chromatin remodeling (ARID1A), and in important growth pathways, specifically epidermal growth factor receptor family (ERBB2) and PIK3CA/MTOR.[21]

Pathology

The gross appearance of gallbladder carcinoma varies, depending on the stage of the disease and extent of spread. Early-stage lesions that have not infiltrated through all layers of the gallbladder wall may be indistinguishable from chronic cholecystitis. Occasionally, a sessile or pedunculated tumor is present and suggests the diagnosis of a gallbladder carcinoma.[22] More advanced gallbladder carcinomas are grossly evident by infiltration into the liver or contiguous organs, such as the duodenum or stomach.[23]

Microscopically, >90% of gallbladder carcinomas are adenocarcinomas, with the remaining cases being adenosquamous, squamous, anaplastic carcinomas, and, rarely, carcinoid tumors or embryonal rhabdomyosarcoma.[8,22] Carcinoma *in situ* is an early lesion, with the malignant cells involving only the mucosal layer of the gallbladder wall. Gallbladder adenocarcinomas generally have a predominant papillary or tubular arrangement of cells.[22] Papillary adenocarcinoma is characterized by an extended stroma covered by columnar cells. The tubular formations of tubular adenocarcinoma may be lined by tall columnar cells or by cuboidal epithelium. Mucin production and signet ring cells can be identified frequently in gallbladder adenocarcinomas.[22] More poorly differentiated carcinomas have solid sheets or nests of small, scattered cells infiltrating into the stroma and destroying the normal gallbladder wall architecture. Vascular, lymphatic, and perineural invasion by the carcinoma can be demonstrated frequently.

Advanced locoregional disease usually is present at the time of diagnosis of gallbladder carcinoma. Only 10% of patients with this disease have cancer confined to the gallbladder wall.[8] Direct extension of the carcinoma into the gallbladder fossa of the liver is present in 69–83% of patients.[23–25] Direct invasion of the liver usually indicates the presence of other regional disease because fewer than 12% of patients with liver involvement have no other sites of regional disease. Direct invasion of the extrahepatic biliary tract occurs in 57% of cases; the duodenum, stomach, or transverse colon is involved in 40%; and the pancreas is involved in 23%. The hepatic artery or portal vein is encased by tumor in 15% of patients. Regional lymph node metastases in the cystic, choledochal, or pancreaticoduodenal lymphatic drainage basins are present in 42–70% of patients.[23] More distant lymph node metastases occur along the aorta or inferior vena cava in approximately 25% of cases. Importantly, lymph node metastases can occur in the absence of liver or other contiguous organ involvement by the gallbladder carcinoma.

The pattern of lymph node metastases from gallbladder carcinoma is predictable on the basis of anatomic studies that have identified three pathways of lymphatic drainage of the gallbladder (Figure 1).[26] The main pathway is the cholecysto-retropancreatic pathway, with lymphatic vessels on the anterior and posterior surfaces of the gallbladder that converge at a large retroportal lymph node. This principal retroportal lymph node communicates

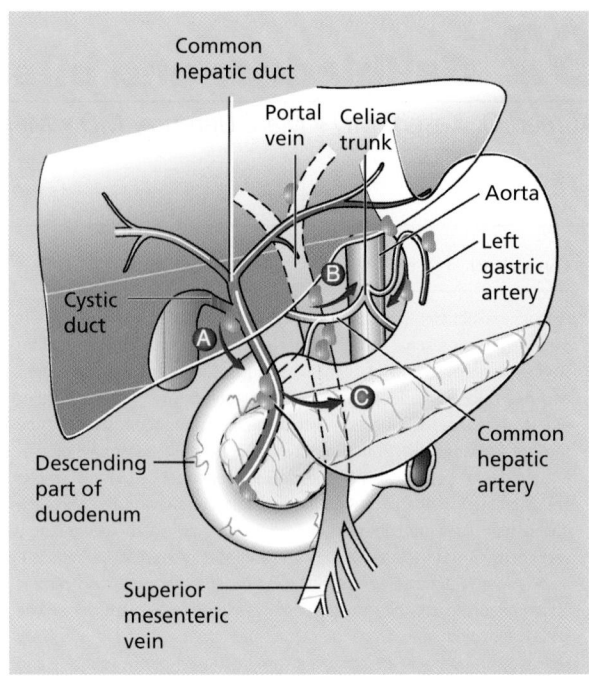

Figure 1 Patterns of lymphatic drainage from the gallbladder. (A) The main pathway of lymphatic drainage and, thus, lymph node metastasis from gallbladder cancer is to the cholecysto-retropancreatic nodes. This pathway drains from the gallbladder to nodes along the cystic duct and common bile duct and then to nodes posterior to the duodenum and pancreatic head. (B) The cholecysto-celiac pathway courses from the gallbladder through the gastrohepatic ligament to celiac nodes. (C) The third lymphatic drainage route is the cholecysto-mesenteric pathway, coursing from the gallbladder posterior to the pancreas to aortocaval lymph nodes.

with the choledochal and pancreaticoduodenal lymph nodes. The cholecysto-celiac pathway consists of lymphatics from the anterior and posterior walls of the gallbladder that run to the left in front of the portal vein and then communicate with groups of pancreaticoduodenal lymph nodes or aorticocaval lymph nodes lying near the left renal vein. The final pattern of spread of gallbladder carcinoma is related to vascular invasion. Noncontiguous liver, pulmonary, and bone metastases have been found in 66%, 24%, and 12% of gallbladder carcinoma patients, respectively.[23]

The staging systems used for gallbladder carcinoma are based on the pathologic characteristics of local invasion by the tumor and lymph node metastases. Before the American Joint Cancer Committee (AJCC) developed a tumor-node metastasis (TNM) staging schema for gallbladder carcinoma, the Nevin and colleagues staging system was used frequently.[27] Studies of gallbladder carcinoma performed in Japan generally apply the staging system of the Japanese Society of Biliary Surgery.[28] Most recent studies stage patients according to the TNM criteria. Carcinoma *in situ* corresponds to a T1aN0M0 tumor in the AJCC staging system. The characteristics of these three staging systems are outlined in Table 1.

Clinical presentation

The most common symptoms and signs in patients with gallbladder carcinoma are nonspecific. Right upper quadrant abdominal pain, which may or may not be exacerbated by eating a fatty meal, is the predominant presenting complaint in 75–97% of patients.[2,8,29] Right upper quadrant abdominal tenderness is present in a slightly smaller percentage of patients. These symptoms and signs usually are ascribed to cholelithiasis or cholecystitis. Nausea, vomiting, and anorexia are present in 40–64% of patients; clinically evident

Table 1 Comparison of the three most commonly used staging systems for gallbladder carcinoma.

Stage	Nevin	JSBS	AJCC-TNM
I	Cancer confined to the mucosa	Cancer confined to subserosal layers	T1aN0M0, T1bN0M0
II	Cancer involves the mucosa and muscularis	Direct invasion of the liver and/or bile duct, porta hepatis lymph node metastases	T2N0M0
III	Cancer extends through the serosa (all three layers of the gallbladder wall involved)	More extensive liver invasion by cancer, more extensive regional lymph node metastases (gastrohepatic, retropancreatic)	T1N1M0, T2N1M0, T3AnyNM0
IV	Tumor extends through all three layers of the gallbladder wall with cystic lymph node metastasis	Liver, peritoneal, and/or distant organ metastases	T4AnyNM0, any TAnyNM1
V	Tumor invades the liver by direct extension and/or metastasis to any distant organ	No stage V	No stage V

Abbreviations: AJCC, American Joint Committee on Cancer; JSBS, Japanese Society of Biliary Surgery; T, primary tumor; Tx, primary tumor cannot be assessed; T1, tumor invades mucosa or muscle layer; T1a, tumor invades mucosa; T1b, tumor invades muscle; T2, tumor invades perimuscular connective tissue, no extension beyond serosa or into liver; T3, tumor invades beyond serosa or into one adjacent organ or both (extension <2 cm into liver); T4, tumor extends >2 cm into liver and/or into two or more adjacent organs (stomach, duodenum, colon, pancreas, omentum, extrahepatic bile ducts); N, regional lymph nodes; Nx, regional lymph nodes cannot be assessed; N0, no regional lymph node metastasis; N1, regional lymph node metastasis; N1a, metastasis in cystic duct, pericholedochal, and/or gastrohepatic lymph nodes; N1b, metastasis in peripancreatic, periduodenal, periportal, celiac, and/or superior mesenteric artery lymph nodes; M, distant metastasis; Mx, presence of distant metastasis cannot be assessed; M0, no distant metastasis; M1, distant metastasis.

jaundice is present in 45%; and weight loss greater than 10% of normal body weight is noted in 37–77%.

Although 45% of patients are jaundiced at presentation, 70% of patients present with a serum bilirubin elevated at least two times greater than normal.[29] Serum alkaline phosphatase levels are elevated in two-thirds of patients with gallbladder carcinoma. Alanine aminotransferase and aspartate aminotransferase levels are elevated in one-third of patients and are consistent with advanced hepatic invasion and metastases. In these patients with TNM stage III or IV disease, the serum CEA level is elevated in >80% of patients.[29] The incidence of elevated serum CEA levels in early-stage disease is not known.

Diagnostic studies

Before ultrasonography and CT (computerized tomography) became widely available, the preoperative diagnosis rate for gallbladder carcinoma was only 8.6–16.3%.[2] Ultrasonography is the primary imaging study for symptomatic patients with presumed cholelithiasis or choledocholithiasis. High-resolution ultrasonography is able to detect early and locally advanced gallbladder carcinoma.[30] An early tumor as small as 5 mm can be recognized as a polypoid mass projecting into the gallbladder lumen or as a focal thickening of the gallbladder wall.[31] In patients with locally advanced gallbladder carcinoma, ultrasonography can demonstrate extrahepatic and intrahepatic bile duct obstruction, porta hepatis lymphadenopathy, direct hepatic extension of tumor, and hepatic metastases. Preoperative ultrasonography may suggest the correct diagnosis in up to 75% of patients with gallbladder carcinoma.[31,32] However, ultrasonography does not accurately detect celiac or paraortic lymphadenopathy or peritoneal tumor dissemination.[33] Blood flow studies with color Doppler ultrasonography are also useful because gallbladder cancers have high-velocity arterial flow in 90% of cases, while benign lesions have minimal flow.[34] Recent advances in endoscopic ultrasonography, including the use of contrast-enhancing agents, may improve the diagnostic accuracy in assessing the T stage of the gallbladder cancer.[35]

CT scans are performed less frequently in patients with presumed benign biliary tract disease. However, if gallbladder carcinoma is suspected, CT findings can correctly predict the diagnosis in 88–95% of patients.[36,37] The CT characteristics of gallbladder carcinoma include diffuse or focal gallbladder wall thickness of greater than 0.5 mm in 95% of patients, gallbladder wall contrast

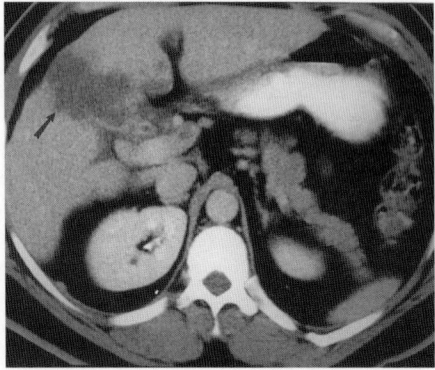

Figure 2 High-resolution, helical CT scan in a patient with gallbladder carcinoma. Direct tumor invasion into the hepatic parenchyma is evident.

enhancement in 95%, intraluminal mass in 90%, direct liver invasion by tumor in 85% (Figure 2), regional lymphadenopathy in 65%, concomitant cholelithiasis in 52%, dilated intrahepatic or extrahepatic bile ducts in 50%, noncontiguous liver metastases in 12%, invasion of contiguous gastrointestinal tract organs in 8%, and intraluminal gallbladder gas in 4%.[36] CT can also demonstrate calcification of the gallbladder wall (Figure 3).

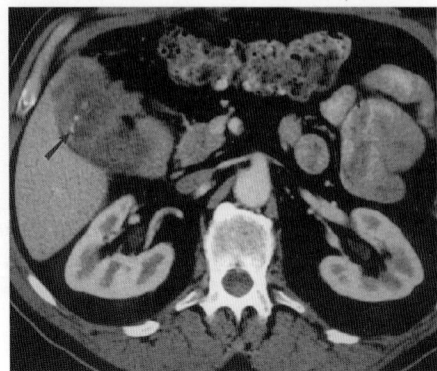

Figure 3 A high-resolution, helical CT scan in another patient with gallbladder cancer. A locally invasive tumor is again noted with areas of calcification (arrow) seen in the thickened gallbladder wall.

Treatment

Resection

The curative resection rates for gallbladder carcinoma range from 10% to 30%.[38] The majority of patients are not candidates for curative resection because of extensive locoregional disease, noncontiguous liver metastases, and/or distant metastases. Although it is clear that long-term survival can be achieved in some patients with resectable lesions, the extent of resection remains a controversial issue.

Simple cholecystectomy is an adequate therapy for gallbladder carcinoma confined to the mucosa (T1aN0M0). The 5-year survival rate for patients undergoing simple cholecystectomy for disease confined to the mucosa ranges from 57% to 100%.[39,40] However, employing simple cholecystectomy as the sole therapy for patients with T1aN0M0 tumors is not universally agreed upon. Some authors recommend that extended cholecystectomy (cholecystectomy, wedge resection of the gallbladder fossa including a 3–5 cm margin of normal liver, and a cystic, pericholedochal, gastrohepatic, pancreaticoduodenal, and paraortic lymphadenectomy) be performed to treat patients with these very early-stage lesions.[41,42]

These authors recommend that all gallbladders be opened at the time of cholecystectomy for frozen section evaluation of any suspicious areas in the mucosa. If an unsuspected gallbladder carcinoma is diagnosed by frozen section biopsy or if a T1aN0M0 gallbladder carcinoma is diagnosed on final pathology, these authors advocate that an extended cholecystectomy be performed. The bias for this aggressive surgical treatment of T1aN0M0 gallbladder carcinoma

is based on the small number of cases of regional lymph node recurrence in patients treated with simple cholecystectomy alone. No rationale is provided for the liver resection because the small number of patients who did fail after simple cholecystectomy developed metastases in the pericholedochal or cystic lymph nodes and not in the liver. Furthermore, the incidence of subsequent lymph node metastases in T1aN0M0 patients was <10% in the small groups of 32 and 36 patients, respectively.[41,42] The incidence of lymph node metastases in 201 patients with gallbladder carcinoma confined to the mucosa was only 2.5% in a study of patients who underwent cholecystectomy and regional lymphadenectomy.[39] The mortality rate for extended resection ranges from 2% to 5%, and major postoperative morbidity occurs in 13–40%.[39,40,43] Therefore, the morbidity and mortality associated with extended cholecystectomy is excessive compared with the potential survival benefit that would occur in <5% of patients with T1aN0M0 lesions.

There is a rationale for performing extended cholecystectomy in patients with T1b tumors or AJCC-TNM stage II and III gallbladder carcinomas (Figure 4). In 165 patients with T1b gallbladder carcinomas, there was a 15.6% incidence of regional lymph node metastasis.[39] Of 867 patients with a T2 primary lesion, 56.1% had regional lymph node metastases.[39] The 453 patients with T3 tumors had a 74.4% incidence of regional lymph node metastases. The 5-year survival rate following extended cholecystectomy for AJCC stage II and III gallbladder carcinoma ranges from 7.5% to 71%.[39,40,43,44] Regional lymph node metastases and/or direct tumor invasion of the hepatic parenchyma are indicators of poor prognosis, with significant reductions in 5-year overall survival rates associated with these pathologic findings.[45,46] Microscopically

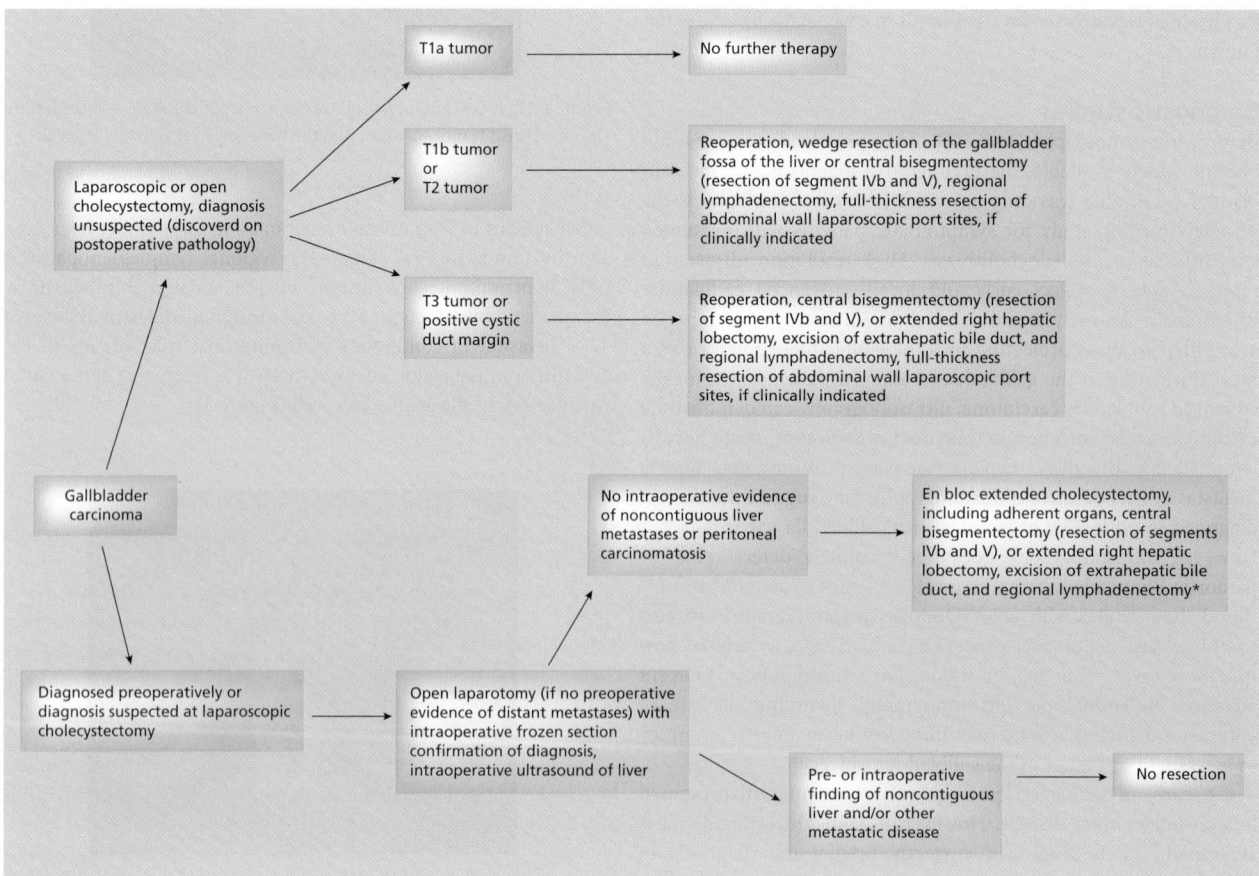

Figure 4 Algorithm to guide surgical decision making for patients with gallbladder cancer. *Regional lymphadenectomy includes complete dissection and removal of the cystic, pericholedochal, pancreaticoduodenal, gastrohepatic, and paraortic lymph nodes.

positive liver resection margins also have a negative impact on survival because these patients had a median survival of 8.9 months compared with 67.2 months for patients with tumor-free margins.[45] Preoperative helical CT scans and intraoperative ultrasonography are used to assess the extent of direct invasion into the hepatic parenchyma, which assists with decision making regarding the extent of liver resection necessary to clear all disease. If adequate tumor-negative resection margins are attained, the radicality of liver resection does not affect survival, as attested by similar long-term survival rates following right lobectomy, extended right lobectomy, right trisegmentectomy, and central bisegmentectomy for gallbladder cancer.[39,40,47–49] T1b patients are classified as stage I in the AJCC system, but, arguably, with a 15.6% incidence of regional lymph node metastases, long-term survival benefit may occur in a significant number of these patients who undergo an extended cholecystectomy (Figure 4).

All authors do not perform an en bloc resection of the extrahepatic bile duct as part of an extended cholecystectomy. Because gallbladder carcinoma is found to invade the extrahepatic bile duct in 57% of cases, with almost all cases occurring in patients with T3 or T4 tumors, an en bloc resection of the proper hepatic and common bile ducts with Roux-en-Y hepaticojejunostomy should be included in an extended cholecystectomy of transmurally invasive tumors. This includes those individuals in whom a clinically unsuspected gallbladder carcinoma is diagnosed pathologically following a simple cholecystectomy with a positive margin at the cystic duct. Gallbladder cancer involving the cystic duct and gallbladder neck frequently grows along the proper hepatic and right bile ducts, necessitating a right or extended right hepatic lobectomy and excision of the extrahepatic ducts to remove all disease.[50]

Extremely radical operations have been proposed for patients with extensive T3N1M0 or T4N01M0 tumors. This includes hepatopancreatic duodenectomy and abdominal organ cluster transplantation for locally advanced gallbladder carcinoma.[39,51,52] The operative mortality rate for these radical procedures is at least 15%, with a greater than 90% incidence of major morbidity. Resection of the portal vein and/or hepatic artery with vascular reconstruction frequently is necessary to resect completely all gross malignant disease. The largest report of patients undergoing hepatopancreatic duodenectomy for gallbladder carcinoma is 150 cases from Japan, with a 5-year survival rate of 14%.[39] The patients who did not die from intraoperative or postoperative complications all succumbed to recurrent and/or metastatic carcinoma.

It is estimated that 80,000 laparoscopic cholecystectomies are performed each year in the United States. On average, gallbladder carcinoma is diagnosed in 2% of patients undergoing cholecystectomy for presumed benign biliary tract disease. Thus, approximately 1600 patients who annually undergo laparoscopic cholecystectomy could suffer inadvertent dissemination of gallbladder carcinoma.[53–56] However, the potential laparoscopic dissemination of tumor cells may not significantly alter the natural history of gallbladder cancer in most patients. A review of our experience at the University of Texas MD Anderson Cancer Center with diagnostic and therapeutic laparoscopy in patients with gastrointestinal malignancies indicated that port site recurrence is a harbinger of widespread metastasis in >95% of patients; thus, it is rarely an isolated site of recurrent malignant disease.[57] Furthermore, a report drawn from the National Cancer Data Base between 1989 and 1995 revealed no change in incidence or survival from gallbladder cancer during the time laparoscopic cholecystectomy supplanted open cholecystectomy as the procedure of choice for gallbladder disease presumed benign.[58] Nonetheless, because of the

large number of cholecystectomies being performed laparoscopically and the small but measurable risk of dissemination of tumor cells, it has been recommended that (1) unless the surgeon feels capable of performing a definitive extended cholecystectomy for gallbladder carcinoma, patients in whom gallbladder carcinoma is suspected preoperatively by clinical or radiologic criteria should be referred without laparoscopy, laparotomy, or percutaneous biopsy, and (2) if gallbladder carcinoma is suspected on visual inspection during an attempted laparoscopic cholecystectomy, either an open definitive operation should be performed or the operation should be terminated without biopsy and the patient referred for appropriate surgical therapy.[53] Patients who underwent laparoscopic cholecystectomy and were then found on pathologic analysis to have gallbladder cancer should still be considered for aggressive surgical treatment because long-term disease-free survival will result in a subset of these patients.[59]

Palliation/chemotherapy

The majority of patients with gallbladder carcinoma are diagnosed at an advanced, unresectable stage of disease. As in patients with hilar bile duct cancer, relief of symptomatic jaundice should be considered. Patients with unresectable gallbladder carcinoma frequently have extensive involvement of the extrahepatic bile duct and may have bulky porta hepatis lymphadenopathy, which makes endoscopic placement of an internal stent difficult. When unresectable gallbladder carcinoma is diagnosed at the time of laparotomy, a surgical biliary bypass, such as an intrahepatic cholangioenteric anastomosis, can be performed and results in significant symptomatic relief in >90% of patients.[60] When the diagnosis is made on the basis of radiographic and percutaneous biopsy findings, jaundice can be relieved by placement of percutaneous transhepatic biliary catheters.

In contrast to patients with hilar bile duct carcinoma, in whom gastroduodenal obstruction is a relatively rare event, between 30% and 50% of patients with advanced gallbladder carcinoma will develop a clinically significant element of gastroduodenal obstruction.[61] This can be treated surgically with a bypass procedure such as gastrojejunostomy, by endoscopic placement of an expandable metal stent, or by placement of a decompressing gastrostomy tube and feeding jejunostomy tube. A percutaneous endoscopic gastrostomy tube can also be used to decompress the obstructed stomach in patients with advanced disease and limited expected survival time.

Chemotherapy studies that describe the results of chemotherapeutic treatment of unresectable or metastatic gallbladder carcinoma suffer from small numbers of patients and inclusion of patients with hilar bile duct carcinoma. In general, primary treatment options for patients with advanced gallbladder carcinoma include a fluoropyrimidine-based or gemcitabine-based chemotherapy regimen. A study of 53 patients with gallbladder carcinoma who received systemic chemotherapy with 5-fluorouracil (5-FU) or 5-FU plus other chemotherapeutic agents showed objective antitumor responses in 12% or less of the patients in each treatment arm.[62] Fluoropyrimidines combined with doxorubicin administered systemically have produced objective response rates of 30–40%.[63,64] A meta-analysis of three randomized studies comparing chemotherapy with gemcitabine alone versus gemcitabine plus platinum agents showed improved median overall survival of 3.8 months ($P < 0.001$) and median progression-free survival of 3.3 months ($P < 0.001$) in patients receiving doublet chemotherapy for advanced gallbladder and biliary tract malignancies.[65] Complete remission is rare and in most studies, median survival is 11 months or less. However, the literature regarding treatment results with specific regimens is limited because most series are small, and many reports consist of a mix of bile duct cancers, gallbladder cancer, and either pancreatic or hepatocellular cancer. More details about systemic treatment options are explained in the cholangiocarcinoma section.

Radiation therapy

Analysis of the patterns of failure after resection of gallbladder carcinoma revealed that local recurrence was the first and, in a significant number of cases, the only site of failure in more than one-half of patients.[66] External beam radiation therapy (EBRT) to a total dose of 45 Gy can produce radiographic evidence of tumor reduction in 20–70% of these tumors and provide temporary relief of jaundice in up to 80% of patients.[67-69] In general, EBRT is a palliative treatment. The median survival for locally advanced gallbladder carcinoma patients treated with radiation therapy is approximately 10 months.[66-69] Occasional long-term survivors are reported following treatment with higher doses of radiation therapy or with administration of radiation-sensitizing chemotherapeutic agents such as 5-FU during EBRT.[66] However, extrahepatic bile duct stricture has been reported in several of the long-term survivors treated with high doses of radiation therapy.[70]

Multidisciplinary approaches

The majority of patients who undergo an extended cholecystectomy or more radical resection for AJCC stage II, III, or IV gallbladder carcinoma develop tumor recurrence and die as a result of their disease. Nonrandomized studies and case reports have suggested that overall survival can be improved by administering adjuvant radiation therapy and/or chemotherapy after resection of stage II, III, or IV tumors.[71-73] Unfortunately, the number of patients who have received postsurgical adjuvant treatment is small, and a variety of treatment regimens have been used. In a nonrandomized study, 9 patients with stage IV gallbladder carcinoma were treated with complete surgical resection alone, while 17 patients were treated with complete resection combined with 20–30 Gy of intraoperative radiation therapy.[74] Ten of these 17 patients also received 36.4 Gy of postoperative EBRT. The surgical procedures performed in both groups of patients included extended cholecystectomy and a variety of more radical procedures, including hepatopancreatic duodenectomy. There were no 3-year survivors among the 9 patients treated with resection alone, but there was a 3-year survivorship of 10.1% in the 17 patients treated with resection and radiation therapy. There is a single report of 18 patients treated with preoperative chemoradiation therapy (4500 cGy, 180 cGy/fraction, 5 days/week, continuous intravenous infusion of 5-FU 350 mg/m² /day on days 1–5 and 21–25) prior to a planned resection of known gallbladder cancer.[75] Thirteen of the 18 patients underwent resection; one patient refused operation, one patient did not complete preoperative chemoradiation, one patient had disease progression after chemoradiation, and two patients had unresectable disease found at laparotomy. The actuarial 5-year survival rate in the 13 resected patients was 57%.

While most additional literature about postoperative therapy comes from single-institution retrospective reviews, a recently reported nonrandomized phase 2 study evaluated the role of adjuvant chemotherapy and concurrent chemoradiotherapy in 79 patients with a pathologic diagnosis of extrahepatic cholangiocarcinoma or gallbladder carcinoma (but not ampullary cancer) after radical resection, with pathologic stage T2-4 or N1 or positive resection margins.[76] Patients received four cycles of gemcitabine (1000 mg/m² on days 1 and 8) and capecitabine (1500 mg/m² /day on days 1–14) every 21 days followed by concurrent capecitabine

(1330 mg/m² /day) and radiotherapy (RT) (45 Gy to regional lymphatics; 54–59.4 Gy to tumor bed). For all patients, the 2-year survival rate was 65%; it was 67% and 60% in R0 and R1 patients, respectively. Median overall survival was 35 months (R0, 34 months; R1, 35 months).

Furthermore, a recent meta-analysis that included 20 studies involving 6712 patients with resected gallbladder or bile duct cancers did show a nonsignificant survival benefit in patients who received adjuvant chemotherapy or chemoradiotherapy, especially in those with lymph-node-positive disease.[71] However, owing to limited clinical trial data, the optimal adjuvant treatment strategy for patients who have undergone surgical resection for gallbladder carcinoma has not been established.

Bile duct cancer

Cholangiocarcinomas are malignant tumors that arise from the epithelium of the intrahepatic or extrahepatic bile ducts. In the United States, approximately 3000 patients are diagnosed with cholangiocarcinoma of both the intra- or extrahepatic biliary system annually.[77] There is only a slight male preponderance of cases of cholangiocarcinoma. Cholangiocarcinomas can arise at any site in the intra- or extrahepatic biliary system, but perihilar tumors comprise two-thirds of the cases of cholangiocarcinoma (Figure 5).[78]

Causative factors

There are distinct differences between the factors associated with cholangiocarcinoma and those associated with HCC (Table 2). Only 10–20% of cholangiocarcinomas occur in cirrhotic patients, compared with the 70–90% of HCCs that arise in cirrhotic livers.[77,79,80] A cohort study in Denmark of 11,605 patients with cirrhosis indicated a 60-fold increased risk of developing hepatocellular cancer and a 10-fold increased risk of cholangiocarcinoma.[80] Frequently, the cirrhosis associated with cholangiocarcinomas is a subacute secondary biliary type that results from the neoplastic obstruction of the bile ducts, indicating that, in some cases, cirrhosis in cholangiocarcinoma patients is the result of the tumor rather than its cause.

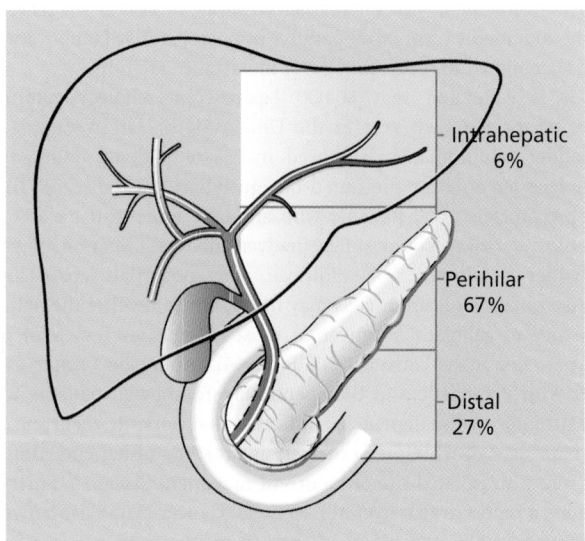

Figure 5 The distribution of 294 cholangiocarcinomas into intrahepatic, perihilar, and distal subgroups. Source: Aretxabala 1999.[75] Reproduced with permission of Elsevier.

Table 2 Factors associated with increased risk to develop cholangiocarcinoma versus hepatocellular carcinoma.

Cholangio carcinoma	Hepatocellular carcinoma
Liver fluke infection	Cirrhosis
Ophisthorchis sinensis	Chronic hepatitis B virus infection
Opisthorchis viverrini	Chronic hepatitis C virus infection
Congenital/chronic cystic dilation	Aflatoxin B1 ingestion of the bile ducts
Choledochal cyst	Chronic ethanol ingestion
Caroli disease	Primary biliary cirrhosis
Hepatolithiasis	Hemochromatosis
Primary sclerosing cholangitis	α-1-Antitrypsin deficiency
Ulcerative colitis	Glycogen storage disease
Thorotrast exposure	Hypercitrullinemia
Cholelithiasis	Porphyrias
Asbestos	Hereditary tyrosinemia
Dioxin (Agent Orange)	Wilson disease
Polychlorinated diphenyls	Hepatotoxin exposure
Nitrosamines	Thorotrast
Isoniazid	Polyvinyl chloride
Methyldopa	Carbon tetrachloride

Cholangiocarcinoma is more prevalent in Southeast Asia than in other parts of the world. The higher incidence in this geographic region is related to parasitic infection with the liver flukes *Opisthorchis sinensis* and *Opisthorchis viverrini*.[81,82] Liver flukes induce hyperplasia, fibrosis, and adenomatous proliferation of human biliary epithelium and are associated with hepatolithiasis. The fluke infestation suggests a direct etiologic role in the subsequent development of cholangiocarcinoma, but this relationship is not established unequivocally.

Several disorders that can produce chronic inflammation of the bile ducts have been associated with an increased risk of developing cholangiocarcinoma. These include polycystic liver disease, choledochal cysts, congenital dilation of the intrahepatic bile ducts (Caroli syndrome), sclerosing cholangitis (occasionally in association with inflammatory bowel disease), hepatolithiasis, and cholelithiasis.[83-88] Hepatolithiasis is not a common disorder, and only 5–7% of patients with documented hepatic stones develop cholangiocarcinoma.[87,88] The reported incidence of cholangiocarcinoma developing in areas of congenital cystic dilation of the bile duct, including choledochal cysts and Caroli disease, ranges from 3% to 30%.[89,90] Patients with primary sclerosing cholangitis are also at increased risk to develop cholangiocarcinoma, with incidence rates ranging from 9% to 40%.[91,92] Patients with ulcerative colitis may also develop sclerosing cholangitis, but cholangiocarcinoma occurs in only 0.4–1.4% of individuals with ulcerative colitis.[91] In patients with sclerosing cholangitis, whether associated with ulcerative colitis or not, radiologic distinction between sclerosing cholangitis and cholangiocarcinoma is often impossible. One study showed that the serum tumor marker CA19-9 had an 89% sensitivity and 86% specificity in diagnosing cholangiocarcinoma in patients with sclerosing cholangitis.[93] Combining serum CA19-9 levels with serum CEA levels may further increase the diagnostic accuracy to detect cholangiocarcinoma in patients with sclerosing cholangitis.[94]

Patients who underwent diagnostic radiography with intravenous injection of Thorotrast (thorium dioxide) are at high risk of developing HCC, angiosarcoma, and cholangiocarcinoma.[95] Cholangiocarcinoma is the most frequent hepatic neoplasm reported in patients who have received Thorotrast. Exposure to several drugs or carcinogens has also been linked to an increased risk to develop cholangiocarcinoma (Table 2). Because cholangiocarcinoma is a relatively rare neoplasm, it has been difficult to prove its pathogenesis related to any of these factors, but it is clear that chronic inflammation of the biliary tree by any cause is associated with an increased risk of developing cholangiocarcinoma.

Chronic inflammation of the biliary system or exposure to genotoxic agents concentrated in bile may produce damage to the DNA of biliary epithelial cells, leading to the development of cholangiocarcinoma. Mutations in the p53 tumor suppressor gene and in the K-*ras* proto-oncogene have been identified in cholangiocarcinoma patients.[96,97] There may be geographic and population-based differences in the mutation rates of these two genes in cholangiocarcinoma, but alterations in p53 and K-ras are observed in significant proportions of patients with any of the identified factors (Table 2) that increase risk to develop cholangiocarcinoma. Overexpression of *c-erbB-2*, a proto-oncogene that encodes a transmembrane protein that is highly homologous to epidermal growth factor receptor (EGFR), has been confirmed in human cholangiocarcinoma cells and in benign proliferative biliary epithelium from patients with hepatolithiasis, primary sclerosing cholangitis, and liver fluke infestation.[98] Alterations in *c-erbB-2* expression may occur early in the chronic inflammation-induced proliferation of biliary epithelium leading to malignant transformation. Chronic inflammation may also produce the overexpression of the *Bcl-2* proto-oncogene observed in cholangiocarcinomas, which may promote tumorigenesis by inhibiting normal apoptotic processes.[99]

Lastly, recent comprehensive genomic profiling has also shown that intra- and extrahepatic cholangiocarcinomas share frequent genomic alterations in cell cycle regulation (CDKN2B) and chromatin remodeling (ARID1A).[21] Intrahepatic cholangiocarcinomas are further characterized by FGFR fusions, IDH1/2 (isocitrate dehydrogenase) substitutions, BRAF substitutions, and MET amplification while extrahepatic cholangiocarcinomas have frequent PIK3CA/MTOR pathway alterations.

Clinical presentation

The clinical features of cholangiocarcinoma are nonspecific and depend on the location of the tumor. The usual clinical presentation of patients with hilar cholangiocarcinoma is painless jaundice. Patients may also report concomitant onset of fatigue, pruritus, fever, vague abdominal pain, and anorexia. The serum liver function tests in patients with hilar cholangiocarcinoma commonly demonstrate obstructive jaundice, with alkaline phosphatase and total bilirubin levels elevated in greater than 90% of patients.[77] Cholangiocarcinomas that arise in peripheral bile ducts within the hepatic parenchyma usually reach a large size before becoming clinically evident. Patients with these large peripheral hepatic tumors usually present with hepatomegaly and an upper abdominal mass, abdominal and back pain, and weight loss.[77] Jaundice and ascites are late and usually preterminal sequelae in patients with large intrahepatic cholangiocarcinomas. Jaundice associated with a large hepatic cholangiocarcinoma is caused by a combination of extension of the tumor to the bifurcation of the left and right hepatic ducts, and by compression of the contralateral bile ducts by the expanding tumor.

Serum alkaline phosphatase levels are elevated in >90% of patients with cholangiocarcinoma.[78] Serum bilirubin also is elevated in the majority of cholangiocarcinoma patients, particularly in those with a tumor arising in the central portion of the liver or the extrahepatic hilar bile ducts.[100] In contrast to HCC, serum α-fetoprotein levels are abnormal in fewer than 5% of cholangiocarcinoma patients.[78] There is an increase in serum CEA levels in 40–60% of cholangiocarcinoma patients.[78,101] Another tumor marker, CA19-9, is elevated in >80% of patients with cholangiocarcinoma.[101]

Pathology

Cholangiocarcinomas originating in the periphery of the hepatic parenchyma usually are solitary and large, but satellite nodules occasionally are present.[102] Gross tumor invasion of the large portal or hepatic veins occurs much less frequently than in HCC. The gross and microscopic appearance of intrahepatic cholangiocarcinomas may have prognostic significance because tumors with periductal infiltration have a higher incidence of lymph node and intrahepatic metastasis.[103] Metastases to the regional lymph nodes, lungs, and peritoneal cavity are more common in cholangiocarcinoma than in HCC. When the tumor causes long-standing biliary obstruction, the liver may show secondary biliary cirrhosis.

Microscopically, low cuboidal cells that resemble the normal biliary epithelium characterize cholangiocarcinomas. Varying degrees of pleomorphism, atypia, mitotic activity, hyperchromatic nuclei, and prominent nucleoli are noted from area to area in the same tumor. Rarely, a clear cell variant of cholangiocarcinoma occurs, which must be distinguished from clear cell renal carcinoma with liver metastasis.[104] Cholangiocarcinomas are mucin-secreting adenocarcinomas, and intracellular and intraluminal mucin often can be demonstrated. The presence of mucin is useful in differentiating cholangiocarcinoma from HCC. The absence of bile production by cholangiocarcinoma can also be useful in distinguishing this tumor from HCC. Immunohistochemical staining that is positive for epithelial membrane antigen and tissue polypeptide antigen may be useful in confirming a diagnosis of cholangiocarcinoma.[105,106] Immunohistochemical staining for cytokeratin subtypes can be helpful in differentiating cholangiocarcinoma from metastatic colorectal carcinoma.[107] Cholangiocarcinomas are usually locally invasive, which spread along nerves or in subepithelial layers of the bile ducts.

Diagnostic studies

Peripheral intrahepatic cholangiocarcinoma is often difficult to distinguish pathologically and radiographically from a deposit of metastatic adenocarcinoma within the liver. Although transabdominal ultrasonography can detect an intrahepatic malignant tumor greater than 2 cm in diameter, ultrasound findings do not differ between cholangiocarcinomas, liver metastases from extrahepatic adenocarcinomas, and multinodular HCC.[108] CT demonstrates a

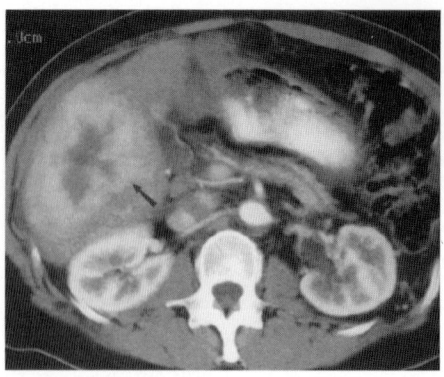

Figure 6 High-resolution, helical CT scan during the arterial contrast phase in a patient with an intrahepatic cholangiocarcinoma. The periphery of the tumor (arrow) has irregular margins and enhances with contrast. A relatively hypovascular area of scar and tumor necrosis is evident in the center of the tumor.

rounded, low-attenuation mass with irregular or lobulated margins (Figure 6). Satellite lesions may be evident, particularly when using helical CT during the optimal period of hepatic contrast enhancement. Calcification within the tumor is present in 25% of cases, and a central scar is observed in 30%.[109] MRI (magnetic resonance imaging) shows a nonencapsulated mass with irregular margins that is hypointense compared with the normal liver on T1-weighted and hyperintense on T2-weighted images. The peripheral rim of the tumor usually enhances following MRI contrast administration. A hyperintense central scar is best seen on T2-weighted images, but the CT and MRI characteristics of intrahepatic cholangiocarcinomas may be present in other types of hepatic tumors.[109]

A diagnosis of hilar cholangiocarcinoma should be suspected in the patient with painless jaundice whose CT scan demonstrates dilated intrahepatic bile ducts with a normal gallbladder and an extrahepatic biliary tree. High-resolution, helical CT scans can provide information on the location of an obstructing biliary tumor and may suggest the extent of involvement of the liver and porta hepatis structures by the tumor (Figure 7). Multiphasic helical CT can correctly identify the level of biliary obstruction by a hilar

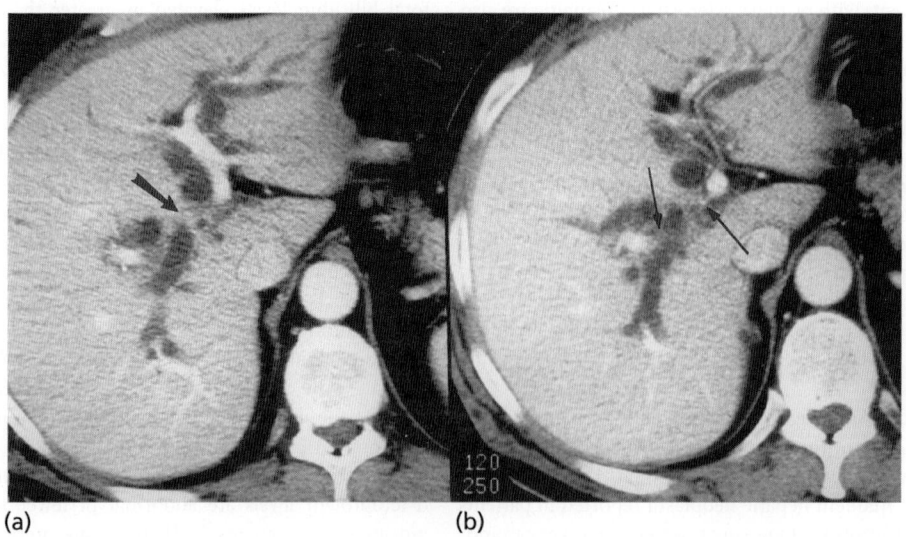

(a)   (b)

Figure 7 High-resolution, helical CT scan in another patient presenting with obstructive jaundice. The tumor mass (a), (large arrow) producing marked intrahepatic biliary duct dilatation is evident. Areas of tumor invasion of the portal vein (b), (small arrows) suggested on the CT scan were confirmed at the time of operation to be tumor invasion of the portal vein.

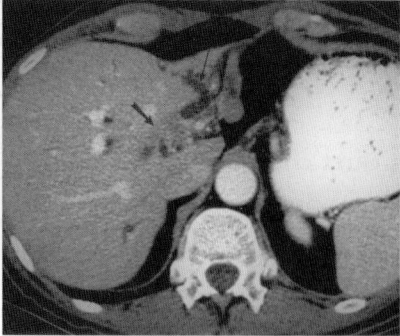

Figure 8 High-resolution, helical CT scan in a patient presenting with several months of increasing pruritus followed by the development of clinically evident jaundice. The relatively hypodense hilar cholangiocarcinoma (large arrow) is evident. Marked atrophy of the left hepatic lobe is noted with dilated intrahepatic bile ducts (small arrow), but little remaining hepatic parenchyma is evident.

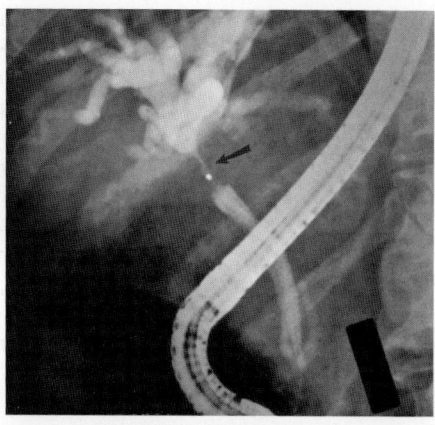

Figure 9 Endoscopic retrograde cholangiopancreatography showing a focal stricture of the proper hepatic bile duct (arrow) with marked dilatation of the intrahepatic bile ducts. This hilar cholangiocarcinoma was completely resected with Roux-en-Y hepaticojejunostomy reconstruction of biliary-enteric continuity.

cholangiocarcinoma in 63–90% of patients.[110,111] Preoperative helical CT is also useful in demonstrating lobar or segmental liver atrophy caused by bile duct obstruction or portal vein occlusion (Figure 8).[111] However, helical CT is not accurate in assessing the resectability of hilar cholangiocarcinomas because of limited resolution in evaluating intraductal tumor spread and significant false-positive and false-negative rates in demonstrating portal vein or hepatic artery involvement by tumor.[110,111]

Like the CT scan, ultrasonography can demonstrate a nondilated gallbladder and common bile duct associated with dilated intrahepatic ducts. In addition, as grayscale ultrasonography has improved, the diagnosis of cholangiocarcinoma is supported by finding a hilar bile duct mass in 65–90% of patients.[112] Ultrasonography and CT scan may be used to demonstrate the presence of intrahepatic tumor due to direct extension or noncontiguous metastases and enlarged periportal lymph nodes, suggesting nodal metastases.[113] Even intraoperative ultrasonography is suboptimal for detecting intraductal spread by hilar cholangiocarcinoma, correctly demonstrating the extent of tumor spread away from the primary biliary tumor in only 18% of cases.[114] Intraoperative ultrasonography can be used to screen for noncontiguous liver metastases from the primary biliary cancer and can accurately detect direct tumor invasion of the portal vein and hepatic artery in 83.3% and 60% of cases, respectively.[114]

Similar to the intrahepatic variety, hilar cholangiocarcinoma usually shows hypointensity on T1- and hyperintensity on T2-weighted MRI. Dilated intrahepatic bile ducts are evident in patients with obstructing tumors, and lobar atrophy is seen in cases of portal venous occlusion. Fast low-angle shot (FLASH) MR with contrast-enhanced coronal imaging has been used to demonstrate intraluminal extension of tumor and to distinguish between blood vessels and bile ducts.[115] Magnetic resonance cholangiopancreatography (MRCP) and MR virtual endoscopy can demonstrate hilar bile duct obstruction by tumor with dilated intrahepatic ducts.[115,116] The advantages of MRCP over direct cholangiography include noninvasiveness and possible visualization of isolated bile ducts.

Cholangiography definitively demonstrates a lesion obstructing the left and right hepatic ducts at the hilar confluence (Figure 9), and percutaneous transhepatic cholangiography (PTC) and endoscopic retrograde cholangiopancreatography (ERCP) are both useful in assessing patients with extrahepatic biliary obstruction. A prospective, randomized comparison of PTC and ERCP in patients with jaundice concluded that the two techniques had similar diagnostic accuracy.[117] PTC was 100% accurate in demonstrating

obstruction at the confluence of the left and right hepatic ducts, while ERCP had an accuracy of 92% in demonstrating these lesions. ERCP has the additional benefit of providing a pancreatogram. A normal pancreatogram helps exclude a small carcinoma of the head of the pancreas as a cause of biliary obstruction. Cytologic specimens can be obtained at the time of PTC and ERCP. The presence of malignant cells in bile or bile duct brushings is confirmed in approximately 50% of patients undergoing PTC or ERCP.[112,117–119]

Drainage of the obstructed biliary tree with partial or complete relief of jaundice and associated symptoms can be achieved with PTC. Improvements in catheter technology led to the development of endoprostheses that can be placed across the malignant obstruction into the duodenum to allow internal drainage.[120] It must be emphasized that providing symptomatic relief for patients by decompressing the biliary tract should not be the primary reason to place these catheters. Prospective, randomized studies have failed to demonstrate a benefit in terms of a decrease in hospital morbidity or mortality by preoperative decompression of biliary obstruction.[121] However, the catheters are useful in identifying and dissecting the hepatic duct bifurcation at the time of operation and aid in the reconstruction of the biliary tract following extirpation of the tumor.[122,123]

Positron emission tomography (PET) is being evaluated as a diagnostic tool in patients with all types of malignant tumors. PET assesses *in vivo* metabolism of positron-emitting radiolabeled tracers like [^{18}F] fluoro-2-deoxy-D-glucose (18FFDG), a glucose analog that accumulates in various malignant tumors because of their high glucose metabolic rates. FDG-PET does not provide anatomic detail to assess resectability of hilar cholangiocarcinomas or intrahepatic malignancies, but it may prove useful in detecting distant metastatic disease that would preclude a curative resection. In patients with primary sclerosing cholangitis, FDG-PET studies may be able to detect small hilar and intrahepatic cholangiocarcinomas and thus may be useful in therapeutic and transplant decision making in these patients.[124] PET has recently been used to aid in the diagnosis and staging of patients with bile duct cancer.[125] PET scan images correctly detected the primary cholangiocarcinoma in 24 of 26 patients (sensitivity 92.3%) and was true negative in 8 patients with benign bile duct disease (adenoma, sclerosing cholangitis, Caroli disease). Distant metastatic disease was diagnosed correctly in 7 of 10 patients with histologically proven metastases, but regional lymph node metastases were identified in only 2 of 15 patients (13.3%).

The role of laparoscopy as part of the diagnostic and staging evaluation of patients with hilar cholangiocarcinoma is being evaluated at our institution. Several patients with seemingly resectable tumors have avoided an exploratory laparotomy when peritoneal tumor implants were found with laparoscopy. In addition, positive cytologic specimens obtained from laparoscopic washings may identify patients at high risk of developing peritoneal carcinomatosis. Finally, laparoscopic ultrasonography can be used to exclude the presence of noncontiguous liver metastases or extensive hilar tumor infiltration in patients with extrahepatic bile duct cancers.[126]

Treatment of intrahepatic cholangiocarcinomas

Resection

Intrahepatic cholangiocarcinomas may be detected in 30–45% of patients before they metastasize or cause jaundice.[127,128] These patients should be considered for operation because long-term survival has been reported in a proportion of the patients undergoing curative liver resection for intrahepatic cholangiocarcinoma.[79,124,128,129] A study of 19 patients who underwent resection of intrahepatic cholangiocarcinoma demonstrated that patients with no porta hepatis lymph node metastases had a 3-year survival rate of 64% compared with 0% for patients with nodal metastases.[124] A larger cohort of 32 patients who underwent resection of intrahepatic cholangiocarcinomas confirmed the negative prognostic impact of regional lymph node metastases and large size (>5-cm diameter) of the primary tumor.[129] The 5-year overall survival rates reported for patients who underwent a margin-negative liver resection for intrahepatic cholangiocarcinoma range from 20% to 48%, with regional lymph node metastases, presence of satellite tumor nodules, portal vein invasion by tumor, and large tumors identified as a poor-prognosis indicator.[124,128,129] Large size of the primary tumor is a poor-prognosis indicator because of the increased frequency of vascular and lymphatic invasion by the tumor as well as growth along neighboring bile duct walls.[130]

Multidisciplinary approaches

As with gallbladder carcinoma, the optimal adjuvant treatment strategy after surgical resection for intrahepatic cholangiocarcinoma has not been determined owing to lack of clinical trial data. Regardless, adjuvant chemotherapy or chemoradiotherapy can be considered in this setting, especially for patients with positive lymph nodes or surgical margins.[71] For patients with unresectable disease, locoregional therapies like radiofrequency ablation (RFA), transarterial chemoembolization (TACE), drug-eluting bead TACE, EBRT, and transarterial radioembolization (TARE) have all been shown to be safe and effective in small retrospective studies.[131] Recently, 79 patients with inoperable intrahepatic cholangiocarcinoma were treated at MD Anderson Cancer Center with high-dose (ablative) RT. RT doses were 35 to 100 Gy (median 58.05 Gy) in 3 to 30 fractions for a median biologic equivalent dose (BED) of 80.5 Gy (range, 43.75–180 Gy).[132] Median overall survival was 30 months. Radiation dose was the single most important prognostic factor and higher doses correlated with an improved local control rate and overall survival. The 3-year overall survival rate for patients receiving BED > 80.5 Gy was 73% versus 38% for those receiving lower doses (P 0.017); 3-year local control rate was significantly higher (78%) after a BED > 80.5 Gy than after lower doses (45%, P 0.04).[132]

In addition, the more traditional approach to unresectable and metastatic disease involves systemic chemotherapy with a fluoropyrimadine or gemcitabine-based regimen. A more detailed discussion of chemotherapy in this setting follows in the treatment section on "Hilar Bile Duct Cholangiocarcinomas".

Hilar bile duct cholangiocarcinoma

In 1890, Fardel first described a primary malignancy of the extrahepatic biliary tract. A report in 1957 described three patients with small adenocarcinomas involving the confluence of the left and right hepatic ducts.[133] Such primary cholangiocarcinomas arising at the bifurcation of the extrahepatic biliary tree are known commonly as Klatskin tumors, following his report in 1965 of a larger series of patients with these lesions.[134]

Prognostic factors

In contrast to reports, the most important factor affecting prognosis is the resectability of the tumor. Patients who undergo curative resection (margin-negative) have 3-year survival rates from 40% to 87% and 5-year survival rates between 10% and 73%.[60,135] The wide range of survival rates is explained by variations in the incidence of factors that portend a poor prognosis in the various series. Significant determinants of improved prognosis in patients undergoing curative resection include well-differentiated tumors, absence of lymph node metastases, absence of direct tumor extension into the liver, papillary histology (vs nodular or sclerotic), serum bilirubin at presentation of <9 mg/dL, and a near-normal or normal performance status. Palliative resection, surgical bypass procedures, and various types of intubation and drainage procedures are associated with 3-year survival rates of 0–4%.[135] Hilar cholangiocarcinomas have a poorer prognosis than do carcinomas arising in the middle or distal thirds of the extrahepatic bile duct, which is related directly to the presentation of hilar tumors at a more locally advanced stage with bilobar liver involvement by tumor and resultant lower rates of curative resection.[136] However, like hilar cholangiocarcinoma, the presence of regional lymph node metastases reduces the 5-year overall survival rate following resection of middle or distal third bile duct cancer to 21% compared with the 65% survival rate in patients with node-negative disease.

Pathologic features of the bile duct cancer are predictors of outcome after resection. Prognosis is affected adversely if the tumor infiltrates the serosa of the bile duct, invades directly into the liver, demonstrates vascular invasion, or has metastasized to regional lymph nodes. Histologic type and grade are also important factors. Patients with the relatively unusual papillary bile duct adenocarcinoma have the most favorable prognosis, with 3-year survival rates up to 75%.[135,137] Patients with the more common nodular or sclerotic types of hilar cholangiocarcinoma have 3-year survival rates of <30%. A pathologic study that correlated gross tumor type with patterns of spread provides evidence that may explain the observed differences in survival outcomes. Papillary and superficial nodular tumors spread predominantly by mucosal extension, rarely invading the deeper layers of the bile duct wall or lymphatic channels, whereas nodular infiltrating or diffuse infiltrating tumors spread by direct or lymphatic extension in the submucosa.[138] The distance of mucosal or submucosal spread away from the gross tumor can be as great as 30 mm, but there were no local or anastomotic recurrences if at least a 5-mm tumor-free margin was attained. Patients with well- or moderately differentiated carcinomas have a 3-year survival rate of up to 51%, whereas no patient with a poorly differentiated carcinoma survived longer than 2 years.[139]

Treatment of hilar bile duct cholangiocarcinomas

Resection

Resection of a hilar cholangiocarcinoma affords the patient the best chance for significant survival; however, 5-year survival rates after resection of hilar cancers are 40% in the most hopeful reports and 10% or less in other accounts. Long-term survival rates after resection of middle or distal common bile duct cholangiocarcinomas, the latter requiring pancreaticoduodenectomy, are generally higher compared with hilar tumors.[78] This is most likely related to higher rates of margin-negative resection with middle or distal extrahepatic bile duct tumors and the absence of direct tumor extension into the liver.

The patterns of failure after curative extrahepatic bile duct resection for hilar cholangiocarcinoma have been described in a few series of patients (Table 3).[139] Locoregional tumor recurrence developed in a high percentage of patients, with failure in the liver (62%), tumor bed (42%), and regional lymph nodes (20%). The caudate lobe is the most frequent site of liver recurrence. Regional lymph nodes include porta hepatis, retroduodenal, and perigastric node groups along the gastrohepatic ligament. Distant metastasis develops in the majority of patients who exhibit a locoregional recurrence; however, it was the site of first failure in only 24%.

Detailed anatomic studies have offered an explanation for the high incidence of liver and local recurrence following resection of a hilar cholangiocarcinoma. In a series of 25 patients undergoing surgery for hilar cholangiocarcinoma, direct invasion of hepatic parenchyma at the hilum was noted in 12 patients (46.2%), with 11 patients (42.3%) also having carcinoma extending into the bile ducts draining the caudate lobe or directly invading the caudate lobe parenchyma.[140] A study of 106 adult human cadavers showed that 97.2% had bile ducts draining the caudate lobe that entered directly into the main left hepatic duct, right hepatic duct, or both. These caudate lobe bile ducts frequently enter the main left or right hepatic ducts within 1 cm of the proper hepatic duct. Thus, a carcinoma arising at the confluence of the right and left hepatic ducts need not be large to extend into the bile ducts draining the caudate lobe.

Because cholangiocarcinoma is known to spread along the wall of the bile ducts and because the caudate lobe and hepatic hilum are frequent sites of tumor recurrence following extrahepatic duct resection, a number of authors now recommend more aggressive resections to include the caudate lobe and hepatic hilar parenchyma.[141-145] An understanding of the Bismuth–Corlette classification of hilar cholangiocarcinoma is useful in planning the extent and site of liver resection (Figure 10).[146] The median survival associated with a more radical surgical approach has varied from 10 to 37 months, with 5-year survival rates of 20–44% and 10-year survival rates as high as 14%.[141-145] Although aggressive surgical resection of hilar cholangiocarcinomas, including hepatic resection, provides the best chance for long-term survival, these operative procedures are associated with significant risk. The operative mortality rate in modern series ranges from 5% to 12%, with postoperative liver failure following an extensive liver resection being the most common cause of death.[141-145] Surgical complications are reported in 25% to 45% of the surviving patients. Infectious complications are the most common postoperative problem, and preoperative placement of biliary stents with resultant contamination of the obstructed biliary tree increases the incidence of infection.[147]

A review of patients with extrahepatic cholangiocarcinoma treated at the University of Texas MD Anderson Cancer Center was reported.[148] Of 91 patients evaluated between 1983 and 1996, 51 (56%) presented with unresectable disease and 40 (44%) underwent resection. The median survival for the resected patients was 22.2 months versus 10.7 months in patients with unresectable disease ($P < 0.0001$). Nine patients, five with hilar and four with distal common duct cholangiocarcinoma, were treated with preoperative chemoradiation therapy (continuous intravenous infusion of 5-FU at 300 mg/m^2/day combined with external beam irradiation). Three of these nine patients had a pathologic complete response to chemoradiation treatment; the remaining six patients had varying degrees of histologic response to treatment. The rate of margin-negative resection was 100% for the preoperative chemoradiation group compared with 54% for the group not

Table 3 Sites of tumor recurrence after curative resection of proximal hilar cholangiocarcinomas.

Site	Frequency (%)
Liver	62
Tumor bed	42
Regional lymph nodes	20
Peritoneum	16
Lungs	71
Bone	31
Skin	7

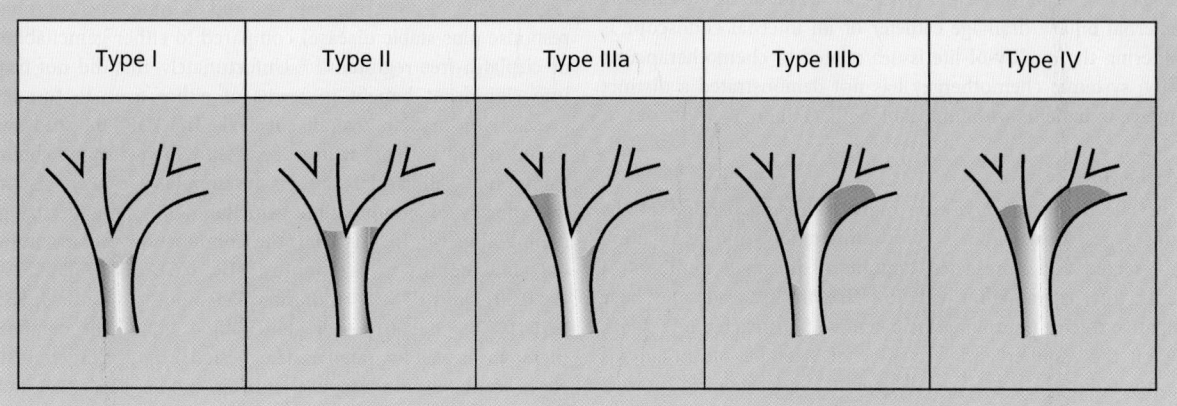

Figure 10 Bismuth–Corlette classification of hilar cholangiocarcinoma. Types I and II can be resected with excision of the extrahepatic bile duct with or without the hilar plate and caudate lobe. Types IIIA and IIIB can be resected with the addition of an en bloc right or left hepatic lobectomy, respectively. Type IV is, by definition, unresectable. Source: Bengmark 1988.[142] Wolters Kluwer Health, Inc.

receiving preoperative treatment ($P < 0.01$). The patients treated with preoperative chemoradiation had no operative or postoperative complications related to treatment. Thus, it appears that neoadjuvant chemoradiation for extrahepatic bile duct cancer can be performed safely, produces significant antitumor response, and may improve the ability to achieve tumor-free resection margins.

Liver transplantation

Total hepatectomy with immediate orthotopic liver transplantation (OLT) has been described in patients with hilar cholangiocarcinoma.[149-154] The 90-day mortality from hemorrhage, sepsis, and graft rejection was 23.1%. Of the patients who survived <3 months following transplantation, the median survival was 11 months in the series prior to 1992 but has improved to 23 months in the recent series. In the older series of patients, the 5-year survival rate was 5.0%. In patients who died 3 months after transplantation, death was due to tumor recurrence in 85.4%. The 5-year survival rate following OLT for extrahepatic cholangiocarcinoma in current studies is 25%, and in the highly selected subset of patients with stage I or II disease, 5-year survival is 73%. Nonetheless, because of the poor results in most reports, many transplantation centers no longer perform liver transplantations in patients with hilar cholangiocarcinoma. Liver transplantation for hilar cholangiocarcinoma should probably be considered only as part of a prospective protocol evaluating multimodality treatment.

Palliation

In general, curative surgical resection is possible in <30% of patients with hilar cholangiocarcinoma.[60,135,136] In patients deemed unresectable on the basis of the findings of diagnostic studies, laparotomy can be avoided by placing percutaneous external drains or endoscopically placed endoprostheses.[155,156] Conventional 10- or 12-French polyethylene endoprostheses have a high rate of occlusion and cholangitis.[156] However, new expandable metal wall stents appear to have improved long-term patency rates and may be used to deliver palliative high-dose rate endoluminal brachytherapy.[157,158] When unresectability is determined at the time of laparotomy, a decision must be made on a surgical bypass versus an operative intubation to provide drainage of the obstructed biliary tree. It is clear that techniques for surgical bypass, operative intubation, and percutaneous external drainage are equivalent in partial or complete relief of jaundice in 70–100% of patients.[60] Seemingly, the only potential advantage to the patient who undergoes surgical bypass instead of operative intubation is the absence of an external drainage catheter in the former group. The advantage of not having an external biliary drainage catheter or an internal endoscope is considering the quality-of-life issues related to chemotherapeutic toxicity; systemic chemotherapy has not demonstrated a distinct advantage in patients with hilar cholangiocarcinoma.

Radiotherapy

RT for bile duct cancer is even more confusing because of the various types, doses, routes of administration, and association with resected and unresected tumors, all in small numbers of patients. Internal radiation with 16 [169]Ir wires or seeds may have a palliative role in improving the patency of obstructed bile ducts; however, the number and frequency of episodes of cholangitis were not reduced, so the overall benefit is uncertain.[159] Internal radiation has been associated with prolongation of survival to an average of 16 months, and occasionally patients with unresectable disease survived >5 years.[160-162] Although the use of EBRT alone to treat patients with unresectable hilar cholangiocarcinoma has

not provided significant differences in overall patient survival, rare long-term survivals have been reported.[163] Intraoperative RT also has been evaluated in association with resectable and unresectable tumors.[164,165] Again, there is a suggestion of a slight prolongation of survival in patients with unresectable tumors, but the most interesting use of intraoperative RT may be as an immediate surgical adjuvant in the resected high-risk tumor bed.

Chemotherapy

Given the high percentage of unresectable hilar and intrahepatic cholangiocarcinomas, various chemotherapeutic regimens and radiotherapeutic regimens have been used in the hope of providing improved palliation and prolongation of survival. One early trial suggested a benefit for chemotherapy over best supportive care alone. The study randomly assigned 90 patients with advanced pancreatic or biliary cancer ($N = 37$) to 5-FU-based systemic chemotherapy versus best supportive care alone and reported a median survival of 6.0 months versus 2.5 months, respectively.[166] Thereafter, single-agent gemcitabine was tested in 23 chemotherapy-naive patients with locally advanced or metastatic biliary tract adenocarcinomas.[167] After a median follow up of 13.4 months, the median time to progression was 8.1 months and overall survival was 13.1 months. This trial supported gemcitabine having clinical benefit in patients with advanced biliary cancers. In general, the more active chemotherapy agents for cholangiocarcinoma now include 5-FU, gemcitabine, capectiabine, cisplatin, and oxaliplatin.[168]

Multiple combination chemotherapy regimens have been tested in the hope of improving response over single agents. 5-FU interferon alpha 2b (IFN-a2b) was tested in 35 patients with biliary tract cancer and reported a 34% partial response (11 of 32 patients), a median time to progression of 9.5 months, and a median survival of 12 months.[169] In a study of 75 patients (45 cholangiocarcinoma, 3 ampulla of Vater, and 27 gallbladder), gemcitabine plus capecitabine combination was well tolerated.[170] The study reported a response rate of 29%, median progression-free and overall survival rates were 6.2 and 12.7 months, respectively. In another study of gemcitabine and oxaliplatin (GEMOX) combination, those who had a good performance status of 0–2, bilirubin <2.5× normal and received GEMOX as first-line chemotherapy ($N = 33$) had a response rate of 33%, a median progression-free survival of 5.7 months, and a median survival of 15.4 months.[171]

A pooled analysis of 104 trials that included 2810 patients receiving different chemotherapy regimens in advanced biliary cancer concluded that the gemcitabine/cisplatin combination offered the highest rates of objective response and of tumor control (objective response plus stable disease) compared to either gemcitabine-free or cisplatin-free regimens.[172] Unfortunately, this did not translate into significant benefit in terms of either time to tumor progression or median overall survival. The ABC-02 study, which included 410 patients with unresectable or metastatic cholangiocarcinoma, gallbladder cancer, or ampullary cancer, also tested the efficacy of combination gemcitabine/cisplatin versus gemcitabine alone.[173] In this trial, the combination therapy improved OS (11.7 months vs 8.1 months; HR, 0.64; 95% CI, 0.52–0.80; $P < 0.001$) and PFS (8.0 months vs 5.0 months; HR, 0.63; 95% CI, 0.51–0.77; $P < 0.001$) over gemcitabine alone. The combination therapy was well tolerated and suggested a significant clinical benefit of combination therapy. Thereafter, another study that included 84 patients with advanced biliary cancer reported similar findings with combination gemcitabine/cisplatin.[174] Because of this, gemcitabine/cisplatin remains the first-line chemotherapy regimen for patients with unresectable of metastatic cholangiocarcinoma or gallbladder cancer. Second-line regimens include 5-FU-based or other gemcitabine-based chemotherapy combinations, which are supported by numerous phase II trials.[175–179]

More recently, several targeted agents have been studied in biliary tract cancers. One study of 42 patients suggested benefit from anti-EGFR by the oral tyrosine kinase inhibitor erlotinib.[180] There were three partial responses and seven patients remained progression-free at 6 months. The latest targeted therapy trial reported on GEMOX with or without cetuximab in 150 patients with advanced biliary cancer.[181] Unfortunately, overall survival and progression-free survival were no different in the treatment arms. Multiple other targeted agents, including sorafenib and panitumumab, have been tested in combination with chemotherapy but have not yielded significantly improved results over chemotherapy alone.[182–186]

Interventional radiology and internal radiotherapy

A combination of external beam plus endoluminal boost irradiation is an attractive treatment program. The favored treatment sequence is to start with external beam irradiation to obtain tumor regression, which provides a better dose distribution from the endoluminal boost irradiation to treat any residual tumor. The use of endoluminal [170]Ir alone for palliative treatment of patients with unresectable hilar bile duct cancers has been reported.[187] Endoluminal doses ranged from 15 to 35 Gy when combined with external beam irradiation (usually 45–50 Gy), or when endoluminal doses of up to 60 Gy were used alone. The dose reference point may vary from 0.5 to 1.0 cm from the central catheter. The total nominal doses of external beam plus endoluminal boost irradiation are between 60 and 70 Gy to the tumor, and although this range exceeds the liver and small intestine tolerance, the highest doses are confined to a small volume of tissue. The median survival for patients treated by this endoluminal method, with or without external beam irradiation, is 15–18 months. Several patients survived for >4 years after treatment; however, the majority of patients had local failure.

Key references

The complete reference list can be found on the Wiley Companion Digital Edition of this title (see inside front cover for login instructions).

9 Khan ZR, Neugut AI, Ahsan H, Chabot JA. Risk factors for biliary tract cancers. *Am J Gastroenterol.* 1999;**94**:149–152.

12 Csendes A, Becerra M, Burdiles P, et al. Bacteriological studies of bile from the gallbladder in patients with carcinoma of the gallbladder, cholelithiasis, common bile duct stones and no gallstones disease. *Eur J Surg.* 1994;**160**:363–367.

14 Albores-Saavedra J, Alcantra-Vazquez A, Cruz-Ortiz H, Herrera-Goepfert R. The precursor lesions of invasive gallbladder carcinoma. Hyperplasia, atypical hyperplasia and carcinoma in situ. *Cancer.* 1980;**45**:919–927.

20 Quan ZW, Wu K, Wang J, et al. Association of p53, p16, and vascular endothelial growth factor protein expressions with the prognosis and metastasis of gallbladder cancer. *J Am Coll Surg.* 2001;**193**:380–383.

23 Fahim RB, McDonald JR, Richards JC, Ferris DO. Carcinoma of the gallbladder. A study of its modes of spread. *Ann Surg.* 1962;**156**:114–122.

26 Ito M, Mishima Y, Sato T. An anatomical study of the lymphatic drainage of the gallbladder. *Surg Radiol Anat.* 1991;**13**:89–104.

44 Groot Koerkamp B, Fong Y. Outcomes in biliary malignancy. *J Surg Oncol.* 2014;**110**:585–591.

53 Fong Y, Brennan MF, Turnbull A, et al. Gallbladder cancer discovered during laparoscopic surgery. Potential for iatrogenic tumor dissemination. *Arch Surg.* 1993;**128**:1054–1056.

62 Falkson G, MacIntyre JM, Moertel CG. Eastern Cooperative Oncology Group experience with chemotherapy for inoperable gallbladder and bile duct cancer. *Cancer.* 1984;**54**:965–969.

65 Yang R, Wang B, Chen YJ, et al. Efficacy of gemcitabine plus platinum agents for biliary tract cancers: a meta-analysis. *Anticancer Drugs.* 2013;**24**:871–877.

69 Kopelson G, Harisiadis L, Tretter P, Chang CH. The role of radiation therapy in cancer of the extra-hepatic biliary system. An analysis of thirteen patients and a review of the literature of the effectiveness of surgery, chemotherapy and radiotherapy. *Int J Radiat Oncol Biol Phys.* 1977;**2**:883–894.

71 Horgan AM, Amir E, Walter T, Knox JJ. Adjuvant therapy of biliary tract cancer: a systemic review and meta-analysis. *J Clin Oncol.* 2012;**30**:1934–1940.

76 Ben-Josef E, Guthrie KA, El-Khoueiry AB, et al. SWOG S0809: a phase II intergroup trial of adjuvant capecitabine and gemcitabine followed by radiotherapy and concurrent capecitabine in extrahepatic cholangiocarcinoma and gallbladder carcinoma. *J Clin Oncol.* 2015;**33**(24):2617–2622.

82 Kurathong S, Lerdverasirikul P, Wongpaitoon V, et al. *Opisthorchis viverrini* infection and cholangiocarcinoma. A prospective, case-controlled study. *Gastroenterology.* 1985;**89**:151–156.

84 Voyles CR, Smadja C, Shands WC, Blumgart LH. Carcinoma in choledochal cysts. Age-related incidence. *Arch Surg.* 1983;**118**:986–988.

86 Wee A, Ludwig J, Coffey RJ Jr, et al. Hepatobiliary carcinoma associated with primary sclerosing cholangitis and chronic ulcerative colitis. *Hum Pathol.* 1985;**16**:719–726.

95 Ito Y, Kojiro M, Nakashima T, Mori T. Pathomorphologic characteristics of 102 cases of thorotrast-related hepatocellular carcinoma, cholangiocarcinoma, and hepatic angiosarcoma. *Cancer.* 1988;**62**:1153–1162.

98 Terada T, Ashida K, Endo K, et al. c-erbB-2 protein is expressed in hepatolithiasis and cholangiocarcinoma. *Histopathology.* 1998;**33**:325–331.

101 Jalanko H, Kuusela P, Roberts P, et al. Comparison of a new tumour marker, CA 19–9, with alpha-fetoprotein and carcinoembryonic antigen in patients with upper gastrointestinal diseases. *J Clin Pathol.* 1984;**37**:218–222.

104 Yamamoto M, Takasaki K, Yoshikawa T, et al. Does gross appearance indicate prognosis in intrahepatic cholangiocarcinoma? *J Surg Oncol Suppl.* 1998;**69**:162–167.

108 Colli A, Cocciolo M, Mumoli N, et al. Peripheral intrahepatic cholangiocarcinoma. Ultrasound findings and differential diagnosis from hepatocellular carcinoma. *Eur J Ultrasound.* 1998;**7**:93–99.

111 Han JK, Choi BI, Kim TK, et al. Hilar cholangiocarcinoma. Thin-section spiral CT findings with cholangiographic correlation. *Radiographics.* 1997;**17**:1475–1485.

114 Kusano T, Shimabukuro M, Tamai O, et al. The use of intra-operative ultrasonography for detecting tumor extension in bile duct carcinoma. *Int Surg.* 1997;**82**:44–48.

119 Tanaka M, Ogawa Y, Matsumoto S, Nakayama F. The role of endoscopic retrograde cholangiopancreatography in preoperative assessment of bile duct cancer. *World J Surg.* 1988;**12**:27–32.

122 Cameron JL, Broe P, Zuidema GD. Proximal bile duct tumors. Surgical management with silastic transhepatic biliary stents. *Ann Surg.* 1982;**196**:412–419.

125 Kluge R, Schmidt F, Caca K, et al. Positron emission tomography with [(18)F]fluoro-2-deoxy-D-glucose for diagnosis and staging of bile duct cancer. *Hepatology.* 2001;**33**:1029–1035.

128 Lieser MJ, Barry MK, Rowland C, et al. Surgical management of intrahepatic cholangiocarcinoma. A 31-year experience. *J Hepatobiliary Pancreat Surg.* 1998;**5**:41–47.

129 Pichlmayr R, Lamesch P, Weimann A, et al. Surgical treatment of cholangiocellular carcinoma. *World J Surg.* 1995;**19**:83–88.

132 Tao R, Krishnan S, Bhosale PR, et al. Ablative radiotherapy doses lead to a substantial prolongation of survival in patients with inoperable intrahepatic cholangiocarcinoma: a retrospective dose response analysis. *J Clin Oncol.* 2015. pii: JCO.2015.61.3778.

134 Klatskin G. Adenocarcinoma of the hepatic duct at its bifurcation within the porta hepatis. *Am J Med.* 1965;**38**:241–248.

136 Burke EC, Jarnagin WR, Hochwald SN, et al. Hilar cholangiocarcinoma. Patterns of spread, the importance of hepatic resection for curative operation, and a presurgical clinical staging system. *Ann Surg.* 1998;**228**:385–394.

138 Ouchi K, Suzuki M, Hashimoto L, Sato T. Histologic findings and prognostic factors in carcinoma of the upper bile duct. *Am J Surg.* 1989;**157**:552–556.

142 Bengmark S, Ekberg H, Evander A, et al. Major liver resection for hilar cholangiocarcinoma. *Ann Surg.* 1988;**207**:120–125.

145 Baer HU, Stain SC, Dennison AR, et al. Improvements in survival by aggressive resections of hilar cholangiocarcinoma. *Ann Surg.* 1993;**217**:20–27.

149 Ringe B, Wittekind C, Bechstein WO, et al. The role of liver transplantation in hepatobiliary malignancy. A retrospective analysis of 95 patients with particular regard to tumor stage and recurrence. *Ann Surg.* 1989;**209**:88–98.

150 Yokoyama I, Sheahan DG, Carr B, et al. Clinicopathologic factors affecting patient survival and tumor recurrence after orthotopic liver transplantation for hepatocellular carcinoma. *Transplant Proc.* 1991;**23**:2194–2196.

159 Meyers WC, Jones RS. Internal radiation for bile duct cancer. *World J Surg.* 1988;**12**:99–104.

166 Glimelius B, Hoffman K, Sjoden PO, et al. Chemotherapy improves survival and quality of life in advanced pancreatic and biliary cancer. *Ann Oncol.* 1996;**7**(6):593–600.

172 Eckel F, Schmid RM. Chemotherapy in advanced biliary tract carcinoma: a pooled analysis of clinical trials. *Br J Cancer.* 2007;**96**(6):896–902. Epub 2007 Feb 27.

173 Valle J, Wasan H, Palmer DH, et al. Cisplatin plus gemcitabine versus gemcitabine for biliary tract cancer. *N Engl J Med.* 2010;**362**(14):1273–1281.

93 Neoplasms of the exocrine pancreas

Robert A. Wolff, MD ▪ Christopher H. Crane, MD ▪ Donghui Li, PhD ▪ Douglas B. Evans, MD ▪ Anirban Maitra, MD ▪ Susan Tsai, MD

Overview

Adenocarcinoma of the pancreas is one of the most morbid and lethal malignancies. Worldwide, it accounts for 330,000 deaths annually. Smoking and obesity are both risk factors for pancreatic cancer and current estimates suggest half of all cases may be preventable. Genetic predisposition to pancreatic cancer is associated with some genetic syndromes to include BRCA1 or BRCA2 germline mutations, Peutz–Jeghers syndrome, and hereditary nonpolyposis colon cancer. Somatic mutations in KRAS, CDKN2A/INK4A, TP53, and SMAD4/DPC4 are common. Pancreatic cancer is often diagnosed when the primary tumor is inoperable or there is metastatic spread rendering the cancer incurable. At present, clinical staging defines the malignancy as resectable (and potentially curable), borderline resectable, locally advanced, or metastatic. Surgery with curative intent is possible for patients with resectable disease and for a subset of patients with borderline resectable disease. While chemotherapy has been proved to prolong survival as a component of adjuvant therapy, and as therapy for locally advanced or metastatic disease, the role of radiation therapy in treatment is less-well defined and not universally accepted. Thus far, molecular targeted therapy has shown no clinically meaningful benefit. Adjuvant and neoadjuvant approaches are employed in patients with resectable and borderline resectable disease. Intense research in the molecular biology of pancreatic cancer continues with increasing interest in the role of the tumor microenvironment in invasion, metastatic potential, and resistance. Novel therapeutic strategies that focus on stromal modification and immunologic manipulation are at the forefront of clinical and translational research efforts.

Introduction

In common parlance, the moniker of "pancreatic cancer" most often refers to the entity known as pancreatic ductal adenocarcinoma (PDAC). This is one of the most lethal and morbid of all solid tumors, notorious for local invasiveness, early spread to regional lymph nodes, and vascular dissemination to distant sites. Cure is possible only in the setting of localized, resectable disease with relapse after surgery occurring in about 80% of patients. PDAC is currently the fourth leading cause of cancer-related death in the United States.[1] In 2015, PDAC will lead to about 40,500 deaths.[1] Worldwide, it is blamed for over 330,000 deaths annually,[2] and by 2020, PDAC is predicted to become the second leading cause of cancer death by 2020.[3]

In this chapter, we will summarize the current literature relevant to the epidemiology, pathology, molecular and cellular biology, and diagnosis and treatment of pancreatic cancer. Future directions in prevention, early detection, clinical management and translational research in genomics, epigenetics, tumor metabolism, and the microenvironment will also be discussed.

Epidemiology

Worldwide, pancreatic cancer is the thirteenth most common type of cancer and the eighth leading cause of cancer-related death.[2] The incidence rates of pancreatic cancer are the highest in industrialized societies and western countries.[4] The age-adjusted incidence rates range from 10 to 15 per 100,000 people in parts of Northern, Central, and Eastern Europe to <1 per 100,000 in areas of Africa and Asia.[5] In the United States, the age-adjusted incidence rate for all races was 13.0 per 100,000 men and 10.3 per 100,000 women per year based on SEER's (Surveillance Epidemiology and End Results) 2001–2005 data.[6] The age-adjusted mortality rate per 100,000 person-years was 15.4 for black men, 12.4 for black women, 12.1 for white men, and 9.0 for white women. The black/white disparity in incidence rate is likely related to environmental influences as the rates are considerably higher in African-Americans than in native Africans.

Most patients are diagnosed between the ages of 60 and 80 years.[4,6] Historically, pancreatic cancer had a male: female ratio of 1.2 : 1, now the incidence is about the same for both sexes.[4]

Etiologic factors

As most other types of human cancers, pancreatic cancer etiology involves both genetic and nongenetic factors (Figure 1).

Hereditary risk factors

Inherited or familial pancreatic cancers represent approximately 5–10% of all pancreatic cancers.[7] At-risk patients for familial pancreatic cancer include those with a minimum of two first-degree relatives with pancreatic cancer.[8] Although the genetic mutations responsible for the majority of clustering of pancreatic cancer in families have not been identified, several pancreatic cancer genes that are associated with either a known cancer syndrome or chronic inflammatory diseases have been identified (Table 1).[7]

PRSS1 and SPINK1

Germ line mutations in *PRSS1* and *SPINK1* genes are associated with hereditary pancreatitis. *PRSS1* gene encodes the cationic trypsinogen protein and premature activation of the trypsinogen results in acute pancreatitis. *SPINK1* gene encodes a trypsin inhibitor and mutation of this gene has been associated with chronic pancreatitis. Individuals with hereditary pancreatitis have been shown to have a 53-fold increased risk for developing pancreatic cancer and a lifetime risk (age 70) of pancreatic cancer of 30–40%.[7]

BRCA1 and BRCA2

Hereditary breast–ovarian cancer syndrome is associated with mutations in *BRCA1* or *BRCA2*. The risk of pancreatic cancer

Holland-Frei Cancer Medicine, Ninth Edition. Edited by Robert C. Bast Jr., Carlo M. Croce, William N. Hait, Waun Ki Hong, Donald W. Kufe, Martine Piccart-Gebhart, Raphael E. Pollock, Ralph R. Weichselbaum, Hongyang Wang, and James F. Holland.
© 2017 John Wiley & Sons, Inc. ISBN: 978-1-118-93469-2

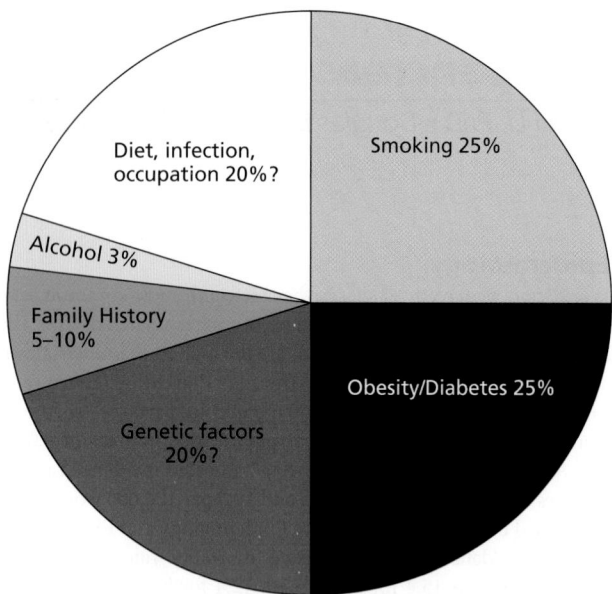

Figure 1 Schematic presentation of known and suspected risk factors for pancreatic cancer.

among *BRCA1* mutation carriers varied between studies.[7] Germ line mutations in the *BRCA2* gene have been found in 10% of patients with familial pancreatic cancer and in 7% of patients with sporadic pancreatic cancer.[9–11] Germ line *BRCA2* mutations represent the most common inherited predisposition to pancreatic cancer and are associated with an up to a 10-fold greater risk of pancreatic cancer than in the general population.[12]

LKB1/STK11

Peutz–Jeghers syndrome, an autosomal dominant trait, is caused by mutations in the *LKB1/STK11* tumor suppressor gene. Individuals with Peutz–Jeghers syndrome have a highly increased risk of pancreatic cancer ranging from 96- to 132-fold higher risk than average risk individuals; the lifetime risk is 5–36%.[13,14] Biallelic inactivation of *the LKB1/STK11* gene has also been found in 4% of patients with resected sporadic PDAC.[15]

CDKN2A (p16)

Germ line mutations of the *CDKN2A (p16)* tumor suppressor gene are mostly related to familial atypical multiple-mole melanoma (FAMMM) syndrome. It has been reported that individuals from FAMMM kindreds have a 13- to 22-fold increased risk of developing

PDAC[16] and individuals who carry *p16/CDKN2A* mutations have a 38-fold increased risk compared with the general population.[17] *CDKN2A* gene is also frequently inactivated in sporadic pancreatic cancer.

HNPCC and FAP

The hereditary nonpolyposis colon cancer (HNPCC, also known as Lynch syndrome), is caused by germ line mutations in several DNA mismatch repair genes.[18] Families with Lynch syndrome have an 8.6-fold increased risk of developing pancreatic cancer.[19] Families with familial adenomatous polyposis (FAP), which is caused by genetic defect in *APC* tumor suppressor gene, have also been reported to have increased risk of PDAC.[20]

PALB2 and ATM

Mutations of the *PALB2* and *ATM* genes have been discovered in familial pancreatic cancer cases.[21–23] PALB2 protein binds with BRCA2 protein stabilizing it in the nucleus, and this complex acts in double stranded DNA repair. ATM is an important regulator of cellular response to DNA damage. It is estimated that PALB2 mutations may account for 1–3% of the familial clustering of pancreatic cancer.[21,22]

A recent study conducted in 727 unrelated familial pancreatic cancer probands has found that the prevalence of deleterious mutations was *BRCA1*, 1.2%; *BRCA2*, 3.7%; *PALB2*, 0.6%; and *CDKN2A*, 2.5%. *BRCA2* and *CDKN2A* account for the majority of mutations in familial pancreatic cancer.[24]

Susceptibility variants

Three genome-wide association studies (GWAS) have been conducted in the United States with a majority of the study population of European ancestry.[25–27] Polymorphic variants of the *ABO*, *NR5A2*, *LINC-PINT*, *PDX1*, *BCAR1/CTRB1/CTRB2*, *ZNRF3*, and *TERT* genes and a nongene chromosome region 13q22.1 have been identified as susceptibility factors for pancreatic cancer with genome-wide significance ($p < 5 \times 10^{-8}$). Two additional GWAS have also been conducted in Chinese[28] and Japanese populations.[29] Post GWAS analyses suggest that genes involved in the pancreas development pathway may play an important role in modifying the risk of pancreatic cancer.[30–32] Initial examination on the interactions of genes with known etiological factors, such as smoking,[33] obesity, and diabetes,[34,35] has generated interesting clues to the genetic factors that predispose individuals with such exposure to pancreatic cancer. Identification of the causal alleles and functional characterization of the genes or variants may involve many genes with modest effect on the phenotype.[36,37]

Table 1 Susceptibility genes for pancreatic cancer.

Gene	Syndrome	Chromosome location	Function
PRSS1	Hereditary pancreatitis	7q35	Trypsinogen, serine protease
SPINK1		5q32	Serine peptide (trypsin) inhibitor
CFTR	Cystic fibrosis	7q31.2	ABC transporter chloride channel
BRCA1	Hereditary breast ovarian cancer	17q21	DNA damage repair
BRCA2		13q12.3	
CDKN2A/P16	Familial atypical multiple mole melanoma	9p21	Cyclin-dependent kinase inhibitor
STK11/LKB1	Peutz–Jeghers syndrome	19p13.3	Serine/threonine kinase
MSH2, MLH1	Hereditary nonpolyposis colorectal cancer	2p21	Mismatch repair
PMS1/2, MGH6		3p21.3	
APC	Familial adenomatous polyposis	5q21	Negative regulator of β-catenin
PALB2	Breast and pancreatic cancer	16p12.2	Partner and localizer of BRCA2
ATM	Ataxia-telangiectasia	11q22–q23	DNA damage response

Tobacco and alcohol

The risk factor most firmly associated with pancreatic cancer is cigarette smoking. It is estimated that approximately 25% of cases of pancreatic cancer are due to cigarette smoking with a 1.5- to 2.0-fold increased risk.[38-41] The risk increases as the amount and duration of smoking increase. Long-term smoking cessation (>10 years) reduces the risk by approximately 30% relative to current smokers.[38,42] Whether smokeless tobacco products, pipe or cigar smoking increases risk remains controversial.[43,44]

The mechanisms of smoking-induced pancreatic cancer involve tobacco carcinogen-induced DNA damage and pancreatic tissue injury.[45] Tobacco carcinogens can be metabolically activated to cause DNA damage and gene mutations.[46,47] Nicotine also plays an important role in tumor promotion and progression via nicotinic acetylcholine receptor and adrenergic receptor-mediated signaling in multifactorial events that lead to pancreatic injury.[45,46,48]

The association between alcohol consumption and PDAC has also been investigated. In general, heavy alcohol consumption (30–40 g alcohol or ≥3 drinks/day) but not light or moderate consumption has been associated with increased risk.[49-52] It appears that alcohol may account for 2–5% of all pancreatic cancer.

Obesity

Similar to tobacco, it has been estimated that obesity accounts for another 25% of the pancreatic cancer cases in the US population.[53] Positive associations between obesity and pancreatic cancer risk have been reported in several large prospective studies and meta-analyses.[54-62] In addition to BMI (body mass index), abdominal fat, a measured by waist to hip ratio, has been related to increased risk of pancreatic cancer, especially in women.[60,61] Obesity at younger age has been associated with a higher risk of pancreatic cancer than weight gain at older age. Furthermore, obesity has been associated with a younger age of disease onset and reduced overall survival (OS).[63]

Biological mechanisms linking obesity to pancreatic cancer are insulin resistance and inflammation.[64] Studies using prediagnostic blood samples have shown positive associations of PDAC risk and markers for hyperglycemia and insulin resistance.[65-68] Insulin and insulin-like growth factors are key regulators for cellular metabolism and growth and their signaling transduction networks play an important role in tumor development and progression.[69-71] The mechanisms driving pancreatic carcinogenesis may have similarities to other inflammatory conditions associated with an increased risk of cancer. Fatty infiltration of the pancreas may lead to steatopancreatitis, suggesting a potential link among obesity, nonalcoholic fatty pancreatic disease, nonalcoholic steatopancreatitis, and PDAC.[72,73]

Diabetes mellitus and antidiabetic medication

Diabetes mellitus has been implicated as both an early manifestation of pancreatic cancer and a predisposing factor.[74] A consistent association of long-term diabetes and risk of pancreatic cancer has been reported from three large-scale meta-analyses[75-77] and three pooled data analyses[68,78,79] with each involved more than 1500 PDAC cases. Of note, PDAC can induce peripheral insulin resistance[80] and type 3c (pancreatogenic) diabetes.[81] It was observed that hyperglycemia could occur 2 years before clinical diagnosis of pancreatic cancer, and one in 125 new-onset diabetics would develop PDAC in 3 years.[82,83] Biomarkers that could help to distinguish type II diabetes mellitus from type 3c diabetes are being pursued.[84,85]

Since the discovery that biguanides, the most commonly used antidiabetic medications, inhibited pancreatic tumor development in experimental animals,[86] the role of antidiabetic therapy in PDAC risk reduction has been intensely studied. Other experimental evidence supports the antitumor effect of metformin.[87,88] Metformin has diverse regulatory effects and the major molecular targets of metformin are the liver kinase B1 (LKB1)-AMP-activated protein kinase (AMPK) signaling and mammalian target of rapamycin (mTOR) pathways, which are central in the regulation of cellular energy homeostasis, cell division, and cell proliferation.[89] Metformin also inhibits the inflammatory response associated with cellular transformation and selectively targets the cancer stem cell.[90,91] In humans, eight cohort studies[92-98] and three case–control studies[99-101] have examined the impact of metformin use on risk of PDAC. Meta-analysis of these studies estimates RR of 0.63.[102] Two additional studies have reported that metformin use in patients with pancreatic cancer and concurrent diabetes is associated with longer survival and reduced risk of death.[103,104]

Pancreatitis and other medical conditions

Chronic pancreatitis is a risk factor for pancreatic cancer, and new onset pancreatitis could be a sign of occult pancreatic cancer.[105] Data pooled from 10 case–control studies with adjustment for obesity and alcohol consumption, demonstrated that the risk of pancreatic cancer was nearly threefold for patients with an interval of >2 years between the pancreatitis and pancreatic cancer diagnoses.[106]

Infectious diseases

Helicobacter pylori may cause subclinical pancreatitis or increased gastrin levels, with resultant trophic effects on the pancreas. Several studies have examined the association between *H. pylori* and pancreatic cancer; with large meta-analyses being showing a weak yet statistically significant association between prior *H. pylori* infection and pancreatic cancer.[107] It has been hypothesized that ABO genotype/phenotype status influences the behavior of *H. pylori* that in turn affects gastric and pancreatic secretory function, and these ultimately influence the pancreatic carcinogenicity of dietary- and smoking-related *N*-nitrosamine exposures, and thus risk of PDAC.[108]

Hepatitis B may also be a risk factor for pancreatic cancer.[109] Subsequent studies were conducted mostly in Asian and a meta-analysis of nine such studies reported that the pooled RR was 1.39 (95% CI: 1.22–1.59) in chronic HBV (hepatitis B virus) carriers and 1.41 (95% CI: 0.06–1.87) in past exposure to HBV.[110] Hepatitis B surface antigen (HBsAg) has been detected in pancreatic and bile juice,[111] and there is evidence of HBV replication in pancreatic cells. HBV results in damage to pancreatic exocrine and endocrine epithelial cells via an inflammatory response.[112,113]

Dietary factors

Various dietary factors have been suspected to play a role in the development of pancreatic cancer. Generally, high intakes of fat or meat increase the risk; whereas high intakes of fruits and vegetables reduce the risk.[5] Less is known about which type of fatty acids pose the greatest risk.[114] Several studies suggest that the method of meat preparation (deep fried, grilled, or barbequed), and subsequent intake of food mutagens may contribute to the development of pancreatic cancer.[115-117]

The associations of dietary carbohydrates, refined sugars, and glycemic index or load with pancreatic cancer have been investigated in many studies but the results are inconsistent. A recent meta-analysis of data from eight prospective cohort studies concluded that there was no association among diets high in glycemic index, glycemic load, total carbohydrates or sucrose, and pancreatic cancer risk.[118]

Decreased pancreatic cancer rates have been associated with the high consumption of vegetables, citrus fruits, fiber, and vitamin C.[5] It remains uncertain whether vitamin D has a protective effect on PDAC.[114]

Occupational exposures

The role of occupational or industrial factors in pancreatic cancer has been investigated extensively. Increased risk of pancreatic cancer has been associated with exposures to some chemicals (e.g., organochlorines, chlorinated hydrocarbons, and formaldehyde) or some specific occupations (e.g., stone miners, cement workers, gardeners, and textile workers).[4,88] The strongest and most consistent occupational risk factors associated with pancreatic cancer to date are chlorinated hydrocarbons and polycyclic aromatic hydrocarbons.[88]

In summary, cigarette smoking and obesity may each be responsible for as many as 25% of the cases of pancreatic cancer implying that half of pancreatic cancer cases may be preventable.[119,120] Conversely, the proportion of pancreatic cancer cases attributable to known inherited pancreatic cancer syndromes is small. Identification of individuals with excessively high risk of pancreatic cancer may allow for focused screening.[121–123] Thus far, proved benefit to screening remains elusive, except in highly selective populations such as high-risk familial pancreatic cancer kindreds.[124] Currently, for those individuals determined to have structural,[124] or blood-based abnormalities,[125] suggesting premalignancy or early stage neoplasm, management remains extremely controversial. Current options range from close observation to aggressive surgical intervention with a variety of approaches in evolution.[126–128]

Prevention of pancreatic cancer

The epidemiology of PDAC described earlier provides strong evidence for the prevention of pancreatic cancer; possibly resulting in a substantial reduction in global pancreatic cancer mortality. Primary prevention strategies expected to significantly reduce the risk of developing pancreatic cancer likely require lifestyle and dietary modifications. In addition, a number of available over the counter agents and widely prescribed medications have potential to reduce the risk of pancreatic cancer (Table 2).[129–132]

Pathology

Histopathology of exocrine pancreatic neoplasms

PDAC accounts for approximately 95% of all neoplasms arising in the pancreas.[133] On histological examination of surgically resected

Table 2 Interventions that may reduce pancreatic cancer risk.

Lifestyle and nutritional factors
Cessation/avoidance of tobacco smoking and smokeless tobacco
Regular exercise
Weight control and weight reduction if needed to BMI < 25 kg/m^2
Healthy diet high in fruits and vegetables
Potential chemopreventive agents
Metformin
Aspirin
Curcumin
Celecoxib
Atorvastatin and other HMG-coenzyme reductase inhibitors
β-Carotene
Vitamins C, D, and E

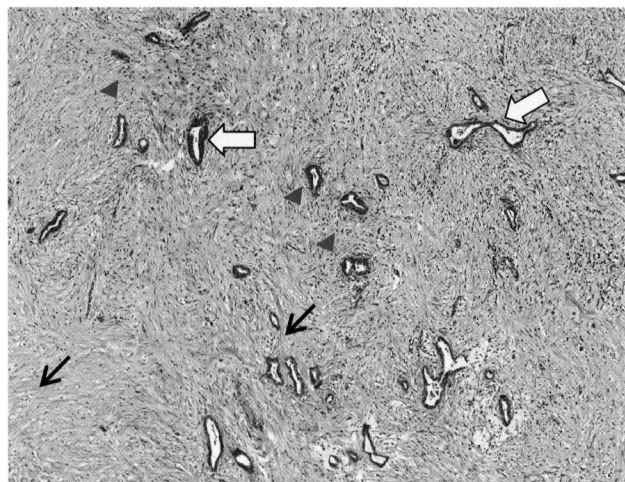

Figure 2 Stromal desmoplasia in pancreatic ductal adenocarcinoma. Infiltrating neoplastic glands (white arrows) are surrounded by a florid host response, comprised spindle-shaped cancer-associated fibroblasts and myofibroblasts (red arrowheads) and extracellular matrix, including collagen 1 (black arrow).

tumors, it is not uncommon to find neoplastic cells infiltrating into lymphatic structures or into the many nerve endings enervating the pancreatic bed, which may explain the pain associated with PDAC. Another defining histological feature of PDAC is an exuberant host stromal reaction to the cancer (desmoplasia), wherein smooth muscle actin expressing myofibroblasts generate abundant extracellular collagen that surrounds infiltrating neoplastic glands (Figure 2).[134] Other components of this host desmoplastic response include secreted glycosaminoglycans (e.g., hyaluronan) that contribute to high interstitial pressures and impede the passive efflux of chemotherapeutics from the circulation into the peritumoral milieu.[135]

PDAC arises through a stepwise histological progression of well-recognized precursor lesions. The most common precursor lesions are microscopic, and known as *pan*creatic *in*traepithelial *n*eoplasia or PanIN, which are almost always present in the pancreatic parenchyma surrounding an invasive cancer. PanINs vary from innocuous low-grade PanIN-1 lesions to the ominous highest grade PanIN-3 (previously known as carcinoma *in situ*), wherein the constituent cells morphologically resemble PDAC, except for their containment within a basement membrane. PanIN-3 lesions share many of the genetic aberrations found in infiltrating cancer. Of note, while PanIN-1 and -2 lesions can occur incidentally (with autopsy studies reporting as many as 50% of elderly individuals with low-grade PanINs in their pancreas),[136] PanIN-3 is essentially never found in the absence of a synchronous PDAC.[137] Thus, the emergence of high-grade PanIN-3 lesions likely represents the critical inflection point in the multistep progression of PDAC. By definition, and in contrast to cystic precursor lesions of PDAC (see below), isolated PanINs are not seen on abdominal imaging, although individuals with germ line mutations or a familial predisposition may have structural pancreatic changes discernible on endoscopic ultrasound (EUS).[128]

Cystic precursor lesions of PDAC comprised two distinct entities—intraductal papillary mucinous neoplasms (IPMNs) and mucinous cystic neoplasms (MCNs).[138] IPMNs arise in either the main duct or one of the side branches of the pancreas and are characterized by broad "finger-like" papillae and secretion of abundant extracellular mucin. MCNs are less common and occur in women with significantly greater propensity than men (9 : 1 ratio). In contrast to IPMNs, MCNs have no communication with the ductal system. Akin to PanINs, the epithelial lining of cystic precursor lesions also demonstrates histological progression from low-grade (adenoma) through high-grade (carcinoma *in situ*) to invasive cancer. Approximately 25–33% of surgically resected cystic lesions are associated with an invasive adenocarcinoma, and the onset of invasion is associated with a significant reduction in median OS.[139,140] The precise timeline of progression from noninvasive cyst to invasive carcinoma is not known, although the median age of presentation for cystic lesions is about a decade earlier than the median age for PDAC, suggesting that this might reflect the period required for progression. Of note, the explosion in the use of abdominal imaging for symptoms not related to the pancreas has led to a veritable "man-made" epidemic of incidentally discovered cystic lesions of the pancreas. As the overwhelming majority of these asymptomatic cysts are not likely to progress to invasive cancer, radiological criteria have been proposed that help distinguish "high risk" from "indolent" cysts.[141,142] Intensive efforts are underway to identify molecular markers from cyst fluid or blood that would further refine this distinction and help prevent unnecessary surgeries and frequent monitoring.[123]

Other uncommon exocrine tumors include (1) acinar cell carcinoma, which bears morphological resemblance to pancreatic acini, wherein the neoplastic cells express acinar enzymes, such as trypsin and chymotrypsin;[143] (2) solid pseudopapillary neoplasm, a cystic tumor of uncertain histogenesis that often arises in the tail of the pancreas in young adults, and typically has a favorable prognosis;[122] (3) serous cystic neoplasm, a cystic tumor characterized by serous (watery) secretion, in contrast to the mucinous contents of IPMN and MCN, and which does not harbor a risk of progression to PDAC;[144] and (4) pancreatoblastoma, the most common pancreatic tumor in children.[145]

Approximately 2% of primary tumors arise from the endocrine compartment (islets of Langerhans) and are known as pancreatic neuroendocrine tumors or PanNETs or "islet cell tumors."[146] PanNETs can be nonfunctional in up to a quarter of cases, or they can express a variety of islet cell hormones such as insulin or glucagon, which may lead to characteristic syndromes owing to systemic hormonal excess. PanNETs do not form glandular structures and are typically not associated with an exuberant host desmoplastic reaction. PanNETs can be readily identified based on expression of neuroendocrine markers such as chromogranin or synaptophysin in tissue sections.

Molecular pathology of exocrine pancreatic neoplasms

The advent of next-generation sequencing technology has enabled considerable advances over the last 5 years in elucidating the genomic landscape of PDAC,[147] as well as that of other variant neoplasms of the exocrine and endocrine pancreas.[148,149] The International Cancer Genome Consortium (ICGC) has sequenced hundreds of PDAC, where the sequencing data is publicly available.[150]

By far, the most common genetic abnormality in the multistep pathogenesis of PDAC happens to be oncogenic mutation of *KRAS*, located on chromosome 12p, which encodes for Ras, a membrane-bound small GTPase.[151] Somatic mutations of *KRAS* are reported in >90% of PDAC cell lines and patient-derived xenografts, although the frequency is somewhat lower (75–90%) in primary tumor samples. The majority of *KRAS* mutations cluster at codon 12, with mutations also found at codons 13 or 61, respectively. Somatic *KRAS* mutations result in constitutive

activation of the GTPase activity of the encoded Ras protein, which, in turn, activates multiple downstream effector pathways.[152] Somatic *KRAS* mutations are present even in the lowest grade PanIN lesions, underscoring its status as an early genetic "hit."[153] In genetically engineered mouse models (GEMMs), expression of a mutant *KRAS* in the pancreas results in preinvasive neoplasia closely recapitulating human PanINs, with a minority of animals progressing to full-fledged invasive cancer.[154] Additional genetic events, such as expression of mutant *p53* or biallelic deletion of the *Ink4a/Arf* locus, significantly accelerate the natural history of Ras-induced pancreatic neoplasia.[155,156] Conversely, in GEMMs with an inducible mutant *KRAS* allele, turning off Ras expression in established PDAC, leads to variable tumor regression.[157,158] Not surprisingly, a multitude of avenues have been explored toward pharmacological inhibition of aberrant Ras activity in PDAC and other *KRAS*-mutant tumors,[159–161] but the clinical results overall have been disappointing. Nonetheless, Ras remains an attractive target, and a large federally funded "RAS Initiative" is currently underway at the National Cancer Institute to identify strategies to block Ras in PDAC and other cancers (http://www.cancer.gov/researchandfunding/priorities/ras).

Somatic inactivation of the *CDKN2A/INK4A* gene, which encodes for the cell cycle regulator p16, is another early genetic event in the multistep progression of PDAC. The p16 protein inhibits the cyclin D1/Cdk-4 complex that normally acts to constrain the retinoblastoma (Rb) protein via phosphorylation.[162] In approximately 95% of PDAC, the *CDKN2A/INK4A* gene is inactivated by one of several mechanisms, including homozygous deletion, the loss of one allele combined with an intragenic mutation in the other allele, or epigenetic inactivation via promoter methylation. A potential therapeutic vulnerability that emerges in the setting of p16 loss pertains to the dependence on Cdk4 activity for unregulated proliferation, which can be targeted using small molecule inhibitors of Cdk4 function.[163]

In the multistep progression model of PDAC, loss of the *TP53*, *SMAD4/DPC4*, and *BRCA2* tumor suppressor genes are considered later genetic events.[164] Somatic mutations of *TP53* are found in approximately 75% of human PDAC, while nuclear accumulation of p53 protein on immunohistochemistry, indicative of an underlying mutation, occurs in the majority of PanIN-3 lesions.[165] The *SMAD4/DPC4* tumor suppressor gene on chromosome 18q21 encodes for an intracellular transducer of the transforming growth factor-β signaling pathway that inhibits cell growth under physiological conditions. The *SMAD4/DPC4* gene is inactivated in approximately 55% of human PDAC through either homozygous deletions or the loss of one allele coupled with an intragenic mutation in the second allele.[166] Epithelial Dpc4 expression is nearly always retained in low-grade PanIN lesions and in noninvasive cystic precursor lesions of PDAC, reiterating that *SMAD4/DPC4* abnormalities generally occur concomitant with progression to invasive cancer.[167,168] Overall, *KRAS*, *CDKN2A/INK4A*, *TP53*, and *SMAD4/DPC4* are the "big four" peaks in the genomic landscape of PDAC, each mutated in over 50% of cases. Patients that harbor in all four genes tend to have a significantly worse OS than those with mutations in 1 or 2 of these genes, underscoring their role in prognosis.[169]

The *BRCA2* gene, which has been discussed in the context of familial predisposition to PDAC, is also somatically mutated in approximately 5% of cancers. The BRCA2 protein plays a critical role in homologous recombination-mediated repair (HRR), and neoplastic cells with *BRCA2* or related gene defects in the HRR pathway are exquisitely sensitive to double-strand breaks induced by agents such as cisplatin or mitomycin C.[170] Another newer class of agents that is being selectively evaluated in tumors with *BRCA2* mutations is PARP ([poly (ADP-ribose) polymerase]) inhibitors, which inhibits a second mechanism of DNA repair in cells already compromised in HRR. The concurrent PARP inhibition in *BRCA2*-mutant PDAC is expected to create a "synthetic lethality" vis-à-vis DNA repair that can be exploited toward a therapeutic advantage.[171]

Although a comprehensive tabulation of genetic abnormalities in PDAC is beyond the scope of this book, significant molecular aberrations are observed within every interrogated cellular component, including DNA methylation, histone marks, coding and noncoding RNAs (latter incorporating both long noncoding RNA and microRNAs), and protein. Many of these abnormalities, such as DNA mutations, aberrant DNA methylation, or deregulated microRNAs, are considered candidate biomarkers for the diagnosis of PDAC in surrogate biospecimens such as blood or pancreatic juice.[172–175] Newly emerging areas of biomarker discovery for early diagnosis of PDAC, and in monitoring for recurrence postresection, include circulating cell-free mutant DNA (cfDNA) and DNA contained within extracellular microvesicles (exosomes),[176,177] which can be detected using ultra-sensitive PCR techniques.[178]

Molecular biology of exocrine pancreatic neoplasms: Translational implications

Below are a few selected examples of recent advances made in understanding the tumor biology of PDAC that have translational relevance within the field of cancer medicine.

A genetic timeline for PDAC progression: The overwhelming majority of PDAC patients present with advanced disease, and early detection remains one of the most promising avenues for improving OS. In a seminal report of PDAC autopsy cases that compared the genomic aberrations present in primary versus synchronous metastatic lesions, investigators calculated that almost two decades might be required for progression from the initial mutant clone(s) to terminal metastatic disease.[179] No more than 2 years of this prolonged genetic timeline occurs during the symptomatic phase of disease, reiterating the importance of elucidating clinically applicable biomarkers that can identify emerging PDAC at a preclinical stage.

PDAC stroma: friend or foe? Traditionally, the cancer-associated myofibroblasts within the exuberant desmoplastic stroma in PDAC have been considered an ally of the invasive cancer.[180,181] One pathway that emerged as particularly relevant in facilitating tumor-stroma crosstalk is the Hedgehog signaling pathway,[182] and depletion of stromal myofibroblasts in PDAC GEMMs using short-term therapy with Hedgehog inhibitors was shown to enhance chemotherapy delivery in preclinical studies.[183] This prompted a randomized clinical trial of an inhibitor of Hedgehog signaling in combination with gemcitabine, but rather unexpectedly, the inhibitor to paradoxical disease progression (www.businesswire.com/news/home/20120127005146/en/Infinity-Reports-Update-Phase-2-Study-Saridegib). A more recent series of studies using both genetic and pharmacological ablation of myofibroblasts in PDAC GEMMs have been instrumental in implicating a tumor-constraining role for stroma.[184–186] Specifically, stromal depletion led to tumor dedifferentiation and increased metastases, with reduced median survival of mice, mimicking the clinical findings. These paradigm-shifting reports have led to a reassessment of the role of stroma in PDAC. One approach that has been proposed in preclinical models is a shift away from stromal ablation to stromal "reprogramming," wherein myofibroblasts are still retained *in situ*, but pharmacological strategies are used to revert their transcriptional profiles to a basal, resting state.[187]

Overcoming immune tolerance in PDAC: Cancer immunotherapy has emerged as one of the most promising therapeutic strategies over the last 5 years with agents known as checkpoint inhibitors resulting in dramatic improvements in survival for patients with melanoma.[188] To date, these successes have not translated to PDAC.[189,190] Some of these failures have been attributed to the unique tumor microenvironment of PDAC. In contrast to certain "immunogenic" cancers such as melanoma, the immunological infiltrate in the PDAC microenvironment is sparse in effector T cells, and populated by cells that dampen tumor rejection, including regulatory T cells, macrophages, and suppressor cells of myeloid origin.[191–193] This immunosuppressive milieu contributes to a state of immune tolerance and facilitates tumor progression. As immunotherapy of PDAC continues to evolve, there is increasing recognition of the importance of combination regimens, such as vaccines to induce an antigen-specific T-cell response in conjunction with blockade of checkpoints,[194] or adoptive therapy using antigen-specific engineered T cells in conjunction with checkpoint inhibitors.[195]

Metabolic vulnerabilities in PDAC: As proposed by Otto Warburg nearly a century ago,[196] cancer cells are known to mostly rely on aerobic glycolysis of exogenous glucose for their energy needs. In addition to glucose, exogenous glutamine is a key elemental fuel for PDAC survival and proliferation.[197] Upon uptake, glutamine is converted by the enzyme glutaminase into glutamate. Not surprisingly, mutant Ras appears to be a critical orchestrator of the intracellular reprogramming. Mutant Ras rewires the metabolic machinery such that glutamate is oxidized via a noncanonical pathway distinct from normal cells, without increasing deleterious intracellular reactive oxygen species levels.[198] In preclinical models, this unique glutamine utilization mechanism is essential for cancer cell survival and has generated enthusiasm about targeting glutaminase or other enzymes of this pathway in PDAC. Second, mutant Ras has been shown to promote dependence on autophagy, a nutrient recycling mechanism wherein lysosomal degradation of damaged proteins, macromolecules, and organelles, generates key intermediates for bioenergetics.[199] Autophagy can be blocked using agents such as chloroquine and has shown promising results in preclinical settings.[200] Finally, mutant Ras leads to profound increase in macropinocytosis, a primitive nutrient uptake mechanism that functions via endocytosis of extracellular fluid and nutrients via the so-called macropinocytic vesicles originating from the cell membrane.[201] Macropinocytosis in PDAC cells enhances uptake of albumin and other extracellular proteins that are catabolized into essential amino acids channeled into various anabolic pathways. Thus, inhibition of macropinocytosis can be leveraged as potential therapeutic avenue. Alternatively, the propensity of PDAC cells to uptake extracellular albumin can be used as a "Trojan horse" strategy, by conjugating therapeutic agents with albumin. In fact, there is some evidence to suggest that the enhanced efficacy of nano-albumin-conjugated paclitaxel might be, at least in part, due to the macropinocytosis-induced uptake of the drug within *KRAS*-mutant cancer cells.

Taken together, these results provide greater understanding of the complexity of PDAC's underlying biology with protracted genomic evolution, a dynamic microenvironment, and distinct differences in metabolism between normal and malignant cells. These insights suggest strategies to modulate the tumor's cellular and extracellular defense mechanisms. A few specific examples translating these recent laboratory-based discoveries to the clinical arena will be discussed in the section titled "Future Directions" at the end of this chapter.

Diagnostic evaluation

The diagnostic work-up of patients ultimately found to have pancreatic cancer can be fragmented and inefficient. Surgeons or subspecialty oncologists may be asked to evaluate a patient at any point in the diagnostic process to include evaluation of abdominal pain, suspicion of a pancreatic mass, or biopsy-confirmed pancreatic cancer with or without complete staging evaluation. Essential clinical information which may have important therapeutic implications can be obtained from a thorough history and physical examination. Some of this information cannot be obtained from imaging studies and includes the assessment of performance status (PS), cardiopulmonary function, evaluation for left supraclavicular or periumbilical adenopathy, or evidence for venous thromboembolism (VTE).

Classification of clinical stage

It is critically important to use standardized, objective radiologic criteria for clinical staging. Modern imaging techniques have revolutionized the clinical staging of pancreatic cancer. Precise and objective anatomic radiographic criteria are used to determine the extent of the tumor–vascular relationship and to categorize clinical staging. The clinical stage of pancreatic cancer can be broadly divided into patients with inoperable disease (metastatic or locally advanced) and localized disease (borderline resectable or resectable); see Table 3 for specific radiographic criteria. The majority of patients will present with metastatic disease, as evidenced by ascites/peritoneal implants, liver, or lung metastases. Confirmation of metastatic disease can be achieved with percutaneous biopsy of the metastatic lesion (preferred) or at the time of endoscopy (EUS-FNA (fine needle aspiration)). In the absence of metastatic disease, the clinical stage is determined by the relationship of the primary tumor to adjacent vasculature. Radiographic findings of a potentially resectable pancreatic cancer (AJCC stages I or II) are (1) the absence of tumor-arterial abutment or encasement and (2) <50% involvement of the superior mesenteric vein (SMV)/portal vein (PV) (Figure 3). As a general rule, any tumor abutment (≤180° tumor-vessel interface) or encasement (>180°) of the celiac axis, common hepatic artery, or superior mesenteric artery (SMA) should be considered a contraindication to immediate surgery. A patient is deemed to have locally advanced, unresectable disease (AJCC stage III) when (1) the tumor encases the SMA or celiac axis, as defined by >180° of the circumference of the vessel (Figure 4), or (2) there is occlusion of the SMPV (superior mesenteric-portal vein) confluence without the possibility for venous reconstruction.

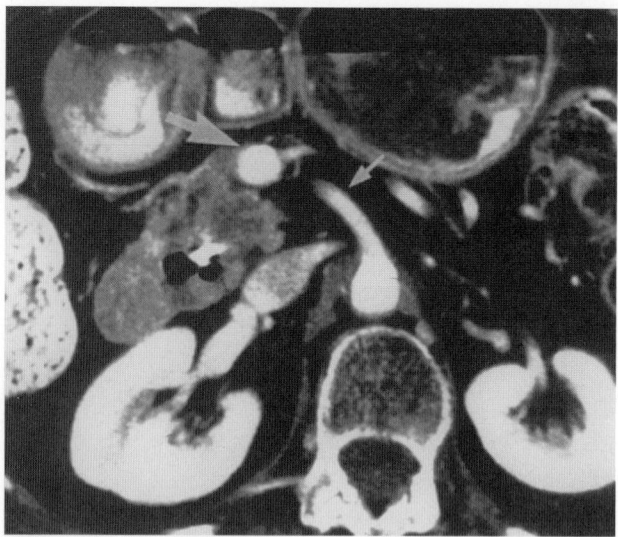

Figure 3 Contrast-enhanced computed tomography scan demonstrating a resectable adenocarcinoma of the pancreatic head. The low-density tumor is easily seen in the pancreatic head. Note the absence of tumor extension to the superior mesenteric artery (SMA) (small arrow); there is a normal fat plane between the low-density tumor and the SMA. However, the tumor (area of low density) does extend to the superior mesenteric vein (SMV) just inferior to the tip of the large arrow. This patient may require venous resection and reconstruction at the time of pancreaticoduodenectomy. This subtle finding would not be apparent on a lesser quality scan. The intrapancreatic portion of the common bile duct contains a stent that was endoscopically placed for biliary drainage.

Patients who have tumor abutment, without encasement, of the SMA or celiac axis, or short segment encasement of the hepatic artery are considered to have borderline resectable pancreatic cancer. In addition, patients with tumors that cause >50% narrowing or short segment occlusion of the SMV/PV that may be amenable to reconstruction are also considered to be borderline resectable. There is emerging consensus that even more subtle tumor-vein abutment may be best considered borderline resectable (especially as neoadjuvant therapy becomes more widely accepted).

Imaging

As accurate characterization of tumor–vascular relationship is critical for clinical staging, interventions such as EUS and ERCP (endoscopic retrograde cholangiopancreatography, which can

Table 3 Radiographic criteria for clinical staging of pancreatic cancer.

Resectable	
Tumor–artery relationship	No radiographic evidence of arterial abutment (celiac, SMA, or hepatic artery)
Tumor–vein relationship	Tumor-induced narrowing ≤50% of SMV, PV, or SMV-PV
Borderline resectable	
Artery	Tumor abutment (≤180°) of SMA or celiac artery. Tumor abutment or short segment encasement (>180°) of the hepatic artery
Vein	Tumor-induced narrowing of >50% of SMV, PV, or SMV-PV confluence. Short segment occlusion of SMV, PV, and SMV-PV with suitable PV (above) and SMV (below) to allow for safe vascular reconstruction
Extrapancreatic disease	CT scan findings suspicious, but not diagnostic of, metastatic disease (e.g., small indeterminate liver lesions which are too small to characterize)
Locally advanced	
Artery	Tumor encasement (>180°) of SMA or celiac artery
Vein	Occlusion of SMV, PV, or SMV-PV without suitable vessels above and below the tumor to allow for reconstruction (no distal or proximal target for vascular reconstruction)
Extrapancreatic disease	No evidence of peritoneal, hepatic, and extra-abdominal metastases
Metastatic	
Evidence of peritoneal or distant metastases	

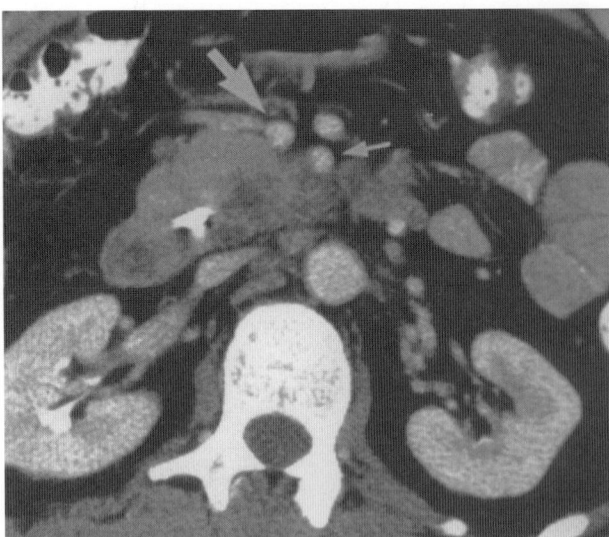

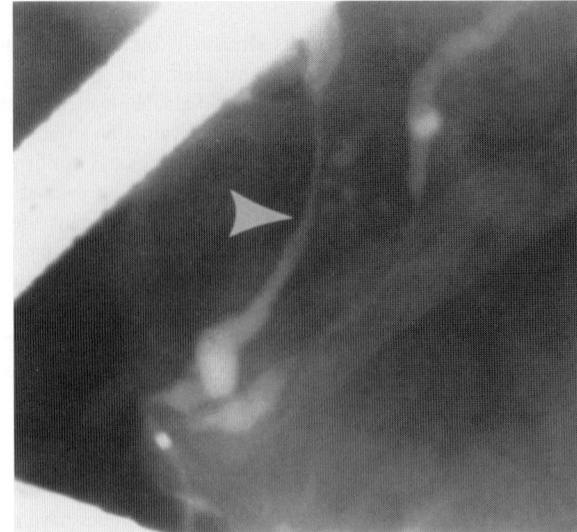

Figure 4 Contrast-enhanced computed tomography scan demonstrating an unresectable adenocarcinoma of the pancreatic head and uncinate process. The low-density tumor is inseparable from the posterior wall of the SMA (small arrow). Direct intraoperative assessment of the extent of retroperitoneal tumor growth in relation to the SMA is not possible until after gastric and pancreatic transection, at which point the surgeon has committed to resection; accurate preoperative imaging of this vital tumor–vessel relationship is thus critical. The large arrow identifies the SMV.

Figure 5 Endoscopic retrograde cholangiopancreatography demonstrating the smooth tapering common bile duct stricture (arrowhead) seen with biliary obstruction secondary to chronic pancreatitis.

induce pancreatitis and interfere with accurate assessment of the extent of disease) should be deferred briefly until high-quality imaging is obtained. The single most important imaging tool for the detection and staging of pancreatic cancer is computed tomography (CT).[202,203] Current multidetector protocols utilize dual-phase technique. A rapid injection of intravenous contrast allows for the maximal enhancement of the pancreas and mesenteric vasculature.[204] The first (arterial) phase is used for visualization of the primary tumor and optimal assessment of the tumor–arterial relationship. The second (venous) phase aids definition of the relationship of the tumor to the surrounding venous structures (SMV, PV, and splenic vein) and may uncover metastases to locoregional lymph nodes and distant organs (particularly to the liver).

If a low-density mass is not seen on CT, the presence of biliary or pancreatic duct obstruction remains concerning for malignancy. Additional imaging with magnetic resonance imaging (MRI) can be considered. Several studies have demonstrated that small pancreatic lesions (<2 cm) are more conspicuous on MRI relative to CT.[205,206] As in CT imaging, the hypovascular nature of pancreatic cancer may make tumors best seen on early phase (arterial) sequences.[204] Ultimately, patients with suspicion of pancreatic cancer without evidence of a mass should undergo EUS. In addition, EUS combined with FNA may provide tissue confirmation of malignancy. Rarely, patients may present with radiographic features concerning for pancreatic cancer without an identifiable mass on CT, MRI, or EUS. If the patient is jaundiced, an ERCP may provide additional radiographic information to include evidence for a double duct sign or smooth tapering more suggestive of sequelae of pancreatitis (Figure 5). In these settings, biliary brushings can provide material for cytologic evaluation. Importantly, pancreatic cancer remains the major diagnostic consideration in patients (without a history of recurrent pancreatitis or alcohol abuse) who have a malignant-appearing stricture of the intrapancreatic portion of the common bile duct or the presence of pancreatic duct dilation without radiographic evidence of a mass. In the presence of an

elevated CA 19-9 level, repeat EUS should be considered and if a cytologic diagnosis cannot be confirmed, upfront surgery would be the obvious next step assuming that the patient is otherwise healthy with no contraindications for major abdominal surgery.

Tissue acquisition

Confirmation of malignancy is required in all patients with locally advanced or metastatic disease before treatment with systemic therapy or radiotherapy. For patients with radiographic evidence of metastatic disease, percutaneous biopsies of the metastatic site can usually be obtained with either US- or CT guidance. For patients with localized disease that may be amenable to surgical resection, we prefer EUS-guided FNA biopsy to minimize the risk of tumor seeding. Furthermore, EUS-guided biopsy is much safer and more accurate than percutaneous CT-guided biopsy for tumors that are smaller or difficult to access using CT guidance.[207] A negative cytology from EUS-guided FNA should not be considered proof that a malignancy does not exist, and repeat EUS-guided FNA may improve diagnostic accuracy.[208] Of note, FNA biopsy should only be performed if a mass is visualized; blind biopsy of the pancreas is inappropriate.

Laparoscopic staging

In the past, laparoscopy was performed in patients who had radiologic evidence of localized pancreatic cancer.[209] However, with the advent of high-quality contrast-enhanced CT, the role of laparoscopy in staging (when performed under a separate anesthesia induction) appears to be decreasing. Moreover, the yield of staging laparoscopy may be improved in those patients with very high levels of serum carbohydrate antigen (CA) 19-9, and acquisition of preoperative CA 19-9 levels is recommended.[210,211] If the suspicion of extra-pancreatic disease is high, or if the patient is a marginal surgical candidate based on medical comorbidities, laparoscopy as a stand-alone procedure may be appropriate.

Biliary drainage

In patients with localized pancreatic cancer, placement of endobiliary stents before surgery relieves the symptoms of biliary obstruction and facilitates the normalization of liver function. The latter is particularly important for patients who will be treated with neoadjuvant therapy, as hyperbilirubinemia prevents the safe delivery of systemic therapy. If neoadjuvant therapy is planned, biliary complications, including stent occlusion and cholangitis, can be minimized with insertion of a short metal stent after cytologic confirmation of cancer.[212] For patients with locally advanced or metastatic pancreatic cancer, an endobiliary self-expandable metal stent has superior long-term patency compared with plastic stents.[213,214]

Certain groups of patients with symptomatic distal bile duct obstruction should not undergo endobiliary metal stent placement. Although covered metal stents can also be removed endoscopically,[215] they should rarely be used to provide temporary biliary decompression in a patient without a tissue diagnosis of malignancy.

Treatment of localized, potentially resectable disease

Surgical considerations
If the primary tumor cannot be resected completely (gross complete resection), surgery for pancreatic cancer (pancreaticoduodenectomy) offers no survival advantage. Patients who undergo a gross incomplete resection have an expected median survival of <1 year.[216] Even microscopically positive surgical margins have a negative impact on OS and the ability to obtain a margin negative resection should be viewed as necessary for long-term survival.[217]

Upfront surgery and adjuvant therapy
Currently, the standard of care for early-stage, resectable disease is surgery followed by adjuvant therapy. Owing to recent advances in operative technique, anesthesia, and critical care, the 30-day in-hospital mortality rate is 2% or less in patients who undergo pancreaticoduodenectomy performed by experienced surgeons.[218–220] Data have also demonstrated that higher hospital volume is associated with lower surgery-related mortality.[221] Upfront surgical resection followed by adjuvant therapy is potentially curative. However, median survival times of 22–24 months have remained stagnant for the last 30 years using this approach.[222,223]

Pancreaticoduodenectomy
The standard surgical procedure for neoplasms of the pancreatic head and periampullary region is pancreaticoduodenectomy. The current technique of pancreaticoduodenectomy has evolved from the procedure first described by Whipple and colleagues in 1935.[224] and incorporates selected aspects of the traditional Whipple procedure and emphasizes the importance of removing all soft tissue to the right of the SMA. The surgical resection is divided into six clearly defined steps (Figure 6); the most oncologically important and difficult part of the operation is step six, during which the pancreas is divided and the specimen is removed from the SMPV confluence and the right lateral border of the SMA.[225]

The high incidence of local recurrence after standard pancreaticoduodenectomy requires particular attention to the SMA margin, the soft tissue margin along the right lateral border of the proximal SMA (Figure 7a).[226] It is critical that this margin be identified for the pathologist and assessed histologically; the residual disease status (termed "R" factor) cannot be determined if the retroperitoneal margin is not assessed histologically.[220,227]

Vascular resection
The goal of vascular resection is to obtain an R0 resection, which requires complete removal of the tumor from the SMV/PV, and exposure of the SMA to allow sharp dissection of the tumor off this artery. Venous resection and reconstruction should be performed for tumors adherent to the SMV or SMPV confluence (Figure 8) or in the presence of short segment occlusion of the SMV/PV with no tumor encasement of the SMA or celiac axis.[220,225]

A very select proportion of patients with locally advanced disease (as currently defined) may be considered for surgery (after neoadjuvant therapy) if (1) tumor encasement of the celiac axis or common hepatic artery can be removed with an Appleby procedure (extended distal pancreatectomy with celiac resection) and (2) there is evidence of radiographic, biochemical (CA 19-9), and physiologic response (improved PS) to preoperative therapy. In these patients, neoadjuvant chemoradiation is recommended and surgical candidacy is reassessed upon the completion of therapy. The most common operation performed for such patients has been a distal pancreatectomy, splenectomy, and en bloc resection of the celiac axis (Appleby procedure). In the small series of patients where resection and arterial reconstruction has been performed, results have been encouraging.[228,229]

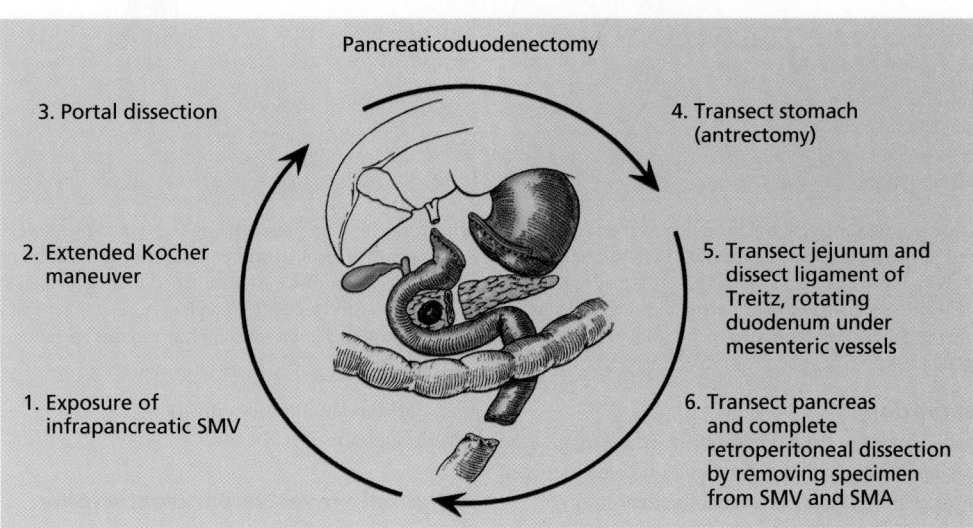

Pancreaticoduodenectomy

3. Portal dissection

4. Transect stomach (antrectomy)

2. Extended Kocher maneuver

5. Transect jejunum and dissect ligament of Treitz, rotating duodenum under mesenteric vessels

1. Exposure of infrapancreatic SMV

6. Transect pancreas and complete retroperitoneal dissection by removing specimen from SMV and SMA

Figure 6 Six surgical steps of pancreaticoduodenectomy.

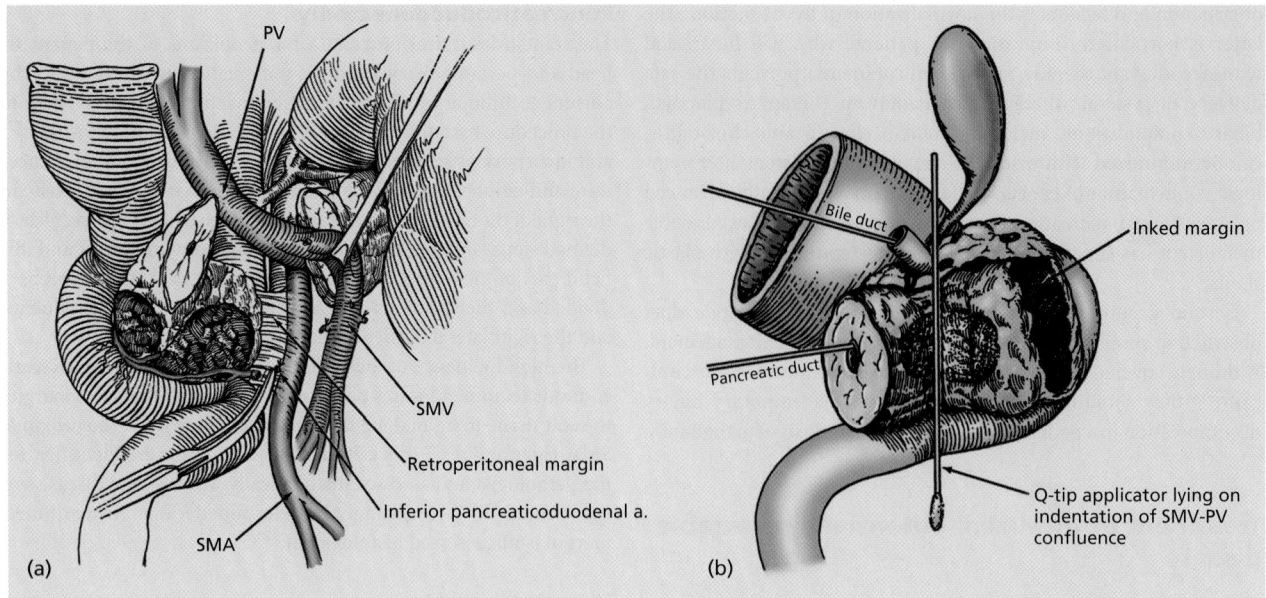

Figure 7 Illustration of the retroperitoneal margin as defined at the time of tumor resection (a). Medial retraction of the SMV and superior mesenteric-portal vein (SMPV) confluence facilitates dissection of the soft tissues adjacent to the lateral wall of the proximal SMA; this site represents the retroperitoneal margin. Complete permanent-section analysis of the pancreaticoduodenectomy specimen requires that it be oriented for the pathologist to enable accurate assessment of the retroperitoneal margin of excision and other standard pathologic variables. The retroperitoneal margin must be identified and inked with the pathologist (b); it cannot be assessed retrospectively. As shown here, a probe is in both the pancreatic duct and the bile duct, and a Q-tip applicator lies on the indentation of the SMPV confluence. One can then ink (for final pathologic assessment) the soft-tissue margin adjacent to the proximal SMA; this represents the retroperitoneal (or mesenteric) margin of excision.

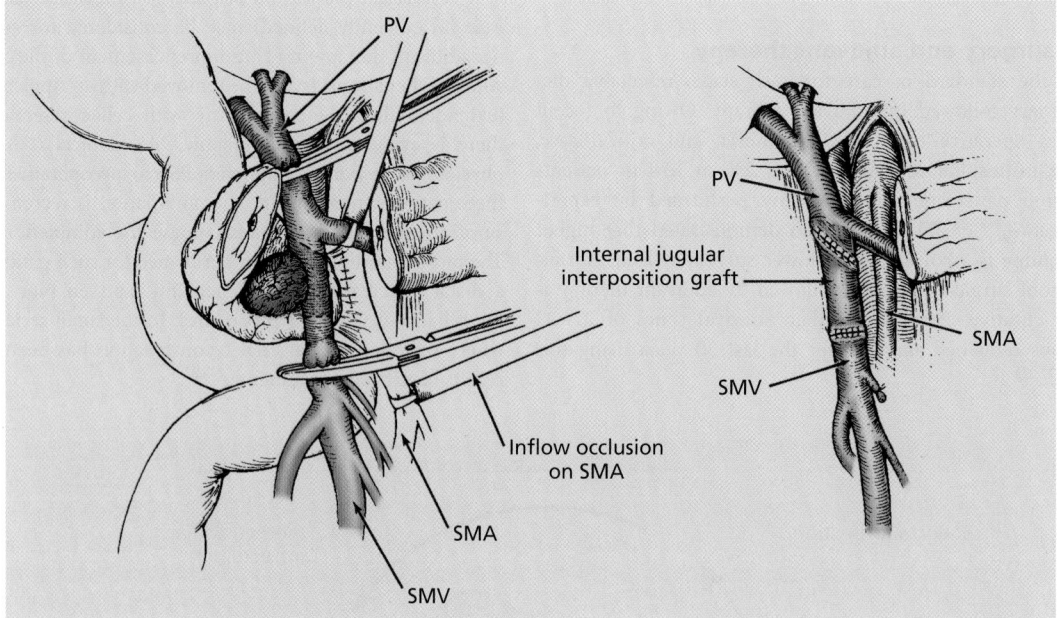

Figure 8 Venous resection/reconstruction. Illustration of resection of the SMV with splenic vein preservation. The intact splenic vein tethers the portal vein (PV), making a primary anastomosis impossible in most cases. Our preferred method of reconstruction of the SMV is to use an internal jugular vein interposition graft. With the splenic vein intact, exposure is inadequate to separate the specimen from the lateral aspect of the proximal SMA. Therefore, the graft can be placed before specimen removal, thereby allowing medial retraction of the reconstructed SMPV confluence, or after separation of the specimen from the SMA posteriorly. Segmental resection of the SMV with splenic vein preservation adds significant complexity to this operation.

Pylorus preservation

Currently, available findings from randomized trials suggest no difference in perioperative factors or patient outcome between standard and pylorus-preserving pancreaticoduodenectomy.[230–232] Most investigators would agree that pylorus preservation should not be performed in patients who have bulky tumors of the pancreatic head or duodenal tumors involving the first or second portions of the duodenum.

Minimally invasive pancreatectomy

Interest in applying minimally invasive techniques to pancreatic resection stems from the hypothesis that open surgical resection is associated with substantial physiologic stress and morbidity. While the advantages and appropriateness of minimally invasive approaches are still controversial, from 1998 to 2009, the rates of minimally invasive pancreatectomy have risen from 2.4% to 7.3%.[233] Minimally invasive procedures include both laparoscopic and robotically assisted procedures.

Laparoscopic distal pancreatectomy is the most common minimally invasive pancreatic operation performed as there is no requirement for anatomic reconstruction after the tumor is removed. Although no prospective trials have been performed comparing open versus laparoscopic distal pancreatectomy, multiple retrospective studies have reported favorable perioperative outcomes, with decreased blood loss, complications rates, and shorter hospital stays associated with the laparoscopic approach.[234,235] The oncologic impact of open versus laparoscopic surgery has been less rigorously reported. Only three studies have described the oncologic outcomes of patients undergoing laparoscopic distal pancreatectomy.[236–238] The largest study was a multicenter, retrospective matched cohort analysis; no differences in R0 resection status (74% vs 66%), lymph nodes examined (14 vs 12), or median OS (16 months vs 16 months) were observed between open and laparoscopic distal pancreatectomy.

In contrast to laparoscopic distal pancreatectomy, which is offered in most major centers, minimally invasive approaches to pancreaticoduodenectomy for pancreatic cancer have not yet achieved widespread acceptance. Few centers have a reported experience with 30 or more patients.[239,240] Among these studies, conversion to an open procedure occurred in approximately 6–10% of cases.

Robotic-assisted pancreaticoduodenectomy has also been reported with perioperative complication rates that appear comparable to the laparoscopic approach.[241–243] Similar to distal pancreatectomy, the oncologic outcomes for minimally invasive pancreaticoduodenectomy are limited. In one of the largest series of minimally invasive pancreaticoduodenectomy for cancer, 108 patients were reported and their survival duration was no different than the larger cohort of patients who underwent an open pancreaticoduodenectomy. The authors suggested that with a minimally invasive approach, more patients may receive adjuvant therapy and in a more timely manner. However, time to the receipt of adjuvant therapy (duration of time from the date of surgery to the start of systemic therapy) has recently been shown to be less important than whether or not the patient receives all intended postoperative therapy.[244]

Pathologic (surgical) staging

The staging system of the AJCC and International Union Against Cancer is given in Table 4. The modifications to the TNM staging system in the sixth edition allow for the accurate staging of patients even if they do not undergo pancreatic resection. The T4 (and stage III) designation is reserved for locally advanced unresectable primary tumors in the absence of distant metastases.[226]

When the (pathologic) pancreaticoduodenectomy specimen is evaluated, the surgeon and pathologist should first evaluate frozen sections of the common bile duct transection margin and the pancreatic transection margin. The SMA margin (the soft tissue margin directly adjacent to the proximal 3–4 cm of the SMA—Figure 7b) is then evaluated on permanent sections by inking the margin and sectioning the tumor perpendicular to the margin.[220] The R status of resection cannot be determined if the SMA margin is not assessed histologically. Most importantly, the surgeon and pathologist should classify this margin after integrating the operative findings and the histologic assessment of this margin. All pancreatic resections should be classified according to the R status: R0, no gross or microscopic residual disease; R1, microscopically positive surgical margins with no gross residual disease; and R2, grossly evident residual disease. The R designation should appear in the final operative report and should be consistent with the pathology report. The final pathologic evaluation of the permanent sections should include a description of the tumor histology and differentiation, gross and microscopic evaluation of the tissue of origin (pancreas, bile duct, ampulla of Vater, or duodenum), and a measurement of the maximum transverse tumor

Table 4 TNM staging system.

Definitions			
Primary tumor (T)			
TX	Primary tumor cannot be assessed		
T0	No evidence of primary tumor		
Tis	*In situ* carcinoma		
T1	Tumor limited to pancreas and 2 cm or less in greatest dimension		
T2	Tumor limited to pancreas and more than 2 cm in greatest dimension		
T3	Tumor extends beyond the pancreas but without involvement of the celiac axis or the superior mesenteric artery		
T4	Tumor involves the celiac axis or the superior mesenteric artery (unresectable primary tumor)		
Regional lymph nodes (N)			
NX	Regional lymph nodes cannot be assessed		
N0	No regional lymph node metastasis		
N1	Regional lymph node metastasis		
Distant metastasis (M)			
MX	Distant metastasis cannot be assessed		
M0	No distant metastasis		
M1	Distant metastasis		
Stage grouping			
Stage 0	Tis	N0	M0
Stage IA	T1	N0	M0
Stage IB	T2	N0	M0
Stage IIA	T3	N0	M0
Stage IIB	T1–3	N1	M0
Stage III	T4	N0/1	M0
Stage IV	T1–4	N0/1	M1

Source: Greene 2002.[226] Reproduced with permission of Springer.

diameter, involved lymph nodes and total lymph nodes examined, and the presence or absence of perineural, lymphatic, and vascular invasion.

Prognostic factors

Investigators have examined pathologic factors of the resected tumor in an effort to establish reliable prognostic variables associated with decreased survival.[218,245] Regional lymph node metastases, poorly differentiated histology, and increased size of primary tumors have all been associated with decreased survival duration. Nevertheless, heterogeneity in patient outcomes remains. For example, in one study of 45 patients with pancreatic adenocarcinoma who underwent complete resection with both negative resection margins and negative regional lymph nodes, median survival was 32 months with a 5-year survival of 40%.[246] However, another group reported on 12 five-year survivors (following complete resection); 4 had poorly differentiated histology, 5 had metastatic disease in regional lymph nodes, 9 had histologic evidence of malignant extrapancreatic soft tissue extension, and 10 had evidence of perineural invasion.[247] Similarly, in a report of actual 5-year survivors, 36% were node positive, and 20% of all node positive patients survived 5 years; this last report utilized preoperative therapy before surgical resection.[248]

Adjuvant (postoperative) therapy

The first report of the beneficial adjuvant therapy was published in 1985 by the Gastrointestinal Tumor Study Group (GITSG).[249] Since that time, several other prospective randomized trials have been conducted and published (Table 5).[250–254]

These assorted trials have posed various questions: whether chemoradiation is better than observation after surgery, whether regimens that contain chemoradiation are superior to those that deliver chemotherapy alone or nothing, whether gemcitabine is superior to 5-FU-based therapy (either as systemic therapy alone, or with additional 5-FU-based chemoradiation).

Two of these studies deserve special mention. CONKO-001, a large, multinational European randomized trial compared gemcitabine with observation after surgery and showed a distinct survival advantage for those patients randomized to receive gemcitabine.[253] In this trial, patients were randomized to receive six cycles of postoperative gemcitabine or observation alone after curative intent surgery. Although the median survival advantage was quite modest for patients randomized to receive gemcitabine (22.8 months vs 20.2 months, $p = 0.005$), the 3- and 5-year survival rates showed the clear superiority of treatment with gemcitabine over observation (26% vs 18% and 20% vs 9%, respectively). This trial provided the best level one evidence that chemotherapy alone improved disease-free and OS compared with surgery alone. ESPAC-3, the largest trial of adjuvant therapy ever conducted, provided additional information.[254] This study enrolled 1088 patients from 159 pancreatic centers in Europe, Australasia, Japan, and Canada. Patients were randomized to receive either 5-FU 425 mg/m^2 and folinic acid (leucovorin) 20 mg/m^2 intravenously × 5 days every 28 days or gemcitabine 1000 mg/m^2 over 30 min weekly × 3 every 28 days. There was no difference in median OS between patients randomized to receive gemcitabine and those randomized to receive 5-FU/folinic acid (23.6 months vs 23.0 months, respectively, $p = 0.42$). However, there was more toxicity leading to serious adverse events caused by 5-FU-based therapy compared with gemcitabine (14% vs 7.5%).

Taken together, CONKO-01 and ESPAC-3 support the use of systemic therapy alone as adjuvant therapy for pancreatic cancer and ESPAC-3 provides further evidence for the use of gemcitabine over 5-FU/folinic acid (based on differences in toxicity, not efficacy). Thus, at present, the standard adjuvant therapy after surgical resection with curative intent is six cycles of gemcitabine, given as three weekly injections every 28 days.

Radiotherapy in adjuvant therapy for pancreatic cancer: No role?

Despite years of investigation, questions still remain as to the possible additional benefits of radiotherapy as a component of adjuvant therapy. Proponents of radiation as a component of adjuvant therapy point to the initial results from the GITSG, single institution reports and data from SEER all showing that postoperative chemoradiation leads to median survival durations similar to those reported in ESPAC-3.[255]

Table 5 Summary of randomized trials of adjuvant therapy in resected pancreatic cancer.

Study (year)	Number of enrolled patients	Patients with R1 resection (%)	Treatment assignment Median survival (months)	Treatment assignment Median survival (months)	p-Value	Local failure rate (%)
GITSG[249] (1985)	49	0	5-FU chemoradiation 21.0	Observation 10.9	0.035	NR
EORTC[250] (1999)	114	19	5-FU chemoradiation 17.1	Observation 12.6	0.09	34
ESPAC-1[251] (2004)	289	18	5-FU chemotherapy 20.1	No chemotherapy 15.5	0.09	60
			5-FU chemoradiation 15.9	No chemoradiation 17.9	0.009	
RTOG 9704[252] (2011)	388 (Head lesions)	≥35	Gemcitabine then 5-FU chemoradiation then gemcitabine 20.5	5-FU then 5-FU chemoradiation then 5-FU 16.9	0.09	26
CONKO 001[253] (2007)	368	19	Gemcitabine 22.8	Observation 20.2	0.005	>35%
ESPAC-3[254]	1088	35	Gemcitabine 23.6	5-FU/Folinic acid 23.0	0.42	NR

Abbreviation: NR, not reported.

In an effort to definitely answer the question about the role of radiotherapy in adjuvant therapy, the Radiation Therapy Oncology Group (RTOG) is conducting a large randomized trial (RTOG 0848), which delivers gemcitabine (with or without erlotinib) to all enrolled patients, and then restages these patients for interval development of metastatic disease.[252] For the subset of patients who do not develop metastatic disease, randomization assigns patients to either two more cycles of gemcitabine alone or one more cycle of gemcitabine followed by 5-FU-based chemoradiation to a total dose of 50.4 Gy to the surgical bed.

Other approaches to adjuvant therapy

Despite negative results using radiation as a component of adjuvant therapy, 5-FU-based chemoradiation remains a cornerstone of completed phase II adjuvant therapy trials. In one study, an intense course of chemoradiation consisting of external-beam radiation therapy (EBRT) at a dose of 45–54 Gy and three-drug chemotherapy: continuous infusion 5-FU, weekly intravenous bolus cisplatin, and subcutaneous interferon alpha (IFNα) reported encouraging survival.[256] With a median follow-up of 31 months, median survival was not reached at the time of the initial report. A subsequent larger study had somewhat less impressive results with a median survival of 24.7 months and significant therapy-related toxicity.[257]

Another novel approach to adjuvant therapy was studied at the Johns Hopkins Hospital (JHH) with a focus on immunotherapy as one component.[258] Investigators there treated a group of 60 patients who had undergone surgical resection of PDAC with an allogeneic pancreatic tumor cell vaccine genetically manipulated to express granulocyte-macrophage colony-stimulating factor (GM-CSF). The first vaccination was administered 8–10 weeks after surgical resection. Subsequently, patients received 5-FU-based chemoradiation. Patients who remained disease free after completion of chemoradiotherapy received further vaccinations. The median OS was 24.8 months. While these results are provocative, larger randomized phase II or III trials will be required to support the incorporation of immunotherapy into standard adjuvant therapy.

Adjuvant therapy for resectable pancreatic cancer: Is this the right strategy?

Adjuvant therapy has been investigated for 30 years; during that time, adjuvant therapy has been refined, not improved. By definition, efforts to advance adjuvant therapy rely on a surgery-first approach. However, upfront surgery for resectable disease has significant drawbacks. First, even when the primary tumor appears technically resectable, positive surgical margins are common and from numerous reports in the literature to include ESPAC-3 show that positive surgical margins are associated with poor survival.[222,254,259–262] Second, pancreatic cancer is a systemic disease, with metastases ultimately present in over 80% of patients who undergo surgical resection. Data from several sources show that approximately 15% of patients who receive preoperative therapy for resectable pancreatic cancer will develop radiographically evident metastases within 6–12 weeks of beginning anticancer therapy.[263–269] It is therefore estimated that in patients who undergo surgery first, the likelihood of having metastatic disease seen on subsequent postoperative imaging is probably at least 20%. Finally, pancreatic cancer surgery is associated with significant morbidity and, in small-volume centers, mortality. Currently, about half of patients who undergo surgery first for pancreatic cancer ultimately receive adjuvant therapy, the other half does not.[270–272]

Given the locally invasive and metastatic properties of PDAC, delivery of multimodal therapy in addition to surgery is required to increase the chances of long-term survival. However, if surgical resection is performed upfront and results in a margin positive resection, any meaningful chance for cure vanishes. Thus preoperative, or neoadjuvant therapy is gaining greater attention as a potentially superior approach to localized disease compared with upfront surgery and postoperative treatment.

Preoperative (neoadjuvant) therapy

There are many practical and theoretical advantages to preoperative treatment of patients with localized pancreatic cancer. Most compelling is the ability to provide immediate systemic therapy for a disease that is systemic at diagnosis in virtually all patients. Moreover, results from a number of institutions suggest that the delivery of chemoradiation as a component of neoadjuvant therapy may aid in the achievement of negative surgical margins at the time of attempted resection.[273] Another important advantage of neoadjuvant therapy is improved patient selection for pancreatic surgery. Using a preoperative strategy, patients with rapidly progressive systemic disease are identified as part of the restaging evaluation performed following neoadjuvant treatment (before planned surgery).

Since 1988, five prospective preoperative trials have been completed at UTMDACC.[263,264,267–269] These trials have had identical eligibility criteria using a CT-based definition of resectable disease (as previously described), a uniform surgical technique for the performance of pancreaticoduodenectomy, and a standardized system for pathologic evaluation of surgical specimens. Our two most recent trials have used a gemcitabine-based preoperative approach. The first trial used rapid-fractionation chemoradiation with seven weekly infusions of gemcitabine. A total of 86 patients were enrolled in this trial.[268] In this trial, 74% of patients underwent successful pancreaticoduodenectomy. Overall, median survival for all 86 patients was 23 months with an actual 5-year survival of 27%. Median survival was 34 months for the 64 patients who completed all therapy to include surgical resection in the form of pancreaticoduodenectomy and 7 months for the 22 patients who did not undergo pancreatic resection (due to disease progression or evolving medical comorbidities). The actual 5-year survival for those who did and did not complete all therapy was 36% and 0%, respectively. In our subsequent gemcitabine-based neoadjuvant trial, we delivered additional systemic therapy before chemoradiation and planned surgery. Preoperative gemcitabine and cisplatin was given every 2 weeks for four doses followed by chemoradiation consisting of four weekly infusions of gemcitabine combined with radiation therapy (30 Gy in 10 fractions over 2 weeks).[269] The study enrolled 90 patients and 79 (88%) completed chemo-chemoradiation. Sixty-two (78%) of 79 patients were taken to surgery and 52 (66%) of 79 underwent pancreaticoduodenectomy. Median survival for the 79 patients who completed Gem-Cis-XRT was 19 months, with a median survival of 31 months for the 52 patients who received all therapy to include surgery and 10.5 months for those patients who did not undergo resection due to disease progression ($p < 0.001$). These results were essentially equivalent to those observed with preoperative gemcitabine-based chemoradiation without induction chemotherapy. Nevertheless, the results from these two preoperative gemcitabine-based chemoradiation trials are sufficiently compelling to justify broader investigation of neoadjuvant treatment for localized stage I/II pancreatic cancer.

Critics have been concerned that the delivery of neoadjuvant therapy may result in local tumor progression, precluding potentially curative surgery. In our studies, local tumor progression has occurred during preoperative therapy, but with rare exception, is accompanied by concurrent metastatic disease. Isolated local tumor progression occurred in <4% of all enrolled patients.

As previously stated, the standard of care in patients with resectable pancreatic cancer is upfront surgery. This strategy results in high rates of R1 resection, rapid onset of metastatic disease in an estimated 20% of patients, and inability to delivery postoperative therapy in almost half the patients. Thus, while neoadjuvant therapy for resectable disease remains investigational, more studies of neoadjuvant therapy are fully justified.

Neoadjuvant therapy in borderline resectable disease

With the advent of MDCT, and better understanding of the implications of positive surgical margins at surgery, tumors that are neither clearly resectable nor clearly unresectable have become increasingly recognized. These tumors are now being described as borderline resectable. While definitions vary, borderline resectable tumors can be broadly defined as tumors which abut but do not encase critical arterial structures such as the SMA, hepatic artery, or celiac axis, or tumors with varying degrees of involvement of the SMV, PV, and SMPV confluence.[274,275] As such, a borderline resectable tumor puts the patient at high risk for a margin-positive resection (R1 or R2) with upfront surgery, an independent predictor of poor survival.[218,259–262] On the basis of results in resectable disease, neoadjuvant chemoradiation leads to low R1 resection rates[267–269] and reduces the risk of an R1 resection compared with upfront surgery.[273] Further support for preoperative chemoradiation comes from our experience showing that approximately 40% of patients with borderline resectable disease can ultimately undergo surgical resection, with a median OS for the subset undergoing surgical resection equal to 40 months. Moreover, an R0 resection was achieved in 96% of resected patients.[276]

Given these lines of evidence, upfront surgery should be discouraged in patients with borderline resectable disease. Preoperative chemotherapy, chemoradiation, or both should be considered as sufficient tumor destruction, particularly at the tumor's periphery, could render a tumor resectable with curative intent (i.e., negative surgical margins).

Current practice guidelines now recommend initial nonoperative (neoadjuvant) multimodality treatment (followed by eventual surgery) for patients with borderline resectable pancreatic cancer.[277–279]

Prospective trials of neoadjuvant therapy for borderline resectable pancreatic cancer are now being reported. Three basic strategies are being investigated: systemic therapy followed by surgical resection, chemoradiation followed by surgery, and induction chemotherapy, subsequent chemoradiation, with surgical resection performed last.[280–282]

The role of radiation in borderline resectable disease

In comparison with adjuvant therapy, radiotherapy may have a better defined role in the preoperative treatment of potentially resectable disease, and as a component of neoadjuvant therapy for those patients who are considered to have borderline resectable disease. Results using preoperative radiation in resectable and borderline resectable PDAC are discussed earlier, with data regarding the role of radiation in borderline resectable cancer beginning to emerge.

Tumors of the pancreatic body and tail

Because adenocarcinomas of the pancreatic body and tail do not obstruct the intrapancreatic portion of the common bile duct, early diagnosis is rare, and most patients present with locally advanced or metastatic disease. The celiac axis or SMA is encased in most patients. Furthermore, peritoneal metastases are more frequent and laparoscopy before laparotomy is advised.[283,284]

Locally advanced pancreatic cancer

In the early 1980s, the delivery of chemoradiation was shown to improve survival compared with radiation alone for patients with locally advanced (unresectable) pancreatic cancer.[285] For over 20 years thereafter, upfront chemoradiation was generally recommended to patients with locally advanced disease. This approach may be partly explained by the lack of active systemic agents for treatment of advanced PDAC at the time. However, after the approval of gemcitabine in 1997 for PDAC, trials that compared gemcitabine alone to chemoradiation showed conflicting results (Table 6). In a French study, patients with LAPC (locally advanced pancreatic cancer) were randomized to receive gemcitabine alone or radiation (total dose 60 Gy) with concurrent 5-FU and cisplatin, followed by gemcitabine.[286] The median OS was higher in the gemcitabine alone arm compared with chemoradiation: 13.0 versus 8.6 months ($p = 0.03$), respectively. Of note, the trial was stopped prematurely owing to poor compliance and toxicity of the chemoradiation regimen.

In contrast, ECOG 4201 showed superiority of gemcitabine-based chemoradiation compared with gemcitabine alone. It compared upfront gemcitabine-based chemoradiation, followed by weekly gemcitabine with standard treatment using gemcitabine alone. Although it closed prematurely after accruing only 74 of a planned 316 patients, a statistically significant median survival benefit was seen in the patients randomized to receive chemoradiation compared with those who received chemotherapy alone, 11.0 months versus 9.2 months, $p = 0.034$. This benefit came at the cost

Table 6 Select trials of chemotherapy, radiation, and chemoradiation in patients with locally advanced pancreatic cancer.

Study (year)	Number of patients	Control arm Median survival (months)	Experimental arm Median survival (months)	*p*-Value
GITSG[285] (1981)	194	XRT 40 Gy (only) 5.5	5-FU + XRT 40–60 Gy 10	<0.01
FFCD/SFRO[286] (2008)	119	Gem alone 13.0	5-FU/Cisplatin + XRT 60 Gy then gem 8.6	0.03
ECOG 4021[287] (2011)	74	Gem alone 9.2	Gemcitabine + XRT 50.4 Gy then gem 11.1	0.017
LAP07[291] (2013)	442 (269 in R2)	Induction gem ± erlotinib (R1) × 4 months if no progression then: gem × 2 months 16.5	Induction gem ± erlotinib (R1) × 4 months if no progression then Capecitabine + XRT 54 Gy 15.3	0.83

Abbreviation: Gem, gemcitabine; XRT, radiation; R1, first randomization; R2, second randomization.

of increased gastrointestinal toxicity (grade 3 or greater gastrointestinal toxicity 38% vs 14% $p = 0.03$) and fatigue, 32% versus 6%.[287] Thus, the addition of radiation to standard chemotherapy resulted in a modest prolongation of median survival at the cost of a modest increase in toxicity that remained manageable.

During this same time period, a shift in the management of LAPC began to occur. In a retrospective analysis conducted at UTMDACC, patients with LAPC who were initially treated with systemic therapy followed by chemoradiation had longer survival times compared with patients who were initially treated with upfront chemoradiation (median survival 11.9 months vs 8.5 months).[288] The authors suggested that systemic therapy acted as a selection mechanism to identify patients with rapidly progressing disease. This was supported by reports from two prospective trials[289,290] that suggested induction chemotherapy followed by chemoradiation led to favorable median OS (15–17 months). Of note, in both trials, approximately 30% of patients progressed on induction systemic therapy delivered for 3–6 months; these patients did not go on to receive subsequent chemoradiation.

Most recently, the trial with the greatest impact on clinical practice is the LAP 07 trial, a multinational trial conducted in Europe. Preliminary data from the LAP 07 trial reveal no clear benefit with the addition of conventional chemoradiation following gemcitabine chemotherapy.[291] Using a 2×2 randomized design, patients received initial gemcitabine with or without erlotinib for 4 months and for those patients who did not developed metastatic disease, a second randomization assigned patients to receive 2 additional months of gemcitabine or capecitabine-based chemoradiation (54 Gy to the gross tumor alone). After a median follow-up of 36 months, there was no difference in median OS between the chemotherapy and chemoradiation groups (15 months vs 14 months, respectively, $p = 0.083$). Further details in regard to the results of LAP 07 are awaited when the manuscript is published.

Chemotherapy alone versus chemotherapy and subsequent chemoradiation: How to select patients?

Similar to the delivery of preoperative therapy before surgical intervention, induction chemotherapy allows an interval of time to uncover unfavorable tumor biology manifest by onset of metastatic disease. Just as resectable patients who develop metastatic disease during preoperative therapy will not benefit from surgery, LAPC patients with aggressive disease that quickly disseminates will not benefit from local therapy in the form of chemoradiation. While LAP 07 did provide a mechanism for identifying patients with aggressive tumor biology with the delivery of 4 months of systemic gemcitabine, it does not provide a mechanism to identify a subset of patients who may benefit from consolidative chemoradiation.

In the future, SMAD4 may be useful to select patients for systemic therapy, of for standard dose or dose-intensified radiation therapy. Currently, the only active clinical trial in the United States for this population has been designed to evaluate the role of radiation after induction chemotherapy with gemcitabine and nab-paclitaxel (RTOG 1201). SMAD4 expression status is a stratification variable and patients are randomized to receive six cycles of chemotherapy alone in the standard arm, four cycles of chemotherapy followed by 50.4 Gy in 28 fractions or four cycles of chemotherapy followed by 63 Gy in 28 fractions using intensity-modulated radiation therapy (IMRT). Concurrent capecitabine will be given with radiation. This trial will evaluate the value of SMAD4 as a predictive marker for chemoradiation decision making and provide further data evaluating the role of chemoradiation in the context of more active chemotherapy.

Gemcitabine-based versus fluoropyrimidine-based chemoradiation

The introduction of gemcitabine was a modest step forward in the treatment of pancreatic cancer. Its value as a systemic agent in pancreatic cancer and discovery of its potent radiosensitizing properties,[292] stimulated the study of combinations of gemcitabine with EBRT for patients with localized pancreatic cancer.[293–297] Most of these studies suggested gastrointestinal toxicity as a dose-limiting factor, but hematologic toxicity has also been observed. At the present time, there is no standard approach for combining gemcitabine and radiation, but several variables appear to be important in predicting the maximum tolerated dose (MTD). These include variations in the size of the radiation portal, the total radiation dose, possibly the dose of radiation per fraction, and whether gemcitabine is administered once or twice weekly.[298]

The best data available data comparing concurrent chemotherapeutic agents in the setting of LAPC come from the SCALOP trial. In a randomized phase II design of 114 patients with locally advanced PDAC, a course of gemcitabine and capecitabine for 12 weeks was followed by chemoradiation with either gemcitabine (300 mg/m^2 weekly) or capecitabine (830 mg/m^2 twice daily on days of radiation). A longer median OS with less toxicity was reported with the use of capecitabine compared to gemcitabine (15.2 months vs 13.4 months, $p = 0.012$).[299]

Radiotherapy technique for patients with locally advanced PDAC

Patients with locally advanced tumors probably do not benefit from regional lymph node irradiation; radiotherapy fields should therefore be confined to the gross tumor. This strategy reduces the gastrointestinal toxicity of chemoradiation. Thus, it is important to identify the pancreatic tumor correctly. On contrast-enhanced CT, pancreatic tumors are typically hypodense compared with the surrounding pancreatic parenchyma. When there is doubt about the location of the primary tumor, CT images should be reviewed with an experienced radiologist. Administration of an oral contrast agent at the time of simulation illuminates the duodenal "c-loop." Endobiliary biliary stents can also be visualized, which facilitates identifying the common bile duct.

The pancreas and duodenum move a median of 1 cm with respiratory excursion.[300] If the gross tumor alone is to be treated, respiratory motion must be either controlled or accounted for in radiotherapy planning. This is commonly accomplished by simply adding an additional margin to the planned radiation fields in the cranial and caudal directions. However, because axial tumor motion is negligible, an additional margin for motion in the axial directions is not necessary. Radiation treatment that is gated to the respiratory cycle (respiratory gating)[301] is a necessary component of radiation dose escalation studies that seek to deliver >60 Gy to the primary tumor while sparing the duodenum. Thus, radiation fields designed to spare the duodenum that are tightly confined to the primary tumor without correction for organ motion could lead to under-dosing of the tumor target, or "marginal miss." A four-field technique is recommended with equally weighted anterior, posterior, and opposed lateral fields. A 2-cm block margin is used in the radial directions, and a 3-cm margin is used in the cranial and caudal directions.

Novel approaches to chemoradiation

Molecular agents as radiosensitizers

Just as molecular agents have been combined with cytotoxic chemotherapy, targeted drugs are being actively investigated as radiosensitizers in solid tumors.[302] In LAPC, none of the currently available inhibitors (gefitinib, erlotinib, panitumumab, or cetuximab) have been evaluated in multi-institutional trials in combination with radiation for pancreatic cancer. Nevertheless, small clinical trials using molecular radiosensitizers have demonstrated encouraging results, particularly those which combine EGFR inhibitors with radiation.[303–305] Unfortunately, as EGFR inhibitors have not significantly improved clinical outcomes for patients with advanced pancreatic cancer when combined with chemotherapy,[306,307] investigation of EGFR inhibition as radiosensitization has stopped as well.

Stereotactic radiation body therapy (SBRT) for pancreatic cancer

Stereotactic body radiotherapy (SBRT) is capable of precisely delivering high doses of radiation to small tumor volumes. The feasibility of SBRT as a pancreatic cancer treatment has been investigated in a phase I and phase II trials of a single fraction of radiation therapy in patients with LAPC.[308,309] On the basis of limited efficacy and significant toxicity, investigation shifted in favor of a five fraction regimen. A multi-institutional trial evaluating SBRT (33 Gy in five fractions in 1 week) has been reported.[310] Results indicate good tolerability and median survivals comparable to chemoradiation at standard fractionation. Thus, it appears that SBRT given in five fractions is perhaps better tolerated and more convenient than standard chemoradiation, with similar efficacy. If long-term survival is the goal, better local tumor control is needed.

Irreversible electroporation in locally advanced pancreatic cancer

Although not a radiotherapeutic intervention, irreversible electroporation (IRE) is being investigated as a local ablative technique receiving increasing attention in oncology.[311] IRE involves the delivery of pulses of high-voltage energy through the placement of electrodes into a solid tumor mass. These pulses lead to the formation of pores in the phospholipid cell membrane, which changes cellular permeability and results in apoptotic cell death. The advantage of IRE over other ablative techniques is the absence of thermal injury to surrounding tissues, specifically vascular and ductal structures.[312] Early experience has been reported using IRE in 27 patients with LAPC.[313] In eight patients, IRE was combined with surgical resection (four head lesions and four left-sided resections) for the purpose of margin accentuation. In the remaining 19, IRE was performed *in situ*. All 27 patients developed elevation of their amylase and lipase, which peaked at 48 h and returned to normal at 72 h postprocedure. Other centers are beginning to report on their experience with IRE to include percutaneous, image-guided localization of the electrodes.[314]

On the basis of current literature, there appears to be growing enthusiasm for this technique, particularly for patients with borderline resectable and locally advanced disease.[315] However, broader multi-institutional experience will be required to develop more refined criteria to select patients and appropriate sequencing of this technique with other therapeutic modalities. As previously emphasized given the systemic nature of PDAC, systemic therapies should precede any local therapeutic intervention (IRE, surgery, or chemoradiation).

Approach to patient with locally advanced pancreatic cancer

Whenever possible, patients with locally advanced disease having a good PS should be treated in the context of a clinical trial. This may involve a predefined course of chemotherapy followed by chemoradiation, or alternatively a program of chemoradiation with a targeted agent, followed by further systemic therapy.

Outside of a clinical trial, systemic therapy may improve both pain control and PS,[316] and avoids the gastrointestinal toxicity associated with chemoradiation.

The role of systemic therapy in pancreatic cancer

While surgery and radiotherapy have important roles in the treatment of pancreatic cancer, these modalities are generally limited to the subset of patients with localized disease. Furthermore, as described earlier in this chapter, radiation therapy may have additional benefits for select patients with locally advanced PDAC. In contrast, systemic therapy has proved benefit as adjuvant therapy after potentially curative surgery,[253] in the treatment of locally advanced PDAC,[291] and as the primary therapy for metastatic disease.[317] Until recently, the mainstay of systemic therapy has been gemcitabine which remains the standard of care as adjuvant therapy and for the treatment of locally advanced PDAC. However, with the advent of FOLFIRINOX and gemcitabine plus nab-paclitaxel (both of which are superior to gemcitabine monotherapy in metastatic disease),[318,319] further investigation of these regimens in earlier stages of disease is certain, with the goal of (1) improving cure rates and survival for those undergoing surgery with curative intent, (2) increasing the proportion of patients with borderline resectable disease undergoing subsequent surgery with curative intent, (3) prolonging survival of patients with borderline resectable disease who are not ultimately surgical candidates, and (4) improving survival for those with locally advanced PDAC.

The evolution of systemic therapy

A history of systemic therapy for pancreatic cancer is beyond the scope of this chapter and is well summarized in a number of review articles published on this subject.

On the basis of the early and more recent trials of systemic cytotoxic agents, several conclusions can be drawn. First, bolus 5-FU has virtually no activity in the setting of advanced PDAC.[316,320] However, both infusional 5-FU and capecitabine have very modest single agent activity in pancreatic cancer of 7–8%.[321,322] Second, gemcitabine monotherapy leads to an objective response rates (RR) of approximately 10%; this has been consistent across studies and time. Third, several gemcitabine doublets lead to improved objective rates compared to gemcitabine alone. However, with the exception of gemcitabine plus nab-paclitaxel, combining gemcitabine with oxaliplatin, cisplatin, bolus 5-FU, or capecitabine has demonstrated no statistically significant improvement in survival compared with delivery of gemcitabine alone (Table 7).[319,323–331] Most importantly, PS remains an important predictor of OS. As early as 1985, PS was observed to have impact on patient survival for patients with all stages of pancreatic cancer.[332] This observation has been supported in the modern era by findings from CALGB 80803[333] and the randomized trial of gemcitabine versus gemcitabine plus nab-paclitaxel.[334]

Table 7 Summary of completed randomized trials of gemcitabine versus a cytotoxic gemcitabine doublet in the treatment of advanced PDAC.

Principal investigator (year)	Number of patients	Patients with metastatic disease (%)	Control arm Median overall survival (months)	Experimental arm Median overall survival (months)	p-Value
Berlin[323] (2002)	322	90	Gem 5.4	Gem + 5-FU 6.7	0.09
Colucci[324] (2002)	107	58	Gem 4.7	Gem + Cisplatin 7.0	0.43
Rocha Lima[325] (2004)	342	80	Gem 6.5	Gem + Irinotecan 6.3	0.79
Louvet[326] (2005)	313	70	Gem 6.0	Gem + Oxaliplatin 9.0	0.15
Heinemann[327] (2006)	195	80	Gem 6.0	Gem + Cisplatin 7.5	0.15
Herrmann[328] (2007)	319	79	Gem 7.2	Gem + Capecitabine 8.4	0.14
Abou Alfa[329] (2007)	349	78	Gem 6.2	Gem + Exatecan 6.7	0.52
Cunningham[330] (2009)	553	71	Gem 6.2	Gem + Capecitabine 7.1	0.08
Colucci[331] (2010)	400	84	Gem 8.3	Gem + Cisplatin 7.2	0.38
Von Hoff[319] (2013)	861	100	Gem 6.7	Gem + nab-paclitaxel 8.5	<0.001

Abbreviation: Gem, gemcitabine.

Table 8 Summary of randomized trials of cytotoxic drugs or drug combinations for advanced or metastatic pancreatic cancer.

Treatment	Burris 1996[316]		Conroy 2011[318] (ACCORD)		Von Hoff 2013[319] (MPACT)	
	Bolus 5-FU	Gem	Gem	FOLFIRINOX	Gem	Gem/nab-P
PS	Karnovsky PS ≥ 50%		ECOG PS 0 or 1		Karnovsky PS ≥ 70%	
Patients with Met Dz (%)	70		100		100	
RR (%)	0	10	9	32	7	23
MS (months)	4.5	5.7	6.8	11.1	6.7	8.5
1-Year survival (%)	2	18	21	48	22	35
Neutropenia (%)	5	25	21	46	27	38
Fatigue (Grades 3–4)	NS	NS	18	24	1	17
Diarrhea (Grades 3–4)	6	2	2	13	1	6
Neuropathy	NS	NS	0	9	7	17

Abbreviations: PS, performance status; Gem, gemcitabine; nab-P, nanoparticle-albumin-bound paclitaxel; MS, median survival; NS, not stated; RR, response rate.

New regimens in metastatic disease: FOLFIRINOX and gemcitabine/nab-paclitaxel

Since the last edition of this text, two new combination regimens have been proved to extend survival of patients with metastatic disease compared with gemcitabine alone (Table 8). FOLFIRINOX was initially shown in a phase 2 trial with 47 patients to generate an objective RR of 26% and a median survival of 10.2 months.[335] It was then investigated in a large randomized phase 3 trial comparing FOLFIRINOX to gemcitabine alone.[318] FOLFIRINOX was superior to gemcitabine in terms of RR (32% vs 9%), progression-free survival (PFS) (6.4 months vs 3.3 months), and OS (11.1 months vs 6.8 months). The hazard ratio for death favored FOLFIRINOX at 0.57, $p < 0.001$. Of note, this trial limited enrollment to chemo-naïve patients with metastatic disease and having an ECOG PS 0 or 1.

Slightly later, nanoparticle, albumin-bound (nab)-paclitaxel was also investigated in pancreatic cancer. At the maximum tolerated dose of nab-paclitaxel (125 mg/m^2) combined with gemcitabine (1000 mg/m^2) administered weekly × 3 weeks followed by 1 week off and repeated, the objective RR was 48%, with a median survival of 12.2 months.[336] This impressive result prompted a larger randomized phase 3 trial comparing gemcitabine plus nab-paclitaxel with gemcitabine alone.[319] The eligibility criteria for this trial allowed for the enrollment of chemo-naïve patients with metastatic disease having a KPS ≥ 70% (roughly equivalent to ECOG PS 0-2). The trial enrolled 861 patients and demonstrated gemcitabine/nab-paclitaxel was superior to gemcitabine alone in RR (23% vs 7%), PFS (5.5 months vs 3.7 months), and survival. Median OS was superior for the doublet at 8.5 months versus 6.7 months for gemcitabine (HR for death, 0.72; $p < 0.001$). Not surprisingly, as seen in prior clinical trials, subsequent analysis revealed that patients with KPS 70–80% had inferior survival compared with those having a KPS 90–100%.[334]

On the basis of these large well-designed clinical trials, both FOLFIRINOX and gemcitabine/nab-paclitaxel represent significant advances in the systemic treatment of metastatic pancreatic cancer. Moreover, the availability of both regimens provides clinical oncologists with some flexibility in choosing frontline therapy as there are differences in the toxicity profiles for these regimens with both regimens sharing a sizable risk for neutropenia.[337]

Molecular agents in pancreatic cancer: Virtually no added value

Attempts to improve pancreatic cancer therapy using modern molecular therapeutics have been disappointing although molecular agents have changed the face of cancer therapy in other gastrointestinal tumors to include hepatocellular carcinoma,[338] advanced colorectal cancer,[339] and more recently gastric cancer.[340] A number of randomized trials have compared the efficacy of gemcitabine or a gemcitabine combination to the same regimen with the addition of a targeted agent.[306,307,333,341–345] Only the combination of gemcitabine and erlotinib has led to a small, statistically significant survival advantage over gemcitabine alone.[306] In a large placebo-controlled, double-blind, phase III trial conducted by the National Cancer Institute of Canada, 569 patients were randomized to receive gemcitabine and erlotinib or gemcitabine plus placebo. The median survival for patients randomized to receive gemcitabine/erlotinib was 6.24 months versus 5.91 months for gemcitabine/placebo; hazard ratio for death 0.82, $p = 0.038$).

More recently, provocative preclinical experiments showed that hedgehog pathway inhibition could modulate the PDAC tumor microenvironment and facilitate enhanced delivery of cytotoxic agents to the tumor mass.[183] This led to the conduct of a placebo-controlled, double-blind, randomized phase 2 trial comparing gemcitabine plus saridegib (a hedgehog inhibitor) with gemcitabine plus placebo in 122 previously untreated patients with metastatic pancreatic cancer. The trial was terminated early based on an interim analysis showing that patients who were randomized to receive the gemcitabine/saridegib arm had inferior survival compared with patients receiving gemcitabine/placebo (www.businesswire.com/news/home/20120127005146/en/Infinity-Reports-Update-Phase-2-Study-Saridegib). Future successful clinical testing of molecular therapeutics for treatment of PDAC will require rigorous and compelling preclinical data, in addition to disciplined clinical trial design. This will be discussed in more detail in section titled "Future Directions."

Systemic therapy for "BRCAness"

Clinicians have recognized for some time that patients with PDAC are heterogeneous and a subset will have a protracted course of disease and survival that significantly exceeds median survival times reported in the literature (for all stages of disease). In addition, the objective responses to chemotherapy can occasionally be quite striking. Such patients likely have underlying germ line or somatic mutations that render the tumors more susceptible to the cytotoxic effects of chemotherapy, particularly DNA damaging agents (oxaliplatin, cisplatin, and mitomycin C) and possibly topoisomerase inhibitors. Genetic testing for germ line mutations in *BRAC1, 2,* and *PALB2* is often negative and cannot explain exquisite sensitivity to these agents. Nevertheless, there appear to be poorly defined subsets of sporadic cancers that may have characteristics suggesting defects in DNA repair pathways with greater sensitivity to treatment with specific cytotoxic agents. Some authors have described these sporadic cancers as having a "BRCAness" phenotype, likely explained by mutations, amplifications, or methylation of the genes regulating DNA repair.[346] There are hints from the clinic to support this notion. A retrospective analysis of patients from JHH who had received cytotoxic therapy with or without a platinum analog suggested that patients with a family history of pancreatic, breast, or ovarian cancer were more likely to benefit from a platinum containing regimen, compared with patients having no such history. Importantly, somatic mutations in *BRCA2* in pancreatic cancer are now being reported in PDAC,[347] and these tumors may also be quite sensitive to DNA damaging chemotherapeutic agents.

In the future, better characterization of BRCAness may identify a broader subset of patients who may benefit from treatment with platinum, mitomycin C, and possibly topoisomerase inhibitors. Of further note, PARP inhibitors, now entering clinical trials in PDAC, may be particularly useful in germ line *BRCA*-mutated patients and/or sporadic tumors considered to have BRCAness.

Approach to the patient with metastatic disease

Options for systemic treatment

On the basis of the data presented earlier regarding the role of cytotoxic therapy in metastatic PDAC, an accurate assessment of a patient's PS is critical to decision making and recommendations for treatment. Systemic therapy for metastatic disease should be actively discouraged in patients with poor PS (ECOG > 2, KPS < 70%) or if significant metastatic tumor burden is present. Whenever possible, patients with good PS should be encouraged to enroll in a clinical trial. When enrollment in a trial is not possible or desired, for ECOG PS 0-1 patients, therapy with FOLFIRINOX or gemcitabine/nab-paclitaxel is appropriate frontline options. In patients with ECOG PS 2 or KPS 70%, gemcitabine/nab-paclitaxel is a valid choice, but should be administered cautiously, with close follow-up and low-threshold for dose/schedule adjustments. For patients who are equivocal candidates for systemic therapy, gemcitabine monotherapy may be considered. The addition of erlotinib in this setting is also reasonable; the anticipated benefits of this drug should not be overstated and it may have decreasing relevance as a component of systemic therapy in the future.[306]

At present, second line therapy should be limited to those patients who are maintaining adequate PS in the face of disease progression and is obviously dependent on prior first line therapy. Supportive care as an alternative to continued anticancer therapy should be thoroughly discussed.

Supportive care and palliation

Metastatic pancreatic cancer is characterized by anorexia, cachexia, and pain. Jaundice may result from the primary tumor or intrahepatic metastases. Local tumor progression can lead to worsening pain, gastric outlet obstruction, or gastroparesis, and patients with peritoneal carcinomatosis may suffer from intractable ascites, intestinal dysmotility, or mechanical obstruction. Constipation is also very common. Patients are also at risk of VTE, but the risk is not clearly higher than that associated with other gastrointestinal tumors.[348] Palliation must always be the primary goal and is facilitated by a multidisciplinary team. Symptomatic relief of biliary obstruction and pain should be addressed before initiation of systemic therapy. For most patients, adequate pain control can be obtained with the use of long- or short-acting narcotics, without excessive sedation.[349] However, if pain is not well controlled with oral or transdermal narcotics or if these agents are poorly tolerated, patients should be evaluated for celiac plexus or splanchnic plexus ablation. Whether EUS-guided neurolytic blocks are superior to fluoroscopic- or CT-guided blocks remains an open question, but EUS-guided neurolysis has been shown to be superior to CT-guided blockade in patients with chronic pancreatitis.[350]

Given the poor prognosis for patients with metastatic disease, biliary obstruction should be relieved with nonsurgical means whenever possible. The use of duodenal stents in patients with mechanical gastric outlet obstruction and poor prognosis is becoming more widely accepted.[351] For patients with intractable symptomatic ascites, paracentesis is generally perceived as most efficacious,[352] but it is not an intervention with durable benefits.

Insertion of an intraperitoneal catheter to control ascites is a preferred alternative to frequent paracenteses, and the overall risk of infection is low.[353]

Prophylactic treatment with low-molecular-weight heparin can reduce the risk of VTE in patients with advanced disease receiving chemotherapy.[354] However, impact on OS with this intervention has yet to be demonstrated.

Future directions

On the basis of evidence presented in other sections of this chapter, progress in the treatment of pancreatic cancer is obviously slow and incremental. With a greater understanding of PDAC tumor biology and microenvironment, coupled with the availability of a broader range of agents designed to kill tumor cells, modulate the tumor microenvironment, or augment the host immune response, better treatment of pancreatic cancer is anticipated. At present, the thrust of ongoing efforts can be partitioned into three categories: (1) improvement in nonimmune killing of tumor cells directly, (2) modulation of the tumor microenvironment to promote cancer cell death, and (3) enhancing immune destruction of PDAC.

Nonimmune killing of tumor cells

Combination cytotoxic chemotherapy

One of the most important lessons from early experience with FOLFIRINOX may be that combination cytotoxic therapy can be more effective than monotherapy or even doublet therapy.[355] Thus, investigation of other triplet combinations is currently underway and includes studies with combinations of gemcitabine, cisplatin and nab-paclitaxel (GAC), and 5-FU, leucovorin, oxaliplatin, and nab-paclitaxel (FOLFOX-A) (www.clinicaltrials.gov).

New cytotoxic drugs: Irinotecan reformulated

MM 398 is a nanoliposomal encapsulation of irinotecan (nal-IRI), which has been reported to have improved pharmacokinetics and tumor biodistribution compared with the parent compound. This drug has been investigated as a single agent in 40 patients with gemcitabine-refractory pancreatic cancer and yielded a RR of 7.5% and median OS of 5.2 months.[356] Subsequently, Napoli-1, a three-armed randomized study comparing nal-IRI alone with nal-IRI plus 5-FU/leucovorin or 5-FU/leucovorin alone, has generated some preliminary results. Nal-IRI plus 5-FU/leucovorin was superior to 5-FU/leucovorin alone in gemcitabine-refractory advanced pancreatic cancer patients (median survival 6.1 months vs 4.2 months, $p = 0.012$).[357] Final results are awaited.

Ruxolitinib

The Janus kinase/signal transducer and transcriptional activator (JAK/Stat)-3 pathway has been reported to be constitutively activated in pancreatic cancer, with inhibition of this pathway abrogating growth of tumor cells *in vitro*.[358] Ruxolitinib is a JAK2 inhibitor recently approved for the treatment of myelofibrosis and other myeloproliferative disorders.[359] This agent has been studied in a group of patients with gemcitabine-refractory pancreatic cancer in a placebo-controlled trial assigning patients to ruxolitinib plus capecitabine or placebo/capecitabine.[360] In a prespecified analysis of enrolled patients with C reactive protein (CRP) levels >13, ruxolitinib/capecitabine prolonged PFS and OS compared with placebo/capecitabine. A larger phase 3 trial of ruxolitinib or placebo with capecitabine is now underway and enrolling patients with CRP levels >10 (www.clinicaltrials.gov).

PARP inhibitors

As discussed previously, a small subset of patients with PDAC harbor germ line mutations of *BRCA1*, *BRCA2*, or *PALB2*. A larger proportion may have somatic mutations of *BRCA1* or *BRCA2* in their tumor cells.[347] These pancreatic tumors are theoretically more susceptible to the effects of PARP inhibition, resulting in synthetic lethality.[361] Investigations of several PARP inhibitors to include olaparib, veliparib, rucaparib, and BMN-673 are now underway in patients with PDAC.[362]

Drugs to modulate the tumor microenvironment

Hyaluronidase

Hyaluronic acid is an important component of the extracellular matrix in which PDAC thrives.[363] Variants of CD44, a transmembrane glycoprotein expressed on the surface of tumor cells, are capable of binding hyaluronic acid, leading to enhanced proliferation and invasion. On the basis of more recent studies, there has been renewed interest in degradation of hyaluronic acid as a means to modulate the tumor stroma and enhance the delivery of cytotoxic chemotherapy.[135,364,365] Early phase clinical investigation of PEGPH20 (PEGylated recombinant human hyaluronidase) has shown promise when combined with single agent gemcitabine.[366] Therefore, a multicenter study is now investigating the addition of hyaluronidase to conventional cytotoxic therapy in an effort to improve the cytotoxic effect of chemotherapy. This trial is currently enrolling patients with previously untreated metastatic disease with the results anticipated in the next 1–2 years (www.clinicaltrials.gov).

Drugs designed to modulate the cellular constituents of PDAC microenvironment

In addition to efforts aimed at manipulating the extracellular matrix of pancreatic cancer, there are now agents becoming available that may modulate the cellular component of PDAC's microenvironment. These include CD40 agonists, which have the capability to release bone marrow-derived elements from primary pancreatic adenocarcinoma tumors based on murine models and clinical investigation.[367] One of these agents, CP-870,893, a monoclonal antibody, is entering clinical investigation and the delivery of such an agent in combination with chemotherapy appears to be safe.[368] However, a clear efficacy signal to suggest augmentation of the cytotoxic effects of chemotherapy or radiation has yet to be established.

Another interesting compound is PF-04136309, a chemokine receptor type 2 (CCR2) antagonist. Activation of CCR2 mobilizes monocytes and macrophages from the bone marrow to infiltrate malignant tumors. These inflammatory monocytes appear to have tumor-promoting properties. Preclinical models have demonstrated that the delivery of PF-04136309 decreases circulating monocytes and reduces the monocytic infiltration of pancreatic adenocarcinomas grown in mice.[369] Furthermore, inhibition of CCR2 resulted in enhanced antitumor immunity, decreased tumor growth, and reduced metastasis. There has been some early clinical investigation of this compound in conjunction with FOLFIRINOX. The drug appears to be safe when delivered in combination with FOLFIRINOX, with early results suggesting improved anticancer effect.[370]

Another approach to modulate PDAC stroma has been proposed by investigators at the Salk Institute. They showed that vitamin D receptor (VDR) is expressed in malignant pancreatic stroma and is associated with markers of inflammation and fibrosis. Treatment with a ligand to the VDR led to transcriptional changes, stromal remodeling, and decreases in markers of inflammation and fibrosis. When calcipotriol (a vitamin D analog) was delivered in conjunction with gemcitabine, they observed increased in intratumoral gemcitabine levels and improved survival in a murine model of pancreatic cancer.[187] Clinical investigation is now adding paricalcitol (a commercially available VDR agonist) to chemotherapy in a neoadjuvant trial (www.ctrc.net/documents/pdf/VonHoff_2015.pdf).

Augmentation of immune response to pancreatic cancer

The entire discipline of immunotherapy in cancer is rapidly changing. Efforts have included the development of more sophisticated and specific vaccination strategies, the delivery of checkpoint inhibitors, the isolation and expansion of T cell subsets from patients for reinfusion, and the molecular manipulation of T cells to enhance cancer cell recognition and immune destruction. Detailed description of such efforts can be found elsewhere in the textbook. Nevertheless, some specific examples of novel immunologic approaches are described in the following sections.

Vaccine therapy

Efforts to enhance the immunologic response to pancreatic cancer using vaccine strategies have been going on for years. The group at JHH has continuously worked to explore the benefit of injecting GM-CSF-secreting allogeneic pancreatic tumor cells (now named GVAX) into patients with pancreatic cancer.[371] Early trials administering GVAX to patients with pancreatic cancer demonstrated the development of specific immune responses and suggested clinically relevant activity.[372] Most recently, in an effort to improve the efficacy of GVAX, a combination of low-dose cyclophosphamide (used to inhibit regulatory T cells) with GVAX and CRS 207 (live-attenuated Listeria monocytogenes-expressing mesothelin) was compared with treatment using low-dose cyclophosphamide (Cy) and GVAX alone in a 2 : 1 randomized phase 2 trial.[373] The trial enrolled 90 patients with metastatic pancreatic cancer (97% previously treated). Patients who received Cy, GVAX, and CRS 207 had longer PFS and OS compared with patients who received only Cy and GVAX. OS was 6.1 months in the Cy/GVAX/CRS 207 arm versus 3.9 months in the Cy/GVAX arm (hazard ratio 0.59; $p = 0.02$). Of further note, in a prespecified per-protocol analysis of patients who received at least three doses (two doses of Cy/GVAX plus one of CRS-207 or three of Cy/GVAX), OS was 9.7 versus 4.6 months in favor of those who received CRS 207. These results are provocative and provide the first strong evidence of a clinical benefit to immune therapy in advanced pancreatic cancer.

Check point inhibition

With the development of checkpoint inhibitors, to include ipilimumab and nivolumab,[188] there has been great interest in the potential for immunotherapy to dramatically augment the current armamentarium of systemic agents used in pancreatic cancer. Unfortunately, early trials of ipilimumab as a single agent in advanced pancreatic cancer have been disappointing.[189] Other checkpoint inhibitors are now being investigated to include nivolumab and MEDI-4736, an anti-PD1 monoclonal antibody.[374] These agents are unlikely to be sufficiently active as single agents to alter the course of pancreatic cancer for most patients, and it can be expected that their future investigation in PDAC will likely involve the delivery of vaccines, cytotoxic drugs, radiotherapy, other molecular agents, or modulated T cells.[375]

Another potentially important target in PDAC is CD47, a cell surface protein expressed by cancer cells. CD47 acts signals macrophages and cytotoxic T cells as a "don't eat me" command. Investigators have synthesized anti-CD47 monoclonal antibodies that can prevent the inhibitory signal of CD47 and promote phagocytosis and subsequent priming of T cells to both recognize and kill cancer cells *in vitro* and in *in vivo* models.[376]

T cells directed against PDAC

A number of groups are intensively working to both decrease the inhibitory signals of regulatory T cells and to amplify the very potent cytotoxic capabilities of tumor-infiltrating lymphocytes (TILs). Much work needs to be done in the fundamental biology and immunology of pancreatic adenocarcinoma, but preclinical and clinical studies are suggesting that these approaches will have the potential to modulate the tumor microenvironment and add to our weaponry in pancreatic cancer.[377]

Discipline, discipline, discipline

Since clinical trials in the treatment of pancreatic cancer began about 50 years ago, some hard lessons have been learned as to the need for greater discipline in clinical trial design and clinical practice for patients with PDAC.

First, as recognized from prior trials in pancreatic cancer, criteria for trial enrollment should include careful assessment of PS, limiting enrollment of patients to those having KPS of at least 70% or ECOG PS > 2. Second, we must use more stringent criteria for protocol entry to segregate patients with distinct clinical stages of PDAC: resectable, borderline resectable, locally advanced, and metastatic disease. Failure to do so hampers rapid-learning and progress in any given disease stage.

Third, we need to be more rigorous in assessing the validity of preclinical models to predict clinical benefit of any given drug or drug combination. Lastly, translational research using innovative imaging, blood-, or tissue-based analyses should be incorporated into virtually every early phase trial seeking to demonstrate tumor cell killing, stromal modification, or other biologic changes deemed relevant for clinical benefit. If we merge our understanding of the fundamental tumor biology with a disciplined approach to preclinical and clinical testing of novel agents and approaches, we are certain to make more significant progress for our pancreatic patients in the near future.

Key references

The complete reference list can be found on the Wiley Companion Digital Edition of this title (see inside front cover for login instructions).

1 Siegel R, Ma J, Zou Z, Jemal A. Cancer statistics, 2014. *CA Cancer J Clin*. 2014;**64**:9–29.

7 Klein AP. Genetic susceptibility to pancreatic cancer. *Mol Carcinog*. 2012;**51**:14–24.

12 Klein AP, Hruban RH, Brune KA, Petersen GM, Goggins M. Familial pancreatic cancer. *Cancer J*. 2001;**7**:266–273.

31 Li D, Duell EJ, Yu K, et al. Pathway analysis of genome-wide association study data highlights pancreatic development genes as susceptibility factors for pancreatic cancer. *Carcinogenesis*. 2012;**33**:1384–1390.

41 Bosetti C, Lucenteforte E, Silverman DT, et al. Cigarette smoking and pancreatic cancer: an analysis from the International Pancreatic Cancer Case–control Consortium (Panc4). *Ann Oncol*. 2012;**23**:1880–1888.

68 Elena JW, Steplowski E, Yu K, et al. Diabetes and risk of pancreatic cancer: a pooled analysis from the pancreatic cancer cohort consortium. *Cancer Causes Control*. 2013;**24**:13–25.

89 Li D. Metformin as an antitumor agent in cancer prevention and treatment. *J Diabetes*. 2011;**3**:320–327.

126 Brand RE, Lerch MM, Rubinstein WS, et al. Advances in counselling and surveillance of patients at risk for pancreatic cancer. *Gut*. 2007;**56**:1460–1469.

134 Feig C, Gopinathan A, Neesse A, Chan DS, Cook N, Tuveson DA. The pancreas cancer microenvironment. *Clin Cancer Res.* 2012;**18**:4266–4276.

147 Jones S, Zhang X, Parsons DW, et al. Core signaling pathways in human pancreatic cancers revealed by global genomic analyses. *Science.* 2008;**321**:1801–1806.

159 Collisson EA, Trejo CL, Silva JM, et al. A central role for RAF—>MEK—>ERK signaling in the genesis of pancreatic ductal adenocarcinoma. *Cancer Discov.* 2012;**2**:685–693.

164 Maitra A, Hruban RH. Pancreatic cancer. *Annu Rev Pathol.* 2008;**3**:157–188.

176 Bettegowda C, Sausen M, Leary RJ, et al. Detection of circulating tumor DNA in early- and late-stage human malignancies. *Sci Transl Med.* 2014;**6**:224ra224.

183 Olive KP, Jacobetz MA, Davidson CJ, et al. Inhibition of Hedgehog signaling enhances delivery of chemotherapy in a mouse model of pancreatic cancer. *Science.* 2009;**324**:1457–1461.

184 Ozdemir BC, Pentcheva-Hoang T, Carstens JL, et al. Depletion of carcinoma-associated fibroblasts and fibrosis induces immunosuppression and accelerates pancreas cancer with reduced survival. *Cancer Cell.* 2014;**25**:719–734.

191 Vonderheide RH, Bayne LJ. Inflammatory networks and immune surveillance of pancreatic carcinoma. *Curr Opin Immunol.* 2013;**25**:200–205.

195 Beatty GL. Engineered chimeric antigen receptor-expressing T cells for the treatment of pancreatic ductal adenocarcinoma. *Oncoimmunology.* 2014;**3**:e28327.

197 Le A, Rajeshkumar NV, Maitra A, Dang CV. Conceptual framework for cutting the pancreatic cancer fuel supply. *Clin Cancer Res.* 2012;**18**:4285–4290.

202 Tamm EP, Balachandran A, Bhosale P, Szklaruk J. Update on 3D and multiplanar MDCT in the assessment of biliary and pancreatic pathology. *Abdom Imaging.* 2009;**34**:64–74.

217 Howard TJ, Krug JE, Yu J, et al. A margin-negative R0 resection accomplished with minimal postoperative complications is the surgeon's contribution to long-term survival in pancreatic cancer. *J Gastrointest Surg.* 2006;**10**:1338–1345.

225 Evans DB, Lee JE, Tamm EP, Pisters PWT. Pancreaticoduodenectomy (Whipple Operation) and total pancreatectomy for cancer. In: Fisher JF, ed. *Mastery of Surgery*, 5th ed. Philadelphia: Lippincott, Williams and Williams; 2007:1299–1317.

227 Verbeke CS. Resection margins and R1 rates in pancreatic cancer – are we there yet? *Histopathology.* 2008;**52**:787–796.

228 Christians KK, Pilgrim CH, Tsai S, et al. Arterial resection at the time of pancreatectomy for cancer. *Surgery.* 2014;**155**:919–926.

233 Tran Cao HS, Lopez N, Chang DC, et al. Improved perioperative outcomes with minimally invasive distal pancreatectomy: results from a population-based analysis. *JAMA Surg.* 2014;**149**:237–243.

244 Valle JW, Palmer D, Jackson R, et al. Optimal duration and timing of adjuvant chemotherapy after definitive surgery for ductal adenocarcinoma of the pancreas: ongoing lessons from the ESPAC-3 study. *J Clin Oncol.* 2014;**32**:504–512.

248 Katz MH, Wang H, Fleming JB, et al. Long-term survival after multidisciplinary management of resected pancreatic adenocarcinoma. *Ann Surg Oncol.* 2009;**16**:836–847.

253 Oettle H, Post S, Neuhaus P, et al. Adjuvant chemotherapy with gemcitabine vs observation in patients undergoing curative-intent resection of pancreatic cancer: a randomized controlled trial. *JAMA.* 2007;**297**:267–277.

254 Neoptolemos JP, Stocken DD, Bassi C, et al. Adjuvant chemotherapy with fluorouracil plus folinic acid vs gemcitabine following pancreatic cancer resection: a randomized controlled trial. *JAMA.* 2010;**304**:1073–1081.

268 Evans DB, Varadhachary GR, Crane CH, et al. Preoperative gemcitabine-based chemoradiation for patients with resectable adenocarcinoma of the pancreatic head. *J Clin Oncol.* 2008;**26**:3496–3502.

274 Varadhachary GR, Tamm EP, Abbruzzese JL, et al. Borderline resectable pancreatic cancer: definitions, management, and role of preoperative therapy. *Ann Surg Oncol.* 2006;**13**:1035–1046.

277 Katz MH, Pisters PW, Evans DB, et al. Borderline resectable pancreatic cancer: the importance of this emerging stage of disease. *J Am Coll Surg.* 2008;**206**:833–846.

291 Hammel P, Huguet F, van Laethem JL, et al. Comparison of chemoradiotherapy and chemotherapy in patients with a locally advanced pancreatic cancer controlled after 4 months of gemcitabine with or without erlotinib: final results of the international phase III LAP 07 study. *J Clin Oncol.* 2013;**31** (suppl):Late Breaking Abstract 4003.

309 Koong AC, Christofferson E, Le QT, et al. Phase II study to assess the efficacy of conventionally fractionated radiotherapy followed by a stereotactic radiosurgery boost in patients with locally advanced pancreatic cancer. *Int J Radiat Oncol Biol Phys.* 2005;**63**:320–323.

313 Martin RC 2nd, McFarland K, Ellis S, Velanovich V. Irreversible electroporation therapy in the management of locally advanced pancreatic adenocarcinoma. *J Am Coll Surg.* 2012;**215**:361–369.

318 Conroy T, Desseigne F, Ychou M, et al. FOLFIRINOX versus gemcitabine for metastatic pancreatic cancer. *N Engl J Med.* 2011;**364**:1817–1825.

319 Von Hoff DD, Ervin T, Arena FP, et al. Increased survival in pancreatic cancer with nab-paclitaxel plus gemcitabine. *N Engl J Med.* 2013;**369**:1691–1703.

334 Tabernero J, Chiorean EG, Infante JR, et al. Prognostic factors of survival in a randomized phase III trial (MPACT) of weekly nab-paclitaxel plus gemcitabine versus gemcitabine alone in patients with metastatic pancreatic cancer. *Oncologist.* 2015;**20**:143–150.

361 Ashworth A. A synthetic lethal therapeutic approach: poly(ADP) ribose polymerase inhibitors for the treatment of cancers deficient in DNA double-strand break repair. *J Clin Oncol.* 2008;**26**:3785–3790.

364 Jacobetz MA, Chan DS, Neesse A, et al. Hyaluronan impairs vascular function and drug delivery in a mouse model of pancreatic cancer. *Gut.* 2013;**62**:112–120.

373 Le DT, Wang-Gillam A, Picozzi V, et al. Safety and survival with GVAX pancreas prime and Listeria Monocytogenes-expressing mesothelin (CRS-207) boost vaccines for metastatic pancreatic cancer. *J Clin Oncol.* 2015;**33**(12):1325–1333.

94
Neoplasms of the small intestine, vermiform appendix, and peritoneum and carcinoma of the colon and rectum

Georgia M. Beasley, MD ▪ Zhifei Sun, MD ▪ Daniel P. Nussbaum, MD ▪ Douglas S. Tyler, MD

Overview

Cancers of the small bowel, large bowel, and appendix compromise a multitude of distinct pathologic entities and clinical presentations. While tumors of the small bowel are uncommon with <3% of all alimentary tract tumors and 0.4% of all malignancies arise in the small bowel, colon cancer is the third most common malignant tumor and the fourth most common cause of cancer death worldwide. Although adenocarcinoma remains the common pathology, many advances have been made regarding our diagnoses and management of carcinoid tumors and even to a larger degree in gastrointestinal stromal tumors. Additional advances include our understanding of genetics, new imaging modalities, and minimally invasive surgeries. This chapter will provide a comprehensive review of the management and treatment of cancers of the small bowel, large bowel, and appendix.

Tumors of the small intestine

The estimated number of new small bowel malignancies in the United States was 9160 in 2014. The small intestine represents 75% of the total length of the gastrointestinal (GI) tract and comprises 90% of its mucosal surface area, yet rarely does this region develop malignant tumors.[1] Recent figures show that <3% of all alimentary tract tumors and 0.4% of all malignancies arise in the small bowel.[2]

Several mechanisms have been postulated to explain the low incidence of neoplastic transformation within the small intestine. The most important of these are the rapid transit of content through the small bowel, which provides a shorter exposure of its mucosa to carcinogens, increased lymphoid tissue in the small intestine with a high level of immunoglobulin A (IgA) expression, and a lower bacterial load in the small bowel that results in a decreased conversion of bile acids into potential carcinogens by anaerobic microorganisms.[3,4] In addition, the liquid contents of the small bowel may cause less mucosal irritation than the more solid contents of the large intestine, and there is the presence in the small intestine of mucosal detoxifying enzymes such as benzopyrene hydroxylase.[5]

Adenocarcinomas comprise 30% to 50% of small bowel malignant tumors, followed by carcinoids (25–30%), lymphomas (15–20%), and, to a lesser extent, sarcomas. Leiomyomas account for 25% of all benign tumors, while others include adenomas and lipomas and rarer neoplasms such as fibromas, fibromyxomas, neurofibromas, ganglioneuromas, hemangiomas, and lymphangiomas.[6]

Clinical presentation

Because the small intestine is relatively inaccessible to routine endoscopy, diagnosis of small intestinal neoplasms is often delayed for months after onset of symptoms. Many small bowel tumors are asymptomatic until late in their course because of their relatively slow growth and the ease with which the liquid contents of the small bowel can pass even a partially obstructing lesion.[6] The remainder are usually found as a result of the symptoms of partial obstruction: nausea and vomiting if the lesion is proximal, as well as crampy abdominal pain, or other nonspecific findings such as weight loss. Hemorrhage is frequently found in those tumors that penetrate beyond the submucosa, but almost always is occult, presenting as microcytic anemia or stool that is positive on guaiac testing. Certain small bowel tumors have more specific presenting symptoms, such as jaundice (ampullary carcinoma) and fever, diarrhea, and weight loss (lymphoma). Endocrine tumors of the gut, the most common of which are carcinoid tumors, may present with their own set of classic symptoms, such as flushing, diarrhea, cyanosis, and intermittent respiratory distress. Only a small proportion of patients with carcinoid tumors have these symptoms, the vast majority being asymptomatic or having symptoms secondary to mass lesion effects.

Eventually, malignant tumors cause enough symptoms for the ensuing medical work-up to reveal the tumor. Unfortunately, some time may pass between the first symptom and diagnosis. In one series, almost one-third of the patients had symptoms for 5 years or more prior to definitive diagnosis.[7] Another study demonstrated a mean duration of symptoms of 7 months prior to diagnosis.[8] Many patients eventually diagnosed with small bowel tumors present as an emergency with either bowel obstruction or perforation.

Diagnostic imaging

Radiographic studies often aid in the diagnosis of these lesions, especially in advanced disease. However, such studies, on many occasions, are not useful for early diagnosis of curable malignancy. Small bowel radiology has undergone dramatic changes in the past 2 decades. Plain films, the small bowel follow-through, and double-contrast modality of enteroclysis may be useful in certain situations but have largely been replaced by cross-sectional imaging techniques (computed tomography (CT) and magnetic resonance imaging (MRI)), which can be used to investigate both extraluminal abnormalities and intraluminal changes. CT scanning with oral contrast has led to nearly 100% recognition of small bowel tumors in some series, although it has limited ability to differentiate among tumor types.[9] This modality appears to be most useful for preoperative staging and metastatic evaluation.[10] In one series, the sensitivity for CT in determining T (tumor) stage was 57%, compared with

Holland-Frei Cancer Medicine, Ninth Edition. Edited by Robert C. Bast Jr., Carlo M. Croce, William N. Hait, Waun Ki Hong, Donald W. Kufe, Martine Piccart-Gebhart, Raphael E. Pollock, Ralph R. Weichselbaum, Hongyang Wang, and James F. Holland.
© 2017 John Wiley & Sons, Inc. ISBN: 978-1-118-93469-2

61% and 42% for colon and gastric cancers, respectively.[11,12] MRI techniques clearly highlight endoluminal, mural, and extramural enteric details and provide vascular and functional information, thereby enhancing the diagnostic value of these techniques in small bowel diseases. MRI offers detailed morphologic information and functional data of small bowel diseases and provides reliable evidence of normalcy, thereby allowing the diagnosis of early or subtle structural abnormalities and guiding treatment and decisions in patient care. MRI has many properties that make it ideal for imaging of the small bowel: the ability to perform real-time imaging, functional imaging, the lack of ionizing radiation, and the improved tissue contrast that can be achieved by using a variety of pulse sequences.[13–15] Magnetic resonance (MR) enteroclysis has yielded a 96.6% accuracy in the detection of small bowel neoplasms.[16,17] In addition to CT and MR, angiography and nuclear scanning may be useful in the case of a bleeding tumor or a suspected hemangioma. Endoscopic ultrasonography (EUS) is used to detect and stage small bowel tumors and allows real-time interventional diagnostic procedures, mainly in the periampullary region. EUS has been shown to be superior to CT and MRI in predicting vascular invasion and overall assessment of T stage of ampullary neoplasms.[18,19] In the past decade, small bowel endoscopy has become increasingly useful as a diagnostic tool. There are three main types of small bowel endoscopy: push enteroscopy, intraoperative or laparoscopically assisted enteroscopy, and, most recently, double-balloon enteroscopy. Push enteroscopy involves an intestinal intubation of a 220- to 250-cm instrument, usually with fluoroscopic assistance, and can be used to examine the jejunum for mean lengths of 120 cm beyond the ligament of Treitz.[20] During intraoperative endoscopy, the surgeon manually manipulates through the small bowel wall with either a push endoscope (anterograde) or a colonoscope (retrograde) to examine the entire small bowel. The surgeon can mark the lesions of interest, usually by suture, and resect at the completion of the enteroscopy. These techniques are particularly useful in prophylactic polypectomy of small bowel large polyps (>15 mm) for conservative approach in management of PJS patients.[21] The recent addition of laparoscopically assisted enteroscopy provides a less invasive technique than interoperative enteroscopy but still requires general anesthesia and both a surgeon and endoscopist.[22] In double-balloon enteroscopy, an endoscope and a soft flexible overtube, each of which has an inflatable balloon attached to its distal end, are employed together. The two tubes are advanced over one another repeatedly using alternating inflation of the balloons to hold position, allowing deep advancement into the small intestine. The entire small intestine can be examined using this method with less discomfort than experienced with the push method.[23] After receiving the Federal Drug Administration (FDA) approval in 2001, a small, swallowable imaging capsule was introduced by Swain and colleagues that is propelled by peristalsis through the intestinal tract and transmits data to a receiver that captures video images.[24] However, the use of capsule endoscopy to evaluate small bowel tumors, particularly submucosal forms, has several limitations.[25,26] Indeed, capsule endoscopy may fail to depict neoplastic disease in as many as 18.9% of cases,[27] and capsule retention occurs in 10–25% of small bowel tumor cases.[27,28]

Treatment

The treatment of small bowel tumors is generally surgical, with simple resection for benign lesions and an aggressive approach for malignant lesions. Overall, the survival for adenocarcinomas, carcinoids, lymphomas, and sarcomas was better in 328 cases from a population-based registry than that for all other organs, except the breast, colon, prostate, and uterus.[29] In rare cases, radiation

or chemotherapy may precede surgery. Duodenal tumors may require pancreaticoduodenectomy if malignant, whereas tumors of the terminal ileum may require right hemicolectomy to ensure complete resection and adequate margins.

Malignant neoplasms of the small bowel

Adenocarcinomas

Adenocarcinomas are the most common malignant tumors in the small bowel, accounting for approximately 30–50% of all malignant small bowel tumors.[30,31] They most commonly arise in the seventh decade of life and are seen slightly more often in men than in women.[32] Cohort studies suggest that increased body mass index and alcohol use may increase risk of small bowel cancer.[33] While primary tumors arise most often in the duodenum (48–52%) and jejunum (23–25%) and less commonly in the ileum (13–16%), the reason for this distribution is unclear.[34,35] Some have postulated that the richness of IgA-secreting cells in the ileum accounts for its relative sparing from adenocarcinoma by neutralizing luminal carcinogens.[4] Others have noted that the abundance of the enzyme benzopyrene hydroxylase may play a protective role by detoxifying potential carcinogens.[36] Adenocarcinoma is staged using the American Joint Committee on Cancer (AJCC) TNM system, and as expected small bowel carcinomas that are well differentiated with only local invasion and no lymph node metastasis tend to have the best prognosis. Unfortunately, little progress has been made in the treatment of small bowel adenocarcinoma. There have been improvements in diagnostic modalities and insights into the molecular basis, but the prognosis is still generally poor.

The histogenesis of small bowel adenocarcinoma most likely follows the adenoma–carcinoma sequence described initially for large bowel cancer.[37] As a result, the single most important risk factor for small bowel adenocarcinoma is preexisting adenoma, either single or multiple, as associated with multiple polyposis syndromes.[38] Small bowel adenocarcinomas have also been associated with alcohol (but not tobacco), nontropical sprue, regional enteritis, celiac disease, and urinary diversion procedures such as ileal conduit.[39–43]

Familial adenomatous polyposis (FAP) is known to be a powerful risk factor for adenocarcinoma, with small bowel cancer being the most common cancer after colon cancer itself.[44] The relative risk (RR) of small bowel carcinoma in these patients has been described as being greater than 100.[45] Other hereditary syndromes associated with small bowel tumors include Peutz–Jeghers (PJ) syndrome (increased incidence of hamartomatous polyps in the jejunum and ileum), Gardner syndrome (adenoma and adenocarcinoma), and von Recklinghausen disease (paraganglioma). Small bowel inflammatory disorders are associated with increased malignancy, including, most notably, Crohn's disease.[46] Crohn's disease is a risk factor for future small bowel adenocarcinoma. An RR of 33 (95% CI: 15.9–60.9) was reported in a 2006 meta-analysis.[47] As with ulcerative colitis (UC) and tumors of the colon, the diagnosis of Crohn's disease precedes small bowel tumors by about 10 years. Several risk factors have been identified in patients with Crohn's disease who develop adenocarcinoma of the small bowel: duration of Crohn's disease, male gender, fistulization, presence of strictures, and surgical creation of blind excluded loops of intestines.[48,49] Other disorders associated with increased risk of malignancy are celiac disease (lymphoma and adenocarcinoma) and immunoproliferative disease (diffuse intestinal lymphoma and immunoproliferative small intestinal disease.[5]

Celiac sprue, while well known to predispose to intestinal lymphoma, is also associated with adenocarcinoma of the small bowel.[40]

The numbers cited in case reports are few, but the presence of disease in otherwise noncharacteristic locations seems to lend credence to the theory that gluten-mediated jejunoileitis is also an independent risk factor for the development of adenocarcinoma of the small bowel as well as lymphomas.[31] Adenocarcinoma of the small intestine, often aggressive, can affect children and is usually associated with degeneration of a PJ hamartoma.[38]

The genetic mechanisms involved in the carcinogenesis of the small bowel remain unknown, most likely because of the small number of cases. Blaker and colleagues from Germany showed that although small intestinal carcinomas reveal complex genetic changes, a significant number of tumors share karyotypic instability and losses of chromosome 18q21-q22. 18q deletions often target the SMAD4 gene and disrupt tumor suppression through TGFβ-signaling.[50] Svrcek and colleagues, using tissue microarray analysis, determined that inactivation of the SMAD4/DPC4 gene is involved in small intestinal adenocarcinoma tumorigenesis and that overexpression of TP53 and abnormal expression of β-catenin are two common events in small intestinal adenocarcinoma.[51] Other pathways include Notch3 signaling associated with MUC5AC expression.[52] There is also recent evidence suggesting DNA mismatch repair genes are involved; the frequency of the dMMR phenotype is variable, ranging from 5% to 35% of cases.[53]

Symptoms of adenocarcinoma of the small bowel range from obstructive symptoms, such as vomiting and jaundice for those with duodenal tumors, to indistinct abdominal pain, weight loss, and anemia for more distal lesions. Weight loss is also common, occurring in more than 50% of patients. Obstruction is found in 40% to 70% of patients prior to presentation. In the collected Mayo series, 71% of patients had either overt or clinical evidence of blood loss.[54] Adenocarcinomas, especially duodenal tumors, usually become symptomatic earlier than other small bowel tumors, allowing for earlier diagnosis and intervention. Despite this, 30–35% of small bowel adenocarcinomas are metastatic at the time of diagnosis.[34,35]

In a recent study conducted by the American College of Surgeons on 5000 small bowel adenocarcinomas, the overall 5-year disease-free survival (DFS) was 30.5%.[55] The median survival in this series was 19.7 months. The primary treatment of adenocarcinomas is wide surgical resection, with removal of lymph nodes and the vascular pedicle. Margins of 5 cm are considered acceptable. Recent reports indicate that even this treatment does not yield good survival rates for node-positive patients. In a recent study examining 217 patients with small bowel adenocarcinoma followed over a 10-year period at MD Anderson Cancer Center, patients with stage IV disease had a shorter 5-year overall survival (OS) than those with I–III disease (5% vs 36%).[35] The 5-year survival was significantly shorter if the positive lymph node ratio (number of positive lymph nodes/number of total lymph nodes) was greater than 75% versus <75% (12% vs 51%).

All attempts should be made to resect the primary lesion to prevent mucosal bleeding. For patients deemed unresectable at the time of laparotomy, some have advocated the use of intraoperative radiation therapy.[56–58] The lack of clinical trials makes this therapy difficult to recommend in a setting other than specialized centers. Data regarding the role of adjuvant chemotherapy are limited, with no evidence of significant benefit in survival in patients with adenocarcinoma of the small intestine treated with adjuvant chemotherapy. An attempted Cochrane review in 2007 failed to find any studies eligible for meta-analysis.[59] Despite this, adjuvant chemotherapy is frequently used because small bowel cancer tends to recur systemically, similar to CRC, and because colon cancers respond to adjuvant therapy. A 2009 retrospective multicenter study suggested that an adjuvant folinic acid, 5-FU, and oxaliplatin (FOLFOX) regimen prolonged OS by around 5 months compared to patients treated with other regimens, but the findings of this small study were not statistically significant.[53] For advanced unresectable disease, a recent phase II study of modified FOLFOX as first-line chemotherapy in advanced small bowel adenocarcinoma reported an objective response rate of 48.5% [95% confidence interval (95% CI): 31–67%], with one complete response in patients with advanced small bowel adenocarcinomas.[60]

Carcinoid tumors

Carcinoid tumors represent approximately 25–30% of malignant tumors of the small bowel.[58,61] Obendorfer used the term "karzinoide" in 1907, but the exact nature of the tumor was not determined until 1928 when Masson described its origin as the chromaffin cell.[62,63] The frequency of carcinoid in large autopsy series, before the era of increased detection by CT and endoscopy, indicated that about 85% were undiagnosed during life.[64] US data show that the incidence of GI carcinoid has increased at a rate of 3%–10% per year over the past three decades.[64,65] The most frequent sites for carcinoids were the GI tract (54.5%) and the bronchopulmonary system (30.1%). Within the GI tract, most occurred in the small bowel (44.7%), rectum (19.6%), and appendix (16.7%). In contradistinction to adenocarcinoma, the carcinoid tends to arise in the distal small intestine rather than in more proximal sites. In the series reported by Moertel, all surgically confirmed, 3% were in the duodenum, 5% in the jejunum, 32% in the proximal ileum, and 60% in the distal ileum.[66] The median age at discovery is 60.9 years, and females constitute 54.2% of patients.[67] The overall 5-year survival rate for patients with GI carcinoid is about 58%, with little change over the past 30 years.[64] However, in the subgroup of patients with well-differentiated carcinoid with distant spread, the 5-year survival rate has improved from 15% to 52% over this time period.[64]

The most useful marker of neuroendocrine cells in tissue sections is chromogranin A (CgA), a glycoprotein stored in secretory granules of neuroendocrine cells. Plasma CgA levels correlate with tumor burden and may be useful for monitoring treatment.[68] Twenty-four-hour measurement of urinary 5-hydroxyindole-3-acetic acid (5-HIAA), the degradation product of serotonin, can also aid in diagnosis. The specificity of 5-HIAA as a marker for these carcinoids is 88%, although tryptophan/serotonin-rich foods (bananas, avocados, plums, eggplants, tomatoes, plantains, pineapples, and walnuts) can provide false elevations, and several drugs can result in increased or decreased 5-HIAA levels.[69] Higher concentrations of 5-HIAA in urine are consistent with a worse prognosis, while persistently low levels predict a more favorable outcome in disseminated disease.[68] Mitotic count and Ki-67 index [a marker of cell proliferation] provide some indication of prognosis.[68]

A unique feature of carcinoid tumors is their ability to produce a variety of protein and peptide products, the most characteristic of which is serotonin. Systemic serotonin is thought to cause most of the symptoms of the carcinoid syndrome, including diarrhea, flushing, wheezing, and right-sided heart disease. Carcinoid syndrome is seen in 5–7% of patients with large tumor burdens and metastatic disease.[54] It is believed that the metastatic component is necessary to ensure drainage of the compounds involved in the syndrome into the systemic circulation and to provide an adequate tumor mass to produce large amounts of peptidergic products.

The clinical manifestations of carcinoid are often vague or absent, and the definitive diagnosis is often not made prior to surgery. Patients with small intestine carcinoid often present at a late stage, and the prognosis is poor once tumors have spread beyond the intestine. In a series of 145 patients with GI carcinoid tumors, only 12 had a proper diagnosis before surgery, and those 12 had definite symptoms of carcinoid syndrome.[54,70] Most often, patients are operated on for signs of bowel obstruction, not by the tumor itself but by a desmoplastic reaction that leads to shrinking of the mesentery as a result of fibrosis and kinking of the bowel.[71] Scintigraphy with radiolabeled octreotide has been successfully used to localize undetected primary and metastatic lesions.[72] Two large European studies show carcinoid lesion detection with a sensitivity of 89% by using this diagnostic tool.[73]

The metastatic potential of a carcinoid tumor correlates closely with its size. In the Moertel series, there were no metastases in tumors <0.5 cm in diameter, 15% in tumors 0.5 to 0.9 cm in diameter, 72% in tumors 1.0 to 1.9 cm in diameter, and 95% metastases in tumors larger than 2 cm.[66] However, small bowel carcinoids may still metastasize when <1 cm. Recent evidence based on 5-HIAA levels suggests that most cases of metastatic carcinoid of unknown primary probably arise from small ileal tumors.[74,75] Extent of disease, which mainly comprises either lymph node (regional) or liver (metastatic) involvement, is a definite predictor of outcome. In Maggard's analysis of 11,427 carcinoids, 5-year survival for localized, regional, and distant disease of the small intestine was 70.4%, 64.1%, and 32.4%, respectively.[65]

Primary surgical resection of the tumor and regional lymph nodes is the only curative treatment for GI NETs; this is usually possible in about 20% of patients. Surgery remains the only approach that allows definitive histopathologic staging, resection of occult lymph node metastasis, and prevention of local complications caused by a desmoplastic resection.[76] Referral for surgical management should not be influenced by the inability to localize the primary tumor. As midgut tumors are difficult to localize on imaging, one study found the primary tumor could be identified intraoperatively in a majority of patients with metastatic NETs, irrespective of preoperative localization status.[77] Careful intraoperative examination is mandatory, because most series report that 30% of these tumors are multicentric.[66] Primary duodenal carcinoids account for only 2.6% of carcinoid tumors in the United States; although they are increasingly recognized with the more widespread use of upper GI endoscopy.[78] Because of the rarity of this disease, management recommendations for duodenal carcinoids have been extrapolated from the experience with midgut and hindgut carcinoids. A recent study by Mullen and colleagues however demonstrated successful margin negative endoscopic resection in six patients with tumors <1.5 cm.[78] Interestingly, this study found lymph node metastases to be present in 54% of patients with duodenal carcinoid, including two patients with tumors smaller than 1 cm and limited to the submucosa. The impact of lymph node metastasis in duodenal carcinoids is uncertain, however, in that no patient developed distant metastases or carcinoid syndrome in this series. In the case of advanced disease, there may be some benefit to debulking procedures, but this remains controversial, because the absolute size of the tumor does not correspond well with the degree of symptoms.[54,79,80] Some authors recommend aggressive treatment even in patients with widely metastatic disease, including resection of all intra-abdominal tumor deposits, segmental liver resection as needed, and hepatic arterial embolization. Cholecystectomy also has been performed to prevent gallbladder necrosis during hepatic embolization. Although it has not been proven whether this aggressive surgical approach increases survival, it has yielded biochemical remission in up to 25% of patients and regression of hepatic metastases for long periods.[69,81] In the MD Anderson experience of 81 patients with carcinoid disease metastatic to the liver who underwent hepatic artery embolization or chemoembolization,

67% experienced a partial response with a mean duration of response of 17 months. Overall, 63% of patients had reduction in their tumor-related symptoms and the OS time was 31 months.[82] Importantly, many patients diagnosed with carcinoid have other malignancies. Using the surveillance, epidemiology, and end results (SEER) database to identify patients diagnosed with small intestine carcinoids between 1973 and 2007, almost one-third of patients with small bowel carcinoid had an associated metachronous primary tumor. The most common sites were prostate (26.2%), breast (14.3%), colon (9.1%), lung/bronchus (6.3%), and bladder (5.3%).[83]

Medical therapy in the form of somatostatin analogues is effective in relieving symptoms of the carcinoid syndrome, though demonstrated tumor regression is rare. Octreotide is an eight amino acid, long-acting somatostatin analogue that binds to receptor subtypes 2, 3, and 5 and has been widely used for both detection and treatment of carcinoid tumors.[84] The currently available SSAs—Sandostatin LAR (octreotide; Novartis) and Somatuline Autogel (lanreotide; Ipsen)—display high-affinity binding for receptor subtypes 2 and 5, low affinity for subtypes 1 and 4, and medium affinity for subtype 3. SOM230 (pasireotide; Novartis), a more recently developed SSA, now in phase III trials, has a wider range of activity against somatostatin receptors and may offer a therapeutic advantage, especially in resistant disease.[85] In one study, octreotide was delivered subcutaneously at a dosage of 150 µg three times a day, showing improved symptoms in 88% of patients and decreased urinary 5-HIAA in 72% of patients.[86] Advances in the understanding of the mechanisms underlying tumor progression have led to the identification of several potential therapeutic targets (including the vascular endothelial growth factor (VEGF) and mammalian target of rapamycin (mTOR) signaling pathways). In a randomized phase 3 trial of everolimus plus octreotide LAR compared with placebo plus octreotide LAR improved progression-free survival in patients with advanced neuroendocrine tumors. However, progression-free survival was still poor at 16.4 (95% CI 13.7–21.2) months in the everolimus plus octreotide LAR group and 11.3 (8.4–14.6) months in the placebo plus octreotide LAR group.[87] Several other agents are being studied, including the use of novel SSTa, VEGF and mTOR inhibitors, and agents that interfere with insulin growth factor 1 receptor and AKT signaling. Another treatment modality is peptide receptor radionuclide therapy. Peptide receptor radionuclide therapy delivers tumoricidal doses of radiation to carcinoid cells highly selectively, with few adverse effects (nausea and occasional bone marrow and renal toxicity). By linking a radioactive isotope (111Indium, 90Yttrium, or 177Lutetium) to a somatostatin analogue, carcinoid cells, with their often high density of somatostatin receptors, may be specifically targeted. Tumor regression rates of up to 50%, with a disease-free response approaching 3 years, have been reported in some studies.[88]

Prognosis of patients with carcinoid disease varies according to several factors. Size of the primary tumor is an important predictor of metastasis and survival. Carcinoid tumors >2 cm in diameter portend a worse prognosis than those <2 cm.[89] In a recent series of 603 patients, lymph node metastasis was also not surprisingly prognostic.[90] In the Maggard series, increased tumor size was associated with a greater likelihood of lymph node involvement.[67] In the carcinoid series at Duke University, a direct correlation was found between size of the primary tumor and extent of disease at presentation.[91] In addition, after controlling for stage of disease, region of origin of primary tumor predicted prognosis in this series of patients. In patients with distant metastases at presentation, those with midgut tumors had markedly better prognosis than did patients with foregut or hindgut tumors. In addition to traditional pathologic determinants, expression of cocaine- and amphetamine-regulated transcript (CART) in small bowel carcinoid tumors is associated with worse survival.[92]

Composite tumors, those that display characteristics of both carcinoid tumors and adenocarcinomas, are well described in the appendix but are less well known in the small intestine. These tumors are relatively rare, with most reports to date encompassing only one or two cases. They are aggressive tumors with a metastatic potential similar to that of adenocarcinoma and should be treated as adenocarcinomas. Lymphatic metastasis appeared histologically to be adenocarcinoma in two cases and carcinoid in one; thus, it seems that these tumors may arise from cells with pluripotential patterns of differentiation.[93]

Gastrointestinal stromal tumors

Gastrointestinal stromal tumor (GIST) is the current nomenclature for a diverse group of benign or malignant GI neoplasms derived from embryonic mesoderm. There are three histologic subtypes of GIST. The spindle cell form is the most common (70%) and consists of uniform, intersecting fascicles with eosinophilic cytoplasm. The epithelioid (20%) and the rare mixed type (10%) forms show more rounded cells with nuclear atypia.[94] Malignant GISTs constitute 15–20% of the malignant tumors found in the small bowel.[95] The annual incidence in the United States is reported to be approximately 5000 cases per year which seems to be rising due to increased awareness and histopathologic diagnosis.[96,97] GISTs affect men and women equally.[98] Most patients diagnosed with GIST are between 40–80 years old with a median age at diagnosis of 60.[99] The most commonly encountered GIST is the sporadic form. Familial GISTs occur and result from a germline mutation in either the KIT or platelet-derived growth factor receptor alpha (PDGFRα) proto-oncogenes.[100,101] The cellular origin of GIST is proposed to be the interstitial cell of Cajal, an intestinal pacemaker cell.[95] GISTs are characterized by mutations in the proto-oncogene C-kit that lead to constitutive activation of its glycoprotein product KIT and the subsequent tyrosine kinase activity.[102] The tyrosine kinase inhibitor, imatinib, has revolutionized the treatment of GIST tumors. More than 95% of GISTs express KIT and biochemical evidence of KIT can be found in almost all GISTs.[103] The most common sites of KIT mutation include exon 11 (70%) and exon 9 (10%) although other regions have been described.[104,105] Other commonly expressed markers include CD34 (70%), smooth muscle actin (30%), and desmin (<5%).[106] Because other malignancies can stain positive for KIT include metastatic melanoma, angiosarcoma, and Ewing's sarcoma, IHC alone is not sufficient for diagnosis.[94] The diagnosis of GIST is based on both morphology and IHC. GIST can also occur in patients with neurofibromatosis type-1 (NF1) and in young women as part of a syndrome that includes, paragangliomas, pulmonary chondromas, and gastric GISTs.[107,108]

GISTs can occur anywhere in the GI tract from the esophagus to the rectum. Stomach represents the most common site (60%), followed by the small bowel (30%), rectum (~5%), and esophagus (~5%).[99] Up to 50% of patients will present with metastatic disease at the time of diagnosis, with the liver and peritoneum being the two most common sites.[109] Most GISTs present as an abdominal mass causing bowel obstruction evidenced as nausea, vomiting and abdominal pain, or as GI bleeding. GISTs usually grow rapidly, with masses 5 cm in diameter or greater being common.[110] This rapid rate of growth explains the propensity for GI blood loss, because these tumors may outgrow their blood supply, become necrotic, and ulcerate. Blood loss is usually chronic, with laboratory studies revealing a microcytic anemia.[110] Fistulas and abscesses are also caused by tumor necrosis. The primary mode of diagnosis and assessment of extent of disease is by contrast-enhanced CT scan of the abdomen and pelvis. Characteristic findings on CT scan include an enhancing, exophytic mass in close association with the stomach or bowel wall. Like other sarcomas, GISTs tend to displace rather than invade adjacent structures. While positron emission tomography (PET) is not used to diagnose GIST, it can be used to assess the response to tyrosine kinase therapy. GIST appears as a submucosal mass on endoscopic evaluation. Endoscopic or percutaneous biopsy is recommended in cases in which neoadjuvant therapy is planned or metastasis is suspected.[111]

The primary treatment of GIST is surgical resection with wide margins. However, there is current debate about the management of tumors <2 cm. Current National Comprehensive Cancer Network (NCCN) guidelines for the management of gastric GISTs <2 cm without high-risk features on EUS include surveillance endoscopy every 6–12 months.[112] For tumors >2 cm, surgical resection included en bloc resection when other organs are involved is advocated. Because lymph node involvement is not common, extensive lymphadenectomy appears to provide no added survival benefit. The role of laparoscopy in the management of patients with GIST continues to expand. Those undergoing laparoscopic resection of GIST up to 8 cm at MSKCC had equivalent perioperative and oncologic outcomes when compared with case-matched controls undergoing open resection.[113] With a median follow-up of 34 months, oncologic outcomes were similar with no positive microscopic margins and one recurrence in each group. Bischof et al. also reported that a minimally invasive approach for gastric GIST was associated with low morbidity, and a high rate of R0 resection, based on their review of nearly 400 patients undergoing surgical resection for GIST.[114] Periampullary GIST tumors of the duodenum represent a more challenging surgical approach. A meta-analysis demonstrated that local resection should be the procedure of choice for duodenal GIST whenever technically feasible, because it is associated with good oncologic outcomes and lower morbidity compared with pancreaticoduodenectomy (PD). The use of imatinib in patients with duodenal GIST may potentially allow a proportion of patients who would otherwise require a PD to undergo local resection instead.[115]

Even after surgical resection, may tumors recur. One study analyzing 200 cases of GIST over a 16-year period found that in patients with primary disease who underwent complete resection of gross disease, the 5-year actuarial survival rate was 54%.[99] Even with complete surgical resection, the majority of tumors recurred, often involving the liver and peritoneal surface. In the largest series of GIST recurrences, the group from Memorial Sloan Kettering Cancer Center retrospectively analyzed 69 such patients.[99] Local recurrence was seen in 76% of patients, of which half had synchronous liver lesions. Surgical resection for recurrent disease was completed in one-third of cases with median survival of 15 months. The advent of tyrosine kinase inhibitors has revolutionized treatment of GIST. Although the mechanism of tumor response was believed to be predominantly inhibition of KIT-driven cells, recent data suggest the immune system contributes substantially to the antitumor effect. Imatinib therapy was shown to induce regulatory T cell apoptosis within the tumor by reducing tumor cell expression of the immunosuppressive enzyme indoleamine 2,3-dioxygenase.[116] This data is critical to devising future treatment strategies that may involve immune modulators to increase response.

Due to high recurrence rates, adjuvant imatinib has been explored in several trials. There have been two American College of Surgeons Oncology Group (ACOSOG) trials looking at the role of adjuvant imatinib mesylate after resection for those patients at intermediate or high risk of recurrence. ACOSOG Z9000 was the first phase II trial studying the efficacy of adjuvant imatinib following complete resection of GIST at high risk of recurrence.[117] Patients underwent complete gross resection of a KIT-expressing primary GIST that was at high risk of recurrence (tumor size >10 cm, tumor rupture, or <5 peritoneal metastases). Following resection, patients received oral imatinib 400 mg/day for 1 year. At a median follow-up of 4 years, the 1-, 2-, and 3-year OS rates were 99%, 97%, and 97%, respectively. The 1, 2, and 3-year recurrence-free survival rates were 94%, 73%, and 61%, respectively. These results compared favorably with historical controls for both recurrence-free survival and OS. ACOSOG Z79001 was a follow-up phase III trial in which patients were randomized to 1 year of oral imatinib or placebo following resection.[118] Imatinib taken once a day for 1 year following surgery for localized, primary GIST (≥3 cm) was compared with placebo in 713 patients. Recurrence-free survival was significantly higher in the imatinib arm (98%) when compared with the control group (83%) while there was no difference in OS. Subsequently, disease survival was found to be longer with 3 years versus 1 year of adjuvant imatinib.[119] However, only a few percent of low-risk patients developed recurrence, and more than 70% of patients appeared to be cured by surgery alone based on recurrence-free survival in the placebo arm. Thus, the value of adjuvant imatinib in patients with resected primary GIST 3 cm should be considered carefully. Risk stratification systems can be used to identify patients who have a low likelihood of recurrence in whom adjuvant therapy is not indicated; risk stratification can also identify patients who should get therapy.[120] For example, patients with KIT exon 11 deletions assigned to 1 year of adjuvant imatinib had a longer regression-free survival.[121] Furthermore, specific mutations have been found to be resistant to imatinib; patients with PDGFRA D842V mutations do not respond to imatinib. Another risk stratification score showed that patients with nongastric GIST with a high mitotic count are at a particularly high risk for recurrence.[121]

The future focus of research for the use of adjuvant imatinib is which patients should be treated and what is the optimal duration.[122] The PERSIST5 trial is an ongoing phase II trial testing 5 years of adjuvant imatinib therapy in patients at moderate to high risk of recurrence (NCT00867113). Expert opinion suggests that currently mutation testing of the tumor should be performed to exclude patients with a PDGFRA D842V mutation or wild-type tumor. In the remaining patients, a discussion should ensue about the goals and current results of adjuvant therapy.[123]

The role of neoadjuvant imatinib in the setting of locally advanced disease has been investigated. Neoadjuvant imatinib mesylate holds much promise because it can lead to marked shrinkage in tumor size, which can frequently be predicted within 2 to 4 weeks of initiating therapy using PET scans. The cytoreductive potential of imatinib in the preoperative setting may enable surgeons to obtain R0 resections with less extensive resections. This is most applicable to GIST tumors near the gastroesophageal junction, ampulla, and in the rectum. Recent results from a phase II trial led by the Radiation Therapy Oncology Group (RTOG) revealed that imatinib is well tolerated in the neoadjuvant setting.[124] The groups were divided into whether disease was locally advanced and >5 cm (Group A) or recurrent/metastatic and >2 cm (Group B). Imatinib administered at 600 mg per day for 8 weeks preoperatively was followed by surgery and an additional 2 years of imatinib. Response rates after 8 weeks of preoperative imatinib were similar between groups A and B (4–7% partial response, 83–90% stable disease, and 4–5% progressive disease).[124] Another phase II trial from MD Anderson Cancer Center investigated either 3, 5, or 7 days of neoadjuvant imatinib in 19 patients.[125] This regimen was tolerated well and response rates by FDG-PET were 69%. The duration of neoadjuvant therapy and

patient selection remain to be defined. Current NCCN guidelines suggest that in patients on neoadjuvant imatinib, once two successive CT scans fail to show any radiographic response, surgical resection should be considered.[112]

In the metastatic setting, there is strong evidence of the effectiveness of imatinib mesylate. Up to 80% of patients with metastatic GIST attain a partial or complete response with imatinib.[118] A recent meta-analysis of two, large, randomized studies[126,127] comparing the efficacy of imatinib given either once (400 mg) or twice daily revealed that the higher dose confers a progression-free survival advantage among patients with exon 9 mutations.[128] The second-line agent for patients with imatinib-resistant disease is sunitinib.[129] Sunitinib targets KIT and PDGFRα, as well as the vascular endothelial cell growth factor receptor (VEGFR). In patients with advanced disease resistant to imatinib, sunitinib is a safe and effective second-line agent.[130] Molecular studies suggest that imatinib is most effective in patients with exon 11 C-kit tyrosine kinase mutations, and sunitinib may be more effective in patients with exon 9 mutations.[128] Other studies have recently been completed examining third-line agents. Regorafenib was shown to significantly improve progression-free survival compared with placebo in patients with metastatic GIST after progression on standard treatments.[131] Although a relatively rare clinical entity, the treatment of GIST is continually evolving and represents an area of active developments.

Lymphoma

Lymphoma accounts for 15–20% of all malignant small bowel tumors.[132] The stomach is the most common site of GI lymphoma (>60%), followed by an equal distribution between the large and small intestines.[133] There is a slight male predominance of approximately 1.5 : 1, and the median age is lower than that of persons with other small bowel tumors (49 years in one large series).[134,135] Lymphomas are the most frequent malignant neoplasms in transplant recipients, appearing on average 20 months after the initiation of cyclosporine.[135] Prognosis is better than for other forms of intestinal lymphomas with two-thirds cured with resection, radiotherapy, acyclovir, and reduction of immunosuppression.[136,137] Small bowel lymphomas also occur in AIDS. Virtually all lesions are B lymphocyte in origin. The prognosis is poor but is dominated by the HIV-related disease such that life expectancy for these patients is not significantly inferior to similar HIV-positive patients without lymphoma.[136]

The clinical presentation of GI lymphoma includes abdominal pain, nausea, vomiting, fatigue, weight loss, and GI bleeding, which may be occult. A mass with bulky adenopathy on CT scan is highly suggestive of abdominal lymphoma.[138] Multiple staging systems have been proposed for GI lymphomas, including the Ann Arbor, Musshoff, and the European–American classification system. Each of these major staging systems recognizes four major stages of small bowel lymphoma: stage I for local disease, stage II for regional involvement, and stages III and IV for advanced disease with metastasis. Imaging is also now included in some staging systems after the 11th International Conference on Malignant Lymphomas (ICML) in 2011.[139]

Resection of small bowel lymphoma is important for local control but rarely eradicates the disease. Disease is often advanced so that fewer than 30% of intestinal tumors are amenable to primary curative resection.[140] Adjuvant therapy is an essential part of the treatment. Surgical resection should be attempted for localized disease and should involve removal of the bowel segments, with wide margins, and the involved mesenteric lymph nodes, if possible. Margins need to be completely clear of tumor since lymphomas may spread for long distances in the submucosal plane. Adjuvant chemotherapy in patients after potential curative resection is advocated.[141] In patients with unresectable lymphoma, radiation therapy and chemotherapy are recommended.[142] Additionally, rituximab, the chimeric monoclonal antibody against the protein CD20, has also shown some promise in B cell lymphomas.[143]

Forty years ago, an unusual immunoproliferative small intestinal disease was reported to be particularly common in the Middle East, especially in southern Iran. This Mediterranean lymphoma is found in children and young adults and carried a poop prognosis.[144] Patients tend to be from lower socioeconomic groups with a background of malnutrition. The tumor progenitor cell is believed to be the perifollicular B cell, which produces IgA. The tumor releases an excess of alpha heavy chains, which are detectable in the serum.[145] However, recent epidemiologic reports from southern Iran suggest that distribution of NHL in the GI tract is similar to Western countries.[146]

Metastatic neoplasms

Metastatic neoplasm involvement of the small bowel is more frequent than primary small intestinal neoplasia. Primary tumors of the colon, ovary, uterus, and stomach involve the small bowel, most often by direct invasion or peritoneal spread. Primaries from the breast, lung, and melanoma metastasize to the small intestine hematogenously. A large review of autopsies from Memorial Sloan Kettering Cancer Center previously found the incidence of GI metastases from metastatic melanoma was 58% small bowel.[147] Within the GI tract, the small bowel is the most frequent site of metastasis of melanoma most likely because of its rich blood supply. A retrospective study of 103 cases of malignant melanoma performed by the Armed Forces Institute of Pathology stated that small bowel involvement by melanoma, even in the absence of a known primary, is usually metastatic.[148] If possible, surgery to remove disease should be offered. Ollila et al. reported on a retrospective review of 124 of 6509 melanoma patients who had GI tract metastases at the John Wayne Cancer Institute from 1971 through 1994.[149] Of these 124 patients, 69 (56%) underwent surgical exploration of the abdomen, of which 46 (67%) had curative resection and 23 (33%) had a palliative procedure only. Almost all (97%) of the 69 surgical patients experienced symptomatic relief postoperatively. The median survival of patients undergoing curative resection was 48.9 months compared with only 5.4 months in patients undergoing palliative procedures and 5.7 months in patients undergoing nonsurgical interventions. Metastatic lesions to the small bowel can be treated with resection in selected cases and/or tumor-specific systemic therapy.

Tumors of the appendix

Neoplasms of the appendix are found in as high as 5% of specimens obtained by appendectomy for acute appendicitis.[150] Most of these lesions are benign, including mucosal hyperplasia or metaplasia, leiomyomas, lipomas, neuromas, and angiomas. Malignancies of the appendix are rare, making up less than 0.5% of all intestinal neoplasms.[151] Among 71,000 appendectomy specimens taken over a 40-year period, Collins found 958 malignant tumors, with an overall incidence of 1.35%.[150]

Broadly, appendiceal malignancies are divided into those of neuroendocrine origin (carcinoid) or epithelial origin. Malignancies of epithelial origin include mucoceles, pseudomyxoma peritonei (PMP), goblet cell carcinomas, and primary adenocarcinomas. In a large series of 5655 appendiceal tumors observed from the SEER database of the National Cancer Institute between 1973 and 2007,

malignant carcinoid comprised of 11% of specimen but had the best 5-year disease-specific survival of 93%.[152]

Tumors of the appendix often present in the setting of appendicitis, which may lead to a pathological diagnoses after appendectomy. However, in the setting of perforated appendicitis complicated by phlegmon or abscess, the paradigm of management has shifted from interval appendectomy towards nonsurgical management. This trend is important because in 2% of patients where nonsurgical management is undertaken, there is an associated underlying cancer diagnoses or Crohn's disease, especially in patients over 40 years old.[153]

Carcinoids

Carcinoids are the most common appendiceal tumors, comprising 32% to 85% of all appendiceal neoplasms, which include both benign and malignant types.[154,155] Malignant carcinoids comprised of 11% of appendiceal malignancies, derived from the SEER study. The SEER study also revealed a sex predominance for appendiceal carcinoids, with tumors from females comprising 68% of the cases. This female predominance may reflect the increased number of pelvic procedures performed in women, leading to more incidental findings, including carcinoids of the appendix. Peak incidence occurs in the third to fourth decades of life, averaging 32 to 42 years in the literature.[156,157]

Most of carcinoids occur in the distal 1/3 of the appendix, where they are unlikely to cause obstruction.[158] Symptoms are more likely with larger tumors and with metastases beyond the regional lymph nodes. Approximately 10% of appendiceal carcinoids are located at the base of the appendix, where they can cause obstruction, leading to appendicitis.[155] Similar to other intestinal carcinoids, appendiceal carcinoids can be vasoactive substances, which are responsible for carcinoid syndrome. Carcinoid syndrome symptoms are rare but indicate metastatic disease, typically to the liver.[159]

In general, metastases from appendiceal carcinoids <2 cm in diameter are uncommon. Moertel and colleagues, in their evaluation of 150 appendiceal carcinoids over a period of 51 years, noted that 4.7% of the cases metastasized but none of the tumors <2 cm exhibited metastatic spread.[160] Extension into the mesoappendix, if present, correlates with nodal metastases and tumor size, and those with high mitoses and Ki67 positivity correlate with tumor aggressiveness.[161,162]

Small (<2 cm) carcinoids at the tip of appendix may be treated with a simple appendectomy.[163] At laparotomy, these tumors appear as small yellow nodules, usually in the distal third of the appendix. Histologically, the cells are small and uniform, and contain a central nucleus with few mitoses. Almost all carcinoids show invasion of the muscular layer of the wall of the appendix, and involvement of lymphatic vessels adjacent to the tumor is essentially universal.[163] Despite this microscopic finding, few patients have regional or distant dissemination of disease. Large (>2 cm) carcinoids and those at the base of appendix require a right colectomy, which removes the draining lymph nodes and any residual disease that might remain at the base of the appendix or in the mesoappendix.

Based on consensus guidelines in 2010 and 2012 from the North American Neuroendocrine Tumor Society (NANETS) and European Neuroendocrine Tumor Society (ENETS), completion colectomy is also recommended for tumors between 1 and 2 cm that also have mesoappendiceal invasion, positive or unclear margins, higher proliferate rate, angioinvasion, and mixed histology consistent with goblet cell carcinoid or adenocarcinoid.[164,165]

In 2010, the AJCC included a TNM staging for appendiceal carcinoid for the first time, which is different from TNM staging systems for carcinoids arising from other intestinal sites and lung. Overall outcomes for early-stage appendiceal carcinoids are optimistic. Based on analysis of 900 appendiceal carcinoid tumors observed from the SEER database, five-year disease-specific survival rates for appendiceal carcinoids were 100% if tumor size <3 cm without regional nodal or distant metastases, 78% if tumor size between 2 and 3 cm with regional nodal metastases or tumor size >3 cm with or without nodal or distant metastases, and 32% if there is distant metastases.[166]

Mucocele

An appendiceal mucocele is any one of a number of lesions that are characterized by dilation of the appendiceal lumen, alteration of the mucosal lining, hypersecretion of mucus, and occasional extension outside of the appendix.[167] The underlying pathology may be a hyperplastic polyp; a benign neoplasm, such as cystadenoma; or a malignant tumor, such as cystadenocarcinoma. Many authors support the use of a system based on histologic findings rather than on the presence of a cystic lesion.[167] In this system, mucoceles of the appendix are classified into simple (obstructive) and mucoceles with proliferative epithelial changes. Benign neoplastic proliferative changes may be localized, as in adenoma of colonic type, or diffuse, as in mucinous adenoma or mucinous cystadenoma. Malignant proliferative groups may be classified as colonic-type adenocarcinoma, mucinous cystadenocarcinoma, and mixed carcinoidadenocarcinoma.[168] The preneoplastic potential of hyperplastic epithelium and the premalignant nature of adenomatous epithelium are seen by the coexistence of hyperplastic, adenomatous, and carcinomatous epithelia all in the same lesion.[168] A consequence of mucoceles of the appendix (cystadenomas and cystadenocarcinomas) is PMP. This lesion, characterized by large quantities of mucus-like material in the peritoneal cavity, is considered to represent dissemination of mucinous cystadenocarcinoma within the peritoneal cavity (see the section on PMP).[169]

Though the diagnosis of appendiceal mucocele is usually an incidental finding at celiotomy, mucinous cystadenomas and cystadenocarcinomas are among the few appendiceal tumors that may be diagnosed preoperatively.[163] CT strongly suggests a mucinous tumor if a mass is present in the right lower quadrant with near water density. Ultrasound shows a diagnostic variable sonographic echogenicity because of the combination of mucin with more anechoic fluid. Although both imaging techniques may be helpful in diagnosing a mucocele, other cystic lesions of the peritoneal cavity, such as ovarian cysts, duplication cysts, mesenteric and omental cysts, or an abscess, may have a similar appearance.[170]

Surgical resection should be pursued, even for a benign-appearing appendiceal mucocele, since lesions that appear to be benign on imaging studies may harbor a cystadenocarcinoma. The extent of resection is dependent on the underlying histology. In the case of hyperplastic polyps or cystadenoma, a simple appendectomy is considered curative. In the series reported by Higa and colleagues, 36 of the 46 patients with mucinous cystadenomas were treated with appendectomy alone with no recurrence.[167] In patients with mucinous cystadenocarcinoma, a substantial number will present with extensive abdominal metastases or PMP. Treatment of the primary lesion includes a formal right hemicolectomy with removal of draining lymph nodes.[171] Stephenson and Brief reviewed 53 appendiceal mucinous cystadenocarcinomas treated by either simple appendectomy or right hemicolectomy. At 10 years, survival was 65% among patients treated with hemicolectomy in contrast to a 37% rate among patients who had received an appendectomy alone.[172] Surgical debulking of metastatic deposits and evacuation of mucus collections are also recommended.

Pseudomyxoma peritonei

PMP is a condition characterized by diffuse collections of gelatinous material in the abdomen and pelvis and mucinous implants on the peritoneal surfaces, originating from ruptured mucinous neoplasms. As the primary tumor grows and occludes the lumen, mucus accumulates leading to appendiceal rupture. The peritoneum is then seeded with mucus-producing cells, which continue to proliferate and produce mucus.[173] Accumulation of intraperitoneal mucus eventually progresses to intestinal obstruction, nausea, vomiting, and starvation, which is fatal. Over the years, the term PMP has begun to be used more generally by clinicians to signify not only intraperitoneal mucinous dissemination from rupture of a benign cystadenoma, but also peritoneal dissemination of mucus-producing adenocarcinomas of the appendix, large and small bowel, as well as lung, breast, pancreas, stomach, bile ducts, gallbladder, and fallopian tubes/ovary.[174,175]

PMP is found incidentally in approximately 2 of 10,000 laparotomies, with a female predominance.[174] The most common presenting symptom in both men and women is increasing abdominal girth; in men the second most common symptom is an inguinal hernia, while for women it is an ovarian mass palpated at the time of a routine pelvic examination.[173] On CT scan, the mucinous material is similar in density to fat and appears heterogeneous. Scalloping of the liver, spleen, and mesentery is found, and calcifications are common. The undersurface of the diaphragm may be greatly thickened by large cystic masses of mucinous tumor. A striking early finding is the characteristic peripheral location of tumor within the abdomen and pelvis and relative sparing and central displacement of the small bowel and mesentery.[173]

Traditionally, treatment for PMP is repeated surgical debulking for symptomatic disease.[174] Debulking is not curative but aims to limit the buildup of mucus and its pressure effect. Invariably, disease recurrence requires repeated and progressively more difficult surgery due to adhesions and fibrosis, with five-year survival of 50%.[176] Cytoreduction and intraperitoneal chemotherapy is a more aggressive approach that includes radical surgical removal of all intra-abdominal and pelvic disease and the administration of intraperitoneal heated chemotherapy. Drug penetration is enhanced by heating the perfusate containing chemotherapy, an approach termed intraperitoneal hyperthermic chemotherapy (IPHC).[177–180] This approach is best suited to patients with minimal residual disease (deposits smaller than 2–2.5 mm) after surgical cytoreduction. It is unlikely that even a heated solution of chemotherapy could penetrate large tumor deposits.

Sugarbaker et al. have written most extensively about treatment of peritoneal surface malignancy with aggressive surgical debulking and IPHC.[179] His group uses four clinical assessments to select patients who are most likely to benefit from combined treatment. First, histopathologic assessment in which noninvasive malignancies such as true PMP or cystic mesothelioma are more likely to be made visibly disease-free through a peritonectomy procedure and are less likely than other invasive histologies to have spread to regional nodes, liver, or other systemic sites. Second, preoperative contrast-enhanced CT of the chest, abdomen, and pelvis not only to exclude liver or other systemic metastases but also to determine if small bowel obstruction or tumor nodules greater than 5 cm are present, which portends a poor prognosis. Two other clinical indices, the peritoneal cancer index (PCI, a quantitative indicator of prognosis derived from the size and distribution of nodules on the peritoneal surface) and the completeness of cytoreduction score (the size of persisting tumor nodules after maximal cytoreduction), are derived intraoperatively. A 2001 report by Sugarbaker and colleagues included 108 patients with PMP treated over a 10-year period (1983–1993) with surgical debulking and intraoperative intraperitoneal heated mitomycin followed by intraperitoneal 5-FU during postoperative days 1 to 6 and three subsequent courses of adjuvant intravenous mitomycin and intraperitoneal 5-FU.[181] Of the 65 patients with true PMP, 5-year survival was 75% and 10-year survival was 68%. Those with carcinomatosis had a poorer outcome with 5- and 10-year survival rates of 26% and 9%, respectively. Morbidity associated with combination of cytoreductive surgery and IPEC is high (37.75%).[182] However, studies have shown that this rate is still acceptable in terms of cost–benefit ratio to patients.[176]

Adenocarcinoma

Primary adenocarcinoma of the appendix is a rare neoplasm, accounting for 4–6% of primary appendiceal neoplasms, arising in preexisting adenomas.[183] The mean age of presentation is 50 years, and a male predominance is noted of anywhere from 4 : 1 to 2.8 : 1.[184–186] The clinical presentation in the majority of patients in the literature is acute appendicitis or an abdominal mass, though the diagnosis is rarely made preoperatively. Perforation may complicate the clinical picture, occurring in up to 40% of cases, but perforation alone has little effect on OS.[187]

Histologically, primary adenocarcinoma is distinguished from an adenoma by invasion of the wall of the appendix by the neoplastic tissue. Lymph node metastases are noted in 25% of cases at presentation.[188] Adenocarcinoma of the appendix has a metastatic potential between that of appendiceal carcinoid and colonic adenocarcinoma, with metastases developing in 20% of patients, often to the ovary.[183] The degree of metastatic involvement varies with the histologic grade; about 30% of the well-differentiated tumors are found to have metastasized, whereas nearly 70% of the poorly differentiated tumors are metastatic at the time of laparotomy.[184,185] The overall 5-year survival rate is 55% and varies with Dukes stage (A 100%, B 67%, C 50%, D 6%).[189]

The literature suggests that surgical treatment of adenocarcinomas should involve more than just an appendectomy. Hesketh reported that the 5-year survival rate was 20% with appendectomy alone compared to 63% with right hemicolectomy.[186] Hopkins et al. reported rates of 20 and 45%, respectively.[190]

Carcinoma of the colon and rectum

Epidemiology

Colorectal cancer (CRC) remains an important global health issue. It is the third most common malignant tumor and the fourth most common cause of cancer death worldwide.[191] CRC is most common in developed nations. In the United States alone, an estimated 130,000 people were diagnosed with CRC in 2014, and approximately 50,000 died from the disease.[192] It is thought that dietary and lifestyle habits, in conjunction with genetic factors, account for the increased incidence in developed countries. Research shows that individuals who migrate from regions where CRC is less common to regions of high incidence will inherit the risk of the host country.[193]

There are disparities in CRC incidence and mortality among genders, races, and ethnic groups. While CRC is the third most common malignancy in the United States for both men and women, and the incidence of colon cancers is similar between the sexes, rectal cancer is more common in men. Right-sided/proximal colon cancers are more common among women compared to distal tumors in men.[191] Moreover, mortality is approximately one-third higher in men.[194] African-Americans have the highest

rates of both incidence and mortality when compared to the White, Asian-American, American Indian, and Hispanic populations.[195] The reasons for the disparities are not entirely known; however it has been postulated that differences in access to high-quality regular screening, timely diagnosis and treatment, dietary and lifestyle factors, and socioeconomic status could play a role.[195,196]

Despite the high prevalence of CRC in the United States, both the incidence and overall mortality from CRC have been declining over several decades. These declines have accelerated recently; as for both males and females, the incidence rates decreased at a rate of approximately 4% between 2008 and 2010, and mortality rates decreased by about 3% over the same time period.[197] Studies have shown that increased screening and detection can reduce the chance of developing or dying from CRC by 10–75%, depending on which screening tests are used and how often they are performed.[198] This increased screening could also be a reason for the shift in anatomic distribution of CRC from rectum and left-sided cancers to more right-sided cancers. Data from the National Cancer Data Base from the years 1988 and 1993 show an increase from 51% to 55% of all CRC to be proximal to the splenic flexure.[199] Multiple studies have confirmed a higher rate of proximal colon cancer rates compared to distal colon or rectal carcinoma rates, both in the United States and globally.[199–202]

Risk factors

Age and racial background

Age is a known risk factor for CRC. The vast majority of cases of CRC occur in people over age 50, with incidence continuing to increase thereafter.[198] In fact, fewer than 10% of all new CRC diagnoses and deaths occur in patients younger than 50.[192] As discussed previously, African-American individuals have a higher incidence and mortality rate of CRC compared to other racial and ethnic populations.[195,198,199].

Personal or family history

Patients with a personal history of adenomatous polyps or previous CRC have an increased risk of developing colon cancer in the future. Size, number, and histology of polyps are important prognostic factors, with size >1 cm, villous or tubulovillous histology, and multiple polyps conferring a greater risk for CRC.[203] Patients with an isolated tubular adenoma of <1 cm do not appear to be at an increased risk of developing CRC.[203] In patients with previous CRC, the incidence of metachronous CRC is 6%, and the incidence of metachronous adenomas is 25%.[204]

Family history of CRC in a first-degree relative increases the risk of developing CRC two- to threefold, while cancer in a second-degree relative increases the risk of CRC by 25–50%.[205,206] In addition, risk increases if there are more than one first-degree relative with colon cancer or if they are diagnosed before age 55.[207] Family history of colonic adenoma also increases the risk of CRC, especially if the adenoma is diagnosed early.

Inflammatory bowel disease

UC and Crohn's disease are well-known risk factors for colorectal carcinoma. For UC, the extent of disease and the duration of disease are the primary prognostic factors. Patients with pancolitis have a 5- to 15-fold increased risk of developing CRC compared to a threefold increased risk with colitis limited to the left colon.[208] The risk also increases the longer the disease is present.[209] Similar characteristics and incidence of CRC have been reported in Crohn's disease.[210–212]

Diet and lifestyle

Westernized dietary habits, including an increased consumption of red meat and fat with a decreased consumption of fruits and vegetables, are associated with CRC. There is conflicting evidence regarding the effect of diets high in fruits and vegetables, but the general consensus is that while there may not be a protection associated with increased consumption, very low consumption does increase risk of developing CRC.[213–215] A high-fat diet containing mixed lipids and saturated fat has been shown to promote colon carcinogenesis.[216,217] Alternatively, high intake of poultry and fish appears to be protective.[218]

Obesity has been associated with an increased risk of CRC in both men and women, and people with a BMI $\geq 30\,\mathrm{kg/m^2}$ appear to have nearly a 20% increased risk of CRC compared to nonobese patients.[219,220] In contrast, physical activity and exercise are correlated with a decreased risk of CRC.[221]

Diabetes mellitus and hyperinsulinemia

There is increasing evidence that diabetes mellitus and insulin resistance are risk factors for CRC. A meta-analysis of 15 studies found the estimated risk of CRC in diabetics was 30% higher than nondiabetics.[222,223] A possible explanation is the hyperinsulinemia associated with diabetes or even chronic insulin treatment for diabetes, resulting in growth signals to colonic mucosal cells via insulin-like growth factor 1.[223,224]

Alcohol and tobacco

Heavy alcohol consumption is correlated with a moderately increased risk of CRC. The association is dose dependent and is irrespective of the type of alcoholic beverage consumed.[225,226] The association between smoking and CRC is not as straightforward, and cigarette smoking may have a greater impact depending on specific somatic polymorphisms.[227]

Genetics

Colorectal tumorigenesis follows a distinct genetic pattern, with accumulation of genomic alterations and progressive waves of clonal expansion of cells that have a growth advantage over their progenitors. Three major categories of genes have been implicated in the development of CRC, namely, oncogenes such as K-*ras*; tumor suppressor genes such as adenomatous polyposis coli (*APC*), deleted in colorectal carcinoma (*DCC*), *p53*, and mutated in colon cancer (*MCC*); and the mismatch repair genes *hMSH2*, *hMLH1*, *hPMS*, and *hPMS2*.

CRC develops from a multistep gene mutation sequence termed loss of heterozygosity (LOH) that can be observed in inherited and sporadic CRC. Fearon and Vogelstein first postulated in 1990 that at least five genes had to be mutated in order to progress in the adenoma to carcinoma sequence.[228] Further studies showed that at least seven genetic alterations take place before the development of cancer. Important genes in the LOH model include *APC*, K-*ras*, *DCC*, and *p53*. An entirely different pathway of cancer development is initiated by defects within the mismatch repair genes. In this case, replication errors (RERs) increase, leading to microsatellite instability and malfunction of the gene. This pathway is referred to as RER and occurs in 20% of all colorectal tumors.[229]

APC gene

The *APC* gene is located on the long arm of chromosome 5 (5q). It is mutated in FAP and Gardner syndrome and in most cases of Turcot syndrome. A mutated *APC* gene is detected in 63% of adenoma and carcinoma, but not in the surrounding tissues,

indicating that this is a somatic mutation. Because *APC* is a tumor suppressor gene, inactivation of the second allele must occur for the cell to lose the tumor-suppressing activity of the APC protein. There is considerable evidence that *APC* mutations occur early and may be the first event in sporadic colorectal mutagenesis.

DCC gene

The *DCC* gene is located on the long arm of chromosome 18 (18q). The gene product is involved in cell–cell adhesion and cell–matrix interactions, which may be important in preventing tumor growth, invasion, and metastasis. In sporadic CRC, *DCC* seems to play a critical role in the ability of a tumor to metastasize.

p53 gene

The *p53* is located on the short arm of chromosome 17 (17p). p53 seems to be the most important determinant of malignancy during colorectal tumorigenesis. As a tetramer, *p53* binds sequences of DNA in the promoter region of other genes to enhance their transcription.[230] Most genes activated by *p53* are thought to be involved in the inhibition of growth. Mutations of *p53* can be found in more than half of all human cancers.[231]

K-ras proto-oncogene

K-*ras* is an oncogene, which acts in a classic dominant fashion and is located on the short arm of chromosome 12 (12p). The K-*ras* protein interacts with putative effector molecules, conveying a growth response. The signal transduction process is perturbed with a mutant K-*ras* protein leading to tumor formation. In sporadic colorectal tumors, K-*ras* mutations have been found in approximately 50% of carcinomas and large adenomas.[232]

Mismatch repair gene

Mismatch repair genes are needed for cells to repair DNA RERs and spontaneous base repair loss. The four DNA mismatch repair genes found in humans are *hMSH2* (chromosome 2p), hMSH6 (chromosome 2p), *hMLH1* (chromosome 3p), *hPMS1* (chromosome 2q), and *hPMS2* (chromosome 7p). They are regarded to contribute to hereditary nonpolyposis syndrome in various percentages.[233]

Inherited syndromes

Even though the vast majority of cases of CRC are sporadic rather than familial, inherited susceptibility results in a dramatic increase in risk of developing CRC. The genetic syndromes are typically inherited in an autosomal dominant fashion and are associated with a very high risk of developing CRC.

FAP is an autosomal dominant process characterized by numerous colonic adenomas which appear during childhood. This syndrome has penetrance approaching 100% with the onset of symptoms and diagnosis generally around age 15 years.[234] If left untreated, FAP will invariably become CRC with a mean age of diagnosis and death of 39 and 42 years, respectively.[235] An attenuated form of APC (AAPC) is a milder variant of FAP with a similar risk for developing CRC. AAPC is characterized by fewer adenomatous polyps and an older average age of diagnosis (usually in the early 50s). Both of these inherited syndromes are caused by different germline mutations in the same *APC* gene, which is located on chromosome 5.[236]

Hereditary nonpolyposis colorectal cancer (HNPCC) is another autosomal dominant inherited syndrome which accounts for 1–5% of all colorectal carcinomas. Also known as Lynch syndrome, this disease is characterized by an early age of onset (some patients can present in their 20s, while the mean age of diagnosis is 48 years), right-sided predominance, multiple synchronous or metachronous colonic tumors, and extracolonic manifestations. The extracolonic neoplasms can include endometrial cancer, renal pelvis and ureter cancer, bladder cancer, small bowel cancer, and skin lesions.[237] As described above, HNPCC is caused by a mutation in one of the mismatch repair genes.[238]

MYH-associated polyposis (MAP) is a recently described autosomal recessive polyposis syndrome associated with a somewhat attenuated phenotype compared to other familial polyposis syndromes.[239] Mutations in *MYH*, a base excision repair gene, are associated with an increased risk of multiple adenomas or polyposis coli.[240] In patients where no *APC* gene mutation is found, especially in those patients with 10–15 or more adenomas, work-up for an *MYH* gene mutation is indicated for diagnosis.[240,241] In addition, these patients are at high risk for synchronous GI cancers.

PJ syndrome is an inherited hamartomatous polyposis syndrome that predisposes to CRC. The two major manifestations of PJ are pigmented mucocutaneous lesions and multiple colonic polyps which have the ability to undergo malignant transformation. PJ is associated with an increased risk of both GI and non-GI malignancies including ovarian, breast, pancreatic, uterine, Sertoli cell, and cervical neoplasms.[242–244] Juvenile polyposis (JP) is another inherited hamartomatous polyposis syndrome that can predispose to CRC. Patients with JP are also at increased risk for gastric, duodenal, and pancreatic cancers.[245,246]

Polymorphisms

Numerous genetic polymorphisms (normal variations in genes) have been found to be associated with developing CRC. Changes in genes such as carcinogen metabolism genes, methylation genes, and tumor suppressor genes can lead to either an increase or decrease in cancer risk. Cytochrome P450 genes, Glutathione-S transferase genes, N-acetyltransferase genes, and tumor suppressor genes have all been implicated in CRC. Cytochrome P450A1 (CYP1A1) is a phase I enzyme which acts on carcinogens found in tobacco smoke.[247] Polymorphisms such as A—>G at Ile462Val, exon 7 in the gene for CYP1A1 puts patients at an increased risk for developing CRC.[248] Patients who smoke cigarettes are especially at risk when they carry a polymorphism in this gene.

Glutathione-S-transferases are phase II enzymes responsible for the detoxification of mutagenic electrophiles, including polyaromatic hydrocarbons.[247] Glutathione-S-transferase Mu (GSTM1) and Theta (GSTT1) have both been discussed in relationship to CRC. In addition, *N*-acetyltransferases are phase II enzymes involved in detoxifying arylamines, which are found in cooked meat.[247] Both GSTT1 and NAT2 rapid acetylator phenotype have been identified as causing an increased risk for CRC.[249]

The most common tumor repressor gene associated with CRC is the *APC* gene. A polymorphism at I1307K, found predominantly in the Ashkenazi Jewish population, confers a twofold increase in CRC risk.[250] Another polymorphism in the *APC* gene, I1317Q, also increases the risk of CRC.[251]

Some polymorphisms have been shown to be protective against CRC. Patients who eat a low-fat diet and who are homozygous for a variant APC gene at codon 1822 have a reduced risk of colon cancer compared to those patients who are wild type and eat a high-fat diet.[252] In addition, variations in a methylation gene for methylenetetrahydrofolate reductase (MTHFR) have been shown to influence CRC risk. Patients who carry the MTHFR 677TT genotype have a reduced risk of CRC.[253]

Presentation, screening, and surveillance

Signs and symptoms

The presentation of large bowel malignancy generally falls into three categories: insidious onset of chronic symptoms, acute onset of intestinal obstruction, or acute perforation. The most common presentation is that of an insidious onset of chronic symptoms (77–92%), followed by obstruction (6–16%), and then perforation (2–7%).[254–256]

Bleeding is the most common symptom of colorectal malignancy.[257] Unfortunately, patient and physician alike often attribute the bleeding to benign conditions. Bleeding may be occult or it may be seen as stool that is black, maroon, or bright red depending on the location of the malignancy.

Change in bowel habits is the second most common complaint, with patients noting either diarrhea or constipation.[257,258] Constipation is more often associated with left-sided lesions because the diameter of the colon is smaller and the stool is more formed than on the right side. Patients may report a gradual change in the caliber of the stool or may have diarrhea if the narrowing has progressed sufficiently to cause obstruction. Carcinomas of the right side of the colon do not typically present with changes in bowel habits, but large amounts of mucus generated by a tumor may cause diarrhea, and large right-sided lesions or lesions involving the ileocecal valve may cause obstruction.

Abdominal pain is as common a presentation as change in bowel habits.[259] Left-sided obstructing lesions may present with cramping abdominal pain, associated with nausea and vomiting, and relieved with bowel movements. Right-sided malignancies may result in vague pain that is difficult to localize. Rectal lesions may present with tenesmus, but pelvic pain is generally associated with advanced disease after the tumor has involved the sacral or sciatic nerves. Less common symptoms include weight loss, malaise, fever, abdominal mass, and symptoms of urinary tract involvement. Bacteremia with *Streptococcus bovis* is highly suggestive of colorectal malignancy.[260,261]

Physical exam is often unrevealing because the abdomen is distended, and masses, primary or metastatic, are not palpable. Tympany, ascites, and distention may be all that is noted on abdominal exam. Rectal exam will only rarely reveal an obstructing tumor. Colorectal malignancy should always be considered when patients present with large bowel obstruction. The diagnosis may be confirmed with contrast enema, rigid or flexible endoscopy, or CT scans of the abdomen and pelvis.

Perforation may result in localized or generalized peritonitis or, if walled off, it may present with obstruction or fistula to an adjacent structure such as the bladder. Perforation occurs in 12–19% of patients with obstruction due to CRC.[262,263] When the perforation occurs proximal to the obstructing lesion, the patients present with diffuse peritonitis and sepsis. Emergent surgical intervention after adequate fluid resuscitation is clearly indicated. However, perforation at the tumor, possibly secondary to tumor necrosis, may follow a more indolent course, and thus may be confused with alternative diagnoses such as appendicitis, diverticulitis, or Crohn's disease.

Screening and surveillance

Cancer screening refers to the testing of a population of apparently asymptomatic individuals to determine the risk of developing CRC. Surveillance refers to the ongoing monitoring of individuals who have an increased risk for the development of the disease. For CRC, surveillance is reserved for patients with inflammatory bowel disease, family cancer syndromes, and those with a previous history of CRC or colorectal adenomas. Various screening and surveillance

Table 1 Screening recommendations, National Comprehensive Cancer Network.

Risk category	Screening and surveillance recommendations
Average risk: Asymptomatic, age 50 or greater; no history of adenoma, sessile serrated polyp, or colorectal cancer	Starting at age 50, colonoscopy every 10 years *or* flexible sigmoidoscopy every 5 years (with interval stool-based testing at 3 years) *or* yearly stool-based testing (guaiac or immunochemical based)
Increased risk without personal history: First-degree relative with CRC or adenomatous polyps at age 60 or greater, two second-degree relatives affected with CRC, or one second-degree relative with CRC at age younger than 50	Colonoscopy every 5 years starting at age 50 or 10 years younger than earliest family diagnosis
First-degree relative with CRC or adenomatous polyps at age younger than 60 or two or more first-degree relative with CRC	Colonoscopy every 3–5 years starting at age 40 or 10 years younger than earliest family diagnosis
Gene carrier or at risk for familial adenomatous polyposis	Flexible sigmoidoscopy or colonoscopy every year beginning at age 10–15
Gene carrier or at risk for hereditary nonpolyposis colorectal cancer	Colonoscopy every 1–2 years beginning at age 25–30 or 2–5 years younger than earliest family diagnosis

modalities are available to detect CRCs and adenomatous polyps. Current screening and surveillance recommendations are listed below (Table 1).

Stool-based screening methods

The advantage of fecal occult blood testing includes availability, convenience, and low cost. Limitations include low sensitivity, low specificity, low compliance, and inability to detect adenomas. Sensitivity is affected by slide storage, ascorbic acid, lesions not bleeding at the time of testing, and degradation of hemoglobin by colonic bacteria. Specificity is adversely affected by exogenous peroxidase activity by red meat and uncooked vegetables and medications that may induce bleeding from noncolonic sources such as aspirin and other nonsteroidal anti-inflammatory drugs. In five large controlled studies including more than 300,000 patients, an increased detection of CRC at earlier stages was demonstrated with the proper use of stool-based screening,[264,265] and testing was also associated with a significant reduction in mortality.[264-268] Stool-based screening techniques include high-sensitivity guaiac-based testing, immunochemical-based testing, and most recently stool DNA tests. DNA testing detects the presence of genomic alterations that are known to occur in CRC oncogenesis; the best tests have demonstrated sensitivities as high as 95%.[269] Currently, DNA tests have not yet been FDA approved, and thus they do not represent a first-line option for screening. As of 2014, high-sensitivity guaiac-based and immunochemical-based stool testing as standalone screening methods are considered appropriate so long as they are performed annually by a healthcare provider and a prescribed diet is followed. Any abnormal test requires follow-up invasive screening. Recently, immunochemical-based testing has proven to have increased sensitivity compared to guaiac-based tests.[270] Stool-based screening is a particularly good option for those who refuse more invasive options.[271]

Flexible sigmoidoscopy

Both rigid and flexible sigmoidoscopies are inexpensive, require no conscious sedation, and afford direct visualization and biopsy of polyps and cancers.[272] The advantage of the flexible sigmoidoscope over the rigid is that it can reach the descending colon and even the splenic flexure. The disadvantage of sigmoidoscopy is that the entire colon is not visualized, and lesions may be missed in the proximal colon. Current National Comprehensive Cancer Network and American Cancer Society Guidelines recommend sigmoidoscopy with or without stool-based screening every 5 years, with subsequent full colonoscopy if adenomatous disease is found.[273]

Barium enema

Barium enema combined with sigmoidoscopy allows for evaluation of the entire colon and rectum. Single-contrast barium enema is significantly less sensitive and specific than double-contrast barium enema (DCBE) and should not be used as a screening tool. DCBE has a sensitivity of 50–80% for polyps <1 cm, 70–90% for polyps >1 cm, and 55–85% for stage I and II carcinomas.[274-276] When combined with sigmoidoscopy, the sensitivity reaches 98% and 99% for carcinomas and adenomas, respectively.[277] Perforation as a result of DCBE has been reported at a rate of 1 per 25,000 studies.[278] Current ACS screening recommendations are for a barium enema every 5 years with subsequent colonoscopy if test results are positive. The NCCN does not include barium enema as a screening option.[273]

Colonoscopy

Examination of the entire colon by colonoscopy is the gold standard screening method. When performed by trained endoscopists, colonoscopy with polypectomy is a safe procedure with a perforation incidence of 0.1%, hemorrhage incidence of 0.3%, and a mortality of 0.01–0.03%. The cecum is visualized in up to 98.6% of patients, and a DCBE may be performed when the cecum is not reached.[279-284] Studies have shown that detecting and removing polyps reduce the incidence of colorectal malignancy, that detecting earlier lesions decreases disease-related mortality, and that fewer carcinomas develop in patients who have colonoscopy and polypectomy.[285,286] Colonoscopy is better than DCBE in detecting lesions <1 cm.[276] Furthermore, a tissue diagnosis or therapeutic intervention may be made at the time of initial evaluation. Colonoscopy also compares favorably with sigmoidoscopy because the entire colon may be directly visualized. In one study, a prevalence of 24% of new adenomas was found when 226 patients underwent colonoscopy within 1 year of flexible sigmoidoscopy. Advanced lesions proximal to the descending colon were found in 6% of these patients.[287] Current ACS screening recommendations are for a colonoscopy every 10 years.

CT colonography

CT colonography (virtual colonoscopy) is an emerging technique that uses three-dimensional reconstruction of the air-distended colon. At the National Naval Medical Center, in 1223 average-risk adults who underwent CT colonography followed by conventional colonoscopy, virtual colonoscopy was as good or better at detecting relevant lesions.[288] However, it may be less accurate in surveillance populations, and subsequent multi-institutional studies have failed to confirm the excellent results from this series. The major limitations include uncertain accuracy, need for full bowel preparation, and follow-up colonoscopy for tissue diagnosis of radiographic abnormalities. CT colonography as the primary method of screening also results in repeated radiation exposure to the patient. Because virtual colonoscopy is considerably time and labor intensive from the standpoint of the radiologist, active investigations into methods of automating the evaluation process are ongoing. Current ACS screening recommendations are for a virtual colonoscopy every 5 years with subsequent colonoscopy if a lesion is found. The NCCN does not include CT colonography as a screening option.[273]

Preoperative work-up and staging

The general physical examination remains a cornerstone in assessing a patient preoperatively to determine the extent of local disease, disclosing distant metastases, and appraising the general operative risk. Special interest should be paid to weight loss, pallor as a sign of anemia, and signs of portal hypertension. In addition, a complete work-up should include routine lab work, colonoscopy, chest X-ray, CT of the abdomen and pelvis, and transrectal ultrasound (TRUS) for those with rectal cancer.

Routine laboratory work

A complete blood count (CBC) may reveal the presence of anemia. Liver function tests (LFTs) may be abnormal in the case of liver metastases. Carcinoembryonic antigen (CEA) levels should be obtained as a baseline against which further values may be compared. Metastatic disease to the liver is often accompanied with very high levels of CEA, and levels surpassing 10 to 20 ng/mL are associated with increased chances of treatment failure.[289]

Colonoscopy

Colonoscopy remains the single most important investigation in the evaluation of colonic diseases. It allows assessment of tumor size, but not depth of invasion, as well as localization in the colon. Further histology from the tumor can be obtained, synchronous tumors are detected, and synchronous polyps may be removed. Synchronous carcinomas occur in 2–7% of patients and synchronous polyps 29.7% of the time.[290] It has been suggested that preoperative colonoscopy alters the operative procedure in 30% of patients.[291]

Radiologic evaluation

A chest X-ray evaluates for pulmonary lesions and serves as a rough guideline for cardiac as well as pulmonary status. The use of CT of the abdomen and pelvis in the preoperative evaluation of patients with colon cancer is controversial. It is our practice to obtain a CT in order to detect involvement of contiguous organs, paraaortic lymph nodes, and the liver. Abnormal LFT's are present in only 15% of patients with liver metastases and may be elevated without liver metastases in up to 40%.[292] Therefore, we do not believe LFT's are a useful screening tool for determining the need for obtaining a CT scan. Abdominal ultrasound can be used in select patient to identify liver metastases, ascites, and gross adenopathy.

PET, and now PET-CT, have emerged as potentially important imaging modalities for CRC. Using the glucose analog fluorodeoxyglucose, metabolically active tissues are visualized. The standardized uptake value can provide a semiquantitative determination to help discriminate benign from malignant disease. Although potentially useful in recurrent cancer, it has not been

helpful in the primary evaluation of patients with colon cancer due to false positive rates and high costs.

TRUS has become an important component of preoperative assessment in patients with rectal cancer. The layers of the rectal wall can be identified and the depth of penetration determined. Sensitivity ranges from 55% to 100% and specificity from 24% to 100% in different studies. The status of lymph nodes also can be predicted in 73–85%.[293] The depth of invasion and lymph node status is especially important if local excision is considered.

More recently, MRI has been utilized for the evaluation of rectal cancers, particularly for preoperative staging purposes. Compared to TRUS, MRI has similar sensitivity in determining depth of invasion within the rectal layers; however, ultrasound is superior in detecting local invasion into perirectal tissues and adjacent organs.[294] MRI and TRUS have highly similar sensitivities in detecting perirectal lymph node metastases, both of which are superior modalities compared to CT.[294] An advantage of MRI, however, is that it can be utilized to evaluate iliac, mesenteric, and retroperitoneal lymph nodes as well.

In addition, MRI has an emerging role in the prognostic risk stratification of patients preoperatively based on the likelihood of having involvement of the circumferential resection margin (CRM). The MERCURY study utilized preoperative MRI to access the relationship of the primary rectal tumor to the mesorectal fascia, choosing a distance of <1 mm to signify potentially involved margins.[295] Patients with potentially involved margins were found to have substantially shorter 5-year OS, DFS, and likelihood of developing local recurrence following resection. In fact, preoperative MRI evaluation of the CRM was found to have superior prognostic ability compared to AJCC TNM staging. Thus, MRI will likely continue to have an increasing role in the preoperative assessment of patients with rectal cancer. In the future, it may also become an integral part of neoadjuvant treatment strategies as a way to evaluate the response to preoperative chemotherapy or chemoradiation therapy.[296]

Staging

Staging systems are important for predicting outcomes, selecting patients for various therapies, and comparing therapies for patients across institutions. For a tumor to be considered as an invasive cancer and staged, it must penetrate through the muscularis mucosa. Malignant cells superficial to this layer are considered carcinoma *in situ*. In 1932, Dukes proposed a classification based on the degree of direct extension along with the presence or absence of regional lymphatic metastases for the staging of rectal cancer. The TNM classification was proposed by the American College of Surgeons' Commission on Cancer to incorporate findings at laparotomy, and over multiple iterations, it has largely replaced Dukes' classification in clinical use (Table 2).

The AJCC has settled on two grading classifications, low grade (well and moderately differentiated) and high grade (poorly and undifferentiated). DNA ploidy assessment is the measurement of the quantum amount of DNA in cells. Diploidy is correlated with good prognosis, while aneuploidy is correlated with poor prognosis. Bowel perforation and elevated preoperative CEA are associated with poorer prognosis.

Lastly, as the genetic determinants of colon cancer become more thoroughly understood, there has been increasing interest in profiling the disease at the genomic level for prognostic purposes. Initially, studies evaluating particular genetic alterations, typically focusing on p53 expression and K-ras mutation status, produced

Table 2 AJCC 7th edition TNM staging system for colorectal cancer.

TX	Primary tumor cannot be assessed
T0	No evidence of primary tumor
Tis	Carcinoma *in situ*, intraepithelial or tumor invades into lamina propria
T1	Tumor invades into submucosa
T2	Tumor invades into muscularis propria
T3	Tumor invades through muscularis propria
T4a	Tumor perforates visceral peritoneum
T4b	Tumor directly invades other structures
NX	Regional lymph nodes cannot be assessed
N0	No regional lymph nodes
N1	1–3 lymph nodes
N1a	1 regional lymph node
N1b	2–3 regional lymph nodes
N1c	Tumor deposits in subserosa, mesentery, or nonperitonealized regional tissue without nodal metastasis
N2	4 or more lymph nodes
N2a	4–6 regional lymph nodes
N2b	7 or more regional lymph nodes
M0	No distant metastases
M1	Distant metastases
M1a	Metastasis confined to one organ or site
M1b	Metastasis in more than one organ or site or within the peritoneal surface

Stage	Depth	Nodal status	Distant metastasis
Stage 0	Tis	N0	M0
Stage I	T1, T2	N0	M0
Stage IIA	T3	N0	M0
Stage IIB	T4	N0	M0
Stage IIC	T4b	N0	M0
Stage IIIA	T1–T2	N1/N1c	M0
Stage IIIB	T1	N2a	M0
	T3–T4a	N1/N1c	M0
	T2–T3	N2a	M0
	T1–T2	N2b	M0
Stage IIIC	T4a	N2a	M0
	T3–T4a	N2b	M0
	T4b	N1–N2	M0
Stage IVA	Any T	Any N	M1a
Stage IVB	Any T	Any N	M1b

Source: Edge 2010.[297] Reproduced with permission of Springer.

conflicting results and were thus unable to add significantly to conventional staging systems.[296] More recently, focus has shifted toward assays that profile many different genes in parallel. Oncotype DX®, for example, is a multigene assay that utilizes polymerase chain reaction (PCR) to quantify the gene expression of 12 genes from an individual tumor to predict disease recurrence following resection.[298] These genes were selected based on an analysis of over 1800 colon cancers (stage II and III) as part of the National Surgical Adjuvant Breast and Bowel Project.[299] Subsequently, two prospective studies have validated the prognostic ability of this platform to predict recurrence risk in patients with stage II and III colon cancer; although they were unable to validate its usefulness in predicting response to chemotherapy.[300,301] As these assays improve, gene profiling will almost certainly become an important part of cancer staging in the near future. Although the role of multigene assays is yet to be determined, a 2014 prospective multicenter study evaluating the effect of providing an Oncotype DX® recurrence score on physician behavior (decision to use adjuvant chemotherapy among patients with stage IIa colon cancer) demonstrated that the score altered the treatment plan in over 40% of the cases.[302] While these results do not confirm any benefit to Oncotype DX in making treatment decisions, they do suggest that there is confidence in the medical oncology community that multigene profiling can provide useful, objective information that may ultimately help guide the need for certain therapies.

Surgical management of CRC

Management of carcinoma in a polyp

Colon cancers that appear to be confined to an adenomatous polyp ("malignant polyps") have their invasion limited to the submucosa. Their propensity for lymph node metastasis appears to be related to a number of histopathologic features, including grade, presence of perineural/perivascular invasion, and overall gross morphology (i.e., sessile vs. pedunculated).

The Haggitt classification system is used to define the depth of involvement of carcinoma into a polyp (Table 3). The risk of lymph node metastasis in Haggitt level 1, 2, and 3 lesions is <1%, and these lesions can usually be managed with complete endoscopic excision and India ink tattooing of the polypectomy site.[303] In these cases, careful colonoscopic surveillance of the polypectomy site is recommended. However, lymphovascular invasion, poor differentiation, or cancer close to the polypectomy resection margin (<2 mm) are usually an indication for a colectomy because of the increased risk of lymph node metastasis. Haggit level 4 lesions have an increased incidence of lymph node metastasis (12–25%) and should be managed with a colectomy.[303] In general, sessile polyps of the colon containing cancer should be managed with a colectomy as they are by definition Haggit level 4.

Most polyps throughout the colon can be removed through the colonoscope using the snare polypectomy technique. The polyp is visualized through the colonoscope and the snare wire is looped

Table 3 Haggitt classification of malignant polyps.

Haggit level	Characteristics
0	Carcinoma *in situ*
1	Carcinoma invading into submucosa but limited to head of polyp
2	Carcinoma invading level of neck of polyp
3	Carcinoma invading stalk
4	Carcinoma invading submucosa below the stalk (above the muscularis propria)

around the polyp and gently tightened while the electric current is applied. Whenever possible the polyp is retrieved for histology. When performed by trained endoscopists, colonoscopy with polypectomy is a safe procedure, with a perforation incidence of 0.3–1% and a hemorrhage incidence of 0.7–2.5%.[304]

Standard resection margins and techniques

Bowel preparation

Despite recent evidence challenging the benefit of mechanical bowel preparation, it remains a cornerstone in modern colorectal surgery. Mechanical cleansing may be accomplished by the use of vigorous laxatives along with repeated enemas until clearing. Until recently, an oral lavage with a polyethylene glycol hypertonic electrolyte solution such as GoLYTELY was used extensively. More recently, oral phospho-soda preparations have become increasingly popular, but their use can be associated with fluid and electrolyte abnormalities.

Antibiotic administration

Perioperative antibiotics can be delivered both orally and intravenously, the former typically employed in combination with mechanical bowel preparation. Intravenous antibiotics are utilized to prevent surgical site infections, which are particularly common among patients undergoing colorectal surgery. Although the exact antibiotic regimen remains debated, it should cover both aerobic and anaerobic bacteria. The enhanced recovery after surgery (ERAS) group recommends a single dose of antibiotics within one hour of surgery, and there is level 1 evidence to support this guideline.[305] While an initial single dose provides equivalent prophylaxis compared to multidose regimens, subsequent dosing may be required in prolonged cases.[305] Oral antibiotics have traditionally been used for two purposes: to act as a cathartic alongside mechanical bowel preparation and to eradicate potentially pathologic intraluminal bacteria. A 2014 Cochrane Review concluded that combined oral and intravenous antibiotic prophylaxis is superior to either intravenous antibiotics alone (HR 0.56) or oral antibiotics alone (HR 0.56). It remains uncertain whether oral antibiotic prophylaxis is necessary if the colon is emptied (complete bowel preparation) prior to surgery.[306]

Right-sided colon cancers

Cancers of the right colon account for up to 30% of primary CRCs.[307] Patients with adenocarcinoma involving the cecum or ascending colon who do not have HNPCC or other synchronous lesions should be treated with a right hemicolectomy (Figure 1a). The ileocolic, right colic, and right branch of the middle colic vessels should be ligated near their origins to assure adequate lymphadenectomy. Approximately 5 to 10 cm of distal small intestine should be resected in continuity with the right colon to assure adequate blood supply at the stapled edge of the small intestine.

Transverse colon cancers

Transverse colon cancers are relatively uncommon, accounting for only 10% of colorectal primaries.[307] Lesions of the proximal and midtransverse colon are usually best managed with an extended right hemicolectomy involving ligation of the ileocolic, right colic, and middle colic vessels (Figure 1b). The ascending colon, hepatic flexure, transverse colon, and splenic flexures are removed with anastomosis of the ileum to the descending colon. It is advisable to avoid an anastomosis between the hepatic and splenic flexure because of concerns over adequacy of blood supply and tension at the anastomosis.

Left-sided colon cancers

Lesions of the splenic flexure and descending colon are also uncommon, accounting for 15% of colorectal primaries.[307] Splenic flexure cancers may be managed with an extended right or left hemicolectomy (Figure 1c). Cancers in the descending colon may be managed with a left hemicolectomy involving division of the left colic artery, preservation of the left branch of the middle colic artery, and anastomosis of the distal transverse colon to the distal sigmoid colon. Alternatively, a left hemicolectomy may be performed with ligation of the inferior mesenteric vessels and an anastomosis between the transverse colon and the upper rectum.

Sigmoid colon cancers

Tumors of the sigmoid colon account for 25% of colorectal primaries.[307] These tumors are usually removed by means of an anterior sigmoid colectomy, which usually involves division of the inferior mesenteric artery either above or below the left colic artery and the superior rectal arteries within the upper mesorectum with anastomosis of the descending colon to the upper rectum (Figure 1d). Large, bulky sigmoid cancers located above the peritoneal reflection but at the level of the pelvic inlet present a unique challenge as their posterolateral borders abut the ureters, hypogastric nerves, and iliac vessels. Proper preoperative planning based on optimal imaging and consideration of ureteral stent placement is essential.

Subtotal colectomy

This resection involves the removal of the entire colon to the rectum with an ileorectal anastomosis (IRA). This procedure is indicated for multiple synchronous colonic tumors that are not confined to a single anatomical distribution for selected patients with FAP with minimal rectal involvement (discussed below) or for selected patients with HNPCC and colon cancer.

Total proctocolectomy

The surgical treatment of FAP depends on the age of the patient and the polyp density in the rectum. Surgical options include proctocolectomy with Brooke ileostomy, total abdominal colectomy with IRA, or restorative proctocolectomy with ileal pouch–anal anastomosis (IPAA). Proctocolectomy with continent ileostomy is rarely performed today. Total abdominal colectomy with IRA has a low complication rate, provides good functional results, and is a viable option for patients with fewer than 20 adenomas in the rectum. These patients must be observed with 6-month proctoscopic examinations to remove polyps and detect signs of cancer. If rectal polyps become too numerous, completion proctectomy, when technically possible, is warranted. The Cleveland Clinic has recently evaluated their registry of patients with FAP who were treated with IRA or IPAA. Prior to the use of IPAA for patients with high rectal polyp burdens, the risk of cancer in the retained rectum

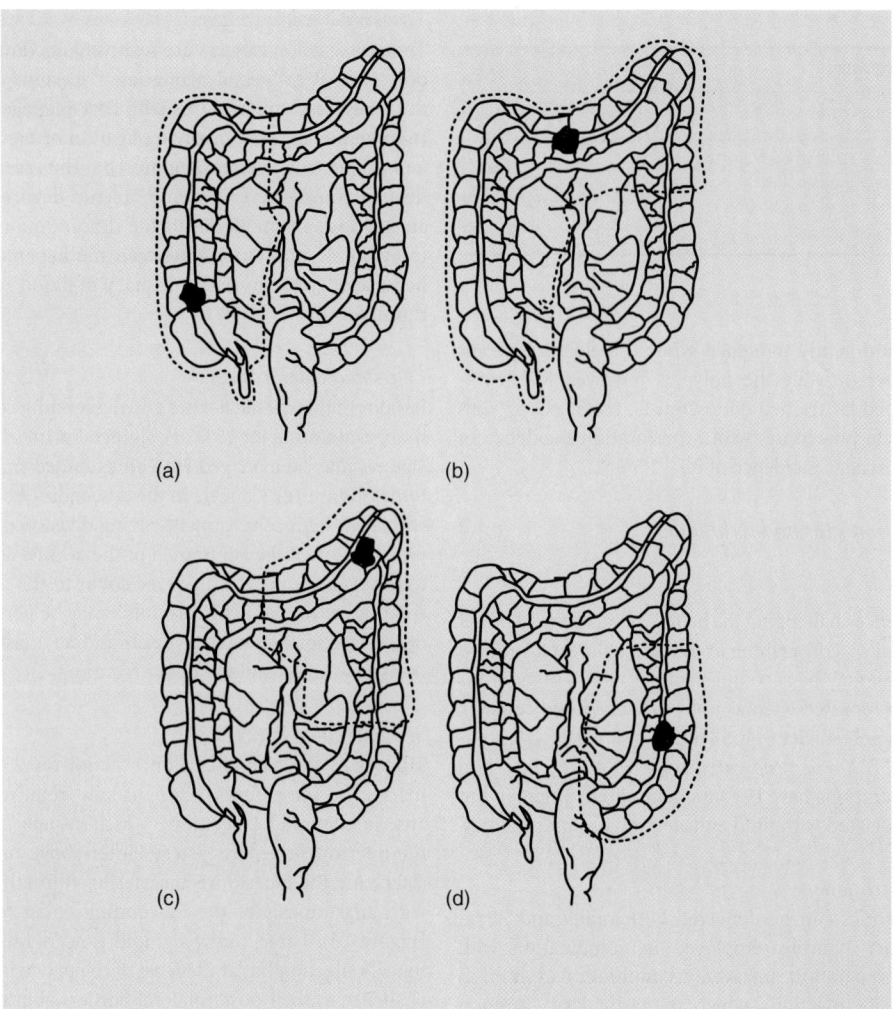

Figure 1 Extent of resection for colon carcinoma: (a) Cecal or ascending colon cancer; (b) transverse colon cancer; (c) splenic fl exure colon cancer; (d) sigmoid colon cancer. Abbreviations: ICA, ileocolic artery; IMA, inferior mesenteric artery; LCA, left colic artery; MCA, middle colic artery; RCA, right colic artery; SA, sigmoidal arteries; SHA, superior hemorrhoidal (rectal) artery.

was 12.9% at a median follow-up of over 17 years.[308] Alternatively, for patients treated with IPAA or the selected use of IRA (for those with small rectal polyp burdens), none developed rectal cancer in the remaining rectum at a median follow-up of 5 years. Restorative proctocolectomy with IPAA has the advantage of removing all or nearly all large intestine mucosa at risk of cancer while preserving transanal defecation. Complication rates are low when the procedure is done in large centers, but morbidity includes incontinence, multiple loose stools, impotence, retrograde ejaculation, dyspareunia, and pouchitis. Approximately 7% of patients have to be converted to permanent ileostomy due to complications from the procedure.[308]

Rectal cancers

The surgical approach to rectal tumors depends upon depth of invasion and distance from the anal verge. The four categories include transanal approaches, transsacral approaches, LAR with total mesorectal excision (TME), and APR.

Local excision

Early studies of local excision have shown up to a 97% local control rate and 80% DFS for properly selected individuals.[309] Local treatment is best applied to T1 rectal cancers within 10 cm

of the anal verge, tumors <3 cm in diameter involving less than one-fourth of the circumference of the rectal wall, highly mobile exophytic tumors, and tumors of low histologic grade. The decision to use local excision alone or to employ adjuvant therapy after local excision is based on the pathological characteristics of the primary cancer and the potential for micrometastases in draining lymph nodes. T1 lesions have positive lymph nodes in up to 18% of cases, whereas the rate for T2 and T3 lesions is up to 38% and 70%, respectively. T2 tumors treated with local resection alone can have recurrence rates of 15% to 44%.[309] It is therefore our practice to treat T1 lesions with poor prognostic features and all T2 tumors with radical surgery.

Local excision of distal rectal cancers can be accomplished by transanal excision, posterior proctectomy (Kraske procedure), or transanal endoscopic microsurgery. Transanal excision is the most straightforward approach and involves using the perirectal fat as the deep plane of dissection to achieve adequate circumferential margins of 1 cm. The Kraske procedure can be used for tumors in the middle and upper rectum and is more suitable for larger rectal lesions than transanal excision. In this procedure, a perineal incision is made just above the anus, the coccyx is removed, fascia divided, and a proctectomy performed. The disadvantage of this procedure is fistula formation and potential to seed the posterior wound with malignant cells. Transanal endoscopic microsurgery provides accessibility to tumors of the middle and upper rectum that would otherwise require a laparotomy or transsacral approach. This approach can be used for selected lesions up to 15 cm from the anal verge. The procedure is technically demanding and requires special equipment, which is expensive and therefore has limited its acceptance in the United States.

Low anterior resection

As surgical treatment for rectal cancer has improved over the past 2 decades, it has become evident that sphincter preservation is feasible without sacrificing oncologic outcomes. The procedure involves removal of the sigmoid colon and the involved rectum, with ligation of the inferior mesenteric artery at its origin. The splenic flexure is routinely mobilized and the reconstruction is performed using the descending colon. The use of the sigmoid colon is discouraged, as the thickened and hypertrophic muscle of the sigmoid is less compliant than the descending colon. The technical feasibility of the LAR was increased with the advent of circular stapling devices, lighted retractors, and the knowledge that distal mucosal margins of resection of 2 cm were adequate. The mesorectal margin, however, should be at least 5 cm distal to the inferior aspect of the tumor or to the end of the mesorectum at the pelvic floor. The technique of TME, which involves sharp excision and extirpation of the mesorectum by dissecting outside the investing fascia of the mesorectum, optimizes the oncologic operation by not only removing draining lymph nodes but also maximizing lateral resection margins around the tumor. Neoadjuvant therapy in properly selected patients is effective in converting probable APRs into sphincter-preserving operations.[310]

Abdominal perineal resection

For patients who have cancers that overlap or abut the sphincter or who are incontinent of stool preoperatively, a combined approach of transabdominal and transperineal dissection is performed to remove the rectal specimen en bloc. Once the rectal specimen is removed via the perineal opening, the perineum is sutured closed and a permanent colostomy is created.

Synchronous and metachronous lesions

The incidence of synchronous colon cancers ranges from 2% to 11%, and incidence of synchronous adenomatous polyps may exceed 30%.[307] For lesions that are widely separated, preservation of colonic length via more than one anastomosis is desirable as long as the adequacy of the required individual cancer resections is not compromised. An alternative to multiple anastomoses is a subtotal colectomy with an ileorectal or ileosigmoid anastomosis. Metachronous colon cancers, defined as those detected more than 6 months following the management of the index lesion, may be managed with either partial or subtotal colectomy as dictated by the location of the lesions.

Lymphadenectomy

An appropriate lymph node dissection should extend to the origin of the primary vessel draining the portion of the colon incorporating the cancer. Resection of a lesion located near two major vessels should involve removal of the two major vessels along with the associated lymph nodes in an en bloc fashion. Apical lymph nodes at the origin of a primary vessel should be removed when feasible and tagged for pathologic analysis. Suspicious lymph nodes outside the field of resection should be sampled and resected when positive. Although not always feasible, efforts should be made by the pathologist to examine a minimum of 12 lymph nodes.[311,312] This allows

for the most accurate staging, which can be used to appropriately select patients for adjuvant therapies.[313] In addition, the absolute number of lymph nodes examined has itself been shown to be associated with survival.[313] Although several series have demonstrated that sentinel node mapping and biopsy is feasible in patients with colon cancer, its true clinical utility in the management of patients with colon cancer awaits further investigation.[314]

Laparoscopic colectomy

Laparoscopic resection of the colon was first described in 1990.[315] The proposed benefits to laparoscopic colectomy include a shorter recovery time and less narcotic use than the traditional open procedure. The technique of a laparoscopically assisted colon resection consists of an intracorporeal approach to explore the abdomen and mobilize the colon. The bowel is then exteriorized through a small incision for extracorporeal resection and anastomosis. There was some initial concerns regarding the ability to achieve an adequate oncologic resection and the frequency of port-site recurrences using the laparoscopic technique for colon cancer.[316] However, the results of several large studies have provided solid evidence demonstrating laparoscopic colectomy in patients with colon cancer provides equivalent oncologic outcomes and superior short-term perioperative morbidity compared to open colectomy.[317-326]

Five prospective randomized trials, Barcelona, Australasian, Clinical Outcomes of Surgical Therapy Study Group (COST), Conventional versus Laparoscopic-Assisted Surgery in Colorectal Cancer (CLASICC), and Colon Cancer Laparoscopic or Open Resection (COLOR), have reported long-term follow-up data on the equivalence of laparoscopic colectomy to open colectomy for colon cancer.[317-322,324,325] The first long-term cancer data from the single-center Barcelona study showed cancer-related survival was significantly higher in the laparoscopically assisted group than in the open surgery group.[317] This was accounted for by the significant improvement in cancer-related survival observed in patients with stage III colon cancer, while there were no differences in patients with stage I or II disease. However, the COST and CLASICC trials showed no such differences between the two groups.[318,319] In a recent follow-up report of the COST trial, 5-year OS, 5-year DFS, recurrence rates, and sites of first recurrence were similar between groups.[324] Similarly, in a recent follow-up report from the CLASICC trial (which also included patients who underwent laparoscopically assisted excision of rectal cancer), there were no differences at 3 years in OS, DFS, or local recurrence between the laparoscopic-assisted surgery group and the conventionally treated (open) group.[325] The COLOR trial demonstrated similar rates of positive surgical margins and number of regional lymph nodes retrieved, as well as equivalent 3-year DFS and OS. Short-term postoperative benefits for laparoscopy included earlier recovery of bowel function, need for fewer analgesics, and shorter hospital stay.[322] The Australasia trial demonstrated similar rates of 5-year OS and and RFS.[323] In all five studies, hospital stay was shorter while operating time for laparoscopically assisted colectomy was longer. The length of ileus was significantly less with laparoscopic colectomy in both the CLASICC and COST trials, while the COST trial also observed significantly less time of use of oral analgesics with laparoscopic colectomy.[318,319] While these short-term patient benefits have been observed, it is unclear if long-term patient benefits exist. In the CLASICC trial, no significant difference in the quality of life (QOL) at 3 years for all scales was observed between the two groups.[325] In a meta-analysis of the four trials which included over 1500 patients, 3-year DFS and OS after laparoscopically assisted or open resection were similar, and disease-free OS rates for stages I, II, and III evaluated separately did not differ between the two treatments.[326] Laparoscopic-assisted colectomy when performed by experienced surgeons has proven to be an equivalent oncologic operation compared to open colectomy for patients with colon cancer.[327]

Future directions in the study of the laparoscopic technique include maturation of more long-term data, appropriate patient selection for laparoscopic versus open procedures, and evaluating the cost-effectiveness of the laparoscopic technique. The rates of conversion to an open procedure from the COLOR, COST, and CLASICC trial were 17%, 21%, and 29%, respectively.[318–320] Patients in the CLASICC trial treated with a converted procedure had higher complication rates making the selection of appropriate patients for laparoscopic surgery important.[319] The cost-effectiveness of the laparoscopic technique given the longer operating time and the advanced surgical training required also requires further evaluation.

The investigational experience with laparoscopic rectal cancer resection is not as complete as the data for laparoscopic colectomy. Surgical resection is an extremely important treatment modality for rectal cancer. The standard for middle and low rectal cancers is precise TME as described by Heald.[328] TME and adequacy of resection margins are associated with low recurrence and optimal survival.[329] Laparoscopic resection of rectal cancer must be able to achieve the same oncologic outcomes. The laparoscopic technique for rectal cancer involves transection of the distal bowel and mesorectum intracorporeally and the division of the remaining mesentery and proximal bowel done extracorporeally. An intracorporeal end-to-end anastomosis is performed by positioning the anvil of the stapler in the descending colon and inserting the circular stapler through the rectum.[330,331] For low rectal cancers requiring laparoscopically assisted APR, the mobilized rectum with mesorectum is retrieved through the perineal incision in the traditional fashion and the perineal wound is closed primarily.[331] Currently, laparoscopically assisted resection of rectal cancer has not been definitely proven to be as oncologically effective as open surgery although currently available data strongly favors such a conclusion.

Several single-center case series of laparoscopically assisted resection of rectal cancer have reported on the safety and feasibility of using the laparoscopic approach.[331–334] There have been several prospective randomized trials comparing laparoscopic and open techniques for resection of rectal and rectosigmoid cancers including the subset of patients in the CLASICC trial.[319,325,330,335] An initial observation in the CLASICC trial was a nonsignificant increase in the rate of positive CRM in patients undergoing laparoscopically assisted anterior resection compared to those undergoing standard open LAR. This difference was not seen in patients undergoing APR. However, in a follow-up report, the higher positivity of CRM did not translate into an increased incidence of local recurrence.[325] This finding may have been a result of small numbers of patients and needs further investigation. Other results from this trial were discussed above in the laparoscopic colectomy section. A 2004 trial of patients with rectosigmoid carcinomas randomized patients to either laparoscopic-assisted or open LAR (APR was not included).[330] Results included no significant differences in 5-year survival, 5-year DFS, or tumor recurrence.[330] Postoperative recovery was significantly better for the laparoscopic group, while the operative time was significantly longer and the cost higher in the laparoscopic group.[330] Most recently and definitively, the Laparoscopic Versus Open Surgery for Rectal Cancer (COLOR II) Trial was a multicenter, randomized, intention-to-treat-based trial comparing short-term perioperative and oncologic outcomes for laparoscopic and open resection for rectal cancers.[335] The trial included over 1100 patients and demonstrated improvements in operative blood loss, return of bowel function, and hospital length of stay. In addition, the two groups had similar rates of complete resection, including CRM positivity. Long-term survival is not yet available from this study, but short-term findings are encouraging that laparoscopic resection of rectal cancers, in appropriately selected patients and among experienced surgeons, can provide equivalent oncologic outcomes compared to traditional open techniques. Two meta-analyses have also been performed.[336,337] Aziz et al. analyzed a total of over 2000 patients and found no significant differences in the proportion of patients with positive radial margins or the number of lymph nodes harvested when considering the laparoscopic rectal cancer surgery, open rectal cancer, laparoscopic APR, and open APR groups.[336] Time to stoma function, first bowel movement, and length of hospital stay were significantly reduced after laparoscopic surgery. In the set of patients undergoing laparoscopically assisted APR, a reduced rate of postoperative wound infection was observed.[336] In the other meta-analysis, short-term outcomes reported included a significantly lower morbidity but longer operating times in the laparoscopically resected group.[337] In addition, there was no difference in wound healing, leakage rates, or positive margins between the two groups.[337] Thus, increasing evidence supports the equality of laparoscopically assisted resection of rectal cancer to traditional open surgery.

In order to establish that laparoscopically assisted resection of rectal cancer is not inferior to open resection, more long-term data on cancer recurrence and survival are needed. Furthermore, similar issues of cost-effectiveness of appropriate patient selection also apply to laparoscopic resection of rectal cancer as conversion rates from the two randomized trials were reported to be 23% and 34%. The laparoscopic procedure also requires longer operating time and advanced technical skill.[325,326] In order to further address concerns about the use of laparoscopically assisted resection of rectal cancer, the American College of Surgery Oncology Group has developed a prospective, randomized phase III trial to determine if laparoscopic surgery is a technically and oncologically safe approach to the resection of rectal cancer (ACSOG-Z6051).[338] The trial has recently been completed, and short-term results are expected soon. As long-term data from this trial become available, a more definitive evaluation of the technique will be established, which can more clearly elucidate the role of laparoscopic surgery for rectal cancer.

Robotic colectomy

There are limited data regarding robotic colorectal surgery, either in comparison to laparoscopic or traditional open surgery. The only randomized data have come from a small study comparing robotic right colectomy to standard laparoscopic right colectomy,[339] which demonstrated equivalent lymph node harvest, margin positivity rate, and need for conversion to open surgery between the two groups. Most other data have come from small, single-institution studies. With regard to retrospective comparative effectiveness studies evaluating robotic versus open colectomy, robotic resections—like laparoscopic resections—have been associated with improvements in perioperative morbidity and other short-term outcomes such as return of bowel function, wound complications, and hospital length of stay.[340–343] However, robotic colectomy has been associated with longer operative times in nearly all studies to date, as well as increased costs of care.[340] These latter two shortcomings may improve as centers develop more experience with the complexities of the robotic system. In comparison to laparoscopic colectomy, robotic resections have been associated with similar lymph node harvest, specimen length, and need for conversion to open surgery.[344] Even compared to laparoscopy, studies to date indicate that robotic colectomy is associated with increased operative room time and increased operating room costs.[344,345] The increase in OR time may be the result of more intracorporeal anastomoses being performed in robotic colectomies, as well as time associated with set-up of the laparoscopic system.[345] Although there is a near complete lack of randomized data, studies to date indicate that there is no difference in short-term oncologic outcomes for robotic colon resections between either laparoscopic or open surgery.

Robotic rectal surgery has several theoretical advantages compared to both traditional open and laparoscopic techniques. In comparison to open surgery, these include a better morbidity profile, as well as improvements in short-term quality metrics such as hospital length of stay and readmission rates. In comparison to laparoscopic rectal resections, robotics may offer lower rates of conversion to open surgery. While there are no randomized studies to date, several single-institutional reviews have demonstrated that robotic rectal resections can be performed safely among experienced surgeons in appropriately selected patients.[342,343,346] In the largest retrospective comparative effectiveness study, robotic LAR has resulted in lower conversion rates and serious complication rates as compared to laparoscopic LAR.[342] Improvements were also appreciated in completeness of the TME. Given the retrospective nature of this study, however, these improvements may be the result of patient selection bias. Currently, the Robotic Versus Laparoscopic Resection for Rectal Cancer (ROLARR) Trial is ongoing, which will provide level 1 evidence as to the perioperative complications, short-term mortality, and 3-year DFS and OS, as well as sexual function assessment for robotic versus laparoscopic rectal resections.[347] Study results are expected in 2016. In the interim, robotic rectal resections should be considered only a technique under investigation, best left to centers and surgeons with experience in advanced minimally invasive surgery.

Perforated colon cancers

Patients with perforated colon cancers often present with peritonitis. In this setting, the goals of surgical management are to remove the diseased segment of colon and prevent ongoing peritoneal contamination. Following resection and thorough irrigation of the peritoneal cavity, options for subsequent management include proximal diversion with creation of a mucous fistula/Hartmann pouch or primary anastomosis with proximal diversion via loop ileostomy. Perforated colon cancer is associated with a high rate of local recurrence and low rate of OS.[348]

Obstructing colon cancers

Cancer is the most common cause of large bowel obstruction.[349] Obstructing right and transverse colon cancers are generally managed with a right hemicolectomy and primary anastomosis. Left-sided colon cancers can be managed with either a single operation or a two-stage procedure.[349] The options for single-stage management include segmental resection or subtotal colectomy with IRA. Subtotal colectomy is attractive because it removes the remaining of the potentially compromised colon, but it is a more extensive operation and may be associated with five to six bowel movements per day. On-table lavage has been used in the setting of segmental resection for obstruction, but postoperative complication rates remain a concern. A two-stage procedure involves first resection of the primary tumor with proximal diversion and then creation of a mucous fistula or Hartmann's pouch. The second stage, performed at a later time, involves reanastomosis of the colon. An alternative two-stage approach in select patients with an obstructing left colon lesion is resection with

Test	Recommendation
History and physical	Every 3–6 months for 5 years; then annually
Serum CEA	Every 3–6 for 5 years
Colonoscopy	Perform 1 year after resection, followed by every 5 years if the first is normal. For patients with rectal cancer who have not received radiation, a rectosigmoidoscopy should be performed every 6 months for 2–5 years
Computed tomography	Annually for 3 years or every 6–12 months in high risk (must include pelvis in patients with rectal cancer)

primary anastomosis and proximal fecal diversion with a loop ileostomy.[349]

Colonic stenting has recently been established as an option for patients with malignant colon obstruction.[350,351] Although it does not represent a long-term solution to the malignant colonic obstruction, stenting is useful in those whose prognosis is limited by the presence of metastatic disease or comorbidities. Stenting has also been used to allow transient relief of obstruction and bowel preparation with or without colonoscopic evaluation of the proximal colon before planned resection.[350,351]

Synchronous distant metastases

The liver is the most common site for colon cancer metastasis, and approximately 17% of patients will present with synchronous liver metastasis.[307] Concomitant resection of colon and liver lesions may be undertaken safely in selected patients. Alternatively, management of liver metastasis may be dealt with at a subsequent operation. Systemic chemotherapy is also an essential component of therapy in these patients and will be discussed below.

Surveillance following resection

The goal of postoperative surveillance following resection of colon adenocarcinoma is identification of asymptomatic recurrences or new primaries that will allow for subsequent early treatment and lead to an improvement in survival. An expert panel assembled by the American Society of Clinical Oncology (ASCO) examined the evidence of supporting the role of various screening tests following resection of CRC (Table 4).[352] Interestingly, CBC, LFTs, FOBT, and CT scanning were not considered essential components of surveillance. With these guidelines in mind, surveillance should be individualized depending on factors unique to a given case, including comorbidities and patient anxiety.

Local recurrence

Local recurrence following resection of colonic adenocarcinoma occurs in approximately 4% of cases with the highest rates in advanced-stage tumors.[353] Although these patients generally have a poor survival, surgical resection of locoregional recurrence can result in long-term survival in up to 15% of patients.[353] Best results are obtained in patients with isolated small recurrences (<5 cm) that can be resected with negative margins.

Adjuvant therapy for CRC

5-Fluorouracil-based regimens

The antifolate 5-FU has been the cornerstone of chemotherapy for CRC since the 1960s. A metabolite of 5-FU, fluorodeoxyuridine monophosphate (FdUMP), inhibits thymidylate synthase (TS) and thus interferes with DNA synthesis.[354] 5-FU is also incorporated into RNA, which disrupts protein synthesis.[354] Studies, however, did not show a survival advantage for adjuvant 5-FU until it was combined with a biomodulator. Leucovorin (LV) (folinic acid), levamisole (an antihelminthic agent), and methotrexate were all explored as modulators of 5-FU.[355-359] LV has been accepted as the standard biomodulator and increases cytotoxicity by stabilizing the FdUMP/TS complex and increasing the intracellular pool of reduced folate.

Multiple prospective trials have shown the clinical benefit of postoperative 5-FU in combination with either LV or levamisole.[355,356,358,359] The National Surgical Adjuvant Breast and Bowel Project C-03 trial showed that 6 months of 5-FU and LV each given weekly at 500 mg/m² for 6 of 8 weeks (Roswell Park regimen) were superior to combination therapy with methyl 1-[2-chloroethyl-3-(4methyl-cyclohexyl)] (CCNU), vincristine, and 5-FU.[359] The incremental increases in DFS from 64% to 73% and in OS from 77% to 84% were proportionally similar to other randomized trials with 5-FU and LV.[359]

There are numerous 5-FU dosing schedules. In the adjuvant setting, these include bolus daily for 5 days every 4 weeks, the so-called Mayo Clinic regimen; weekly for 6 of every 8 weeks, or Roswell Park regimen; and infusional schedules. Unlike the metastatic setting, continuous infusion 5-FU (CIFU) has not shown superiority over bolus-type adjuvant regimens. There was no difference in DFS or OS, but there was a suggestion that it may have an improved toxicity profile.[360,361]

The convenience of oral therapy and the prospect of avoiding long-term intravenous access complications, such as thrombosis and infection, have stimulated development of oral fluoropyrimidines. Capecitabine is a fluoropyrimidine carbamate that is converted to 5-FU in a three-step enzymatic cascade. Preclinical studies had shown that capecitabine exhibits selectivity for neoplastic cells because the final enzymatic conversion involves thymidine phosphorylase, which is preferentially expressed in tumor as opposed to normal tissues.[362,363] Twice-daily oral administration simulates continuous infusion of 5-FU without the costs and inconvenience of a pump.

The X-ACT trial showed that capecitabine was at least equivalent to bolus 5-FU in the adjuvant setting.[362] This noninferiority trial randomized 1987 patients with resected stage III colon cancer to 6 months of adjuvant capecitabine 1250 mg/m² twice daily for 2 weeks of a 3-week schedule or to bolus 5-FU 425 mg/m² and LV 20 mg/m² daily days 1 through 5 of a 28-day cycle (Mayo regimen). The 3-year DFS was 64.2% in the capecitabine arm compared with 60.6% in the bolus 5-FU arm. With a hazard ratio of 0.87% and a $p < 0.001$, this study met its primary endpoint of equivalent DFS. The side-effect profiles are slightly different, with capecitabine having an increased risk for hand–foot syndrome but markedly improved reductions in neutropenia and stomatitis seen in the bolus regimen.[362]

Oxaliplatin-based regimens

Oxaliplatin is a third-generation platinum compound that cross-links DNA and induces apoptosis. Oxaliplatin has properties that are distinct from other platinum compounds such as cisplatin and carboplatin. The preclinical models showed both activity in cisplatin-resistant CRC cell lines and synergism when combined with 5-FU.[364] Oxaliplatin causes little nephrotoxicity, ototoxicity, and alopecia but shares bone marrow suppressive properties and has its own sensory neuropathy that is typically reversible, cumulative, and exacerbated by exposure to cold.[364-367]

Oxaliplatin was quickly moved to the adjuvant setting after initial studies showed its efficacy in the metastatic setting. The MOSAIC

trial randomized 2246 stage II (node negative) and stage III patients to receive either oxaliplatin, folinic acid, and 5-FU (FOLFOX-4) combination or infusional 5-FU/LV.[364,366,367] The infusional 5-FU was given every 2 weeks on a 28-day cycle as LV 200 mg/m² over 2 h followed by bolus 5-FU 400 mg/m² and then a 22-h infusion of 5-FU at 600 mg/m² on days 1 and 2. FOLFOX-4 included the same regimen of 5-FU/LV with addition of oxaliplatin at 85 mg/m² over 2 h every 2 weeks of a 28-day cycle.[364] The probability of being free of disease at three years was 78.2% in the FOLFOX-4 arm compared with 72.9% in the infusional 5-FU/LV arm. Subgroup analysis revealed that stage III patients derived more benefit as evidenced by 3-year DFS (72% receiving FOLFOX-4 vs. 65% receiving 5-FU/LV, $p = 0.0002$) than stage II patients (87% receiving FOLFOX-4 vs 84% receiving 5-FU/LV, $p = $ ns). Oxaliplatin regimens are still restricted by its dose-limiting toxicity of neuropathy, which seriously affected 12% of patients during the trial but the percentage of patients affected dropped to 0.5% after 18 months.[364,366] In 2009, long-term results from the MOSAIC trial were published, which demonstrated statistically significant improvements in 5-year DFS (73.3 vs 67.4%).[368] Among patients with stage III disease, there was a corresponding improvement in 6-year OS (72.9 vs 68.7%); however, there was no statistically significant difference in OS for patients with stage II disease. Furthermore, a subgroup analysis of the MOSAIC trial demonstrated that elderly patients (70–75 years old) with both stage II and III disease did not benefit from the addition of oxaliplatin to 5-FU/LV (hazard ratio 1.1 for OS).[369] The benefit of oxaliplatin does not appear to be dependent on the schedule of 5-FU/LV. NSABP C-07 randomized 2407 patients with stage II/III colon cancer to bolus weekly 5-FU/LV (Roswell Park regimen) or to FLOX (the same 5-FU/LV regimen with biweekly oxaliplatin).[365] The improvement in the hazard ratios and DFS was similar to that seen in the MOSAIC trial. The probability of being alive and free of disease at 3 years was 76.5% in the oxaliplatin arm compared with 71.6% in the control arm.[365] Although the efficacy of FLOX looked similar to the infusional 5-FU used in the MOSAIC trial, it does appear to be slightly more toxic, with increased diarrhea and dehydration.

Irinotecan-based regimens

Irinotecan is a camptothecin derivative that inhibits topoisomerase I by stabilizing DNA breaks that arise in DNA uncoiling for transcription and replication.[370] Two randomized controlled trials showed improved survival in patients receiving irinotecan along with 5-FU/LV, compared with 5-FU/LV alone, as first-line therapy in metastatic disease.[371,372] Despite the proven benefit in advanced disease, preliminary results from three large trials do not support the use of irinotecan in the adjuvant setting. CALGB C89803 compared a bolus version of irinotecan with 5-FU/LV (IFL) with 5-FU/LV alone and found an increase in grade III–IV toxicities (neutropenia, neutropenic fever, and death on treatment) without an improvement in DFS.[373] PETACC-3 and Accord02/FFCD9802 compared the addition of irinotecan with infusional 5-FU and also found increased toxicities in the experimental arm with no improvement in DFS in patients with stage III cancer.[374] On the basis of these trials, irinotecan-based regimens cannot be recommended in the adjuvant setting.[373,374]

Irinotecan is hydrolyzed in the liver to its active metabolite, SN-38, which in turn is glucuronidated to an inactive form by uridine diphosphate glucuronosyltransferase isoform 1A1 (UGT1A1).[370] The adverse events associated with irinotecan, including diarrhea, bone marrow suppression, and nausea or vomiting, have been shown in retrospective studies to correlate with polymorphisms of UGT1A1.[370] A diagnostic test has been approved by the FDA, and several current trials include adjustment of irinotecan dosages on the basis of genetic profiles (pharmacogenomics) of these metabolic enzymes.[370]

Biologic agents

The two most recent FDA-approved therapies in metastatic colon cancer are "targeted," "biologic" agents rather than standard cytotoxic drugs. Both agents are monoclonal antibodies. Bevacizumab targets the VEGF pathway and cetuximab is directed against the epidermal growth factor receptor (EGFR) pathway.

Bevacizumab is a humanized recombinant monoclonal antibody directed against VEGF. By binding ligand and preventing signaling of the VEGF receptor, bevacizumab is thought to interfere with the recruitment and growth of tumor-feeding blood vessels. Two phase III trials have shown an improvement in both DFS and OS after the addition of bevacizumab to 5-FU-based regimens combined with either oxaliplatin or irinotecan in the metastatic setting.[375,376] Side effects seen in these trials thought to be due to the addition of bevacizumab included reversible hypertension and proteinuria, as well as rare serious, but not statistically significant, side effects including GI perforation, wound dehiscence, bleeding, and clotting.[375,376] The AVANT trial compared FOLFOX4, FOLFOX4 plus bevacizumab, and XELOX plus bevacizumab in patients with stage III or high-risk stage II colon cancers.[377] This trial found that the addition of bevacizumab to oxaliplatin-based adjuvant chemotherapy did not improve DFS and suggested that its addition may in fact result in decreased OS. The NSABP C-08 trial compared the addition of bevacizumab to modified FOLFOX6 versus modified FOLFOX6 alone in patients with resected stage II and III colon cancers and also found that the addition of bevacizumab did not increase 3-year DFS.[378]

Cetuximab is a monoclonal antibody directed against EGFR, which is involved with multiple growth signaling pathways. Cetuximab received FDA approval for treatment of irinotecan-resistant metastatic disease in 2004. In irinotecan refractory disease, a 22% response rate was reached in patients treated with cetuximab/irinotecan compared with an 11% response rate with cetuximab as a single agent in a randomized phase II trial.[379] The side effects of cetuximab are relative mild, with an acneiform rash over the face, chest, and back occurring in most patients.[379] Allergic reactions also occur as cetuximab, unlike bevacizumab, is not fully humanized.[379] The US Intergroup N0147 trial comparing FOLFOX-4 with and without cetuximab for patients with resected stage III colon cancer found no difference in 3-year DFS for either patients with wild-type or mutant KRAS.[380] Moreover, grade 3 adverse events and failure to complete 12 cycles of therapy were significantly higher in patients treated with cetuximab.

Summary recommendations

The magnitude of benefit from adjuvant therapy appears to be proportional to the risk of relapse on the basis of pathologic stage. For stage III (node positive) patients, the evidence supports the use of adjuvant chemotherapy for 6 months following resection.[381,382] FOLFOX-4 has the most convincing efficacy data but is associated with increased toxicities compared with 5-FU/LV alone. Capecitabine is a reasonable alternative to intravenous 5-FU/LV. Irinotecan-based regimens cannot be recommended in the adjuvant setting nor can the addition of bevacizumab and cetuximab to established adjuvant regiments. For stage II (node negative) patients, the absolute benefit appears to be real but much smaller. The current trials were not powered to see a difference in this subgroup, so the role of adjuvant treatment for stage II patients is controversial.[381,382] Following the NCCN practice guidelines, FOLFOX-4 or 5-FU is

often considered if the pathology displays high-risk features such as poor differentiation, lymphatic or vascular invasion, bowel obstruction, inadequate staging (<12 lymph nodes removed), perforation, or direct extension into other organs.[382] For stage II patients with no high-risk features, observation or enrollment in a clinical trial is recommended.[382]

The role of adjuvant chemotherapy in older patients remains controversial, particularly regarding the addition of oxaliplatin to 5-FU-based therapies. While the MOSAIC trial failed to demonstrate a benefit in adding oxaliplatin to 5-FU/LV,[369] pooled analysis of three randomized clinical trials suggested that efficacy of adjuvant 5-FU-based chemotherapy was maintained in the elderly (defined as 70 years of age and older), and that toxicity was similar to younger patients except for an increase in leucopenia in one study.[383,384]

Neoadjuvant and adjuvant therapy for rectal cancer

As in colon cancer, surgical resection remains the cornerstone of the curative approach. However, unlike colon cancer, there is significant tendency for local failure after potentially curative resection. Improvements in the initial surgical procedure by performing a TME have reduced but not eliminated the risk of local recurrence. Salvage surgical procedures are technically difficult, often unsuccessful and fraught with morbidity. Therefore the major difference in the adjuvant treatment paradigm for rectal as compared with colon cancer is the addition of radiation therapy to reduce the risk of local failure.

Adjuvant chemotherapy and radiation

Studies in the 1980s and 1990s solidified the superiority of postoperative chemoradiation over surgery alone and surgery followed by radiation without chemotherapy. Chemoradiation reduced the risk of local failure, distant failure, and the risk of death.[385-387] In these studies, chemoradiation involved the use of seumustine (methyl-CCNU) in addition to 5-FU. Semustine carries a small but real risk of acute myeloid leukemia and is no longer used in adjuvant regimens for rectal cancer.[388] The North American Intergroup trial confirmed the lack of additional benefit of semustine in addition to 5-FU and has established the role of continuous infusion 5-FU with radiation.[389] Comparing continuous infusion 5-FU ($225 \, mg/m^2$ per day for 5 weeks) to bolus 5-FU ($500 \, mg/m^2$ days 1–3 and days 36–39) at 4 years, the time to relapse was improved from 53% to 63%, and survival was improved from 60% to 70%. Unlike colon cancer, biomodulation with LV or levamisole has not increased the efficacy of 5-FU in rectal cancer. Intergroup study 0144 compared continued systemic therapy with infusional 5-FU during radiation, bolus 5-FU 4 weeks before and after radiation, and combined bolus and continued infusional 5-FU during radiation. The study found no difference in relapse-free survival or OS between the three groups.[390] A 2012 trial comparing capecitabine-based chemoradiotherapy ($2500 \, mg/m^2$ days 1–14, repeated day 22, followed by 50.4 Gy plus capecitabine $1650 \, mg/m^2$ days 1–38, followed by three cycles of capecitabine) with 5-FU-based radiotherapy (two cycles of bolus 5-FU $500 \, mg/m^2$ days 1–5, 29, followed by chemoradiation with 50.4 Gy and infusional 5-FU, followed by two additional bolus cycles of 5-FU) in patients with stage II–III rectal cancer found that capecitabine was noninferior to 5-FU in terms of 5-year OS, 3-year DFS, and local recurrence.[391] Distant metastasis was less common in the capecitabine group. Adverse reactions differed between the two arms, with leukopenia more common in patients receiving 5-FU and hand–foot skin reactions, fatigue, and proctitis more common in the capecitabine group. Capecitabine is thus a reasonable alternative to 5-FU in adjuvant chemoradiation regimens. In general, adjuvant therapy is recommended for any tumor that is T3 or greater in size or is node positive. Radiation therapy should be directed at the tumor bed, including a 2–5 cm margin as well as the presacral nodes and the internal iliac nodes. If an APR was performed, the perineal wound should be included in the radiation field.[392]

Neoadjuvant chemotherapy and radiation

The neoadjuvant approach is particularly attractive in rectal cancer because downstaging may increase ease and rates of respectability, allow potential sphincter preservation, and increase compliance by avoiding long postoperative recoveries. The Swedish Rectal Cancer Trial was the first to show that a short-term regimen of high-dose preoperative radiotherapy decreased the rate of local recurrence and improved survival compared with surgery alone.[393] The German phase III EORTC 22921 study was the first study to complete accrual in comparing neoadjuvant therapy with combined 5-FU/radiation to postoperative adjuvant 5-FU/radiation.[394] Patients with tumor extending through the muscle wall (T3) or with positive nodes (N1) were randomized to preoperative or postoperative chemoradiation. In both arms, the radiation (5040 GY in 28 fractions) was combined with 5-FU (1000 mg/m^2 over 120 h during the first and fifth week). All patients received additional systemic 5-FU for 4 months. The study failed to see an improvement in OS, but preoperative therapy was associated with an improved rate of local control at 5 years (6% failure compared to 13%), reduced acute and chronic toxicity, increased compliance, and an increased rate of sphincter preservation in patients with low-lying tumors.[394] Interestingly, posttreatment pathology results proved to be highly prognostic with patients who showed marked regression or negative nodes having improved DFS.[394] In 2012, long-term results from the German trial became available. At 10 years, preoperative chemoradiation therapy was associated with improved local control compared to postoperative therapy; however, there remained no difference in OS.[395] There are several theoretical benefits of neoadjuvant as opposed to adjuvant chemoradiation therapy. First, there is the increased possibility of ultimately performing a sphincter-sparing resection. While two studies have demonstrated higher rates of sphincter preservation,[394,396] other large meta-analyses have disputed these findings.[397,398] During resection, adhesions can result in bowel that becomes fixed in the pelvis. By administering radiation in the preoperative versus postoperative period, daily radiation to the same segment of fixed bowel can be avoided. A third hypothetical benefit is the presence of intact vasculature prior to resection, which may result in greater tissue oxygenation and better response to radiation.

Short-course radiation

Short-course radiation (e.g., Swedish or European approach) refers to 25 Gy of radiation without chemotherapy over a 5-day time period. Initially, the Swedish Rectal Cancer Trial demonstrated improved rates of local recurrence and OS for short-course preoperative radiotherapy compared to surgery alone.[393] However, a later analysis of this study population demonstrated that patients treated with short-course radiation had higher rates of GI morbidity following surgery, most notably, bowel obstructions.[399] In a large randomized trial of more than 1,300 patients, short-course preoperative radiation without any adjuvant therapy was compared to postoperative chemoradiation therapy in patients with a positive circumferential margin.[400] Short-course radiation was associated with improved local recurrence rates and DFS, although there was no detectable difference in OS. More recently, the TME trial

comparing patients treated with short-course radiation to patients who underwent TME alone demonstrated improvements in local recurrence (5 vs 11%) without a corresponding increase in OS.[401] While OS was significantly improved among stage III patients treated with short-course RT who had a negative circumferential margin, among node-negative patients with negative margins, the improvement in CRC-specific mortality was countered by an increase in other causes of death. Only one randomized trial has directly compared short-course high-dose radiotherapy to conventional preoperative chemoradiation, which showed no improvement in local recurrence, RFS, or OS.[402] Short-course radiation therapy appears to result in equivalent local control compared with traditional long-course chemoradiation therapy; however, improvements in OS have not been appreciated, and concerns about increased perioperative toxicity remain.

Summary recommendations

Neoadjuvant chemoradiation therapy has been shown to result in tumor downstaging in approximately half of patients, with a pathologic complete response in up to 20%.[403] Thus, although no survival benefit has been proven with preoperative compared to postoperative chemoradiotherapy, it is suggested that preoperative chemoradiotherapy be the preferred treatment for patients with locally advanced rectal cancer, given that it is associated with a superior overall compliance rate, an improved rate of local control, reduced toxicity, improved function, and perhaps an increased rate of sphincter preservation in patients with low-lying tumors.[382] Although no trial has demonstrated conclusively that additional postoperative adjuvant 5-FU-based chemotherapy improves outcomes in patients who have undergone neoadjuvant chemoradiotherapy, guidelines from the National Comprehensive Cancer Network recommend that all such patients receive 5-FU-containing chemotherapy even if they have a pathologic complete response to neoadjuvant therapy.[382]

Chemotherapy for hepatic metastasis

Conversion therapy

Selected patients with initially unresectable liver metastases may become eligible for resection if the response to chemotherapy is sufficient. This approach has been termed "conversion therapy" to distinguish it from "neoadjuvant therapy" which applies to preoperative chemotherapy given to patients who present upfront with apparently resectable disease. The key parameter for selecting the specific regimen in this scenario is not survival or improved QOL but instead response rate. The NCCN currently recommends any chemotherapeutic regimen that is active in the metastatic setting, as the goal of conversion therapy is not to treat occult disease but rather to obtain the tumor regression necessary to convert unresectable metastases to a resectable state.[404] Regimens studied include FOLFIRI,[405] FOLFOX,[406] FOLFOXIRI.[407,408] Between 12% and 40% of patients with isolated but initially unresectable CRC liver metastases have a sufficient downstaging response to permit a subsequent complete resection.[404–408] Following resection, 5-year survival rates average 30–35%, results that are substantially better than expected using chemotherapy alone. In the largest study, 138 (12.5%) of 1104 patients with initially unresectable CRC liver metastases were able to undergo resection after induction chemotherapy that consisted mainly of 5-FU/LV combined with either oxaliplatin (705), irinotecan (7%), or both (4%).[409] Overall 5- and 10-year survival was 33% and 23%, respectively. Targeted and biologic agents have been tested in combination with established chemotherapy regimens in the conversion setting. The addition of cetuximab (an EGFR inhibitor) may substantially increase resectability in patients with wild-type *KRAS*; however, the effect on OS remains controversial.[410–412] Most recently, bevacizumab has been tested in combination with established chemotherapies in the setting of unresectable disease.[413–415] While there may be a modest improvement in conversion rates using bevacizumab in combination with irinotecan-based therapies,[413,414] the same benefit has not been observed with oxaliplatin-based therapies.[415] In summary, chemotherapy alone is not curative in this setting with the majority of radiographic completely responding lesions containing viable tumor. Thus, even in the setting of a complete clinical response, resection is still needed.

Neoadjuvant therapy for hepatic metastasis

There is evidence that perioperative chemotherapy improves both progression-free survival and DFS among patients with initially resectable hepatic metastases; however, its effect on OS remains unproven.[416] Whether patients benefit most from pre- or post-operative therapy remains unclear. The theoretical benefits of neoadjuvant chemotherapy for patients with resectable hepatic metastases include the guarantee that these patients will receive systemic therapy (vs patients who are unable to tolerate post-operative therapy), as well as an earlier initiation of systemic therapy compared to those who receive adjuvant chemotherapy. The EORTC trial randomly assigned 364 patients with up to four metastases without prior exposure to oxaliplatin to liver resection with or without perioperative FOLFOX-4 chemotherapy.[417] Six cycles of chemotherapy were administered prior to surgery, and six cycles were administered postoperatively. Sixty-seven of the 182 patients assigned to chemotherapy had an objective response, while 11 progressed, eight of whom were no longer considered resectable. Overall, 83% of patients were successfully resected, similar to the number who were successfully resected in the surgery alone group, 84%. The postoperative complication rate, however, was significantly higher in the chemotherapy group (25% vs 16%). Patients receiving perioperative chemotherapy had higher rates of hepatic failure, biliary fistulas, and intra-abdominal infection. Postoperative mortality was similar between groups. There is increasing evidence that for patients with resectable hepatic metastases, the use of preoperative chemotherapy is associated with hepatic steatosis, vascular injury, and nodular regenerative hyperplasia, particularly among patients treated with irinotecan or oxaliplatin-containing regimens.[409,418,419] Moreover, there is evidence that among patients who have complete radiographic responses to neoadjuvant therapy, most sites of metastasis nonetheless harbor viable cancer cells.[420] This presents a substantial challenge with regard to operative planning following the cessation of neoadjuvant therapy.

Adjuvant therapy after hepatic resection

Adjuvant chemotherapy is commonly recommended following resection of hepatic colorectal metastasis despite the lack of data to support its use. There are many unknowns, including the timing of resection, optimal drug combination, schedule, and duration of therapy. Because the presence of hepatic metastasis confers stage IV disease, either FOLFOX-4 or folinic acid, 5-FU, and irinotecan (FOLFIRI) for 4 to 6 months is often used.[421] A targeted biologic agent may be considered despite the lack of data supporting use in stage II/III disease. Because of the risk of wound complications and other issues, it is recommended that bevacizumab be discontinued 8 weeks before or after major surgical procedures.[422]

Summary recommendations

There are no widely accepted guidelines for determining which patients with CRC liver metastases should undergo immediate surgery and when neoadjuvant chemotherapy is indicated. However, the increasing reports of liver injury following neoadjuvant chemotherapy have prompted most physicians to recommend initial surgery for low-risk (medically fit with four or fewer lesions), potentially resectable patients, followed by adjuvant chemotherapy.[423] On the other hand, neoadjuvant chemotherapy is reasonable for those who are higher risk or have borderline resectable or unresectable liver metastases. However, the duration should be limited, radiographic response assessment performed frequently, and surgery undertaken as soon as the metastases become clearly resectable.

Metastatic CRC

The last two decades have seen unprecedented advances in the treatment of metastatic CRC, and these improvements serve as a model for the treatment of many additional solid tumors for which progress has been less rapid. In the era when 5-FU was the sole active agent, OS was approximately 11 to 12 months. Currently, the average median survival duration has doubled, with patients routinely living longer than 2 years. This increase has been mainly driven by the availability of new active agents. There are now three different classes of primary chemotherapies with significant antitumor activity (fluoropyrimidines, irinotecan, and oxaliplatin), as well as multiple targeted and biologic therapies with an emerging role in the treatment of CRC (e.g., cetuximab, bevacizumab, panitumumab, and regorafenib). For most patients, the goal of treatment will be palliative and not curative, with the treatment goals being to prolong OS and maintain QOL for as long as possible. For the vast majority of patients with noncurable metastatic CRC, rationally designed doublet combinations, such as FOLFOX or FOLFIRI should be considered the standard chemotherapy backbone for first-line palliative therapy. These regimens have well-documented activity and a tolerable toxicity profile. Other appropriate therapies include XELOX, 5-FU/LV, capecitabine, and FOLFOXIRI.

FOLFOX

The first large size, randomized phase III trial comparing 5-FU and LV versus FOLFOX-4 included 420 patients.[367] Patients received exactly the same regimen of a 2-h infusion of 200 mg/m² of LV followed by a bolus of 400 mg/m² and a 22-h infusion of 600 mg/m² of 5-FU. All drugs were repeated for 2 consecutive days every 2 weeks. Half of the patients were assigned to receive 85 mg/m² of oxaliplatin as a 2-h infusion on day 1 only.[367] Patients allocated to receive FOLFOX-4 had significantly longer PFS (median 9.0 vs 6.2 months; $p = 0.0003$) and better response rate (50.7% vs 22.3%; $p = 0.0001$) when compared with the control arm. However, although a trend could be seen, the improvement in OS did not reach statistical significance (median, 16.2 vs 14.7 months, $p = 0.12$).[367] The lack of survival benefit in this European trial delayed FOLFOX acceptance in the United States. Shortly after, the NCCTG and the American Intergroup conducted the N9741, a phase III trial with three arms.[424] The control arm received IFL regimen, and oxaliplatin was included in the two experimental arms. It was combined at 85 mg/m² with 200 mg/m² of irinotecan in the irinotecan and oxaliplatin (IROX) regimen, or with 5-FU and LV, following the FOLFOX-4 regimen described above.[424] The final results showed a median time to progression of 8.7 months, response rate of 45%, and median survival time of 19.5 months for those patients assigned to FOLFOX-4. These results were significantly superior to those observed for IFL (6.9 months, 31%, and 15.0 months, respectively) or for IROX (6.5 months, 35%, and 1.4 months, respectively).[424] FOLFOX-4 was generally well tolerated but it was associated with a significantly higher rate of sensory neuropathy as described above. More recently, modified FOLFOX6 has emerged as the preferred dosing schedule for the FOLFOX regimen.[425]

Capecitabine/XELOX

Capecitabine, an orally active fluoropyrimidine, allows for the attractiveness of oral dosing and the potential for eliminating the need for a central venous catheter and ambulatory infusion pump. At least five randomized phase III trials have directly compared XELOX (capecitabine, oxaliplatin) versus FOLFOX for first-line or second-line chemotherapy in metastatic CRC.[426,427] None showed that XELOX was inferior to FOLFOX-type regimens in terms of response rate, PFS, or OS. However, in nearly all cases, the PFS and OS curves for XELOX trailed beneath the curves for FOLFOX. In no case was this effect statistically significant or clinically meaningful. Thus, the available evidence supports the view that XELOX can be considered as a noninferior substitute for FOLFOX in palliative therapy.

FOLFIRI

The effectiveness of irinotecan was initially demonstrated in a randomized phase III trial conducted to evaluate irinotecan with or without standard bolus 5-FU and LV versus a standard regimen of bolus 5-FU and LV.[372] The combination regimen became known as the IFL regimen and included 5-FU 500 mg/m^2, LV 20 mg/m^2, and irinotecan 125 mg/m^2 given weekly for 4 weeks every 6 weeks. Irinotecan alone was given at 125 mg/m^2 weekly for 4 weeks every 6 weeks, and the 5-FU/LV was given using the standard Mayo regimen as described above.[372] The three drug regimen was superior to either 5-FU and LV or to irinotecan alone, and the latter produced similar results as the 5-FU/LV regimen. In a comparison of IFL and the Mayo regimens, the median PFS improved from 4.3 months to 7.0 months, and the median OS improved from 12.6 months to 14.8 months.[372] FOLFIRI is a variation of IFL using infusional 5-FU, LV, and irinotecan. There are several variations of FOLFIRI, but one of the favored regimens combines 180 mg/m^2 of irinotecan given on day 1 weekly, 400 mg/m^2 bolus LV weekly, 400 mg/m^2 bolus 5-FU weekly, and followed by a 46 h infusion of 2400 mg/m^2 of 5-FU. The entire cycle is repeated every 14 days. A European trial compared the use of FOLFIRI versus FOLFOX as a first-line therapy for metastatic CRC.[425] Although it has been criticized for its relatively small size, this trial was important because it showed similar response rates and median survivals for FOLFOX and FOLFIRI. However, these data are supported further by the 2005 multicenter trial from the Gruppo Oncologico Dell'Italia Meridionale, in which 360 patients were randomized to FOLFIRI versus FOLFOX4.[428] There were no differences in response rates, time to progression, duration of response, or OS between arms.

While XELOX may be regarded as a valid substitute for FOLFOX, the situation is different for combinations of capecitabine with irinotecan (XELIRI) as an alternative to FOLFIRI. Capecitabine and irinotecan have partially overlapping toxicity profiles, particularly with regard to diarrhea. The potential for greater toxicity reduces the therapeutic advantage of an irinotecan/capecitabine combination and makes the selection of appropriate doses and schedules for this combination difficult.[403]

FOLFOXIRI

There have been two recent trials comparing FOLFOXIRI to FOLFIRI among patients with metastatic CRC.[407,429] The GONO trial randomized 244 treatment-naïve patients with metastatic, unresectable CRC to receive either FOLFOXIRI or FOLFIRI.[407] FOLFOXIRI was dosed every two weeks, with irinotecan (165 mg/m^2), oxaliplatin (85 mg/m^2), and LV (200 mg/m^2) given on day one and 5-FU administered as a 48-h continuous infusion starting on day 1. Partial response rates were higher in the FOLFIRI arm (44 vs 66%); however, there was no difference in complete response. Patients in the FOLFOXIRI arm were more likely to undergo a complete resection of their hepatic metastases (12 vs 36%). Most importantly, both PFS and OS were significantly improved in the FOLFOXIRI arm (7 vs 10 months and 17 vs 23 months, respectively). The HORG trial also compared FOLFOXIRI to FOLFIRI, although the FOLFOXIRI dosing regimen was slightly different.[429] In this trial, no differences in OS, time to disease progression, or response rates were appreciated between groups. Moreover, FOLFOXIRI was associated with a higher rate of treatment toxicity, including alopecia, diarrhea, and neurotoxicity.

Bevacizumab

CRC was the first malignancy for which clear evidence for efficacy of an anti-VEGF strategy was obtained in randomized trials. In a pivotal early trial, the addition of bevacizumab to the bolus IFL regimen significantly improved response rates from 35% to 45%; PFS was extended from 7.1 months to 10.4 months, and more importantly, the OS improved from 15.6 to 20.3 months.[375] The adverse events in this trial were similar among the treatment with some notable exceptions. Patients receiving bevacizumab had an 11% incidence of grade 3 hypertension and a 1.5% incidence of bowel perforations. No patients in the IFL arm presented with such problems.[375] The ECOG 3200 trial compared the use of FOLFOX to combination therapy of bevacizumab and FOLFOX.[376] The median survival for combination therapy was 12.5 months versus 10.7 months for FOLFOX alone. This confirmed that bevacizumab does significantly add potency to oxaliplatin-based regimens. Since 2004, the majority of patients with metastatic CRC have received bevacizumab as a component of first-line therapy regardless of the specific regimen chosen for chemotherapy backbone (FOLFOX, XELOX, FOLFIRI). With regard to the addition of bevacizumab to established regimens in the advanced setting, FOLFOXIRI/bevacizumab appears to have increased progression-free survival and response rates compared to FOLFIRI/bevacizumab among patients who have not received prior adjuvant therapy.[430] FOLFOXIRI/bevacizumab was also found to be superior to FOLFOX/bevacizumab in the conversion setting for patients with hepatic metastases (rate of R0 resection 49 vs 23%).[431]

Anti-EGFR monoclonal antibodies

The benefit of cetuximab added to first-line or second-line irinotecan-containing therapy has been addressed in the CRYSTAL trial and CALGB 80203.[432,433] In the CRYSTAL trial, 1198 previously untreated patients were randomly assigned to FOLFIRI with or without cetuximab.[433] Although the addition of cetuximab significantly improved PFS, the incremental gain was only 0.9 months. The addition of cetuximab also improved the response rate but only by 8%.[433] Early results from the phase II CALGB 80203 trial, which randomly assigned 283 patients to FOLFOX or FOLFIRI with or without cetuximab as first-line therapy, provided confirmatory data supporting the results of the CRYSTAL trial.[432] In a preliminary report, there was a clear demonstration of increased response rate with cetuximab in conjunction with both FOLFOX and FOLFIRI, while the impact on PFS was inconclusive.[432] Furthermore, a retrospective analysis of the CRYSTAL trial investigating the role of KRAS mutation status on PFS and response rate showed that in the KRAS wild-type population, the 1 year PFS rate for those who received cetuximab and FOLFIRI was 43% versus 25% for those who received FOLFIRI alone, and the risk of progression was decreased by 32% in the combination treatment arm.[434] In the KRAS mutant population, however, there was no difference in PFS between the two arms. Long-term results from this study should be available shortly. Most recently, a meta-analysis of 14 trials comparing standard therapies with or without the use of anti-EGFR monoclonal antibodies was performed, which found an increase in progression-free survival only among patients with wild-type KRAS.[435] In this analysis, patients with KRAS mutations demonstrated no clinical benefit from anti-EGFR therapies. KRAS genotyping is now recommended among all patients with metastatic CRC.[404] Other trials evaluating both cetuximab and panitumumab have confirmed a clear benefit for anti-EGFR therapy among patients with wild-type KRAS.[436-438] It is recommended that anti-EGFR therapies not be used among patients with KRAS mutations. Finally, several randomized trials have compared the addition of bevacizumab versus anti-EGFR therapy to established chemotherapies among patients with metastatic wild-type KRAS CRC.[438-440] These data remain inconclusive as to a superiority benefit for either combination. At present, either anti-EGFR therapy or bevacizumab as an addition to a first-line regimen is an acceptable choice of therapy for patients with metastatic CRC with wild-type KRAS.

Summary recommendations

Initial combination therapy is preferred for patients with nonoperable metastatic CRC, in whom the palliative treatment strategy should aim to maximize the number of patients exposed to all active agents. This is best achieved by using well-established combination doublets (i.e., FOLFOX, XELOX, or FOLFIRI) as the chemotherapy backbone, which would then only require one additional step to have all three active agents included in the treatment algorithm for second-line therapy (e.g., FOLFOX followed by FOLFIRI, or FOLFIRI followed by FOLFOX, or FOLFOXIRI). Bevacizumab should be considered a component of first-line therapy regardless of which regimen is chosen. Cetuximab in patients with wild-type KRAS is a reasonable alternative to bevacizumab in combination with established chemotherapy regimens.

Key references

The complete reference list can be found on the Wiley Companion Digital Edition of this title (see inside front cover for login instructions).

17 Van Weyenberg S, Meijerink MR, Jacobs MA, et al. *MR enteroclysis in the diagnosis of small-bowel neoplasms. Radiology.* 2010;**254**(3):765–773.

21 Torroni F, Romeo E, Rea F, et al. *Conservative approach in Peutz-Jeghers syndrome: single-balloon enteroscopy and small bowel polypectomy. World J Gastrointest Endosc.* 2014;**16**(6):318–323.

33 Boffetta P, Hazelton WD, Chen Y, et al. *Body mass, tobacco smoking, alcohol drinking and risk of cancer of the small intestine—a pooled analysis of over 500,000 subjects in the Asia Cohort Consortium. Ann Oncol.* 2012;**23**(7):1894–1898.

52 Eom D, Hong SM, Kim J, et al. *Notch3 signaling is associated with MUC5AC expression and favorable prognosis in patients with small intestinal adenocarcinomas. Pathol Res Pract.* 2014;**210**:501–507.

53 Zaanan A, Meunier K, Sangar F, et al. *Microsatellite instability in colorectal cancer: from molecular oncogenic mechanisms to clinical implications. Cellular Oncology.* 2011;**34**:155–176.

60 Xiang X, Liu YW, Zhang L, et al. *A phase II study of modified FOLFOX as first-line chemotherapy in advanced small bowel adenocarcinoma. Anticancer Drugs.* 2012;**23**(5):561–566.

77 Bartlett E, Roses RE, Gupta M, et al. *Surgery for metastatic neuroendocrine tumors with occult primaries. J Surg Res.* 2013;**184**(1):221–227.

83 Amin S, Warner RR, Itzkowitz SH, Kim MK. *The risk of metachronous cancers in patients with small-intestinal carcinoid tumors: a US population-based study. Endocr Relat Cancer.* 2012;**19**(3):381–387.

87 Pavel M, Hainsworth JD, Baudin E, et al. *Everolimus plus octreotide long-acting repeatable for the treatment of advanced neuroendocrine tumours associated with carcinoid syndrome (RADIANT-2): a randomised, placebo-controlled, phase 3 study. Lancet.* 2011;**378**(9808):2005–2012.

96 Demetri GD, Antonia S, Benjamin RS, et al. *Soft tissue sarcoma. J Natl Compr Canc Netw.* 2007;**5**(4):364–399.

113 Karakousis G, Singer S, Zheng J, et al. *Laparoscopic versus open gastric resections for primary gastrointestinal stromal tumors (GISTs): a size-matched comparison. Ann Surg Oncol.* 2011;**18**(6):1599–1605.

114 Bischof D, Kim Y, Dodson R, Carolina Jimenez M, et al. *Open versus minimally invasive resection of gastric GIST: a multi-institutional analysis of short- and long-term outcomes. Ann Surg Oncol.* 2014;**9**:2941–2948.

115 Chok A, Koh YX, Ow MY, et al. *A systematic review and meta-analysis comparing pancreaticoduodenectomy versus limited resection for duodenal gastrointestinal stromal tumors. Ann Surg Oncol.* 2014;**11**:3429–3438.

116 Balachandran V, Cavna MJ, Zeng S, et al. *Imatinib potentiates antitumor T cell responses in gastrointestinal stromal tumor through the inhibition of Ido. Nat Med.* 2011;**17**(9):1094–1100.

119 Joensuu H. *Twelve versus 36 months of adjuvant imatinib (IM) as treatment of operable GIST with a high risk of recurrence: final results of a randomized trial. J Clin Oncol.* 2011;**29**(suppl; abstract LBA1).

122 Corless C, Ballman KV, Antonescu CR, et al. *Pathologic and molecular features correlate with long-term outcome after adjuvant therapy of resected primary GI stromal tumor: the ACOSOG Z9001 trial. J Clin Oncol.* 2014;**32**(15):1563–1570.

139 Barrington S, Mikhaeel NG, Kostakoglu L, et al. *Role of imaging in the staging and response assessment of lymphoma: consensus of the International conference on malignant lymphomas imaging working group. J Clin Oncol.* 2014;**53**:5229.

146 Geramizadeh B, Keshtkar Jahromi M. *Primary extranodal gastrointestinal lymphoma: a single center experience from southern iran—report of changing epidemiology. Arch Iran Med.* 2014;**17**(9):638–639.

165 Pape UF et al. *ENETS consensus guidelines for the management of patients with neuroendocrine neoplasms from the jejuno-ileum and the appendix including goblet cell carcinomas. Neuroendocrinology.* 2012;**95**(2):135–156.

176 Andreasson H et al. *Outcome differences between debulking surgery and cytoreductive surgery in patients with Pseudomyxoma peritonei. Eur J Surg Oncol.* 2012;**38**(10):962–968.

273 National Comprehensive Cancer Network (2014) *NCCN Clinical Practice Guidelines in Oncology (NCCN Guidelines®): Colorectal Cancer Screening.* Version 1.2014. May 19, http://www.nccn.org/professionals/physician_gls/pdf/colorectal_screening.pdf (accessed 24 March 2016).

295 Taylor FG, Quirke P, Heald RJ, et al. Magnetic resonance imaging in rectal cancer European equivalence study group. Preoperative magnetic resonance imaging assessment of circumferential resection margin predicts disease-free survival and local recurrence: 5-year follow-up results of the MERCURY study. *J Clin Oncol.* 2014;**32**(1):34–43.

299 O'Connell MJ, Lavery I, Yothers G, et al. Relationship between tumor gene expression and recurrence in four independent studies of patients with stage II/III colon cancer treated with surgery alone or surgery plus adjuvant fluorouracil plus leucovorin. *J Clin Oncol.* 2010;**28**(25):3937–3944.

300 Gray RG, Quirke P, Handley K, et al. Validation study of a quantitative multigene reverse transcriptase-polymerase chain reaction assay for assessment of recurrence risk in patients with stage II colon cancer. *J Clin Oncol.* 2011;**29**(35):4611–4619.

301 Yothers G, O'Connell MJ, Lee M, et al. Validation of the 12-gene colon cancer recurrence score in NSABP C-07 as a predictor of recurrence in patients with stage II and III colon cancer treated with fluorouracil and leucovorin (FU/LV) and FU/LV plus oxaliplatin. *J Clin Oncol.* 2013;**31**(36):4512–4519.

302 Srivastava G, Renfro LA, Behrens RJ, et al. Prospective multicenter study of the impact of oncotype DX colon cancer assay results on treatment recommendations in stage II colon cancer patients. *Oncologist.* 2014;**19**(5):492–497.

335 van der Pas MH, Haglind E, Cuesta MA, et al. Laparoscopic versus open surgery for rectal cancer (COLOR II): short-term outcomes of a randomised, phase 3 trial. *The Lancet Oncology.* 2013;**14**(3):210–218.

336 Aziz O, Constantinides V, Tekkis P, et al. Laparoscopic versus open surgery for rectal cancer: a meta-analysis. *Ann Surg Oncol.* 2006;**13**:413–424.

337 Gao F, Cao Y, Chen L. Meta-analysis of short-term outcomes after laparoscopic resection for rectal cancer. *Int J Colorectal Dis.* 2006;**21**:652–656.

339 Park JS, Choi GS, Park SY, Kim HJ, Ryuk JP. Randomized clinical trial of robot-assisted versus standard laparoscopic right colectomy. *Br J Surg.* 2012;**99**(9):1219–1226.

340 Luca F, Ghezzi TL, Valvo M, et al. Surgical and pathological outcomes after right hemicolectomy: case-matched study comparing robotic and open surgery. *Int J Med Robot.* 2011;**7**:298–303.

342 Baik SH, Kwon HY, Kim JS, et al. Robotic versus laparoscopic low anterior resection of rectal cancer: short-term outcome of a prospective comparative study. *Ann Surg Oncol.* 2009;**16**(6):1480–1487. doi:10.1245/s10434-009-0435-3.

343 Kim CW, Kim CH, Baik SH. Outcomes of robotic-assisted colorectal surgery compared with laparoscopic and open surgery: a systematic review. *J Gastrointest Surg.* 2014;**18**:816–830.

369 Tournigand C, André T, Bonnetain F, et al. Adjuvant therapy with fluorouracil and oxaliplatin in stage II and elderly patients (between ages 70 and 75 years) with colon cancer: subgroup analyses of the Multicenter International Study of Oxaliplatin, Fluorouracil, and Leucovorin in the Adjuvant Treatment of Colon Cancer trial. *J Clin Oncol.* 2012;**30**(27):3353–3360.

371 Douillard J, Cunningham D, Roth A, et al. Irinotecan combined with fluorouracil compared with fluorouracil alone as first-line treatment for metastatic colorectal cancer: a multicentre randomized trial. *Lancet.* 2000;**255**:1041–1048.

392 National Comprehensive Cancer Network (2014) *NCCN Clinical Practice Guidelines in Oncology (NCCN Guidelines®): Rectal Cancer. Version 1.2015,* http://www.nccn.org/professionals/physician_gls/pdf/rectal.pdf (accessed 24 March 2016).

394 Sauer R, Becker H, Hohenberer W, et al. German rectal cancer study group: preoperative versus postoperative chemoradiotherapy for rectal cancer. *N Engl J Med.* 2004;**351**:1731–1740.

400 Sebag-Montefiore D, Stephens RJ, Steele R, et al. Preoperative radiotherapy versus selective postoperative chemoradiotherapy in patients with rectal cancer (MRC CR07 and NCIC-CTG C016): a multicentre, randomised trial. *Lancet.* 2009;**373**(9666):811–820.

401 van Gijn W, Marijnen CA, Nagtegaal ID, et al. van de Velde CJ; Dutch Colorectal Cancer Group. Preoperative radiotherapy combined with total mesorectal excision for resectable rectal cancer: 12-year follow-up of the multicentre, randomized controlled TME trial. *Lancet Oncol.* 2011;**12**(6):575–582.

402 Ngan SY, Burmeister B, Fisher RJ, et al. Randomized trial of short-course radiotherapy versus long-course chemoradiation comparing rates of local recurrence in patients with T3 rectal cancer: trans-Tasman radiation oncology group trial 01.04. *J Clin Oncol.* 2012;**30**(31):3827–3833.

403 Das P, Skibber JM, Rodriguez-Bigas MA, et al. Predictors of tumor response and downstaging in patients who receive preoperative chemoradiation for rectal cancer. *Cancer.* 2007;**109**(9):1750–1755.

404 National Comprehensive Cancer Network (2014) *NCCN Clinical Practice Guidelines in Oncology (NCCN Guidelines®): Colon Cancer. Version 2.2015,* http://www.nccn.org/professionals/physician_gls/pdf/colon.pdf (accessed 24 March 2016).

95 Neoplasms of the anus

Bruce D. Minsky, MD ▪ Jose G. Guillem, MD

Overview

Although an uncommon tumor, the incidence of anal cancer has increased over the past few decades. This increase may be due to sexual transmission of human papillomavirus virus as well as the impact of human immunodeficiency virus. Chemoradiation therapy (CMT) involving pelvic radiation and concurrent chemotherapy (5-FU combined with either mitomycin-C or cisplatin) has resulted in 5-year survival rates of approximately 80% while maintaining sphincter preservation for most patients. Surgery is reserved for selected patients with T1M0 disease who can undergo resection with acceptable functional outcomes or an abdominoperineal resection (APR) for salvage following CMT.

Gross anatomy

There are three regions where anal cancers occur; the perianal skin or anal margin, the anal canal, and the lower rectum. The anal canal is 3–4 cm long and extends from the anal verge to the pelvic floor.[1] Cancers of the anal canal and the anal margin have different natural histories. The literature is confusing because of the various definitions of the anal canal and the anal margin. For example, some define the distal limit of the anal canal as the dentate line and all tumors below this as anal margin cancers,[2,3] others consider the distal extent of the anal canal as the anal verge,[4,5] while another definition of anal margin tumors are those tumors that arise within 5 cm of the anal verge.[6]

The incidence of anal margin and anal canal cancers is dependent on the anatomical boundaries. When the anal verge is defined as the distal margin of the anal canal, 15% of tumors arise from the anal margin, but this number increases to 30% when the dentate line is used as the distal limit. To clarify this issue, the American Joint Committee on Cancer (AJCC) and the Union Internationale Contra le Cancer (UICC) formed a consensus that the anal canal extends from the anorectal ring (dentate line) to the anal verge.[7,8] These two organizations agree that anal margin tumors behave in a similar manner to skin cancers and therefore are classified and treated as skin tumors.

There is an extensive lymphatic system for the anus with many connections. The three main pathways include (1) superiorly from the rectum along the superior hemorrhoidal vessels to the inferior mesenteric lymph nodes, (2) from the upper anal canal and superior to the dentate line along the inferior and middle hemorrhoid vessels to the hypogastric lymph nodes, and (3) inferior from the anal margin and anal canal to the superficial inguinal lymph nodes.

Epidemiology

In the United States, cancers of the anal region account for 1–2% of all large bowel cancers and 4% of all anorectal carcinomas. Since 1997, the incidence of carcinoma *in situ* (CIS) and squamous cell cancer (SCC) anus have dramatically increased. However, more men are more likely to be diagnosed with CIS.[9] In 2014, a total of 7210 cases of cancers of the anal region are estimated to occur in the United States, including 2660 men and 4550 women.[10] It is estimated that there will be 950 deaths.

Etiology

HPV infection

Squamous cell carcinoma is closely correlated with HPV (human papillomavirus), most commonly types 16 and 18. In a population-based case–control study from Scandinavia of 417 patients with anal canal cancers, a variety of behavioral factors such as sexual activity and venereal infection, tobacco consumption, and anal inflammatory lesions were examined.[11] A positive correlation was found by both univariate and multivariate analysis for the number of sexual partners and the risk of anal cancer. An association between venereal infection in both men and women was also noted.

Anal intraepithelial neoplasia (AIN) is rare in heterosexual men, whereas the incidence is 5–30% in men who have sex with men (MSM) who are HIV-negative (human immunodeficiency virus). These changes are rare among HIV-negative women. AIN is linked to HPV and is common in MSM and immunosuppressed patients, especially those who are HIV positive.[12,13] In a report from Surawicz et al.[14] of 90 MSM to anal cancer with an abnormal examination of the anal canal, 89% had HPV-associated changes. A recent metatanalysis of 53 trials examining the relationship of HPV infection in MSM revealed that anal HPV and anal SCC precursors were very common.[15] The pooled prevalence of HPV-16 was 35% in HIV positive versus 13% in HIV negative patients. However, the rate of progression to cancer was substantially lower than that reported for cervical precancerous lesions.

HIV (human immunodeficiency virus)

There is a clear association between HIV and anal canal cancer. Cross-referencing US databases for AIDS with those for cancer, the relative risk of anal cancer in homosexual men compared to men in the general population at the time of or after AIDS diagnosis was 84.1.[16] The relative risk of anal cancer for up to 5 years before AIDS diagnosis was 13.9.

Anal canal carcinoma and AIN are associated with condylomata.[13] HPV-16 infection has a strong association with high-grade

Holland-Frei Cancer Medicine, Ninth Edition. Edited by Robert C. Bast Jr., Carlo M. Croce, William N. Hait, Waun Ki Hong, Donald W. Kufe, Martine Piccart-Gebhart, Raphael E. Pollock, Ralph R. Weichselbaum, Hongyang Wang, and James F. Holland.

AIN and a risk of anogenital malignancy. However, HPV infection alone may be insufficient for malignant transformation, as many patients with HPV-positive cytology do not develop either AIN or anal cancer.[17]

Molecular factors

Overexpression of p53 protein has been studied in patients receiving CMT. In an analysis involving approximately 20% of patients entered on both arms of the Radiation Therapy Oncology Group (RTOG) protocol 87-04, there was a trend toward adverse outcome (decreased local control and survival) in patients over expressing p53.[18] In one study of 55 patients, MIB-1 murine monoclonal antibody measurement of Ki 67 failed to predict outcome for patients treated with radiation, with or without chemotherapy.[19] Patel el al proposed that activation of AKT, possibly through the PI3K-AKT pathway, is a component of the development of SCCs.[20] In a cohort of 142 Danish patients with SCC of the anal canal treated with CMT, p16 positivity was an independent prognostic factor for disease specific and overall survival.[21] Williams et al reported that elevated serum SCC antigen in 174 patients with SCC of the anal margin and canal were associated with a decreased chance of achieving a clinical complete response (cCR), local control, or longer survival.[22] Fraunholz reported that EGFR expression correlates with outcome.[23] A systematic review of 29 biomarkers in 21 published trials reported that p53 and p21 were the only markers found to be prognostic in more than one trial.[24]

Other factors

The relationship between anal cancer and fistulas is conflicting. In one study, 41% of anal canal carcinomas were preceded by benign anorectal disease for at least 5 years.[25] However, two studies reveal only a temporal relationship but no evidence of causation.[26,27] In a separate study, homosexual males with a history of anal fissure or fistula had an elevated risk of anorectal squamous cell carcinoma (RR, 9.1).[28] Overall, the incidence of anal canal cancers in patients with Crohn's disease is low.[29] Immunosupressed renal transplant patients have a 100-fold increase in anogenital tumors compared with the general population.[30] In a series of 3595 patients undergoing a solid organ transplant, the incidence of anal cancer was 0.11%.[31]

Pathology

A variety of histologic cell types may occur in the anal area.[32] The majority of these (75–80%) are squamous cell carcinomas[33] and 15% are adenocarcinomas. In addition to the more common types seen in Table 1, other rare histologic entities can arise, such as small cell carcinomas[35] and lymphoma. Melanomas constitute 1–2% of all anal cancers.[36]

Squamous tumors may arise from the entire length of the anal canal as well as from the anal margin. Basaloid carcinomas, which

Table 1 Histologic types of anal cancer.

Type	%
Squamous cell	63
Transitional (cloacogenic)	23
Adenocarcinoma	7
Basal cell	2
Melanoma	2
Pagets disease	2

Source: Peters 1983,[34] Reproduced with permission of MacMillan Publishing Group.

are a variant of squamous carcinoma, are commonly referred to as cloacogenic carcinomas. Adenocarcinomas arise from the glands at the dentate line. Small cell carcinomas are of neuroendocrine origin and are rare.

Tumors of the anal margin include squamous carcinoma, basal cell carcinoma, Bowen's disease (squamous CIS), Paget's disease (adenocarcinoma *in situ*), verrucous carcinoma, and Kaposi's sarcoma. Malignant melanomas may arise from either location but more commonly from below the dentate line.

Squamous cell tumors are divided into those with and without keratinization,[37] and nonkeratinizing tumors are further subdivided into basosquamous, basaloid, and cloacogenic carcinomas. With the exception of melanoma and sarcoma, most clinicians conclude that prognosis is more dependent on stage rather than histology and treat all histologic varieties the same.[38,39] In contrast, using a multivariate analysis, Das and associates reported a higher distant metastasis rate for patients with basaloid histologies.[40]

Studies of flow cytometric analysis are conflicting and have reported both high proliferative index but near-diploid peaks[41] as well as an aneuploid pattern.[42] In a multivariate analysis by Shepard et al, the depth of penetration, inguinal node involvement, and DNA ploidy were of independent prognostic significance.[43]

Natural history

The most common route of spread is by local extension proximally to involve other organs in the pelvis. Hematogenous spread occurs more often from tumors that arise at or above the dentate line.[44] This pattern of spread allows tumor cells into the portal system resulting in liver and lung metastases in 5–8% of patients[44] and bone in 2%.[45] Distant metastases occur with equal frequency independent of the histologic cell type involved. Distant metastases are rarely seen with anal margin tumors.

Lymphatic spread is common and involves the inguinal, pelvic, and mesenteric nodes. Inguinal lymph nodes are positive in 15–63% of cases.[46,47] The incidence of synchronous positive inguinal nodes is 15%.[44,48] In a series of 96 patients, Metachronous positive inguinal nodes appeared in 25% with a median time to presentation of 12 months. Pelvic nodes are less commonly involved and mesenteric nodes are more likely to be involved if the tumors are proximal (50%) than distal (14%).[49] Positive mesenteric nodes in anal margin tumors are rare.

Historic surgical series report survivals of 0–20% following lymph node dissection with synchronous positive nodes.[50,51] Modern CMT has substantially improved this. Patients who undergo lymph node dissection for metachronous lesions have more favorable survivals with rates as high as 83%.[50,52] The majority of these recurrences occur by 2 years but may present as late as 8 years.[49]

Diagnosis

The initial and most common symptom is bleeding, which occurs in over 50% of patients. Other common symptoms include pain, tenesmus, pruritus, change in bowel habits, abnormal discharge, and less commonly, inguinal lymphadenopathy.[49,53,54] Most of these symptoms are associated with benign conditions of the anus including fissure, fistula-in-ano, hemorrhoids, anal pruritus, and anal condyloma. Benign perianal conditions may coexist in 60% of anal margin tumors and in 6% of anal canal tumors.[55]

The most common physical finding is an intraluminal mass that can be misdiagnosed as a hemorrhoid.[45,46] Endoscopically, the tumors may appear as flat or slightly raised lesions, as raised lesions

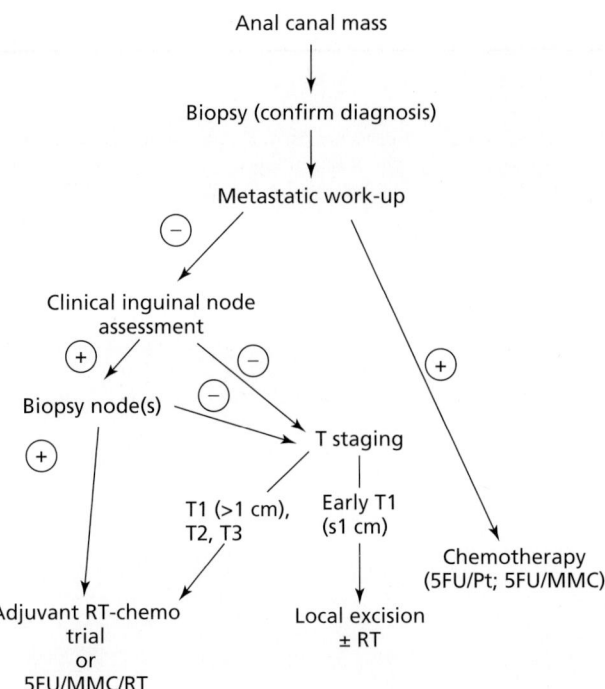

Anal canal mass

↓

Biopsy (confirm diagnosis)

↓

Metastatic work-up

(−)

Clinical inguinal node assessment

(+) (−) (+)

Biopsy node(s)

(+)

T staging

T1 (>1 cm), T2, T3   Early T1 (≤1 cm)

Chemotherapy (5FU/Pt; 5FU/MMC)

Adjuvant RT-chemo trial or 5FU/MMC/RT   Local excision ± RT

Figure 1 Treatment schema for squamous cell cancer of the anal canal.

with indurated borders, or as polypoid lesions (Figure 1). The use of transrectal ultrasound is required and allows for the determination of depth of penetration and involvement of adjacent organs.[56]

An incisional biopsy is recommended for diagnosis. Excisional biopsies should be limited to small superficial lesions. Clinically palpable inguinal lymphadenopathy should be aspirated for cytological examination. A formal inguinal lymph node dissection is not recommended owing to the associated morbidity, failure to have an impact on outcome, and the high control rates with CMT. In a report by Garcia and associates of 46 HIV+ patients, anal brush cytology was more sensitive and specific for external compared with internal lesions.[57] High-resolution anoscopy is helpful in detecting both high-grade intraepithelial and invasive lesions in HIV+[58] and HIV−[59] patients.

Although a metastatic work-up is commonly negative, it includes computed tomography (CT) of the abdomen and pelvis to evaluate the primary tumor and exclude liver metastases. A chest X-ray or chest CT is required.

Most studies reveal a benefit of positron emission tomography (PET) for staging.[60–63] In a series of 41 patients, [18]flourodeoxyuridine glucose positron emission tomography ([18]FDG-PET) detected 91% of nonexcised primaries compared with 59% with CT alone.[64] In addition, 17% of inguinal nodes negative by CT and physical exam were positive by PET. Sveistrup et al.[62] performed a retrospective analysis of 28 patients with SCC and found that compared with transrectal ultrasound, PET/CT upstaged disease in 14% and changed the treatment plan in 17%. Bannas et al.[65] reported that compared with either PET or CT alone, radiation field design was changed in 23% of patient who underwent a combined PET-CT.

Although feasible, the benefit of sentinel inguinal lymph node biopsy is variable and its role remains controversial.[66–68]

Staging

A common staging system was developed in 1997 by the AJCC and the UICC. This staging system accounts for the fact that anal canal

carcinoma is primarily treated by CMT and abdominoperineal resection (APR) is reserved for treatment failure. The TNM classification is clinical. The primary tumor is assessed for size and for invasion of local structures such as the vagina, urethra, or bladder. The seventh edition of the AJCC staging system is seen in Table 2.[69]

Prognostic factors

As with most gastrointestinal cancers, the most important prognostic factors in anal cancer are T and N stage. In patients treated with radiation with or without chemotherapy, the most striking difference in results is seen when comparing T1-2 primary cancers (≤5 cm) versus T3-4 primary cancers (>5 cm). The local failure rates with T3-4 primary cancers are approximately 50% following CMT. When a complete response is achieved, the local failure rate is 25%.

Peiffert et al.[70] reported an increase in local failure with T-stage (T1: 11%, T2: 24%, T3: 45%, and T4: 43%) and a corresponding decrease in 5-year survival (T1: 94%, T2: 79%, T3: 53%, and T4: 19%). A similar decrease in 5-year colostomy-free survival with T1-2 tumors versus T3-4 tumors was reported by Gerard et al.[71] (T1: 83% and T2: 89% vs T3: 50% and T4: 54%).

In contrast to T stage, the impact of positive lymph nodes is less clear. Unlike rectal cancer, inguinal lymph nodes in anal cancer are considered nodal (N) metastasis rather than distant (M) metastasis and patients should be treated in a potentially curative manner. Cummings et al reported that patients with negative nodes who received CMT had a higher 5-year cause specific survival compared with those with positive nodes (81% vs 57%).[72]

The RTOG 87-04 trial (Table 3) reported a higher colostomy rate (which is an indirect measurement of local failure) in N1 versus N0 patients (28% vs 13%).[73] In node negative and possibly node positive patients, the addition of mitomycin-C decreased the overall colostomy rates. The EORTC randomized trial (Table 3) of 45 Gy ± 5-FU/mitomycin-C also reported that patients with positive nodes experienced significantly higher local failure (p = 0.035) and lower survival (p = 0.038) rates compared to those with negative nodes.[76]

Allal et al. reported that, by multivariate analysis, the only variable for which there was a possible impact was overall treatment time (p = 0.09).[80] In the EORTC randomized trial, multivariate analysis identified that positive nodes, skin ulceration, and male gender were independent negative prognostic factors for local control and survival.[76] Goldman et al.[81] also found that women had a more favorable outcome than men. The multivariate analysis of 167 patients by Das et al.[40] revealed that higher T and N stage correlated with increased local failure, N stage, and basaloid histology was associated with distant failure and N stage and HIV+ predicted for lower survival. Other authors have reported that T stage, radiation dose, and percent hemoglobin were significant. In the Intergroup RTOG 98-11 trial (Table 3), multivariate analysis revealed that male gender (p = 0.04), clinically N+ (p < 0.0001), and tumor size >5 cm (0.005) were independent prognostic factors for disease free survival.[77]

The histologic cell type for squamous cancers of the anal canal (squamous versus cloacogenic) has not been found to be of major prognostic significance. In some series, cloacogenic carcinomas have been considered to have a slightly better prognosis.[38,82] However, in a series of 243 patients with resectable anal canal tumors, there was a worse prognosis for nonkeratinizing and basaloid carcinoma versus keratinizing lesions.[83] Small cell carcinomas of the anus are rare and, similar to extra pulmonary small cell cancers in other parts of the body, appear to have a worse prognosis and a high incidence of metastatic disease.[35,84] Location has modest

Table 2 AJCC TNM staging system for anal canal cancer (seventh edition).

Primary tumor (T)			
TX	Primary tumor cannot be assessed		
T_0	No evidence of primary tumor		
T_{is}	Carcinoma *in situ*		
T_1	Tumor ≤ 2 cm in maximum diameter		
T_2	Tumor > 2 cm but ≤ 5 cm in maximum diameter		
T_3	Tumor > 5 cm in maximum diameter		
T_4	Tumor of any size, which invades an adjacent structure(s) (involvement of the sphincter muscle(s) alone is not classified as T4)		
Regional lymph nodes (N)			
N_X	Regional lymph nodes cannot be assessed		
N_0	No regional lymph node metastasis		
N_1	Perirectal lymph node metastasis		
N_2	Unilateral internal iliac and/or inguinal node metastasis		
N_3	Perirectal and inguinal node, and/or bilateral internal iliac and/or inguinal node metastasis		
Distant metastasis (M)			
M_X	Distant metastasis cannot be assessed		
M_0	No distant metastasis		
M_1	Distant metastasis		
Stage groupings			
Stage			
0	T_{is}	N_0	M_0
I	T_1	N_0	M_0
II	T_{2-3}	N_0	M_0
IIIA	T_4	N_0	M_0
	T_{1-3}	N_1	M_0
IIIB	T_4	N_1	M_0
	T_{1-4}	N_{2-3}	M_0
IV	T_{1-4}	N_{0-3}	M_1

Note: Anal margin cancers are classified as skin cancers.
Note: Additional descriptors: Although they do not impact the stage grouping, additional prefixes are used, which indicate the need for additional analysis:

Suffix	Reason
m	The presence of multiple primary tumors in a single site and is recorded in parenthesis: pT(m)NM
y	When classification is performed during or following initial radiation and/or chemotherapy and is based on the amount of tumor present at the time of the examination, and not an estimate of tumor before therapy: ycTNM or ypTNM
r	Indicates recurrent tumor: rTNM
a	Indicates the stage at autopsy: aTNM
Lymphatic vessel invasion (L)	
Lx	Cannot be assessed
L0	No lymphatic vessel invasion
L1	Lymphatic vessel invasion present
Venous invasion (V)	
Vx	Cannot be assessed
V0	No venous Invasion
V1	Microscopic venous Invasion present
V2	Macroscopic venous invasion present

Source: Edge 2010.[69] Reproduced with permission of Springer.

prognostic importance with anal margin tumors having a better outcome than those in the anal canal.

Three studies have examined DNA content (diploid vs nondiploid). Two found no prognostic impact of this factor,[42,43] while in one multivariate analysis of 184 patients,[84] DNA ploidy was an independent prognostic factor for survival. In a separate study,[42] grade was a significant prognostic factor, with low-grade tumors resulting in a 5-year survival of 75% compared with only 24% for high-grade tumors. Data from the Princess Margaret Hospital suggest that the DT-diaphorase mutation is not a strong determinant of treatment outcome in patients who fail CMT.[85]

Tanum and Holm[86] reported p53 expression in 34% of patients with anal cancer. Pretreatment biopsies from 80 patients treated on the CMT arm of the Intergroup RTOG 87-04 randomized trial were examined by immunohistochemistry for p53 expression.[87] For the total group, p53 protein was overexpressed in 47% of tumors. By multivariate analysis, the 4-year local disease-free survival was significantly decreased in those patients whose tumors overexpressed p53 (64% vs 88%, $p = 0.027$). However,

significant differences were not seen in overall disease free or overall survival.

In a retrospective analysis from the Princess Margaret Hospital, p53 was measured by immunohistochemistry in 49 patients who received CMT.[88] The incidence of p53 expression was 82%. By univariate analysis, p53 expression $\geq 5\%$ was a poor prognostic factor for 5-year survival (78% vs 90%) compared with $< 5\%$. It was an independent poor prognostic factor for disease-free survival ($p = 0.01$).

Treatment for primary disease

General principles

Local excision

Local excision has been used in selected patients with tumors that are <2 cm, well differentiated, or tumors found incidentally at

Table 3 Randomized trials of combined modality therapy for anal cancer.

Trial	Number of points	Initial treatment	Assessment/treatment of residual	Arm	% CR	% With colostomy	% Local crude	Control—actuarial	% CFS	Survival—overall
Intergroup[73] RTOG 8704 ECOG 1289	291	45 Gy 5-FU —Vs.— 45 Gy 5-FU/MMC	Residual Positive[a] / Boost 9 Gy +5-FU CDDP / Negative Observe	RT/5-FU / RT/5-FU/ MMC	85 / 92	22 / * / 9	— / — / —	— / —	59 / * / 71	70 (4-year) / 75 (4-year)
ACT I[74,75]	585	45 Gy —Vs.— 45 Gy 5-FU/MMC	≥50% CR[a] 15–20 Gy EBRT or brachytherapy / <50% CR Salvage surgery	RT / RT/5-FU/ MMC	— / —	— / —	41 / * / 64	34 (5-year) * / 59 (5-year)	20 / 30	33 (5-year) / 28 (5-year)
EORTC[76]	110	45 Gy —Vs.— 45 Gy 5-FU/MMC	PR/CR[a] 15–20 Gy EBRT or brachytherapy / < PR Salvage surgery	RT / RT/5-FU/ MMC	54 / 80	— / —	55 / * / 73	50 (5-year) * / 68 (5-year)	40 (5-year) / * / 72 (5-year)	52 (5-year) / 57 (5-year)
Intergroup[77,78] RTOG 98-11 ECOG 1289	598	45 Gy 5-FU/MMC —Vs.— 45 Gy 5-FU/CDDP	Positive[b] 5-FU/CDDP or MMC / Negative Observe	5-FU/CDDP 10–14 Gy / 5-FU/MMC MMC	—	20 / 10	26 / 33	20 / 26	65 / * / 74 (5-year)	71 (5-year) / 78 (5-year)
ACT II[79]	940	50.4 Gy 5-FU/CDDP ± maintenance 5-FU/MMC —Vs.— 50.4 Gy 5-FU/MMC ± maintenance 5-FU/MMC	— / —	5-FU/CDDP 90 / 5-FU/MMC 91						72 PFS (3-year) / 73 PFS (3-year)

CFS, Colostomy free survival; *, statistically significant ($p \leq 0.05$); MMC, Mitomycin-C; CDDP, cisplatin; LN+, lymph node positive; CR, complete response; PFS, progression free survival; EBRT, external beam radiation therapy. The ACT I trial included 23% anal margin cancers.

[a]Biopsy at 6 weeks.
[b]Biopsy at 8 weeks.

the time of hemorrhoidectomy. Of 188 patients with anal canal carcinoma treated at the Mayo Clinic, a subset of 19 were treated with local excision.[35] For the 12 patients with tumors confined to the epithelium and subepithelial connective tissues, 11 had tumors <2 cm and 1 patient had two lesions. The survival was 100%. One of 12 patients recurred, and this patient was without evidence of disease 5 years after salvage APR. Patients with tumors penetrating into muscle who refused a colostomy had a higher recurrence rate. These patients often can be salvaged with an APR or CMT.

In summary, local excision alone is reasonable for those cancers found incidentally following hemorrhoidectomy for T1 tumors, which can be excised while maintaining sphincter continence. They require close follow-up and local recurrences can subsequently be treated with CMT.

Brachytherapy

In contrast with treatment programs in North America where patients receive CMT, patients treated in selected European centers, most commonly France, receive external beam radiation therapy alone, with or without brachytherapy. The nonrandomized data suggest that the results of radiation therapy alone are comparable to CMT; however, the radiation-related toxicity is higher.[89] Brachytherapy techniques commonly involve afterloading ^{192}Ir. A frequent treatment approach is external beam for the first 45 Gy followed by an additional 15–20 Gy with a perineal boost or brachytherapy.

Ortholan and associates treated 66 patients with T1/TIS tumors with brachytherapy with or without small field external beam radiation.[90] With a median follow-up of 50 months, there were only six local failures of which four occurred outside of the radiation field.

Abdominoperineal resection

APR is reserved for salvage in patients who have failed radiation or in patients who have received prior pelvic radiation therapy. The results will be discussed later.

Chemoradiation therapy

The conventional treatment for anal canal cancer was APR until the late 1970s. This standard was challenged by Nigro et al in his initial report of three patients with SCC of the anal canal who, following preoperative treatment with 30 Gy plus concurrent 5-FU and mitomycin-C, were found to have a pathologic complete response at the time of surgery.[91]

Since that time, many single-arm phase II studies have indicated that initial CMT yields an 80–90% complete response rate with APR reserved for salvage. Even in patients with large (≥5 cm) primary cancers, although the complete response rates are lower (50–75%), the majority of patients may be spared a colostomy and have an excellent overall survival.

Chemotherapy

Results of two prospective randomized trials (Table 3) from Europe of CMT versus radiation alone (EORTC[76] and UKCCCR ACT 1[74]) support the use of CMT. With 13-year follow-up of the UKC-CCR ACT 1 trial, patients who received CMT versus radiation alone had a significant improvement in both local control (59% vs 34%) and colostomy free survival (30% vs 20%). However, the improvement in overall survival (33% vs 28%) did not reach statistical significance.[74] In the EORTC trial, CMT resulted in a higher complete response rate (80% vs 54%) and a significantly higher 5-year actuarial local control rate (68% vs 50%) and colostomy-free

survival rate (72% vs. 40%) but no significant difference in survival 57% vs 52%).[76] Although neither trial revealed a significant overall survival advantage, given the improvement in local control and colostomy-free survival, they helped to establish CMT as the standard of care.

Results and controversies

In the North America, CMT has been well established and randomized trials have focused on defining the ideal regimen. The role of mitomycin-C as a necessary component of CMT was confirmed by the Intergroup trial RTOG 87-04.[73] Patients were randomized to 45 Gy plus continuous infusion 5-FU with or without mitomycin-C. At 6 weeks following the completion of treatment patients with less than a complete response had an additional 9 Gy to the primary tumor plus concurrent 5-FU/cisplatin as salvage therapy. If there was still less than a complete response 6 weeks after the completion of this salvage therapy, an APR was performed. Patients who received mitomycin-C had a higher complete response rate (92% vs 85%) and a significantly lower colostomy rate (9% vs 22%) and a corresponding significant increase in colostomy-free survival (71% vs 59%) (Table 3). There was little difference in overall 4-year survival (75% vs 70%). Early grade 4+ toxicity was significantly increased in the mitomycin-C arm (23% vs 7%). Although overall survival was not significantly increased given the advantage in colostomy-free survival, mitomycin-C is considered a necessary component of CMT.

Mitomycin-C versus cisplatin

For patients who receive mitomycin-C-based regimens, rates of complete response are 84% (81–87%), local control is 73% (64–86%), and 5-year survival rate is 77% (66–92%). For patients with T1-2 disease, the complete response rates are >90% with ultimate local control rates following surgical salvage of 80–90%. In patients with T3-4 disease, approximately 50% of patients will require a salvage APR. If they achieve a complete response following the completion of CMT, then only 25% will require salvage APR.

Although the results of 5-FU, mitomycin-C, and concurrent 45 Gy are impressive, there is room for improvement, especially in patients with T3-4 disease. A variety of treatment approaches have been tested. These include the use of 5-FU and cisplatin (as induction therapy and/or concurrently with radiation) and intensifying the radiation dose beyond 45 Gy using external beam or brachytherapy. The combination of 5-FU plus cisplatin is an attractive regimen: (1) patients who have failed 5-FU/mitomycin-C still respond to 5-FU/cisplatin and (2) cisplatin is a radiation sensitizer.

The Intergroup randomized trial RTOG 98-11 was developed to compare conventional CMT with 5-FU/mitomycin-C versus induction 5-FU/cisplatin chemotherapy followed by CMT with 5-FU/cisplatin (Table 3).[78] A total of 682 patients with stages T2-4 squamous (86%), basaloid, or cloacogenic carcinoma of the anal canal were randomized. Patients were stratified by gender, clinical node status, and tumor size and the primary endpoint was disease-free survival. Overall, 27% had tumors >5 cm, 35% had T3-4 tumors, and 26% were clinically node positive.

Treatment details by arm were as follows. Conventional CMT arm: 5-FU (1000 mg/m^2 days 1–4 and 29–32) plus mitomycin (10 mg/m^2 days 1 and 29) and radiation (45–59 Gy). Induction arm: 5-FU (1000 mg/m^2 days 1–4, 29–32, 57–60, and 85–88) plus cisplatin (75 mg/m^2 on days 1, 29, 57, and 85) and radiation (45–59 Gy beginning day 57).

Radiation doses and techniques were the same for both arms. The whole pelvis received 30.6 Gy (1.8 Gy/fx) followed by a 14.4 Gy cone down to the true pelvis. For N0 patients, the inguinal nodes were excluded after 36 Gy. For patients with T3-4 and/or N+ disease or for those T2 lesions with residual disease after 45 Gy, a second cone down of 10–14 Gy to the gross disease or nodal disease was performed.

Palpable inguinal nodes were biopsied before treatment, and a full thickness biopsy was optional 8 weeks following completion of CMT if any palpable residual abnormality was present in the inguinal node region. Local regional failure was defined as the present of disease in the radiation field at the 8-week follow-up.

With long-term follow-up, patient who received mitomycin-C-based treatment had a significant improvement in 5-year disease-free survival (68% vs 58%, $p = 0.006$), 5-year colostomy-free survival (72% vs 65%, $p = 0.05$), and overall survival (78% vs 71%, $p = 0.026$). Although local-regional failure was lower (20% vs 26%), it did not reach statistical significance. There was no difference in Grade 3+ long-term toxicity (13% vs 11%). Consistent with other reports, a separate analysis revealed that higher T and N category had a significant negative impact on outcomes including local regional failure, distant metastasis, colostomy-free survival, disease-free survival, and overall survival.[92]

Similar results were reported in the UKCCR ACT II trial. This four-arm trial compared cisplatin versus mitomycin-C-based CMT (50.4 Gy) with a secondary randomization to maintenance 5-FU/cisplatin versus observation.[79] A total of 940 patients (81% anal canal, 15% anal margin, 43% T3-4, and 62% N+) were randomized. Compared with mitomycin-C-based CMT, patients who received cisplatin-based CMT had no significant differences in the CR rate at 6 months (90% vs 91%), grade 3+ toxicity (72% vs 71%), or 3-year progression-free survival with maintenance (72% vs 73%) or without maintenance chemotherapy (74% vs 73%).

In summary, mitomycin-C-based conventional CMT remains the standard of care. Despite these results, a number of investigators still advocate the use of cisplatin-based CMT based on single institution series.[93] New CMT approaches including the use of cytotoxic agents such as capecitabine, oxaliplatin, and cetuximab have been investigated.[94,95] To date, these approaches, as well as the use of 3 drug regimens,[96] have not shown benefits compared with 5-FU/Mitomycin-C-based CMT.

Dose intensification

Conventional external beam

In an attempt to improve local control and survival, two parallel pilot trials of radiation dose intensification were performed. In both trials, patients received 36 Gy to the pelvis (30.6 whole pelvis plus 5.4 Gy to the true pelvis) and following a 2-week break, received an additional 23.4 Gy to the primary tumor with a 2–3 cm margin for a total dose of 59.4 Gy. The main differences between the two trials were the type of chemotherapy. The RTOG 9208 trial[97] used 5-FU and mitomycin-C, whereas the ECOG 4292 trial(2297) used 5-FU and cisplatin.

The RTOG 9208 trial reported similar results to the standard regimen of 45 Gy plus 5-FU/mitomycin-C used in RTOG 87-04 except for a higher 2-year colostomy rate (30% vs 7%). Similarly, the ECOG 4292 trial did not reveal a benefit compared with conventional treatment.[98] Long-term follow-up of the ECOG 4292 trial revealed a 5-year PFS of 55% and a 5-year overall survival of 69%, which is consistent with other cisplatin-based trials.[99] One retrospective series revealed improved local control and survival with doses >60 Gy.[100] The RTOG 98-11 trial allowed a boost of 10–14 Gy; however, a dose–response analysis has not been presented.[77]

The four-arm UNICANCER ACCORD 03 randomized trial examined the role of both induction chemotherapy and dose escalation. A total of 307 patients received 5-Fu/cisplatin CMT + 45 Gy with or without induction 5-FU/cisplatin. This was followed by a brachytherapy or external beam boost of wither 15 or 25 Gy.[101] Neither induction chemotherapy (77% vs 75%) nor the boost (78% vs 74%) had a significant improvement in 5-year colostomy-free survival.

Brachytherapy

Brachytherapy is an ideal method by which to deliver conformal radiation while sparing the surrounding normal structures. In most series, patients received 30–55 Gy of pelvic radiation with or without chemotherapy followed by a 15–25 Gy boost with Ir192 afterloading catheters. Most use low dose rate, but some investigators have advocated high dose rate.[102–104]

Combining the series, the mean results include a complete response rate of 83% (73–91%), local control rates of 81% (73–89%), and a 5-year survival rate of 70% (60–84%). The primary concern is anal necrosis and reports vary from 2% to as high as 76%[103] with an average of 5–15%. Although a retrospective analysis from Hannoun-Levi et al.[105] revealed an improvement in local control with a brachytherapy versus external beam boost and in another series from France revealed a toxicity benefit from a brachytherapy boost versus no boost,[106] the randomized UNICANCER ACCORD 03 trial discussed earlier did not confirm a local control benefit.[101]

Intensity-modulated radiation therapy

IMRT is a method to deliver pelvic radiation therapy with lower acute and long-term toxicity. By identification of the dose-limiting tissues surrounding the primary tumor and pelvic nodes and using multiple radiation fields to avoid them, IMRT allows for dose escalation with less toxicity. Salama and associates treated 53 patients with IMRT-based CMT.[107] Patients received 45 Gy whole pelvis followed by a boost to a median of 51.5 Gy. Acute grade 3 toxicities were 15% GI and 28% skin. Acute grade 4 toxicities included 30% leucopenia and 34% neutropenia. With a median follow-up of 15 months, freedom from failure included local (84%) and distant (93%) and survivals were colostomy free:84% and overall: 93%. Other investigators have reported similar reductions in acute toxicity.[108–110]

The RTOG 0529 phase II trial examined IMRT in a cooperative group setting.[111] A total of 63 patients were treated with 5-FU/mitomycin-C plus IMRT based on stage (T2N0: 50.4 Gy primary PTV and 42 Gy nodal PTV, T3-4N0-3: 54 Gy primary PTV and 45 Gy nodal PTV). Compared with RTOG 98-11, patients who received IMRT had fewer treatment breaks (49% vs 62%) and lower acute toxicity (grade 2+ heme [73 vs 85, $p = 0.032$], grade 3+ GI [21% vs 36%, $p = 0.0082$], and grade 3+ skin [23% vs 49%, $p < 0.0001$]). Another finding was the steep learning curve for IMRT planning. Although institutions were required to be IMRT certified, 81% of the plans required initial modification and 46% required a second revision. Contouring guides are now routinely available.[112] On the basis of both single institution and RTOG data, IMRT has become the standard of care for CMT treatment of anal cancer.

Radiation therapy alone

Radiation therapy alone with either external beam or combined with brachytherapy may yield comparable local control and survival rates to CMT. However, as it is associated with an increase in anal necrosis even in experienced hands, it should be used with caution.

Is biopsy necessary at 6 weeks?

There is considerable controversy as to the need for the first biopsy at 6 weeks following initial treatment. Data from the Princess Margaret Hospital suggest that SCCs regress slowly and continue to decrease in size for 3–12 months after the completion of CMT.[72] The ACT II trial reported a clinical CR rate of 66% at 11 weeks following CMT, which increased to 84% at 26 weeks.

On the basis of these data, an increasing number of investigators advocate a more conservative approach and do not recommend a posttreatment biopsy. In the RTOG 87-04 trial, of the 25 patients with biopsy proven residual disease after 45 Gy and 5-FU/mitomycin-C who then received salvage therapy with 9 Gy plus 5-FU/cisplatin, 55% achieved a complete response 6 weeks later (a total of 12 weeks following the completion of the initial 45 Gy).[73] It is unclear if the complete response was a result of the "salvage" therapy or was due to an additional 6 weeks of tumor regression following initial therapy.

At many institutions, if there is residual disease at the 6 week posttreatment evaluation, patients do not receive the 1 week of "salvage" therapy. The patients are examined every 6 weeks and providing the tumor continues to decrease in size, no salvage therapy is performed. However, if there is progression of disease or no response at 6 weeks following initial therapy, APR is necessary. In addition to careful physical exam, anal ultrasound may be helpful in following the tumor. In the Intergroup phase III anal canal cancer protocol RTOG 98-11, biopsy at 6 weeks following the initial 45 Gy was optional.

Treatment of the HIV-positive patient

In general, HIV+ patients have received lower doses of radiation and chemotherapy owing to a concern that standard therapy may not be tolerated.[16] With a better understanding of the immunological deficiencies seen in HIV-positive patients, more recent reports have recommended therapy based on clinical and immunological parameters such as a history of prior opportunistic infections and CD4 counts.[113–115] Patients with a CD4 count >200 μL who receive effective doses of antiviral therapy have outcomes similar to non-HIV patients and should be treated as aggressively.[116] CMT can result in prolonged decreased CD4 counts one series reports an increase in late deaths,[117] whereas another series report no increased HIV-related morbidity up to 6 years following CMT.[118] For those patients with a CD4 count <200 μL or who have signs or symptoms of other HIV-related diseases, attenuated doses of radiation and/or chemotherapy are recommended.

Toxicity of treatment

As seen with other cancer therapies, pelvic radiation is associated with acute and long-term toxicity. The acute toxicity is due to a combination of chemotherapy and radiation therapy. These include leukopenia, thrombocytopenia, proctitis, diarrhea, cystitis, and perineal erythema. Long-term toxicity is primarily increased urgency and fecal incontinence.[119,120] This is due to both the impact of radiation on the sphincter and the fact that when the tumor responds it is replaced by fibrotic tissue rather than new sphincter muscle. Acute toxicity is lower with IMRT versus conventional 3D radiation[107–111,121]; however, long-term toxicity data are not yet available.

There are limited reports of functional outcome in the anal cancer literature. One series reports that full function was maintained in 93% of patients[122] and a second series, which used anorectal manometry, reported complete continence in 56%.[123] Another

reported good to excellent function in 93% of patients with a minimum of 1-year follow-up.[124]

Treatment of anal margin cancer

Anal margin cancers are considered to be skin cancers. In brief, a reasonable approach is to recommend a local excision for smaller tumors (≤4 cm), which are not in direct contact with the anal verge. If the patient would require an APR due to anatomic constraints, or if a local excision would compromise sphincter function, or if the tumor is >4 cm and/or node positive, then nonoperative treatment is an appropriate alternative. On the basis of the randomized trial from the UKCCCR (which included 23% of patients with anal margin cancers), CMT is recommended. In a report from Erlangen, 5-year colostomy-free (69%) and overall survival (54%) rates of anal margin tumors treated with CMT were lower than anal canal tumors. However, this may have been due to the higher T stages.[125]

Follow-up after treatment

Patients treated for anal cancer need to be followed carefully as those with local failure are amenable to salvage APR and can achieve long-term survival. Patients should be examined by physical exam and anoscopy every 6 weeks until a complete response is achieved then every 3 months for a total of 2 years. Follow-up examinations can then be decreased to every 6 months for the next 3 years and then yearly after 5 years. When failure of CMT occurs, 95% of the time it occurs within 3 years.[126]

The usefulness of CT of the abdomen and pelvis or FDG-PET for follow-up is unclear. Christensen and colleagues reported that sensitivity for detecting recurrences was 1.0 for 3D ultrasound combined with physical exam versus 0.86 for 3D ultrasound alone versus 0.57 for 2D ultrasound.[127] Goh et al examined MRI in 35 patients 6–8 weeks after CMT and found that it was not helpful in predicting future clinical outcome.[128] As the most common site of failure is at the primary tumor site, there is no substitute for physical exam.

Management of inguinal nodes

When examining the impact of positive lymph nodes on local control and survival, it is important to identify the site of nodal disease and differentiate synchronous versus metachronous nodal disease. Unfortunately, most series do not separate N1 versus N2 versus N3 disease. However, there are data examining synchronous versus metachronous nodal disease.

There are conflicting reports as to the prognosis of patients with synchronous nodal disease who are treated with CMT. Compared with node negative patients, Allal et al report a higher rate of local failure (N1-3: 36% vs N0:19%),[129] and the Intergroup RTOG 87-04 trial reported a higher colostomy rate (N1: 28% vs N0: 13%).[70] Although Cummings and associates reported a local failure rate of only 13% in node positive patients, 5-year cause-specific survival was lower (N1-3: 57% vs N0: 81%).[72] By multivariate analysis, the EORTC randomized trial reported that positive nodes were an independent negative prognostic factor for local failure and survival.[76]

In contrast, in the CMT plus brachytherapy series from Gerard et al.,[71] patients with N1 versus N0 disease had similar 5-year disease specific and overall survival rates. Similarly, complete response rates in the primary tumor are not affected by the presence of nodal disease. Doci and associates report similar rates in patients receiving cisplatin-based therapy (N1-3: 92% vs N0: 100%)[130] and in a separate series of patients receiving mitomycin-C-based therapy, all eight patients with N1-3 disease achieved a complete response.[131] Overall, external beam radiation alone[1,132–134] can control positive nodes in 65% of patients, and CMT[1,73,75,76] can achieve nodal control in approximately 90%.

Patients with T2N0 disease should receive prophylactic radiation. In a retrospective review of patients with stages T1N0 and T2 N0 disease in whom the inguinal nodes were excluded from the radiation field, the inguinal failure rate was 2% and 13%, respectively.[135]

The current treatment recommendations for patients with suspicious positive inguinal nodes include needle aspiration or at the most limited surgical sampling for confirmation of cancer followed by CMT with a boost of 45–50.4 Gy to the involved groin. Although inguinal node dissection should not be performed as part of the initial therapy, it may be done for isolated inguinal recurrence in carefully selected patients as the morbidity from such an approach is significant.

The development of unilateral metachronous inguinal lymph nodes is not associated with such an ominous prognosis. After therapeutic groin dissection, the 5- to 7-year survival rates exceed 50% in two series,[48] but there were no long-term survivors in a small series reported from the Mayo Clinic.[6] Current strategies in patients with metachronous isolated inguinal node metastases after CMT include a formal groin dissection followed by chemotherapy. The use of radiation in this setting depends on prior dose and fields.

Residual or recurrent cancer

1. Anal margin: Locally recurrent anal margin cancers are more successfully controlled by local excision than are recurrences of anal canal cancer.[136,137] A series of recurrent tumors included 16 of 48 patients who, following a local excision, recurred locally,[11] in the inguinal nodes,[4] or both.[1138] There were no visceral failures. The median time to recurrence was 26 months. Ten of the patients with local recurrences underwent repeat local excision and only one required an APR. Nine of these patients survived more than 5 years. All four patients with inguinal node recurrences had inguinal lymphadenectomies, and two were long-term survivors. Although there is little reported experience with radiation therapy or CMT for patients with local recurrence after a local excision, it is a reasonable option for those who would otherwise require an APR, dependent on prior radiation dose, if any.
2. Anal canal. The standard treatment is APR.

Treatment of metastatic disease

Given the low incidence of anal cancer and the high success of CMT, the number of patients who develop metastatic disease is small. Single agent trials of doxorubicin (adriamycin) and cisplatin resulting in limited responses have been reported by several investigators.[139,140] Combination chemotherapy with cisplatin and 5-FU has a response rate of approximately 50% using both systemic and regional (hepatic-arterial) routes.[141–143] Retreatment with 5-FU/mitomycin-C is an alternative. There is limited experience with newer agents such as irinotecan and cetuximab.[144]

A small series of six patients with metastatic disease limited to the para-aortic nodes recommends CMT with an extended radiation field to include the nodes.[145]

Other histologies

Melanoma

Anorectal melanomas are relatively rare, accounting for less than 1% of all anal canal tumors. The presenting stage, defined by the tumor thickness and nodal status, is the primary determinant of survival. Distant metastasis is common.[146–151]

Despite a better local control rate with APR, most series have not shown a clear survival advantage for patients who have had an APR compared with patients having wide local excision.[146,147,152–154]

A retrospective analysis of the SEER database of 126 patients treated from 1973 to 2001 with a variety of therapies was reported by Podnos et al.[155] The 5-year survival based on disease status at presentation included local (32%), local/regional (17%), and distant (0%).

The inability to show a survival benefit for APR compared with wide local excision can be attributed to the small numbers of patients involved in the studies, selection bias, and the lack of randomized data. Any relative advantage of adjuvant immunotherapies, chemotherapy, and radiation therapy is similarly obscured and difficult to interpret. A histologic margin of at least 3 mm should be obtained if local excision is to be used. In view of possible higher local control rates, APR is still a reasonable option.[147–150,156,157]

Adenocarcinoma

Primary adenocarcinoma of the anal canal arising from the anal glands is rare. Most adenocarcinomas in the canal represent rectal cancer with distal spread. In general, they should be treated like adenocarcinomas of the rectum. If T3 and or N+, then preoperative CMT followed by surgery and 4 months of postoperative adjuvant therapy is appropriate. However, the radiation fields should include the inguinal nodes. In a series of 13 patients, Beal and associates recommended the combination of CMT and APR and reported a 2-year actuarial survival of 62%.[158] Adenosquamous cancers of the anus are also rare and have a poor prognosis.[159] Given the squamous component, it is reasonable to treat these patients with combined 5-FU/mitomycin-C and concurrent radiation therapy with APR for salvage.

Sarcoma

Few cases of leiomyosarcoma of the anus have been reported. The optimal treatment for this neoplasm is not known. The standard surgical approach is APR. Using a technique well established for management for sarcomas of the extremities, one approach is local excision and Iridium-192 brachytherapy in an attempt to preserve the anal sphincter.[160–162] This technique may be an alternative to APR in selected patients.

Others

Bowen's disease, Paget's disease, and Kaposi's sarcoma are commonly treated with surgery. Is settings where this could compromise sphincter function there are rare reports of treatment with CMT.

Key references

The complete reference list can be found on the Wiley Companion Digital Edition of this title (see inside front cover for login instructions).

10 Siegel R, Ma J, Zou Z, et al. Cancer Statistics, 2014. *CA Cancer J Clin.* 2014;**64**:9–29.
15 Machalek DA, Poynten M, Fairley CK, et al. Anal human papillomavirus infection and associated neoplastic lesions in men who have sex with men: a systematic review and meta-analysis. *Lancet Oncol.* 2012;**13**:487–500.
16 Melbye M, Cote T, Kessler L, et al. AIDS/Cancer Working Group. High incidence of anal cancer among AIDS patients. *Lancet.* 1994;**343**:636–639.

21 Serup-Hansen E, Linnemann D, Skovrider-Ruminski W, et al. Human papillomavirus genotyping and p16 expression as prognostic factors for patients with American Joint Committee on Cancer stages I to III carcinoma of the anal canal. *J Clin Oncol.* 2014;**17**:1812–1817.

24 Lampejo T, Kavanagh D, Clark J, et al. Prognostic biomarkers in squamous cell carcinoma of the anus: a systematic review. *Br J Cancer.* 2010;**103**:1858–1869.

58 Nahas CS, Lin O, Weiser MR, et al. Prevalence of perianal intraepithelial neoplasia in HIV-infected patients referred for high-resolution anoscopy. *Dis Colon Rectum.* 2006;**49**:1581–1586.

61 Bhuva NJ, Glynne-Jones R, Sonoda WL, et al. To PET or not to PET? That is the question. Staging in anal cancer. *Ann Oncol.* 2012;**23**:2078–2082.

62 Sveistrup J, Loft A, Berthelsen AK, et al. Positron emission tomography/computed tomography in the staging and treatment of anal cancer. *Int J Radiat Oncol Biol Phys.* 2012;**83**:134–141.

68 De Nardi P, Carvello M, Canevari C, et al. Sentinel node biopsy in squamous-cell carcinoma of the anal canal. *Ann Surg Oncol.* 2011;**18**:365–370.

72 Cummings BJ, Keane TJ, O'Sullivan B, et al. Epidermoid anal cancer: treatment by radiation alone or by radiation and 5-fluorouracil with and without mitomycin-C. *Int J Radiat Oncol Biol Phys.* 1991;**21**:1115–1125.

73 Flam M, John M, Pajak T, et al. Role of mitomycin in combination with fluorouracil and radiotherapy, and salvage chemoradiation in the definitive nonsurgical treatment of epidermoid carcinoma of the anal canal: results of a phase III randomized intergroup study. *J Clin Oncol.* 1996;**14**:2537–2539.

74 Northover J, Glynne-Jones R, Sebag-Montefiore D, et al. Chemoradiation for the treatment of epidermoid anal cancer: 13-year follow-up of the first randomised UKCCCR Anal Cancer Trial (ACT I). *Br J Cancer.* 2010;**102**:1123–1128.

75 UKCCCR Anal Cancer Trial Working Party. Epidermoid anal cancer: results from the UKCCCR randomised trial of radiotherapy alone versus radiotherapy, 5-fluorouracil, and mitomycin. *Lancet.* 1997;**348**:1049–1054.

76 Bartelink H, Roelofsen F, Eschwege F, et al. Concomitant radiotherapy and chemotherapy is superior to radiotherapy alone in the treatment of locally advanced anal cancer: results of a phase III randomized trial of the European Organization for Research and Treatment of Cancer radiotherapy and gastrointestinal cooperative groups. *J Clin Oncol.* 1997;**15**:2040–2049.

78 Gunderson LL, Winter KA, Ajani JA, et al. Long-term update of U.S. Intergroup RTOG 98–11 phase III trial for anal canal carcinoma: survival, relapse, colostomy failure with concurrent chemoradiation involving fluorouracil/mitomycin versus fluorouracil/cisplatin. *J Clin Oncol.* 2012;**35**:4344–4351.

79 James RD, Glynne-Jones R, Meadows HM, et al. Mitomycin or cisplatin chemoradiation with or without maintenance chemotherapy for treatment of squamous-cell carcinoma of the anus (ACT II): a randomized, phase 3, open-label, 2x2 factorial trial. *Lancet Oncol.* 2013;**14**:516–524.

91 Nigro ND, Vaitkevicius VK, Considine B. Combined therapy for cancer of the anal canal: a preliminary report. *Dis Colon Rectum.* 1974;**17**:354–358.

92 Gunderson LL, Moughan J, Ajani JA, et al. Anal carcinoma: impact of TN category of disease on survival, disease relapse, and colostomy failure in US gastrointestinal intergroup RTOG 98–11 phase III trial. *Int J Radiat Oncol Biol Phys.* 2013;**87**:638–645.

98 Martenson JA, Lipsitz SR, Wagner H, et al. Initial results of a phase II trial of high dose radiation therapy, 5-fluorouracil, and cisplatin for patients with anal cancer (E4292): an Eastern Cooperative Oncology Group study. *Int J Radiat Oncol Biol Phys.* 1996;**35**:745–749.

99 Chakravarthy AB, Catlano PJ, Martenson JA, et al. Long-term follow-up of a phase II trial of high-dose radiation with concurrent 5-fluorouracil and cisplatin in patients with anal cancer (ECOG E4292). *Int J Radiat Oncol Biol Phys.* 2014;**81**:e607–e613.

101 Peiffert D, Tournier-Rangeard L, Gerard JP, et al. Induction chemotherapy and dose intensification of the radiation boost in locally advanced anal canal carcinoma: final analysis of the randomized UNICANCER ACCORD 03 trial. *J Clin Oncol.* 2012;**30**:1941–1948.

102 Gerard JP, Mauro F, Thomas L, et al. Treatment of squamous cell anal carcinoma with pulsed dose rate brachytherapy. Feasibility study of a French cooperative group. *Radiother Oncol.* 1999;**51**:129–131.

105 Hannoun-Levi JM, Ortholan C, Resbeut M, et al. High-dose split-course radiation therapy for anal cancer: outcome analysis regarding the boost strategy (CORS-03 study). *Int J Radiat Oncol Biol Phys.* 2011;**80**:712–720.

107 Salama JK, Mell LK, Schomas DA, et al. Concurrent chemotherapy and Intensity-modulated radiation therapy for anal cancer patients: a multicenter experience. *J Clin Oncol.* 2007;**25**:4581–4586.

110 Kacknic LA, Tsai HK, Coen JJ, et al. Dose-painted intensity-modulated radiation therapy for anal cancer: a multi-institutional report of acute toxicity and response to therapy. *Int J Radiat Oncol Biol Phys.* 2012;**82**:153–158.

112 Ng M, Leong T, Chander S, et al. Australasian gastrointestinal trials group (AGITG) contouring atlas and planning guidelines for intensity-modulated radiotherapy in anal cancer. *Int J Radiat Oncol Biol Phys.* 2012;**83**:1455–1462.

118 Fraunholz I, Haberl A, Klauke S, et al. Long term effects of chemoradiotherapy for anal cancer in patients with HIV infection: oncological outcomes, immunological status, and the clinical course of the HIV disease. *Dis Colon Rectum.* 2014;**57**:423–431.

121 Das P, Cantor SB, Parker CL, et al. Long-term quality of life after radiotherapy foe the treatment of anal cancer. *Cancer.* 2010;**116**:822–829.

135 Tomaszewski JM, Link E, Leong T, et al. Twenty-five-year experience with radical chemoradiation for anal cancer. *Int J Radiat Oncol Biol Phys.* 2012;**83**:552–558.

158 Beal KP, Wong D, Guillem JG, et al. Primary adenocarcinoma of the anus treated with combined modality therapy. *Dis Colon Rectum.* 2003;**46**:1320–1324.

162 Grann A, Paty PB, Guillem JG, et al. Sphincter preservation of leiomyosarcoma of the rectum and anus with local excision and brachytherapy. *Dis Colon Rectum.* 1999;**42**:1296–1299.

96 Renal cell carcinoma

Earle F. Burgess, MD ▪ Stephen B. Riggs, MD ▪ Brian I. Rini, MD, FACP ▪ Derek Raghavan, MD, PhD, FACP, FRACP, FASCO

Overview

Renal cell carcinoma occurs in 64,000 new patients each year in the United States and results in about 14,000 deaths. For localized disease, cure is achieved by nephrectomy. Meticulous surgical staging is crucial. With improved imaging techniques, active surveillance has become an option for small, asymptomatic renal masses. Modifications in surgical technique, including laparoscopic and robotic approaches, have contributed to reduced morbidity. In more advanced disease, with locoregional or metastatic spread, immune response is a governor of outcome and survival, and immune modulation via interleukin-2 or PDL-1 inhibition results in sustained responses. Cytotoxic chemotherapy has negligible activity, but targeted therapies, such as tyrosine kinase and mammalian target of rapamycin inhibitors, often cause dramatic regressions. Uncommon cancers of the kidney represent about 10% of incident cases, and a general approach to their management is reviewed in this chapter.

Introduction

The incidence of renal cell carcinoma (RCC) is estimated at approximately 64,000 cases with 14,000 deaths in the United States annually.[1] The reported incidence of RCC has increased over time, largely but not entirely owing to an increase in the number of asymptomatic tumors incidentally detected with abdominal imaging obtained for other indications.[2,3]

Many advances in RCC have been made in recent years. Novel approaches to treating localized renal masses that emphasize less invasive and nephron-sparing approaches have been developed. Further, the biology underlying RCC has been elucidated, and agents targeting relevant biologic pathways have demonstrated robust clinical effect in the metastatic setting. This chapter details these advances and summarizes the epidemiology, pathology, staging, and treatment of RCC.

Epidemiology

RCC commonly presents in the sixth to seventh decade of life and develops in men twice as frequently as in women. Tobacco exposure is an established risk factor for RCC with a relative risk of approximately two- to threefold.[4] Obesity is also a risk factor although specific dietary associations are not well defined.[5] Hypertension, but not likely antihypertensive medicine, is associated with RCC development.[6] Acquired polycystic disease also predisposes to the development of RCC.[7] A small percentage of patients (2–3%) will have one of several autosomal dominant syndromes that predispose patients to various RCC histologic subtypes that are detailed subsequently. One Australian study suggested that analgesic abuse is associated with RCC, although more commonly this association is found for cancer of the renal pelvis.

Clinical presentation

In contemporary series, more than 50% of RCC patients present without initial symptoms as a result of abdominal CT scans or ultrasounds performed for an unrelated indication.[8–11] This has changed over the years as evidenced by the fact that in the 1970s, 10% of RCCs were discovered incidentally, compared to 60% in 1998.[3,12]

The most common local symptoms of RCC include hematuria, flank pain and a palpable mass, although this classic triad is currently observed infrequently. Other local presentations include left scrotal varicoceles that may be observed in up to 11% of men because of obstruction of the gonadal vein by tumor in the left renal vein to which it directly empties. Venous involvement can also cause lower extremity edema, ascites, hepatic dysfunction, and pulmonary emboli. Pain or dysfunction of specific organs may be the presenting feature of the patient with metastatic disease.

Systemic symptoms of paraneoplastic syndromes may also be an initial manifestation of RCC. Hypercalcemia is the most common paraneoplastic syndrome in RCC manifesting in 13–20% of patients. This is mediated by tumor production of parathyroid hormone (PTH) or PTH-related peptide. Polycythemia occurs in 1–8% of cases and is postulated to be mediated by elevated erythropoietin levels; anemia is far more common and can be quite severe. Iron studies are suggestive of anemia of chronic disease. Stauffer's syndrome is hepatic dysfunction in the setting of RCC without liver metastases. Corticosteroid-insensitive polymyalgia rheumatica can occasionally occur and often resolves following nephrectomy. Endocrine abnormalities including elevated HCG and ACTH have also been reported. Other systemic manifestations including constitutional symptoms such as fever, weight loss, and fatigue are common.

Pathology

The World Health Organization classification of renal neoplasms published in 2004 categorized malignant parenchymal renal cell neoplasms into three main and several other rare subtypes.[13] The most common RCC histology is the conventional clear cell subtype accounting for 75–80% of all RCCs. The remaining subtypes including papillary (10–15%), chromophobe (5–10%), medullary (<1%), and collecting duct carcinoma (CDC) (<1%). Recently, several new entities, including RCC associated with Xp11.2/TFE3 translocation and mucinous tubular and spindle cell carcinoma, have also been described, in addition to less common variants beyond the scope of this review.

Holland-Frei Cancer Medicine, Ninth Edition. Edited by Robert C. Bast Jr., Carlo M. Croce, William N. Hait, Waun Ki Hong, Donald W. Kufe, Martine Piccart-Gebhart, Raphael E. Pollock, Ralph R. Weichselbaum, Hongyang Wang, and James F. Holland.

Conventional clear cell renal cell carcinoma (ccRCC) arises from the proximal convoluted tubule and has clear cytoplasm on routine microscopic sections. The most common genetic alteration in ccRCC is a highly specific abnormality involving silencing of chromosome 3p [the von Hippel Lindau (*VHL*) gene] that occurs in approximately 35–50% of sporadic cases.[13] Noninherited ccRCC tends to present with larger, unilateral tumors. The inherited VHL syndrome (1/36,000 births) is a highly penetrant autosomal dominant disorder in which patients inherit a *VHL* gene defect on chromosome 3p25 and develop ccRCC and/or a constellation of cysts and tumors in the central nervous system and abdominal viscera.[14] CNS lesions include retinal hemangioblastomas, endolymphatic sac tumors, and craniospinal hemangioblastomas. The visceral lesions in these patients include ccRCCs, pheochromocytomas, pancreatic neuroendocrine tumors, epididymal cystadenomas, and broad ligament cystadenomas. In addition to *VHL* genetic aberrations, comprehensive genomic analysis of more than 400 ccRCC specimens by The Cancer Genome Atlas research network revealed that mutations in components of the PI3K/Akt pathway are common, in addition to chromatin remodeling genes, implicating epigenetic dysregulation in ccRCC tumorigenesis.[15] Well-defined intratumoral heterogeneity,[16,17] suggests that molecular characterization may require a multiplicitous effort, especially when performed for clinical purposes.

Papillary RCCs arise from the distal convoluted tubule and are composed of tubulopapillary structures with hemosiderin deposition and foamy histiocytes within the fibrovascular cores. They are subdivided into type 1 and type 2 papillary RCCs based on the morphology of the tumor cells lining the papillary structures.[13] Papillary carcinomas do not have *VHL* gene inactivation but have trisomy of chromosomes 7, 17 and loss of Y chromosome as the most frequent genetic alterations. Papillary tumors tend to have a multifocal nature and may present with bilateral kidney involvement. Hereditary papillary renal carcinoma (HRPC) is characterized by c-Met proto-oncogene activation (chromosome 7q31-34) and the development of type 1 papillary RCC. Hereditary leiomyomatosis renal cell carcinoma (HLRCC) involves abnormalities of the fumarate hydratase gene (chromosome 1q42-43) and development of type 2 papillary RCC, leiomyomas of skin and uterine leiomyomas and leiomyosarcomas.[18]

Chromophobe RCC arises from the intercalated cells of the kidney and is characterized by large solid sheets of cells with pale or eosinophilic cytoplasm, a thick and distinct cell membrane, and pleomorphic nuclei with an irregular nuclear membrane and perinuclear clearing.[13] The most frequent genetic alterations are a combination of loss of heterozygosity in chromosomes 1, 2, 6, 10, 13, 17, 21 and hypodiploidy. Patients with chromophobe histology tend to present with early stage disease with <5% of patients presenting with metastases.[19,20] Patients with Birt–Hogg–Dube syndrome have a high proportion of RCCs with chromophobe-predominant histology. They possess loss of function mutations in the BHD gene on chromosome 17p, have prominent cutaneous manifestations (fibrofolliculomas), and are predisposed to pneumothoraces from rupture of pulmonary cysts.[21] More recently, comprehensive whole-genome analysis has identified prevalent genomic rearrangements within the promoter region of the TERT gene, the catalytic subunit of telomerase, leading to increased TERT expression.[22] Thus, enhanced telomerase expression via structural promoter rearrangements may be an early pathogenic event in the development of chromophobe RCC.

Prognostic features

Grade

In patients with localized RCC, nuclear Fuhrman grade and TNM stage are consistently the most important prognostic factors.[23] The Fuhrman grading system scores the nuclear grade of RCCs on a scale of 1 (least aggressive) to 4 (most aggressive) based on nuclear and nucleolar size, shape, and content.[24] Higher nuclear grade is associated with a worse 5-year overall survival. Five-year cancer-specific survival rates for localized grade 1, grade 2, and grade 3 or 4 tumors after nephrectomy are 89%, 65%, and 46%, respectively.[23] Fuhrman grading is not useful for chromophobe RCC.[24]

Staging

In a patient with a suspected RCC, staging investigations including a CT of the chest and CT of the abdomen and pelvis are required to define the extent of the disease. The most common sites of metastases include the lungs, abdominal and mediastinal lymph nodes, liver, and bone. Unless a patient has symptoms suggestive of bone or brain metastases, initial bone scans and brain imaging tend to produce relatively low yield.

The 2010 American Joint Committee on Cancer (AJCC) and TNM staging system has been reported in detail previously[25] and reflects the extent of tumor (T), lymph node involvement (N), and presence of metastases (M).

Treatment of localized RCC

A number of treatment options exist for small (<4 cm) renal masses. These include surgical excision, radiofrequency ablation (RFA) or cryotherapy (collectively called thermal ablation), or active surveillance with delayed intervention in very select populations. Surgical resection remains the cornerstone of the treatment of localized stage I and II RCC and usually obviates the need for a renal biopsy. Partial nephrectomy is preferred whenever feasible, especially in a patient with limited renal function, bilateral tumors and/or a patient with a solitary kidney. Although nephron sparing is currently recommended as treatment for small renal masses, its absolute benefit compared to radical nephrectomy (in the elective setting) has come into question.[26] Laparoscopic partial nephrectomy is less invasive and appears to have similar outcomes to that of an open approach. Often the laparoscopic approach is performed with robotic assistance helping to overcome some of the inherent technical demands.[27]

The preferred treatment of large tumors (>7 cm) and locally advanced tumors is a radical nephrectomy, either with a laparoscopic or open procedure. This involves ligation of the renal vasculature, excision of the kidney, Gerota's fascia, and the ipsilateral adrenal grand if it appears involved by tumor on preoperative imaging. Laparoscopic radical nephrectomy is currently widely performed and has decreased postoperative pain to allow for shorter hospitalization and quicker recovery.

Thermal ablative options such as cryoablation and RFA are additional options for selected patients, often being performed in a percutaneous manner. Recent retrospective data, with limited follow-up from a cohort of more than 1400 patients, suggests that the use of percutaneous ablative therapies may result in similar local recurrence-free survival as compared to partial nephrectomy.[28] Unfortunately, randomized controlled trials comparing these noninvasive approaches to traditional surgical treatment are not available, and partial nephrectomy has the perceived advantage of complete pathologic evaluation as well as reduced follow-up with contrasted studies. In general, percutaneous ablation is favored in patients with smaller tumors (<4 cm) desiring an option other than surgery or who are not candidates for invasive operations.

Active surveillance is an emerging approach to small renal masses understanding that 50–60% will be indolent based on size and grade. Mean growth rate is around 0.3 cm per year with a 1–3% metastatic rate.[29-32] However, it should be emphasized that data from published series has been limited with regards to follow-up, so firm conclusions are lacking.[33] Importantly, utilization of percutaneous renal biopsies is evolving. Historically fraught with inconclusive results, more contemporary studies suggest nondiagnostic biopsies to occur less than 10% of the time.[34] Unfortunately, grade accuracy remains intermediate (50–70%).[34-37]

Stage III disease involves the, perinephric tissues, lymph nodes and/or invasion of the renal vein or inferior vena cava. The procedure of choice for these individuals is an open radical nephrectomy for curative intent. Lymph node dissection should be carried out in patients with evidence of enlarged lymph nodes. In patients with no suspected nodal metastases, a routine extended lymph node dissection is controversial.[38]

Although preoperative treatment with targeted molecular therapies may be safe,[39] a role for these agents in the nonmetastatic setting has not been established. Retrospective case series suggest that use of currently available targeted agents before nephrectomy does not result in frequent down-sizing of primary tumors[40,41] and exposes patients to the risk of progression[42] and increased complexity of ensuing surgical management. In patients with inferior vena cava tumor thrombi, neoadjuvant-targeted therapies have also failed to show significant cytoreductive effect on tumor thrombus burden and should not be routinely utilized to influence surgical decision making.[43,44]

Therapeutic intervention for local and/or oligometastatic recurrences may improve patient outcomes, underscoring the importance of detecting recurrences early. An ideal surveillance strategy following definitive management of primary renal tumors should balance the risk of recurrence against the desire to avoid unnecessary diagnostic testing. Individual risk-based surveillance guidelines have been proposed,[45,46] although an optimal surveillance strategy remains to be defined.

Metastatic disease

Prognostic factors

The most widely used prognostic factors for metastatic renal cell carcinoma (mRCC) were developed in the era when patients with mRCC were treated primarily with immunotherapy. The Memorial Sloan Kettering Cancer Center (MSKCC) criteria were developed via multivariable analysis in patients being treated for mRCC.[47] A clinical scoring system was developed and classifies patients into favorable, intermediate, and poor prognosis categories based on the number of adverse risk features present. Significant treatment heterogeneity existed in patients from the original cohort is used to establish these criteria, so updated analysis of additional patients treated with IFN only defined the median overall survival for each prognostic category as 30, 14, and 5 months, respectively (Table 1).[48]

New prognostic factors have been developed for contemporary patients being treated with molecular-targeted therapy described below. Retrospective, multicenter analysis of 645 patients with mRCC treated with sunitinib, sorafenib, or bevacizumab led to the development of a revised prognostic model consisting of three

Table 1 Prognostic criteria for metastatic RCC.

Memorial Sloan Kettering Cancer Center (MSKCC) criteria. Data from Ref. 48
Adverse prognostic factors
- Karnofsky performance status < 80%
- Diagnosis to treatment interval < 1 year
- Hemoglobin < lower limit of normal
- Serum corrected calcium > 10 g/dL
- LDH > 1.5x upper limit of normal

Risk categories and clinical outcome
- 0 prognostic factors (good risk): PFS: 8.3 m OS: 30 m
- 1–2 prognostic factors (intermediate risk): PFS: 5.1 m OS: 14 m
- 3–5 prognostic factors (poor risk): PFS: 2.5 m OS: 5 m

International Metastatic Renal Cell Carcinoma Database Consortium (IMDC) criteria. Data from Ref. 49
Adverse prognostic factors
- Karnofsky performance status < 80%
- Diagnosis to treatment interval < 1 year
- Hemoglobin < lower limit of normal
- Serum corrected calcium > upper limit of normal
- Neutrophil count > upper limit of normal
- Platelet count > upper limit of normal

Risk categories and clinical outcome
- 0 prognostic factors (good risk): OS: 43 m
- 1–2 prognostic factors (intermediate risk): OS: 23 m
- 3–6 prognostic factors (poor risk): OS: 8 m

Abbreviations: OS, overall survival; PFS, progression-free survival.

risk groups (Table 1).[50] External validation by an international mRCC database consortium (IMDC) supports the routine use of this prognostic model with current standard therapies and illustrates survival improvements that have resulted from the evolution of treatment paradigms, as the observed median overall survival for patients in the favorable, intermediate, and poor risk groups, respectively, was 43, 23, and 8 months, respectively.[49] IMDC risk stratification also has prognostic value in patients with metastatic non-ccRCC[51] and may facilitate decision making regarding cytoreductive nephrectomy[52] as discussed in the following section.

Surgery in patients with metastatic disease

Radical nephrectomy is also indicated in many patients with mRCC. Results from two phase III studies demonstrated that cytoreductive nephrectomy before IFN improved overall survival. In a combined analysis of these trials, median survival was 7.8 months in patients treated with interferon-alpha alone versus 13.6 months for patients who underwent cytoreductive nephrectomy initially.[53-55] A greater survival advantage was observed in patients with better performance status. The cytoreductive paradigm remains predominant even though supporting data are primarily empiric and have not been proven in combination with the newer targeted agents. A phase III trial assessing the benefit of nephrectomy before sunitinib in patients with clear cell mRCC is ongoing, although retrospective analysis of the IMDC prognostic criteria in a cohort of 1658 patients has suggested that cytoreductive nephrectomy may benefit patients with at least a 12-month life expectancy and less than four IMDC risk factors.[52] The role for cytoreductive nephrectomy in patients with nonclear cell mRCC remains unproven.[56]

While cytoreductive nephrectomy appears to benefit many patients with clear cell mRCC, it is not curative and should not be performed indiscriminately. Patients who are most likely to benefit from cytoreduction include those with (1) substantial tumor burden (e.g., >75%) in the involved kidney, (2) good performance status, and (3) no central nervous system or liver metastases (with rare exceptions).[57] Other considerations pertain to surgical resectability, particularly, the potential for morbidity if there is proximity to vital structures, encasement of the renal hilum or other complicating factors.

Patients with mRCC with solitary metastases may be considered for metastasectomy, although they represent only 2–3% of cases. Favorable prognostic factors include a long interval between initial diagnosis and development of metastases, solitary metastatic site and ability to achieve a complete resection of known metastatic disease.[58] Patients with favorable features can anticipate up to a 40% 5-year survival with metastasectomy, and thus surgical resection of metastases should be considered in highly selected RCC patients.

Systemic therapy for metastatic disease

Immunotherapy

As early trials employing chemotherapy did not produce any significant benefit,[59,60] immunotherapy had long been the standard of care for the treatment of mRCC in an attempt to harness the innate immune response of RCC tumors based on occasional spontaneous regression of metastatic lesions.[61] IFN and high-dose IL-2 have produced response rates of 10–20% with modest prolongation of overall survival.[62,63] Of note, there were significant side effects including capillary leak syndrome, which necessitated intensive monitoring and occasional vasopressor support. Phase III trials of high-dose IL-2 failed to demonstrate significant benefits for the cohort versus alternative, low-dose cytokine regimens.[64,65] Thus, cytokine-based immunotherapy remains relevant in mRCC owing to the small percentage of patients who may dramatically benefit with a complete response, although attempts to predict the responding group have been uniformly unsuccessful.

Combination of the autologous tumor cell vaccine AGS-003 with sunitinib resulted in possibly prolonged survival relative to historical control in patients with unfavorable risk factors in a small phase II trial,[66] serving as the basis for the ongoing ADAPT phase III randomized trial. Cytotoxic T cell activation through modulation of the inhibitory PD-1/PD-L1 axis has also demonstrated striking antitumor activity.[67–69] Results from ongoing phase III trials of these new immunomodulatory agents are eagerly anticipated.

Targeted therapy

New treatment approaches have resulted from a better understanding of the biology and genetics of RCC. As noted previously, most ccRCCs demonstrate an abnormality of the *VHL* gene (Figure 1). When inactivated, the *VHL* gene product cannot regulate the degradation of the transcription factor hypoxia inducible factor (HIF) alpha, thus resulting in the transcription of numerous hypoxia-regulated genes including vascular endothelial growth factor (VEGF) and platelet-derived growth factor (PDGF). These growth factors promote angiogenesis and tumor growth through binding with their respective receptor tyrosine kinases (RTKs).[14] Activation of RTKs can induce signaling through the PI3K/Akt pathway and further downstream through the mammalian target of rapamycin (mTOR) pathway promoting cell proliferation and survival through regulation of mRNA translation. These intricate pathways have been identified as key therapeutic targets for the treatment of mRCC (Table 2).

VEGF ligand-directed therapy

Bevacizumab is a recombinant monoclonal antibody that binds and neutralizes circulating VEGF. The activity of this agent in the first-line setting for advanced RCC has been established by two randomized phase III clinical trials. The AVOREN study randomized untreated patients with clear cell mRCC and prior nephrectomy to receive the combination of IFN (three times per week at a dose of 9 MIU for up to 1 year) plus bevacizumab (10 mg/kg IV every 2 weeks) or placebo until disease progression.[81] The addition of

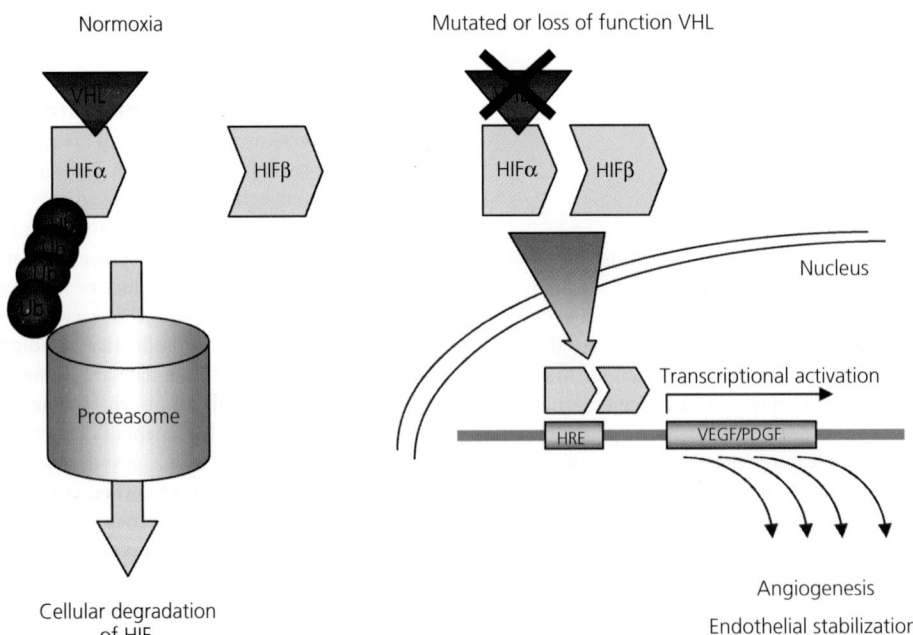

Figure 1 Normal function of VHL in the normoxic state compared to the aberrant VHL state/hypoxia. Under normal conditions, VHL binds to HIFα and polyubiquinates it to mark it for destruction in the cellular proteasome. In conditions of hypoxia or when VHL function is lost, HIFα binds HIFβ and then translocates into the nucleus to activate HIF responsive elements (HRE). This results in transcriptional activation of genes important in angiogenesis and endothelial stabilization such as VEGF and PDGF.

Table 2 Selected clinical trials of targeted agents in metastatic renal cell carcinoma.

Agent	Mechanism	Efficacy			
		Population and trial arms	RR	PFS (months)	OS (months)
Sunitinib[70,71]	Tyrosine kinase inhibitor of VEGF and related receptors	First line *sunitinib* versus *IFN*	47%	11	26.4
			12% $p < 0.001$	5 $p < 0.001$	21.8 $p = 0.051$
Pazopanib[72,73]	Tyrosine kinase inhibitor of VEGF and related receptors	First line *pazopanib* versus *sunitinib*	31%	8.4	28.3
			25% $p = 0.03$	9.5	29.1 NS
Sorafenib[74,75]	Tyrosine kinase inhibitor of VEGF and related receptors	Treatment refractory, second line *sorafenib* versus *placebo*	10%	5.5	17.8
			2% $p < 0.001$	2.8 $p < 0.01$	15.2 $p = 0.146$
Axitinib[76]	Tyrosine kinase inhibitor of VEGF and related receptors	Treatment refractory, second line *axitinib* versus *sorafenib*	19%	8.3	20.1
			11% $p = 0.0007$	5.7 $p < 0.0001$	19.2 NS
Temsirolimus[77]	mTOR inhibitor	Poor risk, first line *temsirolimus* versus *IFN*	8.6%	N/A	10.9
			4.8% NS	N/A	7.3 $p < 0.008$
Everolimus[78]	mTOR inhibitor	Treatment refractory, second line *everolimus* versus *placebo*	1.8%	4.9	14.8
			0%	1.9 $p < 0.001$	14.4 NS
Bevacizumab[79, 80][a]	VEGF ligand-binding antibody	First line *bevacizumab + IFN* vs *placebo + IFN*	31%, 25%	10.2, 8.5	23.3, 18.3
			13%, 13% $p < 0.0001$	5.4, 5.2 $p < 0.0001$	21.3, 17.4 NS

IFN, interferon; N/A, not available or data not yet mature; NS, not statistically significant; p values for PFS are based on hazard ratios.

[a] The results of two phase III bevacizumab trials are shown.

bevacizumab to IFN significantly increased PFS (10.2 vs 5.4 mo) (HR = 0.63; $p = 0.0001$) and objective tumor response rate (31% vs 13%; $p = 0.0001$). A trend toward improved OS was observed with the addition of bevacizumab.[79] A CALGB phase III trial of similar design confirmed a PFS benefit (8.5 vs 5.2 months $p < 0.0001$) and ORR benefit (25% vs 13%, $p < 0.0001$) with the addition of bevacizumab to IFN.[82] OS also trended toward improvement in the bevacizumab arm,[80] although high rates of second-line therapy confounded survival analysis in both trials. Common toxicities included hypertension and proteinuria with rare but serious toxicity including bowel perforation, arterial ischemic events, and bleeding. It is unknown whether bevacizumab must be given in combination with interferon owing to the absence of a bevacizumab monotherapy arm in the phase III trials. Combined use with mTOR inhibition does not improve efficacy,[83] whereas concurrent use with additional VEGF targeted agents is associated with unacceptable risk of thrombotic microangiopathy.[84] Use in patients after prior treatment with other targeted agents remains unproven.

VEGF receptor tyrosine kinase inhibitors

RTKs play an integral role in the signaling cascade of VEGF and PDGF.[85] RTKs have an extracellular domain that binds their respective ligand, which activates oncogenic intracellular signaling cascades through protein phosphorylation events regulated by a cytoplasmic kinase domain. Targeting RTKs with small molecule inhibitors has proven to be an effective therapeutic strategy in mRCC and has led to regulatory approval of multiple agents in this class as detailed below.

Sunitinib is an oral multikinase inhibitor that blocks VEGFR-1, 2 and 3, PDGFR-B, and related RTKs.[86] A pivotal phase III randomized trial[70] in untreated mRCC patients compared first-line sunitinib (50 mg daily four out of 6 weeks) with interferon and demonstrated a significant advantage in objective response rate (ORR) (47% vs 12%; $p < 0.001$), PFS (11 vs 5 months, HR = 0.54; $p < 0.001$), and OS (26.4 vs 21.8 months, HR = 0.82; $p = 0.051$).[71]

Of note, most patients enrolled (94%) had favorable or intermediate risk MSKCC prognostic criteria. Common toxicities included fatigue, hand-foot syndrome, diarrhea, mucositis, and hypertension. This agent has become a standard of care for the first-line treatment of mRCC on the basis of these results. Efforts to improve the toxicity profile by altering dose and schedule of administration have been unsuccessful or remain investigational.[87,88]

Pazopanib is a second-generation oral TKI that inhibits VEGFR-1, -2 and -3, PDGF-A and -B, and c-kit.[89] A randomized phase III trial comparing pazopanib to placebo in patients with mRCC previously untreated or following cytokine failure demonstrated that pazopanib improved PFS (9.2 vs 4.2 months, HR = 0.46; $p < 0.0001$) and ORR (30% vs 3%, $p < 0.001$).[90] Common toxicities included hypertension, diarrhea, nausea, anorexia, and hair depigmentation. Hepatic toxicity is more frequently observed with this agent than others in the class and may be associated with UGT1A1 gene polymorphisms.[91] A large, noninferiority randomized phase III trial compared outcomes and tolerability of pazopanib and sunitinib in previously untreated patients with mRCC with a clear cell component and found that pazopanib resulted in a similar PFS (8.4 vs 9.5 months, HR = 1.05; 95% CI 0.90–1.22), higher ORR (31% vs 25%, $p = 0.03$), and similar OS (28.3 vs 29.1 months, $p = 0.24$).[72,73] Similar drug discontinuation rates were observed, although patients receiving pazopanib reported better quality of life scores including fatigue and hand-foot syndrome. Improved tolerability of pazopanib compared to sunitinib was also demonstrated in the PISCES trial in which patients were randomized in a double-blind manner to receive treatment with one agent for 10 weeks followed by cross-over.[92]

Sorafenib inhibits a broad repertoire of kinases including BRAF, CRAF, VEGFR-2, -3, PDGFB, Flt-3, p38, and c-kit.[93] In the treatment naïve setting, sorafenib has not demonstrated superior antitumor activity compared to IFN and therefore does not have a proven role in this setting.[94] However, in previously treated patients, sorafenib is superior to placebo. The treatment approaches in renal cancer global evaluation trial (TARGET) enrolled 903 patients with previously treated metastatic ccRCC and randomized patients to oral sorafenib 400 mg twice daily versus placebo.[74,75] All patients enrolled had favorable or intermediate risk MSKCC prognostic criteria and over 80% had been previously treated with cytokine therapy. PFS was prolonged in the sorafenib group (5.5 vs 2.8 months, $p < 0.01$). ORR was minimal (10% investigator assessed), and OS was similar to the placebo group (17.8 vs 15.2 months, $p = 0.146$), although an OS benefit could have been obscured from placebo patients being allowed to cross-over and receive sorafenib at progression.

Subsequent development of axitinib, a second-generation inhibitor of VEGFR-1, -2 and -3 of greater potency than earlier agents,[95] resulted in this newer agent largely supplanting sorafenib as a standard second-line choice. In the AXIS trial, over 700 patients with clear cell mRCC previously treated with one line of systemic therapy [cytokines (35%), sunitinib (54%), bevacizumab (8%), or temsirolimus (3%)] were randomized to receive axitinib (5 mg twice daily) or sorafenib (400 mg twice daily).[96] Notably, one-third of enrolled patients had MSKCC poor risk criteria. Median PFS favored the axitinib group (8.3 vs 5.7 months, $p < 0.0001$), although OS (20.1 vs 19.2 months, $p = 0.3744$) and patient reported outcomes were similar between arms.[76] On the basis of these results, many consider axitinib preferable to sorafenib in patients who have failed one prior line of therapy. Axitinib has not been proven superior to sorafenib in the first-line setting.[97] Results from a first-line dose escalation study suggest a possible role for axitinib dose titration, especially in normotensive patients, although the optimal approach remains investigational.[98]

mTOR inhibition

The "mTOR" kinase is regulated by Akt and PI3 Kinase, both downstream of VEGFR, and promotes tumor growth and proliferation through regulation of mRNA translation. Temsirolimus is an FDA-approved mTOR inhibitor that binds to FKBP-12 to create a complex that directly inhibits mTOR. A phase III trial[77] included 626 previously untreated patients with poor prognostic criteria and randomized them to temsirolimus 25 mg IV weekly, interferon alpha 18 MU 3x/week or temsirolimus 15 mg IV weekly + IFN 6 MU 3x/week. Patients were required to have three or more of the following adverse risk features: Karnofsky performance status < 80%, lactate dehydrogenase > 1.5x laboratory upper limit of normal, hemoglobin < laboratory lower limit of normal, serum calcium corrected for albumin > 10 mg/dL, time from first diagnosis of RCC to start of therapy of <1 year and three or more metastatic sites. Of note, 19% of enrolled patients had nonclear cell histology. Temsirolimus monotherapy demonstrated an overall survival advantage compared to interferon alpha (10.9 vs 7.3 months, $p = 0.008$). On the basis of these results, temsirolimus has become a first-line standard of care for patients with poor risk mRCC. In the second-line setting following progression with sunitinib, results of the INTORSECT phase III study[99] showed that temsirolimus confers a similar PFS as sorafenib though inferior OS (12.3 vs 16.6 months, $p = 0.01$) and thus should not be used in VEGF TKI eligible patients this setting.

Everolimus is an oral mTOR inhibitor with US FDA approval for use in patients with mRCC after sunitinib or sorafenib failure on the basis of results from the RECORD-1 randomized phase III trial comparing everolimus to placebo.[78,100] Everolimus demonstrated an improved PFS (4.9 vs 1.9 months, $p < 0.001$) although no OS benefit, owing in part to the high cross-over rate of patients in the placebo arm. Whether the findings of the INTORSECT trial described above are applicable to the use of everolimus is unknown, as studies comparing everolimus to a VEGFR TKI in the second-line setting have not been reported, and the use of a placebo

comparator in the RECORD-1 trial is no longer considered an appropriate control arm given the efficacy of axitinib and sorafenib in this setting. The optimal sequencing of everolimus with a VEGFR TKI has been studied in the RECORD-3 trial.[101] In this randomized phase II noninferiority trial, treatment naïve patients received either everolimus followed by sunitinib at progression or the reverse sequence. The median PFS and OS for first-line everolimus were inferior to first-line sunitinib, providing further support that everolimus should not be used before a VEGFR TKI.

Uncommon cancers of the kidney

A detailed discussion of the biology and management of uncommon variants is beyond the scope of this truncated chapter, in accordance with editorial directions, but has been covered in detail elsewhere.[102,103] However, we will address one variant that appears to have been reported more frequently in the recent past and for which there have been changes in systemic care.

Collecting duct carcinoma

CDC represents less than 1% of kidney cancer,[103–105] although there has been an increasing proliferation of case reports in the past few years. It was originally thought to derive from distal tubular epithelium, but more recently has been show to arise in the collecting ducts.[102,104] CDC, which is usually found in the renal medulla, ranges in size from small to greater than 10 cm and often has an irregular margin with evidence of local infiltration. Often surrounded by desmoplastic stroma, CDC has a variable tubular-papillary pattern of growth, with high-grade nuclei and high mitotic activity. Mucin and sarcomatoid changes may be seen. There is no classical immunohistochemical appearance.

CDC is an aggressive tumor, often presenting at advanced stage.[102,104,105] Common features include hematuria, flank pain, or abdominal pain, and there are frequently metastases at first presentation, including lung, liver, bone, adrenals, or lymph nodes. There is a 2:1 male predominance, with a broad age range of presentation. The appearance on CT scan is not specific and consists mainly of a centrally arising infiltrative lesion without much contrast enhancement.

The diagnosis of CDC is usually made at surgery, which remains the definitive treatment for localized disease. However, this is one of the aggressive variants of renal cancer and thus is often associated with early metastasis. There is little evidence that immunotherapy has any significant utility, and thus most reports of treatment of metastatic disease have involved the use of systemic chemotherapy, mostly predicated on cisplatin-containing regimens.[106,107] Unfortunately, remissions are relatively infrequent and of short duration. It has been suggested that the combination of cisplatin and gemcitabine has sustained activity.[106] More recently, a small series from France reported substantially sustained and long-term remissions from the combination of bevacizumab, gemcitabine, and cisplatin,[107] although it is important to note that the added impact of bevacizumab has not been proven. This work suggests that there may be an additive effect from the combination of chemotherapy and targeted therapy in this disease, and confirmatory evidence will be required before this can be viewed as a standard.

Conclusion

RCC incidence is increasing worldwide. Surgery remains a mainstay of treatment for localized tumors and is part of multimodality therapy in the metastatic setting. An enhanced understanding of the biology of RCC has led to the clinical development of a number of targeted therapies that have substantially altered the therapeutic landscape. Future investigative endeavors include further refinement of the approach to the small renal mass, a better understanding of the biology of response and resistance to targeted therapy, clinical testing of combinations and sequences of targeted therapy in mRCC and the development of novel immunotherapeutic approaches.

Key references

The complete reference list can be found on the Wiley Companion Digital Edition of this title (see inside front cover for login instructions).

1 Siegel R, Ma J, Zou Z, Jemal A. Cancer statistics, 2014. *CA Cancer J Clin.* 2014;**64**(1):9–29.

3 Pantuck AJ, Zisman A, Belldegrun AS. The changing natural history of renal cell carcinoma. *J Urol.* 2001;**166**(5):1611–1623.

8 Lee CT, Katz J, Fearn PA, Russo P. Mode of presentation of renal cell carcinoma provides prognostic information. *Urol Oncol.* 2002;**7**(4):135–140.

9 Luciani LG, Cestari R, Tallarigo C. Incidental renal cell carcinoma-age and stage characterization and clinical implications: study of 1092 patients (1982–1997). *Urology.* 2000;**56**(1):58–62.

12 Nguyen MM, Gill IS, Ellison LM. The evolving presentation of renal carcinoma in the United States: trends from the Surveillance, Epidemiology, and End Results program. *J Urol.* 2006;**176**(6Pt 1):2397–2400; discussion 2400.

14 Cohen HT, McGovern FJ. Renal-cell carcinoma. *N Engl J Med.* 2005;**353**(23):2477–2490.

15 Cancer Genome Atlas Research Network. Comprehensive molecular characterization of clear cell renal cell carcinoma. *Nature.* 2013;**499**(7456):43–49.

19 Cheville JC, Lohse CM, Zincke H, Weaver AL, Blute ML. Comparisons of outcome and prognostic features among histologic subtypes of renal cell carcinoma. *Am J Surg Pathol.* 2003;**27**(5):612–624.

23 Tsui KH, Shvarts O, Smith RB, Figlin RA, deKernion JB, Belldegrun A. Prognostic indicators for renal cell carcinoma: a multivariate analysis of 643 patients using the revised 1997 TNM staging criteria. *J Urol.* 2000;**163**(4):1090–1095; quiz 1295.

24 Fuhrman SA, Lasky LC, Limas C. Prognostic significance of morphologic parameters in renal cell carcinoma. *Am J Surg Pathol.* 1982;**6**(7):655–663.

26 Van Poppel H, Da Pozzo L, Albrecht W, et al. A prospective, randomised EORTC intergroup phase 3 study comparing the oncologic outcome of elective nephron-sparing surgery and radical nephrectomy for low-stage renal cell carcinoma. *Eur Urol.* 2011;**59**(4):543–552.

30 Crispen PL, Wong YN, Greenberg RE, Chen DY, Uzzo RG. Predicting growth of solid renal masses under active surveillance. *Urologic Oncol.* 2008;**26**(5):555–559.

32 Rosales JC, Haramis G, Moreno J, et al. Active surveillance for renal cortical neoplasms. *J Urol.* 2010;**183**(5):1698–1702.

33 Chawla SN, Crispen PL, Hanlon AL, Greenberg RE, Chen DY, Uzzo RG. The natural history of observed enhancing renal masses: meta-analysis and review of the world literature. *J Urol.* 2006;**175**(2):425–431.

38 Blom JH, van Poppel H, Marechal JM, et al. Radical nephrectomy with and without lymph-node dissection: final results of European Organization for Research and Treatment of Cancer (EORTC) randomized phase 3 trial 30881. *Eur Urol.* 2009;**55**(1):28–34.

39 Chapin BF, Delacroix SE Jr, Culp SH, et al. Safety of presurgical targeted therapy in the setting of metastatic renal cell carcinoma. *Eur Urol.* 2011;**60**(5):964–971.

40 Abel EJ, Culp SH, Tannir NM, et al. Primary tumor response to targeted agents in patients with metastatic renal cell carcinoma. *Eur Urol.* 2011;**59**(1):10–15.

44 Cost NG, Delacroix SE Jr, Sleeper JP, et al. The impact of targeted molecular therapies on the level of renal cell carcinoma vena caval tumor thrombus. *Eur Urol.* 2011;**59**(6):912–918.

45 Donat SM, Diaz M, Bishoff JT, et al. Follow-up for clinically localized renal neoplasms: AUA guideline. *J Urol.* 2013;**190**(2):407–416.

47 Motzer RJ, Mazumdar M, Bacik J, Berg W, Amsterdam A, Ferrara J. Survival and prognostic stratification of 670 patients with advanced renal cell carcinoma. *J Clin Oncol.* 1999;**17**(8):2530–2540.

49 Heng DY, Xie W, Regan MM, et al. External validation and comparison with other models of the International Metastatic Renal-Cell Carcinoma Database Consortium prognostic model: a population-based study. *Lancet Oncol.* 2013;**14**(2):141–148.

54 Flanigan RC, Salmon SE, Blumenstein BA, et al. Nephrectomy followed by interferon alfa-2b compared with interferon alfa-2b alone for metastatic renal-cell cancer. *N Engl J Med.* 2001;**345**(23):1655–1659.

55 Mickisch GH, Garin A, van Poppel H, et al. Radical nephrectomy plus interferon-alfa-based immunotherapy compared with interferon alfa alone in metastatic renal-cell carcinoma: a randomised trial. *Lancet.* 2001;**358**(9286):966–970.

57 Rini BI, Campbell SC. The evolving role of surgery for advanced renal cell carcinoma in the era of molecular targeted therapy. *J Urol.* 2007;**177**(6):1978–1984.

62 Coppin C, Porzsolt F, Awa A, Kumpf J, Coldman A, Wilt T. Immunotherapy for advanced renal cell cancer. *Cochrane Database Syst Rev.* 2005;**1**:CD001425.

67 Brahmer JR, Tykodi SS, Chow LQ, et al. Safety and activity of anti-PD-L1 antibody in patients with advanced cancer. *N Engl J Med.* 2012;**366**(26):2455–2465.

71 Motzer RJ, Hutson TE, Tomczak P, et al. Overall survival and updated results for sunitinib compared with interferon alfa in patients with metastatic renal cell carcinoma. *J Clin Oncol.* 2009;**27**(22):3584–3590.

73 Motzer RJ, Hutson TE, McCann L, Deen K, Choueiri TK. Overall survival in renal-cell carcinoma with pazopanib versus sunitinib. *N Engl J Med.* 2014;**370**(18):1769–1770.

78 Motzer RJ, Escudier B, Oudard S, et al. Phase 3 trial of everolimus for metastatic renal cell carcinoma : final results and analysis of prognostic factors. *Cancer.* 2010;**116**(18):4256–4265.

79 Escudier B, Bellmunt J, Negrier S, et al. Phase III trial of bevacizumab plus interferon alfa-2a in patients with metastatic renal cell carcinoma (AVOREN): final analysis of overall survival. *J Clin Oncol.* 2010;**28**(13):2144–2150.

80 Rini BI, Halabi S, Rosenberg JE, et al. Phase III trial of bevacizumab plus interferon alfa versus interferon alfa monotherapy in patients with metastatic renal cell carcinoma: final results of CALGB 90206. *J Clin Oncol.* 2010;**28**(13):2137–2143.

82 Rini BI, Halabi S, Rosenberg JE, et al. Bevacizumab plus interferon alfa compared with interferon alfa monotherapy in patients with metastatic renal cell carcinoma: CALGB 90206. *J Clin Oncol.* 2008;**26**(33):5422–5428.

90 Sternberg CN, Davis ID, Mardiak J, et al. Pazopanib in locally advanced or metastatic renal cell carcinoma: results of a randomized phase III trial. *J Clin Oncol.* 2010;**28**(6):1061–1068.

96 Rini BI, Escudier B, Tomczak P, et al. Comparative effectiveness of axitinib versus sorafenib in advanced renal cell carcinoma (AXIS): a randomised phase 3 trial. *Lancet.* 2011;**378**(9807):1931–1939.

101 Motzer RJ, Barrios CH, Kim TM, et al. Phase II randomized trial comparing sequential first-line everolimus and second-line sunitinib versus first-line sunitinib and second-line everolimus in patients with metastatic renal cell carcinoma. *J Clin Oncol.* 2014;**32**(25):2765–2772.

103 Raghavan D. A structured approach to uncommon cancers: what should a clinician do? *Ann Oncol.* 2013;**24**(12):2932–2934.

106 Dason S, Allard C, Sheridan-Jonah A, et al. Management of renal collecting duct carcinoma: a systematic review and the McMaster experience. *Curr Oncol.* 2013;**20**(3):e223–232.

107 Pecuchet N, Bigot F, Gachet J, et al. Triple combination of bevacizumab, gemcitabine and platinum salt in metastatic collecting duct carcinoma. *Ann Oncol.* 2013;**24**(12):2963–2967.

97 Urothelial cancer

Derek Raghavan, MD, PhD, FACP, FRACP, FASCO ▪ *Richard Cote, MD, FRCPath, FCAP* ▪ *Earle F. Burgess, MD* ▪ *Stephen B. Riggs, MD* ▪ *Michael Haake, MD*

Overview

Urothelial malignancy is one of the most common cancers in Western society and involves the bladder, urethra, ureters, and renal calyces. It is predominantly associated with smoking, industrial dyes, schistomiasis, radiation exposure, and certain geographical locations. Well-defined molecular prognosticators have been identified and, in combination with improved staging techniques, have led to improved outcomes. Patients with nonmuscle invasive urothelial malignancy are best managed by surgical resection, often in combination with intravesical immunotherapy or chemotherapy. Muscle invasive disease is best managed by neoadjuvant cisplatin-based chemotherapy followed by cystectomy; less robust patients are often effectively treated by cisplatin-based chemoradiation. Patients with metastatic disease achieve response rates of up to 70% with MVAC (methotrexate, vinblastine, doxorubicin, and cisplatin) or GC combination chemotherapy but are infrequently cured. New approaches to the management of systemic disease are predicated on recent data reflecting the importance of unblocking checkpoints for immune function and correlate with expression of PD-L1 (programmed death-ligand 1).

Introduction and epidemiology

Bladder cancer is one of the most common malignancies in Western society, with an annual incidence of about 16 cases/100,000 males per year and 5 cases/100,000 females.[1] In the United States, this translates into about 75,000 new cases per year, with approximately 16,000 deaths per year.[2] An additional 3000 cases of upper tract malignancy present each year, and additional cases are found throughout the urothelial lining. This is one of the malignancies for which the incidence and mortality figures have not changed significantly in the past 50 years, although possibly the incidence figures in males are beginning to plateau, reflecting the reduction in cigarette smoking. This is predominantly a disease of older aged males, with a median age at presentation of 60–65 years. There are geographical variations in incidence with increased rates in the Great Lakes region of the United States, in the littoral basin of the Middle East, and in regions with an increased incidence of schistosomiasis (most often squamous carcinoma). In the Balkan region, endemic familial interstitial nephropathy is associated with a 100- to 200-fold increase in upper tract tumors. Urothelial cancer occurs more often in Caucasians than in Asian or African American populations.[2]

The etiology is well-defined, with the most common association being cigarette smoking, and other factors including exposure to dyes and industrial reagents, motor exhaust, reduced intake of fluids (controversial), and analgesic (phenacetin) abuse.[1] Other associations include prior treatment with cyclophosphamide and other oxazophorine cytotoxics, high fat diet, chronic urinary infection, paraplegia, and prior pelvic irradiation. Family history is also relevant, especially for patients with Lynch syndrome, and for upper tract tumors.

Pathobiology and molecular determinants

Bladder cancer consists predominantly of urothelial carcinoma (UC), formerly known as transitional cell cancer.[1,3] This type of cancer can occur anywhere along the urothelial tract and may be multifocal in origin, with identical tumor histology irrespective of site of origin. About 90% of incident cases are UC, with about 5–10% being squamous cell carcinoma, 4–5% being adenocarcinoma, and the remainder consisting of rare cancers, such as small cell anaplastic cancer, sarcoma, melanoma, or lymphoma. Occasionally, other tumors metastasize to the bladder.

Increasingly, bladder cancer is believed to arise from cancer stem cells[4] and that the cancer stem cells have the ability to differentiate along different pathways. Thus, not surprisingly, intermixed histological patterns will be found, although usually UC predominates in such situations. These tumors are associated with a field defect of the urinary mucosa, probably due to antecedent carcinogenic stimuli, and thus can occur at multiple sites.

UC presents as either noninvasive or invasive disease. In the former pattern, two distinct histological subtypes are known, papillary versus flat carcinoma *in situ* (CIS). Noninvasive papillary carcinoma is the single most common presentation for bladder cancer, comprising more than 60% of incident cases. This can be classified according to grade of disease, ranging from tumors generally considered benign (papilloma) to high-grade tumors with a high risk of developing invasion (grades 3 and 4). Grading systems are generally restricted to noninvasive papillary neoplasms, as CIS is high grade by definition, and virtually all invasive tumors are high grade as well.[3]

Grade 1 (well-differentiated) papillary neoplasms show a well-organized pattern similar to the organization of normal urothelium, including polarity of the urothelial cells and the presence of an umbrella cell layer. A fibrovascular stalk is often seen. In grade 2 tumors, there is a higher nuclear to cytoplasmic ratio, and prominent nucleoli, with loss of urothelial orientation and at least partial loss of the umbrella cell layer. Grade 3 (high grade) disease is characterized by poorly differentiated or undifferentiated tissues that are increasingly disorganized and manifest a high mitotic index, with complete loss of the umbrella cell layer. The latest WHO (World Health Organization) nomenclature combines tumor differentiation into only low and high grades, based on the finding that tumor behavior is more accurately reflected in a dichotomized system.[3,5] Although the bladder is heavily invested by fat and muscle, this is not the case in the upper tracts, and thus, the barriers to spread, and patterns of spread, are somewhat different.

Holland-Frei Cancer Medicine, Ninth Edition. Edited by Robert C. Bast Jr., Carlo M. Croce, William N. Hait, Waun Ki Hong, Donald W. Kufe, Martine Piccart-Gebhart, Raphael E. Pollock, Ralph R. Weichselbaum, Hongyang Wang, and James F. Holland.
© 2017 John Wiley & Sons, Inc. ISBN: 978-1-118-93469-2

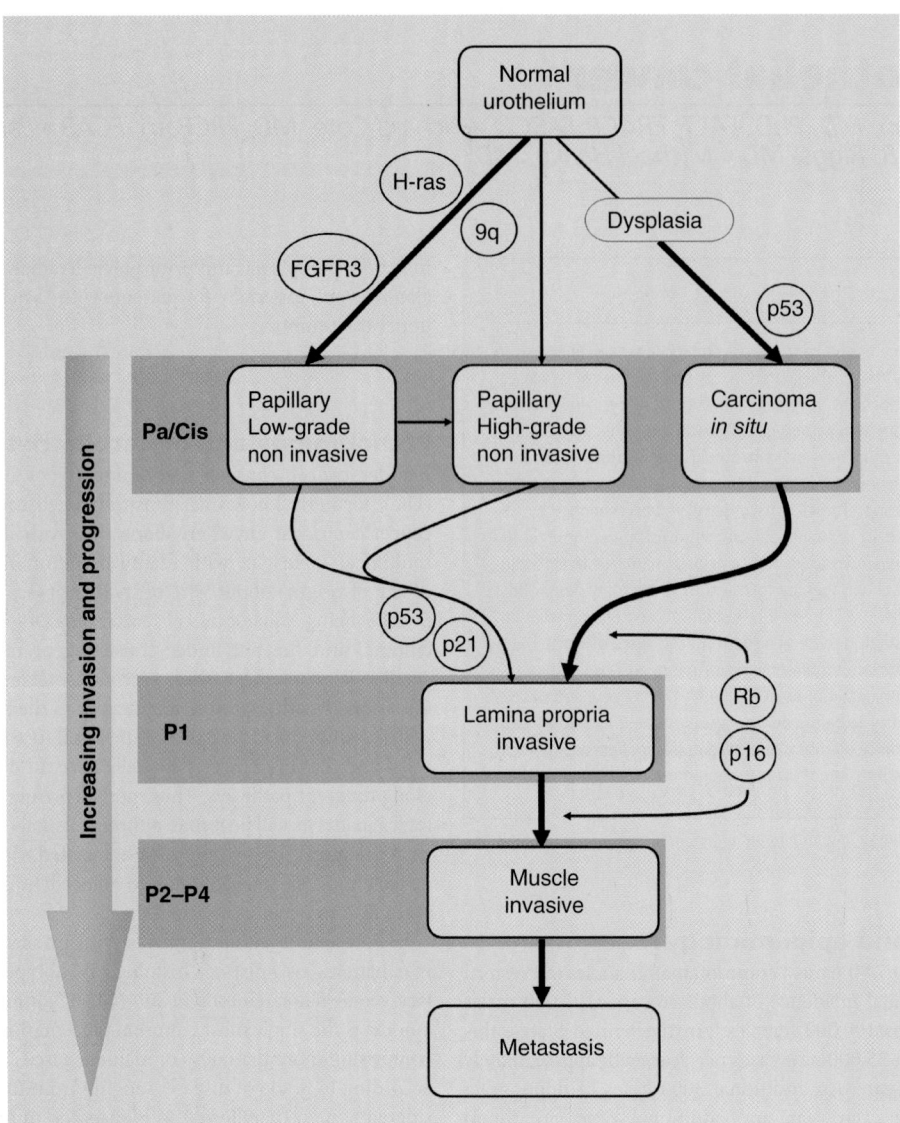

Figure 1 Proposed model for urothelial tumorigenesis and progression. Superficial and invasive tumors have unique molecular profiles and arise from distinct pathways. The locations of molecules indicate events that pose a risk for progression of a particular phenotype. The rare papillary carcinomas that invade are more likely to have genetic alterations at crucial loci. The thickness of arrows represents the relative frequency of occurrence. Source: Mitra 2006. Reproduced with permission of the American Society of Clinical Oncology.

Because the different morphologic subtypes of bladder cancer have long been recognized to have different biologic behavior, these subtypes became the focus of molecular analysis.[5] The earliest cytogenetic studies in bladder cancer demonstrated alterations in chromosomes 9, 11, and 17, reflecting the possible presence of tumor suppressor genes in these areas.[5,6] On the basis of consistent and frequent genetic defects in bladder tumors, it has become clear that there are at least two distinct molecular pathways involved in bladder cancer tumorigenesis and progression (Figure 1), as reviewed elsewhere.[5,6] Papillary tumors frequently show alterations in chromosome 9, particularly at the INK4a/p16 locus. Further, these tumors frequently show constitutive activation of the receptor tyrosine kinase–Ras pathway, exhibiting activating mutations in the HRAS and fibroblast growth factor receptor 3 (FGFR 3) genes. In contrast, flat CIS and invasive tumors frequently show alterations in the p53 gene and protein (TP53) and the retinoblastoma (RB) gene. Similar molecular changes are found in upper tract tumors, and added abnormalities in chromosomes 5q, 1p, 14q, and 8p have been identified.

The RAS–MAPK signal transduction pathway is also important in noninvasive papillary tumors. Most noninvasive papillary UC's show activation of this pathway, generally through the activation of FGFR3, and potentially presenting a target for novel therapies. Other receptor tyrosine kinases are also involved, such as epidermal growth factor receptor (EGFR) and Her2-neu, as reviewed previously.[5]

Cell cycle regulation has clearly been shown to be a critical pathway in flat CIS and invasive UC. A central molecule in this pathway is the p53 tumor suppressor protein, encoded by the *p53* gene. Patients showing alterations in two or three out of the three critical genes (p53, p21, RB) in this pathway have much poorer outcomes than patients with tumors showing alterations in none or only one of these determinants (Figure 1).

Tumor angiogenesis and epigenetic alterations are also important in the genesis and control of UC. Comprehensive whole genome sequencing efforts have now confirmed the prevalence of mutations in chromatin remodeling genes, underscoring the potential importance of epigenetic dysregulation in UC carcinogenesis. Genes

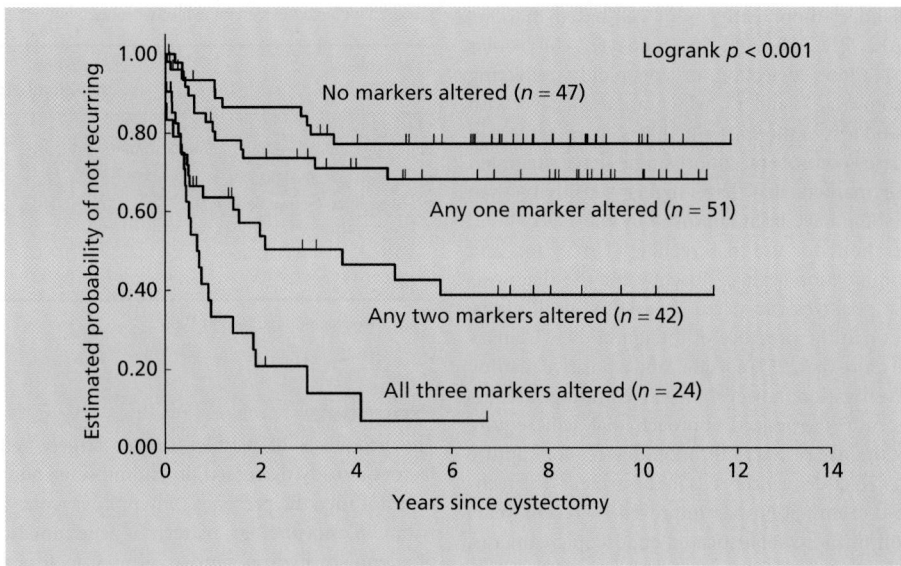

Figure 2 Probability of recurrence-free survival in 164 bladder cancer patients, who underwent radical cystectomy, based on alterations in p53, p21, and/or RB expression. The combined analysis shows an increased risk of recurrence with increasing number of deregulated molecules (logrank $p < 0.001$). Source: Chatterjee 2004. Reproduced with permission of the American Society of Clinical Oncology.

known to be affected by methylation in UC include RASSF1A, DAPK, and INK4A.[5]

Multiplex genome-wide expression analysis has become increasingly important in the analysis of UC and other cancers, leading to more detailed molecular profiles with histogenetic, prognostic, therapeutic targeting, and predictive implications (Figure 2).[5,6]

Clinical presentation

The presentation of bladder cancer usually reflects the extent of disease, with somewhat different patterns associated with non-muscle-invasive tumor, invasive disease, metastases, and the nonmetastatic manifestations of malignancy.[1,8] Patients with noninvasive tumors may present with asymptomatic hematuria (diagnosed on urinalysis), visible hematuria, and irritative patterns such as frequency, dysuria, burning, or nocturia. In patients with a prior history of non-muscle-invasive bladder cancer and prior transurethral resections (TURs), irritative bladder symptoms may be more prominent. Invasive tumors have a similar pattern of presentation, although more advanced tumors may be associated with pelvic pain, slowing of urinary stream, dyspareunia, and occasionally pneumaturia or fecal incontinence. Occasionally, tumors involving the trigone will cause obstruction of ureters, with concomitant flank pain. Flank pain or more generalized abdominal pain occasionally reflects the presence of an upper tract tumor, although usually such features are associated with more advanced local disease.

The presenting features of metastatic disease usually reflect the site(s) of involvement. Common sites include distant lymph nodes, lung, liver and bone, and less commonly brain, skin, other viscera. In the present era of aggressive imaging, many metastases will first be detected upon routine follow-up scans. Pulmonary involvement will classically be associated with cough and dyspnea and occasionally with hemoptysis or chest pain. Liver involvement may present with right upper quadrant pain or shoulder tip pain, and occasionally disruption of function, most commonly manifested by jaundice. Osseous metastases are often associated with bone pain, and less commonly with pathologic fracture, with common

sites of involvement including spine, ribs, pelvis, and skull. Brain metastases may be suggested by the development of headache, confusion, or other motor features. A computed tomography (CT) or magnetic resonance imaging (MRI) brain scan will usually reveal the problem, although rarely a spinal tap will be required to diagnose carcinomatous meningitis in a patient with a normal scan (especially in a patient with suspicious symptoms who has received extensive prior chemotherapy for metastatic disease). Skin metastases are uncommon but usually are manifest by an infiltrative pattern or isolated cutaneous or subcutaneous nodules.

The nonmetastatic manifestations of malignancy consist predominantly of serological syndromes, although occasional patients will present with the thromboembolic syndromes classically associated with advanced adenocarcinomas of the gastrointestinal (GI) tract. Bladder cancer is occasionally associated with the production of granulocyte-macrophage colony-stimulating factors or other cytokines, and a greatly elevated white blood cell count may reflect this phenomenon, rather than underlying infection. Tumors with squamous differentiation may sometimes be associated with hypercalcemia, owing to excess production of immunoreactive parathyroid hormone (PTH)-like substance. In general, these syndromes should be taken in context and generally do not require specific management unless causing clinical problems—for example, severe hypercalcemia and significant thrombotic episodes.

Investigation and staging

The specifics of the presentation will usually govern the nature of the investigations. Presentation with hematuria or other urinary symptoms will usually lead to urinalysis and assessment of possible infection or urinary calculi. The absence of these conditions or the presence of sterile pyuria is usually grounds for assessing urinary cytology and/or progressing to cystoscopic examination. In some clinical practices, to improve upon the sensitivity of urine cytology and to reduce the need for periodic cystoscopy in the follow-up of patients with non-muscle-invasive bladder cancer, novel biomarker dipstick assays have been developed, based on soluble bladder tumor antigens or cell-based markers (NMP22, BTA-TRAK, BLCA-4, and Immunocyt).[9] Molecular analysis (Urovysion) allows detection of aneuploidy reflecting changes in chromosomes 3, 7, and 17, which are associated with high-grade tumors, and loss of the 9p21 site that is characteristic of low-grade disease. Case–control and cohort studies have suggested that several of these markers may have higher sensitivity than urine cytology, and some have been approved by the FDA (Food and Drug Administration) for use in screening (UroVysion and NMP-22) and in combination with cystoscopy for the diagnosis of recurrence.[9] False positives can occur in cystitis, urolithiasis, bowel interposition, or in the presence of foreign bodies. Urinary cytology is said to be more than 95% specific, and a positive reading mandates further investigation; however, negative findings are less helpful. A more recently introduced approach that will require further validation is the use of microfiltration devices for capture and characterization of bladder cancer cells in the urine.[10] The technology of endoscopic examination has improved in recent years with the introduction of more sophisticated endoscopic cameras, high-resolution videography, fluorescence cystoscopy, and narrow banding imaging cystoscopy, leading to improved specificity and sensitivity.[11,12] This has also facilitated instrumentation of the upper tracts.

There is no specific serological workup for bladder cancer. Routine hematological and biochemical testing may reveal chronic anemia of chronic disease or from blood loss, renal dysfunction (from obstruction or the underlying cause of the cancer), and occasionally evidence of metastases, such as raised alkaline phosphatase or liver function tests. No tumor markers have been shown to be specific to bladder cancer, although occasional elevation of HCG, CEA, CA 19-9, or CA125 will be seen, the latter particularly in the presence of elements of adenocarcinoma.

Imaging of the urinary tract may be carried out before or after cystoscopy. A relatively standard approach is to obtain an excretory urogram to delineate the anatomy of the urinary tract, including the presence of tumors of the bladder and upper tracts or hydronephrosis.[8] CT urography is more commonly used in the current era, based on its ability to evaluate the renal parenchyma in addition to the urothelium, and it is performed more rapidly than excretory urography. MRI may also be helpful to define the local anatomy and the extent of an invasive tumor, while also providing staging information about involvement of lymph nodes and distant sites. However, the sensitivity and specificity of non-muscle-invasive pelvic imaging are somewhat limited. Also of importance, CT and MRI scans performed soon after transurethral resection of bladder tumor (TURBT) will often suffer from the artifact of apparently increased depth and invasion owing to the impact of postresection inflammatory infiltrate. The role of the positron emission tomography (PET) scan is limited, although we occasionally use this modality to assist in defining potential metastatic sites for further investigation, with a "positive" result being investigated further and a negative result having limited implications.

Definitive investigation involves TUR with the usual goals of complete tumor eradication and accurate staging. Bimanual examination at the time of TUR allows assessment of tumor stage and the presence of extravesical disease. In the setting of high-grade cancer, the existence of detrusor muscle invasion is important to determine. Unless cystectomy is planned, repeat TUR (in patients with non-muscle-invasive disease) within 4–6 weeks shows upstaging in 30% of patients with muscle identified in the original specimen and 60% of patients in whom no muscle was present initially.

Table 1 Risk factors in metastatic bladder cancer.

Variable	Statistical significance (*p*)	Risk ratio
Three variables		
Visceral metastases (yes/no)	0.0001	1.99
Karnofsky PS (</≥80%)	0.0001	2.05
Hemoglobin (normal/abnormal)	0.0103	1.41
Two variables		
Visceral metastases (yes/no)	0.0001	2.10
Karnofsky PS (</≥80%)	0.0001	2.20

Source: Adapted from Bajorin 1999.

Prognosis

The prognosis of bladder cancer largely reflects several of the factors already discussed, including stage and grade of the tumor, multifocality, the presence of lymphovascular invasion, association with CIS, morphology, pattern of gene mutation, and the presence of anemia or hydronephrosis. Similar factors govern the prognosis of upper tract tumors, including grade, stage, the presence of lymphovascular invasion, aneuploidy, EGFR expression, location of tumor (ureters with worse prognosis than renal pelvis), and the presence of residual disease after surgery.[1]

The AJCC (American Joint Committee on Cancer) Staging Classification[13] generally correlates well with outcome. Although the bladder is heavily invested by fat and muscle, this is not the case in the upper tracts, and thus the barriers to spread and patterns of metastasis are somewhat different from tumors in the bladder.

In addition, Bajorin et al.[14] have developed an algorithm for estimating risk and prognosis for patients with advanced disease, focused on the presence of visceral metastases, performance status, and anemia; this has recently been focused and updated to increase the precision of prediction.[15] Several modifications have been proposed, including prognostic criteria for second line and salvage chemotherapy, but they have not led to improved survival figures, although they may have contributed to avoidance of futile chemotherapy (Table 1).

Management of non-muscle-invasive bladder cancer

The key to effective management of non-muscle-invasive bladder cancer involves cystoscopy and resection of visible bladder tumor(s),[16,17] sometimes followed by postoperative use of intravesical therapy (immunological or cytotoxic reagents) to reduce the risk of recurrence.[8,16,17] As bladder cancer is associated with a field defect, multiple random biopsies of apparently normal urothelium should be performed to identify occult CIS if urine cytology is positive or in the presence of high-grade disease when bladder conservation is contemplated. Usually, endoscopic resection is repeated within 4 weeks of the initial resection in patients with high-grade disease and/or T1 tumors, as up to 50% will have evidence of invasive bladder cancer into muscularis propria on rebiopsy.

The grade and stage of the tumor will dictate subsequent management. Patients with non-muscle-invasive, low-grade papillary bladder cancer are at low risk of progression to invasive disease, although the risk of recurrence may be as high as 60–80%. Patients at increased risk for recurrence on the basis of tumor size, multifocal tumors, or prior recurrent tumors are often given adjuvant intravesical therapy (usually weekly instillations for 6–8 weeks) following resection, mostly with bacillus Calmette Guerin (BCG), which reduces the risk of recurrence by up to around 40%.[14] The mechanism of action of BCG is based on local immunological stimulation, perhaps with alteration of suppressor-helper T cell ratios. Effectively, such treatment allows the bladder to "reject" implantation and recurrence of bladder cancer. This may be a harbinger of the apparent utility of PD-1 targeting, which releases the brake on T cell function, for invasive and metastatic disease.

Randomized trials suggest that BCG is superior to other intravesical agents at preventing tumor progression,[17] and an initial bladder preservation strategy involving intravesical BCG is associated with long-term outcomes similar to early cystectomy for low-grade tumors.[17] Maintenance BCG is associated with a reduction in tumor recurrence and reduced requirement for cystectomy, compared to a single 6-week induction regimen. The optimal schedule of BCG administration has not been defined, and, similarly, the optimal commercial preparations and the ideal duration of administration remain controversial.

The side effects of all the intravesical agents in common use include irritative symptoms and hematuria. BCG may also cause a flu-like syndrome and, because it is an attenuated mycobacterium, it can produce local, regional and systemic TB (tuberculosis)-like infections. Granulomatous infections can occur at extravesical sites, including the prostate, epididymis, testes, kidney, liver, and lungs. BCG sepsis is the most serious complication, and can be life threatening, and should usually be treated with triple-antituberculous therapy.

In some centers, cytotoxic agents such as mitomycin C or gemcitabine[18] are preferred because of purportedly reduced toxicity, although the certainty of this is not substantiated. For patients who refuse cystectomy for relapsed non-muscle-invasive disease, several lines of immunological or cytotoxic intravesical therapy may be feasible and may delay recurrence and progression.

After completion of treatment, patients should be monitored closely with periodic cystoscopy and selective urine cytology and/or tumor marker evaluation at 3–6 months intervals to detect recurrence early. Patients with high-risk non-muscle-invasive bladder cancer (high-grade Ta, T1, or CIS) have at least a 50% risk of developing invasive bladder cancer and a 35% risk of dying from bladder cancer. Moreover, those with persistent or recurrent high-grade disease after one or two courses of intravesical therapy will develop muscle invasion and progression in 80% of cases. Thus, we advocate timely radical cystectomy with urinary diversion for relapsed high-risk disease, particularly for patients with long life expectancy.[19,20] Cure rates approach 90% in this setting, but when cystectomy is delayed, deeply invasive disease may develop and is associated with diminished survival.[19]

Management of invasive bladder cancer

Definitive surgery

Over the past 20 years, radical cystectomy with bilateral pelvic lymphadenectomy has been viewed as the standard treatment for clinically localized invasive bladder cancer.[1,8,20,21] Traditionally, this requires the en bloc removal of the anterior pelvic organs, which include the bladder, prostate, and seminal vesicles in men and the bladder, urethra, uterus, ovaries, and vaginal cuff plus anterior vaginal wall in women.[20] A urinary diversion is formed by the connection of the ureters to detubularized intestinal reservoir. Continent reservoirs, such as the Indiana pouch and orthotopic neobladder, are now standard approaches because they offer improved continence without the need for an external collecting bag. The orthotopic neobladder involves creation of an intestinal reservoir that is attached to the urethra and enables the patient to void normally without self-catheterization.

Radical cystectomy, without adjuvant therapy, is curative in up to 60% of patients with invasive bladder cancer,[20,21] depending on stage and other prognostic factors. The 5-year overall survival rates in large series of patients with T2–T3 disease range from 40% to 65%. Relapse rates reflect stage, grade, the presence of lymphovascular invasion, and expression of adverse molecular prognosticators. Radical cystectomy alone has been reported to be curative in 20–40% of patients with regional metastasis to pelvic lymph nodes, and the outcome is influenced by the primary tumor stage, number of involved lymph nodes, and the presence of extranodal extension.[1,8,20,21] Extended template node dissection may improve cure rates.[20,21] However, this may reflect the case selection bias, surgical skill, or support and salvage techniques available in centers of excellence.

Advances in instrumentation

Laparoscopic radical cystectomy, with or without robotic assistance, has been reported in modest series from centers experienced in laparoscopic surgery.[22,23] The cystectomy and lymph node dissection are commonly performed laparoscopically and the urinary diversion is carried out through a midline incision smaller than is usual for conventional surgery. The potential advantages include reduced blood loss, less postoperative pain, and shorter convalescence, although most of the data have been derived from nonrandomized series, carried out by technically superb surgeons, with careful case selection and relatively short follow-up. More recently, Bochner et al.[24] have reported preliminary outcomes of a randomized trial, which suggested much higher cost for laparoscopic cystectomy, with equivalent toxicities. As this was an early report focused on acute morbidity, long-term outcomes are not yet available.

Another innovation has been the use of prostate-sparing cystectomy, with the intent of ameliorating the extent of mutilation and late effects, although this has not yet been validated by randomized trials. This approach is not useful for patients with extension of tumor into the prostate or with incidental prostate adenocarcinoma.

Role of radiotherapy

For patients with invasive, clinically nonmetastatic bladder cancer who are not surgical candidates, by their choice, technical considerations, or physical fitness, radiation is the treatment of choice.[25–27] There have been no well-designed, randomized studies comparing radiation with surgery in patients with similar characteristics. The optimal technique of dose delivery, either conformal or IMRT (intensity-modulated radiotherapy), remains controversial.[25] Favorable prognostic features for use of radiotherapy include small, localized, T2 tumors, absence of hydronephrosis, normal renal function, maximum debulking by TUR, and absence of anemia.[1,26,27]

A relatively standard radiotherapy approach is to deliver more than 65–70 Gy over 6–7 weeks, with 40 Gy delivered to the bladder, and the highest doses confined to the tumor plus a reasonable margin, as defined by diagnostic scans. Mapping is done at the time of TURBT with CT simulation films in the prone position.[26,27] It is less common today for radiotherapy to be delivered in isolation than for it to be administered in combination with systemic chemotherapy, based largely on the studies of the RTOG (Radiation Therapy Oncology Group) and a randomized trial conducted by the National Cancer Institute of Canada.[28] These studies have shown significantly improved local control from chemoradiation, although a statistically significant survival benefit remains unproved. In the United Kingdom, a randomized trial of chemoradiation with 5-fluorouracil and mitomycin C versus radiation alone showed a significant increase in local control and a strong trend toward a survival benefit from the combination.[29]

Toxicities of radiation include cutaneous inflammation, proctitis occasionally complicated by bleeding and/or obstruction, cystitis or bladder fibrosis, impotence, incontinence, and development of secondary malignancies in the region surrounding the radiation field. Importantly, if radiotherapy fails, salvage surgery is much more complex because of the formation of fibrosis in the irradiated field.

Several innovations in radiation planning and treatment have been introduced in recent years, including devices for tracking physiological movement of the tumor tissue and adjusting the radiation beam, and particle therapy, such as proton beam, with more focused beams and potentially less normal tissue toxicity. No level 1 evidence supports the use of proton beam therapy for bladder cancer, which remains investigational.

Combined modality strategies

Neoadjuvant (preemptive) chemotherapy

We first studied pre-emptive or neoadjuvant systemic chemotherapy plus local treatment more than 30 years ago,[30] based on the rationale that chemotherapy might reduce the extent of local tumor while controlling occult metastases. Our preliminary studies showed that this can shrink primary bladder cancers and result in downstaging, sometimes achieving a complete clinical and pathological remission.[30] However, initial randomized trials did not confirm a survival benefit for single agent regimens. The introduction of multidrug chemotherapy regimens, such as methotrexate, vinblastine, doxorubicin, and cisplatin (MVAC), and cisplatin, methotrexate, and vinblastine (CMV), adapted from use in metastatic disease into neoadjuvant protocols yielded survival benefit, confirmed by randomized clinical trials (Table 2).[31–33]

Thus, the consensus is now that neoadjuvant MVAC or equivalent chemotherapy affords an absolute survival benefit of 7–8%, with an increase in median survival of up to 3 years, when added to radical cystectomy. A statistically significant survival benefit has not been proved when the primary treatment is radiotherapy. Recent national surveys of patterns of practice have indicated that most patients do not receive such treatment, suggesting that change has come slowly in this area of clinical work.[34,35]

To date, no multidrug cytotoxic regimen has been shown to be superior or even equivalent to the MVAC or CMV regimens for neoadjuvant chemotherapy. However, the newer gentle regimens, such as gemcitabine-cisplatin or gemcitabine-carboplatin, are being used increasingly for neoadjuvant therapy. This may be reasonable for the older or frail patients, but may lead to a greater risk of death from cancer for the more robust patient without intercurrent medical disorders. Ideally, a well-powered, randomized clinical trial would be needed to resolve this issue.

The importance of dose-dense MVAC, as initially developed and tested by the European Organization for Research and Treatment of Cancer (EORTC) in the metastatic setting, remains unclear and controversial. Toxicity may be reduced by this approach, but whether long-term results are equivalent is unclear, despite the imprimatur of the NCCN (National Comprehensive Cancer Network) guidelines.

Adjuvant chemotherapy

Chemotherapy administered after radical cystectomy for patients with T3–T4 tumors and/or lymph node involvement improves *disease-free* survival, as one would expect for any effective chemotherapy.[36–41] However, in the randomized trials reported to date, most of which have been flawed by poor design, a disease-free statistical target, or inadequate sample size, a statistically significant improvement in total survival has never been demonstrated, as previously discussed.[42] An Italian group tested the use of adjuvant gemcitabine-cisplatin and demonstrated a statistically nonsignificant inferior survival in the chemotherapy arm.[41] An attempt was made to address these problems in the EORTC international randomized trial that had been in progress for several years, and which suffered from poor accrual, leading to premature closure. This study confirmed a disease-free survival benefit, the largest benefit counterintuitively in patients without node metastases, but no overall survival benefit.[43] This suggests that the adjuvant chemotherapy may have compensated for inadequate definitive surgery.

Although meta-analysis can sometimes help to resolve the failure of small trials to resolve an issue, the study published by the Cochrane group was flawed.[44] It grouped a heterogeneous set of small trials that were poorly designed, poorly executed, or which did not actually compare adjuvant chemotherapy with chemotherapy at relapse and thus confused the issue. However, understanding the significant limitations of historical controls and poorly executed randomized trials, our group has concluded that a survival benefit from adjuvant chemotherapy is still possible, and a survival deficit is unlikely; thus, we sometimes offer this approach to carefully selected otherwise healthy, postcystectomy patients with high-risk disease. A well-powered randomized chemotherapy trial is unlikely to ever answer this question.

Table 2 Results of clinical randomized trials of neoadjuvant chemotherapy for invasive bladder cancer, stages T1–T4.

Series	Neoadjuvant regimen	Definitive therapy	Median survival with/without neoadjuvant therapy (months)	Actuarial long-term survival with/without neoadjuvant therapy
Neoadjuvant				
MRC-EORTC	CMV	RT/cystectomy	44/37.5	35%/30% at 10 years
Intergroup	MVDC	Cystectomy	77/46	42%/35% at 10 years
Nordic 1 trial	DC	Cystectomy	Not reached/72	59%/51% at 5 years
Adjuvant				
EORTC	MVDC	Cystectomy	81/55	44%/39% at 5 years
Stanford	CMV	Cystectomy	63/36	42%/38% at 5 years
USC	CDCy	Cystectomy	52/30	44%/39% at 5 years
Cognetti	GC	Cystectomy	38/58	44%/44% at 6.5 years

Abbreviations: C, cisplatin; D, doxorubicin; M, methotrexate; Cy, cyclophosphamide; V, vinblastine; G, gemcitabine; MRC-EORTC, Medical Research Council/European Organization for Research and Treatment of Cancer; RT, radiotherapy.

Metastatic bladder cancer

Chemotherapy is the first-line treatment of choice for patients with metastatic bladder cancer. The single agent activity of 5-fluoruracil, methotrexate, the vinca alkaloids, doxorubicin, and cisplatin was demonstrated between the 1960s and early 1980s.[45] The combination of methotrexate, vinblastine, and cisplatin, with[46] or without[47] doxorubicin, first produced objective responses in more than 60% of cases, with a median survival of 1 year. Investigators in the United States, Canada, and Australia proved the utility of the MVAC regimen in a randomized trial against single agent cisplatin and confirmed that the benefit persisted with a median follow-up beyond 6 years.[48] The major limitation of the MVAC regimen was substantial toxicity, including grade 3–4 GI effects, stomatitis, and myelosuppression, as well as occasional cases of renal dysfunction and cardiotoxicity.[46,48] Attempts were made to improve the regimen, and Sternberg et al.[49] demonstrated, in a randomized trial, that a dose-intense variant of MVAC yielded higher response rates and reduced toxicity compared to the original regimen, but without achieving a major increment in median survival. However, at 5 years, the number of surviving patients was greater than for standard-dose MVAC but did not reach statistical significance.

Single agent response rates of around 20–30% have been reported for paclitaxel, gemcitabine, docetaxel, ifosfamide, and pemetrexed.[45] The combination of these agents with other standard or investigational drugs has resulted in response rates of 50–80%, sometimes with less toxicity than the conventional-combination MVAC regimen, but median survival figures have remained in the range of 12–20 months, and cure rates for patients with visceral metastases have not exceeded 10–15%.[45] After initial studies with the combination of gemcitabine and cisplatin revealed apparently equivalent response rates and substantially less toxicity than the MVAC regimen,[50] a randomized trial comparing gemcitabine-cisplatin versus MVAC confirmed these observations and showed that survival was similar.[51] Consequently, an international consortium added paclitaxel to this doublet for patients with previously untreated metastatic UCs in an effort to improve cure rates, but without major survival impact in a randomized trial.[52] Several other doublets and triplets have been assessed in phase I–II trials, but none has emerged as a major advance.

An important caveat in interpreting modern clinical trial data is that stage migration has occurred in the management of advanced bladder cancer, largely due to the increased use of aggressive post-surgical imaging via CT, MRI, and PET scans, and there has been increased use of systemic chemotherapy to treat patients with small volume, asymptomatic metastases. This should be borne in mind when considering the utility of novel combinations, such as the ITP regimen (ifosfamide, paclitaxel, and cisplatin), which yields a median survival of about 18 months, which is similar to outcomes in the current use of the MVAC regimen. Before novel regimens can be accepted into routine clinical practice, their safety and efficacy should be defined in randomized trials against accepted current standards. Despite modest progress in the past two decades, the majority of patients with metastases still die of progressive tumor. It is particularly important, in an era of increasing cost awareness and focus on the value proposition, that the aims of chemotherapy are detailed clearly, and that patients unlikely to secure life prolongation or improved quality of life are referred either into Hospice programs or, if still sufficiently fit, into clinical trials of novel approaches. Focal radiotherapy for symptomatic local or metastatic disease may also confer a palliative benefit for such patients.

Because cytotoxic chemotherapy regimens have not improved the cure rate dramatically, alternative approaches are being investigated.

In the past decade, we have focused on novel compounds that target the genes and proteins that control cellular growth, differentiation, and apoptosis. Agents that modulate the function of EGFR and other tyrosine kinase inhibitors have been studied as monotherapy and in combination with chemotherapy. The ability to identify expression of the *HER-2/neu* oncogene, EGFR, and other molecular predictors of response allows some tailoring of treatment. Hussain et al.[53] have assessed herceptin, in combination with a regimen of chemotherapy, against bladder cancers expressing the *HER 2/neu* gene, and showed a response rate of 70%; however, the median survival of 14 months did not suggest that this was a major advance; in this study, a higher response rate was seen in tumors expressing EGFR.

The tyrosine kinase inhibitor, sunitinib (*see* **Chapter 97**), can cause partial remissions in heavily pretreated bladder cancer but of only relatively short duration.[54] Although this suggests some utility of the targeting of anti-angiogenesis pathways in bladder cancer, other studies have shown lack of activity of this group of agents against bladder cancer, and this approach is not gaining traction.

However, two novel approaches appear more promising. Recent data indicate that the MET gene is heavily expressed in urothelial cancer and prostatic adenocarcinoma. Early trials showed significant activity against prostate cancer, and a more recent study has suggested similar anti-cancer efficacy against advanced urothelial cancer.[55]

Preliminary studies have shown substantial expression of programmed death-ligand 1 (PD-L1) in urothelial malignancy, and phase I trials have suggested substantial anti-tumor effect from PD-L1 inhibitors, such as MPDL3280A.[56] Phase II trials are in progress. Despite early promise, such agents, because of their uncertain long-term impact and very high cost, should be validated against established standards before introduction into routine clinical practice.

Another approach that is being investigated anew is the use of surgery to consolidate remissions achieved from chemotherapy.[57] This approach was pioneered in bladder cancer by Alan Yagoda more than 20 years ago. The rationale is based on the high relapse rate observed at responding sites of disease and is supported by the 33% incidence of viable cancer found within resected specimens after complete clinical response. Five-year survival rates, as high as 30–40%, have been reported in patients following complete resection of metastatic sites after cisplatin-based chemotherapy, these represent very heavily selected cases, dominated by single metastases.

Uncommon histologic variants

A detailed discussion of the management of adenocarcinoma, squamous carcinoma, small cell carcinoma, and sarcoma of the bladder is beyond the scope of this brief review and has been detailed elsewhere.[58,59] However, certain principles of management can be noted.[60] All of the uncommon variants tend to be more resistant to chemotherapy than are the pure UCs, and thus a greater emphasis is placed on surgical resection or definitive radiotherapy when possible. Where unusual histologic patterns are noted, it is also important to ensure that the diagnosis is confirmed by an expert tumor pathologist and also to exclude the diagnosis of a metastatic second primary cancer. In general, we recommend referral to a center of excellence at least for confirmation of the diagnosis and a second opinion regarding management.[60]

The prognosis of metastatic tumors of non-transitional type reflects the sites of involvement, growth characteristics, and bulk of disease. As the yield from chemotherapy is less impressive than for urothelial cancer,[48,58,59] consideration of context (age, anticipated active life expectancy, intercurrent disease, sites of metastases) is important when planning the approach to chemotherapy.[60]

As a general rule, squamous carcinomas are sensitive to combinations that include a platinum complex, paclitaxel, and gemcitabine, and occasional responses have been reported after treatment with methotrexate, bleomycin, and ifosfamide. We have shown that the MVAC regimen is not especially useful for squamous carcinoma of the bladder.[48] Patterns of practice vary with the combinations of gemcitabine, ifosfamide, and cisplatin or paclitaxel, gemcitabine, and cisplatin, occasionally producing long-term survival for metastatic disease. Adenocarcinomas tend to respond transiently to regimens used for cancers of the GI tract, such as combinations involving oxaliplatin, irinotecan, and fluoropyrimidines, such as 5-fluorouracil or capecitabine, although there is a paucity of data from well-structured phase II or phase III clinical trial data.

Investigators at the MD Anderson Cancer Center have reported a substantial experience with metastatic small cell anaplastic cancer of the bladder, revealing anticancer efficacy but few cures.[59] The regimens with most utility resemble those used for small cell cancers of the lung and generally involve combinations that include a platinum complex, etoposide, doxorubicin, a taxane, and an oxazophorine. However, there is a general consensus that these tumors are more resistant to chemotherapy than are bronchogenic small cell tumors, and there is thus a greater emphasis on the role of surgical extirpation in the control of the primary tumor. In the metastatic setting, this is less relevant. In addition, there is good level-2 evidence that chemotherapy adds to the survival impact of surgical resection for clinically nonmetastatic disease.

Upper tract tumors

The approach to upper tract urothelial cancers is very similar to that employed for cancers of the bladder, with the caveat that the extent of surrounding fat and muscle is less, thus constituting less obstruction to metastasis. In addition, the phenomenon of "drop metastasis" may occur, in which tumor deposits from the upper tract(s) may seed to the urothelium of the bladder; whether this is the only mechanism of metachronous tumors, or whether this reflects the presence of field defect remains unclear. Details regarding etiology, epidemiology, clinical presentation, and investigation have been addressed in the relevant sections earlier.[61-63]

Surgical treatment

The surgical approach to upper tract tumors is quite different from that employed for the bladder.[64-67] The standard treatment for localized upper tract UC is radical nephroureterectomy, with complete removal of the kidney, surrounding fat and Gerota's fascia, removal of the affected ureter, and the en bloc resection of a bladder cuff. We believe that ipsilateral node dissection or extensive sampling should be performed for prognostication purposes, although there is no level 1 evidence to prove a therapeutic impact from the procedure.

Increasingly, laparoscopic radical nephroureterectomy is being considered as a viable alternative to open surgery, although long-term outcome equivalence has yet to be proven. Nonrandomized series appear to indicate that the results are comparable with respect to tumor control and possibly with less operative morbidity.[65,66]

Nephron-sparing surgery is considered for settings such as bilateral disease, solitary kidney, impaired renal function, or significant comorbid medical conditions. This can be achieved by partial nephrectomy, partial ureterectomy, partial resection of renal pelvis, and percutaneous resection of a renal pelvic tumor. The decision to take this approach is essentially a cost-effectiveness choice, and one which must take into consideration the likely outcome of tumor management versus the morbidity of treatment and its impact on the comorbid state. Low grade tumors, in particular, may be treated safely and effectively by endoscopic means.[67] Case selection is of critical importance, and recurrence rates reflect surgical experience and technique, instrumentation employed, and the prognostic determinants of the tumors being treated.

Radiotherapy and chemotherapy

There is remarkably scanty levels 1–2 information to support the use of radiotherapy for upper tract tumors, beyond palliation for inoperable cases. Dosing is limited by the sensitivity of the normal tissues to the impact of radiotherapy. Furthermore, those tumors with sufficiently poor prognosis to require consideration of radiotherapy for local control actually have a high chance of synchronous or metachronous distant nodal or metastatic involvement, thus vitiating the true role of radiotherapy. In structured trials, adjuvant radiotherapy has not been shown to have a major survival impact for upper tract tumors.[68,69]

The efficacy of intravesical therapy for bladder cancer led investigators to use these agents in upper urinary tract tumors. The most common approach has been to place bilateral ureteral stents followed by instillation of cytotoxic agents (usually BCG) via a urinary catheter, as for bladder cancer; however, uncertainty remains as to how well the agents are being delivered upstream. Alternatively, there have been reports of transcutaneous insertion of flexible catheters into the ureters, followed by infusion of agents. Anecdotal data suggest that tumor regression occurs in response to topical delivery of chemotherapy or immunotherapy.

The use of adjuvant intravesical instillation of BCG, doxorubicin, and mitomycin C after endoscopic treatment has been reported, with evidence of anti-cancer effect on tumors in the upper tracts.[70] These agents have also been delivered via nephrostomy tube after percutaneous treatment. The quality of the data, including length of follow-up, has been variable, but the overall consensus is that relapse and progression can be reduced by this type of treatment. Approximately 30% of patients with upper tract urothelial cancer will develop a recurrence in the bladder, thus requiring long-term cystoscopic surveillance of the bladder for patients with upper tract UC.[71]

The considerations for systemic chemotherapy for upper tract urothelial cancers are essentially identical to those pertaining to urothelial bladder cancer.[45-52] In the past, upper tract tumors were considered to be less responsive than those arising in the bladder. However, there is little evidence to support this, and the international randomized study of MVAC versus cisplatin confirmed similar response rates and survival.[48] Thus, systemic chemotherapy is covered in detail in the section on chemotherapy for bladder cancer.

Summary

Significant progress has been made in the management of bladder cancer over the past 30 years, with refinement of our understanding of the underlying biology, relevance of gene expression and stem cell function, molecular prognostication, improvement in the nature of surgery, reduction in morbidity of surgery, and rationalization of the role of chemotherapy for advanced disease. There is also a place for bladder conservation via chemoradiation. Despite progress, many patients with metastatic disease

die of their disease, and this has led to the search for new systemic therapies, including novel cytotoxics and the assessment of targeted therapies,
with agents targeting the MET gene and PD-L1 currently appearing most
promising. New agents should be compared against standard regimens
in well-structured trials before introduction into routine clinical practice.

Key references

*The complete reference list can be found on the Wiley Companion Digital Edition of this
title (see inside front cover for login instructions).*

1 Raghavan D, Shipley WU, Garnick MB, Richie JP, Russell PJ. Biology and management of bladder cancer. *N Engl J Med*. 1990;**322**:1129–1138.

2 Fleshner N, Kondylis F. Demographics and epidemiology of urothelial cancer of
the urinary bladder. In: Droller M, ed. *American Cancer Society Atlas of Clinical
Oncology: Urothelial Tumors*. London, Hamilton: BC Decker; 2004:1–16.

3 Cote RJ, Mitra AP, Amin MB: Bladder and urethra. In: Weidner N, Cote RJ, Suster
S, Weiss LM eds. *Modern Surgical Pathology*, 2nd ed. Philadelphia, PA; Saunders;
2009, pp. 1079ff, Chapter 31.

4 Brown JL, Russell PJ, Philips J, Wotherspoon J, Raghavan D. Clonal analysis of a
bladder cancer cell line: an experimental model of tumor heterogeneity. *Br J Cancer*.
1990;**61**:369–376.

5 Mitra AP, Cote RJ. Molecular screening for bladder cancer: progress and potential.
Nat Rev Urol. 2010;**7**:11–20.

6 Chatterjee SJ, Datar R, Youssefzadeh D, et al. Combined effects of P53, P21, and PRb
expression in the progression of bladder transitional cell carcinoma. *J Clin Oncol*.
2004;**22**:1007–1013.

7 Mitra AP, Datar RH, Cote RJ. Molecular pathways in invasive bladder cancer:
new insights into mechanisms, progression, and target identification. *J Clin Oncol*.
2006;**24**:5552–5564.

8 Raghavan D, Huben R. Management of bladder cancer. *Curr Probl Cancer*.
1995;**19**:1–64.

11 Grossman HB, Gomella L, Fradet Y, et al. A phase III multicenter comparison of
hexaminolevulinate fluorescence cystoscopy and white light cystoscopy for the
detection of superficial papillary lesions in patients with bladder cancer. *J Urol*.
2007;**178**:62–67.

13 American Joint Committee on Cancer. Bladder cancer. In: Edge SB, Byrd DR,
Compton CC, Fritz AG, Greene FL, Trotti A, eds. *AJCC Cancer Staging Handbook*,
7th ed. New York: Springer; 2010:569–577.

14 Bajorin DF, Dodd PM, Mazumdar M, et al. Long-term survival in metastatic
transitional-cell carcinoma prognostic factors predicting outcome of therapy. *J Clin
Oncol*. 1999;**17**:3173–3181.

15 Apolo AB, Ostrovnaya I, Halabi S, et al. Prognostic model for predicting survival of
patients with metastatic urothelial cancer treated with cisplatin-based chemotherapy. *J Natl Cancer Inst*. 2013;**105**:499–503.

16 Cookson MS, Herr HW, Zhang ZF, et al. The treated natural history of high risk
superficial bladder cancer: 15-year outcome. *J Urol*. 1997;**158**:62–67.

19 Herr HW, Sogani PC. Does early cystectomy improve the survival of patients with
high risk superficial bladder tumors? *J Urol*. 2001;**166**:1296–1299.

20 Stein JP, Lieskovsky G, Cote R, et al. Radical cystectomy in the treatment of invasive
bladder cancer: long-term results in 1054 patients. *J Clin Oncol*. 2001;**19**:666–675.

23 Kader AK, Richards KA, Krane LS, Pettus JA, Smith JJ, Hemal AK. Robot-assisted
laparoscopic vs open radical cystectomy: comparison of complications and perioperative oncological outcomes in 200 patients. *BJU Int*. 2013;**112**:E290–E294.

24 Bochner BH, Sjoberg DD, Laudone VP, et al. A randomized trial of robot-assisted
laparoscopic radical cystectomy. *N Engl J Med*. 2014;**371**:389–390.

25 Sondergaard J, Holmberg M, Jakobsen AR, Agerbaek M, Muren LP, Hoyer M. A
comparison of morbidity following conformal versus intensity-modulated radiotherapy for urinary bladder cancer. *Acta Oncol*. 2014;**53**:1321–1328.

28 Coppin C, Gospodarowicz M, James K, et al. Improved local control of invasive
bladder cancer by concurrent cisplatin and preoperative or definitive radiation.
The National Cancer Institute of Canada Clinical Trials Group. *J Clin Oncol*.
1996;**14**:2901–2907.

29 James ND, Hussain SA, Hall E, et al. Radiotherapy with or without chemotherapy
in muscle-invasive bladder cancer. *N Engl J Med*. 2012;**366**:1477–1480.

30 Raghavan D, Pearson B, Duval P, et al. Initial intravenous cis-platinum therapy: improved management for invasive high-risk bladder cancer? *J Urol*.
1985;**133**:399–402.

31 Grossman HB, Natale RB, Tangen CM, et al. Neoadjuvant chemotherapy plus cystectomy compared with cystectomy alone for locally advanced bladder cancer. *N
Engl J Med*. 2003;**349**:859.

33 Griffiths G, Hall R, Sylvester R, Raghavan D. International phase III trial assessing neoadjuvant cisplatin, methotrexate, and vinblastine chemotherapy for
muscle-invasive bladder cancer: long-term results of the BA06 30894 trial. *J Clin
Oncol*. 2011;**29**:2171–2177.

35 Raj GV, Karavadia S, Schlomer B, et al. Contemporary use of perioperative
cisplatin-based chemotherapy in patients with muscle-invasive bladder cancer.
Cancer. 2011;**117**:276–282.

36 Skinner DG, Daniels JR, Russell CA, et al. The role of adjuvant chemotherapy following cystectomy for invasive bladder cancer: a prospective comparative trial. *J
Urol*. 1991;**145**:459–467.

37 Freiha F, Reese J, Torti FM. A randomized trial of radical cystectomy plus cisplatin,
vinblastine and methotrexate chemotherapy for muscle invasive bladder cancer. *J
Urol*. 1996;**155**:495–500.

39 Stockle M, Wellek S, Meyenburg W, et al. Radical cystectomy with or without
adjuvant polychemotherapy for non-organ-confined transitional cell carcinoma
of the urinary bladder: prognostic impact of lymph node involvement. *Urology*.
1996;**48**:868–875.

41 Cognetti F, Ruggeri EM, Felici A, et al. Adjuvant chemotherapy with cisplatin and
gemcitabine versus chemotherapy at relapse in patients with muscle-invasive bladder cancer submitted to radical cystectomy: an Italian, multicenter, randomized
phase III trial. *Ann Oncol*. 2011;**23**:695–700.

42 Raghavan D, Bawtinhimer A, Mahoney J, Eckrich S, Riggs S. Adjuvant chemotherapy for bladder cancer – why does level 1 evidence not support it? *Ann Oncol*.
2014;**10**:1930–1934.

43 Sternberg CN, Skoneczna I, Kerst JM, et al. Immediate versus deferred chemotherapy after radical cystectomy in patients with pT3–pT4 or N+M0 urothelial carcinoma of the bladder (EORTC 30994): an intergroup, open-label, randomised phase
3 trial. *Lancet Oncol*. 2015;**16**:76–86.

48 Saxman SB, Propert K, Einhorn LH, et al. Long-term follow up of phase III intergroup study of cisplatin alone or in combination with methotrexate, vinblastine, and
doxorubicin in patients with metastatic urothelial carcinoma: a cooperative group
study. *J Clin Oncol*. 1997;**15**:2564–2569.

51 von der Maase H, Sengelov L, Roberts JT, et al. Long-term survival results of
a randomized trial comparing gemcitabine plus cisplatin, with methotrexate,
vinblastine, doxorubicin, plus cisplatin in patients with bladder cancer. *J Clin
Oncol*. 2005;**23**:4602–4608.

52 Bellmunt J, von der Maase H, Mead GM, et al. Randomized phase III study comparing paclitaxel/cisplatin/gemcitabine and gemcitabine/cisplatin in patients with
locally advanced or metastatic urothelial cancer without prior systemic therapy:
EORTC Intergroup Study 30987. *J Clin Oncol*. 2012;**30**:1107–1113.

53 Hussain MA, MacVicar GR, Petrylak DP, et al. Trastuzumab, paclitaxel, carboplatin, and gemcitabine in advanced human epidermal growth factor
receptor-2/neu-positive urothelial carcinoma: results of a multicenter phase
II National Cancer Institute trial. *J Clin Oncol*. 2007;**25**:2218–2224.

56 Powles T, Eder JP, Fine GD, et al. MPDL3280A (anti-PD-L1) treatment
leads to clinical activity in metastatic bladder cancer. *Nature*. 2014;**515**:
558–562.

57 Lehmann J, Suttmann H, Albers P, et al. Surgery for metastatic urothelial carcinoma with curative intent: the German experience (AUO AB 30/05). *Eur Urol*.
2009;**55**:1293–1299.

58 Sternberg CN, Swanson DA. Non-transitional cell bladder cancer. In: Raghavan D,
Scher HI, Leibel SA, Lange PH, eds. *Principles and Practice of Genitourinary Oncology*. Philadelphia: Lippincott-Raven; 1997:315–330.

59 Siefker-Radtke AO, Czerniak BA, Dinney CP, Millikan RE. Uncommon cancers
of the bladder. In: Raghavan D, Blanke CD, Johnson DH, et al., eds. *Textbook of
Uncommon Cancer*, 4th ed. Wiley-Blackwell: Hoboken; 2012:23–33.

60 Raghavan D. A structured approach to uncommon cancers: what should a clinician
do? *Ann Oncol*. 2013;**24**:2932–2934.

63 Munoz JJ, Ellison LM. Upper tract urothelial neoplasms: incidence and survival
during the last 2 decades. *J Urol*. 2000;**164**:1523–1525.

98 Neoplasms of the prostate

Christopher J. Logothetis, MD ▪ Jeri Kim, MD ▪ John W. Davis, MD, FACS ▪ Brian F. Chapin, MD ▪ Deborah Kuban, MD, FACR, FASTRO ▪ Eleni Efstathiou, MD, PhD ▪ Ana Aparicio, MD

Overview

Cancer of the prostate is the most commonly diagnosed nonskin neoplasm and the second leading cause of cancer-related mortality in men in the United States. Considerable advances have been made in screening, diagnosis, and therapy options, particularly in advanced disease, but controversies about the diagnosis and management of prostate cancer, especially in the areas of screening and choice of therapy, continue to evolve. Controversies in advanced disease states have shifted from prognostication to prediction, and current treatment considerations are focused on optimization of sequence or combinations of therapy, determining the role of local control and bone targeting. It is anticipated that addressing these knowledge gaps will lead to an integrated and more effective treatment strategies. Further advances in therapy can be achieved by development of new agents with unique mechanisms of action and rational integration into combination therapies.

Prostate cancer awareness, clinical application of improved biopsy schemes, and advances in imaging combined with the widespread use of prostate-specific antigen (PSA) have resulted in increased detection of prostate cancer. The evolving use of the serum PSA concentration and its change over time have not been paralleled by studies that tested the relevance of those findings until the results of the European Randomized Study of Screening for Prostate Cancer (ERSPC) and the Prostate, Lung, Colorectal, and Ovarian (PLCO) Cancer Screening Trial were first published in 2009.[1] Though many of the apparent discrepancies between these trials can be accounted for by trial design and patient cross-contamination, they brought to the forefront the dilemma of overdiagnosis and overtreatment and the urgent need to improve the accuracy of clinically significant prostate cancer. It is hoped that replacement of the current morphologic and anatomic classification of prostate cancer with one based on improved understanding of biology will lead to molecular classification and bring closer a personalized management of this complex disease.

Salient features that distinguish prostate cancer from other malignancies and that frame the dilemmas surrounding it are its striking age-dependent incidence, with progressively increasing frequency with increasing age; the variable lethality of morphologically identified cancers; the central role of androgen signaling; and the preponderance of bone-forming metastases on its lethal progression. The important advances made in each of these areas will, in the near future, modify the approaches currently used to prevent, prognosticate, and treat prostate cancer.

Biology of prostate cancer

Normal anatomic and histologic features of the prostate

The prostate gland sits in the pelvis, surrounded by the rectum posteriorly and the bladder superiorly, and it is anchored to the bladder pelvic floor; the urethra communicates between the bladder and the prostate into the penis (Figure 1). The prostate is composed of stromal, ductal, and luminal epithelial cells and is organized around branching ducts and individual glands lined with secretory epithelial cells and basal cells.[2] The secretory epithelial cell is the major cell type in the gland. These androgen-regulated cells produce PSA and prostatic acid phosphatase (PAP). The central role of androgen signaling in prostate cancer biology likely accounts for the utility of PSA and PAP in determining disease status clinically. The vast majority of prostate cancers have cells that share properties with the secretory epithelial cells. Unlike the epithelial cells, the basal cell layer is not directly controlled by androgen signaling. Investigators have suggested that the basal cell population contains the prostate stem cells from which the epithelial cells develop. If correct, this view has obvious implications for the prevention and treatment of all stages of prostate cancer.

As in other human tissues, cells belonging to the neuroendocrine system are also present within the prostate. Neuroendocrine cells contain secretory granules and extend dendrite-like processes between adjacent epithelial cells or toward the acinar or urethral lumina.[3,4] A variety of secretory products can be found within the granules, including serotonin, calcitonin, gastrin-releasing peptide, and somatostatin.[3,4] Neuroendocrine cells are commonly identified immunohistochemically by the presence of markers such as chromogranin A or synaptophysin in the cytoplasm. They are terminally differentiated cells that are thought to regulate the growth, differentiation, and function of coexisting prostatic cells, but their exact role remains to be fully understood.

The view that the prostate has a lobar pattern has been challenged. McNeal et al.[5] conducted detailed studies of the normal and pathologic anatomy of the prostate and introduced the transforming concept of anatomic zones rather than lobes to describe the gland. There are four major zones within the normal prostate: peripheral, central, transition (constituting 70%, 20%, and 5% of the glandular tissue, respectively), and anterior fibromuscular stroma (Figure 2). The peripheral zone, which extends posterolaterally around the gland from the apex to the base, is the most common site for the development of prostate carcinomas. The central zone surrounds the ejaculatory duct apparatus and makes up the majority of the prostatic base. The transition zone constitutes two small lobules that abut the prostatic urethra and is the region where benign prostatic hypertrophy (BPH) primarily originates. Some reports suggest that transition zone cancers have a lower malignant potential, but other studies report no difference in outcome compared with those originating in the peripheral zone, when controlled for grade and stage.[6,7]

Surrounding the gland is stroma, which includes fibroblasts, smooth muscle, nerves, and lymphatic tissue. The roles of stromal–epithelial interactions in prostate physiology and cancer development are being elucidated. Recent insights suggest that these interactions are critical in normal function, and increasing

Holland-Frei Cancer Medicine, Ninth Edition. Edited by Robert C. Bast Jr., Carlo M. Croce, William N. Hait, Waun Ki Hong, Donald W. Kufe, Martine Piccart-Gebhart, Raphael E. Pollock, Ralph R. Weichselbaum, Hongyang Wang, and James F. Holland.
© 2017 John Wiley & Sons, Inc. ISBN: 978-1-118-93469-2

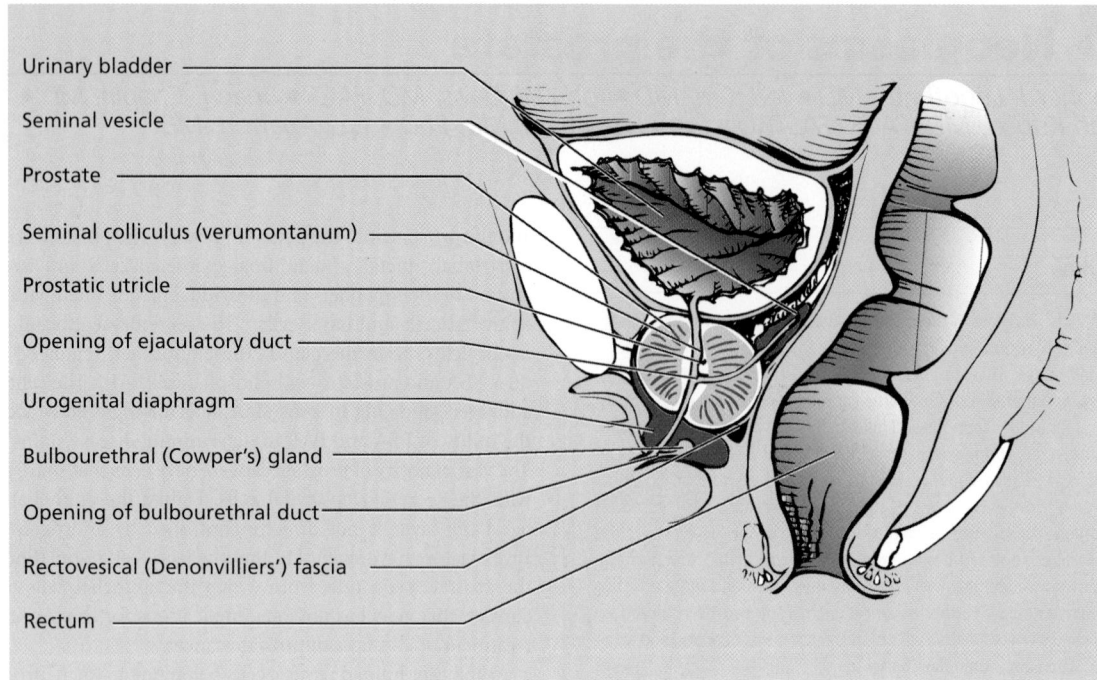

Urinary bladder
Seminal vesicle
Prostate
Seminal colliculus (verumontanum)
Prostatic utricle
Opening of ejaculatory duct
Urogenital diaphragm
Bulbourethral (Cowper's) gland
Opening of bulbourethral duct
Rectovesical (Denonvilliers') fascia
Rectum

Figure 1 Normal prostate anatomy.

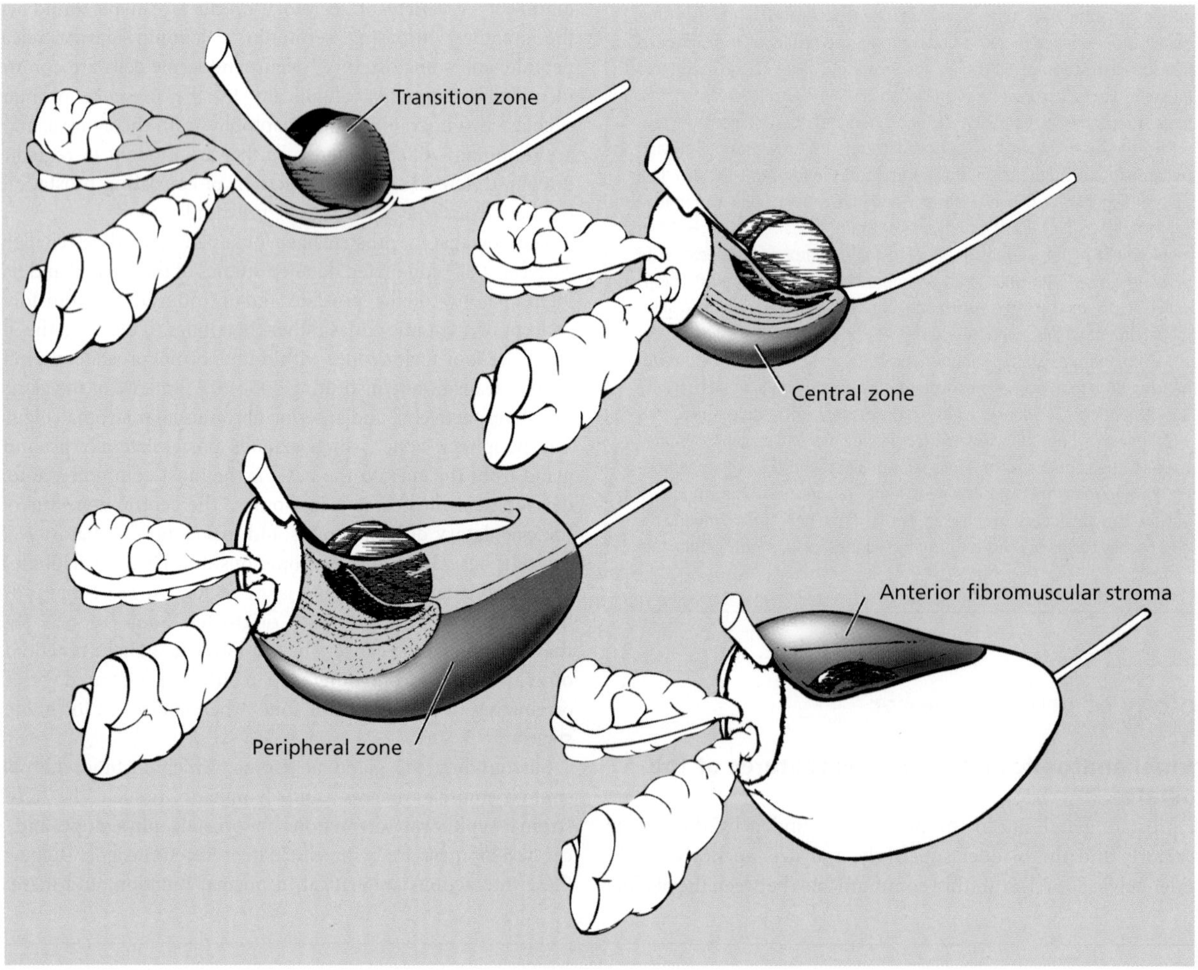

Transition zone

Central zone

Peripheral zone

Anterior fibromuscular stroma

Figure 2 Zonal anatomy of the prostate: the three glandular zones of the prostate and the anterior fibromuscular stroma.

evidence implicates them in prostate carcinogenesis as well. The stromal–epithelial interactions may exert both tumor-promoting and carcinogenesis—and progression—inhibitory effects. Furthermore, the stromal–epithelial interacting pathways implicated in the development of the tumor microenvironment in prostate cancer progression may be those that are shared by the prostate and bone in their normal development and function.[8]

There are varying distinct anatomic barriers surrounding the prostate. The smooth muscle of the prostatic stroma gradually extends into fibrous tissue that then ends in loose connective and adipose tissue. Of particular relevance is the absence of any semblance of a capsule at the gland's apex and anteriorly. This understanding of anatomic detail allows clinicians to determine the adequacy of prostate surgery by accurately defining the surgical margin with increasing confidence. It also allows the surgical delineation of disease as "organ confined" or "specimen confined." The organ-confined cancers do not extend beyond the confines of the prostate, whereas specimen confined indicates that the cancer does not extend beyond the cut margins. The distinction between these two terms is important because they are used to determine the adequacy of surgery and inform the use of postoperative radiation therapy in selected patients.

A final anatomic note about the prostate is that Walsh and Donker[9] described the presence of two neurovascular bundles that pass adjacent to the gland posterolaterally. The neurovascular bundles are essential for normal erectile function, and defining their presence outside of the posterior–lateral prostatic fascia allowed Walsh to develop a "nerve-sparing" radical retropubic prostatectomy procedure that improves the odds of preserving potency.[10]

Premalignant prostatic lesions

Paradigms that are used to explain the progression of other solid tumors may not apply to prostate cancer.[11] Extensive information about the genetic and epigenetic phenomena associated with prostate cancer progression has been developed recently but has yet to pass the threshold of clinical utility to be truly useful. Many clinicians accept that premalignant lesions existing in the prostate may precede the development of cancer by many years. But given the lack of knowledge about the nature or rate of their progression, the morphologic identification of premalignant lesions on biopsy specimens only serves to provide rationale for close monitoring of patients.

Morphologically heterogeneous lesions are included under the single term prostatic intraepithelial neoplasia (PIN) (Figure 3).[12] PIN is defined as the presence of cytologically atypical or dysplastic epithelial cells within architecturally benign-appearing glands and acini. Although three different grades have been described, 1 (mild), 2 (moderate), and 3 (severe), grades 2 and 3 PIN are often combined as "high grade" and worthy of note. PIN is presumed to be a premalignant lesion because it is commonly present adjacent to prostate adenocarcinomas.[13] The finding of PIN is associated with the existence of cancer in sites not sampled on biopsy and implies increased risk of developing a morphologic cancer although the risk of progression has not been established or quantified.

Prospective studies have been small but have reinforced the hypothesis that PIN is the morphologic manifestation of a precursor lesion to morphologic prostate cancer. The data have suggested that the presence of high-grade PIN predicts the subsequent development of cancer, perhaps through a multistep carcinogenesis process. However, close clinical follow-up remains the standard of care after diagnosis of high-grade PIN alone.

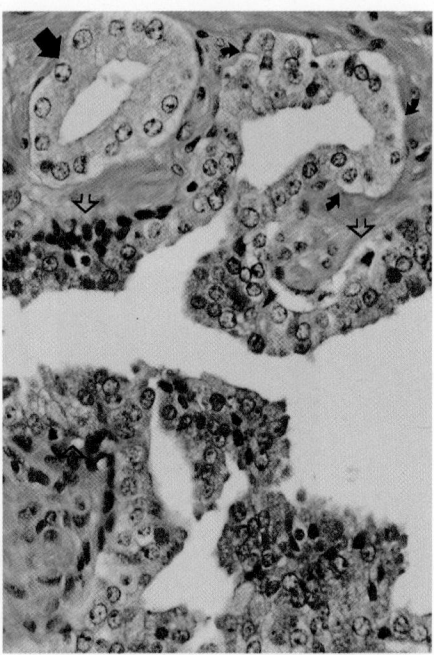

Figure 3 Photomicrograph of high-grade prostatic intraepithelial neoplasia (PIN) with basal cell layer (open arrows) with budding microacinus lacking basal cells (curved solid arrows). A microacinus of invasive Gleason pattern 3 adenocarcinoma is seen in the adjacent stroma (straight solid arrow). Hematoxylin and eosin × 160. Source: Courtesy of Thomas M. Wheeler, MD.

Another lesion that may represent a premalignant change is atypical adenomatous hyperplasia (AAH), although existing data on this are scantier than they are for PIN. The characteristic appearance with AAH is the fulfillment of the architectural criteria for malignancy, with disruption of the basal cell layer, mainly in the transition zone, but without the cytologic changes diagnostic of cancer.[14] Some authors have suggested that a prostatic lesion composed of focal areas of epithelial atrophy associated with chronic inflammation (called proliferative inflammatory atrophy, or PIA) is a precursor of PIN and eventually prostate cancer.[15] Evidence for this hypothesis includes the observation that PIA often occurs adjacent to areas of PIN and prostate cancer[16] and that somatic genetic abnormalities seen in PIA often resemble those seen in prostate carcinoma.[17] Of particular relevance is that PIA implicates inflammation in the progression of prostate cancer.[18] If this hypothesis is confirmed and causally implicated with greater confidence in prostate cancer progression, that finding may lead to more effective prevention strategies.

Histologic features of prostate cancer

Cancers that arise in the epithelium account for >95% of prostate cancers (Figure 4).[19] The reported low frequency of histologic variants may reflect the fact that frequency determinations of variants are principally derived by the examination of primary cancers, among which the more common forms may be overrepresented. However, less common histologic varieties have been described, including mucinous or signet ring tumors, adenoid cystic carcinomas, carcinoid, large prostatic duct carcinomas (including the endometrial type), adenocarcinomas, and small-cell undifferentiated cancers. These unusual subtypes are reported to occur in low frequencies. Because the histologic variants often present with advanced disease clinically, they are not subjected to surgery as often as the more common forms of prostate cancer. In addition, they occasionally manifest only in metastases during progression,

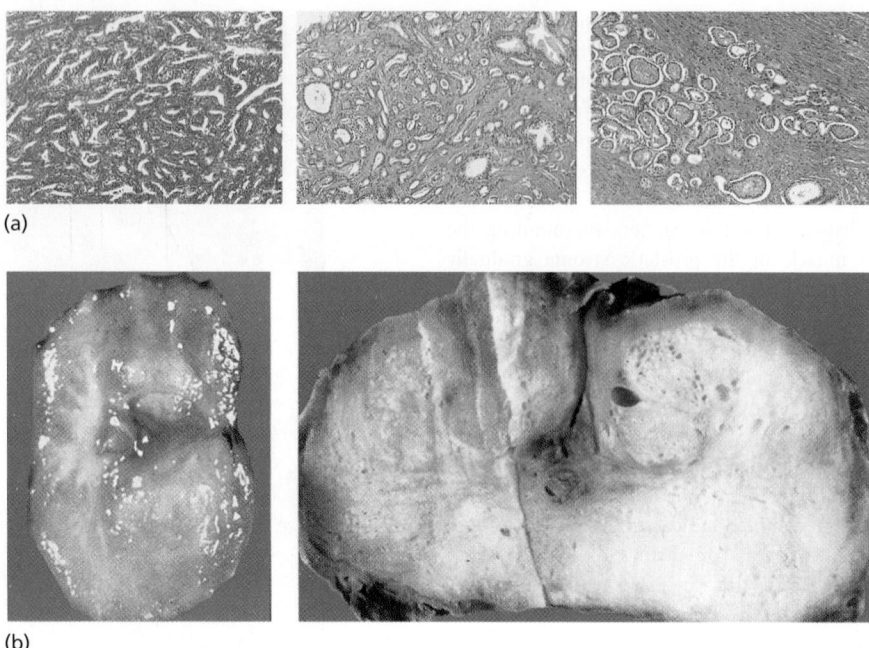

(a)

(b)

Figure 4 (a) Microscopic histologic appearance of prostate adenocarcinoma. (b) Gross histologic appearance of prostate adenocarcinoma.

thus in sites not often sampled. As a consequence, we may be underestimating their frequency because of their manifestation. This fact may be particularly important when attempting to estimate the true frequency of small-cell carcinomas of the prostate, which have been reported with increasing frequency.[20] Nonetheless, it is important to recognize these unusual variants of prostate cancer because standard hormonal therapies may be less effective in their treatment while they may be more responsive to chemotherapy than the more common type.[17,21]

Tumors with a neuroendocrine appearance (i.e., carcinoid and small-cell undifferentiated types) may arise from Kulchitsky cells, which are found in the basal regions of the prostatic epithelium.[22] Small-cell carcinomas of the prostate share histologic and clinical features with other extrapulmonary small-cell carcinomas. These cancers have been described as a histologic continuum, perhaps in some instances reflecting progression of acinar adenocarcinomas.[23] Thus, these "neuroendocrine" cancers of the prostate are likely to be a mechanistically and clinically heterogeneous grouping. Of importance is that they predict a specific pattern of anatomic progression: nonosseous visceral spread with lytic bone metastases and the probability of responsiveness to chemotherapy. These are recognized as a unique and aggressive variant of prostate cancer that account for a significant portion of far advanced prostate cancers.

Transitional cell carcinomas involving the substance of the prostate may also be mistaken for prostate adenocarcinoma. It may be difficult to distinguish a transitional cell carcinoma arising in the transitional epithelium of the distal prostatic ducts from a tumor arising in the bladder epithelium and spreading into the contiguous prostatic ducts.

Study findings have confirmed the primary prognostic importance of the degree of histologic differentiation of prostate adenocarcinoma. The degree of this differentiation is typically determined by patterns of gland formation and, less importantly, by cytologic detail. The most widely accepted grading scheme for adenocarcinoma of the prostate is that developed by Gleason (Figure 5).[25] Gleason created a system for classifying prostate

tumors based on two levels of scoring that recognize the heterogeneous nature of prostate carcinomas. The primary pattern of differentiation is assigned a Gleason grade of 1 to 5 according to the dominant morphologic features of the specimen and its departure from normal appearance; the next most common pattern is also assigned a grade. This results in a two-digit score; for example, $3 + 4 = 7$. The Gleason system has been criticized for inadequately recognizing the proportion of the tumor that is composed of the secondary pattern as well as for lacking adequate distinction between good and poor prognoses in patients whose cancers have Gleason scores of 5–7 (most patients). However, the reproducibility and reliability of Gleason grading between pathologists have consistently been shown to be excellent. Gleason's original work demonstrated a clear association between a higher score and a higher mortality rate, which others have since confirmed.[26] Many other predictors of the clinical behavior of prostate cancer have been explored, but the Gleason score still remains the most broadly applicable and prognostically useful histologic grading system.

Molecular pathogenesis

Unlike the case of breast cancers, in which clinically relevant subsets of cancer have been identified on the basis of molecular profiles, the morphologic characterization of prostate cancer remains the standard.[27] Prostate cancer cells harbor a number of somatic mutations, and in advanced disease, additional alterations accumulate. Alterations that affect the development and progression of prostate cancer include those in the hormonal and growth factor milieu, in hormonal and growth factor receptors, in intracellular signaling pathways, and in cell cycle regulation and apoptosis. The identification of chromosome 8q24 as a susceptibility locus supports the hypothesis that a significant portion of prostate cancers have genetic origins.[28]

Technological advances in genome sequencing made possible to identify germline mutations that have been linked to increased risk of prostate cancer. The *HOXB13 G84E* variant is the first *bona fide* prostate cancer susceptibility gene to be identified. In a study of 94 unrelated patients, the *HOXB13 G84E* variant was associated with

Gleason grading system

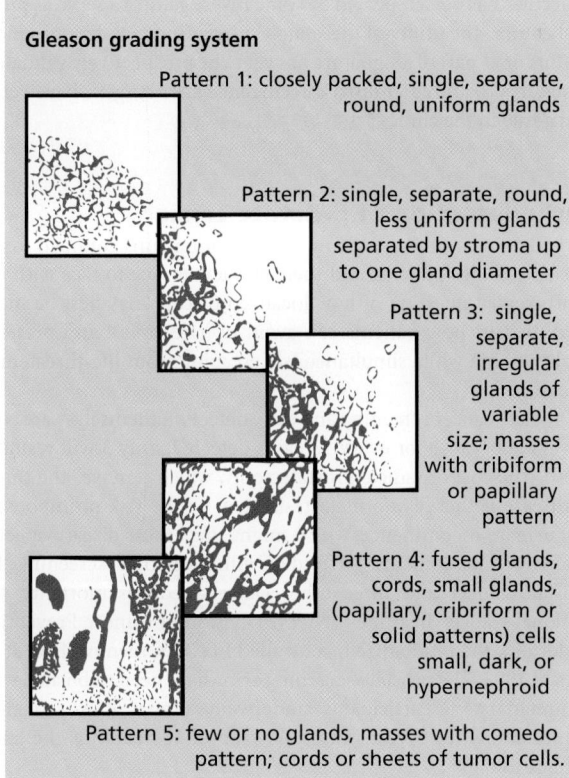

Pattern 1: closely packed, single, separate, round, uniform glands

Pattern 2: single, separate, round, less uniform glands separated by stroma up to one gland diameter

Pattern 3: single, separate, irregular glands of variable size; masses with cribiform or papillary pattern

Pattern 4: fused glands, cords, small glands, (papillary, cribriform or solid patterns) cells small, dark, or hypernephroid

Pattern 5: few or no glands, masses with comedo pattern; cords or sheets of tumor cells.

Figure 5 Histologic grading scheme for adenocarcinomas of the prostate. Source: Kattan 2007.[24] Reproduced with permission of Nature Publishing Group.

Table 1 Growth factors implicated in prostate cancer.

Transforming growth factor beta
Fibroblast growth factor
Epidermal growth factor
Insulin-like growth factor
Platelet-derived growth factor
Vascular endothelial growth factor
Neurotensin
Endothelins
Colony-stimulating factors

a significant risk of early-onset hereditary prostate cancer.[29] Additionally, germline *BRCA1* and *BRCA2* mutations confer high risk of prostate cancer and prognostic of more aggressive prostate cancer.[30] However, these germline mutations have not yet translated into therapeutic relevance.

The hormonal and growth factor milieu to which the prostate is exposed has been consistently associated with the pathogenesis of cancer. In population-based studies, two hormones have been implicated: testosterone and insulin-like growth factor I (IGF-I). The association between testosterone and prostate cancer progression is well known. Several lines of evidence also suggest that IGF may be important in prostate cancer growth. First, several prostate cancer cell lines and prostate xenograft models express both IGFs I and II and their receptors.[31,32] Second, Chan et al.[33] reported on the relationship between plasma IGF-I concentration and prostate cancer, citing a relative risk of 4.3 for men in the highest quartile, compared with men in the lowest quartile. Moreover, a higher incidence of prostate cancer has been noted in patients who had relatively high IGF-I concentrations in plasma samples that had been obtained 5 years prior to the cancer diagnosis,[34] supporting the concept that IGF-I may be important early in the development of prostate cancer. Although this observation has yet to be confirmed, it does implicate IGF-I signaling in prostate cancer progression. It is likely that growth factor and other stromal–epithelial interacting pathways cooperate in prostate cancer progression. Thus, a simple model centered on a single pathway is unlikely to lead to the understanding of human prostate cancer. Other growth factors—including epidermal growth factor, vascular endothelial growth factor (VEGF), platelet-derived growth factor

(PDGF), and transforming growth factor beta (TGF-β)—may also be dysregulated in the development of prostate cancer (Table 1).[35]

The central role of androgen signaling in an endocrine fashion has dominated the understanding of the pathway in prostate cancer. It is clear that androgens are a major mediator of progression, though their role in prostate cancer susceptibility remains poorly understood. In fact, several hormonal receptors are altered in prostate cancer cells. Perhaps the best example is alterations in the androgen receptor (AR). In early cancer, AR mutations are relatively uncommon,[36] but germline variation (CAG repeats) in the *AR* gene has been shown to be a predictor of cancer aggressiveness[37] and may play a role in the frequency and aggressiveness of prostate cancer in African-Americans.[38] It is interesting that AR mutations are more commonly seen in androgen-independent (castrate-resistant) prostate cancer,[36,39] arguing that the AR gene remains central in the growth and survival of prostate cancer even after the need for the ligand (androgens) has been mitigated. Several theoretical frameworks have been proposed for the development of androgen independence, most of which still postulate a cancer cell that depends on a functional *AR* but one that is amplified, oversensitive, promiscuous, or activated by upregulated coactivators or downregulated by corepressors.[40] For example, in LNCaP prostate cancer cells, an *AR* mutation, T877A, which is a substitution of alanine for threonine at position 877, results in an AR that is activated by other steroid hormones and by the androgen antagonist flutamide.[41] This *AR* mutation could help explain the "antiandrogen withdrawal syndrome." However, *AR* mutations occur too infrequently to account for the eventual evolution of most metastatic prostate cancers to a castrate-resistant state.

AR splice variants have been identified in prostate cancer. AR splice variants lacking the ligand-binding domain (ARVs), originally isolated from prostate cancer cell lines derived from a single patient, are detected in normal and malignant human prostate tissue, with the highest levels observed in the late stage, castrate-resistant prostate cancer (CRPC). Approximately 20 AR splice variants have been identified to date, and they are not exclusively found on prostate tissue. The first AR splice variant was identified in the placenta. "The most studied variant (called AR-V7 or AR3) activates AR reporter genes in the absence of ligand and therefore, could play a role in castration resistance." Correlative studies have associated the presence of ARV7 in prostate cancer-infiltrated bone marrow biopsies and circulating tumor cells from patients with metastatic CRPC who have primary resistance to novel androgen signaling inhibitors abiraterone acetate (CYP17 inhibitor) and enzalutamide (second-generation antiandrogen).[42,43]

Recent observations support the view that "intracrine" production of androgens acting in both autocrine and paracrine fashion are implicated in the progression of prostate cancer. Several lines of evidence support the concept that CYP17 lyase is implicated in remodeling the prostate cancer tumor microenvironment: androgens in the microenvironment are at a higher concentration than they are in the serum, CYP17 expression occurs in stage-dependent cancer progression, and tumor regression occurs clinically in castrate-resistant cancers. These data support the hypothesis that androgen signaling can be considered a stromal–epithelial interacting pathway. Difficulty in measuring the concentration of androgens in the local microenvironment continues to plague this concept, and although it is appealing, it remains unproven.

True androgen independence is likely to arise from alternative stromal–epithelial interacting or other signaling pathways. Several bone and prostate development pathways have been noted to be involved in prostate cancer progression and to be associated with higher-grade cancers.[44] This attractive hypothesis could account for the bone-homing and bone-forming phenotype of prostate cancer and for its resistance to therapy in an organ-specific manner.

Molecules that alter intracellular signaling pathways also may be important in the pathogenesis and progression of prostate cancer to a castrate-resistant state. The clearest example to date is the tumor suppressor gene *PTEN*. This gene encodes for a phosphatase that is important in modulating the signal generated by activated growth factor receptors. Somatic mutations in *PTEN* occur at high frequency in prostate carcinoma cells, suggesting this as a frequent target for inactivation. One study documented a 60% rate of *PTEN* mutations; most of these were found in cell lines from metastatic disease, although mutations were also seen in primary cancers.[45] In fact, another group demonstrated higher rates of *PTEN* loss or mutation in tumors of advanced stage and grade.[46] Another pathway that may be inappropriately activated in prostate cancer is the hedgehog pathway. Normal hedgehog signaling is important in early development and patterning of the prostate epithelium. Recent work by Karhadkar et al.[47] demonstrated that activation of the hedgehog pathway distinguishes prostate cancer from normal prostate cells and, further, metastatic prostate cancer from localized cancer. Moreover, they demonstrated that hedgehog pathway inhibition results in PC3 xenograft regression. Both the PTEN and hedgehog pathways are therefore attractive targets for drug development.

Small-cell prostate carcinomas, which often emerge during the progression of CRPC, have garnered much attention in recent times as a model of primary and possibly secondary resistance to AR-directed therapies. Most small-cell prostate carcinomas lack markers of prostatic luminal differentiation such as AR, PSA, PSAP, PSMA, and p501s.[48–56] Instead of these, they often express markers that are characteristic of neural progenitor cells, such as ASCL1, POU4F2, and MYCN.[50,57–59] A decrease in the expression of RE-1-silencing transcription factor (REST), a master repressor of neuronal differentiation, has been proposed as a mechanism involved in this transdifferentiation.[60,61] In addition, small-cell prostate carcinomas are characterized by high Ki67 staining and high levels of expression of genes involved in cell cycle and mitosis, including AURKA, AURKB, PLK1, and UBE2C.[58,60,62] It is noteworthy that concordant AURKA and MYCN amplification has been found in approximately 40% of small-cell prostate carcinomas[58] and that REST knockdown resulted in a derepression of cell cycle genes in prostate cancer models[61] supporting a connection between the aberrant neural development and mitotic programs. Finally, small-cell prostate carcinomas have also been shown to bear frequent Tp53 mutations[49–51,63–65] as well as RB1 and PTEN losses and a high rate of copy number alterations.[50,58,62,63,65,66]

Finally, alterations in molecules that regulate the cell cycle and apoptosis offer promising avenues for further investigation. TP53, p27, p21, and Rb have been studied, and the results have provided variable levels of evidence that they participate in the pathogenesis of prostate cancer.[67] Of particular relevance is that each of these

molecules has been reported by some investigators to serve as prognosticators. The utility of these molecules as independent prognosticators or as part of a signature has yet to be prospectively validated. Signatures that predict disease recurrence after surgery have yet to find a role in the clinic.[68]

Early detection of prostate cancer

Early detection of prostate cancer, when it remains confined to the prostate, brings patients and their physicians face to face with the controversial question of how localized disease may best be managed, that is, how patients can avoid overtreatment and preserve quality of life while simultaneously escaping from life-threatening disease.

Prostate cancer screening and early detection themselves are controversial because for every 18 cases detected, only 3 will result in death. The cost of radical prostatectomy, which removes the threat of disease if there is no metastasis, may be the risk of impotence and urinary incontinence, which might affect these disease-specific quality-of-life domains.[69] To determine whether screening for prostate cancer and three other cancers reduces mortality, the National Cancer Institute's (NCI's) Division of Cancer Prevention undertook the randomized, controlled PLCO Screening Trial at 10 sites in 1993. The prostate screening arms have been published with commentary.[1,70] Participants underwent annual PSA screening examinations for 6 years and follow-up of 13 years for the latter publication.[71,72]

With a sample size of 76,685 men allocated to intervention (38,340) or control (38,345), the extended follow-up diagnosed 4250 cancers in the intervention arm and 3815 in the control. These events corresponded to 158 deaths in the intervention arm and 145 in the controls. The key conclusion was that PSA screening increased detection but did not affect mortality. A common critique of this study as echoed by Smith[70] was significant contamination in the arms in the form of noncompliant screening in the intervention arm and opportunistic screening in the control arm.

Also launched in the 1990s was the ERSPC, which is also testing whether screening saves lives. It was published along with the PLCO trial in 2009. Updated results truncated at 11 years and at 13 years.[71,73] In this trial, there was significantly less contamination of the arms. The ERSPC's results showed a significant relative reduction in prostate cancer mortality by 21% and 29% after adjustment for noncompliance.[74] To prevent one death, the number needed to be screened was 1055 and to detect was 37. The additional follow-up time improved the screening metrics as expected. The authors caution that all-cause mortality was not affected and that overdetection/overtreatment remains a problem with PSA screening.[75] The trial is often criticized in its design as not a unified multicenter study but rather a merger of several screening studies with differences in methodology and outcomes. As a result, the US Preventive Services Task Force (USPSTF) has issued a "D" rating for PSA screening (discourage the use of this service), yet this remains highly controversial.[76,77]

Identifying early disease using PSA and PSAV

Strategies to manage the diagnosis of localized prostate cancer include watchful waiting, radical prostatectomy, and radiotherapy and will result in superior recurrence-free outcomes at earlier stages of intervention. The early detection of prostate cancer debate has centered around using absolute PSA cutoffs versus prostate-specific antigen velocity (PSAV) or PSA isomers. The PSAV, one measure used in monitoring patients with localized disease, has been scrutinized as a tool for use in the diagnosis and prediction of outcomes.

It is calculated using the log slope of at least three PSA values calculated over at least 2 years with no less than 6 months between measures.[78] Conceived as a way to capture the variability of prostate cancer or its progression, PSAV measures are used preoperatively and postoperatively. Researchers sometimes rely on measures taken closer together, consider fewer than three measures, and reduce the longitudinal period to less than 2 years.

Prostate cancer screening can be oversimplified into an algorithm in which all patients with a certain threshold of PSA (e.g., 2.5 or 4.0 ng/mL) or abnormal digital rectal exam (DRE) findings are referred to a urologist for evaluation and possible biopsy. However, patients' overall interests are better served if a more comprehensive evaluation takes place that considers whether they are at increased risk of having prostate cancer because of ethnicity (e.g., African-Americans are at increased risk), age, and/or family history and whether a prostate cancer diagnosis would be likely to affect their overall survival because of a younger age and fewer competing comorbid conditions. A comprehensive PSA history may be beneficial for calculating PSAV, and the complexed PSA test may be useful as a frontline screening tool because it has slightly better specificity than total PSA in the total PSA range of 2.5–4.0 ng/mL.[79]

The PSA blood test has been described as a test that "neither excludes benign disease nor wholly predicts meaningful malignancies."[78] Ian Thompson, principal investigator of the Prostate Cancer Prevention Trial (PCPT), and his colleagues studied 8575 men from the study's placebo group to estimate the receiver operating characteristic (ROC) curve for PSA and concluded that no absolute cutoff value had the high degree of sensitivity and specificity simultaneously required for identification of a risk-free value.[80] Instead, they endorsed viewing all PSA values as a continuum of risk for prostate cancer.[80]

Single measures of PSA performed on blood samples taken decades before a patient's diagnosis have been statistically associated with levels of risk and have garnered great attention because of their apparent simplicity and efficiency and their ability to stratify patients for screening, but their reliability awaits verification.[81,82] These studies relied on blood samples drawn from 21,277 men in Sweden from 1974 to 1986 and on Sweden's cancer registry. From among these samples, prostate cancer diagnoses and blood samples were ascertained for 462, who were matched to controls. The median PSA level was about 0.6 ng/mL in the low-risk group. These investigators' most recent work bases prediction of cancer risk on a single PSA test before age 40.[82] Although the USPSTF recommended against PSA-based screening for prostate cancer in 2012, under the Affordable Care Act, for men over age 50 with Medicare PSA, the test is covered every 12 months.

More widely investigated have been measures of PSAV, a calculation of rising PSA level that was introduced in the early 1990s as a marker of prostate cancer development, a means to reduce unnecessary biopsies, and a way to improve the specificity of PSA testing. However, current standards that shorten the minimum longitudinal monitoring period for calculating PSAV and push ever lower the levels of PSAV considered worrisome (now 3.5 ng/mL/year in men with a PSA <4 ng/mL in one algorithm) actually increase the likelihood of biopsy.[83–86] Cautious investigators[85] argue that to use PSAV to monitor men with a PSA <4 ng/mL, it is necessary to have evidence that such measures ensure that enough cases will be detected within the "window of curability" to make them worthwhile and that the financial and emotional costs of overdiagnosis will not undermine other advances. They also point out that relying on findings about PSAV in undiagnosed cases, which have been largely lacking, would be very different from relying on posttreatment PSAV findings and applying them to the detection setting. They and others have said that prospective studies are needed.[85,87]

An early study on the PSAV was one of men enrolled in a geriatric trial. Carter et al.[83] concluded that in men with PSA values <4 ng/mL, a PSAV <0.75 µg/mL/year indicated absence of prostate cancer and a PSAV ≥0.75 µg/mL/year indicated its presence. In a work published 15 years later, Krejcarek et al.[88] reported that in the undiagnosed patients they studied who had PSAV values <1.0 ng/mL/year, only 6% of those younger than 70 years with cT1c disease had high-grade cancer; however, they found that a median PSAV value of 2.71 ng/mL/year, age, and clinical T stage were significantly related to high-risk disease (Gleason score 4 + 3). Because these subjects had undergone radiotherapy, the findings are not generalizable to patients treated with other therapeutic modalities. The study by Krejcarek et al. was a retrospective evaluation in 358 men to identify those at higher risk, so they could improve outcomes by adding androgen-suppression therapy to radiotherapy and by improving the selection of radiotherapy fields.

A prospective trial conducted at the Royal Marsden Hospital and reported in 2008 studied 237 patients enrolled in an active surveillance trial who had a median PSA level of 6.5 ng/mL at the outset and a median pretreatment PSAV of 0.44 ng/mL/year.[89] The investigators determined that PSA density was a statistically significant independent determinant of PSAV in untreated patients: those with a PSA density measure >0.185 ng/mL had a median PSAV of 0.92 ng/mL/year, and those with a PSA density measure <0.185 ng/mL had a median PSAV of 0.35 ng/mL/year. Because PSA density is a measure available at the outset of diagnosis and does not require longitudinal data collection, it will be a more efficient marker than PSAV is if others confirm this finding.

As a recent commentary by Vickers et al.[90] points out, the use of PSAV in prostate cancer early detection and management of clinically localized disease is questioned. The main arguments against PSAV are lack of clinical utility that it does not add to established predictors of prostate cancer diagnosis, methodologic variability, and it being a poor prognosticator for mortality after conservative management and after prostatectomy.

Staging of prostate cancer

Staging of cancer, which is integral to the treatment decisions that follow, comprises initial clinical staging based on findings from physical examination of the patient and diagnostic tests and pathologic staging based on findings at surgery and on subsequent pathologic study of the removed prostate gland and other tissues. Less definitive than pathologic staging, clinical staging relies on palpation of the prostate; imaging studies, which for patients at low and intermediate risk are sometimes omitted; and needle biopsy results. Physicians can combine the clinical staging with two other significant prognostic factors, the Gleason score and the preoperative PSA value, to classify the case according to the D'Amico system, as low, intermediate, or high risk.[91] This system was first described in 1998 in the report of a retrospective study in which D'Amico et al. evaluated 1872 men with prostate cancer who had been treated with radical prostatectomy, external beam radiotherapy, or radioactive implant with or without neoadjuvant androgen-deprivation therapy. In that study, clinical staging was based on DRE findings alone (American Joint Committee on Cancer tumor stage[92]). The researchers found that with that system, men who had been classified as being at low or intermediate risk had outcomes that were not statistically significantly different from others within their class. Most of this reliability is probably attributable to the Gleason score and the PSA level.

In the staging of prostate cancer, physicians rely on the tumor, node, and metastasis (TNM) system of the American Joint Committee on Cancer to classify cases[92] (Table 2). It reports the extent of the tumor (T), the presence or absence of disease in the regional lymph nodes (N), and the extent of metastasis (M). In a second step of the staging process, the Gleason score is combined with the TNM classification, and cases are identified as stage I, II, III, or IV, progressively representing advances in the extent of disease[92] (Table 3).

Prostate cancer is the most commonly diagnosed cancer in US men, with the exception of skin cancers and in situ cancers.[94] About 3/4 of US men report having been screened at least once, and early prostate cancer, because it has no symptoms, is often diagnosed in outpatient settings. Distinguishing between high- and low-risk localized prostate cancer, maximizing disease control and survival, and avoiding overtreatment, especially in men likely to die of comorbidities, are challenges physicians who treat these men face daily.[95]

The American Urological Association has characterized localized disease into three risk categories[96] (Table 4). Low-risk disease is generally characterized by a PSA value ≤ 10 ng/mL, a Gleason score ≤ 6, a lack of symptoms, and absence of both diseases in the lymph nodes and metastases (i.e., clinical stage T1c or T2). Disease is nonpalpable on DRE, but evidence of tumor may be detected by a transurethral resection of the prostate (TURP) performed because of what was thought to be BPH or by needle biopsy prompted by a high PSA level. PSA values >10 ng/mL but ≤20 ng/mL and/or a Gleason score of 7 (3 + 4 or 4 + 3) are associated with intermediate risk. PSA values >20 ng/mL and/or Gleason scores of 8–10 indicate high-risk cases.

Table 3 Prostate cancer stages.

Stage	TNM classification and Gleason score
I	T1a, N0, M0, Gleason score 1
II	T1a, N0, M0, Gleason score 2, 3–4
	T1, T1b–T2, N0, M0, any Gleason score
III	T3, N0, M0, any Gleason score
IV	T4, N0, M0, any Gleason score
	Any T, N1, M0, any Gleason score
	Any T, any N, M1, any Gleason score

Source: Edge 2010.[93] Reproduced with permission of Springer.

Table 4 Risk stratification for localized prostate cancer.

Risk level	PSA level (ng/mL)		Gleason score		Clinical stage
Low	≤10	and	≤6	and	T1c or T2a
Intermediate	>10–20	or	7	or	T2b but not qualifying for high risk
High	>20	or	8–10	or	T2c

Source: Thompson 2007.[96] Reproduced with permission of Elsevier.

It is noteworthy that there is intense interest in further staging prostate cancer with endorectal coil magnetic resonance imaging (MRI) with multiparametric (mp) techniques.[97] Studies have shown that a suspicious lesion on MRI is an independent risk factor for adverse pathology after radical prostatectomy.[98] On the other hand,

Table 2 TNM clinical and pathologic staging of prostate cancer.

	Clinical stage		Pathologic stage
Primary tumor			
TX	Primary tumor cannot be assessed		
T0	No evidence of primary tumor		
T1	Clinically inapparent tumor neither palpable nor visible by imaging		
T1a	Tumor incidental histologic finding in 5% or less of tissue resected		
T1b	Tumor incidental histologic finding in more than 5% of tissue resected		
T1c	Tumor identified by needle biopsy (e.g., because of elevated PSA)		
T2	Tumor confined within prostate[a]	pT2[b]	Organ confined
T2a	Tumor involves one half of one lobe or less	pT2a	Unilateral, involving one-half of one lobe or less
T2b	Tumor involves more than one-half of one lobe but not both lobes	pT2b	Unilateral, involving more than one-half of one lobe but not both lobes
T2c	Tumor involves both lobes	pT2c	Bilateral disease
T3	Tumor extends through the prostate capsule[c]	pT3	Extraprostatic extension
T3a	Extracapsular extension (unilateral or bilateral)	pT3a	Extraprostatic extension[d]
T3b	Tumor invades seminal vesicle(s)	pT3b	Seminal vesicle invasion
T4	Tumor is fixed or invades adjacent structures other than seminal vesicles: bladder neck, external sphincter, rectum, levator muscles, and/or pelvic wall	pT4	Invasion of bladder, rectum
Regional lymph nodes			
NX	Regional lymph nodes were not assessed	pNX	Regional nodes not sampled
N0	No regional lymph node metastasis	pN0	No positive regional nodes
N1	Metastasis in regional lymph node(s)	pN1	Metastasis in regional nodes
Distant metastasis[e]			
MX	Distant metastasis cannot be assessed (not evaluated by any modality)		
M0	No distant metastasis		
M1	Distant metastasis		
M1a	Nonregional lymph nodes		
M1b	Bone(s)		
M1c	Other site(s) with or without bone disease		

[a]Tumor found in one or both lobes by needle biopsy, but not palpable or reliably visible by imaging, is classified as T1c.
[b]There is no pathologic T1 classification.
[c]Invasion into the prostatic apex or into (but not beyond) the prostatic capsule is classified not as T3 but as T2.
[d]Positive surgical margin should be indicated by an R1 descriptor (residual microscopic disease).
[e]When more than one site of metastasis is present, the most advanced category (pM1c) is used.
Source: Edge 2010.[93] Reproduced with permission of Springer.

a normal lesion or one of low suspicion on mpMRI has a high negative predictive value for clinically insignificant disease.[99] Neither MRI nor any other imaging modality is incorporated into the clinical risk groups for localized disease, nor staging of the primary tumor.

Validated pretreatment nomograms that combine PSA, Gleason score, and clinical stage have been developed to give estimates of pathologic stage, which may be valuable to clinicians planning treatment.[100-103] In a 2007 update of the Partin tables, Makarov et al.[103] analyzed 5730 men who had undergone prostatectomy between 2000 and 2005 at Johns Hopkins Hospital and confirmed that, as these researchers had previously shown, clinical stage contributes significantly to the prediction, as do PSA level and Gleason score, and that cumulatively they are better predictors than any one alone. No patient's disease was clinically staged higher than T2c, and at prostatectomy, almost 75% had disease confined to the prostate. None of the 123 of 164 patients with a clinical Gleason score ≥ 8 who had a workup was found to have metastatic disease. In their series, as in others, the proportion of men presenting with organ-confined disease has been increasing: 54% in 1993,[100] 48% in 1997,[101] 64% in 2001,[102] and 73% in 2007 (year of publication).[103] New in this series was the absence of Gleason scores of 2 to 4, reflecting pathologists' belief that such scores represent sampling error.[104] Among patients with higher clinical stage, the authors reported a trend toward more accurate staging in their 2007 report over that in 2001 and perhaps indicating a broader need for surgery in those patients with higher clinical stage and Gleason scores. A 2013 update to the tables confirms a similar distribution of pathologic stage, updated Gleason scoring, and a more contemporary prognosis.[67,68]

Following up on previous work to improve the accuracy of identifying cases of low-volume, low-grade disease,[105,106] researchers at The University of Texas M.D. Anderson Cancer Center have refined a nomogram specifically for identifying men for active surveillance.[107] This nomogram includes age, PSA density, and tumor length in a biopsy core. The low number of factors, the ease in ascertaining their values with only laboratory tests and extended biopsy, and their nonsubjective nature combined with an area under the curve (AUC) measure indicating good discriminatory power (i.e., 0.727) make this nomogram attractive. The authors admitted that they cannot explain why their analysis indicates that older age would reduce the probability of low-volume, low-grade cancer and that younger men with values appropriately low in the other categories would be good candidates for surveillance. Nonetheless, their work offers for validation a new, practical tool for identifying these low-risk men.

Including a molecular marker as a predictor is another way investigators have attempted to improve a nomogram's accuracy. PCA3, a prostate-specific noncoding mRNA, is readily detected in urine when prostate cancer is present because it is overexpressed 60- to 100-fold 90% of the time.[108] Deras et al.[108] undertook a prospective, multisite study of 570 men immediately before they underwent prostate biopsy and found PCA3 to be reliably sensitive and specific across PSA values <4 and >10 ng/mL and across various values of prostate volume and number of prior biopsies. Overall, PCA3 sensitivity was 54% (95% CI 0.49–0.59) and specificity was 74% (95% CI 0.71–0.77).

Staging is meant to refine the risk of oncologic end points and can be augmented with commercialized genomic prognostic biomarkers taken from biopsy specimens. Cuzick et al.[109] reported a panel of cell cycle progression (CCP) genes known from breast cancer studies and validated them in a cohort of patients managed conservatively. The CCP score, a numerical representation of average CCP gene expression compared to a housekeeping gene panel, was statistically superior in predicting 10-year mortality rates compared to clinical features. Another panel of genes was validated by Klein et al.[110] that mixed several pathways (stromal response, androgen signaling, proliferation, and organization) and linked elements in a small sample of a prostate biopsy with long-term radical prostatectomy outcomes. The development and validation efforts have created a genomic score that estimates adverse pathology (Gleason ≥ 4 + 3 and/or pT3 stage) at radical prostatectomy, from patients with favorable biopsy findings (Gleason 3 + 3 to 3 + 4). Both biomarkers have strong statistical validation but need additional studies on clinical utility impact such as changing recommendations between active surveillance and immediate treatment and correlating such decisions with superior oncologic and quality-of-life outcomes. The theme of disease prognosis from genomics can continue into the postradical prostatectomy space, CCP score in this setting will predict for biochemical recurrence rates along with clinical features, and another genomic classifier (commercialized as Decipher, GenomeDx, San Diego, CA) specifically estimates early metastatic progression from patients with known high-risk pathology. Table 5 compares key clinical end points, clinical utility, and cost.

Imaging of prostate cancer

Although bone and CT scan are standard imaging tools to establish metastatic disease, the staging and detection tasks have been only modestly assisted with T2 weighted MRI. Recently, the addition of novel imaging sequences such as diffusion weighted imaging and dynamic contrast-enhanced imaging together with the T2 weighted images can combine to form an "mp" sequence. There is renewed interest in the MRI for the purposes of either advanced screening (i.e., prior negative biopsy with rising PSA) or enhanced staging (i.e.,

Table 5 Comparison of key features of three commercialized genomic tests for prostate cancer.[111]

	Decipher	Oncotype DX	Prolaris
Tissues tested	RP for high risk—pT3, positive margin, PSA rise	Biopsy—for NCCN very low to intermediate risk	Biopsy or RP
Clinical end points	Early regional nodes or bone metastasis	Risk of unfavorable pathology—pT3 and/or ≥ Gleason 4 + 3	Biopsy—10-year mortality with conservative management RP—biochemical recurrence risk
Clinical utility	Adjuvant/salvage therapy	Active surveillance or immediate therapy	Biopsy—active surveillance or immediate therapy RP—adjuvant/salvage therapy
Cost (USD)	4250	3825	3400

RP, radical prostatectomy; pT3, pathologic stage with extraprostatic extension and/or seminal vesicle invasion; PSA, prostate-specific antigen; NCCN, National Comprehensive Cancer Network; USD, United States Dollar equivalent.

estimating if a patient with low-volume/low-grade disease is likely to be harboring undiagnosed higher-grade/volumes of disease).[112]

Novel software/hardware packages are commercially available that allow the biopsying physician to "fuse" MRI suspicious lesions with the otherwise normal ultrasound images.[113] These additional "targeted" biopsies lead to novel metrics in prostate detection such as increase in tumor upgrading and/or volume measurement per core of tissue. MRI/fusion biopsies, however, do not appear sensitive enough to omit standard extended core biopsies, consisting of random sampling by zone: right and left apex, mid, base, and lateral horns for at least 10–12 cores. Although these systematic biopsies appear necessary to detect some MRI invisible lesions, the targeted cores are more likely to detect higher-grade tumor and omit low-grade detection. In a recent prospective cohort study of 1003 men undergoing both MR/fusion biopsy and standard (sextant) biopsy, targeted biopsy detected 30% more high-risk (Gleason score $\geq 4 + 3$) and 17% fewer low-risk prostate cancer.[114]

Although these conclusions are exciting in the field, the technique and standardization of the imaging have a way to go before being standard. As Emberton[115] commented more than a million biopsies are performed annually in Europe, and if each one would be MRI driven, there would be significant logistical needs to build out proper equipment, technique, and training. In addition, the standardization of reporting is newly reported and ongoing in clinical adoption.[116,117] The current state-of-the art programs are selecting patients for active surveillance or prior negative biopsy/rising PSA for MRI/fusion biopsy and combining teams of dedicated uroradiologist and urologists to advance this exciting new field. The significance will be fewer patients with false negative biopsies and few patients incorrectly selected for active surveillance. Additionally, further prospective studies are needed to evaluate predictive value of this technology for clinical outcomes (e.g., disease reclassification in active surveillance, prostate cancer specific mortality).

Therapy options and applications

Active surveillance

In the pre-PSA era, "watchful waiting" implied an alternative to active treatment and described a period when patients were monitored but not treated until the disease progressed and/or symptoms developed. With the advent of PSA testing, a paradigm shift occurred, in which we now diagnose considerably more early prostate cancers, including those destined to remain clinically insignificant. New strategies are needed for managing select cases of low-risk prostate cancer without imposing immediate therapy. Such an approach has been called different terms, including "watchful observation with selective delayed intervention"[118] and "active surveillance."[119] This new strategy is to forego immediate treatment but closely follow patients with low-risk prostate cancer, pursuing early detection of tumor progression when the disease is still curable and initiating definitive therapy appropriately. For this strategy to fulfill its promise, two clinical tools are mandatory: a method of identifying a priori patients harboring small low-grade, indolent tumors and a surveillance strategy that reliably detects tumor progression when the disease is still curable. Data supporting conservative management of cases with clinically localized prostate cancer can be gleaned from population-based studies[120,121] and a meta-analysis.[122] These pre-PSA era studies had a preponderance of older patients and patients with clinically evident cancers; therefore, their results cannot be directly extrapolated to the PSA-screened population. Other problems included the way patients had been diagnosed—many had not undergone

a full workup for metastasis, and for many, diagnosis was based on fine-needle biopsy results[121]—and the fact that the researchers did not centralize pathology review.[120] Despite their limitations, these observational studies showed that men with low-grade prostate cancer have a protracted course of indolent disease and a very small risk of disease-specific death, even after 20 years of follow-up.[123]

In contrast, the risk of death from disease progression is higher for men with Gleason scores of 7–10. Watchful waiting and prostatectomy were compared prospectively in an important study by Swedish investigators who followed up their initial report with further analyses 3 years later and an estimated 15-year results.[81,124,125] The researchers studied 695 men with T0d, T1b, T1c, or T2 disease who were randomly assigned to undergo radical prostatectomy ($n = 347$) or watchful waiting ($n = 348$). Two-thirds had palpable tumors, but fewer than half in each group—43.8% of those undergoing prostatectomy and 39.7% of those assigned to watchful waiting—had symptoms. In the recently reported extended 23.2 years of follow-up analysis,[82] the investigators observed statistically significant differences at 18 years of follow-up between those who underwent prostatectomy and those who were not treated until androgen-deprivation therapy was used [42.5% vs 67.4%, RR 0.49 (95% CI 0.39 to 0.60; $P < 0.001$)], distant metastasis developed [26% vs 38.3%, RR 0.57 (95% CI 0.44 to 0.75; $P < 0.001$)], and disease-specific mortality occurred [17.7% vs 28.7%, RR 0.56 (95% CI 0.41 to 0.77; $P = 0.001$)]. The benefit from prostatectomy was confined to men younger than 65 years of age. Also, it is important to note that a large proportion of men in the watchful waiting arm did not require any palliative treatment. Whether these findings would be replicable in a US study population is unknown because prostate cancer is typically diagnosed earlier here than it is in Sweden.[126] The Prostate Cancer Intervention versus Observation Trial[127] conducted in the United States compared prostatectomy with watchful waiting in 731 of mostly screened men with localized prostate cancer and life expectancy of at least 10 years. At median follow-up of 10 years, there was no significant statistical difference in all-cause mortality and prostate cancer-specific mortality between the two groups. There was trend toward lower prostate cancer-specific mortality with surgery among men with PSA levels >10 ng/mL and subgroups with higher-risk cancers. In fact, for men with low-risk prostate cancer, there was nonstatistically significant increase in prostate cancer-specific mortality by 15%. Two of the longest-running prospective cohort studies have examined the feasibility of active surveillance, or expectant management. Additionally, there are other large cohort prospective studies underway.[128] Carter et al.[129] studied 81 men believed to have T1c low-volume prostate cancer for a median of 23 months (range 12–58 months). Their median age was 65 years (range 52–73 years). At baseline, all men had a PSA density ≤ 0.15 ng/mL/cm³ and a Gleason score of <7. Free PSA in the men was a median of 17% (range 4.3–37%). Every 6 months, subjects underwent PSA measurement (both free and total) and DRE. Every 12 months, patients underwent transrectal ultrasound-directed biopsy, including evaluation of at least 12 cores. After at least 1 year in the study, 56 (69%) of the men were free of progression and still on surveillance. The other 25 men (31%) met the criteria of progression, which were adverse findings on prostate needle biopsy, including a Gleason score ≥ 7, any Gleason pattern of 4 or 5, more than two cores with cancer involvement, or 50% cancer involvement in any core. Their median time to disease progression was 14 months (range 12–52 months). The researchers found that in men who experienced progression by their definition, the PSA density was statistically significantly higher and the free PSA value statistically significantly lower than those values in men who did not experience progression.

In a larger phase II study, Klotz[130] reported findings on 299 men who at baseline had prostate cancer of grade T2b or lower, a PSA of <15 ng/mL, and a Gleason score ≤ 7. All subjects were older than 70 years. Surveillance included PSA measures, serial bone scans, transrectal sonography (every 6 months for first 2 years and then annually thereafter), and biopsy within 1.5 or 2 years of entering the trial. Criteria for progression were that patients demonstrate PSA, clinical, and histologic disease progression. PSA progression was defined as having a PSA doubling time of <2 years (measured at least three times during a minimum of 6 months), a final PSA of >8 ng/mL, and a regression analysis of ln (PSA) on time $P < 0.05$. Clinical progression was defined as one of the following: doubling of the product of the maximum perpendicular diameters of the primary lesion (measured digitally), TURP necessitated by local progression, ureteral obstruction, or clinical or radiologic evidence of distant metastasis. Histologic progression was defined as a Gleason score ≥ 8 at subsequent biopsy. At 55 months, 60% remained on surveillance; at 96 months, disease-specific survival was 99%, and overall survival was 85%. Thirty-five percent had a PSA doubling time of >10 years (median doubling time 7.0 years). Reasons for abandoning surveillance included patient preference (16%), rapid biochemical progression (12%), clinical progression (8%), and histologic progression (4%). In a recently published update of the study with the median follow-up time of 6.4 years from the first biopsy (range 0.2–19.8 years), Klotz et al.[131] reported the prostate cancer-specific mortality in AS of 1.5%. The risk of dying of another cause was 9.2 times greater than the likelihood of dying from prostate cancer. As AS methods move toward integration of novel imaging and biomarkers, investigators are challenged with including more men with early prostate cancer, minimizing risk of cancer progression, and maximizing quality of life.

Prostate Testing for Cancer and Treatment (ProtecT) will compare active surveillance with active therapies.[132] Investigators of ProtecT, begun in 2001, expect to enroll more than 1500 men in the United Kingdom and to randomize them to treatment with conformal radiotherapy, prostatectomy, or active surveillance. Results are expected in 2016. This trial should offer investigators more information about localized disease detected through PSA screening, helping physicians and patients understand the risks and benefits better and collaborate better in decision-making.

Curative therapy: an anatomic discussion of the challenges of disease control and minimizing side effects

The patient with early disease has the option to pursue one of a number of definitive therapeutic options, each with its own variations in technique. Fundamentally, the options are a radical prostatectomy or dose-escalated radiation therapy. Both treatment categories aim to treat the entire gland by surgical removal or radiation-based destruction. Alternative treatments have also emerged, such as cryotherapy and high-intensity focused ultrasound, that treat all or a portion of the gland. All treatments are associated with a risk of treatment recurrence and varying degrees of quality-of-life side effects specific to prostate cancer treatments: erectile dysfunction, urinary incontinence, urinary irritation and/or obstruction, and bowel dysfunction. The desire to diminish side effects and treatment recurrences has left the field with numerous updates in technique, entirely new technologies, and numerous comparisons. For each question involving treatment

efficacy and side effects, the patient and practitioner want to know both the average results expected and any contributing features that help predict whether an individual patient will experience the favorable or unfavorable end of the range of results. In addition, studies have shed light on whether a particular procedure is reproducible across the range of treatment centers.[133–135] Most patients diagnosed today are very much aware of the potential for side effects and the concept that a practitioner's experience may affect outcomes.

The selection of patients for treatment is often derived by considering the slow natural history of prostate cancer, the life expectancy of the aging man, and the personal wishes of the patient. The most commonly accepted recommendation is that a patient may benefit from treatment if he has 10 or more years of life expectancy. However, this estimation may be a moving target because death from cardiac disease is declining with better treatments. Men should not be denied treatment on the basis of age alone,[136] but the study by Albertsen et al.[121] demonstrated significantly reduced prostate cancer-related death when the disease was diagnosed at age 70 and higher, especially for men with Gleason scores <7. The recent update of the Bill-Axelson study that randomized radical prostatectomy and watchful waiting has been highly beneficial in decision-making.[82] The majority of survival benefit in the radical prostatectomy cohort was observed in men < age 65; however men ages 65–75 had secondary benefits in reduced hormonal therapy, palliative therapy, and metastatic progression.

Radical prostatectomy: a model for the treatment dilemmas concerning therapy for early prostate cancer

The challenges of treating early prostate cancer can be illustrated by an anatomic tour of a radical prostatectomy operation and by using the steps of the operation to highlight what the surgeon and radiotherapist must consider in achieving cancer control with minimal side effects. Refer to Figure 6 as we narrate our way through the intricate anatomy surrounding the prostate gland.

The radical prostatectomy operation involves complete removal of the prostate gland, seminal vesicles, and distal vas deferens. Conceptually, the prostate gland can be thought of as a conical structure with open ends—the bladder neck and the urethra. The sides of the cone have a capsular structure (although not a true histologic capsule) and are surrounded by endopelvic fascia laterally and by Denonvilliers fascia posteriorly. At its apex, the prostate is surrounded by the rhabdosphincter muscle and the dorsal vein complex, which is narrow over the urethra and then spreads into an apron-like structure as it traverses over the midprostate, base of the prostate, and then over the bladder. Regardless of approach and technique, the removal of the prostate requires an intimate understanding of the intricate anatomic structures to be encountered, and a set of allowed surgical motions can be defined.

Access to the prostate

The prostate gland is among the more difficult structures to access for surgery. It is covered anteriorly by the pubic arch, distally by the dorsal vein complex and rhabdosphincter, inferiorly by the rectum, inferolaterally by the nerve bundles, and superiorly by the bladder. The prostate can be exposed with a lower midline abdominal incision from the pubic bone to the umbilicus, and the exposure progresses through extraperitoneal spaces. Alternative approaches include minilaparotomy, laparoscopic access via 5 or 6 ports in the lower abdomen (extraperitoneal or transperitoneal), and perineal access. The minilaparotomy incision is generally 8–10 cm rather than the 15–20 cm long needed for the standard

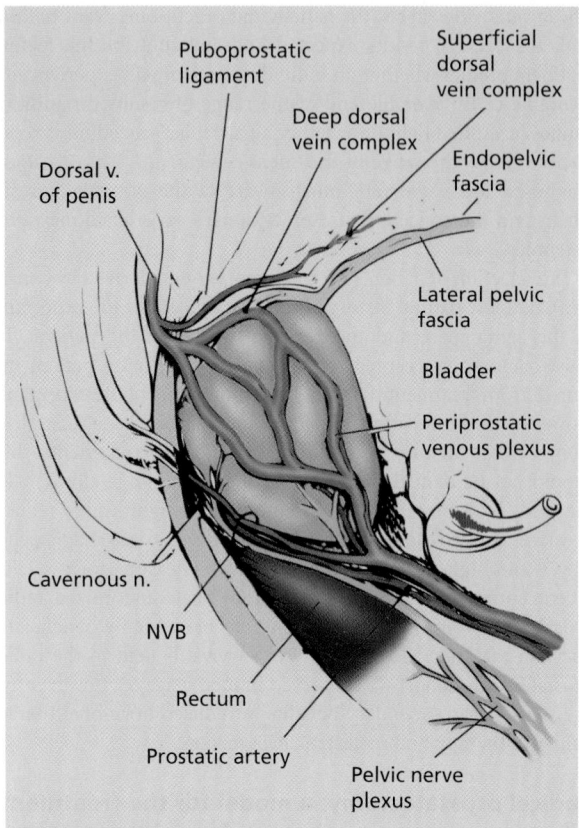

Puboprostatic ligament

Superficial dorsal vein complex

Deep dorsal vein complex

Endopelvic fascia

Dorsal v. of penis

Lateral pelvic fascia

Bladder

Periprostatic venous plexus

Cavernous n.

NVB

Rectum

Prostatic artery

Pelvic nerve plexus

Figure 6 Surgical anatomy of the prostate in relationship to the deep dorsal vein complex, neurovascular bundle (NVB), and other surrounding periprostatic structures (lateral view).

laparotomy. Visualization of the prostate is similar in the two open abdominal approaches, but in the minilaparotomy, the surgeon will rely more on instrument dissection than on manual dissection. The laparoscopic approach has become increasingly popular with the availability of robotic surgical systems to increase the laparoscopic surgeon's dexterity with instruments, with seven degrees of motion and three-dimensional camera view.

The choice of surgical approach depends on both the surgeon's training and the patient's characteristics. The retropubic approach has been taught in most residency programs worldwide; it provides access to the prostate and lymph nodes and entails a familiar transabdominal orientation. The perineal approach may be associated with less pain, and the scar is certainly less visible. There may be an advantage to this procedure in the circumstances of morbid obesity. However, the lymph nodes are not accessible, and this approach may be difficult for larger prostates, for example, those >60 g. The laparoscopic approach requires a steep learning curve of more than 100 cases, whereas the robot-assisted laparoscopic approach requires fewer.[137–139] Differences in postoperative pain and hospital discharge are not reliably seen between open retropubic and laparoscopic approaches[140,141] but may be decreased with the perineal approach.[142] Both perineal and laparoscopic approaches are associated with less bleeding, but in expert hands the transfusion rates are probably not significantly different.[143] Results from nonrandomized comparisons show increased transfusion rates in retropubic prostatectomy if the rates for this group are more than 10–15%.[144]

Moving forward with this discussion, we will discuss only the open retropubic and laparoscopic (both manual and robot-assisted types) operations. However, it is worth noting that although historic

discussions on the perineal operation suggest that the outcomes may increase positive margin rates, decrease potency rates, and cause de novo rectal incontinence,[145] several high-volume centers have published very competitive outcomes,[142,146] and there is arguably a cost savings relative to the use of robotic approaches.[147,148]

Alternative treatments must also consider access to the prostate in their application. Brachytherapy is a form of whole-gland radiation treatment in which radioactively labeled seeds are inserted into the prostate by transperineal access using transrectal ultrasound for guidance. In cases of BPH, the anterior portion of the prostate may extend around the pubic bone's arch, creating a form of interference to needle placement. Thus, in the application of brachytherapy and cryotherapy (another transperineal access ablative therapy), the prostate must be of a certain size (generally <60 g) and shape to allow for access. In contrast, modern external beam radiation treatments can handle a broader range of prostate sizes and shapes. The intensity-modulated radiation therapy (IMRT) technique, for example, uses multiple beams from different angles to boost the dose to the prostate while limiting the dose to surrounding organs such as the bladder and the rectum. Proton beam radiation has recently become popular as another way to limit the dose to normal tissue.

Exposure and dissection of the apex

The anterior and lateral surfaces of the prostate are covered by endopelvic fascia. This fascia can be cut sharply or by using cautery, with care to avoid or ligate varying networks of veins that course along the prostate and often penetrate the apex at 11 and 1 o'clock. The pubovesical ligaments are cut by most surgeons to allow distal ligation of the dorsal vein complex. Mistakes in this region can cause significant blood loss in the open operation, although less so in the laparoscopic and/or robotic approaches because of the positive pressure of the CO_2 pneumoperitoneum.

The rhabdosphincter surrounds the urethra distally, and the apex of the prostate has no capsule-like structure. Therefore, there is tremendous potential for mistakes in this region, and this may be the step of the operation that improves the most with experience. In essence, the surgeon must control the dorsal vein complex with proximal and distal sutures and then make a tangential cut that is as close to the apex as possible to avoid damaging the rhabdosphincter complex yet avoid a positive apical margin. Numerous technique descriptions are available and cannot be fully catalogued, but the objectives of cancer control (i.e., negative surgical margins) and urinary control are strongly influenced by this step.

Alternatives to surgery must also completely treat the apical region while avoiding side effects. Dose-escalated external beam and brachytherapy will inevitably reach both the apex and surrounding rhabdosphincter. However, because those structures are not specifically disrupted, stress incontinence results significantly less often than with surgery. Cryotherapy techniques include temperature monitors at the sphincter to avoid freezing outside of the apex.

Exposure and dissection of the bladder neck

Dissection of the bladder neck is by comparison much easier than that of the apex in the open operation. The Foley catheter can be used as a guide, and electrocautery can be used safely. Care must be taken to preserve the posterior plate of the bladder neck and divide it away from the ureteral orifices. The bladder neck-sparing technique has been reported as possibly beneficial in avoiding urinary continence but is possibly associated with an increased incidence of positive margins.[149] A nonbladder neck-sparing plane can be reconstructed with sutures to match the urethral size for the anastomosis.

Alternatives to surgery must completely treat the base of the prostate while avoiding damage to the bladder. In conventional-dose radiation to the pelvis, the surrounding dose to the bladder and rectum was always a dose-limiting factor. Dose-escalation techniques, however, whether IMRT, proton therapy, or brachytherapy, effectively increase the dose to the prostate while holding down the dose to the bladder. Nevertheless, some of the dose does affect the bladder, accounting for the differing distribution of urinary side effects, including irritation, frequency, and hematuria.

Exposure and dissection of the seminal vesicles

The seminal vesicles present their own surgical challenges. These structures lie immediately posterior to the bladder, with their tips coursing laterally. The vesicles are surrounded by several small arterial branches that must be controlled with clips or sutures. If uncontrolled, these branches may cause significant postoperative bleeding, which may require a second surgery. However, electrocautery must be avoided if possible because the tips of the vesicles lie immediately medial to the neurovascular bundles. Some researchers have reported the concept of leaving the tips intact to avoid nerve damage.[150] Laparoscopic surgeons may address this challenge by dissecting the seminal vesicles posterior to the bladder through the pouch of Douglas. For the radiotherapist, the seminal vesicles cannot be adequately treated by implant therapy but can be targeted by external technique. MRI with an endorectal coil can be used to stage the seminal vesicles for deciding whether to include them in the treatment plan—the trade-off being increased bladder toxicity.

Neurovascular bundle dissection

The technique for neurovascular bundle dissections is usually retrograde (apex to base) for open surgery and anterograde (base to apex) for laparoscopic surgery. For the retrograde approach, the dorsal vein and urethral division steps are completed, and the plane posterior to the Denonvilliers fascia is developed with blunt finger dissection. The bundles on each side can then be palpated. Visually, the neurovascular bundles blend well into the sides of the prostate through a series of lateral fascial layers. A triangle of fascia exists, with its borders being the prostatic fascia medially, the endopelvic fascia laterally, and the Denonvilliers fascia posteriorly. Regardless of the technique, the nerve bundle must be released at two junctions: the anterolateral junction of the prostatic fascia and levator fascia and the medial posterior junction of the Denonvilliers fascia.

During the course of neurovascular bundle dissection, the use of electrocautery must be avoided or the thermal transmission may produce irreparable nerve damage. The portion of the bundle from middle to apex has mostly parallel vessels and a few perforating veins that can be controlled with clips or just transected and left to clot. In contrast, the portion of the bundles near the base gives off perforating arteries to the prostate that must be controlled with clips to avoid hemorrhage. Alternative coagulation devices have been described that produce less thermal discharge, but the nerve bundles are very sensitive to heat, and an athermal technique is preferable. Two different planes of nerve-sparing dissection have been described: intrafascial and interfascial. Surgeons must use judgment in this area because although the closer margin obtained from the intrafascial approach may improve postoperative potency, it moves the inked margin of the resection closer to the prostate gland.[151]

Surgeons may choose to sacrifice the nerve bundles depending on the estimated risk of extraprostatic extension, as determined from pretreatment parameters such as PSA, clinical stage, biopsy Gleason score, number of biopsies with cancer, and volume of cancer on biopsies, and possibly by imaging with sonography or endorectal coil MRI. Nomograms may assist with arriving at this estimate,[103,152,153] but the surgeon's intuition and experience always play a role that is difficult to measure. In general, most patients prefer to have a nerve-sparing operation as long as cancer control can be maintained.

The proximity of the nerve bundle and the prostate capsule also relates to radiotherapy planning. With brachytherapy, the dose delivered can be quite high within the peripheral zone of the prostate but will steeply drop off outside the gland. As a result, intermediate- to high-risk disease may not be adequately treated when there is higher risk of microscopic extraprostatic extension. Many centers will recommend either radiotherapy, as the dose planning can be driven outside of the capsule, or a combination of brachytherapy and radiotherapy. Cryotherapists can also customize treatment in this region by either driving the ice ball extraprostatically if there is a concern or warming the neurovascular bundle region and thus protect it from the ice ball if no cancer is present on a given side.

Urethral division

The urethra must be divided close to the prostate apex, essentially right near the verumontanum. The surrounding rhabdosphincter should be preserved, and excessive trauma from urethral dilators and catheters should be avoided.

Anastomosis

Both running and interrupted suture lines have been described, the latter more popular and feasible with the laparoscopic approaches. The objective is to approximate the bladder to the urethra so that the anastomosis is watertight and the mucosal surfaces are in contact. Excessively large urethral bites that may shorten the functional urethral length should be avoided. Anastomoses that leak or separate may lead to a higher rate of scarring and contracture.[154]

Technical modifications for high-risk disease

A shift has been observed toward selecting more surgical patients with higher-risk disease.[155] This requires additional surgical skill to obtain negative margins while maximizing feasible neurovascular bundle preservation and adding additional staging information with an extended pelvic lymph node dissection. As reviewed by Yuh et al.,[156] the incidence of nerve sparing in high risk varies, and positive lymph nodes may be observed in one-third of patients.

Outcomes of treatment for early disease

Cancer control

Most modern studies use PSA recurrence-free survival as an end point because the data can be collected in a 5- to 10-year time frame rather than the 15- to 20-year time frame needed for longer end points such as disease-specific and overall survival rates. However, as the AUA guidelines[96] stress, PSA recurrence is inconsistently defined and does not directly correlate with longer survival. The most commonly used definition of PSA failure for surgery is a PSA level >0.2 ng/mL, and for radiation, the updated American Society for Therapeutic Radiology and Oncology (ASTRO) recommendation is PSA nadir plus 2 ng/mL.[157] Definitions of risk stratification also vary in different studies. The AUA guidelines recommend the D'Amico criteria and the options for each[91]:

- Low risk: PSA ≤ 10 ng/mL, a Gleason score ≤ 6, and clinical stage cT1c–cT2a.

- Intermediate risk: PSA > 10–20 ng/mL or a Gleason score ≤ 7 or clinical stage T2b.
- High risk: PSA > 20 ng/mL or a Gleason score ≤ 8–10 or clinical stage T2c.

According to these risk groupings, the expected cancer control outcomes of brachytherapy, external beam radiotherapy, and radical prostatectomy in terms of PSA recurrence-free survival are seen in Figure 7.[96] For each modality, the 5-year range of outcomes are low risk, 75–95%; intermediate risk, 70–90%; and high risk, 30–80%. At 10 years, the ranges are low risk, 60–90%; intermediate risk, 40–80%; and high risk, 20–60%. On the basis of the limitations of lack of standardized reporting, different definitions of failure, and lack of head-to-head randomized controlled trials, the AUA panel stated that there are insufficient data to conclude that one treatment is superior to another. For patients choosing radiation therapy, the panel cited two randomized controlled clinical trials showing that higher-dose radiation may decrease the risk of a PSA recurrence.[158,159]

The topic of neoadjuvant and/or adjuvant androgen deprivation was also addressed by the AUA panel. Randomized clinical trials of neoadjuvant androgen deprivation plus radical prostatectomy showed no benefit in terms of PSA recurrence-free survival.[160,161] However, for intermediate-risk patients treated with radiotherapy, one trial showed that neoadjuvant and concurrent androgen deprivation for 6 months may prolong survival after radiotherapy.[162] For high-risk patients treated with radiotherapy, trials demonstrated a survival benefit for a longer duration of adjuvant androgen deprivation,[163] in the 2- to 3-year range. However, it is noteworthy that

the radiotherapy used in these trials was conventional and not dose escalated.

In summary, the AUA guidelines list active surveillance, brachytherapy, radiotherapy, and radical prostatectomy as treatment options for low-, intermediate-, and high-risk disease. For radiotherapy, randomized controlled trials are cited regarding dosages and androgen deprivation use. For the high-risk patient, it is noted that recurrence rates are high and that patients should consider "clinical trials examining new forms of therapy, including combination therapies, with the goal of improved outcomes." It is also worth noting that the AUA panel concluded that first-line hormonal therapy is "seldom indicated in the patients with localized prostate cancer."[164]

The European Association of Urology has also issued a guideline statement on prostate cancer, in which it cites many of the same randomized clinical trials regarding watchful waiting, surgery, and radiotherapy.[165] Additional recommendations based on lower levels of evidence are also cited. Some selected recommendations regarding early disease are as follows:

- Brachytherapy "may be proposed to patients cT1-T2a, Gleason score <7 (or 3 + 4), PSA ≤ 10 ng/mL, prostate volume ≤ 50 mL, without a previous TURP and with a good IPSS (International Prostate Symptom Score) (level of evidence: 2b)."
- Cryotherapy "has evolved from an investigational therapy to a possible alternative treatment method for CaP (prostate cancer) in patients unfit for surgery or in those with a life expectancy <10 years (grade C recommendation)."

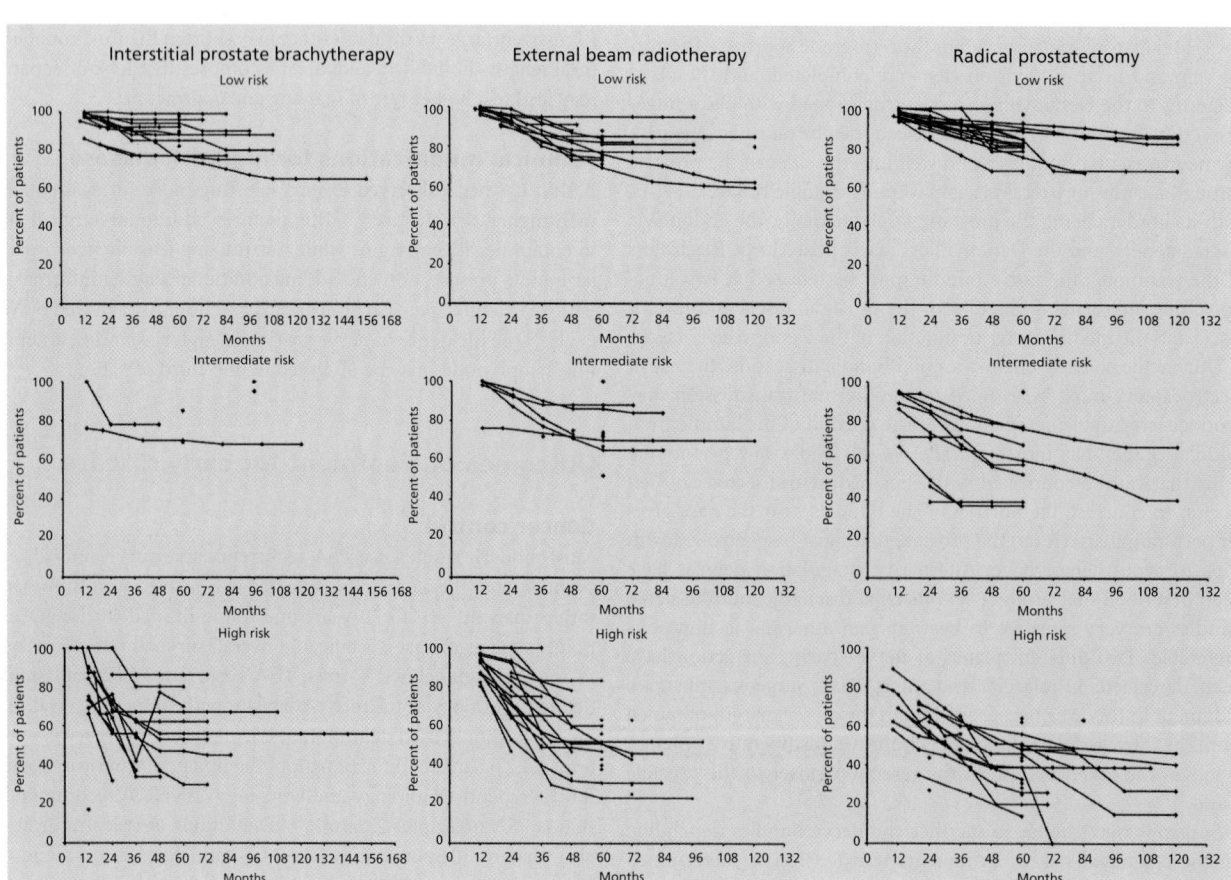

Figure 7 Prostate-specific antigen (PSA) recurrence-free survival in patients with low-, intermediate-, and high-risk prostate cancer treated with interstitial prostate brachytherapy, external beam radiotherapy, or radical prostatectomy.

- "All other minimally invasive treatment options, such as HIFU (high-intensity focused ultrasound), RITA (radiofrequency interstitial tumor ablation), microwaves, and electrosurgery, are still experimental or investigational. For all of these procedures, a longer follow-up is mandatory to assess their true role in the management of CaP (grade C recommendation)."

Another large-scale effort to summarize the state of the literature was prepared for the Agency for Healthcare Research and Quality and published in the *Annals of Internal Medicine*.[166] Again, the researchers met with difficulties because of variations in reporting and definitions, and only three randomized controlled trials compared the effectiveness between primary treatments (none with patients "primarily detected with PSA testing"), so, essentially stated, no conclusions could be drawn.

Complications of treatment

General

As a general statement, radical prostatectomy results in more urinary incontinence than radiotherapy or active surveillance do.[166] Brachytherapy and radiotherapy are associated with more bladder irritation and/or hematuria side effects and less incontinence. Radiotherapy has the higher risk of bowel urgency. All treatments have sexual side effects: although the pattern with radical prostatectomy is one of early loss with gradual improvement, the pattern with brachytherapy or radiotherapy is one of more gradual and delayed loss of function. Younger age and better preexisting function will predict better outcomes from all treatments.

However, there are numerous sources of bias and variability in comparisons, and there is no evidence that any one therapy "has a more significant cumulative overall risk of complications."[164] Although patients often request a single statistic, such as an incontinence rate or potency rate, it is accepted that more accurate quality-of-life research will result from the use of (1) validated instruments that ask multiple questions and offer a range of potential answers; (2) an instrument that is administered by someone other than the treating practitioner; (3) a prospective longitudinal design, including a pretreatment baseline measurement; and (4) an instrument that maintains response rates at >70% throughout the study period. The recent multicenter study by Ferrer et al.[167] evaluated the three standard treatments (radical prostatectomy, brachytherapy, and radiotherapy) with such an ideal method (except for treatment randomization). In the absence of comparisons of side effects in randomized controlled trials, various categories of studies can assist with our understanding of side effects: (1) results from multicenter community or academic series (i.e., voluntary reporting of what goes on in the community), (2) single-surgeon high-volume series (i.e., idealistic results), and (3) Medicare- or claims-based studies (i.e., involuntary outcome reporting).

Multicenter studies

Penson et al.[168] reported the results from the Prostate Cancer Outcomes Study, which is a community-based cohort study conducted at six centers where men underwent radical prostatectomy in 1994 and 1995. In this study, the only relevant predictive information was that the men underwent a radical prostatectomy in the community, that is, no description of technique or quality analysis of the surgeon and/or surgery was given. Among the 1288 patients studied, frequent urinary leakage occurred in 3% at baseline, in 19% at 6 months, in 13% at 1 year, in 9% at 2 years, and in 11% at 5 years. At 5 years, the urinary control level was described as having total control in 35%, occasional leakage in 51%, frequent leakage in 11%, and no control in 3%.

Additional data were presented regarding pad use, irritative symptoms, and bother. Urinary bother started as no problem in 87% at baseline; at 5 years, 45% reported no problem, 42% reported a slight problem, and 13% reported a moderate to great problem. The percentages of patients who reported experiencing erections sufficient for intercourse were 81% at baseline, 9% at 6 months, 17% at 1 year, 22% at 2 years, and 28% at 5 years. Although urinary function and bother scores improved between 2 and 5 years, the percentages of men with no sexual activity were 15% at baseline, 44% at 1 year, and 46% at 5 years. Bilateral nerve sparing predicted a better return of erections at 5 years: 40% for bilateral compared with 23% for unilateral and 23% for nonnerve sparing. Age was also a predictor: in the most favorable group, 61% of men 39–54 years old reported erections.

Sanda et al.[69] reported on a multi-institutional cohort from nine university-affiliated centers, with surgery completed with open, laparoscopic, and robotic-assisted techniques. In theory, this group of surgeons has a high volume, but again, specific technique was not reported. Using the 100-point Expanded Prostate Cancer Index Composite (EPIC) scale, patients who underwent radical prostatectomy had a baseline score for urinary continence of just 90; the score dropped to 50 at 2 months, improved to 70 at 6 months, and plateaued at 80 at 12–24 months.

However, as the results from these two large studies demonstrate, the literature contains varying definitions of incontinence. Sexual function was adversely affected by both radical prostatectomy and radiotherapy. Among patients who underwent radical prostatectomy, potency was better preserved with nerve-sparing techniques. Among patients who underwent radiotherapy, however, potency was better preserved in patients treated with monotherapy than in those given a combination with hormonal therapy (even after a short duration of 6 months). Bowel function was most affected by radiotherapy and brachytherapy even after 1 year—9% with distress related to bowel function.

The AUA guideline panel review[96,164] reported a range of 3–74% for urinary incontinence and suggested that there are insufficient data to provide an overall assessment of urinary outcomes. Those AUA guidelines also provide a large-scale review of published results of erectile dysfunction after radical prostatectomy without details of surgical technique and experience. Rates of erectile dysfunction after 1 year are as high as 90%, and nerve-sparing techniques are helpful.

Expert series

The nerve-sparing operation was initially described by Walsh et al. in the early 1980s,[169] and it became increasingly popular and oncologically safe after the introduction of PSA screening. As one can imagine, patient demand for Walsh's services and the services of other surgeons dedicated full time to this operation became quite high. Walsh et al. published a validated quality-of-life survey study that demonstrated the return of urinary control at 1 year in 93% of patients and a potency rate of 86% at 18 months.[170] A high-volume robot-assisted prostatectomy series also demonstrated excellent results: 1032 of 1110 patients (93%) wore one or no pads per day at 1 year, and potency was reported in 79.2%.[171] Although other studies have looked closely at factors affecting urinary control or potency rates, a recent trend has been to estimate the odds of achieving the "trifecta" of desired outcomes: cancer control, urinary control, and potency. The group from Memorial Sloan Kettering Cancer Center has published the concept as a nomogram.[172]

Expert comparisons have extended across technique choices. Touijer et al.[173] performed a single-institution study involving two high-volume surgeons, one of whom performed laparoscopic and the other, open surgeries. There was an unexpected finding of better return of continence (defined as patient reports of no leakage or not requiring a pad) in the open-surgery group: at 12 months, 75% versus 48%. Descriptions of the surgical techniques were cited, but the true difference that affected outcomes was not described. Those authors suspected the result was due to the apical dissection in the laparoscopic approach and stated that further prospective analysis is needed.

Thus, a clear need in outcomes research in early disease is to better link technique to outcome. An example is seen in the study by Masterson et al.[174] which demonstrated that a specific technical improvement in nerve sparing can be described and the results measured. In the standard technique, the apex is dissected starting with the dorsal vein complex, cutting the urethra and then bluntly mobilizing the posterior plane before releasing the posterolateral neurovascular bundles. In the modified technique, the sequence starts with dissection of the entire neurovascular bundle off the lateral aspect of the prostate from apex to seminal vesicle before the urethra is cut and posterior dissection performed. This avoids excessive traction applied to the neurovascular bundles. The 6-month recovery of erections improved from 40% with the standard technique to 67% with the modification. Such analogies can be seen in the literature on brachytherapy, in which the D90 analysis of the implant quality is a significant predictor of long-term biochemical disease-free interval.[175]

Variations in outcomes and Medicare databases

In multicenter studies and expert series, researchers voluntarily submit their own results and therefore have the ability to decide whether to participate. In the case of other studies, accessible data are used without such a decision to participate from each physician. Even among expert surgeons, complications vary.[135] The Medicare database and the Surveillance, Epidemiology, and End Results (SEER) registries are common sources for data from studies such as these. The advantages of these studies include their large numbers of patients and the opportunity they offer for studying a more average community cohort of patients. Their limitations include sampling only patients over age 65 and that their data end points are designed for billing purposes more than for research and can be incomplete in their assessment of the outcomes.

Quality-of-life data seen in such databases appear quite different from those in expert series. Benoit et al.[176] found urethral stricture in 19.5%, urinary incontinence in 21.7%, and erectile dysfunction in 21.5%. Begg et al.[177] looked at morbidity after radical prostatectomy in the SEER–Medicare Linked Database and found significant trends in the association between surgeon volume and complications and between hospital volume and complications. Recently, Hu et al.[178] analyzed a Medicare sample of patients who underwent minimally invasive radical prostatectomy versus open radical prostatectomy. The trends demonstrated fewer perioperative complications and shorter hospital stay for those who had a minimally invasive radical prostatectomy, although they had higher rates of salvage therapy and anastomotic strictures. However, the unfavorable outcomes with the minimally invasive radical prostatectomy procedure decreased significantly with increasing surgeon volume.

PSAV as a predictor after diagnosis

Researchers have also relied on PSAV to predict disease progression, relapse, and outcomes. In a retrospective study of 102 men who underwent radical prostatectomy,[179] researchers found a statistically significant association between a PSAV of 2 ng/mL/year in the year before diagnosis and tumor volume, which was 2.55 cm^3 in men with biochemical recurrence and 0.94 cm^3 in men who were disease free 5 years postsurgery ($P < 0.05$). The median PSAV in the men who experienced relapse was almost twice that of men who did not (1.98 ng/mL/year vs 1.05 ng/mL/year). Although these results help identify those at high risk, they may also help physicians identify patients whose tumors are more likely eradicable.

The results of two studies published in 2005 revealed associations between PSAV and outcomes. D'Amico et al.[180] studied PSAV in the year before diagnosis in 1095 men with localized prostate cancer to identify those most at risk of death from prostate cancer. They determined that a PSAV of >2.0 ng/mL/year was related to a statistically significantly shorter time to death from prostate cancer ($P < 0.001$) and to death from any cause ($P = 0.01$); those outcomes were also influenced by PSA level, tumor stage, and Gleason score at diagnosis. Factors that predicted time to death from prostate cancer were a clinical tumor stage of T2; a Gleason score of 8, 9, or 10; and an increasing PSA level at diagnosis.

In an even larger study with a follow-up of more than 7 years, Sengupta et al.[181] also found a significant association between increased risk of death from prostate cancer and both preoperative PSAV and PSA doubling time. In 2290 men who underwent radical prostatectomy, 460 with a PSAV of >3.4 ng/mL/year had a greater than sixfold increase in risk of prostate cancer death [hazard ratio (HR) 6.54; 95% CI 3.51–12.91] compared with those with lower PSAV values. In addition, the 506 men whose PSA doubling time was <18 months had a similar increased risk (HR 6.22; 95% CI 3.33–11.61) compared with those with lower PSA doubling times. The authors said that their findings that PSAV is a better predictor than PSA doubling time of biochemical progression while PSA doubling time is a better predictor than PSAV of clinical progression and death conform to the notion that prostate cancer growth follows an exponential rather than a linear model.[181]

In a study in a group of 379 men with prostate cancer who experienced biochemical recurrence after radical prostatectomy, Freedland and colleagues found that PSA doubling time along with pathologic Gleason score and time from surgery to recurrence were statistically significant risk factors for prostate cancer-specific mortality[182]; in a separate study in a cohort with a PSA doubling time of <15 months, the same investigators found that 90% of deaths could be attributed to prostate cancer.[183] In studies of PSAV and PSA doubling time, those same investigators found no relationship between those variables and adverse pathologic findings or biochemical recurrence after radical prostatectomy.[184]

Furthermore, though African-American men are at higher risk for prostate cancer than men of other races, researchers found no relationship between PSAV or PSA doubling time and race among whites, blacks, Hispanics, and Asians. As might be predicted, no relationship was found between PSAV and prostate volume.[179]

Prostate cancer chemoprevention: Large trials

The PCPT involved 18,882 men randomized to treatment with finasteride (a 5α-reductase inhibitor) or placebo.[185] PCPT ended more than a year earlier than planned because its Data Safety and Monitoring Committee determined that the trial had met its primary objective. Prostate cancer prevalence during the 7-year treatment period was 24.8% lower in men taking finasteride than in men taking placebo (95% CI 18.6–30.6; $P < 0.001$). This good news was tempered, however, by the finding that tumors detected in those taking

Table 6 PSA and identification of significant and insignificant tumors.

Tumor type for which at risk	PSA value (ng/mL)			
	0–1.0	1.1–2.5	2.6–4.0	4.1–10.0
Significant tumors	15.6%	37.9%	49.1%	52.4%
Insignificant tumors	51.7%	33.7%	17.8%	11.7%

Source: Thompson 2007.[189] Reproduced with permission of Elsevier.

finasteride were 1.67 times more likely to be of a higher grade (Gleason score 7–10) than were those in subjects taking placebo (37.0% of graded tumors vs 22.2%; $P < 0.001$).

Newer studies of the PCPT data have reassured physicians that finasteride's ability to reduce cancer is clinically significant, explained why the initial results found high-grade disease more frequently in the finasteride arm, and endorsed its use. Taken together, the new results ease the concern that finasteride caused the rate of aggressive cancers to rise in the treated group and encourage physicians to offer finasteride to more men.[186]

According to other reevaluations of the PCPT data, a continuum of risk began at a PSA of even <4.0 ng/mL,[187] and new pathologic studies were undertaken of the PCPT prostate biopsy specimens on which data were available (finasteride, 519 patients; placebo, 716 patients) after results were initially reported to determine whether these tumors were clinically insignificant.[188] Results confirmed that the risk of clinically significant tumors rises with increasing PSA value and that of insignificant tumors falls (Table 6); nonetheless, 62% of cancers in men with Gleason scores ≤ 6 were deemed clinically significant, as were 75% of all cancers detected.[188]

In another reevaluation of the PCPT findings, Pinsky et al.[190] used a statistical model to tackle the problem of determining misclassification rates among the pathology findings in each arm and identifying a "true" relative risk for high-grade disease. They determined that misclassification from low- to high-grade disease from specimens at biopsy to those at radical prostatectomy is a function of the true ratio of low- to high-grade disease and misclassification rates. Although the results were not statistically significant in comparison with those for the placebo arm, the true rate of high-grade disease was lower in the finasteride arm (RR 0.84; 95% CI 0.68–1.05); also in the finasteride arm, the true rate of low-grade disease was both lower and significant (RR 0.61; 95% CI 0.51–0.71) compared with that in the placebo arm. The authors explained this paradox of similarly upgraded rates in both arms despite the finasteride group's having less misclassification as being the result of finasteride's decreasing the ratio of true low-grade to high-grade disease.

In response to evidence reported after the initial analysis of the PCPT[187,189] and to understand the effect of uncovered biases affecting that analysis, Redman and her colleagues[191] undertook a reanalysis, including evaluable patients omitted from the final analysis, estimating the true prevalence of cancer grade using the highest standard (radical prostatectomy), and studying the sensitivity of biopsy for prostate cancer. These reanalyses included one for selection bias and another that included grading information on radical prostatectomy in 500 cancer-diagnosed participants. Both produced greater risk-reduction estimates than the original study analysis had and attributed to finasteride no increased risk of high-grade cancer. In the first of those reanalyses, risk reduction was increased to 30% (RR 0.70; 95% CI 0.64–0.76; $P < 0.0001$), and prostate cancer rates were 21.1% in the placebo group (4.2% high-grade disease) and 14.7% (4.8% high-grade disease) in the finasteride group, with the 14% increase in high-grade disease nonsignificant (RR 1.14; 95% CI 0.96–1.35; $P = 0.12$). In the second

reanalysis by Redman, risk reduction was increased to 27% (RR 0.73; 95% CI 0.56–0.96; $P = 0.02$), and risk of high-grade disease was lower in the finasteride group (placebo 8.2%; finasteride 6.0%). A third reanalysis found that biopsy sensitivity could significantly affect risk ratio estimates. The authors' conclusion was that men had no reason to worry about increased risk of high-grade cancer when they are treated with finasteride.[191]

Earlier reevaluations of the PCPT data helped to explain how detection bias introduced by finasteride increased the sensitivity of PSA level for the end points of prostate cancer and high-grade disease (Gleason score 7–10) and how finasteride increased the sensitivity of the DRE (finasteride 21.3%; placebo 16.7%; $P = 0.015$).[187,189] Detection of high-grade disease by DRE was also found to be more sensitive than the PSA, but the difference was not statistically significant.[189]

Before these new analyses were published, principal investigator of the PCPT Ian Thompson et al.[187] had answered in part the question their own research had posed when they demonstrated that finasteride's ability to increase the sensitivity of the PSA for prostate cancer and high-grade prostate cancer introduced detection bias for these end points. When their end-of-study biopsy findings failed to demonstrate the increased detection of high-grade tumors in the finasteride arm that had been shown in the for-cause biopsies prompted by high PSA values or abnormal DRE findings, the researchers had a reason to suspect that finasteride might not have caused the changes. Thus, Thompson et al.[187] used AUC studies to demonstrate that the AUC for finasteride was significantly greater than that for placebo for cancer detection overall and for high-grade disease, whether the Gleason score was ≥ 7 or ≥ 8. Additionally, the 18-year long-term follow-up of the PCPT study confirmed that finasteride has no significant effect on the overall survival or survival after the prostate cancer diagnosis.[192]

Thompson et al.[187] performed another analysis of PSA in the PCPT data, estimating the ROC curve for PSA, and found that there was no cut point for PSA with both high sensitivity and specificity for monitoring healthy men for prostate cancer; rather, there was a continuum of prostate cancer risk at all PSA levels. The ROC curve was better for high-grade than for overall prostate cancer risk, but as subsequent analysis showed, there is a substantial risk of biopsy-detected prostate cancer and high-grade disease in men with PSA levels <4 ng/mL, which is generally thought to be in the normal range. Although PSA values <4 ng/mL are related to prostate cancer risk, it is not clear how this information should be applied to clinical decision-making. These data illustrate (1) the need for improved biomarkers of risk and prognosis of prostate cancer and (2) the value of biopsy-proven negative controls for assessing prostate cancer risk, biology, and prevention.

Another important NCI-supported chemopreventive randomized, placebo-controlled trial is called Selenium and Vitamin E Cancer Prevention Trial (SELECT). The study evaluated the effects of selenium and vitamin E, separately and combined, against those of placebo in preventing prostate cancer.[193] Paradoxically, the investigators reported a statistically nonsignificant increase in prostate cancer risk in the vitamin E alone group in their first report, which became significant with longer follow-up and more prostate cancer events.[194,195] The serial collection of biospecimens from all SELECT study participants will enable the construction of risk models to help determine which men are most likely to develop prostate cancer and to help identify those most likely to benefit from selenium and vitamin E chemopreventive therapy.

Specimens from the other landmark NCI initiative for prostate cancer prevention, the PCPT, were recently released, making them available to researchers whether they are supported by NCI grants or not.[196]

Putative chemopreventive agents other than finasteride that have been studied or are in development include celecoxib, sulindac, toremifene, soy isoflavones, lycopene, and doxercalciferol. Additionally, novel preventive strategies such as immunotherapy and mechanistically based drug combinations are being explored.[197] Currently under way are molecular epidemiologic studies of diet and prostate cancer risk as well as basic research into the carcinogenicity of specific diet-derived compounds such as heterocyclic amines. Statins have also been of interest. In 2003, the NCI's Division of Cancer Prevention awarded $42 million to fund a consortium made up of six programs headed by experienced cancer prevention principal investigators at six major institutions. Members were charged with becoming national leaders in prevention research and in initiating trials on agents of interest, including some of the agents named earlier.

Algorithm for therapy: future directions

Future studies will affect therapy most dramatically if they address limitations reported in current reviews of the literature. These studies must (1) use a randomized design, including an untreated control group, (2) use standard definitions of cancer control and quality-of-life outcomes, (3) link specific techniques to outcome, and (4) demonstrate that a specific technique can be reproduced by multiple practitioners and produce an effect that is similar across settings in the same way that prescribing a drug produces similar effects across patient groups in different settings. After scientific standards are met, the study design should incorporate measures that will make progress possible by resolving questions, both large and small, posed by other works or by producing data that eliminate potential explanations that could undercut conclusions.

Using current knowledge, investigators can outline an algorithm for patients with localized disease as follows: make a determination about treatment, follow an evidence-based guideline or enroll the patient in a clinical trial if treatment is the option of choice, and incorporate molecular signatures to address tumor heterogeneity. First, patients and their physicians must cooperatively decide whether to pursue treatment. As described earlier, expectant management, also called watchful waiting or active surveillance, permits patients with localized disease to forgo treatment, and national organizations, including the National Comprehensive Cancer Network, have created guidelines for management[138]; however, in some active surveillance studies, as many as 75% of men electing expectant management have been found to pursue therapy within 5 years, mostly because of rising PSA values.[198] Advances in better identification of low-risk cases with refined arrays of prognostic factors, including molecular markers, and closer surveillance may change that trend.

Critical to efforts in the future to spare patients with localized disease the side effects of unnecessary definitive therapy will be better tools for differentiating aggressive from indolent disease. Such tools, some of which are in development, may take the form of nomograms such as those described earlier, of a combination of one or more molecular markers added to PSA values, of genetic variants, or of discriminating molecular signatures.[199–201] With these combinations, we may be inspecting findings not for one specific value but for patterns of values within each collection of factors, and we may be able to obtain this information not only preoperatively but also before biopsy. Furthermore, predictions achieved this way may encompass not only therapeutic response but also natural disease progression.[200]

Locally advanced disease

Clinical presentation

Locally advanced prostate cancer is heralded by disease extension outside the prostate capsule (T3a) or into the seminal vesicles (T3b). The tumor may grow laterally into the pelvic sidewall, centrally into the urethra, superiorly into the bladder neck and trigone, interiorly into the base of the penis, or posteriorly into the rectum. Although patients may be relatively asymptomatic when they are first seen, complaints are related to the direction of spread.

Common symptoms can be similar to those seen with BPH and vesicle outlet obstruction, such as urinary urgency, frequency, and hesitancy, nocturia, dysuria, and decreased stream. Invasion of the bladder or urethra can produce hematuria, and ureteral obstruction can lead to renal impairment. hematospermia can be seen as well. Although Denonvilliers fascia is usually an effective barrier to tumor spread, rectal invasion produces symptoms similar to those seen in primary rectal cancer, such as hematochezia, constipation and obstruction, reduced stool caliber, and pelvic pain. Tumor extension inferiorly into the urogenital diaphragm or corporal bodies may result in perineal pain, priapism, or impotence.

In addition to DRE, the use of pelvic CT scanning or MRI, transrectal ultrasonography, cystoscopy, and rectosigmoidoscopy can help to better define the extent of disease and the adjacent organs involved. The PSA level is usually high in these patients, sometimes markedly so, although very high tumor grade, anaplastic tumors, and ductal variants may produce little PSA, and in these cases, the PSA level is disproportionate to the amount of disease present. In PSA-producing tumors, the PSAV is an important consideration because it is a measure of the growth rate and aggressiveness of the disease. A PSAV >2 ng/mL/year before treatment (prostatectomy or radiation) has been shown to relate to a higher rate of cancer-specific death.[202] A rapid PSA doubling time can also be an early indication of metastatic disease. Laboratory work related to the local extent of the tumor may show a low red blood cell count secondary to chronic bleeding or elevated blood urea nitrogen and creatinine values secondary to ureteral obstruction and renal impairment.

To assess potential disease outside the pelvis, abdominal CT or MRI, bone scanning, and chest X-ray are also indicated.

Therapy options and applications

According to the results of a patient care evaluation completed by the American College of Surgeons in 1990, the most common treatment for locally advanced prostate cancer at that time was radiation or hormone therapy. Combination treatment was used in just 12% of patients.[203] Poor outcomes and subsequent reports of superior results achieved with combined radiation and androgen-deprivation therapy[163,204–206] led to a planned multimodality approach as the mainstay of treatment for these patients. Although surgery may be used selectively for locally advanced disease, it is usually combined with postoperative adjuvant radiation or with chemohormonal therapy or molecular targeting agents in a clinical trial.

Radiation and hormone therapy

Because radiation alone does not successfully eradicate the bulky local disease burden in patients with locally advanced disease (<50% chance) and this modality does not address the significant risk for metastasis in these patients, combined radiation and androgen deprivation has become the standard of care. The results of four randomized clinical trials—RTOG 85-31, EORTC 22863, RTOG 86-10, and RTOG 92-02—with 10 years of follow-up provide compelling supportive evidence for the use of combined therapy.[207] Patients with locally advanced tumors comprised the study group in the Radiation Therapy Oncology Group (RTOG) trials, and the European Organisation for Research on the Treatment of Cancer (EORTC) trial patients had either T3 or T4 tumors or high-grade disease. The radiation dose in all of these trials was low by today's standards, 65–70 Gy. In all of those trials, the main drug was a luteinizing hormone-releasing hormone (LHRH) agonist.

In RTOG 85-31, hormone therapy was given indefinitely beginning after radiation, and in the EORTC trial, it was given concomitantly with radiation and then continued for 3 years. The results from both of these trials revealed a significant benefit in biochemical and clinical end points (local recurrence, distant metastasis, and disease-free survival) as well as in disease-specific and overall survival rates for the patients who received radiation and hormone therapy, as compared with those who received radiation alone.[163,204] In RTOG 85-31, subset analysis showed that this advantage was largely driven by patients with Gleason scores of 7 or higher.[204]

RTOG 86-10 compared the effects of 4 months of hormone therapy, started 2 months before radiation, with those of radiation therapy alone. Patients benefited more from the combined radiation and hormone therapy in the end points of biochemical failure, distant metastasis, and disease-free and disease-specific survival.[205,208] The latest report revealed that just 4 months of adjuvant androgen-deprivation therapy had a profound effect on disease-specific survival[208]: one-third of the patients treated with radiation alone died as a result of prostate cancer within 9 years, whereas it took an additional 9 years for the same number of patients to die of their disease when hormone therapy had been added. However, there still was no significant difference in the overall survival rate.

RTOG 92-02 compared 4 months of hormonal therapy plus radiation (as in the combined treatment arm in RTOG 86-10) with radiation plus 28 months of hormone therapy (hormone therapy for 2 months before and 2 months during radiation followed by 24 more months). Similar to the results from the other studies, there was a between-group difference in all end points except overall survival, for which only patients with Gleason scores of 8–10 benefited from the longer duration of hormone therapy.[206,209]

These study results taken in conglomerate suggest that a longer duration of hormone therapy in conjunction with radiation better addresses not only local disease but also distant dissemination in patients who have a significant local tumor burden, especially in patients with high Gleason scores.

A study by D'Amico et al.[210] included a mixture of patients at intermediate and high risk (T1b–T2b or low risk with T3 by endorectal MRI, PSA 10–40 ng/mL, or Gleason score 7–10). Patients were randomized to receive 70 Gy to the prostate and seminal vesicles alone or 70 Gy combined with 6 months of total androgen blockade starting 2 months before radiation treatment began. This study also showed an advantage in prostate cancer-specific mortality in patients receiving the combination therapy: 2% versus 8% at 8 years after treatment. Additionally, overall survival was 74% versus 61% in favor of the group treated with combination therapy. Of note, however, is that although the survival benefit was of even greater magnitude in patients who had no or minimal comorbidity (90% vs 64%), there was no benefit in patients with moderate or severe comorbidity. In the group with moderate or severe comorbidity, the survival rate was higher than it was in the group treated with radiation alone, although the difference was not statistically significant. D'Amico et al.[211] suggested

that hormone therapy increases the risk of myocardial infarction in this cohort.

In another randomized trial in men with locally advanced (T2b–T4) disease, that of the Trans Tasman Radiation Oncology Group (96.01), the addition of 6 months of total androgen blockade begun 5 months before radiation to a dose of 66 Gy significantly reduced biochemical, local, and distant failure and improved prostate cancer-specific survival.[212] The benefit of adding hormone therapy appeared to increase as the PSA and Gleason score became indicative of higher-risk disease. Although the current trend is to try to decrease the use of hormone therapy or at least limit its duration, because of the recent reports of cardiac morbidity, metabolic syndrome, and bone density effects,[211,213] the ideal duration of hormone therapy has yet to be determined on the basis of a maximal therapeutic ratio.[213]

A follow-up EORTC trial, 22961, was designed to prove the non-inferiority of 6 months of hormone therapy and radiation compared with 3 years of hormone therapy and radiation in men with locally advanced prostate cancer (T2c–T4) and those with T1c–T2b N1–2 disease. The trial closed early after accrual of 990 patients, however, because an interim analysis showed the futility of trying to prove this hypothesis. Five-year PSA and clinical progression-free survival as well as overall survival rates were all lower in the patients who received 6 months of hormone therapy: 78% versus 59%, 82% versus 69%, and 85% versus 81%, respectively.[214] The most recently reported trial (PCS IV) compared 18 months to 36 months of androgen deprivation with moderate-dose radiation. With a median follow-up of 6.5 years, no statistically significant differences were seen in overall and disease-specific survival.[215] Additionally of note is the fact that current standard radiation doses are higher than those used previously, and this has been shown to both decrease local failure and subsequently affect distant metastasis.[216,217] Thus, we must continue to test the most therapeutically beneficial combinations of androgen deprivation and radiation.

Radiation and chemotherapy

Because the results of combined hormone therapy and radiation leave ample room for improvement, combinations with chemotherapy are being tested in clinical trials. In RTOG 99-02, patients with high-risk disease were randomized to treatment with radiation plus 2 years of androgen ablation or to treatment with the same combination followed by treatment with paclitaxel, estramustine, and etoposide for four cycles beginning 8 weeks after radiation.[218] This study was closed prematurely because of excessive thromboembolic toxicity. A follow-up study, RTOG 05-21, has completed accrual and has the same design as RTOG 99-02 but uses docetaxel and prednisone for six cycles after radiation as the adjuvant agents. Future analysis will give some indication as to the efficacy of these agents delivered adjuvantly with radiation. Similar to trials for metastatic disease, attention has turned to the newer targeted agents and the possible combination with radiation.

Radical prostatectomy

Although prostatectomy has been used to treat patients with locally advanced prostate cancer, the reported studies are usually qualified by including patients with less-extensive, resectable disease and lower-grade tumors than have been included in radiation trials. With prostatectomy, PSA disease-free outcome has been in the 50–60% range 5–10 years after treatment, and 60–80% of patients have required adjuvant and/or salvage radiation or hormone ablative therapy postoperatively.[219–222] Unlike the combined approach with radiation, the use of short-course androgen deprivation has not resulted in significant improvement in PSA disease-free progression when combined neoadjuvantly with prostatectomy.[161,223]

To date, surgery has not yielded results superior to those obtained with radiation plus hormonal therapy. A randomized trial comparing 8 weeks of treatment with diethylstilbestrol (DES) and either radiation or radical prostatectomy in patients with T2b–T3 tumors showed similar results with regard to biochemical, clinical progression-free, and cause-specific survival.[224] The dose of radiation used was only in the 60–70 Gy range, and the treatment-related morbidity was treatment specific, as might be expected.

Although several phase II studies have proven that various chemotherapeutic agents and hormonal therapy can be combined neoadjuvantly with surgery with an acceptable level of toxicity, a significant decrease in cancer progression or improvement in survival has yet to be seen.[225–227] The recently opened Cancer and Leukemia Group B (CALGB) 90203 trial randomizes patients to receive either six cycles of neoadjuvant docetaxel plus prednisone and androgen deprivation followed by radical prostatectomy or radical prostatectomy alone.

A series of studies conducted at M.D. Anderson Cancer Center expanded the concept of local control with surgery to more advanced disease states as part of an integrated treatment strategy for patients with more advanced cancers. Although the patients did not meet accepted criteria for prostatectomy, they were at risk for pelvic and urinary outlet obstructive symptoms. No attempt has been made to date to establish the efficacy of this approach in large patient groups. A benefit of this approach is that it has provided relevant human prostate cancer to generate or test new hypotheses. The preoperative platform adds to the evidence that sonic hedgehog signaling is a therapy target for prostate cancer and can be therapeutically modulated in vivo.[228] These findings have prompted the further study of agents that inhibit sonic hedgehog signaling in the therapy of prostate cancer. In addition, we suggest that stromal–epithelial interacting pathways implicated in prostate cancer progression within the primary tumor are also those central to its progression in the bone.[8] The clinical reasoning used to integrate surgery in patients with locally advanced cancers has been extended to patients with castrate-sensitive disease, primarily in the case of prostates with "oligometastatic" cancer.[229] Taken together, these clinical observations establish feasibility.

Several population-based studies have analyzed the effect of local therapy in the metastatic setting and have demonstrated improved survivals for those men receiving radiation or surgery to the primary.[230,231] This influence may be directly related to symptomatic local progression and subsequent complications, but more interestingly local therapy may disrupt the process of metastases and therefore alter tumor biology. The feasibility of radical prostatectomy in the metastatic setting was demonstrated by one study, which showed acceptable morbidity with surgery.[232] Concomitantly, two clinical trials are evaluating the role of local therapy in M1, castrate-sensitive patients. The STAMPEDE trial in Europe has included evaluating the use of radiation to the primary tumor in M1 patients.[233] Meanwhile, a trial out of M.D. Anderson Cancer Center is assessing the integration of best systemic therapy with or without local therapy (surgery or radiation) in castrate-sensitive disease (NCT10751438). While the concept of local therapy in metastatic disease is intriguing, widespread adoption of this practice should not occur until we have more definitive data. These trials will help to identify the subset of patients likely to benefit from an integrative strategy incorporating local therapy in the metastatic setting.

Postprostatectomy radiation

The results of three randomized trials have shown similar benefit for adjuvant radiation after prostatectomy for the indications of extracapsular extension, seminal vesicle involvement, and positive surgical margins, the latter being the most significant predictor of the benefit of radiation.[234–236] All three of these studies have now demonstrated a benefit of at least 20% points in PSA disease-free survival with 10 years of follow-up. The EORTC and the SWOG trials also a reported decrease in local recurrence rates and clinical progression.[237] At the latest update, with a median follow-up of 11.5 years, the SWOG trial has now shown a statistically significant difference in metastasis-free survival, which was the primary study end point.[235] At 15 years after treatment, 54% of the men treated with adjuvant radiation had developed metastatic disease or died, compared with 62% treated with prostatectomy alone; this is a hazard reduction of 25% in favor of the use of adjuvant radiation. Significant improvement in overall survival in the irradiated group was also seen.[235]

As the radiation dose is increased, targeting is improved, and candidates for prostatectomy are chosen more carefully by using newer imaging techniques to rule out metastatic disease, it is likely that the benefit of adjuvant radiation will only increase in the future.

Castrate-resistant locally advanced disease

Bulky tumor located within the prostate is especially problematic in patients with castrate-resistant disease. An evaluation of men progressing to castrate-resistant disease identified patients with an untreated primary tumor as having a significantly increased risk of subsequent local symptoms (20% post-RP vs 46.7% EBRT vs 54.3% with an intact prostate).[238] In men with retained primaries, hormonal therapy will often not debulk the tumor to achieve the desired response with radiation. Additionally, recent data would suggest that androgen deprivation is coupled to DNA repair enzymes and that tumors which demonstrate early androgen insensitivity may be less susceptible to radiation therapy.[239] In patients with metastatic disease, radiation alone can serve the purpose of palliation, relieving symptoms such as hematuria or recurrent urinary obstruction. In patients with greater expected longevity, chemotherapy may be used as a debulking agent prior to or in conjunction with radiation, although the duration and degree of response has not been well documented. Alternatively, prostatectomy may be feasible and will provide symptomatic relief in many of these patients.[240]

Recently, "anaplastic features" identified as clinical features that portend a poor prognosis, but increased chemotherapy responsiveness, have been identified. Of these seven clinical features, the authors found that bulky primary tumors were a significant predictor of worse survival, while neuroendocrine features were not predictive of survival or response to systemic chemotherapy.[241] While late palliative local therapy is possible for retained primaries, it is often in the form of aggressive surgical procedures (cystoprostatectomy and pelvic exenteration).[242] While providing relief for many patients, these procedures are often fraught with significant risk of complications and necessary reoperations making these late interventions less appealing. Clinical trials at M.D. Anderson Cancer Center have incorporated further evaluation of early progressors on initial systemic androgen ablation in an attempt to identify "anaplastic" carcinomas at a time when local therapy is possible to further evaluate its potential impact on disease progression (NCT10751438).

Algorithm for therapy: future directions

To apply the most appropriate treatment strategy, it is critical that physicians use diagnostic imaging, pathology review, PSA kinetics, and tumor markers to their fullest extent in assessing the tumor and individualizing therapy. The current emphasis is on exploring combined therapies that will not only eradicate local disease but will prevent or treat distant micrometastases as well. Trials using molecular targeting agents such as tyrosine kinase inhibitors and antiangiogenic agents in combination with radiation or prostatectomy are currently under way. The doses and toxic effects of these agents must be explored, along with their molecular effects in tissue. Ideally, in the future, molecular markers will enable more precise individualized therapy, predicting tumor growth and dissemination patterns (locoregional vs distant) so that treatment can be designed to effect the best response. The molecular targets of new agents and their effects on tissue—both tumor and stroma—must be defined in detail so that therapy can be matched to the tumor's molecular characteristics. It is in this manner that an individualized, multidisciplinary approach will provide the best strategies for both local and distant disease controls as we move forward.

Metastatic prostate cancer

Among the leading causes of cancer-related deaths worldwide, metastases from adenocarcinoma of the prostate possess a highly conserved clinical phenotype, characterized by osteoblastic bone metastases. Although morbidity and mortality from advanced disease correlate with the volume of bone metastases, notable phenotypic variants observed in approximately 10% of patients include lymph node-dominant metastases, visceral-dominant (liver or lung) metastases, and locally advanced manifestations without bone metastases. Outgrowth of neuroendocrine or small-cell carcinoma is a particular phenomenon associated with prostate cancer at the initial visit or, more commonly, after lengthy periods of hormonal therapy.

At the time of diagnosis of prostate cancer, overt radiologic evidence of metastatic disease varies from 10% to 15% of men from populations among which screening for the disease is commonplace to ≥70% of men from unscreened populations. After therapy directed toward localized disease, the earliest presentation of *micrometastatic disease* is most commonly a rising PSA serum level. Given that approximately ¹⁄₃ of patients treated for localized prostate cancer will experience treatment failure, it has been estimated that nearly 70,000 men are diagnosed yearly with the *rising PSA disease state*, and the prevalence in the United States may be as high as 1 million.[243]

Biochemical recurrence of prostate cancer may be defined variably after surgery,[244] that is, time to PSA ≥0.2 ng/mL with the confirmatory value of >0.2 ng/mL, or radiation therapy,[245] that is, time to PSA nadir + 2 ng/mL. Such working definitions can assist in annotating and harmonizing reportable outcomes from therapy. It is important to recognize that a rise in PSA is not an absolute indicator of malignancy, an absolute indication for therapy, or fully predictive of disease progression or disease-specific mortality. The reasons for this are as follows: (1) benign explanations for PSA rise include incomplete prostatectomy or PSA bounces after radiation therapy, (2) the disease is capable of exceptional indolence, (3) early therapy has no established efficacy in improving overall survival or quality of life, and (4) comorbidities are common in aging men (the median age at diagnosis of the rising PSA disease state is 70 years), and alternative causes of death are incrementally dominant among lower-risk rising PSA disease states.

The *long natural history* of the disease after radical prostatectomy for localized adenocarcinoma of the prostate has been described as a median time to metastases of 8 years and a median life expectancy of 13 years.[246] The investigators of one randomized study of radical

prostatectomy versus watchful waiting in 695 men reported a 19% cumulative incidence of metastases at 12 years in men with clinically localized disease who had undergone surgery at the time of diagnosis, compared with a 26% incidence of metastases in men who had undergone watchful waiting, without an observable plateau.[247] Foci of disseminated but apparently dormant cancer cells may persist for long periods in suitable microenvironmental niches such as within the bone marrow. These clones are thought to remain clinically undetectable in dormant nonproliferative states or in balanced proliferative–apoptotic states before emerging from a dormant state as clinically detectable metastases.[248]

Using PSA doubling time, time to biochemical failure from surgery, and the histologic Gleason grade, for instance, different metastasis-free and overall survival outcomes can be estimated. For example, men with high-grade disease (Gleason score 8–10) and evidence of biochemical failure within 2 years of surgery have a 70% probability of developing metastases in 5 years,[246] and those with PSA doubling times of <3 months have a probability of prostate cancer-specific mortality of nearly 50% within 5 years.[182] In contrast, men with very long PSA doubling times (≥15 months) have prostate cancer-specific mortality rates of no greater than 10% at 10 years.[182] The PSA doubling time are a useful tool to estimate time to meaningful progression and the knowledge deploy therapy in a "risk-adapted manner" and design clinical trials.

The median age at diagnosis of men who have the rising PSA and comorbidities influences timing of therapeutic intervention. Standardized approaches that integrate prognostic markers with age and medical comorbidity will need to be developed to guide future therapy.[249,250] Biomarkers that can link the heterogeneous phenotype of metastatic disease to specific therapeutic strategies are required.

Diagnosis

A diagnosis of metastatic prostate cancer may be suspected with the emergence of symptoms or signs of the disease or with a rapidly rising and/or markedly elevated PSA concentration.

Symptoms and signs of metastatic disease

The emergence of bone pain is perhaps the most common symptom of metastatic prostate cancer. Correctly diagnosing the cause of the pain is critical. A change in the character, location, and severity of preexisting "arthritis" pain, for example, should arouse suspicion. Malignant bone pain is usually unremitting and worsens over time. Base-of-skull syndromes can manifest as occipital pain or cranial nerve palsy; the sixth and twelfth nerves are frequently affected. Mental neuropathy presents as chin numbness related to unilateral or bilateral mandibular infiltration and compression of the vulnerable inferior alveolar nerve. A concomitant finding of exquisite sternal tenderness caused by replacement of the bone marrow with high-volume disease is reminiscent of acute leukemia. Referred pain from malignant nerve-root impingements can mimic benign disease; for example, L2 pain can be mistaken for degenerative disease of the hips and lower thoracic root impingement, as an acute abdomen. The Lhermitte sign may signal spinal cord impingement. Back pain can result from bulky retroperitoneal adenopathy rather than from spinal metastases. On bone scans, benign disease such as vertebral compression fractures from osteoporosis, severe degenerative disease, and Paget's disease of the bone can mimic malignant progression.

The emergence of cough, shortness of breath, and interstitial perihilar infiltrates on chest X-ray suggests lymphangitic spread of disease; infection caused by *Pneumocystis carinii* is rare in men with prostate cancer, even those with long-term steroid exposure. Lung metastases are rarely the sole manifestation of distant disease; lung nodules and pleural effusions are other pulmonary manifestations. High-volume lung metastases, although unusual, should raise the suspicion of concomitant brain metastases. Liver metastases usually remain asymptomatic. High-volume liver metastases, lytic bone disease, and brain metastases can imply the presence of neuroendocrine or small-cell carcinoma.

Local progression in the intact or irradiated prostate may be the dominant manifestation of advancing disease, and DRE is a surprisingly neglected diagnostic tool. Late emergence of irritative or obstructive urinary symptoms after radiation, rectal urgency, a change in stool caliber, or perineal pain suggests failure of local control and invasion of local structures. Lymphedema results from infiltration of regional lymphatics and can be particularly debilitating. Invasion of the base of the bladder can result in obstruction of the bladder outlet or ureter (with resultant hydronephrosis and renal failure), hematuria, and recurrent infections. Penile and scrotal metastases are less common.

Radiologic studies

Radiologic studies that are most useful for staging metastatic disease include radionuclide bone scanning and CT of the abdomen and pelvis. A chest X-ray can identify less common pulmonary manifestations, and CT of the chest is occasionally useful to further characterize small pulmonary nodules, the presence of mediastinal lymphadenopathy, or lymphangitic disease. CT-guided needle biopsies are occasionally required to diagnose indeterminate lesions, but sampling errors and false negatives such as with small bone lesions remain a problem; follow-up is usually required to properly resolve the diagnostic question. MRI is useful for defining the presence of metastatic disease in bony lesions that are indeterminate on bone scans or plain X-rays, screening for suspected spinal cord compression or brain metastases, and evaluating the extent of infiltrative locally advanced disease in the pelvis. Positron emission tomography and indium-labeled capromab pendetide (ProstaScint, Cytogen Corporation, Princeton, NJ) imaging require further development with respect to sensitivity and specificity for metastatic disease and cannot be routinely recommended at this time.

Pathologic studies

Pathologic studies to confirm a diagnosis of metastatic disease may include immunohistochemical testing for PSA and PAP expression; for example, PSA expression may be lost with androgen-deprivation therapy. In the future, molecular evidence of characteristic fusion genes may help resolve indeterminate cases. Men who have a markedly elevated serum PSA concentration (e.g., >100 ng/mL) and a typical metastatic phenotype such as osteoblastic bone metastases at diagnosis rarely require a biopsy to confirm the presence of metastatic disease.

Currently used therapies

Hormonal therapy

Since the discovery of the hormonal biology of prostate cancer,[251] hormonal therapy has been the mainstay in the control of advanced disease. Current therapies are directed toward lowering the concentrations of circulating androgens by surgical or medical castration therapy or by pharmacologic blockade of the binding of androgens to their receptor in target tissue[252] (Figure 8). A combination of surgical and medical castration and AR blockade, referred to as combined androgen blockade, may yield additional benefits[253] in

subsets of patients still to be defined. Data supporting the integration of 5α-reductase inhibitors, which inhibit the conversion of testosterone to dihydrotestosterone, with combined androgen blockade, referred to as triple androgen blockade, are similarly limited. More effective antagonism of the AR such as with an avidly binding antagonist lacking partial agonist activity (e.g., MDV3100) or more selective and potent inhibitors of androgen synthesis (e.g., abiraterone acetate) is an example of novel hormonal approaches currently being investigated in phase I–III clinical trials.

In men with the rising PSA disease state, there is no evidence that the early application of hormonal therapy—before the emergence of metastases—improves overall survival or quality of life. The demonstration of improved survival with the integration of hormonal therapy and radiation therapy for high-risk localized disease[163,254] likely relates to improved local control and a decrease in a late wave of metastases from the primary[255] tumor rather than to the control of micrometastatic disease. In contrast, in a small study of immediate adjuvant versus deferred hormonal therapy for node-positive disease after radical prostatectomy, poorer than expected outcomes with hormonal therapy in the deferred therapy arm[256] suggested that as in the antecedent Medical Research Council trial of immediate versus deferred hormonal therapy in metastatic disease,[257] late application of hormonal therapy results in inferior outcomes in some studies. There is a critical dearth of high-quality studies examining the role of hormonal therapy in the high-risk postoperative adjuvant setting or the rising PSA disease state in the overall survival and quality-of-life end points.

Complications of hormonal therapy[258] include hot flashes, weight gain, diminished libido and energy level, insomnia, mood and intellectual impairment, osteoporosis, sarcopenia, and acceleration of the metabolic syndrome or cardiovascular disease. Some parts of these complications attributed to hormonal therapy, such as neurocognitive effects, may also relate to aging and the debilitating effects of advanced disease.[259] Monotherapy with nonsteroidal antiandrogens (e.g., high-dose bicalutamide) may yield survival outcomes equivalent to those produced by medical castration in low-risk disease[260] but with lesser effects on bone mass, muscle strength, and libido.[261] Intermittent castration therapy with LHRH agonists reduces the cost and morbidity of therapy with no known adverse (or beneficial) effects in terms of duration of disease control; mature results from several randomized phase III trials are awaited.[262]

In men with either the rising PSA disease state or metastatic disease, the decline in PSA with castration therapy yields a nadir value that may be prognostically useful.[263,264] A nadir PSA >4 ng/mL in men with metastatic disease after 7 months of hormonal therapy was associated with a median overall survival of 13 months in contrast to a median survival of 75 months with a nadir PSA of ≤0.2 ng/mL.[264] These data suggest that a lethal phenotype can be identified in this manner for early intervention with experimental strategies.

To date, randomized studies in newly diagnosed metastatic disease have not identified a survival or quality-of-life benefit for early versus deferred introduction of chemotherapy combined with hormonal therapy.[265] Thus, the use of chemohormonal therapy in this setting remains experimental.

Nonhormonal therapy

No convincing evidence supports the value of chemotherapy in treating hormone-naive prostate cancer. A range of nonhormonal therapeutic agents, including vaccines, immunomodulators, angiogenesis and signal-transduction inhibitors, and differentiation agents have been legitimately studied in the rising PSA disease state and in asymptomatic metastatic disease. These settings have

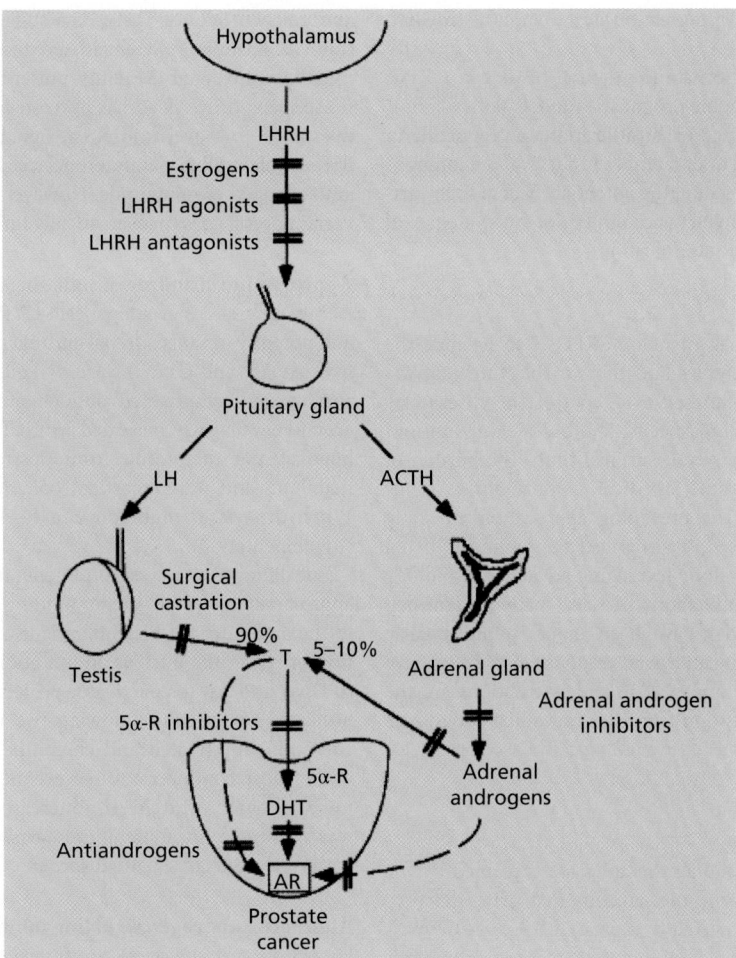

Figure 8 Hormonal axis and therapeutic agents in prostate cancer. Abbreviations: LHRH, luteinizing hormone-releasing hormone; LH, luteinizing hormone; ACTH, adrenocorticotropin; AR, androgen receptor; DHT, dihydrotestosterone; 5α-R, 5-alpha-reductase. Source: Miyamoto 2004.[252] Reproduced with permission of John Wiley and Sons.

particular trial design challenges, including the lack of validated early surrogate end points for survival. To date, there is no evidence that a nonhormonal therapy has a major influence on the natural history of the disease.

Castrate-resistant disease

Durations of hormonal control vary from 6 years in men without metastases[265] to 18 months in men with metastatic disease.[266] When evidence of progressive disease emerges in the context of low serum concentrations of testosterone, by consensus <50 ng/dL,[267] the term *CRPC* may be preferable to "hormone-refractory" or "androgen-independent" prostate cancer.[268] These tumors are often responsive to alternative hormonal therapeutic agents and hence are not strictly hormone refractory. Because persistent signaling via a "supersensitive" AR may occur despite the serum levels of testosterone after castration, they are often not truly androgen independent, either.

Prognosis

Few study reports have described the prognosis for men with CRPC defined by a rising PSA concentration alone. Observations from the placebo arm of a randomized controlled trial of zoledronic acid (201 men with castrate levels of serum testosterone, rising PSA values, and no evidence of bone metastases) demonstrated the potentially lengthy time to the development of bone metastases, particularly in

men with low PSA values and long PSA doubling times.[269] Overall, the risk of bone metastases in this cohort was 33% at 2 years, and the median bone metastasis-free interval was 30 months. More than 50% of the men with PSA doubling times of <6 months developed bone metastases within 18 months, whereas only 40% of those with PSA doubling times of >18 months had developed bone metastases within 3 years.

Although the median overall survival time in asymptomatic CRPC without metastases is 4 years, the prognosis of men with metastatic CRPC varies between symptomatic[270,271] and asymptomatic[272] disease and ranges from 9 to 23 months, respectively. Several predictive nomograms incorporate a range of easily determined clinical and biochemical parameters to predict 12- and 24-month overall survival rates.[273–275] A model that incorporated PSA doubling time, time to PSA progression after initiation of castration therapy, and presence of metastatic disease at the time of CRPC transition defined three prognostic groups to predict clinical progression or event-free survival (EFS)[275]: a low-risk group defined solely by a PSA doubling time of >10 months (median EFS 96 months); an intermediate-risk group with a PSA doubling time of <10 months and a time to PSA progression of >13 months (median EFS 33 months); and a high-risk group defined by a PSA doubling time of ≤10 months, the presence of metastatic disease at progression from androgen-dependent prostate cancer to CRPC transition, and a time to PSA progression of ≤13 months (median EFS 6 months).

Given these evident variations in the natural history of CRPC, there is clearly a need for reliable prognostic models both for routine clinical practice and for accrual stratification and reporting in clinical trials. Interpretations of differences in survival outcomes in clinical trials must take into account the potential effect of such variations, which may be incompletely accounted for by strategies of randomization and prognostic stratification.

Management of CRPC
A key principle in the management of CRPC is to balance the limitations of benefit of therapies and the variable threat of the disease. Current therapies can serve to control the disease by improving symptoms, reducing specific morbidity, and improving quality of life as well as overall survival time. The burden of androgen-deprivation syndrome, medical comorbidities, influences therapeutic choices. The prevailing approach is to apply therapeutics sequentially based on prognostication and predicted tolerance. Future direction will be leveraging advances in biology to apply more effective combinations in select patient identified by predictive markers. Strides have been made in molecularly classifying patients likely to be androgen responsive[42,43,276] or have aggressive variants.[241] These observation and associations are the foundational studies to transition from the prevailing prognostic model for allocation of therapies[277] to a biologically based predictive model.[278]

Secondary hormonal therapy
Responses to secondary hormonal therapies are explained by the incompletely defined endocrine mechanisms that drive the progression of CRPC via the persistently expressed AR or AR bypass pathways. In general, the median duration of progression-free survival for an unselected population treated with secondary hormonal therapy is <6 months with first-generation androgen signaling inhibitors.[279,280] Men with short durations of primary hormonal control and with suboptimal PSA nadir response and rapid PSA doubling times are less likely to experience a prolonged response to secondary hormonal therapies. On a practical level, the choice of a secondary hormonal therapy in CRPC is influenced by details of prior hormonal therapy, comorbidity, and the risk of drug interactions.

A small but significant fraction of men with progressive CRPC given concurrent antiandrogen therapy will experience a 50% drop in PSA and objective regression of disease with *antiandrogen withdrawal* alone; this phenomenon has been described across the broad spectrum of steroidal and nonsteroidal antiandrogen agents. Estimates of the frequency and duration of the antiandrogen withdrawal response (AAWR) have varied, but the single largest prospective study of nonsteroidal antiandrogen agent (bicalutamide, flutamide, or nilutamide) withdrawal (*n* = 132) demonstrated a PSA decline by half in 11%, an objective response in 2%, and a median time to PSA progression of 6 months.[281] In the main they are modest benefit and the interest has been supplanted with the new evidence of efficacy for the improved androgen signaling targeting the AR (enzalutamide) or androgen biosynthesis inhibition (abiraterone acetate). The retained interest is based principally due the biologic significance of AAWR. The finding points to the clinical relevance of the emerging knowledge of the alterations in AR alteration and androgen biosynthesis in prostate cancer progression.[282] Mutations of the AR were found in 10% of bone metastases, and these did not correlate with the AAWR.[283] Withdrawal responses have also been described with steroidal antiandrogens, including the progestins

and glucocorticoids. These data suggest that the AAWR observation has yet to be fully elucidated and may be more complex than initially anticipated. Recently presence of AR splice variants and more specifically ARV7 has been strongly associated with primary resistance to novel androgen signaling inhibitors, namely, the irreversible inhibitor abiraterone acetate and the second-generation antiandrogen enzalutamide. However it is not clear whether splice variant presence is mechanistically linked to resistance.[42,43,284]

Approved novel androgen signaling inhibitors in mCRPC
Abiraterone is a steroidogenesis CYP17 inhibitor that selectively and potently inhibits adrenal androgen synthesis by inhibiting 17-α hydroxylase and C17,20 lyase.[285] Following two positive phase III studies in chemotreated and chemonaive mCRPC, abiraterone acetate is currently indicated in mCRPC.[286,287] Hypertension and hypokalemia that result from upstream accumulation of pregnenolone and adrenocorticotropic hormone as a result of the 17a hydroxylase inhibition can be suppressed with prednisone supplementation.

Enzalutamide is a second-generation antiandrogen that has approximately fivefold higher binding affinity for the AR compared to the antiandrogen bicalutamide. Enzalutamide blocks translocation of AR to the nucleus and in addition prevents binding of AR to DNA and AR to coactivator proteins. Enzalutamide is currently indicated in mCRPC following two positive phase III studies in chemotherapy-treated and chemotherapy-naive mCRPC. Fatigue is the most common adverse events. In the chemotherapy-naive mCRPC trial[288] (PREVAIL), increased incidence of hypertension was reported. Enzalutamide administration has been associated with rare events of seizure disorder.

Alternative androgen signaling inhibitors
High doses of the azole antifungal agent *ketoconazole* (400 mg, 3 times daily) may function to enhance the effects of castration by ablating synthesis of adrenal androgens, themselves weak ligands of the AR but also a source of testosterone. Glucocorticoid replacement is required for ketoconazole-induced adrenal insufficiency. Adverse effects and complications include fatigue, nausea, hepatotoxicity, and drug interactions with agents metabolized by the cytochrome P450 system. This agent has largely been replaced by the more effective and less toxic irreversible CYP17 inhibitor abiraterone acetate.

Estrogens possess some activity in prostate cancer, due at least in part to their castration effects. In the control of advanced disease, DES has demonstrated efficacy equal to that of LHRH agonist therapy, but DES has come into disrepute because of its well-documented thrombotic and cardiac complications, particularly with daily doses >3 mg. The efficacy of oral DES 1 to 3 mg daily in mCRPC[289,290] has been described without clear evidence of a dose–response relationship. The mechanism of action of DES has not been fully established. Thrombotic complications of DES persist even with low doses; concomitant therapy with low-dose warfarin and enteric-coated aspirin or low molecular weight heparin may offer prophylactic benefit. DES-related gynecomastia can be particularly troublesome, and prophylactic breast irradiation is recommended prior to initiation of therapy.

Glucocorticoids as single agents have modest activity in CRPC. The different glucocorticoids have not been compared directly, but low-dose dexamethasone has arguably the highest single-agent activity reported.[291] Many mechanisms may account for the effects of glucocorticoids such as suppression of the hypothalamic–pituitary axis, direct effects via steroid receptors, or modulation of the tumor microenvironment. Cushingoid side effects, weight gain, hyperglycemia, osteoporosis, sarcopenia, insomnia, and mood disturbance are all important considerations with prolonged use of glucocorticoids.

The rationale for *continued castration therapy* in men treated with an LHRH agonist is unsettled. Although select retrospective data suggest the potential for inferior survival outcomes without persistent castration,[292] no randomized prospective data demonstrate an advantage to this approach. A consensus statement from the Prostate-Specific Antigen Working Group for the purpose of harmonizing the conduct of clinical trials in CRPC recommended maintenance of a castrate level of testosterone of <50 ng/dL.[267] The role of more complete suppression of androgen signaling in prostate cancer progression is no longer debated given the efficacy of androgen signaling inhibition in the context of castrate-resistant progression.[286,287]

Serum testosterone levels of >50 ng/dL in men treated with optimal doses of LHRH agonist therapy or after orchiectomy are usually associated with low levels of free serum testosterone. However, rare instances of acquired LHRH agonist resistance have been described, likely related to immunologic mechanisms; these cases emphasize the need for periodic monitoring of serum testosterone concentration. Recent studies have applied methodologies that determine lower concentration of testosterone and establish the clinical relevance of "paracrine/intracrine" concentration of androgens (<50 ng/dL of testosterone).[293]

In contrast to these considerations, PSA decreases and objective responses to *testosterone therapy* in prostate cancer have been described, a further reminder that a deeper understanding of the steroid-regulated biology of prostate cancer is necessary.[294]

Nonhormonal therapy

As is the case with hormone-naive metastatic disease, various nonhormonal therapeutic agents are being evaluated in clinical trials for use in asymptomatic or lower-risk CRPC in lieu of secondary hormonal therapy or chemotherapy. Experimental therapeutic agents in lower-risk settings are justified given the demonstrably limited benefits of standard chemotherapy.

Chemotherapy

Although there has been long-standing nihilism with regard to the role of chemotherapy in CRPC,[11] in the last few years, the results of randomized controlled clinical trials have demonstrated the *overall-survival*[295–297] and/or *quality-of-life*[271,296] advantages of chemotherapy in men with metastatic CRPC.

Mitoxantrone plus prednisone (MP) therapy with 12 mg/m^2 of mitoxantrone at 3-week intervals and 5 mg of prednisone given twice daily was approved for use in the United States by the Food and Drug Association on the basis of greater pain relief with that regimen than with that achieved using prednisone monotherapy in symptomatic CRPC; however, a survival advantage for MP therapy was not shown in this 160-patient randomized trial.[270,271] In a 770-patient study, the SWOG used treatment with 60 mg/m^2 of docetaxel given every 21 days plus 280 mg of estramustine given three times daily for 5 consecutive days and compared that regimen with treatment with MP; the results demonstrated an increase in progression-free survival from 3 to 6 months and an improvement in median survival by 2 months with the docetaxel–estramustine regimen.[295] However, the toxic effects attributed to estramustine were clinically significant, and the patients' quality of life was not improved.

In the multinational 1006-patient TAX 327 trial, a regimen of 10 mg of prednisone daily plus 30 mg/m^2 of docetaxel given weekly for 5 of 6 weeks and a regimen of 10 mg of prednisone daily plus 75 mg/m^2 of docetaxel given every 3 weeks were compared with a regimen of 10 mg of prednisone daily plus 12 mg of mitoxantrone given every 3 weeks.[296] A statistically significant improvement in median survival time similar to that in the SWOG trial (i.e., 2 months) was described for the every 3-week schedule of docetaxel compared with the MP regimen[298] (Figure 9). Similar improvement in PSA decline rates, pain response, and global quality of life were reported for the two dosing schedules of docetaxel compared with those resulting from the MP regimen; in contrast, objective responses were infrequent and no different in the three groups. Progression-free survival outcomes for the individual arms were not described.

The results from these studies prompted the US Food and Drug Administration to approve a regimen of daily prednisone plus 75 mg/m^2 of docetaxel given every 3 weeks for the treatment of CRPC.

More recently, cabazitaxel, a novel tubulin-binding taxane with activity in preclinical models resistant to paclitaxel and docetaxel,[300] was compared to MP for the treatment of men with metastatic CRPC whose disease had progressed during or after treatment with

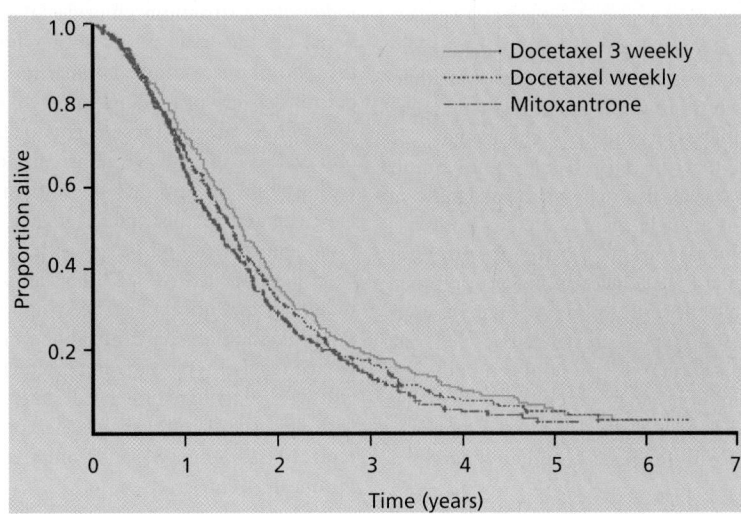

Figure 9 Updated results from TAX 327. Survival benefits are modest with docetaxel chemotherapy: median survival remains under 2 years, and an understanding of biologic subsets that benefit from therapy is required. Source: Eble 2004.[299] Reproduced with permission of World Health Organization.

a docetaxel-containing regimen.[297] In this 775-patient randomized clinical trial, 25 mg/m^2 of cabazitaxel given intravenously every 3 weeks resulted in an improvement of 2.4 months in median overall survival, compared to the MP regimen. Pain palliation was similar in both groups.[301] These findings provided the necessary impetus for the further development of systemic chemotherapeutic regimens for CRPC to affect patients' overall survival time and quality of life.

When should patients with CRPC be offered chemotherapy? The optimum timing of initiation of chemotherapy in men with CRPC is still undetermined. Given its relative ease of administration and cost, secondary hormonal therapy is a reasonable choice for use in asymptomatic or minimally symptomatic patients, those with low burdens of metastatic disease, and those with rising PSA concentrations with adverse kinetics. Observation alone is reasonable for men with indolent PSA kinetics and/or no evidence of metastatic disease. In men with symptomatic CRPC, though, docetaxel or cabazitaxel chemotherapy is preferable to existing secondary hormonal therapeutic agents, given the data demonstrating the survival and quality-of-life benefits of docetaxel. When a single site of disease is dominant and symptomatic in a threatened area such as the spinal column or weight-bearing bone, the use of palliative radiation therapy is reasonable to secure this area before the initiation of chemotherapy. Asymptomatic patients with widespread disease should also be considered for taxane-based chemotherapy.

The *optimal duration* of chemotherapy in CRPC is also undetermined. Continued treatment to two cycles beyond the best response followed by observation is reasonable and commonly used because cumulative fatigue is common with docetaxel-based therapy. Intermittent chemotherapy with a view toward retaining control and providing interrupted therapy for quality-of-life purposes has been described,[302] but the drug holidays become progressively shorter as drug resistance invariably emerges. In addition, the role of maintenance chemotherapy in patients with a stable response is uncertain, and its use must be balanced against emergent toxicity.

The *limits of benefit* of chemotherapy are clear with docetaxel, cabazitaxel, and with all other cytotoxic agents reported to date. Improvements in survival are tangible, but though comparable to those obtained in breast cancer, they remain modest. Another limitation is that therapeutic agents can be expensive and toxic, and the disease is still incurable, with few long-term survivors beyond 5 years.

Third-line therapy, used after treatment with cabazitaxel failures, has not been standardized, and for such patients, participation in a clinical trial should be strongly considered.[303] When assessing therapeutic options for a patient whose disease is taxane resistant, unexplored secondary hormonal maneuvers should be considered.

Consistent with the data that the *microtubule* is an important target in CRPC, *paclitaxel* has also demonstrated significant activity when given weekly as a single agent as well as in several estramustine-containing combinations.[304-306] MP therapy was considered the de facto standard after docetaxel failures, prior to the approval of cabazitaxel, but the results observed were discouraging, with 50% PSA decreases of approximately 20%.[307,308] Data for the role of MP following cabazitaxel have not been published to date. Oral cyclophosphamide given in chronic schedules has demonstrable activity in CRPC and is an alkylator-based approach, distinct from the approaches with the taxanes and anthracyclines described to date.[309,310]

In an effort to build on the taxane experience and the increased understanding of the biology of the disease, a number of randomized phase III clinical trials were conducted in the last decade to test the contribution of various targeted agents (including the endothelin receptor antagonist atrasentan,[311] the multitargeted antiangiogenic receptor tyrosine kinase inhibitor sunitinib,[312] the Src-kinase inhibitor dasatinib,[313] the VEGF inhibitors bevacizumab[314] and aflibercept,[315] the endothelina A receptor antagonist zibotentan,[316] and high-dose calcitriol[317]). Although many of these combinations resulted in a prolongation of progression-free survival over single-agent docetaxel, none resulted in improvements in overall survival.

Carboplatin[318] has also been evaluated in various combination regimens in phase II studies in CRPC[306,319-322] more recently with an emphasis on the treatment of aggressive variants of the disease sharing clinical and phenotypic features with the small-cell neuroendocrine carcinomas of the prostate[241,323] based on the hypothesis that the shared clinical features should predict for shared sensitivity to platinum-based chemotherapy.[20] It has been proposed that platinum sensitivity may be a distinguishing feature of a biologically distinct subset of CRPC and prospective studies are ongoing to test this hypothesis.

Bone-targeting therapy

The specific epithelial–stromal interactions that define the typical metastatic phenotype of prostate cancer are of critical interest. A mechanistic definition of the pathways to bone metastases, including epithelial–stromal interactions[324] (Figure 10) may yield a therapeutic approach that can successfully modulate the natural history of the disease. Given that the dominant morbidity and mortality from the disease can be traced to bone metastases, an organ-targeting strategy has long been of interest to the field. The hallmark pathologic feature of advanced disease in bone is carcinoma cells nested in woven bone with adjacent functionally active osteoblasts. These morphologic features correspond to the characteristic feature of bone-forming metastases that dominate clinical picture of men with advanced prostate cancer. There is intense research interest in modeling the early events of disease progression, including understanding the components and determinant physiologic characteristics of a putative metastatic niche in bone.

The principles of selective uptake in bone and prolonged retention of radiopharmaceutical agents at sites of increased bone mineral turnover guided initial studies of bone targeting in advanced prostate cancer. The natural affinity of the *radioisotope* strontium chloride Sr 89 (half-life 50 days) for the bone, on the basis of its strong homology with calcium, and the phosphonate-coupled samarium Sm 153 (half-life 1.9 days) permit delivery of medium-energy β emitters to the tumor–bone matrix interface.[325] These agents offer a palliative option,[326] and observations of a survival benefit in CRPC with consolidative radioisotope therapy after the initial response to chemotherapy[327] have sparked further interest in an organ-directed approach. A more effective radioisotope with favorable toxicity profile has been developed. RAD 223, an alpha-emitting and bone-homing radiopharmaceutical, has been approved for use in men with symptomatic prostate cancer bone metastases because it demonstrated relief of symptoms and prolongation of survival in men with CRPC.[328] Ongoing studies will determine its role in combination with newer antiandrogens or chemotherapy. RAD 223 has largely replaced strontium 89 and samarium in the United States and European countries.

Evidence of increased markers of bone resorption in cases of CRPC with bone metastases has justified the study of osteoclast-inhibitory bisphosphonates.[329] A large randomized

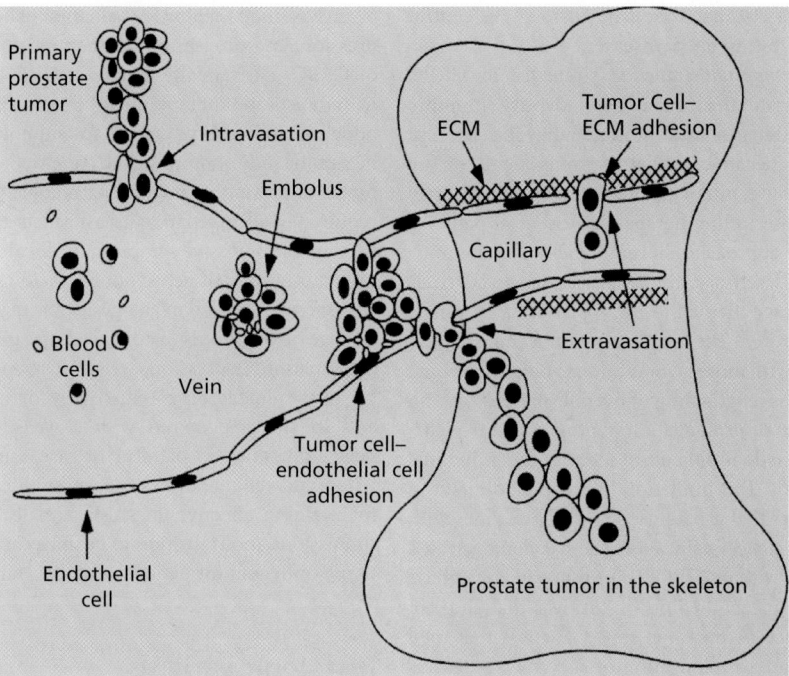

Figure 10 The multistage process of metastases: the pathophysiology of early events in the metastatic cascade, undetected dormant micrometastatic disease, and proliferative disease in the bone microenvironment are likely regulated by distinctive events with differing implications for therapy. Source: Chung 2001.[324] Reproduced with permission of Springer.

phase III trial evaluating zoledronic acid in men with CRPC receiving concomitant chemotherapy demonstrated a reduction in bone pain and "skeletal-related events" with the use of this highly potent bisphosphonate.[330] The receptor activator of nuclear factor κB (RANK) ligand antibody denosumab has demonstrated promising activity in reducing bone lysis markers in men with progressive CRPC treated with zoledronic acid. In a phase III study of 1904 patients comparing zoledronic acid and denosumab in CRPC, denosumab was superior in preventing skeletal-related events.[331] A prospective study of denosumab in men with nonmetastatic CRPC did not meaningfully delay the onset of bone metastases in men at high risk for bone progression.[332,333]

Several lines of evidence implicate the platelet-derived growth factor receptor (PDGFR) in the progression of disease in the bone. Preclinical studies with the PDGFR inhibitor imatinib mesylate in combination with taxane chemotherapy yielded promising results in an orthotopic lytic-dominant model of prostate cancer bone metastases.[334] However, the results from a randomized study of docetaxel with and without imatinib suggested potent inhibition of bone lysis markers without detectable clinical benefit.[335] Cabozantinib, a potent c-Met/VEGFR2, demonstrated striking efficacy in men with bone metastatic CRPC.[336] Surprisingly the efficacy in the phase II setting did not to translate into a survival benefit in met with treatment refractory CRPC in the phase III setting. The failure of these phase III studies points to the challenges faced by investigators to prioritize and apply laboratory observation(s) clinically and transition from phase II to phase III.

Future directions
The substantial limits of the efficacy of contemporary cytotoxic or available bone-targeting therapies in CRPC are known or predictable. It is highly unlikely that novel combinations, doses, or schedules of these agents will meaningfully transform the outcome of prostate cancer in patients. A deeper understanding of the molecular pathways involved in disease progression is now the

necessary basis for reassessing our perspectives about the disease and for advancing the exploration of novel therapeutic approaches. In this regard, novel strategies need to exploit the unique biology of the malignant epithelial cell—its angiogenic, inflammatory, and immunologic microenvironment—and the physical and chemical components of the inorganic matrix that determine survival and progression of disease.

Current perspectives targeting the epithelial cell are centered on androgen dependent pathways that may activate downstream androgen signaling independent of the androgen receptor or entirely independent of the androgen signaling.[40] Evidence that tissue androgens exist and AR signaling occurs despite medical castration[337] has justified continued AR targeting in castrate-resistant disease.[338] AR inactivation, whether by reducing or eliminating ligand synthesis, blocking the ligand–receptor interaction, enhancing degradation of the receptor, inhibiting AR nuclear translocation, or interfering with the interaction between the AR and androgen-response elements,[310] may spare putative AR-negative stem cells that perpetuate the disease.[40] Autopsy series have demonstrated the heterogeneity of AR expression with 40% of metastatic sites expressing <10% AR by immunohistochemistry.[339] The frequent inactivation of the PTEN tumor suppressor in high-grade disease with activation of the *PI3-kinase/Akt signaling and downstream cell survival and proliferation pathways* is currently a dominant theme in the framework of defining the lethal molecular phenotype.[340] Therapeutic agents targeting the AR and PI3-kinase/Akt signaling pathways are currently in trials. A high frequency of *novel gene fusions* in primary prostate cancer specimens was reported in 2005.[341] A 5′ untranslated region of a TMPRSS2 gene is fused to a 3′ ETS-1 family member in most specimens studied to date. These and other novel fusion genes have thus far been found only in malignant epithelial cells across all Gleason grades. The fusions appear nonrandom and are largely exclusive within each individual tumor across all tumor foci. The 5′ TMPRSS2 region contains an androgen-responsive promoter element, which also suggests that this gene fusion is a central biologic event in the progression of the disease.

The broad scope of *immunotherapeutic* strategies in CRPC includes efforts to integrate the innate and adaptive immune response using vaccine strategies and immune adjuvant. The use of agents that can block negative regulatory components of the physiologic immune response, tumor-associated angiogenesis, may modulate the host response to the therapeutic benefit of patients. Although current vaccine approaches have not yielded major anti-tumor activity in phase II settings, the results of phase III trials indicate a survival advantage that led to the approval of Provenge, a prostate cancer vaccine.[342,343] The lengthening of overall survival was greatest in the subset with more favorable (less volume) cancers. The perplexing finding was lengthening of overall survival with no observed tumor regression or prolongation of progression free survival. This outcome has made it difficult to identify the individual patients who derive benefit. This limitation has made it difficult to develop predictive markers that can be used to apply vaccines with greater precision. Immune checkpoint blockade has demonstrated effectiveness in selectmen with mCRPC. This finding led to a phase III study[344] demonstrating lengthening of survival that did not meet statistical significance. A post hoc subset analysis that men with favorable features had a prolongation of survival whereas as the with unfavorable features did not.[344] The lower-volume, more favorable patients not exposed to chemotherapy are the subject of an ongoing prospective randomized study. Overall vaccines and immune checkpoint blockade have demonstrated benefit in subsets of men in the more favorable groups with metastatic CRPC and show great promise for the future.

Summary perspectives

Advances in the understanding of the biology of prostate cancer in general and including CRPC has increased dramatically; we have access to technologies that allow us to characterize clinical prostate cancer in great detail; model systems that reflect the complexities of prostate cancer have been characterized, and multiple new therapies have been added to our clinical armamentarium.[345] These advances have created optimism and elevated the expectations of patients, physicians, and researchers. *The heterogeneity of virtually all known therapeutic targets* indicates that assessing biologic subsets with disproportionate benefit to specific interventions and understanding subsequent emergent resistance remain a preeminent challenge in experimental design. Progress toward achieving these goals has been made; for example, predictors of benefit or resistance to androgen inhibition have been proposed, and the characterization of variants that may benefit most for chemotherapy has been accomplished. These two groups may account for up to sixty percent of men with advanced prostate cancer and therefore serve as the solid foundation for the reclassification of prostate cancer. Acquisition of informative biomarkers is difficult, given the unique distribution of heterogeneous disease to bone; the phenotype of circulating tumor cells may vary substantially from those embedded in a metastatic environment under distinctive paracrine influences. The development of new methods to acquire relevant specimens and apply technologies to characterize them has demonstrated the potential of these strategies. These include enumeration or characterization of circulating tumor cells, bone marrow tumor cells, organoids, cytokine profile, and steroid metabolome.[293,346]

Palliative care

At no time in the management of CRPC is a focus on symptom control inappropriate. The selective and strategic use of external beam *radiation therapy* for palliation of bone pain, spinal cord compression, and prevention of fracture is critical in the management of CRPC. Early in the course of CRPC, external beam radiation or radioisotope therapy must be used sparingly, however, because bone marrow reserve critical for support of systemic therapy may be significantly compromised. *Palliative surgery* on the spine or long bones to prevent or manage pathologic fractures is less commonly required in CRPC than in breast cancer or myeloma. Surgical extirpation of progressive symptomatic localized CRPC can prevent the grievous burden of pelvic floor invasion. The services of a *palliative care specialist* skilled in analgesic pharmacy and the management of a range of symptoms of advanced disease such as anorexia, nausea, constipation, depression, weight loss, insomnia, and delirium can be very valuable. The rediscovery of methadone as an effective and inexpensive opioid with a well-defined safety margin has been influential on patterns of care, and it is the rare patient for whom indwelling devices such as epidural pumps are necessary for maintaining effective analgesia. Finally, facilitation of end-of-life discussions and transition to hospice care at the appropriate time is of major benefit for patients and their families.

Histologic variants

Markers

The WHO histological classification of tumors of the prostate[299] lists more than 30 histologic variants of tumors besides acinar adenocarcinoma that can affect the prostate (Table 7). This section describes the three most common of those variants.

Ductal adenocarcinomas

Of the epithelial tumor variants, the most common are the ductal adenocarcinomas, originally described by Melicow and Pachter[347] as endometrial carcinoma of the prostatic utricle. Once thought to arise from the verumontanum, a müllerian duct remnant, their prostatic origin has been firmly established, but the more recent controversy is centered on whether they truly represent a separate category of prostatic adenocarcinomas with a distinct biology, as opposed to a "mere morphological variant of prostatic adenocarcinoma."[348,349] Ductal adenocarcinomas of the prostate have been reported to constitute 0.13%[350] to 6.3%[351] of all prostate carcinomas. They are characterized by duct-like structures lined by single layer or pseudostratified tall columnar cells with abundant eosinophilic to amphophilic cytoplasm displaying a papillary, cribriform, solid, or glandular architecture.[349] Up to 20% present as pure ductal adenocarcinomas, but most cases are mixed with elements of acinar adenocarcinomas.[351-353] Ductal adenocarcinomas do not express any specific markers that differentiate them from acinar adenocarcinomas. They are strongly positive for PSA and PAP and often express alpha-methylacyl coenzyme A racemase (AMACR) and occasionally carcinoembryonic antigen (CEA).[354-356] Approximately 30% of these tumors demonstrate residual basal cells, as demonstrated by positive staining for high molecular weight cytokeratin (HMWCK or 34betaE12) and p63.[356]

Sarcomatoid carcinomas

Carcinomas of the prostate with spindle cell differentiation, also known as carcinosarcomas or sarcomatoid carcinomas, are rare tumors (with only approximately 100 cases described in the literature[357]) that are characterized by the presence of both malignant high-grade epithelial and mesenchymal components. The epithelial component consists most commonly of acinar adenocarcinoma

Table 7 WHO histologic classification of tumors of the prostate.

Tumor class	Tumor type	Tumor subtype
Epithelial	Glandular neoplasms	Adenocarcinoma (acinar)
		Atrophic
		Pseudohyperplastic
		Foamy
		Colloid
		Signet ring
		Oncocytic
		Lymphoepithelioma-like
		Carcinoma with spindle cell differentiation (carcinosarcoma, sarcomatoid carcinoma)
		Prostatic intraepithelial neoplasia (PIN)
		PIN, grade III (PIN III)
		Ductal adenocarcinoma
		Cribriform
		Papillary
		Solid
	Urothelial tumors	Urothelial carcinoma
	Squamous tumors	Adenosquamous carcinoma
		Squamous cell carcinoma
	Basal cell tumors	Basal cell adenoma
		Basal cell carcinoma
Neuroendocrine tumors		Endocrine differentiation within adenocarcinoma
		Carcinoid tumor
		Small-cell carcinoma
		Paraganglioma
		Neuroblastoma
Prostatic stromal tumors		Stromal tumor of uncertain malignant potential
		Stromal sarcoma
Mesenchymal tumors		Leiomyosarcoma
		Rhabdomyosarcoma
		Chondrosarcoma
		Angiosarcoma
		Malignant fibrous histiocytoma
		Malignant peripheral nerve sheath tumor
		Hemangioma
		Chondroma
		Leiomyoma
		Granular cell tumor
		Hemangiopericytoma
		Solitary fibrous tumor

but may consist of ductal adenocarcinoma or contain elements of small-cell or squamous cell carcinoma.[358–360] In approximately two-thirds of the cases, the mesenchymal component is a nonspecific malignant spindle cell proliferation, but in one-third, it displays specific mesenchymal elements such as those of osteosarcoma, chondrosarcoma, or rhabdomyosarcoma.[359] The adenocarcinoma components are positive for keratin, and the sarcomatoid elements are positive for vimentin. The adenocarcinoma components are also positive for PSA in approximately 75% of the cases.[358]

Neuroendocrine tumors

Of the nonepithelial variants of prostate cancers, neuroendocrine tumors are the most frequently encountered. The WHO classification includes focal neuroendocrine differentiation, carcinoid tumors, and small-cell neuroendocrine carcinoma under this name.[299] Focal neuroendocrine differentiation, when defined as immunohistochemical staining for neurosecretory products such as chromogranin A, serotonin, or synaptophysin, is encountered to some extent in almost all cases of acinar adenocarcinoma[361] and appears to increase during treatment with androgen deprivation.[362,363]

Small-cell carcinomas

Only 0.5–2% of clinical prostate tumor specimens contain small-cell carcinomas, but 12–20% of cases in autopsy series have revealed small-cell carcinoma in the context of acinar adenocarcinoma.[339,364,365] Between 42% and 75% of the clinical cases are preceded by a diagnosis of acinar adenocarcinoma, and mixed elements of high-grade acinar adenocarcinoma are present in 33–74% of the cases.[20,53,54,366,367]

Small-cell carcinomas of the prostate are characterized by small round to spindle-shaped malignant cells displaying scanty cytoplasm, with hyperchromatic nuclei, coarse (salt-and-pepper) chromatin, nuclear molding, and absent or inconspicuous nucleoli. These cells are arranged in sheets with frequent necrosis and a high mitotic rate.[368] Most but not all small-cell carcinomas stain positively for cytokeratin AE1/AE3 and CAM 5.2 (with a characteristic cytoplasmic dot-like pattern), as well as for neuroendocrine markers such as synaptophysin, chromogranin A, neuron-specific enolase, bombesin, and CD56.[52,53,367–369] They are also often positive for TTF-1 and P504S, occasionally positive for CEA, but rarely positive for PSA, PAP, or AR.[368,370]

Clinical presentations

Ductal adenocarcinomas

Ductal adenocarcinomas commonly manifest with symptoms of urinary obstruction and/or hematuria. Cystoscopic examination frequently reveals infiltration of the prostatic urethra and occasional polypoid or villous intraurethral projections arising at or near the verumontanum.[351,354] These tumors are typically high volume and locally advanced at diagnosis, with a 55–93% incidence of extraprostatic extension and a 20–47% incidence of positive margins reported in radical prostatectomy series.[352,353] In most instances, PSA levels are relatively high in patients with advanced disease,[352,371] although some cases manifest with serum PSA levels that are low relative to the tumor burden: in one series of 23 patients with metastatic disease, three patients (13%) had values <4 ng/mL.[372] Most prostatic ductal adenocarcinomas metastasize to the bone and lymph nodes, as acinar adenocarcinomas do, but they have also been found to metastasize to unusual sites such as the penis, testis, and visceral organs.[372,373]

Sarcomatoid carcinomas

Sarcomatoid carcinomas of the prostate typically manifest as large prostatic masses with local invasion, resulting in pelvic or perineal pain, lower abdominal mass, and symptoms of urinary obstruction with low serum PSA levels.[358,360,374] In more than half the cases, the diagnosis is preceded by a history of acinar adenocarcinoma treated with androgen-deprivation or radiation therapy, with the time between the original diagnosis of acinar adenocarcinoma and the diagnosis of sarcomatoid carcinoma ranging from 2 months to 16 years.[358,359,375,376] Both the carcinomatous and sarcomatous elements can metastasize, and metastatic disease is often present at the time of diagnosis, with the most common sites of nonlymph node metastases being the lung, bone, and brain.[358]

Small-cell carcinomas

Most patients with primary small-cell carcinomas have advanced-stage disease at their first visit, with large primary masses leading to lower urinary tract symptoms, bladder outlet obstruction, pelvic pain, ureteral obstruction, and/or hematuria.[54,366] Metastases are present in 75% of patients at the time of diagnosis of small-cell carcinoma.[54] When preceded by a diagnosis of acinar adenocarcinoma of the prostate, the time between that original diagnosis and the diagnosis of small-cell carcinoma can range between 1.5 months and 10 years.[20,54,366,367] Metastases are most often located in pelvic lymph nodes, liver, lungs, and bones,[54,366] although bony metastases are often osteolytic instead of osteoblastic, as would be typical for acinar adenocarcinoma.[52,367] Metastases to uncommon sites, such as the epididymis,[369] subcutaneous tissue,[20] pericardium,[52] or omentum,[366] have been described. Brain metastases occur in up to 20% of patients during the course of the disease, so MRI of the brain or contrast-enhanced CT should be performed as part of the staging workup.[54,367] Serum PSA and PAP levels are often within normal ranges, but serum CEA and lactic acid dehydrogenase levels have been found to be higher than normal in 53–65% and 39–76% of patients, respectively.[20,367] Elevated levels of circulating bombesin, calcitonin, adrenocorticotropic hormone, and somatostatin have also been observed.[367] As is the case for small-cell carcinomas of the lung, a number of paraneoplastic syndromes have been described in association with small-cell carcinomas of the prostate, including hypercalcemia,[369] elevated adrenocorticotropic hormone,[377] syndrome of inappropriate antidiuretic hormone,[52] myasthenic syndrome,[366] and hyperglucagonemia.[378]

Therapy options and applications

Ductal adenocarcinomas

The natural history of ductal adenocarcinomas is debated. Some series describe cases with indolent courses and prolonged survival,[371,373,379,380] whereas others describe cases with aggressive courses and relatively low 5-year survival rates.[351–354] Some authors have proposed that the pure ductal adenocarcinomas have a more indolent behavior, and the prognosis of the more common mixed ductal adenocarcinomas is dictated by the acinar component, which is frequently high grade.[371] Much like acinar adenocarcinomas, most ductal adenocarcinomas are sensitive to both radiation and hormone-deprivation therapies.[350] No published data support the use of chemotherapeutic treatments in this disease other than standard regimens for acinar adenocarcinomas.

Sarcomatoid carcinomas

The prognosis of prostatic sarcomatoid carcinomas is poor, regardless of the histologic type of the sarcomatous elements.[358,359,374] In a 21-patient series with a median follow-up of 10 months (range 1–107 months), 18 patients died of their tumor within the follow-up period,[358] and in a more recent 32-patient series, the actuarial risk of death at 1 year was estimated at 20%.[359] Androgen-deprivation therapy is usually administered to target the malignant epithelial component, and the use of chemotherapy drugs typically administered for the treatment of sarcomas, such as ifosfamide and doxorubicin, has been reported.[360,374] However, among the nine patients given chemotherapy containing docetaxel, estramustine, carboplatinum, or cisplatinum in the series of Hansel et al.,[358] three died within 1 year of the diagnosis, and in five the cancer was unresponsive to chemotherapy. Given the morbidity caused by the local invasion of the primary tumors, palliative surgery (which often will need to involve anterior exenterations with urinary diversion) with or without adjuvant radiation may be appropriate. It is noteworthy that the only long-term survivor described by Dundore et al.[357] was treated by pelvic exenteration and resection of lung metastases. Two other patients in their series, who survived 89 and 107 months, were treated with intratumoral iodine 125 (^{125}I) before dying of carcinosarcoma.

Small-cell carcinomas

Although chemotherapeutic agents are active in the treatment of small-cell carcinomas of the prostate, the prognosis remains poor, with reported median survival times ranging from 5 to 17.5 months.[20,52,366,367] In a recent 83-patient retrospective series, patients with nonmetastatic disease at their initial visit appeared to do slightly better (median disease-specific survival 17.1 months vs 12.5 months in patients with metastatic disease at the initial visit), although only 20% of the patients with nonmetastatic disease received local therapy in addition to systemic therapy.[54] Since these are radiosensitive tumors[381] and at least one patient was apparently cured by surgical excision,[382] it is clear that the role of local therapies deserves further investigation in this patient population. In a 21-patient series described by Amato et al.,[366] four of eight patients responded to a combination of vincristine, doxorubicin, and cyclophosphamide. In a 38-patient phase II study of doxorubicin, etoposide, and cisplatin in patients with histologically proven small-cell carcinoma of the prostate (either pure or mixed with adenocarcinoma), the response rate in patients with measurable disease was 61%, and 84% of symptomatic patients experienced pain reduction.[367] However, there were no complete responses, and the median time to progression and median overall survival were short, at 5.8 months and 10.5 months, respectively. It was concluded that the addition of doxorubicin to the standard etoposide–cisplatin regimen increased the toxic effects without any apparent increase in efficacy. It is also noteworthy that none of the 13 patients subjected to antiandrogen withdrawal in this study responded to that maneuver.[367] It should be noted that even though small-cell carcinomas do not appear to respond to androgen-deprivation therapies, a large proportion of cases have shown coexisting components of acinar adenocarcinoma, so it is recommended that hormonal therapy accompany chemotherapy in the treatment of this disease.[20,52]

Algorithm for therapy: future directions

The main question about these histologic variants is whether they represent true biologic variants with different responses to standard treatments for prostate acinar adenocarcinomas that would require different therapeutic approaches, although differences in prognosis as treatment response profiles between the extremes of morphologic groupings (small-cell vs acinar adenocarcinoma) are obvious. However these are rare subsets and are often insufficient discriminators to make decisions in the majority of patients. Aparicio et al. noted that a group of men with CRPC and clinical features of small-cell cancers had heterogeneous morphologies but shared chemotherapy response profiles, prognosis, and shared biology in experimental model systems. These clinicopathologically identified variant prostate cancers with aggressive feature were dubbed "anaplastic prostate cancer." The report highlights to the inadequacy of morphological characterization in predicting benefit to specific therapies and the urgent need to add molecular classification that reflects "driver biology."

For all three variants, the role of local therapies remains to be determined, and in the case of small-cell carcinoma, it is reasonable to ask whether prophylactic brain irradiation should be offered to patients whose systemic disease is otherwise controlled.

Key references

The complete reference list can be found on the Wiley Companion Digital Edition of this title (see inside front cover for login instructions).

2 McNeal JE. Normal histology of the prostate. *Am J Surg Pathol.* 1988;**12**:619–633.

8 Logothetis CJ, Navone NM, Lin SH. Understanding the biology of bone metastases: key to the effective treatment of prostate cancer. *Clin Cancer Res.* 2008;**14(6)**:1599–1602.

10 Walsh PC. Anatomic radical prostatectomy: evolution of the surgical technique. *J Urol.* 1998;**160(6 pt 2)**:2418–2424.

15 De Marzo AM, Marchi VL, Epstein JI, Nelson WG. Proliferative inflammatory atrophy of the prostate: implications for prostatic carcinogenesis. *Am J Pathol.* 1999;**155**:1985–1992.

19 Bostwick DG. The pathology of early prostate cancer. *CA Cancer J Clin.* 1989;**39**:376–393.

20 Papandreou CN, Daliani DD, Thall PF, et al. Results of a phase II study with doxorubicin, etoposide, and cisplatin in patients with fully characterized small-cell carcinoma of the prostate. *J Clin Oncol.* 2002;**20(14)**:3072–3080.

25 Gleason DF. Classification of prostatic carcinomas. *Cancer Chemother Rep.* 1966;**50**:125–128.

33 Chan JM, Stampfer MJ, Giovannucci E, et al. Plasma insulin-like growth factor-I and prostate cancer risk: a prospective study. *Science.* 1998;**279**:563–566.

35 Ware JL. Growth factors and their receptors as determinants in the proliferation and metastasis of human prostate cancer. *Cancer Metastasis Rev.* 1993;**12(3–4)**:287–301.

39 Taplin ME, Bubley GJ, Shuster TD, et al. Mutation of the androgen-receptor gene in metastatic androgen-independent prostate cancer. *N Engl J Med.* 1995;**332**:1393–1398.

72 Lilja H, Cronin AM, Scardino PT, Dahlin A, Bajartel A, Berglund G. A single PSA predicts prostate cancer up to 30 years subsequently, even in men below age 40. *J Urol.* 2008;**179(206**:abstract 589. Presented 18 May 2008 at the American Urological Association's Annual Meeting in Orlando, Florida).

74 Schroder FH, Denis LJ, Roobol M, et al. The story of the European Randomized Study of Screening for Prostate Cancer. *BJU Int.* 2003;**92(Suppl 2)**:1–13.

75 Thompson I, Tangen C, Paradelo J, et al. Adjuvant radiotherapy for pathologically advanced prostate cancer: a randomized clinical trial. *JAMA.* 2006;**296(19)**:2329–2335.

80 Thompson IM, Ankerst DP, Chi C, et al. Operating characteristics of prostate-specific antigen in men with an initial PSA level of 3.0 ng/ml or lower. *JAMA.* 2005;**294(1)**:66–70.

85 Etzioni RD, Ankerst DP, Weiss NS, Inoue LY, Thompson IM. Is prostate-specific antigen velocity useful in early detection of prostate cancer? A critical appraisal of the evidence. *J Natl Cancer Inst.* 2007;**99(20)**:1510–1515.

91 D'Amico AV, Whittington R, Malkowicz SB, et al. Biochemical outcome after radical prostatectomy, external beam radiation therapy, or interstitial radiation therapy for clinically localized prostate cancer. *JAMA.* 1998;**280(11)**:969–974.

96 American Urological Association. *Guideline for the Management of Clinically Localized Prostate Cancer: 2007 Update.* Linthicum, MD: American Urological Association Education and Research, Inc.; 2007.

101 Partin AW, Kattan MW, Subong EN, et al. Combination of prostate-specific antigen, clinical stage, and Gleason score to predict pathological stage of localized prostate cancer. A multi-institutional update. *JAMA.* 1997;**277(18)**:1445–1451.

104 Epstein JI. Gleason score 2–4 adenocarcinoma of the prostate on needle biopsy: a diagnosis that should not be made. *Am J Surg Pathol.* 2000;**24(4)**:477–478.

105 Ochiai A, Troncoso P, Chen ME, Lloreta J, Babaian RJ. The relationship between tumor volume and the number of positive cores in men undergoing multisite extended biopsy: implication for expectant management. *J Urol.* 2005;**174(6)**:2164–2168.

119 Parker C. Active surveillance: an individualized approach to early prostate cancer. *BJU Int.* 2003;**92**:2–3.

120 Johansson JE, Holmberg L, Johansson S, Bergstrom R, Adami HO. Fifteen-year survival in prostate cancer: a prospective, population-based study in Sweden. *JAMA.* 1997;**277**:467–471.

121 Albertsen PC, Hanley JA, Gleason DF, Barry MJ. Competing risk analysis of men aged 55 to 74 years at diagnosis managed conservatively for clinically localized prostate cancer. *JAMA.* 1998;**280**:975–980.

130 Klotz L. Active surveillance with selective delayed intervention: using natural history to guide treatment in good risk prostate cancer. *J Urol.* 2004;**172**:S48–S51.

140 Wood DP, Schulte R, Dunn RL, et al. Short-term health outcome differences between robotic and conventional radical prostatectomy. *Urology.* 2007;**70(5)**:945–949.

149 Marcovich R, Wojno KJ, Wei JT, Rubin MA, Montie JE, Sanda MG. Bladder neck-sparing modification of radical prostatectomy adversely affects surgical margins in pathologic T3a prostate cancer. *Urology.* 2000;**55(6)**:904–908.

157 Roach M III, Hanks G, Thames H Jr, et al. Defining biochemical failure following radiotherapy with or without hormonal therapy in men with clinically localized prostate cancer: recommendations of the RTOG-ASTRO Phoenix Consensus Conference. *Int J Radiat Oncol Biol Phys.* 2006;**65**:965–974.

158 Pollack A, Zagars GK, Starkschall G, et al. Prostate cancer radiation dose response: results of the M. D. Anderson phase III randomized trial. *Int J Radiat Oncol Biol Phys.* 2002;**53**:1097.

161 Gleave ME, Goldenberg SL, Chin JL, et al. Randomized comparative study of 3- versus 8-month neoadjuvant hormonal therapy before radical prostatectomy: biochemical and pathological effects. *J Urol.* 2001;**166**:500–506.

163 Bolla M, Collette L, Blank L, et al. Longterm results with immediate androgen suppression and external irradiation in patients with locally advanced prostate cancer (an EORTC study): a phase III randomised trial. *Lancet.* 2002;**360**:103–108.

164 Thompson I, Thrasher JB, Aus G, et al. Guidelines for the management of clinically localized prostate cancer: 2007 update. *J Urol.* 2007;**177(6)**:2106–2131.

180 D'Amico AV, Chen MH, Roehl KA, Catalona WJ. Preoperative PSA velocity and the risk of death from prostate cancer after radical prostatectomy. *N Engl J Med.* 2004;**351(2)**:125–135.

187 Thompson IM, Chi C, Ankerst DP, et al. Effect of finasteride on the sensitivity of PSA for detecting prostate cancer. *J Natl Cancer Inst.* 2006;**98(16)**:1128–1133.

188 Lucia MS, Darke A, Goodman PJ, et al. Pathologic characteristics of cancers detected in the Prostate Cancer Prevention Trial: implications for prostate detection and chemoprevention. *Cancer Prev Res.* 2008;**1(3)**:167–173.

201 U.S. National Institutes of Health. *Finasteride in Treating Patients Undergoing Surgery for Stage II Prostate Cancer.* J Kim, principal investigator. Bethesda, MD: U.S. National Institutes of Health; 2008, http://clinicaltrials.gov/ct2/show/NCT00438464.

208 Roach M III, Bae K, Speight J, et al. Short-term neoadjuvant androgen deprivation therapy and external-beam radiotherapy for locally advanced prostate cancer: long-term results of RTOG 8610. *J Clin Oncol.* 2008;**26**:585–591.

216 Kuban D, Tucker S, Dong L, et al. Long-term results of the M. D. Anderson randomized dose-escalation trial for prostate cancer. *Int J Radiat Oncol Biol Phys.* 2008;**70**:67–74.

223 Aus G, Abrahamson P, Ahlgren G, et al. Three-month neoadjuvant hormonal therapy before radical prostatectomy: a 7-year follow-up of a randomized controlled trial. *BJU Int.* 2002;**90**:561–566.

225 Pettaway C, Pisters L, Troncoso P, et al. Neoadjuvant chemotherapy and hormonal therapy followed by radical prostatectomy: feasibility and preliminary results. *J Clin Oncol.* 2000;**18**:1050–1057.

246 Pound CR, Partin AW, Eisenberger MA, et al. Natural history of progression after PSA elevation following radical prostatectomy. *JAMA.* 1999;**281**:1591–1597.

254 Pilepich MV, Winter K, Lawton CA, et al. Androgen suppression adjuvant to definitive radiotherapy in prostate carcinoma—long-term results of Phase III RTOG 85-31. *Int J Radiat Oncol Biol Phys.* 2005;**61**:1285–1290.

257 The Medical Research Council Prostate Cancer Working Party Investigators Group. Immediate versus deferred treatment for advanced prostatic cancer—initial results of the Medical Council Research Trial. *Br J Urol.* 1997;**79**:235–246.

265 Millikan RE, Wen S, Pagliaro LC, et al. Phase III trial of androgen ablation with or without 3 cycles of systemic chemotherapy for advanced prostate cancer. *J Clin Oncol.* 2008;**26(36)**:5936–5942.

271 Tannock IF, Osoba D, Stockler MR, et al. Chemotherapy with mitoxantrone plus prednisone or prednisone alone for symptomatic hormone-resistant prostate cancer: a Canadian randomized trial with palliative endpoints. *J Clin Oncol.* 1996;**14(6)**:1756–1764.

274 Halabi S, Small EJ, Kantoff PW, et al. Prognostic model for predicting survival in men with hormone-refractory metastatic prostate cancer. *J Clin Oncol.* 2003;**21**:1232–1237.

329 Smith MR. Osteoclast targeted therapy for prostate cancer: bisphosphonates and beyond. *Urol Oncol.* 2008;**26**:420–425.

99 Tumors of the penis and the urethra

James F. Holland, MD, ScD (hc) ▪ Raymond S. Lance, MD ▪ Donald F. Lynch, Jr., MD

Overview

Carcinoma of the penis, predominantly squamous, some related to human papilloma virus, is rare in the developed world and among circumcised men, but of major importance elsewhere. Surgery early can be curative. Other modalities are less robust. Voluntary adult circumcision to diminish susceptibility to human immunodeficiency virus infection is being observed as possibly preventive. Urethral cancer, rare, usually of transitional epithelium, is often detected too late for cure.

Squamous carcinoma of the penis is a largely preventable disease, dependent on early circumcision, personal hygiene, access to healthcare, and avoidance of human papilloma virus (HPV). Because the disease is rare in the developed world, the efficacy of HPV immunization will likely be determined in the developing world. Early recognition of tumor lesions correlates with lower staging and more effective treatment with better organ sparing and lower mortality.

Cancer of the penis is an unusual disease in the United States (<2000/year) and Europe, but is a major health problem in Africa, Asia, and South America. Approximately 95% of primary penile cancers are squamous cell carcinomas (SCCs) (Figure 1). Other cancers involving the penis are verrucous carcinoma, alternatively known as giant condyloma or Buschke-Lowenstein tumor, a variant of squamous carcinoma which does not metastasize, but which spreads aggressively by local extension and destroys surrounding tissue (Figure 2).[1] Epidemic Kaposi's sarcoma associated with acquired immunodeficiency syndrome (AIDS) is now uncommon (Figure 3). Melanoma and basal cell carcinoma very rarely involve the penis. A scaly red clearly demarked intraepithelial squamous carcinoma *in situ* (CIS) is denominated Bowen's disease when it involves the base of the penis and the scrotum. When CIS involves the glans or prepuce, it appears as shiny red velvet and is known as erythroplasia of Queyrat (Figure 4). Carcinomas *in situ* have the potential to develop into invasive squamous carcinoma in about 20%. Biopsy is required to establish a diagnosis. Leukemias and lymphomas can present as priapism. Diagnosis and therapy for them are systemic.

Epidemiology and etiology

In countries where infant circumcision is common, such as Israel and the United States, the incidence of squamous carcinoma of the penis is low. Circumcision later in life has not conferred protection, perhaps because it was done for cause such as phimosis and balanitis.[2] Proper hygiene is made difficult by phimosis, perpetuating chronic inflammation of the glans penis and preputial tissue. Inexpensive adult circumcision as a protective measure against human

immunodeficiency virus (HIV) infection, recently practiced in Africa, may alter this information.[2]

An association between cervical cancer in women whose partners have penile cancer has been observed, and squamous carcinoma of the penis and of the cervix has been associated with human papilloma viruses (HPV [16,18,31]).[3] The foreskin of 9% of uncircumcised preadolescent boys contained HPV, attesting to the ubiquity of this virus.[4] Uncircumcised men are three times more likely to harbor HPV than circumcised men, and female partners of circumcised men are less likely to develop cervical cancer.[5,6] HPV shedding may occur in asymptomatic carriers, in those with unrecognized intraurethral lesions, or men with condyloma accuminata, exposing their partners of either sex. Tobacco smoking is correlated with increased HPV infection and cancer of the penis and cervix.[5]

Diagnosis

Early invasive tumors may be small and largely unremarkable, sometimes resembling small abrasions (hair cuts) or calloused thickenings of penile skin. The initial lesion of squamous carcinoma most commonly presents on the glans or prepuce. It varies from a small, velvety, reddened, raised maculopapule to an ulcer, hyperkeratotic area, or exophytic papillary tumor. Biopsy is required to make the diagnosis and should include contiguous normal skin for comparison.[1] More advanced lesions may be exophytic or ulcerated, and very advanced cancers may completely destroy the penile shaft. Metastases to the inguinal lymph nodes may produce large ulcerations in the groin late in the course of the disease. Well-differentiated tumors tend to metastasize infrequently, while more poorly differentiated tumors have a high propensity for early metastasis. Several studies have confirmed that higher tumor grade increases the likelihood of inguinal nodal metastases.[7]

Metastasis

Invasive squamous carcinoma of the penis follows a predictable pattern of metastasis. Lesions of the glans, coronal sulcus, prepuce, and distal shaft spread to the deep inguinal nodes, while lesions of the proximal shaft and base of the penis spread to the more lateral and superficial inguinal nodes. Subsequent spread to the external iliac, obturator, and iliac chains follows.[8] Metastases to distant sites are infrequent and occur late in the course of disease. Left untreated, penile cancer progresses, causing the deaths of the majority of those untreated within 3 years.

Because primary lesions may be infected or chronically inflamed, secondary inflammation of the inguinal nodes is often present which may be difficult to distinguish from metastatic disease. Careful re-examination of the inguinal nodes following a 4–6-week course of broad-spectrum antibiotic therapy may help to differentiate inflammation from cancer.

Holland-Frei Cancer Medicine, Ninth Edition. Edited by Robert C. Bast Jr., Carlo M. Croce, William N. Hait, Waun Ki Hong, Donald W. Kufe, Martine Piccart-Gebhart, Raphael E. Pollock, Ralph R. Weichselbaum, Hongyang Wang, and James F. Holland.
© 2017 John Wiley & Sons, Inc. ISBN: 978-1-118-93469-2

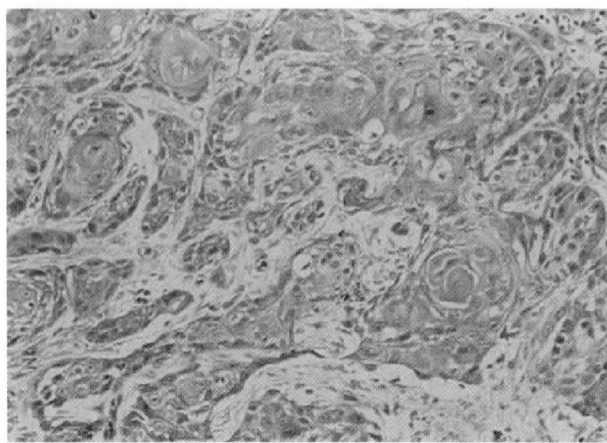

Figure 1 Microscopic squamous cell carcinoma, moderately well differentiated, with characteristic keratin pearl formation.

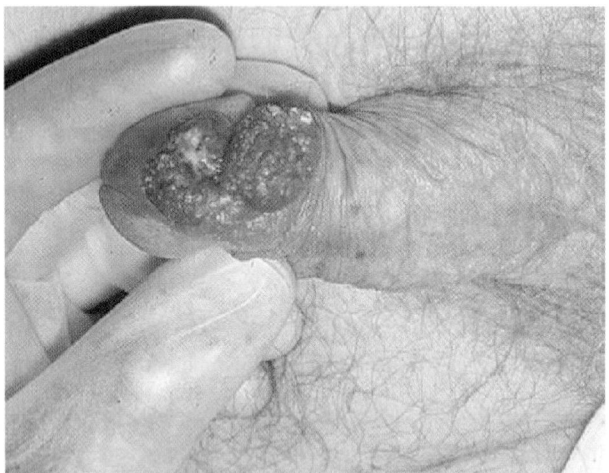

Figure 2 Verrucous carcinoma (Buschke-Lowenstein tumor).

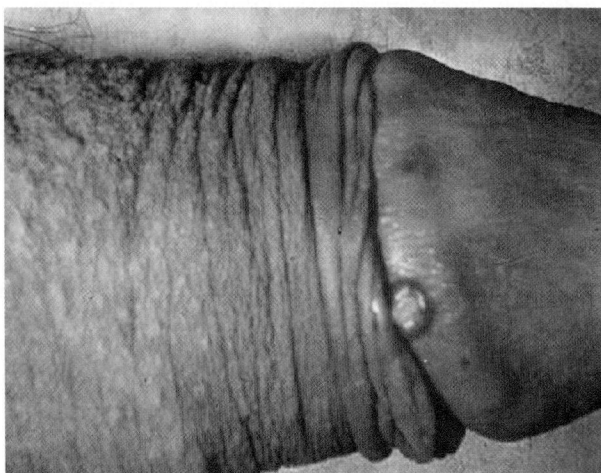

Figure 3 Lesion of epidemic (AIDS-related) Kaposi sarcoma involving glans. Courtesy of Dr. Victor Marcial.

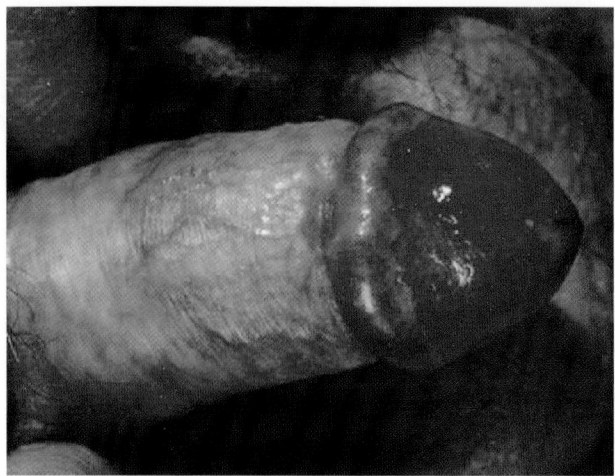

Figure 4 Erythroplasia of Queyrat of glans.

Tumor staging

Once the diagnosis of squamous carcinoma is established, complete staging is undertaken. Inguinal nodes are carefully palpated. Additional studies should include chest X-ray, computerized tomography (CT) of the pelvis and inguinal regions, and possibly magnetic resonance imaging (MRI).[9] Positron emission tomography-computerized tomography (PET-CT) and MRI are superior to palpation for detection of suspicious nodal enlargement. Lymph angiography is no longer used as a staging procedure. MRI provides good discrimination of penile structures and may identify corpora cavernosal or spongiosal invasion.

The American Joint Committee on Cancer (AJCC) Tumor, Nodes, Metastases (TNM) system, seventh edition, is the accepted staging system for penile cancer (Table 1).

Surgical treatment

Treatment of penile cancer is based on the extent of the primary tumor and its tumor grade, established by biopsy of the lesion. Antibiotic therapy is begun before biopsy and continued throughout surgical treatment and from 4 to 6 weeks afterward. Lymph node metastasis is assessed. Once the tissue diagnosis is confirmed, small superficial tumors may be treated successfully with local surgical excision, LASER surgery,[11] Mohs' micrographic surgery,[12] or superficial radiation therapy.

Larger tumors with invasion may sometimes be managed with organ-sparing surgery or radiotherapy (RT), but deeply invasive cancers, particularly those that deform the glans or that involve the shaft structures, may not be amenable to conservative measures. These lesions, which involve the distal shaft or glans, are usually managed by partial penectomy providing that a 2-cm margin can be achieved and still leave enough penile length to allow voiding while standing and to permit intercourse.[13,14] More advanced cancers that involve the base of the penis are best managed by total penectomy with creation of a perineal urethrostomy.[14] Extensive lesions that involve the base of the penis and the bulbar urethral portion may require cystoprostatectomy or even anterior or total pelvic exenteration with urinary diversion.

Inguinal or pelvic lymph node metastasis constitutes an important factor predicting survival in men with SCC of the penis. The superficial inguinal lymph nodes receive lymphatic drainage from the penile shaft and base. The deep inguinal lymph nodes receive

Table 1 AJCC (2010) TNM staging of penile cancer.

Primary tumor (T)	
TX	Primary tumor cannot be assessed
T0	No evidence of primary tumor
Tis	Carcinoma *in situ*
Ta	Noninvasive verrucous carcinoma[a]
T1a	Tumor invades subepithelial connective tissue without lymph vascular invasion and is not poorly differentiated (i.e., grades 3–4)
T1b	Tumor invades subepithelial connective tissue with lymph vascular invasion or is poorly differentiated
T2	Tumor invades corpus spongiosum or cavernosum
T3	Tumor invades urethra
T4	Tumor invades other adjacent structures

Regional lymph nodes (N)
Clinical stage definition[a]

cNX	Regional lymph nodes cannot be assessed
cN0	No palpable or visibly enlarged inguinal lymph nodes
cN1	Palpable mobile unilateral inguinal lymph node
cN2	Palpable mobile multiple or bilateral inguinal lymph nodes
cN3	Palpable fixed inguinal nodal mass or pelvic lymphadenopathy unilateral or bilateral

Anatomic stage/prognostic groups

Stage 0	Tis	N0	M0
	Ta	N0	M0
Stage I	T1a	N0	M0
Stage II	T1b	N0	M0
	T2	N0	M0
	T3	N0	M0
Stage IIIa	T1–3	N1	M0
Stage IIIb	T1–3	N2	M0
Stage IV	T4	Any N	M0
	Any T	N3	M0
	Any T	Any N	M1

ICD-O-3 topography codes	
C60.0	Prepuce
C60.1	Glans penis
C60.2	Body of penis
C60.8	Overlapping lesion of penis
C60.9	Penis, NOS

[a]Clinical stage definition based on palpation, imaging.
Source: Edge et al.[10] Reproduced with permission of Springer.

drainage from the glans, prepuce, and distal shaft. There is crossover of the lymphatic channels at the base of the penis so that a lesion on one side of the penis may metastasize to the contralateral inguinal nodes. The deep inguinal nodes drain to the external iliac and obturator chains and, subsequently, to the common iliac nodes and the retroperitoneal nodes surrounding the aorta and inferior vena cava.[15]

A meticulous inguinal node dissection is curative in 40–60% of cases. Traditional node dissection carries with it a high likelihood of morbidity: flap necrosis, wound infection, chronic lymphangitis, lymphocele, and chronic lower limb edema. A modified, less extensive dissection has been adopted by many surgeons, which has reduced some of the adverse sequelae of groin dissection.[16] Nonetheless, inguinal node dissection should not be undertaken lightly, and clinical and imaging assessment should be made. Inguinal lymph nodes are palpable in 50–82% of patients at initial diagnosis. In only about half these cases is cancer found on lymph node dissection.[17] Lymphadenectomy may be indicated if palpable nodes remain after 4–6 weeks of antibiotic therapy. PET-CT and MRI should be done at that time. Sentinel node biopsy may

be helpful. About 25% of patients with impalpable nodes have metastatic disease and should undergo a node resection.[18] For those with impalpable nodes and negative imaging studies, close and continued follow-up is essential with repeated imaging and examination.[19,20] Patients with metastases to the groin who do not undergo appropriate node dissection usually die of their disease within 3 years.

Tumor grade

Tumor grade as well as stage is important in assessing the risk of nodal metastases. Patients with grade I well-differentiated tumors that are limited to the skin and superficial tissues of the penis are unlikely to have tumor metastases to inguinal nodes. Patients with moderately or poorly differentiated lesions with any degree of invasion of the deeper penile structures are at significant risk of groin metastasis.[19] Contemporary practice supports early surgery if higher grade tumor and more than superficial invasion are documented on biopsy.

Pelvic lymphadenectomy

Patients found to have inguinal node metastases should undergo pelvic lymphadenectomy on the affected side.[21] This can be done extraperitoneally via a midline incision or through a modified groin incision at the time of inguinal node dissection, although at some centers the procedure is staged several weeks later. Patients with three or less lymph nodes below the bifurcation of the external and internal iliac vessels often do well, but metastases above the bifurcation have usually been fatal.

Radiotherapy

Primary RT of penile cancer is used more widely in Europe than in the United States but may be appropriate for small superficial lesions or for selected larger lesions when organ preservation is the goal, or when patients refuse surgery.[22] Tissue preservation may not be feasible in more advanced lesions, however. Concurrent chemotherapy may enhance the effectiveness of RT. RT can be delivered either as external beam administered with wax block delivery or as brachytherapy with a mold or with Iridium[192] wires. Iridium[192] or Cesium[137] may be used to boost dosages in bulky or extremely cornified tumors. The normal dose is 30–50 Gy given over 3–5 weeks. Boosts to 65–70 Gy utilizing various brachytherapy techniques may follow if clinically indicated. RT is often the treatment of choice in symptomatic lesions of Kaposi's sarcoma. RT may be used as primary therapy in a select group of men presenting with localized penile cancer.[23] This group is small but includes young men with small superficial noninvasive lesions located on the distal penis and those who refuse to have surgery as initial treatment. In addition, RT is used for men with inoperable tumors.

Acute radiation reactions—edema, tissue inflammation, skin irritation, tenderness, and dysuria—are common. Such symptoms usually subside promptly when therapy is completed. Long-term effects of radiation may include telangiectasia, hyperpigmentation, diminished sensation, scarring, and atrophy of the treated tissues. Fibrotic change and fistulization may occur in large lesions where significant tissue damage has occurred before the RT. Late recurrences in radiated sites may occur up to a decade after definitive treatment, affirming that close follow-up is essential.

Randomized trials comparing RT to surgery have not been reported. In one study of clinically localized penile cancer, local regional relapse occurred in 56% of those treated with definitive primary radiation therapy compared to 13% of those treated by surgery. Of the RT failures, 73% were salvaged with surgery.[24]

RT to the groin following inguinal surgery increases complications. Some studies have suggested benefit from such treatment, while others show no improvement when compared with patients treated by surgery alone. RT to bulky unresectable lymph node metastases is rarely effective, except as a palliative measure, usually in concert with systemic chemotherapy.

Chemotherapy

Chemotherapy is used in treating penile cancer as an adjuvant to definitive surgical or radiation therapy or as a radiosensitizer. Experience with various treatment protocols is limited by the relative rarity of the disease. Combination chemotherapy with vincristine, bleomycin, and methotrexate (VBM) has been successful in rendering patients with fixed nodal metastases resectable.[25] Extensive experience with cisplatin or carboplatin in combination with fluorouracil, paclitaxel, or docetaxel has caused regression in SCCs of esophagus, head and neck, and anus. Many of these cancers are also related to HPV. The recognition that the molecular characteristics of SCCs are more relevant than their organs of origin supports the use of these agents in SCC of the penis. Neoadjuvant chemotherapy can reduce tumor burden under direct observation.[26] Postoperative adjuvant chemotherapy requires a randomized series to establish its definitive value. Although used simultaneously with radiation, adjuvant chemotherapy has been used after surgery on the presumption of its importance by analogy with proven effectiveness in other sites. Where positive nodes have been excised, there are many data to support adjuvant chemotherapy. In patients where SCCs of the penis have been totally removed, who do not have inguinal metastases on biopsy, or even on the basis of clinical and imaging negativity, the use of adjuvant chemotherapy is still controversial.

Prognosis

Left untreated, squamous carcinoma of the penis is invariably lethal, killing most of those afflicted within 3 years. Outcome is directly related to the extent of the disease at diagnosis and the presence or absence of inguinal metastases. Disease-related survival for localized tumor is approximately 80%, for regional nodal disease about 50%, and for pelvic metastases about 10%. In a retrospective study of men with positive pelvic lymph nodes, adjuvant chemotherapy resulted in a median survival of 22 months versus 10 months in its absence.[27] In a prospective study of cisplatin, fluorouracil, and a taxane for men with N2 or N3 M0 disease, disease-free survival at 2 years was only 37%.[26]

Carcinoma of the urethra

Male urethral carcinoma

The male urethra averages some 18 cm in length and is subdivided into the penile urethra, the membranous urethra, and the prostatic urethra. Beginning distally, the penile urethra is composed of the meatus and fossa navicularis, which is lined with stratified squamous epithelium. The pendulous urethra extends from the proximal fossa navicularis to the suspensory ligament of the penis, where it then becomes the bulbar urethra between the ligament and the urogenital membrane. These areas are lined with stratified or pseudo-stratified columnar epithelium as is the short (1.5 cm)

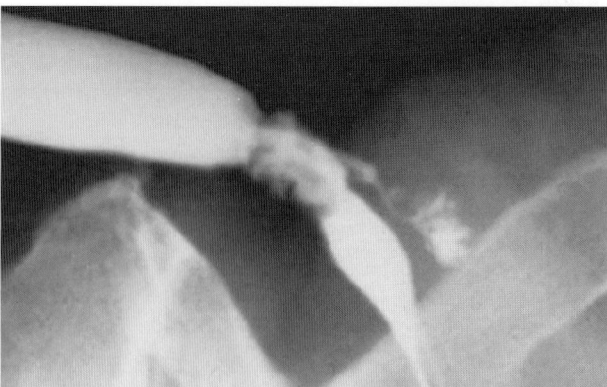

Figure 5 Retrograde urethrogram demonstrating squamous cell carcinoma of bulbous urethra associated with a stricture.

membranous urethra. This contains the external sphincter, which is composed of striated muscle fibers. The prostatic urethra passes through the prostate and is lined with transitional cell epithelium.

From 50% to 75% of male urethral cancers arise in the bulbar urethra (Figure 5). The remainder occurs predominantly in the fossa navicularis. About 90% of male urethral tumors demonstrate SCC histology.[28] Stricture of the urethra is often a result of the cancer. Transitional cell or undifferentiated carcinomas usually predominate at the bladder neck and within the prostatic urethra. Poorly differentiated transitional cell carcinomas often exhibit squamous characteristics. Adenocarcinoma can arise in the glands of Littre or the prostatic utricle but are rare. Metastasis to the penis from other organ sites is also rare.

Obstructive symptoms are common in proximal lesions, while urethral bleeding and a palpable mass characterize cancers of the penile urethra. In general, the more proximal a tumor, and the longer its delay in diagnosis, the higher the stage is.

If the urethra is retained following cystectomy for bladder cancer, urethral tumors if they develop are usually transitional cell carcinomas. If urethrectomy is a component of cystectomy for bladder cancer, the entire structure, including the fossa navicularis, must be excised.[29]

Lymphatic draining of the distal urethra is similar to that of penile tumors. Tumors of the fossa and pendulous urethra drain to the superficial inguinal lymph nodes, whereas tumors of the bulbar, membranous, and prostatic urethral segments drain to the iliac obturator and presacral node groups. Crossover metastasis may occur at the prepubic lymphatic plexus.

Staging

The AJCC staging system for urethral carcinoma is given in Table 2. In the older terminology, anterior and posterior tumors were delineated at the suspensory ligament.

Surgical management

Low-grade, low-stage tumors of the urethra are uncommon but can be managed by transurethral resection or laser fulguration. Biopsy is essential to establish histopathology and the depth of the neoplasm. Partial penectomy with at least a 2 cm margin may be adequate if the tumor does not involve the corpus spungiosum or the corpora cavernosa.[30] Advanced or more proximal lesions usually require total penectomy and creation of a perineal urethrostomy. Anterior exenteration and radical cystoprostatourethrectomy may be required for carcinomas of the membranous or prostatic urethra.

Table 2 AJCC (2010) TNM staging of urethral cancer.

Primary tumor (T) (male and female)	
TX	Primary tumor cannot be assessed
T0	No evidence of primary tumor
Ta	Noninvasive papillary, polypoid, or verrucous carcinoma
Tis	Carcinoma *in situ*
T1	Tumor invades subepithelial connective tissue
T2	Tumor invades any of the following: corpus spongiosum, prostate, and periurethral muscle
T3	Tumor invades any of the following: corpus cavernosum, beyond prostatic capsule, and anterior vagina bladder neck
T4	Tumor invades other adjacent organs

Regional lymph nodes (N)	
NX	Regional lymph nodes cannot be assessed
N0	No regional lymph node metastasis
N1	Metastasis in a single lymph node 2 cm or less in greatest dimension
N2	Metastasis in a single node more than 2 cm in greatest dimension or in multiple nodes

Anatomic stage/prognostic groups			
Stage 0a	Ta	N0	M0
Stage 0is	Tis	N0	M0
	Tis pu	N0	M0
	Tis pd	N0	M0
Stage I	T1	N0	M0
Stage II	T2	N0	M0
Stage III	T1	N1	M0
	T2	N1	M0
	T3	N0	M0
	T3	N1	M0
Stage IV	T4	N0	M0
	T4	N1	M0
	Any T	N2	M0
	Any T	Any N	M1

Source: Edge et al.[10] Reproduced with permission of Springer.

Metastases to superficial or deep inguinal lymph nodes often lead to pelvic and systemic metastases.[31] Attentive clinical and imaging assessment is crucial in the follow-up of urethral cancer. Inguinal node dissection is critical if metastatic adenopathy is suspected based on MRI, PET/CT, or clinical examination. Deep pelvic adenectomy is also indicated for positive nodes, although the success of such surgery in extending survival is uncommon.

Adjuvant therapy

Because most urethral cancers carry a poor prognosis from surgery alone, if they are not superficial and local, chemotherapeutic regimens appropriate for the tumor type have been used as adjuvant treatment. Radiation therapy is also used. Clinical reports endorse these efforts, although prospective studies with controls have not been reported. Neoadjuvant chemotherapy or chemoradiotherapy for patients with T3 disease or clinically positive inguinal adenopathy had superior surgical outcome compared to those who underwent primary surgery without adjuvant participation.[32]

Female urethral carcinoma

The female urethra is largely contained within the anterior vaginal wall. In the adult, it is 2–4 cm in length. It is lined distally with stratified squamous epithelium changing to columnar epithelium proximally. At the bladder neck, transitional cell epithelium is found. A urethral diverticulum in the distal urethra may be a remnant of Wolffian or ectopic cloacal epithelium.

The histopathology of female urethral cancer depends on the cell of origin. Squamous carcinoma is the most frequent, comprising about 50% of tumors. Transitional cell carcinoma and adenocarcinoma are about 25% each. Tumor grade apparently does not influence metastasis and prognosis as much as in men. Mixed tumors, undifferentiated carcinomas, melanoma, cloacogenic carcinoma, and clear cell adenocarcinomas are rare but do occur.

Urethral carcinomas spread first by local extension and then metastasize by lymphatic channels and hematogenously. Lymphatic drainage of the distal urethra and the labia leads to the superficial and deep inguinal nodes. Proximal urethral drainage leads to iliac, obturator, presacral, and preaortic nodes. Palpable adenopathy is present at presentation in up to half the patients and almost always represents metastatic cancer.[33] Adenocarcinomas more commonly metastasize to distant sites hematogenously, including liver, lung, brain, and skeleton.

Staging

The AJCC TNM staging system is presented in Table 2. The entire length of the female urethra is often involved.

Surgical management

Most urethral tumors in women present with bleeding or dysuria because of a urethral mass. Distal urethral lesions generally are diagnosed early at a low stage. Local excision, partial urethrectomy, RT, and laser ablation have all been employed with some success. Higher stage more extensive urethral carcinomas can be managed with cystourethrectomy and an ileal pouch, or when bladder preservation is possible, interposition of the amputated vermiform appendix as a conduit to the surface (the Mitrofanoff procedure). Proximal lesions present later and at higher stage than distal lesions. Obstructive symptomology is the hallmark of proximal urethral lesions. Extensive lesions that involve the bladder or the vaginal wall may necessitate cystectomy or even anterior exenteration with urinary diversion. Local recurrence is common. Positive inguinal nodes by clinical or imaging techniques and proximal urethral carcinomas require deep pelvic node adenectomy.

References

1 Barnholtz-Sloan JS, Maldonado JL, Powsang J, Guiliano AR. Incidence trends in primary malignant penile cancer. *Urol Oncol.* 2007;**25**:31–367.

2 Albero G, Castellsagué X, Lin HY, et al. Male circumcision and the incidence and clearance of genital human papillomavirus (HPV) infection in men: the HPV Infection in men (HIM) cohort study. *BMC Infect Dis.* 2014;**14**:75.

3 Martinez I. Relationship of squamous cell carcinoma of the cervix uteri to squamous cell carcinoma of the penis among Puerto Rican women married to men with penile cancer. *Cancer.* 1969;**24**:777.

4 Balci M, Tuncel A, Baran I, et al. High-risk oncogenic human papilloma virus infection of the foreskin and microbiology of smegma in prepubertal boys. *Urology.* 2015;**86**(2):368–372.

5 Daling JR, Madeleine MM, Johnson LG, et al. Penile cancer: importance of circumcision, human papillomavirus and smoking in *in situ* and invasive disease. *Int J Cancer.* 2005;**116**:606–615.

6 Castellsague X, Bosch FX, Munoz N, et al. Male circumcision, penile human papillomavirus infection, and cervical cancer in female partners. *N Engl J Med.* 2002;**346**:1105–1112.

7 Ornellas AA, Correia AL, Marota A, Seixas ALC. Surgical treatment of invasive squamous cell carcinoma of the penis: retrospective analysis of 350 cases. *J Urol.* 1994;**151**:1244–1247.

8 Srinivas V, Morse MJ, Herr HW, Sogani PC, Whitmore WF Jr. Penile cancer: relation of extent of nodal metastasis to survival. *J Urol.* 1987;**137**:880.

9 Scardino E, Villa G, Bonoma G, et al. Magnetic resonance imaging combined with artificial erection for local staging of penile caner. *Urology.* 2004;**63**:1158–1162.

10 Edge, S., Byrd, D.R., Compton, C.C., Fritz, A.G., Greene, F.L., Trotti, A. (Eds.). *AJCC Cancer Staging Manual.* Springer New York, 2010.

11 Blastein LM, Finkelstein LH. Laser surgery for treatment of squamous cell carcinoma of the penis. *J Am Osteopath Assoc.* 1990;**90**:338.

12 Mohs FE, Snow SN, Messing EM, Kuglitsch MG. Microscopically controlled surgery in the treatment of carcinoma of the penis. *J Urol.* 1985;**133**:961–966.

13 Bevan-Thomas R, Slayton JW, Petaway CA. Contemporary morbidity from lymphadenectomy for penile squamous cell carcinoma: the MD Anderson experience. *J Urol.* 2002;**167**:1638–1642.

14 Culkin DJ, Beer TM. Advanced penile carcinoma. *J Urol.* 2003;**170**:359–365.

15 Ravi R. Correlation between the extent of nodal involvement and survival following groin dissection for carcinoma of the penis. *Br J Urol.* 1993;**72**:817–819.

16 Ravi R. Morbidity following groin dissection for penile carcinoma. *Br J Urol.* 1993;**72**:941–945.

17 Fraley EE, Zhang G, Manivel C, Niehans GA. The role of ilioinguinal lymphadenectomy and significance of histological differentiation in treatment of carcinoma of the penis. *J Urol.* 1989;**142**:1478.

18 Theodorescu D, Russo P, Zhang ZF. Outcomes of initial surveillance of invasive squamous cell carcinoma of the penis and negative nodes. *J Urol.* 1996;**155**:1626–1631.

19 Horenblas S, Van Tinteren H. Squamous cell carcinoma of the penis IV: prognostic factors of survival, analysis of tumor, odes, and metastasis classification system. *J Urol.* 1994;**147**:153–158.

20 D'Ancona CA, de Lucena RG, Querne FA, et al. Long-term followup of penile carcinoma treated with penectomy and bilateral modified inguinal lymphadenectomy. *J Urol.* 2004;**174**:498–501.

21 Lynch DF. Commentary on: Svinivas SV. Relation of extent of nodal metastasis to survival. *Semin Urol Oncol.* 1997;**15**:136–139.

22 Gerbaulet A, Lambin P. Radiation therapy of cancer of the penis. *Urol Clin North Am.* 1992;**19**:325–332.

23 Jakosbsen JK. A urologist's contemporary guide to penile cancer. *Scand J Urol.* 2015;**14**:1–6.

24 Ozsahin M, Jichlinski P, Weber DC, et al. Treatment of penile carcinoma: to cut or not to cut? *Int J Radiat Oncol Biol Phys.* 2006;**66**:674–679.

25 Tana S. Up-to-date management of carcinoma of the penis. *Eur Urol.* 1997;**32**:5–15.

26 Nicolai N, Sangalli LM, Necchi A, et al. A combination of cisplatin and 5-fluorouracil with a taxane in patients who underwent lymph node dissection for nodal metastases from squamous cell carcinoma of the penis: treatment outcome and survival analyses in neoadjuvant and adjuvant settings. *Clin Genitourin Cancer.* DOI: 10.1016/i, eigc, 2015.07.009, PMID 26341040 [ePub ahead of Print].

27 Sharma P, Djajadiningrat R, Zargar-Shoshtari K, et al. Adjuvant chemotherapy is associated with improved overall survival in pelvic node-positive penile cancer with lymph node dissection: a multi-institutional study. *Urol Oncol.* 2015;**33**:e17–e23.

28 Ray B, Canto AR, Whitmore WF Jr. Experience with primary carcinoma of the male urethra. *J Urol.* 1977;**117**:591–594.

29 Varol C, Thalmann GN, Burkhard FC, Studer UE. Treatment of urethral recurrence following radical cystectomy and ileal bladder substitution. *J Urol.* 2004;**172**:937–942.

30 Zeidman EJ, Desmond P, Thompson IM. Surgical treatment of carcinoma of the male urethra. *Urol Clin North Am.* 1992;**19**:359–372.

31 Gakis G, Morgan TM, Efstathiou JA, et al. Prognostic factors and outcomes in primary urethral cancer: results from the international collaboration on primary urethral carcinoma. *World J Urol.* 2015;**34**(1) 97–103. PMID: 25981402, [Epub ahead of print].

32 Gakis G, Morgan TM, Daneshmand S, et al. Impact of perioperative chemotherapy on survival in patients with advanced primary urethral cancer: results of the international collaboration on primary urethral carcinoma. *Ann Oncol.* 2015;**8**:1754–1759.

33 Dimarco DS, Dimarco CS, Zincke H, Webb MJ, Slezak JM. Surgical treatment for local control of female urethral carcinoma. *Urol Oncol.* 2004;**22**:404–409.

100 Testis cancer

Christian Kollmannsberger, MD, FRCPC ▪ Craig R. Nichols, MD ▪ Siamak Daneshmand, MD ▪ Eric K. Hansen, MD ▪ Christopher L. Corless, MD, PhD ▪ Bruce J. Roth, MD ▪ Lawrence Einhorn, MD

Overview

Cancer of the testis is a relatively uncommon disease, accounting for approximately 1% of all cancers in males. However, it represents a highly curable neoplasm, the incidence of which is focused on young patients at their peak of productivity. Curative treatment of disseminated nonseminomatous germ cell tumors often combines surgery and chemotherapy. The goal of initial therapy is never palliation or prolongation of survival, but cure.

Epidemiology

Incidence

Age-related incidence of testicular cancer reveals a bimodal distribution.[1] The major peak occurs between ages 15 and 35 years, owing almost exclusively to tumors of germ cell origin, which account for approximately 95% of all testicular cancer. Embryonal carcinoma represents the predominant histopathologic diagnosis up to the age of 35 years, after which seminoma is more common. From 2001 to 2005, the median age at diagnosis for cancer of the testis was 34 years of age.[2]

The incidence of testicular cancer varies based on geographic distribution. The incidence is highest in northern Europe and North America and lowest in Asia and Africa. There is also a striking influence of race, with the incidence among black and Hispanic males worldwide far less than that for their white counterparts.[3,4] In the United States, estimates of the incidence ratio between white and African-American patients range from 4 to 5 : 1. Testicular cancer appears to be increasing among young white males in the Scandinavian countries, the United Kingdom, and the United States.[5] Standardized incidence rates increased annually 2–5%, with marginal differences between seminomas and nonseminomas. In the United States, the annual percentage change from 1989 to 2005 was 0.8%. It is estimated that 8090 cases of testicular cancer were diagnosed in the United States in 2008, with approximately 380 persons dying of the disease.[6]

Risk factors

Cryptorchidism is the major identifiable risk factor associated with the development of testicular cancer, with a risk ratio reported between 2.5 and 14 in case–control studies.[7] The location of the maldescended testicle appears to be an important cofactor, because those patients with intra-abdominal retention have a fourfold higher incidence of malignancy than those with the testicle retained in the inguinal canal. It seems unlikely that maldescent alone represents the initiating event in the development of germ cell tumors (GCTs): Only 10% of testicular tumors are associated with cryptorchidism, whereas 10–20% of the malignancies in patients with cryptorchidism occur in the contralateral, normally descended testicle; prepubertal orchiopexy fails to prevent the subsequent development of malignancy in the undescended testicle; and first-degree male relatives of patients with testicular cancer exhibit an increased incidence of cryptorchidism, hydroceles, and inguinal hernias, as well as testicular cancer.[8,9] These data suggest that some genetic predisposition and/or in utero environmental event may result in several genitourinary developmental abnormalities, including maldescent and germ cell neoplasia. An increase in the frequency of cryptorchidism has been observed and appears to parallel the timing and magnitude of the increase in incidence of testicular cancer. Brothers of men with testicular germ cell tumors (TGCTs) have an 8-fold to 10-fold risk of developing TGCT, whereas the relative risk to fathers and sons is approximately fourfold. This familial relative risk is much higher than that for most other types of cancer. A genome-wide linkage search yielded evidence for a testicular cancer susceptibility gene on chromosome Xq27 that may also predispose to undescended testes.[10]

TGCTs occur at increased frequency in men with human immunodeficiency virus (HIV). In one multicenter study, 35 patients with HIV-related GCTs were identified. The median age at GCT diagnosis was 34 years (range, 27–64 years). The median CD4 cell count was 315/mm³ (range, 90–960/mm³). There were seminoma in 26 patients (74%) and nonseminomatous germ cell tumor (NSGCT) in nine patients (26%). Twenty-one patients (60%) had stage I disease and 14 patients had metastatic disease. Overall, six patients relapsed, three died from GCT, and seven died from HIV, resulting in a 2-year overall survival rate of 81%. HIV-related seminoma occurred more frequently than in the age-matched and sex-matched HIV-negative population, with a relative risk of 5.4 (95% confidence interval [CI] = 3.35–8.10); however, NSGCT did not occur more frequently, and there was no change in the incidence of GCT since the introduction of highly active antiretroviral therapy. The authors concluded that testicular seminoma occurs significantly more frequently in HIV-positive men than in the control population. Patients with HIV-related GCTs present and should be treated in a similar manner to those in the HIV-negative population. Most of the mortality relates to HIV infection.[11]

An additional predisposition is the association of mediastinal NSGCTs with Klinefelter's syndrome. Approximately 10% of all patients with mediastinal nonseminoma have Klinefelter's syndrome, and there does not appear to be an increased incidence in patients with testicular or retroperitoneal primary tumors.[12]

An association of dysplastic nevus syndrome and testicular cancer has been observed.[13] A twofold higher incidence of multiple atypical nevi, and the attendant risk of melanoma, has been noted.

Holland-Frei Cancer Medicine, Ninth Edition. Edited by Robert C. Bast Jr., Carlo M. Croce, William N. Hait, Waun Ki Hong, Donald W. Kufe, Martine Piccart-Gebhart, Raphael E. Pollock, Ralph R. Weichselbaum, Hongyang Wang, and James F. Holland.
© 2017 John Wiley & Sons, Inc. ISBN: 978-1-118-93469-2

Patients with a history of unilateral testicular cancer are at risk of developing cancer in the other testicle. In a large series, 2.7% of 2338 patients developed a contralateral testicular tumor during the period of follow-up.[14-16] Investigators at the Royal Marsden Hospital reported a similar rate of 2.75% for developing contralateral tumors among 760 men in an interval as long as 15 years.[17]

Between 1950 and 2001, 3984 patients with testicular cancer were treated at Memorial Sloan Kettering for GCT. A total of 58 patients with bilateral TGCTs were identified. Median follow-up was 60 months. Ten of the 58 patients (17%) had synchronous tumors, while the other 48 (83%) had metachronous tumors. Overall, seminoma was the most common histology of the synchronous and metachronous tumors. Most patients in the synchronous and metachronous tumor groups presented with low-stage disease. Of the 58 patients, 52 (89%) had no evidence of disease, and 6 (11%) were dead of disease at the last follow-up. Treatment of the second tumor appeared to be influenced by therapy for the first tumor in 16.7% of cases.[18]

Some clinicians recommend routine biopsy of the contralateral testis for patients diagnosed with unilateral testicular cancer. Fossa and colleagues evaluated the risk of contralateral testicular cancer and survival in a large population-based cohort of men diagnosed with testicular cancer before age 55 years using Surveillance, Epidemiology, and End Results (SEER) data. From 29,515 testicular cancer cases reported to the SEER Program of the National Cancer Institute (NCI), from 1973 through 2001, estimates of prevalence of synchronous contralateral testicular cancer, the observed-to-expected ratio (O/E), 15-year cumulative risk of metachronous contralateral testicular cancer, and the 10-year overall survival rate of both synchronous and metachronous contralateral testicular cancer were made. A total of 175 men presented with synchronous contralateral testicular cancer; 287 men developed metachronous contralateral testicular cancer (O/E = 12.4 [95% CI = 11.0-13.9%]; 15-year cumulative risk = 1.9% [95% CI = 1.7-2.1%]). In the multivariable analysis, only nonseminomatous histology of the first testicular cancer was associated with a statistically significantly decreased risk of metachronous contralateral testicular cancer (hazard ratio [HR] = 0.60; 95%

CI = 0.46-0.79%; $p < 0.001$). Increasing age at first testicular cancer diagnosis was associated with decreasing risk of nonseminomatous metachronous contralateral testicular cancer (odds ratio (OR) = 0.90; 95% CI = 0.86-0.94%). The 10-year overall survival rate after metachronous contralateral testicular cancer diagnosis was 93% (95% CI = 88-96%), and that after synchronous contralateral testicular cancer was 85% (95% CI = 78-90%). The low cumulative risk of metachronous contralateral testicular cancer and favorable overall survival of patients diagnosed with metachronous contralateral testicular cancer is in accordance with the current US approach of not performing a biopsy on the contralateral testis.

These observations underscore the importance of continued long-term follow-up of patients with TGCTs.

Pathology

Origin and molecular genetics

Testicular tumors fall into several broad groups (Table 1). Classification of the GCTs has been based on morphology, but recent molecular studies have yielded a more ontological scheme consisting of five distinct subtypes that differ in their proposed cell of origin.[19] Accordingly, teratomas and yolk sac tumors arising in neonates and young children derive from primordial germ cells or very early gonocytes distributed along the gonadal ridge or in the testis/ovary. These tumors retain most of the genomic imprinting from both parental genomes. The teratomas remain diploid, while the yolk sac tumors show gains of chromosomes 1q, 12p13-14, and 20q, and losses of 1p, 4, and 6q.[19]

Spermatocytic seminoma is a second, distinct subtype of GCT thought to derive from postpubertal spermatogonia/spermatocytes. Accordingly, these tumors have a paternal pattern of genomic imprinting and show variable ploidy, sometimes with a gain of chromosome.[10]

Two of the other five proposed subtypes of GCT do not occur in the testis. Dermoid cysts of the ovary, which are thought to arise from oogonia/oocytes, are diploid/tetraploid and show maternal

Table 1 Primary tumors of the testis.

Type	Relative frequency	Genotype/comments
Germ cell tumors		
Infants and children	~1% of all testis tumors	
Yolk sac tumor	65–80% of prepubertal	Aneuploid
Teratoma	20–35% of prepubertal	Diploid; mature elements; benign
Adolescents and adults	95% of all testis tumors	
ITGCNU	>90% of postpubertal	Aneuploid (near triploid)
Seminoma	~45% of postpubertal	Aneuploid (near triploid); iso12p
Nonseminomatous (NSGCT)	~55% of postpubertal	Aneuploid (near triploid); iso12p
Embryonal carcinoma	~75% of NSGCT	
Yolk sac tumor	~50% of NSGCT	
Teratoma	~50% of NSGCT	Malignant (even mature elements)
Choriocarcinoma	~10% of NSGCT	
Adults (usually >50 years)		
Spermatocytic seminoma	<1% of postpubertal	Variable ploidy; gain of chromosome 9
Spermatocytic seminoma with sarcoma	Very rare	
Sex cord-stromal tumors		
Leydig cell tumor	~3% of all testis tumors	7–10% metastasis (postpubertal)
Sertoli cell tumor	<1% of all testis tumors	
Granulosa cell tumor		
Adult type	Very rare	
Juvenile type	Uncommon	Infants <6 months
Mixed/indeterminate	Rare	
Mixed germ cell/sex cord-stromal tumors		
Gonadoblastoma	Very rare	

Table 2 Markers of testicular germ cell tumors.

Morphologic subtype	Serum	Immunohistochemistry	FISH
ITGNCU		PLAP, KIT, OCT3/4	
Seminoma	HCG (low)	PLAP, KIT, OCT3/4	Excess 12p
Embryonal carcinoma	HCG (low)	CD30, OCT3/4, PLAP	Excess 12p
Yolk sac tumor	AFP	AFP, PLAP	Excess 12p
Choriocarcinoma	HCG (high)	HCG	Excess 12p
Teratoma			Excess 12p

Abbreviations: AFP, α-fetoprotein; FISH, fluorescence *in situ* hybridization; HCG, human chorionic gonadotropin; PLAP, placental/germ cell alkaline phosphatase.

genomic imprinting. Hydatidiform mole (gestational trophoblastic disease) is a placental-derived neoplasm that contains a purely paternal genome as a result of fertilization of an empty ovum.

The fifth subtype of GCT consists of seminoma and the NSGCT patterns that, together, account for 95% of primary testicular neoplasms (Table 1). Variants of this GCT subtype also occur in the ovary (dysgerminoma), anterior mediastinum, and midline brain (germinoma). It is suggested that seminoma and NSGCT are derived from gonocytes that have lost their genomic imprinting as a result of being later in their development than those that give rise to infantile teratomas and yolk sac tumors. These gonocytes are polypoid (triploid or tetraploid), probably because of meiotic arrest. Depending on exactly when this arrest occurs during fetal development, the affected cells may be distributed to one or both testes, accounting for the bilateral GCTs observed in 2–3% of patients.

Seminomas and NSGCT share a common precursor lesion called intratubular germ cell neoplasia, unclassified (ITGCNU). Growing *in situ* within seminiferous tubules, ITGCNU cells express markers shared with embryonic stem cells, including the transcription factors OCT3/4 and NANOG.[20,21] These factors are essential to the development of embryonic stem cells in mice, but are not expressed in normal spermatogonia in mice or humans. Their presence in ITGCNU supports the theory that a pluripotent gonocyte is the cell of origin for both seminoma and NSGCT. In addition, OCT3/4 serves as a highly specific immunohistochemical marker in the diagnosis of extra-TGCTs (Table 2).[20,22]

Progression of ITGCNU to an invasive GCT is accompanied by a number of common events.[23] One is the acquisition of excess genetic material from the short arm of chromosome 12. In 80% of cases, this is accomplished through loss of 12q and reduplication of 12p (isochromosome 12p), while in 20%, the additional 12p sequences are distributed among other derivative chromosomes. Interestingly, the embryonic stem cell gene *NANOG* is on 12p. Fluorescence *in situ* hybridization (FISH) for 12p is used in paraffin sections as a diagnostic marker for GCTs and also for nongerm cell derivatives.

Additional events associated with malignant progression of ITGCNU include loss of expression of the homeobox gene *NKX3.1*,[24] loss of the tumor suppressor PTEN,[25] and decreased expression of the cell cycle regulator p21.[26] Mutations of *TP53* are rare in postpubertal GCTs, but the effects of this important tumor suppressor may be by *MDM2* overexpression[26] or downregulation of *LATS2* by microRNAs mi-R372 and mi-R373. A genetic screen implicates miRNA-372 and miRNA-373 as oncogenes in TGCTs.[27]

Although seminoma and NSGCT share a common origin, they are clinicopathologically distinct cancers. Little is known of what determines their differences, but oncogenic mutations in KIT (a receptor tyrosine kinase) are found in 25% of seminomas and are essentially absent in NSGCT. These mutations may occur very early in seminoma tumorigenesis, as they are present in ITGCNU,[28] and in dysgerminoma/germinoma of the ovary, mediastinum, and

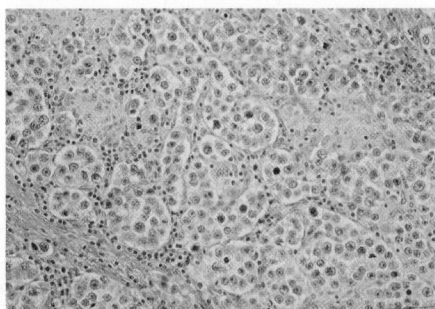

Figure 1 Small nests of seminoma are separated by a lymphoid infiltrate and a focal granulomatous reaction.

brain. Based on studies in mice, *KIT* gene function is essential to the development of primordial germ cells and to normal spermatogenesis; therefore, constitutive activation of this kinase may favor the seminoma pathway. Unfortunately, KIT kinase inhibitors such as imatinib are not likely to be of benefit to seminoma patients harboring *KIT*-mutant tumors, because most of the published mutations are inherently resistant to the available drugs.

Seminoma

Approximately 45% of all postpubertal TGCTs are pure seminoma ("classic" seminoma). The incidence is increased to 60% in cryptorchid testes. On gross examination, such tumors are generally homogeneous and well demarcated. Distinct lobulation may be apparent, with the nodules separated by dense fibrous bands. Areas of necrosis and hemorrhage are usually discrete. Microscopically, there is a monotonous distribution of uniform, rounded cells with large, centralized nuclei and nucleoli. The cytoplasm may be either clear or granular and will frequently stain for glycogen, lipid, and/or placental/germ cell alkaline phosphatase (PLAP). Stromal elements include an infiltrate rich in T lymphocytes and containing occasional granulomas (Figure 1). These features may mimic granulomatous orchitis.

Seminoma presents most commonly in the fourth and fifth decades, usually as an enlarging, painless testicular mass. Approximately 70% of patients present with stage I disease, 20% with stage II, and only rarely with disease above the diaphragm. Lymphatic spread is to the para-aortic (PA) lymph nodes and then to the mediastinal or supraclavicular lymph nodes. Hematogenous dissemination to the lung, liver, bone, or adrenal is a late occurrence. Seminomas contain syncytiotrophoblastic giant cells that stain for human chorionic gonadotropin (HCG). Low-level HCG elevation is seen in 5–10% of patients with pure seminoma and likely reflects syncytiotrophoblastic elements present within the tumor (Table 2). Seminoma does not secrete α-fetoprotein (AFP).

Nonseminomatous germ cell tumors

The most common postpubertal GCTs of the testis are composed of one or more elements that are collectively known as "nonseminomatous." Four morphologic patterns are recognized among this group. In most cases, these patterns are intermixed in varying proportions, often subtly merging from one to the next. Areas of seminoma may be included (termed "mixed GCTs" by some), but the prognosis is determined by the presence of the other elements and is less favorable, overall, than for pure seminomas.

Embryonal carcinoma

Embryonal carcinoma is present in up to 90% of NSGCT cases. Macroscopically, it forms a soft, fleshy, inhomogeneous mass with areas of necrosis and hemorrhage. Direct invasion of the spermatic cord, epididymis, and tunica albuginea occurs.

The microscopic appearance is extremely variable and may include papillary, solid, tubular, and glandular patterns, frequently interrupted by geographic necrosis (Figure 2). Large polygonal cells with indistinct cytoplasmic borders (unlike seminoma) are the rule, with pale granular cytoplasm, large nuclei, and one or more centrally placed nucleoli. Mitotic figures and multinucleated cells are common. Clinically, these are aggressive tumors with lymph node metastases present in two-thirds of patients.

Yolk sac tumor

Yolk sac tumor, formerly called endodermal sinus tumor, is present in approximately half of NSGCT cases, but is rare in pure form in the postpubertal patient.[29] The most readily recognized pattern consists of a cluster of tumor cells surrounding a small central blood vessel (Schiller–Duval body) (Figure 3). The morphologic spectrum is broad, including microcystic (lacelike), micropapillary, solid, and hepatoid patterns. The tumor cell nuclei are smaller than those of embryonal carcinoma. Cytoplasmic globules are common and stain for AFP, which accounts for the serum elevations characteristically present in patients with this tumor (Table 2).

In its pure form, yolk sac tumor is the most common testicular neoplasm in infants and young children (Table 1). Despite morphologic similarity to the subtype observed in postpubertal NSGCT, the pediatric tumor is an oncogenetically distinct entity and carries a better prognosis.

Choriocarcinoma

Choriocarcinoma is an uncommon element in NSGCT (15%) and is rare as a pure tumor. On gross examination, areas of choriocarcinoma are characteristically hemorrhagic. Microscopically, the diagnosis requires a combination of cytotrophoblasts and syncytiotrophoblasts (Figure 4). Stroma is sparse but tends to be highly vascular.

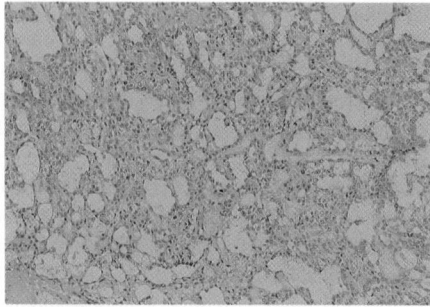

Figure 2 Yolk sac tumor. Numerous microcysts occur in the most common pattern of yolk sac tumor.

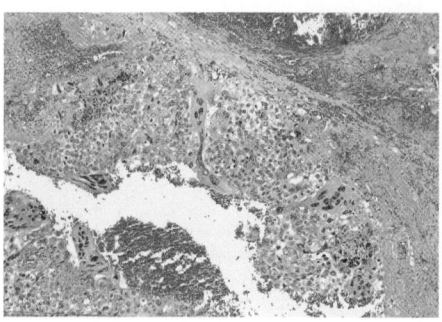

Figure 3 Choriocarcinoma. Syncytiotrophoblastic cells "cap" islands of mononucleated cytotrophoblast. Note the hemorrhagic background.

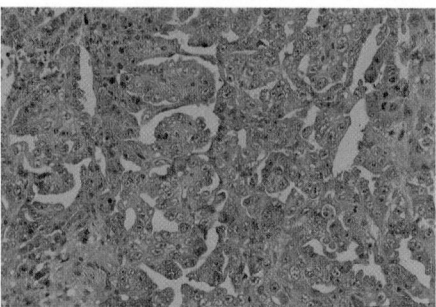

Figure 4 Embryonal carcinoma. Irregularly shaped glands and papillae are lined by pleomorphic cells with vesicular, crowded nuclei and poorly defined cytoplasmic membranes.

Choriocarcinoma of the testis represents the most aggressive subtype of NSGCT, often presenting with large-volume visceral metastases and/or brain metastases. Extreme elevations of serum HCG levels are characteristic.

Teratoma

Teratoma is defined as a tumor that contains elements of all three germ layers present with varying degrees of differentiation. Teratomatous elements are recognized in approximately half of NSGCT cases, but are not usually pure. Macroscopically, teratomas tend to be large and have multiloculated cysts containing serosanguineous fluid as well as cartilaginous solid areas. Microscopically, all manner of tissue elements may be present, including cysts with squamous, respiratory, or intestinal-type linings, mature cartilage, muscle, and fibroblastic stroma (Figure 5). Areas that are less well differentiated ("immature teratoma") are often intermixed (Figure 6). Regardless of the degree of differentiation, all teratomas in the postpubertal setting are regarded as malignant. In postchemotherapy specimens teratoma is the most common residual element. The presence of nonteratomatous NSGCT may be an indication for additional therapy.

A pure form of mature teratoma is common among pediatric patients under the age of 4 years. Although morphologically similar to mature areas of teratoma within NSGCT, these lesions arise through a different pathway and are essentially benign[30] (Table 1). Rarely, a nonteratomatous element is identified and may give rise to metastases.

Nongerm cell cancers arising from germ cell tumors

Given the pluripotent nature of the gonocytes from which seminomas and NSGCT are thought to arise, a nongerm cell element may emerge and become the dominant pattern in advanced

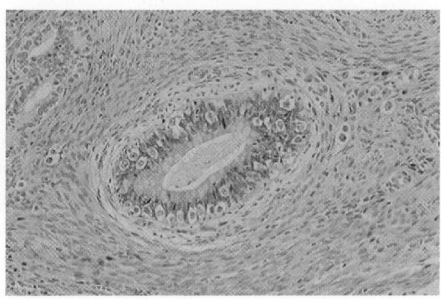

Figure 5 Mature teratoma. There are mature-appearing small glands, a portion of a pilosebaceous unit, and bundles of smooth muscle.

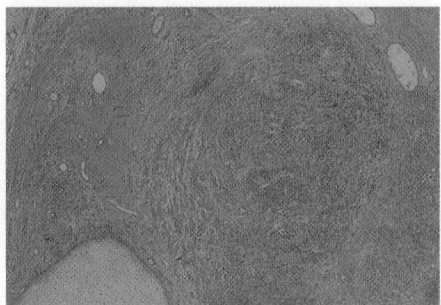

Figure 6 Immature teratoma. An island of immature neuroepithelium is present adjacent to a nodule of hyaline cartilage.

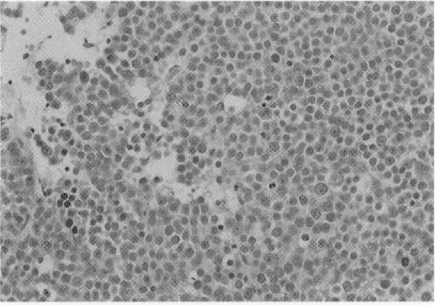

Figure 7 Spermatocytic seminoma. There is a diffuse sheetlike arrangement of neoplastic cells that vary in size.

cases of postpubertal testicular cancer. Among these are cancers morphologically resembling embryonal rhabdomyosarcoma, adenosquamous carcinoma, leiomyosarcoma, Wilms' tumor, glioblastoma multiforme, and primitive neuroectodermal tumor (PNET), all of which are associated with resistance to chemotherapy.[31] Myelodysplasia and leukemia may also evolve from NSGCT.[32]

Spermatocytic seminoma

Spermatocytic seminoma accounts for 1–2% of TGCTs. On gross examination, it has a grayish appearance and tends to be softer than classic seminoma. Microscopically, these tumors tend to form tubular clusters and are composed of round cells of highly variable size that bear resemblance to the cellular stages of normal spermatogenesis (Figure 7). In contrast to classic seminoma, stromal lymphocytic infiltration is not a feature of spermatocytic seminoma. This tumor tends to occur over the age of 50, with a median age of 65 years. The prognosis following surgery is excellent, as there are only anecdotal reports of metastases.

Sex cord-stromal tumors

Tumors arising from stromal tissue account for only 4% of all adult testicular tumors but represent almost 20% of childhood testicular tumors. These tumors are thought to arise from primitive gonadal mesenchyme and are subcategorized as Leydig cell tumor, Sertoli cell tumor, gonadoblastoma, granulosa cell tumor, and mixed/indeterminate types (Table 1).

Leydig cell tumor

Leydig cell tumor represents about 3% of all testicular tumors, and although they may be seen in children, the median age of appearance is 60 years. Histologically, they are typified by cells with abundant oncocytic cytoplasm and round, regular nuclei. Clinical symptoms are usually related to the production of both androgens and estrogens by tumor cells, leading to precocious puberty in a child and gynecomastia in the adult. Approximately 10% of Leydig cell tumors metastasize, but this occurs only in the postpubertal patient. In patients with metastatic disease, treatment with radiation or chemotherapeutic agents has generally been ineffective. Retroperitoneal lymph node dissection (RPLND) is an important staging procedure. The therapeutic role of RPLND in low-volume metastatic retroperitoneal disease is unclear, but waiting to resect higher-volume tumor is ineffective. A prophylactic RPLND should, therefore, be considered in patients with clinical stage I tumors.

Sertoli cell tumor

Sertoli cell tumor shows no age predilection, presenting as a testicular mass that may be accompanied by gynecomastia or impotence secondary to estrogen production. Microscopically, these lesions are composed of rounded cells growing in cords and sheets in a fibrous background. Therapy is primarily directed at resection of the primary lesion, with a staging work-up to include abdominal computed tomography (CT) scan and chest radiography. RPLND is controversial in clinical stage I disease. Large primary tumors with frequent mitoses or necrosis may prompt an RPLND. Sertoli cell tumors can respond to platinum combination chemotherapy.

Clinical presentation

Most patients seek medical attention because of a swollen testis. Accompanying symptoms include a sensation of heaviness or aching in the affected gonad. Severe pain is rare, unless there is associated epididymitis or bleeding in the tumor. Because testicular cancer is commonly associated with low sperm counts, patients may present during an infertility work-up.

Approximately 25% of patients with disseminated disease present with symptoms from metastatic disease.[33] Severe back pain from metastasis to the retroperitoneum is the most frequent and is the presenting symptom in patients with primary retroperitoneal GCTs. Shortness of breath, chest pain, and hemoptysis are usually manifestations of advanced lung metastases. Primary mediastinal GCTs are an exception, in that these tumors (if malignant) present with symptoms of mediastinal compression with pain, dysphagia, shortness of breath, and superior vena cava syndrome. Teratomas of the mediastinum produce few symptoms and are commonly discovered on routine chest film obtained for minor chest complaints.

Diagnosis

Understanding the diagnosis and staging of TGCTs depends on understanding the anatomy of the vascular and lymphatic drainage of the testis as well as the likely sites of metastatic spread of the disease. The spermatic cord contains the lymphatic and vascular supply of the testis. The lymphatic and vascular supply diverges medially when the spermatic vessels cross ventral to the ureter. The landing zones for the lymphatic drainage of the right testis are the interaortocaval nodes below the renal vasculature and the ipsilateral distribution of nodes, especially the paracaval and preaortic nodes. The primary landing zone for a left-sided primary tumor includes in the PA nodes below the left renal vessels and the PA and preaortic nodes. Ipsilateral common iliac nodes are uncommonly involved unless large-volume disease is present.

Unusual patterns of disease can be seen (or created) in patients who have had prior pelvic surgeries including herniorrhaphy, abdominal orchiopexy, or scrotal violations.[34] The proper and only diagnostic procedure in this setting is a radical inguinal orchiectomy. Transscrotal procedures can disrupt predictable patterns of lymphatic metastases and should not be done.

Tumors of the testis can present with a discrete nodular density or as diffuse infiltration of the entire testis (particularly seminoma and lymphoma). The other testis serves as a useful reference standard. If a testicular mass is suspected, transscrotal ultrasonography should be performed. The presence of a hypoechoic mass represents a testicular neoplasm, and a radical inguinal orchiectomy is required to make a diagnosis and to ensure local control of a primary testicular cancer.

Extragonadal germ cell tumors (EGCTs) arising within the retroperitoneum or mediastinum require specialized management. A diagnosis may be made on the basis of significantly elevated tumor markers in a patient with a mass in the anterior mediastinum or retroperitoneum. If there is no marker elevation, tissue confirmation is required. Chemotherapy is the primary treatment; attempts at debulking or total removal of mediastinal GCTs as initial management are inappropriate. Primary retroperitoneal GCTs may be associated with an occult testicular primary. Such patients should have a thorough evaluation of the gonads, including the use of testicular ultrasonography. If a previously unsuspected testicular tumor is found, orchiectomy can serve as the diagnostic procedure. Otherwise, fine-needle aspiration of the abdominal mass or exploratory laparotomy is required. In addition, an i(12p) chromosomal abnormality is diagnostic for GCT in a patient who presents with undifferentiated cancer.

A transscrotal biopsy should never be performed. If, at the time of scrotal orchiectomy, the surgeon identified the tumor and removed the testis in toto, then the inguinal portion of the spermatic cord must be removed. If a testicular biopsy was performed, management of the hemiscrotum depends on the primary treatment modality. Patients who are receiving primary chemotherapy do not need hemiscrotectomy. Inguinal lymphadenectomy is reserved for patients with palpable inguinal lymphadenopathy. For patients with early-stage seminoma who have had a scrotal violation, approximately 5–10% will experience local failure. Extending the field to include the groin and scrotum diminishes these prospects but is associated with increased infertility.

Tumor markers

Serum HCG and AFP have significant value in the diagnosis, prognosis, and management of patients with GCTs. AFP is derived from the yolk sac or embryonal carcinoma elements of germ cell cancers. Elevation of AFP is not seen in normal adults. The half-life of this protein in the serum is approximately 5 days. In germ cell cancers, syncytiotrophoblastic components elaborate HCG. The protein comprises an alpha subunit and a beta subunit, each of which is antigenically distinct. The serum half-life of the entire protein is 18–30 h.

Serum HCG and AFP are elevated in 85% of patients with disseminated NSGCTs. AFP alone is elevated in 40% of patients, and HCG alone is elevated in 50–60% of patients with disseminated nonseminomatous testicular cancer. Elevated lactic acid dehydrogenase (LDH) is less specific and is mainly a correlate of disease bulk.

Pure seminoma is most frequently associated with normal AFP and HCG, but approximately 10% of all cases, and up to 30% of patients with advanced disease, may have low levels (usually <100 mIU/mL).[35] Any elevation of AFP in patients with seminoma must be viewed as evidence of nonseminomatous disease, and management should proceed accordingly.

AFP and HCG should be determined before and after orchiectomy, but the absence of marker elevation should not influence the decision to undertake the procedure. Likewise, normalization of serum markers after orchiectomy does not ensure that all disease has been removed, although persistence of marker elevation implies residual disease.

The rate of disappearance of elevated tumor markers is very useful in determining response to chemotherapy. HCG is the most useful in this regard; a 10-fold decrease in the HCG level over a 3-week period is consistent with potentially curative chemotherapy. Less steep declines of HCG levels may correlate with the emergence of drug resistance. Likewise, the reappearance of markers often predates the radiographic appearance of recurrent disease.

The presence of tumor markers also can lead to errors in clinical management. First, HCG determination can be nonspecific, and there is some cross-reactivity in the radioimmunoassay with luteinizing hormone. Also, HCG can be falsely elevated in patients who use marijuana. HCG determination should be repeated to ensure that the elevation is not a laboratory error. If the level is still high, the patient should be queried regarding drug usage. Testosterone should be given in a dose of 300 mg intramuscularly to ensure that a hypogonadal state with resultant high levels of luteinizing hormone is not interfering with the determination of HCG. If the level remains increased, restaging procedures and investigation of sanctuary sites (brain and contralateral testis) are in order. A retrospective review by Zon and colleagues evaluated management problems in patients with very high HCG levels.[36] Forty-one patients with an HCG >50,000 mIU/mL were included. All patients received cisplatin-based chemotherapy. Two of these 41 patients had normal HCG levels at the time of the fourth course of chemotherapy. Eight additional patients had normalized the HCG within 1 month of completion of the fourth course of therapy. Of these ten patients, seven remain continuously free of disease, and three are currently disease-free with salvage therapy. Thirty-one patients still had an abnormal HCG more than 1 month after completing the fourth course of primary chemotherapy. Fifteen of these patients are continuously disease-free, despite no further treatment. A subset of patients with very high HCG levels do not have a consistent predictable decline of HCG with treatment. Absolute dependence on predicted patterns of decline in these patients would have resulted in overtreatment. Our strategy has been to wait for a rising serum HCG before considering salvage therapy.

False-positive elevation of AFP is quite rare. Differential considerations include laboratory error, other tumor types (such as hepatocellular carcinoma), and liver inflammation from cirrhosis or hepatitis. An occasional patient may have baseline elevation of AFP (usually <100 ng/mL) that remains static over time and does not reflect active disease. Some individuals have familial, hereditary, mildly elevated serum AFP levels in the range of 15–30 ng/mL. Patients with clinical stage I disease, normal imaging, normal contralateral testicle, and a minimally elevated AFP level (<25 ng/mL) should be observed and only be treated if there is a clear AFP increase and/or development of metastases.[37]

Staging

GCTs are typically categorized as stage I, referring to tumors confined to the testis; stage II, indicating metastatic disease to the nodes of the periaortic or vena caval zone without pulmonary or visceral involvement; and stage III, which denotes metastasis above the diaphragm or involving other viscera. The AJCC and World Health Organization (WHO) classification is the international standard classification (Table 3).[39]

Standard procedures to establish clinical stage include physical examination, abdominal and chest CT scans, and serum levels of AFP, βHCG, and LDH. Brain imaging and bone scans should be performed only when clinically indicated (e.g., clinical symptoms and/or poor-risk disease). The role of positron emission tomography (PET) remains investigational in the initial staging of patients with GCTs and is not considered a standard staging procedure. PET scan will not reliably detect teratoma or microscopic carcinoma. PET scan has been investigated in patients with residual masses after chemotherapy for seminoma, and the persistence of PET avidity is associated with risk of recurrence, but a PET scan cannot differentiate between residual teratoma and necrosis.[40]

Therapy

Carcinoma *in situ*

Carcinoma *in situ* (CIS) or tubular intraepithelial neoplasia (TIN) is a true premalignant condition leading to both seminomatous and nonseminomatous invasive GCTs in up to 50% of untreated cases (Figures 8 and 9).[41] Management is controversial. Observation after diagnosis of TIN offers the best chance of retained fertility but requires a compliant patient and risks the possible requirement for more intensive treatment of invasive disease. Low-dose radiotherapy (18–20 Gy in 1.5–2.0 Gy fractions) will eradicate the TIN with high probability of decreased or eliminated fertility without affecting potency.[41,42] Total orchiectomy will obviously eliminate TIN in the effected testicle, as well as all germ cells and Leydig cells within that testicle. It may be the favored option in some patients with TIN in one testicle and a normal contralateral testicle. Partial orchiectomy alone is ill advised because TIN is typically a diffuse process within the effected testicle. Chemotherapy is not indicated for TIN.[43]

Nonseminoma: Early stage

Knowledge of the natural history of testicular primary lesions and their lymphatic drainage patterns is key to understanding the therapeutic options. Testicular lymphatics arise in proximity to the embryonic origin of the testicle, in the genital ridge in the high lumbar region. Although the afferent lymphatic channels accompany testicular descent into the scrotum, draining lymph nodes remain in the retroperitoneum.

In 1910, Jamieson and Dobson demonstrated that the drainage pattern for testis tumors differed according to the side of the primary lesion, with right-sided lesions draining to the paracaval, interaortocaval, and preaortic nodes and left-sided lesions to the PA and preaortic nodes.[44]

Table 3 AJCC staging.

TNM clinical classification

T:	*Primary tumor:* The extent of the primary tumor is classified after radical orchiectomy (see pT). If no radical orchiectomy has been performed, TX is used
N:	*Regional lymph nodes*
NX	Regional lymph nodes cannot be assessed
N0	No regional lymph node metastasis
N1	Metastasis with a lymph node mass ≤2 cm in greatest dimension or multiple lymph nodes, not >2 cm in greatest dimension
N2	Metastasis with a lymph node mass >2 cm but not >5 cm in greatest dimension, or multiple lymph nodes, any one mass >2 cm but not >5 cm in greatest dimension
N3	Metastasis with a lymph node mass >5 cm in greatest dimension
M:	*Distant metastasis*
MX	Distant metastasis cannot be assessed
M0	No distant metastasis
M1	Distant metastasis
M1a	Nonregional lymph node or pulmonary metastasis
M1b	Distant metastasis other than to nonregional lymph node and lungs

pTNM pathologic classification

pT:	*Primary tumor*
pTX	Primary tumor cannot be assessed (if no radical orchiectomy has been performed, TX is used)
pT0	No evidence of primary tumor (e.g., histologic scar in testis)
pTis	Intratubular germ cell neoplasia (carcinoma *in situ*)
pT1	Tumor limited to testis and epididymis without vascular/lymphatic invasion; tumor may invade tunica albuginea, but not tunica vaginalis
pT2	Tumor limited to testis and epididymis with vascular/lymphatic invasion, or tumor extending through tunica albuginea with involvement of tunica vaginalis
pT3	Tumor invades spermatic cord with or without vascular/lymphatic invasion
pT4	Tumor invades scrotum with or without vascular/lymphatic invasion
pN:	*Regional lymph nodes*
pNX	Regional lymph nodes cannot be assessed
pN0	No regional lymph node metastasis
pN1	Metastasis with a lymph node mass ≤2 cm in greatest dimension and ≤5 positive nodes, none >2 cm in greatest dimension
pN2	Metastasis with a lymph node mass >2 cm but not >5 cm in greatest dimension; or >5 nodes positive, not >5 cm; or evidence of extranodal extension of tumor
pN3	Metastasis with a lymph node mass >5 cm in greatest dimension
pM:	*Distant metastasis*
	The pM category corresponds to the M category
S:	*Serum tumor markers*
SX	Serum marker studies not available or not performed
S0	Serum marker study levels within normal limits LDH, HCG, and α-fetoprotein
S1	<1.5.N and <5000 and 1000
S2	1.5–10.N or 5000–50,000 or 1000–10,000
S3	>10.N or >50,000 or >10,000

N, the upper limit of normal for the lactate dehydrogenase assay.
Source: Edge 2010.[38] Reproduced with permission of Springer.

Stage I nonseminoma

The cure for patients with stage I nonseminoma is close to 100%. Three therapeutic options exist—primary RPLND, adjuvant chemotherapy, and active surveillance—all of which result in a similarly excellent outcome. Attention has therefore been focused on the reduction in toxicity. The accurate diagnosis of clinical stage I disease is critical. Following inguinal orchiectomy and the diagnosis of nonseminoma, serum levels of β-HCG and AFP must return to normal (if elevated before orchiectomy), and abdominal CT, chest radiography, and/or chest CT must all be negative before a patient can be labeled as having clinical stage I disease. In this clinical

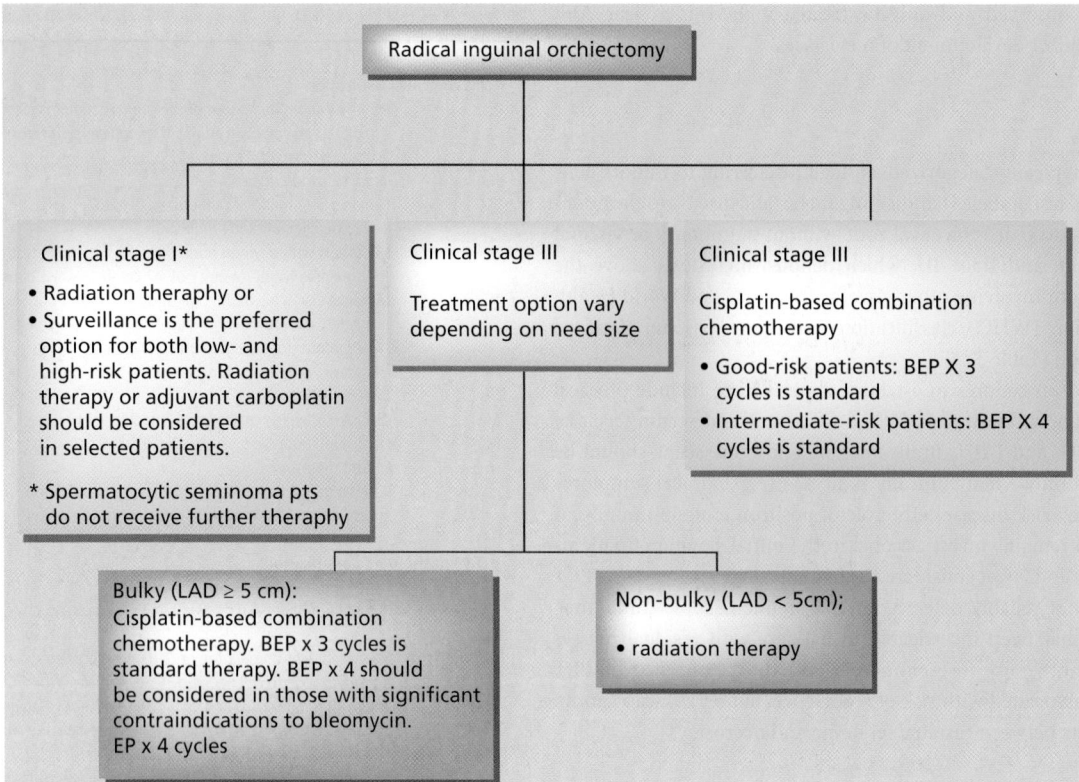

Figure 8 Treatment of seminoma.

setting, approximately 30% of patients will suffer a relapse if no other therapy is administered, with the retroperitoneum remaining as the area at highest risk. Approximately 8–10% of patients will develop metastases outside of the retroperitoneum, mostly in the lungs.[45]

Freedman and colleagues developed a mathematical model on the basis of the four identified prognostic factors and were able to identify a subset of patients with a 58% relapse rate at 2 years.[46] These four factors included invasion of testicular veins, invasion of testicular lymphatics, absence of yolk sac elements, and presence of undifferentiated tumor. Pathologic T-stage higher than 1, the presence of components of embryonal carcinoma, and percent of the primary tumor occupied by teratoma have also been described.[46–48] The importance of vascular invasion as the most dominating independent risk factor has been emphasized. Clinically, the presence of vascular invasion in the primary tumor specimen discriminates the "high-risk" patients with a risk of relapse of approximately 50% from the "low-risk" patients without lymphovascular invasion and an approximately 15–20% risk of relapse.

There is an ongoing controversy regarding the optimal management of patients with clinical stage I nonseminoma. All three options—RPLND, adjuvant chemotherapy, and active surveillance—are discussed later.

Retroperitoneal lymph node dissection

Based on a predictable lymphatic pattern of spread of testicular tumors, RPLND emerged as a treatment option for testicular cancer as early as 1907.[49–51] In the United States, primary RPLND became the conventional approach for patients with clinical stage I NSGCTs. In Europe and Canada, consensus guidelines do not currently advocate primary RPLND in early-stage disease.[52,53] Nevertheless, RPLND does provide the most accurate method of detecting retroperitoneal nodal disease, which account for more

than 90% of the first site of metastatic spread. RPLND alone can be curative in 50–80% of clinical stage I disease who are found to have limited nodal disease at surgery (pN1). More than five metastatic lymph nodes, diseased nodes measuring more than 2 cm, and any extranodal extension (pN2–pN23) are virtually all cured following two cycles of adjuvant chemotherapy.[54] Primary RPLND also has the advantage of removing retroperitoneal teratoma, which is chemoresistant, virtually eliminating the risk of late relapse of teratoma.[55] However even in pure teratomas, only 20% of patients will harbor occult retroperitoneal lymph node metastases at the time of diagnosis.[56] Relapses in the retroperitoneum are exceedingly rare in patients who undergo RPLND by experienced surgeons. The overall relapse rate for patients with disease limited to the testicle is approximately 10%, with the great majority of relapses occurring in the lungs.

Radical lymphadenectomy via a thoracoabdominal (extraperitoneal) approach was described in 1950 [57] and popularized by Skinner in the 1980s,[58] while reports of pure abdominal (anterior) approaches dominated the 1970s,[59,60] with each approach having intrinsic advantages. The thoracoabdominal approach is associated with significantly higher morbidity including pain and chest complications albeit lower rates of small bowel obstruction.[58] To reduce morbidity Donohue and colleagues described the midline anterior approach, and since the incidence of suprahilar metastases in clinical stage I disease was shown to be rare, the technique evolved to include only infrahilar RPLND.[61] The thoracoabdominal incision has largely been replaced by the anterior midline approach.

In experienced hands, the classic bilateral RPLND is associated with minimal perioperative morbidity and virtually no mortality.[62] A major side effect is the loss of antegrade ejaculation, with resultant need for assisted reproductive technology in over 90%

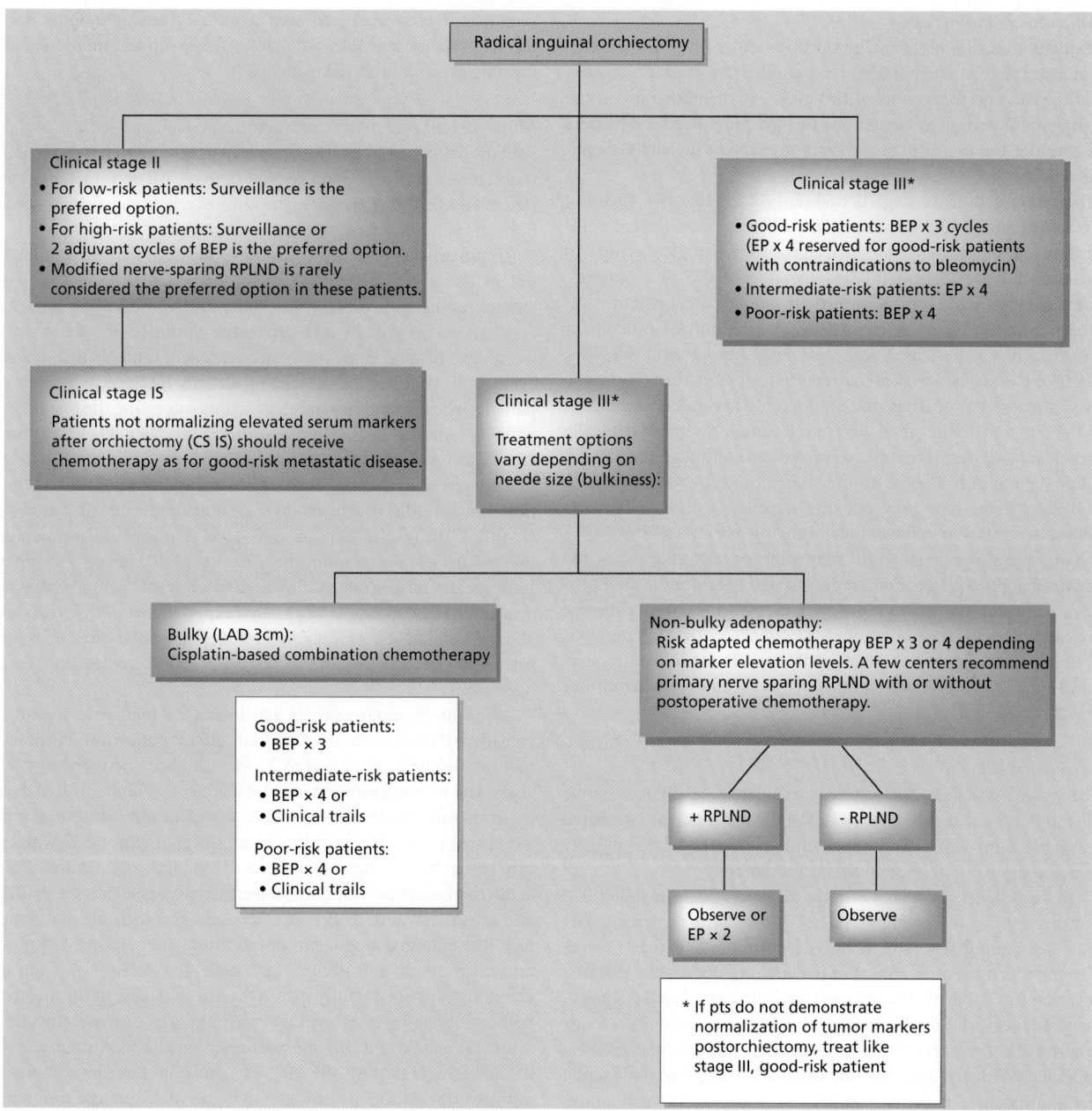

Figure 9 Treatment of nonseminoma.

of patients. An improved understanding of the nerves and pathways responsible for seminal emission and ejaculation along with meticulous anatomic studies of the distribution of right-sided and left-sided tumors led to further modification of the surgical "templates" for RPLND.[63,64] Several nerve-sparing modifications of the classic node dissection have now been described.[65–67] Any template used must adhere to strict principles of thoroughly resecting all interaortocaval lymph nodes and ipsilateral lymph nodes from the level of the renal hilum down to the bifurcation of the ipsilateral common iliac artery. Dissection is minimized on the contralateral side particularly below the level of the inferior mesenteric artery (IMA). To minimize retroperitoneal recurrence, some advocate bilateral infrahilar dissections only sparing the contralateral nodes below the IMA.[68] Modified template nerve-sparing RPLND is now considered standard for patients undergoing surgery for clinical stage I disease. Meticulous preservation of the postganglionic sympathetic fibers arising from the sympathetic chain and the

hypogastric plexus results in uniformly high rates of preservation of ejaculatory function (96–100%) while maintaining more than 99% cure rate.[59,66,69]

To further reduce the morbidity of surgery, laparoscopic techniques for RPLND have been used.[70] Although operating room times are longer, long-term follow-up in over 550 patients has shown no difference in relapse rates compared with traditional open RPLND. However, the vast majority (>90%) of the patients with positive nodes have received adjuvant chemotherapy raising the question of the true efficacy of this approach.

Radiotherapy

Although previously utilized in stage I nonseminoma, radiotherapy is no longer used based on the overwhelming success of combination chemotherapy, the safety of active surveillance, as well as the limited efficacy of radiotherapy in nonseminomas.

Adjuvant chemotherapy

The definition of a high-risk group by vascular invasion, the efficacy and safety of chemotherapy for good-risk metastatic disease, and the near-perfect results of two cycles of chemotherapy in the setting of fully resected stage II disease have prompted investigators to consider the use of primary chemotherapy in high-risk stage I disease.

Based on data from stage II trials suggesting that two cycles of bleomycin, etoposide, and cisplatin (BEP) may be sufficient adjuvant treatment, the MRC designed a prospective study offering two cycles of BEP to patients with high-risk stage 1 NSGCTT[71] to evaluate the efficacy and long-term toxicity of adjuvant chemotherapy. One hundred and fourteen patients were treated and followed up for a median of 4 years. The 2-year recurrence-free survival was 98%. The 95% CI excluded a true recurrence rate of more than 5%. Of the two patients who recurred, one was found to have adenocarcinoma of the rete testis rather than a germ cell tumor. No major clinically significant long-term toxicities were observed, although the median follow-up was only 4 years. Adjuvant chemotherapy with two cycles of BEP achieves a near-universal cure in patients with stage I disease with relapse rates in various studies ranging from 0% to 2%.

Two cycles of adjuvant BEP were subsequently adopted as the standard approach to patients with vascular invasion for the European consensus guidelines, whereas patients with low-risk disease are candidates for active surveillance.[52]

Recent data suggest that 1 cycle of BEP results in similar outcome and 1 cycle of BEP is now recommended as the adjuvant chemotherapy of choice.[72,73]

Active surveillance

The main rationale for active surveillance is that systemic chemotherapy is highly effective and thus patients who are cured by orchiectomy alone can be spared the treatment-related toxicity of a primary RPLND or adjuvant chemotherapy.

An early large prospective study of surveillance included 373 patients with a median follow-up of 5 years.[74] The recurrence rate was 27% and of these 80% recurred within the first year. Overall cure rate for the entire cohort of patients exceeded 98%. Vascular invasion was confirmed as the most important prognostic factor. A large data set including 1139 stage I nonseminoma patients recently confirmed active surveillance as an excellent and safe management modality. With a recurrence rate of 19% (44% in lymphovascular invasion-positive patients and 14% in negative patients) and a disease-specific survival of 99.7% on long-term follow-up, this series of surveillance underlines the efficacy of the approach.[75]

There are now reports of more than 3000 patients worldwide with clinical stage I disease who have had no other therapy administered following orchiectomy with relapse rates and survival remarkably similar between trials, regardless of the size of the study or country of origin.[76] Almost all patients on active surveillance relapse within 2 years after diagnosis with IGCCCG good-prognosis disease.[74,77] Only 2–3% of relapses occur beyond 2 years.[75] Thus careful surveillance plus chemotherapy at the earliest sign of recurrence is an effective management approach to patients with stage 1 NSGCTT. Active surveillance has been adopted as the standard of care for patients with low-risk disease by the European consensus guidelines and for patients with both low-risk and high-risk disease by the Canadian consensus guidelines.[52]

Based on a randomized prospective trial, a sufficient follow-up schedule for vascular invasion-negative patients consists of tumor markers and clinical examination every 2 months for the first 2 years and every 4–6 months for years 3–5. Chest X-rays are done every 4 months for the first 2 years and then every 6 months thereafter until year 5.[78] CT scans are performed at 3, 12, 24, and 56 months. Various surveillance schedules with closer follow-up and more frequent imaging exist for high-risk patients.

Management preferences in stage 1 NSGCTT

Patients with stage 1 NSGCTT, especially those at high risk of recurrence, have a choice of management options. All options, when carried out meticulously, result in the same excellent survival prospects but with different shortcomings.

Arguments for retaining primary surgery are that when done in one of the few high-volume centers in the United States or elsewhere, results are excellent, infertility and complication rates are very low, and essentially such procedure eliminates the abdomen as a source of relapse. However, even in excellent centers, preoperative evaluations routinely fail to reliably identify the seventy percent of patients who are pathological stage I, thus subjecting the majority of patients to major surgery without therapeutic benefit. In addition, 25–35% of patients will require additional two cycles of BEP due to extensive retroperitoneal disease. Most importantly, RPLND does not eliminate the risk of recurrence outside the retroperitoneum (8–10%). The results of community-level primary surgical management of stage I nonseminoma have demonstrated not only a numerically greater relapse rate as compared to adjuvant chemotherapy but also an increased number of patients experiencing both scrotal and abdominal relapses, strongly suggesting that primary RPLNDs performed by less experienced urologists result in inadequate cancer operations.[72]

Adjuvant chemotherapy, in particular for high-risk disease, is considered the standard of care in many countries. While the recurrence rate is decreased to 2–4%, adjuvant chemotherapy will also result in overtreatment in at least 50% of patients.[76] All of these patients will experience hair loss; a significant disruption from work, school, and life; exposure to significant neutropenia with the rare risk of fatal complications; risk of vascular complications; rare acute chemotherapy reactions; at least temporary effects on fertility; and the anxiety and fears that all patients receiving chemotherapy face. The potential long-term complications are currently unknown and relapses can still occur. Thus, patients treated with adjuvant chemotherapy are not fully spared the fear of relapse or the inconvenience of ongoing imaging. Expert groups are now recommending one cycle of adjuvant BEP for high-risk stage I nonseminoma.[73,79]

Concerns regarding the lack of compliance are an argument against surveillance, in particular in high-risk CSI nonseminoma.[76] There is no evidence that the level of compliance across varying geographies materially impacts survival.[76,80,81] Survival rates consistently approach 100% even in series with reported "unsatisfactory" compliance. Educating patients is crucial and emphasizing that later identification of disease might well lead to more complicated and complex therapies is fully warranted. Concerns about the undissected retroperitoneum leading to a significant number of late refractory cancer or late recurrence of teratoma have not been realized in this and other studies.[76,80,82,83]

On surveillance, only patients who relapse will receive treatment. Treatment of these patients will be slightly longer than adjuvant BEP (6 vs. 9 weeks).[84] In our opinion, there is only a small difference in toxicity between two and three courses of chemotherapy. However, there is a major difference between no chemotherapy and two courses. Active surveillance completely spares 70–75% of patients the burden of any active treatment.

Clinical stage II

Tumor marker-positive disease and/or large-volume abdominal disease (>2 cm on abdominal CT, stage IIB) should be treated with primary chemotherapy. Standard treatment is three cycles of BEP for IGCCCG good-prognosis disease.[84] Only in the case of significant contraindication to bleomycin four cycles of etoposide and cisplatin (EP) can be considered.[85] Most patients with stage IIA/B will achieve a clinical complete remission with resolution of all lymph node metastases and normalization of tumor markers (80–90% in stage IIA and 65–85% in stage IIB).[84,85] Only patients with persistent retroperitoneal residual disease on the postchemotherapy CT scan should undergo RPLND. The relapse rate with this strategy is 4–9% for stage IIA and 11–15% for stage IIB.[86–88] Tumor marker-negative stage IIA (lymph nodes ≤2 cm) represents a particular problem. Some of these patients will have benign lymph node enlargement; however, some will have teratoma, pure embryonal carcinoma, or mixed tumors. There is currently no diagnostic tool to determine the nature of these masses reliably. Management options include primary RPLND or a surveillance period with repeat imaging after 6–8 weeks. If the lesions shrink, no further therapy is required; for stable or growing lesions, most centers would consider primary chemotherapy, with a few selected centers considering primary RPLND.

Seminoma: Early stage

Orchiectomy and postoperative radiation therapy constituted the standard of care for early-stage seminoma patients during most of the twentieth century.[89–91] A radical orchiectomy by an inguinal approach is highly effective therapy for controlling disease at the primary tumor site. Occult or gross PA lymphatic tumor deposits can be eradicated with high probability after low doses of radiation therapy (20–25 Gy), owing to the extreme radiosensitivity of seminoma. Trials have investigated surveillance in stage I seminoma. With a large majority of patients experiencing prolonged disease-free survival in early-stage seminoma, long-term quality of life will assume, increasing significance in evaluating management options.

Stage I seminoma: Primary and adjuvant therapy

Stage I disease comprises 85% of all seminoma cases.[92] Surveillance studies demonstrated that an orchiectomy is curative approximately 80–85% of the time. Chemotherapy and/or radiation can be given as salvage therapy or as prophylaxis. Regardless of the elected management method, disease-specific survival at 5 years is over 99%.[93–96] The treatment of relapsed treatment-naïve disease appears to be as curable as it is at first presentation.

Four major series demonstrated that surveillance is a viable option.[93–95,97–100] Their combined experience was pooled to better identify candidates for treatment or surveillance.[94] In the entire group of 638 patients, six patients (0.9%) died of disease or complications of treatment of relapse. The overall 5-year and 10-year relapse-free rates were 82.3% and 78.7%, respectively. The majority (68.6%) of relapses occurred within 2 years, but still 7% of recurrences occur after 6 years. The two most important prognostic factors were tumor size and rete testis invasion. Patients with tumors >4 cm in diameter were twice as likely to relapse as those with smaller tumors. The rete testis is a communicating network of seminal channels traversing the mediastinum (or hilum) of the testis. Rete testis invasion was seen in 37% and defined as extension of the tumor into the testicular mediastinum without necessarily involving the tubular lumens. For patients with large tumor size and rete testis invasion, the rates of recurrence were as high as 33%. For patients without these factors, the recurrence rates were as low as 13%. This analysis could not be validated in a subsequent, recently published analysis from the two groups using an independent data set, although tumor size as a linear variable is associated with risk.[101,102]

The schedule for surveillance testing is in flux and in general the previous intense schedules are being revised downward.[75] Many centers concentrate observations into the highest period of risk and use progressively less CT scans in follow-up. Many schedules in seminoma are recommending a 3–2–1 with 3 abdominal/pelvic CTs the first year, 2 the second, and 1 the third with no CTs thereafter. Thus, although surveillance is a very attractive option, the frequency of follow-up imaging and tests cannot be reduced in any given patient. Therefore, patients who elect surveillance need to be compliant and reliable.

Patients with stage I seminoma have been successfully treated with orchiectomy and adjuvant radiation for over 60 years with overall survival rates now above 99%. Adjuvant PA radiation results in a 3–4% rate of relapse with most of those being salvageable with additional radiation and/or chemotherapy. Analogous to the movement for surveillance is a simultaneous drive to reduce the toxicity of initial adjuvant therapy by reducing radiation dose and volume treated.

Radiation dose has been gradually reduced to 20–25.5 Gy in 1.5–2 Gy fractions in current practice. The MRC TE18/EORTC 30942 trial addressed whether the radiation dose could be safely lowered from 30 to 20 Gy.[103] Most patients received only radiation to the PA nodes, and they were randomized to 30 Gy in 15 fractions versus 20 Gy in 10 fractions. The 0.7% absolute difference in relapse rates was statistically insignificant, and the lower dose was associated with less lethargy and inability to carry out normal work at 1 month.

Similarly, radiotherapy volume has been reduced.[104] Ipsilateral pelvic lymph node irradiation did not significantly improve the 96% relapse-free survival at 3 years obtained with PA node field only radiation. However, four of nine of the patients who had been treated with PA node radiation had pelvic node involvement as a component of their relapse. Thus, patients who receive PA node radiation alone must still be followed with CT scans of the pelvis. Current practice is to treat the PA nodes from the top of T11 or T12 to the bottom of L5. Ipsilateral pelvic lymph node irradiation is still recommended, however, for patients who have had prior pelvic or inguinal surgery as this can disrupt normal lymphatic flow. PA node radiation alone is sufficient for patients with an undisturbed testicular lymphatic drainage.

Postorchiectomy chemotherapy

A large randomized trial was conducted by the EORTC/MRC in which patients with well-staged clinical stage I seminoma were randomly allocated to standard prophylactic radiation therapy (primarily PA radiation at 20–30 Gy) or treatment with single-course single-agent carboplatin (AUC 7).[105,106] This trial was designed to exclude an absolute increase in relapse at 2 years of 3%. In a 1 : 2 randomization scheme, 560 patients were assigned to single-agent carboplatin, and 885 were assigned to standard radiation therapy. With median 4-year follow-up, the 3-year relapse-free survival rate was 95.9% for radiation compared with 94.8% for carboplatin ($p = 0.31$), the majority of relapses on the carboplatin arm occurring in the abdomen and almost all of the recurrences in the radiation arm occurring outside the radiation portal. There were fewer new second primary TGCTs with carboplatin (two patients) versus radiotherapy (10 patients). The authors' conclusions were that single-agent carboplatin was a safe and effective adjuvant treatment of clinical stage I seminoma, but follow-up longer than 4 years is necessary. Criticisms of the study were that the pattern of abdominal relapse with the carboplatin-treated patients may necessitate abdominal imaging in follow-up and that short follow-up may underestimate the true incidence of relapse. This trial was updated,[106] and with median 6.5 year follow-up, there remains no significant difference in 5-year relapse-free survival between carboplatin (95%) and radiotherapy (96%). The rate of new second primary GCTs was lower with carboplatin (two patients) versus radiotherapy (15 patients).

Consensus guidelines in Europe and in Canada reflect the collected work of experienced radiation oncologists, medical oncologists, and urologists. The European consensus statement favors surveillance for all patients independent of the individual risk for relapse. Only if surveillance is not applicable, the equally effective alternatives are either adjuvant radiation or adjuvant carboplatin. A risk-adapted strategy with selection of adjuvant treatment according to individual risk is currently being investigated and is still experimental.[107]

Stage II seminoma

Several different staging systems have defined stage II seminoma, depending on how the distinctions are made for nodal size. Regardless of the specific staging system used, the potential for supradiaphragmatic involvement increases with the size of the subdiaphragmatic disease. At most centers, the arbitrary cutoff for systemic chemotherapy is 5 cm, while patients with nodal masses <5 cm can be treated with radiation alone. Unlike with stage I, surveillance is not an option, and the expected 5-year relapse-free survival drops to 89–95% for patients treated with radiation alone.[108–110] The overall survival still remains around 97–99% because of the effectiveness of salvage therapy. For patients with stage II seminoma, the standard radiation field incorporates the PA and ipsilateral pelvic lymph nodes. The treatment of stage II seminoma with radiation has also evolved. Historically for a patient with stage II seminoma, radiation was delivered to the PA nodes, to the pelvic lymph nodes, and prophylactically to the mediastinum. This practice, although effective at limiting supradiaphragmatic failures, became associated with cardiac morbidity. Chemotherapy is now favored for patients who are at significant risk of supradiaphragmatic involvement.

There is also an increasing experience with chemotherapy as primary management of small- to moderate-volume stage II seminoma.[111] A Spanish collaborative study entered 72 patients at 26 participating centers. Eighteen patients had stage IIA disease, and 54 patients had stage IIB disease. Eighty-three percent of patients achieved complete response (CR), and 17% achieved partial response (PR) with residual mass. After a median follow-up of 71.5 months, six patients with stage IIB disease experienced relapse, and one of these died of seminoma. Three patients experienced nonseminoma-related deaths. The estimated 5-year progression-free survival rates for patients with stage IIA or IIB disease were 100% and 87% (95% CI, 77.5–97%), respectively. Five-year progression-free and overall survival rates for the whole group were 90% (95% CI, 82–98%) and 95% (95% CI, 89–100%), respectively; mild to moderate emesis, stomatitis, and diarrhea were the most common nonhematologic effects. Such experiences strongly suggest that primary chemotherapy may be an effective alternative to abdominal radiation.

Therapy for disseminated disease

Chemotherapy: pre-cisplatin

A broad spectrum of chemotherapeutic agents were tested from 1952 to 1972 in disseminated GCTs. In the early 1960s, the vinca alkaloids were tested. Vinblastine induced complete remissions in 4 of 30 treated patients.[109] Although these were of short duration, they provided investigators with a rational component of subsequent combination regimens.

Several antitumor antibiotics were also found to have single-agent activity, including actinomycin D. In 1970, bleomycin was reported to induce complete remissions.[112,113]

An early combination regimen described in 1960, which contained methotrexate, actinomycin D, and chlorambucil, remained popular throughout the rest of the decade.[114] Li reported an objective response rate of 52%, with more than half of those being CR. These were the first durable remissions, with five patients alive at 9–39 months after treatment.

A further advance occurred when vinblastine and bleomycin were used in combination.[115] This regimen resulted in 65% of patients achieving a complete remission, including some durable responses.

The most important event in the development of curative therapy for disseminated disease was the 1965 report by Rosenberg and colleagues of the antibacterial effect of platinum coordination compounds.[116] One of these compounds, cis-diamminedichloroplatinum (II) (cisplatin) was found also to have significant antitumor activity. Preclinical studies revealed testicular atrophy as a side effect in the dog model, prompting some investigators to predict activity for this compound against human testicular malignancies in the clinical setting. Cisplatin was soon reported to be the single most active agent against TGCTs, with response rates of 70% and complete remission rates of 50%.[114] Thirty years later, it remains the most active drug in GCTs.

Indiana University studies

In 1974, investigators at Indiana University began studies using vinblastine (PVB) in patients with disseminated testicular cancer. The initial study remains a landmark study in modern oncology.[117] This study incorporated principles of combination chemotherapy, as well as the concept of surgically resecting residual disease after the completion of chemotherapy. Induction chemotherapy was brief (three to four courses), and maintenance chemotherapy was given for 2 years after induction therapy. Thirty-three of 47 patients (70%) obtained a complete remission with chemotherapy. Of the remaining 14 patients, five obtained a complete remission with resection of residual disease. Six of the patients attaining remission relapsed.

The initial study proved that PVB was remarkably effective, and yet there was substantial toxicity. The next study was designed to compare the original PVB program with a similar regimen with a lower dose of vinblastine (0.3 mg/kg vs. 0.4 mg/kg).[118] Seventy-eight patients were entered into this study, with 70% of all patients remaining continuously free of disease with equivalent results with the different vinblastine dosages. As expected, however, the reduction in the vinblastine dose led to less sepsis and granulocytopenic fever. Thus, the lower dose of vinblastine, along with cisplatin and bleomycin, became the standard regimen for PVB.

Confirmation of the results of these trials was obtained in a large EORTC trial.[119] This trial tested the contribution of high-dose vinblastine (0.4 mg/kg) versus lower-dose vinblastine (0.3 mg/kg) and the value of maintenance vinblastine. The trial of 214 patients failed to demonstrate any advantage for patients assigned to high-dose vinblastine therapy or for those assigned to maintenance vinblastine.

A third-generation study was begun at Indiana University in 1978 in conjunction with the Southeastern Cancer Study Group (SECSG).[120] The previous studies had used maintenance therapy with monthly vinblastine for 2 years after the completion of induction therapy. This trial tested the contribution of maintenance

Table 4 International germ cell consensus classification.

Good prognosis
Nonseminoma testis or retroperitoneal primary and no nonpulmonary visceral
    metastases and α-fetoprotein <1000 ng/mL, βHCG <5000 IU/L, and LDH <1.5
    upper limit of normal
Seminoma of any primary site and no nonpulmonary visceral metastases and
    normal α-fetoprotein, any βHCG, and any LDH
Intermediate prognosis
Nonseminoma testis or retroperitoneal primary and no nonpulmonary visceral
    metastases and α-fetoprotein >1000 ng/mL and <10,000 ng/mL or βHCG
    >5000 IU/L and <50,000 IU/L or LDH >1.5 normal and <10 normal
Seminoma of any primary site and nonpulmonary visceral metastases and normal
    α-fetoprotein, any βHCG, and any LDH
Poor prognosis
Nonseminoma with mediastinal primary, nonpulmonary visceral metastases, or
    α-fetoprotein >10,000 ng/mL or βHCG >50,000 IU/L, or LDH >10 upper limit of
    normal

Abbreviations: LDH, lactate dehydrogenase; βHCG, β-human chorionic
gonadotropin.

chemotherapy. Patients with disseminated testicular cancer received
four courses of induction chemotherapy with PVB. Patients obtaining a complete remission with chemotherapy, or after resection of
teratoma, were randomized to receive maintenance vinblastine or
no further therapy. This study failed to demonstrate an advantage
to the maintenance therapy arm.

The next study was a randomized trial comparing cisplatin plus
bleomycin and either PVBs or etoposide (BEP).[121] Two hundred
sixty-one patients with disseminated germ cell cancer were entered,
and 244 were evaluable for response. Of these, 123 were randomly
allocated to receive BEP, and 83% achieved a disease-free status.
One hundred twenty-one patients were assigned to receive PVB,
and 74% attained a disease-free status. In the combined subgroups
of patients with minimal or moderate disease by the Indiana classification system, 90% achieved a disease-free status, with no difference between the two treatment arms. However, PVB patients
experienced significantly more paresthesias, myalgias, and abdominal cramping. Because BEP had substantially less neuromuscular
toxicity with equal or superior therapeutic results, cisplatin, etoposide, and bleomycin became and remain a standard regimen.

Prognostic classifications

An international consortium collected clinical data on patients
receiving platinum-based therapy for metastatic GCT to develop
a new prognostic model for disseminated disease.[122] Data on
5202 patients with NSGCT and 660 patients with seminoma
were analyzed. Independent predictors of outcome in univariate analysis were mediastinal primary site for nonseminomatous
tumors, degree of AFP, HCG, and LDH elevation, and the presence of nonpulmonary visceral metastasis. Good-risk patients
with nonseminomatous disease were those with testicular or
retroperitoneal primary, favorable markers, and no nonpulmonary
visceral metastases (anticipated progression-free survival 90%).
Poor prognosis included those patients with mediastinal primary
nonseminoma, those with nonpulmonary visceral metastases, or
those with unfavorable elevation of tumor markers (anticipated
progression-free survival 40%). An intermediate group had an
anticipated progression-free survival rate of 75%. For seminoma,
only good-risk and intermediate-risk groups were identified by the
absence or presence of nonpulmonary visceral metastases (Table 4).
This classification should be the standard classification system for
comparing results of clinical studies done at various institutions.

Treatment of good-risk disseminated germ cell tumors

Patients with good-risk disease constitute approximately 56% of
patients presenting with disseminated disease. The IGCCC for
good-risk disease suggests that more than 90% of patients in this
category enjoy long-term disease-free survival.

Because virtually all these patients achieve complete remission
with standard chemotherapy, additional trials addressed the possibility of reducing the amount of chemotherapy (thus decreasing
acute and chronic toxicity) while maintaining the excellent cure rate.
Approaches included shortening of the duration of therapy, use of
chemotherapeutic agents with less single-agent toxicity, and a reduction in the number of agents.

The SECSG performed a trial in which patients with good-risk
disease were randomized to receive either three or four courses of
BEP.[123] There was no difference in the percent of patients achieving complete remission, and 92% of patients on both arms were
disease-free with a median follow-up of 19 months. On the basis
of these results, three courses of BEP (cisplatin 20 mg/m² plus
etoposide 100 mg/m² intravenously [IV] days 1–5, repeated every
3 weeks, with bleomycin 30 units IV weekly) are the standard
therapy at Indiana University for patients with good-risk disease.

ECOG completed a trial randomizing patients with minimal or
moderate disease to receive three courses of either BEP or EP alone
to eliminate the inconvenience (and possible pulmonary toxicity)
of weekly bleomycin.[124] However, patients receiving bleomycin
had superior survival. EORTC conducted a trial comparing four
cycles of EP with or without bleomycin in patients with good-risk
NSGCT.[125] Complete remission rate (95% vs. 89%) favored the
bleomycin-containing arm, but relapse rates were similar. Another
trial randomized good-risk patients to receive VP-16 (etoposide),
combined with either cisplatin for four cycles (standard arm) or
carboplatin.[126] In addition, the MRC/EORTC compared etoposide
and bleomycin with either cisplatin or carboplatin in good-risk
patients.[127,128] The advantages of carboplatin are its relative lack of
nephrotoxicity and neurotoxicity and the ability to administer on an
outpatient basis without aggressive prehydration. However, inferior
survival was seen in patients receiving carboplatin in these trials.
Toner and colleagues reported inferior survival with four cycles of
a dose-reduced version of BEP in comparison with standard BEP
for three cycles.[129] In summary, analysis of all trials attempting
to further reduce toxicity by the elimination of bleomycin or the
substitution of carboplatin for cisplatin has shown therapeutic
inferiority.

A final attempt to eliminate bleomycin from chemotherapy for
good-risk regimens comes from the French collaborative study.[130]
The trial enrolled 257 patients who were randomly allocated to
three cycles of BEP or four cycles of EP (both regimens used
5-day schedules with 500 mg/m² of etoposide per cycle). At the
time of trial initiation, an older prognostic classification was used.
The trial was underpowered for survival, but using the original
prognostic classification system and when patients were reclassified
by the IGCCCC system, there were more unfavorable outcomes
and more deaths in the EP. A definitive trial would require a very
large patient population to prove equivalence of the two regimens.
Toxicity was not substantially different between the two arms with
the exception of more skin and neurologic toxicity in the BEP arm
and more neutropenia and thrombocytopenia in the EP arm. There
were no therapy-related deaths in either arm and no difference in
pulmonary toxicity. The authors concluded that BEP at standard
"American" BEP represented standard therapy for good-risk disseminated GCTs. They also concluded that further testing of this
concept was not likely to be fruitful and that there was very little

chance that four cycles of EP could be proven superior. European and Canadian consensus statements also endorse BEP × 3 as the standard regimen for IGCCC good-risk disseminated disease.

Further reductions in the amount of therapy are unlikely to reduce toxicity significantly, but have the potential to reduce the cure rate in this stage of disease. Alternative schedules of BEP have also been reported. De Wit and colleagues report the results of a study from the EORTC and the MRC in which patients received either three cycles of BEP with etoposide given as 100 mg/m² days 1–5 or 165 mg/m² days 1–3, cisplatin given as either 20 mg/m² days 1–5 or 50 mg/m² on days 1 and 2 only, and weekly bleomycin. There was some mild increase in ototoxicity and gastrointestinal side effects with the 3-day schedule, and long-term quality of life parameters and late toxicities are not available. These two versions of the BEP regimen yielded no significant difference in 2-year overall survival, with a 98% cure rate in patients with HCG < 1000.[131]

Treatment of patients with "intermediate-risk" disseminated disease

Intermediate-risk disease was defined by the IGCCCG classification in 1995; very few studies are available. An EORTC randomized study comparing EP plus either bleomycin (BEP) or ifosfamide (VIP) in an intermediate prognosis group found comparable response rates as well as similar long-term survival rates of 83% in the BEP and 85% in the VIP arm.[132] The VIP regimen was associated with more acute hematologic toxicity. The study was prematurely discontinued when data became available from a competing study in poor-risk patients that showed no improvement in outcomes with VIP but rather very similar results to BEP.[133] In a subsequent study a combination of paclitaxel plus BEP (T-BEP) was compared to BEP alone.[134] The study was closed early due to slow accrual and failed to show an overall survival benefit. No other large studies are currently available in the intermediate-risk group, and four cycles of BEP or 4 cycles of VIP remain the standard of care.

Treatment of patients with "poor-risk" disseminated disease

Patients with disseminated testicular cancer who present with poor prognostic features remain a therapeutic challenge. One approach is the exploration of chemotherapy dose intensification.

Preclinical models, as well as dose-intensity analysis of clinical trials, suggest a steep dose–response relationship for cisplatin. This has been tested in several clinical trials of intensive cisplatin in patients with poor-prognosis germ cell cancer. Ozols and colleagues reported the results of a randomized trial of aggressive, high-dose cisplatin therapy versus PVB in poor-risk testicular cancer patients.[135] There was a 2 : 1 randomization of 52 poor-risk patients to receive an aggressive arm with cisplatin, 40 mg/m² (double the standard dose) on days 1–5 with vinblastine, bleomycin, and etoposide in standard doses versus classic PVB with cisplatin given at 20 mg/m² on days 1–5. Of the patients receiving the aggressive arm, 88% had a CR, as compared with 67% of the patients receiving PVB. The PVB arm had a high incidence of relapse, with 41% of the patients having disease recurrence, as compared with 17% of the patients receiving high-dose cisplatin, bleomycin, and VP-16 (PVeBV). Overall, 68% of the group were randomized to the aggressive treatment remained disease-free, as compared with only 33% of the patients receiving standard therapy. Unfortunately, there was a substantial increase in toxicity including myelosuppression and hearing loss in the patients receiving the high-dose cisplatin. Whether the apparent superiority of the high-dose regimen was

attributable to the high-dose cisplatin, the inclusion of etoposide, or other factors, was not clear.

Rigid testing of the impact of high-dose cisplatin therapy in disseminated germ cell cancer was accomplished in a trial of the SECSG and SWOG in advanced germ cell cancer.[136] This trial enrolled only patients with advanced disease by the Indiana classification system. Patients were assigned at random to receive standard doses of etoposide and bleomycin and either standard-dose cisplatin (20 mg/m² daily for 5 days) or high-dose cisplatin (40 mg/m² daily for 5 days). One hundred fifty-nine patients with advanced disseminated germ cell cancer were enrolled. Of these, 153 were evaluable for toxicity and response. Among 76 patients assigned to high-dose therapy, 52 (68%) became disease-free with chemotherapy alone or subsequent surgery. Among 77 patients on the standard-dose arm, 56 (73%) became disease-free with chemotherapy alone or surgical resection of residual disease. Overall, 74% of the patients receiving the high-dose cisplatin are alive, and 63% are continuously free of disease, as compared with 74% alive and 61% continuously free of disease on the standard-dose arm. The high-dose arm was associated with significantly more ototoxicity, neurotoxicity, gastrointestinal toxicity, and myelosuppression. In contrast to the NCI study, this large randomized trial found no therapeutic benefit of dose escalation of cisplatin.

In a follow-up to the SECSG trial of cisplatin dose intensity, ECOG conducted a trial testing the substitution of ifosfamide for bleomycin.[136] Three hundred four patients with advanced-stage disseminated germ cell cancer by the Indiana classification system were entered into this trial, which randomized patients to either four standard courses of BEP or to four courses of VIP with etoposide (75 mg/m² daily for 5 days), ifosfamide (1.2 g/m² daily for 5 days), and cisplatin (20 mg/m² daily for 5 days). Two hundred ninety patients were fully evaluable for toxicity, and 286 were evaluable for response. The rates for complete remission (VIP 37%, BEP 31%), favorable response (VIP 63%, BEP 60%), failure-free at 2 years (VIP 64%, VIP 60%), and 2-year survival (VIP 74%, BEP 71%) were not statistically different between the two treatments. Grade 3 or greater toxicity, primarily hematologic, was significantly greater on the VIP arm ($p < 0.0001$). There were five therapy-related deaths on each arm. This analysis failed to demonstrate benefit for VIP relative to standard therapy with BEP.

A similar trial evaluating the role of ifosfamide in poor-risk patients with GCT was reported by EORTC and MRC.[137] Patients were randomized to BEP/EP or intensively scheduled bleomycin, vincristine, and cisplatin followed by VIP-B. There were no differences in time to progression or overall survival. Grade 3 or 4 myelosuppression and weight loss were more pronounced in the bleomycin, Oncovin (vincristine), and prednisone (BOP)/VIP-B arm. The authors concluded that the intensive BOP/VIP-B therapy was more toxic, but without therapeutic advantage.

Another dose-dense regimen including cisplatin, cyclophosphamide, doxorubicin, vinblastine, and bleomycin (CISCA-VB) was compared to BEP in a randomized trial including intermediate- and poor-risk patients. No improved outcome but more toxicity was observed in the dose-dense arm.[138]

A recently published randomized trial by the GETUC group tested the concept of unfavorable tumor marker decline within the first cycle of BEP chemotherapy. Patients with slower than predicted marker decline were randomized to either standard BEP or a dose-dense intensification regimen including bleomycin, paclitaxel, oxaliplatin, cisplatin, ifosfamide, and etoposide.[139]

Three-year progression-free survival was improved in the dose-dense group (59% vs. 48%; $p = 0.05$).

High-dose chemotherapy as primary treatment of poor-risk disease

Investigators in Germany attempted to intensify therapy for poor-risk patients by incorporating growth factors and peripheral blood progenitor cell support to give high-dose, repetitive chemotherapy cycles. Patients with poor-risk disseminated GCTs were given repetitive cycles of cisplatin $25-30 \, mg/m^2$ on days $1-5$, etoposide $100-250 \, mg/m^2$ on days $1-5$, and ifosfamide $2 \, g/m^2$ on days $1-5$ every 22 days for four cycles.[140] At the highest dose levels, support with growth factors and peripheral blood progenitor cells was required. With these supportive care techniques, this high-dose therapy was tolerated with no dose-limiting myelosuppression, mucositis, renal toxicity, or neurotoxicity. However, three of the 32 patients at the highest dose levels died of causes related to therapy. Of the 23 evaluable for response, 20 (87%) attained disease-free status, and three relapsed.

A trial of 115 patients randomized poor-risk patients to conventional therapy with cisplatin, vinblastine, etoposide, and bleomycin versus similar therapy followed by a single cycle of high-dose cisplatin, etoposide, and cyclophosphamide.[141] This trial failed to demonstrate an advantage for the high-dose arm.

A large-scale trial has been conducted for poor-risk patients that compared two courses of standard therapy (BEP) followed by two cycles of very high-dose carboplatin, etoposide, and cyclophosphamide versus BEP × 4.[142] Two hundred nineteen patients were randomly assigned to standard BEP × 4 ($n = 108$) or BEP × 2 followed by two high-dose cycles of carboplatin, etoposide, and cyclophosphamide with stem cell rescue with each high-dose cycle. There were 10 deaths on treatment (six on high-dose arm and four on standard BEP). Toxicity was more severe on the high-dose arm. The 1-year durable complete remission rate was 52% on the high-dose arm and 48% on the standard BEP arm ($p = 0.53$), that is, no significant difference between the two arms.

A European trial comparing high-dose VIP to standard therapy in poor-risk GCTs was conducted based on the promising phase 1/2 trial reported by Schmoll and colleagues.[143] Two hundred twenty-one patients with either Indiana "advanced disease" ($n = 39$) or IGCCCG "poor-prognosis" criteria ($n = 182$) received one cycle of VIP followed by three to four sequential cycles of high-dose VIP plus stem cell support every 3 weeks, at six consecutive dose levels. After 4-year median follow-up, progression-free survival and disease-specific survival rates in the poor-prognosis subgroup were 69% and 79% at 2 years and 68% and 73% at 5 years, with 76% for gonadal/retroperitoneal versus 67% for mediastinal primaries. Severe toxicity included treatment-related death (4%), treatment-related acute myeloid leukemia (1%), long-term impaired renal function (3%), chronic renal failure (1%), and persistent grade $2-3$ neuropathy (5%).

Postchemotherapy surgery

Introduction

Surgical resection of residual masses following chemotherapy for disseminated disease is a vital component of the multimodality treatment of testis cancer. Twenty–fifty percent of patients who undergo induction chemotherapy for metastatic germ cell cancer have significant residual retroperitoneal disease requiring resection for cure. The presence of large residual masses around vital structures and the resultant severe desmoplastic reaction following chemotherapy often make surgery challenging. These operations should ideally be performed by experienced surgeons in high-volume centers.

Indications for postchemotherapy RPLND (PC-RPLND)

Postchemotherapy surgery should be considered only if serum tumor markers have normalized or reached a plateau. Typically postchemotherapy RPLND (PC-RPLND) is indicated if there is radiographic evidence of residual disease postchemotherapy, although the indications are different for seminomas than nonseminomas. Patients who have normalized their markers and have complete resolution of retroperitoneal adenopathy are considered at low risk of relapse and generally do not require surgery.[144] Some authors however advocate PC-RPLND in all cases of nonseminoma due to the increased presence of teratoma and viable GCT even in patients with complete radiographic and serologic response.[145] PC-RPLND should be performed $4-6$ weeks following the last round of chemotherapy in order to allow patients to recover. Imaging must include CT scan of the chest, abdomen, and pelvis which should be performed reasonably close to time of surgery to ascertain persistence of residual disease in the retroperitoneum.

Nonseminoma

Although most authors advocate resection of "residual" masses following chemotherapy for NSGCT, there is no consensus on nodal size criteria. It is often difficult to measure the exact size of residual nodal tissue, since nodes are often matted together. The definition of a "normal" CT scan following chemotherapy for testis cancer varies.[146] Investigators have reported that up to one-third of small retroperitoneal postchemotherapy masses measuring ≤2 cm in diameter contain residual teratoma or GCT.[147] There are currently no reliable imaging techniques or prediction models to accurately identify patients who have residual teratoma or viable GCT postinduction chemotherapy.[148] The utility of 18-fluorodeoxyglucose positron emission tomography (FDG-PET) scan is limited in the decision-making analysis of postchemotherapy residual masses in NSGCT since it cannot distinguish fibrosis from teratoma. Although a positive PET scan is highly suggestive of residual viable tumor, false-negative rates of up to 40% have been reported.[149] Most experts agree that PC-RPLND is indicated when there are residual radiographically detectable lesions following first-line chemotherapy. Patients with teratoma present in the orchiectomy specimen are at increased risk of residual teratoma and should be considered for PC-RPLND when there is any residual mass.[147] Patients who have an increased serum AFP, teratoma in the primary tumor, and a postchemotherapy cystic mass in the retroperitoneum may also be candidates for PC-RPLND rather than salvage chemotherapy. Beck *et al.* confirmed that cystic teratomas contain variably elevated levels of HCG and AFP and postulated that a leak into the bloodstream could explain the elevated tumor markers in this situation.[150] Teratomas can rarely invade the vena cava and present with a tumor thrombus, and this should not be mistaken for a deep venous thrombosis.[151]

Seminoma

Following induction chemotherapy, the presence of distinct residual masses is uncommon. CT scans often reveal a sheetlike distribution of tissue around the IVC and/or aorta that resolves over a prolonged period.[152] Viable cancer is present in approximately 20% patients with residual masses >3 cm and almost no patients with residual masses <3 cm.[153] Since there is no concern about residual teratoma in pure seminomas, routine PC-RPLND for residual disease postchemotherapy will result in overtreatment in approximately 80% of patients. PC-RPLND in this setting is one of the most challenging surgical scenarios that urologists encounter, and rates of adjunctive surgery and complications tend to be higher.[154] To reduce the morbidity of surgery, a number of investigators have evaluated the role of FDG-PET. In a multicenter study ("SEMPET" trial), 56 PET scans were evaluated in 51 patients with CT-documented residual masses measuring 1–11 cm after adequate chemotherapy for bulky seminoma. All 19 cases with residual lesions >3 cm, and 35 of the 37 cases with residual lesions ≤3 cm were correctly predicted by PET scan. The sensitivity, specificity, and positive predictive values of PET in determining residual viable disease were 80%, 100%, and 100%, respectively.[155] Not all studies have confirmed the reliability of PET, and a number of false positives have been documented.[156,157] Nevertheless, PET scans may be the best noninvasive test to predict the presence of viable residual tumor in patients with postchemotherapy residual masses. Resection of postchemotherapy masses in seminoma remains controversial, and management should be individualized. Further management of patients with positive PET scans may include surveillance, biopsy, resection, or radiation.

Extent of surgery

PC-RPLND is a technically demanding operation. The boundaries of surgical resection remain controversial. Although modified nerve-sparing templates may be appropriate for lower-stage disease, several investigators have demonstrated the presence of tumor outside these templates in advanced disease. In 113 patients with initial bulky retroperitoneal tumors, if the residual mass was removed accompanied by a modified RPLND, nine patients (8%) would have tumor left in the retroperitoneum. The outcomes of limited versus full bilateral PC-RPLND in 62 patients based on frozen section analysis of the resected mass were investigated. In patients with necrosis on frozen section (37 patients), a limited dissection was performed, and for those with teratoma or viable cancer, a full bilateral template was utilized. After a median follow-up of 6 years, there was one relapse of teratoma seen in the retroperitoneum in the group who underwent a limited dissection. The concordance between frozen section and final pathology was 89%.[158] In a study of 50 PC-RPLND specimens, all low-volume left-sided primary tumors followed a predictable pattern of spread to a modified left-sided template, whereas right-sided primaries had about a 20% crossover rate. After a mean follow-up of 53 months, there were no infield recurrences.[159] Carver et al. reviewed their experience with 532 patients who underwent PC-RPLND for metastatic NSGCT and found that 7–32% patients had evidence of extratemplate retroperitoneal disease. Interestingly 2/24 (8%) patients with residual masses <1 cm had extratemplate metastases.[160] Therefore, it appears that the most prudent approach would be a full bilateral dissection in the postchemotherapy setting, although a limited template can be considered in low-volume left-sided primaries.

The surgical approach should be adapted to the size and location of the mass. Most masses can be accessed via a midline approach, whereas larger masses and those requiring suprahilar dissections are best approached through a thoracoabdominal incision or a midline incision extended to the costochondral junction. Thoracoabdominal approaches afford the possibility of surgical resection of ipsilateral lung lesions. Adjunctive surgery is required in about 20% of patients undergoing PC-RPLND. The most common adjunctive procedure includes a left nephrectomy and occasionally en bloc vena caval and/or aortic resection with graft placement.[161] Although simultaneous PC-RPLND and thoracic resections are feasible, more complex mediastinal masses are probably best approached in a staged manner to reduce complications. Findings of fibrosis in the retroperitoneal specimen should not preclude thoracic resections since up to 20% of patients can have teratoma or viable cancer in the chest.[162]

Complication rates following PC-RPLND performed at high-volume centers are higher than for primary RPLND ranging from 7% to 30% with a mortality rate of about 1%.[163,164] The most significant source of morbidity in this postchemotherapy group is pulmonary toxicity related to prior bleomycin. Retrograde ejaculation remains a significant morbidity although patients with smaller masses are candidates for nerve-sparing approaches with about an 80% probability of preservation of ejaculatory function.[165,166]

Pathology

The histopathologic findings in postchemotherapy surgical specimens determine the need for further treatment and surveillance protocol. The incidence of persistent cancer is decreasing most likely due to optimized chemotherapy regimens and better selection of patients for surgery. Pathologic findings in patients with advanced NSGCT after induction therapy are approximately: necrosis in 40–50%, teratoma in 35–40%, and viable carcinoma in 10–15% of specimens.[167] Following salvage chemotherapy, the finding of viable carcinoma increases to about 50%.[168] Patients with viable disease resected at postchemotherapy surgery are generally recommended to receive two postoperative cycles of cisplatin-based therapy, with two-thirds remaining disease-free in the long term.[136] Patients with completely resected very-low-volume disease may be observed. However, patients with unresectable disease, partial resection, or elevated tumor markers should be considered for full salvage chemotherapy.

"Desperation" RPLND

Patients with elevated or rising tumor markers following induction chemotherapy who have progressed after salvage chemotherapy and have resectable retroperitoneal disease may be candidates for "desperation PC-RPLND." These patients often have chemotherapy-resistant disease and surgery may afford the only chance for cure. PC-RPLND in this setting is technically arduous, often involving removal of adjacent organs and/or great vessels, and is usually associated with significantly lower survival rates. Despite elevated markers, up to 50% of patients will harbor mature teratoma or necrosis/fibrosis in the surgical specimen.[169] In patients with viable germ cell cancers in the resected specimen, up to one-third will have long-term disease-free survival.[170] Incomplete resection portends a poor prognosis.

Chemotherapy of seminoma

Modern chemotherapy series involving patients with bulky stage II or stage III disseminated seminoma report cure rates of more than 90%.[62] When compared with earlier studies of radiotherapy in this setting where cure rates ranged from 20% to 60%, cisplatin-based chemotherapy is the treatment of choice. Standard initial therapy remains cisplatin combinations.

Patients with disseminated seminoma and nonpulmonary visceral involvement do less well and are classified as intermediate risk.[126] Good-risk patients usually receive BEP × 3 and intermediate-risk patients receive BEP × 4.

The management of patients with residual radiographic abnormalities after completion of cisplatin-based combination chemotherapy is controversial. Motzer and colleagues report results of 41 patients with bulky stage II, stage III, or stage IV disease treated with cisplatin-based combination chemotherapy.[171]

Twenty-three patients had significant residual radiographic abnormalities, including 14 patients with masses ≥3 cm in size. Of these 23 patients, 19 underwent surgical exploration, and five had significant findings other than fibrosis (four viable seminomas and one teratoma). The authors recommend biopsy of residual radiographic abnormalities after chemotherapy for seminoma if the residual disease measures ≥3 cm.

A different policy has also been adopted. Surgery in this setting is extremely difficult because of a dense desmoplastic reaction. Also, these patients are older, sometimes have had abdominal radiotherapy as well as chemotherapy, and, as in several series, are prone to operative mortalities.[171] A review of seminoma from Indiana reports only a 10% incidence of relapse in the setting of residual radiographic disease >3 cm postchemotherapy.[172] There was no evidence in this series that risk of recurrence was related to the diameter of the residual mass. At Indiana University, close observation is recommended in this setting.

The use of PET scans to predict viable tumor in postchemotherapy residuals of patients with pure seminoma >3 cm remains controversial.[173] A widely endorsed conservative policy is to base evaluations and subsequent therapy on size and biopsy findings. Patients who have <3 cm residual mass after systemic chemotherapy are observed. Patients with 3 cm or greater residual masses are submitted to PET scanning. PET-negative masses are observed without intervention. Patients with large PET-positive masses undergo surgical biopsy or resection, and subsequent approaches are defined by pathological findings.

Radiation therapy for postchemotherapy residual masses had been considered; however, very few of these masses contain seminoma. Furthermore, the curability with radiation is questionable if chemotherapy does not cure the patient. In addition, the risk of long-term complications, including leukemia, is increased when both chemotherapy and radiation are employed. Therefore, radiation for residual masses should not be performed.[40]

Salvage chemotherapy

Twenty–thirty percent of GCT patients will not achieve durable complete remission with first-line therapy.[174] These individuals, as well as those who relapse from complete remission, are candidates for salvage chemotherapy. The decreased efficacy and increased toxicity of second-line chemotherapy requires the expertise of individuals well versed in the intricacies of careful assessment of patients with GCTs and of therapeutic options for this stage of testicular cancer.

Patient selection

There are several clinical situations that may mimic persistent, progressive, or recurrent disease. One involves the appearance of nodular lesions in the chest at the end of chemotherapy or soon after completion.[1] These nodules can represent bleomycin-induced pulmonary injury and are characteristically located in a subpleural region. This possibility should be considered in a patient who is otherwise responding serologically or radiographically and has new abnormalities in the lungs in separate sites from the original disease.

Another clinical situation frequently mistaken for progressive disease is growing teratoma.[175] Radiographically enlarging metastatic lesions during chemotherapy concurrently with normal or normalizing serologic markers often represent teratoma. Appropriate management is surgical resection of residual radiographic abnormalities rather than salvage chemotherapy.

A conservative policy is to reserve salvage therapy until there is a clear demonstration of rising markers on serial determinations. The

vagaries of interpretation of low-level marker elevation makes such a policy necessary to ensure that patients are not treated with intensive salvage chemotherapy on the basis of a false-positive marker elevation.

Occult central nervous system (CNS) metastasis should be considered in the setting of systemic sustained remission and elevation of serum tumor markers. CT scans or MRI should be performed, along with evaluations for a testicular sanctuary site. The CNS evaluation should proceed even in the absence of clinical signs or symptoms if the only evidence of progressive disease is a rising marker.

The other important sanctuary site from chemotherapy is the testis. In most settings, the primary in the testis has been removed in the initial diagnostic process. However, in some patients presenting with advanced disease, chemotherapy is initiated without a tissue diagnosis. In such cases, the testis must be removed at the completion of chemotherapy, even if the primary tumor is no longer evident. The possibility of a metachronous contralateral testicular primary should also be entertained.

Prognostic factors in the salvage situation

The importance of clinical prognostic factors in the second-line situation has been increasingly recognized.[176,177] Outcomes vary between the different conventional and high-dose regimens reported to date caused by the heterogeneity of the patient population. Patients with gonadal primary tumor sites, cisplatin-sensitive disease, and relapse after CR to first-line therapy are more likely to achieve a favorable treatment outcome with conventional-dose salvage therapy than patients with cisplatin-refractory disease, an incomplete response to first-line therapy, or a mediastinal primary tumor site.[178] Einhorn et al.[179] recently reported refractory disease, advanced initial tumor stage, and the timing of high-dose chemotherapy (third or subsequent chemotherapy) as adverse prognostic factors. These risk factors discriminated a good-, intermediate-, and poor-prognosis group with a long-term survival of approximately 80%, 60%, and 40%, respectively. The International Prognostic Factor Study Group developed a prognostic classification for relapsed patients similar to the IGCCCG classification for treatment-naïve patients, which included individual data from almost 2000 relapsed patients collected at high-volume centers around the world.[180] Based on seven significant factors on multivariate analysis including histology (seminoma vs. non-seminoma), primary tumor site (mediastinal vs. retroperitoneal vs. gonadal), response to first-line chemotherapy (CR vs. PR vs. others), progression-free interval following first-line chemotherapy, AFP and HCG level at diagnosis of relapse, and the presence of nonpulmonary visceral metastases, the model is able to differentiate five distinct risk groups ranging from very low to very high. Due to the large, international, and multicenter patient population included, this model is widely applicable and is now considered the new standard prognostic model for relapsed patients.

Standard salvage therapy

Patients relapsing after cisplatin-based first-line chemotherapy have a less favorable prognosis than patients at initial diagnosis, primarily because of the paucity of active single agents in patients refractory to cisplatin. During the three decades since the introduction of cisplatin, only a few new agents including etoposide (VP-16), ifosfamide, paclitaxel, gemcitabine, and oxaliplatin have demonstrated activity in platinum-refractory patients. The rate of patients responding favorably to conventional salvage chemotherapy is approximately 50% and thus substantially lower than after first-line treatment. Long-term remissions are only achieved in 20–30% of patients.

The salvage chemotherapy regimen that serves as a basis for comparison is the regimen of vinblastine, ifosfamide, and cisplatin (VeIP).[181] One hundred thirty-five patients who had not progressed during cisplatin-based therapy received VeIP as initial salvage chemotherapy. Toxicity of the regimen in this pretreated population was significant, with 71% developing granulocytopenic fever. Transfusions of platelets (27%) and red blood cells (49%) were common. Renal insufficiency (serum creatinine >4 mg%) was observed in 7% of patients. Three patients died of causes related to treatment. Despite the formidable toxicity, the therapeutic results were gratifying. Fifty-six patients (45%) achieved a disease-free status with either chemotherapy alone (34 patients, 25%) or by resection of teratoma (15 patients, 12%) or of viable carcinoma (7 patients, 6%). Thirty-two (24%) of these patients are continuously disease-free, and 42 (32%) are currently disease-free (minimum follow-up of 5 years). Among the patients with extragonadal primaries, only six of 31 attained disease-free status, and only one is continuously disease-free. These results have been confirmed by other investigators.[182]

Investigators from Memorial Sloan Kettering Cancer Center evaluated paclitaxel plus ifosfamide plus cisplatin (TIP) as second-line therapy for patients with favorable prognostic features, but relapsed testicular cancers.[183] Twenty-three of 30 patients (77%) achieved a CR to chemotherapy alone, and an additional patient achieved a durable partial remission with normal markers. Only two patients relapsed and treatment was generally well tolerated. This study underscores the importance of patient selection. TIP has evolved into a widely used standard conventional-dose salvage regimen.[184,185]

Recurrent seminoma may be uniquely sensitive to salvage chemotherapy. Miller and colleagues reported the results of VeIP in patients with seminoma recurring after primary cisplatin/etoposide-based treatment.[186] Of these 23 patients, 19 (83%) achieved disease-free status, and 13 (56%) are continuously free of disease.

High-dose chemotherapy as initial salvage therapy

High-dose chemotherapy has been studied as initial salvage chemotherapy. Barnett and colleagues reported the results of 18 patients with recurrent or persistent germ cell cancer after cisplatin-based primary therapy who were given conventional induction chemotherapy with cisplatin, etoposide, vincristine, and bleomycin on a weekly schedule or vinblastine, ifosfamide, and cisplatin combinations.[187] Consolidation with high-dose chemotherapy was given with autologous bone marrow support. Patients received high-dose carboplatin, etoposide, and either cyclophosphamide or ifosfamide. There were two toxic deaths, it was too early to evaluate two patients, and eight of 14 patients remained free of progression.

Siegert and colleagues reported the results of high-dose carboplatin, etoposide, and ifosfamide.[188] Patients received two induction courses of conventional-dose cisplatin, etoposide, and ifosfamide before receiving escalated therapy. Seventy-four patients received treatment with conventional therapy, followed by carboplatin 1500–2000 mg/m^2, etoposide 1200–2400 mg/m^2, and ifosfamide 0–10 g/m^2. Two patients (3%) died of causes related to treatment. Responses included 21 patients (28%) with complete remission with chemotherapy alone or with adjunctive surgery and 14 (19%) patients with marker-negative partial remission. Twenty-five of these patients (34%) maintained their response from 31 to 261 months.

A randomized trial looking at the concept of a single consolidating high-dose chemotherapy cycle after conventional induction chemotherapy was conducted in patients with favorable prognostic criteria. Most patients included had primary gonadal or retroperitoneal GCTs, and all had previously achieved a complete or partial remission from platinum combination chemotherapy. Patients were randomized to either four cycles of VIP or VeIP or three cycles of VIP followed by one high-dose cycle consisting of carboplatin, etoposide, and cyclophosphamide. The 1-year event-free survival and 3-year survival rates (35% vs. 42% in favor of high-dose chemotherapy) were disappointingly low in particular for the high-dose arm.[189]

With the development of peripheral stem cell transplantation, sequential high-dose chemotherapy utilizing two or three high-dose chemotherapy cycles became feasible. Motzer et al.[190] reported a 41% long-term disease-free rate in 37 patients with cisplatin-resistant disease and unfavorable prognostic criteria after two cycles of conventional TIP chemotherapy followed by three cycles of high-dose carboplatin and etoposide.

Sequential high-dose chemotherapy consisting of one cycle of VIP followed by three cycles of high-dose carboplatin and etoposide was compared with three cycles of VIP followed by a single high-dose cycle of carboplatin, etoposide, and cyclophosphamide.[191] No difference in survival probabilities between single high-dose and sequential high-dose chemotherapy arm was observed. The trial was underpowered to ascertain whether one of the two high-dose regimens should be used as salvage treatment in any particular patient population. However, morbidity and mortality of sequential high-dose chemotherapy with a 2-drug regimen was lower compared to the single 3-drug regimen, and 10% of patients with cisplatin-refractory disease achieved long-term survival.

At Indiana University, 184 patients have been treated with salvage tandem high-dose chemotherapy since 1989. One hundred and seventy patients received two consecutive courses of high-dose carboplatin and etoposide, and 110 of the 184 patients underwent 1–2 cycles of cytoreductive conventional chemotherapy with vinblastine, cisplatin, and ifosfamide prior to high-dose chemotherapy. All patients underwent aggressive resection of residual masses after chemotherapy whenever technically feasible. Overall, the long-term disease-free rate was 63%. Eighteen of 40 patients with progressive metastatic disease and tumors that were refractory to platinum remained disease-free after a median of 49 months, confirming that high-dose chemotherapy is able to overcome cisplatin resistance in a substantial number of patients.

A second large retrospective analysis was performed by the International Prognostic Factor Group and included 1594 patients treated with either SCD-CT or SHD-CT. A significant advantage in favor of SHD-CT was seen across all subgroups.[192]

In summary, high-dose chemotherapy yields excellent results in patients with relapsed germ cell cancer and carries an acceptable morbidity and low mortality in young and fit patients. While high-dose chemotherapy is an established treatment option for patients with unfavorable prognostic criteria, its role in patients with favorable prognostic criteria remains controversial. However, given the low morbidity and mortality, as well as the excellent results, high-dose chemotherapy serves as an alternative to conventional salvage therapy in this setting. Due to the complexity of the disease and therapeutic situation as well as the necessity of close multidisciplinary cooperation between medical oncologists, urologists, and radiation oncologists, all relapsed patients should be referred to a specialized center.

Treatment of multiply recurrent germ cell cancer

High-dose chemotherapy for multiply recurrent germ cell cancer

Investigations into the use of high-dose carboplatin (CBCDA) and etoposide (VP-16) with autologous bone marrow support began in 1986. Initial investigations were on patients who were heavily pretreated and for whom no other curative therapeutic options existed.

The initial phase 1/2 dose escalation study examined the use of two courses of high-dose CBDCA and VP-16 in patients with GCTs refractory to cisplatin (defined as progression after or within 4 weeks of the last cisplatin dose) or recurrent after primary therapy with cisplatin-based therapy and a salvage therapy with an ifosfamide–cisplatin combination.[193] Overall, seven (21%) of 33 patients died as a consequence of the treatment. Deaths were primarily caused by infection, although one patient died of veno-occlusive disease of the liver. This was a very heavily pretreated patient population; more than half the patients have received three or more prior chemotherapy regimens, and 67% of patients were cisplatin-refractory. Eight patients obtained a complete remission, and six had a partial remission, for an overall response rate of 44% (95% CI, 27–63%). Of the eight patients attaining complete remission, three are long-term disease-free survivors, and a fourth patient died at 22 months, free of germ cell cancer, from a therapy-related acute myeloid leukemia.[194] An overview of the experience at Indiana University with 49 patients with multiply relapsed and refractory germ cell cancer treated with double autologous transplantation demonstrated a 45% long-term disease-free survival after a median of 46-month follow-up.

Other investigations

Other investigators have reported similar results using high-dose chemotherapy in patients with multiply relapsed testicular cancer. Several conclusions can be drawn. First, high-dose chemotherapy can cure 15–20% of patients experiencing multiple cisplatin-refractory/relapses of germ cell cancer and should be the treatment of choice after failure of ≥2 conventional regimens. Second, outcomes after SHD-CT in the third- or later-line setting are substantially worse than for SHD-CT in the second-line setting. Third, therapy-related mortality in this heavily treated patient population is now <5%, and there is no standard high-dose salvage regimen, but all are based on etoposide/carboplatin. Lastly, patients with mediastinal nonseminomatous primary tumors fare particularly poorly and represent a group of patients who do not benefit from high-dose chemotherapy.

Salvage ("desperation") surgery

Some patients in the salvage setting are best approached with salvage surgery rather than chemotherapy. This is especially true for late relapsers or patients with relapsed disease confined to a single anatomic site. Indiana University performed a retrospective review of all patients who felt to have chemotherapy-refractory disease and were submitted to surgery for attempts at curative resection.[195] All patients had serologic or other evidence of progressive cancer. A total of 48 patients were reviewed, the majority of whom underwent isolated retroperitoneal lymphadenectomy (33 patients). Of these, 38 (79%) were rendered free of gross disease by surgery, and 29 (60%) attained a serologic remission. Ten patients (21%) remain continuously free of disease with follow-up ranging from 31 to 89 months. Clinical benefit was obtained only in that group of completely resected patients with a solitary site of disease

at the time of surgery. Patients with multiple sites of metastasis, although resectable, were not cured. Albers et al. also reported a high long-term disease-free rate after salvage surgery for patients with persistently elevated tumor markers.[196] In carefully selected patients with chemotherapy-incurable disease, salvage surgery offers a significant prospect of long-term disease-free survival. Such decisions about surgeries should be made at centers with significant experience in GCT management. In general, selection to attempt desperation surgery includes slowly increasing tumor markers after an initial CR to either first-line or second-line chemotherapy, radiographic respectable residual disease in one or two sites, and increasing markers with resectable disease after exhausting all chemotherapy options.[197]

New agents

The development of new active compounds offers the best hope of truly changing the prospect for cure in recurrent or resistant GCTs, as well as better therapy for patients presenting with poor-risk features. Several drugs have demonstrated single-agent activity, including oxaliplatin,[198] paclitaxel, and gemcitabine. A phase 2 study from ECOG evaluated the combination of paclitaxel and gemcitabine in 30 patients with refractory GCTs.[199] The overall response rate was 21.4%, including three patients with complete remissions. Two patients remain continuously disease-free for 15+ and 25+ months. Oxaliplatin plus gemcitabine was investigated in three studies with response rates of 16%, 32%, and 46%.[200–202] All of these studies reported long-term survivors, in particular when chemotherapy was followed by resection of residual lesions. Targeted agents are currently explored within clinical studies.

Special situations

Late relapse

Relapses in patients with disseminated testicular cancer who achieve a complete remission occur the first year following therapy, and the overwhelming majority within 2 years. A late relapse in this disease is generally accepted to be one that appears after a disease-free interval of more than 24 months after initial cisplatin-based chemotherapy. Late relapses following complete remission occur in 2–3% of cases, with recurrences as late as 32 years following complete remission. Those patients who have had recurrences with isolated mature teratoma in general have done well following excision, whereas those with marker-positive carcinoma, disseminated disease, and/or transformation seem to have an unfavorable prognosis. Chemotherapy-naïve patients, for example, relapsing from active surveillance or from primary RPLND, have a very good prognosis with cisplatin-based chemotherapy even if they relapse beyond 3 years.[75]

At Indiana University, 81 patients were analyzed retrospectively who had recurrence of GCT after 2 or more years of being disease-free.[203] Sixty percent had recurrences after >5 years (maximum was 32 years). Serum marker elevation was seen, with 56% of patients having an elevated AFP and 27% of patients an elevated HCG. Fifteen patients (19%) had a recurrence of teratoma, eight are continuously free of disease, and four patients are currently free of disease after further surgery (271–1021 months). Seven patients experienced recurrence with sarcomatous elements (with or without teratoma); four are currently disease-free. Fifty-nine patients had germ cell carcinoma as their initial late recurrence. Only 10 of these patients (17%) are continuously disease-free (101–781 months). Nine other patients are currently disease-free. Aggressive surgery was required in almost all these patients. Overall, 65 patients received cisplatin-based chemotherapy, and 17 (26%) achieved a disease-free status with chemotherapy with or without adjunctive surgery. Twelve of the 17 have relapsed. Only two patients treated with chemotherapy alone are continuously free of disease (neither of these patients had received previous chemotherapy). A second series of 77 additional patients demonstrate similar findings.[204]

Sharp and colleagues reviewed 75 patients for management of late relapse of GCT. In this modern series, the median time to late relapse was 6.9 years (range, 2.1–37.7 years). Overall, 56 patients (75%) had recurrence in the retroperitoneum. The 5-year cancer-specific survival was 60% (95% CI, 46–71%). Patients who underwent complete surgical resection at time of late relapse ($n = 45$) had a 5-year cancer-specific survival of 79% versus 36% for patients without complete resection ($n = 30$; $P < 0.0001$). The 5-year cancer-specific survival for chemotherapy-naive patients was significantly greater than patients with a prior history of chemotherapy as part of their initial management (5-year cancer-specific survival, 93% vs. 49%, respectively). As this was a series of patients referred at the time of late relapse, it is unknown how representative these results are for the late relapsing population as a whole. Nonetheless, these and other data suggest that such patients can obtain long remissions or cures after late relapse. Patients who are chemotherapy naïve often are rendered disease-free with standard approaches including cisplatin-based chemotherapy coupled with postchemotherapy surgery. A consistent feature of such studies is that for patients with regional confined disease who have late presentations with atypical yolk sac findings, elevated AFP and prior chemotherapy are best served by aggressive primary surgery.

Although the appearance of late relapses is relatively rare (1–3% beyond 2 years), these data support current recommendations for continued lifetime follow-up.

Long-term toxicity of chemotherapy

Since the mid-1970s, the majority of testicular cancer patients with disseminated disease have been cured with combination chemotherapy with or without adjunctive surgery or radiation. Late complications of curative therapy have been seen in other malignancies, most notably Hodgkin's disease (e.g., sterility, therapy-related second malignancies). Concerns about similar late effects of cisplatin-based therapy have been raised, and information is now available on a significant number of patients with follow-up of more than 10 years.

Nephrotoxicity

The acute effects of cisplatin on both renal glomerular and tubular functions are well documented, with decreases in both glomerular filtration rate (GFR) and effective renal plasma flow (ERPF) accompanied by magnesium wasting and elevated levels of β2-microglobulin, indicative of proximal tubule dysfunction. Most investigators reported that the acute decreases in GFR and ERPF do not deteriorate further during the months to years following completion of chemotherapy; however, long-term subclinical impairment is frequently found.[205–207]

Vascular toxicity

Raynaud's phenomenon is the most common vascular toxicity seen in patients following chemotherapy for testicular cancer. Although anecdotally reported after therapy with single-agent bleomycin, it is much more common following combination therapy. Vogelzang and colleagues reported a 21% incidence of this

phenomenon in patients treated with vinblastine plus bleomycin, as compared with 41% when cisplatin was added to these two drugs.[208] Studies employing provocative testing suggest that even asymptomatic individuals may exhibit an exaggerated vasospastic response to cold stimuli.[208] Symptoms persist indefinitely, with 49% of patients in one series reporting continued symptoms at a median of 8.5 years from completion of therapy. The vasospasm has, in general, been refractory to therapy, although some success has been reported with the calcium channel blocker nifedipine.[209] The replacement of vinblastine by VP-16 in combination therapy with cisplatin and bleomycin has not reduced the incidence of Raynaud's phenomenon.[210]

The relationship of cisplatin-based chemotherapy to large-vessel ischemic events is less clear. There are case reports of myocardial ischemia and infarction, as well as cerebrovascular accidents, following vinblastine administration as a single agent or combined with bleomycin. Several anecdotal reports of major cardiovascular events in young men receiving chemotherapy for testicular cancer suggested a causal association between chemotherapeutic treatments and these events.[122,211,212] Weijl and colleagues identified patients with liver metastases or those receiving high-dose corticosteroids to be at high risk of developing thromboembolic complications.[213] Questionnaires to assess cardiovascular toxicity were distributed to all participants in the Testicular Cancer Intergroup Study, and toxicity reviews from the chemotherapy flow sheets were conducted.[213] Patients with pathologic stage I testicular cancer were registered and observed after retroperitoneal lymphadenectomy. Patients with pathologic stage II disease were randomized to receive two postoperative courses of adjuvant cisplatin-based chemotherapy or observation. Any patient who experienced a recurrence after observation or adjuvant therapy was given four cycles of cisplatin-based chemotherapy.

A review of toxicity of treatment in those patients receiving adjuvant chemotherapy ($n = 97$) or chemotherapy for recurrent disease ($n = 83$) revealed no cases of acute cardiovascular toxicity. When the median follow-up after study enrollment was 5.1 years, 459 questionnaires were mailed, and 270 were returned. The percentage of returns was equal among the observed, adjuvant, and recurrent groups (59%, 54%, and 64%, respectively). There was a significant increase in the incidence of extremity paresthesias in the two groups receiving chemotherapy. Fatal myocardial infarction was reported in two patients in the observation group, and one nonfatal infarct was reported in the adjuvant treatment group. No patient in any group reported stroke. Three patients in the observation group and one patient in the recurrent group experienced a thromboembolic event.

In contrast, other population-based studies highlight a substantial increase in risk in cardiovascular disease particularly in patients who have received high cumulative doses of cisplatin. Fossa and colleagues identified 38,907 patients, who were 1-year survivors of testicular cancer within 14 population-based cancer registries in North America and Europe.[214] They calculated standardized mortality ratios (SMRs) for noncancer deaths and evaluated associations between histology, age at testicular cancer diagnosis, calendar year of diagnosis, and initial treatment and the risk of noncancer mortality. A total of 2942 deaths from all noncancer causes were reported after a median follow-up of 10 years, exceeding the expected number of deaths from all noncancer causes in the general population by 6% (SMR = 1.06, 95% CI = 1.02–1.10); the noncancer SMRs did not differ statistically significantly between patients diagnosed before and after 1975 when cisplatin-based chemotherapy came into widespread use. Compared with the general population, testicular cancer survivors had higher mortality from infections (SMR = 1.28,

95% CI = 1.12–1.47) and from digestive diseases (SMR = 1.44, 95% CI = 1.26–1.64). Mortality from all circulatory diseases was statistically significantly elevated in men diagnosed with testicular cancer before age 35 years (1.23, 95% CI = 1.09–1.39) but not in men diagnosed at older ages (SMR = 0.94; 95% CI = 0.89–1.00). Men treated with chemotherapy (with or without radiotherapy) in 1975 or later had higher mortality from all noncancer causes (SMR = 1.34, 95% CI = 1.15–1.55), all circulatory diseases (SMR = 1.58, 95% CI = 1.25–2.01), all infections (SMR = 2.48, 95% CI = 1.70–3.50), and all respiratory diseases (SMR = 2.53, 95% CI = 1.26–4.53). Testicular cancer patients who were younger than 35 years at diagnosis and were treated with radiotherapy alone in 1975 or later had higher mortality from all circulatory diseases (SMR = 1.70, 95% CI = 1.21–2.31) compared with the general population. In longer follow-up, hypertension, glucose intolerance, unfavorable lipid profiles, and vascular events often arose.[215] The development of metabolic syndrome is well described in association with testicular cancer and cisplatin-based chemotherapy.[216]

Haugnes and colleagues examined this question in a Nordic national follow-up study (1998–2002). Patients >60 years were excluded, leaving 1135 patients eligible who were divided into four treatment groups (surgery ($n = 225$), radiotherapy ($n = 446$)) and two chemotherapy groups (cumulative cisplatin dose 850 mg ($n = 376$) and cisplatin dose >850 mg ($n = 88$)). A control group consisted of 1150 men from the Tromsø Population Study. Metabolic syndrome was defined according to a modified National Cholesterol Education Program definition. Both chemotherapy groups had increased odds for metabolic syndrome compared with the surgery group, highest for the cisplatin >850 group [OR 2.8, 95% CI 1.6–4.7]. Also, the cisplatin >850 group had increased odds (OR 2.1, 95% CI 1.3–3.4) for metabolic syndrome. The association between metabolic syndrome and the cisplatin >850 group was strengthened after adjusting for confounding variables.

Patients with testicular cancer should be followed indefinitely. They need good medical management with weight reduction, smoking cessation, lipid profile monitoring, and appropriate blood pressure management. Patients and their treating physicians should remain cognizant of a persisting unfavorable cardiovascular risk profile in long-term survivors.[217,218]

Neurotoxicity

Peripheral neuropathy and ototoxicity observed in treated testicular cancer patients are attributable primarily to cisplatin, with a somewhat lesser contribution in older studies by vinblastine. The peripheral effects became manifest clinically as a distal sensory neuropathy, with paresthesias and dysesthesias, disturbances of position and vibratory sensation, and relative sparing of motor units.[219] Subjectively, these symptoms may be present for prolonged periods, with 43% of patients in one study reporting persistent symptoms 6–12 years after completion of therapy.[220] Objective studies confirmed the irreversibility of the neuropathy and suggest that the dorsal root ganglion represents the primary target of cisplatin-induced damage.

The ototoxicity associated with cisplatin is primarily high-frequency hearing loss and is related to the cumulative dose of cisplatin.[221,222] Other risk factors for ototoxicity include a serum creatinine level higher than 1.5 mg/dL, increased age, and preexisting hearing impairment.

Second malignancies

Second primary cancers are a leading cause of death among men with testicular cancer.[223] Travis and colleagues reviewed 14 population-based tumor registries in Europe and North America (1943–2001) and identified 40,576 patients who were 1-year

survivors of testicular cancer. A total of 2285 second solid tumors were reported in the cohort. The relative risk and excess annual risk decreased with increasing age at testicular cancer diagnosis ($P < 0.001$); the excess annual risk increased with attained age ($P < 0.001$), but the excess relative risk decreased. Among 10-year survivors diagnosed with testicular cancer at age of 35 years, the risk of developing a second solid tumor was increased (RR = 1.9, 95% CI = 1.8–2.1). Risk remained statistically significantly elevated for 35 years (RR = 1.7, 95% CI = 1.5–2.0; $P < 0.001$). Cancers of the lung (RR = 1.5, 95% CI = 1.2–1.7), colon (RR = 2.0, 95% CI = 1.7–2.5), bladder (RR = 2.7, 95% CI = 2.2–3.1), pancreas (RR = 3.6, 95% CI = 2.8–4.6), and stomach (RR = 4.0, 95% CI = 3.2–4.8) accounted for almost 60% of the total excess. Overall patterns were similar for seminoma and nonseminoma patients, with lower risks observed for nonseminoma patients treated after 1975. Statistically significantly increased risks of solid tumors were observed among patients treated with radiotherapy alone (RR = 2.0, 95% CI = 1.9–2.2), chemotherapy alone (RR = 1.8, 95% CI = 1.3–2.5), and both (RR = 2.9, 95% CI = 1.9–4.2). For patients diagnosed with seminomas or nonseminomatous tumors at age of 35 years, cumulative risks of solid tumors 40 years later (i.e., to age of 75 years) were 36% and 31%, respectively, compared with 23% for the general population.

Treatment with high-dose etoposide can result in a unique secondary leukemia. Nichols and colleagues reviewed records of patients with germ cell cancer entering clinical protocols using etoposide at Indiana University.[194] Between 1982 and 1991, 538 patients entered serial clinical trials, with planned etoposide doses from 1500 to 2000 mg/m^2 in combination with cisplatin plus either ifosfamide or bleomycin. Of these, 348 patients received an etoposide combination as initial chemotherapy, and 190 patients received etoposide as part of salvage treatment. In all, 315 patients are alive, and 337 patients have been followed up beyond 2 years. The median follow-up for patients still alive is 4.9 years. Two patients (0.37%) developed leukemia. One patient developed acute undifferentiated leukemia with a t(4:11)(q21:q23) cytogenetic abnormality 2.3 years after starting etoposide-based chemotherapy, and one patient developed acute myelomonoblastic leukemia with normal chromosome studies 2 years after beginning chemotherapy. During this period, a number of patients were seen outside clinical trials, and we are aware of several hematologic abnormalities in this group, including one patient with acute monoblastic leukemia with a t(11:19)(q13:p13) abnormality. However, this low incidence of secondary leukemia does not alter the risk–benefit ratio of etoposide-based chemotherapy for germ cell cancer.

Fertility

Gonadal dysfunction is common in patients with a history of testicular cancer even when managed by orchidectomy alone. Fertility and sexual functioning have been evaluated in cross-sectional studies of long-term survivors of testicular cancer. In total, 680 patients treated between 1982 and 1992 completed the EORTC Qly-C-30 (qc30) questionnaire, the associated testicular cancer-specific module, and a general health and fertility questionnaire. Patients were subdivided according to treatment: orchidectomy either alone (surveillance [S] $n = 169$), with chemotherapy (C, $n = 272$), radiotherapy (R, $n = 158$), or both chemotherapy and radiotherapy (C/RT $n = 81$). In the surveillance group, 6% of patients had an elevated LH, 41% an elevated FSH, and 11% a low (<10 nmolL^{-1}) testosterone. Hormonal function deteriorated with additional treatment, but the effect in general was small. Low testosterone was more common in the C/RT group (37% $P = 0.006$), FSH abnormalities were more common after chemotherapy (C 49%, C/RT 71%

both $P < 0.005$) and LH abnormalities after radiotherapy (11%, $P < 0.01$) and chemotherapy (10%, $P < 0.001$). Baseline hormone data were available for 367 patients. After treatment, compared to baseline, patients receiving chemotherapy had significantly greater elevations of FSH (median rise of 6 (IQR 3–9.25) iu L^{-1} compared to 3 (IQR 1–5) iu L^{-1} for S; $P < 0.001$) and a fall (compared to a rise in the surveillance group) in median testosterone levels (−2 [IQR −8.0 to −1.5] vs. 1.0 [IQR −4.0 to 4.0] $P < 0.001$). Patients with low testosterone (but not elevated FSH) had lower quality of life scores related to sexual functioning on the testicular cancer-specific module and lower physical, social, and role functioning on the EORTC Qly-C-30 (qc30) questionnaire. Patients with a low testosterone also had higher body mass index and blood pressure. Treatment was associated with reduction in sexual activity, and patients receiving chemotherapy had more concerns about fathering children. In total, 207 (30%) patients reported attempting conception of whom 159 (77%) were successful and a further 10 patients were successful after infertility treatment with an overall success rate of 82%. There was a lower overall success rate after chemotherapy (C 71%; CRT 67% compared to S 85% ($P = 0.028$)). Elevated FSH levels were associated with reduced fertility (normal FSH 91% vs. elevated 68% $P < 0.001$).

Before the effects of therapy on fertility are examined, it must be recognized that up to 80% of testicular cancer patients will be oligospermic prior to the initiation of any therapy.[224] Although the etiology of this oligospermia is not fully understood, several mechanisms have been proposed, including an autoimmune process or a primary endocrine dysfunction resulting in impaired spermatogenesis.[225,226]

The chemotherapy administered for testicular cancer has acute effects on both spermatogenesis and Leydig cell function; most patients remain azoospermic with elevated serum gonadotropins for the first 12 months following therapy. These toxic effects are reversible in a significant number of patients, however, as approximately 50% will see a return of both spermatogenesis and Leydig cell function during the second year after completion of therapy.[227,228] Several factors decrease the likelihood of the return of spermatogenesis, including age over 30 years, treatment duration of more than 6 months, and prior abdominal radiotherapy.[229,230] In the Indiana University experience, at least one-third of patients treated with chemotherapy alone have been able to father children without congenital anomalies. Two cycles of adjuvant cisplatin-based chemotherapy given to patients with high-risk stage I GCTs do not adversely affect fertility or sexual activity.[231] In an analysis of 170 patients, the probability of spermatogenesis increased after orchiectomy and cisplatin-based chemotherapy to 48% by 2 years and to 80% by 5 years.[232]

Pulmonary toxicity

Bleomycin is solely responsible for the pulmonary toxicity observed in chemotherapy-treated testicular cancer patients. Pulmonary fibrosis develops in approximately 5% of individuals and can be fatal.[233] Toxicity is related to cumulative dose, with a significant increase above 450 units. The earliest physical finding is an inspiratory lag and should prompt immediate discontinuation of the drug. Subsequent signs and symptoms include bibasilar rales, nonproductive cough, and exertional dyspnea. Laboratory abnormalities include decreases in diffusing capacity and late changes, including hypoxia and hypercapnia. Radiographic abnormalities include subpleural-based nodules, visible on the chest radiograph or chest CT scan.

The risk of developing symptomatic bleomycin-induced lung disease increases with age >70 years, prior or concomitant chest

radiotherapy,[113,234] decreased renal function,[235] and high concentrations of inspired oxygen. Because the mortality for this condition approaches 50% and therapeutic interventions, such as corticosteroids, are ineffective, early diagnosis of asymptomatic patients and subsequent discontinuation of the drug are particularly important. The incidence of clinically significant bleomycin toxicity is negligible, however, with three cycles of BEP.

Long-term toxicity of radiation therapy

Toxicity of radiation

Acute

Acute radiation toxicity is dependent on what organs are irradiated, the radiation dose, and the volume. MRC TE10 trial randomized patients to PA only or PA with an ipsilateral pelvic field (dogleg [DL]).[104] The acute toxicity of nausea/vomiting was similar but slightly higher in the DL arm. As expected the DL field would not include much more small bowel than the PA area ($p = 0.08$). Nevertheless, both groups experienced nausea requiring medication in 25–30% of patients treated. Since DL treats much more bone marrow, the rates of mild leukopenia were almost twice as high when compared with the PA field alone. Nineteen percent experienced clinically detectable leukopenia for the PA arm versus 42% for the ipsilateral pelvic field arm ($p < 0.0001$). Diarrhea was reported in 7% of the PA arm only, but 14% in the ipsilateral pelvic field arm ($p = 0.013$).

In the MRC TE18 trial comparing 30 Gy with 20 Gy, patients were asked to complete a daily symptom diary in addition to their physician-recorded symptoms.[103] The patients who received 20 Gy tended to have less significant nausea than the patients who received the higher dose ($p = 0.06$). Leukopenia was also less ($p = 0.02$). Significantly more patients receiving 30 Gy reported moderate or severe lethargy (20% vs. 5%) and an inability to carry out their normal work (46% vs. 28%). But by 12 weeks, the two groups were similar. The lower doses and smaller fields in these trials reduced the acute toxicity without compromising treatment and may lower the chronic and late sequelae of radiation.

Approximately 50% of patients diagnosed with seminoma have some degree of impairment in spermatogenesis with lower than average fertility.[235] Consequently, before adjuvant radiation, appropriate counseling, baseline fertility testing, and semen cryopreservation should be considered in patients considering having children in the future. Exposure of the remaining testis to internal radiation scatter from adjuvant radiotherapy to the PA or PA and ipsilateral pelvic nodes after orchiectomy may further impair fertility. The degree of fertility impairment is dose dependent, and temporary azoospermia may occur at dose levels as low as 40–50 cGy (0.4–0.5 Gy).[236,237] Permanent sterility occurs after 2–3.5 Gy. For a patient who is concerned about fertility, the radiation dose can be lowered to below the threshold where permanent spermatogenesis is affected. The difference in testicular dose depending on the treated field is illustrated by the MRC TE10 trial comparing the DL and PA field with the PA field alone. The median time to the first "normal" posttreatment sperm count was 13 months for PA patients and 20 months for DL patients, despite the fact that scrotal shielding was used in 63% of the DL patients and only 3% of the PA patients.[104] Testicular shielding with a clamshell reduces the dose to the testes by approximately 3–10-fold. For patients treated with PA and DL or PA radiation fields with gonadal shielding, the average testicular dose per fraction is 1.48 and 0.65 cGy, respectively.[238] Therefore, for men treated with testicular shielding, the cumulative testicular dose is approximately 0.5–2% of the prescription dose, and the majority of men will recover to their baseline sperm concentrations.[104,236,238] Hormonal changes require much higher doses and are not detectable based on testosterone. Subtle Leydig cell dysfunction, as measured by serum FSH and LH concentrations, may occur, which are also dose and field dependent. Temporary mild elevation of FSH and LH (in the normal range) may occur with resolution to normal by 3 years with PA and DL fields, while minimal increase in FSH but not LH may occur after PA field only.[239]

Chronic

The avoidance of chronic toxicity or permanent late effects has raised the profile of surveillance as a preferred treatment option for many young patients with seminoma. Because radiation for seminoma historically incorporated a mediastinal field, cardiac toxicity developed in many patients. At MD Anderson Cancer Center, of 477 men with stage I or II testicular seminoma treated between 1951 and 1999[240] with a median follow-up of 13.3 years, the cardiac-specific SMR was 1.61, while the cancer-specific SMR was 1.91. Both toxicities were only evident after 15 years of follow-up. Fifteen years may represent the latency period for chronic toxicity to develop, but it may also demonstrate that radiation treatment doses and fields prior to 1990 are more toxic versus modern practices.

The risk of second malignancies for patients treated with historical methods was quantified in a large international population-based cancer registry study.[221] More than 40,000 survivors of testicular cancer were identified, having been diagnosed from as early as 1943 up to 2001. The risk of developing a second solid tumor among 10-year survivors was almost twice that of the general population (RR = 1.9). Overall patterns were similar for seminoma and nonseminoma patients, with lower risks observed for nonseminoma patients treated after 1975. Significantly increased risks of solid tumors were observed among patients treated with radiotherapy alone (RR = 2.0, 95% CI = 1.9–2.2), chemotherapy alone (RR = 1.8, 95% CI = 1.3–2.5), and both (RR = 2.9, 95% CI = 1.9–4.2). For patients given radiotherapy alone, risks were 1.1, 1.5, and 2.0 in the follow-up periods of 1–4, 5–9, and 10 or more years. Relative risks tended to be highest among patients treated with radiation alone in typical infradiaphragmatic sites: stomach (RR = 4.1), pancreas (RR = 3.8), kidney (RR = 2.8), bladder (RR = 2.7), colon (RR = 1.9), and rectum (RR = 1.8). However, there was also increased risk of second malignancy in supradiaphragmatic sites as well, likely related to the supradiaphragmatic radiotherapy fields frequently applied in the past. The cumulative risk of solid tumors at age 75 for men diagnosed at age 35 was 36% for seminoma and 31% for nonseminomatous tumors compared with 23% for the general population. These results are difficult to extrapolate to current practice that uses smaller radiotherapy fields and lower doses.

Sanctuary sites and CNS metastases

It is quite uncommon for testicular cancer patients to present with CNS metastasis,[52,53] making CNS prophylaxis inappropriate for any subset of patients with advanced germ cell cancer. In patients with advanced hematogenous metastases or large-volume choriocarcinoma, however, clinical suspicion should be heightened, and careful investigation of even minor CNS symptoms is warranted.

Patients with CNS involvement should be approached with curative intent. All patients require systemic therapy. Resection should be considered for superficial solitary metastasis. Patients with multiple brain metastases or CNS disease accompanying advanced

systemic involvement should receive whole-brain radiotherapy (30–50 Gy in 3–6 weeks at <2 Gy per fraction) along with appropriate systemic chemotherapy.[52,53,241,242] Patients relapsing with a solitary CNS metastasis without involvement of other sites undergo resection followed by CNS radiotherapy and two postoperative courses of "adjuvant" cisplatin-based chemotherapy.

The other important sanctuary site from chemotherapy is the testis. In most settings, the testicular primary was removed in the initial diagnostic process. However, in some patients presenting with advanced disease, chemotherapy is initiated without a tissue diagnosis. In such cases, the testis must be removed at the completion of chemotherapy even if the primary tumor is no longer evident. If there is an intact primary, one must consider this as a possibility as a source of persistent or increasing marker elevation during and after treatment.

The possibility of a metachronous contralateral testis primary must, at times, be entertained. In the setting of complete radiographic remission of systemic disease and a persistent or new elevation of serum tumor markers, the remaining testicle should be carefully examined and testicular ultrasonography be performed to rule out an occult primary. For patients with a metachronous contralateral testis lesion, organ-sparing surgery is now a viable option to preserve fertility.[243]

Extragonadal germ cell tumors (EGCTs)

An important subset of GCTs are extragonadal in origin. Overall, approximately 5–10% of all germ cell cancers arise in nongonadal sites, particularly in the mediastinum and retroperitoneum. EGCTs have also been described in the pineal and sacrococcygeal region and rarely in the prostate, vagina, orbita, liver, and gastrointestinal tract.

EGCTs were once thought to represent metastasis from an occult gonadal primary. Autopsy findings in 20 patients with extragonadal mediastinal GCTs found only one case of a testicular primary and one patient with a testicular scar.[244] Both these cases were associated with clinically occult lower retroperitoneal involvement. Primary retroperitoneal GCTs are more commonly associated with an occult testicular primary site, especially when the tumor is not midline in origin. EGCTs more likely represent malignant transformation of germinal elements distributed to these sites without a testicular focus.

In adults, the mediastinum is the most common extragonadal site for the development of GCTs.[245,246] The most frequent symptoms at initial presentation include dyspnea (25%), chest pain (23%), and cough (17%), followed by fever (13%), weight loss (11%), vena cava occlusion syndrome, and fatigue/weakness (6%).[247] The most common tumor in this site is mature teratoma,[248] suggested by the presence of a large circumscribed anterior mediastinal mass with normal serum HCG and AFP. Management of mature teratoma is surgical, and there is no role for chemotherapy or radiotherapy. Although these tumors histologically are benign, removal is often difficult. The tumors are commonly adherent to adjacent structures, such as the pericardium, lung, and great vessels. Nonetheless, excellent outcome is the rule.[249] In a series from the Mayo Clinic, 64 of 69 patients were long-term survivors. Four of the remaining patients died as the result of surgical complications.

The principles of management of extragonadal NSGCTs parallel those of testicular germ cell cancer. The diagnosis should be considered in any young person with a poorly differentiated cancer arising in midline structures. Serum tumor markers should be obtained, and, if the clinical condition is stable, a biopsy also should be obtained. In most settings, surgical debulking should not be considered part of primary management. Cisplatin-based chemotherapy should be given as with testicular germ cell cancer. However, cure rates for NSGCTs of mediastinal origin are significantly inferior compared with those of testicular origin. An international analysis of 635 patients with EGCTs demonstrated an almost 90% chance of cure with pure seminoma irrespective of the primary site, but only 45% survival at 5 years for patients with mediastinal nonseminomatous tumors.[247] High-dose chemotherapy with autologous stem cell support is not recommended outside of clinical trials.

Patients with residual radiographic abnormalities after completing chemotherapy for nonseminomatous EGCTs should be considered for surgical extirpation of residual disease whenever feasible even if elevated tumor markers have normalized. Vuky and colleagues report the surgical results of 32 patients with nonseminoma GCTs arising from the mediastinum who underwent adjunctive surgery following chemotherapy.[250] Viable tumor was discovered in 66% of patients and teratoma in 22%.

Several important biologic associations with mediastinal NSGCTs include a high frequency (up to 20%) of Klinefelter's syndrome.[12,251]

Approximately 10% of patients with mediastinal NSGCTs develop associated malignant hematologic dyscrasias. Between 1976 and 1989, of the 40 patients with mediastinal NSGCTs at Indiana University, six developed a hematologic malignancy.[32] In addition, 11 other patients were referred to Indiana University, or a case material was forwarded for evaluation of this association. Of this group of patients, six developed acute megakaryoblastic leukemia, five had acute nonlymphocytic leukemia (not M7), two developed a virulent myelodysplastic syndrome, two were found to have extramedullary megakaryocytic myelosis, and two presented with massively elevated platelet counts and cytogenetic abnormalities or excess blasts in the marrow. The median time to the development of the hematologic abnormalities was 6 months, with five of the patients having simultaneous presentations of the two disorders. Thirty-three similar patients have been reported in the literature. The median interval between the two diagnoses in this review was 5 months, with 13 cases presenting simultaneously. A retrospective review of 287 patients with nonseminomatous mediastinal GCTs revealed 17 patients with hematologic disorders with a median time of onset occurring 6 months after the diagnosis of GCT and a median survival of only 5 months after the diagnosis of the hematologic disorder.[252]

Careful clinical and cytogenetic analyses of these cases suggest that these tumors do not arise as a consequence of therapy for GCTs, but represent a unique and biologically important association between these disorders. Similar cases are not found among those patients with testicular or retroperitoneal germ cell cancer treated with identical chemotherapy. Most compelling, however, is the finding of the most common karyotypic abnormality of germ cell cancer, isochromosome 12p, in a mediastinal GCT and in the leukemic blasts of one of these patients.[31] This implies that the mediastinal GCT and the hematologic malignancy arose from a common progenitor cell.

Patients with EGCTs, particularly those with retroperitoneal or nonseminomatous tumors, are at an increased risk of metachronous testicular cancer.[253] The cumulative risk 10 years after a diagnosis of EGCT was approximately 14% for patients with retroperitoneal or nonseminomatous EGCTs.

Associations of mediastinal NSGCTs with other nonhematologic non-GCTs are unproven. Ulbright and colleagues found 269 cases of teratoma-containing material, including 209 testicular, 28 retroperitoneal, and 32 mediastinal primary sites.[254] Among this group of patients, 11 demonstrated malignant nongerm cell elements, including embryonal rhabdomyosarcoma, adenosquamous carcinoma, leiomyosarcoma, Wilms' tumor, and glioblastoma multiforme. They were identified prior to the initiation of therapy in 10 of the 11 cases. In patients with multiple samples available, histologic progression was often identified, moving from atypical features to overt nongerm cell elements. The authors suggested that these malignant nongerm cell elements are derived from the teratomatous elements within the tumor. Three of the 11 cases were patients with mediastinal primaries (27%), whereas mediastinal primaries made up only 12% of cases reviewed. In contrast, no association between nonhematologic non-GCTs and EGCTs was found in the largest series of EGCTs to date.[255]

Unrecognized germ cell tumor syndrome

On occasion, a patient will present with a clinical picture compatible with an EGCT, but without corroborating serologic or histopathologic evidence of a GCT. Greco and colleagues suggest that such patients should undergo a thorough histopathologic evaluation and, in some cases, receive empiric cisplatin-based chemotherapy.[168] The clinical features of the "unrecognized GCT syndrome" include patients younger than 50 years of age; tumor primarily involving the midline (mediastinum or retroperitoneum), lungs (in the form of multiple pulmonary nodules), or lymph nodes; an elevated βHCG or AFP; or clinical evidence of rapid tumor growth. Seventy-one prospectively identified patients fitting this description were classified as having poorly differentiated carcinoma or poorly differentiated adenocarcinoma and one or more of the above clinical features. Results of serologic investigation revealed normal AFP and HCG in 51 of these patients. Thirteen had elevation of one marker, and five had elevation of both markers. Light microscopy revealed poorly differentiated carcinoma in 48 patients (68%), poorly differentiated adenocarcinoma in 18 patients (25%), and poorly differentiated large cell carcinoma in five patients (7%). Electron microscopy resulted in a change in the histologic diagnosis in 17 (52%) of the 33 patients with poorly differentiated carcinoma undergoing this procedure, with neuroendocrine tumors being the most frequent new diagnosis. Sixty-eight of the patients were treated, with 62 patients receiving cisplatin-based treatment. Fifteen patients (23%) had CR, and 18 patients (29%) had PR. Patients obtaining a response were generally young, were male, and had midline involvement of the retroperitoneum, mediastinum, or cervical lymph nodes. All 15 had the light microscopic diagnosis of poorly differentiated carcinoma. A series of 41 patients with poorly differentiated carcinoma of unknown primary were evaluated at Memorial Sloan Kettering Cancer Center.[107] Thirty percent were found to have tumors containing i(12p), increased copies of 12p, or a deletion of the long arm of chromosome 12. Seventy-five percent of patients demonstrating chromosomal abnormalities responded to cisplatin-based chemotherapy versus 18% in patients for whom no diagnosis could be made.

These results suggest that poorly differentiated carcinomas of unknown primary are responsive to chemotherapy and may even be curable. A subset of these patients probably represents histologically and serologically atypical germ cell cancers. Patients with metastatic poorly differentiated carcinoma should be investigated to identify a primary site. Serum HCG and AFP should be measured. Patients with a dominant pulmonary or mediastinal mass should have fiber-optic bronchoscopy. Thorough investigations with light microscopy, immunoperoxidase staining, and cytogenetics should be carried out to further characterize the tumor. Patients should receive a trial of cisplatin-based chemotherapy.

Key references

The complete reference list can be found on the Wiley Companion Digital Edition of this title (see inside front cover for login instructions).

6 Jemal A, Thomas A, Murray T, Thun M. Cancer statistics, 2002. *CA Cancer J Clin.* 2002;**52**:23–47.

13 Raghavan D, Zalcberg JR, Grygiel JJ, et al. Multiple atypical nevi: a cutaneous marker of germ cell tumors. *J Clin Oncol.* 1994;**12**:2284–2287.

17 Sokal M, Peckham MJ, Hendry WF. Bilateral germ cell tumours of the testis. *Br J Urol.* 1980;**52**:158–162.

20 Jones TD, Ulbright TM, Eble JN, et al. OCT4 Staining in testicular tumors: a sensitive and specific marker for seminoma and embryonal carcinoma. *Am J Surg Path.* 2004;**28**:935–940.

22 Cheng L. Establishing a germ cell origin for metastatic tumors using OCT4 immunohistochemistry. *Cancer.* 2004;**101**:2006–2010.

30 Brosman S. Testicular tumors in prepubertal children. *Urology.* 1979;**13**:581–588.

36 Zon RT, Nichols C, Einhorn LH. Management strategies and outcomes of germ cell tumor patients with very high human chorionic gonadotropin levels. *J Clin Oncol.* 1998;**16**:1294–1297.

41 Dieckmann KP, Skakkebaek NE. Carcinoma in situ of the testis: review of biological and clinical features. *Int J Cancer.* 1999;**83**:815–822.

47 Hoskin P, Dilly S, Easton D, Horwich A, Hendry W, Peckham MJ. Prognostic factors in stage I nonseminomatous germ-cell testicular tumors managed by orchiectomy and surveillance: implications for adjuvant chemotherapy. *J Clin Oncol.* 1986;**4**:1031–1036.

53 Krege S, Beyer J, Souchon R, et al. European consensus conference on diagnosis and treatment of germ cell cancer: a report of the second meeting of the European Germ Cell Cancer Consensus Group (EGCCCG): part II. *Eur Urol.* 2008;**53**:497–513.

59 Donohue JP. Retroperitoneal lymphadenectomy: the anterior approach including bilateral suprarenal-hilar dissection. *Urol Clin North Am.* 1977;**4**:509–521.

67 Richie JP. Clinical stage 1 testicular cancer: the role of modified retroperitoneal lymphadenectomy. *J Urol.* 1990;**144**:1160–1163.

76 Groll RJ, Warde P, Jewett MA. A comprehensive systematic review of testicular germ cell tumor surveillance. *Crit Rev Oncol Hematol.* 2007;**64**:182–197.

80 Colls BM, Harvey VJ, Skelton L, et al. Late results of surveillance of clinical stage I nonseminoma germ cell testicular tumours: 17 years' experience in a national study in New Zealand. *BJU Int.* 1999;**83**:76–82.

84 Mead G. for the IGCCCG. International germ cell consensus classification: a prognostic factor-based staging system for metastatic germ cell cancers. International Germ Cell Cancer Collaborative Group. *J Clin Oncol.* 1997;**15**:594–603.

89 Boden G, Gibb R. Radiotherapy and testicular neoplasms. *Lancet.* 1951;**2**:1195–1196.

95 Schmoll H-J, Souchon G, Bokemeyer C. European consensus on diagnosis and treatment of germ cell cancer: a report of the European Germ Cell Cancer Consensus Group (EGCCCG). *Ann Oncol.* 2004;**15**:1377–1399.

99 von der Maase H, Specht L, Jackobsen GK, et al. Surveillance following orchidectomy for stage I seminoma of the testis [comment]. *Eur J Cancer.* 1993;**29A**:1923–1924.

106 Oliver RT, Mead GM, Fogarty PJ, Stenning SP, MRC TE19 and EORTC 30982 trial collaborators. Radiotherapy versus carboplatin for stage I seminoma: updated analysis of the MRC/EORTC randomized trial (ISRTN27163214). *J Clin Oncol.* 2008;**26**:May 20 suppl:abstr 1.

112 Warwick OH, Alison RE, Darte JM. Clinical experience with vinblastine sulfate. *Can Med Assoc J.* 1961;**85**:579–583.

118 Einhorn L, Donahue J. Cis-diamminedichloroplatinum, vinblastine, and bleomycin combination chemotherapy in disseminated testicular cancer. *Ann Intern Med.* 1977;**87**:293–298.

121 Einhorn L, Williams SD, Troner M, Birch R, Greco FA. The role of maintenance therapy in disseminated testicular cancer. *N Engl J Med.* 1981;**305**:727–731.

124 Einhorn LH, Williams SD, Loehrer PJ, et al. Evaluation of optimal duration of chemotherapy in favorable-prognosis disseminated germ cell tumors: a Southeastern Cancer Study Group protocol. *J Clin Oncol.* 1989;**7**:387–391.

128 Horwich A, Sleijfer DT, Fossa SD, et al. Randomized trial of bleomycin, etoposide, and cisplatin compared with bleomycin, etoposide, and carboplatin in good-prognosis metastatic nonseminomatous germ cell cancer: a Multi-institutional Medical Research Council/European Organization for Research and Treatment of Cancer Trial. *J Clin Oncol.* 1997;**15**:1844–1852.

135 Ozols RF, Ihde DC, Linehan WM, et al. A randomized trial of standard chemotherapy v a high-dose chemotherapy regimen in the treatment of poor prognosis nonseminomatous germ-cell tumors. *J Clin Oncol.* 1988;**6**:1031–1040.

140 Kaye SB, Mead GM, Fossa S, et al. Intensive induction-sequential chemotherapy with BOP/VIP-B compared with treatment with BEP/EP for poor-prognosis metastatic nonseminomatous germ cell tumor: a Randomized Medical Research Council/European Organization for Research and Treatment of Cancer study. *J Clin Oncol.* 1998;**16**:692–701.

145 Sheinfeld J. Risks of the uncontrolled retroperitoneum. *Ann Surg Oncol.* 2003;**10**:100–101.

148 Vergouwe Y, Steyerberg EW, Foster RS, et al. Validation of a prediction model and its predictors for the histology of residual masses in nonseminomatous testicular cancer. *J Urol.* 2001;**165**:84–88; discussion 88.

151 Moore CJ, Daneshmand S, Kondagunta GV, et al. Management of difficult germ-cell tumors. *Oncology (Williston Park).* 2006;**20**:1565–1570, 1575; discussion 1575–1576.

156 Ganjoo KN, Chan RJ, Sharma M, et al. Positron emission tomography scans in the evaluation of postchemotherapy residual masses in patients with seminoma. *J Clin Oncol.* 1999;**17**:3457–3460.

160 Carver BS, Shayegan B, Eggener S, et al. Incidence of metastatic nonseminomatous germ cell tumor outside the boundaries of a modified postchemotherapy retroperitoneal lymph node dissection. *J Clin Oncol.* 2007;**25**:4365–4369.

164 Baniel J, Sella A. Complications of retroperitoneal lymph node dissection in testicular cancer: primary and post-chemotherapy. *Semin Surg Oncol.* 1999;**17**:263–267.

169 Beck SD, Foster RS, Bihrle R, et al. Post chemotherapy RPLND in patients with elevated markers: current concepts and clinical outcome. *Urol Clin North Am.* 2007;**34**:219–225; abstract ix–x.

172 Friedman EL, Garnick MB, Stomper PC, et al. Therapeutic guidelines and results in advanced seminoma. *J Clin Oncol.* 1985;**3**:1325–1332.

177 Nichols CR. Treatment of recurrent germ cell tumors. *Semin Surg Oncol.* 1999;**17**:268–274.

184 Kondagunta GV, Bacik J, Bajorin D, et al. Etoposide and cisplatin chemotherapy for metastatic good-risk germ cell tumors. *J Clin Oncol.* 2005;**23**(**36**):9290–9294.

191 Lorch A, Kollmannsberger C, Hartmann JT, et al. Single versus sequential high-dose chemotherapy in patients with relapsed or refractory germ cell tumors: a prospective randomized multicenter trial of the German Testicular Cancer Study Group. *J Clin Oncol.* 2007;**12**(**19**):2778–2784.

198 Kollmannsberger C, Beyer J, Liersch R, et al. Combination chemotherapy with gemcitabine plus oxaliplatin in patients with intensively pretreated or refractory germ cell cancer: a study of the German Testicular Cancer Study Group. *J Clin Oncol.* 2004;**22**(**1**):108–114.

204 Meijer S, Mulder NH, Sleijfer DT, et al. Influence of combination chemotherapy with cis-diamminedichloroplatinum on renal function: long-term effects. *Oncology.* 1983;**40**:170–173.

209 Cantwell BMJ, Mannix KA, Roberts JT, et al. Thromboembolic events during combination chemotherapy for germ cell malignancy. *Lancet.* 1988;**2**:1086–1087.

214 Haugnes HS, Aass N, Fossa SD, et al. Components of the metabolic syndrome in long-term survivors of testicular cancer. *Ann Oncol.* 2007;**18**(**2**):241–248.

220 Reddel RR, Kefford RF, Grant JM, et al. Ototoxicity in patients receiving cisplatin: importance of dose and method of drug administration. *Cancer Treat Rep.* 1982;**66**:19–23.

224 Morrish DW, Venner PM, Siy O, et al. Mechanisms of endocrine dysfunction in patients with testicular cancer. *J Natl Cancer Inst.* 1990;**82**:412–418.

229 Bohlen D, Burkhard FC, Mills R, et al. Fertility and sexual function after orchiectomy and two cycles of chemotherapy for stage I high-risk nonseminomatous germ cell cancer. *J Urol.* 2001;**165**:141–144.

Overview

Vulvar and vaginal carcinomas are uncommon diseases that generally affect post-menopausal women, although 19% of vulvar carcinomas occur in women >50 years old. Risk factors for vulvar cancer include human papilloma virus and chronic inflammation. Vulvar intraepithelial neoplasia can often be managed with wide local excision, but several other modalities have been utilized. Most vulvar malignancies are squamous cell carcinomas that are managed by surgical excision and radiotherapy. Sentinel lymph node biopsy has been used to spare the morbidity observed after regional lymph node dissection. For more advanced lesions, chemo-radiotherapy with agents such as 5-FU, cisplatin, and mitomycin C is utilized. Other vulvar malignancies include Bartholin gland carcinomas, basal cell carcinomas, verrucous carcinomas, and melanomas. Carcinomas of the vagina are most frequently squamous cell, but clear cell adenocarcinomas have been seen in younger women. In the past, clear cell carcinomas were associated with prenatal exposure to diethyl-stibestrol. Vaginal melanomas can occur, as well as endodermal sinus tumors, rhrabdomysarcomas, and fibroepithelial vagina polyps.

Cancer of the vulva

Incidence and epidemiology

Vulvar cancer accounts for about 4% of cancers in the female reproductive organs and 0.6% of all cancers in women. It is the fourth most frequent gynecologic cancer.[1] The American Cancer Society estimated that in 2014, about 4850 cancers of the vulva were diagnosed in the United States and about 1030 women die of this cancer.[2]

Risk factors include cigarette smoking, human papillomavirus (HPV), vulvar or cervical intraepithelial neoplasia, chronic immunosuppression, chronic vulvar inflammatory diseases (e.g., lichen sclerosis and lichen planus), and northern European ancestry.[3] Most vulvar carcinomas occur in older women, with more than 50% of the patients being 60–79 years of age. Kumar et al. found that younger patients with vulvar cancer are increasing with frequency, and through evaluation of the SEER database found that 19.3% of patients diagnosed with vulvar cancer are <50 years old. In addition, there is a striking survival difference between the younger and older women with squamous cell vulvar cancer (Figure 1).[4]

This increased frequency in younger patients may be attributed to an increase in HPV, specifically HPV-related vulvar intraepithelial neoplasia that progresses to cancer.

Vulvar cancer is thought to develop through two types of pathways, the first related to HPV infections and the second related to a chronic inflammatory process.[5] Several epidemiologic studies suggest a sexually transmitted origin for carcinoma of the vulva. Condyloma acuminatum associated with HPV has been noted in many patients with premalignant and malignant vulvar disease. It

has been estimated that in the United States, over 1 million women each year develop perineal warts and that as many as 10% are infected with HPV.[6] Currently, HPV types 6 and 11 are most frequently found in benign vulvar warts, and HPV types 16, 18, 31, 33, and 45 are more frequently associated with intraepithelial neoplasia or invasive carcinoma.[6–8] HPV can be found in approximately 50% of vulvar carcinomas; the tumors are often multifocal and associated with vulvar dysplasias. HPV-negative tumors are often found in older women.[9,10] These can be associated with chronic inflammatory disease as seen with vulvar dystrophies.

Although epidemiologic evidence strongly suggests a viral cause, other associations have been implied as well. Factors such as granulomatous diseases of the vulva, diabetes, hypertension, and obesity also have been associated with vulvar carcinoma, but perhaps this is because of the usually advanced age of patients. A case–control study by Mabuchi et al.[11] found that domestic servants, or those working in laundry or cleaning plants, have an increased risk of vulvar carcinoma, thus suggesting an environmental component.

The association of carcinoma *in situ* (CIS) with invasive carcinoma of the vulva indicates a continuum from preinvasive to invasive carcinoma. Jones et al.[12] evaluated 405 cases of vulvar intraepithelial neoplasia (VIN) 2–3, they found that 3.8% of patients that are treated will progress to cancer, and 10 patients who did not undergo treatment progressed in 3.9 years (mean). Progression, however, may differ between younger and older patients. Some authors suggest that the multifocal CIS of women in their thirties or forties is less likely to progress compared to older women.[13–15]

Vulvar intraepithelial neoplasias

In 2004, The International Society for the Study of Vulvar Disease developed the current classification system for VIN (Table 1). Previous classification included VIN 1, 2, and 3 according to the degree of abnormality. Currently, only high-grade disease is defined as VIN and hence would take that nomenclature. It has been shown that VIN 1 is not a cancer precursor and therefore is not described as VIN. In 2004, they developed two categories to describe VIN: VIN, usual type (includes former VIN 2 and 3 of warty or basaloid and mixed types), and VIN, differentiated type (associated with lichen sclerosis).[16] In addition, the College of American Pathologists and the ASCCP confirmed a two-tier system with the recent Lower Anogenital Squamous Terminology (LAST) terminology project.[17] American College of Obstetrics and Gynecology (ACOG) and the American Society for Colposcopic and Cervical Pathology (ASCCP) issued a committee opinion on treatment of VIN cases given that there has been such an increase over the past 30 years, confirming agreement with International Society for the Study of Vulvovaginal Disease (ISVDD) nomenclature of VIN differentiated type and usual type, and discussing treatment recommendations. Of note, many pathologists and practitioners still use the old classifications.

Holland-Frei Cancer Medicine, Ninth Edition. Edited by Robert C. Bast Jr., Carlo M. Croce, William N. Hait, Waun Ki Hong, Donald W. Kufe, Martine Piccart-Gebhart, Raphael E. Pollock, Ralph R. Weichselbaum, Hongyang Wang, and James F. Holland.
© 2017 John Wiley & Sons, Inc. ISBN: 978-1-118-93469-2

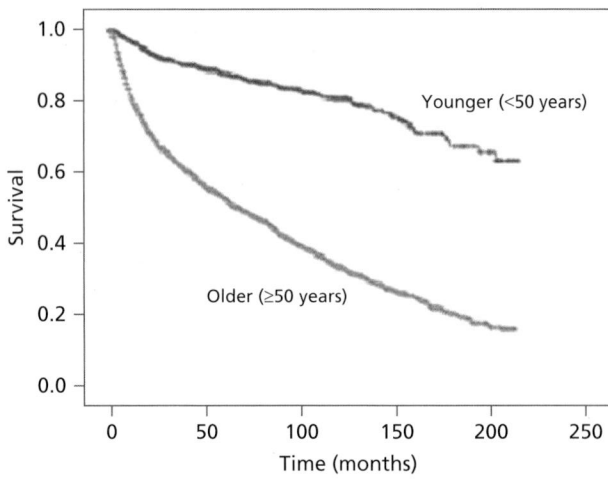

Figure 1 Comparison of survival of younger patients (<50 years; blue line) with that of older patients (≥50 years; green line) with squamous cell cancer of the vulva, 1988–2005. Log-rank $p = 0.001$. Source: Kumar 2009.[4] Reproduced with permission of Elsevier.

Table 1 Classifications of vulvar dysplasias.

Old classifications
Intraepithelial dysplasia
Mild dysplasia (VIN I)
Moderate dysplasia (VIN II)
Severe dysplasia (VIN III)
Current classifications (ISSVD 2004)
VIN-differentiated (associated with vulvar dermatologic conditions)
VIN-usual type (including warty, basaloid, and mixed VIN, associated with HPV)

Abbreviations: VIN, vulvar intraepithelial neoplasia; HPV, human papillomavirus.

VIN can present with a variety of symptoms. The most common is irritation or itching; however, 20% of patients are asymptomatic.[18] Grossly, the lesions can be flat, raised (maculopapular), or verrucous. In color, they may be brown (hyperpigmented), red (erythroplastic), white, or discolored.

White lesions can appear to have a whitish, thickened keratin layer (leukoplakia) or a diffuse, white, brittle, paperlike appearance (lichen sclerosus) (Figure 2). Areas of squamous hyperplasia (hyperplastic dystrophy) and dysplasia can also have a white appearance. Unlike lichen sclerosus, however, the tissue often is thickened, and the process tends to be focal or multifocal rather than diffuse.[15] It is important to biopsy lichen sclerosis as there may be an underlying vulvar carcinoma.[19,20]

Microscopically, atypical changes in the vulvar epithelium consistent with preinvasive lesions usually are marked by loss of maturation of the squamous epithelium. There are increased mitotic activity and an increase in the nuclear cytoplasmic ratio.

There is suggestion that there are two distinct causes of vulvar dysplasia leading to vulvar cancer. The first type is seen in younger patients and is related to HPV infection and smoking. This type presents itself as a "warty" dysplasia. The more common type is in elderly patients and is unrelated to smoking or HPV. This group is more related to lichen sclerosis adjacent to the tumor. Approximately 20% of vulvar cancer has been reported to have vulvar dysplasia.

The best method of establishing a diagnosis is a high index of suspicion and early biopsy. Several methods also can be used to help assess these lesions. Cytology, colposcopy, acetic acid, and

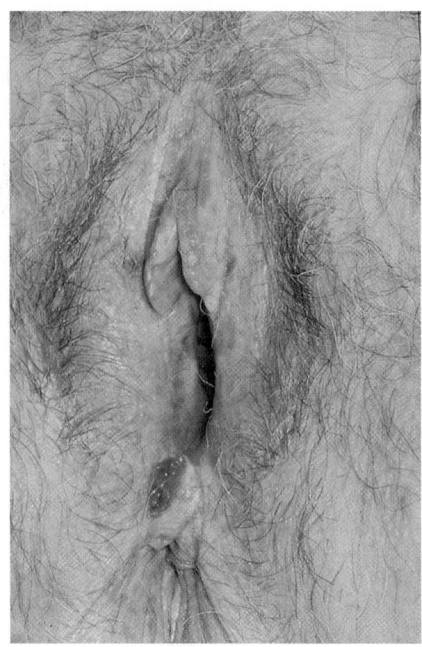

Figure 2 White, brittle paperlike appearance or lichen sclerosus of the vulva.

toluidine blue O can be used cautiously before biopsy. In general, however, cytologic evaluation of the vulva has not been helpful as a screening examination because the vulvar skin often is thickened and keratinized. Colposcopic examination of the vulva is difficult because unlike cervical lesions, the changes are difficult to recognize. Therefore, colposcopic examination is not used for routine vulvar examination; rather, it is primarily employed for patients who are being evaluated or followed for vulvar atypia or intraepithelial malignancies. The toluidine blue O test is nonspecific and stains nuclei in the superficial part of the epithelium. Colposcopy is performed after applying a 1% aqueous solution of toluidine blue O to the vulva for 1 min and decolorizing the tissue with 1% acetic acid. Areas that retain the stain are biopsied. A positive test, however, does not always indicate a premalignant condition because 20% of benign areas on the vulva stain positively.[19]

To obtain the entire thickness of the skin for a definitive diagnosis, a biopsy of the vulva usually is done with a Keyes dermal punch. Occasionally, a larger biopsy is needed, in which case a larger field can be locally anesthetized with lidocaine and a small scalpel or cervical biopsy punch used to obtain a specimen.[21]

Once the correct diagnosis has been established by biopsy, appropriate therapy can be undertaken. For lichen sclerosis, local measures, for example, wearing cotton underclothes and avoiding strong soaps and detergents, often are used to diminish irritation. Topical fluorinated corticosteroids applied twice daily for 1–2 weeks are helpful in controlling pruritus, but prolonged use of these steroid preparations can lead to vulvar atrophy or contracture. If long-term therapy is needed, a nonfluorinated compound such as 1% hydrocortisone is used. Some patients with lichen sclerosus have severe contracture in the area of the posterior fourchette. Treating these areas surgically with plastic repair of the fourchette has been suggested.[22,23]

VIN can be treated by a variety of methods, and many authors have reported successful control of the disease by wide local excision.[10,22] Adequate margins must be obtained with wide excision; however, this often may be difficult because of the multifocal nature of the disease. Wallbillich et al.[24] found that positive margins increased recurrence from 11% to 32%, and recurrence was associated with smoking and a large lesion size.

Other modalities also have been reported in the treatment of VIN. Carbon dioxide laser vaporization and photodynamic therapy[25] of the vulva to a depth of 3 mm have been used, and current evidence indicates that laser therapy is as effective as surgical excision for the control of this disease. Before lasering the vulva, however, it is necessary to ascertain by histologic confirmation that invasive disease does not exist. Leuchter et al.[26] treated 142 patients with CIS of the vulva. Of those treated by laser, 17% had a recurrence, a result that is similar to that in lesions treated by local excision.

Imiquimod has been used also for conservative medical treatment. A systematic review that included two randomized control trials found a complete response rate of 51%.[27] 5-Fluorouracil (5-FU) cream has been used successfully to treat CIS of the vulva, and application of this has been reported to be successful in 75% of cases. With continuous application, however, this treatment causes edema and pain. Most recently, a multicenter, randomized, phase 2 trial between cidofovir and imiquimod for treatment of VIN3 showed a response rate of approximately 46% for both groups treated.[28]

Paget disease

Paget disease is a rare intraepithelial disorder of the vulvar skin that is seen in postmenopausal women.[29–31] Unlike VIN, the intraepithelial neoplastic cells are glandular rather than squamous. The lesion primarily occurs in Caucasians of an average age of 65 years. Grossly, it appears as a reddish, eczematoid lesion. Microscopically, this type of lesion is characterized by large pale cells that often occur in nests and infiltrate the epithelium. Once the diagnosis is made, it is important to rule out the presence of an underlying cancer. Invasive vulvar Paget disease occurs in approximately 10% of Paget disease.[20] If the anal area is involved, one needs to consider an anal carcinoma. A review by Lee et al.[30] reported a total of 75 cases of Paget disease of the vulva: 16 (22%) of the patients had underlying invasive carcinoma of the adnexal structures and 7 (9%) had adnexal CIS.

Paget disease of the vulva often spreads in an occult manner, with margins extending beyond the normal appearance of the lesion.[31] If there is no evidence of an underlying malignant neoplasm, a wide local excision or total vulvectomy usually is performed.[32] If a wide local excision is performed, a slightly deeper excision is needed to remove the epidermis down to the level of the underlying fat to ensure removal of adnexal skin structures. Because this lesion extends subepithelially, a frozen section in the operating room may assist in ensuring complete removal.

Bergen et al. evaluated 14 patients with Paget disease of the vulva that was treated by vulvectomy, skinning vulvectomy with a graft, or hemivulvectomy.[32] With a median follow-up of 50 months, all patients were free of disease; however, three patients had locally recurrent disease. Other modalities (topical 5-FU cream, laser) have not been used for treatment of this disease. Because both local and distant recurrence is a major risk, close follow-up is required.

Invasive vulvar carcinomas

The International Federation of Gynecology and Obstetrics (FIGO) adopted a new surgical staging system in 2009 (Table 2). This surgical staging has been modified once prior, in 1995, after it became a surgically staged cancer in 1989. The most recent staging system addresses lack of predictive value seen in the previous stages with regard to the size of the lesion, and number and size of lymph node metastasis.[32] Specifically, in the new system, there was an addition of three pathologic groupings within stage III (A, B, and C): this identifies the number of positive node, the size of each node, and

extracapsular spread. In addition, many centers use the tumor, node, and metastasis (TNM) classification.

Vulvar cancer can spread by direct extension, lymphatic embolization, or hematogenous dissemination. Metastasis to the femoral nodes without inguinal node involvement has been reported but is uncommon. The direct lymphatic pathways from the clitoris to the pelvic nodes have been described but are not of clinical significance. The overall incidence of lymph node metastasis is approximately 30%. Pelvic node metastasis is uncommon with an overall frequency of 9%. Approximately 20% of patients with positive groin nodes have positive pelvic nodes.[33,34]

Squamous cell carcinoma

Squamous cell carcinomas comprise approximately 90% of primary vulvar malignancies. Grossly, these carcinomas usually appear as ulcerated or polyploid masses on the vulva. Biopsy reveals the characteristic histologic appearance: the tumor appears in nests and cords of squamous cells infiltrating the stroma, often with islands of keratin. On physical examination, there is usually an ulcerated lesion or wart-like lesion. Recently, there has been an increased incidence of warty carcinoma accounting for 20% of all cases.

Different clinical results have been reported with this definition. Spread to regional lymph nodes has varied from 0% to 10% in tumors with less than a 5 mm depth of invasion.[35–40] For example, Hoffman et al.[38] reported no nodal metastases in 43 patients whose tumor invaded <2 mm. Lesions that were at risk of spreading to inguinal nodes included tumors with confluent tongues rather than those with individual tongues merely extending into the stroma. Depth of invasion of the stroma to ≤1 mm is associated with a risk of lymph nodes metastasis of <1%, hence no need for patient with <1 mm stromal invasion to undergo an inguinal lymph node dissection. Tumors with a depth of invasion of 1.1–3.0 mm are associated with lymph node metastasis of 6–12%, and this rate increases to 15–20% with a depth of invasion of 3.1–5 mm.[41]

The risk of nodal involvement may be decreased when CIS is present in the lesion. Rowley et al.[39] noted that only 1 of 35 cases with adjacent CIS had nodal metastases. By contrast, 5 of 27 had positive lymph nodes when superficial stage I lesions penetrating 2.1–5.0 mm did not have adjacent CIS.

Sentinel inguinal lymph node biopsy

Sentinel lymph node biopsy (SLNB) is being used in vulvar cancer. In patients with a clinically negative groin examination, an SLNB is an alternative to inguinofemoral lymphadenectomy. SLNB results in less morbidity without compromising detection for lymph node metastases. The Gynecologic Oncology Group (GOG 173) compares SLNB to inguinofemoral lymphadenectomy in 452 women with squamous cell vulvar cancer, for tumors with a depth >1 mm, and size between 2 and 6 cm.[42] The sensitivity of the SLNB is 92%, and the negative predictive value is 96% in this study. Another multicenter observational study GROnigen INternational Study on Sentinel nodes in Vulvar cancer (GROINSS-V) analyzed 623 groins from 403 patients, confirming a decrease in short- and long-term morbidities.

Patients undergoing an SLNB report less treatment-related morbidity compared to inguinofemoral lymphadenectomy without compromising the overall quality of life.[43] The results of the observational study GROINSS-V II, evaluating and performing a full inguinofemoral lymph node dissection in the setting of a positive SLNB and observation only of a negative SLNB, are still pending.

The above-mentioned studies are all based on surgeons with "vast experience" performing SLNBs. It is still recommended that

Table 2 TNM classification and staging of vulvar carcinoma.

TNM classification	
T	Primary tumor
Tis	Preinvasive carcinoma (CIS)
T1	Tumor confined to the vulva and/or perineum; 2 cm or less in diameter
T2	Tumor confined to the vulva and/or perineum; more than 2 cm in diameter
T3	Tumor of any size with adjacent spread to the urethra, vagina, or anus
T4	Tumor of any size infiltrating the bladder mucosa, the rectal mucosa, or both, including the upper part of the urethral mucosa, or fixed to the anus
N	Regional lymph nodes
N0	No nodes palpable
N1	Unilateral regional lymph node metastases
N2	Bilateral regional lymph node metastases
M	Distant metastases
M0	No clinical metastases
M1	Distant metastases (including pelvic lymph node metastases)

FIGO staging (2009)		
IA	T1aN0M0	Tumor confined to the vulva and/or perineum: 2 cm or less in greatest dimension, ≤1 mm stromal invasion, no nodal metastasis
IB	T1aN0M0	Tumor confined to the vulva and/or perineum: 2 cm or greater in greatest dimension, >1 mm stromal invasion, no nodal metastasis
II	T2	Tumor of any size with extension to adjacent perineal structures (1/3 lower urethra, 1/3 lower vagina, anus) with negative nodes
IIIA	T1 or T2, N1a or N1b, M0	Tumor of any size with or without extension to adjacent perineal structures (1/3 lower urethra, 1/3 lower vagina, and anus) and positive inguinofemoral lymph node, (1) 1–2 lymph node metastasis (<5 mm) or (2) 1 lymph node metastasis ≥5 mm
IIIB	T1 or T2, N2a or N2b, M0	Tumor of any size with or without extension to adjacent perineal structures (1/3 lower urethra, 1/3 lower vagina, and anus) and positive inguinofemoral lymph node, (1) 3 or more lymph node metastaisis (<5 mm) or (2) 2 or more lymph node metastasis ≥5 mm
IIIC	T1 or T2, N2c, M0	Positive node with extracapsular spread
IVA		Tumor invades any of the following: upper urethra, bladder mucosa, rectal mucosa, pelvic bone, and/or bilateral regional node metastasis
IVB		Any distant metastasis including pelvic lymph nodes

Abbreviations: FIGO, International Federation of Gynecology and Obstetrics; TNM, tumor, node, and metastasis.
Source: Adapted from Barakat 2013.

in the setting of lack of expertise with SLNB, an inguinofemoral lymphadenectomy is done, which is common in the setting of vulvar cancer, which is overall a rare cancer.

Treatment

Clinical stage IA

Tumors showing a depth of the stroma 1 mm or less have minimal risk for lymphatic dissemination. They do not require an inguinofemoral lymph node dissection because the risk of lymph node metastases in this setting is very low risk. These lesions are usually treated with a wide radical excision. These patients have a high cure rate; however, surveillance is needed to rule out recurrence.

Clinical stage I/II

The recommendation for a clinical stage I or II vulvar cancer is a wide radical excision with unilateral or bilateral SLNB versus an inguinal femoral lymphadenectomy (depending on size, location, and institution) for both staging and therapeutic purposes. Margins need to include at least a 2 cm margin lateral of normal tissue, with the deep margin to the deep perineal fascia. The laterality of the lesion determines the need for bilateral versus unilateral inguinofemoral lymph node dissection (or SLNB). A subanalysis of GOG 173 shows that a bilateral lymph node dissection is required except when the tumor is located more than 2 cm or greater from the midline. For both stages I and II, surgical resection usually leads to excellent long-term survival and local control.

The pattern of spread for this carcinoma relates to the intricate lymphatic drainage of the vulva (Figure 3). Tumors located in the middle of either labium initially drain to the ipsilateral inguinal femoral nodes, whereas midline perineal tumors can spread to either the left or right side. Using technetium-99 m colloid, Iversen and Aas showed that when radioactivity was injected to one side of the vulva, 98% of it localized in the ipsilateral nodes and <2% in the contralateral nodes.[34] Tumors along the midline in the clitoral or urethral areas may spread to either groin. From the inguinal-femoral nodes, lymphatic spread continues to the deep pelvic iliac and obturator nodes. Although there has been concern in the past that tumors in the clitoral–urethral area could spread directly to the deep pelvic nodes, current evidence indicates that this is rare.

Stages I, II, and III invasive carcinoma

The prognosis of a patient with vulvar carcinoma relates to the stage of disease (Figure 4). The presence of carcinoma in the regional lymph nodes correlates with the size and thickness of the primary lesion, the degree of tumor differentiation, and the involvement of vascular spaces by the tumor as seen in Table 3, which comes from a classic study by Sedlis et al.[44] In 272 women with invasive vulvar carcinoma reported by the GOG, regional nodes were involved in 8.9% of stage I, 25.3% of stage II, and 31.1% of stage III lesions.[45,46] With larger lesions, 4 mm or greater in thickness, 31% of nodes were positive. Hacker et al.[47] reported an actuarial 5-year survival rate of 96% in those with negative nodes survival decreased to 94% with one positive node, 80% with two positive nodes, and 12% with three or more nodes involved by tumor.

Not only is the number of nodes important but there also appears to be a correlation with the size of the metastases. Hoffman et al.[48] noted that 14 of 15 patients with inguinal lymph node metastases measuring <36 mm survived free of disease for 5 years compared with 12 of 29 patients whose tumor metastases measured >100 mm.

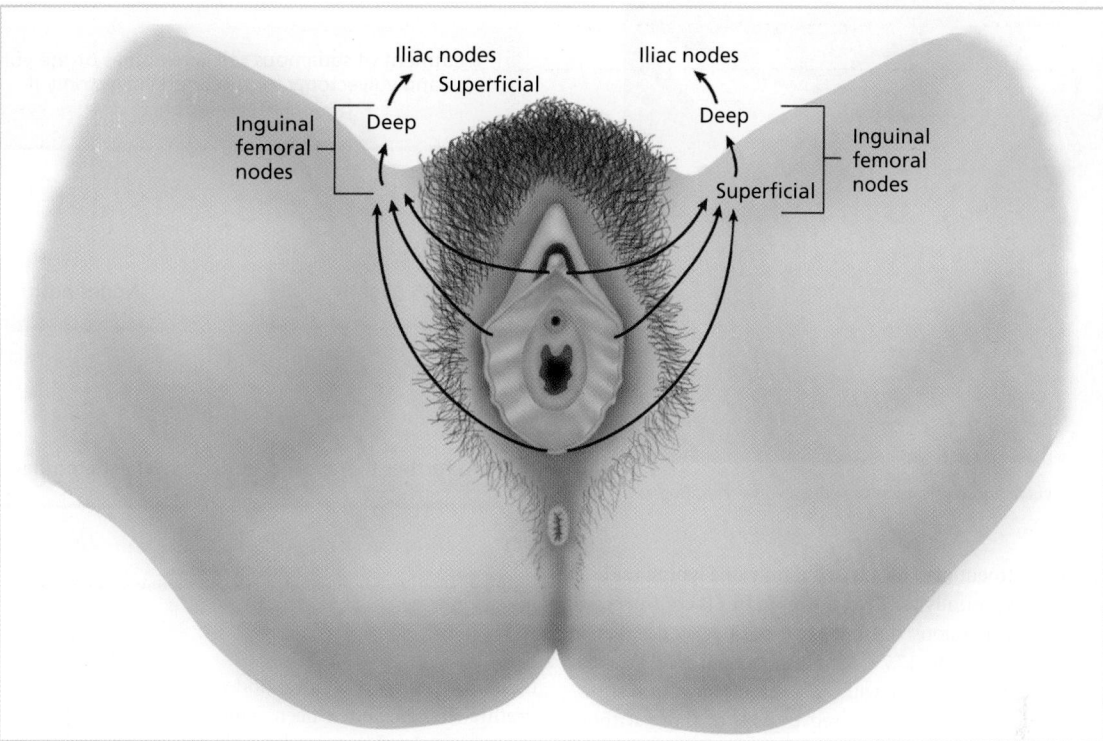

Figure 3 Lymphatic drainage of the vulva.

Percent of cases by stage

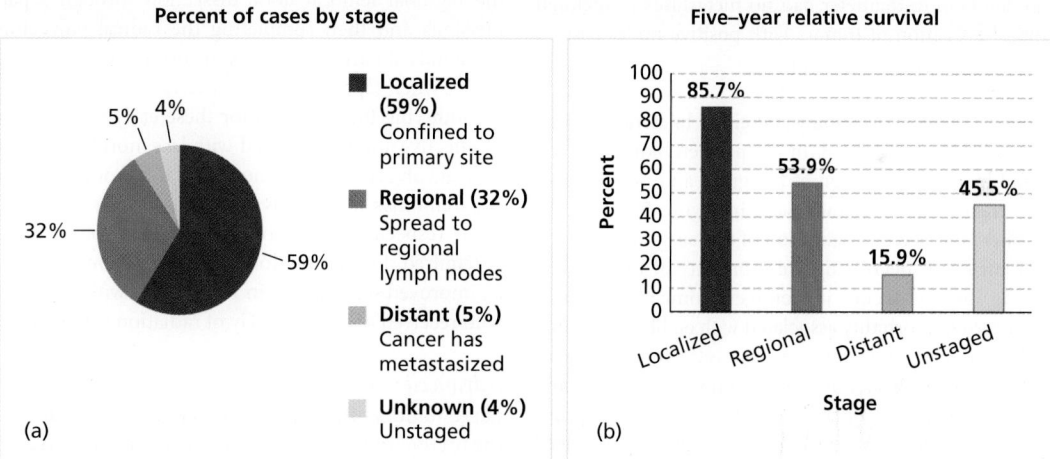

- **Localized (59%)** Confined to primary site

- **Regional (32%)** Spread to regional lymph nodes

- **Distant (5%)** Cancer has metastasized

- **Unknown (4%)** Unstaged

(a)

Five–year relative survival

(b)

Figure 4 (a) Percent of cases and (b) 5-year relative survival by stage at diagnosis: vulvar cancer. Source: National Cancer Institute, Surveillance, Epidemiology, and End Results Program (SEER) 2011. Stat Fact Sheets: Vulvar Cancer (reproduced from http://seer.cancer.gov/statfacts/html/vulva.html, accessed 12 Feb 2015).

Table 3 Prognostic factors of stage, grade, and tumor thickness associated with positive regional nodes.

Stage	Positive nodes (%)	Grade	Positive nodes (%)	Tumor thickness (mm)	Positive nodes (%)
I	8.9	1	0	<1	3.1
II	25.3	2	8.0	2	8.9
III	31.1	3	24.6	3	18.6
IV	62.5	4	47.7	>4	31.0

Source: Sedlis 1987.[44] Reproduced with permission of AJOG.

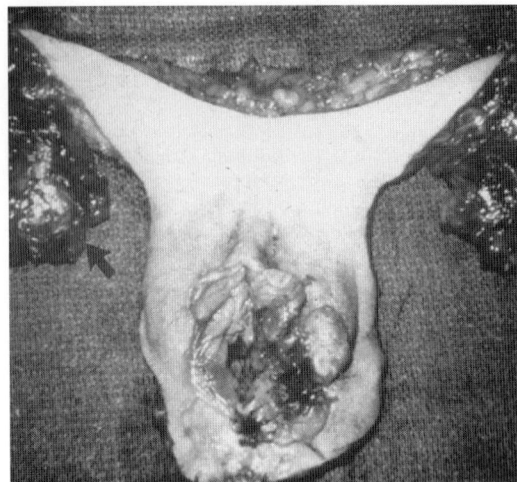

Figure 5 Gross vulvectomy specimen showing a vulvar carcinoma.

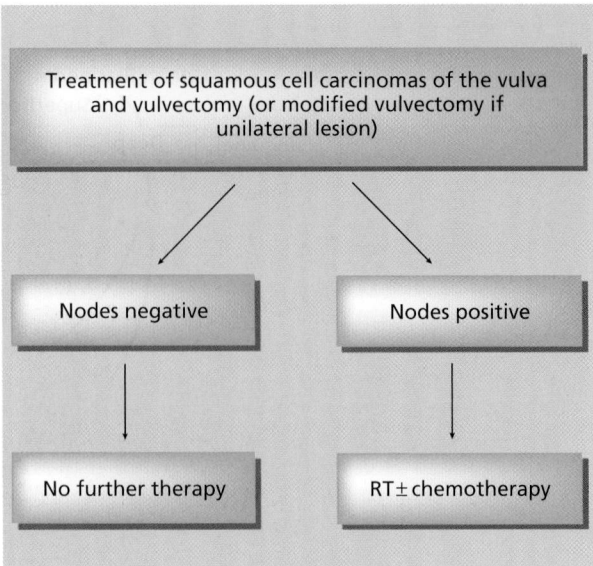

Figure 6 Treatment of squamous cell carcinomas of the vulva. RT, radiation therapy.

No additional treatment may be advised if only one lymph node in the groin in microscopically positive; however, this is controversial. Patients with stage 1 lesions did not have positive nodes, yet in patients with stage 4 lesions, 47.7% of nodes were positive. Vascular space involvement is prognostic with 72% vascular invasion showing regional node metastasis compared to 34% of those without vascular invasion. Nodal involvement also correlates with the location of the primary lesion.[49] Lesions on the labia are associated with 7.4% positive nodes, whereas clitoral lesions have a higher incidence of positive nodes (27.4%).[50] Boyce et al.[51] reported that six tumors under 1 cm in diameter had no metastases to regional nodes but that the fraction of tumors with positive nodes rose to 55% for 29 cases with lesions over 4 cm.

Therapy for stages I and II and early stage III vulvar carcinoma is accomplished with radical vulvectomy and either bilateral inguinal femoral node dissection[52] or SLNB. In the past, en bloc of radical vulvectomy and bilateral dissection of the groin and pelvic nodes were standard treatments (specimen seen in Figure 5). Over the past 30 years, there has been modification of this surgical approach through triple incisions, decreasing the morbidity of the surgery. Since often, the disease occurs in younger women with small tumors and concern of morbidity associated with en bloc resection. The deep pelvic nodes are rarely removed unless the inguinal nodes are involved. Most oncologists now remove only the inguinal and femoral nodes at the time of operation and treat the deep pelvic nodes with external radiation if superficial nodes are involved with tumor.

A wide variety of management options of the primary lesion have been proposed. Management of patients with small lesions should be individualized. Since the early 1980s, radical local excision has been advocated in patients with small tumors. The literature indicates that the incidence of local invasive recurrence is similar with local excision and more radical approaches. Radical local excision is most appropriate for unilateral, isolated lesions. This approach has been used for risk factors such as large tumor sites, positive capillary-lymphatic space invasion, or surgical margins that are <8 mm.

Different surgical approaches to invasive vulvar carcinoma have been evaluated. Classically, an en bloc dissection has been performed. Radical vulvectomy and groin dissection have been carried out through a single suprapubic incision that extends between the left and right anterior iliac spines (Figure 5). This operation removed the entire vulva, including the clitoris, subcutaneous tissue, and inguinal femoral nodes. If the lesion involved the distal urethra, this has often been removed without the loss of urinary continence. In this procedure, the major complication has been wound breakdown and infection (occurring in 50% of the patients). Modifications have been introduced to decrease the incidence of wound breakdown. These modifications include performing the inguinal femoral node dissection through separate inguinal incisions and then completing the radical vulvectomy, which is the standard currently. Tumor recurrences rarely occur in the skin bridge when separate groin incisions are used.[46,53]

Modifying the approach for these early-stage lesions appears to be effective and is associated with less morbidity than the standard radical vulvectomy. If the nodes are free from tumor in stages I and II carcinomas of the vulva, no further therapy is required. If the nodes (especially the femoral nodes) are involved, pelvic irradiation is required. From a randomized study, Homesley et al.[45] reported an improved survival rate in 118 patients with positive lymph nodes who received 4500–5000 cGy of radiation (Figure 6).

Advanced vulvar tumor

Large tumors of the vulva encroaching on the anorectal area and the urethra require more extensive treatment than a radical vulvectomy. Depending on location and ability for resection, approaches can include a radical surgery versus neoadjuvant chemoradiation followed by resection. A radical surgery may leave larger defect that could require skin grafts such as gracilis myocutaneous grafts. If the nodes are negative, a 5-year survival rate of 50% has been reported.[49,54]

A combination of preoperative radiation and surgery is usually the standard depending on location and need for extensive radical surgery. External radiation using newer techniques such as intensity-modulated radiotherapy (IMRT) often is given to reduce the size of the tumor before surgical removal by radical vulvectomy, with or without regional lymph node dissection. Approximately 4000–4500 cGy is delivered to the pelvis and inguinal nodes, the operation being performed 5 weeks after the completion of radiation. This approach may obviate a urinary or fecal diversion. Boronow et al.[55,56] reported a 5-year survival rate of 80% in 26 patients with primary carcinoma of the vagina and vulva who were treated with this technique. Rotmensch et al.[57] recently reported 16 patients with advanced vulvar lesions who were treated with preoperative radiation to the vulva and achieved an overall 5-year survival rate of 45%. Recurrences were more likely if the resection margins were within 1 cm of the tumor. Complications have included stenosis of the introitus and urethra as well as rectovaginal fistula.

The approach has been to not only administer preoperative radiation for advanced lesions but also add chemotherapy. Commonly, agents such as 5-FU, cisplatin, and mitomycin C have been used, producing up to 46% reduction in tumor with chemoradiation; in previous studies, the most common toxicities were acute cutaneous and wound complications.[58] The GOG performed a phase II trial (GOG 101), which enrolled locally advanced T3 or T4 tumors not amenable to surgical resection via radial vulvectomy, and treated them with radiation aplus weekly cisplatin followed by surgical resection of residual tumor. They found a 64% complete response rate.[59] Because the vulvar skin is prone to radiation dermatitis, fibrosis, and ulceration, radiation as the sole therapy has been less than desirable. However, if the patient is inoperable because of medical conditions, radiation can be used as the primary treatment of a vulvar carcinoma.[60]

Recurrent vulvar cancer

Recurrences may be local or distant. More than 80% of recurrences occur in the first 2 years after therapy. The risk of recurrence of vulva carcinoma increases as the stage of disease increases. In an analysis of 502 patients, the majority of recurrences were local; 53.4% were located in the perineal region.[61] Other areas included the inguinal regional, 19% and then distant recurrences in pelvis and beyond, 6% and 8%, respectively.

Different modalities have been used to treat local recurrences. Both radiation therapy and resection of local vulvar recurrence provide effective control and a 5-year survival rate of approximately 60% if local.[61] Local vulvar recurrences can be further excised. However, if recurrence is located in the inguinal region, survival drops dramatically, with a 5-year survival of 27%. The combination of chemotherapy and radiation therapy has been used to treat recurrent disease and some large primary vulvar carcinomas. Disseminated disease requires chemotherapy, but, unfortunately, no chemotherapy has been successful in this situation. There are no prospective trials in this patient population and much of the data that exists is extrapolated from metastatic cervical cancer. Therefore, most metastatic recurrences are treated with a platinum-based regimen, usually carboplatin and paclitaxel, second to better tolerance to cisplatin plus paclitaxel seen in a cervical cancer trial. Palliative care is recommended for patients who cannot tolerate chemotherapy. Overall prognosis is poor for this population (Figure 7).

Bartholin gland carcinoma

Primary carcinoma of Bartholin gland accounts for 5% of all vulvar cancers, and over 200 cases have been reported[62]; approximately 50% of those tumors are nonepidermoid in nature. Bartholin gland carcinomas can be squamous if they originate near the orifice of the duct or papillary if they arise from the transitional epithelium of the duct, or they can be adenocarcinomas if they arise from the gland itself. An enlargement of Bartholin gland in a postmenopausal female should raise the suspicion of malignancy. These tumors are treated similarly to primary squamous cell carcinomas of the vulva by radical vulvectomy and bilateral inguinal femoral lymphadenectomy. The overall 5-year survival rate of approximately 70% is below that reported for all carcinomas of the vulva and probably relates

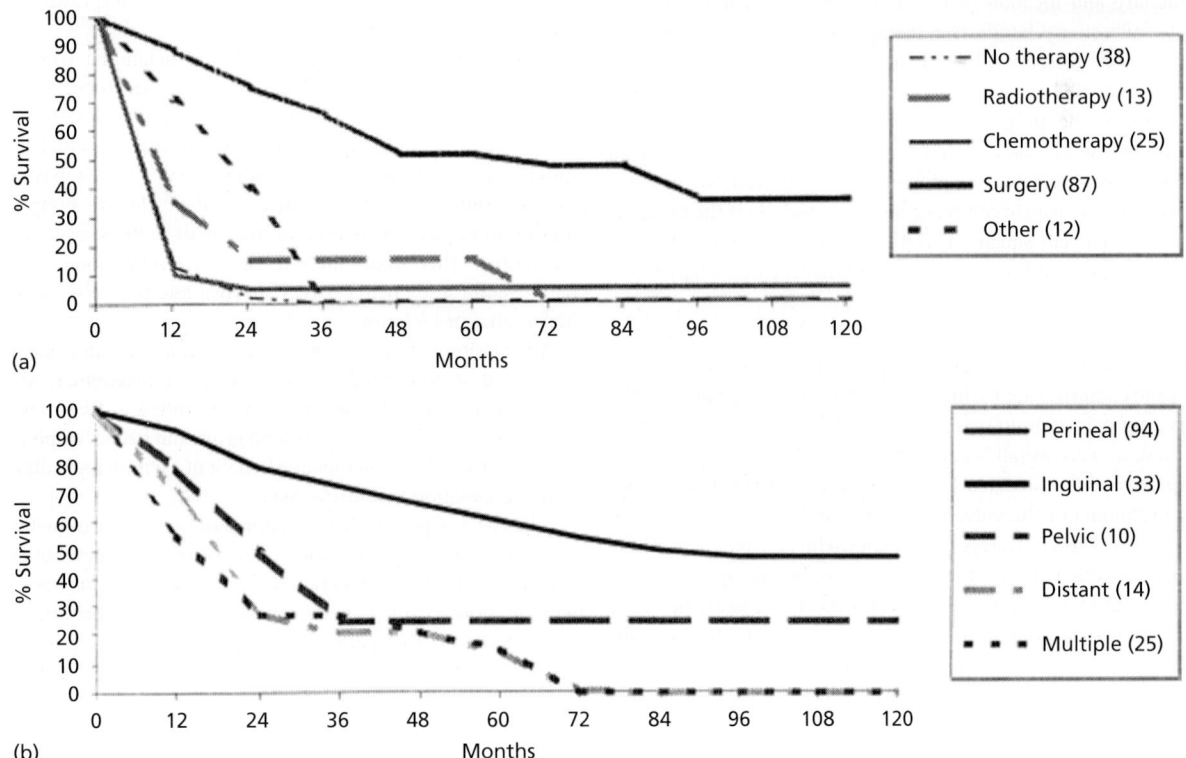

Figure 7 (a) Survival rate after vulvar carcinoma recurrence by type of therapy. The number of cases is shown in parentheses. There was a statistical difference between surgery and other forms of treatment (p, 0.000001). (b) Survival rate of patients with disease recurrence according to the site of the recurrence (the number of patients is shown in parentheses). Source: Maggino 2000.[61] Reproduced by permission of John Wiley and Sons.

to a delay in diagnosis. A Bartholian gland carcinoma of the vulva is classified if the tumor is in the correct anatomic position, deeply located in the labium majora, the underlying skin is intact, and there is some normal gland present.

The adenoid cystic variety of Bartholin gland carcinoma invades locally and rarely metastasizes. It is slow growing with a tendency to recur locally and invade the periocular tissue. It usually requires only wide local excision for adequate therapy. Rosenberg et al.[63] reported five cases of adenocystic carcinoma of Bartholin's gland, with four patients alive and free of disease 28–57 months after treatment.

Basal cell carcinoma

Basal cell carcinoma is rarely encountered in the female genital tract. Such lesions are usually locally invasive, nonmetastatic tumors that are commonly found on the labium majus. Metastasis to the regional lymph nodes is uncommon. Therapy consists of wide local excision of the lesion. If the surgical margins are free of tumor, the disease is cured.

Verrucous carcinoma

Verrucous carcinoma of the vulva is a variant of epidermoid carcinoma. Clinically, it appears as large, condylomatous lesions. They are locally aggressive, nonmetastatic, fungating tumors that gradually increase in size, pushing into rather than invading the underlying structures. Histologically, they consist of mature squamous cells with extensive keratinization. To establish the diagnosis, adequate biopsy is important because biopsy of a large verrucous carcinoma often can lead to an incorrect diagnosis of condyloma acuminatum.

These tumors tend to grow slowly and invade locally, rarely spreading to regional lymph nodes. In 24 cases of verrucous carcinoma, Japaze et al.[64] found no lymph node metastases. Depending on the size and location of the tumor, a wide local excision or simple vulvectomy is effective therapy; radical vulvectomy with inguinal node dissection or radiation therapy is not indicated as treatment for this entity. Radiation therapy is ineffective and can even worsen the prognosis, causing malignant changes within the tumor. The 17 cases treated surgically by Japaze et al. had an excellent 5-year survival rate of 94%. Close long-term follow-up is needed because disease can recur locally, especially if the tumor is large. If concurrent squamous cell carcinoma is found within the verrucous carcinoma, local excision is an inadequate therapy.[65]

Melanoma

Melanoma is the most frequent nonsquamous cell malignancy of the vulva and comprises approximately 5% of primary carcinomas of the vulva. Approximately 400 cases of melanoma of the vulva have been reported, with an overall 5-year survival rate of approximately 33%, irrespective of the therapeutic modality used. Patients with malignant melanoma of the vulva vary widely in age, ranging from 10 to 96 years, with an average age of approximately 60 years. These lesions most often affect the labia minora or the clitoris.[66]

For vulvar melanomas, the FIGO classification usually has been used. This classification is not, however, as good a prognostic indicator as is the depth of invasion. A system for vulvar melanoma analogous to that used by Clark for cutaneous melanoma has been adopted (Table 4). New prognostic factors have been described to predict survival. These include the primary tumor thickness, ulceration, number of metastatic lymph nodes, micrometastatic disease in the sentinel lymph node, and the site of distant metastasis. Levels I–V have been identified based on the Clark classification. The

Table 4 Classification of melanomas of the vulva.

Clark level	
I	Intraepithelial
II	Extension to papillary dermeis
III	Filling the dermal papillae
IV	Invasive of collagen in reticular dermis
V	Extension into subcutaneous fat
Breslow depth of invasion	
I	<0.75 mm from skin surface
II	0.76–1.4 mm from skin surface
III	>1.5 mm from skin surface

level of invasion correlates with survival, which varies from 100% for level II to 83% for level IV and 28% for level V.[67]

Two varieties of melanoma have been described: nodular and superficial spreading melanoma.[68] The superficial spreading melanoma is more common and has a better prognosis, with a 5-year survival rate of 71%. Nodular melanoma has a worse prognosis, and this directly relates to its potential for vertical growth. The 5-year survival rate for nodular melanoma, which is more invasive, is only 38%.

The thickness of the tumor also may be useful in evaluating this lesion. Breslow[69] reported a classification using depth of invasion as measured from the skin surface. In his classification, Breslow reported the overall prognosis as excellent and the spread to regional nodes as unlikely for melanomas with a thickness of <0.76 mm, measured from the surface to the deepest point of penetration.

Wide local excision has been recommended for Clark level I and II disease when no palpable regional nodes are present.[70] In a report of 36 melanoma cases, Rose et al.[71] noted that wide excision was as effective as radical vulvectomy. Prognosis was better for younger patients, presumably because most had superficial spreading rather than nodular melanomas.

A reasonable approach is to excise a melanoma with a 2 cm margin and without node dissection for cases that are <2 mm thick. However, others would recommend a radical local excision with 1–2 cm margins from the primary lesions and an ipsilateral inguinofemoral lymphadenectomy. This is based on a multi-institutional nonrandomized trial of elective lymph node dissection versus obstruction for intermediate thickness cutaneous melanoma. This study showed elective lymph node dissection had a significantly better 5-year survival rate than observation for melanomas of 1–4 mm.

An excision with a 2–3 cm margin combined with node dissection could be performed for more advanced melanomas. An alternative approach for lesions that have extended to Clark levels III, IV, and V is radical vulvectomy with groin and pelvic lymphadenectomy;[72] although the therapeutic benefit of a lymph node dissection in this population is controversial.

It has been reported that melanoma of the vulva can metastasize to pelvic nodes, bypassing the inguinal femoral nodes, but current evidence indicates that pelvic node involvement does not occur without prior inguinal node involvement. A further therapeutic consideration is that patients with melanoma whose pelvic nodes are involved with tumor usually do not survive their disease.

Long-term results generally are not available for large series of melanomas. Most series of malignant melanoma report an overall survival rate of approximately 50%.[73] For lesions that correspond to Clark level I or II (lesions 0.76 mm thick) and are treated by wide local excision, the 5-year survival rate is in the vicinity of 100%. Prognosis becomes poorer with melanomas more than 3 mm thick.

If the regional nodes are negative, the survival rate is approximately 60%; if the regional nodes are involved with tumor, survival is only 30%.

The role of chemotherapy for distant metastasis has not been well established. Regressions, but not cures, have been reported with various multiagent cytotoxic programs, including chemotherapy and/or immunotherapy. These patients should be encouraged to enroll in clinical trials if available.

Sarcoma

Sarcomas of the vulva are rare. Leiomyosarcomas appear to be the most frequently encountered sarcomas in this group of patients[74] and surgical removal by wide local excision is the recommended initial treatment of choice. The 5-year survival rate is reported to be approximately 100%. Locally recurrent lesions are similarly treated. Chemotherapeutic considerations are the same as for those sarcomas in other sites of the female genital tract.[75]

Cancer of the vagina

Primary vaginal cancers are rare, constituting about 3% of all gynecologic malignancies.[2,76-78] It is estimated that 3170 cases of vaginal cancer had been diagnosed in the United States in 2014 and 880 of those women died of this cancer.

Carcinoma of the vagina is defined as a primary carcinoma arising in the vagina and not involving the external os of the cervix superiorly or the vulva inferiorly. The majority of vaginal tumors are secondary to metastasis from other sites. Approximately 30% of primary vaginal cancers have *in situ* or invasive cervical cancers previously treated.

The most common symptom of vaginal carcinoma is abnormal painless bleeding or discharge. With advanced tumors, pain or urinary frequency occasionally occurs, especially in cases of anterior wall tumors. Constipation or tenesmus has been seen with tumors involving the posterior vaginal wall. These tumors usually are diagnosed by direct biopsy of the tumor mass, and abnormal cytologic findings often will lead to diagnosis of a vaginal cancer.

The staging criteria for vaginal carcinomas according to the FIGO are given in Table 5.

Premalignant vaginal disease

Premalignant disease of the vagina is generally detected on cytologic screening. Once an abnormal cytology is obtained, a biopsy directed by colposcopic examination is required to verify the severity of the changes. Because vaginal intraepithelial neoplasia is often multifocal, it is necessary to inspect the entire vaginal canal.[79]

Most lesions occur at the vaginal apex. Audet-Lapointe et al.[80] noted that 61 of 66 cases of vaginal intraepithelial neoplasia

Table 5 FIGO staging classification for vaginal carcinoma.

Stage	
0	CIS
I	Carcinoma limited to vaginal wall
II	Carcinoma involves subvaginal tissue without extension to pelvic sidewall
III	Carcinoma extends to pelvic sidewall
IV	Carcinoma extends beyond true pelvis or involves mucosa of bladder or rectum
	IVA Spread to adjacent organs and/or direct extension beyond the true pelvis
	IVB Spread to distant organs

Abbreviations: CIS, carcinoma *in situ*; FIGO, International Federation of Gynecology and Obstetrics.
Source: Adapted from Barakat 2013.

occurred in the upper third of the vagina. These lesions usually can be excised locally. Other modalities often are preferred, however, because of the multifocal nature of this disease or the necessity of excising large areas, requiring skin grafting.[81]

Nonsurgical approaches for treating these lesions include laser ablation and 5-FU cream for widespread multifocal disease. Carbon dioxide laser frequently has been used and, if carried to a depth of 2–4 mm, allows for vaporization of abnormal tissue. Preliminary results reported by Petrilli et al.[82] with this modality have shown a success rate of approximately 90%. Radiation currently is not recommended for the treatment of noninvasive disease because of the proximity of the bladder and rectum and the availability of newer modalities.

Another approach to treating vaginal intraepithelial neoplasia is the use of 5% 5-FU cream for approximately 7 days, repeated every 3–4 weeks if the vaginal intraepithelial neoplasia persists. Hyperkeratotic lesions appear to be less sensitive to treatment because of their thickness and parakeratosis. Krebs[83] reported on the use of 5% 5-FU daily for 10 days and noted that 17 of 20 patients with vaginal condylomas responded to this therapy. Petrilli et al.[82] and Ballon et al.[84] reported success rates of 80–90% for vaginal intraepithelial neoplasia after multiple cycles of therapy. Another approach is the use of imiquimod as described for treatment of vulvar dysplasias (as seen above in vulvar sections), there have been retrospective studies describing response, however the use considered off label.

Invasive carcinomas of the vagina

Squamous cell carcinomas of the vagina may appear grossly as either ulcerated or fungating tumors or they may be exophytic and protrude through the vaginal canal. They are the most common vaginal malignancy and account for 90% of primary vaginal cancers. The disease occurs primarily in women over 50 years of age. Most squamous cell carcinomas occur in the upper third of the vagina. In examining the patient, it is important to visualize the entire vagina because lesions on the posterior wall can be concealed by the speculum.[85] Microscopically, these tumors have the classic findings of invasive squamous cell carcinoma. They have pleomorphic squamous cells with occasional keratin pearls.

The location of the tumor determines the areas of lymphatic spread (Figure 8).[86] The lymphatics of the middle and upper vagina communicate superiorly with the lymphatics of the cervix and drain into the pelvic nodes of the obturator, internal, and external iliac chains. The lymphatics of the distal third of the vagina drain to the inguinal and pelvic nodes, with a pattern of drainage similar to that of the vulva. The posterior wall lymphatics drain to the rectal lymphatic system. Positive inguinal nodes are present in 31.6% of disease in the lower vagina. The treatment for vaginal cancer is individualized.

Depending on the location, both radiation including high dose rate brachytherapy and surgery have been used effectively in treating these lesions (Table 6). Treatment is often individualized, depending on the size, stage, and location of the tumor.[84,87]

If the tumor is <2 cm thick, some investigators advocate using only local radiation.[88,89] If the carcinoma is <0.5 cm thick, intracavitary irradiation with a vaginal cylinder to deliver 8000 cGy to the mucosa will give over 90% tumor control.[90] Spirtos et al.[91] studied 23 stage I patients and noted only two local recurrences, and both of these had tumor doses of <7500 cGy. For larger lesions, external radiation is used, with a concomitant reduction in the local vaginal component of primary tumor treatment.[92] Implants, however, often cannot be used in patients with larger stage III or IV carcinomas. If such is the case, only external beam radiation is used, and a

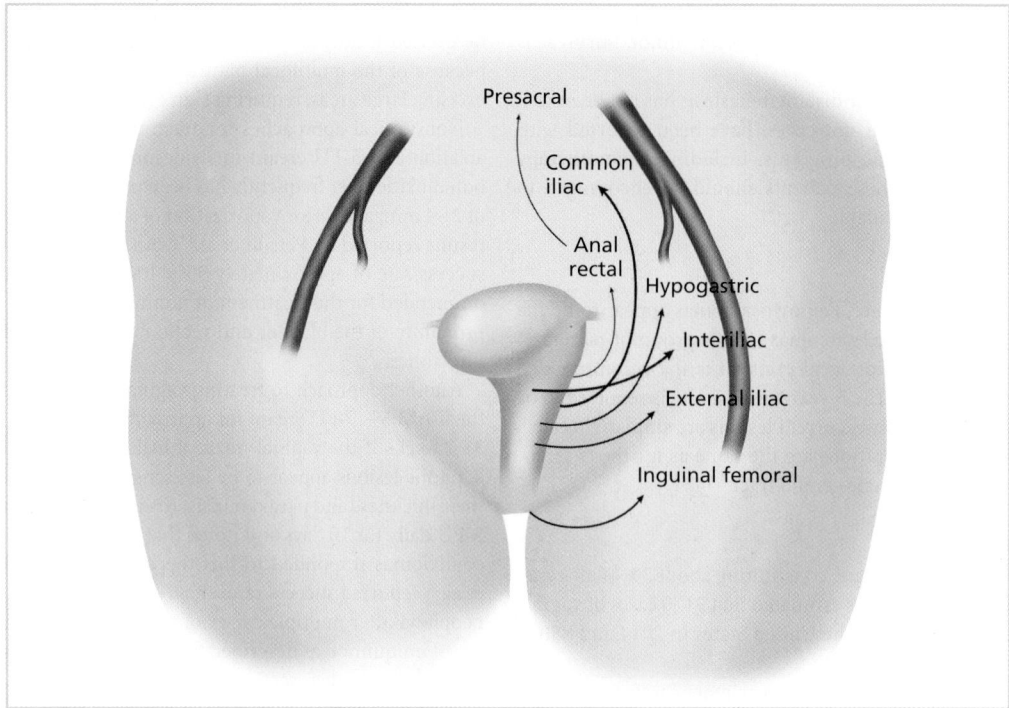

Figure 8 Lymphatic drainage of the vagina.

Table 6 Treatment scheme for vaginal carcinoma.

Stage	External therapy (cGy)	Implant (interstitial) cGy
I		
∑, small tumors (<2 cm)	—	6000–7000
∑, all others	Whole pelvis (4000)	3000–4000 cGy
II	Whole pelvis (4000–5000)	3000–4000 cGy
III	Whole pelvis (5000)	2000
IV	Whole pelvis (5000; an additional 1000–2000 through reduced field if implant not possible)	2000 (if possible)

1 cGy = 1 rad.
Source: Adapted from Nori et al.[90] Reproduced with permission from Elsevier.

central boost is given after an initial whole-pelvis dose of 5000 cGy radiation.[93]

Small tumors located in the upper third of the vagina often can be excised.[94,95] In patients with these, a radical hysterectomy, partial vaginectomy, or pelvic lymphadenectomy usually is effective. Surgery has been preferred in younger patients.

If distant metastasis occurs, effective cis-platinum-based chemotherapy for recurrent squamous cell carcinoma of the vagina has not been developed.[96] For squamous cell carcinoma, a variety of regimens using multiagent chemotherapy similar to those for cervical carcinoma have been employed.

The overall survival rate for patients with primary carcinoma of the vagina is related to the stage of the disease.

Clear cell adenocarcinoma of the vagina

Clear cell adenocarcinomas have been seen more frequently in young women since 1970 because of the association with intrauterine exposure to diethylstilbestrol.[97,98] Three predominant histologic patterns are found with clear cell carcinoma; they have been described as tubulocystic, solid, and papillary patterns.[99,100]

Most clear cell carcinomas of the vagina are polypoid or nodular, with a reddish color.

Clear cell carcinomas can spread locally and by the lymphatic and hematogenous routes. Metastases to regional pelvic nodes have been found in approximately one-sixth of stage I cases. Spread to regional pelvic nodes becomes more frequent in higher-stage tumors.

Clear cell adenocarcinomas are staged as other carcinomas of the vagina are by the FIGO. Some 80% have been diagnosed as stage I or II.

Several prognostic factors have been identified. Older patients (i.e., >19 years of age) have a more favorable prognosis than younger patients.[101] This difference has been associated with the presence of a more favorable tubulocystic pattern of clear cell adenocarcinoma, which is the most frequent histologic pattern found in older patients. In addition, smaller tumor diameter and superficial depth of invasion correlate with improved patient survival. Survival also depends on the stage of the disease. In 547 patients treated for clear cell adenocarcinoma of the vagina, the 5-year survival rate for those in stages I, II, III, and IV has been 93%, 83%, 37%, and 0%, respectively (Table 7).[101]

Because of the young age of these patients, surgery often is the primary therapy. For stage I and early stage II disease (Figure 9), radical hysterectomy, partial or complete vaginectomy, pelvic lymphadenectomy, and replacement of the vagina with a

Table 7 Survival at 5 and 10 years for 547 patients with clear cell adenocarcinoma of the vagina and cervix.

Stage	Survival (%)	
	5 years	10 years
I	93	87
IIA	80	66
IIB	58	49
II (vagina)	83	67
III	37	12
IV	0	0

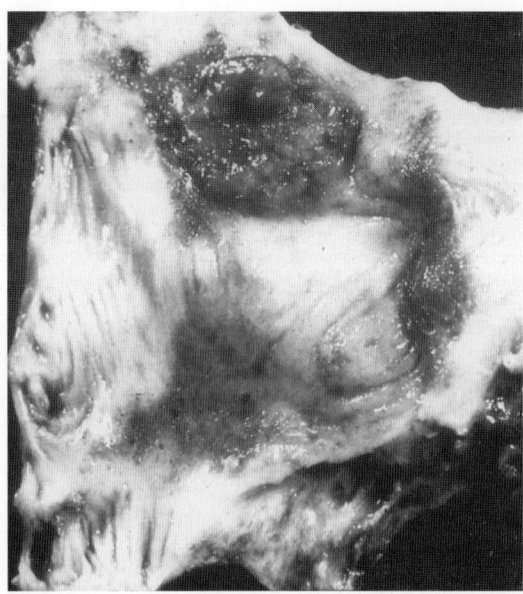

Figure 9 Clear cell adenocarcinoma of the anterior wall, with vaginal adenosis on the posterior wall at the edge of the tumor.

split-thickness skin graft have been the approaches most frequently used.[102]

In patients with small stage I tumors of the vagina, efforts have been made to preserve fertility. The tumor has been excised with retroperitoneal lymph node dissection, followed by local radiation. Senekjian et al.[102] reported that the survival rate of patients with small vaginal tumors treated with such an approach compares favorably with that of patients treated with conventional therapy. In their series, eight pregnancies were reported in five patients who were treated locally.

Larger tumors have been treated with whole-pelvis radiation in addition to intracavitary implant. For tumors >2 cm, whole-pelvis radiation of 4000–5000 cGy has been given, with an additional implant of 3000–4000 cGy.[103] In a few instances, exenterative surgery has been performed for larger tumors; however, this procedure usually has been applied to central recurrences following primary radiation therapy.[104]

If there is a recurrence, therapy consists of additional radical surgery, often requiring exenteration or extensive radiation localized to the pelvis. Systemic chemotherapy has been used in cases of metastatic disease. Cisplatin (75–100 mg/m^2) with a continuous infusion of 5-FU (1 g/m^2 for 3–5 days every 3–4 weeks) is currently recommended. However, no single agent or combination of chemotherapeutic agents has emerged as the most effective.[105] Prolonged follow-up is necessary because recurrences, especially in the lungs and supraclavicular areas, have been reported as long as 19 years after primary therapy.

Vaginal melanomas

Malignant melanomas of the vagina are rare; they constitute <1% of all melanomas occurring in females. The age distribution of the neoplasm has ranged from 26 to 98 years,[53] with a median age of 70 years. Most patients are postmenopausal and present with vaginal bleeding, discharge, or a mass. Tumors may vary from 0.5 to 7.5 cm in diameter, with approximately 30% being 2 cm or less in diameter. Most of these tumors develop in the distal third of the vagina, commonly on the anterior wall. Primary vaginal melanomas presumably arise from vaginal melanocytes that are present in approximately 3% of normal females. Histologically, this neoplasm is similar to other

melanomas found elsewhere and tends to be deeply invasive in the vagina.

The prognosis is worse than that of vulvar melanomas. Chung et al.[106] reported a 5-year survival rate of only 21% in a series of 19 patients. Reid et al.[107] reported a 5-year survival rate of 17.4% in 15 cases, but the prognosis was improved for those tumors that were small and <3 cm in diameter. More recently, Borazjani et al.[108] reported improved survival for cases in which there were fewer than six mitoses/10 high-power fields. The best prognostic factor is the size of the lesion.

Optimal treatment has not been established. Treatment usually consists of radical surgery or wide excision of the vagina and dissection of the regional lymph nodes, depending on the location of the lesion. Recently, a more conservative approach has been used for wide local excision followed by pelvic radiation. Because of the poor prognosis, adjunctive radiation and chemotherapy have been used as local recurrences, and distant metastases with this disease are common. If possible, these patients should enroll in a clinical trial.

Rare vaginal tumors in young females

Endodermal sinus tumor is a rare germ cell malignancy that is usually found in the ovary.[109] This tumor secretes alphafetoprotein, which often is a useful tumor marker for monitoring patients with this neoplasm. It is usually found in infants and children under the age of 3.[110,111] Patients generally present with complaints of bleeding or spotting from the vagina. On physical examination, there is a friable red to pinkish-white polypoid tumor. This tumor is aggressive, and most patients have died. Therapy has involved surgery, radiation, and chemotherapy. Young and Scully[112] reported six patients who were disease free from 2 to 9 years after local therapy with operation, irradiation, or both, followed by systemic chemotherapy with vincristine, actinomycin D, and cyclophosphamide (VAC).[112] Copeland et al.[113] reported similar results using the combination of chemotherapy and excision,[113] and Collins et al.[114] recently noted the regression of tumor with chemotherapy alone.[115] In this report, a 5-month-old patient had regression of the tumor after VAC therapy.

Another rare tumor found in the vaginas of young females is sarcoma botryoides, or embryonal rhabdomyosarcoma.[116] This tumor is usually found in children <8 years of age. As with endodermal sinus tumor, the most common symptom has been vaginal bleeding. In 58 cases reviewed by Hilgers,[50] the average age at onset of symptoms was 38.3 months. This tumor resembles clusters of grapes and forms multiple polypoid masses that are believed to begin in the subepithelial layers of the vagina and to rapidly expand, filling the vagina. Histologically, these tumors are identified by the presence of rhabdomyoblasts that may contain cross-striations. Because of infiltration of the tumor under the vaginal epithelium, there is often a distinct subepithelial zone, called the cambium layer. The 5-year survival rate of these tumors in the past has ranged from 10% to 35%, and exenterative procedures have often been used.[117] Hilgers reviewed the literature on pelvic exenterations in 21 cases of embryonal rhabdomyosarcoma and found that this form of therapy was ineffective in curing these patients.[118] Effective control with less radical surgery has been achieved using multimodal treatment consisting of multiagent chemotherapy, VAC, combined with operation or radiation.

Hayes et al.[119] recently reported 21 patients with vaginal rhabdomyosarcoma who received chemotherapy.[119] In their series, seven relapsed, with five of these seven having had residual disease following incomplete resection. In 17 of 21 patients who received chemotherapy before surgery, a subsequent delayed excision could be performed. Data regarding the long-term survival of a large number of patients are not available, but such a combined approach appears to result in effective therapy with less mutilating surgery.

A rare, benign, fibroepithelial vaginal polyp that resembles sarcoma botryoides can be found in the vaginas of infants or pregnant women.[68,120,121] Although large a typical cells are present microscopically, epithelial infiltration, a cambium layer, and strap cells are absent. Grossly, these polyps do not resemble the grape-like appearance of sarcoma botryoides. These hormonally stimulated hyperplastic lesions are called pseudosarcoma botryoides, and treatment by local excision is effective.

Key references

The complete reference list can be found on the Wiley Companion Digital Edition of this title (see inside front cover for login instructions).

1 Whitcomb BP. Gynecologic malignancies. *Surg Clin North Am.* 2008;**88**:301–317.

10 Stroup AM. Demographic, clinical, and treatment trends among women diagnosed with vulvar cancer in the United States. *Gynecol Oncol.* 2008;**108**:577–583.

11 Mabuchi K, Bross DS, Kessler II. Epidemiology of cancer of the vulva: a case control study. *Cancer.* 1985;**55**:1843–1848.

13 Chafe W, Richards A, Morgan L, Wilkinson E. Unrecognized invasive carcinoma in vulvar epithelial neoplasia (VIN). *Gynecol Oncol.* 1988;**31**:154.

19 Raspollini MR, Asirelli G, Taddei GL. Analysis of lymphocytic infiltrate does not help in prediction of vulvar squamous cell carcinoma arising in a background of lichen sclerosus. *Int J Gynaecol Obstet.* 2008;**100**:190–191.

20 Armes JE, Lourie R, Bowlay G, Tabrizi S. Pagetoid squamous cell carcinoma in situ of the vulva: comparison with extramammary paget disease and nonpagetoid squamous cell neoplasia. *Int J Gynecol Pathol.* 2008;**27**:118–124.

21 Mulvany NJ, Allen DG. Differentiated intraepithelial neoplasia of the vulva. *Int J Gynecol Pathol.* 2008;**27**:125–135.

25 Campbell SM, Curnow A. Extensive vulval intraepithelial neoplasia treated with a new regime of systemic photodynamic therapy using meta-tetrahydroxychlorin (Foscan). *J Eur Acad Dermatol Venereol.* 2008;**22**:502–503.

29 Helwig EP, Graham JH. Anogenital (extramammary) Paget's disease. *Cancer.* 1963;**16**:387.

30 Lee SC, Roth LM, Ehrlich C, Hall JA. Extramammary Paget's disease of the vulva—a clinicopathologic study of 13 cases. *Cancer.* 1977;**39**:2540.

34 Iversen T, Aas M. Lymph drainage from the vulva. *Gynecol Oncol.* 1983;**16**:179.

37 Hacker NF, Nieburg RK, Berek JS, et al. Superficially invasive vulvar cancer with nodal metastases. *Gynecol Oncol.* 1983;**15**:65.

39 Rowley KC, Gallion HH, Donalson ES, et al. Prognostic factors in early vulvar cancer. *Gynecol Oncol.* 1988;**31**:43.

40 Berman ML, Soper JT, Creasman WT, et al. Conservative surgical management in superficially invasive stage I vulvar carcinoma. *Gynecol Oncol.* 1989;**35**:352.

46 Landrum LM, Lanneau GS, Skaggs VJ, et al. Gynecologic Oncolgy Group risk groups for vulvar carcinoma: improvement in survival in the modern era. *Gynecol Oncol.* 2007;**106**:521–525.

51 Boyce J, Fruchter RG, Kasambilides E, et al. Prognostic factors in carcinoma of the vulva. *Gynecol Oncol.* 1985;**20**:364.

52 Le T, Elsugi R, Hopkins L, Faught W, Fung-Kee-Fung M. The definition of optimal inguinal femoral nodal dissection in the management of vulva squamous cell carcinoma. *Ann Surg Oncol.* 2007;**14**:2128–2132.

53 Christopherson W, Buchsbaum HJ, Voet R, Lifschitz S. Radical vulvectomy and bilateral groin lymphadenectomy utilizing separate groin incisions: report of a case with recurrence in the intervening skin bridge. *Gynecol Oncol.* 1985;**21**:247.

54 Blotti F, Zullo MA, Angioli R. Incontinence after radical vulvectomy treated with Macroplastique implantation. *J Minim Invasive Gynecol.* 2008;**15**:113–115.

55 Boronow RC. Combined therapy as an alternative to exenteration of locally advanced vulvar vaginal cancer. *Cancer.* 1982;**49**:1085.

56 Boronow RC, Hickman BT, Reagan MT, et al. Combined therapy as an alternative to exenteration for locally advanced vulvovaginal cancer. *Am J Clin Oncol.* 1987;**10**:1711.

57 Rotmensch J, Rubin SJ, Sutton HG, et al. Preoperative radiotherapy followed by radical vulvectomy with inguinal lymphadenectomy for advanced vulvar cancer. *Gynecol Oncol.* 1990;**36**:181.

58 Moore DH, Thomas GM, Montana GS, et al. Preoperative chemoradiation for advanced vulvar cancer: a phase II study of the Gynecologic Oncology Group. *Int J Radiat Oncol Biol Phys.* 1998;**42**:1317–1323.

63 Rosenberg P, Simonsen E, Risberg B. Adenoid cystic carcinoma of Bartholin's gland: a report of 5 new cases treated with surgery and radiotherapy. *Gynecol Oncol.* 1989;**34**:145.

67 Phillips GL, Twiggs LB, Okagaki T. Vulvar melanoma: a microstaging study. *Gynecol Oncol.* 1982;**14**:80.

69 Breslow A. Thickness, cross-sectional areas, and depth of invasion in the prognosis of cutaneous melanoma. *Ann Surg.* 1970;**172**:908.

73 Podratz KC, Gaffey TA, Symmonds RE, et al. Melanoma of the vulva: an update. *Gynecol Oncol.* 1983;**16**:153.

75 Lieb SM, Gallousis S, Greedman H. Granular cell myoblastoma of the vulva. *Gynecol Oncol.* 1979;**8**:12.

80 Audet-Lapointe P, Body G, Vauclair R, et al. Vaginal intraepithelial neoplasia. *Gynecol Oncol.* 1990;**36**:232.

85 Gupta N, Mittal S, Dalmia S, Misra R. A rare case of primary invasive carcinoma of vagina associated with irreducible third degree uterovaginal prolapse. *Arch Gynecol Obstet.* 2007;**276**:563–564.

87 Beriwal S, Heron DE, Mogus R, Edwards RP, Kelley JL, Sukumvanich P. High dose rate brachytherapy (HDRB) for primary or recurrent cancer in the vagina. *Radiat Oncol.* 2008;**3**:7.

88 Andersen ES. Primary carcinoma of the vagina: a study of 29 cases. *Gynecol Oncol.* 1989;**33**:317.

89 Otton GR, Nicklin JL, Dickie GJ, et al. Early-stage vaginal carcinoma—an analysis of 70 patients. *Int J Gynecol Cancer.* 2004;**14**:304–310.

91 Spirtos NM, Doshi BP, Kapp DS, Teng N. Radiation therapy for primary squamous cell carcinoma of the vagina: Stanford University experience. *Gynecol Oncol.* 1989;**35**:20.

93 Prempree T, Viravathana T, Slawson RG, et al. Radiation management of primary carcinoma of the vagina. *Cancer.* 1977;**40**:109.

95 Basaran A, Ayhan A. Cancer of the vagina treated with wide local excision and modified Martius (labial) flap interposition. *Gynecol Oncol.* 2008;**108**:455–456.

96 Samant R, Lau B, Choan E, Le T, Tam T. Primary vaginal cancer treated with concurrent chemoradiation using Cis-platinum. *Int J Radiat Oncol Biol Phys.* 2007;**69**:746–750.

97 Herbst AL, Scully RE. Adenocarcinoma of the vagina in adolescence. *Cancer.* 1970;**25**:745.

102 Senekjian EK, Frey KW, Anderson D, Herbst AL. Local therapy in stage I clear cell adenocarcinoma of the vagina. *Cancer.* 1987;**60**:1319.

103 Senekjian EK, Frey KW, Herbst AL. Pelvic exenteration in clear cell adenocarcinoma of the vagina and cervix. *Gynecol Oncol.* 1989;**34**:413.

102 Neoplasms of the cervix

Anuja Jhingran, MD ▪ Ana M. Rodriguez, MD, MPH, FACOG

Overview

Cervical cancer is the third most common cancer among women world-wide and the fourth leading cause of cancer deaths in females, with an estimated 529,800 new cases and 275,100 deaths in the year 2008. The incidence is declining in the United States with 12,900 new cases and 4100 deaths in 2015. Squamous cell carcinoma is the most common histology with the human papilloma virus (HPV) being the most common etiology. Cervical cancer can be easily prevented with pap smears, HPV testing, and hopefully the HPV vaccine. Early stage cervix cancer can be treated with surgery including now fertility sparing surgery and there are high cure rates. Local advance cervical cancer is treated with combination of chemotherapy and radiation therapy with high survival rates but there is room for improvements with advancing stage. Systemic chemotherapy can be used for treatment of both recurrent and metastatic disease, but careful attention should be paid to balancing benefit and toxicity. The key to success will be the transportation of success seen in the developing countries to success in areas of the world where advanced-stage invasive cervical cancer is most common.

Epidemiology

Incidence and mortality

Cervical cancer is the third most common cancer among women worldwide and the fourth leading cause of cancer deaths in females, with an estimated 529,800 new cases and 275,100 deaths in the year 2008.[1] The incidence of cervical cancer in developing countries remains nearly twice that in developed countries, with the highest rates observed in Africa, South-Central Asia, and South America (29 per 100,000 per year) and the lowest in Western Asia, Australia/New Zealand, and North America (7.5 per 100,000 per year).[2] In the United States, it is estimated that there will be 12,900 new cases of cervical cancer in 2015, with 4100 related deaths.[3] Cervical cancer is frequently seen in the Hispanic population (10.5% of all cases of cervical cancer) followed by the African-American population (10.2%), American Indians (9.5%), whites (7.1%), and Pacific Islanders/Asian (6.4%).[3]

In the past 40 years, primarily because of the introduction of screening with the Pap smear, the incidence and mortality rates for cervical cancer have declined in most developed countries.[4] In the United States; incidence rates have declined nearly by 70% during this period. Rates of invasive cancer per 100,000 females have declined from 10.2 in 1998 to 8.5 in 2002.[5] In developing countries, however, cervical cancer continues to be a significant health problem owing to suboptimal screening programs and a lack of therapy for precancerous conditions.

There are no reliable data on the prevalence and incidence of precancerous cervical lesions. In the United States, the National Cancer Institute (NCI) estimates that each year approximately 300,000 women are found to have premalignant cervical lesions, whereas the American Cancer Society reported that in 2001, an estimated 65,000 women were found to have carcinoma *in situ* (CIS) of the cervix. From the SEER data, the overall incidence of squamous cell CIS among whites is 41.4 per 100,000 woman-years from 1991 to 1995.[6]

Risk factors for cervical neoplasia

Human papillomavirus and other sexually transmitted agents
Epidemiologic evidence has long suggested a sexually transmitted etiology for cervical neoplasia. Supporting this hypothesis, several measures of sexual behavior (including multiple sexual partners, early age at first sexual intercourse, and sexual habits of male partners) have consistently been associated with an increased risk of cervical neoplasia.[7] In the mid-1970s, the hypothesis of a causal relationship between human papillomavirus (HPV) and cervical neoplasia was first proposed.[8] Since then, a large body of experimental, clinical, and epidemiologic research has accumulated supporting an etiologic role for some types of HPV.[9]

Of the more than 78 types of HPV that have been described, in excess of 35 types are associated with anogenital disease, and 30 or more are associated with cancer.[10] Similarly, HPV DNA has been detected by polymerase chain reaction (PCR) in up to 94% of women with preinvasive lesions [cervical intraepithelial neoplasia (CIN)] and in up to 46% of women with cytologically normal tissue.[9,11]

HPV types classified as intermediate and high risk have been identified in about 77% of high-grade squamous intraepithelial lesion s (HGSILs) (CIN 2 and 3) and in 84% of invasive lesions.[12] In the series studied by Bosch and colleagues, HPV types 16, 18, 31, and 45 were detected in approximately 80% of the cases.[13] HPV 16 is by far the most prevalent HPV type in women with cervical neoplasia, present in up to 50% of HGSILs and invasive lesions, and it is the most common HPV type identified in cytologically normal women.[12,14,15]

The association between cervical neoplasia and HPV is independent of study population, study design, and HPV detection method.[13] Higher risk has been associated with specific HPV types (16, 18, 31, 33, 35, and 45), increasing viral load, and concurrent infection with multiple HPV types.[16,17] An increased risk of high-grade CIN ranging from 16- to 122-fold has been reported among women whose test results were positive for HPV of any type.[17] The percentage of cases of CIN attributed to HPV has been estimated to range from 60% to 92%.[11] In addition, adjustment for HPV status appears to account for most of the associations between cervical neoplasia and number of sexual partners and other characteristics of sexual behavior.[11,16,17]

Holland-Frei Cancer Medicine, Ninth Edition. Edited by Robert C. Bast Jr., Carlo M. Croce, William N. Hait, Waun Ki Hong, Donald W. Kufe, Martine Piccart-Gebhart, Raphael E. Pollock, Ralph R. Weichselbaum, Hongyang Wang, and James F. Holland.
© 2017 John Wiley & Sons, Inc. ISBN: 978-1-118-93469-2

Although a strong and consistent association between HPV and cervical neoplasia has been clearly established, the discrepancy between HPV prevalence and the incidence of cervical neoplasia suggests that other cofactors are necessary for the development and progression of the disease.

Numerous studies have addressed the association between HIV and cervical neoplasia.[7] The Centers for Disease Control and Prevention added invasive cervical cancer to the list of conditions related to AIDS in 1993.[15] HIV-positive women have been reported to have higher rates of cervical abnormalities, larger lesions, higher grade histology, and higher recurrence rates than HIV-negative women. In addition, HIV-positive women have been reported to have higher HPV prevalence and HPV persistence rates than HIV-negative women. A meta-analysis by Mandelblatt and colleagues concluded that HIV is a cofactor in the association between HPV and cervical neoplasia, and this association seems to vary with the level of immune function.[18]

Other molecular markers

Other specific genetic abnormalities may also play an important role in carcinogenesis and the aggressiveness of cervical tumors, although, to date, the role of most of these genetic abnormalities in cervical cancer does not appear as important as the role of HPV. Most studies report a 32–34% incidence of c-*myc* activation in cervical cancers, predominantly through amplification.[19,20] Amplification has been related to tumor size and nodal status as well as a risk factor for relapse.[21] Mutations have been reported in the *K-ras* and *H-ras* genes in cervical cancer at a rate of only 10–15%.[22] One report found that increased ras p21 expression correlated with risk of lymph node metastasis.[23]

Epidermal growth factor receptor (EGFR) is expressed not only in a large proportion of cervical carcinomas but also in normal and premalignant epithelia. The prognostic role of EGFR in cervical carcinoma remains controversial, although two studies found EGFR prognostic for overall survival (OS) and disease-specific survival (DSS) in patients with invasive cervical cancer.[24,25]

The apoptosis inhibitor Bcl2 prevents apoptosis. Two studies have shown that Bcl2 is overexpressed in 61–63% of all cervical cancer and correlates inversely with OS,[26,27] whereas other studies have found no correlation with survival.[28]

Angiogenesis is critical for the progression of most cancers. One angiogenic factor, VEGF, has recently been associated with cervical cancer,[29,30] but the precise role that angiogenic factors play in the development and progression of cervical cancer requires further elucidation.

Sexual behavior

Although previous studies report a strong and consistent association between cervical neoplasia and some characteristics of sexual behavior of women and their male sexual partners, a weaker association has been found in more recent studies in which HPV infection has been taken into account.[16,31] This, characteristics of sexual behavior may be only a proxy measurement for infection with HPV and other infectious agents that may be causally related to cervical neoplasia.

The association between early age at first sexual intercourse and increased risk has been less consistent. After controlling for HPV and other risk factors, a statistically significant association between age at first sexual intercourse and cervical neoplasia has remained in some studies, but in others, no association has been observed.[16,17,32] The association between cervical neoplasia and early age at sexual intercourse may indicate a period of higher susceptibility of the cervical tissue, a higher likelihood of exposure, or a longer period of exposure to carcinogenic factors. Establishing age at first sexual intercourse as an independent effect is, however, difficult because of its high correlation with number of sexual partners.

An association between factors related to male sexual partners and an increased risk of cervical neoplasia has also been suggested.[33] Among men, the prevalence of HPV has been associated with the number of sexual partners and sexual contact with prostitutes.[34] In addition, higher HPV prevalence has been reported among males in geographic areas with higher rates of cervical cancer incidence than among males in geographic areas with lower rates, which supports a possible contribution of male partners to cervical carcinogenesis in their female sex partners.[34] Male circumcision has been associated with a reduced risk of penile HPV infection and, in the case of men with a history of multiple sexual partners, a reduced risk of cervical cancer in their current female partners.[35]

Reproductive factors

No consistent relationships have been established between cervical neoplasia and menstrual or reproductive characteristics, including age at menarche or menopause, parity, number of spontaneous or induced abortions, age at first pregnancy, first live birth, or last birth, and number of vaginal deliveries or Cesarean sections. There is an association among increased risk of cervical neoplasia and higher parity, early age at first birth, higher number of live births, and vaginal deliveries.[16,17,35,36] Repeated trauma to the cervix during childbirth could be an etiologic factor.[35]

Smoking habits

Several epidemiologic studies have provided evidence supporting an approximately twofold increased risk among smokers and a dose–response relationship with duration and intensity of smoking.[37,38] Some support an independent effect of smoking, whereas others do not.[16,17,39] High levels of nicotine, cotinine and tobacco-specific *N*-nitrosamines have been detected in the cervical mucus of active and passive smokers. DNA damage has been found in cervical tissue and exfoliated cells of women smokers. The local cell-mediated immune response is impaired in smokers. Furthermore, reduction of cervical lesion size has been documented among women participating in smoking cessation intervention.[40] Although the mechanism of smoking-induced carcinogenesis in cervical tissue is not fully understood, current biologic, epidemiologic, and clinical studies suggest that cigarette smoking may be a risk factor for cervical neoplasia.

Risk factors for cervical adenocarcinoma

Adenocarcinoma of the cervix accounts for more than 20% of all cervical cancers. However, in most developing countries, the incidence is increasing, particularly among younger women. Between the early 1970s and mid-1980s, the incidence of adenocarcinoma more than doubled among women under 35 years of age.[41] Adenocarcinoma is associated with a higher likelihood of HPV-16 and HPV-18, which is present in more than 80% of cases. HPV 18 accounts for approximately 50% of adenocarcinoma of the cervix but only 15% of squamous cell carcinoma.[42] Adenocarcinoma has been linked to several other risk factors more commonly associated with endometrial cancer, including obesity[43] and nulliparity.[6]

Summary

Cervical neoplasia continues to be a major health problem worldwide. Higher incidence and mortality rates are observed in developing countries. Among more developed countries, a significant decline in incidence and mortality has been observed in the past 50 years, which has been attributed to the introduction of screening programs. Current epidemiologic data support a strong role for HPV infection in the etiology of cervical neoplasia. This association satisfies all criteria for causality in epidemiologic research: strength, consistency, and specificity of the association; dose–response and temporal relationship; and biologic plausibility.[11] HPV infection appears to explain many of the established risk factors for cervical neoplasia, including sexual behavior and cigarette smoking. Nonetheless, the high prevalence of HPV infection in young healthy women compared with the low incidence of cervical neoplasia and the low progression rate of untreated CIN lesions support the existence of other cofactors in cervical carcinogenesis.[44] Future epidemiologic studies will need to further assess the role of these cofactors and their interaction with HPV. In addition, the role of viral factors such as HPV persistence and HPV variants in the progression of cervical neoplasia as well as of the determinant factors of HPV persistence will require further evaluation.[45] Similarly, the impact of recent trends in environmental factors such as smoking, exogenous hormones, and dietary factors deserves further attention.[7]

Histologic classification of epithelial tumors

The histologic classification of epithelial tumors of the uterine cervix by the World Health Organization (WHO) separates them into three main groups: squamous cell carcinomas, adenocarcinomas, and other epithelial tumors (Table 1).[46,47]

Table 1 Modification of the WHO histologic classification of epithelial tumors of the uterine cervix.

Squamous cell carcinoma
Microinvasive squamous cell carcinoma
Invasive squamous cell carcinoma
Verrucous carcinoma
Warty (condylomatous) carcinoma
Papillary squamous cell (transitional) carcinoma
Lymphoepithelioma-like carcinoma
Adenocarcinoma
Mucinous adenocarcinoma
Endocervical type
Intestinal type
Signet-ring type
Endometrioid adenocarcinoma
Endometrioid adenocarcinoma with squamous metaplasia
Clear cell adenocarcinoma
Minimal-deviation adenocarcinoma
Endocervical type (adenoma malignum)
Endometrioid type
Serous adenocarcinoma
Mesonephric carcinoma
Well-differentiated villoglandular adenocarcinoma
Other epithelial tumors
Adenosquamous carcinoma
Glassy cell carcinoma
Mucoepidermoid carcinoma
Adenoid cystic carcinoma
Adenoid basal carcinoma
Carcinoid-like tumor
Small cell carcinoma
Undifferentiated carcinoma

Source: Reproduced with permission from Carcinoma and other tumors of the cervix. In: *Blaustein's Pathology of the Female Genital Tract*, 4th ed.

Squamous cell carcinoma

The majority of cervical carcinomas are squamous cell carcinomas, which are classified as either large cell nonkeratinizing or large cell keratinizing. Nonkeratinizing carcinoma is characterized by squamous cells with somewhat hyperchromatic nuclei and a moderate amount of cytoplasm growing in discrete nests separated by stroma (Figure 1). In the center of some of the nests, the squamous cells appear to differentiate and degenerate. Keratinizing carcinoma is characterized by cells with very hyperchromatic nuclei and densely eosinophilic cytoplasm growing in irregular invasive nests. Many of these nests have central "pearls" that contain abundant keratin. The average age of patients with squamous cell carcinoma is 51.4 years. Selected variants of squamous cell carcinoma are described in the following paragraphs.

Verrucous carcinoma

Verrucous carcinomas are exophytic with frond like papillae and macroscopically resemble condylomas. They rarely metastasize, but local invasion can be extensive. Death usually occurs because of ureteral obstruction, infection, or hemorrhage.

This tumor rarely goes to the nodes, therefore, for early-stage disease, the treatment of choice is a type II modified radical hysterectomy without lymphadenectomy.

Papillary squamous cell carcinoma

Papillary squamous cell carcinomas of the uterine cervix with transitional or squamous differentiation often resemble transitional cell carcinomas of the urinary tract (Figure 2). Urinary tract transitional cell carcinomas have a cytokeratin profile strongly positive for cytokeratin 20, whereas primary genital tract transitional cell carcinomas stain positive for cytokeratin 7.[48] Invasive papillary transitional cell carcinomas of the uterine cervix are potentially aggressive carcinomas. It is important to distinguish these carcinomas from benign squamous papillomas and condyloma acuminata.[49] Biopsy material must include the underlying stroma to permit identification of invasion.

Lymphoepithelioma-like carcinoma

Lymphoepithelioma-like carcinomas are histologically similar to lymphoepitheliomas arising in the nasopharynx and salivary glands (Figure 3). These carcinomas are usually well circumscribed and composed of undifferentiated cells. The cancer cells are surrounded by inflammatory infiltrates composed of lymphocytes, plasma cells, and eosinophils.[50] Hasumi and colleagues reported 39 cases

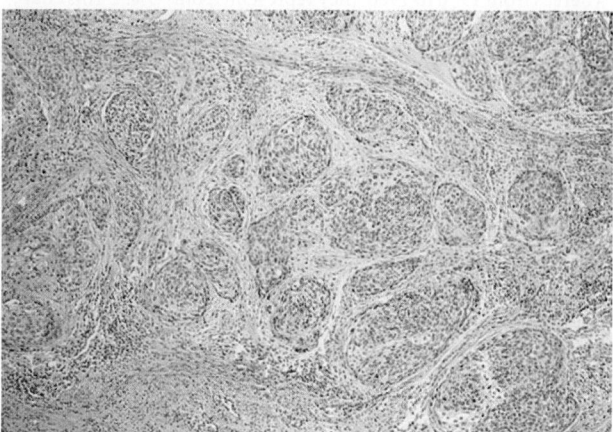

Figure 1 Squamous cell carcinoma, nonkeratinizing.

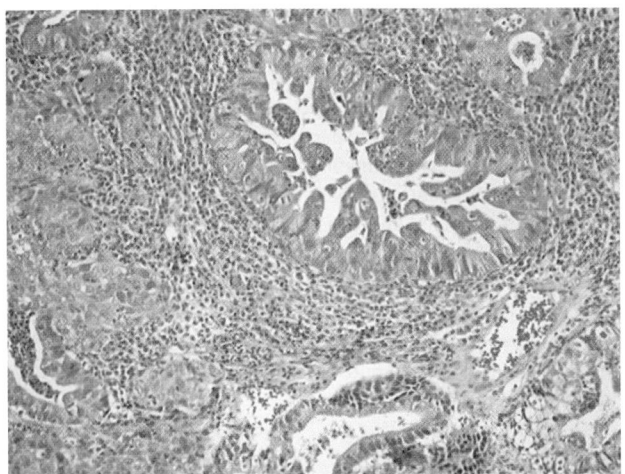

Figure 2 Papillary squamous cell (transitional) carcinoma.

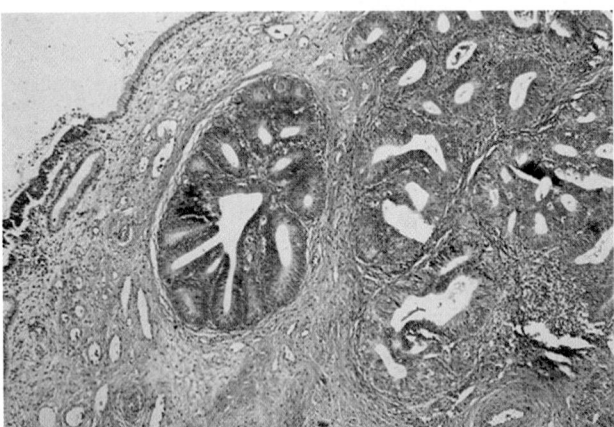

Figure 3 Lymphoepithelioma-like carcinoma.

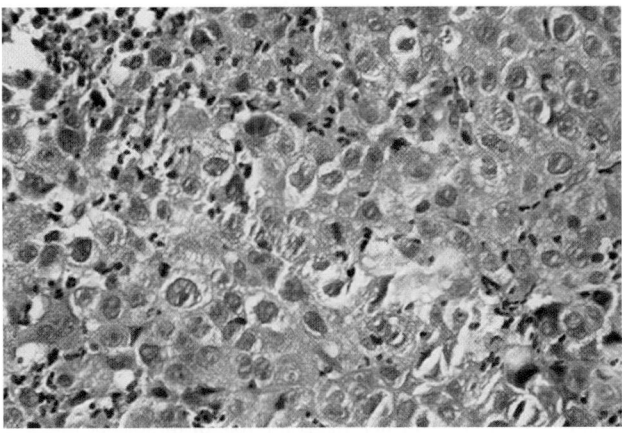

Figure 4 Mucinous adenocarcinoma, endocervical type.

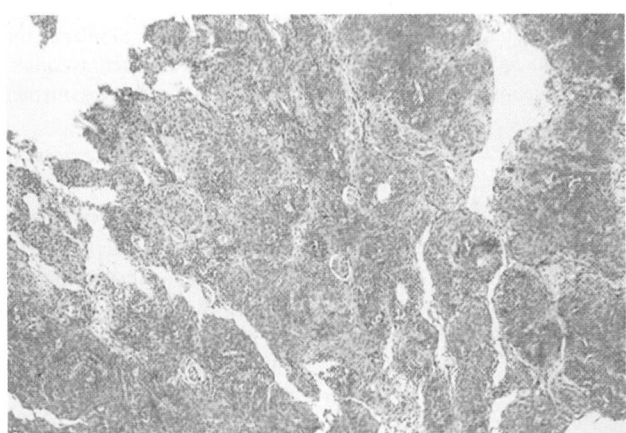

Figure 5 Endometrioid adenocarcinoma.

from the Cancer Institute Hospital in Tokyo. Their patients, 72% of whom were younger than 50 years of age, were treated with radical hysterectomy and pelvic lymphadenectomy. Two patients had positive lymph nodes. At the time of the report, 38 of the 39 patients were alive. The single death occurred 5 months after surgery and was due to serum hepatitis.

Adenocarcinoma

Adenocarcinomas represent 20–25% of cervical carcinomas today, whereas from 1950 to 1960, they represented only 5%.[51] This change in prevalence is a worldwide phenomenon.[52] The mean age at diagnosis for patients with invasive adenocarcinoma is between 47 and 53 years. Selected variants of adenocarcinoma are described in the following paragraphs.

Mucinous adenocarcinoma is the most common type of cervical adenocarcinoma.[53] In the WHO classification, the first type of mucinous adenocarcinoma is composed of cells that resemble the columnar cells of the normal endocervical mucosa and is referred to as the endocervical type (Figure 4). The second type is termed the intestinal type because it is composed of cells similar to those present in adenocarcinomas of the large intestine. A third type is composed of signet-ring cells and designated the signet-ring type. Frequently, mucinous adenocarcinomas are a mixture of these cell types.

Endometrioid adenocarcinoma is the second most common type of primary endocervical tumor, accounting for 30% of all primary

endocervical tumors. Endometrioid adenocarcinomas resemble typical endometrioid adenocarcinoma arising from the endometrial cavity (Figure 5). Identification of the site of origin (i.e., whether the primary tumor is in the endocervix or endometrium) may be difficult, but proper identification is important as the site or origin significantly influences therapy.

Adenoma malignum is difficult to distinguish cytologically from normal endocervical glands (Figure 6) and is referred to as minimal-deviation adenocarcinoma. A distinguishing feature of

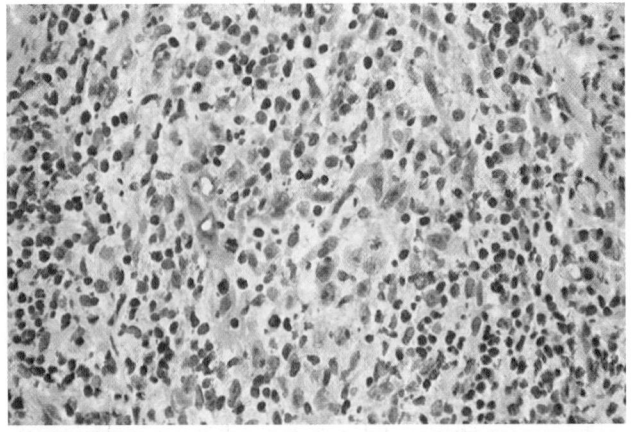

Figure 6 Mucinous adenocarcinoma, endocervical type (adenoma malignum).

adenoma malignum is a bizarre and irregular glandular branching pattern. These irregular glands invade deeply into the stroma, and diagnosis requires a large tissue specimen from a cone biopsy or hysterectomy specimen. Adenoma malignum is extremely rare and is sometimes associated with Peutz–Jegher syndrome.[54] The survival rate is poor if the well-differentiated pattern leads to under treatment.

Other epithelial tumors

Adenosquamous carcinoma is defined as a cancer that contains an admixture of histologically malignant squamous and glandular cells.[55] Adenosquamous carcinomas account for 5–25% of the cervical carcinomas in some series.[56,57] These carcinomas are similar in their clinical presentation, epidemiology, and pattern of spread to squamous cell carcinomas and adenocarcinomas. The poorly differentiated form of adenosquamous carcinoma can be made up of large uniform polygonal cells with a finely granular cytoplasm of the ground-glass type, hence the term "glassy cells" (Figure 7). Similar to other undifferentiated tumors, glassy cell carcinomas spread early and are aggressive.[57] The mucoepidermoid carcinoma, also placed in this category, contain large cell nonkeratinizing or focally keratinizing squamous carcinoma, which stains positive for mucin but lacks recognizable glands. The mucinous component includes goblet or signet-ring-type cells localized in a nest of squamous cells. These carcinomas represent 20% of the carcinomas in some series if mucin is measured.

Small cell neuroendocrine carcinoma contains small anaplastic cells with scant cytoplasm (Figure 8). These highly aggressive

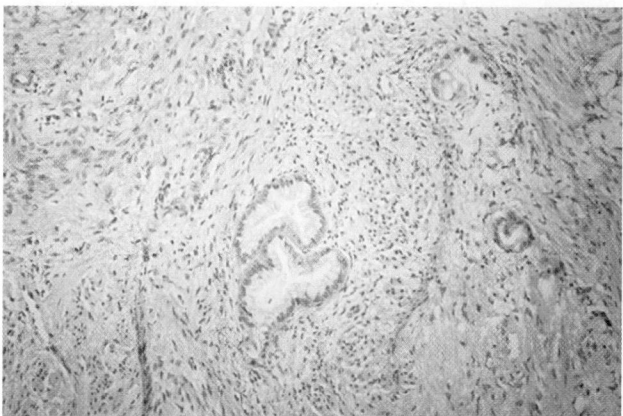

Figure 7 Glassy cell carcinoma.

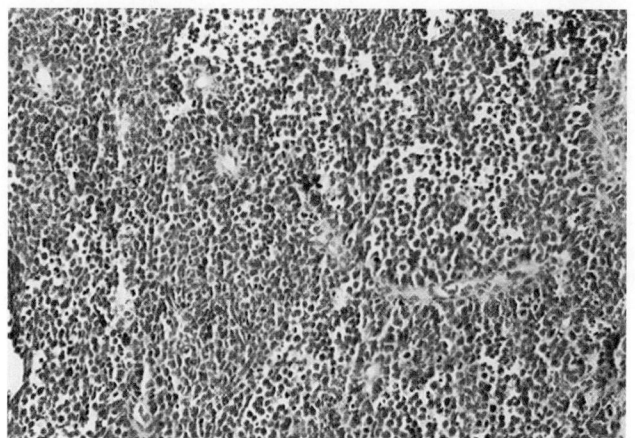

Figure 8 Small cell carcinoma.

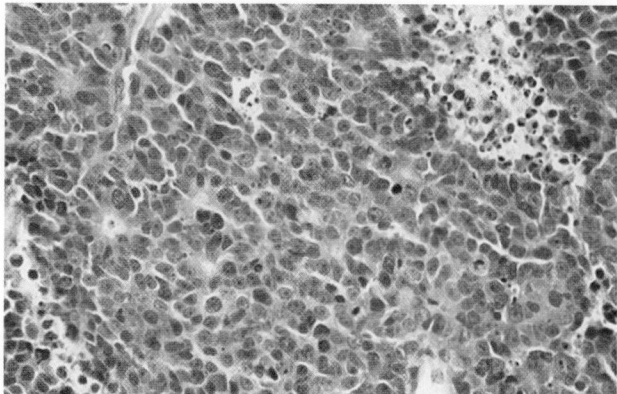

Figure 9 Non-small-cell neuroendocrine carcinoma.

cancers diffusely infiltrate the cervical stroma.[58] Staining reveals neuroendocrine markers in most cases. Women with small cell carcinoma are likely to be 10 years younger than those with squamous cell carcinoma. Small-cell carcinomas are frequently associated with widespread metastasis to multiple sites, including bone, liver, skin, and brain. These tumors should not be confused with small squamous cell carcinomas, which are associated with a better prognosis. Efforts to treat these cancers with approaches typically used for small cell carcinomas of the lung have had mixed results.

Non-small cell neuroendocrine carcinoma

Nonsmall cell neuroendocrine carcinomas of the cervix have been reported, but they are not listed in the current WHO classification of cervical tumors.[59] The tumors contain intermediate to large cells, high-grade nuclei, and eosinophilic cytoplasmic granules of the type seen in neuroendocrine cells. A trabecular pattern is frequently evident, with or without glandular differentiation (Figure 9). Tumors are usually immunoreactive for chromogranin. Reported survival rates for patients with these aggressive carcinomas are similar to those for patients with small cell carcinoma.

Diagnosis and treatment of precancerous lesions

The most recent guidelines for screening for cervical cancer are listed in Figure 10.[60] CIN is an increasingly common finding among sexually active young women. Since the introduction of the Bethesda system, the proportion of Pap smears identified as having low-grade cytologic abnormalities, minimal or ambiguous cytologic changes classified as atypical squamous cells of undetermined significance (ASCUS), or low-grade squamous intraepithelial lesions (LGSIL)s has increased.[44] Approximately 50 million Pap smears are done yearly in the United States, and 5–10% of these smears are reported as having low-grade cytologic abnormalities. Although near consensus exists regarding the evaluation and management of HGSILs and carcinoma detected on Pap smears, controversy continues regarding appropriate management of ASCUS and low-grade abnormalities.[61] Issues include the risk of progression of the disease, the anxiety caused to the patient, the risk of overtreating patients with minor disease, and, more recently, the financial implications of prompt intervention and treatment.[62]

As more studies of women with mildly atypical Pap smears were published, data showed that 5–20% of women presenting with a single mildly atypical Pap smear were at risk of HGSILs or other more severe lesions.[63] In addition, it has recently been estimated that more than one-third of the HGSIL cases in a routine screening

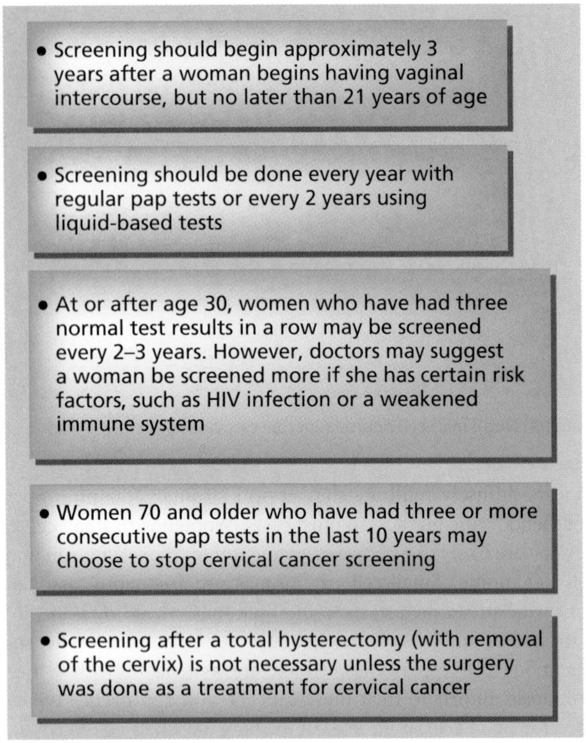

- Screening should begin approximately 3 years after a woman begins having vaginal intercourse, but no later than 21 years of age

- Screening should be done every year with regular pap tests or every 2 years using liquid-based tests

- At or after age 30, women who have had three normal test results in a row may be screened every 2–3 years. However, doctors may suggest a woman be screened more if she has certain risk factors, such as HIV infection or a weakened immune system

- Women 70 and older who have had three or more consecutive pap tests in the last 10 years may choose to stop cervical cancer screening

- Screening after a total hysterectomy (with removal of the cervix) is not necessary unless the surgery was done as a treatment for cervical cancer

Figure 10 Screening guidelines for the early detection of cervical cancer.

population are proceeded by a cytologic diagnosis of ASCUS.[64] This has led some clinicians to suggest that it is safer and more expeditious to perform colposcopy in women with a finding of ASCUS.[65] However, given the relatively high frequency of low-grade cytologic

abnormalities in the absence of significant disease and the high financial and emotional cost of colposcopy, some have argued that these women should be evaluated by repeat cytology rather than colposcopy. The American College of Obstetricians and Gynecologists and a NCI consensus panel have acknowledged that managing a single mildly atypical Pap smear by repeating the test is an acceptable practice.[61,66]

The main goal in managing ASCUS and low-grade cytologic abnormalities is to identify those women at higher risk of HGSILs, primarily women more than 25 years old who cannot be relied on to return for long-term follow-up, who are suspected of having or known to have a history of abnormal cytologic findings or treatment of cervical neoplasia, who may be promiscuous, and who have no history of adequate screening.[67] Currently, two strategies are recommended for managing these lesions: the physician may repeat the Pap smear and perform a colposcopic evaluation, or, for patients with an ASCUS cytologic diagnosis or LGSILs without clinical evidence of cervical disease and without risk factors, the physician may repeat the Pap smear without performing colposcopy (Figure 11).[61,67] The American Society for Colposcopy and Cervical Pathology (ASCCP) also emphasizes HPV testing when triaging with ASCUS or LGSIL PAPs (Papanicolaous).

Management of low-grade cytologic abnormalities

Low-grade cytologic abnormalities are usually treated first with antibiotics and repeating the smear several months later. If the smear result regressed to normal, the patient is scheduled for an annual Pap smear screening, whereas patients whose smears remained abnormal are referred for colposcopic evaluation, and Pap test every 4–6 months for 2 years. After three consecutive negative smears in the 2-year follow-up period, patients can be monitored using a routine cervical cancer screening protocol.[68,69] For patients with clinical suspicion of cancer or persistent abnormal

Management of women with no lesion or biopsy-confirmed cervical intraepithelial neoplasia—grade 1 (CIN1) preceded by "lesser abnormalities"* ∞

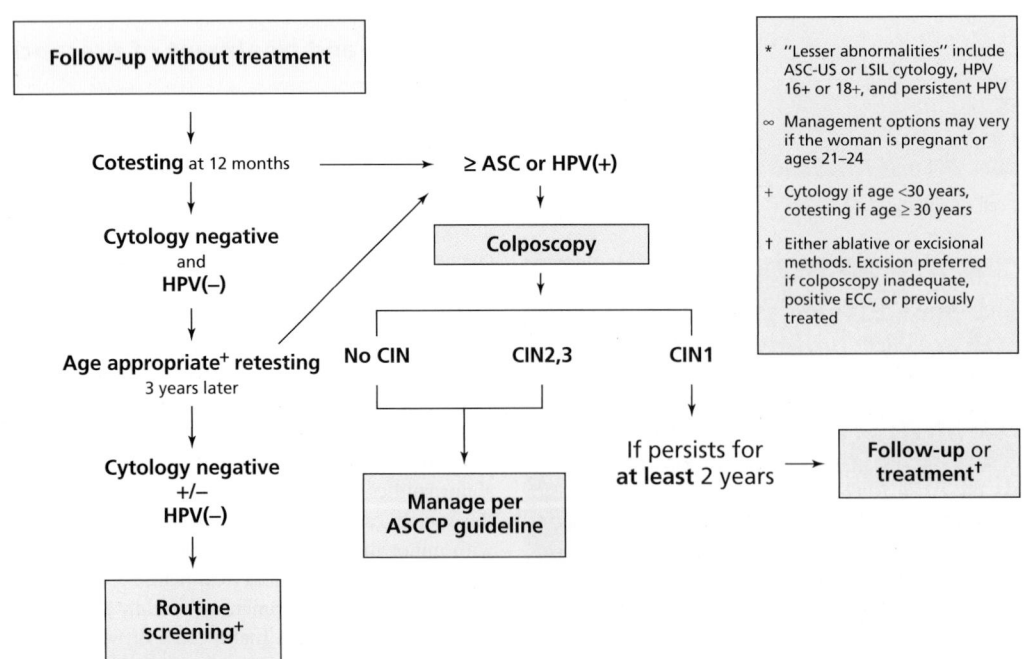

Figure 11 Management of women with biopsy-confirmed cervical intraepithelial neoplasia-grade 1 (CIN 1). Source: Massad et al. 2013.[67] Reproduced with permission of the American Society for Colposcopy and Cervical Pathology.

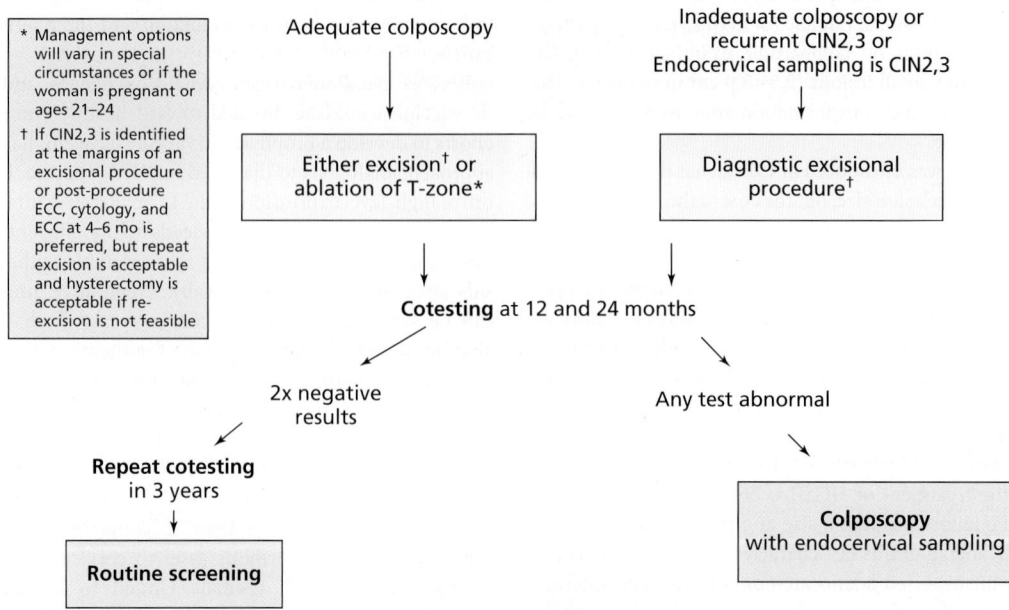

Management of women with biopsy-confirmed cervical intraepithelial neoplasia—
grade 2 and 3 (CIN2,3)*

Figure 12 Management of women with biopsy-confirmed cervical intraepithelial neoplasia grades 2 and 3 (CIN 2.3). Source: Massad et al. 2013.[67] Reproduced with permission of the American Society for Colposcopy and Cervical Pathology.

Pap smears during the 2-year follow-up, colposcopic evaluation is recommended. Recommended management form ASCCP for women with ASCUS or LGSIL Paps is based on age. For women aged 21–24 years with ASCUS or LGSIL, the recommendation is to repeat cytology at 12 months. For older women with LGSIL Pap and no HPV testing or positive HPV testing, recommendation is to proceed with colposcopy (Figure 12).[67]

In view of the costs, both emotional and economic, associated with evaluating women with low-grade cytologic abnormalities, considerable interest has arisen in developing novel cost-effective triage strategies for these patients. HPV DNA testing, automated cytology screening, and cervicography are being evaluated as adjunct methods in the assessment and triage of patients with low-grade cytologic abnormalities. Most research has focused on the assessment of HPV testing.

Several researchers have assessed the value of HPV DNA testing as a specific and economical alternative for triage of low-grade cytologic abnormalities and as an adjunct to cervical cytology in primary screening.[70–73] With second-generation HPV DNA detection methods, including PCR-based methods and the hybrid capture HPV DNA assay, both of which have a higher sensitivity and detect a broader range of HPV types with high oncogenic risk than earlier methods, results have been more consistent, supporting the role of HPV typing in the triage of patients with low-grade cytologic abnormalities and as an adjunct to cytology in primary screening.[70–73]

New data on HPV primary screening from the ATHENA trial were presented to the FDA in the spring of 2014 supporting the evidence that HPV testing alone is an excellent alternative screening strategy.[74] More experience and data analysis pertaining to this new strategy will permit a more formal ACS evaluation in the future.

The preferences of clinician and patient and cost considerations should dictate the choice of treatment of CIN, but proper management of LGSILs is expected to remain a fiercely debated

question. Although management guidelines have increasingly included nontreatment of LGSILs as an option for patients who may be reliable for long-term follow-up, concerns over legal responsibility for progressive lesions continue to drive intensive follow-up protocols, particularly in the United States, that may not be cost-efficient.[75] Guidelines recently published may be helpful to follow.

Management of high-grade cytologic abnormalities

Optimal management of HGSILs includes colposcopic evaluation and biopsy or in women older than 24 years of age to proceed to a loop electrical excision procedure (LEEP) without performing colposcopic evaluation. The consensus is that HGSILs should be treated once diagnosed.[76] For biopsy-proven HGSILs with negative findings on endocervical curettage (ECC), a satisfactory colposcopy examination, and congruent Pap smear and biopsy results, ablation of the transformation zone has been the standard of care for several decades. Three outpatient therapies are used in the United States for treating these lesions: cryotherapy, laser ablation, and LEEP. For patients with unsatisfactory colposcopic examination findings, a Pap smear result more severe than the biopsy findings, the presence of an adenomatous component, suspicion of invasive cancer, or positive findings on ECC, a cone biopsy is indicated. Cone biopsies (talked about later in the chapter) remove tissue to a depth of 20–30 mm and up to 30 mm in diameter, including the transformation zone.

The three outpatient therapies of cryotherapy, laser vaporization, and LEEP have been the focus of controversy. Safety, efficacy, and cost issues have dominated the debate. Cryotherapy, introduced in 1972, was the first outpatient treatment of CIN and remains a dependable treatment because of its reliability, low complication rate, ease of use, and low cost.[77] Another advantage of cryotherapy is that leaving a large dead viral HPV load within disrupted cells may improve the immune response to the causative agent of CIN. Major disadvantages include lack of ability to tailor treatment to the size of the lesion, lack of a tissue specimen, and the risk of treatment of undetected invasive lesions. Eligible for cryotherapy are patients with satisfactory findings on colposcopic examination, negative findings on ECC, and small lesions (2.5–3.0 cm in diameter) that allow the entire lesion and transformation zone to be covered by the cryotherapy probe.

Laser vaporization was introduced in 1977. It has the advantage of being easily tailored to lesion size, but the cost of the equipment and the lack of a tissue specimen are major disadvantages.[77] In addition, laser vaporization requires more training and skills than the other two procedures and is associated with more serious safety issues (eye injuries and inadvertent burns). Candidates for this procedure are patients with large CIN lesions, young women with suspicious or invasive lesions or adenocarcinoma *in situ* in whom preservation of fertility is desired, and patients unwilling to undergo LEEP under local anesthesia.

LEEP was introduced in 1989, and it is currently the technique of choice for the treatment of HGSILs. LEEP is reliable and easy to use. It can be tailored to lesion size and provides a tissue specimen.[77] The advantage of this last characteristic is underscored by the finding of unsuspected adenocarcinoma *in situ* and microinvasive squamous cell carcinoma in 2–4% of LEEP specimens.[67,77] LEEP, however, has the potential to result in unintentional removal of excessive cervical stroma and removal of disease-free tissue (more frequent when LGSILs are treated). Other disadvantages include its high cost and the increased risk of bleeding and infection. Bleeding after LEEP has been reported in 2–7% of cases.[77] The high rates of overtreatment observed with LEEP have been related to misdiagnosis of abnormality and multiple punch biopsies of small lesions before treatment.[67] The use of LEEP in see-and-treat protocols has been shown to improve patient compliance with treatment when patient selection is adequate. This strategy has been suggested as having the greatest potential benefit for populations with poor treatment compliance.[67]

No statistically significant differences in success rates (based on recurrence and persistence) between cryotherapy and laser vaporization have been reported, but variability in these rates from study to study is striking.[77,78]

Prevention

Chemopreventative management

One of the more exciting research areas in therapy for CIN is the use of chemopreventative agents. These therapies involve ingestion of an agent that reverses precancerous changes, returning the tissue to normal. Laboratory data have shown that retinoids can induce apoptosis in dysplastic cervical cells, suggesting that these compounds may be active in cell-cycle control.[79] Women with HGSIL and colposcopically evident lesions are the target population for chemoprevention studies because they have a higher risk of persistent disease or progression to cancer. α-Difluoromethylornithine and retinoids (vitamin A derivatives) are two drugs currently receiving attention in the United States and China.[80,81]

Vaccine development

Papillomaviruses are epitheliotropic agents that induce benign papillomas of the skin and mucous membranes. In contrast to hepatitis B virus (HBV), there are more than 100 HPV genotypes (types). A subset of HPV types that are almost always transmitted sexually is the main cause of human cervical cancer. Infection with these HPV types is a strong risk factor for cervical cancer, and HPV DNA from one or more of these types is found in virtually all cervical tumors.[82,83] The virus encodes oncoproteins that appear to be required for both the induction and the maintenance of the cancer.

Because papillomaviruses contain oncogenes, and a prophylactic vaccine would be directed toward healthy young individuals, efforts to develop a prophylactic vaccine have emphasized a subunit approach, analogous to that used for HBV vaccine. Indeed, constitutive high-level expression of the L1 major structural viral protein, even in nonmammalian cells, leads to its efficient self-assembly into virus like particles (VLPs) that resemble authentic viral capsids structurally and antigenically. Preparative amounts of VLPs can be synthesized in insect cells or yeast. Such VLPs are suitable immunogens that, as is true of authentic virions, possess the immunodominant conformational epitopes capable of raising high titers of neutralizing antibodies.

Two vaccines have been developed: Gardasil, a quadrivalent vaccine targeting HPV 6, 11, 16, and 18,[84] and Cervarix, a bivalent vaccine that targets HPV 16 and 18.[85] These vaccines are now licensed in more than 55 countries worldwide and are expected to be an enormous asset to cervical cancer prevention efforts. The FUTURE (Female United to Unilaterally Reduce Endo/Ectocervical Disease) II study group performed a randomized, double-blind, placebo-controlled trial in order to evaluate a quadrivalent vaccine (Gardasil) against HPV types 6, 11, 16, and 18 for the prevention of high-grade cervical lesions associated with HPV 16 and 18. After 3-year follow-up from the first dose of the vaccine, the efficacy of the vaccine in preventing the primary endpoint was 98% in the per-protocol susceptible population and 44% in an intention-to-treat population of all women who had undergone randomization. The study concluded that the quadrivalent vaccine was highly effective in preventing HPV 16- and 18-related high-risk cervical lesions, and that widespread immunization of girls may result in a substantial decrease in cervical cancer resulting from infection with HPV 16 and 18.[84]

The interim analysis of the randomized double-blind-controlled trial of the Papilloma Trial against Cancer In young Adults (PATRICIA) looking at the efficacy of prophylactic administration of bivalent vaccine against infection with HPV 16 and 18 was published in June 2007.[85] This vaccine has also shown evidence of cross-protection against HPV 45 and 31. The vaccine had an efficacy of 90.4%, and there were no significant safety profile differences between the study groups.[85]

HPV vaccines are presently recommended for all 11–12-year-old girls, though vaccination can be started as early as 9 years, and women between the age of 13 and 26 should also be vaccinated if they are not yet sexually active. Recent data from the United States suggest that HPV vaccination and biennial cervical screening from the age of 24 years will reduce the annual total PAP test volume by 43% and result in the reduction in the workload at sexually transmitted disease clinics.[86] The Markov model of incorporation of the HPV vaccination into a UK national cervical screening program predicts a 76% reduction in cervical cancer deaths and 66% reduction in high-grade lesions.[86] However, there are problems in world widespread distribution of the vaccinations including price of the vaccine, accessibility of the vaccines in countries due to lack of immunization infrastructure, and opposition by conservative groups to the vaccination of young girls against what is perceived to be an sexually transmitted disease.[87]

Diagnosis and treatment of invasive lesions patterns of spread

During the transition from *in situ* to invasive carcinoma, tumor cells penetrate the epithelial basement membrane and enter the underlying cervical stroma. Once the cervical stroma is invaded, the lymphatics and blood vessels are accessible, and dissemination beyond the cervix is possible.

The cervical, vaginal, and uterine lymphatic channels coalesce to form major drainage pathways. The major lymphatic trunks are the utero-ovarian (infundibulopelvic), parametrial, and presacral, which drain into the paracervical, obturator, hypogastric, external iliac, common iliac, inferior gluteal, presacral, and lower aortic lymph nodes. A series studying the incidence and distribution pattern of retroperitoneal lymph node metastases in 208 patients with stages 1B, IIA, and IIB cervical carcinomas who underwent radical hysterectomy and systemic pelvic node dissection reported that 53 patients (25%) had node metastasis.[88] The obturator lymph nodes were the most frequently involved, with a rate of 19% (39 of 208), and the authors proposed them as sentinel nodes for cervical cancers. In fact, finding negative obturator nodes may be an indication that the pelvic lymph node dissection can be limited.

Cervical cancers of similar size may have very different metastatic potentials, depending on their intrinsic aggressiveness and histologic cell type. Cervical carcinomas also invade directly. As the cancer grows, disease may extend to the lateral pelvic walls, into the bladder or rectum, or into the vagina.

The incidence of lymph node metastasis at diagnosis for each of the squamous cell carcinoma stages designated by the International Federation of Gynecology and Obstetrics (FIGO) has been well defined by surgical series.[89-91] Pelvic node involvement occurs in 10–25% of stage I carcinomas, 25–30% of stage II carcinomas, and 30–45% of stage III and IV carcinomas. Stage I carcinomas are more likely to metastasize to nodes once they reach 3 cm.[92,93] Because most patients with large bulky adenocarcinomas are treated with radiation therapy, the incidence of positive nodes by tumor size is not as well defined for adenocarcinoma as it is for squamous cell carcinoma. The incidence of positive nodes for poorly differentiated squamous cell carcinoma and for poorly differentiated adenocarcinoma is higher than that for the better-differentiated carcinomas.

Carcinoma of the cervix spreads in an orderly manner. Nodes adjacent to the cervix are usually the first to be involved, and "skip" metastases are uncommon. Patients with positive para-aortic nodes usually have positive pelvic nodes. The incidence of positive para-aortic nodes in 978 patients with stage IB and IIA carcinoma whose aortic nodes were sampled before radical hysterectomy was 4.7% and 8.4%, respectively. The incidence of positive nodes in patients with adenocarcinomas is probably equal to that in patients with squamous cell-carcinomas when cancer size, histologic differentiation, and extent of tumor or FIGO stage are similar. Many large series report poorer survival rates for patients with adenocarcinomas than for patients with squamous cell carcinomas, especially those who have bulky lesions.[94,95] Small cell carcinoma and some of the carcinomas classified as other epithelial tumors are particularly aggressive. Carcinomas of the cervix, regardless of histology and size of the primary tumor, may contain highly malignant clones of cells that can prove unpredictable and spread extensively.

Clinical symptoms

The clinical symptoms of carcinoma of the cervix are vaginal bleeding, discharge, and pain. The growth pattern of the carcinoma plays a role in the development of symptoms. Exophytic carcinomas bleed earlier in a sexually active patient (because of contact) than lesions that expand the cervix. Lesions that expand the endocervix in a barrel-shaped configuration may leave the squamous epithelium of the exocervix intact until the lesions exceed 5 or 6 cm in transverse diameter; therefore, carcinomas with this growth pattern may be silent and grow large before the patient bleeds. Cytologic findings may be negative unless the endocervix is sampled with a brush device. Ulcerative lesions that destroy the exocervix bleed early, and necrosis and infection induced by the cancer's outgrowing its blood supply result in a foul-smelling vaginal discharge.

Severe pelvic pain experienced during the pelvic examination may indicate salpingitis. Tubal infections require management before radiation therapy. Patients with an adnexal mass need surgical treatment before radiation therapy is started.

Paracervical extension of a carcinoma may remain silent until fixation to the pelvic wall occurs. Fixation with or without nodal involvement may obstruct a ureter. Ureteral encroachment is usually a silent process. Patients may present with bilateral ureteral obstruction with impending renal failure and report no history of urinary system complaints. Direct invasion of branches of the sciatic nerve roots causes back pain, and encroachment on the pelvic wall veins and lymphatics causes edema of a lower extremity. The triad of back pain, leg edema, and a nonfunctioning kidney is evidence of an advanced carcinoma with extensive pelvic wall involvement.

The anatomic position of the bladder, so closely adjacent to the cervix, favors contiguous spread from the cervix to the bladder. Urinary frequency and urgency are early manifestations of such spread; patients with advanced disease may present with hematuria or incontinence, suggesting direct extension of tumor to the bladder. Cystoscopy and biopsy should confirm the cause of hematuria or incontinence.

In contrast, posterior extension to the rectum and disruption of the rectal mucosa is an unusual pattern of disease spread in untreated patients. The deep cul-de-sac provides anatomic separation of the rectum and cervix. In patients who present with rectal mucosal involvement, there is usually extensive involvement of the posterior vaginal wall with direct extension to the rectum. For staging and treatment planning, cystoscopy and sigmoidoscopy are essential.

Metastatic carcinoma in para-aortic nodes may extend through the node capsule and directly invade the vertebrae and adjacent nerve roots. Back pain owing to involvement of the lumbar vertebrae and psoas muscles may be a manifestation of massive nodal disease; however, hematogenous spread to the lumbar vertebrae and involvement of the psoas muscle without significant nodal disease may occur.

Diagnosis

The diagnosis of cervical carcinoma is made by pathologic examination of a tissue specimen. A biopsy sample taken from the periphery of a tumor is more likely to contain morphologically intact neoplastic cells that are best able to represent the tumor pathologically. A biopsy specimen taken from the center of a tumor mass may include necrotic tumor debris; the result of hypoxia induced by the tumor's outgrowing its blood supply. Therefore, to rely on these dead and distorted cells is to compromise the accuracy of the histologic interpretation.

The endocervix should be curetted if no lesion is visible or if the cervix is enlarged, nodular, or hard. Older patients with adenocarcinoma require an endometrial biopsy. It may be difficult to distinguish an endocervical primary tumor from an endometrial primary tumor involving the lower uterine segment.

Table 2 Relapse rates for patients with stage IIB or III cervical cancer.

Hemoglobin (gm/dL)	Patients (number)	Relapse rate (%)		
		Local	Distant	Total
<10	29	46	18	49
10–11.9	319	29	24	47
12–13.9	578	20	16	33
≥14	129	20	18	33

Relapse rates for patients with stage IIB or III cancer of the cervix according to average hemoglobin level during radiation therapy. p Values: p = 0.002 (local), p = 0.1 (distant), p = 0.0007 (total).
Source: Bush 1986.[96] Reproduced with permission of Elsevier.

Patients with an abnormal Pap smear and no visible lesion require colposcopy and biopsy. The tissue specimen may be a simple colposcopy-directed biopsy specimen, an endocervical specimen obtained with a curette, or a conization specimen.

It is the current recommendation of FIGO to classify as stage IA any invasive cancer that can be identified only with a microscope. All gross lesions, even with superficial invasion, are at least stage IB cancers. Vascular space involvement, either venous or lymphatic, should not alter staging. Many clinicians prefer to use the term microinvasion and use criteria recommended by the Society of Gynecologic Oncologists instead of using the FIGO staging system. Microinvasion is invasion limited to 3 mm in depth, is measured from the base of the squamous or glandular epithelium of origin, and does not encompass lymphatic or vascular space involvement. A simple punch biopsy is inadequate for making the diagnosis of microinvasion: a conization specimen, containing the entire neoplastic process, is necessary. Additional tissue is required from patients with positive cone margins because an occult, frankly invasive carcinoma may lie adjacent to a positive margin.

Evaluation and staging

Successful therapy planning requires detailed evaluation of the patient's general medical condition and the size and extent of the carcinoma. Medical illness must be stabilized and anemia must be corrected before treatment commences. Patients with anemia,

which has been extensively studied, have a higher local relapse rate than patients with a normal hemoglobin (Table 2).[96,97] The patient's surgical history is important, and operative notes may describe the status of the abdominal organs as well as report abdominal and pelvic operations. Diagnoses of importance to therapy planning include ulcerative bowel disease, diverticulitis, and pelvic inflammatory disease. Such inflammatory conditions induce adhesions and fix loops of the intestines to each other, the adjacent organs, and the peritoneal surfaces.

Patients with small stage I carcinomas should undergo chest radiography, a complete blood count, urinalysis, and blood chemistry analysis before treatment. Patients with advanced carcinomas require cystoscopy and proctoscopy. It is important to apply the FIGO rules for clinical staging (Table 3).[98] It is clearly stated in the FIGO guidelines that for staging purposes, the following examinations are permitted: cystoscopy, inspection, colposcopy, ECC, hysteroscopy, proctoscopy, intravenous pyelography, chest radiography, and skeletal radiography.[99] Findings from examinations such as lymphangiography, laparotomy, laparoscopy, computed tomography (CT), magnetic resonance imaging (MRI), and other examinations unnamed by FIGO should not be the basis for changing the clinical stage, despite the fact that such examinations or procedures can provide valuable information for planning therapy. The tumor-nodes-metastasis (TNM) staging categories have also been accepted by FIGO.[100] Lymph node status is not addressed in the FIGO staging system for carcinoma of the cervix, but three radiologic imaging techniques are available to evaluate lymph node status: CT, MRI, and fluorodeoxyglucose-positron emission tomography (FDG-PET) detect abnormal lymph nodes more lymphangiography.

The best radiologic imaging technique for detecting lymph node metastases is unclear. CT and MRI are good in identifying enlarged nodes; however, the accuracy of these techniques in the detection of positive nodes is compromised by their failure to detect small metastases, and many enlarged nodes are not due to metastases, but inflammation associated with advanced disease. The accuracy of MRI in the detection of lymph node metastases (72–93%) is similar to that of CT; however, when compared with surgical findings, MRI is superior to CT, clinical examination, and sonography in the

Table 3 Modified FIGO staging.

Stage	Description
I	The carcinoma is strictly confined to the cervix (extension to the corpus should be disregarded)
IA	Invasive cancer identified only microscopically. All gross lesions, even with superficial invasion, are stage IB cancers. Invasion is limited to measured stromal invasion with a maximum depth of 5 mm and a width no >7 mm
IA1	Measured invasion of stroma ≤3 mm in depth and ≤7 mm in width
IA2	Measured invasion of stroma >3 and ≤5 mm in depth and ≤7 mm in width
IB	Clinical lesions confined to the cervix or preclinical lesions larger than stage IA
IB1	Clinical lesions ≤4 cm
IB2	Clinical lesions >4 cm
II	The carcinoma extends beyond the uterus but has not extended onto the pelvic wall or to the lower third of vagina
IIA	Involvement of up to the upper 2/3 of the vagina. No obvious parametrial involvement
IIA1	Clinical visible lesion ≤4 cm
IIA2	Clinical visible lesion >4 cm
IIB	Obvious parametrial involvement
III	The carcinoma has extended onto the pelvic wall. On rectal examination, there is no cancer-free space between the tumor and the pelvic wall. The tumor involves the lower third of the vagina. All cases with hydronephrosis or a nonfunctioning kidney should be included unless they are known to result from another cause
IIIA	No extension onto the pelvic wall but involvement of the lower third of the vagina
IIIB	Extension onto the pelvic wall or hydronephrosis or nonfunctioning kidney
IV	The carcinoma has extended beyond the true pelvis or has clinically involved the mucosa of the bladder or rectum
IVA	Spread to adjacent organs
IVB	Spread to distant organs

Abbreviation: FIGO, International Federation of Gynecology and Obstetrics.
Source: From Ref. 98.

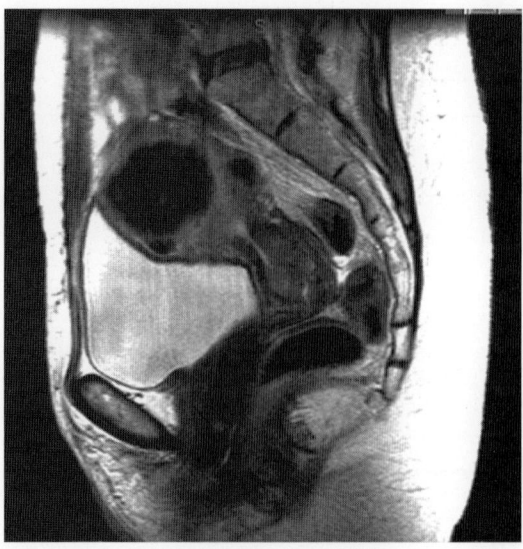

Figure 13 Magnetic resonance image of a patient with cervical tumor.

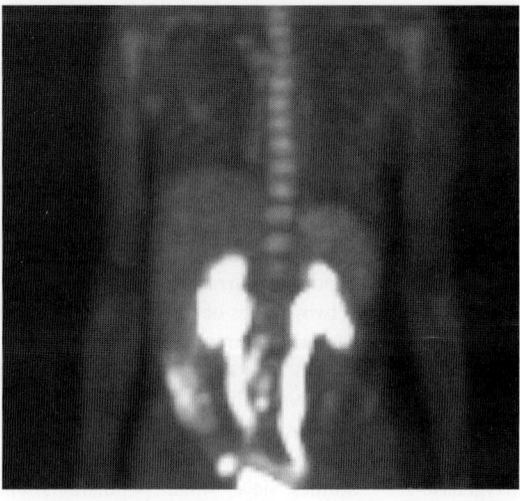

Figure 14 Positron emission tomography scan of a patient with cervical tumor showing positive nodes.

evaluation of tumor location, tumor size, depth of stromal invasion, vaginal extension, and parametrial extension of cervical cancer.[101–104] Furthermore, studies suggest that MRI is a cost-effective method of evaluating cervical cancers.[104] Figure 13 shows an MRI of a patient with a cervical tumor.

PET or PET/CT is the rapidly expanding modality in oncologic imaging (Figure 14). In a study of 101 patients with carcinoma of the cervix, Grigsby and colleagues reported that CT demonstrated enlarged pelvic lymph nodes in 20% and enlarged para-aortic lymph nodes in 7%, while PET demonstrated abnormal FDG uptake in pelvic lymph nodes in 67%, abnormal FDG uptake in para-aortic lymph nodes in 21%, and abnormal FDG uptake in supraclavicular lymph nodes in 8%.[105] The 2-year progression-free survival rate (PFS), based solely on para-aortic lymph node status, was 64% in CT-normal and PET-normal patients, 18% in CT-normal and PET-abnormal patients, and 14% in CT-abnormal and PET-abnormal patients. The authors concluded that often CT and that the findings on PET are a better predictor of survival than those on CT in patients with carcinoma of the cervix. Further studies are needed to confirm these results and determine if PET

imaging is better than surgical staging particularly for determining if patients have positive para-aortic nodes.

In some patients, surgical examination of the lymph nodes is warranted. The risk of occult para-aortic metastases is highest in patients with grossly involved pelvic nodes, and these patients may be the best candidates for operative exploration. These patients also may benefit from removal of the grossly enlarged nodes, which may be difficult to control with radiation alone.[106] When lymph node metastases are sought surgically, the extraperitoneal approach is currently the preferred technique.[107] It is preferred because high complication rates resulted from using a transperitoneal approach followed by radiation therapy.[108] Lymph node exploration and dissection may also be performed using a laparoscopic approach, which is associated with a shorter postoperative recovery time and probably less late radiation morbidity than open transperitoneal staging.[109]

Prognostic factors

FIGO stage correlates with survival and control of pelvic disease in patients with cervical cancer; however, prognosis is also influenced by other factors, including tumor characteristics and patient characteristics that are not included in the FIGO staging system.

Tumor size and local extent

Tumor size is one of the most important predictors of local recurrence and death in patients with cervical cancer treated with surgery or radiation therapy (Figure 15). The FIGO staging classification for stage I disease was recently modified to include tumor diameter (i.e., ≤4 cm, stage IB1; >4 cm, stage IB2).[98] For patients with more advanced disease, other estimates of tumor bulk that correlate with prognosis include presence of medial versus lateral parametrial involvement in FIGO stage IIB disease and unilateral versus bilateral pelvic wall involvement in FIGO stage IIIB disease.[111,112]

In patients who have had a radical hysterectomy, histologic evidence of extracervical spread (≥10 mm) and deep stromal invasion (>70% invasion) are associated with a poorer prognosis, as is parametrial extension, which is associated with higher rates of lymph node involvement, local recurrence, and death from cancer.[91,113–115] Uterine body involvement is associated with an increased rate of distant metastases in patients treated with radiation or surgery.[116]

Lymph node involvement

Lymph node metastasis is another important prognostic factor for survival that is not part of the FIGO staging system. In several surgical series, after a radical hysterectomy, patients with positive pelvic lymph nodes had a 35–40% lower 5-year survival rate than patients with negative nodes.[89,91] However, recent studies suggest that post-operative chemoradiation improves these results.[117] Several authors have reported a correlation between size of the largest node involved or higher number of nodes involved and decreased survival rates. Patients with positive para-aortic nodes have a survival rate that is about half that of patients with similar-stage disease and negative para-aortic nodes.[89,91,114,118,119] With extended-field radiation therapy, patients with early-stage disease and positive para-aortic nodes have a cure rate of approximately 40–50%.

There is a strong correlation between positive lymph nodes in patients with cervical neoplasms and positive lymph-vascular space invasion (LVSI) in the tumor specimen. However, LVSI may be an independent predictor of prognosis, as a number of large series of patients treated with radical hysterectomy have demonstrated.[113,114,120,121] Roman and colleagues reported a

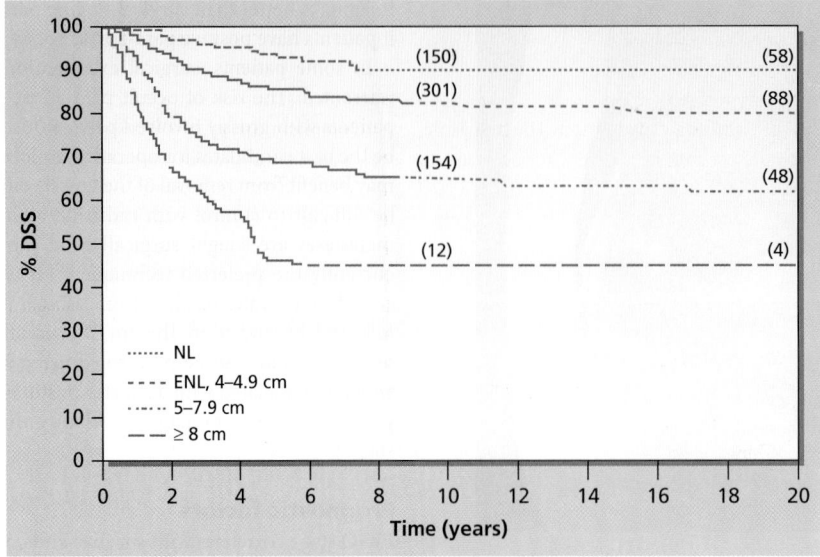

Figure 15 Disease-specific survival (DSS) is indicated for patients grouped according to size of cervix (NL, cervix of normal size; ENL, enlarged cervix, 4–4.9 cm). Source: Lai et al. 1999.[110] Reproduced with permission of Wolters Kluwer Health.

correlation between the percentage of histopathologic sections containing LVSI and the incidence of lymph node metastasis.[122] In patients with adenocarcinoma of the cervix, there is a strong correlation between LVSI and outcome.[123,124]

Histologic type

There is controversy regarding whether adenocarcinomas of the cervix are associated with outcome similar to that seen with squamous carcinomas of the cervix. In several retrospective studies, investigators found that patients with adenocarcinomas of the cervix had outcome similar to that of patients with squamous carcinoma of the cervix treated with radiation therapy.[125,126] However, other investigators have come to an opposite conclusion. Among patients treated surgically, they found that patients with adenocarcinoma had unusually high relapse rates compared with the rates in patients with squamous cell carcinoma and among patients treated with surgery or irradiation, they found that patients with adenocarcinoma had poorer survival rates than the rates seen in patients with squamous cell carcinoma.[110,127,128] Eifel et al.,[127] in an analysis of 1767 patients treated with radiation for FIGO stage IB disease, reported that patients with adenocarcinoma had a significantly higher risk of recurrence and death from disease. This finding was independent of age, tumor size, and tumor morphology. There was no difference in the rate of pelvic recurrence between patients with bulky adenocarcinoma (≥4 cm) and patients with squamous cell carcinoma; however, the rate of distant metastasis was almost twice as high in patients with adenocarcinoma as in patients with squamous cell carcinoma. Although the prognostic significance of histologic grade for squamous carcinomas has been disputed, there is a clear correlation between the degree of differentiation and the clinical behavior of adenocarcinomas.[123,124,129]

Other tumor factors

Pretreatment SCCAg levels have been shown to correlate with tumor bulk, stage, histology, grade, type of tumor (i.e., exophytic vs infiltrative), microscopic depth of invasion, and risk of lymph node metastases in patients with early-stage disease.[130–132] The most important property of the pretreatment SCCAg level, however, is its ability to predict clinical outcome. Several authors have

reported significantly lower survival rates in patients with very elevated values compared with patients with normal baseline levels, independent of stage.[132–135] Monitoring of tumor response using SCCAg needs further investigation, especially studies designed to determine how often SCCAg measurement should be done, the level of SCCAg that is significant, which patients would benefit from this monitoring and the cost-effectiveness of using SCCAg as a tool for monitoring patients after treatment.[136]

Several authors have reported a correlation between HPV subtype and prognosis.[137–139] In two studies of patients with histologically negative lymph nodes, investigators reported higher rates of disease recurrence when findings on PCR assay of the lymph nodes were strongly positive for HPV DNA.[140,141]

Other molecular markers that have recently been evaluated for predictive power in cervical carcinoma are EGFR and cyclooxygenase-2.[142] Studies have small populations and are presently too difficult to interpret. Other biologic features that have been investigated for their predictive power, with variable results, include inflammatory response in cervical stroma, peritoneal cytology, tumor vascularity, and DNA ploidy or S-phase fraction.[143,144]

Patient factors

Several investigators have reported correlations between low hemoglobin level before or during treatment and poor prognosis.[111,145] It has been speculated that the poor prognosis of anemic patients is cause in part by hypoxia-induced radiation resistance. Other patient-related factors that have been shown to correlate with prognosis include age, platelet count, socioeconomic status, and smoking.[93,146–150] Kucera et al.[149] reported that smokers with cervical cancer had a poorer 5-year survival rate than nonsmokers, and this relationship was statistically significant in patients with stage III disease (5-year survival rate 20.3% vs 33.9%, $p < 0.01$).

Surgical treatment options

Sentinel lymph nodes

A biopsy of sentinel lymph node was originally a process meant to simplify the surgical procedure and decrease morbidity by removing just one or a few nodes instead of systematic lymphadenectomy. However, the concept may have other advantages including a more reliable detection of key nodes in atypical localizations, detection of small metastasis, and intraoperative triage of patients, thanks to identification of key nodes for pathologic evaluation. The first large, multicenter study on sentinel lymph nodes for cervical cancer was published in 2008 and found a sensitivity of only 77%, which was a major setback for this procedure in cervical cancer.[151] However, there were multiple problems with this study including the size of tumors included, lack of surgeon proficiency assessment, and pathologic ultrastaging. Subsequent studies have shown a very high sensitivity in women with small tumors undergoing lymphatic mapping including a recent large French SENTICOL study that has reported a sensitivity of 92% and a negative predictive value of 98%.[152] Presently, sentinel lymph node biopsies is a useful intraoperative triage for patients with small tumors where the false-negative rate is lower.

Cervical conization and LEEP

Cervical conization is a procedure that removes or destroys the transformation zone and can be diagnostic, therapeutic, or both. A conization specimen is conical, as the name implies, and its size varies according to the area in question. The cone is shallow when an exocervical lesion is removed. The cone is deeper when the endocervix is being investigated. Patients requiring conization usually have one of the following: normal colposcopy findings and an abnormal Pap smear or positive ECC specimens; abnormal colposcopy findings in the form of failure to visualize the entire squamocolumnar junction or failure to define the extent of the lesion; microinvasive carcinoma in a biopsy specimen; adenocarcinoma *in situ* in a biopsy or ECC specimen; or a lack of correlation between cytologic (Pap smear), colposcopic, and histologic interpretations.

Cone biopsy is designed to completely remove the squamocolumnar junction and the lower portion of the endocervical canal in women with very small cervical cancers. The surgical specimen should include the entire lesion, as this permits measurement of both depth of invasion and extent of lateral spread.

Another surgical technique that can be used for conization is LEEP. In LEEP, a thin wire loop electrode is used to excise the lesion in patients with HGSIL. LEEP is an outpatient procedure. Although destructive techniques (such as laser ablation and cryotherapy) can provide effective treatment of suspicious lesions; the preferred technique is one that provides an appropriate histologic specimen, such as cervical cold knife conization (CKC) LEEP, or laser conization. Recently, Linares and colleagues compared CKC, laser conization, and LEEP and found that LEEP was associated with fewer complications and a shorter operating time than the other two procedures.[153] The only drawback of the LEEP procedure was a slightly shorter cone depth and a slightly higher risk of lesion recurrence.[153]

Patient selection

Conization as sole treatment of early cervical cancers is a relatively recent concept. For women who have very limited risk of lymph node spread and who have a strong desire to maintain fertility, conization may be an option.[154,155] MD Anderson Cancer Center recommends that conization be considered only for patients with squamous cell lesions that invade <3 mm, have no LVSI, and have uninvolved resection margins.[156] There is very little information on which to base a recommendation regarding the use of conization as therapy for women with nonsquamous cervical cancer.[157]

Complications of CKC include hemorrhage, pelvic cellulitis, cervical stenosis, and incompetent cervix.[158] In addition, because this procedure requires general anesthesia, there is the additional burden of possible complications and cost of anesthesia.

Complications of LEEP are similar to but not the same as those of CKC: Infection, bleeding, burns to the vagina, cervical stenosis, cervical incompetence, and recurrence of dysplasia. With LEEP, however, stenosis is rare (occurring in 1% of patients) and is seen primarily in nulliparous, perimenopausal, or postmenopausal patients. Cervical incompetence is usually only a complication of multiple procedures. The other advantage of LEEP is that it does not require general anesthesia. As mentioned earlier, when three conization techniques (CKC, laser conization, and LEEP) were compared, LEEP was associated with fewer complication as well as decreased operative time.[153]

Radical trachelectomy

Recently, for early stage disease, several groups have tried to preserve the uterus and child-bearing capability by treating patients with a radical vaginal trachelectomy. This technique involves a laparoscopic pelvic lymphadenectomy followed by vaginal resection of the cervix, the upper 1–2 cm of the vaginal cuff, and the medial portions of the cardinal and uterosacral ligaments. The cervix is transected at the lower uterine segment, and a prophylactic cerclage is placed at the time of surgery. Several investigators recommend that this procedure be limited to patients with a tumor not exceeding 2 cm.[159,160]

Extrafascial hysterectomy

The extrafascial technique permits removal of the intact uterine fundus and cervix, leaving the parametrial soft tissues and a portion of the upper vagina. Extrafascial hysterectomy can be accomplished through an abdominal incision, transvaginally, or using a combination of laparoscopic and transvaginal techniques.

Simple extrafascial hysterectomy is the standard definitive treatment option for women with stage IA1 cervical cancers and is sometimes performed following radiation therapy for bulky endocervical carcinomas. For patients with stage IA2 disease, there is some controversy regarding the most appropriate surgical procedure. These patients have 3–5% incidence of lymph node metastases and a higher rate of vaginal recurrence than patients with IA1 disease. So, although some data suggest that these IA2 lesions can be effectively resected with extrafascial hysterectomy, many American gynecologic oncologists limit this operation to women with IA1 tumors.[161,162] There is uniform consensus that conization-only therapy should not be offered to women with stage IA2 disease.

Radical hysterectomy

Radical hysterectomy involves the en bloc removal of the uterus, cervix, parametrial tissues, and upper vagina. In the early twentieth century, Wertheim of Vienna described the radical hysterectomy for the treatment of cervical cancer. In the 1940s, Meigs of the United States championed the procedure, to which he added a pelvic lymphadenectomy. Today, radical hysterectomy with pelvic lymphadenectomy is the standard treatment in the management of stage IA2-IIA tumors.

The type II (modified radical) hysterectomy is a less extensive version of the type III (radical) hysterectomy. The primary indication for type II hysterectomy is early invasive carcinoma, tumors <2 cm diameter. The type II operation ensures an adequate paracervical specimen and a vaginal cuff of 2–3 cm. In the type II operation, the medial half of the parametrium and upper one-third of the vagina are included in the surgical specimen. This is accomplished by exposing the ureters and taking the medial half of the cardinal and uterosacral ligaments instead of taking these ligaments where they attach to the pelvic wall and pelvic floor. The posterior approach is the surgeon's choice. The incidence of bladder and ureteral complications is lower with the type II operation than with a type III procedure. The type II hysterectomy can be performed with a modified or complete pelvic lymphadenectomy.

The type III (radical) hysterectomy is the classic Wertheim-Meigs radical hysterectomy. This operation is reserved for patients with stage IB and selected stage IIA carcinomas. The vaginal extension for stage IIA patients should be limited to no more than 1 cm. The parametrium, cardinal, and uterosacral ligaments are severed at the pelvic wall, and half of the vagina is removed. The uterine vessels are taken at their origin from the internal iliac vessels. The ureters are taken out of their tunnel and reflected laterally. This dissection of the distal ureters sacrifices the blood supply from the uterine and superior vesicle arteries. Reflection of the ureters clears the way for applying instruments across the parametrium along the pelvic wall. Complete removal of the cardinal ligaments and the rectal pillars and uterosacral ligaments at their base results in a greater risk of bladder atony, and loss of the distal-ureter blood supply results in a greater risk of fistulae. This operation produces an excellent cure rate in properly selected patients. In young patients, the ovaries are spared.

Intraoperative and immediate postoperative complications of radical hysterectomy include blood loss (average, 0.8 L), ureterovaginal fistula (occurring in 1–2% of patients), vesicovaginal fistula (<1%), pulmonary embolus (1–2%), small bowel obstruction (1–2%), and postoperative fever secondary to deep vein thrombosis, pulmonary infection, pelvic cellulitis, urinary tract infection, or wound infection (25–50%).[163] Subacute complications include lymphocyst formation and lower extremity edema, the risk of which is related to the extent of the node dissection. Lymphocysts may obstruct a ureter, but hydronephrosis usually improves with drainage of the lymphocyst.[164] The risk of complications may be increased in patients who undergo preoperative or postoperative irradiation.

Although most patients have transient decreased bladder sensation after radical hysterectomy, with appropriate management severe long-term bladder complications are infrequent. However, chronic bladder hypotonia or atony occurs in approximately 3–5% of patients despite careful postoperative bladder drainage.[165] Bladder atony probably results from damage to the bladder's innervation and may be related to the extent of the parametrial and paravaginal dissection.[166] Radical hysterectomy may be complicated by stress incontinence, but reported incidences vary widely and may be influenced by the addition of postoperative radiation therapy.[167] Patients may also experience constipation and, rarely, chronic obstipation after radical hysterectomy.

Criteria for selecting patients who are appropriate candidates for radical hysterectomy include factors affecting the patient's suitability for major surgery as well as tumor characteristics, including tumor volume and lymphatic involvement. Patient factors play a very important role in the selection of primary radical surgery versus primary radiation therapy in patients with early-stage disease. The ability to preserve ovarian function as well as a more pliable vagina is important to young women facing this decision. Just as important, for women with significant medical problems, including obesity, primary radiation therapy may be the better treatment option.

Table 4 5-Year survival rates for stage IB-IIA cervical cancer patients after radical hysterectomy and bilateral pelvic lymphadenectomy.

First author (references)	Stage	Year	n	Survival (%)
Sall[169]	IB-IIA	1979	219	90.0
Kenter[170]	IB-IIA	1989	213	87.3
Lee[171]	IB-IIA	1989	343	87.2
Ayhan[90]	IB-IIA	1991	270	80.7
Hopkins[129]	IB	1991	213	92.5
Alvarez[172]	IB	1991	401	85
Averette[89]	IIB-IIA	1993	726	90.1
Landoni[163]	IB-IIA	1997	172	83

Abbreviation: N, number of patients.

In patients with early-stage (IA-IB1) disease, tumor characteristics play a very important role in treatment selection. Patients with high-risk factors may benefit from up-front definitive radiation therapy plus possible chemotherapy. Multiple studies have found that morbidity increases in patients who receive both radical surgery and radiation therapy.[168] High-risk tumor characteristics include large tumor size, which is associated with lymph node spread, increased chance of recurrence, and decreased survival rates. Eifel et al.[164] found that DSS decreased significantly in patients with stage IB carcinoma if the tumor diameter was >5 cm (88% vs 69%, $p < 0.0001$). Other high-risk factors include lymph node metastases, parametrial involvement, and positive surgical margins.

Outcomes after surgical treatment

Reported 5-year survival rates for women with stage IB cervical cancer treated with radical hysterectomy and pelvic lymphadenectomy are approximately 80–90% (Table 4).[89–91,168–176] Patients with positive surgical margins or positive lymph nodes are at the highest risk of recurrence and poor outcome. Delgado et al.,[91] in a large prospective study, reported 3-year DSS rates of 85.6% in patients with negative nodes and 50–74% in patients with positive nodes. In the group with positive nodes, increasing number of positive nodes and involvement of common iliac nodes correlated with decreased survival. A randomized study showed that postoperative chemoradiation improved survival in patients with positive lymph nodes, positive surgical margins, or tumor present in the parametrium.[117]

Radiation therapy

The management of invasive carcinoma of the cervix with primary radiation therapy involves a combination of external beam radiation therapy (EBRT) plus either low dose rate (LDR) or high dose rate (HDR) intracavitary irradiation. The goal of treatment is to balance these two elements in a way that optimizes the ratio of tumor control to treatment complications. The required dose varies according to the tumor burden in the cervix, paracervical sites, and regional nodes. Factors that influence the tolerable dose of radiation include the patient's vaginal and uterine anatomy, the degree of tumor-related tissue destruction and infection, and patient characteristics (e.g., body habitus, comorbid illnesses, and smoking habits).

Treatment options EBRT

EBRT is used as initial treatment in patients with bulky tumors. The usual plan is to give 40–45 Gy to the whole pelvis. This gives a homogeneous distribution to the central mass plus the regional lymph nodes. Such treatment reduces the primary tumor and any regional lymph nodes harboring disease, and it destroys microscopic foci in lymph-vascular spaces adjacent to the tumor. The shrinkage of the primary tumor allows better dose distribution from intracavitary irradiation.

High-energy photons (15–18 MV) are usually preferred for pelvic treatment because they spare superficial tissues that are unlikely to be involved with tumor. Simulation films, as well as CT, MRI, PET scan, and lymphangiography, guide the radiation oncologist in selecting boundaries for the portals. Typical radiation therapy fields are shown in Figure 16. A standard course of

radiation therapy is 40 to 45 Gy given with external beam radiation therapy (EBRT). Patients with grossly positive pelvic nodes within the 40- to 45-Gy field require a boost with a small field (Figures 16 and 17). The dose to the boost area is 8–10 Gy. The total dose to the positive nodes, including a 1–2 cm margin, is 60–66 Gy, which includes the contributions from brachytherapy intracavitary systems. Intensity-modulated radiation therapy (IMRT) may be used to boost the dose to large pelvic nodes (up to approximately 66 Gy) in a very tightly defined volume.

There has been a recent interest in using IMRT in the treatment of cervical carcinoma. Unlike standard treatment, IMRT

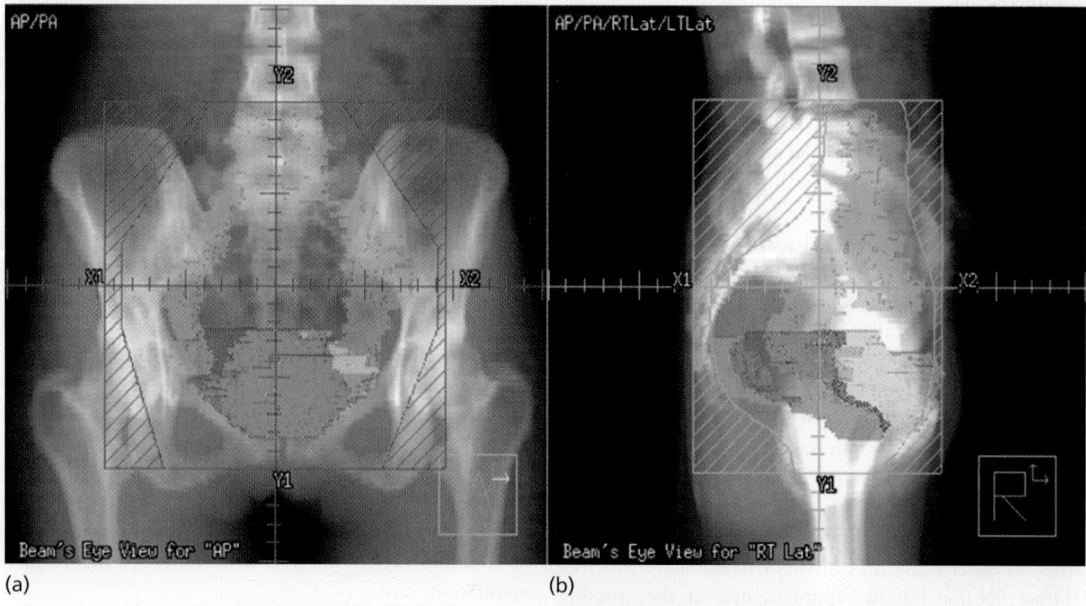

Figure 16 Typical radiation fields for a patient with cervical cancer. (a) Anterior field; (b) lateral field.

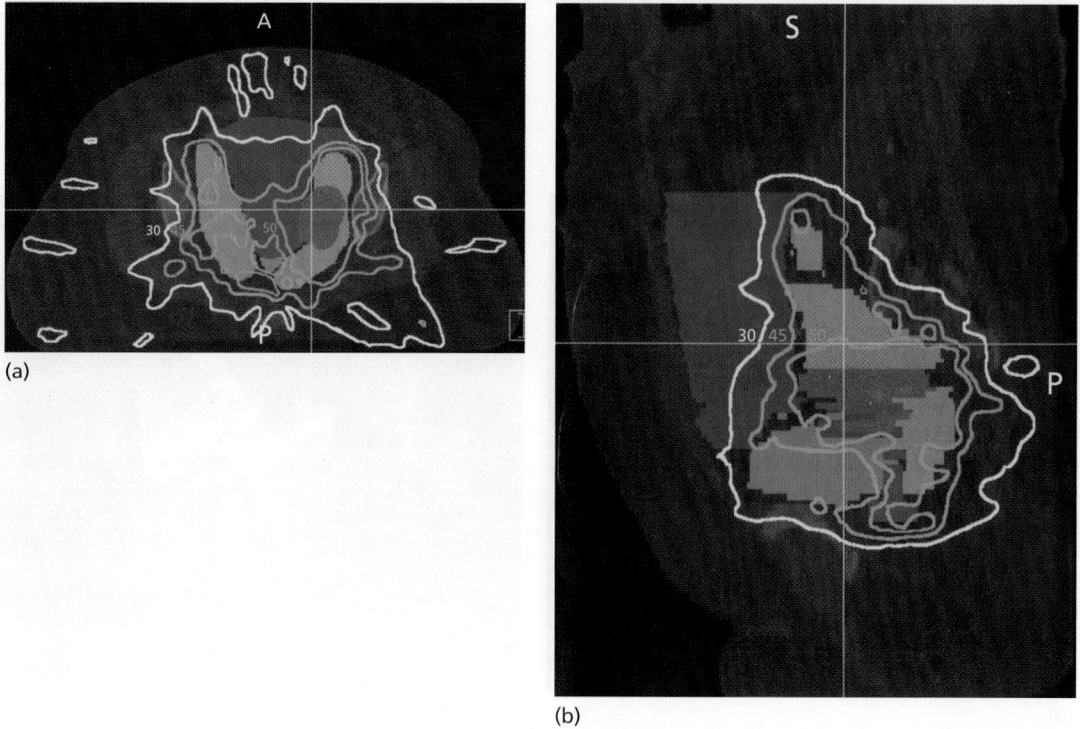

Figure 17 Dose distribution of a typical intracavitary system; it is important to note how quickly the dose falls off the further one gets from the system. (a) Anterior view; (b) lateral view.

allows one to dose paint tissues in the area of treatment, that is, allowing higher doses to tumor, while giving less dose to normal tissues especially small bowel (Figure 17). Mundt et al.[177] have published reports showing a decrease in both acute and chronic[178] bowel toxicities in patients with endometrial or cervical carcinoma treated postoperatively to the pelvis with IMRT compared to standard treatment. However, the highly conformal dose distributions achieved by IMRT also increases the room of error. In particular, great attention needs to be given to internal organs motion (especially the bladder and the rectum) and tumor regression, and therefore at this time IMRT is still considered the investigation therapy, especially in the field of intact cervix. Several multi-institutional trials are underway evaluating the use of IMRT for cervical cancer.

Intracavitary radiation therapy (ICRT)

The importance of ICRT (intracavitary radiation therapy) for cervical cancer should not be underestimated because, although EBRT plays a critical role in sterilizing pelvic wall disease and improving tumor geometry, too much reliance on external beam irradiation will compromise the chance for central disease control and increase the risk of complications.

Brachytherapy is usually delivered using afterloading applicators that are placed in the uterine cavity and vagina. Ideal placement of the intrauterine tandem and vaginal ovoids produces a pear-shaped radiation distribution, delivering a high radiation dose to the cervix and paracervical tissues and a reduced dose to the rectum and bladder. Several systems have been used throughout the world to determine dose rates and doses for cervical cancer. In the United States, the paracentral doses are most frequently expressed at a single point, point A, which is defined earlier. Point A bears no consistent relationship with the tumor or target volume but lies approximately at the crossing of the ureter and uterine artery. Other systems of dose specifications include the International Commission on Radiation Units and Measurements (ICRU) reference points based on ICRU Report 38 (1985) and the mg-h system. Whichever system of dose specification is used, emphasis should always be placed on optimizing the relationship between the intracavitary applicators and the cervical tumor and other pelvic tissues. Source,

strength, and position should be carefully chosen to provide optimal tumor coverage with exceeding safe doses to normal tissue (Figure 18).

In the past, clinicians regarded the radiobiological advantages of LDR intracavitary treatment (usually delivery of 40–60 cGy/h to point A) as a major factor contributing to the success of cervical cancer treatment. These LDRs permit repair of sublethal cellular injury, preferentially sparing normal tissues and optimizing the therapeutic ratio. During the past two decades, computer technology has made it possible to deliver brachytherapy at very HDRs (<100 cGy/min) using a high-activity cobalt 60 or iridium 192 source and remote afterloading. HDR intracavitary therapy is now become the standard of care in most parts of the world. Clinicians have found this approach attractive because it does not require that patients be hospitalized and may be more convenient for the patient and the physician. Multiple randomized and nonrandomized studies have suggested that survival rates and complications rates with HDR treatment are similar to those with traditional LDR treatment.[179] In 2012,[180] the American Brachytherapy Society suggested guidelines for the use of HDR brachytherapy for carcinoma of the cervix. The group emphasized the importance of factors that were already considered critical to successful LDR treatment—optimized applicator position, balanced use of external beam therapy and brachytherapy, compact overall treatment duration, and delivery of an adequate dose to tumor while respecting normal tissue tolerance limits.

Image-based brachytherapy is becoming increasingly common, particularly in Europe. Institutions are using MRI-based treatment planning to plan their doses to tumor as well as doses to avoid structures such as the bladder and rectum; however, large prospective studies and careful analysis will be needed before this becoming standard of care.

Interstitial brachytherapy

Several groups have advocated the use of interstitial perineal template brachytherapy in patients with poor anatomy or parametrial or pelvic sidewall disease. These implants are usually placed transperineally, with placement guided by a Lucite template that encourages parallel placement of hollow needles that penetrate the cervix

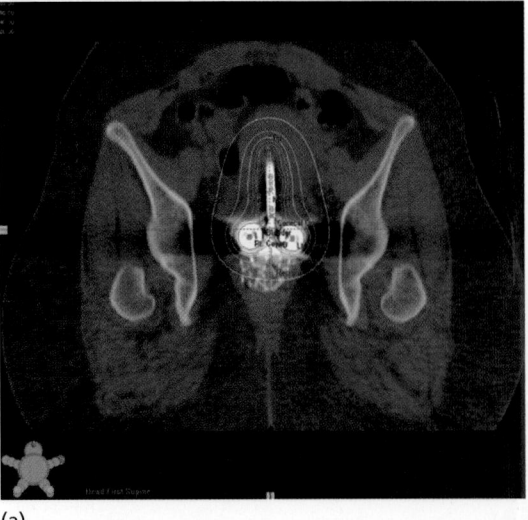

(a)

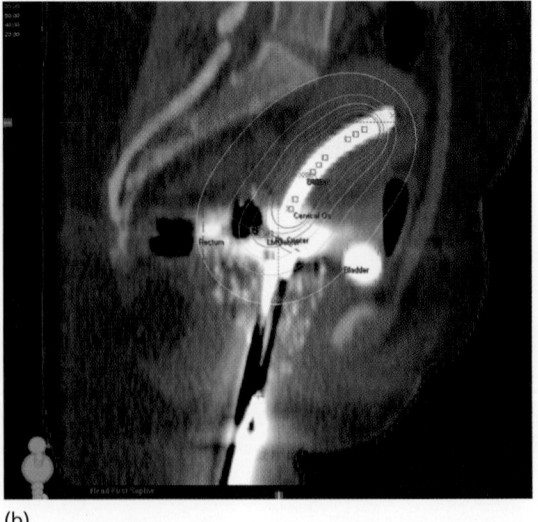

(b)

Figure 18 A patient with cervical cancer being treated with radiation therapy after a hysterectomy. The areas that need to be covered are the nodes and vagina. This is an IMRT plan that conforms to the area that needs to be covered while sparing the small bowel. Most of the small bowel receives <30 Gy.

and paracervical spaces and are usually loaded with iridium 192. Advocates state that the advantages of this method are the ease of inserting implants in patients whose uterus is difficult to probe, the ability to place sources directly into the parametrium, and the relatively homogeneous dose. Recent updates report poor survival rates and higher rates of major complications for patients with stage IIB and IIIB disease.[181,182] Outside of an investigational setting, interstitial treatment of primary cervical cancers should probably be limited to patients who cannot accommodate intrauterine brachytherapy and patients with distal vaginal disease that requires a boost with interstitial brachytherapy.

Patient selection

For patients with IB1 tumors, the choice between surgery and radiation therapy is based primarily on patient preference, anesthetic and surgical risks, physician preference, and understanding of the nature and incidence of complications of radiation therapy and hysterectomy. In general, surgery is often chosen for younger patients in the hope of preserving ovarian function and hopefully reducing vaginal shortening, while radiation therapy is often selected for older postmenopausal women to avoid the morbidity of a major surgical procedure. Patients with stage IB2 disease can be treated with either surgery followed by radiation therapy or definitive radiation therapy. The biases are so large that the Gynecologic Oncology Group (GOG) could not complete trial randomizing patients with stage IB2 disease between surgery followed by chemoradiation therapy and definitive radiation therapy. Radiation therapy is the primary local therapy for most patients with stage IIB-IVA disease.

Outcomes

Stage IB-IIA disease

Radical radiation therapy achieves excellent survival and pelvic disease control rates in patients with stage IB-IIA cervical cancer. Eifel et al.[164] reported 5-year DSS rates of 90%, 86%, and 67% in patients with stage IB tumors with cervical diameters of <4, 4–4.9, and >5 cm, respectively. The 5-year survival rates of patients with stage IIA disease range from 70% to 85% and, like survival rates in patients with stage IB disease, are strongly correlated with tumor size.[112,183,184] Studies suggest that results for patients with bulky tumors may be improved further by concurrent administration of chemotherapy.[185,186]

Stage IIB-IVA disease

Five-year survival rates of 65–75%, 35–50%, and 15–20% have been reported in patients who received radiation therapy alone for stage IIB, IIIB, and IV tumors, respectively (Table 5).[111,112,184,187] The addition of cisplatin-containing regimens may further improve local control and survival.[186,188,189]

Complications

Acute side effects

Acute side effects of pelvic irradiation include symptoms related to the bowel, bladder, rectum, and vagina. Most patients experience mild fatigue and mild to moderate diarrhea that usually is controllable with antidiarrheal medication and dietary modifications. Less frequently, patients may complain of bladder or urethral irritation. These symptoms may be treated with Pyridium or antispasmodics after urinalysis and urine culture have ruled out a urinary tract infection. Patients treated with extended-field radiation may have nausea, gastric irritation, and mild depression of peripheral blood

Table 5 Pelvic disease control and survival rates[a].

FIGO stage	Patients (n)	Control rate (%)	Survival rate (%)
I	229	93	89
IIA	315	88	85
IIB	314	80	62
IIIA	266	63	62
IIIB	216	57	50
IV	43	18	20

[a]Pelvic disease control rates and survival rates of 1383 patients with carcinoma of the intact uterine cervix treated with irradiation alone, according to the Fletcher guidelines: a French cooperative study.
Source: Barillot et al. 1997.[112] Reproduced with permission of Elsevier.

cell counts. Acute symptoms may be increased in patients receiving concurrent chemotherapy. Unless the ovaries have been transposed, all premenopausal patients who receive pelvic radiotherapy experience ovarian failure by the completion of treatment.

Fatal or life-threatening complications of ICRT are rare. Thromboembolic events, uterine perforation, fever, vaginal laceration, and the usual risk of anesthesia are other less serious complications associated with ICRT.[190]

Problems after therapy

For patients with cervical cancer, overall estimates of the risk of major complications of radiation therapy usually range between 5% and 15%.[191,192] The risk of experiencing a late complication is greatest within the first 3 years after treatment; however, major complications have been reported as late as 30 years or more after treatment. Most complications occurring after radiation involve the rectum, bladder, or small bowel. During the first 3 years after treatment, rectal complications are most common and include bleeding, stricture, ulceration, and fistula. The average onset of major urinary tract complications tends to be somewhat later than that of intestinal complication, with an actuarial risk of hematuria requiring transfusion of 2.6% at 5 years.[191] The overall risk of developing a gastrointestinal or urinary tract fistula was 1.7% at 5 years with an increased risk of patients who underwent adjuvant hysterectomy or pretreatment transperitoneal lymphadenectomy. The risk of small bowel obstruction is strongly correlated with a number of patient characteristics and treatment factors including type of surgery, history of pelvic infection, history of smoking, and body habitus.[150,191,192]

Patients who are treated with radiation for cervical cancer tend to have varying degrees of atrophy, telangiectasia, or scarring of the upper third of the vagina. However, more severe shortening can occur. Changes may be greater in patients with very extensive tumors and in patients who are elderly, sexually inactive, or hypoestrogenic.[192,193] Regular intercourse and use of vaginal dilators may help prevent vaginal shortening.

Current practice by disease stage

CIS and stage IA1 disease

Treatment of HGSILs is rapidly changing. LEEP is one effective therapy for HGSILs. Other techniques such as cryosurgery and laser ablation have also proven effective. Regardless of the technique used, HGSILs should be entirely visible by colposcopy, the entire transformation zone should be visualized, and the ECC specimen should be negative. Conization with a knife is preferred when the ECC specimen is positive. All margins must be clear of intraepithelial lesions.

Stage IA1 (microinvasive) squamous cell carcinomas that invade the stroma <3 mm and have no LVSI are usually not visible to the unaided eye, and cytology is abnormal. The diagnosis requires cone biopsy, which yields a specimen adequate for diagnostic purposes. Conization alone is also potentially a low-risk therapy for patients who wish to retain fertility and who have invasion <3 mm in depth with no LVSI. It is important to remember that the margins of a cone specimen must be negative. When the conization specimen has a positive margin, a second tissue specimen must be obtained because foci of frankly invasive carcinoma may lie adjacent to the positive margin. Patients should be informed that the conservative approach carries a small risk. There is very little current information on which to base a recommendation regarding the use of conization as therapy for women with nonsquamous cervical cancers.[155] Patients who elect conization therapy must be willing to be monitored closely for the development of residual or recurrent cervical neoplasia.

The most conventional treatment of stage IA1 disease is a type 1 (simple extrafascial) hysterectomy. If the patient is young, the ovaries are left in place. Patients can also be treated with radiation therapy alone, usually consisting of intracavitary therapy alone. The 10-year disease control rate with radiation therapy alone is 95–100%.[194]

Stage IA2 disease

Small lesions that invade 3–5 mm have an average risk of lymph node metastasis of about 5%. The standard treatment of patients with this stage of disease is type II (modified radical) hysterectomy and pelvic node dissection.

Recently, a number of studies have explored less radical surgical options for early-stage cervical cancer, including simple hysterectomy, simple hysterectomy, simple trachelectomy, and cervical conization with or without sentinel lymph node biopsy and pelvic lymph node dissections especially in patients who wish to preserve fertility. Such options may be available for patients with low-risk early-stage cervical cancer including patients with any histology except neuroendocrine tumor, tumor size <2 cm, stromal invasion <10 mm, and no LVSI. Presently, three international trials are underway looking at this option for patients with early-stage disease.

If surgery is contraindicated, these patients can be treated with radiation alone, usually with pelvic radiation therapy plus brachytherapy. However, in special situations, brachytherapy alone may be sufficient in controlling disease.

Stage IB1 and small-stage IIA disease

Treatment of invasive carcinoma or carcinoma of FIGO stage IB or greater is determined on the basis of tumor size and the presence or absence of lymph node metastases (Figure 5).

Stage IB1 tumors, which are <4 cm in size, are considered small; however, they are associated with a significant risk of microscopic paracervical extension or lymph node metastasis. In a prospective study in patients treated with radical hysterectomy who had clinically estimated maximum tumor diameter <3 cm, the GOG reported that 16% of the patients (42 of 261) had lymph node metastasis.[195] Landoni et al.[163] found a 25% incidence of positive nodes (28 of 114 patients) in patients treated with radical hysterectomy for stage IB-IIA tumors that measured 4 cm or less on initial clinical examination. Therefore, for patients with stage IB1 or small IIA (<4 cm diameter) disease, the treatment is either type III (radical) hysterectomy plus bilateral pelvic lymphadenectomy or radical radiation therapy. The goal of both of these treatment options is to destroy malignant cells in the cervix, paracervical tissues, and regional lymph nodes.

OS rates for patients with stage IB1 or small IIA disease treated with either surgery or radiation therapy are usually in the range 80–90%, suggesting that the two treatments are equally effective. However, only one prospective randomized trial has compared the two treatments directly.[163] There were no significant differences in the rates of relapse or survival between the two arms, but the overall rate of grade 2 and 3 complications was greater for patients treated with hysterectomy. Therefore, for patients with stage IB1, the choice of treatment is based on patient preference, anesthetic and surgical risks, physician preference, and an understanding of the nature and incidence of complication with radiation therapy and hysterectomy. The role of pelvic radiation therapy after radical hysterectomy is still being defined. The GOG, in a prospective trial, randomized patients with intermediate risk of recurrence after radical hysterectomy for stage IB carcinoma to pelvic irradiation or no further treatment.[196] The preliminary analysis showed a 47% reduction in the risk of recurrence when postoperative irradiation was given (15% vs 28%, $p = 0.008$). An update of this study published in 2006 showed a statistically reduction in the risk of recurrence and PFS however no statistical difference in OS with the addition of postoperative radiation therapy. The conclusion by the authors was that pelvic radiotherapy after radical surgery significantly reduced the risk of recurrence and prolongs PFS in women with stage IB cervical cancer, particularly in patients with adenocarcinoma or adenosquamous histologies.[197] The Southwest Oncology Group reported the results of a randomized trial of patients treated with radical hysterectomy followed by radiation therapy versus radiation therapy plus cisplatin-based chemotherapy in patients with high risk factors including pelvic lymph node metastases, parametrial involvement, and or positive margins. The authors found that patients who received radiation therapy plus chemotherapy had a significant improvement in survival compared with the survival of patients treated with radiation alone.[117]

Stage IB2 disease

Patients with tumors >4 cm in diameter whose para-aortic lymph nodes are found to be free of disease have excellent survival rates when treated with whole-pelvis EBRT plus brachytherapy. However, these tumors appear on clinical examination to be technically resectable, and the ideal management of these tumors is a subject of considerable controversy. The approach to these tumors differs widely between centers, and the biases are so large that the GOG closed a trial early owing to a lack of accrual that compared surgery plus chemoradiation versus chemoradiation alone.

Although radiation therapy is effective for many patients with stage IB2 disease, central disease recurrences occur in at least 8–10% of patients with bulky endocervical cancers.[167,183,184] The literature contains numerous reports on the use of an adjunctive hysterectomy for patients with bulky endocervical carcinomas treated with primary radiation therapy. However, in 1999, the GOG concluded from a study that evaluated adjunctive hysterectomy, that adjunctive hysterectomy did not improve local control or survival but did increase toxicity when added to chemoradiation therapy in patients with stage IB2 disease.[185]

Several investigators recommend treating these tumors with initial surgery followed by postoperative radiation therapy or chemoradiation depending on the pathology findings. In a randomized trial by Landoni et al.,[163] patients with stage IB2 tumors were randomized to initial surgery versus definitive radiation therapy. In this trial, even though the survival was similar in both arms, 84% of the patients treated with initial surgery required postoperative radiation therapy, which contributed to a higher complication rate in that arm.

Several trials have been initiated to study the role of induction chemotherapy before surgical exploration in patients with bulky lesions who would otherwise be poor candidates for radical hysterectomy.[198,199] A meta-analysis[200] collected individual patient data (IPD) from 21 randomized trials of neoadjuvant chemotherapy in locally advanced cervical cancer. This analysis included data from comparison of the benefits of neoadjuvant chemotherapy followed by radical radiotherapy versus radical radiotherapy alone (2074) and for comparison of neoadjuvant chemotherapy followed by surgery (±radiotherapy) versus radical radiotherapy alone (872 patients). They found that the group of trials using cycles lasting longer than 14 days showed a significant 25% increase in the relative risk of death with neoadjuvant chemotherapy, representing an absolute 8% reduction in 5-year survival compared to shorter chemotherapy cycle lengths, where there was a significant 17% decrease in the relative risk of death, representing an absolute improvement in 5-year survival of 7%. They also found a significant 35% increase in the risk of death for trials that used <25 mg/m^2 cisplatin per week, reducing absolute 5-year survival by 11%; however, the results for the higher dose-intensity group were less clear, with only a trend toward increased survival. The second comparison of patients treated with neoadjuvant chemotherapy and surgery versus radiation therapy only showed that patients treated with neoadjuvant chemotherapy had a highly significant 35% reduction in the risk of death ($p = 0.0004$) that translated into a 14% absolute increase in 5-year OS.[201] Unfortunately, this meta-analysis only included trials before 1999, when radiotherapy alone was still the standard treatment. Ultimately, however, this approach may need to be compared with optimized chemoradiation to determine the most effective, least toxic therapy for these patients. The EORTC (European Organisation for Research and Treatment of Cancer) completed a trial addressing this specific question. Patients with IB2 cancers are being randomized to neoadjuvant chemotherapy followed by radiation or current chemotherapy and radiation.

Two prospective randomized trials[185,186] indicate that patients who are treated with radiation for bulky central disease benefit from concurrent administration of cisplatin-containing chemotherapy. A third study suggests that patients who require postoperative radiotherapy because of findings of lymph node metastasis or involved surgical margins also benefit from concurrent chemoradiation.[117] These studies are discussed in more detail in the section titled "Concurrent Chemoradiation," later in this chapter.

Stage IIB-IVA disease

Radiation therapy is the primary local treatment of most patients with locoregionally advanced (stages IIIB-IVA) cervical carcinoma. The success of treatment depends on a careful balance between EBRT and brachytherapy that optimizes the dose to tumor and normal tissues and on the overall duration of treatment. In the French Cooperative Group study of 1875 patients treated with radiation therapy according to Fletcher guidelines, Barillot et al.[112] reported 5-year survival rates of 70%, 45%, and 10% for patients with stage IIB, IIIB, and IVA tumors, respectively.

Local and distant disease recurrences continue to be a problem for patients with locally advanced disease. Neoadjuvant chemotherapy has produced excellent tumor responses; however, randomized trials have failed to demonstrate improvements in survival. Other approaches that have been used to try to improve outcome in these patients, including neutrons, hyperbaric oxygen, and hypoxic cell sensitizers, have also produced disappointing results.

Concurrent chemoradiation

In 1999, five prospective randomized trials, involving patients with locoregionally advanced cervical cancer,[117,185,186,188,189] provided compelling evidence that the addition of concurrent cisplatin-containing chemotherapy to standard radiotherapy reduces the risk of disease recurrence by as much as 50% and thereby improves the rates of pelvic disease control and survival (Table 6).

In two studies,[188,189] the GOG randomly assigned patients with stages IIB-IVA disease to receive either hydroxyurea or cisplatin-containing chemotherapy during external beam irradiation. All three of the cisplatin-containing regimens in these trials produced local control and survival rates superior to those for the control (hydroxyurea and radiation). In a third study,[185] patients with stage IB tumors measuring at least 4 cm in diameter were randomly assigned to receive radiation alone or radiation plus weekly cisplatin before an extrafascial hysterectomy. Patients who received cisplatin were more likely to have a complete histologic response and were more likely to be disease free at the time of preliminary analysis. A fourth study,[117] sponsored by the Southwest Oncology Group and the GOG, randomized patients after a radical hysterectomy pelvic radiation therapy or pelvic radiation therapy plus chemotherapy if they had high risk factors. The trial found improvement of survival of chemotherapy and radiation therapy compared to radiation therapy alone at 5 years; however, the benefit of the chemotherapy to the radiation therapy in a univariate analysis was less significant in tumors size <2 cm and patients with only one node positive.[205] The absolute improvement in 5-year survival for adjuvant chemotherapy in patients with tumors ≤2 cm was only 5% (77% vs 82%), while for those with tumors >2 cm, it was 19% (58% vs 77%). Similarly, the absolute 5-year survival benefit was less evident among patients with one nodal metastasis (79% vs 83%) than when at least two nodes were positive (55% vs 75%).[205]

During the same interval, the Radiation Therapy Oncology Group (RTOG)[186] conducted a trial in which radiotherapy alone was compared with pelvic irradiation (including prophylactic para-aortic irradiation) plus concurrent cisplatin and 5-FU. This study demonstrated a significant improvement in outcome for patients with stages III or IV disease as well as for patients with stages IB2 or II cervical cancer with concurrent chemotherapy.[194] An update of this trial, with a median follow-up period of 6.6 years for the surviving patients,[206] reported that the OS rate for patients treated with chemotherapy and radiation therapy compared to radiation therapy was still significantly better (67% vs 41% at 8 years, $p = < 0.0001$) and the conclusion by the authors was that chemotherapy with radiation therapy significantly improved the survival rate of women with locally advanced cervical cancer without increasing the rate of late treatment-related side effects.[206] Only one large randomized trial has failed to demonstrate a significant advantage from concurrent cisplatin-based chemotherapy in cervical cancer patients. Pearcey et al.[202] published this trial in 2002. The authors suggest that difference in technique could explain the difference between their results and the results of the five earlier trials, although the survival rate in their control arm indicated that the margin for improvement was smaller than that in the earlier trials. This trial was also the smallest of the six trials.

Taken together, the randomized trials provide strong evidence that the addition of concurrent cisplatin-containing chemotherapy to pelvic radiotherapy benefits selected patients with locally advanced cervical cancer. It remains to be resolved whether or not 5-FU plays a significant role. The combination of cisplatin plus

Table 6 Prospective randomized trials: role of concurrent radiotherapy and cisplatin-containing chemotherapy[a].

First author (references)	Eligibility	Patients (numbers)	CT: investigational arm	CT: control arm	Relative risk of recurrence (90% CI)	p Values
Rose[188]	FIGO IIB–IVA	526	Cisplatin 40 mg/m² /week (up to 6 cycles)	HU 3 g/m² (2×/week)	0.57 (0.42–0.78)	<0.001
			Cisplatin 50 mg/m²; 5-FU 4 g/m²/96 h; HU 2 g/m² (2×/week) (2 cycles)	HU 3 g/m² (2×/week)	0.55 (0.40–0.75)	<0.001
Morris[186]	FIGO IB–IIA (≥5 cm); IIB–IVA or pelvic nodes involved	403	Cisplatin 75 mg/m²; 5-FU 4 g/m²/96 h (3 cycles)	None[a]	0.48 (0.35–0.66)	<0.001
Keys[185]	FIGO IB (≥4 cm)	369	Cisplatin 40 mg/m²/week (up to 6 cycles)	None[b]	0.51 (0.34–0.75)	0.001
Whitney[189]	FIGO IIB–IVA	368	Cisplatin 50 mg/m²; 5-FU 4 g/m²/96 h (2 cycles)	HU 3 g/m² (2×/week)	0.79 (0.62–0.99)	0.03
Peters[117]	FIGO I–IIA after radical hysterectomy with nodes, margins, or parametrium positive	268	Cisplatin 50 mg/m²; 5-FU 4 g/m²/96 h (2 cycles)	None	0.50 (0.29–0.84)	0.01
Pearcey[202]	FIGO IB–IIA (≥5 cm), IIB–IVA or pelvic nodes involved	259	Cisplatin 40 mg/m²/week (up to 6 cycles)	None	0.91 (0.62–1.35)[c]	0.43
Wong[203]	FIGO IB–IIA (>4 cm), IIB–III	220	Epirubicin 60 mg/m², then 90 mg/m² q4 weeks for 5 more cycles[d]	None	~0.65	0.02
Lorvidhaya[204]	FIGO IB–IVA	926	Mitomycin-C 10 mg/m² day 1 and 29 Oral 5-FU 300 mg/day days 1–14 and 29–42	None	0.001	—

Abbreviations: CI, confidence interval; FU, follow-up; HU, hydroxyurea; PA, para-aortic; RT, radiotherapy.

Results from prospective randomized trials that investigate the role of concurrent radiotherapy and cisplatin-containing chemotherapy for patients with locoregionally advanced cervical cancer.

[a]Patients in control arm had prophylactic para-aortic irradiation.

[b]All patients had extrafascial hysterectomy after radiotherapy.

[c]Survival.

[d]Chemotherapy was begun on day 1 and continued every 4 weeks throughout and after radiation therapy.

[e]This study had four arms: arm 1, conventional radiation therapy (RT); arm 2, conventional RT with adjuvant chemotherapy consisting of 5-FU orally at 200 mg/day given for 3 courses of 4 weeks, with a 2-week rest every 6 weeks; arm 3, conventional RT with concurrent chemotherapy; and arm 4, conventional RT with concurrent and adjuvant chemotherapy. The addition of adjuvant therapy did not affect recurrence, but there was a significant difference in the recurrence rate between the conventional RT and the conventional RT plus concurrent chemotherapy arms.

FU was tested in four of the trials [RTOG 90-01, GOG 85, GOG 120, and Southwest Oncology Group (SWOG) 8797]. In GOG 120, the frequency of grade 3 and 4 leukopenia was significantly higher in the arm with cisplatin/5-FU and hydroxyurea compared to the arm with cisplatin and hydroxyurea alone, with equal effectiveness. Therefore, it was felt that cisplatin alone was equally effective as cisplatin-5-FU and less toxic, although there has been no adequately powered direct randomized comparison of these two regimens without hydroxyurea.

A meta-analysis of 18 trials[207] with concurrent chemotherapy and radiation (4580 patients) in patients with cervical cancer concluded that concomitant chemotherapy and radiotherapy improved overall and PFS and reduced local and distant recurrence in selected patients with cervical cancer. Concomitant chemotherapy and radiation therapy produced a 12% absolute increase in survival with greater evidence of benefit in the trials using platinum-based chemotherapy than in those with nonplatinum-based chemotherapy.[207] More recently, a systematic review and meta-analysis based on IPD[208] has documented a 7% absolute improvement in 5-year survival. The benefits were similar in the trials using platinum and nonplatinum chemoradiotherapy.[208] In this analysis, there is a suggestion that the magnitude of benefit with chemoradiotherapy varies according to stage, but not to other patients characteristics, suggesting a greater benefit in patients with early-stage disease compared to stage III and IV disease.[208]

In 2012, Duenas-Gonzales published a large phase III study that randomized patients with locally advanced cervical cancer to cisplatin plus radiation versus cisplatin plus gemcitabine and radiation therapy.[209] Women assigned to treatment with the combination regimen also received additional systemic therapy after chemoradiation was complete. With a median follow-up of 3 years, women who received cisplatin plus gemcitabine had a 32% reduction in disease progression and a higher rate of PFS at 3 years compared with those treated with cisplatin alone (74% vs 65%, respectively). In addition, cisplatin plus gemcitabine resulted in a 32% survival advantage. However, there were methodological problems with follow-up in this study and a second publication by the authors purported no benefit in various subgroups.[210] Despite these results, there are reports from other investigators that the combination of cisplatin, gemcitabine, and pelvic irradiation results in unacceptable toxicity[211] and presently is not commonly used in the United States.

These studies raise other interesting questions that will undoubtedly be the subjects of future studies. Although North American studies have emphasized cisplatin-containing regimens, investigators in Southeast Asia have reported improved outcome when radiation was combined with epirubicin[203] or mitomycin and 5-FU.[204] Other drugs that are being studied for their radiosensitizing effects in patients with advanced disease are paclitaxel,[212] carboplatin,[213] nedaplatin,[214] topotecan,[215] and multiple biologic response modifiers. RTOG just published results of a phase II study evaluating the combination of bevacizumab with cisplatin in combination with radiation therapy and found results that were promising with 3-years OS, DFS, and LRF of 81.3%, 68.7%, and 23.3%, respectively, in 49 patients.[216] Another potential pathway is the inhibition of ribonucleotide reductase (RNR). Elevated RNR levels are associated with an increased risk of an incomplete response to chemoradiation and an increased risk of disease recurrence.[217] Therefore, targets that inhibit RNR may be of potential value in combination with RT. One such agent, 3-aminopyridine-2-carboxaldehyde thiosemicarbazone, has been evaluated in a single-institution phase 2 trial and with a median follow-up of 20 months; clinical responses were observed in 24 of 25 patients with suggested metabolic complete responses noted in 23 of 24 patients evaluated by PET/CT at 3 months.[218] These encouraging results have prompted a larger, multi-institutional, randomized phase II study as well as a possible phase III through NRG. Other potential targets/pathways that are being investigated include EGFR expression and inhibition of poly (adenosine diphosphate-ribose) polymerase (PARP).

Para-aortic metastasis

Metastatic cancer in the para-aortic lymph nodes can be confirmed with fine-needle aspiration, laparoscopy, or extra-peritoneal laparotomy. Laparoscopy and laparotomy, using the extra-peritoneal approach, allows the removal of positive nodes and sampling of other para-aortic nodes, which may enhance control with radiation therapy and help design the treatment field.

The superior boundary of the extended EBRT portal provides a margin of 3 cm above the most cephalad of the positive nodes. The superior boundary limit is the T12 vertebra. Currently, patients with positive pelvic nodes or low common iliac nodes may have the field extended to the L1–L2 interspace.

Patients with para-aortic lymph node involvement can be treated effectively with extended-field irradiation. Five-year survival rates range from 25% to 50%.[219,220] The value of prophylactic extended-field irradiation was tested in two randomized trials and both trials found no advantage in the use of prophylactic para-aortic radiation.[221,222]

The role of concurrent chemotherapy with extended-field irradiation has been evaluated in several phase II studies.[223] Although, side effects are greater when treatment fields are enlarged, combined therapy may be tolerable if careful consideration is given to the chemotherapy regimen, volume of tissue irradiated, and other factors that might increase the risk of serious toxicity. In conclusion, it is tempting to extrapolate from the results achieved with combinations of pelvic radiation and chemotherapy; however, patients need to be informed that the cost-benefit ratio of concurrent chemotherapy and extended-field irradiation has not been formally tested but this is where IMRT may be a benefit in reducing acute toxicity.

Unsuspected invasive cancer discovered after simple hysterectomy

Sometimes the pathologist discovers unsuspected invasive cervical carcinoma in the tissue specimen in patients who undergo hysterectomy for what is presumed to be a benign pelvic condition. Many factors can lead to such an event.[224]

Patients with unsuspected invasive cervical carcinoma detected after simple hysterectomy have been classified in five groups according to the amount of disease and presentation: (1) microinvasive cancer, (2) tumor confined to the cervix with negative surgical margins, (3) positive surgical margins but no gross residual tumor, (4) gross residual tumor by clinical examination documented by biopsy, and (5) patients referred for treatment more than 6 months after hysterectomy (usually for recurrent disease).[225] The therapy plan is based on the amount of residual disease. Patients with minimal invasion and no residual disease require at most brachytherapy to the vaginal apex; patients with gross disease at the specimen margin require full-intensity therapy. Patients with minimal or no known gross residual disease (groups 1–3) have excellent 5-year survival rates (59–79%), whereas rates for patients with gross residual disease (groups 4 and 5) are poorer (in the range of only 41%).[226]

Recurrent disease

Prognostic factors

Various clinicopathologic features have been associated with adverse outcomes in patients with recurrent cervical carcinoma in the pelvis; however, the relatively small numbers of patients and the heterogeneity of clinical and treatment parameters in most series preclude detailed statistical analysis of these factors. Two clinical factors commonly correlated with the probability of the success of salvage therapy are the location (central vs side wall involvement) and the size of the recurrent pelvic tumor.[227] The presence of nodal disease in conjunction with pelvic relapse portends a dismal outcome; other unfavorable clinical variables include nonsquamous histologies (particularly adenocarcinomas) and a higher FIGO stage at the time of diagnosis of the primary tumor.[228] Controversial factors include the interval between primary therapy and relapse and symptomatic versus asymptomatic pelvic failures.[172,228,229]

Radical hysterectomy

In rare, carefully selected patients initially treated with primary radiation therapy, radical hysterectomy for salvage may be a feasible alternative to exenterative surgery. Coleman et al.[230] reported 50 patients who underwent radical hysterectomy for persistent or recurrent disease after definitive radiation therapy. The 5- and 10-year survival rates were 72% and 60%, respectively. Severe complications were noted in 64% of patients, and 42% of patients had permanent complications. The authors concluded that radical hysterectomy was an alternative to exenteration in patients with small, centrally recurrent cervical cancer, but that it should be used only in carefully selected patients.[230]

Pelvic exenteration

Pelvic exenteration is a potentially curative procedure for patients who, following radiation therapy, have a central pelvic recurrence or a new primary tumor in the irradiated field.[231–233] Advances in surgical technique, anesthesia, and postoperative care have decreased intraoperative and postoperative complications, and thus have greatly reduced operative mortality.[224,232,233] Advances in ostomy appliances and care have given patients the opportunity to live a nearly normal life and to be able to meet their personal needs and responsibilities after surgery. The type of exenteration is determined by the anatomical site of the cancer (Figure 19).

Anterior exenteration

Anterior exenteration encompasses the removal of the uterus, adnexa, bladder, urethra, and vagina. Patients selected for this operation have cancers that are sufficiently anterior to allow clearance of the rectum and do not extend to involve the vaginal apex or the posterior vaginal wall. Vaginal reconstruction is performed as indicated.

Posterior exenteration

In posterior exenteration, the uterus, adnexa, anus, rectosigmoid colon, levator muscles, and vagina are removed. Many gynecologic oncologists leave a portion of the anterior vaginal wall

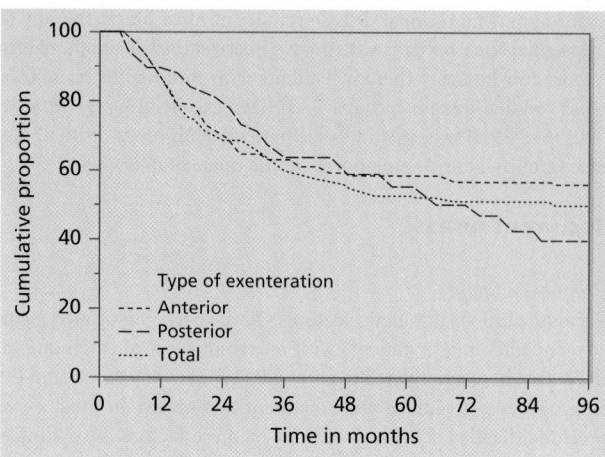

Figure 19 Survival curves are shown to compare the three types of exenterations performed in an MD Anderson series (1955–1984). Although the curves are similar, it should be noted that posterior exenteration is performed more frequently than the other procedures for vulvar and anorectal cancer and is associated with more local cancer recurrences. Source: Rutledge 1987.[231]

to support the urethra, and this can lessen postoperative urinary incontinence. This procedure is performed in patients with lesions confined to the posterior vaginal wall and rectovaginal septum.

Total pelvic exenteration

In total pelvic exenteration, the uterus, adnexa, bladder and urethra, vagina, rectosigmoid colon, levators, and anus are all removed. Patients treated with this procedure usually have lesions that are central or involve the upper half of the vagina. Contiguous extension to the base of the bladder and rectovaginal septum leaves no opportunity to perform a less extensive operation. Vaginal reconstruction is performed for functional purposes and to aid in the reconstruction of the pelvic floor. An omental pedicled graft is required to aid in reconstruction of the pelvic floor, and this technique for bringing in a new blood supply has been a major factor in reducing postoperative complications.[234] In both anterior and total pelvic exenteration, a continent urinary conduit can be constructed.

Total pelvic exenteration is widely used, and 5-year survival rates of 40–50% can be expected. At MD Anderson, a total of 448 exenterations were done from 1955 to 1984 and reported by Rutledge.[231] The 5-year survival rates for patients treated with exenteration are shown in Figure 19.

Radiation therapy

Patients who have an isolated pelvic recurrence after initially being treated with a radical hysterectomy should be treated with radical radiation therapy. A literature review by Lanciano found disease-free survival rates ranging from 20% to 50% following radiation therapy for locoregional failures. More favorable outcomes were reported in patients with small-volume disease and a central pelvic relapse location.[227] In most patients, treatment consisted of EBRT with or without brachytherapy. Patients who have isolated central recurrences without pelvic wall fixation or regional metastasis can be cured in up to 60–70% of cases.[229] The prognosis is much poorer when the pelvic wall is involved (usually 10–20% of patients survive 5 years after radiation therapy).

Treatment of stage IVB or recurrent disease

Chemotherapy

Single-agent chemotherapy

Using chemotherapy to treat metastatic or recurrent carcinoma of the cervix is relatively ineffective. Median survival ranges between 4 and 8 months. The most active single agents include cisplatin, paclitaxel, topotecan, vinorelbine, and ifosfamide. Cisplatin is regarded as the most active agent in cancer of the cervix. The response rate (RR) is 17–21%.[235,236] Doses used range from 50 to 100 mg/m^2. Bonomi and colleagues compared 50–100 mg/m^2 and noted that the higher dose was associated with a better partial RR (31% vs 21%) and a slightly better complete RR (13% vs 10%). Response duration, PFS, and survival measures failed to improve with the higher dose.[236] Carboplatin given at 340–400 mg/m^2 every 28 days to 175 patients induced a complete response in 10 (5.7%).[237] The total RR for carboplatin from a number of studies is 19%.

Paclitaxel has consistently demonstrated clinical activity, even in patients who received prior platin therapy with RRs of 17–31% and median survival of about 7 months, including those patients with nonsquamous histology. The other three—topotecan, vinorelbine, and ifosfamide[238–240]—have also shown substantial responses and are being used in combination therapy in phases II and III trials.

Combination chemotherapy

Nineteen single agents have activity against cervical cancer, defined as the ability to induce a 15% RR when used as a single-agent (Table 7), but survival rates have not been improved by adding other drugs to cisplatin. Numerous reports describe a higher RR with combination therapies accompanied by an increase in toxicity. Ifosfamide has received the most interest until recently. Several

Table 7 Single-agent chemotherapy for cervical cancer.

Agent	Response (%)
Alkylating agents	
Cyclophosphamide	38/251 (15)
Chlorambucil	11/44 (25)
Melphalan	4/20 (20)
Ifosfamide	35/157 (22)
Mitolactol	16/55 (29)
Heavy metal complexes	
Cisplatin	190/815 (23)
Carboplatin	27/175 (15)
Antitumor antibiotics	
Doxorubicin	45/266 (17)
Bleomycin	19/176 (11)
Mitomycin	5/23 (22)
Antimetabolites	
Fluorouracil	29/142 (20)
Methotrexate	17/96 (18)
Hydroxyurea	0/14 (0)
Plant alkaloids	
Vincristine	10/55 (18)
Vinblastine	2/20 (10)
Etoposide	0/31 (0)
Miscellaneous agents	
Altretamine	12/64 (19)
Irinotecan (CPT-11)	36/192 (19)
Paclitaxel	14/74 (19)
Docetaxel	1/13 (8)
Topotecan	8/43 (19)
Hexamethylmelamine	12/64 (19)
Razoxane	5/28 (18)

Source: Data from Refs 235–240.

small phase II studies evaluated treatment with combinations of ifosfamide and either cisplatin or carboplatin in patients who had not received radiotherapy. RRs for these combinations ranged between 50% and 62%.[241–244]

Combinations of cisplatin and continuous infusion 5-FU,[245–247] cisplatin and paclitaxel,[248,249] cisplatin and vinorelbine,[250] and cisplatin and gemcitabine[251,252] also produce high response in previously untreated patients. The combination of carboplatin and liposomal doxorubicin has shown modest activity in this clinical setting.[253] Again, RRs decrease significantly if patients have had previous irradiation.[246,252]

A GOG-randomized phase III trial reported that combining topotecan with cisplatin had a better RR than cisplatin alone.[254] The RR was 13% in the cisplatin arm and 27% in the combination arm. There was also an improvement in median survival by 3 months as well as a slight improvement in quality of life as determined by the functional assessment of cancer therapy-cervical (FACT-CX). They found the previous radiosensitizing chemotherapy and interval from diagnosis predicted for response. Response was more frequent in nonirradiated sites (70% vs 23%). This has led the GOG to their next prospective trial for primary stage IVB or recurrent/persistent carcinoma of the cervix. In this trial, patients were randomized between four arms: arm 1, paclitaxel and cisplatin (PC); arm 2, vinorelbine and cisplatin (VC); arm 3, gemcitabine and cisplatin (GC); and arm 4, topotecan and cisplatin (TC). This study was closed early due to futility. However, in 513 patients, VC, GC, or TC was not superior to PC in terms of OS, but the trend in RR, PFS, and OS favored PC.[255] In a separate report, health-related quality of life outcomes for this study showed no difference between the four arms except that PC had a higher rate of neuropathy, but the final conclusion was that PC should be the standard of care for recurrent or metastatic cervical cancer.[256]

Recently, however, a major step forward in the treatment of patients with recurrent or metastatic cervical cancer was achieved with the result of GOG 240, which randomly assigned patients to treatment with 1 of 2 chemotherapy regimens (cisplatin plus paclitaxel vs paclitaxel plus topotecan) and to bevacizumab versus no bevacizumab.[257] There was no difference in outcomes noted between the chemotherapy regimens. However, when compared with chemotherapy alone, the addition of bevacizumab significantly improved OS (17 months vs 13.3 months), PFS (8.2 months vs 5.9 months), and RR (48% vs 36%) without a significant deterioration in health-related quality of life.[258] Major treatment-related toxicities included fistula (3%), thromboembolism (8%), and easily managed hypertension (25%).[258] Since this publication, cisplatin-paclitaxel-bevacizumab triplet has been listed as Category 2A in the National comprehensive Cancer Network (NCCN) Clinical Practice Guidelines for Cervical Cancer.[259]

Despite the result of GOG 240, the prognosis of patients with recurrent or metastatic cervical cancer remains poor and represents an urgent unmet need worldwide. Therefore, better alternatives need to be explored including determining prognostic factors, administration of novel agents that may improve the therapeutic index of definitive chemoradiation and various immunotherapeutic approaches. Moore et al.[260] evaluated 428 patients enrolled in three GOG trials and determined 5 prognostic factors including race, performance status, pelvic disease, prior radiosensitizer, and time interval from diagnosis to the first recurrence <1 years, that may have utility in clinical practice to identify women who are not likely to respond to standard cisplatin-based regimens and that may benefit from investigational trials.

The rationale for immunotherapy in cervical cancer is based on the causative role of HPV infection in the disease. HPV infection invokes cellular immune response, and regulatory T cells appear to play a role in local immune suppression in HPV-associated tumors. New agents that interrupt the mechanisms involved in cancer immune evasion have soon promising results. Basu presented final results of a randomized phase II trial involving 110 women from India with recurrent/refractory cervical cancer who were randomized to receive live attenuated *Listeria monocytogenes* vaccine with or without cisplatin at the 2014 Annual Meeting of the American Society of Clinical Oncology.[261] The final 12-month OS was 36% and 18 month OS was 28%.[261] The overall RR was 11% and included 6 complete responders and 6 partial responders. [321]The addition of cisplatin did not significantly improve OS or RR.[261] These promising results have led to a trial in the United States using the same live-attenuated vaccine under the auspices of the NRG (GOG 265/NCT01266460).

Other pathways including regulatory pathways that limit the immune response to cancer including the upregulation of cytotoxic T lymphocyte-associated molecule-4 (CTLA-4) and PD-1 are increasing being well characterized. In addition, the role of adoptive immunotherapy using tumor-infiltrating lymphocytes represents another potential useful approach for patients with advanced or metastatic disease. In this technology, the tumor is excised and enriched for tumor-infiltrating lymphocytes, which are expanded after selection and reinfused to patients after lymphodepletion. On the basis of the responses noted in tumors such as malignant melanoma, this approach is being evaluated in an ongoing trial at the NCI for patients with recurrent or refractory metastatic cervical cancer (NCT01266460).

Signaling pathways affected by HPV are also an area where novel targeted drugs may be a benefit in the fight against cervical cancer. Genomic data have documented KRAS and P13KCA mutations and are now awaiting proof of concept by demonstration that these pathways are both turned on and necessary for the cervical cancer success. Endpoints including showing purposeful activations of MEK/ERK and AKT proliferation, invasion and survival pathways would provide justification for testing active agents targeting these pathways. Potential new agents include cetuximab, gefitinib, erlotinib, and selumetinib. Irradiation is a major cause of DNA damage. Therefore, inhibition of PARP provides another potential target for the treatment of cervical cancer. Two trials currently are being conducted among patients with cervical cancer through NRG (GOG 127W/NCT0101266447and GOG76HH/NCT01282852).

Summary

In patients with recurrent cervical cancer, it is important first to determine if the patient is a candidate for definitive surgery or radiation therapy. Five-year survival rates range from 20% to 50% if one of these therapies can be administered. Systemic chemotherapy can be used for treatment of both recurrent and metastatic disease, but careful attention should be paid to balancing benefit and toxicity. Further research is needed to determine the impact of chemotherapy on quality of life and the sensitivity to chemotherapy of patients who received prior chemotherapy as part of chemoradiation therapy as well as the importance of biological and immunotherapy agents. The key to success will be the transportation of success seen in the developing countries to success in areas of the world where advanced-stage invasive cervical cancer is most common.

Key references

The complete reference list can be found on the Wiley Companion Digital Edition of this title (see inside front cover for login instructions).

4 Coleman MP, Esteve J, Damiecki P, et al. Trends in cancer incidence and mortality. *IARC Sci Publ.* 1993;**121**:1–86.

7 Brinton LA. Epidemiology of cervical cancer—overview. In: Munoz FB, Bosch FX, Shah KV, Meheus A, eds. *The Epidemiology of Human Papillomavirus and Cervical Cancer.* Oxford (UK): Oxford University Press; 1992:3–23.

11 Munoz N, Bosch FX. Cervical cancer and papillomavirus: epidemiological evidence and perspective for prevention. *Salud Publica Mex.* 1997;**39**:274–282.

13 Bosch FX, Manos MM, Munoz N, et al. Prevalence of human papillomavirus in cervical cancer: a worldwide perspective. International biological study on cervical cancer (IBSCC) study group [comments]. *J Natl Cancer Inst.* 1995;**87**:796–802.

70 Cox JT, Lorincz AT, Schiffman MH, et al. Human papillomavirus testing by hybrid capture appears to be useful in triaging women with a cytologic diagnosis of atypical squamous cells of undetermined significance. *Am J Obstet Gynecol.* 1995;**172**:946–954.

74 US Food and Drug Administration. *Cobas HPV Test-P10020/S008.* Parsippany. NJ: US Food and Drug Administration; 2014. Accessdata.fda.gov/scripts/cdrh/cfdocs/cfTopic/pma/pma.cfm?num=P1000203008 (accessed 1 October 2014).

75 Cullen AP, Reid R, Campion M, et al. Analysis of the physical state of different human papillomavirus DNA's in intraepithelial and invasive cervical neoplasm. *J Virol.* 1999;**65**:606–612.

77 Mitchell MF, Tortolero-Luna G, Cook E, et al. A randomized clinical trial of cryotherapy, laser vaporization, and loop electrosurgical excision for treatment of squamous intraepithelial lesions of the cervix. *Obstet Gynecol.* 1998;**92**:737–744.

85 The HPV PATRICIA Study Group. Efficacy of a prophylactic adjuvanted bivalent L1 virus-like-particle vaccine against infection with human papillomavirus types 16 and 18 in young women: an interim analysis of a phase III double-blind, randomized controlled trial. *Lancet.* 2007;**369**:2161–2170.

87 Rogers LJ, Eva LJ, Luesley DM. Vaccines against cervical cancer. *Curr Opin Oncol.* 2008;**20**:570–574.

92 Piver MS, Chung WS. Prognostic significance of cervical lesion size and pelvic node metastases in cervical carcinoma. *Obstet Gynecol.* 1975;**46**:507–510.

93 Mitchell PA, Waggoner S, Rotmensch J, et al. Cervical cancer in the elderly treated with radiation therapy. *Gynecol Oncol.* 1998;**71**:291–298.

105 Grigsby PW, Siegel BA, Dehdashti F. Lymph node staging by positron emission tomography in patients with carcinoma of the cervix. *J Clin Oncol.* 2001;**19**:3745–3749.

117 Peters WAI, Liu PY, Barrett R, et al. Cisplatin, 5-fluorouracil plus radiation therapy are superior to radiation therapy as adjunctive therapy in high-risk, early-stage carcinoma of the cervix after radical hysterectomy and pelvic lymphadenectomy. Report of a phase III intergroup study. *Gynecol Oncol.* 1999;**72**:443.

152 Lecuru F, Mathevet P, Querleu D, et al. Bilateral negative sentinel nodes accurately predict absence of lymph node metastasis in early cervical cancer: results of the SENTICOL study. *J Clin Oncol.* 2011;**29**:1686–1691.

161 Lohe KJ, Burghardt E, Hillemanns HG, et al. Early squamous cell carcinoma of the uterine cervix. II. Clinical results of a cooperative study in the management of 419 patients with early stromal invasion and microcarcinoma. *Gynecol Oncol.* 1978;**6**:31–50.

185 Keys HM, Bundy BN, Stehman FB, et al. Cisplatin, radiation, and adjuvant hysterectomy for bulky stage IB cervical carcinoma. *N Engl J Med.* 1999;**340**:1154–1161.

186 Morris M, Eifel PJ, Lu J, et al. Pelvic radiation with concurrent chemotherapy compared with pelvic and paraaortic radiation for high-risk cervical cancer. *N Engl J Med.* 1999;**340**:1137–1143.

188 Rose PG, Bundy BN, Watkins J, et al. Concurrent cisplatin based chemotherapy and radiotherapy for locally advanced cervical cancer. *N Engl J Med.* 1999;**340**:1144–1153.

189 Whitney CW, Sause W, Bundy BN, et al. A randomized comparison of fluorouracil plus cisplatin versus hydroxyurea as an adjunct to radiation therapy in stages IIB–IVA carcinoma of the cervix with negative para-aortic lymph nodes: a Gynecologic Oncology Group and Southwest Oncology Group study. *J Clin Oncol.* 1999;**17**:1339–1348.

195 Delgado G, Bundy BN, Fowler WC, et al. A prospective surgical pathological study of stage I squamous carcinoma of the cervix: a Gynecologic Oncology Group study. *Gynecol Oncol.* 1989;**36**:314–320.

196 Sedlis A, Bundy BN, Rotman MZ, et al. A randomized trial of pelvic radiation therapy versus No further therapy in selected patients with stage IB carcinoma of the cervix after radical hysterectomy and pelvic lymphadenectomy: a Gynecologic Oncology Group study. *Gynecol Oncol.* 1999;**73**:177–183.

197 Rotman M, Sedlis A, Piedmonte MR, et al. A Phase III randomized trial of postoperative pelvic irradiation in stage IB cervical carcinoma with poor prognostic features: follow-up of a Gynecologic Oncology Group Study. *Int J Radiat Oncol Biol Phys.* 2006;**65**:169–176.

198 Sardi JE, Giaroli A, Sananes C, et al. Long-term follow-up of the first randomized trial using neoadjuvant chemotherapy in stage Ib squamous carcinoma of the cervix: the final results. *Gynecol Oncol.* 1997;**67**:61–69.

199 Eddy G, Bundy B, Creasman W, et al. Treatment of "bulky" stage IB cervical cancer with or without neoadjuvant vincristine and cisplatin prior to radical hysterectomy and pelvic/para-aortic lymphadenectomy: a phase III trial of the gynecologic oncology group. *Gynecol Oncol.* 2007;**106**:362–369.

200 Neoadjuvant Chemotherapy for Cervical Cancer Meta-Analysis Collaboration. Neoadjuvant chemotherapy locally advanced cervical cancer: a systematic review and meta-analysis of individual patient data from 21 randomised trials. *Eur J Cancer.* 2003;**39**:2470–2486.

201 Tierney JF, Vale C, Symonds P. Concomitant and neoadjuvant chemotherapy for cervical cancer. *Clin Oncol.* 2008;**20**:401–416.

202 Pearcey R, Brundage M, Drouin P, et al. Phase III trial comparing radical radiotherapy with and without cisplatin chemotherapy in patients with advanced squamous cell cancer of the cervix. *J Clin Oncol.* 2002;**20**:966–972.

204 Lorvidhaya V, Chitapanarux I, Sangruchi S, et al. Concurrent mitomycin C, 5-fluorouracil, and radiotherapy in the treatment of locally advanced carcinoma of the cervix: a randomized trial. *Int J Radiat Oncol Biol Phys.* 2003;**55**:1226–1232.

205 Monk BJ, Wang J, Im S, et al. Rethinking the use of radiation and chemotherapy after radical hysterectomy: a clinical-pathologic analysis of a Gynecologic Oncology Group/Southwest Oncology Group/Radiation Therapy Oncology Group Trial. *Gynecol Oncol.* 2005;**96**:721–728.

206 Eifel PJ, Winter K, Morris M, et al. Pelvic irradiation with concurrent chemotherapy versus pelvic and para-aortic irradiation for high-risk cervical cancer: an update of radiation therapy oncology group trial (RTOG) 90-01. *J Clin Oncol.* 2004;**22**:872–880.

207 Green JA, Kirwan JM, Tierney JF, et al. Survival and recurrence after concomitant chemotherapy and radiotherapy for cancer of the uterine cervix: a systematic review and meta-analysis. *Lancet.* 2001;**358**:781–786.

209 Duenas-Gonzalez A, ZarbaJJ PF, et al. Phase III, open label, randomized study comparing concurrent gemcitabine plus cisplatin and radiation followed by adjuvant gemcitabine and cisplatin versus concurrent cisplatin and radiation in patients with stage IIB to IVA carcinoma of the cervix. *J Clin Oncol.* 2011;**29**:1678–1685.

223 Varia MA, Bundy BN, Deppe G, et al. Cervical carcinoma metastatic to para-aortic nodes: extended field radiation therapy with concomitant 5-fluorouracil and cisplatin chemotherapy: a Gynecologic Oncology Group study. *Int J Radiat Oncol Biol Phys.* 1998;**42**:1015–1023.

227 Lanciano R. Radiotherapy for the treatment of locally recurrent cervical cancer. *J Natl Cancer Inst Monogr.* 1996;**21**:113–115.

231 Rutledge FN. Pelvic exenteration: an update of the U. T. M. D. Anderson Hospital experience and review of the literature. In: Rutledge FN, Freedman RS, Gershenson DM, eds. *Gynecologic Cancer: Diagnosis and Treatment Strategies.* Austin (TX): University of Texas Press; 1987:7.

254 Long HJ 3rd, Bundy BN, Grendys EC Jr, et al. Randomized phase III trial of cisplatin (P) vs cisplatin plus topotecan (T) vs MVAC in stage IVB, recurrent or persistent carcinoma of the uterine cervix: a Gynecologic Oncology Group study [abstract 9]. *Gynecol Oncol.* 2004;**92**:397.315.

255 Monk BJ, Sill MW, McMeekin DS, et al. Phase III trial of four cisplatin-containing doublet combinations in stage IVB, recurrent or persistent cervical carcinoma: a Gynecology Oncology Group study. *J Clin Oncol.* 2009;**27**:4649–4655.

256 Cella D, Huang HQ, Monk BJ, et al. Health-related quality of life outcomes associated with four cisplatin-based doublet chemotherapy regimens for stage IVB recurrent or persistent cervical cancer: a Gynecology Oncology Group study. *Gynecol Oncol.* 2010;**119**:531–537.

257 Tewari KS, Sill MW, Long HJ, et al. Improved survival with bevacizumab in advanced cervical cancer. *N Engl J Med.* 2014;**370**:734–743.

258 Penson RT, Huang HQ, Wenzel LB, et al. Bevacizumab for advanced cervical cancer: patient-reported outcomes of a randomized, phase 3 trial (NRG Oncology-Gynecologic Oncology Group protocol 240). *Lancet Oncol.* 2015;S1470–S2045.

259 NCCN (2014) Clinical Practice Guidelines in Oncology (NCCN guidelines). Cervical Cancer Version 1. NCCN.org.

260 Moore DH, Tian C, Monk BJ, et al. Prognostic factors for response to cisplatin-based chemotherapy in advanced cervical carcinoma: a Gynecologic Oncology Group study. *Gynecol Oncol.* 2010;**116**:44–49.

261 Basu P, Mehta AO, Jain MM, et al. ADXS11-001 immunotherapy targeting HPV-E7: final results from a phase 2 study in Indian women with recurrent cervical cancer. *J Clin Oncol.* 2014;**325s**(**suppl;abstr5610**).

103 Endometrial cancer

Jamal Rahaman, MD ▪ Karen Lu, MD ▪ Carmel J. Cohen, MD

Overview

Endometrial carcinoma is the most frequent gynecologic cancer in the United States with over 50,000 new cases diagnosed per year. Over 80% have Type I cancers with the classic estrogen-dependent endometrioid histology and a favorable prognosis. Type II cancers have a different molecular profile associated with more virulent disease and diminished survival and include uterine serous papillary carcinomas (UPSC) and clear cell carcinomas. The Cancer Genome Atlas (TCGA) has recently defined four molecular subtypes of endometrial cancer based on somatic mutations, copy number alterations, and microsatellite instability status. Over 75% of patients are present with irregular or postmenopausal bleeding. Surgical staging includes a total hysterectomy, bilateral salpingo-oophorectomy, and pelvic and para-aortic lymph node sampling, which can be performed via a laparotomy, laparoscopy, or robotic surgery. Surgery, where possible, constitutes the definitive primary treatment for most patients with endometrial carcinoma. Primary radiation therapy and primary hormonal therapy are alternatives for inoperable patients. Adjuvant therapy for Stage I disease is determined by age, depth of myometrial invasion, lymphovascular space invasion, and tumor grade. For patients with advanced and recurrent disease, radiation therapy, chemotherapy, and hormonal therapy are utilized. Paclitaxel (T), carboplatin (C), cisplatin (P), and doxorubicin (A) are the most active single agents with TC and TAP being the most effective combination of chemotherapy regimens. Hormonal therapy includes oral progestins, the progesterone-containing intrauterine device, tamoxifen, gonadotropin-releasing hormone analogs, and aromatase inhibitors. Emerging biologic agents with activity include bevacizumab and mTOR inhibitors. Tumor molecular profiling, minimal invasive surgery, sentinel lymph node assessment, and integration of novel biologic therapies will likely play a greater role in the future.

Epidemiology

In 2015, approximately 54,870 new cases of uterine corpus cancer will be diagnosed in the United States and 10,170 women will die from this cancer.[1] Since 1991, the death rate from endometrial cancer in the United States has exceeded that of cervical cancer, although cervical cancer is the most prevalent gynecologic cancer in less developed countries, causing the most gynecologic cancer deaths worldwide.[1,2] After declining between the mid-1980s and 1990, the incidence rates for endometrial cancer increased by about 0.6% per year from 1988 to 1999. Norway, Czechoslovakia, and other northern European countries also reported significant increases in the incidence of endometrial cancer. Despite an increase in incidence, early stage disease has an excellent prognosis.[2] Results from FIGO show that 85% to 91% of Stage I patients are alive at 5 years, and patients in the SEER database with localized disease have 96% 5-year survival.[2,3]

While black women have a lower incidence of endometrial carcinoma than white women, their mortality is higher.[1,4] Hicks and colleagues observed that black women were diagnosed with less favorable histologies, more advanced stages of disease, and more poorly-differentiated tumors than were white women.[4] Black women were treated surgically less frequently, and the surgically-treated patients with advanced-stage disease received adjuvant radiotherapy (RT) less often and chemotherapy more often than did white patients. Five-year survival was poorer for black women, even for those with stage I disease who were treated surgically.[1,4]

Risk factors

Risk factors include larger body size, obesity, diabetes, nulliparity, history of colon and/or breast carcinoma, ovulatory failure, increased endogenous estrogen exposure, and exposure to exogenous oral estrogens. Peripheral aromatization of estrogen precursors in body fat results in a higher level of circulating estrogen explaining, in part, the risk from obesity. Nulliparity, compared with multiparity of five or more births, menopause after age 53 years, and 50 pounds of excess weight are all important risk factors, increasing a woman's probability for endometrial cancer by 5–10 times compared with patients without these risk factors.

Pathologic conditions increasing the risk of endometrial cancer often include increased levels of endogenous estrogen or the requirements for exogenous estrogen supplementation.[5] Gusberg and Kardon reviewed the endometrial histology from 115 patients with theca-granulosa cell ovarian tumors and found that 21% developed endometrial carcinoma and 43% had precancerous hyperplasia.[5] Others have not found the same incidence of adenocarcinoma but have identified a high incidence of atypical hyperplasias.[6,7] Patients with polycystic ovary syndrome usually do not ovulate and, thus, are exposed to endogenous unopposed estrogen production. When endometrial carcinoma occurs in women younger than 45 years of age, it is often in patients with polycystic ovary syndrome[8,9] and is most frequently surrounded by atypical hyperplasia histologically. Finally, patients who are treated for ovarian dysgenesis by oophorectomy and unopposed estrogen replacement develop endometrial carcinoma in the residual uterus.[10] This association of continuous unopposed exposure to endogenous estrogens or exogenous oral estrogens and endometrial carcinoma has been widely reported.[11–19]

The Centers for Disease Control and Prevention reported that oral contraceptive use for at least 12 months diminished the risk of endometrial cancer by 50% compared with the risk for women who had never used oral contraception. Nulliparous women seemed to benefit most, and the protection lasted for a decade following the discontinuation of oral contraceptive use.[20] Brinton and Hoover's study observed that previous oral contraceptive use did not protect women from increased relative risk of endometrial cancer when they employed unopposed estrogen in postmenopausal hormone

Holland-Frei Cancer Medicine, Ninth Edition. Edited by Robert C. Bast Jr., Carlo M. Croce, William N. Hait, Waun Ki Hong, Donald W. Kufe, Martine Piccart-Gebhart, Raphael E. Pollock, Ralph R. Weichselbaum, Hongyang Wang, and James F. Holland.
© 2017 John Wiley & Sons, Inc. ISBN: 978-1-118-93469-2

replacement therapy, suggesting that the role of the progestogen in the combination oral contraceptive pills is essential in protecting against endometrial carcinoma.[12]

For more than 20 years, tamoxifen has been used to treat breast cancer, following the observation that it causes regression of metastatic tumor, diminishes the incidence of cancer in the contralateral breast, delays time to recurrence, and improves survival in subsets of patients.[21] Clinically, tamoxifen diminishes serum cholesterol, increases sex hormone-binding globulin,[22] preserves bone density in the lumbar spine,[23] thickens the vaginal epithelium in some patients,[23,24] and is associated with the enlargement of uterine fibroids, the growth of endometrial polyps, and the development of endometrial neoplastic change. These are all estrogen-like functions. Paradoxically, the same drug is associated with the production of vaginal atrophy, the onset of vasomotor symptoms, and the development of clinical dyspareunia. These are features of estrogen deprivation.

The action of tamoxifen may be organ specific, just as it is known to be species specific in its association with hepatic neoplasia in laboratory animals. When immortalized breast cancer and endometrial cancer cell lines were implanted in athymic mice, both cancers grew well in the same animal. When tamoxifen treatment was given, the breast cancers were inhibited and the endometrial cancers continued to grow.[25] Several investigators have described an increase in the incidence of endometrial cancers among patients with breast cancer who were treated with tamoxifen.[26-31] Killackey and colleagues were the first to report endometrial carcinoma occurring in three breast cancer patients receiving antiestrogens.[28] The strongest initial data implicating tamoxifen use in the subsequent development of endometrial carcinoma were reported by Fornander and colleagues, who reviewed the frequency of new primary cancers in the Swedish Cancer Registry for a group of 1,846 postmenopausal women with early breast cancer.[26] There was a 6.4-fold increase in the relative risk of endometrial cancer in the 931 tamoxifen-treated (40 mg/day) patients compared with controls. The National Surgical Adjuvant Breast and Bowel Project (NSABP) described observations on 3,863 patients studied prospectively.[27] In the B-14 protocol, 2,843 patients with node-negative, ER-positive breast cancer received either tamoxifen (20 mg/day) or placebo. An additional 1,020 patients taking tamoxifen were registered in this project. The relative risk calculated for the tamoxifen-treated group compared with the placebo group was 7.5, with an annual hazard rate of 0.2 per 1,000 for the placebo group and 1.6 per 1,000 for the randomized tamoxifen-treated group. More recently, in the Breast Cancer Prevention Trial (P-1) of the NSABP, 13,388 women were randomly assigned to receive placebo (6,707) or 20 mg/day of tamoxifen (6,681) for 5 years.[32] The rate of endometrial carcinoma was increased in the tamoxifen group (risk ratio = 2.53); this increase occurred primarily in women aged 50 years or older. All endometrial carcinomas in the tamoxifen group were stage I, and no endometrial cancer deaths have occurred in this group.

A prospective longitudinal study in Canada on 304 women with breast cancer receiving tamoxifen found that routine surveillance with ultrasonography was not useful in asymptomatic patients.[33] In another study, Barakat and colleagues evaluated 159 tamoxifen-treated patients by serial office endometrial biopsies obtained at the start of tamoxifen therapy and at 6-month intervals for 2 years, followed by three additional annual biopsies.[34] Although the procedure was feasible, significant pathology requiring hysterectomy was observed in only three patients, and the authors concluded that the utility of routine endometrial biopsy for screening in tamoxifen-treated women is limited. None of these studies provide strong support for screening with ultrasonography

Table 1 Clinical and molecular features of endometrial carcinoma.

Features	Type I	Type II
Clinical37		
Risk factors	Unopposed estrogen	Age
Race	White > black	White = black
Degree of differentiation	Well differentiated	Poorly differentiated
Histology	Endometrioid	Nonendometrioid
Stage	I/II	III/IV
Prognosis	Favorable	Unfavorable
Molecular		
K-ras overexpression	Yes	Yes
HER2/neu overexpression	No	Yes
TP53 overexpression	No	Yes
PTEN mutations	Yes	No
Microsatellite instability	Yes	No

or endometrial biopsy.[35] Prompt evaluation of any vaginal bleeding is mandated. However, clinicians should not be reluctant to obtain endometrial biopsies or vaginal ultrasound in patients with multiple risk factors.

In 1980, Bokhman first proposed the concept of a Type II endometrial cancer as distinct from the classic Type I estrogen-dependent endometrioid endometrial cancer. (Table 1). These women have a distinct phenotype and now are recognized to also have a different molecular profile associated with more virulent disease and diminished survival.[36,37] Type I cancers are associated more frequently with tamoxifen therapy and unopposed estrogen use.

Pathology

Endometrial hyperplasia

When Gusberg and colleagues introduced the term "adenomatous hyperplasia" to describe the pattern of hyperplastic glands noted in association with, and often prior to, the development of endometrial adenocarcinoma, they included all of the variants of precursor histology. These ranged from a mild arrangement of densely crowded glands with eosinophilic cytoplasm through the spectrum of more disordered arrangements, characterized by intraluminal tufting and an increase in mitosis, pseudopalisading, and bizarre nuclei.[38] Similarly, Hertig and Sommers studied preinvasive changes in the endometrium and described three intensities of abnormality which they called "adenomatous hyperplasia," "atypical hyperplasia," and "carcinoma in situ."[39] Kurman and colleagues followed 170 patients with endometrial hyperplasia for a minimum of 1 year; the mean follow-up time was 13.4 years.[40] They established criteria for distinguishing lesions on the basis of architectural abnormalities and cytologic abnormalities. Only 1.6% of patients without cytologic atypia progressed to cancer compared with 23% of those with atypical cytology. Architectural abnormalities were not prognostically important. Table 2 presents the details of Kurman and colleagues' classification and observations. Their classification of simple or complex hyperplasia, with or without atypia, is now accepted for describing these lesions.

Endometrioid adenocarcinoma

Endometrioid adenocarcinoma is the most common of the endometrial cancer histologies. It is characterized by the disappearance of stroma between abnormal glands that have infoldings of their linings into the lumens, disordered nuclear chromatin distribution,

Table 2 Comparison of follow-up of 170 patients with simple and complex hyperplasia and simple and complex atypical hyperplasia.

	No of patients	Regressed n (%)	Persisted n (%)	Progressed to carcinoma n (%)
Simple hyperplasia	93	74[41]	18[19]	1[1]
Complex hyperplasia	29	23[41]	5[17]	1[3]
Simple atypical hyperplasia	13	9[42]	3[23]	1[8]
Complex atypical hyperplasia	35	20[43]	5[14]	10[29]

Source: Adapted from Kurman et al. 1985.[40] Reproduced with permission from John Wiley and Sons.

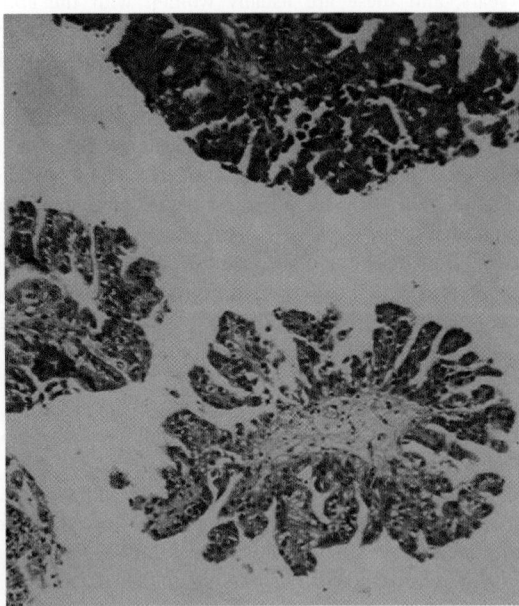

Figure 1 Uterine papillary serous carcinoma. Broad stalks supporting papillary fronds, appearing like papillary ovarian carcinoma. Courtesy of Diane Deligdisch, MD, Mount Sinai School of Medicine. A four-color version of the figure is available on the CD-ROM. a Correlation of the Federation Internationale de Gynecologie d'Obstetrique (FIGO), Unio Internationale Contre Cancrum (UICC), and American Joint Committee on Cancer (AJCC) nomenclatures.

nuclear enlargement, and a variable degree of mitosis, necrosis, and hemorrhage. This classic variety accounts for 80–95% of the adenocarcinomas.

Adenosquamous carcinoma

Adenosquamous cancer has malignant elements from both its squamous component and its adenomatous component. It usually accounts for 7% or less of the adenocarcinomas of the endometrium. It is suggested that adenosquamous cancer will not behave differently from endometrioid adenocarcinomas of the same stage and grade.

Uterine papillary serous carcinoma

Described by Hendrickson and colleagues in 1982, uterine papillary serous carcinoma (UPSC) comprises 5 to 10% of stage I endometrial carcinomas and is characterized by expansive papillary architecture with a fibrovascular matrix, marked cytologic atypia, bizarre nuclei, and widespread nuclear pleomorphism (Figure 1).[44,45] The features are suggestive of papillary serous cystadenocarcinoma of the ovary. The lesion is highly virulent, usually found with deep myometrial penetration at the time of diagnosis, often extrauterine in location in patients with clinical early-stage disease, and almost always incurable when the disease has spread beyond the uterus.[45–48]

Endometrial papillary adenocarcinoma

Endometrial papillary adenocarcinomas must be distinguished from UPSC because of their different behavior. Histologically, they are characterized usually as being well-differentiated endometrioid adenocarcinomas composed of very slender papillations, orderly neoplastic epithelial cells, few mitoses, and less cellular disorder than UPSC. The distinction between these two groups has been carefully detailed by Chen and colleagues.[49] The endometrial carcinomas with papillary features behave identically to the endometrioid adenocarcinomas.

Clear cell carcinoma

Kurman and Scully described clear cell cancers in detail.[50] Histologically, although there are a variety of patterns, a presentation of polygonal or flattened cells with clear cytoplasm accounts for more than half of the cells. This group constitutes approximately 6% of endometrial carcinomas and occurs more frequently in older women. The 5-year overall survival rate is approximately 40%,[51] but this may be a result of the older age of the patients and the fact that clear cell carcinomas are generally found in patients with higher stages of cancer. Clear cells often appear in histologic mixtures when tumors are assigned to a different category on the basis of the prevalent cell type, and their presence usually confers a diminished prognosis.[52]

Genomic alterations

The Cancer Genome Atlas (TCGA) has recently provided a comprehensive mapping of DNA, RNA and protein alterations in endometrioid and serous endometrial cancers.[53] In the decades leading up to the TCGA, individual genes and proteins had been implicated in the pathogenesis of endometrial cancer. Based on these molecular alterations, and clinical features, endometrial cancers have been classically divided into Type I and Type II (Table 1). Type I tumors include low to moderate grade endometrioid tumors and demonstrate high estrogen and progesterone receptor (PR) positivity and PTEN mutations. Type II tumors include high grade endometrioid and serous histologies and are characterized by a high mutational rate of TP53. This dual classification, while oversimplified, still holds some clinical utility.

The PI3K pathway is the most common dysregulated pathway in endometrial cancer, with mutations seen in multiple key members. Loss of PTEN (phosphate and tensin homolog deleted on chromosome 10) occurs in approximately 75–85% of tumors of the endometrioid histology[54] and results in unopposed activation of the PI3K pathway. Mutations account for the majority of PTEN loss, and may occur early in endometrial carcinogenesis. However, other mechanisms including gene methylation and destabilization of the protein may also contribute to PTEN loss. Mutations have also been found in other components of the PI3K pathway, including PIK3CA, PIK3R1 and AKT ().[55] A key downstream effector of the PI3K pathway is mTOR, which stimulates protein synthesis and entry into the G1 phase of the cell cycle. Therapies that target mTOR, AKT and PIK3CA are currently being tested in endometrial cancer patients with advanced and recurrent disease.

The Ras/Raf/MEK/ERK pathway is also frequently dysregulated in endometrial cancer. K-ras mutations occur in approximately 18–20% of endometrioid endometrial cancers. Mutations in the FGFR2 receptor tyrosine kinase occur in approximately 12% of endometrioid endometrial cancers, and do not co-occur with tumors that have K-ras mutations. Among early stage endometrioid endometrial cancer patients, K-ras mutations are associated with a more favorable prognosis and FGFR2 mutations are associated with a worse prognosis.[56] Therapies that target FGFR2 have shown limited efficacy.[57] Therapies that target the Ras/Raf/MEK/ERK pathway are currently being studied in combination with PI3K pathway inhibitors. ARID1A has been shown to be mutated in approximately 25% of low grade and 44% of high grade endometrioid cancers.[58] The WNT pathway is another important dysregulated pathway in endometrioid endometrial cancer, with beta-catenin or CTNNB1 mutations occurring in approximately 10–28% of cases.[59]

Microsatellite instability occurs in approximately 35% of endometrioid endometrial cancers.[56] The MSI phenotype results primarily from somatic silencing of MLH1 through promoter methylation. In a minority of cases, MSI results from germline mutations in the Lynch syndrome genes, including MLH1, MSH2, MSH6 or PMS2. MSI status has not been found to have prognostic significance in endometrioid endometrial cancer patients.

TP53 mutations occur in the majority of serous cancers. In addition to mutations, stabilization of the protein can also lead to p53 overexpression. Similar to high grade serous ovarian cancer, TP53 mutations occur early in the pathogenesis of uterine serous cancers. Other alterations that have been reported in uterine serous cancers include mutation in PPP2R1A, amplification and overexpression of ERBB2 or Her2/neu, mutations in FBXW7 and overexpression of cyclin E.[43,60–63]

Rather than through a single gene approach, the TCGA performed a large scale, integrated genomic analysis of both endometrioid and serous endometrial cancers.[53] Four molecular subtypes of endometrial cancer were defined, based on somatic mutations, copy number alterations, and microsatellite instability status. These four groups are: (1) POLE ultramutated; (2) hypermutated/microsatellite unstable; (3) copy number low/microsatellite stable, and (4) copy number high (serous-like). The first group, called POLE "ultramutated" tumors, includes the clinically most favorable tumors with endometrioid histology. POLE refers to DNA polymerase epsilon, which is involved in DNA replication and harbors numerous hotspot mutations in tumors in this category. There are few copy number abnormalities in tumors of the POLE subtype, but a very high number of mutations. Mutations in PTEN, PIK3R1, PIK3CA, and KRAS are common. The second group, called MSI "hypermutated" tumors, includes endometrioid tumors with microsatellite instability due to MLH1 promoter methylation, few copy number abnormalities, and mutation rates lower than the "ultramutated" POLE group but higher than the copy number low/MSS group. Mutations in KRAS and PTEN are frequent. The third group is the copy number low/MSS group which has PTEN and PIK3CA mutations, but is characterized by frequent beta catenin mutations. The fourth group is the copy number high (serous-like) tumors with extensive copy number abnormalities. In addition to most of the serous tumors, approximately one quarter of the grade 3 endometrioid patients fall in this category. Validation of these four subtypes is needed, as is defining its clinical utility. Another classification of endometrioid endometrial cancers has also been proposed, also based on TCGA gene expression data. In

this classification, presence of beta catenin mutations in low grade endometrioid tumors was associated with a poor prognosis.[64] Our ultimate goal is to integrate known clinical and pathologic features with molecular data to develop a useful classification to better guide patient care.

Diagnosis

The median age for patients with adenocarcinoma of the endometrium is 61 years, with the highest prevalence during the sixth decade. Only 5% develop adenocarcinomas before the age of 40 years, and these are usually women with the abnormal syndromes discussed previously. Eighty percent of patients are post-menopausal. Irregular or postmenopausal bleeding is the presenting symptom in at least 75% of patients, and at the time of diagnosis, 75% of patients have disease confined to the uterus. Thus, it is obvious that irregular bleeding is a critical symptom, and by explaining it histologically, one has an opportunity to identify endometrial cancer when it is highly curable by relatively uncomplicated therapy.

The traditional technique for diagnosis has been fractional dilation and curettage of the uterus, with careful sampling of both the endometrial cavity and the endocervical canal. Once a procedure for the hospital operating room, this is now performed as an office procedure with greater than 95% accuracy.[65,66] There will always be patients who require general anesthesia in a hospital setting, however, either because of very low pain thresholds, cervical stenosis, or other intercurrent ailments.

Hysteroscopy, either by direct observation or with video-camera amplification, allows direct assessment of the topography of the endometrial cavity with the possibility for more selective sampling and the assurance of not missing any occult lesions. Many reserve this procedure as an accompaniment to formal dilation and curettage under anesthesia. However, caution should be exercised because hysteroscopic dissemination of malignant cells has been described in the literature.[67,68]

Imaging

Noninvasive radiographic imaging techniques, such as magnetic resonance imaging[69] and ultrasonography,[70] are not cost-effective for screening. For diagnosis and documenting recurrence, these techniques and CT scan and PET scan can achieve an accuracy rate above 80%.[42,71–76]

Staging

Historically, endometrial cancer staging was a clinical exercise, based on physical examination, noninvasive radiographic testing, and measurement of the depth of the uterine cavity. In 1988, the International Federation of Gynecology and Obstetrics (FIGO) introduced the requirement for surgical staging of patients with endometrial carcinoma following the GOG 33 study that demonstrated that 9.6% of 843 patients in clinical stage I had lymph node metastasis on comprehensive surgical staging.[77–80]

In 2009, FIGO updated the surgical staging classification for endometrial cancers as indicated in Table 2.[41] In addition, in 2009 uterine carcinosarcomas were to continue to be staged using the 2009 FIGO staging for endometrial cancer and new specific Staging Classifications were developed for leiomyosarcomas, endometrial stromal sarcomas and uterine adenosarcomas (Table 3).

Surgical staging requires the performance of total hysterectomy, bilateral salpingo-oophorectomy, and washings for cytologic examination. Lymph node sampling from the pelvic and para-aortic lymph nodes is preferred for those patients whose cancers are other than well-differentiated with greater than minimal myometrial

Table 3 Staging—endometrial carcinoma.

TNM categories	FIGO[a] stages	Definition
Primary tumor (T)		
TX		Primary tumor cannot be assessed
T0		No evidence of Primary Tumor
Tis[b]		Carcinoma in situ (preinvasive carcinoma)
T1	I	Tumor confined to the corpus uteri
T1a	IA	Tumor limited to the endometrium or invades less than one-half of the myometrium
T1b	IB	Tumor invades one-half or more of the myometrium
T2	II	Tumor invades stromal connective tissue of the cervix but does not extend beyond the uterus[c]
T3a	IIIA	Tumor involves serosa and/or adnexa (direct extension or metastasis)[d]
T3b	IIIB	Vaginal involvement (direct extension or metastasis) or parametrial involvement[d]
	IIIC	Metastasis to pelvic and/or para-aortic lymph nodes[d]
T4	IVA	Tumor invades bladder mucosa and/or bowel (bullous edema is not sufficient to classify a tumor as T4)
Regional Lymph Nodes (N)		
NX		Regional lymph nodes cannot be assessed
N0		No regional lymph node metastasis
N1	IIIC1	Regional lymph node metastasis to pelvic lymph nodes (positive pelvic nodes)
N2	IIIC2	Regional lymph node metastasis to para-aortic lymph nodes, with or without positive pelvic lymph nodes
Distant Metastasis (M)		
M0		No distant metastasis
M1	IVB	Distant metastasis (includes metastasis to inguinal lymph nodes, intra-peritoneal disease or lung, liver or bone. It excludes metastasis to para-aortic lymph nodes, vagina, pelvic serosa or adnexa)

[a]Either G1, G2, or G3.
[b]Note: FIGO no longer includes Stage 0 (Tis).
[c]Endocervical glandular involvement only should be considered as Stage I and no longer as Stage II.
[d]Positive cytology has to be reported separately without changing the stage.
Data from Pecorelli 2009[41] and Edge 2010.[81]

penetration. While the tradition has been to perform this surgery abdominally (typically through a vertical midline incision), minimally invasive techniques have increasingly been integrated into the forefront with conventional or robotic-assisted laparoscopy.[82] There has been investigational assessment of the role of sentinel lymph node identification with colorimetric and fluorescent imaging to minimize the impact of extensive lymph node dissection.[83,84]

Initially, the adoption of a surgical staging system created controversy regarding what constitutes an adequate staging procedure, which patients should be surgically staged, and whether extensive staging or lymphadenectomy has therapeutic value.[79]

Prognostic factors

Several factors have been identified in large prospective surgical-pathologic staging studies conducted by the GOG[77,80] that are predictive of extrauterine spread of disease at the time of initial diagnosis and ultimate survival. Surgical stage and age are highly-significant prognostic features that maintain their significance in each of the analyses performed in the various reports.

Histologic type

Whereas 80–95% of endometrial cancers are classic endometrioid adenocarcinomas, the remainder constitute a series of histologic types with a more unfavorable prognosis. These include serous papillary adenocarcinoma and clear cell, undifferentiated, and squamous cancers. These cell types confer an unfavorable prognosis independent of other known prognostic factors (Table 1).[85]

Tumor grade

Within classic endometrioid adenocarcinomas, tumor grade is highly significant as an independent prognostic factor (Table 4). In addition, numerous studies have demonstrated that, in general, there is a greater tendency for the less differentiated tumors to be associated with other poor prognostic factors, including deep

Table 4 Histopathology: degree of differentiation.

G1:	5% or less of a nonsquamous or nonmorular solid growth pattern.
G2:	6% to 50% of a nonsquamous or nonmorular solid growth pattern.
G3:	More than 50% of a nonsquamous or non-morular solid growth pattern.

myometrial penetration, vascular space invasion, and increasing stage.[80,86,87] Salvesen and colleagues showed that morphometric nuclear grade was a stronger prognostic factor than subjective histologic grade.[88]

Myometrial invasion

The depth of myometrial penetration is a very important independent prognostic factor for outcome in stage I disease. Deeper penetration is associated with higher probabilities of tumor recurrence and death.[80,86,89] Although increasing depth of invasion correlates with increasing grade of tumor, depth appears to be a more significant prognostic factor and predicts for the presence of extrauterine disease as detected at surgical staging procedures.[77] Regardless of grade, however, only 1% of patients with disease confined to the endometrium have extrauterine disease compared with patients with deep muscle invasion, for which the incidence of pelvic node invasion rises to 25% and para-aortic nodal involvement rises to 17%.[77] DiSaia and colleagues found that patients with only endometrial involvement had an 8% recurrence rate compared with 12% if there was superficial or intermediate myometrial invasion versus 46% if there was involvement of the outer third of the myometrium.[89]

Capillary lymphatic space invasion

Vascular space invasion is a significant risk factor for recurrence, but it is not as important as the grade and depth of myometrial penetration. Approximately 15% of endometrial adenocarcinomas have capillary-like space invasion and is associated with a five-fold increase rate of positive pelvic (27%) and para-aortic lymph (19%) node involvement.[77,90]

Positive peritoneal cytology

Positive peritoneal cytology as the sole upstaging factor was dropped in the 2009 FIGO staging revisions as a stage-defining characteristic.[41] The presence of positive peritoneal cytology in washings is associated with an increased risk of relapse.[80] Approximately 15% of patients have positive peritoneal cytology[80] and this is often related to other poor prognostic factors, such as high grade or deep myometrial penetration. Thus, it is not surprising that it is also associated with an increased risk of metastases to pelvic (25%) and paraaortic (19%) lymph nodes. Opinions and data in the literature conflict with respect to interpreting the independent prognostic significance of peritoneal cytology. Approximately 5% of patients with positive peritoneal cytology have no evidence of extrauterine disease,[77] but approximately one-third of patients with extrauterine disease do have positive cytology. In a review of the literature, Wethington categorized patients into groups based on low-risk uterine features (grade 1–2, <50% depth of invasion, no lymphovascular space invasion) with positive peritoneal cytology. In this group, positive cytology occurred in 11% of cases and had a recurrence rate of 4%. Patients with higher-risk features plus positive cytology had a 32% risk of recurrence.[91]

Race

Liu and colleagues reviewed the treatment patterns, risk factors, and survival of 219 patients treated surgically for endometrial cancer between 1990 and 1993.[92] In this study, black women, when compared with white women, had a higher incidence of unfavorable histology (38% vs 12%), advanced-stage disease (51% vs 19%), poor differentiation (49% vs 18%), and poor survival.

Hormone receptor status

The presence of cytoplasmic ER- and PR- binding proteins has been quantitatively associated with better histologic differentiation,[93] favorable histologic subtype, and response to therapy.[94–96] Ligand binding to ER and PR was higher in well-differentiated lesions and was significantly lower in grade 3 lesions and the nonendometrioid carcinomas.[96] Alterations in receptor expression, receptor assembly and activation, response element recognition, and/or receptor degradation are among the possible explanations for loss of hormone binding. In addition, recent evidence suggests that promoter site hypermethylation might account in part for the loss of ER.[97] Likewise, differential expression of the PR-alpha (PRA) and PR-beta (PRB) have been reported.[98] PRA appears to down-regulate ER action and PRB is the primary activator of the progesterone responsive gene, and the loss of either would theoretically result in an unopposed estrogen effect. Clinically, reduced levels of ligand interaction with the ER, PR or both in endometrial cancer samples significantly (p < .01) correlate with recurrence and death from disease.[95,96]

Treatment of primary disease

Surgery

The initial surgical staging procedure, outlined earlier (see Figure 2), is the standard therapeutic procedure as well. When there is disease outside the uterus and in the retroperitoneal nodes, there is no reason to believe that aggressive cytoreductive efforts might not help

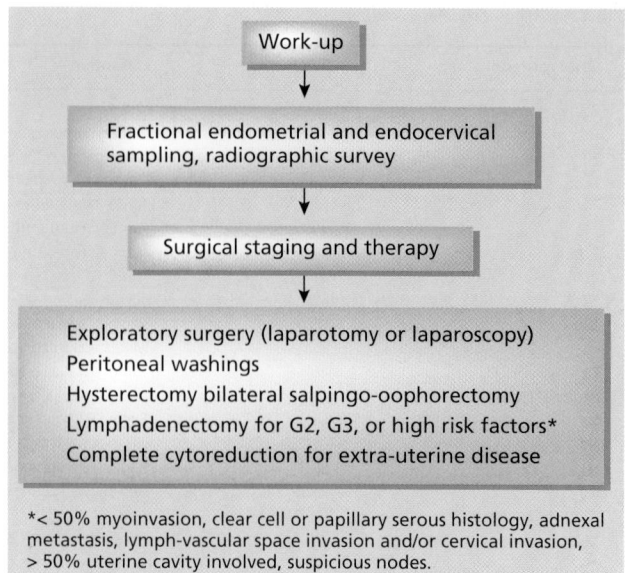

Figure 2 Surgical management of endometrial carcinoma.

in presenting a reduced tumor burden during adjunctive therapy, despite the absence of a clinical trial suggesting efficacy.

There are occasions when, at the time of staging laparotomy, cervical or parametrial invasion is detected and a radical (Wertheim) hysterectomy with pelvic and aortic lymphadenectomy is performed to achieve clearance of all disease. However, the addition of tailored external beam RT following surgery has largely eliminated the routine performance of such procedures.[99]

Surgery for recurrent disease is generally confined to those patients who have symptoms of intestinal or urinary tract obstruction, isolated regional recurrence, or isolated lung metastases that have not responded to cytotoxic or hormonal therapy. For such patients, surgery may be useful to correct functional deficits or to excise isolated recurrences or resistant metastatic deposits.

After several years of debate and discussion, minimally invasive techniques have been integrated into the management of endometrial cancer as a standard of care.[100] Techniques utilized in the initial treatment of endometrial cancer include laparoscopic assisted vaginal hysterectomy (LAVH),[101–105] total laparoscopic hysterectomy (TLH),[106–108] and robotic hysterectomy[82] with pelvic and paraaortic nodal dissection to stage patients. Minimally invasive staging techniques include transperitoneal and extraperitoneal assessment of nodes,and may be done at the time of hysterectomy or at a later time to re-stage patients following incomplete surgical staging. Robotic surgery may represent the next step forward in minimally invasive surgery. Since FDA approval for hysterectomy and myomectomy procedures in 2005, there has been an increasing utilization of robotic surgery within gynecologic oncology.[82,109–113]

The role of Sentinel Lymph Node (SLN) mapping for endometrial cancer staging is currently being evaluated, however, there is no randomized trial reported yet. According to current NCCN guidelines, SLN may be considered (category 3) during surgical staging of apparent uterine confined cancer when there is no metastasis demonstrated by imaging studies and no obvious disease at exploration. The expertise of the surgeon and attention to technical detail is critical.[83,84,114]

Radiation therapy (RT)

Although surgery, where possible, constitutes the definitive primary treatment for most patients with endometrial carcinoma, it is clear that RT is the second most effective modality in its management.

Definitive irradiation for inoperable patients

Modern surgical techniques and improved postoperative care have diminished the number of patients considered inoperable. Nevertheless, because endometrial cancer is frequently a disease of the elderly (over 65 years of age), who are often obese and sometimes diabetic with other co-morbidities, surgery is not always possible. Several relatively large series have demonstrated pelvic RT as effective definitive management of endometrial cancer without initial surgery.[115-119]

The proportion surviving depends on tumor grade, just as for patients treated surgically; those with grade 1 tumors have better survival rates than do those with grade 3.[115] Significant numbers of patients die of causes unrelated to their primary carcinoma.[119] Inoperable patients who did not die from comorbidities had a median 5-year survival rate that approached that of operable patients.[119]

Some patients with small uteri may be cured by intracavitary radiation only, but usually, definitive management consists of both external beam and intracavitary irradiation because of more favorable radiation dosimetry. Complication rates are acceptable (usually less than 10%). After definitive irradiation, the pattern of failure in contrast to that following surgery, consists mainly of central failure in the uterus. This observation is important for developing treatment strategies for patients with stage II disease. Removal of the uterus at some point in treatment provides better overall central control than that achieved by radiation alone. Three series indicate 5-year survival rates of approximately 50% for patients with Stage II disease who received RT as definitive therapy.[99,115,120,121]

Kucera and colleagues reported their experience with high-dose iridium-192 intracavitary brachytherapy without additional external beam radiation in 228 patients.[122] At 5 years, the overall survival rate was 59.7%. In clinical stage IA disease, the survival rate was 88.6% at 5 years and 82.7% at 10 years—significantly different in comparison with 80.2% and 63.4%, respectively, in stage IB disease. Others have also reported high–dose-rate brachytherapy with or without external beam radiation,[123,124] and the American Brachytherapy Society published guidelines and recommendations.[124,125]

Adjuvant RT for stage I disease

The present recommendation to give postoperative RT in surgical stage I is dependent on prognosis as defined by the histologic features of the primary tumor within the endometrium. Extensive staging studies have identified that several of the aforementioned factors predict for the presence of clinically occult extrauterine disease.[80]

Although patients considered to be at high risk of recurrence (e.g., those with grade 2 or 3 disease with penetration of the outer 50% of the myometrium) have generally been treated with postoperative adjuvant RT, there is only one randomized trial addressing the benefit of adjuvant RT in surgically staged patients (GOG-99).[126] There are three randomized clinical trials in patients who had incomplete surgical staging (Aalders,[86] Portec-1,[127] and Portec-2[128]).

The GOG-99 study stratified risk and validated pelvic radiation therapy (RT) for improved recurrence free survival in the high intermediate risk (HIR) group. The HIR subgroup of patients was defined (as an increased recurrence rate of 25% at 5 years based on GOG 33) as those with[1] moderately to poorly differentiated tumor, the presence of lymphovascular invasion, and outer third myometrial invasion;[2] age 50 years or greater with any two of the risk factors listed

above; or[3] age of at least 70 years with any risk factor listed above. The treatment difference was particularly evident among the HIR subgroup (2-year cumulative incidence of recurrence in NAT vs RT: 26% vs 6%; RH = 0.42). Overall, radiation had a substantial impact on pelvic and vaginal recurrences (18 in NAT and 3 in RT),[126] but did not achieve a significant difference in overall survival.

Vault irradiation

On a theoretic basis, the patient who undergoes thorough staging, ideally with a bilateral pelvic and lower para-aortic lymphadenectomy, might be at low risk of a pelvic side wall recurrence in the absence of lymph node metastasis. Other occult pelvic side wall disease not found at surgery, such as in the lymphatic channels in the parametrium or in parametrial lymph nodes, occurs infrequently and is an unlikely source of recurrence. The major site for possible recurrence within the pelvis for these patients would be the vaginal vault, which is amenable to brachytherapy with a lower morbidity.[129,130] There are several retrospective studies which have demonstrated rare pelvic recurrences in high-risk patients (stage IB, grade 3 and stage IC) who undergo therapeutic pelvic lymphadenectomy and either no RT[131,132] or vault brachytherapy[132] alone in the absence of lymph node metastasis.[130,133-137] In addition the prospective data from PORTEC-2 supports this hypothesis for vaginal brachytherapy alone in unstaged patients with HIR features by the PORTEC definition (where intermediate risk factors were outer-half invasion, grade 3, or greater than 60 years of age, but excluded deeply invasive high-grade tumors, and where patients were deemed HIR with two of the three factors). At a median follow-up of 45 months, the estimated 5-year vaginal recurrence rates were 1.8% for brachytherapy alone and 1.6% for external irradiation. The nodal failure rate was significantly different at 3.8% for the brachytherapy-alone arm and 0.5% for external beam irradiation. Distant metastases, disease-free survival, and OS were similar in both arms.[128]

Stage III

The 2009 FIGO surgical staging for endometrial cancer includes patients with metastases to pelvic and/or para-aortic lymph nodes as stage IIIC. The current staging classification covers a broad spectrum of prognostic groups that have diverse outcomes after standard surgery with or without adjuvant pelvic irradiation. Unfortunately, many of the published series include patients with microscopic extension to the adnexa (stage IIIA), those with malignant ascites (stage IIIA), and those with gross pelvic side wall disease (stage IIIA or IIIC) without distinction, resulting in widely variable survival data.

Treatment recommendations at this time for patients with stage III disease must be made on an individual basis. Those in whom appropriate surgical staging has been completed without evidence of disease beyond the ovaries should be considered for adjuvant postoperative pelvic irradiation, although the importance of microscopic adnexal invasion in patients without other risk factors is unclear. For those who have had surgical staging and who have pelvic but not para-aortic nodal involvement, it may be appropriate to offer postoperative adjuvant irradiation confined to the pelvis. Disease-free survival rates between 35% and 60% have been reported for patients receiving 45–50 Gy of external beam irradiation to the paraaortic nodes, usually with pelvic irradiation. In almost no case is macroscopic para-aortic nodal disease curable with RT without complete cytoreduction first.[65,70,80,138-148] Retrospective data from Johns Hopkins Hospital suggest that in patients with stage IIIC endometrial carcinoma, complete resection of macroscopic nodal disease and the administration of adjuvant

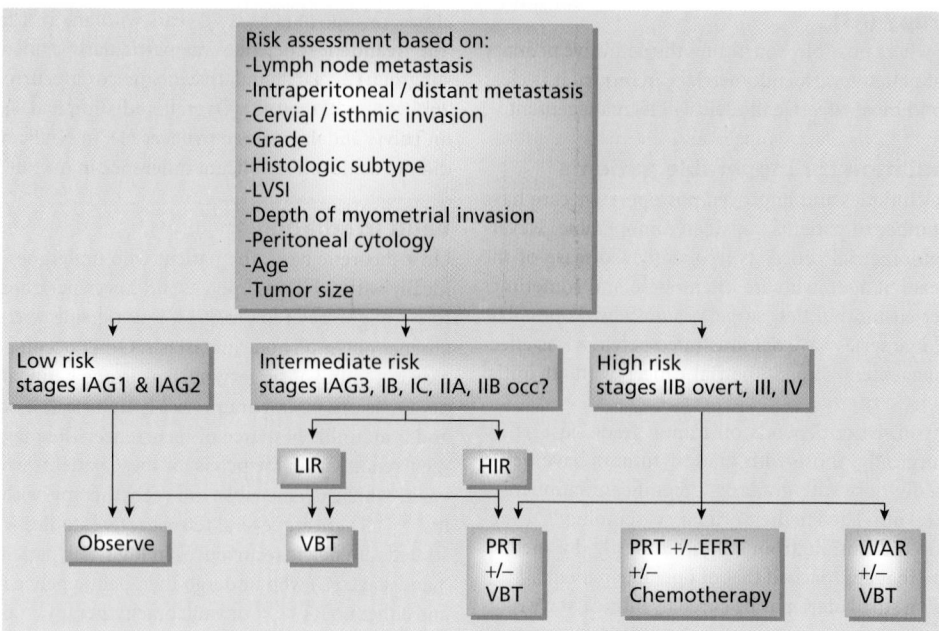

Figure 3 Postoperative management of endometrial carcinoma. EFRT = extended field radiation therapy; PRT = pelvic radiation therapy; VBT = vaginal brachytherapy; WAR = whole abdominopelvic radiotherapy; LIR = low intermediate risk; HIR = high intermediate risk based on Gynecologic Oncology Group 99: age <50, 50–70, >70, LVSI = lymph–vascular space invasion, outer third invasion, grade 2 or 3 (see text).

chemotherapy, in addition to directed RT, are associated with improved survival (Figure 3).[149]

Some subsets of Stage III endometrial cancer patients may be candidates for cytotoxic chemotherapy with or without RT and two Phase III trials are currently evaluating this concept (GOG 258 and Portec 3).

Adjuvant chemotherapy for high risk early stage disease

Stringer et al[150] studied 31 patients with high risk stage I endometrial cancer and 2 patients with occult stage II disease. Postoperatively, the patients were treated with cisplatin, 50 mg/m2, doxorubicin, 50 mg/m2, and cyclophosphamide, 500 mg/m2, (CAP) every 4 weeks for six cycles. The 2-year progression-free interval rate was 79%, and the 2-year survival was 83%. The median survival time for patients was not reached at 45 months. These results were considered superior to those of historical controls from the same institution.

The GOG randomized patients with high risk clinical stage I and stage II disease to postoperative whole-pelvis irradiation with or without doxorubicin and found no difference in PFI and OS.[151]

The Japanese GOG was designed to address the relative efficacy of CAP chemotherapy versus WPRT in Stage IC to III. Although there was no difference in PFS or OS in the entire cohort, a subgroup analysis of 120 HIR patients reported improved PFR and OS.[152]

GOG 249 is the phase III trial that examined vaginal cuff brachytherapy followed by three cycles of Paclitaxil / carboplatin (TC) chemotherapy versus external beam RT in patients with high risk uterine confined endometrial carcinoma. The preliminary results presented at SGO 2014 suggest no significant difference in survival outcomes between the groups.

In a study of 74 patients with Stage I UPSC, Kelly et al have demonstrated that all patients with residual disease (including disease confined to the endometrium) have improved PRI and OS with adjuvant platinum based chemotherapy. There were no vaginal recurrences in those receiving vaginal brachytherapy.[45,153] Because clear cell carcinoma behaves like UPSC, despite the absence of data they should be treated in a similar fashion with TC chemotherapy and vaginal brachytherapy.[45,52]

Treatment of recurrent disease

Radiotherapy
Patients who develop isolated vaginal recurrences without previous radiation can expect a salvage rate of 80% with RT.[154] Those who develop a component of extra pelvic recurrence will require systemic therapy.

In the patient who has had initial adjuvant postoperative pelvic irradiation, there may rarely be a role for interstitial therapy at relapse if there is isolated central pelvic failure. For some, systemic therapy may be applicable. For patients with other sites of disease or bony, cerebral, or nodal metastases, short courses of palliative irradiation may be useful in relieving the symptoms of disease. Similarly, palliative irradiation may be used for the uncommon patient (approximately 3% of those at presentation) who has stage IV disease.

Surgery
Unlike ovarian carcinoma, little is known regarding the role of secondary cytoreduction in recurrent endometrial carcinoma.[155] In a report from an Italian group, 20 women with recurrent endometrial adenocarcinoma were treated with maximal cytoreductive surgery.[156] Sixty-five percent of patients had complete resection of their tumor. Women with no residual tumor had a significantly increased progression-free and overall survival compared with women with residual tumor; however, there was a 10% perioperative death rate in this series. The role of pelvic exenteration was examined in a four-institution retrospective review of 31 patients.[157] Twenty patients underwent exenteration with curative intent, all of whom had received pelvic irradiation previously. The 5-year disease-free survival rate was 45%.

Cytotoxic chemotherapy

Cytotoxic chemotherapy for patients with endometrial cancer was rarely administered before 1980. In his 1974 literature review, Donovan reported only 126 patients who had been treated with 16 different agents.[158] In 1977, Muggia and colleagues reported that doxorubicin (Adriamycin, 37.5 mg/m2) in combination with cyclophosphamide (500 mg/m2) intravenously (IV) every 21 days in 11 patients with recurrent endometrial cancer resulted in five objective responses.[159] The GOG studied single-agent doxorubicin at a dose rate of 60 mg/m2 IV every 3 weeks and reported a 37% response rate in 43 patients.[160] Although the most frequent adverse effect was on the hematopoietic system, cardiac toxicity occurred in 12%, and there was one cardiotoxic death in a patient who had received more than 500 mg/m2 of drug. This study was important because it clearly established the value of doxorubicin as a single agent in the chemotherapy of endometrial cancer. Studies by GOG and The Eastern Cooperative Oncology Group demonstrated no benefit from adding cyclophosphamide (Table 6).[175,176]

The GOG found no efficacy for cisplatin alone in heavily-pretreated patients[177]; however, Trope observed four responses (36%) in 11 chemotherapy-naive patients given cisplatin, 50 mg/m2.[178]

A combination of cisplatin and doxorubicin in advanced or recurrent endometrial cancer produced response rates of 33–80%, depending on the proportion of patients treated previously with either chemotherapy or radiation.[146,147]

If one selects only drugs that have achieved at least a 20% response rate in studies including at least 20 patients, the list is small (Table 5). Paclitaxel is an active drug in recurrent endometrial adenocarcinoma. The GOG studied paclitaxel in patients with advanced or recurrent adenocarcinoma of the endometrium.[144] Among 28 evaluable patients, four complete responses and six partial responses were observed, for an overall response rate of 35.7%. Similarly, Lissoni and colleagues evaluated paclitaxel in 19 patients with advanced endometrial adenocarcinoma previously treated with cisplatin, doxorubicin, and cyclophosphamide.[145] Two complete responses and five partial responses were achieved, for an overall response rate of 37%.

Our best information on combination chemotherapy comes from the randomized phase III trials listed in Table 6. The randomized trials that have included hormonal therapy are listed in Table 7.

Table 6 lists the randomized trials that compared single agents with one or two different combinations. In the European Organisation for Research and Treatment of Cancer (EORTC) study reported by van Wijk and colleagues, a survival advantage was demonstrated with a response rate of 43% for the doxorubicin and

cisplatin combination versus 17% for single-agent doxorubicin (p < 0.001).[148] The GOG found no difference when doxorubicin and cisplatin were administered in a circadian fashion compared with a standard fashion.[179]

The GOG also conducted a phase III study of doxorubicin plus cisplatin versus doxorubicin plus 24-hour paclitaxel in primary stage III or IV or recurrent endometrial carcinoma. This study found no difference in response rate, progression-free survival, or overall survival.[180]

The next phase III prospective randomized GOG study (Protocol 177) compared standard doxorubicin (60 mg/m2) and cisplatin (50 mg/m2), that is, AP against TAP (Taxol 160 mg/m2/3 h), doxorubicin (45 mg/m2), and cisplatin (50 mg/m2).[181] Two hundred sixty-six patients were randomized, and the results indicated that TAP produced a significant improvement in response rate (57% vs 34%; p < 0.01), progression-free survival (median 8.3 vs 5.3 months; p < 0.01) and overall survival (median 15.3 vs 12.3 months; p = 0.037). Neurologic toxicity was worse for those receiving TAP, with 12% grade 3 and 27% grade 2 peripheral neuropathy.

The GOG followed up with GOG Protocol 209 which randomly assigned patients with advanced (stage IVB) or recurrent disease to either TAP or TC (paclitaxel and carboplatin). Trial data presented in 2012 demonstrated similar oncologic outcomes but the toxicity and tolerability profile favored TC.[186]

In patients with surgical bulk reduction (to residual < 2 cm) for stage III to IVA disease, a randomized phase III trial, GOG Protocol 122, demonstrated that chemotherapy with doxorubicin (60 mg/m2) and cisplatin (50 mg/m2) had superior progression-free survival (0.71; 95% confidence interval [CI] = 0.55–0.91; p < 0.01) and overall survival (0.68; 95% CI = 0.52–0.89; p < 0.01)[150] compared with whole-abdomen radiation.[187]

Hormone therapy

Kelly and Baker, in 1961, described six objective responses in 21 patients that lasted from 9 months to 4.5 years.[188] Since then, numerous reports described treatment with a variety of progestational drugs: most commonly 17-hydroxyprogesterone caproate, medroxyprogesterone acetate (MPA), and megestrol acetate (MA). Reifenstein analyzed 992 patients treated with hydroxyprogesterone caproate by 113 investigators.[189] He studied the records of 314 patients in detail and found that there was little response before 7 weeks of treatment, that the longest remissions were achieved with a minimum of 12 weeks of initial therapy, and that there was no relationship between clinical response and patient

Table 5 Single-agent cytotoxic chemotherapy for endometrial cancer.

Agent	Reference	N	Prior treatment	No CR + PR	(%)
Paclitaxel	144	28	No	4 + 6	36
Paclitaxel	145	19	Yes	2 + 5	37
Cisplatin	161,162	75	No	3 + 18	28
Carboplatin	163–165	76	No	5 + 18	28
Doxorubicin	160,166,167	280	No	31 + 49	29
Epirubicin	168	27	No	2 + 5	26
Fluorouracil	169	34	NS	7	21
HMM	170	30	No	10	33
Docetaxel	171	35	No	3+4	21
Topotecan	172,173	42	No	3+5	20

Note: Reported series with at least 20 patients with a response rate of at least 20%.
HMM = Hexamethylmelamine.
CR = complete response; PR = partial response. NS = Not stated.
Data from Muss,[174] Thigpen.[166]

Table 6 Randomized trials of combination chemotherapy regimens for endometrial cancer.

Author	Year	Regimen	Number evaluable	RR %	Median PFS (months)	Median overall survival (months)
Thigpen[176]	1994	A	132	22	3.2	6.7
		AC	144	30	3.9	7.3
Thigpen[166]	2004	A	150	25	3.8	9.2
		AP	131	42*	5.7*	9.0
Aapro[167]	2003	A	87	17	7.0	7.0
		AP	90	43*	8.0	9.0*
Gallion[179]	2003	AP standard	169	46	6.5	11.2
		AP circadian	173	49	5.9	13.2
Fleming[180]	2004	AP	157	40	7.2	12.6
		AT	160	43	6.0	13.6
Fleming[181]	2004	AP	129	34	5.3	12.3
		TAP	134	57*	8.3*	15.3*

PFS = Progression Free Survival;
RR = response rate = complete response + partial response;
C = cyclophosphamide;
A = doxorubicin (Adriamycin); P = cisplatin; F = 5-fluorouracil.
T = Paclitaxel * = Significant difference.

Table 7 Randomized trials of combination chemotherapy + hormonal therapy for endometrial cancer.

Author	Year	Regimen	Number evaluable	RR %
Horton[182]	1982	CA + MA	55	27
		CAF + MA	56	16
Cohen[183]	1984	F- Mel + MA	126	38
		CAF + MA	131	36
Ayoub[184]	1988	CAF	20	15
		CAF + MPA/TAM	23	43[a]
Cornelison[185]	1995	APE + MA	50	54
		F-Mel + MPA	50	48

RR = response rate = complete response + partial response; C = cyclophosphamide;
A = doxorubicin (Adriamycin); P = cisplatin; F = 5-fluorouracil; Mel = melphalan.
MA = Megestrol acetate; MPA = Medroxyprogesterone acetate.
TAM = Tamoxifen.
[a] = Significant difference.

age when correction was made for tumor differentiation. Kauppila reviewed 1,068 patients treated in 17 different trials with either MPA (Provera), MA, or hydroxyprogesterone caproate and found an overall response rate of 34%.[190] The duration of response was approximately 20 months and the average survival time was approximately 25 months.

The optimum dose for progestational treatment has not been determined and the doses employed in the most recent GOG studies were based on dose-seeking studies by Kohorn and Thigpen.[191,192] There is no evidence that lower doses are not equally effective and there is no advantage for the parenteral route[190]; therefore, selecting lower doses in special circumstances may be permissible in order to avoid complications.

Ramirez and colleagues,[193] in reviewing the literature, found that the majority of patients with well-differentiated endometrial adenocarcinoma who undergo conservative treatment for primary uterine cancer (in lieu of hysterectomy) with a progestational agent respond to treatment (62 of 81 = 76%). When an initial response is not achieved or when disease recurs after an initial response (15 of 62 = 24%), carcinoma extending beyond the uterus is rare. In addition, Montz and colleagues[194] described the feasibility of using a progesterone-containing intrauterine device to treat presumed FIGO stage IA, grade 1 endometrioid cancer in women at high risk of perioperative complications.

In summary, the following generalizations can be made concerning progestational therapy:[1] the response rate for patients with advanced or recurrent endometrial carcinoma ranges from 10–30%, probably relating to the receptor level in the tumor;[2] well-differentiated cancers respond best;[3] the PR level diminishes sharply as the grade of the tumor increases;[4] clinical responses may not occur before 7–12 weeks of therapy;[5] two-thirds of patients will not respond;[6] there is no published evidence that progestational agents employed in an adjuvant mode offer any benefit;[7] appropriate oral doses based on GOG studies are 160 mg/day of megestrol or 200 mg/day of MPA; however, lower doses can be individualized; and[8] oral progestins and the progesterone-containing intrauterine device are alternatives to consider for primary treatment of selected cases of early-stage, low-grade endometrial cancer.

Tamoxifen

Hormonal therapy by agents other than progestogens has been studied by many researchers. Extrapolating from the experience with breast cancer, investigators employed tamoxifen in doses of 20–40 mg daily for patients with advanced or recurrent endometrial carcinoma. In a review of eight published studies, Moore and colleagues[195] described an overall response rate of 22%. As one might predict, there is a wide spectrum of reported responses, ranging from 0–53%.[196] This variation may be explained by the report of Edmonson and colleagues,[197] who found a 21% response rate in patients naive to hormone therapy and no response in patients who had failed progesterone treatment. Not unlike the progestin experience, it would seem that tamoxifen is more likely to be effective in patients with low-grade tumors, receptor positivity, and either no previous hormone therapy or a previous response to progestin therapy.

Because progestins ultimately down-regulate PRs, and because tamoxifen induces these receptors in target tissues, the notion of the combined administration of these hormones has been examined by the GOG with two different strategies. In Whitney and colleagues' report, tamoxifen citrate 40 mg/day combined with alternating weekly cycles of MPA 200 mg/day in 58 patients with recurrent or measurable advanced endometrial carcinoma resulted in a 33% response rate (10.3% complete response and 23.4% partial response), with a median progression-free interval of 3 months and a median overall survival of 13 months.[198] In the Fiorica study, alternating 3-week courses of MA (160 mg/day) and tamoxifen citrate (40 mg/day) in 56 patients with recurrent or measurable advanced endometrial carcinoma produced a 27% response rate (21.4% complete response and 5.4% partial response), with a median progression-free interval of 2.7 months and a median overall survival of 14.0 months.[199]

The combination of tamoxifen, progestin, and chemotherapy has also been tested. Ayoub and colleagues studied 46 patients with metastatic endometrial cancer, randomly assigning them to receive monthly cycles of cyclophosphamide, adriamycin (doxorubicin), and 5-fluorouracil (CAF) or CAF plus MPA, 200 mg daily for 3 weeks, followed cyclically by tamoxifen, 20 mg daily for 3 weeks.[184] Objective responses of 15% and 43% were seen, respectively, with CAF and CAF plus hormonal therapy (p = 0.05). Because progestational agents have not improved the response to chemotherapy in previously cited studies,[200] it is reasonable to attribute this difference to the addition of tamoxifen. Pinelli and colleagues evaluated sequential cyclical hormone therapy (MA and tamoxifen citrate) plus the single agent carboplatin.[201] Of 13 evaluable patients, 4 patients had a complete response and 6 had partial responses, for an overall response rate of 77%. The median progression-free interval was 14 months for complete responders. The median survival was 11 months for all patients and 33 months for complete responders.

Other hormones

Gonadotropin-releasing hormone analogues have been tested in small phase II trials of patients with recurrent endometrial carcinoma, with response rates varying from 0% to 35%.[202–204] Aromatase inhibitors have been tested in a limited fashion. The GOG phase II trial had a 9% response rate (2 partial responses of 23) with anastrozole,[205–207] whereas the Canadian National Cancer Institute study reported a 9.4% response rate (2 partial responses of 28) with letrozole.[208]

Biologic therapies

New molecular and biologic therapies for recurrent or metastatic endometrial cancer are being evaluated in clinical trials. In a phase II trial of 52 evaluable patients (with up to two prior chemotherapy regimens), bevacizumab demonstrated a 13.5% response rate and an overall survival of 10.5 months.[209] Preliminary results of a phase II trial of the mTOR inhibitor temsirolimus in chemo-naïve patients with recurrent or metastatic endometrial cancer were encouraging with 5 (27%) partial responses out of 19 evaluable patients.[210] A phase II trial of the mTOR inhibitor everolimus combined with an aromatase inhibitor letrozole demonstrated a 32% response rate (n = 35; nine complete responses and two partial responses) in patients with recurrent endometrial cancer.[211]

The future

Efforts must continue to expand information about molecular characteristics to better define patient susceptibilities and therapeutic possibilities. From a surgical standpoint, laparoscopy and robotic surgery are now accepted as standard techniques, but the role of sentinel lymph node assessment is still incompletely defined. For patients with early disease and poor prognostic features, further randomized studies comparing RT with systemic therapy are required. For patients with advanced or recurrent disease, better systemic therapy including biologic agents must be identified. It is obvious that with a cure rate in the United States of approximately 80%, it will be essential that patients with poor prognostic features or recurrent or metastatic disease be entered into collaborative trials to maximize the opportunities for improving survival.

Key references

The complete reference list can be found on the Wiley Companion Digital Edition of this title (see inside front cover for login instructions).

18 Gusberg SB. Precursors of corpus carcinoma, estrogen and adenomatous hyperplasia. *Am J Obstet Gynecol.* 1947;**54**:905–27.

30 Cohen CJ, Rahaman J. Endometrial cancer. Management of high risk and recurrence including the tamoxifen controversy. *Cancer.* 1995;**76(10 Suppl)**:2044–52.

32 Fisher B, Costantino JP, Wickerham DL, et al. Tamoxifen for prevention of breast cancer: report of the National Surgical Adjuvant Breast and Bowel Project P-1 Study. *J Natl Cancer Inst.* 1998;**90(18)**:1371–88.

36 Bokhman JV. Two pathogenetic types of endometrial carcinoma. *Gynecol Oncol.* 1983;**15(1)**:10–7.

40 Kurman RJ, Kaminski PF, Norris HJ. The behavior of endometrial hyperplasia. A long-term study of "untreated" hyperplasia in 170 patients. *Cancer.* 1985;**56(2)**:403–12.

41 Pecorelli S. Revised FIGO staging for carcinoma of the vulva, cervix, and endometrium. *Int J Gynaecol Obstet.* 2009;**105(2)**:103–4. Epub 2009/04/16.

43 Tashiro H, Isacson C, Levine R, Kurman RJ, Cho KR, Hedrick L. p53 gene mutations are common in uterine serous carcinoma and occur early in their pathogenesis. *Am J Pathol.* 1997;**150(1)**:177–85.

44 Hendrickson M, Ross J, Eifel P, Martinez A, Kempson R. Uterine papillary serous carcinoma: a highly malignant form of endometrial adenocarcinoma. *Am J Surg Pathol.* 1982;**6(2)**:93–108.

45 Boruta DM 2nd, Gehrig PA, Fader AN, Olawaiye AB. Management of women with uterine papillary serous cancer: a Society of Gynecologic Oncology (SGO) review. *Gynecol Oncol.* 2009;**115(1)**:142–53. Epub 2009/07/14.

50 Kurman RJ, Scully RE. Clear cell carcinoma of the endometrium: an analysis of 21 cases. *Cancer.* 1976;**37(2)**:872–82.

51 Christopherson WM, Alberhasky RC, Connelly PJ. Glassy cell carcinoma of the endometrium. *Hum Pathol.* 1982;**13(5)**:418–21.

52 Olawaiye AB, Boruta DM 2nd. Management of women with clear cell endometrial cancer: a Society of Gynecologic Oncology (SGO) review. *Gynecol Oncol.* 2009;**113(2)**:277–83. Epub 2009/03/03.

53 Cancer Genome Atlas Research N, Kandoth C, Schultz N, et al. Integrated genomic characterization of endometrial carcinoma. *Nature.* 2013;**497(7447)**:67–73.

54 Djordjevic B, Hennessy BT, Li J, et al. Clinical assessment of PTEN loss in endometrial carcinoma: immunohistochemistry outperforms gene sequencing. *Mod Pathol : an official journal of the United States and Canadian Academy of Pathology, Inc.* 2012;**25(5)**:699–708.

58 Mao TL, Ardighieri L, Ayhan A, et al. Loss of ARID1A expression correlates with stages of tumor progression in uterine endometrioid carcinoma. *Am J Surg Pathol.* 2013;**37(9)**:1342–8.

65 Cohen CJ, Gusberg SB, Koffler D. Histologic screening for endometrial cancer. *Gynecol Oncol.* 1974;**2(2–3)**:279–86.

77 Creasman WT, Morrow CP, Bundy BN, Homesley HD, Graham JE, Heller PB. Surgical pathologic spread patterns of endometrial cancer A Gynecologic Oncology Group Study. *Cancer.* 1987;**60(8 Suppl)**:2035–41.

80 Morrow CP, Bundy BN, Kurman RJ, et al. Relationship between surgical-pathological risk factors and outcome in clinical stage I and II carcinoma of the endometrium: a Gynecologic Oncology Group study. *Gynecol Oncol.* 1991;**40(1)**:55–65.

82 Boggess JF, Gehrig PA, Cantrell L, et al. A comparative study of 3 surgical methods for hysterectomy with staging for endometrial cancer: robotic assistance, laparoscopy, laparotomy. *Am J Obstet Gynecol.* 2008;**199(4:360)**:e1–e9. Epub 2008/10/22.

83 Abu-Rustum NR. Sentinel lymph node mapping for endometrial cancer: a modern approach to surgical staging. *J Natl Compr Canc Netw.* 2014;**12**(2):288–97. Epub 2014/03/04.

86 Aalders J, Abeler V, Kolstad P, Onsrud M. Postoperative external irradiation and prognostic parameters in stage I endometrial carcinoma: clinical and histopathologic study of 540 patients. *Obstet Gynecol.* 1980;**56**(4):419–27.

91 Wethington SL, Barrena Medel NI, Wright JD, Herzog TJ. Prognostic significance and treatment implications of positive peritoneal cytology in endometrial adenocarcinoma: Unraveling a mystery. *Gynecol Oncol.* 2009;**115**(1):18–25. Epub 2009/07/28.

96 Mariani A, Sebo TJ, Webb MJ, et al. Molecular and histopathologic predictors of distant failure in endometrial cancer. *Cancer Detect Prev.* 2003;**27**(6):434–41. Epub 2003/12/04.

100 Walker JL, Piedmonte MR, Spirtos NM, et al. Recurrence and survival after random assignment to laparoscopy versus laparotomy for comprehensive surgical staging of uterine cancer: Gynecologic Oncology Group LAP2 Study. *J Clin Oncol.* 2012;**30**(7):695–700. Epub 2012/02/01.

106 Obermair A, Manolitsas TP, Leung Y, Hammond IG, McCartney AJ. Total laparoscopic hysterectomy for endometrial cancer: patterns of recurrence and survival. *Gynecol Oncol.* 2004;**92**(3):789–93. Epub 2004/02/27.

107 Nezhat F, Yadav J, Rahaman J, Gretz H, Cohen C. Analysis of survival after laparoscopic management of endometrial cancer. *J Minim Invasive Gynecol.* 2008;**15**(2):181–7. Epub 2008/03/04.

116 Grigsby PW, Kuske RR, Perez CA, et al. Medically inoperable stage I adenocarcinoma of the endometrium treated with radiotherapy alone. *Int J Radiat Oncol Biol Phys.* 1987;**13**(4):483–8.

125 Nag S, Erickson B, Parikh S, Gupta N, Varia M, Glasgow G. The American Brachytherapy Society recommendations for high-dose-rate brachytherapy for carcinoma of the endometrium. *Int J Radiat Oncol Biol Phys.* 2000;**48**(3):779–90. Epub 2000/10/06.

126 Keys HM, Roberts JA, Brunetto VL, et al. A phase III trial of surgery with or without adjunctive external pelvic radiation therapy in intermediate risk endometrial adenocarcinoma: a Gynecologic Oncology Group study. *Gynecol Oncol.* 2004;**92**(3):744–51.

127 Creutzberg CL, van Putten WL, Koper PC, et al. Surgery and postoperative radiotherapy versus surgery alone for patients with stage-1 endometrial carcinoma: multicentre randomised trial. PORTEC Study Group Post Operative Radiation Therapy in Endometrial Carcinoma. *Lancet.* 2000;**355**(9213):1404–11. Epub 2000/05/03.

128 Nout RA, Smit VT, Putter H, et al. Vaginal brachytherapy versus pelvic external beam radiotherapy for patients with endometrial cancer of high-intermediate risk (PORTEC-2): an open-label, non-inferiority, randomised trial. *Lancet.* 2010;**375**(9717):816–23. Epub 2010/03/09.

152 Susumu N, Sagae S, Udagawa Y, et al. Randomized phase III trial of pelvic radiotherapy versus cisplatin-based combined chemotherapy in patients with intermediate- and high-risk endometrial cancer: a Japanese Gynecologic Oncology Group study. *Gynecol Oncol.* 2008;**108**(1):226–33. Epub 2007/11/13.

153 Kelly MG, O'Malley DM, Hui P, et al. Improved survival in surgical stage I patients with uterine papillary serous carcinoma (UPSC) treated with adjuvant platinum-based chemotherapy. *Gynecol Oncol.* 2005;**98**(3):353–9. Epub 2005/07/12.

154 Huh WK, Straughn JM Jr, Mariani A, et al. Salvage of isolated vaginal recurrences in women with surgical stage I endometrial cancer: a multiinstitutional experience. *Int J Gynecol Cancer.* 2007;**17**(4):886–9. Epub 2007/02/21.

166 Thigpen JT, Brady MF, Homesley HD, et al. Phase III trial of doxorubicin with or without cisplatin in advanced endometrial carcinoma: a gynecologic oncology group study. *J Clin Oncol.* 2004;**22**(19):3902–8.

167 Aapro MS, van Wijk FH, Bolis G, et al. Doxorubicin versus doxorubicin and cisplatin in endometrial carcinoma: definitive results of a randomised study (55872) by the EORTC Gynaecological Cancer Group. *Ann Oncol.* 2003;**14**(3):441–8.

181 Fleming GF, Brunetto VL, Cella D, et al. Phase III trial of doxorubicin plus cisplatin with or without paclitaxel plus filgrastim in advanced endometrial carcinoma: a Gynecologic Oncology Group Study. *J Clin Oncol.* 2004;**22**(11):2159–66.

186 Miller DFV, Fleming G, et al. Randomized phase III noninferiority trial of first line chemotherapy for metastatic or recurrent endometrial carcinoma: A Gynecologic Oncology Group Study. SGO. *Gynecol Oncol.* 2012;**125**:771.

187 Randall ME, Filiaci VL, Muss H, et al. Randomized phase III trial of whole-abdominal irradiation versus doxorubicin and cisplatin chemotherapy in advanced endometrial carcinoma: a Gynecologic Oncology Group Study. *J Clin Oncol.* 2006;**24**(1):36–44. Epub 2005/12/07.

193 Ramirez PT, Frumovitz M, Bodurka DC, Sun CC, Levenback C. Hormonal therapy for the management of grade 1 endometrial adenocarcinoma: a literature review. *Gynecol Oncol.* 2004;**95**(1):133–8. Epub 2004/09/24.

198 Whitney CW, Brunetto VL, Zaino RJ, et al. Phase II study of medroxyprogesterone acetate plus tamoxifen in advanced endometrial carcinoma: a Gynecologic Oncology Group study. *Gynecol Oncol.* 2004;**92**(1):4–9. Epub 2004/01/31.

199 Fiorica JV, Brunetto VL, Hanjani P, Lentz SS, Mannel R, Andersen W. Phase II trial of alternating courses of megestrol acetate and tamoxifen in advanced endometrial carcinoma: a Gynecologic Oncology Group study. *Gynecol Oncol.* 2004;**92**(1):10–4. Epub 2004/01/31.

104 Epithelial ovarian, fallopian tube, and peritoneal cancer

Jonathan S. Berek, MD, MMS, FASCO ▪ *Michael L. Friedlander, MD, MBChB, PhD* ▪ *Robert C. Bast Jr., MD*

Overview

Ovarian cancer is one of the most treatable solid tumors, as the majority will respond temporarily to surgery and cytotoxic agents. The disease, however, frequently persists and recurs in 70% of cases, having the highest fatality-to-case ratio of all the gynecologic cancers.[1,2] Ovarian cancer is neither a common nor a rare disease, with a lifetime risk of 1 in 70 and a prevalence in the postmenopausal population in the United States of 1 in 2500, which impact strategies for early detection and prevention. Germ line mutations of BRCA1 and BRCA2 are associated with 10–15% of ovarian cancers and increase the risk of ovarian cancer dramatically. Factors that contribute to persistent ovulation increase the risk in women with sporadic disease, whereas use of oral contraceptives decreases the risk of disease post menopause. While epithelial ovarian cancers have been thought to arise from the ovarian surface epithelium or in the lining of inclusion cysts beneath the ovarian surface, many high-grade serous "ovarian" carcinomas as well as peritoneal cancers are now believed to arise in the fimbriae of fallopian tube, rather than the ovary or peritoneum.[3–10] Epithelial ovarian cancers can exhibit serous, endometrioid, mucinous, or clear cell histotypes. Low-grade type I ovarian cancers grow slowly, can evolve from tumors of low malignant potential, bear Ras mutations in a majority of cases, express wild type TP53, often are detected in early stage (I–II), and respond less frequently to platinum- and taxane-based therapy. High-grade type II ovarian cancers grow rapidly, arise from precursors with TP53 mutations, are driven by DNA copy number changes, are diagnosed in late stage (III–IV), and frequently respond to combination chemotherapy. Owing to a lack of specific symptoms or an effective screening strategy, more than 70% of ovarian cancers are diagnosed in an advanced stage (III–IV). Primary treatment of epithelial ovarian cancer involves cytoreductive surgery and 6–8 cycles of carboplatin and paclitaxel. For those women with small volumes of disease after surgery, intraperitoneal administration of chemotherapy improves survival. Recurrent disease cannot be cured with currently available agents, but survival can be prolonged with combinations of cytotoxic agents including retreatment with paclitaxel and carboplatin. Palliative agents include liposomal doxorubicin, gemcitabine, topotecan, bevacizumab, pemetrexed, and etoposide. Experimental therapy for low-grade cancers involves MEK inhibitors, whereas trials of PI3K pathway inhibitors and PARP inhibitors are underway in patients with high-grade epithelial ovarian cancers. Combinations of targeted agents will be required.

65 years. Less than 1% of epithelial cancers are found in women younger than 30 years of age, and most ovarian malignancies in these younger patients are germ cell tumors (GCTs) (*see Chapter 105*).[2] The prevalence of ovarian cancer among postmenopausal women in the United States is 40 per 100,000 or 1 in 2500. The lifetime risk for a woman to develop ovarian cancer in the United States is approximately 1 in 70 (1.4%), compared to 1 in 8 or 9 for breast cancer. The prevalence of ovarian cancer in the general population impacts substantially on strategies for prevention and early detection. In the absence of better markers for increased risk, strategies for prevention must have few, if any, serious adverse effects and screening strategies must be highly specific. A strong hereditary component contributes to development of the disease in at least 10% of cases with inherited germ line mutations in *BRCA1* and *BRCA2* being the most common with only a small percentage of cases related to mutations in mismatch repair (MMR) genes or p53.

In 2015, in the United States, almost 22,000 new cases of ovarian cancer and more than 14,000 deaths are expected.[1] There is a trend toward improved survival for ovarian cancer.[1,2] On the basis of Surveillance, Epidemiology, and End Results (SEER) data in the United States, the 5-year survival for all stages combined increased from 33.6% in 1975 to 45.9% in 2003 to 2011.[2] Using statistical models for analysis, rates for new ovarian cancer cases have been falling on average 1% per year over the past 10 years. Death rates have been falling on average 1.6% per year over the same period. The death rate decreased 22% from 10 per 100,000 women per year in 1976 to 7.8 per 100,000 per women per year in 2010.[2] Ovarian cancer rates are highest in women aged 55–64 years (median age 63 years), and deaths are highest in people aged 75–84 years (median age 71 years).[2]

The incidence of ovarian cancer varies in different geographic locations throughout the world. Western countries, including the United States and the United Kingdom, have an incidence of ovarian cancer that is 3–7 times greater than in Japan, where epithelial ovarian tumors are considered rare.[10,11] In Asia, the incidence of GCTs of the ovary appears to be somewhat higher than in the West. Japanese immigrants to the United States, however, exhibit a significant increase in the incidence of epithelial ovarian cancer at a rate approaching that of white women from the United States. The incidence of epithelial tumors is about 1.5 times greater in whites than in blacks.

Incidence, etiology, and epidemiology

Incidence

Ovarian, fallopian tube, and peritoneal cancers are predominantly diseases of postmenopausal women, with only 10–15% of all cases diagnosed premenopause.[1–3] The median age for diagnosis of epithelial cancers from these three sites ranges between 60 and

Etiology and epidemiology

In the past, most epithelial ovarian cancers were thought to arise from a single layer of epithelial cells that covers the ovarian surface or from the epithelial cells that line "inclusion cysts" immediately beneath the ovarian surface. Over the past decade, this view has been modified. Of all epithelial ovarian cancers, approximately 10–15% arise in women with germ line mutations of BRCA1 and

Holland-Frei Cancer Medicine, Ninth Edition. Edited by Robert C. Bast Jr., Carlo M. Croce, William N. Hait, Waun Ki Hong, Donald W. Kufe, Martine Piccart-Gebhart, Raphael E. Pollock, Ralph R. Weichselbaum, Hongyang Wang, and James F. Holland.
© 2017 John Wiley & Sons, Inc. ISBN: 978-1-118-93469-2

BRCA2 and most of these are high-grade serous neoplasms. Up to 80% of these high-grade serous "ovarian cancers" associated with BRCA1/2 mutations are derived from the fimbriae of the fallopian tube, accounting for at least 10% of all epithelial ovarian cancers. Some 20% of high-grade serous cancers coat the ovary rather than grow from it and have been termed "primary peritoneal carcinomas." Most of these high-grade serous primary peritoneal cancers are likely to arise from fimbriae of the fallopian tube, although some may be derived from developmental remnants of the secondary Müllerian system.[12] Primary peritoneal carcinoma explains how "ovarian cancer" can arise in a patient whose ovaries, but not fallopian tubes, were surgically removed many years earlier.[13–15] Thus, at least a third, and possibly a majority of high-grade serous cancers arise from the fallopian tube, although the remainder are still of ovarian origin. High-grade serous cancers of the ovary, fallopian tube carcinomas, and peritoneal carcinomas should be regarded as a single disease entity and managed with a common approach. In this regard, fallopian tube cancer is now included in the same FIGO (International Federation of Gynecology and Obstetrics) staging system with ovarian cancer, as discussed in the following paragraph.[4]

The causes of ovarian cancer are not well understood.[16,17] Cigarette smoking has been linked to mucinous ovarian cancers but not to the more common serous carcinomas.[17] Case–control studies have also pointed to an association of white race, high-fat diet, and galactose consumption with a higher incidence of the disease.[16,18] Prior reproductive history and the number of ovulatory cycles are associated with development of the disease, with low parity, infertility, early menarche, and late menopause increasing the risk.[16,19,20] Fertility-enhancing drugs, such as clomiphene citrate, and gonadotropins used for ovulation induction have been thought to increase the risk of ovarian cancer (ROC), but the data have not been consistent and have not adequately distinguished the influence of infertility per se from the use of fertility-stimulating agents.[21–24] A pooled analysis of eight case–control studies that included 5207 cases and 7705 controls found an association of fertility-stimulating drugs with serous borderline tumors but not with invasive ovarian cancers.[24] Many case–control and cohort studies have failed to link hormone replacement therapy to an increased risk of epithelial ovarian cancer.[25] A large cohort study had reopened controversy regarding this issue.[26] Among 44,241 postmenopausal women in the Breast Cancer Detection Demonstration Project, 329 developed ovarian cancer. Women who had received estrogen replacement therapy only for more than 10 years without progestin were at increased risk of developing ovarian cancer. By 20 years, the relative risk (RR) was 3.2-fold. This is supported by a recent meta-analysis, which included individual data from just over 12,000 postmenopausal women, 55% of whom had used hormone therapy, who developed ovarian cancer. Among women last recorded as current users, risk was increased even with <5 years of use (RR 10.43, 95% confidence interval [CI] 10.31–10.56; $p < 00.0001$). Combining current-or-recent use resulted in a RR of 10.37 (95% CI 10.29–10.46; $p < 00.0001$); this risk was similar in European and American prospective studies and for estrogen-only and estrogen–progestagen preparations but differed across the four main histological subtypes, being definitely increased only for the two most common types, serous (RR 10.53, 95% CI 10.40–10.66; $p < 00.0001$) and endometrioid (10.42, 10.20–10.67; $p < 00.0001$). The authors concluded that the increased risk may be causal and that women who use hormone therapy for 5 years from around age 50 years have about one extra ovarian cancer per 1000 users.[27]

Prevention

As parity is inversely related to the ROC, having at least one child reduces the RR by 30–40% and use of oral contraceptives for 5 or more years reduces the risk by 50%.[21] Women who have had two children and have used oral contraceptives for 5 or more years have as much as 70% reduction in risk. To date, oral contraceptive medication is the only documented method of chemoprevention for ovarian cancer, and it can be recommended to women for this purpose. When counseling patients regarding birth control options, this important benefit of oral contraceptive use should be emphasized. This is also important for women with a strong family history of ovarian cancer in the absence of BRCA1 or BRCA2 mutation.[28] Surgical prevention is important, but its use depends critically on identifying women at sufficient risk to justify prophylactic salpingo-oophorectomy with or without total abdominal hysterectomy.

Genetic predisposition

Hereditary ovarian cancer
The ROC is significantly higher than that of the general population in women with a family history of breast or ovarian cancer as well as in families with Lynch syndrome.[29–45] Although most epithelial ovarian cancer is sporadic, at least 10–13% of patients with epithelial ovarian cancer have a germ line mutation in either BRCA1 or BRCA2.[42]

BRCA1 and BRCA2
Most hereditary ovarian cancer results from mutations in the BRCA1 gene, which is located on chromosome 17, with a smaller fraction of familial ovarian cancers associated with mutations in BRCA2, which is located on chromosome 13. Both genes mediate DNA repair. BRCA1-associated ovarian cancers generally occur in women approximately 10 years earlier than those with non-hereditary tumors.[36,42] As the median age of epithelial ovarian cancer is 62–63 years, a woman with a first- or second-degree relative who had early onset ovarian cancer may have a higher probability of having a BRCA1 or BRCA 2 mutation. There is, however, no significant family history in 44% (95% CI, 35.8–52.2%) of mutation-positive women, which underscores the importance of offering mutation testing to all women with high-grade serous ovarian cancer diagnosed under the age of 70 irrespective of family history, and this is reflected in current guidelines.[44]

There is a higher carrier rate of BRCA1 and BRCA2 mutations in women of Ashkenazi Jewish descent, Icelandic women, and in other ethnic groups.[35,36] There are three specific founder mutations that are carried by the Ashkenazi population: 185delAG and 5382insC on BRCA1, and 6174delT on BRCA2. The carrier rate of at least one of these mutations for a patient of Ashkenazi Jewish descent is 1 in 40 or 2.5%, which is considerably higher than the general Caucasian population. The increased risk is a result of the *founder effect*—that is, a higher rate of mutations that have occurred within a specific population group that was geographically or culturally isolated in the past in which one or more of the ancestors carried the mutant gene.

A combined analysis of 22 studies unselected for family history has found that women who have a germ line mutation in the BRCA1 gene have a lifetime ROC of 39% (18–54%), and the risk has been calculated to be 11% (2.4–19%) in women with a BRCA2 mutation.[45] Women with a BRCA1 or BRCA2 mutation have a risk of breast cancer as high as 65% and 45%, respectively. The breast cancers typically occur at a young age and may be bilateral. There is a higher incidence of triple-negative (ER-, PR-, HER2-) breast cancers in women with *BRCA1* mutations. A large consortium found genetic risk modifiers on 4q32.2 and 17q21.31 that significantly increased the risk of developing ovarian cancer in *BRCA1*-mutation carriers, which may explain the variable risks that have been reported.[46]

Lynch syndrome

There are other less common genetic causes of ovarian cancer. Lynch syndrome, which is also known as the *hereditary nonpolyposis colorectal cancer (HNPCC) syndrome*, confers increased risk for colorectal cancer and a wide range of other malignancies (e.g., endometrial, ovarian, and gastric cancer) as a result of a germ line MMR genetic mutation.[39] The mutations that have been associated with this syndrome are *MSH2*, *MSH6*, *MLH1*, *PMS1*, and *PMS2*. The risk of endometrial cancer equals or exceeds that of colorectal cancer in women with Lynch Syndrome. The diagnosis of gynecologic cancer precedes that of colorectal cancer in over half the cases, making gynecologic cancer a "sentinel cancer" for Lynch syndrome. The lifetime ROC in women with Lynch Syndrome has been estimated at approximately 6–12%. The mean age at diagnosis is 42.7–49.5 years. There is a higher risk of endometrioid and clear cell subtypes, and the majority of cases are diagnosed in stage I or II.

The management of women at high risk for ovarian cancer

The management of a woman with a strong family history of epithelial ovarian cancer must be individualized and will depend on her age, reproductive plans, and the estimated level of risk. A thorough pedigree analysis is important. A geneticist should evaluate the family pedigree for at least three generations. Decisions about management are best made after careful study of the pedigree and, whenever possible, verification of the histologic diagnosis of the family members' ovarian cancer as well as the age of onset and other tumors in the family. Although recommended by the National Institutes of Health Consensus Conference on Ovarian Cancer[47], the value of screening with transvaginal ultrasonography and CA125 has not been established in women at high risk. The findings of two prospective studies of annual transvaginal ultrasonography and CA125 screening suggest a very limited benefit, if any, of screening high-risk women.[48,49]

Data derived from a multi-institutional consortium of genetic screening centers has suggested that the use of oral contraceptives is associated with a lower ROC in women who have a *BRCA1* or *BRCA2* mutation,[50] but this has not been confirmed.[51] Tubal ligation may also decrease the ROC in patients with a *BRCA1* but not *BRCA2* mutation, but the protective effect is not nearly as strong as risk-reducing bilateral salpingo-oophorectomy (BSO).[52]

The value of prophylactic risk-reducing BSO in these patients has been well documented.[53–58] Occult ovarian/fallopian tube cancers detected at the time of risk-reducing BSO have been reported in many studies with wide variability in reported prevalence ranging from 2.3% to 23%. The performance of a prophylactic salpingo-oophorectomy reduces the risk of BRCA-related gynecologic cancer by 96%.[56] There remains a small risk of subsequently developing a peritoneal carcinoma. The risk of developing peritoneal carcinoma was 0.8% and 1%, respectively, in two series.[54,55] As discussed earlier, many so-called ovarian cancers arise from the fallopian tube, and it is essential that women having prophylactic surgery have their fallopian tubes removed as well and that these

are carefully assessed by the pathologist as it is easy to miss small cancers or precursor lesions, particularly in the fimbrial end of the fallopian tube.[6] Prophylactic salpingo-oophorectomy in premenopausal women also reduced the risk of developing subsequent breast cancer by 50–80%.[54,55]

Grann et al.[59] reported the application of Markov modeling—that is, quality-adjusted survival estimate analysis—in a simulated cohort of 30-year-old women who tested positive for *BRCA1* or *BRCA2* mutations. The analysis predicted that a 30-year-old woman could prolong her survival beyond that associated with surveillance alone by 1.8 years with *tamoxifen*, 2.6 years with prophylactic salpingo-oophorectomy, 4.6 years with both *tamoxifen* and prophylactic salpingo-oophorectomy, 3.5 years with prophylactic mastectomy, and 4.9 years with both prophylactic surgeries. Quality-adjusted life expectancy was estimated to be prolonged by 2.8 years for *tamoxifen*, 4.4 years with prophylactic salpingo-oophorectomy, 6.3 years for *tamoxifen* and prophylactic salpingo-oophorectomy, 2.6 years with mastectomy, and 2.6 years with both operations. This has been supported by a study of women with *BRCA1* and *BRCA2* mutations which found that risk-reducing mastectomy was associated with a lower risk of breast cancer, risk-reducing BSO was associated with a lower ROC, and that there was an improvement in all-cause mortality, breast cancer-specific mortality as well as ovarian cancer-specific mortality.[60]

The survival of women who have a *BRCA1* or *BRCA2* mutation and develop ovarian cancer is longer than that for those who do not have a mutation. In one study, the median survival for mutation carriers was 53.4 months compared with 37.8 months for those with sporadic ovarian cancer from the same institution.[61] These findings have recently been confirmed in a population-based study from Israel in which Chetrit et al.[62] reported that among Ashkenazi women with ovarian cancer those with *BRCA1* and *BRCA2* mutations had an improved long-term survival (38% vs 24% at 5 years). This may result from intrinsic growth properties or from a better response to chemotherapy.

Recommendations

Current recommendations are that all women under the age of 70 with a nonmucinous epithelial ovarian, fallopian tube, or peritoneal cancer should undergo testing for *BRCA*1 to *BRCA*2 mutations.[63] The recommendations for management of women at high risk for ovarian cancers are summarized as follows[40,41,47,51–59,64]:

1. Women who appear to be at high risk for ovarian and or breast cancer should undergo genetic counseling; if there is a probability of 10% or greater of having a *BRCA* mutation, they should be offered genetic testing for *BRCA1* and *BRCA2*.

2. Women who wish to preserve their reproductive capability or delay prophylactic surgery should undergo periodic screening by transvaginal ultrasonography and CA125 every 6 months, although the efficacy of this approach has not been established and is not based on evidence that this reduces mortality.

3. Oral contraceptives should be recommended to young women at increased risk.

4. Women who do not wish to maintain their fertility or who have completed their family should undergo PBSO. In women who have a strong family history of breast or ovarian cancer, annual mammographic and magnetic resonance imaging (MRI) breast screening should be performed commencing at age 30 years, or younger if there are family members with documented very early onset breast cancer.

5. Women with a documented Lynch syndrome should be counseled about prophylactic hysterectomy and oophorectomy after

childbearing, in view of the risk of both endometrial and ovarian cancer. Although there are no definitive studies to support screening, endometrial sampling and transvaginal ultrasound of the ovaries may be considered from ages 30 to 35. Colonoscopy is recommended every 1–2 years starting from ages 20 to 25 or 10 years younger than the youngest person diagnosed in the family.[39,65,66]

Molecular, cellular, and clinical biology

Similar to most epithelial cancers, more than 90% of epithelial ovarian cancers arise from the progeny of a single cell, that is, ovarian cancer is generally a clonal disease.[67] Despite origin from a single cell, ovarian cancers are markedly heterogeneous at a molecular, cellular, and clinical level. A number of genetic abnormalities are observed in ovarian cancers (Table 1)[68] that activate or inactivate different genes. The function of several tumor suppressor genes has been lost (Table 2)[68] by deletion, loss of heterozygosity, inactivating mutation (BRCA1, BRCA2, and TP53), promoter methylation (ARHI), histone modification, or loss of processed miRNAs. Abnormalities in miRNA processing with decreases in Dicer and Drosha have been found in 60% and 51% of ovarian cancer associated with a poor outcome.[69] Oncogenes have been amplified, transcriptionally overexpressed and/or mutationally activated (Table 3).[68] At a cellular level, the fraction of proliferating cells can vary from 1% to 90%.[70] Ovarian cancers vary in histotype exhibiting the serous, endometriod, mucinous and clear cell variants described in the following paragraphs, related at least in part to the aberrant expression of HOX genes associated with normal gynecologic development.[71]

Biologically and clinically, there is a major distinction between low-grade (type I) and high-grade (type II) epithelial ovarian cancers.[72] Low-grade serous cancers (comprising <10% of ovarian epithelial malignancies) are thought to develop from borderline tumors, to present in early stage (I–II) and to depend on mutations of Ras (>50%), PIK3CA (30%), and PTEN (10%), as well as upon expression of the insulin-like growth factor receptor (IGFR), which responds to IGF produced by the tumor stroma. High-grade serous cancers (comprising 60% of all ovarian epithelial malignancies) are thought to develop from histologically normal ovarian and fallopian tube epithelial cells, to present in late stage (III–IV), and to depend on amplification of multiple wild-type oncogenes and the functional loss of tumor suppressor genes. While *TP53* is rarely mutated in low-grade type I cancers, it is mutated in nearly all high-grade serous type II cancers. When germ line and somatic mutations of BRCA1/2 are associated with epithelial ovarian cancer, the cancers are generally high grade. Defects in homologous recombination DNA repair deficiency (BRCAness) are associated with up to half of high-grade cancers, but few, if any, low grade cancers, possibly accounting for the fact that high-grade cancers are more sensitive to platinum-based chemotherapy than low-grade cancers. Current strategies are being developed to exploit this deficiency using PARP inhibitors in the presence and absence of BRCA1/2 mutations. The PI3-kinase pathway is a potential target in both type I and type II cancers and is activated in at least half of high-grade cancers.[73]

The Tumor Cancer Genome Atlas (TCGA) project has sequenced DNA from more than 300 high-grade serous ovarian cancers and aside from *TP53* (98%) and *BRCA1/2* (15–20%) only a few genes are mutated more than 1% of the time (NF1, RB1, CSMD3, and CDK12).[74] Consequently, low-grade cancers are driven by mutations and high-grade cancers by DNA copy number abnormalities.

Clear cell ovarian cancers have mutations of ARID1A (49%),[75] a chromatin-processing enzyme and PP2R1A (6%), a phosphatase. Endometriod ovarian cancers also have mutations of ARID1A (30%). Among the nonepithelial ovarian cancers, 97% of granulosa cell tumors (see the following discussion) exhibit a characteristic mutation, 402C→G (C134W) in FOXL2, a gene encoding a transcription factor known to be critical for granulosa-cell development.[76]

Ascites formation results from increased leakage of proteinaceous fluid from capillaries under the influence of vascular endothelial growth factor/vascular permeability factor (VEGF/VPF) produced by ovarian cancers and from inhibition of fluid outflow through diaphragmatic lymphatics that have been blocked by metastatic disease.[77] Studies of the immunobiology of the peritoneal cavity suggest that it may function as an immunoprivileged site, with elevated levels of suppressive molecules and growth factors. Angiogenesis in ovarian cancer has been shown to depend on multiple factors including VEGF and IL-8. The presence of multiple angiogenic factors can explain, in part, development of resistance to bevacizumab therapy. Autophagy and tumor dormancy are regulated by ARHI (DIRAS3) an imprinted tumor suppressor gene that is downregulated in 60% of ovarian cancers of low and high grade.[78,79] The upregulation of ARHI and high prevalence of autophagy in dormant, drug-resistant cancer cells in positive second look specimens after primary surgery and chemotherapy, suggest that autophagy could be a target in ovarian cancer.[80]

Upregulation and aberrant glycosylation of extracellular mucins have provided markers for monitoring disease. MUC-1 is a mucin expressed by more than 80% of ovarian cancers.[81] In transformed cells, aberrant glycosylation exposes peptide determinants recognized by murine monoclonal antibodies that have been used for serotherapy. CA125 is also a mucin (MUC16) associated with cells that line the coelomic cavity during embryonic development. CA125 is shed from 80% of epithelial ovarian cancers[82,83] and can be measured using the murine monoclonal antibody OC125.

Table 1 Genetic and epigenetic abnormalities in epithelial ovarian cancer.

Activating events	
Amplification by CGH	1q22 (RAB25), 3q26 (PKCiota, EVI1, PIK3CA), 5q31 (FGF-1), 8q24 (MYC), 19q (PI3Kp85, AKT2), 20p, 20q13.2 (BTAK)
Mutation[a]	K-Ras, BRAF, CTNNB1, CDKN2A, PIK3CA, KIT, MADH
Hypomethylation	BORIS, CLDN-4, IGF2, MCI, SAT2, SNCG
Histone modification	cyclin B1, GATA4, GATA6, p21/WAF1
miRNA	BAP1, DLK1, MSX2, PTEN, SIP1, VEGFA, ZEB1/2
Inactivating events	
Deletion by CGH	4q, 5q, 16q, 17p, 17q; Xp, Xq
LOH	(>50 %): 17p13, 17q21 (>30 %): 1p, 3p, 5q, 5q, 6q, 7q, 8q, 9p,10q,11p, 13q, 18q, 19p, 20; Xp
Mutation	ARID1A, TP53, Rb1a, APC, BRCA1, BRCA2, CDK12, NF1, PTEN, PP2R1A
Promoter methylation	APC, ARHI, ANGPTL, ARLTS1, BRCA1, DAPK, FBX032, H-CADHERIN, hMLH1, HOXA10, HOXA11, Hsulf-1, ICAM-1, LOT-1, MCJ, MUC2, MYO188, OPCML, PACE-4, PALP-B, PAR-4, PEG3, p16, p21, RASSF1, SOCS1, SOCS2, SPARC, TMS/ASC, TUBB3, 14-3-3σ
Histone modification	Adam 19, GATA4, GATA6, RASSF1
miRNA	BCL2, FGF2, MMP13, PAR8, c-SRK, VEGFA
Inhibition of growth by chromosome transfer	2, 3, 7, and 22

[a] www.Sanger.ac.uk

Table 2 Putative tumor suppressor genes in epithelial ovarian cancer.

Gene	Chromosome	Downregulated or inactivated	Mechanisms of downregulation	Function
ARHI (DIRAS3)	1p31	60% of all histotypes	Imprinting; LOH; promoter methylation; transcription downregulated by E2F1 and E2F4	26 kDa GTPase; inhibits proliferation and motility; induces autophagy and dormancy; upregulates p21; inhibits Cyclin D1, PI3K, Ras-MAP, Stat3
ARID1A	1p35.5	49% of clear cell and 30% of endometrioid histotypes	Mutation	Chromatin remodeling
RASSF1A	3p21	—	Hypermethylation	Inhibits proliferation and tumorigenicity in many different cancers. Interacts with Ras inhibiting downregulating cyclin D and signaling through JNK, stabilizes microtubules, and regulates spindle checkpoint and fas- and TNF-induced apoptosis
DLEC1	3p22.3	73%	Promoter hypermethylation and histone hypoacetylation	166 kDa cytoplasmic protein that inhibits anchorage-dependent growth
SPARC	5q31	70–90% decreased expression; 9% lost	Transcription, hypermethylation	32 kDa Ca++ binding protein; prevents adhesion
DAB-2 (DOC2)	5q13	58–85% lost	Transcription	105 kDa protein binds GRB2 preventing Ras/MAP activation, prevents c-fos induction and decreases ILK activity, contributing to anoikis and inhibiting proliferation and anchorage-independent growth and tumorigenicity
LOT-1 (ZAC1)	6q25	39%	Imprinting; hypermethylation LOH; transcription downregulated by EGF, TPA	55 kDa nuclear zinc finger protein inhibits proliferation and tumorigenicity
RPS6KA2	6q27	64%	Monoallelic expression in ovary; LOH	90-kDa ribosomal S6 serine threonine kinase that inhibits growth, induces apoptosis, decreases pERK and cyclin D1, and increases p21 and p27
PTEN (MMAC-1)	10q23	3–8% mutated; expression lost in 27%, particularly in endometrioid and clear cell histotypes	Promoter methylation; LOH; mutation	PI3 phosphatase; decreases proliferation, migration, and survival; decreases cyclin D and increases p27
OPCML	11q25	56–83%	Promoter methylation; LOH; mutation	GPI-anchored IgLON family member; induces aggregation; inhibits proliferation and tumorigenicity
BRCA2	13q12-13	3–6%	Mutation; LOH	Binds RAD51 in repair of DNA double-strand breaks (DSBs)
ARLTS1	13q14	62%	Promoter methylation	ADP ribosylation factor induces apoptosis
WWOX	16q23	30–49%, particularly in mucinous and clear cell histotypes	LOH; mutation	Decreases anchorage-independent growth and tumorigenicity; mouse homolog required for apoptosis
TP53	17p13.1	50–70% overall; 96% of high-grade serous histotype	Mutation	53-kDa nuclear protein induces p21 with cell cycle arrest promoting DNA stability; induces apoptosis
OVCA1	17p13.3	37%	LOH	50 kDa protein; decreases proliferation and clonogenicity; decreased Cyclin D1
BRCA1	17q21	6–8%	Mutation; LOH; promoter methylation	E3 ubiquitin ligase that participates directly in repair of DNA DSBs through homologous recombination; regulates c-Abl; induces TP53, androgen receptor, estrogen receptor and c-Myc
PEG3	19q13	75%	Imprinting; LOH; promoter methylation; transcription	Induces TP53-dependent apoptosis
PPP2R1A	19q13.44	7% of clear cell histotype	Mutation	Protein phosphatase 2 regulatory subunit inhibits proliferation

Candidate tumor suppressor genes with preliminary reports in the literature also include APC, BRMS1, CTGF, EPB41L3, MAP2K4, MKK4, RNF43, RP36RA7, PINX1, SFRP4, SLIT2, SOX11, TUSC3, and 53BP1.

Table 3 Oncogenes associated with epithelial ovarian cancer.

Oncogenes	Chromosome	Amplified (%)	Overexpressed (%)	Mutated (%)	Function
Rab25	1q22	54	80–89	—	Cytoplasmic GTPase/apical vessel trafficking
Evi-1	3q26	—	—	—	Transcription factor
eIF-5A2	3q26	—	—	—	Elongation factor
PKCi	3q26	44	78	—	Cytoplasmic serine-threonine kinase
PIK3CA (PI3K p110α)	3q26	9–80	32	8–12	Cytoplasmic lipid kinase
FGF-1	5q31	—	51	—	Growth factor for cancer and angiogenesis
Myc	8q24	20	41–66	—	Transcription factor
EGFR	7p12	11–20	9–28	<1	Tyrosine kinase growth factor receptor
Notch-3	9p13	20–21	62	—	Cell surface growth factor receptor
K-Ras	12p11-12	5–53	30–52	2–24	Cytoplasmic GTPase
HER-2	17q12-21	6–11	4–12	—	Tyrosine kinase growth factor receptor
p85 PI3K	19q	—	—	—	Cytoplasmic lipid kinase
Cyclin E	19q12	12–53	42–63	—	Cyclin
AKT2	19q13.2	12–27	12	—	Cytoplasmic serine-threonine Kinase
BTAK/Aurora A	20q13	10–15	48	—	Nuclear serine-threonine kinase/activates telomerase

Additional targetable genes with low or high gain of copy number in >20% of high-grade serous ovarian cancers include *AKT1*, *AKT3*, *CDK2*, *IL8RB*, *EPCAM*, *ERBB3*, *FGFR2*, *HDAC4*, *HSP90AB1*, *HSP90B1*, *IGF1*, *IGFR1*, *LPAR3*, *MAP3K6*, *MAPK15*, *MAPKAPK2*, *MAPKAPK5*, *MECOM*, *MSTN*, *MTOR*, *NCAM1*, *NOS1*, *NOS3*, *PIK3CD*, *POLB*, *POLE*, *RHEB*, *RICTOR*, *PPS6KC1*, *RAPTOR*, *SKI1*, *STAT1*, *STAT4*, *TERT*, *TGFB1*, *TGFB2*, *TGFBR3*, *TNFRSF9*, and *VEGFA*.

Regression and progression of disease tend to correlate well with falling or rising CA125 levels. The precise function of the glycoprotein is unknown,[84–86] but knockout of murine MUC16 does not affect the development or fertility of mice.[87] In cancer cells, CA125 expression is upregulated transcriptionally and 80% of the CA125 is cleaved and shed. Interaction of CA125 is with mesothelin at the peritoneal surface and is likely to be the first point of contact for ovarian cancer cells metastasizing within the peritoneal cavity.

Classification and pathology

Primary ovarian cancers are classified according to the structures of the ovary from which they are derived.[88] As noted above, most have thought to be derived from the epithelial cells that cover the ovarian surface or that line inclusion cysts, although, as described earlier, this concept has recently been challenged by recognition that many high-grade serous cancers arise from the fimbriae of fallopian tubes. These cells are ultimately derived from the coelomic epithelium of mesodermal origin and share cytologic markers with mesothelium. Germ cell malignancies constitute the next most common group and the least common tumors are derived from ovarian stromal cells (*see **Chapter 105***). Granulosa-Theca tumors are derived from the specialized connective tissue of the ovary and are the least common (*see **Chapter 105***).

Epithelial malignancies account for 85–90% of ovarian cancers. The majority of epithelial lesions are seen in patients who are 40 years of age or older. Under the age of 40 years, epithelial malignancies are uncommon, and most malignancies seen in women under the age of 30 years are of germ cell origin. The histologic types of the epithelial tumors are listed in Table 4. The majority of lesions, about 75%, are of the serous type, followed by the mucinous, endometrioid, clear cell, mixed, Brenner, and undifferentiated histologies.[11]

Invasive histotypes

Serous carcinomas may have a complex admixture of cystic and solid areas with extensive papillations, or they may contain a predominantly solid mass with areas of necrosis and hemorrhage (Figure 1). The poorly differentiated tumors may have some areas with a papillary pattern, but other portions may be indistinguishable from the other histologic patterns described in the following paragraphs (Figure 2). Stage I or II lesions are most frequently

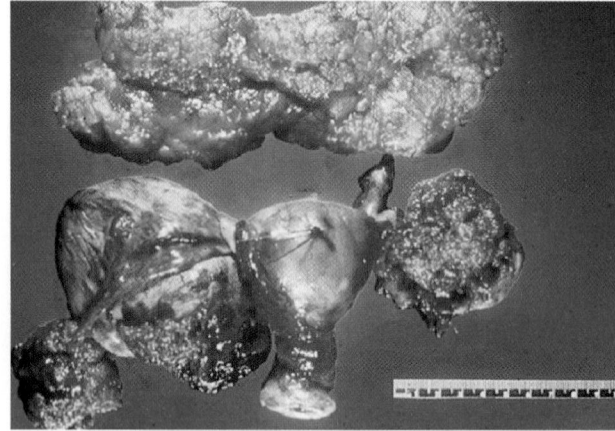

Figure 1 Serous cystadenocarcinoma gross with omentum.

unilateral, with about 10–20% involving both ovaries. Conversely, about 50–70% of stage III serous carcinomas are bilateral.[11]

Mucinous tumors tend to be large, with many masses over 20 cm in diameter (Figure 3). The histologic pattern resembles uterine endocervical glands. The lesions frequently contain areas of hemorrhage, necrosis, and various quantities of mucin. These tumors are bilateral in 10–20% of cases. Occasionally, mucin is secreted into the peritoneal cavity and produces a condition known as pseudomyxoma or myxoma peritonei. A mucocele of the appendix may also be seen in conjunction with this tumor.

Endometrioid carcinomas of the ovary resemble typical carcinomas of the endometrium. These tumors may be seen with synchronous endometrial carcinoma, and when they are, both lesions may be of low stage. Rarely, endometrioid carcinomas may arise in conjunction with pelvic endometriosis, resulting from malignant transformation of a benign process (Figure 4).[11] Similar to previous endometrial cancers, endometrioid ovarian cancers are associated with inactivating mutations of *PTEN* with consequent activation of PI3 kinase signaling. Bilaterality is seen in 10–15% of stage I and II disease and in about 30% of stage III.

Ovarian clear cell carcinomas have abundant intracellular glycogen that is removed during histopathologic processing. About one-fourth of clear cell tumors are associated with endometriosis. Clear cell tumors are only rarely bilateral.[11]

Table 4 Epithelial ovarian tumors.

Histologic type	Cellular type
1. Serous	Endosalpingeal
(a) Benign	
(b) Borderline	
(c) Malignant	
2. Mucinous	Endocervical
(a) Benign	
(b) Borderline	
(c) Malignant	
3. Endometrioid	Endometrial
(a) Benign	
(b) Borderline	
(c) Malignant	
4. Clear cell "mesonephroid"	Müllerian
(a) Benign	
(b) Borderline	
(c) Malignant	
5. Brenner	Transitional
(a) Benign	
(b) Borderline (proliferating)	
(c) Malignant	
6. Mixed epithelial	Mixed
(a) Benign	
(b) Borderline	
(c) Malignant	
7. Undifferentiated	
(a) Anaplastic	
8. Unclassified	
(a) Mesothelioma	
(b) Other	

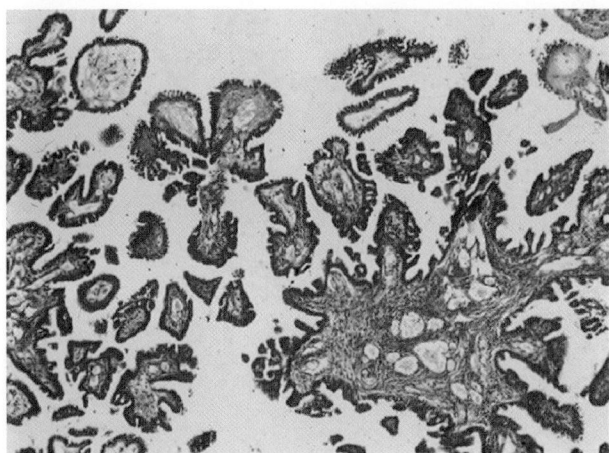

Figure 2 Poorly differentiated serous carcinoma of ovary.

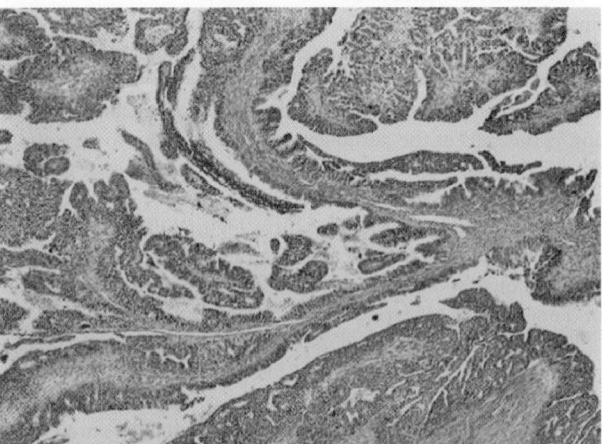

Figure 3 Mucinous cystadenocarcinoma.

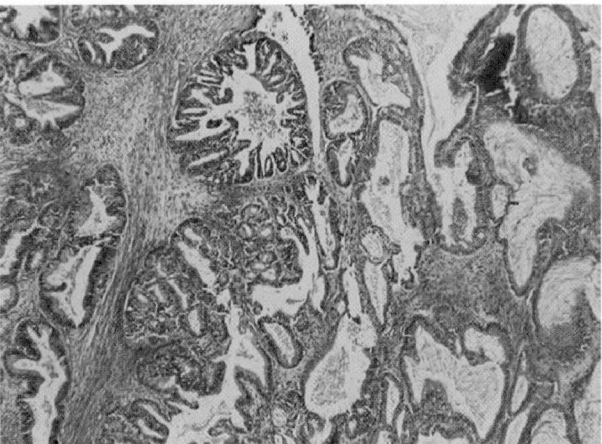

Figure 4 Endometrioid carcinoma.

Brenner tumors are uncommon, representing less than 1% of all epithelial malignancies. Mixed epithelial tumors may contain small areas of Brenner tumor histology, which have a histologic pattern similar to that of transitional cell. Malignant Brenner tumors are unilateral.[11]

Borderline tumors

Borderline tumors, or those of low malignant potential, are important to differentiate from those that are frankly invasive. The treatment and prognosis for borderline lesions are considerably different from those for invasive malignancies. Borderline tumors tend to remain confined to a single ovary at the time of diagnosis and also tend to occur in younger, premenopausal women (Figure 5). They may be confused with a well-differentiated invasive ovarian cancer, and the treatment for the two may be different. Thus, in a young patient who has a lesion confined to the ovary, which is suspected of being an epithelial ovarian cystadenocarcinoma, a borderline tumor must be excluded because bilateral oophorectomy, hysterectomy, and chemotherapy are unnecessary in these patients. In women under the age of 40 years, about 60–70% of nonbenign ovarian neoplasms are borderline, whereas in women over 40 years, only 10% are borderline.[11,89] Histologic criteria for borderline tumors include (1) the presence of epithelial cell proliferation with

a "piling up" of cells, the so-called pseudostratification; (2) cytologic atypia, but with rare mitoses; and (3) no evidence of stromal invasion. Borderline tumors tend to remain confined to the ovary but may be associated with peritoneal disease, which represents either dissemination or the multifocal evolution of the disease. In those rare patients with peritoneal involvement, death can occur by progressive intestinal obstruction.

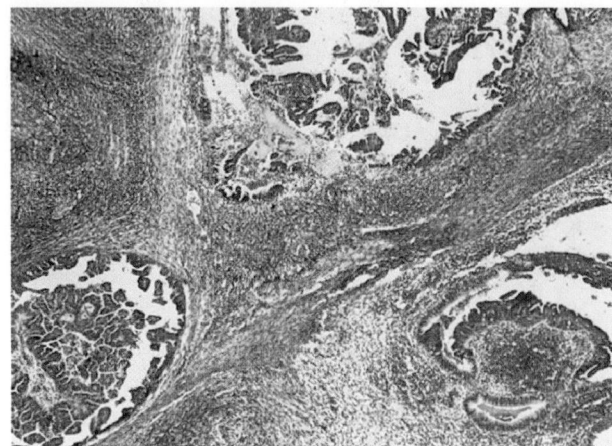

Figure 5 Borderline serous tumor.

Peritoneal carcinomas

Epithelial malignancies that coat the surface of the ovary and peritoneum are referred to as peritoneal carcinomas.[14] These cancers are distinct from the very rare peritoneal mesotheliomas that exhibit a different natural history, as well as response to chemotherapy.[90] The cells of the peritoneum have the ability to recapitulate any of the histologic patterns seen in ovarian cancers, although serous carcinomas occur most frequently and the other histologic types are rarely seen. Many of these high-grade serous primary peritoneal cancers are likely to arise from fimbriae of the fallopian tube, although some may be derived from developmental remnants of the secondary Müllerian system.[12]

Recognition of peritoneal carcinomas explains the occurrence of ovarian cancer after oophorectomy.[91] In addition, peritoneal cancers can involve the surface of the ovaries without ovarian enlargement. Thus, ovaries can be innocent bystanders in a process originating in the peritoneal cavity. Therapeutically, peritoneal malignancy should be treated as one would manage an epithelial ovarian cancer.

Patterns of spread

Ovarian epithelial tumors spread primarily by direct exfoliation and implantation of cells throughout the peritoneal cavity but also metastasize via the lymphatic and hematogenous routes. GCTs (*see* **Chapter 105**) have a greater predilection for spread via the retroperitoneal lymphatics, which must be evaluated carefully when staging those tumors that appear to be confined to the ovary.[11,92]

Exfoliated ovarian cancer cells spread directly to the pelvic and abdominal peritoneal surfaces and tend to follow the path of circulation of peritoneal fluid from the right pericolic gutter cephalad to the right hemidiaphragm. At primary surgery, the parietal and visceral peritoneum can be studded with dozens to hundreds of metastatic nodules. The intestinal mesenteries can become involved by peritoneal metastases. Adhesions form between loops of small intestine producing mechanical obstruction, even though involvement of the lumen of the intestine by direct extension is uncommon. The intestinal dysfunction can also result from involvement by tumor of the myenteric plexus, the autonomic innervation of the intestine that is found in the mesentery. This condition has been referred to as "carcinomatous ileus." Large pelvic masses can compress the rectum producing colonic obstruction.

Spread via the lymphatics is common in epithelial ovarian cancer. Apparent stage I and II tumors have retroperitoneal lymphatic dissemination in about 5–10% in most series, whereas lymphatic dissemination in stage III has been reported to be as high as 42–78% in carefully explored patients.[93] Most of these lymph nodes are not enlarged but are microscopically positive for malignant cells. Spread through the retroperitoneal and diaphragmatic lymphatics can result in metastasis to the supraclavicular lymph nodes on the left and right, respectively. Bloodborne metastasis of ovarian cancer is uncommon at diagnosis and is often a late finding in the disease. Hematogenous dissemination at the time of diagnosis to the parenchyma of the liver or lung is seen in a minority of patients. In advanced recurrent disease, parenchymal metastases are seen more frequently in the parenchyma of the lung and even of the brain.

Clinical symptoms

Some patients with ovarian cancers confined to the ovary are asymptomatic, but the majority will have nonspecific symptoms that do not necessarily suggest an origin in the ovary. In one survey of 1725 women with ovarian cancer, 95% recalled symptoms before diagnosis, including 89% with stage I/II disease and 97% with stage III/IV disease.[94] Seventy percent had abdominal or GI symptoms, 58% pain, 34% urinary symptoms, and 26% pelvic discomfort. At least some of these symptoms could have reflected pressure on the pelvic viscera from the enlarging ovary. Goff et al. have developed an ovarian cancer symptom index and reported that symptoms associated with ovarian cancer were pelvic/abdominal pain, urinary frequency/urgency, increased abdominal size or bloating, and difficulty eating or feeling full when they were present for less than 1 year and occurred >12 days a month. The index had a sensitivity of 56.7% for early ovarian cancer and 79.5% for advanced-stage disease.[95] Interestingly, a population-based study from Australia found that there did not appear to be a significant difference in the duration of symptoms or the nature of symptoms in patients with early as opposed to advanced-stage ovarian cancer.[96,97]

Metastatic ovarian cancer is rarely asymptomatic. In addition to the GI and urinary symptoms noted in early-stage disease, formation of ascites can produce an increase in abdominal girth. Pleural effusion may lead to dyspnea as the first complaint. Acute symptoms, such as those of adnexal rupture or torsion, are uncommon. Vaginal bleeding is also an uncommon symptom in postmenopausal women, although premenopausal patients may present with irregular or heavy menses. Detection of an adnexal mass by pelvic examination can permit the early diagnosis of ovarian cancer. As malignancy is rare and the majority of palpable adnexal masses are benign, an enlarged ovary discovered on pelvic examination is not likely to be an ovarian malignancy. In premenopausal women, ovarian cancer is uncommon and represents less than 7% of all adnexal masses.[11] Even in postmenopausal women, 70–80% of adnexal tumors are benign. In some patients who complain primarily of abdominal symptoms, however, a pelvic examination frequently is omitted and the tumor missed. Signs of advanced disease include abdominal distention and a fluid wave consistent with ascites. These signs are nonspecific and can be associated with many conditions arising in the abdominal cavity, especially malignancies of other primary sites or carcinomatosis from metastatic tumors of the GI tract and breast.

Diagnosis

The diagnosis of ovarian cancer is usually made at laparotomy, but occasionally at laparoscopy. If a pelvic mass is suspicious and the most likely diagnosis is ovarian cancer, surgery should not be unnecessarily delayed. In premenopausal patients, however, simple cystic ovarian lesions can be observed over a period of 1–2 months. Lesions that are essentially mobile, are unilateral, and have a smooth contour are much less likely to be neoplastic, and are unlikely to be malignant. In premenopausal patients with cystic lesions of less than 8 cm, attempted suppression with oral contraceptives is indicated. In women who are definitely postmenopausal, cystic masses larger than 5 cm should be removed unless they represent a chronic finding. Those masses that regress in size can be managed with continued observation, whereas those that persist or enlarge must be evaluated surgically. Conversely, patients whose lesions are irregular, predominantly solid, and somewhat immobile should undergo an exploratory laparotomy.

The preoperative evaluation of patients can be aided by the use of blood biomarkers. Three algorithms have been developed for distinguishing malignant from benign pelvic masses. Ultrasound, CA125, and menopausal status have been combined to create a risk of malignancy index (RMI) that has achieved a sensitivity of 71–88% with a reciprocal specificity of 97–74% for predicting the presence of ovarian cancers in women with pelvic masses.[98] An OVA1 panel including CA125, apolipoprotein A1, transthyretin, transferrin, and B2-microglobulin combined with imaging and menopausal status provides 92% sensitivity at 42% specificity in postmenopausal women and 85% sensitivity at 45% specificity for premenopausal women.[99] The negative predictive value for women judged at low risk is 94%–96%. Similar sensitivity and higher specificity have been attained with a risk of malignancy index (ROMA) calculated from CA125 and HE4 values combined with menopausal status alone, without imaging.[100] In an initial trial of patients referred to academic centers, the sensitivity for predicting a malignant pelvic mass was 93%, specificity 75%, and negative predictive value 94%. In a subsequent community-based trial, a sensitivity of 94%, specificity of 75%, and negative predictive value of 99% were attained.[101] The ROMA has been shown superior to the RMI.[100] Both the OVA1 and the ROMA panels have been approved for use by the US FDA. Utilization of these panels could assure that women with ovarian cancer receive optimal surgery. At present, less than half of women in the United States with ovarian cancer have their initial operation with a gynecologic oncologist trained to perform optimal cytoreductive surgery.

Ultrasonographic signs of malignancy include an adnexal pelvic mass with areas of complexity, such as irregular borders; multiple echogenic patterns within the mass; and dense, multiple irregular septae. Bilateral tumors are more likely to be malignant, although the individual characteristics of the lesions are of greater significance. Transvaginal ultrasonography may have a somewhat better resolution than transabdominal ultrasonography for adnexal neoplasms. Newer techniques using Doppler color-flow imaging may enhance the specificity of ultrasonography for demonstrating findings consistent with malignancy.

Radiographic techniques, including abdominal radiographs, computed tomography (CT) scans, PET-CT (positron emission tomography) scans, and nuclear MRI, are not useful before the surgical diagnosis of ovarian cancer. The preoperative evaluation of patients who have a suspicious pelvic mass can omit these studies when blood chemistries and enzymes suggest normal hepatic and pancreatic function. In patients with ascites and no pelvic mass, however, a CT or MRI may be useful in identifying other potential sites of origin. Paracentesis is not recommended because of the frequency of metastatic implantation and growth in the needle tract.

Liver–spleen scans, brain scans, and bone scans are unnecessary unless specific symptoms suggest metastasis to these sites.

In premenopausal women, radiographic studies of the intestines are not required unless there is the finding of occult blood in the rectum or there are symptoms indicating upper or lower intestinal obstruction. A barium enema or endoscopy is appropriate in postmenopausal patients. Mammography should be performed to exclude primary breast cancer, which can coexist with ovarian cancer or spread to the ovaries. Cervical cytology should be performed, although ovarian cancer cells are unlikely to exfoliate through the uterus to the cervix. In patients with irregular or heavy menses, an endometrial biopsy should be performed to exclude primary endometrial pathology.

The differential diagnosis of an adnexal mass includes a variety of functional changes of the ovary, benign neoplasms of the reproductive tract, and inflammatory lesions of these organs. A hydrosalpinx, endometriosis, and pedunculated uterine leiomyomata can simulate an ovarian neoplasm. Nongynecologic diseases, such as inflammatory processes of the colon and rectum, must be excluded.

Screening

There is no well-established strategy for early detection of ovarian cancer. Discovery of a pelvic mass on routine physical examination can lead to surgery before the dissemination of a malignancy, but conventional diagnosis detects less than 20% of patients in stage I. Given the prevalence of ovarian cancer in the postmenopausal population, any screening strategy must be highly specific (>99.6%) as well as highly sensitive for early-stage disease (>75%) to achieve a PPV of 10% (i.e., 10 laparotomies for each case of ovarian cancer detected). Two approaches have been evaluated for early detection of ovarian cancer: ultrasonography and serum tests such as CA125.

Ultrasonography

Transvaginal sonography (TVS) has proved superior to transabdominal sonography (TAU) for the detection of a pelvic mass. In three large studies that screened 66,620 women with TVS, 565 operations were performed to detect 45 ovarian cancers, 34 of which were invasive.[102–104] Overall, the sensitivity for early-stage disease was 78%, but the specificity fell just short of that required for a PPV of 10% with 12 operations per case of ovarian cancer detected. The most promising single study achieved a PPV of 9.9%. Confirmatory tests with Doppler ultrasound have not proved consistent, but additional studies with 3-D power Doppler are underway to improve specificity in distinguishing malignant from benign ovarian abnormalities.

CA125

CA125 is elevated in 50–60% of patients with stage I and in 90% with stage II ovarian cancer.[105] CA125 levels can rise 10–60 months before diagnosis with an average estimated lead time of 1.9 years before diagnosis of disease in all stages.[106] In the Prostate, Lung, Colorectal and Ovarian (PLCO) screening trial, 37,500 postmenopausal women had an annual CA125 and TVS for 3 years.[107] If either were abnormal, women were referred to a gynecologist. CA125 alone had a PPV of 3.7%; TVS alone had a PPV of 1%. If both were abnormal, the PPV rose to 23.5%, but 60% of the invasive ovarian cancers would have been missed. Thus, the specificity for a single determination of CA125 or a single TVS is not adequate to screen a population at average risk, but specificity can be improved with a two-stage strategy that utilizes CA125 followed by ultrasound in a subset of women with elevated CA125. Use of CA125 to trigger ultrasound has been evaluated in trials in Sweden and in the United Kingdom.[108,109] The latter randomized 22,000 women to conventional surveillance or to annual CA125 with TAU if the value were elevated. When TAU was abnormal, surgery was undertaken. Among 10,985 women screened, 29 operations were performed to detect 6 cancers, providing a PPV of 21%. During 7 years of follow-up, 10 more cancers were diagnosed in the screened group. Over the same intervals, 21 ovarian cancers were diagnosed in the control group. Median survival in the screened group (72.9 months) was significantly greater ($p = 0.0112$) than that in the control group (41.8 months).

Risk of ovarian cancer (ROC) algorithm

A rising CA125 is a more specific indicator of ovarian cancer. Analyzing serum samples stored from screening studies in Stockholm and in the United Kingdom with an improved CA125 II assay, it has been possible to improve the specificity of CA125 as a screening tool by following the values of an individual over time.[110,111] Elevated CA125 levels in women without ovarian cancer remain static or decrease with time, whereas levels associated with ovarian malignancy tend to rise. This finding has been incorporated into an algorithm that uses age, rate of change of CA125, and absolute levels of CA125 to calculate an individual's "risk of ovarian cancer" (ROCA, risk of ovarian cancer algorithm). Patients at sufficient risk undergo TVS. Over the past 15 years, a trial has been conducted with the ROCA in the United States coordinated by the MD Anderson SPORE in Ovarian Cancer. Some 18 patients have undergone surgery based on the algorithm. Six have had benign disease, two have had borderline tumors (stage I) and ten have had invasive ovarian cancers with seven in early stage (I–II) and three in stage III. Only three operations have been required to detect each case of ovarian cancer.[112] Currently, accrual to a larger trial has been completed in the United Kingdom that includes 200,000 postmenopausal women who were randomized to three groups: a control group (~100,000) that has been followed with conventional pelvic examinations; a second group (~50,000) that had annual TVS; and a third group (~50,000) that had CA125 determined at least annually. On the basis of the ROCA, patients in the third group were referred for TVS and/or surgery. Women were screened for 3 years and followed for 7 years. Results from the initial 3 years of the "prevalence phase" of accrual suggested that a higher fraction of early stage disease could be detected (48%) with the ROCA and that no more than 3–4 operations would be required for each case detected.[113] Results of the study will become available in late 2015, but it is already apparent that use of the ROCA doubled the number of screen-detected ovarian cancers compared to use of an arbitrary threshold for CA125.[114] Results from the first year of screening suggest that the ROCA followed by TVS will have substantially higher specificity and no less sensitivity than annual TVS, but data in subsequent years will be required to determine whether screening improves survival.

Whatever the outcome of the current trial in the United Kingdom, strategies based on CA125 alone are not likely to exceed a sensitivity of 80%, as CA125 is not expressed by 20% of epithelial ovarian cancers. Greater sensitivity might be attained through the use of multiple serum markers in combination, provided that specificity was not compromised. Two other biomarkers—HE4 and CA72.4—detect a fraction of patients (15%) missed by CA125. Autoantibodies against TP53 can also detect 18% of patients missed by CA125 and provide 13–33 months of lead time.

Current recommendations for screening women at average risk

The application of screening techniques other than pelvic examination for ovarian cancer in the entire female population is unwarranted at this time. The sensitivity and specificity of ultrasound or CA125 alone are inadequate. Use of annual CA125 followed by TVS appears more promising, but application of this approach outside of a research study will depend on the outcome of the UKCTOCS trial. If a significant improvement in survival and mortality are observed, the MD Anderson trial has shown that this approach is feasible in the United States.

Current recommendations for screening women at high risk

Although ultrasound and CA125 screening have been advocated for women at increased genetic ROC, the efficacy of surveillance to reduce mortality or detect cancers at an earlier stage is unproved. Many of the occult cancers found after PBSO (prophylactic bilateral salpingo-oophorectomy) have been in the fimbrial end of the fallopian tube, and this consistent finding suggests that ultrasound of the ovaries is unlikely to detect cancers at an early stage in women at high genetic risk. Screening can be problematic because this high-risk population generally includes premenopausal women who have a higher incidence of false-positive CA125 elevations and ultrasound abnormalities. In these high-risk populations, initial screening trials using ultrasound alone or in combination with color-flow Doppler were associated with high false-positive rates (2.5–4.9%). The current trend among those who support screening is to combine ultrasound every 6–12 months with CA125 every 3–6 months.

There are five prospective studies where combined screening has been undertaken in high-risk populations.[33,115–118] In three screening programs involving a total of 1228 women with a family history of ovarian cancer, no invasive ovarian cancer was detected and false-positive rates have ranged from 0.4% to 3.9%.[33,48,49,115–119] In one of the remaining two studies, one case of ovarian cancer was detected on screening 137 high-risk women with a false-positive rate of 0.7%; in the other study, nine ovarian cancers were detected in screening 180 women with a false-positive rate of 3.9%.[117,118] The findings of two prospective studies of annual transvaginal ultrasound and CA125 screening in 888 *BRCA1* and *BRCA2* mutation carriers in the Netherlands and 279 mutation carriers in the United Kingdom are not encouraging and suggest a very limited benefit of screening in high-risk women.[48,49] Therefore, it is unlikely that annual screening will reduce mortality from ovarian cancer in *BRCA1/2* mutation carriers. Women in the high-risk population who request screening should be counseled about the current lack of evidence for the efficacy for either CA125 or sonography as well as the associated false-positive rates. Many will still opt for screening despite the risks and limitations of the available strategies.

Staging

Ovarian, fallopian tube and peritoneal malignancies are staged according to the new FIGO system of 2014 (Table 5) that is based on the findings at surgical exploration. A preoperative evaluation should exclude the presence of extraperitoneal metastases. A thorough surgical exploration is important because subsequent treatment will be determined by the stage of disease. In patients whose exploratory laparotomy does not reveal any macroscopic evidence of disease by inspection and palpation of the entire intra-abdominal space, a careful search for microscopic spread must be undertaken. In an earlier series in which patients did not

Table 5 FIGO staging of ovarian, fallopian tube, and peritoneal cancer (2014).

Stage I: Tumor confined to ovaries or fallopian tube(s)	T1-N0-M0
IA: Tumor limited to one ovary (capsule intact) or fallopian tube; no tumor on ovarian or fallopian tube surface; no malignant cells in the ascites or peritoneal washings	T1a-N0-M0
IB: Tumor limited to both ovaries (capsules intact) or fallopian tubes; no tumor on ovarian or fallopian tube surface; no malignant cells in the ascites or peritoneal washings	T1b-N0-M0
IC: Tumor limited to one or both ovaries or fallopian tubes, with any of the following	
IC1: Surgical spill	T1c1-N0-M0
IC2: Capsule ruptured before surgery or tumor on ovarian or fallopian tube surface	T1c2-N0-M0
IC3: Malignant cells in the ascites or peritoneal washings	T1c3-N0-M0
Stage II: Tumor involves one or both ovaries or fallopian tubes with pelvic extension (below pelvic brim) or primary peritoneal cancer	T2-N0-M0
IIA: Extension and/or implants on uterus and/or fallopian tubes and/or ovaries	T2a-N0-M0
IIB: Extension to other pelvic intraperitoneal tissues	T2b-N0-M0
Stage III: Tumor involves one or both ovaries or fallopian tubes, or primary peritoneal cancer, with cytologically or histologically confirmed spread to the peritoneum outside the pelvis and/or metastasis to the retroperitoneal lymph nodes	T1/T2-N1-M0
IIIA1: Positive retroperitoneal lymph nodes only (cytologically or histologically proven):	
IIIA1(i) Metastasis up to 10 mm in greatest dimension	
IIIA1(ii) Metastasis more than 10 mm in greatest dimension	
IIIA2: Microscopic extrapelvic (above the pelvic brim) peritoneal involvement with or without positive retroperitoneal lymph nodes	T3a2-N0/N1-M0
IIIB: Macroscopic peritoneal metastasis beyond the pelvis up to 2 cm in greatest dimension, with or without metastasis to the retroperitoneal lymph nodes	T3b-N0/N1-M0
IIIC: Macroscopic peritoneal metastasis beyond the pelvis more than 2 cm in greatest dimension, with or without metastasis to the retroperitoneal lymph nodes (includes extension of tumor to capsule of liver and spleen without parenchymal involvement of either organ)	T3c-N0/N1-M0
Stage IV: Distant metastasis excluding peritoneal metastases	
Stage IVA: Pleural effusion with positive cytology	
Stage IVB: Parenchymal metastases and metastases to extra-abdominal organs (including inguinal lymph nodes and lymph nodes outside of the abdominal cavity)	Any T, any N, M1

FIGO, International Federation of Gynecology and Obstetrics.

undergo careful surgical staging, the overall 5-year survival for patients with apparent stage I epithelial ovarian cancer was only about 60%.[4] Survival rates of 90–100% have been reported for properly staged patients found to have stage IA or IB disease.[4]

Metastases in clinically apparent stage I or II epithelial ovarian cancer are common. About 30% of patients whose ovarian epithelial cancers appear to be confined to the pelvis have occult metastatic disease in the upper abdomen or in the retroperitoneal lymph nodes.[120] Histologic grade was a significant predictor of occult metastasis, that is, 16% of patients with grade 1 lesions were upstaged, compared to 34% with grade 2 and 46% with grade 3 disease.

Although the literature has emphasized the importance of thorough surgical exploration in patients with disease apparently localized to the ovaries, scant recognition is made of the semantic difficulty presented by the concept of extension to other pelvic (i.e., stage II) or abdominal (i.e., stage III) organs. No problem exists when the surgeon encounters discrete implants, or seeds, separate from the primary tumor, or when solid tumor is found growing into adjacent structures. A more common situation, however, is the apparently benign adherence of the tumor to adjacent structures in the absence of metastatic implants or obvious direct tumor extension. There is a considerable body of evidence that such benign adherence, when it is dense, is associated with a relapse risk equivalent to stage II, and that these patients should not be included in stage I but rather in stage II.[120] Adherence is considered dense when sharp dissection is required to mobilize the tumor, when a raw area is left at the site of adherence, or when rupture of a cyst results from dissecting free the adhesions. It is the practice at most North American centers to advance the stage of densely adherent tumors to stage II, and this was done in a recent multicenter study of stage I and II disease.[120]

After a comprehensive staging laparotomy, less than 25% of women are found to have local or regional disease (FIGO stages I and II). Although accounting for only 15–20% of all cases, approximately one-third to one-half of all cured patients are derived from stage I, highlighting its importance. An in-depth understanding of the management of stage I is hampered by the small fraction of patients with limited disease, as well as by their excellent long-term prognosis (over an 80% 5-year relapse-free rate). Consequently, phase III randomized trials are difficult to conduct with this group owing to their small numbers and relatively low rate of recurrence and death.

Prognosis

The prognosis of epithelial ovarian cancer can be correlated with numerous clinical and biologic factors. Tumor stage, grade, and size of metastatic disease after resection correlate best with outcome.[121,122] As discussed in the following text, among patients with low-stage disease, tumor grade correlates with prognosis (i.e., patients with stage I high-grade lesions have a higher risk of recurrence and shorter survival than do those of low-grade lesions).[122] In patients with advanced-stage disease, the size of residual disease after surgery correlates most clearly with survival.[123] Complete removal of all visible tumor has the best prognosis. The rapidity with which disease regresses during chemotherapy also correlates with survival. A short apparent half-life of the serum tumor marker CA125 has correlated with improved survival in more than a dozen studies.[124] Normalization of CA125 by the third course of chemotherapy has been associated with a favorable prognosis. The presence of malignant ascites has been shown to also adversely impact on prognosis.

Treatment of early-stage epithelial cancer

The treatment of early-stage epithelial ovarian and fallopian tube cancer must be individualized. Thorough surgical exploration and staging are indicated for all patients with early-stage disease. Adjuvant treatment with chemotherapy is appropriate for those women at highest risk of recurrence.

Surgery

The initial treatment for invasive stage I epithelial ovarian cancer is surgical, that is, the performance of a total abdominal hysterectomy, BSO, and surgical staging. In certain circumstances, a unilateral salpingo-oophorectomy may suffice, as discussed in the following sections.

Adjuvant chemotherapy

The GOG reported the results of a randomized study comparing three cycles of carboplatin and paclitaxel with six cycles in 457 patients with early-stage ovarian cancer.[125] An unexpectedly large number of patients (126, 29%) had incomplete or inadequately documented surgical staging in this study. The recurrence rate for six cycles was 24% lower (hazard ratio [HR] 0.76 CI 0.5–1.13 $p = 0.18$) for six cycles versus three cycles, but this was not statistically significant. The estimated probability of recurrence at 5 years was 20.1% for six cycles and 25.4% for three cycles. They concluded that three cycles of adjuvant carboplatin and paclitaxel was a reasonable option for women with high-risk early-stage ovarian cancer, particularly in women with nonserous cancers although many oncologists would recommend six cycles, if chemotherapy is given to early-stage patients with high-grade serous. Two large parallel randomized phase 3 clinical trials were conducted on women with early-stage disease: the International Collaborative Ovarian Neoplasm Trial 1 (ICON1) and the Adjuvant Chemotherapy Trial in Ovarian Neoplasia (ACTION).[126,127] When the data from the two trials were combined and analyzed,[128] a total of 465 patients was randomized to receive platinum-based adjuvant chemotherapy and 460 to observation until disease progression. After a median follow-up of more than 4 years, the overall survival was 82% in the chemotherapy arm and 74% in the observation arm (HR = 0.67, $p = 0.001$). Recurrence-free survival was also better in the chemotherapy arm: 76% versus 65% (HR = 0.64, $p = 0.001$). The results of this analysis must be interpreted with caution because most of the patients did not undergo thorough surgical staging, but the findings suggest that platinum-based chemotherapy should be given to patients who have not been optimally staged.

Management of invasive early-stage low-risk disease (stages IA and IB, low grade)

In patients who have undergone a thorough staging laparotomy where there is no evidence of spread beyond the ovary, the performance of an abdominal hysterectomy and BSO is appropriate therapy. The uterus and contralateral ovary can be preserved in women with stage IA diploid lesions who wish to preserve fertility. These women should be followed carefully with periodic pelvic examinations and CA125 levels. Generally, the other ovary and uterus are removed at the completion of childbearing. In a recent report by Guthrie et al.,[129] the outcome of 656 patients with early-stage epithelial ovarian cancer was studied. No patients who had a properly documented stage I, grade 1 cancer died of their disease; that is, there was a 100% survival in this condition when patients were surgically staged, and thus adjuvant chemotherapy is unnecessary in patients with low-risk low-stage ovarian cancer.

Management of invasive early-stage high-risk disease (stage IA and IB, high grade, stage IC and stage II)

High-risk stage I is defined as stage IA or IB, grade 3, stage IC, or clear cell carcinomas. In patients whose disease is more poorly differentiated or in whom there are malignant cells either in ascitic fluid or in peritoneal washings, additional therapy is indicated. Patients with grade 2 and grade 3 tumors, with densely adherent tumors, with large-volume ascites, and/or with positive peritoneal cytology, have a relapse risk of 20–45%, and postoperative treatment is warranted. Regrettably, it would appear that thorough staging with negative findings, including random peritoneal biopsies and lymph node sampling, does not eliminate the risk of relapse in patients with these characteristics. Patients with early-stage high-risk epithelial ovarian cancer have been treated with single-agent carboplatin or a combination of carboplatin and a taxane. Given a risk of recurrence and death of >20%, it is recommended that six cycles of chemotherapy with carboplatin (area under the curve [AUC] 5–6) and paclitaxel be considered in patients with high-risk low-stage ovarian cancer.

Management of early-stage borderline tumors

The principal treatment for borderline ovarian tumors is the surgical resection of the primary tumor. There is no evidence that either subsequent chemotherapy or radiation therapy improves survival. After performing a frozen section and determining that the histology is borderline, premenopausal patients who desire preservation of ovarian function may be managed with a conservative operation, such as a unilateral salpingooophorectomy. Thus, hormonal function and fertility can be maintained. In patients in whom an ovarian cystectomy has been performed and a borderline tumor is documented in the permanent pathology, no additional surgery is warranted.

There has been considerable controversy regarding the optimum treatment of patients with localized borderline ovarian tumors. This has been due, in part, to lack of unanimity regarding the histopathologic criteria for borderline tumors. For all stages of ovarian cancer, borderline tumors have a more favorable natural history than have invasive tumors. There is no evidence to suggest any benefit of adjuvant chemotherapy for patients with stage I or stage II borderline tumors. In a large GOG trial, a total of 51 patients were reclassified as having borderline tumors. In these carefully staged patients, there have been no deaths directly attributable to cancer. While a substantial number of patients did receive adjuvant chemotherapy in these trials, there is no evidence that it was necessary or beneficial. If, after careful histologic review of multiple slides sectioned at 1-cm intervals, no evidence of stromal invasion is found, patients with localized borderline tumors should not receive adjuvant chemotherapy.

Treatment of advanced stage epithelial cancer

A scheme for the management of patients with advanced-stage epithelial cancer is shown in Figure 6. The components of this approach are discussed in the following sections.

Cytoreductive surgery

Patients who have advanced-stage epithelial ovarian cancer documented at initial exploratory laparotomy should undergo cytoreductive surgery to remove as much of the tumor and its metastases as possible in order to facilitate the effectiveness of subsequent therapies. The operation usually includes the performance of a total abdominal hysterectomy and BSO, a complete

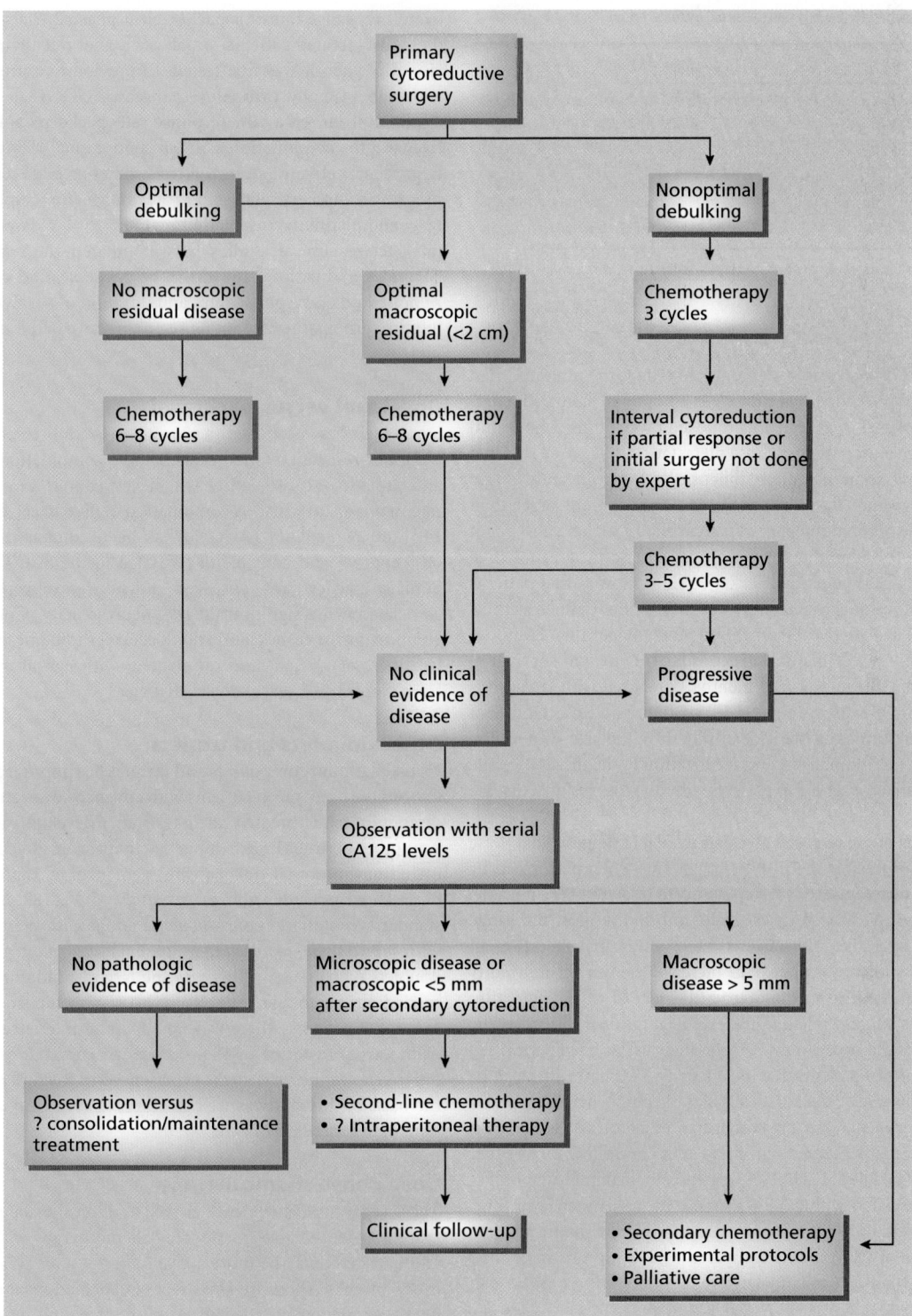

Figure 6 Treatment scheme for patients with advanced-stage ovarian cancer.
*Perform in a research setting where treatment will be based on outcome. Source: Berek 2015. Reproduced with permission of Wolters Kluwer Health.

omentectomy, and resection of metastatic lesions on the peritoneal surfaces or from the intestines. In addition, the pelvic tumor may directly involve the rectosigmoid colon, the terminal ileum, and the cecum. In some patients, most or all of their disease is confined to the pelvic viscera and the omentum, so that removal of these organs results in the extirpation of all gross tumor and patients with no macroscopic residual disease, a situation that is associated with a reasonable chance of complete response.

The rationale for cytoreductive surgery relates to the following three general theoretical considerations: (1) potential physiologic benefits from excising the tumor; (2) improved tumor perfusion and increased growth fraction, which may increase the likelihood of a response to chemotherapy or radiation therapy; and (3) enhanced immunologic competence of the patient.[131,132]

The principal goal of cytoreductive surgery is to remove all of the primary cancer and, if possible, its metastases. If resection of

Table 6 Nomenclature for patient status-residual ovarian cancer.

Residual disease		Status
None	Pathologic	Complete remission
Microscopic disease	Only	Microscopic
Macroscopic disease	<5 mm	Minimal residual
Macroscopic disease	<1–2 cm	Optimal residual
Macroscopic residual disease	>1–2 cm	Suboptimal
Macroscopic disease	>2–3 cm	Bulky residual

Nomenclature for status of patient based on the extent of residual ovarian cancer before treatment.

all metastases is not feasible, the goal is to reduce the tumor burden by resection of all individual tumors to an optimal status. The definition of "optimal" was initially proposed by Griffiths, who found that the survival of patients whose metastatic disease was resected to less than 1.5 cm in maximum dimension was significantly longer than the survival of those whose residual lesions were larger than 1.5 cm.[133] The optimal category of patients had a higher subsequent response rate to chemotherapy and longer disease-progression-free interval (PFI). Subsequently, Hacker et al.[134] showed that patients whose largest residual lesions were less than 5 mm (defined as minimal residual disease [MRD]) survived much longer than did those with larger nonresectable tumor deposits. The median survival of patients in this category was 40 months, compared with 18 months for patients whose disease was >1.5 cm (Figure 6). Resectability of the metastatic tumor is often determined by the size of nodules, the extent of carcinomatosis, and the location of the disease.[135] The greatest benefit is observed in patients with no gross residual disease (Table 6).

An analysis of the retrospective data available suggests that these operations are feasible in 70–90% of patients when performed by gynecologic oncologists.[131,134-143] Complete resection is achievable, however, in only 30% of cases. Major morbidity is in the range of 5% and operative mortality is 1%.[136] Intestinal resection in these patients does not appear to increase the overall morbidity of the operation. The median survival and PFI of patients after cytoreductive surgery relate to the extent of residual disease at the completion of the laparotomy. A meta-analysis has been performed with 81 cohorts of patients that included 6885 women with stage III or stage IV disease.[143] A statistically significant positive correlation was found between percent maximal cytoreduction and log median survival time that remained significant after controlling for all other variables ($p < 0.001$). Each 10% increase in maximal cytoreduction was associated with a 5.5% increase in median survival time. Cohorts with 25% or less maximal cytoreduction had a median survival time of 22.7 months compared to 33.9 months in cohorts with greater than 75% maximal cytoreduction.

Adjuvant chemotherapy with platinum compounds and taxanes

Systemic chemotherapy is the standard primary treatment for advanced epithelial ovarian cancer.[144-169] A variety of regimens containing combinations of cytotoxic drugs have been tested in the treatment of advanced epithelial ovarian cancer. Combination chemotherapy has been shown to be superior to single-agent therapy in most adjuvant studies in patients with advanced epithelial ovarian cancer.

Meta-analyses have suggested that cisplatin and carboplatin are equally effective against epithelial ovarian cancer.[164] Paclitaxel was shown to be a very active agent against ovarian cancer.[144,145] The overall response rates for paclitaxel in phase 2 trials were 36% in previously treated patients, which is a higher rate than was seen for cisplatin when it was first tested. In previously untreated patients with suboptimally cytoreduced disease (GOG132), single agent cisplatin produced a 70% response rate, paclitaxel a 42% response rate, and the combination a 70% response rate.[148] Two of the three large, prospective randomized trials demonstrated an overall and progression-free survival (PFS) advantage for combining paclitaxel and platinum over platinum alone.[146,147,160] Two randomized, prospective clinical studies have compared the combination of paclitaxel and carboplatin to that of paclitaxel and cisplatin.[157,158] In both studies, response rates and duration of survival are similar, but the carboplatin-containing regimens have had more acceptable toxicity.

Docetaxel versus paclitaxel

Docetaxel has produced a 23–28% overall response rate in platinum-resistant ovarian cancer, and a combination of docetaxel and cisplatin or carboplatin has achieved a 66-81% overall response rate in phase 2 trials.[168] A combination of *docetaxel* (75 mg/m² over 1 h) and *carboplatin* (AUC 5) has been compared to *paclitaxel* (175 mg/m²) and *carboplatin* (AUC 5) in the SCOTROC trial.[169] Similar efficacy was observed, but docetaxel/carboplatin was associated with significantly less neurotoxicity. Consequently, a combination of carboplatin and docetaxel should be considered for treatment of ovarian cancer in patients with significant neuropathy from comorbid disease such as diabetes.

Other doublets and triplets

Use of platinum compounds and taxanes has improved median and OS, but the outcome in patients with advanced ovarian cancer is still disappointing. Ultimately, drug resistance develops in the majority. A number of drugs have exhibited activity against recurrent disease including liposomal doxorubicin, gemcitabine, topotecan, navelbine, and etoposide. A five-arm study, GOG-182, compared the standard combination of *carboplatin* and *paclitaxel* in combination with *gemcitabine, topotecan,* or *liposomal doxorubicin* in sequential doublets or triplets.[170] This was the largest randomized trial ever carried out in women with advanced ovarian cancer and recruited over 4000 patients. There was no apparent difference between any of the arms in terms of PFS or median survival, but there were differences in the side effects experienced in the different arms. On the basis of this study as well as others, carboplatin and paclitaxel remain the standard of care.

Dose-dense chemotherapy

There is preclinical evidence as well as clinical evidence to suggest that dose-dense, dose-fractionated chemotherapy with carboplatin and paclitaxel may be more active than the same treatments given every 3 weeks. There are a number of explanations for this, including an antiangiogenic effect of weekly metronomic paclitaxel, as well as decreasing the accelerated repopulation of cancer cells between cycles, and reducing the acquisition of drug resistance.[171,172]

A phase III study by the Japanese Gynecologic Oncology Group (JGOG) randomized 637 women with FIGO stage II to IV ovarian cancer to receive either weekly paclitaxel at a dose of 80 mg/m² in combination with three-weekly carboplatin (AUC 6) or three-weekly dosing of both drugs (carboplatin AUC 6 and paclitaxel 180 mg/m²).[173] After a median follow-up of 29 months, they reported that the median PFS was 17.2 months in the standard three-weekly paclitaxel arm, compared to 28 months in the weekly paclitaxel arm (HR 0.71; 95% CI 0.58–0.88, $p = 0.0015$) and the 3-year OS (at 42 months follow-up) was 65.1% and 72.1%, respectively (HR 0.75; 95% CI 0.57–0.98, $p = 0.03$) (Figure 11.19). The median PFS in patients with residual disease at least 1 cm was 17.6 months in the dose-dense arm compared to 12.1 months in the conventional arm. The median PFS in the patients with residual disease <1 cm was not statistically different between the two arms. The median overall survival in the patients with residual disease at least 1 cm was better in the dose-dense arm compared to the conventional arm (51.2 months vs 33.5 months).

They concluded that dose-dense treatment offered better survival than conventional treatment and was a potential new standard of care for first-line chemotherapy for patients with advanced epithelial ovarian cancer. The improvements in PFS and overall survival exceed any benefits seen previously in any phase III trial in ovarian cancer. It is unclear whether these benefits relate to pharmacogenomic or pharmacodynamic differences in the Japanese population. This and other studies have suggested that Asian patients with ovarian cancer have a significantly better survival than do Caucasian patients.[174] A GOG phase III study of patients with advanced-stage ovarian cancer (Protocol 218) revealed that the overall survival was significantly higher in Asian patients when adjusted for age, stage, residual disease, performance status, and histology.[175]

It is essential that the JGOG study be confirmed in a predominantly Caucasian population. An Italian trial (MITO-7; NCT00660842) investigated a different schedule of weekly carboplatin (AUC 2 mg/mL/min) plus weekly paclitaxel (60 mg/m^2) compared with carboplatin (AUC 6 mg/mL/min) and paclitaxel (175 mg/m^2) administered every 3 weeks. The weekly regimen did not significantly improve PFS compared with the conventional regimen (18.8 months vs 16.5 months; $p = 0.18$), but was associated with better quality of life and fewer toxic effects.[176] The GOG 262 study was presented recently.[177] The design of GOG 262 was similar to the JGOG 3016 trial, the main difference being that patients could be treated also with IV bevacizumab 15 mg/kg every 3 weeks in both arms. The decision to receive bevacizumab was dependent on the treating doctors and patient wishes. The vast majority of patients (84%) received bevacizumab until progression. The population of patients included a large fraction with gross residual disease (63%) and 13% of patients received neoadjuvant chemotherapy. Only 24% had microscopic residual disease. The median PFS was the same in both arms and was just over 14 months. Only 112 patients did not have bevacizumab, with approximately equal numbers in both arms and interestingly, the median PFS was 14.2 months with dose-dense paclitaxel and only 10.3 months with three-weekly scheduling of paclitaxel. This was a subset analysis and definitive conclusions are difficult to draw.

Intraperitoneal chemotherapy

As cancer spreads over the surface of the peritoneum and often recurs at this site, investigators have evaluated intraperitoneal (IP) administration of chemotherapy that can achieve high local concentrations of drug. A randomized, prospective trial performed by the Southwest Oncology Group (SWOG) and the GOG compared IP cisplatin (100 mg/m^2) to intravenous (IV) cisplatin (100 mg/m^2), each given with II cyclophosphamide (600 mg/m^2), in patients with disease less than 2 cm in diameter.[178] The IP cisplatin arm had a significantly longer overall median survival than the intravenous arm, 49 months versus 41 months ($p = 0.03$). In the patients with the least residual disease (<0.5 cm maximum residual), however, there was not a statistically significant difference in median survival between the two treatments, 51 months versus 46 months ($p = 0.08$).

Results of this randomized trial became available as paclitaxel was being incorporated into clinical practice. In a follow-up trial conducted by the GOG, a standard regimen of IV cisplatin (75 mg/m^2) and IV paclitaxel (135 mg/m^2 over 24 h) was compared to a dose-intense regimen that was initiated by giving moderately high-dose carboplatin (AUC = 9) for two induction cycles followed by IP cisplatin 100 mg/m^2 and IV paclitaxel (135 mg/m^2 over 24 h).[179] The dose-intense arm produced slightly better progression-free median survival (27.6 months vs 22.5 months, $p = 0.02$), but there was not a statistically significant difference in overall survival (52.9 months vs 47.6 months, $p = 0.056$).

A pivotal landmark randomized prospective GOG study[180] compared IP cisplatin and paclitaxel with IV cisplatin and paclitaxel and was reported in late 2006. Four hundred and twenty-nine patients were randomly assigned and 415 were eligible. The median PFS was 23.8 months in the IP arm versus 18.3 months in the IV arm ($p = 0.05$). The median overall survival was 65.6 months in the IP group and 49.7 months in the IV group ($p = 0.03$)—90% of patients in the IV arm received the six planned cycles of therapy, whereas only 42% of patients received the assigned six cycles of IP therapy with the remainder switching to IV therapy. The reasons for discontinuing were primarily for catheter-related problems, but there were also significantly more side effects in the IP group with more patients experiencing severe fatigue, abdominal pain, hematological toxicity, nausea and vomiting, as well as metabolic and neurotoxicity. In all likelihood, the toxicity can be reduced with more experience, appropriate dose modifications, and better antiemetics. The results of this study together with the previous studies led to an NCI Clinical Announcement recommending that women with optimally cytoreduced stage III ovarian cancer be considered for IP chemotherapy, and this is widely used in the United States.

There has been a *Cochrane Review* as well as a separate meta-analysis that concluded that IP chemotherapy was associated with better outcomes than IV chemotherapy.[181,182] The meta-analysis included six randomized trials with a total of 1716 ovarian cancer patients. The pooled HR for PFS of IP cisplatin as compared to IV treatment regimens was 0.792 (95% CI = 0.688–0.912, $p = 0.001$), and the pooled HR for OS was 0.799 (95% CI: 0.702–0.910, $p = 0.0007$). The authors conclude that these findings strongly support the incorporation of an IP cisplatin regimen to improve survival in the frontline treatment of stage III, optimally debulked ovarian cancer. Similar conclusions were reached in the Cochrane Review. The reviewers concluded that their analysis establishes the benefit of IP chemotherapy and that it is associated with an increased overall survival and PFS in patients with optimally debulked stage III advanced ovarian cancer. However, they also commented on the potential for catheter-related complications and increased toxicity with IP therapy and concluded that the optimal dose, timing, and mechanism of administration should be addressed in the next phase of clinical trials. The role of IP chemotherapy, however, is still contentious with some arguing that the trials to date were not pure tests of IP therapy and were flawed, and, in addition, they have raised concerns about the technical difficulties as well as increased toxicity of IP therapy.[183] Although decisions regarding primary therapy must be individualized, IP therapy should be seriously considered for all optimally cytoreduced patients with ovarian cancer, given the difference in overall survival. This is underscored by the recent updated survival results reported from GOG172. The median survival with IP therapy was 61.8 months (95% CI, 55.–69.5), compared with 51.4 months (95% CI, 46.0–58.2) for intravenous therapy. IP therapy was associated with a 23% decreased risk of death (adjusted HR 0.77; 95% CI, 0.65–0.90; $p = 0.002$). Survival improved with increasing number of IP cycles.[184]

Neoadjuvant chemotherapy

Some authors have suggested that, for patients with suboptimal stage III and stage IV disease, chemotherapy may be given in lieu of cytoreductive surgery. A series performed at Yale by Schwartz et al.[185] suggested that the survival of patients treated with "neoadjuvant" or cytoreductive chemotherapy was comparable to those patients treated historically with cytoreductive surgery followed by conventional chemotherapy in the same institution. However, two or three cycles of chemotherapy before cytoreductive surgery may be helpful in patients with massive ascites or large pleural effusions. Chemotherapy may eliminate the effusions, improve the patient's performance status, and decrease postoperative morbidity, particularly within the chest. Bristow et al.[186] reported the results of a systemic overview of neoadjuvant chemotherapy and concluded that neoadjuvant chemotherapy represents a viable alternative management strategy for the limited number of patients felt to be optimally unresectable by an experienced ovarian cancer surgical team; however, currently available data suggest that the survival outcome achievable with initial chemotherapy is inferior to successful upfront cytoreductive surgery.

A prospective randomized study of "interval" cytoreductive surgery was reported by the European Organization for the Research and Treatment of Cancer (EORTC) in 1995. Interval surgery was performed after three cycles of platinum-combination chemotherapy in patients whose primary attempt at cytoreduction was suboptimal. Patients in the surgical arm of the study demonstrated a survival benefit when compared with those who did not undergo interval debulking.[187] In a 10-year follow-up analysis, the risk of mortality was reduced by more than 40% in the group that was randomized to the debulking arm of the study.[188] A prospective phase III study of interval cytoreductive surgery conducted by the GOG[189] failed to confirm these findings: The median survival of the 216 women who underwent interval cytoreduction was 32 months, compared with 33 months for the 209 women who did not undergo cytoreduction. This analysis reflected the fact that all patients had been operated on initially by a gynecologic oncologist, so they had already undergone a maximal attempt at tumor resection.[190]

Several investigators suggested that neoadjuvant chemotherapy followed by an interval cyto-reduction might be appropriate in women whose performance status was poor.[185,191,192] In 2010, Vergote et al.[193] reported the results of a randomized EORTC-NCIC (National Cancer Institute of Canada) study of primary debulking surgery (PDS) versus three cycles of neoadjuvant chemotherapy followed by interval debulking surgery in 670 patients with stages IIIC–IV epithelial ovarian, fallopian tube, and peritoneal cancer. All the patients were reported to have had extensive stage IIIC or IV disease. Just over 60% had metastatic lesions that were larger than 10 cm in diameter, and 74.5% had lesions larger than 5 cm. Patients were randomly assigned either to PDS followed by at least six courses of platinum-based chemotherapy or to three courses of neoadjuvant platinum-based chemotherapy followed by interval debulking surgery in all patients whose disease has responded or is stable, followed by at least three additional courses of platinum-based chemotherapy. The median overall survival was 29 months in the primary-surgery group and 30 months in the neoadjuvant chemotherapy group. The median PFS in both groups was 12 months suggesting that the study included a relatively poor prognostic subset of patients. There was lower postoperative morbidity and mortality reported in the group that received neoadjuvant chemotherapy.

Complete tumor resection was the strongest independent predictor of overall survival in both groups. The results of this study have been widely debated and the findings criticized by a number of authors.[194–197] In an analysis of this study, Du Bois et al.[194] noted that the patients recruited to this study had a poorer performance status than those in most upfront randomized trials, and that the complete resection rates varied considerably from country to country and were considered to be low. In the PDS group, only about 20% of patients were completely cytoreduced to no residual disease, which is much lower than what would be expected in experienced centers. Indeed, there were very different optimal debulking rates reported in different countries, ranging from 62% in Belgium to 3.9% in the Netherlands suggesting highly variable surgical expertise. The median OS was only 30 months, which is considerably less than the 60+ months expected with optimal cytoreduction followed by chemotherapy, suggesting that the study included a poor performance status cohort of patients with very advanced disease.

There have been two other randomized trials of neoadjuvant chemotherapy that have completed enrollment. The first study is the chemotherapy or upfront surgery (CHORUS) trial, which had a similar design to the EORTC trial, was conducted in the United Kingdom and was reported recently.[198] The CHORUS study had very similar findings to the EORTC study. Five hundred and fifty-two patients were randomized to receive either neoadjuvant chemotherapy followed by interval debulking and then three additional cycles or PDS followed by six cycles of platinum-based chemotherapy. The optimal debulking rate was only 16% in the PDS group, compared to 40% following neoadjuvant chemotherapy. The median duration of surgery was only 120 min in both groups, which is clearly not long enough for aggressive debulking surgery. There was a 5.6% postoperative mortality rate in the PDS group, which is much higher than expected and may reflect patient selection. The median PFS was 12 months, which is clearly not long enough for aggregroup compared to the primary chemotherapy group and the median overall survival was 22.6 months in the primary-surgery group versus 24.1 months in those who had primary chemotherapy. The HR for death was 0.87 in favor of primary chemotherapy, with the upper bound of the one-sided 90% CI 0.98 (95% CI 0.72–1.05). There were more serious adverse events and deaths within 28 days of surgery in the primary surgery group, and the authors concluded that in women with stage III or IV ovarian cancer, survival with primary chemotherapy was noninferior to primary surgery and a reasonable option in selected patients.

There remain very divergent views regarding the place of neoadjuvant chemotherapy. A survey of SGO members found that 82% felt there was not enough evidence to justify the use of neoadjuvant chemotherapy.[199] In contrast, 70% of ESGO members felt there was sufficient evidence to recommend neoadjuvant chemotherapy. On the basis of the above-mentioned considerations, the performance of a debulking operation as early as possible in the course of the patient's treatment should be considered the standard of care.[200] Neoadjuvant chemotherapy followed by interval cytoreduction should be reserved for patients with a poor performance and nutritional status, as these patients will usually have decreased postoperative morbidity if chemotherapy is given before cytoreduction.

Bevacizumab adjuvant therapy

Inhibition of angiogenesis with drugs such as bevacizumab has demonstrated activity and benefit in women with recurrent ovarian cancer and in view of this there are two large randomized trials investigating the impact of the addition of bevacizumab to standard carboplatin and paclitaxel for adjuvant therapy in patients with advanced ovarian cancer. There is evidence in other tumor types such as colon cancer and lung cancer that the addition of beva-cizumab to chemotherapy increases response rates and PFS and also survival in some studies.[201,202]

Two large phase III studies (GOG 218 and ICON 7) have investigated the role of bevacizumab in the first-line setting. The GOG 218 trial was a three-arm randomized study that recruited 1873 patients with stage III–IV ovarian, fallopian tube, and peritoneal cancer.[203] Patients with stage III disease were required to have macroscopic residual disease. The patients were randomly assigned to one of the following: (1) a control group that received 6 cycles of carboplatin and paclitaxel chemotherapy with concurrent placebo in cycles 2 through 6, followed by placebo alone every 3 weeks for a total of 22 cycles; (2) a group that received standard chemotherapy for 6 cycles in combination with bevacizumab (15 mg/kg) in cycles 2 through 6, followed by placebo alone for a total of 22 cycles; and (3) a group that received standard chemotherapy for 6 cycles with bevacizumab in cycles 2 through 6, followed by the continuation of bevacizumab alone, for a total of 22 cycles. At a median follow-up of 17.4 months, the hazard of progression or death was the same in the bevacizumab with chemotherapy group compared with the control group (HR, 0.908; $p = 0.16$) and significantly lower in the bevacizumab with chemotherapy and maintenance group (HR, 0.717; $p < 0.001$). In an analysis of PFS, in which patients with an elevated CA-125 were censored, the median PFS was 12 months in the control group but 18 months in the bevacizumab maintenance group (HR, 0.645; $p = 0.001$). This was confirmed in a recent analysis on independent radiologic review of all patients in GOG 218. To date, there does not appear to be any significant difference in OS, and this may be due to many patients receiving multiple subsequent regimens at relapse, including crossover to bevacizumab or other anti-VEGF agents that could potentially influence overall survival.

The ICON7 trial had a similar design and enrolled 1528 patients with high risk (clear cell or grade 3 tumors).[204] Patients with stage I and II ovarian, fallopian tube, or peritoneal cancer, as well as stages III and IV, were included. They were randomized to six cycles of chemotherapy alone or 6 cycles of chemotherapy plus bevacizumab (7.5 mg/kg), followed by 12 cycles of maintenance bevacizumab every 3 weeks. With a median follow-up of 19.4 months, the median PFS was 17.3 months in the control group and 19 months in the bevacizumab group (HR, 0.81; $p = 0.004$). The improvement in PFS with bevacizumab was maintained with a median follow-up of 28 months. An exploratory OS analysis showed a significant improvement in survival in the high-risk subgroups (stage III with >1 cm residual and stage IV [HR, 0.64; $p = 0.002$]). This was confirmed in a recently presented update of the survival data, which showed that there was a 4-month improvement in median survival from 35 to 39 months in the high-risk subgroup.[205] However, there

was no survival advantage found between the two arms in ICON7. Bevacizumab was associated with an increase in toxicity, which included bleeding (mainly grade 1 mucocutaneous bleeding), grade 2 or higher hypertension (18% with bevacizumab vs 2% with standard therapy), grade 3 or higher thromboembolic events (7% with bevacizumab vs 3% with standard therapy), and gastrointestinal perforations (occurring in 10 patients in the bevacizumab group vs 3 patients in the standard-therapy group).

In contrast to the GOG 218 study, the ICON7 study enrolled patients with advanced-stage cancer with no visible residual disease, as well as patients with high-risk early-stage disease. In the ICON7 study, a lower dose of bevacizumab was used (7.5 mg/kg vs 15 mg/kg in GOG 218) for a shorter maintenance period (12 cycles vs 16 cycles). In both studies, PFS curves converged a few months after bevacizumab was discontinued, suggesting that antiangiogenic treatment may delay, but not prevent, disease progression. This raises the issue of the advisability of patients with high-risk disease continuing treatment indefinitely. This is currently under investigation but has significant cost-benefit implications. There are still no good biologic markers to identify which patients are most likely to benefit from the incorporation of bevacizumab into the first-line setting. The optimal dose is also unclear.

Management of advanced invasive ovarian cancer

The treatment of choice for patients with advanced invasive epithelial ovarian cancer is cytoreductive surgery followed by six to eight cycles of chemotherapy with a combination of carboplatin (AUC 5-6) and paclitaxel (175 mg/m^2 over 3 h) every 3 weeks (Table 7). As discussed earlier, a dose-dense regimen or IP regimen are both evidence-based options as is the addition of bevacizumab, and the choice of treatment should be individualized. In patients at risk for severe neuropathy, diabetics, for example, a combination of docetaxel (75 mg/m^2) and carboplatin (AUC 5) provides an alternative that is less neurotoxic. In women who cannot tolerate the toxicity of taxanes, carboplatin alone (AUC 5-6) is a reasonable option.

Management of advanced borderline tumors

The place of chemotherapy in patients with advanced-stage borderline tumors is uncertain and controversial. The GOG is evaluating the use of chemotherapy in patients with advanced-stage borderline tumors who have recurrent disease after initial surgery. Until the results of this trial are known, the current approach to treatment is primarily surgical. Patients should undergo cytoreductive surgery and observation. Borderline tumors, even in advanced stage, have a favorable prognosis. The first symptomatic recurrence may be several years after diagnosis. In contrast to the 20–25% survival

Table 7 Chemotherapy for advanced epithelial ovarian, fallopian tube, and peritoneal cancer: recommended regimens.

Drugs	Dose	Administration (h)	Interval	Number of treatments
Standard regimens				
Carboplatin Paclitaxel	AUC = 5–6 175 mg/m^2	3	Every 3 weeks	6–8 cycles
Carboplatin Paclitaxel	AUC = 5 80 mg/m^2	3	Every 3 weeks Every week	6 cycles 18 weeks
Carboplatin Docetaxel	AUC = 5 75 mg/m^2	3	Every week Every 3 weeks	6 cycles
Cisplatin Paclitaxel	75 mg/m^2 135 mg/m^2	3 24	Every 3 weeks	6 cycles
Carboplatin (single agent)[a]	AUC = 4–6	3	Every 3 weeks	6 cycles, as tolerated

[a]In patients who are elderly, frail or poor performance status.
AUC, are under the curve dose by Calvert formula.
Source: Reproduced from Berek *et al.*, 2015, p. 510.[130]

rates for advanced epithelial invasive carcinoma of the ovary, the survival rate for patients with stage III borderline tumors is over 60%. Consequently, secondary cytoreductive surgery frequently will lead to another prolonged interval of symptom free survival. Chemotherapy can be administered to the patients in whom cytoreductive surgery is no longer feasible, although its efficacy is uncertain and response rates very low.

Assessment of response in patients who are clinically free of disease

Many patients who have undergone optimal cytoreductive surgery and subsequent therapy for epithelial ovarian cancer will have no evidence of disease at the completion of treatment. Tumor markers and radiologic assessments have proved to be too insensitive to exclude accurately the presence of subclinical disease.[206–208] A technique used to evaluate residual disease has been the second-look operation, which is no longer routinely used[209,210] because second-look laparotomies have not been shown to influence patient survival with currently available chemotherapy; they should be done only in a research setting, to test second-line or salvage therapies that are likely to be affected by the volume of disease, such as immunotherapies or antiautophagic therapies.

Maintenance chemotherapy

The optimal management of patients who do achieve a clinical complete remission after induction chemotherapy remains to be determined. Even patients who achieve a surgically confirmed complete remission have a 30–50% recurrence rate. Some investigators have suggested that second-look laparotomy should be performed to identify patients who may be candidates for IP therapy.[211] There is no evidence, however, that the routine sequential administration of IP chemotherapy after IV induction chemotherapy prolongs survival.

Clinical trials have been performed to determine whether maintenance chemotherapies are of benefit in patients who achieve a surgically confirmed clinical complete remission. A study conducted by the GOG and SWOG compared 3 and 12 monthly cycles of "consolidation" chemotherapy with paclitaxel (135–175 mg/m^2 IV over 3 h) for patients who had achieved a clinical remission following primary paclitaxel and carboplatin chemotherapy.[212] PFI was 21 and 28 months in the 3-cycle and 12-cycle paclitaxel arms ($p = 0.035$), respectively. Consequently, 9 months of additional chemotherapy provided an additional 7 months of PFS. To date, there is no difference in OS between the two arms. Two placebo-controlled randomized trials have been performed in Europe using consolidation with four cycles topotecan given to patients in clinical remission following chemotherapy with carboplatin and paclitaxel, and in both trials, there was no improvement in survival compared with placebo.[213,214]

Follow-up examinations

The optimal frequency of follow-up examinations is unknown, but for those patients who have completed chemotherapy and who are in clinical remission, a pelvic examination and a CA125 every 3 months for 1–2 years is reasonable. An elevated CA125 (>35 U/mL) can provide lead time of approximately 3–6 months before there are clinical signs or symptoms of recurrence. The Gynecologic Cancer Inter Group (GCIG) developed a standard definition for CA125 progression, which is now widely used in clinical trials. Patients with elevated CA125 pretreatment and subsequent normalization of CA125 must show evidence of CA125 greater than or equal to 2× the upper normal limit on two occasions at least 1 week apart, or patients with elevated CA125 pretreatment that never

normalizes must show evidence of CA125 greater than or equal to 2× the nadir value on two occasions at least 1 week apart.

A rising CA125 may prompt the performance of a CT scan. The role of PET scanning in this setting has not been defined. A recent review concluded that PET has a sensitivity of 90% and a specificity of 85% approximately for the detection of recurrent ovarian cancer and that it appears to be particularly useful for the diagnosis of recurrence when CA125 levels are rising and conventional imaging is inconclusive or negative, although the value of this is debatable. Combined ^{18}fluorodeoxyglucose (FDG)-PET/CT devices, which perform contemporaneous acquisition of both ^{18}FDG-PET and CT images, may be more valuable to detect recurrent ovarian cancer; this technique may be useful for the selection of patients with late recurrent disease who may benefit from secondary cytoreductive surgery.[215]

A rising CA125 level in the absence of changes on physical examination or CT scan in a patient in initial remission poses a dilemma. At present, additional cytotoxic therapy is not recommended based on a rising CA125 alone in the absence of clinical symptoms or radiologic evidence of recurrence. Treatment with tamoxifen or anastrozole has sometimes been given and although stabilization or a fall in CA125 may be observed in approximately 20% of patients, the value of this intervention is uncertain. The GOG has compared tamoxifen to thalidomide in patients with a rising CA125 without other evidence of disease recurrence. Similar efficacy was observed, although tamoxifen was less toxic. There are also trials using a rising CA125 to evaluate a paradigm to evaluate the activity of novel cytostatic targeted drugs. As more effective salvage therapy becomes available, serum markers such as CA125 may have greater utility. In patients whose disease was never found to be metastatic to the chest or who never had a pleural effusion, chest radiograph surveillance is not mandatory. In the absence of a rising CA125, follow-up CT or MRI scans should be used with discretion during the first 3 years after chemotherapy.

Treatment of recurrent epithelial cancer

The majority of women who relapse will be offered further chemotherapy with the likelihood of benefit related in part to the initial response and the duration of response. The goals of treatment include improving control of disease-related symptoms, maintaining or improving quality of life, delaying time to progression, and possibly prolonging survival, particularly in women with platinum-sensitive recurrences. Many active chemotherapy agents (platinum, paclitaxel, topotecan, liposomal doxorubicin, docetaxel, gemcitabine, pemetrexed, and etoposide) as well as targeted agents (bevacizumab) are available and the choice of treatment is based on many factors, including likelihood of benefit, potential toxicity, and patient convenience.[216,217] Women who relapse >6 months after primary chemotherapy are classified as "platinum-sensitive" and usually receive further platinum-based chemotherapy with response rates ranging from 27% to 65% and a median survival of 12–24 months.[218,219] Patients who relapse within 6 months of completing first-line chemotherapy are classified as "platinum-resistant" and have a median survival of 6–9 months and a 10–30% likelihood of responding to chemotherapy. Patients who progress while on treatment are classified as having "platinum-refractory" disease. Objective response rates to chemotherapy in patients with platinum-refractory ovarian cancer are very low, typically less than 10%.[216]

Platinum-sensitive disease

In general, randomized trials have shown that response rates, median PFS, and overall survival rates are superior for platinum-based combination chemotherapy compared to single-agent platinum chemotherapy. The use of combination *platinum plus paclitaxel* chemotherapy versus *single-agent platinum* has been tested in two multinational randomized phase III trials[220] and a randomized phase II study.[221] In a report of the ICON4 and AGO-OVAR-2.2 trials, 802 women with platinum-sensitive ovarian cancer who relapsed after being treatment free for at least 6–12 months were randomized to platinum-based chemotherapy (72% carboplatin or cisplatin alone; 17% CAP; 4% carboplatin plus cisplatin; and 3% cisplatin plus doxorubicin) or paclitaxel plus platinum-based chemotherapy (80% paclitaxel plus carboplatin; 10% paclitaxel plus cisplatin; 5% paclitaxel plus both carboplatin and cisplatin; and 4% paclitaxel alone). The AGO-OVAR-2.2 trial did not accrue its planned number of patients. In both trials, a significant proportion of the patients had not received paclitaxel initially. Combining the trials for analysis, there was a significant survival advantage for the paclitaxel-containing therapy (HR = 0.82), with a median follow-up of 42 months. The absolute 2-year survival advantage was 7% (57% vs 50%), and there was a 5-month improvement in median survival (29 months vs 24 months). PFS was better with the paclitaxel regimen (HR = 0.76); there was a 10% difference in 1-year PFS (50% vs 40%) and a 3-month prolongation in median PFS (13 months vs 10 months). The toxicities were comparable, except there was a significantly higher incidence of neurologic toxicity and alopecia in the paclitaxel group, whereas myelosuppression was significantly greater with the non-paclitaxel-containing regimens.

Two randomized trials have compared *carboplatin alone* to *carboplatin and gemcitabine* or *carboplatin and liposomal doxorubicin*.[222,223] There was a higher response rate with the combination therapy and a longer PFS, but the studies were not powered to look at overall survival. In the GCIG study comparing carboplatin and gemcitabine with carboplatin alone, the response rate was 47.2% for the combination and 30.9% for carboplatin, with the PFSs being 8.6 and 5.8 months, respectively. A SWOG study of carboplatin versus carboplatin and liposomal doxorubicin was closed early because of poor accrual, but with 61 patients recruited, the response rate was 67% for the combination and 32% for carboplatin. The PFS was 12 months versus 8 months; intriguingly, the overall survival was 26 months compared to 18 months (p = 0.02).[224] A phase II study from France confirmed the high response rate of 67% with carboplatin and liposomal doxorubicin in patients with platinum-sensitive recurrent ovarian cancer.

A large GCIG study (CALYPSO) comparing carboplatin and liposomal doxorubicin (CD) with carboplatin and paclitaxel (CP) recruited almost 1000 patients. With a median follow-up of 22 months, PFS for the CD arm was statistically superior to the CP arm (HR, 0.821; 95% CI, 0.72–0.94; p = 0.005); median PFS was 11.3 months versus 9.4 months, respectively. Overall, severe non-hematologic toxicity (36.8% vs 28.4%; p = 0.01) leading to early discontinuation (15% vs 6%; p = 0.001) occurred more frequently in the CP arm. More frequent grade 2 or greater alopecia (83.6% vs 7%), hypersensitivity reactions (18.8% vs 5.6%), and sensory neuropathy (26.9% vs 4.9%) were observed in the CP arm; more hand–foot syndrome (grade 2 to 3, 12% vs 2.2%), nausea (35.2% vs 24.2%), and mucositis (grade 2 to 3, 13.9% vs 7%) in the CD arm. This trial demonstrated superiority in PFS and better therapeutic index of carboplatin and liposomal doxorubicin compared to carboplatin and paclitaxel, and this regimen is now widely used.

Some researchers have hypothesized that treating patients with nonplatinum drugs to prolong the platinum-free interval will allow the tumor to again become more platinum sensitive over time.[225] However, there are no data to support the hypothesis that the interposition of a nonplatinum agent will result in an increase in platinum sensitivity because of a longer interval since the last platinum treatment.

Nonplatinum regimens have been investigated as second-line therapy,[226,227] including a large phase III trial of *trabectedin plus liposomal doxorubicin* compared to *liposomal doxorubicin alone*.[228] This trial included patients with platinum-resistant as well as platinum-sensitive recurrent disease. In patients with "platinum-sensitive" recurrence, response rates were higher for the combination of trabectedin plus liposomal doxorubicin (35% vs 23%) and the median PFS was 9.2 months versus 7.5 months, respectively (HR, 0.73; 95% CI, 0.56–0.95; p = 0.0170).[228] The authors did not report on the response rates to subsequent platinum-based chemotherapy in patients with either platinum-sensitive or platinum-resistant disease and whether there was any apparent increased likelihood of response to platinum as a result of increasing the platinum-free interval.

OCEANS is a randomized trial of bevacizumab in 484 women with platinum-sensitive recurrent ovarian cancer. Patients with recurrence ≥6 months after first-line platinum-based therapy and measurable disease were randomly assigned to *carboplatin and gemcitabine* plus either *bevacizumab or placebo* for 6–10 cycles. Bevacizumab or placebo was then continued until disease progression. The primary end point was PFS by RECIST. The PFS for the bevacizumab arm was superior to that for the placebo arm (HR, 0.484; 95% CI, 0.388–0.605; p < 0.0001). The median PFS was 12.4 months in the bevacizumab arm compared to 8.4 months in the placebo arm. The objective response rate (78.5% vs 57.4%; p < 0.0001) and duration of response (10.4 months vs 7.4 months; HR, 0.534; 95% CI, 0.408–0.698) were also significantly improved with the addition of bevacizumab. Quality of life was not assessed but there were no new or unexpected toxicities observed. There are no data regarding the impact on overall survival. The findings of this study support the role of bevacizumab in selected patients with platinum-sensitive recurrent ovarian cancer.

Other forms of antiangiogenic therapy are being evaluated in clinical trials.[229] *VEGF Trap* (aflibercept) functions as a soluble decoy receptor soaking up ligand before it can interact with its receptor and is being evaluated in phase 2 trials in patients with recurrent ovarian cancer. There are also a number of other oral agents that target angiogenesis through tyrosine kinase inhibition.

Platinum-resistant/refractory disease

In platinum-refractory patients—defined as those progressing on treatment—the response rates to second-line chemotherapy are less than 10% (Table 7). The management of women who are platinum-resistant (i.e., progressing within 6 months of completion of chemotherapy) is complex and these patients should be offered clinical trials if available. However, the Aurelia trial recently demonstrated the added benefit of *bevacizumab to chemotherapy*, and this is likely to change the standard of care as the FDA recently approved the use of bevacizumab in patients with platinum-resistant ovarian cancer based on the results of Aurelia.[230]

All randomized trials of combination versus single-agent chemotherapy in resistant/refractory ovarian cancer have failed to show superiority of combination chemotherapy over single-agent treatment. There are a variety of potentially active single agents, the most frequently used being *paclitaxel, docetaxel, topotecan, liposomal doxorubicin, gemcitabine, ifosfamide, trabectedin, oral etoposide, tamoxifen, pemetrexed,* and *bevacizumab*.[226,227,231–234]

Almost 200 patients with platinum-resistant ovarian cancer were randomized to receive either *gemcitabine* or *liposomal doxorubicin*. In the gemcitabine and liposomal doxorubicin groups, median PFS was 3.6 months versus 3.1 months, median overall survival was 12.7 months versus 13.5 months, and overall response rate was 6.1% versus 8.3%, respectively. In the subset of patients with measurable disease, overall response rate was 9.2% versus 11.7%, respectively. None of the efficacy end points showed a statistically significant difference between treatment groups. The liposomal doxorubicin group experienced significantly more hand–foot syndrome and mucositis, whereas the gemcitabine group had significantly more constipation, nausea and vomiting, fatigue, and neutropenia.[235]

These findings are similar to the results of a large randomized phase III trial comparing *patupilone* to *liposomal doxorubicin* in 829 patients with platinum-refractory/resistant ovarian cancer.[236] Patupilone is a microtubule-stabilizing agent that induces cell-cycle arrest and apoptosis after binding to its molecular target, β-tubulin, and has been reported to have a 16% overall response rate in patients with platinum-refractory and platinum-resistant recurrent ovarian cancer. The primary endpoint of the study was overall survival. There was no difference in patient outcomes between the two treatments. The median PFS was 3.7 months in both arms, and the overall survival was 13.2 months in the patupilone arm and 12.7 months in the liposomal doxorubicin arm; 20% of patients in the experimental arm discontinued treatment because of toxicity. Frequently observed adverse events of all grades were common and included diarrhea (85%) and peripheral neuropathy (39%) in the patupilone arm and stomatitis/mucositis (43%) and hand–foot syndrome (41.8%) in the liposomal doxorubicin arm. The majority of patients in this trial had platinum resistant, not platinum-refractory disease. Furthermore, almost all had a WHO performance status of 0 or 1, so this selected population is not necessarily representative of the large group of women with platinum-resistant/refractory ovarian cancer. The results highlight the poor prognosis of these patients, and underscore the importance of symptom benefit and quality-of-life considerations. Arguably, these should be the primary aim of chemotherapy and should be used as coprimary end points, along with traditional endpoints such as PFS and OS in clinical trials.

Single-agent paclitaxel has shown objective responses in 20–30% of patients in phase II trials of women with platinum-resistant ovarian cancer.[237–242] The main toxicities have been asthenia and peripheral neuropathy. Weekly paclitaxel is more active than three-weekly dosing and is also associated with less toxicity. In a study of 53 women with platinum-resistant ovarian cancer, weekly paclitaxel (80 mg/m^2 over 1 h) had an objective response of 25% in patients with measurable disease, and 27% of patients without measurable disease had a 75% decline in serum CA125 levels.[240]

Docetaxel also has some activity in patients with platinum-resistant disease.[243–245] The GOG studied 60 women with platinum-resistant ovarian or primary peritoneal cancer.[245] Although there was a 22% objective response rate, the median response duration was only 2.5 months, and therapy was complicated by severe neutropenia in three-quarters of the patients.

Topotecan is an active second-line treatment for patients with platinum-sensitive and platinum-resistant disease.[246–259] In a study of 139 women receiving topotecan 1.5 mg/m^2 daily for 5 days, response rates were 19% and 13% in patients with platinum-sensitive and platinum-resistant disease, respectively.[246] The predominant toxicity of topotecan is hematologic, especially neutropenia. With the 5-day dosing schedule, 70–80% of patients have severe neutropenia and 25% have febrile neutropenia, with or without infection.[246,251] In some studies, regimens of 5 days produce better response rates than regimens of shorter duration,[246–256] but in others, reducing the dose to 1 mg/m^2/day for 3 days is associated

with similar response rates but lower toxicity. In a study of 31 patients, one-half of whom were platinum-refractory,[259] topotecan 2 mg/m^2/day for 3 days every 21 days had a 32% response rate. Continuous infusion topotecan (0.4 mg/m^2/day for 14–21 days) had a 27–35% objective response rate in platinum-refractory patients.[252] Weekly topotecan administered at a dose of 4 mg/m^2/week for 3 weeks with a week off every month produced a response rate similar to the 5-day regimen with considerably less toxicity. Therefore, this is now considered the regimen of choice for this agent.

Liposomal doxorubicin (Doxil in the United States and Caelyx in Europe) has activity in platinum- and taxane-refractory disease. Its predominant severe toxicity is the hand–foot syndrome, also known as palmar–plantar erythrodysesthesia or acral erythema, which is observed in 20% of patients who receive 50 mg/m^2 every 4 weeks.[260,261] Liposomal doxorubicin does not cause neurologic toxicity or alopecia. It is administered every 4 weeks, which makes it convenient, and it is relatively well tolerated at the lower dose of 40 mg/m^2, which is widely used. In a study of 89 patients with platinum-refractory disease, including 82 paclitaxel-resistant patients, liposomal doxorubicin (50 mg/m^2 every 3 weeks) produced a response in 17% (one complete and 14 partial response). In another study, an objective response rate of 26% was reported, although there were no responses in women who progressed during first-line therapy.[262]

There have been two randomized trials comparing *liposomal doxorubicin with either topotecan or paclitaxel*. In a study of 237 women who relapsed after receiving one platinum-containing regimen, 117 of whom (49.4%) had platinum-refractory disease, liposomal doxorubicin 50 mg/m^2 over 1 h every 4 weeks was compared with topotecan 1.5 mg/m^2/day for 5 days every 3 weeks. The two treatments had a similar overall response rate (20% vs 17%), time to progression (22 weeks vs 20 weeks), and median overall survival (66 weeks vs 56 weeks). The myelotoxicity was significantly lower in the liposomal doxorubicin–treated patients. In a second study comparing liposomal doxorubicin with single-agent paclitaxel in 214 platinum-treated patients who had not received prior taxanes,[263] the overall response rates for liposomal doxorubicin and paclitaxel were 18% and 22%, respectively, and median survivals were 46 and 56 weeks, respectively. Neither was significantly different. In practice, most patients are treated with a starting dose of 40 mg/m^2 of liposomal doxorubicin every 4 weeks because dose reduce is common when 50 mg/m^2 is used initially.

Gemcitabine is a nucleoside analog of cytidine and has been reported to have response rates of 10–20% in patients who have platinum-resistant disease and 6% in those with platinum-refractory disease.[231–233,264,265] The principal toxicities are myelosuppression and gastrointestinal.

The most common toxicities with *oral etoposide* are myelosuppression, nausea, and vomiting. Grade 4 neutropenia is observed in approximately one-fourth of patients, and 10–15% have severe nausea and vomiting.[234] Although an initial study of intravenous etoposide reported an objective response rate of only 8% among 24 patients,[234] a subsequent study of oral etoposide given for a prolonged period (50 mg/m^2 daily for 21 days every 4 weeks) had a 27% response rate in 41 women with platinum-resistant disease, three of whom had durable complete responses. In 25 patients with platinum- and taxane-resistant disease, eight objective responses (32%) were reported. Oral etoposide should be considered in patients with paclitaxel- and platinum-resistant disease.

Immmunotherapy

There is considerable interest in the use of check-point inhibitors in ovarian cancer. The results of anti-PD1 and anti-PDL1 antibodies in melanoma and in lung cancer-stimulated trials in ovarian cancer.

Hamanishi and colleagues from Kyoto, Japan, presented a phase II study using *nivolumab* (anti-PD1 antibody) in which there was an objective response rate of 17% in patients who were heavily pre-treated and had platinum-resistant disease, including a complete response in a patient with an ovarian clear cell carcinoma.[266] Other reports in solid tumors including ovarian cancer are encouraging.[267] Cell-based therapy using genetically engineered CAR T cells is being developed against several targets, including mesothelin and ESO-NY.[268]

Hormonal therapy

Epithelial ovarian tumors frequently contain elevated levels of estrogen and androgen receptors, particularly in low-grade cancers. Some patients with epithelial ovarian tumors have had responses to endocrine therapy, although it appears that the overall response rate in high-grade cancer is approximately 10–20%. Progestational agents, tamoxifen, aromatase inhibitors, and GNRH agonists have been used either alone or in combination with cytotoxic chemotherapy in patients with advanced disease.[269–272] In a study of patients with advanced, largely high-grade epithelial ovarian cancer, tamoxifen exhibited only a 13% partial response rate, but disease progression was delayed in 30%. Higher response rates have been reported in small studies with aromatase inhibitors in recurrent low-grade ovarian cancers with strong ER expression.

Targeted therapy and PARP inhibitors

With the exception of bevacizumab that has exhibited a 20% objective response rate and a 40% 6 month PFS, a variety of single targeted drugs (sorafenib, tensirolimus, gefitinib, imatinib, mifepristone, enzastaurin, lapatinib, and vorinostat) have produced less than a 10% objective response and <25% 6-month PFS in patients with recurrent epithelial ovarian cancer. Current research is focused on identifying combinations of drugs that might exhibit synthetic lethality.

The concept of synthetic lethality is deceptively simple and explains the selective and targeted effect of PARP inhibitors in cells with dysfunction in the homologous repair pathway. Loss of function of BRCA 1 or 2 results in increased sensitivity to inhibition of PARP1 due to accumulation of unrepaired single-strand DNA breaks in proliferating cells which results in collapse of replication forks and, consequently, to double-strand DNA breaks (DSBs).[273] These DSBs are not repaired in BRCA 1 or 2 tumour cells, which are deficient in homologous repair and this leads to genetic instability and cell death. The synthetic lethal interactions between PARP1 and BRCA 1 or 2 have been confirmed *in vitro* as well as in a number of phase 1 and 2 clinical trials in women with recurrent ovarian cancer.[274,275] The initial phase I trial of olaparib (AZD2281) reported an impressive clinical benefit rate (CBR) of 63% in women with BRCA mutations and recurrent ovarian cancer.[275] This led to the enrollment of an expanded cohort of 50 patients with *BRCA1/2* mutations, which confirmed activity in a heavily pretreated group of patients with recurrent ovarian cancer with a CBR of 46%.[276] A Response Evaluation Criteria in Solid Tumors (RECIST) radiological response or GCIG CA125 response was seen in 40% of patients. There was a correlation between response to olaparib and platinum sensitivity; platinum-sensitive patients had a 69% CBR compared with 46% and 23% in platinum-resistant and refractory patients, respectively.[276] These findings led to a number of randomized phase 2 trials and a large amount of interest in the role of PARP inhibitors to treat not only women with BRCA mutations but also those with "sporadic" ovarian cancer. The molecular heterogeneity of high-grade sporadic serous ovarian cancer is now better appreciated and it is apparent that at least 50% of these tumors have dysfunction of the homologous repair DNA repair pathway and may also be sensitive to PARP1 inhibition.[277] The challenge is to

be better able to identify which tumors have impaired homologous repair and are, therefore, most likely to respond to PARP inhibition and there are a number of pharmaceutical companies developing companion diagnostic tests to help identify patients most likely to respond or benefit from PARP inhibitors.

The maintenance studies with PARP inhibitors have been particularly interesting. Ledermann et al.[278] reported significant prolongation in PFS in patients with platinum-sensitive recurrent ovarian cancer randomized to maintenance olaparib or placebo after responding to chemotherapy. The benefit was much greater in women with BRCA mutations (HR = 0.18; 95% CI 0.11, 0.31; $p < 0.00001$; median PFS 11.2 months vs 4.3 months).[279] In view of the results of this study, large confirmatory trials have been carried out with olaparib as well as a number of other PARP inhibitors. It seems likely that PARP inhibitors will play an increasingly important role in the management of women with BRCA-related ovarian cancer as well as in patients with HRD in the near future. There are studies combining PARP inhibitors with chemotherapy as well as with angiogenesis inhibitors, and this is a very active area of research with at least five different PARP inhibitors being investigated by different pharmaceutical companies. The recent report by Liu et al of extraordinary high response rates with olaparib and cediranib of 79% as well as very impressive increase in PFS compared with olaparib alone (17.7 months vs 9 months) have led to new studies with the hope that these novel treatments may be used instead of chemotherapy in the future.[280]

In a multi-institutional phase III, randomized placebo-controlled trial of maintenance niraparib in patients with platinum-sensitive, recurrent ovarian cancer, a progression-free survival advantages were observed: 21 vs. 5.5 mos in women who carry germ-line mutations in BRCA1-2, 12.9 months vs. 3.8 months in those with homologous-recombination defects (HDR), and 9.3 months vs. 3.9 months in BRCA1-2 negative (all significant differences p < 0.001).

Palliative radiotherapy

Radiotherapy as a palliative modality in ovarian cancer may be very useful if the sole dominant symptomatic problem for the patient is localized to a site and volume that may be safely encompassed in a limited radiation field. For example, a fixed pelvic mass eroding the vaginal mucosa causing bleeding, pain, or bowel or bladder dysfunction may occur without obvious disseminated symptomatic peritoneal disease. Localized masses in the retroperitoneal nodes or in extra abdominal sites such as the supraclavicular or inguinal node regions or bony or brain metastases may benefit from palliative irradiation as would painful hepatomegaly from hepatic capsular distention. An objective and subjective response rate of patients treated with radiation for recurrent ovarian cancer after resistance to available chemotherapeutic agents has been reported. A study from Memorial Sloan-Kettering Cancer Center documented subjective or objective responses in 70% of patients who had platinum-refractory disease.[281] While the optimal dose for palliation has not been established, it is clear that durable palliation may be achieved with local radiotherapy for ovarian cancer recurring after chemotherapy even in the presence of chemoresistant disease. Palliative whole brain irradiation is indicated for documented cerebral metastases in those whose life expectancy is several weeks to months.

Key references

The complete reference list can be found on the Wiley Companion Digital Edition of this title (see inside front cover for login instructions).

1 Siegel R, Ma J, Zou Z, et al. Cancer statistics. *CA Cancer J Clin.* 2015;**65**:5–29.

2 SEER Cancer Statistics Factsheets. *Ovary Cancer.* Bethesda, MD: National Cancer Institute; 2005. http://seer.cancer.gov/statfacts/html/ovary.html.

9   Erickson BK, Conner MG, Landen CN. The role of the fallopian tube in the origin of ovarian cancer. *Am J Obstet Gynecol.* 2013;**209**:409–414.

27   Collaborative Group on Epidemiological Studies of Ovarian Cancer, Beral V, Gaitskell K, et al. Menopausal hormone use and ovarian cancer risk: individual participant meta analysis of 52 epidemiological studies. *Lancet.* 2015;**385**:1835–1842.

35   Struewing JP, Hartge P, Wacholder S, et al. The risk of cancer associated with specific mutations of BRCA1 and BRCA2 among Ashkenazi Jews. *N Engl J Med.* 1997;**336**:1401–1408.

47   Moyer VA. U.S. Preventive Services Task Force. Screening for ovarian cancer: U.S. Preventive Services Task Force reaffirmation recommendation statement. *Ann Intern Med.* 2012;**157(12)**:900–904.

55   Rebbeck TR, Lynch HT, Neuhausen SL, et al. Prophylactic oophorectomy in carriers of BRCA1 or BRCA2 mutations. *N Engl J Med.* 2002;**346**:1616–1622.

56   Haber D. Prophylactic oophorectomy to reduce the risk of ovarian and breast cancer in carriers of BRCA mutations. *N Engl J Med.* 2002;**346**:1660–1661.

60   Domchek SM, Friebel TM, Singer CF, et al. Association of risk-reducing surgery in BRCA1 or BRCA2 mutation carriers with cancer risk and mortality. *JAMA.* 2010;**304(9)**:967–975.

63   Genetic Testing for Heritable Mutations in the BRCA1 and BRCA2 Genes EVIQ Guidelines Cancer Institute NSW November 2013. https://www.eviq.org.au

68   Bast RC Jr, Romero I, Mills GB. Molecular pathogenesis of ovarian cancer. In: Mendelsohn J, Howley PM, Israel MA, Gray JW, Thompson CB, eds. *The Molecular Basis of Cancer,* 4th ed. Philadelphia, PA: Elsevier Health; 2015:531–547.

69   Merritt WM, Lin YG, Han LY, et al. Dicer, drosha and outcomes in patients with ovarian cancer. *N Engl J Med.* 2008;**359**:2641–2650.

70   Bast RC Jr, Hennessy B, Mills GB. The biology of ovarian cancer: new opportunities for translation. *Nat Rev Cancer.* 2009;**9**:415.

72   Kurman RJ, Shih IM. Molecular pathogenesis and extraovarian origin of epithelial ovarian cancer – shifting the paradigm. *Hum Pathol.* 2011;**42**:918.

74   Cancer Genome Atlas Research Network. Integrated genomic analyses of ovarian carcinoma. *Nature.* 2011;**474**:609.

82   Bast RC Jr, Klug TL, St. John E, et al. A radioimmunoassay using a monoclonal antibody to monitor the course of epithelial ovarian cancer. *N Engl J Med.* 1983;**309**:883–887.

83   Bast RC Jr, Feeney M, Lazarus H, et al. Reactivity of a monoclonal antibody with human ovarian carcinoma. *J Clin Invest.* 1981;**68**:1331–1337.

86   Bast RC, Spriggs DR. More than a biomarker: CA125 may contribute to ovarian cancer pathogenesis. *Gynecol Oncol.* 2011;**121**:429–430. PMID: 21601106.

95   Goff BA, Mandel LS, Drescher CW, et al. Development of an ovarian cancer symptom index: possibilities for earlier detection. *Cancer.* 2007;**109(2)**:221–227.

98   Jacobs I, Oram D, Fairbanks J, Turner J, Frost C, Grudzinskas JG. A risk of malignancy index incorporating CA 125, ultrasound and menopausal status for the accurate preoperative diagnosis of ovarian cancer. *Br J Obstet Gynaecol.* 1990;**97(10)**:922–929.

99   Ueland FR, Desimone CP, Seamon LG, et al. Effectiveness of a multivariate index assay in the preoperative assessment of ovarian tumors. *Obstet Gynecol.* 2011;**117**:1289–1297.

101   Moore RG, Miller C, Disilvestro P, et al. Evaluation of the diagnostic accuracy of the risk of ovarian malignancy algorithm in women with a pelvic mass. *Obstet Gynecol.* 2011;**118**:280–288.

112   Lu KH, Skates S, Hernandez MA, et al. A two-stage ovarian cancer screening strategy using the risk of ovarian cancer algorithm (ROCA) identifies early stage incident cancers and demonstrates high positive predictive value. *Cancer.* 2013;**119**:3454–3461.

113   Menon U, Gentry-Maharaj A, Hallett R, et al. Sensitivity and specificity of multimodal and ultrasound screening for ovarian cancer, and stage distribution of detected cancers: results of the prevalence screen of the UK Collaborative Trial of Ovarian Cancer Screening (UKCTOCS). *Lancet Oncol.* 2009;**10**:327–340.

114   Menon U, Ryan A, Kalsi J, et al. Risk algorithm using serial biomarker measurements doubles the number of screen-detected cancers compared with a single-threshold rule in the United Kingdom Collaborative Trial of Ovarian Cancer Screening. *J Clin Oncol.* 2015;**33**:2062–2071.

130   Berek JS, Friedlander ML, Hacker NF. Epithelial ovarian, fallopian tube, and peritoneal cancer. In: Berek JS, Hacker NF, eds. *Berek & Hacker's Gynecologic Oncology,* 6th ed. Philadelphia: Lippincott Williams & Wilkins; 2015:464–529.

133   Griffiths CT. Surgical resection of tumor bulk in the primary treatment of ovarian carcinoma. *Natl Cancer Inst Monogr.* 1975;**42**:101–109.

146   McGuire WP, Hoskins WJ, Brady MF, et al. Cyclophosphamide and cisplatin compared with paclitaxel and cisplatin in patients with stage III and stage IV ovarian cancer. *N Engl J Med.* 1996;**334**:1–6.

147   Piccart MJ, Bertelsen K, James K, et al. Randomized intergroup trial of cisplatin–paclitaxel versus cisplatin–cyclophosphamide in women with advanced epithelial ovarian cancer: three year results. *J Natl Cancer Inst.* 2000;**92**:699–708.

148   Muggia F, Braly PS, Brady MF, et al. Phase III randomized study of cisplatin versus paclitaxel versus cisplatin and paclitaxel in patients with suboptimal stage III or IV ovarian cancer: a Gynecologic Oncology Group study. *J Clin Oncol.* 2000;**18**:106–115.

157   Swenerton K, Jeffrey J, Stuart G, et al. Cisplatin-cyclophosphamide versus carboplatin-cyclophosphamide in advanced ovarian cancer: a randomized phase III study of the National Cancer Institute of Canada Clinical Trials Group. *J Clin Oncol.* 1992;**10**:718–726.

158   Ozols RF, Bundy BN, Greer B, et al. Phase III trial of carboplatin and paclitaxel compared with cisplatin and paclitaxel in patients with optimally resected stage III ovarian cancer. *J Clin Oncol.* 2003;**21**:3194–3200.

160   The International Collaborative Ovarian Neoplasm (ICON) Group. Paclitaxel plus carboplatin versus standard chemotherapy with either single agent carboplatin or cyclophosphamide, doxorubicin and cisplatin: in women with ovarian cancer: the ICON3 randomised trial. *Lancet.* 2002;**360**:505–515.

164   Aabo K, Adams M, Adnitt P, et al. Chemotherapy in advanced ovarian cancer: four systematic meta analyses of individual patient data from 37 randomized trials. Advanced Ovarian Cancer Trialists' Group. *Br J Cancer.* 1998;**78**:1479–1487.

169   Vasey PA, Paul J, Birt A, et al. Docetaxel and cisplatin in combination as first-line chemotherapy for advanced epithelial ovarian cancer. Scottish Gynaecological Cancer Trials Group. *J Clin Oncol.* 1999;**17**:2069–2080.

170   Bookman MA, Brady MF, McGuire WP, et al. Evaluation of new platinum-based treatment regimens in advanced-stage ovarian cancer: a Phase III Trial of the Gynecologic Cancer Intergroup (GOG182). *J Clin Oncol.* 2009;**27**:1419–1425.

178   Alberts DS, Liu PY, Hannigan EV, et al. Intraperitoneal cisplatin plus intravenous cyclophosphamide versus intravenous cisplatin plus intravenous cyclophosphamide for stage III ovarian cancer. *N Engl J Med.* 1996;**335**:1950–1955.

179   Markman M, Bundy B, Benda J, et al. Randomized phase III study of intravenous cisplatin/paclitaxel versus moderately high dose intravenous carboplatin followed by intraperitoneal paclitaxel and intraperitoneal cisplatin in optimal residual ovarian cancer: an Intergroup trial (GOG, SWOG, ECOG). *J Clin Oncol.* 2001;**19**:921–923.

180   Armstrong D, Bundy B, Wenzel L, et al. Intraperitoneal cisplatin and paclitaxel in ovarian cancer. *N Engl J Med.* 2006;**354**:34–53.

187   van der Burg MEL, van Lent M, Buyse M, et al. The effect of debulking surgery after induction chemotherapy on the prognosis in advanced epithelial ovarian cancer. *N Engl J Med.* 1995;**332**:629–634.

201   Cohen MH, Gootenberg J, Keegan P, Pazdur R. FDA drug approval summary: bevacizumab (Avastin) plus Carboplatin and paclitaxel as first-line treatment of advanced/metastatic recurrent nonsquamous non-small Cell lung cancer. *Oncologist.* 2007;**12(6)**:713–718.

203   Burger RA, Brady MF, Bookman MA, et al. Gynecologic Oncol ogy Group. Incorporation of bevacizumab in the primary treatment of ovarian cancer. *N Engl J Med.* 2011;**365(26)**:2473–2483.

204   Perren TJ, Swart AM, Pfisterer J, et al. A phase 3 trial of bevacizumab in ovarian cancer. *N Engl J Med.* 2011;**365(26)**:2484–2496.

222   Pfisterer J, Plante M, Vergote I, et al. Gemcitabine plus carboplatin compared with carboplatin in patients with platinum-sensitive recurrent ovarian cancer: an intergroup trial of the AGO-OVAR, the NCIC CTG, and the EORTC GCG. *J Clin Oncol.* 2006;**24**:4699–4707.

223   Alberts DS, Liu PY, Wilczynski SP, et al. Randomized trial of pegylated liposomal doxorubicin (PLD) plus carboplatin versus carboplatin in platinum-sensitive (PS) patients with recurrent epithe- lial ovarian or peritoneal carcinoma after failure of initial platinum- based chemotherapy (Southwest Oncology Group Protocol S0200). *Gynecol Oncol.* 2008;**108**:90–94.

224   Pujade-Lauraine E, Wagner U, Aavall-Lundqvist E, et al. Pegylated liposomal doxorubicin and carboplatin compared with paclitaxel and carboplatin for patients with platinum-sensitive ovarian cancer in late relapse. *J Clin Oncol.* 2010;**28(20)**:3323–3329.

230   Poveda AM, Selle F, Hilpert F, et al. Bevacixumab combined with weekly paclitaxel, pegylated liposomal doxorubicin, or topotecan in platinum-resistant recurrent ovarian cancer: analysis by chemotherapy cohort of the fandomized phase III AURELIA Trial. *J Clin Oncol.* 2015;**63**:1408.

235   Mutch DG, Orlando M, Goss T, et al. Randomized phase III trial of gemcitabine compared with pegylated liposomal doxorubicin in patients with platinum-resistant ovarian cancer. *J Clin Oncol.* 2007;**25**:2811–2818.

275   Fong PC, Boss DS, Yap TA, et al. Inhibition of poly(ADP-ribose) polymerase in tumors from BRCA mutation carriers. *N Engl J Med.* 2009;**361(2)**:123–134.

276   Fong PC, Yap TA, Boss DS, et al. Poly(ADP)-ribose polymerase inhibition: frequent durable responses in BRCA carrier ovarian cancer correlating with platinum-free interval. *J Clin Oncol.* 2010;**28(15)**:2512–2519.

278   Ledermann J, Harter P, Gourley C, et al. Olaparib maintenance therapy in platinum-sensitive relapsed ovarian cancer. *N Engl J Med.* 2012;**366(15)**:1382–1392.

281   Mizra MR, Monk BJ, Herrstedt J, et al. Niraparib Maintenance Therapy in Platinum-Sensitive, Recurrent Ovarian Cancer. *NEJM.* DOI: 10.1056/NEJMoa1611310.

105 Nonepithelial ovarian malignancies

Jonathan S. Berek, MD, MMS, FASCO ▪ Michael L. Friedlander, MD, MBChB, PhD ▪ Robert C. Bast Jr., MD

Overview

Compared with epithelial ovarian cancers, nonepithelial ovarian tumors are uncommon, constituting <10% of all ovarian malignancies.[1,2] They include germ cell malignancies, sex-cord–stromal tumors, carcinomas metastatic to the ovary, and a variety of extremely rare ovarian cancers, including sarcomas and lipoid cell tumors. Although there are many similarities in the presentation, evaluation, and management of patients, these tumors also have unique features that require special approaches to management.[1–5] Germ cell malignancies are derived from primordial germ cells of the ovary and can be distinguished by histotype and expression of the biomarkers alpha-fetoprotein (AFP) and/or human chorionic gonadotropin (hCG). They include dysgerminomas (AFP–hCG–), embryonal carcinomas (AFP+hCG+), immature teratomas (AFP–hCG–), endodermal sinus (yolk sac) tumors (AFP+hCG–), and ovarian choriocarcinomas (AFP–hCG+). Germ cell tumors occur in premenarchal girls and young women, grow rapidly, and can present with a symptomatic pelvic mass. As preservation of fertility is often an important priority, unilateral salpingo-oophorectomy can often be performed followed by adjuvant platinum-based therapy. Among the germ cell tumors, dysgerminomas can be bilateral in 10–15% of cases and are associated with gonadal dysgenesis in 5% of cases. Metastatic germ cell cancers can be quite sensitive to chemotherapy and the long-term survival rate is high, even in advanced stages. At some institutions, young patients with stage IA germ cell tumors are followed carefully after resection and chemotherapy given only if there is recurrence with excellent outcomes. Sex-Cord-Stromal tumors include Granulosa-Stromal tumors, Juvenile Granulosa tumors, and Sertoli–Leydig cell tumors. Granulosa-Stromal tumors can occur at all ages and produce estrogen resulting in pseudoprecocious puberty in a small fraction of girls, amenorrhea in pre-menopausal women, and endometrial hyperplasia in postmenopausal adults. Granulosa-Stromal tumors are indolent and often confined to one ovary where surgery can cure stage I disease in more than 75% of cases. Adjuvant chemotherapy is generally not given after complete resection. Late recurrence has, however, been observed. Persistent or recurrent disease has responded to platinum based and hormonal therapy, including progestational agents, luteinizing hormone-releasing hormone agonists, and aromatase inhibitors. Inhibin B has been a useful biomarker. Sertoli–Leydig cell tumors generally present in the third or fourth decade, produce androgens, and induce virilization in more than 70% of patients. As many Sertoli–Leydig cell tumors are in early stage and rarely bilateral, unilateral salpingo-oophorectomy is often performed with 70–90% 5-year survival.

Germ cell malignancies

Germ cell tumors are derived from the primordial germ cells of the ovary and occur with only about one-tenth the incidence of malignant germ cell tumors of the testis. Although they can arise in extragonadal sites such as the mediastinum and the retroperitoneum, the majority of germ cell tumors arise in the gonad from undifferentiated germ cells. The variation in the site of these cancers is explained by the embryonic migration of the germ cells from the caudal part of the yolk sac to the dorsal mesentery before their incorporation into the sex cords of the developing gonads.[1,2]

Germ cell tumors are a model of a curable cancer. The management of patients with ovarian germ cell tumors has largely been extrapolated from the much greater experience of treating males with the more common testicular germ cell tumors. There have been many randomized trials for testicular germ cell tumors, which have provided a strong evidence base for treatment decision making.[6,7] The outcome of patients with testicular germ cell tumors is better in experienced centers, and it is reasonable to suggest that the same will be true for the less common ovarian counterparts. The cure rate is high, and attention is now being directed at reducing toxicity without compromising survival. There are still a small number of patients who die from the disease, and studies are in progress to try to improve the outcome for this high-risk, poor-prognostic subset.[6,7]

In one of the largest reported series, which included 113 patients with advanced ovarian germ cell tumors treated with cisplatin-based chemotherapy, Murugaesu et al.[8] reported that stage and elevated tumor markers were independent poor prognostic indicators. These findings are important because they identify similar prognostic factors for ovarian and testicular germ cell tumors, and are in accordance with the clinical observation that testicular and ovarian germ cell tumors behave similarly. This is relevant for the management of patients with ovarian germ cell tumors because it may help to identify a poor prognostic subset of patients who require more intensive treatment.[8]

Histology and biomarkers

A histologic classification of ovarian germ cell tumors is presented in Table 1.[1,10] Both alpha-fetoprotein (AFP) and human chorionic gonadotropin (hCG) are secreted by some germ cell malignancies. An elevated AFP and β-hCG can be clinically useful in the differential diagnosis of patients with a pelvic mass and in monitoring patients after surgery. Placental alkaline phosphatase (PLAP) and lactate dehydrogenase (LDH) are elevated in up to 95% of patients with dysgerminomas, and serial monitoring of serum LDH levels may be useful for monitoring the disease. PLAP is more useful as an immunohistochemical marker than as a serum marker. The classification of germ cell tumors is based both on histologic features and the expression of tumor biomarkers (Figure 1).[12,13]

In this scheme, embryonal carcinoma, which is composed of undifferentiated cells that synthesize both hCG and AFP, is the progenitor of several other germ cell tumors.[4,13] More differentiated germ cell tumors—such as the endodermal sinus tumor (EST), which secretes AFP, and choriocarcinoma, which secretes hCG—are derived from the extraembryonic tissues; immature teratomas are derived from the embryonic cells and do not secrete

Holland-Frei Cancer Medicine, Ninth Edition. Edited by Robert C. Bast Jr., Carlo M. Croce, William N. Hait, Waun Ki Hong, Donald W. Kufe, Martine Piccart-Gebhart, Raphael E. Pollock, Ralph R. Weichselbaum, Hongyang Wang, and James F. Holland.
© 2017 John Wiley & Sons, Inc. ISBN: 978-1-118-93469-2

Source: Adapted from Serov 1973.[9] Reproduced with permission of WHO.

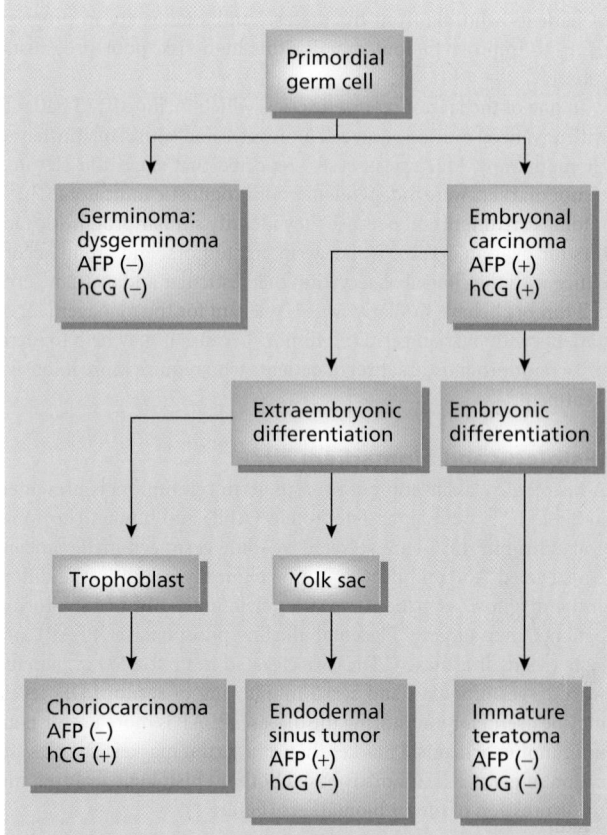

Figure 1 Relationship between examples of pure malignant GCTs and their secreted substances. Abbreviations: AFP, α-fetoprotein; hCG, human chorionic gonadotropin. Source: Berek 2015.[11] Reproduced with permission of Wolters Kluwer Health.

hCG, but may be associated with an elevated AFP. Elevated hCG levels are seen in 3% of dysgerminomas and the level is typically less than 100 International Unit. AFP is never elevated in pure dysgerminomas.[1]

Epidemiology

Although 20–25% of all benign and malignant ovarian neoplasms are of germ cell origin, they account for only about 5% of all malignant ovarian neoplasms.[1] In Asian and Black societies where epithelial ovarian cancers are much less common, they may account for as many as 15% of ovarian cancers. In the first two decades of life, almost 70% of ovarian tumors are of germ cell origin, and one-third of these are malignant.[1,2] Germ cell tumors account for two-thirds of the ovarian malignancies in this age group. Germ cell cancers also are seen in the third decade, but thereafter they become quite rare.

Symptoms

In contrast to the relatively slow-growing epithelial ovarian tumors, germ cell malignancies grow rapidly, and often are characterized by subacute pelvic pain related to capsular distention, hemorrhage, or necrosis. The rapidly enlarging pelvic mass may produce pressure symptoms on the bladder or rectum, and menstrual irregularities also may occur in menarchal patients. Some young patients may misinterpret the symptoms as those of pregnancy, and this can lead to a delay in diagnosis. Acute symptoms associated with torsion or rupture can develop. These symptoms may be confused with acute appendicitis. In more advanced cases, ascites may develop, and the patient may present with abdominal distention.[3]

Signs

In patients with a palpable adnexal mass, the evaluation can proceed as outlined earlier for epithelial cancers. Some patients with germ cell tumors will be premenarchal. If the lesions are principally solid, or a combination of solid and cystic on an ultrasonographic evaluation, a neoplasm is probable and a malignancy is possible. The remainder of the physical examination should search for signs of ascites, pleural effusion, and organomegaly.

Diagnosis

Adnexal masses measuring 2 cm or more in premenarchal girls or complex masses 8 cm or more in premenopausal patients will usually require surgical exploration. In young patients, preoperative blood tests should include serum hCG, AFP, LDH, and CA125 levels, a complete blood count, and liver function tests. A radiograph of the chest is important because germ cell tumors can metastasize to the lungs or mediastinum. A karyotype should ideally be obtained preoperatively on all premenarchal girls because of the propensity of these tumors to arise in dysgenetic gonads, but this may not be practical.[3,14] A preoperative computed tomographic (CT) scan or magnetic resonance imaging (MRI) may document the presence and extent of retroperitoneal lymphadenopathy or liver metastases, but unless there is very extensive meta-static disease, is unlikely to influence the decision to operate on the patient initially. If post-menarchal patients have predominantly cystic lesions up to 8 cm in diameter, they may undergo observation or a trial of hormonal suppression for two cycles.[15]

Dysgerminomas

Dysgerminomas are the most common malignant germ cell tumor, accounting for approximately 30–40% of all ovarian cancers of germ cell origin.[2,12] They represent only 1–3% of all ovarian cancers, but represent as many as 5–10% of ovarian cancers in patients younger than 20 years of age. Seventy-five percent of dysgerminomas occur between the ages of 10 and 30 years, 5% occur before the age of 10 years and they rarely occur after age 50.[1,4] They typically occur in

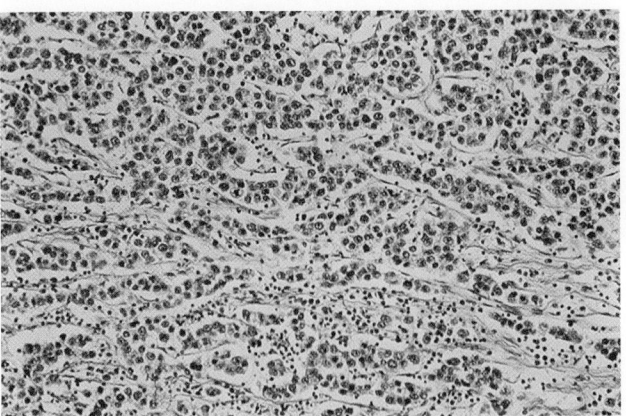

Figure 2 Dysgerminoma.

young women and 20–30% of ovarian malignancies associated with pregnancy are dysgerminomas.

Association with abnormal ovaries

Approximately 5% of dysgerminomas occur in phenotypic females with abnormal gonads.[1,14] Dysgerminomas can be associated with patients who have pure gonadal dysgenesis (46XY, bilateral streak gonads), mixed gonadal dysgenesis (45X/46XY, unilateral streak gonad, contralateral testis), and the androgen insensitivity syndrome (46XY, testicular feminization). Therefore, in premenarchal patients with a pelvic mass, the karyotype should be determined, particularly if a dysgerminoma is considered as the likely diagnosis (Figure 2).

In most patients with gonadal dysgenesis, dysgerminomas arise in a gonadoblastoma, which is a benign ovarian tumor composed of germ cells and sex-cord stroma. If gonadoblastomas are left *in situ* in patients with gonadal dysgenesis, more than 50% will subsequently develop ovarian malignancies.[16]

Approximately 65% of dysgerminomas are stage I at diagnosis.[1,3,5,17–21] Eighty-five to ninety percent of stage I tumors are confined to one ovary, while 10–15% are bilateral. All other germ cell tumors are rarely bilateral. In patients whose contralateral ovary has been preserved, a dysgerminoma can develop in 5–10% of them over the next 2 years.[1] This figure includes patients who have not received systemic chemotherapy, as well as patients with gonadal dysgenesis.

Pattern of spread

In the 25% of patients who present with metastatic disease, the tumor most commonly spreads via the lymphatics, particularly to the higher para-aortic nodes.[19] They can also spread hematogenously or by direct extension through the capsule of the ovary with exfoliation and dissemination of cells throughout the peritoneal surfaces. Metastases to the contralateral ovary may be present when there is no other evidence of spread. An uncommon site of metastatic disease is bone, and when metastasis to this site occurs, the metastases are seen typically in the lower vertebrae. Metastases to the lungs, liver, and brain are rare and seen most often in patients with long-standing or recurrent disease. Metastasis to the mediastinum and supraclavicular lymph nodes is also usually a late manifestation of disease.[17,18]

Treatment

The treatment of patients with early dysgerminoma is primarily surgical, including resection of the primary lesion and limited surgical staging–washings, omental biopsy, careful palpation of all peritoneal surfaces and retroperitoneal nodes, and biopsy of anything suspicious. Chemotherapy is administered to patients with metastatic disease. Because the disease principally affects young women, special consideration must be given to the preservation of fertility.[19,22] A comparison of outcomes based on treatment at the Norwegian Radium Hospital clearly demonstrates the superiority of chemotherapy over radiation. Survival was better and morbidity was lower in the group treated with chemotherapy.[22]

Surgery

The minimum operation for ovarian dysgerminoma is unilateral oophorectomy.[20,23] If there is a desire to preserve fertility, as is usually the case, the contralateral ovary, fallopian tube, and uterus should be left *in situ* even in the presence of metastatic disease because of the sensitivity of the tumor to chemotherapy. If fertility preservation is not required, it may be appropriate to perform a total abdominal hysterectomy and bilateral salpingo-oophorectomy in patients with advanced disease,[5] although this will be appropriate in only a very small minority of patients. In patients whose karyotype contains a Y chromosome, both ovaries should be removed, although the uterus may be left *in situ* for possible future embryo transfer. Cytoreductive surgery is of unproven value, but bulky disease that can be readily resected (e.g., an omental cake) should be removed at the initial operation. It is important not to undertake surgery that is potentially morbid and may delay the initiation of chemotherapy.

In patients in whom the dysgerminoma appears on inspection to be confined to the ovary, a careful staging operation should be undertaken to determine the presence of an occult metastatic disease. These tumors often metastasize to the para-aortic nodes around the renal vessels. Peritoneal washings should be taken for cytology, and a thorough exploration made of all peritoneal surfaces and retroperitoneal lymph nodes, with biopsy or resection of any noted abnormalities. The contralateral ovary should be carefully inspected because dysgerminoma is the only germ cell tumor that tends to be bilateral, and not all of the bilateral lesions have obvious ovarian enlargement. Therefore, careful inspection and palpation of the contralateral ovary and excisional biopsy of any suspicious lesion are desirable.[5,20,21,23] If a small contralateral tumor is found, it may be possible to resect it and preserve some normal ovary.

Many patients with a dysgerminoma will have a tumor that is apparently confined to one ovary and will be referred after unilateral salpingo-oophorectomy without surgical staging. The options for such patients are (1) repeat laparotomy for surgical staging, (2) regular pelvic and abdominal CT scans, or (3) adjuvant chemotherapy.[19] Because most dysgerminomas are confined to the ovary at presentation and are rapidly growing tumors, the author's preference is to offer regular and close surveillance to such patients.[24,25]

Radiation

Loss of fertility and second malignancies are important late effects of radiation therapy, so it is no longer used for primary treatment.[22] Radiation can be used selectively to treat recurrent disease.[5,21,22] Dysgerminomas are very sensitive to radiation therapy, and doses of 2500 to 3500 cGy may be curative; however, it is uncommonly used because these tumors are very sensitive to platinum-based chemotherapy and have a high likelihood of cure.

Chemotherapy

Chemotherapy is regarded as the treatment of choice.[23,26–35] The obvious advantage is the preservation of fertility in most patients, and the reduced risk of second malignancies compared with radiation.[23,36–40] The most frequently used chemotherapeutic regimen

Table 2 Combination chemotherapy for GCTs of the ovary.

Regimens and drugs	Dosage and schedule[a]
BEP	
Bleomycin	30 IU weekly to a maximum of 12 weeks
	15 U/m^2/week × 5; then on day 1 of course 4
Etoposide	100 mg/m^2/day × 5 days every 3 weeks
Cisplatin	20 mg/m^2/day × 5 days, or 100 mg/m^2/day × 1 day every 3 weeks

[a]All doses given intravenously.

is BEP (bleomycin, etoposide, and cisplatin). In the past, VBP (vinblastine, bleomycin, and cisplatin) and VAC (vincristine, actinomycin, and cyclophosphamide) were commonly used but are now rarely prescribed (Table 2).[23,26–30]

The Gynecologic Oncology Group (GOG) studied three cycles of EC (etoposide plus carboplatin): Etoposide (120 mg/m^2 intravenously on days 1, 2, and 3 every 4 weeks) and carboplatin (400 mg/m^2 intravenously on day 1 every 4 weeks) in 39 patients with completely resected ovarian dysgerminoma, stages IB, IC, II, or III.[33] The results were excellent, and GOG reported a sustained disease-free remission rate of 100%. For patients with advanced, incompletely resected germ cell tumors, the GOG studied cisplatin-based chemotherapy on two consecutive protocols.[27] In the first study, patients received four cycles of vinblastine (12 mg/m^2 every 3 weeks), bleomycin (20 unit/m^2 intravenously every week for 12 weeks), and cisplatin (20 mg/m^2/d intravenously for 5 days every 3 weeks). Patients with persistent or progressive disease at second-look laparotomy were treated with six cycles of VAC. In the second trial, patients received three cycles of BEP initially, followed by consolidation with VAC, which was later discontinued in patients with dysgerminomas.[27] VAC does not appear to improve the outcome following the BEP regimen and is no longer used.

A total of 20 evaluable patients with stages III and IV dysgerminoma were treated in these two protocols and 19 were alive and free of disease after 6–68 months (median = 26 months). Fourteen of these patients had a second-look laparotomy, and all findings were negative. A study at MD Anderson Hospital[30] used BEP in 14 patients with residual disease, and all patients were free of disease with long-term follow-up. In another series of 26 patients with pure ovarian dysgerminomas who received BEP chemotherapy, 54% of whom had stage IIIC or IV disease, 25 (96%) remained continuously disease free following three to six cycles of therapy.[35]

These results indicate that patients with an advanced-stage, incompletely resected dysgerminoma have an excellent prognosis when treated with cisplatin-based combination chemotherapy.[34–39,41] The optimal regimen is three to four cycles of BEP based on the data from testis cancers[40–42] with the number of cycles depending on the extent of disease and the presence or absence of visceral metastases. If bleomycin is contraindicated or omitted because of lung toxicity, consideration should be given to four cycles of cisplatin and etoposide rather than three cycles of BEP.

There is no need to perform a second-look laparotomy in patients with dysgerminomas.[43–45] The role of surgery to resect residual masses following chemotherapy for dysgerminomas is not clear, as the vast majority of these patients will only have necrotic tissue and nonviable tumor. In general, these patients should be closely monitored with scans and tumor markers. A positron emission tomography (PET–CT) scan should be considered in patients who have bulky residual masses larger than 3 cm more than 4 weeks after

chemotherapy. A positive PET–CT scan appears to be a sensitive predictor of residual seminoma in males in these circumstances,[46] with residual disease being evident in 30–50% of patients. If the PET–CT is positive or if there is a suggestion of progressive disease on scans, ideally there should be histologic confirmation of residual disease before embarking on salvage therapy.[47]

Recurrent disease

Although recurrences are uncommon, 75% will occur within the first year after initial treatment,[1–4] with the most common sites being the peritoneal cavity and the retroperitoneal lymph nodes. These patients should be treated with either chemotherapy or radiation, depending on the location of disease and the primary treatment. Patients with recurrent disease who have had no therapy other than surgery should be treated with chemotherapy. If previous chemotherapy with BEP has been given, an alternative regimen such as TIP (paclitaxel, ifosfamide, and cisplatin), a commonly used salvage regimen in testicular germ cell tumors,[48] may be tried.

These treatment decisions should be made in a multidisciplinary setting with the input of physicians experienced in the management of patients with germ cell tumors. Consideration may be given to the use of high-dose chemotherapy with peripheral stem cell support in selected patients. A number of high-dose regimens have been used in phase II studies, and the choice depends on the previous chemotherapy, the time to recurrence, and the residual toxicity from the previous therapy.[49,50] It is unclear whether high-dose chemotherapy is superior to conventional dose chemotherapy as first-line salvage therapy for patients with relapsed disease. The only randomized trial, conducted by the European Group for Blood and Marrow Transplantation (EBMT)-IT-94, did not demonstrate superiority for three cycles of VIP or vinblastine, ifosfamide, and cisplatin (VeIP) followed by high-dose chemotherapy compared with four cycles of conventional dose chemotherapy. An international randomized trial (TIGER) plans to randomize 390 patients with recurrent germ cell tumors to four cycles of conventional dose cisplatin-based chemotherapy with TIP, compared with two cycles of paclitaxel-ifosfamide followed by three cycles of high-dose carboplatin and etoposide with autologous stem-cell support (TICE).[50]

Radiation therapy may be considered in selected patients with dysgerminomas with a localized recurrence, but this has the major disadvantage of causing loss of fertility if pelvic and abdominal radiation is required and may also compromise the ability to deliver further chemotherapy if unsuccessful.[22]

Pregnancy

Because dysgerminomas tend to occur in young patients, they may coexist with pregnancy. When a stage IA cancer is found, the tumor can be removed intact and the pregnancy continued. In patients with more advanced disease, continuation of the pregnancy will depend on gestational age. Chemotherapy can be given in the second and third trimesters in the same dosages as given for the nonpregnant patient without apparent detriment to the fetus.[36,51] Relatively few patients have been treated with BEP during pregnancy and some fetal malformations and complications have been reported, underscoring the importance of ensuring that only patients who definitely require chemotherapy during pregnancy should be treated.[52]

Prognosis

In patients with stage IA dysgerminoma, unilateral oophorectomy alone results in a 5-year disease-free survival rate of greater than

95%.[5,21] The features that have been associated with a higher tendency to recurrence include tumors larger than 10–15 cm in diameter, age younger than 20 years, and microscopic features that include numerous mitoses, anaplasia, and a medullary pattern.[1,12]

Kumar et al.[53] abstracted data on malignant ovarian germ cell tumors from the Surveillance, Epidemiology, and End Results (SEER) program from 1988 to 2004. There were a total of 1296 patients with dysgerminomas, immature teratomas, or mixed germ cell tumors, 613 (47.3%) of whom had lymphadenectomies. Lymph node metastases were present in 28% of dysgerminomas, 8% of immature teratomas, and 16% of mixed germ cell tumors ($p < 0.05$). The 5-year survival for patients with negative nodes was 95.7% compared to 82.8% for patients with positive nodes ($p < 0.001$). The same group updated the results recently and reported on 1083 patients with ovarian germ cell tumors who had surgery and who were believed to have disease clinically confined to the ovary.[54] This included 590 (54.5%) who had no lymphadenectomy and 493 (45.5%) who had a lymphadenectomy. Of the latter, 52 (10.5%) were upstaged to FIGO (International Federation of Gynecology and Obstetrics) stage IIIC owing to nodal metastases. The 5-year survival was 96.9% for patients who did not have a lymphadenectomy, 97.7% for those who did, and 93.4% for patients who were found to have stage IIIC disease after lymphadenectomy. These survivals were not statistically different and underscore the excellent prognosis for patients with dysgerminomas.[26–39]

Immature teratoma

Immature teratomas typically contain immature neuroepithelium and may be pure immature teratomas or occur in combination with other germ cell tumors as mixed germ cell tumors. The pure immature teratoma accounts for fewer than 1% of all ovarian cancers, but it is the second most common germ cell malignancy and represents 10–20% of all ovarian malignancies seen in women younger than 20 years of age.[1] Approximately 50% of pure immature teratomas of the ovary occur between the ages of 10 and 20 years, and they rarely occur in postmenopausal women.

Semiquantification of the amount of neuroepithelium correlates with survival in ovarian immature teratomas and is the basis for the grading of these tumors.[55–57] Those with less than one lower-power field[4] of immature neuroepithelium on the slide with the greatest amount of immature neuroepithelium (grade 1) have a survival of at least 95%, whereas greater amounts of immature neuroepithelium (grades 2 and 3) appear to have a lower overall survival (~85%).[57] This may not apply to immature teratomas of the ovary in children because they appear to have a very good outcome with surgery alone, regardless of the degree of immaturity. These findings are from an era when not all patients would have received platinum-based chemotherapy.[58,59]

Some pathologists have recommended a two-tiered grading system, suggesting that immature teratomas be categorized as either low grade or high grade because of the significant inter- and intraobserver difficulty with a three-grade system,[55] which is the author's current practice.

Immature ovarian teratomas may be associated with gliomatosis peritonei, which has a favorable prognosis if composed of completely mature tissues. Recent reports have suggested that these glial "implants" are not tumor derived, but represent teratoma-induced metaplasia of pluripotential müllerian stem cells in the peritoneum.[58,60,61] The researchers have exploited a unique characteristic of ovarian teratomas. The latter typically contain a duplicated set of maternal chromosomes and are therefore homozygous at polymorphic microsatellite loci,

while DNA (deoxyribonucleic acid) from matched normal tissue contains genetic material of both maternal and paternal origin, so exhibits heterozygosity at many of these same polymorphic microsatellite loci.

Malignant transformation of a mature teratoma is a rare event. Squamous cell carcinoma is the most frequent subtype of malignancy, but adenocarcinomas, primary melanomas, and carcinoids may also rarely occur (see the following discussion).[32] The risk is reported to be between 0.5% and 2% of teratomas and usually occurs in postmenopausal patients.

Diagnosis

The preoperative evaluation and differential diagnosis are the same as for patients with other germ cell tumors. Some of these tumors will contain calcifications similar to mature teratomas, and this can be detected by a radiograph of the abdomen or by ultrasonography. Rarely, they are associated with the production of steroid hormones and can be accompanied by sexual pseudoprecocity.[4] AFP may be elevated in some patients with a pure immature teratoma but hCG is not elevated.

Surgery

In a premenopausal patient where the tumor appears confined to a single ovary, unilateral oophorectomy and limited surgical staging should be performed. In the rare postmenopausal patient with an immature teratoma, a total abdominal hysterectomy and bilateral salpingo-oophorectomy may be performed. Contralateral involvement is rare, and routine resection or wedge biopsy of the contralateral ovary is unnecessary.[2] Any suspicious lesions on the peritoneal surfaces should be sampled and submitted for histologic evaluation. The most frequent site of dissemination is the peritoneum and, much less commonly, the retroperitoneal lymph nodes. Bloodborne metastases to organ parenchyma such as the lungs, liver, or brain are uncommon. When present, they are usually seen in patients with late or recurrent disease and most often in tumors that are high grade.[4]

It is unclear whether debulking of metastases improves the response to combination chemotherapy.[62,63] Cure ultimately depends on the ability to deliver chemotherapy promptly. Any surgical resection that may be potentially morbid and therefore delay chemotherapy should be resisted, although surgical resection of any residual disease should be considered at the completion of chemotherapy.

Chemotherapy

Patients with stage IA, grade 1 tumors have an excellent prognosis, and no adjuvant therapy is required. In patients with high-grade, stage IA immature teratomas, adjuvant chemotherapy has commonly been given, although this has been questioned, as excellent results have also been reported with close surveillance and treating only patients who have a recurrence.[19,22,28–30,44,59,64–78]

The most frequently used combination chemotherapeutic regimen in the past was VAC,[72–74] but a GOG study reported a relapse-free survival rate in patients with incompletely resected disease of only 75%.[74] The approach over the past 20 years has been to incorporate cisplatin into the primary treatment of these tumors, and most of the experience has been with the VBP in the past and BEP more recently.[67]

The GOG prospectively evaluated three courses of BEP therapy in patients with completely resected stage I, II, and III ovarian germ cell tumors. Overall, the toxicity was acceptable, and 91 of 93 patients (97.8%) with nondysgerminomatous tumors were clinically free of disease. In nonrandomized studies, the BEP regimen is superior to the VAC regimen in the treatment of completely resected nondysgerminomatous germ cell tumors of the ovary. Some patients can progress rapidly postoperatively, and, in general, treatment should be initiated as soon as possible after surgery, preferably within 7–10 days, in those patients who require chemotherapy.

The switch from VBP to BEP has been prompted by the experience in patients with testicular cancer, where the replacement of vinblastine with etoposide has been associated with a better therapeutic index (i.e., equivalent efficacy and lower morbidity), with less neurologic and gastrointestinal toxicity, and improved outcomes.[67,68] Furthermore, the use of bleomycin appears to be important in this group of patients. In a randomized study of three cycles of etoposide plus cisplatin (EP) with or without bleomycin (EP vs BEP) in 166 patients with germ cell tumors of the testes, the BEP regimen had a relapse-free survival rate of 84% compared with 69% for the EP regimen ($p = 0.03$).[40]

Cisplatin is superior to carboplatin in metastatic germ cell tumors of the testis. One hundred and ninety-two patients with good prognosis germ cell tumors of the testes were entered into a study of four cycles of EP versus four cycles of EC. There were three relapses with the EP regimen versus seven with the EC regimen.[42] A German group randomized patients to (1) a BEP regimen of three cycles at standard doses given days 1–5 versus (2) a CEB regimen of carboplatin [target AUC of 5 (mg/dL/min) on day 1], etoposide 120 mg/m² on days 1–3, and bleomycin 30 mg on days 1, 8, and 15.[79] Four cycles of CEB were given, with the omission of bleomycin in the fourth cycle so that the cumulative doses of etoposide and bleomycin in the two treatment arms were comparable. Fifty-four patients were entered on the trial; 29 were treated with BEP and 25 with CEB chemotherapy. More patients treated with CEB relapsed after therapy (32% vs 13%). Four patients (16%) treated with CEB died of disease progression in contrast to one patient (3%) after BEP therapy. The trial was terminated early after an interim analysis. The inferiority of carboplatin was confirmed in a larger randomized trial reported by Horwich et al.[80] In view of these results, BEP is the preferred treatment regimen.[67,81–83] The 3-day schedule has been found to be equivalent to a 5-day schedule for BEP chemotherapy. A cycle of BEP consisted of etoposide 500 mg/m², administered at either 100 mg/m² days 1–5 or 165 mg/m² days 1–3, and cisplatin 100 mg/m², administered at either 20 mg/m² days 1–5 or 50 mg/m² days 1 and 2. Bleomycin 30,000 International Unit is administered on days 1, 8, and 15 during cycles 1–3.

Recurrent disease

The principles and approach are identical to the management of recurrent dysgerminoma, as discussed earlier.

Second-look laparotomy

Second-look operation for ovarian germ cell tumors[44,45] is not indicated in patients who have received adjuvant chemotherapy (i.e., stage IA, grades 2 and 3). However, surgery should be considered in patients with metastatic immature teratomas who have residual disease at the completion of chemotherapy because they may have residual mature teratoma and are at risk of growing teratoma syndrome, a rare complication of immature teratomas.[84–86] Furthermore, cancers can arise at a later date in residual mature teratoma, and it is important to resect any residual mass and exclude persistent disease, as further chemotherapy may be indicated.

The principles of surgery are based on the much larger experience of surgery in males with residual masses following chemotherapy for germ cell tumors with a component of immature teratoma.[87]

Mathew et al.[88] reported their experience of laparotomy in assessing the nature of postchemotherapy residual masses in ovarian germ cell tumors. Sixty-eight patients completed combination chemotherapy with cisplatin regimens, of whom 35 had radiologic evidence of residual masses. Twenty-nine of these 35 patients underwent laparotomy, and 10 patients (34.5%) had viable tumor, including 7 cases (24.2%) of immature teratoma. Nineteen patients (65.5) had no evidence of malignancy, including 3 (10.3%) cases showing mature teratoma, and 16 (55.2%) showing necrosis or fibrosis only. None of the patients with a dysgerminoma or embryonal carcinoma and a radiologic residual mass of less than 5 cm had viable tumor present, whereas all patients with primary tumors containing a component of teratoma had residual tumor, strengthening the case for surgery in patients with metastatic immature teratoma and any residual mass.[88,89]

Prognosis

The most important prognostic feature of the immature teratoma is the grade of the lesion.[1,55] In addition, the stage of disease and the extent of tumor at the initiation of treatment also have an impact on prognosis.[4] Overall, the 5-year survival rate for patients with all stages of pure immature teratomas is 70–80%, and it is 90–95% for patients with surgical stage I tumors.[11,44,55,64]

The degree or grade of immaturity generally predicts the metastatic potential and prognosis. The 5-year survival rates have been reported to be 82%, 62%, and 30% for patients with grades 1, 2, and 3, respectively,[55] but many of these patients were treated in an era before optimal chemotherapy was available, and these figures do not match current experience and more recently published data.[69] For example, Lai et al.[90] reported on the long-term outcome of 84 patients with ovarian germ cell tumors, including 29 immature teratomas, and the 5-year survival was 97.4%.

Occasionally, these tumors are associated with mature or low-grade glial elements that have implanted throughout the peritoneum. Such patients have a favorable long-term survival.[4] Mature glial elements can grow and mimic malignant disease and may need to be resected to relieve pressure on surrounding structures.

Endodermal sinus tumor

ESTs have also been referred to as yolk sac carcinomas because they are derived from the primitive yolk sac.[1] They are the third most frequent malignant germ cell tumor of the ovary. ESTs have a median age of 18 years at diagnosis.[1–3,91,92] Approximately one-third of the patients are premenarchal at presentation. Abdominal or pelvic pain occurs in approximately 75% of patients, whereas an asymptomatic pelvic mass is documented in 10% of patients.[11] Most ESTs secrete AFP and rarely may also elaborate detectable alpha-1-antitrypsin (AAT). There is a good correlation between the extent of disease and the level of AFP, although discordance also has been observed. The serum level of AFP is useful in monitoring the patient's response to treatment, as well as in follow-up.[91–98]

Surgery

The treatment of an EST consists of surgical exploration, unilateral salpingo-oophorectomy, a frozen section for diagnosis, and limited surgical staging. A hysterectomy and contralateral salpingo-oophorectomy should not be done.[4,94,95] Conservative surgery and adjuvant chemotherapy allow fertility preservation as with other germ cell tumors.[23] In patients with metastatic disease, all gross disease should be resected if possible. At surgery, the tumors tend to be solid and large, ranging in size from 7 to 28 cm (median 15 cm) in the GOG series. Bilaterality is not seen in EST, and the other ovary is involved with metastatic disease only when there are other metastases in the peritoneal cavity. Most patients have early-stage disease: 71% stage I, 6% stage II, and 23% stage III.[95,99]

Chemotherapy

All patients with ESTs should be treated with chemotherapy shortly after recovering from surgery. Before the routine use of combination chemotherapy, the 2-year survival rate was approximately 25%. After the introduction of the VAC regimen, the survival rate improved to 60–70%, which highlights the chemosensitivity of the majority of these tumors.[73,74] All patients should be treated with a cisplatin-based regimen such as BEP, which is considered the standard of care. The chance of cure now approaches 100% for patients with early-stage disease and is at least 75% for patients with more advanced-stage disease.[95]

The optimal number of treatment cycles has not been established in ovarian germ cell tumors, but it is reasonable to extrapolate from the much larger experience in testicular germ cell tumors where three cycles of BEP are considered optimal for good prognosis, low-risk patients, and four cycles for patients with intermediate to high-risk tumors.[100] In patients for whom bleomycin is omitted or discontinued because of toxicity, four cycles of cisplatin and etoposide are recommended. An alternative approach is to use VIP (etoposide, ifosfamide, and cisplatin) in patients with more advanced disease in whom bleomycin is contraindicated. Four cycles of VIP are equivalent to four cycles of BEP, but it is more myelotoxic and requires growth-factor support.[6,7,101] These patients should only be treated by clinicians experienced in the management of germ cell tumors as the outcomes of patients in inexperienced hands are compromised.

Neoadjuvant chemotherapy followed by fertility-sparing surgery may also be a reasonable option for patients with advanced ovarian germ cell tumors not suitable for optimal cytoreduction, as shown in a recent study of 21 patients from India.[102]

Embryonal carcinoma

Embryonal carcinoma of the ovary is an extremely rare tumor that is distinguished from a choriocarcinoma of the ovary by the absence of syncytiotrophoblastic and cytotrophoblastic cells. The patients are very young, their ages ranging between 4 and 28 years (median 14 years) in two series.[103] Older patients have been reported.[104] Embryonal carcinomas may secrete estrogens, with the patient exhibiting symptoms and signs of precocious pseudopuberty or irregular bleeding.[1] The presentation is otherwise similar to that of the EST. The primary lesions tend to be large, and approximately two-thirds are confined to one ovary at the time of presentation. These lesions frequently secrete AFP and hCG, which are useful for following the response to subsequent therapy.[96] The treatment of embryonal carcinomas is the same as that for ESTs.[57]

Choriocarcinoma of the ovary

Pure nongestational choriocarcinoma of the ovary is an extremely rare tumor. Histologically, it has the same appearance as gestational choriocarcinoma metastatic to the ovaries.[105] The majority of patients with this cancer are younger than 20 years. The presence of hCG can be useful in monitoring the patient's response to

Table 3 POMB/ACE chemotherapy for GCTs of the ovary.

POMB		
Day 1	Vincristine 1 mg/m² IV; methotrexate 300 mg/m² as a 12-h infusion	
Day 2	Bleomycin 15 mg by 24-h infusion, folinic acid rescue started 24 h after the start of methotrexate in a dose of 15 mg every 12 h for 4 doses	
Day 3	Bleomycin 15 mg by 24-h infusion	
Day 4	Cisplatin 120 mg/m² as a 12-h infusion, given together with hydration and 3 mg magnesium sulfate supplementation	
ACE		
Days 1–5	Etoposide (VP16) 100 mg/m², days 1 to 5	
Days 3–5	Actinomycin D 0.5 mg IV, days 3, 4, and 5	
Day 5	Cyclophosphamide 500 mg/m² IV, day 5	
OMB		
Day 1	Vincristine 1 mg/m² IV; methotrexate 300 mg/m² as a 12-h infusion	
Day 2	Bleomycin 15 mg by 24-h infusion; folinic acid rescue started at 24-h	
Day 3	Bleomycin 15 mg by 24-h infusion	

The sequence of treatment schedules is two courses of POMB followed by ACE. POMB is then alternated with ACE until patients are in biochemical remission as measured by hCG and AFP, PLAP, and LDH. The usual number of courses of POMB is three to five. Following biochemical remission, patients alternate ACE with OMB until remission has been maintained for approximately 12 weeks. The interval between courses of treatment is kept to the minimum (usually 9–11 days). If delays are caused by myelo-suppression after courses of ACE, the first 2 days of etoposide are omitted from subsequent courses of ACE.

treatment. In the presence of high hCG levels, isosexual precocity has been seen, occurring in approximately 50% of patients whose tumors appear before menarche.[106,107]

There are only a few limited reports on the use of chemotherapy for these nongestational choriocarcinomas, but complete responses have been reported to the MAC regimen (methotrexate, actinomycin D, and cyclophosphamide) as described for gestational trophoblastic disease.[105] These tumors are so rare that no good data are available, but the options also include the BEP or POMB-ACE regimens (Table 3). The prognosis for ovarian choriocarcinomas has been poor. The majority of patients have metastases to organ parenchyma at the time of initial diagnosis, and they should be managed as high-risk germ cell tumors.

Polyembryoma

Polyembryoma of the ovary is another extremely rare tumor, which is composed of "embryoid bodies." This tumor replicates the structures of early embryonic differentiation (i.e., the three somatic layers: endoderm, mesoderm, and ectoderm).[1,12] They occur in very young, premenarchal girls with signs of pseudopuberty, and AFP and hCG levels are elevated. Women with polyembryomas confined to one ovary may be followed with serial tumor markers and diagnostic-imaging techniques to avoid cytotoxic chemotherapy. In patients who require chemotherapy, the BEP regimen is appropriate.[73]

Mixed germ cell tumor

Mixed germ cell malignancies of the ovary contain two or more elements of the tumors described earlier. In one series, the most common component of a mixed germ cell tumor was dysgerminoma, which occurred in 80%, followed by EST in 70%, immature teratoma in 53%, choriocarcinoma in 20%, and embryonal carcinoma in 16%. The most frequent combination was a dysgerminoma and an EST.

The mixed germ cell tumors may secrete either AFP or hCG—or both or neither—depending on the components.

These tumors should be managed with combination chemotherapy, preferably BEP. The serum marker, if positive initially, may become negative during chemotherapy, but this may reflect regression of only a particular component of the mixed lesion. Therefore, a second-look laparotomy may be indicated if there is residual disease following chemotherapy, particularly if there was an immature teratomatous component in the original tumor.

The most important prognostic features are the size of the primary tumor and the relative percentage of its most malignant component.[74] In stage IA lesions smaller than 10 cm, survival is 100%. Tumors composed of less than one-third EST, choriocarcinoma, or grade 3 immature teratoma also have an excellent prognosis, but it is possibly less favorable when these components comprise the majority of the tumor.

Surveillance for stage I ovarian germ cell tumors

Surveillance is a common approach to the management of young men with apparent stage I testicular germ cell tumors. There is a large body of evidence to support this approach, as well as guidelines on what constitutes appropriate surveillance.[6,7] Although as many as 20–30% of patients will relapse, almost all will be cured with salvage chemotherapy with BEP, and the potential adverse effects of chemotherapy can be avoided in most patients.

Although this is a very common approach in young men, it has not been widely adopted in females with ovarian germ cell tumors. However, some data are now available to support surveillance in selected patients whose disease is confined to the ovary. Cushing et al.[108] reported a study of 44 pediatric patients with completely resected ovarian immature teratomas who were followed carefully for recurrence of disease with appropriate diagnostic imaging and serum tumor markers. Thirty-one patients (70.5%) had pure ovarian immature teratomas with a tumor grade of 1 ($n = 17$), 2 ($n = 12$), or 3 ($n = 2$). Thirteen patients (29.5%) had an ovarian immature teratoma plus microscopic foci of yolk sac tumor. The 4-year event-free and overall survival for the ovarian immature teratoma group and the ovarian immature teratoma plus yolk sac tumor group was 97.7% (95% confidence interval, 84.9–99.7%) and 100%, respectively. The only yolk sac tumor relapse occurred in a child with ovarian immature teratoma and yolk sac tumor who was then treated and salvaged with chemotherapy.[108]

The Charing Cross Group initially reported a prospective study of 24 patients with stage IA ovarian germ cell tumors who were also enrolled in a surveillance program. The group consisted of nine patients (37.5%) with dysgerminoma, nine (37.5%) with pure immature teratoma, and six (25%) with ESTs (with or without immature teratoma). Treatment consisted of surgical resection without adjuvant chemotherapy, followed by a surveillance program of clinical, serologic, and radiologic review. A second-look operation was performed, and all but one patient were alive and in remission after a median follow-up of 6.8 years. The 5-year overall survival was 95%, and the 5-year disease-free survival was 68%. Eight patients required chemotherapy for recurrent disease or a second primary germ cell tumor. This included three patients with a grade II immature teratoma, three patients with a dysgerminoma, and two patients with dysgerminoma who developed a contralateral dysgerminoma 4.5 and 5.2 years after their first tumor. All but one, who died of a pulmonary embolus, was successfully salvaged with chemotherapy.[109]

The same group updated its experience and reported on the safety of the ongoing surveillance program of all stage IA female germ cell tumors.[25] Thirty-seven patients (median age 26, range 14–48

years) with stage I disease were referred to Mount Vernon and Charing Cross Hospitals between 1981 and 2003. Patients underwent surgery and staging followed by intense surveillance, which included regular tumor markers and imaging. The median period of follow-up was 6 years. Relapse rates for stage IA nondysgerminomatous tumors and dysgerminomas were 8 of 22 (36%) and 2 of 9 (22%), respectively. In addition, one patient with mature teratoma and glial implants also relapsed. Ten of these 11 patients (91%) were successfully cured with platinum-based chemotherapy. Only one patient died from chemoresistant disease. All relapses occurred within 13 months of initial surgery. The overall disease-specific survival of malignant ovarian germ cell tumors was 94%.

More than 50% of patients who underwent fertility-sparing surgery went on to have successful pregnancies. They concluded that surveillance of all stage IA ovarian germ cell tumors was safe and feasible, and that the outcome was comparable with testicular tumors. They questioned the need for potentially toxic adjuvant chemotherapy in all patients with nondysgerminomas who have greater than 90% chance of being salvaged with chemotherapy if they relapse.

This strategy is appealing and is supported by a larger pediatric literature, but there is much less experience in adults. It deserves further study, but this will require international collaboration. If a surveillance program is to be instigated, it is essential that the protocols used by the Charing Cross group are closely adhered to and that patients understand that the data for adults are limited.

The surveillance policy is very strict and includes a CT scan of chest, abdomen, and pelvis after surgery, if not done preoperatively. At 12 weeks following surgery, a repeat MRI/CT of the abdomen and pelvis or a second-look laparoscopy should be performed if there has been inadequate initial staging. If all of these are negative, MRI/CT imaging should be repeated at 12 months. Patients are reviewed monthly in year one, every 2 months in year two, every 3 months in year three, and so on until year five, after which they are seen every 6 months for another 5 years. A pelvic ultrasound and chest X-ray should be done on alternate visits. Tumor markers including AFP, β-hCG, CA125, and LDH measurements should be done every 2 weeks for 6 months and then monthly for 6 months, every other month in year two, every third month in year three, and so on until year five when they are repeated every 6 months for 5 years.[25,109]

Late effects of treatment of malignant germ cell tumors of the ovary

Although there are substantial data regarding late effects of cisplatin-based therapy in men with testicular cancer, much less information is available for women with ovarian germ cell tumors. The toxicity of BEP chemotherapy has been well documented in men and includes significant pulmonary toxicity in 5% of patients, with fatal lung toxicity in 1%; acute myeloid leukemia or myelodysplastic syndrome in 0.2–1% of patients; neuropathy in 20–30%; Raynaud phenomenon in 20%; tinnitus in 24%; and high-tone hearing loss in as many as 70% of patients. In addition, late effects occur on gonadal function, there is an increased risk of hypertension and cardiovascular disease, and some degree of renal impairment occurs in 30% of patients.[110,111] These side effects underscore the importance of limiting BEP to three cycles for low-risk and to four cycles for high-risk patients, and emphasize the need for these patients to be referred to major referral centers.[89,112]

Gonadal function

An important cause of infertility in patients with ovarian germ cell tumors is unnecessary bilateral salpingo-oophorectomy and hysterectomy. Although temporary ovarian dysfunction or failure is common with platinum-based chemotherapy, most women will resume normal ovarian function, and childbearing is usually preserved.[14,21,23,36–40] In one representative series of 47 patients treated with combination chemotherapy for germ cell malignancies, 91.5% of patients resumed normal menstrual function, and there were 14 healthy live births and no birth defects.[23] Factors such as older age at initiation of chemotherapy, greater cumulative drug dose, and longer duration of therapy all have adverse effects on future gonadal function.[37,89,112–114]

A large study of reproductive and sexual function after platinum-based chemotherapy in ovarian germ cell tumor survivors was recently reported by the GOG, and 132 survivors were included in the study. Surprisingly, only 71 (53.8%) had fertility-sparing surgery; of these, 87.3% were still having regular menstrual periods. Twenty-four survivors had 37 offspring after cancer treatment.[82,115]

Secondary malignancies

An important cause of late morbidity and mortality in patients receiving chemotherapy for germ cell tumors is the development of secondary tumors.[89] Etoposide in particular has been implicated in the development of treatment-related leukemias.

The chance of developing treatment-related leukemia following etoposide is dose related. The incidence of leukemia is approximately 0.4–0.5% (representing a 30-fold increased likelihood) in patients receiving a cumulative etoposide dose of less than 2000 mg/m^2[116] compared with as much as 5% (representing a 336-fold increased likelihood) in those receiving more than 2000 mg/m^2[117] In a typical three- or four-cycle course of BEP, patients receive a cumulative etoposide dose of 1500 or 2000 mg/m^2, respectively.

Despite the risk of secondary leukemia, risk–benefit analyses have concluded that etoposide-containing chemotherapy regimens are beneficial in advanced germ cell tumors; one case of treatment-induced leukemia would be expected for every 20 additionally cured patients who receive BEP as compared with PVB (cisplatin, vinblastine, and bleomycin). The risk–benefit balance for patients with low-risk disease, or for high-dose etoposide in the salvage setting, is less clear.[117]

Sex-cord–stromal tumors

Sex-cord–stromal tumors of the ovary account for approximately 5–8% of all ovarian malignancies.[1–4,118–123] They are derived from the sex cords and the ovarian stroma or mesenchyme, and are usually composed of various combinations of elements, including the "female" cells (i.e., granulosa and theca cells) and "male" cells (i.e., Sertoli and Leydig cells), as well as morphologically indifferent cells. A classification of this group of tumors is presented in Table 4.[10,124]

Granulosa-stromal cell tumors

Granulosa–stromal-cell tumors include granulosa cell tumors, thecomas, and fibromas. The granulosa cell tumor is a low-grade malignancy. Thecomas and fibromas are benign but rarely may have morphologic features of malignancy and then may be referred to as fibrosarcomas.[1,125]

Granulosa cell tumors, which may secrete estrogen, are seen in women of all ages and are classified as either Adult Granulosa Cell tumors or Juvenile. Five percent of cases are found in prepubertal girls; the others are distributed throughout the reproductive and

Table 4 Sex cord–stromal tumors.

A. Granulosa-stomal cell tumors
  1 Granulosa cell tumor
  2 Tumors in the thecoma-fibroma group
    a. Thecoma
    b. Fibroma
    c. Unclassified
B. Androblastomas: Sertoli–Leydig cell tumors
  1 Well differentiated
    a. Sertoli cell tumor
    b. Sertoli–Leydig cell tumor
    c. Leydig cell tumor; hilus cell tumor
  2 Moderately differentiated
  3 Poorly differentiated (sarcomatoid)
  4 With heterologous elements
C. Gynandroblastoma
D. Unclassified

Source: Adapted from Serov 1973.[9] Reproduced with permission of WHO.

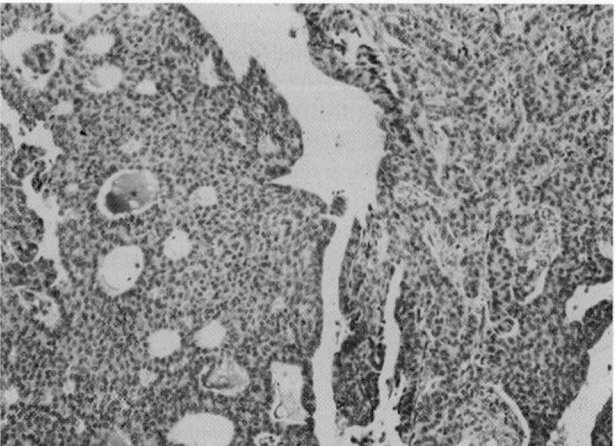

Figure 3 Granulosa cell tumor.

postmenopausal years.[122,123,126,127] They are bilateral in only 2% of patients (Figure 3).

Of the rare prepubertal lesions, 75% are associated with sexual pseudoprecocity because of the estrogen secretion.[123] In the reproductive age group, most patients have menstrual irregularities or secondary amenorrhea. In postmenopausal women, abnormal uterine bleeding is frequently the presenting symptom. Endometrial cancer occurs in association with granulosa cell tumors in at least 5% of cases, and 25–50% are associated with endometrial hyperplasia.[1,120,122,123,126] Rarely, granulosa cell tumors may produce androgens and cause virilization.

The other symptoms and signs of granulosa cell tumors are nonspecific and the same as most ovarian malignancies. Ascites is present in approximately 10% of cases, and rarely a pleural effusion.[122,123] Granulosa tumors tend to be hemorrhagic; occasionally, they rupture and produce a hemoperitoneum.

Granulosa cell tumors are usually stage I at diagnosis but may recur 5–30 years after initial diagnosis.[121] The tumors may also spread hematogenously, and metastases can develop in the lungs, liver, and brain years later. Malignant thecomas are extremely rare, and their presentation, management, and outcome are similar to those of the granulosa cell tumors.[125,127]

A somatic missense point mutation in the gene encoding the forkhead box protein L2 (FOXL2) has been found to be present in all adult-type granulosa cell tumors of the ovary. FOXL2 402 CG leads to a gain or change of function and is believed to be a driver mutation for adult granulosa cell tumors. There is an effort to see if it can be targeted.[128-130]

Diagnosis

Inhibin is secreted by granulosa cell tumors and is a useful tumor marker for diagnosis and surveillance.[131-135] It is a polypeptide hormone secreted primarily by granulosa cells and is an inhibiter of pituitary FSH secretion. Inhibin decreases to nondetectable levels after menopause. However, certain ovarian cancers (mucinous epithelial ovarian carcinomas and granulosa cell tumors) produce inhibin, which may predate clinical recurrence.[136-138] An elevated serum inhibin level in a premenopausal woman presenting with amenorrhea and infertility is suggestive of a granulosa cell tumor.

In the past, inhibin assays could not distinguish between the two inhibin subunits, inhibin A and B, and total inhibin has been measured. However, there are now specific immunoassays for inhibin A and B. Inhibin B is the predominant form of inhibin secreted by granulosa cell tumors and has been reported to reflect disease status more accurately than inhibin A. Measurement of serum inhibin B concentrations rather than total inhibin or inhibin A may be better for the follow-up of granulosa cell tumors.[134,139]

Antimüllerian hormone (AMH), also called Müllerian inhibitory substance (MIS), is produced by granulosa cells and is emerging as a potential marker for these tumors.[135] An elevated AMH level appears to have high specificity. The test is commercially available, and its role in the management of granulosa cell tumors is being investigated.[140] An elevated estradiol level is not a sensitive marker of this disease.[137]

The histologic diagnosis can be facilitated by staining for markers of ovarian granulosa cell tumors (e.g., inhibin, CD99, and AMH).[131,132] Antibodies against inhibin appear to be the most useful, but they are not specific.[128] In one report, positive staining for inhibin was present in 94% of granulosa cell tumors and in 10–20% of ovarian endometrioid tumors and metastatic carcinomas to the ovary.[135] The latter demonstrated significantly weaker staining. Molecular testing for a mutation in FOXL2 is now available to help with the diagnosis if it is in doubt.[129,130]

Treatment

The treatment of granulosa cell tumors depends on the age of the patient and the extent of disease. For most patients, surgery alone is sufficient primary therapy, with radiation and chemotherapy reserved for the treatment of recurrent or metastatic disease.[122,123,126,127]

Surgery

Because granulosa cell tumors are bilateral in approximately 2% of patients, a unilateral salpingo-oophorectomy is appropriate therapy for stage IA tumors in children or in women of reproductive age.[119] At the time of laparotomy, if a granulosa cell tumor is identified by frozen section, then a limited staging operation is performed, including an assessment of the contralateral ovary.[141-144] As with germ cell malignancies, staging is limited to washings, omental biopsy, careful palpation of the peritoneal surfaces and retroperitoneal nodes, and biopsy of any suspicious lesions. If the opposite ovary appears enlarged, it should be biopsied. If there is metastatic disease, an effort should be made to resect all disease because these tumors are typically slow growing and do not respond well to chemotherapy. In perimenopausal and postmenopausal women for whom ovarian preservation is not important, a hysterectomy and bilateral salpingo-oophorectomy should be performed. In premenopausal patients in whom the uterus is left *in situ*, a dilation and curettage of the uterus should be performed because of the possibility of a coexistent adenocarcinoma of the endometrium.[122]

Radiation

There is no evidence to support the use of adjuvant radiation therapy for granulosa cell tumors, although pelvic radiation may help to palliate isolated pelvic recurrences.[121,122,138] Radiation can induce clinical responses and occasional long-term remission in patients with persistent or recurrent granulosa cell tumors, particularly if the disease is surgically cytoreduced.[138,145,146] In one review of 34 patients treated at one center for more than 40 years, 14 (41.2%) were treated with measurable disease.[145] Three (21%) were alive without progression for 10–21 years following treatment.

Chemotherapy

There is no evidence that adjuvant chemotherapy in patients with stage I disease will prevent recurrence. Patients with metastatic granulosa cell tumors have been treated with a variety of different anti-neoplastic drugs over the years. There has been no one consistently effective regimen, although complete responses have been reported anecdotally in patients treated with the single agents cyclophosphamide and melphalan, as well as the combinations VAC, PAC (cisplatin, doxorubicin, and cyclophosphamide), PVB, and BEP.[4,119,147-158] More recently, carboplatin and paclitaxel[138] as well as bevacizumab[159] have shown benefit.

The rarity of these tumors has made it impossible to conduct well-designed randomized studies for patients with stages II to IV disease. In retrospective series, postoperative chemotherapy has been associated with a prolonged progression-free interval in women with stage III or IV disease,[138,149] but an overall survival benefit has not been shown.[150] Despite the absence of data supporting a survival benefit, some experts recommend postoperative chemotherapy for women with completely resected stage II to IV disease because of the high risk of disease progression and the potential for long-term survival after platinum-based chemotherapy.[138,151-154] Acceptable options include BEP, EP, PAC, and carboplatin and paclitaxel.[138]

For patients with suboptimally cytoreduced disease, combinations of BEP have produced overall response rates of 58–83%.[138,151,155] In one study, 14 of 38 patients (37%) with advanced disease undergoing second-look laparotomy following four courses of BEP had negative findings.[151] With a median follow-up of 3 years, 11 of 16 patients (69%) with primary advanced disease and 21 of 41 patients (51%) with recurrent disease were progression free. This regimen was associated with severe toxicity and two bleomycin-related deaths. Carboplatin and etoposide,[156] PVB,[122,157] and PAC[147,158] have also been reported to have relatively high response rates.

There is a need to develop less toxic and equally active regimens for this older group of patients. Paclitaxel is an active agent, and the combination of platinum with a taxane has been reported to have a response rate of 60%, which makes it a more attractive alternative.[160-162]

Recurrent disease

The median time to relapse is approximately 4–6 years after initial diagnosis.[119,121,142,154] There is no standard approach to the management of relapsed disease. A common site of recurrence is the pelvis, although the upper abdomen may also be involved. Further surgery can be effective if the tumor is localized, but diffuse intra-abdominal disease is difficult to treat. Chemotherapy or radiation may be useful in selected patients.

Approximately 30% of these tumors are estrogen receptor-positive and 100% are progesterone receptor-positive on immunostaining.[163,164] The use of hormonal agents such as progestins or luteinizing hormone-releasing hormone (LHRH) agonists has been suggested, but there are limited available data.[137] LHRH agonists have been reported to have a 50% response rate in 13 patients from small clinical series and case reports,[164-166] whereas four of five patients (80%) were reported to respond to a progestational agent.[167] Freeman recently reported two patients with recurrent adult granulosa cell tumors who had received multiple treatment modalities, including chemotherapy, and had previously progressed on leuprolide. Both patients were treated with anastrozole. Inhibin B levels normalized, as did clinical findings. Both were maintained on treatment for 14 and 18 months, respectively.[168]

The numbers are too small to draw any conclusions, and it is likely that there has been significant publication bias, with more reports of responses to treatment.[169]

Prognosis

The prognosis for granulosa cell tumor of the ovary depends on the surgical stage of disease.[121,123,138,170-173] Most granulosa cell tumors are indolent and are confined to one ovary at diagnosis; the cure rate for stage I disease is 75–92%.[123,144,154,173] However, late recurrences are not uncommon.[119,121,123] In one report of 37 women with stage I disease, survival rates at 5, 10, and 20 years were 94%, 82%, and 62%, respectively. The survival rates for stages II to IV at 5 and 10 years were 55% and 34%, respectively.[138]

In adult tumors, cellular atypia, mitotic rate, and the absence of Call-Exner bodies are the only significant pathologic predictors of early recurrence.[153] Neither an abnormal tumor karyotype nor p53 overexpression appears to be prognostic.[174] The DNA ploidy of the tumors has been correlated with survival. Holland et al.[148] reported DNA aneuploidy in 13 of 37 patients (35%) with primary granulosa cell tumors. The presence of residual disease was found to be the most important predictor of progression-free survival, but DNA ploidy was an independent prognostic factor. Patients with no residual disease and DNA diploid tumors had a 10-year progression-free survival of 96%.

Juvenile granulosa cell tumors

Juvenile granulosa cell tumors of the ovary are rare and make up less than 5% of ovarian tumors in childhood and adolescence.[156] Approximately 90% are diagnosed in stage I and have a favorable prognosis. The juvenile subtype behaves less aggressively than the adult type. Advanced-stage tumors have been successfully treated with platinum-based combination chemotherapy (e.g., BEP).[138]

Sertoli–Leydig cell tumors

Sertoli–Leydig tumors occur most frequently in the third and fourth decades, with 75% of the lesions seen in women younger than 40 years. They account for less than 0.2% of ovarian cancers.[13] Sertoli–Leydig cell tumors are most frequently low-grade malignancies, although poorly differentiated tumors may behave more aggressively.

The tumors typically produce androgens, and clinical virilization is noted in 70–85% of patients.[175,176] Signs of virilization include oligomenorrhea followed by amenorrhea, breast atrophy, acne, hirsutism, clitoromegaly, a deepening voice, and a receding hairline. Measurement of plasma androgens may reveal elevated testosterone and androstenedione, with normal or slightly elevated

dehydroepiandrosterone sulfate.[1] Rarely, the Sertoli–Leydig tumor can be associated with manifestations of estrogenization (i.e., isosexual precocity, irregular or postmenopausal bleeding).[176]

Treatment

Because these low-grade tumors are bilateral in less than 1% of cases, the usual treatment is unilateral salpingo-oophorectomy and evaluation of the contralateral ovary in patients who are in their reproductive years.[176] In older patients, hysterectomy and bilateral salpingo-oophorectomy are appropriate.

There are limited data regarding the utility of chemotherapy in patients with persistent disease, but responses in patients with measurable disease have been reported with cisplatin in combination with doxorubicin or ifosfamide or both[176] as well as the regimens mentioned earlier for granulosa cell tumors. Because of their rarity, most series have included them with granulosa cell tumors.[152] Pelvic radiation can also be used for recurrent pelvic tumor but with limited responses.

Prognosis

The 5-year survival rate is 70–90%, and recurrences thereafter are uncommon.[1,2,176] The majority of fatalities occur with poorly differentiated lesions.

Uncommon ovarian cancers

There are several varieties of malignant ovarian tumors, which together constitute only 0.1% of ovarian malignancies. These lesions include lipoid (or lipid) cell tumors, primary ovarian sarcomas, and small cell ovarian carcinomas.

Lipoid cell tumors

Lipoid cell tumors are thought to arise in adrenal cortical rests that reside in the vicinity of the ovary. More than 100 cases have been reported, and bilaterality has been noted in only a few.[1] Most are associated with virilization and occasionally with obesity, hypertension, and glucose intolerance, reflecting glucocorticoid secretion. Rare cases of estrogen secretion and isosexual precocity have been reported.

The majority of these have a benign or low-grade behavior, but approximately 20% develop metastatic lesions in the peritoneal cavity, or rarely at distant sites. The primary treatment is surgical, and there are no data regarding radiation or chemotherapy for this disease.

Sarcomas

Malignant mixed mesodermal sarcomas of the ovary are usually heterologous, and 80% occur in postmenopausal women.[177-183] The lesions are biologically aggressive, and their presentation is similar to that of most epithelial ovarian malignancies.

Such patients should be treated by cytoreductive surgery and postoperative platinum-containing combination chemotherapy. Silasi et al.[184] reported their experience with 22 patients from Yale, all but two of whom presented with advanced-stage disease. The median survival for the entire cohort was 38 months. The median survival was 46 months for 18 optimally debulked (<1 cm) patients and 27 months for four suboptimally debulked (>1 cm) patients. After optimal cytoreduction, six patients were treated with cisplatin and ifosfamide; they had a median progression-free interval of 13 months and a median survival of 51 months. The combination of

carboplatin and paclitaxel was administered to four patients following optimal cytoreduction; their median progression-free interval
was 6 months, and median survival was 38 months. The difference
in survival between the cisplatin and ifosfamide group and the
carboplatin and paclitaxel group was not statistically significant
($p = 0.48$). First-line cisplatin and ifosfamide or carboplatin and
paclitaxel can achieve survival rates comparable to those observed
in epithelial ovarian cancer.

Leiser et al.[185] reported the Memorial Sloan-Kettering experience
with platinum and paclitaxel in 30 patients with carcinosarcomas
of the ovary. Twelve patients (40%) had a complete response, seven
(23%) a partial response, two (7%) stable disease, and nine (30%)
progression of disease. The median time to progression for responders was 12 months; with a median follow-up of 23 months, the
median overall survival was 43 months for survivors. The 3- and
5-year survival rates were 53% and 30%, respectively.

Small cell carcinomas

This rare tumor occurs at an average age of 24 years (range 2 to 46
years).[186] The tumors are all bilateral. Approximately two-thirds of
the tumors are accompanied by paraneoplastic hypercalcemia. This
tumor accounts for one-half of all of the cases of hypercalcemia associated with ovarian tumors. Approximately 50% of the tumors have
spread beyond the ovaries at the time of diagnosis.[1,2]

Management consists of surgery followed by platinum-based
chemotherapy. Radiation therapy may be considered in selected
patients. In addition to the primary treatment of the disease, control of the hypercalcemia may require aggressive hydration, loop
diuretics, and the use of bisphosphonates.

In a collaborative Gynecologic Cancer Intergroup study, data
were collected for 17 patients treated in Australia, Canada, and
Europe.[187] The median follow-up was 13 months for all patients
and 35.5 months for surviving patients. Ten patients (58.8%) had
FIGO stage I tumors, six (35.3%) stage III, and in one patient,
stage was unknown. All underwent surgical resection and adjuvant
platinum-based chemotherapy. Seven received adjuvant pelvic,
whole-abdominal, or extended-field radiation. The median survival
for stage I tumors was not reached, whereas it was 6 months for
stage III tumors. For the 10 patients with stage I tumors, 6 also
received adjuvant radiotherapy, with 5 alive and disease-free; 4
received no adjuvant radiotherapy, with 1 alive and disease-free.
Of the seven patients with stage III or unknown tumor stage,
all but one have died. The only long-term survivor was treated
with platinum-based chemotherapy (BEP) followed by para-aortic
and pelvic radiotherapy. Recurrences were most frequent in the
pelvis and the abdomen. Patients receiving salvage treatment with
chemotherapy and radiotherapy did poorly.

Although the optimal approach to management is not known,
in view of these findings, the authors advocate a multimodality
treatment approach, including surgical resection of gross disease,
chemotherapy with carboplatin and paclitaxel or cisplatin and
etoposide, and the addition of various fields of pelvic radiotherapy either sequentially or concurrently. Others have advocated
high-dose chemotherapy with stem cell support and have reported
a number of long-term survivors.[188,189]

Metastatic tumors

Approximately 5–6% of ovarian tumors are metastatic from other
organs, most frequently from the female genital tract, the breast,
or the gastrointestinal tract.[190–207] The metastases may occur from
direct extension of another pelvic neoplasm, by hematogenous
spread, by lymphatic spread, or from transcoelomic dissemination,
with surface implantation of tumors that spread in the peritoneal
cavity.

Gynecologic primary

Nonovarian cancers of the genital tract can spread by direct extension or metastasize to the ovaries.[1] Under some circumstances, it is
difficult to know whether the tumor originates in the fallopian tube
or in the ovary when both are involved, especially because many
high-grade serous carcinomas that were thought to be primary ovarian malignancies are now believed to actually arise in the fallopian
tube, as discussed earlier.[208] Cervical cancer spreads to the ovary
only in rare cases (<1%), and most of these are at an advanced clinical stage or are adenocarcinomas. Although adenocarcinoma of the
endometrium can spread and implant directly onto the surface of
the ovaries in as many as 5% of cases, two synchronous primary
tumors probably occur with greater frequency. In these cases, an
endometrioid carcinoma of the ovary is usually associated with the
adenocarcinoma of the endometrium.[209]

Nongynecologic primary

The frequency of metastatic breast carcinoma to the ovaries
varies according to the method of determination, but is relatively
common, particularly in patients with estrogen receptor positive
metastatic breast cancer. In autopsy data of women who die of
metastatic breast cancer, the ovaries are involved in 24% of cases,
and 80% of the involvement is bilateral.[190–196] Similarly, when
ovaries are removed as treatment for metastatic breast cancer in
premenopausal women, approximately 20–30% of patients have
evidence of ovarian metastases, 60% bilaterally. The involvement of
ovaries in early-stage breast cancer is considerably lower, but precise
figures are not available. In almost all cases, ovarian involvement is
occult but in some patients, a pelvic mass is discovered after other
metastatic disease becomes apparent.

Krukenberg tumor

Krukenberg tumors account for 30–40% of metastatic cancers to
the ovaries, and are characterized by mucin-filled, signet-ring cells
in the ovarian stroma.[200,201] The primary tumor is most frequently
the stomach but less common primaries include the colon, breast,
or biliary tract. Rarely, the cervix or the bladder may be the primary
site. Krukenberg tumors can account for approximately 2% of ovarian cancers, and they are usually bilateral. The tumors are usually
not discovered until the primary disease is advanced, and therefore,
most patients die of their disease within a year. In some cases, a primary tumor is never found.

Other gastrointestinal tumors

In other cases of metastasis from the gastrointestinal tract to the
ovary, the tumor does not have the classic histologic appearance
of a Krukenberg tumor; most of these are from the colon and, less
commonly, the small intestine. One to two percent of women with
intestinal carcinomas will develop metastases to the ovaries during
the course of their disease.[192,197–199,202,203] Before exploration for an
adnexal tumor in a woman more than 40 years of age, a colonoscopy
or gastroscopy should be performed to exclude a primary gastrointestinal carcinoma with metastases to the ovaries if there are any
gastrointestinal symptoms.

Metastatic colon cancer can mimic a mucinous cystadenocarcinoma of the ovary histologically, and the histologic distinction
between the two can be difficult.[202–206] Tumors that arise in

the appendix may also be associated with ovarian metastasis and have frequently been confused with primary ovarian malignancies, especially when associated with pseudomyxoma peritonei.[202,206] When the ovaries are involved with metastasis, a bilateral salpingo-oophorectomy should be performed at the time of surgery for colon cancer.[197,207]

Melanoma

Rare cases of malignant melanoma metastatic to the ovaries have been reported,[210] and must be distinguished from the rare case of a melanoma arising in an ovarian teratoma.[211] In cases of metastatic disease, the melanomas are usually widely disseminated. Removal would be warranted for palliation of abdominal or pelvic pain, bleeding, or torsion.

Carcinoid

Metastatic carcinoid tumors represent fewer than 2% of metastatic lesions to the ovaries.[212] Conversely, only some 2% of primary carcinoids have evidence of ovarian metastasis, and only 40% of these patients have the carcinoid syndrome at the time of discovery of the metastatic carcinoid.[213] In perimenopausal and postmenopausal women explored for an intestinal carcinoid, it is reasonable to remove the ovaries to prevent subsequent ovarian metastasis. Furthermore, the discovery of an ovarian carcinoid should prompt a careful search for a primary intestinal lesion.

Lymphoma and leukemia

Lymphomas and leukemia can involve the ovary. When they do, the involvement is usually bilateral.[214–217] Approximately 5% of patients with Hodgkin disease will have lymphomatous involvement of the ovaries, but this occurs typically with advanced-stage disease. With Burkitt lymphoma, ovarian involvement is very common. Other types of lymphoma involve the ovaries much less frequently, and leukemic infiltration of the ovaries is uncommon.

Sometimes, the ovaries can be the only apparent sites of involvement of the abdominal or pelvic viscera with a lymphoma—in this circumstance, a careful surgical exploration may be necessary. An intraoperative consultation with a hematologist–oncologist should be obtained to determine the need for such procedures if frozen section of a solid ovarian mass reveals a lymphoma. In general, most lymphomas no longer require extensive surgical staging, although enlarged lymph nodes should generally be biopsied. In some cases of Hodgkin disease, a more extensive evaluation may be necessary. Treatment involves that of the lymphoma or leukemia in general. Removal of a large ovarian mass may improve patient comfort and facilitate a response to subsequent radiation or chemotherapy.[216]

Key references

The complete reference list can be found on the Wiley Companion Digital Edition of this title (see inside front cover for login instructions).

1 Scully RE, Young RH, Clement RB. Tumors of the ovary, maldeveloped gonads, fallopian tube, and broad ligament. In: *Atlas of Tumor Pathology: 3rd series, Fascicle 23*. Washington, DC: Armed Forces Institute of Pathology; 1998:169–498.

2 Chen LM, Berek JS. Ovarian and fallopian tubes. In: Haskell CM, ed. *Cancer Treatment*, 5th ed. Philadelphia, PA: WB Saunders; 2000:900–932.

11 Berek JS, Friedlander ML, Hacker NF. Germ cell and nonepithelial ovarian cancer. In: Berek JS, Hacker NF, eds. *Berek & Hacker's Gynecologic Oncology*, 6th ed. Wolters Kluwer: Philadelphia, PA; 2015:530–559.

19 Lu KH, Gershenson DM. Update on the management of ovarian germ cell tumors. *J Reprod Med.* 2005;50:417–425.

29 Williams SD, Blessing JA, Liao S, et al. Adjuvant therapy of ovarian germ cell tumors with cisplatin, etoposide, and bleomycin: a trial of the Gynecologic Oncology Group. *J Clin Oncol.* 1994;12:701–706.

30 Gershenson DM, Morris M, Cangir A, et al. Treatment of malignant germ cell tumors of the ovary with bleomycin, etoposide, and cisplatin. *J Clin Oncol.* 1990;8:715–720.

54 Mahdi H, Swensen RE, Hanna R, et al. Prognostic impact of lymphadenectomy in clinically early stage malignant germ cell tumour of the ovary. *Br J Cancer.* 2011;105(4):493–497.

66 Mann JR, Raafat F, Robinson K, et al. The United Kingdom Children's Cancer Study Group's second germ cell tumor study: carboplatin, etoposide, and bleomycin are effective treatment for children with malignant extracranial germ cell tumors, with acceptable toxicity. *J Clin Oncol.* 2000;18:3809–3818.

95 de La Motte RT, Pautier P, et al. Prognostic factors in women treated for ovarian yolk sac tumour: a retrospective analysis of 84 cases. *Eur J Cancer.* 2011;47(2):175–182.

112 Matei D, Miller AM, Monahan P, et al. Chronic physical effects and health care utilization in long-term ovarian germ cell tumor survivors: a Gynecologic Oncology Group study. *J Clin Oncol.* 2009;27:4142–4149.

113 Zhang R, Sun YC, Zhang GY, et al. Treatment of malignant germ cell tumors and preservation of fertility. *Eur J Gynaecol Oncol.* 2012;33:489–492.

114 Monahan PO, Champion VL, Zhao Q, et al. Case–control comparison of quality of life in long-term ovarian germ cell tumor survivors: a Gynecologic Oncology Group Study. *J Psychosoc Oncol.* 2008;26(3):19–42. PMID: 19042263.

115 Gershenson DM, Miller AM, Champion VL, et al. Reproductive and sexual function after platinum-based chemotherapy in long-term ovarian germ cell tumor survivors: a Gynecologic Oncology Group Study. *J Clin Oncol.* 2007;25:2792–2797.

120 Boyce EA, Costaggini I, Vitonis A, et al. The epidemiology of ovarian granulosa cell tumors: a case control study. *Gynecol Oncol.* 2009;115:221–225.

124 Roth LM. Recent advances in the pathology and classification of ovarian sex cord-stromal tumors. *Int J Gynecol Pathol.* 2006;25:199–215.

128 Zhao C, Vinh TN, McManus K, et al. Identification of the most sensitive and robust immunohistochemical markers in different categories of ovarian sex cord-stromal tumors. *Am J Surg Pathol.* 2009;33:354–366.

129 Shah SP, Köbel M, Senz J, et al. Mutation of FOXL2 in granulosa-cell tumors of the ovary. *N Engl J Med.* 2009;360:2719–2729.

130 Köbel M, Gilks CB, Huntsman DG. Adult-type granulosa cell tumors and FOXL2 mutation. *Cancer Res.* 2009;69:9160–9162.

131 Lappohn RE, Burger HG, Bouma J, et al. Inhibin as a marker for granulosa-cell tumors. *N Engl J Med.* 1989;321:790–793.

138 Schumer ST, Cannistra SA. Granulosa cell tumor of the ovary. *J Clin Oncol.* 2003;21:1180–1189.

139 Chang HL, Pahlavan N, Halpern EF, et al. Serum Müllerian Inhibiting Substance/anti-Müllerian hormone levels in patients with adult granulosa cell tumors directly correlate with aggregate tumor mass as determined by pathology or radiology. *Gynecol Oncol.* 2009;114:57–60.

140 Geerts I, Vergote I, Neven P, et al. The role of inhibins B and anti-müllerian hormone for diagnosis and follow-up of granulosa cell tumors. *Int J Gynecol Cancer.* 2009;19(5):847–855.

142 Brown J, Sood AK, Deavers MT, et al. Patterns of metastasis in sex cord-stromal tumors of the ovary: can routine staging lymphadenectomy be omitted? *Gynecol Oncol.* 2009;113:86–90.

143 Abu-Rustum NR, Restivo A, Ivy J, et al. Retroperitoneal nodal metastasis in primary and recurrent granulosa cell tumors of the ovary. *Gynecol Oncol.* 2006;103:31–34.

144 NCCN (2013) *National Comprehensive Cancer Network (NCCN) Guidelines*, www.nccn.org (accessed 15 May 2013).

161 Brown J, Shvartsman HS, Deavers MT, et al. The activity of taxanes in the treatment of sex cord-stromal ovarian tumors. *J Clin Oncol.* 2004;22:3517.

169 Sommeijer DW, Sjoquist KM, Friedlander M. Hormonal treatment in recurrent and metastatic gynaecological cancers: a review of the current literature. *Curr Oncol Rep.* 2013;15(6):541–548.

173 Auranen A, Sundström J, Ijäs J, et al. Prognostic factors of ovarian granulosa cell tumor: a study of 35 patients and review of the literature. *Int J Gynecol Cancer.* 2007;17:1011–1018.

176 Tomlinson MW, Treadwell MC, Deppe G. Platinum based chemotherapy to treat recurrent Sertoli-Leydig cell ovarian carcinoma during pregnancy. *Eur J Gynaecol Oncol.* 1997;18:44–46.

184 Silasi DA, Illuzzi JL, Kelly MG, et al. Carcinosarcoma of the ovary. *Int J Gynecol Cancer.* 2008;18:22–29.

185 Leiser AL, Chi DS, Ishill NM, et al. Carcinosarcoma of the ovary treated with platinum and taxane: The Memorial Sloan-Kettering Cancer Center experience. *Gynecol Oncol.* 2007;105:657–661.

187 Harrison ML, Hoskins P, du Bois A, et al. Small cell of the ovary, hypercalcemic type—analysis of combined experience and recommendation for management. A GCIG study. *Gynecol Oncol.* 2006;100:233–238.

188 Pautier P, Ribrag V, Duvillard P, et al. Results of a prospective dose-intensive regimen in 27 patients with small cell carcinoma of the ovary of the hypercalcemic type. *Ann Oncol.* 2007;18:1985–1989.

189 Nelsen LL, Muirhead DM, Bell MC. Ovarian small cell carcinoma, hyper-calcemic type exhibiting a response to high-dose chemotherapy. *S D Med.* 2010;**63**(**11**):375–377.

193 Moore RG, Chung M, Granai CO, et al. Incidence of metastasis to the ovaries from nongenital tract tumors. *Gynecol Oncol.* 2004;**93**:87–91.

196 Yada-Hashimoto N, Yamamoto T, Kamiura S, et al. Metastatic ovarian tumors: a review of 64 cases. *Gynecol Oncol.* 2003;**89**:314–317.

197 Ayhan A, Guvenal T, Salman MC, et al. The role of cytoreductive surgery in non-genital cancers metastatic to the ovaries. *Gynecol Oncol.* 2005;**98**:235–241.

204 Seidman JD, Kurman RJ, Ronnett BM. Primary and metastatic mucinous adeno-carcinomas in the ovaries: incidence in routine practice with a new approach to improve intraoperative diagnosis. *Am J Surg Pathol.* 2003;**27**:985–993.

208 Levanon K, Crum C, Drapkin R. New insights into the pathogenesis of serous ovarian cancer and its clinical impact. *J Clin Oncol.* 2008;**26**:5284–5293.

211 Davis GL. Malignant melanoma arising in mature ovarian cystic teratoma (dermoid cyst): report of two cases and literature analysis. *Int J Gynecol Pathol.* 1996;**15**:356–362.

213 Robbins ML, Sunshine TJ. Metastatic carcinoid diagnosed at laparoscopic excision of pelvic Endometriosis. *J Am Assoc Gynecol Laparosc.* 2000;**7**:251–253.

216 Azizoglu C, Altinok G, Uner A, et al. Ovarian lymphomas: a clinicopathological analysis of 10 cases. *Arch Gynecol Obstet.* 2001;**265**:91–93.

106 Molar pregnancy and gestational trophoblastic neoplasia

Donald P. Goldstein, MD ▪ *Ross S. Berkowitz, MD* ▪ *Neil S. Horowitz, MD*

Overview

Gestational trophoblastic neoplasia (GTN) is among the rare human malignancies that can be cured in the presence of widespread metastases. GTN includes a spectrum of interrelated tumors, including hydatidiform mole, invasive mole, choriocarcinoma, placental-site trophoblastic tumor (PSTT), and epithelioid trophoblastic tumor (ETT), which has varying propensities for local invasion and metastasis. With the exception of PSTT and ETT, all GTNs arise from the cytotrophoblast and syncytial cells of the villous trophoblast and produce abundant amounts of human chorionic gonadotropin (hCG). Measurement of hCG levels serves as a reliable tumor marker for diagnosis, monitoring of treatment response, and follow-up to detect recurrence. PSTT and ETT originate from the intermediate cells of extravillous trophoblast and produce hCG sparsely, making its use as a tumor marker that is less reliable. Although GTN most commonly follows a molar pregnancy, it may follow any gestational event, including therapeutic or spontaneous abortion and ectopic or term pregnancy. Before the development of effective chemotherapy in 1956, the majority of patients with GTN localized to the uterus were cured with hysterectomy, but metastatic disease was almost always fatal. Most women can now be cured and their reproductive function preserved if treated early and according to well-established guidelines. GTN patients are categorized using a prognostic scoring system into low- and high-risk disease based on response to single-agent chemotherapy. Low-risk GTN generally responds to monotherapy while high-risk disease requires multiagent regimens to achieve remission. Despite chemotherapy, subsequent pregnancy outcomes are similar to the general population.

Molar pregnancy and gestational trophoblastic neoplasia (GTN) comprise a group of interrelated diseases that includes complete hydatidiform (CHM) and partial hydatidiform (PHM) mole, invasive mole, choriocarcinoma (CCA), placental site trophoblastic tumor (PSTT), and epithelioid trophoblastic tumor (ETT). Molar pregnancy and GTN produce a distinct tumor marker, human chorionic gonadotropin (hCG), which can be used for diagnosis, monitoring the effects of therapy, and follow-up to detect relapse. Complete and partial moles are noninvasive, localized tumors that develop as a result of an aberrant fertilization event that leads to a proliferative process. The other trophoblastic tumors which as a group are referred to as GTN represent malignant disease because of their local invasion and metastases. GTN most commonly develops from a molar pregnancy but can rise *de novo* after any gestation. Although these tumors are rare, it is important for medical oncologists to understand their natural history and management because of their life-threatening potential in reproductive-age females and their high degree of curability with preservation of reproductive function if treated early and appropriately.[1,2] Despite the advances made in the management of GTN over the past 60 years, patients with protracted delays in diagnosis, particularly after nonmolar pregnancies, still present with extensive tumor burdens and are at substantial risk for treatment failure and death.

Incidence

The reported incidence of molar pregnancy and GTN varies substantially in different regions of the world.[3] The incidence of complete and partial molar pregnancy in North America and Europe is approximately 1 : 1250 and 1 : 650, respectively, whereas the incidence in Asian countries is 3–10 times greater.[4,5] Variations in the incidence rates of molar pregnancy throughout the world may result from differences between reporting hospital-based versus population-based data.

The incidence of GTN is also difficult to establish with certainty because accurate epidemiologic data is not available in most countries. Approximately 50% of GTN cases arise from molar pregnancy, 25% from miscarriages or tubal pregnancies, and 25% from term or preterm pregnancy.[6] GTN which develops after a non-molar pregnancy is usually due to CCA, whereas PSTT and ETT occur rarely. The incidence of GTN following a non-molar pregnancy in Europe and North America is estimated at 2–7 per 100,000 pregnancies, whereas in Southeast Asia and Japan, the incidence is higher at 50–200 per 100,000 pregnancies, respectively.[7,8]

Risk factors

The two main risk factors for molar pregnancy and GTN are extremes of maternal age (especially over 35 and under 16) and a history of previous mole.[9-13] Parazzini et al.[11] noted that the risk for CHM was increased twofold for women older than age 35 years and 7.5-fold for women older than age 40 years. Ova from older women may be more susceptible to abnormal fertilizations. Most cases of molar disease and GTN occur in women under 35 because of the greater number of pregnancies in this age group. The risk for PHM has not been associated with maternal age.

Histopathologic classification of GTN

Hydatidiform mole may be categorized as either complete or partial based on gross morphology, histopathology, and karyotype.[14,15] CHM is characterized by hydropic villi with trophoblastic hyperplasia. Embryonic or fetal tissues are not identifiable. Partial moles are characterized by the presence of two populations of chorionic villi, some appearing normal and some exhibiting focal swelling and focal trophoblastic hyperplasia. Fetal and embryonic tissues are commonly present. Locally invasive or metastatic GTN that develops after either a complete or partial mole can have the histologic features of either molar tissue or CCA.

Holland-Frei Cancer Medicine, Ninth Edition. Edited by Robert C. Bast Jr., Carlo M. Croce, William N. Hait, Waun Ki Hong, Donald W. Kufe, Martine Piccart-Gebhart, Raphael E. Pollock, Ralph R. Weichselbaum, Hongyang Wang, and James F. Holland.
© 2017 John Wiley & Sons, Inc. ISBN: 978-1-118-93469-2

CCA does not contain chorionic villi but is composed of sheets of both anaplastic cyto- and syncytiotrophoblasts. Although CCA is most commonly preceded by a CHM, it may develop after any gestation. After a non-molar pregnancy, persistent GTN usually has the histologic pattern of CCA but rarely can be present as PSTT or ETT. CCA is a highly vascular tumor that disseminates via the blood stream initially to the lungs. Distant sites such as the brain, liver, kidney, gastrointestinal tract, and spleen are usually late manifestations of the disease in patients where there has been delayed diagnosis.

PSTT and ETT are uncommon variants of CCA, which are composed almost entirely of mononuclear intermediate trophoblast and do not contain chorionic villi.[16,17] Both PSTT and ETT tend to infiltrate the myometrium and, in contrast to CCA, metastases are a late manifestation of the disease. These tumors display a wide clinical spectrum and when metastatic can be difficult to control even with surgery and chemotherapy. They are characterized by low hCG levels so a large tumor burden may be present before the disease is diagnosed.

Clinical presentation and diagnosis

Post-molar GTN

Complete moles develop uterine invasion or metastasis in about 15% and 4% of patients, respectively.[18] Approximately 1–4% of patients with PHM develop persistent tumor, which is generally non-metastatic.[19] After molar evacuation, all patients must be monitored for the development of post-molar GTN, defined as those patients who develop persistently elevated hCG levels, require chemotherapy and/or excisional surgery, or have evidence of metastases. According to the International Federation of Gynecology and Obstetrics (FIGO) criteria, the presence of post-molar GTN should be diagnosed if the following is present: (1) serum hCG values that plateau (decline of <10% for at least four values over 3 weeks); (2) serum hCG levels rise (increase more than 10% over 2 consecutive weeks); and (3) persistence of detectable serum hCG for more than 6 months after molar evacuation.[20]

Patients on rare occasion present with a false positive elevation in their serum hCG concentration owing to a number of factors other than GTN. The differential diagnosis of an elevated hCG value includes (1) pregnancy, (2) germ cell tumor of the ovary or other site, (3) non-trophoblastic gonadotropin-producing tumor (e.g., hepatoma), or (4) phantom hCG caused by heterophilic antibody.[21] Post-menopausal women have also been reported to have detectable low hCG levels of pituitary origin, which can be suppressed by hormone replacement therapy.[22]

Non-metastatic GTN

Locally invasive GTN also occurs infrequently after non-molar pregnancies.[18] These patients may present with persistently elevated hCG levels, irregular vaginal bleeding, uterine subinvolution, or asymmetric uterine enlargement. Theca lutein ovarian cysts are rare in the absence of high levels of hCG (>100,000 mIU/mL). The trophoblastic tumor may erode into uterine vessels, causing vaginal hemorrhage, or may perforate through the myometrium, producing intra-abdominal bleeding. Bulky necrotic tumors in the endometrial cavity may also serve as a nidus for sepsis, causing pelvic pain and purulent discharge.

Metastatic GTN

Metastases develop in approximately 4% of patients after complete mole and infrequently after other gestations.[18] When metastases occur, the pathology is usually CCA because this tumor has a propensity for early vascular invasion and dissemination. The presenting signs and symptoms in these patients depend on the sites of metastasis: hemoptysis from lung lesions, acute neurologic deficits from intracranial hemorrhage, and so on.

The most common site of metastasis *is* the lung. Eighty percent of patients with metastatic GTN have pulmonary involvement on chest radiographs or computed tomography (CT). Because respiratory symptoms and radiographic findings may be striking, the patient may be thought to have a primary pulmonary process. Pulmonary hypertension can develop as a result of pulmonary arterial occlusion by trophoblastic emboli. The development of early respiratory failure requiring intubation is associated with a dismal outcome.[23] Gynecologic symptoms may be minimal or absent even when the patient has extensive metastases. *The diagnosis of GTN should be considered in any woman in the reproductive age group with unexplained pulmonary or systemic symptoms.*

Vaginal metastases are present in 30% of patients with metastatic GTN. Because these lesions are highly vascular, they may hemorrhage if biopsied.[18]

Hepatic and cerebral metastases occur in approximately 10% of patients with metastatic GTN. Hepatic and cerebral lesions invariably have the histologic pattern of CCA and usually follow a non-molar pregnancy. These patients characteristically have protracted delays in diagnosis and extensive tumor burdens. Virtually, all patients with hepatic and cerebral metastases have concurrent pulmonary or vaginal involvement.[24,25]

Staging and risk assessment

An anatomic staging system for GTN was adopted by the FIGO in 1982[20]:

Stage I: Lesion confined to uterus.

Stage II: Lesion outside uterus but confined to vagina and pelvis.

Stage III: Lung metastases with or without evidence of uterine or pelvic disease.

Stage IV: Distant metastatic sites such as the brain, liver, kidney, gastrointestinal tract, and spleen.

In addition to anatomic staging, the World Health Organization (WHO) has adopted a prognostic scoring system (Table 1) that reliably predicts the risk of drug resistance and assists in selecting the appropriate chemotherapy.[20,27] Prognostic scores <7 are associated with a low risk of resistance to single agent chemotherapy. When the prognostic score is 7 or greater, the patient is considered to be at high risk of developing drug resistance to single agent therapy and requires intensive combination chemotherapy. Patients with stage I GTN usually have a low-risk score and those with stage IV disease generally have a high-risk score. Therefore, the distinction between low and high risk mainly applies to patients with stages II and III disease. The FIGO stage is designated by a Roman numeral and is followed by the modified WHO prognostic score designated by an Arabic number separated by a colon (e.g., II:6).

Data from Charing Cross Hospital indicate that only 30% of low-risk patients with a WHO prognostic score of 5–6 can be cured with monotherapy, which suggests that a multidrug regimen should be administered initially. These patients characteristically present with pre-treatment hCG levels >100,000 mIU/mL and ultrasound evidence of a large tumor burden.[28]

Table 1 Scoring system for gestational trophoblastic tumors based on prognostic factors.

	Score[b]			
	0	1	2	4
Age (years)	<39	>39	—	—
Antecedent pregnancy	Mole	Abortion	Term	—
Interval[a]	<4	4–6	7–12	—
hCG (IU/L)	<10^3	10^3–10^4	10^4–10^5	—
ABO groups (female × male)	—	O × A	B	—
		A × O	AB	—
Largest tumor, including uterine tumor	—	3–5 cm	5 cm	—
Site of metastases	—	Spleen, kidney	Gastrointestinal tract and liver	Brain
Number of metastases identified	—	1–4	4–8	>8
Prior chemotherapy	—	—	Single drug	Two or more drug

[a]Interval is the time (months) between end of antecedent pregnancy and start of chemotherapy.
[b]The total score for a patient is obtained by adding the individual scores for each prognostic factor. Total score: <7 = low risk; and ≥7 = high risk.
Source: Data from Matsui et al. 2004.[26]

Management of GTN

Pretreatment evaluation and staging of GTN

Patients with GTN must undergo a thorough evaluation in order to determine their stage and risk status, which will guide the clinician in selecting the appropriate treatment (Figure 1). The physical examination should always include a vaginal speculum examination to detect implants, which can hemorrhage. Radiographic evaluation should include a pelvic ultrasound to look for evidence of retained trophoblastic tissue in the uterine cavity, myometrial invasion, and to evaluate the pelvis for local spread. Chest imaging is also required, as the lungs are the most common site of metastases. Although chest CT scans are more sensitive than a chest X-ray, they are not included in staging as detection of occult pulmonary metastases does not affect outcome. Pulmonary metastases can be detected by chest CT in up to 40% of patients with a negative chest X-ray.[29] In the absence of pulmonary and vaginal metastases, involvement of distant organs such as the brain and liver is rare. As long as the clinical picture is compatible with GTN, metastases need not be biopsied because of their vascularity and the risk of hemorrhage.

Management of low-risk GTN

Primary therapy of low-risk GTN

Low-risk GTN includes patients with both stage I (non-metastatic) and stages II and III (metastatic) GTN whose prognostic score is <7. In patients with stage I GTN, the selection of primary therapy is based on the patient's desire to preserve fertility. If the patient has completed her childbearing, hysterectomy should be considered.[30] At the time of surgery, we recommend the administration of one course of adjuvant single-agent chemotherapy, either methotrexate (MTX) or actinomycin D (ACTD) for treatment of occult metastases.

Single-agent chemotherapy with sequential MTX/ACTD is the preferred treatment in patients with stage I GTN who desire to retain fertility, as well as in patients with low-risk metastatic GTN. MTX with folinic acid (MTX-FA) *is* the preferred single-agent regimen at the New England Trophoblastic Disease Center (NETDC).[31] MTX-FA induced complete remission in 147 (90.2%) of 163 patients with stage I GTN and in 15 (68.2%) of 22 patients with low-risk stages II and III GTN. One course of MTX-FA induced remission in 132 (81.5%) of these patients. ACTD is used as primary therapy in those patients with pre-existing hepatic dysfunction, who develop hepatic toxicity to MTX, or sequentially in those patients who prove resistant to MTX.[32]

Single-agent chemotherapy with either MTX or ACTD has achieved excellent and comparable remission rates in both non-metastatic (80–90%) and low-risk metastatic (60–70%) GTN.[2,18,32] Several protocols using MTX and ACTD have been used effectively in the treatment of GTN, but until recently, there has been no prospective randomized study comparing all of these regimens (Table 2).[32] Single-agent chemotherapy should be administered at a fixed time interval. A decline in the hCG level less than a one log indicates that the patient's tumor is relatively resistant to that drug, and an alternative agent is substituted.

Salvage therapy of low-risk GTN

Patients with low-risk GTN who develop resistance to sequential single-agent chemotherapy can usually achieve remission with combination chemotherapy consisting of MTX, ACTD, cyclophosphamide, etoposide, and Oncovin[R] (EMA/CO) (etoposide, methotrexate, actinomycin D, cyclophosphamide, vincristine) (Table 3).[33] The use of etoposide, particularly in patients with low-risk GTN, has been of concern because of a report by Rustin et al.[34] that its use was associated with an increased risk of secondary malignancies. A more recent report from the same institution on a larger number of patients has shown that the risk is limited.[35] If the disease is resistant to both single-agent and combination chemotherapy, hysterectomy or local resection (if the patient wants to preserve fertility) may be considered. Ultrasonography, MRI (magnetic resonance imaging) scan, pelvic arteriography, and/or PET (positron emission tomography) scan may aid in identifying the site of resistant uterine tumor when local resection is planned. The administration of three additional courses of the last effective agent reduces the risk of relapse in patients with low-risk disease.[36]

Management of high-risk GTN, stages II and III

Primary therapy

Women with FIGO stages II and III and a WHO score of 7 or higher are at high risk for developing chemotherapy resistance and disease recurrence and should be treated with primary combination chemotherapy with EMACO, which is associated with complete remissions in 76–86% of patients.[37–39]

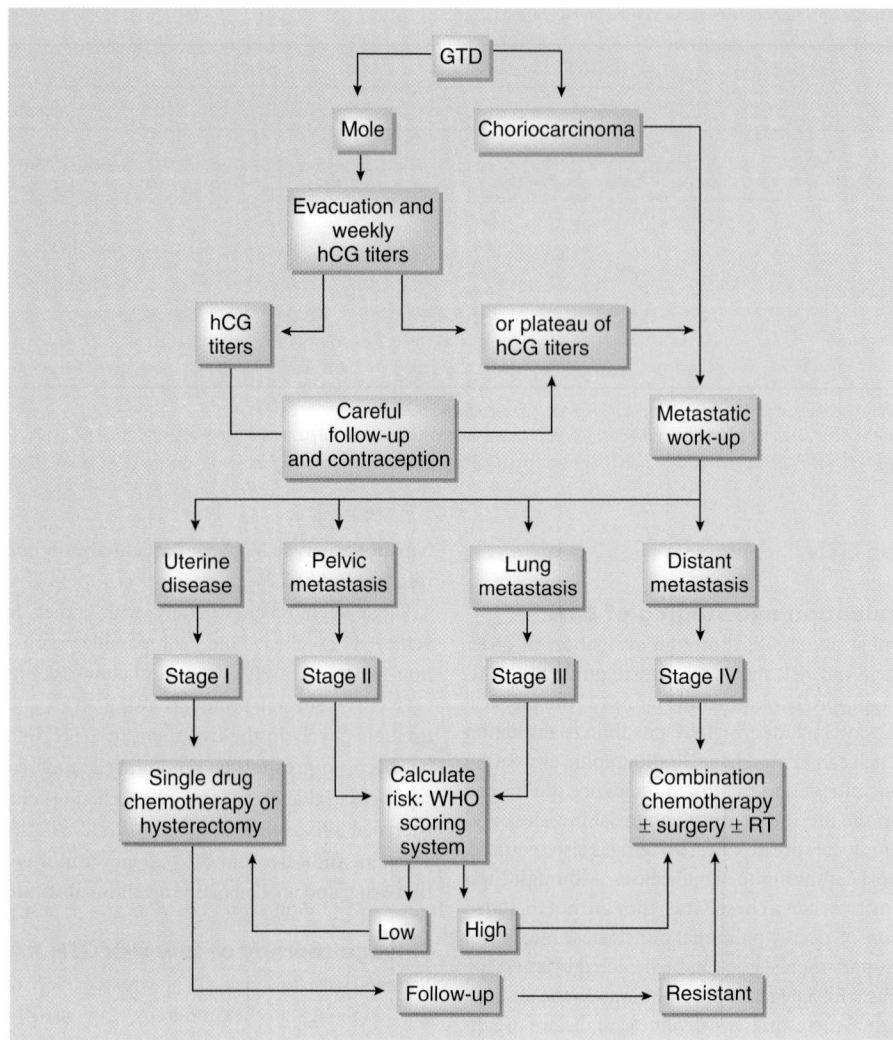

Figure 1 Algorithm for the management of gestational trophoblastic disease (GTD).

Table 2 Single-agent regimen.

Methotrexate treatments

MTX-FA
   MTX 1.0 mg/kg IM on days 1, 3, 5, and 7
   FA 0.1 mg/kg IM or po on days 2, 4, 6, and 8
5-day MTX
   MTX 0.4 mg/kg/day IV or IM daily for 5 days
Pulse MTX
   MTX 50 mg/m^2 IM weekly

Actinomycin D treatments

5-day Act-D
   Act-D 12 µg/kg/day IV for 5 days
Pulse Act-D
   Act-D 1.25 mg/m^2 IV every 2 weeks

Abbreviations: FA, folinic acid; IM, intramuscular; and IV, intravenous.

Table 3 EMACO regimen.

Time	Treatment
Day 1	Etoposide 100 mg/m^2 by IV infusion in 200 mL of saline over 30 min
	Act-D 0.5 mg IV push
	MTX 100 mg/m^2 IV push
	MTX 200 mg/m^2 by IV infusion over 12 h
Day 2	Etoposide 100 mg/m^2 by IV infusion in 200 mL of saline over 30 min
	Act-D 0.5 mg IV push
	FA 15 mg IM or po every 12 h for 4 doses beginning 24 h after starting MTX
Day 8	Cyclophosphamide 600 mg/m^2 IV in saline Oncovin (vincristine) 1.0 mg/m^2 IV push

Abbreviations: Act-D, actinomycin D; FA, folinic acid; IM, intramuscular; IV, intravenous; MTX, methotrexate; and po, per os (by mouth).

Salvage therapy

Patients with disease resistant to EMACO may be treated by modifying that regimen by substituting cisplatin and etoposide (EMA/CE) on day 8.[33] Combination chemotherapy is administered at 2–3 week intervals, toxicity permitting, until the patient attains *three* consecutive weekly undetectable hCG levels, after which at least three additional courses of chemotherapy should be administered to reduce the risk of relapse.

Management of stage IV GTN

Patients with stage IV disease *include patients who* are the highest risk *of developing* rapidly progressive disease and chemoresistance. The use of primary combination chemotherapy in conjunction with the selective use of radiation and surgical treatment has resulted in significantly improved survival. At the NETDC, before 1975, only 30% of patients with stage IV disease survived. After 1975, when the concept of early intensive multi-agent treatment was introduced, complete sustained remission was achieved in 80% of patients.

Table 4 EMACE regimen.

Time	Treatment
Day 1	Etoposide 100 mg/m^2 by IV infusion in 200 mL of saline over 30 min Act-D 0.5 mg IV push MTX 100 mg/m^2 IV push MTX 1,000 mg/m^2 by IV infusion over 12 h
Day 2	Etoposide 100 mg/m^2 by IV infusion in 200 mL of saline over 30 min Act-D 0.5 mg IV push FA 30 mg IM or PO every 12 h for 6 doses beginning 32 h after starting MTX
Day 8	Cisplatin 60 mg/m^2 IV with prehydration etoposide 100 mg/m^2 by IV infusion in 200 mL of saline over 30 min

Abbreviations: Act-D, actinomycin D; FA, folinic acid; IM, intramuscular; IV, intravenous; MTX, methotrexate; and po, per os (by mouth).
Source: Bagshawe 1976.[1] Reproduced with permission of Wiley.

All patients with stage IV GTN are managed with primary combination chemotherapy with EMA/CO. When CNS metastases are present, the MTX dosage in the infusion is increased to 1 g/m^2.[40] Patients who develop resistance to EMA/CO should then be treated with EMA/CE (Table 4). A number of other salvage regimens have been reported to achieve remission in small series of patients. Second-line therapy with etoposide in combination with cisplatin and bleomycin (BEP) or vinblastine in combination with cisplatin and bleomycin (PVB) have also been shown to be effective in patients with resistant GTN.[41–44]

The potential role of autologous bone marrow transplantation or stem cell rescue in GTN has yet to be defined. However, individual cases have been reported where ultra-high-dose chemotherapy with autologous bone marrow or stem cell support has induced complete remission in patients with refractory disease.[45,46]

Despite the efficacy of well-recognized regimens, efforts continue to identify new agents effective in treating resistant disease. Although ifosfamide and paclitaxel have been used successfully, further studies are needed to define their potential role in either primary or second line therapy.[47,48] Osborne et al.[49] have reported that a novel 3-drug doublet regimen consisting of paclitaxel, etoposide, and cisplatin (TE/TP) induced complete remission in two patients with relapsed high-risk GTN. Wan et al.[50] demonstrated the efficacy of floxuridine (FUDR)-containing regimens in drug-resistant patients. Matsui et al.[26] found that 5FU (5-fluorouracil) in combination with ACTD could also be used effectively as salvage therapy.

Role of surgery
Surgery is performed to either treat complications or excise sites of resistant tumor.[51] Hysterectomy may be necessary to control uterine hemorrhage or sepsis or to reduce the tumor burden and thereby limit the need for chemotherapy. Bleeding from vaginal metastases may be managed by packing, wide local excision, or arteriographic embolization of the hypogastric arteries.[52] Thoracotomy may be performed to excise persistent viable tumor despite intensive chemotherapy.[53] However, fibrotic nodules may persist indefinitely on chest roentgenograms after complete gonadotropin remission is attained. An extensive metastatic survey should be undertaken to exclude other sites of persistent tumor. A PET scan may be useful to identify occult sites of viable tumor.[54] Hepatic resection may be required to manage bleeding metastases although embolization has also been utilized in this setting.[55] Craniotomy may be necessary to provide acute decompression or to control bleeding, in addition to its role in the primary resection of solitary metastatic disease.[32]

Role of radiation therapy
When cranial metastases are identified whole-brain irradiation and systemic chemotherapy are promptly instituted at the NETDC to reduce the risk of cerebral hemorrhage. Yordan et al.[56] reported that deaths as a result of cerebral involvement occurred in 11 (44%) of 25 patients treated with chemotherapy alone, but in none of 18 patients treated with brain irradiation and chemotherapy. Excellent results have also been achieved in selected cases with local resection, particularly when the tumor is solitary and located peripherally.[32,40,51]

Excellent cure rates have also been reported in patients with cerebral metastases with intensive chemotherapy alone. Newlands et al.[40] have documented excellent remission rates in patients with brain involvement who were treated with chemotherapy alone. Intensive combination chemotherapy including high-dose intravenous and intrathecal MTX induced sustained remission in 30 (86%) of 35 patients with cerebral lesions. The patients with superficial solitary brain metastases underwent craniotomy at the start of therapy.

Craniotomy may also be necessary to provide acute decompression or control bleeding. Craniotomy should also be performed to manage life-threatening complications thereby providing an opportunity to control the disease with chemotherapy. Infrequently cerebral metastases may be resectable when they become resistant to chemotherapy. Athanassiou et al.[57] reported that four of five patients undergoing craniotomy for acute intracranial complications were ultimately cured. Fortunately, most patients with cerebral metastases who achieve remission have no residual neurological deficit unless a bleed has occurred.

However, we have observed rare cases of significant dementia and progressive memory loss in patients who received whole head irradiation. Although the controversy regarding the optimal treatment protocol for cerebral metastases has not been resolved, Neubauer et al.[58] have reported that multimodal therapy including chemotherapy, surgical resection, and radiation therapy(whole brain or stereotactic) has improved overall survival from 46% to 64%.

Management of PSTT and ETT
Patients with PSTT and ETT require special consideration because of the unique nature of their disease. We believe that the primary therapy of all patients with non-metastatic PSTT and ETT should be hysterectomy without adjunctive chemotherapy because this variant of CCA is relatively resistant to chemotherapy.[16,59,60] If deep myometrial involvement is present, it is our policy to also perform a pelvic lymphadenectomy. Unlike CCA, these tumors tend to remain localized in the uterus for long periods of time before metastasizing. Once metastases occur both PSTT and ETT have a high mortality rate. Kingdon et al.[61] in their review of deaths from GTN found that 30% of those dying from GTN had PSTT histology. In the absence of demonstrable metastases, no further treatment is required.

Although universally accepted guidelines on how to manage PSTT and ETT are not available because of their rarity, given their aggressive clinical behavior the use of multimodal therapy with surgery, radiation and chemotherapy has improved survival. The use of EMA/EP in PSTT has been shown to be curative in patients with metastases.[62] Papadopoulos et al.[62] reported that a long interval from the antecedent pregnancy to clinical presentation was the most important prognostic factor. While all 27 patients survived when the interval was <4 years, all seven patients died when the interval exceeded 4 years. Although not applicable to the majority of patients, fertility-sparing surgery has also been employed successfully.[63,64]

Results of therapy

Stage I GTN

Between July 1965 and December 2013, 624 patients with stage I GTN were treated at the NETDC and all attained remission. 478 out of 582 patients (82%) who were treated with primary single-agent chemotherapy achieved remission with sequential MTX/ACTD. All 35 patients managed with primary hysterectomy and adjuvant single-agent chemotherapy achieved remission with no further treatment. Seven patients with high-risk scores achieved remission with primary combination chemotherapy. The remaining 104 patients resistant to primary treatment were treated successfully with either combination chemotherapy or surgical intervention.

Stages II and III GTN

Complete remission was achieved at the NETDC in all 37 patients with stage II GTN and in 225 out of 226 patients with stage III GTN. Single-agent chemotherapy induced remission in 16 (76.2%) of 21 patients with low-risk stage II disease and in 113 (73.3%) of 154 patients with low-risk stage III disease. All patients with disease resistant to single-agent chemotherapy attained remission with combination chemotherapy. Sixteen patients with high-risk stage II and 12 (92.3%) of 13 patients with high-risk stage III GTN achieved remission with combination regimens. There was one death in the high-risk stage III group.

Stage IV GTN

Before 1975, only 6/20 patients (30%) with stage IV GTN achieved remission at the NETDC. However, after 1975, 25 (75.5%) of 33 patients with stage IV disease attained remission. This dramatic improvement in survival resulted from the use of intensive multimodal therapy early in the course of treatment. While brain irradiation is commonly employed in the United States for cerebral metastases, excellent remission rates have been reported in patients with cerebral metastases who were treated with chemotherapy alone.[40] Recently, Alifrangis et al.[65] reported that the use of induction chemotherapy with low-dose etoposide and cisplatin resulted in improved survival in patients with high-risk GTN and large tumor volumes.

hCG follow-up and relapse

All patients with stages I, II, and III GTN are followed with weekly hCG values until undetectable for three consecutive weeks and then monthly until undetectable for 12 months. Patients with stage IV GTN are followed monthly for 24 months because they are at greater risk for late relapse. All patients must be encouraged to use effective contraception during the entire interval of monitoring. Relapse rates at the NETDC are as follows: stage I, 2.9%; stage II, 8.3%; stage III, 4.2%; and stage IV, 9.1%. The mean time to recurrence from the last nondetectable hCG level was 6 months, and this did not differ among the four stages.[66]

When relapse occurs, the patient should be restaged, and appropriate therapy begun with a new regimen not previously utilized in this patient. All relapsed patients in the series with stages I, II, and III achieved remission, whereas both patients with relapsed stage IV GTN died.

Quiescent GTN

A rare cause of persistent (at least 3 months) low-level hCG is quiescent GTN (range 0.5–200 mIU/mL) that most commonly follows a molar pregnancy. Quiescent GTN is thought to be due to the presence of highly differentiated, non-invasive syncytiotrophoblast cells. This condition is characterized by the following: (1) foci of disease are not readily identifiable clinically; and (2) hCG level unresponsive to therapy, presumably because the growth cycle of these cells is comparable to normal cells. Patients with quiescent GTN should not be treated with chemotherapy, but close follow-up is indicated because 6–10% will eventually develop active GTN requiring treatment. The presence of low levels of hyperglycosylated hCG indicates the presence of quiescent GTN. Increasing levels of hyperglycosylated hCG indicate the development of active GTN that requires treatment.[21]

Subsequent pregnancies

Patients with complete and partial mole can anticipate normal reproduction in the future.[67] However, these patients are at increased risk of developing molar pregnancy in later conceptions. Patients treated for GTN with chemotherapy can also expect normal reproduction in the future.[68] Importantly, the frequency of later major and minor congenital malformations is not increased. Data from the NETDC and 10 other centers have been reported concerning the outcome of 3191 pregnancies after chemotherapy.[67] These subsequent pregnancies resulted in 2342 (73.4%) live births, 89 (4.7%) premature deliveries, 40 (1.3%) stillbirths, and 457 (14.3%) spontaneous abortions. Although the frequency of stillbirths appears to be somewhat increased, congenital malformations were noted in only 46 (1.6%) infants, which is consistent with the general population. Woolas et al.[68] noted that there was no difference in either the conception rate or pregnancy outcome between women treated with single-agent MTX and those receiving combination therapy. Furthermore, only 7% of women who wished to become pregnant failed to conceive.

Because the risk of a repeat molar pregnancy is increased 10-fold, an obstetrical ultrasound should be obtained in the late first trimester of subsequent pregnancies to confirm normal fetal development. In addition, an hCG test should be performed 6 weeks after completion of any subsequent pregnancy to rule out occult GTN. Later products of conception should also be evaluated by a pathologist following any spontaneous miscarriage or therapeutic abortion.

Key references

The complete reference list can be found on the Wiley Companion Digital Edition of this title (see inside front cover for login instructions).

1 Bagshawe KD. Risks and prognostic factors in trophoblastic neoplasia. *Cancer.* 1976;**38**:1373–1385.

2 Goldstein DP, Berkowitz RS. *Gestational Trophoblastic Neoplasms: Clinical Principles of Diagnosis and Management.* Philadelphia: WB Saunders; 1982:1–301.

4 Palmer JR. Advances in the epidemiology of gestational trophoblastic disease. *J Reprod Med.* 1994;**39**:155–162.

12 Elias KM, Goldstein DP, Berkowitz RS. Complete hydatitdform mole in women older than age 50. *J Reprod Med.* 2010;**55**:208–212.

13 Elias KM, Shoni M, Bernstein MR, et al. Complete hydatidiform mole in women aged 40-49 years. *J Reprod Med.* 2012;**57**:254–258.

16 Feltmate C, Genest DR, Wise L, et al. Placental site trophoblastic tumor: a 17-year experience at the New England Trophoblastic Disease Center. *Gynecol Oncol.* 2001;**82**:415–419.

19 Berkowitz RS, Goldstein DP. Presentation and management of molar pregnancy. In: Hancock BW, Newlands ES, Berkowitz RS, eds. *Gestational Trophoblastic Disease.* London: Chapman and Hall; 1997:127–142.

20 Kohorn EI. The new FIGO 2000 staging and risk factor scoring system for gestational trophoblastic disease: Description and critical assessment. *Int J Gynaecol Cancer.* 2001;**11**:73–77.

21 Cole LA, Khanlian SA, Giddings A, et al. Gestational trophoblastic diseases: 4. Presentation with persistent low positive human chorionic gonadotropin test results. *Gynecol Oncol.* 2006;**102**:165–169.

23 Bakri YN, Berkowitz RS, Khan J, et al. Pulmonary metastases of gestational trophoblastic tumor: risk factors for early respiratory failure. *J Reprod Med.* 1994;**39**:175–178.

24 Newlands ES, Holden L, Seckl MJ, et al. Management of brain metastases in patients with high risk gestational trophoblastic tumours (GTT). *J Reprod Med.* 2002;**47**:465–471.

25 Bakri YN, Subhi J, Amer M, et al. Liver metastases of gestational trophoblastic tumor. *Gynecol Oncol.* 1993;**48**:110–113.

27 World Health Organization. *Trophoblastic diseases: technical report series 692.* Geneva: WHO; 1983.

28 McGrath S, Short D, Harvey R, et al. The management and outcome of women with post-hydatidiform mole 'low-risk' gestational trophoblastic neoplasia, but hCG levels in excess of 100,000 IU/L. *Br J Cancer.* 2010;**102**:810–814.

29 Garner EIO, Garrett A, Goldstein DP, Berkowitz RS. Significance of chest computed tomography findings in the evaluation and treatment of persistent gestational trophoblastic neoplasia. *J Reprod Med.* 2004;**49**:411–414.

30 Clark RM, Nevadunsky NS, Ghosh S, et al. The evolving role of hysterectomy in gestational trophoblastic neoplasia at the New England Trophoblastic Disease Center. *J Reprod Med.* 2010;**55**:194–198.

31 Berkowitz RS, Goldstein DP, Bernstein MR. Ten years experience with methotrexate and folinic acid as primary therapy for gestational trophoblastic disease. *Gynecol Oncol.* 1986;**23**:111–118.

32 Seckl M, Sebire N, Berkowitz RS. Gestatioanl trophoblastic disease. *Lancet.* 2010;**376**:717–729.

33 Newlands ES, Bower M, Holden L, et al. Management of resistant gestational trophoblastic tumors. *J Reprod Med.* 1998;**43**:111–118.

34 Rustin GJS, Newlands ES, Lutz JM, et al. Combination but not single-agent methotrexate chemotherapy for gestational trophoblastic tumors increases the incidence of second tumors. *J Clin Oncol.* 1996;**14**:2769–2773.

35 Savage PM, Cook R, O'Nions J, et al. The effects of chemotherapy treatment for gestational trophoblastic tumours on second tumour risk and early menopause. XVII World Congress on Gestational Trophoblastic Diseases, 2014;71-2. (Abstract).

36 Lybol C, Sweep FC, Harvey R, et al. Relapse rates after two versus three consolidation courses of methotrexate in the treatment of low-risk gestational trophoblastic neoplasia. *Gynecol Oncol.* 2012;**125**:576–579.

37 Newlands ES, Bagshawe KD, Begent RH, et al. Results with the EMA/CO (etoposide, methotrexate, actinomycin D, cyclophosphamide, vincristine) regimen in high risk gestational trophoblastic tumours, 1979 to 1989. *Br J Obstet Gynaecol.* 1991;**98**:550–556.

40 Newlands ES, Holden L, Seckl MJ, et al. Management of brain metastases in patients with high risk gestational trophoblastic tumor. *J Reprod Med.* 2002;**47**:465.

44 Lurain JR, Schink JC. Importance of salvage therapy in the management of high-risk gestational trophoblastic neoplasia. *J Reprod Med.* 2012;**57**:219–224.

49 Osborne R, Covens A, Merchandani DE, Gerulath AS. Successful salvage of relapsed high-risk gestational Trophoblastic neoplasia patients using a novel paclitaxel-containing doublet. *J Reprod Med.* 2004;**49**:655–658.

51 Lurain JR, Singh DK, Schink JC. Role of surgery in the management of high-risk gestational troph0blastic neoplasia. *J Reprod Med.* 2006;**51**:773–777.

53 Fleming EL, Garrett L, Growdon WB, et al. The changing role of thoracotomy in gestational trophoblastic neoplasia at the New England Trophoblastic Disease Center. *J Reprod Med.* 2008;**53**:493–498.

54 Dhillon T, Palmieri C, Sebire NJ, et al. Value of whole body 18 FDG-PET to identify the active site of gestational trophoblastic neoplasia. *J Reprod Med.* 2006;**51**:879–883.

57 Athanassiou A, Begent RHJ, Newlands ES, et al. Central nervous system metastases of choriocarcinoma: 23 years' experience at Charing Cross Hospital. *Cancer.* 1983;**52**:1728–1735.

58 Neubauer NL, Latif N, Kalakota K, et al. Brain metastasis in gestational trophoblastic disease: an update. *J Reprod Med.* 2012;**57**:288–292.

59 Palmer JE, Macdonald M, Wells M, et al. Epithelioid trophoblastic tumor: a review of the literature. *J Reprod Med.* 2008;**53**:465–475.

61 Kingdon SJ, Coleman RE, Ellis L, Hancock BW. Deaths from gestational trophoblastic neoplasia. Any lessons to be learned? *J Reprod Med.* 2012;**57**:293–296.

62 Papadopoulos AJ, Foskett M, Seckl MJ, et al. Twenty-five years clinical experience of placental site trophoblastic tumors. *J Reprod Med.* 2002;**47**:460–464.

65 Alifrangis C, Agarwal R, Short D, et al. EMA/CO for high-risk gestational trophoblastic neoplasia:good outcome with induction low-dose etoposide-cisplatin and genetic analysis. *J Clin Oncol.* 2013;**31**:280–286.

66 Goldstein DP, Zanten-Przybysz I, Bernstein MR, Berkowitz RS. Revised FIGO staging system for gestational trophoblastic tumors; recommendations regarding therapy. *J Reprod Med.* 1998;**43**:37–43.

67 Vargas R, Barroilhet L, Esselen K, et al. Subsequent pregnancy outcomes in patients with molar pregnancy and persistent gestational trophoblastic neoplasia: updated results. *J Reprod Med.* 2014;**59**:188–194.

68 Woolas RP, Bower M, Newlands ES, et al. Influence of chemotherapy for gestational trophoblastic disease on subsequent pregnancy outcome. *Br J Obstet Gynecol.* 1998;**105**:1326–1327.

107 Gynecologic sarcomas

Jamal Rahaman, MD ▪ Carmel J. Cohen, MD

Overview

Sarcomas are extremely rare and account for less than 1.5% of gynecologic cancers. Carcinosarcoma and leiomyosarcoma each account for 35–40% of uterine sarcomas, with endometrial stromal sarcoma (ESS) accounting for 10–15% and other sarcomas including adenosarcomas comprising 5–10%. Uterine carcinosarcoma should be classified as a metaplastic carcinoma of the uterus. Most adenosarcomas and ESSs have good prognosis and respond to hormonal therapy. Undifferentiated endometrial sarcoma (UES) and adenosarcomas with sarcomatous overgrowth are rare and have poor prognosis and require chemotherapy. ESS are histologically and clinically distinct from UES and each have distinct gene rearrangements. More than 50% of Stage I leiomyosarcomas (LMSs) and carcinosarcomas patients will recur. Chemotherapy is required for advanced or recurrent disease. In LMSs, the active drugs are doxorubicin, ifosfamide, gemcitabine, and docetaxel. For uterine carcinosarcomas, the drugs of choice are ifosfamide, cisplatin/carboplatin, and paclitaxel. Adjuvant radiation therapy may provide locoregional control in select cases of uterine carcinosarcomas. Hormonal therapy, including progestational agents, GnRH analogues, and aromatase inhibitors, has a role in the treatment of advanced or recurrent low-grade ESSs and adenosarcomas.

Historical perspective

Sarcomas (including mesenchymal and mixed epithelial–mesenchymal malignancies) of the vulva, vagina, cervix, uterus, and ovaries account for less than 1.5% of the cancers of these organs. Classification of these cancers was a taxonomic dilemma until Ober, in 1959,[1] proposed a classification which Kempson and Bari[2] revised in 1970 and the World Health Organization[3] and the College of American Pathologist[4] reclassified in 2003 (Table 1). Uterine carcinosarcomas are not classified as a uterine sarcoma any longer and should be classified as a metaplastic carcinoma of the uterus[5] but is discussed in this chapter.

Incidence and epidemiology

The most common site for sarcoma in the female pelvis is the uterus comprising only 4–9% of uterine cancers, with an annual incidence rate of less than 20 per million females.[6,7] Overall incidence for Blacks is twice that of Whites, but there were no differences in survival for women receiving similar therapy.[6,7] Risk of carcinosarcoma increases sharply with age. Incidence rate per million women per year is 8.2 for carcinosarcomas, 6.4 for leiomyosarcomas (LMSs), 1.8 for endometrial stromal sarcomas (ESSs), and 0.7 for unclassified sarcomas.[6,7] Authors have reported that carcinosarcoma and LMS each account for 35–40% of uterine sarcomas, ESS accounting for 10–15%, and other sarcomas comprising 5%.[7]

Risk factors

Epidemiologic risk factors for uterine sarcoma are undefined except for radiation exposure[8,9] and previous tamoxifen use.[10,11]

Pathology

The uterus is the most common site of gynecologic sarcomas arising from the endometrium only (ESS), the myometrium only (LMS), or contributions from both (carcinosarcomas).[1,12] The homologous tumors include carcinoma plus a sarcoma indigenous to the uterus, while the heterologous tumors includes a sarcoma resembling tissue from some extrauterine source (bone, cartilage, striated muscle). Müllerian adenosarcomas are mixed müllerian tumors composed of malignant stroma and benign epithelium.[3,13,14]

Endometrial stromal lesions

Endometrial stromal nodules (ESN) are rare. They are characterized by a well-defined noninfiltrating border without evidence of myometrial or vascular invasion. Two-thirds are found as isolated lesions within the myometrium with no apparent connection to the endometrium.[3]

ESS is low grade with metastatic potential. Like ESN, they are composed of uniform cells that mimic proliferative endometrium. However, they exhibit myometrial and/or vascular invasion.[3] Histologically, they are characterized by densely uniform stromal cells with minimal cellular pleomorphism, mild nuclear atypia, and rare mitotic figures. Of note, an isolated finding of increased mitotic figures does not confer an adverse prognosis in an otherwise typical low-grade ESS.[15]

The diagnosis of ESS may be complicated by variant morphologic features (Table 1).[3] In tumors with focal smooth muscle differentiation, the tumor is categorized as ESS if the smooth muscle component involves <30% of the total tumor volume. Tumors composed of a larger smooth muscle component are designated as mixed endometrial stromal and smooth muscle tumors.[3,16]

Undifferentiated endometrial sarcoma (UES—previously referred to as high-grade ESSs) is characterized by marked cytologic atypia, nuclear pleomorphism, high mitotic activity, and extensive invasion. In addition, UES usually show destructive myometrial invasion.[3]

Molecular and genetic alterations

The following molecular features are characteristic of ESS and are also found in ESN: The majority are immunoreactive for the estrogen receptor (ER) and progesterone receptor (PR). They are typically immunohistochemically positive for CD10 and negative for desmin

Holland-Frei Cancer Medicine, Ninth Edition. Edited by Robert C. Bast Jr., Carlo M. Croce, William N. Hait, Waun Ki Hong, Donald W. Kufe, Martine Piccart-Gebhart, Raphael E. Pollock, Ralph R. Weichselbaum, Hongyang Wang, and James F. Holland.
© 2017 John Wiley & Sons, Inc. ISBN: 978-1-118-93469-2

Table 1 Classification of uterine sarcomas. College of American Pathologist Classification of Uterine Sarcomas.

Histologic type (select all that apply)
Leiomyosarcoma
Low-grade endometrial stromal sarcoma#
Low-grade endometrial stromal sarcoma with:
• Smooth muscle differentiation
• Sex cord elements
• Glandular elements
Other (specify): _____
High-grade endometrial stromal sarcoma
Undifferentiated uterine/endometrial sarcoma
Adenosarcoma
Adenosarcoma with:
• Rhabdomyoblastic differentiation
• Cartilagenous differentiation
• Osseous differentiation
• Other heterologous element (specify): _____
Adenosarcoma with sarcomatous overgrowth
Other (specify): _____

Low-grade endometrial sarcoma is distinguished from benign endometrial stromal nodule by infiltration into the surrounding myometrium and/or lymphovascular invasion. Minor marginal irregularity in the form of tongues <3 mm (up to 3) is allowable for an endometrial stromal nodule. This protocol does not apply to endometrial stromal nodule.
Data from Tavassoli[3] and Otis.[4]

and h-caldesmon and loss of heterozygosity of PTEN, and deregulation of the Wnt signaling pathway.[5,17,18]

UES shows increased staining for proliferation markers (Ki67, p16, and p53) and does not generally exhibit immunoreactivity against ER, PR, desmin, or smooth muscle antigen (SMA).[5] UES also expresses the receptor tyrosine kinase CD117 (c-KIT),[19] cyclin D1,[20] and human epidermal growth factor receptor 2 (HER2 or ERBB2), which are not typically found in ESS.[5]

Gene rearrangements have been described and validated in patients with ESSs with at least 75% having a gene rearrangement.[21,22] The t(7;17) translocation resulting in the *JAZF1-SUZ12* gene fusion is the most common translocation found in approximately 35–50% of ESSs.[22] Other noted gene fusions are *JAZF1-PHF1, EPC1-PHF1, JAZF1* only, and *PHF1* only.[21–25]

UESs lack these *JAFZ1*-based rearrangements but instead appear to frequently harbor the *YWHAE-FAM22A/B* genetic fusion,[26–29] which may be specific to these tumors as this rearrangement was not detected in 827 other cases representing 55 tumor types.[27]

Patterns of spread

Uterine sarcomas are spread by lymphatic, hematogenous, local extension, and peritoneal dissemination.[30–38]

Rose et al.[30] studied the autopsy findings of 73 patients with uterine sarcoma, including 43 patients with carcinosarcoma, 19 with LMS, 9 with ESS, and 2 with endolymphatic stromal myosis. The peritoneal cavity and omentum were the most frequently involved sites (59%), followed by lung (52%), pelvic (41%) and paraaortic (38%) lymph nodes, and liver parenchyma (34%). Of note, the presence of lung metastasis was often a sole metastatic site.

Lymph node metastasis in adult soft-tissue sarcomas is <3%, with some variation among histologic subtypes.[39] The risk of lymph metastasis in LMS overall was approximately 6.4% in a series of 357 patients.[40] However, the rate of occult lymph node metastasis in clinically normal nodes and disease clinically confined to the uterus was only 3.5% among 57 surgically staged patients with LMS.[35]

Carcinosarcomas have a higher rate of both overall (25%)[41] and occult (18%)[35] lymph node metastasis. The rate of overall and occult lymph node metastasis in ESS is 16% and 6%, respectively.[42] Deep myometrial invasion and extensive lymph–vascular space invasion (LVSI) further increase the risk of occult metastasis.[32,43] The rate of lymph node metastasis in adenosarcomas is approximately 3%.[44]

Clinical profile

Uterine endometrial stromal tumors

Patients with endometrial stromal tumors are commonly perimenopausal with irregular vaginal bleeding. The tumor tissue may protrude through the cervical overall survival (OS) and may grow large without penetrating through the uterine wall. The diagnosis is usually made by endometrial sampling.[16,45,46]

LMS

LMS commonly occurs during the fourth and fifth decades of life, with a peak incidence at 45 years, after which there is a gradual decline in incidence until the eighth decade. The lesion is frequently associated with benign leiomyomas, although among leiomyomas, sarcoma is found less than 1% of the time.[47] There is debate over whether the lesion "develops" from a benign leiomyoma or occurs independently. Ferenczy et al.[48] were unable to demonstrate a developmental relationship, whereas Spiro and Koss[49] found intermediate changes in leiomyomas and proposed malignant transformation. Often LMSs are discovered by chance at the time of myomectomy or hysterectomy.[47,50]

Carcinosarcoma

The incidence of carcinosarcoma increases at 50 years and plateaus after age 75 years. Vaginal bleeding, heavy discharge, and abdominal pain are characteristic. Endometrial sampling is more often diagnostic than in LMS because LMS invades the endometrial cavity infrequently.

Tumor biomarkers

Goto et al. reported that serum lactate dehydrogenase (LDH) was elevated in a small series of LMS and was useful in combination with dynamic MRI. The positive predictive value was 91% using the combined assessment compared to 39% for LDH alone and 71% for MRI alone.[51]

Imaging studies

ESS has a nonspecific appearance on ultrasound.[52] The characteristic pattern of ESS consists of worm-like tumor projections along the vessels or ligaments, which are best visualized on MRI with diffuse-weighted imaging.[53] There are few studies describing the characteristic appearance of UES.[54]

Kurjak et al.[55] evaluated the role of transvaginal color Doppler ultrasonography in differentiating uterine sarcomas from leiomyomas. Computed tomography will identify extrauterine spread, and magnetic resonance imaging can assess the depth of myometrial invasion. Imaging studies are performed preoperatively to characterize the uterine mass and evaluate for lymph node involvement and other metastases but cannot reliably differentiate between a uterine sarcoma and other uterine findings. There are few data suggesting the best choice of imaging.[54,56] The FDG-PET showed a better detection rate than the abdominal CT scan for extrapelvic metastatic lesions.[57–59]

Diagnosis

Of patients with uterine sarcomas, 75–95% present with abnormal vaginal bleeding.[60,61] Pelvic pain, discharge, and aborting tissue occur frequently. Endometrial biopsy may confirm carcinosarcoma in the majority of cases[62]; however, LMS and ESS are missed in at least 40% and 20% of cases, respectively.[34,63,64]

TNM and FIGO staging classification

Uterine sarcomas require surgical staging. The International Federation of Gynecology and Obstetrics (FIGO) did not have a sarcoma-specific system until recently and the Endometrial Staging criteria were applied until 2009. FIGO devised a uterine sarcoma-specific staging system in 2009 for LMS, EES, and UES and another specific for adenosarcoma (Tables 2 and 3).

Carcinosarcomas are to be staged using the 2009 revised FIGO Staging for endometrial carcinomas (*see* **Chapter 103**).

Prognostic factors and prognosis

Prognostic factors differ for the three major types of uterine sarcomas. Major and colleagues reported the GOG clinicopathologic study of clinical stage I and II uterine sarcoma, which included 59 patients with LMS and 301 patients with carcinosarcoma.[35] Of the 453 patients eligible for analysis, 430 underwent complete surgical

Table 2 STAGING—Leiomyosarcoma, endometrial stromal sarcoma, and undifferentiated uterine sarcoma.

TNM categories	FIGO stages	Definition
Primary tumor (T)		
TX		Primary tumor cannot be assessed
T0		No evidence of Primary Tumor
T1	I	Tumor is limited to the uterus
T1a	IA	Tumor is 5 cm or less (≤5 cm) in greatest dimension
T1b	IB	Tumor is greater than 5 cm (>5 cm) in greatest dimension
T2	II	Tumor extends beyond the uterus, but is within the pelvis (tumor extends to extrauterine pelvic tissue)
T2a	IIA	Tumor involves the adnexa
T2b	IIB	Tumor involves other pelvis tissue
T3	III	Tumor invades abdominal tissues (not just protruding into the abdomen)
T3a	IIIA	Tumor invades abdominal tissues at one site
T3b	IIIB	Tumor invades abdominal tissues at more than one site
T4	IVA	Tumor invades bladder mucosa and/or rectum
Regional lymph nodes (N)		
NX		Regional lymph nodes cannot be assessed
N0		No regional lymph node metastasis
N1	IIIC	Regional lymph node metastasis to pelvic lymph nodes
Distant metastasis (M)		
M0		No distant metastasis
M1	IVB	Distant metastasis (excluding adnexa, pelvic and abdominal tissues) Specify site(s), if known: _____

Data from Otis[4] and D'Angelo and Prat.[5]

Table 3 STAGING—Uterine adenosarcoma.

TNM categories	FIGO stages	Definition
Primary tumor (T)		
TX		Primary tumor cannot be assessed
T0		No evidence of primary tumor
T1	I	Tumor limited to the uterus
T1a	IA	Tumor is limited to the endometrium/endocervix without myometrial invasion
T1b	IB	Tumor invades less than or equal to 50% (≤50%) total myometrial thickness
T1c	IC	Tumor invades greater than 50% (>50%) total myometrial thickness
T2	II	Tumor extends beyond the uterus, but is within the pelvis (tumor extends to extrauterine pelvic tissue)
T2a	IIA	Tumor involves the adnexa
T2b	IIB	Tumor involves other pelvis tissue
T3	III	Tumor invades abdominal tissues (not just protruding into the abdomen)
T3a	IIIA	Tumor invades abdominal tissues at one site
T3b	IIIB	Tumor invades abdominal tissues at more than one site
T4	IVA	Tumor invades bladder mucosa and/or rectum
Regional lymph nodes (N)		
NX		Regional lymph nodes cannot be assessed
N0		No regional lymph node metastasis
N1	IIIC	Regional lymph node metastasis to pelvic lymph nodes
Distant metastasis (M)		
M0		No distant metastasis
M1	IVB	Distant metastasis (excluding adnexa, pelvic and abdominal tissues) Specify site(s), if known: _____

Modified from Otis[4] and D'Angelo and Prat.[5]

staging that included lymphadenectomy. The median survival was 62.6 months for homologous carcinosarcoma, 22.7 months for heterologous carcinosarcoma, and 20.6 months for LMS. The overall recurrence rate for homologous carcinosarcoma was 56%.

In patients with LMS, lymph vascular space involvement and involvement of the cervix and isthmus were common, whereas lymph node metastases, adnexal metastases, and positive peritoneal cytology were infrequent findings. The only surgicopathologic finding that correlated with progression-free interval was the mitotic index.[2,35,37,65] While there were no treatment failures among the three women who had less than 10 mitoses per 10 high-power fields, 61% of women with 10–20 mitoses per 10 high-power fields and 79% of women with greater than 20 mitoses per 10 high-power fields developed recurrences.

In contrast to patients with LMS, surgicopathologic factors of carcinosarcoma that related to progression-free interval included adnexal spread, lymph node metastasis, histologic cell type (heterologous vs homologous), and the grade of sarcoma. Of note, patients with carcinosarcoma had high rates of nodal and adnexal metastases and positive peritoneal cytology. Pelvic nodes were involved twice as often as aortic nodes (15% vs 7.8%), and both nodal groups were involved in 5% of the patients.[35]

Morcellation

In patients undergoing laparoscopic hysterectomy for a presumed uterine sarcoma, power morcellation should not be attempted.

Wright (2014) used a large insurance database to identify 36,470 women undergoing minimally invasive hysterectomy with power morcellation performed to demonstrate that the prevalence of uterine cancers was 27 per 10,000 (99 cases).[66] In addition to this cohort, 26 cases of other gynecologic malignancies were found (a prevalence of 7/10,000), 39 uterine neoplasms of uncertain malignant potential (11/10,000), and 368 cases of endometrial hyperplasia (101/10,000).[66]

LMS

Morcellation of a uterine leiomyosarcoma is associated with a worsened outcome.[67] Park et al.[68] reported a series in which the 5-year disease-free survival (DFS) was 40% in women who underwent tumor morcellation and were subsequently diagnosed with leiomyosarcoma, compared to 65% in those with leiomyosarcoma who had not undergone morcellation ($p = 0.04$). Similarly, the 5-year OS was 46% after morcellation compared to 73% in those not morcellated ($p = 0.04$).[68]

ESS

In one study, tumor morcellation in women with ESS was associated with a lower 5-year DFS compared with those who did not have a morcellation (55% vs 84%, respectively, odds ratio 4.03, 95% CI 1.06–15.3).[69] However, no significant impact on OS was reported.

Surgical treatment

The initial therapy for sarcomas of the gynecologic tract is surgical except for embryonal rhabdomyosarcomas. Patients with uterine sarcoma require total abdominal hysterectomy and careful staging including pelvic and paraaortic lymph node sampling. In patients with carcinosarcoma limited to the uterus by pathologic staging, the cytologic presence of malignant cells in the peritoneal washings is a poor prognostic factor.

The ovaries could be retained in premenopausal patients with LMS because this appears to improve their prognosis.[12,64,70,71] However, a bilateral salpingo-oophorectomy should be performed in all other patients, including those with low-grade ESS,[72,73] because these tumors may be hormone dependent or responsive and have a propensity for extension into the parametria, broad ligament, and adnexal structures.

For carcinosarcoma, a high percentage of patients with clinical stage I or II disease is upstaged at the time of laparotomy[74,75]; thus, it appears reasonable to surgically stage these patients. There is a paucity of data regarding the role of lymph node sampling in patients with LMS and ESS, but it appears that almost all patients with these sarcomas who have lymph node metastases also have evidence of intraperitoneal disease spread.[47]

Unlike other gynecologic malignancies, there is a role for thoracotomy or video-assisted thoracoscopy in patients with uterine sarcoma metastatic to the lung. Levenback and colleagues reviewed 45 patients whose pulmonary metastases from uterine sarcoma were resected at Memorial Sloan-Kettering Cancer Center, the majority of which were LMS (84%).[76] The mean survival of patients with unilateral disease (39 months) was significantly greater than that of patients with bilateral disease (27 months). Recurrent or metastatic low-grade ESS may also be amenable to surgical excision of pelvic disease or pulmonary metastases.

Postsurgical therapy for gynecologic sarcomas

Although complete surgical removal is the ideal initial therapy for patients with sarcoma of the gynecologic tract, there is no randomized study proving that surgical cytoreduction influences OS for patients with advanced or recurrent disease. Similarly, the therapeutic benefit of lymphadenectomy has not been proven but is rational. For patients with sarcoma of the uterus or ovary, no formal trial has evaluated the role of lymphadenectomy in addition to hysterectomy and bilateral salpingo-oophorectomy.

For patients with uterine sarcoma, there is no definitive evidence from prospective trials that adjuvant therapy of any type leads to overall improvement in survival. To review the currently understood role of radiotherapy and chemotherapy in sarcomas, LMS is separated from the remaining homologous and heterologous carcinosarcomas because the patterns of relapse for the former are somewhat different from those of the latter group.

Radiation oncology

Radiation therapy for LMS

In contrast to other sarcomas, patients with LMS confined to the uterus appear to have a dominant pattern of failure outside the pelvis and abdominal cavity (65%) with a minority of patients with a first recurrence confined to the abdomen and/or pelvis (28%).[77–79] Thus, in LMS, although the rate of failure in the pelvis is not insubstantial, little is to be potentially gained by delivering pelvic irradiation as a postoperative adjuvant treatment insofar as two-third of patients have some component of distant disease at first recurrence. Radiation treatment is reserved for isolated pelvic relapse only.

Radiation therapy for carcinosarcoma

Historically, pre- or postoperative pelvic irradiation has been used as an adjunct to surgery for carcinosarcoma. Many retrospective reviews illustrate this common use.[60,75,80–86] In several reports for carcinosarcoma, the pelvic recurrence rate was 56%, while the distant metastasis rate was 45%. This represents a higher risk of pelvic recurrence than that seen in patients with LMS.[60,80–82,86] It also demonstrates that surgery alone, even for disease apparently confined to the uterus, is inadequate for control of disease in the pelvis. Some but not all studies have shown benefit from postoperative irradiation,[87,88] especially in local control.[60,84,88–93] Rates of distant metastases in series of patients treated with or without adjuvant pelvic irradiation are similar, in the order of 35–45%.[60,81,84]

There has been only one randomized clinical trial evaluating the role of adjuvant pelvic radiotherapy in stage I and II Uterine Sarcomas. The EORTC enrolled 224 patients(103 LMS, 91 carcinosarcoma, and 28 ESS) from 1998 to 2001 and demonstrated an improved local control rate for patients with carcinosarcoma (24% recurrence in RT vs 47% in observation) but no survival benefit. There was no improvement in local control for LMS (20% local recurrence in RT vs 24% in observation group).[93]

The morbidity associated with pelvic recurrence in uterine sarcomas may be substantial; therefore, it is reasonable to offer adjuvant pelvic irradiation to patients with carcinosarcoma to improve locoregional control rates. The doses of radiation have not been standardized; however, it is probable that doses should be at least 50 Gy, fractionated over 5 weeks.

The GOG[94] also conducted a phase III study of whole-abdomen irradiation (WAI) versus three cycles of cisplatin-ifosfamide and mesna (CIM) in 206 eligible patients with optimally debulked

Table 4 Single-agent activity in uterine sarcomas.

Drug	Prior chemotherapy	Schedule	Response, n (%)			References
			CS	LMS	ESS	
Ifosfamide	No	1.5 g/m²/d + mesna, 0.3 g/m²/d, d 1–5 q 4 weeks	9/28 (32)	6/35 (17)	7/21 (33)	97–99
Cisplatin	No	50 mg/m² q 3 weeks	12/63 (19)	1/33 (3)	—	100
	Yes	50 mg/m² q 3 weeks	5/28 (18)	1/19 (5)	—	101, 102
	No	75–100 mg/m² q 3 weeks	5/12 (42)	—	—	103
Doxorubicin	No	60 mg/m² q 3 weeks	4/41 (10)	7/28 (25)	—	96
	No	50–90 mg/m² q 3 weeks	0/9 (0)	—	—	104
Liposomal doxorubicin	No	50 mg/m² q 4 weeks	—	5/32 (16)	—	105
Etoposide	Yes	100 mg/m²/d, d 1–3 q 4 weeks	2/31 (6)	3/28 (11)	—	106
	Yes	50 mg/m²/d, d 1–21 q 4 weeks	—	2/29 (7)	—	107
	No	100 mg/m²/d, d 1–3 q 3 weeks	—	0/28 (0)	—	108
Mitoxantrone	Yes	12 mg/m² q 3 weeks	0/17 (0)	0/12 (0)	—	109
Paclitaxel	No	175 mg/m² q 3 weeks	—	3/34 (9)	—	110
Paclitaxel	Yes	170 mg/m² q 3 weeks	8/44 (18.)	—	—	111
Topotecan	No	1.5 mg/m²/d, d 1–5 q 3 weeks	—	3/36 (8)	—	112
Gemcitabine	Yes	1000 mg/m² d 1, 8, 15 q 4 weeks	—	9/44 (20.5)	—	113
Trabectedin	No	1.5 mg/m2 q 3 weeks	—	2/20 (10)	—	114
Docetaxel	No	100 mg/m² q 3 weeks	—	0/16 (0)	—	115

Abbreviations: ESS, endometrial stromal sarcoma; LMS , leiomyosarcoma; CS, carcinosarcoma.

stage I–IV carcinosarcoma. Although there was no significant advantage, the observed difference favored the use of chemotherapy. The adjusted recurrence rate was 21% lower for CIM patients and the adjusted death rate was 29% lower. Moreover, there was a significant increase in late adverse events in the WAI patients.[95]

Primary pelvic irradiation has been employed rarely in patients with sarcoma deemed inoperable. Literature reports suggest that in approximately half or two-thirds of patients, pelvic disease could be controlled with standard fractionated irradiation; a small proportion of patients are cured with such treatment.[60,80–82]

Finally, radiation may be useful as a palliative measure for recurrent or uncontrolled pelvic tumor causing pain or bleeding.

Chemotherapy

Two characteristics of uterine sarcomas increase the likelihood that systemic therapy will be required: a recurrence rate of at least 50% even in stage I disease and a tendency to recur at distant sites. Nevertheless, the amount of meaningful data on the use of systemic therapy is limited by the low incidence of these lesions. Studies by the GOG first identified the differential sensitivity of carcinosarcoma and LMS to drug therapy.[96] Because these two cell types respond differently to chemotherapy, they are discussed separately.

Single-agent therapy

Several drugs have been studied in advanced or recurrent carcinosarcoma and/or LMS (Tables 3 and 4), including cisplatin,[101,100,103,102] ifosfamide,[97–99] doxorubicin,[96,104] liposomal doxorubicin,[105] etoposide,[106–108] mitoxantrone,[109] paclitaxel,[110,111] topotecan,[112] gemcitabine,[113] trimetrexate,[116] and docetaxel.[117,115]

Carcinosarcoma

Ifosfamide is the most active single agent in the treatment of advanced or recurrent carcinosarcoma of the uterus with a 32.2% overall response rate in chemo-naïve patients.[97] Paclitaxil[111] and cisplatin[100] are the two other very active single agents with overall response rates of 18.2% and 18%, respectively.

Leiomyosarcoma

Of the single agents that have been tested in patients with LMS (Table 4), the most active are doxorubicin,[96] gemcitabine,[113] and ifosfamide[98] with response rates of 25%, 20.5%, and 17.2%, respectively.

Endometrial stromal sarcoma

There are few data in the gynecologic literature regarding the use of chemotherapy for ESS.[34,63,118] Ifosfamide[99] had an overall response rate of 33.3% in 21 women with metastatic ESS.

Combination chemotherapy

Leiomyosarcoma

The most active combination is Gemcitabine 900 mg/m² intravenously on days 1 and 8 plus docetaxel 100 mg/m² intravenously on day 8, with granulocyte colony-stimulating factor subcutaneously on days 9–15. The GOG conducted two phase II studies with this regimen with gemcitabine at a fixed dose rate of 10 mg/m²/min as first-line and second-line therapy for metastatic LMS. As initial therapy for metastatic uterine leiomyosarcoma, this combination achieved a 36% response rate among 42 patients and an additional 26% with stable disease.[119] This doublet achieved a 27% response rate in the second-line study among the 48 patients with an additional 50% with stable disease (median duration 5.4 months).[120]

The other very active combination is Adriamycin and ifosfamide. The GOG[121] reported a 30% response rate in 33 patients treated as first line with conventional doses of ifosfamide. Leyvraz et al.[122] achieved a 49% response rate in 37 patients treated with a dose-intensive regimen with ifosfamide, 10 g/m² as a continuous infusion over 5 days, plus doxorubicin intravenously, 25 mg/m²/day for 3 days.

Carcinosarcoma

In uterine carcinosarcoma, three randomized clinical trials have defined the best combination chemotherapy regimens. GOG-0108 evaluated the combination of ifosfamide-mesna with or without cisplatin as first-line therapy in patients with advanced, persistent, or recurrent uterine CS. The combination regimen demonstrated a significantly improved overall response rate (54%) when compared to the single-agent regimen (36%) but no survival advantage.

In the GOG-0161, there was a 31% decrease in the adjusted hazard of death and a 29% decrease in the adjusted hazard of progression in those patients receiving paclitaxel-ifosfamide/mesna-growth factor relative to ifosfamide alone for uterine CS.[123] Thus, paclitaxel/ifosfamide became the standard arm for future GOG studies testing combination chemotherapy for uterine CS.

The GOG Phase II trial (GOG-0232B) formally tested the efficacy of paclitaxil and carboplatin (T/C) in 55 patients with advanced uterine CS. The proportions of patients with confirmed complete and partial responses were 13% and 41%, respectively, resulting in a total overall response rate of 54% with a median progression-free survival of 7.0 months and median survival was 14.4 months.[124] Thus, the GOG current Phase III trial for uterine CS (GOG 261) was designed as a noninferiority trial to test the efficacy of T/C compared to paclitaxel/ifosfamide. The trial has completed accrual and it is expected that it will confirm paclitaxel and carboplatin to be the best backbone chemotherapy regimen for carcinosarcoma.

Adjuvant chemotherapy for limited disease

LMS
The role of adjuvant chemotherapy following complete resection of early stage uterine leiomyosarcoma is still under investigation but preliminary results of studies of adjuvant systemic chemotherapy are promising. The only randomized trial (GOG Protocol 20) of adjuvant chemotherapy in early stage uterine sarcomas to date assigned patients to either doxorubicin 60 mg/m² every 3 weeks for eight cycles or no further therapy. There were only 48 patients in the LMS subset and with these small numbers it was underpowered to assess a significant difference in recurrence or survival.[125]

The Sarcoma Alliance for Research through Collaboration conducted a phase II, multicenter study of four cycles of adjuvant fixed-dose-rate gemcitabine docetaxel followed by four cycles of doxorubicin in 47 patients with uterus-limited leiomyosarcoma. Although 78% of the patients remained progression free at 2 years, this dropped to 50% at the 3-year follow-up.[126] A phase III multicenter randomized trial (GOG 277) comparing gemcitabine and docetaxel followed by doxorubicin to the current standard approach of observation is currently being conducted.

Carcinosarcoma
The GOG also reported a study (GOG Protocol 117) of adjuvant ifosfamide, mesna, and cisplatin in 65 patients with completely resected stage I or II carcinosarcoma of the uterus in which no postoperative radiotherapy was allowed. Progression-free survival and OS rates, respectively, were 69% and 82% at 24 months and 54% and 52% at 84 months. The overall 5-year survival rate was 62%.[127] As more than half of the recurrences involved the pelvis, the study suggested that a combined sequential approach with chemotherapy and radiotherapy might be beneficial for this group of patients.

Hormone and biologic therapy
Receptors for estrogen and progesterone are identified in patients with uterine sarcoma.[45,128] Sutton and colleagues studied 43 patients with various uterine sarcomas and found ERs in 55.5% of the tumors and PRs in 55.8%.[128] The presence of receptors was not influenced by stage or grade, but levels were much higher and more prevalent in

patients with ESS of low grade, and this group of tumors frequently responds to progestational hormone treatment.[45,46,118,129–131] The cessation of estrogen replacement therapy and tamoxifen is also advised.[45,132]

Recent use of aromatase inhibitors[59,133] and gonadotropin-releasing hormone analogues[134] has been described in ESS, with dramatic and prolonged responses.[45,132,135] The addition of bevacizumab to fixed-dose rate gemcitabine-docetaxel failed to improve overall response rate, PFS, or OS in a GOG phase III trial of 102 chemo-naïve patients with metastatic uterine leiomyosarcoma.

Mullerian adenosarcomas
The term "mullerian adenosarcoma" was coined in 1974 for a distinctive uterine tumor characterized by a malignant, usually low-grade, stromal component, and a generally benign, but occasionally atypical, glandular epithelial component.[13] Most adenosarcomas arise in the endometrium and, rarely, in the endocervix, lower uterine segment, and myometrium.[14,136,137] In a Gynecologic Oncology Group study in 1993, adenosarcomas accounted for 7% of uterine sarcomas.[35] Uterine adenosarcoma occurs in all age groups but is most common in women after the menopause. In the largest reported series, the peak incidence was in the eighth decade with 38% occurring in patients aged below 50 years.[136] The most common presenting symptom is abnormal vaginal bleeding but some patients present with pelvic pain, an abdominal mass, or vaginal discharge.

Grossly, the majority are solitary polypoid masses with a spongy appearance secondary to the presence of small cysts.[14,136] Minimal histologic criteria were described by Clement and Scully[136] in a review of 100 cases of adenosarcoma published in 1990. They include at least one of the following: two or more stromal mitoses per 10 HPF, marked stromal hypercellularity, and significant stromal cell atypia. A minority of cases have "sarcomatous overgrowth," when more than 25% of the tumor is composed of pure sarcoma. In these cases, the sarcoma is typically high grade and the lesions are aggressive.[14,138] Most adenosarcomas without stromal overgrowth express ER and PR in the sarcomatous component and this may be used for therapeutic purposes. However, hormonal receptors are negative in adenosarcomas with stromal overgrowth.[14,139,140] Besides stromal overgrowth, the only other histopathological feature associated with decreased survival is myometrial invasion.[14,44,136,138,140]

Müllerian adenosarcomas have been described in extrauterine sites including the ovary and areas of endometriosis in the vagina, rectovaginal-septum, gastrointestinal tract, urinary bladder, pouch of Douglas, peritoneum, and liver.[14,137,140–142] Ovarian adenosarcomas are much more likely to exhibit malignant behavior than their uterine counterparts, probably owing to the lack of an anatomic barrier to peritoneal dissemination.[14,142]

Nonuterine gynecologic sarcomas

The vulva
Fewer than 500 patients with vulvar sarcoma have been described in the literature. LMS, rhabdomyosarcoma, and fibrosarcoma are the most frequently diagnosed vulvar tumors.[143] The clinical behavior of these tumors is related to their grade, mitotic count, histology, and stage.[143,144] For the lowest grade tumors, wide local excision should suffice. However, for the more aggressive histologic patterns, radical vulvectomy with lymphadenectomy followed by cytotoxic

chemotherapy should be considered, although the role of adjuvant chemotherapy has not been studied in these tumors.[144]

The vagina

Sarcomas represent 3% of primary vaginal cancers.[145] LMSs are the most common vaginal sarcoma in adults and present most commonly with vaginal bleeding in a patient above the age of 40. Although[146] this tumor is highly virulent, survivors are among those treated by hysterectomy, oophorectomy, and vaginectomy.

Embryonal rhabdomyosarcomas (RMS), formerly termed sarcoma botryoides, occur most frequently in children and have a typical grape cluster-like appearance. The disease was once uniformly fatal, provoking radical extirpative surgery that resulted in exenteration for young girls. Pediatric embryonal RMS of the vagina is best approached with induction multiagent-combination therapy, such as VAC, followed by local resection with or without brachytherapy, with radical surgery being reserved for those with persistent or recurrent disease.[147]

The ovary

Most types of sarcomas described in the vagina, vulva, or uterus have been found in the ovary as well.[148,149] Ovarian carcinosarcomas are rare and aggressive tumors, associated with a poor prognosis and accounts for only 1–4% of all ovarian cancer.[150] The mainstay of treatment remains maximal cytoreductive surgical effort for metastatic disease followed by platinum-based chemotherapy. Survival is better for patients with early stage disease and those whose tumors have homologous stromal elements.[150]

The fallopian tube

The fallopian tube is the least frequent site of primary sarcomas in the gynecologic tract. The most common histologic type is carcinosarcoma,[151,94,152–154] with treatment identical to ovarian carcinosarcomas with maximal cytoreduction for metastatic disease followed by platinum-based chemotherapy.[151]

Key references

The complete reference list can be found on the Wiley Companion Digital Edition of this title (see inside front cover for login instructions).

2 Kempson RL, Bari W. Uterine sarcomas. Classification, diagnosis, and prognosis. *Hum Pathol.* 1970;**1**(3):331–349.

3 Tavassoli FA, Devilee P. Tumors of the uterine corpus. In: *World Health Organization Classification of Tumours. Pathology and Genetics of Tumours of the Breast and Female Genital Organs.* Lyons: IARC Press; 2003:217–258.

4 Otis COAC, Nucci MR, McCluggage WG. Protocol for the Examination of Specimens from Patients with Sarcoma of the Uterus. College of American Pathologists 2013 [cited 2015 01/04/2015]; Available from: http://www.cap.org/apps/docs/committees/cancer/cancer_protocols/2013/UterineSarcomaProtocol_3000.pdf.

5 D'Angelo E, Prat J. Uterine sarcomas: a review. *Gynecol Oncol.* 2010;**116**(1):131–139. Epub 2009/10/27.

6 Harlow BL, Weiss NS, Lofton S. The epidemiology of sarcomas of the uterus. *J Natl Cancer Inst.* 1986;**76**(3):399–402.

13 Clement PB, Scully RE. Mullerian adenosarcoma of the uterus. A clinicopathologic analysis of ten cases of a distinctive type of mullerian mixed tumor. *Cancer.* 1974;**34**(4):1138–1149. Epub 1974/10/01.

14 McCluggage WG. Mullerian adenosarcoma of the female genital tract. *Adv Anat Pathol.* 2010;**17**(2):122–129. Epub 2010/02/25.

21 Chiang S, Ali R, Melnyk N, et al. Frequency of known gene rearrangements in endometrial stromal tumors. *Am J Surg Pathol.* 2011;**35**(9):1364–1372. Epub 2011/08/13.

30 Rose PG, Piver MS, Tsukada Y, Lau T. Patterns of metastasis in uterine sarcoma. An autopsy study. *Cancer.* 1989;**63**(5):935–938.

35 Major FJ, Blessing JA, Silverberg SG, et al. Prognostic factors in early-stage uterine sarcoma. A Gynecologic Oncology Group study. *Cancer.* 1993;**71**(4 **Suppl**):1702–1709.

44 Arend R, Bagaria M, Lewin SN, et al. Long-term outcome and natural history of uterine adenosarcomas. *Gynecol Oncol.* 2010;**119**(2):305–308. Epub 2010/08/07.

45 Amant F, Floquet A, Friedlander M, et al. Gynecologic Cancer InterGroup (GCIG) consensus review for endometrial stromal sarcoma. *Int J Gynecol Cancer.* 2014;**24**(9, **Suppl. 3**):S67–S72. Epub 2014/07/18.

46 Rauh-Hain JA, del Carmen MG. Endometrial stromal sarcoma: a systematic review. *Obstet Gynecol.* 2013;**122**(3):676–683. Epub 2013/08/08.

47 Leibsohn S, d'Ablaing G, Mishell DR Jr, Schlaerth JB. Leiomyosarcoma in a series of hysterectomies performed for presumed uterine leiomyomas. *Am J Obstet Gynecol.* 1990;**162**(4):968–974; discussion 74-6.

51 Goto A, Takeuchi S, Sugimura K, Maruo T. Usefulness of Gd-DTPA contrast-enhanced dynamic MRI and serum determination of LDH and its isozymes in the differential diagnosis of leiomyosarcoma from degenerated leiomyoma of the uterus. *Int J Gynecol Cancer.* 2002;**12**(4):354–361. Epub 2002/07/30.

65 Gadducci A, Cosio S, Romanini A, Genazzani AR. The management of patients with uterine sarcoma: a debated clinical challenge. *Crit Rev Oncol Hematol.* 2008;**65**(2):129–142. Epub 2007/08/21.

66 Wright JD, Tergas AI, Burke WM, et al. Uterine pathology in women undergoing minimally invasive hysterectomy using morcellation. *JAMA.* 2014;**312**(12):1253–1255. Epub 2014/07/23.

68 Park JY, Park SK, Kim DY, et al. The impact of tumor morcellation during surgery on the prognosis of patients with apparently early uterine leiomyosarcoma. *Gynecol Oncol.* 2011;**122**(2):255–259. Epub 2011/05/14.

69 Park JY, Kim DY, Kim JH, Kim YM, Kim YT, Nam JH. The impact of tumor morcellation during surgery on the outcomes of patients with apparently early low-grade endometrial stromal sarcoma of the uterus. *Ann Surg Oncol.* 2011;**18**(12):3453–3461. Epub 2011/05/05.

70 Aaro LA, Symmonds RE, Dockerty MB. Sarcoma of the uterus. A clinical and pathologic study of 177 cases. *Am J Obstet Gynecol.* 1966;**94**(1):101–109.

71 Garg G, Shah JP, Liu JR, et al. Validation of tumor size as staging variable in the revised International Federation of Gynecology and Obstetrics stage I leiomyosarcoma: a population-based study. *Int J Gynecol Cancer.* 2010;**20**(7):1201–1206. Epub 2010/10/14.

75 Silverberg SG, Major FJ, Blessing JA, et al. Carcinosarcoma (malignant mixed mesodermal tumor) of the uterus. A Gynecologic Oncology Group pathologic study of 203 cases. *Int J Gynecol Pathol.* 1990;**9**(1):1–19.

93 Reed NS, Mangioni C, Malmstrom H, et al. Phase III randomised study to evaluate the role of adjuvant pelvic radiotherapy in the treatment of uterine sarcomas stages I and II: an European Organisation for Research and Treatment of Cancer Gynaecological Cancer Group Study (protocol 55874). *Eur J Cancer.* 2008;**44**(6):808–818. Epub 2008/04/02.

95 Wolfson AH, Brady MF, Rocereto T, et al. A gynecologic oncology group randomized phase III trial of whole abdominal irradiation (WAI) vs. cisplatin-ifosfamide and mesna (CIM) as post-surgical therapy in stage I-IV carcinosarcoma (CS) of the uterus. *Gynecol Oncol.* 2007;**107**(2):177–185.

96 Omura GA, Major FJ, Blessing JA, et al. A randomized study of adriamycin with and without dimethyl triazenoimidazole carboxamide in advanced uterine sarcomas. *Cancer.* 1983;**52**(4):626–632.

114 Monk BJ, Blessing JA, Street DG, Muller CY, Burke JJ, Hensley ML. A phase II evaluation of trabectedin in the treatment of advanced, persistent, or recurrent uterine leiomyosarcoma: a Gynecologic Oncology Group study. *Gynecol Oncol.* 2012;**124**(1):48–52.

119 Hensley ML, Blessing JA, Mannel R, Rose PG. Fixed-dose rate gemcitabine plus docetaxel as first-line therapy for metastatic uterine leiomyosarcoma: a Gynecologic Oncology Group phase II trial. *Gynecol Oncol.* 2008;**109**(3):329–334. Epub 2008/06/07.

120 Hensley ML, Blessing JA, Degeest K, Abulafia O, Rose PG, Homesley HD. Fixed-dose rate gemcitabine plus docetaxel as second-line therapy for metastatic uterine leiomyosarcoma: a Gynecologic Oncology Group phase II study. *Gynecol Oncol.* 2008;**109**(3):323–328. Epub 2008/04/09.

122 Leyvraz S, Zweifel M, Jundt G, et al. Long-term results of a multicenter SAKK trial on high-dose ifosfamide and doxorubicin in advanced or metastatic gynecologic sarcomas. *Ann Oncol.* 2006;**17**(4):646–651. Epub 2006/02/28.

123 Homesley HD, Filiaci V, Markman M, et al. Phase III trial of ifosfamide with or without paclitaxel in advanced uterine carcinosarcoma: a Gynecologic Oncology Group Study. *J Clin Oncol.* 2007;**25**(5):526–531.

124 Powell MA, Filiaci VL, Rose PG, et al. Phase II evaluation of paclitaxel and carboplatin in the treatment of carcinosarcoma of the uterus: a Gynecologic Oncology Group study. *J Clin Oncol.* 2010;**28**(16):2727–2731. Epub 2010/04/28.

125 Omura GA, Blessing JA, Major F, et al. A randomized clinical trial of adjuvant adriamycin in uterine sarcomas: a Gynecologic Oncology Group Study. *J Clin Oncol.* 1985;**3**(9):1240–1245.

126 Hensley ML, Wathen JK, Maki RG, et al. Adjuvant therapy for high-grade, uterus-limited leiomyosarcoma: results of a phase 2 trial (SARC 005). *Cancer.* 2013;**119**(8):1555–1561. Epub 2013/01/22.

130 Cheng X, Yang G, Schmeler KM, et al. Recurrence patterns and prognosis of endometrial stromal sarcoma and the potential of tyrosine kinase-inhibiting therapy. *Gynecol Oncol*. 2011;**121**(2):323–327. Epub 2011/02/01.

136 Clement PB, Scully RE. Mullerian adenosarcoma of the uterus: a clinico-pathologic analysis of 100 cases with a review of the literature. *Hum Pathol*. 1990;**21**(4):363–381. Epub 1990/04/01.

142 Eichhorn JH, Young RH, Clement PB, Scully RE. Mesodermal (mullerian) adenosarcoma of the ovary: a clinicopathologic analysis of 40 cases and a review of the literature. *Am J Surg Pathol*. 2002;**26**(10):1243–1258. Epub 2002/10/03.

144 Curtin JP, Saigo P, Slucher B, Venkatraman ES, Mychalczak B, Hoskins WJ. Soft-tissue sarcoma of the vagina and vulva: a clinicopathologic study. *Obstet Gynecol*. 1995;**86**(2):269–272. Epub 1995/08/01.

147 Raney RB Jr, Gehan EA, Hays DM, et al. Primary chemotherapy with or without radiation therapy and/or surgery for children with localized sarcoma of the bladder, prostate, vagina, uterus, and cervix. A comparison of the results in Intergroup Rhabdomyosarcoma Studies I and II. *Cancer*. 1990;**66**(10):2072–2081. Epub 1990/11/15.

148 Oliva E, Egger JF, Young RH. Primary endometrioid stromal sarcoma of the ovary: a clinicopathologic study of 27 cases with morphologic and behavioral features similar to those of uterine low-grade endometrial stromal sarcoma. *Am J Surg Pathol*. 2014;**38**(3):305–315. Epub 2014/02/15.

149 Lan C, Huang X, Lin S, Cai M, Liu J. Endometrial stromal sarcoma arising from endometriosis: a clinicopathological study and literature review. *Gynecol Obstet Invest*. 2012;**74**(4):288–297. Epub 2012/09/19.

150 del Carmen MG, Birrer M, Schorge JO. Carcinosarcoma of the ovary: a review of the literature. *Gynecol Oncol*. 2012;**125**(1):271–277. Epub 2011/12/14.

151 Yokoyama Y, Yokota M, Futagami M, Mizunuma H. Carcinosarcoma of the fallopian tube: report of four cases and review of literature. *Asia Pac J Clin Oncol*. 2012;**8**(3):303–311. Epub 2012/08/18.

108 Neoplasms of the breast

Hope S. Rugo, MD ▪ Melanie Majure, MD ▪ Anthony Dragun, MD ▪ Meredith Buxton, PhD ▪ Laura Esserman, MD, MBA

Overview

Breast cancer in women remains a major medical problem with significant public health and societal ramifications, including issues related to screening, risk factors, prevention, diagnosis, treatment, and survival following diagnosis. Major advances have markedly improved the understanding of clinical phenotypes, as well as the biologic pathways that drive tumor growth and resistance. This research has led to dramatic changes in treatment that have contributed to a significant reduction in breast cancer mortality over the last two decades, and is the basis of ongoing clinical research. Molecular profiling has provided insights into the heterogeneity of breast cancer subtypes; combining biology and tumor burden has allowed stratification of both risk and treatment to begin the process of individualizing screening, prevention, and treatment. As new information accumulates, new paradigms of management become the standard of care reflected in international guidelines. Our challenge is to apply new formation and treatment appropriately and effectively, and to understand both response and resistance. Information obtained from molecular, biologic, and pathologic investigations and clinical trials provides the major focus of this chapter.

Epidemiology

Breast cancer is the most common malignancy in North American women and in women throughout the industrialized world. In the United States, breast cancer accounts for 29% of all cancers in women. The American Cancer Society (ACS) estimated 231,840 women to be diagnosed with breast cancer in 2015.[1]

The lifetime risk for a woman being diagnosed with breast cancer is 1 in 8 or 12%.[2] Age-specific probabilities of developing breast cancer are provided in Table 1. This risk is even higher for women with certain risk factors, such as a strong family history or known genetic mutations. These figures exclude the 64,640 expected cases of in situ breast cancer. In addition, 2350 men are expected to be diagnosed with breast cancer.

The incidence of breast cancer increased about 30% between 1980 and the late 1990s in Western countries, with a marked decline between 2002 and 2003. This increase in diagnosis was attributed to increased screening, as well as to increased use of postmenopausal hormone replacement therapy (HRT) and changes in reproductive factors. In 2002, the first results of the Women's Health Initiative Trial were published, revealing a significant increase in the risk of breast cancer in postmenopausal women undergoing HRT. These results led to a major decrease in the use of HRT, and correspondingly between 2002 and 2003, breast cancer rates dropped 7%, primarily affecting Caucasian women aged 55 and higher.[4,5] Since 2004, the incidence of breast cancer in the United States has been relatively stable.[2,3] It varies significantly by race and ethnicity, as described in Table 2. However, rates between white and African–American women in the United States are now converging (see below).[3]

Breast cancer is the most frequently diagnosed cancer in women worldwide. In 2012, it was estimated that 1.7 million cases would be diagnosed, accounting for 25% of all cancer cases in women.[6] The rates vary by geographic region, with about one-half of the incidences occurring in more developed countries, with generally higher rates found in Northern America, Australia/New Zealand, and Northern and Western Europe. By contrast, the rates are intermediate in Central and Eastern Europe, Latin American, the Caribbean, and Western Asia, and low in most of Africa and Southern and Eastern Asia. The cumulative risk of developing breast cancer in less developed areas is a 3.3% (until age 74) compared to an 8% risk in more developed areas. The variation in international incidence rates is likely due to differences in risk factors as well as the availability of early detection methods.[7] The incidence of breast cancer has been increasing in many countries in Asia, South America, and Africa, possibly because of changes in lifestyle, including reproductive patterns, diet, obesity, and physical activity.[6,8]

The mortality rate from breast cancer in the United States slowly increased by 0.4% from 1975 to 1990, then decreased by 34% from 1990 to 2010.[3] This decrease has been attributed to improvements in treatment as well as early detection,[9] with the largest decrease in women below 50 years of age (an annual decrease of 3.1% vs 1.9% in those aged 50 years and higher). Breast cancer is the second leading cause of cancer-related deaths in women in the United States (after lung cancer) and the leading cause of cancer death in those between the ages of 20 and 59. The ACS estimated 40,290 deaths of women from breast cancer in 2015, representing 6.8% of all cancer deaths in the United States. Mortality rates vary by race and ethnicity with African-American women experiencing the highest annual breast cancer death rate, despite having a lower incidence rate than white women. This difference has been attributed to variations in biologic subtype, later stage of disease at diagnosis, and poorer survival by stage, driven in large part by differences in socioeconomic status. Death rates declined in almost all racial and ethnic groups from 2001 to 2010, with a much higher reduction in white than African-American women.

A majority of breast cancers are diagnosed at an early stage, with 61% diagnosed when the disease is localized to the breast; another 32% are diagnosed after the cancer has spread to the regional lymph nodes and only 6% have metastasized at the time of initial diagnosis. Five year survival rates depend on the stage of tumor detection, with 98.6% alive when diagnosed at a localized stage, 84.9% alive when the tumor has spread to regional lymph nodes, and only 26% when diagnosed with distant spread of disease.

Risk factors

Although breast cancer is common, the risk of developing the disease varies depending on a number of factors, with female gender

Holland-Frei Cancer Medicine, Ninth Edition. Edited by Robert C. Bast Jr., Carlo M. Croce, William N. Hait, Waun Ki Hong, Donald W. Kufe, Martine Piccart-Gebhart, Raphael E. Pollock, Ralph R. Weichselbaum, Hongyang Wang, and James F. Holland.
© 2017 John Wiley & Sons, Inc. ISBN: 978-1-118-93469-2

Table 1 Age-specific probabilities of developing invasive breast cancer (cancers diagnosed in females of all races between 2008 and 2010).

Current age	Probability of developing breast cancer in the next 10 years (%)	Corresponding to a risk of
20	0.06	1 in 1732
30	0.44	1 in 228
40	1.45	1 in 69
50	2.31	1 in 43
60	3.49	1 in 29
70	3.84	1 in 26
Lifetime risk	12.29	1 in 8

Source: DeSantis 2014.[3] Reproduced with permission of Wiley.

and increasing age being the most important ones. Germline mutations in DNA repair genes markedly increase the lifetime risk of developing breast and other cancers and increase the risk at younger ages. Other lifestyle-related factors have a more modest impact on risk, and the effect of altering modifiable factors on an individual's risk of developing breast cancer is largely unknown.[10] The risk factors associated with the development of breast cancer are clearly defined in Table 3.

Gender

The incidence rate of age-adjusted breast cancer is more than 100-fold higher in women than in men in the United States, a ratio that is similar worldwide. Male breast cancer represents less than 1% of all cancer in men and about 1% of all breast cancer. Germline mutations in BRCA1 and BRCA2 are the best understood risk factors for breast cancer in men, with a range of lifetime risk of just over 1% (BRCA1) to almost 7% (BRCA2). Worldwide, mortality has decreased less in men than women, and clinical trials have been unsuccessful to date because of low accrual. An international consortium has recently started collaborative clinical trials focusing on male breast cancer.

Age

The median age of breast cancer diagnosis in women in the United States is 61, with the majority of cases diagnosed in women between the ages of 55 and 64. In other parts of the world, where life expectancy is shorter, the median age of development of breast cancer is 10–15 years younger. Age-related mortality rates parallel this pattern.

Socioeconomic class

Breast cancer is diagnosed more frequently in women of higher economic class and educational status.[10,11] This finding is likely related to lifestyle factors such as diet, age at first childbirth, exogenous hormonal use, and alcohol consumption. However, mortality is higher in women of lower socioeconomic classes, correlating with observed differences including higher stage at diagnosis, more aggressive tumor biology, and reduced access to care.

Ethnicity

The incidence and mortality rates of breast cancer vary considerably by ethnicity and race, as outlined in Table 2. In the United States,

from 2010 to 2012, the risk of being diagnosed with and dying from breast cancer was 12.64% and 2.66% for whites, 11.14% and 3.26% for blacks, 10.25% and 1.74% for Asian/Pacific Islanders, 9.81% and 2.08% for Hispanics, and 8.15% and 1.66% for American Indians/Alaskans.[1] Studies of migrant populations showed that when people living in low-risk geographic areas move to high-risk areas (e.g., a move from Asia to the United States), their incidence of breast cancer increases, approaching the rates of the host population within one to two generations, suggesting an important role of lifestyle in determination of risk even within ethnic and racial groups.[12]

Family history and genetic mutations

Family history is a significant risk factor for breast cancer, but existing data are complicated by associations established before routine genetic testing (see below).[13] In general, compared with a woman with no affected relatives, a single affected first-degree relative approximately doubles the risk. Two first-degree relatives triple the risk, and three or more quadruples the risk. A first-degree relative affected at an early age increases risk further to about threefold, twofold, and 1.5-fold if diagnosed below 40 years, from 40 to 59 years, and from 50 to 60 years of age, respectively. There is little impact from breast cancer diagnosed at older ages unless multiple family members are diagnosed.

Individuals inheriting a germline mutation in either BRCA1 or BRCA2 have a markedly higher lifetime risk of breast and ovarian cancers than the general population. The risk of developing breast cancer is estimated to be 50–85% in women and is often at a younger age of onset.[14] There is also an increased risk of second primary breast cancers, estimated to be about 40–60%. These mutations are inherited by autosomal dominant transmission, and more than 2000 different mutations, polymorphisms, and variants have been reported in BRCA1 on chromosome 17 and BRCA2 on chromosome 13.[15,16] There is clearly a higher risk of carrying a mutation in populations with homogeneous ethnicity, such as those with Ashkenazi Jewish heritage, with associated characteristic BRCA1 (185delAG, 5382insC) and BRCA2 (6174delT) mutations; the combined frequency of these genes in the general population exceeds 2%.[17–19] Similar "founder" mutations have been identified in Belgium, Denmark, Finland, France, Holland, Hungary, Iceland, Norway, Russia, and West Africa, among other ethnic communities.[20] The BRCA genes encode DNA repair enzymes that play a major role in double-stranded DNA repair through the homologous recombination pathway. The resulting defect in DNA repair in cells with dysfunctional BRCA activity has been currently used to design specific therapies such as PARP inhibitors that further damage DNA, leading to tumor cell death (see treatment sections).

Familial breast cancer accounts for less than 10% of all breast cancers, and BRCA1- and BRCA2-related familial breast cancers appear to be responsible for only about two-thirds of these cases. A number of other genes have been identified, which increase the risk of developing breast and other cancers, including TP53 (Li–Fraumeni syndrome), PTEN (Cowden syndrome), ATM, CHECK2 and PALB2, as well as others.[21–25] A large number (>75) of more common risk variants (>5%) have been identified by

Table 2 Rates by race or ethnicity: United States, 2007–2011.

	Non-Hispanic White	African-American	Hispanic-Latino	American Indian/Alaskan Native	Asian/Pacific Islander
Incidence rates (per 100,000)	127.6	123.0	86	91.7	86.0
Mortality rates (per 100,000)	22.2	31.4	14.5	15.2	11.3

Source: Siegel 2015.[1] Reproduced with permission of Wiley.

Table 3 Risk factors associated with the development of breast cancer.

Major increase
Mutations in *BRCA1, BRCA2*, tp53 (Li–Fraumeni syndrome)
Increasing age
Developed countries
Family history of breast or ovarian cancer in first-degree relatives
Atypical hyperplasia, LCIS before the age of 45
Exposure to ionizing radiation
Moderate increase
Prior diagnosis of breast cancer
Early menarche
Late menopause
Nulliparity or delayed first full-term pregnancy (above age 30)
High socioeconomic status
Alcohol intake
Atypical hyperplasia, LCIS over the age of 45
Obesity (postmenopausal women only)
High breast density
Diagnosis of soft-tissue sarcoma in son or daughter
Prior diagnosis of uterine, ovarian, or colon cancer
Modest increase
Benign breast disease with hyperplasia (no atypia)
Oral contraceptives (for longer than 10 years)
Postmenopausal estrogen replacement therapy
Questionable increase (no evidence to support)
Interrupted first pregnancy
High-fat diet
Complex fibroadenoma
Decrease
Full-term pregnancy before age 20
Multiple pregnancies
Ovariectomy before age 45
Regular exercise, particularly during adolescence and early adulthood
Breast-feeding
No effect
Breast reduction

genome-wide association studies (GWAS) over the last decade and validated by large consortia[26,27] that have a moderate impact on risk [relative risk (RR) < 1.5].[28] While being individually associated with a modest effect on breast cancer, in combination they can contribute substantially to overall risk.

Interestingly, certain breast cancer phenotypes have been associated with specific mutations, although all phenotypes have been reported. Triple-negative [estrogen receptor (ER) and progesterone receptor (PR) and HER2/neu nonamplified] tumors occur more frequently in women with BRCA1 mutations, hormone receptor-positive (HR+) tumors in those with mutations in BRCA2 or CHEK2, and HER2/neu and HR+ in those with the Li–Fraumeni syndrome.[29,30] Importantly, many of the common risk alleles are more strongly associated with the development of HR+ breast cancer.[28,31] A total of seven variants are associated with the more aggressive hormone receptor-negative (HR−) disease,[32] with four new loci recently identified.[33] Multigene testing panels are now widely available and have the potential to detect an additional 4% of individuals with potentially deleterious mutations, for whom counseling and testing may be of value.[34]

The National Comprehensive Cancer Network® (NCCN®) recommends that patients with a personal history of breast cancer and one or more of the following should be tested for germline mutations: A family history of a deleterious mutation in BRCA1 or BRCA2, diagnosis at age ≤45, diagnosis at age ≤50 with an additional primary cancer, ≥1 close blood relative with breast cancer at any age, an unknown or limited family history, or diagnosis at age ≤ 60 with triple-negative breast cancer (TNBC). Additional criteria include patients diagnosed at any age with breast cancer and ≥1 close blood relative with breast cancer diagnosed ≤50 or

ovarian cancer, ≥2 close blood relatives with breast cancer or with pancreatic cancer and/or prostate cancer at any age. Patients with a personal history of ovarian cancer, male breast cancer, as well as several other criteria are also included in this recommendation. In general, testing should first be performed on the affected family member with testing for those without a cancer diagnosis reserved for situations when the affected family member is not available for testing.[378] One recent series of more than 200 patients with TNBC found BRCA mutations in 15.4%; this rate increased to 18.3% in those meeting NCCN Clinical Practice Guidelines In Oncology (NCCN Guidelines®) for screening; rates vary based on age, ethnicity, and race.[35]

Additional criteria for genetic screening include diagnosis at any age with breast cancer; a close blood relative with ovarian cancer, pancreatic cancer, or prostate cancer; or any male relative with breast cancer. Those with ethnicities associated with higher mutation frequency should always be considered for testing. Indeed, one trial found that approximately 12% of breast cancers in Ashkenazic women could be attributed to mutations in BRCA1 or BRCA2.[17]

Identification of germline mutations in women with breast cancer, and in women at risk for mutations, is extremely important. Screening and risk-reducing surgery have been found to reduce mortality from cancer.[36-39] Educating people about these strategies as well as the mechanism of identifying tumors is critical.

Endocrine and reproductive risk factors

Duration and extent of exposure to estrogen and progesterone clearly affects the risk of developing breast cancer, regardless of subtype. Longer duration of ovulation, as indicated by earlier age of menarche, and later age at menopause are associated with an annual increase of 3–4% in the risk of breast cancer.[11] Younger age at first childbirth decreases the risk of breast cancer about 3% per year from age 30 to 20, with multiparity having a lesser protective effect. Women having their first child at age >30 years have a higher risk of breast cancer than nulliparous women, particularly within the first 5 years after delivery. The possible mechanism for this apparent enhancement in risk might be the stimulatory effect of pregnancy (and its altered hormonal environment) on an otherwise involuting epithelium. Prolonged breast-feeding appears to reduce risk, with short durations providing little impact and with higher protection when lactation is at younger ages.[40] In a recent meta-analysis, each birth decreased the RR of breast cancer by 7%, and each year of breast-feeding decreased the RR by an additional 4.3%.[41]

Exogenous hormones

Although controversial for many years, results from the large Women's Health Initiative randomized controlled trial provided definitive evidence of the risks associated with postmenopausal HRT with combined estrogen and progesterone. In this study, 16,608 postmenopausal, otherwise healthy, women were randomly assigned to conjugated estrogen plus medroxy progesterone acetate or placebo.[42] The combined estrogen and progesterone arm was stopped in July 2002 after a median 5.6 years of follow-up, because health risks exceeded health benefits. There were a 29% increase in coronary heart disease, 26% increase in breast cancer, 41% increase in stroke, and 13% increase in pulmonary embolism associated with HRT. Simultaneously, there were a 47% reduction in colorectal cancer and 34% reduction in hip fractures among women on hormonal replacement. No protective effect was found for memory loss or other measures of intellectual function. Although risk decreased right after stopping HRT, the overall increased risk persisted during long-term follow-up. The Million Women Study and the HERS II study reached similar conclusions.[43-45]

The United States Preventive Services Task Force (USPSTF) concluded that the harmful effects of combined estrogen and progestin exceed the prevention of chronic disease effects in most women. Although short-term use of HRT might be beneficial for control of vasomotor symptoms related to menopause, long-term use is not indicated.

The use of oral contraceptives has long been associated with a slight increased risk of breast cancer. A recent large study of a US health care delivery system in women between the ages of 20 and 49 years has found increased risk in recent users taking high-dose estrogen preparations, but not in those taking low-dose estrogen contraceptives.[46] Risk does not appear to be sustained after cessation of use.

Exercise and obesity

There is convincing evidence that lack of physical activity is a risk factor for postmenopausal breast cancer and that active women have a relative reduction in breast cancer risk.[47,48] This benefit is clearly modified by weight, with little to no benefit from exercise seen in obese women. In the Women's Health Initiative, women engaging in regular strenuous exercise at age 35 had a 14% relative decrease of risk of breast cancer. Even 1.25–2.5 h per week of brisk walking was associated with an 18% relative decrease in breast cancer risk compared with sedentary women, with a slightly higher risk reduction in those who reported an additional 10 h of brisk walking or equivalent exercise per week.[49]

A high body mass index (>25 kg/m^2), particularly when associated with weight gain after menopause and abdominal obesity, has been clearly associated with an increased risk of postmenopausal breast cancer.[10,50–52] The RR for postmenopausal women is about 1.5 for those with a body mass index > 25 and 2 for those who are obese (body mass index > 30). In the Women's Health Initiative trials, obesity was also associated with an increased risk of HR+ breast cancer and more advanced disease at diagnosis.[53] The data in premenopausal women are more complicated, without a clear relationship between weight and risk of breast cancer.[54]

Higher physical activity and reduced body mass index have been associated with lower relative levels of estradiol and estrone as well as serum insulin levels, which may in part explain the impact of exercise on breast cancer risk.[55–57] The ACS has published guidelines on exercise and nutrition to reduce cancer risk.[58,59] Adherence to these guidelines has been associated with lower risk of breast cancer.[54]

Metformin and diabetes mellitus

In the Women's Health Initiative, use of metformin in diabetic women reduced the risk of breast cancer.[60] Metformin is known to increase insulin sensitivity and reduce hyperinsulinemia, and hyperinsulinemia has been associated with carcinogenesis and proliferation in preclinical models.[61] In addition, signaling through expression of the insulin-like growth factor receptor is related to both proliferation and therapeutic resistance in breast cancer, and metformin may inhibit downstream signaling through the mammalian target of rapamycin (mTOR).[62–65] Diabetes mellitus has been associated with a higher risk of breast cancer in some studies, but not in others; however, it is more clearly shown to worse outcome after diagnosis of breast cancer.[52,66–69] Metformin is currently being tested in women with early-stage breast cancer (ESBC) in a multicenter clinical trial.[70,71]

Breast density

Breast density is a common and significant risk factor for breast cancer across ethnicities and is inversely associated with age and body mass index.[72–76] Numerous state laws require reporting of breast density information to women at the time of screening mammography.[75] The highest quartile of breast density appears to have significantly elevated risk, with a 4.5- to 5-fold higher risk than those with the least dense breast tissue. Using the density reported on standard mammography (1, 2, 3, and 4 relating to fatty, scattered fibroglandular, heterogeneous, and homogeneous densities, respectively), studies reproducibly show strong correlation with breast cancer risk. The impact of breast density is modified by individual risk factors, as measured by the Breast Cancer Surveillance Consortium (BCSC) 5-year risk model, where women at moderate or high risk for breast cancer using this model and extremely high density had the highest risk for interval cancer.[76] The hazard ratio for interval cancer cases was 1.62 for those with high or very high BCSC 5-year risk and extremely dense breasts, rising to 3.45 in those aged 70–74 years. A risk model has been developed for this purpose combining the BCSC risk model and breast density and benign breast disease (BBD), which can assist in accurately identifying high-risk women who might be eligible for primary prevention.[70] The Gail Risk model for estimating 5-year and lifetime risks for breast cancer has also been modified by using a multiplier of breast density and Gail model risk, with a modest impact on breast cancer risk assessment.[77,78] In addition, these patients could possibly be referred for additional imaging, although to date there have been no definitive data that alternate imaging modalities will provide better information and improve cancer detection, stage at diagnosis or breast cancer specific survival.

Alcohol

Numerous studies suggest that alcohol increases the risk of breast cancer. This is thought to be due to increased serum and tissue concentrations of estradiol mediated by the impact of ethanol on hepatic clearance. Alcohol was associated with a modest increase in risk of breast cancer in the Women's Health Initiative observational study, with the maximum increase observed with the highest daily consumption. This impact appeared to be subtype specific.[79] When compared with women who never drink, those who were reported to consume more than seven drinks per week had almost a twofold increased risk of invasive lobular cancer (hazard ratio 1.82 with a 95% confidence interval (CI) of 1.18–2.81), but there was no difference in the risk of invasive ductal cancer, even when both subtypes were HR+.

Radiation exposure

Exposure to ionizing radiation is a known risk factor for breast cancer. Atomic bomb survivors and patients treated in the past with irradiation for postpartum mastitis, acne, hirsutism, or arthritic conditions and repeated fluoroscopic chest radiography used to monitor tuberculosis have an increased incidence of breast cancer, even after low or moderate radiation doses.[80,81] Survivors of Hodgkin's disease who received radiation therapy to the chest in adolescence or at a young age, particularly when the radiation was combined with chemotherapy, have a marked increase in breast cancer risk.[82] The latency period between radiation exposure and development of breast cancer is long, with a median of 30 years although this time is shorter in those treated with both radiation and chemotherapy. The risk of developing breast cancer as a result of common diagnostic radiologic procedures is minimal, and radiology technicians do not have an increased incidence of breast cancer.[83] Recent evidence has suggested that therapeutic radiation administered to treat primary breast cancer modestly increases (~30%) the risk of developing contralateral breast cancer more than 5 years after treatment.[84]

Table 4 Relative risk[a] of invasive breast carcinoma based on histologic examination of breast tissue without carcinoma.

No increased risk (no proliferative disease)
Adenosis
Apocrine change
Duct ectasia
Mild epithelial hyperplasia of usual type
Slightly increased risk (1.5–2 times) (proliferative disease without atypia)
Hyperplasia of usual type, moderate, or florid
Papilloma (probably)
Sclerosing adenosis
Moderately increased risk (4–5 times) (atypical hyperplasia or borderline lesion)
Atypical ductal hyperplasia
Atypical lobular hyperplasia
High risk (8–10 times) (carcinoma in situ)[b]
Lobular carcinoma in situ—both breasts
Ductal carcinoma in situ (noncomedo)—unilateral, local

[a]Women in each category are compared with women matched for age who have had no breast biopsies for the risk of invasive breast cancer during the ensuing 10–20 years. These risks are not lifetime risks.
[b]Only smaller examples of noncomedo ductal carcinoma have consistently been assessed as risk indicators after biopsy only.
Source: Dupont 1985.[86]

Benign breast disease

Most forms of BBD appear to be unrelated to an increased breast cancer risk, and the majority of women with lumpy breasts and most of those with BBD do not have a significantly increased risk of breast cancer.

However, a number of studies, including a recent meta-analysis, suggest that the presence (or history) of BBD, particularly in those with a previous biopsy for benign disease, is associated with an increase in breast cancer risk.[85] This association is generally limited to biopsy-proven lesions with histologic atypia or proliferation (atypical ductal or lobular hyperplasia) (Table 4).[87,88] When compared with women who never had a breast biopsy, women with BBD without hyperplasia had an odds ratio of developing breast cancer of 1.5, women with hyperplasia without atypia had an odds ratio of 1.9, and women with hyperplasia and atypia had an odds ratio of 2.6–5.3, and this increased to 11 in women with both atypia and family history.[86,89] A study from Mayo Clinic on 9087 women with BBD suggested that the combination of young age (<45 years) and atypia had a hazard ratio of 6.99 for developing breast cancer.[88] The importance of identifying this risk factor is the ability to significantly reduce risk using chemoprevention with hormone therapy and to use a risk-based screening approach.[87,88]

Other

Bisphosphonates

The use of oral bisphosphonates has been associated with a reduced risk of invasive breast cancer, particularly the incidence of HR+ disease.[90–92] Osteoporosis may be a marker for lower postmenopausal exposure to estrogen and has been associated with lower breast cancer risk, and hence the possibility of interaction between this variable and the cancer-inhibiting effects of bisphosphonates exists.[93,94] A recent meta-analysis suggested a 15% RR reduction in any breast cancer and 32% RR reduction in invasive disease, with the benefit seen in patients who used bisphosphonates for more than 1 year compared with nonusers.[95]

Calcium and vitamin D

Although previous studies supported a possible role of vitamin D and calcium in reducing breast cancer incidence, subsequent studies have failed to find an association between risk of breast cancer and dietary intake.[96] A large study showed a lower breast density in younger women taking supplemental vitamin D, and another demonstrated a possible impact in women with the highest mammographic breast density.[93,94]

Other dietary factors

A diet high in animal fat and low in fruits and vegetables has been associated with a higher risk of breast cancer. However, this is closely related to additional factors such as exercise and body fat. A primary prevention trial was conducted in more than 48,000 postmenopausal women without a history of breast cancer.[97] Women in the intervention group were assigned to a diet with low total fat intake (20% of energy) and consumption of five to six servings of vegetables, fruits, and grains daily. At 8 years of follow-up, there was no reduction in invasive breast cancer risk, but a trend toward decreased risk in the most adherent group was shown. Given that this diet is also associated with reduction in a number of other comorbid conditions and that a longer intervention might have more impact, this seems a reasonable and easily applied lifestyle modification.

Breast cancer risk assessment models

Statistical models can be used to estimate a woman's risk of breast cancer. Some models predict the risk of developing breast cancer framing both short-term and lifetime risk. The models are highly dependent on the age of the person; thus, a very low short-term risk for a young woman may be accompanied by a high lifetime risk. The Gail Risk Assessment model[98–100] and the Claus model[101] are the most frequently used models to predict a woman's risk of breast cancer.[102] Other models such as BRCAPRO,[103] Frank,[104] and Couch[105] predict the risk or probability of carrying a genetic mutation. These models should be used to guide decisions to perform genetic testing for the presence of cancer-causing mutations in *BRCA1* or *BRCA2*. They do not identify the risk of developing cancer; rather, prediction will depend on the results of the test aiming at determining inherited predisposition for breast cancer. The interpretation of the results of genetic testing depends on knowing whether the proband (person with a cancer) is the one being tested and whether a known cancer-causing mutation is present in the family. Over the past 5 years, new models have emerged that include breast density, exposures, family history, and single nucleotide polymorphisms such as the Breast Cancer Surveillance Consortium model has been validated in over 1 million women.[106]

Gail model

The Gail Risk Assessment model is the most commonly used statistical model for estimating the risk of developing breast cancer in women undergoing annual screening. Gail and colleagues used data from 284,780 predominantly white women in 28 participating centers of the Breast Cancer Detection Demonstration Project to develop the model. This is an unconditional logistic regression model based on the relationship between risk in a woman with specified risk factors and the risk in a woman with no risk factors. Risk factors used in this model include age, age at menarche, age at first live birth, number of first-degree relatives with breast cancer (mother, sisters, or daughters only), number of breast biopsies, and breast pathology exhibiting atypical hyperplasia.

The Gail model is applicable to the largest number of women. A score of 1.67 (which is the average 5-year Gail score for a 60-year-old woman) was used as the minimum risk criterion to join the National Surgical Adjuvant Breast and Bowel Project (NSABP) P-01 prevention trial in the United States. The Gail Risk model has been currently used widely for clinical decision making for individual patients, with many forms of access (National Cancer Institute's Web site, handheld, and computer applications). It is good at predicting the risk for a population, but a cutoff of 1.67 does not show high discriminatory power.[107] Ozanne and colleagues developed improved methods for incorporating Gail Risk by comparing a woman's Gail Risk in context with other women. Being able to show women that they are in the highest quartile or decile of risk is much more discriminatory and much more helpful in identifying truly high-risk women.[108] A limitation of the model is the treatment of family history: neither paternal family history of breast cancer nor age at onset in affected relatives is accounted for in the model. As described earlier, a multiplier can be used to incorporate breast density with subsequent improvement in predictive performance of the model.[74,109]

The BCSC model, a similar tool that incorporates BI-RADS breast density, exhibited a better risk discrimination and calibration than the Gail model in a multiethnic cohort of more than one million American women.[74] Neither Gail nor BCSC incorporates modern knowledge of genetic risk factors. The addition of polygenic risk (76 single nucleotide polymorphisms) improved the performance of the BCSC model, including density and polygenic risk. Other models have also been developed to include multiple risk factors, including family history, more comprehensive genetic factors, and exposures.[100,103,184-186]

Hereditary models

Models such as BRCAPRO,[101] Frank,[102] and Couch[103] are designed to predict the chance of carrying a BRCA1 or BRCA2 mutation based on an autosomal dominant pattern of inheritance and the incidence of mutations within high-risk populations, and the BRCAPRO model also predicts the risk for developing breast and ovarian cancer as a separate output. The models are based on multiple variables in both maternal and paternal cancer history, including age of diagnosis, multiple primary cancers, bilateral breast cancer, Ashkenazi Jewish ancestry, and the number of first-, second-, and third-degree relatives with breast cancer. The BRCAPRO model also includes ovarian and pancreatic cancers. This high-risk category rarely occurs.

The hereditary models are used clinically for women with a positive family history of breast cancer and are discriminatory and well calibrated for predicting the presence of a *BRCA* mutation. It is predicted that at most, 10–15% of diagnosed breast cancers are in women with either *BRCA1* or *BRCA2* GENE mutations. BRCAPRO performs well in predicting mutations in families of African-American descent similarly to Caucasian families. It has been suspected that approximately 20% of breast cancers are caused by unidentified hereditary factors. Indeed, the use of clinical genetic testing with panels of multiple genes known to be associated with hereditary breast or ovarian cancer is identifying patients who carry a mutation in one of these less common genes. This, in turn, increases the percentage of breast cancers that are related to hereditary factors. The remaining 70% are thought to be sporadic or nonhereditary cancers.

Biomarkers

Germline mutations such as BRCA1 and BRCA2 (BRCA1/2) predict lifetime risk and risk at a younger age. However, there are no tests that are predictive for a specific age of onset, or the short-term risk of developing breast cancer. Understanding individual risk at specific time points will help design effective screening and prevention strategies and will also provide markers for the effectiveness of preventive strategies. These markers would need to be modifiable

like risk factors. Potential modifiable risk factors include atypia and breast density. The presence of atypia has also been shown to predict a higher benefit from the use of tamoxifen, with a risk reduction of up to 89% in the NSABP P-1 study.[110] Multiple investigators are conducting biomarker studies to determine whether these markers are reliable surrogate markers that change in response to interventions.[111] How would these biomarkers then be used to test prevention interventions? Agents such as selective estrogen modifiers or aromatase inhibitors (AIs) that are known to target ER-positive disease can be used to treat women with cytologically documented atypia and the impact of the intervention measured by reduction in atypia. Change in breast density can also be measured over the course of the treatment (6–12 months) and used as a surrogate to better define those populations most likely to benefit from preventive interventions. Other modifiable risks include exercise, diet, and weight. The use of frameworks for communicating risk and shared decision making for risk reduction is critical.[112-114]

Regulation of breast cancer growth

Understanding the basis for the development and regulation of breast cancer growth provides us with a foundation for developing strategies for breast cancer prevention and treatment. The adult female breast is composed of epithelial lactiferous ducts terminating in secretory alveoli embedded in a fibrous tissue framework and fat. Normal breast growth and development are regulated by the complex interaction of many hormones and growth factors, some of which are secreted by the mammary cells themselves and may have autocrine functions. Estradiol regulates the expression of several genes corresponding to peptides and proteins involved in mammary cell growth control mechanisms. Binding to specific receptors triggers effects of these growth factors and hormones. Polypeptide hormone receptors are typically located on the cell membrane, whereas receptors of the steroid hormone family are found mostly in the nuclear compartment of the cell.[115,116] However, steroid hormone receptors can also be found localized to the cell membrane. The interaction of growth factors, cytokines, and hormones with specific membrane receptors triggers a cascade of intracellular biochemical signals, resulting in the activation and repression of various subsets of genes. Several of these hormones have been shown to play an active role in breast epithelial cell growth and development and in lactation. Because these hormones and their receptors regulate normal breast tissue, it is not surprising that malignant cells arising from breast tissue might also express receptors for many of these hormones and might retain some degree of hormonal dependence.

Genetic aberrations in growth factor signaling pathways, for the most part acquired, are inextricably linked to developmental abnormalities and to a variety of chronic diseases, including cancer. Malignant cells arise as a result of a stepwise progression of genetic events that include the unregulated expression of growth factors or components of their signaling pathways.

Growth regulation of breast cancer cells by hormones and growth factors is shown schematically in Figure 1. The biological role of estrogens is mediated through high-affinity binding to ER by molecules belonging to a family of ligand-inducible nuclear receptors that have steroid and thyroid hormones and vitamins as known ligands.[114]

Breast cancer cells under estrogen control can synthesize and secrete their own growth factors that could auto stimulate breast cancer cells or adjacent stromal tissues through autocrine or paracrine mechanisms.[117] Aromatase is abundantly expressed in

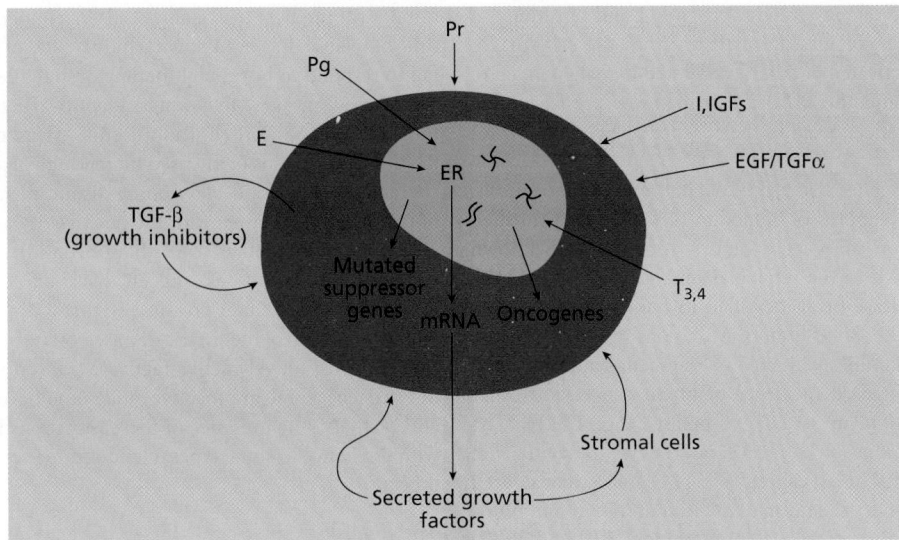

Figure 1 Growth regulation of breast cancer by hormones and growth factors. *Abbreviations*: E, estrogen; EGF, epidermal growth factors; I, insulin; IGFs, insulin-like growth factors; Pg, progesterone; Pr, prolactin; T3,4, thyroid hormones; TGF-α, transforming growth factor alpha; TGF-β, transforming growth factor beta.

many breast cancers, providing the malignant cell with the ability to synthesize its own major growth factor, estrogen. Stromal tissues may also secrete IGF-1 and IGF-2 that can stimulate breast cancer cells. The identified potential autocrine/paracrine growth factors include epidermal growth factor (EGF), TGF-α, IGF-2, platelet-derived growth factor, and fibroblast growth factor (FGF). EGF, TGF-α, IGF-1, and IGF-2 have been found to be expressed and secreted by cultured breast cancer cells and human breast cancer tissue specimens.[118] They are potential mitogens for the epithelial (malignant) component of the tumor. Platelet-derived growth factor and FGF are secreted by breast cancer cells and may be responsible for the proliferation of the mesenchymal stromal component evident in many breast cancers.

Human breast cancer cells also secrete several peptides that may have autocrine inhibitory activity. TGF-β is a family of growth factors that inhibit the proliferation of epithelial tissues and stimulate the proliferation of stromal tissues.[50] Studies suggest that ER-negative breast cancer cells are more sensitive to TGF-β than cells expressing ER. The malignant potential of breast cancer is likely to depend, in part, on the balance between growth stimulators and growth inhibitors produced by the tumors. The epithelial and/or stromal cells within the tumor also secrete proteases, such as the cathepsins, stromelysins, gelatinases, or urokinase plasminogen activator, which may participate in tumor invasiveness and metastatic potential.

In ER-positive breast cancer cells, expression and secretion of certain autocrine growth factors, such as TGF-α and IGF-2, are stimulated by estrogen and inhibited by antiestrogens. In ER-negative breast cancer cells, secretion of these factors is not estrogen regulated. Investigators have hypothesized that changes in the expression of these secreted factors may mediate to some extent the growth effects of estrogens and antiestrogens. Estrogens and antiestrogens have a variety of other effects on breast cancer cells. Estrogen stimulates RNA, DNA, protein synthesis, and the activity of key regulatory enzymes. Antiestrogens have the opposite effects in most tissues. Estrogens ultimately regulate movement of the cells through the cell cycle and mitosis.

Disturbance of normal growth control mechanisms within a cell can result in uncontrolled cell division and the development of cancer. Such cellular transformation occurs through the activation

of oncogenes, loss or mutation of tumor suppressor genes, or both. The normal counterparts of oncogenes, termed proto-oncogenes, function as growth regulators in normal cells. Alterations of proto-oncogenes are associated with the initiation, promotion, and/or maintenance of tumors in animals and humans. The products of oncogenes are frequently growth factors, growth factor receptors, molecular switching, or transcription factors. Oncogenes often found overexpressed in human breast cancer tissue include members of the *myc* and *ras* family (*c-myc*, *Ha-ras-1*), *int-2*, which is involved in mouse (and, presumably, human) mammary gland carcinogenesis, and the members of the epidermal growth factor receptor (EGFR, *erbB*) family, including *erbB-2* (also known as *HER2* or *neu*), *HER3*, and *HER4*. Overexpression and mutation of growth factor receptors often lead to constitutive activation of these receptors (i.e., signaling in the absence of their cognate ligands). Growth-promoting signals may be continuously transmitted into the cells, resulting in activation of multiple intracellular signal transduction pathways and unregulated cell growth. Genes normally involved in cell cycle control, particularly members of the cyclin D and E families, may also function as oncogenes. Overexpression of these oncogenes may contribute to the initiation and maintenance of the malignant phenotype. Tissue-specific expression of *myc*, *ras*, and *HER2* in mammary glands of transgenic mice has been shown to result in an increased incidence of both benign and malignant breast pathology. Altered expression of these otherwise normal genes can have profound effects on growth homeostasis of breast epithelium. Recent studies have shown that blockade of these growth factor receptors or pathways has therapeutic implications.[68] Monoclonal antibodies to *HER2* have dramatic antitumor effects, and they downregulate the phosphatidyl inositol 3-kinase (PI3K) signaling pathway. Furthermore, these antibodies have synergistic interactions with cytotoxic agents, such as the anthracyclines, the platinum analogs, vinorelbine, and the taxanes. The EGFR, when overexpressed, confers an adverse prognosis to patients with EGFR-overexpressing tumors. However, EGFR does not seem to be a critical driver of malignant behavior in breast cancer, and monoclonal antibodies against this target have had only marginal success in clinical trials.

Quantification of the expression of these oncogenes in human breast cancer specimens has been shown to provide valuable information on tumor aggressiveness, prognosis, and sensitivity to therapy.[69] Signaling molecules downstream from the cell surface receptors are often activated or otherwise altered in malignant cells. The PI3K pathway and the MAP kinase pathway are frequently activated in breast cancer, even in the absence of EGFR or HER2 overexpression.

Tumor suppressor genes also play a role in breast carcinogenesis. Loss of the normal "suppressor" function of these genes through mutations or deletion may cause cancer. Alterations in known suppressor genes, such as the retinoblastoma gene (*RB1*) and the human *TP53* gene, have been identified in human breast cancer cells, as well as in other solid tumors. Mutations in the *TP53* gene have been found in families with the Li–Fraumeni syndrome, who have a markedly increased incidence of breast cancer and other neoplasms. In addition, up to 50% of breast cancers have been shown to have mutations in the *TP53* gene. The two mutated genes associated with familial breast cancer, *BRCA1/2*, are also considered tumor suppressor genes. The normal function of the protein products of these genes is to control cell proliferation (*RB1* and *TP53*) or facilitate/mediate DNA repair (*TP53*, *BRCA1/2*). Mutations lead to mutated proteins and thus to dysregulated transit of cells through the cell cycle. Recognition that mutational inactivation of suppressor genes is associated with breast cancer could lead to early recognition of high-risk families, as well as to new treatment strategies to reverse the malignant phenotype by introducing normal gene copies through gene therapy or by treatment with the normal suppressor protein itself. Such strategies are under active investigation, both in the laboratory and early clinical trials.

Estrogen and progesterone receptors

ERs are members of the nuclear hormone receptor superfamily and have several functional domains. There are two subtypes, with each subtype having several isoforms and splice variants. The ERα (alpha) gene has been mapped to the long arm of chromosome 6 (6q24-q27), whereas the ERβ (beta) gene is located on band q22-24 of chromosome 14. There are at least three PR subtypes. Other estrogen-induced proteins regulate events leading to cell proliferation. When receptors are bound to antiestrogens, such as tamoxifen, transcription of growth-promoting genes is blocked, although other genes might be activated by tamoxifen.

Nuclear localization of ER leads to its genomic effects. Upon binding its ligand, the ER–ligand complex binds to the estrogen responsive element and initiates transcription of estrogen-driven genes. In its cell membrane localization, ER mediates the nongenomic effects of ligand binding, mostly through cross talk with peptide growth factor receptors (EGFR and HER2). Upon development of antiestrogen resistance, there is marked increase in the nongenomic effects of ER.

The most important application of the ER assay is the selection of appropriate patients for endocrine therapy. Approximately 50–60% of patients with ER-positive tumors benefit from endocrine therapy. This percentage includes patients with metastatic disease who achieve a major objective remission (partial or complete) and those who derive long-term (>6 months) stability of the disease with endocrine therapy; both groups have equivalent survival expectations. The ER status predicts equally well for all modalities of endocrine therapy. Patients with no detectable ER or PR in their tumors do not benefit from endocrine therapy; however, breast cancers with very low but detectable ER and/or PR respond, albeit infrequently, to endocrine therapy (see systemic therapy sections).

Tumor ER and PR status can change over time or with intervening therapy; thus, repeat biopsies of accessible tissue may be helpful in selecting sequential therapies. However, ER status on the primary tumor still predicts reasonably well for endocrine response at the time of relapse. It is not known why 40–50% of ER-positive tumors fail to respond to hormonal therapy despite the presence of receptor. Clearly, an assay that would identify truly hormone-sensitive tumors would be more clinically useful. At least one multigene assay, the Oncotype DX, is being used increasingly in the United States to characterize the risk of developing distant metastases after 5 years of tamoxifen for women with ER-positive disease.[119]

Variant and/or mutated ERs have been identified in breast cancer tissue.[120] Current data suggest that the frequency of mutations in ESR1 increases under pressure, so that it is increasingly common with progression of metastatic diseases. Some of these altered receptors are constitutively active (activate transcription in the absence of estrogen), some are inactive, and some have predominant negative activity. The presence of these mutations has been associated with resistance to some types of endocrine therapy, but response to others.

Pathology

Histologic types

Pathologic classifications of mammary carcinoma are frequently confusing to the individual who is not a specialist in breast disease. Table 5 lists the distribution of various histologic types of invasive breast cancer.

Epithelial neoplasms of the breast

Tumors arising from ductal epithelium may be found only within the lumen of the ducts of origin; that is, the carcinomas are intraductal and do not penetrate the basement membrane or invade surrounding stroma. Most frequently, such tumors arise from large ducts and may present as several types. If they grow into the ducts with a papillary configuration, they are recognized as papillary carcinomas (Figure 2). Such lesions are rare, accounting for only 1% of breast cancers. Histologically, pleomorphic duct epithelial cells with disturbed polarity can be demonstrated, as can their "heaping up" into papillae. Difficulty may be encountered in differentiating a papillary carcinoma from a benign atypical papilloma. Papillary carcinomas rarely invade the surrounding stroma. A survival rate approaching 100% may be anticipated upon complete excision of

Table 5 Distribution of histologic types of invasive breast cancers 2008–2012, selected.

Histologic type	No.	%
Adenocarcinoma	287,384	97.4
Infiltrating duct carcinoma	216,104	73.2
Lobular carcinoma	26,726	9.1
Mixed ductal and lobular carcinoma	27,371	9.3
Inflammatory adenocarcinoma	1003	0.3
Mucinous adenocarcinoma	5737	1.9
Tubular adenocarcinoma	1850	0.6
Papillary adenocarcinoma	1754	0.6
Paget disease	1259	0.4
Other adenocarcinomas	3336	1.1
Adenocarcinoma, NOS	2176	0.7
Epidermoid carcinoma	145	0
Other specific carcinomas	2415	0.8
Medullary adenocarcinoma	815	0.3
Other	1600	0.5
Unspecified, carcinoma, NOS	3356	1.1

Abbreviation: NOS, not otherwise specified.
Source: Howlader 2015.[2]

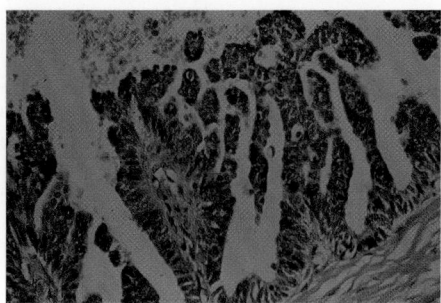

Figure 2 Papillary carcinoma of the breast. This uncommon tumor, <1%, rarely infiltrates and has a favorable prognosis.

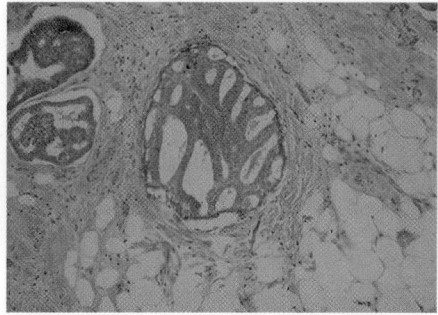

Figure 3 Ductal carcinoma in situ (DCIS), cribriform type. Duct spaces are completely involved by a proliferation of ductal cells with relatively uniform nuclei, arranged in back-to-back (cribriform) glands. The glands are almost uniform in size and shape and exhibit rigid inner borders (so-called cookie-cutter appearance). Source: Courtesy of Dr. Ira Bleiweiss, Mount Sinai School of Medicine.

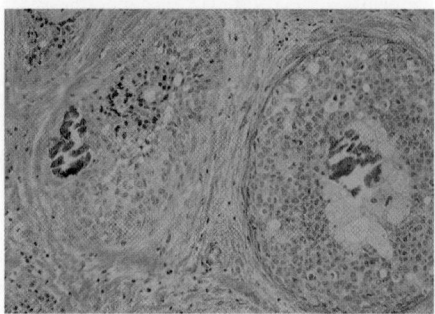

Figure 4 Ductal carcinoma in situ (DCIS), comedo type. Two duct spaces contain tumor cells with high nuclear grade, focal necrosis, and calcifications. The combination of high-grade nuclei and central necrosis is diagnostic of comedocarcinoma. Source: Courtesy of Dr. Ira Bleiweiss, Mount Sinai School of Medicine.

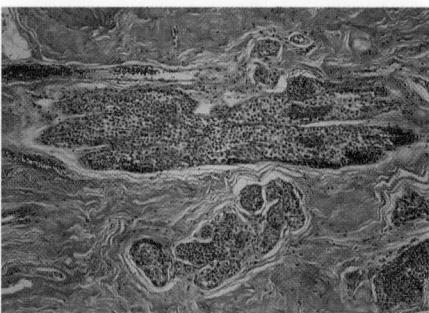

Figure 5 Lobular carcinoma in situ (LCIS). Terminal ducts and acini are completely filled and dilated by a uniform small cell proliferation. Source: Courtesy of Dr. Ira Bleiweiss, Mount Sinai School of Medicine.

such tumors. When these tumors do invade surrounding tissue, they grow rather slowly and attain considerable bulk. Skin and fascial attachments are unusual, and axillary node involvement is a late feature. Clinically, noninvasive tumors are found to be movable, circumscribed lesions that have a soft consistency not unlike that of fibroadenomas.

The noninvasive variety of ductal carcinoma, referred to as intraductal carcinoma or ductal carcinoma in situ (DCIS), is a proliferation of a subgroup of epithelial cells confined to the mammary ducts without light microscopic evidence of invasion through the basement membrane into the stroma. The histologic diagnosis of DCIS poses certain problems. It is often difficult to distinguish between benign but highly atypical hyperplasia and DCIS, and it is sometimes difficult to identify small foci of stromal invasion. Occasionally, it is difficult to distinguish between DCIS and lobular carcinoma in situ (LCIS), as the former may extend into breast lobules and the latter may involve extralobular ducts. Some lesions may be intermediate between the two. A variety of histologic patterns of DCIS has been recognized. The most frequently encountered are comedo, cribriform, solid, papillary, and micropapillary (Figure 3). The different histologic patterns have been associated with differences in biologic behavior. The proliferative rate has been found to vary according to the histologic characteristics of DCIS. A high proliferative rate has been observed with comedo DCIS, and a low proliferative rate with cribriform, papillary, and solid DCIS. A type of carcinoma known as comedocarcinoma is characterized by ducts that are dilated and filled with carcinoma cells. These are necrotic and can be expressed as semisolid necrotic plugs. Such cancers are not usually regarded as a separate cell type, but they rather represent a descriptive variant of intraductal carcinoma. Patients whose DCIS exhibits comedo features have been shown to have increased rates of local recurrence and may progress more rapidly to invasive breast cancer than other types (Figure 4). Human EGF-receptor 2 (HER2/neu or HER2) protein overexpression has been observed in solid and comedo types of DCIS, but not in papillary or cribriform types.

Lobular carcinoma arises from the small end ducts of the breast. The noninvasive variety—the so-called LCIS—is characterized by small cells of low nuclear grade that fill and expand lobules without penetration of the basement membrane (Figure 5). When this lesion extends beyond the boundary of the lobule or terminal duct from which it arises, it is known as invasive lobular carcinoma. Often the small cells interdigitate between collagen bundles in a single line, the so-called "Indian file." At other times, lobular carcinoma may be almost indistinguishable from the conventional invasive ductal carcinoma (Figure 6). Noninvasive mammary carcinomas comprise almost 22% of all neoplastic lesions of the female breast, and LCIS accounts for about 60% of these, or 12% of all tumors. Whereas DCIS often accompanies invasive ductal carcinoma, and may well

be its usual precursor, LCIS may be followed by invasive ductal or invasive lobular carcinomas in either breast. Thus, LCIS is more a systemic marker than a local precursor. With the increased use of mammography, a much higher proportion of noninvasive cancers is being detected.

Invasive ductal carcinomas in which no special type of histologic structure is recognized are designated "not otherwise specified" (NOS) and are the most common duct tumors, accounting for almost 80% of breast cancers (Figure 7). They are characterized clinically by their stony hardness to palpation. When they are transected, a gritty resistance is encountered, and the tumor

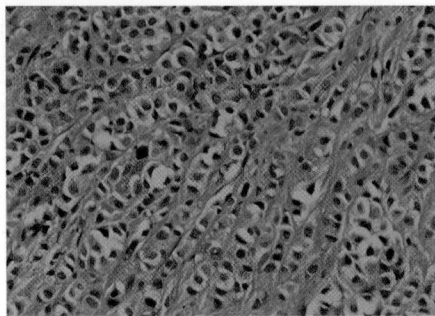

Figure 6 Infiltrating lobular carcinoma. Tumor cells with relatively uniform nuclei invade in a single file or linear pattern (so-called Indian file). Source: Courtesy of Dr. Ira Bleiweiss, Mount Sinai School of Medicine.

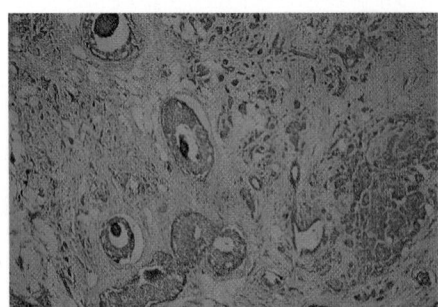

Figure 7 Infiltrating ductal carcinoma of the breast, not otherwise specified (NOS). Approximately 80% of breast cancers exhibit this histology, about one-third of the time with additional types of differentiation.

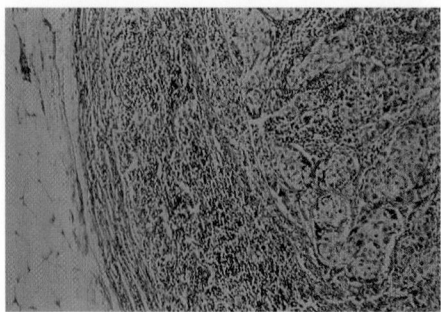

Figure 8 Medullary carcinoma of the breast accounts for approximately 5–7% of breast cancers. Despite its relatively poor differentiation, this tumor has a better prognosis than does infiltrating ductal carcinoma.

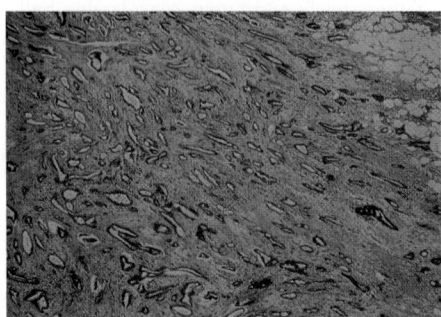

Figure 9 Tubular carcinoma of the breast. This tumor is rare in its pure form, <1%, but has a better prognosis than infiltrating duct carcinoma not otherwise specified (NOS). Partial tubular differentiation is seen in 20% of infiltrating duct carcinomas NOS.

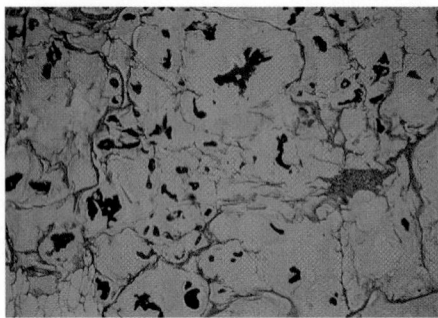

Figure 10 Mucinous or colloid carcinoma of the breast. This tumor is uncommon (~2%), but has a rather favorable prognosis.

retracts below the cut surface. Yellowish chalky streaks that represent necrotic foci are observed. Histologically, varying degrees of fibrotic response are present. They frequently metastasize to axillary lymph nodes, and their prognosis is the poorest of the various tumor types. More than half (52.6%) of breast cancers are pure invasive ductal lesions (NOS).

Several other types of invasive carcinomas arise from large ducts, and each has its own distinct histopathologic image. Medullary carcinoma, comprising 3–6% of all mammary carcinomas, often attains large dimensions (Figure 8). This tumor is formed by cells of relatively high nuclear grade, and it usually exhibits an extensive infiltration of the tumor by small lymphocytes. Medullary carcinomas have a relatively well-circumscribed border, sometimes described as a "pushing" border, in contrast to the NOS tumors in which small nests of cells tend to infiltrate the adjacent stroma more extensively. A study of medullary cancer using 336 typical and 273 atypical medullary breast cancers from 6404 patients enrolled in various stage I and stage II NSABP trials indicated that the survival of patients with typical medullary cancers was higher than those with NOS invasive ductal carcinomas. Survival was comparable for those with atypical medullary and NOS types.[121]

Tubular carcinoma is an invasive carcinoma in which tubule formation is highly prominent. This tumor represents 1–2% of breast cancers and has a low nuclear grade with some cell polarity (Figure 9). Its prognosis is favorable, and, when combined with small size, it is a curable tumor.

Mucinous or colloid carcinoma, which comprises about 1–2% of all mammary carcinomas, is characterized on microscopy by nests and strands of epithelial cells floating in a mucinous matrix. It usually grows slowly and can reach bulky proportions. When the tumor is predominantly mucinous, the prognosis tends to be good (Figure 10).

Two entities represent special manifestations of mammary carcinoma. Paget disease of breast occurs in 1–4% of all patients with breast cancer. Clinically, the patient presents with a relatively long history of eczematoid changes in the nipple, with itching, burning, oozing, and/or bleeding. The nipple changes are associated with an underlying carcinoma in the breast that can be palpated in about two-thirds of the patients. The subjacent tumor may be either intraductal or of the invasive duct type. Prognosis is related to the invasiveness and histologic type of the associated tumor. Histologically, the nipple epithelium contains nests of carcinoma cells.

Inflammatory breast cancer (IBC), or "dermal lymphatic carcinomatosis" of the breast, is characterized clinically by skin redness, warmth, edema (peau d'orange), visible erysipeloid margin, induration of the underlying breast, and rapid evolution, usually less than 3 months from first sign to diagnosis. These features must be present at the time of primary diagnosis. Biopsies of the erythematous areas and adjacent normal-appearing skin

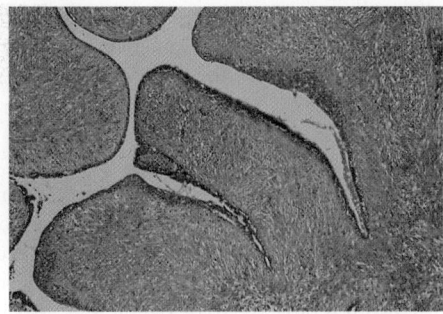

Figure 11 Phyllodes tumor (cystosarcoma phyllodes). Leaf like projections, lined by benign epithelium, contain a hypercellular stroma.

often but not always reveal poorly differentiated cancer cells filling and obstructing the subdermal lymphatics. Inflammatory cells are rarely present. Patients typically have signs of advanced cancer, including palpable axillary nodes, supraclavicular nodes, and/or distant metastases. IBC represents about 1–2% of breast cancers in the United States and Western Europe, although its incidence is reportedly higher in North Africa and the Middle East.

Several other histologic types of mammary carcinomas have been described but are rarely (<1%) encountered. Adenocystic carcinoma, carcinosarcomas, pure squamous cell carcinoma, basal cell carcinomas, and the so-called lipid-rich carcinomas have been observed. Because of their rarity, clinical correlates are practically nonexistent. Metaplastic cancers, previously rare, are increasingly recognized as a distinct and poor prognosis subset of TNBCs.

Nonepithelial neoplasms of the breast

A variety of nonepithelial neoplasms of the breast have been described. Fibrosarcomas, leiomyosarcomas, rhabdomyosarcomas, and angiosarcomas are all infrequent.[122] Non-Hodgkin lymphomas can have their initial onset in the breast and can also occur as a focus of generalized disease. These usually have a B-cell phenotype. Some cases resemble carcinoma on routine histology; immunohistochemistry (IHC) is often helpful in resolving this issue. Only a few cases of Hodgkin disease and leukemia have been reported with initial manifestation in the breast.

Phyllodes tumor (cystosarcoma phyllodes) is a rare biphasic neoplasm that is partially epithelial and partially mesenchymal (Figure 11). Phyllodes tumors may achieve a large size and, not infrequently, demonstrate some invasion of adjacent breast tissue. They are best managed by local excision with a rim of normal breast tissue. Phyllodes tumors are classified as benign, borderline or indeterminate, and malignant. Malignant phyllodes tumors can metastasize and are highly resistant to therapy, with no known effective therapy. High mitotic rate, cellular atypia, stromal overgrowth, infiltrative margins, hemorrhage, and necrosis are considered features of malignancy; however, these findings are extremely rare. Although it is difficult to determine from clinical or histologic appearance the tumors that behave malignantly and metastasize, malignant histology and stromal overgrowth are predictive of metastasis.[123]

Prognostic factors

Tumor size

In addition to being a determinant for optimal local therapy, tumor size has prognostic significance in the determination of additional therapy. As the size of the tumor increases, the risk of recurrence

(ROR) or metastasis also increases, for both lymph node-negative and node-positive tumors. Because the risk of treatment failure is already high for patients with node-positive breast cancer, increasing tumor size adds relatively little prognostic value. However, tumor size is often the main prognostic indicator in node-negative breast cancer. This variable is particularly important to decide whether to use or not adjuvant systemic therapy in patients with node-negative breast cancer. Tumor size refers only to the invasive component and hence should be determined in all three dimensions by the pathologist. Approximately 25–30% of patients with negative lymph nodes and a primary tumor less than 2 cm in diameter will experience a recurrence within 20 years of follow-up.[124] Patients with tumors ≤1 cm in diameter have an excellent prognosis, with <15% recurring at 10 years without effective adjuvant therapy. The largest database demonstrating the relationship among tumor size, lymph node status, and breast cancer survival comes from the Surveillance, Epidemiology, and End Results (SEER) program.[1] Less than 2% of patients with tumors under 1 cm and negative nodes died of breast cancer within 5 years, and only 4% at 10 years.[125] Considering the excellent prognosis for this group of patients with very small tumors, as well as the expense and toxicity of treatment, routine use of chemotherapy is not indicated. The combination of poor nuclear grade and lymphatic vessel invasion identifies a small subset (~10%) of patients with T1a, b N0 M0 breast cancer with a significant risk of relapse, up to 30%, that warrants systemic adjuvant therapy.[126]

Axillary lymph node involvement

Involvement of the ipsilateral axillary lymph nodes is still the most reliable and reproducible prognostic indicator for primary breast cancer. In general, 50–70% of patients with positive lymph nodes have a relapse, whereas only 15–45% of patients with all lymph nodes negative for metastatic disease have a relapse after locoregional treatments only. The risk of tumor recurrence in a patient with primary breast cancer is a continuum related to the number of positive axillary lymph nodes.[127] With each additional positive lymph node found, the ROR and metastasis increase by a few percentage points. Thus, patients with 4–10 positive lymph nodes have a higher risk than those with one to three positive nodes, and those with 10 or more positive nodes have a higher risk than 80% probability of recurrence and metastasis.

Both macro- and micrometastases within the lymph nodes have prognostic significance.[128] Recent data suggest that micrometastases (N1mic) result in an intermediate risk compared with macrometastases, although this remains controversial.[129,130] By contrast, isolated tumor cells (ITC, <0.2 mm) appear to be without prognostic significance.[131]

In recent years, primary breast cancer has been diagnosed in earlier and mostly localized stages. A classic axillary lymph node dissection (ALND) has no therapeutic benefit for patients with a node-negative axilla and is associated with considerable short- and long-term morbidity. An alternative (diagnostic) staging procedure for these patients is the sentinel lymph node biopsy (SLNB)[132] that markedly limits the extent of the surgical procedure in the axilla and, for the high majority of patients with negative axillary lymph nodes, precludes the need for formal axillary dissection while providing similar (and in some cases superior) diagnostic and prognostic information. The identification of a single (or only a few) sentinel node also permits the pathologist to perform a more detailed assessment to detect micrometastases by combining light microscopy, IHC, and even more sensitive molecular techniques. The finding of ITCs does not convey prognostic impact and should not be used to direct either local or systemic therapy. Randomized trials comparing axillary dissection with SLNB have demonstrated that the latter is associated with significantly reduced morbidity. Because of these results, SLNB has replaced classic axillary dissection for early localized breast cancer in a substantial percentage of patients with clinically negative axillae.

Although axillary lymph node status is still the most powerful prognostic indicator, 15–45% of patients whose lymph nodes do not contain metastases still experience a recurrence and die. Because of this limitation, other prognostic markers have been developed to improve prognostic accuracy, particularly in the group of patients with node-negative tumors. Molecular tests based on gene expression suggest that biology of the tumor may be more important than its stage. Women with node-positive breast cancer who were determined to be of low risk based on the MP gene assay had excellent recurrence-free survival regardless of whether chemotherapy was administered or not. This contrasted with the recurrence-free survival of those with a high-risk score, whose outcome was significantly poorer, but appeared to be moderated by chemotherapy.[133] A similar finding has been seen with the Oncotype DX gene assay.[134] This will continue to be an important area of research, and molecular analysis of tumors is already a major tool for determining therapy.

Histologic type

Several histologic variables have been reported to have prognostic significance.[120] The prognoses of ductal and lobular carcinomas are sufficiently similar to prompt the same treatment modalities. Several less common cancers, including pure tubular carcinoma, mucinous or colloid carcinoma, papillary carcinoma, and all noninvasive breast cancers, have substantially better prognoses, particularly when found in a node-negative stage.[135] The more favorable prognosis of these histologic types often justifies omission of adjuvant systemic treatment, particularly for small tumors (<3 cm). Because most of these special types have small dimensions when diagnosed, and are node negative, regional treatment is usually all that is required.

Histologic grade or differentiation

Tumor grade has been shown to be an important prognostic indicator. In general, tumors expressing features that indicate a high degree of tumor differentiation are associated with the most favorable prognosis. Multiple studies have shown that higher grade is associated with higher rates of recurrence and metastases and poorer survival. These correlations are independent of tumor size and lymph node involvement. High tumor grade is also associated with HR– and increased response to cytotoxic therapy. Conversely, low grade is associated with hormonal sensitivity and lower response to chemotherapy.

The clear definition of various histologic differentiation grades led to the recognition that those grades had reproducible prognostic significance. A similar finding can be observed for nuclear grade, although some find that histologic grade is a more reliable prognostic indicator as it includes cellular and tissue-related criteria. Nuclear grade can be determined in cytologic specimens.

The most frequently used grading system is the Elston–Ellis modification of the Scarff–Bloom–Richardson system.[136] In this system, invasive ductal breast cancers are categorized into three histologic grades, depending on their degree of tubular and/or gland formation, cellular pleomorphism, and the number of mitoses per high-power microscopic field. Within each of these categories, a score of 1–3 is assigned, with 1 representing the most favorable findings (e.g., prominent gland formation, little cellular pleomorphism, and low mitotic rate) and 3 indicating the least favorable ones. The scores for each of these categories are added together.

Grade 1 carcinoma (well differentiated or low grade) is defined as having a total of 3–5 points, grade II (moderately differentiated or intermediate grade) 6–7 points, and grade 3 (poorly differentiated or high grade) 8–9 points.

Tumor necrosis

Tumor necrosis of varying degrees was encountered in 60% of 1539 patients with invasive breast cancer in NSABP protocol B-04. Necrosis, particularly when observed to be of marked degree, was positively correlated with increased rates of treatment failure. Although necrosis was observed to be significantly associated with a number of clinical and histopathologic features purportedly related to worse prognosis in this disease, it was not correlated with pathologic nodal status, and multivariate analysis revealed it to influence treatment failure independently of tumor size in lesions less than 5 cm in their highest diameter. It is likely that tumor necrosis is a marker of proliferation and not a unique prognostic factor.

Lymphatic and blood vessel invasion

Lymphatic and blood vessel invasion has been associated with poor prognosis in numerous clinical reports. One-third of NSABP patients exhibited extension into lymphatics within the predominant mass, and the remaining 23% were considered questionable (Figure 12). Such a finding was associated with other unfavorable characteristics. Blood vessel invasion was observed in only 5% of patients and was associated with the finding of four or more positive axillary nodes, lymphatic invasion, and certain other unfavorable findings (Figure 13).

Multicentricity

Many breast cancers are multicentric in origin. In an examination of 904 NSABP cases, either invasive or noninvasive cancers regarded as independent were found in 13.4% patients. The frequency of

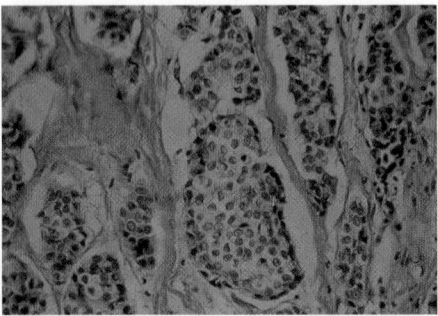

Figure 12 Lymphatic invasion by breast cancer. The vessel walls are thin and lined with endothelial cells.

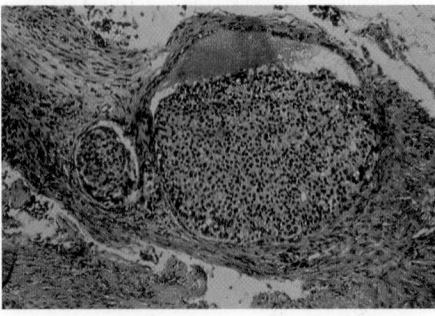

Figure 13 Blood vessel invasion by breast cancer. The vessel wall structure is recognizable, together with erythrocytes in the vessel.

invasive and noninvasive multicentric cancers was 4.1% and 9.3%, respectively. Increased utilization of magnetic resonance imaging (MRI) of the breast for preoperative assessment of the extent of disease indicated that multicentricity is more common than that it was previously determined by mammography.

Despite the significant incidence of multifocal lesions in both breasts in a woman with a primary breast cancer, two or more clinically overt primary cancers in the primary breast are uncommon. Similarly, synchronous bilateral tumors are uncommon, and the incidence of a second asynchronous primary tumor in the uninvolved or opposite breast (~4–6% in 10 years) fails to approach the incidence predicted by the number of occult lesions detected by random biopsy, autopsy, or MRI.

Markers of proliferative capacity

Measurement of the proliferation rates of malignant tissues found high prognostic values for several types of cancer, including breast cancer. Several techniques are used to evaluate the proliferative capacity of the malignant cell, including mitotic indices, thymidine-labeling indices (TLIs) and S-phase fraction (SPF). The mitotic index is determined by counting mitotic figures using light microscopy on a tumor specimen stained with hematoxylin and eosin. It has been validated by both univariate and multivariate analyses. Many proteins play a role in the control of the cell cycle or are expressed at higher levels during certain phases of the cell cycle. Ki-67 and proliferating cell nuclear antigen (PCNA) are additional markers for the proliferation rate of malignant tumors.[92,93] Of these, Ki-67 has been more extensively studied, and it correlates strongly with the results of SPF determination and, therefore, long-term prognosis. This technique can be performed on fresh or frozen tissues and archival paraffin-embedded material. A low value indicates a more slowly proliferating tumor and is associated with a lower rate of recurrence, regardless of axillary nodal status. A high Ki-67 fraction is strongly correlated with other adverse prognostic factors, such as high histologic and cytologic grades, aneuploidy, and a negative steroid receptor status. Not surprisingly, the predictive molecular assays that have emerged are driven in part by genes that regulate proliferation.

Immunologic factors

Tumor-infiltrating lymphocytes[137] have been associated with improved outcome in aggressive breast cancer subtypes, such as TNBC. Preliminary data demonstrating efficacy of immune checkpoint inhibitors in breast cancer have highlighted the need to better understand the individual immune environment in individual tumor cases.

Diagnosis and screening

Historically, the primary presenting symptom of breast cancer was a palpable mass, often first detected by the patient. At present, the increasing use of mammography, particularly in screening programs, has resulted in many cancers being found at a preclinical stage. A simple discussion of the signs and symptoms of breast cancer without consideration of these preclinical manifestations would be incomplete. To some extent, this indicates a higher complexity in selecting for biopsy patients who are suspected of having carcinoma. The clinical and mammographic signs and symptoms are best understood against the background knowledge of the anatomy and biology of breast cancer—how it grows and extends locally.

Patient history

The patient's history should include standard epidemiologic and reproductive information to assess the RR factors. Information about lumps, pain, or any changes in the breast should be obtained and correlated with physical findings. Although pain is probably the most frequent breast complaint, it is uncommonly the presenting factor in cancer. Breast cancer, particularly in its early stages, is usually painless. Most breast pain is related to hormone stimulation and swelling of breast tissue (although these symptoms may draw attention to a mass that proves to be cancer). Careful questioning of the patient usually reveals that the pain is cyclic, beginning any time between ovulation and the onset of menstruation, and that commonly it is most intense a few days before menstruation. Pain usually disappears in the first or second day of the menstrual period, only to return in the next cycle. Cyclic pain is present at a mild level in more than 50% of women of childbearing age. Less frequently, the pain can reach intense proportions. Some patients report that, during the worst days, it is too painful even to take a shower.

The most effective treatment is explanation and reassurance, although some patients who are extremely symptomatic and incapacitated by the pain may require treatments with hormones or hormone-blocking drugs. There are occasional reports that caffeine limitation or low-fat diets help, but relief seems to be individual, and these reports are not supported by persuasive clinical trials.

A patient who reports a lump or any other physical change in her breast needs careful attention. The history should describe any change in the character or size of the lump and whether or not it has been tender. Pain should be described with respect to its timing in the menstrual cycle. Lumpy changes associated with a fibrocystic process may wax and wane, but it is distinctly unusual for a carcinoma to do anything but increase in size. If the physician is unsure, the patient should be reexamined after the menstrual period.

Other descriptive changes, such as skin thickening or discoloration, the presence of axillary masses, or nipple discharge, should be elicited. Nipple discharge may be serous, watery, or milk-like. It may be clear or have a yellow or greenish hue, or it may be sero sanguineous or bloody. Although the latter may indicate a neoplasm, this is most commonly an intraductal papilloma, which is benign. It is possible, but rare, for such a discharge to signal an intraductal papillary carcinoma; all bloody discharges require further investigation.

Clear or serous discharge, particularly if it involves more than one major duct opening on a nipple, is likely to be benign. Nonbloody discharge that is not spontaneous but requires manual compression to elicit is also likely to be benign. In an apocrine system such as the breast, there are always some cell desquamation and liquefaction and, therefore, some fluid present in the duct system. If this is not well absorbed, it can make its way through the collecting ducts to the nipple and present as a discharge. Similarly, if the duct is blocked by fibrosis or inspissated material, the pressure of secretion can cause dilation and cyst formation. Cytologic examination of the discharge is less accurate and not very useful.

Physical examination

The patient should be examined, first in a sitting and then in a supine position. When the patient is sitting erect, more useful information is obtained visually than by palpation. When the arms are raised and stretched upward, the contour of the skin is pulled tight, allowing for easier detection of contour abnormalities in the upper half of the breast. This position also emphasizes dimpling, particularly in the lower half of the breast. Because much of the breast tissue coalesces in the sitting position, it is very difficult when palpating to appreciate true masses and often easy to be confused by confluent tissue. The axilla is palpated by relaxing and adducting the patient's arm, but this is best done with the patient in the sitting position.

With the patient supine and the arm raised such that the hand is behind the head and the elbow lies flat on the pillow, the breast tissue can be spread across the chest wall, allowing for proper palpation. The patient should be slightly turned to the contralateral side to aid this process. It is important to proceed in a pattern, but whether it be performed by quadrants or strips is up to the examiner. Skin changes such as dimpling, peau d'orange (edema), erythema, or areas of fixation and ulceration suggest advanced cancer that has invaded the skin or the immediate subcutaneous tissue. Skin retraction is often more easily detected when the patient is sitting with the arms raised or when the patient is leaning forward. Retraction or asymmetry of the nipple is another worrisome sign unless the patient reports that this has been present all her life. A subtle reddish thickening of the nipple and areola or flaking of the superficial epithelium may suggest Paget disease.

The examination is concluded with a search for axillary, infraclavicular, and supraclavicular nodes and palpation of the liver to detect enlargement. Although palpably enlarged axillary nodes increase the probability of metastases, careful studies have shown that clinical judgment is highly inaccurate. In a study conducted by the NSABP, a group of cancer patients were judged by their clinicians to have normal axillary nodes, where 38% showed histologic evidence of metastatic tumor when the specimens were examined pathologically.[120] Conversely, in 25% of such cases, nodes that appeared enlarged and were judged to contain cancer were found to be normal. Evaluation should include axillary ultrasound, with a fine-needle aspiration (FNA) of abnormal-appearing nodes.

The most difficult clinical decision is differentiating between a pathologic mass and physiologic density associated with fibroglandular (or fibrocystic) changes. A true lump has definite margins. Whether these are smooth, as in a gross cyst or fibroadenoma, or somewhat irregular, as in carcinoma, they delineate a discrete mass that requires further investigation. Invasive ductal carcinomas are usually hard, and predominant in the breast, in contrast to multiple firm masses that may exist in BBD. Lobular carcinomas are not usually so hard and thus are more difficult to recognize.

It is important to measure the size of a tumor so that subsequent examinations can more accurately establish any change in size. Advanced cancers may be fixed, but early palpable lesions will certainly be mobile with respect to skin or fascia and muscle of the chest wall. There is, however, a subtle difference in mobility (better called "movability") characteristic of cysts or fibroadenomas, which have capsules and move much more easily within the surrounding breast tissue. Carcinoma, on the contrary, which has no capsule and is surrounded by an infiltrating desmoplastic process, tends to move with the neighboring breast tissue rather than within it, because the process "locks" it into the stroma and surrounding glandular tissues, even when it is not fixed to surrounding structures, such as the skin or muscle. Even an experienced examiner could fail to distinguish correctly between benign and malignant lesions.

Imaging

For almost 30 years, annual mammograms for women over 40 years of age have been a cornerstone of the strategy to reduce mortality from breast cancer. Advances in our understanding of breast cancer biology, and screening in general, have led to revise and improve our screening strategy.[138] In 2009, the USPSTF introduced changes to screening guidelines, recommending that annual mammograms for all women of age 40–75 years be replaced by biennial screening for women of age 50–75 and that screening between 40 and

Table 6 International screening strategies.

Country	Start age	Stop age	Frequency
USA	40	NA	Annually
Sweden	40	74	Biennially
UK	50	70	Triennially
The Netherlands	50	70	Biennially
France	50	74	Biennially
Italy	50	70	Biennially
Germany	50	70	Biennially

50 years of age should be individualized by considering patient context, including the patient's values regarding specific benefits and harms. The 2015 update further supported these recommendations (http://www.uspreventiveservicestaskforce.org/). The ACS revised its mammography screening guidelines in October 2015.[139] Screening was still strongly recommended, but the age at its start was modified. Annual screening was recommended for women aged 45 between 54 years, and women of age ≥ 55 years could transition to screen every other year. However, the ACS also noted that women should have the opportunity of annual screening and should continue to screen as long as they have a life expectancy of at least 10 years or more. It also recommended that women between the 40 and 44 years of age should have the opportunity of annual screening, if advised (Table 6).

Screening recommendations continue to spark debate, and scientific opinion on the effectiveness of annual screening is greatly divided. One side argues that annual mammograms starting at 40 reduce interval cancers, but others believe that annual screening results in more false positives with unnecessary treatment and that a more targeted approach could result in fewer false negatives and less overdiagnosis without increasing interval cancers. For most women, the discomfort and inconvenience of the annual mammogram is offset by the belief that it is one of the best ways to find cancers at an earlier, more curable stage. Unfortunately, cancers that are most likely to present at a more advanced stage or have a worse prognosis are those that are most likely to develop in between screening or are less likely to be visualized by standard radiographic tests. The reduced screening frequency recommended by the 2009 USPSTF was meant to balance benefits and harms and is more in line with policies of most other Western nations.

An increasingly vocal group questions the effectiveness of screening altogether. The 25-year follow-up results of the Canadian National Breast Screening Study (CNBSS), one of the early pivotal trials of screening, were published in February 2014 when they concluded (confirming their previous findings from 10- to 15-year follow-ups) that annual mammograms do not reduce deaths versus simple clinical breast exams.[140] Switzerland has recommended ending mammography screening altogether because of lack of evidence that the benefits outweigh the harms.[141] Editorials and perspectives regularly feature opposing viewpoints,[142–144] highlighting the broad disagreement over screening guidelines.

The annual screening approach to mammography, which is still the current standard, has its roots in the large randomized screening trials of the 1980s.[145] The overview of the Swedish trials showed a relative reduction in breast cancer mortality of 21%, with the maximum benefit for women in their 60s. The screening interval in the Swedish trials ranged from 18 to 33 months. Much has changed since these initial studies. Most of the effective systemic therapies used today were not available at the time when these screening studies were initiated, but currently have a clear role in reducing breast cancer mortality.[146] At present, systemic therapy has been thought to constitute up to two-thirds of the reduction in mortality and mammography about one-third.[9,147] Importantly, the extensive use and effectiveness of endocrine therapy[148,149] may mitigate the impact of finding some cancers later.

The potential harm caused by mammographic screening that is most familiar to women is the "false-positive." With each mammogram, a woman's risk of receiving a false-positive increases, and with it, the risk of a biopsy that turns out to be benign. After 10 years of annual screening, over half of all women will receive a false-positive recall, and 7–9% will have a false-positive biopsy.[150] In general, the specificity of mammography is approximately 90%, indicating a 1/10 probability of occurrence of a false-positive result. However, only approximately 5 in 1000 women actually have breast cancer when they are screened, so the majority of abnormal mammograms are false-positives.[151] These affect women in several ways. A recent systematic review has shown that psychological distress can endure for up to 3 years, reducing adherence to subsequent screening.[152] Similarly, a study from Holland showed 93% of women return after negative screens, but after one false-positive, only 56% return, and after two false-positive recalls, only 44% return.[153] Biennial screening, relative to annual screening, was shown in the BCSC to reduce the false-positive rate by 50%, with only a small but statistically insignificant increase of late-stage cancer diagnoses.[154]

Another potential harm of breast screening comes from "overdiagnosis."[155] Two decades of research has shown us that breast cancer is a spectrum of disease, spanning indolent lesions of epithelial origin (IDLE)[156] to aggressive disease. Screening, by nature, is more likely to identify slow growing and IDLE tumors[136] as highlighted by the 25-year follow-up results of the CNBSS. Half of the mammography-detected cancers that would not otherwise have been found by regular breast examination were deemed to be clinically insignificant.[138] A recent meta-analysis estimated that 20% of all cancers (up to 50% of screen-detected cancers) fall into the category of overdiagnosis.[157] Data suggest that a woman has a greater chance of being overdiagnosed than of having her life saved by screening.[158] Similar results were obtained when molecular markers were used to identify ultralow-risk disease.[159,160]

Most precancerous breast lesions and DCIS likely qualify as overdiagnosis. DCIS was rarely diagnosed before screening was adopted but increased 500-fold afterward.[161] The tumor cells comprising DCIS are morphologically similar to those of invasive cancer, and hence it has been assumed that DCIS ultimately progresses to invasive cancer. Because routine care for DCIS is mastectomy or lumpectomy and radiation, the natural history of DCIS is unclear.[162,163] Epidemiologic evidence suggests that only a subset progresses to invasive disease over a lifetime.[164] Furthermore, unlike cervical cancer, where the removal of precancerous lesions caused a sharp decline in invasive cervical cancer, after a decade of removing DCIS lesions from more than 50,000 women per year, there has been no decline in incidence of invasive cancers[162] (there was a short period of decline, but it was due to the sharp reduction in HRT after results of the Women's Health Initiative study were released).[4,165] Molecular markers are now available that identify a low risk form of DCIS whose 5-year risk for developing breast cancer is about the same as that of an average 65-year-old woman (2.5%)[166,167] Yet DCIS diagnoses result in >20,000 mastectomies per year, many of which are bilateral.[168,169]

Research to improve screening is ongoing, focusing on identifying the populations of patients who are most likely to benefit and developing molecular signatures to identify cancers with an extremely low risk of progressing.[156,170,171] Criteria and threshold for recall after an abnormal scan and biopsy are being actively evaluated and improved. The BI-RADS[172] recommends biopsy with a score of 4, which has a >2–95% chance of being either invasive cancer or DCIS. BI-RADS 4A (low suspicion <10%), 4B (intermediate 10–50%), and 4C (moderate >50%, but <95% risk of cancer) categories could help better refine biopsy thresholds.[173]

However, reducing the burden of overdiagnosis and false-positive recall could perhaps be best accomplished by modernizing our screening approach by incorporating our improved understanding of individual breast cancer risk.

The idea of risk-stratifying screening recommendations has been attracting attention recently.[174] The Institute of Medicine has advocated for technology integration and biology and risk stratification in the development of breast-screening models. They noted that personalization—more frequent screening of those at highest risk—could improve the positive predictive value of the screening test and potentially lead to fewer unnecessary interventions.[175,176] Because most people have a relatively low risk, personalized screening will result in the majority of the population getting less-frequent examinations, reducing false-positive recalls and biopsy rates.[154] This was also the conclusion of the USPSTF following their comprehensive review of mammography in 2009[155] that the balance of benefits and harms of screening depends on individual risk factors for women in their 40s and comorbidities for women over 74 years of age.[177] Women in their 40s with twice the average risk were thought to obtain the same benefits from screening compared with women in their 50s.[178] As such, the decision whether to screen women in their 40s should be based on individual risk factors. The USPSTF urged clinicians to discuss the pros and cons of screening with their patients in the context of their individual risk. For women of ages 50–74, USPSTF found that screening every other year would preserve benefits and minimize risks compared with annual screening.

The USPSTF guidelines have met resistance[179-181] and the medical community has failed to reach consensus on the issue. Women have also been reluctant to believe that less screening could somehow be beneficial, which, on the surface, is understandable.[177] Finally, USPSTF guidelines did not state how to integrate risk assessment into practice. Thus, while we have witnessed major advances in the diagnosis, prognosis, and treatment of breast cancer, our approach to screening has not fundamentally changed since the 1980s. It is imperative to move beyond the current debate and test new approaches to breast cancer screening to maximize the benefits and minimize the harms to women. Clearly, this means new studies to help us understand screening in the context of modern adjuvant therapies. However, it also indicates using three decades of knowledge on the natural history of breast cancer and the factors that contribute to an individual's personal risk of developing and/or dying from the disease. Just as our approach to treatment has evolved from one-size-fits-all to more individualized, patient-centered, evidence-based treatment, so too must our approach toward screening.[147]

In the last decade, concomitant advances in our understanding of disease mechanisms and analytical capabilities have given us the ability to treat disease with a higher degree of precision than ever before. In breast cancer, this is reflected in how we select specific therapies based on measured characteristics of an individual's disease.[117,168,182,183] On the contrary, we largely approach breast cancer screening as if everyone is the same. A more risk-adapted approach has the potential to benefit patients, providers, and payors. The Patient-Centered Outcomes Research Institute (PCORI), established as part of the Affordable Care Act, has recently funded a randomized trial to test personalized screening versus annual screening, in an effort to focus forward on how to make screening better for women and their providers (wisdomstudy.org). The proposed pragmatic trial seeks to resolve this controversy by comparing an updated individualized approach to breast screening with annual screening. Despite our vastly improved understanding of breast cancer risk, the only criterion used to establish a woman's screening recommendations is her age (and BRCA status if known). However, currently, there have been models that incorporate family history and breast density, endocrine exposures, gene mutations, and atypia to assess breast cancer risk,.[100,103,184–186] Most recently, certain common gene variants have been confirmed predictors as well.[187] Advances in breast cancer biology, risk assessment (genomics), and imaging (density) have provided us with all the tools and knowledge required to implement a personalized model; one that provides recommendations on when to start, when to stop, and how often to screen, depending upon well-characterized measures of their personal risk. The study is being conducted by the University of California-wide Athena Breast Health Network. The potential benefits of risk-based screening to health care payers are numerous and enormous. Our current breast cancer screening costs $8–10 billion and results in 600,000 benign biopsies annually. If we compare the costs of the most widely adopted annual screening practice of women of age 40–80, with the USPSTF recommendations, the difference in cost would be approximately $6.3 billion—a figure larger than the NCI's annual budget.[188,189]

MRI screening

MRI is increasingly being used in the management of breast cancer. MRI has the advantages of providing a three-dimensional (3D) view of the breast, performing with high sensitivity in dense breast tissue, and using nonionizing radiation. MRI has the following drawbacks as well: high cost, variability in performance, and moderate specificity that in combination with high sensitivity often leads to unnecessary workup.[190]

MRI is not appropriate as a general screening tool. It is at least 10 times costlier than mammography. MRI should be reserved for those situations where there is a high prior probability of identifying a cancer (high risk) and very high sensitivity is preferred and where other less expensive, robust screening tools (e.g., mammography) are known to be less sensitive,[156,191] such as BRCA1 or BRCA2 mutation carriers, which have an 85% lifetime risk of developing breast cancer. Although an average 35-year-old woman would have a 1/10,000 chance of having a cancer, a mutation carrier would have a risk in the range of 1 to 5/100, and MRI would be much more sensitive in this population than mammography. Women with a very high 5-year Gail risk and very dense breast tissue may also fall into this category. Use of a density-modified Gail Risk score,[52] which combines both risk and breast density as recorded on a mammogram (BI-RADS density), enables the identification of women both at high risk and at risk for false-negatives with mammography. The density-modified Gail risk is calculated by multiplying the lifetime Gail risk by 0.59, 1.00, 1.41, or 1.94 for a BIRADS of 1, 2, 3, or 4, respectively. Women with a lifetime risk of >50%, as calculated by the density-modified Gail model, are recommended for MRI screening. Consideration can be given to women with a 35–49% lifetime risk using this tool, although there has been no current evidence to support the addition of annual MRI screening.

The true measure of a screening test is not whether it finds more cancers, but whether finding the cancers decreases mortality and morbidity from breast cancer. No study has yet shown that cancers found by MRI decrease mortality from breast cancer. However, two large studies have shown that screening using MRI is more sensitive in high-risk women, with remarkably similar results.[192,193] If tumor size and lymph node involvement are used as surrogates for outcome, MRI does improve the stage at which tumors are identified in women in the highest risk cohort. In the Netherlands study, the cancers found in the 1909 women screened with mammography and MRI were compared with two appropriate control groups of mutation carriers and high-risk patients, none of whom had access to MRI screening. In the highest risk group (50–85% estimated lifetime risk), 63% of mutation carriers with screened cancers had negative nodes when screened with MRI compared with 47% with negative nodes in the controls. In the moderate-risk group (15–30% estimated lifetime risk), only 12% had lymph node involvement and 87% had negative nodes (compared with 52–56% positive nodes and 44–48% negative nodes in the control groups). Therefore, MRI appears to be capable of finding cancers at an earlier stage. However, the rate of detection of cancer is also important, and MRI should be used where that rate is high and significantly higher than that in the usual screened group. Of note, the cancer detection rates were 26.5, 5.4, and 7.8 per 1000 woman years for the mutation carriers, high-risk group, and moderate-risk group, respectively. This should be compared with the detection rate of 5 to 7/1000 women where mammography is most cost-effective, in women aged 50–70 years. The only group that had a higher rate of cancer development was the highest risk group, the mutation carriers, and we should be careful to restrict the use of MRI for those women.

Screening comes at a price, both financial and psychological. In the Netherlands study of 1909 women screened for 10 years, 1200 extra procedures were performed. In the process of finding the 45 cancers, MRI led to twice as many extra procedures (420) compared with mammography (207) and three times as many unnecessary biopsies, 24 versus 7 for MRI and mammography, respectively.[190] It is common to recommend 3- or 6-month follow-up studies after an abnormal imaging test. However, MRI examinations cost US $1000–2000, so it is inappropriate to order these tests unless there truly is a situation where the likelihood of finding an abnormality is much higher than in the general population and where mammography would be unlikely to be effective. The two key messages are that we need to find ways of stratifying risk to appropriately tailor the use of technology and MRI screening should be undertaken only in facilities that have the capability of investigating MRI abnormalities, both with ultrasound and MRI-guided biopsy, if necessary. The Blue Cross/Blue Shield technology assessment concluded in 2003, which showed that MRI screening was justified in women who carry an inherited predisposition to breast cancer. The studies conducted in the Netherlands and Canada[190,194] strengthened this conclusion. The moderate- and high-risk women probably gain less overall because the risk is not as high, suggesting that MR must become more specific and follow-up of abnormalities easier before we implement widespread screening of intermediate risk women.

Not all MRI exams are alike. There is a great deal of variability in technique, sequences, interpretation, and capability for follow-up and biopsy. Although the use of breast MRI has proliferated rapidly, standards have not. Clinicians ordering breast MRIs need to know that technique, time of menses (midcycle is optimal 4–14 days after starting menses[190]), and the skill in interpretation affect results. Interpreting images performed in different institutions is also a challenge because of the relative inability to transfer and view images electronically. Each of these areas is under active investigation, and further research and technological improvements will substantially improve our ability to appropriately integrate MRI into breast cancer management.

MRI has also been used after a diagnostic test reveals an abnormality. The most definitive study on the performance characteristics of MRI for the evaluation of mammographic abnormalities and palpable masses is the multi-institutional International Breast MRI Consortium (IBMC) study. High sensitivity and moderate specificity were confirmed in this study. Diagnostic characterization of lesions by MRI is improving, but it is not sufficiently specific to substitute a biopsy. MRI after an abnormal diagnostic mammogram significantly increases false-positives. Currently, there has been no role for MRI in the diagnosis of breast cancer unless suspicious mammographic findings cannot be evaluated or localized or unless there is another compelling reason to order MRI (e.g., if a patient is a mutation carrier or has a very high risk of cancer and very dense breast tissue).

Perhaps, the most important role for MRI is the staging of known cancer in the breast and monitoring the response to therapy.[190] MRI reveals that tumors form distinct patterns in the breast, and different types of tumors, such as lobular and inflammatory cancers, are more commonly associated with distinct patterns. Initial imaging characteristics identify women likely to have a particularly poor response, such as diffuse tumors with large volumes.[195]

Risk and prevention

If we can reduce the frequency of screening at those with lower risk, in accordance with the recommendations of the USPSTF, those at lower risk to develop breast cancer will be screened less, thus reducing false-positive results. The process of callbacks and biopsies from false-positives is extremely stressful, characterized by increased anxiety and changes in screening choices that have been shown to persist long after the issue is resolved.[152,193] Personal risk-assessment may improve the general understanding of their *personal* breast cancer risk. At present, only one in 10 women has accurate perceptions of her personal risk, while four in 10 have never discussed their personal breast cancer risk with a doctor.[196] They are not aware that some tumors grow rapidly and present between screens (interval cancers) and need attention regardless of a prior normal screen.[197] There are effective, viable prevention options available to the estimated 2 million American women who are at high risk, yet many are completely unaware of their predisposition[198] and so cannot benefit from them. There are three level I studies that have demonstrated the ability of endocrine risk-reducing agents. The NSABP P-01 study of over 13,000 women with a Gail Risk of at least 1.67, randomized to tamoxifen versus placebo, showed that risk of developing invasive cancer or DCIS could be reduced by 50% and more (85%) in the setting of atypia.[199] This has been confirmed by the IBIS trial,[200] and furthermore, younger women (below 50 years of age) had more to gain, and benefits continued for 10 years, even when therapy was stopped after 5 years. The STAR trial compared tamoxifen with raloxifene, and a selective estrogen receptor modulator (SERM) was developed to improve breast density, but noted to reduce hormone-positive breast cancer in postmenopausal women and reduce fracture risk in the MORE study.[201] Raloxifene does not stimulate the endometrial lining and has fewer endometrial side effects including bleeding and endometrial cancer, and although the risk-reducing impact was not quite as high as tamoxifen, it is considered the better choice for postmenopausal women.[202] This is supported by the long-term follow-up of the IBIS 2 trial,[203] which showed an increased risk of death from endometrial cancer in postmenopausal women on tamoxifen. Finally, a prevention study (MAP.3) using the AI exemestane showed a 60% reduction in the risk of hormone-positive invasive breast cancer in postmenopausal women compared with those on tamoxifen.[204] There has been a poor uptake of endocrine risk reduction in the United States and worldwide. This is likely from a combination of a failure to automate or integrate risk assessment into primary care, a failure to appreciate

the benefits of risk reduction, a failure to assess whether a woman receives specific benefit. Cholesterol, for example, is a measure that is used to demonstrate the lowering of cardiac risk. Breast density has been proposed as a possible dynamic measure of risk, where women on tamoxifen who demonstrate a reduction in breast cancer density are the ones who derive the risk reduction benefit.[205,206] This is an important point of study and is likely incorporated into future prevention studies. Furthermore, we know that communicating individual risk can motivate increased screening uptake[207] and that women are more motivated to use preventive interventions when they understand they are high risk[112] and specifically stand to benefit.

Biopsy

When a woman presents with diagnostic abnormality, a decision to intervene should be made in the context of the likelihood of the lesion being invasive cancer or in situ cancer, as well as the age, underlying health condition, and life expectancy of the patient. A decision about which type of biopsy to perform is made by thinking about the need for future procedures. The goal should be to minimize the total number of procedures (including definitive cancer surgery), discomfort and scarring, and diagnostic wait time and anxiety and to enable the optimal timing of procedures.

A number of options are available for the diagnosis of masses and mammographic abnormalities. For palpable lesions, the options include FNA, core biopsy, or excisional biopsy. Minimally invasive techniques, core biopsy, and FNA are quite accurate in experienced hands and when the "triple assessment" is used. Triple assessment is the consideration of the imaging, clinical, and pathologic findings. If there is significant discordance, further evaluation should be pursued. In general, excisional biopsy is not the optimal diagnostic procedure. Minimally invasive biopsy techniques can be performed immediately in the office and facilitate a rapid diagnosis and discussion of options and full evaluation of the extent of disease in the breast before definitive surgery. FNA or core biopsies can also be used to confirm the suspicion of multicentric disease and thereby avoid multiple trips to the operating room and in general allow the optimal sequencing of interventions.

The type of biopsy performed should depend on the expertise at a given institution. FNA is highly accurate, with sensitivity and specificity of 98% and 99%, respectively. FNA both for palpable and mammographic lesions has been used extensively and successfully in Sweden and the United Kingdom, where it is the standard diagnostic tool. This technique requires practitioners who have training and experience in sampling the lesion (the aspect prone to the highest error), preparing the slides, and interpreting cytology.[208] The advantage is that it can be performed right away and yields results within a day. Both FNA and core biopsy are preferred when there is a high suspicion of invasive cancer and the anticipation that a sentinel lymph node dissection (SLND) will be performed. When an SLND is performed, the type of biopsy performed affects the accuracy of the SLND. Core biopsy and FNA have a lower false-negative rate than excisional biopsy when a subsequent sentinel node dissection is performed: 8% compared with 14% for incisional biopsy and 15% for excisional biopsy. In the setting of a patient with a large obvious tumor, FNA can facilitate the rapid confirmation of a diagnosis and a discussion of options, including neoadjuvant therapy and clinical trials. For patients who opt for surgical management, no further test is needed. For those who opt for neoadjuvant therapy, a core biopsy should be obtained for histology to confirm invasive disease, to save for future studies in the event of complete pathologic response and potentially for clinical trials. In the event that cytology expertise does not exist in a given institution, a core biopsy can also be rapidly performed in the office setting.

Recall for mammographic abnormalities is common, and the likelihood of cancer being diagnosed from a mammographic biopsy (cancer to biopsy rate) is highly variable, from 10% to 40%. A low cancer to biopsy rate is not necessary for high sensitivity, and in fact, the most experienced and highly trained mammographers find more cancers and order fewer biopsies for what turns out to be benign.[116] Cancer to biopsy rates decline over time in settings where quality improvement and feedback on performance are the rule. Several ways exist to avoid biopsies of noncancerous tissue. The first is to take the extra time to get old mammograms for comparison. Circumscribed mass lesions that have been stable for over 2 years will be converted to probably benign and not require a biopsy. If an experienced mammographer has not read the films, a second opinion can always be obtained.

In the event that a biopsy is recommended, it is important to make sure that the lesion is not palpable. If it is, and particularly if the lesion is suspicious for cancer, an FNA not only establishes the diagnosis but also confirms that the palpable mass is indeed the cancer, avoiding the need for wire localization at the time of lumpectomy. An attempt to locate nonpalpable suspicious mammographic masses with ultrasound will enable diagnostic and definitive procedures to be ultrasound-guided, which is more comfortable for patients. In the event that a mammographic lesion can only be seen on mammogram, a stereotactic biopsy can be performed using digital images to locate the lesion and direct the core biopsy. The sensitivity of this procedure is as high as 98% by experienced practioners.[206] A specimen radiograph is obtained to confirm that the target has been obtained (usually calcifications). If there is a risk that all calcifications will be removed, it is then critical to leave a clip to localize the area later.

It is important to perform procedures in the context of their value to the overall management of the patient. If cancer is not present, an adequate sampling of the calcifications or lesions should be performed. If cancer is present, the minimal amount to establish the diagnosis is sufficient. At this point, the diagnostic procedure is not definitive and wide excision is needed. Some radiologists take over 30 core biopsy samples. This is not necessary and can create hematomas, distortion of tissue, and difficulty assessing the true extent of the lesion. It is also unpleasant for the patient.

Some mammographic lesions cannot be biopsied using stereotactic techniques because either the lesion is too close to the chest wall or the breast compresses to less than 3 cm in the direction the biopsy needle would be placed. In this case, an excisional biopsy must be performed. A wire is placed by the radiologist to guide the surgery, with the tip of the wire just under or at the level of the calcifications or mass. The surgeon should use the radiologist's estimate for the likelihood of malignancy to determine the extent of resection. For lesions more likely to be cancer, the lesion and a 1-cm rim of tissue should be taken. For less-suspicion lesions, a smaller volume of tissue can be taken. In order to avoid taking unnecessary tissue, an incision should be made near the tip of the wire or the expected location of the abnormality. Starting the excision at the insertion site of the wire only leads to excessive tissue being removed and usually results in a close margin at the end of the wire. Making the incision over the lesion is helpful in locating the biopsy cavity in the event that an additional resection is necessary. All specimens need to be sent to mammography or evaluated using a Faxitron to assure the surgeon that the target lesion has been removed. Mammographers routinely recommend a biopsy of any lesion that is a BI-RADS 4 or higher. However, a BI-RADS classification of 4 includes lesions that have a risk of as low as 3% or as high as 75% for being malignant. The

lesion may be suspicious for either in situ or invasive cancer—no distinction is implied by the categorization of a BI-RADS 4. The surgeon should understand both the type of lesion suspected and a more specific estimate of risk, because they may make a difference in how the patient is evaluated. An older woman with several comorbidities and a mammogram with a BI-RADS 4, if she has a lesion that is approximately 90% likely to be benign and 10% likely to be DCIS, may not need a biopsy. This is the type of lesion that could be followed on mammography. In general, we recommend that a minimally invasive biopsy be used to establish a diagnosis, but excisional biopsy may be the procedure of choice for a woman who has a confined cluster of linear calcifications that are highly suspicious for high-grade DCIS. In this situation, a core biopsy would likely reveal DCIS, and a negative biopsy would be discordant and require wire localization and excision. If the likelihood of associated invasive cancer is low, a sentinel node dissection or axillary sampling will not be necessary, and therefore, there is little value in starting with a stereotactic biopsy.

Ductal carcinoma in situ

DCIS is defined by cytologically malignant epithelial cells within the ductal system of the breast that have not invaded through the basement membrane into the breast parenchyma. Figure 3 shows a histological example of DCIS.

Before the advent of screening, DCIS comprised about 3% of breast cancers detected. As the interest in finding smaller cancers increased, and targeted calcifications rather than only masses, we began to identify DCIS more frequently. DCIS now accounts for approximately 20–25% of screen-detected breast cancers. The cells that comprise DCIS appear similar to invasive cancer both pathologically and molecularly, and therefore the presumption was made that these lesions were the precursors of cancer and that early removal and treatment would reduce cancer incidence and mortality. However, long-term epidemiology studies have amply demonstrated that the removal of 50,000 to 60,000 DCIS lesions annually has not been accompanied by a reduction in the rate of occurrence of invasive breast cancers.[209] This is in contrast to the experience with the removal of colonic polyps and cervical intraepithelial neoplasia (CIN) lesions of the cervix, where the removal of precursor lesions has led to a decrease in the incidence of colon and cervical cancer, respectively.[164] For low-grade DCIS, there is no evidence from SEER that women have the same survival whether they have any intervention or not. Of the 57,222 women diagnosed with DCIS, 2% (1169) had observation only. In women with low-grade DCIS, survival was identical at 10 years with and without surgery (98.6% vs 98.8%, respectively).[210]

From the results of a large observational study of >100,000 women diagnosed with DCIS, Narod and colleagues showed that the risk of dying from breast cancer is extremely low.[211] Less than 1% of patients in this 20-year study died of breast cancer (compared with 5% of patients who died of other causes). Using the Kaplan–Meier method, the breast cancer-specific mortality rate is 3.3% at 20 years, almost similar to the statistic listed by ACS as the chance that breast cancer will be responsible for a woman's death (ACS.org).

Two ongoing therapeutic questions related to the treatment of DCIS concern the use of radiation and hormonal therapy. While radiation decreases the chance of an invasive breast cancer occurrence, and a recurrence of DCIS, radiation after lumpectomy for DCIS does not result in a reduction in breast cancer mortality. This has been shown consistently.[212] While some reports suggest that low-grade DCIS with wide margins (>10 mm) recur in as few as 3% of cases with surgery only without radiotherapy. Two large prospective studies by the Dana-Farber Cancer Institute and the Eastern Cooperative Oncology Group (ECOG) encountered local recurrence rates of 12.5% and 7% in low- and intermediate-grade DCIS, respectively.

One of the leading proponents of treating favorable DCIS with lumpectomy only has been Silverstein and colleagues, who, in 1995, developed the Van Nuys Prognostic Index (VNPI) to help define selection criteria for cases with low recurrence risk.[136] The original VNPI classes were determined from the retrospective analysis of 333 patients treated at two institutions between 1979 and 1995. Patients received 1–3 points for three factors: tumor grade and the presence or absence of necrosis (combined into one category), tumor size, and margin status. Over two-thirds of the patients had an intermediate-risk VNPI (cumulative score of 5–7), and, similar to the randomized data, radiation reduced the probability of breast cancer recurrence in this cohort (32% vs 15%; $p = 0.17$).[160] Less than one-third of their patients had small, low-grade disease with widely negative surgical margins, and the breast cancer recurrence rate was low after breast conservation surgery (BCS) only (3% breast cancer recurrence rate among 76 patients treated without radiation). Subsequently, this group has also incorporated patient age into their prognostic index. Similar data were subsequently reported from a population-based cohort study of 1036 women ≥40 years of age in San Francisco treated with lumpectomy only for DCIS. This study found overall a relatively high recurrence rate (20% and 10% for all recurrence and invasive recurrence, respectively, at 5 years) but reported that the subset of patients with mammographically detected low-grade disease treated with surgery that achieved widely negative margins had a lower ROR after surgery only.[137]

Using an expansion of this original cohort, Silverstein and colleagues reanalyzed their data, focusing on the importance of margin status for patients treated with DCIS. In this analysis,[138] they reported that 93 patients with a margin width of 10 mm or more had an 8-year local recurrence rate of only 3%. This rate was found to be much higher after treatment with lumpectomy without radiation when the margin width was 1–10 mm (recurrence rate 20%) and margins were under 1 mm (58%). When this study was updated and expanded to include 212 patients with margin widths of ≥10 mm, the breast recurrence rate in this cohort increased to 14%.[139] In addition, the low recurrence rate noted in the setting of 10-mm margins could not be confirmed in a single-arm prospective trial conducted at the Dana-Farber/Harvard Cancer Center. In this study, 157 patients with grade 1 or 2 DCIS, ≤2.5 cm, underwent wide local excision only with achievement of negative margins of ≥1 cm.[142] The trial was closed early because the recurrence rate met predefined stopping rules, with an estimated 5-year local recurrence rate of 12.5% (invasive cancer occurrence of 6%). The authors concluded that even in this highly selected group of patients, there was a substantial local recurrence rate. The ECOG has also conducted a prospective study of 711 patients with DCIS treated with surgery plus/minus tamoxifen without radiation. Two different patient strata were enrolled: (1) low- or intermediate-grade DCIS, size < 2.5 cm, and (2) high-grade DCIS, size < 1 cm. All patients were required to have a negative post lumpectomy mammogram and negative margins of 3 mm or more. The 5-year risk of in-breast tumor recurrence (IBTR) was 7% in the low- and intermediate-grade stratum and 14% in the high-grade stratum.[141] Given the success of salvage therapies and the low risk of cancer-associated death with surgical-only treatment, it is reasonable to inform patients about the available data and have them participate in their locoregional treatment decisions.

At present, a debate has been ongoing regarding the overdiagnosis and subsequent overtreatment of pure DCIS in the modern era, given the technologic improvements in breast screening over the past decade. At the same time, long-term combined follow-up of the NSABP B-17 and B-24 trials shows that an *invasive* recurrence after surgery only for DCIS increases the risk of breast cancer-related death and that radiation reduces this risk of invasive recurrence by more than half (19.4% vs 8.9%).[211] Although the VNPI and ECOG studies cited above provide guidance in terms of identification of a low-risk subgroup of DCIS, they do not hold the same weight as a prospective randomized trial.

In 1998, the RTOG initiated such a trial for selected women with low-/intermediate-grade DCIS ≤ 2.5 cm in the highest extent with ≥3-mm margins, originally designed for 1800 patients.[213] Unfortunately, the study was ended in 2006 because of poor accrual; however, in the 636 patients enrolled, radiation reduced the local failure rate from 6.7% to 0.9% at 7 years ($p < 0.001$). The clinical impact of this statistical benefit is up for discussion, and patients must be counseled regarding the trade-offs of toxicity and inconvenience of adjuvant radiation versus the higher risk of a (possibly invasive) recurrence and need for subsequent salvage therapy. An emerging clinical tool to counsel patients and tailor adjuvant recommendations for DCIS may be genomic sequencing. In a tissue analysis of over 300 patients treated on the abovementioned phase II ECOG trial, the 21-gene Oncotype DX assay (see section on adjuvant therapy) was used to score patients according to the risk of invasive recurrence and was found to be predictive, independent of clinical factors.[165] It remains to be seen whether such a strategy provides cost-effective utility over the currently used clinical selection factors.

Radiation has small but real risks.[214] Given the lack of mortality benefit, it is appropriate to consider reserving external beam radiation for breast conservation when invasive cancer occurs in the setting of DCIS with many high-risk features. Many invasive lesions do not require radiation in the postmenopausal setting,[215–217] and hence certainly it should not be a surprise that there is no benefit of radiation in the noninvasive setting.

The second major area of research and controversy regarding the management of DCIS concerns the use of hormonal therapy. After completion of the B-17 trial, the NSABP conducted the B-24 trial, which randomized 1802 patients treated with lumpectomy and radiation to receive either tamoxifen or placebo for 5 years.[218] The eligibility of this trial differed from B-17 in that it included patients with positive surgical margins, which ended up being present in 25% of the study population. In addition, the primary end point of the study was not ipsilateral breast recurrence, but rather the probability of having an ipsilateral recurrence or developing a contralateral breast cancer. Therefore, this trial was designed to investigate the combined therapeutic benefit of tamoxifen against the index DCIS and the chemopreventive benefit of tamoxifen in reducing subsequent independent breast cancers.

The results of the B-24 trial indicated that patients treated with tamoxifen, surgery, and radiation had a 5-year rate of noninvasive or invasive breast cancers of 8.2% compared with 13.4% for those treated only with surgery and radiation.[142] Clearly, a component of this benefit was the chemoprevention effects of tamoxifen. In B-24, the use of tamoxifen resulted in a 41% reduction in the 5-year incidence of contralateral breast cancers. These data are consistent with the reduction in second primary breast cancers seen in the adjuvant tamoxifen trials and the NSABP P-1 trial, which found that tamoxifen decreased breast cancer development in women at increased risk for breast cancer by 49%.[110] In a subsequent retrospective analysis of ER expression from stored tumor material from 628 patients

(327 placebo, 301 tamoxifen), it was found that the benefit of tamoxifen was limited to 482 patients (77%) with ER-positive disease. In this cohort, tamoxifen was associated with a significant reduction in both ipsilateral breast recurrence and the development of contralateral breast cancer. There was no apparent benefit of tamoxifen in those with ER-negative tumors, but the sample size precluded, detecting a small benefit.

The UK/ANZ trial provides additional information concerning the interaction of radiation and tamoxifen after lumpectomy in patients with DCIS.[219] In this study, use of tamoxifen decreased the rate of DCIS recurrence, but not invasive recurrence for patients who did not receive radiation. However, in patients treated with radiation after lumpectomy, tamoxifen provided no benefit in ipsilateral breast events. Unlike the B-24 trial, this study required all patients to have negative surgical margins after lumpectomy and did not include the development of a contralateral breast cancer as an event in their primary outcome measure.

These data suggest that, for patients treated with an adequate lumpectomy that achieves negative surgical margins and subsequently receive radiation, the therapeutic benefits of tamoxifen are likely to be very low in reducing ROR in the ipsilateral breast, but there will be a protective benefit in the contralateral breast. Interestingly, a survey found that 56% of US practitioners routinely recommend tamoxifen for women with DCIS compared with only 22% of European practitioners.[146] Despite the lack of clarity concerning the therapeutic benefits of tamoxifen in DCIS, for patients with ER-positive disease, the addition of tamoxifen is likely to have chemopreventive effects and minimize the risks of subsequent new breast cancers. NSABP B = 35 is a phase III trial that compared the effects of 5-year tamoxifen use to the AI anastrozole in 3104 postmenopausal women diagnosed with DCIS.[220] With a median follow-up of 9 years, there was an absolute difference of 4.3% in breast cancer-free interval favoring anastrozole. This difference was magnified in women under the age of 60, where the absolute difference was 6.7%. Consistent with prior studies, no difference in overall survival (OS) was observed; less uterine cancers and more osteoporotic fractures were observed in patients treated with anastrozole.

Among DCIS patients, breast cancer-specific mortality is associated with age at diagnosis, ethnicity, and DCIS characteristics such as ER status, grade, size (>5 cm), and comedonecrosis. Despite their significance in a multivariable analysis, high-risk characteristics, such as ER-negativity and high grade, often overlap. Only a small minority of patients will have one or more of these high-risk characteristics. For young women (<40 years of age) who present with symptomatic DCIS, about 5% of the population, we should be cognizant that this is a different disease than the average DCIS. In addition, African-American women who are more likely to be at risk for hormone-negative breast cancer and women with hormone-negative or human epidermal growth factor receptor-2 positive (HER2+) breast cancer may be those that should continue to be treated according to the current aggressive standards. In total, these groups probably constitute about 20% of the population of DCIS.

There are uncommon cases where DCIS is associated with a higher risk than has been appreciated. When DCIS is diagnosed before the age of 35 or even 40, some of these lesions do pose an increased risk of breast cancer-specific mortality. DCIS diagnosed before the age of 40 is likely different, as it would present as a symptomatic event (e.g., a mass or bloody nipple discharge), as screening before the age of 40 is rare.

It has always been assumed that DCIS indicates a higher local risk—but the similarity of the ipsilateral and contralateral invasive breast cancer risk (5.9% and 6.2%) with long-term follow-up[211] suggests that DCIS may behave more as a risk factor like atypia. Oncotype DCIS, a gene expression score obtained on formalin-fixed tissues, demonstrated that low-risk lesions simply excised appear to carry the risk equivalent to a Gail Risk of 2.5[167] A unilateral recurrence of DCIS or contralateral DCIS event has no effect on mortality. However, an invasive cancer does: 18-fold for unilateral and 13-fold for contralateral, suggesting that all risk depends on the probability of the occurrence of an invasive cancer. DCIS may best represent an opportunity to alter the environment of the breast and approach using standard risk reduction or endocrine risk reduction. For premenopausal women, tamoxifen is a good choice for HR+ DCIS. For postmenopausal women, AIs have been shown to have a higher impact on risk reduction. If AIs produce adverse side effects, raloxifene is a good alternative. Tamoxifen should probably not be used for DCIS in postmenopausal women given the risks reported with longer duration hormone therapy in IBIS 2.[203]

High-risk lesions (e.g., HER2+, <40, ER−, large size) should be aggressively treated, but the Narod analysis suggests that our current approach of surgical removal and radiation may not suffice for the rare cases that lead to breast cancer mortality and new approaches need to be investigated. In a study characterizing the immune environment of high-risk lesions that are most likely to recur, we found that the tumor microenvironment associated with recurrence was replete with activated macrophages and a paucity of activated T cells.[221]

Treatment of early-stage breast cancer

Staging and classification

The purposes of staging are to (1) plan a therapeutic strategy that is most appropriate for the patient, (2) allow for more intelligent projection of outcome based on the disease status of the patient, and (3) permit comparison of therapeutic results obtained from different sources by different means. The common staging methods are clinical and pathologic, but newer methods involving biologic assessments are under development and validation. Regardless of the staging method used, it is important to remember that the stage represents the state of disease or biologic potential of a patient's tumor. The benefits of a particular staging method must be judged against its accuracy in performing this task.

The tumor node metastasis (TNM) classification devised by the Union for International Against Cancer (UICC) and accepted by the American Joint Committee on Cancer Staging is of world standard.[222] The TNM is based on the clinical features of tumor (T), the regional lymph nodes (N), and the presence or absence of distant metastases (M) (Table 7).

In general, clinical staging systems underestimate the extent of disease. The inclusion of pathologic information improves staging accuracy and is the basis for most modern clinical trials. In all cases, it is wise to remember that the goal is to define the biologic activity of the tumor. Cox regression statistical models demonstrate that the presence of nodal metastases are the most important factor, and the number of nodes involved can be used to further subset the prognostic groups. It is generally acknowledged that nodal metastases that penetrate the capsule and extend into adjacent perinodal tissue carry a worse prognosis.

In a regression analysis model, tumor size is found to be closely related to axillary lymph node involvement.[84,223] Tumor size is not an important discriminant within axillary node groups, except for patients with more than four involved nodes. Thus, size, which can be a function of either time or growth rate, is less useful than

Table 7 TNM stage definitions.

Primary tumor (T)

TX	Primary tumor cannot be assessed
T0	No evidence of primary tumor
Tis	Carcinoma in situ
Tis (DCIS)	Ductal carcinoma in situ
Tis (LCIS)	Lobular carcinoma in situ
Tis (Paget's)	Paget disease of the nipple with no tumor
T1	Tumor 2.0 cm or less in highest dimension
T1mic	Microinvasion 0.1 cm or less in highest dimension
T1a	Tumor more than 0.1 but not more than 0.5 cm in highest dimension
T1b	Tumor more than 0.5 cm but not more than 1.0 cm in highest dimension
T1c	Tumor more than 1.0 cm but not more than 2.0 cm in highest dimension
T2	Tumor more than 2.0 cm but not more than 5.0 cm in highest dimension
T3	Tumor more than 5.0 cm in highest dimension
T4	Tumor of any size with direct extension to (1) chest wall or (2) skin, only as described below
T4a	Extension to chest wall, not including only pectoralis muscle adherence/invasion
T4b	Edema (including peau d'orange) and/or ulceration of the skin of the breast and/or satellite skin nodules confined to the same breast
T4c	Both T4a and T4b
T4d	Inflammatory carcinoma

Regional lymph nodes (N)

NX	Regional lymph nodes cannot be assessed (e.g., previously removed)
N0	No regional lymph node metastasis
N1	Metastasis to movable ipsilateral axillary lymph node(s)
N2	Metastasis in ipsilateral axillary lymph node(s) fixed or matted, or in clinically apparent ipsilateral internal mammary nodes in the absence of clinically evident axillary lymph node metastasis
N3	Metastasis in ipsilateral infraclavicular lymph node(s) with or without axillary lymph node involvement, or in clinically apparent ipsilateral internal mammary lymph node(s) and in the presence of clinically evident axillary lymph node metastasis, or metastasis in ipsilateral supraclavicular lymph node(s) with or without axillary or internal mammary lymph node involvement

Pathologic classification (pN)

pNX	Regional lymph nodes cannot be assessed (previously removed or not removed for pathologic study)
pN0	No regional lymph node metastasis identified histologically; isolated tumor cell (ITC) clusters are no higher than 0.2 mm, single tumor cells, or a cluster of fewer than 200 cells in a single histologic cross section, detected by histology or immunohistochemistry (IHC)
pN0(i-)	No regional lymph node metastasis histologically, negative IHC
pN0(i+)	Malignant cells in regional lymph node(s) no higher than 0.2 mm
pN0(mol-)	No regional lymph node metastases histologically, negative molecular findings by RT-PCR
pN0(mol+)	Positive molecular findings by RT-PCR, but no regional LN metastases detected by histology or IHC
pN1	Micrometastases, or metastases in 1–3 axillary lymph nodes, and/or in internal mammary nodes with metastases detected by sentinel lymph node biopsy, but not clinically detected
pN1mi	Micrometastases (>0.2 mm and/or more than 200 cells, but none higher than 2.0 mm)
pN1a	Metastases in 1–3 axillary lymph nodes, at least one metastasis higher than 2.0 mm
pN1b	Metastases in internal mammary nodes with micrometastases or macrometastases detected by sentinel lymph node biopsy, but not clinically detected
pN1c	Metastases in 1–3 axillary lymph nodes and in internal mammary nodes with micrometastases or macrometastases detected by sentinel lymph node biopsy, but not clinically detected
pN2	Metastases in 4–9 axillary lymph nodes, or in clinically apparent internal mammary lymph nodes in the absence of axillary lymph node metastasis
pN2a	Metastases in 4–9 axillary lymph nodes; or in clinically detected lymph nodes in the absence of axillary lymph node metastases
pN2b	Metastases in clinically detected internal mammary lymph nodes in the absence of axillary lymph node metastases
pN3	Metastasis in 10 or more axillary lymph nodes; or in infraclavicular lymph nodes; or in clinically apparent ipsilateral internal mammary lymph nodes in the presence of 1 or more positive level 1, II axillary lymph nodes; or in more than 3 axillary lymph nodes and in internal mammary lymph nodes with micrometastases or macrometastases detected by sentinel lymph node biopsy, but not clinically detected; or in ipsilateral supraclavicular lymph nodes
pN3a	Metastases in 10 or more axillary lymph nodes (or at least one tumor deposit higher than 2.0 mm), or metastases to the infraclavicular lymph nodes
pN3b	Metastases in clinically detected ipsilateral internal mammary lymph nodes in the presence of one or more positive axillary lymph nodes, or in more than 3 axillary lymph nodes and in internal mammary lymph nodes with micrometastases or macrometastases detected by sentinel lymph node biopsy but not clinically detected
pN3c	Metastases in ipsilateral supraclavicular lymph nodes

Distant metastasis (M)

MX	Presence of distant metastasis cannot be assessed
M0	No distant metastasis
M1	Distant metastasis present

(continued overleaf)

Table 7 (*Continued*)

AJCC stage groupings	
Stage 0	Tis, N0, M0
Stage IA	T1, N0, M0
Stage IB	T0, N1mi, M0
	T1, N1mi, M0
Stage IIA	T0, N1, M0
	T1, N1, M0
	T2, N0, M0
Stage IIB	T2, N1, M0
	T3, N0, M0
Stage IIIA	T0, N2, M0
	T1, N2, M0
	T2, N2, M0
	T3, N1, M0
	T3, N2, M0
Stage IIIB	T4, N0, M0
Stage IIIC	T4, N1, M0
	T4, N2, M0
	Any T, N3, M0
Stage IV	Any T, Any N, M1

Source: Edge 2010.[222] Reproduced with permission of Springer.

axillary node involvement, which is a more specific indicator of biologic aggressiveness. Some patients with large masses may have slow-growing tumors, which have not metastasized. By contrast, patients are also diagnosed with small but aggressive tumors found by screening mammography, in whom distant metastases are already present. These patients may die rapidly despite the initial favorable local clinical features. A biologic classification would identify these women more accurately than does the TNM system; this is the goal of future modifications to current staging.

Surgery

Over the past three decades, revolutionary changes have occurred in the locoregional management of primary breast cancer. As a result, radical and extended radical mastectomy has been relegated to the archives of surgical history. The publication of a series of randomized controlled clinical trials comparing radical mastectomy to less-extensive surgical interventions led a National Institutes of Health (NIH)-sponsored consensus development conference (1990) to recommend that breast preservation is the preferable treatment for women with stages I and II breast cancer, because it provides survival figures equivalent to those of total mastectomy and axillary dissection while, at the same time, preserving the breast.[224]

Information from various sources indicates that many patients with breast cancer have disseminated disease by the time a clinical diagnosis is established. This is not surprising, because a breast tumor of 1 cm has already progressed through 30 of the theoretical 40 doublings that result in a tumor of approximately 1 kg, a size that could be lethal to the patient. However, at present, we know that breast cancer is a heterogeneous disease, and that some patients have tumors with a low potential for metastatic spread, and that some, even when small and confined to the breast, have a high risk for metastatic spread.[86,89] Molecular profiling is likely to add much to our ability to distinguish these types of tumors and tailor treatment accordingly.

Treatment failed in three of four patients with positive axillary nodal involvement and in almost nine of 10 patients with four or more involved nodes 10 years after radical mastectomy without adjuvant chemotherapy for what were considered clinically "curable" breast cancers. These findings emphasize the systemic nature of some breast cancers and indicate the inadequacy of extensive local and regional surgery when used as sole modalities of treatment in those women at high risk to develop metastases.

Breast-conserving treatments

The goal of breast conservation is to remove the tumor and a rim of normal tissue while preserving the contour and shape of the breast. Tumor left at a margin will increase the ROR. Recht and colleagues, in a study of 533 patients, showed that recurrence risk depends on the amount of tumor left at the margin: grossly positive margins, focally positive margins, and close margins were associated with a recurrence risk of 27%, 14%, and 7%, respectively. Close margins did not materially change the recurrence risk in this study where all women received radiation therapy. The presence of extensive intraductal carcinoma, once thought to be a contraindication to breast conservation, has now been shown not to be associated with higher risk of local recurrence if all of the DCIS has been excised. After breast conservation, 90% of all in-breast recurrences, in the first decade after diagnosis, are in the same quadrant and genetically identical to the primary breast cancer. Long-term follow-up studies of BCS versus mastectomy, however, show that there is an ongoing risk for developing new cancers in the breast after 10 years, but these often occur in other quadrants.

With the advent of lumpectomy, there was a need to adopt a two-stage approach to biopsy and then to definitive surgery. Preoperative core needle biopsies, either clinically or radiologically directed, should be considered standard, so that the surgeon has a definite diagnosis before any surgery takes place and can better plan the operation. A detailed algorithm describing an optimal surgical strategy for the management of primary breast cancer has been described and is presented in Figure 14.

If an open breast biopsy must be carried out, it should be done as if a lumpectomy were being performed. Attention must be focused toward ensuring that specimen margins are likely to be free of tumor should a malignancy be encountered. In all circumstances where breast conservation is feasible, the operation carried out to establish the definitive diagnosis of a breast lesion becomes the definitive

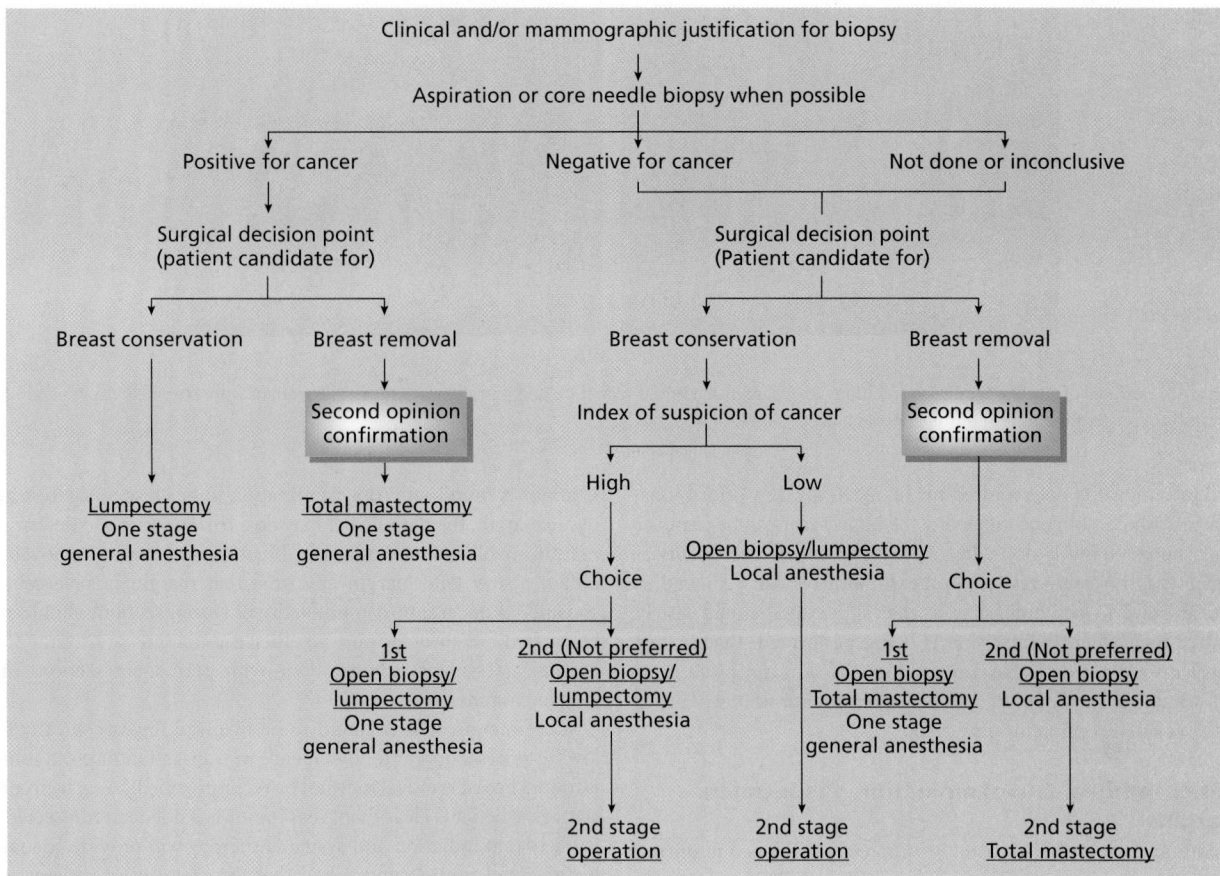

Figure 14 Recommended surgical strategy for management of primary breast cancer.

treatment, regardless of the time at which axillary surgery was performed. Most breast cancer operations—biopsy, lumpectomy, axillary dissection, and even mastectomy—can be performed as outpatient procedures with comparable low levels of surgical complications and equal or better personal and social adjustment to the procedure.

Technique and cosmetic considerations

In order to achieve the best cosmetic results, incision should be planned based on the extent of tumor in the breast, the location of the tumor, and the original shape of the breast. Many options now exist for patients who require breast surgery. The extent of resection of tissue depends on breast size. Plastic surgery techniques can be used to improve symmetry, both with and without cosmetic surgery on the contralateral breast. Once breast tissue is removed, undermining the breast tissue at the level of the fascia provides the opportunity to arrange the closure of the breast tissue in a medial to lateral direction, thereby avoiding the displacement of the nipple either superiorly or inferiorly. Mastopexy or reduction can be performed on the contralateral breast to improve symmetry. If there is a significant degree of ptosis in the breast, a partial mastectomy can be accomplished by performing a breast reduction, thereby combining a cosmetic enhancement with the oncologic procedure of removing the breast tissue (Figure 15). In a breast reduction procedure, more than half of the breast tissue can be removed; thus, this technique can be used for larger tumors or when there is scattered in situ disease in a single quadrant. Figure 15a and b

shows a patient with significant discomfort from her large breast, who had always wanted to undergo breast reduction surgery.

Clear margins were easily obtained by removing over a quadrant of the breast tissue, leaving medial and lateral flaps of at least 1 cm, and achieving a very nice cosmetic result. Preoperative MRI can be very useful for planning the surgical approach. High-resolution scans should be used to maximize the anatomic detail provided by MRI. When breast surgery is required, it provides an opportunity to change the shape and size of the breast, which, if desired by the patient, may make the surgical resection easier and turn an unpleasant procedure to a more tolerable one.

In order to perform a satisfactory lumpectomy, it is essential that the incision be placed directly over the tumor. The use of a circumareolar incision for removing a lesion that is not in proximity to the areola is not optimal, nor is tunneling through breast tissue to remove a lesion that is not beneath the incision. Tumor-free specimen margins are difficult and often impossible to obtain when such an incision is made. Reexcision of the tumor site to obtain free margins through such an incision is equally difficult. If there is concern that a mastectomy may eventually be necessary, the incision should be made with some thought as to what type of incision would be made if a mastectomy were required. In instances where lumpectomy cannot be carried out because of the inability to obtain tumor-free margins, mastectomy incisions can be modified to accommodate the lumpectomy incision. Preoperative diagnosis with needle biopsy can be of significant importance in planning the incision and should be the standard.

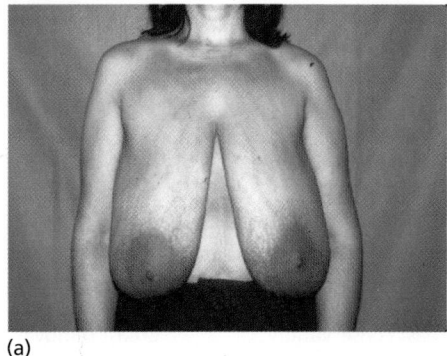 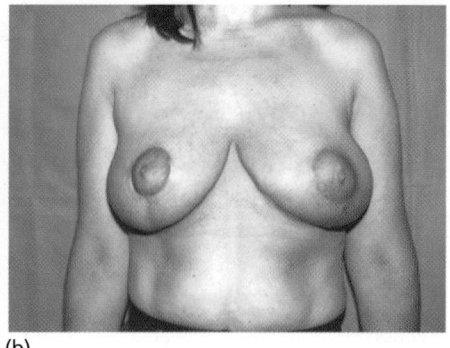

(a)   (b)

Figure 15 Example of a breast reduction technique to accomplish a breast reduction and partial mastectomy in a woman with extremely large, pendulous breasts. (a) Preoperative and (b) postoperative images.

Skin removal is not required for lumpectomy. If a prior biopsy was performed, skin encompassing the biopsy scar can be removed when lumpectomy is done, but it is not essential. The quality of cosmesis is inversely related to the amount of skin removed. A special point to be emphasized is that skin edges should not be undermined when the excision is being performed, that is, thin skin flaps are not desirable. Undermining of skin can result in an unfavorable cosmetic result, and hence removal of skin may be the better cosmetic option in some cases.

Tumor removal and examination of specimen margins

The tumor is removed so that it is completely enveloped in normal fat and/or breast tissue. This procedure does not necessitate the removal of a predefined amount of normal tissue around the lesion, just the amount adequate to achieve specimen margins grossly free of tumor. Orienting the specimen is particularly important. Adopting a standard procedure to orient and ink specimens in your institution will improve communication among pathologists, surgeons, and radiation oncologists. A typical standard is to use a long stitch for the lateral margin and short stitch for the superior margin, secured to a piece of Telfa posteriorly to improve orientation. This is particularly beneficial for specimens requiring specimen radiography, by preserving the shape and improving the chance to identify and further resect a specific margin that may be close to the radiographic lesion (Figure 16).

If a prior excisional biopsy was performed and margins were not evaluated, it is obligatory that, at the time of node dissection, a resection be performed to ensure tumor-free margins.

The specimen is immediately delivered to the pathologist, who must confirm or establish the diagnosis of cancer (if a needle biopsy was not done), aid the surgeon in deciding intraoperatively whether the specimen margins are grossly free of tumor, and take an aliquot of tumor for any special studies.

The pathologist receives the specimen and carefully orients it by means of the suture tags that the surgeon has placed. After measurement, the uncut specimen is inspected for gross margin involvement. If there is evidence that the tumor has been transected, the surgeon is immediately apprised of the precise location of the margin involvement so that additional tissue can be removed from that area while the pathologist is completing inspection of the specimen. The pathologist then coats the entire surface of the specimen with India ink, blots it dry, and then bisects the tumor and specimen transversely. Some pathologists use multiple colors (e.g., for the posterior, anterior superior half, and the anterior inferior half) to improve the ability to pinpoint the location of an involved margin.

If tumor is found on gross examination to be close to the resected tissue margin, the pathologist may do a frozen section to determine margin involvement. Additional breast tissue can be removed to obtain a new true margin any time that margin involvement is considered uncertain. A multiplicity of frozen sections should not be carried out to determine whether the margins are tumor free. Margin assessment is better done with permanent sections in a detailed manner.

If the margin is later found to be involved microscopically following re-resection and no evidence of transaction of gross tumor is found, breast removal may not be recommended. In such circumstances, when it is clear that gross tumor has not been transected, it is likely that radiation and systemic therapy will provide adequate locoregional tumor control and that the majority of patients will remain free of local recurrence. An update on their series of reports on margin control from the Joint Center in Boston demonstrates that recurrence rates are the same for focally positive margins as for true negative ones.[225] Similarly, when a breast tumor recurrence occurs following lumpectomy, it is likely that tumor control will be obtained by repeat lumpectomy if such tumors are small and can be removed with tumor-free specimen margins.

Pathologic criteria used for making a decision about whether the tumor involves specimen margins can vary. Many pathologists infer margin involvement by such subjective designations as tumor "very

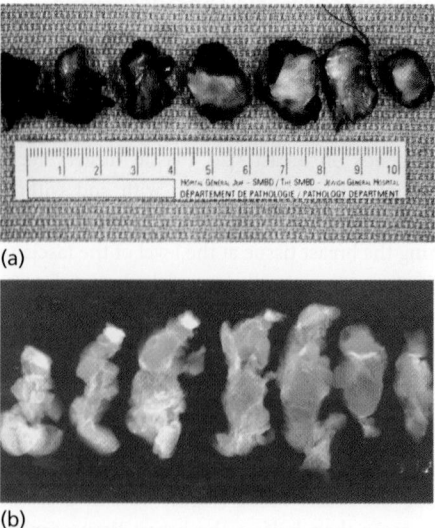

(a)

(b)

Figure 16 (a) Image of gross specimen. (b) Radiograph of gross specimen showing calcifications.

close" to margin. A review of cases showed that there was residual cancer in only 12% of total mastectomy specimens removed because the margin was close. Thus, it is most appropriate to regard lines of resection as involved only when cancer is transected.

For mammographically detected carcinomas requiring radiographic guidance, one or more wires are placed in the breast to either bracket calcifications or pinpoint the center of the lesion or calcifications. Specimen mammography is required once the lesion is removed to confirm the presence of the lesion as well as the location of the mammographic abnormality relative to the margins. Whenever possible, nonpalpable lesions that can be identified using ultrasound should be localized using that technique, because these procedures are better tolerated by patients and do not use compression required for mammographic localization. Some surgeons are being trained to use ultrasound as it can better improve the targeted excision of solid lesions in the operating room. This reduces the need and time for communication between the operating room and radiology suite. However, it requires that surgeons be specially trained, very skilled in the technique, and able to determine which lesions they can accurately identify to avoid missing the lesion intraoperatively.

Mastectomy

Patients who undergo mastectomy can opt reconstruction or not. Cosmetic considerations are important, regardless of a woman choosing reconstruction. It is important to try to leave a flat surface on the chest wall so that wearing a prosthesis is possible and comfortable. Avoiding skin folds in the axillary line can be accomplished through fishtail incisions at the axillary portion of the axilla or contouring the incisions in the axilla using plastic surgery techniques to avoid excess skin.

Immediate reconstruction has been shown to be safe,[226] even in the setting of locally advanced disease (Figure 17), when appropriate multimodal therapy is used. Therefore, any woman considering mastectomy should also be told about options for reconstruction, both immediate and delayed. Complications after reconstruction are common and should be expected by both the surgeon and patient. Expectations about outcomes should be appropriately set, and women should be prepared for the possibility of multiple surgical procedures to optimize the reconstructive outcome.

If the decision to use chemotherapy does not require additional tissue or definitive resection of the primary tumor, and if chemotherapy if going to be part of multimodal treatment for a given woman, and if she is strongly considering mastectomy, based on the extent of disease or patient preference, neoadjuvant chemotherapy should be recommended (see systemic adjuvant therapy: neoadjuvant therapy). Sequencing the surgery and reconstruction after systemic therapy minimizes the risk that a complication would delay adjuvant therapy and gives women much more time to consider surgical options and adjust to the diagnosis. Neoadjuvant systemic therapy increases breast conservation rates. In a recent study of carboplatin and bevacizumab added to anthracycline- and taxane-based chemotherapy, treatment before surgery led to a conversion rate of 42% from ineligible to eligible for breast conservation therapy.[227] Breast conservation was successful in 93% of those who chose it. However, about 30% of women who were eligible for breast conservation chose mastectomy. Neoadjuvant chemotherapy allows many patients with large breast tumors to have clinically meaningful tumor reduction, indicating response that would affect ability to undergo breast conservation. However, response varies by imaging and tumor subtypes. In the ISPY-1

trial, concordance between tumor size on MRI and surgical pathology was higher in well-defined tumors, particularly those with a triple-negative subtype, and was lower in HR+ diffuse tumors.[228]

For women who are ambivalent about reconstruction, delayed reconstruction may be optimal. However, cosmetic outcomes are better when reconstruction is performed immediately, and scars can be minimized and tailored to the type of reconstruction that has been chosen. It is difficult to make reconstruction decisions within days, and women who are deciding should be reassured that an extra week or two to study their options and make good decisions would not affect their survival outcome. They will likely live for decades with the consequence of this decision, and hence the investment of a few weeks, if necessary, to ensure that they are comfortable with their decision is important.

Two basic types of reconstruction can be offered: implant reconstruction and autologous tissue reconstruction. Implants can be placed as expanders or permanent implants. Expanders are the most commonly used form of reconstruction. They are placed under the pectoralis muscle and the pocket is gradually expanded until is it larger than the desired breast size. Then the expander is exchanged for a permanent implant and the breast shape is contoured. The entire process can take 6–8 weeks. An alternative technique, used in conjunction with skin-sparing mastectomy (SSM), is the placement of permanent implants. The majority of implants used for reconstruction are saline. Although silicone implants were pulled off the market because of a concern that they increased the risk for developing autoimmune disease, several large studies have failed to show a definitive connection; as a result, silicone implants are again being used.[128] There are specific instances where silicone products may be preferred (e.g., if a permanent implant is placed immediately, but the ability to expand the implant is desired). Autologous tissue flaps include TRAM, DIEP, or latissimus dorsi flaps (Figures 18 and 19).

Decision about the type of reconstruction depends largely on patient preference, although treatment considerations can also play an important role. If radiation is anticipated, complications are less if autologous tissue is used. There is controversy about whether TRAM flaps can tolerate radiation, and several published reports suggest that radiation causes significant deleterious effects on the

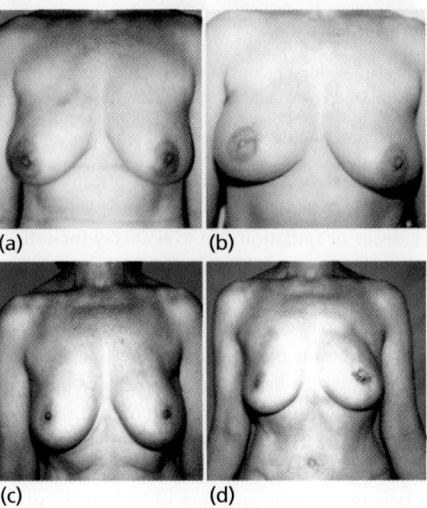

(a) (b)

(c) (d)

Figure 17 Preoperative and postoperative images of a skin-sparing mastectomy with immediate reconstruction with TRAM flap delayed nipple reconstruction in a 37-year-old women (a, b) and 65-year-old woman (c, d). Postoperative images at 12 weeks (b) and 8 weeks (d) show appearance 5 days after nipple reconstruction.

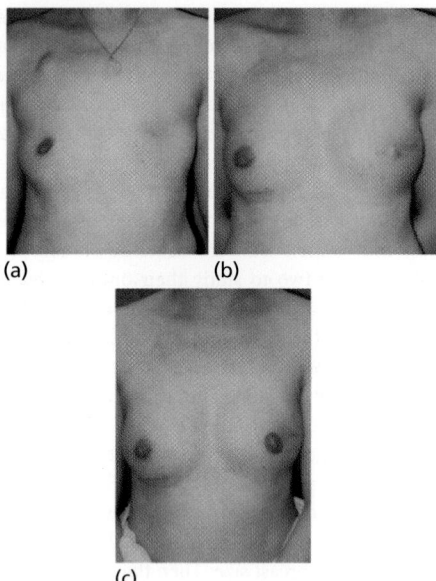

(a)   (b)

(c)

Figure 18 Examples of total skin-sparing technique combined with various reconstruction techniques. (a) Placement of immediate implant using mastopexy incision and contralateral mastopexy. Mastectomy is on left; images are 3 weeks postoperative. (b) Bilateral mastectomy with placement of immediate implants in a woman at high risk after recurrence subsequent to prior lumpectomy for subcentimeter DCIS. Preoperative MRI demonstrated single small focus of lateral recurrence. (c) Mastectomy on right followed by immediate reconstruction using TRAM flap.

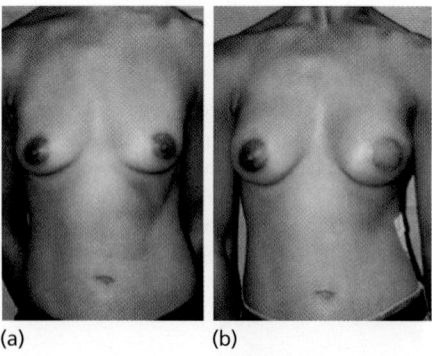

(a)   (b)

Figure 19 Latissimus dorsi reconstruction with bilateral augmentation in a 39-year-old woman. Pre- (a) and (b) 12-week postoperative image.

flap. It may be that free flaps, requiring an anastomosis, tolerate radiation as well as pedicle flaps, or more likely, institutions that use higher doses of radiation (up to 6500 Gy including the boost) may experience more complications. An institution from Dundee, Scotland, that limits radiation to the chest wall to 4500–5000 Gy recently reported excellent results in a large series of patients.

A new technique for mastectomy is the total skin sparing mastectomy (TSSM), which has become a standard procedure in many centers.[229,230] This technique removes all of the breast tissue, including the tissue of the areola and nipple, but preserves the overlying dermis. A report of 171 cases shows that over time, the technique has become reliable and that various incisions can be used to achieve excellent results. This technique results in 99% preservation of nipple and areola skin. Although follow-up is limited, early results show that the local recurrence rate is extremely low (<2%), and we anticipate that the total skin sparing technique will not affect recurrence risk. The key is the complete removal of the nipple duct

tissue (Figures 18 and 19). This technique can be combined with any reconstructive technique except the use of permanent implants. The immediate expansion of the skin significantly increases the risk of skin necrosis. This exciting development in technique, while challenging, offers safety associated with the removal of all of the breast tissue combined with superior cosmetic results. The opportunity to use TSSM is particularly important when considering prophylactic mastectomy for women at highest risk and may enable them to feel comfortable about the cosmetic result to undergo the surgery.

Axillary dissection

Axillary dissection is not used with the intent of enhancing curability, because regional lymph nodes are regarded as indicators of distant metastatic disease rather than instigators of such tumor.

The incision for axillary dissection should be separate from that used for the removal of tumor in the breast. A longitudinal incision placed along the posterolateral margin of the pectoralis major muscle or a transverse incision just below the axillary hairline may be used. At present, an axillary dissection includes nodes from axillary levels I and II. Anatomic delineation of this dissection is the latissimus dorsi muscle laterally, the axillary vein superiorly, and the medial border of the pectoralis minor muscle medially. Removal of the pectoralis minor muscle is not required. The nerves to the serratus anterior and latissimus dorsi muscles should be identified and preserved. The axillary vein should be visualized and followed under the pectoralis minor muscle to the medial border. These are the minimal limits for the dissection. The average number of nodes removed is about 15. Although the lumpectomy site in the breast is not drained, a suction drain is present in the axilla for several postoperative days.

The management of the axilla has changed significantly since the introduction of sentinel node dissection. This procedure limits considerably the extent of surgical procedure in the axilla and, for majority of patients with negative axillary lymph nodes, precludes the need for formal axillary dissection while providing similar (and in some cases superior) diagnostic and prognostic information. The identification of a single (or a few) sentinel node(s) also permits the pathologist to perform a more detailed assessment of multilevel sections of the sentinel node. The detection of micrometastases is significantly increased by combining light microscopy, IHC, and even more sensitive molecular techniques. However, the prognostic significance of identifying isolated metastatic cells in histologically negative lymph nodes by more sensitive techniques is still undetermined; therefore, at this time, it is not considered sufficient to constitute stage 2 disease. Sentinel node biopsy and assessment are under extensive evaluation by large cooperative research groups, including the NSABP and ACOSOG. ACOSOG Z-010 trial required clinicians not to use immunohistochemical analysis in their hospital, so that all nodes could be centrally stained and the results blinded to assess the prognostic significance of microscopic metastases to the lymph nodes. NSABP B-32 randomized 5611 women with negative sentinel lymph node (SLN) to either SLN biopsy only or SLN biopsy followed by ALND. Women who were found to have positive SLN also proceeded to full ALND. The strength of the study is that it is the largest randomized trial of SLND and that it is representative of a cross section of surgeons across the country with 232 surgeons participating across 80 centers. Although longer-term outcomes, regional control, and survival are not yet known, the technical results are. On average, three SLNs were removed per patient; the SLN identification rate was 97.2% and improved with surgeon experience, and 26% of patients had a positive sentinel node. In 61.5% of patients with a positive sentinel node, the additional nodes were negative (38.5% had additional positive nodes). The false-negative rate (axillary node involvement when the SLN was negative) was 9.7%, which did not change with experience, but was significantly affected by the type of biopsy used for diagnosis; the false-negative rates were 8.0%, 14.3%, and 15.2% for FNA/core, incisional biopsy, and excisional biopsy, respectively. The number of SLNs identified also affected SLN false-negative rates. The confidence in a negative result is higher if more than one SLN is identified, or if the prior probability of having a negative node is high, but may be less for the woman with a higher prior probability of having a positive node.

Sentinel lymph node dissection

The use of radiotracer material or visible blue dyes to locate and remove the SLN (the node that drains the tumor site most directly) is becoming a standard technique for evaluating the axilla. This technique was initially described for melanoma and then studied in breast cancer patients and has a high degree of accuracy once the operator has become proficient with the technique. The ability to identify a sentinel node ranges from 85% to 97%. The ACOSOG, in selecting surgeons to participate in a sentinel node registry trial as well as a trial to determine if full node dissection after SLN removal was beneficial, required proof that the sentinel node could be identified in 90% of cases and that the false-negative rate for SLN was less than 5%. Lymphedema rates after SLND are reported to be <7% compared with 17–25% with ALND.[231] SLND has been shown to exhibit similar performance after neoadjuvant chemotherapy[232]; although the identification of the SLN may be somewhat lower, the false-negative rate is very similar. Although still somewhat controversial, the potential benefits of using SLND after neoadjuvant therapy are that the patient is spared an additional operation before starting chemotherapy—they may avoid an axillary dissection as tumor in the nodes may disappear with chemotherapy—and that the information about the presence of tumor in the nodes after chemotherapy is beneficial in predicting local recurrence rates and determining the need for radiation therapy.[151] Intraoperative frozen section has not been as accurate in detecting nodal metastases as is specific analysis done later in the laboratory. Imprint cytology has recently been reported to have a very low false-negative rate, but the sensitivity is not as high as frozen section. In NSABP B-32, cytology was found to indeed have a low false-positive rate, 0.4%, but a sensitivity of 61.5%. Intraoperative detection of LN metastases is beneficial as it enables the surgeon to proceed to a full axillary dissection at the time of SLND, thereby avoiding a second procedure. Clinicians should use the technique in their own institution that yields the lowest false-positive rate to avoid further surgery.

Radioisotope injection with a gamma isotope-labeled colloid and scanning with a handheld probe is replacing blue dye injection, which provides a visible clue of blue lymphatics, leading to the blue sentinel node. Although some authors strongly favor one or the other of these, the majority of reports indicate that the combination of both results in the highest level of successful identification of the sentinel node. In NSABP B-32, the radioisotope had a higher SLN identification than blue die. There is a small but real risk (<1%) of anaphylaxis with Lymphazurin blue dye. The risk of severe anaphylaxis was shown to be 0.2% in NSABP B-32. Anesthesiologists should be aware of this possibility if blue dye is used.

Need for axillary dissection

It is frequently asked whether all lumpectomy patients require axillary staging. If the need for systemic therapy, as well as the type of systemic therapy, can be determined by patient and tumor characteristics other than the status of the axillary nodes, then the need for axillary staging becomes less clear. Furthermore, if all node-negative and node-positive patients were to be given the same systemic adjuvant therapy, as is the case in trials of preoperative chemotherapy, there would seem to be no reason to know the nodal status, except for predicting patient outcome. The Early Breast Cancer Trialists' Collaborative Group (EBCTCG) overview suggests that adjuvant chemotherapy benefits women with node-negative and node-positive cancers and that the proportionate reduction in risk of treatment failure is the same for both groups, and many oncologists offer adjuvant chemotherapy to all women except those that have such a low proportionate reduction as to be of little real gain. However, modified decision-making tools such as adjuvantonline.com, a well-validated tool for predicting absolute benefit of chemotherapy,[233] or molecular tools that provide a recurrence score (RS) such as the Oncotype DX[234] have increased the ability of oncologists to refine recommendations for systemic therapy. The molecular characteristics of the tumor may be more important than stage in determining whether to perform adjuvant therapy and which type to use. Two molecular tests used in the United States (trial assigning individualized options for treatment (TAILORx) trial) and Europe microarray in node-negative disease may avoid chemotherapy (MINDACT) are in clinical trials to better answer these questions. As these data mature, the roles of sentinel node dissection and axillary dissection will need to be clarified. In the molecular age, there are still situations where removal of all possible locoregional tumor may be very important: for those women in whom surgical excision is the primary treatment, for example, in a setting with a low predicted ROR, or for women who have undergone neoadjuvant chemotherapy and have residual disease and possibly resistant to best available therapies. In the setting of complete pathologic response after neoadjuvant therapy, the probability of performing surgery may be low, and the increasing use of sentinel node dissection after neoadjuvant chemotherapy in women with clinically N0 disease, regardless of nodal status pretreatment, is an example of modifying the extent of surgical treatment to response to therapy. The need for axillary dissection may also be questioned, particularly in elderly women with ER-positive disease who are planning to undergo adjuvant hormonal therapy. In this setting, the status of the axillary nodes would not likely alter the decision about administration of adjuvant therapy. In almost all cases with clinically negative axilla, however, sentinel node dissection is a standard part of staging and surgical management and can be successfully performed in most women with very low morbidity. In the setting of positive sentinel nodes, level I and II axillary dissections are considered standard management. Although it is generally accepted that axillary dissection provides optimal local control of the axilla, a randomized trial comparing total mastectomy with and without axillary dissection suggested that not all patients (∼50%) with positive axillary lymph nodes would develop an axillary recurrence in the absence of an axillary dissection.

The multicenter ACOSOG Z011 trial randomized women having breast-conserving surgery with a positive sentinel node to either full axillary dissection or not.[235] The target accrual was 1900; 991 were actually enrolled. There was no difference between the two arms between 5-year axillary or in-breast recurrence, and most importantly, there was no difference in either disease-free or OS. These important results have already had a significant impact on standard management of the axilla, sparing many women from the potential long-term toxicities of a full axillary dissection. Management of the axilla in women undergoing mastectomy with a positive sentinel node still mandates further axillary sampling unless radiation is planned for the primary tumor.

Since the routine use of mammographic screening, the vast majority of patients diagnosed with invasive breast cancer have T1 or T2 primary tumors that are amenable to a breast-conserving locoregional treatment. Breast conservation therapy has currently been firmly established as an appropriate standard of care for women with early-stage breast disease. This therapy consists of three important components: removal of the tumor with achievement of negative margins (often called a lumpectomy, tylectomy, or a segmental mastectomy), surgical assessment of axillary lymph nodes with either a sentinel lymph node surgery and/or a level I/II ALND, and breast irradiation. Most women treated with modern breast conservation approaches achieve excellent outcomes. When combined with systemic therapy, the annual local recurrence rate after appropriate breast conservation treatments has been reported to be less than 0.5% for women with favorable disease.[236,237] Furthermore, the complication rates of breast conservation therapy are very low and continue to improve with advances in surgical and radiotherapy techniques.

Despite these facts, breast conservation remains underutilized in the United States. In a recent multinational randomized trial comparing two hormonal therapies for women with early stage disease, the rate of breast conservation in the United States was only 49%.[238] By contrast, the rate of breast conservation in the United Kingdom was 58%, and even higher rates were observed in Sweden, Germany, or Australia/New Zealand. Previous data had also indicated that the use of breast conservation varies within regions of the United States, with Southern and Midwestern women less likely to be treated with breast conservation than those from either the East or West Coast.[239] The reasons for the underuse of breast conservation are likely multifactorial. Unfortunately, some women undergo mastectomy based on a misperception that mastectomy is likely to achieve a superior outcome. It is critical, therefore, that breast cancer providers understand the data concerning breast conservation, so that patients with newly diagnosed disease can be given the option of this treatment if appropriate.

Breast conservation therapy versus mastectomy
Breast conservation has been studied as an alternative locoregional treatment to mastectomy for over 40 years. After initial successful results were obtained in single institutions, a number of phase III clinical trials were initiated, which directly compared the outcome of patients treated with breast conservation versus those of patients treated with mastectomy.[240-242] The NSABP B-06 study was one of the most important trials.[234] This trial began in 1976 and enrolled 1843 women. Patients with T1 or T2, N0, or N1, M0 breast tumors of 4 cm or less were randomly assigned to one of the following three treatment groups: (1) modified radical mastectomy, (2) lumpectomy and axillary dissection, and (3) lumpectomy, axillary dissection, followed by radiation therapy. With 20 years of follow-up, this trial demonstrated that breast conservation therapy provides survival equivalent to mastectomy.

Contraindications for breast conservation therapy
Selected patients with ESBC are not suitable for breast conservation therapy, because the primary tumor cannot be successfully removed with a lumpectomy. For example, patients presenting with diffuse suspicious calcifications that cannot be resected with a lumpectomy that leaves an acceptable aesthetic result are best treated with a mastectomy. Similarly, patients in whom repeated attempts of BCS did not achieve negative surgical margins are best managed with a mastectomy. Increasingly, however, women who present with stage II and III cancers can be treated with neoadjuvant chemotherapy or hormone therapy, and over 50% have sufficient shrinkage of the primary tumor to enable breast conservation. A second reason why some patients are not candidates for breast conservation is that

they are at high risk for radiation complications. Specific examples of such patients include those previously treated with radiation, women who are pregnant, and patients with certain connective tissue diseases. For women early in the course of their pregnancy, internal radiation scatter from irradiation of the intact breast can reach lethal and teratogenic dose levels.[243] Certain collagen vascular diseases, such as systemic scleroderma, polymyositis, dermatomyositis, lupus erythematosus, and mixed-connective tissue disorders have been associated with significant risks, including breast fibrosis and pain, chest wall necrosis, and brachial plexopathy.[244]

Radiation therapy
For more than 100 years, radiation has had a vital function in the effective treatment of breast cancer. From its crude and early history as the first adjuvant therapy to radical surgery to its role as the vehicle that drove the breast conservation revolution of the 1970s, radiation oncologists and surgeons formed the first "multidisciplinary" cancer teams. Radiation therapy is a component of care for the overwhelming majority of breast cancer patients at some point during the course of their disease. Therefore, it is crucial that radiation oncologists become involved at the time of diagnosis to collaborate with medical oncologists and breast surgeons in the prospective design of each patient's care path. At present, radiation therapy has been in the midst of a technological renaissance, creating challenges and controversies in the balance of evidence-based medicine and personalized, modified therapy.

Role of radiation in BCS for early-stage invasive disease
Defining the role of radiation in breast conservation therapy has been the focus of numerous randomized prospective clinical trials conducted over the past 30 years.[241,242] In conclusion, these trials have demonstrated that radiation after breast-conserving surgery significantly improves local control, minimizes the risk of subsequent distant metastases, and decreases breast cancer death rates.

Benefits of adjuvant radiation
The NSABP B-06 trial was one of the first randomized studies to evaluate the benefit of radiation after lumpectomy. This trial showed that for patients treated with breast conserving surgery, whole-breast radiation therapy (WBRT) offered significant clinical benefits. After 20 years, the recurrence rates in the breast were 40% and 14% for those treated with lumpectomy only and lumpectomy plus WBRT, respectively. The almost two-thirds reduction in the ROR was very similar to reductions observed in other similarly designed trials.[234] The data from NSABP B-06 and the other prospective clinical trials assessing the role of radiation for patients with invasive disease treated with breast conservation have been analyzed by the EBCTCG. In this important meta-analysis, the individual patient data from 7300 women were studied. Breast irradiation after lumpectomy reduced the 10-year rate of in-breast recurrence from 29% to 10% for patients with negative lymph nodes and from 47% to 13% for patients with positive lymph nodes. More importantly, radiation use significantly decreased the 15-year risk of dying from breast cancer. For patients with negative lymph nodes, breast cancer mortality decreased from 31% to 26% and for patients with positive lymph nodes, it decreased from 55% to 48%.[242]

Use of a "boost" after WBRT
A strategy to reduce local recurrence after WBRT even further is dose escalation via an additional boost of radiation to the tissue

at the highest risk in the postoperative tumor bed. The first randomized trial investigating the impact of a 1000-cGy boost following 5000-cGy WBRT was performed in Lyons, France. The use of a boost led to a small but statistically significant reduction in the rates of local recurrence at 5 years (3.6% vs 4.5%, $p = 0.04$).[245] Subsequently, the EORTC completed a much larger trial that randomized over 5000 patients to 5000-cGy WBRT with or without an additional tumor bed boost of 1600 cGy. This trial again demonstrated a reduced breast recurrence rate in patients treated with a boost (10.2% vs 6.2% at 10 years; $p < 0.001$).[246] In a subset analysis, this benefit was noted across all ages but most pronounced in younger women.

Omission of radiation for selected patients

Although the data are conclusive that radiation is beneficial for the majority of patients treated with breast-conserving surgery, there remains an interest as to whether subsets of patients may do well with surgery only. Therefore, some trials have selected patients with more favorable disease characteristics to investigate the omission of radiation. An early trial conducted in Milan, Italy, randomized patients who underwent quadrantectomy and axillary clearance for tumors ≤2.5 cm to undergo WBRT versus no further therapy. The 10-year results from this trial showed that radiation reduced the breast recurrence rate from 24% to 6% ($p < 0.001$).[247] For patients with even smaller primary tumors (stage I), separate randomized trials in Sweden and Finland showed that radiation reduced the 5-year breast recurrence rate from 18% to 2% ($p < 0.0001$) and from 14.1% to 6.2% ($p = 0.029$), respectively.[248,249]

Data from early trials have also indicated that the use of systemic treatment (either chemotherapy or tamoxifen) does not require breast radiation. In the aforementioned NSABP B-06 trial, chemotherapy was used in patients with lymph node-positive disease, and the 20-year breast recurrence rate for these patients was 44% when no radiation was used versus 9% when radiation was used.[234] A trial from Scotland that required systemic treatment for all of the 589 enrolled patients yielded a 6-year breast recurrence rate of 6% in the surgery, systemic therapy, and radiation arm versus 25% in patients randomized to forego radiation.[250]

Four more modern trials conducted among very low-risk subgroups of patients diagnosed in the mammographic era have further refined the selection criteria.[215,216,251,252] In all four of these studies, radiation achieved a statistically significant reduction in breast recurrence rate, although the absolute benefit for some subcategories of patients treated with surgery only was relatively small. The NSABP B-21 trial enrolled only patients with lymph node-negative breast cancers whose primary tumors measured ≤1.0 cm. All patients underwent lumpectomy and ALND and were randomized to tamoxifen only, radiation only, or tamoxifen plus radiation.[249] A contemporary Canadian trial had very similar eligibility criteria and results. Finally, two trials recently tested the omission of radiation for older women with early stage, biologically favorable disease. Long-term results of the CALGB study showed that for patients over the age of 70, the 10-year recurrence rates were 10% and 2% in the tamoxifen only and tamoxifen plus radiation arms, respectively.[215] Furthermore, there were no differences in the rates of salvage mastectomy, distant metastases, or OS between the two groups. The similarly structured Scottish PRIME II trial enrolled over 1300 patients with early-stage disease of age ≥65 and found 5-year local recurrence rates of 4% and 1% for those on tamoxifen only and tamoxifen plus radiation ($p = 0.0002$), respectively.[216]

In conclusion, almost all of the clinical studies to date have indicated that breast radiation reduces local recurrences following BCS and therefore should be considered a standard component of treatment for all women with early-stage invasive disease. Thus far, most attempts to define favorable subsets of ESBC patients who may not require radiation have been unsuccessful with the exception of older women with biologically favorable disease planning to undergo hormonal adjuvant therapy. In this cohort, the ROR is low, the overall benefit is small, and hence the addition of radiation should be based on the patients' life expectancy and personal preferences.

Radiation as a substitute for radical axillary surgery in early-stage node-positive patients

In the era of mammographic diagnosis, ubiquitous systemic therapy, and SLNB, there has been an enormous interest in reducing the use of axillary dissection for not only node-negative patients but also low-volume node-positive patients. The interest in eliminating radical axillary surgery is particularly important for patients in whom radiation is planned, as the risk of lymphedema and its impact on quality of life (QOL) are higher when these modalities are combined. The previously referenced ACOSOG Z0011 trial showed that for patients undergoing BCS with WBRT for early-stage disease with one to two positive nodes, the addition of axillary dissection to SLNB did not improve disease-free or OS at 5 years.[233] The EORTC 10981-22023 (AMAROS) analyzed a similar patient population, including patients with more than two positive nodes (5%) and patients who had undergone mastectomy (18%).[253] Over 1400 patients with a positive SNLB were randomized to receive either axillary dissection or axillary irradiation, and at 6 years there was no statistical difference in axillary recurrence. Although the trial was underpowered because of the low overall number of events, the rate of upper extremity lymphedema was significantly higher for patients who underwent dissection. These two trials taken together have had a broad, practice-changing effect on the locoregional treatment of early-stage node-positive patients, directing therapy away from radical surgery. Given that axillary recurrences are rare events, typically occurring within 2 years,[234,254] longer-term follow-up of these two trials is unlikely to alter their significant impact on clinical practice.

Role of radiation after mastectomy for locally advanced disease

A strong rationale exists for combining the beneficial effects of radiation and mastectomy for selected women with locally advanced breast cancer, in whom areas of subclinical disease extend beyond the operative field. The initial studies that investigated radiation after mastectomy began in the 1950s and represented some of the first controlled clinical trials in oncology history. After five decades of study, there still remain controversies over the selection criteria and value of postmastectomy radiation therapy (PMRT), mainly due to two factors: the late-term morbidity of early radiation techniques and the addition of systemic therapy as a routine component of care. In general, however, as PMRT techniques have improved and systemic therapies decrease the competing risk of distant metastases, improvements in locoregional control gained by radiation have had a consequential positive effect on survival.

Modern data supporting PMRT

There have been several meta-analyses conducted to quantify the value and risk of PMRT, the most comprehensive and important being the work of the EBCTCG. This group was able to obtain the raw data from every randomized prospective trial of PMRT, including nearly 10,000 randomized to radiation versus observation following mastectomy and axillary clearance. For node-positive patients, PMRT reduced the risk of locoregional recurrence threefold (29–8%), which led to a 5% absolute decrease in breast cancer mortality (60% vs 55%) at 15 years. For patients with node-negative disease, the locoregional benefit was smaller (8–3%) and not associated with a difference in survival.[242] Overall, data from this meta-analysis suggested that a long-term survival benefit was only manifested in the trials where there was a ≥10% improvement in 5-year locoregional control.[242] As such, there is a clear indication that the role of PMRT in eradication of persistent postsurgical microscopic disease is to prevent the development of a subsequent local source for distant metastasis, which eventually can lead to death.

The three PMRT randomized trials that most heavily influenced the EBCTCG meta-analysis all involved relatively modern radiation techniques and the judicious use of systemic therapy. The Danish Breast Cancer Cooperative Group (DBCCG) 82b trial, perhaps the most important study, randomized 1708 premenopausal women with stage II or III breast cancer to mastectomy and CMF-based chemotherapy with or without PMRT.[255] The majority of patients entered in this trial had one to three positive lymph nodes; however, the median number of axillary lymph nodes resected was only seven, rather than a formal level I/II axillary dissection. Patients randomized to PMRT had an improved OS rate at 10 years (54% vs 45%, $p < 0.001$), likely a consequence of decreased locoregional recurrence (9% vs 32%, $p < 0.001$). Simultaneously, investigators in Vancouver, British Columbia, conducted a similar, albeit smaller, trial in which 318 premenopausal women with lymph node-positive disease were randomized to receive mastectomy and CMF with or without PMRT.[256] The results were nearly identical with PMRT providing a 10% absolute benefit in long-term OS (20-year rates: 47% vs 37%, $p = 0.03$) and an even higher benefit in locoregional control (87% vs 61%; $p < 0.0001$).

Finally, the DBCCG 82c randomized 1300 postmenopausal patients to mastectomy and tamoxifen with or without PMRT.[257] The stage of disease and extent of axillary surgery were also very similar to the 82b trial. The magnitude of benefits in OS and local control was similar to the two previous studies in terms of 10-year OS (45% vs 36%, $p = 0.03$) and locoregional control (92% vs 65%; $p < 0.001$). At almost 20 years of follow-up, updates of the DBCCG 82b and 82c combined data continue benefits of PMRT for both locoregional control (86% vs 51%, $p < 0.0001$) and distant metastasis-free survival (47% vs 36%, $p < 0.0001$).[258]

Current indications for postmastectomy radiation

The American Society of Clinical Oncology (ASCO) consensus guidelines for PMRT, published almost 15 years ago, recommended treatment for patients with stage III disease (defined by T3 with involved lymph nodes, T4 primaries, or four or more involved lymph nodes)[259] after mastectomy, standard axillary dissection, and chemotherapy due to the magnitude of survival benefit for these locally advanced patients. However, the landmark publication left the role of PMRT for patients with stage II disease with one to three positive nodes unsettled and hence controversial. The reason for this is that although most of the patients in the Danish and British Columbia trials had one to three positive lymph nodes, the benefit of PMRT for this subset has been inquired by surgeons who indicate the inadequate clearance of the axilla in the standard arm of the larger Danish trial. Indeed, the long-term locoregional recurrence rate for these patients in the Danish trials, who were treated without PMRT, was 41% versus 21% in similar patients who underwent a more complete axillary clearance in the British Columbia trial.[256,260] It is important to note that inadequate axillary surgery may have led to an underestimation of the true number of positive lymph nodes and that many of these patients would likely have had four or more lymph nodes who already underwent more extensive surgery.

The findings and critiques of the Danish and Canadian Studies heavily influenced the ASCO consensus guidelines for PMRT (published in 2001), which in turn have guided clinical practice patterns for over a decade. More recently, a meta-analysis by the EBCTCG published in 2014 has sought to clarify the utility of PMRT for the most controversial patients, those with small primary tumors and one to three positive nodes.[258] Data from 22 randomized trials including over 3700 patients treated with PMRT after axillary dissection to at least level II were analyzed for differences in 10-year locoregional recurrence and 20-year survival. For patients with one to three positive nodes in whom systemic therapy was followed ($n = 1133$), PMRT significantly reduced locoregional recurrence by more than three-quarters (20% vs 4%; $p < 0.0001$) and improved breast cancer-specific mortality by approximately 8% (50% vs 42%; $p = 0.01$). Interestingly, the magnitude of benefit in this controversial subgroup was nearly the same as that for patients with four or more positive nodes for both locoregional recurrence (32% vs 13%; $p < 0.00001$) and breast cancer mortality (80% vs 70%; $p = 0.04$).

Therefore, there should remain no doubt regarding the utility of PMRT for all patients with positive lymph nodes and a >10-year life expectancy. In addition to the number of positive lymph nodes, other adverse pathologic features such as the volume of nodal disease, the presence of extra nodal extension, and the percentage of nodes involved should be used to guide clinical decision making. In conclusion, the EBCTCG update,[261] together with the aforementioned AMAROS trial,[253] indicated a trend of expanding the application of PMRT at a time when the role of axillary dissection is diminishing. It is likely that a more complete understanding of tumor biology and genomic profiling will play a role in further guiding clinical practice in the not-to0-distant future.

Integrating PMRT with breast reconstruction

Two trends on a collision course over the last decade have been the expanding indications for PMRT, particularly in younger patients, versus the increasing use of elective mastectomy combined with reconstruction in this population.[262] While breast reconstruction, both implant- and tissue flap-based, poses certain challenges for the treating radiation oncologist, it should never be considered a contraindication to PMRT. While plastic surgery practice patterns are highly variable and guided more by experience than randomized trials, there are certain common principles that have developed over time. In general, immediate reconstruction (in a patient requiring PMRT) is best accomplished with a tissue expander (TE)/implant-based technique.[259] This is the most popular modality as it consolidates surgical procedures and allows full-tissue expansion through the month long course of adjuvant chemotherapy. The TE may be swapped for the permanent implant before PMRT[263] or left in place through the course of PMRT, allowing its deflation to improve radiation dosimetry.[264] Alternatively, autologous flap techniques are the procedures of choice for delayed reconstruction, where vascularized tissue is brought into the irradiated field for improved wound healing and cosmetic results.[262] While breast reconstruction after mastectomy proves vital to many patients in terms of QOL posttreatment, it is important that patients not short change their oncologic therapy for fear of consequences that are cosmetic and rectifiable.

Role of radiation after neoadjuvant chemotherapy

Modified radical mastectomy followed by adjuvant chemotherapy and PMRT has been the historical standard locoregional therapy for patients with locally or regionally advanced primary tumors. However, over the past three decades, the use of neoadjuvant chemotherapy (chemotherapy before surgery) has significantly increased in patients with advanced disease. This strategy was first adopted for patients with unresectable or marginally resectable disease, and the initial clinical data from such patients indicated that chemotherapy achieved high rates of tumor response. Subsequently, this approach has also been investigated in patients with large, resectable breast cancers at diagnosis.

Breast conservation after neoadjuvant chemotherapy

One of the original main reasons to investigate sequencing chemotherapy before surgery was to determine whether breast conservation could be offered to selected patients with larger primary tumors whose residual disease would then be amenable to a breast-conserving operation. In order to investigate this, the NSABP and EORTC independently conducted clinical trials that compared neoadjuvant chemotherapy with adjuvant chemotherapy for patients with stage II or III breast cancer. Although both trials found that breast conservation rates were higher in the neoadjuvant chemotherapy arms,[265,266] the NSABP study showed that this increase was largely due to a near tripling of breast conservation use for patients with T3 disease postchemotherapy (22% vs 8%).[264]

The goal of breast conservation therapy for patients with advanced disease is to achieve an aesthetically acceptable cosmetic outcome and a low risk of breast recurrence. Accordingly, for patients with large initial primaries, resection must be directed at the postchemotherapy tumor bed rather than the initial volume of residual disease. However, one concern with resecting only the postchemotherapy volume of residual disease is that some advanced breast cancers do not shrink concentrically to a solitary nidus in response to neoadjuvant chemotherapy, but rather break up into nests of residual disease over the initially involved volume.[193] In such cases, surgery directed at the primary core may exert more pressure of microscopic disease around the tumor bed site, which may theoretically be associated with higher rates of breast cancer recurrence.

In the NSABP B-18 trial, the overall rate of breast cancer recurrence did not statistically differ in the patients treated with neoadjuvant chemotherapy compared with those treated with adjuvant chemotherapy (16-year rates of 13% vs 10%, respectively).[267] However, breast cancer recurrence rate was higher in patients with large primary tumors in whom a response to neoadjuvant chemotherapy permitted a breast conserving surgery. In this subset of patients treated with neoadjuvant chemotherapy, the breast recurrence rate at 8 years was 16%, which was more than twice the rate in the patients with smaller tumors who were treated with breast-conserving surgery first.[264] Other multicenter series have also shown relatively high breast cancer recurrence rates in patients who receive neoadjuvant chemotherapy.[268,269]

In contrast to these data, single-institution studies with careful selection criteria and a high degree of multidisciplinary coordination have reported excellent rates of local control. Investigators at the University of Texas MD Anderson Cancer Center have recently published the results of one of the largest studies investigating breast conservation after neoadjuvant chemotherapy.[267] In this study, 340 carefully selected patients who had a favorable response to chemotherapy were treated with breast-conserving surgery and radiation. Despite the fact that 72% of patients in the study had clinical stage IIB or III disease, the 5- and 10-year breast cancer recurrence rates were only 5% and 10%, respectively. Four tumor-related factors were associated with breast cancer

recurrence and locoregional recurrence: clinical N2 or N3 disease, lymphovascular space invasion, a multifocal pattern of residual disease, and residual disease higher than 2 cm in diameter.[270] These investigators subsequently developed a prognostic index from these factors and found that for patients with 0 or 1 index, breast conservation will offer similar excellent outcome as mastectomy and radiation. However, mastectomy and radiation were associated with a lower risk of locoregional recurrence in the patients with three or more adverse factors.[271]

PMRT after neoadjuvant chemotherapy

While data indicate that breast conservation therapy is appropriate for patients with advanced primary tumors that have a favorable response to neoadjuvant chemotherapy, much less is known about the indications for and efficacy of PMRT for such patients. As previously discussed, for patients treated with up-front mastectomy, the decision to administer radiation therapy is made based on the pathological extent of disease. It is clear that neoadjuvant chemotherapy changes the extent of pathological disease in 80–90% of cases, and this may hold implications for locoregional recurrence.[268] Therefore, both the pretreatment clinical stage and the extent of pathologically defined residual disease need to be considered when assessing the risk of locoregional recurrence in patients treated with neoadjuvant chemotherapy and mastectomy. Indeed, in an analysis of the patients treated with neoadjuvant chemotherapy, mastectomy, and no radiation, a multivariate analysis of locoregional recurrence predictors found that both pre- and posttreatment factors were independent predictors.[272] One large retrospective study of PMRT after neoadjuvant chemotherapy compared outcomes of 579 patients who received radiation following neoadjuvant chemotherapy and mastectomy with 136 patients who were treated with neoadjuvant chemotherapy and mastectomy only.[273] Despite the fact that the PMRT cohort had more extensive disease than those treated without radiation, irradiated patients had a significantly lower locoregional recurrence rate at 10 years (8% vs 22%, $p = 0.001$). In the subgroup of patients with clinical T4 tumors, clinical stage IIIB/C disease, and in those with four or more positive lymph nodes after chemotherapy, the absolute improvement in locoregional recurrence risk was approximately 30–40%. The use of radiation in these same subgroups was associated with an approximately 15–20% improvement in overall and cause-specific survival. In a subsequent analysis from this group that focused only on patients who achieved a pathologic complete response (pCR), the locoregional recurrence rate for them with clinical stage III disease was improved with radiation therapy (33% vs 7%, $p = 0.04$).[274]

Whether to use PMRT for patients with clinical stage II disease who have positive lymph nodes after chemotherapy remains less clear. A report of 132 patients with clinical stage II disease who did not receive radiation therapy after neoadjuvant chemotherapy and mastectomy indicated that patients with clinical T3N0 disease or four or more positive lymph nodes had high rates of locoregional recurrence.[275] The 5-year local recurrence rates in the remaining patients were less than 10%. In the patients with clinical stage II disease who had one to three positive lymph nodes after neoadjuvant chemotherapy, the 5-year rate of locoregional recurrence was 8%. It is important to recognize that this study had a small sample size and that the studied population was prone to selection biases, in that they represented only those patients for whom the treating physicians elected not to use radiation.

On the basis of the available data, it is reasonable to recommend PMRT for all patients with clinical stage III disease at initial presentation. It is also reasonable to infer that patients with clinical stage

I or II disease who have four or more positive lymph nodes after chemotherapy or a primary tumor size >5 cm should receive radiation. The role of PMRT is currently controversial for patients with clinical stage I or II disease who have one to three positive lymph nodes after neoadjuvant chemotherapy[276] and node-positive disease at diagnosis, but proceed toward a pCR. Fortunately, these clinical conundrums are the subjects of two ongoing complementary prospective randomized trials in the United States. The NSABP B-51 trial is open to pathologically confirmed node-positive patients who convert to node-negative after neoadjuvant chemotherapy. Patients are then randomized to WBRT with or without regional nodal irradiation (postlumpectomy) or PMRT versus observation (postmastectomy).[277] The Alliance A011202 trial randomizes similar patients who remain node-positive after chemotherapy to axillary dissection versus PMRT.[278]

Details of radiation treatment

The planning and design of the treatment fields and the delivery of radiation treatments for breast cancer are of critical importance and require modern equipment and attention to detail. It is clear that radiation treatments can have serious normal tissue consequences and even cause life-threatening radiation injuries, which can be avoided or minimized with modern treatment techniques.

There have been a number of recent advances in the field of radiation oncology that directly benefit breast cancer patients. One of these major advances has been the use of 3D imaging to assist in field design. Computed tomography (CT)-based simulation allows radiation oncologists to design treatment fields on CT images acquired from patients in their treatment positions, thereby permitting better visualization of the targeted regions and the normal tissues that one wishes to avoid, such as the heart. An example of a field design for a stage I left breast cancer treatment after lumpectomy is shown in Figure 20. In this image, the tumor bed has been contoured on individual CT slices and reconstructed for the image. The breast is treated with a medial tangentially oriented beam, with a deep edge that enters near the midline and transverses the anterior thorax to exit near the midaxillary line. This field is opposed with a lateral tangent beam to match the decrease of dose as the beam travels through the breast and ultimately provides a homogeneous dose distribution. Other regions of interest, such as lymph nodes in the axilla, internal mammary chain, or supraclavicular fossa, can similarly be contoured to visualize their anatomical location with respect to treatment field borders. Figure 21 shows a "beam's eye view" of a medial tangent beam used to treat the breast (including the tumor bed), the upper internal mammary lymph nodes, and level I and a portion of level II of the axilla.

A second major advance has been the development of 3D dose calculation systems, which more accurately calculate and display the dose on the CT images throughout the 3D treatment volume. Finally, the currently used modern treatment tools also allow the dose to be modulated in three dimensions. The goal of such modulation is to provide a homogeneous dose distribution, which minimizes the risk of normal tissues and targeted areas receiving more than and less than the prescribed dose, respectively.

The treatment planning process is the initial critically important step in radiation treatments of breast cancer. Patients are conventionally immobilized in a supine position with the ipsilateral arm abducted and externally rotated. They then undergo a CT scan that acquires the image set used for treatment planning. Reference marks are placed on the patient's skin of the breast. The planning process, in which the fields are designed and the dose distribution optimized typically takes 2–3 days and does not require the patient to be present. Following completion of planning, daily treatments

begin, which typically require 15 min each day in the treatment room. The therapy is painless and the patients' experience slightly differs from that of a diagnostic X-ray treatment. A number of alternative positioning[279] and respiratory management[280] techniques have recently been developed to improve dosimetry in large-breasted patients and further minimize heart exposure for left-sided cancers.

The most common course of treatment entails 25–28 treatments of 180–200 cGy per day to the breast or chest wall with or without inclusion of lymphatic regions at risk (total dose 4500–5040 cGy). This course is typically followed by five to eight supplemental treatments of 180–200 cGy per day to the tumor bed region (often called a tumor bed or chest wall boost) for an additional 1000–1600 cGy. In total, treatments are given 5 days a week for approximately 6–6.5 weeks. This strategy of delivering the lowest biologically effective daily dose over a protracted number of weeks is appropriate for patients in the postlumpectomy or postmastectomy setting, with or without inclusion of the regional lymph nodes and is referred to as conventionally fractionated radiation therapy (CFRT).

New radiation treatment approaches for early-stage breast cancer

Some patients treated for breast cancer fail to receive recommended radiation and a number of patients who are excellent candidates for breast conservation therapy elect to be treated with mastectomy to avoid radiation.[281,282] A major factor that contributes to both of these scenarios concerns the inconvenience and expense associated with 5–7 weeks of CFRT. This schedule is particularly burdensome for patients who have significant home or work responsibilities, patients in rural areas who need to travel for access to the nearest radiation facility, and patients who rely on public transportation. In addition, worldwide, there are too few radiation oncologists, facilities, and equipment to offer this type of treatment schedule to all patients with breast cancer who will benefit from radiation.

For these reasons and others, a number of strategies have been developed to shorten the radiation treatment schedule and lessen the burdens of time and out-of-pocket expense. The simplest strategy is called hypofractionated radiation therapy (HFRT), where the amount of radiation delivered per treatment is increased to decrease the overall treatment course by about one-half. As the amount of radiation per fraction increases, the total dose delivered

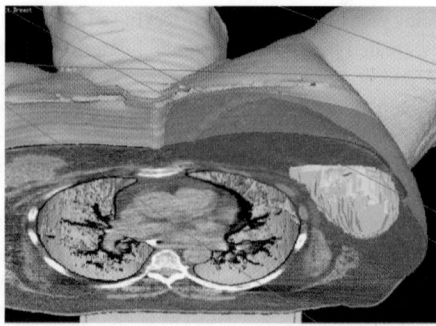

Figure 20 Cross-sectional image of radiation fields used for the treatment of left-sided invasive breast cancer. The red-shaded areas represent the volume included within the fields. The solid yellow object represents the tumor bed, which was reconstructed by contouring this region on sequential computed tomography slices. Two opposed treatment fields are used: a medial tangent that obliquely enters the medial breast and exits the lateral breast and an opposed lateral tangent field. The fields are opposed to match the falloff of radiation dose that occurs as beams travel through tissue.

Table 8 Outcomes for selected randomized clinical trials comparing conventionally fractionated radiotherapy (CFRT) to hypofractionated radiotherapy (HFRT).

Trial	Median follow-up (years)	N	Dose (cGy)	# fractions	IBTR[a] (%)	LRR[a] (%)	DFS[a] (%)	OS[a] (%)	Cosmesis[a] (% good or excellent)	Acute toxicity[a] (% ≥ grade 3)
Canada[283]	10	612	5000	25	6.7	—	—	84	71.3	3.0
		622	4250	16	6.2	—	—	85	69.8	3.0
Royal Marsden[284]	10	470	5000	25	12	—	—	—	71	—
		466	4290	13	9.6	—	—	—	74	—
		474	3900	13	15	—	—	—	58[b]	—
START A[285,286]	9	749	5000	25	6.7	7.4	77	80	—	0.3
		750	4160	13	5.6	6.3	77	82	—	0.0
		737	3900	13	8.1	8.8	76	80	—	0.0
START B[286,287]	10	1105	5000	25	5.2	5.5	78	81	—	1.2
		1110	4050	15	3.8	4.3	82[c]	84[c]	—	0.3

Abbreviations: N, number of patients; FRAC, fractions; IBTR, in-breast tumor recurrence; LRR, locoregional recurrence; DFS, disease-free survival; OS, overall survival.

[a]All statistical p values are nonsignificant in the comparison of CFRT to HFRT, unless otherwise specified.

[b]Measure found to be statistically inferior to CFRT ($p < 0.05$).

[c]Measure found to be statistically superior to CFRT ($p < 0.05$).

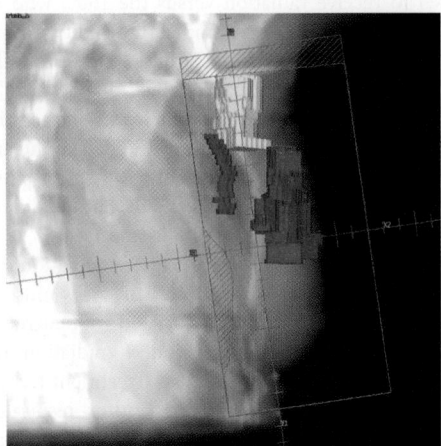

Figure 21 A beams' eye-view of a medial tangent radiation treatment field designed to cover the breast, low axilla, and upper internal mammary lymph node chain. The reconstructed contours of a tumor bed (red), upper internal mammary lymph node region (blue) and the low axilla (yellow) are shown.

is commensurately adjusted downward to provide radiobiologic equivalence to CFRT dosing. Results of large randomized trials of HFRT are shown in Table 8.

In 1986, a clinical trial was initiated at the Royal Marsden Hospital, which included approximately 1500 patients randomized to receive CFRT versus one of two HFRT schedules, 3900–4290 cGy in 13 fractions over 5 weeks.[284] The results were promising and led to the establishment of the UK Standardisation of Breast Radiotherapy (START) Trialists' Group, which developed two randomized trials comparing CFRT and HFRT for approximately 4500 women with ESBC. In the HFRT arms of the START A trial,[285] patients received either 4160 cGy or 3900 Gy in 13 fractions over 5 weeks, and in START B,[287] patients received a dose of 4050 cGy in 15 fractions over 3 weeks. Long-term follow-up at 10 years in the START trials showed that HFRT is a safe and effective treatment for ESBC, equivalent in every way to CFRT.[284,286,288] During the same period of time in Canada, Whelan and colleagues initiated a randomized trial evaluating HFRT (4256 cGy in 16 fractions) in more than 1000 patients with early-stage node-negative breast cancer. After 10 years of follow-up, patients in both arms were noted to have equivalent cosmetic outcomes and recurrence and survival rates.[283,287]

A second strategy, called accelerated partial breast irradiation (APBI), shortens the total treatment time to only 1 week by both increasing fraction size and minimizing the volume of breast tissue being irradiated. The rationale is that 80% of patients who undergo lumpectomy for small primary tumors have no residual disease after lumpectomy or disease that is within 2 cm of the index cancer.[289] Most of the APBI outcome data with a follow-up of ≥5 years have been from studies that investigated interstitial brachytherapy as a method to deliver the radiation dose. For this procedure, patients have brachytherapy catheters surgically implanted around (multi-catheter technique) or directly into (balloon catheter technique) the lumpectomy cavity. Subsequently, high-dose rate radioactive seeds are temporarily placed within the catheters in two sessions per day for 5 days. To date, the 10-year outcome data for highly selected patients with favorable disease characteristics using this approach in small prospective and randomized have been excellent.[290,291] However, others have noted higher rates of clinical fat necrosis and poorer efficacy than conventional breast external beam radiation.[292,293] The outcome data using balloon brachytherapy is also favorable, with the largest study of approximately 1500 patients on the American Society of Breast Surgeons (ASBS) registry showing a 4% risk of breast recurrence at 5 years.[294] Because the placement of brachytherapy catheters at a separate surgical procedure carries with it its own logistical difficulties and risks, other methods of APBI radiation have been developed. Three-dimensional conformal external beam APBI uses sophisticated external beam planning to replicate the favorable dosimetry of brachytherapy with a noninvasive technique.[295]

Taken together, these data suggest that APBI warranted additional study in a large randomized prospective trial with rigid quality assurance to assure proper standardization and volumetric target coverage. In order to address this, the NSABP and RTOG were combined a decade ago to sponsor a phase III trial (NSABP B-39/RTOG 0413) of over 4000 patients with stage 0, I, or II breast cancer randomized to undergo CFRT or APBI (brachytherapy or external beam).[21] This study closed to enrollment in 2013 after reaching its accrual goal, and it may be the most effective breast radiotherapy study in decades.

Another strategy of APBI that has already been compared to CFRT in a phase III trial uses specialized equipment to deliver a single large fraction of radiation directly into the tumor bed in the operating room at the time of lumpectomy. The largest phase III APBI trial published to date (TARGIT-A) randomized over 2200 postmenopausal women with early breast cancer to receive CFRT or single-dose intraoperative radiotherapy (2000 cGy to the tissue–applicator interface).[296] At 4 years, the same risk of local recurrence was observed in each arm (1%), although 15% of intra-operative patients received additional breast irradiation because of adverse pathologic findings after surgery. The favorable results seen for selected early-stage patients treated with intraoperative APBI in such a well-controlled large study may be an early indication of what may ultimately be expected from NSABP B-39/RTOG 0413. Considering this, ASTRO developed consensus criteria for the use of APBI to aid in the selection of patients currently appropriate for one of these options.[297] While not perfect, the guidelines serve as a stopgap compilation of the best available evidence for this popular strategy until the results of B-39 become available.

In the mean time, investigators have been developing even more novel techniques such as stereotactic ablative radiotherapy to expand the limits of APBI, making it less invasive with even fewer treatments.[298,299] It is likely that as the future unfolds, APBI in one of its many forms will be a method increasingly available for the modified treatment of selected ESBC.

Morbidity of radiation treatments for breast cancer

Modern radiation treatments for breast cancer are well tolerated and have low rates of acute toxicity and long-term morbidity. Acute effects typically occur during or immediately after treatment and are mostly self-limited. The usual acute effects associated with breast therapy or PMRT include treatment-related fatigue and radiation dermatitis. These effects are usually relatively mild and most women can continue to work and their usual daily routines.

Late effects following treatment are also relatively unusual, particularly for patients treated after breast-conserving surgery for ESBC or DCIS. For these patients, the most common late effect is a change in breast aesthetics. The cosmetic results after lumpectomy and breast irradiation are influenced by technique, patient body habitus, use of systemic therapy, and the extent of surgery. Approximately 70–85% of women treated with breast-conserving surgery and radiation consider their aesthetic outcome (comparing the treated to the untreated breast) as good or excellent.[300,301]

The other more common complication from locoregional therapy is lymphedema. Irradiation of the supraclavicular fossa and axillary apex after a level I–II dissection can double the rate of lymphedema from 8–10% (surgery only) to 15–20%. Rates can increase further if level III dissections have been performed and in cases with unresected involved lymph nodes in the infra- or supraclavicular fossa, which necessitate higher radiation doses to this region. Other patient-related factors that contribute to lymphedema include obesity and subsequent injury or infection of the ipsilateral arm.

Breast cancer patients treated with radiotherapy are also at theoretical risk for development of pulmonary toxicity, as standard tangential fields skim a small percentage of ipsilateral lung tissue because of the natural curvature of the thorax and arrangement of the breast in the supine position. It is generally accepted that lung tissue is sensitive to radiation exposure, and even the smallest doses exceed tolerance.[302] Therefore, the strategy has generally been to use 3D planning, intensity modulation, and/or prone positioning to minimize the volume of exposed lung to the prescription dose. In the modern era of radiation planning and technique, the development of radiation pneumonitis or consequential clinically significant fibrosis after whole breast irradiation is extraordinarily uncommon.[300,303]

Injury to the brachial plexus is of theoretical concern for the treatment of locally advanced breast cancer, where regional nodal irradiation is required. With CFRT, doses to the brachial plexus (typically 4500–5000 cGy) remain well below the theoretical dose threshold that imparts a 5% risk of injury at 5 years (6000–6500 cGy). In cases where patients have gross disease present in the supraclavicular fossa, dose escalation approaching or exceeding this threshold may be necessary, and careful attention to the location and dosimetry of the brachial plexus is important. However, in such cases, the risk of tumor-induced brachial plexopathy by direct invasion far exceeds that of iatrogenic injury.

Cardiovascular morbidity has been the most significant long-term concern associated with breast cancer radiation. It is clear that the early cruder radiation techniques used for breast cancer treatment have been associated with premature cardiac events in long-term survivors, largely the result of unnecessary, and in the past, unquantifiable, dose delivered to underlying cardiovascular structures.[304] Modern radiation treatments for breast cancer are associated with less cardiovascular morbidity and mortality than earlier radiation techniques. In the Danish PMRT trials, an electron beam technique was exclusively used in treating the chest wall to minimize dose to the cardiac structures. After a median follow-up of 117 months, there was no increase in mortality or cardiac-related hospitalizations in the approximately 1500 patients randomized to receive radiation versus the 1500, who were randomized to no radiation.[305] A similar morbidity and mortality analysis was performed in Canada, where long-term follow-up of 2128 patients treated with radiation failed to show a difference in cardiovascular morbidity between women with left- or right-sided breast cancer.[306] A US report analyzing SEER data found an increase in cardiovascular deaths for irradiated breast cancer patients with left- versus right-sided tumors in the 1970s, but the difference was not found in patients treated in the 1980s and 1990s.[307]

In summary, there is no true "safe" cardiac radiation dose in the treatment of breast cancer patients, and the risks must be placed in context with the cardiotoxicity associated with current systemic cytotoxic and targeted therapies. Modern radiation treatments should be considered safe and effective. Treatment technique and equipment, prone patient positioning and/or respiratory management when appropriate, and mindfulness on the part of the radiation oncologist are all important to assure minimization of radiation-associated morbidities.

Systemic therapy for early stage breast cancer

Breast cancer is a complex heterogeneous disease with variable clinical presentations and outcomes. After a patient is diagnosed with ESBC, she should receive multidisciplinary care that aims for cure. Unfortunately, 20–30% of women with a diagnosis of ESBC will develop recurrent disease with distant metastases.[308]

After a patient is diagnosed with ESBC, decisions regarding treatment are influenced by clinicopathologic variables. Clinical factors such as age, menopausal status, size of tumor, and nodal status, as well as pathologic factors such as tumor grade, biomarkers, and proliferation rate are used to determine aggressiveness of a cancer and select treatment options. Tumor biomarkers as determined by IHC and in situ hybridization (ISH) are utilized to stratify breast cancer into three primary types that are prognostic and strongly predict response to specific therapies. The primary types are HR+, HER2+, and TNBCs.

HR+ breast cancers express ERs and PRs for which the current standard assay is IHC. The ER, a ligand-modulated transcription factor, is the primary driver of oncogenesis in HR+ breast cancer through its effects on cellular proliferation. ER and PR bind estrogen with high affinity, leading to conformational changes and entry into the nucleus. This hormone–receptor complex binds to estrogen-specific response elements to activate or repress gene expression. When ER or PR is bound by antiestrogens, growth-promoting genes are blocked. The presence of ER or PR is associated with responsiveness to endocrine therapy.

IHC can be performed on tissue or cytology specimens that are fresh or archived. ER and PR concentration varies for different tumors. The ASCO/College of American Pathologists (CAP) Guideline Recommendations define HR+ as ≥1% staining of tumor cells for ER or PR, as patients with carcinoma cells expressing ER or PR as low as 1% have had significant clinical responses to hormone therapy.[309] A proportion of 60–80% of breast cancer specimens express ER.

A proportion of 15–20% of breast cancers overexpress HER2, of which approximately 50% are also HR+. The HER2 oncogene encodes a transmembrane glycoprotein receptor with intracellular tyrosine kinase activity. The HER2 receptor is a member of the EGFR family of receptors, which are involved in the activation of signal transduction pathways that regulate growth and differentiation of normal and malignant breast epithelial cells. HER2 overexpression is prognostic and predictive of response to specific chemotherapies and HER2-directed therapies.

The most recent ASCO/CAP guidelines for HER2 testing have recommended that all patients with ESBC or metastatic breast cancer (MBC) have HER2 status assessed by a validated HER2 test.[310] Expression of HER2 is determined with IHC for the HER2 membrane protein or with ISH [fluorescent in situ hybridization (FISH), chromogenic ISH, or dual in situ hybridization (DISH)] to quantify HER2 gene amplification. FISH can be performed using either a single probe for HER2 or dual probe for HER2 and centromere 17 (CEP17).

A breast cancer is defined as HER2+ by IHC when circumferential membrane staining is 3+ (complete and intense membrane staining in ≥10% of tumor cells).[308] IHC of 0–1 is HER2 negative (HER2−), while IHC of 2+ is equivocal, and reflex FISH should be performed. A breast cancer is defined as HER2+ by FISH when the ratio of HER2 to CEP17 is >2.0 or <2.0 plus an average HER2 copy number of >6.0 signals/cell. A FISH ratio of <2 and/or an average HER2 copy number <4 signals/cell is negative, while a FISH ratio of <2 and/or an average HER2 copy number of 4.0–6.0 signals/cell is equivocal, and reflex IHC should be performed. Repeat testing should be considered if results seem discordant with other histopathologic findings.

By definition, TNBC lack IHC staining for ER, PR, and HER2 and HER2 amplification by FISH. The ASCO/CAP panel guidelines define HR− as <1% staining of tumor cells by IHC in the presence of appropriately stained extrinsic and intrinsic controls.[311] The ASCO/CAP guidelines define HER2 negativity as 0–1+ by IHC or FISH nonamplified.[308]

The annual hazard rates for breast cancer recurrence are highest within the first few years after primary therapy, peaking at approximately 3–5 years and decreasing to a steady state by 7 or 8 years. However, patterns of recurrence vary significantly by breast cancer subtype. Up to 50% of distant recurrences from HR+ ESBC occurs in the first 5 years after diagnosis, but rates of recurrence and/or death from 0.5% to 3% per year extend for another 15 years. In comparison, the ROR of TNBC is highest within the first 3 years of diagnosis, but the magnitude of risk declines rapidly thereafter, with only rare recurrences after 5 years. Even with adjustment for age, race, stage, tumor size, nodal status, race, and treatment, TNBC is associated with a significantly worse OS than HR+ BC (HR 2.72, CI 2.39–3.10, $p < 0.0001$).[309] HER2+ ESBC is associated with a more aggressive clinical course with shorter time to relapse and OS than HER2− ESBC. Its natural history dramatically improved with the advent of the HER2-targeted monoclonal antibody trastuzumab, which resulted in a 50% reduction in recurrence rates and an approximately 30% increase in OS. However, the outcome of HER2+ ESBC is also dependent on hormone receptor status, as

demonstrated by a reduced response to endocrine-based therapies in HR+/HER2+ ESBC.

Optimal management of ESBC includes a combination of local and systemic therapy. Systemic therapy is used primarily to decrease risk of distant recurrence in patients with invasive disease, but hormone therapy is highly effective in reducing both local recurrence and contralateral new cancers. HR+ disease is treated with one of the several classes of agents, including the SERM tamoxifen, the AIs, and gonadotropin-releasing hormone agonists (GnRHa) to suppress ovarian function in premenopausal women, either with or without chemotherapy. Chemotherapy is the primary systemic treatment for TNBC and is used together with trastuzumab for HER2+ disease.

Targeted biologic therapy is being actively studied in the treatment of ESBC. In general, these agents have demonstrated high efficacy together with standard therapy compared with standard therapy only in the treatment of MBC. Classes of agents include monoclonal antibodies and oral tyrosine kinase inhibitors directed to HER2, cyclin-dependent kinase 4/6 (CDK 4/6) inhibitors or PI3K inhibitors combined with hormone therapies, and immunotherapies that reverse tumor immune tolerance. Details on these trials are available at http://www.cancer.gov/about-cancer/treatment/clinical-trials/search.

Standard treatment recommendations for ESBC are generally applied to specific risk groups, based on biologic subtypes, extent of disease, and patient-related factors. Variable outcomes within these risk groups suggest that different molecular pathways underlie this phenotypic diversity. The rapid evolution in biomedical research and technology over the last two decades has led to an increasing understanding of the molecular pathways that drive cancer growth, affecting both prognosis and response to therapy. Current technologies allow determination of prognosis and help to predict the benefit of chemotherapy in HR+ breast cancer, but unfortunately do not predict which chemotherapy regimen or combination is most effective—leading primarily to overtreatment. New tests facilitate the determination of patients who are at a higher risk for late recurrence. Hopefully, ongoing research will identify combinations of biomarkers or gene signatures that will help to individualize therapy and allow appropriate use of new targeted biologic therapy for the patients who need it most.

The practice of breast oncology is rapidly evolving and oncologists are encouraged to stay informed of such changes through review guidelines and consensus statements provided through national and international organizations. The NCCN Guidelines® provide statements of evidence and consensus with frequent updates and are available at NCCN.org. The St. Gallen International Expert Consensus on the Primary Therapy of Early Breast Cancer has been recently updated and is available at http://www.oncoconferences.ch/mm//mm001/Ann_Oncol-2015-Coates-annonc_mdv221.pdf. The Institute for Quality in the ASCO has created practice guidelines based on review of the best available evidence by expert panels and are available at http://www.instituteforquality.org/practice-guidelines.

Prognosis and prediction

There have been multiple attempts to integrate prognostic information into standardized prognostic indices. The University of Nottingham index is based on tumor grade, axillary lymph node involvement, and hormone receptor status.[312,313] It has been validated prospectively and confirmed by an independent center, but still has limited applications in the determination of individual prognosis. The Adjuvantonline program (Figure 22) (https://www.adjuvantonline.com/index.jsp) is a prognostic index that was in extensive use until the development and widespread use of gene expression assays (see below). This is a free online software that

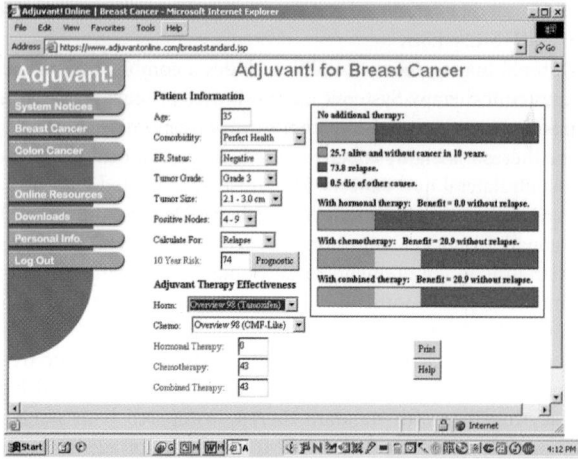

Figure 22 Online prognostic software that predicts 10-year probability of recurrence and mortality, as well as the probability of benefit from various systemic adjuvant treatment options based on individual patient and tumor characteristics.

uses patient age, comorbid conditions, tumor size, grade, number of positive axillary nodes, and ER status to calculate the 10-year probability of relapse and death for an individual patient.[231] Using this estimated risk level, the program also calculates the absolute benefit the patient would derive from adjuvant tamoxifen, AIs, and various chemotherapy regimens. Investigators from British Columbia recently validated the program, with observed results <2% of those predicted. Unfortunately, Adjuvantonline was developed before routine testing for HER2, and recurrence includes both local and distant risk. For this reason, benefits of chemotherapy in particular may be either amplified or reduced inappropriately.

Intrinsic breast cancer subtypes

Gene expression profiling allows for the simultaneous examination of multiple genetic alterations and the measurement in activity of thousands of genes within a single breast cancer cell, providing a more accurate classification of tumors. In 2000, Perou et al.[314] used this technology to evaluate 189 breast cancer samples, of which 122 contained expression patterns with significant gene clusters. These clusters were determined to represent four distinct intrinsic breast cancer subtypes: luminal A and B, HER2 enriched, and basal-like. Retrospective studies demonstrated that these subtypes are associated with prognosis and predict treatment outcomes.

The luminal subtypes of breast cancer involve genes associated with the luminal epithelial cells of normal breast tissue and clearly overlap with HR+ breast cancers, the majority (90–95%) of which are of the luminal subtype.[315] The luminal A subtype, which carries the best prognosis, is found in approximately 40% of breast cancers and is associated with high expression of ER-related genes, but low expression of the HER2 and proliferation-related gene clusters. By contrast, the luminal B subtype is found in about 30–40% of all breast cancers and is associated with reduced expression of several luminal-related genes, low expression of the HER2 gene, and higher expression of the proliferation cluster. Regardless of systemic therapy, luminal B cancers have a worse baseline 5- and 10-year distant recurrence-free survival than luminal A cancers.

The HER2-enriched subtype is associated with high expression of HER2 and proliferation-related genes, and a higher frequency of genomic mutations than other breast cancers.[313] Interestingly, some HER2- breast cancers are identified as HER2-enriched.

The basal-like subtype is associated with high expression of proliferation-related gene clusters, such as EGFR, and low expression of ER- and HER2-related genes and is thus generally negative for the ER, PR, and HER2.[313] However, the basal-like subtype is not synonymous with TNBC and is associated with the expression of proteins within the basal layer of the breast duct epithelium. Breast cancers with the basal-like subtype have a poor prognosis with an increased risk for relapse within the first 5 years of diagnosis, but after which the risk rapidly declines. Subsequent studies evaluating variable outcomes with neoadjuvant chemotherapy for TNBC revealed seven additional subtypes: basal-like 1 and 2, immunomodulatory, mesenchymal, mesenchymal stemlike, luminal androgen receptor (AR), and unstable.[316,317]

Multigene assays

Several multigene assays that were developed over the last two decades, including Oncotype DX, MammaPrint (MP), Prosigna, the Breast Cancer Index (BCI), and EndoPredict (EP), are commercially available to provide risk assessment for patients with ESBC and in some cases predict benefit of adjuvant therapies. Most importantly, these assays permit rational individualization of treatment by predicting outcome with hormone therapy only for HR+ disease, or alternatively predicting benefit of chemotherapy. The most commonly used assays with the largest supportive data are Oncotype DX and MP.

The Oncotype DX assay, commercially available since 2004, was originally intended as a tool to assess prognosis and predict chemotherapy benefit for women with node-negative, HR+ ESBC, a category of patients for whom the utility of adjuvant chemotherapy is difficult to define when utilizing traditional clinical factors only.[117,181] More recently, the assay was validated for use in patients with node-positive disease.[134] This multigene assay quantifies the expression of 21 genes through a quantitative reverse transcriptase polymerase chain reaction (qRT-PCR) platform applied to a single formalin-fixed paraffin-embedded (FFPE) breast cancer tissue sample.[117] The assay is only available through a central laboratory. The 21-gene signature is composed of 16 breast cancer-related genes associated with proliferation, ER regulation, and the HER2 pathway as well as five reference genes for normalization. Expression levels of the 21 genes are applied to an algorithm that calculates the RS, which determines a patient's 10-year ROR after taking 5 years of adjuvant tamoxifen only, as well as her 10-year ROR after adjuvant chemotherapy followed by 5 years of adjuvant tamoxifen. The RS is a continuous variable that ranges from 0 to 100 and falls into one of three categories: low risk (RS <18), intermediate risk (RS 18–30), and high risk (RS >30). Patients with low risk have no benefit from chemotherapy, whereas those with high risk have a significant benefit. The benefit of adjuvant chemotherapy for patients in the intermediate-risk category is less clear and currently under investigation (see below; the TAILORx trial).

The developers of the Oncotype DX assay selected 250 genes from genomic databases and tested their expression on tumor samples from several clinical trials, including the tamoxifen-only arms of NSABP B-14 and NSABP B-20.[117] A final panel of 21 genes was selected from these tests and used to calculate the RS of each tumor sample. The initial validation of the prognostic utility of the Oncotype DX assay was performed by evaluating fixed tissue samples from a subset of patients on the tamoxifen-only arm of the NSABP B-14 clinical trial, which included women with HR+ and node-negative ESBC and compared tamoxifen with placebo for 5 years after primary surgery. A total of 668 fixed samples were analyzed and given an RS. The 10-year rate of distant recurrence was split into three groups: 6.8% (95% CI, 4.0–9.6) for low risk (RS

<18), 14.3% (95% CI, 8.3–20.3) for intermediate risk (RS 18–30), and 31% (95% CI, 23.6–37.4) for high risk (RS >30). The ROR was significantly lower with the low RS than high RS group ($p < 0.001$).

Several studies have demonstrated the ability of Oncotype DX to predict the benefit of chemotherapy for the different RS groups. Paik et al. measured the RS for a subset ($n = 651$) of tumor samples from NSABP B-20, a clinical trial of postmenopausal women with HR+ node-negative ESBC.[181] NSABP B-20 randomized 2363 patients to receive either tamoxifen or adjuvant CMF or MF followed by tamoxifen.[318] Paik et al. observed a statistically significant interaction between the benefit of chemotherapy and the RS ($p = 0.038$), with a large benefit for patients with a high RS [RR, 0.26; 95% CI, 0.13–0.53] and a mean absolute decrease in 10-year distant recurrence rate of 27.6% (SE, 8.0%). In comparison, minimal benefit from chemotherapy was observed in patients with a low RS (RR, 1.31; 95% CI, 0.46–3.78) and no decrease in 10-year distant recurrence rate (−1.1%; SE, 2.2%).

Albain et al.[134] performed a retrospective analysis of the association between RS and disease-free survival (DFS) for a subset of postmenopausal women with HR+ node-positive ESBC enrolled in the phase III clinical trial, SWOG-8814, that compared adjuvant tamoxifen versus adjuvant cyclophosphamide, adriamycin, and 5-FU (CAF) followed by tamoxifen. An RS was assessed for 40% of the 927 patients enrolled in the parent trial. The RS was prognostic of DFS in the tamoxifen-only group (HR 2.64, 95% CI 1.33–5.27; $p = 0.006$). Patients with a low RS observed no benefit from CAF (log-rank $p = 0.97$; HR 1.02, 0.54–1.93), while those with a high RS had a statistically significant improvement in DFS (HR 0.59, 95% CI, 0.35–1.01; log-rank $p = 0.033$).

The benefit of adjuvant chemotherapy for patients with node-negative disease with an intermediate-risk Oncotype DX RS is poorly defined and is currently under evaluation in two randomized phase III clinical trials. TAILORx (NCT00310180) evaluates patients with a node-negative HR+ breast cancer with an RS between 12 and 30. The study was initiated in 2006 with a total of 10,273 patients enrolled in it.[319] Patients with an RS between 11 and 25 ($n = 6897$) were randomized to receive either adjuvant chemotherapy followed by endocrine therapy or endocrine therapy only. Patients with an RS between 26 and 30 were all treated with combined chemotherapy followed by hormone therapy, and those with a score <11 were treated with hormone therapy only. Standard local therapy was recommended. The final data collection was planned to occur in December 2017, but outcome data from the low-risk secondary study group was published in 2015.[320] A total of 1626 patients with a median age of 58 were treated with a median tumor size of 1.5 cm; 59% had intermediate grade histology and a median age of 58. More than half of the patients were treated with an AI (59%). The 5-year invasive disease-free survival (IDFS) rate was 93.8%, and the 5-year distant recurrence-free interval (DRFI) was 99.3% with a 98% OS. Recurrence risk was not significantly affected by age, tumor size, or histologic grade. These data support the clinical utility of gene expression assays in determining breast cancers at very low risk that clearly do not require chemotherapy. The data from the intermediate risk group are eagerly anticipated.

The SWOG Rx for POsitive Node, Endocrine Responsive BC (RxPONDER S1007) clinical trial (NCT01272037) is a prospective study evaluating the noninferiority of endocrine therapy to chemotherapy followed by endocrine therapy in patients with HR+/HER2− node-positive (one to three lymph nodes) breast cancer with an RS of ≤25.[321] A total of 4000 patients will be randomized to receive either chemotherapy followed by endocrine therapy or endocrine therapy only. Each patient's adjuvant therapy will be chosen by the treating physician according to standard treatment options. The estimated date of completion of this study is February 2022.

The MP 70-gene breast cancer recurrence assay is intended as a prognostic test for women under 62 years of age with node-negative or positive (one to three lymph nodes), HR+ or HR−, ESBC with a primary tumor no larger than 5 cm.[322] DNA microarray technology is used to measure the mRNA expression levels of 70 specific genes in a breast tumor sample. The test was originally designed for fresh frozen samples but has since been validated for use on FFPE. Expression levels of the 70-genes are used to place patients into low- or high-risk groups. Patients with low-risk are estimated to have a 13% chance of developing metastasis at 10 years without adjuvant therapy compared with high-risk patients associated with a 56% chance.

The assay was developed at the Netherlands Cancer Institute using tumor tissue samples from 78 women with node-negative breast cancer, who did not receive systemic adjuvant therapy and for whom outcomes were documented.[323] The entire genome of each of these tumor samples was evaluated with microarray technology to identify genes most associated with recurrence risk. The 70 genes most predictive of recurrence were selected for the MP assay. The assay was later validated retrospectively in its ability to distinguish between low- and high-risk patients with node-negative HR+ breast cancer using several different tissue banks. One study applied the assay to 307 tissue samples from women with HR+ node-negative ESBC, with a significant difference in prognosis between high- and low-risk groups (HR = 2.32).[167] Subsequent data validated the prognostic value of MP in node-positive disease as well.[324,325]

The MINDACT trial is a prospective multicenter trial within the Breast International Group (BIG) that is evaluating the MP 70-gene profile in both node-negative and one to three node-positive diseases.[133] MINDACT has enrolled 6600 patients, classified as high- and low-risk groups by MP and clinicopathologic risk through Adjuvant!Online. Patients with concordant high risk are offered adjuvant chemotherapy, and those with concordant low risk do not receive chemotherapy.[326] Patients with discordant risk are randomized to receive adjuvant chemotherapy based on either MP or Adjuvant!Online. Patients receiving chemotherapy are also randomized to two different chemotherapy regimens, and those receiving hormone therapy are randomized to two different adjuvant endocrine therapy approaches. The first efficacy results are expected in 2016.

The Prosigna® score is intended to estimate the 10-year risk of distant recurrence for postmenopausal women with HR+ breast cancer, either node-negative (stage I or II) or node-positive (stage II only). The Prosigna score, also known as ROR score, is calculated with a proprietary algorithm that combines a patient's intrinsic breast cancer subtype, as determined by the Predictor Analysis of Microarray 50 (PAM-50), with gross tumor size. PAM-50 is a 50-gene subset derived from the larger gene set used by Perou et al. in 2000 to define the intrinsic breast cancer subtypes. PAM-50 was applied to banked tissue samples to assess prognosis of 761 patients who did not receive any systemic therapies for their ESBC. Results from PAM-50 and associated primary tumor size are used to calculate an ROR score, which is then used to stratify patients with HR+ breast cancer into low-, medium-, and high-recurrence-risk subsets. The selected 50 genes and associated intrinsic subtypes remained significant when evaluated with multivariable analyses that included standard parameters.

Gnant et al.[327] performed an independent, retrospective validation study that demonstrated level 1 evidence of the increased prognostic reliability of the PAM-50-derived ROR score compared with standard clinical predictors. The study cohort included 1478 patient tissue samples from the ABCSG-8 clinical trial, which randomized 3091 women with HR+ ESBC not treated with adjuvant chemotherapy to either 2 years of adjuvant tamoxifen followed by 3 years of adjuvant anastrozole or 5 years of adjuvant tamoxifen. The ROR score added statistically significant prognostic information in comparison to standard clinical predictors ($p < 0.0001$). Samples assigned to the luminal A subgroup had a significantly lower ROR at 10 years than those in the luminal B subgroup.

The BCI, the combination of a two-gene ratio (HOXB13:IL17BR; H/I) and a five-gene (BUB1B, CENPA, NEK2, RACGAP1, and RRM2) molecular grade index (MGI), was developed using a cohort of tamoxifen-treated patients from the randomized prospective Stockholm trial and has been shown to provide an individual risk of distant breast cancer recurrence based on a continuous risk model.[328,329] BCI has been shown to significantly predict 0- to 10-year ROR beyond standard clinicopathologic factors and to predict late distant recurrence.[330] A subset analysis of tumor samples from the extended adjuvant hormone therapy MA. 17 trial suggested that H/I could identify a high-risk group in the 5-year tamoxifen group and found that patients with a high H/I score who received letrozole after 5 years had a decreased probability of distant recurrence.[331]

EP is an RNA-based multigene score including eight cancer-related and three reference genes that predicts the likelihood of distant recurrence in patients with early-stage, ER-positive, and HER2− breast cancer treated with adjuvant endocrine therapy only.[332,333] EP is also combined with nodal status and tumor size into a comprehensive risk score, EPclin.

Hormone therapy for HR+ breast cancer

The role of estrogen in the development and progression of breast cancer was demonstrated over a century ago when a subset of unselected patients with advanced breast cancer were treated with surgical oophorectomy resulting in transient disease control. Throughout the mid-twentieth century, premenopausal women with a history of resected ESBC underwent ovarian ablation through radiation or surgery and were subsequently found to have reduced disease recurrence.[334] Such outcomes led researchers to evaluate systemic endocrine therapies for the treatment of advanced breast cancer as well as for the prevention of disease recurrence in ESBC.

Systemic hormone-based therapy for HR+ ESBC was not available for general use until tamoxifen was approved for postmenopausal women in 1985 and later for premenopausal women in 1990. As a SERM, tamoxifen competitively inhibits estrogen from binding ER, with subsequent antagonist and agonist effects depending on the target tissue. Although incompletely understood, these differential effects are presumptively due to variable interactions with coactivator and corepressor proteins involved in ER-mediated gene regulation.

Tamoxifen was first evaluated as an adjuvant therapy in the Nolvadex Adjuvant Trial Organisation (NATO) clinical trial, which was initiated in 1977 and randomized 1285 women with ESBC to tamoxifen 10 mg bid for 2 years or no further treatment. At a maximum follow-up of 8 years, patients treated with tamoxifen had a 36% reduction in recurrence ($x^2 = 17.69$, $p = 0.0001$) and 29% reduction in all-cause risk of death ($x^2 = 7.48$, $p = 0.0062$).[335] The initial trials of 5 years of adjuvant tamoxifen demonstrated a small gain in 5-year survival, but a longer follow-up demonstrated that the mortality reduction persisted beyond 5 years with an absolute reduction in mortality three times higher at 15 years after diagnosis. The mortality reductions during years 5–9 and 10–14 were each equivalent to the mortality reduction in years 0–4. A meta-analysis

by the EBCTCG published in 1988 included 28 trials evaluating adjuvant tamoxifen and clearly established that tamoxifen reduces 5-year mortality for all patients, but with a greater effect in women ≥50 years than those <50 years.[336] The 2011 EBCTCG meta-analysis of endocrine therapy reported that in the trials of tamoxifen for 5 years versus placebo, at a median follow-up of 13 years, tamoxifen resulted in a significant reduction in breast cancer recurrence at 15 years (RR 0.61, 95% CI 0.57–0.65) and in breast cancer mortality at 15 years (RR 0.70, 95% CI 0.64–0.75).[337] Use of adjuvant tamoxifen for 5 years reduces the annual breast cancer recurrence by almost 40% and death by 31%, independent of age, chemo, LN, and menopausal status. Unfortunately, the ROR does not decrease over time, and over 50% of recurrences and two-thirds of deaths occur over 5 years after diagnosis.

Although of great benefit with regard to the reduction of breast cancer recurrence and OS, tamoxifen is not without troublesome side effects, including some infrequent but serious adverse events (AEs). Antagonistic effects on the central nervous system (CNS) lead to dysfunctional thermoregulation experienced as hot flashes by almost 80% of patients on tamoxifen that is most significant in premenopausal women. Agonistic activity on uterine tissue can facilitate endometrial hyperplasia with a subsequent development of fibroids, polyps, and malignant tumors. The EBCTCG overview analysis of individual patient data from trials of tamoxifen versus placebo demonstrated a 2.4-fold increase in endometrial cancer, but without an adverse effect on mortality.[338] Patients who were diagnosed with endometrial cancer were almost exclusively >50 years. Long-term follow-up has demonstrated a very small increased incidence of uterine sarcoma that generally presents at an advanced stage, 2–5 years after initiation of tamoxifen therapy. Several pooled analyses have demonstrated an increase in venous thromboembolic events of two- to threefold with tamoxifen, an effect observed primarily seen in women with age ≥55 years and higher body mass index. Additional side effects include vaginal discharge, sexual dysfunction, menstrual irregularities, and cataracts.

AIs were initially evaluated in and approved for postmenopausal women with advanced breast cancer and were later studied as an alternative to tamoxifen for adjuvant therapy in postmenopausal women. Aromatase converts androgens to estrogen in peripheral tissues. AIs inhibit this enzymatic activity with a rapid decrease in circulating estrogen. They do not block the secretion of estrogen from ovarian tissue and are therefore not appropriate for premenopausal women with intact ovarian function.

The first and second generations of AI were too toxic for further development, but the third generation of AI—exemestane, anastrozole, and letrozole—was safer and better tolerated. Anastrozole and letrozole are nonsteroidal agents that bind reversibly to aromatase as opposed to exemestane, a steroidal agent that binds irreversibly to aromatase. Side effects and symptoms of AI are discussed below. AIs are associated with an increased risk of osteoporosis, fractures, musculoskeletal symptoms of arthralgias, joint stiffness and bone pain, hot flashes, and sexual dysfunction.

Adjuvant hormonal therapy for postmenopausal women

The development of third-generation AIs challenged and later replaced tamoxifen as the primary adjuvant hormonal therapy in postmenopausal women with HR+ ESBC. Several pivotal phase III clinical trials were initiated in the 1990s to demonstrate the superiority of AIs over tamoxifen for the reduction of their recurrence risk and the improvement of OS of postmenopausal women. Other studies examined the optimal time course of adjuvant hormonal therapy to optimize risk reduction while limiting toxicities. Preclinical data demonstrating tamoxifen resistance in breast cancer cell lines as well as large clinical trials reporting toxicities associated with long-term tamoxifen therapy led investigators to evaluate switching patients to an AI after 2–3 years of adjuvant tamoxifen, known as sequential adjuvant therapy. Extended adjuvant therapy, treatment with tamoxifen for 10 years or tamoxifen for 5 years followed by an AI for 5 years, was explored in an effort to further reduce late recurrence risk in HR+ ESBC.

The Arimidex, Tamoxifen, Alone or in Combination (ATAC) study was the first clinical trial to demonstrate the efficacy of an AI over tamoxifen.[336,339,340] All 9241 randomized participants were postmenopausal and had completed primary treatment with surgery as well as radiation and/or chemotherapy as needed. Patients were not excluded according to hormone receptor status, and 84% were HR+. The three study arms consisted of 5 years of either anastrozole 1 mg daily, tamoxifen 20 mg daily, or a combination of both. The initial analysis, performed with a median follow-up of 33.3 months, demonstrated a 3-year DFS in the anastrozole arm of 89.4% and in the tamoxifen arm of 87.4%, which was statistically significant with an HR of 0.83 (95% CI 0.71–0.96, $p = 0.013$). The combination and tamoxifen arms were similar with an HR of 1.02 (CI 0.89–1.18, $p = 0.8$). Anastrozole was better tolerated with respect to endometrial cancer ($p = 0.02$), vaginal bleeding or discharge ($p < 0.0001$), cerebrovascular events and venous thromboembolic events ($p = 0.0006$ for both), and hot flashes ($p < 0.0001$). However, arthralgias and fractures were significantly less frequent in the tamoxifen than anastrozole arm ($p < 0.0001$ for both). At the 10-year follow-up, anastrozole remained more efficacious in comparison to tamoxifen and the combination arm with regard to DFS (HR 0.91; 95% CI, 0.83–0.99; $p = 0.04$) and time to recurrence.

BIG 1–98 study was a phase III double-blinded clinical trial of postmenopausal women with ESBC that was designed to compare adjuvant monotherapy with letrozole versus tamoxifen for 5 years as well as sequential therapy with letrozole given before or after tamoxifen.[341] A total of 8010 patients were randomized after surgical treatment to one of the four arms: letrozole 2.5 mg daily for 5 years, tamoxifen 20 mg daily for 5 years, letrozole for 2 years followed by tamoxifen for 3 years, and tamoxifen for 2 years followed by letrozole for 3 years. A protocol amendment in 2005 allowed for crossover from tamoxifen to letrozole because of a significant DFS benefit. At a median follow-up of 8.7 years, letrozole monotherapy was significantly better than tamoxifen monotherapy with regard to DFS and OS, whether assessed with intention to treat or inverse probability of censoring weighting (IPCW), which accounts for selective crossover to letrozole from tamoxifen. At a median follow-up of 8 years, no statistically significant difference was appreciated between the sequential arms.

A meta-analysis published in 2011 reported a cohort of patients ($n = 9856$) from the ATAC and BIG 1–98 trials, who were randomized to receive an AI (anastrozole or letrozole) for 5 years or tamoxifen for 5 years, demonstrating an absolute decrease in recurrence of 2.9% (SE = 0.7%) in those treated with an AI. Recurrences in the AI group were 9.6% compared to 12.6% with tamoxifen ($2p < 0.00001$), with a nonsignificant absolute decrease in breast cancer mortality of 1.1% (SE = 0.0%).

The Intergroup Exemestane Study (IES) randomized 4742 postmenopausal patients with HR+ ESBC who remained disease free after 2–3 years of tamoxifen therapy to either switch to exemestane or remain on tamoxifen for a total of 5 years of adjuvant hormonal therapy.[342] At a median follow-up of 30.6 months, a significant improvement in DFS was noted in the exemestane switch arm

(unadjusted HR 0.68, 95% CI, 0.56–0.82; $p < 0.001$) with an absolute benefit of 4.7% at 3 years after randomization. At a median follow-up of 91 months, this gain was not lost, but no additional benefit was observed (HR, 0.94; 95% CI, 0.80–1.10; $p = 0.60$).[343] However, an improvement in OS was observed (HR 0.86; 95% CI, 0.75–0.99; $p = 0.04$). Subgroup analyses illustrated a benefit in patients with node-positive or -negative disease and ER+ disease irrespective of PR status. An increase in osteoporosis (9.2% vs 7.2%, $p = 0.01$) and fracture (7% vs 4.9%, $p = 0.003$) was also observed, as expected.

A recent meta-analysis presented by Forbes et al. at ASCO in 2014 including approximately 37,000 women further supported the use of AIs in postmenopausal women.[344,345] In trials comparing AI to tamoxifen with a total of 22,533 postmenopausal women with HR+ ESBC, there was a significant reduction in recurrence during years 0–1 (RR 0.66; 95% CI 0.54–0.80) and 2–4 (RR 0.75, 95% CI 0.64–0.88). The meta-analysis also reported on sequential adjuvant therapy. In clinical trials in which women were assigned to sequential tamoxifen followed by an AI versus 5 years of tamoxifen, there was a significant reduction in recurrence (RR 0.84, 95% CI 0.73–0.97) that was lowest during years 2–4 (RR 0.56, 95% CI 0.46–0.67). Furthermore, there were fewer breast cancer-related deaths with sequential adjuvant therapy than tamoxifen only (RR 0.84, 95% CI 0.73–0.97). In trials comparing AI and sequential treatment ($n = 12,799$) using tamoxifen followed by an AI, the recurrence risk was lower for the former than the latter during years 0–1 (RR 0.75, 95% CI 0.75–0.89), but similar during years 2–4 (RR 0.99, 95% CI 0.85–1.15). The similarity during years 2–4 was thought most likely due to the fact that the patients in the sequential group were likely transitioned to AI during that time frame.

Knowing that AIs were more efficacious than tamoxifen in the postmenopausal ESBC setting, clinical trials were developed to evaluate extended AI therapy. MA.17 was a phase III clinical trial that randomized 5187 postmenopausal women with ESBC who previously received 5 years of tamoxifen followed by 5 years of either letrozole or placebo. At a median follow-up of 64 months, a significant benefit in DFS (HR 0.68; 95% CI 0.45–0.61) and OS (HR 0.51, 95% CI 0.42–0.61) was apparent. These results led to the approval of extended adjuvant treatment with tamoxifen followed by letrozole. Patients who were randomized to placebo were allowed to take letrozole after publication of the trial results and patients were unblinded. Those patients who chose to take letrozole still experienced an increase in DFS, despite a substantial lapse in time between therapies with a median of 2.8 years.

Two large, multinational clinical trials evaluated the extended use of adjuvant tamoxifen and presented similar outcomes. The Adjuvant Tamoxifen: Longer Against Shorter (ATLAS) clinical trial randomized 12,894 patients with ESBC who had completed 5 years of tamoxifen to continue tamoxifen for a total of 10 years or stop at that point of time. More than half of the participants (53%) were known to have ER+ disease, for whom allocation to tamoxifen resulted in a significant benefit with regard to breast cancer recurrence (18% vs 21%, $p = 0.002$) and overall mortality (639 deaths vs 722 deaths, $p = 0.01$).[346] The reduction in recurrence became more significant over time with the recurrence rate ratio of 0.9 (95% CI 0.79–1.02) during years 5–9 and 0.75 (95% CI 0.62–0.90) in later years. The cumulative risk of endometrial cancer during years 5–14 was 31% for patients randomized to continue tamoxifen versus 16% for controls with an absolute mortality increase of 0.2%.

The Adjuvant Tamoxifen—To Offer More (aTTom) clinical trial randomized 6953 women with ESBC who had completed >4 years of tamoxifen to either an additional 5 years of tamoxifen

Table 9 Comparative efficacy of adjuvant hormonal therapies.[337,349]

	Recurrence rate ratio			15-Year recurrence risk difference	15-Year breast cancer mortality rate ratio
	years[a] 0–4	years 5–9	years 10–14		
TAM[b] (5 years) vs observation	0.53 (2p < 0.00001)	0.68 (2p < 0.00001)	0.97	13.2% (RR 0.61 95% CI 0.57–0.65; 2p < 0.00001)	0.70 (p < 0.00001)

	Recurrence rate ratio			10-Year recurrence risk difference	10-Year breast cancer mortality rate ratio
	Years 0–1	Years 2–4	Year 5 and beyond		
AI[c] (5 years) vs TAM (5 years)	0.64 (95% CI 0.52–0.78; p < 0.00001)	0.80 (95% CI 0.68–0.93; p < 0.00001)	NSE[d] (minimal f/u after year 10)	3.6% (95% CI 1.7–5.4)	0.85 (95% CI 0.75–0.96; 2p = 0.009)
AI (5 years) vs TAM (2–3 years) -> AI (to year 5)	0.74 (95% CI 0.62–0.89; 2p = 0.002)	0.99 (95% CI 0.85–1.15)	NSE (minimal f/u after year 7)	NSE (2p = 0.045)	0.89 (95% CI 0.78–1.03; 2p = 0.11)
TAM (2–3 years) -> AI (to year 5) vs TAM (5 years)	NSE (in part due to timing of data collection)	0.56 (95% CI 0.46–0.67; p < 0.0001)	NSE (minimal f/u after year 10)	2.0% (95% CI 0.2–3.8)	0.84 (95% CI 0.72–0.96; 2p = 0.015)

[a]Years, years postsurgery.
[b]TAM, tamoxifen.
[c]Aromatase inhibitor.
[d]NSE, no significant effect.

or placebo.[347] At a median follow-up of 4.2 years, an insignificant reduction in recurrence in the extended therapy arm (RR = 0.94, 95% CI 0.81–1.09, p = 0.4). At a median follow-up of 5 years, a significant time-dependent reduction in recurrence was observed with continued tamoxifen (rate ratio 0.99 during years 5–6 [95% CI 0.86–1.15], 0.84 during years 7–9 [95% CI 0.73–0.95], and 0.75 thereafter [95% CI 0.66–0.86]).[348] It is important to note that 61% of patients did not have hormone receptor status tested. The rate of endometrial cancer doubled with 10 years of tamoxifen, but with no associated increase in death.

The EBCTCG recently published a patient-level meta-analysis of AI versus tamoxifen in HR+ ESBC that included 31,920 post-menopausal women.[349] Recurrence rate ratios in patients treated with 5 years of AI versus 5 years of tamoxifen were significant from years 0–1 (RR 0.64, 95% CI 0.52–0.78) and years 2–4 (RR 0.80, 0.68–0.93), but was no longer significant in the following years. Mortality at 10 years was lower with AI than tamoxifen (RR 0.85, 95% CI 0.75–0.96; 2p = 0.009). Results of studies comparing 5 years of AI or 5 years of tamoxifen with 2–3 years of tamoxifen followed by AI to year 5 showed a recurrence rate ratio favoring AI only during the time that the treatments differed. However, breast cancer mortality and all-cause mortality were reduced with AI throughout the study, regardless of the similar or different treatment methods. AEs were as expected, with 10-year endometrial cancer incidence increased with tamoxifen in comparison to AI (1.2% vs 0.4%) and with 5-year risk of bone fractures increased more with AI than with tamoxifen (8.2% vs 5.5%). Comparative efficacies of various hormone therapies evaluated in the 2011 and 2015 EBCTCG meta-analyses are provided in Table 9.

The 2014 ASCO Clinical Practice Guideline Focused Update for adjuvant endocrine therapy recommended that postmenopausal women with HR+ ESBC receive a minimum of 5 years of AI or sequential tamoxifen followed by AI.[350] They should be offered a total of 10 years of therapy. The 2015 St. Gallen Consensus on Primary Therapy stated that some postmenopausal women can be treated with 5 years of tamoxifen but that higher risk patients should receive an AI at some point.[345] Furthermore, patients with node-positive HR+ ESBC should receive 10 years of endocrine-based therapy, regardless of menopausal status.

Adjuvant hormonal therapy for premenopausal women

The incidence of HR+ breast cancer in premenopausal women has increased in the last two decades, most likely in the context of diet and lifestyle. Tamoxifen was classified as the standard adjuvant hormonal therapy for premenopausal women with HR+ EBC in 1995. A subsequent EBCTCG meta-analysis in 2001 demonstrated that 5 years of tamoxifen reduced the recurrence rate by 50% and BC-related mortality by 31%, regardless of age.[351] The role of other therapies, such as ovarian suppression, chemotherapy, or other hormonal therapies such as AIs, remained quite unclear.

INT 0101 (E5188) was a phase III randomized clinical trial of premenopausal with node-positive, HR+ ESBC. Patients were randomized to receive either CAF only, CAF followed by goserelin, or CAF followed by goserelin with tamoxifen.[352] The combination of CAF followed by goserelin and tamoxifen was associated with a significant improvement in time to recurrence and DFS compared with the combination of CAF plus goserelin, with a median follow-up of 11.5 years. Retrospectively, benefit was skewed toward women <40 years of age, possibly because they are most likely to regain ovarian function. Unfortunately, the study design did not include a CAF followed by tamoxifen arm, as this sequence was not believed to be of benefit at the time of study design. The inclusion of goserelin was associated with more weight gain, development of diabetes mellitus, and hot flashes.

INT 0101 (E5188) was the first clinical trial to assess the role of LHRH agonists as an adjuvant treatment for premenopausal women. Cuzick et al.[353] performed a meta-analysis of 16 randomized clinical trials evaluating the use of LHRH agonists as adjuvant treatment for premenopausal women with HR+ breast cancer in 2007. Included trials assessed LHRH only, LHRH in combination with tamoxifen, LHRH in combination with chemotherapy, or the combination of LHRH, chemotherapy, and tamoxifen. None of the included trials compared chemotherapy with tamoxifen versus chemotherapy with LHRH. Trials of LHRH only demonstrated a statistically insignificant reduction in RR and death but lacked statistical power. The primary finding was that LHRH plus chemotherapy with or without tamoxifen resulted in a significant benefit in women of ≤40 years of age. Notably, the meta-analysis was underpowered to assess many important questions, such as the role of tamoxifen in premenopausal women and furthermore, none of the chemotherapy regimens were taxane-based and only a few were anthracycline-based.

The Austrian Breast and Colorectal Cancer Study Group 12 (ABCSG-12) clinical trial randomized 1803 women with HR+ ESBC who were receiving a 3-year course of goserelin to receive anastrozole or tamoxifen, with or without zoledronic acid over 3 years.[354] At a median follow-up of 48 months, no DFS benefit was seen for women randomized to ovarian suppression plus AI (HR 1.10, 95% CI 0.78–1.53).

The SOFT/TEXT clinical trials have been proved as the most effective adjuvant endocrine therapy for premenopausal women with HR+ ESBC. TEXT and SOFT were phase III randomized clinical trials initiated in 2003 by the International Breast Cancer Study Group (IBCSG) in collaboration with the BIG and the North American Breast Cancer Group.[355] The Tamoxifen and Exemestane Trial (TEXT) compared the use of adjuvant tamoxifen plus ovarian suppression and exemestane plus ovarian suppression over a 5-year period. A total of 2672 patients were randomized after surgery and received chemotherapy. By contrast, the Suppression of Ovarian Function Trial (SOFT) involved three arms comparing ovarian suppression plus tamoxifen, ovarian suppression plus exemestane, and tamoxifen only over 5 years. A total of 3066 women were randomized to the above arms after completing surgery and/or chemotherapy and were required to remain premenopausal before trial initiation. More than half of the study participants (53%) received chemotherapy. Bisphosphonates were not allowed in either trial unless patients had osteopenia or osteoporosis.

The original statistical analysis plans for TEXT and SOFT were to compare DFS between treatment groups within each trial separately, but because of fewer events occurring in this relatively

low-risk population, trial amendments in 2011 allowed for a combined analysis of the TEXT and SOFT arms comparing exemestane plus ovarian suppression to tamoxifen plus ovarian suppression. The TEXT/SOFT combined analysis of 4960 patients was reported at a median follow-up of 68 months in July 2014.[356] The 5-year DFS in the exemestane plus ovarian suppression arm was 91.1% and in the tamoxifen plus ovarian suppression group was 87.3% with no difference in overall survival. AE rates were similar to those seen in prior studies of postmenopausal women, at 30.6% and 29.4% with exemestane and tamoxifen, respectively. The results suggest that patients with HR+ ESBC with higher-risk disease may achieve a greater reduction in distant recurrence with ovarian suppression plus AI. However, the data are not fully mature and over 50% of expected recurrence events have not yet occurred, suggesting that the current conclusions be accepted with caution.

Analysis of the addition of tamoxifen to ovarian suppression as addressed by SOFT was announced at the San Antonio Breast Cancer Symposium in December 2014. At a median follow-up of 67 months, the 5-year DFS was 86.6% in the ovarian suppression plus tamoxifen arm compared with 84.7% in the tamoxifen-only arm (HR 0.83; 95% CI, 0.66–1.04; $p = 0.10$).[357] However, a higher treatment effect with tamoxifen plus ovarian suppression was appreciated in patients who had received chemotherapy (HR 0.78; 95% CI, 0.60–1.02) compared with those who received chemotherapy and tamoxifen only. This effect was also noted in patients who had received chemotherapy followed by exemestane plus ovarian suppression (HR 0.65; 95% CI, 0.49–0.87) compared with chemotherapy followed by tamoxifen only. Results from SOFT and TEXT are provided in Table 10.

Comparison of the combined TEXT/SOFT results and ABCSG-12 is difficult given differences in trial design. Only 5% of patients in the ABCSG-12 study received chemotherapy, fewer patients were

Table 10 Summary of results from the TEXT and SOFT clinical trials.

TEXT/SOFT primary analysis at a median follow-up of 68 months (n = 4690)[355]				
	5-Year DFS	**5-Year BC[a]-free survival**	**5-Year distant BC recurrence-free survival**	**5-Year overall survival**
TAM[b]/ovarian suppression	87.3%	88.8%	92.0%	96.9%
EXE[c]/ovarian suppression	91.1%	92.8%	93.8%	95.9%
	5-Year DFS (HR[d] for recurrence, new cancer, or death)	**5-Year BC-free survival (HR for recurrence)**	**5-Year distant BC recurrence-free survival (HR)**	**5-Year OS (HR for death)**
TAM/ovarian suppression vs EXE/ovarian suppression	0.72 ($p < 0.001$)	0.66 ($p < 0.001$)	0.78 ($p = 0.02$)	Insignificant
SOFT primary analysis at a median follow-up of 67 months (n = 3066)[357]				
	5-Year DFS	**5-Year BC-free survival**	**5-Year BC-free survival (chemo[e])**	**5-Year overall survival (chemo[e])**
EXE/ovarian suppression	Not reported	90.9%	87.8%	Not reported
TAM/ovarian suppression	86.6%	88.4%	84.8%	94.5%
TAM	84.7%	86.4%	83.6%	90.9%
	5-Year DFS (HR for recurrence, new cancer, or death)	**5-Year BC-free survival (HR for recurrence)**	**5-Year OS (chemo[e]) (HR for death)**	
TAM/ovarian suppression vs TAM	0.83 (95% CI 0.66–1.04; $p = 0.10$)	0.81 (95% CI 0.63–1.03; $p = 0.09$)	0.64 (95% CI 0.42–0.96)	
Within the subset of SOFT participants <35 years of age (n = 350), 233 were included in the primary analysis, 94% of whom received chemotherapy				
	EXE/ovarian suppression	**TAM/ovarian suppression**	**TAM**	
BC-free survival at 5 years	83.4%	78.9%	67.7%	

[a]BC, breast cancer.
[b]TAM, tamoxifen.
[c]EXE, exemestane.
[d]HR, hazard ratio.
[e]Subset of patients who received chemotherapy.

enrolled, ovarian suppression was given for only 3 years, and the addition of zoledronic acid may have abrogated the effect of AI, resulting in no significant difference between study arms.

The 2014 ASCO Clinical Practice Guideline Focused Update for adjuvant endocrine therapy recommended that premenopausal women with HR+ ESBC receive 5 years of tamoxifen.[350] The guidelines state that tamoxifen should be extended to a total of 10 years if a patient remains pre- or perimenopausal after the initial 5-year period. If a woman is postmenopausal after 5 years of tamoxifen, she should be offered continuation of tamoxifen or a switch to an AI for 5 additional years. The 2015 St. Gallen Consensus on Primary Therapy recommends that ovarian suppression plus either tamoxifen or an AI be considered for premenopausal women with high risk of HR+ ESBC.[345] High-risk patients were defined as those ≤35 years, premenopausal, status postchemotherapy, and with multiple positive nodes.

Adjuvant chemotherapy for HR+/HER2− ESBC

The first demonstration that the natural history of breast cancer could be altered with systemic therapy involved patients who were randomized to undergo radical mastectomy plus 3 days of thiotepa starting at the time of surgery or placebo.[358] A significant improvement in 5-year survival for premenopausal women with at least four positive axillary lymph nodes treated with thiotepa in comparison to placebo was reported in 1968, findings that persisted after 10 years of follow-up. A second generation of clinical trials in the 1960s provided further evidence that a disease-free interval could be prolonged with systemic therapy. A clinical trial conducted jointly by the NSABP and the ECOG showed that L-phenylalanine mustard (L-PAM) administered orally for 24 months to patients with node-positive ESBC treated initially with radical mastectomy could prolong the disease-free interval of patients.[354] Extended follow-up for more than 20 years showed not only a significant prolongation of DFS but also a significant benefit in the OS of premenopausal patients with the use of this single agent. A similar trend, initially observed in postmenopausal women, was not sustained.

The single-agent regimens examined in the aforementioned early clinical trials showed that systemic chemotherapy could improve outcomes and served as an impetus to design multiple-drug regimens. A third generation of clinical trials from the 1970s introduced regimens that are in use to date. Bonadonna et al. initially reported the Milan Study in 1976, which evaluated the combination of cyclophosphamide 100 mg/m^2 daily for 14 days, methotrexate 40 mg/m^2 iv days 1 and 8, and fluorouracil 600 mg/m^2 iv days 1 and 8 (CMF) given on a 4-week schedule for 12 cycles versus observation after radical mastectomy in women with node-positive ESBC.[359] The study showed a significant reduction in treatment failure (5.3% vs 24%; $p < 10^{-6}$) in all subgroups of patients treated with CMF. Two-thirds of patients experienced various toxicities, including nausea, vomiting, anorexia, alopecia, cystitis, and amenorrhea. A median follow-up of 19.4-year results from the Milan trial continued to indicate a benefit in premenopausal, but not postmenopausal women.[360] Although CMF was initially reported as less beneficial in postmenopausal women, longer follow-up suggested that older women were more likely to have had dose reductions and that the benefit was similar across age-groups when similar doses were provided.[361]

CMF was broadly used as the primary chemotherapeutic regimen of choice in the 1980s and continues to serve as reasonable adjuvant chemotherapy for a select group of patients. However, subsequent regimens containing anthracyclines and later taxanes were clearly defined as the standard adjuvant chemotherapy at the beginning of the twenty-first century.

Treatment combining doxorubicin (Adriamycin) and cyclophosphamide (AC) was reported as effective and safe for patients with MBC in 1975.[362] A large number of prospective trials evaluating various combinations of the anthracyclines doxorubicin and epirubicin were then conducted to determine optimal combinations as well as treatment frequency and length.

NSABP B-15 was designed to evaluate the benefit of a short course of chemotherapy, AC (doxorubicin 60 mg/m^2 iv and cyclophosphamide 600 mg/m^2 iv) given every 3 weeks for four cycles, over the more time-intensive CMF regimen, given every 4 weeks for six cycles.[363] The study randomized 2194 women with node-positive tamoxifen-nonresponsive ESBC treated with primary surgery to either AC or CMF. (Tamoxifen-nonresponsive ESBC was defined as ESBC in all women ≤49 years of age and women 50–59 years with PR disease). With a median follow-up of 3 years, no significant difference in DFS or OS was observed. However, NSABP B-15 suggested that AC was preferable to CMF given its shorter treatment duration. Similar outcomes were noted in NSABP B-16, which included women with tamoxifen-responsive ESBC. Further analysis of existing randomized trials indicated that anthracycline-containing regimens that included three or more drugs (e.g., FAC, CAF, and FEC) had superiority over CMF.

Contemporary adjuvant chemotherapy for HR+/HER2− breast cancer have used taxanes in combination with anthracyclines. Several clinical trials, including CALGB 9344, NSABP B-28, BCIRG 001, and E1199, demonstrated the efficacy of such combinations.

CALGB 9344 had several aims, one of which was to evaluate the addition of paclitaxel to AC.[364] A total of 3121 patients with node-positive ESBC were randomized to AC (with varying doses of doxorubicin, described in detail below), with or without four cycles of paclitaxel 175 mg/m^2 iv every 3 weeks. At a median of 5 years, the DFS for AC only was 65% and for AC plus paclitaxel was 70%, with an HR for recurrence with the addition of paclitaxel of 17%. OS for patients receiving AC only was 77% and for AC plus paclitaxel was 80%, with an HR for death with the addition of paclitaxel of 18%. The addition of paclitaxel resulted in an absolute improvement of DFS and OS at 5 years of 5% and 3%, respectively. These results led to the approval of paclitaxel in sequence with AC as adjuvant chemotherapy for ESBC in 2005.

NSABP-28 opened in 1995 and enrolled a total of 3060 women with node-positive resected operable breast cancer who were then randomized 1:1 to receive either four cycles of standard AC followed by four cycles of paclitaxel 225 mg/m^2 every 3 weeks (AC/T) or four cycles of standard AC only.[365] All patients received concurrent tamoxifen. At a median follow-up of 64.6 months, DFS was 76% in the AC/T arm and 72% in the AC only arm with a statistically significant reduction in the RR of disease recurrence (RR 0.83; 95% CI 0.72–0.95; $p = 0.006$). Although the addition of paclitaxel to AC clearly improved DFS, no improvement in OS was appreciated with a 5-year OS of 85% in both groups.

Breast Cancer International Research Group (BCIRG) 001, a phase III clinical trial, was initiated in 1997 and compared six cycles of FAC to six cycles of docetaxel 75 mg/m^2 iv plus AC (TAC) every 3 weeks.[366] A total of 1491 women with node-positive ESBC were randomized to the two arms. At a median follow-up of 55 months, the TAC arm was associated with a reduction in the risk of relapse (HR 0.72, 95% CI 0.59–0.88, $p = 0.001$) and death (HR 0.70, 95% CI 0.53–0.91; $p = 0.008$). Benefits in relapse risk and OS were maintained at a median follow-up of 124 months with HR 0.80 (95% CI 0.68–0.93; log-rank $p = 0.0043$) and HR 0.74 (95% CI 0.61–0.90; log-rank $p = 0.020$), respectively.[367] Benefits were independent of the number of positive nodes, hormone receptor status, and HER2 status. BCIRG 001 clearly showed a role for docetaxel in the adjuvant setting.

The E1199 clinical trial was designed to compare the taxanes paclitaxel and docetaxel, as well as schedules of weekly or every 3 weeks, using a 2×2 factorial design.[368] A total of 4950 women with operable, node-positive or high-risk node-negative ESBC were randomized after primary surgery followed by four cycles of AC given every 3 weeks to one of the following arms: (1) paclitaxel 80 mg/m^2 iv weekly (infused for 1 h) for 12 weeks, (2) paclitaxel 175 mg/m^2 iv (infused for 3 h) every 3 weeks for four doses, (3) docetaxel 35 mg/m^2 iv (infused for 1 h) weekly for 12 weeks, or (4) docetaxel 100 mg/m^2 iv (infused for 1 h) every 3 weeks for four doses. At a median follow-up of 63.8 months, no differences were observed in the primary comparisons between taxane type and schedule. However, the weekly paclitaxel arm was associated with a significant improvement in DFS (HR, 0.79; $p = 0.006$) and OS (HR, 0.76; $p = 0.01$) as a prespecified secondary comparison to paclitaxel given every 3 weeks. These results led the NCCN to recommend weekly paclitaxel followed by AC as a preferred adjuvant regimen for ESBC.[369] With a median follow-up of 12.1 years, DFS was still significantly improved, but quantitatively less pronounced in the weekly paclitaxel arm (HR 0.84; $p = 0.011$), whereas OS was only marginally improved (HR 0.87, $p = 0.09$).[370] In addition, the arm with docetaxel given every 3 weeks was found to have a significant improvement in DFS (HR 0.79, $p = 0.001$) and a marginal improvement in OS (HR 0.86; $p = 0.054$) compared with every 3-week paclitaxel.

With a clear description that both anthracyclines and taxanes were strongly beneficial for the treatment of ESBC, researchers sought to optimize the benefit of a regimen while concurrently limiting its toxicity by evaluating various doses and intensities. Dose density improved outcomes, but increasing doses of doxorubicin were not more effective.

CALGB 8541 randomized 1572 women with node-positive breast cancer to one of three arms that varied the dose or frequency of cyclophosphamide in CAF.[371] The arms were cyclophosphamide 400 mg/m^2 iv plus doxorubicin 40 mg/m^2 iv every 28 days plus fluorouracil 400 mg/m^2 iv twice every 28 days for six cycles, cyclophosphamide 600 mg/m^2 iv plus doxorubicin 60 mg/m^2 iv every 28 days plus fluorouracil 600 mg/m^2 iv twice every 28 days for four cycles, and cyclophosphamide 300 mg/m^2 iv plus doxorubicin 30 mg/m^2 iv every 28 days plus fluorouracil 300 mg/m^2 iv twice every 28 days for four cycles. Thus, the first two groups received the same total dose, but with a higher intensity in the second group, while the third group received half the total dose of the other groups, but at the same intensity as the first group. At a median follow-up of 3.4 years, patients treated with a higher or moderate dose intensity had a statistically significantly longer DFS and OS, suggestive of a dose–response effect, and resulting in the selection of cyclophosphamide 600 mg/m^2 as the standard dose for adjuvant AC in ESBC.

The second aim of CALGB 9344 (described above) was to assess whether increasing doses of doxorubicin provided additional benefit.[364] All patients enrolled on the CALGB 9344 received AC with doxorubicin at one of three doses (60, 75, or 90 mg/m^2 iv) plus standard cyclophosphamide (600 mg/m^2 iv) every 3 weeks for four cycles, followed by either paclitaxel for four cycles (as described above) or no additional chemotherapy. No benefit was observed with higher doses of doxorubicin as demonstrated by a DFS of 69%, 66%, and 67% for patients who received 60, 75, and 90 mg/m^2 iv of doxorubicin, respectively.

Preclinical studies revealed that a given dose of chemotherapy kills a certain fraction of cancer cells rather than a specific number.

Breast cancers grow with nonexponential Gompertzian kinetics, but regrowth after cytoreduction is in fact more rapid than in exponential models.[372] Several researchers hypothesized that more frequent administration of cytotoxic chemotherapy would provide more effective disease control than increasing doses. An initial limitation to studying this hypothesis was the increased risk of myelosuppression. The development of filgrastim, a recombinant human granulocyte colony-stimulating factor (CSF) that reduces neutropenia, however, allowed for the evaluation of dose-intensified regimens.[373]

CALGB 9741 was the pivotal clinical trial that demonstrated that dose density, the administration of chemotherapy with a shortened intertreatment time interval, improved clinical outcomes.[374] The study additionally evaluated whether sequential or concurrent administration of chemotherapy agents would provide more benefit, with the hypothesis that higher dose density would be achieved with sequential therapy, which would additionally minimize toxicity. This study enrolled 2005 women with node-positive ESBC to one of four arms: (1) sequential doxorubicin (A) 60 mg/m^2 iv $\times$ four doses followed by paclitaxel (T) 175 mg/m^2 iv for four doses, followed by cyclophosphamide (C) 600 mg/m^2 iv for four doses, with all doses given every 3 weeks; (2) sequential ACT as above, with all doses given every 2 weeks with filgrastim; (3) concurrent AC for four cycles every 3 weeks followed by T for four cycles, with all doses given every 3 weeks; and (4) concurrent AC for four cycles followed by T for four cycles, with all doses given every 2 weeks with filgrastim. Drugs were provided with the same dose in all arms. At a median follow-up of 36 months, the dose-dense regimens (every 2 weeks) showed a clear improvement in DFS (risk ratio 0.74; $p = 0.010$) and OS (risk ratio 0.69; $p = 0.013$). The 4-year DFS was 82% for the dose-dense regimens and 75% for the less-dense regimens. No difference was observed between concurrent and sequential schedules. Patients on the dose-dense regimens experienced less-severe neutropenia than other regimens.

With results from CALGB 9741, CALGB 9344, and BCIRG 001, dose-dense AC plus a taxane became the standard of care for node-positive and high-risk node-negative breast cancers. Such regimens are associated with significant toxicity however, with short- and long-term risks. Myelosuppression was initially a more frequent complication that improved with the development of G-CSF. Anthracyclines are associated with increased cardiotoxicity (odds ratio 5.43, 95% CI 2.34–12.62) and is a dose-limiting side effect. Researchers therefore sought less toxic, equally efficacious treatment regimens for women with lower-risk ESBC. US Oncology Research Trial 9735, a phase III clinical trial, randomized 1016 patients with resected operable ESBC to either docetaxel 75 mg/m^2 iv plus cyclophosphamide 600 mg/m^2 iv (TC) every 3 weeks for four cycles or standard AC with no prophylactic G-CSF allowed.[375] A proportion of 16% of the study participants were $\geq$65 years of age, a population that was poorly represented in many of the pivotal trials of ESBC. Older women were more likely to have node-positive disease than their younger counterparts. At a median of 5.5 years, 86% of the TC group remained disease-free, in comparison to 80% of the AC group (HR 0.67, 95% CI 0.50–0.94; $p = 0.015$) with no OS benefit appreciated. This benefit was persistent at a median of 7 years of follow-up (HR 0.74, 95% CI 0.50–0.97, $p = 0.033$). In addition, a benefit in OS was recognized with 87% of the TC group alive in comparison to 82% of the AC group (HR 0.69; 95% CI, 0.50–0.97; $p = 0.032$).[376] The DFS and OS benefit was independent of age, nodal status, or receptor status. Toxicities varied by regimen, with an increase in myalgias, arthralgias, edema, and febrile neutropenia in the TC group in comparison to an increase in nausea

Table 11 Preferred and alternative neoadjuvant and adjuvant chemotherapy regimens for early-stage breast cancer, by subtype.

Preferred neoadjuvant/adjuvant chemotherapy regimens	
HER2− ESBC	Dose-dense doxorubicin + cyclophosphamide (ddAC)/dose-dense paclitaxel (ddT)
	dose-dense doxorubicin + cyclophosphamide (ddAC)/weekly paclitaxel (T)
	docetaxel + cyclophosphamide (TC)
HER2+ ESBC	Doxorubicin + cyclophosphamide (AC)/paclitaxel + trastuzumab (TH) ± pertuzumab
	docetaxel + carboplatin + trastuzumab (TCH) ± pertuzumab
Alternative neoadjuvant/adjuvant chemotherapy regimens	
HER2− ESBC	Dose-dense doxorubicin + cyclophosphamide (ddAC)
	doxorubicin + cyclophosphamide (AC)
	fluorouracil + doxorubicin + cyclophosphamide (FAC)
	fluorouracil + epirubicin + cyclophosphamide (FEC)
	docetaxel + doxorubicin + cyclophosphamide (TAC)
	cyclophosphamide + methotrexate + fluorouracil (CMF)
HER2+ ESBC	Paclitaxel + trastuzumab (TH)
	FEC/taxane + trastuzumab ± pertuzumab
	AC/taxane + trastuzumab ± pertuzumab

Source: Network NCCN 2015. Adapted with permission from the NCCN Clinical Practice Guidelines in Oncology NCCN Guidelines® for Breast Cancer V.3.2015. © National Comprehensive Cancer Network, Inc 2015. All rights reserved. Accessed [September 15, 2015]. To view the most recent and complete version of the guideline, go online to NCCN.org. NATIONAL COMPREHENSIVE CANCER NETWORK®, NCCN®, NCCN GUIDELINES®, and all other NCCN Content are trademarks owned by the National Comprehensive Cancer Network, Inc.

and vomiting in the AC group. Febrile neutropenia was not more frequent in older patients.

CALGB 40101 (Alliance) was designed to evaluate whether single-agent paclitaxel was noninferior to AC in an effort to identify a regimen that provided benefit to women with lower-risk node-positive (one to three lymph nodes) or node-negative ESBC.[377] A total of 3871 patients were enrolled and randomized to four arms based on a 2×2 factorial design. The arms were standard AC every 3 weeks for four or six cycles and paclitaxel weekly for 12 or 18 weeks. The study accrued slowly, however, and the two longer duration arms were closed, with further randomization restricted to the two remaining arms. The study was closed early in July 2010 because of failure to achieve the planned accrual target of 4646 patients. At a median follow-up of 6.1 years, HR of 1.26 and 1.27 for DFS and OS, respectively, favored treatment with AC, failing to provide evidence that paclitaxel was noninferior to AC. As expected, more neuropathy was present in the paclitaxel arms, while more hematologic toxicities were observed in the AC arms; paclitaxel was felt overall to be less toxic.

Given the improvement in treatment efficacy for ESBC with combined chemotherapies, such as with AC/T, TAC, and TC, other regimens that were initially evaluated in MBC were evaluated in the adjuvant setting. As of 2015, no additional adjuvant chemotherapy regimens have added benefit to HR+/HER2− ESBC. Preferred and alternative adjuvant (and neoadjuvant) chemotherapy regimens for ESBC are listed in Table 11. Addition of capecitabine or gemcitabine did not improve outcomes.

Single-agent capecitabine, the prodrug form of 5-fluorouracil, is associated with a response rate up to 30% in patients with MBC. Unlike other chemotherapies, capecitabine is administered orally, which is preferable for many patients. Capecitabine was first evaluated in the setting of ESBC as part of the CALGB 49907 clinical trial.[379] The study focused on elderly patients, as it was felt an oral therapy would be better tolerated. CALGB 49907 randomized 633 patients ≥65 years with resected primary operable breast cancer to capecitabine daily for 14 days on a 21-day cycle or to oncologists' choice of CMF or AC. At a median follow-up of 2.4 years, the rates of relapse and death in the capecitabine arm were twice as high as in the standard therapy arm, with a recurrence HR of 2.09 ($p < 0.001$).

The FINXX clinical trial evaluated the addition of capecitabine to anthracycline/taxane-based therapy.[380] Patients were randomized to receive docetaxel with capecitabine for three cycles followed by cyclophosphamide, epirubicin, and capecitabine (TX/CEX) for three cycles or three cycles of docetaxel followed by CEF for three cycles (T/CEF). At a median follow-up of 59 months, no significant difference in recurrence-free survival was demonstrated, with an HR of 0.79 (95% CI, 0.60–1.04; $p = 0.087$).

Given its efficacy in MBC, gemcitabine was evaluated as an adjuvant therapy in combination with an anthracycline and taxane. The tAnGo phase III clinical trial randomized patients with high-risk ESBC to receive either epirubicin 90 mg/m^2 iv and cyclophosphamide 600 mg/m^2 iv (EC) every 3 weeks for four cycles followed by gemcitabine 1250 mg/m^2 iv (days 1 and 8) and paclitaxel 175 mg/m^2 iv (day 1) (GT) for four cycles every 3 weeks or EC followed by paclitaxel only (EC/T).[381] A total of 3152 patients were enrolled, of which 55% were ≤50 years, 77% were node-positive, 41% were ER+, and 26% were HER2+. A preplanned interim analysis at 30 months was notable for no difference in DFS (HR 1.0, 95% CI 0.8–1.2, $p = 0.96$) or OS (HR = 1.1, 95% CI 0.9–1.4, $p = 0.35$) between the two treatment groups, suggesting no benefit from the addition of gemcitabine.

A clear majority of the 2015 St. Gallen panel members agreed that luminal A-like ESBC was generally less responsive to chemotherapy.[345] The panel agreed that luminal B-like ESBC with low-risk scores based on Oncotype DX, MP, and Prosigna should not receive chemotherapy. Relative indications for chemotherapy in luminal-like ESBC were grade 3 histology, ≥4 positive LN, high Ki-67, and extensive lymphovascular invasion.

Chemotherapy for HER2+ ESBC

Retrospective analyses of several of the pivotal adjuvant chemotherapy trials revealed that the greatest benefits were observed in subsets of patients with overexpression of HER2. CALGB 8869 was designed to determine whether molecular markers could predict a patient's response to adjuvant chemotherapy in CALGB 8541.[382] A total of 442 tumor samples were randomly selected from the CALGB 8541 clinical trial. Patients with tumors that had ≥50% overexpression of c-erbB-2 were found to have a significantly longer DFS and OS after receiving the high-dose CAF regimen, and no benefit was seen in those without HER2 overexpression.

As described earlier, CALGB 9344 assessed the effect of escalating doses of doxorubicin as well as the addition of a taxane to anthracycline-based chemotherapy on DFS and OS for women with node-positive ESBC.[364] In a retrospective analysis of tumor samples from CALGB 9344, Hayes et al.[383] assessed whether additional benefit was seen in patients with HER2+ ESBC. Approximately 50% of the study participants were randomly selected and their tumor samples were centrally assessed with IHC and/or FISH for HER2 status. As stated elsewhere, no benefit was seen when patients were treated with doses of doxorubicin above 60 mg/m^2; consistent with these earlier findings, no benefit was seen with higher doxorubicin dosing in the subset of patients with HER2+ tumors. However, the addition of paclitaxel resulted in a significant benefit for patients with HER2+ disease with an HR for recurrence of 0.59 ($p = 0.01$). Little benefit was appreciated in those patients with HR+/HER2− ESBC.

Hugh et al. assessed prognostic significance and predictive response of tumor subtypes to adjuvant chemotherapy for over 90% of tumor samples from participants in BCIRG 001.[384] BCIRG 001, described in detail above, compared TAC with FAC in patients with operable node-positive breast cancer. Tumor subtypes were defined by IHC for ER, PR, HER2, and Ki-67. Patients were subdivided into triple-negative (14.5%), HER2 (8.5%), luminal B (61.1%), and luminal A (15.9%). Three-year DFS p values were calculated with luminal B as referent. Patients with ER−/PR−/HER2+ observed only a marginally significant benefit in DFS with HR 0.50 (95% CI, 0.29–1.83).

The recognition that a significant benefit was appreciated with anthracycline- and taxane-based chemotherapy in patients with HER2+ ESBC led to the general recommendation that patients with HER2+ breast cancer receive adjuvant chemotherapy.

Trastuzumab-based therapy

The development of anti-HER2 antibody trastuzumab resulted in a dramatic improvement in the outcomes of women with HER2+ breast cancer, with a significant reduction in the development of recurrent breast cancer. Trastuzumab is a humanized monoclonal antibody that suppresses growth, proliferation, and survival of HER2 overexpressing cancer cells. The antibody is targeted against the extracellular region of HER2, preventing dimerization with other HER2 molecules. Scientists have proposed several mechanisms to explain the cellular and molecular activity of trastuzumab. A compelling hypothesis is that trastuzumab activates antibody-dependent cellular cytotoxicity through immunologic targeting of HER2+ tumor cells. In vitro studies have demonstrated that removal of the Fc portion of the trastuzumab antibody destroys trastuzumab activity, while enhancement of the Fc receptor results in increased activity in mouse HER2 enriched tumor models.[385,386] An alternative proposal is that after trastuzumab binds HER2, natural killer cells are triggered and facilitate apoptosis. A well-accepted mechanism is that trastuzumab interferes with cell signaling along the MAPK and PI3K/Akt pathways that are involved in cell growth and proliferation.[387] Binding of HER2 by trastuzumab prevents HER2 from dimerizing, which is necessary for Akt phosphorylation, blocking tyrosine kinase Src signaling.

Toxicities of trastuzumab

Trastuzumab is generally well tolerated, but cardiac toxicity is a rare but serious adverse effect. Cardiac toxicity was an unexpected finding in the original trastuzumab studies that were conducted in the MBC setting. Cardiac dysfunction due to trastuzumab is defined as a reduction in left ventricular ejection fraction (LVEF) of ≤5% with symptoms of congestive heart failure or ≤10% in the absence of symptoms.[388] A meta-analysis by Seidman et al. of cardiotoxicity in clinical trials of trastuzumab reported that the use of an anthracycline with concurrent trastuzumab resulted

in unacceptable cardiotoxicity (27%).[389] Cardiotoxicity was less significant in patients who received trastuzumab only (3–7%) or trastuzumab plus paclitaxel (13%). In comparison, 8% of patients receiving anthracyclines without trastuzumab developed cardiotoxicity. Holding of trastuzumab results in reversal of cardiotoxicity in most patients, at which time trastuzumab therapy can be resumed. Optimal monitoring of LVEF in patients on trastuzumab is not well defined, and recommendations vary from every 3 to 6 months.

Historic trials of trastuzumab (B3-1, N9831, BCIRG-006, and HERA)

Trastuzumab was approved as an adjuvant HER2-directed therapy in 2006, in the context of four large clinical trials evaluating over 13,000 women that consistently reported a reduction in 3-year recurrence risk of approximately 50%. Four studies were initiated around 2000 and asked several questions with slight variations in design.

NSABP B-31 enrolled 2030 women with node-positive HER2+ breast cancer who were all to receive standard AC followed by paclitaxel, given either every 3 weeks or weekly.[390] Patients were randomized to receive trastuzumab, starting with paclitaxel, for a total of 52 weeks, or to receive paclitaxel only. A second study, North Central Cancer Treatment Group (NCCTG) N9831, enrolled 3506 women, also with node-positive HER2 ESBC, that had two arms identical to those of NSABP B-31 as well as a third arm that received trastuzumab for 52 weeks, but only after the completion of AC/T (XX). A combined analysis of NSABP B-31 and the first two arms of NCCTG N9831 at a median 2-year follow-up demonstrated a significantly longer DFS in the trastuzumab-containing arms (HR 0.48; 95% CI 0.39–0.59, $p < 0.001$) with an absolute difference in DFS of 12% at 3 years. Trastuzumab arms were associated with a 53% reduction in risk of distant recurrence (95% CI 0.37–0.61, $p < 0.0001$) and a reduction in mortality by one-third, in comparison to the control arms (95% CI 0.48–0.93, $p = 0.015$).

BCIRG006 was a global, multicenter clinical trial that randomized 3222 women to three arms: two arms similar to the NSABP B-31 and NCCTG N9831 studies [standard AC followed by docetaxel with trastuzumab (AC/TH)] and a third, nonanthracycline-containing arm with docetaxel, carboplatin, and trastuzumab (TCH).[387] At a median 2-year follow-up, a clear improvement in DFS was appreciated in the trastuzumab-containing arms, with a 51% reduction in risk of relapse in the AC/TH arm ($p < 0.0001$) and a 39% reduction in the risk of relapse ($p = 0.0002$) in the TCH arm. No comparisons of efficacy could be drawn between the AC/TH and TCH arms due to study design. A nonstatistically significant trend toward survival benefit was observed in the trastuzumab-containing arms.

The Herceptin Adjuvant (HERA) phase III clinical trial enrolled 5090 women with HER2+ ESBC who had completed four cycles of adjuvant (or neoadjuvant) chemotherapy and radiation (if indicated) to one of three arms: observation, 1 year of trastuzumab, or 2 years of trastuzumab.[391] The first interim analysis reported an absolute benefit in DFS of 8.4% at 2 years when comparing 1 year of trastuzumab versus observation. Event-free patients in the observation arm were allowed to cross over to receive trastuzumab.[392] Even so, intention-to-treat analysis of 4-year DFS with 1 year of trastuzumab in comparison to observation was significant (78.6% vs 72.2%; HR 0.76; 95% CI 0.66–0.87, $p < 0.0001$). No difference in OS was appreciated. Outcomes associated with 1 years versus 2 years of trastuzumab are discussed below.

NSABP B-31, NCCTG N9831, BCIRG 006, and HERA demonstrated a significant benefit in DFS with the addition of trastuzumab to adjuvant chemotherapy for HER2+ ESBC. The NCCN Guidelines for Breast Cancer that were updated in 2015 state that patients with HER2+ ESBC with a primary tumor >0.5 cm or positive lymph nodes should receive adjuvant chemotherapy with trastuzumab.[395] Preferred and alternative adjuvant (and neoadjuvant) chemotherapy regimens for HER2+ ESBC are listed in Table 11. The guidelines state that the benefit of trastuzumab in patients with node-negative T1a (≤0.5 cm) or T1b (0.5–1.0 cm) is uncertain and must be carefully weighed with its known toxicities. This question was recently addressed in the APT clinical trial that is described in detail below.

The NCCN Guidelines currently recommend that adjuvant trastuzumab be administered with taxane-based chemotherapy and then as a single agent to complete a total of 1 year (or 52 weeks).[393] This duration was selected arbitrarily in the above clinical trials of trastuzumab. NSABP B-31, NCCTG N9831, and BCIRG 006 only evaluated 1 year of trastuzumab, but HERA evaluated both 1 and 2 years of trastuzumab. At a median follow-up of 8 years, no significant difference was observed in the DFS of patients randomized to 1 or 2 years of trastuzumab (HR 0.99, 95% CI 0.85–1.14, $p = 0.86$).[394] Furthermore, grade 3–4 AEs and LVEF dysfunction were more frequent in patients who received trastuzumab for 2 years (20.4% and 7.2%, respectively) than 1 year (16.3% and 4.1%, respectively).

Given the toxicities and costs associated with trastuzumab, researchers investigated whether a shortened course of trastuzumab (9 weeks, 3 months, or 6 months) would be noninferior to the recommended 52-week course. To date, shorter regimens have not proven equivalent in efficacy to the standard 52 weeks of trastuzumab.

The Finland Herceptin (FIN-HER) clinical trial evaluated the efficacy of a short course of trastuzumab to limit cardiotoxicity.[392] This phase III clinical trial enrolled 1010 women with node-positive or high-risk node-negative breast cancer to receive either docetaxel for three cycles, followed by FEC, or vinorelbine for three cycles, followed by FEC. A total of 232 participants had HER2+ disease and were additionally randomized to receive or not to receive 9 weeks of trastuzumab during cycles of docetaxel or vinorelbine. The 3-year DFS was improved in the trastuzumab-containing arms (HR for recurrence or death 0.42, 95% CI, 0.21–0.83; $p = 0.01$). No reductions in LVEF or cardiac failure events were observed.

The Protocol for Herceptin as Adjuvant therapy with Reduced Exposure (PHARE) phase III clinical trial enrolled 3384 patients with HER2+ ESBC who had already completed primary surgery, at least four cycles of chemotherapy, and 6 months of trastuzumab.[395] Patients were randomized to continue trastuzumab for an additional 6 months (for a total of 12 months) or to discontinue trastuzumab (for a total of 6 months) in an attempt to demonstrate noninferiority. At a median follow-up of 42.5 months, the DFS was 87.8% and 84.9% in the 12- and 6-month arms, respectively, and OS was 95% and 93.1%, thus failing to show noninferiority in the shorter arm.

The Hellenic Oncology Research Group recently reported on a phase III clinical trial that randomized 481 women with node-positive or high-risk node-negative HER2+ ESBC to undergo either 12 or 6 months of trastuzumab in combination with adjuvant chemotherapy.[396] In particular, after primary surgery, all patients received dose-dense FEC followed by docetaxel 75 mg/m² every 14 days for four cycles with concurrent trastuzumab, which was then extended for either a total of 12 or 6 months. The 3-year DFS for the 12- and 6-month arms was 95.7% versus 93.3% respectively (HR = 1.57; 95% CI 0.86–2.10; $p = 0.137$), failing to show noninferiority for the 6-month arm.

The Short-HER phase III clinical trial (NCT00629278) compared 3 and 12 months of trastuzumab.[397] The study aimed to randomize 2500 women with node-positive or high-risk node-negative HER2+ ESBC to receive four cycles of anthracycline-based chemotherapy, followed by four cycles of taxane-based chemotherapy with concurrent trastuzumab followed by a total of 18 cycles of every 3-week trastuzumab or three cycles of every 3-week docetaxel in combination with trastuzumab, followed by three cycles of FEC with no additional trastuzumab. The study was completed in 2010, but no results have been released as of August 2015.

The Synergism or Long Duration (SOLD) study was a phase III clinical trial (NCT00593697) sponsored by the Finnish Breast Cancer Group to evaluate 9 weeks versus 52 weeks of trastuzumab.[398] A total of 2168 women with HER2+ ESBC were randomized to receive either three cycles of every 3-week docetaxel with concurrent trastuzumab (TH) followed by FE75C for three cycles or the same regimen followed by every 3-week trastuzumab for a total of 52 weeks. The study was completed in November 2014, but no results have been released as of August 2015.

The Persephone phase III clinical trial aimed to enroll 4000 patients with HER2+ EBSC to compare 6 months of trastuzumab to the 12-month standard. The study was started in 2007, and 3166 patients had been randomized as of 2014.[399] The first planned interim analysis of noninferiority is expected in mid-2016.

The preceding clinical trials demonstrated the importance of HER2-directed therapy with trastuzumab for women with node-positive or high-risk node-negative HER2+ ESBC. Women with small node-negative HER2+ ESBC were not included in these studies, and proper management of such disease is unclear. An NCCN database of 520 patients with HR-/HER2+ ESBC with tumors ≤1 cm has reported a median 5-year DFS of 94% (T1bN0), 93% (T1aN0), and 94–96% (T1a-bN0).[400] The Adjuvant Paclitaxel and Trastuzumab (APT) clinical trial was a single-arm multicenter investigator initiated clinical trial to develop an efficacious regimen that limited toxicities for patients with small node-negative HER2+ ESBC as such patients are expected to have generally favorable prognosis.[401] All patients received paclitaxel 80 mg/m² iv weekly for 12 weeks and 12 weeks of trastuzumab for 9 additional months. A total of 410 patients were enrolled, with 87.7% completing study treatment. The study demonstrated that a combination of weekly paclitaxel with trastuzumab only was appropriate. The 3-year DFS was 98.7% (95% CI 97.6–99.8), better than historic controls. AEs included 13 patients with one episode of grade 3 neuropathy and 13 patients with asymptomatic declines in ejection fraction from which all but two patients recovered.

Pertuzumab adjuvant and neoadjuvant studies

Pertuzumab, a humanized monoclonal antibody, is a first-in-class HER heterodimer inhibitor that binds to the HER2 dimerization domain and prevents interaction of HER2 with other HER family members. Unlike trastuzumab, which prevents only HER2 homodimerization, pertuzumab inhibits HER2:HER3 binding, which is the most active HER complex.[402] Pertuzumab was approved by the Food and Drug Administration (FDA) in 2012 for use in patients with MBC based on the results from the CLEOPATRA clinical trial, which demonstrated that the combination of docetaxel, trastuzumab, and pertuzumab was superior to docetaxel plus trastuzumab only. Results from the NeoSphere clinical trial, which evaluated neoadjuvant pertuzumab in combination with docetaxel and trastuzumab, led to its approval in the neoadjuvant setting in 2014. The Adjuvant Pertuzumab and Herceptin IN IniTial TherapY of Breast Cancer (APHINITY) clinical trial (NCT01358877) was designed to determine whether pertuzumab, when given in combination with standard adjuvant chemotherapy and trastuzumab, resulted in an increased efficacy.[403] A total of 4810 patients with node-positive HER2+ ESBC were randomized in a double-blind manner to one of two arms in a 1 : 1 ratio. All patients received six to eight cycles of adjuvant chemotherapy with either an anthracycline–taxane or taxane–platin regimen based on investigator's choice. The investigational arm included concurrent trastuzumab and pertuzumab that extended for 1 year, whereas the comparator arm included concurrent trastuzumab and placebo that extended for 1 year. Initial results are expected in 2016.

Pertuzumab is not yet approved in the adjuvant setting. However, the most recent NCCN Guidelines for Breast Cancer state that patients with pathologic stage ≥ T2N1, HER2+ ESBC who did not receive a neoadjuvant pertuzumab-containing regimen can receive adjuvant pertuzumab.[395]

Investigational studies of new adjuvant therapies for HER2+ ESBC

Lapatinib is an oral small-molecule dual tyrosine kinase inhibitor of HER2 and EGFR. Lapatinib was approved in combination with capecitabine for patients with HER2+ MBC who had progressed on trastuzumab.[404] Although generally well tolerated, lapatinib is associated with mild to moderate diarrhea, rash, and mild, transient increases in liver transaminases. The Tykerb Evaluation After CHemotherapy (TEACH) trial evaluated the efficacy and safety of lapatinib as an adjuvant therapy for patients who had received chemotherapy for HER2 ESBC without trastuzumab.[405] This multinational, double-blinded phase III clinical trial randomized 3147 patients to receive lapatinib or placebo, to be started at any time after completion of adjuvant chemotherapy. At a median follow-up of 47.4 months in the lapatinib group and 48.3 months in the placebo group, no significant difference in the occurrence of DFS events was appreciated (13% vs. 17%, HR = 0.83, 95% CI 0.70–1.00; $p = 0.053$). However, central assessment of HER2 status showed that only 79% of the study participants were HER2+ and that the DFS benefit was marginal. The study authors concluded that lapatinib might be an appropriate adjuvant therapy for women with HER2 ESBC who are unable to receive adjuvant trastuzumab.

The Adjuvant Lapatinib and/or Trastuzumab Treatment Optimization (ALTTO) clinical trial randomized 8381 patients with HER2+ ESBC to receive 1 year of lapatinib plus trastuzumab (L + T), 1 year of trastuzumab, and 1 year of lapatinib or trastuzumab only as adjuvant therapy.[406] ALTTO was a companion study to the NEOALTTO clinical trial (described in neoadjuvant section) that demonstrated a doubling in the pCR rate with L + T in comparison to trastuzumab only.[407] The initial results of the ALTTO clinical trial were announced at ASCO in 2014. An insignificant improvement was observed in the 4-year DFS with L + T (88%) versus trastuzumab (86%) (HR 0.84, 97.5% CI, 0.70–1.02; $p = 0.048$) and with trastuzumab followed by lapatinib (87%) versus trastuzumab (86%) (HR 0.93, 97.5% CI, 0.76–1.13; noninferiority $p = 0.044$). The initial results from ALTTO were both surprising and disappointing in the context of the NEOALTTO results, leading researchers to question the utility of pCR.

Neratinib is an oral multityrosine kinase inhibitor of HER2, HER4, and EGFR. This novel drug was initially studied in a phase II clinical trial of patients with HER2+ MBC in combination with trastuzumab and paclitaxel, which demonstrated an improvement in progression-free survival (PFS).[408] Positive results in the metastatic and neoadjuvant setting led to the evaluation of neratinib as an extended adjuvant therapy for HER2+ ESBC. The ExteNET clinical trial was a double-blind, placebo-controlled, phase III clinical trial evaluating the efficacy of 12 months of neratinib following standard chemotherapy with trastuzumab.[409] The study randomized 2840 patients with HER2+ ESBC who had completed primary surgery and standard adjuvant chemotherapy

with trastuzumab to receive neratinib or placebo for 1 year. At a 2-year median follow-up, the neratinib arm was demonstrated to improve DFS in comparison to placebo (93.9% vs. 91.6%; HR 0.67; $p = 0.0046$). The most frequently observed AE in the neratinib arm was diarrhea, with grade 3 diarrhea experienced by 40% of patients.

The ATEMPT phase II clinical trial (NCT01853748) is evaluating the use of single agent ado-trastuzumab emtansine (T-DM1) as an adjuvant therapy with a goal to avoid the toxicity associated with chemotherapy while reducing the risk of disease recurrence, building upon the outcomes from the APT study.[401] T-DM1 is an antibody–drug conjugate linking trastuzumab to the cytotoxic agent DM1. T-DM1 was approved by the FDA as a second-line therapy for HER2+ MBC in 2013 based on results from the EMILIA clinical trial (described in the MBC section). ATEMPT was started in May 2013 with an intention to enroll 500 women with stage I HER2+ breast cancer. Patients are randomized in a 3 : 1 ratio to T-DM1 given every 3 weeks for 51 weeks with weekly paclitaxel given in combination with weekly trastuzumab for 12 cycles followed by 9 months of trastuzumab monotherapy to complete 1 year of trastuzumab therapy. The estimated final data collection for the primary outcome measure of DFS is estimated for May 2017.

Triple-negative breast cancer

No targeted therapies are available for the treatment of TNBC, in contrast to HR+ and HER2+ ESBC that have endocrine- and HER2-based therapies, respectively. For this reason, chemotherapy is the singular adjuvant therapy for patients with TNBC. A majority of the retrospective analyses of tumor subtypes in the pivotal adjuvant chemotherapy trials failed to specify outcomes for TNBC. However, the available analyses have clearly demonstrated significant benefits with taxane-based regimens for TNBC.

The E1199 clinical trial, described in detail above, compared the efficacies of paclitaxel and docetaxel, as well as treatment frequency (3 weeks vs. weekly) in patients with operable, node-positive, or high-risk node-negative ESBC who had already undergone primary surgery followed by four cycles of standard AC.[366] An exploratory analysis of the 1025 patients with TNBC at a median follow-up of 12.1 years demonstrated that weekly paclitaxel was associated with a significant improvement in DFS and OS when compared to every 3-week paclitaxel (DFS HR 0.69; $p = 0.001$; OS HR 0.69; $p = 0.019$).[368] These findings showed that patients with TNBC, who are treated with AC followed by weekly paclitaxel, experience a 10% absolute improvement in DFS and OS at 10 years. US Oncology Research Trial 9735, described in detail above, demonstrated that four cycles of TC were superior to four cycles of standard AC with regard to DFS and OS in patients with TNBC.[374]

Several phase III clinical trials of bevacizumab, a humanized monoclonal antibody against vascular endothelial growth factor (VEGF), suggested some benefit in patients with metastatic TNBC when studied in combination with chemotherapy. The adjuvant bevacizumab-containing therapy in TNBC (BEATRICE) clinical trial randomized 2591 patients with operable primary TNBC to chemotherapy with or without bevacizumab at a dose equivalent to 5 mg/kg weekly for 1 year.[410] TNBC status was centrally confirmed. At a median follow-up of approximately 32 months, the 3-year invasive DFS and OS were similar in both arms.

Several neoadjuvant clinical trials (discussed elsewhere) of platinum agents have demonstrated an improved pCR in patients with BRCA1 ESBC, the majority of which are TNBC. No study specifically evaluating platinum regimens for TNBC in the adjuvant setting has been reported.

Table 12 Potential benefits of using neoadjuvant chemotherapy in breast cancer.

Benefits
Improves the ability for patients presenting with inoperable disease or inflammatory breast cancer to undergo surgery
Increases the rate of breast conservation surgery
Improves the cosmetics of breast conservation if more limited surgery can be performed after response to therapy
May allow early identification of resistance, allowing ineffective therapy to stopped earlier
May allow less extensive postsurgical radiation fields
Response to neoadjuvant chemotherapy is prognostic, particularly when minimal or no invasive cancer is found at the time of surgery. Treatment in the neoadjuvant setting is an invaluable research tool to:
Compare the effectiveness of two systemic regimens, or the addition of a targeted agent to standard therapy
Study biological factors that influence chemotherapy sensitivity/resistance
Identify patients at high risk for recurrence despite standard treatment for participation in clinical studies of new agents
Allow early regulatory approval of treatments that have been demonstrated to improve response to standard therapy while waiting for larger adjuvant studies to be completed

Neoadjuvant chemotherapy: sequencing surgery and chemotherapy

Breast cancer treatment historically started with surgical removal followed by chemotherapy, radiation therapy, and hormone therapy, as needed. However, an increasing percentage of breast cancer patients are being treated with chemotherapy before definitive surgery. Preoperative (or neoadjuvant) chemotherapy was initially used in women with inflammatory or inoperable breast tumors in an attempt to render the disease operable. Subsequently, neoadjuvant chemotherapy was investigated as a strategy to permit breast conservation therapy for patients with larger T2 or T3 disease. Even more recently, neoadjuvant chemotherapy has been explored as a treatment option to allow for early evaluation of the effectiveness of systemic therapy and thus provide an opportunity to test promising new agents earlier in the course of the disease. As a result, these treatment philosophies have permitted the majority of breast cancer patients to be eligible for neoadjuvant chemotherapy. Table 12 reviews some of these potential benefits.

Over the years, numerous studies have been conducted to assess the worth of preoperative chemotherapy for primary operable breast cancer. The NSABP B-18, a randomized trial comparing the preoperative and postoperative administration of four cycles of doxorubicin and cyclophosphamide (AC) in patients with operable breast cancer,[411] found no difference in DFS and OS in the preoperative chemotherapy group compared with the postoperative adjuvant therapy group. The EORTC completed a confirmatory trial of very similar design, with results quite similar to those obtained in NSABP B-18.[365]

One unanswered question that arose from B-18 concerned the need for further therapy following initial treatment, and this was addressed in the Aberdeen trial.[412] In this small study, 162 patients received four cycles of doxorubicin, cyclophosphamide, vincristine, and prednisolone (CVAP), and responders were randomized to receive four more cycles of CVAP or four cycles of docetaxel (100 mg/m^2) and nonresponders received four cycles of docetaxel. Improvement in response rates was seen in those who received docetaxel and translated into longer relapse-free and OS rates. This study confirmed that improvements in pCR rate are associated with improvement in relapse-free survival (RFS) and OS. The MD Anderson[413] and NSABP B-27[414] studies both also confirmed that treatment with a noncross-resistant regimen was associated

with a trend toward improved RFS and OS compared with those continuing with the doxorubicin regimen.

NSABP B-27 also confirmed that the rate of pCR-predicted RFS and validated the use of pCR as a surrogate marker of long-term benefit from treatment. Therefore, pCR was identified as a useful tool for comparing treatment options.

The response to preoperative chemotherapy became a prognostic marker for DFS and survival. Thus, response to preoperative chemotherapy can be used as an intermediate end point in testing new regimens or the additional effect of new drugs administered after well-established regimens, without having to wait for several years until DFS and survival end points can be compared. With the demonstration that preoperative chemotherapy is equivalent to postoperative chemotherapy for DFS and survival, new chemotherapeutic regimens can be tested in this setting without fear of putting patients at a disadvantage.

As a result, numerous preoperative (or neoadjuvant) treatment studies have followed, which have studied choice of chemotherapy and scheduling consideration. Anthracycline-based regimens concurrently or sequentially including a taxane have shown an increased response rate in the neoadjuvant setting than nontaxane-containing regimens.[364,401–412,415–417]

Neoadjuvant studies have examined chemotherapy, endocrine therapy, and biologic therapy (e.g., HER2-targeted therapy). Studies have shown that certain chemotherapy regimens can benefit specific tumor subtypes.

For patients with TNBC, platinum-based therapies have shown benefit in the metastatic setting; therefore, carboplatin has been studied in combination with NACT and have shown that carboplatin may improve pCR rates.[418,419] Carboplatin in combination with a PARP-inhibitor has also shown early promise.[420]

For patients with HER2+ breast cancer, HER2-directed therapies have been shown to be beneficial in improving pCR rates and longer-term outcomes. The benefit of trastuzumab has been shown in several studies, most notably the NOAH study[421,422], which showed that standard neoadjuvant chemotherapy plus trastuzumab (with the continuation of trastuzumab after surgery) increased pCR [trastuzumab (38%) vs no trastuzumab (19%) ($p = 0.001$)] and EFS rate compared to patients with standard chemotherapy only. The addition of pertuzumab with NACT and trastuzumab showed increased benefit as compared with controls (NACT plus trastuzumab) in both the NeoSphere[379] and TRYPHAENA[423] studies. On the basis of these results and the fact that the confirmatory adjuvant trial APHINITY (NCT01358877) had completed accrual, FDA granted accelerated approval to the addition of pertuzumab to chemotherapy and trastuzumab in the neoadjuvant setting. Lapatinib has not met with similar success as pertuzumab, with several studies showing no increase in benefit when substituted for trastuzumab and limited benefit when administered together.[404,424,425] Additional HER2-directed therapies are under study and have shown some initial promise in phase II studies.[426]

Neoadjuvant studies also have looked at response-adjusted schedules, that is, a set number of cycles of therapy are followed by the same or noncross-resistant therapy based on depending on clinical assessment of response or lack thereof, respectively.[427] While these studies have not shown evidence of increased benefit, this study design is an interesting step toward tailoring and individualizing treatment based on early response.

Table 13 summarizes details of several key neoadjuvant chemotherapy studies.

Studies of endocrine therapy are more limited and have focused predominately on postmenopausal women.[431] The use of endocrine therapy in postmenopausal women may be equivalent to that of

Table 13 Summary of selected neoadjuvant trial results.

Breast cancer subtype	Study	Chemotherapy backbone	Comparator	pCR rates (95% confidence intervals)	Summary
HER2 positive; HER2 negative[422]	NOAH	Doxorubicin, paclitaxel, cyclophosphamide, methotrexate, and fluorouracil	+/– Trastuzumab (H)	HER2 positive: H (38%) versus no H (19%) (p-value 0.001); 3-year EFS: with H 71% [61–78%] versus without 56% (46–65%), hazard ratio 0.59 (0.38–0.900; p=0.013)	H + neoadjuvant chemotherapy (and continuation of H after surgery) increased pCR and EFS rate compared to chemotherapy
HER2 positive[425]	CALGB 40601	Paclitaxel (T)	Trastuzumab (H); Lapatinib (L); H + L	TH: 46% (37–55%); TL: 32% (22–45%); THL: 56% (47–65%)	L arm discontinued early due to lack of efficacy; addition of L to H did not increase pCR
HER2 positive[424]	NSABP B-41	Doxorubicin plus cyclophosphamide (AC) followed by paclitaxel (T)	Trastuzumab (H); Lapatinib (L); H + L	H: 49.4% (41.8–56.5%); L: 47.4% (39.8–54.6%); H+L 60.2% (52.5–67.1%); HR-negative H (58.2%), L (54.9%), H+L (69.8%)	L or L + H did not show an increased benefit above H alone
HER2 -positive[407]	NeoALTTO	Paclitaxel (T)	Trastuzumab (H); Lapatinib (L); H + L	H 36.49% (25.60–48.49); L 33.78% (23.19–45.72); L + H 61.33% (49.38–72.36)	L + H showed a higher pCR rate than H or L alone
HER2 positive[428]	GeparQuinto	Epirubicin and cyclophosphamide (EC) followed by docetaxel (D)	Trastuzumab (H) or lapatinib (L)	ECH-DH: 30.3% (25.2–35.8%); ECH-DL: 22.7% (18.2–27.8%)	Chemotherapy + H resulted in higher pCR rate than chemotherapy + L; associated with less serious adverse events
HER2 positive[358]	NeoSphere	Trastuzumab (H) + docetaxel (D)	Group A: H+D; Group B: pertuzumab (P)+H+D; Group C: P+H; Group D: P+D	Group A (H+D): 29.0% (20.6–38.5%); Group B (P+H+D): 45.8% (36.1–55.7%); Group C (P+H): 16.8% (10.3–25.3%); Group D (P+D): 24.0% (15.8–33.7%)	P+H+D (group B) showed a significantly higher pCR rate compared to H+D
HER2 positive[423]	TRYPHAENA	5-fluorouracil Epirubicin and Cyclophosphamide (FEC), Docetaxel (D), Carboplatin (Carbo) + Trastuzumab (H), and Pertuzumab (P)	Arm A: FEC+H+Px3→D+H+Px3; Arm B:FECx3→T+H+Px3; Arm C: TCarboH+P × 6	Arm A: 54.7% (42.7–66.2%); Arm B: 56.2% (44.1–67.8%); Arm C: 63.6% (51.9–74.3%)	Study of cardiac tolerability and efficacy of anthracycline with H+P. Concurrent anthracycline with H+P was well tolerated but did not increase pCR
HER2 positive or TNBC[418]	GeparSixto; GBG 66	Paclitaxel (T) + liposomal A HER2 positive: trastuzumab (H) + lapatinib (L) TNBC: bevacizumab	+/– Carboplatin (Carbo)	no Carbo: 36.9% (31.3–42.4%); Carbo: 43.7% (38.1–49.4%)	The addition of Carbo increased pCR rate for those with TNBC
TNBC[419]	CALGB 40603	Paclitaxel (T) followed by doxorubicin/cyclophosphamide (AC)	Carboplatin (Carbo); Bevacizumab (Bev)	Carbo: 54% (48–61%); No Carbo: 41% (35–48%); Bev: 52% (45–58%); No Bev: 44% (38–51%)	Addition of Carbo to standard neoadjuvant chemotherapy increased pCR
All[266]	NSABP B-18	Doxorubicin/cyclophosphamide (AC)	Order of therapy (surgery followed by 4 cycles of AC vs. 4 cycles of AC followed by surgery)	Comparison of outcome between postoperative versus preoperative AC by hazard ratio; DFS: 0.99, DDFS: 0.70, OS: 0.83	DFS and OS were no different in the preoperative chemotherapy group from the postoperative adjuvant therapy group
All[265]	EORTC 10902	5-Fluorouracil, epirubicin, and cyclophosphamide (FEC)	Order of therapy (surgery followed by 4 cycles of FEC vs. 4 cycles of FEC followed by surgery)	OS (hazards ratio, 1.16; P = 0.38), PFS (hazards ratio, 1.15; P=0.27), time to LRR (hazard ratio, 1.13; P=0.61)	Preoperative chemotherapy and postoperative chemotherapy yield similar results in terms of DFS, OS, and local control

(continued overleaf)

Table 13 (Continued)

Breast cancer subtype	Study	Chemotherapy backbone	Comparator	pCR rates (95% confidence intervals)	Summary
All[414]	NSABP B-27	Doxorubicin/cyclophosphamide (AC) followed by docetaxel (D)	Group 1: 4 cycles of preoperative AC followed by surgery; Group II: 4 cycles of AC followed by four cycles of D followed by surgery; Group III: 4 cycles of AC followed by surgery and then four cycles of D.	pCR: Group 1: 12.9% Group II: 26.1% Group III: 14.5%	Addition of 4 cycles of preoperative D after 4 cycles of preoperative AC significantly increased the pCR rate compared to AC alone
All[427]	GeparTrio	Docetaxel (D) + doxorubicin/cyclophosphamide (AC) - 2 cycles	4 cycles of DAC or 6 cycles of DAC (for 1390 patients whose tumor decreased by >50%)	8 cycles (23.5%) versus 6 cycles (21%); adjusted odds ratio 1.27 (0.90–1.81)	8 cycles of DAC did not result in a higher pCR rate than 6 cycles
HR negative or HR positive and clinically node positive[429]	GeparQuattro	Epirubicin and cyclophosphamide (EC) followed by docetaxel (D)	D + capecitabine (DX), or D followed by X (D-X)	D: 22.3%, DX: 19.5%, D-X: 22.3% pCR +/- D: 2.8% -(2.4–8.0%); EC + DX v EC plus D-X: 2.8% (-8.0–2.4%)	No difference in breast conservation or pCR; no difference in pCR with concomitant or sequential X
All[420,426,430]	I-SPY 2 Trial	Paclitaxel (T) followed by doxorubicin/cyclophosphamide (AC)	Veliparib and carboplatin (VC)	pCR estimates (95% probability intervals): VC versus control for TNBC: 51% (35–69%) 26% (11–40%)	**Adaptive randomization in multiarmed trials efficiently identifies responding tumor subtypes.** VC + standard therapy is highly likely to improve pCR rates in TNBC
			Neratinib (N)	N versus control for HER2+/HR-: 56% (37–73%): 33% (11–54%)	N + standard therapy is highly likely to improve pCR in HER2+/HR- breast cancer
			MK-2206+/- trastuzumab (H)	MK-2206 versus control for HER2+/HR-: 67.5% versus 36%; HR- 49.5% versus 26.2%; HER2+: 52.6% versus 29.0%	The three signatures for MK-2206 (HER2+/HR-, HR- and HER2+) indicate activity in both HR- and HER2+ disease
			T-DM1 (ado-trastuzumab emtansine) + pertuzumab (P)	TDM1+ P versus control (TH): HER2+: 52% versus 22% HER2+/HR-: 64% versus 33% HER2+/HR+: 46% versus 17%	T-DM1 + pertuzumab graduated in all HER2+ signatures, including HR+ and HR- subsets
			Pertuzumab (P) + trastuzumab (H) (6 other investigational agents being tested to date)	THP versus control (TH): HER2+: 54% versus 22% HER2+/HR-: 74% versus 33% HER2+/HR+: 44% versus 17%	THP → AC substantially improves pCR rates over standard TH → AC and graduated in all 3 HER2+ signatures, including HR+ and HR- subsets

pCR: pathologic complete response; TNBC: triple-negative breast cancer; EFS: event-free survival; DFS: disease-free survival; OS: overall survival; DDFS: distant disease-free survival; HR: hormone receptor.

chemotherapy, although the evidence is limited and more studies are needed.[432,433] Studies of different endocrine treatments have demonstrated superior efficacy with AIs compared with tamoxifen in clinical trials among postmenopausal women, with improvement in breast conserving surgery, which is related to duration of exposure.[434-436] Among AIs, there do not appear to be differences in clinical response.[437] Ki-67 and a scoring system that takes into account residual tumor as well as proliferation are being studied as a marker for early response or resistance to neoadjuvant hormone therapy.[438,439] Current strategies have been evaluating the addition of a number of targeted biologic therapies that have showed improvement in disease control in advanced disease to neoadjuvant hormone therapy with AIs.[440] These include PI3K and CDK 4/6 inhibitors, among others.[441] The mTOR inhibitor everolimus was first studied in the neoadjuvant setting before being tested in a registration trial in the second-line metastatic setting. It was not possible to identify markers of response and resistance in that initial study, and this goal has proved to be elusive in neoadjuvant endocrine trials.[442]

There has been a growing interest in studying neoadjuvant endocrine therapy in a broader cohort of HR+ breast cancers in both pre- and postmenopausal women; however, pCR does not appear to be a good surrogate end point of response. Currently, we do not have good early markers of response in HR+ breast cancer. Thus, neoadjuvant therapy can provide the platform to aid in the understanding of the biology of different breast cancers and the response to therapy and help target our effort to improve response and outcome.

Neoadjuvant setting as a registration end point for novel agents

The I-SPY 2 Trial uses an innovative model (an adaptive design that allows you to "learn as you go") to accelerate the testing and identification of new investigational agents in combination with NACT.[443] The trial has demonstrated the ability of multiple companies to collaborate in a trial that uses a common chemotherapy backbone (master trial), where new agents are introduced as amendments. The goal of the study is to promote the testing of new agents with phase I and Ib (in combination with paclitaxel) safety data in the primary disease setting in patients with high risk for early recurrence, to learn for which tumor subtype agents were most effective, and to increase the chance of success of confirmatory phase III trials. Agents "graduate" from the trial if their ability to increase pCR (in comparison to control) for one or more disease subtypes predicts that there will be an 85% likelihood of success in a confirmatory phase III trial. In this way, the most effective agents can be chosen to forward phase III trials, thereby improving 10–30% success rate seen in phase III trials in oncology.[444] The FDA agreed that the neoadjuvant setting would serve as an opportunity to improve the efficiency of testing novel agents.[445] The FDA has shown its support of neoadjuvant clinical trials by confirming the evidence base for pCR as a surrogate end point for event-free survival (EFS), conducting a meta-analysis of 12 international trials.[446] Their main objectives included establishing an association between pCR and EFS and OS to determine if pCR is best correlated with long-term survival in certain subtypes and finally if an increase in frequency in pCR predicts EFS and OS. Their findings established the best definition of pCR. Eradication or absence of tumor in both breast and lymph nodes, ypT0 ypN0 or ypT0/is ypN0 (vs breast only, ypT0/is), was better associated with EFS and OS [(EFS HR: ypT0 ypN0: 0.44; ypT0/is ypN0: 0.48 vs. ypT0/is: 0.60) and (OS HR: ypT0 ypN0 0.36; ypT0/is ypN0: 0.36 vs ypT0/is: OS 0.51)]. They also found that the association between pCR and long-term

outcomes was strongest in patients with TNBC (EFS: HR 0.24, 95% CI 0.18–0.33; OS: 0.16, 0.11–0.25) and in those with HER2+/HR− tumors who received trastuzumab (EFS: 0.15, 0.09–0.27; OS: 0.08, 0.03, 0.22).

The FDA then issued guidance on the use of pathologic response as an end point for accelerated approval.[447] Regular approval of new drugs in ESBC usually requires trials to show clinical benefit in improvement in DFS or OS. The FDA can grant accelerated approval based on a surrogate end point that has been shown to reasonably approximate clinical benefit, and thus the FDA has proposed the use of pCR rate as a surrogate for DFS and OS for HER2+, triple-negative, and more proliferative hormone-positive disease. Importantly, accrual must be completed for the EFS end point (either in the neoadjuvant setting or as a separate adjuvant trial) before accelerated approval can be granted.[448] If demonstration of an improvement in DFS or OS is not shown in confirmatory trials, the neoadjuvant indication would be removed from the labeling. One randomized trial could support accelerated approval based on the improvement in pCR rate followed by confirmation of the clinical benefit with improvements shown in DFS and OS. The neoadjuvant setting provides a forum to rapidly design and test new treatment strategies and accelerate drug development.

There was concern that the nonconcordant results of the ALTTO[449] and NeoALTTO[404] studies would cast doubt on the use of pCR as a surrogate end point. However, the HR of 0.86 observed in ALTTO with lapatinib and trastuzumab was in fact predicted by NeoALTTO, but the number of events was not sufficient to make it statistically significant, AC was given postoperatively rather than preoperatively in NEOALTTO, and the patient population in the ALTTO study was at lower risk (smaller tumors and less node-positive patients) than those in the NEOALTTO study.[450] These studies also showed the importance of using the same populations for the pCR assessment and EFS assessment, which is the goal of the I-SPY 3 international trial. A new meta-analysis is being planned for the HER2-targeted neoadjuvant studies, once the results are finalized.

Treatment for advanced breast cancer

Role of radiation for recurrent and metastatic breast cancer

The role of palliative radiotherapy is well established in the treatment of symptomatic MBC, but also continues to evolve as a complement to systemic cytotoxic, targeted, and hormonal therapies. Painful bony metastases and simple pathologic fractures of nonweight-bearing bones respond well to short courses of directed radiotherapy. However, local radiotherapy is no substitute for proper orthopedic fixation in highly diseased weight-bearing bones. A phase III randomized trial from RTOG compared single fraction of 800 cGy versus the standard 3000 cGy in 10 fractions found equivalent results for control of bony metastases.[451] Although multiple fraction therapy may be appropriate for complicated bone metastases involving adjacent soft tissue, the single treatment approach minimizes time in treatment and is certainly appropriate in most clinical situations. For patients with widespread osseous disease, modern intravenous pharmaceuticals, such as samarium-153 lexidronam, provide excellent pain relief and improved functionality without the severe and irreversible bone marrow suppression of earlier agents.[452]

In terms of the treatment of brain metastases, treatment with radiotherapy is quite standard and preferable to surgical treatment in the presence of widespread, poorly controlled systemic metastases. The generally accepted course of palliative whole-brain irradiation for multiple lesions is 3000–3750 cGy in 10–15 fractions, particularly for widespread intracranial disease.[453] The optimal therapy for solitary or limited brain metastasis, particularly in patients with well-controlled extracranial disease, is moving away from whole-brain radiation and toward stereotactic radiosurgery (SRS) to avoid neurocognitive toxicity.[454] In such patients, the toxicity associated with whole-brain treatment may be reserved for those with multiple brain metastases or recurrent metastases after SRS.

For patients with oligometastatic disease (three or fewer sites of gross tumor), there is emerging evidence that focal radiotherapy may be an important supplement to systemic therapy, even in the asymptomatic patient.[455] A current phase II/III trial is currently evaluating the benefit of adding stereotactic body radiotherapy or surgical resection of limited metastases to standard systemic therapy.[456] Finally, for patients with locally recurrent disease, even those who have undergone prior radiotherapy, directed radiation and modern reirradiation can be safely integrated with surgery and systemic therapy and are crucial to providing durable local control and improving QOL.[457,458]

Systemic therapy for metastatic breast cancer

The incidence of MBC is not formally monitored, but estimates predict that approximately a quarter of all patients diagnosed with ESBC will ultimately develop recurrent disease with distant metastases.[459] A proportion of 5% of all women diagnosed with breast cancer are found to have de novo MBC, characterized by the presence of distant metastasis at initial diagnosis. In general, recurrences peak 3–5 years after primary therapy for ESBC and then decrease to a steady state by 8 years. Women with HR+ ESBC remain at risk for recurrence for up to 20 years, although 50% of distant recurrences occur within the first 5 years after diagnosis. In comparison, recurrences of TNBC generally occur within the first 3 years with a dramatic reduction in risk thereafter. HER2+ breast cancers historically had a poor clinical outcome and recurred along a timeline similar to TNBC, but as stated in the adjuvant section, HER2-directed therapies have dramatically improved ROR and OS.

As addressed in the adjuvant section of this chapter, clinicopathologic factors—such as age; menopausal status; the size, grade, histology, and biomarker status of a tumor; and nodal status—affect ROR. However, the frequent development of recurrent disease in patients with small node-negative tumors who completed optimal adjuvant therapy clearly demonstrates that clinicopathologic factors only do not fully explain risk. Regardless of adjuvant therapy, patients with the luminal B intrinsic subtype have worse recurrence-free survival at 5–10 years after diagnosis than those with the luminal A intrinsic subtype.[313] Patients with the basal-like subtype have worse outcomes than those with luminal B subtype at 5 years after diagnosis, but these survival curves in fact cross after 10 years.

As with timing of recurrence, the location and extent of metastatic disease are generally associated with specific cancer subtypes. HER2+ breast cancers have a more aggressive biology and tropism for developing visceral and CNS metastasis. TNBC tends to recur locoregionally as well as in the lung or brain, but less commonly in bone.[309] HR+ breast cancers typically involve bone and soft tissue and follow an indolent course, but in some cases present more aggressively with visceral involvement.

The median survival of patients with MBC is 2–3 years. Long-term prognosis is determined by tumor biology, growth rate, disease burden, organ localization, duration of treatment response, and resistance or sensitivity to interventions. Most patients with overt distant metastases are presently incurable. However, among those who achieve a complete remission after standard chemotherapy, a few remain progression-free for extended periods of time, occasionally exceeding 10 years. PFS is generally longer for those patients who present with low-volume metastases to the skin, lymph nodes, or bone and shorter for patients with multiple organ involvement, particularly those patients with metastases to the liver, brain, and lung. Survival is longer for patients with HR+ tumors and those who achieve a complete remission with chemotherapy compared with patients with TN or HER2+ tumors and those who fail to respond to systemic treatment.

For the majority of patients with MBC, treatment is strictly palliative, with a goal to delay the progression of disease while concurrently improving QOL through the alleviation of symptoms due to disease and treatment. Patients who are diagnosed with MBC should be informed that their disease is incurable but treatable and encouraged that patients can live with metastatic disease for many years. Given the considerable heterogeneity of MBC, individualized treatment plans should be guided by a multidisciplinary group that includes, but is not limited to medical, surgical, and radiation oncologists, palliative care specialists, psycho-oncologists, specialized oncology nurses, social workers, and patient navigators.[460]

When a patient has symptoms or physical exam findings suspicious for disease recurrence, evaluation should include radiologic evaluation of the chest, abdomen, pelvis, and bones.[409,458] This assessment can be achieved with either a CT of the chest, abdomen, and pelvis in combination with a bone scan or PET/CT. Imaging of the brain should not be performed routinely in asymptomatic patients. In addition, laboratory studies should include a complete blood count and a comprehensive metabolic panel. If the serum tumor markers CA 15–3, CA 27.29, and CEA are elevated at baseline, then they can be assessed monthly in combination with physical examination and radiologic imaging to follow treatment response.

On the basis of findings from this baseline assessment, every effort should be made to obtain pathologic confirmation of metastatic disease.[409,458] ER, PR, and HER2 must be reassessed on the pathology specimen with high-quality assays, as discordance between primary tumor and metastasis is not uncommon. Discordance occurs in 10–30% of cases in the ER and 20–50% of cases in the PR, while higher concordance is observed in HER2.[461] In the unusual circumstance that tumor tissue cannot be obtained, patient and tumor characteristics are helpful to determine whether a tumor is likely to respond to hormonal manipulation. Older postmenopausal patients with a history of HR+/HER2− ESBC with a disease-free interval exceeding 3 years and small-volume metastatic disease located predominantly in soft tissue and/or bone are more likely to respond to endocrine therapy than patients with opposite characteristics. In the case of an indolent clinical course, a negative ER assay should prompt a repeat assay to ensure a false-negative result does not preclude potentially beneficial endocrine therapy.

A clear association exists between the use of treatment guidelines and improvement in survival. Several guidelines exist for the management of MBC. Guidelines developed at the Second International Consensus Conference for Advanced Breast Cancer (ABC2) in Lisbon, Portugal, in November 2013 were a joint effort between the European School of Oncology (ESO) and the European Society for Medical Oncology (ESMO).[458] ASCO's Clinical Practice Guidelines provide evidence-based recommendations that are developed by a multidisciplinary group of experts using a systematic review of phase III trials as well as clinical experience. Several ASCO Clinical Practice Guidelines exist for MBC and can be found at http://www.instituteforquality.org/practice-guidelines.[462–465]

Systemic therapies for HR+/HER2− MBC

Most patients with a new diagnosis of HR+/HER2− MBC are initially treated with endocrine-based therapy. Chemotherapy should be reserved for those patients with threatened or existing end-organ dysfunction, for whom a rapid reduction in tumor burden is essential. Only a few clinical trials have compared endocrine-based therapy with chemotherapy in patients with HR+/HER2− MBC. A Cochrane meta-analysis published in 2003 evaluated 10 relevant studies and reported that although chemotherapy resulted in a more rapid response rate (RR 1.25; 95% CI, 1.01–1.54; $p = 0.04$), no difference in OS was observed (HR 0.94; 95% CI, 0.79–1.12; $p = 0.5$).[466] The included trials were conducted several decades ago, evaluated variable hormone therapies, and failed to adequately assess QOL. Given the goals of treatment, most guidelines recommend that patients with HR+/HER2− MBC are initially treated with hormone therapy, except with rapid progression.[409,458]

Endocrine-based treatment options for patients with HR+/HER2− MBC include tamoxifen, the non-steroidal aromatase inhibitors (NSAIs) anastrozole and letrozole, the steroidal AI exemestane, and fulvestrant, as well as less-commonly used therapies such as megestrol acetate and estradiol. When choosing treatments, one must consider prior endocrine therapy in the adjuvant setting and the amount of time that elapsed between adjuvant therapy and recurrence. Side effect profiles and logistics associated with drug administration should also be considered on an individualized basis.

Approximately 50% of patients will respond to treatment with first-line hormone-based therapy. Patients who completed adjuvant hormonal therapy and achieved a long disease-free interval are likely to respond to first-line hormonal therapy. The time to maximal response with endocrine therapy can be quite prolonged, and treatment should not be abandoned prematurely. Patients should be continued on a therapeutic trial of a specific hormone therapy for at least 6–12 weeks in the absence of progressive disease before switching to other therapies. Patients without clinical response or with progressive disease after two sequential lines of hormone therapy should transition to chemotherapy. Patients who respond to hormone therapy often can continue on several sequential hormone therapy lines until either no further lines are available or upon development of visceral crisis.

Virtually all patients with HR+/HER2− MBC will eventually develop secondary resistance to hormone therapy. Over the last decade, molecularly targeted drugs have been developed in combination with first- and second-line hormone therapies to overcome or prevent hormone resistance. Several of these combinations have resulted in improved PFS, further delaying transition to chemotherapy.

Endocrine-based therapies for premenopausal HR+/HER2− MBC

Premenopausal women with MBC were historically treated with bilateral oophorectomies, suppressing serum estrogen to postmenopausal levels. The LHRH agonists goserelin and leuprolide became available for use in MBC in the 1980s, providing similar clinical benefits without surgical intervention.[467] Tamoxifen was not initially studied as a single agent for premenopausal breast cancer, but rather in combination with LHRH agonists. Klijn et al.[468] published a meta-analysis in 2001 that reviewed four phase II clinical trials evaluating LHRH agonists with or without tamoxifen with a total of 506 women with MBC. The combination arms resulted in increased RR, PFS, and OS in comparison to LHRH agonists only. No published trials have compared tamoxifen with or without LHRH agonists.

Both the ABC2 consensus guidelines and the NCCN Guidelines recommend ovarian suppression or ablation in combination with endocrine-based therapy as the first treatment for premenopausal women with HR+/HER2− MBC.[409,458] The initial endocrine-based therapy should be tamoxifen, unless metastases developed within 12 months of adjuvant tamoxifen. If tamoxifen resistance is proven or after a patient progresses on first-line tamoxifen with or without an LHRH agonist, then the same treatment sequences recommended for postmenopausal women can be followed, but with continued use of LHRH agonist.

Endocrine-based therapies for postmenopausal HR+/HER2− MBC

Tamoxifen was approved for use in postmenopausal women with MBC in 1977 and remained the primary therapy for HR+ MBC for over two decades. Early clinical trials compared tamoxifen with available hormonal therapies, such as diethylstilbestrol, ethinyl estradiol, megestrol acetate, and fluoxymesterone. Tamoxifen was found in many cases to have response rates as high as 50% in patients with HR+ MBC and more tolerable side effects.[469]

Several multicenter phase III clinical trials published in 2000 and 2001 demonstrated that third-generation nonsteroidal AI were either superior or equivalent to tamoxifen as the first-line therapy for postmenopausal women with MBC.[470–472] The largest was a phase III study that randomized 907 postmenopausal women with HR+ (or hormone receptor status unknown) MBC to either letrozole 2.5 mg daily or tamoxifen 20 mg daily.[469] Patients on the letrozole arm experienced a higher clinical benefit rate (CBR) (49% vs 38%; $p = 0.001$) and a significantly longer TTP (41 weeks vs 26 weeks; HR 0.70; 95% CI, 0.60–0.82; $p = 0.001$) than those patients on the tamoxifen arm. A meta-analysis by Mauri et al.[473] in 2006 evaluated trials comparing AI with tamoxifen and other hormonal therapies and demonstrated a statistically significant survival benefit from third-generation AI in the first-line setting (11% relative hazard reduction; 95% CI, 1–19%; $p = 0.03$). The side effects and toxicities associated with tamoxifen and AI are discussed in the adjuvant hormonal therapy section. Incomplete cross-resistance exists between steroidal and nonsteroidal AI.[474] Studies have clearly demonstrated that patients who progress on one AI can reach a clinically meaningful benefit with an agent from the other class.[475,476]

Fulvestrant is a first-in-class pure ER antagonist that competitively inhibits binding of ER by estradiol, leading to accelerated degradation of ER and inhibition of estrogen signaling through the ER.[477] In comparison to the estrogenic effects of tamoxifen, fulvestrant has fewer noxious side effects and adverse toxicities. On the basis of phase III clinical trial results demonstrating similar response rates and time to progression (TTP) as anastrozole, fulvestrant was approved by the FDA in 2002 to be administered as a monthly intramuscular injection. Initial approval was based on a dose of fulvestrant 250 mg intramuscularly (IM) monthly, but the subsequent COmparisoN of Faslodex In Recurrent or Metastatic breast cancer (CONFIRM) trial, as described below, demonstrated that fulvestrant 500 mg IM monthly with a loading dose was superior.[478]

North American Trial 0021 was a phase III, double-blind, double-dummy clinical trial that randomized 400 postmenopausal women with HR+ MBC to receive fulvestrant 250 mg IM monthly or anastrozole 1 mg daily.[481,479] Approximately 96% of patients had received tamoxifen as adjuvant or metastatic therapy. At a median follow-up of 16.8 months, no statistically significant differences were appreciated in TTP (HR 0.92; 9.14% CI, 0.74–1.15; $p = 0.42$), CBR, overall response (OR), or AEs.

The randomized, double-blind, double-dummy, phase III clinical Evaluation of Faslodex versus Exemestane Clinical Trial (EFECT) compared fulvestrant with exemestane in women with HR+ MBC who had progressed or recurred after treatment with a nonsteroidal AI.[480] A proportion of 60% of the 693 women enrolled in this study had received at least two prior endocrine therapies. Fulvestrant was given with a loading dose of 500 mg IM on day 0, followed by 250 mg on days 14 and 28 and 250 mg every 4 weeks thereafter, whereas exemestane was administered orally at 25 mg daily. Similar to Trial 0021, no statistically significant difference was appreciated. The median TTP was 3.7 months in both groups (HR 0.963; 95% CI, 0.819–1.133; $p = 0.6531$). ORR (7.4% vs 6.7%; $p = 0.736$) and CBR (32.2% vs 31.5%; $p = 0.853$) were similar between fulvestrant and exemestane, respectively. Both treatments were well tolerated in a meaningful proportion of patients.

The phase III CONFIRM trial was designed to determine whether a higher dosing regimen of fulvestrant would increase treatment efficacy, as suggested by preclinical and clinical phase II results.[476] A total of 736 postmenopausal women with HR+ MBC were randomized to receive fulvestrant 500 mg IM (on days 0, 14, 28, and every 28 days thereafter) or 250 mg IM (every 28 days). All participants had prior antiestrogen or AI treatment in either the adjuvant or metastatic setting. A prolonged PFS (HR 0.80; 95% CI, 0.68–0.94; $p = 0.006$) was demonstrated with fulvestrant 500 mg IM versus 250 mg IM. AEs such as injection site pain, nausea, and bone pain occurred with similar incidence and severity between the two groups. These results led to the FDA approval of fulvestrant 500 mg IM in September 2010.

The Fulvestrant fIRst-line Study comparing endocrine Treatments (FIRST) was a phase II open-label clinical trial that randomized 205 women with HR+ MBC to fulvestrant 500 mg IM (on days 0, 14, 28, and every 28 days thereafter) or anastrozole 1 mg daily.[477] Patients had not received endocrine therapy for advanced disease, and <30% received adjuvant endocrine therapy that had been completed >12 months before randomization. Follow-up analysis after 79.5% of patients had discontinued treatment showed a median TTP of 23.4 months on the fulvestrant arm compared with 13.1 months on the anastrozole arm (HR 0.66; 95% CI, 0.47–0.92; $p = 0.01$).[482] Recently, Robertson et al. have reported a significant benefit in median OS for fulvestrant 500 mg versus anastrozole (HR 0.70; 95% CI, 0.50–0.98; $p = 0.041$), with a median difference of 5.7 months between the two arms[483]

The phase III SoFEA clinical trial evaluated the role of combination endocrine therapy in postmenopausal women with HR+ MBC who had progressed or recurred on an NSAI.[484] A total of 723 women were randomized to receive fulvestrant plus anastrozole, fulvestrant with placebo, or exemestane with placebo. No difference in PFS was appreciated in the fulvestrant plus anastrozole arm versus the fulvestrant plus placebo arm, or the exemestane arm versus the fulvestrant plus placebo arm. However, the study used a suboptimal fulvestrant dose of 250 mg IM.

Additional endocrine-based therapies exist for patients who progress on hormone therapies, but have a low-tumor burden with minimal symptoms or are poor candidates for chemotherapy, such as ethinyl estradiol and megestrol acetate. Preclinical studies have demonstrated that HR+ breast cancer cells undergo estradiol-induced apoptosis after prolonged estrogen deprivation. A phase II clinical trial by Ellis et al. randomized 66 women with HR+ MBC who had progressed on AI to receive estradiol 30 mg daily or 6 mg.[485] A CBR of approximately 30% was demonstrated in both arms, but fewer serious AEs were observed in the low-dose arm. Megestrol acetate is a progestational agent with activity in HR+ MBC. Early studies demonstrated a response rate of 25%

and median PFS of 15 months to megestrol acetate 40 mg four times daily in MBC.[486] The benefit of megestrol acetate after treatment with an AI has not been assessed. Notable side effects include weight gain, fluid retention, vaginal bleeding, venous thromboembolic disease, and poor QOL.

Active endocrine-based therapy trials

Several ongoing clinical trials have been evaluating the optimal sequence of standard hormone therapies as well as new antiestrogens. Positive safety and efficacy results from the phase II FIRST study led to the design of the Fulvestrant and AnastrozoLe COmpared in hormonal therapy Naïve advanced breast cancer (FALCON) clinical trial (NCT01602380).[487] This randomized, double-blind, multicenter phase III clinical trial enrolled 450 postmenopausal women with HR+ locally advanced or MBC who did not undergo prior endocrine-based therapy in the adjuvant or metastatic setting. Patients are randomized to receive fulvestrant 500 mg IM (on day 1, 14, and 28, followed by every 28 days thereafter) or anastrozole 1 mg daily. A press release in mid-2016 stated that the FALCON trial had met its primary endpoint of improved PFS with fulvestrant compared to anastrozole. Results will be presented in the fall of 2016.

Other studies evaluating endocrine-based therapies are focused on novel hormone agents, such as ER-degrading agents, androgen antagonists, and AR inhibitors. Details on these trials are available at http://www.cancer.gov/about-cancer/treatment/clinical-trials/search.

Endocrine-based therapy in combination with targeted drugs

Hormone-based therapy is an effective and generally well-tolerated treatment option to control disease while delaying the transition to chemotherapy in patients with HR+/HER2− MBC. Unfortunately, all patients will ultimately develop disease that is resistant to endocrine-based therapies. Patients who relapse within the first 2 years of starting adjuvant endocrine therapy, within 12 months of completing adjuvant endocrine therapy, or progress <6 months after starting endocrine therapy for MBC have secondary or acquired resistance.[458] Molecular mechanisms involved in the acquisition of primary and secondary resistance are complex. Preclinical studies have recognized the presence of adaptive cross talk between the ER and various growth factor receptor and intracellular signaling pathways. Putative mechanisms that allow breast cancer cells to escape the inhibitory effects of hormone-based therapy include mutations in the ER gene (ESR), enhanced signaling through upregulation of growth factor pathways, induction of estrogen-independent growth, hypersensitivity to low estrogen concentrations, and cyclin D1 overexpression. An improvement in the understanding of mechanisms of hormone resistance through preclinical models led to the development of clinical trials that aim to delay or revert endocrine resistance by combining traditional hormone-based therapy with drugs that selectively target tumor biology. Table 14 lists many of the investigational therapeutics, their mechanism of action and molecular target, and breast cancer subtype of interest.

Endocrine-based therapy and antiangiogenic agents

Angiogenesis plays a well-defined role in the development of breast cancer. Preclinical studies suggest that VEGF, which is secreted by HR+ breast cancer cells, drives tumor proliferation through neoangiogenesis. Elevated levels of VEGF are associated with early recurrence and hormone therapy resistance. The

Table 14 Investigational drugs, associated molecular targets, and breast cancer subtypes of interest in ongoing clinical trials.

Molecular targets	Investigational drug	Mechanism(s) of action	Breast cancer subtypes under investigation and if tested as single agent or in combination
Fibroblast growth factor (FGF) pathway	Lucitanib	FGF receptor inhibitor; VEGF receptor inhibitor; PDGF receptor inhibitor	Any subtypes with FGFR mutation (single agent)
Insulin-like growth factor (IGF) pathway	Cixutumumab (IMC-A12)	Anti-IGF-1 receptor monoclonal antibody	Any subtype (with temsirolimus) HER2+ (with cytotoxic agent and lapatinib)
JAK/STAT pathway	Ruxolitinib (INCB-18424)	JAK1/2 inhibitor	HER2+ (with trastuzumab) HER2− (with cytotoxic agents) Any subtype (with cytotoxic agents)
MAPK pathway	Selumetinib (AZD6244, ARRY-142886)	MEK inhibitor	HR+ (with EBT[a])
PI3K/Akt/mTOR pathway	Alpelisib (BYL719) Taselisib (GDC-0032)	Alpha-specific PI3K inhibitor	HR+/HER2− (with EBT) HER2+ (with HER2-directed therapies) TNBC (with enzalutamide)
	Buparlisib (BKM120) Pictilisib (GDC-0941)	Pan-class 1 PI3K inhibitor	HR+/HER2− (with EBT; ribociclib; with cytotoxic agent) TNBC (with cytotoxic agent)
	MK-2206 Triciribine (BML-EI332) AZD5363	Akt inhibitor	Any subtype (with cytotoxic agent) HR+/HER2− (with EBT)
	Temsirolimus	mTOR inhibitor	HR+/HER2− (with EBT) TNBC (with cytotoxic agent; bevacizumab)
	Sapanisertib (MLN0128)	mTORC1/2 inhibitor	HR+/HER2− (with EBT)
Cyclin-dependent kinases (CDK)	Abemaciclib (LY2835219) Dinaciclib (SCH727965) Ribociclib (LEE-001)	CDK 4/6 inhibitor	HR+/HER2− (with EBT)
Colony-stimulating factor (CSF)-1 receptor	PLX3397	CSF-1R inhibitor; KIT inhibitor	TNBC (with cytotoxic agent)
Glycoprotein NMB (gpNMB)	Glembatumumab vedotin (CDX-011)	Anti-gpNMB antibody–drug conjugate	TNBC (single agent)
Heat shock protein 90 (HSP90)	Ganetespib (STA-9090)	HSP90 inhibitor (a novel small molecule inhibitor)	HR+/HER2− (with cytotoxic agent) Any subtype (single agent)
HER2	Neratinib (HKI-272)	Dual HER2/EGFR tyrosine kinase inhibitor	HER2+ (single agent) HER2+ (with cytotoxic agent) HER2+ (with trastuzumab) HER2 equivocal (with cytotoxic agent)
	Margetuximab	Fc-optimized anti-HER2 monoclonal antibody	HER2+ (single agent; with cytotoxic agent)
	MM-302	HER2-targeted liposomal doxorubicin (a novel antibody–drug conjugate)	HER2+ (single agent)
	ONT-380 (ARRY-380)	HER2-specific inhibitor (a novel small molecule inhibitor)	HER2+ (single agent)
HER3	Patritumab (U3-1287)	Anti-HER3 monoclonal antibody (a novel agent)	HER2+ (with cytotoxic agent; with trastuzumab)
Histone deacetylase (HDAC)	Entinostat Vorinostat Panobinostat	HDAC inhibitor	HR+/HER2− (with EBT; with immunotherapy) HER2+ (with cytotoxic agent; with trastuzumab) All subtypes (single agent)
PARP	Olaparib Veliparib (ABT-888)	PARP1/2 inhibitor	TNBC (single agent; with cytotoxic agent)
	Talazoparib (BMN-673)	PARP1/2 inhibitor, PARP1/2 trapper	gBRCA (single agent)
PD-1 and PD-L1	Pembrolizumab (MK-3475)	Anti-PD-1 monoclonal antibody	TN (with cytotoxic agents) HR+/HER2− (with HDAC inhibitor; with EBT)
	Atezolizumab (MPDL3280A)	Anti-PD-L1 monoclonal antibody	TNBC (single agent) HER2+ (with cytotoxic agent; with trastuzumab)
SRC	Dasatinib	SRC inhibitor	HER2+ (with trastuzumab and cytotoxic agents)
Steroid hormones	Bazedoxifene	Selective estrogen receptor modifier	HR+ (with CDK 4/6 inhibitor)
	Enobosarm (GTx-024)	Selective androgen receptor modifier	TN/AR+ (single agent) ER+/AR+ (single agent)
	Bicalutamide	Antiandrogen	HR+ or HR−/AR+ (with CDK 4/6 inhibitor)
	Enzalutamide	Androgen receptor inhibitor	HR+/HER2− (with EBT) TNBC (single agent; with PI3K inhibitor)

[a]EBT, endocrine-based therapy.

Letrozole/Fulvestrant and Avastin (LEA) study was the first phase III clinical trial evaluating the combination of hormone therapy with the anti-VEGF monoclonal antibody bevacizumab as a first-line therapy for patients with HR+/HER2− MBC.[488] The study randomized 380 patients to receive endocrine therapy (either letrozole or fulvestrant) in combination with bevacizumab 15 mg/kg iv every 3 weeks or endocrine therapy only. Approximately one-half of the study participants received endocrine therapy in the adjuvant setting, of which only 20% received an AI. At a median follow-up of 23.7 months, the median PFS was 19.3 months in the bevacizumab-containing arm and 14.4 months in the control arm (HR 0.83; 95% CI, 0.65–1.06; $p = 1.26$). Time to treatment failure and OS were similar in both arms, whereas toxicities were more significant in the bevacizumab-containing arm.

Initial results from CALGB 40503 (Alliance), a large phase III clinical trial evaluating the combination of first-line letrozole with bevacizumab in patients with HR+ MBC, were reported by Dickler et al. at ASCO 2015.[489] At a median follow-up of 39 months, 258 PFS events had been observed, with a median PFS of 20 months in the combination arm in comparison to 16 months in the letrozole-only arm (HR 0.74; 95% CI, 0.58–0.95; $p = 0.016$). ORR ($p = 0.004$) and CBR ($p = 0.005$) were significant in the bevacizumab-containing arm, but no difference in OS was appreciated. A significant increase in toxicity was appreciated in the combination arm with 50% of those patients reporting high-grade AEs in comparison to only 14% of patients on the control arm.

Endocrine-based therapy and PI3K/Akt/mTOR pathway inhibitors

The PI3K/Akt/mTOR pathway has critical roles in cellular proliferation, metabolism, and survival. Hyperactivation of the PI3K/Akt/mTOR pathway leads to increased downstream signaling with ligand-independent activation of the ER. The PI3K/Akt/mTOR pathway is frequently dysregulated in approximately 50% of HR+ MBC, and inappropriate upregulation is associated with poor outcomes and resistance to hormonal therapies. Preclinical studies of mTOR inhibitors in combination with endocrine therapy demonstrated synergistic inhibition of HR+ breast cancer cell lines. The addition of the mTOR inhibitor everolimus to second-line hormone therapy with exemestane for patients with MBC more than doubled PFS with a numerical but nonsignificant improvement in OS, leading to regulatory approval of everolimus in this setting.[488] Toxicity was significantly increased, including stomatitis.[489] Ongoing trials are evaluating the use of everolimus as well as other inhibitors of the PI3K pathway in various disease settings. Inhibitors of the alpha-specific subunit of PI3K have already provided encouraging early results, with different and possibly more favorable toxicity outcomes.

The Breast Cancer Outcomes with Everolimus (BOLERO-2) clinical trial was a double-blinded, randomized, phase III study that evaluated the addition of everolimus, an mTOR inhibitor, to exemestane in women with HR+/HER2− MBC who had progressed on an NSAI.[490] At a median follow-up of 18 months, the median PFS was 7.8 months in the everolimus plus exemestane arm in comparison to only 3.2 months in the placebo plus exemestane arm, respectively.[491] These significant PFS results were the basis for the FDA approval of everolimus in combination with exemestane in patients who had progressed on NSAI. A final analysis at 39 months showed a 4-month benefit in OS (HR 0.89; 95% CI, 0.73–1.10; $p = 0.14$) that was insignificant.[492] Everolimus is associated with many class-specific AEs that are dose-limiting and can cause significant morbidity, including stomatitis, rash, and noninfectious pneumonitis. Several ongoing

studies have been evaluating everolimus in the neoadjuvant, adjuvant, and metastatic settings. Details on these trials are available at http://www.cancer.gov/about-cancer/treatment/clinical-trials/search.

HORIZON was a randomized, placebo-controlled phase III clinical trial that randomized 1112 postmenopausal women with HR+ MBC to receive the mTOR inhibitor temsirolimus 30 mg daily (5 days every 2 weeks) plus letrozole 2.5 mg daily or placebo plus letrozole in the first-line setting.[493] Approximately 60% of these patients did not receive endocrine-based therapy in the adjuvant setting. No improvement in PFS was seen in the overall patient population (HR 0.90; 95% CI, 0.76–1.07; $p = 0.25$) or among those patients who received prior adjuvant endocrine-based therapy (HR 0.84; 95% CI, 0.66–1.08; $p = 0.17$). Discrepancies between the BOLERO-2 and HORIZON results are in part attributed to variations in pharmacokinetics, dosing schedules, and study populations.

Endocrine-based therapy and CDK 4/6 inhibitors

CDK are a class of serine/threonine kinases with a key role in the regulation of cell replication and division. CDK 4/6 forms a complex with cyclin D to inactivate the retinoblastoma protein (Rb), permitting activation of gene transcription. Dysregulation of CDK can lead to excessive cell proliferation, complicated by tumor growth and resistance. Preclinical studies have demonstrated that inhibitors of CDK 4/6 induce cell growth arrest and apoptosis of breast cancer cell lines and that a synergistic effect occurs when ER+ breast cancer cells are exposed to CDK 4/6 inhibitors plus endocrine-based therapies.[494] CDK 4/6 inhibitors are a novel class of small-molecule therapeutics that are administered orally. Their primary toxicity is a self-limited, uncomplicated neutropenia. Several CDK 4/6 inhibitors are actively investigated in clinical trials with promising outcomes.

Palbociclib is an oral CDK 4/6 inhibitor with promising results in both phase II and III settings. In the first-line setting, a phase II trial showed doubling in PFS with the addition of palbociclib to letrozole, without an improvement in OS.[495] These data led to accelerated FDA approval of palbociclib in combination with letrozole as first-line therapy for metastatic HR+ breast cancer, with final approval dependent on results from a phase III trial, which should be available in 2016. In the second-line setting, the addition of palbociclib to fulvestrant also more than doubled PFS, and OS data are immature.[496] The primary toxicity from palbociclib is self-limited, uncomplicated neutropenia.

PALOMA-1/TRIO-18 was an international, randomized, open-label, phase II clinical trial evaluating the addition of palbociclib, a CDK 4/6 inhibitor, to letrozole in the first-line setting of HR+/HER2− MBC.[493] A total of 165 postmenopausal women were randomized to palbociclib 125 mg, taken once daily for 21 days of a 28-day cycle, plus letrozole 2.5 mg daily or to letrozole only. Approximately 50% of patients had de novo MBC and therefore no prior treatment. The median PFS for the letrozole-only arm was 10.2 months, while the palbociclib-containing arm was 20.2 months (HR 0.488; 95% CI, 0.319–0.748; one-sided $p = 0.0004$). The study was not powered to assess OS. Grade 3–4 neutropenia was present in 54% of patients on the palbociclib-containing arm versus only 1% of patients on the letrozole-only arm. No cases of febrile neutropenia or neutropenia-related infections occurred during the study. These results published in February 2015 led to the accelerated approval by the FDA of palbociclib in combination with letrozole for the initial hormone-based treatment of HR+/HER2− MBC.[497]

The PALOMA-2 phase III clinical trial is an ongoing, confirmatory study with a similar design to PALOMA-1 (ClinicalTrials.gov identifier NCT 0201740427). Over 650 patients were randomized with a 3:1 ratio to palbociclib plus letrozole or placebo plus letrozole. Initial results are expected in 2016.

PALOMA-3 was a phase III clinical trial evaluating the combination of fulvestrant with palbociclib in patients with HR+/HER2− MBC who had progressed or relapsed on prior hormonal therapy.[494] A total of 521 patients were randomized in a 2:1 ratio to palbociclib plus fulvestrant or placebo plus fulvestrant. The study allowed for enrollment of premenopausal women on ovarian suppression with goserelin. The median PFS was 9.2 months in the palbociclib-containing arm in comparison to 3.8 months in the placebo arm (HR for progression or death 0.42; 95% CI, 0.32−0.56; $p < 0.001$).

Palbociclib has been the only approved CDK4/6 inhibitor to date, but ongoing clinical trials are investigating the CDK 4/6 inhibitors ribociclib and abemaciclib in the metastatic as well as neoadjuvant and adjuvant settings.

Ribociclib and abemaciclib

MONALEESA-1 is a randomized phase II clinical trial evaluating the biologic activity of ribociclib (LEE-001), a CDK 4/6 inhibitor, in the neoadjuvant setting (ClinicalTrials.gov identifier NCT01919229). The study is completed and initial results are expected in 2016. MONALEESA-2 is a double-blinded, placebo-controlled, phase III clinical trial evaluating the combination of letrozole 2.5 mg daily and ribociclib 600 mg daily (taken once daily for 3 weeks followed by 1 week off in 4-week cycles) in an estimated 500 patients with HR+/HER2− MBC who have received no prior therapy for advanced disease (ClinicalTrials.gov identifier NCT01958021). A press release in mid-2016 announced that MONALEESA-2 had met its efficacy endpoint. Data is expected later in 2016.

Abemaciclib (LY2835219) is a CDK 4/6 inhibitor with less hematologic, but more gastrointestinal toxicity than other class members. MONARCH-1 is a phase II clinical trial evaluating single-agent abemaciclib (LY2835219) in patients with HR+/HER2− recurrent, locally advanced, or MBC who have progressed on both hormone therapy and chemotherapy in the metastatic setting (ClinicalTrials.gov identifier NCT02102490). Data was presented by Dickler et al. at the ASCO meeting in 2016, demonstrating an overall response rate of 19.7%, with a clinical benefit rate of 42.4%. MONARCH-3 is a randomized, double-blinded phase III clinical trial enrolling an estimated 450 postmenopausal women with HR+/HER2− MBC to receive an NSAI plus abemaciclib or NSAI plus placebo in the first-line setting (ClinicalTrials.gov identifier NCT02246621). Final data collection for PFS is expected in June 2017. A phase II study evaluating the efficacy and safety of abemaciclib in patients with HR+/HER2− breast cancer involving brain metastases is also ongoing (ClinicalTrials.gov identifier NCT02308020).

Endocrine-based therapy and androgen receptor inhibitors

Expression of the AR is quite variable across breast cancer subtypes, with approximately 84–95% of HR+ breast cancers also expressing AR, in comparison to only 10–43% in HR− breast cancers.[498] Preclinical data suggest that the AR is involved in the development of resistance to AI. A multicenter, double-blinded, phase II clinical trial that randomized 247 patients with HR+/HER2− MBC to exemestane plus enzalutamide 160 mg daily or placebo is ongoing (ClinicalTrials.gov identifier NCT02007512).

Endocrine-based therapy and PI3K inhibitors

Several ongoing phase II and III clinical trials are evaluating oral PI3K inhibitors, such as the class I pan-PI3K inhibitor buparlisib (BKM120) and the alpha-selective PI3K inhibitors alpelisib (BYL719) and taselisib, as first- and second-line therapies for MBC. BELLE-2 was a randomized, double-blinded, placebo-controlled, phase III clinical trial evaluating the combination of fulvestrant 500 mg IM (on days 0, 14, 28, and every 28 days thereafter) with buparlisib 100 mg daily in postmenopausal women with HR+/HER2− MBC who have progressed on an AI (ClinicalTrials.gov identifier NCT01610284). Data was presented by Baselga et al. at the San Antonio Breast Cancer meetings in 2015, demonstrating a minimal benefit in PFS and significant toxicity. Interestingly, circulating cell free DNA was evaluated in a small subset of patients, and demonstrated a greater benefit in patients with demonstrated mutations in PIK3CA. This interesting hypothesis generating data is encouraging, but the little benefit in PFS and toxicity make it highly unlikely that further development of buparlisib will be pursued. BELLE-3 is the only ongoing trial with buparlisib, a randomized, placebo-controlled phase III clinical trial evaluating the combination of fulvestrant 500 mg IM (on days 0, 14, 28, and every 28 days thereafter) with buparlisib 100 mg daily in postmenopausal women with HR+/HER2− MBC who have progressed on an mTOR inhibitor in combination with endocrine therapy (ClinicalTrials.gov identifier NCT01633060). This study will help determine whether an alternative drug targeting the PI3K/Akt/mTOR pathway is beneficial after progression on an mTOR inhibitor.

Although the results of buparlisib were discouraging, two PIK3CA alpha targeted agents are in phase III trials, based on encouraging data from earlier phase studies. Both trials are comparing fulvestrant with placebo or with the targeted agent in postmenopausal women with HR+ HER2- MBC. SOLAR-1 is evaluating alpelisib (NCT02437318), and SANDPIPER is evaluating taselisib (NCT02340221).

The combination of endocrine therapy and PI3K inhibitors is also under investigation in the neoadjuvant setting. NEO-BELLE, a randomized, double-blinded phase II clinical trial in post-menopausal women with HR+ HER2− ESBC comparing the combination of letrozole 2.5 mg daily with the alpha specific PI3K inhibitor (alpelisib) or letrozole plus placebo, (ClinicalTrials.gov identifier NCT01923168). Patients randomized to the experimental arm will receive alpelisib 300 mg daily. Treatment will continue for 24 weeks, unless unacceptable toxicity or progression occurs, at which time the patients will undergo surgery. The trial originally included buparlisib; following the disappointing results of BELLE-2, this arm was discontinued.

Many ongoing studies are evaluating drugs that target the PI3K/Akt/mTOR pathway in ESBC and MBC. Details on these trials are available at http://www.cancer.gov/about-cancer/treatment/clinical-trials/search.

Endocrine-based therapy and HDAC inhibitors

Preclinical models of entinostat, a novel inhibitor of class 1 histone deacetylases (HDAC), demonstrated restoration of hormone sensitivity through downregulation of growth factor signaling pathways, normalization of ER levels, and increases in aromatase level.[499] ENCORE301 was a randomized phase II clinical trial that randomized 130 postmenopausal women with HR+/HER2− MBC who had progressed on an NSAI to receive exemestane 25 mg daily plus entinostat 5 mg po weekly or exemestane plus placebo.[500] Intention to treat analysis showed an improved PFS in the entinostat-containing arm with a PFS of 4.3 months versus 2.3 months in the control arm

Table 15 Commonly used single-agent and combination chemotherapy regimens for HER2− and HER2+ metastatic breast cancer.

HER2− MBC	Single agent	Paclitaxel (weekly)
		Docetaxel (every 3 weeks)
		Nab-paclitaxel
		Doxorubicin
		Pegylated liposomal doxorubicin
		Epirubicin
		Capecitabine
		Eribulin
		Ixabepilone
		Vinorelbine
		Gemcitabine
		Carboplatin
		Cisplatin
	Combination	Docetaxel + capecitabine
		Gemcitabine + paclitaxel (or docetaxel)
		Gemcitabine + carboplatin (or cisplatin)
HER2+ MBC	Paclitaxel (or docetaxel) + trastuzumab + pertuzumab	
	T-DM1	
	Lapatinib + capecitabine	
	Paclitaxel + trastuzumab	
	Vinorelbine + trastuzumab	

(HR 0.73; 95% CI, 0.50–1.07; one-sided $p = 0.055$). Median OS was evaluated as an exploratory end point and notably improved in the entinostat-containing arm (28.1 months) in comparison to the control arm (19.8 months) (HR 0.59; 95% CI, 0.36–0.97; $p = 0.036$). These results led to the designation of entinostat as a breakthrough therapy by the FDA in 2013. E2112, a phase III clinical trial that compares exemestane with or without entinostat, aims to enroll 600 patients with HR+/HER2− MBC (ClinicalTrials.gov identifier NCT02115282).

The pan-HDAC inhibitor vorinostat is currently under investigation with the immune checkpoint inhibitor pembrolizumab to assess the response of hormone therapy-resistant MBC to epigenetic immune priming. Pembrolizumab is discussed in detail below. This phase II clinical trial aims to enroll 58 patients with HR+ MBC with prior hormone therapy in the metastatic setting to receive tamoxifen 20 mg daily, vorinostat 400 mg daily (5 days on, 2 days off weekly, on a 21-day cycle), and pembrolizumab 200 mg iv every 3 weeks (ClinicalTrials.gov identifier NCT02395627). Patients are randomized to start pembrolizumab at the start of either cycle 2 or cycle 4.

Guidelines and recommendations for treatment of HR+/HER2− MBC

The ABC2 consensus guidelines state that the preferred first-line endocrine therapy for postmenopausal women with HR+/HER2− MBC is either an AI or tamoxifen, depending on type and duration of adjuvant therapy.[458] Fulvestrant high dose is also included as a first-line option. Second, the guidelines state that patients with HR+/HER2− MBC who experience disease progression after treatment with an NSAI should be considered for treatment with everolimus plus exemestane. The NCCN Guidelines are in agreement with these statements from the ABC2.[409]

Chemotherapy for MBC

Decisions regarding the use of chemotherapy in MBC depend in large part on the subtype of a patient's disease. Chemotherapy is the only treatment available for metastatic TNBC and is generally combined with HER2-targeting agents in HER2+ MBC. As stated earlier, chemotherapy for HR+/HER2− MBC should

be reserved for the rapid management of visceral crisis, de novo hormone resistance, or when patients develop irreversible resistance to endocrine-based therapies. Table 15 includes commonly used single-agent and combination chemotherapy regimens used in MBC.

Chemotherapy can be administered as a single agent or as a more intensive regimen of two or more drugs in combination. Historically, combination regimens were selected over single-agent chemotherapy as the increased RR and TTP associated with combined regimens were presumed to improve OS as well. A meta-analysis by Carrick et al. in 2009 reviewed 43 trials of chemotherapy for MBC, involving 9742 patients to assess outcomes associated with single-agent versus combination chemotherapy.[501] A proportion of 55% of trial participants included in this meta-analysis received first-line therapy. Combination regimens were not only superior with regard to RR, PFS, and OS (HR for OS 0.88; 95% CI, 0.83–0.94; $p < 0.0001$) but also were associated with a statistically significant increase in toxicity. A subsequent meta-analysis by Dear et al.[502] in 2013 evaluated 12 trials, including nine different treatment comparisons, to evaluate benefits of combination chemotherapy versus sequential use of the same agents. The meta-analysis demonstrated no difference in OS (HR 1.04; 95% CI, 0.93–1.15; $p = 0.45$) between combination and sequential chemotherapy. However, combination chemotherapy was associated with increased tumor response (RR 1.16; 95% CI 1.06–1.28; $p = 0.001$) and decreased risk of progression (HR 1.11; 95% CI 0.99–1.25; $p = 0.08$) in comparison to sequential single-agent chemotherapy.

Maintenance chemotherapy is the continuation of a treatment beyond the achievement of best response. In 2011, Gennari et al. reported a meta-analysis of randomized clinical trials comparing first-line therapies given over a prespecified duration or continued as maintenance therapy.[503] This meta-analysis included 11 trials with 2269 patients and showed that maintenance chemotherapy was associated with an improved OS (HR 0.91; 95% CI 0.84–0.99; $p = 0.046$) and PFS (HR 0.64; 95% CI 0.55–0.76; $p < 0.001$). The role of maintenance chemotherapy was more recently assessed in a multicenter phase III clinical trial in South Korea.[504] A total of 324 patients with MBC were enrolled and received six cycles of paclitaxel plus gemcitabine in the first-line setting. The 231 patients who achieved disease control were then randomized to the maintenance paclitaxel plus gemcitabine arm or observation off any treatment. Median PFS was significantly longer in the maintenance arm than in the observation arm (7.5 months vs 3.8 months, respectively; $p = 0.026$). In addition, median OS was significantly longer in the maintenance arm than in the observation arm (32.3 months vs 23.5 months, respectively; $p = 0.047$). Not surprisingly, maintenance chemotherapy was associated with increased myelosuppression and neuropathy. The study included patients with metastatic TNBC and HR+ MBC. Patients with HR+ MBC on the observation arm did not receive maintenance hormone therapy, and only 20% had received any prior endocrine therapy. Subset analyses demonstrated that the PFS benefit was primarily seen in those patients with the TN subtype. Maintenance endocrine therapy after achieving best response with induction chemotherapy has not been studied in clinical trials, but is a reasonable option.[458]

A majority of patients will respond to first-line therapies. No clinical trials have demonstrated an improvement in OS using a specific chemotherapy in comparison to another in the first-line setting for MBC. In general, anthracyclines and taxanes are considered as the most effective classes of chemotherapy for breast cancer and are commonly used therapies in the first-line setting. However, treatment choice should be individualized, with consideration of prior adjuvant chemotherapy regimens, timing of relapse, total lifetime anthracycline exposure, and comorbidities.

Single-agent chemotherapy

The taxanes paclitaxel and docetaxel, compounds that stabilize microtubules and thereby induce cell cycle arrest, are among the most effective and best tolerated chemotherapies for the treatment of breast cancer. The FDA originally approved single-agent paclitaxel in 1994 at a dose of 175 mg/m^2 iv every 3 weeks, given as a 1- to 3-h infusion. CALGB 9840 was a phase III clinical trial that randomized 585 patients with MBC to receive paclitaxel at either 80 mg/m^2 iv given 3 weeks a month or paclitaxel 175 mg/m^2 iv given every 3 weeks as first- or second-line chemotherapy.[505] A combined analysis, which included an additional 158 patients treated with every 3-week paclitaxel 175 mg/m^2 on the CALGB 9342 study, demonstrated a significant improvement in OS of 24 months on the weekly arm in comparison to 12 months on the every 3-week arm (HR = 1.28; $p = 0.0092$). RR (42% vs 29%) and median TTP (9 months vs 5 months) were also significantly increased. Grade 3 neuropathy was more common on the weekly than every 3-week arm (24% vs 12%; $p = 0.0003$), whereas higher rates of myelosuppression and infectious complications were noted on the every 3-week arm.

Docetaxel is generally administered at a dose of 75–100 mg/m^2 every 3 weeks as a 1-h infusion. Several small phase II and III clinical trials have compared weekly docetaxel at 35–40 mg/m^2 with every 3-week docetaxel between 75 and 100 mg/m^2 iv, and a meta-analysis by Mauri et al. in 2010 demonstrated no significant difference in ORR, PFS, or OS between these docetaxel schedules.[506–509] However, the weekly schedule resulted in less myelosuppression and neuropathy, but more frequent nail changes and epiphora.

A phase III clinical trial has compared docetaxel 100 mg/m^2 iv every 3 weeks with paclitaxel 175 mg/m^2 iv every 3 weeks in patients with MBC who had progressed on anthracycline-containing therapy. Of the 372 patients randomized, those on the docetaxel arm experienced a longer TTP than those on the paclitaxel arm (5.7 months vs 3.6 months; HR 1.64; 95% CI, 1.33–2.02; $p < 0.0001$) as well as longer OS (15.4 months vs 12.7 months; HR 1.41; 95% CI, 1.15–1.73; $p = 0.03$).[510] However, the preferred regimens of

weekly paclitaxel and every 3-week docetaxel have not been compared in a head-to-head trial. Docetaxel and paclitaxel are not completely cross-resistant and many patients derive clinical benefit from treatment with one taxane after developing resistance to the other.[511,512]

Nanoparticle albumin-bound paclitaxel (nab-paclitaxel) was developed to avoid the infusion reactions associated with the solvents used with paclitaxel and docetaxel, Cremophor EL and Polysorbate 80, respectively. The FDA approved nab-paclitaxel in 2005 based on its superior efficacy in comparison to every 3-week paclitaxel in a phase III clinical trial.[513] In particularly, 454 women with MBC were randomized to receive nab-paclitaxel 260 mg/m^2 iv every 3 weeks or paclitaxel 175 mg/m^2 every 3 weeks. Approximately 40% of study participants had not received prior chemotherapy in the metastatic setting. Patients on the nab-paclitaxel arm had significantly higher ORR (33% vs 19%; $p = 0.001$) and longer TTP (23.0 weeks vs 16.9 weeks; HR 0.75; $p = 0.006$) than those on the paclitaxel arm. Grade 4 neutropenia was less common on the nab-paclitaxel arm than the paclitaxel arm (9% vs 22%; $p < 0.001$), while grade 3 sensory neuropathy was more common on the nab-paclitaxel than the paclitaxel arm (10% vs 2%; $p < 0.001$), but most episodes resolved with treatment interruption and dose reduction. No corticosteroids or antihistamines were used on the nab-paclitaxel arm and no hypersensitivity reactions occurred. No study has compared weekly nab-paclitaxel with the preferred weekly paclitaxel regimen.

A phase II randomized clinical trial compared several schedules of nab-paclitaxel and every 3-week docetaxe.[514] In this study, 300 patients with treatment naïve MBC were randomized to nab-paclitaxel 300 mg/m^2 iv every 3 weeks, 100 mg/m^2 the first 3 of every 4 weeks, 150 mg/m^2 the first 3 of every 4 weeks, or docetaxel 100 mg/m^2 every 3 weeks. The nab-paclitaxel arm at 150 mg/m^2, the first 3 of every 4 weeks, was associated with the highest RR, PFS, and OS.[515] Rates of peripheral neuropathy due to nab-paclitaxel are fairly similar to paclitaxel and docetaxel, but rates of neutropenia are lower.

Anthracyclines are a reasonable first-line chemotherapy for MBC, but evaluation of a patient's cardiac risk factors and lifetime anthracycline exposure (doxorubicin 450–550 mg/m^2 and epirubicin 900 mg/m^2) is critically important to reduce risk of cardiotoxicity. Doxorubicin is typically given as 60–75 mg/m^2 every 3 weeks or 20 mg/m^2 weekly. Epirubicin can be given as 75–100 mg/m^2 every 3 weeks or 20–30 mg/m^2 weekly. Pegylated liposomal doxorubicin (PLD) is an enhanced form of doxorubicin that is encapsulated in liposomes to minimize adverse effects, while maintaining treatment efficacy. Several phase III clinical trials comparing PLD and doxorubicin have demonstrated equivalent efficacy with a significantly lower risk of cardiotoxicity, allowing for anthracycline-based retreatment in the metastatic setting.[516–518] PLD is also associated with less alopecia and nausea, but more hand-foot syndrome and mucositis.

A randomized controlled trial of first-line doxorubicin versus paclitaxel every 3 weeks, with crossover allowed at progression, found a higher RR and PFS with first-line doxorubicin, but no statistically significant difference in OS.[519] Doxorubicin resulted in more toxicity, but better control of cancer-related symptoms. By contrast, the single-agent arms of doxorubicin and paclitaxel every 3 weeks in the E1193 clinical trial showed equivalent RR, time to treatment failure, OS, and QOL.[520] A meta-analysis of three clinical trials, including 919 patients who were randomized to single-agent anthracycline versus every 3-week taxane, demonstrated similar RR (33% and 38%, respectively; $p = 0.08$) and OS (HR 1.01; 95% CI, 0.88–1.16; $p = 0.90$), but an increase in PFS with anthracyclines

(HR 1.19; 95% CI, 1.04–1.36; $p = 0.011$).[521] No clinical trials have compared anthracyclines with weekly paclitaxel in the first-line setting.

Capecitabine is an orally administered third-generation fluoropyrimidine carbamate that is preferentially converted in tumor tissue to its active metabolite 5-fluorouracil by thymidine phosphorylase, thus allowing for more selective cytotoxicity with fewer toxic side effects. Several phase II clinical trials have demonstrated that single-agent capecitabine has activity in patients with MBC with prior exposure to anthracyclines and taxanes with RR of 15–29% and OS of 10.1–15.2 months.[522–525] The FDA approved capecitabine for use in patients with MBC in 1998, as a single agent in patients with MBC refractory to anthracycline and taxanes, and in combination with docetaxel in 2001, as described below. Both the FDA approval and the capecitabine package insert recommend capecitabine starting dose of 1250 mg/m² twice daily for 2 weeks followed by a 7-day rest period. However, lower starting doses of 1000 mg/m² twice daily for 2 weeks, followed by a 1-week rest period are associated with similar efficacy, but less palmar-plantar erythrodysesthesia and diarrhea.[526]

Eribulin, a novel synthetic inhibitor of tubulin polymerization, was approved for use in patients with MBC who had received two prior chemotherapies in the metastatic setting by the FDA in 2010 in the context of significant results from the EMBRACE study, a phase III clinical trial of heavily pretreated patients with MBC.[527] In this open-label study, 762 patients were randomized in a 2 : 1 ratio to receive eribulin 1.4 mg/m² iv on days 1 and 8 of a 21-day cycle or physician's choice chemotherapy. Median OS was significantly improved in the eribulin arm (13.1 months; 95% CI, 11.8–14.3) in comparison to the physician's choice arm (10.6 months; 95% CI, 9.3–12.5; HR 0.81, 95% CI, 0.66–0.99; $p = 0.041$). Peripheral neuropathy led to the discontinuation of eribulin in 5% of patients.

The effects of eribulin and capecitabine on both OS and PFS were compared in a phase III clinical trial in an attempt to identify a standard therapy for use in patients with MBC that had progressed on both anthracycline- and taxane-based therapies.[528] A total of 1102 women with MBC were randomized to receive eribulin or capecitabine as their first-, second- or third-line chemotherapy. Eribulin was not superior to capecitabine with regard to OS (15.9 months vs 14.5 months; HR 0.88; 95% CI, 0.77–1.00; $p = 0.56$) or PFS (4.1 months vs 4.2 months; HR 1.08; 95% CI, 0.93–1.25; $p = 0.30$). No difference in objective RR was observed with 11.0% for eribulin and 11.5% for capecitabine. QOL scores were also similar, with a majority of AEs of grades 1 or 2.

Ixabepilone is an epothilone, a novel class of antimicrotubule agents developed to overcome taxane and anthracycline resistance. Phase II studies of ixabepilone 40 mg/m² iv every 3 weeks in heavily pretreated patients with MBC demonstrated objective RR of approximately 12% and stable disease in 40–50% of participants.[529,530] Transient peripheral neuropathy, myelosuppression, alopecia, and fatigue were common toxicities in these studies. Its approval by the FDA in 2007 was based on a phase III clinical trial evaluating the combination of ixabepilone and capecitabine, but labeling allows for monotherapy. Ixabepilone is currently only available in the United States.

The semisynthetic vinca alkaloid vinorelbine has been evaluated extensively for the treatment of MBC and used in clinical practice for several decades, but has never gained regulatory approval by the FDA. Phase II clinical trials of single-agent vinorelbine dosed at 30 mg/m² on days 1 and 8 of a 21-day cycle have demonstrated RR of 40–50% in the first line and 20–35% in second line for patients with MBC.[531,532] Vinorelbine is well tolerated with myelosuppression as the main side effect.

Some chemotherapy treatments used in MBC are approved as single agents, but more commonly used in combinations, as described below. Gemcitabine is a pyrimidine antimetabolite that inhibits DNA synthesis through a unique mechanism of action. It has been studied as a first-, second-, and third-line treatment for patients with MBC with average RRs of 37%, 26%, and 13%, respectively.[533–535] Given its limited toxicity as well as unique mechanism of action, it is often combined with other chemotherapy treatment methods, such as taxanes and platinums. In 2004, the U.S. FDA approved gemcitabine in combination with paclitaxel for use in patients with MBC who had progressed on prior anthracycline treatment. Cisplatin and carboplatin are DNA cross-linking agents with similar activity in previously untreated MBC, with objective response rates between 8% and 35%.[536–538]

The preferred single-agent chemotherapies for recurrent MBC according to the NCCN Guidelines are doxorubicin, PLD, paclitaxel, capecitabine, gemcitabine, vinorelbine, and eribulin.[409]

Combination chemotherapy regimen

Several regimens of combination chemotherapy are available for when a more rapid tumor response is needed to improve cancer-associated symptoms or in the context of a life-threatening visceral crisis. However, such regimens are generally more toxic and their use should be carefully assessed/weighed. Some combination regimens approved for use in the adjuvant or neoadjuvant setting have also been demonstrated as effective in the metastatic setting, such as an anthracycline plus cyclophosphamide with or without fluorouracil, and CMF. Non-anthracycline-containing taxane-based regimens include paclitaxel or docetaxel combined with gemcitabine, docetaxel plus capecitabine, and paclitaxel plus either cisplatin or carboplatin. Available combination regimens for patients who progress on both anthracyclines and taxanes include gemcitabine plus carboplatin. Suggested combination regimens are found within the NCCN Guidelines for Breast Cancer, which are available at NCCN.org.[395,409]

The phase III Intergroup E1193 randomized clinical trial compared single-agent doxorubicin, single-agent paclitaxel, and doxorubicin plus paclitaxel, with allowance for crossover between single-agent arms after progression, in patients with MBC.[518] Response rates and TTP were statistically superior in the combination arm at 47% and 8 months, respectively, than in either of the two single-agent arms (36% and 5.8 months with doxorubicin; 34% and 6.0 months with paclitaxel). However, no benefit in OS was observed in the combination arm in comparison to sequential single-agent therapy. Global QOL measurements were similar in all arms.

Combination chemotherapy regimens typically are based on preclinical evidence of synergy between two agents with distinct mechanisms. Taxanes enhance the activity of capecitabine through the upregulation of thymidine phosphorylase, and early phase I studies clearly demonstrated synergy between docetaxel and capecitabine. A phase III clinical trial reported by O'Shaughnessy et al.[539] in 2002 randomized 511 patients with anthracycline-resistant MBC to receive capecitabine 1250 mg/m² po twice daily on days 1–14 plus docetaxel 75 mg/m² iv on day 1 of a 21-day cycle or docetaxel 100 mg/m² iv every 21 days. The combination arm was associated with a significant increase in ORR (42% vs 30%; $p = 0.006$), median TTP (6.1 months vs 4.2 months; HR 0.652; 95% CI, 0.545–0.780; $p = 0.001$), and OS (14.5 months vs 11.5 months; HR 0.75; 95% CI, 0.634–0.947; $p = 0.0126$). This clinical trial was the first to demonstrate improved OS with a docetaxel-containing combination. However, more patients in the combination arm than the single-agent arm (20% vs 7%) received sequential single-agent docetaxel after completion of the study, complicating interpretation of OS.

A phase III clinical trial that randomized 170 patients to receive gemcitabine 1000 mg/m^2 iv on days 1 and 8 of a 21-day cycle plus docetaxel 75 mg/m^2 iv on day 8 or docetaxel 175 mg/m^2 iv every 3 weeks demonstrated an increase in TTP with the combination arm (HR 0.77; 95% CI, 0.59–1.01; log-rank = 0.06), but no difference in RR or OS.[540] However, few patients enrolled in this study received second- or third-line treatment. A global phase III clinical trial randomized 529 patients with MBC who had received an anthracycline in the adjuvant setting to receive gemcitabine 1250 mg/m^2 iv on days 1 and 8 plus paclitaxel 175 mg/m^2 iv on day 1 every 21 days or paclitaxel only.[541] TTP was longer (6.14 months vs 3.98 months; log-rank $p = 0.0002$) and RR was increased (41.4% vs 26.2%; $p = 0.0002$) in the combination arm in comparison to paclitaxel only. However, the trial did not use the optimal weekly schedule of paclitaxel. These results led to the FDA approval of gemcitabine in combination with paclitaxel as a first-line treatment for patients with MBC in 2004. A phase III clinical trial evaluated gemcitabine plus paclitaxel or docetaxel with every 3-week or weekly schedules.[542] In this study of 240 patients, similar TTP and OS were demonstrated between the various arms. Similar ORRs were observed with the different taxanes, but weekly schedules were favored over every 3-week schedules. The combinations of docetaxel with either gemcitabine or capecitabine have been compared in several phase III clinical trials. A pooled analysis of these studies has shown no difference in OS, PFS, or ORR.[543]

Preclinical studies have demonstrated synergy between gemcitabine and platinum agents, and subsequent clinical trials demonstrated that this combination has moderate activity in patients with prior exposure to anthracyclines and taxanes. A multicenter phase II clinical trial that treated 39 patients with heavily pretreated MBC with gemcitabine 1000 mg/m^2 iv on days 1 and 8 and carboplatin AUC 4 on day 1 every 3 weeks reported an ORR of 31% (95% CI, 17–48%) and a median TTP of 5.3 months (95% CI, 2.6–6.7 months).[544] A multicenter phase II clinical trial that treated 33 patients with heavily pretreated MBC with gemcitabine 1000 mg/m^2 iv and cisplatin 30 mg/m^2 iv on days 1 and 8 of a 21-day cycle reported an ORR of 25.8% (95% CI, 17–48%) and a median TTP of 4 months (95% CI, 2.15–5.85 months).[545]

Antiangiogenic agents plus chemotherapy in MBC

As mentioned in the adjuvant section, neoangiogenesis plays an important role in the development of breast cancer, and several antiangiogenic agents have been evaluated in the metastatic setting. The FDA approved the monoclonal antibody bevacizumab in combination with chemotherapy for the first-line treatment of MBC in 2008. This approval was based on results from the phase III E2100 clinical trial that randomized 722 patients with MBC to weekly paclitaxel with or without bevacizumab (10 mg/kg iv every 2 weeks).[546] The bevacizumab-containing arm was associated with a significant benefit in PFS (11.8 months) in comparison to the control arm (5.9 months; HR 0.6), but with no difference in OS ($p = 0.16$). Subsequent phase III studies of bevacizumab in combination with first-line chemotherapy demonstrated a less-significant PFS improvement and no effect on OS, leading to withdrawal of the FDA approval of bevacizumab for MBC in 2011.

The phase III AVastin And DOcetaxel (AVADO) clinical trial randomized 736 patients with MBC to docetaxel 100 mg/m^2 iv plus bevacizumab at 7.5 or 15 mg/kg iv or docetaxel plus placebo every 3 weeks.[547] At a median follow-up of 25 months, PFS was superior in both bevacizumab-containing arms, most notably with a PFS of 10.1 months in the bevacizumab (15 mg/kg)-containing arm in comparison to 8.2 months in the control arm. The phase III RIBBON-1 clinical trial randomized 1237 patients with HER2− MBC to investigator's choice first-line chemotherapy with or without bevacizumab 15 mg/kg, and found a statistically significant improvement in median PFS when bevacizumab was given in combination with capecitabine, taxanes, or anthracyclines. A meta-analysis of E2100, AVADO, and RIBBON-1, published in 2012 by Rossari et al.,[548] demonstrated a significant improvement in 1-year OS in bevacizumab containing arms, but no difference in median OS (HR 0.97; 95% CI, 0.86–1.08, $p = 0.056$).

Many additional phase II and III clinical trials have evaluated the addition of bevacizumab to first-, second-, and subsequent-line chemotherapies. The phase III RIBBON-2 clinical trial evaluated the combination of bevacizumab with investigator's choice second-line chemotherapy, and found a statistically significant improvement in median PFS from 5.1 to 7.2 months with the addition of bevacizumab to either capecitabine, taxanes, gemcitabine, or vinorelbine.[549] Similar to other studies, no significant effect on OS was appreciated. In addition to the absence of a survival benefit, bevacizumab in combination with chemotherapy is associated with an increased risk of grade 3–4 hypertension (4.4%), thromboembolic disease (3.2%) proteinuria (1.7%), and hemorrhage (1.4%).[550] The ongoing global, double-blinded, phase III MERiDiAN clinical trial is evaluating first-line weekly paclitaxel with or without bevacizumab in patients with HER2− MBC.[551] The study will assess PFS in all patients as well as the subgroup of patients with high-baseline VEGF-A concentrations as a predictive marker of treatment benefit.

Other types of antiangiogenic agents have been evaluated for the treatment of MBC. Sunitinib, a small molecule multitargeted TKI that inhibits the VEGF receptor, was studied in combination with capecitabine in a phase III clinical trial of patients with anthracycline- and taxane-resistant MBC.[552] The study randomized 442 patients with up to two prior regimens for MBC to capecitabine 2000 mg/m^2 with or without sunitinib 37.5 mg po daily. ORR, PFS, and OS were similar between the two arms.

Ramucirumab, a humanized monoclonal antibody against VEGF receptor-2, was studied in combination with docetaxel in the phase III ROSE/TRIO-12 clinical trial.[553] This double-blinded study randomized 1144 patients with HER2− MBC to receive first-line docetaxel 75 mg iv with ramucirumab 10 mg/kg iv or placebo every 3 weeks. No statistically significant difference in median PFS (HR 0.88; $p = 0.077$) or OS (HR 1.01; $p = 0.915$) was detected, while toxicities such as fatigue, hypertension, hand-foot syndrome, and stomatitis were significantly higher in the ramucirumab-containing arm. No antiangiogenic agents are approved for the treatment of MBC as of 2015, but many remain under evaluation and can be found at www.clinicaltrials.gov.

Systemic therapies for HER2+ MBC

In the absence of HER2-targeted therapy, patients with HER2+ breast cancer experience shortened OS because of aggressive tumor behavior.[554] The approval of trastuzumab in combination with paclitaxel for the first-line treatment of HER2+ MBC in 1998, and later for ESBC in 2006, dramatically improved outcomes for these patients. Unfortunately, 15% of patients with HER2+ ESBC will develop incurable metastatic disease after completing 1 year of adjuvant trastuzumab, and 30–50% of patients treated with trastuzumab in the metastatic setting will progress within 1 year. The development and FDA approval of three additional HER2-directed therapies, lapatinib, pertuzumab, and T-DM1, has further improved the survival of patients with HER2+ MBC. Many novel HER2-directed therapies are currently under evaluation and described below.

Pivotal trials of trastuzumab in HER2+ MBC

The early clinical trials of trastuzumab in patients with HER2+ MBC evaluated first- and second-line trastuzumab monotherapy and trastuzumab in combination with chemotherapy. A single-arm study of first-line trastuzumab monotherapy in 114 women with HER2+ MBC showed an RR of 26% and CBR of 38%.[555] In comparison, a study of trastuzumab monotherapy in 222 patients with HER2+ MBC and progression after one or two chemotherapy regimens resulted in an ORR of 15% and median duration of response of 9.1 months.[556]

The FDA approval of trastuzumab was based on the pivotal phase III trial by Slamon et al., which randomized 469 women with HER2+ MBC to standard chemotherapy (an anthracycline plus cyclophosphamide, or paclitaxel) plus trastuzumab versus chemotherapy only in the first-line setting.[557] Trastuzumab was given with a loading dose of 4 mg/kg iv followed by 2 mg/kg iv weekly. The addition of trastuzumab to chemotherapy was associated with a longer TTP (7.4 months vs 4.6 months; $p < 0.001$), higher ORR (50% vs 32%; $p < 0.001$), longer duration of response (9.1 months vs 6.1 months; $p < 0.001$), and longer OS (25.1 months vs 20.3 months; $p = 0.046$) in comparison to chemotherapy only. The primary toxicity associated with trastuzumab was a reduction in LVEF, which was most prominent in patients receiving the combination of anthracycline and cyclophosphamide plus trastuzumab (27%), in comparison to paclitaxel plus trastuzumab (13%), anthracycline and cyclophosphamide only (8%), or paclitaxel only (1%). This increased toxicity led to the general recommendation that anthracyclines not be combined with trastuzumab in the metastatic setting.[409,464]

Several other phase II and III clinical trials of single-agent chemotherapy plus trastuzumab in the first-line setting have been performed. In a multinational phase II clinical trial that was reported by Marty et al. in 2005, 186 patients with HER2+ MBC were randomized to docetaxel 100 mg/m² iv every 3 weeks with or without trastuzumab until disease progression.[558] The addition of trastuzumab to docetaxel was associated with an increased median TTP (11.7 months vs 6.1 months; $p = 0.0001$), ORR (61% vs 34%, $p = 0.0002$), and OS (31.2 months vs 22.7 months; $p = 0.0325$) in comparison to the control arm. Patients in the control arm who crossed over to single-agent trastuzumab at the time of progression had an OS similar to those on the docetaxel plus trastuzumab arm (30.3 months vs 31.2 months, respectively), clearly demonstrating the effectiveness of trastuzumab in the second-line setting.

Several single-arm phase II clinical trials reported ORRs of 63–78% with the combination of vinorelbine plus trastuzumab in patients with HER2+ MBC, a regimen that is generally well tolerated with primary AEs of neutropenia and neuropathy.[559-561] Essentially all other studies combining trastuzumab with chemotherapy have demonstrated safety and efficacy, although the majority are single-arm trials. In many countries, the combination of trastuzumab with chemotherapy has become the standard of care for patients with HER2+ MBC, regardless of the type of chemotherapy used and its efficacy.[562]

Preclinical studies demonstrated synergy between platinum agents, taxanes, and trastuzumab, and subsequent clinical trials attempted to further improve clinical benefit by combining these drugs.[563] A multicenter phase III clinical trial randomized 196 women with HER2+ MBC and without prior treatment in the metastatic setting to six cycles of trastuzumab and paclitaxel 175 mg/m² iv every 3 weeks with or without carboplatin AUC 6 iv, followed by weekly maintenance trastuzumab.[564] Patients in the carboplatin-containing arm were found to have increased ORR (52% vs 36%; $p = 0.04$) and PFS (10.7 months vs 7.1 months; HR 0.66; 95% CI, 0.59–0.73; $p = 0.03$), as well as increased grade 4 neutropenia. A prespecified subset analysis of patients with HER2+ IHC 3+ (in comparison to 2+) demonstrated an even higher ORR (57% vs 36%; $p = 0.03$) and PFS (13.8 months vs 7.6 months; HR 0.55; 95% CI, 0.46–0.64; $p = 0.005$). No improvement in OS was observed.

BCIRG 007 was a multicenter phase III clinical trial that evaluated the addition of carboplatin to docetaxel and trastuzumab in the first-line setting.[565] A total of 263 women with untreated HER2+ MBC were randomized to eight cycles of trastuzumab plus docetaxel 100 mg/m² iv every 3 weeks, or trastuzumab, carboplatin AUC 6 iv and docetaxel 75 mg/m² iv every 3 weeks, with maintenance trastuzumab thereafter. In comparison to the above study by Robert et al., no significant differences were appreciated in TTP, RR, OS, or toxicity. The lack of any benefit with the addition of carboplatin was thought in part because of use of a higher dose of docetaxel in the control arm. The addition of carboplatin to a taxane and trastuzumab has not become a standard first- or second-line regimen, due in large part to the development of additional HER2-directed agents, which have resulted in improved PFS and OS, as described below.

Few studies have compared trastuzumab monotherapy with trastuzumab plus chemotherapy. A phase III study of first-line trastuzumab and docetaxel versus trastuzumab monotherapy, followed by trastuzumab plus docetaxel at the time of progression resulted in a significant improvement in median PFS (HR 4.24; $p < 0.01$) and OS (HR 2.72; $p = 0.04$) with upfront combination therapy.[566] A majority of the 112 patients in this study had visceral metastases and multiple metastatic sites. A similar phase II study in 101 patients compared first-line docetaxel plus trastuzumab with single-agent trastuzumab, followed by single-agent docetaxel upon progression.[567] The two arms had similar PFS, but there was an improved RR and a statistically insignificant improvement in OS with the combination. This trial design does not reflect the current clinical practice of continuing trastuzumab together with chemotherapy after progression, the use of which was confirmed to improve outcome in the German Breast Group (GBG) 26 / BIG 03–05 study clinical trial, as designed below.

Before the FDA approvals of lapatinib and T-DM1, the optimal second-line therapy for patients who had progressed on first-line taxane plus trastuzumab was unknown. Some researchers theorized that progression was due to chemotherapy resistance, and that trastuzumab should therefore be continued at the time of progression.[568,569] The GBG 26/BIG 03-05 study was a phase III clinical trial that randomized patients with HER2+ MBC who had progressed on first-line taxane plus trastuzumab to receive second-line capecitabine plus continued trastuzumab versus capecitabine only.[570] GBG 26/BIG 03-05 closed early after accruing only a third of its target, in part due to the approval of lapatinib with capecitabine for the second-line setting. Despite this, continuation of trastuzumab with capecitabine rather than capecitabine only was associated with a statistically significant improvement in ORR (48.1% vs 27.0%; $p = 0.0115$) and TTP (8.2 months vs 5.6 months, $p = 0.0338$), although the numerical improvement in OS was not significant (24.9 months vs 20.6 months, $p = 0.73$) as the study was underpowered. Other attempts were made to study the continuation of trastuzumab after progression, but GBG 26/BIG 03-05 is the only prospective study to demonstrate its effectiveness.

Trastuzumab is either given with a loading dose of 4 mg/kg iv followed by 2 mg/kg iv weekly or with a loading dose of 8 mg/kg iv followed by 6 mg/kg iv every 3 weeks.[409] A subcutaneous formulation of trastuzumab was recently developed as a cost-effective alternative to the standard iv formulation.[571] The enHANced treatment with NeoAdjuvant Herceptin (HannaH), multinational, open-label, randomized phase III clinical trial has recently demonstrated that trastuzumab 600 mg subcutaneous (sc) every 3 weeks was noninferior to standard intravenous trastuzumab in the neoadjuvant setting with regard to pCR.[572] Participants on the subcutaneous arm suffered more frequent infections. The fixed-dose sc formulation of trastuzumab has been recently approved in the European Union as a patient-preferred alternative because of shorter administration times and less discomfort. An ongoing phase III clinical trial, Preference for Herceptin SC or IV Administration (PrefHER), evaluates both patient and physician preference as well as cost savings associated with the subcutaneous formulation (ClinicalTrials.gov Identifier, NCT01401166).

Beyond trastuzumab: additional HER2-directed therapies

Approximately 30–50% of patients with trastuzumab-naïve HER2+ MBC do not achieve an objective response to trastuzumab plus chemotherapy in the first-line setting, and subsequently experience shorter TTP (7–17 months) and OS (22–38 months).[557,560] Furthermore, acquired resistance to trastuzumab ultimately develops in all patients. Proposed mechanisms for de novo and acquired trastuzumab resistance include intrinsic molecular changes to HER2, upregulation of parallel compensatory signaling pathways, defects in antibody-dependent cellular cytotoxicity, and alterations in apoptosis.[573,574] An intense interest in the development of alternative approaches to block downstream effects of the HER2 pathway has led to significant improvements in outcomes, as outlined below.

Lapatinib for HER2+ breast cancer

Lapatinib is an oral, small-molecule TKI that targets the intracellular kinase domain of HER2 and is active against trastuzumab-resistant HER2-overexpressing breast cancer cells. The FDA approved lapatinib in combination with capecitabine in 2007 in the context of a phase III clinical trial of patients who had progressed on regimens containing a taxane plus trastuzumab. A total of 324 patients with HER2+ MBC were randomized to lapatinib 1250 mg po daily plus capecitabine 2500 mg/m^2 po daily (days 1–14 of a 21-day cycle) or capecitabine only.[402] A significant improvement in independently assessed PFS was observed on the lapatinib-containing arm in comparison to the control arm (8.4 months vs 4.4 months; HR 0.49; 95% CI, 0.34–0.71; $p < 0.001$). The final analysis demonstrated a survival advantage in the lapatinib-containing arm in comparison to the capecitabine arm (75.0 weeks vs 64.7 weeks).[575] No case of reduced LVEF or cardiomyopathy was observed. Diarrhea (60% vs 39%; $p \leq 0.001$) was more common in the combination arm than in the control arm, but most cases were grade 1 or 2, and rates of grade 3 diarrhea were similar (12% vs 11%). Fewer cases of CNS metastasis were observed in the lapatinib-containing arm (4 patients vs 11 patients), but this finding was not statistically significant.[402] From 2007 to 2012, lapatinib plus capecitabine was considered an appropriate second-line therapy for HER2+ MBC after progression on a taxane plus trastuzumab therapy.[576]

Preclinical studies have demonstrated synergy as well as lack of cross-resistance between lapatinib and trastuzumab. EGF104900 was a phase II clinical trial that randomized 296 patients with heavily pretreated HER2+ MBC to lapatinib plus trastuzumab or lapatinib only.[577] Participants had received a median of three prior trastuzumab-containing regimens. The combination of lapatinib plus trastuzumab was superior to lapatinib only with regard to PFS (HR 0.74; 95% CI, 0.58–0.94, $p = 0.011$), CBR, and OS (14.5 months vs 9.5 months; HR 0.74; 95% CI, 0.57–0.97; $p = 0.026$).[578] Rates of diarrhea were higher in the combination arm (60% vs 48%; $p = 0.03$) than in the lapatinib arm, but rates of grade 3 diarrhea were the same (7%).

NCIC CTG MA.31 was an international, open-label phase III clinical trial that randomized 652 women with treatment naïve HER2+ MBC to receive 24 weeks of a taxane in combination with either lapatinib or trastuzumab, followed by the same HER2-directed monotherapy.[579] The combination of lapatinib and a taxane was inferior with regard to both PFS (9.1 months vs 13.6 months; $p < 0.001$) and OS in comparison to trastuzumab and a taxane, providing clear evidence that trastuzumab is superior to lapatinib in the first-line setting.

HER2+ breast cancers exercise a tropism for the CNS. Unfortunately, trastuzumab cannot cross the blood–brain barrier. An estimated 10–15% of patients with HER2+ MBC develop brain metastasis after treatment with trastuzumab despite control of systemic disease. This high frequency of CNS metastases is likely due to multiple factors, but the extension of life through systemic control afforded by trastuzumab likely increases the likelihood that CNS metastases will become clinically apparent. As stated earlier, Geyer et al. reported a statistically insignificant trend of fewer cases of CNS metastasis with the combination of lapatinib plus capecitabine versus capecitabine only.[402] Several investigations have subsequently evaluated the ability of lapatinib to prevent or treat CNS metastasis.

Patients treated with single-agent lapatinib after receiving radiotherapy for progressive brain metastases achieved ORR of only 6%, but in combination with capecitabine ORR were more pronounced at 21–31.8%.[580–582] The phase II LANDSCAPE clinical trial treated patients with HER2+ untreated brain metastases with lapatinib plus capecitabine, and showed a CNS ORR of 65.9%, TTP of 5.5 months, and OS of 17.0 months.[583]

CEREBEL was a multicenter, open-label, phase III clinical trial designed to evaluate the effect of lapatinib plus capecitabine on the development of CNS metastasis as first site of progression.[584] A total of 540 patients with HER2+ MBC were randomized to lapatinib 1250 mg/mg daily plus capecitabine 2000 mg/m^2 twice a day (days 1–14 of a 21-day cycle) or every 3-week trastuzumab plus capecitabine 2500 mg/m^2 twice a day (days 1–14 of a 21-day cycle). The study was terminated early because of the absence of difference in the incidence of CNS metastases as first site of relapse with 3% on the lapatinib-containing arm and 5% on the trastuzumab-containing arm. Furthermore, patients on the trastuzumab-containing arm exhibited higher PFS (HR 1.30; 95% CI, 1.04–1.64) and OS (HR 1.34; 95% CI, 0.95–1.64).

Pertuzumab for HER2+ MBC

Pertuzumab, as described in the adjuvant section, is a humanized monoclonal antibody that prevents HER2 dimerization by binding a different epitope than trastuzumab.[585,586] The combination of pertuzumab and trastuzumab leads to a more comprehensive blockade of the HER2 signaling pathway, and strongly enhances antitumor activity in comparison to single-agent activity in preclinical studies.[587] A phase II clinical trial compared single-agent pertuzumab with the combination of pertuzumab and trastuzumab in patients with HER2+ MBC who had progressed on trastuzumab plus chemotherapy.[588] While pertuzumab only had minimal antitumor activity, the combination therapy resulted in a CBR of 50%, ORR of 24.2%, and PFS of 5.5 months with minimal additional toxicity.

The Clinical Evaluation of Pertuzumab and Trastuzumab (CLEOPATRA) study was an international, multicenter, clinical trial that led to the FDA approval of pertuzumab in combination with docetaxel and trastuzumab in 2012.[589] The study randomized

808 patients with HER2+ MBC and no prior treatment in the metastatic setting to receive trastuzumab plus docetaxel 75 mg/m^2 iv with either pertuzumab or placebo every 3 weeks. Pertuzumab was given with a loading dose of 840 mg followed by 420 mg every 3 weeks. Trastuzumab plus either pertuzumab or placebo were continued after discontinuation of chemotherapy in responding patients until tumor progression or death. Less than 50% of the participants had received treatment in the adjuvant setting and approximately 10% had received adjuvant trastuzumab.

The CLEOPATRA study demonstrated that the addition of pertuzumab led to a 6.3-month improvement in investigator-assessed PFS (18.7 months vs 12.4 months; HR 0.68; 95% CI, 0.51–0.75; $p < 0.001$) and 15.7-month improvement in OS (56.5 months vs 40.8 months; HR 0.68; 95% CI, 0.58–0.80; $p < 0.001$) in comparison to the control arm.[590] The ORR was 80.2% in the pertuzumab group and 69.3% in the control group.[591] The median number of docetaxel cycles per patient was eight in both the control group (1–41 cycles) and pertuzumab group (1–35 cycles). The addition of pertuzumab did not lead to increased rates of cardiac dysfunction, but was associated with more frequent diarrhea (66.8% vs 46.3%) and rash (33.7% vs 24.2%) than those in the control arm.

The incidence of CNS metastasis as first site of disease progression was similar between the pertuzumab and control groups (13.7% vs 12.66%).[589] However, the median time to development of CNS metastasis was prolonged in the pertuzumab group (15.0 months) compared with the control group (11.9 months; HR 0.58; 95% CI, 0.39–0.85; $p = 0.0049$). OS in patients with CNS metastases as the first site of disease progression was associated with a statistically insignificant trend in favor of the pertuzumab group (34.4 months vs 26.4 months).

Several predictive biomarkers were appreciated in the CLEOPATRA clinical trial. Elevated serum HER2 protein levels, serum HER2 and HER3 mRNA levels, and low-serum HER2 extracellular domain (sHER2) were associated with a significantly better prognosis ($p < 0.05$).[592] Patients with wild-type PIK3CA had a longer median PFS than those with mutant PIK3A in both the control (13.8 months vs 8.6 months) and pertuzumab groups (21.8 months vs 12.5 months).

Several ongoing clinical trials have been evaluating combinations of trastuzumab and pertuzumab with various chemotherapies in the settings of both ESBC and MBC. Details on these trials are available at http://www.cancer.gov/about-cancer/treatment/clinical-trials/search.

T-DM1 for HER2+ MBC

The novel antibody drug conjugate T-DM1 allows for intracellular delivery of the highly potent antimicrotubule cytotoxic agent emtansine directly to HER2+ breast cancer cells. T-DM1 was discussed in the adjuvant section, but originally investigated in the metastatic setting. In 2013, the FDA approved T-DM1 for use in patients with HER2+ MBC who had progressed after a trastuzumab-containing taxane regimen in the metastatic setting. The approval of T-DM1 was based on the EMILIA study, an international, multicenter, open-label phase III clinical trial that randomized 991 patients with HER2+ MBC to T-DM1 or lapatinib plus capecitabine, the standard option at that time for patients who had progressed on trastuzumab-based therapy.[593] Enrolled patients had progressed on trastuzumab and a taxane. T-DM1 resulted in a significantly improved median PFS (9.6 months vs 6.4 months; HR 0.65; 95% CI, 0.55–0.75; $p < 0.001$) and median OS (30.9 months vs 25.1 months; HR 0.68; 95% CI 0.55–0.85; $p < 0.001$) in comparison to lapatinib plus capecitabine. Furthermore, T-DM1 was better tolerated with lower overall toxicity. The most common grade 3–4

AEs with T-DM1 were thrombocytopenia (12.9%) and elevated transaminases (2.9–4.3%).

Additional evidence for the efficacy of T-DM1 was shown in TH3RESA, an international, randomized, open-label phase III clinical trial that evaluated T-DM1 in patients with HER2+ MBC who had progressed on two or more HER2-targeted regimens.[594] Participants of this study were heavily pretreated, with approximately 50% having four previous lines of chemotherapy for MBC. A total of 602 patients were randomized in a 2 : 1 ratio to T-DM1 or physician's treatment of choice. Treatment with T-DM1 was associated with a 2.9-month increase in median PFS over the control arm (6.2 months vs 3.3 months; HR 0.528; $p < 0.001$), as well as an increase in interim median (HR 0.552; $p = 0.0034$, efficacy stopping boundary not crossed). Safety results were similar to those in EMILIA.

The phase III MARIANNE clinical trial compared the use of single-agent T-DM1, T-DM1 plus pertuzumab, and trastuzumab with chemotherapy in the first-line setting for HER2+ MBC.[595,596] The study was designed before the approval of pertuzumab plus trastuzumab in combination with docetaxel and therefore did not include the current first-line standard of care for HER2+ MBC. Approximately 31% of the enrolled patients had received neoadjuvant or adjuvant HER2-directed therapy, while 37% were treatment naive in the context of de novo HER2+ MBC. Initial results were presented at ASCO 2015, and although the TDM-1-containing arms were noninferior in PFS (HR 0.91; 97.5% CI, 0.73–1.13; $p = 0.31$) in comparison to trastuzumab plus chemotherapy, they failed to demonstrate superiority in PFS.

Treatment recommendations for HER2+ MBC

The optimal sequence of all known HER2-directed therapies is unknown. The available chemotherapy regimens in combination with HER2-directed therapies for HER2+ MBC are listed in Table 15. Results of CLEOPATRA, EMILIA, and TH3RESA were used to generate the most recent guidelines published by ABC2, ASCO, and NCCN.[409,458,464] In general, the combination of trastuzumab, pertuzumab, and a taxane is the preferred first-line treatment option for HER2+ MBC. A common and appropriate clinical practice is to discontinue the taxane, while continuing the biologic therapy after completion of eight cycles of this first-line regimen. T-DM1 is the preferred second-line treatment (in comparison to lapatinib plus capecitabine), and is also preferred for a later cycle (in comparison to treatment of physician's choice) if not provided in the second-line setting. Use of pertuzumab beyond its combination with trastuzumab and chemotherapy in the first line is not supported; however, if a patient has not received pertuzumab, it can be used beyond the first-line.

Almost 50% of patients with HER2+ breast cancer also have HR+ disease, which is associated with biologic characteristics that confer a relative resistance to endocrine therapy in comparison to HR−/HER2+ disease. Patients with HR+/HER2+ disease are generally classified as the luminal B intrinsic subtype group.[313] Preclinical and clinical trials have demonstrated that resistance to hormone-based therapies in part can be overcome by HER2-directed therapy, suggesting a cross talk between the ER and HER2 pathways. Patients with nonvisceral, indolent disease, and comorbidities that limit chemotherapy options are appropriate candidates for combined hormone therapy and HER2-targeted agent.[458]

The phase III Trastuzumab and Anastrozole Directed Against ER+ HER2+ Mammary Carcinoma (TAnDEM) clinical trial randomized 207 postmenopausal women with HR+/HER2+ MBC to anastrozole with or without trastuzumab.[597] Patients on the trastuzumab-containing arm were found to have a significant improvement in PFS in comparison to the anastrozole arm (4.8 months vs 2.4 months; HR 0.63; 95% CI, 0.47–0.84; $p = 0.0016$), but no difference in OS. The international, open-label, phase III eLEcTRA clinical trial randomized postmenopausal women with HR+/HER2+ MBC to letrozole only or letrozole plus trastuzumab in the first-line setting.[598] The study closed early after enrolling only 57 out of a planned 370 patients because of poor accrual. The median TTP was shorter in the letrozole arm than in the combination arm (3.3 months vs 14.1 months (HR 0.67; $p = 0.23$), with a reduced CBR (39% vs 65%; odds ratio; 95% CI, 1.01–8.84). Although not statistically significant, these findings are similar to those in the TAnDEM clinical trial. Although chemotherapy in combination with HER2-targeting agents is generally selected for most patients with HR+/HER2+ MBC, those patients who receive endocrine therapy over chemotherapy should receive it in combination with HER2-targeting agents given the PFS benefit showed in the TAnDEM clinical trial.[458]

Somatic mutations of HER2 in HER2− breast cancer

Cancer genome sequencing studies have demonstrated the presence of HER2 somatic mutations in patients with HER2− breast cancer. A study by Bose et al. evaluated 25 such patients and identified 13 activating mutations that presumptively drive oncogenic transformation.[599] Breast cancer cells bearing these activating mutations treated with neratinib were potently inhibited. An ongoing multicenter phase II clinical trial has been currently evaluating the use of neratinib in patients with solid tumors and HER2 somatic mutations (ClinicalTrials.gov Identifier NCT01953926). A second, ongoing phase II clinical trial evaluates the use of neratinib with or without fulvestrant in patients with HER2− MBC and HER2 somatic mutations (ClinicalTrials.gov Identifier NCT01670877).

HER2-directed therapy in combination with targeted drugs

As described earlier, bevacizumab has been evaluated in combination with hormone therapy to reverse hormone resistance in HR+ MBC and also in combination with chemotherapy, but remains unapproved for breast cancer in the United States. VEGF is upregulated in HER2-overexpressing breast cancer cells, and antiangiogenic agents are also of great interest in HER2+ MBC. The combination of bevacizumab, trastuzumab, and capecitabine was associated with an ORR of 73% and PFS of 14.4 months in a small, phase II clinical trial. The phase III AVEREL clinical trial randomized 424 patients with HER2+ MBC to docetaxel plus trastuzumab with or without bevacizumab in the first-line setting.[600] An independent assessment demonstrated a statistically insignificant clinical benefit with the addition of bevacizumab, with PFS in the control arm versus bevacizumab-containing arm (13.9 months vs 16.5 months; HR 0.0162) that failed to meet the protocol-specified primary end point. No unexpected AE occurred with the combination of trastuzumab and bevacizumab. Interestingly, higher concentrations of plasma VEGF-A were associated with poorer outcome, but also a larger bevacizumab treatment effect.

Trastuzumab resistance is associated with loss of the tumor suppressor gene PTEN, alterations in the PI3K pathway, and increased activation of mTOR.[601,602] Several phase III clinical trials have investigated the use of the mTOR inhibitor everolimus in combination with chemotherapy for HER2+ MBC, but failed to demonstrate a benefit. In the BOLERO-3 clinical trial, 569 women with HER2+ MBC were randomized to receive everolimus 5 mg/daily or placebo, with all participants receiving weekly vinorelbine plus trastuzumab.[603] Patients who recurred during or within 12 months of adjuvant trastuzumab or progressed during or within 4 weeks of trastuzumab in the MBC setting were considered trastuzumab-resistant. PFS was modestly prolonged at 7 months in the everolimus arm compared with 5.78 months in the control arm (HR 0.78; 95% CI, 0.65–0.95; $p = 0.0067$), and OS has not yet been reported. Subgroup analyses demonstrated more benefit from everolimus in patients <65 years and with nonvisceral HR−/HER2+ MBC. As experienced in other trials and in clinical practice, everolimus was associated with significant toxicity. An exploratory analysis of archived tumor tissue showed significant benefit derived from the addition of everolimus in patients with a low PTEN concentration than in those with a high PTEN concentration (HR 0.40; 95% CI, 0.20–0.82; p-interaction = 0.01), and in patients with a high pS6 concentration than in those with low pS6 concentration (HR 0.48; 95% CI, 0.24–0.96; p-interaction = 0.04). PIK3CA mutations did not seem to predict benefit (HR 0.65; 95% CI, 0.21–1.45; p-interaction = 0.32).

Everolimus was also evaluated as a first-line treatment for HER2+ MBC in the phase III BOLERO-1 clinical trial that randomized 719 treatment naïve patients in a 2 : 1 ratio to paclitaxel plus trastuzumab with either everolimus 10 mg daily or placebo.[604] Initial results were presented at SABCS 2014 by Hurvitz et al., which showed no improvement in PFS (14.95 months vs 14.49 months; HR 0.89, 95% CI, 0.73–1.08; $p = 0.1166$). The PFS of participants with HR−/HER2+ on the everolimus-containing arm was notable, but it failed to meet prespecified significance as designated by protocol. The safety profile was similar to that reported in BOLERO-3 and other everolimus-based trials. With the combined data from BOLERO-3 and -1, everolimus does not play any therapeutic role in the treatment of HER2+ MBC.

Novel targeted agents in HER2+ MBC

MM-302 is a pegylated liposomal antibody–drug conjugate that delivers doxorubicin particularly to HER2+ breast cancer cells and thereby limits exposure of healthy tissues to chemotherapy. A phase I clinical trial demonstrated both the safety and antitumor activity of MM-302 in combination with trastuzumab in HER2+ MBC.[605] HERMIONE is an ongoing, international, multicenter, open-label, randomized phase II clinical trial that evaluates the effectiveness of MM-302 30 mg/m² iv every 3 weeks plus trastuzumab in comparison to physician's choice of chemotherapy (e.g., vinorelbine, capecitabine, or gemcitabine) plus trastuzumab in patients with anthracycline naïve HER2+ MBC that have progressed on pertuzumab and T-DM1 (ClinicalTrials.gov identifier NCT02213744).[606] Margetuximab is a chimeric monoclonal antibody similar to trastuzumab with an Fc fragment engineered to promote increased binding to CD16A and subsequently preserve the antiproliferative effects of trastuzumab. Preclinical studies demonstrated superiority of margetuximab over trastuzumab, and a phase I trial revealed that margetuximab was well tolerated. An active phase II trial evaluates margetuximab in patients with MBC with HER2 equivocal by IHC and negative by FISH (ClinicalTrials.gov Identifier NCT01838021). A planned phase III clinical trial SOPHIA aims to randomize 528 patients with HER2+ MBC who have progressed on trastuzumab, pertuzumab, and T-DM1 to receive chemotherapy with either margetuximab or trastuzumab (ClinicalTrials.gov Identifier NCT02492711). These and other investigational HER2-directed drugs are presented in Table 14.

ONT-380, previously known as ARRY-380, is an orally active, reversible, and selective small molecule HER2 inhibitor. There are two ongoing phase Ib trials with ONT-380 in patients with HER2+

MBC. The first trial is designed to evaluate ONT-380 in combination with T-DM1 in patients previously treated with a taxane and trastuzumab (ClinicalTrials.gov Identifier NCT01983501). The second trial is designed to evaluate ONT-380 in combination with capecitabine and/or trastuzumab in patients previously treated with trastuzumab and T-DM1 (ClinicalTrials.gov Identifier NCT02025192). Interim analyses of both studies demonstrated that ONT-380 was well tolerated and provided clinical benefit.[607,608]

Many small-molecule TKI have been evaluated in the setting of MBC. Neratinib, a potent irreversible TKI of HER1, 2, and 4 described in the adjuvant section, overcame trastuzumab resistance in HER2+ breast cancer cells in preclinical studies. A phase I clinical trial evaluated neratinib in combination with weekly paclitaxel and trastuzumab in patients with HER2+ MBC previously treated with HER2-directed therapy and a taxane demonstrated an ORR of 38%, CBR of 52%, and PFS of 3.7 months.[405] A phase II clinical trial failed to demonstrate superiority of neratinib monotherapy over lapatinib plus capecitabine in patients with HER2+ MBC, who were treated with at least two prior trastuzumab-containing regimens.[609] A multinational, open-label, phase I/II clinical trial evaluated the safety and efficacy of neratinib in combination with capecitabine in patients with trastuzumab-pretreated HER2+ MBC.[610] The ORR was 64% in lapatinib-naive patients and 57% in patients with prior lapatinib exposure, and median PFS was 40.3 and 35.9 weeks, respectively. The most common toxicities were diarrhea (88%) and hand-foot syndrome (48%). In the ongoing phase II NEfERTT clinical trial, 479 patients with HER2+ MBC were randomized to first-line paclitaxel with either neratinib or trastuzumab (ClinicalTrials.gov Identifier NCT00915018). A press release in November 2014 reported similar PFS between the two treatment arms, but fewer brain metastases in those treated with neratinib versus trastuzumab (7.4% vs 15.6%; $p = 0.006$).[611] Toxicity was increased with neratinib, with grade 3 diarrhea experienced in 30% and 4% of patients receiving neratinib and trastuzumab, respectively. The NEfERTT clinical trial did not use prophylactic antidiarrheal therapy, and several trials have reported a marked reduction in diarrhea with the use of prophylaxis. The ongoing phase III NALA study aims to randomize 600 patients with HER2+ MBC who have progressed on ≥2 HER2-directed regimens in the metastatic setting to neratinib plus capecitabine versus lapatinib plus capecitabine (ClinicalTrials.gov Identifier NCT01808573).

A phase I clinical trial evaluates the combination of the alpha-selective PI3K inhibitor alpelisib (BYL719) in combination with T-DM1 in patients with HER2+ MBC, who have progressed on prior trastuzumab- and taxane-based treatment (ClinicalTrials.gov identifier NCT02038010). A phase Ib clinical trial currently evaluates the PI3K inhibitor taselisib (GDC-0032) in combination with several currently approved HER2-directed therapies (ClinicalTrials.gov identifier NCT02390427). A class I pan-PI3K inhibitor pilaralisib (SAR245408) will be combined with trastuzumab and paclitaxel in a phase I/II clinical trial of patients with trastuzumab refractory HER2+ MBC.[612]

Systemic therapies for triple-negative MBC

Chemotherapy remains the mainstay of treatment for all stages of TNBC. As described in the neoadjuvant section, TNBC is quite sensitive to anthracyclines and taxanes. Several clinical trials evaluating the addition of carboplatin to standard chemotherapy in the neoadjuvant setting have showed pCR rates of 22–53% in TNBC.[416,613] Long-term outcomes of PFS and OS are not yet available, however, and platinum agents are not yet the standard of care for early-stage TNBC.

Platinum agents have also been evaluated in the setting of metastatic TNBC, with initial results from the first phase III clinical trial comparing first-line carboplatin to docetaxel reported at SABCS 2014.[614] The multicenter TNT study randomized 376 women with untreated metastatic TNBC to carboplatin AUC 6 iv every 3 weeks or docetaxel 100 mg/m² iv every 3 weeks with an option for crossover at the time of progression. At a median follow-up of 11 months, the ORR and PFS rates were similar in both groups. A prespecified subgroup analysis of the 43 trial participants with germline BRCA1/2 mutations demonstrated a statistically significant increase in ORR in the carboplatin arm compared with the docetaxel arm (68% vs 33%; $p = 0.03$).

Primary tumor samples from participants in the TNT study were analyzed for homologous recombination deficiency (HRD) with an HRD Assay developed by Myriad Genetics.[615] Patients with germline or somatic BRCA mutations tended to have high HRD scores. No significant difference in PFS or OS was observed between the two treatment arms in patients with high HRD scores, or in those with low HRD scores.

Approximately 75% and 50% of BRCA1/2-associated breast cancers, respectively, are triple-negative. BRCA1/2 are tumor suppressor genes with products that play key roles in the repair of double-stranded DNA breaks through homologous recombination. When the remaining wild-type BRCA allele in a tumor precursor cell is lost in patients with a germline BRCA1/2 mutation, genomic instability ensues because of reduced efficiency of HR. This impaired DNA repair mechanism is thought to confer increased sensitivity to platinum agent, as shown in the TNT trial.

Poly(adenosine diphosphate-ribose) polymerase (PARP) recognizes and repairs single-stranded DNA breaks through base excision repair. PARP inhibitors prevent the repair of single-stranded DNA and are highly selective for BRCA-mutant tumor cells. While a single mutated gene product may be compatible with cell viability, additional mutations in related genes are more likely to lead to cell death. This concept of synthetic lethality is a critical genetic concept that has directed the evaluation of PARP inhibitors for the treatment of BRCA-associated and BRCA-like TNBC.

Proof of the activity of PARP in BRCA-associated cancers was demonstrated in an international, multicenter, phase II clinical trial that treated 54 women with BRCA-associated MBC and at least one prior chemotherapy regimen with single-agent olaparib.[616] An RR of 41% and median PFS of 5.7 months were achieved when participants received olaparib 400 mg twice daily. A phase I clinical trial currently evaluates the combinations of olaparib with either buparlisib (BKM120, a novel class I pan-PI3K inhibitor) or alpelisib (BYL719, a novel alpha-selective PI3K inhibitor), in patients with TN MBC (ClinicalTrials.gov Identifier NCT01623349).

Several other PARP inhibitors are under investigation as monotherapy or in combination with other targeted therapies or chemotherapy, including veliparib (ABT-888), talazoparib (BMN-673), iniparib, niraparib, and rucaparib. A phase 1 dose escalation study of the PARP inhibitor veliparib (ABT-888) in combination with carboplatin in patients with metastatic TNBC or a germline BRCA1/2 mutation in HER2− MBC is ongoing (ClinicalTrials.gov Identifier NCT01251874). A phase III clinical trial of carboplatin and paclitaxel in combination with veliparib (ABT-888) or placebo in patients with BRCA-associated HER2− MBC is ongoing (ClinicalTrials.gov Identifier NCT02163694). The study aims to enroll 270 patients with an estimated primary completion date of January 2017.

Preclinical studies of talazoparib have demonstrated that this PARP inhibitor has much higher potency that other class members.[613] The phase II ABRAZO clinical trial evaluates talazoparib in patients with BRCA1/2 mutations and MBC who have either progressed more than 8 weeks after their last platinum agent dose or who have received more than two regimens in the metastatic setting, but no platinum agents (ClinicalTrials.gov identifier NCT020234916). The international, multicenter, phase III EMBRACA clinical trial evaluates single-agent talazoparib in patients with germline BRCA mutations and locally advanced or MBC.[617] A planned 429 patients with no more than two prior chemotherapy regimens in the metastatic setting will be randomized 2 : 1 to talazoparib 1.0 mg daily in 21-day cycles or physician's choice treatment (capecitabine, eribulin, gemcitabine, or vinorelbine) with a primary end point of PFS. Talazoparib Beyond BRCA (TBB) is a single-arm phase II clinical trial evaluating talazoparib in patients with metastatic TNBC who are BRCA1/2 wild-type, but with a HRD as determined by the HRD assay developed by Myriad® (ClinicalTrials.gov identifier NCT02401347).

Recent clinical trials in metastatic TNBC

Approximately 10–32% of TNBC express the AR, and agents that block AR signaling are under active investigation in the setting of MBC.[314] Monotherapy with the nonsteroidal antiandrogen bicalutamide was evaluated in a phase II clinical trial of patients with AR positive (AR+)/HR− MBC.[618] Out of 424 patients with HR− MBC screened, 12% were deemed to have AR+ tumors with >10% AR+ by IHC. The 6-month CBR was 19% (95% CI, 7–39) and median PFS was 12 weeks (95% CI, 11–22), clearly demonstrating proof of principle. Traina et al. reported the results of an open-label phase II clinical trial evaluating single-agent enzalutamide, a potent AR inhibitor, in patients with AR+ metastatic TNBC at ASCO 2015.[619] Out of 404 patients screened for AR positivity by IHC, 79% had AR > 0% and 55% had AR ≥ 10% by IHC. A total of 118 patients were treated with enzalutamide 160 mg daily. Gene profiling was used to develop an androgen-related gene signature, and patients with the signature had a superior median PFS (32 weeks) to those without the signature (9 weeks). An ongoing phase Ib/II clinical trial is evaluating the effect of the PI3K inhibitor taselisib (GDC-0032) in combination with enzalutamide in patients with metastatic AR+ TNBC (ClinicalTrials.gov identifier NCT02457910). These and other investigational agents are listed in Table 14.

The reversal of immune tolerance in MBC through immunotherapy has attracted research attention recently. Immune tolerance to tumor cells can occur through engagement of tumor surface ligands, such as programmed cell death ligand 1 (PD-L1), with inhibitory receptors of anti-tumor T-cells, such as programmed cell death protein 1 (PD-1) and B7.[620,621] PD-L1 is expressed in approximately 20% of TNBC, significantly higher than in other types of breast cancer.[622] Preclinical studies of monoclonal antibodies against PD-L1 and PD-1 have demonstrated restoration of tumor-specific T-cell immunity, particularly in the metastatic TNBC setting. Initial results of two phase 1b expansion studies of anti-PD-1 and anti-PD-L1 antibodies were reported at SABCS 2014. Single-agent treatment with the highly selective anti-PD-1 antibody pembrolizumab (MK-3475) was evaluated in 32 heavily pretreated women with TN MBC, 58% of whom expressed PD-L1.[623] Disease stabilization was appreciated in 25.9% of patients, and disease response in 18.5%. The anti-PD-L1 antibody atezolizumab (MPDL3280A) was evaluated in 21 patients with heavily pretreated, PD-L1-positive metastatic TNBC, of whom 19% had an ORR, including two complete responses and two partial responses. The 24-week PFS was 27% (95% CI, 7–47).[624]

Many novel agents are under investigation in the setting of metastatic TNBC, including macrophage inhibitors, biologics, and FGFR inhibitors (Table 14). PLX3397 is a novel oral tyrosine kinase inhibitor that potently inhibits CSF-1 receptor kinase, which plays a key role in the regulation of tumor-associated macrophages. A phase Ib/II clinical trial of PLX3397 in combination with eribulin in patients with metastatic TNBC is ongoing (ClinicalTrials.gov Identifier NCT01596751). CDX-011 (glembatumumab vedotin) is an antibody–drug conjugate that binds to glycoprotein (gp) NMB. The phase II METRIC clinical trial aims to randomize 300 patients with gpNMB overexpressing TN MBC to CDX-011 or capecitabine to assess the safety and efficacy of CDX-011 (ClinicalTrials.gov Identifier NCT01997333). Approximately 25% of breast cancers have aberrant FGF signaling.[625] Lucitanib is a novel oral inhibitor of fibroblast FGF receptors 1 and 2 and VEGFR1-3 with activity against breast cancer cells in preclinical studies. Lucitanib monotherapy in patients with FGF-aberrant MBC was associated with an ORR of 50% in a phase I clinical trial. A dose-finding phase II clinical trial with a similar design is currently underway in patients with FGF-aberrant MBC, including those with TNBC.[626]

Management of CNS metastasis in MBC

Overall, CNS metastases occur in a small percentage of patients with MBC, but in metastatic TNBC and HER2+ MBC, the incidence is significant at 30–45%.[627–630] The management of parenchymal brain metastases often involves a coordinated effort between neurosurgeons, radiation oncologists, and medical oncologists. Patients with a single or limited number of potentially resectable brain metastases should be treated with surgery or radiosurgery. Leptomeningeal carcinomatosis is a overwhelming complication of MBC and often heralds the final stages of a patient's cancer. Treatment for leptomeningeal carcinomatosis may include intrathecal chemotherapy, radiation, and supportive care. As stated earlier, the incidence of brain metastases in patients with HER2+ BC treated with trastuzumab has increased over the last two decades. This trend is most likely due to an overall improvement in OS in patients treated with trastuzumab, and the failure of trastuzumab to penetrate the CNS.[651] As stated earlier, lapatinib showed a statistically insignificant trend toward decreased development of CNS metastases as the first site of progression.[402] Lapatinib, neratinib, and other therapies targeted toward CNS metastases are under evaluation.

Liver-targeted therapy in MBC

No prospective randomized clinical trial data, including PFS and OS, exist for the focal management of liver lesions. However, many locoregional techniques exist. Local therapy of liver metastases should only be attempted in highly selected patients after a thorough discussion with a multidisciplinary tumor board.[458]

Bone-targeted therapies in MBC

Bone is the most common site of metastasis with up to 80% of patients with MBC developing osseous metastases during their clinical course. Osseous metastases are the most frequent source of morbidity and disability related to breast cancer with complications of pain, fracture, spinal cord compression, and hypercalcemia. Bone-targeted agents are an important aspect of systemic management alongside antineoplastic therapy, whereas localized treatment with radiation or surgery can be used for more acute management of impending or active fractures. Orthopedic assessment of metastatic lesions in major weight-bearing sites (e.g., hips, femora, humera, and shoulders) is recommended to prevent pathological fractures that would lead to disability or death. Radiotherapy to painful sites of bone metastasis or impending fracture sites in weight-bearing bones is commonly used in association with systemic treatments.

Bone-modifying therapy should start at the first evidence of osteolytic bone metastases. Bisphosphonates are effective inhibitors of osteoclast activation. In several phase III clinical trials, the bisphosphonate zoledronic acid was found to reduce the risk of a skeletal-related event (SRE), mean time to SRE, and annual skeletal morbidity in comparison to pamidronate as well as placebo.[631,632] In a large phase III trial, denosumab significantly delayed time to first and subsequent SRE compared with zoledronic acid; there were no differences in OS, DFS, and serious AEs.[633] Denosumab causes more hypocalcemia and is more costly but is associated with a quicker administration time, fewer acute-phase reactions, and fewer renal side effects. The two classes of agents appear to have similar rates of osteonecrosis of the jaw.

Special topics

Contralateral prophylactic mastectomy

Patients with unilateral breast cancer treated with mastectomy often consider undergoing contralateral prophylactic mastectomy to decrease the risk of contralateral breast cancer. Several large institutional and geographic studies of patients with unilateral breast cancer treated with mastectomy in the United States have demonstrated an increase in contralateral prophylactic mastectomy over the past two decades.[374,634-636] This has not been associated with a decrease in breast cancer mortality. However, in patients who have a high risk of developing contralateral breast cancer, such as those with BRCA1/2 mutations, contralateral prophylactic mastectomy has improved long-term survival and is cost-effective.[637-639] Younger age and family history have been associated with higher risks of contralateral breast cancer, and there are emerging data that this may be due to polygenic causes.[640]

Factors that have been associated with the pursuit of contralateral prophylactic mastectomy include patient age <50 years, Caucasian race, a family history of breast cancer, BRCA mutation testing, invasive lobular histology, preoperative MRI, breast reconstruction, and treatment at an NCI-designated cancer center.[634,641-643] Together with the increase in contralateral prophylactic mastectomy over the past 15 years, mastectomy techniques that spare the nipple–areola complex (NAC) skin, such as nipple-sparing mastectomy (NSM) and TSSM that require immediate breast reconstruction, have been increasingly used[229,644-648]

Many studies have demonstrated an increased risk of contralateral breast cancer in patients with BRCA1/2 mutations, and contralateral prophylactic mastectomy improves long-term survival in these patients.[637,638,642,649,650] In a study comparing BRCA1/2-negative families and BRCA1/2-positive families, the 25-year risk of contralateral breast cancer was 44.1% for BRCA1 mutations, 33.5% for BRCA2 mutations, and 17.2% for no mutations identified.[651]

A recent study evaluating the pursuit of contralateral prophylactic mastectomy in patients with access to TSSM and immediate breast reconstruction showed an increasing percentage of patients who underwent contralateral prophylactic mastectomy between 2006 and 2013, which is consistent with prior reports.[374,634,635,642] In this study, 50% of patients underwent contralateral prophylactic mastectomy: 45% of patients without known deleterious mutations and 100% with deleterious mutations. These proportions are significantly higher than that previously reported.[374,635,642] This is likely due to the inherent selection biases of having patients who were mostly Caucasian, relatively young, and treated at an NCI-designated cancer center with access to surgeons who performed TSSM with immediate breast reconstruction.[642,643]

The range of patients who test negative for genetic mutations but still undergo contralateral prophylactic mastectomy (in women who elect mastectomy) is 27–58%.[642,652,653] Within this group, there is an increasing trend of contralateral prophylactic mastectomy related to younger patient age, younger age of relatives diagnosed with breast or ovarian cancer, and increasing number of family members with breast or ovarian cancer. Previous studies have reported that increasing number of relatives with breast cancer is correlated with an increasing risk of contralateral prophylactic mastectomy in BRCA1/2-positive families[654] In patients from BRCA1/2-negative families, the 25-year risk of contralateral breast cancer was 28.4% for those who were younger than 40 years at their first breast cancer diagnosis, which approaches 33.5% observed in patients with BRCA2 mutations.[649] These findings suggest that patients diagnosed at younger ages or with strong family histories may perceive an increased risk of contralateral breast cancer that could not be measured. There is evidence that a polygenic risk score may assess inherited risk of contralateral breast cancer and identify patients who have risks of contralateral breast cancer equivalent to BRCA carriers.[640] The choice of contralateral prophylactic mastectomy is made more frequently in patients with risk factors for contralateral breast cancer and in those with tumors of lower pathologic stages[651] suggests that women with tumors of higher pathologic stage may be concerned about the higher risk of ipsilateral recurrence compared with the development of contralateral breast cancer. Examination of the pathology of prophylactic mastectomy specimens shows that only 2.2–4.7% of them exhibited pathologic abnormalities, including DCIS, LCIS, and mucinous carcinoma.[651,655,656]

However, women should know that additional contralateral prophylactic mastectomy procedures may lead to a small but increased risk of postoperative complications in patients. Contralateral prophylactic mastectomy was associated with double the risk of superficial nipple necrosis and implant exposure. It was also associated with increased risks of wound breakdown and infections requiring oral antibiotics, but these RR estimates were <2. Contralateral prophylactic mastectomy was not associated with an increased risk of implant loss in patients who had implant-based reconstruction. These results are consistent with other studies which have found that contralateral prophylactic mastectomy increases complications by 1.5–2.1 times compared with unilateral mastectomy.[657-660]

Several studies have demonstrated that patients who feel the benefits of reducing the risk of contralateral breast cancer, decreased screening, and better aesthetic results after reconstruction may outweigh the increased risk of postoperative complications with contralateral prophylactic mastectomy, even in the absence of any data that it will reduce mortality. Those who chose contralateral prophylactic mastectomy have expressed a subjective fear of developing cancer, have a family history of breast cancer, and/or wish to maintain or improve breast cosmesis.[661-665] Their subjective sense of vulnerability may be much higher than their actual risk of contralateral breast cancer.[666] Some European authors have suggested that an increased fear of cancer and the acceptability of plastic surgery have contributed to the rising use of contralateral prophylactic mastectomy in the United States.[667] A patient-reported outcome study showed that those who underwent contralateral prophylactic mastectomy had higher satisfaction with their breasts and overall reconstructive outcomes than those who did not have contralateral prophylactic mastectomy.[668]

Management of isolated locoregional recurrence

If an isolated chest wall or regional lymph node recurrence is detected, biopsy confirmation and surgical resection are recommended. If not irradiated earlier, radiotherapy to the chest wall and involved regional lymph node-bearing area is indicated, and hormone therapy should be used for HR+ disease. An open-label trial (the CALOR trial) randomized patients with surgically resected locoregional recurrence with or without chemotherapy.[455] Patients with HR+ disease received adjuvant endocrine therapy, and radiation was required for microscopically involved surgical margins. The trial included only 162 patients, but at a median follow-up of 4.9 years, DFS events were significantly less frequent in those receiving chemotherapy compared with those who did not (28% vs 44%). Chemotherapy was significantly more effective in those with HR− disease, but the numbers are too small to draw a definitive conclusion.

On the basis of these data, patients with locoregional recurrence should receive available treatments based on disease subtype and prior therapy, including radiation therapy, hormone therapy, and chemotherapy.

Breast cancer in pregnancy

Approximately 1–2% of women with breast cancer are pregnant at the time of diagnosis, at an average age of 35 years. Nonpregnant breast cancer patients with an equivalent stage of disease as a pregnant patient have similar prognoses. Unfortunately, diagnosis is often delayed in pregnant patients because of physical examination changes associated with pregnancy, and their prognosis is often worse due to a higher stage at diagnosis.[669]

In general, radiographic assessments should be performed only when results would modify disease management.[670] Ultrasound is often the initial imaging study performed in a pregnant woman.[671] Mammography is not contraindicated and radiation exposure to the fetus is minimal, but abdominal shielding is recommended. Sensitivity of a mammogram in a pregnant or lactating patient is reduced, however, because of increased breast density in pregnancy. MRI with contrast is contraindicated as no data exist with regard to the effect of gadolinium on the fetus.[672]

Treatment recommendations for the management of breast cancer in pregnancy must be based on detailed discussions between the patient's surgeon, medical oncologist, and obstetrician. Furthermore, a patient's belief and value system must be considered. Treatment options for women who develop breast cancer during their pregnancy are similar to those options available to nonpregnant patients. However, the timing and sequence of treatment depends on the trimester of pregnancy at diagnosis as well as whether the disease is locally advanced or not.[670] Although rarely warranted, pregnancy termination should be considered, particularly when diagnosed in the first trimester. If diagnosis of a low-risk breast cancer occurs late in pregnancy, it is generally appropriate to delay treatment until after delivery. Mastectomy is appropriate at any point during pregnancy with minimal risk to the fetus, whereas radiation therapy is clearly contraindicated and delayed until after delivery.[673–675]

Chemotherapy can cause teratogenesis and must be avoided in the first trimester. A single prospective and several retrospective clinical trials have evaluated the use of chemotherapy in pregnancy, and a consensus is that doxorubicin-based therapy is appropriate in the second and third trimesters with minimal maternal, fetal, or neonatal toxicity.[676–679] A retrospective study in 2012 demonstrated no significant differences in birth weight, gestational anomalies, or neutropenia in patients receiving every 3-week doxorubicin and cyclophosphamide (AC) or dose-dense AC with pegfilgrastim,[680] and other studies have demonstrated similar findings. Insufficient data exist to support the use of other chemotherapies or biologics, whereas tamoxifen is clearly associated with miscarriage and congenital malformations.

Male breast cancer

The most common presenting symptoms of male breast cancer include breast mass, bloody nipple discharge, nipple retraction, axillary mass, and local or distant pain. Male patients often present with more advanced disease because of the lack of awareness of the diagnosis. Evaluation and diagnosis are similar to that performed in women. Most men with early-stage disease are treated with simple mastectomy and SLND, and those with locally advanced disease should first be offered neoadjuvant therapy. Adjuvant radiation follows the same practice patterns as those for women.

Because of the rarity of breast cancer in men, no randomized clinical trial of systemic therapy specific to men with breast cancer has been performed. Adjuvant therapy options for male breast cancer are similar to those for women. A retrospective study by Giordano et al. in 2005 reported the outcomes of 156 men with breast cancer treated at a single institution.[681] A total of 135 men had ESBC and 85% of the study population had HR+ disease. OS was significantly higher in those who received hormone-based therapy (HR 0.45, 0.01). Tamoxifen is preferred over AI. A retrospective analysis of hormonal therapy in 257 men with ESBC demonstrated a higher risk of death with AI over tamoxifen (HR 1.55, 95% CI 1.13–2.13, $p = 0.007$). Poor adherence to tamoxifen is common in men and clearly associated with worse 10-year rates of DFS (42% vs 80%, $p = 0.007$) and OS (50% vs 80%, $p = 0.008$) in comparison to high adherence.[682]

Retrospective studies have demonstrated a response rate of up to 80% in male patients with HR+ breast cancer. Experience with other hormone-based therapies as well as newer targeted therapies is quite limited. In general, chemotherapy has similar efficacy in men as women with MBC.

Inflammatory breast cancer

IBC is an aggressive, locally advanced form of breast cancer that constitutes up to 2% of newly diagnosed breast cancers in the United States. The prognosis of patients with IBC is poor and before the advent of systemic chemotherapy, the 5-year survival rate after optimal locoregional therapy was <5%.[683] Although multidisciplinary approaches have improved outcomes, a population-based study using SEER data from 2004 to 2007 demonstrated that patients with IBC have a 43% increased risk of death from breast cancer than locally advanced non-IBC (HR 1.43; 95% CI 1.10–1.86, $p = 0.008$).[684]

IBC is a clinical diagnosis characterized by a physical examination notable for erythema and edema (peau d'orange) involving at least one-third of the skin of the breast and present for no longer than 6 months.[685] Dermal lymphatic involvement is not necessary to support the diagnosis, and a core biopsy of the breast generally provided a definitive diagnosis. A palpable underlying mass is frequently absent, and IBC is often mistaken as mastitis and treated with antibiotics.

The standard approach to IBC is neoadjuvant chemotherapy, and the use of regimens containing both anthracyclines and taxanes is recommended.[409,683] Patients with HER2+ IBC should be administered neoadjuvant regimens identical to their HER2+ non-IBC counterparts. Most cases of IBC respond dramatically to chemotherapy, and >90% of patients are generally rendered free of locoregional disease. Locoregional treatment after neoadjuvant chemotherapy should include both mastectomy and radiation therapy. Some centers have used breast-conserving surgery after a complete response to neoadjuvant chemotherapy, but this practice pattern is not recommended by international consensus committees. Furthermore, SSM is contraindicated in IBC.[683]

Treatment of the elderly

The fastest growing segment of the US population is that aged ≥65 years. At present, this group represents 12% of the population, but 50% of breast cancers occur in this group. As life expectancy of US women is 80 years, and as our elders are healthier even today, the life expectancy of most breast cancer patients exceeds 10 years. Few studies have been carried out to clearly define the management of elderly women with breast cancer.[686,687] The definition of "elderly" may be based on chronologic age, physiologic age, or life expectancy. Increasingly, therapeutic decisions in this group are made based on comorbid conditions that usually limit life expectancy to a much greater extent than breast cancer. Treatment methods should not vary between different age-group patients. The presence of important comorbid conditions changes life expectancy and hence the expected benefits from all our interventions for breast cancer. The standard treatment for elderly patients with ESBC should be lumpectomy, SLNB, and radiotherapy, with adjuvant systemic treatment defined based on prognostic factors, ER, PR, and HER2. Increasingly, molecular profiles that predict tumor behavior will aid us in tailoring treatment. Results of a recent study on the impact of MP on women >60 years of age at intermediate risk by Adjuvant!Online provided additional information not predicted by clinical data only.[688] In the future, we will describe the use of molecular tests to define a population of patients where we can test the impact of less intervention.

At present, the use of AIs or tamoxifen has become standard therapy for the management of women with HR+ tumors, regardless of age. Endocrine therapy is not indicated for patients with HR− tumors. It should be noted that in CALGB 9343, women over 70 years of age with ER-positive tumors treated with tamoxifen or tamoxifen plus radiation were much more likely to die of other disease. At 8 years, death from breast cancer was 3% and death from other causes was 21%.

When the risk of breast cancer is sufficiently high to provide chemotherapy and the benefits of this treatment exceed risks, full-dose chemotherapy should be given to elderly patients.[689] The use of less than full-dose chemotherapy will usually be ineffective, at the cost of unnecessary toxicity. In a CALGB study, however, women who received doxorubicin in a CAF regimen at a dose of 30 mg/m² four times every 4 week did as well as those who received 60 mg/m² four times or 40 mg/m² six times if their HER2/neu assay was negative. Prospective validation of these results is needed. Recently, there has been interest in devising protocols to evaluate new drugs that may be less toxic in such patients. A phase III clinical trial compared single-agent oral capecitabine with classical CMF or AC in the adjuvant treatment of patients >65 years of age. Capecitabine was clearly inferior to the standard regimens in DFS, and standard chemotherapy was well tolerated.[690]

Symptom management and survivorship

The ACS estimated that there were more than 3 million breast cancer survivors as of 2014.[1] Approximately 72% of breast cancer survivors (>2 million women) are aged ≥60 years; fewer than 10% are <50. Understanding the issues facing both young and old survivors is critical to supporting QOL and appropriate risk reduction and monitoring.

Standard posttreatment follow-up care for survivors of ESBC should include surveillance for cancer recurrence or new primary breast cancers and prevention of secondary cancers. Patients should be assessed for late psychosocial and physical affects and provided with interventions for the consequences of treatment, such as new medical problems, symptoms, and psychological distress. Finally, both primary care providers and cancer specialists should jointly manage the coordination of survivorship care.

During the first 3 years after completion of combined modality therapy for primary breast cancer, patients should be visited every 3–6 months with a careful history and complete physical examination at each visit.[409] For the subsequent 2 years, patients should be visited every 6–12 months and annually thereafter. Patients who have undergone breast-conserving surgery should undergo a mammogram 6 months after completion of radiation therapy, 1 year after the initial mammogram, and annually thereafter. Imaging studies should be performed only if warranted by symptoms or physical findings. Complete blood counts, comprehensive metabolic panels, tumor markers, and imaging are not recommended outside of symptoms or physical findings, as early detection of MBC provides no advantage to OS. Active areas of research include monitoring of circulating cell-free DNA as an early marker of disease recurrence.

The transition from provider-intense cancer treatment to a posttreatment program with less-frequent visits can be difficult for many patients, particularly in resource-poor, low- and middle-income settings. Patients should be educated with regard to recognizing signs and symptoms of disease recurrence, management of short- and long-term physical and psychosocial symptoms, and the importance of healthy lifestyle modifications to maintain a healthy weight through physical activity.[692,693] At this time, the general recommendation is that cancer survivors achieve 150 min of moderate-intensity activity a week. Additional survivorship concerns include fertility, fatigue and depression, cognitive dysfunction, pain, lymphedema, sexual dysfunction, sleep disorders, bone health, cardiac toxicity, and healthy lifestyle choices. Some of these issues are reviewed in detail in the NCCN Guidelines for Survivorship Version 1.2016.[691]

Obesity and diabetes in breast cancer

Patterson et al.[692] evaluated the effect of comorbid medical conditions on breast cancer outcomes for 2542 women with ESBC followed for a median of 7.3 years. Most notably, patients with diabetes had over twice the ROR (HR 2.1, 95% CI 1.3–3.4) and mortality (HR 2.5, 95% CI 1.4–4.4). A meta-analysis by Sparano et al. in 2012 demonstrated that obesity was associated with inferior DFS (HR 1.24, 95% CI 1.06–1.46, $p = 0.0008$) and OS (HR 1.37; 95% CI 1.13–1.67; $p = 0.002$) in patients with HR+ breast cancer, but not other subtypes.[694]

Several clinical trials have evaluated various interventions for weight loss and nutrition in an effort to improve outcome. The WINS study was a phase III clinical trial initiated in 1994 that randomized 2437 women with ESBC in a 60:40 ratio to receive a low-fat eating plan guided by registered dieticians versus observation. Long-term analysis was presented at SABCS 2014.[42] At a median follow-up of 5 years, patients in the intervention arm achieved reductions of 9.2% in fat calories and 6 pounds in weight. Recurrence was 24% lower in the intervention arm over a mean of 60 months of follow-up. The maximum benefit from the intervention was observed in women with HR− ESBC who achieved a 54% decrease in mortality, whereas no benefit was appreciated in women with HR+ ESBC. However, the Women's Healthy Eating and Living (WHEL) randomized clinical trial, which compared a low-fat diet high in vegetables and fruits with observation in 3088 women, showed no effect on breast cancer events or mortality at 7.3 years of follow-up.[695]

Fertility management

Women of reproductive age constitute 15% of invasive breast cancer worldwide.[459] These women often experience premature ovarian failure or infertility after receiving chemotherapy, which can damage ovarian reserve.[696] The ASCO Clinical Practice Guidelines for fertility preservation for patients with cancer recommend that fertility preservation be discussed with all patients of reproductive age before initiation of therapy, if infertility is a potential risk.[697] Patients who are ambivalent or desire fertility preservation should be referred to reproductive specialists. Embryo and oocyte cryopreservation are the only established methods of fertility preservation. Emerging data suggest that the risk of ovarian failure might be reduced with the use of goserelin during adjuvant chemotherapy in patients with HR− ESBC.[698]

The Prevention of Early Menopause Study (POEMS)/S0230 clinical trial was a phase III clinical trial that assessed the development of ovarian failure in premenopausal women with HR− ESBC who were treated with chemotherapy plus goserelin.[698] Unfortunately, the study failed to reach its target enrollment of 416 patients because of early closure for loss of funding. A total of 257 women were randomized to standard cyclophosphamide-containing chemotherapy with or without goserelin. Results of the study were available for only 218 women at a median follow-up of 4.1 years. Ovarian failure occurred in 8% of the patients in the goserelin arm, in comparison to 22% in the control arm (odds ratio, 0.30; 95% CI, 0.9–0.97; two-sided $p = 0.04$). The rate of pregnancy was higher in women in the goserelin arm than the control arm (21% vs 11%, $p = 0.03$). The authors concluded that although data were missing, goserelin, when administered in combination with chemotherapy in women with HR− ESBC, appeared to reduce the risk of early menopause as well as improve maintenance of fertility.

As premenopausal patients with HR+ ESBC undergo adjuvant endocrine therapies for several years, they have delayed childbirth. Such patients often consider oocyte or embryo cryopreservation before the initiation of therapy but are theoretically at increased risk of accelerated tumor growth because of ovarian stimulation and increasing estrogen levels. Oktay et al.[696] have recently described an ovarian stimulation protocol for patients with HR+ ESBC that uses letrozole in combination with follicle-stimulating hormone to limit the increase of estrogen levels. In the study, 131 women with ESBC underwent ovarian stimulation with concurrent letrozole 5 mg/day before chemotherapy and cryopreservation. The live birth per embryo transfer rate in the study population was 51.5%, similar to the US national mean for women without cancer.

Alopecia

Hair loss due to chemotherapy is emotionally traumatic for many women with breast cancer and is often ranked as the most feared side effect of treatment. Devices to facilitate scalp cooling and prevent chemotherapy-induced alopecia have been studied and widely used throughout Europe and Canada for decades, with recent studies in the United States demonstrating efficacy with common chemotherapy regimens for ESBC. The Dutch Scalp Cooling Registry of almost 1500 women who underwent scalp cooling during chemotherapy reported efficacy in 50% of patients and no cases of scalp metastasis at 5 years of follow-up.[699] Several small clinical trials over the last few years using newer systems such as the Penguin cold cap, the Digni-Cap, and PAXMAN Orbis scalp cooler have reported higher degrees of efficacy with reports of ≤25% hair loss in 65–75% of users. Ongoing clinical trials in the United States have continued to evaluate the safety and efficacy of these systems (NCT01831024, NCT01986140).

Lymphedema

Lymphedema of the arm is characterized by regional swelling because of accumulation of protein-rich fluid within body tissues, leading to disfigurement and decreased mobility and function.[700]

It affects approximately 21% of breast cancer survivors with variable incidence depending on the type of surgery. In addition to decreased functionality, patients experience paresthesias, pain, and psychologic distress, resulting in a reduced QOL. Early physiotherapy, including manual lymph drainage, massage of scar tissue, and shoulder exercises, starting within days of surgery results in a lower incidence of lymphedema. Treatment options for lymphedema include physical therapy to optimize range of motion, progressive resistance training with compression garments, weight loss, and properly fitted compression garments.[691] Patients should be referred to a lymphedema specialist when available. Operative therapies are considered a last option and remain under investigation.

Hot flashes

A proportion of 65–80% of ESBC survivors develop hot flashes that may occur with chemotherapy-induced ovarian suppression or antiestrogen therapies. Several randomized controlled trials have demonstrated that pharmacologic intervention with either venlafaxine, gabapentin, or clonidine (SSRI) reduced the frequency of hot flashes more effectively than placebo.[701] The effectiveness of nonpharmacologic interventions including acupuncture and cognitive behavioral therapy is less clear, in part due to methodologic issues regarding sham interventions.

Bone health

Estrogen deprivation results in bone resorption with rapid bone loss. Women treated with AIs are therefore at increased risk of bone density loss and subsequent adverse skeletal events. Patients on AIs should undergo a fracture risk assessment with a dual-energy X-ray absorptiometry (DEXA) scan as well as review of clinical factors such as age, prior fracture history, low body mass index, and tobacco and alcohol use. Bone density should be repeated every 1–2 years. In addition, patients should be encouraged to take calcium and vitamin D. Patients who develop osteopenia or osteoporosis while on AI therapy should be considered for either a bisphosphonate or denosumab.

Adjuvant bisphosphonate therapy to reduce the risk of distant recurrence in women with ESBC has been evaluated for several decades with variable results. A meta-analysis of individual patient data from randomized studies of adjuvant bisphosphonate therapy has been recently published by the EBCTCG.[702] A total of 18,766 women were enrolled in trials of bisphosphonate therapy for 2–5 years. The reduction in bone recurrence was significant (HR 0.83, 95% CI 0.87–1.01; $2p = 0.004$). A clear reduction in recurrence, distant recurrence, bone recurrence, and breast cancer mortality was observed in postmenopausal patients.

Key references

The complete reference list can be found on the Wiley Companion Digital Edition of this title (see inside front cover for login instructions).

1 Siegel RL, Miller KD, Jemal A. Cancer statistics, 2015. *CA Cancer J Clin.* 2015;**65**:5–29.
14 Mavaddat N, Peock S, Frost D, et al. Cancer risks for BRCA1 and BRCA2 mutation carriers: results from prospective analysis of EMBRACE. *J Natl Cancer Inst.* 2013;**105**:812–822.
42 Chlebowski RT, Rohan TE, Manson JE, et al. Breast cancer after use of estrogen plus progestin and estrogen alone: analyses of data from 2 Women's Health Initiative randomized clinical trials. *JAMA Oncol.* 2015;**1**:296–305.
98 Gail MH. Twenty-five years of breast cancer risk models and their applications. *J Natl Cancer Inst.* 2015;**107**.
119 Paik S, Shak S, Tang G, et al. A multigene assay to predict recurrence of tamoxifen-treated, node-negative breast cancer. *N Engl J Med.* 2004;**351**:2817–2826.

138 Esserman LJ, Thompson IM, Reid B, et al. Addressing overdiagnosis and overtreatment in cancer: a prescription for change. *Lancet Oncol.* 2014;**15**:e234–e242.

139 Oeffinger KC, Fontham ET, Etzioni R, et al. Breast cancer screening for women at average risk: 2015 guideline update from the American Cancer Society. *JAMA.* 2015;**314**:1599–1614.

146 Early Breast Cancer Trialists' Collaborative Group (EBCTCG). Effects of chemotherapy and hormonal therapy for early breast cancer on recurrence and 15-year survival: an overview of the randomised trials. *Lancet.* 2005;**365**:1687–1717.

148 Dowsett M, Cuzick J, Ingle J, et al. Meta-analysis of breast cancer outcomes in adjuvant trials of aromatase inhibitors versus tamoxifen. *J Clin Oncol.* 2010;**28**:509–518.

199 Fisher B, Costantino JP, Wickerham DL, et al. Tamoxifen for the prevention of breast cancer: current status of the National Surgical Adjuvant Breast and Bowel Project P-1 study. *J Natl Cancer Inst.* 2005;**97**:1652–1662.

204 Goss PE, Ingle JN, Ales-Martinez JE, et al. Exemestane for breast-cancer prevention in postmenopausal women. *N Engl J Med.* 2011;**364**:2381–2391.

235 Giuliano AE, Hunt KK, Ballman KV, et al. Axillary dissection vs no axillary dissection in women with invasive breast cancer and sentinel node metastasis: a randomized clinical trial. *JAMA.* 2011;**305**:569–575.

241 Morris AD, Morris RD, Wilson JF, et al. Breast-conserving therapy vs mastectomy in early-stage breast cancer: a meta-analysis of 10-year survival. *Cancer J Sci Am.* 1997;**3**:6–12.

242 Early Breast Cancer Trialists' Collaborative Group. Favourable and unfavourable effects on long-term survival of radiotherapy for early breast cancer: an overview of the randomised trials. Early Breast Cancer Trialists' Collaborative Group. *Lancet.* 2000;**355**:1757–1770.

267 Rastogi P, Anderson SJ, Bear HD, et al. Preoperative chemotherapy: updates of National Surgical Adjuvant Breast and Bowel Project Protocols B-18 and B-27. *J Clin Oncol.* 2008;**26**:778–785.

337 Early Breast Cancer Trialists' Collaborative Group, Davies C, Godwin J, et al. Relevance of breast cancer hormone receptors and other factors to the efficacy of adjuvant tamoxifen: patient-level meta-analysis of randomised trials. *Lancet.* 2011;**378**:771–784.

342 Coombes RC, Hall E, Gibson LJ, et al. A randomized trial of exemestane after two to three years of tamoxifen therapy in postmenopausal women with primary breast cancer. *N Engl J Med.* 2004;**350**:1081–1092.

345 Coates AS, Winer EP, Goldhirsch A, et al. Tailoring therapies-improving the management of early breast cancer: St Gallen International Expert Consensus on the Primary Therapy of Early Breast Cancer 2015. *Ann Oncol.* 2015;**26**:1533–1546.

350 Burstein HJ, Temin S, Anderson H, et al. Adjuvant endocrine therapy for women with hormone receptor-positive breast cancer: American Society of Clinical Oncology clinical practice guideline focused update. *J Clin Oncol.* 2014;**32**:2255–2269.

364 Henderson IC, Berry DA, Demetri GD, et al. Improved outcomes from adding sequential Paclitaxel but not from escalating Doxorubicin dose in an adjuvant chemotherapy regimen for patients with node-positive primary breast cancer. *J Clin Oncol.* 2003;**21**:976–983.

365 Mamounas EP, Bryant J, Lembersky B, et al. Paclitaxel after doxorubicin plus cyclophosphamide as adjuvant chemotherapy for node-positive breast cancer: results from NSABP B-28. *J Clin Oncol.* 2005;**23**:3686–3696.

366 Martin M, Pienkowski T, Mackey J, et al. Adjuvant docetaxel for node-positive breast cancer. *N Engl J Med.* 2005;**352**:2302–2313.

367 Mackey JR, Martin M, Pienkowski T, et al. Adjuvant docetaxel, doxorubicin, and cyclophosphamide in node-positive breast cancer: 10-year follow-up of the phase 3 randomised BCIRG 001 trial. *Lancet Oncol.* 2013;**14**:72–80.

371 Wood WC, Budman DR, Korzun AH, et al. Dose and dose intensity of adjuvant chemotherapy for stage II, node-positive breast carcinoma. *N Engl J Med.* 1994;**330**:1253–1259.

374 Citron ML, Berry DA, Cirrincione C, et al. Randomized trial of dose-dense versus conventionally scheduled and sequential versus concurrent combination chemotherapy as postoperative adjuvant treatment of node-positive primary breast cancer: first report of Intergroup Trial C9741/Cancer and Leukemia Group B Trial 9741. *J Clin Oncol.* 2003;**21**:1431–1439.

404 Geyer CE, Forster J, Lindquist D, et al. Lapatinib plus capecitabine for HER2-positive advanced breast cancer. *N Engl J Med.* 2006;**355**:2733–2743.

405 Goss PE, Smith IE, O'Shaughnessy J, et al. Adjuvant lapatinib for women with early-stage HER2-positive breast cancer: a randomised, controlled, phase 3 trial. *Lancet Oncol.* 2013;**14**:88–96.

457 Aebi S, Gelber S, Anderson SJ, et al. Chemotherapy for isolated locoregional recurrence of breast cancer (CALOR): a randomised trial. *Lancet Oncol.* 2014;**15**:156–163.

460 Cardoso F, Costa A, Norton L, et al. ESO-ESMO 2nd international consensus guidelines for advanced breast cancer (ABC2). *Breast.* 2014;**23**:489–502.

466 Wilcken N, Hornbuckle J, Ghersi D. Chemotherapy alone versus endocrine therapy alone for metastatic breast cancer. *Cochrane Database Syst Rev.* 2003;**2**:CD002747.

471 Mouridsen H, Gershanovich M, Sun Y, et al. Superior efficacy of letrozole versus tamoxifen as first-line therapy for postmenopausal women with advanced breast cancer: results of a phase III study of the International Letrozole Breast Cancer Group. *J Clin Oncol.* 2001;**19**:2596–2606.

479 Osborne CK, Pippen J, Jones SE, et al. Double-blind, randomized trial comparing the efficacy and tolerability of fulvestrant versus anastrozole in postmenopausal women with advanced breast cancer progressing on prior endocrine therapy: results of a North American trial. *J Clin Oncol.* 2002;**20**:3386–3395.

490 Baselga J, Campone M, Piccart M, et al. Everolimus in postmenopausal hormone-receptor-positive advanced breast cancer. *N Engl J Med.* 2012;**366**:520–529.

495 Finn RS, Crown JP, Lang I, et al. The cyclin-dependent kinase 4/6 inhibitor palbociclib in combination with letrozole versus letrozole alone as first-line treatment of oestrogen receptor-positive, HER2-negative, advanced breast cancer (PALOMA-1/TRIO-18): a randomised phase 2 study. *Lancet Oncol.* 2015;**16**:25–35.

496 Turner NC, Ro J, Andre F, et al. Palbociclib in hormone-receptor-positive advanced breast cancer. *N Engl J Med.* 2015;**373**:209–219.

502 Dear RF, McGeechan K, Jenkins MC, et al. Combination versus sequential single agent chemotherapy for metastatic breast cancer. *Cochrane Database Syst Rev.* 2013;**12**:CD008792.

503 Gennari A, Stockler M, Puntoni M, et al. Duration of chemotherapy for metastatic breast cancer: a systematic review and meta-analysis of randomized clinical trials. *J Clin Oncol.* 2011;**29**:2144–2149.

504 Park YH, Jung KH, Im SA, et al. Phase III, multicenter, randomized trial of maintenance chemotherapy versus observation in patients with metastatic breast cancer after achieving disease control with six cycles of gemcitabine plus paclitaxel as first-line chemotherapy: KCSG-BR07-02. *J Clin Oncol.* 2013;**31**:1732–1739.

520 Sledge GW, Neuberg D, Bernardo P, et al. Phase III trial of doxorubicin, paclitaxel, and the combination of doxorubicin and paclitaxel as front-line chemotherapy for metastatic breast cancer: an intergroup trial (E1193). *J Clin Oncol.* 2003;**21**:588–592.

557 Slamon DJ, Leyland-Jones B, Shak S, et al. Use of chemotherapy plus a monoclonal antibody against HER2 for metastatic breast cancer that overexpresses HER2. *N Engl J Med.* 2001;**344**:783–792.

565 Valero V, Forbes J, Pegram MD, et al. Multicenter phase III randomized trial comparing docetaxel and trastuzumab with docetaxel, carboplatin, and trastuzumab as first-line chemotherapy for patients with HER2-gene-amplified metastatic breast cancer (BCIRG 007 study): two highly active therapeutic regimens. *J Clin Oncol.* 2011;**29**:149–156.

589 Baselga J, Cortes J, Kim SB, et al. Pertuzumab plus trastuzumab plus docetaxel for metastatic breast cancer. *N Engl J Med.* 2012;**366**:109–119.

593 Verma S, Miles D, Gianni L, et al. Trastuzumab emtansine for HER2-positive advanced breast cancer. *N Engl J Med.* 2012;**367**:1783–1791.

631 Rosen LS, Gordon D, Kaminski M, et al. Long-term efficacy and safety of zoledronic acid compared with pamidronate disodium in the treatment of skeletal complications in patients with advanced multiple myeloma or breast carcinoma: a randomized, double-blind, multicenter, comparative trial. *Cancer.* 2003;**98**:1735–1744.

633 Stopeck AT, Lipton A, Body JJ, et al. Denosumab compared with zoledronic acid for the treatment of bone metastases in patients with advanced breast cancer: a randomized, double-blind study. *J Clin Oncol.* 2010;**28**:5132–5139.

681 Giordano SH, Perkins GH, Broglio K, et al. Adjuvant systemic therapy for male breast carcinoma. *Cancer.* 2005;**104**:2359–2364.

109 Malignant melanoma

Justin M. Ko, MD, MBA, FAAD ▪ Susan M. Swetter, MD ▪ Jonathan S. Zager, MD ▪ Vernon K. Sondak, MD
▪ Scott E. Woodman, MD, PhD ▪ Kim A. Margolin, MD

Overview

Melanoma comprises a wide variety of malignant cell types arising from the skin, the mucous membranes, and the pigmented cells of the eye. While these tumors are all classified as melanoma and share a common molecular biology of pigmentation and biological resemblance to cells of neural crest origin, important distinctions in other molecular characteristics and patterns of exposure to ultraviolet light as a carcinogen determine their clinical natural history, including the response to therapeutic interventions. While the majority of melanomas are diagnosed at an early stage and curable with minimal surgery, melanoma has the potential for early and widespread dissemination via lymphatic and hematogenous routes. Surgery remains the mainstay of therapy for primary, regional, and many cases of single- or oligo-metastatic disease, but systemic therapies have dramatically improved the prognosis for metastatic melanoma, particularly immunotherapies that enhance existing cellular immunity. The rapid discovery of new molecular targets, immunotherapy combinations (including the use of radiotherapy), and understanding of the mechanisms of therapeutic resistance are likely to lead to even greater improvements in the prognosis for patients with melanoma in the near future.

Dermatologic principles in melanoma

Epidemiology and etiology

Melanoma incidence and mortality rates continue to rise worldwide, driven by increased ultraviolet (UV) light exposure (both natural and artificial sources) and differences in prognosis according to age and sex. In the United States, 76,380 new cases of invasive cutaneous melanoma will be diagnosed and approximately 10,130 deaths will occur in 2016.[1] Incidence has been increasing steadily for the past 30 years, and since 2004, Caucasians have experienced an increase in incidence by 3% each year, faster than that of nearly all cancers.[2] Western states with increased ultraviolet radiation (UVR) have a greater incidence.[3] Incidence rates are rising more than twofold among young women (ages 15–39) and increasing even more sharply among middle-aged and older men.[3,4]

The increase in melanoma incidence has been attributed to factors including increased intermittent UVR exposure in fair-skinned populations, higher rates of skin biopsies and screening resulting in the detection of thinner, more favorable lesions, and potential changes in the histologic interpretation of early evolving lesions from atypical melanocytic hyperplasia or severely dysplasia to melanoma *in situ*.[5,6] However, continued increases in the incidence rates of thicker tumors, including steep rises among individuals of lower socioeconomic status, points to a true increase in potentially fatal cases and lack of screening as a critical factor accounting for recent melanoma incidence trends.[7]

Risk factors

Environmental factors

The risk of developing melanoma is related to acute, intense, and intermittent exposure to UV light, but the relationship between UV exposure and melanomagenesis is not straightforward. Melanomas frequently occur in locations often covered by clothing, and indoor workers have been shown to have a higher incidence of melanoma on sun-exposed sites, observations that provide support for the notion that melanomas arise through different molecular pathways.[8,9] Melanoma incidence rates on sun-exposed and less exposed body areas also have different age peaks,[10] around 55 years for melanomas on intermittently exposed sites such as the trunk and proximal extremities, which probably reflects a period of vulnerability to UV radiation early in life and a latency to full melanomagenesis followed by a decline in the incidence of melanomas attributable to those mechanisms.[11] Conversely, melanomas on chronically exposed sites such as the face and distal extremities continue to rise with age. Signature DNA mutations induced by UV are found commonly in driver mutations identified in melanoma[12] but not as often as in nonmelanoma skin cancers that are more directly related to chronic sun exposure, so alternate sources of mutagenesis are likely. Nevertheless, a randomized study in Australia showed that consistent daily application of both UVA- and UVB-filtering broad-spectrum sunscreen (compared with discretionary or nonuse) resulted in a decreased incidence of melanoma.[13] Indoor tanning is now proven to be a major contributor to the increasing incidence of cutaneous melanoma among young women, with greater melanoma risk proportional to measures of tanning practices, including increasing years, hours, and sessions of indoor tanning.[14,15] Alarmingly, 76% of melanomas in fair-skinned participants were attributed to tanning bed use at young ages. A strong association of tanning bed use with recreational drugs,[16] suggesting a common genetically mediated addiction, is consistent with animal studies showing sunlight-seeking behaviors mediated by opioid-related substances through endorphin receptors.[17]

Host factors

Although the process by which normal melanocytes transform into melanoma cells is not entirely understood, it is believed to involve progressive genetic mutations that alter cell proliferation, differentiation, and death and impact cellular susceptibility to the carcinogenic effects of UVR.

Melanoma is largely a disease of individuals of fair complexion, including those with red or blond hair and fair skin, who burn easily or have a history of severe sunburn, or who are unable to tan.[18] Caucasians with an increased number of nevi or a tendency to freckle are also at increased risk for developing melanoma.[19] The risk of cutaneous melanoma in the presence of increased numbers

Holland-Frei Cancer Medicine, Ninth Edition. Edited by Robert C. Bast Jr., Carlo M. Croce, William N. Hait, Waun Ki Hong, Donald W. Kufe, Martine Piccart-Gebhart, Raphael E. Pollock, Ralph R. Weichselbaum, Hongyang Wang, and James F. Holland.
© 2017 John Wiley & Sons, Inc. ISBN: 978-1-118-93469-2

of common/typical nevi, large nevi, and/or clinically atypical nevi (CAN) on the body was confirmed in a pooled analysis of melanocytic nevus phenotype, even at different latitudes.[20] Both prior personal history and family history are important risk factors for the development of melanoma.[21] Solid-organ transplant populations are at far greater risk of squamous cell carcinomas and also develop more melanomas compared to the general population.[22]

Genetic predisposition and familial melanoma

The majority of melanomas appear to be sporadic, with only 5–10% of cases attributable to an identified familial predisposition.[23] Familial melanoma is characterized by an increased risk of developing melanoma, a higher incidence of multiple primary melanomas, and typically an earlier age at onset.[24] Specific genetic alterations have been implicated in the pathogenesis of familial melanoma. Mutations at the CDKN2A locus on chromosome 9p21, which codes for the tumor suppressor p16 and p14/ARF, account for about one-third of familial cases. Additional melanoma risk occurs in CDKN2A mutation carriers who express variants of the melanocortin receptor gene MCR1, which is associated with red hair, fair skin, and freckling. As mutations of either of these genes are present in only a subset of familial melanoma kindreds, other melanoma susceptibility genes likely exist. Formal recommendations for p16 mutation testing have been proposed in patients with a personal or family history of 3 or more invasive melanomas or cancer "events," defined as 2 invasive melanomas and 1 pancreatic cancer in the patient or family members, or vice versa, which conveys a >20% risk of carriage.[25] However, owing to the low frequency of mutations even among high-risk individuals and the lack of implications for dermatologic surveillance, genetic testing other than for research purposes is generally not recommended.

Atypical mole syndrome/phenotype

The presence of numerous CAN, also termed "dysplastic nevi," is the most important clinical risk factor for melanoma. Compared with the general population, patients with CAN have a 2- to 15-fold elevated risk of developing melanoma, and risk increases with the number of CAN and/or personal or family history of melanoma.[26] An atypical mole phenotype is characterized by numerous (>50–100) common nevi along with multiple (generally >5), large (>6–8 mm) nevi with color variegation, border irregularity, and asymmetric shape. Melanomas seldom arise in association with pre-existing atypical nevi, and over 70% of melanomas in patients with any type of melanocytic nevus (common, atypical, or congenital) are believed to develop de novo, although CAN with severe histologic dysplasia may more often be true melanoma precursors.[27] Melanomas associated with atypical/dysplastic nevi are generally thin superficial spreading type, possibly due to increased skin surveillance in affected individuals.

Congenital melanocytic nevi (CMN)

Congenital melanocytic nevi (CMN) are evident in 1–6% of neonates and uncommonly transform into melanoma.[28] Patients with "large or giant" congenital nevi (lesions >20 cm in diameter in an adult, >6 cm on the body of an infant, or >9 cm on the head of an infant) have a less than 5% lifetime risk of developing a melanoma[29–32] with about half arising during the first few years of life.[33] The risk of melanoma arising within small-sized (<1.5 cm) and medium-sized CMN is low and virtually nonexistent before puberty.[34] Management of CMN hinges on many variables including ease of monitoring and potential psychosocial benefits and harms of surgical procedures.

Melanoma risk assessment

Several risk assessment tools have been used to target individuals at high risk for melanoma, in particular Caucasian men over 65 and individuals of lower socioeconomic status—two groups with the highest melanoma mortality.

Current risk assessment tools are derived from a large case–control study of 718 non-Hispanic white patients and 945 controls that involved inspection of the back for suspicious moles and asked two questions about complexion and history of sun exposure.[35] Mild freckling and light complexion were demonstrated as risk factors for both men and women. In addition, >17 small moles and ≥2 large moles in men or ≥12 small moles on the backs of women were also significant risk factors. These data led to the Melanoma Risk Assessment Tool, which is available from the National Cancer Institute (http://www.cancer.gov/melanomarisktool/). The tool calculates absolute risk of melanoma over the next 5 years up to age 70.

Prognostic factors

A number of clinical factors affect patient prognosis including age, gender, and anatomic location of the primary tumor. In general, men, older age individuals, and those with melanoma on the head and neck tend to fare worse. A population-based study in France during 2004–2008 showed that male patients had thicker and more frequently ulcerated tumors. Older patients had thicker and more advanced melanomas, with more frequent head and neck location.[36]

While newer concepts in the taxonomy of melanoma suggest distinct molecular, genetic, anatomic, and UV-exposure-linked characteristics, growth kinetics of certain histological subtypes also appear to play a role in prognosis. The rapidly growing nodular subtype of melanoma tends to elude early detection based on clinical characteristics alone. Nodular melanoma (NM) comprises <15% of subtyped melanoma cases in the United States and Australia, but accounts for a disproportionate number of thicker tumors (>2 mm) and melanoma deaths compared with other histologic subtypes.

Newer molecular techniques such as gene expression profiling may soon assist in identifying thin melanomas with more aggressive behavior.[37]

Clinical presentation

Cutaneous melanoma can occur anywhere but is most common on the lower extremities and back in women and on the trunk in men. From a clinical standpoint, a new or changing "mole" or skin lesion is the most-common warning sign for melanoma. The so-called "ABCDEs" of early diagnosis pioneered by Rigel et al.[38] are an easy mnemonic to improve recognition of the classic early signs of melanoma (Table 1). To simplify further, Weinstock[39] succinctly focused the message by emphasizing that the most important warning sign is a new or changing skin lesion. The "ugly duckling" warning sign refers to a pigmented or clinically amelanotic lesion that looks different from the rest, which may be of value to identify melanomas that lack the classic ABCD criteria (e.g., nodular, amelanotic, or desmoplastic subtypes).[40,41]

As histologic features of a primary melanoma are critical for melanoma staging and prognostication, proper initial biopsy of a suspicious lesion is paramount. An excisional biopsy with narrow clinical margins (1–3 mm) of normal-appearing skin around the pigmented lesion is preferred when possible to provide accurate diagnosis and histologic microstaging. An important exception to this rule is the lentigo maligna (LM) subtype of melanoma in situ, in which the risk of misdiagnosis is high if small or partial biopsy specimens are taken. The best diagnostic biopsy technique in this

Table 1 ABCDEs: clinical features of melanoma.

A	Asymmetry—the two halves of the lesion do not match each other
B	Border irregularity—may appear ragged, notched or scalloped
C	Color variation—color is not uniform or lesion may be many colors displaying shades of tan, brown, or black. White, reddish, or blue-gray discoloration is of particular concern
D	Diameter—usually >6 mm (roughly the diameter of a pencil eraser) although melanomas may be smaller in size; any growth in a nevus warrants an evaluation
E	Evolving lesion—changes in size or color; critical for nodular or amelanotic melanoma, which may not exhibit the ABCD criteria above

case is often a broad shave biopsy that extends into at least the papillary dermis, provides the opportunity to exclude microinvasive melanoma, and allows for optimal histopathologic interpretation of the tumor.

Pathologic features

With the exception of NM, the growth patterns of the other clinicopathologic subtypes are characterized by a preceding in situ (radial growth) phase that lacks the biologic potential to metastasize and may last from months to years before dermal invasion (vertical growth) occurs.

Dermal invasion confers metastatic potential, although the greatest risk occurs in the setting of a vertical growth (tumorigenic) phase.[42] Immunohistochemical staining for lineage [S-100, human melanoma black 45 (HMB-45), melan-A/Mart-1] or proliferation markers (Ki67) may be helpful in some cases for histologic differentiation from melanoma simulators such as melanocytic nevi, Spitz nevi, cellular blue nevus, clear cell sarcoma, or malignant peripheral nerve sheath tumor.[43] A study of melanoma biomarker expression in melanocytic tumor progression examined differential expression of melanoma biomarkers between nevi, primary melanoma, and metastases.[44] Approaches combining Ki67/Anti-MART-1 (Melan-A) and HMB-45/MITF immunostains have also been shown to hold promise in the diagnosis of melanoma.[45]

A pathology report for melanoma should include cytomorphology and architecture, along with tumor thickness (Breslow depth), presence of ulceration, dermal mitotic rate (measured as number per mm^2), and microsatellites and lymphovascular invasion, if present. Anatomic level of invasion (Clark's level) has less prognostic significance and is now considered optional in pathology reporting.

Atypical melanocytic lesions in children and adolescents in particular may be difficult to distinguish from true melanoma, including atypical Spitz tumors and Spitz or melanocytic tumors of uncertain malignant potential (STUMPs or MelTUMPs, respectively). As such, molecular techniques such as comparative genomic hybridization (GGH) and fluorescence in situ hybridization (FISH) have been utilized to assist in the determination of malignant versus benign behavior.[46-49] Newer gene expression profiling techniques may be of further value of molecular testing for challenging atypical melanocytic neoplasms and to aid in prognosis and risk stratification,[50-53] and some of these findings may yield prognostic data sufficiently robust to support their inclusion in future melanoma staging systems.

Clinicopathologic subtypes

The four major classical "histogenetic" subtypes of primary cutaneous melanoma are based on histopathologic findings, anatomic site, and degree of sun damage. These include superficial spreading melanoma, NM, lentigo maligna melanoma (LMM), and acral lentiginous melanoma. In addition, there are other rarer variants (<5% of melanomas), which include (1) desmoplastic/neurotropic melanoma, (2) mucosal (lentiginous) melanoma,[53] (3) blue nevus-like melanoma, (4) melanoma arising in a giant/large congenital nevus, and (5) melanoma of soft parts (clear cell sarcoma).

Superficial spreading melanoma

Superficial spreading melanoma accounts for nearly 70% of cutaneous melanoma, commonly displays the ABCDE signs, and is the most-common subtype in individuals aged 30–50 years, as well as those with atypical/dysplastic nevi. It is most common on the trunk in men and women and on the legs in women.

Nodular melanoma

NM is the next most-common melanoma subtype, and occurs in 15–30% of patients, most commonly on the legs and trunk in men and women. It typically presents as a dark brown-to-black papule or dome-shaped nodule with rapid growth over weeks to month, which may ulcerate and bleed with minor trauma. This subtype is responsible for most thick melanomas at diagnosis.[54,55]

Lentigo maligna melanoma

LMM incidence is rising in the United States.[56] It is typically located on chronically sun-damaged skin (head, neck, and arms) of fair-skinned older individuals (average age 65 years), slowly growing over years to decades. The in situ precursor lesion termed LM is typically a longstanding large >1–3 cm flat (macular) lesion, demonstrating pigmentation ranging from dark brown to black, although white or hypopigmented areas are common within LM. Dermal invasion denoting progression to LMM is characterized by the development of raised brown-black nodules within the in situ lesion.

Acral melanoma

Acral melanoma is the least-common subtype of melanoma in white persons (2–8% of melanoma cases), although the most-common subtype of melanoma in darker-complexioned individuals (i.e., African American, Asian, and Hispanic persons), representing 29–72% of melanoma cases in these populations. Because of delays in diagnosis, it may be associated with a worse prognosis.[57,58] Acral lentiginous melanoma occurs on the palms, soles, or beneath the nail plate (subungual melanoma), which may manifest as diffuse nail discoloration or a longitudinal pigmented band (melanonychia striata) within the finger or toenail. Pigment spread to the proximal or lateral nail folds is termed the Hutchinson sign, which is a hallmark for subungual melanoma.

Less-common subtypes

Desmoplastic melanoma is a less common but important melanoma subtype, given its predilection for older age individuals, clinical features similar to nonmelanoma (keratinocytic) skin cancer, and potential indication for adjuvant radiation therapy following wide excision (depending on tumor thickness, perineural invasion, and margin status). Amelanotic melanoma (<5% of melanomas) can occur with any subtype and often mimics basal cell or squamous cell carcinoma, dermatofibroma, or a ruptured hair follicle. It occurs most commonly in the setting of the nodular or desmoplastic subtype or melanoma metastasis to the skin, presumably because of the inability of these poorly differentiated cancer cells to synthesize melanin pigment.

Genetics and molecular pathology

Significant complexity exists in the clinical and histopathological presentation, cells of origin (epithelium associated versus nonepithelium associated), causative relationship to UV radiation, age of onset, somatic mutations, and germline genetic predisposition. Melanoma is not a homogeneous disease but instead is composed of biologically distinct subtypes, the phenotype of which is driven by underlying genetic alterations.[59]

One growth factor pathway that has garnered considerable attention as related to melanoma is the RAS–RAF–MAPK–ERK (mitogen-associated protein kinase, MAPK) signaling cascade. A unique mutation at position 1799 of the gene for the serine–threonine kinase BRAF in the MAPK pathway—occurring in about half of cutaneous melanomas—results in a substitution of glutamine (about 75–80% of cases) or lysine for valine (most of the remaining cases) at position 600 which confers constitutive activity, resulting in hyperproliferation and resistance to apoptosis among cells driven by this oncogenic mutation.[60] The biology of melanoma in cells dependent on a BRAF mutation is also impacted by coexisting mutations or other alterations of gene expression in linked pathways, particularly the PTEN/AKT/PI3K/mTOR pathway that is critical in the control of metabolic sensors and the cancer/microenvironment nutrient balance. Activating mutations of NRAS, as well as less-common oncogenes such as c-kit (covered in greater detail below), result in downstream activation of both of these pathways.

Most BRAF-mutated melanomas arise in intermittently sun-exposed skin, while melanomas from chronically sun-exposed areas have a lower incidence of BRAF mutations and occasionally carry a mutation or amplification of c-KIT, a receptor tyrosine kinase that[61,62] may be altered in about 15–20% of acral and mucosal melanomas.[61–63] Activation of c-kit results in the stimulation of both the MAPK and PI3K–AKT pathways, producing both proliferative and survival advantages.[64]

The observation that *BRAF* mutations noted in benign melanocytic nevi[65] typically arising by early adolescence occurred with the same frequency as in non-CSD melanoma led Bastian and colleagues to propose that patients with acquired nevi and non-CSD melanomas may have a particular susceptibility for developing *BRAF*-mutated melanocytic neoplasms at relatively low doses of UV radiation. This concept was supported in subsequent studies that demonstrated a germline variation in the melanocortin receptor 1 (MC1R) to significantly contribute to this susceptibility.[66,67] More specifically, variants of MC1R were shown to strongly increase the risk for non-CSD melanomas with *BRAF* mutation.

None of the oncogenes or tumor suppressor genes identified in melanoma are thought to be solely responsible for melanoma pathogenesis, and some appear to be mutually exclusive due to overlapping downstream functions. For instance, NRAS, as mentioned above, activates Raf kinases in response to growth factor receptor activation and harbors activating mutations in 15–20% of melanomas, but almost never occurs with a BRAF mutation.[67] The

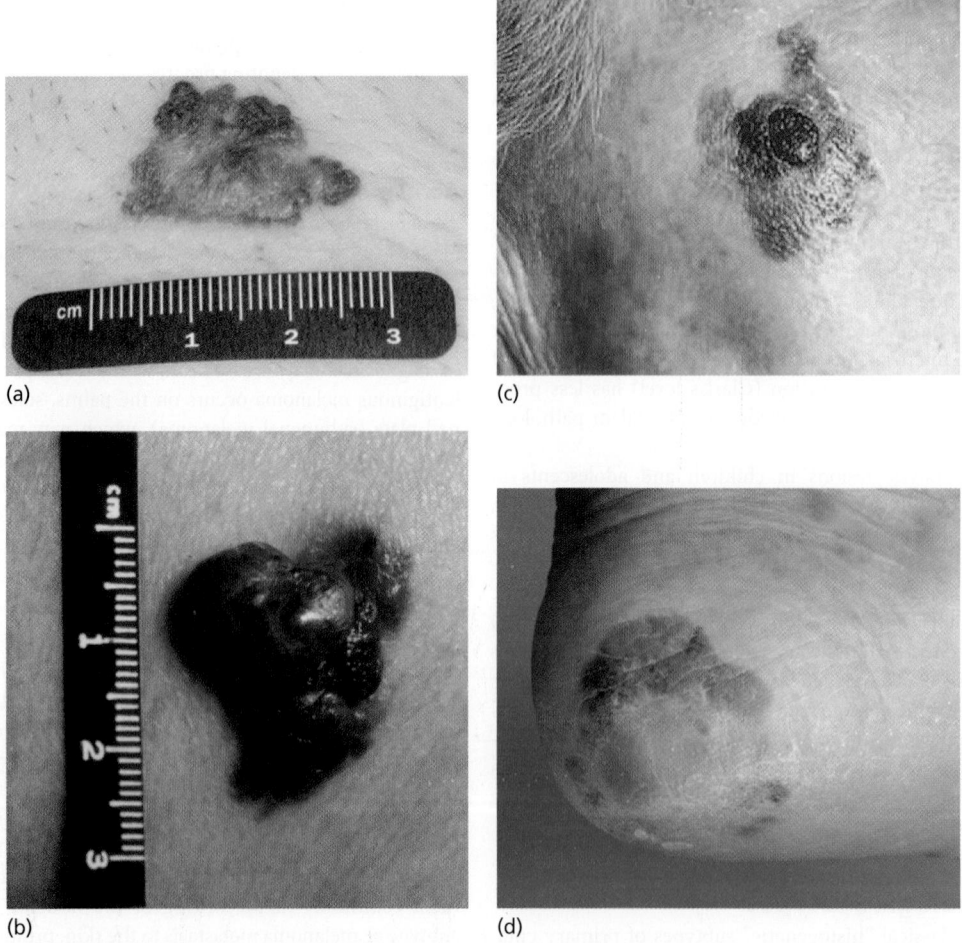

Figure 1 (a) Superficial spreading melanoma. Note the irregular borders, a variegation in color, and size >6 mm. (b) Nodular melanoma. (c) LMM with a nodular area of accelerated growth. (d) Acral lentiginous melanoma of heel. Source: Courtesy of Jeffrey E. Gershenwald, MD.

loss of the p16 tumor suppressor is a relatively frequent event in melanoma, and there is significant overlap with BRAF mutation.[68] PTEN mutations and deletion have been described in a minority of melanomas and appear to coincide with BRAF mutation (Figure 1).[69]

Surgical management of melanoma

Management of primary cutaneous melanoma

Surgery remains the mainstay of treatment for primary cutaneous melanoma, and the specific recommendations have not changed significantly over the last decade. Primary melanoma is treated by wide excision with a defined margin of adjacent normal-appearing skin. The margin of resection is dependent on the Breslow depth of the tumor and the site of the primary. Margin widths are measured from the biopsy scar or residual pigment at the time of surgery; it is not expected to equate to a histopathologic measurement on the resection specimen. A histologically negative margin, however, is always the goal in excising the primary tumor. Current recommendations for width of the excision in invasive melanoma (Table 2) are supported by randomized trials, summarized in Table 3.[71–74] For melanoma *in situ*, the recommended margin is 0.5–1 cm.[75] For invasive melanomas ≤1 mm in depth, 1 cm margins are recommended and are associated with low rates of local recurrence. For melanomas between 1 and 2 mm, 1–2 cm margins are recommended, taking into consideration cosmetic or functional outcome. For melanomas >2 mm, 2 cm margins are recommended, whenever feasible.[75] A meta-analysis found that margins >2 cm are unnecessary even for thick primaries, and margins should not be <1 cm for any invasive melanoma.[76]

Management of the regional lymph nodes

The role of sentinel lymph node biopsy

The presence of occult tumor deposits within clinically negative lymph nodes (defined by the AJCC staging system as "microscopic" disease) is a key predictor of outcome in clinical stage I and II melanoma,[77] and evidence suggests even tiny nodal micrometastases have clinical relevance.[78,79] Melanoma micrometastases in the regional lymph nodes cannot reliably be detected by any imaging modality including PET–CT[80,81] or ultrasonography.[82,83] Sentinel lymph node biopsy (SLNB) can identify micrometastases with low morbidity.[84] In 2012, an evidence-based assessment of the

Table 2 Recommended margins of wide excision for cutaneous melanoma based on primary tumor thickness and location.

Breslow thickness	Primary site	Recommended excision margin (cm)
Melanoma *in situ*	Anywhere on the skin	0.5–1
0.01–1.00 mm	Anywhere on the skin	1
1.01–2.00 mm	Head/neck, distal extremity[a]	1
	Trunk or proximal extremity[b]	2
>2.00 mm	Head/neck, distal extremity[a]	1
	Trunk or proximal extremity	2

[a]Subungual primary tumors may require distal digital amputation.
[b]If a skin graft would be required to reconstruct the excision defect, it is acceptable to take a 1 cm excision margin.
Note: Local anatomic constraints and specific patient factors may justify minor deviations from the standard margin recommendations.
Adapted from Sondak and Gibney 2014.[70]

Table 3 Summary of ASCO-SSO recommendations for sentinel lymph node biopsy in melanoma.

- SLNB is recommended for patients with cutaneous melanomas with Breslow thickness of 1 to 4 mm at any anatomic site;
- SLNB may be recommended for staging purposes and to facilitate regional disease control for patients with melanomas that are >4 mm in Breslow thickness;
- There is insufficient evidence to support routine SLNB for patients with melanomas that are <1 mm in Breslow thickness, although it may be considered in selected high-risk patients;
- Completion lymph node dissection is recommended for all patients with a positive SLNB.

SLNB, sentinel lymph node biopsy.
Adapted from Wong et al, 2012.[85]

indications for SLNB in melanoma was issued jointly by ASCO and the Society of Surgical Oncology (SSO) (Table 4).[85]

The panel found that the strongest evidence supported SLNB for patients with intermediate-thickness melanomas, based on interim results from the prospective randomized Multicenter Selective Lymphadenectomy Trial I (MSLT-1).[77] Key ASCO–SSO SLNB recommendations are summarized in Table 3. The mature results of MSLT-1 (Table 5)[86] and retrospective institutional series[89–92] also support SLNB for patients with clinically node-negative thick melanomas (>4 mm). Controversy remains regarding the use of sentinel node biopsy in patients with thin melanomas (<1 mm), which were not adequately assessed in the MSLT-1 study nor included in the prospective but nonrandomized Sunbelt Melanoma Trial.[93–95]

Today, the majority of newly diagnosed cutaneous melanomas are T1 lesions (≤1 mm in thickness), with a low overall risk of nodal metastasis or death from melanoma.[96] Recommending sentinel node biopsy for all patients with T1 melanomas is not cost-effective.[95] ASCO–SSO recommends that SLNB for thin melanoma be considered in selected cases with "high-risk" features (Table 6).[85]

On the basis of the large retrospectively collected registry data, SLNB seems well justified for many patients with melanomas 0.76–1.00 mm, but not for the majority of patients with melanomas <0.76 mm in thickness.[96] In addition, patient age, preference, and comorbidities need to be considered in the decision regarding SNLB.

A few other clinical situations pertaining to the use of SLNB deserve mention. Desmoplastic melanomas in general appear to have a lower risk of nodal metastases,[97,98] and some authors advocate abandoning SLNB in this histologic type.[99] In recent series, the risk of nodal metastases has been shown to be high enough to justify routine consideration of SLNB in all patients with desmoplastic melanomas ≥1 mm in thickness.[99] Pediatric melanoma patients have a higher incidence of nodal metastases, yet an apparent better overall prognosis compared to adults, and the role of SLNB in these patients remains controversial, especially for the so-called atypical melanocytic proliferations of childhood.[100–103]

Completion lymphadenectomy for sentinel node-positive disease

NCCN guidelines,[75] strongly supported by decades of clinical experience, call for routine performance of a therapeutic lymphadenectomy in all melanoma patients with clinically positive nodes and no radiographic evidence of distant metastases. The routine use of completion lymphadenectomy after a positive SLNB is more controversial,[104] although it is recommended by the ASCO/SSO guidelines as standard of care in the absence of clinical

Table 4 Summary of selected final results of the Multicenter Selective Lymphadenectomy Trial 1 (MSLT-1).

	Result	Comment
Feasibility	At least one sentinel node was identified in 99.5% of patients undergoing SLNB	SLNB highly feasible in a worldwide experience
Yield and false-negative rate	The sentinel node was positive in 19% of patients with melanomas ≥1.2 mm: 16% for melanomas 1.2–3.5 mm and 33% for melanomas >3.5 mm	SLNB is an effective staging procedure with an acceptable false-negative rate
	Nodal recurrence occurred in 5.9% of patients with a negative sentinel node: 4.8% for melanomas 1.2–3.5 mm and 10.3% for melanomas >3.5 mm	
Prognostic significance	A positive sentinel node was associated with ~2.5-fold increases in disease recurrence and death from melanoma for melanomas 1.2–3.5 mm; 10-year melanoma-specific survival was 85% for patients with a negative sentinel node versus 62% for patients with a positive sentinel node	Sentinel node status is the strongest known prognostic indicator in clinically node-negative intermediate-thickness melanoma
Survival impact of SLNB	There was a nonsignificant 3% increase in 10-year melanoma-specific survival for intermediate-thickness melanoma patients randomized to SLNB versus observation	SLNB does not significantly affect survival for all patients subjected to the procedure
Relapse-free survival impact	Patients randomized to SLNB had a statistically significant improvement in relapse-free survival compared to observation	SLNB significantly reduces melanoma recurrence for intermediate and thick melanomas, mostly by decreasing subsequent nodal relapse
Impact on node-positive patients	Patients with intermediate-thickness melanoma and positive nodes who were randomized to SLNB (with completion lymphadenectomy) had statistically significantly improved distant metastasis-free survival and melanoma-specific survival compared to observation arm patients who failed clinically in the regional nodal basin; there were no significant differences for patients with thick melanomas and positive nodes between the SLNB and observation arms	Early treatment of intermediate-thickness node-positive melanoma by radical lymphadenectomy improves outcomes significantly; patients with thick node-positive melanomas may be at such high risk of distant disease that timing of lymphadenectomy loses importance

SLNB, sentinel lymph node biopsy.
Adapted from Sondak and Gibney 2014.[70] Original data from Morton.

Table 5 High-risk features for selecting T1 melanomas for sentinel lymph node biopsy.

High-risk criterion	Impact on likelihood of finding a positive node	Comment
Thickness 0.76–0.99 mm	In a registry series of 1250 patients with melanomas ≤1 mm selected by a wide variety of criteria to undergo SLNB, metastases were detected in 6.3% of 891 melanomas ≥0.76 mm but in only 2.5% of 359 melanomas ≤0.75 mm. No metastases were detected in sentinel nodes from patients with melanomas <0.5 mm.[87] In a large contemporary single-institution experience from a center where SLNB was routinely offered to patients with melanoma ≥0.76 mm without requiring any other high-risk feature to be present, 8.4% of patients had a positive sentinel node[86]	Most patients with thin melanomas and a positive sentinel node are found in this upper end of the T1 thickness spectrum; very few unselected patients with melanomas <0.76 mm are at sufficient risk of nodal metastasis to justify SLNB
Ulceration	18.3% of patients in a registry series[87] and 23.5% of patients in a single-institution series[88] who had ulcerated T1 melanomas had a positive sentinel node	Relatively rare finding in T1 melanomas (present in <10% of cases) but perhaps the highest risk factor for sentinel node positivity in thin melanoma
Mitotic count	Mitotic count ≥1/mm² was not predictive of nodal metastases in a registry series[87] but was predictive in a single-institution series[88]	Presence of even one dermal mitosis in a T1 melanoma upstages the tumor from T1a to T1b in the current AJCC staging system. It remains unclear whether the presence of dermal mitoses is sufficient to justify SLNB, especially in melanomas <0.76 mm
Patient age	—	Younger patients have a higher risk of positive sentinel nodes across all tumor thickness categories as well as more years at risk for nodal recurrence
Clark level	Clark level was a significant predictor of sentinel node status in a registry series[87] but not in a single-institution series[88]	Clark level IV melanomas are more likely to be at the thicker end (≥0.76–1.00 mm) of T1 where most nodal metastases are encountered. The value of SLNB for Clark IV melanomas <0.76 mm has not been demonstrated

SLNB, sentinel lymph node biopsy.
Data from Han 2012[87] and Han 2013.[88]

trial participation.[85] The MSLT-1 trial showed that outcomes for patients with intermediate-thickness melanoma undergoing completion lymphadenectomy were superior to those for patients who recurred in the nodal basin,[86] but by the nature of the trial, the contribution of the completion lymphadenectomy over and above removal of the sentinel node could not be assessed. Nonsentinel nodes are only found to have tumor involvement in a minority of cases,[107] and at least some sentinel node-positive patients do well for an extended period of time even without undergoing completion lymphadenectomy.[86] The morbidity of lymphadenectomy, especially severe lymphedema, has been shown to be less for completion lymphadenectomy after a positive SLNB than for therapeutic lymphadenectomy after nodal recurrence.[109] A prospective randomized trial comparing ultrasound surveillance of the lymph

Table 6 Summary of follow-up guidelines for patients with completely resected melanoma from various national and international organizations. These guidelines have not been prospectively validated and hence should only be considered as recommendations.

Stage	Physical examination	Imaging
Stage I	Every 3–12 months × 5 years with annual follow-up beyond 5 years as clinically indicated	No imaging needed unless clinically indicated
Stage II	Every 3–6 months × 2 years, then every 3–12 months for an additional 3 years with annual follow-up beyond 5 years as clinically indicated[a]	Cross-sectional body imaging considered for higher risk patients: CT and/or PET/CT, to screen for recurrent disease. Consider brain MRI annually[b]
Stage III–IV	Every 3–6 months × 2 years, then every 3–12 months for an additional 3 years with annual follow-up beyond 5 years as clinically indicated[c]	Cross-sectional body imaging should be considered for higher risk patients: CT and/or PET/CT, to screen for recurrent disease. Consider brain MRI annually[b]

[a]Consider more frequent and longer follow-up in high-risk stage II patients with thick and/or ulcerated primary tumors.
[b]Ultrasonography can be considered to evaluate regional nodal basins.
[c]Consider more frequent and longer follow-up in high-risk stage IIIb/c patients.
Abbreviations: CT, computed tomography; CXR, chest X-ray; PET/CT; positron emission tomography/computed tomography.
Adapted from Fields and Coit 2011.[145]

node basin to immediate completion lymphadenectomy for sentinel node-positive patients, MSLT-2, recently completed accrual with results pending (clinicaltrials.gov NCT00297895).

Radical lymphadenectomy for macroscopic nodal disease
In contrast to the situation for SLNB identified microscopic disease, a therapeutic radical lymph node dissection is virtually always indicated for clinically evident, resectable nodal metastasis; systemic therapy and/or radiation is not an adequate substitute for surgical treatment of the clinically positive nodal basin.[75]

Management of in-transit and locoregional recurrent melanoma
Wide excision is indicated for biopsy-proven local, satellite, or in-transit recurrence in the absence of distant disease. Full radiographic staging (with PET/CT or CT and brain MRI or CT) should be performed before curative-intent excision of the recurrent tumor.

Intra-arterial regional perfusion therapies
Hyperthermic isolated limb perfusion (HILP) and isolated limb infusion (ILI) are methods by which an extremity with unresectable locally recurrent or in-transit metastatic melanoma is isolated from systemic circulation and high-dose chemotherapy administered intra-arterially with limited systemic exposure. HILP is performed by directly dissecting and cannulating the major vessels of the extremity and circulating chemotherapy via a cardiopulmonary bypass machine, which allows increased temperature and an oxygenated perfusate. HILP can achieve concentrations within the limb 15–25 times higher than would be tolerated systemically, with limb temperatures reaching 39–41°C. By virtue of the increased concentration and the potential synergistic effects of hyperthermia, drugs such as melphalan, with little or no activity if administered systemically, become highly effective regional agents.[110,111] Response rates in the range of 80–90% with complete response (CR) rates as high as 60–70% have been reported.[111–114] Melphalan is the

most-common agent used in the United States, while melphalan plus tumor necrosis factor alpha (TNF-α) is often used in Europe.[115] The value of TNF-α has not been clearly demonstrated, as a large multicenter randomized trial found no statistically significant differences in either overall or CR rates or survival and the addition of TNF-α was associated with significantly higher regional toxicity.[114]

Isolation of the limb during HILP substantially minimizes the risk of systemic toxicity from the high-dose chemotherapy; however, significant morbidity may still occur. The most-common morbidity is lymphedema and has been reported to occur in 12–36% of patients. Severe regional toxicities including compartment syndrome in up to 5% of cases as well as limb loss in up to 3.3% of cases have been described.[115,116]

ILI is the less-invasive counterpart to HILP and is a low-flow infusion conducted in a mildly hyperthermic, acidotic, and hypoxic environment. Catheters are percutaneously placed into the artery and vein of the uninvolved limb and advanced into the vessels of the involved limb proximal to the extent of disease, avoiding the need for open surgical cannulation with its attendant morbidity. The chemotherapy is manually circulated for 30 min.[117] Regional CR rates after ILI are in the range of 23–44% with partial response (PR) rates in the range of 27–56%.[117,118] Although these results are lower than reported after HILP, the two techniques have not been prospectively compared in a head-to-head manner in a clinical trial setting. In a recent retrospective comparison of HILP and ILI (ILI = 94, ILP = 109), the overall response rate was 53% for ILI versus 80% for ILP ($p > 0.001$). Median overall survival (OS) was 46 months for ILI versus 40 months for ILP ($p = 0.31$). There were no differences in age, sex, or N stage between groups; however, BOD was higher for the ILI group (high BOD 58 vs. 44%, $p = 0.04$).[119] Importantly, ILI can be readily repeated if necessary and appears to have less regional toxicities than HILP (erythema and edema of the skin are among the most-common side effects with tissue loss seen <1% of the time) and virtually no systemic toxicities.[116–119]

There is some debate regarding whether ILI or HILP should be employed first in the treatment of in-transit melanoma, and this decision is based in part on the presence of nodes requiring node dissection or a high burden of disease in the limb, both of which might be better addressed with HILP, although the data are lacking to support this theory. In view of the relative morbidities and effectiveness, HILP is usually reserved as a salvage procedure for patients who progress rapidly after ILI without any evidence of distant metastasis. Repeat ILI can be attempted in patients who had a good initial response to ILI but eventually progressed.

Intralesional and topical therapies
Intralesional therapy in melanoma has several advantages over regional or systemic therapy. Local drug administration allows for delivery of an increased concentration of the agent and reduced regional and systemic exposure, potentially increasing efficacy and lowering toxicity. Moreover, alterations in the tumor microenvironment can be immunogenic and induce local immune responses that result in the "bystander effect," where uninjected distant lesions exhibit a response, as has been reported with multiple different types of intralesional therapies.

Bacille Calmette-Guèrin (BCG) was one of the first intralesional therapies used for in-transit metastases. In that initial landmark series, 90% of injected cutaneous lesions regressed and 17% of patients also had regression of uninjected lesions. Some patients remained disease free for years after completion of the BCG injections.[120] Interleukin-2 (IL-2) has also been used for intralesional injection in melanoma; the toxicity profile of IL-2 appears to be better than that of BCG. There is a risk of local reactions, and flu-like symptoms following injections are very common (85%).[121] Intralesional treatment with IL-2 is relatively expensive. PV-10 is a 10% solution of rose bengal, a water-soluble xanthine dye used for decades as an intravenous diagnostic agent for assessing hepatic function and topically by ophthalmologists, making it a potentially low-cost treatment that has shown efficacy when "repurposed" for intralesional administration.[122] Responses have been reported in patients refractory to previous systemic ipilimumab, anti-PD1 and vemurafenib, with evidence of bystander effects in uninjected lesions.[123]

Talimogene laherparepvec (TVEC, previously known as OncoVEX), is a genetically modified oncolytic herpes virus incorporating the coding sequence for human granulocyte-macrophage colony-stimulating factor (GM-CSF). Oncolytic viruses are designed to selectively replicate in tumors, thereby infecting and destroying cancer cells and inducing immune responses that target the cancer cell. Expression of the GM-CSF gene (GM-CSF) in tumor cells is expected to recruit and activate antigen-presenting cells and immune effectors that mediate potent antitumor T cell cytotoxicity. Tumor destruction in this fashion may also induce T cells capable of circulating and exerting antitumor effects in nearby and distant uninjected metastases. The phase III OPTiM study included 436 patients randomized in a 2 : 1 manner to intralesional TVEC or subcutaneous GM-CSF alone, respectively. There was a 26.4% objective response rate for TVEC compared to a 5.7% for GM-CSF ($p < 0.001$). There was a statistically significant increase in the primary endpoint of durable response rate (DRR), defined as a partial or CR lasting for 6 months or more. DRR was 16.3% for TVEC and 2.1% for GM-CSF ($p < 0.001$). Overall survival results also favored TVEC, although without statistical significance.[126] This promising form of viral-mediated immune gene therapy is now being tested in combination with immune checkpoint blockers and other immunomodulatory interventions, and other oncolytic viruses with or without transgenes are also under investigation for melanoma and other malignancies.[124]

Imiquimod and diphencyprone (DPCP) are topically applied, rather than injected intralesionally. This approach is particularly appealing for patients with multiple small cutaneous nodules. Topical application of imiquimod, with or without additional agents such as topical 5-fluorouracil, resulted in regression of up to 90% of treated superficial lesions.[125,126] DPCP is a contact sensitizer that induces contact hypersensitivity; in a cohort of 50 patients treated with DPCP, 23 patients (46%) achieved a CR and an additional 19 patients (38%) showed a PR. The side effect profile of DPCP is tolerable, with skin reactions such as blistering and irritation being the most-common side effects.[127]

Radiation therapy

In patients with in-transit or regional recurrence, radiation may offer a benefit. Treatment protocols are not well defined but the potential for symptom control makes radiation an option for selected patients with unresectable locoregional melanoma[128] and is now under active investigation as an immunomodulator, detailed later in this chapter.

Surgical metastasectomy for stage IV melanoma

Patients with isolated, resectable distant metastatic melanoma are candidates for surgical management aimed at removing all known sites of disease. Identifying which patients will benefit from metastasectomy requires good clinical judgment and a thorough preoperative staging that includes PET–CT of the body and MRI of the brain to rule out occult sites of metastasis.[129]

There has been only one prospective (albeit nonrandomized) trial evaluating surgery for patients with stage IV melanoma, the S9430 trial conducted by the Southwest Oncology Group.[130] Patients with stage IV melanoma were enrolled as soon as the determination of potential resectability was made, before actually undergoing surgery. This allowed the investigators to estimate resectability rate and define relapse-free and overall survival after complete resection. Among the 77 study patients, 3 patients had no evidence of melanoma in the resected specimen (the suspected metastatic deposit was either a second primary malignancy or a benign finding) and 2 patients had only stage III disease. An additional 8 patients were not able to have all disease resected. Therefore, 64 patients (88.9%) were in fact resected to a disease-free state. After a median follow-up of 5 years, all but 6 (9.4%) had recurred, with a median relapse-free survival (RFS) of approximately 5 months. Median overall survival was 21 months with an estimated 12-month survival of 75% and survival at 4 years was 31%.[130] Although small, this prospectively derived and with otherwise unselected patients, the resectability and survival rates reported in S9430 are the most representative data available for comparing surgical and nonsurgical approaches to stage IV melanoma. It is possible that using the more sensitive current imaging methods to find patients with resectable single or oligometastases would lead to more favorable outcomes if the study were done now. However, new systemic therapy approaches to metastatic melanoma are becoming so effective that a reconsideration of the role of surgery in front-line management may be appropriate, and of great importance is the investigation of the potential for neo-adjuvant therapies from among the molecularly targeted agents and the new immunotherapies, particularly PD-1 blocking agents that work relatively quickly and may render a formerly unresectable lesion more amenable to surgery.

The role of adjuvant therapy for stage II and III disease

Immunotherapy

Immunotherapy has been the adjuvant treatment approach evaluated most extensively in melanoma, and the most extensively evaluated adjuvant immunotherapy has been interferon-α (IFN-α), in a variety of doses, schedules, and formulations. High-dose IFN-α is a 1-year adjuvant therapy regimen involving two components: a 1-month "induction" phase administering 20 million units of IFN-α2b/m^2 of body surface area intravenously 5 days per week for 4 weeks, followed by an 11-month "maintenance" phase administering 10 million units/m^2 subcutaneously three times a week. Three randomized trials have demonstrated that high-dose IFN-α is associated with improved RFS, and two trials showed improved OS as well.[131,132] In the United States, high-dose IFN-α is approved for use in the adjuvant therapy of thick, node-negative and node-positive melanoma. To date, no studies of high-dose IFN-α have defined subsets of patients that clearly respond better or worse to treatment. The relative importance of the induction and maintenance phases has not been adequately defined, but it does appear that the 4-week induction phase alone is inadequate.[133]

Adjuvant IFN-α regimens involving lower doses of IFN-α (3–10 million units administered three times a week not adjusted for body surface area and without the initial intravenous component) have also been tested. Low-dose IFN-α is approved for adjuvant use in some European countries and has been advocated for use in intermediate-thickness, node-negative melanoma as well.[134] In the absence of direct comparisons between high- and low-dose IFN-α regimens, meta-analyses have been performed to assess the overall and comparative efficacy of adjuvant IFN-α therapy. Meta-analysis results clearly support that IFN-α therapy delays recurrence, with an overall RFS improvement of 17% (hazard ratio for recurrence 0.83) in the latest analysis, but do not identify clear differences between high- and low-dose regimens in efficacy. Meta-analysis results also show a statistically significant improvement in OS for adjuvant IFN-α, with a 9% (hazard ratio for survival 0.91) improvement seen.[135]

Pegylated IFN-α was approved in the United States as an alternative adjuvant treatment for stage III melanoma in 2011, based on the results of a single randomized trial.[136] This trial demonstrated a statistically significant improvement in RFS, in keeping with trials of standard IFN-α, but did not show an OS benefit. An interesting observation was made, however, that the subset of patients with sentinel node-positive melanoma from an ulcerated primary showed a dramatic survival benefit (41% improvement) when treated with pegylated IFN-α. Although some other IFN-α trials have seen a similar benefit in this subset,[137,138] this is best considered an unproven but provocative finding pending definitive replication. Pegylated IFN-α has not been directly compared to high-dose IFN-α, but appears to have fewer serious side effects with pharmacologic properties that might make it a more favorable agent for the maintenance phase. Unlike high-dose IFN-α, pegylated IFN-α is intended to be given subcutaneously for 5 years (3 mcg/kg/week), and the 1-month intravenously administered induction phase is replaced with a 2-month long subcutaneously administered induction phase at a higher dose (6 mcg/kg/week).

Other adjuvant systemic therapies under investigation

The availability of new agents with documented survival benefits in unresectable metastatic melanoma has spurred trials of these agents in the adjuvant setting. It remains to be seen if these agents will be equally or more effective than available IFN-α regimens, and how the toxicities of these new drugs will be tolerated by patients who are disease free and possibly cured at the time of treatment. Nonetheless, it is likely that the advances in understanding melanoma biology and the regulators of the antitumor immune response that have profoundly changed treatment for stage IV melanoma will eventually translate into new, more effective and hopefully less toxic approaches to the prevention of recurrence by adjuvant therapy.

A multiagent biochemotherapy regimen consisting of IFN-α, IL-2, dacarbazine, vinblastine, and cisplatin was compared to high-dose IFN-α in a randomized trial showing a statistically significant RFS advantage but no difference in OS.[139] Although this is the first randomized trial to ever show a statistically significant advantage over high-dose IFN-α, the toxicity of this regimen limits its use, and the lack of an OS advantage argues against this becoming a new standard for the adjuvant treatment of melanoma.

Ipilimumab has been shown to improve survival in stage IV melanoma (detailed later in this chapter), with less toxicity than is associated with biochemotherapy, making it a logical candidate to evaluate in the adjuvant setting. Preliminary data from a randomized trial comparing ipilimumab at 10 mg/kg (a dose higher than that approved for use in the treatment of unresectable metastatic melanoma) to placebo showed statistically significantly improved RFS relapse for the ipilimumab arm.[140] Unfortunately, the toxicity of the regimen was unexpectedly severe. Data regarding the impact of this adjuvant ipilimumab regimen on OS are pending. Importantly, the relative impact of adjuvant ipilimumab over that provided by IFN-α is currently unknown. Given the toxicity

encountered with adjuvant ipilimumab at 10 mg/kg, there is also a need to assess the risk–benefit ratio relative to the standard 3 mg/kg ipilimumab dose. A randomized trial has been conducted to evaluate ipilimumab at 10 and 3 mg/kg compared to high-dose IFN-α (E1609, NCT01274338). This trial has completed accrual and results are eagerly awaited. The safety and tolerability of anti-PD1 antibodies appear to be superior to both IFN-α and ipilimumab, making these antibodies ideal candidates for evaluation as adjuvant therapy. The results of completed but not yet mature randomized trials of ipilimumab versus nivolumab (Checkmate 238, NCT 02833906) and of pembrolizumab versus placebo (EORTC Keynote 054. NCT 02362594) will likely define future adjuvant systemic therapy recommendations.

Additional trials investigating the activity of adjuvant BRAF inhibitors alone or in combination with MEK inhibitors have completed accrual and await outcome data. Legitimate concerns have been raised about the tolerability of these agents in the adjuvant setting, particularly considering the potential for rapid development of resistance and for secondary malignancies to arise in patients taking these agents, and their routine use is not recommended in the adjuvant setting.[141]

Adjuvant radiation to the resected nodal basin

Criteria for identifying patients at high risk of regional recurrence in the resected nodal basin after radical lymphadenectomy include multiple (≥4) or matted tumor-involved lymph nodes, the presence of extranodal extension of tumor in at least one node, and large size (≥3 cm) of any one lymph node. In a prospective trial, 217 eligible patients possessing at least one of these criteria were randomized to observation or postoperative nodal basin irradiation after lymphadenectomy.[108] After a median follow-up of 40 months, nodal basin relapse occurred in 34 of 108 patients (31.5%) in the observation arm, confirming the high risk of regional recurrence in these patients. Nodal basin relapse was significantly reduced in the adjuvant radiotherapy group compared with the observation group, but no differences were noted for RFS when all sites of relapse were included or for OS.[108] This confirmed the ability of postoperative radiation to significantly decrease recurrence within the nodal basin in patients at high risk of such recurrence, and radiation should be considered for selected high-risk cases. It will also be important to study the interaction of adjuvant locoregional radiotherapy with immune checkpoint blockade in the adjuvant therapy of high-risk melanoma.

Surveillance for high-risk melanoma patients

A variety of algorithms have been proposed regarding the frequency and nature of the follow-up evaluation of melanoma patients after surgical treatment.[142–144] To date, no studies have documented that surveillance of patients after surgical treatment of melanoma with any imaging or laboratory studies (including chest X-rays, PET/CT, or MRI scans) are cost-effective. One study evaluating the results of follow-up after surgery in stage melanoma III patients found that half of all recurrences were detected by patients, and that "neither more intense nor more frequent follow-up is associated with discovery of resectable first relapses."[142] While most proposed follow-up algorithms involve more frequent follow-up in the initial years after surgery, the conditional probability of recurrence of stage I and II melanoma is actually fairly constant over the first decade after surgery.[144] Education is key and should be focused on both the patient and family as well as the primary care physicians, dermatologists, and surgeons alike, and melanoma centers may want to train and even "certify" providers in their catchment area. Patients should be willing to return to the melanoma center for evaluation of suspected recurrence, because properly diagnosing recurrence (e.g., documenting nodal recurrence by needle aspiration cytology instead of open biopsy) is important to successful treatment. Importantly, we need to individualize the follow-up, identifying which patients are best suited to have the bulk of their surveillance outside the melanoma center and which ones should return more frequently.

Table 6 summarizes the follow-up guideline for patients with completely resected melanoma from various national and international organizations. These guidelines have not been prospectively validated and hence should only be considered as recommendations. (Adapted from Fields and Coit.[142])

Uveal melanoma and rare melanomas of the eye

Uveal melanoma (UM) is the most-common primary intraocular cancer of the eye in adults and represents 5% of all melanomas. The term "UM" is used for melanomas that arise within the uveal tract (i.e., iris, ciliary body, or choroid), while the broader term "ocular" melanoma includes such sites as conjunctiva and eyelid, which behave like cutaneous melanoma. UMs are further designated as anterior (iris) or posterior (ciliary body and/or choroid) chamber tumors. Anterior chamber UM is rarer (<10% of UMs) and tends not to metastasize, whereas approximately half of patients diagnosed with posterior chamber UM will develop metastases.

Local therapy for UM employs radioactive plaque, proton therapy, or enucleation of the primary UM tumor. In a randomized study comparing ^{128}I plaque brachytherapy with enucleation, 85% of patients receiving radiation retained their eye, and 37% had visual acuity over 20/200 in the irradiated eye 5 years after therapy. No survival difference was seen between the radioactive plaque and enucleation groups.[145] Thus, a radiotherapeutic approach has become the strategy of choice for primary UM treatment, with enucleation reserved for the remaining <10% of cases in which radiotherapy is not possible (e.g., bulky disease, technically difficult tumor location, patient preference). Because most patients do not undergo enucleation, fine-needle aspiration techniques are now often used to obtain the pathologic and molecular diagnostic information that is critical to prognosis.

UM metastases are hematogenous, because the uveal tract does not appear to contain clear lymphatic channels with draining lymph nodes. The liver is ultimately involved in 95% of metastatic UM cases and is the sole site of metastatic UM in approximately 50% of patients. The most common other sites of metastatic UM are lung (24%), bone (16%), and skin (11%). Unlike cutaneous melanoma, UM infrequently metastasizes to lymph nodes or brain. The clinical course of patients with UM is highly dependent on disease progression in the liver. The median survival after diagnosis of patients with liver metastases is approximately 4–6 months with a 1-year survival of approximately 10–15%. Patients with metastases limited to extrahepatic sites have a median survival of approximately 19–28 months with a 1-year survival of approximately 76%. Thus, hepatic-versus extrahepatic-only disease may represent distinct biological entities.[146]

Approximately 90% of UM harbor activating, mutually exclusive, recurrent mutations in the g-protein alpha q (*GNAQ*) or 11 (*GNA11*) subunit genes. Nearly all *GNAQ/11* gene mutations localize to a hotspot in exon 5 (Q209), although a small number localize to exon 4 (R183). *GNAQ/11* gene mutations are early tumorigenic events that are insufficient to initiate metastatic disease, but some

of the downstream pathways in UM resulting from additional molecular aberrations, such as protein kinase C and others, may be targetable with investigational agents in development.[147] Additional recurrent missense mutations in *SF3B1* (altering the R625 amino acid position in most cases) or *EIF1AX* (exons 1 or 2) genes occur in equal proportion in approximately 40% of UM tumors and are essentially mutually exclusive with each other. Truncating and nontruncating mutations are observed in the nuclear ubiquitin carboxy-terminal hydrolase *BAP1* gene located on chromosome 3p21.1. Genetic aberrations in *BAP1* tend to co-occur with monosomy 3, resulting in the loss of heterozygosity of BAP1. Both *BAP1* gene mutations and monosomy 3 tend not to co-occur with *SF3B1* or *EIF1AX* gene mutations, and the former are associated with a high risk of developing metastatic UM.[148] Consistent with *BAP1* mutations leading to loss of tumor suppression, there have been multiple reports of germline *BAP1* mutations within families that result in a high incidence of UM.[149] Another recurrent chromosomal aberration observed in UM is 8q copy number gain (often with 8p loss), which tends to accompany monosomy 3 and is associated with a shorter time to relapse. Conversely, 6p copy number gain (often with 6q loss) is usually present in tumors that lack monosomy 3 or 8q copy number gain and is associated with a low risk of metastasis. Less-frequent chromosomal aberrations, such as 1p and/or 16q loss, have also been described. With the exception of *BAP1*, the identification of specific genes that correlate functionally with these chromosomal aberrations is less clear.[150]

Multiple anatomic, histologic, and molecular features within primary tumors are associated with poor prognosis: (1) location in ciliary body (poorer) > choroid ≫ iris (rarely metastasize); (2) greater tumor size; (3) extrascleral invasion; (4) epithelioid > spindle cell histology; (5) higher mitotic rate; (6) presence of monosomy 3 ± chr 8q gain; and (7) class 2 ≫ class 1b ≫ class 1a gene expression profile (a 15-gene expression profile that accurately predicts outcome and does not require chromosomal analysis). However, the strongest risk factors for metastasis are copy number profile (e.g., presence of monosomy 3/chr 8q gain) and/or a class 1b/2 gene expression profile.[151,152]

Metastatic UM has proven essentially recalcitrant to traditional chemo- and immunotherapeutic approaches. Given the current inability to therapeutically target the aforementioned molecular aberrations characteristic of UM, there has been a major focus on targeting the "effector" molecules associated with these genetic alterations. The most successful systemic approach to date has been to target the MEK–MAPK pathway that is clearly activated by *GNAQ/11* mutations. A phase II randomized clinical trial showed that treatment of metastatic UM patients with single-agent selumetinib (a small molecule MEK inhibitor) resulted in tumor regression in 50% and RECIST responses in 15% of cases. A significant difference in median progression-free survival following treatment with selumetinib (15.9 weeks) compared to dacarbazine (7 weeks) was shown, although without an improvement in overall survival.[153] Targetable effectors of mutant *BAP1*/monosomy 3 are still under investigation. Retrospective analyses of metastatic UM patients from multiple centers treated with ipilimumab suggest that long-term tumor response was observed in a subset (~5%), as well as prolonged stable disease (SD) in a slightly larger subset of advanced disease patients.[154] More recently, therapy of metastatic uveal melanoma with antibodies blocking PD-1 or PD-L1 was reported from a multi-institution retrospective series and also showed very low activity,[155] further evidence that the successful therapy of this melanoma variant requires strategies that focus on its unique molecular biology and targets in its immune tumor microenvironment.

For patients with liver-only or -dominant metastatic UM, multiple therapies specifically directed at the liver have been explored: isolated or percutaneous hepatic perfusion of chemotherapy, transarterial chemoembolization (TACE), radioembolization or cryoembolization, or selective internal radiation therapy (SIRT). Liver-directed therapy studies tend to have low patient numbers, but when taken in aggregate, suggest relatively high tumor response, prolonged time-to-progression, and/or survival in the population of patients upon whom they have been employed. Nine studies (totaling 209 patients) using TACE (mostly cisplatin-based) reveal a 2% CR, 24% PR, and 33% SD rate when taken in aggregate. Eight pooled studies (totaling 277 patients) show hepatic intra-arterial chemotherapy (mostly employing either a fotemustine or melphalan-based regimen) to have a 9% CR, 22% PR, and 29% SD rate to this approach. Finally, four studies (totaling 59 patients) treated with hepatic arterial perfusion reveal an 8% CR, 44% PR, and 10% SD rate (reviewed in Ref. 156).

There may be a role for surgical resection of metastatic UM if there is a relatively stable and safely resectable solitary lesion(s). In a study in which 61 patients had surgical resection in addition to chemotherapy, a 22-month median overall survival was observed among patients who could undergo resection with curative intent compared to 10 months among those who could not. Variations in patient referral and selection criteria are important factors in all of these outcomes, which must be validated by performing well-controlled prospective randomized trials.

With one of the most predictive sets of molecular markers of metastatic risk, the relatively recent identification of clear genetic drivers within primary UM tumors, and a wide spectrum of clinically relevant approaches (molecular inhibitors, immunotherapies, radiation and surgery) now available, there is tremendous excitement that truly effective therapies for UM in both the adjuvant and advanced settings are within practical reach.

Melanoma of the conjunctival surface of the eye is rare and may complicate primary acquired melanosis. Recent reports demonstrating the presence of typical activating BRAF mutations in 29% and NRAS mutations in 18% of a cohort of 78 conjunctival melanomas provide further evidence of the close relationship of melanomas in this site to cutaneous melanomas, with case reports of clinical responses to vemurafenib that corroborate the importance of BRAF as an oncogenic driver in conjunctival melanoma.[157,158]

Biology and therapy of advanced melanoma

The diagnosis of metastatic melanoma may be triggered by new symptoms or signs in a patient with a history of melanoma (about half of the presentations) or a new but asymptomatic finding on radiographic surveillance scans, based on guidelines and practice that take into account the initial stage, time-dependent risk of relapse, and likelihood that intervention will change the natural history of the disease. Skin and soft tissue are more common sites of initial metastatic disease than visceral sites, and a minority of patients have widespread metastatic disease secondary to hematogenous spread, such as is common with mucosal melanomas.

Uncommonly, advanced melanoma may present as a solitary or multiple metastases—even in the central nervous system—without a known history or evidence of a concurrent new primary melanoma. It has been postulated that immune-mediated control or regression of a missed primary controlled by a local immune response explains this phenomenon, which also has a slightly more favorable prognosis than matched cases with a known primary.[159] Melanoma spreads widely and spares few organs or sites, with a particular affinity for the brain, where it is often the immediate or major contributing cause of death due to bleeding and edema. Other sites of melanoma metastasis that are rare for other cancers include the small and large intestine and even the heart. Characteristics of primary melanoma that pose increased propensity to specific sites of metastasis are under investigation. For example, the CCL25 and CCR9 chemokine: chemokine receptor interaction has been reported in intestinal metastases[160] and increased activity of the phosphatase and tensin homolog (PTEN)-related pathway is associated with a higher rate of eventual metastasis to the brain (reviewed in Ref. 161). Many other molecular alterations, most recently the expression of a variant CD44v6 molecule, a receptor for hyaluronic acid that is highly expressed by brain,[162] have been reported to impact the risk and/or the biological behavior of established brain metastases (reviewed in Ref. 163).

Molecularly targeted therapy for melanoma

Metastatic melanoma is divided into three substages based on modest differences in the survival curves for M1a, limited to skin and soft tissue; M1b, involving lung with/without skin/soft tissue; and M1c, metastatic to any visceral organ and/or with elevation of the serum lactate dehydrogenase (LDH) above the institutional upper limit of normal.[94] The differences among these subsets are being eclipsed by a rapid growth in understanding of the molecular basis of different melanomas such as detailed by Bastian's group.[61] However, except for notable examples such as the melanomas that carry actionable oncogenic driver mutations (BRAF, c-kit, NRAS) and UM, which is routinely excluded from most clinical trials of immunotherapy, clinical trials for advanced melanoma have included unselected patients, with prestratification in some instances for known prognostic variables such as the LDH and the performance status.

Melanoma, together with lung cancer, has the highest frequency of mutations per cell among all human malignancies, which is largely attributable to frequent $C \rightarrow T$ transitions resulting from solar UV exposure.[12] A few mutations result in "driver" oncogenes (such as activating BRAF v600^E or v600^K mutations or NRAS mutations at G12, G13 or Q61) and/or important "passenger" alterations that collaborate to varying degrees in oncogenesis (such as PTEN loss of function, which occurs in at least 20–30% of melanomas, often in association with BRAF mutations,[164] and many others such as TP53 and p16INK4a and p14ARF[12]). Simultaneous mutation of BRAF and NRAS is rarely found in primary melanomas untreated with BRAF inhibitors. The importance of the PTEN pathway and its downstream mediators of a wide variety of proliferative, metabolic and antiapoptotic functions is illustrated by a large number of mechanisms for pathway activation, including hypermethylation of the PTEN promoter and rare mutations of AKT or PI3kinase isoforms (reviewed in Ref. 165).

The molecular drivers currently targetable by therapeutic agents approved for melanoma are limited to BRAF-activating mutations, which are tested by either pcr-based or gene sequencing methods[166] for the mutations encoding BRAF v600^E or one of the less-common activating mutations at residue 600 of the BRAF serine–threonine kinase. BRAF v600^E has a change from valine to glutamic acid ($V \rightarrow E$) and accounts for approximately 75% of cases, while the next most common is valine to lysine ($V \rightarrow K$) in about 17%. Other amino acid substitutions account for the small number of remaining cases.[167] Tumors carrying V600^K are associated with more advanced age, chronic sun damage, and a somewhat less favorable outcome even with BRAF inhibition.[168] There are many assays available for next generation genomic sequencing that detect

Table 7 Antitumor activity and toxicities of molecularly targeted agents[a]

DRUG (References)	Vemurafenib[178]	Vemurafenib[177]	Dabrafenib[176]	Trametinib[179]	Dab + Tram[176]	Dab + Tram[177]	Vemu + Cobimetinib[h 178]
Patient number	239	352	212	214	211	352	254
Objective response (%)	45	51	51	22	67	64	68
CR (%)	4	8	9	2	10	13	10
Progression-free survival (median, mo)	6.2	7.3	8.8	4.8	9.3	11.4	9.9
TOXICITIES[c]							
All grade 3 (%)	49	57	34	Grade 3 or 4	32	48	49
All grade 4 (%)	9	1.4	3	8	3	1	13
Fever	22	21	28	—	51	53	26
Fatigue	31	—	35	26	35	—	32
Headache	—	—	29	—	30	—	—
Nausea or emesis	24	15	26	18	30	29	10
Chills	—	8	16	—	30	31	—
Arthralgia	40	51	27	—	24	24	32
Diarrhea	28	38	14	43	24	32	17
Rash	35	43	22	57 (acneiform 19)	23	22	17
Hypertension	—	—	14	15	22	—	—
Peripheral edema	—	—	5	26	14	—	—
Increased transaminase	18	—	5	—	11	—	18
Photosensitivity	15	22	—	—	—	4	28
Hyperkeratosis	29	25	32	—	9	4	10
Keratoacanthoma	20	KA or SCC	21	—	—	KA or	1
Squamous cancer	11	18	9	—	—	SCC 1	3
Alopecia	—	26	26	17	—	—	2
Hand-foot syndrome	—	25	27	—	5	4	—
Decreased LVEF	—	—	2	—	4	8	—

[a]From randomized trials.

[b]Thirty percent of patients had asymptomatic grade 1–2 creatinine phosphokinase elevation.

[c]Reversible transient drug-induced retinopathy, rarely reported.

additional alterations with therapeutic implications, for example, activating c-kit mutations in about 20% of mucosal and 15% of acral melanomas with occasional responsiveness to imatinib[170–172] and related tyrosine kinase inhibitors, and NRAS mutations, which have shown responsiveness to MEK and cyclin-dependent kinase (CDK) 4/6 inhibitors inhibitors although not as sensitive as BRAF-mutated melanoma[172] These assays are also valuable for discovery of new mechanisms of resistance, especially when performed sequentially on biopsies before and during therapy. Also of interest is the recent observation of BRAF gene fusions with several other molecular species in Spitzoid nevi that provide unique targets for several agents already in testing.[173]

Disease regression occurs in the majority of patients treated with single-agent BRAF or MEK inhibitors (Table 7) and can be improved with the combination of inhibitors, which have shown survival benefit over single-agent BRAF inhibition. As some of the toxicities of BRAF inhibitors occur via paradoxically-enhanced signaling from upstream pathways that also activate MEK,[174] these effects are less prominent during combined therapy; furthermore, the secondary low-grade cutaneous proliferations (keratoacanthoma and squamous cancers) attributed to mutant HRAS activation upstream of MEK[175] are also reduced during combination therapy. Such combinations also yield higher response rates and additional disease regression, as shown on the "waterfall" plots of maximum regression in individual subjects. Longer progression-free and overall survival has also been reported with these combinations over BRAF inhibition alone.[176–179] Toxicities of single-agent therapy with either BRAF or MEK inhibitors are generally tolerable but may require dose reduction, brief drug holiday, or a switch in agent(s). They are briefly summarized in Table 7, but further management guidelines are available from recent experience[181,182] and will undoubtedly emerge with more experience, particularly since the regulatory approval of these agents has led to their more widespread use.

Acquired resistance to single MAPK inhibitors occurs after a median of 6 months and somewhat later (median 8–11 months) with combined MAPK inhibitors (Table 7), although a fraction of patients may enjoy prolonged control.[183] The mechanisms of resistance as well as protection against resistance are becoming evident from the many clinical trials that provide tissue for analysis before therapy and during therapy or at the time of progression. Reactivation of MEK signaling occurs in most cases of acquired resistance to MAPK inhibition, via alterations in BRAF (gene amplification or truncation mutations); secondary mutations in NRAS with the downstream consequence of increased CRAF heterodimerization with blocked mutant BRAF to reactivate downstream signaling; rare MEK mutations or related (COT1) activation; and several receptor kinase alterations (Figure 2) that also activate the PI3kinase/AKT pathway.[182,183] An earlier-onset form of therapy resistance, termed "adaptive" by Kugel and Aplin, involves shifts in metabolic or receptor tyrosine kinase signaling that confer growth advantage or resistance to apoptosis and may also be targetable with small molecule inhibitors or antibodies but have been less extensively studied than acquired mechanisms.[184] Therapeutic trials to delay or prevent the emergence of resistance will be critical, as established resistance is difficult to overcome with any form of targeted therapy. For example, the activity of combination MEK plus BRAF inhibitor after BRAF inhibition fails is modest (only 15% response, PFS <4 months[185]), and current efforts are focused on preventing or delaying resistance by improving front-line therapy and molecular typing. The use of intermittent dosing, based on strong preclinical data[188] and clinical anecdotes, is also under investigation (clinicaltrials.gov NCT02196181).

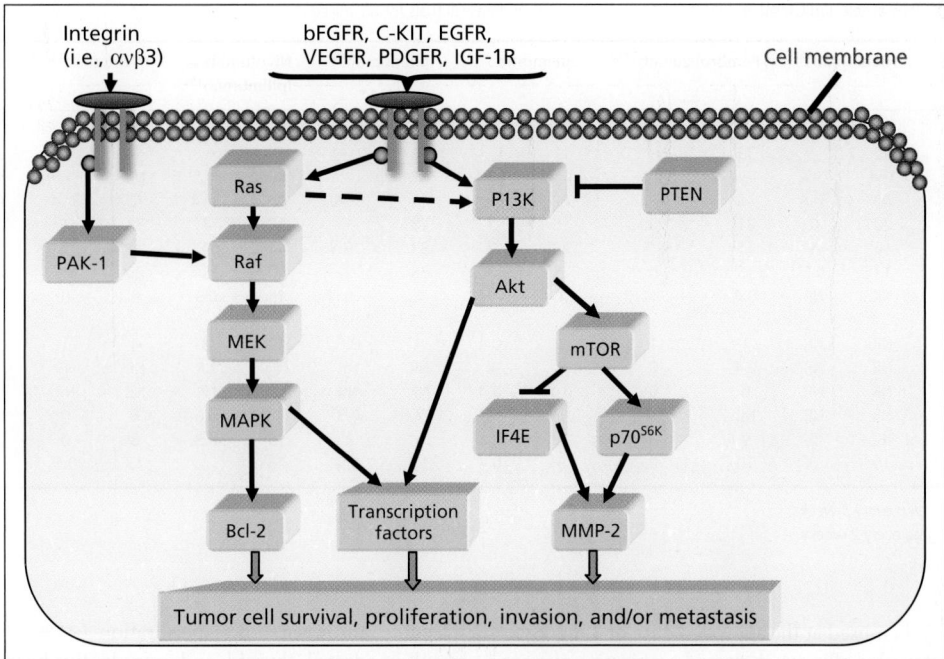

Figure 2 Multiple molecular pathways, such as the RAF/MEK/MAPK and PI3K/AKT pathways, have been found to support melanoma proliferation and survival. Understanding these pathways will enable the development of targeted therapies for melanoma.

The choice between immunotherapy and targeted agents for the first-line therapy of patients whose melanoma carries a BRAF activating mutation remains unclear, as the kinetics of benefit are so different. MAPK inhibitors work quickly and relieve symptoms within days to weeks, while immunotherapy responses may require weeks to months, particularly ipilimumab, which has shown several patterns of response, including both delayed responses after objective progression as well as the appearance of new lesions before an overall objective response.[189] Until the completion of planned drug-sequencing trials (see below) to answer this question, it is generally recommended that patients with a BRAF-mutated melanoma and rapidly growing, symptomatic or very high tumor burden be treated first with combination MAPK inhibitors. This critical question is being tested in a large U.S. cooperative group trial (NCT02224781). Patients with advanced melanoma carrying an activating BRAF mutation are randomized to initial therapy with dabrafenib plus trametinib versus ipilimumab plus nivolumab. Upon progression, patients are crossed over to the opposite treatment. The trial results will define the optimal initial therapy and sequence among these patients, as well as important predictors (which may range from simple clinical tests such as serum LDH to complex immunologic parameters in blood or tumor) of benefit from each regimen. Additional unresolved questions include whether and how to continue targeted agents in patients requiring palliative radiotherapy (which can interact to enhance skin and liver toxicities) or surgery for single sites of symptomatic progression during disease control in other sites.

Immunotherapy for advanced melanoma

Interleukin-2 and other cytokines
IL-2 is an immunomodulatory cytokine with pleiotropic effects on immune effectors that has activity against melanoma when given at high pharmacologic doses. Most recent data show a 15–25% rate of objective response and an RFS plateau of 20%.[190] To date, clinical criteria for safety and the availability of an expert team to administer high-dose IL-2 and the associated supportive care are used to select patients for this form of treatment; although many dose and schedule alterations and the addition of a variety of toxicity modulators have been studied, no modification of the original regimen has improved its unfavorable therapeutic index. The toxicities of high-dose IL-2 result from a generalized capillary leak syndrome mediated by small molecule vasoactive agents such as nitric oxide and a reversible systemic inflammatory response syndrome with multiorgan dysfunction that may also be attributed to the effects of IL-2-induced inflammatory mediators such as tumor necrosis factor and interferon-γ. Studies are now underway to identify immunologic or genetic predictors of benefit (clinicaltrials.gov NCT01288963) that will potentially complement those under investigation for selection of other immunotherapies (detailed below) as single agents or, more likely, in combination or carefully sequenced strategies. Other trials test the activity of regimens that combine or sequence IL-2 with immune checkpoint blockers as well as the potential role for newer cytokines, particularly those that stimulate cytotoxic T cells but, unlike IL-2, do not also stimulate regulatory T cells or activation-induced cell death. The importance of collecting blood and tumor tissue before and, whenever possible, during therapy for the elucidation of biomarkers of response and resistance (and possibly of toxicity) has emerged as a critical element likely to lead to better selection criteria for first and subsequent therapies.

Immune checkpoint inhibitors in advanced melanoma
Ipilimumab is a fully human antibody to CTLA4, a molecule that provides an "immune checkpoint" on activated effector T cells by engaging with the ligand B7.1 on tumors or on dendritic cells and removing it from the activating receptor CD28. In the presence of anti-CTLA4, activation is restored, and a pre-existing but ineffective immune response against tumors is enhanced. CTLA4 blockade also promotes homing of effector T cells to tumor and elimination

Table 8 Activity and toxicities of selected CTLA4 and PD-1 blocking antibodies from Phase III trials for advanced melanoma.

Drug (references)	Nivolumab[194]		Pembrolizumab[195,a]		Ipilimumab[195]		Ipilimumab[196]		Nivolumab + Ipilimumab[196]		Nivolumab[196]		Pembrolizumab[197,b]	
Patient number	206		277		256		315		314		316		178	
ORR (%)	40		33		12		19		58		44		38	
Overall survival	1-yr	79%	1-yr	74%	1-yr	58%	NR		NR		NR		NR	
Toxicity (%)[c], grades	All	3–4	All	3–4	All	3–4	All	3–4	All	3–4	All	3–4	All	3–4
Fatigue	20	0	21	0	15	1	28	1	35	4	34	1	21	1
Colitis/diarrhea	16	1	17	2.5	23	3	33	6	44	9	19	2	8	0
Dermatitis/pruritus/rash	17	0.5	15	0	25	1	35	2	40	5	26	0.6	21	0
Hypophysitis/other endocrinopathy[c]	NR	NR	0.4	0.4	1	2	4	0	15	0.3	9	0	5	0
Hepatitis	NR	NR	1	1	1	0.4	4	0.6	18	8	4	1	NR	NR
Pneumonitis	NR	NR	0.4	0	0	0	NR	NR	NR	NR	NR	NR	NR	NR
Nephropathy	NR	NR	0	0	0.4	0.4	NR	NR	NR	NR	NR	NR	NR	NR
Fever	NR	NR	NR	NR	NR	NR	7	0.3	18	0.6	6	0	NR	NR
Arthralgia	6	0	9	6	5	0.8	6	1	10	0.3	8	0	7	1
Nausea	16	0	10	0	9	0.4	16	0.6	26	2	13	0.6	4	0

[a]Pembrolizumab 10mg/kg every 3 weeks.
[b]Pembrolizumab 2mg/kg every 2 weeks.
[c]NR = not reported

of Treg cells.[190,191] When used at the approved dose of 3 mg/kg × 4 doses at 3-week intervals, ipilimumab provides objective response in 10–15% of patients, with less than partial regressions or disease stabilization in another 10–15%.[192] The survival appears to plateau after 2.5 years at about 20%, so these patients may be cured by a durable and effective immune response (reviewed in Ref. 193). Likely as a result of additional mechanisms of action, the patterns of response to CTLA4 blockade may be atypical and delayed, making it more difficult to know when to switch a patient to second-line therapy upon the appearance of progression. However, with the advent of new checkpoint blocking agents particularly antibodies that block the PD-L1/PD-1 interaction (see below and Table 8, Refs 194–197), practical recommendations for the use of single-agent ipilimumab are evolving rapidly. For melanoma and some other malignancies, the role of combined or optimally-sequenced CTLA4 and PD-1 or PD-L1 blockade are now the most critical clinical questions. Remaining questions include the survival benefit and safety/tolerability use of adjuvant ipilimumab (covered earlier in this chapter) and the therapeutic index of higher doses and more prolonged dosing schedules of CTLA4 blockade as well as novel combinations with other immunomodulatory agents (see Figure 3). For example, the addition of GM-CSF (daily for 2 weeks of every 3) to a 10 mg/kg dose of ipilimumab, given every 3 weeks × 4 and then every 12 weeks, was recently shown to both enhance survival and reduce ipilimumab's toxicities,[192] an intriguing result that warrants further study for both advanced disease and in the adjuvant setting. Although the BRAF mutation has been associated with a higher likelihood of relapse and slightly more aggressive metastatic disease,[199] it does not appear to impact the activity of ipilimumab in melanoma.[200]

Hypofractionated or other schemes of radiation may also overcome resistance to ipilimumab and other immunomodulatory therapies via multiple mechanisms that include enhanced antigen and MHC expression, reduction of suppressive cells and molecules, and induction of inflammatory substances that promote dendritic cell function, which in turn enhances tumor antigen-specific responses, and many clinical trials have been initiated to study these effects in melanoma and other tumors.[201–203] Important interactions among these modalities are shown in Figure 3.

Ipilimumab's toxicities are immune-based and include pruritus, rash, fatigue, and diarrhea (about 1/3 to half of patients), while colitis requiring intervention is less common (7–10%) but can cause bleeding and even bowel perforation (<1%). Hypophysitis may result in adrenal, thyroid, and reproductive hormone insufficiency requiring replacement hormone therapy and sometimes a brief course of therapeutic glucocorticosteroid for local inflammation, especially if vision is compromised by compression of the optic chiasm by the inflamed pituitary. Immune-related hepatitis and rare cases of other organ involvement such as neuropathy have been reported. The first line of therapy for most immune-related adverse events is generally a brief course of therapeutic glucocorticoids followed, if necessary, by anti-tumor necrosis factor antibody (for rare cases of steroid-resistant hepatitis, mycophenolate mofetil is preferred) (reviewed in Ref. 204). While an association between autoimmune reactions and tumor regression has been reported for CTLA4 antibody therapy,[205] and the generation during therapy of a higher circulating lymphocyte count has also correlated with therapeutic benefit, these associations are imperfect and do not provide insight into *pretreatment* biomarkers that can be used to foresee the likelihood or either benefit or toxicity. However, a recent report details the presence in pretreatment melanoma biopsies of common exomic mutation sequences creating immunogenic MHC class I-binding tumor neoepitopes from the tumors of patients who benefited from CTLA4 blockade.[206] This report, along with others that demonstrate benefit associated with antigen-specific immune responses to melanoma in patients benefiting from ipilimumab,[207] lends support to the concept that immune checkpoint inhibition exploits existing antitumor immune responses, which in many cases are now believed to be tumor-specific mutations, presumably derived from the damage induced by carcinogens of known importance in tumorigenesis.[208] Thus, combinations with other immunomodulators that provide costimulation, reduce negative signaling in the tumor microenvironment, or enhance the functions of antigen-presenting cells are under investigation. Insights from further study of pre- and posttreatment tumor and circulating cells and their gene expression and patterns of activation may also lead to better selection criteria for initial therapy in individual patients.

PD-1 (for programmed death), has two important ligands, PD-L1 (expressed on a wide variety of cells and variably inducible in tumors, generally by cytokines produced by infiltrating lymphocytes) and PD-L2 (predominantly expressed on hematopoietic cells). Ligand engagement of PD-1 triggers negative signaling in effector T cells, rendering them unresponsive to further antigen stimulation and eventualy apoptotic, a cascade that, in the case

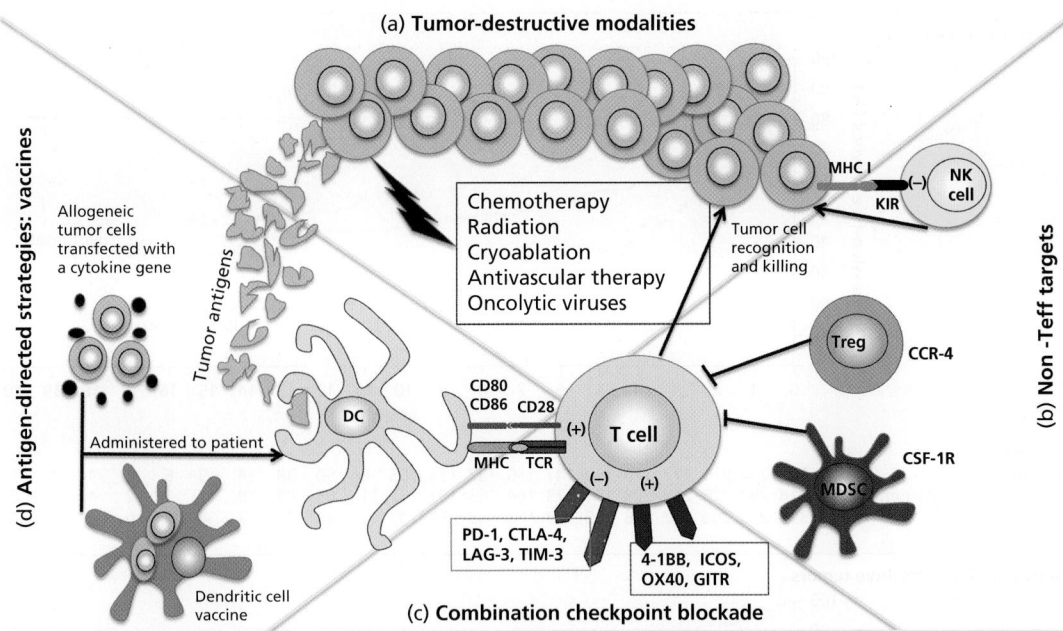

Figure 3 Combination strategies with cytotoxic T-lymphocyte-associated antigen 4 (CTLA-4) blockade—(a) conventional and novel therapies may efficiently destroy tumor and liberate tumor-associated antigens (TAAs), thereby enhancing antigen presentation and tumor-specific adaptive immunity; (b) novel-targeted agents may inhibit the suppressive effects of regulatory T cells (Treg) and myeloid-derived suppressor cells (MDSCs) or enhance innate immunity via natural killer (NK) cell-killer immunoglobulin-like receptor (KIR) activity; (c) immune checkpoints and costimulatory receptors can be targeted in combination with CTLA-4 to enhance T-cell function; (d) adaptive immunity to known TAAs can be enhanced via vaccine strategies employing peptides, whole proteins, whole cells, DNA, or virus-based vectors. CSF-1R, colony-stimulating factor 1 receptor; DC, dendritic cell; GITR, glucocorticoid-induced tumor necrosis factor receptor (TNF) receptor-related protein; ICOS, inducible T-cell costimulator; LAG-3, lymphocyte activation gene 3; MHC, major histocompatibility complex; PD-1, programmed cell death 1; TCR, T-cell receptor; Teff, effector T cell; TIM-3, T-cell immunoglobulin and mucin-containing domain 3. Source: Funt et al. 2014.[198] Reproduced with permissions of UBM Medica.

of tumor expressing PD-L1, may be one mechanism of tumor resistance to immune control. This may be of particular importance in "adaptive resistance," a term used to describe the induction of PD-L1 on tumor cells by γ-interferon produced by infiltrating CD8 lymphocytes, which may set the stage for effective immunotherapy by PD-1 or PD-L1 blocking antibodies.[209–211] Such antibodies, fully human or extensively humanized, have recently been studied in patients with advanced melanoma and several other malignancies, and the results of these studies, which showed objective responses in about 25–30% of patients previously treated with ipilimumab and, if BRAF mutant, with a BRAF inhibitor, led to the approvals of pembrolizumab and nivolumab in late 2014 for advanced pretreated melanoma. However, the randomized trial that demonstrated a dramatic progression-free and overall survival benefit of nivolumab over dacarbazine (hazard ratio for death 0.42, 1-year survival 73% vs 42%) in the first randomized study for patients with untreated BRAF wild-type melanoma[194] (Figure 4), quickly led to the routine use of these antibodies in the first-line setting, even for patients with BRAF mutant melanoma.

The toxicity data for PD-1 blocking antibodies have demonstrated the expected superior therapeutic ratio over single-agent ipilimumab, which has lower benefit and higher immune-related side effects (data summarized in Table 8). Most toxicities affect the same tissues targeted by ipilimumab's immune-related adverse effects but appear to be less frequent and severe; unique toxicities such as pneumonitis, nephritis, and neuritis have been reported in occasional patients on PD-1 axis blockade, and rare case reports describe other unusual events likely to represent loss of immune tolerance resulting from this form of checkpoint blockade. However, also shown in Table 8, while the combination of CTLA4 and PD-1 blockade has shown higher response rates and progression-free

survival over single-agent ipilimumab (further detailed below), the toxicities of the combination are much more frequent, of higher grade, and include events not reported previously for either agent alone. The advantage of combined blockade over PD-1 blockade alone is also under intense investigation, as the retrospective subset analyses of this ground-breaking study suggested that for high PD-L1-expressing tumors, the benefits of single agent nivolumab are comparable to those of combined therapy, while for tumors without PD-L1 expression, the optimal therapy may require both agents. It has been postulated that blocking PD-L1 rather than PD-1 would leave intact the immune tolerance dependent on PD-L2:PD-1 interactions. Two PD-L1 antibodies currently under investigation in melanoma and other malignancies (Atezolizumab and Durvalumab) have demonstrated preliminary activity and may be combinable with other agents of interest in melanoma, including bevacizumab (antivascular endothelial factor, which has immunopotentiating properties), MAPK inhibitors, and other immunomodulatory agents that costimulate cytotoxic cells or inhibit local suppressive cells or molecules in the tumor microenvironment.

Combination therapy with concurrent ipilimumab and nivolumab showed particularly dramatic antitumor effects confirmed in a phase III study comparing the combination with each of the single agents in untreated advanced melanoma.[197] Several recent reports have described potential biomarkers of benefit from PD-1/PD-L1 antibodies in both melanoma and non-small-cell lung cancer, including the expression of PD-L1 on tumor and/or stromal cells, the presence of a brisk CD8 lymphocyte infiltrate, and oligoclonality of the T-cell receptors among the tumor-infiltrating CD8 cells in melanoma,[215,216] and the explosion of clinical settings in which these agents are now undergoing evaluation is certain to reveal additional insight into predictive factors and mechanisms

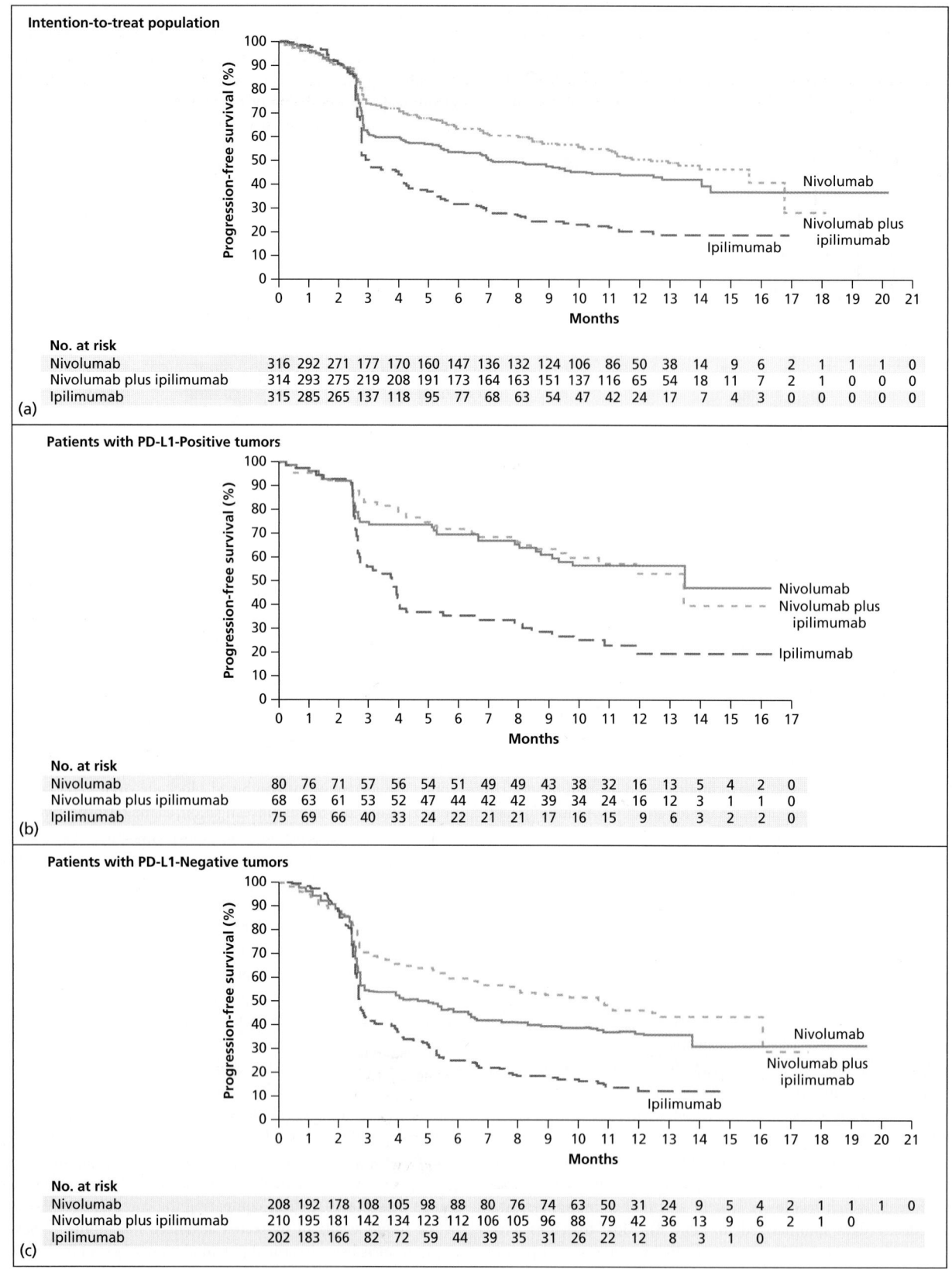

Figure 4 PFS, nivolumab plus ipilimumab versus either single agent. (a) Kaplan–Meier curves for progression-free survival in the intention-to-treat population. The median progression-free survival was 6.9 months (95% CI, 4.3 to 9.5) in the nivolumab group, 11.5 months (95% CI, 8.9 to 16.7) in the nivolumab-plus-ipilimumab group, and 2.9 months (95% CI, 2.8 to 3.4) in the ipilimumab group. Significantly longer PFS was observed for nivolumab plus ipilimumab than for ipilimumab (hazard ratio for death or disease progression, 0.42; 99.5% CI, 0.31 to 0.57; P < 0.001) and for nivolumab versus ipilimumab (hazard ratio, 0.57; 99.5% CI, 0.43 to 0.76; P < 0.001). (b) PFS for patients with PD-L1-positive tumors, and (c) PFS for patients with PD-L1-negtive tumors. Source Larkin et al 2015.[196] Reproduced with permission of the New England Journal of Medicine.

of activity and failure. Other checkpoint blocking antibodies and related immunomodulatory agents also hold promise in melanoma, including agonistic antibodies that costimulate T cells through ligands associated with activation (agonistic anti-CD137, anti-OX40, anti-CD40, anti-CD27) and dendritic cells (Toll receptor ligands and tumor vaccines antigens bound to dendritic cell-targeting antibodies). Other strategies include the inhibition of other immunosuppressive signals in the tumor microenvironment, such as indoleamine dioxygenase or signaling receptors on suppressive tumor-associated macrophages.

Sequential or simultaneous administration of molecularly targeted and immunotherapeutic agents

The data from retrospective series suggested that patients with BRAF-mutated melanoma who started with targeted therapy and then received ipilimumab at the time of progression had more unfavorable outcomes than patients who started with immunotherapy and crossed over to targeted therapy at the time of treatment failure.[217,218] While this outcome may have resulted from a true treatment-sequence effect, it may also reflect the assignment of patients with more aggressive disease to targeted therapy first, and patients with less aggressive tumor to immunotherapy first. An ongoing randomized clinical trial to test this question of optimal sequence, comparing the two combination regimens with the highest reported activity in melanoma (detailed below) as first-line therapy with a crossover to the alternative therapy at progression, will answer this critical question of the optimal first-line therapy and sequence of therapies for these patients, who comprise approximately half of those with advanced melanoma arising in common cutaneous sites (clinicaltrials.gov NCT 02224781). Concurrent therapy with MAPK inhibitors while initial combination therapy with vemurafenib and ipilimumab proved excessively toxic,[219] many other combinations of molecularly targeted therapy with immunotherapy are under investigation, based in part on promising data supporting the importance of BRAF mutation in resistance to immunotherapy and its inhibition in promoting immune response (reviewed in Ref. 220).

Cytotoxic agents and combinations with immunotherapy for advanced melanoma

Until the advent of high-dose IL-2, therapy for metastatic melanoma was of very limited benefit, with low rates of objective response to single-agent cytotoxic therapies and limited response durations for both IL-2 and cytotoxic agents or combinations. The standard and only FDA-approved drug was dacarbazine, with response rates in the 10–12% range, and an oral equivalent of this drug, temozolomide, has often been used with similar outcomes but better tolerance.[221] Although expectations were high for temozolomide as treatment for patients with brain metastases due to its central nervous system penetration and its widespread use in primary brain tumors, the low activity of dacarbazine and temozolomide in melanoma tempered enthusiasm, and it is now used predominantly for patients who have failed or cannot tolerate the other agents detailed above. Alternative multiagent regimens have been more toxic and without proven benefit despite reports of higher response rates, particularly to "biochemotherapy" combinations with at least 3 cytotoxic agents and 2 immunotherapies, usually IL-2 and IFN-α.[222] Nanoparticle-albumin-bound paclitaxel or unmodified paclitaxel as a single agent or in combination with carboplatin are cytotoxic regimens with modest activity against melanoma but have not demonstrated survival benefit in prospective trials.[223]

Melanoma metastatic to the brain

Melanoma has the highest propensity of any adult solid tumor to spread hematogenously to the brain, and due to its vascular nature and its high growth rate in many cases, it poses serious threats to the survival and well-being of patients. Surgical resection may be required for diagnosis and is often necessary for immediate relief of the complications of edema, bleeding, and rapidly progressive neurologic deficits. The impact of whole-brain radiation given in standard or alternative dose and fractionation schedules has been minimal and cannot be distinguished from the benefits of simply treating patients with glucocorticosteroids.[224] Stereotactic radiotherapies (SRS) have the most favorable outcomes despite the lack of randomized, controlled comparisons,[225] with the maximum size and number of lesions amenable to treatment varying by center and type of modality (gamma-knife or cyberknife). Whole-brain radiotherapy is of limited palliative benefit and may be offered to patients with numerous lesions or failure of prior therapy, including systemic agents, which are increasingly showing activity against melanoma brain metastases (molecularly targeted agents[226] and ipilimumab[227]). Ongoing investigations test double MAPK inhibition for melanoma metastatic to the brain, including preoperative therapy of resectable disease to allow post-therapy analysis of responding and nonresponding metastases (clinicaltrials.gov NCT01978236). Despite the lack of direct penetrance of the intact BBB by these therapies,[228] their level of activity against melanoma brain metastases is in the range reported outside of the central nervous system, probably due to several factors, including the loss of BBB integrity resulting from tumor growth and inflammation as well as, in the case of immunotherapies, peripherally activated lymphocytes that gain access and migrate to the melanoma metastasis in the CNS.[229,230] Further understanding of the process of brain metastasis for the prevention and selection of optimal therapies will depend on factors that include the molecular characteristics of the primary site as well as changes occurring as melanoma cells experience other metastatic niches before the brain. Investigation of earlier-stage disease has provided limited and heterogeneous insights, but recent reports suggest the importance of the PTEN/AKT/PI3 kinase pathway either intrinsically or via signals from nearby astrocytes.[163] It will be important to study the effects of other checkpoint inhibitors such as PD-1 and PD-L1 antibodies in patients with melanoma metastatic to the brain, and such studies are ongoing (clinicaltrials.gov NCT02085070 and NCT02320058).

Tumor-infiltrating lymphocyte (TIL) therapy in melanoma

The ability to isolate, expand, and infuse large numbers of autologous tumor-derived cytotoxic T lymphocytes, usually derived from dissected fragments of excised tumor and expansion of predominantly CD8 lymphocytes in IL-2-containing medium into patients with advanced melanoma, has been under investigation for over 20 years and appears to be improving. Using regimens that include lymphodepleting high-dose chemotherapy and, in some cases, total body irradiation to provide homeostatic cytokines and high-dose IL-2 to stimulate *in vivo* expansion and survival of antitumor effector cells, response rates in the range of 50% with durable complete remissions in 20% of patients have been reported among patients experiencing adequate TIL (tumor-infiltrating lymphocyte) growth and able to complete the entire course of therapy.[231] Further manipulations have included pretreatment with BRAF inhibitors, "young" TIL cells, and immune checkpoint blockers, and it is likely that the need for HDIL-2 in these regimens will be replaced by more tolerable factors to expand and maintain the infused cytotoxic cell product. Recent observations regarding the immunobiology of TIL cells in melanoma are consistent with the findings detailed earlier for effective melanoma immunotherapy with PD-1 checkpoint blockade, including the presence of multiple immune checkpoints (PD-1, LAG3, TIM3) and costimulatory molecules (4-1BB, ICOS) on CD8 effector T cells and oligoclonality of T-cell receptor beta gene sequences on CD8 cells with antigen specificity for tumor-specific mutations.[232]

The recent advent of multiple new targeted agents and immune checkpoint inhibitors will provide ample opportunities to study the role of TIL cell therapies both for patients who fail to achieve durable benefit from the former agents and as part of multicomponent strategies for optimal therapy of advanced melanoma. While advanced melanoma will continue to be a lethal disease for a fraction of patients, the rapid emergence of highly active molecularly targeted therapies and immunotherapies with mechanisms of action and resistance that are more successfully probed and manipulated promise to counter the threat of this constellation of diseases and to continue to lead the way in new therapeutic discoveries.

originating from cells with molecular features predisposing them to traffic to and thrive in the brain, is still an important cause of melanoma death despite some responsiveness to targeted and immunotherapies and remains under intense investigation.

Summary

Melanoma is rising in incidence and mortality in a pattern reflecting exposure to ultraviolet light (both natural and artificial) and other carcinogens that have not been fully elucidated. Familial risk factors include rare mutations of cyclin kinase genes and more common polymorphisms of genes such as the melanocortin receptor that control pigmentation of the skin and hair. Other risk factors include large numbers of moles or atypical nevi. Among the clinicopathologic subtypes, nodular melanoma has the most unfavorable prognosis owing to more rapid growth, the absence of an initial noninvasive radial growth phase, and a propensity to be nonpigmented, resulting in thicker tumors at diagnosis. Surgical excision guidelines include the need for adequate margins around the primary site to reduce the probability of local relapse; sentinel node biopsies guided by lymphoscintigraphic- and lymphatic-tracking dyes at the time of wide local excision; and completion lymph node dissection for patients with one or more involved sentinel nodes. Imaging guidelines are often tailored to the calculated risk of relapse using the 2009 AJCC staging system based on Breslow thickness, ulceration, mitotic rate, and number and size of nodal metastases. Metastasis occurs via predominantly hematogenous spread for uveal and mucosal melanoma and some cutaneous melanomas, while lymphatic spread is also common with cutaneous melanomas. Surgical management of metastatic melanoma depends on the number and location of metastases but can be associated with prolonged relapse-free survival. Metastatic melanoma is divided by prognosis into skin/soft tissue only, lung, and visceral metastasis and/or elevation of serum lactate dehydrogenase. Metastasis to the brain is more common in melanoma than any other malignancy and carries the most unfavorable prognosis, although improvements have resulted from stereotactic radiosurgery, and new molecularly targeted therapies as well as immunotherapies have shown activity against brain metastases. Melanoma is an immunogenic tumor that has been successfully treated with high-dose interleukin-2, *ex vivo* expanded tumor-infiltrating lymphocytes, and antibodies that block the CTLA4 and PD-1/PD-L1 immune checkpoints. Combinations with radiation therapy have also shown promise through multiple modulations of suppressive factors in the tumor immune microenvironment. Molecularly targeted agents, particularly those that inhibit sequential steps in the mitogen-activated protein kinase pathway in melanomas carrying an oncogenic activating mutation of BRAF, have also improved survival, and new agents to prevent or overcome resistance as well as to target other molecular drivers are under investigation. The challenge of brain metastases, likely

Key references

The complete reference list can be found on the Wiley Companion Digital Edition of this title (see inside front cover for login instructions).

12 Hodis E, Watson IR, Kryukov GV, et al. A landscape of driver mutations in melanoma. *Cell.* 2012;**150**:251–263.

26 Choi JN, Hanlon A, Leffell D. Melanoma and nevi: detection and diagnosis. *Curr Probl Cancer.* 2011;**35**:138–161.

28 Price HN, Schaffer JV. Congenital melanocytic nevi-when to worry and how to treat: Facts and controversies. *Clin Dermatol.* 2010;**28**:293–302.

37 Abbas O, Miller DD, Bhawan J. Cutaneous malignant melanoma: update on diagnostic and prognostic biomarkers. *Am J Dermatopathol.* 2014;**36**:363–379.

55 Demierre MF, Chung C, Miller DR, Geller AC. Early detection of thick melanomas in the United States: beware of the nodular subtype. *Arch Dermatol.* 2005;**141**:745–750.

61 Curtin JA, Fridlyand J, Kageshita T, et al. Distinct sets of genetic alterations in melanoma. *N Engl J Med.* 2005;**353**:2135–2147.

84 Valsecchi ME, Silbermins D, de Rosa N, et al. Lymphatic mapping and sentinel lymph node biopsy in patients with melanoma: a meta-analysis. *J Clin Oncol.* 2011;**29**:1479–1487.

85 Wong SL, Balch CM, Hurley P, et al. Sentinel lymph node biopsy for melanoma: American Society of Clinical Oncology and Society of Surgical Oncology joint clinical practice guideline. *J Clin Oncol.* 2012;**30**:2912–2918.

86 Morton DL, Thompson JF, Cochran AJ, et al. Sentinel node biopsy or nodal observation in melanoma: final trial report. *N Engl J Med.* 2014;**370**:599–609.

88 Han D, Zager JS, Shyr Y, et al. Clinicopathologic predictors of sentinel lymph node metástasis in thin melanoma. *J Clin Oncol.* 2013;**31**:4387–93.

94 Balch CM, Gershenwald JE, Soong S-j, et al. Final version of 2009 AJCC melanoma staging and classification. *J Clin Oncol.* 2009;**27**:6199–6206.

106 Wong SL, Morton DL, Thompson JF, et al. Melanoma patients with positive sentinel nodes who did not undergo completion lymphadenectomy: a multi-institutional study. *Ann Surg Oncol.* 2006;**13**:809–816.

108 Burmeister BH, Henderson MA, Ainslie J, et al. Adjuvant radiotherapy versus observation alone for patients at risk of lymph-node field relapse after therapeutic lymphadenectomy for melanoma: a randomised trial. *Lancet Oncol.* 2012;**13**:589–597.

114 Cornett WR, McCall LM, Petersen RP, et al. Randomized multicenter trial of hyperthermic isolated limb perfusion with melphalan alone compared with melphalan plus tumor necrosis factor: American College of Surgeons Oncology Group Trial Z0020. *J Clin Oncol.* 2006;**24**:4196–4201.

119 Dossett LA, Ben-Shabat I, Olofsson Bagge R, Zager JS. Clinical Response and Regional Toxicity Following Isolated Limb Infusion Compared with Isolated Limb Perfusion for In-Transit Melanoma. *Ann Surg Oncol.* 2016;**23**:2330–5.

124 Andtbacka RH, Kaufman HL, Collichio F, et al. Talimogene laherparepvec Improves durable response rate in patients with advanced melanoma. *J Clin Oncol.* 2015;**33**:2780–2788.

130 Sosman JA, Moon J, Tuthill RJ, et al. A phase II trial of complete resection for stage IV melanoma: results of Southwest Oncology Group (SWOG) clinical trial S9430. *Cancer.* 2011;**117**:4740–4746.

136 Eggermont AM, Suciu S, Testori A, et al. Long-term results of the randomized phase III trial EORTC 18991 of adjuvant therapy with pegylated interferon alfa-2b versus observation in resected stage III melanoma. *J Clin Oncol.* 2012;**30**:3810–3818.

140 Eggermont AM, Chiarion-Sileni V, Grob JJ, et al. Adjuvant ipilimumab versus placebo after complete resection of high-risk stage III melanoma (EORTC 18071): a randomised, double-blind, phase 3 trial. *Lancet Oncol.* 2015;**16**:522–530.

143 Romano E, Scordo M, Dusza SW, et al. Site and timing of first relapse in stage III melanoma patients: implications for follow-up guidelines. *J Clin Oncol.* 2010;**28**:3042–3047.

151 Harbour JW. A prognostic test to predict the risk of metastasis in uveal melanoma based on a 15-gene expression profile. *Methods Mol Biol.* 2014;**1102**:427–440.

174 Solit DB, Rosen N. Towards a unified model of RAF inhibitor resistance. *Lancet Oncol.* 2014;**15**:323–332.

176 Long GV, Stroyakovskiy D, Gogas H, et al. Combined BRAF and MEK inhibition versus BRAF inhibition alone in melanoma. *N Engl J Med.* 2014;**371**:1877–88.

177 Robert C, Karaszewska B, Schachter J, et al. Improved overall survival in melanoma with combined dabrafenib and trametinib. *N Engl J Med*. 2015;**372**:30–39.

178 Larkin J, Ascierto PA, Dréno B, et al. Combined vemurafenib and cobimetinib in BRAF-mutated melanoma. *N Engl J Med*. 2014;**371**:1867–1876.

188 Payne R, Glenn L, Hoen H, et al. Durable responses and reversible toxicity of high-dose interleukin-2 treatment of melanoma and renal cancer in a Community Hospital Biotherapy Program. *J Immunother Cancer*. 2014:**14**:13.

194 Robert C, Long GV, Brady B, et al. Nivolumab in previously untreated melanoma without BRAF mutation. *N Engl J Med*. 2015;**372**:320–330.

196 Larkin J, Chiarion-Sileni V, Gonzalez R, et al. Combined nivolumab and ipili-mumab or monotherapy in untreated melanoma. *N Engl J Med*. 2015;**373**:23–34.

202 Demaria S, Pilones KA, Vanpouille-Box C, et al. The optimal partnership of radi-ation and immunotherapy: from preclinical studies to clinical translation. *Radiat Res*. 2014;**182**:170–81.

212 Topalian SL, Sznol M, McDermott DF, et al. Survival, durable tumor remission, and long-term safety in patients with advanced melanoma receiving nivolumab. *J Clin Oncol*. 2014;**32**:1020–1030.

110 Other skin cancers

William G. Stebbins, MD ▪ Eric A. Millican, MD ▪ Victor A. Neel, MD, PhD

Overview

Several more common types of nonmelanoma skin cancer are presented with attention to etiology and current treatment options.

The skin is a heterogeneous organ, consisting of elements of ectodermal, endodermal, and mesodermal origin. Such a diverse group of tissues gives rise to a wide variety of benign and malignant tumors. Many of these tumors are rare and will not be discussed in this chapter. Table 1 lists the more common premalignant and malignant tumors, which we discuss in detail. These are tumors relevant to the oncologist because they have the capacity to metastasize and cause serious medical harm. We also touch on several tumor syndromes that may present with unusual benign skin tumors that, if recognized, should prompt the clinician to conduct a detailed search for an internal malignancy. Melanoma, Kaposi sarcoma, the malignant histiocytoses, and the cutaneous lymphomas are discussed elsewhere in this book.

The incidence of nonmelanoma skin cancer (NMSC), which includes squamous cell carcinoma (SCC) and basal cell carcinoma (BCC), is increasing (Table 2). In the United States, approximately 480,000 persons were diagnosed with NMSC in 1983,[1] over 1 million in 2008,[2] and an estimated >3.5 million in 2014.[3] The ratio of BCC to SCC among whites in the United States, Australia, and the United Kingdom is about 4:1.[1,4,5] Together, these two tumors account for approximately 90% of all skin cancers. In recent years, the role of the sun in the causation of these common skin tumors has received much attention.[6]

Ultraviolet radiation in the pathogenesis of skin cancers

In the past several decades, research on the relationship between the sun and skin cancer has escalated principally because of fear of the consequences of increased ultraviolet B (UVB) radiation on the earth's surface as a result of ozone depletion in the stratosphere. There is now general consensus over the role of sunlight in the etiology of NMSC.[7,8] Chuang and colleagues[9] reported a 45-fold increase in NMSC in the Japanese population in Kauai, Hawaii, as compared with the Japanese population in Japan. Another study showed the incidence of SCC, but not BCC, in a group of Caucasian fishermen in Maryland correlated directly with the amount of sun exposure.[10] A population-based study on nearly 12,000 patients also demonstrated the close correlation between chronic cumulative sun exposure and SCC.[11] Geographically, the incidence of skin cancer in whites increases toward the equator, further supporting the role of sunlight in carcinogenesis.

UVB imprints a unique signature on the DNA it damages. Cellular attempts to repair this damage can lead to CC>TT mutations or C→T transitions. UVA can also induce these mutations, though likely indirectly through the creation of reactive oxygen species.[12,13] In the precursors of SCC (known as actinic keratoses), inactivating mutations of the tumor suppressor *P53* harbor these UV-induced errors.[14] Because *P53* is involved in the transcriptional regulation of DNA repair genes, cell-cycle control genes, and the induction of cell death, damage to this important regulator by UV irradiation is one mechanism that allows for the overgrowth of damaged cells.

In addition to natural sun exposure, indoor tanning is increasingly recognized as carcinogenic. According to a meta-analysis, patients who reported ever using a tanning bed had a 67% increased risk of developing SCC and a 29% increase risk of BCC.[15] Two independent case–control studies also found a greater than 60% increase in the risk of early-onset (younger than age 50) BCC.[16,17] Overall, more than 419,000 cases of skin cancer in the United States are attributable to indoor tanning annually.[18] These and other similar findings led the International Agency for Research on Cancer to classify UV tanning devices as Group 1 carcinogens.[19] More recently, the United States FDA reclassified tanning devices as class II (moderate-to-high risk) devices, and several states have passed legislation limiting their use among minor children. UVB and UVA (320–400 nm) also have direct and indirect effects on the cutaneous immune system, lowering cell-mediated immunity, and inducing T-suppressor cell production.[20] Loss of local immunity is thought to be another factor influencing carcinogenesis.

Tumors arising from the epidermis

Actinic keratosis

Definition

Actinic keratosis, also known as solar keratosis, is a very common lesion occurring in susceptible persons as a result of prolonged and repeated solar exposures. The action of ultraviolet radiation results in damage to the keratinocytes and produces single or multiple, discrete, dry lesions with adherent scale. These premalignant lesions may, in time, progress to SCCs.

Epidemiology

Actinic keratosis affects predominantly the sun-exposed areas of fair-skinned people. The incidence in elderly whites may approach 100% in some populations.[1] Actinic keratosis may appear at a much younger age (under 30 years) in individuals with an outdoor

Holland-Frei Cancer Medicine, Ninth Edition. Edited by Robert C. Bast Jr., Carlo M. Croce, William N. Hait, Waun Ki Hong, Donald W. Kufe, Martine Piccart-Gebhart, Raphael E. Pollock, Ralph R. Weichselbaum, Hongyang Wang, and James F. Holland.
© 2017 John Wiley & Sons, Inc. ISBN: 978-1-118-93469-2

Table 1 Common premalignant and malignant neoplasms of the skin.

	Premalignant	Malignant
Epidermis	Actinic keratosis	Keratoacanthoma
	Arsenical keratosis	Basal cell carcinoma
	HPV-induced premalignant papules (epidermodysplasia verruciformis, bowenoid papulosis)	Merkel cell carcinoma
	Mucosal leukoplakia	Squamous cell carcinoma
Dermal		Dermatofibrosarcoma protuberans
		Malignant fibrous histiocytoma
		Angiosarcoma
Appendageal	Nevus sebaceous	Sebaceous carcinoma
		Extramammary Paget disease
Benign cutaneous tumors associated with cancer syndromes		
Trichilemmomas → Cowden disease (breast/visceral tumors)		
Sebaceous tumors → Muir–Torre syndrome (GI/GU tumors)		
Mucosal neuromas → MEN type IIB (thyroid carcinoma/pheochromocytoma)		

Abbreviations: GI, gastrointestinal; GU, genitourinary; HPV, human papillomavirus; MEN, multiple endocrine neoplasia.

Table 2 Nonmelanoma skin cancer statistics (U.S. 2014).

	BCC and SCC	Merkel cell carcinoma
Magnitude of the problem (yearly)	>3,500,000 new patients	1000-1500 new patients
Severity of the problem (yearly)	2% deaths from SCC	300-500 deaths
	Disfigurement	Incidence increasing
	Disability	

Source: http://www.skincancer.org/skin-cancer-information/skin-cancer-facts, accessed September 2, 2014

occupation, such as farmers, ranchers, and sailors, or an outdoor lifestyle. The lesions are more common in transplant recipients[21] and albinos.[22] It is rare in darker-skinned individuals, and almost never affects blacks, East Indians, or other Asians.

Clinical features

The onset of actinic keratosis is typically insidious and therefore often passes unnoticed for some time. The characteristic lesion is rough and gritty to palpation, similar to the feel of coarse sandpaper. Lesions are usually skin-colored or yellow brown, often with a reddish tinge, and round-to-oval, often <1 cm in diameter. They may be flat to papular, as in the hypertrophic variety of actinic keratosis (Figure 1). There may be single or multiple scattered discrete lesions, typically limited to sun-exposed areas. A pigmented variant, named spreading pigmented actinic keratosis, is a brown, slowly growing, slightly scaly lesion that tends to appear on the face and may be larger than 1.5 cm in diameter, making it difficult to distinguish from lentigo maligna.

Diagnosis

The diagnosis of actinic keratosis is usually based on clinical examination alone. The hypertrophic variant may sometimes be confused with early SCC. Suchniak and colleagues[23] demonstrated histologically the presence of *in situ* or invasive SCCs in 50% of lesions diagnosed clinically as hypertrophic actinic keratoses.

Treatment

Flat actinic keratosis lesions are most easily treated with cryotherapy.[24] Brief applications of liquid nitrogen with a cotton tipped swab or spray gun will suffice in the majority of cases. Retreatment may be necessary for more stubborn lesions. It is not necessary to freeze to the point of blistering. Curettage and electrodesiccation of the lesions are equally effective, but carry a slightly greater risk of scarring and dyspigmentation. The hypertrophic lesions are best evaluated by biopsy to rule out invasive SCC.

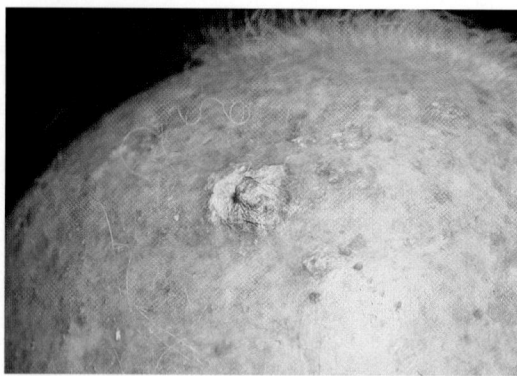

Figure 1 Actinic keratosis. Multiple discrete lesions on the scalp. These lesions are "gritty" to palpation. The largest lesion in the center of the picture represents the hypertrophic variant. This must be differentiated from a squamous cell carcinoma in situ.

Where large areas of skin are involved, 5-fluorouracil preparations may be applied twice a day to the affected areas for up to 4 weeks. This results in a brisk reaction in the treated areas, ranging from redness, soreness, and weeping, to shallow ulceration and crusting (Figure 2), which gradually subsides after discontinuation of the cytotoxic cream. Newer formulations containing 0.5% 5-fluorouracil used once daily for 4 weeks may cause less skin irritation.[25]

Multiple additional topical approaches are available. 5% imiquimod cream has been used twice weekly for 16 weeks for nonhypertrophic, actinic keratoses of the face/scalp in immunocompetent individuals. Side effects include redness, itch and/or burning, and hypopigmentation at the local site. Imiquimod works via upregulation of inflammatory cytokines through stimulation of toll-like receptor 7 (TLR7). Topical 3% diclofenac gel has been reported to be efficacious for actinic keratoses.[26] The product is used twice daily for 60–90 days. The frequency of complete

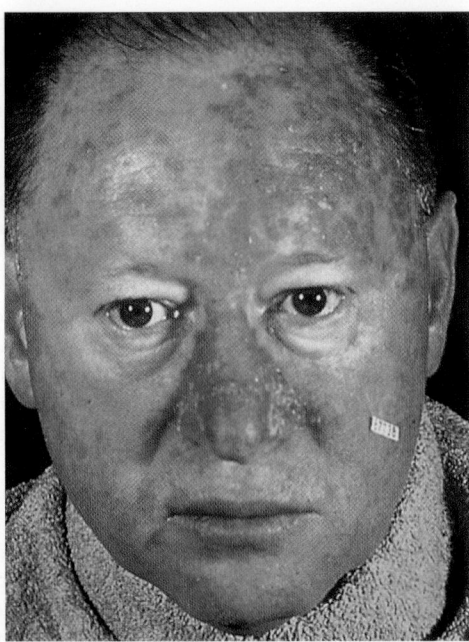

Figure 2 Actinic keratosis. Extensive actinic keratosis on the face. Note that the right half has been used as control and the left half of the forehead and the nose were treated with 5% 5-fluorouracil cream for 14 days.

response seems lower than with 5-fluorouracil or imiquimod, and skin irritation can result from treatment. The FDA recently approved another topical medication, ingenol mebutate, which works via induction of direct cell death as well as nonspecific inflammation. This medication has demonstrated comparable results to other topically applied therapies with the advantage of a being administered over a shorter 2–3 day course.[27]

Lastly, photodynamic therapy (PDT) employs a topically applied photosensitizer, aminolevulinic acid, which is preferentially absorbed by the premalignant cells and photoactivated upon exposure to blue or red light. PDT results in clearance of up to 90% of actinic keratoses in patients with extensive actinic keratoses of the face and scalp.[28] Stinging of the treated skin occurs during light exposure. A sunburn-like reaction follows therapy.

Course and prognosis

The lesions of actinic keratosis may disappear spontaneously, but, in general, they persist if not treated. There is modest lifetime risk (<10%) of an individual actinic keratosis transforming into SCC. Marks and colleagues[29] reported that 60% of SCCs arise from pre-existing solar keratoses.

Keratoacanthoma

Definition

Keratoacanthoma is a common, rapidly growing low-grade tumor that may involute spontaneously, even if untreated. It is believed to originate from the hair follicles.

Epidemiology

Few studies have been done on the incidence of keratoacanthoma.[30] Chuang and colleagues[31] reported an incidence rate of 103.6 per 100,000, based on the small population in Kauai, Hawaii. It is most common between the ages of 60 and 65 years and is rare in persons younger than the age of 20 years. In contrast to SCC and BCC, there is no increase in frequency in old age. It is uncommon in blacks or

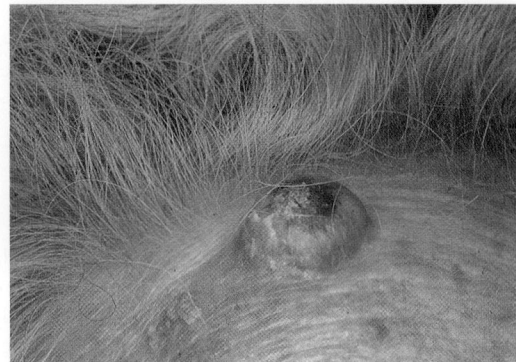

Figure 3 Keratoacanthoma. A pink, dome-shaped lesion with a central core of keratin. This rapidly growing lesion is located on the mid-forehead. Source: Courtesy of P.L. McCarthy, MD.

Japanese, and is approximately two to three times more common in males. The majority of patients have a solitary lesion.

Sun exposure and exposure to chemical carcinogens such as tar are thought to be etiologic factors. The possibility of a viral etiology is still being debated. The presence of HPV has been demonstrated by DNA hybridization and polymerase chain reaction (PCR) studies.[32] The possibility of a genetic defect has also been proposed because these tumors are more common in patients with the Muir–Torre syndrome than in the general population.

Clinical features

Keratoacanthomas characteristically arise on hair-bearing skin. The most common areas are the central parts of the face: cheeks, nose, ears, lips, eyelids, and forehead, as well as the dorsa of the hands, wrists, and forearms. The trunk and scalp are uncommon sites. Typically, the lesion presents as a solitary, rapidly growing, firm, dome-shaped, flesh-colored to slightly pink lesion with a plug of keratin in the central crater (Figure 3). The evolving lesion typically grows rapidly for 2–4 weeks to a size of up to 2 cm in diameter. The mature lesion involutes spontaneously after a few months, leaving a scar. The complete cycle of growth to spontaneous resolution takes 4–6 months.[33] Multiple or recurrent lesions may occur, particularly in cases associated with tar exposure. Multiple lesions associated with defects in cell-mediated immunity and with multiple internal malignant neoplasms and sebaceous adenomas, as part of Muir–Torre syndrome, have been noted. There is no evidence that the solitary type is associated with internal malignancy.

Diagnosis

The main differential diagnosis is to distinguish keratoacanthoma from SCC. The rapid evolution and spontaneous involution, the characteristic dome shape with a central plug of keratin, and the relatively young age of the patient are all clues to the diagnosis. In most cases, a wedge biopsy is essential to exclude an invasive SCC.

Treatment

Keratoacanthomas may resolve spontaneously. Surgical excision of the lesion will produce better cosmetic results and provide tissue for histopathologic diagnosis. Radiotherapy[34] has been used successfully in lesions that cannot be distinguished from SCCs, as well as the so-called giant aggressive keratoacanthomas.[35,36] The dosage used, 4000–6000 cGy, is the same as the tumoricidal dosage used for SCCs. A biopsy of the lesion to rule out SCC prior to treatment may be prudent.

Course and prognosis

Keratoacanthoma is a low-grade tumor that carries a very good prognosis. Reports of malignant transformation or metastasizing lesions are probably misdiagnosed SCCs.

Squamous cell carcinoma

Definition

SCC is a malignant tumor arising from epidermal or appendageal keratinocytes or from squamous mucosal epithelium. There is often a history of damage by exogenous agents acting as carcinogens, such as sunlight, ionizing radiation, local irritants, or arsenic. The tumor cells have a tendency toward keratin formation. Variants include Bowen disease, an *in situ* SCC; verrucous carcinoma, a low grade SCC with a clinicopathologically distinct warty appearance; Buschke–Loewenstein tumor, the subset of verrucous carcinoma found on the genitals; oral florid papillomatosis, which involves the oral cavity; and epithelioma cuniculatum which involves the plantar surface.

Epidemiology

The incidence of cutaneous SCC varies greatly for different parts of the world, different races, and different life habits and occupations. The incidence was reported as 41.4 cases per 100,000 in 1983,[1] and is increasing.[2] Over the past three decades, SCC incidence has increased over 200% in the United states, and >700,000 cases are diagnosed annually.[37]

As previously mentioned, mutations in the *P53* tumor-suppressor gene have been found in a number of SCCs.[38] Phototherapy patients who received broadband UVB or psoralen plus ultraviolet A (PUVA) for the treatment of skin diseases, such as psoriasis or mycosis fungoides (cutaneous T-cell lymphoma), are also at increased risk.[39,40] The incidence of SCC is much higher in immunosuppressed patients, and these patients should be followed very carefully. Many dermatology departments now have dedicated clinics for immunosuppressed and transplant patients.[41] Depending on the dose of immunosuppressive drugs and previous sun exposure, transplant patients have up to a 65-fold increased risk of developing SCC.[42] The SCC to BCC ratio also reverses from 0.25 to 1 in the general population to 1.5–3 to 1 in transplant patients. Tumors in such patients tend to behave more aggressively.[39,43]

Verrucous carcinoma of the skin is a rare tumor, with more than 100 reported cases.[44] Approximately 80–90% of patients are male, with a mean age of 52–60 years. The Buschke–Loewenstein tumor is a verrucous carcinoma of the anogenital mucosa. Penile Buschke–Loewenstein tumor is the most common, with an incidence between 5% and 24% of all penile cancers. Vaginal, cervical, perianal, and perirectal Buschke–Loewenstein tumors are less common than penile ones. The etiology of these tumors is linked to HPV, particularly to HPV serotypes 6 and 11.[44]

The incidence of Bowen disease has not been extensively investigated. The incidence has been reported as 14 per 100,000 population in Rochester, Minnesota,[45] and 142 per 100,000 population in Kauai, Hawaii.[46]

Progress has been made in the identification of heritable risk factors in NMSC.[47] Polymorphisms of the melanocortin-1 receptor, which are linked to an increased risk of melanoma, segregate with patients at an elevated risk for both SCC and BCC.

Clinical features

SCC often arises in skin that is damaged or has been subjected to chronic irritation. Thus, the skin adjacent to the carcinoma may show evidence of solar damage, such as actinic keratoses, wrinkling, dryness, telangiectasias, and irregular pigmentation. Alternatively, there may be features of radiodermatitis from previous radiation therapy,[48] a sinus tract associated with an underlying osteomyelitis, or scarring from a burn ("Marjolin ulcer").[49] Chronic venous ulcers of the lower extremities are also associated with increased risks of developing SCC.[50] Chronic ulcers that show features of proliferation beyond the expected granulation process should raise the suspicion of malignant transformation.

SCC usually evolves faster than BCC, but not as rapidly as keratoacanthoma. The earliest lesion, the intraepidermal SCC or carcinoma *in situ*, typically appears as a scaly, erythematous plaque on sun-exposed areas, often with a sharply demarcated but irregular outline (Figure 4). Bowen disease is clinically identical to SCC *in situ*. Bowen disease on the glans penis is also known as erythroplasia of Queyrat.

Invasive SCC (Figure 5) almost always arises from a preexisting premalignant lesion or an *in situ* carcinoma, although *de novo* SCC has been reported.[51] The lesion is typically an erythematous, indurated papule, plaque, or nodule, which may be polygonal, oval, round, or verrucous in shape (Figures 6 and 7). The tumor tends to increase both in elevation and diameter with time. A hallmark of SCC is its firmness on palpation. The late lesion is often eroded, crusted, and ulcerated with an indurated margin. The ulcer is often covered with a purulent exudate and bleeds easily (Figure 7). Early ulceration is often a marker for anaplastic lesions. Regional lymphadenopathy may be present either as a response to infection of the ulcer or from metastases. The latter tend to be rubbery and more irregular, and may be fixed to adjacent tissues.

Verrucous carcinoma of the skin is most commonly found on the soles of men.[44] Typically, it presents as a slowly enlarging cauliflower-like mass. It is locally aggressive and may grow to a significant size. The ball of the foot is involved in more than 50% of cases. Other locations include the face, buttocks, oral cavity, trunk, and extremities. The bulk of the tumor is soft and may be foul-smelling. If left untreated, the tumor will eventually penetrate the underlying soft tissue and bone. However, metastasis is rare.

The Buschke–Loewenstein tumor most commonly affects the penile glans and prepuce of uncircumcised males, presenting as a cauliflower-like, fungating, foul-smelling tumor on the coronal sulcus. In women, it may be present on the vagina, cervix, or vulva. The Buschke–Loewenstein tumor has a tendency to infiltrate deeply, causing destruction of underlying tissues.

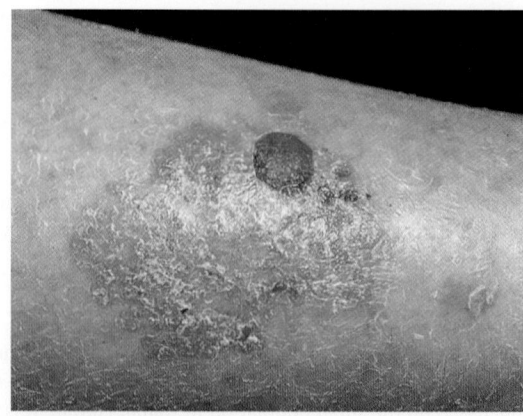

Figure 4 Squamous cell carcinoma (SCC) arising in SCC in situ. A nodule of invasive SCC on the lower leg arising within the well-demarcated, erythematous scaly plaque of SCC in situ.

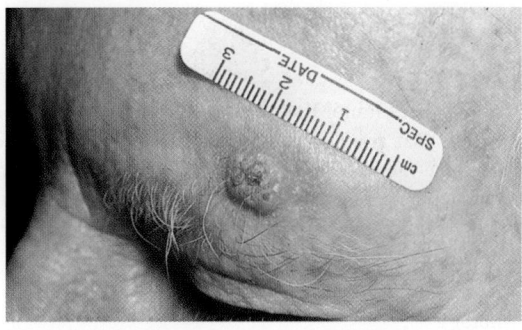

Figure 5 Invasive squamous cell carcinoma. Erythematous, hyperkeratotic nodule on the forehead resembling a keratoacanthoma (see Fig. 112–3). An incisional or excisional biopsy is necessary to distinguish the two lesions.

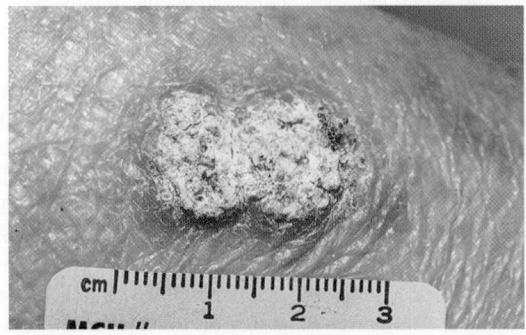

Figure 6 Invasive squamous cell carcinoma. A hyperkeratotic, crusty plaque on the forearm. Note the evidence of sun damage in the surrounding skin: wrinkling, bruising, and a lackluster appearance.

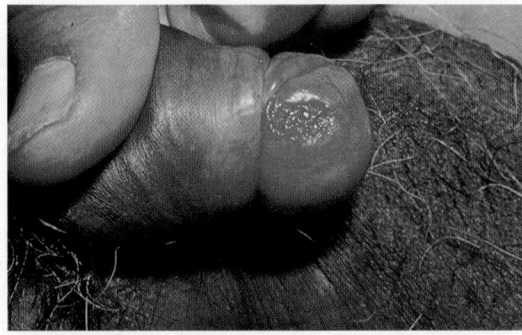

Figure 7 Invasive squamous cell carcinoma. An ulcerated lesion on the glans penis with an indurated margin. The ulcer typically bleeds easily.

SCC of the lip may arise from an area of leukoplakia or actinic cheilitis, and almost always occurs on the lower lip. This tumor is typically much more aggressive than those on glabrous skin and has a higher rate of metastasis.

Carcinomas arising in longstanding radiation dermatitis tend to be histologically anaplastic and extremely aggressive, with a high rate of metastasis.[52]

Treatment

The choice of treatment modality depends on the degree of differentiation of the tumor and the presence or absence of metastasis. The size, shape, location of the tumor, and the predisposing factors should also be considered. In the case of a localized, well-differentiated tumor with no evidence of metastasis, the goal should be complete eradication of the lesion. In the presence of

lymph node metastases or unresectable tumors, palliative treatment may be considered. The variety of modalities available for consideration include electrodessication and curettage (ED&C), excisional surgery, Mohs surgery, cryosurgery, electrosurgery, and radiation therapy.[34,53–55]

Electrodessication and curettage

ED&C is an option for SCC *in situ*, particularly on the trunk. The primary drawback is the lack of histologic confirmation of clear tumor margins, but in properly chosen patients the recurrence rate is similar to excisional surgery.[56] Invasive SCC and tumors with high-risk features have a higher risk of recurrence, however, and the preferred treatment for these tumors would allow for proper margin assessment. The larger, circular scar left from the ED&C procedure is also a deterrent for some patients.

Excisional surgery

Surgical excision with primary closure or repair with skin graft or flap is the treatment of choice for relatively small lesions with distinct borders. There should be an adequate margin of clearance of 3–5 mm to minimize the risk of recurrence. Brodland and Zitelli[57] reported that margins of 4 mm were required to achieve a 95% tumor clearance rate. For invasive or large tumors (>2 cm in diameter), or tumors on high-risk areas such as the scalp, ears, nose, eyelids, or lips, Mohs micrographic surgery is the preferred approach.

Prophylactic lymph node dissection is not recommended because of the relatively low rate of metastasis. Sentinel lymph node biopsy is an emerging approach for high-risk tumors, though the specific indications remain undefined. Tumors that have metastasized to regional lymph nodes are best treated with excision, lymph node dissection, and chemoradiation.

Mohs surgery

Mohs micrographic surgery is a technique wherein a single physician excises the tumor and performs a histologic examination of 100% of the surgical margin. This technique has the lowest local recurrence rate of all treatment modalities while also allowing maximum conservation of surrounding healthy tissue, allowing for an optimal cosmetic result.[57] It is the treatment of choice for tumors on cosmetically or functionally sensitive areas, as well as for recurrent tumors. It is also indicated for immunocompromised patients, tumors in previously irradiated skin, or tumors with high-risk features including poor differentiation, breslow depth ≥2 mm, diameter ≥2 cm, or perineural invasion. Appropriate use criteria for Mohs surgery have been published.[57,58]

Cryosurgery

Treatment of SCC by freezing with liquid nitrogen is best restricted to the carcinoma *in situ* on areas that are not cosmetically sensitive. This modality has the advantage of simplicity with a high cure rate when employed in the proper situation.[54,59]

Radiation therapy

Radiation therapy is an option for patients who cannot tolerate other more invasive treatment modalities. The treatment schedule is determined by the treatment modality, size, depth, and location of the tumor and the particular time-dose-fractionation schedule used. A fractionated dose provides the best cure rate and the lowest risk of adverse events, but fractionation schedules vary from 5 to 30 fractions.[34] Most radiation for skin cancers in the United States is delivered using electron beam or superficial X-ray therapies with a dose between 4000 and 6000 cGy. The reported 5-year control rates for these approaches are 89% and 68% for primary and recurrent SCC, respectively.[60] While reasonable, these are significantly below the 5-year cure rates for excisions or Mohs micrographic surgery. More recently, high-dose rate electronic brachytherapy has become a popular treatment approach, but 5-year control data is lacking.[61] Postoperative radiation therapy can also be considered as an adjuvant treatment for certain high-risk tumors including those with perineural invasion or other high risk features (see AJCC high-risk features in the following).

Patient and tumor site selection are critical for all radiation therapy. Good cosmetic results can be obtained for carefully selected small lesions of the nose, lip, eyelid, and canthus, though these may deteriorate with time. Lesions on the dorsum of the hand and those over bony and cartilaginous structures should not be treated with radiation because of the risk of radiation necrosis. Lesions in younger patients should be approached with caution given the risk of tumors arising secondary to the treatment. Tumors that do arise in areas of chronic radiation dermatitis should not be treated with further radiation.

Chemotherapy

The use of oral acitretin has decreased the incidence of SCC when given as a chemopreventive agent. The benefit from such long-term use has to be weighed against the toxicity, which includes hypertriglyceridemia, arthralgias, mucocutaneous xerosis, and alopecia. In organ transplant recipients, where the risk of developing skin cancer and risk of death from SCC is increased, chronic use of retinoids may be justified.[62]

Course and prognosis

The risk factors correlated with local recurrence and metastatic rates include treatment modality, prior treatment, location, size, depth, histologic differentiation, histologic evidence of perineural involvement, precipitating factors other than ultraviolet light, and host immunosuppression. SCC in skin carries an overall metastatic rate of 3–6%.[63] Those arising from sun-damaged skin typically have a low risk for metastasis whereas those arising from chronic osteomyelitic sinus tracts, irradiated areas, and burn scars have a much higher metastatic rate (31%, 20%, and 18%, respectively). Carcinoma on the lower lip, although mostly sun induced, has a metastatic incidence of about 15%. Tumor arising in areas such as the glans penis (see Figure 7), the vulva, and the oral mucosa also have a high rate of metastasis. It is estimated that as many as 8,800 patients died of SCC in 2012.[37]

The seventh edition of the American Joint Committee on Cancer (AJCC) staging system for SCC was released in 2010, and includes high-risk features of tumor diameter ≥2 cm, tumor thickness >2 mm or Clark level ≥IV, poor differentiation, perineural invasion, invasion into cranial bone, and anatomic location on the ear or lip.[64] Although this is an improvement over the sixth edition staging system, some have proposed alternative staging systems that may more accurately stratify high-risk tumors into different prognostic groups.[65]

With proper treatment, the overall 5-year remission rate is 90%, including SCC of the lip.[63] Frankel and colleagues[66] recommended follow-ups at least every 3 months for a year after treatment of SCC, and semiannually thereafter for up to 4 years.

Basal cell carcinoma

Definition

BCC is a malignant tumor that very rarely metastasizes. It is composed of cells that arise from the epidermis and the appendages which resemble the basal layer of the epidermis and is associated with a characteristic stroma. It tends to grow slowly and invade locally over many years. Eventually it can ulcerate, hence its archaic name "rodent ulcer."

Epidemiology

BCCs account for more than 75% of NMSC diagnosed in the United States each year.[67,68] Incidence varies from 422 per 100,000 general population in Kauai, Hawaii,[30] to 146 per 100,000 in Rochester, Minnesota.[69] BCC is the most common form of skin cancer in whites,[1] and is rare in darkly pigmented people. It most frequently occurs in persons older than 40 years of age. The frequency is slightly higher in males. Other risk factors include geographic locations with high solar intensity, exposures to inorganic trivalent arsenic, ionizing radiation, and immunosuppression. Phototherapy patients receiving UVB or PUVA for treatment of certain dermatoses, such as psoriasis or mycosis fungoides, are also at increased risk.[39] Recent studies suggest a correlation between BCCs and exposures to sunlight in early life and intense intermittent (recreational) sun exposures.[70,71] This is contrary to the previous belief that BCCs result from cumulative lifetime sunlight exposures. Genetic studies show that loss-of-function mutations in the tumor-suppressor gene patched, or gain-of-function mutations in the smoothened gene, lead to the formation of sporadic basal cell tumors.[72,73] Germline mutations in these genes lead to Gorlin or basal cell nevus syndrome.

Clinical features

BCC is characteristically slow-growing over months to years. It is usually asymptomatic unless ulceration occurs, and then there is bleeding. It most frequently occurs on sun-exposed areas such as the face and upper trunk, and is not seen on the palms and soles.

Early lesions are round-to-oval papules or nodules, firm to palpation, often with an umbilicated center that may be ulcerated. The color is pink to red and often has a translucent or pearly quality (Figure 8). If left untreated, the lesion enlarges slowly and is destructive to neighboring structures by direct invasion. Long-standing lesions are ulcerated as a rule (Figure 9). The surrounding skin often shows telangiectasias and other evidence of solar damage, such as actinic keratoses, atrophy, wrinkling, dryness, and irregular pigmentation. Some BCCs are pigmented and may exhibit a bluish hue.[74] These may be confused with malignant melanoma (Figure 10). The so-called superficial-type BCC usually presents on the trunk as an irregular, atrophic plaque with a slightly raised border and can be mistaken for psoriasis or dermatophytic infection (Figure 11). Infiltrative-type BCCs can be difficult to detect. They are often ivory-white, and may resemble morphea and are therefore called morphea-form BCCs. This type of lesion usually occurs on the face and has a more aggressive behavior.[75]

Treatment

The choice of therapy depends on the type and size of the lesion, the location, the general condition of the patient, the cosmetic considerations, and, not least, the experience and skill of the operator.[67] Morphea-form BCCs usually have indistinct borders clinically and may result in underestimation of the extent of the tumor. Lesions situated in the nasolabial crease, around the eye, and behind the ear

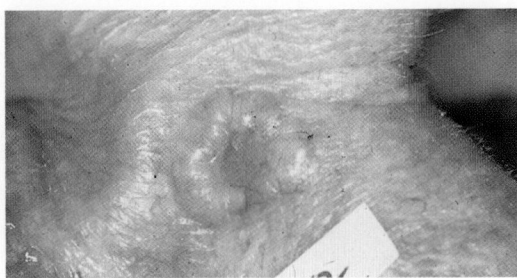

Figure 8 Basal cell carcinoma. A pearly nodule with an umbilicated, ulcerated center and telangiectasia.

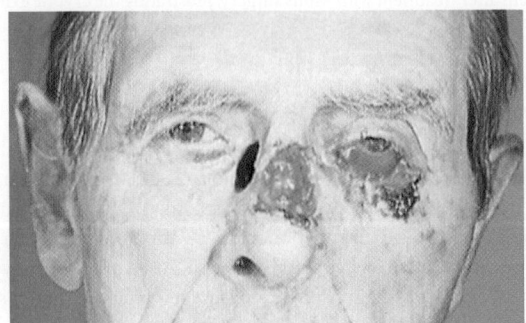

Figure 9 Basal cell carcinoma. Note the erosive nature of such a long-standing lesion.

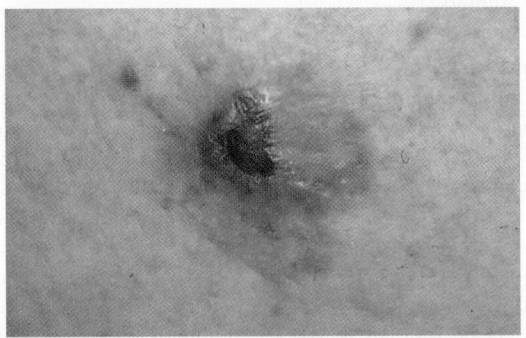

Figure 10 Pigmented basal cell carcinoma. A pink, irregular plaque with dark-blue to black pigmentation at the center that mimics a superficial spreading melanoma. The shiny quality is one clue to the diagnosis.

also tend to undermine deeply and extend far beyond the clinical border (Figure 12). Lesions that ulcerate early tend to be more aggressive. Knowledge of the behavior of the different clinical and pathologic types of BCC is essential in determining the choice of therapy. Treatment of BCCs should be aimed at a cure in the first instance. Under-treatment will result in recurrence and deep invasion.

Electrodesiccation and curettage

ED&C can be a reasonable option for small (<1 cm) tumors in low-risk areas that lack high aggressive histologic features. In carefully selected patients, the recurrence rate is similar to excision, but in less appropriate lesions the recurrence rate can exceed 20%.[76] Primary drawbacks include the lack of histologic confirmation and the appearance of a round, hypopigmented scar.

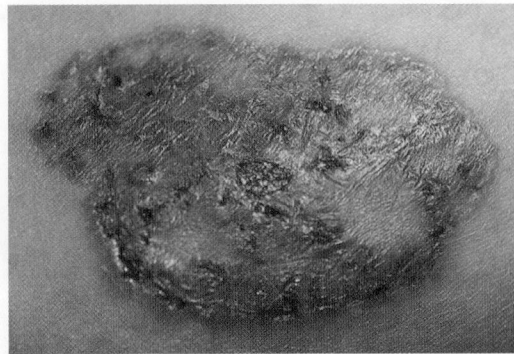

Figure 11 Superficial basal cell carcinoma. A large, 5-cm lesion on the abdomen. The pearly, string-like border is the clue to the clinical diagnosis.

Surgical excision

Surgical excision of the tumor with 4 mm margins followed by primary closure produces good cosmetic results and allows the surgical margins to be examined by the pathologist to confirm adequate margins.[77] Tumor present at the lateral excision margins will result in marginal recurrences, which tend to present early and may be reexcised with relative ease. Inadequate deep margins result in recurrences which tend to present late, together with invasion of deep structures. For lesions without aggressive histologic features on the trunk or extremity the recurrence rate is less than 5%.[77]

Mohs surgery

Mohs micrographic surgery offers the lowest recurrence rate of all treatment options while allowing maximum conservation of healthy surrounding tissue (see Figure 12). According to the appropriate use criteria published in 2012, Mohs surgery is indicated for tumors with aggressive histologic features including morpheaform, infiltrative, metatypical, and micronodular patterns. It is also indicated for nearly all recurrent tumors, lesions on the head, neck, genitals, pretibial legs, hands, and feet as well as nodular tumors >2 cm on the trunk.[58] Advantages include complete margin assessment of the tumor and maximal tissue preservation. Disadvantages include cost and, in some areas, limited availability of trained Mohs surgeons.[78]

Radiation therapy

Treatment with ionizing radiation is an option in selected patient populations, in particular, elderly or fragile patients who cannot tolerate invasive procedures. Electron beam and superficial X-ray therapies yield 5-year control rates of 95% and 86% in primary and recurrent BCCs.[60] Electron beam brachytherapy has been used with early success in BCC, but large studies and 5-year data are lacking.[61] Lesions >5 cm have higher recurrence rates than smaller tumors.[79] The treatment schedule is chosen according to the type, location, size, and depth of the tumor, the total dose of radiation, and the number of fractions that will be given. Atrophy, necrosis, and scarring may be kept to a minimum when the total dose, typically in the range of 4000–6000 cGy, is divided into several smaller fractions over several weeks. Hypo-fractionated schedules with 5–8 treatments have been suggested, particularly with high-dose rate brachytherapy, to minimize patient inconvenience. However, these may have more adverse events and poorer cosmesis compared to traditional 20–30 fraction regimens.[80]

Chemotherapy

Topical applications of 5% 5-fluorouracil cream to the tumor twice a day for several weeks is best suited only for small, superficial tumors in elderly patients who cannot tolerate other more

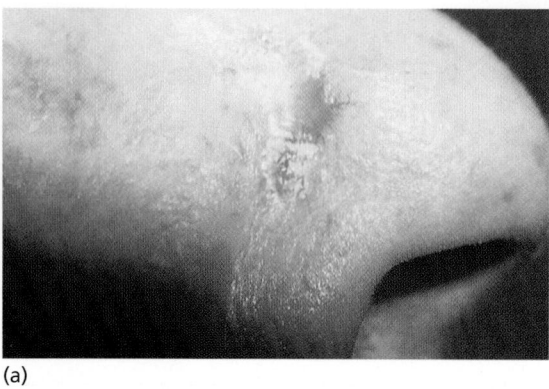 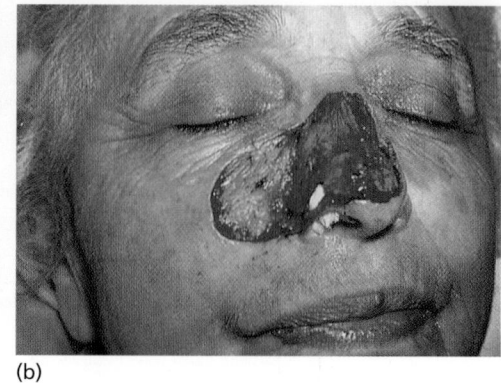

(a)   (b)

Figure 12 (**a**) Basal cell carcinoma. The lesion is quite limited clinically. (**b**) Same patient after treatment with Mohs surgery, illustrating the cryptic extension far beyond the clinically evident border.

aggressive forms of treatment. The rate of recurrence, however, is considerably higher. Intralesional 5-fluorouracil has also been tried in nodular lesions.[81,82] Five percent imiquimod cream five times per week for 6 weeks has been shown to be effective therapy for the majority of biopsy-proven superficial BCCs in immunocompetent individuals. Lesions >2.0 cm or lesions not located on trunk, neck, or extremities (other than hands and feet) are excluded in the FDA indications.

In 2012 the FDA approved vismodegib for metastatic or "locally advanced" BCC. Vismodegib inhibits the transmembrane protein smoothened, blocking the hedgehog signaling cascade. In the pivotal phase 2, nonrandomized trial, 30% of patients with metastatic disease and 43% of patients with locally advanced (inoperable) disease showed at least a partial response. The median response duration was 7.6 months.[83] Adverse events are almost universal, and they include muscle spasm, dysgeusia, alopecia, diarrhea, and amenorrhea.[84]

Course and prognosis

BCCs are slow growing as a rule. However, if left untreated, they may reach a large size, with consequent extensive tissue destruction. In a comprehensive review of recurrence rates for primary BCCs, the results are highly comparable for the various treatment modalities.[78] Most studies reported a 95% or higher cure rate.[76,85] A lower 5-year recurrence rate has been reported with Mohs surgery than with other commonly used modalities. Metastasis, although rare, may occur, particularly in large or recurrent lesions.[86] In such cases, the prognosis is usually poor, with a 1-year survival rate of less than 20%, and a 5-year survival rate of approximately 10%. In general, the 5-year occurrence rate of new BCCs developing in patients with a previous BCC may be as high as 45%.[87]

Merkel cell carcinoma

Definition

The Merkel cell was first described by Merkel in 1875. It is a nondendritic, nonkeratinocytic epithelial clear cell normally found in the epidermis and dermis of mammals and humans. Merkel cell carcinoma (MCC) was first described by Toker in 1972, and is thought to arise from the cutaneous Merkel cell. It is a high-grade malignant tumor, with a high rate of local recurrence and metastasis. Mortality of 33% at 3 years exceeds that seen in cutaneous melanoma.

Epidemiology

MCC is a relatively uncommon neoplasm. Data from SEER show a 3-fold increase in incidence from 1996 to 2001, which had quadrupled by 2006 (0.15–0.6 per 100,000 annually).[88,89] This is partially because of improved diagnostic accuracy with the advent of targeted immunostains such as cytokeratin 20 (CK20). Approximately 1500 cases of MCC were diagnosed in 2007 and it is believed that this incidence has remained fairly consistent in recent years. The median age at diagnosis is 69 years, and 90% of patients are older than 50 years. There is a slight male predominance. Higher rates of MCC are seen in patients with HIV, CLL, or solid organ transplantation. A previously unknown polyoma virus was recently identified in 80% of MCC tumors.[90]

Clinical features

The most common sites of involvement are head and neck (49%), extremities (38%), with the lower extremities more frequently involved than the upper extremities, and trunk (13%), mainly lower back and buttocks. The lesions present as papules or nodules, pink to red to violet, often with overlying telangiectasia. Typically, the tumors are <2 cm in size. MCC can be suspected based on the mnemonic AEIOU (asymptomatic/lack of tenderness, expanding rapidly, immune suppression, older than 50 years, UV-exposed site on a person with fair skin).[88] CK20 immunostaining (perinuclear dot pattern) has greatly assisted diagnosis of MCC.

Treatment

Wide local excision is the standard treatment modality.[91] Alternatively, local excision with margin control by frozen-section histology (Mohs surgery) may be of value.[92] Studies have shown that sentinel lymph node biopsy is predictive of nodal involvement.[93] Postoperative adjuvant radiation therapy remains controversial in patients with a negative sentinel node biopsy. However, it has been shown to improve local and regional control in patients with positive sentinel nodes, and is strongly recommended in patients with bulky regional disease and multiple metastatic lymph nodes.[89] It also may be beneficial for either local recurrences or for local control after node dissection.[94] Chemotherapy regimens have not been shown to extend life.

Course and prognosis

Overall mortality by 3 years is approximately 33% for patients with MCC. Outcome is based on primary tumor size and stage of disease. Sentinel node biopsy is of value in identifying patients with disease in the nodes (stage III). In 2010, The AJCC instituted a 4-stage classification for MCC (stage I—tumor < 2cm; stage II—tumor ≥ 2 cm; stage III—regional nodal metastases; stage IV—distant metastases).[89] Immunosuppressed patients have a higher mortality than immunocompetent patients.[95]

Tumors arising from dermis

Dermatofibrosarcoma protuberans

Definition
Dermatofibrosarcoma protuberans (DFSP) is a locally malignant, slow-growing tumor originating in the dermis. The tumor cells resemble fibroblasts with various degrees of atypia.

Epidemiology
DFSP is an uncommon tumor that typically presents during early to mid-adult life, and rarely in children. Males are affected 4 times as often as females. It may be more common in blacks than in whites. Associations with arsenic exposure, burn or surgical scar, acanthosis nigricans, and rapid growth during pregnancy have been reported.

Clinical features
DFSP is most commonly situated on the trunk and proximal extremities. It typically presents as a solitary, slow-growing nodule with multiple palpable surface irregularities.[96] The early lesion may resemble a dermatofibroma, keloid scar, or SCC (see Figure 13). The lesion is firm to palpation and varies from flesh color to reddish to yellow. The center may be ulcerated. The tumor can achieve an enormous size with multiple satellite nodules, if untreated. The characteristic irregular surface on a firm, plaque-like base may suggest the diagnosis. A biopsy will provide confirmation. The average size at the time of surgery is approximately 5 cm.

Recently, DFSPs were shown to harbor chromosomal translocations that fuse the collagen type I alpha gene with the gene for platelet-derived growth factor B.[97] The presence of this specific t(17;22) translocation permits the diagnosis of DFSP in equivocal cases.

Treatment
DFSP has a high recurrence rate after conventional surgical excision, with a range of 30–50%.[98] Lateral surgical margins of at least 3 cm excised through the deep fascia are the current recommendation for conventional excision. In one large series, this yielded a recurrence rate of approximately 10%. Because of the potential for deforming surgical defects, Mohs surgery, which permits microscopic control of the excision margins, is the treatment of choice. This allows the subclinical margins to be mapped at the time of surgery, and, consequently, the surgical margins more precisely determined. Prophylactic lymph node dissection is not recommended because of the low initial risk of metastasis. Recently, the receptor tyrosine kinase inhibitor imatinib has been used with success in treating multiply recurrent and metastatic cases of DFSP.[99]

Course and prognosis
In a review of 136 cases of DFSP treated with Mohs surgery, a local recurrence rate of 6.6% was determined, although smaller studies have shown fewer recurrences.[100] The experience of the Mohs surgeon is critical in preventing tumor recurrence. Historically, late recurrences are frequent, thus long-term follow-up is recommended.

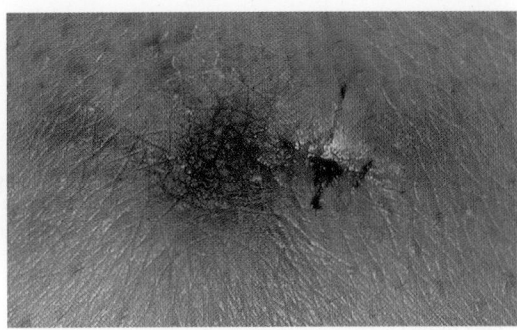

Figure 13 Dermatofibrosarcoma protuberans on the back of the neck. Firm papule resembling a dermatofibroma. Source: Courtesy of R.A. Johnson, MD.

Cutaneous angiosarcoma

Definition
Angiosarcoma (AS) is an aggressive malignancy of endothelial cells, arising in the setting of chronic lymphedema, chronic radiation dermatitis or on the face and scalp of the elderly patients.

Epidemiology
Cutaneous AS affects elderly men more often than women. Sun does not appear to be an important factor because the tumor often appears under cover of hair.[101] AS developing in areas of chronic lymphedema (so-called Stewart–Treves syndrome) is an infrequent complication of mastectomy, axillary node dissection for melanoma, lymphedema secondary to filarial infection and chronic idiopathic lymphedema. Unfortunately, up to 0.5% of women undergoing mastectomy and lymph node dissection develop AS within 1–30 years. Radiation-induced AS is a rare iatrogenic complication of radiation that develops in or near the irradiated site. The incubation period may be up to 40 years in some cases.

Clinical features
In all three presentations, the clinical features can be similar. Bruise-like macules, papules, and nodules develop and tend to enlarge quickly. Ulceration can occur in advanced lesions. On the face, facial edema can be the presenting sign. In all cases, the lesions extend beyond the clinical borders.

Treatment
Treatment for AS is not promising. One problem is that by the time a diagnosis is made the tumors have spread several centimeters beyond the clinically appreciated borders. AS of the face and scalp is rarely less than 10 cm in diameter at presentation. Wide surgical resection followed by radiotherapy is the mainstay of treatment. In a study of 24 patients with AS of the face and scalp, local control was obtained in 57%. However, of those patients, 47% developed distant metastases.[102] In surgically unresectable tumors, radiation therapy and adjuvant chemotherapy with intralesional recombinant interleukin-2 and interferon-α-2b[103] or liposomal doxorubicin[104] may extend the life of some patients. Targeted biologic therapies such as imantinib mesylate and bevacizumab are also being investigated.[105]

Course and prognosis
Survival at 5 years is approximately 12%.[101]

Tumors arising from appendages

Sebaceous carcinoma

Definition
Frequently arising on the eyelid, sebaceous carcinoma is a malignant adnexal neoplasm.

Epidemiology
Sebaceous carcinoma is the second most frequent malignancy of the eyelid next to BCC.

Clinical features
Misdiagnosis of sebaceous carcinoma is frequent. The tumor usually appears as a painless, flesh-colored papule, or nodule on the upper or lower eyelid where it is easily dismissed as a chalazion or chronic blepharitis. Ulceration is often the feature that stimulates clinical suspicion and biopsy. Focal loss of eyelashes and a yellowish hue are other diagnostic clues. Sebaceous tumors are frequently associated with the Muir–Torre syndrome, as described later in this chapter.

Treatment
In a recent evidence-based review on the management of eyelid malignancies, Mohs micrographic surgery and excision with frozen-section control were shown to be superior to other modalities, including radiation therapy.[106]

Course and prognosis
A study of 18 patients with sebaceous carcinoma treated with the Mohs technique reported an 11% recurrence rate after an average follow-up of 37 months.[107] One patient had metastatic disease (5.6%). This compared favorably to other published rates of recurrence and metastasis, which had been as high as 30% and 22%, respectively.

Extramammary Paget disease

Definition
Extramammary Paget disease (EMPD) is a neoplasm of apocrine glands that clinically resembles Paget disease of the breast, but occurs in areas rich in apocrine glands, including the perineum and axilla.

Epidemiology
More frequent in women and whites, EMPD usually strikes after the fifth decade.

Clinical features
EMPD is a scaly, sharply marginated plaque, most commonly found in the vulva. Because itching and burning are common symptoms, it is often mistaken for intertrigo or flexural eczema, and the diagnosis is delayed. Progressive enlargement of the plaque in the face of topical steroid or antifungal medications is a diagnostic clue.

Treatment
Evaluation to identify the presence of underlying malignancy is crucial. Surgical excision is the treatment of choice for primary EMPD. Although conventional surgery can yield a recurrence rate of more than 40%, microscopically controlled excision (Mohs surgery) appears to yield at least as good results while sparing tissue loss. High-dose (4000 cGy) radiotherapy produced local regression in one small study. Ablative carbon dioxide laser treatment is palliative, as recurrence rates are very high. More recently, topical imiquimod 5% cream has been used with some success as either monotherapy or in combination with other treatments.[108]

Course and prognosis
When EMPD is associated with an adenocarcinoma, the prognosis is poor. However, even primary EMPD can eventually ulcerate and become locally invasive and spread to lymph nodes, with depth of invasion >1 mm being an important prognostic factor. Even after wide excision, local recurrence still approaches 25%.

Benign cutaneous tumors associated with cancer syndromes

Trichilemmoma (in Cowden disease)

Definition
Trichilemmoma is a tumor that exhibits features of outer root sheath differentiation of hair. In Cowden disease, multiple trichilemmomas are associated with multiple hamartomatous neoplasms of ectodermal, mesodermal, and endodermal origin, the most important include fibrocystic disease and carcinoma of the breast, adenoma and follicular adenocarcinoma of the thyroid, gastrointestinal polyps, and lipomas.[109]

Epidemiology
Cowden disease is a rare autosomal dominant condition with variable expressivity. Fewer than 100 cases are reported to date. Male patients slightly exceed females among all the cases reported. All reported patients are white, except for one Japanese and two black patients. The age span is between 4 and 75 years, with the median age being 39 years.

Clinical features
In Cowden disease, trichilemmomas present as small lichenoid, skin-colored to yellow-tan papules with a smooth surface. They are concentrated on the face, especially around the orifices and the ears. Similar papules may appear on the extremities, including palmoplantar surfaces, and the oral cavity, particularly on the gingiva and the tongue (Figures 14 and 15). The presentation of these papules usually precedes the appearance of breast cancer and, therefore, can serve as a marker of associated cancer.

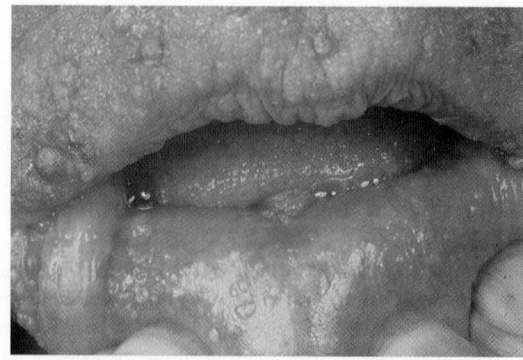

Figure 14 Cowden disease. Multiple trichilemmomas on the upper lip. Similar papules are present on the mucosal surface of the lower lip.

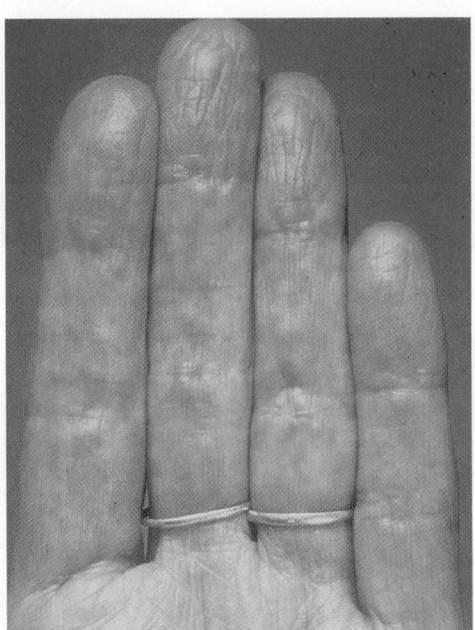

Figure 15 Cowden disease. Translucent keratotic papules on the palmar surface. Source: Courtesy of R.A. Johnson, MD.

Genetics

Germ line mutations in the protein tyrosine phosphatase *PTEN* have been linked to multiple families with Cowden disease.[110]

Treatment

Therapies are directed toward achieving good cosmetic appearance and treatment of the various associated benign and malignant tumors, as indicated. In view of the high incidence of breast cancer in female patients, which may be as high as 50%, frequent breast examination and mammography are indicated.

Sebaceous adenoma (in Muir–Torre syndrome)

Definition

Sebaceous adenoma is a rare, benign tumor consisting of incompletely differentiated sebaceous lobules within the dermis. In Muir–Torre syndrome, multiple sebaceous adenomas, carcinomas and keratoacanthomas are associated with multiple visceral malignant neoplasms, most commonly carcinoma of the colon and carcinoma of the ampulla of Vater. These sebaceous tumors are rare enough that the presence of a single lesion in an otherwise healthy patient warrants an investigation for internal neoplasms.

Epidemiology

Solitary sebaceous adenoma is a rare tumor that occurs in elderly patients of both sexes. The multiple type, associated with Muir–Torre syndrome, is familial, with more than 50% of reported patients having an immediate family member with a history of internal cancer, most frequently of the colon.[111]

Clinical features

Sebaceous adenoma typically appears as a firm, flesh-colored to waxy-yellow papule or pedunculated lesion, usually less than 1 cm in size. The surface may be smooth or verrucous. Older lesions may be plaque-like or ulcerated. It is usually located on the face or scalp and is usually slow growing.

Genetics

The DNA mismatch repair gene *HMSH2* has been identified as one of the genes disturbed in Muir–Torre syndrome.[112] Mismatch repair gene immunohistochemistry (IHC) of sebaceous neoplasms can be helpful as part of the workup of patients with suspected Muir–Torre syndrome, although sensitivity and specificity are fairly poor when used as a screening tool.[113]

Treatment

The treatment of choice is surgical excision. The tumor is also radiosensitive.

Multiple mucosal neuromas (multiple endocrine neoplasia 2B, MEN2B)

Definition

Mucosal neuromas present as small, discrete and coalescing, painless nodules, usually involving the lips, and sometimes studding the margins of the tongue. The association of multiple mucosal neuromas, medullary thyroid carcinoma and pheochromocytoma has been established as a familial syndrome.

Epidemiology

Discrete mucosal neuromas are common and often result from direct trauma, as in the typical bite neuroma. More than 150 cases of multiple neuromas associated with endocrine tumors have been described in the literature.[114]

Clinical features

In MEN2B, diffusely enlarged lips are an early feature. Diffuse and symmetric fleshy papules and nodules occur on the tongue by the end of first decade. Any mucosal surface may be involved. Patients often develop a Marfanoid habitus. Most importantly, medullary thyroid carcinoma may develop in early adulthood. These tumors produce calcitonin and can stimulate parathyroid hyperplasia. Pheochromocytomas are frequently present as well.

Genetics

In all cases studied to date, mutation in the protooncogene *RET*, a receptor tyrosine kinase, has been uncovered.[115]

Course and prognosis

Medullary thyroid carcinoma is often the cause of death. Routine screening for this tumor with ultrasonography and by measuring serum calcitonin levels is useful, but current recommendations suggest prophylactic thyroidectomy in cases where a *RET* mutation is documented.[116]

Metastatic tumors to the skin

Cutaneous metastases of internal cancers are uncommon. In a report of 7316 non-melanoma cancer patients,[117] only 1% of patients had cutaneous metastases at the time of diagnosis. In a study of 2298 patients reported as having died of visceral carcinoma, only 2.7% had evidence of cutaneous metastases.[118] In a more recent retrospective study of 4020 patients with metastatic carcinomas and melanoma, 10% had cutaneous metastases. In general, the incidence of the various cancers metastatic to the skin correlates well with the incidence of the particular primary tumor.[119]

The spectrum of metastatic tumors differs slightly between the two sexes.[119] In one study, the most common primary sources of metastatic carcinoma to the skin in males were malignant melanoma (32%), lung (12%), large intestine (11%), carcinoma of the oral cavity (9%) and larynx (5.5%), and kidney (5%). In females, breast is by far the most common source (70%), followed by melanoma (12%), and ovary (3%), and large intestine, lung, and oral cavity, each accounting for 1.3–2.3% of the cases.[119] In females, the incidence of lung carcinoma has increased dramatically in recent years, resulting in a corresponding rise in the incidence of cutaneous metastatic lung carcinoma deposits. Other carcinomas that metastasize to the skin include thyroid, pancreas, liver, gallbladder, urinary bladder, endometrium, prostate, and testis. However, these are quite rare.

Typically, metastatic cancer presents as multiple, firm, nonulcerated nodules. When solitary, they may be misdiagnosed as primary skin tumors. Inflammatory skin metastases mimicking cellulitis may occur in 10% of metastases from breast cancer. The most common sites for skin metastases are chest and abdomen, followed by head and neck; metastasis to the extremities is rare. Metastases in the scalp can be associated with alopecia ("alopecia neoplastica"). Dissemination may be via the bloodstream or via the lymphatics. Carcinomas of the breast and of the oral cavity tend to spread through the lymphatics, whereas others tend to spread hematogenously. Lymphatic dissemination may explain the observation that skin metastases tend to be close to the site of the primary tumor: chest in lung carcinoma, abdominal wall in gastrointestinal tumors, and lower back in renal cell carcinoma.

The prognosis for patients with cutaneous metastases is generally poor. In Lookingbill and colleagues,[119] the average time from diagnosis of skin metastases to death for the various primary tumors varies from 1 to 34 months. The variability in prognosis may be the result of advances in cancer therapy during the past decades. Some patients with metastatic melanoma to skin as the sole site of metastasis may have prolonged disease-free survival.

Key references

The complete reference list can be found on the Wiley Companion Digital Edition of this title (see inside front cover for login instructions).

2 Cancer Facts & Figures. In: Society AC, editor. Atlanta: American Cancer Society; 2008:2008.
7 Weinstock MA. Death from skin cancer among the elderly: epidemiological patterns. *Arch Dermatol.* 1997;**133**(10):1207–1209.
9 Chuang TY, Reizner GT, Elpern DJ, Stone JL, Farmer ER. Nonmelanoma skin cancer in Japanese ethnic Hawaiians in Kauai, Hawaii: an incidence report. *J Am Acad Dermatol.* 1995;**33**(3):422–426.
11 Franceschi S, Levi F, Randimbison L, La Vecchia C. Site distribution of different types of skin cancer: new aetiological clues. *Int J Cancer.* 1996;**67**(1):24–28.
20 Clydesdale GJ, Dandie GW, Muller HK. Ultraviolet light induced injury: immunological and inflammatory effects. *Immunol Cell Biol.* 2001;**79**(6):547–568.
21 Ramsay HM, Fryer AA, Hawley CM, Smith AG, Harden PN. Non-melanoma skin cancer risk in the Queensland renal transplant population. *Br J Dermatol.* 2002;**147**(5):950–956.
22 Lookingbill DP, Lookingbill GL, Leppard B. Actinic damage and skin cancer in albinos in northern Tanzania: findings in 164 patients enrolled in an outreach skin care program. *J Am Acad Dermatol.* 1995;**32**(4):653–658.
23 Suchniak JM, Baer S, Goldberg LH. High rate of malignant transformation in hyperkeratotic actinic keratoses. *J Am Acad Dermatol.* 1997;**37**(3 Pt 1):392–394.
24 Drake LA, Ceilley RI, Cornelison RL, et al. Guidelines of care for actinic keratoses. Committee on Guidelines of Care. *J Am Acad Dermatol.* 1995;**32**(1):95–98.
25 Gupta AK, Weiss JS, Jorizzo JL. 5-fluorouracil 0.5% cream for multiple actinic or solar keratoses of the face and anterior scalp. *Skin Therapy Lett.* 2001;**6**(9):1–4.
26 Jarvis B, Figgitt DP. Topical 3% diclofenac in 2.5% hyaluronic acid gel: a review of its use in patients with actinic keratoses. *Am J Clin Dermatol.* 2003;**4**(3):203–213.
32 Hsi ED, Svoboda-Newman SM, Stern RA, Nickoloff BJ, Frank TS. Detection of human papillomavirus DNA in keratoacanthomas by polymerase chain reaction. *Am J Dermatopathol.* 1997;**19**(1):10–15.
39 Katz KA, Marcil I, Stern RS. Incidence and risk factors associated with a second squamous cell carcinoma or basal cell carcinoma in psoralen + ultraviolet a light-treated psoriasis patients. *J Invest Dermatol.* 2002;**118**(6):1038–1043.
40 Nijsten TEC, Stern RS. The increased risk of skin cancer is persistent after discontinuation of psoralen+ultraviolet A: a cohort study. *J Invest Dermatol.* 2003;**121**(2):252–258.
41 Christenson LJ, Geusau A, Ferrandiz C, et al. Specialty clinics for the dermatologic care of solid-organ transplant recipients. *Dermatol Surg.* 2004;**30**(4 Pt 2):598–603.
42 Jensen P, Hansen S, Möller B, et al. Skin cancer in kidney and heart transplant recipients and different long-term immunosuppressive therapy regimens. *J Am Acad Dermatol.* 1999;**40**(2 Pt 1):177–186.
43 Martinez J-C, Otley CC, Stasko T, et al. Defining the clinical course of metastatic skin cancer in organ transplant recipients: a multicenter collaborative study. *Arch Dermatol.* 2003;**139**(3):301–306.
44 Schwartz RA. Verrucous carcinoma of the skin and mucosa. *J Am Acad Dermatol.* 1995;**32**(1):1–21.
46 Reizner GT, Chuang TY, Elpern DJ, Stone JL, Farmer ER. Bowen's disease (squamous cell carcinoma in situ) in Kauai, Hawaii. A population-based incidence report. *J Am Acad Dermatol.* 1994;**31**(4):596–600.
51 Lebwohl M. Actinic keratosis: epidemiology and progression to squamous cell carcinoma. *Br J Dermatol.* 2003;**149**(Suppl 66):31–33.
52 Maalej M, Frikha H, Kochbati L, et al. Radio-induced malignancies of the scalp about 98 patients with 150 lesions and literature review. *Cancer Radiother.* 2004;**8**(2):81–87.
62 De Graaf YG, Euvrard S, Bouwes Bavinck JN. Systemic and topical retinoids in the management of skin cancer in organ transplant recipients. *Dermatol Surg.* 2004;**30**(4 Pt 2):656–661.
63 Cherpelis BS, Marcusen C, Lang PG. Prognostic factors for metastasis in squamous cell carcinoma of the skin. *Dermatol Surg.* 2002;**28**(3):268–273.
68 Hoy WE. Nonmelanoma skin carcinoma in Albuquerque, New Mexico: experience of a major health care provider. *Cancer.* 1996;**77**(12):2489–2495.
70 Kricker A, Armstrong BK, English DR. Sun exposure and non-melanocytic skin cancer. *Cancer Causes Control.* 1994;**5**(4):367–392.
72 Johnson RL, Rothman AL, Xie J, et al. Human homolog of patched, a candidate gene for the basal cell nevus syndrome. *Science.* 1996;**272**(5268):1668–1671.
73 Lam CW, Xie J, To KF, et al. A frequent activated smoothened mutation in sporadic basal cell carcinomas. *Oncogene.* 1999;**18**(3):833–836.
81 Newman MD, Weinberg JM. Topical therapy in the treatment of actinic keratosis and basal cell carcinoma. *Cutis.* 2007;**79**(4 Suppl):18–28.
88 Heath M, Jaimes N, Lemos B, et al. Clinical characteristics of Merkel cell carcinoma at diagnosis in 195 patients: the AEIOU features. *J Am Acad Dermatol.* 2008;**58**(3):375–381.
90 Feng H, Shuda M, Chang Y, Moore PS. Clonal integration of a polyomavirus in human Merkel cell carcinoma. *Science.* 2008;**319**(5866):1096–1100.
91 Allen PJ, Zhang ZF, Coit DG. Surgical management of Merkel cell carcinoma. *Ann Surg.* 1999;**229**(1):97–105.
92 O'Connor WJ, Roenigk RK, Brodland DG. Merkel cell carcinoma. Comparison of Mohs micrographic surgery and wide excision in eighty-six patients. *Dermatol Surg.* 1997;**23**(10):929–933.
93 Messina JL, Reintgen DS, Cruse CW, et al. Selective lymphadenectomy in patients with Merkel cell (cutaneous neuroendocrine) carcinoma. *Ann Surg Oncol.* 1997;**4**(5):389–395.
95 Skelton HG, Smith KJ, Hitchcock CL, McCarthy WF, Lupton GP, Graham JH. Merkel cell carcinoma: analysis of clinical, histologic, and immunohistologic features of 132 cases with relation to survival. *J Am Acad Dermatol.* 1997;**37**(5 Pt 1):734–739.
97 Wang J, Hisaoka M, Shimajiri S, Morimitsu Y, Hashimoto H. Detection of COL1A1-PDGFB fusion transcripts in dermatofibrosarcoma protuberans by reverse transcription-polymerase chain reaction using archival formalin-fixed, paraffin-embedded tissues. *Diagn Mol Pathol.* 1999;**8**(3):113–119.
98 Parker TL, Zitelli JA. Surgical margins for excision of dermatofibrosarcoma protuberans. *J Am Acad Dermatol.* 1995;**32**(2 Pt 1):233–236.
99 Maki RG, Awan RA, Dixon RH, Jhanwar S, Antonescu CR. Differential sensitivity to imatinib of 2 patients with metastatic sarcoma arising from dermatofibrosarcoma protuberans. *Int J Cancer.* 2002;**100**(6):623–626.
100 Snow SN, Gordon EM, Larson PO, Bagheri MM, Bentz ML, Sable DB. Dermatofibrosarcoma protuberans: a report on 29 patients treated by Mohs micrographic surgery with long-term follow-up and review of the literature. *Cancer.* 2004;**101**(1):28–38.
102 Sasaki R, Soejima T, Kishi K, et al. Angiosarcoma treated with radiotherapy: impact of tumor type and size on outcome. *Int J Radiat Oncol Biol Phys.* 2002;**52**(4):1032–1040.
103 Ulrich L, Krause M, Brachmann A, Franke I, Gollnick H. Successful treatment of angiosarcoma of the scalp by intralesional cytokine therapy and surface irradiation. *J Eur Acad Dermatol Venereol.* 2000;**14**(5):412–415.

104 Wollina U, Füller J, Graefe T, Kaatz M, Lopatta E. Angiosarcoma of the scalp: treatment with liposomal doxorubicin and radiotherapy. *J Cancer Res Clin Oncol.* 2001;**127**(**6**):396–399.

107 Spencer JM, Nossa R, Tse DT, Sequeira M. Sebaceous carcinoma of the eyelid treated with Mohs micrographic surgery. *J Am Acad Dermatol.* 2001;**44**(**6**):1004–1009.

109 Gustafson S, Zbuk KM, Scacheri C, Eng C. Cowden syndrome. *Semin Oncol.* 2007;**34**(**5**):428–434.

110 Liaw D, Marsh DJ, Li J, et al. Germline mutations of the PTEN gene in Cowden disease, an inherited breast and thyroid cancer syndrome. *Nat Genet.* 1997;**16**(**1**):64–67.

111 Pettey AA, Walsh JS. Muir-Torre syndrome: a case report and review of the literature. *Cutis.* 2005;**75**(**3**):149–155.

115 Santoro M, Carlomagno F, Romano A, et al. Activation of RET as a dominant transforming gene by germline mutations of MEN2A and MEN2B. *Science.* 1995;**267**(**5196**):381–383.

116 Sanso GE, Domene HM, Garcia R, Pusiol E. de M, Roque M, et al. Very early detection of RET proto-oncogene mutation is crucial for preventive thyroidectomy in multiple endocrine neoplasia type 2 children: presence of C-cell malignant disease in asymptomatic carriers. *Cancer.* 2002;**94**(**2**):323–330.

111 Bone tumors

Timothy A. Damron, MD, FACS

Overview

Bone tumors are uncommon lesions that affect all ages of patients and may involve any bone in the body. Bone lesions may be benign neoplasms or reactive lesions, primary bone sarcomas, metastatic carcinomas to bone, myeloma, or lymphoma. The benign bone lesions, which predominate in children and young adults, may behave in an inactive, active, or aggressive fashion, and the latter may simulate malignancy. Primary bone sarcomas have a bimodal distribution, whereas metastatic disease, myeloma, and lymphoma of bone predominate in adults. Despite the broad spectrum of bone tumors, each individual entity has a distinct clinical and radiographic presentation, with a predilection for specific locations, which lends itself to narrowing the differential diagnosis and selecting appropriate management.

Bone sarcomas account for less than 0.2% of all cancers. During 2014, approximately 3020 new cases of primary bone sarcomas were diagnosed, and approximately 1460 deaths occurred. The three most common bone sarcomas are osteosarcoma, chondrosarcoma, and Ewing sarcoma. However, the most common primary malignancy of bone is myeloma, and the most common cancer that involves bone is metastatic carcinoma.

The pathologic classification of bone tumors continues to evolve. To a large extent, classification continues to be according to the cell of origin or tissue type. Primary bone tumors may derive from cartilage cells, bone cells, and vascular cells, among others, but for some tumors, the cell of origin is unknown. The most widely accepted pathologic classification system to date is that of the World Health Organization.

Introduction

As a group, bone tumors are uncommon lesions arising from a wide array of cells, affecting all ages of patients, and involving any bone in the body. They include benign lesions, primary bone sarcomas, metastatic carcinomas to bone, myeloma, and lymphoma. The benign bone lesions may behave in an inactive, active, or aggressive fashion. Despite the broad spectrum of bone tumors, each individual entity has a distinct clinical and radiographic presentation, with a predilection for specific locations, which lends itself to narrowing the differential diagnosis and selecting appropriate management.

Bone sarcomas account for less than 0.2% of all cancers.[1] During 2014, approximately 3020 new cases of primary bone sarcomas were diagnosed, and approximately 1460 deaths occurred. The three most common bone sarcomas are osteosarcoma (45%), chondrosarcoma (36%), and Ewing sarcoma (18%).[2] However, the most common primary malignancy of bone is myeloma, and the most common cancer that involves bone is metastatic carcinoma. Malignancies of bone as a group are only the tip of the iceberg, as the vast majority of bone lesions are benign.

The pathologic classification of bone tumors continues to evolve. To a large extent, classification continues to be according to the cell of origin or tissue type. Primary bone tumors may derive from cartilage cells such as chondrocytes (enchondromas, periosteal chondromas, chondroblastomas, chondromyxoid fibromas, chondrosarcomas), bone cells such as osteoblasts and osteocytes (osteoma, osteoid osteoma, osteoblastoma, osteosarcoma), and vascular cells (hemangioma and angiosarcoma), among others, but for some tumors, the cell of origin is unknown. The most widely accepted pathologic classification system to date is that of the World Health Organization (WHO), and their terminology is used to a large degree in this chapter, although some tumors, such as benign fibrous tumors, are grouped differently.[3] The WHO classification of bone tumors has been updated since the last publication of this text (Table 1).

The introductory sections of this chapter deal with the pretreatment phase (evaluation, staging, and biopsy), the middle sections with surgical treatment (surgical margins through reconstructive options), radiation therapy, and medical management, and the final sections with the specific benign and malignant bone tumors as well as congenital syndromes related to bone tumors.

Evaluation

Crucial information about bone lesions is derived from the history, physical examination, and radiographic features. The goal of evaluation of any bone lesion is to arrive at a narrow differential diagnosis which will guide subsequent action. In some cases, a specific diagnosis may be determined, and, depending upon the diagnosis, the action may include observation (e.g., nonossifying fibroma, enchondroma), biopsy confirmation (e.g., aneurysmal bone cyst (ABC), chondroblastoma, giant cell tumor, osteosarcoma), irrigation/debridement (e.g., osteomyelitis), aspiration/injection (e.g., unicameral bone cyst), radiofrequency ablation (RFA) (e.g., osteoid osteoma), excision (e.g., osteochondroma), or prophylactic stabilization (e.g., established metastatic carcinoma, myeloma). In other cases, the lesion may only be categorized according to a general category of biologic behavior: latent, active, or aggressive. Latent bone tumors may be observed. Active lesions often require biopsy and curettage with or without grafting. Aggressive bone tumors almost always require biopsy confirmation prior to treatment and include both benign aggressive lesions (e.g., ABC, chondroblastoma, and giant cell tumor of bone) and malignancies (e.g., primary bone sarcomas, metastatic carcinoma, myeloma, lymphoma).

Important historical features are the patient's age and the means by which the lesion was discovered. Age divisions are particularly helpful when the patient is less than 5 years old, where metastatic neuroblastoma has its peak occurrence and sarcomas are rare, and when the patient is older than 40, where the differential diagnosis, in order of decreasing frequency, includes metastatic carcinoma, myeloma, lymphoma, and primary bone sarcomas such

Holland-Frei Cancer Medicine, Ninth Edition. Edited by Robert C. Bast Jr., Carlo M. Croce, William N. Hait, Waun Ki Hong, Donald W. Kufe, Martine Piccart-Gebhart, Raphael E. Pollock, Ralph R. Weichselbaum, Hongyang Wang, and James F. Holland.
© 2017 John Wiley & Sons, Inc. ISBN: 978-1-118-93469-2

Table 1 Classification of bone tumors by 4th edition of WHO classification on bone and soft-tissue tumors.[3]

Chondrogenic tumors
Osteochondroma
Chondromas: enchondroma, periosteal chondroma
Chondromyxoid fibroma
Osteochondromyxoma
Subungual exostosis and bizarre parosteal osteochondromatous proliferation
Synovial chondromatosis
Chondroblastoma
Chondrosarcoma (grades I–III) including primary and secondary variants and
    periosteal chondrosarcoma
Dedifferentiated chondrosarcoma
Mesenchymal chondrosarcoma
Clear cell chondrosarcoma
Osteogenic tumors
Osteoma
Osteoid osteoma
Osteoblastoma
Low-grade central osteosarcoma
Conventional osteosarcoma
Telangiectatic osteosarcoma
Small cell osteosarcoma
Parosteal osteosarcoma
Periosteal osteosarcoma
High-grade surface osteosarcoma
Fibrogenic tumors
Desmoplastic fibroma of bone
Fibrosarcoma of bone
Fibrohistiocytic tumors
Nonossifying fibroma and benign fibrous histiocytoma of bone
Ewing sarcoma
Hematopoietic neoplasms
Plasma cell myeloma
Solitary plasmacytoma of bone
Primary non-Hodgkin lymphoma of bone
Osteoclastic giant cell-rich tumors
Giant cell lesion of the small bones
Giant cell tumor of bone
Notochordal tumors
Benign notochordal cell tumor
Chordoma
Vascular tumors
Hemangioma
Epithelioid hemangioma
Epithelioid hemangioendothelioma
Angiosarcoma
Myogenic, lipogenic, and epithelial tumors
Leiomyosarcoma
Lipoma
Liposarcoma
Adamantinoma
Tumors of undefined neoplastic nature
Aneurysmal bone cyst
Simple bone cyst
Fibrous dysplasia
Osteofibrous dysplasia
Langerhans cell histiocytosis
Erdheim–Chester disease
Chondromesenchymal hamartoma
Rosai–Dorfman disease

category is the painful bone lesion, and this includes a wide variety of active and aggressive bone lesions. Pathologic fractures may be divided into those preceded by pain, which are usually associated with active or aggressive bone tumors, and those not preceded by pain, which are more commonly latent lesions. Pathologic fractures preceded by pain should usually be biopsied, whereas those not preceded by pain may often be observed at least until the fracture heals, although exceptions exist.

Plain radiographs are standard for the radiologic evaluation of any bone tumor. These should be evaluated for location (epiphyseal, metaphyseal, diaphyseal, surface, or intracortical), lesional border characteristics (type 1 (geographic), type 2 (moth eaten), or type 3 (permeative)), bone response to the lesion (periosteal reaction), and matrix mineralization pattern (cartilaginous, osseous, ground glass) when present (Table 2). Classification of the type 1 border can be broken down into three specific subtypes.[5] Type 1A is characterized by a thick, sclerotic margin and usually represents a benign lesion. Type 1B is still well defined but lacks the thick, sclerotic margin, as these lesions potentially have a slightly faster growth pattern and in unusual cases may actually represent low-grade malignancies. Type 1C begins to blend with the moth-eaten pattern, representing a more aggressive pattern, including cortical destruction. Type 1C is characteristic of giant cell tumor of bone or lymphoma.[6] Hyaline cartilage tumors are one exception to the general rule that benign lesions usually have a sclerotic rim, as most benign enchondromas lack a 1A border. Putting these radiographic features together with the clinical features will often yield a narrow differential diagnosis.

Bone scans help to determine whether the lesion shows uptake of the Tc[99] radionuclide, indicating an active or aggressive lesion, and whether the lesion is solitary or only one of numerous lesions. Myeloma deposits in bone serve as an exception to the rule, often being cold on bone scan. Some aggressive lesions, such as renal carcinoma metastases, may not be hot on bone scan if tumor destruction outpaces the bone's ability to form bone in response.

Positron emission tomography (PET) has come to play an increasing role in evaluation and staging of bone lesions.[6] On average, PET avidity is greater for malignant bone tumors than for benign bone tumors. However, 18F-FDG PET avidity has been shown to be nonspecific for malignancy, and many benign tumors, ranging from nonossifying fibroma to osteoid osteomas, also show this finding, albeit with greater variability. PET scans have come to play an increasing role in staging for malignant bone tumors, but they are less sensitive than routine chest computerized tomography (CT) for pulmonary metastases.[6]

Magnetic resonance imaging (MRI) of bone tumors is indicated when the diagnosis is not evident from the plain radiographs and for determining the local extent of bone sarcomas. Specific bone tumors that may be confirmed with MRI include simple bone cysts (rim enhancement of a fluid-filled lesion) and ABCs (septations separating multiple loculated areas filled with blood, as indicated by fluid-fluid levels). Perilesional edema is common surrounding bone sarcomas but may also be seen in certain benign conditions, including osteomyelitis, osteoid osteoma, chondroblastoma, Langerhans cell histiocytosis (LCH), and chondromyxoid fibroma. CT is indicated to find the radiolucent nidus of an osteoid osteoma within the surrounding reactive bone, to assess for endosteal scalloping in a cartilage tumor to distinguish enchondroma from chondrosarcoma, to find the pattern of lesional mineralization when it is unclear, and to supplement MRI in difficult anatomic locations such as the sacrum, pelvis, and scapula.

as chondrosarcoma, secondary osteosarcoma, malignant fibrous histiocytoma of bone, and fibrosarcoma.

The means of discovery of a bone lesion is variable. Bone lesions discovered incidentally during evaluation for other reasons are usually latent lesions that require nothing further than observation. In adult patients, the most common lesion discovered incidentally is an enchondroma; in pediatric patients, it is a nonossifying fibroma. Painless bony masses are usually osteochondromas, but other surface bone lesions may present in this fashion. The broadest

Table 2 Classic examples of bone tumors fitting specific patterns of lesional borders, bone response, and lesional matrix on plain radiographs.

Radiographic category	Type	Classic examples[a]		
Lesional border	Geographic (well defined)	1A	Nonossifying fibroma	
			Unicameral bone cyst	
		1B	Aneurysmal bone cyst	
			Chondroblastoma	
		1C	Giant cell tumor	
			Lymphoma	
	Moth eaten (blurred)	Metastatic carcinoma		
		Myeloma		
		Lymphoma		
		Osteomyelitis		
	Permeative (poorly defined)	Osteosarcoma		
		Ewing sarcoma		
		Metastatic carcinoma		
		Lymphoma		
Bone response	Marginal sclerosis	Nonossifying fibroma		
		Fibrous dysplasia		
	Cortical thickening	Osteoid osteoma		
		Osteomyelitis		
	Laminar periosteal response	Stress fracture		
	Endosteal expansion and scalloping	Low- to intermediate-grade chondrosarcoma		
	Periosteal rimming	Aneurysmal bone cyst		
		Giant cell tumor of bone		
	Codman's triangle Cumulus cloud reaction	Osteosarcoma		
	Onion-skinning periosteal response	Ewing sarcoma		
Lesional matrix	Punctate rings and arcs	Hyaline cartilage tumors (enchondromas/chondrosarcomas)		
	Ground-glass appearance	Fibrous dysplasia		
	Osteoblastic	Osteoid osteoma		
		Osteoblastoma		
		Osteosarcoma		
		Metastatic carcinoma (prostate, breast)		
		Lymphoma		

[a]None of the radiographic findings here are specific, and there is considerable overlap; hence, those lesions listed may be considered classic but by no means the only ones that may present with such findings.
Source: Damron 2008.[4] Reproduced with permission of Wolters Kluwer Health.

Staging

Staging of bone sarcomas requires assessment of both the primary site and distant disease. For assessment of the primary site, radiographs and MRI of the entire involved bone should be obtained in order to check for other "skip" lesions. The two most common sites of metastases from bone sarcomas are lung followed by bone. Hence, the most crucial staging studies to obtain are chest radiograph and CT to evaluate the lungs as well as a total body bone scan or PET scan to evaluate the rest of the skeleton.

Traditionally, the staging system most commonly used for musculoskeletal sarcomas was that originally described by Doctor William Enneking and adopted by the Musculoskeletal Tumor Society (MSTS) (Table 3). Variables incorporated into the MSTS staging system include the presence or absence of metastases, grade (high or low), and local extent of the tumor (intraosseous or with extension into the soft tissues). The typical chondrosarcoma is low grade and intracompartmental (confined to the bone), so it is usually stage IA. The conventional high-grade osteosarcoma usually extends into the soft tissue, and since 80% without evidence of distant metastases, the typical stage is IIB. Evidence of metastases equates to a stage III in this system.

The current most widely accepted staging system for bone sarcomas is that of the American Joint Committee on Cancer (AJCC)[8] (Table 4). This system has more well-documented prognostic significance (Figure 1). Variables incorporated into the AJCC system include presence or absence of metastases (with multiple/discontinuous bone tumors separated from distant metastases), grade (grade 1 or 2 vs. grade 3 or 4), and size (8 cm or smaller vs. larger than 8 cm). This system is similar to the MSTS system in

Table 3 Musculoskeletal Tumor Society staging system.

Stage	Grade	Local extent	Metastases
I	Low	A – intracompartmental	None
		B – extracompartmental	
II	High	A – intracompartmental	
		B – extracompartmental	
III	Any	Any	Present

Source: Enneking 1980.[7] Reproduced with permission from the Association of Bone and Joint Surgeons.

separating stage I from II based on grade, but the A–B designation is based upon size here. For osteosarcoma and Ewing sarcoma, stage IIB patients have higher rates of metastases than stage IIA patients. Patients with "skip lesions" (discontinuous lesions in the same bone) are designated as stage III. Distant metastases in this system are stage IV, but since metastases to sites other than the lung (such as bone) carry a worse prognosis than lung metastases patients alone, a separate designation is reserved for those two groups (IVA and IVB). Hence, for a less than 8 cm low-grade chondrosarcoma, the typical staging would be stage IA. For a larger than 8 cm high-grade osteosarcoma without skip lesions or metastases, the typical staging is stage IIB. There were no changes in the AJCC staging between the 2002 and 2012 versions.[10]

Biopsy

Biopsy of bone tumors is indicated when a specific benign diagnosis cannot be determined based by radiographic evaluation

Table 4 American Joint Committee on Cancer staging system for bone sarcomas.

Primary tumor [T]	
TX	Primary tumor cannot be assessed
T0	No evidence of primary tumor
T1	Tumor 8 cm or less in greatest dimension
T2	Tumor more than 8 cm in greatest dimension
T3	Discontinuous tumors in the primary bone site
Regional lymph nodes [N]	
NX[a]	Regional lymph nodes cannot be assessed
N0	No regional lymph node metastasis
N1	Regional lymph node metastasis
Distant metastasis [M]	
MX	Distant metastasis cannot be assessed
M0	No distant metastasis
M1	Distant metastasis
M1a	Lung
M1b	Other distant sites
Histologic grade [G]	
GX	Grade cannot be assessed
G1	Well differentiated—low grade
G2	Moderately differentiated—low grade
G3	Poorly differentiated—high grade
G4	Undifferentiated—high grade

Stage	Tumor [T]	Node [N]	Metastasis [M]	Grade [G]
Stage IA	T1	N0	M0	G1, 2 low grade
Stage IB	T2	N0	M0	G1, 2 low grade
Stage IIA	T1	N0	M0	G3, 4 high grade
Stage IIB	T2	N0	M0	G3, 4 high grade
Stage III	T3	N0	M0	Any G
Stage IVA	Any T	N0	M1a	Any G
Stage IVB	Any T	N1	Any M	Any G
	Any T	Any N	M1b	Any G

[a]Because of the rarity of lymph node involvement in sarcomas, the designation NX may not be appropriate and could be considered N0 if no clinical involvement is evident. Ewing sarcoma is classified as G4.

Source: Edge 2010.[9] Reproduced with permission from Springer.

alone. When the clinicoradiographic diagnosis of a latent lesion such as nonossifying fibroma, unicameral bone cyst, or enchondroma can be made, biopsy is generally unnecessary. Some active lesions, such as fibrous dysplasia, intraosseous lipoma, and osteochondroma do not always require biopsy if the diagnosis can be established radiographically. For most other active and all aggressive lesions, biopsy should be done to determine or confirm the diagnosis. Suspected high-grade sarcomas should be biopsied prior to initiating treatment neoadjuvant.

Careful consideration must be given when metastases are suspected, because the treatment of metastatic carcinoma to bone differs dramatically from that of a primary bone tumor. Hence, even for patients with a history of a known carcinoma with predilection to bone (breast, prostate, lung, renal, thyroid), the first bone metastases should generally be established by biopsy unless the clinical situation represents a terminal state (known wide metastases to other sites). When dealing with suspected metastatic disease requiring a biopsy, reamings are not the best way to submit a biopsy specimen, because once the intramedullary canal to and through the lesion has been breached, all associated bone and soft tissue has been potentially contaminated with tumor. If the pathology shows sarcoma, rather than metastatic disease, unnecessary contamination of previously uninvolved tissue will have already occurred.

There are four general biopsy techniques applicable to bone tumors: (1) fine needle biopsy, (2) core needle biopsy, (3) incisional open biopsy, and (4) excisional biopsy. Fine needle aspiration (FNA) biopsy provides only cells for cytology and is usually done by interventional radiologists. An FNA is useful in two general clinical situations where bone tumors are involved: (1) when the diagnosis of a bone lesion is strongly suspected (metastatic carcinoma, recurrent sarcoma) and (2) for difficult-to-access lesions (spine, pelvis, scapula). Core needle biopsies allow for interpretation of the tissue architecture in addition to the cytological detail. For bone lesions, core biopsies may be done in the same situations as FNA and for bone lesions with soft-tissue extension. Incisional open biopsy is the workhorse biopsy tool for bone lesions, as it provides adequate tissue for histological interpretation. However, there are numerous pitfalls to open biopsy which must be considered, and for most incisional biopsies, the surgeon who will be doing the definitive surgery, no matter what the final diagnosis, is the person who should do the biopsy.[11,12] Excisional biopsy is usually only used for bone tumors such as osteochondromas, where the radiographic features establish the diagnosis, the morbidity of excision is small, and the surface location of the lesion lends itself to excision.

Surgical margins

Surgical margins depend upon the type of excision done, and the appropriate type of excision varies according to bone tumor type. There are four types of excisions: (1) intralesional, (2) marginal, (3) wide, and (4) radical.[13] For most benign bone lesions, an intralesional excision by way of a curettage is appropriate. When necessary, metastatic bone lesions undergoing surgery for stabilization may be

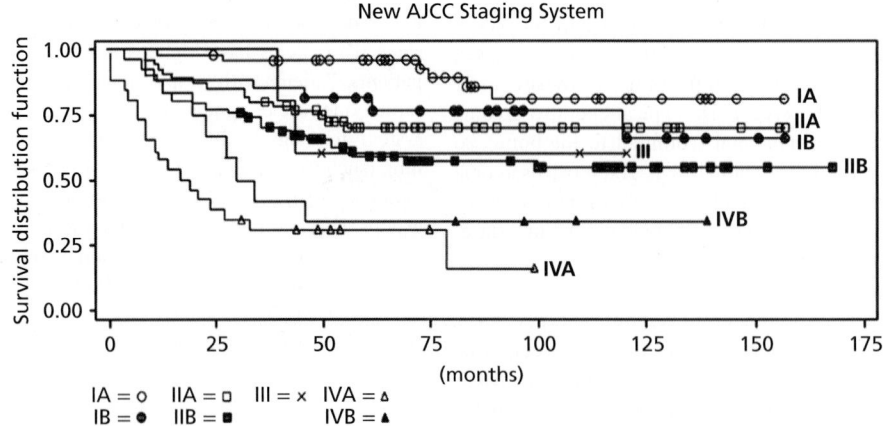

New AJCC Staging System

IA = o   IIA = □   III = x   IVA = △
IB = ●   IIB = ■   IVB = ▲

Figure 1 Survival according to staging by the new American Joint Committee on Cancer staging system for bone sarcomas. Source: ACS 2014.[1] Reproduced with permission of The American Cancer Society.

treated by curettage. For aggressive benign lesions (ABC, chondroblastoma, and giant cell tumor), an extended intralesional curettage is indicated. This differs from a simple curettage in that it utilizes mechanical (high-speed burr, pulsatile lavage) and adjunctive (phenol, laser, liquid nitrogen, argon beam coagulation) techniques to extend the margin into normal bone. Recent trends suggest that most extremity low-grade chondrosarcomas may also be treated in this way. Marginal en bloc excision (through the pseudocapsule surrounding the tumor) is appropriate for osteochondromas, but wide resection (excision with a cuff of normal tissue) is indicated for most bone sarcomas.

Limb salvage versus amputation

Two issues must be considered in making the decision regarding limb salvage versus amputation: oncologic safety and function. First and foremost, in order for a patient to be a candidate for limb salvage, the oncologic procedure should not lower the expected survival beyond that which could be achieved with an amputation. This question has been addressed prospectively, and—in properly selected patients—survival is no less with limb-sparing surgery when compared to amputation.[14,15] However, this decision still needs to be made carefully for each patient. Oncologic safety considers two variables: response to chemotherapy (when applicable) and surgical margin. The poorer the response to chemotherapy, the greater the likelihood of local recurrence for any given margin achieved intraoperatively. Hence, for a poor response to chemotherapy (tumor progression), limb salvage surgery is a relatively strong contraindication. A wide surgical margin is the goal of bone sarcoma surgery, and it can almost always be achieved with the appropriately planned level of amputation but not always with limb-sparing surgery. If vital structures (major vessels and nerves) are encased by the soft-tissue extent of the sarcoma, necessitating their resection along with the tumor, limb salvage is contraindicated and amputation is preferable.

As with oncologic safety, if limb salvage is to be done, the expected function of the planned reconstruction should be at least equivalent to that of a comparable level amputation. In the lower extremity, function with a below-knee amputation is generally thought to be better than a distal tibial reconstruction, so a distal tibial location is a relative indication for amputation. In the upper extremity, it is preferable to be able to preserve 2 of the 3 major nerves (radial, ulnar, median) for limb salvage. Tumor encasement of more than one major upper extremity nerve and/or the axillary or brachial vessels is an indication for amputation.

Operative management of metastatic carcinoma, myeloma, and lymphoma

There are four settings that potentially require operative management for patients with bone lesions from metastatic carcinoma, myeloma, and lymphoma: (1) biopsy to establish diagnosis, (2) prophylactic stabilization of impending pathologic fracture, (3) operative fixation of pathologic fracture, and (4) en bloc resection of isolated lesions. Biopsy issues have been previously discussed but cannot be emphasized enough: the diagnosis should be established before embarking upon an operative treatment plan. Prediction of impending fracture risk is evolving. Currently, fractures are predicted based upon clinical and radiographic criteria. A rating system devised by Mirels has been devised based upon four variables[16] (Tables 5 and 6). The Mirels system is valid across experience

Table 5 Mirels scoring system for predicting risk of pathologic fracture in metastatic disease.

	One point	Two points	Three points
Site	Upper extremity	Lower extremity	Peritrochanteric
Size	<1/3	1/3–2/3	>2/3
Nature	Blastic	Mixed	Lytic
Pain	Mild	Moderate	Functional

Source: Mirels 1989.[16] Reproduced with permission from Wiley.

Table 6 Mirels definitions, fracture risk, and treatment recommendations based upon point totals.

Definition	Points	Fracture risk (%)	Recommendation
Nonimpending	≤7	<10	Observe
Borderline	8	15	Consider fixation
Impending fracture	9	33	Prophylactic fixation
Impending fracture	≥10	>50	Prophylactic fixation

Source: Mirels 1989.[16] Reproduced with permission from Wiley.

levels, but it still has a low specificity of approximately 33%.[17] Evaluation of CT-based biomechanical analyses for this purpose are under study.[18]

When pathologic fractures occur in the setting of disseminated malignancies, they usually warrant operative fixation in order to improve function since these patients have limited life expectancy. Exceptions include moribund immediately preterminal patients, those who cannot tolerate operative intervention, and fractures that are usually managed by nonoperative means. In order for the patient to benefit from the procedure, life expectancy should be longer than the expected time required to recover from any proposed procedure.

The principles of operative fixation for fractures in this clinical situation differ from those of standard fracture fixation. Since later lesions may develop elsewhere in the bone, intramedullary nail fixation, as opposed to plate/screw fixation, is preferred in the long bones in order to protect the remainder of the bone. Immediate stability is the goal in order to avoid prolonged recovery that diminishes patient function, so bone cement is much more commonly used to supplement fixation in this situation. Fracture healing in the setting of metastatic carcinoma and myeloma is notoriously slow, so the fixation should be planned assuming there will be no fracture healing. Postoperative radiotherapy has been shown to improve function and reduce reoperation rates.[19]

Reconstructive alternatives

Benign bone tumors

The defects created after curettage of benign bone tumors can be filled with autologous bone graft, allograft bone, synthetic filler material, or bone cement.[20] Bone cement is usually reserved for defects created after extended intralesional curettage of giant cell tumors of bone. Bone cement provides immediate stability that allows full weight bearing, solidifies with an exothermic reaction that extends the margin, and provides a clear radiographic border to facilitate diagnosis of local recurrence. In cases where large lesions have been curetted, prophylactic stabilization with pins or plates/screws may be used to minimize the chance of fracture.

Primary bone sarcomas

Following resection of bone sarcomas, numerous alternatives are available to reconstruct the large bone and associated soft-tissue deficits that result. Selection of the appropriate reconstruction in each instance requires consideration of the patient age and expectations, prognosis, adjuvant treatments, type of resection, and anatomic site. In general, reconstructive techniques include endoprostheses, structural allografts, allograft–prosthetic composites, and vascularized bone grafts. Over time, the use of endoprosthetic and allograft–prosthetic composite reconstructions following resections that include a joint has increased, while the indications for structural allografts have continued to decline. Apart from allograft–prosthetic composite reconstructions, the main role for structural allografts has been for intercalary reconstructions (when the joints above and below the diaphyseal segment can be preserved). The most frequent type of resection for sarcomas is intra-articular (removal of the bone up to and including the joint surface), requiring reconstruction of the joint surface, usually with a joint replacement. When the tumor invades the joint, an extra-articular resection (removal of both sides of the joint) is indicated, and this is often better reconstructed with a joint fusion using intervening allograft bone.

Patient age is a major consideration, since skeletally immature patients will develop limb length discrepancy unless the reconstruction accommodates the loss of growth on the operative side. For patients less than 8 years old, the potential limb length discrepancy is so profound that standard means of reconstruction is generally contraindicated. In these difficult situations, amputation, rotationplasty, and vascularized fibula grafting with open growth plates are viable alternatives.[21–27] Rotationplasty in the lower extremity after resection of a tumor around the knee involves fixing the foot and ankle in a position rotated 180 degrees from normal so that the heel points forward and the ankle is situated at the level of and functions as the patient's knee. In this situation, the patient is able to function as a below-knee amputee rather than having to settle for a higher above-knee amputation. In patients older than 8 years old, expandable endoprosthetic reconstructions are available.[28–32] In recent years, the availability of such growing prostheses with a noninvasive mechanism has increased their attraction.[31] However, the complication rates have proven to be high, and their durability once the patient reaches skeletal maturity has been less than optimal.[33]

Upper extremity

For reconstructions following bone sarcoma resection about the shoulder, function is most dependent on whether the deltoid muscle may be preserved during resection of the tumor.[34,35] If a tumor of the proximal humerus extends into the deltoid and the deltoid has to be removed to achieve a wide margin, function of the shoulder will be poor regardless of the reconstruction. When the deltoid can be preserved, consideration is often given to using an allograft–prosthetic composite reconstruction.[36] In this way, the patient's remaining rotator cuff tendons can be repaired to the allograft tendons, and there is potential for improved function. If an osteoarticular allograft reconstruction is chosen, there is an increased risk of nonunion of the allograft–host junction, fracture, and subchondral collapse. The scapula and all portions of the humerus may be reconstructed with an endoprosthesis. The distal upper extremity is an unusual site for bone sarcomas.

Lower extremity

Following limb-preserving bone sarcoma resection of the pelvis (internal hemipelvectomy), no reconstruction is needed when the hip joint is able to be preserved (e.g., anterior pubic/ischial rami and supra-acetabular iliac resections), and some surgeons do not reconstruct even following resection of the acetabular portion of the pelvis. The numerous reconstructive alternatives for the acetabulum and hip joint following internal hemipelvectomy are fraught with complications.[37,38] For the proximal femur, reconstruction is often done with either an endoprosthetic hemiarthroplasty (replacing the femoral head side but without a cup in the pelvis) or an allograft–prosthetic composite.[39–41] The latter reconstruction allows attachment of the patient's hip abductors to the allograft tendon, which may improve stability and gait.

Most reconstructions of the distal femur utilize a distal femoral replacement endoprosthetic total knee reconstruction. Because of the attachment of the extensor mechanism through the patellar tendon to the tibial tuberosity, resection of the proximal tibia necessitates consideration of extensor mechanism reconstruction. Here, the primary alternatives are endoprosthetic proximal tibial total knee reconstruction or allograft–prosthetic composite reconstruction. For both reconstructions, the medial head of the gastrocnemius muscle is often used both to cover the allograft and/or prosthesis and to reconstruct the extensor mechanism. With an allograft–prosthetic composite reconstruction of the proximal tibia, the patient's remaining patellar tendon may be sutured to the allograft tendon, further augmenting the extensor mechanism reconstruction.

Complications

Complications after resections and reconstructions for bone sarcomas are numerous and frequent. Infection is a concern with all reconstructions, particularly considering the large dead space created following these procedures, the prolonged wound healing while receiving adjuvant treatments, and the prevalence of chemotherapy-induced neutropenia. However, certain complications are associated with specific anatomic sites and types of reconstructions. The proximal tibia is an anatomic site particularly prone to infection and wound breakdown given the paucity of soft-tissue coverage. For endoprosthetic reconstructions of the shoulder and hip, joint instability and frank dislocation are relatively common complications. All endoprosthetic reconstructions are prone to loosening, but prosthetic survival is acceptable (proximal femur (90%), distal femur (60%), proximal tibia (50%)).[42] Exciting new developments in alternative compliant means of fixation other than those commonly used with joint arthroplasties have been reported and warrant continued close follow-up.[43] Reports of their use around the knee show 80% 10-year survivorship.[44] Allografts, particularly when used alone, are prone to nonunion at the allograft–host junction and to fracture.

Radiotherapy for bone tumors

Radiotherapy plays a limited role in the treatment of primary tumors of bone, but it is a mainstay of local treatment for bone lesions resulting from metastatic carcinoma, myeloma, and lymphoma. Radiotherapy should generally be avoided in the treatment of benign bone tumors, but low-dose radiotherapy has been advocated in recalcitrant symptomatic spine cases of LCH.[45] For bone sarcomas, radiotherapy may be considered for the treatment of Ewing sarcoma, but it is not part of standard treatment for osteosarcoma or chondrosarcoma.

Potential complications of bone irradiation include postradiation sarcoma, spontaneous and fragility fracture, osteonecrosis, and—in pediatric patients—growth arrest or angular deformities. Postradiation sarcomas typically occur at a minimum of 3 years following the radiation exposure and after mean doses of 50 Gy.[46]

Risk factors for postradiation fracture include periosteal stripping, neoadjuvant chemotherapy, femoral location, higher-dose irradiation, and circumferential irradiation.[47] Postradiation fractures are gaining increasing attention because of their difficulty in management, prolonged healing times and high nonunion rates (45–67%), and the frequent need for surgical treatment, multiple operations, radical bone resection/reconstruction, and/or amputation.[47]

Medical management of bone tumors

The roles for medical management of bone tumors continue to expand. As a rule, high-grade bone sarcomas warrant chemotherapy to address systemic microscopic disease. Chemotherapy for bone sarcomas is usually initiated prior to (neoadjuvant chemotherapy) and completed after local surgical or radiation treatment. Hence, the treatment of both conventional high-grade osteosarcoma and Ewing sarcoma begins with neoadjuvant chemotherapy. There is no established role for chemotherapy in the treatment of low-grade chondrosarcoma.

Use of bisphosphonates to inhibit osteoclast-mediated bone destruction has become standard of care for myeloma and many metastatic carcinomas, including breast, prostate, and lung.[48] Recently, bisphosphonate drugs have also been used off-label for specific benign bone lesions, including fibrous dysplasia and giant cell tumor, but their efficacy has not been established. Of concern, however, is the risk of bisphosphonate-related osteonecrosis of the jaw and atypical subtrochanteric proximal femur fractures.[48,49]

Specific benign bone tumors

Cartilage tumors

Cartilage tumors can be divided into those that derive from mature hyaline cartilage (chondromas and osteochondromas) versus those that derive from immature cartilage (chondroblastoma and chondromyxoid fibroma).

Chondromas

The WHO classification lists enchondromas and periosteal chondromas under the general heading of "Chondromas."[3] Enchondromas are the intramedullary variety of these benign hyaline cartilage tumors, and periosteal chondromas are the variety that

reside on the bone surface. Enchondromatosis (multiple enchondromas/Ollier's disease and Maffucci's syndrome) is discussed under the section titled "Congenital syndromes." The latter represents multiple enchondromas combined with hemangiomas.

Enchondromas are relatively common among primary bone tumors, representing up to 17% overall. They likely represent residual rests of hyaline growth plate cartilage left behind during skeletal immaturity. Most of these lesions are asymptomatic and incidentally noted on imaging studies done for other causes of pain.[50] Enchondromas represent the most common bone lesion seen in the small bones of the hands and feet. In the long bones, they are most commonly located in the femur (where they are frequently picked up on X-rays of patients with hip or knee pain) and the humerus (where they are picked up during radiologic evaluation of patients with common causes of shoulder pain). Solitary enchondromas of the flat bones are rare, and the possibility of chondrosarcoma needs to be considered when a cartilage lesion occurs there. Because the radiographic characteristics of hyaline cartilage are fairly typical, the primary challenge is distinguishing enchondromas from chondrosarcomas.

The natural history of enchondromas is that they become more calcified over time. Hence, mature lesions in adults almost always display a characteristic punctate pattern of calcified arcs and rings which is so distinctive as to often allow the diagnosis to be confirmed radiographically without biopsy (Figure 2). They can be associated with some endosteal scalloping. However, when they have periosteal reaction, expansion of the surrounding bone, more extensive cortical destruction, or soft-tissue extension, they have to be considered chondrosarcomas. MRI characteristics of enchondromas are a lobular pattern of organization which is dark on T1-weighted (T1W) images and bright on T2-weighted (T2W) images. Increased uptake on bone scan is typical of enchondromas and should not be considered to be a sign of malignancy; it is likely due to ongoing remodeling of the surrounding bone.

Under the microscope, enchondromas are comprised of benign, sparsely cellular hyaline cartilage, but the degree of cellularity and atypia is variable. In certain locations, such as the fingers and other small bones, the histologic features often appear more aggressive despite their benign behavior.

The vast majority of enchondromas, especially when they present as asymptomatic lesions with typical radiological findings, can simply be observed to ensure that they do not progress. However, when either the radiographic features or associated pain cast doubt on the

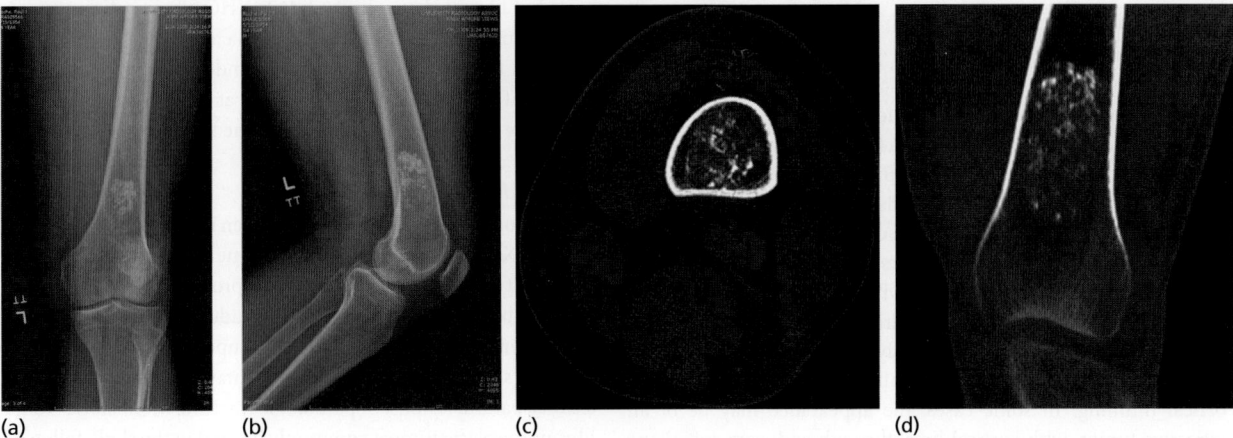

(a)   (b)   (c)   (d)

Figure 2 Enchondroma. Anteroposterior (a) and lateral (b) distal femur radiographs as well as axial (c) and coronal (d) CT scans show the characteristic punctate arcs and rings of hyaline cartilage without prominent endosteal scalloping or cortical destruction to suggest features of chondrosarcoma.

diagnosis, the lesion may require a complete curettage and complete histological review to differentiate from chondrosarcoma. Cartilage lesions rarely recur after curettage.

Periosteal chondromas, by contrast, are distinctly unusual benign hyaline cartilage lesions. They more commonly present as a bump on a digit or as a low-grade painful lesion elsewhere. Radiographically, they usually show a typical "saucerization" of the underlying cortex of this surface lesion. They need to be distinguished from periosteal chondrosarcoma. Smaller lesions (less than 7 cm) are usually chondromas. Depending upon the location, periosteal chondromas may be removed by curettage or en bloc excision.

Chondroblastoma

This immature cartilage-derived tumor is an uncommon benign process that typically presents with joint pain, is difficult to diagnosis, and occurs in the epiphysis of the long bones.[51] The vast majority of cases occur in skeletally immature patients, and their presentation with joint pain (due to their location at the end of long bones), mimicking symptoms of far more common processes, and their initially subtle radiographic findings may lead to a prolonged course prior to diagnosis. Although they may occur in numerous bones, their most common locations are the proximal humerus, distal femur, and proximal tibia.

Radiograph appearance can be subtle, since its immature cartilage usually does not cause the calcification seen so characteristically with hyaline cartilage lesions. Furthermore, the subtle epiphyseal round radiolucency of chondroblastoma is not usually surrounded by a very obvious sclerotic rim. Easier to recognize on MRI, chondroblastoma is dark on T1W and bright on T2W images and shows extensive perilesional edema. Bone scans are hot at the site of the lesion.

Chondroblastoma histology shows a preponderance of rounded cells with distinct folded "coffee-bean" nuclei arranged in a pseudolobulated "cobblestone" pattern of organization. Giant cells and chondroid matrix may also be seen.

Treatment of chondroblastoma must take into account the fact that while it usually behaves only as an active lesion, it may also behave in an aggressive fashion. An extended intralesional curettage remains the classic treatment of choice, but more recently RFA has been employed in selected lesions with considerable success.[52] When RFA is used for large lesions beneath weight-bearing articular surfaces, the risk of collapse must be considered.[52] Chondroblastoma is also one of two benign bone lesions (along with giant cell tumor) that carry the potential to develop pulmonary metastases, so initial screening and subsequent surveillance of the lungs should be considered.

Chondromyxoid fibroma

Like chondroblastoma, chondromyxoid fibroma is a benign tumor of immature cartilage.[53] Unique from chondroblastoma, however, is the metaphyseal eccentric location in long bones, often immediately adjacent to the growth plate. It is a rare tumor, representing less than 1% of bone tumors. The most common long bone involved is the tibia. One-third of these tumors occur in flat bones. Chondromyxoid fibromas usually present with pain.

Radiographic features of chondromyxoid fibroma include its eccentric metaphyseal location, lytic lobulated, soap-bubble appearance usually without matrix mineralization, and associated cortical thinning. In some cases, the appearance may be of an aggressive tumor, with cortical breakthrough and even soft-tissue extension (Figure 3). Under the microscope, the tumor is arranged in lobules which are more cellular around the periphery than the sparsely cellular myxoid center. The characteristic cells are "stellate" in shape.

Treatment is typically by curettage and grafting. Local recurrence rates range from 15% to 25%. Chondromyxoid fibromas do not metastasize.

Osteochondroma

The most common tumor of bone, osteochondroma, is an exophytic growth of physeal cartilage away from the growth plate and joint but paralleling the temporal course of long bone growth.[54] As the cartilage grows, it leaves behind either a sessile or pedunculated bony prominence. These tumors form and grow during the period of skeletal immaturity, cease growing at or around the time of skeletal maturity, and remain throughout a patient's life unless excised. They may present as a painless mass or with pain. Pain is usually from irritation of the overlying soft tissues or bursitis but may also result from fracture of the stalk or malignant degeneration. Malignant degeneration is rare in solitary osteochondromas, but it occurs somewhat more commonly in patients with the hereditary form, multiple hereditary exostoses (see section titled "Congenital syndromes").

Osteochondromas may be diagnosed radiographically with confidence. They are an exophytic metaphyseal projection characterized by continuity of the cortical and underlying medullary bone. When they have a stalk, the cap of the osteochondroma is directed away from the nearest joint. MRI is sometimes used to assess the thickness of the cartilage cap, which may be up to 3 cm in children. In adults, however, the cap should be less than 1.5 cm; thicker caps should cause suspicion for chondrosarcoma arising from the underlying osteochondroma. Under the microscope, osteochondromas have a benign hyaline cartilage cap overlying normal trabecular bone.

Treatment of osteochondromas is based on symptoms and clinical presentation. When they are asymptomatic, they may be observed. When they are painful in children, they may be excised, but the older the child and the farther away from the growth plate, the lower the risk of recurrence. In adults, any symptomatic or enlarging osteochondroma should be investigated further with an MRI to make sure that it has not developed into a chondrosarcoma.[54]

Fibrous tumors

These three lesions are grouped together based on their histologic similarity in giving the light microscopic appearance of being comprised of fibrous tissue. In the latest WHO classification system for bone lesions, however, fibrous dysplasia and osteofibrous dysplasia are listed together under "tumors of undefined neoplastic nature." "Nonossifying fibromas" are classified as "fibrohistiocytic tumors" under the current WHO outline of bone tumors.[3]

Fibrous dysplasia

The etiology of fibrous dysplasia has been identified to be a mutation of the GNAS gene, creating a developmental anomaly of bone formation. It is a relatively common bone process which has its onset in children but may also be diagnosed in adults. The spectrum of clinical presentation is broad and depends upon age, number of lesions, and site(s) of involvement. Patients may present with incidental lesions, painful lesions, or pathologic fracture. Monostotic (solitary) fibrous dysplasia is most commonly located in the skull, followed by the femur, tibia, and ribs. Polyostotic lesions (less common than the monostotic form) most often involve the femur, pelvis, and tibia.

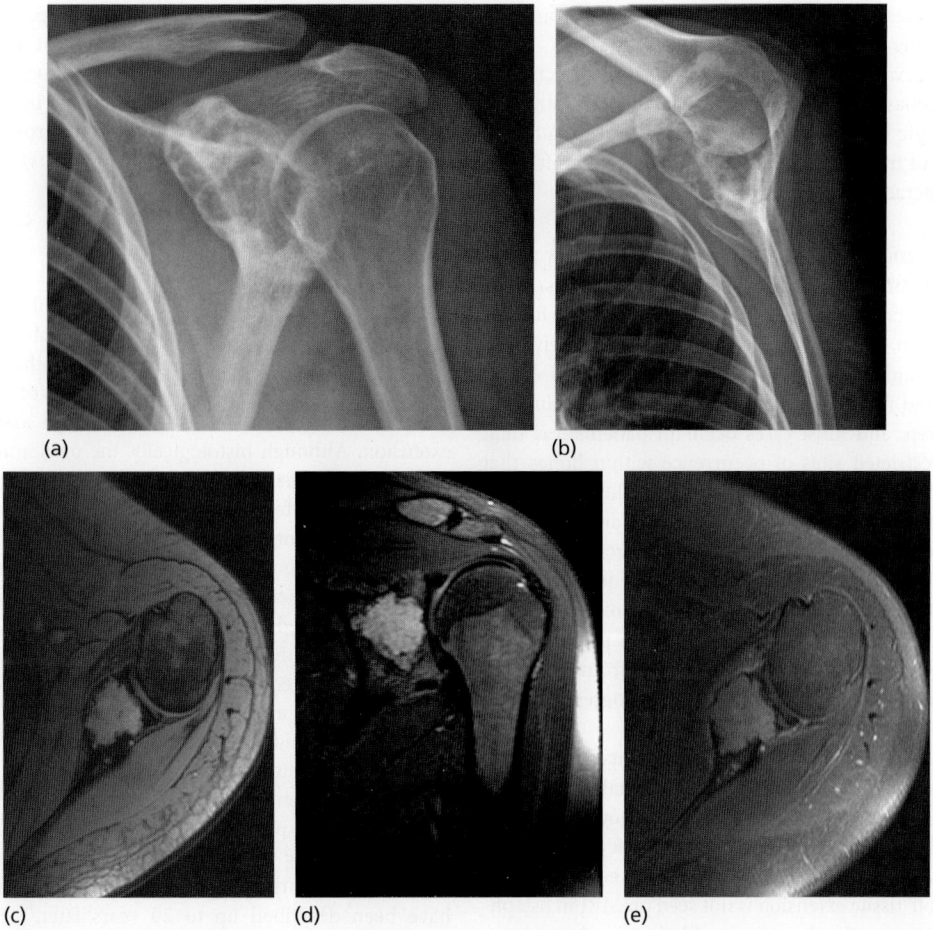

Figure 3 Chondromyxoid fibroma. Anteroposterior shoulder (a) and scapular-Y (b) radiographs, T2-weighted axial (c) and coronal (d) and proton-density axial (e) MRI images show the features of a chondromyxoid fibroma, in this case involving a flat bone, the scapula. Note the cortical thinning and focal cortical destruction that characterizes aggressive behavior and may lead to confusion with chondrosarcoma.

The polyostotic form may also present as McCune–Albright syndrome (see section titled "Congenital syndromes") or Mazabraud's syndrome (associated intramuscular myxomas).

Radiographically, lesions of fibrous dysplasia usually present as geographic lytic lesions. In long bones, they are frequently described as "long lesions in long bones." They affect any portion of the bone (epiphysis, metaphysis, or diaphysis) and have a characteristic "ground-glass" appearance of the matrix. In the proximal femur, extensive involvement may lead to a "shepherd's crook" deformity. Uptake on Tc99 bone scan is usually intense. Under the microscope, immature woven bone classically described as taking the form of "Chinese characters" lacks the osteoblastic rimming seen with osteofibrous dysplasia and is surrounded by bland-appearing fibroblasts.

Treatment is based upon age, location, and symptoms. When the radiographic appearance is classic, symptomatic lesions may be observed. For some symptomatic lesions, curettage and grafting may be done, but structural bone graft is usually preferred, as particulate graft materials are usually resorbed. Prophylactic stabilization is often considered in the proximal femur, where the disorganized trabecular bone of fibrous dysplasia predisposes to stress fracture and remodeling. For symptomatic patients with polyostotic fibrous dysplasia, bisphosphonates have been used with some success.[55,56]

Nonossifying fibroma and fibrous cortical defect

Nonossifying fibromas and fibrous cortical defects are variants of a spectrum of developmental abnormalities of skeletally immature bone.[57] Fibrous cortical defects are smaller and generally confined to the cortex, while nonossifying fibromas are larger, extending into the medullary canal. They are so common as to almost be considered variants of normal. Fully 1/3 of children seen in the emergency room for knee injuries will show evidence of one or more of these lesions. They are almost always an incidental, asymptomatic finding. In the rare instance where they are discovered after a fracture has occurred through one, the characteristic history is the absence of pain leading to the time of fracture. This absence of pain underscores their latent nature without active features. The metaphysis of long bones is affected most frequently, particularly around the knee.

These lesions may be diagnosed with confidence on plain X-rays in nearly all cases. Their characteristic features are an at least partially intracortical, eccentric metaphyseal position, a soap-bubble lytic geographic appearance, and a thin rim of sclerotic bone around the periphery of the lesion. MRI, when necessary, shows a low signal center on both T1W and T2W sequences that is also characteristic. Perilesional edema is absent in the absence of fracture. Rarely, biopsy is needed to establish the diagnosis, and in those instances, the histopathology features a storiform, whirling background of fibroblasts with scattered giant cells.

Treatment of the vast majority of fibrous cortical defects and nonossifying fibromas should be observed alone. The unusual associated pathologic fracture should be treated according to the location and type of fracture, combining curettage and grafting of the lesion when operative management is indicated.

Osteofibrous dysplasia

In the past, osteofibrous dysplasia has been referred to as ossifying fibroma and Campanacci's disease.[57] It is unique among fibrous tumors in its location (anterior tibial shaft almost exclusively) and histology (bone islands surrounded by osteoblastic rimming and separated by a bland fibrous background). It is almost exclusively a tumor of children, and most cases occur in patients less than 8 years old. Its restricted sites of occurrence within bones that have a relatively superficial location (tibia, fibula, ulna, radius) are distinctive, as is the fact that it may be bilateral and multifocal within a single bone. It should be distinguished from adamantinoma, a bone sarcoma that also occurs most frequently in the anterior aspect of the tibia. Clinical presentation of osteofibrous dysplasia is variable, with some patients noticing a painless lump over the tibia, others presenting with episodic pain from associated stress fractures, and rare patients developing progressive tibial bowing.

Radiographically, osteofibrous dysplasia presents most commonly in the tibia within the middle or proximal third in an eccentric anterior position with a lytic, soap-bubble, or saw-toothed appearance. In older patients, there is radiographic overlap with adamantinoma, from which it must be distinguished. Unlike in adamantinoma, soft-tissue extension is not seen on MRI in osteofibrous dysplasia. As an active lesion, osteofibrous dysplasia shows increased uptake on bone scan. Under the microscope, osteofibrous dysplasia must be distinguished from both fibrous dysplasia and adamantinoma. While both osteofibrous dysplasia and fibrous dysplasia have woven bone islands within a sea of benign fibrous tissue, only osteofibrous dysplasia has osteoblastic rimming around those islands. The distinction from adamantinoma is that osteofibrous dysplasia does not show islands of epithelioid cells seen in the more aggressive condition.

Treatment of osteofibrous dysplasia varies according to age, symptoms, and radiographic appearance. Prior to closure of the growth plate, an asymptomatic and radiographically classic lesion may be observed. If stress fractures occur, bracing should be considered. When the radiographic features are atypical, biopsy should be undertaken to establish the diagnosis. Surgical excision with or without grafting is only indicated for progressive deformity or in symptomatic patients after skeletal maturity. Some authors have suggested that due to the high incidence of recurrence after curettage and grafting, an extraperiosteal resection should be performed in all cases.[58]

Giant cell tumors

Giant cell tumor of bone is a relatively common (5–10% of all bone tumors) benign tumor of bone characterized by its distinct histology and behavior.[59] In the current WHO classification system, it is classified as an "osteoclastic giant cell-rich tumors." It is one of four benign bone tumors (along with ABC, chondroblastoma, and osteoblastoma) that have the potential to behave in an aggressive fashion. In addition, along with chondroblastoma, it is unique in its potential to create pulmonary metastases despite its benign designation. Because giant cell tumor typically behaves in an active or aggressive fashion, it presents clinically with pain, swelling, and limited range of motion at the associated joint and sometimes with pathologic fracture. It is a tumor of adulthood, peaking in young adults aged 20 to 40, and it is very unusual in skeletally immature patients. The most common locations are around the knee (distal femur and proximal tibia), wrist (distal radius), sacrum, and shoulder (proximal humerus).

Radiologically, giant cell tumor has its epicenter within the metaphysis of the long bones but almost always extends to involve the epiphysis, creating an eccentric radiolucency typically with geographic type 1C borders that abuts the subchondral bone of the adjacent joint. In skeletally immature patients, however, the lesion is usually metaphyseal. It is purely lytic without matrix mineralization, and it may show radiographic signs of aggressive behavior complete with cortical destruction and an associated soft-tissue extension. Although histologically, the predominate feature is the multinucleated giant cell, it is the background stromal cell with identical nuclear features which is the true neoplastic cell.

Local treatment of giant cell tumor depends upon location. In expendable locations, such as the proximal fibula or distal ulna, en bloc excision is appropriate. For most sites, however, the recommended treatment is extended intralesional curettage and either grafting or cementing of the defect. Extended curettage involves mechanical removal (curettes) combined with a high-speed burr and additional means of extending the margin (e.g., phenol, liquid nitrogen, or laser). The local recurrence rate for intralesional curettage of giant cell tumor varies from 30% to 47% after simple curettage but is less than 25% with extended curettage. An integral part of the care of patients with giant cell tumor is assessment for potential pulmonary metastases and extended follow-up for early diagnosis of local recurrence. Recurrences have been described up to 20 years later.[59] For "unresectable" giant cell tumors, options include radiotherapy, embolization, or denosumab. Denosumab is a Rank ligand inhibitor which inhibits the ability of the background stromal cells in giant cell tumor from coalescing to form giant cells.[60] Although early results have been promising, questions remain regarding its role in long-term use and complications that may be associated with such application.[61]

Hemangioma of bone

The most common benign bone tumor of the spine, hemangioma of bone is a proliferation of blood vessels that may rarely be seen in other locations. The vast majority of hemangiomas of bone, particularly in the spine, are asymptomatic incidental findings, and the true source of any presenting symptoms should be sought apart from this tumor. Rarely, they may cause expansion of the bone or pathologic fracture. In the spine, these problems may cause neurologic compromise.

In the spine, the radiographic characteristics of hemangioma of bone are so typical that in the majority of cases, no biopsy is needed for confirmation. Radiographs show "jailbar" vertical striations. Axial CT and MRI scans show a "polka-dot" pattern. On T2W MRI images, hemangiomas show high signal; after contrast administration, these lesions enhance markedly. When radiographic features are atypical, biopsy will usually show variably sized benign blood vessels, but numerous histologic subtypes have been described. In nonspinal sites, appearances are variable, and biopsy is often needed.

Since most hemangiomas are asymptomatic, management in the majority should simply be observation. For the rare truly symptomatic, "atypical," or "aggressive" lesion, consideration may be given to excision, radiotherapy, embolization, and sclerosing therapy.[62]

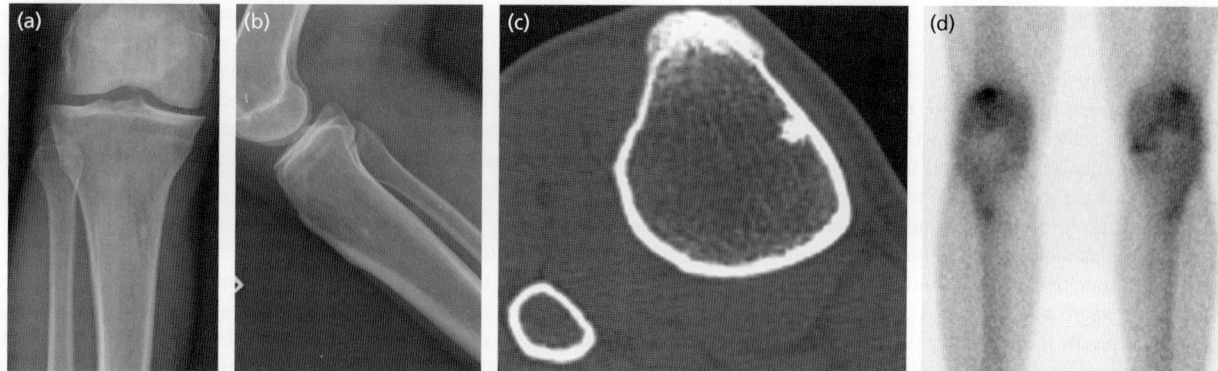

Figure 4 Enostosis (bone island). Anteroposterior (a) and lateral (b) radiographs of the knee show an incidental small radiodense bone lesion. Axial CT (c) shows the characteristic radiating spicules that extend from the periphery of the sclerotic bone island and interdigitate with the surrounding bone trabeculae. As in this case (d), there is usually absence of uptake on bone scan.

Osteogenic tumors

Enostosis

Enostosis, or bone island, is a localized region of dense lamellar bone within cancellous bone of the medullary canal.[63] Enostoses are uniformly benign latent lesions that are incidental asymptomatic findings during radiographic evaluation of other problems. They are most concerning when they occur in adults as part of the autosomal dominant condition osteopoikilosis, where they present as multiple lesions and must be distinguished from osteoblastic metastatic disease.

On plain radiographs and CT scans, enostoses are densely sclerotic areas within medullary bone that are distinguished by the lack of a central nidus (as seen in osteoid osteoma), presence of radiating spicules emanating from the periphery of the lesion, and absence of uptake on bone scan (except in giant enostoses) (Figure 4). They usually do not require biopsy, but under the microscope, the histology is that of mature lamellar bone.

No treatment is necessary. Once the diagnosis is established, nothing more than observation is warranted.

Osteoid osteoma

A benign bone-forming condition that typically presents with a unique and distinctive pain pattern, osteoid osteoma is most common in adolescents and young adults.[64] The pain pattern is that of pain that is worse at night and relieved (in 70% of patients) dramatically and completely over a very short time course (20–30 min) with nonsteroidal anti-inflammatory drugs (NSAIDs). Relief with NSAIDs is theorized to be due to the beneficial effect these agents have on lowering the elevated prostaglandin levels known to be present within the nidus of osteoid osteoma. Osteoid osteomas occur with greatest frequency in the femur and tibia, but they are also one of the three most common tumors of the posterior elements of the spine (along with osteoblastoma and ABC). In the spine, they may cause painful scoliosis, where they are located in the concavity of the curve. In juxta-articular locations, they may cause an arthropathy, with associated effusion and synovitis.

The characteristic radiographic finding in an osteoid osteoma is the radiolucent nidus, which is less than 2 cm in diameter and usually surrounded by dense sclerotic reactive bone. The lesion is usually intracortical, appearing eccentrically in the bone, so the reactive bone may extend both into the medullary canal and also cause expansion of the bone externally. The reactive bone may be so dense that the nidus is only evident on CT or MRI evaluation. On MRI, the extensive perilesional edema associated with osteoid osteoma is characteristic. Osteoid osteomas are always intensely hot on bone scan. Histologically, the nidus of an osteoid osteoma is characterized by irregularly arranged seams of variably mineralized osteoid surrounded by both osteoblasts and osteoclasts within a highly vascular fibrous stroma.

Treatment of osteoid osteoma has evolved considerably over time. The mainstay of operative treatment currently is RFA.[65] Success of first-time RFA in eliminating symptoms is approximately 90%. When RFA is not feasible (spinal lesions close to nerve roots, juxta-articular or difficult to access sites), surgical excision of the nidus will eliminate the symptoms. However, the nidus is sometimes difficult to localize intraoperatively, and numerous techniques have been described. The third option is medical management with NSAIDs, but the mean duration of treatment needed before the lesion ceases to cause symptoms is 2.5 years.

Osteoblastoma

Osteoblastoma shares a great deal of similarity with osteoid osteoma, and to a large degree, the primary distinguishing feature of osteoblastoma is the larger size of its nidus.[64] Similarities include their peak occurrence in adolescent and young adult patients, predilection for the posterior elements of the spine, and their underlying histology. Differences include the absence of the typical pain pattern of osteoid osteoma, the potential for aggressive behavior, and a nidus of larger than 2 cm in osteoblastoma. In addition, a much higher proportion of osteoblastomas (up to 70%) are located in the spine, making the long bones an unusual site.

Radiological features are similar to osteoid osteoma but with a larger nidus that typically shows some faint calcifications. The microscopic appearance overlaps considerably with that of osteoid osteoma, showing irregularly arranged seams of variably mineralized osteoid surrounded by both osteoblasts and osteoclasts within a highly vascular fibrous stroma.

Because of its larger size and potential for more aggressive behavior than osteoid osteoma, treatment of osteoblastoma involves excision, usually by extended intralesional curettage. Recurrence rates range from 10% to 30%. Radiation should be reserved for recurrent lesions in difficult locations such as the spine.

Cysts and other tumors

Aneurysmal bone cyst

ABC may occur as a primary or a secondary lesion.[66] Primary ABCs are neoplastic proliferations characterized by gene rearrangements involving the oncogene USP6 and the promoter CDH11.[67,68] Secondary ABCs occur in association with other primary bone lesions and do not carry the same chromosomal abnormalities.[68] Along with chondroblastoma, giant cell tumor, and osteoblastoma, ABC is one of the four benign bone tumors that have the potential to behave in an aggressive manner. Peak age range is from 1 to 20 years. They typically present with pain and sometimes with swelling and/or pathologic fracture. Anatomic distribution is predominately within the long bones, with the femur and tibia being the most common, but ABC is also one of the three most common tumors of the posterior elements of the spine (along with osteoid osteoma and osteoblastoma).

Radiographically, the classic appearance of an ABC is that of an eccentric, osteolytic, aneurysmal-like "blown-out cortex" surrounded only by an "eggshell thin rim" of reactive bone. However, these features are not present in all cases, and the plain films may show an appearance that overlaps with other benign conditions such as simple bone cyst, nonossifying fibroma, and fibrous dysplasia (Figure 5). In those cases, MRI of ABC will often show septations separating loculated regions filled with blood, manifest as fluid–fluid levels. The radiographic presence of these characteristic findings, however, does not clinch the diagnosis, and underlying primary lesions should be sought. Biopsy is indicated to establish the diagnosis and to distinguish from telangiectatic osteosarcoma, which has an overlapping radiographic appearance. The microscopic appearance of ABC is that of blood-filled lakes separated by bland fibroblastic septa with evidence of hemosiderin deposition and scattered giant cells.

Because of its potential for aggressive local behavior and its highly vascular tissue, treatment of ABC is challenging, and the natural history is sometimes difficult to predict.[69] In most cases, an initial thorough curettage is preferred in order to allow complete histologic examination that may reveal other underlying primary lesions and to distinguish from telangiectatic osteosarcoma. Before curettage, consideration should be given to preoperative embolization, particularly for central lesions that do not lend themselves to intraoperative tourniquet control of bleeding. Intraoperative bleeding may be life threatening. Some authors have suggested embolization or aspiration/injection as definitive treatments, but these options do not allow complete histologic review.[70] Local recurrences do not always progress in an aggressive fashion, so these may sometimes be observed closely. Low-dose irradiation should be reserved for incompletely excised, aggressive, recurrent lesions in difficult-to-access locations such as the spine.

Simple bone cyst

In contrast to ABC, simple (or unicameral) bone cyst is usually an inactive lesion and at worst an active lesion. Without a prior fracture, it is a single cavity within bone filled with serous or serosanguinous fluid. Most simple bone cysts are diagnosed during childhood and are located in the proximal humerus, proximal femur, or calcaneus. In young adults, they are more common in the calcaneus and ilium. Simple bone cysts are usually asymptomatic until fracture, and many present with pathologic fracture following minimal trauma.

Radiographically, simple bone cysts are usually centrally located within the metaphysis or metadiaphysis of a long bone, are purely radiolucent in the absence of prior fracture, lack prominent marginal sclerosis, thin and sometimes slightly expand the surrounding cortex, and may rarely demonstrate the pathognomonic "fallen fragment sign" after fracture. The fallen fragment (or leaf) sign is a thin wafer of cortical bone that is situated at the caudad aspect of the bone cyst because it passed through the fluid in the cyst to reach that position. MRI of simple bone cyst shows homogeneous fluid signal within the lesion, dark on T1W and bright on T2W sequences. Peripheral rim enhancement without any central enhancement is the norm. In some cases after fracture, blood products mixed with the serous fluid may produce a single low fluid–fluid level, but the lack of septations and numerous fluid–fluid levels should distinguish a simple bone cyst. When aspirated, clear serous fluid is obtained unless there has been a fracture, in which case, the fluid can be bloody. After curettage, histologic findings reveal only a bland fibrous membrane with scattered histiocytes.

Treatment of simple bone cysts depends upon location, age, and presentation. In the proximal humerus, pathologic fractures should be allowed to heal first. Approximately one of seven simple bone cysts will heal after fracture (Figure 6). If the cyst does not heal with fracture healing, then definitive treatment options usually employ some form of aspiration and injection. Various agents have been

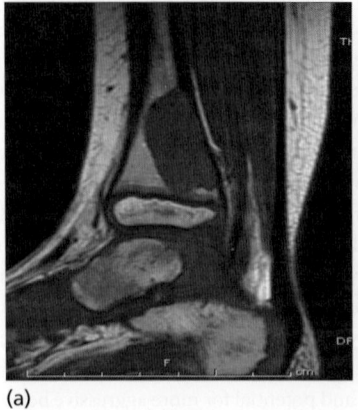 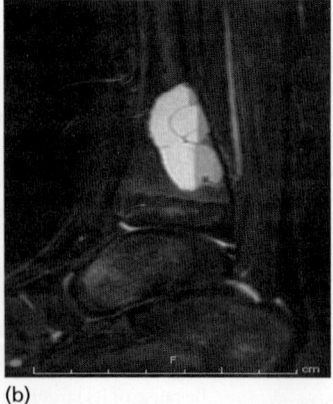 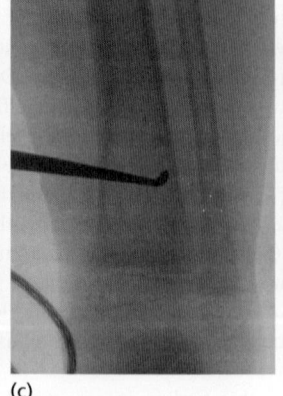 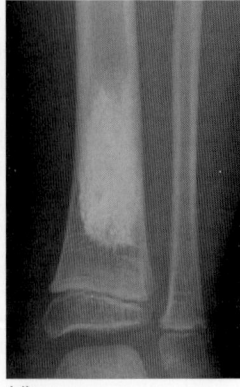

(a) (b) (c) (d)

Figure 5 Aneurysmal bone cyst. Magnetic resonance images of this radiolucent bone lesion that presented with pain in a 4-year-old show fluid signal characteristics on T1-weighted sagittal images (a), but the septations and fluid–fluid levels characteristic of aneurysmal bone cyst are best seen in this case on the T2-weighted sagittal images (b). Intraoperative fluoroscopic images (c) show that this lesion does not show aggressive features seen with many aneurysmal bone cysts (ballooned-out cortex). This lesion was curetted completely and filled with synthetic graft material (d).

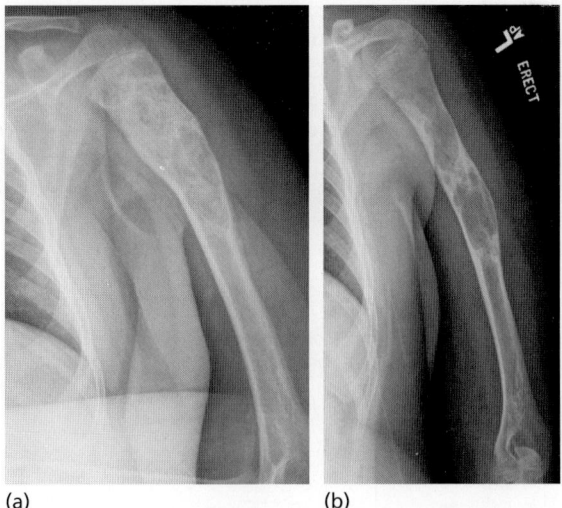

(a)   (b)

Figure 6 Unicameral bone cyst (simple bone cyst). Plain radiographs of the left humerus of a 9-year-old (a) who has incurred two prior fractures with minimal trauma through this lytic geographic proximal humeral bone lesion abutting the proximal humeral growth plate. At this point, there is evidence of healing within the cyst, which occurs in approximately 1/7th of simple bone cysts after fracture. However, 2 years later (b), the cyst shows signs of recurrence, with increased radiolucency in the mid-diaphysis. Note that the proximal humeral growth plate has grown away from the bone cyst. These lesions are only active during skeletal immaturity.

used in the injection, including methylprednisolone, demineralized bone matrix, bone marrow, and combinations of agents. In the only level I study comparing bone marrow with steroid injection, the steroid was superior to bone marrow alone in radiographic evidence of healing.[71] In the proximal femur, the risk of fracture through unicameral bone cysts is higher, and the consequences are potentially more devastating, so consideration should be given to open curettage and grafting here in order to prevent fracture. When a proximal femoral simple bone cyst has caused a pathologic fracture, open reduction and internal fixation of the fracture should be accompanied by curettage and grafting. In some locations, such as the calcaneus and ilium, observation may be elected if the cyst is asymptomatic, since pathologic fractures in these sites are very unusual. Regardless of the means of treatment, approximately 60% respond with progressive healing of the lesion. Partial healing may occur in another 30%, but 10% persist or recur. The natural history of simple bone cyst must always be borne in mind, as those in the typical locations resolve after skeletal maturity. Hence, the closer the patient is to skeletal maturity, the less aggressive the approach should be.

Langerhans cell histiocytosis

Langerhans cell histiocytes, the cells of origin of this disease entity, are a component of the reticuloendothelial system involved in phagocytizing foreign debris and originating in the bone marrow.[45] The group of disease entities encompassed by LCH classically includes solitary eosinophilic granuloma, Hand–Christian–Schüller disease (may include classic triad of multifocal bone lesions, exophthalmos, and diabetes insipidus), and Letterer–Siwe disease (disseminated, often fatal form). The younger the patients at clinical presentation, the more likely they are to have disseminated disease, with most disseminated disease patients being less than 2 years and most patients with eosinophilic granuloma being between 5 and 20 years of age. Current classifications of LCH include involvement of "nonrisk" organs, including

the bone, skin, and lymph node, "risk" organs (liver, spleen, lung, and bone marrow), and "CNS-risk" areas (orbit, mastoid, and temporal skull), the latter due to the risk for development of diabetes insipidus, other endocrine abnormalities, and brain lesions. Isolated nonrisk involvement is generally considered a benign disease.[72] Solitary eosinophilic granuloma is more common in flat bones such as the skull, pelvis, ribs, and vertebral bodies; in the long bones, it occurs as a diaphyseal or metaphyseal lesion. In multifocal disease, the skull and jawbones as well as bones of the hands and feet are more commonly involved.

Clinical presentation varies depending upon the stage of the disease. Patients with solitary or isolated multifocal bone disease often present with pain localized to the site of involvement or a limp with involvement in the lower extremity, but the bone lesions may also be asymptomatic and discovered as incidental findings. Systemic manifestations of this disease spectrum may include diabetes insipidus, exophthalmos, fevers, infections, hepatosplenomegaly, lymphadenopathy, and papular rash, among others.

Radiological presentation is variable, and hence bone lesions in LCH are "great mimickers" (along with osteomyelitis), often simulating more aggressive processes including sarcomas (Figure 7). They typically show a lytic appearance with permeative margination and soft-tissue extension, and they are often mistaken for Ewing sarcoma. In the spine, they create a "vertebra plana" appearance, with profound flattening of the vertebral body. On MRI, these lesions will also show considerable perilesional edema. Bone scan has a 30% false-negative rate, so a skeletal survey should always be performed in patients with any form of LCH. Because of the overlap in clinical presentation with other entities, including Ewing sarcoma and lymphoma, biopsy is indicated in order to establish the diagnosis. Under the microscope, the characteristic Langerhans histiocyte (large, basophilic, coffee-bean-shaped nucleus) predominates, often accompanied by numerous eosinophils.

Treatment of biopsy-proven LCH depends upon the stage and the symptoms, location, size, and number of bone lesions. Systemic involvement involving "risk" organs warrants consideration of chemotherapy. Low-dose radiotherapy is sometimes employed for vertebral lesions at risk for collapse. Surgical treatment for isolated bone involvement may involve curettage alone, curettage and grafting, prophylactic stabilization, and corticosteroid aspiration/injection. Patients with solitary eosinophilic granuloma generally do well with little treatment, and in some cases, the bone lesions resolve after biopsy alone. Patients with systemic disease have prognosis inversely proportional to age at presentation and extent of involvement.

Primary bone sarcomas

Adamantinoma

An epithelial neoplasm, adamantinoma is a rare primary bone sarcoma of low grade that is thought to be derived from ectopic rests of epithelial cells.[73] It represents approximately 0.4% of all bone tumors. Older children and young adults are most commonly affected, and 95% affect the tibia, particularly the anterior aspect, or both the tibia and fibula. The most common presentation is of progressive pain and swelling localized to the middle third of the lower leg.

Radiographically, adamantinoma is an eccentric destructive lytic process that usually destroys the anterior cortex of the mid-tibia and leads to an associated soft-tissue mass. The medullary border usually has a rim of sclerotic reactive bone surrounding the radiolucent areas. On MRI, the lesion is dark on T1W and bright

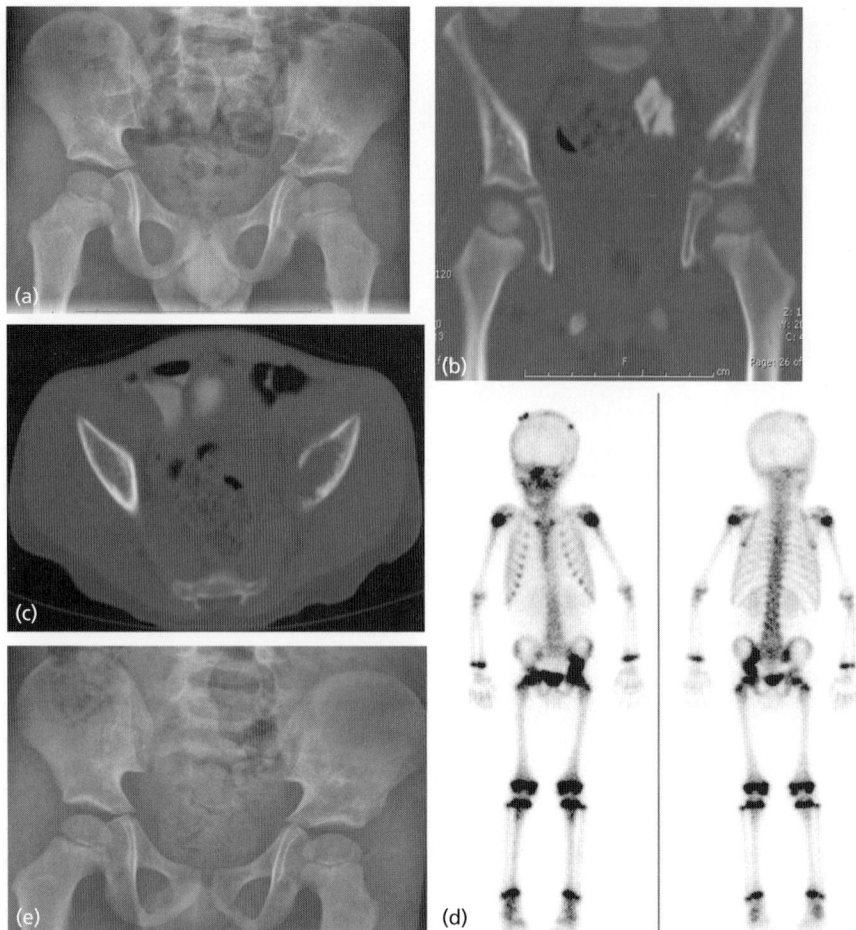

Figure 7 Langerhans cell histiocytosis (eosinophilic granuloma). This anteroposterior pelvis radiograph (a) of a 4-year-old boy shows a left supra-acetabular lytic bone lesion with moth-eaten borders. Cortical destruction seen on coronal (b) and axial (c) CT scans causes concern for metastatic neuroblastoma or Ewing sarcoma, but biopsy showed sheets of Langerhans cells interspersed with eosinophils. Bone scan (d) showed increased uptake in this lesion, and a skeletal survey was done to exclude other lesions that might not show up on bone scan. In this case, there were only a solitary lesion and no visceral involvement. One year after biopsy and curettage, the lesion is less apparent on radiograph (e), and the patient remains asymptomatic.

on T2W sequences with soft-tissue extension commonly and sometimes multifocal disease. Under the microscope, it shows a biphasic arrangement with epithelial groups of cells often forming glandular structures and surrounded by a background of fibrous tissue.

Treatment of adamantinoma is surgical and involves achieving a wide surgical resection of all involved bone and soft tissue with a margin of uninvolved tissue. Although cure is achieved in 85% of cases, long-term follow-up is necessary, as these tumors may recur or metastasize years later.

Chondrosarcoma

Chondrosarcomas derive from chondrocytes, the cartilage cells that are crucial to bone growth and development.[74–77] Among bone tumors, they are relatively common, representing the second most common bone sarcoma after osteosarcoma. The vast majority of chondrosarcomas are low-grade tumors arising in adults in a wide variety of anatomic sites. The most common locations are the pelvis, followed by the femur, ribs, humerus, scapula, and tibia. Chondrosarcomas are often painful, and this symptom often leads to their discovery. Because of the prevalence of cartilage neoplasms of bone and the overlap in clinical, radiographic, and even histologic appearance between benign and malignant, one of the most difficult challenges is the differentiation enchondromas from chondrosarcomas.

Chondrosarcomas may be classified in other ways than grade. Specific histologic subtypes (clear cell, dedifferentiated, and mesenchymal) other than conventional low-grade chondrosarcoma are discussed individually below. Conventional low-grade chondrosarcomas may arise de novo as "primary chondrosarcomas" or in association with preexisting benign cartilage lesions (enchondromas and osteochondromas) as "secondary chondrosarcomas" (Figure 8). Further, chondrosarcomas that arise within the medullary bone are "central," whereas those arising on the surface of the bone (periosteal/juxtacortical chondrosarcoma or secondary chondrosarcoma arising within a preexisting osteochondroma) are "peripheral."

On plain radiographs, conventional chondrosarcomas usually show the same sort of hyaline cartilage mineralization in the forms of arcs and rings that typify enchondromas. However, a number of features that accompany this mineralization pattern point toward a malignant diagnosis. These include cortical destruction with soft-tissue extension, progressive enlargement over time, cortical expansion and >50% endosteal scalloping, enlarging regions of radiolucency, and periosteal reaction. MRI may be more sensitive at showing soft-tissue extension and perilesional edema, but the pattern of being dark on T1W images and bright on T2W images holds true for both benign and malignant cartilage tumors. CT scan is often best at delineating the degree of scalloping and

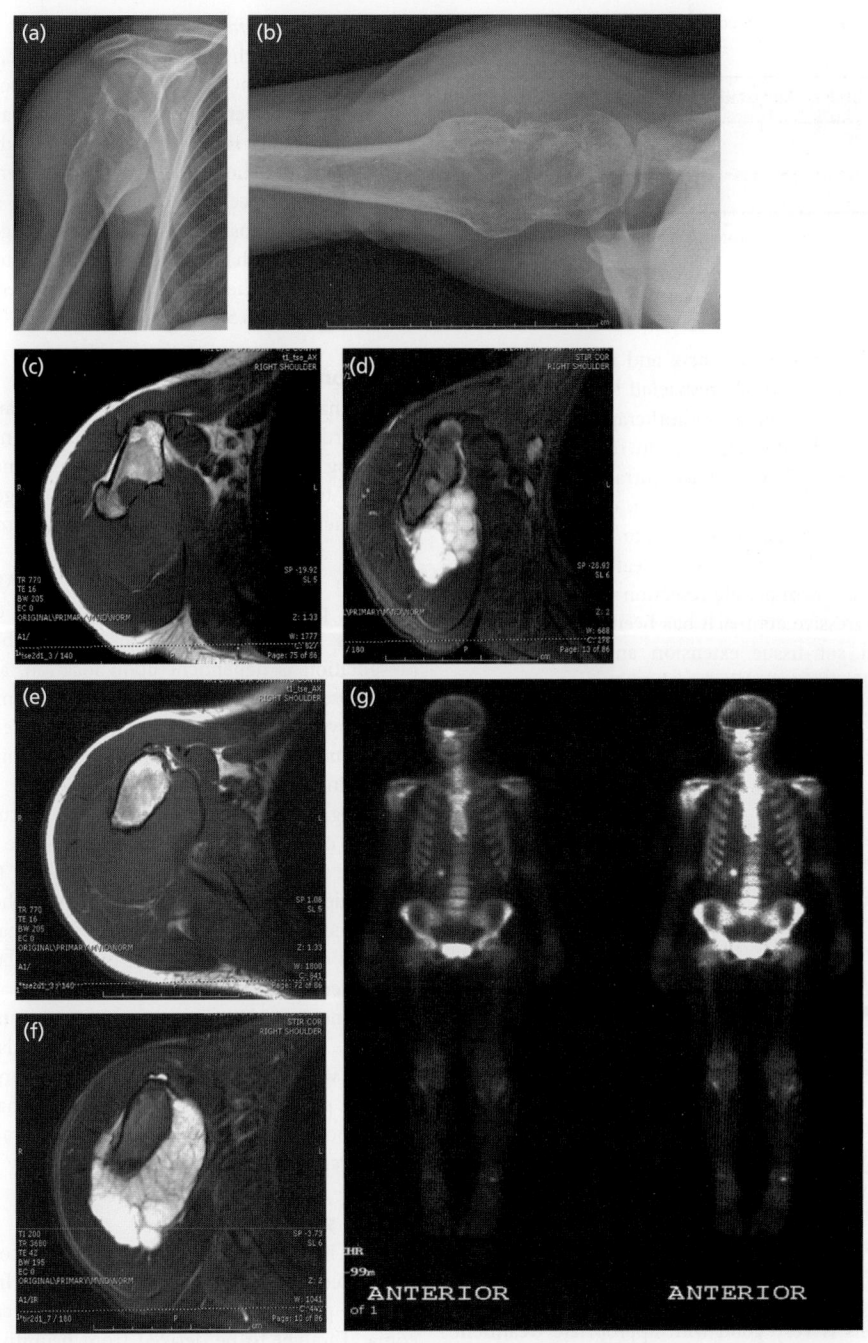

Figure 8 Secondary peripheral chondrosarcoma. This 26-year-old woman with underlying multiple osteochondromatosis developed pain and swelling in her right shoulder. Anteroposterior (a) and axillary lateral (b) right shoulder radiographs show numerous osteochondromas arising from the proximal humeral metaphysis but also a large soft-tissue shadow associated with the bone. In addition, particularly on the lateral view, there is cortical irregularity. Magnetic resonance axial T1-weighted (c, e) and T2-weighted (d, f) images show that there is a cartilage cap measuring more than 2 cm thick, indicative of a chondrosarcoma arising from the underlying osteochondroma and extending into the underlying bone as well. (g) Uptake is noted in the right proximal humerus on bone scan. This patient underwent proximal humeral resection and prosthetic reconstruction.

cortical destruction. Bone scans usually show increased uptake in any hyaline cartilage tumor, so they do not play a major role in distinguishing benign from malignant cartilage tumors. The classic histologic distinction between enchondromas and chondrosarcomas is the presence of "encasement" (hyaline cartilage lobules isolated and surrounded by rimming reactive bone) in enchondromas compared to "permeation" (cartilage tumor permeating around preexisting bone trabecular) in chondrosarcomas. In addition, increased cellularity, cytologic atypia, and binucleation

favor chondrosarcoma. The anatomic site has to be considered as well. The histologic appearance of enchondromas arising in the hand or in the setting of Ollier's disease may have a malignant histologic appearance but nonetheless have a benign course. Overall, the histologic distinction between benign and low-grade malignant cartilage tumors is fraught with difficulty, and this process should always take into account the clinical presentation and radiographic features. In many hyaline cartilage tumors, a firm diagnosis may be established based largely on clinical and radiographic grounds.

Table 7 Chondrosarcoma survival, metastatic potential, and local recurrence rates according to grade.

Type	5-Year survival (%)	Metastatic potential (%)	Recurrence rate
Grade I	90	0	Low
Grade II	81	10–15	Intermediate
Grade III	29	>50	High

Source: Damron 2008.[81] Reproduced with permission from Wolters Kluwer Health (Table 6.3-4, p. 201).

Because of the large amount of matrix and relatively low cellularity, current treatment is usually restricted to surgical means. There is no standard role for either radiotherapy or chemotherapy in most low-grade chondrosarcomas. In recent years, there has been a shift to performing extended intralesional curettage with local adjuvants (phenol, liquid nitrogen, or laser) followed by bone grafting or cementation for grade I intramedullary chondrosarcomas rather than the classic treatment recommendation, which was to perform a wide resection of the tumor.[78–80] However, this less aggressive approach has been limited to chondrosarcomas without soft-tissue extension and generally does not apply to grade II or grade III chondrosarcomas. Prognosis for chondrosarcoma is closely related to grade (Table 7). As with other predominately low-grade tumors, long-term follow-up is recommended.

Clear cell chondrosarcoma

Similar to conventional chondrosarcoma in being a low-grade sarcoma, clear cell chondrosarcoma has a distinctive location (the epiphysis of long bones) and histology (large cells with abundant clear cytoplasm in a cartilage matrix). The most common locations of this rare tumor are the proximal epiphyses of the femur, tibia, or humerus. Peak ages are 20 to 40 years. Pain is the usual presenting symptom.

Given its epiphyseal location, clear cell chondrosarcoma should be considered in the differential diagnosis of chondroblastoma but in older patients (since most chondroblastomas are in skeletally immature patients). On plain radiographs, clear cell chondrosarcoma is seen as a radiolucent lesion that extends to subchondral bone and can have an appearance very similar to that of giant cell tumor of bone. The large clear cells are distinctive under the microscope, and the permeative pattern belies its malignant behavior.

Wide en bloc resection is the standard of care for clear cell chondrosarcoma. Prognosis is very good with appropriate treatment. Overall recurrence rate is approximately 15%.

Dedifferentiated chondrosarcoma

Among chondrosarcomas, dedifferentiated chondrosarcoma is the most aggressive and carries the worst prognosis. By definition, it consists of a conventional low-grade chondrosarcoma adjacent to a region of high-grade sarcoma, often osteosarcoma. The most common locations are the femur, pelvis, humerus, ribs, and scapula. Radiographically, a lytic region developing within an otherwise typical chondrosarcoma may signify a dedifferentiated chondrosarcoma. Treatment for chondrosarcoma should be directed at the high-grade component, but the role for chemotherapy remains to be established, and prognosis is uniformly poor, with a 10–15% 5-year survival rate.[74,82,83] A recent report showed a survival advantage with ifosfamide-based chemotherapy compared to standard non-ifosfamide chemotherapy when combined with surgery in one series.[82]

Mesenchymal chondrosarcoma

The rarest of all chondrosarcomas of bone, mesenchymal chondrosarcoma is a highly aggressive chondrosarcoma which predominately affects teenagers and young adults. The most common locations are in the axial skeleton, and the tumor is usually eccentric. Under the microscope, mesenchymal chondrosarcomas show nodules of cellular chondroid tissue surrounding vascular spaces. As with most chondrosarcomas, surgery is the mainstay of treatment, although recent reports continue to explore the potential benefits of chemotherapy.[75] Prognosis has been reported as ranging from <30% to 52% 5-year survival.[2]

Chordoma

Chordoma is a low-grade malignancy arising from vestigial notochordal remnants that exist in the midline of the spine. Following the distribution of those remnants, chordoma is a midline tumor involving the sacrococcygeal, spheno-occipital, and other mobile spine regions. Chordoma predominately involves adults, and in the adults, the sacrum is the most common location. It is very rare in African-Americans. In younger patients, the skull is the most common location. It accounts for only 3–4% of all primary bone tumors. Clinical presentation is dependent upon location, although pain is usually a presenting symptom. In the sacrum, bowel, bladder, or sexual symptoms may be present. In the skull, cranial nerve deficits may be present. In the mobile spine, back or leg pain predominates.

Radiographs of chordoma may be difficult to interpret as the findings of lytic destruction are often subtle in these anatomically complex sites. Only CT or MRI will show the extensive anterior soft-tissue mass that usually accompanies the bone destruction in chordoma. Under the microscope, chordoma is composed of nests or cords of physaliferous cells, distinctive large cells with bubbly vacuolated cytoplasm.

Treatment of chordoma involves wide surgical resection when possible, but irradiation improves the disease-free interval in patients with marginal or contaminated margins.[84] Chemotherapy does not play a role in this low-grade malignancy. Local recurrence is common (up to 70%), and overall survival drops from 75–85% at 5 years to 40–50% at 10 years.

Ewing sarcoma

Overall, Ewing sarcoma is the third most common bone sarcoma after osteosarcoma and chondrosarcoma.[2] In patients 5–30 years old (the peak ages for Ewing), Ewing is second only to osteosarcoma. Thought to be derived from primitive mesenchymal cells, Ewing sarcoma is a poorly differentiated malignant small round blue cell tumor closely related to other tumors within the Ewing family of tumors.[85] The Ewing family of tumors includes Ewing sarcoma, primitive neuroectodermal tumor (PNET), and Askin's tumor, all of which have translocations involving the EWS gene on chromosome 22. The most common locations are the femur and pelvis, but vertebral body and rib involvement is also relatively common. Presenting symptoms usually include both pain and swelling, but in approximately 20%, the symptoms may be accompanied by fever and malaise. In 10%, pathologic fractures are present at diagnosis. Increased ESR is common, and some patients may also have anemia and leukocytosis.

Radiographically, Ewing sarcoma has a varied presentation depending upon the location. Within the long bones, it has a predilection of diaphyseal involvement, and onion-skinning periosteal reaction (numerous layers of reactive new bone a few millimeters apart formed as the periosteum is lifted off by the expanding tumor and repetitively forms reactive bone) is frequent, accompanied by permeative poorly defined borders, cortical destruction, and usually an associated soft-tissue mass. The radiographic pattern is almost always lytic. Under the microscope, Ewing sarcoma is a prototypical small round blue cell tumor and is difficult to distinguish from other such entities (such as lymphoma and metastatic neuroblastoma) without special studies. Immunohistochemistry is positive for CD-99 (the MIC2 protein) in 95% of cases. The most definitive test is demonstration of the t(11;22)(q24;q12) or similar translocation (t(21;22)) by fluorescent *in situ* hybridization (FISH). Resulting fusion proteins that result from these translocations are EWS-FLI1 and EWS-ERG.

Treatment of Ewing sarcoma involves neoadjuvant multiagent chemotherapy for systemic disease and either wide surgical resection or irradiation for local disease.[85] Active chemotherapeutic agents in Ewing sarcoma include adriamycin, vincristine, cytoxan (cyclophosphamide), and actinomycin D. It has been the chemotherapy that has led to the greatest improvement in survival. The latest trend is for increased surgical resection in sites that previously would have received radiotherapy, but historically Ewing sarcoma has been considered a radiosensitive tumor. Radiotherapy is still utilized for unresectable central locations (some pelvic tumors, sacrum, spine, cranium), for metastatic disease, and as a surgical adjuvant if margins of resection are close or microscopically positive. Surgical resection has evolved from being used initially only for expendable bones (iliac wing, rib, fibula, proximal radius, distal ulna) to now being used more frequently for most reconstructable anatomic sites (femur, tibia, humerus). The pelvis remains a controversial site for local treatment of Ewing sarcoma, where surgery has been used with increasing frequency and acceptable results.[86] However, there have been no randomized studies comparing radiotherapy to surgical resection in Ewing patients, and retrospective studies suffer from selection bias, as radiotherapy has traditionally been used for the worst centrally located tumors. Currently, some trials have suggested that the prognosis is as good as 65–70% 5-year survival, but based on minimum 5-year follow-up for 3225 Ewing sarcomas collected in the National Cancer Database, 5-year survival was only 50.6% for Ewing sarcoma.[2]

Osteosarcoma

The most common bone sarcoma, osteosarcoma comprises a somewhat heterogeneous group of sarcomas that are predominately high grade but with three low- to intermediate-grade variants (Table 8). The common thread is that they are felt to be derived from the osteoblast cell line and are bone-forming sarcomas.[87,88] Ninety percent of osteosarcomas are conventional high grade. Classically, the age distribution has been described as bimodal, but the peak age is during the second and third decades of life; cases in older adults usually occur in the setting of Paget's disease (Pagetoid

osteosarcoma) or following irradiation (postradiation osteosarcoma). Clinical presentation almost always involves progressively worsening pain and sometimes associated swelling. The most common locations reflect the most active areas of growth in skeletally immature patients—the distal femur followed by the proximal tibia and proximal humerus. Overall, there is a 1.5 : 1 male to female ratio.

Radiographically, osteosarcomas in general are bone-forming, relatively poorly defined metaphyseal tumors that frequently have associated soft-tissue extension accompanied by cumulus cloud-type bone formation (Figure 9). Some histologic subtypes, especially the fibroblastic and telangiectatic osteosarcomas, form radiolucent tumors without the classic bone formation. Telangiectatic osteosarcoma, due to its blood-filled lakes, can closely resemble a benign ABC on imaging studies, so this tumor should always be considered in the differential diagnosis of an apparent ABC. On MRI, the typical osteosarcoma is dark on T1W and bright but heterogeneous on T2W sequences, usually shows soft-tissue extension, and may show skip lesions within the medullary canal. They show increased uptake on bone scan. Under the microscope, there is some variation, particularly between the low- and high-grade variants, but the key element is malignant osteoid production. The most common histologic subtype is osteoblastic, followed by chondroblastic, fibroblastic, and—rarely—telangiectatic.

Treatment depends upon grade and extent of the tumor. For all high-grade variants, neoadjuvant multidrug chemotherapy is key, and this involves adriamycin, ifosfamide, cisplatin, and methotrexate.[89] The advantage of neoadjuvant chemotherapy is that it allows determination of percent tumor necrosis after resection and often reduces the size of the soft-tissue extension of the tumor, facilitating surgical resection. Tumor necrosis >95% is strongly predictive of disease-free and overall survival. Drug resistance is sometimes seen due to the P-glycoprotein membrane-bound pump (coded for by the MDR-1 gene), which pumps the chemotherapeutic agents out of the cell. Local disease is addressed by wide surgical resection. There is no role for radiotherapy in standard treatment of osteosarcoma. For low-grade central and parosteal osteosarcoma (the low-grade variants), treatment only involves wide surgical resection; neither chemotherapy nor radiotherapy plays a role.

Features unique to the various clinicopathologic subtypes will be presented later.

Conventional osteosarcoma

As the classic osteosarcoma, conventional high-grade osteosarcoma has the typical radiographic appearance of a metaphyseal tumor most common in the distal femur, proximal tibia, and proximal humerus. It usually demonstrates a cloud-like bone formation with permeative borders on plain radiographs and often has cortical breakthrough with an associated soft-tissue extension bordered by Codman's triangles (reactive bone formed by the bordering periosteum as it is lifted away from the bone surface by the expanding tumor) (Figure 9).

Histologically, osteosarcoma is comprised of pleomorphic cells with frequent mitoses forming lacelike pink osteoid. Conventional osteosarcoma may show a predominance of bone formation (osteoblastic), chondroid matrix (chondroblastic), fibrous background (fibroblastic), or blood-filled pools (telangiectatic). Differentiation of chondroblastic osteosarcoma from chondrosarcoma and fibroblastic osteosarcoma from fibrosarcoma is based upon the presence of malignant osteoid.

Table 8 Osteosarcoma variants according to grade.

Low grade	Intermediate grade	High grade
Low-grade intramedullary Parosteal	Periosteal	Conventional High-grade surface Secondary Pagetoid Postradiation Small cell

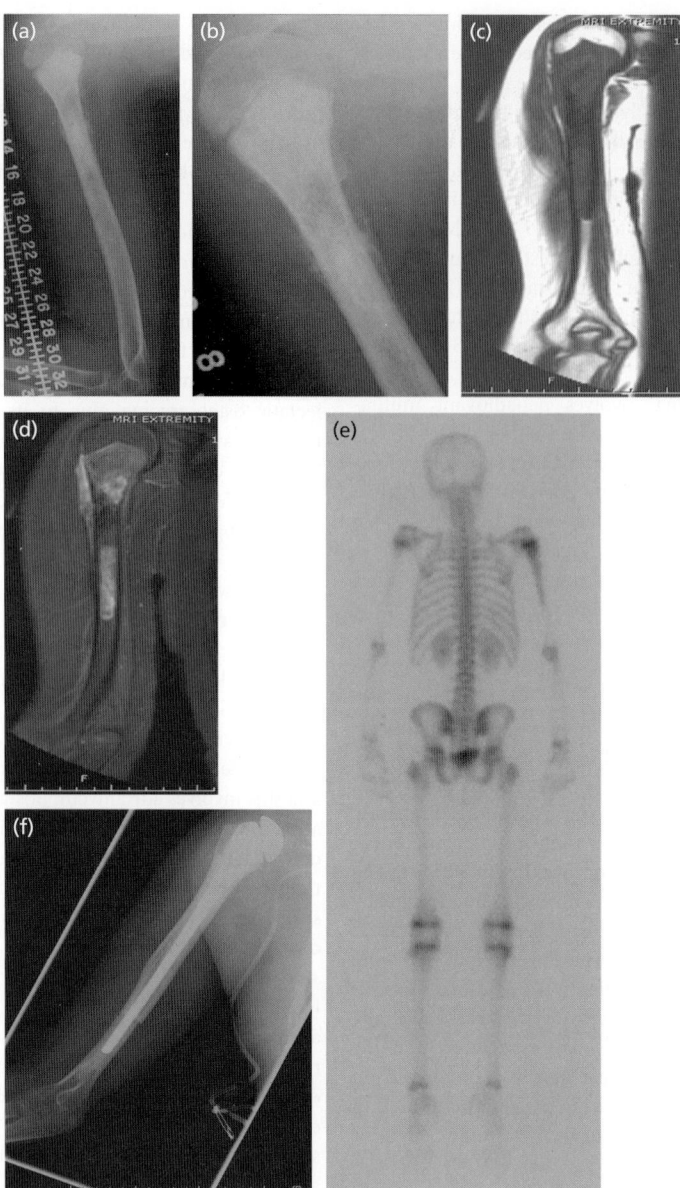

Figure 9 Conventional osteosarcoma. A 13-year-old girl with right shoulder pain and swelling has shoulder radiographs (a, b) showing a radiodense proximal humeral metaphyseal lesion with permeative borders and Codman triangle periosteal reaction and soft-tissue extension. Coronal T1-weighted (c) and T2-weighted (d) MRI images show the soft-tissue extension and extent of the tumor within the medullary canal. Bone scan (e) shows increased uptake in the proximal humerus. In a young patient, these features are nearly diagnostic of osteosarcoma, and a biopsy confirmed the diagnosis of high-grade osteosarcoma. After neoadjuvant chemotherapy, the patient underwent wide resection and proximal humeral allograft–prosthetic reconstruction (f).

Prognosis for osteosarcoma has improved considerably over the years due primarily to the use of multiagent chemotherapy. Clinical trials involving patients with nonmetastatic disease report actuarial 5-year survival rates of 75–80%. For all comers, including all ages and those with metastatic disease, data from the National Cancer Database of the American College of Surgeons suggests a less optimistic outlook.[2] Based upon 8104 osteosarcomas cases with a minimum 5-year follow-up from 1985 to 1998, the relative 5-year survival rate for high grade was 52.6%. For osteosarcoma patients younger than 30 years, the relative 5-year survival rate was 60%; for those aged 30 to 49 years, it was 50% and for those aged 50 years or older it was 30%. For the approximately 20% of patients with osteosarcoma that present with metastases, aggressive treatment leads to 5-year survival in 30–40%, but for patients who develop metastases after treatment, 5-year survival is only 15–20%.

High-grade surface

Although the other two surface osteosarcomas (parosteal and periosteal) are low or intermediate grade, this surface variant is defined by its more aggressive radiographic and histologic appearance and clinical behavior. Otherwise, the clinical presentation, demographic features, pathology, and treatment are identical to those of conventional high-grade osteosarcoma.

Low-grade intramedullary

Along with parosteal osteosarcoma, low-grade central intramedullary osteosarcoma is the only other low-grade osteosarcoma. In contrast to the two other low- to intermediate-grade osteosarcomas (parosteal and periosteal, respectively), this one is not a surface tumor; conversely, this is the only intramedullary low-grade osteosarcoma. A rare tumor, it represents only 1–2% of all

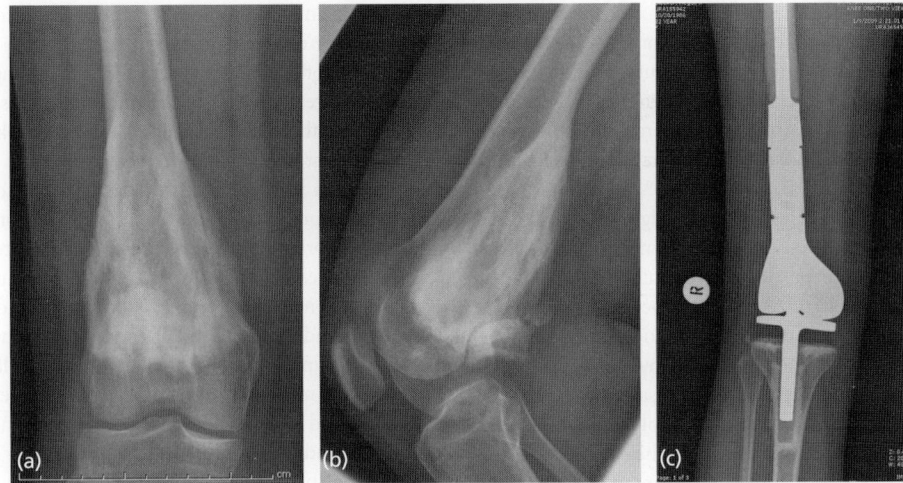

Figure 10 Low-grade central osteosarcoma. This 26-year-old woman was diagnosed with low-grade central osteosarcoma after a prolonged course with pain and swelling over several years. Plain anteroposterior (a) and lateral (b) radiographs show a sclerotic predominately intramedullary lesion of the distal femoral metaphysis. Biopsy showed streaming osteoid separated by a relatively bland fibrous background. Following wide surgical resection, the distal femur was reconstructed with a distal femoral replacement total knee arthroplasty (c).

osteosarcomas. Clinical presentation usually involves pain. The typical patient is slightly older than classic osteosarcoma, often being in the third decade of life.

Radiographically, the well-demarcated radiodensity that characterizes low-grade intramedullary osteosarcoma is often confused with fibrous dysplasia (Figure 10). Under the microscope, the appearance is distinctly different from high-grade conventional osteosarcoma. Like parosteal osteosarcoma, low-grade central osteosarcoma is comprised of broad bands of osteoid separated by a hypocellular fibroblastic stroma with minimal atypia and rare mitoses.

As for both of the low-grade osteosarcomas, low-grade intramedullary osteosarcoma is treated by wide surgical resection alone without chemotherapy or radiotherapy. Overall prognosis is quite good, with local recurrences in only approximately 5% following appropriate surgery and a 90% 5-year survival rate which drops slightly to 85% at 10 years. In rare cases, dedifferentiation may occur by way of an adjacent high-grade sarcomatous component.

Parosteal

The low-grade surface osteosarcoma, parosteal osteosarcoma is a distinct clinical, radiographic, and pathologic entity that accounts for 5% of osteosarcomas. Similar to its intramedullary counterpart, the peak age is in the third decade of life. Females are affected more commonly than males (M : F 1 : 2). Parosteal osteosarcoma has a strong predilection for the posterior aspect of the distal femur (80% of cases); the proximal tibia and proximal humerus are other relatively common locations. It usually presents as a painless posterior distal thigh mass that may decrease knee range of motion.

Radiographically, parosteal osteosarcoma usually shows a lobulated, fairly densely ossified mass that has the appearance of being "stuck on" the underlying bony cortex. In unusual cases, the tumor may encircle the bone, and the underlying cortex may show reactive changes. Under the microscope, parosteal osteosarcoma looks like low-grade central osteosarcoma, with a sparsely cellular fibroblastic stroma between broad bands of osteoid.

Treatment for parosteal osteosarcoma involves wide surgical resection alone; there is no established role for chemotherapy or radiotherapy. In rare instances, dedifferentiated areas may arise. Overall prognosis is 86% 5-year survival.[2]

Periosteal

Another surface tumor, periosteal osteosarcoma accounts for only 1–2% of osteosarcomas. Clinical presentation and peak age are the same as for conventional osteosarcoma, but it has a predilection for the tibial diaphysis and the femoral diaphysis. Radiographically, in addition to its diaphyseal surface predilection, periosteal osteosarcoma is characterized by mineralization, which may present as a sunburst periosteal reaction or patchy calcification reflecting its often chondroblastic histology. Under the microscope, periosteal osteosarcoma is similar to conventional osteosarcoma except for being intermediate grade and usually having a chondroblastic pattern. Treatment usually employs conventional neoadjuvant chemotherapy followed by wide surgical resection. Prognosis is intermediate between parosteal and conventional osteosarcoma.

Secondary

Secondary osteosarcomas have a peak age in older patients, have the worst prognosis of all osteosarcomas, and arise within the setting of a predisposing condition, either Paget's disease of bone or previous irradiation. Osteosarcoma arising as the high-grade component of a dedifferentiated chondrosarcoma is discussed in the chondrosarcoma section.

Pagetoid

Sarcomatous degeneration within Paget's disease occurs in a small percentage (1–15%) of patients with this metabolic bone condition characterized by rapid bone turnover. Peak age is in 55–85 years old. Clinical presentation is usually heralded by a change in the patient's baseline pain and/or a new soft-tissue mass or swelling. Due to the prevalence of Paget's disease in flat bones, Paget's osteosarcoma has a predilection for the scapula, pelvis, and ribs. Radiographic presentation is usually of an aggressive osteoblastic or osteolytic area arising within Pagetoid bone. Treatment involves chemotherapy—if the patient can tolerate it—and wide surgical resection. The benefits of chemotherapy in this group remain unproven. Prognosis is poor, with 5–18% 5-year survival.[2]

Postradiation

The criteria for defining postradiation sarcoma are that the sarcoma arises within a previously irradiated area without a preexisting sarcoma of the same histologic type and that a latent period of at least 3–4 years has elapsed since the initial radiotherapy and the development of the sarcoma. Postradiation osteosarcoma arises within previously irradiated bone and represents 70% of postradiation bone sarcomas. Other pathologies include malignant fibrous histiocytoma and fibrosarcoma. Clinical presentation is that of swelling and pain arising within the previously irradiated region. Radiographically, postradiation sarcomas of bone appear as an aggressive lesion within the previously irradiated field. Under the microscope, they may show the histology of high-grade conventional osteosarcoma, malignant fibrous histiocytoma, or fibrosarcoma. Treatment is by surgical resection and adjuvant chemotherapy when the patient can tolerate it, although the benefits of chemotherapy in this group are unproven.[90] Prognosis is extremely poor, ranging from 5% to 30% 5-year survival.

Small cell

Other than their histologic appearance, small cell osteosarcomas resemble high-grade conventional osteosarcomas. Under the microscope, the only feature that distinguishes this tumor—comprised predominately of small round blue cells with indistinct cytoplasm—from Ewing sarcoma is the presence of osteoid, which is sometimes difficult to identify on biopsy. Treatment and prognosis are as for conventional osteosarcoma.

Vascular sarcomas

There are two major subtypes of vascular sarcomas in the current WHO classification which may involve bone: epithelioid hemangioendothelioma and angiosarcoma.[91–93] Hemangiopericytoma, which has previously been included in this category, has been reclassified as a solid fibrous tumor in the latest WHO schema.[94] These tumors represent a spectrum of disease, with hemangioendothelioma at the less aggressive end of the spectrum and angiosarcoma at the aggressive end. These are rare tumors, as a group representing less than 1% of bone sarcomas. Clinically, they have a broad age range but are most common in middle-aged and older adults. As with most bone sarcomas, presenting symptoms include pain and swelling. Rarely, pathologic fracture may occur, more commonly with angiosarcoma. One-third of patients with vascular sarcomas will have multifocal disease, either "skipping joints" in a single limb or involving disseminated sites throughout the body. Any bone may be affected, but long bones predominate.

Radiographically, these tumors are typically lytic and destructive, but a combination of osteolysis and sclerosis may be seen. Soft-tissue extension is not usually seen in these tumors. Under the microscope, each tumor has a characteristic appearance with some evidence of rudimentary vascular channels. Treatment of vascular sarcomas may involve wide surgical resection or radiotherapy. Epithelioid hemangioendothelioma is a particularly radiosensitive tumor and may be treated primarily with radiotherapy. The role of chemotherapy for this group of tumors is not well established. For extensive or multifocal disease, radiotherapy has efficacy.

Metastatic disease to bone

The most common malignancy to affect bone is metastatic carcinoma. It is far more common than bone sarcoma or myeloma. The most common "osteophilic" primary tumors to affect bone arise from primaries of the breast, prostate, lung, kidney, and thyroid. Patients with breast and prostate cancer have usually had their primary cancer treated and then develop delayed metastatic disease to bone. Patients with metastatic lung carcinoma more commonly present with metastatic bone disease as the presenting symptom of their lung cancer. Patients with kidney and thyroid cancer may present with either concurrent or delayed metastatic disease. For a primary carcinoma metastatic to bone in a patient with no history of cancer, the most common sources are lung and kidney primaries. Metastatic carcinoma to bone most commonly involves patients older than 40 years. In patients less than 5, metastatic neuroblastoma predominates, and in older pediatric patients, rhabdomyosarcoma is the most common primary source. Presenting symptoms may involve pain, swelling, or pathologic fracture, but in some cases, the bone lesions are asymptomatic and are discovered on routine staging studies. In the spine, neurologic symptoms and even paraplegia may be seen. The most common sites are the spine, proximal femur, pelvis, ribs, sternum, proximal humerus, and skull. Metastases distal to the elbow and knee are unusual, and when they are present, the most common source is lung carcinoma.

Evaluation of bone lesions suspected of being due to metastatic disease involves a comprehensive physical examination, laboratory parameters, and a radiographic evaluation of common sites of primary disease. Since myeloma is often in the differential diagnosis of metastatic carcinoma in adults, serum and urine protein electrophoresis is often requested. Lactate dehydrogenase may be elevated in lymphoma, although it is nonspecific. Prostate-specific antigen is usually elevated in prostate cancer. Renal cell carcinoma may cause hematuria. Standard radiographs of any involved bone, a total skeleton bone scan, and CTs of the chest, abdomen, and pelvis comprise the classic radiographic evaluation. Increasingly, PET-CTs are being utilized in this setting.

Radiographically, metastatic carcinoma may have a myriad of appearances. Some tumors, such as prostate metastases, are typically osteoblastic. Breast cancer metastases usually show a combination of osteolysis and sclerosis. Metastases from lung, kidney, and thyroid cancer are usually purely osteolytic. Bone scans usually show increased uptake at multiple sites, but solitary metastatic lesions are not uncommon, and certain very aggressive bone metastases, such as those from renal or thyroid carcinoma, may not show increased uptake. Pathology often falls into a general descriptive category, such as adenocarcinoma, squamous cell carcinoma, or poorly differentiated carcinoma. In these cases, immunohistochemistry markers are of greater importance in identifying the source (Table 9). Some tumors have specific histopathology patterns, such as clear cell carcinoma of the kidney, well-differentiated follicular carcinoma of the thyroid, and metastatic pigmented malignant melanoma of the skin.

Treatment of metastases can be viewed as systemic and local. Systemic treatment is directed both at the primary tumor (discussed in other chapters throughout the text) and at the mediator of bone destruction, the osteoclast. Bisphosphonates have become widely accepted in the setting of metastatic bone disease to inhibit the osteoclastic bone destruction. Operative management of metastatic

Table 9 Examples of immunohistochemistry markers for evaluation of metastatic disease to bone.

Immunohistochemistry marker	Primary tumor source
Prostate-specific antigen (PSA)	Prostate carcinoma
Thyroid transcription factor (TTF-1)	Lung carcinoma
Leukocyte common antigen (LCA)	Lymphoma

Table 10 Common primary tumors metastatic to bone: Frequency of bone involvement and survival after metastases.

Primary tumor	Percentage of patients that develop metastatic disease	Fraction of patients with mets who have bone involvement clinically (%)	Median survival after diagnosis of mets (months)	Mean 5-year survival (%)
Breast carcinoma	65–75	—	24	20
Prostate carcinoma	65–75	30–40	40	25
Lung carcinoma	30–40	20–40	<6	<5
Renal carcinoma	20–25	15–25	6	10
Thyroid carcinoma	60	20–40	48	40

Source: Damron 2008.[95] Reproduced with permission from Wolters Kluwer Health.

carcinoma, myeloma, and lymphoma has been discussed in a previous section. Once bone metastases are diagnosed, prognosis is poor, but survival varies according to the underlying primary tumor (Table 10).

Myeloma

Myeloma represents the most common primary bone malignancy. As it is covered elsewhere in this text, only the details related to bone will be presented here. Myeloma predominately affects adults aged 50 to 80 and has a propensity to affect blacks greater than Caucasians by a ratio of 2:1. Clinical presentation may involve pain, pathologic bone fracture, bone marrow failure (manifesting as fatigue and weakness from anemia, bruising and bleeding from thrombocytopenia, recurrent infections from neutropenia), renal failure, or hypercalcemia. A solitary plasmacytoma in the bone does not clinch the diagnosis of myeloma. Diagnostic criteria for myeloma include at least 10% plasma cells in the bone marrow, monoclonal protein in the serum (monoclonal gammopathy on serum protein electrophoresis) or urine (Bence-Jones proteins on urine protein electrophoresis), and end-organ failure (hypercalcemia, renal insufficiency, anemia, or bone lesions).

Radiographic manifestations of myeloma include single or multiple "punched-out" small lytic lesions sometimes coalescing into much larger lesions. Since 80% of myeloma bone lesions do not show increased uptake on bone scan, a skeletal survey should be considered to search for other lesions during the initial evaluation. Under the microscope, myeloma is comprised of sheets of plasma cells with large round, clockface, eccentric nuclei and perinuclear clearing.

Bone lesions from myeloma are very sensitive to radiotherapy, but for large lesions or those with pathologic fracture, surgical fixation is warranted. For surgical management of myeloma bone manifestations, please refer to the earlier section.

Bone lymphoma

Primary lymphoma of bone was first described as "reticulum cell sarcoma" and is comprised of malignant lymphoid infiltrate within bone in the absence of concurrent lymph node or visceral involvement. Just about any age may be affected, and the most common locations are the femur, ilium, and ribs. Clinical presentation may include pain, an associated soft-tissue mass, or pathologic fracture. Unlike diffuse lymphoma, these patients rarely have systemic symptoms.

Radiographically, lymphoma may be diaphyseal or metaphyseal and typically has a permeative, poorly defined border on plain films. Many cases are osteolytic, but in some cases a sclerotic appearance may simulate osteosarcoma. Under the microscope, primary lymphoma of bone is a small round blue cell tumor which requires immunohistochemistry in order to distinguish it from Ewing sarcoma. Ninety percent of primary bone lymphomas are large B-cell type. Immunohistochemical markers for B cells include CD19 and CD20.

Treatment of primary bone lymphoma requires a multidisciplinary approach. Chemotherapy is the primary treatment modality, with surgery reserved for biopsy, fracture fixation, and prophylactic fixation of impending fractures. Chemotherapy often involves cyclophosphamide, doxorubicin, vincristine, and prednisone (CHOP) and rituximab (monoclonal antibody against CD20). Although local radiotherapy is often employed in addition to chemotherapy, recent reports are beginning to question its benefits to overall survival, particularly in light of its adverse effects on bone fragility and fracture healing.

Congenital syndromes

A number of congenital syndromes either involve bone lesions, predispose to development of bone malignancies, or both. Some of these syndromes are covered in this section.

Enchondromatosis

Enchondromatosis may involve simply multiple enchondromas (Ollier's disease) or the combination of multiple enchondromas with multiple soft-tissue hemangiomas (Maffucci's syndrome). Both syndromes occur sporadically. Neither has a known cause. They are uncommon and are typically diagnosed in childhood. Radiographically, the enchondromas individually are not different than those of solitary disease. The most important distinguishing feature of these two syndromes is the risk of developing malignancy.

Ollier's disease

Multiple enchondromatosis carries up to a 20–30% risk of developing one or more chondrosarcomas. Hence, these patients should be followed on an annual basis for surveillance. The most common locations for chondrosarcomas in Ollier's disease are the pelvis, proximal femur, and proximal humerus.

Maffucci's syndrome

Patients with Maffucci's syndrome are also at risk of developing chondrosarcomas, but they are at increased risk of developing numerous other types of malignancies as well. In fact, the risk of malignancy in Maffucci's patients approaches 100%. Common primaries include acute lymphocytic leukemia, astrocytoma, and gastrointestinal malignancies. Vigilant surveillance is essential for early diagnosis of these tumors.

Familial adenomatous polyposis

The early onset of multiple colorectal polyps characterizes this autosomal dominant condition caused by a mutation in the adenomatous polyposis coli (APC) gene. The only bone lesion associated with familial adenomatous polyposis (and the related Gardner syndrome) is osteoma. These lesions do not require specific treatment, nor do they predispose to bone malignancy. The only malignancy associated with this familial adenomatous polyposis is colon cancer.

Polyostotic fibrous dysplasia, McCune–Albright syndrome, and Mazabraud's syndrome

While most fibrous dysplasia lesions occur in a single location (monostotic), some involve multiple bones (polyostotic fibrous dysplasia). In addition, polyostotic fibrous dysplasia may be accompanied in 30–50% of cases by distinctive pigmented cutaneous markings with a "coast-of-Maine" irregular border, precocious puberty, or endocrinopathies, a syndrome named McCune–Albright (or Albright's syndrome). Rarely, fibrous dysplasia may occur in the setting of soft-tissue myxomas (Mazabraud's syndrome). The common etiologic thread for these conditions is the presence of activating mutations of the GNAS1 gene. Usually these patients are diagnosed in childhood or adolescence either with manifestations of their underlying bone disease (pain, limp, swelling, angular deformity, limb length discrepancy, or craniofacial abnormalities), the characteristic skin lesions, precocious puberty, or one of numerous endocrinopathies (hyperparathyroidism, hyperthyroidism, Cushing's syndrome, acromegaly, diabetes, rickets, osteomalacia, hyperprolactinemia).

Radiographically and histologically, the individual fibrous dysplasia lesions are the same as those described previously for solitary fibrous dysplasia. Treatment should address any associated condition (particularly the endocrinopathy) as well as the bone manifestations. Since polyostotic fibrous dysplasia is more often associated with progressive deformity, particularly in the proximal femur, more aggressive prophylactic treatment—including both surgical intervention and bisphosphonate therapy—should be considered. Malignancy in these conditions is rare and usually preceded by radiotherapy.

Multiple osteochondromatosis

An autosomal dominant condition attributable to mutation of either the EXT1 or EXT2 gene, multiple osteochondromatosis (multiple hereditary exostoses) is rare compared to the solitary occurrence of osteochondromas, the most common benign bone tumors. The condition is usually diagnosed in early childhood between ages 2 and 10. Typical manifestations include "knobby" protuberances near joints, short stature, shortened limbs, coxa valga, genu valgum, radial head dislocation, and pain. Radiologic features consist of multiple osteochondromas, each of which has the characteristic features of a solitary osteochondroma. As for solitary osteochondromas, excision is only recommended for symptomatic tumors. Risk of malignant degeneration has been estimated at between 3% and 10% and typically involves a low-grade chondrosarcoma (Figure 11).

Retinoblastoma syndrome

Patients with a germline mutation of the RB1 gene are predisposed to develop not only retinoblastoma but also—via a "second-hit" somatic mutation—other malignancies, the most common of which is osteosarcoma. Hence, this syndrome has also been referred to as "retinoblastoma/osteogenic sarcoma syndrome." Patients with

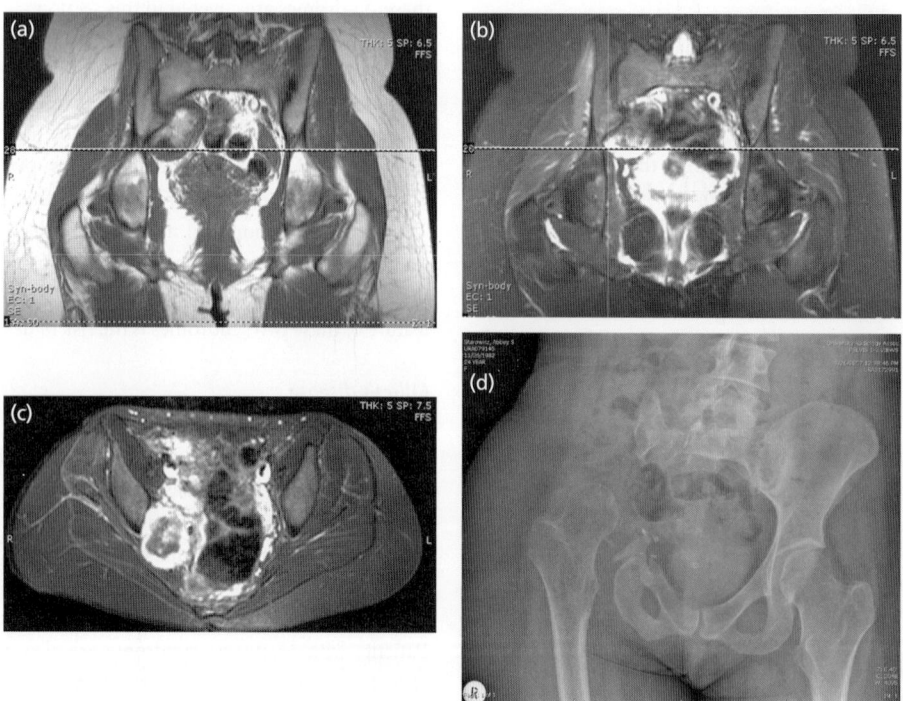

Figure 11 Secondary chondrosarcoma in osteochondromatosis. A 23-year-old woman with known multiple hereditary exostoses developed pelvic pain. Radiographs were not revealing, but MRI images (a–c) revealed a mass arising from a small osteochondroma on the inner table of the pelvis beginning at the level of the sacroiliac joint and extending to the sciatic notch. Biopsy confirmed low-grade chondrosarcoma. The patient underwent internal hemipelvectomy without reconstruction (d). The pelvis is a common location for development of chondrosarcomas in osteochondromatosis, and regular screening in these patients is advisable.

retinoblastoma are usually diagnosed before age 3, and the potential for osteosarcoma peaks in the adolescent age range. Radiographic presentation, histology, and treatment of the osteosarcoma are the same as for conventional high-grade osteosarcoma, discussed previously.

Rothmund–Thomson syndrome

This rare syndrome is important in the context of bone tumors because of its predisposition for development of osteosarcoma. An autosomal recessive genetically transmitted syndrome attributable to mutation in the RECQL4 helicase gene on chromosome 8, Rothmund–Thomson syndrome is usually diagnosed within the first 6 months of life based on a characteristic sun-sensitive erythematous rash that eventually leaves a hyper- and hypopigmented poikiloderma. Genetic testing confirms the disorder in a substantial number of cases, but related conditions such as Werner syndrome and Bloom syndrome should be excluded. Other orthopedic-associated manifestations include osteoporosis, clavicular hypoplasia, syndactyly, patellar aplasia, genu valgum, and benign osseous lesions. There is no specific treatment for Rothmund–Thomson syndrome. High vigilance should be maintained to diagnosis of musculoskeletal malignancies such as osteosarcoma.

Werner syndrome

A syndrome related to Rothmund–Thomson syndrome by gene homology and clinical overlap, Werner syndrome (adult progeria) is another autosomal recessive disorder and is caused by mutation in the WRN gene on chromosome 8. The resultant RecQ helicase deficiency predisposes to development of a wide variety of malignancies, including osteosarcoma, although soft-tissue sarcomas, thyroid cancer, and melanomas are much more common. Diagnosis is not usually made until adulthood due to manifestations of premature aging (scleroderma, premature graying and alopecia, nonsenile cataracts, calcific valvular deposits, atherosclerosis, diabetes, and hypogonadism) confirmed by genetic testing and elevation of urinary hyaluronic acid level. Orthopedic-associated conditions include osteoporosis, muscle wasting, calcific deposits, and pes planus. For patients with an established diagnosis of Werner syndrome, vigilance should be maintained for the early diagnosis of malignancy.

Key references

The complete reference list can be found on the Wiley Companion Digital Edition of this title (see inside front cover for login instructions).

1 American Cancer Society. *American Cancer Society: Cancer Facts and Figures 2014.* Atlanta: American Cancer Society, http://www.cancer.org/acs/groups/content/@research/documents/webcontent/acspc-042151.pdf; 2014.
2 Damron TA, Ward WG, Stewart A. Osteosarcoma, chondrosarcoma, and Ewing's sarcoma: National Cancer Data Base Report. *Clin Orthop Relat Res.* 2007;**459**:40–47.
3 Fletcher CDM, Bridge JA, Hogendoorn P, Mertens F (eds). *WHO Classification of Tumours of Soft Tissue and Bone,* 4th ed. Lyon, France: WHO Press; 2013.
4 Damron TA (ed.). *Orthopaedic Surgery Essentials: Oncology and Basic Science.* Philadelphia, PA: Lippincott, Williams and Wilkins; 2008.
5 Davies AM, Sundaram M, James SJ (eds). *Imaging of Bone Tumors and Tumor-Like Lesions: Techniques and Applications.* Berlin: Springer Science & Business Media; 2009.
7 Enneking WF, Spanier SS, Goodman MA. A system for the surgical staging of musculoskeletal sarcoma. *Clin Orthop Relat Res.* 1980;**153**:106–120.
10 AJCC. Bone sarcoma. In: *AJCC Cancer Staging Manual,* 7th ed. New York, NY: Springer; 2010.
12 Mankin HJ, Mankin CJ, Simon MA. The hazards of the biopsy, revisited. Members of the Musculoskeletal Tumor Society. *J Bone Joint Surg Am.* 1996;**78**:656–663.

16 Mirels H. Metastatic disease in long bones. *Clin Orthop Relat Res.* 1989;**249**:256–264.
17 Damron TA, Morgan H, Prakash D, Grant W, Aronowitz J, Heiner J. Critical evaluation of Mirel's rating system for impending pathologic fractures. *Clin Orthop Relat Res.* 2003;**415S**:S201–S207.
18 Snyder BD, Hauser-Kara DA, Hipp JA, Zurakowski D, Hecht AC, Gebhardt MC. Predicting fracture through benign skeletal lesions with quantitative computed tomography. *J Bone Joint Surg Am.* 2006;**88**:55–70.
19 Townsend PW, Smalley SR, Cozad SC, Rosenthal HG, Hassanein RE. Role of postoperative radiation therapy after stabilization of fractures caused by metastatic disease. *Int J Radiat Oncol Biol Phys.* 1995;**31**(1):43–49.
22 Hanlon M, Krajbich JI. Rotationplasty in skeletally immature patients. Long-term follow-up results. *Clin Orthop Relat Res.* 1999;**1**(358):75–82.
29 Eckardt JJ, Kabo JM, Kelley CM, et al. Expandable endoprosthesis reconstruction in skeletally immature patients with tumors. *Clin Orthop Relat Res.* 2000;**1**(373):51–61.
32 Hoffman C, Hillmann A, Krakau H, et al. Functional results and quality of life measurements in patients with multimodal treatment of a primary bone tumor located in the distal femur. Rotationplasty versus endoprosthetic replacement. *Med Pediatr Oncol.* 1998;**31**:202–203.
33 Cipriano CA, Gruzinova IS, Frank RM, Gitelis S, Virkus WW. Frequent complications and severe bone loss associated with the repiphysis expandable distal femoral prosthesis. *Clin Orthop Relat Res.* 2014;**473**(3):831–838.
35 Damron TA, Rock MG, O'Connor MI, et al. Functional laboratory assessment after oncologic shoulder joint resections. *Clin Orthop Relat Res.* 1998;**348**:124–134.
36 O'Connor MI, Sim FH, Chao EY. Limb salvage for neoplasms of the shoulder girdle. Intermediate reconstructive and functional results. *J Bone Joint Surg Am.* 1996;**78**(12):1872–1888.
37 O'Connor MI, Sim FH. Salvage of the limb in the treatment of malignant pelvic tumors. *J Bone Joint Surg.* 1989;**71A**:481–494.
42 Malawer MM, Chou LB. Prosthetic survival and clinical results with use of large-segment replacements in the treatment of high-grade bone sarcomas. *J Bone Joint Surg Am.* 1995;**77**:1154–1165.
44 Healey JH, Morris CD, Athanasian EA, Boland PJ. Compress knee arthroplasty has 80% 10-year survivorship and novel forms of bone failure. *Clin Orthop Relat Res.* 2013;**471**(3):774–783. doi: 10.1007/s11999-012-2635-6.
45 Azouz EM, Saigal G, Rodriguez MM, et al. Langerhans' cell histiocytosis: pathology, imaging and treatment of skeletal involvement. *Pediatr Radiol.* 2005;**35**:103–115.
46 Sheppard DG, Libshitz HI. Post-radiation sarcomas: a review of the clinical and imaging features in 63 cases. *Clin Radiol.* 2001;**56**(1):22–29.
47 Cannon CP, Lin PP, Lewis VO, Yasko AW. Management of radiation-associated fractures. *J Am Acad Orthop Surg.* 2008;**16**(9):541–549.
48 Body JJ. Bisphosphonates for malignancy-related bone disease: current status, future developments. *Support Care Cancer.* 2006;**14**(5):408–418.
49 Shane E, Burr D, Abrahamsen B, et al. Atypical subtrochanteric and diaphyseal femoral fractures: second report of a task force of the American Society for Bone and Mineral Research. *J Bone Miner Res.* 2014;**29**(1):1–23. doi: 10.1002/jbmr.1998. Epub 2013 Oct 1.
50 Levy JC, Temple HT, Mollabashy A, et al. The causes of pain in benign solitary enchondromas of the proximal humerus. *Clin Orthop Relat Res.* 2005;**431**:181–186.
51 Springfield DS, Capanna R, Gherlinzoni F, et al. Chondroblastoma: A review of seventy cases. *J Bone Joint Surg Am.* 1985;**67**:748–755.
53 Wu CT, Inwards CY, O'Laughlin S, et al. Chondromyxoid fibroma of bone: a clinicopathologic review of 278 cases. *Hum Pathol.* 1998;**29**:438–446.
56 Chapurlat RD. Medical therapy in adults with fibrous dysplasia of bone. *J Bone Miner Res.* 2006;**21**(**Suppl 2**):P114–P119.
58 Lee RS, Weitzel S, Eastwood DM, et al. Osteofibrous dysplasia of the tibia. Is there a need for a radical surgical approach? *J Bone Joint Surg (Br).* 2006;**88**(5):658–664.
59 O'Donnell RJ, Springfield DS, Morwani HK, et al. Recurrence of giant cell tumors of the long bones after curettage and packing with cement. *J Bone Joint Surg Am.* 1994;**76**(12):1827–1833.
61 Xu SF, Adams B, Yu XC, Xu M. Denosumab and giant cell tumour of bone-a review and future management considerations. *Curr Oncol.* 2013;**20**(5):e442–e447. doi: 10.3747/co.20.1497.
64 Greenspan A. Benign bone-forming lesions: osteoma, osteoid osteoma, and osteoblastoma. Clinical, imaging, pathologic, and differential considerations. *Skeletal Radiol.* 1993;**22**:485–500.
65 Rimondi E, Bianchi G, Malaguti MC, et al. Radiofrequency thermoablation of primary non-spinal osteoid osteoma: optimization of the procedure. *Eur Radiol.* 2005;**15**:1393–1399.
66 Ramirez AR, Stanton RP. Aneurysmal bone cyst in 29 children. *J Pediatr Orthop.* 2002;**22**(4):533–539.

71 Wright JG, Yandow S, Donaldson S, Marley L, Simple Bone Cyst Trial Group. A randomized clinical trial comparing intralesional bone marrow and steroid injections for simple bone cysts. *J Bone Joint Surg Am*. 2008;**90**(**4**): 722–730.

72 Allen CE, McClain KL. Langerhans cell histiocytosis: a review of past, current and future therapies. *Drugs Today (Barc)*. 2007;**43**(**9**):627–643.

78 Verdegaal SH, Brouwers HF, van Zwet EW, Hogendoorn PC, Taminiau AH. Low-grade chondrosarcoma of long bones treated with intralesional curettage followed by application of phenol, ethanol, and bone-grafting. *J Bone Joint Surg Am*. 2012;**94**(**13**):1201–1207. doi: 10.2106/JBJS.J.01498.

85 Weber KL. Current concepts in the treatment of Ewing's sarcoma. *Expert Rev Anticancer Ther*. 2002;**2**(**6**):687–694.

112 Soft tissue sarcomas

Robert G. Maki, MD, PhD, FACP ▪ Chandrajit P. Raut, MD, MSc, FACS ▪ Brian O'Sullivan, MD, FRCPI, FRCPC

Overview

The management of soft tissue sarcomas is driven by the anatomic site and histology of the primary and is increasingly affected by the specific genetics of the sarcoma. In this chapter, we focus on the principles of management of this group of over 50 cancer subtypes to highlight commonalities and differences from anatomical constraints of surgery to specifics of adjuvant radiation to identification of systemic therapeutics that are appropriate for each histology.

We will discuss in this chapter the etiology, presentation, diagnosis, staging, and multidisciplinary management of patients with sarcomas of soft tissue. Surgery remains paramount to achieve cure for the vast majority of sarcomas. Radiation therapy is used for larger tumors in the appropriate clinical context. The evolution of increasingly sophisticated radiation techniques is highlighted in this chapter. As pertains to systemic therapy, this chapter is written at a time in which first-line therapies for soft tissue sarcomas may change, raising anew some questions of adjuvant therapy that remain incompletely answered. Where appropriate, we attempt to link specific histologies or molecular changes to therapeutic suggestions, with the understanding and hope that novel agents will supplant the medications that are available but that have not materially affected outcomes for few diagnoses other than GIST in the past several years.

Sarcomas of nonosseous tissues, known traditionally as soft tissue sarcomas (STS), comprise a group of rare malignancies that exhibit tremendous diversity of anatomic site, specific genetic alterations, and histopathologic characteristics. These tumors share a common embryologic origin, arising primarily from mesodermal tissues. The notable exceptions are sarcomas of the neural tissues [such as malignant peripheral nerve sheath tumors (MPNST)] and possibly the Ewing sarcoma/primitive neuroectodermal tumor (PNET) family of tumors, which are believed to arise from ectoderm and angiosarcomas, which are derived from endoderm. Despite the fact that the somatic nonosseous tissues account for as much as 75% of total body weight, primary neoplasms of these connective tissues are comparatively rare, accounting for <1% of adult malignancies and 15% of pediatric malignancies. About 12,000 people receive a diagnosis of STS in the United States each year, with approximately 5000 deaths annually.[1] An understanding of these cancers is important because patients' outcomes will be compromised if initial management is not thoughtful. Furthermore, biologic insights about sarcomas are providing new strategies for the detection, treatment, and prevention of more common malignancies.

This chapter reviews current concepts in the diagnosis, staging, and multidisciplinary management of patients with sarcomas of nonosseous tissues. The evolving contributions of molecular biology and basic scientific principles underlying the varied differentiation and clinical behavior of these tumors will also be reviewed. Although histopathologic aspects of sarcomas are increasingly important in categorizing these tumors, the anatomic site of primary disease remains an important variable on which treatment and outcome may depend. Extremity sarcomas account for approximately 50% of all sarcomas and are the primary focus of the therapy sections of this chapter. Special topics such as retroperitoneal sarcomas (RPS), gastrointestinal stromal tumors (GISTs), and dermatofibrosarcoma protuberans (DFSPs) are addressed separately later in this chapter. Sarcomas at other anatomic sites are not discussed because of their rarity. Throughout the chapter, the emphasis is on identifying what is known from definitive data and what requires additional research.

Etiology

Most sarcomas are believed to arise spontaneously, as may be increasingly understood for many cancers in general.[2] The conceptual frameworks that address the neoplastic transformation of mesenchymal stem cells are in rapid evolution owing to new insights from the molecular analysis of sarcomatous and normal tissues from STS patients and family members. Genetics and environmental factors appear to play a role in the neoplastic transformation of soft tissues into sarcomas.[3]

It has been recognized for more than 30 years that sarcomas can arise in persons with certain genetic predispositions to cancer development. One of the earliest observations of familial cancer development (i.e., genetically transmitted predisposition to malignancy) was the development of sarcoma and other tumor types (such as breast cancer) in certain families.[4] This autosomal dominant genetic predisposition has now become known as the Li–Fraumeni syndrome, and it has been characterized at the molecular level as a germline mutation of the *TP53* gene, which presumably acts in this context as a faulty tumor suppressor.[5,6]

Other genetic disorders are also associated with an increased risk of developing specific sarcomas. The best-studied example of this is the predilection of patients with neurofibromatoses to develop (MPNSTs, also referred to as neurofibrosarcomas or malignant schwannomas).[7,8] Type 1 neurofibromatosis (von Recklinghausen disease) is an autosomal dominant disease that can disrupt the function of the *NF1* gene, located on chromosome 17q11.2. The endogenous function of the *NF1* gene product, neurofibromin, remains incompletely understood, but it appears to act as a tumor suppressor via stimulation of guanosine triphosphatase activity. Common mutations in *NF1* include truncations, with loss of function leading to uncontrolled signaling through *ras* pathways, which impact on therapeutic options.[9,10] *NF1* loss appears to be a fundamental process that facilitates the development of MPNSTs over time in patients with neurofibromatosis. Patients with type 1 neurofibromatosis have up to a 10% cumulative lifetime risk of developing sarcoma (usually MPNST); it is unclear why the risk is

Holland-Frei Cancer Medicine, Ninth Edition. Edited by Robert C. Bast Jr., Carlo M. Croce, William N. Hait, Waun Ki Hong, Donald W. Kufe, Martine Piccart-Gebhart, Raphael E. Pollock, Ralph R. Weichselbaum, Hongyang Wang, and James F. Holland.
© 2017 John Wiley & Sons, Inc. ISBN: 978-1-118-93469-2

not greater, given the protean effects of *ras* activation; other factors such as inactivation of epigenetic regulators in the PRC2 complex may contribute to the neoplastic phenotype.[11–13]

Survivors of childhood retinoblastoma have also been noted to have an increased risk of sarcoma development later in life.[14,15] These data provide another model of a dysfunctional or deleted tumor suppressor genetic element (in this case, the product of the *Rb* gene on chromosome 13q14). The risk of STS in retinoblastoma patients and their families is accompanied by the risk of developing several other types of neoplasms, including osteosarcomas, breast cancer, and lung cancer. No reasons have been convincingly posited for the development of one type of malignancy over another in patients with *Rb* mutations, and this remains an important question to be addressed by future research on mechanisms of neoplastic transformation.

Gardner syndrome represents an important genetic connection between dysfunctional regulation of epithelial and mesenchymal cells. Gardner syndrome represents a subset of familial adenomatous polyposis disorders of the bowel (usually the colon); patients with the syndrome also have extracolonic abnormalities such as epidermoid cysts and osteomas. The molecular lesion has been identified as a defect within the *APC* (adenomatous polyposis coli) gene on chromosome 5q21. Patients with Gardner syndrome are at much increased risk of developing mesenteric and intraperitoneal desmoid tumors.[16,17] Desmoid tumors are mesenchymal cells proliferating in a pattern of aggressive fibromatosis, characterized by bland cells that—although histologically benign—act in a malignant manner with uncontrolled proliferation and infiltration of vital structures; spontaneous desmoid tumors more commonly demonstrate the β-catenin gene, *CTNNB1*, which is in the same signaling pathway as APC.[18,19] It remains poorly understood why some patients with Gardner syndrome develop desmoid tumors whereas others do not, and the lifetime risk of developing desmoid tumors has been estimated at approximately 10–20%, representing a nearly 1000 times greater risk than that of the general population.

Certain environmental exposures have also been associated with the development of sarcomas. One of the most important is ionizing radiation. Radiation-associated sarcoma is most often a late effect of radiotherapy (RT) given to treat another condition (often a prior malignancy). Sarcomas have been noted as a late effect of RT for breast cancer, Hodgkin lymphoma, non-Hodgkin lymphomas, and other tumor types.[20] The radiation dose appears to be correlated with the later development of sarcoma, with a very low risk in patients who received <10 Gy. The molecular mechanisms may be complex, as it has been noted clinically that sarcomas appear at the margins of prior RT fields. This suggests that the mutagenic effect may be maximal at the edges of prior RT where scatter radiation leads to a dose sufficient to induce mutations but insufficient to kill the mutated cells. Traditionally, radiation-associated sarcomas were thought to arise with a median of ~9 years following RT, although RT-associated sarcomas are observed earlier in some patients. MPNSTs, angiosarcomas, osteosarcomas, and undifferentiated pleomorphic sarcomas (UPS) comprise the majority of radiation-associated sarcomas. Clinical outcomes are worse in patients with radiation-associated sarcomas compared to histology-matched controls. Radiation-associated sarcomas should be approached as new primary disease and treated appropriately to optimize the patient's outcomes.

Certain chemical exposures have also been weakly linked to sarcomagenesis, although chemical-induced development of sarcomas in animal models is one of the more reliable models of studying neoplastic transformation in the laboratory. Hepatic angiosarcomas are associated with exposure to several classes of chemicals, such as polyvinyl chloride and arsenic compounds.[21] The relationship between exposure and development of sarcoma is more tenuous for other compounds, including dioxins (such as Agent Orange and other phenoxyacetic acid-based herbicides) and chlorophenols used in wood preservatives.[22]

Chronic irritation or inflammation of tissues is a controversial potential cause of sarcomas. Certainly, there is an increased sarcoma risk in the lymphedematous arms of women who have undergone radical mastectomy (the Stewart–Treves syndrome), often with the additional complicating variable of prior RT.[23,24] Limited data, typically case reports only, suggest that other sources of chronic tissue irritation and inflammation might be associated with sarcomagenesis.[25] Although a history of trauma is not infrequently elicited from patients with STSs, the impact of such trauma on sarcoma development is dubious.

Severe and chronic immunosuppression following solid organ transplantation represents yet another risk factor for the development of sarcomas. Sarcomas represent a disproportionate percentage of tumors (10%) in patients following solid organ transplantation, with Kaposi sarcoma comprising the majority of these.[26,27]

Screening

Given the rarity of sarcomas in the general population, no general screening is indicated beyond routine health care surveillance. However, it is important for physicians to be aware of the predisposing genetic tendencies and environmental exposures that might increase patients' risk of sarcoma development. A complete family history should reveal clues about genetic predispositions, including a family history of polyposis, neurofibromatosis, retinoblastoma, any cancer at a young age in first-degree relatives, or sarcomas. Genetic counseling is appropriate to discuss issues relating to these predispositions, in particular given the finding of Li–Fraumeni-like families that lack canonical *TP53* mutations.[28] In patients at increased risk of sarcoma, a more detailed clinical evaluation might be required at a lower threshold of intervention than one might use in general practice. Rapidly growing masses, especially symptomatic ones, in patients with neurofibromatosis should be considered for surgical removal to rule out the potential of sarcomatous transformation of a neurofibroma. Similarly, any superficial or deep abnormalities of skin or soft tissues in patients with a history of prior RT should be evaluated very thoroughly.

Clinical presentation, classification, and diagnosis

Sites of origin

Sarcomas of nonosseous tissues have been noted to arise at virtually all anatomic sites. The anatomic sites and site-specific histologic subtypes of more than 5113 sarcomas treated at a single referral institution are outlined in Figure 1. Approximately one-third to one-half of all sarcomas of nonosseous tissues occur in the lower extremities, where the most common histopathologic subtypes have traditionally been noted to include liposarcomas and the entity "UPS", formerly termed malignant fibrous histiocytoma (MFH). With improved pathologic tools to categorize sarcomas (e.g., immunohistochemistry, DNA, and RNA analyses), it is increasingly recognized that UPS may have some features in common with poorly differentiated liposarcomas or leiomyosarcomas, as well as other histologic subtypes.[29] RPSs comprise 15–20%

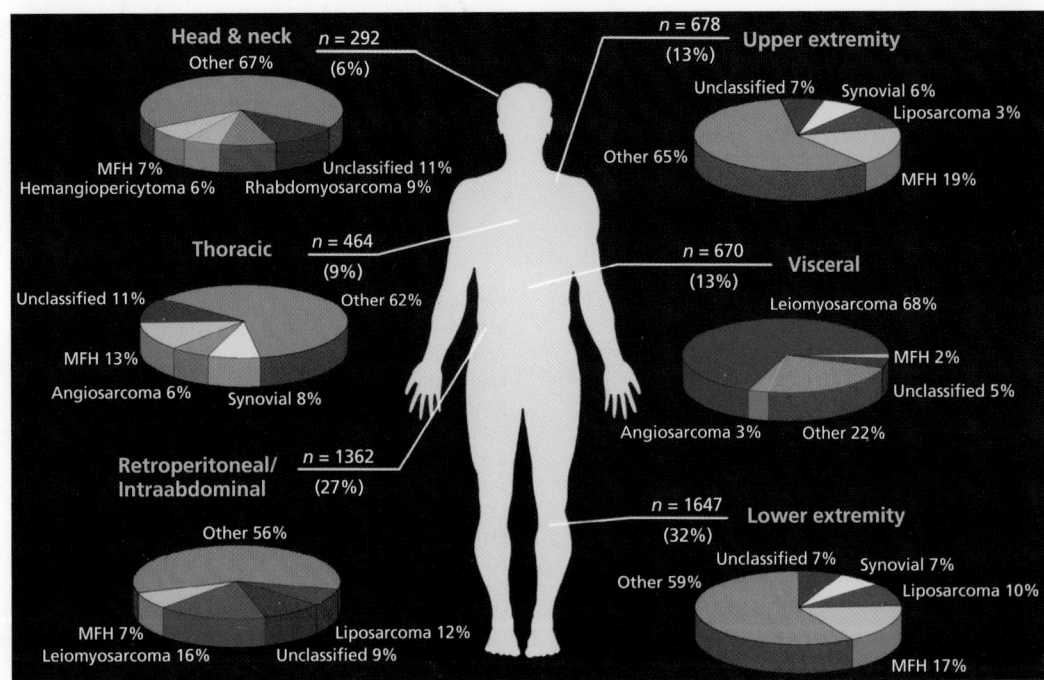

Figure 1 Anatomic distribution and site-specific histologic subtypes of 5113 consecutive STSs seen at the University of Texas MD Anderson Cancer Center Sarcoma Center. Source: Data from MDACC Sarcoma Database, June 1996 to June 2005.

of all STSs, with well-differentiated/dedifferentiated liposarcoma and leiomyosarcoma being the predominant histologic subtypes. Visceral sarcomas make up an additional 24%, and the head and neck sarcomas approximately 4% of sarcomas.

Clinical presentation

The majority of patients with nonosseous sarcomas present with a painless mass, although pain is noted at presentation in up to one-third of cases.[30] Delay in diagnosis of sarcomas is common, with the most common incorrect diagnosis for extremity and trunk lesions being hematoma or "lipoma." Late diagnosis of RPS is extremely common, as tumors in this area can grow to massive size before causing any symptoms (such as abdominal distention or psoas irritation with back or groin discomfort) or functional compromise such as hydronephrosis from ureteric obstruction.

Physical examination should include an assessment of the size and mobility of the mass. Its relationship to the fascia (superficial vs deep) and nearby neurovascular and bony structures should be noted. A site-specific neurovascular examination and assessment of regional lymph nodes should also be performed. Sarcomas rarely metastasize to lymph nodes, with those that do being limited to a few specific histopathologic subtypes. Presence of true nodal metastases should prompt the clinician to investigate whether the diagnosis of sarcoma is accurate.

Histopathologic classification

Methods of classification
In broad terms, sarcomas can be classified as neoplasms arising in bone versus those arising from the nonosseous or periosseous soft tissues. Sarcomas of nonosseous tissues can be further grouped into those that arise from the viscera (e.g., gastrointestinal or gynecologic organs) and those that originate in nonvisceral soft tissues such as muscle, tendon, adipose tissue, pleura, synovium, and other connective tissues.

The most universally applied classification scheme for STS is based on histogenesis, as outlined in the recently updated WHO (World Health Organization) sarcoma classification system.[31] This classification system is reproducible between pathologists for the better differentiated tumors. However, as the degree of histologic differentiation declines, the determination of cellular origin becomes increasingly difficult. For example, pathologists may vary in their criteria to consider a tumor a UPS versus a poorly differentiated leiomyosarcoma; the use of specific DNA tests and ready availability of an increasing battery of immunohistochemical markers have improved consistency in diagnosis. Nonetheless, the lack of familiarity with sarcomas in general leads to misdiagnosis in up to 20% of outside cases reviewed at reference centers.

Difficulties in establishing the specific cellular origin of STS have occasionally been viewed as having limited clinical importance because clinical investigators have not had sufficient data to tie the histologic subtype directly to biologic behavior or to specific therapeutic interventions. Important exceptions to this generalization include epithelioid sarcoma, clear cell sarcoma, angiosarcoma, and embryonal rhabdomyosarcoma, all of which have a greater risk of regional lymph node metastasis.[32,33] In a single-institution study, the overall rate of nodal metastasis at the time of presentation was only 2.7%; however, the rate was much higher for specific histologic subtypes: angiosarcoma (13%), embryonal rhabdomyosarcoma (14%), and epithelioid sarcoma (17%).[32] Thus, treatment strategies may differ for these. For the remaining histologic subtypes, biologic behavior appears to be determined more by histologic grade than by histologic subtype. However, as the fundamental biologic and molecular understanding of the mechanisms of malignant transformation in sarcomas increases, in-depth categorization may well prove to have important clinical ramifications. The tools required to categorize or subclassify sarcomas at the molecular level are now increasingly available for many sarcoma subtypes, including GIST, synovial sarcoma, liposarcoma,

Table 1 Selected cytogenetic aberrations in nonosseous sarcomas.

Histologic subtype	Cytogenetic finding	Genes
Myxoid liposarcoma	t(12;16)	*FUS-DDIT3*
Well-differentiated liposarcoma	Rings and giant markers	Amplified 12q13–15
		HMG1C
		CDK4
		HDM2
Lipoma (minimal atypia)	12q abnormalities	Amplified 12q13–15
Lipoma	12q14-15 abnormalities	
	6p abnormalities	
Synovial sarcoma	t(X;18)	*SS18-SSX1, SSX2* or *SSX4*
Ewing's family/PNET	t(11;22) and others	*EWSR1-FLI1* and others
Rhabdomyosarcoma	t(2;13) or t(1;13)	*PAX3(or 7)-FOXO1* (alveolar)
Clear cell sarcoma	t(12;22)	*EWSR1-ATF1*
Extraskeletal myxoid chondrosarcomas	t(9;22)	*EWSR1-NR4A3*
	t(9;17)	*TAF15-NR4A3*
Dermatofibrosarcoma protuberans	t(17;22)	*COL1A1-PDGFB*
Endometrial stromal sarcoma (low grade)	t(7;17)	*JAZF1-SUZ12*
Desmoplastic small round-cell tumor	t(11;22)	*EWSR1-WT1*
Alveolar sarcoma of soft parts	t(X;17)	*ASPSCR1-TFE3*

Abbreviation: PNET, primitive neuroectodermal tumors.

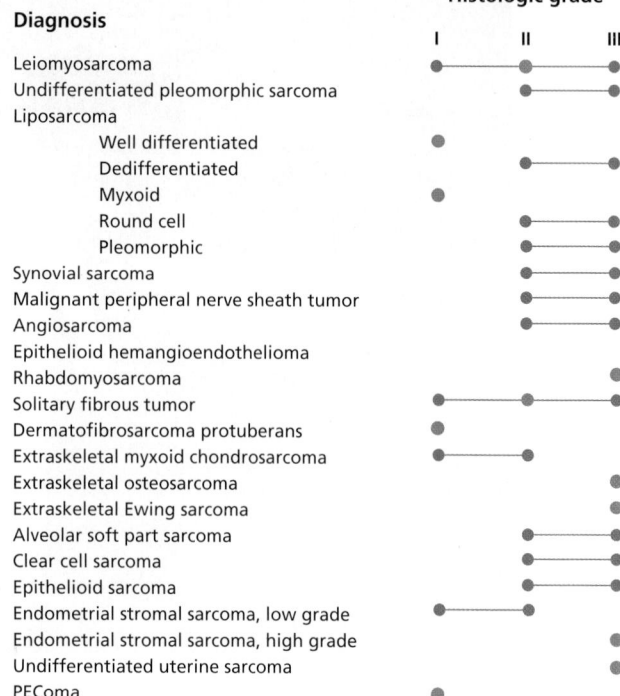

Figure 2 Spectrum of grades observed among histologic subtypes of STS. Source: From Ref. 35. Adapted from Enzinger FN and Weiss SW, editors. Soft tissue tumors. 5th ed. Mosby-Year Book Inc; 2008.

Ewing sarcoma/PNET, and rhabdomyosarcomas (Table 1). Future clinical trials will need to take histologic and molecular characteristics into account in a more sophisticated manner than in the past three decades of research when markers were not so readily available.

Histologic grade

Biologic aggressiveness can often be predicted based on histologic grade.[34] The spectrum of grades varies among specific histologic subtypes (Figure 2). In careful comparative multivariate analyses, histologic grade has been the most important prognostic factor in assessing the risk of distant metastasis and tumor-related death.[34,36] Several grading systems have been proposed, but there is no consensus regarding the specific morphologic criteria that should be employed in the grading of STS.

Two of the most commonly employed grading systems, both first published in 1984, are the US National Cancer Institute (NCI) system developed by Costa and colleagues and the system developed by the Federation Nationale des Centres de Lutte Contre le Cancer (FNCLCC) Sarcoma Group.[29,30,37] The NCI system is based on the tumor's histologic subtype, location, and amount of tumor necrosis, but cellularity, nuclear pleomorphism, and mitosis count are also to be considered in certain situations. The FNCLCC system employs a score generated by the evaluation of three parameters: tumor differentiation, mitotic rate, and amount of tumor necrosis. In a retrospective comparison of these two grading systems, in a population of 410 adult patients with nonmetastatic STS, univariate and multivariate analyses suggested that the FNCLCC system has a slightly better ability to predict distant metastasis and tumor-related death.[38] Significant discrepancies in assigned grade were observed in one-third of cases. An increased number of grade 3 tumors, reduced number of grade 2 tumors, and better correlation with overall and metastasis-free survival were observed in favor of the FNCLCC system. The FNCLCC system is the best presently

available grading system and is employed as part of the AJCC/UICC STS staging system, with the caveat that several new diagnostic categories have been identified since 1984 whose histological grades are undefined by FNCLCC criteria.

In discussing grade, it is important to note well-described characteristics of sarcomas. First, there is often substantial intratumoral heterogeneity within individual sarcomas. Therefore, diagnoses based on very limited amounts of tumor may be inaccurate [e.g., diagnoses based only on fine-needle aspiration (FNA) biopsy specimens]. This is particularly true for such histopathologic subtypes as dedifferentiated liposarcomas, where one area of the tumor might have a relatively low-to-intermediate-grade appearance and another area within the same tumor might have high-grade components more evident. Any discussion of the clinical relevance of grading must take into account this variability inherent in the diagnostic process, which will add to the clinical variability in outcomes among patients with any given grade of sarcomas.

Second, the grade of tumors may evolve over time. This process is best described in the evolution of dedifferentiated liposarcoma arising in conjunction with well-differentiated liposarcoma in the same patient. Additional examples include the round-cell liposarcoma growing from what was previously myxoid liposarcoma and fibrosarcomatous degeneration that will occasionally accompany multiply recurrent DFSPs.

Imaging

Optimal imaging of the primary tumor is dependent on the anatomic site. For soft tissue masses of the extremities, trunk, and occasionally head and neck, magnetic resonance imaging (MRI) generally has been regarded as the imaging modality of choice

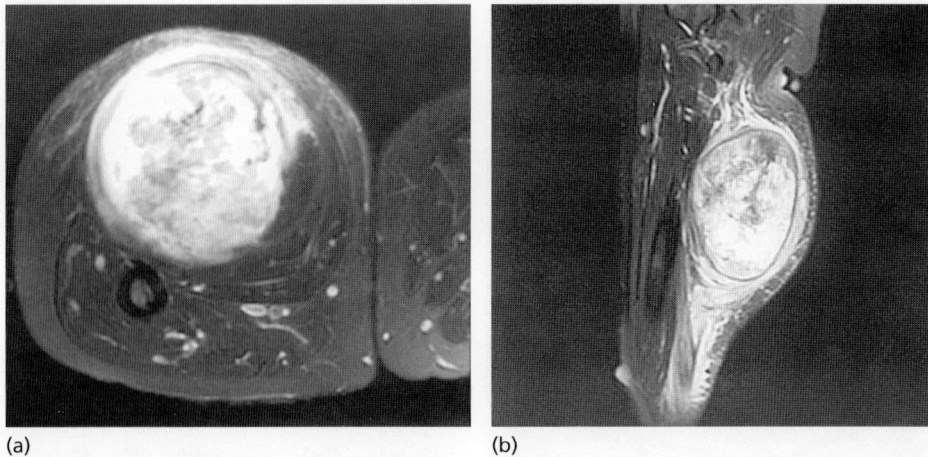

(a)   (b)

Figure 3 (a) Weighted T2-fat-saturated magnetic resonance image of a TNM T2b high-grade sarcoma in the posterior thigh compartment of a 55-year-old woman. Note the containment by the superficial fascia overlying the posterior thigh muscles, where there is a "strip" of peritumoral edema. Anteriorly, the lesion can be seen to be separate from the femur, but the edge of the tumor is less clearly defined than its superficial component, presumably because of muscle infiltration. (b) Sagittal MRI of the same patient. The main lesion manifests a well-defined border. However, a clear zone of peritumoral edema is evident tracking proximally toward the head of the femur, seen at the top of the figure. Inferiorly, the edema seems to be even more pronounced as evidenced by the triangular signal enhancement pointing inferiorly. Whether the zone of edema harbors microscopic disease is uncertain, and this uncertainty can complicate accurate treatment planning (see text).

(Figures 3 and 4) because MRI enhances the contrast between tumor and muscle and between tumor and adjacent blood vessels and provides multiplanar definition of the lesion.[39] However, a study by the Radiation Diagnostic Oncology Group that compared MRI and computed tomography (CT) in patients with malignant bone ($n = 183$) and soft tissue ($n = 133$) tumors demonstrated no specific advantage of MRI over CT.[40] That said, although it may be true that the diagnostic evaluation is equally served by both modalities, surgery and RT planning may require additional information provided by the multiplanar capability of MRI and the ability to perform MRI/CT image fusion.[41,42] For pelvic lesions or evaluation of specific fixed organs, such as the rectum or the liver, the multiplanar capability of MRI may provide superior single-modality imaging (Figure 4), whereas in the retroperitoneum and abdomen, CT usually provides satisfactory anatomic definition of the lesion. Occasionally, MRI with gradient sequence imaging can better delineate the relationship of a tumor to midline vascular structures, particularly the inferior vena cava and aorta (Figure 5). More invasive studies such as angiography or cavography are rarely used in evaluation of STS.

Cost-effective imaging to exclude the possibility of distant metastatic disease is dependent on the size, grade, and anatomic location of the primary tumor. In general, patients with low- and intermediate-grade tumors or high-grade tumors 5 cm or less in diameter require only a chest radiograph for satisfactory staging of the chest. This directly reflects the comparatively low risk of presentation with pulmonary metastases in these patients.[43,44] However, patients with high-grade tumors larger than 5 cm (T2) should undergo more thorough staging of the chest by CT owing to the increased risk of presentation with established metastatic disease in this group.[44,45] Patients with RPS and intra-abdominal visceral sarcomas should undergo imaging of the liver to exclude the possibility of synchronous hepatic metastases; the liver is a more common site of first metastasis from these lesions. CT is usually adequate in these patients to assess the liver, although the increased sensitivity of MRI of the liver may be valuable if any questionable findings are noted on initial CT.

Positron emission tomography (PET) scans may be used selectively to look for extent of disease, particularly when evaluating an ambiguous lesion that could represent a potential metastasis noted on other imaging. However, PET scans are not routinely utilized in staging work-up of STS.

Biopsy

Biopsy of the primary tumor is essential for most patients presenting with soft tissue masses. In general, any soft tissue mass in an adult that is enlarging (even if asymptomatic), is larger than 5 cm, or persists beyond 4–6 weeks should be biopsied. The preferred biopsy approach is generally the least invasive technique required to allow a definitive histologic diagnosis, assessment of grade. In most centers, core-needle biopsy provides sufficient tissue for diagnosis and results in substantial cost savings compared with open surgical biopsy.[46,47] When core-needle biopsy yields insufficient tissue for diagnosis, incisional biopsy is considered to yield optimal amounts of tissue to assess histopathology over a larger area of tumor volume, given the known heterogeneity of sarcomas, as well as to provide sufficient material for detailed molecular and cytogenetic assays. Direct palpation can be used to guide needle biopsy of most superficial lesions, but less accessible sarcomas often require imaging-guided biopsy for safe percutaneous sampling of the most radiographically suspicious area(s) of the mass. Tumor recurrences within the needle track after percutaneous biopsy are exceedingly rare but have been reported, leading some physicians to advocate tattooing the biopsy site for subsequent excision. FNA generally does not provide sufficient material for initial diagnosis, but can be used to confirm recurrence or metastatic disease. Exceptions to this idea exist; endoscopic ultrasound-guided FNA for visceral sarcomas such as GISTs may provide enough tissue for diagnosis while minimizing risk of tumor rupture; in this scenario, it is not feasible to assess mitotic rate. The need for sufficient tissue to conduct more specific molecular testing is a final major rationale for use of core-needle biopsy over FNA. Another major limitation of FNA (compared to core-needle biopsy) is that there is no semblance

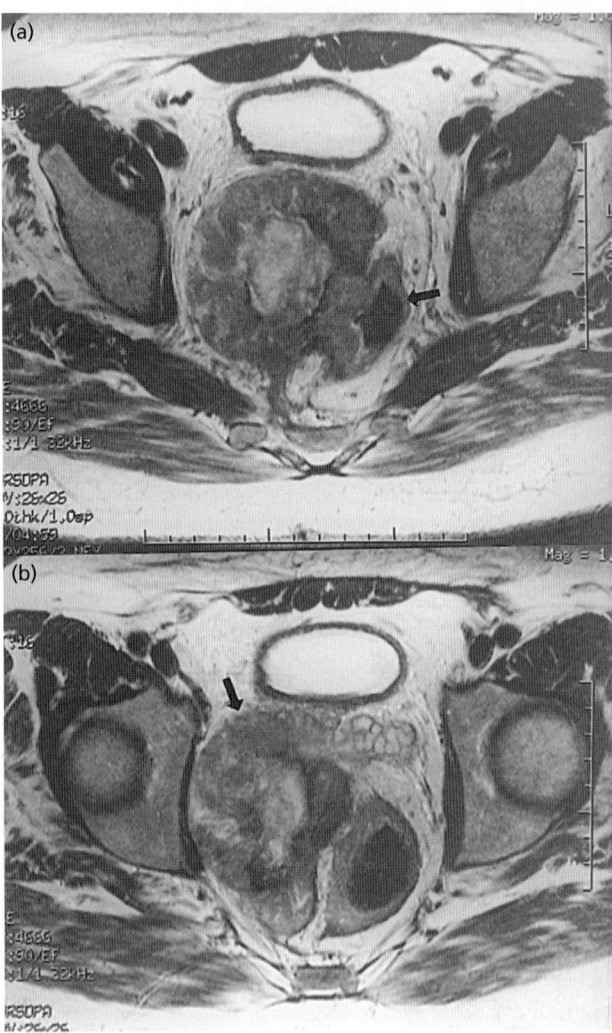

Figure 4 A 57-year-old man with T2 pelvic leiomyosarcoma. (a) Axial T2-weighted fast spin-echo MRI reveals a heterogeneous mass involving the rectum (arrow, air in rectal lumen). (b) Note that the mass abuts right seminal vesicle (arrow).

of preserved tissue architecture to evaluate characteristics such as degree of tissue necrosis.

A practical approach for biopsy and staging of the patient who presents with a primary extremity soft tissue mass is outlined in Figure 6. Small (<5 cm) superficial lesions on an extremity where the morbidity of excisional biopsy is minimal (i.e., remote from joints, tendons, and neurovascular structures that would compromise the surgical margin) are easily biopsied by excisional biopsy with microscopic assessment of surgical margins. For extremity lesions, incisions used for excisional biopsies should be oriented longitudinally along the length of the limb. T2 lesions, T1 lesions located beneath the investing fascia of the extremity, or superficial T1 lesions situated in proximity to joints, tendons, or neurovascular structures are best biopsied by percutaneous core-needle biopsy.

Staging and prognostic factors

Staging

The relative rarity of STS, the anatomic heterogeneity of these lesions, and the presence of more than 50 recognized histologic subtypes of variable grades have made it difficult to establish a

Table 2 American Joint Committee on cancer staging system for STSs, 7th edition.

TX	Primary tumor cannot be assessed					
T0	No evidence of primary tumor					
T1	Tumor 5 cm or less in greatest dimension					
T1a	Superficial tumor					
T1b	Deep tumor					
T2	Tumor more than 5 cm in greatest dimension					
T2a	Superficial tumor					
T2b	Deep tumor					
N1	Regional lymph node metastasis					
G1	Well differentiated					
G2	Moderately differentiated					
G3	Poorly differentiated					
G4	Poorly differentiated or undifferentiated (four-tiered systems only)					
Stage I	T1a, 1b, 2a, 2b	N0	M0	G1–2	G1	Low
Stage II	T1a, 1b, 2a	N0	M0	G3–4	G2–3	High
Stage III	T2b	N0	M0	G3–4	G2–3	High
Stage IV	Any T	N1	M0	Any G	Any G	High or low
	Any T	N0	M1	Any G	Any G	High or low

Source: Edge et al. 2010.[49] Reproduced with permission of Springer.

functional system that can accurately stage all forms of this disease. The staging system (7th edition) of the American Joint Committee on Cancer (AJCC) and the Union for International Cancer Control is the most widely employed staging system for STS (Table 2).[49] The system is designed to optimally stage extremity tumors but is also applicable to torso, head and neck, and retroperitoneal lesions; a separate staging system is provided for GISTs.

A major limitation of the present staging system is that it does not take into account the anatomic site of STS. Anatomic site, however, has been recognized as an important determinant of outcome.[50,51] Therefore, although site is not a specific component of any present staging system, outcome data should be reported on a site-specific basis, when feasible. Furthermore, the staging system also fails to include histology, a critical prognostic factor.

Conventional prognostic factors

A thorough understanding of the clinicopathologic factors known to impact outcome is essential in formulating a treatment plan for the patient with STS. Several multivariate analyses of prognostic factors for patients with localized sarcoma have been reported.[52–54] However, with few exceptions, most studies have analyzed fewer than 300 patients.

The largest studies established the clinical profile of what is now accepted as the high-risk patient with extremity STS: the patient with a large (≥5 cm), high-grade, deep lesion. In addition, unappreciated prognostic significance includes specific histologic subtypes, for example, MPNST, and the increased risk of adverse outcome associated with a microscopically positive surgical margin or presentation with locally recurrent disease. The type of microscopically positive surgical margins also appears important. Patients with low-grade liposarcomas have a relatively low risk of local recurrence (LR), as do those patients in whom the positive margin is planned before surgery to preserve critical structures and RT can sterilize the small amount of residual disease. However, patients with two categories of positive margin remain at relatively higher risk of LR. These include patients who underwent "unplanned" excision and still have positive margins on re-excision and those with unanticipated positive margins after primary resection.[55] An "unplanned excision" is defined as an excisional biopsy or resection carried out without adequate preoperative staging or consideration of the need to remove normal tissue around the tumor.

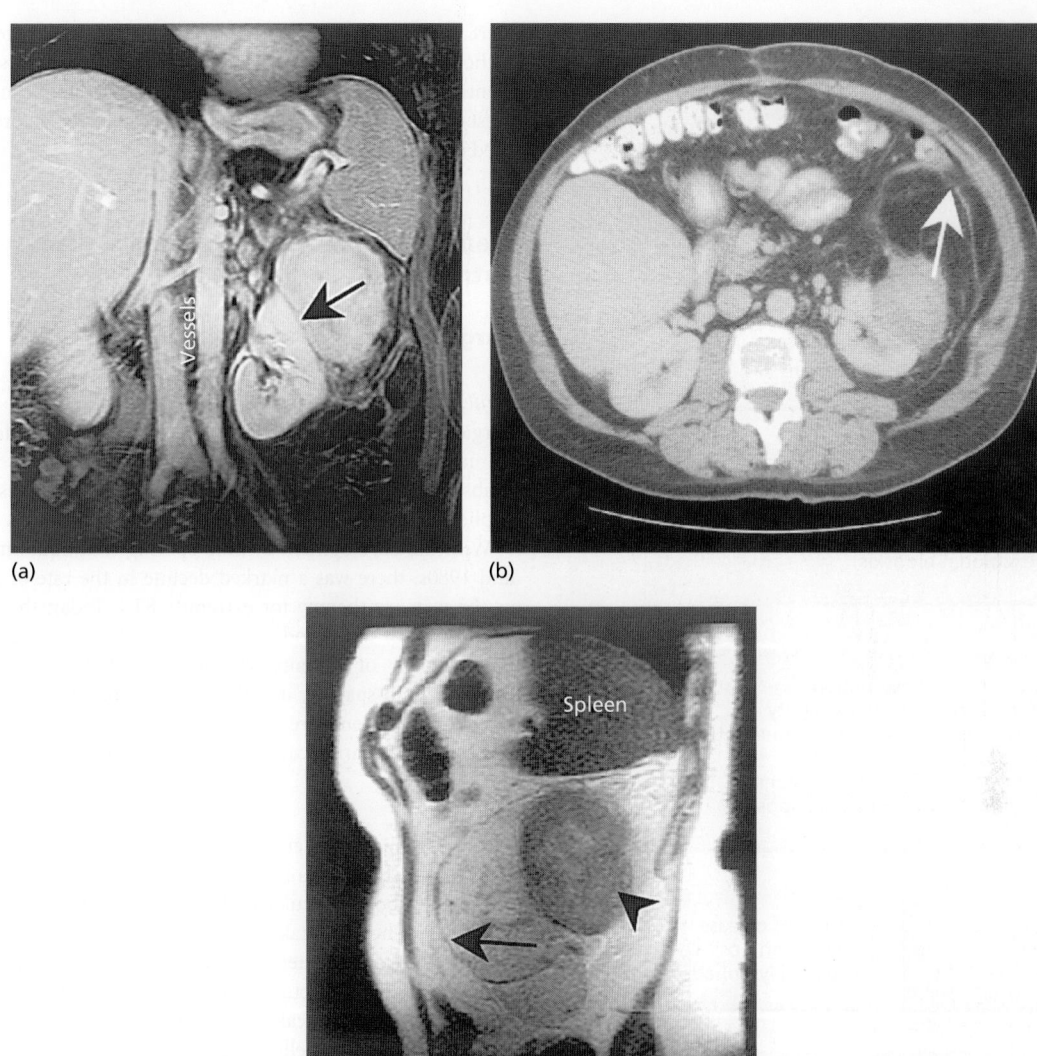

Figure 5 (a) Coronal fat-saturated gadolinium-enhanced MRI showing a solid liposarcoma, 8.3 cm × 6.6 cm, adjacent to and compressing the upper pole of the left kidney. The mass lies below the spleen and is separate from the kidney (line of demarcation, arrow), but is part of a larger fatty tumor. The midline vessels are well visualized. (b) CT image of the same lesion. The mass can be seen adjacent to the kidney, as before. An additional mass of fatty attenuation with gray areas of edema, inflammation, or increased cellularity can be seen bounded by a rim anteriorly (arrow). This mass has the appearance of abnormal fat, which must be considered in treatment planning. Note the displacement of the bowel containing contrast. (c) Sagittal MR image of the same case but without gadolinium. The potential advantage of MR imaging in separating the anterior edge of the retroperitoneal sarcoma (long arrow) from the normal fat anteriorly is seen. The more solid component can also be seen (arrowhead) inferior to the spleen. In addition, these images can be exported digitally to a three-dimensional RT treatment planning workstation or CT simulator workstation where the MR images can be fused to the CT planning slices. This can provide more accurate demonstration of tumor in selected cases for contouring the GTV and clinical target volume than may be possible with CT images alone. This is particularly helpful in situations where CT as well as MRI does not show tumor.

Unlike for other solid tumors, the adverse prognostic factors for LR of an STS are distinct from those that predict distant metastasis and tumor-related death.[52] In other words, patients with a constellation of adverse prognostic factors for LR are not necessarily at increased risk of distant metastasis or tumor-related death. Therefore, staging systems that are designed to stratify patients for risk of distant metastasis and tumor-related death will not necessarily stratify patients for risk of LR.

Kattan and colleagues from the Memorial Sloan-Kettering Cancer Center (MSKCC) have utilized a database of over 2000 prospectively followed adult patients with STS to predict the probability of sarcoma-specific death by 12 years.[51] The results have been used to construct and internally validate a nomogram to predict sarcoma-specific death (Figure 6); this and similar nomograms have been validated in a variety of clinical situations, for example, RPS, or for disease-specific contexts, for example, liposarcoma, for individual patients.[56-59] These tools may be used for patient counseling, follow-up scheduling, and clinical trial eligibility determination.

Potential molecular prognostic factors

Specific molecular parameters evaluated for prognostic significance in STS have included *TP53* mutation, *MDM2* amplification, Ki-67 status, altered expression of the RB gene product in high-grade sarcomas, and histologic grade, but not *SS18-SSX* fusion type, which appears to be an important prognostic factor in patients with synovial sarcoma.[60] Complete discussion of the extensive literature on

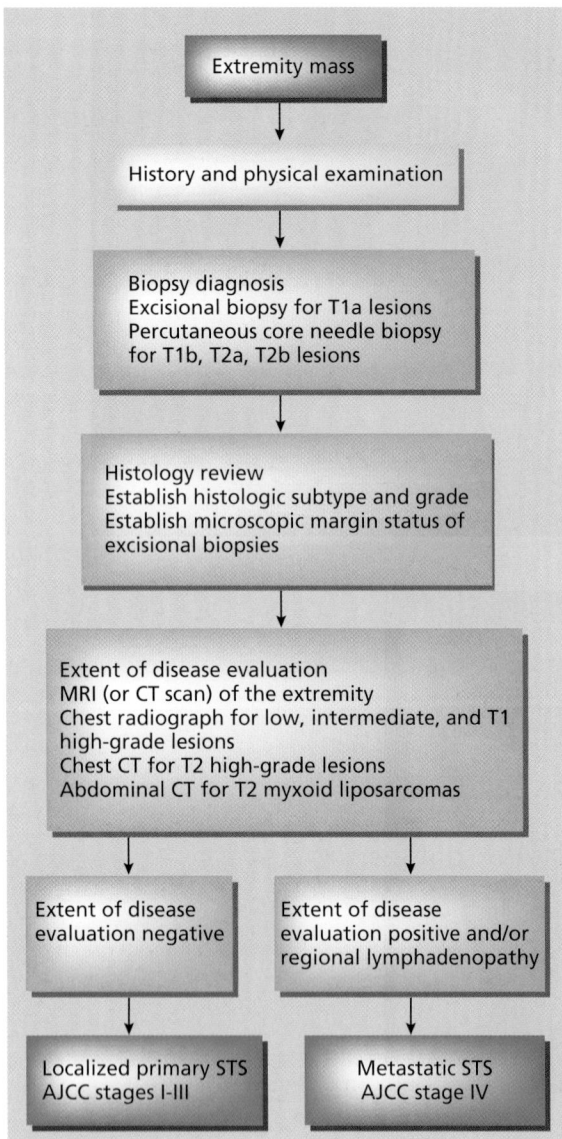

Figure 6 Approach for pretreatment evaluation and staging of the patient presenting with a primary extremity soft tissue mass. AJCC, American Joint Committee on Cancer. Source: Pisters 1998.[48] Reproduced with permission of Springer.

molecular prognostic factors in sarcoma is beyond the scope of this chapter. Readers are referred to more detailed reviews.[61,62]

As an example of the difficulty of using even the most commonly recognized markers as prognostic factors, one needs to look no further than Ki-67, an antigen expressed throughout the majority of the cell cycle. Ki-67 is used as a measure of the fraction of cells undergoing division. Preliminary reports of series of heterogeneous sarcomas in adults suggested that Ki-67 nuclear staining correlated with histologic grade, but was not an independent prognostic factor when histologic grade was taken into account.[63] Conversely, additional studies in larger numbers of patients indicated that Ki-67 status was an independent prognostic factor for clinical outcomes.[64] It is only with the development of consensus guidelines regarding the nature of Ki-67 immunohistochemistry and its interpretation that we can expect to see more careful accurate assessment of this biomarker in sarcoma outcomes.[65] It is also with the inconsistencies in the Ki-67 data that one can extrapolate the difficulty of using

increasingly available genetic markers for outcome determination. Although specific protein, DNA, and RNA parameters have been identified as having independent prognostic significance, there is presently no consensus on how these prognostic factors should be used in clinical practice.

Treatment of localized primary disease of the extremities

Surgery

General issues
Surgical resection remains the cornerstone of therapy for localized primary STS. The discussion that follows focuses on STSs in the limbs, the most common site of origin, but the principles are equally applicable to sarcomas of other primary anatomic sites.

With the development of limb-sparing techniques in the 1970s and 1980s, there was a marked decline in the rate of amputation as the primary therapy for extremity STS. Today, the widespread application of multimodality treatment strategies means that the vast majority of patients with localized STS of the extremities undergo limb-sparing, usually function-sparing treatment; fewer than 10% of patients presently undergo amputation.[66,67] In selected patients, limb sparing can be approached with surgery alone.

Amputation
Most surgeons consider definite major vascular, bony, or nerve involvement by STS as relative indications for amputation. Complex en bloc bone, vascular, and nerve resections with interposition grafting can be undertaken, but the associated morbidity is high. Therefore, for a few patients with critical involvement of major bony or neurovascular structures, for example, in the foot, amputation remains the only surgical option, but offers the prospect of prompt rehabilitation with excellent local control and survival rates. Other indications for amputation include tumor fungating through the skin or associated with a pathologic fracture with lack of reasonable salvage option.

Combined-modality limb-sparing treatment
Currently, at least 90% of patients with localized extremity sarcomas can undergo limb-sparing procedures. The use of limb-sparing multimodality treatment approaches for extremity sarcoma stems from phase 3 trial from the NCI published in 1982, in which patients with extremity sarcomas amenable to limb-sparing surgery were randomly assigned to receive amputation or limb-sparing surgery with postoperative RT.[68] The arms of this trial included postoperative chemotherapy with doxorubicin, cyclophosphamide, and methotrexate. With over 9 years of follow-up, this study established that for patients for whom limb-sparing surgery is an option, limb-sparing surgery combined with postoperative RT and chemotherapy yielded disease-related survival rates comparable to those for amputation while simultaneously preserving a functional extremity.

Satisfactory local resection involves resection of the primary tumor via a longitudinally oriented incision with a margin of normal tissue. Dissection along the tumor pseudocapsule (enucleation) is associated with LR rates in one-third to two-third of patients. In contrast, wide local excision with a margin of normal tissue around the lesion is associated with LR rates in the range of 10–31%, as noted in the control arms (surgery alone) of randomized trials evaluating postoperative RT and in single-institution reports.[69]

Table 3 Phase 3 trials of adjuvant radiotherapy for localized extremity and trunk sarcoma stratified by grade.

Histologic grade	First author/institution (references)	Treatment group	Radiation dose, Gy	Number of patients	Number of local failure (%)	LRFS (%)	OS (%)
High grade	Pisters/MSKCC[69]	Surgery + BRT	42–45	56	5(9)	89	27
		Surgery	—	63	19(30)	66	67
	Yang/NCI[70]	Surgery + EBRT	45 + 18 (boost)	47	0(0)	100	75
		Surgery	—	44	9(20)	78	74
Low grade	Pisters(/MSKCC[69]	Surgery + BRT	42–45	22	8(36)	73	96
		Surgery	—	23	6(26)	73	95
	Yang/NCI[70]	Surgery + EBRT	45 + 18 (boost)	26	1(4)	96	NR
		Surgery	—	24	8(33)	63	NR

Abbreviations: BRT, brachytherapy; LRFS, local recurrence-free survival; MSKCC, Memorial Sloan-Kettering Cancer Center; NCI, National Cancer Institute; NR, not reported; OS, overall survival; EBRT, external-beam radiotherapy.

In the modern era, a discussion of limb-preserving approaches must be linked to a discussion of the role of adjuvant therapies, most commonly RT. Several randomized controlled trials have addressed issues surrounding the use of adjuvant therapy and collectively have established important milestones in the evolution of the local management of STS. With a single exception, these trials have focused on extremity lesions and the themes of surgery and adjuvant RT.

Yang et al.[70] randomized 91 patients with high-grade extremity lesions following limb-sparing surgery to receive adjuvant chemotherapy alone or concurrent chemotherapy and RT. An additional 50 patients with low-grade tumors were to receive adjuvant RT or no further treatment following limb-sparing surgery. The local control rate for those who received RT was 99% compared with 70% in the no-RT group ($p = 0.0001$). The results were similar for high- and low-grade tumors (Table 3).

Adjuvant RT was also evaluated in a randomized trial of 126 cases treated between 1982 and 1987 (Table 3).[69] Brachytherapy (BRT) was administered postoperatively, via an iridium-192 implant that delivered 42–45 Gy over 4–6 days. At 5 years, the local control rate for high-grade tumors was 91% with BRT compared with 70% in surgery-alone controls ($p = 0.04$). Of note, no improvement in local control with BRT was evident for the low-grade tumors (the local control rate was 74% with surgery alone and 64% with BRT). The full explanation for grade-specific differences in local control with BRT remains unresolved, although one suggestion implicates the relatively long cell cycle of low-grade tumors: low-grade tumor cells may not enter the radiosensitive phases of the cell cycle during the relatively short BRT time. Additional discussion of the pros and cons of BRT compared to external beam radiotherapy (EBRT) is included in the section on "Methods of Radiotherapy Delivery".

Satisfactory surgical margins to omit radiotherapy

There are no randomized data to define what constitutes a satisfactory gross resection margin for a sarcoma. In general, every effort should be made to achieve a wide margin (2 cm is often an arbitrary choice) around the tumor mass, except in the immediate vicinity of functionally important neurovascular structures, where, in the absence of frank neoplastic involvement, dissection is performed in the immediate perineural or perivascular tissue planes. Technical details of the surgical approach to extremity sarcomas are beyond the scope of this chapter, but are reviewed elsewhere.[71] The principle remains that adequate clearance of potential tumor-bearing tissues can be achieved if there is sufficient distance between the surgical margin and the edge of any grossly evident tumor (e.g., at least 2 cm for the closest margin), or where an intact barrier to tumor spread is excised en bloc with the tumor. In such cases, there is little evidence that RT is required even when potential adverse prognostic

factors, such as large high-grade tumors are present. The exception in cases of "unplanned" excision where significant contamination of surrounding tissues may have taken place and the precise extent of the tumor is essentially unknown. Depending on the histology, margins of <2 cm are reasonable when an appropriate biological barrier (such as muscle fascia) constitutes that margin. Histologies with infiltrative borders, such as myxofibrosarcoma, may require wider margins or resection. On the other hand, tumors with good prognoses, such as well-differentiated liposarcoma/atypical lipomatous tumor, may be managed by a more limited, marginal resection.

Management of regional lymph nodes

Given the low (2–3%) prevalence of lymph node metastasis in adults with sarcomas, there is no role for routine regional lymph node dissection in most patients.[32] However, patients with angiosarcoma, embryonal/alveolar rhabdomyosarcoma, and epithelioid sarcoma have an increased incidence of lymph node metastasis and should be carefully examined for lymphadenopathy. These patients may benefit from the inclusion of lymph node regions electively in adjuvant RT fields.

For patients with STS, lymph node metastasis has been regarded as a particularly adverse finding conferring similar risk to distant metastasis in the TNM (tumor–nodes–metastasis) stage classification. Nevertheless, therapeutic lymph node dissection results in a 34% actuarial survival rate, and thus the rare patients with regional nodal involvement who have no evidence of extranodal disease should undergo therapeutic lymphadenectomy.[32] Although formerly classified as being as prognostically as adverse as distant metastasis in the TNM staging classification, isolated lymph node metastasis (as opposed to synchronous distant metastasis), if treated intensively, appears to have a prognosis similar to patients with stage III tumors (i.e., those with high-grade, deep lesions, and lesions larger than 5 cm). The impact of isolated nodal disease was adjusted in the AJCC/UICC staging system by moving N1 disease alone into the stage III group.[49] The validity of including N1 disease into stage III was questioned in a follow-up manuscript, in which survival for N1 patients more closely parallels survival with stage IV than node negative AJCC stage III disease.[72]

Radiotherapy

Rationale for combining radiotherapy with surgery

The use of RT in combination with surgery for STS is supported by two phase 3 clinical trials (Table 3) and is based on two premises: microscopic nests of tumor cells can be destroyed by RT, and less radical surgery can be performed when surgery and RT are combined.[69,70] Although the traditional belief was that STSs were resistant to RT, radiosensitivity assays performed on sarcoma cell lines grown *in vitro* have confirmed that the radiosensitivity of sarcomas is similar to that of other malignancies; this confirmation supports the first premise.[73,74] The second premise stresses the philosophy of preservation of form (including cosmesis where possible) and function as a goal for many patients with extremity, truncal, breast, and head and neck sarcomas.[75–77] Similar principles govern the frequent use of RT for sarcomas at problematic sites such as, for example, RPS, high-risk sarcomas of the head and neck with skull base invasion, or spinal canal invasion by paravertebral lesions. While the efficacy of RT has been confirmed through prospective randomized clinical trials for extremity sarcomas, it has not been confirmed for other sites. Currently, there is an ongoing phase III trial evaluating preoperative RT for primary RPS.

Visceral sarcomas are not ordinarily managed with RT, in part because of the mobile nature of these structures within the pelvic, abdominal, or thoracic compartments. After resection of visceral sarcomas, accurate identification of the field at risk of residual disease is particularly problematic. Contaminated loops of the bowel or mesentery may relocate remotely within the abdominal cavity after surgery, and pleural contamination and mediastinal shift may occur following intrathoracic resections. Fixed tumors in the pelvis or tumors attached to internal truncal walls may occasionally be suited to preoperative or postoperative RT. Typically, however, the vast size of the radiation fields needed to cover entire body cavities, coupled with the limited RT doses that can be safely administered to the organs within the cavities, and the overwhelming risk of distant rather than LR, confines adjuvant RT for the investigational setting.

Essential elements in treatment planning of external beam radiotherapy

Accurate tumor localization is the first essential for RT planning. It primarily uses CT for dosimetric reasons, but MRI can provide complementary information about the tumor extent and can be assimilated in the computer planning workstation through image fusion technology.[41,42] Further essential information is obtained from the pathology and operative reports, and metallic clips placed at the time of surgery may also help define the tumor bed.

It is usually helpful to secure the targeted area to minimize setup variations and eliminate movement during treatment. Simple maneuvers such as comfortable limb positioning or fashioning of customized thermoplastic molds for immobilization will facilitate reliable and consistent treatment setups. RT of superficial tissues, including the scar following definitive resection, with appropriate application of tissue-like bolus material should be considered, but with the recognition that fibrosis, atrophy, and telangiectasias may result. Traditionally, dose uniformity within irregular volumes was optimized using beam segmentation, compensators, or wedge filters. However, this has now largely been replaced by the use of intensity-modulated radiotherapy (IMRT), which addresses issues that include the size, shape, and location of targets and the nature of the normal tissues surrounding them including their contour and width. IMRT is particularly useful in situations where the target volume is adjacent to critical normal tissues as found at the skull base or within the abdomen. Whenever possible, the entire limb circumference, whole joints, or pressure areas (e.g., elbow or heel) should not be treated with what is considered to be a full RT dose, as this may adversely affect limb function and cause distal edema.

It is also prudent to assess baseline function before initiating RT. This is especially important with paired organs, such as eyes or kidneys, if the functional ablation of one organ by RT is expected and is a frequent problem in treating RPS. If right sided or of great size, an RPS may infiltrate the liver capsule or be "hooded" by the liver,

making RT access to an appropriate tissue volume surrounding the tumor extremely difficult. This area may be particularly appropriate for IMRT approaches because of the exquisite conformality that is possible with this approach and permits the liver and the other normal tissue to be excluded from the irradiated volume.[78,79] Fortunately, although the tolerance of the entire liver to radiation is low, part of the liver may be safely treated to much higher doses. In these instances, if a subsequent liver resection is needed because of tumor infiltration or adherence to the capsule, detailed consultation between the surgical and radiation oncology teams is needed to ensure that an adequate volume of nonirradiated liver remains *in situ*.

Dose fractionation issues

Total radiation doses administered postoperatively for sarcoma depend on the tumor grade and involvement of the surgical margin.[70,80,81] Typical total doses are 60 Gy for low grade and 66 Gy for high-grade tumors, respectively. When RT is given preoperatively, the total dose used in most institutions is approximately 50 Gy in daily fractions administered over 5 weeks.[81,82] However, data regarding radiation dose response are very limited and based on underpowered retrospective studies. On the basis of the current data, higher doses of RT are probably indicated in the postoperative setting (compared with preoperative RT), but the search for an alternative lower dose postoperative schedule seems desirable. These are discussed below in relation to the volumes to be used and the consequences of using different doses in terms of potential morbidity.

The fraction size used in conventional fractionation schemes varies (usually 1.8 or 2.1 Gy).[81,83] Absence of late effects can be expected with smaller fraction size; this tissue is particularly important when critical structures are irradiated. Several altered fractionation schemes have been described including hyperfractionated, hypofractionated, and accelerated schedules.[84–87] Most recently, preoperative hypofractionated RT for extremity and trunk wall STS was recently evaluated in a series of 272 patients. RT was delivered preoperatively for 5 consecutive days in 5 Gy per fraction. The LR rate was higher (19%) with the hypofractionated schedule compared to many contemporary series.[88] Longer follow-up of this novel strategy is warranted. Neither hyper- nor hypofractionation regimens are likely to replace conventional daily fractionation in the near future, for a combination of reasons that include the small nonrandomized nature of studies, resources needed for some protocols, concerns about efficacy and toxicity, and the fact that modern targeting techniques with IMRT may offset some of the potential benefits that underpin the choice of altered fractionation protocols.

Radiation dose and target volumes

Guidelines have recently been published on how to address the technical design of the radiation volumes and should be discussed for additional detail regarding this topic.[89]

Many STS respect barriers to tumor spread in the axial plane of the extremity, such as bones, interosseous membranes, or major fascial planes. Consequently, extremity STS tend to spread longitudinally within the specific muscle groups of the extremity. Therefore, the margins of the RT volume must be wide in the cephalocaudal direction. In the cross-section, there may be much greater security in defining nontarget structures, especially those delimited by an intact barrier to tumor spread. Bone, interosseous membranes, and fascial planes are considered barriers to tumor spread in the axial direction, and, therefore, descriptions of radiation margins employed are principally in the cephalocaudal direction.

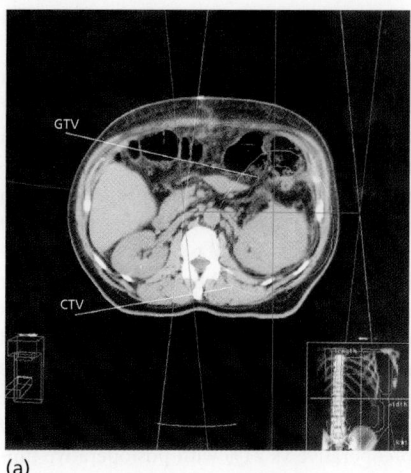 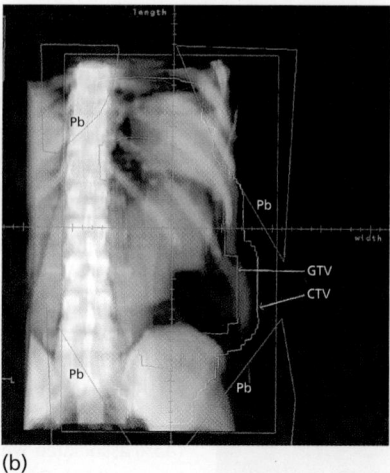 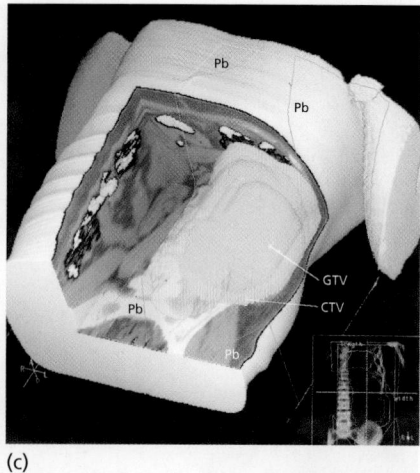

(a)   (b)   (c)

Figure 7 (a) The GTV has been contoured on a CT simulator workstation (red outline). This includes the anterior abnormal fat shown earlier (Figure 5b,c). This process is performed with many thin CT slices to permit reconstruction of the image later for three-dimensional treatment planning. The CTV is outlined in yellow to account for potential microscopic spread beyond the GTV. An additional margin will also be added to account for setup variation and organ motion. Note the displacement of the bowel loops by the tumor mass. The straight lines show the path of the beam for a conventional setup with opposed anterior and posterior fields. (b) The contoured GTV and CTV information displayed in a beam's eye view (BEV) using a digitally reconstructed radiograph created by the CT simulator. Shielding (Pb) can be placed once the path of the beam within the target areas defined is seen on the BEV. One can also discern the opaque tumor partially displacing the bowel from target area. (c) A three-dimensional reconstruction with the GTV, CTV, and areas to be shielded (Pb) shown with abdominal wall and anterior structures cut away. Generally, these "cut-away" images are most useful for visualizing the edge of the target volume adjacent to critical anatomy that must be protected and when the spatial relationship cannot be verified precisely with conventional imaging.

For nonextremity lesions, the preferred direction of spread is also along the direction of the involved musculature, but care must be taken to ensure that the fascial planes are appropriately recognized and encompassed in the radiation target volume.

Earlier, this chapter summarized principles concerning anatomic planes and the preferential pathways for sarcomas to spread within tissues. This information facilitates the design of target areas for RT. The basic elements in RT planning are to first define a gross tumor volume (GTV) and then place a margin around it to encompass tissues at risk of harboring microscopic residual disease [clinical target volume (CTV)] (Figures 7a–c and 8).[90] Generally, RT is phased so that an initial volume (phase 1) around the risk zone is treated to doses that are capable of sterilizing microscopic amounts of tumor cells (e.g., 45–50.4 Gy in 1.8 or 2.0 Gy fractions). When delivering RT postoperatively, it is customary to have at least one field reduction to permit an augmented dose to a smaller volume surrounding the highest risk zone (phase 2). This dose is usually 15–16 Gy but can be higher if there is gross residual disease. For the phase 1 volume, the surgical bed is expanded with a 1.5-cm radial margin and a 4-cm craniocaudal margin to encompass microscopic disease in the surrounding tissues; the boost is applied to the original sarcoma localization with a 1.5-cm radial margin and a 2-cm craniocaudal margin. In preoperative RT, historically more recent but potentially the most prevalent approach used today, the GTV is treated to a dose of 50 Gy in 25 fractions over 5 weeks with surgery following 4–6 weeks later. In general, the CTV encompasses the GTV with a 4-cm craniocaudal and a 1.5–2.0 cm radial margin for microscopic disease coverage. CTV should also include peritumoral edema as it may harbor tumor cells at some distance from the GTV.[91] Following preoperative RT, a postoperative "boost" has traditionally been used but is generally restricted to patients who received preoperative RT and have margin-positive disease at surgery. This is because the local control rate for margin-negative cases is in excess of 90% even when a boost is not provided.[81,92,93] A positive margin is declared when the tumor reaches the inked surface of the specimen, and clear margins can be declared if the tumor does not reach the ink irrespective of how close it is.[81]

The need for a radiation therapy boost following preoperative RT and surgery with positive resection margins has been questioned in a retrospective review of 216 ESTS (extremity soft tissue sarcomas) patients; 52 received preoperative RT (50 Gy) alone and were compared to 41 who received preoperative RT with a postoperative boost (generally 16 Gy). A portion of the population did not receive RT at all, or received postoperative RT and were excluded (123 of 216). The postoperative boost cohort had lower 5-year LR-free rates (74% vs 90% for preoperative RT only) indicating that a postoperative boost provides no obvious advantage.[94] A similar study ($n = 67$) yielded almost identical results.[95] These results suggest that a benefit from a delayed postoperative boost following preoperative RT and surgery is at best debatable, and the increased risk and challenges of managing later RT morbidity (e.g., radiation-induced fractures) resulting from the higher radiation doses involved should be considered when treating STS.

The defined external beam volumes for extremity STS reflect those of the prospective Canadian Sarcoma Group randomized clinical trial discussed later.[96] However, the recently completed UK postoperative phase III randomized "VORTEX" trial (NCT NCT00423618) compared a 5-cm longitudinal margin from GTV in the standard arm to a 2-cm margin and results are awaited.[97] A completed RTOG-0630 trial (NCT NCT00589121) addressing the role of IMRT defined slightly smaller preoperative RT volumes (longitudinal 3 cm), although its results may be less easily interpreted owing to its nonrandomized nature.[98] In any event, the size of the RT volume margins is not appreciably smaller than the 4-cm longitudinal margin noted above and further outcome reports will be needed in the future to guide practice if target volumes are being reduced in the interest of normal tissue protection.

Despite the variations noted in target volume coverage, the local control rates reported for extremity STS using combinations or surgery and RT are approximately 90% and may suggest that the zone of microscopic involvement may be less than that was

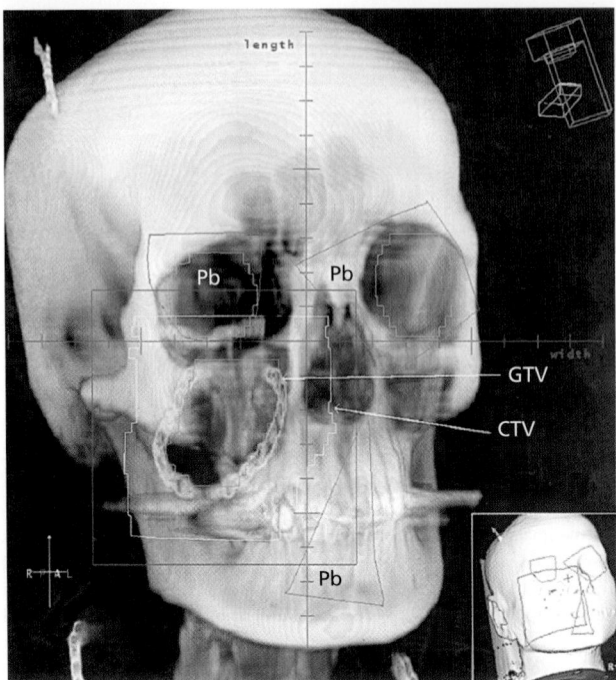

Figure 8 A digitally reconstructed radiograph of the head and neck of a young woman with an STS of the right cheek. Because of the proximity to the right eye, preoperative radiotherapy has been chosen because of its ability to permit maximal restriction of the CTV to the local environment of the tumor. The same process was followed using a CT simulator as described in Figure 6. The GTV on the cheek can be seen with the surrounding CTV. Shielding (Pb) is also evident. A hair clip, which the patient was wearing during the CT slice acquisition, is evident in the right parietal area; one can also see her necklace. The smaller inset shows a three-dimensional image of the patient with potential beams applied.

previously realized. Recent improvements in surgical technique may lessen the degree of intraoperative tumor dissemination, and irradiation of all surgically handled tissues, scars, and drain sites may be unnecessary. This seems particularly relevant for major centers where surgery is performed by teams with extensive experience in sarcoma management. One must also consider the possibility that case selection factors may explain apparent variations in practice between BRT and external beam RT approaches.

Sequencing of radiotherapy and surgery

The two most common methods of EBRT delivery are preoperative and postoperative RT. Preoperative RT is delivered to an undisturbed and potentially better oxygenated tumor site, which may be one reason why lower preoperative radiation doses do not appear to compromise local control.[99] Nielsen et al.[100] repeated RT planning in patients who had undergone preoperative RT and surgery and observed that the field size and number of joints irradiated in preoperative RT were significantly less than if the treatment had been administered postoperatively. Another advantage of preoperative RT is that it promotes collaboration between the surgical and radiation oncologists and facilitates the formulation of a coordinated management plan before any treatment.

The Canadian Sarcoma Group SR2 clinical trial represents the only prospective randomized comparison of preoperative versus postoperative RT.[96] As was anticipated, the trial showed that preoperative RT results in an increased rate of acute wound complications (WCs). On the other hand, as also anticipated, the trial

also showed that postoperative delivery is associated with increased limb fibrosis, edema, joint stiffness, and bone fractures.

Long-term follow-up of patients treated in the Canadian Sarcoma Group NCIC trial (SR2) showed that, of 129 patients evaluable for late toxicity, 48% in the postoperative group compared to 32% in the preoperative group had grade 2 or greater fibrosis ($p = 0.07$).[101] Edema was more frequently seen in the postoperative group (23% vs 16%), as was joint stiffness (23% vs 18%). Patients with these complications had lower function scores (all p values <0.01) on the Toronto Extremity Salvage Score and the Musculoskeletal Tumor Society Rating Scale. Field size predicted greater rates of fibrosis ($p = 0.002$) and joint stiffness ($p = 0.006$), and marginally predicted edema ($p = 0.06$). Acute wound-healing complications were twice as common with preoperative compared to postoperative RT. The increased risk was almost entirely confined to the lower extremity (43% associated with preoperative vs 21% with postoperative timing; $p = 0.01$). Of interest, additional reports, including one from the University of Texas M.D. Anderson Cancer Center, using the same criteria for classifying WCs as were used in the Canadian NCI trial, found almost identical results.[66]

The influence of time interval between preoperative EBRT and surgery on the development of WC in extremity sarcoma has also been studied. While the interval had little influence, the data still suggested that the optimal interval to reduce potential WC was 4 or 5 weeks between RT and surgery.[67]

In the initial report of the SR2 trial with 3.3 years median follow-up, an improvement in overall survival (OS) ($p = 0.048$) in the preoperative RT arm was noted and partially explained by increased deaths in the postoperative RT unrelated to sarcoma.[96] The local failure rate was identical in the 2 arms (7%) (Figure 9). However, updated results were recently presented and the preliminary survival difference had dissipated.[101] The 5-year results for preoperative versus postoperative, respectively, were local control, 93% versus 92%; metastatic relapse-free, 67% versus 69%; recurrence-free survival, 58% versus 59%; OS, 73% versus 67% ($p = 0.48$); and cause-specific survival, 78% versus 73% ($p = 0.64$). Cox modeling showed only resection margins as significant for local control. Tumor size and grade were the only significant factors for metastatic relapse-free, OS, and cause-specific survival. Grade was the only consistent predictor of recurrence-free survival.

For the present, decisions about preoperative versus postoperative RT for extremity soft tissue sarcoma should be individualized, taking into account tumor location, tumor size, RT volumes needed, comorbidities, and risks. In general, preoperative RT provides some advantages over postoperative RT, but exposes the patient to significantly increased risks of serious postoperative WCs. A summary of the relative indications that can be used to select patients for preoperative RT is provided in Table 4. In addition, although much of the discussion about preoperative RT is focused on extremity lesions, patients with RPS tolerate preoperative RT substantially better than postoperative RT. This is because the tumor acts as a tissue expander to exclude the bowel from the RT volume (Figure 7a–c). This is discussed in detail later in the section titled "Retroperitoneal Sarcomas."

Methods of radiotherapy delivery

In general terms, the most generally accepted methods of delivering RT include EBRT and BRT. The former also includes the controversy about its scheduling (preoperative vs postoperative) discussed earlier and in conventional terms also needs attention to the potential role of IMRT that was also mentioned earlier. No randomized trials directly comparing external beam RT and BRT have been undertaken, but both forms of RT have been compared with surgery alone.

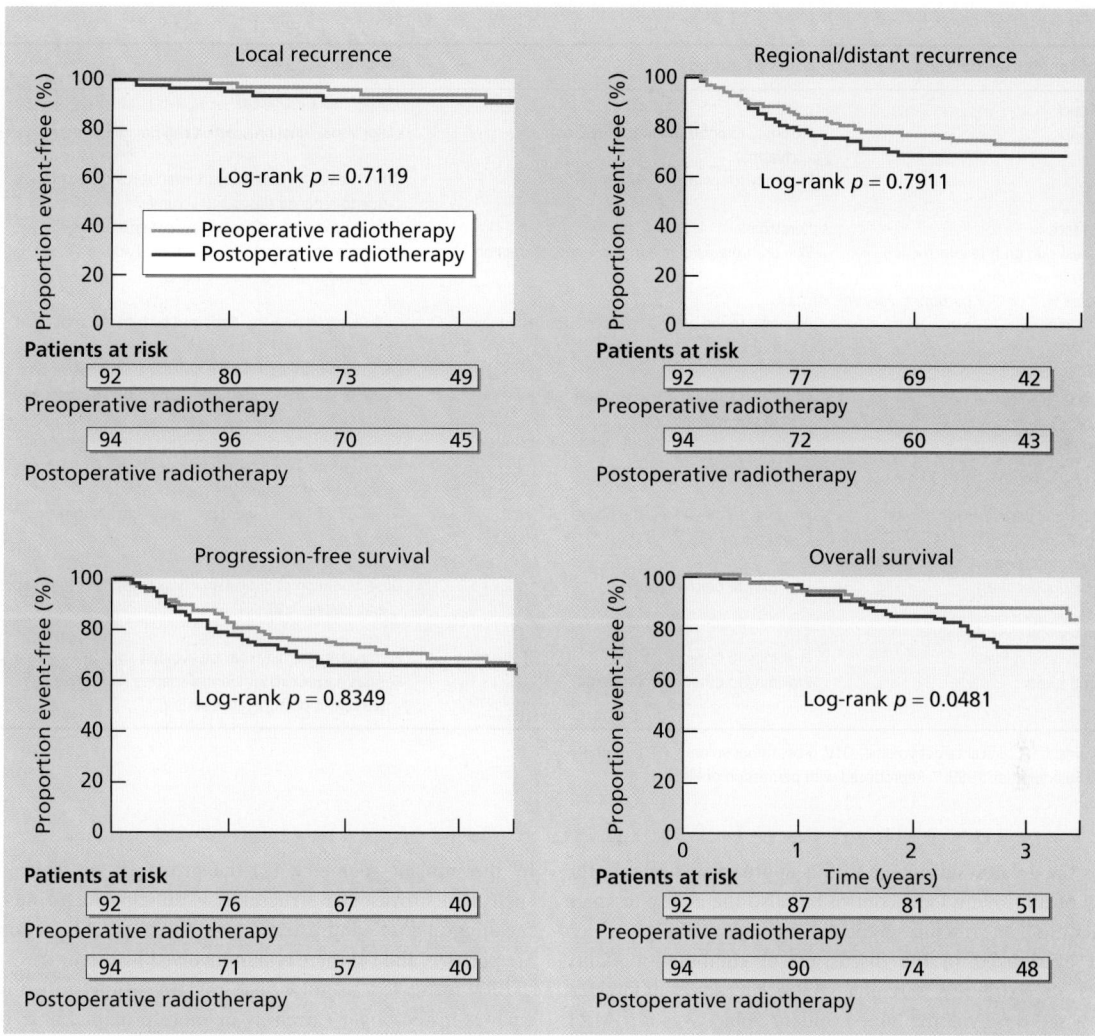

Figure 9 Kaplan–Meier plots for probability of local recurrence, metastasis (local and regional recurrence), progression-free survival, and overall survival in the Canadian Sarcoma Group randomized trial of the NCI of Canada Clinical Trials Group comparing preoperative and postoperative radiotherapy. Source: O'Sullivan et al. 2002.[96] Reproduced with permission of Elsevier.

There also have been no randomized trials addressing IMRT but two prospective phase II trials exist and institutional data are emerging.

Intensity-modulated radiotherapy

Target coverage and protection of normal tissues from high-dose areas appear to be superior for IMRT compared to traditional techniques in ESTS.[102] A recent retrospective review spanning noncoincident treatment time periods compared surgery combined with either IMRT ($n = 165$) or conventional EBRT ($n = 154$). Allowing for known limitations associated with studies involving treatments deployed over different eras, IMRT showed significantly reduced LR for primary ESTS (7.6% LR for IMRT vs 15.1% LR for conventional RT; $p = 0.02$).[103]

Two prospective phase II trials [from Princess Margaret (NCT00188175) and the Radiation Therapy Oncology Group (RTOG 0630: NCT00589121)] investigated if preoperative image-guided radiotherapy (IGRT) using conformal RT/IMRT could reduce RT-related morbidities.[98,104] The characteristics of the Princess Margaret (PMH) and RTOG 0630 trials differed in several ways, particular relating to the exclusion of upper extremity lesions in the PMH trial, the use of a boost following preoperative RT in RTOG 0630 as well as the potential to use chemotherapy in

the RTOG trial, and some aspects of the choice of target coverage mentioned below. The two trials also differed regarding their primary endpoints.

The PMH trial showed reduced wound-healing complication (WC) rates (31%) in lower extremity compared to the 43% risk in the previous Canadian Sarcoma Group NCIC SR2 trial that only used 2D and 3D RT.[96] The need for tissue transfer, RT chronic morbidities, and subsequent secondary operations for WCs were reduced while maintaining good limb function and local control (93%). The RTOG-0630 trial reported a significant reduction of late toxicities in comparison to the NCIC-SR2 trial (11% vs 37% in SR2), which is very similar to the IGRT PMH trial. Importantly, both the PMH and RTOG-0630 trials defined the CTV differently (longitudinal margin of 3 cm from the gross tumor for high-grade lesions and 2 cm for low-grade lesions versus 4 cm longitudinal margins in the PMH trial). Potentially, the reduction in CTV margins of this degree could explain the improvement in limb function with comparable local control, although an alternative possibility is the reduction in normal tissues receiving the target dose in all dimensions, which is shared by both studies. In the end, it also seems that IMRT is capable of conforming the dose more suitably to the desirable target volume compared to traditional conformal techniques.

Table 4 Relative indications for preoperative RT, despite concerns related to wound complications.

Treatment context/sarcoma site	Issues of concern	Comments
Head and neck		
Paranasal sinus	Proximity to optic apparatus (eye, orbit, chiasma)	Major visual functional deficit can be minimized
Skull base	Proximity to spinal cord, brain stem	Other "lesser" morbidities (dental, xerostomia) may also be less due to reduced doses and volumes
Cheek and face	Xerostomia	Early caries or loss of teeth, loss of sense of taste
Split thickness skin graft reconstruction (especially lower limb)	Skin graft breakdown and consequent infection	Many months to years of recreational and/or vocational disability may occur during healing (rare)
Large volume GTV or CTV occupying coelomic cavities		
Retroperitoneum	Proximity to the bowel, the liver, and the kidney	Critical organs may be displaced by tumor or not fixed or adherent as is likely in postoperative setting
		Entire tumor treated before possible contamination of cavity
Some small bowel lesions	Proximity to critical anatomy, especially intestine with side wall adherence	Contamination of abdominal cavity renders postoperative RT unsuitable
Thoracic wall/pleura	Proximity to the lung or the cardiac structures	The lung may be displaced by the chest wall or pleural tumor and can be avoided with preoperative RT, or permits GTV to be treated before operative contamination
Abdominal trunk walls, pelvic side wall	Proximity to the kidney, the bowel, the liver, and the ovaries	Avoid CTV encroachment on vulnerable anatomy
GTV adjacent to dose limiting critical anatomy		
Thoracic inlet/upper chest	Proximity to brachial plexus	Dose limitation of critical anatomy lends itself to preoperative wall low neck RT.
Additional volume considerations		
Medial thigh (young male)	Proximity to testes	Permanent infertility may be avoided
Central limb tumor	Proximity to other compartments	Permits partial circumferential sparing, which would not be feasible in postoperative setting

Abbreviations: CTV, clinical target volume; GTV, gross tumor volume; RT, radiotherapy.
Source: O'Sullivan et al. 1999.[77] Reproduced with permission of Elsevier.

Perhaps the greatest advantage to this approach is not only the possibility of improving local control but also the ability to spare bone toxicity and late fractures by achieving bone avoidance, which are often overlooked in the discussion of combined-modality treatments of extremity sarcoma. A recent study addressed evidence-based dose volume bone avoidance objectives for IMRT planning in 230 patients (176 lower and 54 upper extremity) with a median follow-up of 41.2 months.[105] The overall risk of fracture was 2% (4/230 patients), which compares favorably to a previous reported incidence of 6%, and suggests that efforts to achieve bone avoidance are appropriate.

Brachytherapy

BRT has some putative advantages over external beam, including a shorter overall treatment time (4–6 days vs 5–6.5 weeks) and quicker initiation of RT after surgery while clonogenic numbers are at a minimum. Because of its brevity, BRT is also more easily integrated into protocols that include systemic chemotherapy than is external beam RT, with its protracted courses. The irradiated volume is also smaller with BRT, which may confer functional advantages. BRT may also have an advantage in situations in which normal tissue tolerance to RT is compromised. One such scenario would be when a postoperative RT boost to the operative bed is desired in patients who received preoperative RT. The use of BRT with surgery in previously irradiated tissues is another situation to achieve limb salvage.[106,107] As noted earlier, no apparent benefit for BRT over surgical excision alone is evident with low-grade lesions, and external beam appears more effective for these tumors (Table 3).[69,70,108] BRT also permits radiation volumes to be mapped according to intraoperative findings. The American Brachytherapy Society Guidelines differ from those for EBRT and also advise that BRT as a sole treatment modality is contraindicated in the following situations: (1) the CTV cannot be adequately encompassed

by the implant geometry, (2) the proximity of critical anatomy, such as neurovascular structures, is anticipated to interfere with meaningful dose administration, (3) the surgical resection margins are positive, and (4) there is skin involved by tumor.[109,110]

BRT seems less useful where implant geometry is not optimal, such as in the upper extremity or more proximal limb regions.[111] The results of the BRT randomized trial were discussed earlier. In addition, BRT was compared retrospectively to IMRT in 134 high-grade ESTS with similar adverse features.[112] The 5-year local control rate was 92% for IMRT compared to 81% for BRT ($p = 0.04$). Unfortunately, while the results of BRT, including its more restrictive criteria for use, suggest lower efficacy compared to EBRT, there is no randomized controlled trial comparing these seemingly effective local adjuvants.

Traditionally BRT studies, including those mentioned above, used low-dose rate techniques. High-dose rate (HDR) BRT has potential logistic advantages including lower radiation staff exposure, outpatient delivery, and optimized dose distributions by varying dwell times. However, wound-healing complications may occur in sarcoma management and caution is also recommended when placing catheters adjacent to neurovascular structures. As yet, no large series evaluating HDR BRT for STS is available nor has it been directly compared to LDR, partly because of technical differences.

Additional approaches to RT delivery

In addition to external beam RT, BRT, and IMRT, several other approaches for RT delivery exist. These include particle beam RT (electrons, protons, pions, or neutrons), intraoperative radiotherapy (IORT) using external beam or BRT approaches, and combinations of other techniques (e.g., hyperthermia) with RT. IORT has been used most often in the management of RPS and will be discussed later. Some reports also describe IORT for extremity sarcomas.[113,114] Formal clinical trials have not compared the relative merits of these approaches, and their use may be governed as much by the availability of an approach at a given center as by any special advantage that it may confer. In the case of proton beam RT, its ability to achieve accurate targeting provides an advantage when tumors lie in proximity to critical structures.[115,116] In general, however, although reports on the use of many of these approaches exist, the problems of selection bias need to be considered in interpreting these small series in which treatments were not randomly assigned.[117,118]

Systemic therapy

Systemic agents, including both traditional cytotoxic chemotherapy drugs and newer small molecule oral kinase inhibitors (SMOKIs), are used widely in the metastatic setting for patients with STSs. The use of chemotherapy in the adjuvant setting remains somewhat controversial. However, if chemotherapy is going to have the same impact as radiation and surgery in the management of sarcomas, more effective drugs must be identified to help improve the cure rate for patients with primary tumors and unseen microscopic metastatic disease. This section will review the use of chemotherapy in the adjuvant and metastatic settings. A brief discussion of chemotherapy combined with radiation therapy is also included in this section.

Adjuvant systemic therapy following primary surgical resection
Although local or local–regional recurrence is a problem for a small subset of patients following primary therapy, the major risk to life in sarcoma patients is uncontrolled systemic disease. The availability of systemic therapy with proven, albeit often limited, ability to induce shrinkage of advanced sarcomas has raised the question of whether the early use of systemic treatment might affect microscopic metastatic disease and yield improvements in OS and disease-free survival (DFS).

Certainly for Ewing sarcoma/PNET, rhabdomyosarcoma, and osteogenic sarcoma, adjuvant or neoadjuvant chemotherapy is an appropriate standard of care.[119–122] However, for more common STSs such as leiomyosarcoma, liposarcoma, and high-grade UPS (formerly known as MFH), the benefit of chemotherapy, if there is one, is small.[123] As adjuvant therapy is utilized by many practitioners for more common diseases where the benefit is a relatively small one, such as stage I breast cancer and stage II colon cancer, this small potential benefit is an issue that needs to be discussed on an individualized basis. Certainly, the lack of available effective agents for metastatic sarcoma has impeded progress in this area, but the utility of imatinib in both the metastatic and adjuvant setting in GIST gives hope that new agents will contribute to the ultimate goal of any type of systemic therapy specifically increasing the cure rate for people with new diagnoses.

There have been over a dozen studies of anthracycline-based adjuvant chemotherapy for STSs that date back nearly as long as the initial development of doxorubicin.[124,125] These will not be reviewed here, as anthracycline/ifosfamide-based therapy constitutes a better standard of care in patients offered adjuvant chemotherapy, and only one of the studies completed by 1992 had used ifosfamide.

In one of the largest combination chemotherapy studies, the Italian Sarcoma Study Group (ISSG) examined patients with primary or recurrent resected STS of the extremity or limb girdle treated or not treated with radiation.[126,127] A total of 104 patients were randomized to receive no chemotherapy or to receive ifosfamide (1800 mg/m^2/day for 5 consecutive days with mesna) and epirubicin (60 mg/m^2 on 2 consecutive days), with filgrastim support. Interim analysis in 1996 led to early conclusion of the trial because the study had reached its primary endpoint, specifically improved DFS. At a median follow-up of 36 months, OS in the chemotherapy arm was

72%, compared with 55% for the control arm ($p = 0.002$). However, with long-term follow-up, the OS difference showed only a trend to statistical significance on an intention-to-treat analysis.[126] This study is the strongest single study in the literature supporting the use of adjuvant chemotherapy for STS. Interpretation of the study is made more difficult with the observation of equivalent distant ± LR rates at 4 years.

Conversely, no survival benefit was observed in an EORTC phase III study of adjuvant chemotherapy versus observation (doxorubicin 75 mg/m^2, ifosfamide 5 g/m^2 per cycle for 5 cycles, with filgrastim support).[128] A total of 351 patients were accrued between 1995 and 2003, and 130 (80%) of the 163 patients receiving chemotherapy completed all 5 cycles. OS was not statistically different between arms (HR 0.94, 95% confidence interval 0.68–1.31 for the treatment arm, $p = 0.72$) and relapse-free survival was also not statistically different (HR 0.91, CI 0.67–1.22, $p = 0.51$). The 5-year OS rate was 67% for the treatment arm and 68% for the control group. The major differences between this study and the ISG study were a lower dose of ifosfamide and use of epirubicin in the ISSG trial, but it is unclear based on data from metastatic disease of the relevance of these differences.

The most recent and comprehensive overview of adjuvant chemotherapy for extremity sarcomas to date was the 2008 meta-analysis of 18 studies encompassing sarcomas of all anatomic sites.[129] In this analysis, 93 potential studies were considered and 18 ultimately selected, constituting 1953 patients with STSs of extremity and nonextremity. Pathology review was not centralized. The results of the meta-analysis, including the actuarial outcome probabilities and the hazard ratios, are summarized in Figure 10 and Table 5.

Study data from the 18 trials were combined without examining individual patient data. Combining all data, LR risk, distant recurrence risk, overall recurrence risk, and OS were superior with chemotherapy. For OS, the relative risk of death was 0.77 with chemotherapy (95% CI, 0.64–0.93), $p = 0.01$, and relative recurrence risk was 0.67 (95% CI, 0.56–0.82), $p = 0.0001$. The absolute risk reduction of any recurrence was 10% and absolute risk reduction for OS was 6%. However, as pointed out in a commentary on a prior meta-analyses,[131] these data have to be interpreted with caution. For example, (1) individual patient data were not reviewed and interrogated, (2) in an older analysis, 18% of patients did not have histology available for review, recognizing the error rate in pathology review at expert centers, (3) ineligibility rates were high, and (4) the largest individual trial was not included (published after the meta-analysis publication). Although the meta-analysis cannot replace a well-designed randomized study, it reinforces many of the findings from smaller studies that local and distant recurrence-free survival is definitely improved, and OS modestly so, at least in unselected patients.

Preoperative (neoadjuvant) chemotherapy
Preoperative chemotherapy has theoretical advantages over postoperative treatment. First, preoperative chemotherapy provides an *in vivo* test of chemotherapy sensitivity. Patients whose tumors show objective evidence of response are presumed to be the subset that will benefit most from further postoperative systemic treatment. In contrast, it is assumed that the population of nonresponding patients will derive minimal or no benefit from further chemotherapy and can therefore be spared its toxicity. On the other hand, it is conceivable that the patients whose tumors respond to chemotherapy may not be those who would derive the most from chemotherapy, because these lesions with favorable biology might be those destined to do well irrespective of any systemic

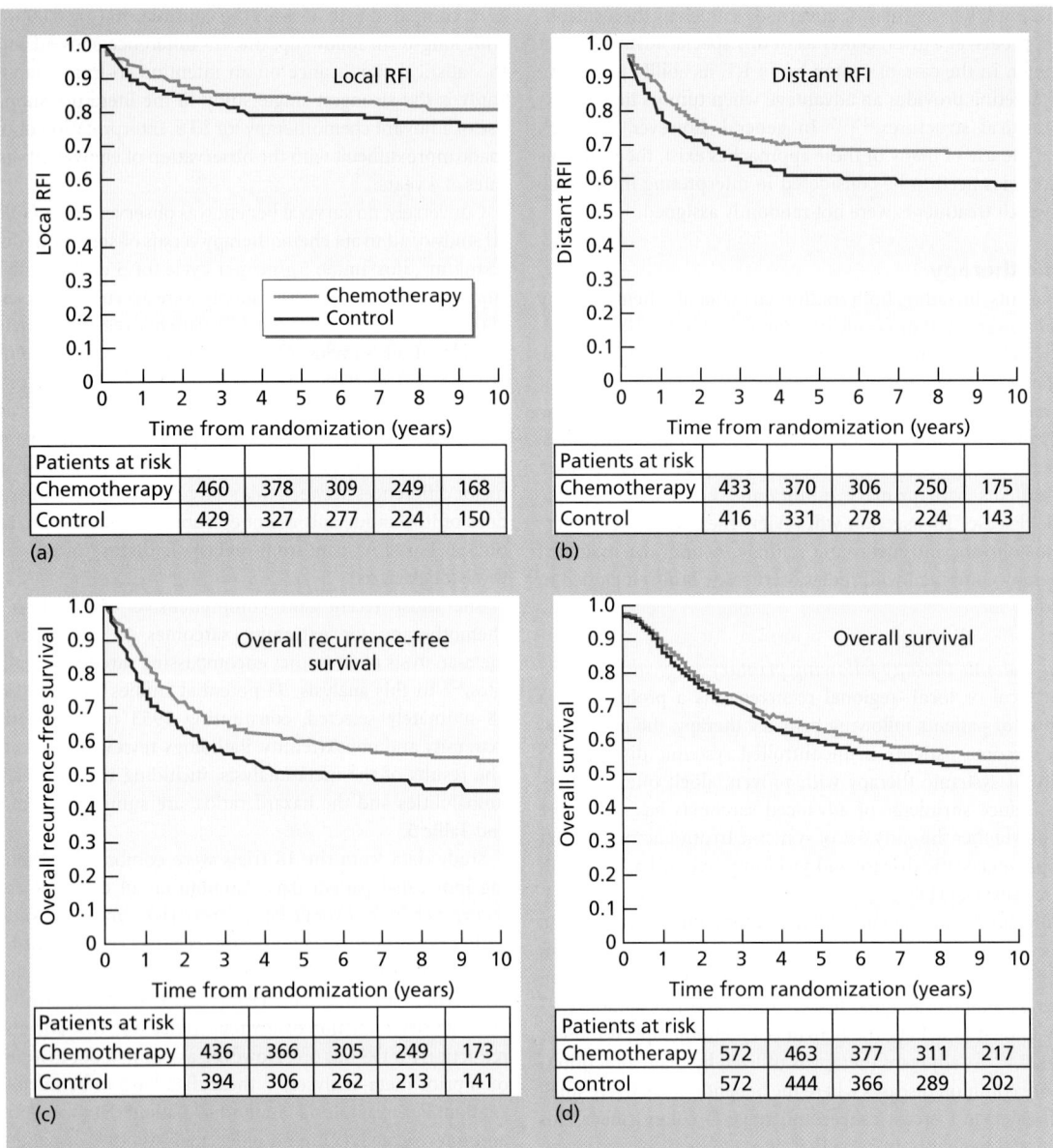

Figure 10 Actuarial curves from individual patient data meta-analysis: (a) local recurrence-free interval (RFI), (b) distant recurrence-free interval, (c) overall recurrence-free survival, and (d) overall survival. Source: O'Bryan et al. 1977.[130] Reproduced with permission of Wiley.

Table 5 Relative risks and 95% confidence intervals for clinical outcomes with adjuvant chemotherapy (2008 meta-analysis).

	Doxorubicin	Doxorubicin–ifosfamide	Combined
Local RFI	0.75 (0.56–1.01)	0.66 (0.39–1.12)	0.73 (0.56–0.94)
Distant RFI	0.69 (0.56–0.86)	0.61 (0.41–0.92)	0.67 (0.56–0.82)
Overall RFS	0.69 (0.56–0.86)	0.61 (0.41–0.92)	0.67 (0.56–0.82)
Overall survival	0.84 (0.68–1.03)	0.56 (0.36–0.85)	0.77 (0.64–0.93)

Source: Pervaiz et al. 2008.[129] Reproduced with permission of Wiley.

treatment. In contrast, those who do not respond may be those with unfavorable disease who could derive the greatest benefit from the discovery of highly effective systemic treatments.

A second potential advantage of preoperative chemotherapy is that it treats occult microscopic metastatic disease as soon as possible after the cancer diagnosis. This may theoretically prevent the development of chemotherapy resistance by isolated clones of metastatic cells or prevent the postoperative growth of microscopic metastases, but given the nature of growth of sarcomas, at most one or two doublings of the tumor would be affected, far fewer than the >35 typically required in the development of a >1-cm tumor. Chemotherapy-induced cytoreduction may permit a less radical and consequently less morbid surgical resection than would have been required initially. In patients with large STS of the extremities, cytoreduction may reduce the morbidity of limb-sparing surgical procedures and possibly even allow patients who might otherwise have required an amputation to undergo limb-sparing surgery.

Investigators from the MD Anderson Cancer Center reported long-term results with doxorubicin-based preoperative chemotherapy for AJCC stages IIC and III (formerly AJCC stage IIIB) extremity STS.[132] In a series of 76 patients treated with doxorubicin-based preoperative chemotherapy, radiologic response rates included complete response, 9%; partial response, 19%; minor response, 13%; stable disease, 30%; and disease progression, 30%. The overall objective major response rate (complete plus partial responses) was

27%. At a median follow-up of 85 months, 5-year actuarial rates of LR-free survival, distant metastasis-free survival, DFS, and OS were 83%, 52%, 46%, and 59%, respectively. The event-free outcomes reported from MD Anderson are similar to those observed with chemotherapy in the phase 3 postoperative chemotherapy trials. Furthermore, comparison of responding patients (complete and partial responses) and nonresponding patients did not reveal any significant differences in event-free outcome. Conversely, only 1/29 patients in a smaller study from Memorial Sloan-Kettering demonstrated WHO defined tumor shrinking after two cycles of doxorubicin-based therapy.[133]

Ifosfamide-containing combinations also have been used in the preoperative setting. Selected patients treated with aggressive ifosfamide-based regimens have had major responses, and preliminary results suggest that response rates may be higher than in historic controls treated with non-ifosfamide-containing regimens.[134] However, as noted above, the randomized phase 2 neoadjuvant study of doxorubicin and ifosfamide chemotherapy showed no benefit for the treatment arm, although the study was not specifically designed to determine a survival advantage.[135]

Regional administration of chemotherapy
It is hypothesized that the antineoplastic action of adjuvant chemotherapy will be improved by modifying factors related to drug delivery. One such modification is administering chemotherapy regionally rather than systemically. Intraperitoneal chemotherapy is used in primary therapy of ovarian cancer or appendiceal carcinoma, where it remains more superficial and accessible to peritoneal chemotherapy compared to other cancers that more commonly form more distinct masses that intraperitoneal chemotherapy cannot penetrate. For a period of time, intraperitoneal chemotherapy was used for GIST and gastrointestinal leiomyosarcomas that spread to the peritoneum, but this approach was abandoned given the access to tyrosine kinase inhibitors for GIST. Perhaps the situation in which regional therapy is most commonly used for sarcoma is intra-arterial chemotherapy used in some centers for osteogenic sarcoma, which provides both a higher concentration of drug locally as well as systemic effects after infusion. In some situations, chemotherapy is administered with radiation (see below).

Other investigators evaluated whole-body or regional hyperthermia to enhance the efficacy of combination chemotherapy, using methods to increase the temperature of the entire body or a specific region alone to 41°C.[136-138] In the 341 patient randomized study of primary and locally recurrent high-risk sarcomas, combination of preoperative hyperthermia and EIA chemotherapy (etoposide, ifosfamide, and doxorubicin) was superior to EIA alone in terms of local control and disease-free survival, although OS was not impacted. The study was criticized for not being able to sort out the contribution of radiation and hyperthermia, and what appeared to be a high frequency of R1 and R2 resections for patients going on study. Concurrent hyperthermia and chemotherapy is an approved treatment in some European countries, but remains investigational in the United States.

Combined preoperative chemotherapy and RT
Data regarding combination chemotherapy and radiation are more developed than hyperthermia and chemotherapy, largely from the commonality of the former being available at various institutions. As with combinations with hyperthermia, the primary putative advantage of preoperative chemotherapy with radiation is the potential to shrink selected lesions resectable only by amputation sufficiently that they become amenable to a limb-sparing approach.

Concurrent chemotherapy and radiation has been employed extensively by Eilber and colleagues at UCLA and has been modified and examined by other groups.[139,140] The first chemotherapy–radiation treatment protocol typically involved intra-arterial doxorubicin with high dose per fraction RT (35 Gy of external beam radiation delivered in 10 daily fractions, which was reduced to 17.5 Gy in 5 daily fractions to minimize local toxicity). Although the intra-arterial route delivers chemotherapy more directly to the tumor, it is more complex, expensive, and prone to complications than intravenous chemotherapy.[141] Indeed, a prospective randomized trial comparing preoperative intra-arterial doxorubicin with intravenous doxorubicin, both followed by 28 Gy of radiation delivered over 8 days and then surgical resection, showed no differences in LR or survival.[140]

The largest study to date directly studying systemic chemotherapy combined with RT examined razoxane as the radiation-sensitizing agent in a randomized study of drug versus no drug in combination with radiation therapy for resectable or unresectable STSs.[142] Acute skin reactions were enhanced in the razoxane arm, but late toxicity was not greater than in the control arm. Although there are imbalances in the arms of the study, for the 82 of 130 evaluable cases examined with gross disease RT (median dose 56–58 Gy) with razoxane (daily oral doses of 150 mg/m² throughout RT) showed an increased response rate (74% vs 49%) and improved local control rate (64% vs 30%; $p < 0.05$) compared with external beam radiation alone.

Either ifosfamide or cyclophosphamide has been routinely combined with radiation therapy as part of the definitive therapy for Ewing sarcoma and rhabdomyosarcoma in an attempt to continue systemic therapy at the same time as maximizing local control.[119] In general, toxicity does not appear to be greater than that seen for radiation alone. However, skin toxicity from the combination was greater in one study than that seen with radiation alone.[143]

An alternative sequential chemotherapy and radiation strategy in patients with localized, high-grade, large (>8 cm) extremity STSs has been examined.[144-146] This treatment protocol involved 3 courses of doxorubicin, ifosfamide, mesna, and dacarbazine (MAID) with two 22-Gy courses of radiation (11 fractions each) for a total preoperative radiation dose of 44 Gy. This was followed by surgical resection with careful microscopic assessment of surgical margins. An additional 16-Gy (8 fraction) boost was delivered for microscopically positive surgical margins. The outcomes of 48 patients treated with this regimen were compared with those of matched historic controls and was superior to that of the historical control patients.[144] The 5-year actuarial local control, freedom from distant metastasis, DFS, and OS rate were 92% versus 86% ($p = 0.1155$), 75% versus 44% ($p = 0.0016$), 70% versus 42% ($p = 0.0002$), and 87% versus 58% ($p = 0.0003$) for the MAID and control patient groups, respectively. Febrile neutropenia was a complication in 25% of patients. Wound-healing complications were substantial and occurred in 14 (29%) patients receiving the chemotherapy/radiation sequential therapy. One patient who received chemotherapy developed late fatal myelodysplasia. Given the favorable results of this study in comparison to historical controls for high-risk extremity STS, the Radiation Therapy Oncology Group conducted a multi-institutional trial, modifying the chemotherapy in an attempt to address the local toxicity issue. The report of the trial suggested combined-modality treatment can be delivered successfully in a multi-institutional setting albeit with some toxicity. Efficacy results are consistent with previous single-institution results.[145,146] The question remains whether this approach in high-risk, extremity STS confers significant survival benefits following and intense regimen of neoadjuvant chemoradiotherapy and surgery, which seems sustained even with long-term follow-up.

Although significant toxicity was observed, local control was improved in the prior studies compared to historical controls, raising the possibility that combined chemotherapy and radiation could be combined safely to decrease local control risk. Pisters et al.[132] examined concurrent doxorubicin and irradiation in the neoadjuvant setting in 27 patients with extremity STS. Preoperative external beam radiation was administered in 25 fractions of 2 Gy each. Doxorubicin was administered in escalating doses with a bolus followed by 4-day continuous infusion weekly. Radiographic restaging was performed 4–7 weeks after chemoradiation. Patients with localized disease underwent surgical resection. The maximum tolerated dose of continuous infusion doxorubicin combined with standard preoperative radiation was 17.5 mg/m^2/week; 7 of 23 (30%) patients had grade 3 dermatologic toxicity at this dose level. Macroscopically complete resection (R0 or R1) was performed in all 26 patients who underwent surgery. In 22 patients who were treated with doxorubicin at the maximum tolerated dose and subsequent surgery, an encouraging 11 patients (50%) had 90% or greater tumor necrosis, including 2 patients who had complete pathologic responses. This approach appears valid with other radiation-sensitizing agents as well, such as gemcitabine.[147] Further studies of combination therapy are also discussed later in the section titled "Retroperitoneal Sarcomas."

Other multicenter trials of adjuvant therapy for STS

It is well recognized that different sarcoma subtypes have different chemotherapy resistance/sensitivity patterns, details of which are discussed in greater detail elsewhere.[61] For example, synovial sarcoma is typically resistant to gemcitabine–docetaxel, and leiomyosarcomas are typically less sensitive to ifosfamide than other forms of sarcoma. Synovial sarcoma and myxoid/round-cell liposarcoma appear to be more sensitive to chemotherapy in the metastatic setting than other subtypes of sarcoma and may well be two subtypes that respond to both anthracyclines and ifosfamide. These data argue that adjuvant chemotherapy should be examined on a subtype-specific basis. Combined nonrandomized data from UCLA and MSKCC showed that adjuvant chemotherapy may indeed be useful in the setting of synovial sarcomas and myxoid/round-cell liposarcoma and argued for the use of chemotherapy in the neoadjuvant setting for all types of STS, based on institutional databases.[148–150] Notably, data of all patients treated or not treated with chemotherapy from MD Anderson and MSKCC indicated in the adjuvant or neoadjuvant setting that there was no statistical difference in OS in the group of patients who received chemotherapy versus those who did not.[151] However, these data are inherently biased in that it is likely that younger, healthier patients with higher risk tumors were those selected to receive chemotherapy. Even though there was no statistically significant difference between the group of patients who received chemotherapy and those who did not, there were still shifts in the frequency of patients with larger sarcomas with a predominance of liposarcoma toward receiving chemotherapy, perhaps representing the selection bias that allowed a group of patients with an inherently poorer outcome to do as well as those with a better outcome.

In summary, for AJCC stage III STS, if there is a benefit to chemotherapy in the adjuvant setting, it appears to be a modest one. There is variation in practice between centers and between practitioners as to who is an appropriate candidate for chemotherapy. Given this situation, it is the authors' practice to attempt to compare benefits and risks of systemic therapy and individualize

the plan of treatment for a given clinical setting. Patients below age 50 may be those who benefit most among this very heterogeneous patient population. Certainly, the finding of 35% or more of STS with specific genetic translocations or mutations brings hope that the benefit seen with GIST and adjuvant imatinib therapy will carry over to the adjuvant setting for a subset of patients with STS of the extremities and trunk when traditional adjuvant cytotoxic chemotherapy is combined with novel therapeutics.

"Pediatric" sarcomas and adjuvant therapy

The standard of care for nearly all sarcomas specific to the pediatric population involves chemotherapy. It is of proved benefit in patients with osteogenic sarcoma, Ewing sarcoma, and rhabdomyosarcoma. A few brief comments on these chemotherapy-responsive tumors follow.

Neoadjuvant chemotherapy is the standard of care for the initial treatment of osteogenic sarcoma.[121] In the era before systemic therapy, cure rates for osteogenic sarcoma, even in the setting of amputation for primary disease, was only on the order of 15%. With chemotherapy, the survival rate is 65–70%. Yet the 30–35% of patients who relapse remain a frustrating problem because the addition of new agents has changed the chance for cure comparatively modestly, and the one agent demonstrating benefit in a randomized trial was not approved in the United States.[120] The outcome of adjuvant chemotherapy (degree of tumor necrosis after chemotherapy) is directly associated with improved clinical outcome and provides the opportunity for changing chemotherapy for a poor initial response. The standard of care for adjuvant chemotherapy is a backbone of cisplatin and doxorubicin, with methotrexate employed in most pediatric and some adult patients. The benefit for methotrexate as part of adjuvant treatment was called into question in a 1997 paper in which the combination of doxorubicin and cisplatin alone was shown equivalent to a more complicated and toxic regimen containing high-dose methotrexate.[152] However, the methotrexate component of neoadjuvant therapy has been observed to be important in a variety of studies and remains an integral part of combination therapy for osteosarcoma.[153] Less questionable is the benefit from nonspecific immune system stimulator muramyl tripeptide (MTP), which was shown in a large pediatric clinical trial to improve OS when used in the adjuvant setting, while there was no benefit in survival seen with the addition of ifosfamide to the standard methotrexate–doxorubicin–cisplatin (MAP) backbone.[120]

Through a series of international clinical studies, the adjuvant program for rhabdomyosarcoma typically involves an induction course of chemotherapy, followed by combination chemotherapy and radiation, followed by the completion of chemotherapy, which will last approximately 48 weeks in pediatric population. The standard of care is the combination of vincristine, dactinomycin, and cyclophosphamide, as this combination was shown as effective as VAI and VIE and less toxic.[119] The addition of doxorubicin to the vincristine, dactinomycin, and cyclophosphamide regimen did not appear to improve OS and is omitted in the treatment of pediatric rhabdomyosarcoma.[154] The frequent dosing of vincristine is extremely difficult to complete for adults and requires dose adjustment or shorter courses of therapy for adults than for children with this diagnosis. Children with this diagnosis appear to fare better than adults with the same diagnosis stage in most studies, as well as in everyday practice.[155,156]

For patients with Ewing sarcoma, in distinction from rhabdomyosarcoma, the addition of additional agents (ifosfamide and etoposide) to an existing backbone of vincristine, doxorubicin, and cyclophosphamide chemotherapy improved outcome for localized disease, with a 2-week schedule superior to a 3-week schedule of treatment;[122] however, not published were data that the 2-week schedule was not beneficial for patients over age 18. This 5-drug regimen is a good standard of care for patients with a new diagnosis of Ewing sarcoma. It is often difficult to administer the 14 cycles of chemotherapy to adults, and abbreviation to the adjuvant therapy program is often necessary. It is also not clear if all 14 cycles are necessary for best outcomes. As with rhabdomyosarcoma, children with Ewing sarcoma fare better than adults with the same diagnosis, all else being equal.[157-159]

Treatment of locally advanced disease

Hyperthermic isolated limb perfusion, isolated limb infusion, and regional hyperthermia
Hyperthermic isolated limb perfusion (ILP), an investigational technique in the United States (although recently approved by regulatory agencies in other parts of the world), has received considerable attention in the treatment of locally advanced, unresectable sarcomas of nonosseous tissues. ILP involves local perfusion of high-dose chemotherapy (most commonly melphalan) and, when available, tumor necrosis factor alpha (TNFα) under hyperthermic conditions. An oxygenated circuit is established by local arterial and venous cannulation on a bypass pump. Systemic circulation is minimized by placement of a tourniquet proximally.

ILP has been evaluated in two settings: (1) attempted limb preservation in cases of locally advanced extremity lesions surgically amenable only to amputation and (2) function extremity preservation for the short survival duration anticipated in cases of locally advanced extremity lesions with synchronous pulmonary metastases (stage IV disease).

A multicenter phase 2 trial evaluated a series of 55 patients with radiologically unresectable extremity STS using HILP with high-dose TNFα and melphalan, and interferon-α in some patients.[160] A major tumor response was seen and limb salvaged in over 80% of patients. Regional toxicity was limited, and systemic toxicity was minimal to moderate. There were no treatment-related deaths. Despite the high rate of complete responses (15–30%) and limb sparing (>80%) achieved by ILP, no randomized trials have compared ILP to aggressive limb-sparing resection with RT for STS. Therefore, ILP should be considered as a potential treatment, when other options are limited or not available, in appropriately selected patients. Eligible patients should be referred to centers where this therapy is available.

Isolated limb infusion (ILI) has been evaluated in extremity STS in a more limited manner, and parallels work done with intra-arterial chemotherapy. Like IPL, ILI relies on circulating high-dose chemotherapy in an isolated extremity. Unlike ILP, ILI is conducted through percutaneously placed catheters and is performed under hypoxic conditions. However, there is limited experience with ILI in extremity STS. Similar to ILP, ILI has not been directly compared to aggressive limb-sparing resection with EBRT in a randomized trial. However, patients under consideration for ILP and ILI are often no candidates for surgery with EBRT at first evaluation, and therefore ILP and ILI may be considered as potential therapies in appropriately selected patients.

Definitive radiation for local control
Apart from patients with some very radiosensitive subtypes of sarcomas, most patients who undergo RT as the sole treatment modality for sarcoma have been deemed to have locally advanced unresectable disease. RT alone is a rare treatment choice that should be done only at centers skilled in the management of sarcomas; medically fit patients with grossly "unresectable" but nonmetastatic disease should always be referred to a specialty center for multidisciplinary management, which may combine surgery, RT, and possibly chemotherapy. For example, proximal inguinal or axillary tumors that encircle major vascular structures in the proximal leg or arm may be resected along with the involved vasculature and the vessels reconstructed. Adjuvant RT is also generally used. Rarely, a patient with truly inoperable locally advanced disease may require RT alone, with either photon or particle (proton, neutron, or pion) beams.[161-163] No formal clinical trials have been performed to compare these strategies with each other, and they are generally administered in an adverse clinical setting. Local control has been reported in 40–70% range.

Treatment of metastatic disease

Clinical problem of metastases
The diagnosis of recurrent or metastatic disease in patients with STSs is often heartbreaking. Patients and physicians are aware that, in general, such a diagnosis is typically fatal. The role of the multidisciplinary sarcoma team in the management of patients with metastatic sarcoma is to recognize opportunities in which multimodality care might still improve important outcomes such as survival or quality of life. Both surgery and systemic chemotherapy can play an important role in improving these outcomes in selected patients. Overall, it is important to recognize that chemotherapy is usually given with the palliative aim of prolonging life and improving quality of life.

The most common site of metastasis from STS of the extremities is the lungs. Indeed, the lungs are the only site of metastasis in approximately 80% of patients with metastases from primary extremity and trunk STS.[61] Primary visceral and gastrointestinal sarcomas such as GIST commonly metastasize to the liver, while other visceral sarcomas may metastasize to lungs as well. Extrapulmonary metastases are uncommon forms of first metastasis from extremity sarcomas and usually occur as a late manifestation of widely disseminated disease. The median survival after development of distant metastases is approximately 12 months (Figure 11),[165] although more contemporary data suggest that median survival may presently be 15–18 months for unselected patients who receive cytotoxic chemotherapy; the optimal treatment of patients with metastatic STS requires an understanding of the natural history of the disease and individualized selection of treatment options based on patient factors, disease factors, and limitations imposed by prior treatment.

The approach to patients with advanced or metastatic sarcomas is changing over time. We increasingly realize clinical trials must be stratified rationally for data of value to be derived. Studies of "sarcomas" without stratification by histology or molecular features will soon seem as naïve as studies of "cancer" without further qualification. These mesenchymally derived diseases lumped under the heading of "sarcomas" can be quite different, and studies need to take that into account. In a similar manner, the consideration of a specific sarcoma histology may be supplemented or even superseded by the genetic profile of the tumor. To generate studies of sufficient size and power, large-scale collaborations on a national and international level will be required. Such collaborations are already in place among the nations of Europe individually and collectively (e.g., the Soft Tissue and Bone Sarcoma Group of the EORTC), Canadian centers, and cooperative trials groups and other clinical trials collaborations such as SARC (Sarcoma Alliance

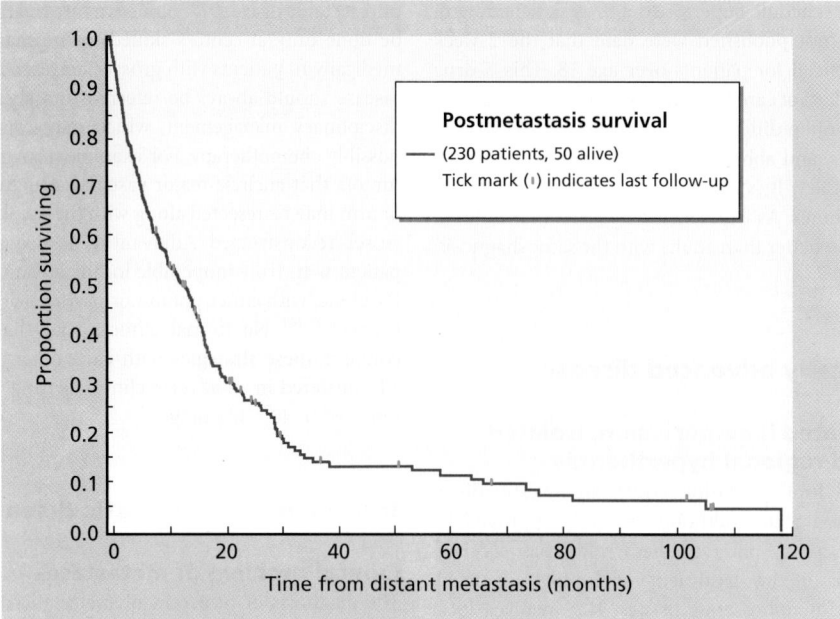

Figure 11 Postmetastasis survival (from time of diagnosis of M1 disease) in a cohort of 230 patients with primary STS of the extremities. The median postmetastasis survival was 11.6 months. Source: Slater et al. 1986.[164] Reproduced with permission of Elsevier.

for Research through Collaboration) in the United States. With these collaborations, it is hoped that further research will rapidly translate research findings into the novel therapeutics that are so desperately required by patients with sarcomas.

Resection of metastatic disease

Many investigators have reported their experience with pulmonary metastasectomy for metastatic STS in adults.[166,167] Three-year survival rates following thoracotomy for pulmonary metastasectomy range from 23% to 54%. As a result, some patients can be resected with curative intent, similar to the situation for osteogenic sarcoma. As the ability to completely resect all metastatic disease is an important determinant of outcome, the reported interinstitutional variability in postmetastasectomy survival rates is partially a function of whether survival was reported for all patients who underwent thoracotomy or only for the subset who underwent complete resection.

It remains difficult to predict which patients with pulmonary metastases will benefit from pulmonary resection. A number of clinical criteria have been evaluated by univariate analysis in this regard, including the disease-free interval, number of metastatic nodules, and tumor doubling time. Multivariate analyses from both the NCI and Roswell Park Cancer Institute confirm that a short disease-free interval and incomplete pulmonary resection are adverse prognostic factors for survival for patients with pulmonary metastases.[166–169] A multivariate analysis from MD Anderson suggested that, in addition, the presence of more than three metastatic pulmonary nodules on preoperative chest CT is an adverse prognostic sign. The most important prognostic factor impacting survival appears to be the ability to completely resect all disease. In the review of postmetastasectomy outcomes in one series, the median survival among patients who were able to undergo complete resection of metastases was 20 months as compared with 10 months among patients who did not have complete resection (Figure 12).[165] In summary, the ability to achieve complete resection and the number of pulmonary nodules present appear to best define the postoperative prognosis for these patients.

Unfortunately, metastasectomy benefits only a fraction of patients who develop pulmonary metastases. This is best illustrated by data from MSKCC, where a population of 716 patients who presented with primary extremity sarcoma were followed for the subsequent development and treatment of pulmonary metastases (Figure 13).[170] Of an initial group of 716 patients, 148 patients (21%) developed pulmonary metastases. Isolated pulmonary metastases occurred in 135 (91%) of these 148 patients. Of the 135 patients with pulmonary-only metastases, 78 (58%) were considered to have operable disease, and 65 (83%) of those taken to thoracotomy were able to undergo complete resection of all of their pulmonary metastatic disease. Thus, 44% of all patients with pulmonary metastases were able to undergo complete metastasectomy. The median survival from the time of complete resection was 19 months, and the 3-year survival rate was 23%. All patients who did not undergo thoracotomy died within 3 years. For the entire cohort of 135 patients developing pulmonary-only metastases, the 3-year survival rate was only 11%.

Several series of repeat pulmonary metastasectomy also have been published. In a series of 43 patients thus treated at the NCI, 72% of patients could be rendered free of disease at the second thoracotomy, with a median survival duration from the time of second thoracotomy of 25 months.[171] In a report from MD Anderson of a series of 39 patients undergoing reoperation for a second pulmonary metastasis after successful initial metastasectomy, factors predicting long-term survival included the presence of a solitary metastasis and the ability to perform a complete resection.[172] Patients with isolated second metastatic sites fared better than those with multiple resected lesions.

The disappointing overall results of treatment of metastatic disease underscore the importance of careful patient selection for resection of pulmonary metastases. The following criteria are generally agreed upon: (1) the primary tumor is controlled or is controllable, (2) there is no extrathoracic disease, (3) the patient is a medical candidate for thoracotomy and pulmonary resection, and (4) complete resection of all disease appears possible. With

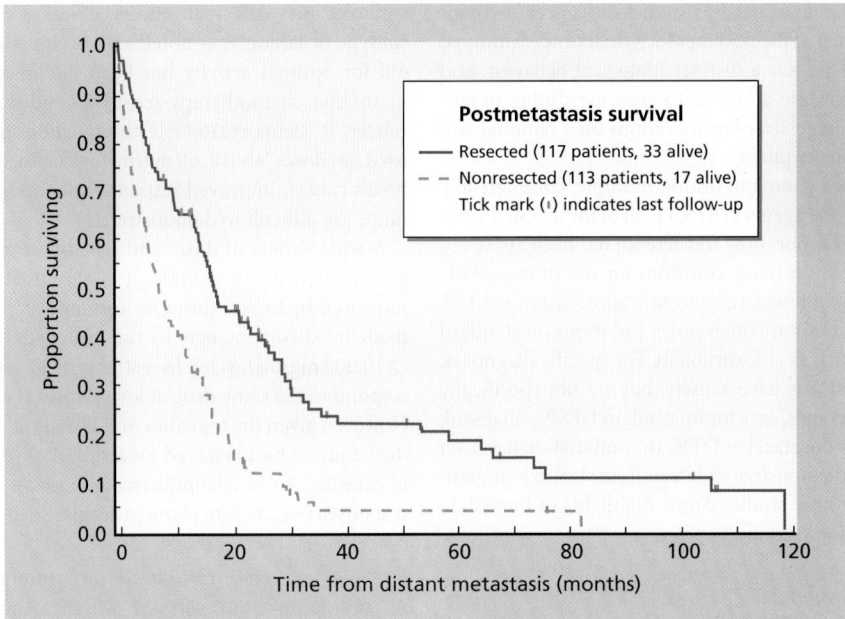

Figure 12 Postmetastasis survival stratified by resection of pulmonary metastatic disease. The median survival among patients undergoing complete resection of pulmonary metastatic disease was 20 months. Source: Billingsley et al. 1999.[165] Reproduced with permission of Wiley.

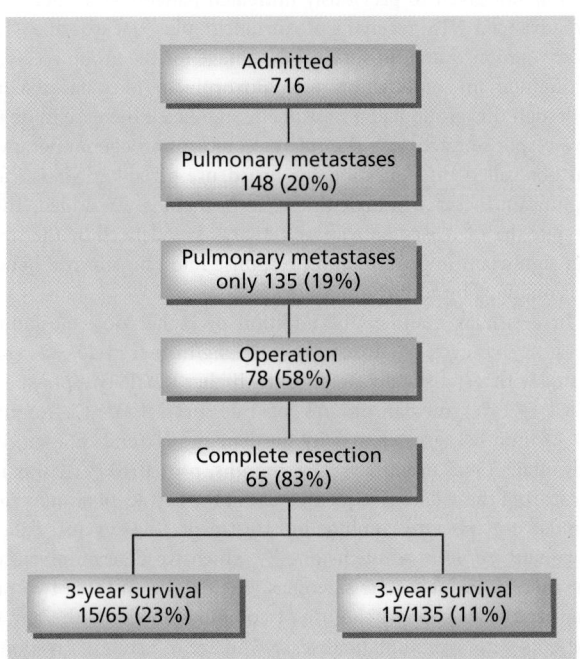

Figure 13 Risk and subsequent management of pulmonary metastases in 716 patients with primary or locally recurrent extremity STS. Source: Brennan 1996.[170] Reproduced with permission of Elsevier.

careful patient selection, the morbidity of thoracotomy (or repeated thoracotomies) can be limited to the subset of patients who are most likely to benefit from this aggressive treatment approach. The potential role of systemic adjuvant chemotherapy following complete metastasectomy is discussed below in the section "Individualized Therapy" on individualizing chemotherapy for metastases.

Chemotherapy for metastatic disease

Natural history of metastases

A good place to begin a discussion of chemotherapy for unresectable metastatic sarcoma is the expected course of the disease. The EORTC contributed greatly to define the expected course of unresectable metastatic sarcoma by publishing its large series of more than 2000 patients with advanced sarcomas of soft tissues to describe prognostic features and the response to anthracycline-based chemotherapy in an era before GIST was recognized as a unique entity.[173] In this study reviewing more than 20 years of experience, the median OS was approximately 1 year. Subsets of patients had longer median survival; such patients were typically those who were younger, had a better performance status, had low-grade sarcoma, had no liver metastases, and had developed metastatic disease following a longer interval from initial diagnosis. Importantly, this study concluded that the variables predicting improved survival were actually different from variables predicting objective response to chemotherapy (the latter variables include such items as high-grade tumor and liposarcoma subtype). Thus, one interpretation that is reasonable is that the most important predictors of survival with metastatic sarcoma are variables dependent on the tumor biology itself, as well as certain patient factors such as age and comorbid disease. These data are critical to understand so that information regarding the impact of new drugs and treatments can be interpreted appropriately, based on a comparison with the correct expectations for the natural or treated history of the disease in past clinical trials.

Individualized therapy

The approach to patients with advanced or metastatic sarcomas is evolving as are new therapeutics, and in this context, the use of therapies directed at specific histologies or DNA alterations is evolving, as are the entirely orthogonal approaches involving immunotherapy. We increasingly recognize that clinical trials must be stratified rationally for data of value to be derived. Studies of "sarcomas" without stratification will soon seem as naïve as studies of "cancer" without further qualification; each of the >50 mesenchymal cancers lumped under the heading "STSs" has a distinct biological behavior, and studies need to take that into account. To generate studies of sufficient size and power, large-scale collaborations on a national and international level will be required.

Tremendous effort has gone into testing multiple, commercially available and experimental agents in STS. Of all of these tested since the common use of ifosfamide, only trabectedin has been approved in Europe and pazopanib in many countries for use in metastatic soft tissue sarcoma; eribulin was also recently approved in the U.S. for liposarcoma; behind this are other novel variations on standard agents being studied, such as aldoxorubicin. For specific diagnoses, imatinib and other SMOKIs have activity, but are not specifically approved for use in sarcomas, save for imatinib in DFSPs. That said, gemcitabine with either docetaxel or DTIC in combination has been shown superior in progression-free and overall survival versus gemcitabine only in randomized studies. Some highlights of these data are noted in the following section.

Anthracyclines and ifosfamide
With the caveat that specific sarcomas demonstrate differential sensitivity to different chemotherapy agents, doxorubicin and ifosfamide remain the most active agents for metastatic sarcoma, with RECIST response rates in the 10–20% range for each drug.[174] Depending on the ratio of sensitive versus less sensitive subtypes of STSs in past studies, the response rate can be significantly higher. For example, synovial sarcoma and myxoid/round-cell liposarcomas are relatively sensitive to ifosfamide (as well as doxorubicin), while GIST, alveolar soft part sarcoma, and extraskeletal myxoid chondrosarcoma appear to be largely resistant to both agents.

It is important to recognize that response rates *per se* increasingly are being criticized as poor surrogates of clinical benefit. Many sarcomas contain acellular desmoplastic stromal tissues. Even when chemotherapy successfully induces significant tumor cell kill *in vivo*, the matrix left behind appears largely unaffected, leading to falsely negative imaging findings of tumor response to chemotherapy. Thus, objective response rates based on imaging may underestimate the antitumor efficacy of chemotherapy. Conversely, simply shrinking a tumor and achieving a nondurable response may not be worth the toxicities of aggressive multiagent chemotherapy. Thus, from both standpoints, RECIST-defined responses may not be an ideal indicator of antitumor efficacy in sarcoma management in general, with GIST a case in point.[175,176] Increasing attention in the field of sarcoma drug development is thus being paid to other important indicators of clinical outcomes, such as progression-free survival duration, percentage survival at a given time point, and OS rate.

Some drugs may slow disease progression and prolong survival even if objective response rates are low, although the clinical data to support those claims must be generated with rigor and careful attention to consistency of follow-up. Nonetheless, despite observations that clinical benefit might be underestimated by RECIST, it remains the yardstick by which radiological responses are measured.

Dose–response relationships
The sensitivity of sarcomas to chemotherapy was first convincingly demonstrated with doxorubicin in the early to mid 1970s.[124] Subsequent studies of doxorubicin in sarcomas have widely been viewed as supporting a dose–response relationship, with doses of 50 mg/m²/cycle or less associated with less antitumor activity than doses of 60 mg/m²/cycle or higher. Although a dose–response relationship is evident, it is important to recognize that other variables may affect antitumor efficacy, such as histopathologic subtype of sarcoma, as noted above. Nonetheless, as a dose threshold for optimal activity has been documented with doxorubicin in another chemotherapy-sensitive solid tumor, specifically breast cancer, it seems reasonable to conclude that doxorubicin is best used at doses above 60 mg/m²/cycle. In addition, analogous to breast cancer, improved response rates above 75 mg/m²/cycle dose range are difficult to demonstrate.

A wide variety of dose- and schedule-ranging studies have been performed with ifosfamide. It is clear that antitumor response is improved by higher doses of ifosfamide.[134,177] This point has been made most convincingly by the responses to high-dose ifosfamide (≥10,000 mg/m²/cycle) in patients who had previously failed to respond to the same drug at lower doses (i.e., ≤6000 mg/m²/cycle). However, given the toxicities of this drug at higher doses, high-dose ifosfamide is best reserved for a subset of patients with disease that is expected to be chemotherapy sensitive to achieve meaningful responses (e.g., before planned surgical extirpation of metastases).

Single-agent versus combination chemotherapy
A continuing controversy is whether the optimal approach to patients with advanced sarcomas is combination chemotherapy regimens or sequential single agents. One of the best prospective randomized trials of combination chemotherapy for advanced disease came from a US intergroup study in which ifosfamide was or was not given to previously untreated patients with metastatic or advanced STS receiving doxorubicin plus dacarbazine. This study demonstrated no survival advantage for the group receiving ifosfamide in combination with doxorubicin plus dacarbazine, although this group had a statistically significant increase in objective response rate.[178,179] The role of combination chemotherapy is further called into question for broad use given the statistically significant increase in toxicities when ifosfamide was added. Thus, despite the increased anticancer activity as evidenced by the small but significant improvement in response rates, no survival benefit was obtained by adding a third drug.

In a similar manner, the addition of higher dose ifosfamide (10 g/m² per cycle) to doxorubicin (75 mg/m² per cycle) was associated with a statistically significantly higher RECIST response rate (26% vs 14%), median progression-free survival rate (7.4 months vs 4.6 months), greater toxicity burden, and a trend to a survival advantage (14.3 months vs 12.8 months, $p = 0.076$).[180] It was not clear from these data if sequential use of the two agents would yield similar outcomes to combination treatment. The survival data in particular serve as a touchstone by which we determine success for therapy in metastatic sarcomas. The data from these two randomized trials support the use of combination chemotherapy for patients with symptomatic disease who are in need of a response; by the same token, it is not unreasonable to use single agents sequentially to minimize patient toxicity for less symptomatic or asymptomatic patients who remain in need of therapy.

Strategies to improve the therapeutic index of chemotherapy

Dose intensification using stem cells
An obvious strategy to increase response rates has been to increase dose intensity, adding stem cell support, as examined in hematological malignancies, breast adenocarcinoma, and other malignancies. This was initially attempted solely with provision of autologous bone marrow support and in the past decade has been significantly facilitated by the availability of hematopoietic cytokines to improve

hematologic tolerance to myelosuppressive chemotherapy. It is clear that peripheral blood progenitor cells can be mobilized and harvested following standard chemotherapy for sarcoma supported by granulocyte colony-stimulating factor.[181] Testing the limits of high-dose therapy, full-dose doxorubicin, ifosfamide, and cisplatin are possible with stem cell support not clearly better than standard dosing in osteogenic sarcoma.[182] Even in chemotherapy-sensitive diseases such as Ewing sarcoma, dose intensification with autologous stem cell support does not appear to be beneficial for improving survival, although contamination of stem cells with tumor cells may be a contributing factor to its lack of efficacy. The use of high-dose chemotherapy with stem cell and cytokine support remains investigational for sarcomas.

Encapsulated anthracyclines

Another strategy to increase the therapeutic index of anthracyclines is to encapsulate the drug within a liposomal vehicle. At least three liposomal preparations of anthracyclines have been tested, and all have shown some efficacy against sarcomas. Notably, the most widely used agent has decreased cardiac risk in comparison to older preparations of larger liposomes containing doxorubicin. Pegylated liposomal doxorubicin (Doxil/Caelyx) is a small liposome with polyethylene glycol anchored within the lipid bilayer, acting as a hydrophilic coating to preserve the circulating half-life of the liposome and prevent degradation within the reticuloendothelial system. This preparation, given at a dose less than that of unencapsulated doxorubicin, is better tolerated than doxorubicin, with substantially less myelotoxicity, cardiac toxicity, and alopecia at the cost of hand–foot syndrome and idiosyncratic reactions to the first dose of therapy; while its dose is lower, it has long half-life in the circulation (30–70 h), leading to an area under the curve for 50 mg/m^2 that is 300 times that of doxorubicin itself. In a randomized phase 2 study, pegylated liposomal doxorubicin demonstrated similar activity to normal doxorubicin (9% vs 10% response rate in the era before GIST was recognized as a separate type of sarcoma); formal noninferiority or equivalence was not determined, but pegylated liposomal doxorubicin was significantly less toxic than doxorubicin.[183] Less toxic anthracycline preparation has yielded a way to extend systemic therapy to patients with poorer performance status and in principle is a novel way of treating very slowly growing connective tissue lesions such as myxoid liposarcomas or desmoid tumors.

Beyond anthracyclines and ifosfamide

Few other agents beyond doxorubicin and ifosfamide demonstrate activity in soft tissue sarcoma, but this is a generalization in an era in which more histology specific data are needed for treatment decision making. It is recognized that dacarbazine (DTIC) has minor activity in STS, and studies have demonstrated that leiomyosarcoma and to a lesser degree solitary fibrous tumor are two diagnoses in which dacarbazine and its orally absorbed relative temozolomide have greatest activity.[184–186] Gemcitabine and docetaxel as a combination was first demonstrated to have activity in uterine leiomyosarcoma, after relatively disappointing phase 2 trials of gemcitabine as a single agent, suggesting true synergy between the two agents.[187,188] Randomized study of gemcitabine and docetaxel showed the combination was superior to gemcitabine alone with respect to both PFS and OS in a group of unselected sarcomas.[189] Notably, responses were most common in UPS and pleomorphic liposarcoma, more than leiomyosarcoma. A randomized study demonstrated the superiority in PFS and OS of gemcitabine and dacarbazine over dacarbazine alone, the second in which gemcitabine combinations were superior to single agents

in important radiological and clinical outcomes.[190] The addition of bevacizumab to the gemcitabine–docetaxel combination did not add to the chemotherapy backbone, and progression-free survival was numerically, although not statistically, inferior to treatment with the two chemotherapy drugs alone.[191] Thus, either the gemcitabine–docetaxel or gemcitabine–dacarbazine combinations are good options after failure of doxorubicin and/or ifosfamide. Indeed, the perception of toxicity of gemcitabine-based therapy versus doxorubicin-based therapy has led to its acceptance in first line in metastatic sarcoma patients in the United States.[192] The author generally employs gemcitabine–dacarbazine for leiomyosarcomas and gemcitabine–docetaxel in UPS, pleomorphic liposarcoma, and pleomorphic liposarcoma, given the responses seen to date on and off trial.

Newer agents

Sarcomas represent a fertile ground for the field of drug development. Doxorubicin was first recognized as an effective agent against sarcomas and subsequently was developed into one of the most widely used anticancer agents ever discovered. Imatinib and its spectacular results in a chemotherapy-resistant diagnosis provided a proof of principle that has since been borne out in other solid tumors with EGFR inhibitors, BRAF inhibitors, and the like. A few of newer agents and their utility in sarcoma are noted below. The next edition of this chapter will no doubt contain much more information on new drug and new targets in a specific histology or molecularly characterized subset of sarcomas, much as is happening across medical oncology.

Trabectedin (ET-743, ecteinascidin)

Trabectedin is a marine-derived drug from the marine tunicate *Ecteinascidia turbinata*. It covalently binds to the minor groove of the DNA and blocks the cell cycle in late S and G2 and affects the transcription in part by prevention of binding of transcription factor NF-Y, thus decreasing expression of a variety of genes, including multidrug resistance genes. After initial promising results in phase 1 studies, multiple phase 2 trials were performed, the most successful of which (a randomized phase II study of two schedules of drug) led to the drug's approval in Europe for refractory STS.[193,194] A follow-up randomized study showed greater activity of trabectedin than dacarbazine.[195]

The randomized phase 2 study of trabectedin in patients with metastatic leiomyosarcoma and liposarcoma compared a weekly schedule of drug with a 24-h infusion schedule.[193] In this 270 patient study, the longer 3-weekly infusion was associated with median time to progression of 3.7 months versus 2.3 months, $p = 0.03$; OS showed a numerically longer median OS for the 3-weekly infusion, 13.9 months versus 11.8 months, $p = 0.19$. Particular activity is noted in myxoid–round-cell liposarcoma, although activity in other histologies has been observed.

In a similar manner, the microtubule-targeted agent eribulin demonstrated activity in a phase 2 study,[196] which led to the conduct of a study similar to that of the trabectedin trial above, in which eribulin was tested against dacarbazine in a phase 3 trial in leiomyosarcoma and liposarcoma. The phase 3 data confirmed the activity seen in phase 2. The OS was not significantly different between trabectedin and dacarbazine in this study (12.4 months vs 12.9 months), there was a significant improvement in PFS with trabectedin over dacarbazine (median 4.2 months vs 1.5 months) in this randomized phase III trial.

Beyond cytotoxics, the most important result to date involves the SMOKI pazopanib. After the demonstration of activity in a phase 2 trial,[197] a phase 3 study termed PALETTE was conducted, involving 369 patients with STS progressing after standard therapy. With a 2:1 randomization for pazopanib 800 mg versus placebo, the pazopanib arm demonstrated statistically superior PFS. Median PFS in the placebo arm was 4.6 months in the pazopanib arm and 4.6 months in the pazopanib arm, with a corresponding HR of 0.35 ($p < 0.001$) as assessed by independent radiology review. Median OS at final analysis was 10.7 months in the placebo arm versus 12.6 months in the pazopanib arm, HR = 0.87, $p = 0.26$.[198] These data were sufficient to obtain broad international approval for pazopanib for metastatic STS worse after standard therapy.

Increasingly, the molecular characteristics of specific sarcomas will dictate therapeutic options. On the basis of the tumor DNA alterations (gene loss, translocation, or mutation), mTOR inhibitors such as sirolimus have activity in perivascular epithelial cell tumors (PEComas),[199] and imatinib and other inhibitors of PDGF receptor and CSF1 receptor have activity in DFSPs[200] and tenosynovial giant cell tumor (TGCT).[201,202] Crizotinib, the ALK inhibitor, is active in *ALK* translocation positive inflammatory myofibroblastic tumor (IMT). There will be increasing numbers of such agents demonstrating activity as targets other than kinases come into focus therapeutically, perhaps including chondrosarcomas with their frequent *IDH1* and *IDH2* mutations, and synovial sarcoma, Ewing sarcoma, and MPNSTs, which appear to have alterations in epigenetic regulators PRC1, LSDs, and BRD4, respectively, each becoming targetable imminently as are other epigenetic regulators such as EZH2.

Management of local recurrence

If an isolated LR is identified, the treatment goals are the same as for patients with primary tumors, namely, optimal local control while maintaining as much function and cosmesis as possible.[107] Early identification of local relapse may improve the chance of successful salvage therapy, and, like newly diagnosed patients, these patients are probably best managed in specialized multidisciplinary sarcoma centers. An approach to the evaluation and management of locally recurrent STS is summarized in Figure 14. The initial evaluation must include a full review of previous therapy because this will have a bearing on the therapeutic options available. Therefore, all prior surgery and pathology reports should be examined, as should reports on previous chemotherapy and previous RT, especially volume treated, dose, and energy of radiation.

Staging should be performed in the same way as for newly presenting patients. The areas adjacent to the original lesion and potentially contaminated by previous surgical interventions should be scrutinized carefully. Both these areas and tissues adjacent to the recurrent tumor, containing potential tumor extensions, should be considered at risk and candidates for resection and/or inclusion in radiation fields.

Several distinct groupings are evident under the rubric of "locally recurrent" disease: (1) cases in which prior treatment did not include RT, (2) cases treated with RT in the past, (3) cases in which distant metastases are also present, and (4) cases in which it is difficult to distinguish between recurrence and secondary tumors induced by RT. Although the therapeutic options available are more limited in recurrent disease and the challenge posed by these cases are much more formidable, a proportion of these patients

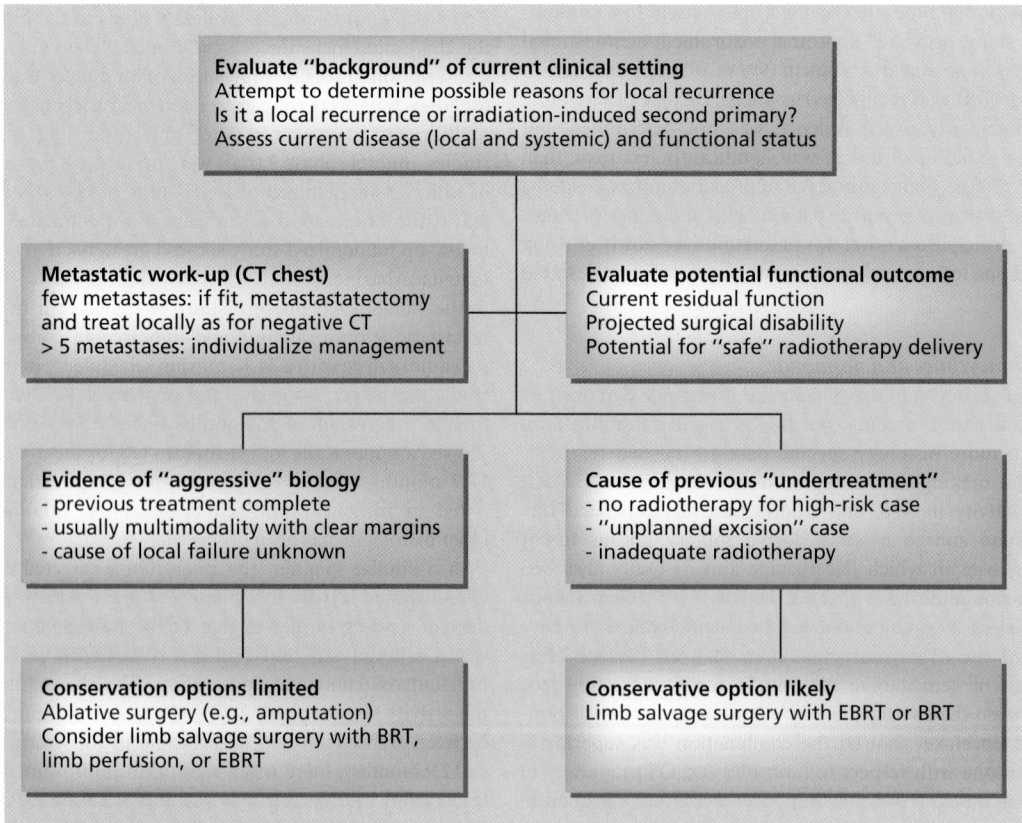

Figure 14 Schema for approaching the patient with local recurrence of STS. The schema is oriented toward extremity lesions but is equally applicable to other anatomic sites (e.g., head and neck and retroperitoneum). *Abbreviations*: BRT, brachytherapy; EBRT, external beam radiotherapy. Source: Catton et al. 1999.[107] Reproduced with permission of Elsevier.

can be cured. Clinical experience is needed to determine which therapeutic options are appropriate in a given case of recurrent disease.

Gastrointestinal stromal tumors

No discussion of sarcomas would be complete without noting the remarkable advances made with one particular sarcoma subtype, GIST, which has changed the way people think about solid tumors. With the recognition of KIT as a good marker for GIST to distinguish it from other sarcomas and the recognition of *KIT* or *PDGFRA* activating mutations that are likely responsible for the constitutive activation of *KIT*,[203] clinical studies followed rapidly and have been done in parallel to studies investigating the biology of GIST. Of note, presence of an immunohistochemical marker cannot be equated with tumor response, as is suggested by companies that purport this to be the case. Ewing sarcomas can mark positive for KIT by immunohistochemistry, but *KIT* is not mutated in these tumors and Ewing sarcomas do not respond to imatinib.

Surgical principles for management of primary GIST differ from those for other sarcomas and visceral adenocarcinomas. In general, resection requires a minimal margin of normal tissue, not the wide margins of other sarcomas or visceral adenocarcinomas. Unlike gastric cancer, GIST do not generally metastasize to local–regional lymph nodes (except in some GIST arising in the pediatric population), rendering lymph node dissection unnecessary in the vast majority of patient. Thus, gastric GISTs can often be removed by simple wedge resections, and large gastric resections are only rarely required, generally due to anatomic constraints. Similarly, GISTs arising in the small intestine, the colon, or the rectum may be resected with minimal margins. Furthermore, patients with GIST undergoing a macroscopically complete resection and with positive microscopic margins are not at increased risk for LR compared to those resected with negative margins.[204]

After the recognition of *in vivo* efficacy of imatinib in a GIST cell line,[203] treatment of metastatic disease has rapidly advanced from treating a single patient to phase 1, 2, and 3 studies for patients with metastatic disease.[205–209] The results have been remarkably consistent. Imatinib is at least 10-fold more active than any agent ever examined for treatment of GIST (formerly called GI leiomyosarcoma). The response rate to imatinib is approximately 50%, 30–35% with stable disease, and ~15% with overt progression on therapy. The US phase 3 data indicate that 400 and 800 mg yield equivalent time-to-progression curves, but the European/Australian phase 3 study indicates that time to progression is improved with the higher dose (800 mg daily) arm.[206] Remarkably, patient kinase genotype determined relative sensitivity to therapy (Figure 15).[210] Patients with *KIT* exon 11 mutation had an 80–90% response rate, while patients with *KIT* exon 9 mutation had a high response rate only one-third to one-half. Patients with no mutation in *KIT* or *PDGFRA* had a much lower response rate, but still higher than that observed for any other chemotherapy drugs. For the time being, regardless of mutation status, imatinib remains the first-line standard of care for metastatic GIST. A dosage of 400 mg daily is a reasonable starting point for most patients, with increase toward 800 mg if there is evidence of progression of disease or the presence of exon 9 mutation.[211] Therapy should not be interrupted if new hypodense lesions appear in the liver; these likely represent occult metastatic disease, as has been borne out with radiological and clinical experience.[176]

The median time to progression for patients with metastatic GIST on imatinib is approximately 2 years. Patients with progression on a lower dose of imatinib can respond further with dose increases. The

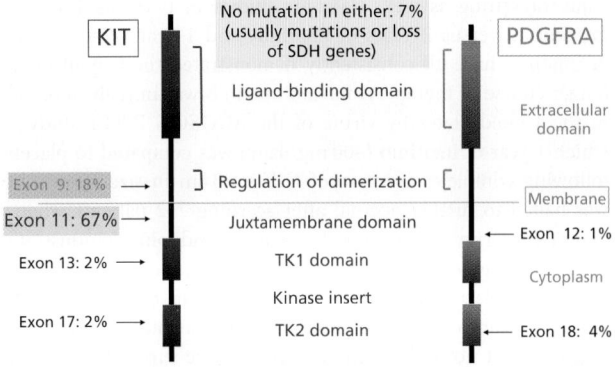

Figure 15 Mutation status of gastrointestinal stromal tumors and location on the KIT or PDGFRA protein.

phase 1 study of imatinib indicated that the maximum tolerated dosage is 800 mg daily (400 mg by mouth bid). Patients with progression of disease have had unusual patterns of progression, the so-called tumor within a tumor, which represents clone(s) with second resistant *KIT* mutations.[160] In some cases, tumor regrowth in an apparently necrotic tumor is observed, and in others only one metastatic deposit is seen to progress instead of the multiplicity of lesions seen in many patients with advanced GIST. As a result some patients have been treated with carefully planned operations to remove problematic individual sites of metastatic disease.

The rationale for consideration of metastasis surgery for patients with responding or stable metastatic disease on imatinib is based on the observations that (1) pathologic complete response to imatinib is very rare (<5%) and many (perhaps most) patients will eventually develop secondary resistance to imatinib owing chiefly to the development of secondary resistance mutations. Reports from high-volume centers demonstrate that carefully selected patients treated by imatinib and subsequent metastasectomy appear to have very favorable progression-free survival rates. Whether this is due to case selection or bona fide clinical benefit related to surgery is unclear.[212,213] Randomized controlled trials of the impact of metastasectomy in patients with stable or responding disease were planned in the United States, Europe, and China. Poor accrual led to the closure of the European and Chinese trials, and the American trial was never started.

The utility of imatinib in metastatic GIST spawned new SMOKIs, some of which have been through phase 3 trials with subsequent regulatory approval. In the setting of imatinib resistance for metastatic disease, the addition of mTOR inhibitor everolimus to imatinib demonstrated minor activity.[214] However, greater activity has been observed with other KIT-targeted SMOKIs. Sunitinib is active in imatinib-resistant GIST and is associated with both significantly improved progression-free survival and OS in comparison to placebo.[215] With the demonstration of activity of sorafenib in GIST,[216,217] regorafenib (a fluorinated form of sorafenib) was found active in phase 3 trial of drug against placebo, in which better attention was paid to the placebo group; in this so-called GRID study, the patients on placebo were crossed over more rapidly to drug than the study involving sunitinib, perhaps accounting for the lack of OS benefit seen in the GRID study.[218] After failure of other agents, some form of SMOKI appears to be indicated for further therapy; use of imatinib was superior to placebo in late stage patients in a randomized trial.[219]

Given the remarkable activity of imatinib in the metastatic setting, it is not surprising that imatinib has been tested in the adjuvant setting as well. Data for studies of 0 versus 1 year of imatinib, 0 versus 2 years of imatinib, and 1 year versus 3 years of imatinib have all consistently demonstrated the benefit of the longer course of therapy. Adjuvant imatinib was initially approved in the United States by virtue of the ACOSOG Z9001 study, in which 1 year of imatinib (400 mg/daily) was compared to placebo following complete resection of GISTs >3 cm in size. This study was halted to further accrual after accruing 762 patients when a planned interim analysis for the primary endpoint demonstrated superior progression-free survival in the imatinib arm (97% vs 83% in the placebo arm).[220] A randomized trial comparing 1 year versus 3 years of adjuvant imatinib subsequently demonstrated improvement not only in the recurrence-free survival but also in the OS, favoring longer duration of adjuvant therapy.[221] Whether longer adjuvant treatment with imatinib for longer periods adds further benefit is uncertain and is the subject of a single-arm 5-year trial of imatinib. At this juncture, the best recommendation that can be made is that 3 years of adjuvant treatment be considered for patients with intermediate- and high-risk resected primary GISTs. Risk is well stratified by clinical, pathological, and molecular features of the primary tumor.[222–224]

Locally aggressive lesions: DFSPs, tenosynovial giant cell tumor (TGCT), perivascular epithelial cell tumor (PEComa) as targets for small molecule oral kinase inhibitors

DFSP is a nodular "protuberant" lesion arising from the dermis with characteristically slow but persistent growth over many years. Although histologically of low grade or borderline malignant potential, DFSP has a propensity for LR after simple excision. A chromosomal translocation t(17;22) and gene fusion product (Table 1) result in the expression of a COL1A1-PDGFB fusion protein that is processed to mature PDGF-B, resulting in apparent autocrine or paracrine interaction with the PDGF-B receptor on the cell surface of DFSP. Notably, imatinib inhibits the PDGF tyrosine kinase receptor in a similar manner that it inhibits the BCR-ABL tyrosine kinase receptor of chronic myeloid leukemia and KIT kinase of GIST. In recurrent DFSP, imatinib has activity, confirming that kinases can be very good targets in solid tumors, even rare ones, if the genetics of the tumor are suggestive.[200,225–227]

For a similar reason, the t(1;2) COL6A3-CSF1 generates a fusion protein that is responsible for the aggressive inflammatory infiltrate of TGCT (formerly termed pigmented villonodular synovitis). Imatinib has activity against CSF1R (FMS, CD115) and can cause recurrent lesions to shrink.[201] More specific SMOKIs or monoclonal antibodies against CD115 can also shrink recurrent TGCT lesions. Finally, PEComa, found in the genetic syndrome tuberous sclerosis, and the related lesion lymphangioleiomyomatosis lack either TSC1 or TSC2, tumor suppressor genes. TOR (target of rapamycin) is activated downstream after TSC1 and TSC2 inactivation, and thus it is not surprising that SMOKI sirolimus and structurally related compounds are active in these conditions, as further proof of principle of blockade of a "driver" kinase in a solid tumor can yield radiological and clinical benefit for patients.[199]

Retroperitoneal sarcomas

RPS comprise about 15% of STS. RPS present late and are located in regions where the administration of both surgery and RT is often compromised (e.g., adjacent to the small bowel and the liver). Consequently, the local control rates achieved with combined-modality treatment of extremity STSs are not seen in RPS.[54,228–232] For example, in a series of 102 RPS patients treated at Princess Margaret Hospital, complete excision was achieved in only 45, gross disease remained in 29, and only a biopsy was possible in 28.[232] The overall local–regional relapse-free rates were 28% and 9% at 5 and 10 years, respectively. RT did not improve survival but appeared to significantly lengthen the time to local–regional relapse, especially with higher doses. Complete tumor resection was the only significant prognostic variable for survival and local–regional and distant failure, similar to other series referenced above. RPS patients should be evaluated in a multidisciplinary clinic before treatment so that patients can benefit from the expertise and investigational approaches available in such centers.

Controversial reports from Europe explored extended surgery termed compartmental resection as a strategy to improve local control for patients with RPS.[233,234] These retrospective reports from France and Italy have suggested that local control may be enhanced by resecting adjacent involved viscera—primarily the kidney and the colon. Interpretation of these reports is complicated by significant selection bias and, as outlined in an editorial that accompanied these papers,[235] no specific therapeutic recommendation could be made based on these data. At this time, there are no clinical trials demonstrating improved local control with more radical surgery that involves resection of adjacent uninvolved viscera.

Pre- and postoperative radiotherapy approaches

A variety of adjuvant RT approaches have been used for RPS. One approach, evaluated in a prospective randomized trial, used an IORT boost (20 Gy) to the tumor bed followed by postoperative external beam (35–40 Gy); this approach was compared with conventional postoperative RT (50–55 Gy). In this study of 35 patients, the incidence of local–regional recurrence was lower in the experimental treatment arm, but no improvement in survival was demonstrated.[236] IORT was associated with a high rate of peripheral neuropathy when large, sometimes overlapping, RT portals were used to cover the sacral plexus region. However, gastrointestinal complications were more common in the control group, in whom higher doses were delivered to the bowel.

Other researchers have investigated strategies employing preoperative RT. Gieschen et al.[237] from the Massachusetts General Hospital reported on 37 patients who underwent preoperative RT, resection, and then, when feasible, electron beam IORT. The grossly complete resection rate was 83%, and the 5-year actuarial OS, DFS, local control, and freedom from distant disease rates were 50%, 38%, 59%, and 54%, respectively. Earlier reports from the same group described a 70% complete resection rate and 81% 4-year local control rate. The more recent report also indicates that complete resection and IORT improved OS and local control rates (74% and 83%, respectively) compared with no IORT (30% and 61%, respectively). However, the study was not randomized, and potentially more favorable and accessible lesions may have been chosen for IORT. Petersen and colleagues at the Mayo Clinic found improved local control, at least of primary tumors, using a similar treatment approach.[238]

The University of Toronto Sarcoma Group described an unusually favorable outcome, especially for primary lesions, in a single-arm prospective trial of preoperative RT (median dose of 45 Gy in 25 fractions) plus postoperative BRT in selected cases.[239] Of interest, acute toxicity resulting from preoperative RT was differentiated prospectively from the effects of other treatments. Although the median radiation volume exceeded 7 L, preoperative external beam RT was associated with extremely low gastrointestinal toxicity scores. Furthermore, no patient was hospitalized for acute toxicity, and there were no treatment interruptions or cessations of treatment because of acute toxicity. The remarkably low toxicity of the preoperative RT with enormous volumes has been attributed to the displacement of the bowel outside the target volume. In contrast, the selective use of postoperative BRT was associated with toxicity, and there was little evidence that BRT contributed to the enhanced tumor outcome reported.

The University of Texas MD Anderson Cancer Center and Princess Margaret Hospital groups combined the data from their phase 2 and pilot studies. This pooled analysis demonstrated very favorable OS rates for patients treated with preoperative radiation combined with surgical resection.[240] However, we again caution against overinterpretation of results that could be explained by surgical technique at major referral centers or by case selection. Similarly, it remains unclear what contribution was provided by the BRT or IORT, which should probably remain protocol based or be reserved for nonstandard use in selected cases. Notably, however, the preoperative RT approach seems to continue to demonstrate favorable local control and OS in very long-term follow-up of the PMH study.

The results of these three reports add credence to the advantages posited for preoperative RT in RPS: (1) the tumor bulk often displaces the small bowel from the high-dose RT region, resulting in a safer and less toxic treatment; (2) the bowel is unlikely to be fixed by surgical adhesions as when RT is given postoperatively, enabling safe delivery of a higher dose to the true area at risk; (3) optimum knowledge of the gross tumor location is possible, permitting better radiation targeting; (4) the tumor is contained by an intact peritoneal covering, providing a physical barrier to immediate tumor dissemination; (5) the risk of intraperitoneal tumor dissemination at the time of surgery may be reduced by the biologic impact of preoperative RT; and (6) using traditional principles of sarcoma RT, the radiation dose believed to be biologically effective is lower in the preoperative setting. Although RT planning for RPS can be complex, the use of conformal techniques or intensity modulation usually permits the RT dosage to be administered safely to the critical organ preoperatively. It is imperative that members of both the surgical and radiation oncology teams be present in the operating room when a significant amount of the liver has been irradiated preoperatively to evaluate the planned residual liver volume. We cannot overemphasize the detailed evaluation of dosimetry and treatment planning films are needed to be certain that a sufficient volume of unirradiated liver is left unresected at the time of surgery.[241]

The only standard that exists at present for RPS treatment is that complete surgery should be performed wherever possible. The adjuvant RT approaches described above should be considered experimental and be the subject of further assessment. Recently, it was also suggested that a more scientifically sound approach to study design should be undertaken in RPS, particularly exploring the role of external beam RT through a randomized controlled trial.[174] The European Organisation for Research and Treatment of Cancer (EORTC) is currently conducting a phase 3 randomized study of preoperative RT plus surgery versus surgery alone (NCT01344018) that is readily on target for completion.[242]

Chemoradiation approaches

Although chemotherapy alone has not been associated with obvious improvements in outcome of RPS, chemoradiation, as in other solid tumors, is a subject of interest as a treatment strategy for RPS. This is especially relevant in high-grade RPS, which have a more adverse prognosis than the more common low-grade lesions.

Pilot studies using concurrent preoperative chemotherapy and external beam radiation have been reported, often in patients with extremely large tumors, with acceptable toxicity and with achievement of local control in patients in whom a negative-margin resection was possible.[141,243] These reports demonstrate that chemoradiation approaches are feasible. Additional phase 2 studies will be necessary to clarify response rates and toxicity profiles and determine whether chemoradiation should be tested in phase 3 trials. As discussed earlier, the Radiation Therapy Oncology Group completed a phase 2 study of preoperative doxorubicin and ifosfamide followed by preoperative RT and then by surgical resection with an intra- or postoperative radiation boost in patients with intermediate- and high-grade RPS. This study demonstrated significant toxicities and event-free outcomes that were considered modest.[144,146]

Additional issues in STS management

Functional outcome and morbidity of treatment

The functional result of extremity sarcoma management has become an important component of outcome assessment. Assessing the functional result is difficult, as it requires methods that are valid and reproducible. Many centers have yet to become experienced in the development and use of these methods, and much of the literature contains significant heterogeneity in patient samples.

Thus far, the variables associated with poorer functional outcome include large tumor size, higher doses and larger volumes of radiation, nerve sacrifice, postoperative fracture, and wound-healing complications.[244,245] To evaluate and compare functional outcome, it is imperative that functional data be reported consistently. Three disease-specific scoring scales have been reported as useful in assessing functional outcome.[246] This area has been discussed in detail by Davis, who observed that "function" has many meanings in the literature.[246] The concepts of impairment, disability, and handicap following extremity STS are likely misunderstood and certainly not used consistently. Davis noted that impairment is a disorder of structure or function whereas disability is a restriction or lack of ability to perform an activity. Handicap results from impairment and disability and prevents or restricts an individual from performing in a role that is normal for the individual. For sarcoma patients, impairments can be manifested as soft tissue fibrosis, loss of motion at a joint, and decreased muscle strength; disability can be manifested as limited mobility and difficulty performing routine self-care and activities of daily living; and handicap can be evident in limitation in family roles, social functioning, and the capacity for employment.

Impairments are the most frequently reported deficits following limb-preserving therapy for extremity STS, and up to 50% of patients appear to experience significant impairments.[246] Disability occurs less frequently, although reports are contradictory. It seems likely that many sarcoma patients learn to accommodate their impairments. Handicap has received little attention in the literature. However, the limited data suggest that up to 50% of patients may experience changes in their employment and vocation status after treatment of extremity STS. The continuing challenge in treating sarcomas is to define the therapeutic ratio for the patient with sarcoma of the extremity. Specifically, the aim of the multidisciplinary team will be to minimize the amount of treatment while maintaining or improving current standards of disease control to reduce treatment morbidity and enhance patient outcome.

Wound complications

Considerable variability in reporting wound-healing complications exists in the literature. WCs have been reported in up to 40% of patients undergoing extremity sarcoma surgery.[85,247–249] Differences in the definition of WCs probably account for some of the variability in reporting. The retrospective data suggest that factors associated with compromised wound healing include advanced patient age, poor nutritional status, lower extremity tumor location, large tumor size, and preoperative adjuvant treatment, especially RT.[247,248,250] Particularly high complication rates were noted with combination preoperative RT and hyperthermia.[117] Although many authors have reported an association of WCs with preoperative RT, reports of high rates of surgical complications without RT or chemotherapy also exist.[251] Most likely, these relate to the risk of major WCs associated with extensive tumor resection, particularly in the lower extremities. The use of vascularized tissue transfers to replace resected tissues and optimize wound closure may decrease the risks of major WCs and allow for more extensive limb-sparing surgical approaches.[250,252,253] As noted earlier, the SR2 trial results have confirmed the adverse effect of preoperative RT on wound healing in a prospective manner, but did not resolve the contribution of tissue transfer for wound reconstruction as its use was determined on an individual basis at the surgeon's discretion.[96]

Molecularly and pathobiologically based sarcoma management

Management of sarcomas is increasingly being driven by the specific nature of the disease entity, most importantly the pathophysiologic subtype. The work of Pasteur and Koch was fundamental for the recognition and definition of pathogenic microbes; similarly, many laboratories today are identifying molecular lesions that will redefine the field of sarcoma research. An example of this work is in the recognition of soft tissue Ewing sarcoma/PNET family of tumors as relatives of their bony primary counterparts by virtue of the same spectrum of translocations in each clinical setting. These tumors should be treated with curative intent using an aggressive multimodality approach that begins with multiagent chemotherapy. If primary surgery has removed measurable disease, adjuvant chemotherapy is definitely indicated, with consideration of adjuvant RT. By adopting similar strategies for PNETs and Askin tumors as for conventional Ewing sarcomas, outcomes improved. The molecular similarities between tumors of this family have led to the current convention of considering them morphologic and clinicopathologic variants of the same underlying molecular disease process.[254,255]

Greater understanding of the biology of translocation gene products points to epigenetic events being important in sarcomagenesis and should impact on the efficacy of chemotherapy. Ewing sarcoma and synovial sarcoma are chemotherapy-responsive STS subtypes. While *TP53* could be posited as a reason that certain sarcomas are chemotherapy sensitive, *TP53* status is not the only factor dictating chemotherapy sensitivity as there are other *TP53* wild-type sarcomas that are far less sensitive to chemotherapy, for example, extraskeletal myxoid chondrosarcoma and alveolar soft part sarcoma. Striking research on the epigenetic mSWI/SNF (BAF) complexes and their role in synovial sarcoma hopefully will shed light on some of the basic mechanistic aspects permitting synovial sarcoma survival, in order to better engender tumor cell death.[256,257]

As a final example, the multiple histopathologic subtypes of liposarcomas are becoming increasingly well researched and well understood, and mechanisms by which some forms acquire their characteristic DNA signature are beginning to become understood.[258] Myxoid and round-cell liposarcomas usually exhibit a characteristic chromosomal rearrangement t(12;16) (q13;p11) *FUS-DDIT3*. These liposarcomas tend to be relatively sensitive to chemotherapy, with trabectedin standing out as most active in this specific diagnosis. Trabectedin appears to inhibit the binding of the FUS-DDIT3 fusion protein to DNA, which then causes liposarcoma cell death or differentiation.[259,260] The rarer pleomorphic liposarcoma subtype has more in common with undifferentiated pleomorphic sarcoma than other liposarcomas. Finally, well-differentiated liposarcomas exhibit ring and giant marker chromosomes on cytogenetic analysis and these karyotypic abnormalities, often involving massive amplification of chromosome 12q, carry through in dedifferentiated liposarcomas. Unraveling the ability of the *CDK4* and *HDM2* loci on 12q to amplify hundreds of times in well-differentiated–dedifferentiated liposarcoma may provide insight on how better to attack these relatively chemotherapy-insensitive sarcomas.[261–263]

Immunotherapy for STS

As of the time of this publication, the examination of the immune system as treatment for sarcoma cannot even be considered in its infancy, but rather in a prenatal state. Immunotherapy is already approved in some countries for osteogenic sarcoma, with the nonspecific immune adjuvant mifamurtide (MTP-PE) improving the cure rate when used as part of adjuvant treatment.[120] While the proof of principle of engineered T-cell therapy in NY-ESO-1-positive sarcomas such as synovial sarcoma already has been demonstrated by Robbins et al.,[264,265] the potential benefit of immune checkpoint blockade is still very much unclear, as no studies were able to be started in sarcomas until 2015. If the hypothesis holds that the cancers with the most DNA mutations and alterations will be most responsive to immunotherapy, then we expect to see undifferentiated pleomorphic sarcoma, leiomyosarcoma, and osteosarcoma among the best responders and much less activity in translocation-associated sarcomas. Conversely, CAR T-cell therapy may be more easily targeted to translocation-associated sarcomas if an appropriate target antigen can be identified.

Summary

It is clear that STS management has improved in the past 10 years. In fewer than three decades, the standard of care has shifted toward coordinated multimodality care in specialty centers, with increased rates of function-sparing surgery and better outcomes for patients. Judicious use of aggressive multimodality approaches shows promise to decrease relapse rates and improve survival rates. The genomic and immunological revolutions in cancer are furthering the fundamental understanding of these unusual diseases and providing novel approaches for diagnostic techniques, which will banish the vagaries and lack of consistency that have plagued this field of clinical investigation and also will provide resources for selecting new targets for therapy. New therapeutic initiatives are attacking the basic mechanisms of sarcomatous transformation of cells in some subtypes of STS, and it is hoped that these initiatives will improve outcomes for patients with less morbidity than current treatments entail. Large collaborative studies should further this work.

Key references

The complete reference list can be found on the Wiley Companion Digital Edition of this title (see inside front cover for login instructions).

3 Thomas DM, Ballinger ML. Etiologic, environmental and inherited risk factors in sarcomas. *J Surg Oncol.* 2015;**111**:490–495.

4 Li FP, Fraumeni JF Jr. Soft-tissue sarcomas, breast cancer, and other neoplasms. A familial syndrome? *Ann Intern Med.* 1969;**71**:747–752.

6 McBride KA, Ballinger ML, Killick E, et al. Li-Fraumeni syndrome: cancer risk assessment and clinical management. *Nat Rev Clin Oncol.* 2014;**11**:260–271.

7 Kolberg M, Holand M, Agesen TH, et al. Survival meta-analyses for >1800 malignant peripheral nerve sheath tumor patients with and without neurofibromatosis type 1. *Neuro Oncol.* 2013;**15**:135–147.

14 MacCarthy A, Bayne AM, Brownbill PA, et al. Second and subsequent tumours among 1927 retinoblastoma patients diagnosed in Britain 1951-2004. *Br J Cancer.* 2013;**108**:2455–2463.

20 Gladdy RA, Qin LX, Moraco N, et al. Do radiation-associated soft tissue sarcomas have the same prognosis as sporadic soft tissue sarcomas? *J Clin Oncol.* 2010;**28**:2064–2069.

28 Mitchell G, Ballinger ML, Wong S, et al. High frequency of germline TP53 mutations in a prospective adult-onset sarcoma cohort. *PLoS One.* 2013;**8**:e69026.

31 WHO. *Classification of Tumours of Soft Tissue and Bone.* Lyon: International Agency for Research on Cancer; 2013.

32 Fong Y, Coit DG, Woodruff JM, Brennan MF. Lymph node metastasis from soft tissue sarcoma in adults. Analysis of data from a prospective database of 1772 sarcoma patients. *Ann Surg.* 1993;**217**:72–77.

34 Brennan MF, Antonescu CR, Moraco N, Singer S. Lessons learned from the study of 10,000 patients with soft tissue sarcoma. *Ann Surg.* 2014;**260**:416–421; discussion 421-412.

36 Lahat G, Tuvin D, Wei C, et al. New perspectives for staging and prognosis in soft tissue sarcoma. *Ann Surg Oncol.* 2008;**15**:2739–2748.

38 Guillou L, Coindre JM, Bonichon F, et al. Comparative study of the National Cancer Institute and French Federation of Cancer Centers Sarcoma Group grading systems in a population of 410 adult patients with soft tissue sarcoma. *J Clin Oncol.* 1997;**15**:350–362.

44 von Mehren M, Randall RL, Benjamin RS, et al. (2015) *NCCN Clinical Practice Guidelines in Oncology: Soft Tissue Sarcoma* (accessed March 01 2015).

49 Edge SB, Byrd DR, Compton CC, Fritz AG, Greene FL, Trotti A III (eds). Soft tissue sarcoma. In: *AJCC Cancer Staging Manual.* New York: Springer; 2010:291–298.

51 Kattan MW, Leung DH, Brennan MF. Postoperative nomogram for 12-year sarcoma-specific death. *J Clin Oncol.* 2002;**20**:791–796.

52 Pisters PW, Leung DH, Woodruff J, Shi W, Brennan MF. Analysis of prognostic factors in 1,041 patients with localized soft tissue sarcomas of the extremities. *J Clin Oncol.* 1996;**14**:1679–1689.

54 Gronchi A, Miceli R, Shurell E, et al. Outcome prediction in primary resected retroperitoneal soft tissue sarcoma: histology-specific overall survival and disease-free survival nomograms built on major sarcoma center data sets. *J Clin Oncol.* 2013;**31**:1649–1655.

61 Brennan MF, Antonescu CR, Maki RG. *Management of Soft Tissue Sarcoma.* New York: Springer; 2013.

62 Dei Tos AP. A current perspective on the role for molecular studies in soft tissue tumor pathology. *Semin Diagn Pathol.* 2013;**30**:375–381.

69 Pisters PW, Harrison LB, Leung DH, Woodruff JM, Casper ES, Brennan MF. Long-term results of a prospective randomized trial of adjuvant brachytherapy in soft tissue sarcoma. *J Clin Oncol.* 1996;**14**:859–868.

70 Yang JC, Chang AE, Baker AR, et al. Randomized prospective study of the benefit of adjuvant radiation therapy in the treatment of soft tissue sarcomas of the extremity. *J Clin Oncol.* 1998;**16**:197–203.

72 Maki RG, Moraco N, Antonescu CR, et al. Toward better soft tissue sarcoma staging: building on american joint committee on cancer staging systems versions 6 and 7. *Ann Surg Oncol.* 2013;**20**:3377–3383.

77 O'Sullivan B, Wylie J, Catton C, et al. The local management of soft tissue sarcoma. *Semin Radiat Oncol.* 1999;**9**:328–348.

78 O'Sullivan B, Ward I, Haycocks T, Sharpe M. Techniques to modulate radiotherapy toxicity and outcome in soft tissue sarcoma. *Curr Treat Options Oncol.* 2003;**4**:453–464.

89 Haas RL, Delaney TF, O'Sullivan B, et al. Radiotherapy for management of extremity soft tissue sarcomas: why, when, and where? *Int J Radiat Oncol Biol Phys.* 2012;**84**:572–580.

96 O'Sullivan B, Davis AM, Turcotte R, et al. Preoperative versus postoperative radiotherapy in soft-tissue sarcoma of the limbs: a randomised trial. *Lancet.* 2002;**359**:2235–2241.

100 Nielsen OS, Cummings B, O'Sullivan B, Catton C, Bell RS, Fornasier VL. Preoperative and postoperative irradiation of soft tissue sarcomas: effect of radiation field size. *Int J Radiat Oncol Biol Phys.* 1991;**21**:1595–1599.

101 Davis AM, O'Sullivan B, Turcotte R, et al. Late radiation morbidity following randomization to preoperative versus postoperative radiotherapy in extremity soft tissue sarcoma. *Radiother Oncol.* 2005;**75**:48–53.

102 Hong L, Alektiar KM, Hunt M, Venkatraman E, Leibel SA. Intensity-modulated radiotherapy for soft tissue sarcoma of the thigh. *Int J Radiat Oncol Biol Phys.* 2004;**59**:752–759.

104 O'Sullivan B, Griffin AM, Dickie CI, et al. Phase 2 study of preoperative image-guided intensity-modulated radiation therapy to reduce wound and combined modality morbidities in lower extremity soft tissue sarcoma. *Cancer.* 2013;**119**:1878–1884.

107 Catton CN, Swallow CJ, O'Sullivan B. Approaches to local salvage of soft tissue sarcoma after primary site failure. *Semin Radiat Oncol.* 1999;**9**:378–388.

112 Alektiar KM, Brennan MF, Singer S. Local control comparison of adjuvant brachytherapy to intensity-modulated radiotherapy in primary high-grade sarcoma of the extremity. *Cancer.* 2011;**117**:3229–3234.

119 Crist WM, Anderson JR, Meza JL, et al. Intergroup rhabdomyosarcoma study-IV: results for patients with nonmetastatic disease. *J Clin Oncol.* 2001;**19**:3091–3102.

120 Meyers PA, Schwartz CL, Krailo MD, et al. Osteosarcoma: the addition of muramyl tripeptide to chemotherapy improves overall survival – a report from the Children's Oncology Group. *J Clin Oncol.* 2008;**26**:633–638.

121 Whelan JS, Bielack SS, Marina N, et al. EURAMOS-1, an international randomised study for osteosarcoma: results from pre-randomisation treatment. *Ann Oncol.* 2015;**26**:407–414.

122 Womer RB, West DC, Krailo MD, et al. Randomized controlled trial of interval-compressed chemotherapy for the treatment of localized Ewing sarcoma: a report from the Children's Oncology Group. *J Clin Oncol.* 2012;**30**:4148–4154.

126 Frustaci S, De Paoli A, Bidoli E, et al. Ifosfamide in the adjuvant therapy of soft tissue sarcomas. *Oncology.* 2003;**65(Suppl 2)**:80–84.

127 Frustaci S, Gherlinzoni F, De Paoli A, et al. Adjuvant chemotherapy for adult soft tissue sarcomas of the extremities and girdles: results of the Italian randomized cooperative trial. *J Clin Oncol.* 2001;**19**:1238–1247.

128 Woll PJ, Reichardt P, Le Cesne A, et al. Adjuvant chemotherapy with doxorubicin, ifosfamide, and lenograstim for resected soft-tissue sarcoma (EORTC 62931): a multicentre randomised controlled trial. *Lancet Oncol.* 2012;**13**:1045–1054.

129 Pervaiz N, Colterjohn N, Farrokhyar F, Tozer R, Figueredo A, Ghert M. A systematic meta-analysis of randomized controlled trials of adjuvant chemotherapy for localized resectable soft-tissue sarcoma. *Cancer.* 2008;**113**:573–581.

141 Eilber F, Eckardt J, Rosen G, Forscher C, Selch M, Fu YS. Preoperative therapy for soft tissue sarcoma. *Hematol Oncol Clin North Am.* 1995;**9**:817–823.

144 DeLaney TF, Spiro IJ, Suit HD, et al. Neoadjuvant chemotherapy and radiotherapy for large extremity soft-tissue sarcomas. *Int J Radiat Oncol Biol Phys.* 2003;**56**:1117–1127.

145 Kraybill WG, Harris J, Spiro IJ, et al. Long-term results of a phase 2 study of neoadjuvant chemotherapy and radiotherapy in the management of high-risk, high-grade, soft tissue sarcomas of the extremities and body wall: Radiation Therapy Oncology Group Trial 9514. *Cancer.* 2010;**116**:4613–4621.

151 Cormier JN, Huang X, Xing Y, et al. Cohort analysis of patients with localized, high-risk, extremity soft tissue sarcoma treated at two cancer centers: chemotherapy-associated outcomes. *J Clin Oncol.* 2004;**22**:4567–4574.

160 Wardelmann E, Merkelbach-Bruse S, Pauls K, et al. Polyclonal evolution of multiple secondary KIT mutations in gastrointestinal stromal tumors under treatment with imatinib mesylate. *Clin Cancer Res.* 2006;**12**:1743–1749.

165 Billingsley KG, Lewis JJ, Leung DH, Casper ES, Woodruff JM, Brennan MF. Multifactorial analysis of the survival of patients with distant metastasis arising from primary extremity sarcoma. *Cancer.* 1999;**85**:389–395.

166 Billingsley KG, Burt ME, Jara E, et al. Pulmonary metastases from soft tissue sarcoma: analysis of patterns of diseases and postmetastasis survival. *Ann Surg.* 1999;**229**:602–610; discussion 610–602.

167 van Geel AN, Pastorino U, Jauch KW, et al. Surgical treatment of lung metastases: The European Organization for Research and Treatment of Cancer-Soft Tissue and Bone Sarcoma Group study of 255 patients. *Cancer.* 1996;**77**:675–682.

173 Van Glabbeke M, van Oosterom AT, Oosterhuis JW, et al. Prognostic factors for the outcome of chemotherapy in advanced soft tissue sarcoma: an analysis of 2,185 patients treated with anthracycline-containing first-line regimens – a European Organization for Research and Treatment of Cancer Soft Tissue and Bone Sarcoma Group Study. *J Clin Oncol.* 1999;**17**:150–157.

176 Choi H, Charnsangavej C, Faria SC, et al. Correlation of computed tomography and positron emission tomography in patients with metastatic gastrointestinal stromal tumor treated at a single institution with imatinib mesylate: proposal of new computed tomography response criteria. *J Clin Oncol.* 2007;**25**:1753–1759.

177 Patel SR, Vadhan-Raj S, Burgess MA, et al. Results of two consecutive trials of dose-intensive chemotherapy with doxorubicin and ifosfamide in patients with sarcomas. *Am J Clin Oncol.* 1998;**21**:317–321.

178 Antman K, Crowley J, Balcerzak SP, et al. An intergroup phase III randomized study of doxorubicin and dacarbazine with or without ifosfamide and mesna in advanced soft tissue and bone sarcomas. *J Clin Oncol.* 1993;**11**:1276–1285.

180 Judson I, Verweij J, Gelderblom H, et al. Doxorubicin alone versus intensified doxorubicin plus ifosfamide for first-line treatment of advanced or metastatic soft-tissue sarcoma: a randomised controlled phase 3 trial. *Lancet Oncol.* 2014;**15**:415–423.

183 Judson I, Radford JA, Harris M, et al. Randomised phase II trial of pegylated liposomal doxorubicin (DOXIL/CAELYX) versus doxorubicin in the treatment of advanced or metastatic soft tissue sarcoma: a study by the EORTC Soft Tissue and Bone Sarcoma Group. *Eur J Cancer.* 2001;**37**:870–877.

187 Hensley ML, Maki R, Venkatraman E, et al. Gemcitabine and docetaxel in patients with unresectable leiomyosarcoma: results of a phase II trial. *J Clin Oncol.* 2002;**20**:2824–2831.

189 Maki RG, Wathen JK, Patel SR, et al. Randomized phase II study of gemcitabine and docetaxel compared with gemcitabine alone in patients with metastatic soft tissue sarcomas: results of sarcoma alliance for research through collaboration study 002 [corrected]. *J Clin Oncol.* 2007;**25**:2755–2763.

190 Garcia-Del-Muro X, Lopez-Pousa A, Maurel J, et al. Randomized phase II study comparing gemcitabine plus dacarbazine versus dacarbazine alone in patients with previously treated soft tissue sarcoma: a Spanish Group for Research on Sarcomas study. *J Clin Oncol.* 2011;**29**:2528–2533.

191 Hensley ML, Miller A, O'Malley DM, et al. Randomized phase III trial of gemcitabine plus docetaxel plus bevacizumab or placebo as first-line treatment for metastatic uterine leiomyosarcoma: an NRG Oncology/Gynecologic Oncology Group Study. *J Clin Oncol.* 2015;**33**:1180–1185.

193 Demetri GD, Chawla SP, von Mehren M, et al. Efficacy and safety of trabectedin in patients with advanced or metastatic liposarcoma or leiomyosarcoma after failure of prior anthracyclines and ifosfamide: results of a randomized phase II study of two different schedules. *J Clin Oncol.* 2009;**27**:4188–4196.

195 Demetri G, Schoffski P, Placeholder P (2015) Trabectedin vs Dacarbazine in L-sarcomas.

196 Schoffski P, Ray-Coquard IL, Cioffi A, et al. Activity of eribulin mesylate in patients with soft-tissue sarcoma: a phase 2 study in four independent histological subtypes. *Lancet Oncol.* 2011;**12**:1045–1052.

198 van der Graaf WT, Blay JY, Chawla SP, et al. Pazopanib for metastatic soft-tissue sarcoma (PALETTE): a randomised, double-blind, placebo-controlled phase 3 trial. *Lancet.* 2012;**379**:1879–1886.

206 Verweij J, Casali PG, Zalcberg J, et al. Progression-free survival in gastrointestinal stromal tumours with high-dose imatinib: randomised trial. *Lancet.* 2004;**364**:1127–1134.

207 Demetri GD, von Mehren M, Blanke CD, et al. Efficacy and safety of imatinib mesylate in advanced gastrointestinal stromal tumors. *N Engl J Med.* 2002;**347**:472–480.

211 Debiec-Rychter M, Sciot R, Le Cesne A, et al. KIT mutations and dose selection for imatinib in patients with advanced gastrointestinal stromal tumours. *Eur J Cancer.* 2006;**42**:1093–1103.

214 Schoffski P, Reichardt P, Blay JY, et al. A phase I-II study of everolimus (RAD001) in combination with imatinib in patients with imatinib-resistant gastrointestinal stromal tumors. *Ann Oncol.* 2010;**21**:1990–1998.

215 Demetri GD, van Oosterom AT, Garrett CR, et al. Efficacy and safety of sunitinib in patients with advanced gastrointestinal stromal tumour after failure of imatinib: a randomised controlled trial. *Lancet.* 2006;**368**:1329–1338.

218 Demetri GD, Reichardt P, Kang YK, et al. Efficacy and safety of regorafenib for advanced gastrointestinal stromal tumours after failure of imatinib and sunitinib (GRID): an international, multicentre, randomised, placebo-controlled, phase 3 trial. *Lancet.* 2013;**381**:295–302.

221 Joensuu H, Eriksson M, Sundby Hall K, et al. One vs three years of adjuvant imatinib for operable gastrointestinal stromal tumor: a randomized trial. *JAMA.* 2012;**307**:1265–1272.

222 Joensuu H, Vehtari A, Riihimaki J, et al. Risk of recurrence of gastrointestinal stromal tumour after surgery: an analysis of pooled population-based cohorts. *Lancet Oncol.* 2012;**13**:265–274.

224 Joensuu H, Rutkowski P, Nishida T, et al. KIT and PDGFRA mutations and the risk of GI stromal tumor recurrence. *J Clin Oncol.* 2015;**33**:634–642.

225 Heinrich MC, Joensuu H, Demetri GD, et al. Phase II, open-label study evaluating the activity of imatinib in treating life-threatening malignancies known to be associated with imatinib-sensitive tyrosine kinases. *Clin Cancer Res.* 2008;**14**:2717–2725.

228 Gronchi A, Miceli R, Allard MA, et al. Personalizing the approach to retroperitoneal soft tissue sarcoma: histology-specific patterns of failure and postrelapse outcome after primary extended resection. *Ann Surg Oncol.* 2015;**22**:1447–1454.

231 Singer S, Antonescu CR, Riedel E, Brennan MF. Histologic subtype and margin of resection predict pattern of recurrence and survival for retroperitoneal liposarcoma. *Ann Surg.* 2003;**238**:358–370; discussion 370–351.

235 Pisters PW. Resection of some – but not all – clinically uninvolved adjacent viscera as part of surgery for retroperitoneal soft tissue sarcomas. *J Clin Oncol.* 2009;**27**:6–8.

238 Petersen IA, Haddock MG, Donohue JH, et al. Use of intraoperative electron beam radiotherapy in the management of retroperitoneal soft tissue sarcomas. *Int J Radiat Oncol Biol Phys.* 2002;**52**:469–475.

245 Stinson SF, DeLaney TF, Greenberg J, et al. Acute and long-term effects on limb function of combined modality limb sparing therapy for extremity soft tissue sarcoma. *Int J Radiat Oncol Biol Phys.* 1991;**21**:1493–1499.

246 Davis AM. Functional outcome in extremity soft tissue sarcoma. *Semin Radiat Oncol.* 1999;**9**:360–368.

254 Antonescu C. Round cell sarcomas beyond Ewing: emerging entities. *Histopathology.* 2014;**64**:26–37.

255 Antonescu CR, Dal CP. Promiscuous genes involved in recurrent chromosomal translocations in soft tissue tumours. *Pathology.* 2014;**46**:105–112.

256 Kadoch C, Crabtree GR. Reversible disruption of mSWI/SNF (BAF) complexes by the SS18-SSX oncogenic fusion in synovial sarcoma. *Cell.* 2013;**153**:71–85.

257 Su L, Sampaio AV, Jones KB, et al. Deconstruction of the SS18-SSX fusion oncoprotein complex: insights into disease etiology and therapeutics. *Cancer Cell.* 2012;**21**:333–347.

258 Garsed DW, Marshall OJ, Corbin VD, et al. The architecture and evolution of cancer neochromosomes. *Cancer Cell.* 2014;**26**:653–667.

259 Di Giandomenico S, Frapolli R, Bello E, et al. Mode of action of trabectedin in myxoid liposarcomas. *Oncogene.* 2014;**33**:5201–5210.

261 Crago AM, Socci ND, DeCarolis P, et al. Copy number losses define subgroups of dedifferentiated liposarcoma with poor prognosis and genomic instability. *Clin Cancer Res.* 2012;**18**:1334–1340.

263 Dickson MA, Tap WD, Keohan ML, et al. Phase II trial of the CDK4 inhibitor PD0332991 in patients with advanced CDK4-amplified well-differentiated or dedifferentiated liposarcoma. *J Clin Oncol.* 2013;**31**:2024–2028.

264 Robbins PF, Morgan RA, Feldman SA, et al. Tumor regression in patients with metastatic synovial cell sarcoma and melanoma using genetically engineered lymphocytes reactive with NY-ESO-1. *J Clin Oncol.* 2011;**29**:917–924.

265 Robbins PF, Kassim SH, Tran TL, et al. A pilot trial using lymphocytes genetically engineered with an NY-ESO-1-reactive T-cell receptor: long-term follow-up and correlates with response. *Clin Cancer Res.* 2015;**21**:1019–1027.

113 The myelodysplastic syndrome

Lewis R. Silverman, MD

Overview

The existence of a hematopoietic disorder characterized by anemia and dyspoiesis preceding the onset of acute myelocytic leukemia (AML) has been recognized since the early part of the twentieth century. Initially designated as preleukemia, the syndrome was ill defined and could only be established with certainty retrospectively. Moreover, the terminology itself conveyed an unwarranted confidence in predicting the outcome that often belied the facts. The more accurately descriptive and appropriate designation as a myelodysplastic syndrome (MDS) was adopted in 1976 by the French–American–British (FAB) study group. The FAB classification permitted the prospective identification of patients within this heterogeneous clonal disorder.

MDS, derived from a multipotent hematopoietic stem cell, is characterized clinically by a hyperproliferative bone marrow, reflective of ineffective hematopoiesis, and is accompanied by one or more peripheral blood cytopenias. Bone marrow failure results, leading to death from bleeding and infection in the majority, while transformation to acute leukemia occurs in up to 40% of patients. The evolution of the disease proceeds in accordance with the multistep pathogenesis theory of carcinogenesis and can thus serve as an important model in furthering our understanding of the processes involved in neoplastic transformation.

This constellation of findings raises the question of whether MDS represents a frank neoplastic state or is merely a preneoplastic condition in transition. The syndrome appears to represent a spectrum where the initial lesion in the genome, though clinically undetectable, subsequently evolves, with the acquisition of additional genetic and epigenetic lesions, to a state of frank neoplasia.

The designation of this disorder as an MDS, rather than preleukemia, permits its distinction from other abnormalities that are known to be associated with the development of acute leukemia. These latter include the classic myeloproliferative syndromes (polycythemia vera, chronic myelocytic leukemia, agnogenic myeloid metaplasia, essential thrombocythemia), aplastic anemia, paroxysmal nocturnal hemoglobinuria (PNH), as well as Fanconi, Bloom, and Down syndromes. These particular "preleukemic states" are beyond the scope of this chapter.

MDS can be further divided into primary and secondary syndromes. The former arise de novo and are of indeterminate etiology, while the latter are induced by identifiable environmental, occupational, or iatrogenic causes.

Estimates of the incidence of MDS range from a frequency equal to that of AML or approximately 14,000 new cases per year in the United States to almost twice that of AML. The SEER database now tracks the disease; thus more accurate data will be available in the future. An estimate based on medical insurance claims indicated a total of 107,000 cases in the observation period from 2009 through 2011. The consensus is that the incidence is increasing owing to a number of factors, including greater awareness, greater diagnostic precision, and the aging of the population.

History

Luzzatto first described a case of chronic anemia associated with bone marrow erythroid hyperplasia, which he designated as "pseudoaplastic anemia."[1] It was not until Rhoads' and Bomford's description of this entity, however, that the designation of the disease as refractory anemia (RA) became generally accepted.[2,3]

In the early 1950s, it became apparent that some patients with RA could develop leukemia, which led to the term preleukemia.[4,5] The designation as "preleukemia" often seemed erroneous, since many patients succumbed as a result of bone marrow failure without developing leukemia. In 1976, the FAB established diagnostic criteria for MDS that would permit prospective diagnosis.[6]

Estimates of the incidence of MDS range from a frequency equal to that of AML or approximately 14,000 new cases per year in the United States to almost twice that of AML.[7,8] The SEER database now tracks the disease; thus more accurate data will be available in the future. An estimate based on medical insurance claims indicated a total of 107,000 cases in the observation period from 2009 through 2011.[8]

Classification

Based[9] on bone marrow cellularity, the syndrome was divided into three groups: acquired sideroblastic anemia, refractory anemia with excess blasts (RAEB), and chronic myelomonocytic leukemia (CMML). In 1982, the FAB group updated and expanded their classification to include five categories of MDS based on morphologic characteristics and the percentage of blasts in the bone marrow and peripheral blood.[6] These included (1) RA, (2) refractory anemia with ringed sideroblasts (RARS), (3) RAEB (>5% to <20% blasts), (4) CMML, and (5) refractory anemia with excess blasts "in transformation" (RAEB-T) (20% to <30% blasts). Concerns that the classification might result in an underdiagnosis of M6 myeloid leukemia (erythroleukemia) led to further revision and refinement in 1985.[10]

Some debate focuses on the category of CMML and whether this truly represents a subgroup of MDS or should more appropriately be considered a subgroup of the myeloproliferative disorders (MPD). Some patients with CMML have features of both MDS and MPD and thus an overlap syndrome with characteristics of both.[9] The biologic behavior appears related most closely to the percentage of blasts in the bone marrow.[11–13]

The International Prognostic Scoring System (IPSS) has been advanced based on the percentage of bone marrow blasts, cytogenetics, and degree of cytopenias.[14] The IPSS has predictive value for both survival and risk of transformation to acute leukemia (Table 1).

Holland-Frei Cancer Medicine, Ninth Edition. Edited by Robert C. Bast Jr., Carlo M. Croce, William N. Hait, Waun Ki Hong, Donald W. Kufe, Martine Piccart-Gebhart, Raphael E. Pollock, Ralph R. Weichselbaum, Hongyang Wang, and James F. Holland.
© 2017 John Wiley & Sons, Inc. ISBN: 978-1-118-93469-2

Table 1 IPSS score.

Prognostic variable	Score value				
	0	**0.5**	**1.0**	**1.5**	**2.0**
Bone marrow blasts (%)	<5	5–10	—	11–20	21–29
Karyotype	Good	Intermediate	Poor	—	—
Cytopenias	0/1	2/3	—	—	—

Scores	Cytogenetics
Low: 0	Good: normal
Intermediate: 1: 0.5–1.0	-y
Intermediate: 2: 1.5–2.0	del (5q)
High: >2.5	del (20q)
	Poor: chromosome 7 abnormalities
	Complex ≥ 3 abnormalities
	Intermediate: other

Source: Adapted from Nazha 2013.[15]

Table 2 International Prognostic Scoring System—revised (IPSS-R) classification of MDS according to prognostic risk subgroups.

International Prognostic Scoring System (IPSS)	Risk of transformation to acute myeloid leukemia (in 25% of patients) (years)	Median survival (years)
Very low	Not reached	8.8
Low	10.8	5.3
Intermediate-1	3.2	3.0
High	1.4	1.6
Very high	0.73	0.8

Source: Adapted from Greenberg 2012.[16]

Table 3 World Health Organization (WHO) classification.

Refractory anemia (RA)
• With ringed sideroblasts
• Without ringed sideroblasts

Refractory cytopenia with multilineage dysplasia (RCMD)
• With ringed sideroblasts
• Without ringed sideroblasts

Refractory anemia with excess blasts
• RAEB-I (6–10% blasts)
• RAEB-II (11–19% blasts)

5q-syndrome
CMML (MDS/MPD)
Myelodysplastic syndrome, unclassifiable

Source: Adapted from Fenaux 2009.[18]

The IPSS was revised (IPSS-R) and now separates patients into five subcategories with greater predictive value and utilizes peripheral blood count values in a more discriminatory manner.[16] The cytogenetic subgroups have also been revised based on further risk assessment. These revisions were based on analyses of 7012 patients compared to 816 for the original IPSS. The IPSS-R is better able to segregate patients into risk groups and is dynamic able to predict prognosis not just for patients newly diagnosed but also patients at anytime during their course of disease. These classifications have been validated and have become, along with the World Health Organization (WHO) classification,[17] the standard classifications (Tables 2 and 3). If cytogenetic data are not available, however, the predictive power of the IPSS models diminish significantly.

In 1999, another classification system was published by a working group of the WHO, not only relying more closely on the FAB system's conventional morphologic criteria but also considering cytogenetic markers (Table 3). Data from 1600 patients with primary MDS were evaluated, expanding the FAB system by two categories for a total of seven, all having a high degree of correlation with prognosis. CMML with WBC $> 13 \times 10^9$/L was eliminated from the WHO categories and included with MPNs, while those with WBC $< 13 \times 10^9$/L are still classified as MDS/MPN. RA was split into pure refractory anemia (PRA) and refractory cytopenia with multilineage dysplasia (RCMD). Some conditions previously classified as RARS were placed in the pure sideroblastic anemia[19] group, while those with additional dysplastic features were put into the RCMD category, along with RAs without ringed sideroblasts. RAEB was divided into RAEB-I and RAEB-II, based on medullary and peripheral blast counts. RAEB-T was included under AML.

Additionally, MDS associated with karyotypic abnormality 5q was separated as a distinct entity, although its relatively benign nature prevails only if the proportion of medullary blasts is less than 5%. The WHO classification has been updated with some modification as noted in Table 3.

Etiology

Although the etiologic agent cannot be identified in the majority of patients with MDS, in some, exposure to ionizing radiation, chemicals, drugs, or other environmental agents can be implicated.

Radiation exposure has been clearly linked to the development of stem cell abnormalities.[20] In addition, the leukemias that developed in survivors of atomic bomb explosions were often preceded by a preleukemic state.[21] Atomic bomb survivors continue to exhibit an increased incidence of genetic instability seen as structural and numerical chromosomal abnormalities long after the initial exposure, which may contribute to the development of MDS and AML.[22]

Chemical injury to the marrow is a well-established phenomenon, and an increased risk of leukemogenesis has been noted among workers exposed to petrochemicals, particularly benzene, and the rubber industry.[23] Many of the initial cases of benzene-induced leukemia were associated with a preleukemic syndrome. Exposure of human cell lines to hydroquinone, a benzene metabolite, is associated with the development of abnormalities of chromosomes 5, 7, and 8 and may be responsible, in part, for the DNA damage associated with the chemical exposure.[24] In patients with or without ringed sideroblasts, exposure to diesel oil fumes ($p < 0.01$), diesel oil liquids ($p < 0.01$), or ammonia ($p < 0.05$) was associated with the development of MDS.[25] A careful history of exposure to environmental and occupational hazards should be an integral part of the work-up of all patients with MDS. Additional environmental factors may include use of hair dye and cigarette smoking.[26]

Therapy-related myelodysplasia and leukemia following treatment with radiation and/or chemotherapy have been recognized, since these were initially observed in patients treated for Hodgkin's disease.[27] Since the initial reports following treatment of Hodgkin's disease, therapy-induced MDS has been reported following treatment of cancers of the breast, lung, ovary, and gastrointestinal tract, non-Hodgkin's lymphomas, seminoma, multiple myeloma, polycythemia vera, chronic lymphocytic leukemia (CLL), as well as nonmalignant conditions.[28-30] The leukemogenic potential is greatest for alkylating agents, nitrosoureas, and procarbazine. The risk associated with exposure to these particular agents is further substantiated by the increased frequency of abnormalities involving chromosomes 5 and 7 in comparison with the much lower frequency of abnormalities involving these chromosomes in patients treated with anthracyclines, which nonetheless carry risk, or antimetabolites.[30] Leukemogenicity appears to be a function of both dose and time of exposure, as observed in patients with ovarian cancer treated with melphalan or chlorambucil. The use of etoposide in combination with cisplatin or other alkylating agents in patients treated for germ cell tumors is associated with an increased risk of MDS or AML.[31] The relationship of the cumulative dose of etoposide or teniposide to development of MDS or therapy-related AML remains to be determined.[32] Abnormalities involving deletions of a portion of the short arm of chromosome 17 (17p) associated with either mutations or overexpression of the TP53 oncogene have also been described related to prior chemotherapy.[19] This has been identified in both patients with lymphoid neoplasms treated with alkylating agents as well as in those with MPNs treated with either hydroxyurea or p. 32. Recently, treatment-related MDS has been reported in association with both fludarabine and cladribine.[20]

It has long been debated whether the increase in leukemogenic potential derives as a direct result of exposure to radiation and/or chemotherapy or more simply reflects a natural predisposition related to the underlying disease. The risk of developing MDS and/or metachronous leukemia has been reported to be increased in association with certain cancers, such as multiple myeloma, lymphoma, carcinoma of the lung, and CLL.[33,34] However, the difference in the rates of developing leukemia after various treatments for polycythemia vera or Hodgkin's disease point to treatment as the most critical etiologic factor. In patients with polycythemia vera, the risk of developing leukemia is significantly elevated in those treated with chlorambucil compared with those treated with phlebotomy alone.[35] Similarly, patients with Hodgkin's disease treated with doxorubicin, bleomycin, vinblastine, and dacarbazine (ABVD) have a much lower incidence of therapy-related leukemia

than those treated with the nitrogen mustard, vincristine, procarbazine, and prednisone (MOPP) regimen.[36] The recognition of this potential risk has led to efforts to develop equally potent but less leukemogenic therapies, particularly in diseases with the potential for long-term survival. In a registry review of patients with chronic neutropenia treated with filgrastim, 9% of patients with congenital neutropenia developed MDS and/or leukemia compared with none of the patients with cyclical or idiopathic neutropenia.[37] The relationship of the use of filgrastim and the development of MDS in these patients is uncertain.

High-dose chemotherapy with stem cell support is being applied as a curative approach in a number of malignancies, non-Hodgkin's lymphoma among them. As noted previously, an increased risk of developing MDS or metachronous leukemia in association with lymphoma has been suggested. Although therapy-induced MDS in patients with non-Hodgkin's lymphoma treated with standard doses of chemotherapy has been identified, MDS has now been recognized as a late complication of treatment with high-dose chemotherapy regimens.[38] The reported actuarial risk ranges from 6.4% up to 18% at 6 years.[39] Strategies currently under study that use high-dose myeloablative treatments earlier in the course of this disease in patients with poor prognosis make the identification of the magnitude of this problem an increasingly important issue. Studies demonstrate that there are multiple abnormal hematopoietic clones in patients with MDS which coexist and can give rise to subclones.[40] These clones can give rise to the leukemic clone in patients who transform to AML.[41]

Pathobiology

Clonal origin

A substantial body of evidence has accumulated that points to a clonal origin for MDSs. The identification of nonrandom chromosomal abnormalities detectable in 30–70% of patients with MDS confirmed the likelihood that these were clonal disorders.[42-47] Evidence that these disorders originate from pluripotent stem cells was suggested by reports of patients developing biphenotypic and lymphoid leukemias following MDS.[42,48]

Analysis of the patterns of inactivation of an X-linked polymorphic enzyme such as glucose-6-phosphate dehydrogenase (G6PD) has proven to be a useful tool in the analysis of the clonal origin of tumors. Raskind et al.[49] have demonstrated that 21 of 24 B lymphoblastoid lines transformed by Epstein–Barr virus expressed a single light chain immunoglobulin and contained only one of the G6PD isoenzymes. In contrast, the T cells expressed both the A and B G6PD isoenzymes. The frequency with which the lymphoid lineage is involved as part of the abnormal clone in MDS is variable, B lymphocytes being involved more regularly than T cells.[50-53] Other studies have found evidence that only cells committed to the myeloid lineage are involved in the clone but that lymphocytes are of polyclonal origin.[50-53] Fluorescent in situ hybridization (FISH) or polymerase chain reaction analysis of loss of heterozygosity has confirmed the involvement of an early stem cell that can give rise to CD34+ cells as well as those of erythroid, megakaryocytic, and myelomonocytic lineage, but not lymphocytes.[54] Subsequently, in a study using combined techniques of immunophenotyping and FISH, B lymphocytes were found to be involved in patients with the 5q-syndrome.[55] Molecular and flow cytometric analysis of T-cell clonality has also suggested involvement of T cells in the MDS clone of some patients. The reason for the discrepant findings is unclear but may reflect the heterogeneity of the disease and interpatient variability. Molecular studies have demonstrated a variety of clones present in MDS patients, a founding clone, and a number of sub-clones bearing recurrent gene mutations and mutations of novel gene pathways.[41]

In vitro progenitor growth characteristics

A variety of abnormalities in the growth of hematopoietic progenitors has been detected in colony assays *in vitro* of both bone marrow and peripheral blood from patients with all categories of MDS.[56] None has proved instructive of clinical response.

Bone marrow microenvironment

Histologic examination of bone marrow trephine biopsies has pointed to abnormalities of the microenvironment.[57] They noted the presence of clusters of immature precursor cells in the central intertrabecular region of the marrow, rather than along the endosteal surfaces. They cited this as evidence of abnormal localization of immature precursors (ALIP). In a series of 40 patients, the presence of ALIP correlated significantly with shortened survival and was associated with an increased risk of transformation to AML. These findings were independent of the FAB subtype and were detected even in patients with RA. However, care must be applied to differentiate true ALIP from pseudo-ALIP. In the latter case, the clusters of cells are either of erythroid or megakaryocytic origin and do not convey the same prognostic information compared with the former, where the immature cells are of myeloid origin. The determination of the immature precursor phenotype by immunohistochemical methods may be helpful in distinguishing pseudo- and true ALIP. ALIP is not, however, specific to patients with MDS and, therefore, not helpful as a diagnostic tool.[58]

Recent data in a mouse model suggest that osteoblasts have a modulating influence on leukemic blasts in the bone marrow microenvironmental niche.[58] Reduction in osteoblasts is associated with leukemic progression and shortened survival.[59] This opens a possibility that osteoblast number could be a drug target in modulating progression of MDS/AML.

Signal transduction

Whether the primary pathophysiologic defects resulting in disordered maturation and function are intrinsic to hematopoietic progenitor cells or derive from their interaction with accessory cells and other microenvironmental factors or a combination thereof is uncertain. Hematopoietic cell defects may relate not only to quantitative abnormalities of progenitors but also reflect abnormalities in signal transduction in response to cytokines or other regulatory molecules that trigger proliferation and differentiation pathways. Hematopoietic cells from MDS patients display impaired responses to a number of cytokines and are unable to respond to external signals owing either to abnormalities in number or function of cytokine receptors or to dysfunctional postbinding signal transduction.

Hematopoietic progenitors have impaired responses to cytokine stimulation with decreased CFU-GM, CFU-GEMM, and BFU-E colony number.[60] Purified blast cells from MDS patients proliferate but do not mature in response to granulocyte colony-stimulating factor (G-CSF) and granulocyte-macrophage colony-stimulating factor (GM-CSF). Purified populations of CD34+ cells from MDS patients also demonstrate impaired responses to G-CSF.[61] Receptor abnormalities in MDS are not commonly observed[62–64] although in some patients their number is either diminished or their structure aberrant. In patients with a truncated erythropoietin receptor progenitor, differentiation to erythropoietin is blocked and cells undergo apoptosis.[65] On the other hand, defects in signal transduction appear to play a larger role in the aberrant response of hematopoietic progenitors to regulatory molecules.[63,64,66] This pertains both to the cytokine signal transduction pathways and factors which regulate apoptosis.[63,64,66] Patients with MDS have defective activation of STAT5 in response to erythropoietin but not IL-3, suggesting a defect in the erythropoietin signaling pathway. Despite the relative impairment, increasing concentrations of cytokines can partially correct the defects.[67,68] Epigenetic changes resulting in transcriptional silencing are another potential mechanism affecting cytokine signaling. Evidence demonstrates aberrant hypermethylation of the SOCS-1 gene in 31% of MDS patients associated with increased activity of the JAK/STAT pathway.[69] Hypermethylation which occurs in other genes such as p15 may be explained in part by the overexpression of DNA methyltransferases 1 and 3A that have been identified in bone marrow of MDS patients.[70]

The majority of patients with MDS have hypercellular bone marrows with evident proliferation of various cellular lineage components. One interpretation of this finding is a compensatory response in the marrow to feedback signals secondary to the peripheral blood cytopenias. Yet, the response does not translate into effective hematopoiesis; a role for increased apoptosis has been suggested.[71–73] A deficiency in cytokines or relative resistance to their effects could explain this phenomenon of ineffective hematopoiesis. In several studies, bone marrow cells from MDS patients have demonstrated increased expression of Fas and Fas ligand. In marrow cultures, strategies that block tumor necrosis factor-mediated (TNF) signals, such as the use of anti-TNF-α antibody, significantly increased the numbers of hematopoietic colonies compared with untreated cells. Additional studies have implicated a dysregulated Fas pathway and TNF-α as contributing to ineffective hematopoiesis.[71–73] Inhibition of the TGF-B signaling pathway, which is overexpressed in some patients, can restore hematopoiesis, suggesting a negative regulatory role for TGF-B.

Increased apoptosis was identified in both mature cells and immature CD34+ cells by assays for annexin V, measurements of mitochondrial membrane potential, and caspase 3 activity from cell lysates in patients with MDS compared with patients with de novo AML. These results demonstrated that the patients with MDS had increased apoptosis in all FAB subcategories, which was distinctive compared with patients with AML and was equally applicable to the RAEB-T alone group.[74]

Cytogenetics

Chromosomal abnormalities, found in 30–70% of MDS patients, are similar to those seen in patients with AML and involve complete or partial deletions, most frequently involving chromosomes 5(-5,5q-), 7(-7,7q-), and 8(8+).[75,76] Certain karyotypic abnormalities that are associated with core binding factor rearrangements, such as t(15;17) in acute promyelocytic leukemia (M3), t(8;21) in AML (M2), and inv 16 in AML (M4), have only rarely been identified in MDS. Moreover, patients with these AML subtypes have good prognoses with potential for cure. Thus, they should be viewed as having AML and should be managed accordingly. Furthermore, abnormalities involving partial deletions of the long arm of chromosome 20 (20q-), seen frequently in MDS, particularly RARS, polycythemia vera, and myeloproliferative syndromes, are usually not seen in patients with de novo AML. Abnormalities are identified most frequently in patients with higher risk. Although specific chromosomal abnormalities have been identified, unlike AML, no specific abnormality has been associated with any specific subcategory. Techniques using FISH have identified additional chromosomal abnormalities in patients beyond those with banding alone and are complementary to standard techniques.[77]

Table 4 Cytogenetics: revised cytogenetic IPSS-R groupings.

Risk group	Cytogenetic groupings	Doublet	Complex	Median overall survival (months)
Very low	Del 11q -Y	—	—	60.8
Low	Normal del (5q) del (12p) del (20q)	Including del(5q)	—	48.6
Intermediate	del 7q +8 i(17p) +19 any other independent clones	Any other	—	26
High	Inv(3)/t(3q)/del(3q) -7	Including -7/del(7q)	3	15.8
Very high	—	—	>3	5.9

Source: Adapted from Schanz 2012.[76]

Many studies have demonstrated that the presence of karyotypic abnormalities is an independent prognostic variable. Furthermore, more complex abnormalities are associated with shortened survival compared with either single clonal abnormality or a normal karyotype. Certain specific clonal subtypes have varying prognostic significance for both survival and the risk of leukemic transformation. Monosomy 7 or 5 and 7q are associated with shortened survival, while deletions of the long arms of chromosome 20 (20q-) and 5(5q-syndrome) and deletion of y[78] as the sole abnormality are associated with longer survival. In the IPSS, cytogenetic findings are an independent prognostic variable classifying patients according to three subgroups: good, intermediate, and poor risk. Further studies have improved our understanding of the cytogenetic risk groups in MDS. Analysis of cases in the German–Austrian and MD Anderson databases demonstrated that cytogenetics was underweighted as a risk factor in the IPSS and suggested that poor-risk cytogenetics was just as poor a risk factor in patients as those with > 20% blasts.[75] This led to a revision of the IPSS cytogenetics group. Nineteen different cytogenetic subgroups were identified among more than 2900 patients. These groups were categorized into five prognostic subgroups including: very good, good, intermediate, poor, and very poor and were incorporated into the revised IPSS (Table 4).[16]

Genetic instability as demonstrated by clonal evolution occurs in a substantial percentage of patients. Around 20–35% have been found to undergo clonal evolution during the course of the disease, independent of karyotypic status at the outset. The significance of clonal evolution with respect to leukemic transformation and survival is contradictory at the outset. In some studies, clonal evolution was associated with a poor prognosis without an increased risk of leukemic transformation. In contrast, Glenn and colleagues have demonstrated karyotypic changes in clinically stable patients.[79] One study of 31 patients evolving to AML from MDS suggests that additional abnormalities involving chromosomes 1, 7, 8, 11, and 17 may contribute to the transformation process.[80] Subclonal evolution suggests genomic instability. Microsatellite instability involving defects in the DNA mismatch repair system has been identified in some MDS patients, particularly those with therapy-related disease.[81] Assessment of the clonal architecture in the marrow of MDS patients demonstrates that there is a founding clone and multiple secondary clones with acquisition of additional mutations leading to clonal evolution.[41]

One particular abnormality involving a deletion of part of the long arm of chromosome 5 (5q-) deserves special note. As originally described, the del 5q-syndrome is associated with a refractory macrocytic anemia, a normal or increased platelet count, giant thrombocytes, dyserythropoiesis, hypolobulated megakaryocytes, female predominance, prolonged survival, and a low rate of leukemic transformation. It is important to differentiate the del 5q-syndrome from instances where this deletion is found in combination with other chromosomal abnormalities or in association with FAB subtypes other than RA that have a more aggressive clinical course associated with shorter survival. Patients with del 5q have been identified to have a deficiency in RPS14 ribosomal RNA as the genetic defect responsible for the bone marrow failure in these patients (see section "Gene mutations and dysregulation").[82]

Patients with MDS secondary to exposure to mutagenic or carcinogenic agents have similar findings in terms of the types and significance of the chromosomal abnormalities. Patients treated with epipodophyllotoxins (etoposide and teniposide) can develop specific translocations involving the breakpoint at 11q23. This leads to transcription of a fusion protein involving the mixed-lineage leukemia (MLL) gene.

Additional techniques have been explored that can detect abnormalities in the genome not identifiable by normal metaphase cytogenetics (MC).[83] Single nucleotide polymorphism arrays (SNP-A) reveal a higher percentage of genetic abnormalities than indicated by MC.

Gene mutations and dysregulation

Alterations in the control and expression of proto-oncogenes in the cellular genome, leading to abnormalities of cellular proliferation and differentiation, are thought to contribute to the molecular basis of neoplastic transformation.[84] Point mutations of the ras family of oncogenes have been identified in association with a number of human tumors, including lung, pancreatic, colorectal, and hematopoietic neoplasms.[85] Activated ras genes with specific point mutations involving codons 12, 13, and 61 have been identified in 20–30% of patients with AML and 9–48% of patients with MDS. These findings have suggested that activation of ras genes either may contribute to the development of MDS or, once established, to the process of transformation of the commonly affected stem cell. Ki-ras with H-ras is involved in only a few cases. CMML was the FAB subtype most frequently associated with a ras mutation. The abnormality was found in 40% of cases.[86–88]

Recently a number of genes have been identified with recurrent somatic mutations in patients with MDS involving a number of different pathways including those involved in epigenetic regulation,

Table 5 Gene mutations in MDS.

Candidate gene	Chromosome	Frequency in MDS (%)	Putative functional significance
Epigenetic pathway			
ASXL1 *612990	20q	11–15	Unknown
IDH1/IDH2*147700/*147650	2q/15q	4–11	Decreased survival
DNMT3A*602769	2p	8	Decreased survival
EZH2*601573	7q	2–6	Decreased survival
TET2*612839	4q	11–26	Unknown
SETBP1	18	—	Unknown
SIGNALING	—	—	—
JAK2*147796	9p	2	Unknown
N/KRAS*164790/*190070	1p/12p	3–6	Increased risk of progression to AML
CBL*165360	11q	1	Unknown
FLT3 ITD*136351	13q	0–2	Decreased survival
Transcription factor			
RUNX1*151385	21q	4–14	Decreased survival; more common in therapy-related MDS
Other			
TP53*191170	17p	10–18	Decreased survival and increased risk of progression to AML
NPM1*164040	5q	2	Unknown
RNA splicing			
SF3B1	—	14	Alternate protein splicing
SRSF2	—	12	Alternate protein splicing
U2AF1	—	7	Alternate protein splicing
ZRSR2	—	3	Alternate protein splicing

RNA splicing, signal activation, and transcription factors (Table 5). Many of these mutations are oncogenic, and there are patterns of association or mutual exclusions in some of these abnormalities. These mutations are not exclusive to MDS but are seen in the myeloid spectrum of disease including AML and the MPNs.[89,90] The data in some of these studies indicate that there are mutations that appear early in the process of MDS, whereas others are later appearing mutations. The presence of some mutations has prognostic significance particularly EZH2, TP53, Runx1, DNAMT3A, and ASLX1.[91] Some of these mutations may lead to an increased propensity to subclonal evolution, and an increased number of mutations appear to be associated with poorer outcome and higher rate of transformation to AML. The functional dysregulation of some such as TET2 or IDH1 and IDH2 mutations results in abnormalities of the hydroxymethylation, but the major impact on pathways of these abnormalities is unknown. These recurring mutations will provide insight into disease mechanism and prognostic information and offer potential for therapeutic targets (Figure 1).

CD34+ progenitors modified to express a mutated N-ras were found to have defective differentiation in response to erythropoietin. This was manifest as reduced proliferation, increased doubling time, and decreased number of cells in S/G2M, leading to a failure to express the differentiation program in the late erythroblast stage. These cells also tended to undergo accelerated apoptosis, suggesting that expression of a mutated N-ras could be partially responsible for the pathophysiology underlying MDS.[92]

Deletion of all or part of chromosome 5 in a substantial number of patients with either de novo or secondary MDS has led to the hypothesis of a tumor suppressor gene located within a short segment of the long arm in the so-called critical region at 5q21–5q34. This region has been the focus of intensive study, and candidate genes either deleted or dysregulated have been identified, narrowing the region of interest. The interferon regulatory factor-1 (IRF-1) is a DNA binding regulatory factor that regulates, in part, expression of interferon and interferon-inducible genes by binding to promoter regions. It functions as an activator, has antiproliferative and antioncogene activity, and can reverse a transformed phenotype. The *IRF-1* gene has been mapped to the 5q31 region. A loss of one or both IRF-1alleles in patients with MDS or AML with a del 5q has been described. *In vitro* studies have suggested that loss of the *IRF-1* gene is associated either with a transformed phenotype and/or with chemo- and radiation-induced apoptosis. Although these data suggest a potential role for the *IRF-1* gene, studies have not confirmed these observations.[93,94] A recent study suggests a role for overexpression of IRF-1 leading to an upregulation of Toll-like receptors, resulting in an activated apoptotic pathway. The lack of identification of a definitive tumor suppressor gene responsible for the disease has led to other approaches investigating the underlying mechanism. Ebert and colleagues used RNA-mediated interference (RNAi) to identify genes that might be involved. They identified a partial loss of function of the ribosomal subunit protein, *RSP14* gene, that was associated with a block in erythroid differentiation in progenitor cells from patients with the del 5q-. Using the RNAi *in vitro*, they were able to recapitulate the phenotype of cells from patients with del 5q-. Overexpression of the *RSP14* gene in cells from patients with del 5q was able to rescue the phenotype and restore normal erythropoiesis, suggesting that this gene is causal for the del 5q- hematopoietic picture. The loss of function of the RSP14 results in reduction in processing of the 18s pre-rRNA levels. This is similar to the mechanism involved in the Diamond–Blackfan anemia, the congenital bone marrow failure state.[82]

Point mutations in the TP53 tumor suppressor gene have been reported in 8% of MDS cases.[95] In one series, patients with secondary myelodysplastic syndrome (sMDS) or therapy-related acute myelocytic leukemia (tAML) were found to have a higher than expected prevalence of TP53 mutations in leukemic, but not germline tissues. Accumulation of TP53 abnormalities with sequential follow-up was identified in patients as they transform to AML.[96] Microsatellite instability was identified and was consistent with a mutator phenotype, suggesting that these patients were at higher risk of developing therapy-related MDS/AML. Patients have been described with a 17p-syndrome characterized by dysgranulopoiesis with pseudo-Pelger–Huët hypolobulation and small vacuoles in neutrophils. In one series, 15 of 16 patients with this deletion had an associated deletion of TP53, suggesting a potential role for loss of a tumor suppressor gene as a contributing factor to the morphologic, cytogenetic, and molecular phenotype of this syndrome. The expression of several other genes, including EVI-1,

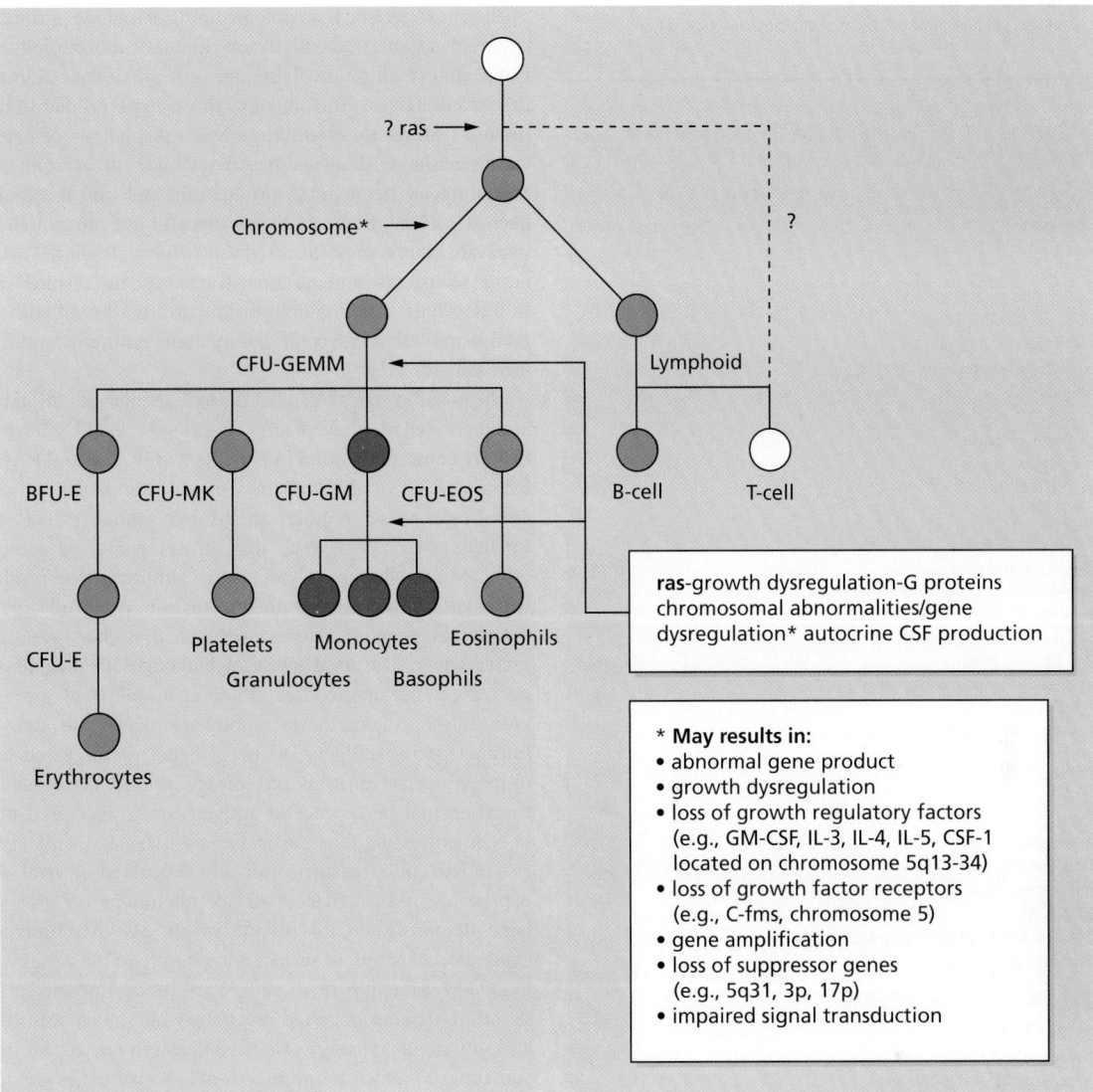

Figure 1 Multiple steps involved in the pathogenesis of MDS affecting a pluripotent hematopoietic stem cell (white circle). Chromosomal abnormalities and ras mutations may occur as early or late events in the pathogenesis of the disease. In younger patients, disease appears to originate in a stem cell committed along a more restricted lineage pathway (●) and is similar to the stem cell origin in some patients with de novo AML. In most patients with MDS, the disease originates from a multipotent stem cell affecting progeny involving multiple hematopoietic lineages (● ●). *May result in abnormal gene product; growth dysregulation; loss of growth regulatory factors (e.g., GM-CSF, IL-3, IL-4, IL-5, CSF-1 located on chromosome 5q13–34); loss of growth factor receptors (e.g., cfms, chromosome 5); gene amplification; loss of suppressor genes (e.g., 5q31, 3p, 17p); impaired signal transduction. *Abbreviations*: IL, interleukin; CSF, colony-stimulating factor.

c-mpl, PDGF, MLL, and the CSF-1 receptor, has recently been described to be dysregulated in some patients with MDS.[97] The EVI-1 gene, located on chromosome 3, has been shown to play a role in both myeloid and erythroid differentiation. Dysregulation of gene expression is associated with blocks in myeloid and erythroid maturation.[97]

The V617F JAK 2 mutation has been described in patients with the MPDs, polycythemia vera, myelofibrosis, and essential thrombocythemia. There is also a small subset of patients with MDS with the mutation. These patients usually have high platelet counts and may have sideroblastic anemia. Some have designated this small subset RARS-T (T = thrombocytosis).

Clinical and laboratory features

The clinical and laboratory picture in patients with MDS is dominated by and derives from the defect involving a multipotent hematopoietic stem cell. Although the disease has occasionally been described in children and adolescents, it is primarily encountered in adults in their sixth decade or older. In most reports, the median age is over 65, and there appears to be a male predominance. The clinical presentation is nonspecific. The symptoms relate primarily to the cytopenias, with those attributable to anemia being most common. These include fatigue, weakness, pallor, dyspnea, angina pectoris, and cardiac failure. Other signs and symptoms encountered less frequently include easy bruising, ecchymosis, epistaxis, gingival bleeding, petechiae, and bacterial infections, particularly respiratory and dermal. Physical findings are nonspecific. Hepatic and/or splenic enlargement is reported in 10–40% of patients and is most commonly found in CMML. Lymphadenopathy and skin infiltration are uncommon. Nontherapy-related MDS has been reported in association with other neoplasms, including lymphoproliferative and plasma cell disorders as well as carcinomas.

Erythrocytes

Morphology
  Anisocytosis
  Poikilocytosis
  Oval macrocytes
  Microcytes
  Basophilic stippling
  Howell–Jolly bodies
  Circulating nucleated red cells
  Megaloblastoid maturation
  Multinucleated precursors
  Nuclear budding
  Karyorrhexis
  Defective hemoglobinization
  Ringed sideroblasts
  Increased stainable iron

Enzymes
  Increased hexokinase
  Decreased pyruvate kinase
  Decreased 2,3-diphosphoglycerate mutase
  Decreased phosphofructokinase
  Increased adenosine deaminase
  Increased pyruvate kinase
Decreases or loss of blood group antigens
Increased fetal hemoglobin
Aberrant globin chain synthesis
Disordered ferrokinetics

Leukocytes

Morphology
  Pseudo-Pelger–Huët cells
  Abnormal chromatin clumping
  Abnormal nuclear bridging
  Monocytosis
  Defective granule formation (hypogranulation)
  Megaloblastoid maturation
  Auer rods
Increased LAP
Decreased myeloperoxidase
Increased muramidase (CMML)
Loss of granule membrane glycoproteins
Inappropriate surface antigens
Lineage infidelity
Decreased adhesion
Defective chemotaxis
Deficient phagocytosis
Impaired bactericidal activity

Megakaryocytes

Morphology
  Micromegakaryocytes
  Hypolobulated nuclei
  Large mononuclear forms
  Circulating megakaryocyte fragments
  Giant thrombocytes
Defective platelet aggregation
Deficiency in thromboxane A2
Bernard–Soulier-like defect

Immune deficiencies
Decreased T-cell IL-2 receptors
Decreased IL-2 production
Decreased NK activity
Decreased NK response to gamma interferon
Decreased response to mitogens
Decreased T4 cells
Immunoglobulin abnormalities
Autoantibodies
Autoimmune phenomenon
Impaired self-recognition

The characteristic hematologic findings include peripheral blood cytopenias associated with dysmyelopoietic morphology and functional abnormalities involving one or more of the cell lines and are detailed in Table 6. The bone marrow is hypercellular in the majority and features the dysmyelopoietic morphology of part or all of the progenitors. Abnormalities involving erythrocyte enzymes, surface antigens, hemoglobin production, and iron metabolism have been described. Some of the changes in enzyme activity, such as pyruvate kinase, may affect red cell survival. Impaired activity of A and H transferase and galactosyltransferase has resulted in changes in blood types. Hemoglobin production is affected with increased fetal hemoglobin, aberrant globin chain synthesis, and disordered ferrokinetics.

The myeloid series often reveals leukopenia with immature forms and increased numbers of large unstained cells (LUC). Neutropenia is more commonly found in patients with RAEB and RAEB-T than RA and RARS.[27] Leukocytosis most often accompanies CMML and, by definition, requires an absolute monocytosis ($>1 \times 10^9$/L) for diagnosis. Monocytosis may, however, also be present in the other MDS subtypes. Cytoplasmic abnormalities result in cells with hypo- or defective granule formation, Auer rods, or abnormal azurophilic granules. Histocytochemical studies reveal cells with increased or decreased levels of leukocyte alkaline phosphatase, decreased myeloperoxidase staining, and loss of granule membrane glycoproteins. Surface antigen analysis has shown loss of lineage-specific antigens, with persistent or increased expression of inappropriate antigens and lineage infidelity. In some instances, the abnormal persistence of antigens or an increased proportion of cells expressing those antigens was associated with an increased risk of leukemic transformation and shortened survival. Abnormal expression of an activated surface phenotype on monocytes has been demonstrated in patients within all FAB subtypes, while expression of activated surface antigens on granulocytes was almost exclusively seen in patients with excess blasts. Impaired granulocyte function includes impaired respiratory burst, deficit in chemotaxis and superoxide release, as well as a defect in neutrophil stimulation signaling.[98,99] Nuclear and functional abnormalities are outlined in Table 6.

Megakaryocytes can be decreased and their morphology is often bizarre (Table 6). Patients with RAEB and RAEB-T more commonly have thrombocytopenia, decreased megakaryocytes, and greater degrees of dysmegakaryopoiesis. Megakaryocyte fragments and giant thrombocytes may circulate in the peripheral blood. Hemorrhagic symptoms in these patients may be due not only to thrombocytopenia but also to functionally defective platelets as well. Dysfunction can result from defective platelet aggregation, deficiencies in thromboxane A2 activity, or the development of a Bernard–Soulier-type platelet defect. This latter defect has developed from a deficiency in the membrane glycoprotein GP Ib-IX complex.

A small percentage of patients present with hypoplastic bone marrows and cytopenias that morphologically may be difficult to distinguish from aplastic anemia.[100] Cytogenetic analysis with or without interphase FISH may be helpful in establishing a diagnosis.

The relationship of MDS to abnormalities of the immune system is of particular interest given the broad range of abnormalities described. There is a decrease in the number of T-cell interleukin-2 (IL-2) receptors, as well as IL-2 production. The latter is due, in part, to a failure of immunoregulatory B cells. NK cell activity and responsiveness to α-interferon are decreased, as is α-interferon production, while total numbers of NK cells are variable. There are decreases in the number of T cells, responsiveness to mitogenic stimulation, the total number of cells, and the T4/T8 ratio. The latter is due predominantly to a decrease in T4 cells.

Immunoglobulin abnormalities manifest as autoantibodies or a positive direct Coombs' test is often present. The relationship of the disease to the immune abnormalities is poorly understood. A general dysregulation of the immune system appears prevalent in many patients. Consistent with this is the finding of altered antibody repertoires of self-reactive IgM and IgG in MDS patients, indicating a disturbance in self-recognition mechanisms. Whether some abnormalities relate, in part, to the number of red cell transfusions or whether they are reversible with effective treatment is unknown. Given the nature of the defect in a multipotent stem cell with potential to differentiate along multiple pathways, the dysregulation of T and B cells should not be surprising.

Establishing a diagnosis

The diagnosis in most patients is readily established with standardized testing, which should include history and physical examination, complete blood count, and review of the peripheral blood smear. The findings of cytopenias in the absence of explanation from biochemical, vitamin deficiency, hemorrhage, toxin/drug, or infectious etiology should lead to a bone marrow aspirate and biopsy. Routine cytogenetic evaluation should be included as well. The diagnosis of MDS is based primarily on morphologic criteria demonstrating dysmorphic features in the peripheral blood and bone marrow precursors (Table 6). Although some of the classification systems include cytogenetic information (IPSS, IPSS-R, and WHO), they are based primarily on bone marrow and peripheral blood morphology. Analysis of the marrow population using flow cytometric analysis has become standard for the diagnosis and subtyping in patients with acute leukemia. It is more routinely being applied to establish a diagnosis of MDS as well. Abnormal populations and skewed antigen expression can be identified. However, comparative studies of bone marrow morphology and flow cytometry results have not been conducted, and thus one cannot be certain if used alone whether flow cytometry results can reliably establish a diagnosis and classification of MDS. Accurate classification according to FAB, IPSS, IPSS-R, or WHO criteria must be based, at least in part, on bone marrow morphology. Thus, flow cytometry should be viewed as a complementary examination but not sufficient to establish the diagnosis and classification. Cytogenetics are abnormal in up to 70% of patients, with abnormalities that are not diagnostic but maybe suggestive of the diagnosis. Gene mutation analyses of genes commonly mutated in myeloid diseases are becoming commercially available and can be used to support a diagnosis of MDS. However, gene mutations have been described in normal patients with no manifestation of a hematologic malignancy and whose significance is uncertain.[101] So gene mutations alone are insufficient to establish a diagnosis.

Diagnostic dilemmas

Some patients with MDS present with features also suggestive of an MPN, representing an "overlap syndrome."[102] In these patients, cytopenias may present simultaneously with elevated white or platelet counts. In some patients, an increased leukocyte count may be accompanied by monocytosis. Under current classification systems, some of these patients will be clearly defined as MPN, while others are still categorized as MDS, depending on the upper limit of WBC permitted in the classification system. Others may have myelofibrosis with or without marked splenomegaly and peripheral blood cytopenias yet also have dysplastic features suggesting MDS.

These patients are more difficult to classify. Those with myelofibrosis with markedly enlarged spleens and a leukoerythroblastic peripheral smear are more likely classic myelofibrosis with myeloid metaplasia, while patients without significant splenomegaly and/or the peripheral leukoerythroblastic picture may be considered to have primary MDS with fibrosis. The presence of V617F Jak2 mutation would favor a diagnosis of an MPN over MDS except in patients with RARS-T.

The hypoplastic MDS variant is often indistinguishable from aplastic anemia and may have many features in common.[103,104] Those patients with increased expression of HLA-DR 15 and the PNH phenotype (decreased expression of CD59), whether MDS or aplastic anemia, may respond to immunomodulatory treatments. Cytogenetic abnormalities, if present, involving chromosomes frequently abnormal in MDS, may suggest the diagnosis of MDS, but do not completely exclude aplastic anemia. In these patients, therapeutic options may be the determinants in the orientation of the diagnosis in the absence of other criteria.

Finally, there are patients who present with severe pancytopenia and bone marrow findings that are nondiagnostic (i.e., minimal, if any, dysmorphic changes; no increase in myeloblasts) and without any cytogenetic abnormalities. Some of these patients may have MDS, and only with continued observation and testing will a diagnosis be unequivocally established. Gene mutations may also suggest MDS. Others may have been exposed to a bone marrow insult (toxin, infectious agent, etc.), which may never be identified, but which may permit eventual complete or partial marrow recovery, which takes months or years. In these latter individuals, in the absence of clear diagnostic evidence, patience, continued observation, and supportive care (SC) are usually the best approaches pending a declarative diagnosis. One other consideration for these patients would be an immune-mediated injury to hematopoietic stem cells. The differential in these patients would include large granular lymphocytic (LGL) leukemia, where T-cell receptor and immunoglobulin gene rearrangement studies and T-cell subsets may be informative.[105]

Pathogenesis and relation to leukemic transformation

Initiation and promotion of an abnormality affecting a multipotent stem cell may be related to a variety of factors, including chemical insult, radiation, or infection, leading to modification of gene expression. Since most patients with MDS are in the sixth, seventh, or eighth decades, cell senescence may also play a role. Once established, the clonal lesion follows the multistep process of oncogenesis and results in the transformation to acute leukemia in up to 40% of patients. It is likely that multiple events occur and lead to evolution of the disease and ultimate emergence of a dominant clone of cells.[106,107] Based on the knowledge of a number of abnormalities that do occur, one may speculate on the possible interrelationship of these events that contribute to the pathogenesis. Mutations of the ras oncogene, either as an early or late event in the development of the disease, may be one of the steps in this process. One model of ras mutation results in impaired growth and differentiation along with impaired response to erythropoietin and increased apoptosis, similar to the response of the *in vivo* phenotype. Such mutations may serve to confer a growth advantage to the mutated cells, resulting in their progressive expansion. As a late event, the selective growth advantage may be sufficient to trigger a leukemic transformation. However, when alteration of the *ras* gene occurs as an early event, it may be insufficient to trigger further progression and may require the concerted action of other factors such as those accompanying chromosomal abnormalities and the attendant gene dysregulation that occurs. The identification of many more somatic mutations involving differing pathways including those involved in epigenetic regulation, signaling, transcription factors, and RNA splicing suggests that the pathogenesis is more complex. Models that will allow the study of the role of these mutations will be critical.[108]

The impaired response of hematopoietic progenitors suggests an underlying abnormality of signal transduction. Mutations of cytokine receptors can result in a signal that is muted or overexpressed. Mutations have been identified of the FLT3 and G-CSF receptor in association with transformation to AML in patients with MDS. Most studies, however, have not identified abnormalities of cytokine receptors, suggesting a defect further downstream from the ligand–receptor interaction.[109,110] The increase in apoptosis in the bone marrow with apparent dysregulation of TNF-α and TGF-β further suggests cytokine dysregulation. Hematopoietic progenitors with impaired cellular response to cytokine signals could behave as though deprived of obligate survival factors and thus undergo accelerated apoptosis. This would be the predominant phenotype until further genetic or growth regulatory changes occurred that would trigger a proliferative advantage and transformation to AML. In patients with severe congenital neutropenia, evolution to an MDS or acute leukemia is usually accompanied by acquired mutations in the G-CSF receptor.[111] Point mutations of the G-CSF receptor gene cause truncation of the C-terminal cytoplasmic region of the receptor. Cells with this defect fail to undergo terminal maturation to granulocytes in response to the G-CSF. In a mouse model, the equivalent G-CSF receptor mutation leads to expansion of the G-CSF receptor-responsive progenitor population. Treatment with G-CSF leads to neutrophilia, accompanied by increased activation of transcription factors and prolonged external cell surface expression owing to defective internalization. Further genetic mutations in the face of clonal expansion can contribute to leukemogenesis.

Karyotypic abnormalities have been described in up to 79% of patients with MDS and appear to be a later phenomenon. This is suggested by the identification of karyotypic abnormalities in cells belonging to already established clones derived from a multipotent stem cell and by their greater frequency in patients with increased bone marrow blasts. The association in some studies of complex karyotypic abnormalities with an increased risk of leukemic transformation further suggests that these anomalies confer a growth advantage to a clone, as well as reflecting underlying genetic instability. This instability, manifest by clonal evolution with the subsequent acquisition of additional chromosomal abnormalities, has also been associated with disease progression, either to a more malignant subtype or to frank AML. Finally, most of the karyotypic abnormalities involve complete or partial deletions of chromosomes and suggest that gene loss may play a role in the pathogenesis. The critical region on the long arm of chromosome 5, in the interstitial region q13–q34, contains genes encoding a number of important proteins, including GM-CSF, IL-3, IL-4, IL-5, CSF-1, and the oncogene *cfms*, which codes for the CSF-1 receptor. Changes in this critical region may result in the production of an abnormal gene product or a point mutation. Deletion or loss of chromosomal material may result in a cell hemizygous for a mutant allele, which can be expressed, or loss of a tumor suppressor gene. Several chromosomal regions that are commonly deleted in patients with MDS have been identified, including del 1q, del 5q, del 17p, and del 3p, and may contain tumor suppressor genes whose loss may contribute to the transformation process.

Dysregulation of the cell cycle may occur and contribute to the leukemic transformation. The cyclin-dependent kinase inhibitor (CDKI) gene p1 5INK4B undergoes aberrant methylation of the CpG islands in up to 50% of patients with MDS studied in one series. Patients with high-risk MDS had the highest frequency of hypermethylation compared to those with low-risk MDS. In addition, hypermethylation became more prominent as disease progressed.

Treatment

For many years, the management of patients with MDS was a frustrating and daunting task, compounded by the age of the patients, their debility secondary to bone marrow failure, comorbidities, and a lack of effective treatments. The mainstay of therapy was primarily SC, consisting of transfusions and antibiotics in an effort to alleviate symptoms, but without impact on the disease outcome. Therapeutic efforts are complicated by the heterogeneity of the disease, which determines individual prognosis. Additional complicating features, including the general lack of randomized trials and the lack of uniform response criteria, made the interpretation of therapeutic results more difficult. The last decade has witnessed an expanded interest in the treatment of MDS, with the identification of new effective therapeutic strategies.

Differentiation-inducing and novel-acting agents

There has been great interest in the potential of differentiation therapy as an antitumor modality since Charlotte Friend and her colleagues first demonstrated that dimethyl sulfoxide (DMSO) could induce differentiation of murine erythroleukemic cells *in vitro*, thus altering their malignant phenotype.[112] The phenomenon although readily achieved *in vitro* is more difficult to demonstrate in the clinical setting. A number of agents that have effectively induced differentiation *in vitro* were tested in MDS without significant success (e.g., cis- and trans-retinoic acid, vitamin D3, butyrate, and hexamethylene bisacetamide [HMBA]).

The hypomethylating agent (HMA) azacitidine (AzaC) has produced significant benefit (Table 7).[113–116] The promoter region of genes that are not expressed is often associated with hypermethylated CpG islands. Aberrant acquired changes in methylation, or epigenetic events, affecting intergenic and intron regions as well result in gene silencing and can have important effects on genes regulating the cell cycle and differentiation programs. A series of experiments by Christman, Acs, Taylor, and Jones and colleagues led to the development of a biochemical model that provided an explanation for the action of AzaC as an inducer of differentiation through its effects on DNA methylation.[117–119] AzaC, once incorporated into DNA, covalently binds to DNA methyltransferase, the enzyme in mammalian cells responsible for methylation of newly synthesized DNA. This binding results in hypomethylated DNA distal to the binding point and leads to transcription of previously quiescent methylated genes. In patients with β-thalassemia,[120] treatment with AzaC resulted in an increase in fetal hemoglobin production, which was associated with hypomethylation in the region of the gamma globin chain gene. Based on this model, two trials testing the efficacy of AzaC in MDS were undertaken by the Cancer and Leukemia Group B (CALGB) which demonstrated a 50% response rate in patients with higher-risk MDS.[115,121] This led to the conduct in the CALGB of a phase III trial of AzaC compared with SC. In the trial design, patients with progression could cross over to treatment after a minimum of 4 months in the SC group. Responses occurred in 60% on the AzaC arm (7% CR, 16% PR, 37% improved) compared with 5% (improved) for SC ($p < 0.0001$). The median time to leukemic transformation or death was significantly delayed for those on AzaC (21 mos. vs. 13 mos. for SC [$p = 0.007$]). Probability of transformation to AML as the first event was lower on AzaC (15%) than SC[116] ($p = 0.001$).

Table 7 Randomized controlled trials in patients with MDS drug versus supportive care ± placebo.

Agent	Response to treatment	Quality of life	Frequency of transformation to AML	Time to progression	Time to AML or death	Survival at 24 months
Cis-retinoic acid	NSSD	—	—	—	—	NSSD
Low-dose cytarabine	Cytarabine	—	NSSD	NSSD	NSSD	NSSD
G-CSF	G-CSF	—	NSSD	NSSD	SC[a]	SC[a]
GM-CSF	GM-CSF	—	NSSD	—	—	NSSD
Azacitidine	Azacitidine[b]	Azacitidine[c]	Azacitidine[b]	Azacitidine[d]	Azacitidine[e]	Azacitidine[f]
Decitabine	Decitabine	Decitabine	NSSD	NSSD	NSSD	NR

[a]Differences are for patients with RAEB. For those with RAEB-T, there was NSSD between G-CSF and SC.

[b]$p < 0.001$.

[c]Fatigue ($p = 0.001$), physical functioning ($p = 0.002$), dyspnea ($p = 0.0014$), and mental health index ($p = 0.0077$).

[d]$p < 0.0001$.

[e]$p = 0.004$.

[f]$p = 0.03$.

Abbreviations: NSSD, no statistically significant difference between agent tested and placebo or supportive care (SC); —, endpoint not assessed in trial; NR, not reported.

The quality of life (QOL) of patients on the AzaC arm was significantly superior to that experienced by individuals in the control group as measured by several test methods. Striking improvement in their QOL ensued. Patients on the AzaC arm experienced significantly greater improvement over time than patients in the SC group in fatigue, physical functioning, dyspnea, psychosocial distress, and positive affect. After crossover to AzaC, significant improvements occurred in fatigue, physical functioning, dyspnea, and general well-being.[122] Median survival for AzaC and SC (analyzed by intent to treat regardless of crossover) was 20 and 14 months, respectively ($p = 0.1$). The probability of survival at 24 months was 41% for AzaC compared with 25% for SC ($p = 0.03$). In order to eliminate the confounding effect caused by including the 49 crossover patients in the survival analysis, a landmark analysis was done in which the survival of three subgroups of patients was compared from a 6-month landmark date. These subgroups were SC patients who never crossed over or who crossed over only after 6 months, SC patients who crossed over before 6 months, and patients who were initially randomized to AzaC. The 36 patients who died before the landmark date were excluded. The additional median survival (after the 6-month landmark date) for these three groups was 11, 14, and 18 months, respectively. The AzaC group was significantly different from the SC subgroup who crossed over late or never ($p = 0.03$). SC patients who crossed over early (subgroup 2) had a longer median survival than the patients who crossed over late or never (subgroup 1), though this did not reach statistical significance ($p = 0.11$). Results demonstrate that patients treated with AzaC had significantly higher response rates, improved QOL, delayed time to progression, improved survival at 24 months, delayed time to leukemic transformation or death, and significantly reduced risk of transformation to AML compared with SC. On crossover to AzaC treatment, the same individuals were evaluated for QOL according to the same serial interviews. Striking improvement in their QOL ensued. Patients on the AzaC arm experienced significantly greater improvement over time in fatigue (EORTC, $p = 0.001$), physical functioning (EORTC, $p = 0.002$), dyspnea (EORTC, $p = 0.0014$), psychosocial distress (MHI, $p = 0.0015$), and positive affect (MHI, $p = 0.0077$) than patients in the SC group. Significant differences persisted after controlling for RBC transfusions. Prior to crossover, the QOL of patients on SC was stable or worsening. After crossover to AzaC, significant improvements occurred in fatigue (EORTC, $p = 0.0001$), physical functioning (EORTC, $p = 0.004$), dyspnea (EORTC, $p = 0.0002$), and general well-being (MHI, $p = 0.016$). Detailed analyses make unlikely placebo or Hawthorne effects as

explanations for improvements in QOL by AzaC. Additional analyses demonstrated that AzaC results in transfusion independence in 45% of patients and is effective in producing responses in patients according to the WHO AML classification (blasts > 20%) with a median survival of 19.3 months, suggesting a potential benefit in this patient population.[123] Thus, AzaC is the only agent other than allogeneic bone marrow transplantation to alter the natural history of MDS. Furthermore, AzaC is not age restricted, as is marrow transplantation. A second randomized controlled trial has confirmed and extended these observations demonstrating a significant survival advantage for patients treated with AzaC compared to a conventional care regimen (a physician-directed choice of either best SC, low-dose cytarabine, or induction chemotherapy with an anthracycline and cytarabine) with median overall survival (OS) for AzaC of 24.4 months compared to 15 months for the conventional care regimen.[18] Time to AML or death was significantly delayed for patients in the AzaC-treated group. Transfusion independence occurred in 45% of patients, and there was a reduction by 33% in the infections requiring intravenous antibiotics in the AzaC-treated patients. Time to initial response is slow, requiring repetitive monthly cycles to see a response, with the median time to response of three cycles—an observation seen consistently across all AzaC studies. Additional analyses suggest that maintenance therapy with AzaC is also beneficial.[124]

AzaC acts via a number of mechanisms. It can be a cytotoxic agent, but *in vitro* data indicate that it also functions as a biologic response modifier, affecting cytokine signal transduction pathways.[125] Another hypomethylating agent, decitabine (2-deoxy-5-AzaC), has also been evaluated.[126–129] Although response criteria are different, decitabine, like AzaC, produces responses. In a North American randomized trial of decitabine compared to SC, decitabine was superior with a response rate of 17% CR + PR compared to 0% for SC. However, there was no difference in the second coprimary endpoint of time to AML or death between the two groups.[129] In a second randomized trial conducted in Europe by the EORTC of decitabine compared to SC in patients with intermediate-2 or high-risk disease, there was no difference in time to AML or death or survival between the two groups.[126] An alternative dosing regimen of 20 mg/m^2/day × 5 days every 4 weeks has yielded response rates that are comparable but maybe less myelosuppressive.[130,131] However, this was not a controlled trial, and the effects on modifying disease outcome are uncertain.[132]

Epigenetic combinations

Single-agent HMAs produce responses in half the patients treated but are not curative. Combination epigenetic therapy with HMAs and a variety of histone deacetylase inhibitors (HDACs) has been explored.[132] *In vitro* combinations of HMAs and HDACs are synergistic in reexpressing epigenetically silenced genes. The effect is sequence dependent with the HMA required to be administered before the HDAC to see the effect, and this observation has led to a series of combination translational trials. AzaC has been combined with entinostat in a randomized trial comparing the single agent to the combination. There was no difference between the combination and AzaC monotherapy in response or OS. Analysis of the methylation differences between the two arms suggests that there was a negative interaction between the combination and monotherapy with reduced hypomethylation in the patients treated with the combination.[133] AzaC combined with vorinostat in phase I–II study demonstrates a response rate up to 75% with an increase in time to AML or death and overall survival in the cohort of AzaC 75 mg/m^2/day 1–7 and vorinostat 200 mg BID days 3–9.[134] The combination studies are associated with GI toxicity, nausea, vomiting, and fatigue being described in many patients. This toxicity can be tolerated by some but may hinder longer-term tolerance among patients and may contribute to an inability to maintain patients on treatment to obtain the full effect. AzaC in combination with mocetinostat has also shown positive clinical response; however, pericardial inflammation was observed and studies were halted.

Signal inhibitors: Multikinase inhibitors

Rigosertib is a Ras mimetic molecule with multikinase inhibitory activity. It is a broad inhibitor of the PI3 kinase/AKT pathway and has been tested alone and in combination in MDS.[135] As a single agent, rigosertib administered IV has shown improvement in peripheral blood counts and a reduction in marrow blast percentage in patients that were predominantly HMA failures.[135] In a randomized phase III study, patients were randomized to either rigosertib or BSC (which could include low-dose cytarabine) with OS as the primary endpoint in patients who were HMA failures. The trend was in favor of rigosertib, 8.2 months versus 5.9 ($p = 0.33$, HR 0.87 [95% CI 0.67–1.14]). Although the trial did not meet the primary endpoint, there were several subgroups that demonstrated a survival benefit.[136] Rigosertib is being tested in a new phase III study. Rigosertib is also being studied in combination with AzaC based on *in vitro* studies which demonstrated synergistic interaction enhancing apoptosis between the two agents. Data from the phase I study of the combination demonstrates the regimen to be well tolerated and yields responses in patients with MDS and AML including those that have failed prior treatment with an HMA.[137]

Retinoic acid and related compounds, highly effective inducers of differentiation *in vitro*, have been disappointing in their lack of efficacy in several clinical trials.[138]

Anti-TNF and the IMIDs. The observations regarding the potential role of TNF in the pathophysiology of MDS (described in the section titled "Signal transduction") have led to therapeutic strategies targeting TNF in small pilot studies. Etanercept, an anti-TNF fusion protein, caused erythroid response of 30% in one trial and a lower response in the other.[139] Thalidomide has not only been tested based on potential anti-TNF activity but also because of effects on vascular endothelial growth factor (VEGF). Responses predominantly in the erythroid lineage ranged from 10% to 19%.[140] Somnolence and neuropathy forced withdrawal of patients from treatment. Lenalidomide, an analog without sedative or neuropathic side effects and with more potent *in vitro* anti-TNF and anti-VEGF effects, was tested in a phase II trial. Of the 148 patients with low and intermediate-1 disease with del 5q either isolated or combined with other cytogenetic abnormalities, 67% patients became red cell transfusion independent.[141] The median duration of transfusion independence was 115 weeks.[141] These data were confirmed in a second study wherein 10 mg/day should be the initial dose. In a second study of low and intermediate-1 disease in patients without a deletion 5q, 26% patients achieved transfusion independence for a median of 41 weeks. Lenalidomide has been combined with AzaC and produced an overall response rate of 67%.[142] The combination was well tolerated but will require more testing to determine if it is better than either agent alone.

Novel fusion proteins for TGFβ superligand family with ligand trap activity toward the activin type 2 receptors are in clinical development in patients with lower risk, red cell transfusion-dependent MDS. In early phase trials, these agents, sotatercept and luspatercept, have reduced transfusion need in some patients and eliminated RBC transfusion requirement in patients with low transfusion burden lower-risk disease.[143] These agents are undergoing further clinical testing.

Hormones

Although used as a nonspecific stimulant of erythropoiesis in aplastic anemia with some benefit, androgens have not proven to be useful in MDS. Initial observations suggesting that treatment with androgens accelerated the disease and was associated with an increased rate of leukemic transformation were not confirmed in subsequent studies, nor was any efficacy identified.[144,145]

Glucocorticoid therapy yielded an overall response rate of only 9%, and furthermore, 24% of nonresponding patients experienced significant deleterious side effects.

Danazol has been reported to produce improvements in the thrombocytopenia and anemia in patients with MDS. Danazol may be helpful in those patients where immune-mediated cell destruction contributes to the deficit.

Chemotherapy

Chemotherapeutic agents, alone and in combination, have been used to treat patients with MDS. These agents have been employed in a variety of regimens ranging from attenuated low-dose schedules[99] to the more conventional antileukemic myelotoxic-type strategies. These have been employed to treat patients at all stages of disease. Antileukemic-type treatments have not substantially altered the outcome of the disease for most patients and have been associated with significant toxicity in many. In a retrospective analysis of chemotherapy induction compared to an HMA, the trend suggested a benefit for the HMA.[15]

The pharmacologic interaction between fludarabine and cytosine arabinoside increases intracellular ara-CTP and has been exploited in a regimen with activity in patients with relapsed AML. Subsequently, the combination with (FLAG) or without (FA) G-CSF has been tested in patients with MDS and de novo AML.[146] The two regimens yielded comparable complete response (CR) rates of 60% and 55%, respectively, with the response rate generally higher in the subgroups of MDS with excess blasts. Overall, 27% of patients (MDS and AML) died during induction. The median projected survival was 29 weeks for FA and 39 weeks for FLAG. These differences were not statistically significant. In patients with deletion of chromosome 5 or 7, FLAG produced a response rate of 64% versus 36% for FA. However, the differences were attributed by the authors to factors other than an effect of treatment. Use of G-CSF was associated with a more rapid recovery of neutrophil count, but this did not translate into decreased rates of infection or infection-related mortality.

Overall, there were no differences in treatment outcome for patients with MDS compared with AML.

Cytosine arabinoside has been extensively tested. In a review of the literature, low-dose cytosine arabinoside was reported to produce 16% CR in 170 patients.[147,148] Median duration of CR was 10.5 months, but achievement of a response appeared to have little effect on overall survival. In a randomized trial conducted by Eastern Cooperative Oncology Group (ECOG) and Southwest Oncology Group (SWOG), patients with MDS were treated with either low-dose cytarabine or SC. Patients in SC who progressed could cross over and receive treatment with cytarabine. There was no significant difference between the cytarabine and SC groups with respect to overall survival, time to progression, or frequency of transformation to AML (Table 7). In a subset analysis in the most recent randomized trial, AzaC compared to a conventional care regimen was superior to low-dose cytarabine improving survival significantly in patients with intermediate-2 and high-risk MDS.[18]

Clofarabine use in varying doses ranging from 15 to 40 mg/m² IV daily × 5 days has yielded responses between 25% and 50% of patients with variable duration of response in both untreated and those that have failed HMA therapy. The role and utility of clofarabine in MDS treatment remain to be determined.[149]

In general, results from earlier studies indicated that responses to treatment of patients with either MDS or AML following MDS are less favorable than treatment of de novo AML. Age appears to influence the rate and duration of response, with younger patients achieving CR more frequently and remaining in remission longer compared with older patients. Achievement of a CR in MDS is associated with improved survival in comparison to nonresponding patients, but the duration of the response is substantially shorter in comparison with patients with de novo AML who achieve response. Treatment prior to the transformation to AML and patients with shorter intervals between the diagnosis of MDS and leukemic transformation are associated with higher response rates. However, aggressive antileukemic-type treatment is associated with high rates of morbidity and mortality, with up to 30% of the patients dying from drug-related complications.

Iron chelation. For patients with lower-risk disease who are red cell transfusion dependent, accumulation of iron leading to iron overload and ultimate tissue damage from hemochromatosis is a long-term problem. Use of chelation is recommended for patients who have received ≥ 20–25 units of lifetime transfused RBC or a serum ferritin > 1000–2000 ng/mL (NCCN Guidelines Version 2.2014). Use of deferasirox has been shown to reduce serum ferritin and labile plasma iron.[150] Some studies have suggested an impact on survival, but there have been no randomized trials and other factors could be at play as well including patient selection bias. However, chelation should be part of the management strategy for lower-risk RBC transfusion-dependent patients. In patients with higher risk, the role of chelation is undetermined. In the absence of effective primary therapy for the MDS, chelation in this patient population is probably not warranted until or unless the patients achieve a hematological response to primary therapy.

Bone marrow transplantation
Results of allogeneic and syngeneic bone marrow transplantation from a series of reports containing small numbers of MDS patients have suggested that 35–40% can achieve durable long-term disease-free remissions when treated with this modality.[151] This has been substantiated with the results from two larger single-institution series. In one large series, 251 patients treated between 1981 and 1996 were evaluated. Appelbaum and colleagues reported an estimated (Kaplan–Meier) 5-year disease-free survival

(DFS) of 40%. Younger age, shorter duration of disease, female gender, and de novo MDS were predictors of better DFS. Patients under the age of 20 years had a 60% DFS rate compared with 40% and 20% for those 20–50 years old or over the age of 50, respectively. Patients with low-risk MDS had a 55% DFS at 6 years compared with only 30% for those with high-risk MDS.[152,153] This difference correlated with a higher rate of relapse among those with more advanced disease. Among patients with low and intermediate-1 risk according to the IPSS score, there were almost no relapses. The 5-year DFS for those in the low and intermediate-1 groups was 60%, 36% for those in intermediate-2, and 28% for those in the high-risk group. Patients undergoing matched unrelated donor (MUD) marrow transplants fare less well. In an analysis of results from the National Marrow Donor Program, patients receiving MUD transplants during the first 4 years of registry data (1986–1990) had a disappointing DFS of only 18% at 2 years and 24% OS at 2 years. In one study, patients with primary MDS demonstrated a survival advantage over those with secondary MDS (56% vs. 27%).

The exact role and timing of bone marrow transplantation remain to be determined, as does the optimal conditioning regimen. A recent analysis of patients with low-risk disease suggests that watchful waiting until evidence of disease progression increases life expectancy compared with immediate transplantation. For patients with high-risk disease, transplantation shortly after diagnosis was associated with better life expectancy.[154] These data were recently updated for patients 60–70 years old and favor transplant for higher-risk patients with some gain in life expectancy, whereas nontransplant approaches are favored for lower-risk patients.[155] For patients 40 years or younger with a compatible related donor, however, transplantation should be favored, since no other therapy thus far is curative. However, selection of transplant candidates for patients under the age of 50 remains problematic. There are some younger patients with low-risk MDS with a median survival greater than 15 years treated with SC alone.[156] Fewer patients over the age of 40 have been transplanted, but limited data for those with related donors suggest that up to 30% may survive disease-free. Transplantation for those without a related donor is a more difficult choice in view of the data noted previously. Given the age of most patients with MDS and the availability of donors, transplantation in the foreseeable future is likely to be of limited value, benefiting only about 5–10% of all patients with MDS.[151]

Because of the age of most MDS patients and the potential toxicity of fully ablative transplantation regimens, interest has developed in reduced-intensity conditioning hematopoietic stem cell transplantation as an alternative. These treatment strategies use conditioning regimens, often fludarabine based, which are better tolerated and not intended to be fully ablative. They permit chimerism to be established with either sibling or volunteer unrelated matched donors. Recent reports demonstrate that this strategy can be used in patients over the age of 60 years with mortality rates ranging from 0% to 21%. Chimerism was established in 83% of patients. Duration of remission and relapse is dependent on the IPSS classification, similar to fully ablative transplantation. Thus, this is a feasible approach that can be extended to older patients, but further studies will be necessary to determine its potential role in therapy.[151,155]

AzaC has been explored as both a bridge to transplant with administration prior to allogeneic transplant and a maintenance strategy postallogeneic transplant.[157,158] Treatment is well tolerated in both the pre- and posttransplant setting, but randomized trials will be required to assess whether AzaC in either the pre- or posttransplant setting positively impacts disease outcome.

The use of high-dose chemotherapy with either autologous bone marrow or peripheral blood stem cell (PBSC) infusion has been used in a limited fashion. The European group reported on 79 patients treated with intensive chemotherapy and autologous bone marrow transplantation in first CR. Fifty-five of the 79 in whom the duration of first CR was known were matched with 110 patients with de novo AML. The 2-year survival for all 79 patients was 39%, and the DFS at 2 years was 28% for the 55 patients with MDS/sAML versus 51% for patients with de novo AML. Relapse rates were 69% for MDS/sAML and 40% for de novo AML ($p = 0.007$).[159,160] Use of PBSC infusion is more problematic given that adequate collection from patients with MDS is obtained in only half the patients.

Growth factors. The hematopoietic growth factors are regulatory glycoproteins that control the proliferation and differentiation of bone marrow stem cells.[161] Several studies have defined the effects of GM-CSF in MDS.[162] In a controlled study, patients were randomized to observation or treatment with rhGM-CSF. Those treated had significant increases in neutrophils, eosinophils, monocytes, and lymphocytes, while the frequency of infections was decreased in comparison with those observed in the absence of this cytokine. There were no differences in platelet count, hemoglobin, or transfusion requirements between the two groups. The risk of leukemic transformation appeared greatest for those patients with greater than 15% blasts in the bone marrow and may be a critical level with respect to leukemic transformation.

Filgrastim (G-CSF) has also been evaluated. In a randomized controlled trial, 102 patients with RAEB or RAEB-T were treated with either G-CSF or SC.[161] No differences in frequency or time to progression to AML were seen between the two groups. There was no difference in survival for those with RAEB-T. However, among patients with RAEB, those in the treatment group had a significantly shortened survival compared with patients in the control group, resulting in early termination of the study.

Erythropoietin has also been studied in patients with MDS, with red cell responses being demonstrated in 20–25% of the patients tested.[77,163,164] Responses were confined to the erythroid lineage. A meta-analysis suggests that efficacy declines as bone marrow failure progresses. Those who have lower serum erythropoietin levels and less transfusion need are more likely to respond. The observation that *in vitro* erythropoiesis improved in patients treated *in vivo* with G-CSF led to two clinical trials of erythropoietin and G-CSF in combination. The response rate ranged from 35% to 40% and appeared to enhance the activity of erythropoietin. Serum erythropoietin levels in these trials, as in others, are of predictive value with few responses in patients with levels above 500 U/L. In another report, the response-enhancing effect of G-CSF was not substantiated. In a series of 191 patients treated with the combination, the overall response was 39%. Low-risk disease was associated with a higher response, and patients achieving a CR had a longer duration of response. An algorithm based on transfusion need and serum erythropoietin levels may be a useful guide for patient selection. Effects of erythropoietin therapy on survival suggest that elimination of a transfusion requirement may be beneficial.[78]

For patients with a variant of MDS characterized by severe hypoplasia and pancytopenia, which may resemble severe aplastic anemia (hypoplastic MDS), administration of antithymocyte globulin produced responses in 11 of 25 patients treated (9 of 14 RA; 2 of 6 RAEB).[79,80] Responses were characterized predominantly by loss of transfusion requirement, and 3 of 25 had normalization of their counts. There were no changes in the dysplastic features or in bone marrow cellularity. In the completed study, 61 patients were treated, with 21(34%) responding. Transfusion requirement was eliminated in 76% of responding patients or 25% overall. The effect may be mediated, in part, through an immunosuppressive effect alleviating a T-cell suppression of hematopoietic progenitors. Patients who

are younger and have more cytopenias, shorter duration of red cell transfusion dependence, and the presence of HLA-DRB1-15 appear more likely to respond.

Clinical management

The management of patients with MDS presents a series of difficult choices (Figure 2). For patients with RA or RARS, low- or intermediate-1-risk groups, who have better prognoses and in whom the disease is manifest predominantly as asymptomatic anemia, observation and SC should be the mainstay. For those who require red cell transfusions, which in and of itself is a negative prognostic variable, a trial of erythropoietin with or without G-CSF appears reasonable.[81] Treatment with lenalidomide or AzaC in patients who fail an ESA or have severe leukopenia or thrombocytopenia is a consideration. Those patients with a karyotypic abnormality (other than the 5q-syndrome, very good risk cytogenetics) have a less favorable prognosis. Such patients warrant closer follow-up and are candidates for investigational studies, particularly if they manifest an increasing number of blasts in the bone marrow or develop significant neutropenia or thrombocytopenia. Patients with low-risk disease who fail therapy with erythropoietin with or without G-CSF for anemia or who have severe cytopenias in other lineages can be considered for treatment with AzaC, which has demonstrated efficacy in low-risk disease with amelioration of symptoms. Single-agent lenalidomide or an HMA can lead to transfusion independence in between 25% (lenalidomide) and 50% (AzaC) of patients. For patients with lower-risk disease that is progressing, who fail lenalidomide and/or HMA and who have a compatible donor, allogeneic bone marrow transplantation should be considered, since it is the only therapy that has so far achieved cures.[154,155]

Patients with higher-risk disease (intermediate-2 or high risk; high risk and very high risk—IPSS-R) have a poorer prognosis and are candidates for treatment with an HMA. Those with RAEB-I (5–10% blasts) without other poor prognostic features (i.e., abnormal karyotype, severe thrombocytopenia or severe neutropenia) could be closely observed to determine the relative stability of the disease. Those with evidence of progression are candidates for immediate intervention.

Patients with higher-risk disease can benefit from treatment with AzaC which should be considered the standard first-line therapy for these patients. It has demonstrated significant benefit compared with SC, induces remission, decreases transfusion requirements, extends survival, and improves the QOL.[116,122] This therapy may now represent the standard of care. Alternatively, they can be treated as part of an investigational program. Stem cell transplantation is a consideration for those patients as a potential curative strategy and should be considered early in the evaluation process after the diagnosis is established, if a donor is available, and if the patient's age and risk classification warrants it. However, the rate of relapse is high, and many centers will not consider these patients as candidates. Strategies aimed at inducing a remission prior to transplantation may be useful.[154,155,165]

For patients who have transformed to leukemia, aggressive antileukemic chemotherapy can be undertaken or an HMA is a consideration for older patients. The CR rate for antileukemic chemotherapy ranges between 30% and 60% but is associated with a high rate of treatment-related morbidity and mortality. Most patients relapse. The HMAs have been used in these patients and may improve survival.[166] Patients with hypoplastic MDS, particularly if younger, may benefit from antithymocyte globulin with or without cyclosporine or other immunomodulatory effects. Patients

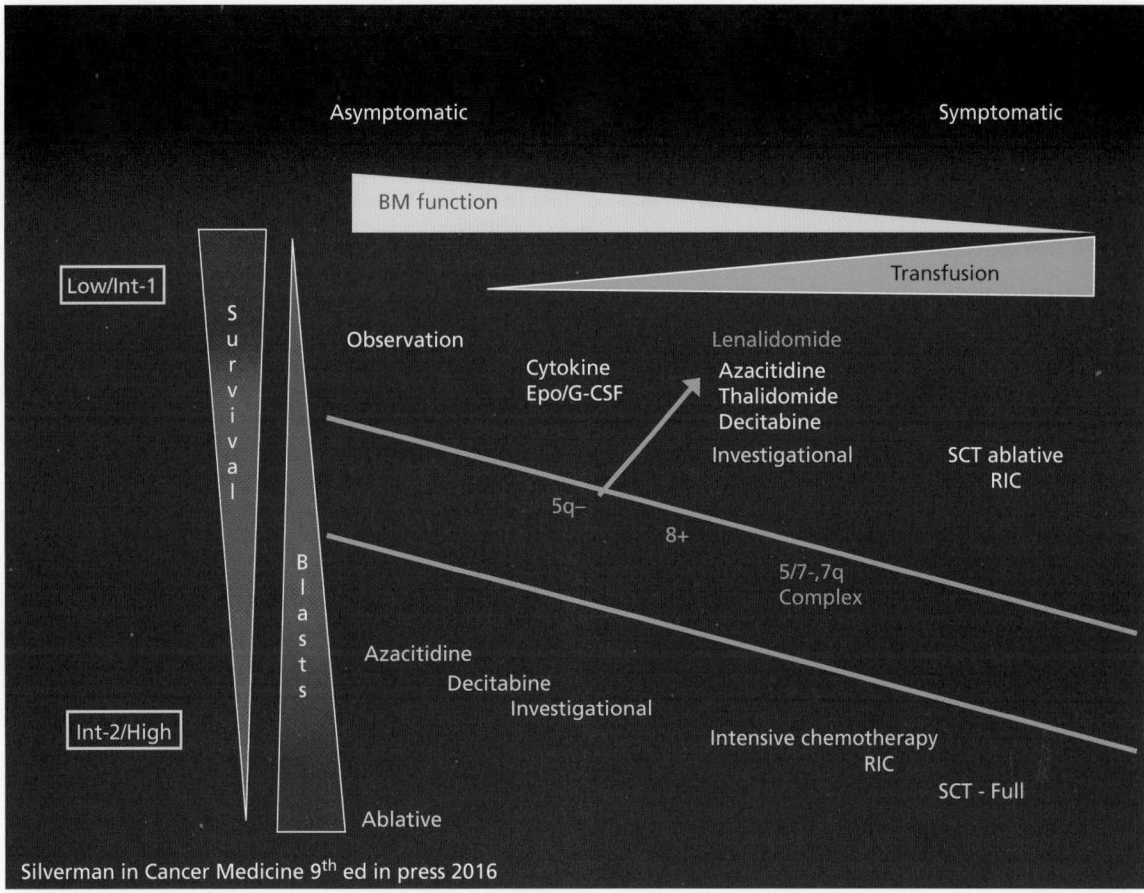

Figure 2 Treatment algorithm for patients with the myelodysplastic syndrome.

who have either primary or secondary HMA failure have a poor prognosis, and an investigational agent should be considered.[167]

Future directions

Progress in the prevention and therapy of MDS depends on a better understanding of the basic biochemical and molecular defects that contribute to the development of this syndrome. Identification of gene mutations and in the epigenome will be informative and will help to individualize therapeutic decisions. Well-designed clinical trials using clearly defined biologic endpoints are critical. Survival is the ultimate goal, but too global a composite to serve as the sole working criterion. QOL assessments have gained favor as useful tools in the measure of the effects of treatment. These assessments should be included routinely in phase II and III studies and help as a critical measure of a palliative treatment. Finally, cost analysis is another useful gauge of treatment efficacy. Pharmacoeconomic studies should also be included in future phase III studies.

In a disease characterized by the development of a progressive uncoupling of cellular maturation and proliferation, induction differentiation is an attractive approach. This has proven to be a highly provocative strategy in the treatment of acute promyelocytic leukemia with trans-retinoic acid. AzaC, which may act in part as a biologic response modifier with effects on the epigenome and gene signaling, may be advantageously combined with other agents such as HDACs.[132] Drugs that interfere with or block abnormal signal transduction (e.g., tyrosine and multikinase inhibitors) may

prove beneficial.[135] Tumor vaccines and the use of immunomodulatory strategies that can stimulate auto- or allogeneic T cells will be explored in the coming years with PD-1/PDL-1 checkpoint inhibitors.

Key references

The complete reference list can be found on the Wiley Companion Digital Edition of this title (see inside front cover for login instructions).

3 Bomford PR, Rhoads CP. Refractory anaemia. I. Clinical and pathological aspects. *Q J Med*. 1941;**10**:175.

4 Block M, Jacobson LO, Bethard WF. Preleukemic acute human leukemia. *J Am Med Assoc*. 1953;**152**:1018.

6 Bennett JM, Catovsky D, Daniel MT, et al. Proposals for the classification of the acute leukaemias. French-American-British (FAB) co-operative group. *Br J Haematol*. 1976;**33**:451–458.

7 Aul C, Gattermann N, Schneider W. Age-related incidence and other epidemiological aspects of myelodysplastic syndrome. *Br J Haematol*. 1992;**82**:358.

10 Bennett JM, Catovsky D, Daniel M-T, et al. Proposed revised criteria for the classification of acute myeloid leukemia. A Report of the French-American-British Cooperative Group. *Ann Intern Med*. 1985;**103**:620–625.

16 Greenberg PL, Tuechler H, Schanz J, et al. Revised international prognostic scoring system for myelodysplastic syndromes. *Blood*. 2012;**120**(12):2454–2465.

17 Harris N, Jaffe E, Diehold J, et al. World Health Organization classification of neoplastic diseases of the hematopoietic and lymphoid tissues: report of the Clinical Advisory Committee Meeting—Airlie House, Virginia, November 1997. *J Clin Oncol*. 1999;**17**:3835–3849.

21 Kamada N, Uchins H. Preleukemic states in atomic bomb survivors. *Blood Cells*. 1976;**2**:57.

25 Farrow A, Jacobs A, West RR. Myelodysplasia, chemical exposure, and other environmental factors. *Leukemia*. 1989;**3**:33.

30 Kantarjian HM, Keating MJ. Therapy-related leukemia and myelodysplastic syndrome. *Semin Oncol*. 1987;**14**:435.

35 Berk PD, Goldberg JD, Silverstein MN, et al. Increased incidence of acute leukemia in polycythemia vera associated with chlorambucil therapy. *N Engl J Med*. 1981;**304**:441.

116 Silverman LR, Demakos EP, Peterson BL, et al. Randomized controlled trial of azacitidine in patients with the myelodysplastic syndrome: a study of the cancer and leukemia group B. *J Clin Oncol*. 2002;**20**:2429–2440.

122 Kornblith AB, Herndon JE 2nd, Silverman LR, et al. Impact of azacytidine on the quality of life of patients with myelodysplastic syndrome treated in a randomized phase III trial: a Cancer and Leukemia Group B study. *J Clin Oncol*. 2002;**20**:2441–2452.

123 Silverman LR, McKenzie DR, Peterson BL, et al. Further analysis of trials with azacitidine in patients with myelodysplastic syndrome: studies 8421, 8921, and 9221 by the Cancer and Leukemia Group B. *J Clin Oncol*. 2006;**24**:3895–3903.

124 Silverman LR, Fenaux P, Mufti GJ, et al. Continued azacitidine therapy beyond time of first response improves quality of response in patients with higher-risk myelodysplastic syndromes. *Cancer*. 2011;**117**:2697–2702.

126 Lübbert M, Suciu S, Baila L, et al. Low-dose decitabine versus best supportive care in elderly patients with intermediate- or high-risk myelodysplastic syndrome (MDS) ineligible for intensive chemotherapy: final results of the randomized Phase III Study of the European Organisation for Research and Treatment of Cancer Leukemia Group and the German MDS Study Group. *J Clin Oncol*. 2011;**29**:1987–1996.

127 Wijermans P, Lubbert M, Verhoef G, et al. Low-dose 5-aza-2′-deoxycytidine, a DNA hypomethylating agent, for the treatment of high-risk myelodysplastic syndrome: a multicenter phase II study in elderly patients. *J Clin Oncol*. 2000;**18**:956–962.

130 Kantarjian H, Oki Y, Garcia-Manero G, et al. Results of a randomized study of 3 schedules of low-dose decitabine in higher-risk myelodysplastic syndrome and chronic myelomonocytic leukemia. *Blood*. 2007;**109**:52–57.

131 Steensma DP, Baer MR, Slack JL, et al. Multicenter study of decitabine administered daily for 5 days every 4 weeks to adults with myelodysplastic syndromes: the alternative dosing for outpatient treatment (ADOPT) trial. *J Clin Oncol*. 2009;**27**:3842–3848.

132 Navada SC, Steinmann J, Lubbert M, et al. Clinical development of demethylating agents in hematology. *J Clin Invest*. 2014;**124**:40–46.

133 Prebet T, Sun Z, Figueroa ME, et al. Prolonged administration of azacitidine with or without entinostat for myelodysplastic syndrome and acute myeloid leukemia with myelodysplasia-related changes: results of the US Leukemia Intergroup Trial E1905. *J Clin Oncol*. 2014;**32**:1242–1248.

134 Silverman LR, Verma A, Odchimar-Reissig R, et al. A phase II trial of epigenetic modulators vorinostat in combination with azacitidine (azac) in patients with the myelodysplastic syndrome (MDS): initial results of study 6898 of the New York Cancer Consortium. *Blood*. 2013;**122**(21):386.

135 Silverman LR, Greenberg P, Raza A, et al. Clinical activity and safety of the dual pathway inhibitor rigosertib for higher risk myelodysplastic syndromes following DNA methyltransferase inhibitor therapy. *Hematol Oncol*. 2015;**33**(2):57–66.

136 Garcia-Manero G, Fenaux P, Al-Kali A, et al. Overall survival and subgroup analysis from a randomized phase III study of intravenous rigosertib versus best supportive care (BSC) in patients (pts) with higher-risk myelodysplastic syndrome (HR-MDS) after failure of hypomethylating agents (HMAs). *Blood*. 2014;**163**: abstract.

137 Navada SC, Garcia-Manero G, Wilhelm F, et al. A phase I/II study of the combination of oral rigosertib and azacitidine in patients with myelodysplastic syndrome (MDS) or acute myeloid leukemia (AML). *Blood*. 2014;**124**: abstract 3252.

166 Kantarjian HM, Thomas XG, Dmoszynska A, et al. Multicenter, randomized, open-label, phase iii trial of decitabine versus patient choice, with physician advice, of either supportive care or low-dose cytarabine for the treatment of older patients with newly diagnosed acute myeloid leukemia. *J Clin Oncol*. 2012;**30**:2670–2677.

167 Prébet T, Gore SD, Esterni B, et al. Outcome of high-risk myelodysplastic syndrome after azacitidine treatment failure. *J Clin Oncol*. 2011;**29**:3322–3327.

114 Acute myeloid leukemia in adults: mast cell leukemia and other mast cell neoplasms

Richard M. Stone, MD ▪ Charles A. Schiffer, MD

Overview

Acute myeloid leukemia (AML) is the most common variant of acute leukemia occurring in adults, comprising approximately 80% of acute leukemia cases diagnosed in individuals of age >20 years. Remarkable advances in transfusion medicine, treatment of infections, development of potent antiemetics, improved chemotherapeutic approaches, and increased use of safer allogeneic transplantation have led to an improved outcome at least in younger patients. Moreover, a more sophisticated understanding of pathophysiology, particularly in the area of genomics, may soon lead to less toxic, patient-specific, and more effective therapies. At present, approximately 80% of younger (age <60 years) adults and 30%–50% of all older patients achieve complete remission (CR) defined as a morphologically normal bone marrow with reasonable neutrophil and platelet counts and no evidence of extramedullary disease. Varying with patient age and other biologic factors, 10–70% of these complete responders can be expected to achieve long-term survival with the likelihood that most of these individuals are cured of their disease. However, AML is largely an intrinsically chemoresistant disease, the outcome in older adults has changed little, and the chemotherapeutic approach has remained stagnant.

Introduction

Acute myeloid leukemia (AML) affects adults of all ages, but is particularly common in older adults. The median age of patients with AML is approximately 70 years (Figure 1). AML can present as either a de novo leukemia without an apparent antecedent illness or an evolution from marrow disorders such as myelodysplasia, myeloproliferative neoplasms, aplastic anemia, and Fanconi anemia, or after the administration of therapy for other types of cancers or nonmalignant disorders.[1–4] AML presenting without prior marrow disease or anti-neoplastic therapy is termed de novo, whereas other types are considered secondary. Such terms may be less important predictors of response to therapy and long-term outcome than the mutational profile reflecting the biological heterogeneity of this condition.[5] Proper care of patients with AML is a multidisciplinary effort, benefiting from a team approach. Expertise in transfusion medicine, infectious disease, placement and care of indwelling catheters, nutrition, and antineoplastic drug pharmacology are required, as well as sophisticated diagnostic laboratory facilities and psychosocial counseling for both patients and their families are needed. Optimally, allogeneic stem cell transplant, currently used in patients up to age 75, should be available. These disciplines are described elsewhere in this book, but their critical importance in the care of the leukemia patient cannot be overestimated.

Pathogenesis and etiology

Pathophysiology

The pathophysiology of AML can be partially explained by the acquisition of genetic changes in hematopoietic stem cells that both promote self-renewal and impair normal hematopoietic differentiation, resulting in an accumulation of immature cells. The genetic landscape of de novo AML has been recently characterized.[6] An average of five mutations are found in an individual's leukemia cells and "only" 30 mutations are recurrent (observed in more than 3% of patients). Of the 30 recurrent mutations, several are relatively common, including gain-of-function mutations, which are targets for therapy in active development. FLT3 is a transmembrane tyrosine kinase, which is mutated in approximately 30% of patients with AML.[7] Approximately three-quarters of these mutations are length or internal tandem duplication (ITD) mutations, in which the protein is elongated in the juxtamembrane region by three to more than 100 amino acids. This type of mutation is associated with an adverse prognosis because of a high relapse rate. Both the ITD mutation and the less common tyrosine kinase domain point mutation (usually D835Y) cause ligand-independent constitutive activation of the receptor. There are several FLT3 inhibitors in active development, both as single agents and in combination with chemotherapy in mutant FLT3 patients. A second common mutation is a point mutation in the NPM1 shuttle protein.[8] Such mutations, particularly if occurring in patients with a normal karyotype without an associated FLT3 mutation, confer a favorable prognosis.[9] Mutations in the Ras guanine nucleotide-binding protein occur in approximately 20% of patients with AML and are associated with increased proliferation.[10] Attempts to inhibit posttranslational modification, a required step for activation of Ras, have been largely unsuccessful in AML.[11] Ras pathway interruption, such as with MEK inhibitors (useful in melanoma and other solid tumors), shows promise.[12] Mutations in the isocitrate dehydrogenase genes IDH1 and IDH2 occur in approximately 20% of patients with AML (~10% for each case).[13] While the prognostic significance of these mutations is unclear, they cause the neomorphic production of 2-hydroxygluterate (2HG) rather than the usual reaction product, alpha-ketogluterate. 2HG levels may correlate with disease activity.[14] Inhibition of IDH1 or IDH2 with small molecules may prove to be a fertile therapeutic intervention. Mutations in transcriptional machinery and mutations in enzymes, which are epigenetically active (posttranslational modification of the DNA) potentially leading to profound effects on gene expression, are common in AML.[6] DNMT3, mutations occurring in approximately 20% of patients with AML,[15] confer an adverse prognosis, although may be associated with a response to dose-intensified daunorubicin during induction.[16] The presence of some of these so-called epigenetic

Holland-Frei Cancer Medicine, Ninth Edition. Edited by Robert C. Bast Jr., Carlo M. Croce, William N. Hait, Waun Ki Hong, Donald W. Kufe, Martine Piccart-Gebhart, Raphael E. Pollock, Ralph R. Weichselbaum, Hongyang Wang, and James F. Holland.
© 2017 John Wiley & Sons, Inc. ISBN: 978-1-118-93469-2

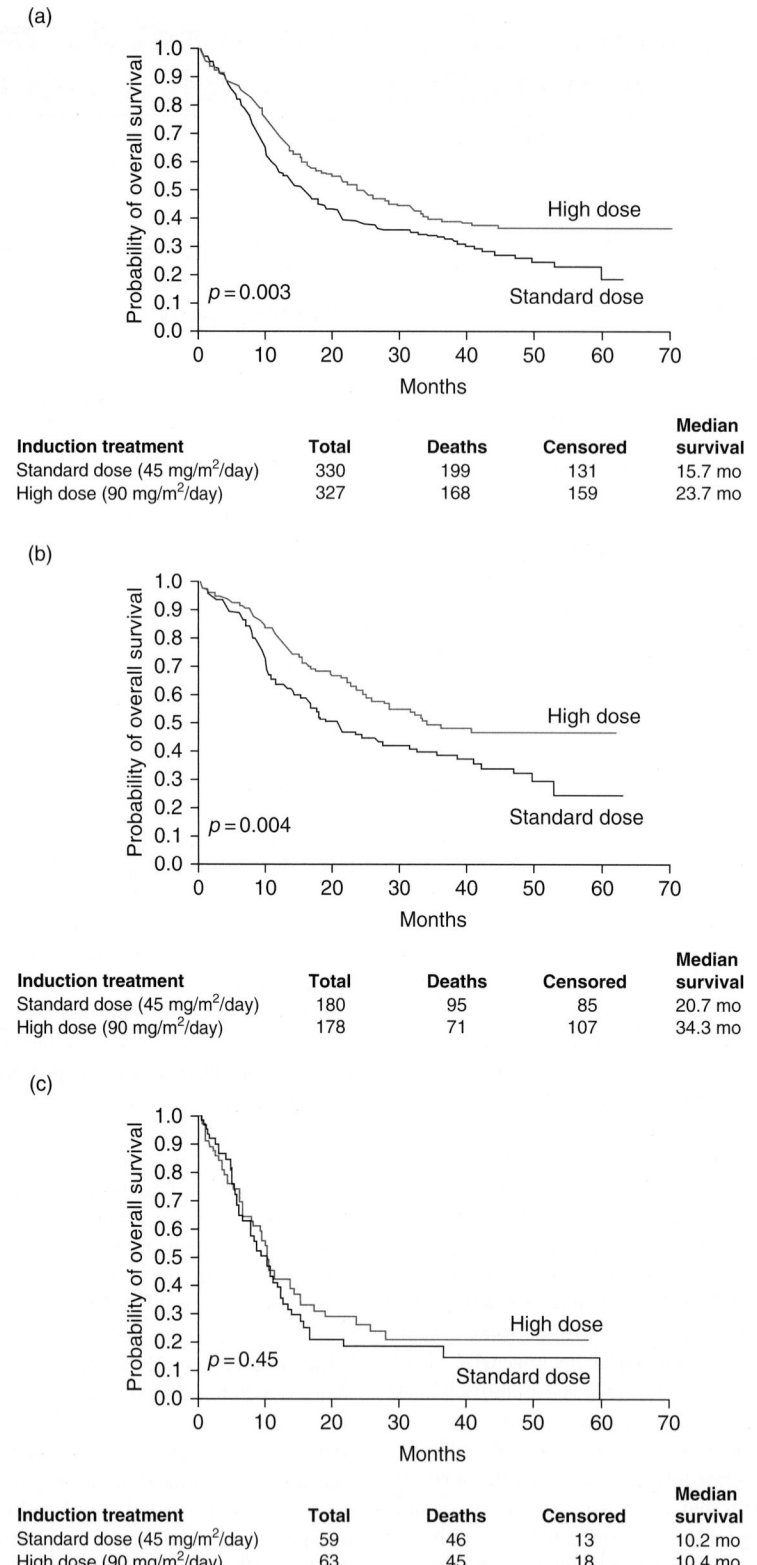

Figure 1 Data from ECOG demonstrating that overall survival in AML patients less than age 60 is approximately 40% and varies according to the cytogenetic risk and daunorubicin dose. Source: Fernandez 2009.[4] Reproduced with permission of NEJM.

modifying enzymes such as ASXL1, EZH2, and TET2 is often associated with AMLs that have arisen from a myelodysplastic syndrome (MDS) prodrome. TP53 mutation confers a bleak prognosis.[17] On the contrary, CEBPα (biallelic) mutations are favorable.[18]

Genetic complexity of AML is an important feature of disordered molecular pathophysiology. The epigenetic profiles[19] of AML can differ widely and perhaps suggest a specific therapy. Specific epigenetic profiles are found in distinct cytogenetic subsets of AML. Moreover, because of either mutations or altered patterns of genome regulation, messenger RNA[20] and indeed microRNA expression patterns offer both pathophysiological insights and prognostic information. For example, microRNA expression patterns, particularly with moieties that control immunological regulation, have been found to play an important role in AML.[21] Integration of the vast potential array of data including genomic lesions, epigenomic changes, and RNA and microRNA expression patterns yield an enormous amount of information and will be the subject of intense research in the future. The overexpression of many specific genes such as BAALC[22] or WT1[23] has been shown to confer an adverse prognosis, but their independent significance remains to be confirmed.

Genetic changes in AML were first recognized by the identification of genes at cytogenetic break points involved in balanced translocations. Many of these chromosomal abnormalities, for example, t(8;21), t(15;17), and inv(16), are associated with specific AML subtypes and are of prognostic importance. The fusion proteins generated by the translocation generally result in disruption of transcription factors, which is believed to be critical in myeloid differentiation.[24-27] Murine experiments indicate that transfection of mutated genes that primarily alter cell differentiation, such as AML1/ETO resulting from the t(8;21) translocation, produces abnormal hematopoiesis, but is not sufficient to generate frank AML.[27] Initial murine experiments suggested a "two-hit" hypothesis, in which mutations affecting both differentiation and proliferative signaling pathways are needed to result in AML.[28] The mechanisms that account for poor prognosis in patients with complex cytogenetics remain to be elucidated. Findings in 5q-MDS suggest a mechanism by which haploinsufficiency can lead to a myeloid malignancy.[29] Many patients with the so-called monosomal karyotype (two monosomes or one monosomal plus one stromal abnormality) have p53 mutations, and this abnormality likely accounts for the dismal prognosis in this disease subset.[17]

Exposure and risk

Although more acquired genetic lesions that lead to leukemia are being defined, DNA damage from a known cause comprises only a small fraction of patients with AML. Leukemia occurs with increased frequency after exposure to nuclear bomb[30] or therapeutic radiation,[31] after certain types of chemotherapy,[32,33] and with heavy and continuous occupational exposures to benzene or petrochemicals.[34,35] There are two types of chemotherapy-related leukemias: (1) the classic alkylating agent-induced type, in which the leukemia is usually preceded by a myelodysplastic prodrome and is characterized by clonal abnormalities, often with loss of chromosome 5 and/or 7[32] and (2) an epipodophyllotoxin/topoisomerase II inhibitor-associated type with a shorter (median 2 years vs 5 years) incubation period, often with myelomonocytic or monocytic differentiation and abnormalities at the 11q23 region.[33] Recent studies have challenged preconceived notions about the origin of therapy-related leukemia: (1) some patients who have been exposed to chemotherapy have genetic[5] or cytogenetic lesions[36] and clinical behavior indistinguishable from de novo AML; (2) preexisting p53 mutant hematopoietic clones due to the "normal" stochastic accumulation of mutations may be selected for survival after genotoxic therapy and thus predispose to the development of AML.[37]

Familial AML

AML is not usually a familial or inherited disorder, which is a fact worth noting to concerned families. There appears to be an increased incidence of acute leukemia in the first 6 months after diagnosis in the identical twin of an affected child.[38] Familial syndromes have been described in which the incidence of leukemia was increased.[39-41] In some of these families, different types of leukemias and other cancers have been found, whereas in other potentially more informative families, such as a large family in which more than or equal to seven cases of erythroleukemia or myelodysplasia developed in three successive generations,[41] the morphologic or clinical characteristics of the leukemia have been similar, suggesting a common, heritable genetic mutation. A family has been described in which three patients with AML had identical inherited mutations in CEBPA,[42] a gene involved in granulocytic differentiation, while another large kindred with a familial platelet disorder with a predisposition toward AML had been shown to be associated with mutations in the gene encoding CBF-α (formerly AML1).[43] Finally, there seems to be a predisposition toward evolution to AML in individuals with inherited polymorphisms in the receptor for granulocyte colony-stimulating factor (G-CSF).[44] AML is also more common in certain inherited conditions identified by an inability to repair DNA damage (e.g., Fanconi anemia)[45] or with defective telomerase machinery.[46]

Prognosis

As noted, AML is a genetic and biological heterogeneous disease; thus, it is not surprising that a patient's prognosis at the time of diagnosis can vary widely from a cure rate of 80–90% in acute promyelocytic leukemia (APL) to virtually zero in those patients with monosomal karyotype and/or p53 mutations in their malignant cells. A reasonably accurate prognosis can be derived from the knowledge of three factors (in addition to the obvious importance of comorbid disease and frailty in the elderly) to estimate the likelihood of long-term favorable outcome in patients with AML: (1) age; (2) cytogenetics; and (3) genetics. In general, the likelihood of remission, the chance of getting through standard remission induction without treatment-related mortality, and the likelihood of not relapsing vary inversely with age.[47] For practical reasons, patients above 55–65 years of age are considered older adults with AML; however, the ability to withstand cytotoxic chemotherapy varies between individuals. The Eastern Cooperative Oncology Group (ECOG) Performance Status scale offers some help in this regard, but there is a trend toward using a more detailed and comprehensive geriatric assessment to determine a patient's ability to withstand chemotherapy.[48] In addition to the increased likelihood of occurrence of comorbid diseases with aging, other considerations are the more limited stem cell reserve in the older population[49] and the inevitable decline in hepatic and renal function. Moreover, the fact that leukemia in older adults tends to be more biologically aggressive with an increased ratio of adverse chromosomal abnormalities to favorable abnormalities[50] and the increased likelihoods of the so-called myelodysplasia-related genetic abnormalities and an antecedent clinical marrow stem cell disorder are associated with a relatively poor outcome. The prognosis is sufficiently adverse that a different treatment approach is generally employed in older adults with AML.

For the last 40 years, we have relied upon chromosomal findings at diagnosis to establish prognosis and in some cases to guide therapy. Numerous studies have divided newly diagnosed younger adults with AML into three prognostic categories.[51,52] Approximately 15% were found to have more favorable prognostic abnormalities (not including APL) including core-binding factor translocations such as t(8;21) and pericentric inversion of chromosome 16. Such patients have a high complete remission (CR) rate and relatively low relapse rate, although at least two-thirds are destined to relapse with an increased likelihood of an adverse outcome in those with an associated mutation in the c-KIT tyrosine

Table 1 Cytogenetics- and genetics-based risk.

Risk group	Features	Approximate 4-year survival (%)	Approximate prevalence (%)
Very high	Monosomal karyotype (two monsomies or one monosomy plus balanced translocation)	10	6
High	Complex (>3 abormalities) or unfavorable (-7, 7q-, -5, 5q-, 3q, or t(6;9)) cytogenetics	20	12
Intermediate	Normal cytogenetics (with *FLT3* mutation or *FLT3*-ITD not present/*NPM1* wild type/*CEBPα* wild type) or other karyotype	35	25
	Inversion 16 or t(8;21) with *c-KIT* mutation	40	5
	Normal cytogenetics (with *FLT3*-ITD not present/*NPM1* mutation)	50	25
Favorable	Normal cytogenetics (with *CEBPα* biallelic mutation)	60	5
	t(8;21) or inversion 16 (with *c-KIT* wild type)	65	10
Very favorable	t(15;17)	85	12

Source: Stone 2013.[59] Reproduced with permission of the American Society of Clinical Oncology.

kinase gene.[53] Approximately 15% had unfavorable chromosomal abnormalities,[50] including complex karyotypes (generally greater than three, although in some classifications five distinct chromosomal abnormalities) or the so-called monosomal karyotype (two monosomies or one monosomy plus one structural abnormality).[54] Patients in this adverse prognostic category taken together have a 15% likelihood of long-term disease-free survival, but those with monosomal karyotype are destined to fare even worse.[55] This is partially explained by high incidence of TP53 gene mutations in this subgroup.[17] About 70% of patients are considered to have an intermediate prognosis with an approximate long-term survival chance of 40%. Some of these patients have well-characterized abnormalities such as trisomy 8 or translocations involving the 11q23 region (the MLL gene) from chromosome 11.

However, the vast majority of the intermediate prognostic group comprised those with a normal karyotype. Significant effort has been made in the last 10–20 years to divide patients with normal karyotypes into prognostic subgroups. At present, the following three genes have been generally used to provide information required for such a classification: CEBPα, NPM1, and FLT3. Patients with biallelic CEBPα mutations in the leukemia cells tend to exhibit a high expected disease-free survival of 80%; however, only a small number of patients have such an abnormality.[18] The presence of FLT3 ITD (ITD) mutation producing variations in the length of this transmembrane tyrosine kinase is considered adverse, while a mutation in the NPM1 nuclear shuttle protein is considered favorable. When considering the possible combinations of these two mutations, only the subgroup of patients with an NPM1 mutation without a concomitant FLT3 ITD mutation are destined to exhibit high survival rates.[9] This is the only patient group within the intermediate chromosomal prognostic category that is recommended to undergo a postremission approach based on chemotherapy only.[9] A recent study suggests that only those with NPM1 mutant and FLT3 ITD wild-type genetic patterns as well as an IDH1/IDH2 mutation had a high overall survival[16] but this remains to be confirmed by other studies. DNMTA3 mutations also imply an adverse prognostics,[15,56] similarly to those who have MDS-associated abnormalities such as EZH2 and ASXL1 mutations.[57]

In older adults, there is a higher incidence of complex or adverse cytogenetic findings. However, a small number of older adults have favorable karyotypes and should be treated with conventional induction and consolidation regimens if their other medical conditions permit.[50] In addition, a large minority of older patients with a normal karyotype at the time of diagnosis who have an NPM1 mutation without an associated FLT3 ITD mutation can be expected to exhibit a higher survival rate than older adults who lack this genetic/chromosomal pattern.[58]

Table 1 depicts a modified European LeukemiaNet (ELN) classification scheme[59] showing the frequency and general prognosis of those younger adults with various combinations of cytogenetic and genetic findings. This list will likely change over time as other genetic abnormalities are introduced into the equation.

Morphologic classification and clinical and laboratory correlates

The diagnosis of AML depends on the examination of well-prepared specimens of peripheral blood and bone marrow. Both bone marrow aspirates and biopsies should be evaluated. Although the biopsy is usually not helpful in identifying individual cells, it provides the best assessment of cellularity, can occasionally identify aggregates of leukemic cells that are not seen on aspirate, and is necessary to evaluate marrow fibrosis. In 1976, a group of morphologists from France, the United States, and Great Britain suggested a classification system designed to standardize definitions of the sometimes clinically and biologically distinct subtypes of AML and acute lymphoblastic leukemia (ALL).[60] This French, American, and British (FAB) classification has been serially modified, initially in 2002,[61] and in 2016[62] by a World Health Organization (WHO)-sponsored undertaking, which represented efforts to improve concordance among different observers and incorporate new findings from immunologic, cytogenetic, and molecular studies.

The diagnosis of AML requires that myeloblasts constitute 20% or more of bone marrow cells or circulating white blood cells (WBC), generally evaluated on Wright or Wright–Giemsa stained smears. The FAB classification required >30% blasts to distinguish AML from myelodysplasia. Although this change was based on a study which showed that the outcome could be based solely on the blast count,[63] it is unclear that this is biologically well founded. The difference in eligibility criteria should be considered when comparing older AML trials with more recent studies. Neoplastic promyelocytes, monoblasts or promonocytes, and megakaryoblasts are included in this percentage, and their presence defines the various morphologic subtypes described below. An assortment of histochemical stains may be used to aid in subclassification and distinguish AML from ALL. Monoclonal antibodies directed against antigen groups [termed cluster designations (CD)] considered to be restricted to cells committed to myeloid differentiation are also helpful in making this diagnostic distinction. Antibodies against CD11b, CD13, CD14, CD33, and C117 are used most commonly.[64] These antigens are found on normal hematopoietic elements, are not leukemia-specific, or unique to different AML FAB subtypes. In general, they do not correlate with prognosis, with the possible exception of CD34 antigen,[65] which is detected on undifferentiated hematopoietic progenitors and can be found on the blasts of patients with either AML or ALL. It is suggested that patients with AML whose blasts strongly express CD34 have an inferior outcome because of chemotherapy-resistant leukemia, particularly in patients with less morphologically differentiated leukemias in which other myeloid-associated antigens are less strongly expressed.[66]

The FAB and WHO nomenclatures classify the subtypes of AML according to the normal marrow elements that the blasts most closely resemble. This does not indicate, however, that the leukemic event exclusively involves the cell lineage that is most prominently represented morphologically. Until recently, the involvement of other hematopoietic lineages could be inferred only by the presence of prominent morphologic abnormalities in these other cell lines. In patients with myelodysplasia or erythroleukemia, there is usually morphologic evidence of trilineage dysplasia with the inference that the initial cell that was malignantly transformed was a hematopoietic precursor with capability of multilineage maturation.[67] Fialkow and colleagues,[68] on their study of female patients with X chromosome-linked polymorphisms of glucose-6-phosphate dehydrogenase, were able to demonstrate involvement of myeloid, but not erythroid or megakaryocytic progenitors in some patients with AML. This first observation was proved prescient; however, at present, we believe that most hematopoietic elements emanate from a disordered stem cell, with multilineage involvement being quite common. Moreover, AML should be considered oligoclonal, rather than monoclonal; clonal heterogeneity exists at diagnosis; and the predominant clone can change with time, given the selective pressure exerted by chemotherapy. For example, there is evidence for persistence of certain subclones at remission as well as the emergence at relapse of clones, which have acquired "progression" mutations (or these mutations were present in very small subclones at diagnosis)[5] and that a small clone at diagnosis could be the one to lead to relapse.

Representative examples of different subtypes of AML are shown in Figures 2–11. The immunologic, cytogenetic, and (where they exist) clinical correlates of these morphologic subtypes are reviewed in Table 2.

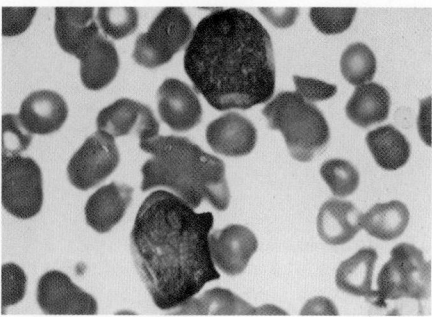

Figure 3 One of the blasts from a patient with M1 acute myeloid leukemia contains a prominent Auer rod.

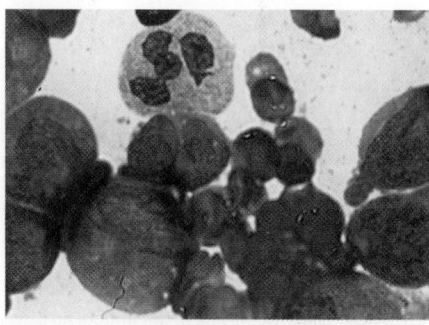

Figure 4 M2. Leukemia is characterized by evidence of continued myeloid differentiation with myelocytes and more mature myeloid elements present.

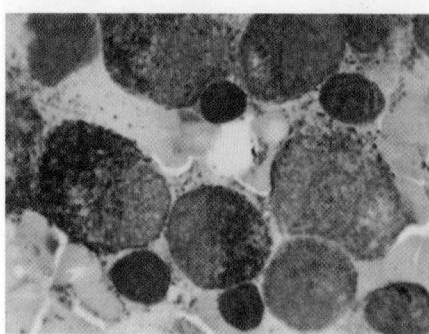

Figure 5 M3. Promyelocytic leukemic cells usually have spherical nuclei with heavily granulated cytoplasm. Extracellular granules are often noted, and blasts with multiple Auer rods (not shown) are common. This leukemia has typical 15;17 translocation and a characteristic clinical picture of disseminated intravascular coagulation.

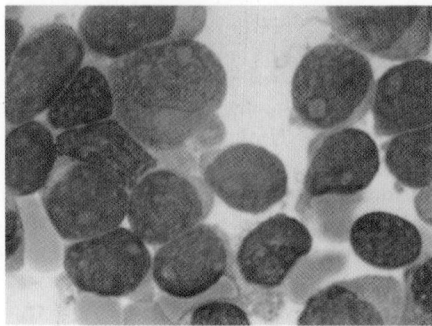

Figure 2 M0. Marrow blasts from patients with this undifferentiated type of acute myelogenous leukemia can have variable amounts of agranular cytoplasm. Cells are peroxidase- and Sudan Black-negative and can be confused with FAB M7 or FAB L2. Myeloid commitment of these blasts can be confirmed by immunophenotyping with antibodies against myeloid antigens and/or demonstration of ultrastructural peroxidase-positive granules using transmission electron microscopy.

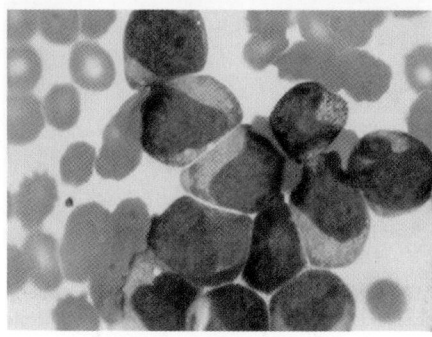

Figure 6 M4. Myelomonocytic leukemia has blasts with both myeloid and monocytoid appearance.

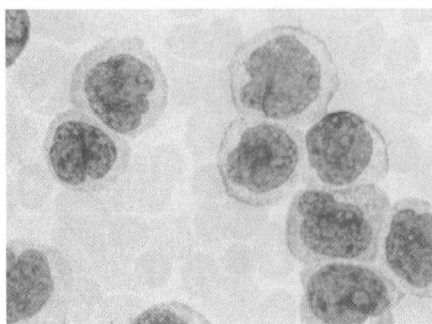

Figure 7 M5. Monocytic leukemia. Prominent nuclei filled with nucleoli in some cells, light granulation, and large amounts of lightly basophilic cytoplasm give these cells the appearance of promonocytes.

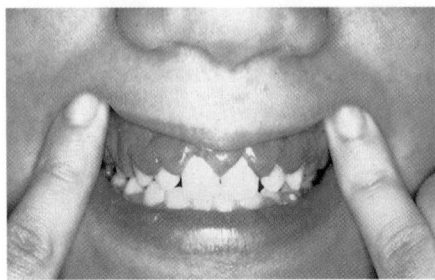

Figure 8 M5. Gingival hypertrophy due to infiltration by leukemic cells in acute monocytic leukemia.

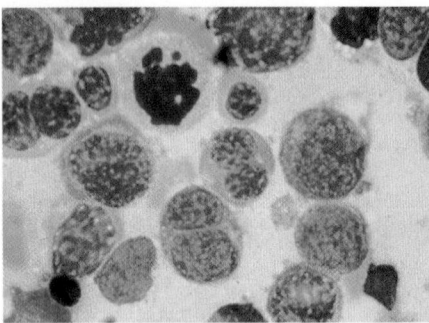

Figure 9 M6. Erythroleukemia is characterized by the presence of bizarre megaloblastic and often multinucleated erythroid precursors. Karyorrhexis is seen in some cells. The somewhat arbitrary distinction between FAB M6 and myelodysplastic syndrome with excess blasts in transformation is made by quantification of the fraction of myeloid blasts.

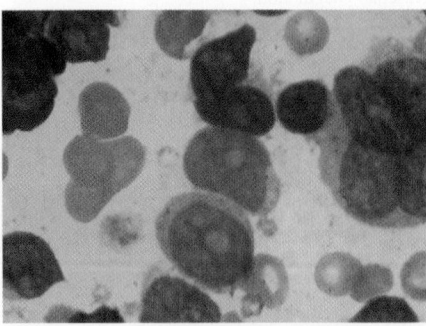

Figure 10 M7. Megakaryocytic leukemia. Blasts in this category are often morphologically undifferentiated. The presence of multinucleated cells, dysplastic micromegakaryocytes, and cytoplasmic budding can be useful diagnostic clues. The diagnosis is confirmed by immunophenotyping or ultrastructural studies.

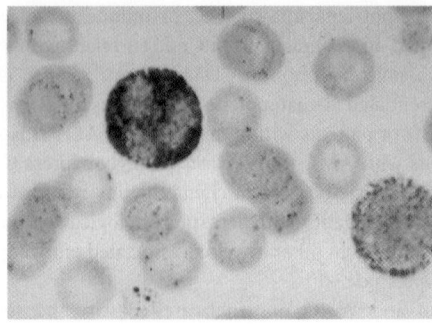

Figure 11 Typical granular staining with Sudan Black B of a blast and a neutrophil from a patient with FAB M1 acute myeloid leukemia.

Peripheral blood

Most patients with AML present with anemia (median hemoglobin 8 g%), thrombocytopenia (median platelet count 40,000–50,000/μL), and leukocytosis (median WBC count 10,000–20,000/μL). The red blood cell morphology is usually relatively normal. Large, sometimes hypogranular, platelets can be observed, and functional defects can contribute to hemorrhagic manifestations. Most patients are neutropenic, and morphologic abnormalities (nuclear hyperlobulation, hypogranulation, Pelger–Huet anomaly) are often noted in the remaining neutrophils. Careful examination can detect blasts in most patients, although it can be difficult to distinguish among leukemia subtypes (or occasionally even to be confident of the diagnosis of acute leukemia) in patients with a low number of circulating blasts. In occasional patients, marked leukopenia at presentation (the so-called aleukemic leukemia) may obscure the diagnosis until a marrow examination is performed.

AML with recurrent genetic abnormalities

Clinical findings associated with t(8;21), inv(16), and t(15;17) have been appreciated for decades and are described in the sections on M2, M4 with eosinophilia, and M3 (APL) later. AML with t(8;21) and inv(16) are referred to as "core binding factor" (CBF) leukemias because of the molecular abnormalities in transcription produced by these translocations. Mutations of the C-KIT tyrosine kinase receptor, which result in a constitutive proliferative signal, are found in approximately 25% of patients with CBF AML with data suggesting a poorer outcome in patients with this additional mutation as well as in whom the protein is overexpressed.[53]

The 2008 WHO classification added inv3(q21;q26.2), t(3;3)(q21; 26.2), and t(1;22) (p13;q13) [RBM15-MLK1] usually found in infants (see M7 later) as well as t(6;9) (p23;q23)[DEK-NUP214] to this group. The translocation t(6;9) is very uncommon, may occur more frequently in younger patients, and can be found in association with a variety of AML morphologies, often with prominent basophilia.[69] FLT3 *ITD* mutations are found in approximately two-thirds of patients with t(6;9).[70] The outcome with chemotherapy only is poor, and allogeneic transplantation should be performed if possible.

AML with MDS-related changes

Addition of this category shows that a substantial fraction of AML, particularly in older patients, evolves from a prior myelodysplastic disorder. This group includes patients with a prior history of MDS, those with >50% dysplasia in at least two cell lines and patients with the so-called "MDS cytogenetics," including, -5, -7, i(17)/t(17p), -13, del 11q, del (12p), del 9q and those with complex karyotypes,

Table 2 Recurring karyotypic and molecular abnormalities in AML.

Cytogenetic abnormality	FAB morphology	Affected genes	Median age	Approximate incidence in de novo AML	Prognostic effects	Comments
t(8;21)	M2	AML1/ETO	30 years	5–7%	Favorable	Auer rods usually present
t(15;17)	M3	PML-RARa	40	5–8%	Favorable—high cure rate with ATRA-based therapy	DIC
t(11;17)	Similar to M3	PLZF/RARa	?	<1%	Poor response to ATRA-based therapy	
abn 16q22	M4 with eosinophilia	CBFA/MYH11	35–40	5%	Favorable	High reinduction rate post relapse
abn11q23	M5	MLL + many partners	>50	3%	Poor except t(9;11)	Hyperleukocytosis, extra medullary disease
+8	Varied		>60	5–10%	Poor	Common in patients with secondary AML, prior MDS
del 5, del 7, 5q-, 7q-, or combinations	Varied; common in FAB M6		>60	15–20%	Poor	
Inv 3	Abnormal megakaryocytes	Ribophorin/EVI1	?	<1%	Poor	Increased platelet count; other abnormalities common (del 5, del 7)
+13	Varied; sometimes undifferentiated		Probably >60	~1–2%	Poor	Higher frequency of hybrid features
t(6;9) (p2;q34)	M2/M4 with basophilia	DEK/CAN	?	<1%	Poor	Prominent basophilia
t(9;22)	Usually M1	BCR/ABL	Probably >50	~1%	Poor	Splenomegaly
t(1;22)	Often M7	MOZ/CBP	Infants	<1%	Poor	Organomegaly
t(8;16)	M4,5	KAT6A/CREBP	?	<1%	Poor	Erythrophagocytosis, often threap-related
Molecular abnormality						
Fms-related tyrosine kinase gene mutations	Varied—most common in CN-AML; can be found with (6;9); t(15;17)	Internal tandem repeat or point mutation of	?	~30% in CN-AML	Adverse	
Nucleophosmin (NPM1)—(5q35) mutation	Varied	Nucleophosmin (NPM1); often found with other mutations	?	~35% of AML, ~50% of CN-AML	Favorable DFS except when associated with mutation	
CEBPα gene	Varied	Mutation results in decreasing levels of CEBPα (CCAAT entamer binding protein)	?	~15% of CN-AML	Favorable when biallic with FLT3 ITD mutation	
Overexpression of BAALC (brain and acute leukemia cytoplasmic) protein	Varied	Overexpression of BAALC	?	Studied most extensively in CN-AML	Adverse—further studies needed	
Partial tandem duplication of MLL (mixed lineage leukemia) gene	Varied	Affects HOX gene function	?	~8% of CN-AML	Unclear—further studies needed	
IDH1, IDH2	varied	isocitrate dehydrogenase	?	IDH1 in 10%, IDH2 in 18%	variable	specific inhibitors in clinical trials
TET2	varied (common in MDS)	DNA methylation	>60	15%	adverse	increased with older age
DNMT3A	varied	DNA methylation	>60	20%	adverse	increased with older age
ASXL1	varied	epigenetic regulation	?	6%	adverse	associated with other mutations

Abbreviations: AML, acute myelogenous leukemia; ATRA, all *trans* retinoic acid; DIC, disseminated intravascular coagulation; FAB, French, American, and British; MDS, myelodysplastic syndrome.

which may include these changes as well as the presence of marker chromosomes.[67] These leukemias seem to arise in a very early hematopoietic stem cell and tend to have low response rates with short durations of response. It seems likely that those patients in this category, only based on morphological abnormalities, may exhibit a variety of oncogenic pathways based on mutational profile and thus may not have a uniformly poor prognosis.[5]

Therapy-related AML

This category includes patients whose AML followed treatment with chemotherapy and/or radiation therapy for other disorders. Morphology and karyotypes are often similar to those observed in MDS with the addition of a group of patients with abnormalities of 11q23 associated with prior treatment with topoisomerase II inhibitors and often with a short interval until the development of AML.[32,33] Therapy-related AML tends to be more resistant to chemotherapy, and allogeneic transplant should be considered in patients who achieve remission. It is important to note that some patients with therapy-related AML can have inv(16), t(8;21), and t(15;17) (APL) or genetics typical of de novo AML and respond well to standard approaches for these subtypes, although perhaps not as well as those with these karyotypes with de novo disease.[5,36]

Extramedullary AML (aka myeloid sarcoma)

Occasionally patients will present for medical attention because of lesions identified to be composed of myeloblasts by histochemical staining, but without apparent bone marrow involvement. Masses can involve the skin, gastrointestinal tract, ovaries, the central nervous system (CNS), and virtually every body organ. There have been only few systematic studies on the management of such patients, although there is a risk of high eventual systemic relapse rate without treatment.[71] Most clinicians consider induction and consolidation in medically fit patients after diagnosis. Despite such "early" treatment, the recurrence rate is high; the role of stem cell transplant is unclear, but it is reasonable to consider transplantation to maintain the remission. Some of these patients have a t(8;21) chromosomal translocation, but in this setting, may not have the same favorable prognostic input as found in more typical t(8;21) AMLs.[72]

AML not otherwise specified

This category includes the large group of patients whose AML does not fall into the previously listed groups.

FAB classification

Although the "old" FAB classification is not used currently, clinical–pathological correlates can be discussed. Wright–Giemsa stained peripheral blood or bone marrow aspirate smears can prefer AML to ALL. In general, the blasts from patients with AML are larger, with more abundant cytoplasm and more prominent, often multiple, nucleoli. The definitive diagnosis depends, however, on the presence of Auer rods, which are linear bundles of myeloid-containing granules. Cytochemical stains, such as myeloperoxidase, which is present in 73% of blasts, can diagnose AML.

M0: Minimally differentiated AML

As shown in Figure 2, some patients have blasts that resemble myeloid blasts, but are negative at the light microscopic level when examined with myeloperoxidase, Sudan Black B, or other histochemical stains. The myeloid nature of these leukemias

can be detected, however, by immunologic means or by election microscopy of peroxidase-stained preparations. Electron micrographs reveal ultrastructural peroxidase-positive granules, whereas immunologic phenotyping shows reactivity with antibodies directed against myeloid antigens and nonreactivity with antibodies that characterize lymphoid differentiation.[73,74] The cells are often reactive with antibodies directed against CD34. In general, terminal deoxynucleotidyl transferase (TdT) is absent, but can sometimes be detected in a minority of blasts.

Approximately 7% of patients with untreated AML have minimally differentiated AML (M0 AML), which is relatively resistant to treatment.[75] This undifferentiated leukemia can easily be confused with ALL, and it is therefore critically important to obtain data of immunophenotyping of blasts from patients with morphologically undifferentiated leukemias. Other than resistance to chemotherapy, this M0 variant does not appear to be associated with specific clinical findings. Many M0 patients have complex karyotypic abnormalities.[75] No distinctive cytogenetic pattern has been noted, except trisomy 13, which has been reported to occur in some patients with morphologically less differentiated leukemias.[76]

M1: Myeloid leukemia without maturation

The blasts from patients with M1 morphology have round nuclei with moderate amounts of sometimes lightly granulated cytoplasm, which can contain Auer rods (Figure 3). In contrast to M2, there is little evidence of myeloid maturation, with <10% of cells beyond the level of the promyelocyte. There is no particular age, gender, clinical feature, or characteristic cytogenetic abnormality associated with this morphologic variant.

M2: Myeloid leukemia with maturation

In contrast to M1, there is obvious continued maturation in the myeloid series with the presence of promyelocytes, myelocytes, and often more mature myeloid elements. Granulation is generally more obvious; Auer rods are often prominent (Figure 4). Approximately 20–25% of patients with M2 AML have a characteristic translocation between chromosomes 8 and 21 [t(8;21)(q22;22)]; this translocation is seen almost exclusively in patients with M2 and Auer rods. Such patients have a lower median age (~30 years), very high initial complete response rate (>85% in most series), lower relapse rate, and increased long-term disease-free survival, particularly when treated with high-dose cytarabine-based consolidation therapy,[77] except for a subset with an activating mutation of *KIT* or adverse gene signature.[78] The incidence of extramedullary granulocytic sarcomas, often in unusual sites, may be increased in patients with t(8;21) M2 AML, whose blasts express the adhesion molecule CD56 on their surface. These can present as discrete tumor masses, sometimes in paraspinal locations, confer a poor prognosis, and are distinct from the gingival and cutaneous involvement found in monocytic leukemia.[71]

M3: Acute promyelocytic leukemia

APL is one of the most distinctive subtypes of AML with regard to morphologic, clinical, cytogenetic features, and response to differentiating agent therapies, such as all-trans retinoic acid (ATRA) and arsenic.[79] In most patients, the morphologic diagnosis is straightforward, with the marrow being replaced by blasts that resemble unusually heavily granulated progranulocytes. The nuclei are spherical, with obvious nucleoli, and the cytoplasm is filled with multiple, large, and often coalesced azurophilic granules (Figure 5). Auer rods are usually observed, and multiple Auer rods (the so-called faggot cells) are frequently noted. In a minority of patients, the blasts are hypogranular, and sometimes granules can only be visualized by an electron microscope.[80] This hypogranular variant often has cells with bilobed or lobulated nuclei, which can sometimes be confused with monocytic variants of AML. In contrast to the typical leukopenic presentation of APL, patients with the hypogranular variant tend to have higher white cell counts. In both types of APL, staining with either Sudan Black B or myeloperoxidase is strongly positive. Class II human leukocyte antigens (HLA DR), which are found on all hematopoietic precursors, are not usually detected on the surface of the malignant progranulocytes. The explanation for and biologic implications of this finding are not known. By contrast, CD33 is consistently strongly expressed.[81]

Patients with APL tend to be somewhat younger, with a median age of 30–40 years, although it is observed in patients of all ages. APL accounts for approximately 10% of AML and may be more prevalent in Latinos[82] and obese people.[83] It is almost uniformly characterized by hypofibrinogenemia, variable depletion of other coagulation factors, elevated levels of fibrin degradation products, and increased consumption of endogenous and transfused platelets. The granules contain potent procoagulants, and the rate of disseminated intravascular coagulation (DIC) is generally increased following lysis of blasts by chemotherapy,[84] often with increased bleeding, although the problem can be rapidly ameliorated with the use of ATRA.[85] In some patients, there is evidence that accelerated fibrinolysis may be the primary event triggering coagulopathy.[86] APL is associated with the highest frequency of hemorrhagic morbidity and mortality, the latter usually related to intracranial hemorrhage, emphasizing the need to initiate ATRA at the first thought of APL.[87] Before DIC is controlled with ATRA, severe hypofibrinogenemia (<100 mg/dL) may require supplementation with cryoprecipitate, and thrombocytopenia should be managed with the aggressive use of platelet transfusions.

Almost all patients with APL have a characteristic translocation involving chromosomes 15 and 17 [t(15;17) (q22;q12)],[88] which may be accompanied by additional cytogenetic abnormalities, such as trisomy 8.[89] Reverse transcription polymerase chain reaction (RT-PCR) can be used to detect the fusion transcript, is useful for assessing minimal residual disease (MRD),[90] and permits the proper classification of a patient with clinically and morphologically typical APL and an apparently normal karyotype. The break point on chromosome 17 is in an intron of the retinoic acid receptor alpha gene. A gene that has been termed *PML*, also with DNA-binding capability, is translocated from chromosome 15, resulting in the formation of a fusion protein that functions in a dominant manner to block transcription of genes controlled by *RAR*-α, probably by nuclear corepressor activity. Retinoic acid treatment relieves the corepressor activity,[91,92] allowing transcription of genes involved in differentiation.[93] There is also interest in the use of histone deacetylase inhibitors in patients with APL as another means of enhancing gene expression.[94] FLT3 *ITD* mutations can be detected in approximately one-third of patients with APL, are associated with higher WBC counts and M3 variant morphology, but unlike the case for non-APL AML, does not always seem to be associated with inferior outcome.[95,96] A group of patients with a leukemia similar in morphology to APL, but with alternate translocations such as t(11;17)(q23;q21) have been described. Although *RAR*-α is rearranged, these patients fail to respond to ATRA. A novel zinc-finger gene termed PZLF from chromosome 11 is translocated to *RAR*-α, rather than the *PML* gene from chromosome 15, creating a fusion protein that does not allow the ATRA-mediated release of transcriptional corepressor activity.[97]

Historically, the remission rate in patients with APL treated with anthracycline-based chemotherapy was quite high. Initial drug resistance was very unusual, and most treatment failures were related to hemorrhagic or infectious deaths. APL is uniquely sensitive to single agent anthracycline therapy, which can produce CR rates >80%.[98] In contrast to other types of AML, remission can be attained with chemotherapy in APL without producing bone marrow aplasia.[99] Posttreatment bone marrows frequently remain cellular with abnormal progranulocytes, with follow-up marrows demonstrating disappearance of these cells and return of normal hematopoiesis without additional chemotherapy. DIC does not reappear despite the persistence of morphologically abnormal cells. Undoubtedly, this unique feature of APL is related sensitivity to agents that have a differentiating and noncytotoxic mechanism of action (see section titled "Therapy of Acute Promyelocytic Leukemia (APL)"), and is now cured in at least 80% of patients with minimal or no chemotherapy with the use of ATRA and arsenic trioxide in combination.[100]

M4: Myelomonocytic leukemia

Myelomonocytic leukemia is characterized morphologically by a mixture of myeloid and monocytic elements and represents approximately 15–20% of newly diagnosed patients with AML. According to the FAB criteria, >20% of the leukemic cells must be monocytic in morphology to distinguish this variant from FAB M1 and particularly from FAB M2. The monocytic elements often resemble partially differentiated monocytes with lightly granulated, grayish cytoplasmic, and folded nuclei, which are frequently seen in the peripheral blood (Figure 6). Monocytic derivation can be confirmed by staining with nonspecific esterases such as α-naphthyl acetate and α-naphthyl butyrate.

There is no distinct clinical picture associated with this variant, perhaps because this classification encompasses a wide spectrum of patients owing to the generous morphologic criteria for inclusion. The median age tends to be somewhat higher, and there may be an increased incidence of hyperleukocytosis and extramedullary leukemic involvement, as can be seen with monocytic leukemia. There is no particular cytogenetic clustering, and it is impossible to accurately predict short- or long-term outcome in patients with M4.

M4EO: Myelomonocytic leukemia with eosinophilia

Approximately 5% of patients with de novo AML have typical morphologic features of myelomonocytic leukemia in the presence of variable numbers of dysplastic eosinophils at various stages of maturation. The distinctive eosinophils usually represent only 5–10% of the cells of the marrow.[101] In general, these cells contain large basophilic granules in addition to typical eosinophilic counterparts. Occasional patients with M2 morphology with eosinophilia have also been described.

M4Eo tends to occur in patients of younger age (median 35–40 years) and is associated with an excellent prognosis.[102] CR rates are high (generally >85%), and failure because of initial drug resistance is unusual. In some series, this variant represents the subtype with the most favorable long-term prognosis. Mutations of the *C-KIT* tyrosine kinase receptor have recently been described in some patients with CBF AML, with data indicating a poorer outcome in this subset.[53,78] In addition to long initial CRs, second remissions, which are often quite sustained, are generally easier to accomplish in patients with FAB M4Eo.[103] Older series indicated the possibility of achieving a high rate of CNS relapse in patients with bone marrow eosinophilia. With more intensive regimens using higher doses of cytosine arabinoside (ara-C), CNS relapse in AML is unusual, and patients with FAB M4Eo do not require prophylactic CNS therapy.

All patients with FAB M4Eo exhibit a cytogenetic abnormality, involving chromosome 16 at band q22. In most patients, the cytogenetic changes involve a pericentric inversion (inv16), although translocations between the two chromosomes 16 with homologous deletions at 16q22 have also been noted.[104] This break point involves a fusion between the CBF-β chain and the gene encoding the smooth muscle myosin heavy chain. The fusion protein thus generated may use nuclear corepressor activity (in the form of histone deacetylase), which prevents transcription of genes required for myeloid differentiation in a manner analogous to the CBF-α ETO fusion in t(8;21) M2 AML.[105] Although it is evident that patients with inv(16) leukemia respond very well to intensive chemotherapy [3-year DFS rate of >60–70% in those receiving high-dose ara-C (HIDAC)],[102] the reason for this is unclear.

M5: Monocytic leukemia

Two variants of monocytic leukemia have been described; in both, >80% of the blasts are of monocytic derivation. Less common is the so-called M5a, in which the monocytic blasts have spherical nuclei and small amounts of sometimes deeply basophilic cytoplasm without evidence of morphologic differentiation. In monocytic leukemia with differentiation (M5b), at least 20% of the blasts resemble promonocytes with folded nuclei and abundant, lightly granulated cytoplasm, generally without Auer rods. The nuclear folding can often be quite marked with rarification of the nuclear chromatin (Figure 7). Phagocytosis of other hematopoietic elements by these cells is frequently noted in bone marrow preparations. These monocytic elements stain prominently with nonspecific esterase that is inhibited by fluoride.

Although observed in patients of all ages, monocytic leukemias are somewhat more common in older adults. Patients with FAB M5 have higher blast counts at diagnosis, and problems with hyperleukocytosis are most common in this morphologic variant (see section titled "Complications").[106] In addition, the incidence of extramedullary leukemia is highest in M5, particularly in those with evidence of morphologic differentiation.[107] For example, it is common for patients to present to the dentist with gingival hypertrophy (Figure 8). Skin infiltration is common at both diagnosis and relapse, and it generally represents the initial site of recurrence, sometimes while the bone marrow is still morphologically normal. Other less common areas of extramedullary involvement include the gastrointestinal tract, conjunctiva, and the CNS. It is likely that extramedullary infiltration is related to active migration of the leukemic promonocytes to these sites. These partially differentiated cells are capable of migration to skin windows in vivo as well as phagocytosis of microorganisms and adherence to nylon fibers in vitro.[108]

Serum levels of lysozyme are elevated in most patients with AML, but are generally much higher in patients with monocytic leukemia.[109] Lysozyme can affect renal tubular function, and severe, symptomatic hypokalemia can occur in patients with FAB M4 and M5 leukemia. This problem generally resolves with cytoreduction, but can also produce hypokalemic side effects of vomiting and diarrhea.

In addition to the initial problems presented by complications of hyperleukocytosis, patients with monocytic leukemia tend to have lower complete response rates related to drug-resistant disease. Although previous studies indicated that CR durations tend to be shorter with very low rates of long-term disease-free survival, an analysis of a large number of patients treated by the ECOG suggested similar outcomes to other morphologic subtypes of AML when other risk factors are taken into account.[110] A variety of cytogenetic abnormalities can be detected, although the most common findings involve abnormalities of chromosome 11 at band q23. This break point, at what has been termed the mixed lineage leukemia (*MLL*) gene, can be involved in leukemias of myeloid or lymphoid origin as well as in those following therapy with epipodophyllotoxins and other drugs directed at topoisomerase II.[111] The *MLL* gene, also called *All-1* or *HRX*, may combine with at least 16 different genes in balanced translocation.[112] *MLL* is homologous to a gene important in the development of *Drosophila* and includes DNA-binding elements. The t(9;11) translocation is relatively common, involving the MLL gene, which may in fact confer a better prognosis than formerly thought, with high initial CR rates.[113,114] There is an association between M5b with extensive erythrophagocytosis and the t(8;16)(p11;p13), a translocation involving the CBP class of translocation factors that are positive regulators of myeloid differentiation.[115]

M6: Erythroleukemia

Erythroleukemia, often called Di Guglielmo syndrome previously, is a variant of AML, in which morphologic abnormalities of erythropoiesis are most prominent.[116] Cases of pure erythroleukemia, in which the predominant malignant cell is clearly identified as a pronormoblast, are rare. Rather, this is a disease of the myeloid stem cell with marked dysplastic changes in all three hematopoietic lines. Together with the increase in myeloid-appearing blasts, there is persistence of morphologic abnormalities in the erythroid series with profound megablastosis, multinuclearity, karyorrhexis, increased number of mitoses, and staining with periodic acid–Schiff (PAS), often in a block pattern (Figure 9). Increased iron stores are usually observed, often with ringed sideroblasts. These changes are morphologically identical to those observed in patients with myelodysplasia, and many observers feel that most cases of erythroleukemia are biologically similar, if not identical, to patients with refractory anemia with excess blasts. This contention is supported by the very poor response to therapy in both groups, the tendency for the disease to occur in patients of older age, and the presence of similar cytogenetic abnormalities (complex karyotypic abnormalities, loss of part, or all of chromosomes 5, and/or 7, and marker chromosomes).[116] Nonetheless, in order to be consistent in terms of protocol entry and reports of clinical trials, the FAB and WHO groups, somewhat arbitrarily distinguished among M6, myelodysplasia (RAEB), and other FAB subtypes with significant numbers of erythroblasts by quantification of the number of erythroblasts and myeloblasts. Most of these patients will now be placed in the "AML with MDS-related Changes" in the most recent WHO iteration. M6 is defined by the presence of >30% blasts among nonerythroid cells when >50% of the marrow nucleated elements are erythroid. Antibodies against glycophorin A are lineage-specific for erythroblasts, but immunologic phenotyping is rarely needed to identify these morphologic subtypes.

M7: Megakaryocytic leukemia

Morphologic abnormalities of megakaryocytopoiesis, usually characterized by the presence of mono- or binucleated micromegakaryocytes, are common in many variants of AML and can be particularly prominent in patients with M6 or myelodysplasia. A minority of these patients have thrombocytosis and abnormalities of chromosome 3 [inv(3) (q21;q26)]. This cytogenetic abnormality is often found in association with other chromosomal deletions, with a variety of primary morphologies (M1, M2, M4), and in patients with a prior background of MDS.[117] These patients have a poor response to initial treatment and low overall survival (OS). Thrombocytosis is present not only in patients with the inv(3) karyotype, but also in those with AML at the time of diagnosis.[118]

The gene at the chromosome 3q21 break point is associated with the activation of EVI1 transcription factor.[119]

Diagnosis of FAB M7 is reserved for patients in whom the predominant leukemic cell is of megakaryocytic lineage.[120] In some patients, there is evidence of megakaryocytic dysplasia or multinucleated cells that strongly point toward principal involvement of the megakaryocyte (Figure 10), whereas in others, the leukemia is undifferentiated morphologically, with variable amounts of agranular cytoplasm, and it is sometimes confused with M1 or ALL. Sudan Black B (Figure 11), myeloperoxidase, and α-naphthyl butyrate stains are negative, whereas PAS and acid phosphatase may be positive, usually in a diffuse, speckled pattern. However, histochemical staining is nondiagnostic and the definitive diagnosis depends on the detection of platelet-specific peroxidase by either ultrastructural techniques or the demonstration of a variety of platelet antigens (usually glycoprotein IIb/IIIa [CD41] or von Willebrand factor) on the surface of the blasts.[121] At times, the diagnosis can be quite difficult to confirm, particularly because of the increased marrow reticulin in most patients, rendering the marrow fibrotic and inaspirable. Careful evaluation of peripheral blood blasts is necessary in such patients. It is likely that most patients with acute myelosclerosis in fact have acute megakaryocytic leukemia, which should not be confused with the late stages of primary myelofibrosis, and, indeed, prominent splenomegaly is not a clinical feature of M7. Although it is an uncommon variant of AML, most series suggest that this subtype is associated with a very poor prognosis. Prolonged aplasia is common following induction chemotherapy, and, because of the marrow fibrosis, it is often difficult to follow the results of therapy with repeated marrow aspirations. There have been relatively few cytogenetic evaluations of this variant, and except for the inv(3) karyotype and cases of t(1;22) (p13;q13) [RBM15/MKL1 gene fusion] found in infants,[122] no consistent abnormality has been identified.

Acute panmyelosis with myelofibrosis

This is a very rare variant of AML felt to derive from the hematopoietic stem cell, in which the marrow demonstrates a marked increase in reticulin fibers with evidence of morphologically abnormal trilineage hematopoiesis and a variable number of blasts with an immature myeloid immunophenotype.[123,124] Patients usually present with pancytopenia and constitutional symptoms. It can sometimes be difficult to distinguish acute panmyelosis with myelofibrosis (APMF) from acute megakaryocytic leukemia or MDSs with myelofibrosis. APMF responds poorly to standard chemotherapy.

Mixed phenotypic leukemia

There are certain cases of acute leukemia that defy easy categorization, because the cells may have features of both lymphoid and myeloid derivation. The WHO 2008 monograph on classification of hematopoietic and lymphoid tissues uses the term "mixed phenotype acute leukemia" (MPAL) to encompass these heterogeneous groups of neoplasms. MPALs are defined by immature cells which display cytochemical or immunophenotypic features of both myeloid and lymphoid lineages (biphenotypic), or there are two different populations of leukemia cells: myeloid and lymphoid (bilineal). The difference between bilineal and biphenotypic cells generally does not alter the diagnostic therapeutic approach. Although prior systems such as the EGIL (European Group for Immunological Characterization of Acute Leukemias) were used,[125] the most recent algorithm is based on the 2008 WHO monograph.[126] Such entities tend to have features of either B-ALL and AML or T-ALL and AML and are called B-myeloid or

T-myeloid diseases, respectively. Entities with evidence of derivation from both lineages are specified if there is a known recurrent genetic lesion such as Philadelphia chromosome-positive leukemia, MLL-rearranged leukemia, or AML-defining balanced translocation such as t(8;21). Technically, MPALs also exclude secondary leukemias, leukemias with FGFR1, mutations, and CML in blast crisis.[127]

The essential features of an MPAL is the specific expression of certain lineage-defining markers in two categories. Although the algorithm is slightly complex, CD3 expression is evidence of T-lymphoid derivation, and CD19 together with one or two other markers indicate B-lymphoid origin. Myeloid origin can be determined by a set of monocytic immunophenotypic markers or most commonly by myeloperoxidase expression. TdT is characteristically seen in ALL; however, because 25% of AML patients express TdT, this is not considered a lineage defining abnormality. It is also important to indicate that many AMLs may have lymphoid antigens detectable by flow cytometry, but do not meet the criteria for biphenotypic leukemia. Such cases should be considered in the AML prognostic and therapeutic rubric.[127]

The literature does not yield clear guidelines for the treatment of MPALs. In particular, patients with BCR/ABL-positive disease should be treated by chemotherapy together with a tyrosine kinase inhibitor. Most other MPALs should be treated with an ALL regimen, although controversy certainly exists particularly if there is prominent expression of myeloperoxidase or even Auer rods. A regimen that combines AML- and ALL-type chemotherapy is also possible, but may be more toxic than a more typical ALL regimen. Given the relatively resistant nature of MPALs, it is reasonable to consolidate any remissions achieved with an allogeneic stem cell transplant.

Presenting signs and symptoms

Patients with AML generally present with symptoms related to complications of pancytopenia, including combinations of weakness, easy fatigability, infections of variable severity, or hemorrhagic findings such as gingival bleeding, ecchymoses, epistaxis, or menorrhagia. Occasionally patients present with prominent extramedullary sites of leukemia usually related to either cutaneous or gingival infiltration by leukemia cells. Bone pain is infrequent in adults with AML, although some individuals describe sternal discomfort or tenderness, occasionally with aching in the long bones, particularly of the lower extremities. In general, it is difficult to determine the time of onset of AML precisely, at least in part because individuals have different symptomatic thresholds for choosing to seek medical attention. It is likely that most patients have had more subtle evidence of leukemia for weeks, to perhaps months, before diagnosis.

The findings on physical examination are variable and generally nonspecific. If fever is present, an infectious site must be vigorously sought and treated empirically with broad-spectrum antibiotics. A large number of patients have fever related solely to the underlying leukemia, which abates with appropriate chemotherapy. Examination of the skin can reveal pallor, infiltrative lesions suggestive of leukemic involvement, cutaneous sites of infection, which may be either primary or embolic, or, most commonly, petechiae or ecchymoses related to thrombocytopenia and/or coagulopathy. Examination of the fundus reveals hemorrhages and/or exudates in the majority of patients (see section titled "Ophthalmic Complications"). The conjunctivae may be pale, according to the magnitude of the anemia. Careful examination of the oropharynx and teeth is important because of the infrequency of leukemic involvement.

Palpable adenopathy is uncommon in patients with AML, and significant lymph node enlargement is rare. Similarly, hepatomegaly and splenomegaly are uncommon and, if found, may suggest the possibility of ALL or chronic myeloid leukemia in blast crisis. None of these findings is a diagnostic of acute leukemia, and the final diagnosis and categorization depends on appropriate evaluation of the peripheral blood and bone marrow.

Because of the rigorous nature of the chemotherapy required for the successful treatment of AML, particular attention should be paid to other medical problems that could complicate management of the patient. A history of congestive heart failure or other heart disease may preclude therapy with anthracyclines and mandates careful monitoring of the large amounts of intravenous fluids, including antibiotics, blood and platelet transfusions, hydration for nephrotoxic antimicrobial agents, and sometimes parenteral nutrition, given during the 3–4 weeks of chemotherapy-induced pancytopenia. Prior transfusion for other disorders or multiple previous pregnancies may presage difficulties with platelet transfusions or herald the occurrence of transfusion reactions after red blood cell or platelet administration. Careful appraisal for possible drug allergies is critical, because virtually every patient will require antibiotic therapy. A history of prior herpes simplex infections (or the presence of an elevated antibody titer) provides justification for prophylactic administration of acyclovir.[128] In premenopausal women, menses should be suppressed with a GNRH agonist or estrogens and/or progestational compounds until thrombocytopenia is resolved. Considerations of fertility preservation should be discussed with selected patients. Sperm-banking in males wishing to have a family should be considered, although many patients are either oligo- or azospermic at the time of diagnosis. GNRH antiagonist therapy, by shutting down the pituitary–ovarian axis during chemotherapy, may preserve fertility in females with childbearing potential.[129]

Once the diagnosis (Table 3) is established, the physician and staff must present the goals of therapy and the side effects of treatment to the patient and his/her family. For almost all patients, this discussion can rightfully emphasize the potential benefits of treatment with regard to both the short- and long-term outcomes. It is appropriate and necessary to repeat this discussion and counsel later during the patient's course of hospital stay. In general, for younger patients, induction therapy followed by postremission treatment with intensive chemotherapy and/or allogeneic transplant is appropriate. For older patients (>60–65 years), there may be merit to the standard, more aggressive approach, but hypomethylating agent therapy should be discussed.

Therapy: general overview

The therapy of AML has traditionally been divided into stages: induction, postremission therapy of varying intensity and duration, and postrelapse therapy. In newly diagnosed patients with AML, the goal of induction therapy is to achieve CR, which then permits the administration of subsequent therapy that for most patients is designed to maximize the rate of disease-free survival and cure. CR is defined primarily on morphologic grounds and includes the development of a bone marrow containing less than 5% blast elements, no signs of extramedullary leukemia, and return of normal neutrophil (>1500/μL) and platelet (>150,000/μL) counts. Even if the bone marrow contains <5% blasts, patients are not considered to be in remission if distinctive morphologic signs of leukemia, such as Auer rods, are noted. Low hemoglobin levels and the presence of symptoms unrelated to leukemia no longer exclude CR, as they are often treatment-related and slow to normalize.

Table 3 Initial diagnostic evaluation.

History and physical examination—In addition to an overall comprehensive evaluation, emphasis should be placed on the following:
- Duration of symptoms
- Menstrual history
- Prior pregnancies, transfusions, history of transfusion reactions
- Drug allergies (antibiotics)
- Sites of infection: rectum, vagina, oropharynx, gingiva, skin
- Signs of hemorrhage
- Signs of extramedullary leukemia—skin, gingiva
- Dentition status

Bone marrow aspirate and biopsy
- Morphologic classification
- Cytochemistry
- Immunophenotyping
- Cytogenetics
- Terminal deoxynucleotidyl transferase
- Genomic studies

Blood chemistries
- Blood urea nitrogen, creatinine, electrolytes, uric acid
- Transaminases, alkaline phosphatase, bilirubin, lactate dehydrogenase, calcium, phosphorus

Coagulation studies
- Prothrombin time, activated partial thromboplastin time, fibrinogen, fibrin split products

Chest radiograph, electrocardiogram, left ventricular ejection fraction if clinically indicated
HLA typing (patient and family); lymphocytotoxic (anti-HLA) antibody screen
Herpes simplex and cytomegalovirus serology
Lumbar puncture (only if symptomatic)

Abbreviation: HLA, human leukocyte antigen.

It has been assumed that CR is accomplished because the cytotoxic chemotherapy markedly decreases the number of cells in the leukemic clone, thereby allowing repopulation of the bone marrow by residual normal progenitors, whose proliferation had been suppressed. This explanation is supported by observations that cytogenetic abnormalities present in the original leukemia cells cannot be detected in patients in remission. However, in some patients, intensive chemotherapy appears to eliminate the block in differentiation such that the apparently normal cells seen in the bone marrow and peripheral blood during a CR are actually progeny of the leukemic clone.[130,131] as determined by X chromosome-linked polymorphisms (glucose-6-phosphate dehydrogenase isoenzyme or restriction fragment-length polymorphisms) or the presence of disease-specific mutations in apparent normal cells at the time of CR.[132] The frequency of such "clonal CRs," the possible association with particular subtypes of AML or remission duration, the mechanism by which this important biologic phenomenon occurs, and a number of important technical issues need to be further defined.

Induction therapy: general principles

Induction therapy is designed to produce rapid clearing of leukemic cells from the peripheral blood with subsequent marrow aplasia. The only exception to this principle occurs in patients with APL (FAB M3), in whom remission can be achieved despite the persistence 2–3 weeks later of what appear morphologically to be viable leukemia cells,[133] although, especially given the use of ATRA/arsenic-based therapies, multiple marrows in APL need not be done. Approximately 1 week after standard induction therapy (the so-called "3 + 7"; 3 days of anthracycline, usually daunorubicin and 7 days of continuous infusion cytarabine) is completed (generally 2 weeks after the initiation of treatment), bone marrow aspirates and biopsies are done to evaluate the magnitude of cytoreduction. If the marrow is profoundly hypoplastic, one waits for count recovery. If the marrow is not hypoplastic and only leukemia cells are noted on the day 14 marrow, then a second course of therapy is generally administered. If high-dose cytarabine-based therapy was used as induction chemotherapy, multiple marrow examinations are not recommended.

At times, particularly if the "day 14" marrow is hypocellular, it can be difficult to distinguish between residual leukemia cells and normal undifferentiated hematopoietic progenitors. In this instance, it is advisable to delay retreatment and perform another marrow aspirate in a few days. If there is no evidence of further maturation, then a second course of treatment is indicated. The presence of erythroid precursors, juvenile megakaryocytes, or increased peripheral blood platelet or neutrophil counts serve as indicators to delay a second course of treatment as normal regeneration is occurring. With standard regimens, approximately 30% of patients with AML require two courses of treatment to enter remission. Despite these guidelines, there remains considerable variability and imprecision as to when a second course of therapy is indicated.

Most trials report results as complete response or no response. It is beneficial, however, to more rigorously classify the causes of failure in investigations of prognostic factors or assessment of the cytotoxic activity of different regimens, to achieve remission. One such classification divides nonresponders into those with apparent chemotherapy-resistant leukemia, those who die with aplastic bone marrows in whom the response to chemotherapy cannot be determined, and those in whom either early death or failure to obtain adequate bone marrow studies before death preclude determination of whether persistent leukemia was present. Patients with drug-resistant leukemia include those who survive treatment and those who die but have morphologic evidence of leukemia in the bone marrow or blood. The criteria for CR are generally reached a median of 30–35 days after treatment has begun, although patients achieve adequate levels of circulating neutrophils (>500/µL) and no longer require platelet transfusion (at counts of ~10–20,000/µL), at least 7–10 days earlier, which may be beneficial in sorting out activity of novel and/or noncytotoxic agents. Other types of responses include PR (50% reduction in marrow blast with adequate count recovery), CRp (same as CR, but platelets are not fully recovered), CRi (same as CR, but with low neutrophil counts), and morphological leukemia-free state (<5% marrow blasts, without mention of normal cell counts). This categorization is relatively simple to perform in most patients and can be beneficial in distinguishing between failures due to drug resistance and inadequacy of supportive care.[2,133]

The overall rate of CR with standard chemotherapy in large cooperative group studies is approximately 65%. Patient age and cytogenetics are the most critical clinical variables, with CR rates of 75–80% in younger patients and approximately 50% in patients >60 years of age. The reasons for treatment failure vary according to patient age. With improved supportive care, it is uncommon for patients <50 years of age to die from complications of treatment, and most of the approximately 25% induction failure rate is a consequence of drug-resistant leukemia. By contrast, in patients >60 years of age, failures are due to drug-resistant leukemia and deaths occurring during marrow aplasia as a consequence of reduced end organ tolerance, occurring at overall frequencies of 40% and 10%, respectively.

Table 4 Representative chemotherapy regimens for acute myeloid leukemia.

	Dose	Route	Days
Induction			
Cytarabine+	100–200 mg/m²	Continuous IV infusion	1–7
Daunorubicin	45–60 mg/m²	IV	1–3
or			
Idarubicin	12 mg/m²	IV	1–3
or			
Mitoxantrone	12 mg/m²	IV	1–3
Postremission			
Cytarabine	3 g/m² q12h (over 3 h)	IV (6 doses)	1, 3, 5
or			
Cytarabine	1.5–2 g/m² q12h (over 1 h)	IV (8 doses)	1–4 (12 doses)
or			
Cytarabine	100 mg/m²	Continuous IV infusion	1–5

See text for details about number of courses and patient selection for different regimens.

Although there have been gradual improvements in the CR rates worldwide in younger adults with AML during the past 25 years, much of this can be attributed to better supportive care and not to changes in therapy. With the exception of the use of ATRA and arsenic for patients with APL (see below), relatively few changes in therapy have been made since the introduction of combined therapy with daunorubicin and ara-C, the so-called "7 and 3" regimen.[134] This two-drug combination was derived from observations of single-agent activity of either compounds. Daunorubicin is generally administered by intravenous push at doses of 45–90 mg/m²/day for 3 days; ara-C is administered at doses of 100–200 mg/m²/day by continuous infusion for 7 days (Table 4). A series of randomized studies[134–140] by the Cancer and Leukemia Group B (CALGB) showed that:

1. Results were superior using the 7 and 3 regimen to 5 days of ara-C and two doses of daunorubicin.
2. The addition of oral 6-thioguanine (DAT regimen) to the 7 and 3 regimen did not increase the CR rate.
3. Continuous infusions of ara-C produced a slightly better outcome than twice-daily short intravenous infusions when combined with daunorubicin.
4. Results were not improved when ara-C was administered by continuous infusion for 10 days compared with 7 days.
5. Substitution of doxorubicin for daunorubicin produced almost identical CR rates, although mucosal toxicity was higher with doxorubicin.
6. There was no overall benefit from doubling the dose of ara-C from 100 to 200 mg/m²/day.

Other modifications of the 7 and 3 regimen

Most attempts to improve the 7 and 3 induction regimen have not led to increase in OS. Alternative anthracyclines or other agents such as mitoxantrone, rubidazone, aclacinomycin, amsacrine, mitoxantrone, and idarubicin have been used in several trials.[141–145] None of these studies showed a survival or disease-free survival advantage with these different agents, perhaps because most are relatively similar in structure and mechanism of action and hence, become susceptible to the same mechanisms of resistance. The largest reported experience has been with idarubicin, where three initial trials showed that induction results are at least equivalent to results achieved with daunorubicin and ara-C.[142,144] An important randomized trial did not show an advantage for idarubicin compared with daunorubicin, in older patients.[146] In addition, the duration of myelosuppression was longer in the idarubicin cohorts, calling into question the equitoxicity of the arms. Therefore, the substitution of these compounds did not have a major impact on the long-term disease-free survival rate of patients with AML.

An Australian trial added etoposide to the 7 and 3 regimen.[147] The CR rate was similar in older patients when compared with daunorubicin and ara-C only with a possibly modest prolongation of CR duration in younger patients receiving etoposide. This was a relatively small study and the overall disease-free survival in the group receiving etoposide during both remission induction and postremission therapy was similar to other larger studies using daunorubicin and ara-C only. Large phase I studies from the CALGB, in which etoposide was added to the 7 and 3 regimen, had outcomes similar to the past experience with only the two drugs.[148]

Because HIDAC is a beneficial postremission therapy (see below), several groups have tested the use of this approach during induction in younger patients. Studies have compared standard 7 and 3 to daunorubicin plus intermediate- or high-dose ara-C ($2-3 \text{ g/m}^2$ for 8–12 doses).[149-151] These studies failed to show an increased CR rate for the recipients of HIDAC, although one study documented a more prolonged duration of CR (but no change in OS) in the patients randomized to HIDAC.[149] The addition of HIDAC to standard daunorubicin/ara-C during induction has also been studied. Although a small trial showed an 87% remission rate in patients <60 years old,[152] a cooperative group trial failed to confirm those positive results.[153] Results seem to be equivalent if HIDAC is used either as part of induction or only as postremission therapy.[154]

New induction strategies

Although it is evident that 3 + 7-based strategies remain the standard of care, new data suggest that many patients (perhaps all of those up to age 65) should be treated with daunorubicin at a dose exceeding the originally used 45 mg/m^2. The ECOG 1900 study randomized patients to 45 mg/m^2 per day of daunorubicin for 3 days versus 90 mg/m^2 for 3 days and found for most subgroups (and even those with high white counts or FLT3 ITD with longer follow-up)[155] that the higher dose resulted in prolonged survival. A study in older adults in Europe with a similar design also suggested that a dose of 90 mg/m^2 per day was better than 45 mg/m^2 at least in those between 60 and 65 years of age.[156] A report from a study conducted in the United Kingdom suggested that 60 mg was equally efficient as 90 mg/m^2.[157] As noted, most studies that have added drugs to the 3 + 7 backbone or substitute HIDAC for standard continuous infusion ara-C in 3 + 7 have not led to an increased OS. However, the Polish Acute Leukemia Study Group showed that the addition of cladrabine to anthracycline/cytarabine was superior to 3 + 7[158]; however, the CR rate in the control group in these younger adults was lower than expected and these results need to be confirmed by additional studies. Continuous infusion of HIDAC and idarubicin has led to favorable results in nonrandomized phase 2 studies at the MD Anderson Cancer Center.[159] Addition of CCNU to the 3 + 7 regimen benefited older adults in a French trial.[160] The FLAG IDA regimen, while quite intensive and toxic, led to a high remission rate and disease-free survival rate.[161] Another agent that could potentially be added to a 3 + 7-type backbone is gemtuzumab ozogamicin (GO), an antibody toxin conjugate directed against the CD33 antigen expressed on blasts from most patients with AML and which was initially approved as a single-agent treatment for older adults with relapsed AML[162] and then withdrawn after randomized trials comparing standard initial induction treatment with or without the addition of GO showed marginal benefit and/or equivocal results.[163] However, trials in France[164] and the United Kingdom[165] have suggested that the addition of relatively small

doses of GO to standard chemotherapy may have a benefit in patients up to age 70 with AML. The drug has still not reentered the market until the time of this writing; confirmatory trials in North America will likely be required to show that it is worth using this drug routinely, although results in those with favorable chromosomal abnormalities are encouraging.[166]

Approach to the older patient and other poor prognostic subgroups

Is it worth administering cytotoxic chemotherapy with a 3 + 7 induction approach to patients who have little chance for long-term benefit? This is still a subject of major debate and controversy relevant to the care of AML patients older than 60–65 years of age and some selected younger patients whose prognosis is very poor based on monosomal karyotype[54] or p53 mutations[17] if known at the time of diagnosis. For younger adults with known adverse prognostic features, there seems to be little recourse at the moment to using a 3 + 7 regimen or similar induction approach followed by postremission therapy followed by allogeneic stem cell transplant if possible. If a sibling donor, matched unrelated donor, or "favorable" partially mismatched unrelated donor is not available, then strong consideration should be made for haploidentical or umbilical cord blood stem cell transplantation (SCT) in these cases. The degree of chemotherapeutic resistance is profound in such cases and the results with allogeneic transplant remain relatively poor, but still may offer a slightly better outcome than[17] a chemotherapy-based postremission approach.

It is possible that some older adults will be better served by using a lower-dose chemotherapy approach to initial therapy than a standard 3 + 7 regimen. For a standard chemotherapy, the daunorubicin dose should be $\geq 60 \text{ mg/m}^2$ in virtually all patients. On the contrary, particularly when adverse prognostic factors are present, at times it may be reasonable to consider lower-dose chemotherapy with drugs such as the hypomethylating agents, azacitidine or decitabine, or in clinical trials, with the slightly more toxic single agent, clofarabine. Although there are many prognostic algorithms for older adults, features that are generally considered to decrease the likelihood of good outcome with 3 + 7-based chemotherapy are those that were used in the clofarabine phase II[167] trial, including age > 70 years, antecedent hematological abnormality, comorbid diseases, nonfavorable cytogenetics. A phase 2 trial using 30 mg/m^2 of clofarabine for 5 days produced a 35% CR rate with a 10% rate of toxic death. In part because of difficulties in defining a group of patients "unfit for intensive therapy," this trial did not result in the Food and Drug Administration (FDA) approval and clofarabine is being evaluated in a large ECOG-led phase III trial comparing clofarabine to 3 + 7 in this age-group.

In Europe, low-dose ara-C is another frequently used option for patients who are deemed not fit or at least "inappropriate" for standard induction chemotherapy. Low-dose ara-C seems to be slightly better than hydrea,[168] but is used little in the United States. Two important trials have compared hypomethylating agent to other therapies for older adults with AML. One such trial compared decitabine to low-dose ara-C or supportive care and yielded a 25% CR rate.[169] Although decitabine is approved for an initial therapy for older AML patients in Europe, it is not approved in the United States, primarily because the pivotal trial did not meet its primary end point of extending OS. A trial reported in preliminary form comparing 5-azacitidine to conventional care regimens for AML patients whose white count was less than 15,000/µL again did not meet its primary end point, but certainly suggested that 5-azacitidine was a viable alternative to low-dose ara-C or supportive care.[170] It should be emphasized, however, that the CR rates are much lower with hypomethylating agents and low-dose ara-C than with standard chemotherapy, and that the less-intensive treatments have largely been evaluated only in patients with less-proliferative forms of AML with the likelihood that results would be even poorer than summarized, should these treatments be used in patients with high circulating blast counts or a high marrow blast infiltration; as such induction with a 3 + 7-based regimen ideally in the context of a clinical trial should be the default therapy for the relatively fit older adult under approximately 75 years of age.

Patients to be treated with a hypomethylating agent should probably be managed in the same manner as those with MDS receiving such agents. The patient should continue to receive the hypomethylating agent every 4–6 weeks until toxicity or obvious progression occurs. It certainly seems that prolonged exposure to these agents is an important factor in achieving relatively good long-term results. If a patient does achieve a very good outcome such as a CR rate in response to a hypomethylating agent, then the older adult in question, if under approximately 75 years of age, could yet be considered for a nonmyeloablative allogeneic transplant.[171] This usually occurs only in people who elect or are given aggressive chemotherapy, but this is nonetheless a consideration even in those who receive a less-intensive chemotherapy.[172]

Postremission therapy

Morphologic assessments of CR are subjective and relatively insensitive. A better quantitation of malignant cells present at the time of CR (MRD) could segregate patients into prognostic subgroups. It is estimated that as many as 10^9 leukemia cells may still be present in patients with apparent morphologic CR. Only few patients can remain in CR for 1–2 years without further treatment, but it is generally accepted that some form of therapy after CR is required to achieve long-term disease-free survival. In a trial conducted by the German Cooperative Leukemia Group, a subset of 37 patients did not receive postremission therapy for a variety of protocol and medical reasons; all of these individuals relapsed.[173] The ECOG reported a randomized study in which patients achieving CR were randomized to either no therapy, lower-dose maintenance therapy, or an intensive postremission program.[174] All of the patients in the no-treatment arm relapsed rapidly, with a median CR duration of 4 months, resulting in early termination of this arm of the trial. Similar results were noted in a smaller randomized study reported by Embury and colleagues.[175] Although timed sequential therapy, in which patients receive additional chemotherapy during the early postinduction recovery phase, has been associated with prolonged remissions in the absence of postremission chemotherapy,[176,177] this treatment regimen is more analogous to consolidation therapy. Thus, it remains a standard practice to administer chemotherapy with or without subsequent SCT after remission is achieved with conventional regimens.

Younger adults are generally treated with curative intent and should receive postremission chemotherapy that includes intensive (or myelosuppressive) "consolidation" chemotherapy and/or SCT. The term "maintenance" is generally referred to lower-dose outpatient therapy administered on an intermittent basis for months to years, patterned on the model successfully used in childhood ALL, but this approach has not been clearly found to be useful in patients with AML.

A variety of agents have been used for postremission therapy, including the agents successfully administered in initial induction, with a particular focus on HIDAC as consolidation, as well as different classes of compounds, some of which have proved activity in AML, and others of which may have had only limited activity. Because a variety of prognostic factors significantly affect

ultimate outcome, independent of the type of therapy administered, good results in small nonrandomized studies may reflect inadvertent patient selection and must ultimately be confirmed by multi-institutional applicability.

Overall, in adults, it can be expected that the administration of some sort of intensive postremission chemotherapy will result in a median CR duration of 12–18 months with approximately 20–25% of complete responders remaining as long-term disease-free survivors (Figure 10). A large review of CALGB patients who achieved CR showed a relatively constant relapse rate of 4.7% per month during the first 6 months following CR. The failure rate decreased in subsequent 6-month intervals (3.5% per month in months 7–12 and 2.4% per month in months 13–18), with a flattening of the curves after 3+ years of CR.[178] In general, patients relapsing earlier have leukemia that is more drug resistant than those who relapse late.[179] Older randomized trials of postremission therapy conducted by the CALGB failed to demonstrate long-term benefits from: (1) an alternate month compared with a monthly schedule of maintenance therapy; (2) 3 years of relatively low-dose maintenance therapy compared with 8 months of a similar program (indeed, there was a modest survival advantage for patients randomized to stop therapy after 8 months); (3) doubling of the dose of ara-C from 100 to 200 mg/m² during maintenance therapy; and (4) addition of nonspecific immunotherapy in the form of methanol-extractable residue of Bacille Calinette Grain (MER) to maintenance therapy. With regard to the role of maintenance chemotherapy, an older ECOG study demonstrated no benefit from the addition of 2 years of maintenance therapy following two courses of postremission treatment with DAT (daunorubicin, ara-C, thioguanine).[180] Studies from Germany reported by Buchner et al.[181,182] suggested a modest prolongation of CR duration when long-term maintenance therapy was administered after a single course of postremission DAT, although with a questionable effect on long-term survival. There was less effect of maintenance in later studies when more intensive postremission consolidation was used before the maintenance.[181,182]

Two important randomized trials have shown that HIDAC in the postremission setting is better than lower doses of the drug in younger patients. In an ECOG study, patients randomized to receive one course of very intensive postremission consolidation with a HIDAC-type regimen had a longer median duration of remission than patients receiving 2 years of lower-dose maintenance therapy.[183] The CALGB randomized 596 AML patients in CR to receive four courses of ara-C administered at three different dose levels [100 mg/m² by continuous intravenous infusion (CIV) for 5 days, 400 mg/m² CIV for 5 days, and 3 g/m² IV for 3 h q12h on days 1, 3, and 5 (total six doses/course)]. There was no benefit from the higher-dose arms in patients >60 years of age with a median duration of CR of approximately 13 months and with only 10–12% long-term disease-free survival.[184] In addition, there was a substantial incidence of CNS neurotoxicity in older patients, manifested primarily as cerebellar dysfunction. Other studies have also failed to show a benefit for higher doses of ara-C in older patients.[185] By contrast, patients <60 years of age benefited substantially from the HIDAC regimen in terms of both relapse-free and OS. The long-term results in patients <40 years of age were similar to those reported with autologous or allogeneic bone marrow transplant (BMT).

These studies strongly support the use of HIDAC-based consolidation programs in younger patients with AML. It is not known how many courses of such therapy are needed, the optimal dose and schedule of HIDAC, and whether the addition of other active agents will improve on these results. It is likely that ara-C incorporated into DNA is maximal at $1-1.5$ g/m^2 per dose and a recently completed randomized study from the United Kingdom has shown identical OS when doses of 1.5 g/m^2 were compared with the original CALGB doses of 3 g/m^2.[186] In another randomized study, the use of other potentially noncross-resistant regimens substituted for HIDAC was not superior to three cycles of HIDAC[187] and studies from the Medical Research Council (MRC) in Britain, which used multiple postremission courses using a variety of different drugs, produced similar overall outcomes.[188,189] The CALGB data suggest that the benefit from HIDAC was most pronounced in patients with favorable cytogenetic findings [t(8;21) and inv (16)] with much less effect in patients with unfavorable karyotypes typically associated with drug resistance.[77] If a chemotherapy-based approach is medically feasible, most clinicians attempt to administer at least three courses of reasonably intensive HIDAC-based therapy postremission regimens. As allogeneic SCT is currently becoming more commonly used, HIDAC-based postremission therapy has been reserved most appropriately for younger patients with inv16, t(8;21) or those with normal cytogenetics with an NPM1 mutation but no FLT3 ITD mutations.[9]

The decision about the type of postremission therapy must consider the patient's medical condition and the possible persistence of infection (particularly with fungal organisms) acquired during induction, as well as the ability to provide adequate platelet transfusion therapy, in an attempt to balance the risk of intensive postremission approaches with the potential benefit. Depending on the intensity of the consolidation program, a 5% mortality rate in CR is to be expected and must be carefully explained to the patient, although the use of myeloid growth factors after consolidation can appreciably shorten the duration of severe neutropenia and potentially make the administration of this therapy safer.[190,191]

An alternative way to administer high-dose chemotherapy in AML is autologous SCT. Cryopreserved autologous bone marrow can rapidly reconstitute recipients of ablative regimens, although marrow recovery may be delayed compared with allogeneic BMT.[192] Experience using cytokine-mobilized peripheral blood stem cells (PBSCs) indicates that the durations of neutropenia and particularly thrombocytopenia are shortened compared with the use of bone marrow.[193] The autologous procedure is well tolerated and can be readily used in patients up to 65 years of age and perhaps older. The major disadvantages include the absence of a graft-versus-leukemia effect, as well as concern that viable leukemic progenitors will be administered with the autologous stem cells. A number of purging techniques have been used including monoclonal antibodies directed against myeloid blasts, as well as incubation with high concentrations of cytotoxic agents[192] that rather remarkably spare hematopoietic progenitors, although delayed marrow reconstitution is not uncommon.[193] It is unknown whether these in vitro manipulations are beneficial. When unpurged autologous BMT was harvested after high-dose consolidation therapy, retrospective comparisons did not suggest an increased rate of relapse. A number of centers and groups have reported relapse-free survival rates >40% following autologous SCT in first CR.[194–196] Historically, syngeneic transplant experience in this situation showed relapse rates of approximately 50%, which is probably the best that can be expected with the autologous approach. Other evidence of the potential of this approach derive from reports of apparent cure rates of 20% in patients transplanted in the second and third remissions of AML.[192]

Allogeneic SCT represents an alternative major therapeutic option for postremission therapy for younger patients, and

increasingly, nonmyeloablative SCT is being considered in selected older patients. Syngeneic SCT, using identical twins as donors,[197] and allogeneic SCT using HLA-identical siblings,[198] were first evaluated in patients with advanced, refractory AML. After demonstrating an approximately 10% rate of long-term disease-free survival in this refractory group of patients and a 40–50% disease-free survival in patients in first remission receiving syngeneic transplants, studies of allogeneic transplantation in first remission AML were conducted.[199] Early small series were promising, demonstrating a low rate of relapse with most of the mortality related to complications of acute and chronic graft-versus-host disease (GVHD). With the current advances in supportive care, particularly the use of novel GVHD prophylactic and active therapies, allogeneic SCT is safer and more commonly used.[200,201]

In the 1990s several large prospective trials "genetically" assigned patients with histocompatible siblings to allogeneic BMT (usually only in those ≤45 years of age) while randomizing the others to either autologous BMT or chemotherapy.[188,202] In the first of these trials which included 422 patients <45 years of age (median 33 years), disease-free survival was similar in patients undergoing allogeneic BMT (55% projected at 4 years) and autologous BMT (48%) and superior to the chemotherapy group (30%), which received a second course of consolidation chemotherapy with intermediate-dose ara-C and m-amsacrine.[202] OS was similar, however, because many patients relapsing after chemotherapy could be successfully re-induced and then undergo SCT in second CR. Many patients did not undergo treatment as randomized, and no information was provided about responses to the three treatments in different cytogenetic risk groups.

Another similarly designed trial performed in France failed to show a benefit for either type of BMT compared with patients receiving intensive postremission chemotherapy.[203] A large study conducted in Germany failed to show a benefit from autologous transplantation given as a component of consolidation therapy. The MRC 10 trial conducted in Great Britain[188] showed that autologous BMT was beneficial. Patients who were not assigned to allogeneic BMT received three cycles of post-CR chemotherapy and were then randomized to nonpurged autologous BMT or observation. The *addition* of the autologous transplant prolonged CR duration, but there was no significant difference in OS between the two groups. Allogeneic BMT was not significantly better than autologous BMT; no modality was clearly better than another in different cytogenetic risk groups. The MRC trials were updated with an intent to treat analysis of results in patients with and without matched sibling donors.[189] Again, there was no apparent survival benefit compared with chemotherapy for patients who had available donors in whom a transplant could have been performed, and no advantage when patients with donors who were and were not transplanted were compared.

The trial conducted by the North American Intergroup[204] found that chemotherapy was at least as good as autologous or allogeneic BMT in leading to cure, based on the intent to treat analysis. As in all the other studies, many patients assigned to either modality of BMT did not receive this therapy for a variety of reasons. Some general conclusions can be drawn concerning the role of allogeneic BMT in the management of patients with AML in first CR:

1. Applicability of the technique is somewhat limited by patient age. Mortality from GVHD increases every decade. Improvements in supportive care and the increased use of reduced intensity transplants using nonmyeloablative conditioning regimens and PBSCs allow increased use of transplantation to older individuals. Early side effects are markedly decreased by the

nonablative approach, which is medically feasible in most older patients.[205] A systematic prospective study showed that because of clinical, administrative, and donor availability issues, only a small fraction of older patients in first CR can in fact proceed to transplantation.[206] Nonetheless, because the results are poor with chemotherapy in older adults and are better (at least with those who make it to transplant (35% disease-free survival) with reduced-intensity alloSCT, it is generally accepted as feasible for adults up to age 75.

2. Less than one-third of potential recipients have suitable HLA-matched family donors. Alternatives include the use of matched unrelated donors, partially mismatched family donors, haploidentical donors, or cord blood preparations. Administrative delays in identifying suitable donors remain problematic despite the availability of millions of HLA-type donors worldwide.[207] This is particularly true for patients from ethnic minority groups with less common HLA types and also indicates that there is considerable selection bias in reports of unrelated donor transplants, because some higher-risk patients relapse while awaiting for a donor to be identified. Nonetheless, with the use of molecular histocompatibility typing, the results following unrelated allogeneic transplant are equivalent to those with matching sibling transplant extending the use of allogeneic transplant for a much larger group of patients with AML in first remission.[208,209] Umbilical cord blood may offer an alternative source of stem cells for those without matched siblings or unrelated donors. The incidence of GVHD is much lower following cord blood transplants despite the fact that many of these transplants use mismatched donors. Engraftment can be delayed, however, and dosage considerations represent an issue for many adult recipients, although the use of double cord transplants has helped to address this problem.[210,211] At present, haploidentical transplantation from partially matched siblings, parents, or children is also available, and hence donors are available for almost all recipients, although the relapse rate may be higher than that with matched donor.[212]

3. Although allogeneic SCT can cure some patients with chemotherapy-resistant disease, there remains an appreciable relapse rate and at least some of the factors predictive of drug resistance and relapse after chemotherapy also apply to SCT recipients.[213,214]

4. The antileukemic effect following BMT correlates with the occurrence and severity of GVHD, presumably as a result of a graft-versus-leukemia effect. Attempts to attenuate GVHD with a variety of immunosuppressive approaches are associated with a decrease in GVHD, but also an increase in the relapse rate.[215] Selective T-cell depletion approaches and other immunologic manipulations of the graft are being evaluated in an attempt to make allogeneic SCT safer without an increased relapse risk.[216,217]

5. As many as 10–20% of surviving patients may have significant symptoms and impairment of performance status because of chronic GVHD. There is also a small increase in the frequency of secondary tumors in long-term survivors.[218]

There seems little controversy about the advisability of using a HIDAC-based postremission approach for those with CBF cytogenetic abnormalities and in using an allogeneic transplantation-based approach for those with adverse prognosis based on molecular or karyotypic findings at diagnosis. However, there still remains controversy about handling intermediate-risk patients, particularly those with normal chromosomes. Meta-analysis have suggested that in general, all patients with nonfavorable cytogenetics should fare slightly better with an SCT approach.[219–221] The only subgroup in the intermediate prognosis group for whom this is not clear-cut is those with normal cytogenetics and an NPM1 mutation but without a FLT3 ITD mutation. Survival rats of patients treated by a chemotherapy-based approach are higher, and it would be reasonable to reserve SCT for second remission for such patients as well as for those with favorable translocations.

Therapy of relapsed and refractory AML

A number of agents with clear-cut activity when used alone or in combination in patients with relapsed or refractory AML are available, including amsacrine, mitoxantrone, diaziquone, idarubicin, fludarabine, 2-chlorodeoxy-adenosine, etoposide, homoharringtonine, topotecan, carboplatin, and clofarabine. There is considerable heterogeneity among relapsed patients, and a number of factors in addition to the specific drugs used influence the outcome of treatment.[222–224] Some consistent trends are evident: (1) Response rates are uniformly low in patients with primary refractory leukemia, in those with short initial CR durations, or in those who relapsed while receiving postremission chemotherapy; (2) leukemias that evolved from a prior hematologic disorder, and patients with poor-risk cytogenetics are particularly resistant to further therapy; and (3) patients in second and subsequent relapses have a poorer prognosis than patients in their first relapse, and the durations of subsequent remissions tend to decrease progressively.

Results from the MRC in Great Britain, which prospectively followed all patients entered on an induction AML trial, are supportive of these conclusions.[224] In another study, patients whose initial remission was more than 18 months had a reinduction rate of 64% (37 of 58) compared with a 29% CR rate in 278 patients with shorter initial remissions. Furthermore, the duration of second CR was longer in the former group (8 months vs 3 months). Patient age and cytogenetic findings are also important prognostic factors, emphasizing the higher effect of patient selection on the results of reported phase II trials. In the absence of comparative trials, differing results may very well be the consequence of patient selection rather than the superiority of a particular regimen.

The type and timing of therapy for relapsed patients should be individualized. Patients with other medical problems who have had poor responses to initial therapy have a small likelihood of sustained benefit from reinduction therapy and, indeed, may have their life shortened by intensive therapy. Some of these patients can be supported for many months, with maintenance of a reasonable quality of life, with a more conservative approach using red blood cell and platelet transfusions and oral hydroxyurea to control elevated WBC counts or symptoms such as bone pain. However, there is no potential for long-term benefit. Conversely, younger patients with longer initial responses may derive prolonged benefit from intensive reinduction therapy, if a remission or at least a good response can be followed by allogeneic stem cell transplant.

Recurrence of leukemia is often detected when the patient is asymptomatic, blood counts are normal, and there is modest marrow infiltration by blasts. Although it is logical to begin reinduction therapy at the earliest sign of relapse, when tumor burden is presumably the lowest, there are no data to demonstrate the validity of this approach except possibly as preparation for subsequent SCT. The drawback of early treatment is that reinduction therapy is often unsuccessful and may result in excessive early morbidity and premature patient death, but if long-term survival is the goal (e.g., an allogeneic stem cell transplant), there is no reason to delay.

There are essentially no comparative trials providing guidance about the choice of agents to be used. The initial decision is generally between reuse of drugs that have previously been effective in a given patient, compared with the use of new drugs, some of which may be investigational. If a patient has relapsed while receiving chemotherapy, it makes little sense to use these same agents for reinduction. The oft-quoted guidance is to repeat the induction regimen if the disease-free intent is >1 year, otherwise a HIDAC-based approach ($2-3$ g/m^2 q12h for $8-12$ doses) is reasonable. There is no proven benefit of postremission chemotherapy in patients achieving second or third remissions. The drawback of postremission chemotherapy in this setting is that one is potentially depriving patients of time when they would be asymptomatic and discharged from hospital by the administration of therapy of variable toxicity, but no proven long-term efficacy.

It is unclear whether SCT should be offered at the time of initial relapse or whether patients should be reinduced and transplanted when a second remission is achieved. Unfortunately, most patients do not achieve second remission, and some develop medical problems during reinduction therapy that preclude subsequent transplantation. Enthusiasm for transplantation in relapse derives from reports from Seattle indicating that the results of allogeneic transplantation in early relapse were equivalent to or better than those achieved in patients transplanted in second or subsequent remissions.[225] It is often a practical problem to identify patients during early relapse and to be able to refer such patients for transplantation rapidly. Nonetheless, it would probably be best to consider allogeneic transplantation for patients in early relapse if a suitable donor is available, particularly in younger patients. Similarly, allogeneic BMT can result in long-term survival in some patients with primary refractory leukemia, and it is advisable to HLA-type patients and their families at diagnosis to allow for this possibility. It is more difficult to use nonrelated donors for these purposes because of delays caused by tissue typing, identification of donors, and stem cell procurement. Currently, most transplant centers have recommended that patients in more florid relapse receive induction chemotherapy first because of poor results with SCT as primary therapy in such patients. Because many patients under 75 years of age have an allogeneic transplant in CR1, many relapses to date have occurred after such a procedure. Relapse after allogeneic SCT are particularly ominous, with a 7% chance of 2-year survival.[226] Selected patients who relapse following BMT can derive benefit from donor lymphocyte infusions[226] or a second BMT[227] and, in general, can receive and tolerate further chemotherapy. Targeted therapies, such as sorafenib in FLT3 ITD mutant AML[228,229] or immune checkpoint inhibitors,[230] produce better results in the post-SCT relapse setting.

Patients who achieve second remission after a first remission in which only chemotherapy or autologous SCT was used probably have a higher chance of long-term survival if transplanted in second remission. Hence, relapsed patients who are candidates for allogeneic transplantation should have donor searches done while they are undergoing reinduction treatment. Patients who respond to reinduction chemotherapy have also identified themselves as affected with more chemotherapy-sensitive disease with predicted better outcomes from allogeneic transplantation.

Therapy of acute promyelocytic leukemia (APL)

Treatment for APL differs substantially from that for other subtypes of AML in that the use of the so-called "differentiation therapy" is included in the former. In theory, if leukemic progenitors could be forced to undergo terminal differentiation in vivo, then the leukemic clone could lose the capacity for self-renewal and be eliminated, with fewer side effects than those occurring with intensive cytotoxic chemotherapy. With the exception of the HL-60 cell line and blasts obtained from patients with APL, it has been difficult to reproducibly induce fresh leukemia cells to differentiate in vitro.

Limited clinical trials evaluating "differentiating" therapies, including vitamin D and low-dose ara-C, produced disappointing results except for some patients with APL who derived transient benefit from treatment with cis-retinoic acid.[231] The differentiation paradigm was verified, however, by dramatic responses in patients with APL reported from China with ATRA administered orally for $30-90$ days.[232] CRs were seen in >80% of both relapsed and previously untreated individuals. Marrow aplasia did not occur and serial bone marrows showed maturation of the abnormal, hypergranulated promyelocytes.[233,234] DIC resolved promptly, with a profound reduction in the requirement for platelet transfusions following ATRA treatment. Although the hemorrhagic complications are decreased, approximately $20-30$% of patients treated with ATRA only develop significant side effects that can include fever, rapidly evolving pulmonary insufficiency, pericarditis, and pleurisy. This syndrome can occur independently of the leukocytosis frequently observed with ATRA therapy and can be fatal. Optimal management includes the prompt administration of corticosteroids at the first signs of the "ATRA" syndrome.[235,236] Resistance to ATRA eventually develops in patients treated in relapse, and virtually all patients treated with ATRA only relapse. Possible pharmacokinetic mechanisms include induction of more rapid metabolism of the ATRA and induction of cytoplasmic retinoic acid-binding protein in normal tissues that bind the ATRA, thereby decreasing the exposure of residual APL cells to the drug.[237]

Once the efficacy of ATRA in APL was recognized, much effort was made to determine the optimal way to use this agent. Trials conducted on both sides of the Atlantic showed that combinations of retinoic acid and anthracycline-based chemo are better than either agent alone both during induction and postremission therapy.[85,238] A risk score based on platelet and white counts at diagnosis derived from results in these trials, notably from successive Spanish (PETHEMA) trials, indicated that those with the poorest long-term outcome are those with a white count >10,000/μL and those with the best long-term outcomes are those with a white count <10,000/μL and platelet count >40,000/μL at the time of diagnosis.[239] Before the introduction of arsenic trioxide, the standard of care could be summarized as anthracyclines plus ATRA, followed by two to three cycles of retinoic acid plus anthracycline as consolidation. Maintenance therapy with oral antimetabolites and ATRA for approximately 1 year after completion of intensive chemotherapy was thought to add an event-free and OS benefit[238] and higher doses of ara-C were felt to be beneficial in those with high-risk disease based on a white count >10,000/μL at diagnosis.[240] Further, disease recurrence could be predicted by development of molecular evidence of disease (PML-RARα) transcripts by PCR measurement ahead of morphologic relapse.[90] Patients who could be rendered molecularly negative with additional therapy could then be salvaged with an autologous transplant,[241] whereas those who remained molecularly positive would be better served by an allogeneic transplant. Some of the late relapses were in the CNS,[242] prompting calls for routine use of prophylactic intrathecal therapy at least in those with high white count at diagnosis and in all patients in relapse after control of the coagulopathy and thrombocytopenia. There was also some question such as whether

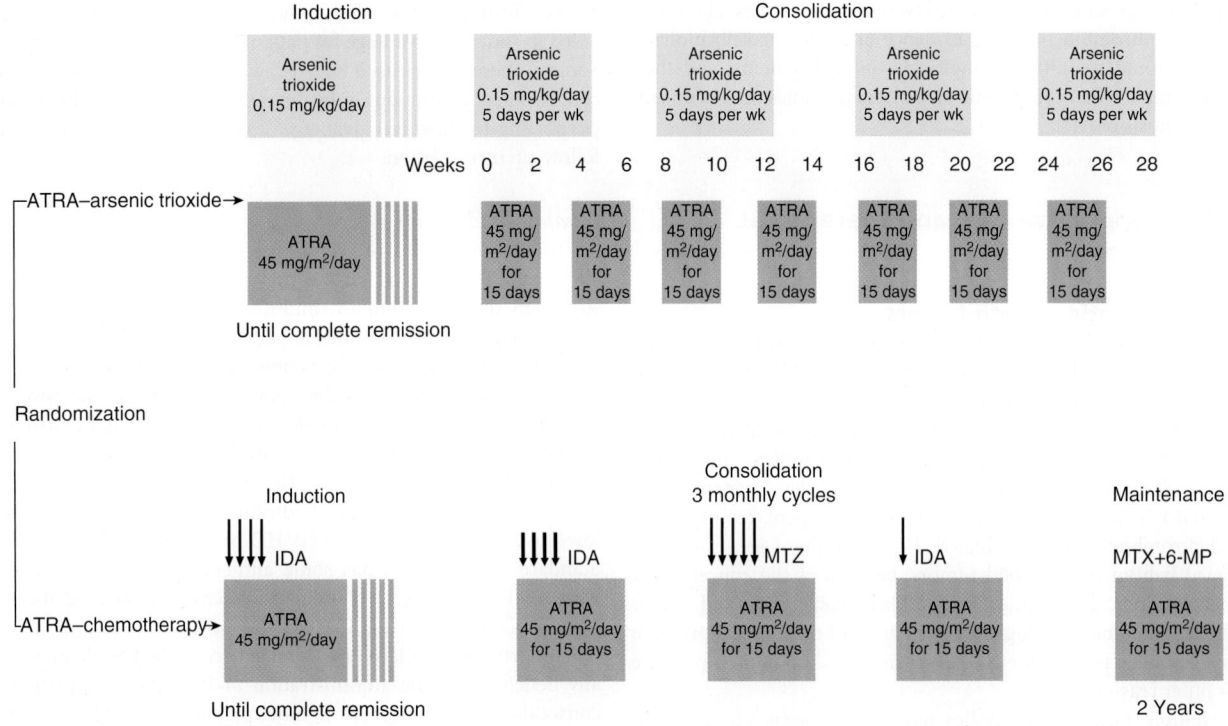

Figure 12 Treatment Groups. In the all-trans retinoic acid (ATRA) – chemotherapy group, the chemotherapy regimen was as follows: idarubicin (IDA) at a dose of $12 \, mg/m^2$ of body surface area per day on days 2, 4, 6, and 8 of the induction phase; IDA at a dose of $5 \, mg/m^2/day$ on days 1–4 of the first cycle of consolidation therapy; mitoxantrone (MTZ) at a dose of $10 \, mg/m^2/day$ on days 1–5 of the second cycle of consolidation therapy; IDA at a dose of $12 \, mg/m^2/day$ on day 1 of the third cycle of consolidation therapy; and intramuscular or oral methotrexate (MTX) at a dose of $15 \, mg/m^2/week$ and oral 6-mercaptopurine (6-MP) at a dose of $50 \, mg/m^2/day$, alternating with ATRA at a dose of $45 \, mg/m^2/day$, for 15 days every 3 months for 2 years. The vertical lines in the induction therapy boxes indicate variability in the duration of remission induction therapy. The arrows indicate the approximate timing and doses of the different chemotherapeutic agents. Source: Lo-Coco 2013.[100] Reproduced with permission of NEJM.

this intensive chemotherapy could lead to MDS and/or secondary leukemias.[243]

The demonstration, again in China, that intravenous arsenic trioxide produces a high rate of CR even in patients with advanced, multiply relapsed disease,[244] spurred a major change in our approach to APL. Although the precise mechanism of action and the explanation for its relative specificity for APL remain to be elucidated, arsenic trioxide serves to accelerate apoptotic cell death in APL.[245] Recently, tetra-arsenic tetra-sulfide has been shown to be very active in both newly diagnosed and relapsed APL patients with the advantage of oral administration.[246] While arsenic trioxide first became the standard therapy for relapsed APL, it is currently routinely used during induction and/or postremission treatment of APL. Investigators from China showed high response rates using ATRA and arsenic as initial treatment,[247] while other studies from India[248] and Iran[249] reported high molecular CR rates, which were durable using arsenic only. Using only ATRA and arsenic in patients not deemed to be candidates for anthracycline-based therapy, with GO added for patients with high WBC or insufficient response, the MD Anderson Group demonstrated a leukemia-free survival (LFS) rate as high as that observed in cooperative trials using more standard therapy.[250,251] The North American Intergroup evaluated the addition of two courses of arsenic as consolidation therapy post remission and showed a survival benefit compared with the standard treatment without arsenic.[252] Patients with high-risk disease (WBC > 10K) fared very well with this approach. Australian investigators also showed the value of a combined chemo/ATRA/arsenic approach.[253]

One of the most dramatic changes in the way we treat APL derived from a Gruppo Italiano Malattie Ematologiche Maligne dell'Adulto (GIMEMA)-led trial which compared a chemotherapy-free based approach (ATRA and arsenic trioxide given together as both induction and post remission therapy) to the aforementioned PETHEMA approach using anthracyclines and retinoic acid (Figure 12)[100] The trial was designed as a noninferiority effort and was restricted to patients <70 years of age whose white count was <10,000/μL at diagnosis. Patients assigned to the ATRA/arsenic arm had a 93% event-free and 95% OS, which was statistically superior to the outcome in patients assigned to the chemotherapy-containing arm. As such, the new standard of care for those with white count <10,000/μL at diagnosis is the regimen of ATRA and arsenic as used in the GIMEMA trial. The standard of care for those patients whose white count >10,000/μL has not yet emerged, but it is reasonable to use CALGB 9710[252] or the EORTC trial[240] approach in such patients as favorable results have been obtained with these regimens in this subgroup. The future of APL therapy certainly involves the minimal use of cytotoxic chemotherapy. It may soon be possible to cure a large majority of patients with this disease by pills, as oral formulations of arsenic trioxide may be able to replace the frequent and relatively cumbersome IV arsenic infusions.

The major remaining problem in the treatment of APL is the prevention of hemorrhagic death, often the consequence of delays in diagnosis and the initiation of therapy with ATRA. APL should be suspected in patients presenting with hemorrhagic symptoms in association with abnormalities of coagulation including hypofibrinogenemia, accompanied by seemingly modest elevations of the prothrombin time and evidence of accelerated fibrinolysis. ATRA should be initiated empirically in such patients and then discontinued when cytogenetic or molecular studies fail to confirm the diagnosis of APL.

Other supportive care and therapeutic approaches

Hematopoietic growth factors

Because of the higher myelosuppression-associated toxicity and mortality, particularly in older adults with AML, the development of hematopoietic growth factors (HGFs) ameliorated such side effects. Granulocyte-macrophage colony-stimulating factor (GM-CSF), G-CSF, and interleukin (IL)-3 as well as the thrombopoietic factors, megakaryocyte growth and development factor (MGDF), IL-11, and the newer thrombopoietic agents (romiplostim and eltrombopag) were evaluated. The use of these agents in AML lagged behind that in solid tumors, because of the concern that pharmacologic doses would lead to blast proliferation and a poor clinical outcome. Although adverse effects of this clinical problem have not been proved, the HGFs have not lived up to their promise for other reasons.

Multiple randomized studies have been completed in which older patients received an HGF or placebo following the completion of initial induction therapy, with the goal of increasing CR rate by reducing infectious complications as a consequence of shortened durations of severe myelosuppression.[254–259] All trials noted a decrease in the order of 2–5 days in the number of days of neutropenia <500/μL, sometimes in association with a smaller 1- to 2-day reduction in the duration of hospital stay, but with the exception of a smaller trial reported by the ECOG,[254] there was no significant difference in the incidence of severe infection, deaths from infections, CR rate, or survival. One randomized trial using G-CSF after induction therapy for older patients with AML showed an increased CR rate for the G-CSF recipients.[258] Unexpectedly, the infectious mortality was similar in the two groups of patients, and the reason for the increased CR rate is unclear. There was no difference in OS.

In conclusion, the benefits of growth factors administered after the completion of induction therapy are modest at best.[260] By contrast, G-CSF following intensive consolidation therapy has appreciably shortened the duration of neutropenia, albeit without improvement in CR duration or survival.[190] Because of the potential for eliminating the need for hospitalization, the use of HGF can be recommended following consolidation therapy. Smaller studies with pegylated thrombopoietin failed to show reduced needs for platelet transfusions during the induction or consolidation treatment of AML.[261] The thrombopoietin agonists romiplostim and eltrombopag, each approved in steroid-refractory ITP, have been used in clinical trials in MDS,[262,263] but evidence suggesting leukemia cell stimulation has precluded use in AML and MDS.

Although in vitro evidence suggests that HGFs can increase the cytotoxic effects of ara-C, at least in part by increasing the fraction of cells in S-phase,[264,265] clinical results with the priming strategy have been disappointing. An early study from the MD Anderson Group suggested that GM-CSF administered before and during chemotherapy produced lower response rates and survival than those observed in a historical control group treated with chemotherapy only.[266] Most subsequent studies that randomized patients to receive GM-CSF/G-CSF or no marrow stimulants,

before, during, and/or after induction chemotherapy[267–269] also failed to show an advantage for patients primed with growth factor. Some of these studies used HIDAC, whereas others evaluated more conventional continuous infusion schedules. One of the studies purporting to show an advantage[270] could not be confirmed in a follow-up investigation.

Immune modulation

A critical component of the therapeutic benefit associated with allogeneic SCT is related to the graft-versus-leukemia effect. Although this is a complex, multifactorial set of events, further studies may enable the rational application of lymphokines to stimulate the appropriate cells in patients treated with chemotherapy only. Circulating natural killer (NK) cells that can be cytotoxic to leukemia cell lines, and autologous leukemia cells in vitro, can be detected after both autologous and allogeneic transplantation, but not after chemotherapy.[271] The numbers of NK cells can be expanded by the posttransplant administration of IL-2,[272] although low-dose IL-2 can ameliorate GVHD by expanding T-reg cells.[273] Standard or high IL-2 has some antileukemic effect in patients with AML in relapse.[274,275] Pilot trials have documented the feasibility of administering IL-2 in the postchemotherapy setting, but unfortunately, a large randomized trial failed to demonstrate any benefit from the administration of IL-2 after completion of consolidation chemotherapy in older patients with AML.[276] A similar trial in younger adults documented a trend toward improved LFS and OS in patients randomized to IL-2, but many patients refused randomization or IL-2 if they are randomized to receive it.[277] Another randomized trial showed that a combination of histamine plus IL-2 was beneficial in the late postremission setting,[278] but has been criticized because of the heterogeneity of the prerandomization chemotherapy. Vaccine-based approaches using dendritic cell fusions to present leukemia-associated antigens, such as WT1 and PR1, engineered T cells, or transducing AML cells to express proteins capable of stimulating immune response, are under development.[279–282]

Circumvention of drug resistance

Drug resistance is conferred by properties of a small fraction of leukemia cells, presumably the fraction capable of efficient self-renewal.[283,284] Investigations of these leukemia "stem cells" have been hampered by difficulties in reliably and repeatedly cloning leukemic cells from individual patients to allow serial studies to be performed. In addition, a potential sampling bias exists in that the in vitro results are a reflection only of the characteristics of cells obtained at a single point in time that can grow in an artificial environment. Nonetheless, there is considerable interest in the development of drugs, which may preferentially target these cells.[285]

The multidrug resistance (MDR) phenotype is associated in most cases with increased amounts of a membrane glycoprotein (p-170), which serves as a pump accelerating the efflux of a wide variety of agents, including the anthracycline antibiotics, vincristine, taxanes, and mitoxantrone.[286] Levels of p-170 can be assessed by flow cytometric studies of individual AML cells, Western blots of cell preparations, and indirectly by mRNA levels and gene expression, and are increased in patients refractory to chemotherapy.[287,288] The MDR phenotype is most common in patients with relapsed or refractory disease, older patients, and those with other adverse prognostic factors.[289,290]

Incubation with a variety of compounds in vitro, including the calcium channel blockers verapamil, quinine, and cyclosporine A, can reverse the effect of p-170.[290] Cardiotoxicity occurs at the doses of verapamil required to produce this effect. Cyclosporine can reverse the MDR phenotype in vitro at drug levels that are likely to be clinically acceptable in terms of toxicity. A randomized trial of the addition of cyclosporin A to an ara-C plus continuous infusion daunorubicin regimen for patients with relapsed AML suggested an OS benefit for adults in the experimental arm.[291] PSC-833 is a more potent nonimmunosuppressive cyclosporine analogue, which has been evaluated in randomized trials as an adjunct to standard therapy. Unfortunately, no improvement in CR rates was observed, with some trials showing increased toxicity in the PSC833 recipients.[292,293] Because of their effects on normal tissues such as the liver and kidney, these modulators also affect the pharmacokinetics of antineoplastic agents, such that the dosage of anthracyclines or etoposide usually has to be attenuated if given with an MDR modulator.[294] Other MDR modulators have been similarly disappointing.[295]

Minimal residual disease (MRD)

A number of techniques can detect residual leukemia cells in patients with morphologic CR, including (in approximate descending order of sensitivity) conventional cytogenetics,[296] Southern blotting for known gene rearrangements, fluorescent in situ hybridization (FISH), multiparameter flow cytometry, and RT-PCR.[297,298] Serial measurement of MRD is an important component of the management of APL, chronic myelogeneous leukemia, and childhood ALL, but is not sufficiently standardized to be used routinely in patients with AML.[299] Technical problems abound, including the requirement for a known and already cloned abnormality when applying molecular techniques and the potential for changes in antigen expression over time when using immunologic monitoring. Only few large prospective studies have been conducted on this topic. Although preliminary data are compatible with the logical premise that persistence of detectable disease presages eventual relapse, false-positive and false-negative rates may be appreciable and could result in incorrect decisions about further treatment. Serial monitoring is cumbersome, and it is hoped that future studies will determine specific time points after completion of therapy when detection of MRD is prognostically significant. It is also likely that different sampling strategies will be needed for different AML subtypes. The key clinical question is whether intervention with further therapy or allogeneic SCT is valuable if applied earlier, before gross relapse. There are no prospective data addressing this issue, but retrospective studies have shown much higher-than-expected relapse rates in allogeneic transplant recipients with detectable MRD. Because of the presence of residual disease, autologous collection and high-dose therapy may be predicted to be of less value in this circumstance.

Small-molecule inhibitors and other novel approaches

While there has not been any newly approved drug in non-APL/AML for many years (not counting GO, which was approved and then withdrawn), many agents are under development. A comprehensive discussion of all such agents is beyond the scope of this chapter; however, it is worth highlighting progress in tyrosine kinase inhibitor therapy as well as a few other interesting agents in developments.

The success of imatinib and other BCR-ABL inhibitors in CML prompted a search for similar gain-of-function mutations in AML, whose inhibition could lead to therapeutic benefit.

Gain-of-function mutations in the FLT3 transmembrane tyrosine kinase occur in approximately 30% of patients with de novo AML, consisting most commonly of an ITD mutation, which elongates the juxtamembrane region by between 3 and 100 amino acids; a smaller number of patients have an activating point mutation in the tyrosine kinase domain.[7] Both types of mutations can cause ligand-independent activation[300] and a myeloproliferative disease in murine models.[301] Several so-called FLT3 inhibitors are under development, although none as of yet has been approved by the FDA. Single-agent trials with midostaurin,[302] lestaurtinib,[303] and sorafenib[304] each showed responses in patients with advanced, mutant FLT3 AML. Sorafenib is approved as a vascular endothelial growth factor receptor inhibitor in patients with advanced renal and hepatocellular carcinomas. Midostaurin can inhibit the growth of cells with a tyrosine kinase domain mutation, while most other agents (except for crenolanib)[305] cannot and are only being developed in the FLT3 population that has the ITD mutation. Quizartinib, a potent and relatively specific FLT3 ITD inhibitor, has shown a relatively high response rate as a single agent[306] and is being compared with chemotherapy in mutant FLT3 ITD patients with AML in relapse; however, an important mechanism of resistance is the outgrowth of clones with an FLT3 TKD mutation.[307]

Given the relatively rare CR and brief duration of response with single-agent FLT3 inhibitor therapy, there has been a major thrust to develop these agents in combination with chemotherapy. A trial testing the addition of lestaurtinib to chemotherapy in relapsed mutant FLT3 ITD patients was negative,[308] but several other clinical trials comparing chemotherapy with or without an FLT3 inhibitor are underway. Moreover, FLT3 inhibitors, particularly sorafenib, seem to be effective in some patients with mutant FLT3 AML who have relapsed after allogeneic stem cell transplant.[228,229]

Given that a sizable minority of patients with favorable chromosome (the so-called CBF translocations) AML have either over of c-kit and/or mutations in the c-kit tyrosine kinase, the c-kit inhibitor dasatinib has been added to chemotherapy in this cytogenetic subset of patients with AML. Preliminary results are encouraging and a randomized trial is ongoing.[309] Another gain-of-function mutation noted in approximately 20% of AML patients occur in the IDH1 or IDH2 genes whose products catalyze the neomorphic production of 2-hydroxygluterate, which epigenetically affects gene expression in a pro-leukemic manner.[310] Preliminary results with IDH1 and IHD2 inhibitors have been encouraging.[311] MEK pathway inhibitors in patients with activating mutation of the RAS oncogene[12] have also led to responses.

In addition to these genomically based therapies, there are a host of other agents under development, which take advantage of potential biologic differences between AML cells and normal stem cells. AML cells in the marrow niche have their survival promoted by factors elaborated by endothelial and other cells in the marrow stroma.[312] Drugs such as the CXCR4 inhibitor, plerixafor, may disrupt the survival signals making AML cells more amenable to killing via cytotoxic agents.[313] ABT199 is a BCL2 inhibitor with significant advantage in CLL,[314] and it may be used alone or in combination with chemotherapy to promote apoptosis in AML cells. Another agent in development is KPT330, a nuclear export protein inhibitor, which works primarily by preventing expulsion of tumor suppressor genes from the nucleus of cancer cells in general, and in AML cells in particular.[315] There are several antibodies and immunoconjugates targeting CD123,[316] believed to be specifically expressed on leukemic stem cells. The developmental pathway for any agent in AML is slightly daunting as it has to be determined if it is going to be useful as a single agent in advanced patients and whether it needs to be added in chemotherapy in patients in earlier stages of the disease. In the latter case, given the relatively high initial response rate to chemotherapy in patients, large trials or trials with a novel design are needed.

Complications

Hyperleukocytosis

Leukemic blasts are considerably less deformable than mature myeloid cells[317] and are "stickier" than lymphoblasts because of the expression of cell surface adhesion molecules. With increasing blast counts, usually at levels >100,000/μL in the myeloid leukemias, blood flow in the microcirculation can be impeded by plugs of these more rigid cells. Local hypoxemia may be exacerbated by the high metabolic activity of the dividing blasts, with endothelial damage and hemorrhage. Red blood cell transfusions can potentially further increase the blood viscosity and make the situation worse and should be either withheld or administered slowly, until the WBC decreases. Coagulation abnormalities, including DIC, further increase the risk of local hemorrhage. Liberal use of platelet transfusions is recommended, particularly because the platelet count is frequently overestimated because of the presence of fragments of blasts on blood smears, which can be mistakenly counted as platelets by automated blood cell counters.[318]

Although pathologic evidence of leukostasis can be found in most organs in patients with extremely high blast cell counts, clinical symptomatology is usually related to CNS and pulmonary involvement.[319,320] Occasionally, dyspnea with worsening hypoxemia can occur following therapy and lysis of trapped leukemic cells. Spurious elevation of serum potassium can occur because of the release from WBCs during clotting, and it is sometimes necessary to measure potassium levels on heparinized plasma. Similarly, pO_2 can appear falsely decreased because of the enhanced metabolic activity of the WBCs, even when the specimen is appropriately placed on ice during transport to the laboratory. Pulse oximetry provides an accurate assessment of O_2 saturation in such circumstances. Hyperleukocytosis is more common in patients with myelomonocytic or monocytic leukemia, and it is possible that the clinical manifestations are exacerbated by the migration of leukemic promonocytes into tissue where further proliferation occurs.

The initial mortality rate for patients with AML and symptomatic hyperleukocytosis is high.[320] If patients survive the initial period, they tend to have somewhat lower remission rates and shorter CR durations. Symptomatic hyperleukocytosis in AML (and rarely in ALL) constitutes a medical emergency, and effort should be made to lower the WBC count rapidly. In most patients, rapid cytoreduction can be achieved by chemotherapy, with either standard induction agents or high doses of hydroxyurea ($3 g/m^2$/day). Some centers also advocate low-dose cranial irradiation, including the retina, to prevent further proliferation of leukemic cells in CNS sites, where drug delivery may theoretically be compromised. This treatment is well tolerated, although there are no comparative studies to determine whether the results are superior to chemotherapy only.

In some patients, it is impossible to initiate chemotherapy immediately because of renal insufficiency, metabolic problems, delays in initiating allopurinol therapy to prevent hyperuricemia, or similar considerations. In such patients, emergency leukapheresis has been used to lower or stabilize the white count.[321,322] Although intensive leukapheresis, with procedure times often lasting many hours, can improve pulmonary and CNS symptomatology, there are theoretic and practical limitations to its benefits. It is difficult, for example, for leukapheresis to affect already established

vascular plugs, particularly if vascular invasion has taken place. In such cases, chemotherapy is the primary modality, although theoretically, leukapheresis could decrease further accumulation of leukocytes at these sites. Furthermore, it is precisely the patient in whom leukostasis is most likely to occur, that is, the patient with high and rapidly rising blasts counts, in whom the technical limitations of leukapheresis are apparent, in that it is often difficult, even with highly efficient cell separators, to reduce the rising count. In such patients with a high proliferative thrust, cycle-specific chemotherapeutic agents are more likely to be most immediately effective. Leukapheresis is also of modest benefit to patients who develop pulmonary problems during cytotoxic treatment, because in some such patients, the symptoms are related at least in part to a local inflammatory response following leukocyte lysis.[323]

Central nervous system leukemia

Involvement of the CNS is considerably less common in patients with AML than in both adults and children with ALL. Most clinicians imply that the incidence has decreased even further in recent years, perhaps because of the use of higher doses of ara-C, which can penetrate into the CNS. The incidence of CNS leukemia has been <5% in large AML clinical trials in recent years.[324] Therefore, diagnostic lumbar punctures are not routinely indicated in the absence of CNS symptoms, and chemotherapy regimens do not include CNS prophylaxis. Symptoms are consequences of increased intracranial pressure and usually consist of a constant headache, sometimes associated with lethargy or other mental changes. Cranial nerve signs (most commonly cranial nerves III or VI) and, occasionally, peripheral nerve manifestations are secondary to nerve root involvement and can be accompanied by headaches or occur alone.[325]

The diagnosis is usually suspected clinically and/or by meningeal enhancement on MRI with gadolinium and confirmed by examination of cytocentrifuge preparations of cerebrospinal fluid (CSF) after lumbar puncture. Cell counts can vary from as few as 5 to >1000/μL. Most patients have moderate elevations in CSF protein with a moderate decrease in glucose. Treatment consists of the administration of intrathecal chemotherapy, with the addition of cranial radiation (usually 2400 cGy), to patients who do not respond fully to chemotherapy or in whom cranial nerve involvement is present.[325] Either methotrexate (15 mg/dose when administered by lumbar puncture) or ara-C (50 mg/dose) can be used as initial therapy, with a crossover to the other agent in the event of refractoriness or relapse. A typical schedule includes treatment twice to thrice a week until the CSF has cleared, generally occurring after a few injections. Treatment is then given at weekly intervals for two more doses to be followed by monthly administration for 1 year. An Ommaya reservoir to permit intraventricular drug administration is frequently needed because of either difficulties in performing repeated lumbar punctures or concern that in some individuals, the CSF flow does not deliver sufficient amounts of the drug from the lumbar space to the entire CNS.[326] Successful therapies with systemically administered agents that penetrate the CNS, such as diaziquone (AZQ), high-dose methotrexate, or HIDAC, have also been reported.[327] Slow-release (depo) preparations of ara-C may be an alternative.[328] Unfortunately, the relapse rate is high, either concomitantly with bone marrow relapse or independently, even after initial successful therapy.

It has been suggested that the incidence of CNS leukemia is higher in patients with FAB M4 E0 morphology and possibly in patients with monocytic leukemia and high circulating blast counts.[329] This may no longer be the case using more contemporary treatment regimens, and prophylactic therapy is not indicated in such individuals. As noted, CNS involvement can occur in patients with APL with high white blood count.

Ophthalmic complications

Essentially every ocular structure can be involved in the leukemias, sometimes dominating the clinical picture in the prechemotherapy era.[330] Leukemia cells can infiltrate the conjunctiva and lacrimal glands, producing obvious masses that may require treatment with radiation therapy. Involvement of the choroid and retina is most common, however. A prospective study of 53 newly diagnosed adults with AML documented retinal or optic nerve abnormalities in 64% of patients.[331] Hemorrhage and cotton wool spots (a consequence of nerve fiber ischemia) were most frequent, and the occurrence of these findings was unrelated to patient age, FAB type, WBC count, or hematocrit. Initial platelet counts were lower in patients with retinopathy. A total of 10 patients had decreased visual acuity, including five with macular hemorrhages. It was felt that many of the cotton wool spots were either a consequence of or exacerbated by ischemia due to anemia. Definite leukemic infiltrate of the retina could not be confirmed. All patients received aggressive chemotherapy and platelet transfusion support; no patient received cranial or ocular irradiation. All ocular findings resolved in patients achieving CR and there was no residual visual deficit in any patient. Infectious ocular problems were not noted and seem to be uncommon, perhaps because the prompt empiric use of antibacterial and antifungal antibiotics has decreased the possibility of hematogenous spread of infections to the eye.

Pregnancy

AML is occasionally diagnosed in pregnancy, either because of clinical manifestations or as an incidental finding during blood count checks. If detected during the first trimester, termination of pregnancy followed by treatment of the leukemia is advisable. The management of patients diagnosed later in pregnancy, such as late in the second trimester or during the third trimester, is more problematic. If the leukemia is relatively indolent, it is sometimes possible to manage patients conservatively with leukapheresis and/or transfusion with induction of labor and delivery of the fetus as soon as possible.[332] There have also been many reports of patients treated with chemotherapy later in their pregnancy.[333,334] The majority of these women have not aborted, and there has been no report of leukemia occurring in children or an increased incidence of abnormalities in infants.

Metabolic abnormalities

Patients receiving therapy for AML can experience a wide range of metabolic problems such as vomiting, diarrhea, impaired nutrition, or renal dysfunction, usually because of side effects from antibiotics, particularly amphotericin B. Some metabolic disorders are related to the leukemic process itself. Hyperuricemia, occasionally accompanied by urate nephropathy with renal insufficiency, is the most frequent metabolic accompaniment of AML. All patients should receive allopurinol ($\geq$300 mg/day) as soon as the acute leukemia is diagnosed, so that chemotherapy can be administered once it is medically appropriate. In most patients, urate nephropathy can be avoided or ameliorated with vigorous hydration and urinary alkalization with systemic or oral administration of sodium bicarbonate. Allopurinol can usually be discontinued within 1 or 2 days after chemotherapy is completed. In occasional patients with markedly elevated levels of uric acid, the use of recombinant urate oxidase, which can rapidly lower levels within a few hours, may be advisable.[335] A single dose is almost always sufficient, and the

decision about subsequent doses depends on serial monitoring of uric acid.[336]

Tumor lysis syndrome occurs more frequently in patients with ALL, although some AML patients experience hyperphosphatemia, hypocalcemia, hyperkalemia, and renal insufficiency because of massive leukemic cell death. The inciting cause seems to be the release of large amounts of phosphate from lysed blasts, which coprecipitates with calcium in the kidneys, leading to hypocalcemia and sometimes to oliguric renal failure. Hyperuricemia further contributes to this problem, which is usually self-limited and responds to judicious hydration.

Despite markedly hypercellular marrows, hypercalcemia is extremely unusual in patients with AML. Severe, occasionally symptomatic, hypokalemia is frequent, particularly in patients with monocytic leukemias. The mechanism appears to be renal potassium loss because of tubular damage induced by the high levels of lysozyme often noted in these patients. Aggressive replacement with parenteral potassium is required; the syndrome usually abates after cytoreduction by chemotherapy. Finally, rare patients have been described in whom lactic acidosis has been a constant metabolic accompaniment of the leukemia both at the time of presentation and relapse.[337] The mechanism is unclear, although anaerobic metabolism by the leukemia cells at sites of leukostasis has been postulated.

Summary

Largely because of improvements in supportive care and the anticipatory management of complications of the treatment and underlying disease, the overall outlook for adults <60 years of age with AML has improved worldwide. It is equally clear, however, that results have leveled off and that new approaches are needed to increase the fraction of patients cured. Dramatic advances in molecular genetics offer promise both because of increased understanding of leukemia biology and the production of small molecules, monoclonal antibodies, cytokines, and HGF with potential clinical utility. Further clarification of mechanisms of drug resistance with the possibility of enhancement of the effectiveness of currently available drugs is also an exciting and achievable prospect. These strategies, as well as clinical trials designed to assess the appropriate use of SCT and newer more specifically targeted drugs, determine that therapy for AML will be both more successful and less empiric in the future.

Mast cell leukemia and other mast cell neoplasms

Mast cell disorders are classified among the myeloproliferative diseases and produce a wide spectrum of clinical findings, ranging from reactive benign syndromes with cutaneous involvement to malignant variants with mast cell infiltration of multiple organs, including the bone marrow.[338,339]

Reactive mast cell hyperplasia

Mast cell hyperplasia frequently occurs in tissues involved in immediate or delayed-type hypersensitivity reactions, such as in the nasal mucosa during allergic rhinitis. Increased numbers of mast cells in the bone marrow have been noted in association with a wide range of malignant disorders, including lymphoproliferative disorders,[340] hairy cell leukemia,[341] and myeloid neoplasms.[342,343] The mast cells in such patients appear to be reactive rather than derived from the malignant clone.

Neoplastic mast cell disease

Urticaria pigmentosa is by far the most common manifestation of neoplastic mast cell proliferation.[344] The typical eruption of urticaria pigmentosa consists of multiple discrete hyperpigmented nodulopapular lesions and portends a benign clinical course, particularly in children. Cutaneous symptoms may include the classic urticarial wheals that result from mast cell degranulation due to mechanical insult (Darier's sign), pruritus, or episodic flushing. A blurred distinction exists between cutaneous mastocytosis (CM)[345] and systemic mast cell disease (SMCD), an indolent disorder in which mast cells may also be found in extracutaneous sites. The level of serum tryptase is higher in SMCD than in CM.[346] Systemic mastocytosis may present with a variety of constitutional and/or gastrointestinal symptoms, each of which can be attributed to excessive elaboration of mast cell mediators. Such symptoms, which may also present to a lesser degree in patients with urticaria pigmentosa, include rhinitis, asthma, nausea, vomiting, diarrhea, syncope, chest pain, bone pain, and rectal discomfort.[347] The bony skeleton, the gastrointestinal tract, and the spleen can also be sites of mast cell infiltration.

Malignant mastocytosis is a more aggressive subset of SCMD characterized by a much less favorable clinical course.[347] Unlike indolent systemic mastocytosis, in which an affected patient has a normal life expectancy, survival beyond 1–2 years after diagnosis of malignant mastocytosis is uncommon. The bone marrow is always involved, eosinophilia and cytopenias are common, and adenopathy and/or organomegaly are frequently noted.[348] In the early 1990s, it was recognized that mast cells from patients with systemic mastocytosis are capable of growing independent of stimulation with C-KIT ligand, the critical mast cell growth factor.[349] Cell lines and patient samples demonstrated that the basis for this growth independence was constitutive activation of C-KIT,[350,351] most often associated with a mutation at codon 816 in the kinase domain, although mutations of the juxtamembrane region have also been described.[352] The ASP-816 VAL mutation has been detected in both B cells and monocytes from patients, suggesting that systemic mastocytosis is a clonal disorder evolving from an early hematopoietic stem cell.[352] By contrast, blasts from patients with mast cell leukemia do not have this mutation, suggesting an alternative derivation of the leukemia.[353]

Mast cell leukemia represents a rare and aggressive subtype of malignant mastocytosis characterized by the presence of large numbers of atypical mast cells in the peripheral blood.[354–356] Patients with mast cell leukemia have a median survival of <6 months, in contrast to those with the nonleukemic type of malignant mastocytosis, who tend to survive for a longer time. The majority of reported cases of mast cell leukemia arise in patients with preexisting malignant mast cell disease. Criteria required for the diagnosis of mast cell leukemia are: (1) the percentage of mast cells in the peripheral WBC differential must be ≥10%; (2) the leukemic mast cells should display features of morphologic atypia; and (3) cytochemical properties of the leukemic cells must be typical of mast cell derivation (the presence of metachromatic granules staining with chloroacetate esterase, but not with peroxidase).[355]

Although bone marrow infiltration with atypical mast cells is always present in mast cell leukemia, hematologic findings at the time of diagnosis can vary widely. A mild to moderate degree of anemia is always present; initial leukocyte count can range from normal to >50,000/μL.[355] The percentage of atypical mast cells (hypogranulated metachromatically staining cells with fragmentation, cytoplasmic tails, and multiple nuclei) may be relatively low (but >10%), but almost always increases substantially with time. Karyotypic studies in several patients with mast cell leukemia have been normal, although the lack of dividing cells for metaphase analysis frequently precludes cytogenetic evaluation. Bone marrow cells from patients with systemic mastocytosis often display cytogenetic abnormalities, such as trisomy 8 and monosomy 7/7q-, 20q-, typical of those with myeloproliferative disorders.[355,356] Particularly in patients with concomitant eosinophilia, it is important to exclude cytogenetic abnormalities affecting platelet-derived growth factor recept (PDGFR, involving chromosome 5q31-32), because such patients can benefit from treatment with imatinib.

Treatment

Treatment of mast cell neoplasms is based on the disease subtype and clinical manifestations. Patients with CM usually require no treatment. SMCD, however, has protean clinical manifestations. For example, those with hematological abnormalities may require supportive care, which could include transfusions or the empiric use of HGFs. Avoidance of mast cell stimulants such as anesthesia, alcohol, aspirin, and morphine may diminish flushing, pruritus, diarrhea, and symptoms that may be histamine-related.[357–359] H1 and H2 antihistamines or disodium chromoglycolate may offer palliative benefit. Radiation therapy may control localized disease without causing histamine release.[360]

Unfortunately, the typical ASP-816 VAL mutation is insensitive to the C-KIT inhibitors imatinib mesylate,[351,361,362] and nilotinib,[363] although in vitro studies suggest that this mutated C-KIT may be sensitive to dasatinib.[364] Preclinical data suggest that the multitargeted kinase inhibitor, PKC412 (midostaurin), may also inhibit the product of this activating mutation, and early reports suggest potential clinical activity.[365,366] Cladribine and alpha interferon exhibit cytoreductive activity in systemic mastocytosis and should be considered in patients with active systemic symptoms.[367,368] Responses are usually transient however, and subsequent therapy for those with malignant mastocytosis or frank mast cell leukemia (activating mutations of c-kit are not believed to occur in this entity) is not at all standardized, although induction therapy with an anthracycline in combination with cytarabine for patients with leukemia could be followed by consolidation with HIDAC. Allogeneic hematopoietic SCT could be considered in specific patients, although there is limited experience with this approach.

Key references

The complete reference list can be found on the Wiley Companion Digital Edition of this title (see inside front cover for login instructions).

1 Leukemia SSFSAM, 2013, www.seer.cancer.gov/statfacts/html/amyl.html (accessed 2 Apr 2016).

2 Cheson BD, Bennett JM, Kopecky KJ, et al. Revised recommendations of the International Working Group for Diagnosis, Standardization of Response Criteria, Treatment Outcomes, and Reporting Standards for Therapeutic Trials in Acute Myeloid Leukemia. *J Clin Oncol.* 2003;**21**:4642–4649.

3 Rowe JM, Tallman MS. How I treat acute myeloid leukemia. *Blood.* 2010;**116**: 3147–3156.

5 Lindsley RC, Mar BG, Mazzola E, et al. Acute myeloid leukemia ontogeny is defined by distinct somatic mutations. *Blood.* 2015;**125**(9):1367–1376.

6 Network TCaGAR. Genomic and epigenomic landscapes of adult de novo acute myeloid leukemia. *N Engl J Med.* 2013;**368**:2059–2074.

7 Kindler T, Lipka DB, Fischer T. FLT3 as a therapeutic target in AML: still challenging after all these years. *Blood.* 2010;**116**:5089–5102.

8 Marcucci G, Haferlach T, Döhner H. Molecular genetics of adult acute myeloid leukemia: prognostic and therapeutic implications. *J Clin Oncol.* 2011;**29**:475–486.

9 Schlenk RF, Dohner K, Krauter J, et al. Mutations and treatment outcome in cytogenetically normal acute myeloid leukemia. *N Engl J Med.* 2008;**358**:1909–1918.

16 Patel JP, Gönen M, Figueroa ME, et al. Prognostic relevance of integrated genetic profiling in acute myeloid leukemia. *N Engl J Med.* 2012;**366**:1079–1089.

17 Rucker FG, Schlenk RF, Bullinger L, et al. TP53 alterations in acute myeloid leukemia with complex karyotype correlate with specific copy number alterations, monosomal karyotype, and dismal outcome. *Blood*. 2012;**119**:2114–2121.

47 Ossenkoppele G, Lowenberg B. How I treat the older patient with acute myeloid leukemia. *Blood*. 2015;**125**:767–774.

48 Hurria A, Lachs MS, Cohen HJ, et al. Geriatric assessment for oncologists: rationale and future directions. *Crit Rev Oncol Hematol*. 2006;**59**:211–217.

50 Frohling S, Schlenk RF, Kayser S, et al. Cytogenetics and age are major determinants of outcome in intensively treated acute myeloid leukemia patients older than 60 years: results from AMLSG trial AML HD98-B. *Blood*. 2006;**108**:3280–3288.

51 Grimwade D, Hills RK, Moorman AV, et al. Refinement of cytogenetic classification in acute myeloid leukemia: determination of prognostic significance of rare recurring chromosomal abnormalities among 5876 younger adult patients treated in the United Kingdom Medical Research Council trials. *Blood*. 2010;**116**:354–365.

54 Slovak ML, Kopecky KJ, Cassileth PA, et al. Karyotypic analysis predicts outcome of preremission and postremission therapy in adult acute myeloid leukemia: a Southwest Oncology Group/Eastern Cooperative Oncology Group Study. *Blood*. 2000;**96**:4075–4083.

62 Vardiman JW, Thiele J, Arber DA, et al. The 2016 revision of the World Health Organization (WHO) classification of myeloid neoplasms and acute leukemia: rationale and important changes. *Blood*. 2009;**114**:937–951.

78 Cairoli R, Beghini A, Grillo G, et al. Prognostic impact of c-KIT mutations in core binding factor leukemias: an Italian retrospective study. *Blood*. 2006;**107**:3463–3468.

100 Lo-Coco F, Avvisati G, Vignetti M, et al. Retinoic acid and arsenic trioxide for acute promyelocytic leukemia. *N Engl J Med*. 2013;**369**:111–121.

133 Dohner H, Estey EH, Amadori S, et al. Diagnosis and management of acute myeloid leukemia in adults: recommendations from an international expert panel, on behalf of the European LeukemiaNet. *Blood*. 2010;**115**:453–474.

157 Burnett AK, Russell N, Hills RK, et al. A randomised comparison of daunorubicin 90 mg/m^2 Vs 60 mg/m^2 in AML induction: results from the UK NCRI AML17 trial in 1206 patients. *Blood*. 2014;**124**:7.

158 Holowiecki J, Grosicki S, Giebel S, et al. Cladribine, but not fludarabine, added to daunorubicin and cytarabine during induction prolongs survival of patients with acute myeloid leukemia: a multicenter, Randomized Phase III Study. *J Clin Oncol*. 2012;**30**:2441–2448.

161 Burnett AK, Russell NH, Hills RK, et al. Optimization of chemotherapy for younger patients with acute myeloid leukemia: results of the medical research council AML15 trial. *J Clin Oncol*. 2013;**31**:3360–3368.

164 Castaigne S, Pautas C, Terré C, et al. Effect of gemtuzumab ozogamicin on survival of adult patients with de-novo acute myeloid leukaemia (ALFA-0701): a randomised, open-label, phase 3 study. *Lancet*. 2012;**379**:1508–1516.

165 Burnett AK, Russell NH, Hills RK, et al. Addition of gemtuzumab ozogamicin to induction chemotherapy improves survival in older patients with acute myeloid leukemia. *J Clin Oncol*. 2012;**30**:3924–3931.

166 Rowe JM, Lowenberg B. Gemtuzumab ozogamicin in acute myeloid leukemia: a remarkable saga about an active drug. *Blood*. 2013;**121**:4838–4841.

179 Breems DA, Van Putten WL, Huijgens PC, et al. Prognostic index for adult patients with acute myeloid leukemia in first relapse. *J Clin Oncol*. 2005;**23**:1969–1978.

183 Cassileth PA, Lynch E, Hines J, et al. Varying intensity of postremission therapy in acute myeloid leukemia. *Blood*. 1992;**79**:1924–1930.

184 Mayer RJ, Davis RB, Schiffer CA, et al. Intensive postremission chemotherapy in adults with acute myeloid leukemia. Cancer and Leukemia Group B. *N Engl J Med*. 1994;**331**:896–903.

202 Zittoun RA, Mandelli F, Willemze R, et al. Autologous or allogeneic bone marrow transplantation compared with intensive chemotherapy in acute myelogenous leukemia. European Organization for Research and Treatment of Cancer (EORTC) and the Gruppo Italiano Malattie Ematologiche Maligne dell'Adulto (GIMEMA) Leukemia Cooperative Groups. *N Engl J Med*. 1995;**332**:217–223.

206 Estey E, de Lima M, Tibes R, et al. Prospective feasibility analysis of reduced-intensity conditioning (RIC) regimens for hematopoietic stem cell transplantation (HSCT) in elderly patients with acute myeloid leukemia (AML) and high-risk myelodysplastic syndrome (MDS). *Blood*. 2007;**109**:1395–1400.

219 Koreth J, Schlenk R, Kopecky KJ, et al. Allogeneic stem cell transplantation for acute myeloid leukemia in first complete remission: systematic review and meta-analysis of prospective clinical trials. *JAMA*. 2009;**301**:2349–2361.

221 Stelljes M, Krug U, Beelen DW, et al. Allogeneic transplantation versus chemotherapy as postremission therapy for acute myeloid leukemia: a prospective matched pairs analysis. *J Clin Oncol*. 2014;**32**:288–296.

226 Schmid C, Labopin M, Nagler A, et al. Donor lymphocyte infusion in the treatment of first hematological relapse after allogeneic stem-cell transplantation in adults with acute myeloid leukemia: a retrospective risk factors analysis and comparison with other strategies by the EBMT Acute Leukemia Working Party. *J Clin Oncol*. 2007;**25**:4938–4945.

240 Ades L, Sanz MA, Chevret S, et al. Treatment of newly diagnosed acute promyelocytic leukemia (APL): a comparison of French-Belgian-Swiss and PETHEMA results. *Blood*. 2008;**111**:1078–1084.

252 Powell BL, Moser B, Stock W, et al. Arsenic trioxide improves event-free and overall survival for adults with acute promyelocytic leukemia: North American Leukemia Intergroup Study C9710. *Blood*. 2010;**116**:3751–3757.

260 Schiffer CA. Hematopoietic growth factors as adjuncts to the treatment of acute myeloid leukemia. *Blood*. 1996;**88**:3675–3685.

289 Leith CP, Kopecky KJ, Godwin J, et al. Acute myeloid leukemia in the elderly: assessment of multidrug resistance (MDR1) and cytogenetics distinguishes biologic subgroups with remarkably distinct responses to standard chemotherapy. A Southwest Oncology Group study. *Blood*. 1997;**89**:3323–3329.

316 Mardiros A, Dos Santos C, McDonald T, et al. T cells expressing CD123-specific chimeric antigen receptors exhibit specific cytolytic effector functions and antitumor effects against human acute myeloid leukemia. *Blood*. 2013;**122**:3138–3148.

322 Röllig C, Ehninger G. How I treat hyperleukocytosis in acute myeloid leukemia. *Blood*. 2015;**125**:3246–3252.

354 Bain BJ. Systemic mastocytosis and other mast cell neoplasms. *Br J Haematol*. 1999;**106**:9–17.

365 Gotlib J, Berube C, Growney JD, et al. Activity of the tyrosine kinase inhibitor PKC412 in a patient with mast cell leukemia with the D816V KIT mutation. *Blood*. 2005;**106**:2865–2870.

115 Chronic myeloid leukemia

Jorge Cortes, MD ▪ Richard T. Silver, MD ▪ Hagop M. Kantarjian, MD

Overview

Chronic myeloid leukemia (CML) was the first malignancy where a unique chromosomal abnormality, the Philadelphia chromosome, was directly linked to it. The further unraveling of the molecular and physiologic consequences of this abnormality, with a fusion gene (BCR-ABL) translating into a chimeric protein with increased tyrosine kinase activity, led to the development of specific tyrosine kinase inhibitors. The use of such agents as initial therapy has resulted in a dramatic change in the natural history of the disease where patients properly managed are expected to have a life expectancy similar to that of the general population. Several treatment options are also available for patients who may not have optimal response to their initial therapy. Current research is focusing on approaches that may increase the probability of successful treatment discontinuation for more patients.

Chronic myeloid leukemia (CML) is a myoproliferative neoplasm affecting a pluripotent progenitor and involving myeloid, erythroid, megakaryocytic, B, and sometimes T, lymphoid cells, but not marrow fibroblasts. It is characterized by the presence of a unique chromosomal abnormality, the Philadelphia chromosome (Ph).

Historical perspective

In 1960, a minute chromosome was identified in patients with CML, an abnormality later identified as a balanced translocation between chromosomes 9 and 22.[1,2] Later studies demonstrated that this translocation resulted in the creation of a chimeric gene, BCR-ABL, that when transfected into mice can induce CML.[3] Translation of this chimeric gene results in a fusion protein with constitutive tyrosine kinase activity.[4] Interferon-alpha was the first therapy to induce the disappearance of the Philadelphia chromosome, establishing complete cytogenetic responses (CCyRs) as the gold standard of response to therapy.[5] The knowledge of the activation of a tyrosine kinase led to the development of tyrosine kinase inhibitors (TKIs), initially imatinib[6] and later second- and third-generation drugs that radically changed the natural history of the disease (Figure 1).[7] Today, patients diagnosed with CML, if properly managed, have a life expectancy similar to that of the general population.

Incidence and epidemiology

CML accounts for 15% of all leukemias.[1,2] The median age of onset of CML is 55–65 years, and the incidence increases with age with a slight male preponderance (ratio 1.8:1).[8] It is estimated that 5980 new cases of CML will be diagnosed in the United States in 2014 with 810 patients dying from their disease.[9] The incidence in the United States has remained constant at about 1.81:100,000. With modern therapy, the annual mortality has decreased from 15–20%

to 2%, and the estimated median survival may exceed 20 years. Thus, the prevalence of CML in the United States in the next three decades may exceed 200,000 cases.[10]

Risk factors

In most patients with CML, a causative factor cannot be identified. Although ionizing radiation is leukemogenic, the most common leukemia following radiation is acute myeloid leukemia. CML has been reported following the atomic bomb catastrophe in Japan in 1945, and in earlier studies in radiologists and in patients with ankylosing spondylitis treated with radiation therapy.[3,4,11,12] No other known risk factors have been recognized.

Pathology

CML typically follows a biphasic or triphasic course with a chronic phase, followed by an intermediate accelerated phase, and eventually a frequently terminal blastic phase.[13] Leukocytosis is common with white cell counts frequently greater than 100×10^9/L. Historically, the median survival for patients in chronic phase was 3–6 years, with an estimated annual risk of transformation to the blastic phase of 5–10% in the first 2 years and 15–20% subsequently. Accelerated phase is characterized by increasing maturation arrest. Different criteria have been used to define accelerated phase. One common classification defines accelerated phase as the presence of any of the following: ≥15% blasts, ≥30% blasts plus promyelocytes, ≥20% basophils, platelets $<100\times10^9$/L unrelated to therapy, or cytogenetic clonal evolution.[14] Other criteria have been proposed, such as the World Health Organization (WHO) proposal, but some of these classifications[7,15] have not been clinically validated.[16] The median survival for patients in accelerated phase was 1–2 years,[8,17] but has greatly improved with the use of TKI.[18] The blastic phase is defined by the presence of ≥30% blasts in the peripheral blood or bone marrow or by the presence of extramedullary disease with immature cells.[19] The WHO proposed this to be changed to ≥20% blasts, but this change is not justified based on clinical data.[10,16] The blastic phase can be classified according to the immunophenotype as myeloid, lymphoid, biphenotypic, or mixed lineage (lymphoblastic–myeloblastic). Lymphoid blastic phase occurs in 20–30% of patients, myeloid in 50%, and undifferentiated in 25%.[11,20] The median survival in blastic phase is 3–6 months. Patients with lymphoid blastic phase have a better prognosis, with a response rate of ≥90% and median survival of >18 months with TKI combined with chemotherapy.[21]

Laboratory features in the chronic phase include leukocytosis with left maturation shift and frequently basophilia and eosinophilia (Figure 2). Thrombocytosis is common but thrombotic phenomena are unusual. Some degree of anemia is common. There is a reduction in leukocyte alkaline phosphatase (LAP) activity and a marked elevation of serum B12 levels.

Holland-Frei Cancer Medicine, Ninth Edition. Edited by Robert C. Bast Jr., Carlo M. Croce, William N. Hait, Waun Ki Hong, Donald W. Kufe, Martine Piccart-Gebhart, Raphael E. Pollock, Ralph R. Weichselbaum, Hongyang Wang, and James F. Holland.
© 2017 John Wiley & Sons, Inc. ISBN: 978-1-118-93469-2

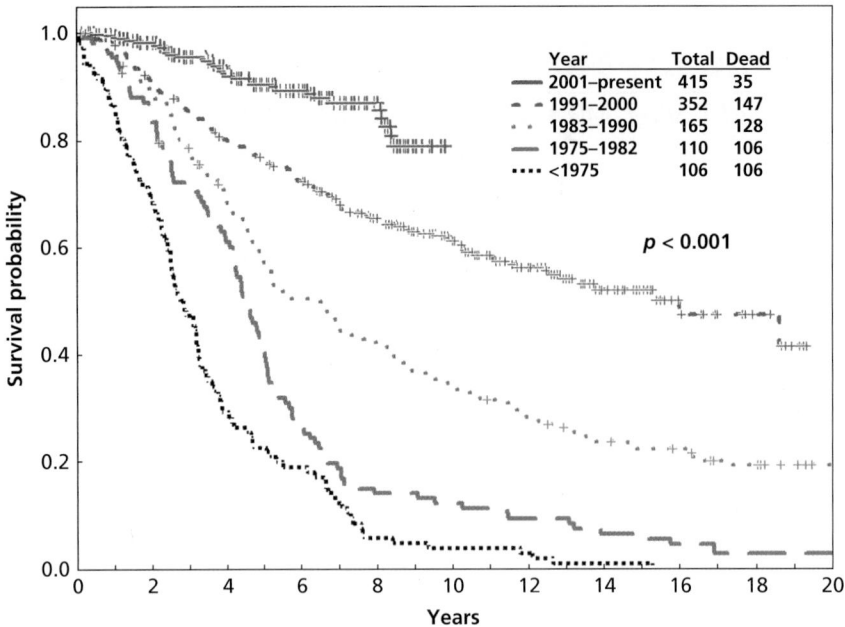

Figure 1 Survival of patients with newly diagnosed CML in chronic phase referred to MD Anderson Cancer Center ($N = 1148$; 1965–2010). Source: Kantarjian et al. 2012.[7] This research was originally published in Blood. © The American Society of Hematology.

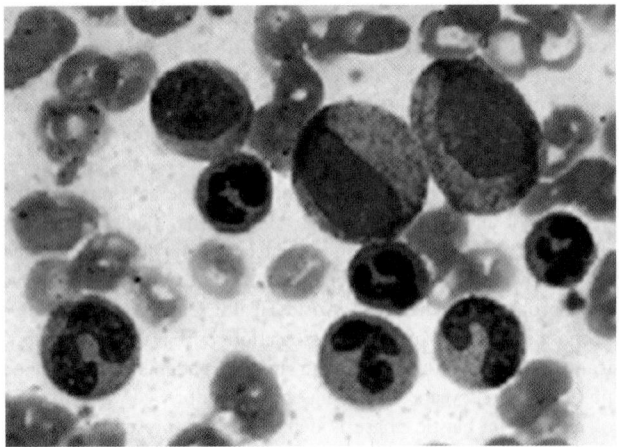

Figure 2 Chronic myeloid leukemia. Leukocytosis with myelocytes, metamyelocytes, band cells, and polymorphonuclear leukocytes are characteristics of the peripheral blood in the chronic phase of this disease.

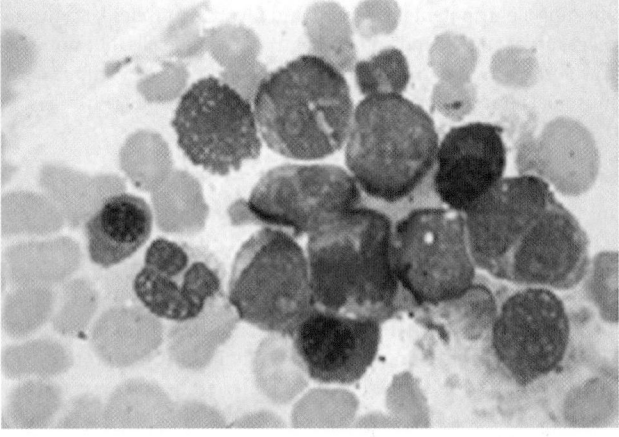

Figure 3 Chronic myeloid leukemia, myeloid blast crisis. The marrow aspiration shows predominance of blast forms, which have a myeloid appearance.

The bone marrow is hypercellular. In chronic phase, all stages of differentiation are present, but the myelocytes predominate, whereas myeloblasts and promyelocytes account for <10% of cells (Figures 3 and 4). Megakaryocytes may be increased, and there might be increased reticulin fibrosis, which may worsen with disease progression, and is reversed with TKI.[22]

In the blastic phase, lymphoid blasts contain terminal deoxynucleotidyl transferase (TdT). Lymphoblasts usually express CD10, CD19, and CD22 or other B-cell markers[20]; T-cell blastic phase is less common. The myeloid blastic phase may mimic acute myeloid leukemia. The myeloblasts stain with myeloperoxidase and express myeloid markers including CD13, CD33, and CD117.

Rarely, patients may be present in lymphoid or myeloid blastic phase without a recognized antecedent chronic phase. The differentiation between this presentation and Ph-positive acute lymphoblastic (ALL) or myeloid (AML) leukemias may be impossible, but the distinction is semantic as the treatment and prognosis are the same. Megakaryoblastic, erythroblastic, and basophilic transformations are uncommon.

Prognostic classification

Prognosis in CML is variable. Risk classifications have been proposed to stratify patients and assist in treatment decisions. The Sokal model is most frequently used[23] and defines three risk groups: low (about 40–50% of all patients), intermediate (about 30%), and high risk (10–20%), with median survivals of 4.5, 3.5, and 2.5 years, respectively, with busulfan or hydroxyurea. The model still predicts response to therapy and progression-free survival with imatinib therapy, although outcomes for all risk groups are significantly better than in the past. Other classifications have been proposed such as the Harford score (more applicable to interferon-treated patients),[24] the simpler but not universally validated EUTOS score (based only on percentage of

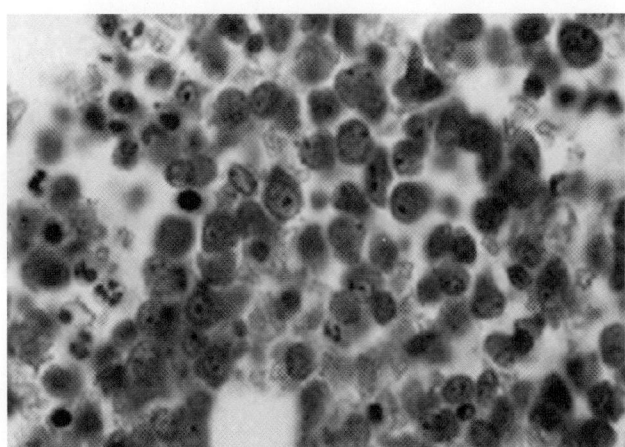

Figure 4 Chronic myeloid leukemia, blast phase. This bone marrow biopsy shows "blasts" with prominent nucleoli comprising about 75% of the marrow cells.

basophils and size of spleen),[25–27] or the Gratwohl score for SCT (stem cell transplant).[20,28] With TKI therapy, the significance of several prognostic factors (older age, marrow fibrosis, deletion of derivative 9q, complex Ph chromosome) has been reduced or eliminated.[21–23,29–32] Interestingly, adolescents and young adults may have a worse outcome, arguably because of poor adherence to therapy.[33]

Pathogenesis

The primary biologic defect in CML is unregulated proliferation with discordant maturation, reduced apoptosis, and defective adherence to the bone marrow stroma.[34–36]

Cytogenetics

The hallmark of CML is the Ph chromosome. This results from a reciprocal translocation between chromosome 9 and chromosome 22, t(9;22)(q34.1;q11.21) that transposes the 3′ segment of the *ABL* gene to the 5′ segment of the *BCR* gene.[2] This abnormality creates the chimeric BCR-ABL oncogene (Figure 5).

The Ph chromosome is found in ~95% of patients with CML. It is also observed in 5% of children and 15–30% of adults with acute lymphoblastic leukemia and in 2% of patients with newly diagnosed acute myeloid leukemia.[37] Some patients have variant translocations, which may be simple (involving chromosome 22 and one additional chromosome other than chromosome 9) or complex (involving chromosomes 22, 9, and at least one other chromosome).[38] These patients historically had an inferior outcome, but with imatinib therapy they have a similar prognosis to patients with the classic Ph chromosome.[31,32]

Progression of CML is frequently accompanied by additional cytogenetic abnormalities. The most common abnormalities include a second Ph chromosome, isochromosome 17, trisomy 8, trisomy 19, and deletion 20q.[39] The molecular consequences of these abnormalities are not known. Mutations or deletions of tumor suppressor genes, such as p16 and TP53, and methylation of ABL, BCR, p15, and cadherin-13 may contribute to transformation.[40–44] Activation of JAK–STAT pathway might be responsible for the survival of the leukemic stem cell.[45,46] In blast phase, granulocyte-macrophage progenitors are the candidate stem cells, and the activation of β-catenin may enhance the self-renewal activity of these cells.[47]

After successful treatment with TKI, chromosomal abnormalities are found in the Ph-negative cells in 10–15% of patients, most frequently trisomy 8, monosomy 7 or 5, and deletion 20q.[48] These may regress spontaneously in some cases, but in rare instances (<1%) may lead to the development of a myelodysplastic syndrome or AML.[40–42,49–51]

Molecular biology

The reciprocal 9;22 translocation results in a chimeric oncogene, BCR-ABL, that codes for a Bcr-Abl oncoprotein with constitutional tyrosine kinase activity.[46,52]

There is some heterogeneity in the breakpoints on chromosomes 9 and 22. On chromosome 9, breaks may occur in a region 200 kb or more in length, resulting in most of the c-*abl* gene being translocated.[46] The breakpoints within the *ABL* gene occur either upstream of exon Ib, downstream of exon Ia, or, more frequently, between exons Ib and Ia. Breakpoints in BCR occur most frequently in the major breakpoint cluster region that includes exons e12–e16

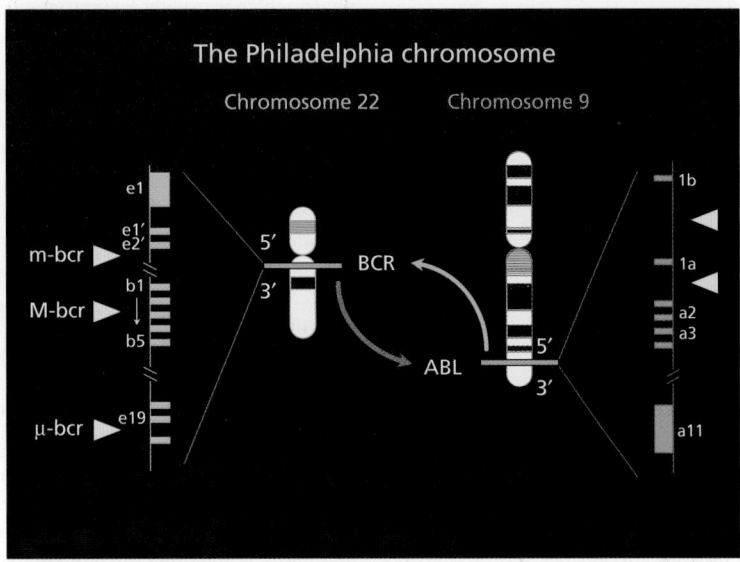

Figure 5 Schematic of 9;22 chromosome translocation.

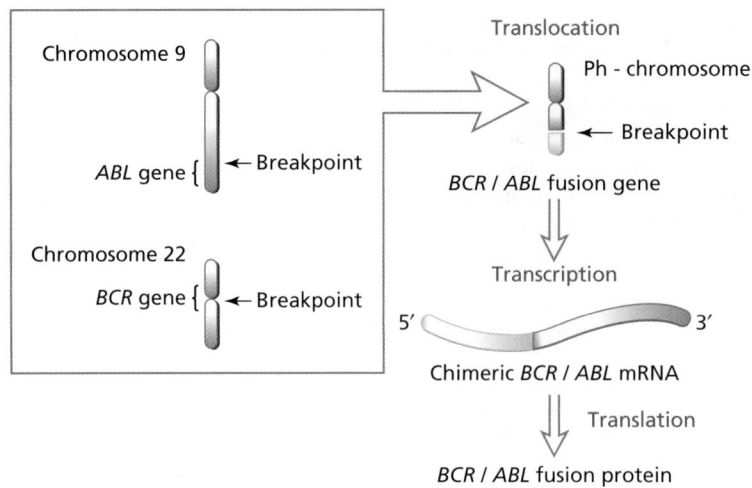

Figure 6 Summary of the cytogenetic and molecular effects of the Ph chromosome.

(formerly b1–b5), resulting in either b2a2 (e13a2) or b3a2 (e14b2) fusion transcripts, both of them generating a 210-kDa protein (p210*BCR-ABL1*). In few patients with CML (but more frequently in Ph-positive ALL), the breakpoint may occur in the minor breakpoint cluster region, resulting in an e1a2 fusion (translated into a 190-kDa protein).[53] Less frequently, the breakpoint may occur in a different, more distal, breakpoint region μ-bcr.

Transcription of the fusion BCR-ABL oncogene results in a chimeric BCR-ABL mRNA that is translated into three fusion proteins of varying sizes p190[Bcr-Abl], p210[Bcr-Abl], and p230[Bcr-Abl], according to the breakpoint on *BCR* (Figure 6). In all instances, the fusion protein has unregulated constitutive tyrosine kinase activity that triggers intracellular signaling pathways such as STAT, RAS, RAF, JUN kinase, MYC, AKT, and BCL-2, which confer the malignant phenotype.[52]

Most patients with typical chronic phase CML express either the b2a2 (e13a2) or b3a2 (e14a2) rearrangements. The clinical features, response to treatment, and prognosis are similar in both groups. Patients with Ph-positive acute lymphoblastic leukemia may express either p210[Bcr-Abl] (30–50%) or p190[Bcr-Abl] (50–70%). Rare patients with CML in chronic phase express e1a2 (p190[Bcr-Abl]) and have a worse prognosis.[53,54] The p230[Bcr-Abl] is associated with a more indolent disease and a phenotype similar to chronic neutrophilic leukemia.

In approximately 5–10% of morphologically typical cases of CML, the Ph chromosome cannot be identified. In one-third of these, the BCR-ABL rearrangement is present. These patients have similar characteristics, response to treatment, and prognosis as Ph-positive CML.[16,55] The other two-thirds lack the BCR-ABL rearrangement (called "atypical CML" in the WHO classification) with different clinical and hematologic features, including lower initial white cell and platelet counts, with progression characterized by progressive cytopenias and organomegaly rather than blastic transformation and a median survival of 18–24 months.[17,56,57] This type of leukemia is not discussed further in this chapter. Reverse transcriptase polymerase chain reaction (RT-PCR) can detect the BCR-ABL transcript with a sensitivity of 10^{-5}.[48,58] BCR-ABL rearrangement has been identified in up to 25–30% of normal adults using RT-PCR approximately 3-log more sensitive (sensitivity $\sim 10^{-8}$) than the one used clinically.[59] This suggests that clonal disease requires escape from immune surveillance and/or a second oncogenic event to become clinically relevant.

A subset of patients treated with TKI develop resistance. Several mechanisms of resistance have been identified; the most common are mutations in the BCR-ABL kinase domain (KD). More than 50 different mutations have been reported and involve many of the domains in the BCR-ABL structure, including the P-loop (the domain where ATP binds), the activation loop, and the catalytic domain, as well as the amino acids where imatinib makes contact with BCR-ABL.[60] Different mutations vary in their sensitivity to different TKI. Some mutations are inhibited by slightly higher concentrations of TKI than that is required to inhibit the wild-type form; others are completely insensitive.[61,62] Mutational analysis is useful in patients with resistance to TKI to identify the TKI predicted to inhibit a given mutation as determined by the IC$_{50}$ for particular agents. For example, F317L and V299L are insensitive to dasatinib, V299L is insensitive to bosutinib, and F359V and E255K/V are insensitive to nilotinib, while T315I is sensitive only to ponatinib (a third-generation TKI effective against all mutations).[63–65]

Diagnosis

Approximately 90% of patients are diagnosed in the chronic phase, which is usually asymptomatic.[13] Symptoms usually develop insidiously and are usually due to splenomegaly (pain, abdominal fullness, early satiety) or anemia (fatigue). Less commonly, patients may be present with gout, anorexia, weight loss, unexplained fever, or signs of platelet dysfunction (e.g., ecchymoses or hemorrhage). Patients with very high WBC may have signs of hyperviscosity (priapism, cerebrovascular accidents, tinnitus, confusion, retinal hemorrhage). Symptoms associated with the accelerated phase may include fever, night sweats, weight loss, or bleeding associated with thrombocytopenia. Occasionally, blood and bone marrow features of accelerated phase occur in patients who are asymptomatic and identified only during routine follow-up. The blastic phase of CML is commonly associated with constitutional symptoms (night sweats, weight loss, fever, bone pain), anemia, an increased risk of infections, and/or bleeding.

When the diagnosis of CML is suspected, a bone marrow aspiration is mandatory. Although the diagnosis of CML can be made in peripheral blood, proper staging and recognition of all features of the disease can only be made with the evaluation of the bone marrow and peripheral blood. The bone marrow aspiration should include the following: (1) cell differential for proper staging; (2) assessment of fibrosis and other characteristics; and (3) cytogenetic analysis by G-banding to confirm the presence of the Ph chromosome and possibly additional chromosomal abnormalities; at least 20 metaphases are required for a proper interpretation of the karyotype and assessment of response. In addition, RT-PCR is recommended at the time of diagnosis. Although the number of BCR-ABL transcripts has no bearing on the prognosis (and is not reliable at baseline when using ABL as the control gene), it permits investigation of unusual transcripts (e.g., e19a2, b2a3, b3a3) not detected by standard PCR.

During the course of treatment, a bone marrow aspiration with cytogenetic analysis should be performed every 6 months until a CCyR is confirmed. Thus, a bone marrow is needed less frequently or perhaps not at all in most patients. It may be appropriate to continue doing karyotype analysis in patients with recognized chromosomal abnormalities in Ph-negative metaphases. FISH can be used to assess achievement of a cytogenetic response, and it can be done in peripheral blood, but it does not provide information on the presence of additional chromosomal abnormalities whether in Ph-positive cells (i.e., clonal evolution) or in Ph-chromosome-negative cells. A bone marrow aspiration should be performed in all patients with unexplained changes in peripheral blood counts or in those with loss of major molecular response (MMR) (and definitely if levels are close to 1% using the international scale). During treatment, patients should also be monitored with RT-PCR at 3, 6, and 12 months after the start of therapy and every 6 months after that.

Assessment for mutations is unnecessary at the time of diagnosis in patients in the chronic phase as mutations have not been found in this setting with the standard methodology. A search for mutations should be done when there is loss of CCyR. Patients who do not meet the recommended response criteria at the given times as per the European Leukemia Net (ELN) recommendations may have a mutation analysis performed, but mutations are more commonly found among patients with secondary resistance (i.e., loss of cytogenetic response) compared to those with primary resistance (i.e., not achieving optimal response).

Staging and prognostic factors

CML has three stages: chronic, accelerated, and blast phases. The features that define each phase are described earlier in the section titled "Pathology". For patients in the chronic phase, risk classifications have been proposed. These include the Sokal,[23] Hasford (Euro),[24] and EUTOS[25] classifications. These classifications are used mostly for prognostic purposes; treatment recommendations generally apply equally to all risk groups. The Sokal score is the most commonly used and is obtained through the formula: exp (0.0116 × (age [years] − 43.4)) + (0.0345 × (spleen size [cm] − 7.51) + (0.188 × ((platelets [10^9/L]/700)^2 − 0.563)) + (0.0887 × (blasts [%] − 2.10)). Based on the score, three risk groups are identified: low (score < 0.8), intermediate (score 0.8 – 1.2), and high risk (>1.2). In the United States, only 10 – 15% of patients have a high-risk score at the time of diagnosis, whereas in other areas of the world, these can represent up to one-third of all patients.

Treatment

Initial treatment for all patients with CML is with TKI. Imatinib mesylate, a selective Bcr-Abl TKI introduced in the 1990s, has changed the natural history of CML.[6,66–70] Patients in the chronic phase at the time of diagnosis treated with TKI have a life expectancy that matches that of the general population.[71]

Imatinib mesylate

Imatinib is a potent inhibitor of Bcr-Abl and few other tyrosine kinases such as c-kit and PDGFR.[6,72] It was first used in CML after failure or intolerance to interferon-alpha.[73,74] Imatinib 400 mg taken orally daily, given to 454 patients, resulted in a CCyR of 57%. The estimated 5-year survival rate was 76%.[73]

The efficacy of imatinib in previously untreated patients was demonstrated in a multicenter randomized trial comparing imatinib to the combination of interferon-alpha and low-dose cytarabine [IRIS (Insulin Resistance Intervention after Stroke) trial].[75,76] With 8 years of follow-up, a CCyR was achieved by 83% of all patients, resulting in an event-free survival of 81%, transformation-free survival of 92%, and overall survival of 85%.[77] The standard starting dose of imatinib in the chronic phase is 400 mg daily. Higher doses of imatinib (600 – 800 mg daily) may result in improved response rates that are achieved earlier.[78,79] It is controversial whether higher doses result in improved long-term outcome of patients.[65,80–82] To date, 400 mg daily remains the standard initial dose. Among patients in chronic phase who progress on imatinib 400 mg daily therapy, dose escalation to 600 or 800 mg daily recaptured some CCyRs.[83,84]

Second-generation tyrosine kinase inhibitors

Dasatinib and nilotinib are second-generation TKI that are approximately 300-fold[85] and 30-fold[86] more potent than imatinib, respectively. They were first investigated and approved for treatment of patients who have experienced resistance or intolerance to imatinib. Subsequently, trials demonstrated that both of these agents resulted in more, deeper and faster responses than those seen with imatinib.[87–89] This translated in a lower rate of transformation to accelerated and blast phase compared to imatinib. Thus, both agents are approved and considered standard for the initial treatment of patients with chronic phase CML.

In the randomized trial of dasatinib versus imatinib, the rate of confirmed CCyR by 12 months was 77% with dasatinib versus 66% with imatinib, and the cumulative rate of MMR by 36 months was 69% versus 55%, respectively. At 3 months, 84% of patients treated with dasatinib achieved BCR-ABL/ABL transcript <10% compared to 64% with imatinib. Transformation to accelerated and blast phase occurred in 3% and 5%, respectively. No difference in event-free or overall survival has been reported up to 4 years of minimum follow-up.[90,91] The standard starting dose of dasatinib for patients with newly diagnosed CML in chronic phase is 100 mg once daily.

A similar randomized trial investigated two different dose schedules of nilotinib (300 mg twice daily and 400 mg twice daily) compared to imatinib. By 12 months, the rate of CCyR was 80% with nilotinib 300 mg twice daily and 78% with 400 mg twice daily compared to 65% with imatinib. By 3 years, the rates of MMR were 73%, 70%, and 53%, respectively. BCR-ABL/ABL levels of <10% were achieved by 91% treated with nilotinib 300 mg twice daily, 89% with nilotinib 400 mg twice daily, and 67% with imatinib; the rates of freedom from progression to accelerated or blast phase at 4 years were 96.7%, 97.8%, and 93.1%, respectively. The 4-year estimated progression-free survivals were 92.7%, 96.3%, and 92%, and overall survivals were 94.3%, 96.7%, and 93.3%.[92,93] Nilotinib 300 mg twice daily is the standard therapy for newly diagnosed CML in chronic phase.

Bosutinib has also been investigated as an initial therapy for CML. There is an increase rate of responses, with deeper and faster responses resulting in fewer transformations to the accelerated and blast phases. However, bosutinib is not currently approved as an initial therapy for CML.[94]

Treatment algorithm

Achievement of a CCyR is associated with near eradication of the risk of transformation to accelerated and blast phases and a significant survival benefit, with a 10-year survival probability of 70–80% equivalent to that of the general population. Achieving molecular responses increases the probability of long-term durable responses although such responses have not resulted in improved survival among patients with CCyR. The 7-year probability of event-free survival for patients that achieve MMR is 95% compared to 86% among those with CCyR but no MMR. There is no difference in survival free from transformation to accelerated or blast phase or in overall survival. Deeper responses may offer the possibility of considering treatment discontinuation, something that today should be considered only through clinical trials.

In addition to the depth of response, the time to response is important to improve long-term outcomes. Patients with BCR-ABL/ABL transcripts <10% at 3 months from the start of therapy have significantly better probability of EFS (approximately 95%) compared to those with >10% transcripts (approximately 80%).[95–98] There is also a significant but smaller difference in the overall survival. This has resulted in recommendations of what is considered optimal response to therapy that include BCR-ABL/ABL <10% by RT-PCR and/or Ph <35% by standard karyotype at 3 months, BCR-ABL/ABL <1% and/or Ph 0% at 6 months, and BCR-ABL/ABL <0.1% at 12 months. Levels above these are defined as warning or failure (Table 1).[99]

Patients who achieve an optimal therapy can continue therapy unchanged. The current algorithm involves therapy to continue indefinitely although studies are ongoing to determine whether treatment may be discontinued in some patients. Those who meet the definition of warning can continue therapy but adherence should be assessed, therapy optimized, and patients monitored rigorously every 3 months with treatment change considered if failure is identified. Once the definition of failure is met, treatment changes should be implemented.[99]

Intolerance is another reason why treatment change may be needed. Despite the excellent overall tolerability of TKI, they all have adverse events that need monitoring and adequate management. With proper management[100] that may include transient treatment interruptions, dose adjustments, medical management of adverse events, and supportive care, most patients can continue therapy as an experience and adequate response. In general, patients should not be changed to a different TKI based on the first occurrence of an adverse event unless this is life threatening (e.g., Stevens–Johnson's, myocardial infarction, stroke). True intolerance to TKI occurs in only approximately 5% of all patients. Suggestions for the management of the most common adverse events are presented in Table 2.

Treatment options after failure of prior TKI

Several TKI are available for the management of patients with resistance (as defined by the ELN[99]) or intolerance to prior TKI. These include dasatinib, nilotinib, bosutinib, and ponatinib. In addition, omacetaxine, a protein-synthesis inhibitor (not a TKI), is also approved for patients who have received at least two prior TKI.

Among patients who have received imatinib as their only prior TKI and experienced resistance or intolerance, dasatinib at a dose of 100 mg once daily induced a CCyR in 44% of patients with resistance and 67% of those with intolerance. A MMR occurred in 37% of patients with resistance or intolerance, with a 6-year probability of progression-free survival of 49% and overall survival of 71%.[101,102] Similarly, nilotinib, at a dose of 400 mg twice daily (the standard dose for second-line therapy), induced CCyR in 41% of patients with resistance to imatinib and 51% of those with intolerance for a 4-year progression-free survival of 57% and overall survival of 78%.[103] Bosutinib is also a second-generation TKI with an activity against Src and Abl, 30–50 times more potent than imatinib against Abl but, in contrast to other TKI used for CML, with minimal inhibitory activity against c-kit or PDGF-R. Bosutinib has also been effective in this patient population inducing a CCyR in 48% of patients with resistance and 52% of those with intolerance to imatinib with MMR in 64% and 65% of those achieving CCyR, respectively. This resulted in a progression-free survival of 73% and 95%, respectively.[104] None of these agents is active in patients with the T315I mutation.

Bosutinib and ponatinib have been investigated among patients who have received two or more TKI. With bosutinib 500 mg once daily, a major cytogenetic response was achieved in 30–35% of 118 patients who had received imatinib and were then resistant or intolerant to dasatinib, or resistant to nilotinib. The corresponding rates of CCyR were 14%, 28%, and 27%, respectively, and 2-year estimates of progression-free survival 65%, 81%, and 77%.[105] Ponatinib is a potent inhibitor of Abl tyrosine kinase activity as well as other kinases including c-kit, FLT3 and VEGFR. Importantly, it has potent inhibitory activity against unmutated BCR-ABL or in the presence of any of the KD mutations tested, including the multiresistant T315I.[106] With ponatinib at a dose of 45 mg daily, among 267 patients of which 93% had received at least two prior TKI (60% had received at least three), a major cytogenetic response was achieved in 56% (complete in 46%) and a MMR in 34%. Major cytogenetic response was sustained for at least 12 months in 91%, and the overall survival was 94% at 12 months. For patients with T315I, the response rates were 70%, 66%, and 56%, respectively, with similar durability of response and overall survival.[107,108] With omacetaxine, 20% of patients treated in chronic phase after resistance to at

Table 1 Suggested management of most common adverse events associated with imatinib.

Adverse events	Management
Nausea/vomiting	Take with food, fluids
	Antiemetics
Diarrhea	Loperamide
	Diphenoxylate atropine
Peripheral edema	Diuretics
Periorbital edema	Steroid-containing cream
Skin rash	Avoid sun exposure
	Topical steroids
	Systemic steroids (early intervention important)
Muscle cramps	Tonic water or quinine
	Electrolyte replacement as needed
	Calcium gluconate
Arthralgia, bone pain	Nonsteroidal anti-inflammatory agents
Elevated transaminases (uncommon)	Hold therapy and monitor closely
	Dose reduction upon resolution
Myelosuppression	
Anemia	Treatment interruption/dose reduction usually not indicated
	Consider erythropoietin or darbepoietin[a]
Neutropenia	Hold therapy if grade ≥3 (i.e., ANC < 1 × 10⁹/L)
	Consider filgrastim[a] if recurrent/persistent, or sepsis
Thrombocytopenia	Hold therapy if grade ≥3 (i.e., platelets <50 × 10⁹/L)
	Consider IL 11[a] 10 mcg/kg 3–7 days/week

[a]The use of erythropoietin, darbepoietin, filgrastim, and interleukin-11 (IL-11) in this setting is not standard and should be considered investigational.

Table 2 Response criteria according to the European Leukemia Net.

Time (mo)	Response		
	Failure	Warning	Optimal
3	No CHR, and/or Ph+ >95%	BCR-ABL >10%, and/or Ph+ 36–95%	BCR-ABL ≤10%, and/or Ph+ ≤35%
6	BCR-ABL >10% and/or Ph+ >35%	BCR-ABL 1–10%, and/or Ph+ 1–35%	BCR-ABL <1%, and/or Ph+ 0%
12	BCR-ABL >1% and/or Ph+ >0%	BCR-ABL >0.1–1%	BCR-ABL <0.1%
Any	Loss of CHR Loss of CCyR Confirmed MMR loss Mutations CCA/Ph+	CCA/Ph– (–7, or 7q–)	BCR-ABL <0.1%

Abbreviations: CHR, complete hematologic response; Ph+, percentage of metaphases with presence of the Philadelphia chromosome (a minimum of 20 required for full assessment); CCyR, complete cytogenetic response; MMR, major molecular response; CCA/Ph+, clonal chromosomal abnormalities in cell with the Philadelphia chromosome. Source: Adapted from Quintas-Cardama et al. 2009. This research was originally published in Blood. © The American Society of Hematology.

least two prior TKI achieved a major cytogenetic response, with a median overall survival of 33.9 months.[109] Responses can be seen regardless of mutation status including patients with T315I.[110] Allogeneic SCT should also be considered in patients who have experienced resistance to TKI.

Stem cell transplantation

Allogeneic SCT may be curative in 40–80% of patients who receive a transplant from an HLA-identical sibling or an unrelated donor.[111] Among patients transplanted in first chronic phase, 3514 from a match-related sibling and 1052 from an unrelated donor, the 5-year survival probability was 63% and 55%, respectively, and the leukemia-free survival was 55% and 50%, respectively. The 5-year cumulative incidence of relapse is 12–14%.[111] However, for patients who have been alive and in continuous complete remission for ≥5 years, the survival rate at 15 years was 88% for those receiving sibling donor cells and 87% from those with unrelated donors, with cumulative incidence of relapse of 8% and 2%, respectively, with relapses documented as late as 18 years after transplant.[112] Patients who were treated with stem cell transplant had a higher probability of death for the first 14 years after transplant compared to individuals in the general population of similar age, sex, and race.[112] The availability of donors has improved in recent years because of the increasingly successful results with transplant using cord blood or haploidentical donors, and the reach has extended to higher age groups with the use of non-myeloablative conditioning regimens. In addition, early mortality rates have decreased with improved supportive care and GVHD (graft-versus-host disease) prophylaxis and management. However, with the availability of TKI, the role of SCT has changed significantly. Several reports have confirmed that previous exposure to TKI does not adversely affect the outcome after SCT although time from diagnosis to SCT remains an important prognostic factor for the outcome after transplant.[113,114] Similarly, patients transplanted in chronic phase have a significantly better outcome than those transplanted in advanced phase.[111] Until the advent of ponatinib and omacetaxine, SCT was the only available therapy for patients with T315I mutation, with 2-year survival probability of 59% for patients transplanted in chronic phase.[115,116]

Patients transplanted in accelerated or blastic phase have significantly worse outcomes, with 5-year survival probabilities of 40% accelerated phase and 10–15% blastic phase. Patients in blastic phase transplanted after achievement of a second chronic phase may have long-term outcomes similar to that of the accelerated phase.[28,117,118]

Treatment recommendations in CML in 2015

The results with imatinib to date have been excellent and durable, and with shorter follow-up, the results with dasatinib and nilotinib appear superior with earlier and deeper responses and with lower rate of transformation, although these outcomes have not translated into a significant difference in event-free or overall survival. The life expectancy of patients treated with TKI is similar to that of the general population, particularly for those patients achieving a CCyR. Based on this, TKIs are standard initial therapy for all patients with CML in chronic phase. Because of the improved outcome with dasatinib or nilotinib in randomized trials compared to imatinib,[90–93] these agents are preferred in many instances. However, imatinib is likely to remain the treatment of choice for a large percentage (perhaps the majority) of patients throughout the world. It should be emphasized that imatinib is also adequate treatment. The most important aspect to offer a patient the best possible long-term outcome is the proper management of the patient. This includes a close follow-up to recognize and manage adverse events. All TKI have adverse events associated with them, but most of these are manageable through transient treatment interruptions, dose adjustments, and/or medical interventions. Very few patients (around 5%) are truly intolerant to a given drug. Until ongoing studies demonstrate a long-term benefit of early change in therapy, patients not having a major cytogenetic response (or not having BCR-ABL/ABL transcripts <10%) at 3 months may continue therapy unchanged but they need to be checked again at 6 months.[99] For patients still not achieving a major cytogenetic response (or still with BCR-ABL/ABL transcripts >10%) after 6 months of therapy treatment change may be considered, although there are also no studies that have shown that change of therapy in this setting alters long-term outcome. Patients need to continue with monitoring at least every 6 months as detailed earlier. A change of therapy is clearly indicated when the criteria for failure is met (as defined by the ELN). In these instances (i.e., failure), randomized trials have demonstrated that a change of therapy from imatinib to a second-generation TKI improves the outcome compared to an increase in the dose of imatinib.[119] A mutation analysis is always indicated when the criteria of failure are met, and a bone marrow aspiration is also needed to determine the cytogenetics and stage of the patient before change. If a mutation is identified, this can guide which TKI is expected to induce a response (e.g., if F317L or V299L identified, consider nilotinib or ponatinib; if F359V, consider bosutinib, dasatinib, or ponatinib; for T315I, ponatinib or omacetaxine may be considered).[61,62] If there is no mutation, or there is a mutation for which there is no available information or no meaningful difference between the various TKI, then other considerations may help in the decision of what drug to use, such as comorbidities that might expose the patient more to adverse events associated with one drug or another, the adverse event profile that might be more acceptable for a given patient, and the dose schedule that a patient might find more convenient or acceptable to optimize adherence. Patients with resistance to at least two TKI can be considered for SCT. SCT may also be considered in other settings where long-term therapy might not be optimal or feasible (e.g., for cost considerations).

Patients with accelerated phase features at the time of diagnosis can be treated with a TKI, particularly dasatinib or nilotinib, as their prognosis in this setting is nearly identical to that of patients in chronic phase.[120] SCT for these patients is not required unless not responding adequately. Patients who progress to accelerated phase while on treatment with TKI for chronic phase should receive a different TKI and considered for SCT.[121] Patients with blast phase CML should receive TKI, usually in combination with chemotherapy,[21,122,123] and SCT should be strongly considered. Although results for SCT in this setting are best with the least residual disease, once the patient achieves a hematologic complete remission transplant can proceed as further chemotherapy may cause comorbidities that may make SCT impossible or of greater risk, and response may not improve further.

Suvivorship and follow-up

Patients with CML should continue therapy and have close follow-up indefinitely. This includes not only monitoring of the status of the disease (with PCR in peripheral blood every 6 months) but also attention to co-morbidities and possible side effects. There is increased awareness of adverse events that will need continued assessment. These include arteriothrombotic events such as ischemic heart disease (including angina and myocardial infarction), ischemic heart disease (including transient ischemic attacks and strokes), and peripheral arterial occlusive disease, particularly with ponatinib and nilotinib. Attention should be paid to monitoring and managing risk factors such as hypertension (frequently caused or aggravated by ponatinib), diabetes (frequently caused or aggravated by nilotinib), hyperlipidemia (also associated with TKI therapy), and others. Recent analyses also suggest there might be an impairment of renal function with TKI, particularly with imatinib. Patients on dasatinib with respiratory symptoms should be evaluated for pleural effusion or pulmonary hypertension. Although most adverse events occur early during the course of the disease, for some (such as pleural effusion or arteriothrombotic events) the incidence is constant and a first event may occur after several years of treatment.

Research is ongoing to explore treatment discontinuation in suitable patients.[124,125] Among patients with sustained undetectable transcripts (with PCR sensitivity of at least 4.5 logs) for at least 2 years, treatment discontinuation yielded a sustained remission in approximately 40% of patients after 3–4 years of follow-up. This approach at the moment should be considered only in clinical trials and patients should continue with close monitoring, at least monthly for the first 6 months, then every 2–3 months for 2 years, and then every 6 months indefinitely.

Conclusion

The outcome of patients with CML has improved significantly since the introduction of TKI. It is expected that a patient with CML diagnosed today may have a life expectancy similar to that of the general population. For a patient to have such favorable outcome, adequate management is important including adequate dose optimization, proper management of adverse events, continued periodic monitoring of disease response, timely intervention

when indicated, and continued support throughout the life of the patient. With this approach, transformation to advanced stages is uncommon and few patients will die of CML.

Summary

Chronic myeloid leukemia (CML) is characterized by the presence of the Philadelphia chromosome. This results in the creation of the BCR-ABL fusion gene, which is in turn translated into a tyrosine kinase with constitutive kinase activity. The disease evolves in three stages: chronic, accelerated, and blast phases. Most patients are diagnosed in the chronic phase and are asymptomatic at the time of diagnosis. Treatment with TKIs has changed the natural history of the disease with a life expectancy that is similar to that of the general population. Imatinib was the first TKI to be used and is still a standard and an effective therapy for frontline therapy. Most patients will achieve a complete cytogenetic response (CCyR) making transformation to accelerated and blast phases very rarely. Higher doses of imatinib have been suggested to provide higher rates of response including deeper molecular responses. Dasatinib and nilotinib are also the approved treatment options for frontline therapy and may improve the rate of complete cytogenetic and major molecular (as well as deeper molecular) responses, with fewer instances of transformation to the accelerated and blast phases, but have not resulted in improved event-free or overall survival compared to imatinib in randomized trials. For patients who experience resistance or intolerance to one TKIs, alternative inhibitors can be used. In this setting, bosutinib and ponatinib are additional options. Overall, approximately 40% of patients with resistance or intolerance to initial therapy might achieve a CCyR with a subsequent TKI. The most common mechanism of resistance is the emergence of mutations of the KD. Different mutations may have differing sensitivities to the various inhibitors, and the presence of such mutations, when present, may allow selection of the most appropriate therapy. Although generally well-tolerated TKIs may have caused adverse events, some of them are potentially serious, which require proper identification and management; this may include the change of therapy in some instances. SCT remains a useful and potentially curative treatment modality for patients who have not experienced adequate response to various lines of therapy. With adequate access to treatment and proper management, patients diagnosed with CML should be able to have a normal life expectancy.

Key references

The complete reference list can be found on the Wiley Companion Digital Edition of this title (see inside front cover for login instructions).

1 Nowell PC, Hungerford DA. A minute chromosome in human chronic granulocytic leukemia. *Science.* 1960;**132**:1497–1501.

7 Kantarjian H, O'Brien S, Jabbour E, et al. Improved survival in chronic myeloid leukemia since the introduction of imatinib therapy: a single-institution historical experience. *Blood.* 2012;**119**(9):1981–1987.

14 Kantarjian HM, Dixon D, Keating MJ, et al. Characteristics of accelerated disease in chronic myelogenous leukemia. *Cancer.* 1988;**61**(7):1441–1446.

23 Sokal JE, Cox EB, Baccarani M, et al. Prognostic discrimination in "good-risk" chronic granulocytic leukemia. *Blood.* 1984;**63**(4):789–799.

31 Quintas-Cardama A, Kantarjian H, Talpaz M, et al. Imatinib mesylate therapy may overcome the poor prognostic significance of deletions of derivative chromosome 9 in patients with chronic myelogenous leukemia. *Blood.* 2005;**105**(6):2281–2286.

33 Pemmaraju N, Kantarjian H, Shan J, et al. Analysis of outcomes in adolescents and young adults with chronic myelogenous leukemia treated with upfront tyrosine kinase inhibitor therapy. *Haematologica.* 2012;**97**(7):1029–1035.

47 Jamieson CH, Ailles LE, Dylla SJ, et al. Granulocyte-macrophage progenitors as candidate leukemic stem cells in blast-crisis CML. *N Engl J Med.* 2004;**351**(7):657–667.

48 Medina J, Kantarjian H, Talpaz M, et al. Chromosomal abnormalities in Philadelphia chromosome-negative metaphases appearing during imatinib mesylate

therapy in patients with Philadelphia chromosome-positive chronic myelogenous leukemia in chronic phase. *Cancer*. 2003;**98**(9):1905–1911.

52 Quintas-Cardama A, Cortes J. Molecular biology of bcr-abl1-positive chronic myeloid leukemia. *Blood*. 2009;**113**(8):1619–1630.

58 Hughes T, Deininger M, Hochhaus A, et al. Monitoring CML patients responding to treatment with tyrosine kinase inhibitors: review and recommendations for harmonizing current methodology for detecting BCR-ABL transcripts and kinase domain mutations and for expressing results. *Blood*. 2006;**108**(1):28–37.

62 Redaelli S, Piazza R, Rostagno R, et al. Activity of bosutinib, dasatinib, and nilotinib against 18 imatinib-resistant BCR/ABL mutants. *J Clin Oncol*. 2009;**27**(3):469–471.

63 Kantarjian H, Schiffer C, Jones D, Cortes J. Monitoring the response and course of chronic myeloid leukemia in the modern era of BCR-ABL tyrosine kinase inhibitors: practical advice on the use and interpretation of monitoring methods. *Blood*. 2008;**111**(4):1774–1780.

69 Druker BJ, Talpaz M, Resta DJ, et al. Efficacy and safety of a specific inhibitor of the BCR-ABL tyrosine kinase in chronic myeloid leukemia. *N Engl J Med*. 2001;**344**(14):1031–1037.

74 Kantarjian H, Sawyers C, Hochhaus A, et al. Hematologic and cytogenetic responses to imatinib mesylate in chronic myelogenous leukemia. *N Engl J Med*. 2002;**346**(9):645–652.

75 Druker BJ, Guilhot F, O'Brien SG, et al. Five-year follow-up of patients receiving imatinib for chronic myeloid leukemia. *N Engl J Med*. 2006;**355**(23):2408–2417.

79 Kantarjian H, Talpaz M, O'Brien S, et al. High-dose imatinib mesylate therapy in newly diagnosed Philadelphia chromosome-positive chronic phase chronic myeloid leukemia. *Blood*. 2004;**103**(8):2873–2878.

82 Hehlmann R, Lauseker M, Jung-Munkwitz S, et al. Tolerability-adapted imatinib 800 mg/d versus 400 mg/d versus 400 mg/d plus interferon-alpha in newly diagnosed chronic myeloid leukemia. *J Clin Oncol*. 2011;**29**(12):1634–1642.

88 Cortes JE, Jones D, O'Brien S, et al. Results of dasatinib therapy in patients with early chronic-phase chronic myeloid leukemia. *J Clin Oncol*. 2010;**28**(3):398–404.

91 Kantarjian HM, Shah NP, Cortes JE, et al. Dasatinib or imatinib in newly diagnosed chronic-phase chronic myeloid leukemia: 2-year follow-up from a randomized phase 3 trial (DASISION). *Blood*. 2012;**119**(5):1123–1129.

92 Kantarjian HM, Hochhaus A, Saglio G, et al. Nilotinib versus imatinib for the treatment of patients with newly diagnosed chronic phase, Philadelphia chromosome-positive, chronic myeloid leukaemia: 24-month minimum follow-up of the phase 3 randomised ENESTnd trial. *Lancet Oncol*. 2011;**12**(9):841–851.

94 Gambacorti-Passerini C, Cortes JE, Lipton JH, et al. Safety of bosutinib versus imatinib in the phase 3 BELA trial in newly diagnosed chronic phase chronic myeloid leukemia. *Am J Hematol*. 2014;**89**(10):947–953.

95 Jain P, Kantarjian H, Nazha A, et al. Early responses predict better outcomes in patients with newly diagnosed chronic myeloid leukemia: results with four tyrosine kinase inhibitor modalities. *Blood*. 2013;**121**(24):4867–4874.

99 Baccarani M, Deininger MW, Rosti G, et al. European Leukemia Net recommendations for the management of chronic myeloid leukemia: 2013. *Blood*. 2013;**122**(6):872–884.

102 Shah NP, Guilhot F, Cortes JE, et al. Long-term outcome with dasatinib after imatinib failure in chronic-phase chronic myeloid leukemia: follow-up of a phase 3 study. *Blood*. 2014;**123**(15):2317–2324.

103 Giles FJ, le Coutre PD, Pinilla-Ibarz J, et al. Nilotinib in imatinib-resistant or imatinib-intolerant patients with chronic myeloid leukemia in chronic phase: 48-month follow-up results of a phase II study. *Leukemia*. 2013;**27**(1):107–112.

104 Gambacorti-Passerini C, Brummendorf TH, Kim DW, et al. Bosutinib efficacy and safety in chronic phase chronic myeloid leukemia after imatinib resistance or intolerance: minimum 24-month follow-up. *Am J Hematol*. 2014;**89**(7):732–742.

107 Cortes JE, Kim DW, Pinilla-Ibarz J, et al. A phase 2 trial of ponatinib in Philadelphia chromosome-positive leukemias. *N Engl J Med*. 2013;**369**(19):1783–1796.

109 Cortes JE, Nicolini FE, Wetzler M, et al. Subcutaneous omacetaxine mepesuccinate in patients with chronic-phase chronic myeloid leukemia previously treated with 2 or more tyrosine kinase inhibitors including imatinib. *Clin Lymphoma Myeloma Leuk*. 2013;**13**(5):584–591.

111 Arora M, Weisdorf DJ, Spellman SR, et al. HLA-identical sibling compared with 8/8 matched and mismatched unrelated donor bone marrow transplant for chronic phase chronic myeloid leukemia. *J Clin Oncol*. 2009;**27**(10):1644–1652.

112 Goldman JM, Majhail NS, Klein JP, et al. Relapse and late mortality in 5-year survivors of myeloablative allogeneic hematopoietic cell transplantation for chronic myeloid leukemia in first chronic phase. *J Clin Oncol*. 2010;**28**(11):1888–1895.

120 Ohanian M, Kantarjian HM, Quintas-Cardama A, et al. Tyrosine kinase inhibitors as initial therapy for patients with chronic myeloid leukemia in accelerated phase. *Clin Lymphoma Myeloma Leuk*. 2014;**14**(2):155–162.

124 Mahon FX, Rea D, Guilhot J, et al. Discontinuation of imatinib in patients with chronic myeloid leukaemia who have maintained complete molecular remission for at least 2 years: the prospective, multicentre Stop Imatinib (STIM) trial. *Lancet Oncol*. 2010;**11**(11):1029–1035.

125 Ross DM, Branford S, Seymour JF, et al. Safety and efficacy of imatinib cessation for CML patients with stable undetectable minimal residual disease: results from the TWISTER Study. *Blood*. 2013.

116 Acute lymphoblastic leukemia

Nitin Jain, MD, MSPH ▪ Stefan Faderl, MD ▪ Hagop M. Kantarjian, MD ▪ Susan O'Brien, MD

Overview

In adults, acute lymphoblastic leukemia (ALL) is a disease with poor prognosis. In the last several years, there have been significant advances in understanding the disease biology, prognostication, and in the development of novel therapies. These include development of monoclonal antibodies, antibody–drug conjugates, tyrosine kinase inhibitors, and more recently, chimeric antigen receptor T-cell therapy. These therapies are beginning to result in improvements in survival of patients with ALL.

Introduction

Acute lymphoblastic leukemia (ALL) is a heterogeneous disease. Identification of cytogenetic-molecular features in ALL has translated into more accurate classification of disease subtypes, institution of risk-adapted therapies, and identification of new drugs. Most impressively, advances in ALL therapy over only a few decades have led to cures for most children with ALL. Adaptation of successful pediatric ALL treatment strategies into therapeutic algorithms for adult ALL have also resulted in significant improvement, although long-term disease-free survival (DFS) rates of around 40% are still inferior. Nonetheless, ongoing molecular dissection of ALL subtypes, refinements of multidrug chemotherapy in combination with the development of new and targeted drugs, comprehension of the kinetics of residual disease, and an increasing grasp of the impact of pharmacogenomic features and drug resistance is expected to contribute to further improvement in the prognosis for adult patients with ALL.

Epidemiology and etiology

ALL is predominantly a disease of children where it constitutes about 80% of all childhood leukemias and 25% of all childhood cancers, peaks between ages 2–5, and is diagnosed at an incidence of 3.5–4/100,000. In contrast, it makes up less than 1% of malignancies in adult patients. The age-adjusted overall incidence of ALL in the United States is about 1.7/100,000, and it is diagnosed annually in approximately 6000 patients in the United States.[1]

ALL is more frequent among Caucasians. Geographic variations in its frequency have been described with higher rates among Hispanic populations in Spain and Latin America.[2] Although there is a slightly higher incidence rate in males than in females among childhood ALL, the rate is much more predominant in males among patients older than 20 years (1.3:1). A higher incidence of ALL has also been observed in industrialized and urban areas giving rise to speculation about socioeconomic factors in the etiology of ALL.[3]

In most cases, no etiology can be established. Among children, only a few cases (<5%) are associated with inherited, predisposing genetic disorders (e.g., Down's syndrome, Bloom's syndrome, ataxia-telangiectasia, Nijmegen breakage syndrome).[4] There is an extensive list of conflicting or isolated papers reporting an increased risk of childhood ALL, based on parental occupation, maternal reproductive history, parental tobacco or alcohol use, maternal diet, prenatal vitamin use, exposure to pesticide or solvents, and exposure to the highest levels (>0.3 or 0.4 μT) of residential, power-line associated magnetic fields.[5,6] Studies have also focused on genetic variability in drug metabolism, DNA repair, and cell cycle checkpoints that might interact with environmental, dietary, maternal, and other external factors to affect leukemogenesis. Genome-wide association studies have identified several genes (such as *ARID5B*, *IKZF1*, *CDKN2A*, *TP63*, *GATA3*) that are associated with increased risk of developing ALL.[7-12]

The peak age for developing childhood ALL of 2–5 years, an association of ALL with industrialized and affluent societies, and the occasional clustering of childhood ALL cases (especially in new towns) have fueled two hypotheses: (1) population-mixing and (2) delayed infection.[13-15] The first hypothesis suggests that clusters of childhood cases result from exposure of susceptible (nonimmune) individuals to a common, fairly nonpathologic infection after mixing naïve hosts with carriers.[13,14] The second hypothesis is based on a two-hit model where susceptible individuals with a prenatally acquired preleukemic clone have had low or no exposure to common infections early in life because of their affluent hygienic environment.[15] Insulation from infection predisposes the immune system of these individuals to aberrant or pathological responses to common infections at an age commensurate with when they encounter pathogens at an age with increased lymphoid proliferation. Indeed, retrospective studies of archived neonatal blood spots and monozygotic twin pairs have identified preleukemic clones and support the notion that additional postnatal transforming events are needed for full leukemic transformation.[16-19]

Clinical presentation

The clinical signs and symptoms of ALL are quite variable. Disease can develop insidiously and persist for months prior to diagnosis, but symptoms occur suddenly in most cases and relate to the expansion of leukemic cells in the marrow, and the involvement of peripheral blood and extramedullary sites such as lymph nodes, liver, spleen, and the central nervous system (CNS). Common symptoms include fatigue, lack of energy, constitutional symptoms (fevers, night sweats, weight loss), easy bruising or bleeding, and dyspnea. Extremity and joint pain may be the only presenting symptoms in children, especially when very young. T-lineage ALL can present with a mediastinal mass, causing stridor, wheezing, pericardial effusions, and superior vena cava syndrome. Testicular involvement occurs with a low frequency predominantly in infant

Holland-Frei Cancer Medicine, Ninth Edition. Edited by Robert C. Bast Jr., Carlo M. Croce, William N. Hait, Waun Ki Hong, Donald W. Kufe, Martine Piccart-Gebhart, Raphael E. Pollock, Ralph R. Weichselbaum, Hongyang Wang, and James F. Holland.
© 2017 John Wiley & Sons, Inc. ISBN: 978-1-118-93469-2

and adolescent boys. Less than 10% of patients have overt CNS involvement at diagnosis, although CNS disease occurs more often in patients with mature B-cell ALL (Burkitt's leukemia/lymphoma). Cranial nerve palsy (especially cranial nerves III, IV, VI, and VII) can lead to double vision, abnormal ocular movements, facial dysesthesias, and facial droop. Nausea and vomiting, headaches, or papilledema may point toward meningeal infiltration and increased intracranial pressure. Chin numbness due to mental nerve involvement may be subtle and can be easily missed unless sought. Diagnosis of CNS involvement is made from cytospin slides from the cerebrospinal fluid (CSF). Although previous guidelines required the presence of >5 WBC/μL of CSF plus identifiable blasts, controversy arose around cases with <5 WBC/μL, with blasts.[20] A more recent approach has been to define three diagnostic scenarios: (1) no detectable blast cells in CSF (CNS 1), (2) <5 WBC/μL and blasts (CNS 2), and (3) ≥5 WBC/μL and blasts or cranial nerve palsies (CNS 3).[21] On physical examination, pallor, ecchymoses, petechiae, generalized lymphadenopathy, and hepatosplenomegaly can be observed. Tumor lysis syndrome is common in patients with mature B-cell ALL, but can also occur in any other subtypes of ALL. Disseminated intravascular coagulation (DIC) is a frequent laboratory finding, but rarely produces clinically significant DIC. Table 1 summarizes the clinical and laboratory characteristics of patients with adult ALL receiving hyper-CVAD chemotherapy as initial treatment presenting to a tertiary referral center.[22]

Diagnosis of ALL

The diagnosis of ALL requires identification of blast cells either in the blood, marrow, or tissue section. A thorough morphologic,

Table 1 Features of adult acute lymphocytic leukemia receiving hyper-CVAD chemotherapy as initial treatment (N = 204).

Characteristic	Variable
Median age (yr)	39.5
Range	16–79
≥60 yr (%)	22
ECOG performance status >2 (%)	7
Organ involvement (%)	1
Lymphadenopathy	32
Splenomegaly	25
Hepatomegaly	16
Median WBC (×10⁹/L)	7.7
WBC >30 × 10⁹/L (%)	26
Chemistry abnormalities (%)	—
↑ Lactic dehydrogenase	59
Creatinine ≥1.3 mg/dL	16
Bilirubin ≥1.3 mg/dL	13
Immunophenotype (%)	—
Precursor B	67
Mature B	9
T cell	12
Other (null, biphenotypic)	12
Myeloid marker positive (%)	54
Karyotype (%)	—
Diploid	22
Ph-positive	16
t(8;14); t(8;2); t(8;22)	4
Hyperdiploid	4
Hypodiploid	5
Risk assignment (%)	—
Standard	22
High	78

Abbreviations: BCM, below costal margin; CNS, central nervous system; ECOG, Eastern Cooperative Oncology Group; LDH, lactate dehydrogenase; ULN, upper limit of normal; WBC, white blood cells.

cytochemical, and immunologic assessment of ALL blasts remains essential in each patient's work up. Identification of distinct cytogenetic-molecular abnormalities has contributed to a more precise classification of the leukemic blasts and thus has enabled a more accurate assessment of the prognosis. Ongoing efforts are focused on genomic profiling leading to a new definition of ALL subtypes and, through it, to the identification of subgroups of patients requiring different treatments and with different prognoses that are only partially distinguished by currently available diagnostic tools.[23,24]

Morphology and cytochemistry

ALL blasts are heterogeneous in size and shape and one of the first attempts to classify ALL was based on this observation. The French American British (FAB) Cooperative Group thus distinguished three subgroups of lymphoblasts: L1 blasts are smaller, have a high nuclear-to-cytoplasmic ratio and inconspicuous nucleoli. The cytoplasm is sparse and variably basophilic. L2 blasts are larger and more pleomorphic, have moderately abundant cytoplasm, a lower nuclear-to-cytoplasmic ratio, and more prominent nucleoli. L1 morphology is more common in children than in adults, whereas L2 morphology is more common in adults. L3 blasts are more homogenous, medium in size, with dispersed chromatin, prominent nucleoli, typically deep blue cytoplasmic basophilia, and sharply demarcated vacuoles. L3 morphology is mostly associated with mature B-cell ALL or Burkitt's lymphoma. Mature B-cell ALL is characterized by a high rate of cell turnover, which is reflected morphologically by the so-called starry sky appearance in marrow biopsy specimens. The distinction into L1, L2, and L3 morphologies has been largely abandoned as with the exception of L3 and its association with mature B-cell ALL, it is no longer prognostically or therapeutically relevant.

Although no cytochemical stain is diagnostic for ALL, the key diagnostic cytochemical feature of ALL is lack of myeloperoxidase (MPO) and nonspecific esterase (NSE) activity. Low-level MPO positivity (3–5%) can occur in patients with lymphoid blast phase of chronic myeloid leukemia and other rare cases.[25,26] Sudan black B staining closely resembles that of MPO itself, but lack of specificity and the ease with which MPO stains can be applied has limited its use. Terminal deoxynucleotidyl transferase (TdT) is a useful marker to distinguish between reactive versus malignant lymphocytosis and is usually positive in ≥40% of ALL blasts. L3 ALL is characteristically TdT-negative.[27]

Immunophenotyping

Immunophenotyping by flow cytometry is an essential step to accurately diagnose ALL, resolve difficult differential diagnoses, and define subtypes further. Although there is no uniformly accepted panel, commonly used markers as listed in Figure 1 are usually sufficient to establish the diagnosis and confirm lineage affiliation in >95% of the cases.

The majority of cases of ALL (75–80%) are of B lineage. Based on their stage of maturation, they can be divided into: (1) pre-pre-B-ALL (pro-B-ALL); (2) early pre-B (common ALL); (3) pre-B-ALL; and (4) mature B-ALL. In their earliest identifiable stage, pre-pre-B-ALL blasts are positive for CD19, CD79a, or CD22, but no other B-cell differentiation antigens. CD19-positive, CD10-negative, cytoplasmic immunoglobulin-negative B-lineage ALL with myeloid marker coexpression is common among infants with ALL, is typically associated with translocation t(4;11) and *MLL* gene rearrangements, and has a poor prognosis. Common ALL (cALL, early pre-B-ALL) represents an intermediate stage in blast

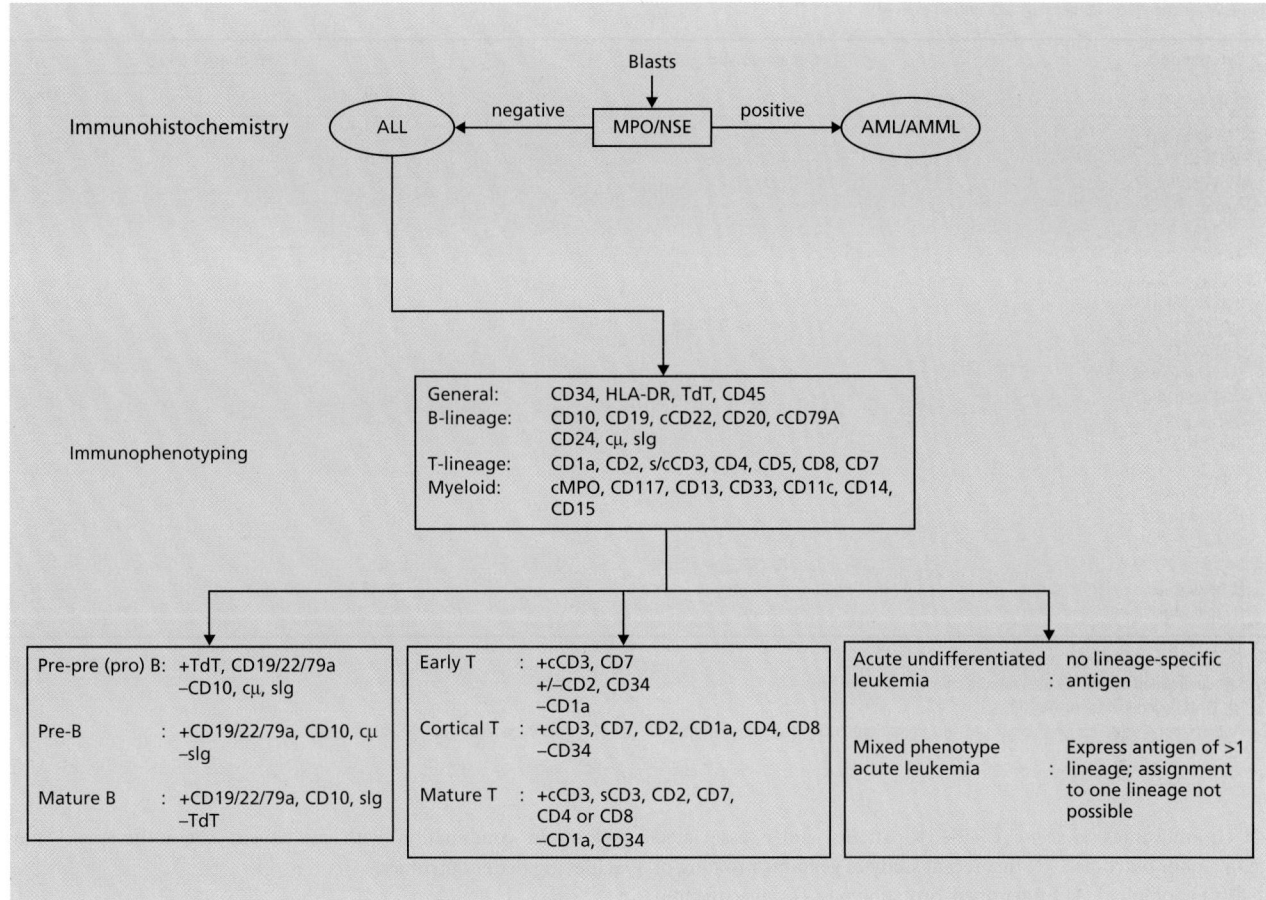

Figure 1 Diagnostic approach to ALL. *Abbreviations*: MPO, myeloperoxidase; NSE, nonspecific esterase; c, cytoplasmic; s, surface.

development and is the most common immunophenotype in adults and children. It is characterized by expression of CD10 (common ALL antigen, CALLA) and is a frequent immunophenotype with Philadelphia chromosome (Ph)-positive ALL. In their more mature stages, pre-B-ALL blasts express TdT, HLA-DR, CD19, CD79a, and cytoplasmic immunoglobulins. A high fraction of pre-B-ALL cases have the translocation t(1;19). Mature B-cell ALL (Burkitt's leukemia) blasts express surface immunoglobulins (sIg, usually IgM), are clonal for κ or λ light chains, and lack expression of TdT. Expression of CD20 is almost ubiquitous in mature B-cell ALL, where as it occurs in only about 40–50% of other ALL subtypes.

T-cell ALL accounts for only 20–25% of cases and similar to B-cell ALL can be further stratified into subtypes based on different stages of intrathymic differentiation. T-cell ALL expresses various levels of CD1a, CD2, CD3, CD4, CD5, CD7, and CD8. CD7 is the most sensitive T-cell marker but lacks specificity because cases of AML or NK-cell leukemia are sometimes CD7-positive. Expression of cytoplasmic CD3 (cCD3) is the most lineage-specific marker for T-cell differentiation. Mature T-ALL expresses both surface CD3 (sCD3) and cCD3, CD2, and either CD4 or CD8 but not both. T-cell ALL of the earlier stages of differentiation expresses cCD3 but not sCD3. Cortical (thymic) T-cell ALL are characterized by expression of CD1a and are double positive for both CD4 and CD8, and are thought to have a favorable outcome.[28] A high-risk subtype of T-cell ALL called early T-cell precursor ALL (ETP ALL) was recently identified and characterized by CD1a negativity, CD8 negativity, weak/absent expression of CD5, and presence of one of

more myeloid markers (CD117, CD34, HLA-DR, CD13, CD33, CD11b, CD65).[29]

Coexpression of myeloid-associated markers is common (15–50% in adult ALL; 5–35% in children), but does not automatically indicate bilineage potential.[30] Myeloid-associated marker expression is more frequent in ALL with translocation t(9;22), t(4;11), and t(12;21), and is generally absent in mature B-cell ALL. Myeloid-associated marker expression has no prognostic significance,[31] but it can be used to distinguish leukemic cells from normal progenitor cells, thereby enabling detection of minimal residual leukemia.

Cytogenetic and molecular abnormalities

Cytogenetic-molecular abnormalities are common in ALL (Table 2).[4,32] Their identification is important as they provide pathobiological insights, serve as targets for drug development, and furnish prognostic information, which has been translated into risk-adapted therapies.[32] Conventional karyotype analysis remains a cornerstone for the detection of chromosome abnormalities. In addition, fluorescence *in situ* hybridization (FISH) and real-time reverse transcriptase polymerase chain reaction (RT-PCR) assays of mRNA are applied to detect minimal residual disease and to monitor patients after therapy.

Numerical abnormalities
Numerical karyotypic abnormalities have an important prognostic impact in ALL. Hypodiploidy defines a karyotype with less than

Table 2 Cytogenetic and molecular abnormalities in ALL.

Cytogenetics	Gene involved	Frequency (%)	
		Adult	Child
t(1;14)(p32;q11)	TAL-1	10–15	5–10
del(5)(q35)	HOX11L2	<2	<2
t(5;14)(q35;q32)	HOX11L2	1	2–3
del(6q), t(6;12)	?	5	<5
del(7p)	?	5–10	<5
+8	—	10–12	2
t(8;14), t(8;22), t(2;8)	c-MYC	5	2–5
t(9;22)(q34;q11)	BCR-ABL	15–25	2–6
del(9)(p21–22)	CDKN2A and CDKN2B	6–30	20
del(9)(q32)	TAL-2	<1	<1
Extrachromosome 9q	NUP214/ABL	<5	?
t(10;14)(q24;q11)	HOX11	5–10	<5
del(11)(q22)	ATM	25–30[a]	15[a]
del(11)(q23)	MLL/AF4	5–10	<5
del(12p) or t(12p)	ETV6-AML1	<1[b]	20–25[b]
del(13)(q14)	miR15/miR16	<5	<5
t(14q11–q13)	TCR α and δ	20–25[c]	20–25[c]
t(14q32)	IGH, BCL11B	5	?
t(1;19), t(17;19)	E2A-PBX1, E2A-HLF	<5	4–5
Hyperdiploidy	—	2–15	10–26
Hypodiploidy	—	5–10	5–10

[a]As determined by loss of heterozygosity.
[b]As determined by polymerase chain reaction.
[c]In T-ALL, overall incidence < 10%.
Abbreviations: IgM, immunoglobulin M; Igκ, immunoglobulin κ; Igλ, immunoglobulin λ; TdT, terminal deoxynucleotidyl transferase.

44 chromosomes, is seen in <5% of patients, and is associated with a poor outcome.[33–36] In a recent study of genomic profiling of >120 hypodiploid ALL identified two subtypes: (1) near-haploid ALL with 24–31 chromosomes harboring alterations targeting receptor tyrosine kinase signaling and *RAS* signaling in majority of the cases and (2) low-hypodiploid ALL with 32–39 chromosomes characterized by alterations in TP53 in >90% of the cases.[36]

Hyperdiploidy is defined by chromosome numbers of more than 46. It is detected more commonly in children than in adults (~25% vs 5%). The range of added chromosomes is not random. Most commonly increased chromosomes are 4, 8, 10, and 21 followed by chromosomes 5, 6, 14, and 17. Gene expression profiles in pediatric patients demonstrated that 70% of the genes that defined this group belonged to either chromosomes X or 21 irrespective of whether or not these chromosomes were increased in the leukemic blasts.[23] Hyperdiploid blasts from patients with ALL have been shown to accumulate more methotrexate and methotrexate polyglutamate, and to be more sensitive to other drugs such as mercaptopurine, thioguanine, cytarabine, and L-asparaginase.[37,38]

Structural abnormalities

Translocation t(9;22)
The translocation between the long arms of chromosome 9 and 22, t(9;22)(q34;q11) Ph is the most common abnormality in adult ALL (15–30%), but is rare in children (<5%).[39] Although $p210^{BCR-ABL}$ is the most frequent oncoprotein in CML, $p190^{BCR-ABL}$ occurs in the majority of patients with Ph-positive ALL. ALL with t(9;22) typically affects older patients, presents with higher white blood cell (WBC) and blast counts at diagnosis, is of a pre-B-cell immunophenotype, and often demonstrates coexpression of myeloid markers.[40] Ph-positive ALL used to be one of the subtypes with the worst long-term DFS, but use of tyrosine kinase inhibitors (TKI; reviewed

below) in combination with multiagent chemotherapy is now achieving better outcomes.

Translocation t(12;21) and del(12p)
Abnormalities of the short arm of chromosome 12 involve *ETV6* (*TEL*) a transcription regulating gene of the Ets family of transcription factors. In translocation t(12;21), *ETV6* is fused to *RUNX1* (*AML1, CBFA2*) on chromosome 21q22.[41] The fusion protein recruits histone deacetylases, induces closure of the chromatin structure, and inhibits transcription, thereby altering both self-renewal and differentiation capacity. The cryptic translocation can be identified in up to 30% of children with ALL using molecular assays making it the most frequent recurring cytogenetic-molecular abnormality in pediatric pre-B-ALL; it is, however, rare in adults.[42] *ETV6-RUNX1*-positve ALL has been associated with an excellent outcome in children, although late relapses may occur.[4] *ETV6-RUNX1*-positive blasts were shown to have suppressed expression of the multidrug resistance-1 (MDR-1) gene have decreased *de novo* purine synthesis and to have suppressed genes involved in purine metabolism.[43]

del(9p21)
Abnormalities of 9p21 occur in up to 15% of patients with ALL.[44] Prognosis in these patients is generally unfavorable, and characterized by higher rates of relapse and shorter survival. The prognostic associations are stronger in childhood ALL and are less well defined in adult ALL.[45,46] Commonly involved genes with del(9p21) include the cyclin-dependent kinase inhibitor genes *CDKN2A* (*MTS1*, *p16*INK4a) and *CDKN2B* (*MTS2*, *p15*INK4b). Using FISH or PCR, heterozygous and/or homozygous deletions of *CDKN2A* have been described in up to 80% of children with T-ALL and 20% of pre-B-ALL.

MLL rearrangements (11q23)

The common denominator of 11q23 abnormalities is involvement of the mixed lineage leukemia gene *MLL (ALL-1, HRX, HTRX1)*. MLL encodes a nuclear protein that maintains the expression of particular members of the *HOX* family and is frequently involved in reciprocal rearrangements with other genes located on chromosomes 4q21, 9p22, 19p13, 1p32, and many others.[47] The fusion of *MLL* with *AF4* on chromosome 4q21 is a frequent abnormality in infant ALL, accounting for up to 85% of the cases, but is detected in only 3–8% of adults.[48] Adults with this translocation tend to be older, have higher WBC counts and organomegaly; sanctuary sites such as the CNS are involved more frequently. CD10-negative, cytoplasmic immunoglobulin-positive pre-B-ALL has a high *MLL* rearrangement rate.[49] Myeloid antigen coexpression is common. Prognosis of *MLL* leukemia is poor in infants and adults but is intermediate in children over 1 year of age.[50]

E2A rearrangements (19p13)

The two known translocations with *E2A* rearrangements on chromosome 19p13 are t(1;19)(q23;p13) and t(17;19)(q21;p13). Translocation t(1;19) is strongly associated with the pre-B-ALL phenotype expressing cytoplasmic immunoglobulin. The translocation juxtaposes *E2A* with the homeobox-containing gene *PBX1*. *E2A-PBX1* functions as a potent transcriptional activator and transforms *in vitro* a variety of cell types including fibroblasts, myeloid progenitors, and lymphoblasts. *E2A-PBX1*-positive ALL rearrangements have a worse prognosis to standard or less aggressive therapy, but does better with more aggressive approaches.[51]

8q24 rearrangements

The *c-MYC* gene, located on 8q24, is involved in one of the three translocations with κ or λ immunoglobulin (Ig) light chain locus in mature B-ALL: (1) the t(8;14)(q24;q32), with a frequency of 80%, is the most common translocation.[52] In this translocation, *c-MYC* is juxtaposed to the immunoglobulin heavy chain (IgH) gene locus on 14q32; (2) the t(8;22)(q24;q11), occurs in about 15% of B-ALL patients and involves the Ig λ gene locus on 22q11; and (3) the t(2;8)(p12;q24)] is the least frequent of translocation and involves the Ig κ gene locus on 2p12.

Other molecular abnormalities

More than 60% of cases of T-cell ALL have activating mutations that involve *NOTCH1*, a gene encoding a transmembrane receptor that regulates normal T-cell development.[53] In fact, activating mutations of *NOTCH1* could be the instigating event in most T-cell leukemias. This genetic abnormality is associated with a favorable prognosis.[54,55] About 2% of childhood ALL cases have intrachromosomal amplification of chromosome 21, which is associated with a B-cell precursor immunophenotype, older age, low leukocyte count and more importantly, an increased risk of relapse.[56]

Gene expression microarrays

Microarray technology is used to establish gene expression profiles that further distinguish subtypes of ALL, stratify patients according to risk and response, and identify genetic markers associated with drug sensitivity and resistance pathways, and yield useful insights into pathogenesis and biology of ALL. Based on gene expression profiling, a new high-risk subtype of B-cell ALL, called Ph-like ALL, has been identified (reviewed in detail below).[57,58]

The therapy of ALL

Combination chemotherapy has been the mainstay of management of both pediatric and adult ALL.[59] The design was based on a combination of all available antileukemia drugs that were delivered in a sequence of extended courses of therapy. The goal was to prevent emergence of resistant leukemic subclones and to rapidly restore normal hematopoiesis. Therapeutic strategies in adult ALL have been patterned after the pediatric regimens, and although various combinations with differences in treatment sequence and choice of agents are being used, the same basic principles apply: induction therapy followed by early intensification and consolidation, specific CNS treatment, and a prolonged maintenance phase.[60,61] Given the high remission rates with these regimens, the focus of current ALL programs is concentrated on improvement of remission duration and survival of adult patients and to improve quality of life of pediatric patients. With this goal in mind, validation of subtype-specific prognostic models and development of risk-adapted and targeted therapy designs have become the major objectives of the clinical trials.

Treatment of newly diagnosed patients

As complex as ALL treatment programs are and as much variations are found in many of its details, an easily recognizable framework is common to all of them and is presented in Figure 2. Because therapy is becoming increasingly subset-specific and depends on proper risk-stratification, the section on prognostic factors is discussed first prior to proceeding to therapy programs in more detail.

Prognostic factors

Efforts to describe risk models for ALL date back to the 1980s and have since experienced continued improvements as a result of the accumulating experience from a sequence of clinical trials. Although remission rates are high with current induction regimens, prognostic models are still useful for risk-directed postremission therapy to improve the DFS rates in adults and children with high-risk ALL and to avoid overtreatment of those with favorable disease. It should be noted that improved treatment has abolished the prognostic impact of many clinical, laboratory, or biological variables. For example, once associated with poor prognosis, T-cell ALL has long-term DFS of over 50% in adults and 80% in children with current therapies including cyclophosphamide and cytarabine, and mature B-cell ALL have complete response (CR) rates of 90% and DFS rates >50% in adults and >80% in children with short-term dose-intense treatment regimens.[59] Information from morphological assessment, immunophenotyping, karyotype analysis, molecular genetics, and, increasingly, measurements of minimal residual disease (MRD) has contributed to a more comprehensive risk stratification of patients. Established adverse risk factors include age >60 years, elevated WBC count at diagnosis [>30,000/μL (B-cell ALL), >100,000/μL (T-cell ALL)], pro-B-cell or early T-cell immunophenotype, the presence of t(4;11)(q21;q23) and other MLL rearrangements, and hypodiploidy or complex karyotype.[39]

Monitoring of MRD after induction and during consolidation has emerged as one of the most powerful predictors of relapse and has been most helpful to further stratify standard-risk patients.[62] The German Multicenter Study Group for Adult ALL (GMALL) prospectively monitored 196 standard-risk ALL patients at up to nine time points in the first year of therapy with quantitative PCR.[63] MRD was predictive for relapse and according to the rapidity of eradication of MRD or persistence of MRD over time, three risk groups could be defined with the 3-year relapse risk varying between 0% (low-risk group) and 94% (high-risk group).

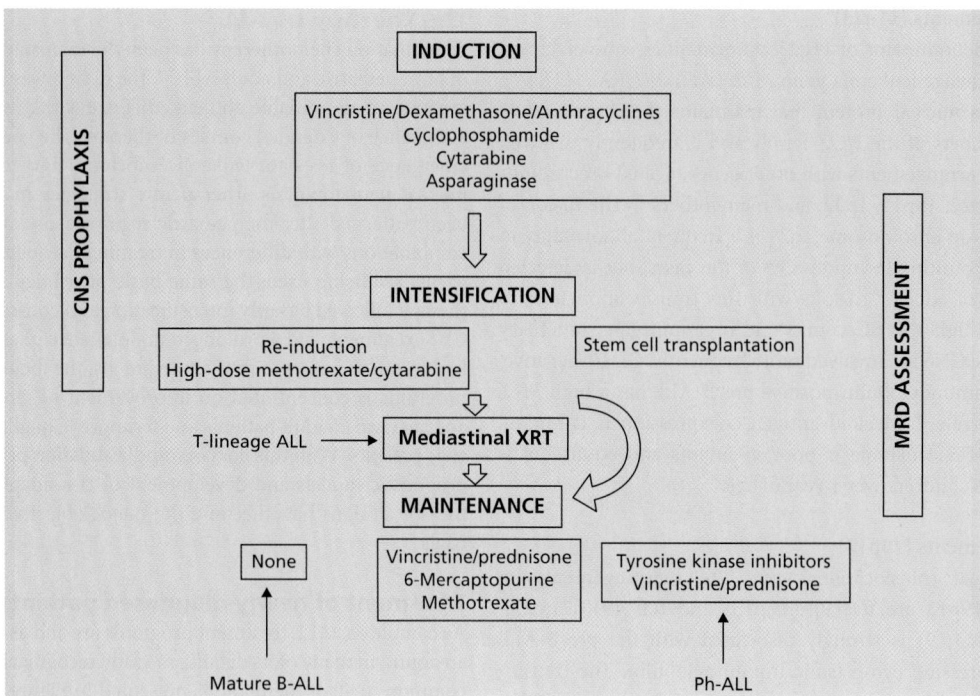

Figure 2 Schematic outline of ALL therapy programs.

Induction therapy

Vincristine, corticosteroids, and a third agent (anthracyclines in adults and asparaginase in children) have long been the backbone of ALL induction therapy.[4] No difference in outcome has been established based on the use of different anthracyclines. Dose intensification of anthracycline during induction has not been shown to definitely improve already high CR rates or to result in significant benefits in DFS.[64,65]

Additional drugs have become part of ALL induction and intensification cycles. These include cytarabine, methotrexate, cyclophosphamide, L-asparaginase, and less frequently etoposide, tenposide, M-amsacrine, or other agents. With CR rates at around 90%, it will be difficult to demonstrate further improvement. Yet, intensification of induction have shown a positive impact on remission duration and survival, and this effect has been most obvious for specific subtypes. Cytarabine and cyclophosphamide have increased response rates and DFS in T-cell ALL.[39] Another important drug has been L-asparaginase. Large randomized pediatric ALL trials have demonstrated improved survival rates where L-asparaginase was given throughout the remission and/or postremission phase.[66–68] L-Asparaginase is a bacterial enzyme, which efficiently depletes serum asparagine. ALL cells require asparagine for protein production, but, in contrast to normal cells, are unable to produce it themselves so that they depend on sufficiently high serum levels for their survival. The most commonly used form of asparaginase is derived from *Escherichia coli,* whose major limitation is development of hypersensitivity and worse tolerability in adults than in children. Pegasparaginase is a modified form of *E. coli* asparaginase with longer serum half-life and reduced risk of hypersensitivity reactions and several studies have been reported in adults.[68,69]

Monoclonal antibodies have been included in adult ALL induction programs. Most experience exists with the anti-CD20 chimeric antibody rituximab [other monoclonal antibodies, including antibody–drug conjugates (ADCs) are reviewed below]. Expression of CD20 has been associated with a higher relapse rate in adult

patients with pre-B-ALL.[70] Several studies have shown improvement in prognosis with chemotherapy plus rituximab combinations especially in mature B-cell ALL.[70,71] A recent update of the modified hyper-cyclophosphamide, vincristine, adriamycin, dexamethasone (hyper-CVAD) regimen from the group at MD Anderson Cancer Center showed that incorporation of rituximab led to very significant improvement in 3-year overall survival (OS) of 75% compared to 47% in the historical controls ($p = 0.003$) in younger patients (<60 years old) with ALL.[70]

Steroids are a standard part of ALL induction and prednisone or prednisolone is the most commonly used steroid, particularly during the maintenance phase. Compared to prednisone and prednisolone, dexamethasone has shown better *in vitro* antileukemic activity and achievement of higher drug levels in the CSF. Using a dose of 6 or 6.5 mg/m^2 throughout therapy, the Children Oncology Group and UK Medical Research Council randomized trials demonstrated a significant reduction in isolated CNS relapse and a significant improvement of event-free survival.[72,73] On the other hand, a smaller study from the Tokyo Children's Cancer Study Group including 231 children with standard- and intermediate-risk ALL showed no difference between dexamethasone (8 mg/m^2 during induction and 6 mg/m^2 during intensifications) and prednisolone (60 and 40 mg/m^2, respectively).[74]

Given the intensity of induction combinations, supportive care has become an important part of ALL therapy. The rationale for hematopoietic growth factors includes shortening of the duration of myelosuppression and therefore associated infectious complications. In addition, a rapid recovery of the marrow function following chemotherapy allows timely administration of dose-intense treatment regimens. Randomized trials have demonstrated advantages of using hematopoietic growth factors such as granulocyte-colony stimulating factor (G-CSF).[75–77] In the double-blinded, randomized Cancer and Leukemia Group B (CALGB) trial 9111, compared to the 102 patients receiving supportive care alone, the G-CSF treated group ($n = 96$) had faster neutrophil recovery to $>1 \times 10^9$/L (16 vs 22 days, $p < 0.001$), platelet recovery (16 vs 19 days, $p = 0.003$), shorter duration of hospital stays ($p = 0.02$), higher CR rates (87% vs 71%, $p = 0.01$), and less mortality (5% vs 11%, $p = 0.04$).[77]

Prophylactic antibiotics including antibacterials (e.g., levofloxacin, ciprofloxacin, trimethoprim–sulfamethoxazole), antifungals (e.g., fluconazole, voriconazole, posaconazole), and antivirals (e.g., acyclovir) should accompany induction therapy until recovery of the neutrophil count to at least 1000/μL in adults. Tumor lysis and, in some cases, DIC should be anticipated in patients with significant leukocytosis and be treated appropriately. Organ involvement and dysfunction may respond to high-dose steroids (e.g., hyperbilirubinemia related to ALL).

Postremission therapy

Postremission therapy consists of an intensified consolidation followed by maintenance therapy and stem cell transplantation (SCT) for some patients. Following the experience from children with ALL, an intensification of postremission therapy has improved outcome, particularly in patients with high-risk disease. There is

no consensus, however, on the optimal type or duration of consolidation. Consolidation programs typically consist of a repetition of the induction sequence or rotational programs including additional agents, which may benefit particular ALL subtypes. As dose, schedule, and combinations of cytostatic drugs vary considerably between studies, it remains difficult to assess the value of the individual components of various programs.

Table 3 details the hyper-CVAD program as one example. During hyper-CVAD, hyperfractionated cyclophosphamide alternates with high doses of cytarabine and methotrexate for eight courses, which equals about 6 months of intensified postremission therapy.[22] Compared to the earlier and less intense VAD program, there has been a significantly better CR rate (91% vs 75%) and survival. In CALGB study 8811, patients underwent early and late intensification courses with eight drugs following a five-drug induction regimen.[60] Maintenance therapy was given until 2 years after diagnosis. The median remission duration was 29 months and the median survival was 36 months, considerably better than the outcome observed with earlier less intense trials.

Table 3 The hyper-CVAD program in ALL.

Component	Drug	Subtype Unspecified	CD20-positive	Mature B cell	T-lineage	Ph-positive
Induction and intensified consolidation						
Hyper-CVAD (cycles 1, 3, 5, 7)	Cyclophosphamide	✓	✓	✓	✓	✓
	Doxorubicin	✓	✓	✓	✓	✓
	Vincristine	✓	✓	✓	✓	✓
	Dexamethasone	✓	✓	✓	✓	✓
	Anti-CD20 Ab (e.g., rituximab)	—	✓[a]	✓	—	✓[a,b]
	TKI (e.g., dasatinib)	—	—	—	—	✓[c]
Methotrexate + HD cytarabine (cycles 2, 4, 6, 8)	Methotrexate	✓	✓	✓	✓	✓
	Cytarabine	✓	✓	✓	✓	✓
	Anti-CD20 Ab (e.g., rituximab)	—	✓[a]	✓	—	✓[a,b]
	TKI (e.g., dasatinib)	—	—	—	—	✓[c]
CNS prophylaxis						
Intrathecal therapy[d]	IT, methotrexate[e]	✓	✓	✓	✓	✓
	IT cytarabine	✓	✓	✓	✓	✓
Pre-maintenance						
Mediastinal XRT	—	—	—	—	✓[f]	—
Nelarabine	Nelarabine	—	—	—	✓[g]	—
Maintenance						
POMP	6-Mercaptopurine	✓[h]	✓[h]	—	✓[h]	—
	Oral methotrexate	✓[h]	✓[h]	—	✓[h]	—
	Prednisone	✓[h]	✓[h]	—	✓[h]	✓[i]
	Vincristine	✓[h]	✓[h]	—	✓[h]	✓[i]
Intensification	Oral methotrexate/ L-asparaginase (months 6 and 18	✓	✓	—	✓	✓
	Hyper-CVAD (months 7 and 19)	✓	✓	—	✓	✓
TKI (e.g., dasatinib)	TKI (e.g., dasatinib)	—	—	—	—	✓[j]

[a]During cycles 1 to 4.
[b]If CD20-positive.
[c]On days 1–14 of the first course; once daily continuously starting cycle 2.
[d]Number of intrathecal therapies depending on risk for CNS disease (4 for low risk, 8 for intermediate risk, 16 for high risk including mature B cell). Two intrathecals are given with each induction/intensified consolidation course).
[e]Dose of intrathecal methotrexate should be reduced by 50% if administered via Ommaya reservoir.
[f]If bulky mediastinal adenopathy (≥7 cm).
[g]Two cycles of 28–35 days each.
[h]Total duration 30 months.
[i]Total duration 24 months.
[j]Continuous administration beyond maintenance.

Most maintenance schedules include 6-mercaptopurine, methotrexate, and monthly pulses of vincristine and prednisone, and extend over 2–3 years. Further intensifications during maintenance are being studied, but remain investigational. Maintenance therapy has become subset-specific. It is of little value in mature B-cell ALL as these patients relapse within the first year of remission and rarely later; TKIs have become an integral component in Ph-positive ALL. Other more T-cell specific drugs such as nelarabine are studied in T-lineage ALL.

SCT has improved outcome for patients with high-risk ALL in first CR.[78–83] Although there has been resistance to apply SCT for standard-risk patients in CR1, recent reports suggest that the benefit of SCT extends also to some standard-risk patients, in some cases possibly based on MRD levels or other features not captured by traditional prognostic markers.[79–81] Studies have also compared the results of allogeneic versus autologous SCT or chemotherapy in patients with ALL in first CR. Unbiased comparisons between treatments remain difficult for several reasons. Most patients lack a matched related sibling and cannot be allocated to allogeneic SCT in the first place. Furthermore, significant heterogeneity exists with regard to transplant preparative regimens, source of stem cells (peripheral blood, marrow), the role of T-cell depletion, and uniform application of prognostic markers.[82,83]

In a French multicenter trial (LALA 87), patients with a matched sibling donor were allocated to receive allogeneic SCT if they were in CR and younger than 40 years ($n = 116$), or were randomized to chemotherapy ($n = 96$) or autologous SCT ($n = 95$) if they were older or had no sibling donor.[84] The 5-year survival rates were not significantly different (48% vs 35%, $p = 0.08$), except for patients with high-risk ALL (Ph-positive ALL, undifferentiated ALL, age > 35 years, leukocyte count > 30×10^9/L, time to CR > 4 weeks), where allogeneic SCT achieved better 5-year survival (44% vs 20%, $p = 0.03$) and DFS (39% vs 14%, $p = 0.01$). In an update of the LALA 87 study, OS rates at 10 years were 44% in the allogeneic SCT arm versus 11% with chemotherapy ($p = 0.009$) in the high-risk group, and 49% and 39%, respectively ($p = 0.6$), for standard-risk patients.[85]

The LALA-94 study focused on a more risk-adapted postremission strategy and the role of allogeneic SCT in ALL.[86] A total of 922 patients were divided into standard-risk, high-risk, Ph-positive, and CNS-positive. All patients received a standard 4-week induction and then divided either postremission chemotherapy (standard-risk group) or allogeneic SCT (all other risk groups) if an HLA-identical sibling was identified. Autologous SCT was offered to patients without donor, or they were randomized between autologous SCT and chemotherapy in the absence of Ph or CNS disease. The study confirmed better DFS for high-risk ALL patients in first CR. On the other hand, autologous transplant did not confer a significant benefit over chemotherapy.

The Groupe Ouest-Est des Leucémies Agiuës et Maladies du Sang (GOELAMS) has evaluated the impact of allogeneic SCT for high-risk patients in first CR versus delayed autologous SCT for patients without matched donors and those older than 50 years.[87] On an intent-to-treat analysis for patients younger than 50 years, 6-year OS was significantly improved with allogeneic SCT compared to autologous stem cell transplant (75% vs 40%, $p = 0.0027$).

The MRC UKALL XII/ECOG E2993 trial was a collaborative effort to address if allogeneic SCT could be beneficial for all suitable adult patients; and if a single autologous SCT could be as effective as postremission chemotherapy.[79] The study enrolled 1929 patients between 15 and 59 years of age. All patients who had an HLA-matched sibling donor were assigned to receive an allogeneic SCT, whereas those who did not or were over age 55 were randomized to receive an autologous SCT versus chemotherapy. Any randomization was preceded by induction chemotherapy and intensification with high-dose methotrexate. High risk was defined as age > 35 years, leukocytosis ($\geq 30 \times 10^9$/L for B-lineage and 100×10^9/L for T-lineage), and Ph-ALL. CR rate was 90% and 5-year survival was 43% for all patients. The following results emerged: (1) survival at 5 years was 53% for Ph-negative patients with a donor versus 45% for those without a donor ($p = 0.02$); (2) 5-year survival for Ph-negative standard-risk patients was superior for patients with a donor compared to those without (62% vs 52%, $p = 0.02$); (3) 5-year survival for high-risk patients was not significantly different whether patients had a donor or not (41% vs 35%, $p = 0.2$). In this group, transplant-related toxicity prevented a better outcome and abrogated the effect of a reduction in relapse rate; and (4) postremission chemotherapy resulted in superior event-free and OS when compared to autologous SCT ($p = 0.02$ and 0.03, respectively).

Although a broader role of allogeneic SCT for patients with ALL in first CR is now emerging, optimal timing remains challenging. Novel therapies (e.g., TKIs for Ph-ALL) may affect outcome requiring a redefinition of SCT in some of the risk groups. Nonmyeloablative SCT has been successfully used in older patients.[83,88,89] The major impediment for SCT remains the fact that less than 30% of patients have a matched sibling donor. Much work is, therefore, invested in improving transplants from partially matched related donors, matched unrelated donors, and umbilical cord blood.[82,83,90,91]

CNS prophylaxis

CNS involvement is rare at diagnosis (<5% in children and <10% in adults).[60,92–94] Nonetheless, in the absence of CNS prophylaxis, CNS disease occurs in 40–50% of the patients and has been a major obstacle to cure.[95] CNS relapse can occur as isolated CNS disease, follow marrow recurrence, or occur concomitantly with a marrow or testicular relapse or both. As CNS relapse confers a poor prognosis, effective CNS prophylaxis is extremely important.[21] CNS prophylaxis should start early and extend through the induction and intensified consolidation phase as delayed CNS prophylaxis has been associated with an increased incidence of CNS disease.

Risk factors for CNS involvement include younger age, T-lineage and mature B-cell ALL immunophenotype, a high WBC count, and the presence of blasts in CSF at diagnosis.[21] Expression of CD7, CD56, and interleukin-15 was found to have prognostic implications with regard to extramedullary manifestations of ALL.[96,97] Elevated serum LDH levels and a high proliferative index (S + G2M >14%) proved to be sensitive predictors of the risk of CNS disease.[98]

Therapeutic modalities for CNS prophylaxis include intrathecal (IT) chemotherapy (methotrexate, cytarabine, steroids), high-dose systemic chemotherapy (methotrexate, cytarabine, L-asparaginase, dexamethasone, 6-thioguanine), and craniospinal irradiation (XRT). Combined triple-modality IT therapy is more effective for CNS control than IT methotrexate alone, but it carries a higher risk of treatment-related CNS morbidity and unexpectedly was associated with an increased risk of bone marrow and testicular relapse in one randomized trial.[99] One explanation for this paradoxical finding is that an "isolated" CNS relapse may in fact be an early manifestation of systemic relapse, and that better CNS control favors leukemic relapse in other sites at a later time. Several studies in children and in adults have demonstrated that IT therapy is equivalent to craniospinal XRT, so that the role of cranial XRT has become controversial.[21] Adverse effects of XRT can be severe and disabling leading to seizures, dementia, and intellectual dysfunction, as well as other complications such as multiple endocrinopathies and growth retardation in children. Patients with cranial nerve root involvement may benefit from selective irradiation to the base of the skull.

Minimal residual disease (MRD)

In children and adults, relapse is thought to result from residual leukemia cells, which persist following achievement of a morphologic and cytogenetic remission, but remain undetectable by conventional methods such as microscopy and cytochemical stains. A number of sensitive techniques have been developed including multicolor flow cytometry and PCR assays. Whatever the assay, detection of residual leukemia cells depends on identification of unique leukemia cell markers. For flow cytometry, aberrant expression of surface marker combinations can be followed, whereas for PCR, leukemia-specific fusions genes (e.g., *BCR-ABL*, *MLL-AF4*, *ETV6-RUNX1*) or patient-specific junctional regions of rearranged immunoglobulin and T-cell receptor genes constitute appropriate markers.[62]

A plethora of studies in both children and adults has provided convincing evidence for the usefulness of MRD monitoring to assess relapse risk.[62,100–105] There is general consensus from pediatric studies that high levels of MRD at the end of induction therapy, persistently high levels during consolidation and maintenance, and continuous increases of MRD levels at any point, are associated with a high risk of relapse.[106] Although more adults have higher levels of MRD at the completion of induction, and the relapse risk is higher even with low levels of MRD compared to children, continuous MRD assessment along several time points has proved predictive for relapse in adult patients as well.[101,102]

Assessment of MRD status has been included in a number of current studies to decide about intensification of postremission therapy. Several questions, however, still remain: (1) what is a clinically relevant threshold of residual disease upon which clinical decisions should be based? (2) which are the most appropriate time points to measure MRD following induction, and how do they change in the context of the specific treatment administered? (3) does intervention based on a molecular relapse improve outcome, and if so, do response criteria upfront need to be modified to include molecular responses? (4) how reproducible are MRD assays across a multitude of laboratories and how reliably can MRD data from different institutions be compared? Beyond being a helpful tool for risk-adapted treatment stratifications, the study of residual disease will hopefully also reveal more about the biology of ALL itself.

Adolescent and young adults (AYA) with ALL

Patients who are in the adolescent and young adult age group (variably defined in clinical studies from 16 years to up to 39 years) could be treated with pediatric-inspired regimens or with adult ALL regimens. Pediatric regimens in general have more intensive treatment with nonmyelosuppressive drugs such as steroids, vincristine, asparaginase, and typically more intensive CNS prophylaxis. Several retrospective and prospective studies have shown better outcomes of this patient population when treated with pediatric regimens versus adult regimens.[107] The group at MD Anderson Cancer recently reported similar outcomes in AYA patients treated with a pediatric regimen (augmented BFM regimen) compared to a historical cohort of patients treated with hyper-CVAD regimen.[108] Recent identification of Ph-like gene signature (see below) in AYA patients with ALL, and its association with poor prognosis, and increase in incidence of Ph-like signature with age adds further complexity to the management of AYA patient population.[24,109]

Salvage therapy

Prognosis of adult patients with relapsed or refractory ALL remains poor. Postrelapse therapies will lead to a second CR in only 30–40% of patients with a 5-year OS of only around 10%. In the MRC UKALL12/ECOG 2993 study, OS at 5 years after relapse was only 7%.[110] Factors predicting for better outcome (indicating 5-year survival rates of 11–12%) included age younger than 20 years and remission durations of more than 2 years. Although there is no standard approach to salvage therapy, there is general consensus, that allogeneic SCT should be first choice in this situation. For most patients, SCT is not an option for lack of a suitable donor, other ongoing comorbid conditions (e.g., infections, poor performance status), or simply uncontrollable disease. Most nontransplant salvage attempts are modeled after patterns familiar from frontline therapy and include: (1) combinations of vincristine, steroids, and anthracyclines; (2) asparaginase and methotrexate combinations; or (3) high-dose cytarabine. Direct comparisons of various regimens are difficult because of differences in patient characteristics, prior drug exposure and sensitivity, number of salvage attempts, variations in dose and schedule of agents, the use of SCT as consolidation in some patients, and not least because of the overall poor outcome. This underscores the need for development of novel therapies for patients with ALL.

Disease subtypes

Ph-positive ALL

Historically, Ph-positive ALL has had the worst survival rates with standard chemotherapy and, being much more frequent in adults than children, was attributed to some degree with the overall worst prognosis for adult patients.[111]

Since the discovery of imatinib and several newer generation TKIs, an array of new treatment possibilities in Ph-positive ALL have become available. Imatinib competitively binds to the ATP binding site of BCR-ABL and inhibits autoactivation of the oncoprotein as well as phosphorylation of downstream intracellular proteins. Imatinib has single-agent activity in Ph-positive ALL with hematologic response rates in the range of 20–30%, but response durations are not maintained and short.[112] Single-agent kinase inhibitor therapy possibly combined with low-intensity therapy (vincristine, steroids) is of particular benefit in elderly and frail patients not considered candidates for more aggressive therapy.[113]

Several studies have successfully combined imatinib with intensive chemotherapy programs.[114–116] The group at MDACC combined imatinib with hyper-CVAD.[114] Imatinib 600 mg was given daily for 14 days with the induction cycle and then continuously thereafter until the dose was again increased to 800 mg for indefinite maintenance therapy. Of the 54 patients with a median age of 51 years (range 17–84 years) treated, 93% achieved a complete remission with a median time to response of 21 days. The molecular response rate based on nested PCR was 52%. Sixteen patients proceeded to allogeneic SCT within a median of 5 months from start of therapy, though survival at 3 years did not seem improved whether or not patients received a SCT (63% vs 56%). Outcome is superior to hyper-CVAD alone: 3-year OS rates were 55% versus 15% ($p < 0.001$). There is a general consensus that imatinib is more effective when started early during induction and when given concurrently with and subsequent to induction and consolidation rather than alternating with chemotherapy.[117]

Dasatinib and nilotinib are two second-generation TKIs, which are many times more potent than imatinib in *in vitro* models, which includes activity against most imatinib-resistant kinase domain mutations. Both have shown activity in imatinib-resistant Ph-positive ALL. The investigators at MD Anderson Cancer Center treated 63 patients with newly diagnosed Ph + ALL with dasatinib in combination with hyper-CVAD chemotherapy.[118,119] A total of 93% patients achieved a major molecular remission and 65% achieved complete molecular remission. The median DFS and OS were 31 and 44 months, respectively. Several studies have confirmed these findings and early TKI therapy is now the standard treatment of Ph + ALL.[39,120–124] Nilotinib has also been combined with multiagent chemotherapy for patients with Ph + ALL.[125] Ponatinib, a third-generation TKI, is currently being investigated in combination with hyper-CVAD chemotherapy as frontline therapy for patients with ALL.[126]

Mature B-ALL (Burkitt's leukemia)

Mature B-cell ALL is a rare entity of ALL and predominates in children. The genetic basis of the disease is the underlying MYC translocation at band 8q24 to either the immunoglobulin heavy chain region on chromosome 14 or less commonly at the λ (22q11) or κ (2p12) loci. Prompt diagnosis and recognition of this entity are essential for optimal treatment outcomes. These patients are at high risk for the development of tumor lysis syndrome. Aggressive hydration and administration of allopurinol and/or rasburicase are important. Intensive chemoimmunotherapy is the standard treatment for these patients.[71,127] Thomas et al. combined hyper-CVAD with rituximab to treat 31 newly diagnosed patients with mature B-ALL or lymphoma and median age of 46 years (29% older than 60 years).[127] The overall CR rate was 86%. The 3-year OS and DFS rates were 89% and 88%, respectively, which was similar in the elderly patients. Younger age and treatment with rituximab were identified as independent favorable factors. Recently, the German ALL study group reported impressive results on 363 patients with Burkitt's leukemia/lymphoma treated prospectively on a chemoimmunotherapy regimen in combination with rituximab.[71] The rate CR, 5-year PFS, and 5-year OS were 88%, 71%, and 80%, respectively.

Ph-like ALL

In 2009, a subgroup of B-cell ALL was identified in children with ALL that had a gene expression profile similar to that of Ph-positive ALL, but these patients lack the Ph.[57,58] These patients, referred as "Ph-like ALL," comprise up to 15% of pediatric B-cell ALL and 20–25% in adolescents and young adults.[24,128] Patients with Ph-like ALL have a very high rate of disease relapse and short overall survival.[24,128–131]

About 50% of Ph-like ALL cases harbor a rearrangement of CRLF2 located at the pseudoautosomal region of Xp22.3/Yp11.3, either as a translocation to the immunoglobulin heavy chain enhancer region at 14q32.33 (IGH-CRLF2), or a focal deletion proximal to CRLF2 resulting in the expression of a P2RY8-CRLF2 fusion transcript.[109,129,132–135]

About 50% of patients with CRLF2 rearrangement have JAK mutations (JAK2, most commonly JAK2R683, and JAK1).[24] Non-CRLF2 rearranged cases have been reported to have fusions of several genes including ABL1, ABL2, JAK2, EPOR, and PDGFRB. These diverse genetic alterations activate signaling pathways, notably ABL1 and PDGFRB (both of which may be inhibited with

the TKI such as dasatinib) and JAK-STAT signaling, which may be inhibited by JAK inhibitor such as ruxolitinib.[109,136]

Harvey et al. evaluated 207 children with "high-risk" B-cell ALL and found that 14% had CRLF2 overexpression.[129] Interestingly, patients with Hispanic ethnicity were more like to have CRLF2 overexpression (35% vs 7% in others, $p < 0.001$).

Early precursor T-cell ALL (ETP ALL)

A subgroup of high-risk T-cell has been identified based on a myeloid gene expression signature.[29] This ALL subset is derived from ETP, cells that recently arrived in the thymus from the bone marrow and retain multilineage differentiation potential. Approximately 10–15% of childhood cases of T-cell ALL and 7–10% of adult cases of T-cell ALL have the ETP phenotype.[29,137] A specific immunophenotype of ETP ALL has been described: (1) CD1a negative; (2) CD8 negative; (3) weak or absent CD5; and (4) presence of one or more of myeloid/stem cell marker such as CD117, CD34, HLA-DR, CD13, CD33, CD11b, and CD65.[29] Patients with ETP ALL have significantly worse outcomes than those with non-ETP T-cell ALL (St Jude's pediatric data—10-year OS, 19% for ETP ALL vs 84% for non-ETP T-cell ALL, $p = <0.0001$; 10-year relapse rate, 72% for ETP ALL vs 10% for non-ETP T-cell ALL, $p = <0.0001$).[29,138] The German ALL study group reported that ETP ALL comprised 7.4% of adult T-cell ALL cases.[137,139,140] They reported a 35% incidence of FLT-3 mutation and a 14% incidence of DNMT3A mutation in patients with ETP ALL.

Novel therapies

A better understanding of the disease biology has led to several novel therapies for patients with ALL (Table 4). A continuous source of active drugs in leukemias is the vast group of nucleoside analogs. Clofarabine is a new generation purine nucleoside modeled after fludarabine and cladribine, but with different mechanisms of action and spectrum of activity.[141] In a phase II trial of clofarabine in 61 pediatric patients with relapsed or refractory ALL, 30% responded.[142] Clofarabine has been approved by the Food and Drug Administration (FDA) for children with

Table 4 New agents in ALL.

Class	Examples
Nucleoside analogs	Clofarabine
	Nelarabine
Liposomal and pegylated compounds	Liposomal vincristine (Marqibo)
	Liposomal doxorubicin
	Pegasparaginase
Monoclonal antibodies	
Unconjugated	Rituximab (CD20)
	Ofatumumab (CD20)
	Epratuzumab (CD22)
	Alemtuzumab (CD52)
Antibody drug/toxin conjugates	Inotuzumab ozogamicin (CD22/calicheamicin)
	SAR3419 (CD19/maytansine)
	Moxetumomab (CD22/Pseudomonas toxin)
Bi-specific antibodies	Blinatumomab (CD19/CD3)
Tyrosine kinase inhibitors	Imatinib
	Dasatinib
	Nilotinib
	Ponatinib
	Ruxolitinib
T-cell immunotherapy	Chimeric antigen receptor T cells

R/R ALL. Kantarjian et al.[143] reported 17% response rate with single-agent clofarabine in adults with relapsed/refractory ALL. The Southwest Oncology Group Study conducted a phase II trial of combination of clofarabine and cytarabine for R/R ALL with a modest response rate of 17%.[144] Nelarabine is a soluble prodrug of 9-β-D-arabinofuranosylguanine (ara-G) with activity predominantly in relapsed T-lineage lymphoid malignancies and is approved by the FDA for this indication.[145–149] Response rates of 33% and up to 41% have been achieved in a group of 121 children and 39 adults with relapsed T-lineage leukemia/lymphoma, respectively.[145,146] Neurotoxicity is the major adverse event of nelarabine, which is both dose and schedule dependent. The MD Anderson group reported 40 patients with newly diagnosed T-cell ALL or T-cell lymphoblastic lymphoma treated with nelarabine in combination with hyper-CVAD chemotherapy.[149] Patients received two cycles of nelarabine at a dose of 650 mg/m² intravenous daily for 5 days both early (after cycles 4 and 5 of hyper-CVAD) and later during the maintenance (replacing cycles 6 and 7 of the maintenance). The overall response rate (ORR) was 97% with 91% patients in CR. The DFS at 3 years was 61% and 3-year probability for OS was 63%. Vincristine is an important component of ALL treatment. Liposomal vincristine facilitates vincristine dose intensification plus enhances target tissue delivery. O'Brien et al. evaluated liposomal vincristine monotherapy in adult patients with Ph-negative ALL in second or greater relapse.[150] Sixty-five patients were treated with a CR/CRi rate of 20% and an ORR rate of 35%. Based on this study, liposomal vincristine has been approved by the FDA for this patient population.

Targeting cell surface receptors

Rituximab, a chimeric monoclonal antibody against the cell surface protein CD20, has a well-established role in B-cell ALL (see above).[70] Ofatumumab targets a different epitope of CD20 and has been found to be more potent than rituximab in promoting complement-dependent cytotoxicity *in vitro* and is currently being studied for patients with ALL.[151,152]

CD19 is expressed uniformly in B-cell ALL. Blinatumomab is a novel antibody (bispecific T-cell engager antibody) designed to target patient's T cells to CD19-expressing tumor cells resulting in a cytotoxic T-cell response.[153] Blinatumomab has been shown to eradicate MRD in a majority of patients with ALL.[154,155] The German ALL study group conducted a phase II trial of blinatumomab in patients with relapsed/refractory B-cell ALL.[156] Blinatumomab was administered by continuous intravenous infusion for 28 days followed by a 14-day treatment-free interval. Responding patients could receive three additional cycles of treatment or proceed to bone marrow transplantation. Of the 36 patients treated, 25 patients (69%) achieved a CR/CRi. The median OS was 9.8 months, and the median relapse-free survival was 7.6 months. In a multicenter international phase II study, 189 patients with R/R ALL were treated with blinatumomab.[157] This study included particularly high-risk patient population [primary refractory or relapsed (first relapse within 12 months of first remission, relapse within 12 months after allogeneic SCT, or no response to or relapse after first salvage therapy or beyond)]. Forty-three percent of patients achieved CR/CRi within two cycles of treatment with blinatumomab. The median overall survival was 6.1 months. Based on these data, blinatumomab is now approved in the United States for treatment of patients with R/R B-cell ALL.

SAR3419 is an ADC that targets CD19. The ADC is created by conjugation of the IgG1 antibody huB4 to the maytansinoid DM4, a potent inhibitor of tubulin polymerization and microtubule assembly. In a phase I study, SAR3419 was administered every 3 weeks in patients with relapsed B-cell lymphoma.[158] The most common drug-related toxicity was ocular toxicity, which was noted in 44% of patients. Of 35 patients evaluable for efficacy, 26 (74%) patients demonstrated a reduction in their tumor size. A second phase I study was conducted to evaluate a once weekly schedule of SAR3419.[159] There was a lower incidence of ocular side effects and 55% of patients noticed tumor shrinkage.

CD22 expression occurs in >90% of patients with ALL. Inotuzumab ozogamicin is a CD22 monoclonal antibody bound to a toxin, calecheamicin, and has shown single-agent activity in relapsed/refractory ALL.[160] In a phase II study, patients were given inotuzumab ozogamicin (1.8 mg/m²) intravenously every 3–4 weeks. Forty-nine patients were treated. The overall response rate was 57% (CR 18%, marrow CR 39%). Based on higher *in vitro* efficacy with more frequent exposure, a weekly schedule (0.8 mg/m² on day 1, and 0.5 mg/m² on days 8 and 15, every 3–4 weeks) has been developed.[161] With the weekly schedule, the overall response rate was 53% with an improved toxicity profile. Inotuzumab ozogamicin in combination with rituximab has been evaluated in patients with R/R NHL.[162] The MTD of inotuzumab ozogamicin in combination with rituximab was 1.8 mg/m² every 4 weeks. The most common grade 3–4 adverse events were thrombocytopenia (31%) and neutropenia (22%). At the MTD, the objective response rates were 87% and 74% in patients with relapsed follicular lymphoma (FL) and diffuse large B cell lymphoma (DLBCL), respectively.

Epratuzumab, an unconjugated monoclonal antibody targeting CD22, has also been studied in ALL. Advani et al.[163] added epratuzumab to the combination of clofarabine and cytarabine in adults with R/R B-cell ALL (Southwestern Oncology Group study S0910). The CR/CRi rate was reported as 52%, significantly higher than their previous trial with clofarabine/cytarabine alone, where the response rate was only 17%.[144] Epratuzumab in combination with vincristine and steroids has also been tested in older patients with R/R ALL with a 20% CR/CRi rate.[164]

Moxetumomab is a recombinant immunotoxin composed of the Fv fragment of an anti-CD22 monoclonal antibody fused to the pseudomonas toxin.[165] In a phase I study in pediatric patients with relapsed/refractory CD22+ B-cell ALL, moxetumomab was administered at doses of ranging from 5 to 40 mcg/kg, every other day for 6 doses.[166] Twenty-one patients were treated. The most common treatment-related adverse events were increased weight, increased transaminases, and hypoalbuminemia. The ORR was 29%. A phase I/II trial of moxetumomab in adult patients with R/R ALL is currently enrolling patients (NCT01891981).

CD52 is expressed on nearly all normal and malignant B lymphocytes and T lymphocytes, monocytes, and macrophages.[167] Alemtuzumab is an unconjugated monoclonal antibody directed against CD52. In a phase I/II CALGB study, alemtuzumab was administered to 24 patients with ALL in CR1 with an intent to eradicate the MRD.[168] Serial assessment of MRD was possible in 11 patients of which 8 patients had a median 1-log decrease in MRD. Alemtuzumab, as a single-agent, has limited activity in relapsed/refractory pediatric and adult patients with ALL.[169,170]

Chimeric antigen receptor (CAR) therapy

Immunotherapy with chimeric antigen receptors (CARs) is an active field of research. CARs are synthetic receptors composed of an antigen-binding domain fused to a transmembrane domain followed by one or more cytoplasmic signaling domains. The resultant receptor is then expressed on autologous or allogeneic T cells. CD19 CARs have shown remarkable activity in B-cell ALL patients with >80% CR rate in a relapsed/refractory patient population.[171–174] Davila et al.[171] reported on 16 patients with relapsed/refractory B-cell ALL who were treated with CD19-directed CAR T cells.

The CR rate was 88%. Maude et al. reported on 30 pediatric and adult patients with R/R ALL treated with CD19-directed CAR T cells.[174] CR was achieved in 27 patients (90%). Six-month event-free survival (EFS) rate was 67% and OS was 78%. Cytokine release syndrome is common after CAR T-cell infusion. Targeting CD19 also leads to B-cell aplasia and these patients require regular immunoglobulin replacement.

T-cell ALL

Unlike B-cell ALL where several therapeutic targets are being investigated, only a limited number of drugs/targets are currently being investigated in T-cell ALL.

Notch inhibition in T-cell ALL

Notch signaling is highly conserved evolutional pathway and is required for commitment of stem cells to T-cell fate.[175,176] Ellisen et al. first reported Notch involvement in T-cell ALL when they described a translocation t(7;9)(q34;q34.3).[177] Weng et al. reported activating *NOTCH1* mutations in 56% of patients with T-cell ALL.[53] Asnafi et al. reported a 72% incidence of *NOTCH1* and *FBXW7* mutations in adult patients with T-cell ALL.[55] Presence of *NOTCH1/FBXW7* mutations is associated with better clinical outcomes.[55,178] A phase I trial of an oral γ-secretase inhibitor MK-0752 in patients with R/R T-cell ALL showed modest clinical activity but with significant gastrointestinal toxicities.[179] Gastrointestinal toxicity is an on-target effect where small bowel epithelial cells are skewed to goblet cell fate instead of enterocytes.[180] A phase I trial with a γ-secretase inhibitor, BMS-906024, given weekly, is currently underway (NCT01363817).

Summary

Progress in the understanding of the biology of ALL and refinements of prognostic systems have led to increasing sophistication of therapy. Patients with mature B-cell ALL do best with short-term dose-intensive therapies, whereas outcome in T-cell ALL has improved with the addition of cyclophosphamide and cytarabine. It is now well established that treatment for Ph-positive ALL should include TKIs, ideally from the start and probably best maintained for many years thereafter. The role of transplantation is modified according to better and more predictable risk stratification. Transplantation should be considered in first remission in any high-risk patients without prohibitively serious comorbidities, or any patients beyond a first remission. Its expansion into standard-risk groups is being discussed, but not a standard approach. As for any other malignancy, the key to improving prognosis of ALL, especially for adult patients, lies in continuously better definitions of the many subtypes of ALL. Ph-like ALL and ETP ALL represent two recently defined high-risk subtypes of ALL and may be targetable with TKIs. Treatment programs in ALL are complex and will continue to be. Development of new drugs such as ADCs and CAR T-cell therapy is very promising. Incorporation of these new agents with the currently established treatment programs remains an ongoing challenge.

Key references

The complete reference list can be found on the Wiley Companion Digital Edition of this title (see inside front cover for login instructions).

9   Mulligan CG, Goorha S, Radtke I, et al. Genome-wide analysis of genetic alterations in acute lymphoblastic leukaemia. *Nature*. 2007;**446**(**7137**):758–764.

22 Kantarjian H, Thomas D, O'Brien S, et al. Long-term follow-up results of hyperfractionated cyclophosphamide, vincristine, doxorubicin, and dexamethasone (Hyper-CVAD), a dose-intensive regimen, in adult acute lymphocytic leukemia. *Cancer*. 2004;**101**(**12**):2788–2801.

24 Roberts KG, Li Y, Payne-Turner D, et al. Targetable kinase-activating lesions in Ph-like acute lymphoblastic leukemia. *N Engl J Med*. 2014;**371**(**11**):1005–1015.

28 Marks DI, Paietta EM, Moorman AV, et al. T-cell acute lymphoblastic leukemia in adults: clinical features, immunophenotype, cytogenetics, and outcome from the large randomized prospective trial (UKALL XII/ECOG 2993). *Blood*. 2009;**114**(**25**):5136–5145.

29 Coustan-Smith E, Mullighan CG, Onciu M, et al. Early T-cell precursor leukaemia: a subtype of very high-risk acute lymphoblastic leukaemia. *Lancet Oncol*. 2009;**10**(**2**):147–156.

36 Holmfeldt L, Wei L, Diaz-Flores E, et al. The genomic landscape of hypodiploid acute lymphoblastic leukemia. *Nat Genet*. 2013;**45**(**3**):242–252.

53 Weng AP, Ferrando AA, Lee W, et al. Activating mutations of NOTCH1 in human T cell acute lymphoblastic leukemia. *Science*. 2004;**306**(**5694**):269–271.

55 Asnafi V, Buzyn A, Le Noir S, et al. NOTCH1/FBXW7 mutation identifies a large subgroup with favorable outcome in adult T-cell acute lymphoblastic leukemia (T-ALL): a Group for Research on Adult Acute Lymphoblastic Leukemia (GRAALL) study. *Blood*. 2009;**113**(**17**):3918–3924.

57 Den Boer ML, van Slegtenhorst M, De Menezes RX, et al. A subtype of childhood acute lymphoblastic leukaemia with poor treatment outcome: a genome-wide classification study. *Lancet Oncol*. 2009;**10**(**2**):125–134.

58 Mullighan CG, Su X, Zhang J, et al. Deletion of IKZF1 and prognosis in acute lymphoblastic leukemia. *N Engl J Med*. 2009;**360**(**5**):470–480.

60 Larson RA, Dodge RK, Burns CP, et al. A five-drug remission induction regimen with intensive consolidation for adults with acute lymphoblastic leukemia: cancer and leukemia group B study 8811. *Blood*. 1995;**85**(**8**):2025–2037.

61 Kantarjian HM, Cortes JE, O'Brien S, et al. Long-term survival benefit and improved complete cytogenetic and molecular response rates with imatinib mesylate in Philadelphia chromosome-positive chronic-phase chronic myeloid leukemia after failure of interferon-alpha. *Blood*. 2004;**104**(**7**):1979–1988.

63 Bruggemann M, Raff T, Flohr T, et al. Clinical significance of minimal residual disease quantification in adult patients with standard-risk acute lymphoblastic leukemia. *Blood*. 2006;**107**(**3**):1116–1123.

70 Thomas DA, O'Brien S, Faderl S, et al. Chemoimmunotherapy with a modified hyper-CVAD and rituximab regimen improves outcome in de novo Philadelphia chromosome-negative precursor B-lineage acute lymphoblastic leukemia. *J Clin Oncol*. 2010;**28**(**24**):3880–3889.

71 Hoelzer D, Walewski J, Dohner H, et al. Improved outcome of adult Burkitt lymphoma/leukemia with rituximab and chemotherapy: report of a large prospective multicenter trial. *Blood*. 2014;**124**(**26**):3870–3879.

79 Goldstone AH, Richards SM, Lazarus HM, et al. In adults with standard-risk acute lymphoblastic leukemia, the greatest benefit is achieved from a matched sibling allogeneic transplantation in first complete remission, and an autologous transplantation is less effective than conventional consolidation/maintenance chemotherapy in all patients: final results of the International ALL Trial (MRC UKALL XII/ECOG E2993). *Blood*. 2008;**111**(**4**):1827–1833.

80 Cornelissen JJ, van der Holt B, Verhoef GE, et al. Myeloablative allogeneic versus autologous stem cell transplantation in adult patients with acute lymphoblastic leukemia in first remission: a prospective sibling donor versus no-donor comparison. *Blood*. 2009;**113**(**6**):1375–1382.

86 Thomas X, Boiron JM, Huguet F, et al. Outcome of treatment in adults with acute lymphoblastic leukemia: analysis of the LALA-94 trial. *J Clin Oncol*. 2004;**22**(**20**):4075–4086.

92 Lazarus HM, Richards SM, Chopra R, et al. Central nervous system involvement in adult acute lymphoblastic leukemia at diagnosis: results from the international ALL trial MRC UKALL XII/ECOG E2993. *Blood*. 2006;**108**(**2**):465–472.

107 Stock W. Adolescents and young adults with acute lymphoblastic leukemia. *Hematol Am Soc Hematol Educ Program*. 2010;**2010**:21–29.

108 Rytting ME, Thomas DA, O'Brien SM, et al. Augmented Berlin-Frankfurt-Munster therapy in adolescents and young adults (AYAs) with acute lymphoblastic leukemia (ALL). *Cancer*. 2014;**120**(**23**):3660–3668.

109 Roberts KG, Morin RD, Zhang J, et al. Genetic alterations activating kinase and cytokine receptor signaling in high-risk acute lymphoblastic leukemia. *Cancer Cell*. 2012;**22**(**2**):153–166.

114 Thomas DA, Faderl S, Cortes J, et al. Treatment of Philadelphia chromosome-positive acute lymphocytic leukemia with hyper-CVAD and imatinib mesylate. *Blood*. 2004;**103**(**12**):4396–4407.

116 Fielding AK, Rowe JM, Buck G, et al. UKALLXII/ECOG2993: addition of imatinib to a standard treatment regimen enhances long-term outcomes in Philadelphia positive acute lymphoblastic leukemia. *Blood*. 2014;**123**(**6**):843–850.

118 Ravandi F, O'Brien S, Thomas D, et al. First report of phase 2 study of dasatinib with hyper-CVAD for the frontline treatment of patients with Philadelphia chromosome-positive (Ph+) acute lymphoblastic leukemia. *Blood*. 2010;**116**(**12**):2070–2077.

120 Bassan R, Rossi G, Pogliani EM, et al. Chemotherapy-phased imatinib pulses improve long-term outcome of adult patients with Philadelphia chromosome-positive acute lymphoblastic leukemia: Northern Italy Leukemia Group protocol 09/00. *J Clin Oncol*. 2010;**28**(**22**):3644–3652.

126 Jabbour E, Kantarjian H, Thomas DA, et al. Phase II study of combination of hyper-CVAD with ponatinib in front line therapy of patients (pts) with Philadelphia Chromosome (Ph) positive acute lymphoblastic leukemia (ALL). *Blood* (ASH Annual Meeting Abstracts). 2013;**122**:2663a.

127 Thomas DA, Faderl S, O'Brien S, et al. Chemoimmunotherapy with hyper-CVAD plus rituximab for the treatment of adult Burkitt and Burkitt-type lymphoma or acute lymphoblastic leukemia. *Cancer*. 2006;**106**(7):1569–1580.

129 Harvey RC, Mullighan CG, Chen IM, et al. Rearrangement of CRLF2 is associated with mutation of JAK kinases, alteration of IKZF1, Hispanic/Latino ethnicity, and a poor outcome in pediatric B-progenitor acute lymphoblastic leukemia. *Blood*. 2010;**115**(26):5312–5321.

130 Harvey RC, Mullighan CG, Wang X, et al. Identification of novel cluster groups in pediatric high-risk B-precursor acute lymphoblastic leukemia with gene expression profiling: correlation with genome-wide DNA copy number alterations, clinical characteristics, and outcome. *Blood*. 2010;**116**(23):4874–4884.

138 Zhang J, Ding L, Holmfeldt L, et al. The genetic basis of early T-cell precursor acute lymphoblastic leukaemia. *Nature*. 2012;**481**(7380):157–163.

143 Kantarjian H, Gandhi V, Cortes J, et al. Phase 2 clinical and pharmacologic study of clofarabine in patients with refractory or relapsed acute leukemia. *Blood*. 2003;**102**(7):2379–2386.

150 O'Brien S, Schiller G, Lister J, et al. High-dose vincristine sulfate liposome injection for advanced, relapsed, and refractory adult Philadelphia chromosome-negative acute lymphoblastic leukemia. *J Clin Oncol*. 2013;**31**(6):676–683.

154 Topp MS, Kufer P, Gokbuget N, et al. Targeted therapy with the T-cell-engaging antibody blinatumomab of chemotherapy-refractory minimal residual disease in B-lineage acute lymphoblastic leukemia patients results in high response rate and prolonged leukemia-free survival. *J Clin Oncol*. 2011;**29**(18):2493–2498.

155 Topp MS, Gokbuget N, Zugmaier G, et al. Long-term follow-up of hematologic relapse-free survival in a phase 2 study of blinatumomab in patients with MRD in B-lineage ALL. *Blood*. 2012;**120**(26):5185–5187.

156 Topp MS, Gokbuget N, Zugmaier G, et al. Phase II Trial of the anti-CD19 bispecific T cell-engager blinatumomab shows hematologic and molecular remissions in patients with relapsed or refractory B-precursor acute lymphoblastic leukemia. *J Clin Oncol*. 2014;**32**(36):4134–4140.

160 Kantarjian H, Thomas D, Jorgensen J, et al. Inotuzumab ozogamicin, an anti-CD22-calecheamicin conjugate, for refractory and relapsed acute lymphocytic leukaemia: a phase 2 study. *Lancet Oncol*. 2012;**13**(4):403–411.

172 Brentjens RJ, Davila ML, Riviere I, et al. CD19-targeted T cells rapidly induce molecular remissions in adults with chemotherapy-refractory acute lymphoblastic leukemia. *Sci Transl Med*. 2013;**5**(177):177ra38.

173 Grupp SA, Kalos M, Barrett D, et al. Chimeric antigen receptor-modified T cells for acute lymphoid leukemia. *N Engl J Med*. 2013;**368**(16):1509–1518.

174 Maude SL, Frey N, Shaw PA, et al. Chimeric antigen receptor T cells for sustained remissions in leukemia. *N Engl J Med*. 2014;**371**(16):1507–1517.

117 Chronic lymphocytic leukemia

Kanti R. Rai, MD ▪ Jacqueline C. Barrientos, MD

Overview

Chronic lymphocytic leukemia (CLL) is an indolent B-cell neoplasia characterized by a progressive accumulation of small functionally incompetent lymphocytes in the blood, marrow, and lymphoid tissues. Given its indolent presentation, initiation of therapy is deferred until patients become symptomatic. CLL primarily affects the elderly population who generally has clinically significant coexisting conditions. The use of traditional chemoimmunotherapy regimens has been historically limited to fit patients able to tolerate the known toxicities from such regimens. A major shift in the management of CLL is currently taking place with the approval of several new targeted agents with unprecedented clinical activity in patients with poor prognostic markers and high-risk disease. New drug combinations are being evaluated with the goal to optimize treatment approaches based on the clinical and biological profile of the CLL patient.

Chronic lymphocytic leukemia

CLL biology: Historical perspective

CLL is a monoclonal CD5+ B-cell lymphoproliferative disorder derived from antigen-experienced B lymphocytes that differ in their level of immunoglobulin heavy chain variable region (IGHV) gene mutations.[1] Table 1 summarizes some of the important differences between the way CLL is defined now and in the past. The pace of research in CLL received a major boost over the past decade with the finding of chromosomal abnormalities and genetic mutations that contribute to the heterogeneity of the clinical presentation and help predict the disease course. Equally important has been the discovery of the role of the microenvironment and of the signaling factors that are necessary to CLL pathogenesis.[2-5] This greater understanding has led to the development of agents that specifically target dysregulated pathways that allow the proliferation and survival of the malignant clone. The recent introduction of therapies with excellent clinical activity in patients previously refractory to chemotherapy is changing the natural history of the disease with long-term survival expectations substantially improved. Despite these rapid advances, the majority of CLL patients who initially achieve a remission eventually relapse. Presently, research is focused on elucidating mechanisms of resistance to the novel targeted agents.

Incidence and epidemiology

CLL is the most prevalent adult leukemia in the Western world accounting for approximately 30% of all leukemias diagnosed in the United States. Approximately 15,720 new cases of CLL and 4600 deaths are expected in the United States in 2014.[6] For the most part, CLL is a disease of the elderly, with a median age of 71 years at diagnosis. The male : female incidence ratio of CLL is approximately 1.5 : 1.[6,7] CLL is more common in Europe, Australia, and North America than in Asia, Africa, or other less developed countries.[8]

Diagnosis of CLL

The World Health Organization (WHO) classification of hematopoietic tumors describes CLL as a leukemic, lymphocytic lymphoma, distinguishable from small lymphocytic lymphoma (SLL) only by its leukemic presentation.[9] In this classification, CLL is always a disease of neoplastic B cells, while the entity formerly known as T-CLL is now called T-cell prolymphocytic leukemia (T-PLL).[10] The International Workshop on CLL (IWCLL) established the diagnosis of CLL as requiring the presence of at least 5×10^9 clonal B lymphocytes/L (5000/µL) in the peripheral blood confirmed by flow cytometry.[11] Peripheral blood smear review reveals small, mature lymphocytes with a narrow border of cytoplasm (Figure 1). Gumprecht nuclear shadows, also known as "smudge cells," can be found as debris. The nuclear chromatin is clumped and exhibits partially aggregated chromatin with up to 55% larger or atypical cells, cleaved cells, or prolymphocytes.[12]

Pathogenesis and causation

Monoclonal B-cell lymphocytosis and familial CLL

The absence of cytopenias, lymphadenopathy, organomegaly, or disease-related symptoms (B symptoms) in the presence of fewer than 5×10^9 clonal B lymphocytes/L in the peripheral blood is defined as "monoclonal B-lymphocytosis" (MBL).[13] Rawstron and colleagues[14] found MBL among 13.5% of normal first-degree relatives of people known to have CLL. That incidence is much higher than the 3.5% that Rawstron and colleagues discovered among adults with normal blood counts without a first-degree relative with CLL.[15] Furthermore, there is an increased incidence of CLL or related disorders among the family members of people known to have CLL.[17,16] Further research is needed to elucidate a putative CLL predisposition gene or a possible CLL carrier state. Similar to Kyle's MGUS data in multiple myeloma,[18] the rate of progression to CLL that requires treatment is 1.1% per year.[19]

Immunobiology and immunophenotype of CLL cells

Morphologically, CLL cells resemble mature lymphocytes in the normal peripheral blood and coexpress the T-cell antigen CD5 with the B-cell surface antigens CD19, CD20, and CD23. The levels of surface immunoglobulin, CD20, and CD79b are characteristically

Holland-Frei Cancer Medicine, Ninth Edition. Edited by Robert C. Bast Jr., Carlo M. Croce, William N. Hait, Waun Ki Hong, Donald W. Kufe, Martine Piccart-Gebhart, Raphael E. Pollock, Ralph R. Weichselbaum, Hongyang Wang, and James F. Holland.
© 2017 John Wiley & Sons, Inc. ISBN: 978-1-118-93469-2

Table 1 B-cell chronic lymphocytic leukemia as viewed then and now.

Previously	Currently
• A clinically heterogeneous disease with a homogeneous cellular origin	• A clinically heterogeneous disease originating from B lymphocytes that may differ in activation and maturation state or cellular subset
• A disease derived from naive B lymphocytes	• A disease derived from antigen-experienced B lymphocytes that differ in the level of immunoglobulin V gene mutations
• Leukemic cell accumulation occurs because of an inherent apoptotic defect involving the entire mass of leukemic cells	• An inherent apoptotic defect involving the entire mass of leukemic cells is unlikely to exist initially. Cell accumulation occurs because of survival signals delivered to a subset of leukemic cells from the external environment through a variety of receptors (e.g., *BCR*, chemokine, and cytokine receptors) and their cell-bound and soluble ligands
• A disease of accumulation	
• Prognostic markers identify patients at low/intermediate/high (Rai) or A/B/C (Binet) risk with an acknowledged heterogeneity (vis-à-vis clinical outcomes) among patients in the low/A and intermediate/B risk categories	• A disease of accumulation with an associated level of proliferation that exceeds that previously appreciated
• Therapy based largely on clinical observations and trial-and-error methods	• Newer molecular and protein markers separate patients within the low/A and intermediate/B risk categories that follow different clinical courses
	• Above-noted newer findings provide clues to discover discrete targets for developing hypothesis-driven and effective therapeutic agents

Table 2 Malignancies of morphologically mature-appearing B lymphocytes.

Chronic lymphocytic leukemia/small lymphocytic lymphoma (CLL/SLL)
B-prolymphocytic leukemia (B-PLL)
Hairy cell leukemia (HCL)
Follicular lymphoma in leukemic phase (FL-L)
Mantle cell lymphoma in leukemic phase (MCL-L)
Splenic lymphoma with villous lymphocytes (SLVL)
Lymphoplasmacytoid lymphoma

Table 3 Phenotypes of lymphoproliferative disorders.

Disease	Typical phenotypes
CLL	CD20 (d), CD19+, CD22 (d), sIg (d), CD23+, FMC-7−, CD5+, CD10−, CD38+/−
Mantle cell lymphoma	CD20 (i), sIg (i), CD23+/−, FMC-7+/−, CD5+, CD10−, cyclin-D1+
B-prolymphocytic leukemia	CD20 (+i), sIg (+i), FMC-7+/−, CD5+/−, CD10−
Marginal zone B-cell lymphoma	CD23−, CD11c+/−, CD103+/−, CD5+/−, CD10−, CD138 (b)
Lymphoplasmacytic lymphoma	CD23(-/d), sIg+/−, cIg+, CD5+/−
Follicular lymphoma	CD20 (+i), CD5−, CD10+, bcl-2+, CD43−
Diffuse large B-cell lymphoma	CD20 (+i), CD5−, CD10+, bcl-2+/−, CD43+/−, CD5+/−
Burkitt's lymphoma	Bcl-2−, CD10 (+b), CD43+, CD5−
Hairy cell leukemia	CD20 (b), CD22 (b), CD11c (b), CD25+, CD103+, sIg (i), CD123+, CD5−

Abbreviations: +, usually positive; −, usually negative; +/−, may be positive or negative; d, dim; i, intermediate; b, bright; sIg, surface immunoglobulin; cIg, cytoplasmic immunoglobulin.

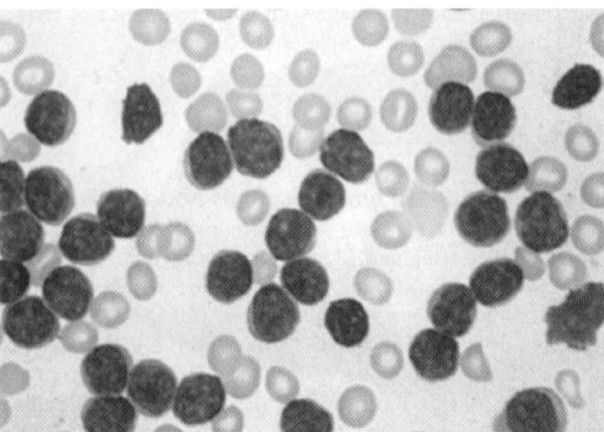

Figure 1 Chronic lymphocytic leukemia morphology in peripheral blood smear. Leukocyte count: 100×10^9/L. Most of the lymphocytes are mature appearing. One smudge cell is present. Platelets are absent in this thrombocytopenic patient (Wright-Giemsa stain; ×100 original magnification).

low compared with those found on normal B cells,[20] with the clones restricted to expression of either kappa or lambda immunoglobulin light chains. Several other malignancies of mature-appearing lymphocytes (Table 2) present with clinical features overlapping those of CLL; hence, flow cytometry is extremely helpful in distinguishing CLL from other diseases (Table 3).[21–23]

Clinical aspects

Patients infrequently present with constitutional symptoms. The classic symptoms are known as "B symptoms": unintentional weight loss of 10% or more, fevers higher than 100.5°F (38°C), or night sweats for more than 1 month without evidence of infection. Fatigue may also be reported.

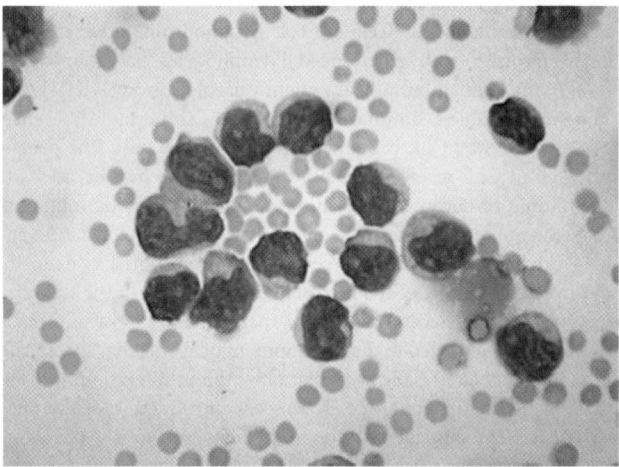

Figure 2 Prolymphocytic leukemia. Peripheral blood smear shows cells with prominent nucleoli and abundant cytoplasm (Wright-Giemsa stain; ×1000 original magnification).

Absolute lymphocytosis in blood

By IWCLL criteria, the presence of at least 5×10^9 B clonal lymphocytes per liter (5000/μL) with the phenotypes CD19+, CD20+, CD23+, and CD5+ is required to diagnose CLL, as lymphocytosis may occur with infections or in other neoplastic conditions (e.g., leukemic phase of lymphomas, hairy cell leukemia (HCL), PLL—Figure 2, and large granular cell leukemia).

Clinical presentation

Upon physical examination, a CLL patient may have enlarged nodes that are firm, rounded, discrete, nontender, and freely mobile upon palpation. The most consistent abnormal finding on physical examination is lymphadenopathy, but splenomegaly or hepatomegaly may also be present. Enlargement may be generalized or localized, and degree can vary widely leading to obstruction of adjacent organs. In addition to palpably enlarged peripheral lymph nodes, liver, and spleen, virtually any other lymphoid tissue in the body—for example, Waldeyer's ring or the tonsils—may be enlarged at diagnosis. In addition, infiltration with CLL cells may occur in any organ or tissue. In contrast to lymphoma, gastrointestinal mucosal involvement is rarely seen in CLL. Similarly, meningeal involvement is extremely unusual.

Radiologic findings

Radiologic examinations are neither required nor recommended as part of an evaluation at the time of initial diagnosis or during routine follow-up. Computed tomography (CT) scans or chest films will often reveal adenopathy not detected on examination, but these findings do not change the clinical Rai or Binet stage. Unless there is a specific clinical question brought up by a new symptom or complaint, we recommend not doing these procedures. The American Society of Hematology embarked on the "Choosing Wisely" campaign to advocate clinical staging and blood monitoring in asymptomatic patients with early-stage CLL rather than performing CT scans. In the setting of a therapeutic research protocol, imaging may be obtained for specific protocol-related purposes.

Laboratory abnormalities

Although the absolute blood lymphocyte threshold for diagnosing CLL was placed at 5×10^9/L, most patients present with considerably higher counts, occasionally even in the hundred-thousand range. Upon examination of a peripheral blood smear, mature-appearing small lymphocytes may be preponderant in the population of leukocytes, ranging from 50% to as much as 100%.

In addition to an increased ratio of mature-appearing lymphocytes in the smears of aspirated marrows, three patterns of infiltration by lymphocytes are recognized in trephine biopsy specimens of the bone marrow (Figure 3): nodular, interstitial, and diffuse. It has been observed that patients with diffuse infiltration tend to have advanced disease and worse outlook. For prognostic purposes, nodular and interstitial patterns, which are associated

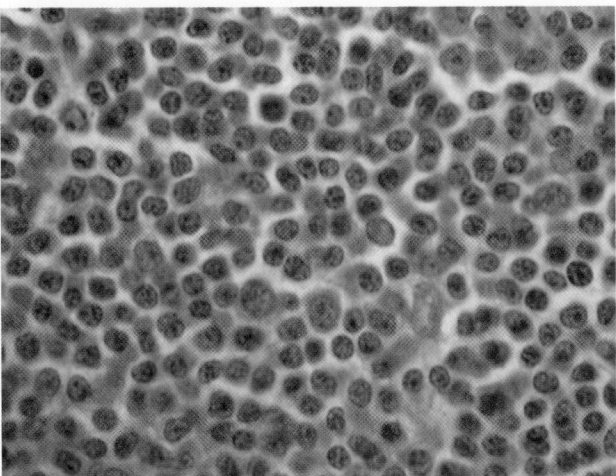

Figure 3 Chronic lymphocytic leukemia (CLL). Marrow biopsy with diffuse infiltration by CLL cells (hematoxylin and eosin stain; ×600 original magnification).

with less-advanced disease and better prognosis, are grouped together and termed "nondiffuse."[24-26]

Asymptomatic anemia and thrombocytopenia may be observed at the time of initial diagnosis, but usually these are of a relatively mild degree. A direct antiglobulin (Coombs) test may be positive in ~25% of cases, but overt autoimmune hemolytic anemia occurs less frequently. In the absence of a reliable test to demonstrate antiplatelet antibodies, autoimmune thrombocytopenia is most often diagnosed on the basis of the presence of adequate numbers of megakaryocytes in the bone marrow with abnormally low platelet counts.

Hypogammaglobulinemia may be present at the time of initial diagnosis, but it becomes clinically significant only later in the course of the disease. All three immunoglobulin classes (IgG, IgA, and IgM) are usually decreased, although in some patients only one or two classes may be reduced. Concurrent hypogammaglobulinemia and neutropenia result in increased vulnerability of CLL patients to severe bacterial, viral, and opportunistic infections. As a large proportion of cells are B lymphocytes, the normal lymphocyte T:B ratio (2:1) is altered. As patients are not immunocompetent, they should avoid inoculation of any live vaccines (varicella, measles, Bacille Calmette-Guérin, etc.). In this immunocompromised population, replication of the virus after administration can be enhanced and live vaccines can actually induce active infection.[27,28]

No abnormalities in blood chemistry are characteristic of CLL, but increased levels of serum lactate dehydrogenase, uric acid, hepatic enzymes [alanine aminotransferase (ALT) or aspartate aminotransferase (AST)], and (rarely) calcium may be observed. Pseudohyperkalemia can occur occasionally in patients with extreme leukocytosis.

Natural history and terminal events

It is a generally held belief that CLL is an indolent disease with a prolonged chronic course and that the eventual cause of death may be comorbidities unrelated to CLL; however, this observation is true for fewer than 30% of all CLL cases. The natural history is heterogeneous in most patients. Many patients live for 5–10 years with an initial course that is relatively benign but that is almost always followed by a terminal phase lasting 1–2 years. During the initial asymptomatic phase, the patients are able to maintain their usual lifestyle, but during the terminal phase, performance status declines rapidly. In patients with progressive disease, the cause(s) of death are directly related to CLL or complications from therapy. Infection is a major cause of mortality in patients with CLL, accounting for 30–50% of all deaths.

Transformations to a high-grade disease are characteristically refractory to usual chemotherapeutic agents.[29] In up to ~10% of CLL patients, a transformation to a diffuse large B-cell lymphoma occurs[30] ("Richter's transformation" or "Richter's syndrome"; Figure 4). Richter's syndrome is associated with a rapidly progressive course, refractoriness to all currently known chemotherapy, and poor overall survival (OS).[31,32] The diagnosis of Richter's syndrome requires histopathologic examination of a lymph node that shows large B cells with high proliferative rate (high Ki-67). In addition, a small proportion of patients with CLL undergo "prolymphocytoid transformation," and peripheral blood morphology reveals the presence of a mixture of small mature CLL cells and prolymphocytes in contrast to typical B-PLL (B-prolymphocytic leukemia) where the circulating cells are monomorphic prolymphocytes.[33] Similar to a Richter's transformation, prolymphocytoid transformation has an aggressive clinical course.

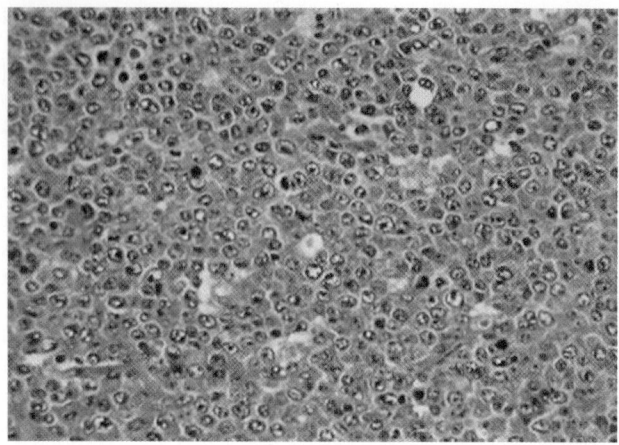

Figure 4 Chronic lymphocytic leukemia, Richter's syndrome. Section of lymph node with immunoblastic proliferation consisting of large cells with prominent nucleoli (hematoxylin and eosin stain; ×600 original magnification).

Table 4 Distribution of cases in various series according to Rai staging.

References	Cases (n)	Series (years)	Stage (% of cases)				
			0	I	II	III	IV
Rai et al.[34]	125	18	23	31	17	11	14
Geisler and Hansen (1981)[35]	102	20	36	19	17	8	31
Baccarani et al. (1982)[36]	188	26.5	26.5	21	9	17	9
Skinnider (1982)[37]	745	19	21	31	16	13	31
MRC CLL-1[a] (1989)	660	28	18	29	10	15	31

[a]The hemoglobin level for stage III in Medical Research Council of Great Britain Chronic Lymphocytic Leukemia Trial I was <110 g/L.

Acute leukemia is observed extremely rarely in the setting of a CLL diagnosis. If it occurs, it is usually myeloid in origin (myelocytic, myelomonocytic, or acute erythroleukemia). Prior therapy with alkylating agents has not been clearly implicated as a cause because a few cases have been observed in treatment-naive patients. The acute leukemia is treated with an acute leukemia regimen, although almost invariably the outcomes are very poor.

Patients with CLL have been found to have over twice the risk of developing another cancer compared to the general population.[31] Skin cancers and other malignancies occur with considerably greater frequency among CLL patients. We recommend that all CLL patients (including treatment-naive) adhere to age-appropriate cancer screening guidelines.

Clinical staging and other prognostic features

Two staging criteria, the Rai[34] system and the Binet[38] system, are widely used in clinical practice owing to their simplicity (only a physical examination and a complete blood count are needed) and accuracy in predicting outcomes.

Method of Rai and colleagues

The Rai system is based on the concept that in CLL, a gradual and progressive increase in the tumor burden of leukemic lymphocytes occurs, resulting in sequential clinical manifestations of the disease. The abnormalities start in the blood followed by the lymph nodes, spleen, and liver; to eventually compromise the bone marrow function. The earliest stage is blood lymphocytosis (clinical stage 0). The later stages (anemia and thrombocytopenia—excluding AIHA and ITP) are explained by progressively increasing bone marrow infiltration by CLL cells.

At the time of initial diagnosis of CLL, approximately 25% of patients are in the earliest clinical stage (stage 0), ~25% are in the advanced stages (stages III and IV), with the remaining 50% in the stage I or II categories. Table 4 shows the stage distributions from various series, revealing a consistent pattern. The median survival times from the time of diagnosis in the Rai series were 150 months for stage 0, 101 months for stage I, 71 months for stage II, 19 months for stage III, and 19 months for stage IV.[34] Although Rai and colleagues noted in their 1975 paper that only three (and not five) distinct actuarial survival patterns emerged

from the data (stage 0, stages I and II combined, and stages III and IV combined), they recommended that the five-stage system be maintained to investigate prospectively whether biologic and clinical differences would emerge between stages I and II and between stages III and IV. In 1987, the Rai staging system was modified to consist of three groups: low (Rai stage 0), intermediate (Rai stages I and II combined), and high (Rai stages III and IV combined) risk categories.[39] The modified Rai staging system was used for risk stratifying patients in the landmark study of chlorambucil against fludarabine in the front-line therapy of CLL conducted in the 1990s that established the superiority of fludarabine.[40] Fludarabine and purine analogs are now part of the combination regimens for frontline therapy in fit patients with no major comorbidities.[41,42]

Method of Binet and colleagues

Binet's method classifies all patients with anemia (defined as hemoglobin below 100 g/L) and/or thrombocytopenia (platelets less than 100×10^9/L), or both, as stage C.[38] All of the remaining (non-C) patients are divided into two groups, depending on the presence of fewer than three (stage A) or three or more (stage B) sites of palpable enlargement of lymphoid organs. This staging takes into consideration five sites: cervical, axillary, and inguinal lymph nodes (whether unilateral or bilateral, each area is counted as one), and the spleen and liver. This system has been found to be of great value in dividing patients into three types of survival curves, with A, B, and C corresponding, respectively, to Rai's low-, intermediate-, and high-risk groups.

Criteria predictive of disease course in the low- and intermediate-risk groups

Virtually, all high-risk group patients (stages III and IV) have a relatively rapid clinical course with an expected shorter survival. The course of disease is not uniform in the other categories. Patients in the low- and intermediate-risk groups (stage 0 and stages I and II, respectively) may have a benign clinical course in which the disease remains indolent and is associated with a long OS measurable in years or even decades. On the other hand, the disease in patients in the low-and intermediate-risk groups may also progress rapidly with relatively short survival times. Major prognostic markers of considerable importance to stratify risk in this heterogeneous disease include chromosomal aberrations, *IGHV* mutation status, CD38, and Zap-70 expression (Table 5). Additional prognostic factors that have been tested and found to be useful in predicting the course of disease include age, gender, comorbidities, complex chromosomal karyotype,[43] genetic mutations,[44] and β-2-microglobulin, among others.

Table 5 Molecular and cytogenetic markers of prognosis in CLL.

	Markers of	
	Good prognosis	**Worse prognosis**
IGHV mutation status	Mutated	Unmutated
ZAP-70	Negative	Positive
CD38	Negative	Positive
FISH cytogenetics	13q del	11q del, 17p del

Major prognostic markers

IGHV gene mutation

Two main subgroups of CLL are recognized based on the presence or absence of mutations in the *IGHV* gene that is expressed by leukemic B cells.[45] Patients with *IGHV*-mutated genes tend to have a milder form of the disease, better progression free, and OS.[46,47] This may be explained in part by the fact that B-cell receptors (BCRs) of unmutated CLL cases transduce stimulatory downstream signals with greater capacity than those of mutated cells.[1,48] Patients with or without *IGHV* mutations may be further subclassified based on other significant findings, such as the presence or absence of mutations in TP53,[49] NOTCH1,[50] SF3B1,[44] ZAP-70 expression,[51] and CD38,[46] all of which have been shown to have an impact on the clinical course of the disease.

Cytogenetics

Cytogenetic analysis of CLL used to be limited because of an inability to induce metaphases in the leukemic cells with conventional banding techniques. Using interphase fluorescence *in situ* hybridization (FISH) technique, chromosomal aberrations can be detected in 82% of cases.[52] A seminal study by Döhner and colleagues found the following common lesions and frequencies in CLL patients: deletion in 13q14 (55%), deletion in 11q (18%), trisomy of 12q (16%), deletion in 17p (7%), and deletion in 6q in 7%. In the same study, normal karyotypes were present in 18% of patients. Among the abnormalities, del(13q), del(11q), and del(17q) were considered to have the greatest significance. Deletion in 13q correlates with the best median OS at 133 months. Patients with deletion of either 11q or 17p have the poorest prognosis with a median OS of 79 and 32 months, respectively. Loss of 11q and 17p are believed to involve alteration of the gene encoding for the ataxia-telangiectasia mutation, and inactivation of the tumor suppressor gene p53, respectively. These high-risk lesions were found to be associated with aggressive disease and resistance to chemotherapy.[53,54] Patients with normal karyotypes and patients with trisomy 12 have similar survival times of 111 and 114 months, respectively.

Zap-70 expression

Zap-70 is an intracellular protein involved in activation signaling normally present in T lymphocytes and natural killer cells (not in normal B lymphocytes).[55] Although ZAP-70 testing can be obtained by flow cytometry, the methodology and reproducibility of these tests have yet to be standardized across centers. Studies demonstrated that its aberrant expression in leukemic B lymphocytes correlates with U-CLL.[51,56] Data show that Zap-70 positivity in CLL as an independent predictor of disease progression and inferior clinical outcome.[55,57] ZAP-70 expression is superior to mutation status in predicting time to treatment.[58,59]

Molecular genetics

A range of genetic mutations has been found to have prognostic implications in CLL. Somatic mutations in the tumor suppressor gene TP53 are one of the most frequent alterations in several human cancers. This mutation is known to be associated with poor prognosis. The German CLL Study Group (GCLLSG) found that 8.5% of previously untreated CLL patients had the p53 mutation, and some of these even in the absence of a 17p deletion.[49] Patients with a p53 mutation have a poor prognosis regardless of whether 17p is deleted, and its presence is associated with poor response to therapy, short progression-free survival (PFS) and OS. Moreover, in a multivariate analysis, TP53 mutations analysis provided prognostic value beyond the recognized adverse genetic factors mentioned earlier in this chapter.[60]

Additional mutations with prognostic significance in CLL include those in NOTCH 1[61] and SF3B1[44] genes. Detailed findings regarding these abnormalities have led some experts to propose the development of a risk algorithm that would incorporate prognostic information regarding gene mutations, chromosomal abnormalities, and changes that take place during clonal evolution in CLL.[62,63]

Treatment

Although early intervention is considered crucial in most malignant diseases, this is not the case in CLL. The lack of evidence that CLL can be cured with currently available modalities[64] has resulted in a "watch and wait" approach for most patients; that is, follow-up approximately every 3–4 months (sooner if there are indications of aggressive disease) with a history, physical exam, and complete blood counts.

The availability of therapeutic agents with significant activity in CLL—namely, purine analogs, monoclonal antibodies, and the most recent introduction of small molecules that target the BCR signaling pathway into our armamentarium—may change the treatment landscape in the future if ongoing early intervention trials demonstrate improved outcomes in asymptomatic high-risk disease. Currently, this approach is not recommended outside of a clinical trial.

Treatment options available for frontline and salvage therapy in CLL are given in Tables 6 and 7, respectively.

IWCLL guidelines to initiate therapy

1. Rai stage I or II (Binet stage B) with disease-related symptoms
2. Rai stage III or IV (Binet Stage C)
3. Massive or rapidly enlarging, symptomatic lymphadenopathy, or splenomegaly
4. Lymphocyte doubling time of <6 months
5. AIHA or thrombocytopenia (or both) that is poorly responsive to corticosteroid therapy.

Enlarging lymph nodes and/or rapid lymphocyte doubling should be assessed cautiously given that such events can be transient. No data exist establishing a particular threshold of lymphocyte count that warrants treatment. Anecdotal evidence suggests that hyperleukocytosis may potentially lead to hyperviscosity symptoms in a minority of patients; thus, therapy may be considered in selected patients at risk.

Goals of therapy

Choosing the optimal treatment for an individual patient depends on the age, functional status, and genetic aberrations. Traditionally, treatment of CLL continued until symptoms resolved or

Table 6 Front-line regimens for chronic lymphocytic leukemia.

Patient population	Treatment options
Patients <70 years of age or older patients without significant comorbidities and without del(17p)	• Fludarabine + cyclophosphamide + rituximab • Bendamustine ± rituximab • Fludarabine + rituximab • Pentostatin + cyclophosphamide + rituximab • Obinutuzumab + chlorambucil • Ofatumumab + chlorambucil • Ibrutinib
Patients aged >70 years or younger patients with comorbidities without del(17p)	• Obinutuzumab + chlorambucil • Ofatumumab + chlorambucil • Ibrutinib • Bendamustine ± rituximab • Cyclophosphamide ± rituximab ± corticosteroids • Fludarabine ± rituximab • Dose reduced fludarabine + cyclophosphamide + rituximab • Chlorambucil
Patients with significant comorbidities unable to tolerate purine analogues	• Obinutuzumab + chlorambucil • Ofatumumab + chlorambucil • Ibrutinib • Chlorambucil
Patients with del(17p)	• Ibrutinib • Idelalisib + rituximab • Alemtuzumab • Clinical trial

Table 7 Salvage therapy for relapsed chronic lymphocytic leukemia.

Patient population	Treatment options
Patients with short response to initial therapy who are younger than 70 years of age or older patients without significant comorbidities and without del(17p)	• Ibrutinib • Idelalisib + rituximab • Fludarabine + cyclophosphamide + rituximab • Pentostatin + cyclophosphamide + rituximab • Bendamustine ± rituximab • Fludarabine + alemtuzumab • Ofatumumab • Lenalidomide ± rituximab • Alemtuzumab ± rituximab • High-dose methylprednisolone + rituximab • R-CHOP • OFAR • Clinical trial
Patients with short response to initial therapy who are aged 70 years or older without del(17p)	• Ibrutinib • Idelalisib + rituximab • Bendamustine ± rituximab • Ofatumumab • High-dose methylprednisolone + rituximab • Alemtuzumab ± rituximab • Clinical trial
Patients with del(17p)	• Ibrutinib • Venetoclax • Idelalisib + rituximab • Alemtuzumab ± rituximab • Clinical trial

troubling lymphadenopathy was controlled. With the advent of the anti-CD20 monoclonal antibody (mAb), rituximab (and its addition to a chemotherapy backbone), came the observation that minimal residual disease-negative (MRD-negative) complete responses improved PFS and OS;[65] therefore, criteria to define complete remission (CR) and MRD negativity were developed.[11]

Nevertheless, creating a clear algorithm for CLL treatment is difficult because of the heterogeneity of the disease and the prevalence of comorbidities in the CLL population. Although a CR and MRD negativity may be desirable endpoints, in some cases, these are not appropriate goals owing to toxicities. Clinicians must match the profiles of the patient to one of the available therapies and set a realistic therapeutic goal.

The introduction of small molecules that target BCR signaling and the microenvironment required a recent update of the previously established response criteria in order to incorporate the "redistribution phenomenon" seen with these novel agents.[66] BCR inhibitors exert their effects by mobilizing CLL cells from the bone marrow and the lymph nodes into the peripheral blood with a resulting lymphocytosis that may be mistaken for progression of disease (PD) or lack of response.

Response criteria to treatment

A CR requires the absence of symptoms attributable to CLL, normal findings on physical examination, a lymphocyte count below 4×10^9/L, neutrophils at 1.5×10^9/L or higher, platelets greater than or equal to 100×10^9/L, and hemoglobin level of 110 g/L or higher. Normalization of serum immunoglobulin levels is not a requirement for complete response. For patients on clinical trials, bone marrow aspirate and biopsy performed at least 2 months after the last treatment should demonstrate a normocellular marrow with lymphocytes making up <30% of nucleated cells for classification of CR. Patients with persistent CLL in the bone marrow are defined as having a partial response (PR). Patients with lymphoid nodules found in the marrow following treatment are categorized as nodular PR. The guidelines recommend that these nodules be further characterized by immunohistochemistry staining to determine if these are CLL cells. Those patients without evidence of CLL but persistent cytopenias after treatment should be considered to be in a CR with incomplete bone marrow recovery (CRi).

Other criteria for strict PR were defined as a reduction in previously elevated lymphocyte counts, enlarged nodes, spleen, or liver by 50% or more. Peripheral blood should also show one of the following: a neutrophil count of 1.5×10^9/or higher, a platelet count of 100×10^9/L or higher, or a hemoglobin level of 110 g/L or higher (or a 50% or better improvement over pretherapy deficits in these counts). These responses must persist for a minimum period of 2 months.[11]

The new concept of "partial response with lymphocytosis" (PRL) require that all PR criteria are met except for the blood lymphocyte count. In the absence of other objective evidence of PD, lymphocytosis alone should not be considered an indicator of PD. Patients with lymphocytosis and no other evidence of PD should continue therapy until they develop definitive signs of PD.[66]

MRD eradication refers to the complete eradication of leukemic cells by either four-color flow cytometry or by allele-specific oligonucleotide PCR. This determination must be made at least 3 months after the completion of therapy in the setting of a clinical trial only.[11] While absence of MRD may indicate a more favorable prognosis in the setting of chemoimmunotherapy, its value as a therapeutic goal remains unclear at this time.

Chlorambucil monotherapy

Despite evidence that chlorambucil monotherapy is associated with lower response rates and shorter remission durations compared to other available agents, chlorambucil remains a widely used agent in frail and older patients given its ease of use and tolerability. Great variability in the dose and schedule of chlorambucil has been observed.[67,68] A CALGB study revealed that chlorambucil is equally effective when given daily or on an intermittent basis.[69] Chlorambucil is usually administered for a period of several weeks until maximum clinical response is reached. Maintenance therapy is uncommon. Recent data seem to suggest combination with a monoclonal antibody targeting CD20 may obtain better results in terms of efficacy with excellent tolerability. The role of monotherapy may change the next few years.

Corticosteroids

Prednisone had been administered to CLL patients in the past as a single agent, usually in an initial dose of 20–60 mg, with dose reductions occurring in a stepwise manner.[67,70] Often, in the first 1–2 months, an increase in the lymphocyte count was followed by a subsequent decline, caused by a shift of lymphocytes from lymph nodes and bone marrow into the blood. Anemia and thrombocytopenia improved in approximately two-thirds of patients. The major side effects were those of chronic corticosteroid therapy and infections. Currently, the major indication for prednisone is for the management of antibody-mediated anemia and thrombocytopenia.

Fludarabine–cyclophosphamide–rituximab (FCR)

FCR remains the standard of care for upfront treatment of medically fit CLL patients. A landmark study done as a single-arm study successfully treated 224 previously untreated patients with fludarabine, cyclophosphamide, and rituximab (FCR).[40,71] The overall response rate (ORR) was 95% with 72% of these patients achieving CR and many achieving MRD negativity. A substantial number of patients remain free of disease more than a decade later. Grades 3–4 neutropenia occurred in over 50%.

A well-designed, phase III trial of 817 previously untreated patients by the GCLLSG evaluated the benefit of adding rituximab to FC establishing FCR's superiority.[41] At a median of 47 months follow-up, a superior PFS was maintained in patients receiving FCR compared with FC (57.9 vs 32.9 months, respectively; $P <$ 0.001).[72] The FCR arm had a greater incidence of neutropenia but not of grade 3 or 4 infections. FCR as well as other purine analog-alkylator-rituximab regimens should all be given with antibiotic prophylaxis against *Pneumocystis*, varicella, and *Candida*. Most recently, FCR was compared with a less toxic regimen (bendamustine and rituximab, BR) but the comparator arm failed to outperform FCR (see section titled "Bendamustine"). A large ongoing US intergroup trial (E1912) is currently accruing patients to evaluate FCR against ibrutinib in combination with rituximab in frontline young CLL patients with no 17p deletion. The primary endpoint of this study is to establish PFS and change in quality of life between the arms.

Bendamustine

The FDA-approved bendamustine in 2008 based on a randomized trial comparing it to chlorambucil in previously untreated CLL patients.[73] Bendamustine, given at a dose of 100 mg/m^2 IV for 2 days every 4 weeks, was found to be superior to chlorambucil in ORR and PFS. Given bendamustine's efficacy and tolerability when combined with rituximab in frontline and relapsed CLL patients,[74,75] the regimen emerged as an attractive approach to improve the early and late toxicities observed with FCR.

The phase III CLL10 trial tested frontline BR compared to FCR in fit patients except 17p deletion patients. Although the ORR was identical in both treatment arms (97.8%), CR was greater in FCR-treated patients and correlated with longer PFS. No difference in OS was observed. Patients receiving FCR experienced significantly greater rates of grade 3/4 adverse events including severe neutropenia, myelosuppression, and infections compared with patients receiving BR. Given the milder toxicity profile of BR, this combination may have a role in the upfront treatment of medically unfit CLL patients.[76]

Ofatumumab

Ofatumumab is a fully human IgG1 anti-CD20 mAb created from transgenic mice that binds a different epitope on CD20 compared with rituximab. It is a type I mAb that has demonstrated greater complement-dependent cytotoxicity in CLL cell lines when compared with rituximab and it is approved as monotherapy for relapsed CLL.[77,78] Ofatumumab has been recently approved for frontline therapy in combination with chlorambucil.[79]

Obinutuzumab

Obinutuzumab is a humanized mAb targeting CD20 indicated in combination with chlorambucil for the treatment of previously untreated patients with CLL. Previously untreated patients with CLL were randomized to receive chlorambucil against chlorambucil plus rituximab against chlorambucil plus obinutuzumab.[80] Goede and colleagues found that, in patients with multiple debilitating coexisting conditions (median age, 73 years), the combination of obinutuzumab with chlorambucil was associated with a significant and clinically meaningful prolongation of PFS, increased CR, and an increased rate of MRD negativity, as compared with the results with a combination of rituximab and chlorambucil. Moreover, treatment with obinutuzumab plus chlorambucil resulted in a significant OS benefit as compared with chlorambucil alone suggesting that the induction of deeper remissions could translate into a survival advantage even in frail patients. Combination studies of this drug with the novel BCR inhibitors are planned.

Ibrutinib

Ibrutinib is an orally bioavailable, small-molecule, irreversible inhibitor of Bruton's tyrosine kinase that has been shown to induce rapid lymph node responses in patients with CLL. As with other kinase inhibitors developed to treat patients with CLL, ibrutinib inhibits several signaling pathways, including BCR, Toll-like receptors, BAFF, and CD40, as well as interfering with the protective effect of stromal cells.[3] In an early phase Ib/II clinical trial, treatment with ibrutinib as monotherapy for patients with relapsed/refractory CLL resulted in a high ORR of 71% and durable remissions (estimated PFS at 26 months: 75%) for all groups of patients tested, including elderly patients and those with high-risk disease.[81] Three-year follow-up indicated long-lasting response to ibrutinib.[82] In the phase III RESONATE trial, ibrutinib was compared with ofatumumab in patients with relapsed/refractory CLL/SLL.[83] The ORRs were 4.1% and 42.6% in patients receiving ofatumumab and ibrutinib, respectively. Outcomes were independent of 17p status and were seen even in patients refractory to purine analogues. Minimal toxicities were reported.

In the largest prospective trial dedicated to the study of del (17p), ibrutinib demonstrated marked efficacy in terms of ORR and PFS, with a favorable risk-benefit profile.[84] At a median follow up of 13 months, 79.3% of patients remained progression-free at 12 months, consistent with efficacy observed in earlier studies.[81] The PFS in this previously treated population compares favorably to that of treatment-naive del 17p CLL patients receiving FCR[42] with a median PFS of 11 months. These results support ibrutinib as an effective therapy for patients with deletion 17p CLL/SLL.

Idelalisib

Idelalisib is a targeted, highly selective oral inhibitor of phosphoinositide 3-kinase delta, an isoform with selective leukocyte expression that promotes the survival and proliferation of malignant B cells. A randomized, double-blind, placebo-controlled phase III trial of rituximab with or without idelalisib in patients was stopped early following recommendations by an independent data and safety monitoring committee with ORR of 81% versus 13% in patients receiving idelalisib plus rituximab compared with placebo rituximab, respectively.[85,86] Subpopulation analysis indicated idelalisib plus rituximab was effective for patients regardless of the presence of 17p, TP53, or *IGHV* mutational status.[87] Combination idelalisib and rituximab also has shown clinical activity in frontline therapy in a small cohort of patients that participated in a phase II trial, including patients with 17p deletion.[88]

Venetoclax

Members of the B-cell lymphoma-2 (BCL-2) protein family are important regulators of intrinsic apoptosis. They are usually overexpressed in CLL cells and contribute to tumor cell survival and drug resistance. Venetoclax is the first-in-class selective and potent inhibitor of BCL2. The drug was recently approved by the US FDA as it induces rapid reduction in CLL disease burden in the blood, lymph nodes, and bone marrow, resulting in a high overall response, including CLL patients with relapsed del(17p). Venetoclax (in combination with rituximab) is currently undergoing evaluation for approval in all patients with relapsed or refractory CLL.

Stem cell transplantation

Although hematopoietic stem cell transplantation (HSCT) is the treatment of choice for many aggressive hematologic malignancies, the role of HSCT in CLL has remained controversial. Autologous stem cell transplantation (SCT) has no clear benefit in CLL.[89] HSCTs should be reserved for very specific cases given the high treatment-related mortality associated with the procedure.

Psychosocial aspects of CLL

A diagnosis of leukemia is a major emotional challenge to patients. Careful explanation of the natural history of the disorder, emphasizing that some patients never need treatment and that early treatment has not been shown to be beneficial, is required at the time of diagnosis. Patients need to be reassured that effective treatments are available when treatment becomes necessary because of progressive disease or symptoms. Knowledge that survival in many early-stage CLL patients is the same as in the age- and gender-matched general population is comforting to patients. Explanation of newer prognostic factors must also be made with care. Favorable markers can reassure that observation is appropriate but many patients have difficulty accepting this initial approach when the markers indicate high risk. Development of a close relationship with patients, particularly those in the early phases of disease, and careful responses to questions raised are important in providing psychological and emotional support to the patient and family. The rapidly increasing range of options for therapy, particularly for younger patients, provides a basis for optimism when treatment becomes necessary.

Unmet needs and future directions

The current goal is to individualize treatment strategies based on the patient's clinical profile when therapy is indicated. As mentioned earlier in this chapter, the exact time to initiate therapy depends on several factors. If the patient has symptoms attributable to CLL, treatment is warranted. The presence of markers of high-risk disease is not an indication for therapy. A gray area exists when no clear symptomatology is present and cytopenias are beginning to manifest. If the patient prefers, it is reasonable to continue observation revisiting the issue before when cytopenias drop to levels of concern.

A purine analog-based regimen such as FCR is still the standard of care in frontline management of young fit CLL patients with no comorbidities. In patients with Coombs positivity or a history of AIHA, avoiding a purine analog may be preferable. For older frail patients with comorbidities who do not carry a 17p deletion, strong consideration should be given to frontline therapy with obinutuzumab plus chlorambucil, BR, ofatumumab and chlorambucil, or ibrutinib; unless a confounding condition exists prohibiting the use of any of these regimens.

There is much expectation that the novel targeted therapies alone or in combination with cytotoxic chemotherapy will impact the clinical outcome of patients with CLL. This is the reason for ongoing large phase III trials comparing frontline chemoimmunotherapy regimens against targeted agents with the potential to change the current standard of care. It is possible that in the future, several patients (including young fit patients) may be treated with relatively nontoxic regimens that do not contain cytotoxic chemotherapy agents. It is also conceivable that the incorporation of the novel targeted agents into chemoimmunotherapy regimens in the frontline may generate deeper responses and longer remissions without increases in toxicity.

The most challenging treatment decision is for patients with symptomatic treatment-naive CLL patients with a deletion 17p. There is no clear consensus among experts as to the best therapy for this group of patients. Cytotoxic chemotherapy regimens are much less effective with suboptimal responses in spite of the addition of monoclonal antibodies. There is encouraging phase I–II data in small cohorts of 17p deletion patients treated with ibrutinib as monotherapy or in combination with rituximab,[90–92] and as such ibrutinib should be definitely considered. Ibrutinib and venetoclax are the only agents approved in the United States for treatment of patients that carry a deletion in chromosome 17. If unable to tolerate ibrutinib or venetoclax, a reasonable choice of therapy would be idelalisib as it has demonstrated clinical activity in 17p deletion patients.[87,88] It is important to mention that stem cell transplant evaluation should be discussed with young fit patients with high-risk disease (17p deletion, failure after a novel targeted agent, short PFS after initial therapy).

Nevertheless, the goals and duration of therapy for CLL are poorly defined. High CR rates with chemoimmunotherapy regimens, as well as the attainability of MRD negativity, had been promising advancements a decade ago, but long-term benefit of these successes remains unproven in patients using a BCR inhibitor. Therefore, MRD negativity should be regarded as a treatment goal only in the setting of a clinical trial.

The recent advances achieved over the past few years—that is, the development of inhibitors of B-cell signal transduction, immunomodulators of the CLL microenvironment, and glycoengineered monoclonal antibodies—have been a breakthrough revolution.[93] The era of targeted therapy in CLL has categorically arrived and we anticipate that progress will continue. We hope that novel therapies and new treatment paradigms will transform the way we manage CLL today.

Acknowledgments

Jacqueline Barrientos' work is supported in part by NIH/NCATS Grant #UL1TR00457 and the 2015 American Society of Hematology-Harold Amos Medical Faculty Development Program (ASH-AMFDP) Fellowship.

Key references

The complete reference list can be found on the Wiley Companion Digital Edition of this title (see inside front cover for login instructions).

1 Chiorazzi N, Rai KR, Ferrarini M. Mechanism of disease: chronic lymphocytic leukemia. *N Engl J Med.* 2005;**352**:804–815.

3 Wiestner A. Emerging role of kinase-targeted strategies in chronic lymphocytic leukemia. *Blood.* 2012;**120**:4684–4691.

9 Jaffe ES, Harris NL, Stein H, et al. Chronic lymphocytic leukemia/small lymphocytic lymphoma. In: Jaffe ES, Harris NL, Stein H, Vardiman JW, eds. *World Health Organization Classification of Tumours: Pathology and Genetics of Tumours of Haematopoietic and Lymphoid Tissues.* Lyon, France: IARC Press; 2001:127–130.

11 Hallek M, Cheson BD, Catovsky D, et al. Guidelines for the diagnosis and treatment of chronic lymphocytic leukemia: a report from the International Workshop on Chronic Lymphocytic Leukemia updating the National Cancer Institute–Working Group 1996 guidelines. *Blood.* 2008;**111**:5446–5456.

18 Rawstron AC, Bennett FL, O'Connor SJ, et al. Monoclonal B-cell lymphocytosis and chronic lymphocytic leukemia. *N Engl J Med.* 2008;**359**:575–583.

31 Apostolia-Maria T, Sijin W, Peter M, et al. Other malignancies in chronic lymphocytic leukemia/small lymphocytic lymphoma. *J Clin Oncol.* 2008. doi: JCO.2008.17.5398.

34 Rai KR, Sawitsky A, Cronkite EP, et al. Clinical staging of chronic lymphocytic leukemia. *Blood.* 1975;**46**:219–234.

38 Binet JL, Auquier A, Dighiero G, et al. A new prognostic classification of chronic lymphocytic leukemia derived from a multivariate survival analysis. *Cancer.* 1981;**48**:198–206.

40 Rai KR, Peterson BL, Appelbaum FR, et al. Fludarabine compared with chlorambucil as primary therapy for chronic lymphocytic leukemia. *N Engl J Med.* 2000;**343**:1750–1757.

41 Keating MJ, O'Brien S, Albitar M, et al. Early results of a chemoimmunotherapy regimen of fludarabine, cyclophosphamide, and rituximab as initial therapy for chronic lymphocytic leukemia. *J Clin Oncol.* 2005;**23**:4079–4088.

42 Hallek M, Fischer K, Fingerle-Rowson G, et al. Addition of rituximab to fludarabine and cyclophosphamide in patients with chronic lymphocytic leukaemia: a randomised, open-label, phase 3 trial. *Lancet.* 2010;**376(9747)**:1164–1174.

44 Wang L, Lawrence MS, Wan Y, et al. SF3B1 and other novel cancer genes in chronic lymphocytic leukemia. *N Engl J Med.* 2011;**365**:2497–2506.

46 Damle RN, Wasil T, Fais F, et al. Immunoglobulin V gene mutation status and CD38 expression as novel prognostic indicators in chronic lymphocytic leukemia. *Blood.* 1999;**94**:1840–1847.

47 Hamblin TJ, Davis Z, Gardiner A, et al. Unmutated IgVH genes are associated with a more aggressive form of chronic lymphocytic leukemia. *Blood.* 1999;**94**:1848–1854.

52 Döhner H, Stilgenbauer S, Benner A, et al. Genomic aberrations and survival in chronic lymphocytic leukemia. *N Engl J Med.* 2000;**343**:1910–1916.

58 Rassenti LZ, Huynh L, Toy TZ, et al. ZAP-70 compared with immunoglobulin heavy-chain gene mutation status as a predictor of disease progression in CLL. *N Engl J Med.* 2004;**351**:893–901.

60 Gonzalez D, Martinez P, Wade R, et al. Mutational status of the TP53 gene as a predictor of response and survival in patients with chronic lymphocytic leukemia: results from the LRF CLL4 trial. *J Clin Oncol.* 2011;**29**:2223–2229.

62 Rossi D, Rasi S, Spina V, et al. Integrated mutational and cytogenetic analysis identifies new prognostic subgroups in chronic lymphocytic leukemia. *Blood.* 2013;**121**:1403–1412.

63 Pflug N, Bahlo J, Shanafelt TD, et al. Development of a comprehensive prognostic index for patients with chronic lymphocytic leukemia. *Blood.* 2014;**124(1)**:49–62.

65 Böttcher S, Ritgen M, Fischer K, et al. Minimal residual disease quantification is an independent predictor of progression-free and overall survival in chronic lymphocytic leukemia: a multivariate analysis from the randomized GCLLSG CLL8 trial. *J Clin Oncol.* 2012;**30(9)**:980–988.

66 Cheson BD, Byrd JC, Rai KR, et al. Novel targeted agents and the need to refine clinical end points in chronic lymphocytic leukemia. *J Clin Oncol.* 2012;**30(23)**:2820–2822.

74 Fischer K, Cramer P, Busch R, et al. Bendamustine in combination with rituximab for previously untreated patients with chronic lymphocytic leukemia: a multicenter phase II trial of the German Chronic Lymphocytic Leukemia Study Group. *J Clin Oncol.* 2012;**30**:3209–3216.

75 Fischer K, Cramer P, Busch R, et al. Bendamustine combined with rituximab in patients with relapsed and/or refractory chronic lymphocytic leukemia: a multicenter phase II trial of the German Chronic Lymphocytic Leukemia Study Group. *J Clin Oncol.* 2011;**29**:3559–3566.

76 Eichhorst B, Fink AM, Busch R, et al. Frontline chemoimmunotherapy with fludarabine (F), cyclophosphamide (C), and rituximab (R) (FCR) shows superior efficacy in comparison to bendamustine (B) and rituximab (BR) in previously untreated and physically fit patients (pts) with advanced chronic lymphocytic leukemia (CLL): final analysis of an international, randomized study of the German CLL Study Group (GCLLSG) (CLL10 study). *Blood.* 2014;**124(21)**:19.

78 Wierda WG, Padmanabhan S, Chan GW, Gupta IV, Lisby S, Österborg A. Hx-CD20-406 Study Investigators. Ofatumumab is active in patients with fludarabine-refractory CLL irrespective of prior rituximab: results from the phase 2 international study. *Blood.* 2011;**118**:5126–5129.

80 Goede V, Fischer K, Busch R, et al. Obinutuzumab plus chlorambucil in patients with CLL and coexisting conditions. *N Engl J Med.* 2014;**370**:1101–1110.

81 Byrd JC, Furman RR, Coutre SE, et al. Targeting BTK with ibrutinib in relapsed chronic lymphocytic leukemia. *N Engl J Med.* 2013;**369**:32–42.

82 O'Brien SM, Furman RR, Coutre SE, et al. Independent evaluation of ibrutinib efficacy 3 years post-initiation of monotherapy in patients with chronic lymphocytic leukemia/small lymphocytic leukemia including deletion 17p disease. *J Clin Oncol.* 2014 (suppl; abstr 7014);**32**:5s.

83 Byrd JC, Brown JR, O'Brien S, et al. Ibrutinib versus ofatumumab in previously treated chronic lymphoid leukemia. *N Engl J Med.* 2014;**371**:213–223.

84 O'Brien S, Jones JA, Coutre S. Efficacy and safety of ibrutinib in patients with relapsed or refractory chronic lymphocytic leukemia or small lymphocytic leukemia with 17p deletion: results from the phase II RESONATE™-17 trial. *Blood.* 2014;**124**:327.

85 Furman RR, Sharman JP, Coutre SE, et al. Idelalisib and rituximab in relapsed chronic lymphocytic leukemia. *N Engl J Med.* 2014;**370**:997–1007.

88 O'Brien S, Lamanna N, Kipps TJ. Update on a phase 2 study of idelalisib in combination with rituximab in treatment-naïve patients ≥65 years with chronic lymphocytic leukemia (CLL) or small lymphocytic lymphoma (SLL). *Blood.* 2014;**124(21)**:1994.

89 Esteve J, Villamor N, Colomer D, et al. Stem cell transplantation for chronic lymphocytic leukemia: different outcome after autologous and allogeneic transplantation and correlation with minimal residual disease status. *Leukemia.* 2001;**15**:445–451.

90 O'Brien S, Furman RR, Coutre SE, et al. Ibrutinib as initial therapy for elderly patients with chronic lymphocytic leukaemia or small lymphocytic lymphoma: an open-label, multicentre, phase 1b/2 trial. *Lancet Oncol.* 2014;**15(1)**:48–58.

91 Farooqui MZ, Valdez J, Martyr S, et al. Ibrutinib for previously untreated and relapsed or refractory chronic lymphocytic leukaemia with TP53 aberrations: a phase 2, single-arm trial. *Lancet Oncol.* 2015;**16(2)**:169–176.

118 Hodgkin lymphoma

Carol S. Portlock, MD ▪ Anita Kumar, MD ▪ James Armitage, MD

Overview

This chapter provides a historical perspective on the marked advances in radiotherapy and chemotherapy that have contributed to significant improvements in the curability of Hodgkin lymphoma (HL) over the past several decades. The classic features and new insights into the epidemiology, biology, and pathologic characteristics of HL are described. With emphasis on the modern clinical approach to the staging, imaging, and treatment of HL, the chapter highlights how current management approaches, such as refined risk stratification, use of PET imaging, and the reduction of radiation field and dose, seek to limit long-term toxicities of therapy while maintaining excellent cure rates. Finally, the authors describe how the development of novel, biologically targeted therapies has contributed to significant changes in the therapeutic landscape for patients with relapsed, refractory HL.

Introduction

Classical Hodgkin lymphoma, cHL, is now potentially curable in at least 80% of patients. Well-defined diagnostic criteria, prognostic factors, improved imaging, emphasis on systemic therapy first, and selective limited field radiotherapy consolidation have all contributed to this outcome. An increased appreciation of curability/quality of survivorship has now added the important goal of reducing the intensity of initial treatment when possible, without compromising cure rates; and, such changes in chemotherapy and radiation dose/field have resulted in reduction of long-term toxicities such as infertility, cardiopulmonary toxicity, and secondary malignancy.

History

In his historic paper of 1832, "On Some Morbid Appearances of the Exorbant Glands and Spleen," Thomas Hodgkin described the clinical history and postmortem findings of massive lymph node and spleen enlargement in patients studied at Guy's Hospital, London.[1] Hodgkin recognized that these patients had suffered from a disease that started in the lymph nodes located along the major vessels in the neck, chest, or abdomen. Sir Samuel Wilks, and later W.S. Greenfield described the microscopic lymph node appearance. Carl Sternberg, in 1898 and Dorothy Reed, in 1902, are credited with the first definitive microscopic descriptions of Hodgkin lymphoma.[2,3] The early treatment of Hodgkin lymphoma with crude X-rays in 1901 followed the discovery of radiographs by Roentgen, radioactivity by Becquerel, and radium by the Curies at the end of the nineteenth century. Before this time, serum and other biologic preparations, arsenic, iodine, and surgery were ineffective in cHL. These first reports of successful X-ray radiograph treatments produced great excitement and premature predictions for the curability of Hodgkin lymphoma.[4,5]

Modern radiation therapy (RT) techniques began in the 1920s with the work of Gilbert, who was one of the first to point out the predictable clinical patterns of cHL. He advocated treatment of apparently uninvolved adjacent lymph node chains that might contain suspected microscopic disease in addition to the involved nodal sites.[6] In 1950, Vera Peters extended this approach, reporting 5- and 10-year survivals of 88% and 79%, respectively, for patients with stage I. [7] However, the concept that early-stage Hodgkin lymphoma might be curable with RT was slow to be accepted. Henry Kaplan developed the linear accelerator and successfully applied this technology to curing cHL. He defined radiation field sizes and doses, refined and improved diagnostic staging techniques, developed models for translating laboratory findings into clinical practice, and, with Saul Rosenberg, promoted early randomized clinical trials in the United States.[8–10]

Advanced-stage cHL was uniformly fatal until the development of combination chemotherapy. Mechlorethamine was shown to be an active drug in the 1940s, and in the mid-1960s Vincent DeVita and colleagues first treated patients with an effective four-drug regimen termed MOPP (mechlorethamine, vincristine, procarbazine, and prednisone).[11] MOPP provided a high rate of complete remission and prolonged survival, resulting in curative outcomes.[12]

Like radiotherapy, randomized trials were also pivotal to the development of combination chemotherapy. These studies demonstrated no benefit of maintenance chemotherapy, established that treatment durations could be relatively short, and, ultimately, showed that ABVD (adriamycin, bleomycin, vinblastine, and dacarbazine) was associated with reduced toxicity and similar efficacy compared to MOPP (or MOPP-containing regimens), thus confirming ABVD as the standard regimen.[13,14]

Epidemiology and etiology

In 2014, there were expected to be 9190 new cases of cHL in the United States. The incidence is 2.7 per 100,000 per year and has remained relatively constant for decades. In the United States, the median age for all new cases is 39 years with 31% occurring between the ages of 20 and 34. Somewhat more men than women (3.1 to 2.4 per 100,000) develop HL.[15] Although a bimodal distribution was previously apparent in economically developed countries, the second peak is less apparent but persistent, as better pathology classification has found many of these cases to be non-Hodgkin lymphomas.

The etiology of Hodgkin lymphoma remains unknown. Epidemiologic data suggests both infectious and genetic components.[16,17]

Holland-Frei Cancer Medicine, Ninth Edition. Edited by Robert C. Bast Jr., Carlo M. Croce, William N. Hait, Waun Ki Hong, Donald W. Kufe, Martine Piccart-Gebhart, Raphael E. Pollock, Ralph R. Weichselbaum, Hongyang Wang, and James F. Holland.
© 2017 John Wiley & Sons, Inc. ISBN: 978-1-118-93469-2

A viral etiology is suggested by an association between cHL in younger patients and childhood factors that decrease exposure to infectious agents at an early age, including increased maternal education, decreased numbers of siblings and playmates, early birth order, and single-family dwellings in childhood for economically developed countries.[18,19] This association has led to the proposal that cHL appears to mimic a viral illness that has an age-related host response to infection (such as seen with polio and infectious mononucleosis). Supporting this theory is the infrequent occurrence of cHL in children younger than 10 years in economically developed countries.

Epstein–Barr virus (EBV) is the leading viral candidate.[16,20,21] EBV is the causative agent in African Burkitt lymphoma, and EBV-associated lymphomas are documented in patients with immune deficiency disorders and following organ transplantation. There is a two- to threefold excess in the incidence of cHL among patients with a prior history of mononucleosis. In addition, there is an altered antibody response pattern to EBV in patients who later develop cHL.

Recent cellular and molecular biology data have provided additional support for the association of EBV and cHL. Through the use of sensitive molecular probes, 30–50% of Hodgkin lymphoma specimens have been found to contain EBV genome fragments in the diagnostic Reed–Sternberg (R–S) cells.[22] EBV genome status appears to be stable over time when studied in initial biopsies and at relapse. EBV genome-positive R–S cells express the so-called type II latency profile, with expression of latent membrane protein (LMP)-1, LMP-2a, EBNA-1, and EBV-encoded ribonucleic acid (EBER). LMP-1 is critical in transformation and acts as an oncogene in transfection studies, whereas EBNA-1 is essential for the replication of the episomal viral genome.

A genetic predisposition is evident with increased incidence among first-degree relatives, in some sibling studies, in monozygotic twins, and among parent–child pairs but not among spouses. In addition, cHL has been linked with certain human leukocyte antigens (HLAs) that are associated with EBV status; and genome-wide association studies have identified, but not proven, non-HLA susceptibility genes.[17]

Immunologic abnormalities in patients

cHL is characterized by functional deficits in cellular immunity and in T-cell-mediated immune responses that exist before treatment. These deficits persist in cured patients[23] and include impairment of delayed cutaneous hypersensitivity, depressed proliferative responses to T-cell mitogen stimulation, enhanced immunoglobulin production, and decreased natural killer cell cytotoxicity. These abnormalities suggest an immunosuppression secondary to chronic overstimulation by cytokines. In patients with active cHL, these findings are consistent with increased cytokine secretion by R–S cells. However, it has been difficult to explain the persistence of these abnormalities in patients after successful treatment.

Treatment-induced immunosuppression returns toward normal after treatment, but has its greatest effect over the first few years.[23] For example, there is an excess of herpes zoster infections, and more than 75% of such cases occur within the first year. Few occur after the third year (6%). The risk of H. zoster appears highest as the intensity of therapy increases.[24]

Unlike the deficits in delayed hypersensitivity, most patients with cHL at diagnosis appear to have relatively normal B-cell number and function which may be adversely affected by treatment.[23] Patients should be encouraged to keep vaccinations up to date.

Pathology

Hodgkin lymphoma is unique among lymphomas for its histologic diversity.[25] Involved lymph nodes contain varying degrees of normal reactive and inflammatory cells, fibrosis, and a scattering of the characteristic malignant cHL cells, the R–S cells, and their mononuclear variants. The typical R–S cell has abundant cytoplasm and 2–3 nuclei, each with a single prominent nucleolus. The large size and unusual appearance of the R–S cell sets it apart from the adjacent smaller background cells. The mononuclear variants have nuclear and cytoplasmic features of R–S cells, but have only a single nucleus. Although the diagnosis of cHL should rarely be made in the absence of R–S cells, the presence of these cells alone is not sufficient to make the diagnosis. R–S-like cells have been found in infectious mononucleosis, non-Hodgkin lymphoma, and in some carcinomas and sarcomas. Thus, criteria for a cHL diagnosis include the presence of the R–S cells and the characteristic background of normal lymphocytes, plasma cells, and eosinophils.

The current pathology classification includes cHL: nodular sclerosis (NSHL), mixed cellularity (MCHL), lymphocyte-rich (LRHL), and lymphocyte depletion (LDHL) subtypes; as well as NLPHL, nodular lymphocyte predominance Hodgkin lymphoma. The subtyping of cHL does not affect clinical management, prognosis, or therapy. Nevertheless, the histologic subtypes are associated with different presentations, distinct natural histories, and variable prognoses. These differences are most evident in NLPHL.

Hodgkin lymphoma subtypes

Two histologic features of NSHL help to differentiate this cHL subtype: a proliferation of collagenous bands dividing the lymph node into circumscribed nodules and these nodules contain a variant R–S cell called the lacunar cell. In formalin-fixed tissue, this cell's abundant pale cytoplasm often retracts and gives the appearance of a cell in space (Figures 1–3). Molecular profiling studies have shown a close relationship between primary mediastinal large B-cell lymphoma and NSHL, rarely a "gray-zone" neoplasm that combines features of both neoplasms may be identified.[26–28]

NSHL is the only subtype of cHL as common in women as in men. It occurs in adolescents and young adults and is unusual in patients older than 50 years. It has a striking propensity to involve lower cervical, supraclavicular, and mediastinal lymph nodes with an orderly pattern of spread.[29] It makes up 60–70% of cHL in economically

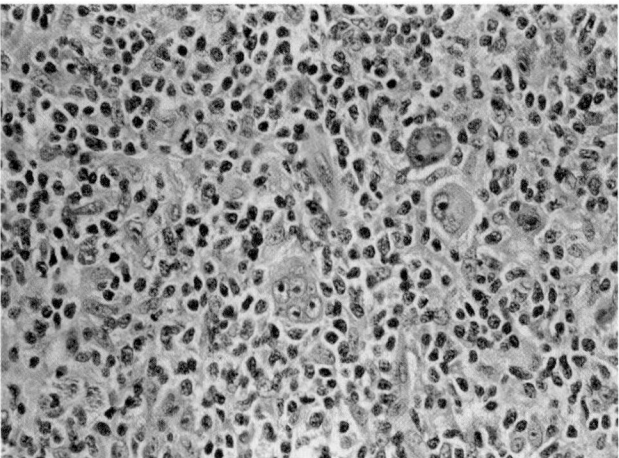

Figure 1 Reed–Sternberg cells and variants in Hodgkin lymphoma of the nodular sclerosis type. Large multinucleated or multilobated cells and a few mononuclear cells with macronucleoli stand apart from cellular background elements.

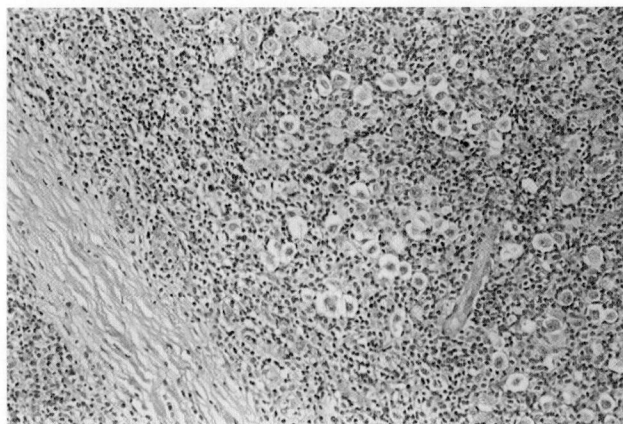

Figure 2 Hodgkin disease, nodular sclerosis. A fibrous band is present in the left lower part of the field. Neoplastic lacunar cells having abundant, clear cytoplasm stand out against the lymphocytic background.

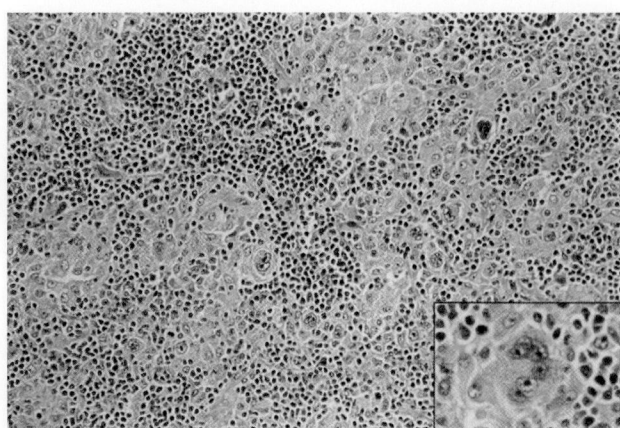

Figure 4 Hodgkin disease, mixed cellularity type. Reed–Sternberg cells in histiocyte-rich cellular background. Inset: Multinucleated Reed–Sternberg cell at higher magnification.

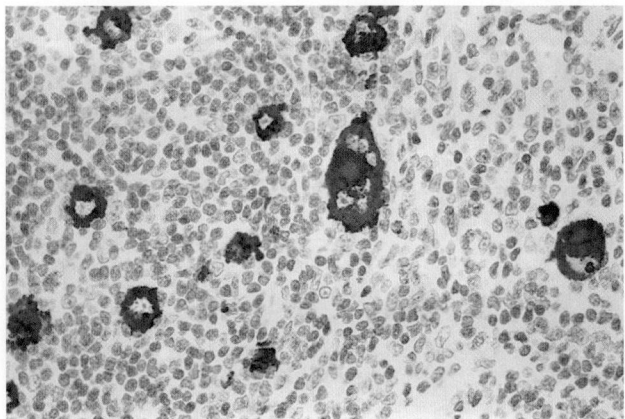

Figure 3 Immunostain for CD15 in Hodgkin disease, nodular sclerosis type. Neoplastic Reed–Sternberg cells and mononuclear Hodgkin cells show positive immunoreactivity.

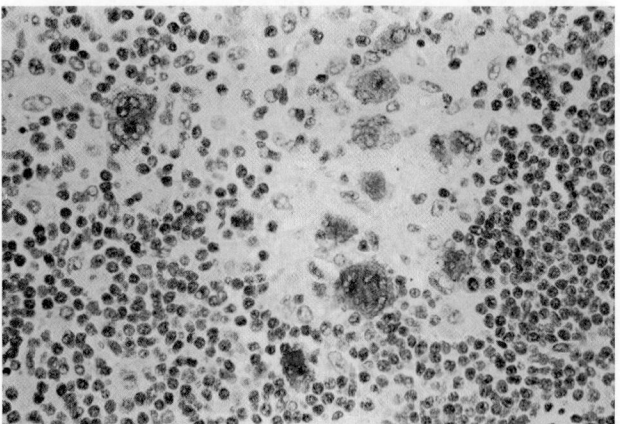

Figure 5 Immunostain for Epstein–Barr virus-latent membrane protein in Hodgkin disease, mixed cellularity type (same biopsy as Figure 4).

developed countries, but is less commonly seen in underdeveloped countries.

MCHL has an inflammatory background abundant in normal cells as well as 5–15 R–S cells and variants per high-power field (Figures 4 and 5). These patients are older, more likely to have B symptoms, and often have abdominal involvement or advanced disease. Approximately 25% with cHL in the United States have MCHL, and it is more common in underdeveloped countries. MCHL can be confused with peripheral T-cell lymphoma, and the antigen PAX5 may be particularly helpful, as it is a B-cell marker.

LRHL may resemble other histologic subtypes and may be nodular or diffuse. R–S cells are relatively rare, and the background is dominated by small mature lymphocytes (Figures 6 and 7). Eosinophils and neutrophils are usually restricted to blood vessels.

LDHL is rarely diagnosed, accounting for less than 1% of cHL in economically advanced countries. Generally, these patients present with advanced disease and B symptoms. R–S cells and "pleomorphic" variant cells are frequent and most cases have only sparse normal lymphocytes.

In NLPHL, the lymph node architecture is usually effaced, although a remnant of normal nodal architecture may remain. Diagnostic R–S cells are not seen, but variant lymphocyte predominance (LP) cells are typical (Figures 8 and 9). These cells often have multilobated nuclei and have been called popcorn cells because of

their resemblance to a popped kernel of corn. Fibrosis is not usually seen. The LP or "popcorn" R–S variants occur in a background of polyclonal B lymphocytes (Figure 9).[30,31] LP cells are usually positive for the B-cell marker CD20, but negative for the cHL markers of CD15 and CD 30 (Figures 10 and 11).[31,32] EBV is rarely detected in NLPHL.[33] The benign disorder, progressive transformation of germinal centers, is often associated with NLPHL. R–S cells and LP variants are absent in this entity. Progressive transformation of germinal centers can also be seen in association with NLPHL in the same or an adjacent node.[32]

NLPHL makes up 5–10% of all Hodgkin lymphoma in the United States. It is often localized to a single peripheral nodal region (high cervical, submandibular, epitrochlear, inguinal, or femoral nodes) and infrequently involves mediastinal or abdominal sites.

Immunophenotype and biology

The R–S cell is of B-lymphocyte origin.[25] These cells may express antigens found on resting or activated lymphocytes, most often B cell: usually positive for PAX5, and infrequently, CD20 or CD79a; and rarely positive for T-cell surface antigens (CD3, CD4, and CD8). The LP cells of NLPHL consistently express B-cell antigens. In cHL, the surface antigens CD30 and CD15 are present on most R–S cells, and nearly all cases are CD30+, and approximately 80% are CD15+,

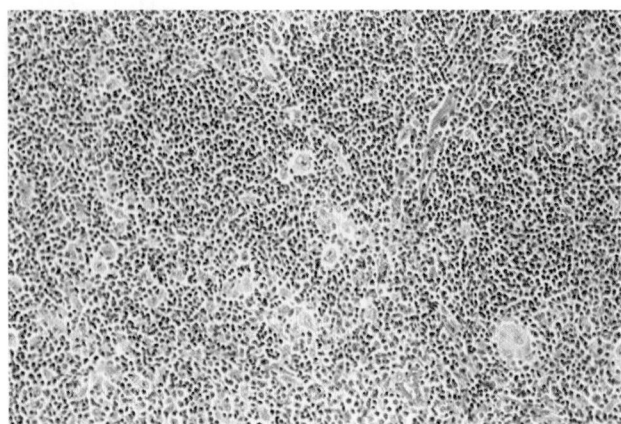

Figure 6 Lymphocyte-rich classic Hodgkin disease. Reed–Sternberg cells and mononuclear Hodgkin cells are relatively rare within the background proliferation of small lymphocytes and histiocytes.

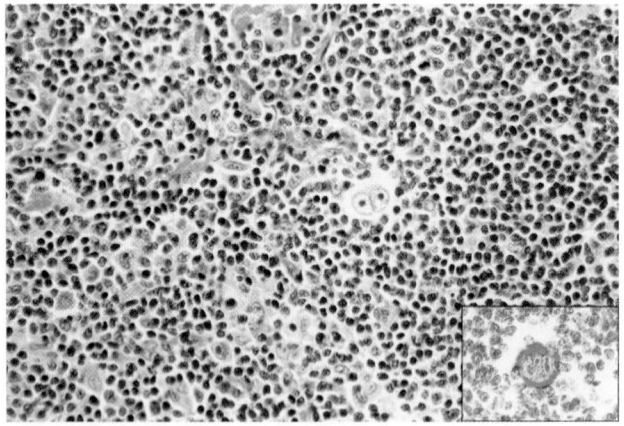

Figure 7 Lymphocyte-rich classic Hodgkin disease. Binucleated Reed–Sternberg cell in center of field. In same biopsy, Reed–Sternberg cells immunostained positively for CD15 (inset).

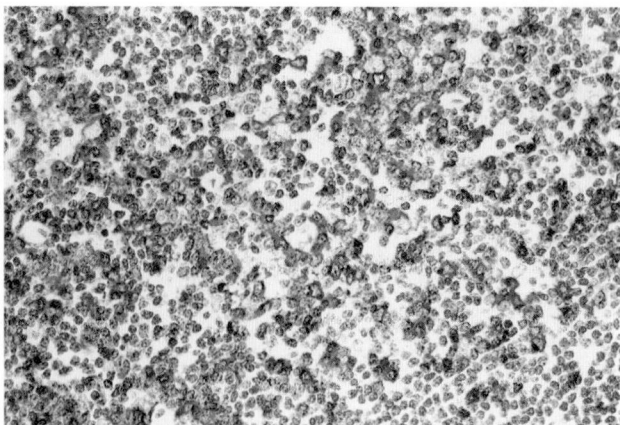

Figure 8 Lymphocyte predominant Hodgkin lymphoma (same biopsy as Figures 9–11). Immunostain for CD57 reveals a marked increase in immunoreactive cells showing localization around nonimmunoreactive L and H cells within a nodule. The CD3 immunostain showed a similar distribution of immunoreactive cells.

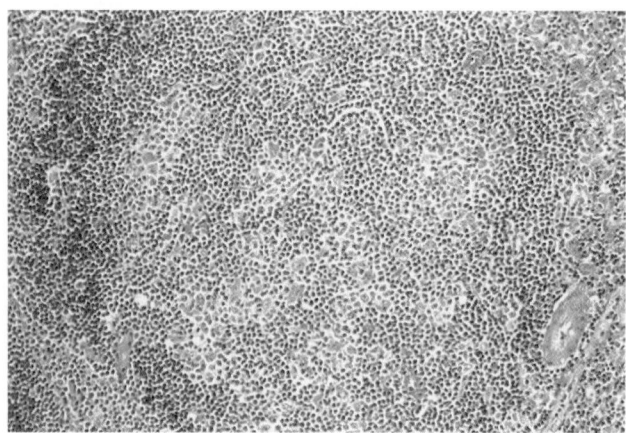

Figure 9 Lymphocyte predominant Hodgkin disease. The vaguely nodular histologic pattern is apparent.

whereas CD45 (leukocyte common antigen) is usually negative. In contrast, the LP cells of NLPHL are CD15 and CD30 negative and CD45 positive.[33]

Microdissection studies of single R–S cells demonstrate clonal immunoglobulin gene rearrangements in the vast majority of cases, confirming the clonality of the cells and establishing their B-cell lineage, despite their aberrant lack of immunoglobulin gene expression.[34,35] Moreover, R–S cells possess somatically mutated V genes, implying a germinal center or postgerminal center origin. The mutational pattern suggests that this may account for the lack of immunoglobulin expression. Other possible mechanisms include epigenetic silencing of heavy chain gene transcription or constitutive expression of Notch 1 and STAT 5.[25] Normal germinal center B cells that lack functional immunoglobulin receptors are usually eliminated within the germinal center via apoptosis; and therefore, R–S cells appear resistant to this usual apoptotic mechanism. This apoptosis pathway via FAS/CD95 is inhibited by c-FLIP, a gene that is constitutively expressed by R–S cells.[36] Several hypotheses have been generated to explain this phenomenon, including activation of the NF-κB pathway, general lineage promiscuity, and Epstein–Barr infection. Evidence favoring the NF-κB pathway includes the observation of constitutive expression of NF-κB in Hodgkin lymphoma-derived cell lines, the finding that suppression of NF-κB impairs tumor growth in severe combined immunodeficient mice and growth of cell lines,[37] and an epidemiology study showing that regular aspirin use is associated with a reduced risk of developing Hodgkin lymphoma, presumably through inhibition of NF-κB transcription.[38] The cause of the constitutive activation of NF-κB may include amplification of the REL gene, mutations in NF-κB inhibition, and somatic mutations in TNFA1P3.[25] LMP-2a expression may substitute for a functional B-cell receptor in EBV-associated cases.

Microdissection studies of LP cells also demonstrate clonal immunoglobulin gene rearrangements, again establishing clonality and confirming B-cell lineage.[34] In addition to demonstrating somatically mutated V genes, intraclonal sequence diversity can also be detected, providing strong evidence that NLPHL is a germinal center lymphoma. In contrast to cHL, the mutations are compatible with functional antigen receptors.

Cytogenetic abnormalities are common in R–S cells; however, no consistent pattern has been described. Rarely, the t(14 : 18) translocation, common in follicular B-cell lymphomas, may be detected. Comparative genomic hybridization studies demonstrate recurrent gains on chromosomal arms 2p (the site of NF-κB, REL, and BCL1 1a), 9p (the site of JAK2), and 12q (the site of MDM2), and amplifications on chromosomal bands 4p16, 4q23–q24, and 9p23–p24

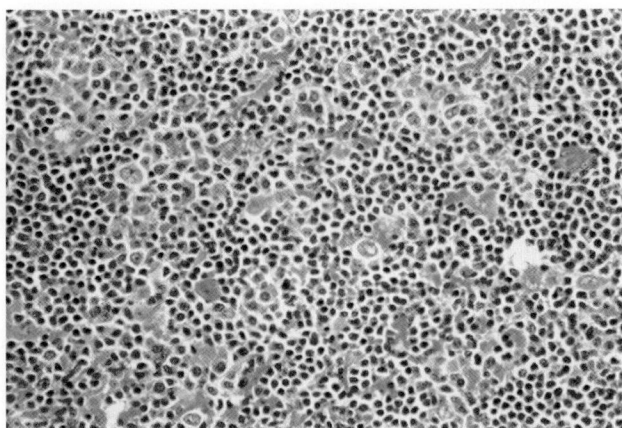

Figure 10 Lymphocyte predominant Hodgkin lymphoma at higher magnification (same biopsy as Figure 9). Within the background of lymphocytes and histiocytes are scattered large lobated cells having a fine chromatin pattern, relatively small nucleoli, and sparse cytoplasm so-called L and H cells.

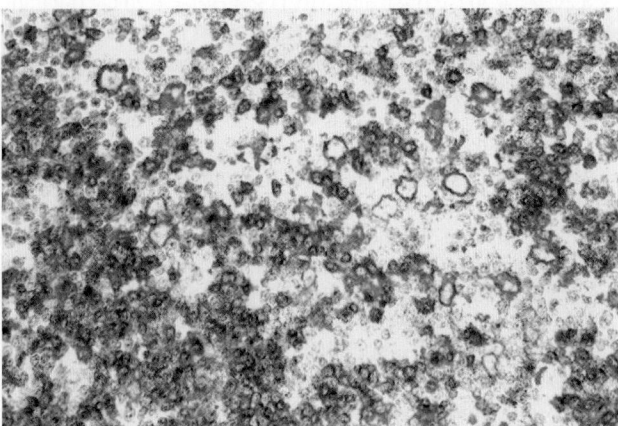

Figure 11 Lymphocyte predominant Hodgkin lymphoma (same biopsy as Figures 9 and 10). Immunostain for CD20 demonstrates positive staining of L and H cells as well as a high percentage of lymphocytes within a nodule.

(associated with high level of PD-L1 protein expression). Recurrent imbalances have been demonstrated in a majority of cHL using genome-wide GeneScan technology.[39]

The tumor microenvironment has been found to have an important role in the pathogenesis, associated manifestations, and prognosis of Hodgkin lymphoma.[40,41] It has been hypothesized that cytokines are responsible for the marked inflammatory component, fibrosis, and diverse histologic patterns of cHL, as well as the associated clinical symptoms of fever, weight loss, and night sweats.[42–44] Many cases are associated with upregulation of tumor necrosis factor receptor (TNFR) and ligand family members, Th2 and to a lesser extent Th1 cytokines, and other chemokines. Necrosis factor receptor (NFR) members may lead to constitutive activation of NF-κB, an important factor in proliferation and survival of B lymphocytes. Preferential expression of Th2 cytokines and chemokines may explain the frequent presence of eosinophils and fibroblasts, as well as local suppression of the cellular immune response. EBV may contribute to the production of cytokines, for example, via LMP-1-induced activation of NF-κB and stimulation of interleukin (IL)-10, a potent inhibitor of cellular immunity. In some cases, specific cytokines may be associated with specific histologic features. For example, transforming growth factor (TGF), a known stimulus

for fibroblast proliferation and collagen formation, is associated with NSHL,[45] and TARC (CCL27), a lymphocyte-directed CC chemokine secreted by Hodgkin cells, may be responsible for the infiltration by CD4+ T cells.[46] Tissue eosinophilia may be due to expression of IL-5, IL-9, CCL11, and CCL28; and IL-13 may play a role in autocrine stimulation of R–S cells.[47]

Staging

Most patients with cHL have a central pattern of lymph node involvement (cervical, mediastinal, and paraaortic) with >80% presenting initially above the diaphragm. In contrast, certain nodal chains (mesenteric, hypogastric, presacral, epitrochlear, and popliteal) are seldom, if ever involved. Spleen involvement is associated with adenopathy below the diaphragm and systemic symptoms. Isolated liver disease is rare; bone and bone marrow involvement is usually focal. Staging has recently been updated with the Lugano classification, incorporating the original Ann Arbor Stage and the later Cotswolds revision (Table 1).[48] PET imaging is now recognized as the most accurate means of identifying all sites of cHL involvement, and routine bone marrow biopsy is no longer recommended. See Table 2 for pretreatment evaluation.

Principles of treatment in classical Hodgkin lymphoma

The initial treatment of cHL is determined by stage at presentation and clinical prognostic category. In general, there are three groups with unique treatment considerations: Early stage, favorable risk; Early stage, unfavorable risk; and Advanced stage.

Radiotherapy

In the earliest years, RT alone was used for treatment, and maximal doses/field sizes were applied. Since then, the RT extent has been dramatically reduced. Several randomized studies confirmed that, in the setting of combined modality therapy (CMT, chemotherapy + radiotherapy), replacing the extended radiation fields (mantle/inverted Y) with involved-field radiotherapy was equivalent, with disease control and survival remaining similar.[49,50] Consolidative RT could be limited to the initial macroscopically involved volume and radiation doses could be reduced.[51] Such reductions in

Table 1 The Lugano classification.[48]

Stage I	A single lymph node or a group of adjacent nodes.
	Stage IE: A single extralymphatic site
	Tonsils, Waldeyer's ring, and spleen are considered nodal tissue
Stage II	Two or more lymph node groups on the same side of the diaphragm
	Stage IIE: Stage I or II nodal extent and limited contiguous extranodal involvement on the same side of the diaphragm
Stage III	Involvement of nodal tissue on both sides of the diaphragm
Stage IV	Noncontiguous extranodal involvement with or without associated lymph nodes
Designations applicable to any disease stage	
A:	No symptoms
B:	Fever (temperature, >38°C [100.4°F]), drenching night sweats, and unexplained loss of >10% of body weight within the preceding 6 months
X:	Bulky disease (a single nodal mass with a maximal dimension of 10 cm or greater, as measured by CT)

Source: Data from Ref. 48.

Table 2 Recommended staging.

> Adequate biopsy reviewed by an experienced hemopathologist (Surgical excisional biopsy is preferred and core needle biopsy may be sufficient in some cases. Fine needle aspiration is inadequate).
>
> History with attention to the presence or absence of systemic symptoms
>
> Physical examination, emphasizing node chains, size of liver and spleen, and Waldeyer ring inspection
>
> Laboratory tests: complete blood count with differential, erythrocyte sedimentation rate, comprehensive metabolic panel including liver function tests, and HIV, hepatitis B and C serologies.
>
> PET scan
>
> Selected CT imaging of neck, chest, abdomen, and pelvis, if required for radiotherapy
>
> No bone marrow biopsy unless PET scan is equivocal and result of biopsy will change treatment
>
> Evaluation of ejection fraction for doxorubicin-containing regimens
>
> Evaluation of pulmonary function for bleomycin-containing regimens
>
> Counseling: fertility preservation

Source: Data from Ref. 48.

dose and volume are expected to lessen late RT effects.[52] Currently, the radiation field can be involved node, INRT (prechemotherapy disease volume with minimal margins requiring excellent prechemotherapy imaging) or involved site, ISRT (initially involved tissue volumes, but requiring more clinical judgment to plan margins, as pretreatment imaging is suboptimal). ISRT has been adopted by many organizations as the standard cHL RT field.[53] Both INRT and ISRT are significantly smaller than involved-field RT.

Chemotherapy

The introduction of combination chemotherapy facilitated the reduction of RT dose/field, and chemotherapy is now the cornerstone of cHL therapy. Prior toxic regimens, such as MOPP, which were associated with infertility and secondary acute leukemia, have been supplanted by the equally efficacious, but less toxic regimen of ABVD.[13] ABVD is the treatment standard in the United States. Many regimens have been developed to further improve outcomes. Dose intensification with escalated BEACOPP (bleomycin, etoposide, doxorubicin, cyclophosphamide, vincristine, procarbazine, and prednisone) led to improved FFTF, but with increased acute and late toxicities and without overall survival benefit.[54–56]

Risk-adapted interim PET

In an effort to optimize outcome and minimize toxicity, early response assessment with an interim FDG-PET (PET) scan is often performed. This PET is done before completion of treatment, often after the second or fourth cycle of chemotherapy. After two cycles of ABVD, interim PET has been found to predict treatment response and clinical outcomes,[57–59] thus leading to the concept of "response-adapted therapy," whereby treatment intensity may be de-escalated with a good early response, or escalated if early response is inadequate.[60]

The cHL criteria for PET response utilize the "five-point scale" (FPS) or Deauville Criteria: baseline and interim PET scans are scored according to uptake in sites initially involved by lymphoma: (1) no uptake, (2) uptake = mediastinal blood pool, (3) uptake = liver, (4) moderately increased uptake > liver, or (5) markedly increased uptake > liver and/or new lesions.[61] A score of 1–3 is usually interpreted as negative for lymphoma, while a score of 4 or 5 is considered positive. In clinical trials, negativity may be more stringently defined as a score of 1–2 in cases where treatment may be substantially reduced for interim PET-negative patients.

Early stage cHL

In early-stage cHL, favorable and unfavorable risk groups have been defined.[62–65] Common unfavorable features include: bulky mediastinal mass, B symptoms, elevated ESR, and involvement of multiple lymph node groups. Bulky disease is variably defined : >1/3 of the mediastinal mass ratio (MMR, maximum width of the mass divided by the maximum intrathoracic diameter), >1/3 of the mediastinal thoracic ratio (MTR, maximum width of the mass divided by the intrathoracic diameter at T5–T6), or any mass >10 cm. Three risk systems have been retrospectively analyzed in early-stage cHL following four cycles of ABVD + IFRT, and the common poor prognostic feature was tumor burden (bulky mass or greater number of nodal sites).[66]

Favorable risk

Many studies in early-stage, favorable risk cHL have focused on reducing late effects without compromising cure. The GHSG HD10 study included 1131 patients with stage IA–IIB disease without any risk features.[67] Four treatment arms were randomized: ABVD × 2 cycles + 30 Gy IFRT, ABVD × 2 cycles + 20 Gy IFRT, ABVD × 4 cycles + 30 Gy IFRT, and ABVD × 4 cycles + 20 Gy IFRT. The 5-year freedom from treatment failure (FFTF) was 91.1% versus 93% for two versus four cycles of ABVD, respectively. Similarly, the 5-year FFTF in the two radiotherapy arms were not significantly different, 92.9% (20 Gy) versus 93.4% (30 Gy). Adverse events and acute toxic effects were more frequent in patients who received ABVD × 4 cycles + 30 Gy of IFRT. The authors recommended two cycles of ABVD followed by 20 Gy IFRT in these favorable patients.

The elimination of radiotherapy altogether in selected early-stage cHL is emerging as a new standard of care. In 2004, MSKCC reported a study of 152 nonbulky cHL patients with stages I, II A or B, and IIIA randomized to six cycles ABVD + RT versus six cycles ABVD alone.[68] At 5 years, FFS and OS for ABVD + RT versus ABVD alone were 86% versus 81% ($P = 0.61$) and 97% versus 90% ($P = 0.08$), respectively. The NCIC and ECOG HD.6 randomized stage IA or IIA nonbulky cHL patients to receive ABVD alone or ABVD + subtotal nodal radiation therapy (sTLI).[69] Patients in the RT group who had a favorable risk profile received sTLI alone, whereas patients with an unfavorable risk profile (any of the following: age older than 39 years, an ESR ≥50 mm/h, mixed cellularity or lymphocyte deplete histology, or ≥4 sites of disease) received two cycles ABVD + sTLI. Patients who received ABVD only received four to six cycles, based on interim CT. At 12 years there was a significant survival benefit favoring ABVD, 94% versus 87% for ABVD + sTLI ($P=0.04$), with excess secondary malignancies in the CMT arm. This study has been criticized, given outdated sTLI, nevertheless it demonstrated the value of ABVD alone and emphasized concerns regarding CMT.

ABVD alone is also being studied with interim PET.[70,71] The UK RAPID study was a randomized noninferiority study including 602 nonbulky stage IA or IIA cHL patients, favorable, and unfavorable risks. All received three cycles ABVD followed by PET imaging. If negative (Deauville 1 or 2), patients were randomized to no further treatment versus one cycle ABVD + 30 Gy IFRT. If interim PET positive, all received one cycle ABVD + 30 Gy IFRT. With median follow-up of 60 months, the 3-year PFS was 94.6% for CMT versus 90.8% for three cycles of ABVD alone, with an absolute risk difference of 3.8 percentage points. The EORTC/LYSA/FIL H10 trial, a randomized noninferiority study of both favorable and unfavorable risk early-stage cHL patients utilizing ABVD and interim PET after two cycles, concluded after a preplanned interim futility analysis that, when compared to CMT, the chemotherapy alone arms should be discontinued. However, the 1-year PFS in the ABVD arms were excellent, approximately 95%, raising the question of whether conclusions were made prematurely. The long-term results of ongoing PET-adapted studies will further clarify whether ABVD alone is an effective strategy for selected early-stage cHL.

Unfavorable risk

The standard of care for patients with early-stage unfavorable risk cHL is combined modality therapy with a 5-year PFS of 80–85%.[50,72] Some with nonbulky unfavorable risk may have good outcome with early-interim PET negativity, and may be candidates for chemotherapy alone.[70] With bulky disease, however, the addition of RT appears particularly important and PET-adapted studies omitting radiotherapy have generally excluded such patients.[73]

Several randomized trials have examined dose and schedule of combined modality therapy in early-stage, unfavorable risk cHL.[50,72,74–76] The GHSG HD11 trial compared 4 CMT regimens in 1570 patients: 4 ABVD + 20 Gy IFRT, 4 ABVD + 30 Gy IFRT, 4 BEACOPP + 20 Gy IFRT, versus 4 BEACOPP + 30 Gy IFRT. Stage IIB was considered advanced stage and excluded. Five-year FFTF was: 81% (4 ABVD + 20Gy), 85% (4 ABVD + 30Gy), 87% (4 BEACOPP + 20Gy), and 87% (4 BEACOPP+30Gy).[72] When combined with 20 Gy IFRT, results favored BEACOPP, however, with 30 Gy, ABVD + RT was equivalent with less toxicity. The authors recommended 4 ABVD + 30 Gy IFRT in early unfavorable cHL.

The GHSG HD14 trial compared four ABVD + 30 Gy IFRT versus two escalated BEACOPP followed by two cycles of ABVD (2 + 2) + 30 Gy IFRT.[76] The "2+2" arm had 5-year FFTF of 94.8% versus 87.7% with 4 ABVD + IFRT ($p = $ <0.001), however, there were significantly increased acute toxicities in the "2+2" arm. At a median follow-up of 43 months, there were no differences in treatment-related mortality or secondary malignancies however.

The Intergroup Trial E2496 compared 6–8 ABVD + 36 Gy IFRT versus Stanford V.[77] For patients with stage I or II bulky disease (bulk defined as MMR of greater than one third on chest radiography or $\geq$ 10 cm on CT), the 5-year FFS was 85% for ABVD + IFRT versus 79% for Stanford V (HR, 0.68; 95% CI, 0.37–1.25), with no significant difference between the two treatment approaches. More patients got IFRT (bulk was defined > 5 cm) with Stanford V and more patients on ABVD received long-course chemotherapy.[75] On the basis of these results, ABVD followed by consolidative RT remains the standard of care for bulky early-stage cHL.

Advanced-stage cHL

The International Prognostic Score (IPS) identifies seven independent prognostic factors associated with inferior progression free and overall survival in advanced cHL: serum albumin less than 4 g/dL; hemoglobin less than 10.5 g/dL; male gender; stage IV disease; age of 45 years or older; white cell count of 15,000/mm^3 or more; lymphocyte count less than 600/mm^3 or 8% of total white cell count.[78] The highest risk group (5 or more risk factors) had a 5-year FFP of 42% as compared to 80% for patients without risk factors. The IPS analyzed data before 1990, prompting a new evaluation. This study included 740 patients treated with ABVD or ABVD-like regimens in the British Columbia Cancer Agency (BCCA) database.[79] The IPS was still found to be prognostically significant, but with a narrower difference between outcomes: 5-year FFP of 70% for patients with > 4 IPS factors compared to 88% with no adverse factors and 5-year OS of 73% and 98%, respectively. These results demonstrate improved outcomes likely due to uniform anthracycline containing chemotherapy (ABVD), growth factor support, improved accuracy of staging, and more accurate pathologic diagnosis.

Treatment

Standard therapy for advanced cHL is six cycles of ABVD. Dose-intensive treatment regimens have been studied. Although phase II trials suggested that Stanford V might have superior efficacy as compared to ABVD, the Intergroup Study for advanced-stage cHL patients found no difference in FFS: 74% for ABVD and 71% for Stanford V at 5 years.[80–82] Moreover, the Stanford V arm was associated with a higher incidence of lymphopenia and neuropathy.

The GHSG-escalated BEACOPP regimen is widely used in Europe, however it has failed to gain popularity in the United States owing to excess toxicities and no clear survival benefit. Three GHSG phase III trials—HD9, HD12, and HD15—have examined BEACOPP.[55,56,83]

In the HD9 study, 1196 patients were randomized: COPP-ABVD, standard-dose BEACOPP, versus escalated BEACOPP.[55] All were eight cycles + RT to initial sites $\geq$5 cm. The 5 and 10-year analyses showed that escBEACOPP was significantly better than BEACOPP or COPP-ABVD with FFTF (82%, 70%, and 64%) and OS (86%, 80%, and 75%). escBEACOPP appeared to have the greatest clinical benefit for IPS scores 4–7, but had greater myelosuppression, infertility and secondary myelodysplasia/acute leukemia.

HD12 compared 8 esc BEACOPP to 4 escBEACOPP + 4 baseline BEACOPP (4+4).[83] Patients were then randomized to no further therapy versus 30 Gy RT consolidation. Five-year FFTF was 86.4% escBEACOPP versus 84.8% 4 + 4, and OS 92% versus 90.3%. The FFTF was better in the RT arm, although OS was not significantly improved.

HD15 trial included 2182 patients: 8 escBEACOPP, 6 escBEACOPP, or eight cycles of a time-intensified standard-dose BEACOPP.[56] RT (30 Gy) was restricted to patients with PET-positive residual sites (2.5 cm or more). Five-year FFTF was 4.4%, 89.3%, and 85.4%; and 5-year OS 91.9%, 95.3%, and 94.5%, respectively. The authors recommended six cycles of escBEACOPP with significantly better outcome, less treatment-related mortality, and fewer secondary cancers.

A subset of cHL is CD20+, with expression of this B-cell antigen on the R–S cell. Phase II studies adding rituximab (anti-CD20 monoclonal antibody) administered weekly for 6 weeks with ABVD in advanced-stage CD20+ cHL have been reported.[84,85] In one study, 5-year EFS and overall survival rates of 83% and 96% were reported and appear promising for this histologic subset.[84]

Risk-adapted interim PET imaging is also being applied in advanced-stage cHL. A phase II study from Israel suggests that risk and response-adapted treatment may be effective. In this study, 45 poor-risk (IPS $\geq$ 3) advanced-stage cHL patients received two cycles of escBEACOPP, followed by a PET scan. If PET was negative, patients were subsequently treated with four cycles of ABVD. For the 31 patients who achieved a negative early-interim PET scan, the 4-year PFS was 87%.[60] Early results from the SWOG S0816 and UK RATHL studies applying interim PET response-adapted treatment strategies in advanced-stage cHL show promise.[86]

Management of relapsed, refractory Hodgkin lymphoma

The standard treatment approach for relapsed, refractory—r/r—cHL is salvage chemotherapy to achieve remission status, followed by myeloablative chemotherapy and autologous stem-cell transplant (ASCT). Various groups have developed prognostic models to predict the outcome of r/r cHL completing ASCT.[87–91] Unfavorable risk factors include: presence of extranodal disease, abbreviated remission duration after frontline therapy (generally < 1 year), and presence of B symptoms. In addition, a powerful independent prognostic factor is pretransplant functional imaging status.[92,93]

In one study with median follow-up of 51 months, patients with a negative PET scan before ASCT had superior outcomes with event-free survival >80% versus 29% for patients with a positive scan.[92]

There are many salvage regimens for r/r cHL including ICE (ifosfamide, carboplatin, and etoposide), DHAP (dexamethasone, high-dose cytarabine, and cisplatin), ESHAP (etoposide, methylprednisolone, high-dose cytarabine, and cisplatin), IGEV (ifosfamide, gemcitabine, and vinorelbine), and GVD (gemcitabine, vinorelbine, and pegylated liposomal doxorubicin).[88,94–97] These regimens have not been prospectively compared, nevertheless, they do appear to have similar efficacy in phase II studies.

The goal of salvage treatment is to achieve a PET-negative remission before consolidative ASCT, as patients with persistent disease at the time of transplant have poor outcomes. This aim may be achieved by one or more salvage regimens, with or without radiotherapy. The potential curative role and significant survival benefit of ASCT in r/r cHL have been established by two large randomized trials comparing chemotherapy alone to chemotherapy followed by ASCT.[98,99]

Novel agents in Hodgkin lymphoma

Approximately 15% of cHL patients will fail both first- and second-line therapy, and require novel therapy. Brentuximab vedotin (BV) was FDA-approved in 2012 for r/r cHL after failure of ASCT or for those not deemed ASCT candidates after failure of at least two multiagent regimens.[100,101] Other agents with demonstrated activity include histone deacetylase inhibitors, PI3-kinase/Akt/Mtor pathway inhibitors, lenalidomide, and bendamustine.[102] Most recently, immune checkpoint inhibitors targeting the programmed death-1 (PD1)-PD1-ligand pathway have shown promise in cHL. The PD1-PD1-ligand pathway dampens immune responses, and inhibition of this pathway results in augmentation of host immune response against tumor cells. Preliminary data (2014 American Society of Hematology) has revealed overall response rates ranging from 50% to 89% for two of these agents, pembrolizumab and nivolumab.[103,104]

Brentuximab vedotin, BV, is an antibody-drug conjugate (ADC) consisting of the chimeric anti-CD30 monoclonal antibody, cAC10, chemically conjugated to monomethyl auristatin E (MMAE).[105,106] MMAE is internalized into the Reed–Sternberg cell, where it is a tubulin inhibitor resulting in cell cycle arrest and apoptosis.[107] The initial phase I study enrolled 45 patients with r/r CD30-positive hematologic malignancies. BV was administered intravenously every 3 weeks at doses ranging from 0.1 to 3.6 mg/kg. Dose-limiting toxicities included grade-4 thrombocytopenia, grade-3 hyperglycemia, and febrile neutropenia. The maximum tolerated dose (MTD) was 1.8 mg/kg every 3 weeks. Promising responses were seen, and a phase 2 study in 102 patients with r/r cHL after ASCT confirmed these results.[101] Patients received 1.8 mg/kg BV every 3 weeks for up to 16 cycles. The overall response rate was 75%, with complete remissions in 34 of 102 (33%). The median PFS was 5.6 months and OS 40.5 months. Moreover, 14 patients remained in durable remission after BV and of these, 9 had not started new therapy and 5 had proceeded to consolidative allogeneic SCT.[108]

BV is now being studied for initial treatment of cHL in combination with AVD: an international phase III study randomizes BV + AVD versus ABVD for advanced-stage cHL. Similar BV combinations regimens are under investigation for early-stage and elderly cHL. Another strategy is BV before ASCT in place of, or in addition to, standard salvage, such as ICE.[109] Post-ASCT, a phase III study of BV maintenance versus placebo demonstrated a significant improvement in median PFS favoring maintenance BV versus placebo (42.9 months vs 24.1 months) in high-risk cHL.[110]

Special populations

NLPHL

This rare subset of lymphoma (see pathology discussion) is now recognized to be highly treatable but likely not curable with standard cHL therapy.[111–113] Management options include excision only, INRT or CMT in early stage; and monitoring, Rituximab alone or with chemotherapy, or palliative INRT for relapsed/advanced-stage disease. Most importantly, survival remains excellent but can be negatively impacted by the late effects of prior therapy. Thus, in this lymphoma, it is important to be mindful of the young age, the intensity of treatment utilized, and the likely good outcome achievable with limited therapy. Like indolent lymphoma, NLPHL is associated with the late development of histologic transformation (T-cell-rich B-cell lymphoma, a subtype of DLBCL, or DLBCL). This may be a life-threatening development and requires a multiagent chemotherapy regimen as in management of DLBCL.

Elderly

In the elderly, the curative aim of cHL treatment remains realistic, although the management approach may be modified for tolerability. ABVD is the standard regimen, although bleomycin may be more lung-toxic, and other regimens are often considered (without adriamycin or bleomycin). Brentuximab vedotin may become a successful substitute for bleomycin in ABVD (see above). Relapsed/refractory cHL may still be approached with salvage chemotherapy/ASCT in selected patients, generally with physiologic age of 70 or less. Without second-line ASCT, most patients do not have a curative option at this time and are managed with phase I–II clinical trials, palliative chemotherapy, and/or RT.

Pregnancy

cHL may occur in young women, and not infrequently, may present during pregnancy. Details of management are discussed elsewhere. Most importantly, cHL is generally a slowly progressive lymphoma and its treatment can often be delayed until delivery, or ABVD can be safely administered during the second and/or third trimesters. Imaging during pregnancy should be minimized with use of MRI, and no PET should be performed.

HIV

cHL may be seen in association with HIV, and in this context the pathology is more likely mixed cellularity or lymphocyte-depleted histologic subtypes, and the stage more advanced with unusual sites such as skin. Treatment regimens remain the same as non-HIV patients, when the CD4 count exceeds 200 and patients receive concurrent cART therapy and prophylactic antibiotics as indicated. A more selective approach is needed in more immunosuppressed patients where infectious complications may be greater.[114]

Post-treatment surveillance

The ability to predict sustained remission and curability has increased with PET imaging. This has raised the important question of when, how frequently, and for how long should surveillance imaging be continued postremission. All agree that in the surveillance setting, PET is too sensitive, identifying excess false positives. Selective CT or MRI imaging can be alternatives when needed. As most relapses occur in the first two years post-treatment, routine imaging after this timeframe is not recommended.[115]

Key references

The complete reference list can be found on the Wiley Companion Digital Edition of this title (see inside front cover for login instructions).

1 Hodgkin's T. On some morbid appearances of the absorbent glands and spleen. *Medico-Chirugical Trans.* 1832;**17**:68–97.

7 Peters M. A study of survivals in Hodgkin's disease treated radiologically. *Am J Roentgenol.* 1950;**63**:299–311.

8 Kaplan H. The radical radiotherapy of regionally localized Hodgkin's disease. *Radiology.* 1962;**78**:553–561.

9 Kaplan HS. Role of intensive radiotherapy in the management of Hodgkin's disease. *Cancer.* 1966;**19**:356.

10 Jacobs C. *Henry Kaplan and the Story of Hodgkin's Disease.* Stanford, CA: *Stanford University Press*; 2010:456. http://www.sup.org/books/title/?id=16764(accessed 9 Jan 2015).

12 DeVita VJ, Simon R, Habbard S, et al. Curability of advanced Hodgkin's disease with chemotherapy: longterm follow up of MOPP-treated patients at the National Cancer Institute. *Ann Intern Med.* 1980;**92**:587–595.

13 Canellos GP, Anderson JR, Propert KJ, et al. Chemotherapy of advanced Hodgkin's disease with MOPP, ABVD, or MOPP alternating with ABVD [see comments]. *N Engl J Med.* 1992;**327**:1478–1484.

14 Bonadonna G, Zucali R, Monfardini S, et al. Combination chemotherapy of Hodgkin's disease with Adriamycin, bleomycin, vinblastine, and imidazole carboxamide versus MOPP. *Cancer.* 1975;**36**:252–259.

16 Vockerodt M, Yap LF, Shannon-Lowe C, et al. The Epstein-Barr virus and the pathogenesis of lymphoma. *J Pathol.* 2015;**235**(2):312–322. doi: 10.1002/path.4459.

17 Kushekhar K, van den Berg A, Nolte I, Hepkema B, Visser L, Diepstra A. Genetic associations in classical Hodgkin lymphoma: a systematic review and insights into susceptibility mechanisms. *Cancer Epidemiol Biomarkers Prev.* 2014;**23**(12):2737–2747.

25 King RL, Howard MT, Bagg A. Hodgkin lymphoma: pathology, pathogenesis, and a plethora of potential prognostic predictors. *Adv Anat Pathol.* 2014 Jan;**21**(1):12–25. doi: 10.1097/PAP.0000000000000002.

29 Mauch PM, Kalish L, Kadin M, et al. Patterns of presentation of Hodgkin's disease. *Cancer.* 1993;**71**:2062–2071.

40 Steidl C, Connors JM, Gascoyne RD. Molecular pathogenesis of Hodgkin's lymphoma: increasing evidence of the importance of the microenvironment. *J Clin Oncol.* 2011 May 10;**29**(14):1812–1826.

41 Steidl C, Lee T, Shah SP, et al. Tumor-associated macrophages and survival in classic Hodgkin's lymphoma. *N Engl J Med.* 2010;**362**(10):875–885.

48 Cheson BD, Fisher RI, Barrington SF, et al. Recommendations for initial evaluation, staging, and response assessment of Hodgkin and non-Hodgkin lymphoma: the Lugano classification. *J Clin Oncol.* 2014 Sep 20;**32**(27):3059–3068.

52 Ng AK, Travis LB. Acute and long-term complications of radiotherapy in Hodgkin lymphoma. In: Specht L, Yahalom J, eds. *Radiotherapy for Hodgkin Lymphoma.* Heidelberg: Springer; 2011:183–196.

53 Specht L, Yahalom J, Illidge T, et al. Modern radiation therapy for Hodgkin lymphoma: field and dose guidelines from the international lymphoma radiation oncology group (ILROG). *Int J Radiat Oncol Biol Phys.* 2014;**89**:854–862.

54 Diehl V, Franklin J, Pfreundschuh M, et al. Standard and increased-dose BEACOPP chemotherapy compared with COPP-ABVD for advanced Hodgkin's disease. *N Engl J Med.* 2003;**348**:2386–2395.

55 Engert A, Diehl V, Franklin J, et al. Escalated-dose BEACOPP in the treatment of patients with advanced-stage Hodgkin's lymphoma: 10 years of follow-up of the GHSG HD9 study. *J Clin Oncol.* 2009;**27**:4548–4554.

57 Gallamini A, Rigacci L, Merli F, et al. The predictive value of positron emission tomography scanning performed after two courses of standard therapy on treatment outcome in advanced stage Hodgkin's disease. *Haematologica.* 2006;**91**:475–481.

61 Gallamini A, Barrington SF, Biggi A, et al. The predictive role of interim positron emission tomography for Hodgkin lymphoma treatment outcome is confirmed using the interpretation criteria of the Deauville five-point scale. *Haematologica.* 2014;**99**(6):1107–1113.

64 Meyer RM, Gospodarowicz MK, Connors JM, et al. Randomized comparison of ABVD chemotherapy with a strategy that includes radiation therapy in patients with limited-stage Hodgkin's lymphoma: National Cancer Institute of Canada Clinical Trials Group and the Eastern Cooperative Oncology Group. *J Clin Oncol.* 2005;**23**:4634–4642.

66 Klimm B, Goergen H, Fuchs M, et al. Impact of risk factors on outcomes in early-stage Hodgkin's lymphoma: an analysis of international staging definitions. *Ann Oncol.* 2013;**24**:3070–3076.

67 Engert A, Plutschow A, Eich HT, et al. Reduced treatment intensity in patients with early-stage Hodgkin's lymphoma. *N Engl J Med.* 2010;**363**:640–652.

68 Straus DJ, Portlock CS, Qin J, et al. Results of a prospective randomized clinical trial of doxorubicin, bleomycin, vinblastine, and dacarbazine (ABVD) followed by radiation therapy (RT) versus ABVD alone for stages I, II, and IIIA nonbulky Hodgkin disease. *Blood.* 2004;**104**:3483–3489.

69 Meyer RM, Gospodarowicz MK, Connors JM, et al. ABVD alone versus radiation-based therapy in limited-stage Hodgkin's lymphoma. *N Engl J Med.* 2012;**366**:399–408.

70 Radford J, Illidge T, Counsell N, et al. Results of a trial of PET-directed therapy for early-stage Hodgkin's lymphoma. *N Engl J Med.* 2015;**372**:1598–1607.

72 Eich HT, Diehl V, Gorgen H, et al. Intensified chemotherapy and dose-reduced involved-field radiotherapy in patients with early unfavorable Hodgkin's lymphoma: final analysis of the German Hodgkin Study Group HD11 trial. *J Clin Oncol.* 2010;**28**:4199–4206.

77 Advani RH, Hong F, Fisher RI, et al. Randomized phase III trial comparing ABVD plus radiotherapy with the Stanford V regimen in patients with stages I or II locally extensive, bulky mediastinal Hodgkin lymphoma: a subset analysis of the North American intergroup E2496 trial. *J Clin Oncol.* 2015;**33**:1936–1942.

78 Hasenclever D, Diehl V. A prognostic score for advanced Hodgkin's disease. International prognostic factors project on advanced Hodgkin's disease. *N Engl J Med.* 1998;**339**:1506–1514.

79 Moccia AA, Donaldson J, Chhanabhai M, et al. International Prognostic Score in advanced-stage Hodgkin's lymphoma: altered utility in the modern era. *J Clin Oncol.* 2012;**30**:3383–3388.

86 Johnson P, McKenzie H. How I treat advanced classical Hodgkin lymphoma. *Blood.* 2015;**125**:1717–1723.

89 Moskowitz CH, Yahalom J, Zelenetz AD, et al. High-dose chemo-radiotherapy for relapsed or refractory Hodgkin lymphoma and the significance of pre-transplant functional imaging. *Br J Haematol.* 2010;**148**:890–897.

92 Moskowitz CH, Matasar MJ, Zelenetz AD, et al. Normalization of pre-ASCT, FDG-PET imaging with second-line, non-cross-resistant, chemotherapy programs improves event-free survival in patients with Hodgkin lymphoma. *Blood.* 2012;**119**:1665–1670.

100 Younes A, Bartlett NL, Leonard JP, et al. Brentuximab vedotin (SGN-35) for relapsed CD30-positive lymphomas. *N Engl J Med.* 2010;**363**:1812–1821.

102 Moskowitz AJ. Novel agents in Hodgkin lymphoma. *Curr Oncol Rep.* 2012;**14**:419–423.

104 Ansell SM, Lesokhin AM, Borrello I, et al. PD-1 Blockade with Nivolumab in relapsed or refractory Hodgkin's lymphoma. *N Engl J Med.* 2015;**372**:311–319.

108 Gopal AK, Chen R, Smith SE, et al. Three-year follow-up data and characterization of long-term remissions from an ongoing phase 2 study of brentuximab vedotin in patients with relapsed or refractory Hodgkin lymphoma. *Blood ASH Annual Meeting Abstracts.* 2013;**122**(21):4382.

109 Moskowitz AJ, Schoder H, Yahalom J, et al. PET-adapted sequential salvage therapy with brentuximab vedotin followed by augmented ifosamide, carboplatin, and etoposide for patients with relapsed and refractory Hodgkin's lymphoma: a non-randomised, open-label, single-centre, phase 2 study. *Lancet Oncol.* 2015;**16**:284–292.

110 Moskowitz CH, Nademanee A, Masszi T, et al. Brentuximab vedotin as consolidation therapy after autologous stem-cell transplantation in patients with Hodgkin's lymphoma at risk of relapse or progression (AETHERA): a randomised, double-blind, placebo-controlled, phase 3 trial. *Lancet.* 2015;**385**: 1853–1362.

113 Shankar A, Daw S. Nodular lymphocyte predominant Hodgkin lymphoma in children and adolescents — a comprehensive review of biology, clinical course and treatment options. *Br J Haematol.* 2012;**159**:288–298.

114 Uldrick TS, Little RF. How we treat classical Hodgkin lymphoma in patients infected with human immunodeficiency virus. *Blood.* 2014 **125**:1226–1235 . pii: blood-2014-08-551598..

115 Ng AK. Current survivorship recommendations for patients with Hodgkin lymphoma: focus on late effects. *Blood.* 2014;**124**(23):3373–3379. doi: 10.1182/blood-2014-05-579193.

119 Non-Hodgkin's lymphoma

Arnold S. Freedman, MD ▪ *Ann S. LaCasce, MD*

Overview

The malignant lymphomas are neoplastic transformations of cells that reside predominantly within lymphoid tissues. Although Hodgkin lymphomas (HLs) and non-Hodgkin lymphomas (NHLs) infiltrate lymphohematopoietic tissues, their biologic and clinical behaviors are distinct. They differ with neoplastic cells of origin, sites of disease, presence of specific symptoms, and response to treatment. Although both are among the most sensitive malignancies to radiation and cytotoxic therapy, their cure rates markedly differ. HLs are cured in nearly 80% of all patients employing both conventional and salvage treatment strategies whereas NHLs are cured in fewer than 50% of patients.

Epidemiology and etiology

Incidence and mortality

In 2014, 70,890 new cases of NHL (non-Hodgkin lymphoma) were diagnosed in the United States[1] with 18,990 deaths predicted. Cases increase steadily with age. There is a slight male predominance and the incidence is higher in Caucasians than in African Americans. Although the rate of increase has slowed since the mid-1990s, the incidence continues to rise by 1.5–2% each year.

The incidence of NHL subtype varies significantly by age. In children, Burkitt's lymphoma (BL), lymphoblastic lymphoma (LBL), and diffuse large B-cell lymphoma (DLBCL) predominate. With increasing age, rates of follicular lymphomas (FLs) and other aggressive lymphomas continue to increase. Small lymphocytic and FLs are most commonly diagnosed in patients over age 60.

Exposures and diseases associated with increased risk of developing NHL

Infectious agents are involved in the pathogenesis of some NHLs (Table 1). Epstein–Barr virus (EBV) has a strong association with development of BL, natural killer cell lymphoma, and human immunodeficiency virus-related (HIV-1) lymphoma.[2,3] About 45–70% of HIV-associated NHLs are EBV related, as are nearly 100% of the primary central nervous system (CNS) lymphomas in HIV-1 positive individuals. Human T-cell lymphotropic virus (HTLV)-1 is responsible for adult T-cell leukemia/lymphoma, endemic to the Caribbean and southern Japan.[4] Gastric marginal zone lymphoma (MZL) is associated with *Helicobacter pylori* infection.[5] Splenic MZL is associated with hepatitis C infection.[6] Chronic hepatitis B infection carries an increased risk of NHL.[7] In Europe, ocular adnexal MZL is linked with *Chlamydia psittaci* infection[8] and MZL involving the skin with *Borrelia burgdorferi*. Immunoproliferative small intestinal disease (Mediterranean lymphoma, alpha heavy chain disease) has been associated with

Campylobacter jejuni.[9] Kaposi sarcoma-associated herpes virus, also known as HHV-8 (human herpes virus-8), has been isolated from the neoplastic cells in patients with primary effusion lymphomas.[10,11]

An increased risk of NHL is associated with a number of exposures and/or disease states. Controversial evidence suggests certain chemical exposures, including the herbicide phenoxyacetic acid, arsenic, pesticides, fungicides, chlorophenols, organic solvents, halomethane, lead, vinyl chloride, or asbestos, increase the risk of NHL.[12-14] Occupational exposures associated with an increased risk include agricultural work, welding, and work in the lumber industry.[15,16]

Diseases of inherited and acquired immunodeficiency and autoimmune diseases are associated with an increased incidence of lymphoma.[17,18] The association between immunosuppression and NHLs is compelling given a percentage of lymphomas will regress with the withdrawal of immunosuppression.[19] Patients undergoing organ transplantation necessitating chronic immunosuppression have a nearly 100-fold risk of NHL, which is greatest in the first-year posttransplant. DLBCL is most common NHL in this setting and is frequently associated with EBV.[20] The rare inherited immunodeficiency diseases such as X-linked lymphoproliferative syndrome, Wiskott–Aldrich syndrome, Chédiak–Higashi syndrome, ataxia telangiectasia, and common variable immunodeficiency syndrome are complicated by highly aggressive lymphomas. An increased risk of NHL has been observed in first-degree relatives with NHL, CLL, and Hodgkin lymphoma (HL).[21]

Pathology, immunobiology, and natural history of NHL

The World Health Organization (WHO) published a new classification of tumors of the hematopoietic and lymphoid tissues (Table 2)[22] that integrate morphology, immunotyping, genetic features, and clinical syndromes. To provide a context for this classification, the large numbers of entities will be grouped into "indolent," "aggressive," and "highly aggressive" categories (Table 2).

Chromosomal translocations and oncogene rearrangements. Given the mechanism of immunoglobulin (Ig) and T-cell receptor (TCR) gene rearrangements in normal lymphoid cells, lymphomas are frequently found to have chromosomal translocations that involve the activation of an oncogene or inactivation of a tumor suppressor gene. The former is more common, whereby a proto-oncogene is brought under the control of a constitutively active promoter, resulting in overexpression of the oncogenic gene and its protein product. Examples include the (8;14)(q24;q32) translocation in BL, involving the *MYC* proto-oncogene and the IgH gene; the (14;18)(q32;q32) translocation in FL, involving the *BCL2* proto-oncogene and the IgH gene; and the (11;14) (q13;q32) translocation in mantle cell lymphoma (MCL), involving the gene encoding cyclin D1 (*CCDN1*)

Holland-Frei Cancer Medicine, Ninth Edition. Edited by Robert C. Bast Jr., Carlo M. Croce, William N. Hait, Waun Ki Hong, Donald W. Kufe, Martine Piccart-Gebhart, Raphael E. Pollock, Ralph R. Weichselbaum, Hongyang Wang, and James F. Holland.
© 2017 John Wiley & Sons, Inc. ISBN: 978-1-118-93469-2

Table 1 Risk factors for the development of lymphoma.

Inherited immunodeficiency states	Acquired immunodeficiency states	Autoimmune and inflammatory disorders	Infectious agents (other than HIV)	Chemicals and drugs
Autoimmune lymphoproliferative disease	HIV-1 infection	Rheumatoid arthritis	Epstein–Barr virus	Herbicides, pesticides, organic solvents
Ataxia telangiectasia	Iatrogenic	Systemic Lupus Erythematosus	HTLV-1	Ionizing radiation
Chediak–Higashi syndrome	Tumor necrosis factor agonists	Sjögren's syndrome	HHV-8	Chemotherapy, radiation therapy
Common variable immunodeficiency		Celiac disease	*Helicobacter pylori*	
Wiskott–Aldrich syndrome		Hashimoto's thyroiditis	*Campylobacter jejuni*	
X-linked lymphoproliferative disease		Inflammatory bowel disease	*Chlamydia psittaci*	
			Borrelia burgdorferi	
			HCV	

HIV-1, human immunodeficiency virus-1; HTLV-1, human T-cell lymphotropic virus-1; HHV-8, human herpes virus-8; HCV, hepatitis C virus.

Table 2 World Health Organization Classification of Lymphoid Neoplasms 2008: selected B- and T-cell neoplasms.

Precursor B- and T-cell neoplasms

    Precursor B-lymphoblastic leukemia/lymphoma
    Precursor T-lymphoblastic leukemia/lymphoma

Mature B-cell neoplasms

    Chronic lymphocytic leukemia/small lymphocytic lymphoma
    B-cell prolymphocytic leukemia
    Lymphoplasmacytic lymphoma
    Splenic marginal zone lymphoma
    Hairy cell leukemia
    Splenic B-cell lymphoma, unclassifiable
    Plasma cell neoplasms
    Extranodal marginal zone lymphoma
    Nodal marginal zone lymphoma
    Follicular lymphoma
    Primary cutaneous follicle center lymphoma
    Mantle cell lymphoma
    Diffuse large B-cell lymphoma (DLBCL)   T-cell/histiocyte-rich large B-cell lymphoma
                                                    Primary DLBCL of the central nervous system
                                                    Primary cutaneous DLBCL, leg type
                                                    EBV-positive DLBCL of the elderly
    DLBCL associated with chronic inflammation
    Lymphomatoid granulomatosis
    Primary mediastinal large B-cell lymphoma
    Intravascular large B-cell lymphoma
    ALK-positive large B-cell lymphoma
    Plasmablastic lymphoma
    Burkitt's lymphoma (BL)
    B-cell lymphoma, unclassifiable, with features intermediate between
        DLBCL and BL
    B-cell lymphoma, unclassifiable, with features intermediate between
        DLBCL and Hodgkin lymphoma

Mature T-cell neoplasms

    T-cell prolymphocytic leukemia
    T-cell large granular lymphocytic leukemia
    Adult T-cell leukemia/lymphoma
    Extranodal NK/T-cell lymphoma, nasal type
    Enteropathy-type T-cell lymphoma
    Hepatosplenic T-cell lymphoma
    Subcutaneous panniculitis-like T-cell lymphoma
    Mycosis fungoides
    Sézary syndrome
    Primary cutaneous CD30+ T-cell lymphoproliferative disorders
    Primary cutaneous peripheral T-cell lymphomas, rare subtypes
    Peripheral T-cell lymphoma, not otherwise specified
    Angioimmunoblastic T-cell lymphoma
    Anaplastic large-cell lymphoma, ALK+
    Anaplastic large-cell lymphoma, ALK-

MALT, mucosal-associated lymphoid tissue; ALK, anaplastic lymphoma kinase; HHV8, human herpes virus-8; NK, natural killer; EBV, Epstein–Barr virus; HIV, human immunodeficiency virus.

and the IgH gene. Less commonly, chromosomal translocations produce fusion genes that encode chimeric oncogenic proteins. Examples of this include the (2;5)(p23;q35) translocation involving the *ALK* (anaplastic lymphoma kinase) and *NPM1* genes in anaplastic large-cell lymphoma (ALCL) and the t(11;18)(q21;q21) translocation involving the *API2* and *MLT* genes in MZL lymphoma. These translocations and rearrangements can be detected by polymerase chain reaction (PCR) using probes that span the chromosomal breakpoints, reverse transcriptase polymerase chain reaction (RT-PCR) to detect the RNA product of the fusion gene, or fluorescence *in situ* hybridization (FISH) using probes to specific chromosomal segments. In cases where the translocation results in expression of a protein or portion of a protein that is never expressed in normal lymphocytes (e.g., ALK kinase), immunohistochemistry can be used to detect the protein.

Indolent lymphomas

The indolent NHLs are generally associated with survival measured in years, even if left untreated, but are typically incurable with conventional treatment. Indolent lymphomas represent 35–40% of the NHLs diagnosed in western countries. The most common subtypes are FL, small lymphocytic lymphoma, and MZL, comprising 22%, 6%, and 5% of all NHLs, respectively. In comparison, lymphoplasmacytic lymphoma, mycosis fungoides/Sézary syndrome, and splenic MZL are rare diseases, comprising 1% or less of all NHLs.

FL is the most indolent NHL and morphologically recapitulates normal germinal centers of secondary lymphoid follicles (Figure 1). The WHO classification includes three grades based on the number of large cells per high power field: grade 1 (0–5) (Figure 2), grade 2,[6–15] and grade 3 (>15). Grade 3 is subdivided into grade 3A, in which centrocytes predominate, and grade 3B, in which there are sheets of centroblasts. Grade 1 and 2 and many cases of grade 3A FLs are approached similarly. FL grade 3B is an aggressive disease and is grouped with DLBCL.

FL and normal follicular center B cells express cell surface antigens including monoclonal immunoglobulin and the B-cell antigens CD19, CD20, CD10, and CD79a, but lack CD5. Cytoplasmic bcl-2 protein is overexpressed in essentially all cases of grade 1–2 disease, whereas nuclear bcl-6 is expressed by at least some of the neoplastic cells. The most common cytogenetic abnormality in FL is t(14;18) that leads to overexpression of the antiapoptotic protein bcl-2 in over 85% of cases (*see **Chapter 8***). Recent sequencing studies

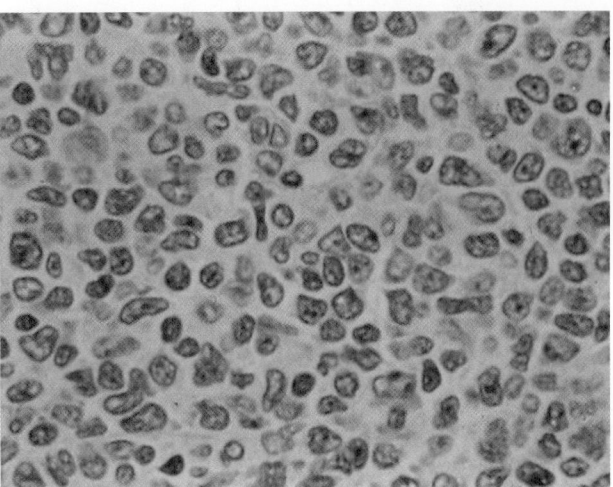

Figure 2 Follicular lymphoma grade I (high power).

have found that the most common mutations in FL (90% of tumors) involve MLL2, a gene encoding a histone H3 methylase. Other less common recurrent mutations involve other genes involving epigenetic modifying genes, such as EZH2, CREBBP, and EP300.[23,24]

FL accounts for about 22% of NHL.[25] Uncommon before the fourth decade, the median age at diagnosis is 60 years. FL is less common in Asians and blacks. Patients usually present with painless peripheral adenopathy, which are often longstanding and may wax and wane. Hilar and mediastinal nodes are often involved, but large mediastinal masses are rare. Patients may present with asymptomatic large abdominal masses. Staging studies usually demonstrates widely disseminated disease with involvement of spleen (40%), liver (50%), and bone marrow (70%). Marrow involvement in FL reveals a unique pattern of paratrabecular infiltration. Few patients present with extranodal extramedullary disease, and only 20% present with B symptoms or lactate dehydrogenase (LDH) elevation. Intestinal-only presentation may occur and has a favorable prognosis.[26] CNS involvement is uncommon although peripheral nerve compression and epidural tumor masses causing cord compression may develop.

FL grade 3 was previously called follicular large-cell lymphoma. BCL6 rearrangements are present in a high fraction of grade 3B cases. Most studies have included both FL grades 3A and 3B, which affects the interpretation of the outcomes. Clinically grade 3B more closely approximates DLBCL.[22,27] In contrast many patients with FL grade 3A have a more indolent disease.

The course of FL is quite variable. Some patients can be observed with waxing and waning disease for 5 years or more without the need for therapy.[28] Others present with more disseminated disease and rapid growth and require treatment due to organ enlargement, lymphatic obstruction, or organ obstruction.

Histologic transformation to aggressive lymphoma, usually DLBCL, occurs in up to 60%, approximately 2–3% per year, of patients with FL and is characterized by rapid progression of lymphadenopathy, extranodal disease, B symptoms, elevated LDH, and often a poor prognosis.[29,30]

Small lymphocytic lymphoma

Small lymphocytic lymphoma and B-cell chronic lymphocytic leukemia are viewed as the same entity by the WHO classification. Although the major population of cells resembles small normal lymphocytes, larger cells resembling those seen in prolymphocytic leukemia are seen in the nodal tissue in areas known as

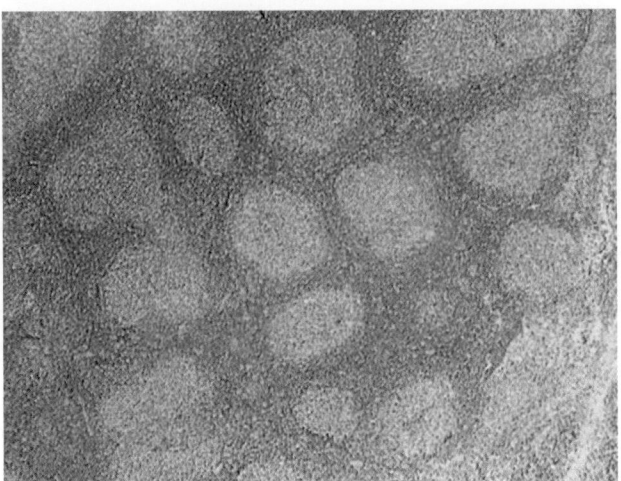

Figure 1 Follicular lymphoma grade I (low power).

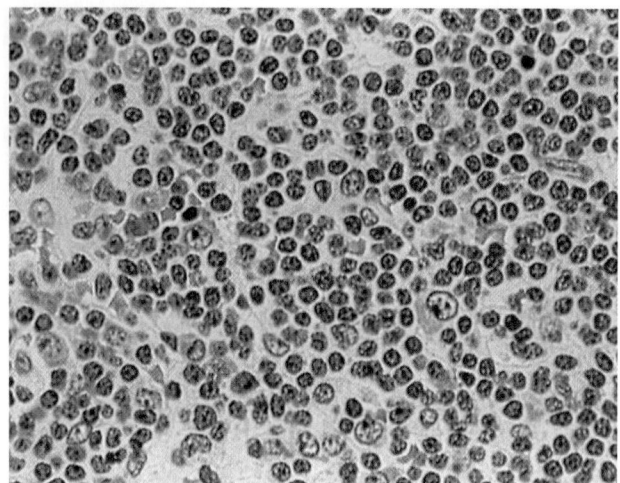

Figure 3 Small lymphocytic lymphoma.

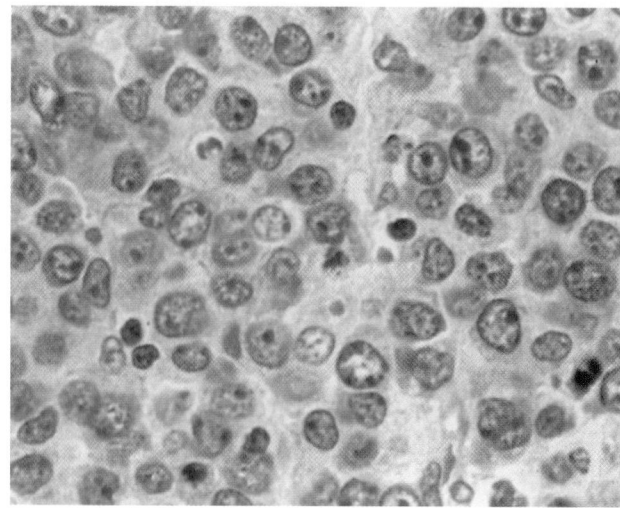

Figure 4 Diffuse large B-cell lymphoma.

proliferation centers (Figure 3 and Figures 2, 3 of *Chapter 116*). The small lymphocytic lymphomas are phenotypically identical to B-cell chronic lymphocytic leukemias but have fewer than 5000 circulating malignant B cells. They express HLA-DR, B-cell antigens CD19, CD20, CD23, weak surface immunoglobulin, and CD5. Cytogenetic abnormalities include trisomy 12 present in about 40% of cases, 13q in 45–55%, 11q abnormalities in 17–20%, and 17p abnormalities in 7–10% of cases. Cases with 13q deletions have the most favorable prognosis, whereas those with 11q or 17p abnormalities have an unfavorable prognosis.[31]

Recent studies suggest that 30–50% of these diseases have non-mutated immunoglobulin variable region genes and correspond to naïve B cells. These cases often express CD38 and the tyrosine kinase ZAP-70 and have a worse prognosis.[32] The remaining 50–70% of cases have mutated immunoglobulin variable region genes, are derived from germinal center or postgerminal center B cells,[33] and have a favorable prognosis.[34] Deep sequencing studies of chronic lymphocytic leukemia have revealed a number of recurrent mutations, including NOTCH1, MYD88, and SF3B1 genes.[35]

Small lymphocytic lymphomas makes up about 6% of all NHLs.[25] The clinical presentation is similar to FL. Unlike B-cell chronic lymphocytic leukemia, the peripheral blood may be normal or reveal only a mild lymphocytosis although the bone marrow is positive in 70–90% of cases. A serum paraprotein is found in about 20% of cases and hypogammaglobulinemia is present in about 40%. Small lymphocytic lymphomas and B-cell chronic lymphocytic leukemia can convert to DLBCL or less commonly HL (Richter syndrome, Figure 4).[36]

Lymphoplasmacytic lymphoma
Lymphoplasmacytic lymphoma is an indolent lymphoma composed of diffuse proliferation of small lymphocytes with evidence of maturation to plasma cells.[37] Evidence of immunoglobulin is seen in these cells by special stains or inclusions. These tumors express B-cell antigens, CD19 and CD20, and surface immunoglobulin M isotype, and in general do not express CD5, CD10, or CD23. Deletions of 6q21 have been identified in 40–60% of patients with lymphoplasmacytic lymphoma and the syndrome associated with this is known as Waldenström's macroglobulinemia. Activating mutations in MYD88, a protein involved in signaling pathways downstream of the Ig receptor, are present in close to 100% of cases.[38]

Lymphoplasmacytic lymphoma represents about 1% of all NHLs. Clinically, this disease is similar to small lymphocytic lymphomas. The median age is early 60s, and virtually all patients have stage IV disease by virtue of bone marrow involvement, and lymph nodes and spleen are commonly involved. B symptoms and elevated serum LDH are rare. A serum M component is common. As with B-CLL, the paraprotein may have autoantibody or cryoglobulin activity. However, most cases with mixed cryoglobulinemia have been shown to be related to concurrent hepatitis C virus (HCV) infection[39] and may respond to therapy directed at hepatitis C. In the WHO clinical study, 5-year overall survival (OS) (58%) and failure-free survival (25%) were identical to that of small lymphocytic lymphomas.

Marginal zone lymphomas
MZLs are a group of distinct entities including nodal MZL; extra-nodal MZL also known as the lymphomas of mucosal-associated lymphoid tissues (MALTs); and the splenic MZL.[40,41] In the nodal MZL, the tumor cells cytologically resemble "normal" monocytoid B cells and often involve lymph node sinuses. Phenotypically, tumor cells express surface immunoglobulin M and B-cell antigens (CD19, CD20). Similar to other indolent lymphomas, MZL can transform into a higher grade lymphoma. The nodal MZLs constitute 1% of all NHLs. Over 70% of patients present with stage III/IV disease and the majority are asymptomatic. Bone marrow involvement is less common than in most indolent lymphomas. The 5-year survival for patients with nodal MZL is 55–79%.

The extranodal MZL tumor cells resemble monocytoid B cells, express CD19, CD20, and surface immunoglobulin M, and are thought to arise from memory B cells. Lymphoepithelial lesions may be seen associated with centrocytes. The disease does not form follicles; rather the malignant cells surround reactive follicles. When extranodal MZL spreads to lymph nodes, the neoplastic cells involve the marginal zones. The most common cytogenetic abnormality is trisomy 3, occurring in up to 60% of cases (particularly the gastric extranodal MZL), and t(11;18), occurring in 25–40% of cases.[42]

Extranodal MZLs constitute about 5% of all NHLs and almost 50% of all gastric lymphomas. B symptoms are uncommon and most patients present with stage I or II disease. There is no age predilection. The gastrointestinal tract (most commonly stomach), lung, dura, lacrimal and salivary glands, skin, thyroid, and breast may be involved. MZL is associated with autoimmune diseases and infections with *H. pylori, B. burgdorferi, C. psittaci, C. jejuni,* and HCV.[43-46] Fewer than 25% of cases have lymph node or bone marrow involvement. Patients can present with peptic ulcer disease, abdominal pain, and sicca syndrome, or a mass at the site of involvement. These lymphomas can disseminate to other MALT sites or bone marrow in about 30% of cases, typically later in the course of the disease. This is more commonly seen in nongastric MZLs.[47] Complete remission rates are high, and OS up to 80% at 10 or more years.[48] Like all indolent NHLs, these can transform to DLBCL.

Splenic MZL constitutes <2% of all NHLs, with a median age of 65, and is uncommon before age 50.[25] Histologically, there is expansion of marginal zones in the spleen. Bone marrow and peripheral blood involvement (referred to as splenic lymphoma with villous or nonvillous lymphocytes) can also be present. In splenic MZL, trisomy 3 is present in 39% of cases. The survival of patients is in excess of 70% at 10 years. Sequencing studies demonstrate recurrent somatic mutations in genes involved in the NOTCH, NF-κB, and B-cell receptor pathways, as well as mutations in TP53.[49]

Aggressive lymphomas

Mantle cell lymphoma

MCL is generally an aggressive disease.[50,51] The neoplastic cells are counterparts of naive "mantle zone" B cells and are medium sized with irregular nuclei. The disease may have either diffuse architecture or a vaguely nodular appearance. Some cases of MCL have a predominance of "blastoid" cells with a high mitotic rate. The cells express B-cell antigens, surface immunoglobulin M with or without immunoglobulin D, CD5, and CD43, but lack CD10 and CD23, respectively, and overexpression of cyclin D1. Approximately 70% of MCLs have t(11;14)(q13;q32) that creates rearrangements of the *bcl-1* (cyclin D1) gene. Eight percent of MCL cases are cyclin D1-negative and overexpress cyclin D2 and 4 or cyclin D3, without chromosomal rearrangements[52] and are clinically similar to cyclin D1-positive cases.[53] Deep sequencing[54] has identified NOTCH1 mutations in a minority of cases, which may be associated with poor prognosis. SOX11 overexpression is also associated with a worse prognosis.[52,55]

MCL constitutes about 7% of all NHLs. About 75% of patients are males, with median age of 63. Approximately 70% of patients have stage IV disease, and B symptoms are observed in approximately one-third of patients. Typical sites of involvement are lymph nodes, spleen, liver, Waldeyer's ring, and bone marrow. Peripheral blood involvement is present in 25–50% of patients at presentation. MCL can involve any region of the gastrointestinal tract, occasionally presenting as multiple intestinal polyposis. The median survival of patients with MCL is 3–6 years and patients with the blastic variant at diagnosis have a median survival of 18 months. Blastic transformation occurs in 35% of patients, with a risk of 42% at 4 years; the median survival is 3.8 months.[56] Mutations and deletions of p53 are also associated with a worse prognosis.[57]

Diffuse large B-cell lymphoma

DLBCL consists of a diffuse proliferation of large cells with a high mitotic rate. The cells have a moderate amount of cytoplasm with either cleaved or noncleaved nuclei often with multiple nucleoli, although there can be great variability in the morphology (Figure 4). DLBCL represents many distinct disease entities.[22] (Table 2) Gene expression profiling has been applied to DLBCL.[58-61] These studies subdivided DLBCL into distinct genetic entities. DLBCLs

correspond to germinal center B cells or activated B cells. The tumor cells generally express B-cell antigens (CD19 and CD20), monoclonal surface immunoglobulin M, and occasionally other heavy chain isotypes. CD5-positive cases are uncommon and may have a worse prognosis.[62] CD10 and bcl-6 support a germinal center origin, whereas expression of MUM1 supports a nongerminal center origin. Approximately 70% express bcl-6 protein, consistent with a germinal center origin.[63]

Several chromosomal abnormalities have been observed in DLBCL. Bcl-6 is associated with chromosomal rearrangements involving 3q27.[64] Rearrangements of the gene occurs in 20–40% of diffuse aggressive lymphomas. t(14;18) has been observed in approximately 30% of patients with DLBCL. Some of these cases may represent histologic transformations of prior FL. By gene expression profile (GEP), the germinal center B-cell (GCB) type is often associated with the t(14;18) and amplifications of the *REL* oncogene on chromosome 2. In contrast, the activated B-cell (ABC) type is associated with loss of 6q21, trisomy 3, gains of 3q and 18q21–22, and mutations of *EZH2*.[65,66] ABC cases also have high-level activation of NF-κB.[67] MYC is rearranged in 10% of DLBCLs, with the partner gene being one of the Ig genes in 60% of cases and alternative genes in 40% of cases. Approximately 20% of MYC-rearranged cases have concurrent BCL2 or BCL6 rearrangements, a combination referred to as "double-hit lymphoma."[68] Amplification and/or overexpression of MYC independent of rearrangements or amplification has also been described and is also associated with a poor prognosis.[69,70]

DLBCL constitutes 31% of all NHLs and is the most common histologic subtype. Patients who are generally middle-aged or older (median age 64 years) present with either nodal enlargement or extranodal disease. DLBCL presents in a localized (stage I or IE) manner approximately 20% of the time and 30–40% of patients will have I or II disease. Stage IV disease is seen in approximately 40% of patients. B symptoms occur in 30% of patients, and unlike most NHLs, LDH is elevated in over half the patients. During the course of the disease, the liver, the kidneys, the lung, the bone, and the peripheral nerves may be involved. Bone marrow involvement is initially found in 10–20% of patients. Extranodal diseases, specifically testicular, bone marrow, paranasal sinus, multiple extranodal sites, and elevated LDH, are other risks for CNS dissemination.[71] Rare cases of DLBCL present with a disseminated intravascular proliferation of large lymphoid cells, involving small blood vessels, without an obvious tumor mass[72-74] most commonly involving the CNS, kidneys, lungs, and skin.

Within the DLBCL group is a distinct clinical entity known as primary mediastinal large B-cell lymphoma (PMLBCL) (7% of all cases of DLBCL).[75] Histologically, the cellular infiltrate is heterogeneous, and sclerosis is frequently present. The immunophenotype includes B-cell antigens (CD19, CD20), but they are often negative for surface and cytoplasmic immunoglobulin. GEP suggests that this is a distinct entity from germinal center or ABC types of DLBCL. Recent studies suggest that the GEP pattern of PMLBCL closely resembles the Reed–Sternberg cells of HL.[76,77] Copy number gains in the region on chromosome 9p containing the genes for JAK2 and programmed cell death ligand 1 and 2 (PDL1 and PDL2) and ligands for the programmed cell death receptor-1 (PD-1), which has a role in suppressing T-cell function, are common.[65] PMLBCL resembles classical HD by GEP.[76] PMLBCL has a female predominance, with a median age of 40. Over 70% of these patients present with stage I/II bulky disease involving the mediastinum. Pleural and pericardial effusions are seen in about one-third of patients. Superior vena cava syndrome is common. Similar to DLBCL, an elevated LDH is present in the majority, whereas bone marrow involvement is infrequent. The prognosis of patients with PMLBCL is similar to patients with DLBCL.

Peripheral T-cell lymphomas

Peripheral T-cell lymphomas (PTCLs) include a large number of entities that constitute 15% of all NHLs in adults.[78] Among these, in decreasing frequency, are PTCL, not otherwise unspecified (NOS); ALCL; angioimmunoblastic T-cell lymphoma (AITL), extranodal NK/T-cell lymphoma, nasal type; and much rarer entities, panniculitis-like T-cell lymphoma, enteropathy-type T-cell lymphoma, and hepatosplenic γ/δ T-cell lymphoma.

PTCLs can be nodal- or extranodal-based diseases. The diffuse cellular infiltrates range from a mixture of small and large cells; infiltrates of pleomorphic cells, often with a background of epithelioid histiocytes, plasma cells, eosinophils, and Reed–Sternberg-like cells; or predominantly large cells. In contrast to B-cell lymphomas, the pattern of expression of T-cell surface antigens is highly variable. The majority express CD2, CD3, and CD4, with a subset of expressing CD8.[79] In most cases, one or more "mature" T-cell antigens, such as CD5 or CD7, are lost. Many cases of PTCL express EBV, especially the extranodal NK/T-cell lymphomas, nasal type.[80] EBV positivity is associated with a poor prognosis.

Abnormal metaphases are seen in 90% of T-cell lymphomas. The most commonly seen translocations in PTCLs are t(7;14), t(11;14), inv(14), and t(14;14). AITL is associated with trisomy 3 and/or 5.[81] These translocations involve genes for the TCR at 14q11, 7q34–35, and 7p15. Young patients with ALCL have t(2;5) and less commonly t(1;2).[82] ALCL in adults generally lack t(2;5). Hepatosplenic γ/δ T-cell lymphomas are associated with isochromosome 7q and trisomy 8.[83]

Patients with PTCL have a similar median age as patients with DLBCL. In contrast, 80% of patients with PTCL have stage III/IV disease and more frequently have B symptoms, hepatosplenomegaly, and extranodal disease, such as the skin. PTCL generally has a worse prognosis than DLBCL.[84,85] A number of uncommon subtypes of PTCL have unique histologic features. AITL, in addition to a pleomorphic heterogeneous cellular infiltrate, displays increased amounts of high endothelial venules, giving a hypervascular appearance. In this subtype, Ig heavy chains may be rearranged in 10% cases, and EBV genomes are detected in most cases and may be in either T or B cells.[86] AITL typically affects older adults who present with the acute onset of generalized lymphadenopathy, hepatosplenomegaly, skin rash, and B symptoms.[86] Immunologic abnormalities are common and include plasmacytosis, polyclonal hypergammaglobulinemia, and a positive Coombs test. The median survival is 30 months. Infection is the most common cause of death, followed by the T-cell lymphoma or development of EBV-positive DLBCL.

ALCL is a T-cell NHL that can present as primary systemic ALCL, ALK-positive; primary systemic ALCL, ALK-negative; and primary cutaneous ALCL. When involving nodes, ALCL characteristically fills the sinusoids of lymph nodes with bizarre large cells. Neoplastic cells derived from patients with ALCL also generally express the phenotype of mature activated T cells (HLA-DR, CD30, CD25). The ALK protein is detected in 40–60% of cases using the ALK1 monoclonal antibody, showing both nuclear and cytoplasmic stainings in cases with the t(2;5).[87] The resulting fusion gene encodes a chimeric NPM-ALK fusion protein with constitutive tyrosine kinase activity. ALK-positive cases are more common in children and younger adults and have a better prognosis than ALK-negative cases.[88]

ALCL constitutes 2% of all NHLs in adults, but is the second most common T-cell lymphoma. The median age of patients with ALCL is 34 with a male predominance. There is a bimodal distribution of this disease, with peaks in childhood, young adults, and late adulthood. In adults, B symptoms, peripheral adenopathy, and retroperitoneal adenopathy are common. Skin is a frequent site of extranodal disease (about 25% of patients), whereas bone marrow involvement is uncommon. An unusual form of ALCL arises within the breast associated with breast implants.[89] The prognosis of adult patients with systemic ALK-positive ALCL is similar to patients with DLBCL.[90] When ALCL, PTCL NOS, and AITL are compared, ALCL has the highest OS, whereas AITL had the lowest.[91]

Gray zone lymphoma

The gray zone lymphomas include B-cell lymphoma unclassifiable with features intermediate between BL and DLBCL (B-UNC/BL/DLBCL) and between DLBCL and cHL (B-UNC/cHL/DLBCL).[22]

In B-cell lymphoma unclassifiable with features intermediate between BL and DLBCL (B-UNC/BL/DLBCL), the neoplastic cells are intermediate to large size, may have a very high Ki67 index, and are CD10+. Cells are more variable in size than BL cells, often BCL2 positive, may be BCL6 negative, and may have a Ki67 index lower than 100%. GEP has shown these to be heterogeneous.[92] Between 30% and 45% cases have chromosomal translocations involving c-myc and bcl-2, known as "double-hit" lymphomas.[68] B-UNC/BL/DLBCL often presents with extranodal disease with high IPI and generally has a poor prognosis. Double-hit lymphomas, with this histology, have a very poor prognosis, with a median OS of 4 months.[93]

B-cell lymphoma, unclassifiable, with features intermediate between DLBCL and classical HL (B-UNC/cHL/DLBCL) has features intermediate between PMBCL and classical HL, or B-UNC/cHL/DLBCL. This rare disease presents commonly in men with a mediastinal mass. Histologically, cells resemble both the Reed–Sternberg cell of classical HL and the large cells of DLBCL or PMLBCL. Fibrous stroma and an inflammatory infiltrate are seen. Malignant cells express CD45, CD20, CD79a, and CD30, but often are CD15(−); other B-cell markers such as PAX5, OCT-2, and BOB1 are often positive. The prognosis of these patients is inferior to both cHL and PMLBCL; the optimal therapy has not been demonstrated.[94]

Highly aggressive lymphomas

Precursor T- or B-lymphoblastic leukemia/lymphoma

LBL and acute lymphoblastic leukemia ALL (*see Chapter 116*) represent two presentations of the same disease with LBL defined as having <25% bone marrow involvement. The neoplastic cells have a high nuclear to cytoplasmic ratio, scant cytoplasm, and nuclei with fine chromatin with multiple small nucleoli and have a high mitotic rate. The nuclei can have folds or convolutions. Typically, nodes involved with LBL are effaced by malignant cells (Figure 5).

The vast majority of LBLs are of T-cell lineage. Several investigators have noted that most T-cell LBLs correspond to stages of thymocyte differentiation (*see Chapter 116*).

Although LBLs represent a major subgroup of childhood NHLs, they are unusual in adults (2% of adult NHLs). Patients are usually males in their 20s or 30s, who present with lymphadenopathy in cervical, supraclavicular, and axillary regions (50%) or with a mediastinal mass (50–75%). This entity may be associated with superior vena cava syndrome, tracheal obstruction, and pericardial effusions. Less commonly, patients present with extranodal disease (e.g., skin, testicular, or bony involvement). More than 80% of patients present with advanced stage disease, almost 50% have B symptoms, and

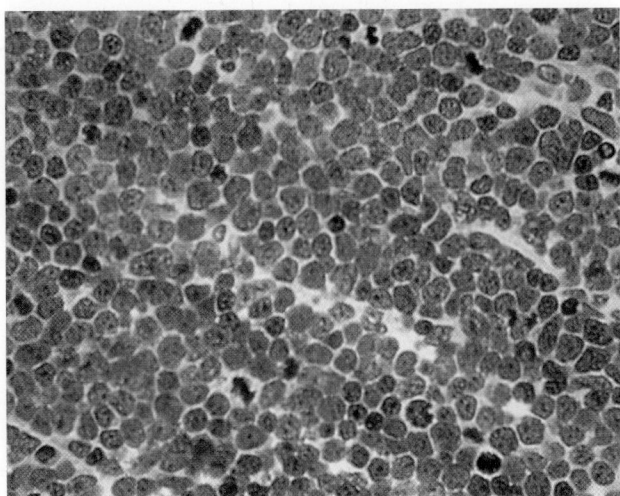

Caribbean basin, Africa, and the southeastern United States. The normal counterparts of the neoplastic cells are activated CD4+ T cells expressing CD2, CD3, CD5, and CD25. The median age of patients is 60.[102] The disease can present as four variants: acute (most common and highly aggressive), lymphomatous, chronic, and smoldering. The median survival of these variants is 6, 10, 24 months, and "not reached," respectively.[103] Patients present with BM and peripheral blood involvement, high white blood cell count, hypercalcemia (owing to PTH-related protein, TGF-β, and RANK ligand), lytic bone lesions, lymphadenopathy, hepatosplenomegaly, skin lesions, and interstitial pulmonary infiltrates.

Differential diagnosis and sites of disease at presentation

More than two-thirds of patients with NHL present with persistent painless peripheral lymphadenopathy. At the time of presentation, differential diagnosis of generalized lymphadenopathy includes infectious etiologies. A firm lymph node larger than 1.5 × 1.5 cm not associated with a documented infection, persisting longer than 4–6 weeks, and progressing should be considered for biopsy. However, lymph nodes in indolent NHLs frequently wax and wane. In teenagers and young adults, infectious mononucleosis and HL should be placed high in the differential diagnosis. Involvement of Waldeyer's ring, epitrochlear, and mesenteric nodes are more frequently observed in patients with NHL than HL. 40% of all patients with NHL present with systemic complaints. B symptoms are more common in patients with aggressive subtypes approaching 50%. Less frequent presenting symptoms, occurring in <20% of patients, include fatigue and malaise.

NHLs also present with thoracic, abdominal, and/or extranodal symptoms. Approximately 20% of patients with NHL present with mediastinal adenopathy. These patients most frequently complain of persistent cough and chest discomfort and rarely display superior vena cava syndrome. Differential diagnosis of mediastinal presentation includes infections, sarcoidosis, HL, and other neoplasms. Involvement of retroperitoneal, mesenteric, and pelvic nodes is common in most subtypes of NHL, and the majority of patients are asymptomatic. Aggressive NHLs can present with primary cutaneous lesions, testicular masses, acute spinal cord compression, solitary bone lesions, and rarely lymphomatous meningitis. Symptoms of primary NHL of the CNS include headache, lethargy, focal neurologic symptoms, seizures, and paralysis.

When NHL presents in an extranodal site, the differential diagnosis is more difficult. NHL uncommonly presents in the lung.[104] Between 25% and 50% of patients with NHLs present with hepatic infiltration, although relatively few have large hepatic masses; these are almost always associated with aggressive lymphoma. Of the advanced stage indolent lymphomas, nearly 75% of patients have microscopic hepatic infiltration at the time of diagnosis. Primary lymphoma of bone occurs in <5% of patients, presenting as a painful bony site, most commonly involving the femur, pelvis, and vertebrae. Approximately 5% of NHLs present as primary gastrointestinal lymphoma. These patients may have hemorrhage, pain, or obstruction as the stomach is most frequently infiltrated followed by the small intestine and the colon, respectively. Most gastrointestinal lymphomas are of the aggressive subtypes, specifically DLBCL, MCL, and the intestinal T-cell lymphoma and may present rarely with bleeding, obstruction, or perforation. The most common site for extranodal MZL is the stomach. A subset of MCLs presents as multiple intestinal polyposis involving any sites in the gastrointestinal tract. Two to fourteen percent of NHL

Figure 5 T-lymphoblastic lymphoma.

the majority have elevated LDH. Although the bone marrow is frequently normal at presentation, virtually all patients develop bone marrow infiltration and a subsequent leukemic phase. Patients with bone marrow involvement have a very high incidence of CNS infiltration. B-cell LBL is a very rare variant, affecting patients with a median age of 39.[95] B-cell LBL presents without a mediastinal mass but instead involves lymph nodes and extranodal sites.

Burkitt's lymphoma
BL cells resemble the small noncleaved cells within normal germinal centers of secondary lymphoid follicles. Because of the high mitotic rate, frequent mitotic figures are seen and, analogous to normal germinal centers, tingible body macrophages are seen, giving the classical "starry sky" appearance. It is generally agreed that the fraction of Ki-67 (proliferating cells) in BL should be 99% or greater.[22]

BL is a tumor of B-lineage derivation identified by the expression of a variety of B-cell-restricted antigens including CD19, CD20, surface immunoglobulin M, CD10, and nuclear bcl-6 protein.[96] The endemic BL is EBV positive, whereas the vast majority of nonendemic BL is EBV negative. BL cells lack bcl-2 protein.

BL involves a translocation of chromosome 8q24 in over 95% of the cases with chromosome 14, 2, or 22.[22] Pathologically identified Burkitt or histologically atypical Burkitt has a GEP that is associated with overexpression of *myc* target genes, differential expression of normal germinal center genes, and decreased expression of MHC class I and NF-κB target genes. These studies will help refine the histologic diagnosis of difficult to classify cases.[92,97,98]

BL, in general, is a pediatric tumor that has three major clinical presentations. The endemic (African) form presents as a jaw or facial bone tumor that spreads to extranodal sites including ovary, testis, kidney, breast, and especially to the bone marrow and meninges. The nonendemic form has an abdominal presentation with massive disease, ascites, renal, testis, and ovarian involvement and, like the endemic form, also spreads to the bone marrow and CNS. Immunodeficiency-related cases more often involve lymph nodes and peripheral blood. BL has a male predominance and is typically seen in patients <35 years of age. These tumors have a high propensity to invade the bone marrow and CNS.

Adult T-cell leukemia/lymphoma
ATLL is a rare disease associated with infection by the HTLV-1 in 100% of cases.[99–101] ATLL is endemic in southern Japan, the

present with renal infiltration, and even less common has localized presentation in the prostate, the testis, or the ovary. The typical histologic subtypes of these sites are DLBCL and BLs. Rare sites of primary lymphoma include the orbit, the heart, the breast, the salivary glands, the thyroid, and the adrenal gland.

Staging and disease detection

The Lugano classification[105] is the currently used staging system. It is derived from the Ann Arbor staging system, which was originally developed for HL in 1971. Table 3 summarizes the essential features of the Ann Arbor system. Because NHLs most frequently disseminate hematogenously, this staging system has proven to be much less useful than for HL. The Lugano modification requires documentation of size of bulk disease.

Systemic "B" symptoms (fever, sweats, and weight loss) are no longer included into the staging system for NHL, because these symptoms are not independent prognostic factors for these patients.

The concept of staging has less impact in NHL than in HL. Multiple studies demonstrate that prognosis is more dependent on lymphoma subtype and clinical parameters than stage at presentation. Staging is undertaken in NHLs to identify the small number of patients who can be treated with local therapy or combined modality treatment and to stratify within subtypes to determine prognosis and assess the impact of treatment.

Diagnosis and initial evaluation

Staging must be undertaken in the context of the histology. After the initial biopsy, blood tests should be obtained, including complete blood count, routine chemistries, renal function, liver function tests, and serum protein electrophoresis to document the presence of circulating monoclonal paraproteins. HIV, hepatitis B (which may reactivate with lymphoma therapy), and hepatitis C serologies should be performed. Serum beta-2 microglobulin can be useful as a surrogate marker of disease burden in indolent NHLs. Serum concentrations of LDH are an important independent predictor of survival. Isolated Waldeyer's ring involvement is associated with intestinal involvement in 20% of cases and endoscopy should be considered. Chest, abdominal, and pelvic computed tomography scan is essential for accurate staging. Unilateral bone marrow biopsies should be performed in most subtypes of lymphoma, as the likelihood of lymphomatous involvement of the marrow is relatively high, especially in most indolent lymphomas. Recently, the role of BM biopsy in DLBCL is being questioned. In a recent analysis of patients with DLBCL undergoing initial staging with PET-CT scanning, the sensitivity and specificity of PET scanning for marrow involvement was 89% and over 99%, respectively. BM biopsy should still be performed in patients with a negative PET scan, but of limited utility in patients with a positive scan showing BM involvement.[106] In patients with aggressive lymphomas with marrow involvement, paranasal sinus involvement, paraspinal masses, testicular, or if clinically indicated, examination of the cerebral spinal fluid (CSF) by lumbar puncture should be performed. Positron emission tomography, PET, using ^{18}F-fluorodeoxyglucose is a highly sensitive and specific scanning modality for detecting NHL in both nodal and extranodal sites. PET scanning is very useful for DLBCL, MCL, and FL and is now recommended in the initial staging of these entities. PET scanning is not as sensitive in SLL and MZL.[107]

The International Harmonization Project has provided consensus recommendations for PET scanning. Among the recommendations are the following: PET should be used for DLBCL and HL; scanning during therapy should still be only part of clinical trials;

Table 3 Revised staging system for primary nodal lymphoma.

Stage	Involvement	Extranodal (E) status
Limited		
I	One node or a group of adjacent nodes	Single extranodal lesions without nodal involvement
II	Two or more nodal groups on the same side of the diaphragm	Stage I or II by nodal extent with limited contiguous extranodal involvement
II bulky*	II as above with "bulky" disease	Not applicable
Advanced		
III	Nodes on both sides of the diaphragm; nodes above the diaphragm with spleen involvement	Not applicable
IV	Additional noncontiguous extralymphatic involvement	Not applicable

*Whether stage II bulky disease is treated as limited or advanced disease may be determined by histology and a number of prognostic factors

and the scan after all therapy is completed can be done at least 3 but preferably 6–8 weeks after chemotherapy and 8–12 weeks after radiation or chemoradiotherapy. There is no evidence that long-term follow-up should include PET scanning.[108] Magnetic resonance imaging is most valuable for evaluation of the brain and spinal cord.

Immunologic and molecular studies

Biologic studies including cell surface markers, cytogenetics, and molecular techniques are used in diagnosis, staging, and minimal disease detection. Monoclonal antibodies directed against cell surface antigens expressed on lymphoid cells and molecular techniques to define immunoglobulin and TCR gene rearrangements are sensitive tools with which to assess tumor cell infiltration. Immunophenotypic and cytogenetic studies can help to determine histologic subtypes of lymphomas. For those NHLs with known chromosomal translocations, it is possible to identify unique chromosomal breakpoints that can be studied with FISH, cytogenetics, and PCR. Studies of minimal disease may provide important prognostic information.

Disease parameters that influence prognosis and assessment of disease response

Prognostic factors in NHL

Aggressive NHLs

Clinical prognostic models have been developed for a number of NHL subtypes. The analysis of a large group (2031 patients) with diffuse aggressive NHLs treated with an anthracycline containing regimen led to the establishment of a prognostic model of predicting outcome known as the International Prognostic Index (IPI) (Table 4).[109] Of a large number of factors examined for all patients, age (≤60 vs >60), serum LDH (≤normal vs >normal), performance status (PS) (0 or 1 vs 2–4), stage (I or II vs III or IV), and extranodal involvement (≤site vs >1 site) were independently prognostic for OS. The 5-year OS rates for patients with scores of 0–1, 2, 3, and 4–5 were 73%, 51%, 43%, and 26%, respectively. The IPI has been adapted following treatment with rituximab and cyclophosphamide, doxorubicin, vincristine, and prednisone (CHOP) therapy for DLBCL. Within that model, the

Table 4 International Prognostic Index (IPI).

International Prognostic Index (IPI)				
Age > 60 years				
LDH > upper limit normal				
ECOG performance status ≥ 2				
Ann Arbor stage III or IV				
Number of extranodal disease sites > 1				
# Factors	Risk group	3-year EFS (%)	3-year PFS (%)	3-year OS (%)
0–1	Low	81	87	91
2	Low-intermediate	69	75	81
3	High-intermediate	53	59	65
4–5	High	50	50	59

Source: Adapted from Ziepert M, Hasenclever D, Kuhnt E, et al. Standard International Prognostic Index remains a valid predictor of outcome for patients with aggressive CD20+ B-cell lymphoma in the rituximab era. *J Clin Oncol* 2010;28:2373.
LDH, lactate dehydrogenase; ECOG, Eastern Cooperative Oncology Group; EFS, event-free survival; PFS, progression-free survival; OS, overall survival.

Table 5 Follicular Lymphoma International Prognostic Index (FLIPI).

Age > 60 years			
LDH > upper limit normal			
Hgb <12 g/dL			
Ann Arbor stage III or IV			
Number of involved nodal areas >4			
# Factors	Risk group	5-year OS (%)	10-year OS (%)
0–1	Low	91	71
2	Intermediate	78	51
3–5	High	52	36

Source: Adapted from Solal-Celigny P, Roy P, Colombat P, et al. Follicular lymphoma international prognostic index. *Blood* 2004;104:1258.
LDH, lactate dehydrogenase; Hgb, hemoglobin; OS, overall survival.

4-year progression-free survival (PFS) is 94%, 80%, and 53% for 0 and 1, 2, and 3 or more risk factors, respectively.[110]

Follicular NHL

A predictive model based on over 4000 patients with FL in the prerituximab era, known as the Follicular Lymphoma International Prognostic Index (FLIPI) score, identified the following prognostic factors: age > 60; stage III/IV; more than four nodal sites; elevated serum LDH concentration; and hemoglobin (Hgb) <12. The 10-year survival rates for patients with 0–1, 2, and 3 or more risk adverse factors averaged 71%, 51%, and 36%, respectively (Table 5).[111] The FLIPI remains clinically relevant with rituximab-based therapy.[112] For other NHLs, prognostic models have been developed from uniformly treated patient populations. The mantle cell lymphoma International Prognostic Index (MIPI) includes age, PS, LDH, and WBC as prognostic factors.[113] The proliferation index alone as well as when incorporated into the MIPI provides additional prognostic utility.[114] Several prognostic models for PTCL NOS have been reported, but generally the IPI provides a reasonable stratification of outcome, with low-risk patients having a 55% 2-year OS and high-risk patients a <15% 2-year OS.[115]

Gene expression profiling as prognostic factors

GEP using DNA microarrays has been used to examine DLBCL to identify prognostic subgroups.[58–60,116] DLBCLs may be subclassified into GCB or ABC types. Patients with GCB DLBCL had significantly better OS than those with the ABC type. On the basis of the findings from gene expression profiling, immunohistochemistry using tissue microarrays has been used for a limited number of gene products as prognostic markers.[116] Germinal center and non-GCB derivation can be determined by expression of CD10 and bcl-6, and MUM1. Using tissue microarrays, 42% of DLBCLs are considered GCB derivation and 58% are non-GCB derivation.

In FL, gene expression profiling has shown that genes associated with the nonmalignant cell infiltrate segregate patients into subgroups with favorable and unfavorable prognoses. Immune response 1 signature (gene associated with certain T-cell and macrophage markers) was favorable, whereas immune response 2 signature (genes highly expressed in macrophages) was unfavorable.[117] Gene expression profiling in MCL patients has identified the proliferation signature and high expression of cyclin D1 as being associated with an unfavorable prognosis.[114]

Therapeutic approaches according to WHO classification

Indolent lymphomas

Therapy of early stage indolent lymphoma

Ten to twenty percent of patients with indolent lymphoma present with stage I/II disease, and patients with all histologic subtypes, should be considered for local radiotherapy (RT) treatment with curative intent. In a study of 177 patients from Stanford (44% stage I and 56% had stage II), the majority of whom were treated with involved or extended field RT[118] experienced OS rates at 10, 15, and 20 years of 64%, 44%, and 35%, respectively. The relapse-free survival rates at 10, 15, and 20 years were 44%, 40%, and 37%, respectively. In a recent report of over 6000 patients with stage I or stage II FL, 34% of whom were initially treated with RT, patients who received initial RT had higher rates of disease-specific survival at 5 (90% vs 81%), 10 (79% vs 66%), 15 (68% vs 57%), and 20 (63% vs 51%) years.[119] A recent retrospective analysis suggested an improved PFS outcome with chemoimmunotherapy or systemic therapy plus RT as compared to RT alone, with no impact on OS.[120] In a small, retrospective study, observation, that is, no immediate treatment, has been reported as an alternative, especially for stage II patients,[121] with a median OS of 19 years. At a median follow-up of 7 years, 63% of patients had not required treatment.

The extranodal MZLs often present with localized disease involving the gastrointestinal tract, salivary glands, thyroid, orbit, conjunctiva, breast, and lung. In patients with *H. pylori*-associated gastric MZL, therapy with antibiotics and a proton pump inhibitor induces disease regression in over 80% of patients with good long-term disease control and OS in a subset.[122–124] The presence of bcl-10 nuclear expression and/or t(11;18) may be useful to prospectively identify those patients with gastric MZL lymphomas who do not benefit from anti-*H. pylori* treatment.[125] Antibiotic therapy (doxycycline) against *Chlamydophila* has been reported with variable results in ocular MZLs.[8] Single-agent rituximab has a overall response rates (RRs) of 87% for treatment naive patients.[130]

For patients with localized disease who progress after antibiotic therapy or are *H. pylori* negative, involved-field RT with or without surgical resection has a 10-year disease-free survival of over 90%.[126,127] For other sites of extranodal MZL, surgery remains a highly effective approach, often with adjuvant involved-field RT, as these diseases tend to remain localized for long periods of time before systemic spread. In a retrospective study of patients with stage IE or IIE MZL, most were treated with involved-field radiation therapy alone.[128] The 5-year disease-free and OS for the entire group was 76% and 96%, respectively. Patients with gastric and thyroid disease had 5-year disease-free survival of 93%, whereas disease-free survival for other sites of involvement was 69% ($p = 0.006$). For MZL, the RR for chemotherapy with alkylating agents, fludarabine or rituximab alone, is high.[129,130]

Treatment of advanced stage indolent NHL

Asymptomatic patients with low-volume disease can be monitored closely without active therapy. The long natural history of indolent NHLs and the lack of symptoms in some patients at diagnosis have fostered close observation as the initial approach to many of these patients. In studies from Stanford and the British National Lymphoma Investigation[131] where asymptomatic patients were randomized either to initial therapy or to deferred treatment until the time of symptoms (usually progressive bulky disease), there was no difference in the actuarial survival between the two groups. In the Stanford study, the median time until therapy was needed was 3 years.[132] "Watchful waiting" versus observation has been studied in the rituximab era. A prospective study compared observation to rituximab alone or rituximab followed by maintenance in previously untreated FL. The median time to next treatment was 34 months in the watch-and-wait patient but was not reached in the rituximab treatment arm. The 3-year PFS was 33%, 80%, and 90% for patients who underwent observation, rituximab alone, and rituximab with maintenance respectively, with 95% OS in all three groups.[133]

The treatment paradigm for treating advanced stage FL has changed with the use of rituximab. Phase III randomized trials have demonstrated a significant improvement in outcome by combining chemotherapy regimens with rituximab.[134–138] All of these studies demonstrated improved RRs, and time to progression in the rituximab containing arms, and improvement in OS.

Other regimens have been compared to rituximab plus cyclophosphamide, doxorubicin, vincristine, and prednisone (R-CHOP) in an effort to improve efficacy and reduce toxicity. Bendamustine-R (BR) was compared to R-CHOP is a phase III randomized trial that included predominantly FL and also mantle cell and MZLs.[139] The median PFS was superior with BR (69.5 months vs 31.2 months) at 45 months without difference in OS. In addition, BR had less toxicity, including lower rates of grade 3/4 neutropenia and leukopenia. Phase II trials employed rituximab alone as initial therapy in patients with indolent lymphoma with overall RRs of 54–73%.[140–142] At a median follow-up of 30 months, median PFS was 34 months in one of the trials. Moreover, extended treatment with rituximab increased event-free survival (EFS) twofold compared to observation.[142] For patients who were treatment naive, 45% were progression free at 8 years with abbreviated maintenance rituximab.[143] Radioimmunotherapy was studied in previously untreated patients with FL. [90]Yttrium-ibritumomab-tiuxetan and 131I tositumomab (no longer available) yield excellent results in phase II studies, but the benefit compared to rituximab has not been evaluated.[144,145] In a randomized trial comparing R-CHOP to CHOP followed by ^{131}I tositumomab, no differences in PFS was seen between the two arms.[146]

Maintenance rituximab after chemoimmunotherapy has been studied in a large phase III trial.[147] In the primary rituximab and maintenance (PRIMA) trial, maintenance rituximab as compared to observation improved PFS, but to date no impact of OS was seen with maintenance in previously untreated FL patients who responded to chemoimmunotherapy [R-CVP, R-CHOP or fluadarabine, cyclophosphamide, mitoxantrone, and rituximab (FCM-R)]

Treatment for other indolent lymphomas

Patients with other indolent NHLs besides FL, including nodal and extranodal MZL, are generally treated similarly to FL. Patients with SLL are treated with chemoimmunotherapy regimens used for chronic lymphocytic leukemia (see **Chapter 117**). In the R-CHOP versus BR study, no difference in PFS was seen for MZLs. For lymphoplasmacytic lymphomas, regimens include dexamethasone, rituximab, cyclophosphamide,[148] BR, bortezomib, and rituximab with or without dexamethasone.[149] For dexamethasone, rituximab, and cyclophosphamide, the overall and complete RRs were 83 and 7%, respectively, and 2-year overall and PFS rates 81% and 67%, respectively. Patients with splenic MZL often benefit from splenectomy with excellent symptom management and improvement in cytopenias.[150] Single-agent rituximab and chemoimmunotherapy have high RRs and 5-year PFS over 90%.[130]

High-dose therapy and autologous stem cell transplantation (ASCT) have been used in first remission for patients with FL[151–156] with an increased risk of second malignancies including MDS/AML and solid tumors. The majority of the randomized trials preceded use of rituximab and reported a significant improvement in PFS, but no OS benefit.[157]

Following relapse, indolent lymphomas continue to be sensitive to single agents including rituximab alone and combination chemotherapy; but the median relapse-free survival with chemoimmunotherapy progressively decreases with each subsequent relapse. A recent update of single-agent rituximab therapy in patients with relapsed FL is from the randomized SAKK trial. Martinelli et al.[143] found that 35% of responders remain in remission at 8 years. However, it remains uncertain as to whether the response data to single-agent rituximab is as high or durable as in patients who received chemotherapy without rituximab as induction therapy.

A phase II trial of rituximab in patients with relapsed indolent NHL[158] yielded overall RR of 40%, with 11% complete remissions and estimated median time to progression of 18 months. Rituximab has been combined with other agents with reasonable results in patients with relapsed/resistant disease. A phase III study in relapsed FL patients who had not previously received an anthracycline or rituximab[159] randomly assigned patients to CHOP versus R-CHOP. Responding patients underwent a second randomization to maintenance rituximab (375 mg/m^2 IV once every 3 months) for a maximum of 2 years or observation. The overall (85% vs 72%) and complete (30% vs 16%) remission rates as well as PFS (33 months vs 20 months) were significantly higher in the R-CHOP. The median PFS from the time of second randomization was longer for those receiving rituximab maintenance (52 months vs 15 months), regardless of induction regimen. Moreover, maintenance rituximab, as compared with observation, also significantly improved 3-year OS (85% vs 77%). A number of phase II trials of other agents plus rituximab associated with high RRs included BR with 90% RR and median PFS of 2 years.[160,161]

Radioimmunoconjugates have been FDA-approved therapies for patients with relapsed follicular NHL. 90-yttrium ibritumomab has an 82% RR with 26% complete responses (CRs) and median duration of response >12 months in patients with relapsed disease.[162] In a phase III study of 143 patients with relapsed or refractory low-grade, follicular, or transformed NHL, the overall RRs to rituximab or the rituximab 90-yttrium ibritumomab tiuxetan combination were 56% and 80%, respectively.[163] As in the upfront setting, the role for radioimmunotherapy in the treatment paradigm of indolent lymphoma remains uncertain. The PI3K delta isoform-specific inhibitor idelalisib was recently approved for used in relapsed follicular and small lymphocytic lymphoma with overall RRs of 57% and median duration of response of 12.5 months.[164]

FL is responsive to low-dose radiation therapy (e.g., total dose of 4 Gy, given as 2 consecutive daily 2 Gy fractions) and can be used for the palliation of patients for an isolated disease site, with CR rates of 57% and overall RR of 82% with respectable durability.[165]

Autologous stem cell transplantation for relapsed indolent NHL

Long-term follow-up of phase II studies suggest that a subset of patients with relapsed FL, with chemosensitive disease, who undergo high-dose therapy and ASCT are long-term survivors with disease-free survival of 48% at 12 years.[71,144,166] A randomized trial compared conventional chemotherapy to ASCT with purged or unpurged bone marrow, referred to as the European CUP trial.[167] In this study, 89 patients with relapsed or progressive FL received three cycles of CHOP. Those patients who achieved a CR or PR, and had <20% bone marrow involvement with FL, were randomized to three further cycles of CHOP chemotherapy or to high-dose therapy and autologous stem cell support with anti-B-cell antibody purging or high-dose therapy and autologous stem cell support without purging. At a median follow-up of 69 months, the overall 5-year survival for all registered patients was 50%, but the median survival had not yet been reached for the subset of patients treated with high-dose therapy and ASCT (either purged or unpurged). Both PFS and OS favored the transplantation arms, but there was no difference between those patients receiving a purged autograft and those receiving an unmanipulated graft.

Allogeneic stem cell transplantation in relapsed FL

Both myeloablative and reduced intensity conditioning (RIC) approaches have been employed for relapsed FL patients. Myeloablative conditioning has a treatment-related mortality of up to 40%; however, the relapse rate is <20%.[168] In contrast, RIC alloSCT has lower treatment-related mortality,[169–171] but some reports suggest that the relapse rate may be higher than conventional myeloablative conditioning. The role of alloSCT versus ASCT for FL remains uncertain. A recent NCCN database retrospective analysis found significantly higher 3-year OS for ASCT versus alloSCT (87% vs 61%).[172] For selected patients, alloSCT remains a potentially curative option for relapsed FL.

Histologic transformation

The prognosis for patients following histologic transformation of indolent NHL is generally poor, particularly in previously treated patients.[173] The median survival of a large series of patients with FL undergoing histologic conversion was 11 months.[174] In a report from Stanford, the median survival for the entire group of patients was only 22 months, except for patients who achieved a CR with treatment who had an actuarial survival of 75% at 5 years.[175] There have been several reports of ASCT in patients after histologic transformation for FL. The DFS is about 40–50%, and patients can relapse with both DLBCL and FL.[176–179] Aggressive therapy with ASCT is a reasonable treatment option for selected patients who have chemosensitive disease.

Aggressive lymphomas

The aggressive lymphomas within the WHO classification include diffuse large B cell, the PTCLs (nonspecified and the specific subtypes), ALCL, and MCL (Table 2).

Therapy of early stage aggressive lymphoma

Fewer than 20% of patients with diffuse large-cell lymphoma have truly localized disease. The recommended treatment for localized disease outside of clinical trials is abbreviated chemotherapy plus involved-field RT, or combination chemotherapy alone. A SWOG randomized trial of patients with localized diffuse aggressive lymphoma compared eight cycles of CHOP to three cycles of CHOP plus involved-field RT. Patients treated with three cycles of CHOP plus RT had a significantly better 5-year PFS and OS than patients treated with eight cycles of CHOP (77% vs 64% for PFS, 82% vs 72% for OS).[180] The benefit of attenuated chemotherapy was largely found in patients over the age of 60. Another randomized trial studied eight courses of CHOP with or without involved-field RT in patients with previously untreated bulky or extranodal stage I or II diffuse aggressive NHL. The disease-free survival was greater for CR patients who received RT (73% vs 56%), although 10-year OS was similar in the two treatment arms (68% vs 65%).[181] The role of radiation therapy remains uncertain in some patients with stage I or II disease. In patients aged 60 or less with low-risk disease, an aggressive regimen (ACVBP) was superior to CHOP plus RT.[182] Similarly, in patients over age 60, the addition of radiation therapy did not improve disease-free or OS for patients who received four cycles of CHOP alone.[183] These studies raise the question of the necessity of RT for patients with early stage disease. A phase II trial of patients with early stage DLBCL with at least one risk factor (age >60; increased serum LDH; stage II disease; or performance status ≥1) utilized three cycles of R-CHOP followed by involved-field radiation therapy.[184] The PFS and OS at 2 and 4 years were 93% and 88%, and 95% and 92%, respectively. A phase III study in patients age 60 or under with IPI score or 0 or 1 compared six cycles of CHOP to R-CHOP, with all patients with bulky disease (masses >7.5 cm) or extranodal sites receiving involved-field radiation. For the patients with IPI score of 0, with no bulk, and includes early stage patients, the 5-year EFS was approximately 90% with R-CHOP alone, suggesting chemoimmunotherapy alone is an option for early stage disease. However, bulky disease, defined as masses >7.5 cm, was associated with inferior outcome. In the MiNT trial of CHOP versus R-CHOP, all patients (IPI 0 or IPI 1) with masses >7.5 cm received 30–40 Gy of involved-field radiation to those sites. Those patients with IPI of 0 and bulk disease had a 10–15% lower PFS than patients without bulk.[185] In the UNFOLDER trial of a similar patient population, early data suggests a benefit for RT after chemotherapy. Presently the most appropriate management of patients with early-stage DLBCL with bulky disease remains controversial.

PMLBCL patients often present with early stage disease, and historically patients have received combined modality therapy. In the MInT trial, 87 patients with PMLBCL[186] received six cycles of R-CHOP, 75% of whom also received radiation therapy; only 7% of patients who received radiation subsequently progressed or relapsed. A recent study of 51 patients treated with dose adjusted EPOCH plus rituximab (DA-EPOCH-R), and no RT, reported an outstanding PFS (93%) and OS (100%).[187] In terms of the needs for radiation, a recent study reported that a negative PET-CT scan at the end of therapy was associated with an excellent outcome in the absence of radiation.[188]

Extranodal NK/T-cell lymphomas present with early stage disease in 97% of cases. The 5-year OS and PFS for patients with stage IE disease were 78% and 63%, respectively, and for stage IIE, the OS and PFS were 46% and 40%, respectively, with no difference between combined modality and RT alone.[189] For patients with stage IE/IIE, early use of RT (50–55 Gy) is critical, whereas chemotherapy initially followed by RT yields inferior results. More recent studies suggest that combined modality treatment may yield more favorable results. Phase II trials of concurrent radiation therapy and weekly cisplatin followed by etoposide, ifosfamide, cisplatin, and dexamethasone reported overall RR of 83% and 3-year PFS and OS of 85 and 86%, respectively.[190,191]

Therapy of advanced stage aggressive lymphoma

The current recommendation for treatment of advanced stage DLBCL or PTCL, outside a clinical trial, is combination chemotherapy with R-CHOP or CHOP, respectively. Recent clinical trials have evaluated the number of cycles and the interval for those cycles. In patients with DLBCL ages 60–80, the GELA group reported that eight cycles of R-CHOP was superior to CHOP alone in terms of PFS, DFS, and OS.[192,193] In a US Intergroup study of CHOP versus R-CHOP in patients over 60,[194] responding patients were randomly assigned to receive either rituximab maintenance therapy or no maintenance. A beneficial impact of rituximab added to CHOP chemotherapy on event-free and OS was observed; however, no benefit was seen for maintenance rituximab following R-CHOP induction. Similarly, in patients <60, R-CHOP with IPI of 0 and 1, the addition of rituximab to CHOP improved time-to-treatment failure and OS. This benefit was greater in the patients with an IPI of 1.[185]

In the RICOVER trial, in patients over age 60, R-CHOP was superior to CHOP given for six or eight cycles (70% vs 57%), and there was no benefit of eight cycles of R-CHOP over six cycles.[195] In another study, R-CHOP given every 21 days (R-CHOP 21) for eight cycles was compared to six cycles of R-CHOP given every 14 days with no difference in PFS or OS.[196] This supports R-CHOP 21 for six cycles as the standard of care. Alternatives to R-CHOP have been examined in phase III trials. The aggressive regimen R-ACVBP followed by consolidation with methotrexate and leucovorin[197] was compared to R-CHOP plus intrathecal methotrexate in patients under age 60 with IPI score of 1. R-ACVBP plus methotrexate and leucovorin led to higher PFS and OS. The benefit was seen in the non-GCB subgroup of patients.[198]

Testicular DLBCL

Historically, the long-term results of treatment of primary testicular DLBCL are worse than predicted by the IPI.[199,200] Current therapy has been defined by a report of 53 patients with untreated stage I or II primary testicular lymphoma treated with six to eight cycles of R-CHOP 21, four weekly doses of intrathecal methotrexate (12 mg), and radiation therapy to the contralateral testis (30 Gy) for all patients and (30–36 Gy) to regional nodes for patients with stage II disease.[199] With a median follow-up of 65 months, the OS and PFS at 5 years were 85% and 74%, respectively.

Prophylaxis for CNS disease in DLBCL is highly controversial.[201] In the prerituximab era, the risk of CNS involvement was 2.8%, with intraparenchymal and intraspinal disease occurring in 66%, and isolated leptomeningeal disease in 26%.[202] Risk factors include the sites of disease (the testis, the ovary, the bone marrow, the breast, the epidural space, the kidneys, the adrenals, and the paranasal sinuses); high-intermediate or high IPI score; multiple extranodal sites; and "double-hit" cytogenetics. With the significant number of parenchymal relapses, intrathecal chemotherapy alone may be inadequate prophylaxis, making high-dose methotrexate a potentially more effective therapy. However, there is no strong evidence that high-dose methotrexate is superior to intrathecal.

The treatment of the subtype of the new WHO entity B-UNC/BL/DLBCL is uncertain.[203,204] There is retrospective evidence that intensive regimens such as modified Magrath regimen with CODOX-M/IVAC (cyclophosphamide, vincristine, doxorubicin, high-dose methotrexate with ifosfamide, cytarabine, etoposide,

and intrathecal methotrexate), HyperCVAD, and DA-EPOCH-R had better outcomes than R-CHOP (ORR 86% vs 57%, 4-year PFS approximately 50–65% vs 0–30%).[205] Those cases with c-myc translocations are associated with a particularly poor prognosis. Data of MYC translocation-positive DLBCL treated with DA-EPOCH-R on the National Cancer Institute phase II studies is promising.[206] This regimen is currently being explored further in BL and MYC translocation-positive DLBCL in a multicenter trial. The entity B-UNC/BL/DLBCL is heterogeneous, but for double-hit lymphomas, many of which are B-UNC/BL/DLBCL, R-CHOP is insufficient.

For PTCL, similar treatment approaches to DLBCL have been taken for patients with localized and advanced stage disease. When patients are stratified by the IPI, the disease-free survival and OS are generally inferior for patients with PTCL than for patients with DLBCL. There is presently no overwhelming evidence to support superiority of different treatment regimens for PTCL.[207] A retrospective subset analysis of a phase III study in PTCL patients of CHOP versus CHOP with etoposide showed a significant improvement in EFS for PTCL patients younger than age 60 with a normal LDH at diagnosis, but there was no difference in OS.[115] ALCL has the most favorable prognosis of the T-cell lymphomas.[91] The prognosis for patients who express the ALK protein is particularly favorable with 5-year OS of 79%.[88] . The anti-CD30 monoclonal-drug conjugate, brentuximab, is being examined in the initial treatment of ALCL given its strong activity in relapsed CD30+ ALCL.

Autologous stem cell transplantation for aggressive NHL in first remission

Several studies have not shown clear evidence for a survival benefit for high-dose therapy and ASCT in first CR/PR for patients with aggressive NHL.[208,209] A meta-analysis of 3079 patients treated in the prerituximab era on 15 randomized trials with either conventional therapy or ASCT in first CR showed no difference in EFS, OS, or treatment-related mortality.[210]

Given the generally inferior prognosis of patients with PTCL, autologous SCT has been investigated in first remission in several phase II studies with encouraging results.[211,212]

Mantle cell lymphomas (MCL)

With the advent of chemoimmunotherapy, the median survival of patients with MCL is now 3–6 years.[213] R-CHOP has been historically the regimen of choice for MCL. A randomized trial comparing R-CHOP to bendamustine plus rituximab (BR) reported superior PFS with BR with less toxicity (35 months vs 22 months).[139] Another study of R-CHOP versus FCR (fludarabine, cyclophosphamide, rituximab)[214] in patients over age 60 yielded similar CR rates, but R-CHOP had less toxicity; the OS at 4 years was 62% versus 47% in favor of R-CHOP.[214] A second randomization of maintenance with interferon-α or rituximab was given until progression. For the patients who received R-CHOP, a survival benefit from maintenance rituximab was observed (OS rate at 4 years of 87% vs 63%).

Autologous transplant for patients <65, in first CR or PR, has shown improvement in PFS as compared to interferon-α maintenance and a nonstatistically significant improvement in OS.[215] Many phase II studies have intensified the induction therapy before ASCT. Incorporation of high-dose cytarabine[216] has given excellent results, with median OS and response duration longer than 10 years and a median EFS of 7.4 years.

HyperCVAD is an intensive regimen, with escalated doses of cyclophosphamide, high-dose methotrexate, and cytarabine. It is an alternative to ASCT for patients in first remission as a way to prolong remissions in MCL. The MD Anderson reported that a median OS was not reached at 8 years, and a median time to failure was 4.6 years.[217] Two multi-institution trials of R-HyperCVAD reported excellent disease control but a significant proportion of patients could not complete the proscribed treatment due to toxicity.[218,219]

The vast majority of patients are with MCL relapse. Three agents are FDA approved for relapsed MCL; bortezomib, lenalidomide, and ibrutinib. Bortezomib has a 29% overall RR (5% CR) with a median duration of 7 months.[220] Lenalidomide, approved for bortezomib failures, has a 26% RR (7% CR) and median duration of response of 17 months.[221] Ibrutinib has a 68% RR (21% CR), with a median duration of 17.5 months.[222] Idelalisib has activity with a 40% RR.[223] ASCT for relapsed MCL patients is of limited benefit.[224] Nonmyeloablative alloSCT can be considered for select relapsed patients. The 3-year PFS and OS are 30% and 40%, respectively.[224]

High-grade lymphomas

Lymphoblastic, Burkitt's lymphomas
The treatment of LBL is detailed in **Chapter 117**.

BL treated with CODOX-M/IVAC, designed for pediatric populations, yields 2-year OS of 82% for low-risk patients and 70% for high-risk patients.[225,226] Similar results have been seen with Hyper-CVAD.[227] A study of DA-EPOCH-R reported excellent results with freedom from progression of 95% and OS of 100%, at a median follow-up of 86 months.[228] There is presently no evidence that first remission autologous transplant is indicated for adult BL.[229]

Adult T-cell leukemia/lymphoma
ATLLs are approached with intensive multiagent chemotherapy regimens.[230] Antiviral therapy with zidovudine and interferon-α should be considered upfront for the smoldering, chronic subtype.[230,231] For the acute leukemia lymphoma type, a phase III randomized trial[232] reported that an intensive regimen (VCAP-AMP-VECP) had a 3-year OS of 24% compared to only 13% with CHOP. With the poor results of chemotherapy, both myeloablative and reduced intensity alloSCT have been applied to ATLL, with limited success.[233,234]

Treatment of recurrent aggressive NHL
The majority of recurrences from chemoimmunotherapy are within the first 2 years after treatment.[235] Following relapse, about 60% of patients' disease remains sensitive to conventional treatment, but <10% of patients with aggressive NHL experience prolonged disease-free survival with second-line treatment regimens. Following relapse, the current curative approach for patients with relapsed NHL involves high-dose therapy and stem cell transplantation.

Conventional salvage therapy
The vast majority of patients with relapsed or refractory DLBCL have limited benefit from conventional salvage regimens with duration of responses and OS of approximately 6 months. Several combination chemotherapy regimens have been compared in randomized trials with equivalent results. Specifically, rituximab plus ifosfamide, carboplatin, and etoposide yield similar results to rituximab plus dexamethasone, cytarabine, and platinum, which is equivalent to rituximab plus gemcitabine, dexamethasone, and platinum.[236–239] The goal is to identify patients with chemosensitive disease who have

the greatest likelihood of benefiting from high-dose therapy and ASCT.

Recurrent PTCL has a very poor prognosis, with a median OS of 6.7 months.[240] Gemcitabine and other conventional chemotherapies have limited benefit.[241] Newer agents for relapsed PTCL, including the antifolate agent pralatrexate, and HDAC histone deacetylase romidepsin and belinostat, all have a 25–30% RR with median durations of response <18 months.[242,243] Nonmyeloablative alloSCT for highly selected patients has a 5-year OS and PFS of 50% and 40%, respectively.[244]

Autologous stem cell transplantation for relapsed aggressive NHL
Disease sensitivity at the time of ASCT has remained the most significant prognostic variable for predicting treatment outcome. Several large series have shown that patients who undergo ASCT with primary refractory disease have less than a 10% probability of disease-free survival. Those relapsed patients whose disease remains sensitive to chemotherapy have a 30–60% probability of long-term disease-free survival. In contrast, only 10–15% of patients with resistant disease are long-term survivors.

ASCT has been compared to conventional salvage therapy for relapsed aggressive NHL in the PARMA trial.[245] Patients with relapsed aggressive NHL (largely DLBCL) received two cycles of cisplatin, cytarabine, and solumedrol and if responsive, were randomized to continued chemotherapy for four additional cycles or high-dose chemotherapy and autologous bone marrow transplantation. With median follow-up in excess of 5 years, patients randomized to the high-dose arm and autologous bone marrow transplantation had superior EFS (46% vs 12%) and OS (53% vs 32%).

Investigators have to date failed to improve on these results with the addition of maintenance therapy post-transplant with rituximab,[246] an anti-CD19 immunotoxin, the oral kinase inhibitor enzastaurin, or adding radioimmunotherapy[247] to the conditioning regimen. For patients with relapsed or refractory DLBCL, high-dose therapy and ASCT remains the treatment of choice for patients with chemosensitive disease. If the recurrence is localized, adjuvant RT either before or after high-dose therapy and ASCT may be beneficial in terms of disease control but may not impact on OS. For patients with chemorefractory disease, clinical trials or palliative therapy, but not stem cell transplantation, should be considered. Several new agents have shown some promise in patients with relapsed DLBCL, including ibrutinib, particularly in the ABC subtype, as well as lenalidomide, and everolimus.

Allogeneic stem cell transplantation in NHL
Allogeneic stem cell transplantation has been applied to patients with relapsed and refractory NHL. Nearly all patients had relapsed disease, many of whom were resistant to conventional dose therapy. In the European Bone Marrow Transplant registry, the recurrence rate after allogeneic transplantation for aggressive NHL was lower than for autologous transplantation without difference in OS, owing to the associated higher transplant-related mortality. The EFS and OS at 5 years was 43%, with treatment-related mortality 25% at 1 year. Patients with recurrent disease following ASCT who have good performance status and chemosensitive disease are considered for alloSCT usually with RIC. Studies have reported 40–60% PFS, at several years, but with treatment-related mortality of 20% for RIC alloSCT and up to 40% for myeloablative transplants.[248,249]

New therapeutic approaches for NHL

Significant improvements have been made in the treatment of NHL, with the major impact in B-cell malignancies. However, less progress has occurred in therapy of many disease entities, such as PTCLs and relapsed and refractory DLBCL. There are a vast number of new, rational targeted agents under evaluation including antibody drug conjugates, kinases inhibitors, and immunotherapies that enhance T-cell cytotoxicity (chimeric antigen receptor T cells and checkpoint blockade antibodies). The most significant advance is our understanding of the genetic events and aberrant pathways driving lymphomagenesis. This knowledge drives the development of agents directed against novel targets, thereby limiting toxicity to normal cells.

Key references

The complete reference list can be found on the Wiley Companion Digital Edition of this title (see inside front cover for login instructions).

22 Swerdlow SH, Campo E, Harris NL, et al. *WHO Classification of Tumours of Haematopoietic and Lymphoid Tissues.* Lyon, France: IARC Press; 2008.

25 Armitage JO, Weisenburger DD. New approach to classifying non-Hodgkin's lymphomas: clinical features of the major histologic subtypes. Non-Hodgkin's Lymphoma Classification Project. *J Clin Oncol.* 1998;**16**(8):2780–2795.

29 Montoto S, Fitzgibbon J. Transformation of indolent B-cell lymphomas. *J Clin Oncol.* 2011;**29**:1827–1834.

31 Grever MR, Lucas DM, Dewald GW, et al. Comprehensive assessment of genetic and molecular features predicting outcome in patients with chronic lymphocytic leukemia: results from the US Intergroup Phase III Trial E2997. *J Clin Oncol.* 2007;**25**(7):799–804.

58 Rosenwald A, Wright G, Chan WC, et al. The use of molecular profiling to predict survival after chemotherapy for diffuse large-B-cell lymphoma. *N Engl J Med.* 2002;**346**(25):1937–1947.

59 Alizadeh AA, Eisen MB, Davis RE, et al. Distinct types of diffuse large B-cell lymphoma identified by gene expression profiling. *Nature.* 2000;**403**(6769):503–511.

60 Monti S, Savage KJ, Kutok JL, et al. Molecular profiling of diffuse large B-cell lymphoma identifies robust subtypes including one characterized by host inflammatory response. *Blood.* 2005;**105**(5):1851–1861.

61 Shipp MA, Ross KN, Tamayo P, et al. Diffuse large B-cell lymphoma outcome prediction by gene-expression profiling and supervised machine learning. *Nat Med.* 2002;**8**(1):68–74.

68 Aukema SM, Siebert R, Schuuring E, et al. Double-hit B-cell lymphomas. *Blood.* 2011;**117**(8):2319–2331.

71 Montoto S, Corradini P, Dreyling M, et al. Indications for hematopoietic stem cell transplantation in patients with follicular lymphoma: a consensus project of the EBMT-Lymphoma Working Party. *Haematologica.* 2013;**98**(7):1014–1021.

78 Rizvi MA, Evens AM, Tallman MS, Nelson BP, Rosen ST. T-cell non-Hodgkin lymphoma. *Blood.* 2006;**107**(4):1255–1264.

91 Sonnen R, Schmidt WP, Muller-Hermelink HK, Schmitz N. The International Prognostic Index determines the outcome of patients with nodal mature T-cell lymphomas. *Br J Haematol.* 2005;**129**(3):366–372.

105 Cheson BD, Fisher RI, Barrington SF, et al. Recommendations for initial evaluation, staging, and response assessment of Hodgkin and non-Hodgkin lymphoma: the Lugano classification. *J Clin Oncol.* 2014;**32**(27):3059–3068.

109 A predictive model for aggressive non-Hodgkin's lymphoma. The International Non-Hodgkin's Lymphoma Prognostic Factors Project. *N Engl J Med.* 1993;**329**(14):987–994.

111 Solal-Celigny P, Roy P, Colombat P, et al. Follicular lymphoma international prognostic index. *Blood.* 2004;**104**(5):1258–1265.

115 Schmitz N, Trumper L, Ziepert M, et al. Treatment and prognosis of mature T-cell and NK-cell lymphoma: an analysis of patients with T-cell lymphoma treated in studies of the German High-Grade Non-Hodgkin Lymphoma Study Group. *Blood.* 2010;**116**(18):3418–3425.

116 Hans CP, Weisenburger DD, Greiner TC, et al. Confirmation of the molecular classification of diffuse large B-cell lymphoma by immunohistochemistry using a tissue microarray. *Blood.* 2004;**103**(1):275–282.

131 Ardeshna KM, Smith P, Norton A, et al. Long-term effect of a watch and wait policy versus immediate systemic treatment for asymptomatic advanced-stage non-Hodgkin lymphoma: a randomised controlled trial. *Lancet.* 2003;**362**(9383):516–522.

133 Ardeshna KM, Qian W, Smith P, et al. Rituximab versus a watch-and-wait approach in patients with advanced-stage, asymptomatic, non-bulky follicular lymphoma: an open-label randomised phase 3 trial. *Lancet Oncol.* 2014;**15**(4):424–435.

136 Marcus R, Imrie K, Belch A, et al. CVP chemotherapy plus rituximab compared with CVP as first-line treatment for advanced follicular lymphoma. *Blood.* 2005;**105**(4):1417–1423.

139 Rummel MJ, Niederle N, Maschmeyer G, et al. Bendamustine plus rituximab versus CHOP plus rituximab as first-line treatment for patients with indolent and mantle-cell lymphomas: an open-label, multicentre, randomised, phase 3 non-inferiority trial. *Lancet.* 2013;**381**(9873):1203–1210.

143 Martinelli G, Schmitz SF, Utiger U, et al. Long-term follow-up of patients with follicular lymphoma receiving single-agent rituximab at two different schedules in trial SAKK 35/98. *J Clin Oncol.* 2010;**28**(29):4480–4484.

147 Salles G, Seymour JF, Offner F, et al. Rituximab maintenance for 2 years in patients with high tumour burden follicular lymphoma responding to rituximab plus chemotherapy (PRIMA): a phase 3, randomised controlled trial. *Lancet.* 2011;**377**(9759):42–51.

164 Gopal AK, Kahl BS, de Vos S, et al. PI3Kdelta inhibition by idelalisib in patients with relapsed indolent lymphoma. *N Engl J Med.* 2014;**370**(11):1008–1018.

167 Schouten HC, Qian W, Kvaloy S, et al. High-dose therapy improves progression-free survival and survival in relapsed follicular non-Hodgkin's lymphoma: results from the randomized European CUP trial. *J Clin Oncol.* 2003;**21**(21):3918–3927.

169 Khouri IF, McLaughlin P, Saliba RM, et al. Eight-year experience with allogeneic stem cell transplantation for relapsed follicular lymphoma after nonmyeloablative conditioning with fludarabine, cyclophosphamide, and rituximab. *Blood.* 2008;**111**(12):5530–5536.

180 Miller TP, Dahlberg S, Cassady JR, et al. Chemotherapy alone compared with chemotherapy plus radiotherapy for localized intermediate- and high-grade non-Hodgkin's lymphoma. *N Engl J Med.* 1998;**339**(1):21–26.

184 Persky DO, Unger JM, Spier CM, et al. Phase II study of rituximab plus three cycles of CHOP and involved-field radiotherapy for patients with limited-stage aggressive B-cell lymphoma: Southwest Oncology Group study 0014. *J Clin Oncol.* 2008;**26**(14):2258–2263.

185 Pfreundschuh M, Trumper L, Osterborg A, et al. CHOP-like chemotherapy plus rituximab versus CHOP-like chemotherapy alone in young patients with good-prognosis diffuse large-B-cell lymphoma: a randomised controlled trial by the MabThera International Trial (MInT) Group. *Lancet Oncol.* 2006;**7**(5):379–391.

187 Dunleavy K, Pittaluga S, Maeda LS, et al. Dose-adjusted EPOCH-rituximab therapy in primary mediastinal B-cell lymphoma. *N Engl J Med.* 2013;**368**(15):1408–1416.

192 Coiffier B, Lepage E, Briere J, et al. CHOP chemotherapy plus rituximab compared with CHOP alone in elderly patients with diffuse large-B-cell lymphoma. *N Engl J Med.* 2002;**346**(4):235–242.

194 Habermann TM, Weller EA, Morrison VA, et al. Rituximab-CHOP versus CHOP alone or with maintenance rituximab in older patients with diffuse large B-cell lymphoma. *J Clin Oncol.* 2006;**24**(19):3121–3127.

195 Pfreundschuh M, Schubert J, Ziepert M, et al. Six versus eight cycles of bi-weekly CHOP-14 with or without rituximab in elderly patients with aggressive CD20+ B-cell lymphomas: a randomised controlled trial (RICOVER-60). *Lancet Oncol.* 2008;**9**(2):105–116.

201 McMillan A, Ardeshna KM, Cwynarski K, Lyttelton M, McKay P, Montoto S. Guideline on the prevention of secondary central nervous system lymphoma: British Committee for Standards in Haematology. *Br J Haematol.* 2013;**163**(2):168–181.

209 Stiff PJ, Unger JM, Cook JR, et al. Autologous transplantation as consolidation for aggressive non-Hodgkin's lymphoma. *N Engl J Med.* 2013;**369**(18):1681–1690.

214 Kluin-Nelemans HC, Hoster E, Hermine O, et al. Treatment of older patients with mantle-cell lymphoma. *N Engl J Med.* 2012;**367**(6):520–531.

217 Romaguera JE, Fayad LE, Feng L, et al. Ten-year follow-up after intense chemoimmunotherapy with Rituximab-HyperCVAD alternating with Rituximab-high dose methotrexate/cytarabine (R-MA) and without stem cell transplantation in patients with untreated aggressive mantle cell lymphoma. *Br J Haematol.* 2010;**150**(2):200–208.

222 Wang ML, Rule S, Martin P, et al. Targeting BTK with ibrutinib in relapsed or refractory mantle-cell lymphoma. *N Engl J Med.* 2013;**369**(6):507–516.

223 Kahl BS, Spurgeon SE, Furman RR, et al. A phase 1 study of the PI3Kdelta inhibitor idelalisib in patients with relapsed/refractory mantle cell lymphoma (MCL). *Blood.* 2014;**123**(22):3398–3405.

224 Fenske TS, Zhang MJ, Carreras J, et al. Autologous or reduced-intensity conditioning allogeneic hematopoietic cell transplantation for chemotherapy-sensitive mantle-cell lymphoma: analysis of transplantation timing and modality. *J Clin Oncol.* 2014;**32**(4):273–281.

228 Dunleavy K, Pittaluga S, Shovlin M, et al. Low-intensity therapy in adults with Burkitt's lymphoma. *N Engl J Med.* 2013;**369**(20):1915–1925.

245 Philip T, Guglielmi C, Hagenbeek A, et al. Autologous bone marrow transplantation as compared with salvage chemotherapy in relapses of chemotherapy-sensitive non-Hodgkin's lymphoma. *N Engl J Med.* 1995;**333**(23):1540–1545.

120 Mycosis fungoides and Sézary syndrome

Richard T. Hoppe, MD ▪ Youn H. Kim, MD ▪ Ranjana H. Advani, MD

Overview

Mycosis fungoides/Sézary syndrome (MF/SS) is the most common cutaneous T-cell lymphoma. It originates in the skin and its presentation may range from very limited patch disease to wide-spread cutaneous tumors. When there is peripheral blood involvement, usually in conjunction with erythroderma, it is known as the SS. Although patients with limited patch disease have a very long natural history, respond to a variety of topical therapies, and even enjoy a survival similar to age-matched control populations, patients who present with cutaneous tumors or extracutaneous disease have a relentless progressive course of disease. Treatments for patients with limited disease are primarily topical and include topical chemotherapy (nitrogen mustard), radiation therapy, and phototherapy. When the disease is advanced, topical therapies are still often needed, but systemic treatment becomes essential. Conventional chemotherapy (single agent or combination) is often not effective. However, systemic biologics such as histone deacetylase inhibitors, the interferons, photopheresis, alemtuzumab, and brentuximab vedotin may achieve responses. Most recently, hematopoietic cell transplant, especially with nonablative conditioning regimens, has shown promising results in a cohort of patients with advanced MF or SS.

Historical perspective

Mycosis fungoides (MF) was first described by the French dermatologist Alibert. MF/SS (mycosis fungoides/Sézary syndrome) is the most common cutaneous T-cell lymphoma (CTCL). Sézary syndrome (SS) is an erythrodermic, leukemic variant of MF.[1]

Incidence and epidemiology

There are <1000 cases in the United States annually.[2] The median age is 55–60 years; however, younger patients may be affected.[3] There is 2:1 male predominance, without racial predilection. The etiology is unknown.[4] There is no evidence to support an association with chemical exposure or any virus.[5,6]

Pathology

Abnormal mononuclear "cerebriform" cells infiltrate the epidermis and upper dermis as single cells or clusters (Pautriermicroabscesses). They have a helper T-cell phenotype (CD4+).[7] Occasional cases are CD8+ (cytotoxic/suppressor T-cell phenotype). Studies indicate monoclonal rearrangements of the T-cell receptors in the skin, lymph nodes, and peripheral blood.[8] Lymph nodes are classified as LN-0–LN-4 depending on the degree of infiltration of atypical cells.[9] Potential involvement with clonal cells may be demonstrated even in lymph nodes with only dermatopathic changes.[10]

Pathogenesis and natural history

MF may present first in a premycotic phase with nonspecific, slightly scaling skin lesions. Later, patches, plaques, tumors, or generalized erythroderma may develop. The disease is often in a "bathing trunk" distribution. Pruritus is a common symptom. Infiltrated plaques may eventually develop into ulcerating or fungating tumors. Infected tumors may lead to sepsis and death.

Patients with erythroderma have intense pruritus. The complex of erythroderma, lymphadenopathy, and circulating abnormal cells in the blood is known as SS.[11] Other presentations include folliculotropic,[12] pagetoid reticulosis,[13] granulomatous,[14] and hypopigmented.[15]

MF is usually indolent,[16,17] but 15–20% develop extracutaneous disease, most commonly those with cutaneous tumors or erythroderma.[18] Regional nodes are the most common site of extracutaneous disease but MF may affect the spleen, liver, lungs, and other organs.[19]

Diagnosis

Immunophenotyping supports routine histology. T-cell receptor gene rearrangements can be detected by Southern blot analysis[20,21] or by methods utilizing polymerase chain reaction (PCR) amplification.[8,22] Flow cytometry studies of the blood may show expansion of the CD4+CD7− population reflective of circulating atypical lymphocytes of Sézary type.[23] PCR methods can be helpful in determination of blood[24] or lymph node involvement.[10]

Patients with limited disease require a good physical examination, careful mapping of skin lesions, complete blood count, Sézary cell detection, screening chemistries, and a chest radiograph. If these are within normal limits, additional studies are unnecessary. Patients with generalized disease should undergo CT (computed tomography) or PET/CT (positron emission tomography and computed tomography) imaging.[25] Enlarged nodes should be biopsied but bone marrow is not routinely sampled.

TNMB staging

The TNMB (tumor, node, metastases, blood) staging system for MF/SS[26] is summarized in Tables 1 and 2.[26]

Prognostic factors and biomarkers

T-classification and presence of extracutaneous disease are the most important prognostic factors for survival (Figure 1).[18] Patients with limited patch/plaque (T1; stage IA) disease have an excellent survival, similar to an age-, sex-, and race-matched control population.[16] Median survival is >33 years and <10% progress to a more advanced stage.

Patients with generalized patch/plaque disease without evidence of extracutaneous involvement (T2; stage IB, IIA) have a median

Holland-Frei Cancer Medicine, Ninth Edition. Edited by Robert C. Bast Jr., Carlo M. Croce, William N. Hait, Waun Ki Hong, Donald W. Kufe, Martine Piccart-Gebhart, Raphael E. Pollock, Ralph R. Weichselbaum, Hongyang Wang, and James F. Holland.
© 2017 John Wiley & Sons, Inc. ISBN: 978-1-118-93469-2

Table 1 Tumor-node-metastasis-blood classification for MF.

T (Skin)	
T1	Limited patch, papules, or plaques covering <10% of the skin surface
T2	Patches, papules, and/or plaques covering ≥10% of the skin surface
T3	One or more tumors (>1 cm in diameter)
T4	Confluence of erythema >80% of body surface area
N (Nodes)	
N0	No clinically abnormal peripheral lymph nodes; biopsy not required
N1	Clinically abnormal peripheral lymph nodes; histopathology Dutch Gr 1 or NCI LN0–2
N2	Clinically abnormal peripheral lymph nodes; histopathology Dutch Gr 2 or NCI LN3
N3	Clinically abnormal peripheral lymph nodes; histopathology Dutch Gr 3–4 or NCI LN4
NX	Clinically abnormal peripheral lymph nodes; no histologic confirmation
M (Viscera)	
M0	No visceral organ involvement
M1	Visceral involvement (must have pathology confirmation and organ involved should be specified)
B (Blood)	
B0	Absence of significant blood involvement: <5% of peripheral blood lymphocytes (PBL) are atypical (Sézary) cells
B1	Low blood tumor burden: >5% of PBLs are atypical (Sézary), but does not meet criteria for B2
B2	High blood tumor burden: >1,000/mcL Sézary cells with positive clone

Source: Olsen et al.[26] Reproduced by permission of the American Society of Hematology.

Table 2 Clinical staging system for MF/SS.

	T	N	M	B
IA	1	0	0	0, 1
IB	2	0	0	0, 1
II	1–2	1, 2	0	0, 1
IIB	3	0–2	0	0, 1
III	4	0–2	0	0, 1
IIIA	4	0–2	0	0
IIIB	4	0–2	0	1
IVA1	1–4	0-2	0	2
IVA2	1–4	3	0	0–2
IVB	1–4	0–3	1	0–2

survival >11 years.[17] Twenty-four percent develop progressive disease and ~20% die from MF. Patients with cutaneous tumors (T3; stage IIB) or generalized erythroderma (T4; stage III) without extracutaneous disease have median survivals of 3–5 years and the majority will die of MF.[27]

Patients with extracutaneous disease in lymph nodes (stage IVA) or viscera (stage IVB) have a median survival of <1.5 years.[28] The presence of Sézary cells in the peripheral blood usually correlates with more advanced T-classification (usually T4) and the presence of extracutaneous disease.[29]

Patients may develop cutaneous tumors with atypical lymphocytes comprising >25% of the dermal infiltrate.[30,31] This is referred to as large cell transformation. These cells may express CD30, have a high proliferation rate, and share a clonal origin with the pre-existing MF.[30,32] These large cells can exhibit variable loss of one or more T-cell-associated antigens.[30,31] These patients may have more rapid disease progression and require more intensive therapy.[33]

Multidisciplinary care

The National Comprehensive Cancer Network (NCCN) has established consensus guidelines for the therapy of MF and the SS.[34] Common skin therapies include corticosteroids, psoralen plus ultraviolet A (PUVA), topical chemotherapy, retinoids, and irradiation. Some patients (10–20%) will require treatment for systemic disease. Treatment selection is based on clinical stage (Figure 2).

Topical chemotherapy

Topical nitrogen mustard (mechlorethamine, HN2) is an effective treatment, especially for T1–2 disease.[35] The mechanism of action may be its alkylating agent properties together with immune mechanisms/interaction with the epidermal cell–Langerhans cell–T-cell axis. HN2 may be applied locally or to the entire skin. It may be mixed in water, but most often is in a gel or an ointment base. Topical HN2 is applied at least once daily during the clearing phase. Skin clearance may require 6 months or longer and is followed by maintenance. The gel preparation is available commercially in a concentration of 0.02% (Valchlor).[36]

If response is particularly slow, the concentration of the ointment-based HN2 may be increased or the frequency of application may be increased. The complete response (CR) rate for T1–T2 disease is ~15% and the partial response (PR) rate is ~50%.[36] The median time to skin clearance is 6–8 months, and response may be maintained for ≥10 months. Treatment is well tolerated. The primary acute complications include cutaneous hypersensitivity,[36] contact dermatitis, skin irritation, and erythema. There is no systemic absorption and it is safe to use even in children.[35]

Topical retinoids

Bexarotene (Targretin) 1% gel is an RXR-selective synthetic retinoid. It is applied thinly to the patches/plaques twice daily. Owing to its irritant effect, it is used to treat only limited areas. Responses are seen in the majority of patients with stage IA–IB disease.[37] The most common toxicity is local irritation, which occurs in most patients. It may be necessary to withhold therapy a few weeks to assess disease activity. Bexarotene gel is approved

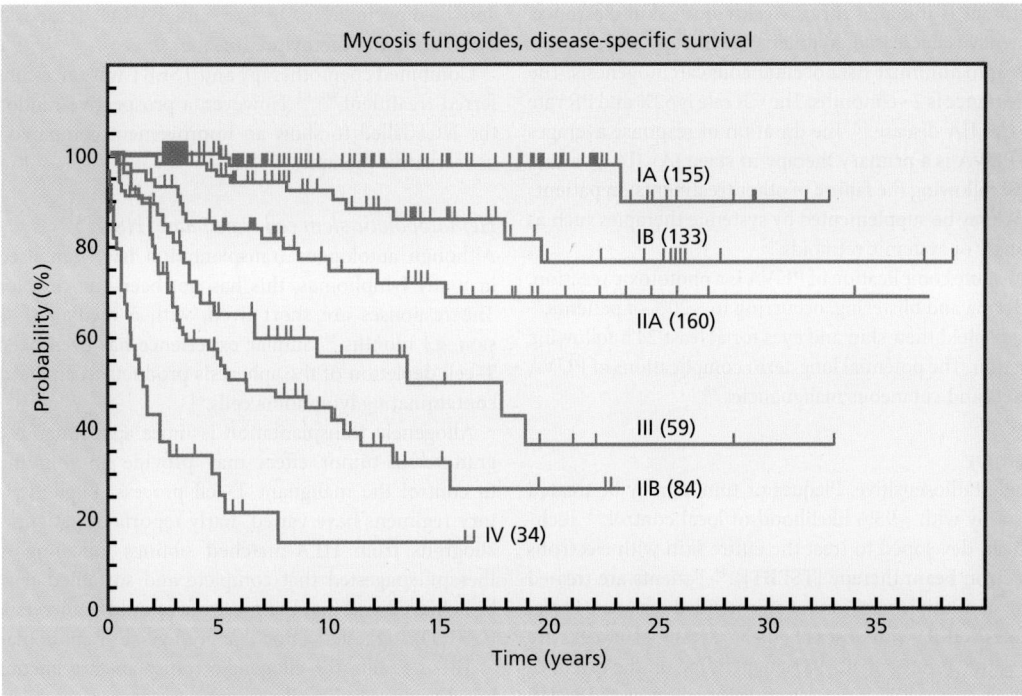

Figure 1 Disease-specific survival by initial disease stage for 525 patients with MF treated at Stanford University.

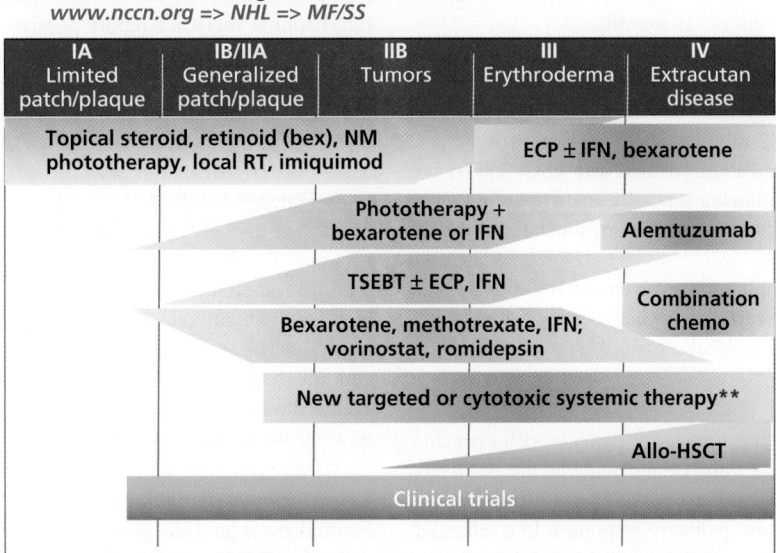

Figure 2 Algorithm for the management of patients with MF/SS.

for patients with stages IA–IB disease who have refractory or persistent disease after other therapies or who have not tolerated other therapies.

Phototherapy

Phototherapy includes ultraviolet (UV) radiation in the UVA or UVB wavelengths. The long-wave UVA has the advantage over UVB in its greater depth of penetration. For limited disease, UVB alone[38] or home UV phototherapy (UVA + UVB)[38,39] may be effective. UVB is initiated daily or three times per week with gradual increase in dose. The frequency is gradually reduced during the maintenance period. Narrow-band UVB (nb-UVB) phototherapy is associated with less toxicity than broadband UVB and achieves

a CR rate of 68% in stage IA–IIA disease.[37] The clinical efficacy of nb-UVB may be superior to broadband UVB.[40]

UVA may be used with a photosensitizing agent, psoralen, as PUVA, referred to as photochemotherapy. In the presence of UVA, psoralen intercalates with DNA, forming monofunctional and bifunctional adducts, which inhibit DNA synthesis. This results in cytotoxic and antiproliferative effects and potential immunomodulatory effects. Patients ingest the psoralen (8-methoxypsoralen) followed by controlled exposure to UVA 1–2 h later. Only the eyes are shielded routinely, but other selected areas can be shielded to minimize undesired photo damage. "Shadowed" areas such as the scalp, perineum, axillae, and other skin folds will not receive adequate exposure.

PUVA treatment is initiated thrice weekly until skin clearance, then the frequency is decreased. Maintenance therapy is discontinued within a year to minimize risks of cutaneous carcinogenesis. The time to skin clearance is 2–6 months. The CR rate is 62% and PR rate 25% in stage IA–IIA disease.[37] The duration of response averages ~12 months. PUVA is a primary therapy in stage IA–IIA or a secondary therapy following the failure of other treatments. In patients with SS, PUVA may be supplemented by systemic therapies such as interferon alpha[41] or systemic retinoids.[42]

The primary acute complication of PUVA is a phototoxic reaction, with erythroderma and blistering, occurring in ~20% of patients.[37] Patients should shield their skin and eyes for at least 24 h following psoralen ingestion. The potential long-term complications of PUVA include cataracts and cutaneous malignancies.[40]

Radiation therapy

MF is extremely radiosensitive. Plaques or tumors may be treated with doses of 8 Gy with ~95% likelihood of local control.[43] Techniques have been developed to treat the entire skin with electrons (total skin electron beam therapy [TSEBT]).[44] Patients are treated while standing in multiple positions at an extended distance. Overall response rates (ORR) with doses of 30–36 Gy in 9–10 weeks are nearly 100%, with CR rates of 40–98%, depending on the extent of skin involvement.[44,45] TSEBT is most useful for patients with IB–IIB disease. In order to reduce toxicity and duration of therapy and to allow repeat application of TSEBT, low-dose (12 Gy) TSEBT programs have been introduced with an ORR of 88% and CR rate 27%.[46] The duration of clinical benefit is >16 months.

The complications of high-dose TSEBT include erythema, desquamation, and temporary epilation. Patients also experience temporary loss of their fingernails and toenails and an impaired ability to sweat for up to 12 months. There is an increased risk of secondary skin malignancy. Patients treated with 12 Gy TSEBT will experience temporary epilation but generally retain their fingernails and toenails, and all other cutaneous effects are much less than with high-dose TSEBT programs.

In patients who have lymph node involvement, traditional megavoltage (4–15 MeV) photon irradiation may be used with doses of 30 Gy in 3–4 weeks to achieve local control.[44]

Systemic chemotherapy

Systemic chemotherapy is appropriate for patients with extracutaneous, advanced, or refractory disease. Virtually, all drugs effective in other lymphomas have been tested in MF/SS. Unfortunately, they often result in only temporary palliative responses. In a retrospective study of 198 patients with MF/SS receiving systemic therapy, the time to next therapy was only 3.9 months, and there were few durable remissions.[47] Following the NCCN published guidelines, it is expected that only a minority of patients with MF (10–20%) require systemic chemotherapy.[48]

In 526 patients reported in single-agent chemotherapy trials, the response rates were 20–80% and the median duration of responses was 3–22 months.[49] Single agents include the anti-folates methotrexate[50–53] and pralatrexate,[54] chlorambucil,[55] the purine analogs,[56–63] pentostatin, 2-CDA, and fludarabine, gemcitabine,[64–67] pegylated liposomal doxorubicin,[68–71] temozolamide,[72,73] and bortezomib.[74,75]

The largest experience with combination chemotherapy is with cyclophosphamide, vincristine, and prednisone with or without doxorubicin.[76,77] CR rates are generally about 25% and response duration 3–20 months.[49] More intensive regimens include etoposide, idarubicin, cyclophosphamide, vincristine, prednisone,

and bleomycin (VICOP-B)[78] and ESHAP (etoposide, high-dose cytarabine, and methylprednisone).[79]

Combined chemotherapy and TSEBT was once considered a preferred treatment.[80–82] However, a prospective randomized trial at the NCI failed to show an improvement compared to sequential conservative therapies.[83,84]

Hematopoietic stem cell transplant (HSCT)

Although autologous transplantation has been used successfully in many lymphomas, this has not been the case for MF/SS.[85–87] The responses are short lived, with a median time to progression <3 months.[85] Similar experience has even been shown with T-cell depletion of the apheresis products in an effort to eliminate contaminating lymphoma cells.[88]

Allogeneic transplantation is more appealing, as an allogeneic graft-versus-tumor effect may provide an immune mechanism to control the malignant T-cell process. Eligibility and preparatory regimens have varied. Early reports of patients who received allografts from HLA-matched siblings following myelo-ablative therapy suggested that complete and sustained remissions could be achieved and that the presence of mild graft versus host disease (GVHD) suggested a possible graft versus lymphoma effect.[89,90]

These results for allogeneic transplant are encouraging, but it has limited applicability owing to transplant-related morbidity and mortality, especially in older patients. More recent data using nonmyeloablative approaches with reduced intensity conditioning regimens are effective and less-toxic than myeloablative regimens.[85] International registries report progression-free survival (PFS) as high as 32% at 5 years and 30% at 7 years.[91–95]

A novel approach is to combine TSEBT, total lymphoid irradiation, and anti-thymocyte globulin as a nonablative preparatory regimen.[96] This regimen has been shown to be associated with a lower risk for GVHD. In a series of 29 patients with stage IIB or IV MF/SS transplanted at Stanford, the incidence of grade II–IV GVHD was 21%.[97] The 2-year PFS was 50% and OS was 76%.

It appears that allogeneic hematopoietic stem cell transplant (HSCT) (especially with reduced intensity conditioning regimens) may result in durable long-term remissions. Larger prospective studies will be required to identify the optimal timing of transplant and the best conditioning regimen. With numerous biological agents showing promising activity and tolerability, there may also be a role for maintenance therapy.

Extracorporeal photopheresis

Photopheresis [extracorporeal photopheresis (ECP)] is a method of delivering PUVA systemically using an extracorporeal technique.[98] The patient's white blood cells are collected via leukapheresis, exposed to a photoactivating drug (8-methoxypsoralen, Uvadex), and then irradiated with UVA. The irradiated cells are then returned to the patient intravenously. The mechanism of action of photopheresis remains unclear but it may induce apoptosis of circulating tumor cells (Sézary cells). The released tumor antigen is then processed by the peripheral dendritic cells leading to the augmentation of systemic antitumor responses.[99] The treatment is most effective for patients with erythroderma (T4).[100] Response rates may be higher when combined with biologic agents such as interferons or retinoids[101–104] or skin-directed therapies such as topical steroids, topical nitrogen mustard, or TSEBT.[48,102] ECP has minimal adverse effects. Some patients may experience nausea, mostly due to the ingested psoralen, and some have a transient low-grade fever or slight malaise after treatment. There are no reports of significant organ damage or bone marrow or immune suppression.[103]

Systemic biologic therapy

IFN-α may be used alone, but more often with other topical or systemic therapies. Reported ORRs when used as monotherapy are 53–74%, with CR rates of 21–35%.[41,104,105] The response rate and duration appear better when combined with phototherapy.[41]

Systemic retinoid therapy with bexarotene may be effective.[106] It may be combined with PUVA (Re-PUVA), IFN-α, or TSEBT. The response rate is 45–55% (10–20% CR).[42,104–111] The most common complications include photosensitivity, xerosis, myalgia, arthralgia, headaches, hyperlipidemia, and central hypothyroidism, as well as possible teratogenic effects. Most toxicities are reversible after cessation of therapy.

Two histone deacetylase (HDAC) inhibitors are useful, Vorinostat (suberoylanilide hydroxamic acid) and romidepsin. Vorinostat, an oral agent, has an ORR rate of 24–30% but only rare CRs.[112,113] The median time to response is 12 weeks, and the median duration of response is 15–26 weeks. Pruritus relief is common. The most common side effects include fatigue, diarrhea, nausea, anorexia, dysgeusia, and thrombocytopenia.

Romidepsin (depsipeptide), an intravenously administered HDAC inhibitor, is associated with an ORR of 34%.[114,115] The primary adverse effects include nausea, vomiting, fatigue, thrombocytopenia, and granulocytopenia.

Alemtuzumab (Campath-1H), a humanized monoclonal antibody directed against CD52, achieves complete and PRs in 32% and 23%, respectively, with a median time to treatment failure of 12 months.[116] Serious infections are a risk, and these patients require antibiotic and antiviral prophylaxis. Modified dose schedules have been introduced that have been associated with less severe toxicities.[117,118] Alemtuzumab is particularly effective in reducing the peripheral blood Sézary count in patients with SS.

Brentuximab vedotin (BV) is an anti-CD30-monomethyl auristatin E anti-tubulin conjugate with potent and selective antitumor activity against CD-30 positive malignancies.[119] Its efficacy in MF, which has variable expression of CD30, has been demonstrated.[120] An objective global response was observed in 73% of patients. The most common adverse events related to BV are peripheral neuropathy, fatigue, nausea, alopecia, and neutropenia.

Lenalidomide is an oral immunomodulatory drug.[121] The ORR is 28%. Primary complications included fatigue, infection, and leukopenia.

Conclusions

MF/SS is a challenging disease. It has a variety of clinical presentations and although often pursues an indolent course, in many patients, it has an aggressive behavior. It responds to topical therapies and systemic biologic treatments, but chemotherapy plays only a minor role in its management. Allogeneic stem cell transplantation may be a curative treatment in selected patients.

Key references

The complete reference list can be found on the Wiley Companion Digital Edition of this title (see inside front cover for login instructions).

1 Kim YH, Hoppe RT. Mycosis fungoides and the Sézary syndrome. *Semin Oncol.* 1999;**26**:276–289.

11 Willemze R, Jaffe ES, Burg G, et al. WHO-EORTC classification for cutaneous lymphomas. *Blood.* 2005;**105**:3768–3785.

18 Kim YH, Liu HL, Mraz-Gernhard S, et al. Long-term outcome of 525 patients with mycosis fungoides and Sézary syndrome at Stanford: clinical prognostic factors and risks of disease progression and second cancer. *Arch Dermatol.* 2003;**139**:857–866.

26 Olsen E, Vonderheid E, Pimpinelli N, et al. Revisions to the staging and classification of mycosis fungoides and Sézary syndrome: a proposal of the International Society for Cutaneous Lymphomas (ISCL) and the cutaneous lymphoma task force of the European Organization of Research and Treatment of Cancer (EORTC). *Blood.* 2007;**110**:1713–1722.

29 Sausville EA, Eddy JL, Makuch RW, et al. Histopathologic staging at initial diagnosis of mycosis fungoides and the Sézary syndrome. Definition of three distinctive prognostic groups. *Ann Intern Med.* 1988;**109**:372–382.

36 Lessin SR, Duvic M, Guitart S, et al. Topical chemotherapy in cutaneous T-cell lymphoma. Positive results of a randomized, controlled, multicenter trial testing the efficacy and safety of a novel mechlorethamine, 0.02%, gel in mycosis fungoides. *JAMA Dermatol.* 2013;**149**:25–32.

37 Heald P, Mehlmauer M, Martin AG, et al. Topical bexarotene therapy for patients with refractory or persistent early-stage cutaneous T-cell lymphoma: results of the phase III clinical trial. *J Am Acad Dermatol.* 2003;**49**:801.

38 Ponte P, Serrao V, Apetato M. Efficacy of narrowband UVB vs. PUVA in patients with early-stage mycosis fungoides. *J Eur Acad Dermatol Venereol.* 2010;**24**:716–721.

43 Thomas TO, Agrawal P, Guitart J, et al. Outcome of patients treat with a single-fraction dose of palliative radiation for cutaneous T-cell lymphoma. *Int J Radiat Oncol Biol Phys.* 2013;**85**:747–753.

44 Hoppe R. Mycosis fungoides: radiation therapy. *Dermatol Ther.* 2003;**16**:347–354.

46 Hoppe RT, Harrison C, Tavallaee M, et al. Low-dose total skin electron beam therapy as an effective modality to reduce disease burden in inpatients with mycosis fungoides: Results of a pooled analysis from 3 phase-II clinical trials. *J Am Acad Dermatol.* 2015;**72**:288–292.

47 Hughes CFM, Khot A, McCormack C, et al. Lack of durable disease control with chemotherapy for mycosis fungoides and Sézary syndrome: a comparative study of systemic therapy. *Blood.* 2015;**125**:71–81.

53 Zackheim HS, Kashani-Sabet M, McMillan AK. Low dose methotrexate to treat mycosis fungoides: a retrospective study in 69 patients. *J Am Acad Dermatol.* 2003;**49**:873–878.

54 Horwitz SM, Kim YH, Foss F, et al. Identification of an active, well-tolerated dose of pralatrexate in patients with relapsed or refractory cutaneous T-cell lymphoma. *Blood.* 2012;**119**:4115–4122.

57 Tsimberidon AM, Giles F, Duvic M, et al. Phase II study of pentostatin in advanced T-cell lymphoid malignancies: update of an M.D. Anderson Cancer Center series. *Cancer.* 2004;**100**:342–349.

71 Dummer R, Quaglino P, Becker JC, et al. Prospective international multicenter phase II trial of intravenous pegylated liposomal doxorubicin monochemotherapy in patients with stage IIB, IVA, or IVB advanced mycosis fungoides: final results from EORTC 21012. *J Clin Oncol.* 2012;**30**:4091–4097.

73 Querfeld C, Rosen ST, Guitart J, et al. Multicenter phase II tri of temozolamide in mycosis fungoides/Sézary syndrome: correlation with O⁶-methylguanine-DNA methyltransferase and mismatch repair proteins. *Clin Cancer Res.* 2011;**17**:5748–5754.

92 Duarte RF, Boumendil A, Onida F, et al. Long-term outcome of allogeneic hematopoietic cell transplantation for patients with mycosis fungoides and Sézary syndrome: a European Society for Blood and Marrow Transplantation Lymphoma Working Party Extended Analysis. *J Clin Oncol.* 2014;**32**:3347–3348.

97 Weng WK, Armstrong R, Arai S, et al. Non-myeloablative allogeneic transplantation resulting in clinical and molecular remission with low non-relapse mortality (NRM) in patients with advanced stage mycosis fungoides (MF) and Sézary syndrome (SS). *Blood.* 2014:2544.

100 Zic JA. The treatment of cutaneous T-cell lymphoma with photopheresis. *Dermatol Ther.* 2003;**16**:337–346.

105 Olsen EA. Interferon in the treatment of cutaneous T-cell lymphoma. *Dermatol Ther.* 2003;**16**:311–321.

106 Apisarnthanarax N, Ha CS, Duvic M. Mycosis fungoides with follicular mucinosis displaying aggressive tumor-stage transformation, successful treatment using radiation therapy plus oral bexarotene combination therapy. *Am J Clin Dermatol.* 2003;**4**:429–433.

107 Duvic M, Martin AG, Kim Y, et al. Phase 2 and 3 clinical trial of oral bexarotene (Targretin capsules) for the treatment of refractory or persistent early-stage cutaneous T-cell lymphoma. *Arch Dermatol.* 2001;**137**:581–593.

113 Olsen EA, Kim YH, Kuzel TM, et al. Phase IIB multicenter trial of vorinostat in patients with persistent, progressive, or treatment refractory cutaneous T-cell lymphoma. *J Clin Oncol.* 2007;**25**:3109–3115.

115 Whitaker SJ, Demierre M-F, Kim EJ, et al. Final results from a multicenter, international, pivotal study of romidepsin in refractory cutaneous T-cell lymphoma. *J Clin Oncol.* 2010;**28**:4485–4491.

118 Querfeld C, Mehta N, Rosen ST, et al. Alemtuzumab for relapsed and refractory erythrodermic cutaneous T-cell lymphoma: a single institution experience from the Robert H. Lurie Comprehensive Cancer Center. *Leuk Lymphoma.* 2009;**50**:1969–1976.

120 Kim Y, Tavallaee M, Sundram U et al. Phase II investigator-initiated study of brentuximab vedotin in mycosis fungoides and Sézary syndrome with variable CD30 expression level: a Multi-Institution Collaborative Project. *J Clin Oncol.* 2015;**33**:3750–3758.

121 Plasma cell tumors

Noopur Raje, MD ▪ Teru Hideshima, MD, PhD ▪ Andrew J. Yee, MD ▪ Kenneth C. Anderson, MD

Overview

Plasma cell disorders have in common a proliferation of monoclonal plasma cells associated with the production of a monoclonal protein. These disorders range from the common, indolent condition of monoclonal gammopathy of undetermined significance to malignancies, such as multiple myeloma, characterized by the presence of hypercalcemia, anemia, renal dysfunction, and/or lytic lesions. Progress in the understanding of the molecular underpinnings of myeloma has led to remarkable advances in its treatment. High-dose melphalan with autologous stem-cell transplant was historically a mainstay of treatment. Now, highly effective and well-tolerated drug classes such as the proteasome inhibitors (e.g., bortezomib and carfilzomib) and immunomodulatory drugs (e.g., lenalidomide and pomalidomide) have rapidly transformed the treatment of myeloma and significantly improved the overall survival. The increasing use of extended treatment strategies such as maintenance therapy and the arrival of newer drug classes such as plasma cell-specific monoclonal antibodies are setting the stage for improving outcomes further.

Multiple myeloma

Multiple myeloma (MM) is a malignant proliferation of plasma cells and plasmacytoid cells in the bone marrow (BM) characterized nearly always by the presence, in the serum and/or urine, of a monoclonal immunoglobulin (Ig) or Ig fragment.[1] This disease has probably been recognized since 1845, when the first patient was noted with bone pain and heat soluble "animal matter" in urine.[2,3] The term MM was coined in 1873, reflecting distinct sites of BM involvement. The plasma cell was discovered in 1890 and MM associated with plasmacytosis shortly thereafter, in 1900. The application of electrophoresis in 1939 and immunoelectrophoresis in 1953 allowed for the identification of monotypic Ig characteristic of MM.[4,5]

Diagnostic criteria

Active MM is both a clinical and a pathological diagnosis that is defined by the presence of a monoclonal protein in the serum and/or urine, with ≥10% plasma cells in the BM, and associated hypercalcemia, renal dysfunction, anemia, and/or bone disease (also known as the "CRAB" criteria, see Figure 1), related to the MM (Table 1).[7,8] *Active* MM must be distinguished from other disorders characterized by monoclonal gammopathies, both malignant and otherwise, in particular monoclonal gammopathy of undetermined significance (MGUS) and smoldering MM. Other conditions associated with a monoclonal protein include Waldenström's macroglobulinemia, non-Hodgkin's lymphoma, primary amyloidosis, idiopathic cold agglutinin disease, essential cryoglobulinemia, and heavy

chain disease. *Smoldering* MM is defined by the presence of a monoclonal protein ≥3 g/dL and/or ≥10% plasma cells in the BM and the absence of end organ involvement (i.e., the CRAB criteria of hypercalcemia, renal insufficiency, anemia, or bone lesions). The International Myeloma Working Group (IMWG) has recently updated the definition of symptomatic myeloma to include any one of the following biomarkers of disease such as ≥60% marrow infiltration with plasma cells, an involved : uninvolved serum free light-chain (FLC) ratio of ≥100, or >1 focal lesion on an MRI.[6]

Monoclonal gammopathy of undetermined significance

MGUS is present in 3.2% of persons 50 years of age or older and 5.3% of persons 70 years of age or older.[9] Patients have <3 g/dL monoclonal Ig, fewer than 10% monoclonal marrow plasma cells, and no bone lesions, anemia, hypercalcemia, or renal dysfunction (CRAB criteria).[8] In a large experience of 1384 patients diagnosed at the Mayo Clinic, 115 patients progressed to MM, IgM lymphoma, primary amyloidosis, macroglobulinemia, chronic lymphocytic leukemia, or plasmacytoma with relative risk of progression of 25.0, 2.4, 8.4, 46.0, 0.9, and 8.5, respectively.[10] The risk of progression of MGUS to MM or related disorders is about 1% per year, and the initial concentration of serum monoclonal protein was a significant predictor of progression at 20 years. Similar results have been published by Cesana et al.[11] Independent prognostic factors associated with MGUS transformation to MM include (1) >5% BM plasmacytosis, (2) Bence Jones proteinuria, (3) decrease in polyclonal serum immunoglobulin, and (4) an elevated erythrocyte sedimentation rate.[11] More recently, risk factors for progression include an abnormal serum kappa : lambda FLC ratio, a high serum monoclonal protein level ≥1.5 g/dL, and non-IgG type monoclonal protein.[12] The risk of progression from smoldering MM to symptomatic disease is related to the proportion of BM plasma cells and serum monoclonal protein level at diagnosis[13] as well as abnormal serum FLC ratio.[14] In some cases, MGUS can be associated with symptomatology requiring therapy. For example, plasma exchange appears to be efficacious in neuropathy associated with IgG or IgA MGUS.[15]

Epidemiology

In addition to MGUS, a potential risk factor for the development of MM includes exposure to irradiation or petroleum products. Unlike leukemia, there is no increased risk of MM with benzene exposure.[16] Families with two or more affected individuals have been reported, suggesting a possible genetic predisposition.[17] MM has also been found to occur with somewhat greater frequency (but less than twofold) in farmers, paper producers, furniture manufacturers, and wood workers.

There are two major misconceptions regarding MM. The first is that MM is a rare disease. MM is the second most common

Holland-Frei Cancer Medicine, Ninth Edition. Edited by Robert C. Bast Jr., Carlo M. Croce, William N. Hait, Waun Ki Hong, Donald W. Kufe, Martine Piccart-Gebhart, Raphael E. Pollock, Ralph R. Weichselbaum, Hongyang Wang, and James F. Holland.
© 2017 John Wiley & Sons, Inc. ISBN: 978-1-118-93469-2

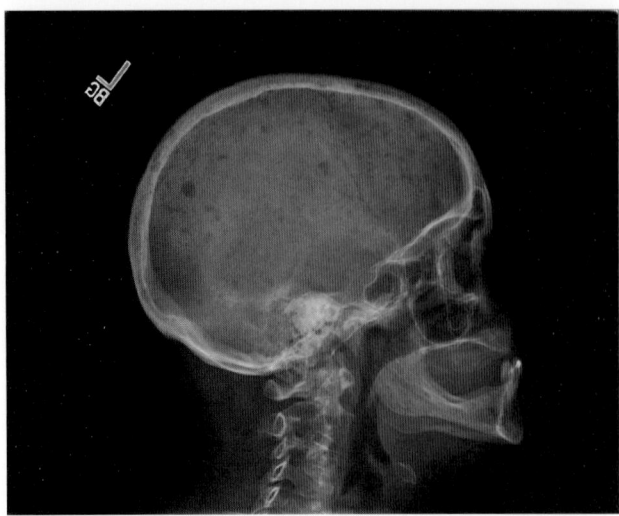

Figure 1 Characteristic lytic bone lesions in multiple myeloma.

Table 1 Classification of monoclonal gammopathies.

Monoclonal gammopathy of unknown significance
<3 g/dL M spike *and*
<10% clonal plasma cells in bone marrow *and*
Absence of CRAB[a] criteria
Smoldering multiple myeloma
≥3 g/dL Monoclonal protein or 10–60% clonal plasma cells in bone marrow
Absence of CRAB criteria
Active multiple myeloma
≥10% plasma cells or biopsy proven plasmacytoma and
Presence of any of the CRAB criteria or *in absence of CRAB criteria*: >1 focal lesion on MRI, ≥ 60% plasma cells in bone marrow; or an abnormal involved:uninvolved FLC ratio of ≥100

[a]CRAB criteria is end organ damage due to the plasma-cell disorder: hypercalcemia (>1 mg/dL higher than the upper limit of normal or >11 mg/dL); renal insufficiency (creatinine clearance <40 mL/min or creatinine >2 mg/dL); anemia (hemoglobin >2 g/dL below lower limit of normal or hemoglobin <10 g/dL); or bone lesions (one or more osteolytic lesions on skeletal radiography, CT, or PET CT).
Source: Rajkumar et al. 2014.[6] Reproduced with permission of Elsevier.

hematologic malignancy, accounting for 24,050 new cancer cases in the United States in the year 2014 and approximately 2% of cancer-related deaths.[18] The highest incidence rates have been reported for African-Americans and Pacific Islanders; Europeans and North American white people have intermediate rates, while generally low rates have been reported for Asians living in Asia and the United States.[19] Although it has been suggested that the incidence of MM is increasing, data from Olmstead County, Minnesota, demonstrate that the incidence of MM has not changed significantly during the past 46 years.[20] A second misunderstanding is that MM is solely a disease of the elderly. In a large Mayo Clinic series, the median age was 66.[21,22] Although 98% of MM patients were 40 years of age or older, 30% of patients were <60 years old. The fact that a significant population of affected individuals is younger than age 70 and therefore can tolerate more aggressive therapeutic approaches influences potential treatment strategies.

Clinical features

The presenting features of 1027 cases of newly diagnosed MM evaluated from 1985 to 1998 are summarized in Table 2.[21] Symptoms

Table 2 Presenting features of multiple myeloma.

Presenting feature	
Anemia (hemoglobin ≤12 g/dL)	73%
Calcium ≥ 11 mg/dL	13%
Creatinine ≥ 2 g/dL	19%
Radiographic abnormality (on plain film)[a]	79%
Bone pain	58%
Fatigue	32%
Weight loss	24%

[a]Lytic lesions present in 67% of patients.
Source: Kyle et al. 2003.[21] Reproduced with permission of Elsevier.

of bone pain and anemia remain the most common presenting features.

Laboratory features

Laboratory evaluation identifies roentgenographic abnormalities in bone and monoclonal Ig in serum and/or urine in the majority of cases. In most series, 50–60% of patients with MM have both serum and urinary monoclonal protein; 20–30% of patients have serum without urinary protein; 15–20% of patients have monoclonal protein in urine only; and only 1–2% of patients do not secrete monoclonal protein in blood and/or urine.[23] IgG or IgA monoclonal proteins are most common, and IgD or IgE are rare. A biclonal process is much more common than previously appreciated, often only documented by immunofixation techniques. Thirty-three percent are IgG and IgA; 24% are IgM and IgG. It appears that patients with biclonal and IgD disease have prognoses similar to those patients with monoclonal disease.[24] Close observation is an appropriate choice for patients with MGUS or smoldering MM, whereas multiple regimens have been employed for therapy of individuals with overt MM. The natural history of MM is a progressive increase in tumor growth. The M protein doubling time, a measure of the MM growth rate, shortens with each relapse. Eventually, marrow failure develops, with sideroblastic anemia, leukopenia, and thrombocytopenia. The median interval from marrow failure to death is 3 (range 1–9) months.[25] Infection and renal failure account for 52% and 21% of deaths, respectively, in patients with MM.[26] Acute myeloid leukemia develops in a small fraction of patients but in excess of the anticipated baseline incidence.[25]

Biology

Cell surface phenotype

B-cell-restricted and associated antigens (Ags) have been utilized to delineate stages of normal and malignant B-cell differentiation.[27] Moreover, antigenic profiles are useful not only to identify stages of malignant B-cell differentiation but also to categorize B-cell tumors. MM cells share cell surface expression of some Ags, for example, CD38 and PCA-1 (prostate cancer antigen-1), which are also present on normal plasma cells, suggesting that the normal cellular counterpart of MM is the normal plasma cell. However, a number of other Ags to date have been described on the surface of MM cells, which in some cases react with B cells at stages of differentiation earlier than the plasma cell and also react with non-B cells.[28–33] Harada et al.[34] have shown that normal plasma cells are CD19+CD56−, whereas no MM cells have this phenotype. The core protein of MUC-1 antigen is expressed on MM cells[35] and its inhibition triggers MM cell death.[36] The expression and function of adhesion molecules on MM cells is described in the following section. This observed heterogeneity in cell surface phenotype has led to controversy as to the cellular origin of MM.

Cellular origin of MM

As is well known, the cells that accumulate in the BM of patients with MM have plasma cell or plasmablast morphology. However, it has been known since the 1970s, based on studies using anti-idiotypic antibodies, that unique idiotypic determinants can identify clones of peripheral blood lymphocytes in patients with macroglobulinemia, MM, MGUS, and chronic lymphocytic leukemia.[37] The presence of idiotypic determinants on cytoplasmic μ-containing pre-B cells in MM BM provided further evidence that the oncogenic event may occur at the pre–B-cell stage. Studies identified B and T cells bearing identical idiotypic determinants, suggesting that target cells for oncogenic transformation could be precursor cells for both B and T cell clones.[38] Aneuploid marrow MM cells can express mRNA for cell surface proteins characteristic of myeloid, erythroid, and platelet lineages, also supporting the view that the malignant clone can extend from an early stage of differentiation.[39] Moreover, monoclonal B lineage cells in peripheral blood of MM patients, which are late-stage B cells (low CD19 and CD20, moderate CALLA and PCA-1, with strong CD45RO antigen expression) are continuously progressing toward the plasma cell stage.[31] However, it remains unclear as to which cell within the malignant clone is "clonogenic" and capable of self-renewal. Some evidence suggests that pre-B and naive B cells migrate from the BM to the lymph node (LN) where antigen recognition, selection, and somatic hypermutation occur. The memory B-cell compartment is thought to contain the cytoplasmic μ-positive precursor cell of MM, which then undergoes Ig class switching in the LN.[40] Ig variable (VH) gene sequence analysis has shown MM tumor cells to be postfollicular, with the mutated homogeneous clonal sequences

indicating no continuing exposure to somatic hypermutation mechanism.[41] VH gene analysis of IgM MM indicates an origin from a memory cell undergoing isotype switch events.[42] Mutated heterogeneous sequences in MGUS suggest that tumor cells remain under the influence of the mutator.[43] Abnormalities of 14q (the location of IgH) are most common in MM. As proto-oncogenes are translocated to this region and overexpressed in B-cell malignancies including follicular lymphoma, Burkitt's lymphoma, and chronic lymphocytic leukemia, they may also play a role in the oncogenesis of MM. In addition, translocations involving switch regions indicate that the final oncogenic molecular event in MM occurs late in B-cell ontogeny.[43] More recently, CD138– cells with a memory B-cell phenotype are thought to be the clonogenic MM "stem" cells, although this concept needs further validation.[44]

Role of adhesion molecules, cytokines, and BM stromal cells in MM

Adhesion molecules mediate both homotypic and heterotypic adhesion of tumor cells to either extracellular matrix (ECM) proteins or bone marrow stromal cells (BMSCs) (Figure 2).[45] Moreover, they play a critical role in pathogenesis of disease progression. After class switching in the LN, adhesion molecules such as CD44, VLA-4 (very late antigen-4), VLA-5, LFA-1 (leukocyte function-associated antigen-1), CD56, syndecan-1 (CD138), and MPC-1 mediate homing of MM cells to the BM.[45–49] Subsequently, binding of MM cells occurs to BMSCs, for example, via VLA-4 to VCAM-1 (vascular cellular adhesion molecule-1), and to ECM, for example, via syndecan to type I collagen and VLA-4 to fibronectin. Such binding not only localizes tumor cells in the BM microenvironment but also stimulates interleukin-6 (IL-6) transcription and secretion from BMSCs with related paracrine growth of MM cells.[50–52] Moreover, triggering via CD40 found on tumor cells induces IL-6 transcription and secretion, with related autocrine MM cell growth

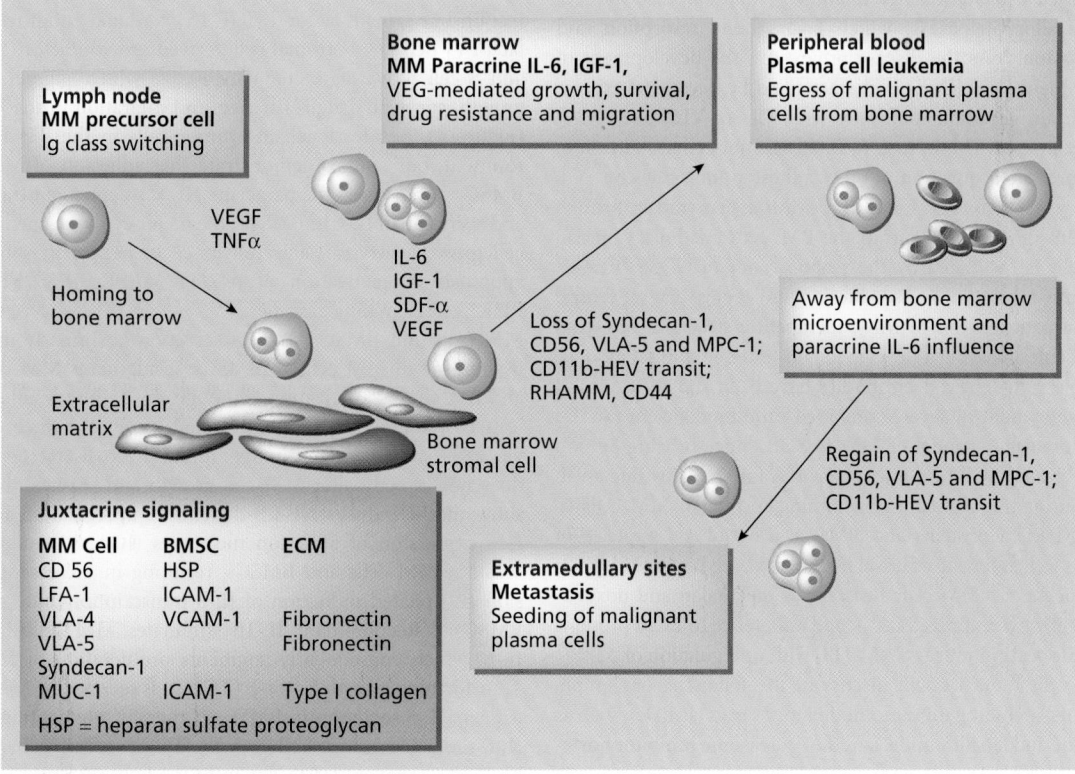

Figure 2 Role of adhesion molecules in myeloma pathogenesis.

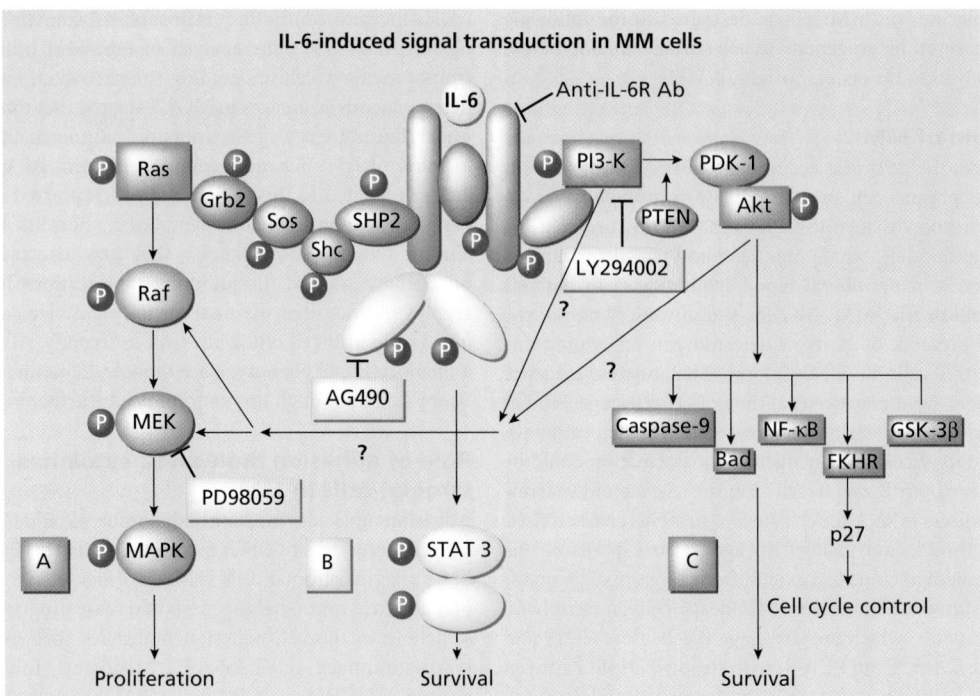

Figure 3 Interleukin-6 signaling cascades.

(Figure 3).[53] TNF-α upregulates adhesion molecules on MM cells and BMSCs, thereby increasing binding and cell adhesion-mediated drug resistance (CAM-DR).[54] Syndecan-1 is a multifunctional regulator of MM cell growth and survival as well as of bone cell differentiation, and elevated serum syndecan-1 correlates with increased tumor cell burden, decreased metalloproteinase-9 activity, and poor prognosis.[55–57] It also mediates decreased osteoclast and increased osteoblast differentiation.[55] Adhesion also induces matrix metalloproteinase-1, which favors bone resorption and tumor invasion.[58] As the disease progresses, the development of plasma-cell leukemia (PCL) is characterized by decreased expression of certain adhesion molecules (e.g., CD56, VLA-5, MPC-1, and syndecan-1), which in turn facilitates tumor cell mobilization. Furthermore, the acquisition of other adhesion molecules on PCL cells, such as CD11b, CD44, and RHAMM, assists transit through endothelium during egress from the BM. Extramedullary spread of MM cells is facilitated by the reappearance of CD56, VLA-5, MPC-1, and syndecan-1. As adhesion molecules play a central role in the pathogenesis of MM, therapeutic strategies targeting these molecules have been developed and tested in animal models; for example, anti-ICAM-1 antibodies have been shown to inhibit tumor development in severe combined immunodeficient (SCID) mice.[59] Moreover, a model of MM in SCID mice bearing human fetal bone grafts (SCID-hu mice) provides for the first time an *in vivo* model for the evaluation of homing of human MM cells to human BM ECM proteins and BMSCs, the biologic sequelae of binding, as well as testing of novel treatments based on interruption of this process.[60,61] MM cells resistant to melphalan and doxorubicin typically overexpress VLA-4, and adherence to ECM proteins such as fibronectin induces CAM-DR, with upregulation of p27^{Kip1} in tumor cells.[62] As we will discuss in the following paragraph, novel agents, including immunomodulatory drugs (IMiDs), such as thalidomide and lenalidomide, and the proteasome inhibitor bortezomib can target both the tumor cell and its BM microenvironment, thereby overcoming CAM-DR.[63–67]

We have characterized the mechanisms whereby MM cells home to the host BM and adhere to BMSCs and ECM proteins, as well as the functional sequelae of this binding, in order to identify targets for novel therapies. Importantly, our past studies have identified those adhesion molecules mediating MM cell binding to fibronectin and BMSCs, as well as the MM cell growth and survival advantage conferred by this binding.[45,52,68–70]

Our studies show that BMSCs secrete cytokines, such as IL-6,[71] insulin-like growth factor-1 (IGF-1),[72] vascular endothelial growth factor (VEGF),[73,74] stromal cell derived growth factor (SDF-1α),[75] and B-cell activating factor (BAFF),[76,77] which augment MM cell growth, survival, drug resistance, and migration in the BM milieu (Figure 4). Besides localizing tumor cells in the BM microenvironment, our studies demonstrate that adhesion of MM cells to BMSCs also triggers the paracrine NF-κB-dependent transcription and secretion of IL-6 in BMSCs, the major cytokine-mediating MM cell growth, survival, and resistance to dexamethasone-induced apoptosis via activation of p42/44 MAPK, JAK2/STAT3, and PI3K/AKT signaling cascades.[50,52,72,78–89] VEGF is secreted by both MM cells and BMSCs, and its secretion is similarly upregulated by binding of MM cells to BMSCs; it augments MM cell growth and BM neovascularization, although the pathophysiologic significance of angiogenesis is undefined.[90,91] VEGF induces migration via PKC signaling.[74] Although tumor necrosis factor-α (TNFα) does not directly alter MM cell growth and survival, our studies show that it induces NF-κB-dependent upregulation in cell surface expression of adhesion molecules (ICAM-1 and VCAM-1) on both MM cells and BMSCs, resulting in increased cell adhesion and related induction of IL-6 transcription and secretion in BMSCs.[54] Recombinant IL-1β stimulates MM cells to produce IL-6, which consequently augments proliferation of MM cells.[92] Transforming growth factor-β (TGF-β) is secreted by MM cells and triggers IL-6 secretion in BMSCs,[93] thereby augmenting paracrine IL-6-mediated tumor cell growth. TGF-β secreted by MM cells likely also contributes to the immunodeficiency characteristic of MM by downregulating B cells, T cells, and natural killer cells,

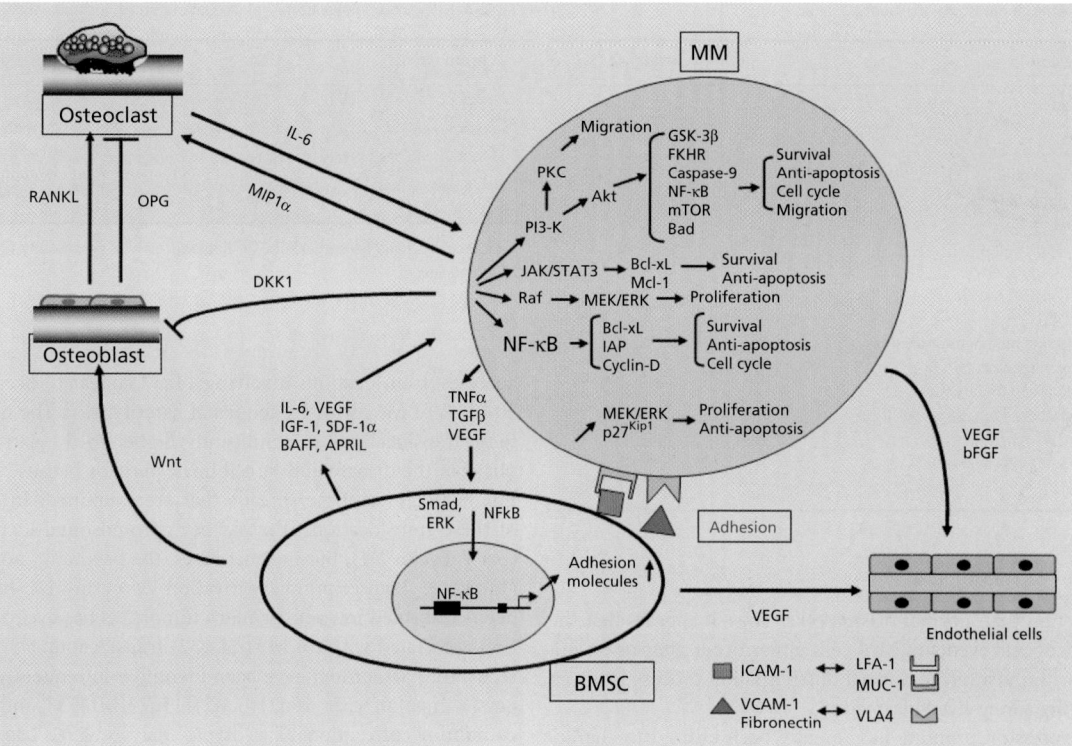

Figure 4 Signaling cascades in the context of the microenvironment.

without similarly inhibiting the growth of MM cells. IL-10 is a proliferation factor, but not a differentiation factor, for human MM cells.[94] IGF-1 has been shown to augment MM cell growth, survival, and drug resistance.[72] Macrophage inflammatory protein-1α (MIP-1α) is an osteoclast stimulating factor in MM.[95,96] BAFF is produced by the BMSCs, and specifically by osteoclasts. It signals through several receptors including BAFF-R, transmembrane activator, calcium modulator, and cyclophilin ligand interactor (TACI), and B-cell maturation Ag (BCMA).[76,77] The level of TACI gene expression in MM cells is associated with microenvironment dependence.[97] This signaling cascade has a prosurvival effect on MM cells. Autocrine growth mediated by IL-15,[98] and most recently IL-21,[99] has been demonstrated in both MM cell lines and patient cells.

Wnt signaling regulates various developmental processes and can lead to malignant formation and has been recently studied in the context of MM. Wnts are a family of secreted glycoproteins that bind to frizzled seven-transmembrane span receptors. Intracellularly, the Wnt signaling cascade blocks degradation of β-catenin in proteasomes, thereby leading to accumulation of β-catenin in the cytoplasm. In MM, a canonical Wnt signaling pathway is activated following treatment with Wnt-3a, associated with accumulation of β-catenin. Wnt-3a treatment further led to significant morphological changes in MM cells, accompanied by rearrangement of the actin cytoskeleton.[100] Derksen et al.[101] demonstrated that MM cells overexpress β-catenin, including its N-terminally unphosphorylated form, consistent with active β-catenin/T-cell factor-mediated transcription. Further accumulation and nuclear localization of β-catenin, and/or increased cell proliferation, was achieved by stimulation of Wnt signaling with Wnt-3a, LiCl, or the constitutively active mutant of β-catenin. Wnt signaling has also been shown as an important regulatory pathway in the osteoblast differentiation of mesenchymal stem cells. Interestingly, MM cells in BM-biopsy specimens contained detectable Dickkopf 1 (DKK1),

a negative regulator of Wnt signaling cascade and a target of the β-catenin/TCF pathway.[102] Moreover, elevated DKK1 levels in BM plasma and peripheral blood from patients with MM correlated with the DKK1 gene-expression patterns and were associated with the presence of focal bone lesions.[103]

Most importantly, adhesion of MM cells to BMSCs induces changes in gene profile: that is, upregulation of growth, survival, and drug resistance genes in tumor cells; upregulation of adhesions molecules on MM cells and BMSCs; and changes in cytokines in BMSCs both in in vitro and in vivo models of human MM in mice.[104–106] Interaction of MM cells with BMSCs activates Notch signaling, which induces melphalan resistance.[107] Induction of proteasome activity when MM cells bind to BMSCs may sensitize them to therapy.

We have shown that IMiDs (e.g., lenalidomide) inhibit VEGF and IL-6, which are known to downregulate antigen-presenting function of dendritic cells in MM.[108] Moreover, lenalidomide directly activates CD28 on T cells, thereby stimulating transcription and secretion of IL-2, with resultant upregulation of T and NK cell anti-MM activity.[108,109] Lenalidomide can upregulate antibody-dependent cellular cytotoxicity (ADCC).[110] IMiDs also affect the cytokine signaling stimulated by the interaction of effector cells with MM cells and BMSCs, and this is via regulation of SOCS1, a member of the suppressor of cytokine signaling (SOCS) genes.[111]

Molecular pathogenesis of MM

The malignant plasma cells in MM are localized to the BM in close association with BMSCs. They are long-lived cells with a very low (1–2%) labeling index (LI) that provides a measure of the proliferative rate of the malignant BMPC predicting survival in patients with newly diagnosed MM. The rearranged Ig genes are extensively somatically hypermutated in a manner compatible with antigen selection, with no evidence that the process of hypermutation is continuing.[41] However, MM cells have a significantly lower rate

Table 3 Myeloma chromosomal alterations.

Genetic lesion	Incidence (%)
Hyperdiploid	60
t(11;14)	20
t(4;14)	15
MAF translocations	5
Del (13q)/monosomy 13	50–60
Del (1p)	7–40
Chr 1q21 amplification	40
Cyclin D dysregulation	80
RAS mutations	30–50
FAM46C, DIS3	10–21
NF-κB activating mutations and CNVs	15–20
IgH *MYC* rearrangements	15
UTX deletions and mutations	30
TP53 inactivations (mutations+del(17p))	10–20
p18 and/or Rb inactivation	<5
p14 promoter methylation	<5
PTEN loss	<2

Table 4 Nonimmunoglobulin sites for illegitimate switch recombination.

Chromosome	Gene	Function
11q13	Cyclin D1	Induces growth
4p16	*FGFR3, MMSET*	Growth factor
8q24	*MYC*	Growth/apoptosis
16q23	c-maf	Transcription factor
6p25	*IRF4*	Transcription factor

Source: Kuel and Bergsagel 2002.[122] Reproduced with permission of Nature Publishing Group.

of Ig secretion than normal plasma cells. Thus, it appears that the critical oncogenic events in MM cells either occur after or do not interfere with most of the normal differentiation process involved in generating a long-lived plasma cell.

Gene expression profiling has recently been utilized to characterize changes associated with the progression from normal plasma cells to MGUS to MM.[112–114] The mRNA profile of MGUS and MM is similar and distinct from that of normal plasma cells.[114] These studies may not only enhance understanding of basic pathophysiology but also identify novel therapeutic targets.

By conventional analyses, karyotypic abnormalities are detected in MM at a frequency of 30–50% in large studies of MM tumors (Table 3).[115–117] The frequency and extent of karyotypic abnormalities correlates with the stage, prognosis, and response to therapy. For example, approximately 20% are abnormal in stage I disease, 60% in stage III patients, and >80% for extramedullary tumor. This analysis is dependent on obtaining reliable metaphase preparations and greatly underrepresents the extent of DNA alterations in these infrequently dividing cell populations. By interphase fluorescence *in situ* hybridization (FISH) analysis, two studies report that at least one chromosome is trisomic in 96% or 89% of MM tumor samples, respectively.[118,119] Although conventional karyotypes are not routinely reported for MGUS, it appears that a substantial fraction of MGUS plasma cells are aneuploid as well. By FISH analysis, the incidence of trisomy for at least one chromosome was 43% and 53% in two studies of MGUS cells; in the former, 61% of the cells had an aneuploid DNA content by image analysis.[118,120] The characteristic numerical abnormalities are monosomy 13 and trisomies of chromosomes 3, 5, 7, 9, 11, 15, and 19. Nonrandom structural abnormalities most frequently involve chromosome 1 with no apparent locus specificity; 14q32(IgH) locus occurs in 20–40%; 11q13(bcl-1 locus) in about 20%, but mostly translocated to 14q32; 13q14 interstitial deletion in 15%; and 8q24 in about 10%, with about half of these involved in a translocation. Importantly, a recent report documents similar translocations in MGUS and MM, including t(4;14)(p16.3;q32) and t(14;16)(q32;q23), without any obvious clinical or biologic correlation.[121]

The hallmark genetic lesion in many B-lymphocyte tumors involves dysregulation of an oncogene as a consequence of a translocation involving the IgH locus (14q32.3); less frequently, variant translocations involve one of the IgL loci (2p12, kappa or 22q11, lambda) (Tables 3 and 4). From conventional karyotypic

analyses, translocations involving 14q32 appear to occur in about 20–40% of MM with an abnormal karyotype.[123] The incidence of these translocations is significantly higher in the extramedullary phase of the disease and in cell lines, perhaps because of a higher number of metaphase spreads that are examined. In about 30% of these translocations, the partner chromosomal locus is 11q13 (bcl-1, cyclin D1), but in most cases, the partner is not identified (14q32+). Transcriptional activation of cyclin D1 has recently been confirmed in some primary tumors, as has cyclin D3 activation associated with t(6;14)(p21;q32) translocation.[121,124,125] Other recurrent partner loci have been identified infrequently, including 8q24(c-myc) in <5%, 18q21(bcl-2), 11q23(MLL-1), and 6p21.1. By combining conventional karyotypic analysis with a comprehensive Southern blot assay, which detects translocations involving IgH switch regions, it has become apparent that most MM cell lines and one primary tumor fully examined have IgH translocations that mainly involve IgH switch regions.[43,126] Recent FISH studies have also shown that IGH gene rearrangements are present in 73% of MM patients.[127] The apparent oncogene dysregulated by t(4;14) is the fibroblast growth factor receptor 3 (*FGFR3*) gene, and it is possible that dysregulated expression of *FGFR3*, as a result of t(4;14), receives an *FGFR3*-mediated signal from FGF produced by stromal cells in the BM microenvironment.[128] In addition to *FGFR3*, the t(4;14) translocation in MM regulates a novel gene, *MMSET*, resulting in IgH/MMSET hybrid transcripts.[129] Ectopic expression of *FGFR3* promotes MM cell proliferation and prevents apoptosis, and its oncogenic potential has been tested in a murine model, confirming its capacity to transform hematopoietic cells.[130,131] Finally, there is evidence that elevated expression of c-myc and selective expression of one c-myc allele may occur frequently in MM, even though structural genetic changes near c-myc have been identified in only 10–20% of tumors.

Ras mutations occur in about 39% of newly diagnosed MM patients, and the frequency of ras mutations increase with disease progression. Mutations of N- and K-ras are rarely detected in solitary plasmacytoma and MGUS, but occur more frequently in MM (9–30%) and in the majority of terminal disease or PCL patients (63–70%).[132,133] Activating mutations of the ras oncogenes may also result in growth factor independence and suppression of apoptosis in MM.

Although translocation (14;18) occurs at a low frequency (0–15%) in MM, an overexpression of Bcl-2 is seen in the majority of MM patients and in MM cell lines.[134,135] High levels of Bcl-2 protein are likely to mediate the resistance of MM cells to apoptosis induced by IL-6 deprivation, staurosporine, or other drugs.[136] In a murine MM cell line, Bcl-XL showed a predominant role in preventing apoptosis in response to cycloheximide treatment or IL-6 withdrawal.[137] Similarly, overexpression of Bcl-2 or Bcl-XL could prevent apoptosis induced by IL-6 withdrawal in the B-9 IL-6-dependent cell line.[138] Mcl-1 is overexpressed in MM cells,

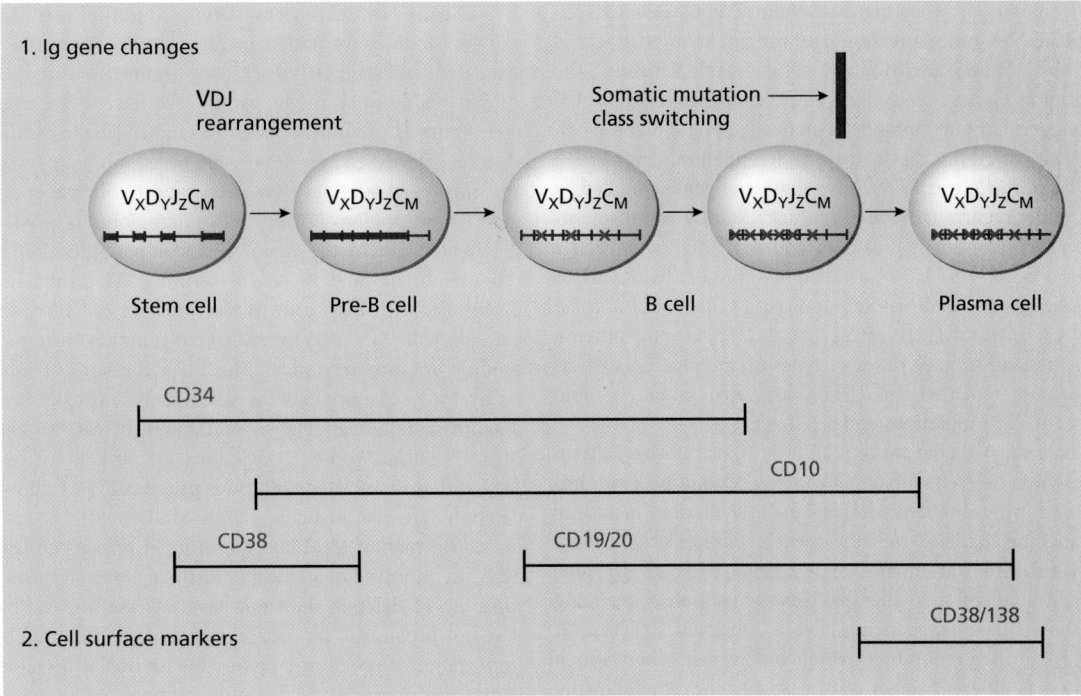

Figure 5 Apoptotic signaling pathways. Source: Adapted from Hideshima et al. 2014.[139]

upregulated by IL-6, and mediates potent resistance to apoptosis, whereas Mcl-1 downregulation triggers apoptosis (Figure 5).[140]

Chromosome 13 deletions are present in over 50% of MM and are associated with poor prognosis.[121,141–143] However, these deletions are also associated with MGUS, and their role in transformation to MM is therefore at present undefined.[121,144,145]

Recent understanding of the molecular pathogenesis of MM has resulted in a new proposed classification of MM.[146,147] Majority of MM tumors have chromosomal abnormalities and are broadly classified into hyperdiploid (HRD) or nonhyperdiploid (NHRD) tumors. Nearly half of MM tumors are HRD, the remaining being categorized as NHRD, which includes tumors that are hypodiploid, pseudodiploid, or subtetraploid. These NHRD tumors have been associated with a poorer prognosis. Five recurrent IgH translocations have been seen in MM including MMSET and FGFR3 (15%), cyclin D3 (3%), cyclin D1 (15%), c-maf (5%), and MAFB (2%) accounting for a prevalence of 40%. Recent evidence suggests that three of these five translocations are predominant in the NHRD tumors.

Deletions of chromosome 17p involving the *TP53* locus are rare in newly diagnosed myeloma (5–10%), but more common in relapsed and refractory cases (20–40%), and are associated with a negative prognosis.[148,149] Regimens containing bortezomib can however overcome this unfavorable prognosis, as shown by the HOVON-65/GMMG-HD4 trial.[150] 1q21 amplification is detected by FISH in about 40% of newly diagnosed and 70% of relapsed myeloma. It can negatively impact overall survival (OS). Possible downstream target genes include *CKS1B*, a protein that regulates cyclin-dependent protein kinases, *PSMD4*, a proteasome subunit modulating response to bortezomib treatment, *MCL1* and *BCL9*.[151–153] In addition, deletions of 1p, present in 7–40% of patients, are linked to reduced PFS (progression-free survival) and OS despite autologous stem-cell transplant.[154–156] *FAM46C* loss or *FAM46C* mutations (evident in 15% of patients) are especially associated with shortened survival (median OS 25.7 months vs 51.3 months, $P = 0.004$).[156,157] The biologic function of FAM46C is unknown, but possibly related to mRNA stabilization. Other abnormalities include *MYC* rearrangements involving unbalanced translocations and insertions, small duplications, amplifications, and inversions on chromosome 8p24[158–161]; homozygous deletions of 11q22 locus resulting in loss of *YAP1*, *BIRC3*, and *BIRC2* genomic region[162–164]; chromosome 4, 14, and 16 aberrations, disrupting *FGFR3*, *WWOX*, and *CYLD*; and deletions or amplifications of chromosome 6 and homozygous deletions of Xp11.2 locus,[165,166] involving *UTX*, a histone H3 lysine 27 (H3K27) demethylase mutated in 10% myeloma.[157,167]

With the advent of cDNA microarrays, an expeditious and comprehensive gene expression profiling is possible to better define disease biology, highlight prognostic factors, and identify potential targets for novel therapies.[124,168] These studies may also identify mechanisms of sensitivity versus resistance to conventional and novel MM therapies.[169,170] Known target antigens likely represent only the tip of the iceberg. Most recently, array comparative genomic hybridization (aCGH) has been correlated with gene profiling to identify chromosomal amplifications and transcript overexpression, respectively.[165] Classical overexpression and knockdown experiments may be done first in cancer models and then in MM models to identify potential novel targets for monoclonal antibody (cell surface) or small molecule inhibitor (intracellular) therapies.

Somatic mutations and interclonal diversity
MM is often preceded by MGUS or smoldering myeloma transforming to overt myeloma,[171,172] characterized by accumulation of mutations conferring growth advantage (driver mutations) or functionally irrelevant mutations (passenger mutations). To date, more than 300 myeloma patient DNA samples have been sequenced using whole-genome-sequencing or whole-exome sequencing approaches.[157,173,174] Frequently mutated genes include *KRAS*, *NRAS*, *FAM46C*, *DIS3*, and *TP53*. Other significant genes are *BRAF* (4% of patients), *TRAF3*, *CYLD*, *RB1*, *PRDM1*, and *ACTG1*. *TRAF3*

and *CYLD* mutations, together with homozygous deletions in *BIRC2/BIRC3*, NIK overexpression, and mutations in other genes (*CARD11* and *MYD88*) contribute to constitutively activating the NF-κB pathway. Genes involved in protein homeostasis, unfolded protein response, or lymphoid/plasma-cell development, such as *PRDM1* involved in plasmacytic differentiation, and *XBP1*, *IRF4*, *LRRK2*, *SP140*, and *LTB* form a cluster of genes mutated in myeloma. Other recurrent mutated genes are *ROBO1*, a transmembrane receptor involved in β-catenin and MET signaling, *EGR1* transcription factor, *FAT3*, a transmembrane protein belonging to cadherin superfamily, and histone-modifying genes (*MLL*, *MLL2*, *MLL3*, *WHSC1/MMSET*, *WHSC1L1*, and *UTX* among others). -PCL patients tend to have different types of aberrancies, such as p14ARF promoter methylation, *PTEN* loss, *RB1* mutations, and higher rates of *TP53* mutations and deletions.[175]

Recent data supports the concept of intratumor heterogeneity in myeloma, where different subclones can emerge and become predominant following different mechanisms of evolution, including linear, branching, parallel, or convergent evolution.[173,176] Clonal diversity similar to Darwinian-like selection favors cancer progression and adaptation to therapy. Next-generation sequencing analyses show that most patients have a subclonal structure at diagnosis, with one predominant clone and several others which can reappear at different stages of disease evolution or following treatment.[173,177,178]

Prognostic factors

Multiple attempts have been made to define clinical and laboratory parameters that have prognostic significance.[7,179–181] The Durie–Salmon system was historically utilized (Table 5).[7] Tumor cell mass for patients in stage I is low at $<0.6 \times 10^{12}$ cells/m², intermediate for patients with stage II disease at 0.6 to 1.2×10^{12} cells/m², and high for patients with stage III disease with $>1.2 \times$ 10^{12} cells/m². In this system, survival duration is 61.2, 54.5, 30.1, and 14.7 months for patients with stage IA, stage IB + IIA + IIB, stage IIIA, and stage IIIB disease, respectively.

Many additional single parameters have been examined for their value as prognostic features. Higher labeling indices, serum IL-6 receptor levels, more ras mutations, more aggressive disease, and shortened survival have been reported in patients with plasmablast morphology.[182] Serum β_2 microglobulin (β2M) represents the light chain of the major histocompatibility complex of the cell membrane, and increased serum β2M results from release by tumors with high growth fraction and cell turnover rates. In patients with MM and normal renal function, rising serum β2M predicts for progression.[183] The LI, a measure of DNA synthesis by MM cells, predicts for survival. It is usually low (<1%) at diagnosis, higher at relapse, and lower in MGUS and indolent MM.[184] Chromosome 13 deletions are present in over 50% of MM and are associated with poor prognosis[141–143]; however, these deletions are also associated with MGUS,[121,144,145] and their role in transformation to MM is therefore at present undefined. HRD MM has improved outcome and distinct clinical features, and chromosome 13 deletion does not have adverse impact.[185] Moreover, it is not prognostic for response to bortezomib, highlighting the importance of prognostic factors for particular therapies.[186] Gene expression profiling will not only define disease pathogenesis but also identify both novel prognostic factors and potential therapeutic targets.[124,130] These studies will also identify mechanisms of sensitivity versus resistance to conventional and novel MM therapies.[169,170] Cyclin D dysregulation has been identified as an early and unifying event in MM. Using gene expression profiling to identify five recurrent translocations, specific trisomies, and expression of cyclin D2 genes, MM can prognostically be divided into eight TC (translocation/cyclin D) groups.[187] Additional molecular classifications have been proposed,[188] with high-risk myeloma defined by deregulated expression of genes mapping to

Table 5 Durie–Salmon staging system and international staging system.

Stage	Durie–Salmon stage	ISS stage	Overall survival by ISS stage

I	All of the following:
	• Hemoglobin value >10 g/dL
	• Serum calcium value normal or ≤12 mg/dL
	• Bone X-ray, 0–1 lesion or solitary bone plasmacytoma only
	• Low M-component production rate:
	  ° IgG value <5 g/dL
	  ° IgA value <3 g/dL
	  ° Urine light-chain M-component on electrophoresis < 4 g/24 h
		Serum β2 microglobulin <3.5 mg/L
		and
		Serum albumin ≥3.5 g/dL
			62 months

II	Neither stage I nor stage III	Serum β2-microglobulin <3.5 mg/L, but serum albumin <3.5 g/dL or Serum β2-microglobulin 3.5 to <5.5 mg/L, irrespective of serum albumin	44 months

III	One or more of the following:
	• Hemoglobin value <8.5 g/dL
	• Serum calcium value >12 mg/dL
	• Advanced lytic bone lesions (≥3 lesions)
	• High M-component production rate
	  ° IgG value >7 g/dL
	  ° IgA value >5 g/dL
	  ° Urine light-chain M-component >12 g/24 h
		Serum β2-microglobulin ≥5.5 mg/L	29 months

Source: Durie and Salmon 1975[7] and Greipp et al.[181]

chromosome 1.[189] Most recently, the first DNA-based classification scheme has been proposed to predict outcome to high-dose therapy (HDT).[165]

Serum IL-6 levels in some studies appear to correlate both with stage of disease and survival.[190,191] IL-6 stimulates hepatocytes to produce acute phase proteins, such as CRP; CRP therefore may reflect the IL-6 level and proliferative status of BM plasma cells. Indeed, CRP levels are significantly lower in patients with MGUS than in those with MM, and survival can be correlated with serum CRP level.[192] High serum soluble interleukin-6 receptor (sIL-6R),[193] hepatocyte growth factor,[194] and syndecan-1[195] levels, as well as low serum hyaluronate levels,[196] are independent prognostic factors predicting poor outcome. The percentage of circulating plasma cells in peripheral blood and their labeling indices are independent prognostic factors for survival in MM after both conventional and HDT.[197,198] Circulating endothelial cells also correlate with disease course and response to thalidomide.[199] Finally, circulating proteasome levels are an independent prognostic factor for survival.[200]

Many of these factors are interrelated and, therefore, of limited independent value. Using multivariate analysis, several groups have found that the best combination of variables to predict outcome was serum β2M, reflecting both the tumor burden and the renal function; and the proliferative activity of plasma cells, evaluated by the LI or number of tumor cells in S-phase. Age and performance status also improves the prognostic assessment.[201,202] An international staging system (ISS) based on serum β2M and albumin has provided a three-stage ISS (Table 5), which is currently the most commonly used staging system and in reporting for clinical trials.[181]

Complications

Complications of MM include bone disease and hypercalcemia, hyperviscosity, recurrent infections, renal failure, and cardiac dysfunction.

Bone disease and hypercalcemia

The presence of osteolytic bone lesions, bone pain, increased risk of pathological fractures, or generalized bone loss (or osteoporosis) is a well-defined feature of myeloma.[203] Myeloma bone disease is characterized by an imbalance between osteoblast and osteoclast activities, with suppression of bone formation by osteoblasts and uncoupled activation of osteoclasts (Figure 6).[204,205] The ligand for receptor activator of NFκB (RANKL) binds to RANK receptor to stimulate osteoclast differentiation, formation, and survival[206]; myeloma cells produce RANKL and upregulate RANKL expression in BMSCs and osteoblasts via direct contact, signal induction,[207–209] or production of IL-7. Moreover, they promote suppression of osteoprotegerin (OPG),[210–212] a decoy receptor that normally prevents RANK–RANKL interaction[213] via soluble factors, integrin $\alpha_4\beta_1$-VCAM1 interaction,[214] production of DKK1,[215] or inactivation by syndecan-mediated internalization into myeloma cells.[216] Interestingly, OPG levels are decreased in the serum of myeloma patients and correlate with the presence of lytic bone lesions[217]; a high RANKL/OPG ratio is associated with a poor prognosis.[218] Recombinant OPG constructs, soluble RANK, OPG peptidomimetics,[211,213,219] and, more recently, an anti-RANKL antibody, denosumab,[220] have been developed to modulate RANKL/OPG axis and reduce osteoclast activity in myeloma. MIP-1α, or chemokine C–C motif ligand, is also produced by myeloma cells and promotes maturation of precursor cells into osteoclasts; MIP-1α signals via CCR1 and CCR5 on osteoclasts

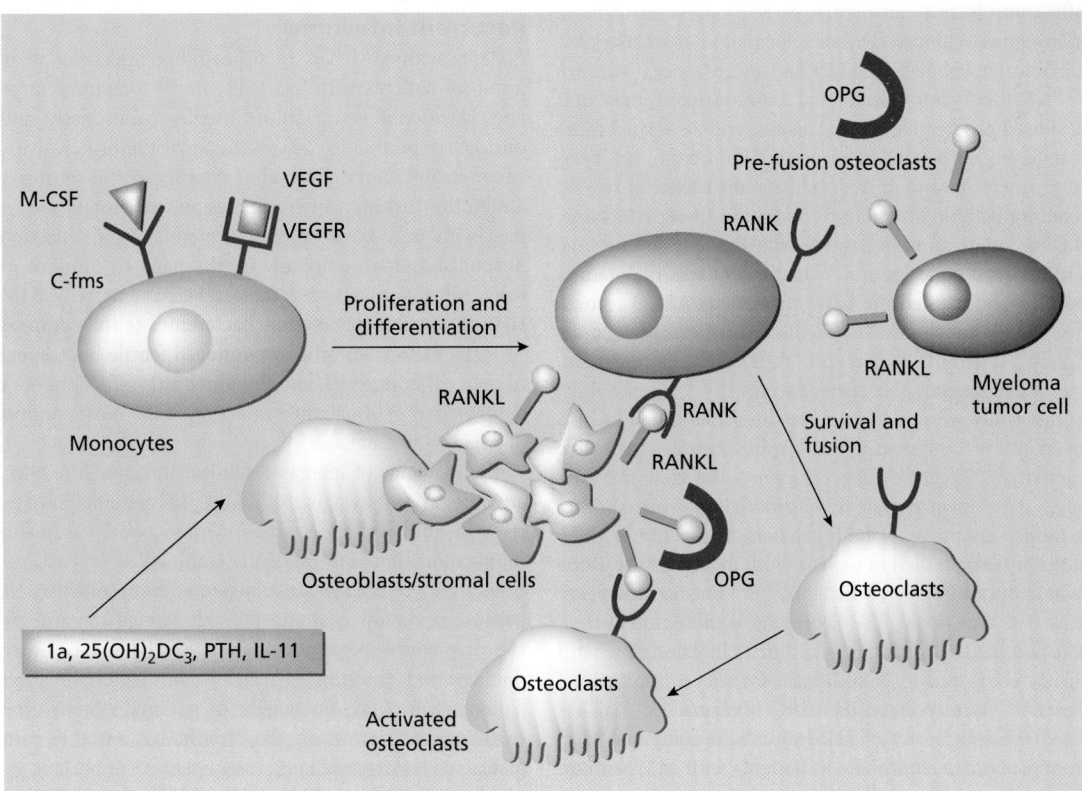

Figure 6 Osteoclastogenesis.

and can further upregulate RANKL in stromal cells.[96,221,222] MIP-1α levels are elevated in myeloma patients,[223] while MIP-1α silencing or blockade of CCR1 reduces bone disease in in vitro or animal models.[96] IL-6,[224] PTHrP,[225,226] annexin II,[227] and ephrinB2/EphB4 axis[228] also promote bone resorption. Osteoblast suppression is another major player in myeloma bone disease: WNT signaling antagonists, including DKK1, frizzled related protein-2 (FRP-2),[229] and sclerostin (SOST),[230] interfere with osteoblast maturation. DKK1 is expressed by myeloma cells and can upregulate RANKL levels in osteoblasts, increasing osteoclast activity.[103,231] DKK1 levels are increased in the serum of myeloma patients,[232] and anti-DKK1 antibodies have been tested in animal studies[233–235] and are currently being studied in clinical trials. Finally, high levels of activin A, a member of TGF-β superfamily, IL-3, and IL-7 via RUNX2/CBFA1 blockade can inhibit bone formation and promote bone reabsorption. Furthermore, the bone niche itself supports myeloma cell survival and prevents TNF-α-mediated apoptosis.[236]

Treatment

Bisphosphonates play a key role in the supportive management of MM by not only blocking osteoclasts and modulate osteoblasts but also have an effect on tumor burden[237]; a similar response is reported with OPG peptidomimetics and RANKL constructs in in vivo xenograft models.[238] Bisphosphonates, especially zoledronic acid, are currently used in the clinic to reduce bone disease,[239,240] but are also associated with an increase in OS when compared to placebo based on a recent meta-analysis.[241] Markers of bone resorption and formation correlate with the extent of osteolytic disease.[242] Specifically, urine levels of pyridinoline (PYD) and deoxypyridinoline (DPD) cross-links and serum levels of tartrate-resistant acid phosphatase isoform 5b (TRACP-5b), a resorption marker only produced by activated osteoclasts and of collagen degradation products, including the N-terminal cross-linking telopeptide of type I collagen (NTX) are elevated in myeloma patients compared with healthy controls and can predict early progression of bone disease in myeloma. Conversely, bone formation markers, such as bone alkaline phosphatase (bALP) and osteocalcin (OC), are reduced.[242] Another randomized trial demonstrated that oral clodronate slowed progressive skeletal disease and associated morbidity but achieved no benefit in survival. Pamidronate has been shown in a prospective randomized trial to reduce skeletal-related events, including pathologic fractures, radiation therapy to bone, and spinal cord compression in patients with Durie–Salmon stage III MM and ≥1 lytic bone lesion.[243] This benefit was maintained until 21 months and formed the basis of previous ASCO recommendations, suggesting that MM patients remain on intravenous bisphosphonates indefinitely to reduce skeletal events and pain, regardless of their response to chemotherapy.[244,245] Interestingly, patients in this study who had failed first-line chemotherapy also had improved survival, suggesting that bisphosphonates may have anti-MM activity.[246] Recent evidence supports the view that bisphosphonates may downregulate IL-6 production from BMSCs as well as induce apoptosis of both osteoclasts and tumor cells. Pamidronate has been studied in patients with indolent MM. Bone turnover was reduced in treated patients,[247,248] but no significant antitumor activity was noted.[249] Zoledronate is more potent than pamidronate and has the advantage of a shorter infusion time with similar efficacy compared to pamidronate for preventing skeletal related events.[250] More recently, the MRC Myeloma IX trial has demonstrated the superiority of zoledronic acid compared with the oral bisphosphonate clodronate in patients with MM with an OS benefit favoring zoledronic acid.[251] A word of caution should however be exercised with the use of bisphosphonate therapy because of reported cases of osteonecrosis of the jaw.[252–254] This newly recognized complication in a small percentage of patients led ASCO to update their guidelines and now recommend discontinuing bisphosphonates after 2 years in patients with very good partial response (VGPR) or better and continuing if response is partial response (PR) or less.[255] Other supportive care measures such as vertebroplasty or kyphoplasty can restore supine stability and relieve pain for patients with localized disease.[256,257]

The treatment of hypercalcemia consists of treatment of the underlying MM, as well as inhibition of osteoclastic bone resorption with corticosteroids, calcitonin, and/or bisphosphonates. Corticosteroids may impair formation of new osteoclasts. Calcitonin and corticosteroids are almost always effective for the short term and useful even in the setting of renal failure. Bisphosphonates bind to the bone surface and inhibit osteoclast activity, and they constitute a mainstay of treatment. Therapeutic recommendations therefore include initial cytotoxic therapy for MM, saline hydration, and bisphosphonate therapy, with the use of calcitonin for nonresponders to these first-line treatments. In a randomized trial of 287 patients with hypercalcemia of malignancy, zoledronate was found to be superior to pamidronate.[258] Hypercalcemia may also be compounded by patient immobility because of bone pain or other reasons.

Hyperviscosity

Hyperviscosity is characterized clinically by spontaneous bleeding with neurologic and ocular disorders. Hyperviscosity occurred in 4.2% of 238 patients with IgG MM and in 22% of 46 patients with serum IgG M components >5.0 g/dL.[259] The IgG3 subclass produces hyperviscosity at lower levels than other IgG paraproteins.[260] The severity of the syndrome is not directly related to the serum viscosity. Clinical findings improve with plasmapheresis, which reduces both MM protein concentration and serum viscosity.

Recurrent infections

Patients with MM had 15 times more infections than a control group of patients with heart disease.[261] *Streptococcus pneumoniae* and Haemophilus infections usually occur early and typically during response to chemotherapy. Gram-negative infections occur in refractory, advancing disease; in the setting of previous antibiotic therapy; instrumentation; immobilization; colonization with hospital flora; and azotemia. Fatal infections may be hospital-acquired, emphasizing the need to minimize indwelling foreign bodies such as catheters in patients with MM. There is lack of correlation between bacteremia (either gram-negative or -positive) and chemotherapy-induced febrile neutropenia. Fungal, herpes, mycobacterial, and Pneumocystis infections are only rarely described in MM patients. Infection is the most common cause of death (20–50% of cases).[26]

The evidence of increased clinical infections in MM has led to attempts at prophylaxis. Although MM patients have normal-fold rises in antibody titers after pneumococcal vaccination, preimmunization titers are markedly diminished.[262] Postimmunization titers are therefore low and considered nonprotective. Nonetheless, because of its low cost and possible benefit to some patients, the use of pneumococcal vaccination has been recommended. In a double-blind randomized trial of gammaglobulin prophylaxis in patients with MM, no benefit of gammaglobulin prophylaxis at reducing infection was noted,[263] although a trial in patients in the plateau phase suggested possible benefit.[264] At present, gammaglobulin is reserved for those patients with recurrent or life-threatening infections and hypogammglobulinemia.

Renal failure

Renal failure in MM can predict for adverse outcome. One series found that 22% of patients had a serum creatinine ≥ 2 mg/dL at diagnosis; renal function normalized with treatment in 48% of those with creatinine <4 mg/dL.[265] The causes of renal failure in MM are often multifactorial and include hypercalcemia; MM kidney, with distal and proximal tubules obstructed by large, laminated casts containing albumin, IgG, and κ and λ light chains surrounded by giant cells; hyperuricemia; toxicity from intravenous contrast; dehydration; plasma-cell infiltration; pyelonephritis; and amyloidosis. The most important predisposing factor is dehydration; aggressive hydration is therefore crucial to avoid irreversible renal dysfunction. Otherwise, treatment is for the underlying disease, along with avoidance of intravenous contrast. The type and quantity of proteinuria can distinguish MM kidney, with larger amounts of light chains and less albuminuria; light-chain deposition disease, characterized by low levels of both light chains and albumin in urine; and amyloidosis, in which large amounts of albuminuria and less light-chain proteinuria occur.[266]

The renal manifestations associated with the production of monoclonal light chains in MM, light-chain deposition disease, and amyloidosis result from the deposition of certain Bence Jones proteins (BJP) as tubular casts, basement-membrane precipitates, or fibrils, respectively.[267–269] For unknown reasons, the severity of the renal manifestations varies greatly from patient to patient. BJP from 40 patients were injected into mice and 26 (65%) were deposited in mouse kidneys as tubular casts, basement-membrane precipitates, or crystals in a pattern similar to those noted in patients.[269] This experimental model has potential value for the identification and differentiation of nephrotoxic or amyloidogenic light chains. The development of progressive kidney damage and MM kidney has been demonstrated in IL-6 transgenic mice, shedding additional insight into the role of IL-6 in the pathogenesis of MM.[270]

Cardiac failure

The mean and median age of patients with MM is approximately 60 years, and affected patients are also frequently at risk of cardiovascular disease. However, patients can be uniquely susceptible to cardiac ischemia and/or congestive heart failure (CHF) because of myocardial infiltration with amyloid, causing dilated or restricted cardiomyopathy, hyperviscosity syndrome, and/or anemia. Rarely, MM patients are also susceptible to high output CHF,[271] mainly in patients with extensive bone disease.[272] This has been attributed to arteriovenous shunting in bone lesions.[273]

Anemia

Anemia in MM can be due to a number of factors, including tumor infiltration of the BM, renal impairment, the myelosuppressive effects of chemotherapy, and a deficient production of erythropoietin (EPO) relative to the degree of anemia. Pilot studies demonstrated efficacy of exogenous EPO administration in MM.[274–276] Osterborg et al.[277] have carried out a randomized study of EPO therapy at 10,000 U/d, a titrated dose of EPO starting with 2000 U/d and escalating stepwise until response, or no EPO for 24 weeks; response was defined as an increase in Hb > 2g/dL and elimination of transfusion need. Sixty percent of EPO-treated groups responded, 72% of those with low EPO levels, and only 20% of those with normal EPO levels. 10,000 units SC three times weekly was the optimal starting dosage, although more recently 40,000 units SC once weekly is a commonly used approach. However, erythropoiesis-stimulating agents such as EPO and darbepoietin are restricted under a risk evaluation and mitigation strategy (REMS) program owing to several trials showing increase in thrombotic risk and adverse effects on survival with these drugs (though this risk has not been as well demonstrated in MM compared to solid tumors).[278,279]

Neuropathies

A variety of malignant and paraproteinemic disorders can be associated with neuropathies.[280] In MM, a symmetric, distal sensory, or sensorimotor neuropathy is most common and is associated with axonal degeneration, with or without amyloid deposition; there is no specific therapy. In some cases, this is associated with monoclonal antibodies directed against peripheral nerve myelin.[281]

Associated diseases

MM has been described in association with both hematologic disorders and solid tumors. Acute leukemia either is induced by leukemogens, such as radiation and alkylating agents, or is part of the natural history of MM. The mean interval from diagnosis of MM to occurrence of acute leukemia is 60 (17–147) months, consistent with either possibility. The occurrence of acute leukemia in untreated MM patients suggests that it may be part of the natural history of the disease.[282] Furthermore, acute leukemia has been reported in 6 of 125 (4.8%) MM patients treated with alkylating agents, which is significantly higher than the incidence of acute leukemia in ovarian cancer patients treated with irradiation and alkylators.[25] Actuarial risk of leukemia in MM patients treated with melphalan and prednisone (MP) or with melphalan, cyclophosphamide, carmustine, and prednisone has been reported to be as high as 17.4% at 50 months from initiation of therapy.[283] Gonzalez et al.[282] described 11 of 476 patients with MM who developed myeloid leukemia or sideroblastic anemia. All had received melphalan–prednisone for a median of 3 years and had major cytogenetic abnormalities. This study suggests that leukemia is predominantly treatment related. Finally, in 628 patients with MM, the incidence and diversity of solid tumors were similar to those observed in otherwise healthy persons of the same age.[284]

Treatment

While MM is not considered curable, its treatments are very effective and very well tolerated, including in the older patient population. The adoption of high-dose melphalan with autologous stem-cell transplant and the introduction of two new drug classes—IMiDs such as lenalidomide and proteasome inhibitors such as bortezomib—have resulted in dramatic improvements in outcomes. A retrospective study comparing patients diagnosed in 1997 and later to those diagnosed before 1997 found a significant improvement in OS, 44.8 months versus 29.9 months, respectively.[285]

An area of active investigation is when to initiate treatment for patients with MM. There is uniform consensus recommending treatment for active MM as defined by the presence of one of the CRAB criteria of end organ involvement.[6] For patients who are asymptomatic, that is, with smoldering MM, the current paradigm recommends close observation. However, the availability of well-tolerated, effective myeloma therapy has now motivated studies examining treatment earlier in the disease, before the onset of symptoms. Recently, the Spanish myeloma group conducted a randomized study of active treatment with lenalidomide and dexamethasone v. observation in patients with high-risk smoldering MM.[286] High risk was defined by the presence of both BM involvement and elevated serum monoclonal protein or flow cytometry criteria and suppressed immunoglobulins (immunoparesis). The study found that 3-year OS was superior in the group undergoing active treatment, 94% versus 80%, and this was the first time this type of benefit was seen in a smoldering MM trial. These results suggest that earlier initiation of therapy may be helpful, and the generalizability of these findings awaits confirmation in further trials as well as identifying the specific patients who are most likely to benefit from early initiation of treatment. Additional strategies in smoldering MM include vaccines, such as with PVX-410, a multipeptide vaccine designed to elicit an immune response against MM cells. This vaccine targets XBP1, CD138, and CS1, which are proteins high expressed in MM cells and involved in MM pathogenesis.[287] PVX-410 is currently in phase I clinical trials and in combination with lenalidomide in order to enhance of the immune response (NCT01718899).[288]

Patients undergoing therapy for MM should have clinical and laboratory assessments to assure both safety and efficacy of treatment. Monoclonal protein in the serum and/or urine should be measured by immunoelectrophoresis and more sensitive immunofixation techniques as well as serum FLCs. The serum FLC assay allows for diagnosis and assessment of patients previously thought to have oligosecretory or nonsecretory disease.[289] A skeletal survey should be done annually, with BM examination reserved for diagnosis and time of subsequent change in clinical status, monoclonal Ig, or hemogram. It is important to remember that reduction of serum or urine M component as objective evidence of tumor response could reflect increased protein catabolism, decreased protein production, or both. Moreover, non-M protein-secreting MM clones may emerge during treatment, so that even a marked reduction in monoclonal Ig may not correlate with decrease in tumor burden.

The Bladé criteria to assess response post-transplant were developed for the European Group for Blood and Marrow Transplant (EBMT), the International BM Transplant Registry (IBMTR), and the Autologous Blood and Marrow Transplant Registry (ABMTR).[290] These criteria include a more sensitive and rigorous definition of complete response (CR), including the absence of paraprotein assayed by immunofixation, and excludes transient responses. More recently, serum free light chain assays have been incorporated into response criteria[291–293] and the IMWG response criteria are now universally used (Table 6). Stricter definitions of complete remission resulted in the inclusion of a category of stringent complete remission in which monoclonal plasma cells are not detectable in the marrow by immunohistochemistry or immunofluorescence and the free light-chain ratio is normal. The previously used near complete remission (only positivity by serum monoclonal immunoglobulin immunofixation) is now included in the new category VGPR and the previously used minor response category was eliminated. Limitations of the new criteria are that response calls are determined by monoclonal immunoglobulin and marrow evaluation. Dynamic changes in skeletal events readily identified by modern imaging techniques such as MRI and FDG PET CT are excluded from response assessments.

Sequencing-based platforms, quantitative PCR (polymerase chain reaction), and multiparametric flow cytometry are now being employed to detect minimal residual disease (MRD) in patients attaining at least a VGPR after primary therapy that may be of significant prognostic value. Martinez-Lopez et al. recently reported the results of sequencing-based BM evaluations on 133 patients in VGPR or better following primary therapy. In patients achieving a CR, the TTP (time to progression) was 131 months for MRD negative patients versus 35 months for MRD positive patients. When stratified by level of MRD, the respective TTP medians were 27

Table 6 Uniform response criteria from the international myeloma working group.

Response subcategory[a]	Response criteria
CR	Negative immunofixation of the serum and urine and disappearance of any soft-tissue plasmacytomas and <5% plasma cells in marrow[b]
sCR	CR as defined above plus Normal FLC ratio and Absence of clonal cells in marrow[b] by immunohistochemistry or immunofluorescence[c]
VGPR	Serum and urine M-protein detectable by immunofixation but not on electrophoresis or 90% or greater reduction in serum M-protein plus urine M-protein <100 mg/24 h
PR	≥50% reduction of serum M-protein and reduction in 24-h urinary M-protein by ≥90% or to <200 mg/24 h
	If the serum and urine M-protein are unmeasurable, ≥50% decrease in the difference between involved and uninvolved FLC levels is required in place of the M-protein criteria
	If serum and urine M-protein are unmeasurable, and serum-free light assay is also unmeasurable, ≥50% reduction in plasma cells is required in place of M-protein, provided baseline marrow plasma-cell percentage was ≥30%
	In addition to the above-listed criteria, if present at baseline, a ≥50% reduction in the size of soft-tissue plasmacytomas is also required
SD	Not meeting criteria for CR, VGPR, PR, or progressive disease

CR, complete response; FLC, free light chain; PR, partial response; sCR, stringent complete response; SD, stable disease; VGPR, very good partial response; M-protein, monoclonal protein.
[a]All response categories require two consecutive assessments made any time before the institution of any new therapy; complete and PR and SD categories also require no known evidence of progressive or new bone lesions if radiographic studies were performed. Radiographic studies are not required to satisfy these response requirements.
[b]Confirmation with repeat marrow biopsy not needed.
[c]Presence/absence of clonal cells is based on the κ/λ of >4:1 or <1:2. An abnormal κ/λ ratio by immunohistochemistry and/or immunofluorescence requires a minimum of 100 plasma cells for analysis.
Note: SD is not recommended for use as an indicator of response; stability of disease is best described by providing the time-to-progression estimates.
Source: Rajkumar et al. 2011.[294]

months for MRD ≥10^{-3}, 48 months for MRD 10^{-3} to 10^{-5}, and 80 months MRD <10^{-5} ($p = 0.003–0.0001$).[295] Although not currently a standard of care, MRD assessment may play an important role in evaluating disease response in the future.

Initial treatment

Oral administration of MP was historically considered a standard form of therapy that produces objective response in up to 50–60% of patients.[296,297] Multiple older studies have examined whether MP is as effective as combination chemotherapy (CCT) (generally with older agents such as vincristine and cyclophosphamide). In an attempt to determine which patients, if any, do better with more aggressive therapy, Gregory et al.[298] examined published reports of 18 randomized controlled trials comparing MP with CCT in the primary treatment of 3814 patients. The overall results suggested that there was no difference in efficacy between these treatment modalities. The studies with a high MP 2-year survival rate showed a survival difference in favor of MP, whereas those with a low rate suggested a difference in favor of CCT. These results imply that, rather than there being no difference between MP and CCT, MP is superior for patients with an intrinsically good prognosis and inferior for those patients with a poor prognosis.

Immunomodulatory drugs

The introduction of thalidomide, an IMiD, was the first in a series of improvements over the MP regimen. The incorporation of thalidomide in combination with MP (MPT, melphalan, prednisone, thalidomide) in newly diagnosed patients with myeloma over the age of 65 years[299] resulted in a 76% complete or PR rate compared to 47% in the MP arm. This translated into a doubling of the 2-year event-free survival (EFS) to 54% versus 27%. On the basis of these data, MPT was the standard of care for transplantation-ineligible patients. However, all studies showed an increase in adverse events in the MPT arm, including infections, neuropathy, and thromboembolism, suggesting that thromboprophylaxis and antimicrobial prophylaxis are required.[300] Melphalan, prednisone, and lenalidomide (MPR) is another effective regimen in this population. Palumbo et al. then went on to evaluate the efficacy and safety of induction therapy with MPR followed by lenalidomide maintenance therapy (MPR-R), as compared with MPR or MP without maintenance therapy, in patients with newly diagnosed MM who were ineligible for transplantation. At a median follow-up of 30 months, the median PFS was 31 months for MPR-R versus 14 months for MPR and 13 months for MP. This benefit was observed in patients 65–75 years of age but not older than 75. Response rates were superior for the lenalidomide-containing regimen 77% for MPR-R and 68% for MPR versus 5% with MP.[301]

Randomized trials with the use of other novel agents such as bortezomib with MP have proven benefits as well. For example, the VISTA trial compared the regimen of bortezomib, melphalan, and prednisone (VMP) MP in patients who were not candidates for autologous stem-cell transplant.[302] OS was significantly improved in the VMP group versus MP group, with 3-year OS of 68.5% versus 54%, respectively.[303]

Most recently, the FIRST trial, a randomized, phase III trial compared continuous lenalidomide with low-dose dexamethasone (Rd) against lenalidomide with low-dose dexamethasone for 18 cycles (Rd18) and MPT for 12 cycles.[304] Median PFS for continuous Rd was 25.5 months versus 20.7 for Rd18 and 21.2 for MPT. The OS at 4 years was 59.4% for Rd versus 55.7% for Rd18 and 51.4% for MPT. In the continuous Rd arm, the ORR was 75.1% (15.1% CR, 28.4% VGPR) versus 73.4 in Rd18 (Cr 14.2%, VGPR 28.5%) and 32.3% MPT (CR 9.3%, VGPR 18.8%). The safety profile with continuous Rd was manageable as hematologic and nonhematologic adverse events were as expected for Rd and MPT. Notably, the incidence of hematological second primary malignancies was lower with continuous Rd than MPT. In newly diagnosed transplant-ineligible patients, the FIRST trial established continuous Rd as the new standard of care. There are ongoing trials looking at three drug combinations including bortezomib, lenalidomide, and dexamethasone at reduced doses and attenuated schedules in this population as well (Table 7).

In the transplant-eligible patients, two studies combined thalidomide with dexamethasone as initial therapy for MM and achieved rapid responses in two-thirds of patients, allowing for successful harvesting of PBSCs for transplantation.[308,309] Thal/dex has been compared with VAD (vincristine, doxorubicin, dexamethasone) and with dex, as initial therapy for patients before collection of autologous stem cells and transplantation. In a case control analysis, Cavo et al.[310] showed that thal/dex achieved higher overall response rates, whereas a randomized phase III (EGOG) trial showed statistically significantly higher response rates for thal/dex than dex-treated patient cohorts.[311] This study provided the rationale for FDA (Food and Drug Administration) approval

Table 7 Novel agent induction for newly diagnosed transplant-ineligible patients.

Study	Regimen	Number of patients	Median follow-up (Mo)	Median OS (Mo)	Median PFS (Mo)
IFM 99-06[305]	MP	196	51.5	33.2	17.8
	MPT	125		51.6	27.5
	MEL100	126		38.3	19.4
IFM 01/01[306]	MPT	113	47.5	44	24.1
	MP	116		29.1	18.5
MM-015[305]	MPR-R	152	30	45.2	31
	MPR	153		NR	14
	MP	154		NR	13
VISTA[307]	VMP	344	60	56.4	N/A
	MP	338		43.1	N/A
FIRST[304]	Rd	536	37	59.4%[a]	25.5
	Rd18	541		55.7%	20.7
	MPT	547		51.4%	21.2

MP, melphalan, prednisone; MPT, melphalan, prednisone, thalidomide; MEL 100, melphalan 100 mg/m²; MPR, melphalan, prednisone, lenalidomide; MPR-R, melphalan, prednisone, lenalidomide induction followed by lenalidomide maintenance; VMP, bortezomib, melphalan, prednisone; Rd, lenalidomide, low-dose dexamethasone continuously; Rd18, lenalidomide, low-dose dexamethasone for 18 cycles; OS, overall survival; PFS, progression-free survival; NR, not reached.
[a]4-year OS.

of this regimen for initial treatment of MM. Moreover, early studies show 91% responses, including 6% complete and 32% near complete/VGPRs to lenalidomide combined with dex.[312] On the basis of these promising results, a phase III trial in the United States headed by ECOG investigated the role of len/dex in newly diagnosed MM. The study design allowed all patients to stay on-study for the first four cycles only for response assessment, after which patients could go off-study to proceed with stem-cell transplant. Safety data from this trial found that combining lenalidomide with the low-dose dexamethasone regimen was preferable to the combination with high-dose dexamethasone, with a reduction in grade 3 or higher nonhematologic adverse events (48% vs 65%), including thromboembolism (12% vs 26%), and infections (9% vs 16%) in the two treatment arms of the trial.[313,314] The low-dose dexamethasone-containing regimen did lead to an increased occurrence of grade ≥3 neutropenia (20% vs 12%). Importantly, the combination with low-dose dexamethasone had a survival benefit over combination with high-dose dexamethasone, with a 1-year OS of 96% and 87%, respectively.[313,314] Prophylaxis against clotting with aspirin, warfarin, or subcutaneous low molecular weight heparin is needed when patients are treated with lenalidomide.[315,316]

Proteasome inhibitors

Richardson et al.[317] examined single agent bortezomib and Jagannath et al.[318] tested bortezomib combined with dex as initial therapy; in both cases, high frequency and extent of response were noted. In a phase I/II trial, Richardson et al.[319] demonstrated the safety and efficacy of the combination of lenalidomide, bortezomib, and dexamethasone (RVD), which showed an unprecedented overall response rate of 100%. Building upon this work, the benefits of combination therapy with RVD as first-line therapy were seen in the results of two-phase II trials—the IFM 2008 trial and the EVOLUTION trial.[320,321] The ORR after induction in the IFM trial was 97% (13% sCR, 16% CR, and 54% ≥VGPR). The EVOLUTION trial was designed to compare RVD with CyBorD (cyclophosphamide, bortezomib, and dexamethasone) in a randomized, multicenter setting. The ORR for the RVD arm after primary treatment followed by maintenance with bortezomib for four 6-week cycles was 85% (24% CR, 51% ≥VGPR).

Table 8 Novel agent induction for newly diagnosed transplant-eligible patients.

Study	Regimen	Number of patients	Cr/nCR (%)	ORR (%)	Outcome
Rajkumar et al.[313]	RD	223	18	79	OS: 87% at 1 year
	Rd	222	14	68	OS: 96% at 1 year
Harousseau et al.[325]	VAD	121	6.4	62.8	PFS 30 months
	Bd	121	14.8	78.5	PFS: 36 months
Reeder et al.[326]	CyBorD	33	39	88	N/A
Richardson et al.[319]	RVD	66	39	100	OS 97% at 18-months
Jakubowiak et al.[323]	CRD	53	62	98	PFS 92% 24-months

RD, lenalidomide, high-dose dexamethasone; Rd, lenalidomide, low-dose dexamethasone; VAD, vincristine, doxorubicin, dexamethasone; Bd, bortezomib, low-dose dexamethasone; CyBorD, cyclophosphamide, bortezomib, dexamethasone; RVD, lenalidomide, velcade, dexamethasone; CRD, carfilzomib, lenalidomide, dexamethasone; OS, overall survival; PFS, progression-free survival; N/A, not available.

Carfilzomib is an epoxomicin analog second-generation proteasome inhibitor that binds to the 20S proteasome in a highly selective and irreversible manner. Given its approval in the treatment of relapsed disease, it is now being studied in the upfront setting.[322] In a dose escalation study conducted by Jakubowiak et al.,[323] the combination of carfilzomib, lenalidomide, and dexamethasone (CRD) has been evaluated where patients received carfilzomib (20, 27, or 36 mg/m^2, days 1, 2, 8, 9, 15, and 16 for 8 cycles then days 1, 2, 15, and 16) with lenalidomide 25 mg days 1–21 and dexamethasone 40 mg weekly cycles 1–4 then 20 mg weekly cycles 5–8 in 28-day cycles. After eight cycles, patients received the regimen every other week for eight cycles. After 24 cycles, maintenance with lenalidomide was recommended off-study. After a median of 12 cycles, 62% achieved at least a near-CR and 42% an sCR. 24-Month PFS was estimated at 92%. The toxicity profile was acceptable and notable for limited peripheral neuropathy.

Doublet and especially triplet regimens of novel drugs in combination with dexamethasone can induce complete remission rates comparable to transplantation regimens,[310,324] as described. Examples of modern regimens in use include doublet combinations of lenalidomide and dexamethasone and bortezomib and dexamethasone, as well as, the triple combination of RVD, CyBorD, and CRD (Table 8).

In patients where stem-cell collection is planned, combinations that include alkylating agents such as melphalan should be avoided as damage to normal hematopoietic stem cells can be incurred, which may render it impossible to collect stem cells for auto-HSCT. Lenalidomide may also hamper the collection of stem cells, although stem cell mobilization with growth factors and chemotherapy may overcome the myelosuppressive effects of lenalidomide.[327–330] The number of cycles of treatment, especially with lenalidomide-containing regimens, is limited to roughly four cycles, as additional cycles may compromise the ability to collect stem cells.[327,331]

Combination therapy with novel drugs achieves complete remission rates comparable to those obtained with auto-HSCT. This has led to the design of ongoing studies that compare novel agents followed by auto-HSCT with novel agents and then auto-HSCT in case of disease relapse. Novel agents seem to be able to overcome some of the cytogenetic adverse prognostic factors such as del 13, t(4;14), and del 17p. It is too early to abandon auto-HSCT as the follow-up

in clinical trials with new agents is too short to determine whether increased complete remission rates translate into durable remissions and EFS and OS. Complete remission rates as a surrogate marker for eventual outcome may prove to be inadequate. The DETERMINATION trial (NCT01208662) is an ongoing phase III, multicenter randomized trial of upfront high-dose melphalan with autologous stem-cell transplant versus transplant at relapse for myeloma patients up to age 65; all patients receive RVD as induction. This trial is designed to address this question of the role of autologous transplant, upfront or at time of relapse, in the context of novel drugs. It is likely that autologous transplant will add to the benefits noted with new drugs.

Radiation therapy

Radiation therapy for MM is used for treatment of localized disease, including plasmacytoma or spinal cord compression syndrome, and is frequently used for palliation. Hemibody radiation therapy has been utilized, either as a consolidation following induction CCT or as salvage therapy for chemotherapy-resistant MM.[332,333] Total body irradiation (TBI) has been used as a component of ablative therapy before hematopoietic stem-cell grafting but is rarely used as high-dose melphalan has equivalent efficacy and less toxicity.[334]

High-dose therapies

The rationale for the administration of alkylating agents (melphalan, cyclophosphamide, and busulfan) in a higher-than-conventional dose with or without TBI, followed by transplantation of syngeneic, allogeneic, and autologous BM or peripheral blood progenitor cells (PBPCs) is as follows: plasma-cell dyscrasias remain uniformly fatal; multiple studies document sensitivity of MM cells to chemotherapy and radiotherapy; and CRs can be obtained with HDT.

Autologous stem cell transplantation

High-dose chemoradiotherapy followed by transplantation of either autologous BM or PBPCs has also achieved high (40%) CR rates, but the median duration of these responses has unfortunately only been 24–36 months.[335,336] Patients with sensitive disease and who are less heavily pretreated have the most favorable outcomes. Most importantly, a national French trial of 200 patients with MM who received two courses of VMCP alternating with VBAP and were then randomized to receive either conventional chemotherapy (eight additional courses of VMCP/VBAP) or HDT (melphalan and TBI) followed by autologous BMT has demonstrated significantly higher response rates, EFS and OS for those patients treated with high dose compared to those receiving conventional therapy.[337] A second randomized trial in MM examined the relative merits of HDT either early versus late as salvage therapy for relapse after conventional therapy.[338] The OS was 64 months in both groups, but the quality-adjusted time without symptoms and toxicity (Q-TWIST) strongly favored the early transplant cohort. The United States Intergroup Trial supports this view.[339] The IFM has conducted a randomized trial comparing high-dose melphalan at 200 mg/m^2 versus melphalan at 140 mg/m^2 plus TBI as ablative therapies.[334] Although response rates and EFS were comparable, toxicity and OS were superior in the high-dose melphalan alone arm, suggesting that TBI should not be considered part of the ablation regimen. A Scandinavian population-based study demonstrated prolonged survival for patients with MM <60 years of age treated with intensive therapy compared with historical controls who received conventional therapy.[340] An additional randomized MRC trial confirmed a 12-month survival benefit in patients receiving high dose compared to conventional therapies.[341] Although these studies are encouraging, it is unlikely that patients are cured after a single

Table 9 Autologous transplantation versus conventional chemotherapy for newly diagnosed myeloma.

Author	Therapy	Patients (n)	CR (%)	EFS (median months)	OS (median months)
Barlogie et al.[342]	Conventional[a]	116	—	22	48
	HDT	123	40	49	62
Lenhoff et al.[340]	Conventional[a]	274	—	—	46% at 48
	HDT	274	34	27	61% at 48
Attal et al.[337]	Conventional	100	5	18	37
	HDT	100	22	27	52% at 60
Fermand et al.[338]	Conventional	96	—	18.7	50.4
	HDT	94	—	24.3	55.3
Blade et al.[343]	Conventional	83	11	34.3	66
	HDT	81	30	42.5	61
Child et al.[341]	Conventional	200	8.5	19.6	42.3
	HDT	201	44	31.6	54.1

CR, complete response; EFS, event free survival; HDT, high-dose therapy; OS, overall survival.

[a] Historical controls.

high dose and stem-cell autografting regimen. In all the studies, the median EFS was prolonged; in four of five studies, transplant led to higher CR rate; and in three of five trials OS was improved (Table 9).

Improving outcome of autografting

Attempts to improve the outcome of HDT followed by autografting include the use of autologous BM or PBPCs either depleted of tumor cells[344–346] or processed to select normal hematopoietic progenitor cells by virtue of CD34 expression.[347,348] These have not translated to improved outcome. Barlogie et al.[349,350] are performing multiple high-dose therapies and stem-cell transplantation. Response rates are higher relative to historically matched controls, but the impact on long-term disease-free survival (DFS) requires further follow-up. A recent comparison of tandem transplant with or without thalidomide has not prolonged OS.[351] In a French-randomized trial comparing a single versus double HDT and stem-cell transplantation, there was no significant difference in the CR rate between single and double transplantation arms, and EFS and OS curves separated only after 3 years.[352] This suggests that only a subset of patients may benefit, and indeed only those patients who did not achieve a CR to the first transplant appeared to benefit from the second.[353] The Bologna 96 study also showed that double autografting mainly benefited patients who did not achieve near CR.[354] The role of tandem transplant is being addressed by the ongoing phase III, multicenter trial of single autologous transplant with or without consolidation therapy versus tandem autologous transplant with lenalidomide maintenance (BMT CTN 0702).

Giralt et al. have reported on the use of cyclosporine to induce GVHD postautografting in an attempt to generate associated autologous graft versus MM effect.[355] It may be possible to stimulate autologous immunity to MM to treat MRD postautografting and thereby improve outcome. We have previously attempted to generate and expand anti-MM-specific autologous T cells *ex vivo* for adoptive immunotherapy of MRD in the patient post-autotransplant. It is now possible to clone the gene for the patient's specific idiotypic protein, identify gene sequences encoding for peptides predicted to be presented within the groove of class I HLA of a given patient's HLA type, and expand peptide-specific T cells *ex vivo*.[356] A similar strategy can be used to expand T cells against peptides within shared antigens that are overexpressed on MM cells, such as the telomerase catalytic subunit (hTERT), MUC-1, or the cytochrome CYP1B1.[35,357,358]

Immunologic responses are also being tested to enhance the immunogenicity of the whole tumor cell. We have shown that MM cells can be fused to DCs and that the use of the MM DC fusion as an antigen-presenting cell presents the entire MM cell as foreign. In a syngeneic murine MM model, vaccinations with MM cell-DC fusions, but not with either MM cells or DCs alone, demonstrate both protective and therapeutic efficacy.[359] Most important, we have shown that patient MM cells can be fused to autologous DCs, which are readily isolated from either patient BM or peripheral blood, and that autologous MM cell-DC fusions can trigger specific cytolytic autologous T-cell responses *in vitro*.[360,361] We are translating these findings into clinical trials of MM-DC fusion vaccines to assess *in vivo* MM-specific T-and B-cell responses, as well as clinical efficacy.[362]

Maintenance therapy

Maintenance regimens have been proposed to extend the duration of complete remission following autologous stem cell transplant. The increased tolerability and efficacy of newer antimyeloma agents has increased the attractiveness and the applicability of this approach; previous attempts at maintenance therapy with older conventional chemotherapy agents such as melphalan or interferon were not beneficial.[363]

A meta-analysis of randomized controlled trials comparing thalidomide maintenance with other regimens after induction chemotherapy that included 2786 patients from six trials, demonstrated that patients receiving thalidomide maintenance had marginally better OS (HR 0.83, $p = 0.07$). The difference was most prominent in groups who receive both thalidomide and corticosteroids (HR 0.70, $p = 0.02$). Thalidomide improved PFS (HR 0.65, $p < 0.01$) but was associated with a higher thrombotic risk (risk difference 0.024, $p < 0.05$) and increased peripheral neuropathy (risk difference 0.072, $p < 0.01$).[364]

Three randomized trials have explored the use of lenalidomide as maintenance therapy, with two of the trials following autologous stem-cell transplant[365,366] and one trial after 9 months of melphalan-based therapy in patients ineligible for high-dose treatment.[301] In all three trials, there was a near doubling in PFS with lenalidomide maintenance, for example, from 27 to 46 months in the CALGB 100104 study.[366] Furthermore, the CALGB study showed an OS benefit with lenalidomide: 15% of the lenalidomide group had died compared to 23% in the placebo group ($p < 0.03$) and at 3 years, the OS was 88% in the lenalidomide group compared to 80% in the placebo group.

A significant concern with maintenance therapy with lenalidomide is the risk of secondary malignancy. The risk of second primary cancers was roughly double in the maintenance group (7–7.7%) compared to the placebo group (2.6–3%). The secondary cancers observed included both hematological malignancies such as acute myelogenous leukemia as well as solid tumors. The risk of a secondary hematologic malignancy appears to be greatest when lenalidomide is given in combination with oral melphalan (HR 4.86, $p < 0.0001$).[367] This increased risk of secondary malignancies and the risk benefit ratio of maintenance therapy should be considered and discussed with the patient when initiating maintenance therapy.

Bortezomib has also been studied as maintenance therapy. In the HOVON-65/GMMG-HD4 study, bortezomib was given every 2 weeks and was associated with increasing the near CR and CR rate from 31% to 49%.[368] Table 10 provides a summary of recent maintenance trials.

Table 10 Maintenance therapies.

Study	Regimen	Number of patients	Outcome
IFM 2005-02[365]	Lenalidomide versus placebo as maintenance following first or second ASCT	614	PFS 41 months versus 23 months
CALGB 100104[366]	Lenalidomide versus placebo as maintenance therapy after ASCT	460	TTP 46 months versus 27 months
HOVON-65/ GMMG-HD4[368]	VAD versus PAD followed by ASCT, then thalidomide or bortezomib as maintenance	827	PFS 28 months versus 35 months

ASCT, autologous stem-cell transplantation; CR, complete response; PAD, bortezomib, doxorubicin, dexamethasone; VAD, vincristine, doxorubicin, dexamethasone; PFS, progression-free survival; TTP, time to progression.

Consolidation therapy

The use of short consolidation treatment after autologous SCT increases the CR rate and relapse-free survival. Ladetto et al.[369] have reported that post-transplant consolidation using the combination of bortezomib, thalidomide, and dexamethasone made it possible to convert 22% of VGPR into full, lasting molecular responses (PCR negative). Enhanced rates of CR, ranging between 10% and 30%, have been reported with post-ASCT (autologous stem-cell transplantation) use of bortezomib and lenalidomide as single agents.[370,371] In the IFM 2008 study, the usefulness and safety of post-transplant consolidation with two cycles of the RVD regimen was evaluated. This study showed that consolidation was feasible, well-tolerated, and effective, resulting in improving the sCR rate from 27% to 40% after consolidation.[372]

Continuous therapy

Recent data in the upfront setting, both in transplant-eligible and -ineligible patients, suggest that continuous therapy may result in improved disease control.[373,374] Several clinical trials have demonstrated superiority of maintenance strategies using thalidomide, lenalidomide, and bortezomib in transplant-eligible patients.

Thus far, the results from lenalidomide trials are perhaps the most convincing. The IFM 2005-02 and CALGB 100104 studies have both demonstrated a doubling of PFS[365,366] although only the CALGB trial has suggested an OS advantage. Lenalidomide certainly fits the requirements of a maintenance drug for continued use in myeloma, as it is administered orally and is generally well tolerated. Most recently, the FIRST trial comparing continuous Rd with Rd for 18 cycles and MPT demonstrated that continuous treatment with lenalidomide is superior to a finite therapy. Median PFS for the continuous Rd arm was 25.5 months versus 20.7 months for Rd18 and 21.2 months for MPT.[304] However, the risk of second primary malignancies, although low, does need to be discussed and balanced in the decision-making process when considering continuous therapy with this agent.

Allogeneic stem-cell transplantation

Syngeneic transplantation has been done infrequently in MM, but some patients reported from Seattle[375] and in European Bone Marrow Transplant Group (EBMT)[376] remain progression free at long intervals post-BMT. The EBMT has reported on allografting in MM.[377-379] Actuarial OS was 32% at 4 years and 28% at 7 years for the 72 (44%) patients who achieved CR after BMT. However, overall PFS was 34% at 6 years, and few patients remain in continuing CR at > 4 years postallograft. Favorable pre-BMT prognostic factors for both response to and survival after BMT were female sex, IgA MM, low serum β2M, stage I disease at diagnosis, one line of previous treatment, and being in CR before BMT. Of major concern is the early 41% transplant-related mortality (TRM; 50% in males) in the EBMT report,[380] which has subsequently been reduced to 20–30% owing to better patient selection, early transplantation, and less pretransplant treatment.[379] In the allografting experience in Seattle, actuarial probabilities of OS and EFS for the 36% patients achieving CR were 50% and 43%, respectively, at 4.5 years.[381] Adverse prognostic factors included transplantation >1 year from diagnosis; serum β2M > 2.5 mg/dL at transplant; female patients transplanted from male donors; having received > eight cycles of chemotherapy; and Durie–Salmon stage III disease at presentation. Again toxicity was common, with 35 (44%) patients dying of transplant-related causes within 100 days of BMT.[381,382] In an attempt to improve the outcome of allografting in MM by avoiding TRM, we carried out T (CD6)-depleted allografting using histocompatible sibling donors in 61 patients with MM whose disease remained sensitive to conventional chemotherapy.[346,383–386] There were 17 (28%) CR and 34 (57%) PR, 2 (3%) NR (not reached), and only 3 (5%) transplant-related deaths. However, DFS after allo BMT was 1 year, with only 20% patients disease free at ≥4 years post-transplant.

Molecular remissions are more common after allografting than after autografting,[387–390] and donor lymphocyte infusions (DLI) can treat relapsed MM postallografting,[391–393] indicating a clinically significant graft-versus MM (GVM) effect. At our center, relapses postautografting versus the higher toxicity and lower relapse rates in allograft recipients result in equivalent long-term outcomes.[394] In an effort to reduce toxicity and exploit GVM, we have utilized CD4+ DLI at 6 months post-CD6-depleted BM allografting in order to enhance GVM and thereby improve outcome.[386] Although prophylactic DLI induces significant GVM responses after allogeneic BMT, only 58% of patients were able to receive DLI despite T-cell-depleted BMT.

The use of nonablative transplantation is an alternative strategy to preserve GVM while avoiding the toxicity of allografting.[395] Melphalan at a dose of 100 mg/m^2 has been used in combination with DLI in high-risk MM patients.[396] Although disease control was achieved in some patients, significant GVHD was noted in this group of patients. Autografting has been performed before nonmyeloablative transplant by several investigators, demonstrating the feasibility of this approach to cytoreduce tumor and then enhance anti-MM immunity.[397,398] For example, Maloney et al.[398] report an overall response rate of 83% with 57% CRs. Chronic GVHD, transplant-related toxicity, and relapse of disease remain a problem. One randomized trial in high-risk MM showed that the combination of autologous stem-cell transplant followed by dose-reduced allogeneic transplant (IFM 99-03) was not superior to tandem autotransplant (IFM 99-04),[399] but a second randomized trial showed superior survival in those patients receiving autologous followed by allogeneic grafts.[400,401] The median OS was 80 months for allografting versus 54 for double autografting. The CR rate after allografting was 55% versus 26% after double autograft. In contrast, a randomized trial in high-risk MM showed that the combination of autologous stem-cell transplant followed by dose-reduced allogeneic transplant (IFM 99-03) was not superior to tandem autotransplant (IFM 99-04).[399] BMT CTN 0102 also evaluated autologous SCT followed by second autologous versus nonmyeloablative allogeneic SCT. In both standard- and high-risk patients, nonmyeloablative allogeneic HSCT after autologous HSCT was not more effective than tandem autologous HSCT.[402] Bjork-strand et al. conducted a prospective study of single or tandem autologous SCT versus reduced-intensity allogeneic SCT based on availability of an HLA-identical sibling. Long-term follow-up of 357 patients who received either autologous SCT (single or double) or auto-allo with HLA-identical sibling matched donor demonstrated that PFS was superior 35% versus 18% ($p = 0.001$) at 60 months for those receiving an auto-allo. Nonrelapse mortality was 12% after auto-allo versus 3% in the auto group ($p < 0.001$), and the incidence of limited to extensive GVHD was 31% and 23%.[403]

The use of allogeneic transplant as salvage therapy, while feasible, is unlikely to be of significant benefit in the heavily pretreated population. The EBMT reported on the outcomes of 229 patients who received reduced-intensity conditioning allogeneic SCT. TRM at 1 year was 22% and 3-year OS and PFS were 41% and 21%, respectively. Twenty-five percent of patients had extensive chronic GVHD.[404] The best outcomes were seen in patients who received a transplant in remission and early in the course of the disease. Adverse OS was associated with chemoresistant disease, more than one prior transplant, and male patients with female donors.

Allografting should only be undertaken in the context of clinical trials, which aim to reduce chronic GVHD, separate GVM from GVHD, and amplify the GVM effect to improve outcome by ameliorating toxicity and maximizing the antimyeloma effect of immunologic effector cells.

Relapsed disease

Almost all patients with MM who initially respond to chemotherapy eventually relapse. In order to overcome resistance to current therapies and improve patient outcome, novel biologically based treatment approaches are needed, which target the mechanisms whereby MM cells grow and survive in BM.[405] To achieve this goal, we have developed systems for studying growth, survival, and drug resistance mechanisms intrinsic to MM cells. Importantly, we have also developed both *in vitro* systems and *in vivo* animal models to characterize mechanisms of MM cell homing to BM, as well as factors (MM cell–BMSC interactions, cytokines, and angiogenesis) promoting MM cell growth, survival, drug resistance, and migration in the BM microenvironment.[73,80,85–87,406–408] These model systems have allowed for the development of several promising biologically based therapies that can target the MM cell and its BM microenvironment, those which target the MM cell only, and those which target only the BM microenvironment (Figure 7).

Immunomodulatory drugs

Drugs that target the MM cell and its BM milieu and thereby can overcome classical drug resistance *in vitro* include IMiDs such as thalidomide, lenalidomide, and pomalidomide[64] and proteasome inhibitors such as bortezomib[66] and carfilzomib. The bench to bedside translation of the IMiD drug lenalidomide has been very rapid. It was shown to target both the MM cell and BM microenvironment *in vitro* and *in vivo* in 2000[64,409]; completed phase I testing which identified an MTD, lack of toxicity, and remarkable anti-MM activity in 2001[410]; and completed phase II testing in 2002.[411]

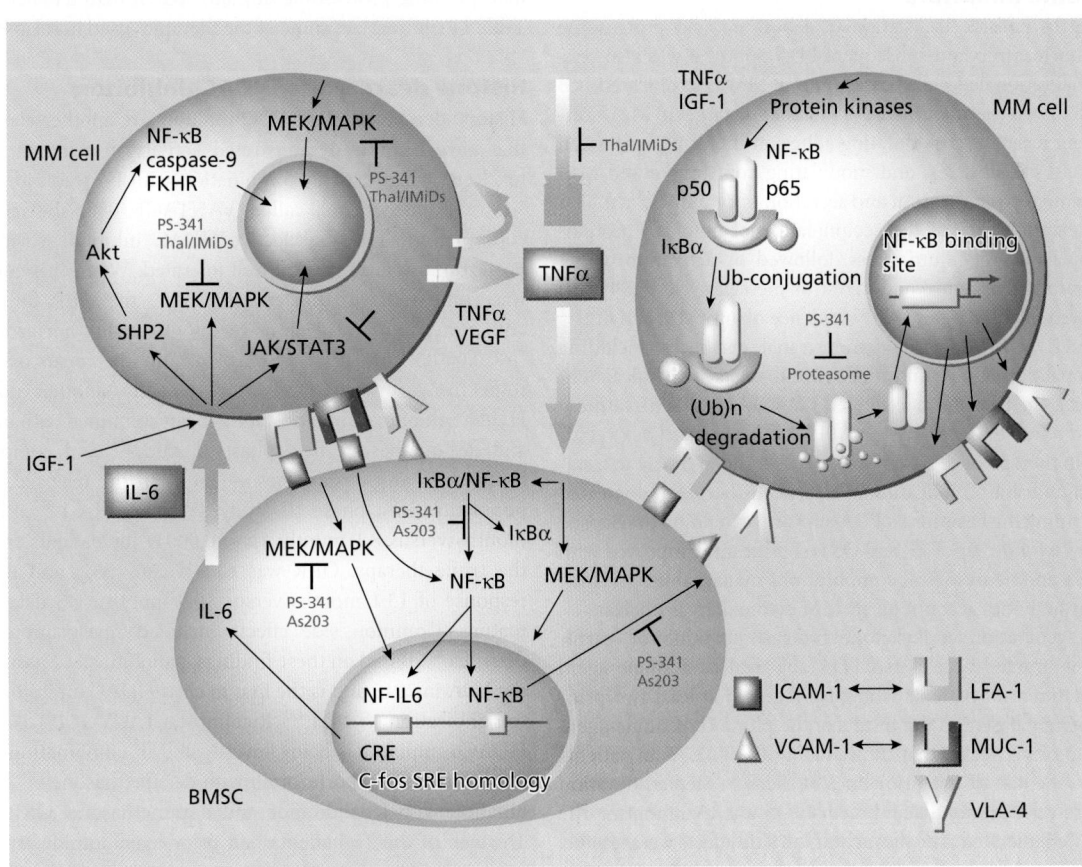

Figure 7 Inhibition of signaling pathways by novel therapeutic agents in multiple myeloma.

Two large phase III trials comparing lenalidomide/dex with dex/placebo were unblinded because of statistically significantly higher response rates, as well as increase in TTP and OS in the lenalidomide/dex treated cohort, providing the basis for its FDA approval to treat relapsed MM after one prior therapy.[412,413] Pomalidomide has also demonstrated potent anti-myeloma effects. Several studies have looked at pomalidomide in combination with low-dose dexamethasone in the relapsed population culminating in the approval of pomalidomide 4 mg orally on days 1–21 of 28-day cycles until progression. The phase II, randomized, open-label study compared pomalidomide and low-dose dexamethasone with single-agent pomalidomide in patients with relapsed, refractory myeloma. Median PFS for the combination arm was 4.2 months versus 2.7 months (HR 0.68, $P = 0.003$). ORR was 33% with combination versus 18% for pomalidomide alone. Median OS was 16.5 months versus 13.6 months, respectively. Refractoriness to lenalidomide and bortezomib did not affect outcomes with pomalidomide and dexamethasone.[414] A phase III study European study comparing pomalidomide and low-dose dexamethasone with high-dose dexamethasone alone showed a longer PFS of 4 months in the combination arm versus 1.9 months for dexamethasone alone (HR, 0.48; $P < 0.0001$). The most common side effects were myelosuppression and infections.[415]

Recently, the mechanism of action of IMiD drugs in MM (as well as their teratogenicity) has been better elucidated, when it was first appreciated that these drugs bind to cereblon (CBN)[416] Binding of IMiD drugs to CBN prevents auto-ubiquitylation of CBN, enhancing CBN-dependent proteasomal degradation of transcription factors IKZF1 (Ikaros) and IKZF3 (Aiolos), which are important to MM proliferation.[417–419]

Proteasome inhibitors

The bench to bedside translation of a boronic acid proteasome inhibitor bortezomib and subsequent FDA approval was also very rapid. Initial rationale to use bortezomib in MM is to block NF-κB activity as NF-κB was identified as a therapeutic target in MM, conferring drug resistance, modulating adhesion molecule expression on MM cells and BMSCs, and modulating constitutive and MM binding-induced transcription and secretion of cytokines.[50] In MM cells, bortezomib leads to the accumulation of unfolded proteins and endoplasmic reticulum stress, followed by activation of the unfolded protein response and arrest of the cell cycle.[420] Phase I trials showed tolerability and early evidence of anti-MM activity.[421] The phase II SUMMIT trial demonstrated responses, including CRs, prolongation of TTP and survival, and associated clinical benefit, forming the basis for accelerated FDA approval for treatment of relapsed refractory MM.[422] The APEX trial compared dex versus bortezomib therapy of relapsed MM was unblinded owing to a statistically significant prolongation in TTP in the bortezomib-treated cohort, forming the basis for its FDA approval extending to relapsed MM.[317] With follow-up, TTP and OS is significantly improved with bortezomib and neurological complications manageable.[423] Which of its many activities account for its MM cytotoxicity is unclear.

A next generation epoxyketone proteasome inhibitor, carfilzomib, was granted accelerated FDA approval as a single agent for the treatment of patients who have received at least two prior lines of therapy based on the results of the phase II of single-agent carfilzomib twice weekly that showed an ORR of 23.7% in patients who had a median of five prior lines of therapy. Median duration of response was 7.8 months and median OS was 15.6 months. The drug was well tolerated. The most common side effects were fatigue, anemia, nausea, and thrombocytopenia with 13.9% reporting peripheral neuropathy (majority of patients had baseline peripheral

neuropathy).[424] Cardiac failure events such as pulmonary edema were seen in 7.2% of patients. The ASPIRE trial recently reported on the results of the combination of carfilzomib with lenalidomide and dexamethasone compared to lenalidomide and dexamethasone in relapsed disease.[425] This combination was well tolerated and afforded a nearly 9 month improvement in PFS underscoring the benefits of combinations even in the relapsed setting.

Oral proteasome inhibitors, ixazomib and oprozomib, are in clinical trials now and will likely gain approval. Ixazomib has already demonstrated safety and efficacy in phase 1 trials in the relapsed, refractory population. Of 60 patients who had received a median of 6 prior regimens including bortezomib (83%), there were 41 evaluable patients. Responses included 1 VGPR, 5 PR, 1 MR, and 15 with SD. Only 10% of patients had drug-related peripheral neuropathy and none ≥grade 3.[426,427] In a phase I/II trial, weekly ixazomib was evaluated in combination with standard dose lenalidomide and dexamethasone in patients with newly diagnosed myeloma. Preliminary results from 58 response evaluable patients demonstrated a 93% overall response rate, with 67% of subjects achieving VGPR or better, including a CR rate of 24%.[426,428] On the basis of these results, ixazomib is being evaluated in combination with lenalidomide and dexamethasone in two large, international phase III trials: TOURMALINE MM1 for relapsed, refractory myeloma patients and TOURMALINE MM2 for newly diagnosed patients. Another oral proteasome inhibitor oprozomib is also under investigation for the treatment of MM.[429] These drugs could significantly impact the treatment of myeloma allowing for completely oral treatment regimens and consequently, completely outpatient care for patients. This could have a measurable quality of life benefit for patients, particularly in the elderly population, and may provide a convenient way of incorporating proteasome inhibitor-based maintenance strategies. Table 11 summarizes some of the therapies used in relapsed disease.

Histone deacetylase (HDAC) inhibitors

Histone deacetylase (HDAC) inhibitors are another class of drugs that have recently demonstrated activity in relapsed, refractory myeloma when used in combination with bortezomib. The phase III, randomized trial, called VANTAGE 088, showed that the combination of a nonselective HDAC inhibitor vorinostat and bortezomib was active and well tolerated. When this combination was compared with bortezomib alone, the ORR for vorinostat and bortezomib was 56.2% versus 40.6% for bortezomib alone ($p < 0.0001$), similarly, PFS was 7.63 months versus 6.83 months, respectively ($p = 0.01$).[431] More recently, another nonselective HDAC inhibitor panobinostat has been combined with bortezomib and dexamethasone in a phase II study[436] and compared with bortezomib and dexamethasone alone in the relapsed, refractory population in a phase III study, PANORAMA-1.[432] PFS was 12 months versus 8.1 months ($p < 0.0001$) for patients treated with the triple therapy. ORR was 61% versus 55% and duration of response of 13.1 months versus 10.9 months. OS data is not yet mature. Common side effects included myelosuppression and diarrhea.[436] Based on these findings, panobinostat was approved by the FDA in 2015 and is the first in class HDAC inhibitor to receive this indication in MM.[432] Ricolinostat (ACY-1215) is a selective HDAC6 inhibitor is being investigated in combination with both lenalidomide and bortezomib with dexamethasone.[437–439] In combination with lenalidomide and dexamethasone, ORR was 69%. Thirteen of the 16 patients had prior lenalidomide and 3/6 were refractory to lenalidomide.[440] In combination with bortezomib and dexamethasone, the ORR was 44%.[441]

Table 11 Novel therapy for relapsed, refractory multiple myeloma.

Trial	Phase	Agent	Number of patients	ORR (%)	OS (Mo)	Outcome (months)
Richardson et al.[317]	Ph3	Bortezomib	669	38	29.8	TTP 6.2 versus 3.5
		Dexamethasone		18	23.7	
Orlowski et al.[430]	Ph3	Bort/PLD	646	44	76%[a]	TTP 9.3 versus 6.5
		Bortezomib		41	65%[a]	
Weber et al.[412]	Ph3	Lenalidomide	353	61	29.6	TTP 11.1 versus 4.7
		Dexamethasone		20	20.2	
Dimopoulos et al.[413]	Ph3	Lenalidomide	351	60	NR	TTP 11.3 versus 4.7
		Dexamethasone		24	20.6	
Richardson et al.[319]	Ph2	RVD	64	64	26	Median TTP 9.5
Siegel et al.[322]	Ph2	Carfilzomib	266	24	15.6	Median PFS 3.7
San Miguel et al.[415]	Ph3	Pom/LoDex	302	31	11.9	Median PFS 4.0 versus 1.9
		HiDex		10	7.8	
Dimopoulos et al.[431]	Ph3	Vor/Bort	637	56	NR	Median PFS 7.6 versus 6.8
		Bort		41	28.1	
San Miguel et al.[432]	Ph 3	Pan/Bort/Dex	768	61	NR	Median PFS 12 versus 8.1
		Bort/Dex		55		
Lokhorst et al.[433]	Ph1/2	Daratumumab	32	42[b]	NR	Median PFS NR
Lonial et al.[434]	Ph2	Elo/Len/Dex	73	92[c]	NR	Median PFS NR[c]
Lentzsch et al.[435]	Ph2	Benda/Len/Dex	29	52	NR	Median PFS 6.1

Bort, bortezomib; PLD, pegylated liposomal doxorubicin; RVD, lenalidomide, bortezomib, dexamethasone; Pom, pomalidomide; Dex, dexamethasone; Lo, low dose; Hi, high dose; Vor, vorinostat; Pan, panobinostat; Elo, elotuzumab; Benda, bendamustine; NR, not reported/reached.
[a]At 15 months.
[b]Of those receiving a dose of ≥4 mg/kg.
[c]Of those receiving dose of 10 mg/kg at 20.8 months.

Monoclonal antibodies

Several monoclonal antibodies are being investigated and demonstrated activity in myeloma. Specifically, novel drugs that target CD38, CS1, and BAFF are in ongoing clinical trials.[427,442] Daratumumab, a monoclonal CD38 antibody, was granted Fast Track Designation and Breakthrough Therapy Designation by the FDA based on results of a phase I/II trial that demonstrated single agent activity in relapsed, refractory myeloma. In the ≥4 mg/kg groups (n = 12), 5 PRs and 3 MRs were observed. Median PFS had not been reached by a data cutoff of 3.8 months.[433] Daratumumab is now being studied in combination with lenalidomide and dexamethasone in relapsed, refractory disease. SAR650984, another CD38 inhibitor, had an ORR of 30.8% as a single agent in the dose-escalation study in RR patients at the MTD.[443] Daratumumab is also being studied in smoldering MM (NCT02316106).

Elotuzumab, a humanized monoclonal IgG1 antibody directed against human CS1 (also known as CD2 subset-1, SLAMF7, CRACC, and CD319), a cell surface antigen glycoprotein that is highly expressed on MM cells and normal plasma cells, has also been granted Breakthrough Therapy Designation by the FDA. In the phase I study, no objective responses were seen, although 26.5% had stable disease (SD) by EBMT myeloma response criteria.[444] In combination with lenalidomide and dexamethasone, objective responses were obtained in 82% (23 of 28) of treated patients. After a median of 16.4 months follow-up, the median TTP was NR for patients in the 20-mg/kg cohort who were treated until disease progression.[445] An ORR of 92% and a median PFS was NR after a median follow-up of 20.8 months at the 10 mg/kg dose, which was the dose used in the ongoing phase III trial, ELOQUENT-2.[434] Phase I results of elotuzumab in combination with bortezomib and dexamethasone are also favorable, with a PR or better in 48% of 27 evaluable patients with relapsed, refractory disease.[446] Elotuzumab in combination with lenalidomide +/− dexamethasone is also being studied in high-risk smoldering MM (NCT02279394).

Tabalumab is a fully human monoclonal antibody designed to have neutralizing activity against both membrane-bound and soluble BAFF and has been combined with bortezomib and dexamethasone in a phase I study. In this study, the ORR was 45.8%.[447] A phase II trial of this combination has been completed and results are forthcoming.

Other treatments

Bendamustine as a single agent or in combination with lenalidomide and dexamethasone is another option for patients with relapsed, refractory myeloma. The combination of bendamustine, lenalidomide, and dexamethasone was evaluated in a phase I/II trial. The median PFS was 6.1 months, PR rate 52%, and VGPR rate 24%.[435] The MTD of bendamustine was 75 mg/m^2 as compared with prior studies using 100 mg/m^2. Toxicity was mainly hematologic arguing in favor of the lower dose, particularly in light of the fact that this population is heavily pretreated.

Other regimens have been explored as well, bortezomib and pegylated liposomal doxorubicin (Doxil) and bendamustine with prednisone and thalidomide.[430,448]

There are currently many new drugs in development that target novel pathways.[449,450] For example, filanesib, a kinesin spindle protein inhibitor, which induces aberrant mitotic arrest and rapid cell death and preferentially acts on MCL-1-dependent cells including myeloma cells, has demonstrated activity in combination with lenalidomide and bortezomib. Several other classes of novel drugs are currently under investigation including the bromodomain inhibitors, cyclin-dependent kinase inhibitors, and inhibitors of the ubiquitin pathway. Data generated from these early studies will provide a better understanding of how these will be incorporated into the continuum of myeloma care.[451–453]

Another area of interest and therapy development is the blockade of interactions between the tumor cells and immune cells. PD-1 and PD-L1 are two targets of interest. PD-1 is a receptor present on T cells that interacts with PD-L1 expressed on tumor cells. Patients with persistent MRD and at relapse have upregulation of PD-L1 and PD-1.[454] There are ongoing clinical trials exploring PD-1 blockade in combination with dendritic cell/myeloma fusion vaccine[362,455] and with, for example, pembrolizumab, lenalidomide, and dexamethasone (NCT02036502).

The choice of therapy for relapsed or refractory patients depends on a number of factors including time since last therapy, prior exposure to novel agents, alone or in combination, and drug-induced comorbidities, for example, neuropathy, renal malfunction, and loss of patient physiologic reserve. In the past decade, there has been a dramatic increase in the number of therapies available to patients with RR myeloma. This is a very dynamic area within oncology and will continue to evolve as more new therapies enter trials and gain approval.

Future directions

Evolution of a new treatment paradigm for MM

Our in vitro and animal model studies have demonstrated the importance of the BM in promoting MM cell growth, survival, drug resistance, and migration in the BM microenvironment and have already derived very promising therapies based on targeting the MM cell in its BM milieu. These studies provide the framework for development of a new treatment paradigm in MM, targeting both the tumor cell and its microenvironment, which is urgently needed as MM remains incurable despite all available therapies.

Identification and validation of novel-targeted MM

Importantly, in our in vitro gene array studies with conventional dex[169] and bortezomib[170] therapies, samples obtained from patients treated on these protocols help to identify in vivo targets and mechanisms of novel drug action on the one hand, versus mechanisms of drug resistance on the other, and also aid in determining whether in vivo targets of these novel therapies correlate with their in vitro anti-MM activities. Excitingly, preclinical studies suggest enhanced activity when these novel agents are combined with conventional agents or with each other. These studies have established a new treatment paradigm targeting the MM cell in its BM microenvironment to further elucidate MM pathogenesis as well as overcome drug resistance and improve patient outcome.

Novel single agents of great promise include new proteasome inhibitor marizomib (NPI-0052), FGFR3 inhibitors,[456,457] MEK inhibitor AZD6244,[458] and Hsp90 inhibitors.[459] Marizomib[460] is a next-generation proteasome inhibitor and active against bortezomib-resistant MM and nontoxic in preclinical models, and is already in clinical trials in relapsed MM. FGFR3 inhibitors are specifically targeting those 15–20% patients with t(4;14) translocation. Hsp90 inhibitors as single agents can achieve responses in relapsed refractory MM.

Profiling of gene and protein expression can also provide the preclinical rationale for clinical protocols combining novel targeted therapies. For example, our studies demonstrate that bortezomib treatment of MM cells in vitro induces death signaling, downregulates survival signaling, and upregulates both ubiquitin/proteasome and stress response gene transcripts.[170] Specifically, bortezomib upregulates Hsp90, which not only is a stress response protein but also plays a major role in protein unfolding required before proteins can be degraded by the proteasome. Our in vitro studies show that Hsp90 inhibitor 17-AAG (KOS953) can block the Hsp90 stress response induced by bortezomib and thereby increase MM cell apoptosis. These gene microarray studies therefore provided the framework for a clinical trial coupling these agents in MM, which shows that Hsp90 inhibitor KOS953 can sensitize to and even overcome resistance to bortezomib,[461] and a phase III clinical trial of bortezomib versus bortezomib with KOS953 in relapsed MM is ongoing.

Proteomic studies can also provide the preclinical basis for clinical application of novel targeted therapies. For example, our in vitro studies demonstrate that exposure of MM cells to bortezomib induces cleavage of DNA repair kinases such as DNA PKcs in a dose- and time-dependent manner.[462] This observation for the first time suggested that bortezomib inhibited DNA repair. Subsequent in vitro studies demonstrated that coupling bortezomib with DNA damaging agents (alkylating agents and anthracyclines) can enhance sensitivity or even restore sensitivity to these agents in resistant MM cells.[463] Already clinical protocols coupling bortezomib with Doxil[464] and with melphalan[463] have demonstrated promising clinical results. Specifically, a large randomized trial of Doxil and bortezomib versus bortezomib in relapsed MM showed significantly increase OR, EFS, and OS in the patients receiving combined therapy, setting the stage for its FDA approval in June 2007.[430]

In order to provide the framework for coupling these novel agents in rational clinical trials, we have also characterized the apoptotic signaling cascades triggered in MM cells by both conventional and these novel agents.[70] For example, use of IMiDs with TRAIL provides dual triggering of caspase 8 death signaling, whereas treatment with IMiDs such as lenalidomide and bortezomib triggers both caspase 8- and caspase 9-mediated MM cell death. The combination of lenalidomide and bortezomib has demonstrated remarkable activity, even in patients resistant to either agent alone.[465]

The mTOR inhibitor rapamycin sensitizes MM cells to both conventional and novel therapies[466,467]; temsirolimus has anti-MM activity in xenograft models.[468] A phase I trial of the combination of the oral mTOR inhibitor everolimus with lenalidomide in relapsed/refractory myeloma was well tolerated and had responses in a heavily pretreated population.[469] Bortezomib inhibits growth (MEK/ERK) and survival (Jak/STAT) signaling, but activates Akt, providing the preclinical rationale for combining bortezomib with the Akt inhibitor perifosine.[470]

Our recent signaling studies have defined the role of the aggresome in degrading ubiquitinated protein in MM, and specifically used the HDAC6 inhibitor tubacin to inhibit its transport to the aggresome for degradation. Blocking the aggresome with tubacin induces a compensatory upregulation of the proteasome; conversely, blocking the proteasome with bortezomib triggers a compensatory upregulation of the aggresome. Importantly, blocking both the proteasome and aggresome with bortezomib and tubacin, respectively, induces synergistic toxicity.[471] The HDAC6 inhibitor ricolinostat (ACY-1215) is currently in clinical trials in combination with lenalidomide, pomalidomide, or bortezomib.[440,441]

It is also possible to combine monoclonal antibodies with novel drugs. Lenalidomide, for example, can markedly augment ADCC induced by anti-CD40 in MM.[110] Finally, gene expression profiling in correlative science studies of patients on clinical protocols will both identify targets of drug sensitivity versus resistance and allow for predicting those patients most likely to respond to conventional and novel targeted therapies. For example, gene expression profiling of patient tumor samples showed genes upregulated in patients responding to bortezomib versus those patients who did not respond. Hsp27 upregulation correlated with intrinsic or acquired bortezomib resistance. Preclinical studies showed that p38MAPK inhibition downregulated Hsp27 expression and restored bortezomib sensitivity in resistant MM cell lines and patient samples,[472] providing the basis for a trial combining these two agents.

Other plasma cell dyscrasias

Plasmacytomas

Clinical characteristics
Plasmacytomas are collections of monoclonal plasma cells originating either in bone (solitary osseous plasmacytoma, SOP) or in soft tissue (extramedullary plasmacytoma, EMP). They comprise <10% of plasma-cell dyscrasias. MM must be excluded before the diagnosis of either SOP or EMP can be made. MRI can be useful to show additional marrow abnormalities consistent with MM.[473] The median age of diagnosis of either SOP or EMP is approximately 50 years, nearly 10 years younger than that for MM.[474–476] Although patients with SOP and EMP can both progress to MM, persons with SOP progress in the majority of cases, in contrast to EMP, where only up to 50% eventually develop MM. The median survival of 86.4 and 100.8 months for patients with SOP and EMP, respectively, is similar; however, PFS is markedly different, 16% for SOP patients versus 71% for EMP patients. The persistence of stable monoclonal Ig in serum and/or urine after primary treatment of plasmacytoma does not necessitate additional therapy, as it does not influence survival or DFS.[474] In contrast, rising monoclonal Ig levels in a patient with a history of either SOP or EMP should trigger a work-up for either recurrent plasmacytoma or MM. It has been suggested, as is true for MM, that serum β2M has prognostic value in patients with SOP. Specifically, 17 of 19 patients with elevated serum β2M had transformation to MM and shorter survival (31 months) than those with normal serum β2M levels.[477]

Treatment
Treatment of SOP and EMP is local therapy, primarily radiotherapy with surgery as needed for structural anatomic support.[474–476] The benefit of chemotherapy, either alone or in combination with radiotherapy and surgery, as primary therapy for SOP or EMP, has not been proven. Moreover, the benefit of adjuvant chemotherapy, given to prevent recurrent disease and/or progression to MM, is also undefined. Disappearance of protein after involved-field radiotherapy predicts for long-term DFS and possible cure.[478]

Immunoglobulin M monoclonal gammopathy

Excess monoclonal IgM in the serum can occur in a variety of diseases. In a Mayo Clinic series of 430 patients in whom a monoclonal IgM protein was identified, 242 (56%) had MGUS, 71 (17%) had Waldenström's macroglobulinemia, 28 (7%) had lymphoma, 21 (5%) had chronic lymphocytic leukemia, 6 (1%) had primary amyloidosis, and 62 (14%) had other malignant lymphoproliferative diseases.[479] The duration of time from the recognition of the M protein to the development of a malignant lymphoid disease ranged from 4 to 9 years, suggesting that long-term follow-up of such patients is necessary.

Waldenström macroglobulinemia

The diagnosis of Waldenström macroglobulinemia (WM) is based on the presence of an IgM monoclonal protein and 10% or more

the BM biopsy showing involvement with small lymphocytes with lymphoplasmacytic features and an immunophenotype characteristic of lymphoplasmacytic lymphoma (see the following discussion).[480] WM corresponds most closely to the lymphoplasmacytic lymphoma (LPA) under the World Health Organization (WHO) classification of lymphoid tumors [LPL/immunocytoma of the Revised European–American (REAL) classification of lymphoma]. WM accounts for approximately 2% of all hematologic malignancies and is more common in men than in women. Its incidence increases with age, and it is more common among whites than among African-Americans.[481,482] Although the etiology of WM is unclear, genetic factors may contribute to the pathogenesis of this disease, as there are reports of families with WM in association with other lymphoproliferative and immunologic disorders.[483] Cytogenetic abnormalities occur in 15–90% of cases, but none are specific for WM.[484,485] The WM B-cell clone demonstrates interclonal differentiation from small lymphocytes with large focal deposits of surface immunoglobulins to lymphoplasmacytic cells and mature plasma cells that contain intracytoplasmic immunoglobulin. This morphologic heterogeneity is reflected by variable expression of phenotypic markers. All WM cells express monoclonal IgM and most cells are CD19, CD20, CD22, and FMC7 positive. High density of CD38 is also detected with variable intensity of the PCA-1 antigen. Predictably, CD45 isoform expression is heterogeneous, probably reflecting ongoing monoclonal B- cell differentiation. In approximately 20% of cases, CD5 and CD23 expression are seen, but their coexpression is uncommon.[486] Circulating clonal B cells in WM increase in patients who fail to respond to therapy or who progress.[487] Recent studies suggest that WM originates from a postgerminal center B cell that has undergone somatic mutations and antigenic selection in the lymphoid follicle and has the characteristics of an IgM-bearing memory B cell.[488–490]

The median age of onset of WM is 61 years. Symptoms are characteristically vague and nonspecific, with the most common being weakness, anorexia, and weight loss. Symptoms due to peripheral neuropathy and Raynaud's phenomenon can precede more serious manifestations. Lymphadenopathy, splenomegaly, and/or hepatomegaly are present in 30–40% of cases, and at least 20–25% lymphoplasmacytoid cells are usually present in the marrow. Visceral involvement of small bowel and peripheral nerves can cause the clinical sequelae of malabsorption and neuropathy, respectively. Hemorrhagic complications may be present, attributable to abnormal bleeding times, decreased platelet adhesiveness, or direct interference by the IgM protein with the release of platelet factor 3 and with coagulation factors. An important part of the differential diagnosis is to exclude the less common entity of IgM MM, which is characterized by lytic bone disease and an absence of organomegaly and/or lymphocytic involvement; rarely, WM can itself progress to IgM MM.[491] Amyloidosis occurs rarely in WM.[492] Hyperviscosity syndrome, described earlier as a rare complication in MM, occurs more commonly in the setting of excess IgM and is characterized by mucosal bleeding and neurologic, ocular, and cardiovascular abnormalities.[259] Therapy with plasmapheresis is more useful to remove excess IgM than it is in the setting of excess IgG monoclonal proteins and related hyperviscosity in MM.

Treatment

The median survival is approximately 50 months, not that dissimilar from the best-reported series of patients with MM. In contrast to persons with MM, however, many individuals with WM have indolent disease requiring no therapy for long periods of time, with survivals in excess of 20 years. Although high-dose therapy with autologous stem-cell support has been shown to be effective in many patients with MM or with low-grade lymphoma, relatively few patients with WM have undergone transplant. Nonetheless, preliminary data suggest that high-dose therapy is associated with a high CR rate and acceptable toxicity, and this approach therefore warrants further investigation, particularly in younger patients with poor prognostic features.[493] Splenectomy has been reported to be effective in chemotherapy-resistant patients with WM and results in a major decrease in monoclonal protein concentration and durable remission.[494,495] Monoclonal antibody therapy with rituximab, a chimeric anti-CD20 monoclonal antibody, produces responses in both treated and untreated patients with low-grade lymphoma. Given that the CD20 antigen is typically present in WM, rituximab has been given to patients and a clinical response was seen in about one-third of previously treated patients in early studies.[496,497] Combinations of rituximab with cyclophosphamide[498] or bortezomib[499] are increasingly used. Rituximab use in WM can be associated with a paradoxical increase in IgM (or flare) with increase in serum viscosity.[500]

Recent evidence suggests the presence of the *MYD88* L265P mutation in the majority of WM patients.[501] Moreover, mutations in the CXCR4 pathway may affect disease presentation.[502] The Burton tyrosine kinase (BTK) is a downstream target of MYD88, an adaptor molecule for Toll-like receptors.[503] Ibrutinib is an oral inhibitor of BTK, and a phase II trial of ibrutinib in 63 patients with previously treated WM demonstrated decrease in monoclonal protein of 50% or better in 73% of patients with a median time to PR of 8 weeks.[504] These findings led to FDA approval of ibrutinib in WM.

Heavy-chain diseases

Since the original description by Franklin et al.[505] of a patient with malignant lymphoma whose serum and urine contained large amounts of the Fc fragment of IgG, the clinical and immunochemical scope of gamma heavy-chain disease (γHCD) has broadened. These diseases are characterized by the presence of a portion of the Ig heavy chain in the serum or urine or both. The median age at diagnosis is similar to that for MM, approximately 60 years.[506] The clinical and laboratory features can be heterogeneous. Most common presenting symptoms are weakness, fatigue, and fever, associated with lymphadenopathy and hepatosplenomegaly. In addition to Ig heavy chain in serum or urine, a lymphoplasmacytic marrow infiltrate is noted in most cases. The clinical course can be fulminant and rapidly progressive; alternatively, the monoclonal heavy chain can persist for years in otherwise asymptomatic patients. Thus, survival is variable, but the median is only 12 months. Treatment options for patients with active disease are similar to those used for lymphoma or MM, whereas patients with indolent disease should be followed expectantly without therapy. Cases of αHCD, μHCD, and δHCD have also been described. HCD is typically associated with non-Hodgkin's lymphoma in the gastrointestinal tract, beginning with plasma cells that produce a heavy chain and aggregate in the intestinal tract and subsequent transformation into a malignant non-Hodgkin's lymphoma of the immunoblastic type, probably arising from the more mature plasma cells.[507] The ideal therapy for heavy-chain disease is not known because of its rarity, but intensive chemotherapy including intravenous cyclophosphamide, doxorubicin, vincristine, and oral prednisone appears to offer some patients long-term remissions.

Amyloidosis

Amyloidosis is relatively rare as a clinically significant disease. It has been classified into five categories. These include (1) primary, with or without plasma cell and lymphoid neoplasms; (2) secondary, associated with chronic infections or autoimmune disease; (3) hereditary, associated with familial Mediterranean fever, Portuguese lower limb neuropathy, and others; (4) amyloidosis associated with aging; and (5) amyloidosis of endocrine glands, with medullary thyroid carcinoma and multiple endocrine neoplasia type 2.[492,508] The amyloid found in most cases of amyloidosis can be assigned to one of two types, according to whether the fibrils consist mainly of the variable region of Ig light chains (AL, or primary amyloidosis) or protein A (AA, or secondary amyloidosis). Protein A has a molecular weight of 8500 Da and consists of 76 amino acids; it is not related to any known immunoglobulin. Establishing the correct diagnosis is key, as monoclonal gammopathy of unknown significance is common, and in a series of 350 patients with suspected AL amyloidosis, 9.7% of patients actually had mutations in the fibrinogen A alpha-chain or transthyretin.[509] Direct classification of the amyloid protein through laser microdissection and mass spectrometry can help improve the accuracy of diagnosis of AL amyloidosis.[510]

In AL amyloidosis, amyloid primarily involves the heart, tongue, gastrointestinal tract, and/or skin, whereas AA primarily results in fibril deposition in liver, kidney, and spleen. A review of 229 patients with AL documented MM in 47 (21%) patients.[508] Initial presenting symptoms were fatigue and weight loss, with pain more common in those who also had MM. Hepatomegaly and macroglossia were present in up to one-third of patients with AL; renal insufficiency was present in one-half of patients, and proteinuria (defined as albuminuria with immune globulin seen, only in MM) was documented in 82% of patients. Nephrotic syndrome, CHF, orthostatic hypotension, carpal tunnel syndrome, and peripheral neuropathy were all more common in those without MM (30–70% of patients studied) than in persons with MM (<20%). Overall median survival was 12 months, 5 months for those with MM in contrast to 13 months for individuals without MM. Although it has been difficult to monitor the distribution and progression of disease, it has been shown that radiolabeled serum amyloid P component, which has specific binding affinity for amyloid fibrils, can be given intravenously and localizes rapidly and specifically in amyloid deposits.[511,512] This technique may therefore facilitate diagnosis and monitoring of the extent of systemic amyloidosis, including the effects of therapeutic interventions.

Treatment

Treatment of AL is making progress. Early studies looked at colchicine or MP or all three, with low response rates.[513] Initial experience with[514,515] dose-intensive melphalan with autologous stem-cell support can achieve CRs, with improvement in performance status and clinical remission of organ-specific disease, guidelines have been developed for patient selection to maximize benefit and minimize TRM and guidelines have been.[516–518] As in MM, patients eligible for high-dose treatments may also do well with chemotherapy.[519] To address this, a randomized trial compared high-dose melphalan and autologous stem-cell transplant with standard melphalan and dexamethasone, and this study did not find a benefit with intensive therapy.[520] A notable limitation of this trial was the high mortality rate in the intensive arm, which has not been seen in other sites, suggesting that the trial may not be generalizable.

Attempts to improve outcomes for patients with symptomatic and advanced multisystem disease may require both solid and stem-cell transplantation, as well as the use of less intensive conditioning regimens. For example, patients with cardiac involvement have unusually high TRM during autologous stem cell mobilization and transplant, and these patients may be managed with a combination of cardiac transplant followed by autologous stem cell transplant.[521] Newer drugs now routinely used in MM are increasingly used in patients with AL amyloidosis, such as the combination of CyBorD, with durable responses.[522]

Key references

The complete reference list can be found on the Wiley Companion Digital Edition of this title (see inside front cover for login instructions).

6 Rajkumar SV, Dimopoulos MA, Palumbo A, et al. International Myeloma Working Group updated criteria for the diagnosis of multiple myeloma. *Lancet Oncol.* 2014;**15**:e538–e548.

7 Durie BGM, Salmon SE. A clinical staging system for multiple myeloma. Correlation of measured cell mass with presenting clinical features, response to treatment and survival. *Cancer.* 1975;**36**:842–854.

9 Kyle RA, Therneau TM, Rajkumar SV, et al. Prevalence of monoclonal gammopathy of undetermined significance. *N Engl J Med.* 2006;**354**:1362–1369.

12 Rajkumar SV, Kyle RA, Therneau TM, et al. Serum free light chain ratio is an independent risk factor for progression in monoclonal gammopathy of undetermined significance. *Blood.* 2005;**106**:812–817.

13 Kyle RA, Remstein ED, Therneau TM, et al. Clinical course and prognosis of smoldering (asymptomatic) multiple myeloma. *N Engl J Med.* 2007;**356**:2582–2590.

21 Kyle RA, Gertz MA, Witzig TE, et al. Review of 1027 patients with newly diagnosed multiple myeloma. *Mayo Clin Proc.* 2003;**78**:21–33.

43 Bergsagel PL, Chesi M, Nardini E, Brents LA, Kirby SL, Kuehl WM. Promiscuous translocations into immunoglobulin heavy chain switch regions in multiple myeloma. *Proc Natl Acad Sci U S A.* 1996;**93**:13931–13936.

45 Teoh G, Anderson KC. Interaction of tumor and host cells with adhesion and extracellular matrix molecules in the development of multiple myeloma. *Hematol Oncol Clin North Am.* 1997;**11**:27–42.

64 Hideshima T, Chauhan D, Shima Y, et al. Thalidomide and its analogues overcome drug resistance of human multiple myeloma cells to conventional therapy. *Blood.* 2000;**96**:2943–2950.

70 Hideshima T, Anderson KC. Molecular mechanisms of novel therapeutic approaches for multiple myeloma. *Nat Rev Cancer.* 2002;**2**:927–937.

90 Singhal S, Mehta J, Desikan R, et al. Antitumor activity of thalidomide in refractory multiple myeloma. *N Engl J Med.* 1999;**341**:1565–1571.

146 Bergsagel PL, Kuehl WM. Molecular pathogenesis and a consequent classification of multiple myeloma. *J Clin Oncol.* 2005;**23**:6333–6338.

150 Neben K, Lokhorst HM, Jauch A, et al. Administration of bortezomib before and after autologous stem cell transplantation improves outcome in multiple myeloma patients with deletion 17p. *Blood.* 2012;**119**:940–948.

157 Chapman MA, Lawrence MS, Keats JJ, et al. Initial genome sequencing and analysis of multiple myeloma. *Nature.* 2011;**471**:467–472.

171 Weiss BM, Abadie J, Verma P, Howard RS, Kuehl WM. A monoclonal gammopathy precedes multiple myeloma in most patients. *Blood.* 2009;**113**:5418–5422.

172 Landgren O, Kyle RA, Pfeiffer RM, et al. Monoclonal gammopathy of undetermined significance (MGUS) consistently precedes multiple myeloma: a prospective study. *Blood.* 2009;**113**:5412–5417.

181 Greipp PR, San Miguel J, Durie BG, et al. International staging system for multiple myeloma. *J Clin Oncol.* 2005;**23**:3412–3420.

188 Zhan F, Huang Y, Colla S, et al. The molecular classification of multiple myeloma. *Blood.* 2006;**108**:2020–2028.

243 Berenson J, Lichtenstein A, Porter L, et al. Pamidronate disodium reduces the occurrence of skeletal events in patients with advanced multiple myeloma. *N Engl J Med.* 1996;**334**:488–493.

251 Morgan GJ, Child JA, Gregory WM, et al. Effects of zoledronic acid versus clodronic acid on skeletal morbidity in patients with newly diagnosed multiple myeloma (MRC Myeloma IX): secondary outcomes from a randomised controlled trial. *Lancet Oncol.* 2011;**12**:743–752.

253 Raje N, Woo SB, Hande K, et al. Clinical, radiographic, and biochemical characterization of multiple myeloma patients with osteonecrosis of the jaw. *Clin Cancer Res.* 2008;**14**:2387–2395.

285 Kumar SK, Rajkumar SV, Dispenzieri A, et al. Improved survival in multiple myeloma and the impact of novel therapies. *Blood.* 2008;**111**:2516–2520.

293 Durie BG, Harousseau JL, Miguel JS, et al. International uniform response criteria for multiple myeloma. *Leukemia.* 2006;**20**:1467–1473.

294 Rajkumar SV, Harousseau JL, Durie B, et al. Consensus recommendations for the uniform reporting of clinical trials: report of the International Myeloma Workshop Consensus Panel 1. *Blood.* 2011;**117**:4691–4695.

295 Martinez-Lopez J, Lahuerta JJ, Pepin F, et al. Prognostic value of deep sequencing method for minimal residual disease detection in multiple myeloma. *Blood.* 2014;**123**:3073–3079.

302 San Miguel JF, Schlag R, Khuageva NK, et al. Bortezomib plus melphalan and prednisone for initial treatment of multiple myeloma. *N Engl J Med.* 2008;**359**:906–917.

304 Benboubker L, Dimopoulos MA, Dispenzieri A, et al. Lenalidomide and dexamethasone in transplant-ineligible patients with myeloma. *N Engl J Med.* 2014;**371**:906–917.

313 Rajkumar SV, Jacobus S, Callander NS, et al. Lenalidomide plus high-dose dexamethasone versus lenalidomide plus low-dose dexamethasone as initial therapy for newly diagnosed multiple myeloma: an open-label randomised controlled trial. *Lancet Oncol.* 2010;**11**:29–37.

317 Richardson PG, Sonneveld P, Schuster MW, et al. Bortezomib or high-dose dexamethasone for relapsed multiple myeloma. *N Engl J Med.* 2005;**352**:2487–2498.

341 Child JA, Morgan GJ, Davies FE, et al. High-dose chemotherapy with hematopoietic stem-cell rescue for multiple myeloma. *N Engl J Med.* 2003;**348**:1875–1883.

366 McCarthy PL, Owzar K, Hofmeister CC, et al. Lenalidomide after stem-cell transplantation for multiple myeloma. *N Engl J Med.* 2012;**366**:1770–1781.

381 Bensinger WI, Buckner CD, Anasetti C, et al. Allogeneic marrow transplantation for multiple myeloma: an analysis of risk factors on outcome. *Blood.* 1996;**88**:2787–2793.

394 Alyea E, Weller E, Schlossman R, et al. Outcome after autologous and allogeneic stem cell transplantation for patients with multiple myeloma: impact of graft-versus-myeloma effect. *Bone Marrow Transplant.* 2003;**32**:1145–1151.

398 Maloney DG, Molina AJ, Sahebi F, et al. Allografting with nonmyeloablative conditioning following cytoreductive autografts for the treatment of patients with multiple myeloma. *Blood.* 2003;**102**:3447–3454.

412 Weber DM, Chen C, Niesvizky R, et al. Lenalidomide plus dexamethasone for relapsed multiple myeloma in North America. *N Engl J Med.* 2007;**357**:2133–2142.

415 San Miguel J, Weisel K, Moreau P, et al. Pomalidomide plus low-dose dexamethasone versus high-dose dexamethasone alone for patients with relapsed and refractory multiple myeloma (MM-003): a randomised, open-label, phase 3 trial. *Lancet Oncol.* 2013;**14**:1055–1066.

425 Stewart AK, Rajkumar SV, Dimopoulos MA, et al. Carfilzomib, lenalidomide, and dexamethasone for relapsed multiple myeloma. *N Engl J Med.* 2015;**372**:142–152.

433 Lokhorst HM, Plesner T, Gimsing P, et al. Phase I/II dose-escalation study of daratumumab in patients with relapsed or refractory multiple myeloma. *ASCO Meeting Abstracts.* 2013;**31**:8512.

434 Lonial S, Jagannath S, Moreau P, et al. Phase (Ph) I/II study of elotuzumab (Elo) plus lenalidomide/dexamethasone (Len/dex) in relapsed/refractory multiple myeloma (RR MM): updated Ph II results and Ph I/II long-term safety. *ASCO Meeting Abstracts.* 2013;**31**:8542.

504 Treon SP, Tripsas CK, Meid K, et al. Ibrutinib in Previously Treated Waldenstrom's Macroglobulinemia. *N Engl J Med.* 2015;**372**:1430–1440.

122

Myeloproliferative neoplasms: essential thrombocythemia, primary myelofibrosis, and polycythemia vera

Ayalew Tefferi, MD

Overview

The chronic myeloid neoplasms are a diverse group of malignant bone marrow conditions that originate in a transformed multipotential hematopoietic progenitor cell. This heterogeneous group of diseases shares an initially indolent clinical course with a variable degree of risk to evolve into overt acute leukemia. Even in the absence of leukemic transformation, the consequences of the cellular excesses or deficiencies characteristic of these disorders are troublesome for patients and all too frequently fatal; some of these disease complications include thrombosis, bleeding, marked hepatosplenomegaly, profound constitutional symptoms, and cachexia.

Under the revised 2008 World Health Organization (WHO) classification system, the broad category of chronic myeloid neoplasms include the myelodysplastic syndromes (MDS, discussed in ***Chapter 113***), myeloproliferative neoplasms (MPN), "MDS/MPN overlap," and a fourth subcategory that is characterized by both prominent blood eosinophilia and a mutation involving either platelet-derived growth factor receptor (PDGFRA or PDGFRB) or fibroblast growth factor receptor 1 (FGFR1).[1,2] The 2008 WHO MPN category includes the four classic "myeloproliferative disorders," which includes chronic myeloid leukemia (CML), polycythemia vera (PV), essential thrombocythemia (ET), and primary myelofibrosis (PMF) as well as chronic neutrophilic leukemia (CNL) chronic eosinophilic leukemia not otherwise specified (CEL-NOS) mastocytosis and MPN, unclassifiable (MPN-U). The "MDS/MPN" category displays features that are characteristic of both MDS (dyserythropoiesis or dysgranulopoiesis) and MPN (peripheral blood granulocytosis, monocytosis, eosinophilia, or thrombocytosis).[3] Included in this category are chronic myelomonocytic leukemia (CMML), juvenile myelomonocytic leukemia (JMML), "atypical chronic myeloid leukemia, *BCR-ABL1*-negative" (aCML), and "MDS/MPN, unclassifiable."[2] "MDS/MPN, unclassifiable" includes the WHO provisional entity of "refractory anemia with ring sideroblasts associated with marked thrombocytosis (RARS-T)."[3]

The first clear descriptions of ET, PV, and PMF were relatively recent; credit for priority is customarily given to Epstein and Goedel (Vienna, 1934) for ET, Vaquez (Paris, 1892) for PV, and Heuck (Heidelberg, 1879) for PMF.[4] Since 1960, CML has been defined by the presence of the Philadelphia chromosome, t(9;22)(q34q11).[5] In the 1980s, the aberrant *BCR-ABL* translocation—the molecular equivalent of the Philadelphia chromosome—was found to be diagnostic of CML and sufficient to cause the disease in a mouse model. Today, CML is the most well-defined and molecularly characterized of Dameshek's original MPD group.[6] This chapter considers the three *BCR-ABL*-negative classic MPN (i.e., ET, PV, and PMF).

Essential thrombocythemia

Epidemiology

ET is an uncommon disorder; estimates of its age- and gender-adjusted incidence range widely, from 0.2 to 2.5 cases per 100,000 persons per year.[7-9] Among younger people (ages 30–50), the disease appears to be more common in women, but this gender imbalance is not as clearly found in other age groups. No clear environmental risk factor has been identified. The incidence of ET (and also of PV and PMF) appears to be increased among Ashkenazi Jews.[10] The median age at diagnosis for all three MPN is approximately 60 years. Familial clustering of ET has been described but is exquisitely rare; some familial cases are associated with mutations in the thrombopoietin (*TPO*) gene that result in increased Tpo production (a megakaryocyte growth factor) with consequent megakaryocyte hyperstimulation.[11,12]

Diagnosis

The chief clinical challenge with respect to ET diagnosis is differentiating genuine autonomous thrombocytosis from the myriad causes of "secondary" or "reactive" thrombocytosis (RT). In more than 80% of routine cases of thrombocytosis, the elevated platelet count is polyclonal and represents a reaction to the presence of a nonmyeloid disorder.[13,14] The thrombocytosis associated with inflammatory, infectious, and malignant conditions is thought to be due to the action of megakaryocyte stimulatory cytokines such as interleukin-6 (IL-6), whereas the peculiar thrombocytosis seen occasionally in iron-deficient states remains poorly understood and may be mediated by erythropoietin (Epo) cross-stimulation of precursor cells committed to platelet production.[15]

The distinction between ET and RT is clinically important because there is an increased risk of thrombosis and bleeding associated with ET, but the risk with RT appears to be much lower.[13] If the presence of RT is not obvious, serum ferritin, and C-reactive protein (CRP—a surrogate marker for IL-6 levels) may be diagnostically useful in excluding iron deficiency and inflammation, respectively.[15] Elevated CRP levels suggest RT and should prompt a more thorough search for an obscure source of reactive cytokines. Of course, an elevated CRP does not strictly rule out ET, for a patient may potentially have ET and a comorbid inflammatory condition, but this is uncommon.[15] Ferritin levels must also be interpreted with caution: although a low value is consistent with iron deficiency, and a high value suggests RT, neither definitively excludes ET.

Holland-Frei Cancer Medicine, Ninth Edition. Edited by Robert C. Bast Jr., Carlo M. Croce, William N. Hait, Waun Ki Hong, Donald W. Kufe, Martine Piccart-Gebhart, Raphael E. Pollock, Ralph R. Weichselbaum, Hongyang Wang, and James F. Holland.
© 2017 John Wiley & Sons, Inc. ISBN: 978-1-118-93469-2

Surgical hyposplenism is usually obvious from a patient's history, but functional hyposplenism due to amyloidosis, celiac sprue, or another cause may not be so blatant.[16] Therefore, examination of a blood smear, searching specifically for Howell–Jolly bodies, should be made during the initial evaluation of each patient with chronic thrombocytosis.

Once these steps have been taken and there is no evidence for RT or hyposplenism, ET increases in likelihood and peripheral blood mutation screening for *JAK2*, *CALR*, and *MPL* mutations might facilitate the diagnosis of an underlying MPN without distinguishing ET from PV or PMF. ET should also be distinguished from other myeloid disorders that may have a very different prognosis and require different therapy. ET look-alike myeloid neoplasms include some cases of MDS, CML, and the other two non-ET classic MPN (i.e., PV and PMF, including the potentially confusing "cellular phase or prefibrotic" PMF). If conventional cytogenetic analysis in a suspected ET patient does not reveal a Philadelphia chromosome, it is prudent to obtain peripheral blood or bone marrow fluorescent *in situ* hybridization (FISH) studies at least once to exclude the possibility of karyotypically occult CML.

Distinguishing ET from PMF is usually not difficult, but there can be exceptions. Mild (grade 1 or 2) reticulin fibrosis can be found in approximately 15% of ET cases.[17] However, cellular phase or prefibrotic PMF, characterized by marrow hypercellularity with florid atypical megakaryocytic hyperplasia but not heavy fibrosis, can mimic ET in presentation and requires careful morphologic examination for distinction.[18] Abnormal megakaryocyte clusters on the bone marrow biopsy are characteristic of all three BCR-ABL-negative PMF. Cytogenetic abnormalities are present in fewer than 10% of patients at diagnosis.[19]

Pathogenesis

As mentioned earlier, clonal myeloproliferation involving the megakaryocytic lineage and sometimes other myeloid lineages (even in cases where the white count and hematocrit are normal) is demonstrable in the majority of female patients with ET via X-chromosome-linked DNA or gene product analysis.[20,21]

In 2005, a *JAK2* gain-of-function mutation (*JAK2*V617F) has been described in the majority of patients with ET as well as those in PMF and PV.[22–25] A much smaller proportion of patients with ET (~5%) carry an *MPL* mutation.[26–29] Most recently in 2013, a third mutation involving the calreticulin gene (*CALR*) was described in about half of the patients with *JAK2*-unmutated ET or PMF.[30] However, the precise pathogenetic contribution of these mutations is not clear.

In ET, megakaryocyte proliferation and platelet production are apparently autonomous, and normal regulatory pathways are apparently defective. The mechanism remains obscure in most cases. Megakaryocytes from ET patients are not inhibited by antibodies against key growth and differentiation cytokines, including IL-3, IL-6, granulocyte-monocyte colony-stimulating factor (GM-CSF), and Tpo.[31,32] Tpo and its receptor, c-Mpl, comprise the major feedback loop controlling megakaryocyte growth and development, but Tpo and c-Mpl dynamics in ET and related disorders appear to be complex. Tpo levels are often normal or elevated in ET despite the increased megakaryocyte mass but are not reproducibly different among normal marrow and ET or RT cases, while c-Mpl expression is often (but not always) markedly down-regulated in ET (Figure 1). However, c-Mpl expression is also down-regulated in other MPNs, so its diagnostic utility for ET is limited.[33,34] The specific cytokines driving megakaryocyte proliferation in ET have not been worked out in detail, but megakaryocyte progenitors from ET patients may display unexplained hypersensitivity to both IL-3 and Tpo.[35,36]

Clinical manifestations

At least half of patients with ET are asymptomatic at presentation; with appropriate therapy many can remain asymptomatic throughout the course of their illness although life expectancy is significantly shorter than the sex and age-matched control population.[37–39] At presentation, microvascular and vasomotor symptoms are found in 25–50% of ET patients. Major thrombosis is seen in 11–25% of patients at diagnosis and 10–22% during follow-up, while major hemorrhage is observed in 2–5% at diagnosis and 1–7% during follow-up.[9,38,40,41] Bleeding complications can be exacerbated by the use of aspirin (ASA) and non-steroidal anti-inflammatory drugs (NSAIDs), which have platelet inhibitory effects. In contrast to other MPN, where splenomegaly is very common, less than 25% of ET patients have palpable splenomegaly at the time of initial presentation.[37]

Vasomotor disturbances (e.g., headaches, lightheadedness, visual symptoms such as blurring and scotomata, palpitations, chest pain, erythromelalgia, and distal paresthesias) are troublesome but not generally life threatening. The proximate cause of such symptoms remains poorly defined; speculation has focused on abnormal platelet-endothelium interactions in the microvasculature, which can be associated with inflammation and transient thrombotic occlusion.[42] Various platelet products such as thromboxane A2 are vasoactive, and some of these probably also play a role in the pathobiology. Erythromelalgia is the most dramatic vasomotor symptom, characterized by erythema, warmth, and pain in distal

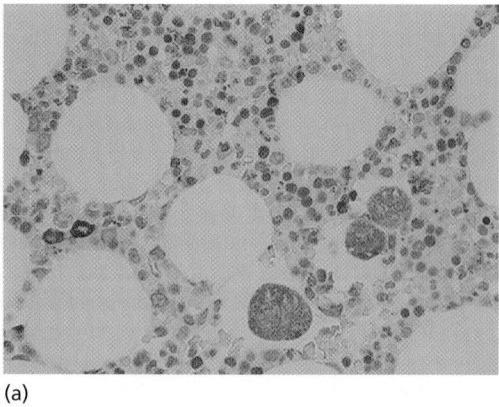

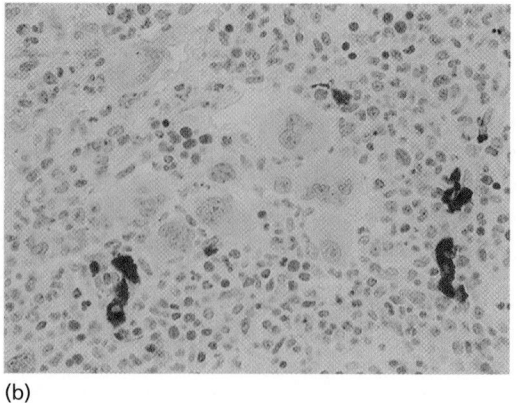

(a) (b)

Figure 1 (a) Normal megakaryocyte c-Mpl immunohistochemical staining and (b) decreased megakaryocyte c-Mpl staining in a myeloproliferative disorder. Source: Tefferi 2001.[37] Reproduced with permission of Elsevier.

extremities; this symptom is rare but not entirely specific for ET.[43] The presence of vasomotor microvessel disturbances does not clearly predict hemorrhage or thrombosis in large vessels.

There are several potentially life-threatening complications of ET: large-vessel thrombosis (both arterial and venous), hemorrhage, and transformation of the disease into either a fibrotic phase resembling PMF or acute myeloid leukemia (AML). Arterial thrombosis can lead to cerebrovascular events, cardiovascular ischemia, organ infarction, and digital gangrene. Venous thrombosis in ET occurs both in sites common to other thrombotic diatheses (e.g., pulmonary embolism and lower extremity deep venous thrombosis) and also in more unusual sites (e.g., cerebral sinus thrombosis, retinal vein thrombosis, and hepatic and portal vein thrombosis).[38]

Mucocutaneous bleeding (epistaxis, gingival bleeding, ecchymoses, and petechiae) can be a major nuisance. This is the most common hemorrhagic problem in ET.[44] Because epistaxis and easy bruising are very common in the general public, it can be difficult to assess the contribution of ET to these symptoms in afflicted patients. If careful control of the platelet count controls the mucocutaneous symptoms, it is reasonable to assume that thrombocytosis was contributory. Serious hemorrhage in ET is most common in the gastrointestinal tract and may be precipitated by ASA or NSAID use.[45] Hemorrhage also occurs in the central nervous system (CNS) and the retina, but such events are, fortunately, uncommon. Paradoxically, patients with extreme thrombocytosis may be at special risk for bleeding, in part related to the development of an acquired von Willebrand factor (vWF) deficiency that is thought to be related to platelet adsorption of large multimers of vWF. This phenomenon can be seen with extreme thrombocytosis of any cause.[46]

Fibrotic and leukemic evolutions of ET are rare events (<5% of patients) during the first 10 years after diagnosis.[37,38]

Prognosis and therapy

When considering therapy for ET, it is important to keep in mind two facts: (1) ET is generally an indolent disorder, with a life expectancy (at least in the first decade of the disease) quite close to that of an age- and gender-matched control population, and (2) no treatment to date has been shown to influence overall survival.[37,47] Therefore, the maxim *primum non nocere* should not be forgotten. Therapy for ET is usually initiated to palliate microvascular symptoms or prevent thrombotic or hemorrhagic complications. Vasomotor disturbances in ET can often be relieved with low dose ASA; 81 mg/day is usually enough. When ASA does not alleviate these symptoms, it is reasonable to add a platelet-lowering agent and this is often successful.

There are only a few randomized trials assessing the most appropriate therapy for diminishing the thrombotic risk in patients with ET, so clinical decisions must usually be based on prospective cohort studies and large retrospective analyses. Therapy should be guided by an individualized assessment of thrombotic risk. Two clinical parameters appear to be quite important in making this judgment: a history of thrombosis and age above 60 years.[41,48] On the basis

Table 1 Risk stratification in polycythemia vera and essential thrombocythemia.

Low-risk	Age below 60 years, and No history of thrombosis, and Platelet count below 1 million/μL
Low-risk with extreme thrombocytosis	Age below 60 years, and No history of thrombosis, and Platelet count above 1 million/μL
High-risk	Age 60 years or older, or A positive history of thrombosis

of the presence or absence of these two risk factors, patients with ET have been grouped into low-, high-, and indeterminate-risk groups and therapeutic decisions have been made accordingly (Tables 1 and 2).[49] This classification has recently been refined with the identification of *JAK2* mutation and cardiovascular risk factors as additional independent risk factors for arterial thrombosis in ET.[50] Accordingly, "low risk," as opposed to "very-low-risk" disease category, is defined by age <60 years and without history of thrombosis, but with either *JAK2* mutation or cardiovascular risk factors. Such patients without *JAK2* mutation or cardiovascular risk factors are assigned a "very-low-risk" disease category. The definition of high-risk disease remains unchanged and includes patients with age ≥60 years or presence of thrombosis history. JAK2V617F allele burden has limited relevance in ET prognosis.

The use of ASA (81–325 mg/day) to decrease thrombotic risk in low- and high-risk ET seems reasonable in view of demonstrated antithrombotic benefit in PV.[51,52] However, patients with very-low-risk disease, as defined earlier, might not require aspirin therapy. The more common approach for high-risk ET patients is to try to lower the platelet count into the normal range. One important randomized trial demonstrated a 20% absolute risk reduction (24–3.6%) in thrombotic events with the use of hydroxyurea (HU) in ET patients in a high-risk group.[53] Other cytoreductive agents have not yet been shown in a randomized manner to reduce thrombotic events. It is not clear precisely how low the goal platelet count should be in the high-risk group—thrombotic events can happen even with a platelet count in the normal range—but <400,000/μL seems to be a reasonable target and is supported by retrospective data.[54,55] For low- and very-low-risk patients, it is not clear that platelet-lowering agents are of any benefit, as thrombotic events are much less common in this group.

HU should be the first cytoreductive drug of choice in high-risk ET because of the high-quality evidence supporting its use. There has been concern about the leukemogenicity of HU, but in two recent studies of HU-treated patients with ET, no cases of leukemia were reported after 5–14 and 2–12 years of therapy.[56,57] Interferon-α2A (IFNα) and, more recently, longer-acting pegylated forms of interferon provide therapeutic alternatives in HU intolerant or refractory cases, but interferon's well-known toxicity limits use as first-line therapy, especially as many high-risk ET patients are elderly and have a difficult time tolerating the necessary doses.[58–60]

Table 2 Proposed risk-adjusted therapy in essential thrombocythemia.

Risk category[a]	Cytoreductive therapy	Aspirin therapy	Childbearing potential[b]
Low	No	Yes	ASA
High	Yes	Yes	Interferon α + ASA
Indeterminate	Sometimes	Yes (unless aVWD)	ASA (unless acquired VWD)

[a]See *Chapter 120* for algorithm regarding risk category assignment.
[b]Suggestions for drug therapy in women of childbearing potential are based on anecdotal evidence of safety.
Abbreviations: ASA, low-dose aspirin; aVWD, acquired von Willebrand disease.

IFNα is the drug of choice for ET patients requiring cytoreduction during pregnancy (see below).

Major bleeding (i.e., enough blood loss to drop hemoglobin level or cause bleeding in a critical organ, like the CNS) occurs in less than 10% of ET patients.[37,38] Extreme thrombocytosis (e.g., platelet count >1 million/μL) appears to be a risk factor for bleeding, in part because of the acquired vWF deficiency described earlier. Therapy designed to lower the platelet count and indirectly raise vWF levels may be indicated in the presence of a substantial reduction in large vWF multimers. In an emergency situation, platelet apheresis is the fastest way to lower the platelet count, but its utility has not been proven conclusively.

Special considerations

Pregnancy in ET is associated with increased risk (~35%) of first trimester spontaneous abortions.[61] There does not appear to be a postpartum thrombosis risk.[62] There is no clear association between the increased risk of spontaneous abortion and the degree of thrombocytosis, nor is there any clear benefit from prophylactic platelet apheresis.[61] High-risk pregnant women with ET (i.e., women with previous thrombosis) require cytoreductive therapy just like other high-risk patients. There is anecdotal evidence of the safety of IFNα in pregnancy but no controlled data. HU and pipobroman are considered teratogenic (FDA pregnancy class D) and anagrelide also crosses the placenta and has unknown effects on the developing fetus (FDA pregnancy class C). The teratogenicity of HU, however, does not appear to be severe enough to justify elective abortion in cases of inadvertent early fetal exposure.[63]

Primary myelofibrosis

Epidemiology

Among the three classic MPN, PMF is the most aggressive. Fortunately, PMF is a rare scourge; the incidence is only 0.4–1.5 cases per 100,000 persons per year, with a median age at diagnosis above 60 years and a slight male predominance.[7,8] PMF has been associated with exposure to ionizing radiation (e.g., in Hiroshima survivors), heavy exposure to petroleum derivatives, and thorium dioxide (Thorotrast) contrast medium, but in the vast majority of cases, there is no such exposure history.[64,65]

Pathogenesis

As with other MPN, myeloid-derived cells in PMF have been shown to be monoclonal by analysis of X-linked genes and gene products.[66] In contrast, the marrow fibroblasts in PMF are polyclonal.[66,67] The florid bone marrow stromal reaction that is so characteristic of PMF includes fibroblast hyperproliferation, a dramatic increase in extracellular matrix proteins such as collagen (mostly type I and type III), increased blood vessel formation (angiogenesis), and increased bone synthesis and osteoblast activity (osteosclerosis).[68,69] Such marrow microenvironmental changes are mediated by a cytokine storm elaborated by the clonal myeloid cells. Indeed, increased cellular and extracellular levels of multiple cytokines with fibrogenic, angiogenic, and/or osteogenic potential have been detected in PMF, lending support to this hypothesis.[70]

There are several murine models in which marrow fibrosis and/or extramedullary hematopoiesis (EMH) have been observed. Mice forced to over-express TPO develop of marrow fibrosis and osteosclerosis, which may be due to hypersecretion of osteoprotegerin, an osteoclast-inhibiting factor.[71,72] Mice that under-express the transcription factor *GATA-1*, which is important in the development and differentiation of hematopoietic cells, suffer impaired megakaryocyte differentiation and diminished platelet production and eventually develop EMH and marrow fibrosis.[73] However, it is not clear to what extent these germ line mouse mutants are faithful models of the neoplastic disorder in humans, where any mutations would be expected to be restricted to hematopoietic cells. Mutations or expression changes in TPO or its receptor (c-Mpl) or *GATA-1* have not been found in human PMF, and mutations in FOG-1, the major GATA-1 cofactor, are also generally absent.[74]

The molecular lesions underlying PMF are beginning to become apparent. Most notable is the 2005 report of a *JAK2* gain-of-function mutation (*JAK2*V617F) that was discovered in the majority of patients with PMF, ET, and PV.[22-25] In 2006 and 2007, other *JAK2* (in PV) and *MPL* (in ET and PMF) mutations were described in *JAK2*V617F-negative cases.[26-29] Most recently in 2013, a third driver mutation in MPN involving the calreticulin (*CALR*) gene has been described and is found in approximately 25% of patients with PMF and is mutually exclusive of *JAK2* or *MPL* mutations.[75] However, the precise pathogenetic contribution of these mutations is not clear. Recurrent karyotypic abnormalities seen in PMF include del(13q), del(20q), trisomy 8, trisomy 9, del(12p), and abnormalities of chromosomes 1 and 7, all of which are found in other chronic myeloid disorders and have no specificity for PMF.[76] About half of patients with PMF have a cytogenetic abnormality at diagnosis, but there is no predominant lesion and no individual cytogenetic abnormality affects more than 15–20% of patients.

Diagnosis

Characteristic features of PMF include a hypercellular marrow with fibrosis; EMH, which is most often manifest as splenomegaly; anemia; and a so-called myelophthisic peripheral blood picture.[70] Marrow fibrosis and a myelophthisic blood picture alone are not diagnostic of PMF, as myelofibrosis is associated with a diverse litany of conditions, including metastatic cancer, other hematologic disorders, and rheumatologic and granulomatous diseases (Table 3). Myelophthisic peripheral blood findings include marked anisocytosis, poikilocytosis, teardrop-shaped red cells (dacryocytes), and left-shifted granulocytopoiesis. The mechanism is unclear. Even EMH is not completely specific for PMF, as it can be observed in other conditions where the bone marrow is replaced (e.g., metastatic cancer) or marrow hematopoiesis is inadequate (e.g., β-thalassemia).[77,78]

Because of hypercellularity and fibrosis, the bone marrow in PMF is often difficult to aspirate, resulting in a dry tap. Core marrow biopsy usually shows heavy collagen fibrosis, osteosclerosis, intra-sinusoidal hematopoiesis, and atypical megakaryocyte hyperplasia. Marrow fibrosis can be difficult to assess on standard hematoxylin and eosin stains and may be better estimated by the use of special stains, such as that for reticulin (a silver impregnation technique that stains a glycoprotein elaborated by stromal cells) or the trichrome stain for collagen. In some cases of PMF, the degree of bone marrow fibrosis may initially be minimal. This finding is often called the "cellular phase" of PMF and can be diagnostically challenging. Fibrosis grading schemes have been developed but are of relatively limited clinical utility.[79]

The bone marrow morphologic features of PMF may sometimes be difficult to distinguish from those of myelodysplastic syndromes with fibrosis (MDS-*f*) and the so-called acute myelofibrosis. The latter entity has substantial overlap with megakaryocytic acute leukemia (AML-M7).[79] Megakaryocytes alone often appear dysplastic in routine cases of PMF, but significant dysplasia in other cell lines favors a diagnosis of MDS-*f*.[79] Acute myelofibrosis (also

Table 3 Causes of bone marrow fibrosis.

Myeloid disorders	Nonhematological disorders	Other hematologic disorders
Myelofibrosis with myeloid metaplasia	Metastatic cancer	Hairy cell leukemia
Chronic myeloid leukemia	Connective tissue disorders (e.g., lupus and systemic sclerosis)	Multiple myeloma
Essential thrombocythemia		Lymphoproliferative disorders
Atypical chronic myeloid disorders	Infections (granulomatous disease, tuberculosis, kala-azar, etc.)	Gray platelet syndrome
Hypereosinophilic syndromes		
Polycythemia vera	Vitamin D deficiency—rickets	
Myelodysplastic syndrome with fibrosis	Renal osteodystrophy	
Malignant histiocytosis	Paget disease	
Systemic mastocytosis	Hyperparathyroidism	
Acute myelofibrosis		
Acute megakaryoblastic leukemia (AML-M7)		
Other acute myeloid leukemias		

[a]See **Chapter 113** for algorithm regarding risk category assignment.
[b]Suggestions for drug therapy in women of childbearing potential are based on anecdotal evidence of safety.
Abbreviations: ASA, low-dose aspirin; aVWD, acquired von Willebrand disease.

known as malignant myelosclerosis or acute myelosclerosis) is suggested when constitutional symptoms are prominent, development of the illness is rapid (i.e., over the course of a few weeks), and the spleen is not palpable. Special stains for megakaryoblasts (e.g., CD61 or vWF) may reveal the presence of an otherwise unrecognized cell population. Sometimes, despite the best efforts of clinicians and pathologists, the diagnosis is simply not clear and patients must be treated expectantly.

Clinical manifestations

About 25% of patients with PMF are asymptomatic at diagnosis. Most patients have anemia and at least some degree of splenomegaly at presentation. The anemia of PMF is multifactorial. Contributing problems include replacement of normal hematopoietic tissue with fibrosis, ineffective hematopoiesis in the remaining myeloid tissue, and hypersplenism. Splenomegaly in PMF may be massive, and the spleen is usually very firm. Spleen and liver enlargement in PMF is secondary to EMH and may be associated with hypercatabolic symptoms (profound fatigue, weight loss, night sweats, and low-grade fever), peripheral edema (from venous compression), diarrhea, early satiety (from gastric compression), and, occasionally, portal hypertension.

Splenomegaly in PMF may be complicated by infarction, an event heralded by moderate to severe pain that may be referred to the left shoulder and often requires opiate analgesics to control.[80] CT imaging in such cases can be unremarkable or may show wedge-shaped or rounded low-attenuation lesions in the spleen. EMH occurs in a great diversity of sites throughout the body. Common sites besides spleen and liver include lymph nodes, skin, pleura, peritoneum, lung, and the paraspinal and epidural spaces. The latter may result in spinal cord and/or nerve root compression, which is a medical emergency requiring corticosteroids to reduce edema and immediate radiotherapy.[81] It is fortunate that localized EMH responds promptly to low doses of gamma irradiation (100–150 cGy).

Red cell transfusion dependence in PMF is widespread. Serum levels of LDH are often elevated, reflecting both ineffective hematopoiesis and injury to the liver by EMH. Hyperuricemia and consequent episodes of gout are not uncommon and reflect ineffective hematopoiesis with high cell turnover. Bone pain is seen and is multifactorial, related to marrow replacement and periostitis. Sweet syndrome (neutrophilic dermatosis) is sometimes associated with PMF, and this lesion must be distinguished from cutaneous EMH since treatment differs.[82]

Death in PMF can come from many directions. Fatal infection and transformation to a resistant myeloid leukemia are common. Overt leukemia occurs in approximately 20% of patients over the first 10 years.[83] Less frequent causes of death include thrombohemorrhagic events and heart failure, often secondary to pulmonary hypertension.

Prognosis

Current risk stratification in PMF is based on eight clinical parameters forming the Dynamic International Prognostic Scoring System (DIPSS)-plus.[84] The eight parameters include unfavorable karyotype (i.e., complex karyotype or sole or two abnormalities that include +8, −7/7q-, i(17q), inv(3), −5/5q-, 12p- or 11q23 rearrangement),[85,86] red cell transfusion need[87,88] platelet count $<100 \times 10^9$/L, age >65 years, hemoglobin <10 g/dL, leukocyte count $>25 \times 10^9$/L, circulating blasts ≥1% and presence of constitutional symptoms.[89] The four DIPSS-plus risk categories based on the aforementioned eight risk factors are low (no risk factors), intermediate-1 (one risk factor), intermediate-2 (two or three risk factors) and high (four or more risk factors) with respective median survivals of 15.4, 6.5, 2.9, and 1.3 years.[84]

Since the publication of DIPSS-plus, several studies that suggest additional prognostic information have been published. For example, a >80% 2-year mortality in PMF was predicted by monosomal karyotype, inv(3)/i(17q) abnormalities, or any two of circulating blasts >9%, leukocytes $≥40 \times 10^9$/L or other unfavorable karyotype.[90] Similarly, inferior survival in PMF has been associated with nullizygosity for JAK2 46/1 haplotype,[91] low JAK2V617F allele burden,[92,93] or the presence of IDH,[94] EZH2,[95] SRSF2,[96] or ASXL1[97] mutations.

Most recently, Tefferi et al. studied 254 patients with PMF and reported mutational frequencies of 58% for JAK2, 25% CALR, 8% MPL, and 9% wild-type for all three mutations (i.e., triple-negative).[98] CALR mutational frequency in JAK2/MPL-unmutated cases was 74%. CALR mutations were associated with younger age, higher platelet count, and lower DIPSS-plus score. CALR-mutated patients were also less likely to be anemic, require transfusions, or display leukocytosis. Spliceosome mutations were infrequent in CALR-mutated patients. In a subsequent international study of 570 patients,[99] the authors reported the longest survival in CALR+ASXL1− patients (median 10.4 years) and shortest in CALR−ASXL1+ patients (median 2.3 years). CALR+ASXL1+ and CALR−ASXL1− patients had similar survival and were grouped together in an intermediate risk category (median survival

5.8 years). Guglielmelli et al.[100] subsequently demonstrated the additional value of the number of prognostically detrimental mutations.

Therapy

Conventional therapy for PMF is largely palliative and has not been shown to improve survival. Patients should be considered for clinical trials of new treatments whenever feasible. Older treatments for anemia include androgen preparations (e.g., oral fluoxymesterone 10 mg two times a day or danazol 400–600 mg/day), which, given the older age of the typical male PMF patient, should be initiated only after ruling out occult prostate cancer.[101] Corticosteroids may also give transient benefit in this setting (e.g., oral prednisone at a starting dose of 30–40 mg/day for first month and then taper off over the second month). Unfortunately, responses to androgens and steroids are uncommon; they occur in less than one-third of PMF patients and are usually of brief duration. In the case of an endogenous Epo level that is less than 100 mIU/mL, it is tempting to consider a brief trial of treatment with erythropoiesis stimulating agents (ESAs).[102] However, such therapy exacerbates PMF-associated splenomegaly, does not work for transfusion-dependent patients, and may be associated with increased risk of leukemic transformation.[103] For symptomatic splenomegaly in PMF, HU is the first choice and ruxolitinib the second drug of choice.[104] An initial dose of 500 mg of HU three times per day typically brings salutary results within 1–2 weeks, and the dose can then be adjusted to optimal effect.

Thalidomide can improve cytopenias and reduce spleen size in PMF.[105] Reported response rates range between 20% and 62% for anemia, 25% and 80% for thrombocytopenia, and 7% and 30% for splenomegaly.[105,106] In conventional doses similar to those used for multiple myeloma (e.g., 200 mg/day and above), thalidomide has been associated with severe myeloproliferative reactions, including accelerated EMH.[107] Lower doses of thalidomide (e.g., 50 mg/day) appear to be better tolerated and responses are often durable.[106,108] The addition of prednisone to the lower dose schedule improves tolerance and may enhance the erythropoietic activity of the drug.[106,108]

Several new drugs have been evaluated in PMF, post-PV/ET MF, and other related MPN, including additional immunomodulators and JAK inhibitors.[109] Pomalidomide, an immunomodulatory drug, improved anemia in 25% of patients when was used alone (2 mg/day) or in combination with prednisone (0.5 or 2 mg/day).[110] In a second phase II study, anemia response was observed only in cases with JAK2V617F mutations (24% vs 0%).[111] Platelet response occurred in 58% of patients, but there was little impact on spleen size. Drug-associated neuropathy or myelosuppression was observed infrequently. Use of doses >2 mg/day failed to increase activity but did produce greater myelosuppression.[112] A phase-3 study comparing pomalidomide with placebo did not demonstrate a significant difference in anemia response, but platelet response was significantly improved with pomalidomide.[113]

A number of JAK inhibitor ATP mimetics have been evaluated in patients with MPN including ruxolitinib (INCB018424), fedratinib (SAR302503), momelotinib (CYT387), lestaurtinib (CEP-701), pacritinib (SB1518), AZD1480, BMS911543, LY2784544, and XL019 (*clinicalTrials.gov*). Ruxolitinib, a JAK1/JAK2 inhibitor, was initially evaluated in a phase I/II study of 153 patients with PMF or post-PV/ET MF.[114] Toxicities included thrombocytopenia, anemia, and a "cytokine rebound reaction" on stopping the drug, with an acute relapse of symptoms and splenomegaly.[115] Improvement in constitutional symptoms and weight gain were seen in the majority of patients and 44% experienced ≥50% decrease in palpable spleen size. Transfusion independence was achieved in 4 of 28 transfusion-dependent patients (14%). A major reduction in proinflammatory cytokines (e.g., IL-1RA, IL-6, TNF-a, and MIP-1b) was measured and correlated with improvement in constitutional symptoms.

Two randomized studies have compared ruxolitinib with either placebo or best supportive care.[116,117] In the COMFORT-1 trial, comparing the drug to placebo (n = 309),[75] ruxolitinib significantly not only improved spleen response (42% vs <1%) and constitutional symptoms (46%) but also produced greater anemia (31% vs 13.9%) and thrombocytopenia (34.2% vs 9.3%). In the COMFORT-2 trial, comparing the drug with "best available therapy" (n = 219),[117] ruxolitinib improved spleen response (28.5% vs 0%) but also worsened thrombocytopenia (44.5% vs 9.6%), anemia (40.4% vs 12.3%), and diarrhea (24.0% vs 11.0%). Long-term follow-up in patients with MF indicated that a high fraction discontinued the drug after a median time of 9.2 months. Severe withdrawal symptoms were observed after stopping the drug with acute relapse of disease symptoms, accelerated splenomegaly, worsening of cytopenias, and occasional hemodynamic decompensation, including a septic shock-like syndrome. In COMFORT-2, 55% of patients discontinued the drug within 3 years. A slight but statistically significant improvement in survival was observed, despite cross-over of the arms. Recent reports have associated ruxolitinib use with serious opportunistic infections.[118]

Fedratinib, a selective JAK2 inhibitor, was initially evaluated in a phase I/II study of 59 patients with PMF or post-PV/ET MF.[119] A >50% decrease in palpable spleen size was observed in 39% and 47% of patients, after 6 or 12 months of treatment, respectively. The majority of patients reported a durable resolution of their symptoms. Side effects included nausea (3%), vomiting (3%), diarrhea (10%), asymptomatic mild increases in serum amylase/lipase (27%), transaminases (27%) or creatinine (24%), thrombocytopenia (24%), and anemia (35%). In general, the presence of JAK2V617F did not correlate with response. A phase-III study (n = 289) comparing fedratinib at two different doses (500 or 400 mg/day) with placebo confirmed the efficacy of the drug in relieving symptoms and reducing the spleen size (49%, 47% and 1%, respectively), but reports of encephalopathy associated with the use of the drug resulted in its withdrawal from further development.[120]

Momelotinib (MMB, GS-0387, and CYT387), a JAK1 and JAK2 inhibitor, has been evaluated in a phase I-II study where response in anemia and spleen size were observed in 59% and 48% of participants, respectively. Decreased transfusion requirement for at least 12 weeks (range 4.7 to >18.3 months) was observed in 70% of 33 patients who were red cell transfused in the month before study entry.[121] Most patients experienced an improvement in constitutional symptoms. Grade 3/4 adverse reactions included thrombocytopenia (32%), hyperlipasemia (5%), elevated liver transaminases (3%), and headache (3%). New-onset treatment-related peripheral neuropathy was observed in 22% of patients (sensory symptoms, grade 1). The study was subsequently expanded to include 166 patients treated at either 150 or 300 mg once-daily, or 150 mg twice-daily for 9 months, with similar results.[122] The drug is currently being compared to ruxolitinib in a phase-III study.

Pacritinib (SB1518) is a JAK2/FLT3 inhibitor that produced an MRI spleen response rate of 32% accompanied by improvement in symptoms but with an anemia response in only 6% of 34 participants in a phase II study.[123] The most common treatment-related adverse events were gastrointestinal, especially diarrhea.

Splenectomy can be considered for patients with refractory splenic pain, disabling constitutional symptoms, symptomatic portal hypertension, and/or a need for frequent red cell transfusions. In one series of 223 PMF patients who underwent splenectomy, durable remissions in constitutional symptoms, transfusion-dependent anemia, portal hypertension, and severe thrombocytopenia were achieved in 67%, 23%, 50%, and 0% of patients, respectively.[124] However, even in experienced centers, the perioperative mortality rate of splenectomy in PMF may be as high as 9%, and overall survival may not be affected; the median postsplenectomy survival is about 2 years.[124] An elevated D-dimer, even in the absence of overt disseminated intravascular coagulopathy, may predict a higher surgical risk. Up to 25% of surgical survivors will develop marked hepatomegaly or extreme thrombocytosis.[124] Presplenectomy thrombocytopenia correlates with the risk of postsplenectomy leukemic transformation, for unclear reasons. Extreme postsplenectomy thrombocytosis is significantly associated with perioperative thrombosis. HU can be used perioperatively to prevent a postsplenectomy rise in platelet count. In poor surgical candidates with symptomatic splenomegaly, the palliative use of splenic irradiation is reasonable, but success is irregular and of brief duration.[125]

The use of allogeneic hematopoietic stem cell transplantation (allo-SCT) in PMF was initially limited because of concerns regarding potential failure of stem cells to engraft in the fibrotic marrow. This concern has not been substantiated. Marrow fibrosis delays post-transplantation platelet recovery by about 3 days and increases platelet transfusion needs slightly, but is not clearly associated with graft failure or other unique transplant-related problems.[126] Interest in allo-SCT in patients with PMF is now growing, but appropriate patient selection and timing remain challenging. While engraftment has not been especially problematic, toxicity continues to be a major issue, even with the newer reduced-intensity "non-myeloablative" conditioning regimens.[127] In one study of allo-SCT in myelofibrosis, the 5-year survival was only 14% for patients older than 44 years, and in another study, the 2-year survival was just 41%.[128,129] Rates of chronic graft-versus-host disease of up to 59% have been reported.[130] Younger patients do somewhat better, with post-transplant survival rates of up to 60%, but the decision to proceed to transplant must only be made after careful deliberation, and patients chosen should be those with particularly limited life expectancy.[128,130]

Polycythemia vera

Epidemiology

The incidence of PV is 0.8–2.6 cases per 100,000 persons per year, with most studies giving figures at the upper end of that range, and this incidence appears to be relatively stable over time.[131,132] As is the case with the other MPN, the incidence of PV increases with age. The median age at diagnosis is approximately 60 years; the disease can also be seen in young people, and 7% of cases are diagnosed before the age of 40.[133,134] There may be a slight male preponderance (on the order of a 1.2:1 male-to-female case ratio), and the disease is more common in Jews, especially Ashkenazi Jews.[10,135] In a few cases, true PV may be familial, but apparently familial erythrocytosis is often proven to be a result of a shared high-oxygen-affinity hemoglobin or a common exposure (e.g., a residence at high altitude or cobalt intoxication).[136,137]

Pathogenesis

X-linked (G6PD) enzyme analysis first demonstrated the clonal nature of hematopoietic cells in PV in 1976.[138] In 2005, a *JAK2* gain-of-function mutation (*JAK2*V617F) that was discovered in the majority of patients with PV.[22–25] In 2007, other *JAK2* mutations were described in *JAK2*V617F-negative cases.[28] *JAK2*V617F is an exon 14G to T somatic mutation. The nucleotide change at position 1849 results in the substitution of valine to phenylalanine at codon 617. *JAK2*V617F is also present in patients with PV, ET, and PMF.[22–25] The mutation has also described in other myeloid neoplasms.[139,140] As of the time of this writing, JAK2V617F has not been reported in lymphoid disorders,[141–144] solid tumor,[145–147] or secondary myeloproliferation.[148,149] In general, mutational frequency is estimated at over 95% in PV, 50% in ET or PMF, 20% in certain other MPNs including refractory anemia with ringed sideroblasts and thrombocytosis (RARS-T) and less than 5% in AML or MDS.[150–153]

*JAK2*V617F induces a PV-like phenotype in murine transplant models.[24,154,155] Mutant allele burden in patients with ET is significantly lower than that seen in patients with either PV or PMF.[156–160] At least in PV, a higher allele burden is the result of *JAK2*V617F homozygosity, which is accomplished by mitotic recombination.[22,23,25] In humans, *JAK2*V617F occurs at a primitive stem cell level and is chronologically an early event.[161–163] Some but not all[164] studies have suggested *JAK2*V617F clonal involvement of NK,[165] T,[166] and B[166] lymphocytes. Regardless, there is evidence to suggest that *JAK2*V617F may not be the initial clonogenic event in either PV or other MPNs and that its presence might not be mandatory for endogenous colony formation.[167–169] The recent demonstration of *JAK2*V617F-negative leukemia clones arising in *JAK2*V617F-positive MPN patients lends further support in this regard.[170,171]

In 2007, a set of *JAK2* exon 12 mutations were described in *JAK2*V617F-negative patients with PV in whom erythrocytosis was the predominant feature.[172] Because of the latter feature, some of the cases were assigned the diagnosis of "idiopathic" erythrocytosis although their serum Epo level was almost always below the reference range and EECs were demonstrated in every instance when tested. The majority of the cases (10 of 11) in the original report[172] were found to harbor one of four exon 12 *JAK2* mutant alleles: N542-E543del (four cases), F537-K539delinsL (three cases), K539L (two cases), H538QK539L (one case). All four exon 12 mutant alleles induced cytokine-independent/hypersensitive proliferation in erythropoietin receptor-expressing cell lines and constitutive activation of JAK-STAT signaling.[172] In addition, *JAK2*K539L induced a PV phenotype in a mouse transplant model. Many other studies have now confirmed the observations from the above-mentioned study[28,173–177] and in the process, most[28,173,174] but not all[175,177] of the studies suggested that exon 12 mutations occurred in virtually all *JAK2*V617F-negative PV cases (i.e., ~3% of all PV cases). Furthermore, several other exon 12 mutation variants were added to the list including R541–E543delinsK, I540–E543delinsMK, V536-I546dup11, F537-I546dup10+547L, and E543-D544del.[174–176]

The erythroid colony-forming progenitor cells (BFU-E and CFU-E) in PV are very sensitive to or independent of normal growth and differentiation signals, including Epo, GM-CSF, stem cell factor, and IL-3.[178,179] Although this finding is characteristic of PV, it is not specific and is also observed in ET and PMF. Serum Epo levels in PV patients are generally very low or inappropriately normal in the setting of erythrocytosis, and excessive Epo-independent BFU-E and CFU-E proliferation leads to an increased red cell mass (RCM).[180,181] As is the case with the Tpo receptor in ET, some families with recurrent PV have been found to harbor Epo receptor mutations, but structural changes in the Epo receptor have been diligently sought in nonfamilial PV but not found.[182,183] Epo receptor expression patterns may be abnormal in PV (e.g., loss of the normal high-affinity Epo receptor) but this finding is not consistent.[184] Cells from patient with PV are consistently observed to by hypersensitive to insulin-like growth factor-1 (IGF-1), which appears to be due to alterations in IGF-1 binding proteins, including increased baseline phosphorylation of the IGF-1 receptor.[185] Decreased activity of the SHP-1 phosphatase (which associates with the receptors for Epo, stem cell factor, and IL-3, and is a negative regulator of signals generated during ligand binding), constitutive activation of STAT-3, increased levels of anti-apoptotic proteins such as Bcl-X_L, and several other biochemical abnormalities have been reported in subsets of patients; their general pathobiologic relevance is yet unclear.[186-188]

Karyotypic abnormalities are found in about 10–20% of untreated patients.[189,190] The lesions seen are those nonspecific abnormalities typical of chronic myeloid disorders, such as trisomy 8, trisomy 9, del(20q), del(13q), loss of the Y chromosome in men, and abnormalities of chromosomes 5 and 7.[190]

Clinical features

Signs and symptoms frequently associated with PV are listed in Table 4. Many of the clinical features of PV are a direct consequence of the increased RCM and are common to all causes of erythrocytosis, but pruritus and splenomegaly strongly suggest PV. Increased RCM can lead to blood hyperviscosity, which leads to a plethora of symptoms and signs. Headaches are frequent, but blurry vision, altered hearing, mucous membrane bleeding, shortness of breath, and malaise are also observed. Hypertension may be a consequence of increased RCM. At least two-thirds of PV patients have splenomegaly, so the combination of splenomegaly and erythrocytosis should strongly suggest PV.[191] Thrombosis occurs in about 40% of patients, most commonly arterial thrombosis.[133] Clots occur at a rate of about 3.9% of patients per year.[133] Arterial thromboses are more likely to be fatal than venous thromboses. As in ET, venous thrombosis can occur in unusual sites, such as mesenteric or hepatic vessels. Bleeding, especially gastrointestinal, is seen in PV but less often than thrombosis.[133] Pruritus is a common and classic PV-associated complaint, which may be provoked by warm water (aquagenic); its pathogenesis is unclear.[192,193] Erythromelalgia (described above under ET) might also trouble patients with PV, as do other vasomotor symptoms; paresthesias and headaches.

Table 4 Polycythemia vera-related clinical and laboratory features.

Symptoms and physical findings	Frequency (%)
Systolic hypertension	72
Splenomegaly	70
Skin plethora (ruddy cyanosis)	67
Conjunctival plethora	59
Headache	48
Weakness	47
Engorged retinal veins	46
Pruritus	43
Dizziness	43
Palpable liver	40
Sweating	33
Diastolic hypertension	32
Visual disturbances	31
Weight loss	29
Paresthesias	29
Dyspnea	26
Joint symptoms	26
Epigastric distress	24

Source: Berlin 1975.[191] Reproduced with permission of Elsevier.

Leukocytosis and thrombocytosis are present in less than half of PV patients.

Diagnosis

The major diagnostic difficulty with respect to PV is distinguishing PV from the many other causes of erythrocytosis (Table 5).

The 1975 Polycythemia Vera Study Group diagnostic criteria[191] were an advancement in their time, but are now chiefly of historical interest.[194,195] These criteria included direct measurement of the RCM, which is a cumbersome procedure that is no longer strictly necessary in most cases. The availability of new diagnostic tools, as well as better appreciation of the tight relationship between hematocrit and RCM, has undermined the use of RCM measurement in the diagnosis of PV.

Because more than 95% of patients with PV carry the *JAK2*V617F mutation, one could initiate the workup of a patient with suspected PV with peripheral blood mutation screening for *JAK2*V617F. In order to minimize the consequences of false-positive or false-negative test results, as well as capture the few cases that are *JAK2*V617F-negative PV, I recommend concomitant measurement of serum Epo level, which is abnormally low in more than 90% of patients with PV.[196] If the results of both tests are suggestive of PV (i.e., mutation-positive and low serum Epo), then the diagnosis is likely and bone marrow examination is encouraged but not essential for making the diagnosis. If the *JAK2*V617F and serum Epo test results are both not consistent with the diagnosis of PV (i.e., mutation-negative and either normal or increased Epo), then further investigation is not advised unless dictated otherwise by the clinical scenario. If there is discrepancy between the molecular test and serum Epo level, one should first repeat both tests and then proceed with bone marrow examination if the results are unchanged. In this regard, the possibility of exon 12 *JAK2* mutations should be entertained in *JAK2*V617F-negative cases with low serum Epo level.

When congenital polycythemia is suspected, initial laboratory testing should include measurement of the oxygen tension at which hemoglobin is 50% saturated (p50). Left-shifted oxygen dissociation curve, suggested by decreased p50, suggests the presence of either high oxygen-affinity hemoglobinopathy (autosomal dominant)[197] or 2,3-bisphosphoglycerate (2,3-BPG) deficiency, usually a consequence of BPG mutase mutation (autosomal recessive).[198] If the p50 is normal, then the possibility of *VHL* mutations should be considered first because they constitute the most frequent mutations in congenital polycythemia. In this regard, Russian ethnic origin would suggest Chuvash polycythemia, which is characterized by increased serum Epo.[199] However, Chuvash-type or other *VHL* mutations have also been described in other ethnic groups and therefore worth considering in the presence of any congenital polycythemia associated with increased serum Epo. There is currently limited information on *HIF-1α* prolyl hydroxylase gene mutation,[200] which incidentally is associated with normal serum Epo level. On the other hand, *EPOR* mutations are well described and should be considered in congenital polycythemia associated with either low or normal serum Epo level.[201]

Prognosis

The median life expectancy for patients diagnosed with PV exceeds 10 years but is worse than a gender- and age-matched control population.[47] Thrombohemorrhagic complications and transformation into AML account for much of the inferior survival.[202] As with ET, older age (>60 years) appears to be a risk factor for thrombosis.[203] Other clearly prognostic factors in PV beyond old age and a history of thrombosis have not been determined. In about 15–20% of cases,

Table 5 Classification of erythrocytosis.

---

1) Apparent Polycythemia
  a) Relative polycythemia due to major fluid shifts
  b) Extreme "high-normal" values
2) True Polycythemia
  a) Polycythemia vera
  b) Secondary polycythemia
    i) Erythropoietin (EPO)-mediated
      (1) Hypoxia-driven
        (a) Central hypoxic process
          (i) Chronic lung disease
          (ii) Right-to-left cardiopulmonary vascular shunts
          (iii) High-altitude habitat
          (iv) Carbon monoxide poisoning and smoker's polycythemia
          (v) Hypoventilation syndromes including sleep apnea
        (b) Peripheral hypoxic process
          (i) Localized
            1. Renal artery stenosis
          (ii) Diffuse
            1. High-oxygen-affinity hemoglobinopathy (*congenital*; *autosomal-dominant*)
            2. 2,3-Diphosphoglycerate mutase deficiency (*congenital*; *autosomal-recessive*)
      (2) Hypoxia-independent (pathologic EPO production)
        (a) Malignant tumors
          (i) Hepatocellular carcinoma
          (ii) Renal cell cancer
          (iii) Cerebellar hemangioblastoma
          (iv) Parathyroid carcinoma
        (b) Non-malignant conditions
          (i) Uterine leiomyomas
          (ii) Renal cysts (polycystic kidney disease)
          (iii) Pheochromocytoma
          (iv) Meningioma
        (c) Abnormally elevated set point for EPO production (congenital)
        (d) Chuvash polycythemia (congenital; abnormal oxygen homeostasis?)
      (3) Intentional EPO doping
    ii) EPO receptor-mediated
      (1) Activating mutation of the erythropoietin receptor
      (2) Some cases of autosomal-dominant congenital polycythemia
    iii) Drug-associated
      (1) Treatment with androgen preparations
      (2) Treatment with novel erythropoietic agents such as CERA
    iv) Unknown mechanisms
      (1) Most cases of autosomal-dominant congenital polycythemia
      (2) Some forms of autosomal-recessive congenital polycythemia
      (3) Post renal transplant erythrocytosis

PV terminates in a "spent phase," a PMF-like state. This transition is usually characterized by worsening anemia and increasing white count and spleen size.

Treatment

As is the case with ET, PV-associated vasomotor symptoms are usually alleviated by low doses of ASA. PV-associated pruritus can be treated with selective serotonin reuptake inhibitors, such as paroxetine.[192] Antihistamines such as hydroxyzine and diphenhydramine are less effective.

The primary goal of treatment in PV is to prevent disastrous thrombotic events without increasing the risk of other life-threatening problems, such as bleeding, or altering the potential for transformation to a fibrotic marrow or acute leukemia. The main tool used to accomplish this goal is therapeutic phlebotomy. The importance of regular phlebotomy as part of a successful treatment program for PV cannot be overemphasized; marrow-suppressing drugs play only a supplementary role. In the first few decades after the disease's description, before aggressive phlebotomy became *de rigueur*, the median survival for patients with PV was on the order of 2 years, and most deaths were due to thrombotic events.[204,205]

Today, most PV-related deaths are still due to thrombosis, but patients treated initially with phlebotomy alone have a median survival of more than 15 years.[133]

On the basis of the studies that have shown an improved cerebral blood flow and normalization of blood viscosity with a hematocrit below 45%, as well as less thrombosis in patients with hematocrits in this range, dropping the hematocrit to below this level and keeping it there should be the goal of phlebotomy-based treatment in PV.[206,207] It has also been widely recommended that females be reduced to a hematocrit of less than 42% because their normal hemoglobin range is lower, but this has not been rigorously tested and whole blood viscosity should not depend significantly on gender.

There has been a long-standing interest in the addition of other therapies to try to further decrease thrombotic risk. Just when these other agents should be added to phlebotomy is controversial. An elevated platelet count does not appear to be a major thrombotic risk factor in PV, and a very elevated platelet count (e.g., >1 million /µL), as in ET, is a risk factor for bleeding in PV.[208] Therefore, young PV patients without a history of thrombosis and with a near-normal platelet count are probably quite safe with phlebotomy alone.

Table 6 Suggested treatment algorithm for patients with polycythemia vera.

Risk category[a]	Age < 60 years	Age ≥ 60 years	Women of childbearing age
Low	Phlebotomy + ASA	Not applicable	Phlebotomy + ASA
Indeterminate	Phlebotomy + ASA if no aVWD	Not applicable	Phlebotomy + ASA if no aVWD
High	Phlebotomy + ASA + HU or IFNα	Phlebotomy + HU + ASA	Phlebotomy + ASA + IFNα

Abbreviations: ASA, low-dose aspirin (if no contraindications); HU, hydroxyurea; IFNα, Interferonα2A; aVWD, acquired von Willebrand disease.
[a]See **Chapter 113** for risk stratification algorithm.

In view of a recent large randomized placebo-controlled study that showed a large reduction in thrombotic events (but not an overall survival improvement) with low-dose aspirin (100 mg/day—a dose not available in the US) aspirin, all patients with PV who do not have a contraindication should receive aspirin.[51] In this trial, the combined endpoint of nonfatal myocardial infarction, nonfatal stroke, or death from cardiovascular causes and the risk of the combined end point of nonfatal myocardial infarction, nonfatal stroke, pulmonary embolism, major venous thrombosis, or death from cardiovascular causes were both reduced (relative risk 0.41 and 0.40 compared with placebo, respectively.) The risk of bleeding at this dose was elevated slightly above those treated with placebo (relative risk 1.6).[51]

There has been interest in myelosuppressive agents in PV for several decades, and opinion about the optimal regimen continues to evolve. In a landmark three-arm-randomized study that originated in the 1960s, two specific agents, oral chlorambucil and intravenous radioactive phosphorus (^{32}P), were each found to decrease the risk of thrombosis when added to phlebotomy.[202] However, overall survival was inferior with either of the additional treatments because of an increased incidence of acute leukemia compared with phlebotomy alone. The incidence of acute leukemia over 13–19 years was 1.5%, 9.6%, and 13.2% for phlebotomy, ^{32}P, and chlorambucil, respectively, and the corresponding median survivals were 12.6, 9.1, and 10.9 years.[202] Several cases of lymphoma were seen in patients treated with chlorambucil, and the incidence of gastrointestinal and skin cancer was also increased.

Other agents have the potential to decrease thrombosis without the same degree of leukemia risk as ^{32}P or alkylators. One of these agents is HU, which decreases thrombotic risk when used as a supplement to phlebotomy, but which appears less leukemogenic than chlorambucil and ^{32}P. In one PVSG study, HU was associated with lower risk of thrombosis in the first 2 years after diagnosis (6.6% vs 14%) when compared to a historical cohort of patients treated with phlebotomy alone, and only 5.9% of patients had transformed to acute leukemia after a median follow-up of 8.6 years.[209] Because the true leukemogenic risk of HU is unknown, it is used most often as a supplement to phlebotomy for groups at especially high risk for thrombosis, such as the elderly and those with prior thrombosis (Table 6).

IFNα2A has salutary effects in PV and is the drug of choice for PV patients who do not tolerate HU or wish to become pregnant because of anecdotal reports of successful maternal and fetal outcomes. This drug controls erythrocytosis in approximately 80% of the patients who can tolerate the necessary dose, which ranges from 4.5 to 27 million units per week (the usual starting dose is 3 million units subcutaneously three times a week), and IFNα2A has a beneficial effect on thrombocytosis.[58,210,211] IFN can also reduce spleen size and frequently gives relief from intractable pruritus. However, at least 20% of patients discontinue therapy because of drug side effects, including fatigue, malaise, fevers, psychological effects, myalgias, and arthralgias.[211] IFNα2A is also more expensive than HU. In addition to women of childbearing potential, it is reasonable to choose IFNα2A for high-risk patients who need a supplement to phlebotomy where the potential benefit of relief from refractory pruritus is desired, or for patients who are particularly concerned about the potential leukemogenicity of HU.

As elaborated earlier, cytoreductive therapy, for prevention of thrombosis, is currently recommended in high-risk (age ≥60 years or presence of thrombosis history) patients with PV based on evidence from controlled studies.[4,5] In this regard, HU is the evidence-based choice for first-line therapy, whereas noncontrolled studies have supported the use of interferon-α and busulfan as second-line drugs of choice.[1] We do not use ruxolitinib in PV, despite its recent FDA approval in HU refractory cases,[20] unless in the presence of severe pruritus or symptomatic splenomegaly that is shown to be refractory to adequate doses of HU, interferon-α, or busulfan.

Key references

The complete reference list can be found on the Wiley Companion Digital Edition of this title (see inside front cover for login instructions).

2 Tefferi A, Vardiman JW. Classification and diagnosis of myeloproliferative neoplasms: the 2008 World Health Organization criteria and point-of-care diagnostic algorithms. *Leukemia.* 2008;**22**(1):14–22.

7 Mesa RA, Silverstein MN, Jacobsen SJ, Wollan PC, Tefferi A. Population-based incidence and survival figures in essential thrombocythemia and agnogenic myeloid metaplasia: An Olmsted County study, 1976–1995. *Am J Hematol.* 1999;**61**(1):10–15.

8 Kutti J, Ridell B. Epidemiology of the myeloproliferative disorders: essential thrombocythaemia, polycythaemia vera and idiopathic myelofibrosis. *Pathol Biol (Paris).* 2001;**49**(2):164–166.

9 Jensen MK, de Nully BP, Nielsen OJ, Hasselbalch HC. Incidence, clinical features and outcome of essential thrombocythaemia in a well defined geographical area. *Eur J Haematol.* 2000;**65**(2):132–139.

11 Kondo T, Okabe M, Sanada M, et al. Familial essential thrombocythemia associated with one-base deletion in the 5′-untranslated region of the thrombopoietin gene. *Blood.* 1998;**92**(4):1091–1096.

20 Elkassar N, Hetet G, Briere J, Grandchamp B. Clonality analysis of hematopoiesis in essential thrombocythemia – advantages of studying T lymphocytes and platelets. *Blood.* 1997;**89**(1):128–134.

21 Fialkow PJ, Faguet GB, Jacobson RJ, Vaidya K, Murphy S. Evidence that essential thrombocythemia is a clonal disorder with origin in a multipotent stem cell. *Blood.* 1981;**58**(5):916–919.

22 Baxter EJ, Scott LM, Campbell PJ, et al. Acquired mutation of the tyrosine kinase JAK2 in human myeloproliferative disorders. *Lancet.* 2005;**365**(9464):1054–1061.

23 Kralovics R, Passamonti F, Buser AS, et al. A gain-of-function mutation of JAK2 in myeloproliferative disorders. *N Engl J Med.* 2005;**352**(17):1779–1790.

29 Scott LM, Tong W, Levine RL, et al. JAK2 exon 12 mutations in polycythemia vera and idiopathic erythrocytosis. *N Engl J Med.* 2007;**356**(5):459–468.

32 Taksin AL, Couedic JPL, Dusanter-Fourt I, et al. Autonomous megakaryocyte growth in essential thrombocythemia and idiopathic myelofibrosis is not related to a c-mpl mutation or to an autocrine stimulation by Mpl-L. *Blood.* 1999;**93**(1):125–139.

39 Tefferi A, Guglielmelli P, Larson DR, et al. Long-term survival and blast transformation in molecularly annotated essential thrombocythemia, polycythemia vera, and myelofibrosis. *Blood.* 2014;**124**(16):2507–2513; quiz 2615. Prepublished on 20 July 2014 as DOI: 10.1182/blood-2014-05-579136.

40 Besses C, Cervantes F, Pereira A, et al. Major vascular complications in essential thrombocythemia: a study of the predictive factors in a series of 148 patients. *Leukemia.* 1999;**13**(2):150–154.

41 Cortelazzo S, Viero P, Finazzi G, D'Emilio A, Rodeghiero F, Barbui T. Incidence and risk factors for thrombotic complications in a historical cohort of 100 patients with essential thrombocythemia. *J Clin Oncol*. 1990;**8**(3):556–562.

43 van Genderen PJ, Michiels JJ. Erythromelalgia: a pathognomonic microvascular thrombotic complication in essential thrombocythemia and polycythemia vera. [Review] [23 refs]. *Semin Thromb Hemost*. 1997;**23**(4):357–363.

50 Tefferi A, Barbui T. New and treatment-relevant risk stratification for thrombosis in essential thrombocythemia and polycythemia vera. *Am J Hematol*. 2015. Prepublished on 16 April 2015 as DOI 10.1002/ajh.24037.

51 Landolfi R, Marchioli R, Kutti J, et al. Efficacy and safety of low-dose aspirin in polycythemia vera. *N Engl J Med*. 2004;**350**(2):114–124.

84 Gangat N, Caramazza D, Vaidya R, et al. DIPSS plus: a refined Dynamic International Prognostic Scoring System for primary myelofibrosis that incorporates prognostic information from karyotype, platelet count, and transfusion status. *J Clin Oncol*. 2011;**29**(4):392–397. Prepublished on 15 Dec 2010 as DOI: 10.1200/JCO.2010.32.2446.

91 Tefferi A, Lasho TL, Patnaik MM, et al. JAK2 germline genetic variation affects disease susceptibility in primary myelofibrosis regardless of V617F mutational status: nullizygosity for the JAK2 46/1 haplotype is associated with inferior survival. *Leukemia*. 2010;**24**(1):105–109.

100 Guglielmelli P, Lasho TL, Rotunno G, et al. The number of prognostically detrimental mutations and prognosis in primary myelofibrosis: an international study of 797 patients. *Leukemia*. 2014;**28**(9):1804–1810. Prepublished on 20 Feb 2014 as DOI 10.1038/leu.2014.76.

110 Tefferi A, Verstovsek S, Barosi G, et al. Pomalidomide is active in the treatment of anemia associated with myelofibrosis. *J Clin Oncol*. 2009;**27**:4563–4569.

113 Tefferi A, Passamonti F, Barbui T, et al. Phase 3 study of pomalidomide in myeloproliferative neoplasm (MPN)-associated myelofibrosis with RBC-transfusion-dependence. *Blood*. 2013;**122**:394.

114 Verstovsek S, Kantarjian H, Mesa RA, et al. Safety and efficacy of INCB018424, a JAK1 and JAK2 inhibitor, in myelofibrosis. *N Engl J Med*. 2010;**363**:1117–1127.

116 Verstovsek S, Mesa RA, Gotlib J, et al. A double-blind, placebo-controlled trial of ruxolitinib for myelofibrosis. *N Engl J Med*. 2012;**366**:799–807. Prepublished on 2 Mar 2012 as DOI 10.1056/NEJMoa1110557.

117 Harrison C, Kiladjian JJ, Al-Ali HK, et al. JAK inhibition with ruxolitinib versus best available therapy for myelofibrosis. *N Engl J Med*. 2012;**366**:787–798. Prepublished on 2 Mar 2012 as DOI 10.1056/NEJMoa1110556.

119 Pardanani A, Gotlib JR, Jamieson C, et al. Safety and efficacy of TG101348, a selective JAK2 inhibitor, in myelofibrosis. *J Clin Oncol*. 2011;**29**:789–796. Prepublished on 12 Jan 2011 as DOI 10.1200/JCO.2010.32.8021.

120 Pardanani A, Harrison CN, Cortes JE, et al. Results of a randomized, double-blind, placebo-controlled phase III study (JAKARTA) of the JAK2-selective inhibitor fedratinib (SAR302503) in patients with myelofibrosis (MF). *Blood*. 2013;**122**:393.

122 Pardanani A, Gotlib J, Gupta V, et al. Update on the long-term efficacy and safety of momelotinib, a JAK1 and JAK2 inhibitor, for the treatment of myelofibrosis. *Blood*. 2013;**122**:108.

141 Melzner I, Weniger MA, Menz CK, Moller P. Absence of the JAK2 V617F activating mutation in classical Hodgkin lymphoma and primary mediastinal B-cell lymphoma. *Leukemia*. 2006;**20**(1):157–158.

142 Lee JW, Soung YH, Kim SY, et al. JAK2 V617F mutation is uncommon in non-Hodgkin lymphomas. *Leuk Lymphoma*. 2006;**47**(2):313–314.

143 Sulong S, Case M, Minto L, Wilkins B, Hall A, Irving J. The V617F mutation in Jak2 is not found in childhood acute lymphoblastic leukaemia. *Br J Haematol*. 2005;**130**(6):964–965.

144 Levine RL, Loriaux M, Huntly BJ, et al. The JAK2V617F activating mutation occurs in chronic myelomonocytic leukemia and acute myeloid leukemia, but not in acute lymphoblastic leukemia or chronic lymphocytic leukemia. *Blood*. 2005;**106**(10):3377–3379.

150 Steensma DP, McClure RF, Karp JE, et al. JAK2 V617F is a rare finding in de novo acute myeloid leukemia, but STAT3 activation is common and remains unexplained. *Leukemia*. 2006;**20**(6):971–978.

151 Renneville A, Quesnel B, Charpentier A, et al. High occurrence of JAK2 V617 mutation in refractory anemia with ringed sideroblasts associated with marked thrombocytosis. *Leukemia*. 2006;**20**(11):2067–2070.

152 Verstovsek S, Silver RT, Cross NC, Tefferi A. JAK2V617F mutational frequency in polycythemia vera: 100%, >90%, less? *Leukemia*. 2006;**20**(11):2067.

163 Delhommeau F, Dupont S, Tonetti C, et al. Evidence that the JAK2 G1849T (V617F) mutation occurs in a lymphomyeloid progenitor in polycythemia vera and idiopathic myelofibrosis. *Blood*. 2007;**109**(1):71–77.

164 Lasho TL, Mesa R, Gilliland DG, Tefferi A. Mutation studies in CD3+, CD19+ and CD34+ cell fractions in myeloproliferative disorders with homozygous JAK2(V617F) in granulocytes. *Br J Haematol*. 2005;**130**(5):797–799.

171 Campbell PJ, Baxter EJ, Beer PA, et al. Mutation of JAK2 in the myeloproliferative disorders: timing, clonality studies, cytogenetic associations, and role in leukemic transformation. *Blood*. 2006;**108**(10):3548–3555.

172 Scott LM, Tong W, Levine R, et al. Somatic mutations of JAK2 exon 12 in polycythemia vera and idiopathic erythrocytosis. *N Engl J Med*. 2007;**365**:459–468.

178 Casadevall N, Vainchenker W, Lacombe C, et al. Erythroid progenitors in polycythemia vera: demonstration of their hypersensitivity to erythropoietin using serum free cultures. *Blood*. 1982;**59**(2):447–451.

179 Dai CH, Krantz SB, Dessypris EN, Means RT Jr, Horn ST, Gilbert HS. Polycythemia vera. II. Hypersensitivity of bone marrow erythroid, granulocyte-macrophage, and megakaryocyte progenitor cells to interleukin-3 and granulocyte-macrophage colony-stimulating factor. *Blood*. 1992;**80**(4):891–899.

Management of Cancer Complications

123 Neoplasms of unknown primary site

John D. Hainsworth, MD ▪ *F. Anthony Greco, MD*

Overview

Cancer of unknown primary site (CUP) is a clinical syndrome accounting for 2–3% of all cancer diagnoses. This heterogeneous group is comprised of patients who have no anatomic primary site identified after a standard clinical evaluation. Complete pathologic evaluation is essential. Accurate prediction of the tissue of origin, based on examination of a biopsy from a metastatic lesion, is now possible in most patients using improved immunoperoxidase stains and molecular gene expression profiling. After completion of clinical and pathologic diagnostic evaluation, approximately 20% of patients with carcinoma of unknown primary site are included in favorable prognosis subsets and require specific treatment as detailed in this chapter. Until recently, the remaining 80% of patients have been treated with empiric combination chemotherapy. However, as therapy for various solid tumors improves and becomes more site specific, empiric chemotherapy is less likely to provide optimal treatment. Site-specific therapy directed by the tissue of origin predicted by molecular profiling or immunoperoxidase staining is now appropriate for these patients. New data supporting the use of site-specific therapy are reviewed.

Cancer of unknown primary site (CUP) is a common clinical entity, accounting for 2–3% of all cancer diagnoses.[1,2] Patients with CUP are heterogeneous with respect to clinical features, pathology, response to treatment, and prognosis. The typical patient develops symptoms at a metastatic site, but routine history, physical examination, imaging studies, and laboratory studies fail to identify a primary site. Biopsy shows carcinoma in most patients; however, histologic examination is insufficient to fully characterize most of these tumors.

Until recently, the major advance in the management of CUP was the identification of several treatable subgroups within this heterogeneous population. Identification of these patients, based on the presence of specific clinical and/or pathologic features, is critical as specific first-line treatment is required for optimal results. For the remainder of CUP patients (about 80%), the development of empiric "broad spectrum" chemotherapy regimens has resulted in modest benefit. However, as treatment improves and becomes more tumor specific in many types of solid tumors, the idea that a single chemotherapy regimen can provide optimum treatment for a heterogeneous group of CUP patients seems increasingly outdated.

In recent years, improved diagnostic techniques, including more precise immunohistochemical (IHC) stains and molecular gene expression tumor profiling (GEP), have enabled accurate prediction of the site of tumor origin in many patients with CUP, even when anatomic primary sites cannot be demonstrated. Although still developing, current data strongly suggest that site-directed treatment based on the predicted site of tumor origin improves treatment outcome as compared to empiric chemotherapy.

Pathologic evaluation

Examination of tumor histology by light microscopy is the critical first procedure in the pathologic evaluation and provides a practical classification system to direct subsequent evaluation. Almost all patients with CUP have carcinoma, which can be divided into five categories by light microscopic evaluation: (1) poorly differentiated neoplasm, (2) poorly differentiated carcinoma, (3) adenocarcinoma, (4) squamous carcinoma, and (5) neuroendocrine carcinoma. Occasionally, melanoma or sarcoma is identified at the initial examination.

As histologic examination rarely results in the identification of the site of tumor origin, additional pathologic evaluation is important in almost every patient with CUP. For this reason, the initial biopsy should be planned so as to yield an adequate amount of tissue for all required pathologic studies; material produced from a fine-needle aspiration biopsy is insufficient in these patients. Close communication between the oncologist and the pathologist is necessary so that the available biopsy material can be "managed" judiciously, ensuring that the most critical studies are obtained.

Poorly differentiated neoplasm

The diagnosis of poorly differentiated neoplasm is made when histologic features do not allow the pathologist to distinguish between carcinoma and other cancers, such as sarcoma, melanoma, and hematopoietic neoplasms. This diagnosis occurs in approximately 5% of CUP patients after standard histologic examination but only rarely after specialized tests (IHC staining, GEP) are performed. Establishing a more precise diagnosis is essential in this group of patients, because highly treatable cancers (e.g., non-Hodgkin lymphoma, poorly differentiated neuroendocrine carcinoma, melanoma) are common.[3–5]

Poorly differentiated carcinoma

Patients with poorly differentiated carcinoma account for approximately 20% of patients with CUP; an additional 10% of patients have poorly differentiated adenocarcinoma. Examination of poorly differentiated carcinoma using routine light microscopy alone is inadequate to assess these tumors optimally. In one series of 87 patients with poorly differentiated carcinoma, other diagnoses were suggested in 16 patients (18%) after IHC studies were done.[6] The use of panels of IHC stains and GEP results in more specific diagnoses in many of these patients.

Adenocarcinoma

Adenocarcinoma is the most frequent light microscopic diagnosis in patients with neoplasms of unknown primary site and accounts for approximately 70% of cases. Because various adenocarcinomas share histologic features, the site of the primary tumor cannot usually be ascertained. Certain histologic features are typically associated with a particular cancer type ("papillary features" with ovarian

Holland-Frei Cancer Medicine, Ninth Edition. Edited by Robert C. Bast Jr., Carlo M. Croce, William N. Hait, Waun Ki Hong, Donald W. Kufe, Martine Piccart-Gebhart, Raphael E. Pollock, Ralph R. Weichselbaum, Hongyang Wang, and James F. Holland.
© 2017 John Wiley & Sons, Inc. ISBN: 978-1-118-93469-2

and thyroid cancer, "signet ring cells" with gastric cancer); however, even these are not specific enough to be used as definitive evidence of the primary site.

In recent years, the ability to accurately predict the site of origin in patients with adenocarcinoma of unknown primary site has improved. The identification of relatively cell-specific proteins by IHC staining allows accurate prediction of the primary site in 35–55% of patients.[7,8] Panels of IHC stains are most useful and are often directed by clinical features (e.g., gender, sites of metastases). In addition, GEP enables prediction of the site of origin in most patients with adenocarcinoma of unknown primary site, including those in which IHC stains are nondiagnostic. Complete evaluation of adenocarcinoma of unknown primary site therefore requires the use of these specialized pathologic techniques.

Squamous carcinoma

Squamous carcinoma accounts for approximately 5% of patients with CUP. The large majority of these patients have specific clinical syndromes for which effective treatment is available. A definitive diagnosis of squamous carcinoma can usually be made by histologic examination.

Neuroendocrine carcinoma

A broad spectrum of neuroendocrine neoplasia is now recognized, owing in part to improved pathologic diagnosis. Approximately 3% of CUP patients have neuroendocrine carcinoma and can be divided into three groups including low-grade tumors (carcinoid/islet cell type), high-grade neuroendocrine tumors (small-cell carcinoma, atypical carcinoid, large-cell neuroendocrine carcinoma), and poorly differentiated carcinoma (neuroendocrine features apparent only with specialized pathologic tests). The distinction between low-grade and high-grade carcinoma is critical in determining treatment.

Immunohistochemical staining

IHC staining is the most widely available adjunctive tool for the classification of neoplasms. Specific IHC staining patterns can usually establish the tumor lineage of poorly differentiated neoplasms (Table 1).[7,9–11] Examples include the distinction between carcinoma and lymphoma, the identification of poorly differentiated neuroendocrine carcinoma, and the occasional identification of melanoma and sarcoma.[5,7,12–14]

When used to evaluate carcinoma of unknown primary site, the accuracy of IHC staining in identifying the tissue of origin has improved. Table 2 shows typical staining patterns for a number of carcinomas. These results must be interpreted in the context of

Table 2 Carcinoma of unknown primary site: IHC staining patterns useful in identifying the tissue of origin.

Specific carcinomas	Immunohistochemical (IHC) staining
Bladder (transitional cell)	CK20 (+), CK5/6 (+), p63 (+), GATA3 (+), urothelin (+)
Breast	CK7 (+), ER (+), PR (+), GCDFP-15 (+), Her2/neu (+), mammaglobin (+), GATA3 (+)
Colorectal	CK20 (+), CK7 (−), CDX2 (+)
Germ cell	PLAP (+), OCT4 (+)
Liver	hepar1 (+), CD10 (+)
Lung: adenocarcinoma	TTF1 (+), CK7 (+), CK20 (−), P63 (+), CK5/6 (+)
Lung: neuroendocrine (small cell/large cell)	TTF1 (+), chromogranin (+), synaptophysin (+)
Lung: squamous	CK7 (+), CK20 (−), P63 (+), CK5/6 (+)
Ovary	CK7 (+), ER (+), WT1 (+), PAX8 (+), mesothelin (+)
Pancreas	CK7 (+), CA19-9 (+), mesothelin (+)
Prostate	PSA (+), CK7 (−), CK20 (−)
Renal	RCC (+), PAX8 (+), CD10 (+), pan-cytokeratin AE 1/3 (+)
Thyroid (follicular/papillary)	thyroglobulin (+), TTF1 (+), PAX8 (+)

clinical and histologic features, as staining patterns overlap and few IHC stains are entirely specific. The prostate-specific antigen (PSA) stain is an exception and is specific for prostate adenocarcinoma.[11] For other carcinomas, panels of IHC stains have been shown to improve specificity; such panels can accurately identify the primary site in approximately two-thirds of biopsies taken from advanced carcinomas of various known primary sites.[15–18] A few classic staining patterns have been described that are usually diagnostic (e.g., CK7+/CK20−/TTF-1+ for lung adenocarcinoma, CK7−/CK20+/CDX2+ for colorectal adenocarcinoma). Four IHC stains (CK7, CK20, CDX2, TTF-1) form the basis of several diagnostic patterns and are appropriate initial stains in the evaluation of most CUP biopsies.

Electron microscopy

The identification of specific ultrastructural features by electron microscopy enables a definitive diagnosis in some poorly differentiated neoplasms. Because it is less widely available, requires special tissue fixation at the time of biopsy, and is relatively expensive, electron microscopy should be reserved for the study of neoplasms whose lineage is unclear after routine light microscopy, IHC staining, and GEP.

Tumor-specific chromosomal abnormalities

Several tumor-specific chromosomal abnormalities are occasionally important in the diagnosis of CUP. Most B-cell and T-cell

Table 1 Poorly differentiated neoplasms: IHC staining patterns useful in determining tumor lineage.

Tumor type	Cytokeratin	Epithelial membrane antigen	Leukocyte common antigen	S-100 protein, HMB45, Melan-A	Vimentin	Desmin	Factor VIII antigen	Chromogranin/ synaptophysin
Carcinoma	+	+[a]	−	−	−	−	−	±
Lymphoma	−	±[b]	+	−	−	−	−	−
Melanoma	−	−	−	+	+	−	−	−
Sarcoma	−	±[c]	−	−	+	+[d]	+[e]	−
Neuroendocrine tumor	+	+	−	−	−	−	−	+

[a] Adenocarcinoma.
[b] Anaplastic large-cell lymphoma (Ki-1 or CD30-positive lymphoma).
[c] Epithelioid sarcoma, synovial sarcoma.
[d] Leiomyosarcoma, rhabdomyosarcoma.
[e] Angiosarcoma.

lymphomas are associated with tumor-specific rearrangements of immunoglobulin genes or T-cell antigen-receptor genes.[19] In the unusual case when the diagnosis of lymphoma cannot be definitively established with either IHC staining or flow cytometric immunophenotyping, the detection of these specific gene rearrangements provides definitive diagnostic information. Specific abnormalities associated with solid tumors include a chromosomal translocation (rcp [11:22][q24; q12]) in all peripheral neuroepitheliomas and most Ewing tumors,[20,21] t(15:19) in children and young adults with carcinoma of midline structures or uncertain histogenesis,[22] and an isochromosome of the short arm or chromosome 12 (i12p) in a large percentage of testicular and extragonadal germ cell tumors.[23] Extragonadal germ cell tumors identified on the basis of i(12p) abnormalities are highly responsive to cisplatin-based chemotherapy.[23] Most of the neoplasms identifiable by specific chromosomal abnormalities can now be identified using methods that are more widely available, including IHC staining and GEP.

Gene expression profiling

Specific gene expression profiles are now recognized in cancers based on their sites of origin, reflecting differences in the gene expression profiles present in their normal tissues of origin.[24] By measuring differential expression of key sets of genes, this method is applicable to many cancer types and is therefore a potentially important diagnostic tool in the evaluation of CUP.

During the last 15 years, a number of assays have been developed for the purpose of predicting the tissue of origin in patients with CUP. Early tests measured only a few gene expression markers, allowing diagnosis of relatively few tumor types.[25-28] More recently, application of either reverse transcriptase polymerase chain reaction (RT-PCR) or gene microarray techniques, coupled with improved bioinformatics systems, has allowed the development of assays capable of detecting more than 40 tumor types/subtypes.[29-37] In the majority of recent studies, one of three commercially available assays has been used: CancerTYPE ID (bioTheranostics, Inc.),[34,35] Cancer Origin Test (Rosetta Genomics),[36,37] or the Tissue of Origin Test (Pathwork, Inc.).[32,33]

In validation studies, tumor biopsies from patients with advanced cancer (primary site known) were assayed in a blinded study; all commercially available assays accurately predicted the tissue of origin in 85–90% of cases.[33,35,37] Accuracy was high regardless of the biopsy site (primary site vs metastasis) or tumor grade (well differentiated vs poorly differentiated).

Accuracy of GEP in predicting CUP tissue of origin

The accuracy of GEP in CUP has been more difficult to assess, as an anatomic primary site is not identified in most patients. However, evidence from several studies strongly suggests that accuracy in CUP is similar to that previously demonstrated in the validation studies using advanced cancers of known primary site. The most direct evidence comes from a study of GEP in patients with CUP who subsequently had primary sites identified during their disease course (9–314 weeks after initial evaluation).[8,38] In 18 of 24 such patients (75%), GEP of the original biopsy specimen resulted in correct prediction of the anatomic primary site. Despite concerns regarding the unique biology of CUP, most of these cancers apparently retain enough of the gene expression profile of their tissues of origin to allow identification with current assays.

GEP has also been evaluated in patients with poorly differentiated neoplasms of unknown primary site who had undefined tumor lineage after standard pathologic evaluation (including a median of 18 IHC stains).[39] Molecular tumor profiling gave a lineage prediction in 25 of 30 patients (carcinoma 10, melanoma 5, sarcoma 8, hematopoietic malignancy 2) and predicted a tissue of origin for all 10 carcinomas. Additional studies and/or response to treatment supported the molecular profiling results in most patients.

Comparisons of IHC versus GEP

Two large studies have compared the accuracy of IHC staining panels versus GEP in the identification of the primary site in patients with metastatic cancer.[40,41] In both studies, pathologists were provided with formalin-fixed biopsy specimens; patient gender and biopsy site were the only clinical details provided. Both methods showed considerable accuracy in these patients with known primary sites. In both studies, GEP provided the correct diagnosis more often than did IHC staining (79% vs 69%; 89% vs 83%, respectively). The accuracy of IHC staining decreased in patients with poorly differentiated histology.[41]

Performing similar comparative studies in patients with CUP is not possible, as the primary site usually remains unknown. In one study, IHC staining suggested a single site of origin in 52 of 149 patients (35%).[8] In these 52 patients, GEP predicted the same site of origin in 77%. However, when IHC did not allow prediction of a single site of origin, the correlation between IHC and GEP predictions was poor. The major findings of this study are diagrammed in Figure 1.

Four smaller studies also demonstrated good correlations between GEP and IHC staining when a single diagnosis is suggested by IHC.[42-45] Overall, 78% of 117 patients reported in these five studies had matching diagnoses when IHC staining predicted a single tissue of origin. However, the ability of IHC staining to make a single diagnosis occurred in <55% of patients in all studies.

Summary and conclusions

Although validation of the accuracy of diagnostic tests is difficult in CUP, data from various studies are generally consistent and have recently been reviewed in detail.[46] Several conclusions are now supported by data:

1. GEP using commercially available assays provides a prediction of the tissue of origin in >90% of patients with CUP. These predictions are accurate in approximately 75% of patients.
2. IHC staining panels predict a single site of origin in 35–55% of patients with CUP. In these patients, IHC and GEP results are usually identical (78% of cases). Oncologists have often been reluctant to make treatment decisions based on IHC predictions; however, this may be a group of patients in whom GEP is not necessary and site-specific therapy can be directed by IHC results.
3. IHC staining results are not helpful unless a single tissue of origin can be predicted. In the remaining patients, GEP greatly increases the chance of accurate prediction of the tissue of origin.

As GEP is incorporated into the diagnostic evaluation of patients with CUP, several potential problems should be considered. First, GEP diagnoses are not 100% accurate, even in the validation studies that used cancers of known primary site. These diagnoses should always be considered in conjunction with clinical features and results of other pathologic studies. Second, several neoplasms have overlapping gene expression profiles, which can occasionally cause a misdiagnosis (e.g., breast, salivary gland, and skin adnexal tumors share similar gene expression profiles). Third, tumor types that are not included in the particular GEP assay being used cannot be diagnosed. When this situation occurs, the tumors are either

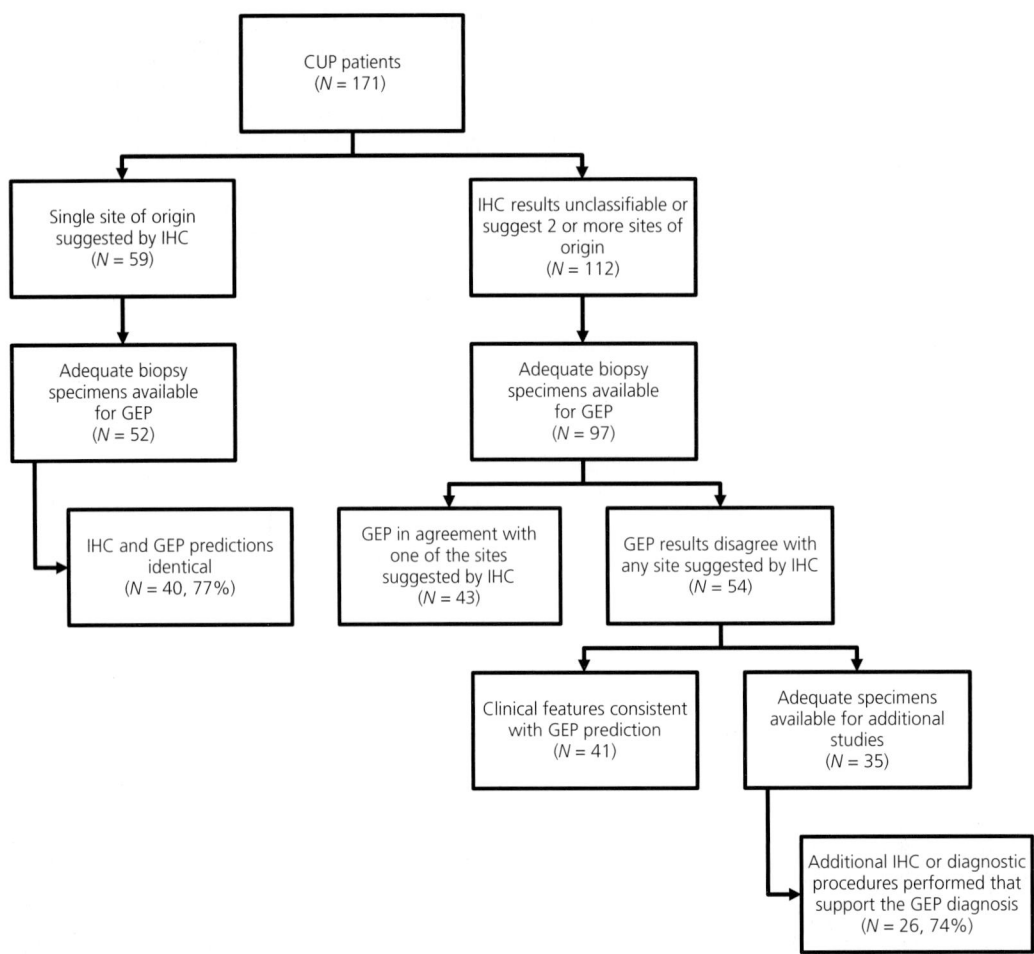

Figure 1 Comparison of IHC and GEP tissue of origin predictions in CUP.

considered unclassifiable or misdiagnosed as a cancer with an overlapping gene expression profile. Finally, performing additional diagnostic studies requires additional biopsy material. The relative priority of available tests should be carefully considered. At times, a repeat biopsy should be considered.

Clinical evaluation

Most patients with CUP develop signs or symptoms at the site of a metastatic lesion and are diagnosed with advanced cancer. Common metastatic sites include the liver, lungs, lymph nodes, and bones; most patients have metastatic tumor at more than one site. The subsequent clinical course is usually dominated by symptoms related to the sites of metastases. During the clinical course, the primary site becomes obvious in only 5–10% of patients.

At autopsy, primary sites can be found in approximately 70% of patients and are usually less than 2 cm in size. Unfortunately, the only large autopsy series were conducted before the routine availability of modern imaging techniques and may therefore not be representative of the current CUP population. The most common primary sites identified in historical autopsy series included the pancreas, hepatobiliary tree, and lung, accounting for approximately 40–50% of all cases.[47,48] Adenocarcinomas of the breast and prostate were identified infrequently, despite being common cancer types.[48]

It is of interest to compare the anatomic primary sites identified at autopsy[48] with the primary sites predicted in a large group of CUP patients recently evaluated with GEP[49] (Table 3). The frequent prediction of primary sites in the gastrointestinal tract (hepatobiliary, pancreas, colon/rectum) and lung by GEP is consistent with autopsy findings. However, the frequent prediction of the urothelium as a primary site and the relatively frequent prediction of breast and ovarian cancers differ from autopsy results. These differences may have practical importance, as breast and ovarian cancers are relatively responsive to treatment.

Adenocarcinoma or poorly differentiated carcinoma

As there is much overlap in the clinical features of patients with adenocarcinoma and those with poorly differentiated CUP, initial clinical evaluations of these two groups are identical (Table 4).

Many of the procedures included in Table 4 (medical history, physical examination, complete blood counts, chemistry profile, computed tomography) are done in the process of arriving at the diagnosis of CUP. Specific signs and symptoms should be evaluated with directed radiologic or endoscopic studies. All men should have a serum PSA level measured. Women with a clinical presentation compatible with metastatic breast cancer should have mammography and breast MRI exams. The role of positron emission tomography (PET) is controversial. Although a number of studies have suggested that PET scanning can identify the primary

Table 3 Sites of origin—Comparison of historical autopsy results and molecular tumor profiling predictions.

Primary site	Molecular tumor profiling predictions[49] (N = 252)	Autopsy results[a][48] (N = 133)
Biliary tract	52 (21%)	0
Urothelium	31 (12%)	0
Lung	28 (11%)	29 (22%)
Colon/rectum	28 (11%)	6 (2%)
Pancreas	12 (5%)	28 (22%)
Breast	12 (5%)	1 (1%)
Ovary	11 (4%)	4 (3%)
Gastric/gastroesophageal	10 (4%)	8 (6%)
Kidney	9 (4%)	8 (6%)
Liver	8 (3%)	16 (12%)
Sarcoma	6 (2%)	0
Cervix	6 (2%)	0
Neuroendocrine	5 (2%)	0
Prostate	4 (2%)	4 (3%)
Skin	4 (2%)	0
Germ cell	4 (2%)	0
Carcinoid, gastrointestinal	3 (1%)	0
Mesothelioma	3 (1%)	0
Other (1 each)	3 (1%)	6 (6%)
Thyroid	2 (1%)	1 (1%)
Endometrium	2 (1%)	0
Melanoma	2 (1%)	0
Skin, basal cell	2 (1%)	0
Unlocated/unclassifiable	5 (2%)	23 (17%)

[a]Three patients who had primary sites located antemortem are included.

Table 4 Recommended initial clinical evaluation.

- Complete medical history—includes detailed review of systems
- Complete physical examination—includes pelvic examination, stool for occult blood
- Laboratory evaluation—complete blood count, comprehensive metabolic panel, lactate dehydrogenase, urinalysis
- Computed tomography—chest, abdomen, and pelvis
- Mammography (women)
- Serum prostate-specific antigen (men)
- Positron emission tomography scan in selected patients
- Pathologic evaluation—includes initial IHC evaluation (CK7, CK20, TTF-1, CDX2)

site in up to 30% of patients,[50] the single prospective study showed no superiority of PET scanning when compared to CT scanning.[51]

Specific features of the initial evaluation, including clinical presentation and pathologic results, should be used to direct further focused evaluation. Several common patient groups, identified by initial clinical and pathologic evaluations, are outlined in Table 5, with recommendations for further evaluation.

Squamous carcinoma

Squamous carcinoma of unknown primary site usually presents with isolated metastases in the cervical or inguinal lymph nodes. As curative therapy is available for many of these patients, the initial clinical evaluation is critical for the purposes of (1) identifying a regional primary site and (2) identifying the extent of local tumor involvement.

The cervical lymph nodes are the most common metastatic site for squamous carcinoma of unknown primary site. Patients are usually middle-aged or elderly, and many have a history of substantial tobacco and alcohol use. Optimal evaluation includes a thorough examination of the oropharynx, hypopharynx, nasopharynx, larynx, and upper esophagus by direct endoscopy, with biopsy

of suspicious areas. Computed tomography of the neck is useful in defining the extent of disease and occasionally in identifying the primary site. PET scanning identifies a primary site in 25% of patients even after other procedures are unrevealing and should be included as a standard diagnostic procedure.[52] When the lower cervical or supraclavicular lymph nodes are involved, a primary lung cancer should be suspected. Fiber-optic bronchoscopy is indicated if computed tomography and head/neck evaluations are unrevealing.

Ipsilateral or bilateral tonsillectomy has been advocated as a diagnostic modality if the primary site remains unidentified after the evaluation described above.[53] In one series, tonsillectomy identified a tonsillar primary site in 23 of 87 patients (26%).[54]

Most patients with squamous carcinoma involving inguinal lymph nodes have a detectable primary site in the genital or anorectal area. In women, careful examination of the vulva, vagina, and cervix is important, with biopsy of suspicious areas. Men should undergo a careful inspection of the penis. Digital examination and anoscopy should be performed in both sexes to exclude lesions in the anorectal area. Identification of a primary site in these patients is important, as potentially curative therapy is available for carcinomas of the vulva, vagina, cervix, and anus even after metastasis to regional lymph nodes.

Metastatic squamous carcinoma in areas other than the cervical or inguinal nodes usually represents metastasis from a primary lung cancer. Computed tomography of the chest and fiber-optic bronchoscopy should be performed if other clinical features suggest the possibility of lung cancer.

Neuroendocrine carcinoma

The initial clinical evaluation of patients with neuroendocrine carcinoma is the same as described in Table 4; however, special consideration is required in determining appropriate treatment.

Low-grade neuroendocrine carcinomas have the histologic appearance of typical carcinoid or islet cell tumors. When presenting with an unknown primary site, these tumors most frequently involve the liver. Some patients have clinical syndromes produced by tumor secretion of bioactive substances. Additional clinical evaluation in these patients should include serum or urine screening for these substances. An octreotide scan and upper and lower gastrointestinal endoscopy should be performed.

High-grade neuroendocrine carcinomas include typical small cell or large cell neuroendocrine carcinomas, as well as poorly differentiated carcinoma that is only recognized as neuroendocrine after IHC staining or GEP. Patients with high-grade neuroendocrine carcinomas usually have multiple metastases at the time of diagnosis and rarely have syndromes mediated by secretion of bioactive peptides. Patients with a history of cigarette smoking should be suspected of having an occult lung primary site, and bronchoscopy should be considered. Patients with IHC staining for thyroid transcription factor-1 (TTF-1) should also be considered for bronchoscopy. Extrapulmonary small cell carcinomas arising from various primary sites (salivary glands, esophagus, pancreas, bladder, prostate, colon/rectum, uterus, cervix) are occasionally identified during clinical evaluation. Patients with IHC staining for CDX2 should be considered for colonoscopy.

The origin of these high-grade neuroendocrine carcinomas remains unclear. Some patients may have small-cell lung cancer with an occult primary site. However, many of these patients have no smoking history, and the absence of pulmonary involvement makes this diagnosis unlikely in most patients. It has been speculated that high-grade neuroendocrine carcinomas share the same origin as low-grade neuroendocrine tumors but represent the

Table 5 Additional evaluation of specific patient subsets identified by initial evaluation.

Patient group	Clinical evaluation	Pathologic evaluation
Women with features of breast cancer (bone, lung, liver metastases; CK7+)	Breast MRI	IHC: ER, GCDFP-15, GATA 3 FISH: HER2 GEP (if necessary)
Women with features of ovarian cancer (pelvic/peritoneal metastases; CK7+)	Pelvic/intravaginal ultrasound	IHC: WT-1, PAX8 GEP (if necessary)
Features of lung cancer (hilar/mediastinal adenopathy; TTF-1+)	Bronchoscopy	IHC: Napsin A FISH: ALK/ROS-1 Mutation: EGFR GEP (if necessary)
Features of colon cancer (liver/peritoneal metastases; CK20+/CK7−, CDX2)	Colonoscopy	Mutation: KRAS GEP (if necessary)
Mediastinal/retroperitoneal mass	Testicular ultrasound Serum HCG, AFP	IHC: OCT4, PLAP FISH: i(12p) GEP (if necessary)
Poorly differentiated carcinoma, with or without clear cell features	—	IHC: chromogranin, synaptophysin, RCC, Hepar-1, HMB-45, Melan-A, serum AFP (if Hepar-1+), octreoscan (if neuroendocrine stains +) Mutation: BRAF (if melanoma stains +) GEP

opposite ends of a "spectrum" of tumor biology. However, it now seems more likely that high-grade neuroendocrine carcinomas have a different oncogenesis; many share the same chromosomal abnormalities commonly seen in small cell lung cancer (deletions of 3p, 5q, 10q, and 17p), while there are no shared molecular abnormalities with the group of carcinoid-type carcinomas.[55,56]

Treatment

Following the initial diagnostic evaluation, several groups of patients emerge. In a few patients, evaluation leads to the identification of an anatomic primary site; these patients no longer have CUP and should be treated appropriately for their defined cancer type. A second group of patients (~20%) fit into various favorable subgroups based on clinical and/or pathologic features, even though an anatomic primary site is not identified (Table 6). The management of each of these subsets is detailed in this section. Finally, the largest group (~80%) consists of patients who do not fit any favorable subset. Empiric chemotherapy has been the treatment standard for this group for many years and will be briefly reviewed. However, increasing evidence supports the use of site-specific therapy for these patients, guided by IHC and GEP predictions of the tissue of origin. These new data will also be reviewed.

Favorable subsets

Women with peritoneal carcinomatosis

In women, adenocarcinoma causing diffuse peritoneal involvement usually originates in the ovary, although carcinomas arising in the gastrointestinal tract or breast can occasionally produce this syndrome. However, peritoneal carcinomatosis also occurs in women with normal ovaries and no other evident primary site. This syndrome has occasionally developed in women from families at high risk for ovarian cancer despite prophylactic oophorectomy[57] and is increased in incidence in women with BRCA1 mutations.[58] Many of these patients have histologic features typical of ovarian carcinoma, such as papillary configuration or psammoma bodies. Clinical features are typical of advanced ovarian cancer, with tumor involvement usually limited to the peritoneal surfaces and elevated serum levels of CA 125 antigen. When histologic features suggest ovarian carcinoma, this syndrome has been termed "multifocal extraovarian serous carcinoma" or "peritoneal papillary serous carcinoma." Rarely, men with peritoneal carcinomatosis, papillary adenocarcinoma, and elevated serum CA 125 levels have also been reported.[59]

Patients with this syndrome often respond well to the chemotherapy regimens effective in the treatment of advanced ovarian carcinoma. Several investigators documented initial response rates

Table 6 Summary of favorable treatment subsets.

Subset	Typical histology	Therapy
Women, isolated axillary LN	Adenocarcinoma	Treat as stage II breast cancer
Women, axillary LN + other metastases	Adenocarcinoma	Treat as metastatic breast cancer
Women, peritoneal carcinomatosis	Adenocarcinoma (often serous) or poorly differentiated carcinoma	Treat as stage III ovarian cancer
Men, blastic bone metastases or high serum PSA or PSA tumor staining	Adenocarcinoma	Treat as metastatic prostate cancer
Colon cancer profile (intra-abdominal metastases + typical histology/IHC)	Adenocarcinoma	Treat as metastatic colon cancer
Single metastatic site	Adenocarcinoma or poorly differentiated carcinoma	Definitive local therapy (resection and/or radiation therapy)
Isolated cervical LN	Squamous carcinoma	Treat as locally advanced head/neck cancer
Isolated inguinal LN	Squamous carcinoma	Definitive local therapy (inguinal node dissection and/or radiation therapy) ± chemotherapy
Extragonadal germ cell syndrome	Poorly differentiated carcinoma	Treat for poor prognosis germ cell tumor
Neuroendocrine carcinoma, low grade	Carcinoid/islet cell features	Treat as advanced carcinoid tumor
Neuroendocrine carcinoma, aggressive	Small cell or poorly differentiated carcinoma	Treat as small cell lung cancer

of 39–66%, with long-term remissions in 15–20% of patients.[60-65] As in ovarian cancer, most long-term remissions occurred in patients who had successful surgical cytoreduction prior to receiving chemotherapy. Optimal management therefore includes initial maximal surgical cytoreduction followed by taxane/platinum chemotherapy.

Women with axillary lymph node metastases

Metastatic breast cancer should be suspected in women who have axillary lymph node involvement with adenocarcinoma.[66] Breast MRI or PET scanning can identify a primary site even when mammography is normal and should be performed.[67,68] Pathologic evaluation of the axillary lymph node biopsy should include measurement of estrogen and progesterone receptors, HER2 expression, and other IHC breast markers (Table 2). When positive, these findings provide strong evidence for the diagnosis of breast cancer.

Women with isolated axillary lymph node metastases are potentially curable and should be managed according to standard guidelines for stage II breast cancer. Primary therapy should include either modified radical mastectomy or axillary lymph node dissection followed by radiation therapy to the breast.[69-71] When mastectomy is performed, an occult breast cancer is identified in 44–82% of patients, even when physical examination and mammograms are normal.[70] Primary tumors are usually less than 2 cm in diameter; in occasional patients, only carcinoma *in situ* is identified in the breast.[72] Selection of adjuvant therapy should follow standard guidelines for node-positive breast cancer.

Women with metastatic sites in addition to axillary lymph nodes may also have metastatic breast cancer. These women should receive a trial of systemic therapy using guidelines for the treatment of metastatic breast cancer, particularly if IHC stains or GEP support a breast cancer diagnosis. Hormone receptor status and HER2 expression should guide therapy, as in patients with metastatic breast cancer.

Men with skeletal metastases

Serum PSA levels should be measured in all men with adenocarcinoma of unknown primary site. Men with elevated serum PSA levels (or positive tumor staining with PSA) should be treated according to guidelines for metastatic prostate cancer, even if clinical features are atypical.[73,74] Osteoblastic bone metastases are also an indication for a trial of prostate cancer treatment, even in the absence of PSA findings.

Colorectal cancer profile

During the last 20 years, the introduction of more effective cytotoxic agents and targeted therapies for the treatment of metastatic colorectal cancer has increased the median survival of these patients from 8 to 24 months.[75] Therefore, the ability to identify these patients from among the heterogeneous group of CUP patients is potentially important, as many of the standard agents used for colorectal cancer are not contained in the empiric chemotherapy regimens used for CUP.

A colon cancer "profile" has recently been defined, which allows prediction of CUP patients likely to have a colorectal site of tumor origin.[76,77] The colon cancer profile includes (1) typical clinical features (liver, peritoneal metastases), (2) histology compatible with lower gastrointestinal tract adenocarcinoma, and (3) typical IHC staining (CK20+/CK7− or CDX2+). In a group of 68 such patients,

treatment according to standard guidelines for metastatic colorectal cancer produced a median survival of 28 months.[77] It is important to note that colonoscopy did not identify an anatomic primary site in any of these patients. Although this approach has not been formally compared to standard empiric CUP therapy, the favorable median survival (as compared to the usual median survival of 8–10 months with empiric chemotherapy) strongly suggests the merit of this approach.

Carcinoma presenting as a single metastatic lesion

Occasionally, only a single metastatic lesion is identified after a complete clinical evaluation. Single lesions have been described in a variety of sites, including lymph nodes, brain, lung, adrenal gland, liver, bone, and skin. The possibility of an unusual primary site (e.g., primary cutaneous apocrine, eccrine, or sebaceous carcinoma) mimicking a metastatic lesion should be considered, but this possibility can usually be excluded on the basis of clinical or pathologic features.

In most of these patients, other metastatic sites become evident within a relatively short time. However, local treatment sometimes results in long disease-free intervals, and occasional patients have prolonged survival.[78] Before initiating local treatment, a PET scan is useful to rule out the presence of other metastatic sites.[79] If no other metastases are detected, the solitary lesion should be resected, if technically feasible. In some instances (e.g., after resection of a solitary brain metastasis), local radiation therapy may also be appropriate to maximize the chance of local control. The role of systemic chemotherapy in addition to definitive local therapy is undefined; however, adjuvant or neoadjuvant chemotherapy should be considered if a sensitive tumor type is suggested by IHC staining or GEP.

Extragonadal germ cell tumor syndrome

A few patients with poorly differentiated carcinoma of unknown primary site have extragonadal germ cell tumors that are unrecognizable by standard histologic criteria.[23,80,81] These patients are usually young males with predominant tumor location in the mediastinum or retroperitoneum. Some also have marked elevations of the serum tumor markers hCG or alpha-fetoprotein. In most of these patients, the diagnosis can be confirmed using IHC, GEP,[39] or identification of the i(12p) chromosomal abnormality specific for germ cell tumors.[23]

These patients should receive treatment for extragonadal germ cell tumor with four cycles of cisplatin-based chemotherapy followed by resection of residual tumor masses. Treatment results are similar to those achieved in the treatment of typical extragonadal germ cell tumors.[23,80]

Squamous carcinoma involving cervical or supraclavicular lymph nodes

Squamous carcinoma of unknown primary site most frequently presents with unilateral involvement of the cervical lymph nodes. The recommended clinical evaluation (previously described) results in the identification of a head and neck primary site in 85% of patients.[82]

When no primary site is identified, patients should be treated according to guidelines for locally advanced squamous carcinoma of the head and neck; approximately 50% have long-term disease-free survival.[83-88] As in patients with known primary sites in the head and neck, extensive involvement in neck nodes and poorly differentiated tumor histology are poor prognostic features.[84,89]

Patients with low cervical or supraclavicular lymph nodes are more likely to have a primary lung cancer, and treatment results are inferior. Nevertheless, patients with no detectable disease below the clavicle should be treated with the same approach as are patients with higher cervical nodes, as occasional patients will have long-term survival.

Squamous carcinoma involving inguinal lymph nodes

Most patients with squamous carcinoma involving inguinal lymph nodes have a detectable primary site in the anogenital area. For the occasional patient in whom no primary site is identified, definitive local therapy with inguinal node dissection or radiation therapy sometimes results in long-term survival.[90] Because combined modality therapy has improved survival of patients with squamous cancer arising in this region (e.g., cervix, anus), the addition of chemotherapy should be considered in patients with an unknown primary site.

Low-grade neuroendocrine carcinoma

Carcinoid or islet cell tumors of unknown primary site usually exhibit an indolent biology, and management should follow guidelines established for metastatic tumors of these types with known primary sites. Treatment with octreotide long-acting release (LAR) lengthens the time to tumor progression with low toxicity.[91] Depending on the clinical situation, appropriate management may also include local therapy (resection of isolated metastasis, radiofrequency ablation, cryotherapy, or hepatic artery chemoembolization). Several cytotoxic agents have some activity (5-FU, streptozocin, capecitabine, temozolomide), and results with targeted agents (sunitinib, everolimus) are promising.

High-grade neuroendocrine carcinoma

This group of patients includes small-cell and large-cell neuroendocrine carcinomas (histologic diagnoses) and patients with poorly differentiated carcinoma recognized to have neuroendocrine carcinoma by IHC staining. These patients should receive treatment with combination chemotherapy used for small-cell lung cancer; high response rates and a minority of long-term survivors (10–15%) have been reported.[92–95]

Poorly differentiated carcinoma

Patients with poorly differentiated carcinoma of unknown primary site form a large and heterogeneous group. The recognition that some of these patients had highly chemotherapy-sensitive neoplasms first occurred in the 1970s.[80,81,96] However, it is likely that currently available diagnostic methods identify the highly responsive patients in this group. The remaining patients with poorly differentiated CUP have a prognosis similar to patients with adenocarcinoma of unknown primary site. These patients should be evaluated using recommendations for adenocarcinoma, with particular attention to determining the tissue of origin using IHC staining and/or GEP.

Empiric chemotherapy for CUP

Approximately 80% of patients with CUP do not fit into any of the favorable subgroups outlined above. For many years, empiric chemotherapy has been the treatment of choice for most of these patients, as their tissue of origin could not be determined. At the time empiric chemotherapy regimens were designed, treatments were poor for many types of solid tumors. In addition, similar cytotoxic agents and regimens were used in the therapy of a variety of cancers. Therefore, it was possible to design "broad spectrum" regimens with reasonable activity against most sensitive tumor types.

Combination regimens containing most of the commonly used cytotoxic agents (taxanes, gemcitabine, topoisomerase I inhibitors, anthracyclines, vinca alkaloids) have been evaluated in the empiric treatment of patients with CUP. Combinations containing a platinum agent and a taxane have been most widely studied and are commonly used.[97–103] Several other combinations (i.e., gemcitabine/platinum, gemcitabine/taxane) have similar activity.[104–106] Several randomized phase II trials have compared various two-drug combinations and have usually yielded similar results.[105,107–111] The addition of a third drug has not improved efficacy.[109,112–115] Although response rates have varied, most trials have reported median survivals within a narrow range of 8–11 months, with 2-year survival rates of 14–24%. In larger trials (containing 100 or more patients), the median survival is consistently about 9 months.[107,112,114,116,117]

Empiric second-line therapy has been evaluated in a few phase II trials. Single-agent gemcitabine and the combinations of gemcitabine/irinotecan, capecitabine/oxaliplatin, and bevacizumab/erlotinib have had modest activity.[118–121]

Although no definitive studies have compared survival with empiric chemotherapy versus best supportive care alone, evidence from several large tumor registries suggests that current treatment results in an improved survival.[122–129] The Swedish Cancer Registry documented an improved median survival for patients with CUP during the years 2001–2008 (6 months) versus 1987–1993 (4 months).[130]

In spite of these modest improvements, the authors are convinced that the era of empiric chemotherapy for CUP is coming to an end. Accurate identification of the tissue of origin is possible in most CUP patients and provides a more rational framework for decisions regarding therapy.

Site-specific treatment directed by the predicted tissue of origin

The tissue of origin can now be accurately predicted in most patients with CUP. Although it is logical to assume that site-specific treatment based on the predicted tissue of origin would be superior to empiric chemotherapy, clinical data to support this assumption have only recently accumulated and remain incomplete. One cause for skepticism regarding a site-specific approach relates to the unique biology of CUP (evidenced by the fact that the primary site does not become apparent). This fundamental clinical difference has led to the speculation that these cancers may also respond differently to systemic therapy. However, increasing evidence indicates that most cancers of unknown primary site retain the characteristics of cancers with known primary arising from the same site.

Several biological and clinical observations now support these similarities. First, gene expression profiles in CUP remain similar to advanced cancers from the same tissue of origin. Second, no unique molecular "signature" common to CUP has been identified. Third, successful treatments for patients in several of the clinically recognized favorable CUP subsets are based on the presumption that they have specific cancer types (e.g., women with axillary nodes are treated for breast cancer and women with peritoneal carcinomatosis are treated for ovarian cancer). Fourth, retrospective studies containing CUP patients predicted to have a colorectal site of origin by either IHC staining[76,77] or molecular tumor profiling[131,132] and treated with standard colorectal cancer therapy

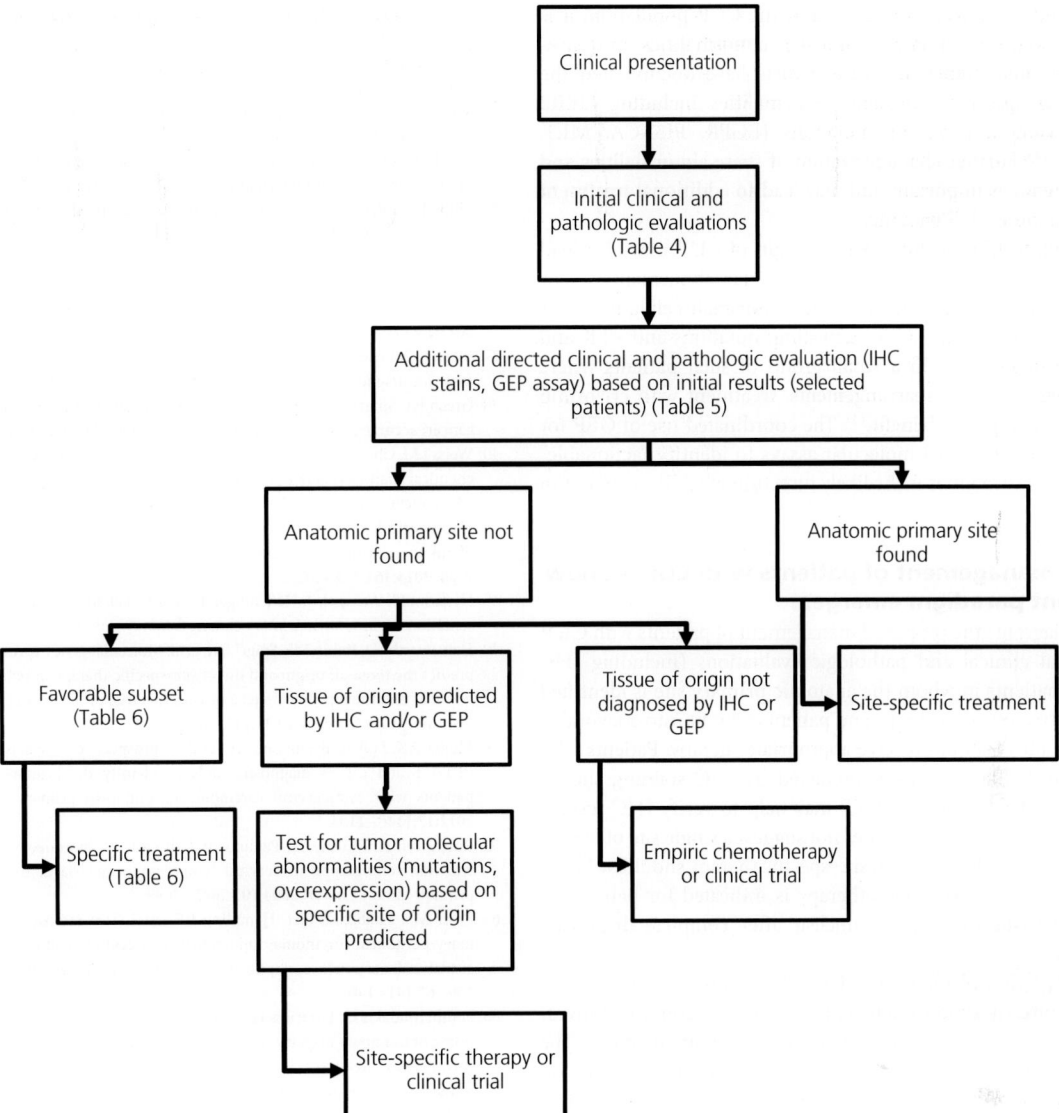

Figure 2 Management of patients with carcinoma of unknown primary site: overview.

documented median survivals >20 months, similar to the survival of patients with metastatic colon cancer.

The strongest support for site-specific therapy comes from a recent large, prospective trial in which previously untreated CUP patients had GEP (92-gene RT-PCR assay[35]). In this trial, a tissue of origin was predicted in 242 of 253 patients (98%). Twenty-six different tissues of origin were diagnosed (Table 3). Patients received site-specific therapy based on the GEP predictions and had a median survival of 12.5 months.[49]

Within this large group, 41% of patients had predicted tissues of origin known to be relatively resistant to standard therapy and were therefore unlikely to benefit much regardless of the treatment used. As predicted, this group did poorly, with a median survival of only 7.6 months. However, the remaining patients (59% of the group) were predicted to have more responsive tumor types and had a median survival of 13.4 months with site-specific therapy ($p = 0.04$). Although the numbers of patients with individual cancer types were small, median survivals within most of these groups were similar to those expected for the predicted tumor types (median survivals, months: ovary 30, breast 28, NSCLC 16, colorectal 13, pancreas 8, biliary tract 7).

In addition to the results from this prospective study, several small retrospective studies and case reports have documented benefits of site-specific treatment directed by the predicted tissue of origin.[133,134] Not all results have been consistent; in one study of 67 CUP patients who had anatomic primary sites identified as part of the initial evaluation, molecular profiling using an early assay predicted the correct primary site in only 35% of patients.[135]

Screening CUP for "actionable" molecular abnormalities

Many new cancer therapies exploit cancer-specific molecular abnormalities critical to cancer cell growth and metastasis. The identification of appropriate patient populations for these agents therefore depends not only on the tumor type but also on the presence of specific targeted molecular abnormalities. Screening of patients with specific cancer types for targeted molecular abnormalities is already a standard part of clinical practice, and screening for broader panels of potentially "actionable" abnormalities is becoming more commonplace.

Limited information currently exists regarding the prevalence of various molecular abnormalities in CUP. However, given the heterogeneity of cancers represented in the CUP population, it is likely that some potentially "actionable" abnormalities are represented. Previous studies and case reports have documented the existence of specific molecular abnormalities including HER2 overexpression and various mutations (EGFR, PI3KCA, MET, others).[136–140] Further characterization of these abnormalities and their frequency is important and may lead to additional treatment options for some CUP patients.

The identification of the tissue of origin of CUP may also lead to directed assessment of specific molecular abnormalities. For example, CUP patients predicted to have nonsmall-cell lung cancer should be evaluated for EGFR-activating mutations and ALK and ROS1 rearrangements. In a small group of such patients where studies identified ALK rearrangements, treatment with crizotinib resulted in therapeutic benefit.[141] The coordinated use of GEP for diagnosis and additional molecular assays to identify "actionable" molecular abnormalities is the likely direction of CUP treatment in the future.

Current management of patients with CUP—A new treatment paradigm emerges

Figure 2 diagrams the proposed management of patients with CUP. After initial clinical and pathologic evaluations (including IHC staining), patients in whom the anatomic primary site is identified should be treated accordingly, and patients who fit into a favorable treatment subset should receive appropriate therapy. Patients who have a single tissue of origin predicted by IHC staining should receive site-specific therapy; GEP may help to verify IHC results. When initial IHC evaluation does not suggest a single site of origin, GEP should be performed, and site-specific therapy should be based on the results. Empiric chemotherapy is indicated for patients in whom the tissue of origin is unclear after complete diagnostic evaluation.

The integration of molecular diagnostics into the management of CUP is already supported by clinical data, but continued investigation is necessary to refine management recommendations. The evolution of improved therapy for CUP patients also depends on improvements in therapy of other cancer types and is linked to the increasing number of precision therapies for these tumors. Optimum and timely integration of new agents into the treatment of patients with CUP will require ongoing efforts to define critical molecular abnormalities as a part of treatment planning for each patient.

Key references

The complete reference list can be found on the Wiley Companion Digital Edition of this title (see inside front cover for login instructions).

5 Horning SJ, Carrier EK, Rouse RV, et al. Lymphomas presenting as histologically unclassified neoplasms: characteristics and response to treatment. *J Clin Oncol.* 1989;**7**:1281–1287.

7 Oien KA, Dennis JL. Diagnostic work-up of carcinoma of unknown primary: from immunohistochemistry to molecular profiling. *Ann Oncol.* 2012;**23**(Suppl 10):271–277.

8 Greco FA, Lennington WJ, Spigel DR, Hainsworth JD. Molecular profiling diagnosis in unknown primary cancer: accuracy and ability to complement standard pathology. *J Natl Cancer Inst.* 2013;**105**:782–790.

11 Oien K. Pathologic evaluation of unknown primary cancer. *Semin Oncol.* 2009;**36**:8–37.

16 Dennis JL, Hvidsten TR, Wit EC, et al. Markers of adenocarcinoma characteristic of the site of origin: development of a diagnostic algorithm. *Clin Cancer Res.* 2005;**11**:3766–3772.

17 Park SY, Kim BH, Kim JH, et al. Panels of immunohistochemical markers help determine primary sites of metastatic adenocarcinoma. *Arch Pathol Lab Med.* 2007;**131**:1561–1567.

18 Anderson GG, Weiss LM. Determining tissue of origin for metastatic cancers: meta-analysis and literature review of immunohistochemistry performance. *Appl Immunohistochem Mol Morphol.* 2010;**18**:3–8.

23 Motzer RJ, Rodriguez E, Reuter VE, et al. Molecular and cytogenetic studies in the diagnosis of patients with poorly differentiated carcinoma of unknown primary site. *J Clin Oncol.* 1995;**13**:274–282.

24 Su AI, Welsh JB, Sapinoso LM, et al. Molecular classification of human carcinomas by use of gene expression signatures. *Cancer Res.* 2001;**61**:7388–7393.

33 Pillai R, Deeter R, Rigl CT, et al. Validation and reproducibility of a microarray-based gene expression test for tumor identification in formalin-fixed, paraffin-embedded specimens. *J Mol Diagn.* 2011;**13**:48–56.

35 Erlander MG, Ma XJ, Kesty NC, et al. Performance and clinical evaluation of the 92-gene real-time PCR assay for tumor classification. *J Mol Diagn.* 2011;**13**:493–503.

37 Meiri E, Mueller WC, Rosenwald S, et al. A second-generation microRNA-based assay for diagnosing tumor tissue origin. *Oncologist.* 2012;**17**:801–812.

38 Greco FA, Spigel DR, Yardley DA, et al. Molecular profiling in unknown primary cancer: accuracy of tissue of origin prediction. *Oncologist.* 2010;**15**:500–506.

40 Weiss LM, Chu P, Schroeder BE, et al. Blinded comparator study of immunohistochemical analysis versus a 92-gene cancer classifier in the diagnosis of the primary site in metastatic tumors. *J Mol Diagn.* 2013;**15**:263–269.

46 Hainsworth JD, Greco FA. Gene expression profiling in patients with carcinoma of unknown primary site: from translational research to standard of care. *Virchows Arch.* 2014;**464**:393–402.

48 Nystrom JS, Weiner JM, Heffelfinger-Juttner J, et al. Metastatic and histologic presentations in unknown primary cancer. *Semin Oncol.* 1977;**4**:53–58.

49 Hainsworth JD, Rubin MS, Spigel DR, et al. Molecular gene expression profiling to predict the tissue of origin and direct site-specific therapy in patients with carcinoma of unknown primary site: a prospective trial of the Sarah Cannon research institute. *J Clin Oncol.* 2013;**31**:217–223.

51 Moller AK, Loft A, Berthelsen AK, et al. A prospective comparison of 18 F-FDG PET/CT and CT as diagnostic tools to identify the primary tumor site in patients with extracervical carcinoma of unknown primary site. *Oncologist.* 2012;**17**:1146–1154.

52 Rusthoven KE, Koshy M, Paulino AC. The role of fluorodeoxyglucose positron emission tomography in cervical lymph node metastases from an unknown primary tumor. *Cancer.* 2004;**101**:2641–2649.

65 Piver MS, Eltabbakh GH, Hempling RE, et al. Two sequential studies for primary peritoneal carcinoma: induction with weekly cisplatin followed by either cisplatin-doxorubicin-cyclophosphamide or paclitaxel-cisplatin. *Gynecol Oncol.* 1997;**67**:141–146.

66 Pentheroudakis G, Lazaridis G, Pavlidis N. Axillary nodal metastases from carcinoma of unknown primary (CUPAx): a systematic review of published evidence. *Breast Cancer Res Treat.* 2010;**119**:1–11.

77 Varadhachary GR, Karanth S, Qiao W, et al. Carcinoma of unknown primary with gastrointestinal profile: immunohistochemistry and survival data for this favorable subset. *Int J Clin Oncol.* 2014;**19**:479–484.

78 Nguyen LN, Maor MH, Oswald MJ. Brain metastases as the only manifestation of an undetected primary tumor. *Cancer.* 1998;**83**:2181–2184.

79 Rades D, Kuhnel G, Wildfang I, et al. Localised disease in cancer of unknown primary (CUP): the value of positron emission tomography (PET) for individual therapeutic management. *Ann Oncol.* 2001;**12**:1605–1609.

84 Grau C, Johansen LV, Jakobsen J, et al. Cervical lymph node metastases from unknown primary tumours. Results from a national survey by the Danish Society for Head and Neck Oncology. *Radiother Oncol.* 2000;**55**:121–129.

90 Guarischi A, Keane TJ, Elhakim T. Metastatic inguinal nodes from an unknown primary neoplasm. A review of 56 cases. *Cancer.* 1987;**59**:572–577.

92 Hainsworth JD, Johnson DH, Greco FA. Poorly differentiated neuroendocrine carcinoma of unknown primary site. A newly recognized clinicopathologic entity. *Ann Intern Med.* 1988;**109**:364–371.

96 Hainsworth JD, Johnson DH, Greco FA. Cisplatin-based combination chemotherapy in the treatment of poorly differentiated carcinoma and poorly differentiated adenocarcinoma of unknown primary site: results of a 12-year experience. *J Clin Oncol.* 1992;**10**:912–922.

97 Briasoulis E, Kalofonos H, Bafaloukos D, et al. Carboplatin plus paclitaxel in unknown primary carcinoma: a phase II Hellenic Cooperative Oncology Group Study. *J Clin Oncol.* 2000;**18**:3101–3107.

104 Pouessel D, Culine S, Becht C, et al. Gemcitabine and docetaxel as front-line chemotherapy in patients with carcinoma of an unknown primary site. *Cancer.* 2004;**100**:1257–1261.

106 Pittman KB, Olver IN, Koczwara B, et al. Gemcitabine and carboplatin in carcinoma of unknown primary site: a phase 2 Adelaide Cancer Trials and Education Collaborative study. *Br J Cancer.* 2006;**95**:1309–1313.

107 Hainsworth JD, Spigel DR, Clark BL, et al. Paclitaxel/carboplatin/etoposide versus gemcitabine/irinotecan in the first-line treatment of patients with carcinoma of

unknown primary site: a randomized, phase III Sarah Cannon Oncology Research Consortium Trial. *Cancer J*. 2010;**16**:70–75.

110 Huebner G, Link H, Kohne CH, et al. Paclitaxel and carboplatin vs gemcitabine and vinorelbine in patients with adeno- or undifferentiated carcinoma of unknown primary: a randomised prospective phase II trial. *Br J Cancer*. 2009;**100**:44–49.

111 Gross-Goupil M, Fourcade A, Blot E, et al. Cisplatin alone or combined with gemcitabine in carcinomas of unknown primary: results of the randomised GEFCAPI 02 trial. *Eur J Cancer*. 2012;**48**:721–727.

117 Lee J, Hahn S, Kim DW, et al. Evaluation of survival benefits by platinums and taxanes for an unfavourable subset of carcinoma of unknown primary: a systematic review and meta-analysis. *Br J Cancer*. 2013;**108**:39–48.

130 Riihimaki M, Hemminki A, Sundquist K, Hemminki K. Time trends in survival from cancer of unknown primary: small steps forward. *Eur J Cancer*. 2013;**49**:2403–2410.

131 Greco F, Lennington W, Spigel DR, et al. Carcinoma of unknown primary site: outcomes in patients with a colorectal molecular profile treated with site-specific chemotherapy. *J Cancer Ther*. 2012;**3**:37–43.

132 Hainsworth JD, Schnabel CA, Erlander MG, et al. A retrospective study of treatment outcomes in patients with carcinoma of unknown primary site and a colorectal cancer molecular profile. *Clin Colorectal Cancer*. 2012;**11**:112–118.

133 Gross-Goupil M, Massard C, Lesimple T, et al. Identifying the primary site using gene expression profiling in patients with carcinoma of an unknown primary (CUP): a feasibility study from the GEFCAPI. *Onkologie*. 2012;**35**:54–55.

140 Gatalica Z, Millis S, Bender R, et al. Molecular profiling cancers of unknown primary: paradigm shift in management of CUP. European Cancer Conference 2013, abstract #LBA39; 2013.

124 Anorexia and cachexia

Takao Ohnuma, MD, PhD

Overview

Cancer cachexia is a wasting syndrome with extensive loss of skeletal muscle mass with or without adipose tissue. It may be contrasted with simple starvation in which fat replaces glucose as the preferred fuel to spare lean body mass. It results from altered metabolism rather than just an energy deficit, and cannot be reversed by conventional nutritional support. The causes of cancer-related cachexia are multifactorial including production of procachectic cytokines and metabolic derangements. European cancer community is credited in developing new definition and classification of cancer cachexia. Recent studies identified anamorelin, an oral ghrelin analogue, as a new agent for the treatment of cancer cachexia.

Introduction

Cachexia is a wasting syndrome that may accompany a plethora of diseases, including cancer, chronic obstructive pulmonary disease, AIDS, and rheumatoid arthritis. It is associated with central and systemic increases of pro-inflammatory factors, and with decreased quality of life, poor responses to pharmacological treatment and shortened survival.[1,2]

Extensive loss of skeletal muscle mass with or without adipose tissue in cachexia may be contrasted with simple starvation in which fat replaces glucose as the preferred fuel to spare lean body mass. Cancer cachexia results from altered metabolism rather than just an energy deficit, and it cannot be reversed by conventional nutritional support.[3,4]

Cachectic patients have a poor tolerance for surgery, chemotherapy, and radiotherapy.[5-8] Cross-sectional images at the level of the fourth lumbar vertebra in patients who underwent surgery revealed that covariate-adjusted mortality increased significantly as lean core muscle area decreased.[7-9]

A lack of universally accepted definitions, diagnostic criteria and classification has impeded progress in both clinical trials and clinical practice. The definition and the classification of cancer cachexia developed in 2010 are shown in Tables 1 and 2.[10]

There is consensus that focus should move from end-stage wasting to supporting patients' nutritional and functional state throughout the course of anticancer treatment. When inadequate nutrient intake predominates (malnutrition), this can be managed by conventional nutritional support. In the presence of systemic inflammation/altered metabolism that characterizes cachexia, a multimodal approach including novel therapeutic agents will likely be required. Three supportive care issues are critical: ensuring sufficient energy and protein intake, maintaining physical activity to maintain muscle mass, and (if present) reducing systemic inflammation. The results of phase II/III trials based on novel drug targets (e.g., cytokines, ghrelin receptor, androgen receptor, and myostatin) are expected by 2016. If effective therapies emerge, early detection of malnutrition and cachexia will be increasingly important.[11]

Etiology and mechanisms

The causes of cancer-related cachexia are multifold and can be grouped into three interrelated categories: anorexia and early satiety, mechanical obstruction of the alimentary tract, and metabolic derangement.

Anorexia in cancer patients can be disease-related, treatment-related and emotional distress-related. Anorexia may result from early satiety, nausea, or dysgeusia, a change in taste. Potential etiologic factors of anorexia and early satiety are presented in Table 3. Abnormalities of taste sensation and olfaction for specific food aromas have been demonstrated in cancer patients.[48]

Cytokines

TNF-α, IL-1, IL-6 [and its subfamily members such as ciliary neurotrophic factor (CNTF) and leukemia inhibitory factor (LIF)], and IFN-γ produced by host immune cells and/or tumor cells have all been implicated as mediators of cancer cachexia.[49-51] These cytokines, called procachectic factors, are characterized in animals by the induction of anorexia, weight loss, an acute-phase protein response, protein and fat breakdown, rises in levels of cortisol and glucagon and falls in insulin level, insulin resistance, anemia, fever, and elevated energy expenditure. Direct interaction may occur with leptin, neuropeptides, or serotonin as mechanisms of induction of cancer anorexia. Anticachectic factors, IL-4, IL-10, IL-12, IL-15, IFN-α, and insulin-like growth factor I (IGF-I), act in opposition to procachectic factors.

Procachectic cytokines are produced by host immune cells including T helper 1 cells, macrophages, and myeloid-derived suppressor cells as part of a persistent inflammatory response. Proteolysis inducing factor (PIF) appears to be produced exclusively by tumors. PIF and TNF-α appear to induce cachexia through a similar pathway, by activating nuclear factor kappa B (NF-κB) transcription factor in muscles.[52,53]

An elevated adrenergic state appears to be similar across tumor types resulting in elevated rates of energy expenditure.[54,55] The primary site of lean body mass depletion is the skeletal muscle, due to an increased protein turnover without equivalent protein synthesis.[54] Available data suggest loss of myosin heavy chain (MyHC) and reduction in fiber size.[54,56] The adenosine triphosphate-ubiquitin-dependent pathway regulating protein breakdown is upregulated in certain cases of cancer cachexia.[54,57]

IL-6 is a multifunctional cytokine involved in a variety of host defenses and pathological processes.[17] IL-6-secreting cells can induce wasting of both muscle and fat stores and ultimately death.[18,19] Serum IL-6 levels were elevated in most experimental models of cachexia. IL-6 was demonstrated to be a sensitive

Holland-Frei Cancer Medicine, Ninth Edition. Edited by Robert C. Bast Jr., Carlo M. Croce, William N. Hait, Waun Ki Hong, Donald W. Kufe, Martine Piccart-Gebhart, Raphael E. Pollock, Ralph R. Weichselbaum, Hongyang Wang, and James F. Holland.
© 2017 John Wiley & Sons, Inc. ISBN: 978-1-118-93469-2

Table 1 Diagnosis of cancer cachexia.

Measurement	Amount	Comments
Weight loss	>5%	In past 6 months (in absence of simple starvation)
or		
Body mass index	<20	If weight loss >2%
or		
Appendicular skeletal muscle index		Consistent with sarcopenia
Dual energy X-ray	Men < 7.26 kg/m² Women < 5.45 kg/m²	If weight loss >2%
Absorptiometry	Men < 32 cm² Women < 18 cm²	Upper arm
Anthropometry	Men <55 cm² Women <39 cm²	Lumbar CT imaging
Bioelectrical impedance	Men <14.6 kg/m² Women <11.4 kg/m²	Unreliable if obese or edematous

Source: Fearon et al. 2011.[10] Reproduced with permission from Elsevier.

Table 2 Stages of cancer cachexia.

Precachexia
Anorexia, metabolic change, weight loss <5%
Cachexia
Weight loss >5% in past 6 months (without starvation)
or
Body mass index <20 and weight loss >2%
or
Anorexia and systemic inflammatory changes and sarcopenia and weight loss >2%
Refractory cachexia
Progressing catabolic state in a cancer usually unresponsive, low performance score and predicted survival < 3 months

Source: Fearon et al. 2011.[10] Reproduced with permission from Elsevier.

Table 3 Possible causes of cancer anorexia.

Name	Character	References
Cytokines	TNFα	12–14
	IL-1	14–16
	IL-6	14, 17–32
Neuropeptides	Dysfunction in the brain circuits	33
Serotonin	Increases in serum and central nervous system (CNS)	34, 35
Serum lactate	Tumor product	36, 37
Glucagon and similar peptides		38, 39
Satietins	Proteins isolated in plasma	40, 41
Hypercalcemia	Occasional paraneoplastic findings	42
Bombesin	Neuropeptide from small-cell lung cancer	43, 44
Toxohormone-L	Lipolytic factor purified from ascitic fluid of patients with hepatoma	45, 46
Anticancer agents (emetogenic)	Cisplatin, doxorubicin, nitrogen mustard, others	47

predictor of weight loss in a number of series, including patients with advanced small-cell lung cancer[20] and colon cancer.[21,22] Elevated IL-6 levels were associated with reduced survival in a variety of cancer types.[23] In addition to IL-6 itself, other IL-6 family cytokines have also been implicated in muscle wasting, including CNTF[24,25] and LIF.[26,27]

IL-6 and related ligands activate signaling by binding to ligand-specific α-receptors (IL-6 receptor-α, also known as gp80) in either membrane-bound or soluble forms.[28] These ligand receptor complexes induce activation of three major pathways: the signal transducers and activators of transcription 1 and 3 (STAT1/3), ERK, and phosphatidylinositol 3-kinase/Akt pathways.[29] These pathways interact with downstream kinases to influence gene expression.[30]

One pathway activated strongly by IL-6 family ligands is the JAK/STAT3 pathway. STAT3 activation was shown to be a common feature of muscle wasting, activated in muscle by IL-6 *in vivo* and *in vitro* and by different types of cancer and sterile sepsis. Moreover, STAT3 activation proved both necessary and sufficient for muscle wasting. Conversely, inhibiting STAT3 pharmacologically with JAK or STAT3 inhibitors reduced muscle atrophy downstream of IL-6. These results indicated that STAT3 was a primary mediator of muscle wasting in cancer cachexia and other conditions of high IL-6 family signaling.[31,32]

Although the underlying mechanisms of muscle cachexia in cancer appear non-overlapping to those in the muscular dystrophies, a dysfunctional dystrophin glycoprotein complex (DGC) appears to be a common link between these two disease states.[58–60]

Tumor-induced alterations in DGC represent a key early event in cachexia.[59] DGC was examined in muscle biopsies. Compared to healthy controls, in 60% of patients with gastrointestinal cancer, dramatic reduction in dystrophin was found, linked with hyperglycosylation of DGC proteins.[59]

While TNF-α induces IL-1, both cytokines exercise their anorectic effect through the brain as well as directly on the gastrointestinal tract, for example, slowed gastric emptying.[12,15] In carcinogen-induced tumors in rats, despite changes in other tissues, IL-1β and its receptor mRNA were the only ones upregulated in the brain, suggesting that they played a major role in this model of cancer-associated anorexia.[16]

Serum levels of circulating TNF-α, IL-1, IL-6 and IFN-γ did not correlate with the anorexia/weight loss syndrome in cancer patients.[13,14] A central mechanism of action in the production of cachexia has been postulated for many cytokines, including IL-1, IL-6, IL-8, TNF-α, IFN-α and other chemokines. Additional comments are pertinent for serotonin and dysfunction of neuropeptidergic circuits. A close relationship between elevated plasma-free tryptophan and anorexia was observed in patients with cancer.[34] Increase in blood tryptophan results in elevated tryptophan levels in the cerebrospinal fluid, inducing increased synthesis of serotonin, a major mediator of cancer anorexia.[35]

Involvement of proteasome activity appears to be a rare event in cancer patients.[54,61] Some findings suggest involvement of the autophagic-lysosomal proteolytic system and cathepsin B during cancer cachexia development in humans.[61,62]

Insulin and ghrelin

Insulin, secreted from the exocrine pancreas, and leptin, produced primarily by adipocytes, both circulate at levels proportional to body fat content. They enter the central nervous system (CNS) in proportion to their plasma levels. As weight increases, insulin secretion is increased both at the basal state and in response to meals. Insulin promotes fat storage and leptin synthesis by fat cells. Leptin has a more important role than insulin in the CNS control of energy homeostasis, for example, leptin deficiency causes obesity with hyperphagia that persists despite high insulin levels, whereas obesity is not induced by insulin deficiency.[63,64] Endogenous control of appetite by the neuropeptide network can be categorized as orexigenic and anorexigenic (Table 4). In cachectic tumor-bearing animals, lower circulating levels of leptin and decreased adipose tissue leptin mRNA content have been

Table 4 Orexigenic (anabolic) and anorexigenic (catabolic) neuropeptides.

Orexigenic molecules
  Neuropeptide Y (NPY)
  Agouti-related protein (AGRP)
  Melanin-concentrating hormone (MCH)
  Hypocretin 1 and 2 (orexins A and B)
  Galanin
  Norepinephrine
  Opioids
  Ghrelin
Anorexigenic molecules
  α-Melanocyte-stimulating hormone (α-MSH)
  Corticotropin-releasing hormone (CRH)
  Thyrotropin-releasing hormone (TRH)
  Cocaine- and amphetamine-regulated transcript (CART)
  Pro-opiomelanocortin (POMC)
  Insulin
  IL-1β
  Urocortin
  Glucagon-like peptide 1 (GLP-1)
  Oxytocin
  Neurotensin
  Serotonin
  Dopamine
  Histamine
  Cholecystokinin
  Bombesin
  Calcitonin-gene-related peptide
  Pituitary adenylate-cyclase-activating polypeptide
  Leptin

Source: Data from Refs. 33 and 63.

described.[65] Similarly, serum leptin levels were reduced in patients with both advanced lung cancer and colon cancer.[66,67] Plasma leptin levels showed gender-dependent associations, and significantly lower levels were found among cachectic women than among cachectic men.[68]

Ghrelin, the "hunger hormone," which functions as a neuropeptide in the CNS, is a peptide produced by ghrelin cells in the gastrointestinal tract. When the stomach is empty, ghrelin is secreted. When the stomach is stretched, secretion stops. Ghrelin acts on hypothalamic brain cells both to increase hunger and to increase gastric acid secretion and gastrointestinal motility in preparation for food intake. The receptors for ghrelin and leptin, with opposing effects, are found on the same brain cells. Ghrelin also plays an important role in regulating reward perception in the ventral tegmental area (a site that plays a role in processing sexual desire and developing addictions) through its interaction with dopamine and acetylcholine.

Ghrelin is encoded by the *GHRL* gene and is produced from the presumed cleavage of the prepropeptide ghrelin/obestatin. Full-length preproghrelin is homologous to promotilin and both are members of the motilin family.

Ghrelin's peculiar structure, consisting of 28 amino acids with a single fatty acid *n*-octanoylated at Ser 3, not only allows binding to the growth hormone (GH) secretagogue receptor but also confers on the molecule a large variety of pleiotropic effects on different metabolic pathways.[69] Two different forms of ghrelin originating from the same precursor are detectable in serum: an unacylated ghrelin (UnAG) and a lower concentration of acylated ghrelin. The acylation of ghrelin is performed mainly in the stomach by the intracellular ghrelin-*O*-acyltransferase, an enzyme only discovered in 2008. Acylated ghrelin, but not UnAG, can bind the growth hormone secretagogue receptor-1a (GHSR-1a), widely expressed in hypothalamic and pituitary regions, mediating GH release, able

to enhance appetite and increase adipose tissue deposits. In a large variety of high-affinity binding sites, UnAG and acylated ghrelin act together, modulating the release of downstream mediators. In addition, novel receptors for UnAG in brain, gut, fat and muscle have been identified, which might promote cell proliferation, differentiation and survival.[70]

Ghrelin's physiological functions include appetite modulation, enhancement of GH release, energy homeostasis, glucose homeostasis, anti-inflammatory action, effects on cardiovascular system, regulation of gastrointestinal tract motility, sexual function, and osteogenesis. GHSR is widely expressed in brain regions controlling body weight, emotional responses, memory, and learning.

The circulating level of ghrelin was reported to be increased in patients with muscle wasting and cancer cachexia. Ghrelin counteracted tumor-induced anorexia in animal systems, and its administration increased food intake and body weight gain.[71–73]

The main molecular mechanisms regulating the cancer anorexia-cachexia syndrome include alterations in brain neurochemistry. In particular, the hypothalamic melanocortin system appears not to respond appropriately to peripheral inputs, and its activity is diverted largely towards the activation of catabolic stimuli promoting metabolism of carbohydrates, lipids, and proteins in peripheral tissues leading to insulin resistance, increased lipolysis, and accelerated muscle proteolysis.[74] Proinflammatory cytokines (TNF-α and IL-1β) and hypothalamic serotonergic neurons have been implicated in the dysfunction of the hypothalamic melanocortin system.[33] Two peptide systems in particular appear to be strongly influential in the control of feeding behavior: these are the orexigenic neuropeptide Y (NPY), and the anorexigenic POMC (pro-opiomelanocortin) systems.[75] Many of these mediators exert their effects through changes in the NPY/POMC systems. Both originate in the hypothalamic arcuate nucleus (ARC) and extend projections widely over the brain.[75] The role of cytokines in cancer anorexia may depend on both the NPY and POMC systems. Hypothalamic IL-1 mRNA has been shown to be significantly increased in methylcholanthrene-induced sarcoma bearing rats. Levels of IL-1 in cerebrospinal fluid of these rats are also increased.[76,77] Injection of IL-1β into the hypothalamus causes significant change in gene expression in skeletal muscle within hours including upregulation of the ubiquitin proteasome pathway. This clearly demonstrates the potential for neural control of muscle protein synthesis and degradation.[78] It has not yet been fully explored in patients with cancer cachexia.[54]

Alimentary tract dysfunction

Abnormalities in perception of taste and smell have been described in cancer patients. Tumors of the mouth, oropharynx, esophagus, stomach, pancreas, liver, and peritoneum may compromise oral intake by mechanical interference. Intestinal obstruction is a common complication of cancer. Malabsorption often occurs secondary to enzymatic insufficiency in pancreas carcinoma or secondary to lymphoma of the intestine or mesentery.[79,80]

Delayed gastric emptying and slowing of peristalsis are pathogenic mechanisms that may contribute to early satiety.[81] Early satiety is common in patients with decreased upper gastrointestinal motility.[82,83]

Biochemical and metabolic derangement

High rates of glucose utilization with production of lactic acid are characteristic features of the neoplastic cell (Warburg effect). Glucose utilization by transplanted tumors in mice was second only to the brain.[84] Hexokinase, which catalyzes the first step of the glycolytic pathway, often highly overexpressed in tumor cells, is a major player in this process. Binding of tumor hexokinase to the outer mitochondrial membrane provides the enzyme with preferential access to ATP generated in the mitochondrion and increases the activity and stability of the enzyme.[85] The end product of the hexokinase reaction, glucose-6-phosphate, serves not only as a source of ATP via glycolysis but is also a key intermediate in the metabolic processes essential for cell growth and proliferation. Lactic acid produced via glucose metabolism may be utilized by other tissues for energy purposes or may be transported to the liver for resynthesis to glucose. The cyclic metabolic pathway, in which glucose is converted to lactic acid by glycolysis in tumor tissue and then reconverted to glucose in the liver, is referred to as the Cori cycle. Conversion of glucose to lactate in cancer cells yields two ATPs, whereas lactate to glucose conversion in the liver requires six ATPs. Thus, a systemic energy losing or futile substrate cycle, involving this interplay of tumor glycolysis and host gluconeogenesis, may be an important cause of cancer cachexia.[86] Assuming that all lactate produced is recycled to glucose, the cancer cell acts as an energy parasite. It may be calculated, however, that if 85% of lactate passes through the gluconeogenic pathway and 15% is oxidized, the host's handling of tumor-produced lactate would be energetically neutral. It has been suggested that the increase in the Cori cycle is insignificant in terms of energy expenditure and that increased glucose catabolism itself is responsible for weight loss and development of cachexia.[87]

Another mechanism of futile cycle is activation of the uncoupling proteins (UCPs) in brown adipose tissues (UCP1) and in skeletal muscles (UCP2 and 3).[88-91] UCPs-3 mRNA levels were higher in the muscle of six patients with gastrointestinal adenocarcinomas with major weight loss than in six similar patients with stable weight and six controls. UCPs-2 mRNA levels did not differ significantly between groups.[90] Elevations in muscle UCPs-3 activity may enhance energy expenditure and this in turn could contribute to tissue catabolism. Other mechanisms of muscle wasting such as mitochondrial dysfunction and activation of PPARγ coactivator-1 may also exist.[92-95]

Recently, extensive re-examination of Warburg effects has been made.[96] Unlike most normal cells, many cancer cells derive a substantial amount of their energy from aerobic glycolysis converting most incoming glucose to lactate even in the presence of oxygen. Although ATP production by glycolysis can be more rapid than by oxidative phosphorylation, it is far less efficient in terms of ATP generated per unit of glucose consumed. This shift therefore demands that tumor cells implement an abnormally high rate of glucose uptake to meet their needs for energy, biosynthesis, and redox. Aerobic glycolysis putatively provides a biosynthetic advantage for tumor cells in that a high flux of substrate through glycolysis allows for effective shunting of carbon to key subsidiary biosynthetic pathways. A key molecule produced as a result of altered cancer metabolism is reduced nicotinamide adenine dinucleotide phosphate (NADPH), which functions as a cofactor and provides reducing power in many enzymatic reactions crucial for macromolecular biosynthesis. NADPH is also an antioxidant and forms part of the defense against reactive oxygen species (ROS) that are produced during rapid proliferation. High levels of ROS can damage macromolecules, inducing senescence and apoptosis. Glutathione (GSH) and thioredoxin (TRX), antioxidant molecules, are maintained in reduced form by NADPH. In addition to the genetic changes that alter tumor cell metabolism, factors of the microenvironment such as hypoxia, pH, and low glucose concentrations play a major role in determining the metabolic phenotype of tumor cells. It has been shown that cancer cells secrete hydrogen peroxide. As a consequence, oxidative stress in cancer-associated fibroblasts drives autophagy, mitophagy, and aerobic glycolysis. This "parasitic" metabolic coupling converts the stroma into a "factory" for the local production of recycled and high-energy nutrients (such as L-lactate) to fuel oxidative mitochondrial metabolism in cancer cells. A loss of stromal Cavolin-1 (Cav-1) is identified as a new biomarker for hypoxia, oxidative stress, autophagy, and the "reverse Warburg effect", leading to early tumor recurrence and poor clinical outcome.[97,98]

Reactive oxygen species (ROS) and oxidative stress

Metabolic reprogramming of distant adipose tissues and muscle occurs in cancer cachexia. Fatty acids are taken up and catabolized by cancer cells to generate ATP and promote tumor growth. Cancer cells frequently invade adipose tissue, inducing the release of free fatty acids from adjacent adipocytes and this release promotes tumor growth.

High levels of free fatty acids in the plasma are a key feature of cancer cachexia and advanced cancer. Fatty acids are the preferred plasma catabolites utilized in cancer cachexia, as measured by comparing plasma disappearance of 14C-labeled palmitate and glucose and measuring generation of 14C-labeled CO_2. Free fatty acids are catabolized to generate acetyl-CoA, ketone bodies, and ATP in tumors. In sum, the catabolic effects exerted by cancer cells on remote adipocytes and myocytes are similar to those that cancer cells exert on fibroblasts adjacent to cancer cells or cancer-associated fibroblasts.

Adipose triglyceride lipase (ATGL) and hormone sensitive lipase (HSL) are key enzymes in the generation of free fatty acids by adipocytes and ultimately in ketogenesis. High ATGL and HSL activity is implicated in cancer cachexia with myocyte apoptosis and loss of muscle mass. Muscle wasting is induced by autophagy and lysosomal degradation in cancer cachexia. ATGL and HSL knockdown studies reveal that they mediate muscle degradation. This highlights the significant reciprocal interactions between metabolism, autophagy, and cachexia.[99]

MicroRNA (miR-), Hormonal Aberration, and Tumor Parasitism, Signaling pathway

Regulation of gene expression has been linked to miR-378 in a human cachexia model.[100,101]

Low levels of testosterone in males with advanced cancer[102,103] and high plasma cortisol values in patients with malignant tumors have been reported.[104,105] These findings may be involved in the increased protein catabolism of skeletal muscles and other organs in cachectic cancer patients.

Signaling pathways involved in cancer cachexia are shown in Table 5.

Signaling pathways involved in muscle atrophy are interdependent. Activation or inhibition of a single pathway may have a cascade of effects on muscle protein balance. No pathway is the sole regulator of the process.[132]

Treatment

The definitive treatment of cancer cachexia is removal of the causative tumor. Short of achieving this goal, various measures have been undertaken with limited success.

Supportive care

Intervention from the stage of precachexia helps. Early nutritional intervention can lead to improvement in nutritional status and

Table 5 Signals involved in cancer-cachexia.

Signals	Expression	Function	References
NF-κB-dependent pathway (IL-1/TNFα/TWEAK (and PIF)↑→ TRAF6 → NF-κB/JNK/p38/ERK → Caspases → MyoD mRNA) (also TWEAK → NF-κB↑ → MuRF1↑ → MyHC loss)	↑	↑Apoptosis Promotes protein degradation	12, 15, 106–108 109–113
Ubiquitin-proteasome pathway (UPP) (muscle-specific ubiquitin ligases MAFbx/atrogin-1↑ and MuRF1↑ → degradation of myofibrillar protein)	↑	Promotes degradation of myofibrillar protein	58, 61[a], 62[a], 114[a], 115–119[a], 120[a], 121–123
Myostatin/activin pathway (myostatin/ActRIIB → SMAD2,3 → UPP, → AKT, → MAFbx and MuRF1)	↑	Negatively regulate myofibrillar protein	60, 124–126
Autophagic-lysosomal pathway (FOXO3A → autophagy → cathepsin B/L)	↑	Promotes protein degradation	61, 62, 127
IL-6, JAK/STAT pathway (IL-6 → gp130 → JAK → STAT3 → pSTAT3)	↑	Promotes protein degradation (myofibrillar and sarcomeric protein)	17–32
Dystrophin glycoprotein complex (DGC) (Defects in myofiber outer membranes and alterations in extracellular matrix proteins → MAFbx/atrogin-1↑ and MuRF1↑)	↑	Muscle membrane damage and muscle wasting	59
Calcium-dependent proteolysis system (IL-1/TNFa → p38/JAK → catepsin → calpains and caspase-3 → apoptosis)	↑	Degrading muscle protein (no precise muscle locations have been reported in cancer cachexia)	61, 120, 128
IGF-1 pathway (IGF-1↓ → PI3K → AKT → mTOR → ↓protein synthesis)	↓	Promotes protein degradation and increased apoptosis Antagonize with MAFbx and MuRF1	129
Mitogen-activated protein kinases (MAPKs), PGC-1α and caspase pathway (p38 MAPKs → PGC-1α → ERK $^1/_2$ → JAK → Caspase 8)	↑	Inhibits thermogenic action, inhibits skeletal muscle	94
Poly(ADP-ribose)polymerase (PARP ↑ → apoptosis↑ → MyoD protein↓)	↑	Muscle DNA fragmentation and apoptosis as well as downregulation of MyoD	130, 131[a]

PIF, proteolysis-inducing factor; MyHC, myosin heavy chain; PGC-1α, PPARγ coactivator-1α; PPARγ, peroxisome proliferator-activated receptor-γ; PARP, poly(ADP-ribose)polymerase.
[a]Animal data are not necessarily reproducible in patients. The references report negative clinical data.

reduction of the inflammatory response.[133] Body weight stabilization during chemotherapy is associated with reduced toxicity and a longer overall survival.[5]

Exercise is effective in preventing cancer,[134] safe during active cancer treatments,[135] and healthy for cancer survivors,[136] improving bone health, muscle strength, quality of life, fatigue, psychosocial distress, depression, and self-esteem.[137] Risk of comorbidities, frequent among cancer survivors, can be significantly reduced through increased physical activity. Moreover, exercise is associated with reduced overall mortality.[138] Physical activity may attenuate the effects of cachexia by modulating muscle metabolism, insulin sensitivity, and inflammation.[137–139] Exercise has been shown to have anti-inflammatory properties, through the upregulation of the anti-inflammatory cytokines both in skeletal muscle and adipose tissue. Exercise should be recommended at the earliest phase of cancer treatment[139] often with the helpful presence of a caregiver or exercise professional during exercise sessions.

Pharmacologic management

Olanzapine is a selective monoaminergic antagonist with a strong affinity for serotonin and dopamine receptors. Low doses of Olanzapine have been well tolerated with promising clinical activity on weight, nutrition, and function in cancer cachexia.[140]

Ghrelin and its analogs, anamorelin, BIM-28131, BIM-28125 and RC-1291.

In 2010, long-term dosing of ghrelin was begun in 17 weight-losing cancer patients with solid gastrointestinal tumors.[141] In a randomized study of high- or low-dose ghrelin, high-dose improved appetite and reduced the loss of whole body fat ($P < 0.04$) and serum GH ($P < 0.05$). No adverse effects were observed. These data led investigators to test the efficacy of a number of synthetic ghrelin analogs including anamorelin, BIM-28125, BIM-28131 (RM-131), L163 255, and RC-1291.

Anamorelin (ONO-7643) (Helsinn Healthcare S.A., Switzerland) is a novel, oral, ghrelin-receptor agonist.

In a short crossover study with placebo in cachectic cancer patients, IGF-1, appetite and weight significantly increased.[142]

In ROMANA 1 and 2, identically designed phase III studies, 484 and 495 patients with inoperable stage III and IV non-small cell lung cancer and cachexia with life expectancy of >4 months were randomly assigned in a 2:1 ratio to receive either anamorelin at 100 mg/day or placebo for 12 weeks. The majority of patients were receiving chemotherapy, and one-eighth were receiving radiotherapy. Cachexia was defined as more than 5% weight loss within the past 6 months or body mass index less than 20 kg/m². Both studies found that patients randomly assigned to placebo continued to lose weight and lean body mass over the 12-week study period, while those assigned to anamorelin gained lean body mass. The differences between the two groups for weight were highly significant at weeks 3, 6, 9, and 12, plus 1.10 and 0.75 kg medians in lean body mass respectively versus minus 0.44 and 0.96 kg in the placebo groups. Body weights increased by an average of 2.2 and 0.95 kg on anamorelin versus 0.14 and 0.57 kg on placebo. Both groups declined in hand grip strength over the course of the study. Quality of life as assessed by the Functional Assessment of Anorexia/Cachexia Therapy (FAACT) also showed a significant difference favoring anamorelin. The most common adverse events were manageable nausea and hyperglycemia (expected as a part of the mechanism of action).[143]

BIM-28125 is another synthetic ghrelin analog with similar actions in experimental models of cancer cachexia.[144] Clinical trials have not yet been reported. Effects of ghrelin and its analogs on cancer cachexia have recently been reviewed.[145,146]

Anabolic androgenic steroids have been used by athletes to promote muscle growth and strength. Randomized clinical trials were carried out to test whether supplements of nandrolone decanoate influenced the outcome of chemotherapy in patients with non-small cell lung cancer.[147,148] Although the treated group experienced less weight loss, response to chemotherapy and survival were comparable. In a three-arm phase III randomized clinical trial for the treatment of cancer anorexia/cachexia, fluoxymesterone, an anabolic steroid, showed significantly less appetite enhancement and did not have as favorable a toxicity profile as megestrol acetate, a progestational agent, or dexamethasone, a corticosteroid.[149]

Enobosarm (GTx-024) is an androgen receptor modulator (SARM) that has tissue-selective anabolic effects in muscle and bone. In 159 cancer patients (stratified by cancer type), once-daily oral enobosarm or placebo was administered for up to 113 days. Significant increases in total lean body mass occurred. The data suggest that enobosarm might lead to improvements in lean body mass, without the toxic effects associated with androgens and progestational agents.[150]

Megestrol acetate and medroxyprogesterone acetate

Significant reduction in serum levels of IL-1a and b, IL-2, IL-6, and TNF-α were observed in cancer patients treated with megestrol acetate which may bear on the mechanism of improved appetite and body weight gain.[151]

In a review of 15 randomized clinical trials including more than 2000 patients, there was a statistically significant advantage for high-dose progestins in regard to improved appetite and gain of body weight.[152] Weight gain produced by megestrol acetate was found to be mainly from increased body fat rather than accretion of lean tissue.[153,154] It has been argued that the gain of adipose tissue as opposed to lean tissue during treatment with megestrol acetate, although suboptimal, should not be disparaged because depletion of body fat is generally an undesirable outcome of cancer.

Megestrol acetate is contraindicated in pediatric cachectic patients, as a significant proportion of such patients developed adrenal insufficiency.[155] Megestrol acetate should also be used with caution in geriatric cancer patients because they are prone to develop deep vein thrombosis because of immobility and increases in serum fibrinogen levels.

Medroxyprogesterone acetate is a more widely used synthetic progestin. Medroxyprogesterone reduced production of cytokines and serotonin.[156] Two placebo-controlled randomized studies have been reported in which increased appetite was described.[157,158] Despite increased appetite, no weight gain was produced in either study.

In advanced cancer patients with delayed gastric emptying or gastroparesis, oral administration of a prokinetic agent, metoclopramide, 10 mg orally four times daily before meals and at bedtime, was shown to be effective in stimulating appetite and relieving other dyspeptic symptoms associated with anorexia.[159,160] A controlled release preparation appears to be more effective than immediate release drug due to its control of nausea associated with advanced cancer even without demonstrated abnormalities of the GI tract.[161]

Dronabinol (delta 9-tetrahydocannabinol, THC) was studied in patients with cancer.[162,163] All patients reported improvements in appetite but all groups nonetheless continued to lose weight. Recently, a randomized study was carried out to compare dronabinol, megestrol acetate, and the combination for palliating cancer-associated anorexia.[164] Megestrol acetate provided superior anorexia palliation among advanced cancer patients, and compared with dronabinol alone. The combination of megestrol and dronabinol did not appear to confer additional benefit.

Marijuana powder and smoke contains many different cannabinoids and reportedly is superior to synthetic dronabinol. Scientific trials have not been done, but with widespread legalization are now possible.

Cancer cachexia is different from simple starvation, in that nutritional support, either enteral or parenteral, has only limited value.

No significant benefit of TPN has been demonstrated in patients undergoing chemotherapy and/or radiotherapy in terms of treatment tolerance, response to chemotherapy or radiotherapy, or in survival.[165,166] Furthermore, other authors have reported that TPN is detrimental. Controversies related to TPN in the treatment of cancer cachexia have been reviewed.[167–169]

From the above discussions, one can speculate that one single therapy may not be successful in the treatment of cachexia. Treatment involving different combinations may be more likely to be useful.[170]

Future directions and summary

It has been realized that diagnosis of cancer cachexia was recognized often too late to reverse by nutritional supplementation. This made early recognition and intervention of cachexia important. Now that it appears nutritional intervention at precachexia is effective, the concept of precachexia is more meaningful. With recognition of precachexia together with the advent of a variety of anticachexia agents, we are at the stage of accomplishing an effective treatment of cachexia.

Physical exercise should be a part of any anticachexia protocol.

Several potentially promising leads beg for well-designed clinical trials. Drugs in need of more clinical studies include GH/insulin,[171] GHRP-2 (growth hormone releasing peptide 2),[172,173] and growth hormone releasing hormone (GHRH) expression plasmids.[174]

The most promising anticachexia agents appear to be ghrelin analogs, such as anamorelin.[143] Additional anticachectic agents potentially useful for supplementation include medroxyprogesterone acetate,[156–158] celecoxib,[175,176] antioxidants,[177,178] olanzapine,[140] native marijuana, and β-hydoxy-β-methylbutyrate/L-arginine/L-glutamine.[179–183]

Investigational drugs of potential benefit include ghrelin mimetics such as BIM-28131,[144] BIM-28125,[144] L163 255,[184] and RC-1291[185]; androgen receptor modulator enobosarm (GTx-024)[150]; anabolic catabolic transforming agents MT-102 and espindrol[186,187]; anti-IL-1α antibody MABp1[188,189]; anti IL-1 receptor antagonist IP-1510[189]; anti-IL-6 antibody ALD518[189–191]; myostatin inhibitors such as Bimagrumab (BYM338)[189] and REGN1033,[189] as well as OHR/AVR118, a broad-spectrum peptide-nucleic acid immunomodulator.[189]

Cachexia has been the major underestimated and unmet medical need. Development of new definition of cancer cachexia and start of anticachexia treatment from precachexia onward should revolutionize treatment of this complex disease with major benefit to all types of cancer therapy.

Key references

The complete reference list can be found on the Wiley Companion Digital Edition of this title (see inside front cover for login instructions).

1 Fearon KCH, Glass DJ, Guttridge DC. Cancer Cachexia: mediators, signaling, and metabolic pathways. *Cell Metab.* 2012;**16**:153–166.

2 von Haehling S, Anker SD. Cachexia as a major underestimated and unmet medical need: facts and numbers. *J Cachexia Sarcopenia Muscle.* 2010;**1**:1–5.

7 Englesbe MJ, Lee JS, He K, et al. Analytic morphomics, core muscle size, and surgical outcomes. *Ann Surg.* 2012;**256**:255–261.

10 Fearon K, Strasser F, Anker SD, et al. Definition and classification of cancer cachexia: an international consensus. *Lancet Oncol.* 2011;**12**:489–495.

11 Aapro M, Arends J, Bozzetti F, et al. Early recognition of malnutrition and cachexia in the cancer patient: a position paper of a European School of Oncology Task Force. *Ann Oncol.* 2014;**25**:1492–1499.

33 Inui A. Cancer anorexia-cachexia syndrome: are neuropeptides the key? *Cancer Res.* 1999;**59**:4493–4501.

54 Johns NA, Stephens KCH, Fearon KC. Muscle wasting in cancer. *Int J Biochem Cell Biol.* 2013;**45**:2215–2229.

59 Acharyya S, Butchbach ME, Sahenk Z, et al. Dystrophin glycoprotein complex dysfunction: a regulatory link between muscular dystrophy and cancer cachexia. *Cancer Cell.* 2005;**8**:421–432.

61 Jagoe RT, Redfern CP, Roberts RG, et al. Skeletal muscle mRNA levels for cathepsin B, but not components of the ubiquitin-proteasome pathway, are increased in patients with lung cancer referred for thoracotomy. *Clin Sci (Lond).* 2002;**102**:353–361.

62 Tardif N, Klaude M, Lundell L, et al. Autophagic-lysosomal patway is the main proteolytic system modified in the skeletal muscle of esophageal cancer patients. *Am J Clin Nutr.* 2013;**98**:1485–1492.

63 Schwartz MW, Woods SC, Porte D Jr, et al. Central nervous system control of food intake. *Nature.* 2000;**404**:661–671.

69 Molfino A, Gioia G, Muscaritoli M. The hunger hormone ghrelin in cachexia. *Expert Opin Biol Ther.* 2013;**13**:465–468.

86 Mathupala SP, Rempel A, Pedersen PL. Glucose catabolism in cancer cells: identification and characterization of a marked activation response of the type II hexokinase gene to hypoxic conditions. *J Biol Chem.* 2001;**276**:43407–43412.

90 Collins P, McCulloch P, Williams G. Muscle UCP-3 mRNA levels are elevated in weight loss associated with gastrointestinal adenocarcinoma in humans. *Br J Cancer.* 2002;**86**:372–375.

94 Puigserver P, Rhee J, Lin J, et al. Cytokine stimulation of energy expenditure through p38 MAP kinase activation of PPARγ coactivator-1. *Mol Cell.* 2001;**8**:971–982.

96 Cainns RA, Harris IS, Mak TW. Regulation of cancer cell metabolism. *Nat Rev Cancer.* 2011;**11**:85–95.

99 Martinez-Outschoorn UE, Lisanti MP, Sotgia F. Catabolic cancer-associated fibroblasts transfer energy and biomass to anabolic cancer cells, fueling tumor growth. *Semin Cancer Biol.* 2014;**25**:47–60.

106 Guttridge DC, Mayo MW, Madrid LV, et al. NF-kappaB-induced loss of MyoD messenger RNA: possible role in muscle decay and cachexia. *Science.* 2000;**289**:2363–2366.

113 Kumar A, Bhatnagar S, Paul PK. TWEAK TRAF6 regulate skeletal muscle atrophy. *Curr Opin Clin Nutr Metab Care.* 2012;**15**:233–239.

114 Op den Kamp CM, Langen RC, Minnaard R, et al. Pre-cachexia in patients with stages I-III non-small cell lung cancer: systemic inflammation and functional impairment without activation of skeletal muscle ubiquitin proteasome system. *Lung Cancer.* 2012;**76**:112–117.

115 Gomes MD, Lecker SH, Jagoe RT, et al. Atrogin-1, a muscle-specific F-box protein highly expressed during muscle atrophy. *Proc Natl Acad Sci U S A.* 2001;**98**:14440–14445.

116 Bodine SC, Latres E, Baumhueter S, et al. Identification of ubiquitin ligases required for skeletal muscle atrophy. *Science.* 2001;**294**:1704–1708.

120 Smith IJ, Aversa Z, Hasselgren P-O, et al. Calpain activity is increased in skeletal muscle from gastric cancer patients with no or minimal weight loss. *Muscle Nerve.* 2011;**43**:410–414.

131 Bossola M, Mirabella M, Ricci E, et al. Skeletal muscle apoptosis is not increased in gastric cancer patients with mild–moderate weight loss. *Int J Biochem Cell Biol.* 2006;**38**:1561–1570.

134 Thompson R. Preventing cancer: the role of food, nutrition and physical activity. *J Fam Health Care.* 2010;**20**:100–102.

136 Rock CL, Doyle C, Demark-Wahnefried W, et al. Nutrition and physical activity guidelines for cancer survivors. *CA Cancer J Clin.* 2012;**62**:243–274.

140 Braiteh F, Dalal S, Khuwaja A, et al. Phase I pilot study of the safety and tolerability of olanzapine (OZA) for the treatment of cachexia in patients with advanced cancer. *J Clin Oncol.* 2008;**26**:196–203.

142 Garcia JM, Friend J, Allen S. Therapeutic potential of anamorelin, a novel, oral ghrelin mimetic, in patients with cancer-related cachexia: a multicenter, randomized, double-blind, crossover, pilot study. *Support Care Cancer.* 2013;**21**:129–137.

143 Temel J, Currow D, Fearon K, et al. Anamorelin for the treatment of cancer anorexia-cachexia in NSCLC: Results from the phase 3 studies ROMANA 1 and 2. ESMO Congress, Barcelona, Spain. Abst 14830-PR. Presented September 27, 2014.

145 Molfino A, Formiconi A, Rossi Fanelli F, et al. Ghrelin: from discovery to cancer cachexia therapy. *Curr Opin Clin Nutr Metab Care.* 2014;**17**:471–476.

146 Argiles JM, Stemmler B. The potential of ghrelin in the treatment of cancer cachexia. *Expert Opin Biol Ther.* 2013;**13**:67–76.

150 Dobs AS, Boccia RV, Croot CC, et al. Effects of enobosarm on muscle wasting and physical function in patients with cancer: a double-blind, randomised controlled phase 2 trial. *Lancet Oncol.* 2013;**14**:335–345.

152 Pascual Lopez A, Roque i Figuls M, Urrutia Cuchi G, et al. Systematic review of megestrol acetate in the treatment of anorexia-cachexia syndrome. *J Pain Symptom Manag.* 2004;**27**:360–369.

153 Loprinzi CL, Schaid DJ, Dose AM, et al. Body-composition changes in patients who gain weight while receiving megestrol acetate. *J Clin Oncol.* 1993;**11**:152–154.

170 Argiles JM, Lopez-Soriano J, Busquets S. Novel approaches to the treatment of cachexia. *Drug Discov Today.* 2008;**13**:73–78.

176 Mantovani G, Macciò A, Madeddu C, et al. Phase II nonrandomized study of the efficacy and safety of COX-2 inhibitor celecoxib on patients with cancer cachexia. *J Mol Med (Berl).* 2010;**88**:85–92.

188 Ma JD, Heavey SF, Revta C, Roeland EJ. Novel investigational biologics for the treatment of cancer cachexia. *Expert Opin Biol Ther.* 2014;**14**:1113–1120.

190 Clarke SJ, Gebbie C, Sweeney C, et al. A phase I, pharmacokinetic (PK), and preliminary efficacy assessment of ALD518, a humanized anti-IL-6 antibody, in patients with advanced cancer. *J Cachexia Sarcopenia Muscle.* 2010;**1**:98.

125 Antiemetic therapy

Patrick M. Forde, MD, MBBCh ▪ *David S. Ettinger, MD, FACP, FCCP*

Overview

Dramatic progress has been made in the prevention and treatment of chemotherapy-induced emesis, especially since the introduction of the 5-HT3 receptor antagonists in the early 1990s and the 2003 introduction of the NK-1 receptor antagonist, aprepitant. Recent surveys indicate the need for heightened awareness of the frequency and severity of acute and, especially, delayed nausea and vomiting from chemotherapy. Fortunately, new agents have been added to the antiemetic arsenal to further enhance the efficacy of antiemetic prophylaxis. Complementary therapies such as acupuncture and mind–body interventions appear promising in controlling nausea, and are being explored further. Appropriate implementation of guidelines for prophylaxis based on the specific chemotherapy agents used will ensure that fewer patients experience these most distressing of side effects.

Overview

Chemotherapy-induced nausea and vomiting (CINV) remains a significant problem for many cancer patients despite recent advances in pharmacologic therapy.[1] It may have a dramatic impact on a patient's quality of life, in addition to physical consequences, including dehydration, nutritional compromise, and metabolic disturbances.[2] Despite the publication of guidelines for preventive antiemetic therapy, some patients continue to receive suboptimal prophylaxis against CINV. Nausea and vomiting occurring after chemotherapy may be more difficult to manage than if the symptoms had been prevented with appropriate pharmacologic intervention. In addition, patients may develop a psychological component to their nausea and vomiting as a result of inadequate management in the past. Thus, optimal control of CINV is a crucial aspect of symptom management among cancer patients.

Historically, approximately 70–80% of all cancer patients receiving chemotherapy experienced emesis,[3] and, fortunately, there have been dramatic improvements since the introduction of effective antiemetic therapy.[1] Studies over the past 25 years have attempted to quantify the impact of chemotherapy side effects on cancer patients. Repeatedly, nausea and vomiting are mentioned as the "major physical," and the "most troublesome and unpleasant" side effects associated with chemotherapy.[4,5] Although there have been recent advances in pharmacologic prevention of CINV, a 1997 study by de Boer-Dennert and colleagues revealed that nausea and vomiting ranked as the first and third most distressing side effects of chemotherapy, despite a decrease in the overall incidence and severity with the introduction of 5-hydroxytryptamine 3 (5-HT3) antagonists.[6] Grunberg and colleagues surveyed patients, medical oncologists, and oncology nurses in 2001–2002 to assess the frequency and provider perception of CINV.[1] Although

improvements in the prevention of acute nausea and vomiting were seen (acute nausea in approximately 35% and acute emesis in 13%), delayed symptoms were seen more frequently (50–60% with nausea and 30–50% with emesis, depending on the chemotherapy used). Strikingly, more than 75% of physicians and nurses underestimated the occurrence of delayed nausea and vomiting. Progress in relieving the symptoms of CINV will only come with greater awareness of the problem and more aggressive use of current medications.

This chapter highlights the pathophysiology of CINV, the emetogenic potential of common chemotherapeutics, classes of antiemetic therapy including complementary therapies, and guidelines for prevention and acute management of CINV.

Pathophysiology of nausea and vomiting

Vomiting is controlled by the central nervous system via a complex pathway of varied afferent inputs and neurotransmitters. In the 1950s, studies by Borison and Wang identified two areas of the brainstem involved in nausea and vomiting: the chemoreceptor trigger zone (CTZ) and the emetic center.[7] The CTZ is located in the area postrema in the floor of the fourth ventricle. Because it lies outside the blood–brain barrier, the CTZ is susceptible to emetogenic stimuli from the bloodstream, such as chemotherapeutic drugs or, more likely, their metabolites.[8] Muscarinic, dopamine D2, serotonin (5-HT3), neurokinin 1 (NK-1) and histamine H1 receptors have been identified in the CTZ. Impulses from the CTZ are then transmitted to the emetic center. In addition to those from the CTZ to the emetic center, afferent pathways from the gastrointestinal tract and pharynx via the vagus and splanchnic nerves are coordinated in the emetic center.[9] Inputs from the cerebral cortex may also be involved, especially in anticipatory emesis. The emetic center receives afferent impulses and coordinates the efferent activities of the salivation center, abdominal muscles, respiratory center, and autonomic nerves that result in vomiting. The emetic center, composed of these indistinct receptor and effector nuclei, is located in the nucleus tractus solitarius of the brainstem.[8]

The most critical neurotransmitters involved in these afferent and efferent pathways are serotonin (5-HT3), dopamine, and substance P. Others include acetylcholine, corticosteroid, histamine, cannabinoid, opiate, and gamma-aminobutyric acid (GABA).[10] Blockade of these neurotransmitters and their receptors forms the basis of action of various antiemetic drugs. The most significant advance in antiemetic therapy came in the early 1990s when the 5-HT3 receptor antagonists became available.[6] Substance P, which binds to the NK-1 receptor, is an emerging target in antiemetic therapy,[11] and one Food and Drug Administration (FDA)-approved NK-1 receptor antagonist, aprepitant, has clinical utility and is in widespread use.[12–14] Drugs such as prochlorperazine, haloperidol, and metoclopramide exert their antiemetic effects by inhibiting dopamine. However, it is not fully known how and where along

Holland-Frei Cancer Medicine, Ninth Edition. Edited by Robert C. Bast Jr., Carlo M. Croce, William N. Hait, Waun Ki Hong, Donald W. Kufe, Martine Piccart-Gebhart, Raphael E. Pollock, Ralph R. Weichselbaum, Hongyang Wang, and James F. Holland.
© 2017 John Wiley & Sons, Inc. ISBN: 978-1-118-93469-2

these pathways chemotherapy and its metabolites have their emetic effects. Metabolites may stimulate the CTZ directly. Serotonin and other neurotransmitters may be released from intestinal cells damaged by chemotherapy. Sensory neurons release substance P, and numerous NK-1 receptors have been identified in both the CTZ and the nucleus tractus solitarius. Despite increasing knowledge of the central nervous system and pathways involved in control of vomiting, no single common pathway has been discovered, and it is unlikely that any single agent will be able to provide complete antiemetic protection from chemotherapy.

Types of nausea and vomiting

Three distinct types of chemotherapy-induced emesis have been identified: acute, delayed, and anticipatory.

Acute emesis is defined as nausea and vomiting within 24 h of chemotherapy. It has its onset within 1–2 h of chemotherapy and peaks in the first 4–6 h without adequate prophylaxis.

Delayed emesis refers to symptoms that start more than 24 h after chemotherapy. It typically peaks at 48–72 h and may last for 6–7 days. Although delayed emesis may be less frequent and severe than acute emesis, it is less well controlled than acute emesis. Cisplatin is most frequently associated with delayed emesis, and it is also seen with carboplatin, cyclophosphamide, and anthracyclines.

Anticipatory emesis is seen in patients who have previously experienced significant nausea and vomiting following chemotherapy. In these patients, symptoms develop as a conditioned response before the chemotherapy is administered. It may be triggered by sights and activities associated with the chemotherapy (e.g., driving to the treatment center). As anticipatory emesis is a conditioned reflex, it is predominantly mediated by the cerebral cortex. As control of CINV has improved, the incidence of anticipatory emesis has declined.[15]

Breakthrough emesis refers to symptoms that occur despite prophylactic treatment and which require rescue therapy. This is a difficult clinical problem to manage and there is little clinical trial data to guide antiemetic selection in this setting.[16,17] Several agents are used empirically, including haloperidol, olanzapine, and lorazepam.[16,17]

Refractory emesis refers to symptoms that occur during a chemotherapy cycle after prophylactic treatment and/or rescue therapy has failed in earlier cycles of chemotherapy.[17]

In addition to chemotherapy-induced emesis, other potential causes of nausea and vomiting in cancer patients include partial or complete bowel obstruction, brain metastases, uremia, electrolyte disturbances (i.e., hyperglycemia, hypercalcemia, hyponatremia), and gastroparesis. Other medications commonly prescribed in cancer patients, such as opiates, may cause emesis as well.

Emetogenic chemotherapy

The severity and frequency of CINV are affected by variables of both the patient and the chemotherapy. Patient-related factors predicting a higher incidence of CINV include a history of chemotherapy, a history of CINV, female sex, younger age, and a history of motion sickness, anxiety, and no/minimal history of alcohol use. Chemotherapy-related factors include the route and rate of administration and drug dosage. The most predictive factor is the specific chemotherapy agent used.[18]

There is no universally accepted classification system of chemotherapy agents by emetogenic potential (Table 1). The most widely accepted, devised by Hesketh and colleagues, divides chemotherapy into five levels of emetogenicity based on the percentage of patients who experience nausea and vomiting following each without any antiemetic prophylaxis. Level 1 drugs result in emesis in less than 10% without antiemetic therapy; level 2, 10–30%; level 3, 30–60%; level 4, 60–90%; and level 5, more than 90% of patients experiencing emesis without prophylaxis.[19] A proposed modification to this classification would classify chemotherapy into four risk categories[20]:

High risk (level 5): more than 90%
Moderate risk (levels 3 and 4): 30–90%
Low risk (level 2): 10–30%
Minimal risk (level 1): <10%

It should be noted that these classification systems were developed with a focus on acute emesis. It is clear from recent data that the frequency and severity of delayed emesis are often underestimated and remain a significant problem for many patients.[1] Adequate antiemetic prophylaxis is required for the duration of days that symptoms are anticipated.

Classes of antiemetics

Our knowledge of the known neurotransmitters involved in the central nervous system pathways that regulate the vomiting response has provided targets for antiemetic therapy (Table 2). In return, successful clinical application of these agents has confirmed the importance of these neurotransmitters and receptors in the vomiting pathway. Neuroreceptors involved in the control of emesis include muscarinic (M1, receptor site for acetylcholine), dopamine (D2, receptor site for dopamine), histamine (H1, receptor site for histamine), 5-HT3 (receptor site for serotonin), NK-1 (receptor site for substance P), and GABA (receptor site for benzodiazepines).[21,22] The most effective and most commonly used antiemetics are the 5-HT3 receptor antagonists, the dopamine antagonists, and corticosteroids. A newer class of agents, the NK-1 receptor antagonists, further expands the repertoire of antiemetic agents.

Serotonin/5-HT3 receptor antagonists

Since the early 1990s, four 5-HT3 receptor antagonists have been approved in the United States: ondansetron, granisetron, dolasetron, and, most recently, palonosetron. These agents revolutionized the antiemetic prophylaxis of highly and moderately emetogenic chemotherapy. Studies of 5-HT3 receptor antagonists used alone demonstrated superior efficacy compared with high-dose metoclopramide alone[23] and equivalence to the combination of high-dose metoclopramide and dexamethasone, the previous standard of care for these patients.[24] However, the combination of 5-HT3 receptor antagonist and dexamethasone was the most effective combination tested.[25] The 5-HT3 antagonists remain the cornerstone of prophylaxis for both highly and moderately emetogenic chemotherapy.

Before 2003, there were three 5-HT3 receptor antagonists approved by the FDA: ondansetron, granisetron, and dolasetron. Numerous subsequent clinical trials demonstrated the clinical equivalence of these three agents, despite differences seen in preclinical models.[26-31] A single-dose prechemotherapy was shown to be as effective as repeat dosing.[32-34] In addition, there was no significant difference whether the agent was given orally or intravenously.[35,36]

In July 2003, a new 5-HT3 receptor antagonist, palonosetron, was approved by the FDA for antiemetic prophylaxis. Palonosetron may have advantages over the other serotonin antagonists because of its higher binding affinity to the 5-HT3 receptor and its longer

Table 1 Emetogenic potential of single antineoplastic agents.

Level	Agent
High risk, level 5 (>90% predicted frequency of emesis without prophylaxis)	Carmustine >250 mg/m² Cisplatin ≥50 mg/m² Cyclophosphamide >1500 mg/m² Dacarbazine Mechlorethamine Streptozocin
Moderate risk, level 4 (60–90% predicted frequency of emesis without prophylaxis)	Amifostine >500 mg/m² Busulfan >4 mg/d Carboplatin Cisplatin <50 mg/m² Cyclophosphamide >750 mg/m² and ≤1500 mg/m² Cytarabine >1 g/m² Dactinomycin Doxorubicin >60 mg/m² Epirubicin >90 mg/m² Melphalan >50 mg/m² Methotrexate >1000 mg/m² Procarbazine (oral dosing)
Moderate risk, level 3 (30–60% predicted frequency of emesis without prophylaxis)	Amifostine >300 mg/m² and ≤500 mg/m² Arsenic trioxide Bendamustine Cyclophosphamide ≤750 mg/m² Cyclophosphamide (oral dosing) Doxorubicin 20 and <60 mg/m² Epirubicin ≤90 mg/m² Ifosfamide Interleukin-2 >12–15 million units/m² Irinotecan Lomustine Methotrexate 250–1000 mg/m² Mitoxantrone <15 mg/m² Oxaliplatin >75 mg/m²
Low risk, level 2 (10–30% predicted frequency of emesis without prophylaxis)	Amifostine ≤300 mg/m² Bexarotene Cytarabine 100–200 mg/m² Capecitabine Docetaxel Doxorubicin (liposomal formulation) Etoposide 5-Fluorouracil <1000 mg/m² Gemcitabine Methotrexate >50 and <250 mg/m² Mitomycin Mitoxantrone Paclitaxel Pemetrexed Temozolomide Topotecan
Minimal risk, level 1 (<10% predicted frequency of emesis without prophylaxis)	Alemtuzumab Asparaginase Bevacizumab Alpha Interferon Bleomycin Bortezomib Cetuximab Chlorambucil (oral dosing) Cladribine Dasatinib Dexrazoxane Denileukin diftitox Erlotinib Fludarabine Gefitinib Gemtuzumab ozogamicin Hydroxyurea Imatinib mesylate Melphalan (low dose, oral dosing) Methotrexate ≤50 mg/m² Pentostatin Rituximab

Table 1 (Continued)

Level	Agent
	Sorafenib Sunitinib Thioguanine (oral dosing) Trastuzumab Valrubicin Vinblastine Vincristine Vinorelbine

Table 2 Classes and recommended doses of selected antiemetics.

Agent	Class	Route	Dose
Ondansetron	5-HT3 receptor antagonist	IV	8–12 mg
—	—	PO	12–24 mg
Granisetron	5-HT3 receptor antagonist	IV	1 mg or 0.01 mg/kg
—	—	PO	2 mg
Dolasetron	5-HT3 receptor antagonist	IV	100 mg or 1.8 mg/kg
—	—	PO	100 mg
Palonosetron	5-HT3 receptor antagonist	IV	0.25 mg
Aprepitant	NK-1 receptor antagonist	PO	125 mg day 1
—	—	—	80 mg day 2, 3
Dexamethasone	Steroid	IV	8–20 mg
—	—	PO	8–20 mg
Prochlorperazine	Dopamine receptor antagonist	IV	10 mg
—	—	PO	10 mg
—	—	Rectal suppository	25 mg
Metoclopramide	Dopamine receptor antagonist	IV	1–2 mg/kg
—	—	PO	20–40 mg
Haloperidol	Dopamine receptor antagonist	IV	1–3 mg
—	—	PO	1–2 mg
Dronabinol	Cannabinoid	PO	5–10 mg

Abbreviations: IV, intravenous; 5-HT3, 5-hydroxytryptamine 3; NK, neurokinin; PO, orally.

half-life. Two phase 3 randomized clinical trials demonstrated the superiority of palonosetron compared with ondansetron and dolasetron, particularly in preventing delayed nausea and vomiting.[37,38] In the first, 592 patients were randomized to receive palonosetron at either 0.25 or 0.75 mg or dolasetron at 100 mg 30 min prior to moderately emetogenic chemotherapy. Less than 5% of patients received concomitant corticosteroids. A statistically significant difference was observed between the palonosetron 0.25 mg and dolasetron arms in complete response (CR), defined as absence of emesis and no rescue medication in the first 24 h). CR rates were 63% in the palonosetron 0.25 mg arm versus 52.9% in the dolasetron arm ($p = 0.049$) and 57% for the palonosetron 0.75 mg arm ($p = 0.412$). For complete control (defined as no emesis, no need for rescue medication, and no symptoms other than mild nausea) of delayed nausea and vomiting (24–120 h), palonosetron 0.25 and 0.75 mg demonstrated statistically significant improvements compared with dolasetron 100 mg (48.1% for palonosetron 0.25 mg compared with 36.1% for dolasetron, $p = 0.027$; 51.9% for palonosetron 0.75 mg, $p = 0.016$). There was no difference among the groups in observed adverse effects, including headache, constipation, and fatigue.[37] In the second study, palonosetron was compared with ondansetron 32 mg. Five hundred and seventy patients receiving moderately emetogenic chemotherapy were randomized to one of two doses of palonosetron (0.25 or 0.75 mg) or ondansetron 32 mg on day 1 of chemotherapy. No patient received corticosteroids. CR rates were superior for the palonosetron 0.25 mg arm compared with the ondansetron group in prevention of both acute (81% vs 68.6%, $p = 0.009$) and delayed (74.1% vs 55.1%, $p < 0.001$) symptoms. Although palonosetron 0.75 mg demonstrated numeric improvement over ondansetron, the results were not statistically significant. Side effects were similar in all groups and included headache, diarrhea, constipation, and fatigue.[38] While palonosetron might be superior to other 5-HT3 agents, particularly in the prevention of delayed symptoms, further studies are needed to evaluate this. All of the 5-HT3 antagonists are well tolerated; the most common adverse effect is headache, occurring in 15–20% of patients. Less common side effects include constipation and dizziness.

More recently, granisetron has been incorporated in a transdermal system (*Sancuso*) for the prevention of CINV. In a phase 3 study, the transdermal granisetron patch was compared to oral granisetron in the management of CINV. The patch formulation contained 34.3 mg of granisetron with the active ingredient being released slowly over 7 days. In a multicenter study involving 641 patients receiving highly or moderately emetogenic chemotherapy, the granisetron patch was not inferior to repeat doses of oral granisetron.[39]

Dopamine receptor antagonists

Three classes of dopamine receptor antagonists are effective in the prevention and treatment of nausea and vomiting: phenothiazines, butyrophenones, and benzamides. In the 1960s, the phenothiazines were the first drugs proved to have efficacy in the prevention of CINV. *Prochlorperazine* is the most commonly used in this class and has efficacy in all classes except the most highly emetogenic chemotherapy.[40] Extrapyramidal effects, including dystonia, may be seen. These are treated with diphenhydramine and cessation of the drug. The butyrophenones, including *haloperidol*, are less frequently used for CINV and have adverse effects similar to those of the phenothiazines. They may be effective in the treatment of breakthrough nausea and vomiting.

Of the benzamides, *metoclopramide* is the best studied and most widely used in CINV. It blocks central and peripheral dopamine (D2) receptors at low doses and exhibits weak 5-HT3 inhibition at high doses. In addition, it speeds gastric emptying and increases sphincter tone at the gastroesophageal junction. Prior to the introduction of the 5-HT3 antagonists, a combination of high-dose intravenous metoclopramide and dexamethasone was the most effective antiemetic prophylaxis for highly emetogenic chemotherapy.[41] Because metoclopramide crosses the blood–brain barrier, side effects, including dystonia and tardive dyskinesia, may be seen, particularly at high doses and in aged patients. Diphenhydramine was commonly given as part of the combination regimen to prevent these adverse effects. This regimen has been replaced by a combination containing a 5-HT3 receptor antagonist because of its improved efficacy and safety profile.[23–25]

Corticosteroids

Corticosteroids, most commonly *dexamethasone*, are effective in preventing nausea and vomiting when used alone or in combination for all emetogenic classes of chemotherapy. For moderately to highly emetogenic chemotherapy, dexamethasone plus a 5-HT3 receptor antagonist +/− an NK-1 receptor antagonist is used.

A meta-analysis of 32 randomized clinical trials including 5613 patients from 1984 to 1998 demonstrated the efficacy of dexamethasone in both moderately and highly emetogenic chemotherapy either alone or in combination with other agents.[42] Later studies revealed the superiority of a combination of 5-HT3 receptor antagonist and dexamethasone compared with either agent alone in highly emetogenic chemotherapy.[43] The site of action of corticosteroids along the vomiting reflex pathway is unknown. Side effects may include insomnia, increased energy, and mood disturbances.

NK-1 receptor antagonists

NK-1 receptors are found in the nucleus tractus solitarius and the area postrema and are activated by substance P.[11] Inhibitors of the NK-1 receptor have demonstrated antiemetic effects and represent a new target for antiemetic therapy. The first approved medication in this class, *aprepitant*, has been shown to prevent both acute and delayed emesis resulting from highly emetogenic chemotherapy.[13,14]

Following promising preliminary data, two randomized phase 3 multicenter trials demonstrated the efficacy of aprepitant for the prevention of both acute and delayed nausea and vomiting. Five hundred and twenty-three patients receiving highly emetogenic chemotherapy (cisplatin >70 mg/m^2) were administered emetic prophylaxis using either aprepitant in combination with 5-HT3 receptor antagonists and dexamethasone (aprepitant 125 mg PO, ondansetron 32 mg IV, and dexamethasone 12 mg PO on day 1, followed by aprepitant 80 mg PO and dexamethasone 8 mg PO on days 2–3 and dexamethasone 8 mg PO on day 4) or a regimen of a 5-HT3 receptor antagonist and dexamethasone alone (ondansetron 32 mg IV plus dexamethasone 20 mg PO on day 1, followed by dexamethasone 8 mg PO twice daily on days 2–4). In the first study, the overall CR (absence of emesis and no need for rescue medication in the first 24 h) was 62.7% in the aprepitant arm versus 43.3% in the standard therapy arm ($p < 0.001$). CR rates for the aprepitant arm and the standard therapy arm, respectively, for acute (82.8% vs 68.4%, $p < 0.001$) and delayed (67.7% compared with 46.8%, $p < 0.001$) symptoms demonstrated the superiority of the aprepitant arm.[13] The second study, which evaluated the same regimens in 521 patients receiving high-dose cisplatin chemotherapy, confirmed these results. Overall CR rates were 72.7% in the aprepitant group versus 52.3% in the standard arm ($p < 0.001$). CR rates in both acute and delayed emesis were also superior in the aprepitant arm (89.2% vs 78.1%, respectively, $p < 0.001$, and 75.4% vs 55.8%, respectively, $p < 0.001$).[14] These data led to the FDA approval of aprepitant in 2003.

Fosaprepitant is a water-soluble phosphoryl prodrug for aprepitant. Fosaprepitant at a dose of 150 mg has been approved by the FDA as a parenteral alternative on day 1 in place of a 3-day, three-drug oral aprepitant regimen.[44]

Aprepitant is a substrate for and moderate inducer and moderate inhibitor of the cytochrome P-450 enzyme 3A4 (CYP3A4).[45] Chemotherapy and other drugs are metabolized by this enzyme, and caution must be used when adding aprepitant in these patients. Docetaxel, paclitaxel, etoposide, irinotecan, ifosfamide, imatinib, vinorelbine, vinblastine, and vincristine are metabolized by CYP3A4. Although, in clinical trials, aprepitant was given to patients receiving these agents without any alteration in dose and no observed adverse effect or decreased efficacy, caution is urged. In addition, aprepitant may interact with other, non-chemotherapy agents. It may induce metabolism of warfarin, leading to reduced levels. Aprepitant appears to increase the active levels of oral dexamethasone and methylprednisolone, and reduced dosing of prophylactic dexamethasone is recommended when used in combination with aprepitant. Other drugs with interactions include oral contraceptives, midazolam, ketoconazole, erythromycin, carbamazepine, rifampin, and phenytoin.

Netupitant is a novel NK-1 receptor antagonist which has a high binding affinity and long half-life (90 h).[46] In a recently reported phase 3 study, 1455 patients receiving moderately emetogenic chemotherapy (AC or EC) were randomized in a 1:1 ratio to either *NEPA,* a single fixed-dose oral combination of netupitant and palonosetron plus standard oral dexamethasone or oral palonosetron plus standard oral dexamethasone.[47] Efficacy endpoints included acute (0–24 h), delayed (25–120 h), and overall (0–120 h) CRs; CR was defined as no emesis and no requirement for rescue medication. The results of this study favored the combination of netupitant and palonosetron for all endpoints with a statistically significant 7–14% absolute increase in CR from 67–75% to 74–84% over the planned four cycles of chemotherapy. Rates of adverse events did not differ significantly between the two arms.

Other classes of antiemetics

Additional classes of antiemetic agents that may be useful in patients include the benzodiazepines, anticholinergics, and cannabinoids. The most commonly used benzodiazepines, lorazepam and alprazolam, block GABA receptors, particularly in the cerebral cortex, and have their greatest utility in the treatment of anticipatory nausea and reduction in the anxiety associated with chemotherapy.[46]

The cannabinoids are likely to become an increasing focus of attention given the legalization of medical marijuana in several parts of the United States. It should be noted that while synthetic cannabinoids have some evidence to support their use for intractable nausea in general, they should be reserved for refractory cases; and further research is required before their use can be recommended on a general basis.[48,49]

Olanzapine, a thiobenzodiazepine, has been found to be effective in preventing acute and delayed emesis.[17,50] It is included in the NCCN guidelines to treat both highly emetogenic and moderately emetogenic chemotherapy-induced emesis.[17]

Anticholinergics such as promethazine or diphenhydramine and, less frequently, transdermal scopolamine may be used for treatment of breakthrough CINV. There are fewer randomized clinical trial data to recommend the use of cannabinoids such as marijuana or its synthetic versions, nabilone and dronabinol,[46] although there is anecdotal evidence to support their use in patients who do not respond to conventional antiemetics.

Complementary and alternative medicine (CAM) therapies

The past decade has witnessed a great interest in complementary and alternative medicine (CAM) therapies, particularly among cancer patients. Various CAM therapies such as acupuncture, hypnosis, massage, and music and herbal supplements such as ginger have been tried to control nausea. Of these, acupuncture and certain mind–body therapies appear promising,[47] but further research is needed before they can be recommended in routine clinical practice.

Acupuncture has been traditionally used in China for symptom management of various conditions, including nausea. A recent meta-analysis involving 11 randomized trials ($N = 1247$), evaluated the effect of acupuncture in controlling CINV among patients who received moderate to high emetogenic chemotherapy.[48] The study found that patients receiving acupuncture had lower acute vomiting than the control group (22% vs 31%, $p = 0.04$). Nonetheless, there was no benefit for delayed CINV. It should be noted that all these studies were done before aprepitant was approved, and thus utility of acupuncture in the current era is not well established.

Mind–body therapies such as *hypnosis, guided imagery,* and *progressive muscle relaxation therapy* (PMRT) have been reported to significantly reduce CINV.[49–52] In a randomized clinical trial in Hong Kong, 71 breast cancer patients receiving antiemetic therapy with metoclopramide and dexamethasone were randomized to progressive muscle relaxation training and imagery (1 h before chemotherapy and then daily for 5 days), versus no intervention. Patients in the intervention arm had decreased duration of CINV ($p = 0.05$) and lower frequency of CINV ($p = 0.07$) as compared to controls. However, the study participants did not receive standard prophylaxis with either 5-HT3 inhibitors or NK-1 inhibitors, limiting the clinical applicability of the study.

Other relaxation therapies such as *music* and *massage* have also been reported to be successful as adjunct antiemetic therapies, in small clinical trials involving about 30 patients.[53,54] These relaxation therapies affect the cerebral cortex, and thus are particularly helpful for decreasing the perception of nausea and in anticipatory nausea.

On the other hand, two trials evaluating efficacy of *ginger* for treatment of CINV were negative.[55,56] A number of clinical trials assessing various CAM therapies are currently under way and would provide further useful information regarding efficacy of these therapies (or lack thereof), facilitating optimal inclusion of these therapies in traditional clinical oncology practice (integrative oncology).[47]

Recommendations for prevention and treatment of chemotherapy-induced emesis

The goal of antiemetic therapy is complete prevention of CINV (Table 3). In patients receiving highly and moderately emetogenic chemotherapy, the period of risk for nausea and vomiting lasts at least 4 days following chemotherapy, and protection with antiemetics is needed throughout this period. The choice of antiemetic prophylaxis is driven by the emetogenic potential of the specific chemotherapy agents as outlined below.[18]

Highly emetogenic chemotherapy

Cisplatin and cyclophosphamide are the most frequently used highly emetogenic chemotherapy agents. Nausea and vomiting are virtually ensured without adequate prophylaxis. Prior to the approval of the NK-1 receptor antagonist aprepitant, the previous recommendation was a combination of a 5-HT3 antagonist and dexamethasone. A regimen of a 5-HT3 receptor antagonist, aprepitant (125 mg PO day 1, 80 mg daily on days 2 and 3) or fosaprepitant 150 mg IV day 1, and dexamethasone (12 mg PO or IV on day 1 and 8 mg PO daily on days 2–4) with oral aprepitant (80 mg PO on days 2–4) or dexamethasone (12 mg PO or IV on day 1, 8 mg PO day 2, then 8 mg BID on days 3 and 4 with fosaprepitant) on days 2–4 is recommended in all patients receiving highly emetogenic chemotherapy. All prophylaxis should begin prior to the administration of chemotherapy.

Moderately emetogenic chemotherapy

A combination of a 5-HT3 receptor antagonist and dexamethasone is recommended in all patients receiving moderately emetogenic chemotherapy. Given recent data and its superior efficacy in preventing delayed symptoms, palonosetron (0.25 mg on day 1 only) is the preferred 5-HT3 receptor antagonist. If others are used, they should be given on day 1 prior to chemotherapy and then repeated

Table 3 Guidelines for prevention of acute and delayed nausea and vomiting in patients depending on emetic risk.

Emetic risk	Acute	Delayed
High (>90%)	Aprepitant + 5-HT3 antagonist + dexamethasone	Aprepitant + dexamethasone
Moderate (30–90%)	5-HT3 antagonist + dexamethasone	Dexamethasone
Low (10–30%)	Dexamethasone or phenothiazine or metoclopramide	None
Minimal (<10%)	None	None

Abbreviations: 5-HT3, 5-hydroxytryptamine 3.

daily on days 2–3. Dexamethasone is given as 12 mg IV or PO on day 1 and then at a daily dose of 8 mg on days 2–3 (either 8 mg daily or 4 mg in divided doses twice daily). In selected patients (those with breakthrough nausea and vomiting despite adequate prophylaxis or those with other patient variables that suggest a higher risk of symptoms), aprepitant (125 mg PO or fosaprepitant 150 mg IV on day 1 followed by 80 mg PO on days 2–3) should be considered. Recent data with netupitant and palonosetron are encouraging; however, netupitant has yet to be approved by the FDA for use in the United States.

Low-risk chemotherapy

Options for antiemetic prophylaxis in patients receiving chemotherapy of low emetogenic potential include dexamethasone (12 mg PO or IV) or prochlorperazine (10 mg PO or IV every 4–6 h) or metoclopramide (20–40 mg PO every 4–6 h or 1–2 mg/kg IV every 3–4 h with diphenhydramine to prevent extrapyramidal symptoms). All prophylaxis should be given prior to the administration of chemotherapy.

Minimally emetogenic chemotherapy

No routine prophylaxis is recommended. If nausea and vomiting do occur, the use of dexamethasone, prochlorperazine, or metoclopramide is recommended. Prophylactic use of these medications should be considered prior to the next cycle of therapy.

Special situations

Breakthrough nausea and vomiting

Ideally, the best treatment for breakthrough nausea and vomiting is to prevent it from occurring at all. At times, despite aggressive prophylaxis, symptoms still occur. The best therapy for breakthrough symptoms is the addition of agents from another class of antiemetics. In addition, an alternative route other than oral, such as intravenous or rectal, may need to be used. These medications work best if taken on a schedule rather than on an as-needed basis. When breakthrough nausea and vomiting occur, the prophylactic regimen should be reevaluated and enhanced prior to the next cycle of therapy.

Anticipatory nausea and vomiting

The key to preventing anticipatory nausea and vomiting is preventing symptoms from occurring with each cycle of chemotherapy. Once the symptoms have developed, agents such as the benzodiazepines may be added to the prophylactic regimen.[57] As outlined above, mind–body therapies such as behavioral therapy, systemic desensitization, and hypnosis have also been proved useful.[49–53]

Multiple-day chemotherapy-induced nausea and vomiting

Patients receiving multiple-day chemotherapeutic regimens to treat a variety of malignancies (e.g., germ cell tumors, lymphoma, multiple myeloma with stem cell transplantation, etc.) are at risk for both acute and delayed nausea and vomiting. Although the NCCN has a section in their guidelines entitled "Principles of managing multiday emetogenic chemotherapy regimens," they state that the antiemetic therapy should be selected based on the chemotherapy drug with the highest emetic risk. The risk of delayed nausea and vomiting will depend on the specific chemotherapeutic regimen used and the emetogenic potential of the last chemotherapeutic drug used in the regimen.

Studies have evaluated the use of repeat dosing of palonosetron in managing multiple-day emetogenic chemotherapy regimens; however, no definitive conclusions can be made and further studies are needed to answer whether a need exists for repeat dosing of palonosetron.[1,2]

With regard to aprepitant, it has been evaluated in the antiemetic management of multiple-drug chemotherapeutic regimens.[3–5] While it may be used in such situations, it is difficult to recommend a specific antiemetic regimen for each day that a multiple drug emetogenic chemotherapeutic regimen is utilized.

The NCCN in their Antiemesis Guideline outlines the general principles for using corticosteroids (dexamethasone), serotonin antagonists (palonosetron), and neurokinin antagonists (aprepitant) in managing multiday chemotherapy regimens.[12]

Radiation-induced nausea and vomiting

Radiation-induced nausea and vomiting (RINV) is seen in nearly all patients receiving total-body irradiation prior to bone marrow transplantation and in more than 80% of those receiving radiation to the upper abdomen.[58] Studies have demonstrated the efficacy of prophylactic 5-HT3 receptor antagonists compared with placebo[59] and the superiority of prophylaxis with 5-HT3 receptor antagonists compared with combinations with metoclopramide and prochlorperazine.[60,61] The recommendation is for all patients undergoing either upper abdominal radiation therapy or total-body irradiation to receive prophylaxis with an oral 5-HT3 receptor antagonist dosed either 2 or 3 times daily with or without oral dexamethasone.[62]

Conclusions

Prevention and treatment of chemotherapy-induced emesis have advanced significantly in recent years. Recent surveys indicate the need for heightened awareness of the frequency and severity of acute and, especially, delayed nausea and vomiting from chemotherapy. Fortunately, new agents have been added to the antiemetic arsenal to further enhance the efficacy of antiemetic prophylaxis. Complementary therapies appear promising in controlling nausea, and are being explored further. Appropriate implementation of guidelines for prophylaxis based on the specific chemotherapy agents used will ensure that fewer patients experience these most distressing of side effects.

Key references

The complete reference list can be found on the Wiley Companion Digital Edition of this title (see inside front cover for login instructions).

1 Grunberg SM, Deuson RR, Mavros P, et al. Incidence of chemotherapy-induced nausea and emesis after modern antiemetics. *Cancer*. 2004;**100**:2261–2268.

2 Mitchell EP. Gastrointestinal toxicity of chemotherapeutic agents. *Semin Oncol*. 1992;**19**:566–579.

6 de Boer-Dennert M, de Wit R, Schmitz PI, et al. Patient perceptions of the side-effects of chemotherapy: the influence of 5HT3 antagonists. *Br J Cancer*. 1997;**76**:1055–1061.

9 Carpenter DO. Neural mechanisms of emesis. *Can J Physiol Pharmacol*. 1990;**68**:230–236.

14 Hesketh PJ, Grunberg SM, Gralla RJ, et al. The oral neurokinin-1 antagonist aprepitant for the prevention of chemotherapy-induced nausea and vomiting: a multinational, randomized, double-blind, placebo-controlled trial in patients receiving high-dose cisplatin—the Aprepitant Protocol 052 Study Group. *J Clin Oncol*. 2003;**21**:4112–4119.

15 Moher D, Arthur AZ, Pater JL. Anticipatory nausea and/or vomiting. *Cancer Treat Rev*. 1984;**11**:257–264.

16 Roila F, Herrstedt J, Aapro M, et al. Group EMGW. Guideline update for MASCC and ESMO in the prevention of chemotherapy- and radiotherapy-induced nausea and vomiting: results of the Perugia consensus conference. *Ann Oncol*. 2010;**21**(Suppl 5):v232–v243.

17 National Comprehensive Cancer Network (2014) *Antiemesis Version 1.2016*, www.nccn.org (accessed 02 May, 2016).

19 Hesketh PJ, Kris MG, Grunberg SM, et al. Proposal for classifying the acute emetogenicity of cancer chemotherapy. *J Clin Oncol*. 1997;**15**:103–109.

20 Koeller JM, Aapro MS, Gralla RJ, et al. A. Antiemetic guidelines: creating a more practical treatment approach. *Support Care Cancer*. 2002;**10**:519–522.

21 Mitchelson F. Pharmacological agents affecting emesis. A review (part I). *Drugs*. 1992;**43**:295–315.

22 Bountra C, Gale JD, Gardner CJ, et al. Towards understanding the aetiology and pathophysiology of the emetic reflex: novel approaches to antiemetic drugs. *Oncology*. 1996;**53**(Suppl 1):102–109.

23 Chevallier B, Cappelaere P, Splinter T, et al. A double-blind, multicentre comparison of intravenous dolasetron mesilate and metoclopramide in the prevention of nausea and vomiting in cancer patients receiving high-dose cisplatin chemotherapy. *Support Care Cancer*. 1997;**5**:22–30.

24 Warr D, Wilan A, Venner P, et al. A randomised, double-blind comparison of granisetron with high-dose metoclopramide, dexamethasone and diphenhydramine for cisplatin-induced emesis. An NCI Canada Clinical Trials Group phase III trial. *Eur J Cancer*. 1992;**29A**:33–36.

25 Heron JF, Goedhals L, Jordaan JP, et al. Oral granisetron alone and in combination with dexamethasone: a double-blind randomized comparison against high-dose metoclopramide plus dexamethasone in prevention of cisplatin-induced emesis. The Granisetron Study Group. *Ann Oncol*. 1994;**5**:579–584.

28 Martoni A, Angelelli B, Guaraldi M, et al. An open randomised cross-over study on granisetron versus ondansetron in the prevention of acute emesis induced by moderate dose cisplatin-containing regimens. *Eur J Cancer*. 1996;**32A**:82–85.

29 Hesketh P, Navari R, Grote T, et al. Double-blind, randomized comparison of the antiemetic efficacy of intravenous dolasetron mesylate and intravenous ondansetron in the prevention of acute cisplatin-induced emesis in patients with cancer. Dolasetron Comparative Chemotherapy Induced Emesis Prevention Group. *J Clin Oncol*. 1996;**14**:2242–2249.

30 Audhuy B, Cappelaere P, Martin M, et al. A double-blind, randomised comparison of the anti-emetic efficacy of two intravenous doses of dolasetron mesilate and granisetron in patients receiving high dose cisplatin chemotherapy. *Eur J Cancer*. 1996;**32A**:807–813.

46 Spinelli T, Calcagnile S, Giuliano C, et al. Netupitant PET imaging and ADME studies in humans. *J Clin Pharmacol*. 2014;**54**(1):97–108.

47 Aapro M, Karthaus, M, Schwartzberg L, et al. (2014) Phase 3 study of NEPA, a fixed-dose combination of netupitant and palonosetron, for prevention of chemotherapy-induced nausea and vomiting during moderately emetogenic chemotherapy cycles. Paper presented at 50th Annual Meeting of the American Society of Clinical Oncology; May 30; Chicago, Il.

48 Hill KP. Medical marijuana: more questions than answers. *J Psychiatr Pract*. 2014;**20**(5):389–391.

49 Einhorn LH, Brames MJ, Dreicer R, et al. Palonosetron plus dexamethasone for prevention of chemotherapy-induced nausea and vomiting in patients receiving multiple-day chemotherapy for germ cell cancer. *Support Care Cancer*. 2007;**15**:1293–1300.

50 Giralt SA, Mangan KF, Maziarz RT, et al. Three palonosetron regimens to prevent CINV in myeloma patients receiving multiple-day high-dose melphalan and hematopoietic stem cell transplantation. *Ann Oncol*. 2011;**22**:939–946.

51 Jordan K, Kinitz I, Voigt W, et al. Safety and efficacy of a triple antiemetic combination with NK-1 antagonist aprepitant in highly and moderately emetogenic multiple day chemotherapy. *Eur J Cancer*. 2009;**45**:1184–1187.

52 Olver IN, Grimison P, Chatfield M, et al. Results of a 7-day aprepitant schedule for the prevention of nausea and vomiting in 5-day cisplatin-based germ cell tumor chemotherapy. *Support Care Cancer*. 2013;**21**:1561–1568.

53 Albany C, Brames MJ, Fausel C, et al. Randomized, double-blind placebo-controlled, phase III cross-over study evaluating the oral neurokinin-1 antagonist aprepitant in combination with a 5HT3 receptor antagonist and dexamethasone in patients with germ cell tumors receiving 5-day cisplatin combination chemotherapy regimens: a Hoosier Oncology Group study. *J Clin Oncol*. 2012;**30**:3998–4003.

54 Sharkey KA, Darmani NA. Parker LA regulation of nausea and vomiting by cannabinoids and the endocannabinoid system. *Eur J Pharmacol*. 2014;**722**:134–146. doi: 10.1016/j.ejphar.2013.09.068.

55 Navani RM, Gray SE, Keir AC, et al. Olanzapine versus aprepitant for the prevention of chemotherapy-induced nausea and vomiting: a randomized phase II trial. *J Support Oncol*. 2011;**9**:188–195.

126 Neurologic complications of cancer

Lisa M. DeAngelis, MD, FAAN

Overview

Neurologic complications of cancer are common and being seen with increased frequency as patients survive longer with better systemic disease control. Metastases can involve the brain, dura, subarachnoid space, spinal cord, roots, and nerve plexus. Chemotherapy can cause acute toxicities, such as encephalopathy from ifosfamide, which impede the delivery of a full course of effective anticancer treatment. In addition, the long-term complications of radiotherapy such as radiation myelopathy, and chemotherapy such as peripheral neuropathy, can markedly impair quality of life. Early identification, treatment, and prevention strategies can reduce these toxicities in our growing population of survivors.

Neurologic complications of cancer can be either metastatic or nonmetastatic (Table 1). Metastatic lesions affect the nervous system by direct invasion (e.g., brachial plexus metastasis), compression [e.g., epidural spinal cord compression (SCC)], or compromise of vascular supply (e.g., sagittal sinus occlusion from skull metastases). Brain metastases are discussed in ***Chapter 77***. Although any tumor can metastasize to the nervous system, certain tumors have a predilection for causing particular central or peripheral nervous system disorders (e.g., leukemias frequently metastasize to the leptomeninges, but rarely to the brain). Prostate cancer commonly causes epidural SCC because of its tendency to metastasize to the vertebral bodies, but leptomeningeal or brain involvement is much less common.[1,2]

Nonmetastatic neurologic complications are often tumor specific. Metabolic derangements are more likely to occur with tumors that metastasize widely to vital organs, such as liver (colon cancer), or that cause changes in fluid and electrolyte balance, such as hypercalcemia (breast cancer) or inappropriate antidiuretic hormone secretion (small-cell lung cancer). Central nervous system (CNS) infections are more common in patients whose cancer is associated with immune suppression, as in Hodgkin disease. Vascular complications are more common in hematologic malignancies than in solid tumors.[7] Paraneoplastic syndromes affecting the nervous system are much more frequent with certain tumors, such as small-cell lung and ovarian cancers.[3] Clinically, identifying the site of neurologic dysfunction by the patient's symptoms and signs will help to determine the diagnosis (Table 2).

Vertebral metastases are common in patients with metastatic cancer, but skeletal complications, including SCC, have been reduced by the use of bisphosphonates.[6] SCC usually results when a vertebral body metastasis extends into the spinal canal or paraspinal tumor invades the epidural space through a neural foramen (Figure 1). Lymphomas may invade the spinal canal through neural foramina without destruction of bone. Epidural lesions may also result when tumors in the colon, kidney, prostate, or head and neck area grow directly into the spinal bony structures. When a metastasis causes the vertebral body to collapse, bone, tumor, and ligament may extend into the spinal canal to compress the spinal cord.

Metastases

Spinal metastases

Metastatic lesions compressing the spinal cord or cauda equina are, after brain metastases, the most common symptomatic neurologic complication of metastatic cancer.[1,2,4] The spinal cord ends at the L-1 or L-2 vertebral body but compression of the cauda equina below that level is usually also considered SCC because the diagnosis and treatment are identical.[1] SCC causes pain and, if untreated, paralysis and incontinence. Patients who become paraplegic as a result of cancer usually die within a matter of months; however, studies indicate that early diagnosis and treatment maintain a patient's independent ambulation and usually result in longer survival.

Approximately 5% of patients dying of cancer have evidence of SCC at autopsy, suggesting 18,000–20,000 new cases of SCC annually in the United States.[1,5] Breast, lung, prostate, and lymphoma are the most common primary cancers causing SCC (Table 3). SCC usually occurs in the late stages of metastatic cancer, but in up to 20% of patients, cancer was unsuspected before the neurologic symptoms.

The thoracic spine is the most common location of SCC, followed by the lumbosacral and cervical spine in a ratio of about 4 : 2 : 1. Two or more contiguous vertebral bodies are involved by metastatic disease in approximately 25% of patients with SCC, but, unlike infection, the intervertebral disc is preserved. As many as 32% of patients have other sites of SCC in addition to the clinically suspected location, emphasizing the importance of imaging the entire length of the spinal canal when evaluating a patient for suspected epidural disease.

Pathophysiology of spinal cord compression

Epidural tumor is found both anterior and posterior to the spinal cord in almost 50% of patients; in approximately 20%, the tumor is circumferential. Histologic studies show that the most common abnormalities are demyelination with infiltration by lipid laden macrophages, interstitial edema, and focal axonal swelling, but infarction is rare, even in patients who develop the sudden onset of paraplegia. Compression of the epidural venous plexus (possibly contributing to spinal cord edema) occurs early in SCC, whereas decreased spinal cord blood flow takes place much later; therefore, venous infarction may contribute to the acute paraplegia, which can happen unpredictably, making SCC a neurologic emergency. The release of potentially neurotoxic substances, including prostaglandins and serotonin, by compressed neural tissue may also play a role in neurologic disability.

Holland-Frei Cancer Medicine, Ninth Edition. Edited by Robert C. Bast Jr., Carlo M. Croce, William N. Hait, Waun Ki Hong, Donald W. Kufe, Martine Piccart-Gebhart, Raphael E. Pollock, Ralph R. Weichselbaum, Hongyang Wang, and James F. Holland.
© 2017 John Wiley & Sons, Inc. ISBN: 978-1-118-93469-2

Table 1 Neurologic complications of cancer.

Metastatic
    Intracranial (usually to brain; see Chapter 70)
    Spinal (usually epidural)
    Leptomeningeal (usually base of brain and cauda equina)
    Cranial nerves (usually from base of skull lesions)
    Peripheral nerves (usually brachial or lumbosacral plexus)
    Muscle (rare)
Nonmetastatic
    Complications of treatment (radiation, chemotherapy)
    Vascular disorders (hemorrhage, infarcts)
    Metabolic, nutritional disorders
    Paraneoplastic syndromes
    Infections

Clinical findings and diagnosis

The symptoms and signs depend on the level of compression (e.g., cervical vs thoracic). Back pain is the first symptom of SCC in virtually all patients (Table 4).[5] The pain may be local (at the involved area of the spine), radicular (radiating into arm, trunk, or leg), or both. Local pain is dull, aching, and progressive and usually localizes to the involved area of the spine. Local pain aggravated by movement implies spinal instability. In the cervical and lumbosacral regions, radicular pain is often unilateral, but in the trunk, it is usually bilateral (band-like), a finding highly suggestive of epidural disease. Pain from SCC is typically worse when the patient is supine, which helps to distinguish SCC from a herniated disc where the pain improves with recumbancy. The pain of SCC is exacerbated by coughing, straining, or valsalva. Pain may be absent in patients whose SCC is identified incidentally on chest or abdominal CT or MRI done to evaluate the patient's primary cancer.

Weakness is the second most common feature of epidural SCC; it usually follows the onset of pain by weeks to months and is most obvious in proximal muscles of the legs. By the time weakness occurs, tone in the lower extremities is usually increased, reflexes are hyperactive, and the plantar responses are extensor. If the SCC occurs below the cord involving the cauda equina, hyporeflexia or areflexia is found. If pain limits strength testing, analgesics should be administered to permit adequate evaluation.

Bowel and bladder dysfunction usually occur late in SCC. However, when the conus medullaris is the site of compression (vertebral lesions from T-10 to L-1), bladder dysfunction may be the first and only sign. The patient may be unaware of urinary retention because bladder sensation is lost; examination reveals a distended bladder, and a postvoid ultrasound reveals urinary retention. The anal sphincter is usually flaccid. Sensory symptoms include numbness and paresthesias that begin in the toes and spread proximally. Except in conus compression, the sacral segments may be spared, even when a sensory level is found on the trunk. In a few patients, gait or truncal ataxia mimicking cerebellar disease may be the only neurologic finding although back pain usually precedes the ataxia. Varicella-zoster eruption may occur at the dermatomal level of epidural metastasis. If it precedes the diagnosis of the spinal metastasis, it can delay recognition of SCC.

None of the clinical symptoms or signs of epidural SCC are specific (Table 5). Some disorders that mimic SCC such as herniated disc or spinal stenosis are common and may confuse the initial evaluation of an individual cancer patient. Others, such as epidural hematomas and abscesses, may be directly related to the cancer or its treatment.

Patients with cancer who develop back pain have SCC until proved otherwise. Evaluation should proceed urgently because

Table 2 Neurologic complications in cancer patients by site.

Site	Usual causes	Typical symptoms and signs
Brain	Metastasis Leptomeningeal metastasis Metabolic/toxic encephalopathy Infection (meningitis, brain abscess) Radiation encephalopathy Cerebral hemorrhage or infarction Paraneoplastic (limbic encephalopathy)	Headache Confusion Hemiparesis Seizures Ataxia
Spinal cord and cauda equina	Epidural metastasis Leptomeningeal metastasis Intramedullary metastasis Epidural abscess or hematoma Radiation myelopathy Myelopathy following intrathecal chemotherapy Paraneoplastic myelopathy	Back pain Paraparesis Sensory level Incontinence
Cranial and peripheral nerves	Extrinsic compression by tumor or other mass (e.g., hematoma) Direct infiltration by tumor Drug toxicity Varicella-zoster infection Radiation plexopathy Paraneoplastic neuropathy	Focal pain Sensory loss Motor weakness Decreased reflexes in nerve distribution (focal lesion) or distally in hands and feet (polyneuropathy)
Neuromuscular junction	Drugs (aminoglycoside antibiotics) Paraneoplastic disorders (Lambert–Eaton myasthenic syndrome, myasthenia gravis)	Weakness without sensory loss Respiratory insufficiency
Muscle	Metastasis Steroid myopathy Cachectic myopathy Paraneoplastic polymyositis or dermatomyositis	Proximal weakness Weakness without sensory loss

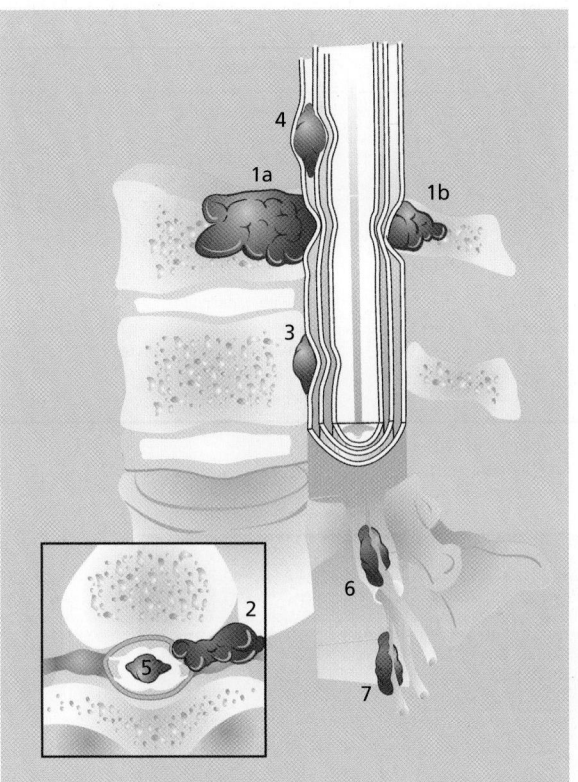

Figure 1 Neoplastic epidural spinal cord compression results from direct extension of a bony metastasis to the vertebral body (1a) or posterior elements (1b), by paraspinal neoplasm infiltrating through neural foramina (2), or a direct metastasis to the epidural space (3). Unusual causes of spinal metastases include subdural metastasis (4), intramedullary metastasis (5), and paraspinal metastasis to the radicular vessels (6) or root (7).

Table 3 Primary cancer causing symptomatic spinal cord compression in 583 patients at Memorial Sloan Kettering Cancer Center (MSKCC).

Primary tumor	No. of patients (%)
Breast	127 (22)
Lung	90 (15)
Prostate	58 (10)
Lymphoreticular	56 (10)
Sarcoma	52 (9)
Kidney	39 (7)
Gastrointestinal	29 (5)
Melanoma	23 (4)
Unknown primary	21 (4)
Head and neck	19 (3)
Miscellaneous	69 (12)
Total	583

Table 4 Symptoms and signs of spinal cord compression in 213 patients at Memorial Sloan Kettering Cancer Center (MSKCC).

	First symptom		Present at diagnosis	
	No.	%	No.	%
Pain	201	94	207	97
Weakness	7	3	157	74
Autonomic dysfunction	0	0	111	52
Sensory loss	1	0.5	112	53
Ataxia	2	0.9	8	4

Treatment

SCC requires urgent therapy directed at reduction of tumor mass and prevention of regrowth.[1,4] Radiation therapy (RT) is the primary treatment for most patients, but surgery and chemotherapy are important modalities in individual patients. The initial treatment for all patients is corticosteroids, which can have an oncolytic effect relieving SCC by shrinking tumors, especially lymphoma, but in most instances, their salutary effects result from the reduction of spinal cord edema. Other treatment is usually started concurrently so the effect of corticosteroids is difficult to evaluate, and the optimal dose has not been determined.

For patients with pain only, dexamethasone at 16 mg every 24 h can be started increasing the dose if pain persists or new symptoms develop. For patients with severe pain, or evidence of myelopathy, an intravenous bolus of 100 mg of dexamethasone should be administered, followed by 100 mg every 24 h in divided doses. The drug should be tapered as the patient is treated with more definitive modalities. Corticosteroids cause side effects, and some may be more prominent in patients with epidural SCC. Perforation of the gastrointestinal (GI) tract may occur in as many as 1% of patients; constipation, a frequent complication of SCC, appears to increase the risk of GI rupture. Thus, a rapid taper, particularly of high initial doses, is essential.

RT is the most common treatment for patients with SCC, many of whom are poor surgical candidates because of advanced cancer or multiple vertebral body metastases.[1,5] RT to a total dose of 3000 cGy (300 Gy × 10 fractions) is administered to the site of compression and one or two vertebral bodies above and below that level. Multiple courses of RT for patients who respond initially but then relapse may be helpful and carry only modest risk.[7] Intensity-modulated stereotactic radiotherapy (IMRT) is effective and safe and can be administered with good results to a previously irradiated site or in place of standard external beam RT.[8-10]

Surgery plays an increasingly important role in SCC treatment. Traditionally, surgery was restricted (1) to patients who developed SCC at sites already irradiated, (2) to patients in whom a diagnosis of cancer had not been established, (3) when epidural defects result from displaced bone or disc fragments, (4) when spinal instability results from bone destruction, and (5) to patients with radio resistant tumors (e.g., renal cancer). However, a prospective phase III trial demonstrated the superiority of surgery plus RT compared to RT alone for SCC.[11,12] Tumor resection that usually required resection of the vertebral body had a superior outcome with significantly better neurologic function for longer, including a greater proportion of patients who regained ambulation and continence. Length of survival was not significantly different between the two groups, but there was a trend toward longer survival with surgery (129 days vs 100 days, $p = 0.08$). These data suggest that surgery should be a consideration in all patients with SCC. However, the patients enrolled in the study were highly selected and it is not

high-grade compression may cause abrupt compromise of the spinal cord and severe neurologic dysfunction. The only necessary diagnostic test for spinal lesions caused by cancer is an MRI (Figure 2). The entire spine should be imaged, but contrast is not necessary to detect spine metastasis or epidural tumor. However, contrast is essential to identify intramedullary or leptomeningeal metastasis (LM). Patients unable to have an MRI (e.g., pacemaker) should be imaged by CT-myelography where full reconstructed images can provide excellent views of the spine in all dimensions.

Table 5 Differential diagnosis of epidural spinal cord compression.

Diagnosis	Example(s)	Diagnostic test
Intramedullary tumor	Glioma	MRI with gadolinium
	Metastasis	
Extramedullary-intradural tumor	Meningioma	MRI with gadolinium
	Neurofibroma	
Leptomeningeal tumor	Metastasis	MRI with gadolinium, CSF cytology
	Primary lymphoma	
Radiation myelopathy	Previous RT to spine	MRI with gadolinium
Arteriovenous malformation	Post-RT cavernous angioma	MRI with gadolinium, myelogram, arteriogram
Transverse myelopathy	Postinfectious myelopathy, multiple sclerosis	MRI with gadolinium
Epidural hematoma	Thrombocytopenia (history of lumbar puncture)	MRI or CT
Epidural abscess	Sepsis, epidural catheter	MRI with gadolinium/culture
Degenerative spinal disorder	Herniated disc, spinal stenosis	MRI
Osteoporosis	Vertebral collapse	MRI/biopsy

Abbreviations: CSF, cerebrospinal fluid; CT, computed tomography; MRI, magnetic resonance imaging; RT, radiation therapy.
Source: Adapted from DeAngelis and Posner, 2008.[1] Reproduced with permission from Oxford University Press.

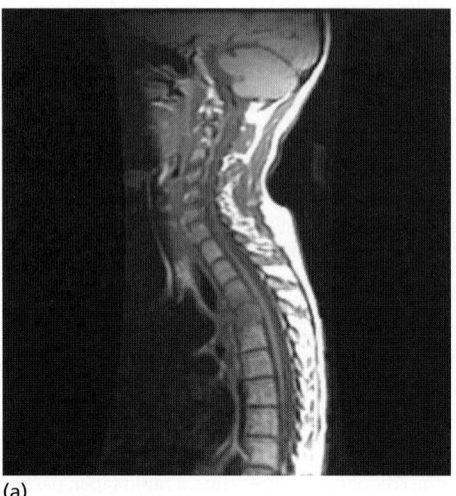
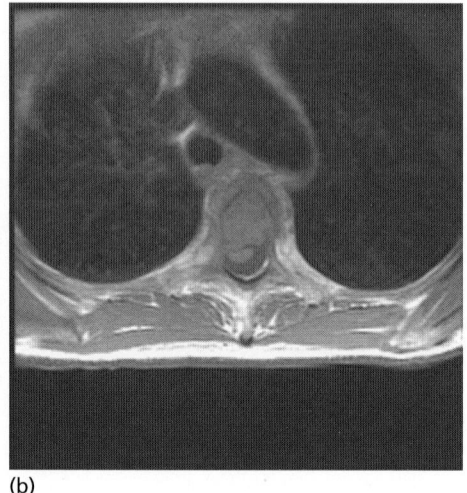

(a)   (b)

Figure 2 MRI demonstrating spinal cord compression from metastatic breast cancer. (a) Tumor in the vertebral body compressing the spinal cord arteriorly. (b) Axial image at the same level demonstrating anterior and lateral compression and distortion of the cord.

clear that the excellent outcome reported can be expected for all patients with SCC. More recently, vertebroplasty and kyphoplasty have proven effective for selected patients with SCC, especially those with vertebral compression fractures and severe pain.[13]

Chemotherapy, with or without RT, is useful in some patients with tumors that are sensitive, especially lymphoma and occasionally other solid tumors.[14] Excellent responses of SCC from chemosensitive tumors to appropriate chemotherapy are seen, but this approach is limited to those who have minimal to no neurologic compromise. If myelopathy is present, RT or surgery must be the primary therapy. Regardless of treatment type, the majority of patients who are ambulatory at the beginning of therapy remain ambulatory. Some paraparetic patients will recover sufficient function to walk again, but only a few who are paraplegic recover useful function.

Leptomeningeal metastasis

LM is less frequent than brain metastasis or SCC but is becoming increasingly common, particularly in patients with small-cell lung, breast, and ovarian cancers. Quality of life and duration of survival are both severely compromised by LM, and fewer than one-half of those treated by currently available therapy receive benefit.

Reliable estimates of the incidence of LM are difficult to obtain, but LM is found in approximately 5% of patients with metastatic cancer. Few studies of LM give incidence figures and the diagnosis is heavily dependent on the diligence with which it is pursued. Recognizing these limitations, the frequency of LM in different cancers varies widely (Table 6).

Pathophysiology

Malignant cells may enter the subarachnoid space by several routes (Figure 3). Subarachnoid invasion can occur via infiltration of the wall of veins and of the marrow trabeculae; malignant cells can attach to leptomeningeal capillaries and move directly into the subarachnoid space. Brain parenchymal lesions can erode into the ventricle or subarachnoid space or be spilled at surgery, causing LM. LM develops in 40% of patients following resection of a cerebellar metastasis, but in only 2–3% of those who had resection of a supratentorial lesion. The choroid plexus is a rare route of entry. Malignant cells may invade the subarachnoid space by direct infiltration along nerve roots, and possibly via epineural lymphatics.

LM causes nervous system dysfunction by several mechanisms:[1] (1) direct infiltration of malignant cells into the brain, spinal cord, cranial nerves, or spinal roots that interferes with neural function, (2) interruption of CSF flow leading to increased intracranial pressure (ICP) with or without hydrocephalus, and (3) infiltration of tumor along the Virchow–Robin spaces may reduce blood supply to the brain causing cerebral infarction.

Table 6 Frequency of leptomeningeat metastases (LM) in various cancers.

Cancer	Percent developing LM	Features
Carcinoma		
Breast	5	Incidence may be increasing, more common with infiltrating lobular carcinoma
SCLC	9–25	Incidence is increasing, risk increases with duration of survival
NSCLC	?	Less common than breast
Melanoma	23	50% at autopsy
Leukemia		
AML	<5	10% without prophylaxis; associated with high WBC count, elevated LDH, extramedullary disease at diagnosis, and monocytic morphology
ALL	11	30% without prophylaxis; associated with T-cell phenotype, Burkitt morphology, and high WBC count
CLL	Rare	May occur during blast crisis
Lymphoma		
NHL	4–10	Associated with diffuse large B-cell and lymphocytic histology, bone marrow involvement
HD	Rare	
Overall	8.6	LM present at autopsy in 56 of 649 brains examined at Memorial Sloan Kettering Cancer Center

Abbreviations: ALL, acute lymphocytic leukemia; AML, acute myelogenous leukemia; CLL, chronic lymphocytic leukemia; HD, Hodgkin disease; LDH, lactic acid dehydrogenase; NHL, non-Hodgkin lymphoma; NSCLC, nonsmall-cell lung cancer; SCLC, small-cell lung cancer; WBC, white blood cell.

Symptoms and signs

LM is strongly suggested by the patient having symptoms or signs at multiple sites of the neuraxis.[1,2] These include (1) headache, particularly early in the morning or posturally induced headache in the absence of brain metastases; (2) cranial nerve palsies, particularly, diplopia or facial weakness; (3) neck pain in the absence of cervical spine metastases; (4) radicular pain in the arms or legs, particularly when accompanied by weakness but without local spine pain; (5) unexplained constipation, impotence, or urinary incontinence or retention; (6) asymmetric leg weakness and diminished reflexes in the absence of pain or sensory changes; and (7) confusion, memory loss, or other cognitive abnormalities.

Diagnosis

The diagnostic gold standard of LM is the demonstration of malignant cells in the CSF. However, imaging is a much more common means of diagnosis currently.[15] A cranial MRI may reveal enhancing cranial nerves or enhancing tumor in cortical sulci; communicating hydrocephalus may suggest LM. A gadolinium-enhanced spine MRI may demonstrate tumor nodules on spinal roots, particularly in the cauda equina, even when symptoms of nerve root dysfunction are absent (Figure 4). The whole neuraxis should be imaged to identify sites of bulky disease. When characteristic findings are identified, this suffices to establish the diagnosis. MRI is 76% sensitive and 77% specific. Occasionally, FDG-PET imaging may identify LM.[16] However, negative imaging does not exclude the diagnosis in a patient with typical features. A lumbar puncture should be performed and the opening pressure, cell count, protein, glucose, and bacterial and fungal studies should be obtained; the cytology specimen should contain at least 10 mL of CSF optimally and should be processed quickly according to the laboratory's protocol.

Malignant cells are found in the initial CSF sample in 50–60% of patients with LM.[1] Cytologic examination is 75% sensitive, but almost 100% specific; additional samples increase the yield, and occasionally cisternal CSF may be positive when lumbar CSF is negative. Likewise, cytology may be positive in ventricular fluid but negative in lumbar fluid or vice versa. Rare cell capture technology may enhance the identification of malignant cells in CSF over routine cytology.[17]

Tumor markers, deoxyribonucleic acid (DNA) studies, and immunocytochemistry may help confirm LM when cytologic studies are negative. In the presence of a normal blood–brain barrier (suggested by a normal CSF protein concentration), the level of tumor antigens, such as carcinoembryonic antigen (CEA), beta human chorionic gonadotropin (βHCG), cancer antigen (CA) 125, CA 27.29, CA 19–9, and prostate-specific antigen (PSA), should be no greater than 1% of the serum level. When that amount is exceeded, and particularly if the CSF level is higher than the serum level, the diagnosis is established, even without a positive cytology. When LM is suspected in patients with lymphoma or leukemia, flow cytometry or molecular markers may demonstrate a clonal excess of cells similar to the systemic neoplasm, suggesting LM.

Treatment

If untreated, LM usually causes relentless progression of neurologic dysfunction and death within weeks. Treatment is not very effective, and it usually does not reverse fixed neurologic deficits. Nevertheless, therapy alters the clinical course in about one-half of patients and often improves symptoms.[1,18] Occasionally, the course may be indolent especially in patients with LM from lymphoma or breast cancer.

The type of primary cancer is the best predictor of response to treatment; the majority of lymphoma and breast cancer patients respond because these tumors are relatively sensitive to RT and systemic and intrathecal chemotherapy. Patients with lung cancer or melanoma respond in about one-third and one-fifth of cases, respectively. Patients with severe neurologic disability from LM are less likely to derive benefit because neural damage is often irreversible. Unlike brain metastases, dexamethasone provides little symptomatic relief unless there is elevated ICP.

Among patients receiving therapy for LM, survival is prolonged only in those whose disease responds to treatment;[1] however, the inability to predict which patients will respond to treatment makes prognostication difficult. In addition to surviving longer (4–6 months median vs 1–2 months median in nonresponders), patients who respond to therapy are less likely to die from their LM than are patients whose disease progresses despite therapy.

Radiation therapy

RT should be administered to symptomatic sites even if subarachnoid tumor is not evident radiographically at the symptomatic location. Entire neuraxis RT is rarely used because of its acute morbidity and myelosuppression that interferes with subsequent chemotherapy. Neuraxis RT is not used even when bulky LM is seen on MRI

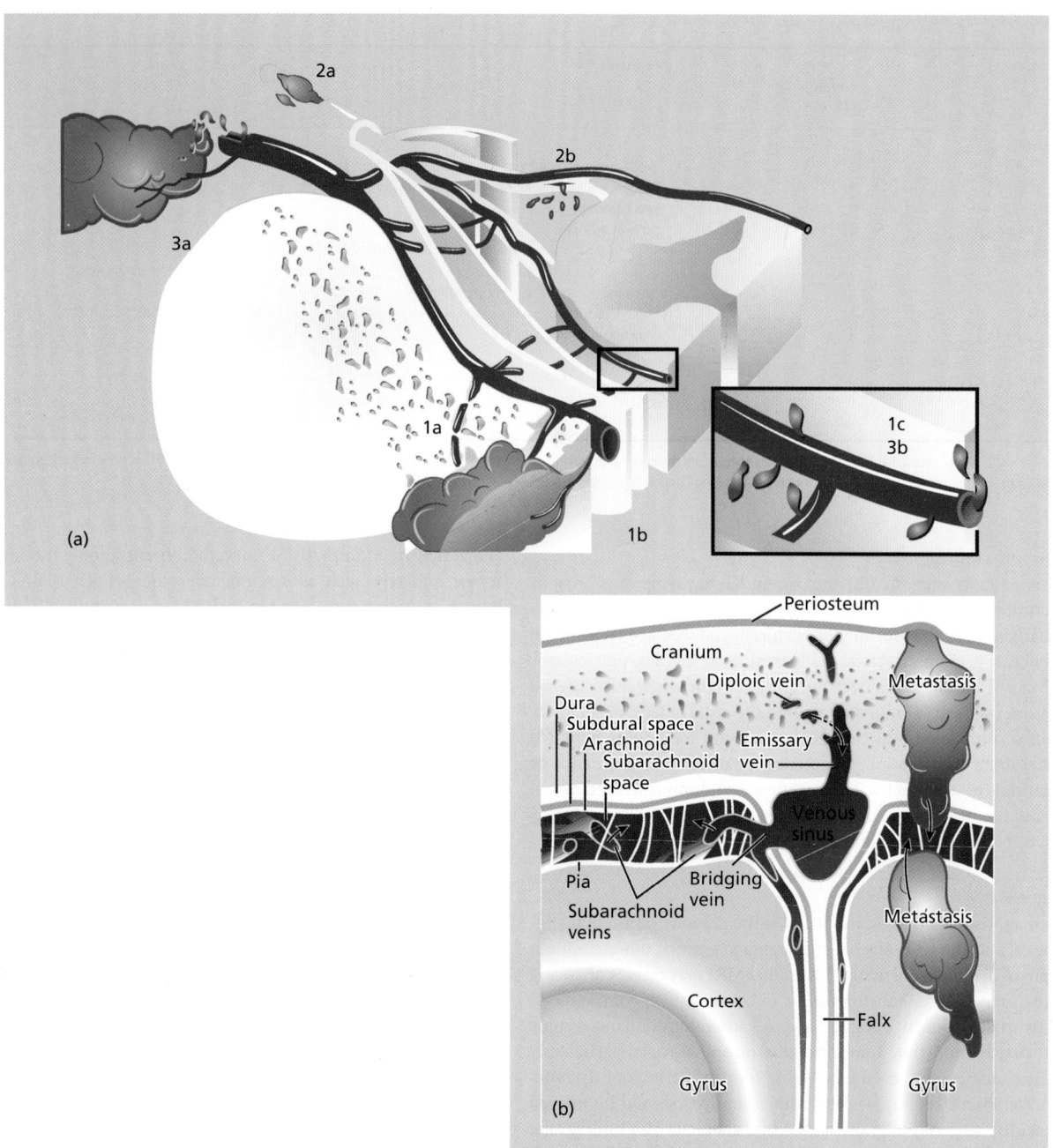

Figure 3 Pathophysiology of leptomeningeal metastases. (a) Mechanisms of tumor cell entry into the spinal subarachnoid space. Tumor may invade the vertebral body (1a) and grow along vertebral veins (1b) into the subarachnoid space (1c). Tumor may invade peripheral nerves or nerve roots outside the vertebral canal (2a) and grow along the nerve sheath into the spinal canal to seed the leptomeninges (2b). The tumor can invade blood vessels outside the central nervous system (3a) and transverse subarachnoid veins into the subarachnoid space (3b). Source: From Ref. 1. (b) Possible mechanisms of tumor entry into the cerebral subarachnoid space. Tumor may enter the cranial subarachnoid space via metastases either to the skull or brain, to the diploic veins of the skull, or directly from subarachnoid veins. The choroid plexus (not shown) is also an occasional site for the formation of leptomeningeal tumor.

along the entire spinal axis. The brain is the most common site to which RT is administered, usually in a dose of 3000 cGy, but the cauda equina also requires RT frequently.

Chemotherapy

Intrathecal chemotherapy is used commonly to treat LM and when it is administered intraventricularly, there is better distribution and greater ease and reliability of delivery than drug administered by lumbar puncture. The most commonly used agent is methotrexate (MTX), which is active against breast cancer, lymphoma, and leukemia, but has poor activity against some of the other common cancers that cause LM. An Ommaya reservoir is usually placed to access the right lateral ventricle. MTX is administered intrathecally to adults in doses of 12–15 mg, diluted in preservative-free saline. With this dose, MTX levels in the CSF exceed the therapeutic concentration of 10^{-6} M and remain above this level for 36–48 h.

Studies of CSF flow dynamics using indium[111]-DPTA (diethylenetriamine penta-acetic acid) cisternography have found impaired CSF flow in a high percentage of patients with LM. Indium[111]

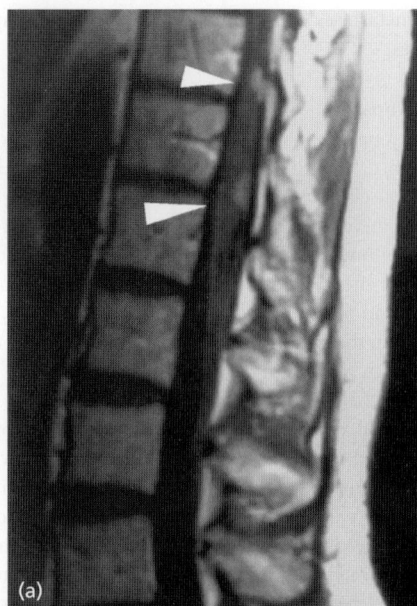

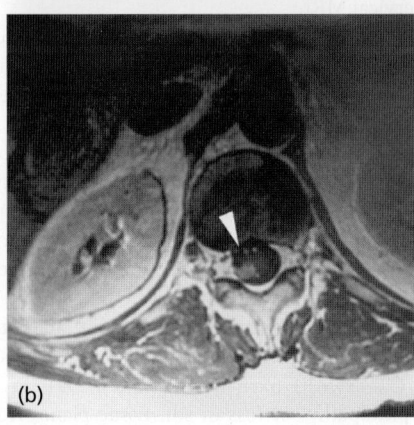

Figure 4 Gadolinium-enhanced MRI demonstrating leptomeningeal metastases from lung cancer. (a) Sagittal and (b) axial images demonstrating enhancing nodules within the thecal sac. This patient had a positive cerebrospinal fluid cytology for malignant cells.

studies predict CSF MTX distribution and indicate that drug reaches all areas of the subarachnoid space unless a complete block is present.[19] Patients with impaired CSF flow have a worse prognosis and increased incidence of leukoencephalopathy. If a patient has symptoms of elevated ICP with or without hydrocephalus, this takes priority and requires placement of a ventriculoperitoneal shunt; no patient with hydrocephalus or a shunt should receive intrathecal chemotherapy, even if a valve can turn off drainage temporarily. Obstruction of CSF flow should be suspected in patients with LM who develop focal leukoencephalopathy around the ventricular catheter track of an Ommaya reservoir (see Methotrexate).

MTX appears in the serum for prolonged periods following intrathecal administration, and myelosuppression and stomatitis may result. Oral leucovorin can avert these complications starting 12 h after MTX injection. Leucovorin does not appear in the CSF, but its active conversion product, 5-methyltetra-hydrofolate (5-methylTHFA), does; however, the CSF levels of 5-methylTHFA are very low after oral leucovorin and are incapable of rescuing tumor cells in the CSF.

Two studies have found that intrathecal MTX as a single agent is equal in efficacy to multiagent intrathecal chemotherapy and has

significantly less systemic toxicity. Patients treated with MTX plus RT respond more often than those treated with either alone. Cytarabine (cytosine arabinoside [ara-C]) and thiotepa may also be useful, particularly in LM from lymphoma, leukemia, or breast cancer. Liposomal cytarabine has a long CSF half-life and can be given every 14 days; it has been reported effective against LM from solid tumors not usually considered sensitive to cytarabine.[20] However, it can cause a severe chemical meningitis and patients must receive prophylactic steroids beginning one day before a dose is administered and continued for at least 2 days following the dose. Intrathecal antibodies such as rituximab and traztusumab have been effective in LM from lymphoma and HER2+ breast cancer, respectively.[21] There are few data to guide decisions regarding the duration of therapy in patients who are clinically stable and whose CSF remains free of malignant cells after 6 months of therapy. Neurotoxicity from intrathecal drug can occur and is discussed later in this chapter.

Because LM disrupts the blood–brain barrier, systemic chemotherapy, particularly when administered in high doses, may also be effective. High-dose intravenous MTX (e.g., 3–8 g/m^2) with leucovorin rescue after 24 h may result in CSF MTX levels that exceed 10^{-6} M and may represent an alternative to intrathecal delivery, particularly in patients with impaired CSF flow. Systemic drugs may also treat bulky LM, whereas intrathecal chemotherapy has insufficient penetration into tumor nodules. Other agents that can reach the CSF or have been reported effective for LM include high-dose cytarabine for hematologic malignancies and capecitabine for breast cancer.[22] Newer agents, including the tyrosine kinase inhibitors and even bevacizumab, have been reported effective in individual patients and should be chosen on the basis of the likely sensitivity of the primary to a given drug.[23,24]

Cranial and peripheral nerve metastases

Lesions of cranial or peripheral nerves often cause severe pain and, depending on the nerve involved, substantial neurologic disability. The frequency of metastatic disease causing cranial and peripheral nerve dysfunction is unknown because only a few studies address this issue in particular tumors. For example, facial nerve paralysis occurs in 5–25% of malignant parotid neoplasms, the lower figure associated with acinous cell carcinomas and the higher with undifferentiated neoplasms. Primary lung cancer arises in the superior sulcus in approximately 3% of patients, the vast majority presenting with pain caused by infiltration of the brachial plexus (Pancoast syndrome). Individual nerves either alone or in combination (mononeuritis multiplex) may be compressed or invaded by tumor.

Pathogenesis

Tumors affect cranial and peripheral nerves either by compression or invasion along perineurial and endoneurial planes. Pancoast tumors and breast carcinoma metastatic to supraclavicular lymph nodes compress the brachial plexus but usually do not invade it, whereas squamous cell carcinoma of the face, certain melanomas, and prostate cancer can be neurotropic, tracking microscopically along the course of a nerve, often reaching the spinal canal or even the brainstem.[25] A blood–nerve barrier similar to the blood–brain barrier may exclude water-soluble chemotherapeutic agents from nerve and provide a "sanctuary" for tumor cells.

Symptoms

The specific symptoms and signs of cranial and peripheral nerve dysfunction depend on the nerves involved and the mechanism of

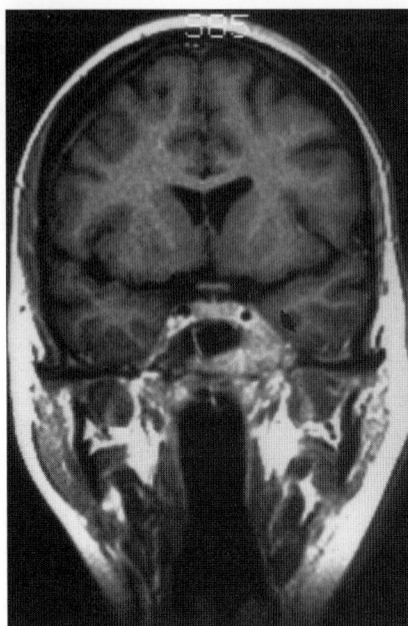

Figure 5 Coronal-enhanced MRI demonstrating a metastasis to the left cavernous sinus (*arrowhead*) from breast carcinoma. Patient presented with retro-orbital pain and had evidence of a partial third, sixth, and V1 palsy.

involvement. With compressive lesions, pain at the site of compression or more distantly in the sensory distribution of the nerve or plexus involved is usually the first symptom. In invasive lesions of nerves, pain and neurologic dysfunction develop simultaneously. In general, when mixed nerves are involved, motor function is affected out of proportion to sensory loss, no matter what the mechanism of nerve involvement is. Compressive lesions of nerves can generally be identified by MRI directed at the area of dysfunction (Figure 5).[1,25] When the lesion is infiltrative, imaging studies may be normal and the diagnosis must be established clinically or by biopsy. Occasionally infiltration of large nerves such as a plexus or root can be imaged by an enhanced MRI or PET.

Cranial and peripheral neuropathies also occur as side effects of radiation, chemotherapy, or as paraneoplastic syndromes. It is frequently difficult to distinguish these nonmetastatic peripheral nerve lesions from those caused by metastases, but in general, the former are usually painless, whereas the latter tend to be painful. Furthermore, most paraneoplastic and drug-induced neuropathies are bilateral and symmetric, whereas metastatic neuropathies are unilateral or at least asymmetric.

Cranial neuropathies

Cranial nerves may be affected by metastases at any point from within the brainstem to their end organ (Table 7). Brainstem metastases occasionally cause isolated cranial nerve dysfunction, but usually other signs reveal the central location of the lesion. LM is a common cause of cranial neuropathies that are often multiple. Base of skull metastases often cause recognizable patterns of cranial nerve dysfunction that localize the lesion.[1,2] Finally, the cranial nerves may be damaged after exiting their foramina.

Evaluation should include an enhanced MRI to visualize the involved cranial nerve along its entire course. Lumbar puncture should be performed even when an appropriately placed skull base metastasis is discovered because LM may coexist. Nonmetastatic causes of cranial neuropathies are also common in cancer patients (Table 8). RT is usually employed for skull base

and orbital metastases. Chemotherapy can be used in appropriate circumstances.

Brachial plexopathy

Brachial plexopathy in cancer patients usually results from metastatic cancer in axillary or cervical lymph nodes, local bony structures (e.g., clavicle), or from superior sulcus lung tumors.[1,2] Because most metastatic tumors compress the plexus from below, the initial symptom is usually pain in the posterior shoulder or pain radiating down the medial aspect of the arm, elbow, and forearm to the fourth and fifth fingers (C-8 or T-1 distribution). Weakness usually begins in the hand and sensory loss begins in the fourth and fifth fingers; both may progress to affect the entire arm. This initial presentation is helpful in distinguishing tumor from the more common cervical disc herniation where pain commonly affects the outer arm and dorsal surface of the forearm, with weakness in the triceps and wrist extensors (C-7 radiculopathy). Tumor masses are occasionally palpable in the axilla or supraclavicular area. When present, an ipsilateral Horner syndrome (ptosis, miosis, and anhydrosis) indicates the tumor has involved the stellate ganglion in the paraspinal region and, therefore, epidural extension must be sought on cervical MRI.

The differential diagnosis includes radiation-induced plexopathy, trauma (e.g., intraoperative positioning, or following central line placement), idiopathic plexopathy, and radiation-induced malignant peripheral nerve sheath tumor. A common diagnostic dilemma is the differentiation of metastatic from radiation-induced plexopathy. Clinical features that distinguish these two conditions include (1) initial symptom of pain in metastatic plexopathy and paresthesias in RT-induced plexopathy; (2) Horner syndrome, which is more consistent with metastatic plexopathy; (3) more rapid progression of symptoms and signs in metastatic plexopathy; (4) supraclavicular fullness in metastatic plexopathy; and (5) lymphedema, which suggests RT-induced plexopathy. CT or MRI may demonstrate a mass in the plexus (metastatic plexopathy) or loss of soft-tissue planes from fibrosis (RT-induced plexopathy). When findings are equivocal, a PET scan may help.

RT is the best available treatment for metastatic plexopathy; chemotherapy may be useful for some previously irradiated patients (e.g., those with breast cancer or lymphoma). There is no satisfactory treatment for radiation-induced plexopathy. Surgical lysis of fibrotic tissue surrounding the nerves has not been helpful, nor has systemic corticosteroid, local steroid injection, hyperbaric oxygen, or bevacizumab. Treatments for pain include carbamazepine, opioids, gabapentin, pregabalin, and neurosurgical ablative procedures.

Lumbosacral plexopathy

The lumbosacral plexus is formed from spinal nerve roots L-2 to S-5. The upper lumbar portion (L-2 to L-4) exits the pelvis mainly as the obturator (adductor muscles) and femoral (quadriceps muscles) nerves, whereas the remainder of the leg is innervated by the sciatic nerve (L-5 to S-1). The bladder, rectum, and anus are innervated by roots S-3, S-4, and S-5. Symptoms are usually unilateral leg weakness and numbness although 25% of metastatic plexopathies may be bilateral. Incontinence requires bilateral loss of innervation and, therefore, its presence suggests central (i.e., cauda equina) or sacral involvement. Clear differentiation requires enhanced spinal MRI and CSF analysis. Local extension of pelvic and abdominal tumors is the predominant cause of metastatic lumbosacral plexopathy. The differential includes herniated lumbar disc, epidural and meningeal metastases to the cauda equina,

Table 7 Metastatic lesions causing cranial neuropathies.

Lesion site	Findings	Comments
Eye	Decreased visual acuity; retinal detachment	Choroidal lesions are more common than retinal: pain, proptosis and diplopia are rare; breast and lung cancer are common causes
Orbit	Pain, proptosis, diplopia; sensory loss V1; decreased visual acuity in one-third of cases, usually late	As common as choroidal metastases; breast and prostate cancer and lymphoma are common causes
Parasellar	Unilateral frontal headache, oculomotor palsies (3, 4, 6), sensory loss V1	Vision rarely affected, no proptosis; lymphoma common
Sella	Diabetes insipidus	Anterior pituitary insufficiency and visual loss are rare; when present, they suggest a primary pituitary tumor. Breast cancer is a common cause
Middle cranial fossa	Facial numbness (V2, 3), VI palsy in some	Lightning-like facial pains (trigeminal neuralgia) rare in patients with neoplastic compression
Jugular foramen	Hoarseness, dysphagia, pain in pharynx (IX, X), sternocleidomastoid weakness (XI), occasionally tongue weakness (XII)	Papilledema may occur if dominant jugular vein is compressed. Glossopharyngeal neuralgia is uncommon
Occipital condyle	Unilateral occipital pain and neck stiffness, unilateral tongue weakness (XII)	Pain may radiate to forehead
Mandible	Unilateral numb chin and gum ("mental neuropathy")	Also results from meningeal or skull base metastases; breast cancer and lymphoma are common causes
Carotid sinus or glosso-pharyngeal nerve	Syncope, pharynx or neck pain on swallowing	Cardioinhibitory, vasodepressor syncope, or both; head and neck cancer, indicates recurrent tumor; may be life-threatening
Left upper mediastinum	Hoarseness, recurrent laryngeal paralysis	Lung, breast and head and neck cancers

Table 8 Nonmetastatic causes of cranial neuropathy in cancer patients.

Cranial Nerve (Symptom)	Causes
II (unilateral vision loss)	Gallium, interferon alpha, RT, temporal arteritis, retinal diseases including hemorrhage
III (diplopia, ptosis)	Diabetes (usually spares pupil), aneurysm, increased intracranial pressure (uncal herniation); myasthenia gravis and Grave disease[a]
IV (jaw pain; facial pain)	Vincristine, trigeminal neuralgia (sudden, lancinating pains without sensory loss)
VI (diplopia)	Vincristine, increased intracranial pressure, head trauma, diabetes, drug toxicity (e.g., narcotics, anticonvulsants), strabismus
VII (facial weakness)	Bell palsy (idiopathic), varicella-zoster infection (Ramsay Hunt syndrome), diabetes
VIII (hearing loss, dysequilibrium)	Cisplatin, aminoglycosides, degenerative disease, acoustic neuroma, RT-induced serous otitis
X (weak phonation, laryngeal paralysis)	Vincristine

[a]Common causes of diplopia, but are not cranial nerve diseases.
Abbreviation: RT, radiation therapy.

radiation-induced plexopathy (usually from brachytherapy for pelvic neoplasms), intraoperative trauma, hematoma, abscess, and diabetic or idiopathic lumbosacral plexopathy. The differential features of metastatic and radiation-induced plexopathy are similar to those for brachial plexopathy. CT or MRI often demonstrates a mass in the region of the lumbosacral plexus. Biopsy is indicated if an abscess or a secondary tumor is suspected. RT is the most commonly employed treatment for metastatic lumbosacral plexopathy. If metastatic disease approaches the spine, epidural disease may be present and should be included in the RT port.

Peripheral neuropathy

Single peripheral nerves are sometimes damaged by metastatic cancer, and more widespread invasion of peripheral nerves, causing either a mononeuritis multiplex or diffuse polyneuropathy, may complicate the course of leukemia or lymphoma; PET imaging of the limbs may be diagnostic.[26] However, when polyneuropathy occurs in cancer patients, it usually results from toxin exposure or paraneoplastic disorders, both of which are discussed below.

Nonmetastatic complications of cancer therapy

Many cancer treatments are neurotoxic (Table 9). Some drugs (e.g., vincristine) cause neurotoxicity even at low doses, whereas others (e.g., cytarabine) cause neurotoxicity only during intensive therapy. Neurologic toxicity is a dose-limiting factor in several cancer treatments, such as RT, and patients may suffer more from these toxicities than from the cancer itself.[1,2,27] The more commonly encountered neurologic toxicities from cancer treatment are discussed in the following section.

Chemotherapy

Vinca alkaloids

Vinca alkaloids cause nerve damage by binding tubulin in peripheral nerves and disrupting the formation of microtubules that mediate fast axonal transport. Neurotoxicity is a dose-limiting side effect of all the vinca alkaloids, but especially of vincristine; vinorelbine can also cause peripheral neuropathy particularly when combined with or following other neurotoxic agents. Central neurotoxicity is

Table 9 Neurotoxicity of agents commonly used in cancer patients.

Acute encephalopathy (delirium)	Headache without meningitis
Corticosteroids	Retinoic acid
Methotrexate (high-dose IV, IT)	Trimethoprim-sulfamethoxazole
Cisplatin	Corticosteroids
Vincristine	Tamoxifen
Asparaginase	Ondansetron
Procarbazine	*Seizures*
5-Fluouracil (± levamisole)	Methotrexate
Cytarabine (high-dose IV, IT)	Etoposide (high-dose)
Nitrosoureas (high-dose or arterial)	Cisplatin
Ifosfamide/mesna	Vincristine
Interferons	Asparaginase
Chronic encephalopathy (dementia)	Nitrogen mustard
Methotrexate	Carmustine
Carmustine	Dacarbazine (intra-arterial or high-dose)
Cytarabine	Busulfan (high-dose)
Fludarabine	
Visual loss	Myelopathy (intrathecal drugs)
Tamoxifen	Methotrexate
Cisplatin	Cytarabine
Interferon alpha	Thiotepa
Cerebellar dysfunction/ataxia	Peripheral neuropathy
Cytarabine	Vinca alkaloids
Phenytoin	Cisplatin
Procarbazine	Oxaliplatin
Aseptic meningitis	Etoposide
Trimethoprim-sulfamethoxazole	Teniposide
IVIg	Paclitaxel
NSAIDs	Suramin
Monoclonal antibodies	Docetaxel
Bortezomib	Bortezomib
Carbamazepine	
Cytarabine (IT)	
Methotrexate (IT)	
Corticosteroids (IT)	

Abbreviations: IV, intravenous; IVIg, intravenous gammaglobulin; IT, intrathecal; NSAID, nonsteroid anti-inflammatory drugs.
Source: Modified from Ref. 1.

rare because vincristine does not penetrate the normal blood–brain barrier. Vinca alkaloids should never be given intrathecally.

Vinca alkaloid neurotoxicity is age (more severe in adults) and dose dependent and appears to be more prominent in patients with hepatic dysfunction, and in those who have received other potentially neurotoxic therapies. Tingling paresthesias develop in the fingertips, and usually in the toes, of virtually all patients treated with vincristine, although clinically detectable sensory loss is often absent. Loss of ankle reflexes is an early and almost universal sign, and with continued therapy, all reflexes may diminish or disappear. Weakness occurs as therapy continues and is of two types: (1) A generalized distal neuropathy that preferentially affects the foot and hand extensors, causing impairment of fine motor function and foot drop. Weakness can become severe enough to render the patient immobile or bed-bound, but the drug should be discontinued before severe weakness. Pre-existing peripheral nerve diseases, especially Charcot–Marie–Tooth neuropathy and probably other neuropathies (e.g., diabetic polyneuropathy), increase the severity of vincristine neuropathy. (2) Some patients develop focal weakness (e.g., unilateral foot drop or cranial nerve palsies, such as ptosis or extraocular muscle, facial, or laryngeal paralysis). Although symptomatic toxicity is usually reversible after discontinuation of the drug, significant weakness may persist in severely affected patients. Autonomic dysfunction, particularly abdominal cramping and constipation, often occurs within hours to days of each dose. Adynamic ileus may result and can be life-threatening; a prophylactic bowel regimen is essential for all patients. Impotence has been reported.

Less common complications of vincristine administration include aching bone pain, sharp stabbing pain in the jaw or throat, or an increase in any pre-existing pain; this typically occurs within hours of injection and subsides over several days. The symptoms appear with the first or second dose and rarely recur with subsequent doses. Hyponatremia from inappropriate secretion of antidiuretic hormone occurs within days of drug administration and may recur with subsequent doses.

Methotrexate

There are several clinically distinct forms of MTX toxicity.[1,2] An acute reaction with meningismus, confusion, fever, and CSF pleocytosis often occurs 4–6 h after intrathecal injection and resolves over several days. This syndrome is frequently confused with infectious meningitis, but the onset is too rapid after the injection for bacterial contamination; antibiotics are unnecessary unless Gram stain or cultures demonstrate organisms. Dexamethasone relieves or prevents some of these symptoms. Mild acute toxicity occurs in as many as 10% of patients, but further doses of intrathecal MTX are usually uneventful.

Paraplegia may follow instillation of MTX or cytarabine by lumbar puncture. The disorder is characterized by weakness and sensory loss in the legs, which evolves over several days to complete transverse myelopathy. Some patients recover, but most remain paraplegic. Extensive necrosis of the spinal cord is found at autopsy. The pathogenesis is unknown, but it appears to be idiosyncratic rather than dose related.

An early delayed reaction follows high-dose systemic MTX in about 4% of patients. The disorder usually occurs 7–10 days after the third or fourth treatment and is characterized by stupor or coma, often associated with lateralizing neurologic signs that change from hour to hour. MRI may show diffusion-positive lesions suggestive of ischemia. Most patients recover completely and the disorder usually does not recur with subsequent doses of MTX. MTX leukoencephalopathy can occur in patients who have received a high cumulative dose of intrathecal or systemic MTX or MTX in combination with cranial RT. In adults, progressive cognitive impairment in the absence of lateralizing signs may be seen in patients who survive >6 months following treatment. Leukoencephalopathy, when clinically present, is always found on neuroimaging, but occasionally it may be found on MRI in asymptomatic patients. The neuropathologic findings consist of multifocal areas of coagulative necrosis and calcification in the white matter, often with a periventricular predominance. Unlike cerebral radionecrosis, fibrinoid necrosis of blood vessels is absent.

Alternatively, focal leukoencephalopathy may develop around an Ommaya reservoir catheter track. When MTX is injected into ventricles with elevated pressure, the drug tracks along the outside of the catheter, producing focal leukoencephalopathy seen on MRI as an enhancing mass (Figure 6); this may resolve on its own or require removal of the catheter.

Platins

Peripheral neuropathy is a dose-limiting toxicity of some platins, particularly cisplatin and oxaliplatin.[1,28] Neuropathic symptoms begin as tingling paresthesias in the toes and fingers; loss of reflexes and reduced vibratory and position sensation are characteristic but pain, temperature sensation, and strength are preserved. Severe, disabling sensory ataxia may result. Symptoms are often mild during treatment but they progress for months before stabilizing, making dose adjustment during treatment difficult. Gradual resolution follows, although some patients are permanently disabled. Lhermitte sign, an electric sensation in the arms, back, or legs upon

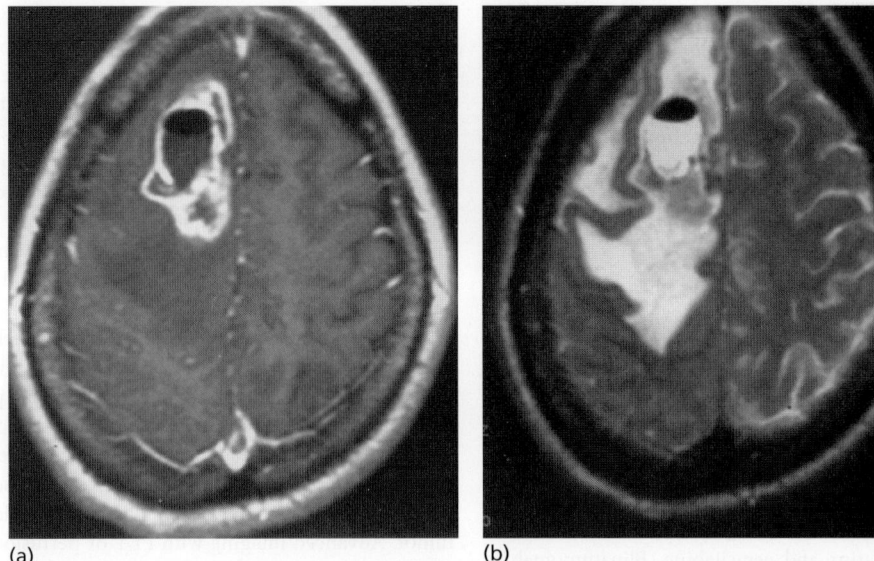

Figure 6 Gadolinium-enhanced T1-weighted (a) and T2-weighted (b) MRIs of focal leukoencephalopathy in a patient with a malfunctioning Ommaya reservoir. This reservoir was obstructed but unrecognized. Multiple courses of methotrexate were instilled into the catheter. The drug dissected around the catheter and into the frontal lobe, causing a region of necrosis with prominent surrounding edema. Air can be seen in the central cavity of the lesion after a recent instillation. The patient presented with seizures and a left hemiparesis, both of which resolved with corticosteroids.

neck flexion, is an occasional manifestation of platin neurotoxicity. Oxaliplatin may cause cold-induced paresthesias either during or shortly after an infusion and may also cause a sensory neuropathy.[28] Magnesium infusions do not prevent oxaliplatin neurotoxicity.[29]

Ototoxicity caused by cisplatin is a result of damage to the organ of Corti. Toxicity severe enough to interfere with speech perception is uncommon, but hearing loss may or may not resolve. Seizures and encephalopathy have been reported in patients receiving cisplatin, independent of the magnesium and calcium wasting commonly caused by the drug. Vascular disease producing neurologic symptoms has been reported as a late delayed effect of cisplatin-based chemotherapy. Many such patients develop Raynaud phenomenon, and a few have developed transient ischemic attacks or cerebral infarctions. Other platinum drugs are less neurotoxic.

Taxanes

Paclitaxel and docetaxel both bind tubulin, stabilizing and promoting microtubular assembly. Both cause a predominantly sensory peripheral neuropathy, beginning with paresthesias of the toes and then fingers.[1,30] More severe sensory impairment and loss of reflexes develop with increasing duration of drug administration. Symptoms usually recover with drug discontinuation. Weakness is seen occasionally, but can be predominantly proximal, mimicking a myopathy, but this is likely secondary to neuropathy. Because taxanes are often used concurrently with or following other neurotoxic agents such as cisplatin, patients may develop significant symptoms with the first few doses because of additive neurotoxic effects. Nab-paclitaxel, the taxane bound to nanoparticles of albumin is less neurotoxic than the standard drug.

5-Fluorouracil

Generalized encephalopathy has been seen in association with severe systemic toxicity during therapy and may indicate an inherited deficiency of dihydropyrimidine dehydrogenase, the enzyme responsible for pyrimidine catabolism.[31] Capecitabine, doubly esterified fluorouracil for oral use, appears to be less neurotoxic than intravenously administered fluorouracil.

Cytosine arabinoside

Intrathecal cytarabine can cause an acute chemical meningitis with confusion, fever, and CSF pleocytosis. This occurs in almost all patients who receive the liposomal preparation (DepoCyt)[20] and requires dexamethasone before and after every DepoCyt injection.

Intravenous high-dose cytarabine (e.g., 3 g/m² every 12 h for six doses) causes neurotoxicity in 10–25% of patients; the risk is increased with older age and poor renal function. Neurotoxicity has been documented with minimum cumulative doses of 18 g/m,[2] but higher cumulative doses (e.g., 30–40 g/m²) are associated with a higher incidence and more severe toxicity. Commonly, a pancerebellar dysfunction starts several days after the initiation of therapy and worsens for several more days. Gradual recovery begins about 2 weeks after onset, but recovery may be incomplete especially in those with severe dysfunction. Pathologic changes include loss of cerebellar Purkinje cells and neurons in the deep cerebellar nuclei. Encephalopathy and seizures also occur, usually in the setting of cerebellar toxicity. A recrudescence of neurologic symptoms may occur with retreatment.

Other drugs

Other commonly used drugs that cause neurotoxicity include bortezomib,[32] suramin, and procarbazine, all of which can cause peripheral neuropathy, although procarbazine does so rarely. Bortezomib neuropathy can be severely painful and predispose to compression neuropathies superimposed on the diffuse neuropathy. A second-generation proteosome inhibitor, carfilzomib, causes less severe peripheral neuropathy. Thalidomide causes peripheral neuopathy, but lenalidomide and pomalidomide are less neurotoxic. High-dose busulfan therapy, used to prepare patients for stem cell transplantation, can cause seizures; at standard doses, the drug is not neurotoxic. Gemcitabine, with or without radiation, has been reported to cause myositis with acute muscle pain and tenderness; it is responsive to steroids.[1,33] Selumetinib, an MEK inhibitor, can cause focal neck extensor weakness causing the dropped head syndrome.[34]

Antibody-mediated neurotoxicity

Ipilumimab can cause hypophysitis with enhancing lesions seen in the hypothalamus on MRI. Chronic rituximab can induce persistant immunosuppression, which may lead to progressive multifocal leukoencephalopathy (PML) owing to reactivation of JC virus in the brain.[35] Restoration of immune function is the only effective therapy of this otherwise lethal disease which presents with confusion and lateralizing signs such as hemiparesis. MRI shows multiple, usually nonenhancing, white matter lesions.

Bevacizumab, and any anti-vascular endothelial growth factor (VEGF) agent, can cause hypertension, which may lead to confusion and seizures from posterior reversible encephalopathy syndrome (PRES).[36] PRES can be identified on MRI by the presence of white matter lesions best seen on MRI FLAIR sequence. PRES warrants immediate attention to blood pressure management. PRES has also been associated with other agents, such as tacrolimus, cyclosporin, and mycophenylate used after allogeneic stem cell transplantation along with many conventional chemotherapeutics such as the platins and gemcitabine. Blinatumomab is a bispecific T-cell receptor-engaging (BITE) antibody used to treat B-cell acute lymphocytic leukemia (ALL). CNS toxicity with encephalopathy, seizures, and ataxia is seen in approximately 20% of patients.[35]

Brentuximab vedotin, a CD30 antibody drug conjugate, can cause a predominantly sensory neuropathy that improves when the drug is held; it can be restarted when the neuropathy has improved.[35] Myalgias are also common with brentuximab vedotin.

Radiation therapy

Despite the fact that cells in the CNS turn over slowly or not at all, the brain, spinal cord, and, to a lesser degree, peripheral nerves are susceptible to damage by ionizing radiation that usually causes symptoms months or years after the radiation has been completed (Table 10).[2] With patients living longer after initial treatment, the problem of delayed radiation damage to the CNS is increasingly important.

Brain toxicity

Acute reactions, occurring within hours of a dose of RT, are rare with current fractionation schedules when patients are pretreated with dexamethasone.[1] Patients with large or multifocal tumors and cerebral edema, especially those with symptoms of increased ICP, are more likely to experience this side effect. Symptoms and signs of acute RT toxicity include worsening of existing deficits, headache, nausea and vomiting, and lethargy. These are usually transient and respond to corticosteroids. The etiology has been ascribed to radiation-induced disruption of the blood–brain barrier with worsening cerebral edema.

Early delayed encephalopathy occurs a few weeks to a few months after RT. Patients being treated for cerebral tumors may develop worsening of lateralizing signs. Symptoms may persist for days to weeks and are often relieved by corticosteroids; complete resolution is usual. Early delayed encephalopathy is often confused with tumor progression and is sometimes called pseudo-progression. MRI reveals an enhancing lesion indistinguishable from progressive tumor. Advanced imaging with PET or perfusion MRI sometimes clarifies the situation; however, gradual resolution of symptoms may be the only confirmation of the cause of the deterioration.[1]

Delayed radiation toxicity is the most serious complication of brain RT, and radionecrosis is its most common manifestation, arising months to years after treatment.[1,2,37] In one study, cerebral radionecrosis occurred in 6% of patients treated with 4500 cGy or more.[37] The total dose is the most important risk factor, and there is a threshold near 6000 cGy above which radionecrosis becomes common. However, high daily fractionation schedules also carry increased risk, and radionecrosis is seen most commonly after stereotactic radiosurgery (SRS) for brain metastases. Headache, focal deficits, and seizures are the usual symptoms. CT/MRI reveals a contrast-enhancing lesion with surrounding edema; PET or perfusion MRI may differentiate tumor that is hypermetabolic and hypervascular from necrosis that is hypometabolic and avascular. However, the differentiation between radionecrosis and tumor is often difficult, and biopsy may be required. Marked symptomatic improvement follows treatment with dexamethasone, and some patients remain well after steroids are discontinued. Surgical

Table 10 Neurologic complications of CNS irradiation.

Complication	Latency	Symptoms and signs	Comments
Brain			
Acute	Hours	Increase in existing deficits, headache, nausea, vomiting, confusion, somnolence	Transient, corticosteroids help
Early	Weeks to months	Increase in existing signs, increased seizures, lethargy	Resolves over days to weeks, steroids help
Delayed			
a. Radionecrosis	6 months to years	Focal mass lesion	Treatment includes steroids and surgery, tumor often coexists
b. Dementia	1 year	Loss of cognitive function	May be subtle
c. Endocrine	Years	Hypothyroidism, amenorrhea/galactorrhea, changes in libido, growth failure	Hypothalamic or pituitary in origin
d. Secondary tumors	10–40 years, earlier if radiated as a child	Symptoms of brain tumor	Meningioma, sarcoma, malignant glioma
e. Stroke	Years	Abrupt onset of neurologic dysfunction	Large or branch vessels
Spinal cord			
Early	Weeks to months	Electric shocks with neck movement (Lhermitte symptom)	Usually transient
Delayed			
a. Myelopathy	Weeks to years	Progressive cord dysfunction, starts with sensory symptoms	Often fatal
b. Lower motor neuron syndrome	Months to years	Focal weakness and atrophy	May improve spontaneously

resection of the necrotic material is often necessary. Reports that anticoagulation or hyperbaric oxygen relieve symptoms require confirmation. Bevacizumab may prove effective.[38]

Radiation may also cause dementia unassociated with necrosis.[1,2] The MRI shows ventricular dilatation, sulcal atrophy, and white matter hyperintensity. Some of these patients respond to ventriculoperitoneal shunting albeit incompletely and temporarily.[1] Cerebral infarction may result from occlusion of cervical or intracranial arteries that have received large doses of RT.[39] Vascular malformations may appear and bleed many years after brain RT. Complicated migraine-like episodes may occur in patients after cranial irradiation called SMART syndrome (stroke-like migaine attacks after RT).[40] Endocrinologic dysfunction may arise years after RT, resulting from either hypothalamic or pituitary failure. Brain tumors may occur decades after cranial RT or radiosurgery administered in adulthood, but latency is often much shorter (median 6 years) in those irradiated in childhood. Radiation-induced brain tumors include meningioma, sarcoma, and malignant glioma.[1]

Spinal cord toxicity

Spinal cord damage caused by RT is uncommon. Transient, electric shock-like sensations following neck flexion (Lhermitte symptom) may occur weeks to months after RT to the cervical cord, including mantle RT for Hodgkin disease.[1] Spontaneous resolution is the rule. Progressive radiation myelopathy, on the other hand, is a devastating complication with onset months to years (median 20 months) following RT. The incidence of radiation myelopathy is affected by the total RT dose and dose per fraction; an estimate of the ED5 (5% incidence of complication) is between 5700 and 6100 cGy for RT delivered in 200 cGy fractions. Symptoms of radiation myelopathy usually begin with sensory changes in the legs and gradually progress to sensory loss, weakness, and sphincter dysfunction. Pain may be present at the level of the cord damage. Unlike SCC, sensory and motor findings are often asymmetric at onset and a Brown-Séquard syndrome is often present. The MRI reveals a normal, enlarged, or atrophic cord that may contrast enhance, but extrinsic compression is absent (Figure 7). Steroids do not reverse the deficits. Anticoagulants and hyperbaric oxygen have been reported to be effective, but this has not been verified, and myelopathy is usually permanent.[1]

Cerebrovascular complications of cancer

Cerebrovascular lesions are the second most common neuropathologic finding, after metastases, in postmortem studies of cancer patients. Hemorrhage into a metastasis is the most common cause of intracranial hemorrhage in cancer patients;[41] it is most common in lung cancer, but occurs proportionately more frequently in melanoma, thyroid, renal, and germ cell metastases. Nonmetastatic intracerebral hemorrhage is seen in patients with leukemia, thrombocytopenia, or coagulopathy.[1] Subdural hemorrhage may occur in association with dural metastases or coagulopathy.[42] A hemorrhage may cause abrupt neurologic symptoms with headache, vomiting, lethargy, and focal deficits or may be unsuspected before obtaining a brain scan. For patients with intracerebral hemorrhage resulting from coagulopathy or thrombocytopenia, the underlying problem should be treated and the patient observed. Subdural hematomas and some hemorrhages into metastases may benefit from surgical evacuation.

Cerebral infarction is as common as hemorrhage.[43,44] Infarctions secondary to accelerated atherosclerosis take place decades following RT that has included cervical or cerebral vessels in the irradiated

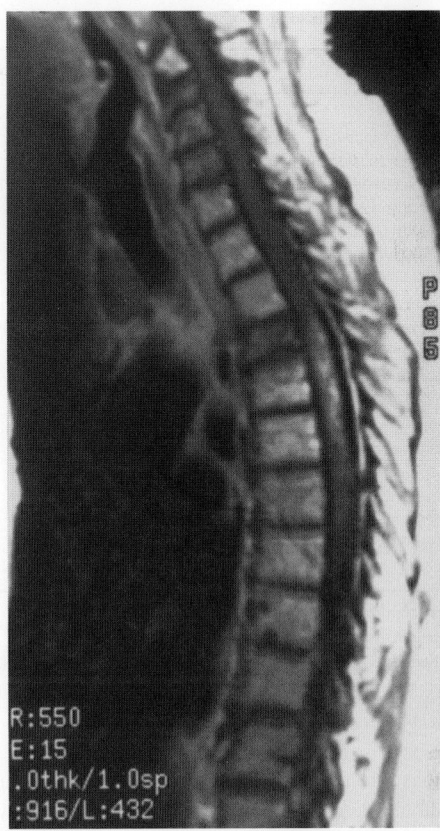

Figure 7 MRI demonstrating radiation myelopathy. The hypodense thoracic vertebral body is the site of a bone metastasis from breast cancer for which the patient was radiated. Some months later, the patient developed a myelopathy, and the contrast-enhancing lesion seen in the spinal cord represents radiation damage.

field. RT for head and neck cancer predisposes to carotid stenosis, and intracranial arterial stenosis with subsequent infarction may occur following cranial RT. Septic cerebral infarction is usually secondary to Aspergillus, Candida, or Mucor. These opportunistic organisms produce a vasculitis, and the infarctions are often multiple and hemorrhagic. Aspergillus is the most common causative agent and is always associated with pulmonary infection. Antifungal therapy is usually unsuccessful, and the outcome is often fatal.

Cerebral venous thrombosis (e.g., superior sagittal sinus thrombosis) may result from compression or invasion of vascular structures by a metastasis, or from a coagulopathy.[112] Clinical features include headache, focal deficits, and seizures. The diagnosis can be made by MRI combined with magnetic resonance venography. Lumbar puncture reveals an elevated opening pressure and frequently red cells in the CSF. Spontaneous resolution usually occurs unless dural metastasis is the cause, in which case RT is required. Anticoagulation is safe and should be considered for progressive neurologic symptoms, even when due to hemorrhage from venous infarction; however, most patients recover fully without treatment.

Cerebral embolism accounts for more than one-half of strokes in patients with cancer.[43,44] It may be cardioembolic, including nonbacterial thrombotic endocarditis (NBTE), which is most common with lung and GI carcinomas. Infarctions in patients with NBTE are often multiple and hemorrhagic. Diffuse encephalopathy and focal deficits usually coexist. Approximately one-third of patients with NBTE also have laboratory evidence of disseminated intravascular coagulation (DIC). Two-dimensional echocardiography is rarely helpful, but transesophageal echocardiography

Table 11 Paraneoplastic neurologic syndromes.

Syndrome	Associated cancer[a]	Clinical features
Brain		
Limbic encephalopathy[b]	SCLC	Depression, memory loss, confusion, abnormal CSF
Brainstem encephalopathy[b]	SCLC	Ataxia, cranial nerve dysfunction, corticospinal dysfunction, abnormal CSF
Subacute cerebellar degeneration	Breast, ovary, SCLC, Hodgkin	Ataxia, dysarthria, nystagmus, normal CSF
Opsoclonus, myoclonus	Lung	Jerky, irregular movements of eyes and skeletal muscles
Optic neuritis, retinal degeneration	SCLC	Painless loss of vision, transient visual obscuration
NMDA receptor encephalitis	Teratoma	Seizures, psychosis, rhythmic movements, impaired cognition
Spinal cord		
Necrotizing myelopathy	SCLC, lymphoma, leukemia	Ascending myelopathy
Subacute motor neuronopathy	Hodgkin and NHL	Patchy weakness, atrophy, and fasciculations
Dorsal root ganglia		
Subacute sensory neuronopathy[b]	SCLC	Dysesthesias, sensory ataxia, areflexia
Peripheral nerve		
Gammopathy associated neuropathy	Myeloma	Sensory loss, weakness, reflex loss
Acute polyradiculitis (Guillain–Barré)	Lymphoma	No cells in CSF; high CSF protein
Neuromuscular junction		
LEMS	SCLC	Proximal weakness, decreased reflexes, ocular muscles spared
Myasthenia gravis	Thymoma	Weakness, ocular muscles often involved
Muscle		
Dermatomyositis, polymyositis	Lung, breast, ovary, GI	Weakness, elevated CPK

[a] The most commonly associated tumors are listed.
[b] Often occur in association with each other.
Abbreviations: CPK, creatine phosphokinase; CSF, cerebrospinal fluid; GI, gastrointestinal; LEMS, Lambert–Eaton myasthenic syndrome, NHL, non-Hodgkin lymphoma; NMDA, *N*-methyl D-aspartate; SCLC, small-cell lung cancer.

may demonstrate the valvular vegetations. Anticoagulation with heparin should be considered; evidence suggests that warfarin is not helpful. It is unknown if agents such as direct thrombin or factor Xa inhibitors are equally effective. DIC alone may result in cerebrovascular thrombosis. Neurologic symptoms usually begin abruptly with diffuse encephalopathy and fluctuating multifocal deficits. Enhanced MRI is typically negative, although small foci of ischemia are seen occasionally on diffusion-weighted sequences. Anticoagulation with heparin may prevent progressive neurologic dysfunction.

Paraneoplastic neurologic syndromes

Paraneoplastic syndromes refer to disorders of unknown etiology that occur with increased frequency in patients with cancer (Table 11).[3] Compared with known complications of cancer, paraneoplastic syndromes are rare, seen in less than 1% of patients with cancer. As paraneoplastic syndromes precede the diagnosis of cancer in about two-thirds of cases, prompt recognition may lead to early diagnosis and cure of the underlying neoplasm. These disorders often debilitate the patient to a greater degree than the malignancy, but some of the syndromes improve with successful treatment of the cancer.

The etiologies of these syndromes are not well understood, but most are suspected to have an autoimmune basis. The strongest evidence for an autoimmune disorder is for the Lambert–Eaton myasthenic syndrome (LEMS), in which autoantibodies inhibit the function of presynaptic calcium channels at the neuromuscular junction, resulting in weakness. Examination demonstrates an increase in muscle power after repetitive muscle contraction (the opposite of myasthenia gravis) and absence of deep tendon reflexes. These findings, along with autonomic and sensory complaints of dry mouth, impotence, and thigh paresthesias, point to a nerve disorder. Several other paraneoplastic syndromes are associated with the presence of specific antibodies, including subacute sensory

neuronopathy, limbic encephalitis, subacute cerebellar degeneration, and gammopathy-associated neuropathies. These specific antibodies serve as markers that not only identify the syndrome as paraneoplastic but also suggest the site of the underlying tumor.[3]

A variety of therapies directed at immunomodulation, including plasmapheresis, corticosteroids, and intravenous immunoglobin, have failed to reverse the neurologic impairment associated with most paraneoplastic disorders. However, some syndromes, such as the LEMS and NMDA receptor encephalitis, respond to immunosuppressive treatments. Some patients with paraneoplastic neurologic disorders have reversal or stabilization of their neurologic dysfunction when the underlying malignancy is treated effectively and this should be a therapeutic priority for all of these patients.

References

1 DeAngelis LM, Posner JB. *Neurologic Complications of Cancer*. New York: Oxford University Press; 2008.
2 Schiff D, Kesari S, Wen PY. *Cancer Neurology in Clinical Practice. Neurologic Complications of Cancer and Its Treatment*. Totowa, New Jersey: Humana Press; 2007.
3 Darnell RB, Posner JB. Paraneoplastic syndromes affecting the nervous system. *Semin Oncol.* 2006;33:270–298.
4 Liu JK, Laufer I, Bilsky MH. Update on management of vertebral column tumors. *CNS Oncol.* 2014;3:137–147.
5 Cole JS, Patchell RA. Metastatic epidural spinal cord compression. *Lancet Neurol.* 2008;7:459–466.
6 Lipton A. Efficacy and safety of intravenous bisphosphonates in patients with bone metastases caused by metastatic breast cancer. *Clin Breast Cancer.* 2007;7(**Suppl 1**):S14–20.
7 Rades D, Evers JN, Bajrovic A, Veninga T, Schild SE. Re-irradiation of spinal cord compression due to metastasis in elderly patients. *Anticancer Res.* 2014;34:2555–2558.
8 Sahgal A, Bilsky M, Chang EL, et al. Stereotactic body radiotherapy for spinal metastases: current status, with a focus on its application in the postoperative patient. *J Neurosurg Spine.* 2011;14:151–166.
9 Katsoulakis E, Riaz N, Cox B, et al. Delivering a third course of radiation to spine metastases using image-guided, intensity-modulated radiation therapy. *J Neurosurg Spine.* 2013;18:63–68.
10 Bydon M, De la Garza-Ramos R, Bettagowda C, Gokasian ZL, Sciubba DM. The use of stereotactic radiosurgery for the treatment of spinal axis tumors: a review. *Clin Neurol Neurosurg*: 2014.

11 Patchell RA, Tibbs PA, Regine WF, et al. Direct decompressive surgical resection in the treatment of spinal cord compression caused by metastatic cancer: a randomised trial. *Lancet*. 2005;**366**:643–648.

12 Bilsky M, Smith M. Surgical approach to epidural spinal cord compression. *Hematol Oncol Clin North Am*. 2006;**20**:1307–1317.

13 Kwok Y, Tibbs PA, Patchell RA. Clinical approach to metastatic epidural spinal cord compression. *Hematol Oncol Clin North Am*. 2006;**20**:1297–1305.

14 Grommes C, Bosl GJ, DeAngelis LM. Treatment of epidural spinal cord involvement from germ cell tumors with chemotherapy. *Cancer*. 2011;**117**:1911–1916.

15 Clarke JL, Perez HR, Jacks LM, Panageas KS, Deangelis LM. Leptomeningeal metastases in the MRI era. *Neurology*. 2010;**74**:1449–1454.

16 Shah S, Rangarajan V, Purandare N, Luthra K, Medhi S. 18F-FDG uptakes in leptomeningeal metastases from carcinoma of the breast on a positron emission tomography/computerized tomography study. *Indian J Cancer*. 2007;**44**:115–118.

17 Nayak L, Fleisher M, Gonzalez-Espinoza R, et al. Rare cell capture technology for the diagnosis of leptomeningeal metastasis in solid tumors. *Neurology*. 2013;**80**:1598–1605.

18 Taillibert S, Laigle-Donadey F, Chodkiewicz C, Sanson M, Hoang-Xuan K, Delattre JY. Leptomeningeal metastases from solid malignancy: a review. *J Neurooncol*. 2005;**75**:85–99.

19 Mason WP, Yeh SD, DeAngelis LM. 111Indium-diethylenetriamine pentaacetic acid cerebrospinal fluid flow studies predict distribution of intrathecally administered chemotherapy and outcome in patients with leptomeningeal metastases. *Neurology*. 1998;**50**:438–444.

20 Glantz MJ, LaFollette S, Jaeckle KA, et al. Randomized trial of a slow-release versus a standard formulation of cytarabine for the intrathecal treatment of lymphomatous meningitis. *J Clin Oncol*. 1999;**17**:3110–3116.

21 Zagouri F, Sergentanis TN, Bartsch R, et al. Intrathecal administration of trastuzumab for the treatment of meningeal carcinomatosis in HER2-positive metastatic breast cancer: a systematic review and pooled analysis. *Breast Cancer Res Treat*. 2013;**139**:13–22.

22 Ekenel M, Hormigo AM, Peak S, Deangelis LM, Abrey LE. Capecitabine therapy of central nervous system metastases from breast cancer. *J Neurooncol*. 2007;**85**:223–227.

23 Ranze O, Hofmann E, Distelrath A, Hoeffkes HG. Renal cell cancer presented with leptomeningeal carcinomatosis effectively treated with sorafenib. *Onkologie*. 2007;**30**:450–451.

24 Vincent A, Lesser G, Brown D, et al. Prolonged regression of metastatic leptomeningeal breast cancer that has failed conventional therapy: a case report and review of the literature. *J Breast Cancer*. 2013;**16**:122–126.

25 Ladha SS, Spinner RJ, Suarez GA, Amrami KK, Dyck PJ. Neoplastic lumbosacral radiculoplexopathy in prostate cancer by direct perineural spread: an unusual entity. *Muscle Nerve*. 2006;**34**:659–665.

26 Zhou WL, Wu HB, Weng CS, et al. Usefulness of 18F-FDG PET/CT in the detection of neurolymphomatosis. *Nucl Med Commun*. 2014;**35**:1107–1111.

27 Kaley TJ, Deangelis LM. Therapy of chemotherapy-induced peripheral neuropathy. *Br J Haematol*. 2009;**145**:3–14.

28 Joseph EK, Chen X, Bogen O, Levine JD. Oxaliplatin acts on IB4-positive nociceptors to induce an oxidative stress-dependent acute painful peripheral neuropathy. *J Pain*. 2008;**9**:463–472.

29 Loprinzi CL, Qin R, Dakhil SR, et al. Phase III randomized, placebo-controlled, double-blind study of intravenous calcium and magnesium to prevent oxaliplatin-induced sensory neurotoxicity (N08CB/Alliance). *J Clin Oncol*. 2014;**32**:997–1005.

30 Argyriou AA, Koltzenburg M, Polychronopoulos P, Papapetropoulos S, Kalofonos HP. Peripheral nerve damage associated with administration of taxanes in patients with cancer. *Crit Rev Oncol Hematol*. 2008;**66**:218–228.

31 Johnson MR, Hageboutros A, Wang K, High L, Smith JB, Diasio RB. Life-threatening toxicity in a dihydropyrimidine dehydrogenase-deficient patient after treatment with topical 5-fluorouracil. *Clin Cancer Res*. 1999;**5**:2006–2011.

32 O'Connor OA, Wright J, Moskowitz C, et al. Phase II clinical experience with the novel proteasome inhibitor bortezomib in patients with indolent non-Hodgkin's lymphoma and mantle cell lymphoma. *J Clin Oncol*. 2005;**23**:676–684.

33 Pentsova E, Liu A, Rosenblum M, O'Reilly E, Chen X, Hormigo A. Gemcitabine induced myositis in patients with pancreatic cancer: case reports and topic review. *J Neurooncol*. 2012;**106**:15–21.

34 Chen X, Schwartz GK, DeAngelis LM, Kaley T, Carvajal RD. Dropped head syndrome: report of three cases during treatment with a MEK inhibitor. *Neurology*. 2012;**79**:1929–1931.

35 Magge R, DeAngelis LM. The double-edged sword: neurotoxicity of chemotherapy. *Blood Rev*. 2014;**29**:93–100.

36 Tlemsani C, Mir O, Boudou-Rouquette P, et al. Posterior reversible encephalopathy syndrome induced by anti-VEGF agents. *Target Oncol*. 2011;**6**:253–258.

37 Ruben JD, Dally M, Bailey M, Smith R, McLean CA, Fedele P. Cerebral radiation necrosis: incidence, outcomes, and risk factors with emphasis on radiation parameters and chemotherapy. *Int J Radiat Oncol Biol Phys*. 2006;**65**:499–508.

38 Boothe D, Young R, Yamada Y, Prager A, Chan T, Beal K. Bevacizumab as a treatment for radiation necrosis of brain metastases post stereotactic radiosurgery. *Neuro Oncol*. 2013;**15**:1257–1263.

39 O'Connor MM, Mayberg MR. Effects of radiation on cerebral vasculature: a review. *Neurosurgery*. 2000;**46**:138–149; discussion 131–150.

40 Black DF, Morris JM, Lindell EP, et al. Stroke-like migraine attacks after radiation therapy (SMART) syndrome is not always completely reversible: a case series. *AJNR Am J Neuroradiol*. 2013;**34**:2298–2303.

41 Navi BB, Reichman JS, Berlin D, et al. Intracerebral and subarachnoid hemorrhage in patients with cancer. *Neurology*. 2010;**74**:494–501.

42 Reichman J, Singer S, Navi B, et al. Subdural hematoma in patients with cancer. *Neurosurgery*. 2012;**71**:74–79.

43 Cestari DM, Weine DM, Panageas KS, Segal AZ, DeAngelis LM. Stroke in patients with cancer: incidence and etiology. *Neurology*. 2004;**62**:2025–2030.

44 Navi BB, Singer S, Merkler AE, et al. Recurrent thromboembolic events after ischemic stroke in patients with cancer. *Neurology*. 2014;**83**:26–33.

127 Dermatologic complications of cancer chemotherapy

Anisha B. Patel, MD ▪ Madeleine M. Duvic, MD

Overview

Dermatologic complications of cancer chemotherapy have become increasingly significant, especially with the continued development of new targeted antineoplastic agents. The frequency of mucocutaneous complications in cancer chemotherapy is often a reflection of the increased proliferative nature of affected tissues, such as the mucous membranes, skin, hair, and nails, which renders them particularly susceptible to the actions of chemotherapeutic drugs. This chapter reviews the specific side effects associated with targeted therapies and the more classic side effects of cytotoxic chemotherapies and their associated drugs.

Diagnosis of cutaneous reactions in the cancer patient is complicated by the degree of their malignancy, concomitant diseases, polypharmacy, and immunosuppression. With the advances in bone marrow transplantation, graft versus host disease (GVHD), opportunistic infections, and malignancies are also being seen more frequently and may mimic and complicate the diagnosis of chemotherapy-induced reactions. The major cutaneous reactions and a variety of miscellaneous reactions are discussed in this chapter and are listed in Table 1. As seen in Table 2, these reactions occur in varying degrees of frequency and severity among the classes of chemotherapeutic drugs. Although dermatologic complications are rarely fatal, it is important to recognize potential reactions as they may result in significant morbidity, chemotherapy cessation or dose reduction, cosmetic disfigurement, and psychological distress. Proper treatment of potentially dose limiting cutaneous toxicity may also allow ideal schedules of chemotherapy administration and optimization of response.

Drug hypersensitivity reactions

"Traditional" drug reactions have been categorized into immunologic and nonimmunologic or toxic. Of the immunologic drug reactions, there are four subtypes, formerly types I–IV, that are outlined in Table 3. The most common reactions are delayed-type, T-cell-mediated drug reactions and include the morbilliform or exanthematous drug eruption. They clinically present as erythematous macules and thin papules on the trunk spreading to the extremities and are usually asymptomatic. When the rash is painful, the differential diagnosis includes erythema multiforme (EM), Stevens Johnsons syndrome (SJS), and toxic epidermal necrolysis (TEN). EM is characterized by targetoid erythematous papules and plaques that tend to start on the extremities, can involve the palms and soles, and, when advanced, form central bullae and spread to the oral and genital mucosa. SJS and TEN, however, start with centrally distributed dusky papules and plaques that coalesce and vesiculate and have severe mucosal involvement. SJS involves <10% of body surface area and TEN involves >30% of body surface area. The mortality rate of SJS is 1–5% and that of TEN is 25–35%.[1]

Drug reaction with eosinophilia and systemic (DRESS) and acute generalized exanthematous pustulosis (AGEP) have unclear pathogeneses. The cutaneous findings in DRESS are not specific; however, the peripheral edema, lymphadenopathy, and liver transaminitis are characteristic. Finally, AGEP presents with abruptly appearing sheets of cutaneous pustules. It usually begins on the face or intertriginous areas, perhaps with burning and itching. It can be accompanied by fever, neutrophilia, and eosinophilia.[2] Ninety percent of cases are drug induced, mostly with antibiotics such as β-lactams, cephalosporins, fluconazole, nystatin, and terbinafine.[1] Other reported triggers include the histone deacetylase inhibitor bryostatin,[3] imatinib, mercury, thallium, iohexol, patch testing, pseudoephedrine, diltiazem, furosemide, and viral infections.[4] These two reactions are less common than the exanthematous eruption and can be more severe.

Targeted cancer therapeutics

These drugs started to emerge in the mid-1990s and we are still delineating all of the side effects. Although the systemic toxicities are decreased, many of the signaling mediators targeted also affect the epithelium, and these effects are much more specific than previous chemotherapy cutaneous reactions. This change is reflected in the literature of even the clinical trials, where adverse events were previously described as a "rash" or "lesion," the descriptions have become more specific, which makes it easier to anticipate and track different reactions.

Numerous targeted therapies are available; however, only those with specific cutaneous reactions occurring at high incidences are discussed below.

Epidermal grown factor receptor (EGFR) inhibitors

Epidermal growth factor receptor (EGFR) has been recognized as a significant regulator of cancer cell proliferation, apoptosis, angiogenesis, and metastasis. Ligand binding to the receptor causes receptor dimerization, which activates the intracellular tyrosine kinase domain.[5] EGFR also plays a significant role in normal skin homeostasis.[6] Activation of EGFR in epidermal keratinocytes promotes cell cycle progression, differentiation, and migration, which are all critical for normal skin function and wound healing.[7] The most common cutaneous side effects for EGFR inhibitors are an acneiform eruption, paronychia, xerosis, eczema, mucositis, and geographic tongue. Acne folliculitis appears on the face and upper trunk 8–10 days after treatment initiation. In phase 1 trials, erlotinib at the maximally tolerated dose induced a pustular acneiform eruption in 50% of cases during the second week

Holland-Frei Cancer Medicine, Ninth Edition. Edited by Robert C. Bast Jr., Carlo M. Croce, William N. Hait, Waun Ki Hong, Donald W. Kufe, Martine Piccart-Gebhart, Raphael E. Pollock, Ralph R. Weichselbaum, Hongyang Wang, and James F. Holland.
© 2017 John Wiley & Sons, Inc. ISBN: 978-1-118-93469-2

Table 1 Major cutaneous reactions associated with chemotherapy.

Drug hypersensitivity reactions (morbilliform, erythema multiforme/Stevens Johnsons/toxic epidermal necrolysis)
Mucosal reactions (stomatitis, aphthae)
Nail reactions (hyperpigmentation, onycholysis, paronychia)
Extravasation reactions (irritant, vesicant)
Pigmentary changes (hyperpigmentation, vitiligo)
Radiation-associated reactions (radiation enhancement, radiation recall, photosensitivity)
Alopecia (anagen effluvium, scarring alopecia)
Acral reactions (acral erythema/toxic erythema of chemotherapy, hand–foot skin reaction)
Neutrophilic dermatoses (Sweet's syndrome, erythema nodosum)
Cutaneous eruption of lymphocyte recovery
Neoplasms (keratoses, squamous cell carcinoma, lentigines, melanoma)

Table 2 Most common mucocutaneous reactions of the major classes of chemotherapeutic drugs.

Alkylating agents	Antibiotics
Hyperpigmentation	Alopecia
Hypersensitivity	Stomatitis
	Chemical cellulitis
	Hyperpigmentation
	Radiation-associated reactions
Vinca alkaloids	**Antimetabolites**
Alopecia	Acral erythema
Chemical cellulitis	Alopecia
Inflammation of keratosis	Hyperpigmentation
Neutrophilic eccrine hidradenitis	Radiation-associated reactions

of therapy.[8] The eruption can be extremely prurituc and EGFR inhibitors have cutaneous side effects that lead to dose alteration in >75% of patients.[9] The presence and severity of acne folliculitis has been correlated with tumor response and survival.[10] This reaction has been reported with cetuximab, panitumumab, nimotuzumab, erlotinib, and gefitinib.[11–13] Oral tetracyclines combined with topical steroids are the gold standard treatment. Retinoids and topical antibiotics have not been proven useful in these patients as the etiology is not follicular plugging and rupture, but epithelial

dysregulation.[11] *Staphylococcus* colonization can worsen the eruption and cultures and antibiotics are recommended if lesions are pustular or crusted (Figure 1).

The human epidermal growth factor receptor (HER)1/2 blockers have the same side effects as EGFR inhibitors, but are milder. Trastuzumab, lapatinib, dacomitinib, and afatinib all have had reported acneiform eruptions.[14–17] Similarly, the vascular endothelial growth factor (VEGF) inhibitors have overlap between the EGFR inhibitors, with mucositis and geographic tongue, and the multikinase inhibitors, with hand–foot skin reaction (HFSR), which is discussed below.[18]

BCR-ABL tyrosine kinase inhibitors

Imatinib mesylate targets the *BCR–ABL* gene and has been used in the treatment of chronic myeloid leukemia and acute lymphoblastic leukemia. It has been shown to frequently cause dose-dependent cutaneous reactions, including facial edema, morbilliform eruption, urticaria, eczematous dermatitis, and AGEP.[19,20] One patient developed an eczematous rash with histologic features of mycosis fungoides.[21]

Second- and third-generation Bcr–Abl-specific TKIs, dasatinib, nilotinib, and ponatinib have been associated with follicular lichenoid eruptions of the scalp, face, and body that can be pruritic and lead to scarring alopecia.[22] This alopecia is irreversible, even upon dose cessation.

Multikinase inhibitors

Sunitinib and sorafenib are the multikinase inhibitors targeting VEGF receptor, platelet-derived growth factor receptor (PDGFR), c-Kit, and FLT-3. Sorafenib also inhibits RAF kinase. They were developed for advanced renal cell carcinoma but have also been used for hepatocellular carcinoma, gastrointestinal stromal tumors, and thyroid cancer. They are most associated with the HFSR as well as mucositis, alopecia, xerosis, and xerostomia. However, because they overlap with multiple groups of targeted therapies, the cutaneous squamous cell carcinoma (SCC) of BRAF inhibitors and the acneiform eruption of VEGF inhibitors can be seen as well.[23]

HFSR appears within 2–4 weeks of starting the therapy and is present in one-fifth to one-third of patients, with sorafenib having a slightly higher incidence. Patients develop a focal keratoderma at points of friction and pressure, which can vesiculate, leading to

Table 3 Immunologically mediated drug hypersensitivity reactions.

IgE-dependent drug reactions (formerly type I)	L-asparaginase, paclitaxel, docetaxel, teniposide, cisplatin (intravesical)	Urticaria
		Angioedema
		Anaphylaxis
Cytotoxic drug-induced reactions (antibody against a fixed antigen; formerly type II)		Petechiae secondary to drug-induced thrombocytopenia
Immune complex-dependent drug reactions (formerly type III)		Vasculitis
		Serum sickness
		Urticaria (certain types)
Delayed-type, cell-mediated drug reactions (formerly type IV) versus undefined	Procarbazine	Exanthematous/morbilliform eruption
	Cytarabine	
	Nucleoside analogues	Fixed drug eruption
	(both can also have IgE-dependent and	Lichenoid drug reaction
	immune-complex-mediated	SJS/TEN
	drug reactions)	AGEP
		DRESS
No reported immunologically mediated reactions	Nitrosoureas	
	Vinca alkaloids	
	Altretamine	
	Dactinomycin	

Source: Adapted from Ref. 1.

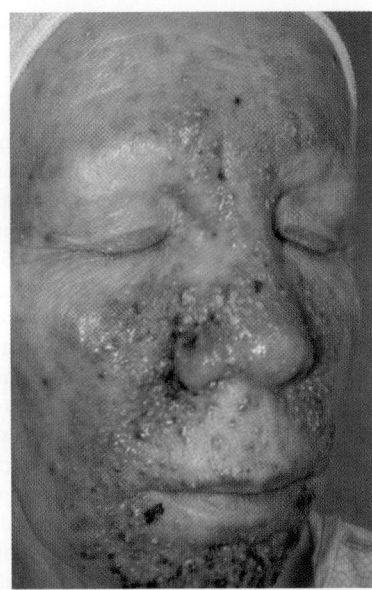

Figure 1 Severe acneiform eruption of the face associated with cetuximab therapy.

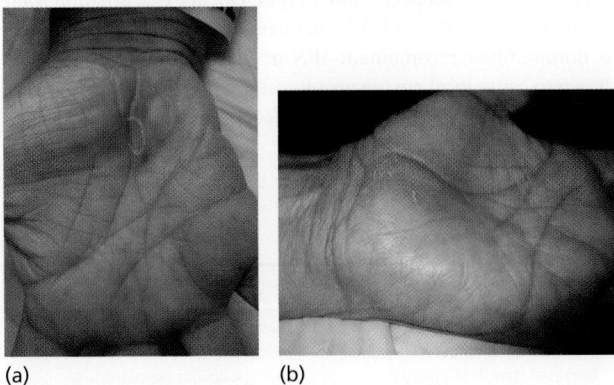

(a)   (b)

Figure 2 Hand–foot skin reaction with sorafenib therapy.

painful blisters (Figure 2). The risk of developing HSFR depends on which drug the patient is on and which cancer type is being treated. The original proposed mechanism was that the VEGFR blocking capabilities of these drugs caused the patients to have a poor response to damage caused by pressure and trauma.[24,25] Most recently, the Fas/Fas ligand response was implicated, proven by blocking the reaction by administering anti-Fas ligand antibody. These are the same mediators of Stevens Johnsons and TEN.[26]

Although more common in multikinase inhibitors such as sorafenib and sunitinib, these lesions have been reported with BRAF inhibitors.[27] These are distinct from the more common hand–foot syndrome/acral erythema (AE)/toxic erythema of chemotherapy seen with cytotoxic chemotherapies. HFSR does not have the diffuse erythema and edema of hand–foot syndrome and also has a longer latency period before appearing (2–4 weeks). HFSR usually self-resolves with continued treatment with the multikinase inhibitors.[28]

mTOR inhibitors

Overlapping with the EGFR signaling pathway is the PI3K/AKT pathway, which activates mammalian target of rapamycin (mTOR). This molecule is associated with cell growth and angiogenesis and sirolimus or rapamycin was the original drug in this category,

followed by everolimus and temsirolimus. All are associated with the papulopustular rash of EGFR inhibitors, which has an incidence of 45.8% in the most recently developed drug, temsirolimus. They all also can induce the more classic morbilliform drug eruption and oral mucositis. As opposed to cytotoxic chemotherapies, individual deeper oral ulcerations more similar to aphthous stomatitis are present as well. Finally, everolimus and temsirolimus also had a population with eczematous dermatitides.[29]

BRAF inhibitors

BRAF inhibitors, first introduced in metastatic melanoma patients, have significant cutaneous side effects that include inflammatory, follicular, and neoplastic eruptions. These side effects lead to dose cessation or reduction in <10% of patients.[30] Of the inflammatory cutaneous toxicities, neutrophilic dermatoses, including acute febrile neutrophilic dermatosis (Sweet's syndrome) and neutrophilic panniculitis, have been attributed to the use of BRAF inhibitors.[30-36]

Two patients with the erythematous pseudovesicular papules and plaques of Sweet's syndrome of the trunk and extremities presenting with systemic symptoms of fever and arthralgias have been reported.[36,37] The patients with neutrophilic panniculitis presented with tender, erythematous nodules of the legs and occasionally arms, and had histology consistent with a neutrophilic lobular panniculitis.[31-34] Vitiligo,[38] cutaneous sarcoidosis,[39] Grover's disease,[40] and hidradenitis suppurativa[41] have been reported less commonly.

Patients on BRAF inhibitors also have increased radiation sensitivity to UV (ultraviolet) light and radiation therapy with quicker and more severe sunburns and acute radiation dermatitis, respectively.[42,43] Further, cases of radiation recall dermatitis have been reported as well.[44,45]

Epidermal and follicular dysregulation contribute significantly to BRAF inhibitor cutaneous side effects. Palmoplantar hyperkeratosis or keratoderma is a thickening of the epidermis without inflammation presenting as thick yellow plaques of the palms and soles similar to a large callus. Most commonly, the keratoderma is seen on the feet in pressure points, without vesiculation.[46] A superficial keratotic plugging of the follicle results in a keratosis pilaris-like eruption. This is seen frequently on the trunk and extremities and is more often asymptomatic than pruritic. It was noted in 5–9% of patients in phase 2 and 3 trials,[47,48] although this may be underreported.[27,49,50]

Neoplastic lesions cause the highest morbidity in these patients. Actinic keratoses (AKs) represent precancerous epithelial lesions typically associated with chronic sun damage. The incidence of AKs is 6–16% in vemurafenib patients[47-49] and 5–10% in dabrafenib patients.[46,51-53] Wart-like keratoses are papillated, hyperkeratotic, well-demarcated papules that are often inflamed and appear in an eruptive nature during BRAF inhibitor therapy. They appear about 3–4 months after therapy.[53] These lesions are not true verruca as human papilloma virus testing has been negative in multiple reports.[54,55] Prompt treatment of both types of lesions with cryotherapy, photodynamic therapy, curettage, and topical 5-fluorouracil (5-FU) helps prevent SCC formation (Figure 3).

Patients with SCC usually present with dome-shaped, well-demarcated, hyperkeratotic, erythematous papules, and nodules. They are quickly growing and more prevalent in older patients with chronic sun damage.[46]

The incidence of SCC is 4–31% in vemurafenib patients[47,48,56] and 6–11% in debrafenib patients.[51,52,57,58] Sosman et al. showed that they are predominantly well-differentiated or keratoacanthoma-type SCC, which are less aggressive than the normal array of

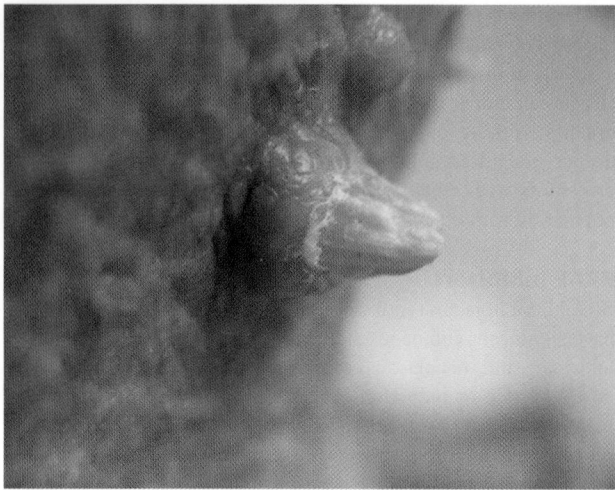

Figure 3 Squamous cell carcinoma with vemurafenib therapy.

sun-induced SCC. The median time to occurrence is 8 weeks. HRAS upregulation has been implicated in a portion of BRAF-induced SCC causing a paradoxical upregulation of the MAP kinase pathway.[47]

Patients have been reported to have involution of nevi as well as new and darkening nevi. The new nevi have shown wild-type BRAF, lack the V600E mutation, and appear in 8–14 weeks.[59] These lesions have been biopsied as common nevi, dysplastic nevi, and new primary cutaneous melanomas. Five of 464 patients in the phase 2 and 3 clinical trials with vemurafenib had a new melanoma.[60]

MEK inhibitors

Selumetinib and trametinib, two new MEK inhibitors, just downstream of BRAF have similar side effects to the EGFR inhibitors.[61] Interestingly, the addition of a MEK inhibitor to a BRAF inhibitor decreases the squamous proliferations seen with the BRAF inhibitor alone, possibly addressing the HRAS mutation as well.

Immunomodulators

With advances in biotechnology, there have been increased developments of cytokines and immunotherapeutic agents, which target cancer at the cellular level. This class of drugs is less specific than the targeted therapies described above and works by enhancing the inflammatory response to metastatic and hematologic tumors. The cutaneous side effects are less specific than those described above, and generally encompass reactive inflammatory processes.

Immune check point inhibitors

Immunomodulatory drugs used for melanoma include ipilimumab and nivolumab or pembrolizumab. Ipilimumab is a monoclonal antibody targeting CTLA4, which inhibits binding of the costimulatory molecule, CD28. Blocking CTLA4 allows unopposed activation of cytotoxic T cells and stimulates the immune response to metastatic melanoma. The main side effects are morbilliform or eczematous eruptions.[62] Similarly, pembrolizumab blocks PD-1, which, when bound to its ligand, decreases the cytotoxic effects of T cells. This molecule is upregulated in tumor cells and is thought

to be a more specific target than CTLA4. The cutaneous side effects are similar to ipilimumab, but also include vitiligo.[63]

Cytokines

Roles have already been established for interleukin 2 (IL-2) as alternative treatment for advanced metastatic melanoma and renal cell cancer and for interferon-α (IFN-α) as standard treatment for chronic myelogenous leukemia, hairy-cell leukemia, cutaneous T-cell lymphoma, melanoma, and Kaposi sarcoma (KS). In addition to significant toxicities (Table 4) such as capillary leak syndrome, there is a 72% incidence of cutaneous reactions reported with IL-2.[64] Commonly, a pruritic diffuse erythroderma occurs 1–3 days after administration and resolves with desquamation 2 days after cessation of therapy (Figure 4).[64] This reaction is clinically similar to toxic shock syndrome and has been associated with staphylococcal sepsis in some patients. Intra-arterial IL-2 also causes hypersensitivity to iodine-containing contrast dyes in up to 30% of patients.[65] Of potential importance, one study of IL-2 for metastatic melanoma has reported a possible correlation between the development of vitiligo and good prognosis.[66] Although IFN-α is relatively less toxic than IL-2, several cutaneous reactions have been reported in the literature. Perhaps one-third of patients will develop a local injection-site reaction. In a study of 1000 patients receiving IFN-α, alopecia and herpes labialis exacerbation were common with 10% and 5% incidence, respectively.[65,67] Similar to nonmodified recombinant IFN-α, pegylated IFN-α has been shown to cause local cutaneous ulcerations at sites of subcutaneous injection.[68] Both IFN-α and IL-2 also induce and/or exacerbate seborrheic dermatitis and psoriasis.[65]

Table 4 Cytokine reactions.

Other INF-α reactions	Other IL-2 reactions
Eosinophilic fasciitis	Erosions in surgical scars
Exacerbation of herpes labialis	Hypersensitivity to iodine contrast dye
Increased growth of eyelashes	Linear IgA bullous dermatosis
Necrotizing vasculitis	Pemphigus vulgaris (de novo, recurrent)
Paraneoplastic pemphigus	Poly/dermatomyositis exacerbation
Psoriasis exacerbation and de novo	Psoriasis exacerbation
Thyroiditis	Staphylococcal infections
	TEN-like bullous desquamation
	Vitiligo

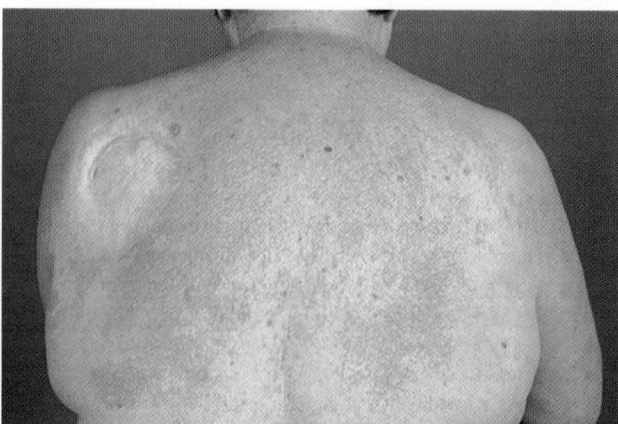

Figure 4 Erythematous rash associated with IL-2 therapy in a melanoma patient.

Table 5 Chemotherapeutic agents associated with alopecia.

Most common or severe		Least common or severe	
Bleomycin	Ifosfamide	Amsacrine	Melphalan
Cisplatin	Interferon-a	Busulfan	Mercaptopurine
Cyclophosphamide	Irinotecan	Carboplatin	Methotrexate
Cytarabine	Mechlorethamine	Carmustine	Mitomycin
Dacarbazine	Nitrosoureas	Chlorambucil epirubicin	Procarbazine
Dactinomycin	Paclitaxel	Gemcitabine	Teniposide
Daunorubicin	Thiotepa	Hydroxyurea	Vinorelbine
Docetaxel	Topotecan		
Doxorubicin	Vinblastine		
Etoposide	Vincristine		
Fluorouracil	Vindesine		
Idarubicin			

Source: Adapted from Ref. 69.

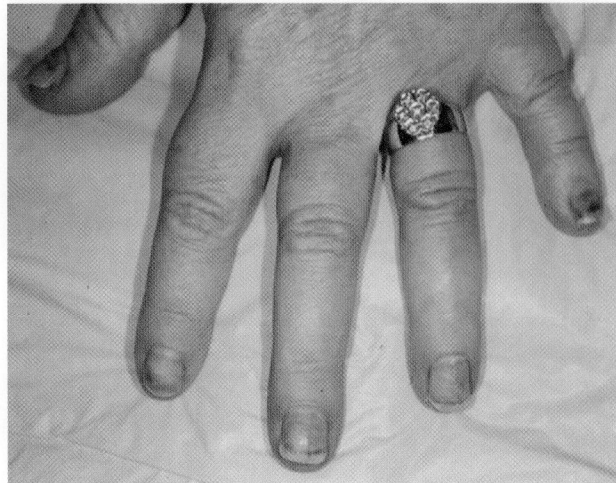

Figure 5 Docetaxel-induced nail hyperpigmentation and onychodystrophy.

Alopecia

Alopecia is the most common dermatologic complication associated with chemotherapy. While most drug-induced alopecias involve a telogen effluvium pattern by inducing normal hairs to synchronize their cycles, the anagen effluvium pattern of hair loss is the most common type of alopecia produced by chemotherapeutic agents (Table 5), with the exception of IL-2 and IFN-α therapy. In chemotherapy, anagen effluvium is caused by the abrupt cessation of the high mitotic activity of hair matrix cells in the anagen phase of hair follicles.[70] Anagen effluvium manifests within 1–2 weeks after the beginning of chemotherapy but is most noticeable 1–2 months later.[71] Hair regrowth can usually be expected 5 months after the end of chemotherapy, although hair color and texture may change.[69] Permanent alopecia has been reported with busulfan/cyclophosphamide therapy.[72]

Hair loss often has emotional impact on patients receiving chemotherapy. Unfortunately, there are currently no widely accepted methods of prevention and treatment for alopecia, although scalp hypothermia, minoxidil, vitamin D3, cyclosporine, and topical doxorubicin monoclonal antibody have been studied.[73,74]

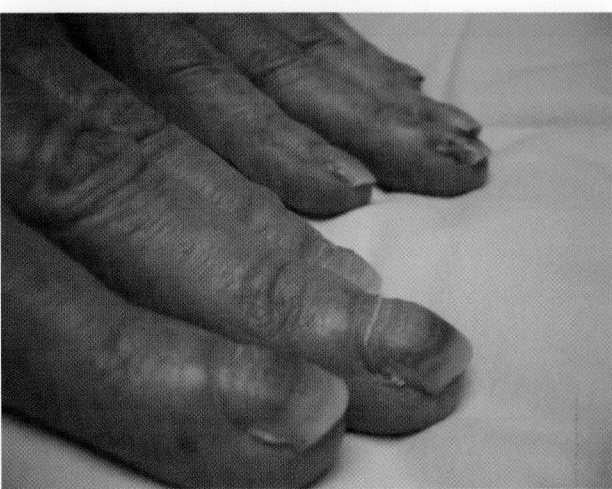

Figure 6 Hyperpigmentation and Beau's lines.

Stomatitis

Stomatitis and other oral complications of cancer chemotherapy are discussed in *Chapter 135* and *Chapter 136*.

Nail reactions

Hyperpigmentation is the most common nail abnormality encountered in patients receiving chemotherapy, particularly in dark-skinned patients.[75] Hyperpigmentation due to chemotherapy-induced melanocyte stimulation should be distinguished from yellow nail syndrome (YNS). YNS nails have increased transverse curvature, absent lunulae, and no cuticle. Suggested etiologies include paraneoplastic process, AIDS (acquired immune deficiency syndrome) association, and drug induction (Figure 5).[76]

Other common nail manifestations include horizontal depressions of the nail plate called Beau's lines (Figure 6), horizontal white discoloration of the entire width of the nail plate called Mees lines, horizontal white discoloration involving partial nail width called leukonychia, onycholysis, and onychodystrophy. Associations between bleomycin and nail loss; hydroxyurea and brittle nails; and etoposide and nail bed pigmentation have also been reported in the literature.[75,77] With the increased use of EGFR inhibitors, paronychia, inflammation of the nail fold, is seen more

commonly and can be extremely painful. Superinfections with *Staphylococcus aureus* and *Candida albicans* are common. Other onychopathies and their associated chemoagents are summarized in Table 6. Patients can be reassured that these nail changes are generally benign and resolve after discontinuation of the causative agent and the affected nails grow out. However, nails damaged by chemotherapy are more susceptible to infection by yeast, dermatophytes, and pseudomonas. Infections may cause lasting damage to the matrix that will not resolve.

Extravasation reactions

Extravasation injury is a well-known adverse event that occurs when offending drugs escape from the veins or intravenous catheters into subcutaneous tissues. Accidental extravasation occurs in approximately 0.1–6% of patients receiving intravenous chemotherapy (Table 7).[78] The cutaneous manifestations of extravasation may range from discomfort and mild erythema to severely painful skin necrosis, ulcerations, and damage to deep tissue structures.

Extravasated cytotoxic agents generally cause two types of local cutaneous reactions: irritant and vesicant reactions. Irritants cause a short-lived and self-limited phlebitis and tender, warm, erythematous reaction along the vein or at the site of intravenous

Table 6 Summary of nail abnormalities and associated chemoagents.

Onychopathy	Associated chemoagents
Beau's lines	Taxanes, bleomycin, cisplatin, doxorubicin, melphalan, vincristine
Transverse leukonychia	Adriamycin
Muehrcke lines	Doxorubicin, cyclophosphamide, vincristine, leucovorin, levamisole, methotrexate
Onycholysis	Taxanes, doxorubicin, fluorouracil, mitoxantrone, bleomycin
Onychomadesis, defluvium unguium	Taxanes, bleomycin, fluorouracil, mercaptopurine, mitoxantrone
Ischemic changes	Bleomycin, taxanes doxorubicin methotrexate nitrogen mustard etoposide cyclophosphamide busulfan melphalan
Melanonychia	Bleomycin, cyclophosphamide, daunorubicin, doxorubicin, fluorouracil, hydroxyurea, aminoglutethimide, busulfan, cisplatin, dacarbazine, docetaxel, idarubicin, ifosfamide, melphalan, methotrexate, mitomycin, and mitoxantrone
Nonmelanotic pigmentation	5-FU
Acute paronychia	Methotrexate taxanes
Pyogenic granuloma	Cetuximab, gefitinib

Table 7 Chemotherapeutic agents associated with chemical cellulitis.

Most common		Least common	
Dactinomycin	Amsacrine	Esorubicin	Plicamycin
Daunorubicin	Bisantrene	Etoposide	Pyrazofurin
Doxorubicin	Bleomycin	Fluorouracil	Streptozocin
Mitomycin	Carmustine	Idarubicin	Vinblastine
	Chlorozotocin	Melphalan	Vincristine
	Cisplatin	Mechlorethamine	Vindesine
	Dacarbazine	Mitoxantrone	Vinorelbine
	Epirubicin	Paclitaxel	

administration. A variant of this local irritation is an erythematous and urticarial hypersensitivity flare reaction that has been associated with the anthracyclines. Vesicants initially cause a similar reaction; however, the irritation may worsen, depending on the amount of drug that has extravasated, leading to nerve and tendon damage and subsequent neurologic deficits, contractures, and joint stiffness. The extent of tissue damage in extravasation largely depends on the concentration, volume, and vesicant nature of the extravasated agent.[78,79]

Paclitaxel can induce an extravasation recall reaction, in which extravasation of the agent at one site has induced a cutaneous reaction, ranging from erythema to ulcerations, at a previous extravasation site.[80] Central lines may dislodge, or venous vessels may be perforated with potentially disastrous consequences, including mediastinitis presenting with fever, severe pleuritic pain, upper extremity and neck swelling, and a widened mediastinum.

Vesicant injury displays poor healing and often continues to worsen, necessitating surgical intervention. Vesicants delay fibroblastic wound contraction and have the ability to bind to DNA, possibly allowing them to be recycled and retained in the tissue to induce damage for a longer duration.[79] One-third of all vesicant extravasations will develop into ulcerations, and vigilant recognition and management of extravasation plays a major role in limiting tissue injury.[81] When extravasation is suspected, prompt discontinuation of the infusion is recommended, followed by aspiration of residual drug and removal of the catheter. Local cold

application and elevation of the affected extremity are commonly used and helpful.[80] Intermittent local cooling alone has an 89.1% success rate in preventing ulceration.[82] For the vinca alkaloids, heat application is recommended instead, as cold application may actually induce ulceration.[81]

The use of antidotes is controversial, and some antidotes such as sodium bicarbonate may be harmful or ulcerative. Sodium thiosulfate (mechlorethamine), hyaluronidase (vinca alkaloids), granulocyte macrophage colony-stimulating factor (doxorubicin), and pyridoxine (mitomycin) have been recommended as local injections.[83–85] The success of locally injected corticosteroids has been variable as few inflammatory cells are involved in extravasation reactions.[85] Whether a local antidote has a specific effect or acts as a diluent is hard to determine. Locally injected saline alone has proven successful in resolving extravasation reactions and preventing ulceration.[86] Although conservative treatment is preferable for most vesicant extravasations, early excision is sometimes favored, especially when the most potent vesicants are involved.[86,87] For topical therapy, the free-radical scavenger dimethyl sulfoxide (DMSO) has shown consistent therapeutic success. In 1995, an analysis of 96 cumulative patients from multiple studies showed that DMSO protected 98.3% of extravasation cases from ulceration.[88]

Pigmentary changes

Hyperpigmentation is a common cutaneous manifestation that may be of cosmetic concern to patients. The skin, mucous membranes, hair, teeth, and nails may be affected, and the reaction may be diffuse or localized. Hyperpigmentation most commonly accompanies use of alkylating agents, antitumor antibiotics, and gemcitabine (Table 8).[77] Among the antimetabolites, methotrexate (MTX) may produce a characteristic hair "flag sign" with horizontal hyperpigmented bands alternating with normal hair color in light-haired individuals.[77] Tegafur can induce hyperpigmentation of the palms, soles, nails, and glans penis in one-third of patients receiving the drug. A flagellate, band-like hyperpigmentation in areas of trauma also occurs with high incidence in 8–20% of patients receiving bleomycin (Figure 7). Busulfan's hyperpigmentation can mimic Addison disease, with symptoms of weakness, weight loss, and diarrhea, but with normal melanocyte stimulating hormone and adrenocorticotropic hormone serum levels.[69] The mechanism of chemotherapy-induced hyperpigmentation reactions is unknown but may involve direct toxicity, melanocyte stimulation, and postinflammatory changes. Although these reactions may occasionally be permanent, in most cases, discoloration will gradually resolve after the discontinuation of the chemotherapy.

Vitiligo, a complete absence of melanocytes resulting in depigmentation, is seen with targeted drug therapies, particularly those used in the treatment of metastatic melanoma (Table 9).[38,62,63] It presents with asymptomatic, depigmented patches, often symmetrical in distribution, not necessarily related to sites of disease. Although speculated to be related to disease response, this has not been proven.

Radiation-associated reactions

Radiation can include environmental exposure to UV rays as well as therapeutic radiation exposure. Three different types of reactions have been noted: enhancement, recall, and photosensitivity (Tables 10, 11).

Table 8 Chemotherapeutic agents associated with hyperpigmentation.

Alkylating agents	Antibiotics Nucleoside analogues	Antimetabolites	Miscellaneous combined regimens
Busulfan	Bleomycin	Fluorouracil	Bleomycin/doxorubicin/vincristine
Cisplatin	Dactinomycin	Methotrexate	Busulfan/cyclophosphamide
Cyclophosphamide	Daunorubicin	Tegafur	Cyclophosphamide/doxorubicin/vincristine/prednisone
Fotemustine	Doxorubicin	Brequinar sodium	Cyclophosphamide/etoposide/carboplatin
Ifosfamide	Mitoxantrone	Docetaxel	Doxorubicin/bleomycin/vinblastine/dacarbazine
Thiotepa	Plicamycin	Hydroxyurea	
Topical carmustine	Gemcitabine	Procarbazine	Ifosfamide/carboplatin/etoposide
Topical mechlorethamine	Troxacitabine	Vinorelbine	Methotrexate/cytarabine/L-asparaginase/daunorubicin/mercaptopurine/ cyclophosphamide

Source: Adapted from Ref. 69.

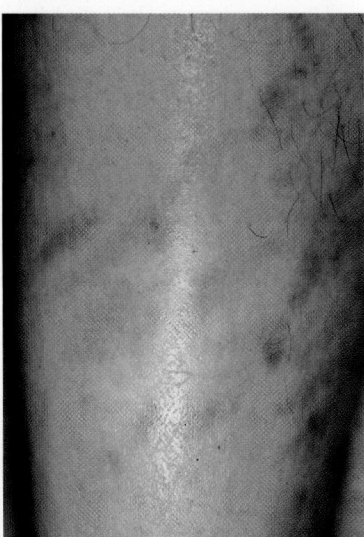

Figure 7 Cutaneous flagellate hyperpigmentation of bleomycin.

Table 10 Chemotherapeutic agents implicated in radiation-associated reactions.

Radiation enhancement	Radiation recall	
Bleomycin	Bleomycin	Hydroxyurea
Camptothecins	Cyclophosphamide	Idarubicin
Chlorambucil	Cytarabine	Lomustine
Cisplatin[a]	Dabrafenib	Melphalan
Cyclophosphamide[a]	Dactinomycin	Methotrexate
Dactinomycin	Daunorubicin	Oxaliplatin
Dabrafenib	Doxorubicin	Paclitaxel
Doxorubicin	Docetaxel	Tamoxifen
Fluorouracil	Edatrexate	Triazinate
Hydroxyurea	Etoposide	Trimetrexate
Interferons	Fluorouracil	Vemurafenib
Mercaptopurine	Gemcitabine	Vinblastine
Methotrexate		
Triazinate		
Vemurafenib		
Vincristine[a]		

[a]Reported only in combination drug regimens.
Source: Adapted from Ref. 69.

Table 9 Chemotherapeutic agents associated with depigmentation/vitiligo.

Vemurafenib	Gefitinib
Dabrafenib	Interferon
Pembrolizumab	IL-2
Imatinib	

Table 11 Chemotherapeutic agents associated with phototoxicity.

Brequinar sodium	Methotrexate
Dabrafenib	Mitomycin C
Dacarbazine	Porphyrins
Dactinomycin	Procarbazine
Doxorubicin	Tegafur
Fluorouracil	Thioguanine
Flutamide	Vemurafenib
Hydroxyurea	Vinblastine
	Vandetanib

Radiation enhancement

Enhancement of radiation therapy may occur when both chemo-therapy and radiation therapy are given within 1 week of each other. Although other organs are also affected in this potentiation, the skin is the most common site of this toxicity. The reaction may appear as dry or moist desquamation, or as erythema and edema. When bullae, erosions, and ulcerations accompany erythema, *Staphylo-coccus* is usually the causative factor.[89] The degree of enhancement of radiation damage depends on, and is inversely related to, the time interval between administration of the drug and radiation. The less time there is between chemotherapy and irradiation, the greater the enhancement effect.[90] Enhancement is also dependent on drug dosage and the pharmacologic mechanism of the drug.[75]

Radiation recall

Radiation recall is an erythematous inflammatory reaction in areas of previously irradiated skin or sunburned skin. This includes

the inflammation of AKs, which are caused by chronic sun exposure. Severe radiation dermatitis can even spread to areas outside the portal as an id reaction. Radiation recall occurs from 8 days up to 15 years after radiation therapy and may also occur in other organs.[77] The radiation dosage and the time interval between radiation and chemotherapy determine the occurrence and severity of recall, respectively.[91] The UV recall reaction is observed with suramin (35% incidence), MTX, vemurafenib, and etoposide/cyclophosphamide therapy, which causes a sunburn reac-tivation if the drugs are administered within 1 week of obtaining a sunburn.[92]

Inflammation of AKs is known as an AK recall reaction and is common in elderly patients with fair complexion and history of sun

Table 12 Chemotherapeutic agents associated with inflammation of actinic keratoses.

Dactinomycin/vincristine/dacarbazine
Docetaxel
Doxorubicin
Doxorubicin/cytarabine/thioguanine
Doxorubicin/vincristine
Fluorouracil
Fluorouracil/cisplatin
Pentaostatin

damage (Table 12). Suramin and cytarabine-induced inflammation of seborrheic keratosis and fludarabine-induced SCC have also been reported. The association between systemic fluorouracil and the irritation of clinical and subclinical AKs is well-known and resembles the effect produced by topical application of 5-FU. AK recall reactions usually appear 1 week following the initiation of drug administration; reactions usually resolve 1–4 weeks following the end of therapy, although they may regress during therapy as well.[93] This recall reaction may be due to a process similar to radiation recall or increased DNA synthesis in AK lesions and consequently higher chemoagent uptake.[93,94] Although these lesions are self-limiting, superficial ulceration and staphylococcal colonization can occur and necessitate antibiotics or corticosteroids. The reaction may or may not recur with drug readministration. Similar to the effect of topical 5-FU on AKs, systemic fluorouracil often clears the affected AKs after the inflammatory reaction resolves.[95]

The mechanism of the recall reaction is currently unknown, although it has been theorized that impaired tissue repair may be a result of inadequate stem cell reserve or mutations in cells that survived radiation.[96]

Generally, the treatment for radiation-associated reactions is symptomatic with an effort to avoid or treat secondary infections with appropriate antibiotics. Severe ulcerative and necrotic reactions may necessitate debridement. Topical mupirocin and systemic corticosteroids are mainstays in the treatment of radiation recall and may even allow continuation of the offending drug without further recall effects.[96]

Photosensitivity

Finally, cutaneous reactions related to chemotherapy and UV light exposure have been well documented, although they are relatively infrequent (Table 11). Generally, most of these reactions involve exogenous phototoxicity with the agents acting as chromophores. Both clinically and histologically, these phototoxic reactions appear as exaggerated sunburns. Phototoxicity has also been reported to affect the nails in the form of mercaptopurine-induced photo-onycholysis, which is tender and usually involves the distal third of the nail.

Another form of photosensitivity is the photoallergy that has been described with flutamide and tegafur, in which the photodistributed cutaneous reaction recurs with readministration of the implicated agent. This has also been observed with vandetanib.[97]

Therapy for photosensitivity reactions is symptomatic with topical corticosteroids and antipruritics. Severe cases may require systemic steroids. Chloroquine and β-carotene have been used for prophylaxis but were not effective in controlled studies.[98] As the agent may remain in the patient's skin for several weeks, patients should be advised to take sun-avoidance measures.

Acral reactions

Two types of acral reactions have been described; the more classical AE and HFSR seen with targeted therapies. AE has many names, including hand–foot syndrome and toxic erythema of chemotherapy (Table 13).

AE was first reported in association with chemotherapy by Zuehlke in 1974.[99] Other names include palmoplantar erythrodysesthesia, palmoplantar erythema, hand–foot syndrome, peculiar AE, and Burgdorf reaction. There is a prodrome of dysesthesia of the palms and soles, evolving into painful, tingling, symmetric, well-demarcated swelling and erythema (Figure 8), followed by a desquamative phase on resolution. Erythema and swelling usually appear on the thenar and hypothenar eminences, lateral aspect of the fingers, and the pads of the distal phalanges. The hands are more often affected than the feet. In its various manifestations, AE may appear as alternating bands of erythema and sparing and may also be accompanied by a mild erythema or a morbilliform eruption on the trunk, neck, chest, scalp, and extremities.[100] MTX and cytarabine can reportedly induce a bullous variant of AE, which may progress to full-thickness epidermal necrosis before resolving.[101]

AE occurs with an incidence of 6–42% in different series and occurs mostly in adults.[102] AE appears to be dose dependent on peak levels and total cumulative dose, as it occurs earlier and more severely after bolus infusions (24 h to 3 weeks), as compared with continuous low-dose administration (2–10 months).[100,103]

Table 13 Chemotherapeutic agents associated with acral erythema.

Most common		Least common	
Capecitabine	Cisplatin	Idarubicin	Paclitaxel
Cytarabine	Cyclophosphamide	Lomustine	Pegylated liposomal doxorubicin
Doxorubicin	Daunorubicin	Melphalan	Floxuridine
Fluorouracil	Docetaxel	Mercaptopurine	Suramin
	Doxifluridine	Methotrexate	Troxacitabine
	Etoposide	Mitomycin	Tegafur
	Hydroxyurea	Mitotane	Vincristine

Source: Adapted from Ref. 69.

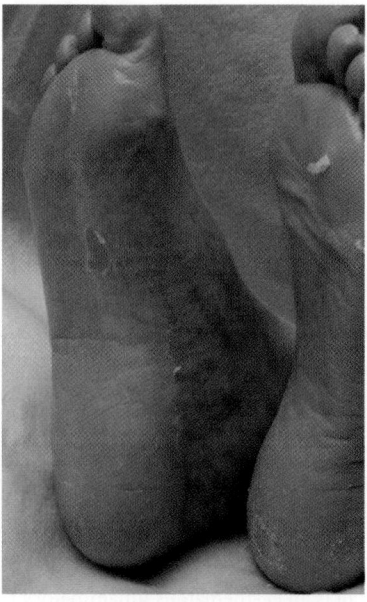

Figure 8 Chemo-induced acral erythema of the palms.

Table 14 Miscellaneous reactions and reactions associated with chemotherapy.

Bullous pemphigoid	Erythema nodosum	Flushing (cont)	Hirsutism (cont)
Dactinomycin/MTX	Busulfan	Plicamycin	Fluoxymesterone
Capillaritis	Diethylstilbestrol	Procarbazine	Tamoxifen
Aminoglutethimide	IL-2	Suramin	Nonmelanoma skin cancer
Cutaneous adherence, acquired	Fixed drug eruption	Tamoxifen	Nitrogen mustard (topical)
Doxorubicin/ketoconazole	Dacarbazine	Teniposide	BRAF inhibitors
Cutaneous ulcers	Hydroxyurea	Trimetrexate	Porphyria
Hydroxyurea	Paclitaxel (bullous)	Folliculitis	Cisplatin
IFN-α, pegylated IFN-α	Procarbazine	Dactinomycin	Porphyria cutanea tarda
IL-2	Flushing	Daunorubicin	Busulfan
Methotrexate	L-Asparaginase	Fluorouracil	Cyclophosphamide
Dermatitis herpetiformis, flare	Bleomycin	Methotrexate	Diethylstilbestrol
Cyclophosphamide/doxorubicin/vincristine	Carboplatin	EGFR inhibitors	Methotrexate
Bleomycin	Carmustine (BCNU)	Furunculosis	Acute intermittent porphyria
Cisplatin	Cisplatin	Fluoxymesterone	Chlorambucil
Vincristine	Cyclophosphamide	Methotrexate	Cyclophosphamide
Dermatomyositis-like reaction	Dacarbazine	Dactinomycin	Pustular psoriasis
Hydroxyurea	Didemnin B	Medroxyprogesterone	Aminoglutethimide
Tamoxifen	Diethylstilbestrol	Procarbazine	Pegylated liposomal doxorubicin
Tegafur	Docetaxel	Vinblastine	Seborrheic dermatitis, flare
Bleomycin	Doxorubicin	Hair color change	Fluorouracil
Docetaxel	Etoposide	Bleomycin	IL-2
Drug-induced SLE	Fluorouracil	Cisplatin	IFN-α
Aminoglutethimide	Flutamide	Cyclophosphamide	Telangiectasia
Diethylstilbestrol	IL-2	Methotrexate	Carmustine (BCNU)
Hydroxyurea	Leuprolide	Tamoxifen	Fluorouracil (topical)
Leuprolide	Lomustine	Hirsutism	Hydroxyurea
Tegafur	Paclitaxel	Diethylstilbestrol	IFN-α
IFN-α			

Abbreviations: EGFR, epidermal growth factor receptor; IFN-α, interferon-α; IgA, immunoglobulin A; IL-2, interleukin-2; MTX, methotrexate; SLE, systemic lupus erythematosus.

AE tends to persist and worsen with further continuation of chemotherapy and may be dose limiting, as the associated pain may progress to become physically and functionally limiting. Cessation of the causative agent will allow resolution of AE in 1–2 weeks, with desquamation and re-epithelialization (Figure 9). AE may or may not recur with readministration. The treatment of AE is symptomatic and aimed at increasing tolerability to allow continued chemotherapy. Corticosteroids have shown variable success. Supportive treatment includes topical wound care, elevation, and pain medication. Similar to the concept of scalp hypothermia for alopecia, the cooling of hands and feet may help prevent AE.[103] Celecoxib, a cyclooxygenase 2 (COX-2) inhibitor, was shown to decrease the incidence of AE in a retrospective study of 67 patients with metastatic colorectal cancer who took capecitabine.[104] Celecoxib also attenuated capecitabine-induced diarrhea, increased tumor response, and increased median time to tumor progression compared with capecitabine alone. Pyridoxine may also reduce dysesthesia and pain to allow continuation of therapy.[105]

The pathogenesis of AE is currently unknown, but it is likely multifactorial. Biopsies of AE appear histologically nonspecific but are consistent with a toxic reaction.[103] In the setting of chemotherapy, diagnosis of AE is a relatively simple matter. However, in bone marrow transplant (BMT) patients, it may be difficult to differentiate from acute GVHD. There is a 35% incidence of AE in BMT patients, which may be due to the use of higher doses of chemotherapy and total body irradiation.[106] Histologically and clinically, AE may resemble acute GVHD in the first 3 weeks: as in AE, the palms are commonly affected in acute GVHD although it usually progresses with involvement of other areas of the body. Since early biopsies of acute GVHD mimic AE, serial biopsies at 3–5-day intervals are helpful in establishing patterns of progression supportive of acute GVHD.[106] Distinguishing AE from acute GVHD is important because the latter requires greater intervention

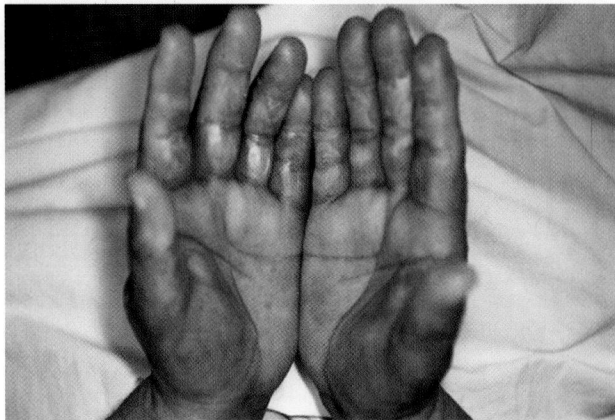

Figure 9 Desquamation phase of hand-and-foot syndrome, secondary to capecitabine.

with further immunosuppression; without treatment, it usually progresses and may be fatal.

HFSR is most commonly seen with multikinase inhibitors, sorafenib and sunitinib. It has also been reported with MEK inhibitors. It is distinguished from AE by the focal nature, overlying calluses, and tendency to vesiculate.

Cutaneous eruption of lymphocyte recovery

The cutaneous eruption of lymphocyte recovery (ELR) may be seen in patients receiving intensive marrow aplasia-inducing chemotherapy.[107] As with ESS, the ELR phenomenon has been observed with various cytotoxic agents but is not associated with a particular agent. Clinically, ELR has the appearance of variably distributed erythematous and pruritic macules, papules, and plaques, which may become confluent and erythrodermic, and is often associated with a couple of days of fever. In the setting of chemotherapy, this reaction has been found to occur 6–21 days after the chemotherapy-induced nadir of the leukocyte count, which correlates with the time of the initial recovery of peripheral lymphocytes. ELR may reflect the return of highly alloreactive immunocompetent lymphocytes to the peripheral circulation and skin.[107] ELR is self-limited and resolves over several days with desquamation and mild residual hyperpigmentation. The differential diagnosis includes acute GVHD, sepsis, viral exanthem, leukemia or lymphoma cutis, eccrine syringosquamous metaplasia, and drug hypersensitivity. Of these types of eruptions, acute GVHD is similar in time of onset to ELR in the setting of bone marrow transplantation. The similarity with ELR is especially true in the case of autologous GVHD, as both involve a lymphocytic recovery in which histocompatibility is present. However, acute autologous GVHD cannot be reliably distinguished from ELR by skin biopsy.[108] As theorized by Horn, GVHD may represent a prolonged form of ELR.[109]

Key references

The complete reference list can be found on the Wiley Companion Digital Edition of this title (see inside front cover for login instructions).

1 Revuz J, Valeyrie-Allanore L. Drug reactions. In: Bolognia J, Jorizzo J, Schaffer J, et al., eds. *Dermatology*, 3rd ed. Philadephia: Elsevier Saunders; 2012, Chapter 21.

2 Sidoroff A, Halevy S, Bavinck JB, et al. Acute generalized exanthematous pustulosis (AGEP)óa clinical reaction pattern. *J Cutan Pathol*. 2001;**28**:113–119.

6 Busam KJ, Capodieci P, Motzer R, et al. Cutaneous side-effects in cancer patients treated with the antiepidermal growth factor receptor antibody C225. *Br J Dermatol*. 2001;**144(6)**:1169–1176.

9 Boone SL, Rademaker A, Liu D, Pfeiffer C, Mauro DJ, Lacouture ME. Impact and management of skin toxicity associated with anti-epidermal growth factor receptor therapy: survey results. *Oncology*. 2007;**72(3-4)**:152–159.

10 Saltz LB, Meropol NJ, Loehrer PJ, Needle MN, Kopit J, Mayer RJ. Phase II trial of cetuximab in patients with refractory colorectal cancer that expresses the epidermal growth factor receptor. *J Clin Oncol*. 2004;**22**:1201–1208.

11 Lacouture ME. Mechanisms of cutaneous toxicities to EGFR inhibitors. *Nat Rev Cancer*. 2006;**6(10)**:803–812.

18 Drucker AM, Wu S, Dang CT, Lacouture ME. Risk of rash with the anti-HER2 dimerization antibody pertuzumab: a meta-analysis. *Breast Cancer Res Treat*. 2012;**135(2)**:347–354.

22 Amitay-laish I, Stemmer SM, Lacouture ME. Adverse cutaneous reactions secondary to tyrosine kinase inhibitors including imatinib mesylate, nilotinib, and dasatinib. *Dermatol Ther*. 2011;**24(4)**:386–395.

23 Balagula Y, Lacouture ME, Cotliar JA. Dermatologic toxicities of targeted anticancer therapies. *J Support Oncol*. 2010;**8(4)**:149–161.

24 Chu D, Lacouture ME, Fillos T, Wu S. Risk of hand-foot skin reaction with sorafenib: a systematic review and meta-analysis. *Acta Oncol*. 2008;**47(2)**:176–186.

25 Chu D, Lacouture ME, Weiner E, Wu S. Risk of hand-foot skin reaction with the multitargeted kinase inhibitor sunitinib in patients with renal cell and non-renal cell carcinoma: a meta-analysis. *Clin Genitourin Cancer*. 2009;**7(1)**:11–19.

27 Boyd KP, Vincent B, Andea A, Conry RM, Hughey LC. Nonmalignant cutaneous findings associated with vemurafenib use in patients with metastatic melanoma. *J Am Acad Dermatol*. 2012;**67(6)**:1375–1379.

29 Balagula Y, Rosen A, Tan BH, et al. Clinical and histopathologic characteristics of rash in cancer patients treated with mammalian target of rapamycin inhibitors. *Cancer*. 2012;**118(20)**:5078–5083.

30 Lacouture ME, Duvic M, Hauschild A, et al. Analysis of dermatologic events in vemurafenib-treated patients with melanoma. *Oncologist*. 2013;**18(3)**:314–322.

31 Infante J, Falchook G, Lawrence D, et al. Phase I/II study to assess safety, pharmacokinetics, and efficacy of the oral MEK 1/2 inhibitor GSK1120212 (GSK 212) dosed in combination with the oral BRAF inhibitor GSK2118436 (GSK436) [abstract 8503]. *J Clin Oncol*. 2011;**29(suppl)**:CRA8503.

32 Zimmer L, Livingstone E, Hillen U, Dömkes S, Becker A, Schadendorf D. Panniculitis with arthralgia in patients with melanoma treated with selective BRAF inhibitors and its management. *Arch Dermatol*. 2012;**148(3)**:357–361.

42 Pulvirenti T, Hong A, Clements A, et al. Acute Radiation Skin Toxicity Associated With BRAF Inhibitors. *J Clin Oncol*. 2014.

46 Anforth R, Fernandez-peñas P, Long GV. Cutaneous toxicities of RAF inhibitors. *Lancet Oncol*. 2013;**14(1)**:e11–e18.

49 Huang V, Hepper D, Anadkat M, Cornelius L. Cutaneous toxic effects associated with vemurafenib and inhibition of the BRAF pathway. *Arch Dermatol*. 2012;**148(5)**:628–633.

57 Trefzer U, Minor D, Ribas A, et al. BREAK-2: a phase IIA trial of the selective BRAF kinase inhibitor GSK2118436 in patients with BRAF (V660E/K) -positive metastatic melanoma. *Pigment Cell Melanoma Res*. 2012;**25**:E2.

58 Hauschild A, Grob J-J, Demidov LV, et al. Dabrafenib in BRAF-mutated metastatic melanoma: a multicentre, open-label, phase 3 randomised controlled trial. *Lancet*. 2012;**380**:358–365.

59 Cohen PR, Bedikian AY, Kim KB. Appearance of New Vemurafenib-associated Melanocytic Nevi on Normal-appearing Skin: Case Series and a Review of Changing or New Pigmented Lesions in Patients with Metastatic Malignant Melanoma After Initiating Treatment with Vemurafenib. *J Clin Aesthet Dermatol*. 2013;**6(5)**:27–37.

61 Curry JL, Torres-cabala CA, Kim KB, et al. Dermatologic toxicities to targeted cancer therapy: shared clinical and histologic adverse skin reactions. *Int J Dermatol*. 2014;**53(3)**:376–384.

62 Lacouture ME, Wolchok JD, Yosipovitch G, Kähler KC, Busam KJ, Hauschild A. Ipilimumab in patients with cancer and the management of dermatologic adverse events. *J Am Acad Dermatol*. 2014;**71(1)**:161–169.

63 Hamid O, Robert C, Daud A, et al. Safety and tumor responses with lambrolizumab (anti-PD-1) in melanoma. *N Engl J Med*. 2013;**369(2)**:134–144.

64 Wolkenstein P, Chosidow O, Wechsler J, et al. Cutaneous side effects associated with interleukin-2 administration for metastatic melanoma. *J Am Acad Dermatol*. 1993;**28**:66–70.

69 DeSpain JD. Dermatologic toxicity of chemotherapy. *Semin Oncol*. 1992;**19**:501–507.

71 Hood AF. Dermatologic toxicity. In: Perry MC, ed. *The chemotherapy source book*, 2nd ed. Baltimore: Williams & Wilkins; 1996:595–606.

74 Dmytriw AA, Morzycki W, Green PJ. Prevention of alopecia in medical and interventional chemotherapy patients. *J Cutan Med Surg*. 2014;**18**:1–6.

77 Susser WS, Whitaker-Worth DL, Grant-Kels JM. Mucocutaneous reactions to chemotherapy. *J Am Acad Dermatol*. 1999;**40**:367–398.

79 Rudolph R, Larson DL. Etiology and treatment of chemotherapeutic agent extravasation injuries: a review. *J Clin Oncol*. 1987;**5**:1116–1126.

89 Hill A, Hanson M, Bogle MA, Duvic M. Severe radiation dermatitis is related to *Staphylococcus aureus*. *Am J Clin Oncol*. 2004;**27**:362–363.

90 Houtee PV, Danhier S, Mornex F. Toxicity of combined radiation and chemotherapy in non-small cell lung cancer. *Lung Cancer*. 1994;**10**:S271–S280.

93 Johnson T, Rapini R, Duvic M. Inflammation of actinic keratoses from systemic chemotherapy. *J Am Acad Dermatol*. 1987;**17**:192–197.

97 Fava P, Quaglino P, Fierro MT, Novelli M, Bernengo MG. Therapeutic hotline. A rare vandetanib-induced photo-allergic drug eruption. *Dermatol Ther*. 2010;**23(5)**:553–555.

103 Baack BR, Burgdorf WHC. Chemotherapy-induced acral erythema. *J Am Acad Dermatol*. 1991;**24**:457–461.

107 Horn TD, Redd JV, Karp JE, et al. Cutaneous eruptions of lymphocyte recovery. *Arch Dermatol*. 1989;**215**:1512–1517.

108 Bauer DJ, Hood AF, Horn TD. Histologic comparison of autologous graft-vs-host reaction and cutaneous eruption of lymphocyte recovery. *Arch Dermatol*. 1993;**129**:855–858.

128 Skeletal complications

Michael A. Via, MD ▪ Ilya Iofin, MD ▪ Jeffrey I. Mechanick, MD

Overview

Metabolic bone disease is highly prevalent among cancer patients, owing to the systemic effects of malignancy, the humoral response, and to commonly prescribed cancer therapies. Surgical approaches to acute fracture can drastically impact quality of life. The use of bone antiresorptive agents can prevent fractures in this population and can reduce bone pain in patients with skeletal metastases.

Introduction

Cancer continues to remain a major public health concern as 44% of American men and 38% of women develop cancer at some point in their lifetime. It is estimated that there will be 1,658,370 new cancer cases in the United States in 2015.[1] As cancer treatments evolve and survival of patients with cancer continues to improve, skeletal complications of cancer are becoming more prevalent. These complications include pain associated with metastases to bone, fractures, and hypercalcemia of malignancy. The skeleton is the most common site of metastatic disease with ~70% of patients dying of cancer having skeletal metastases detected on autopsy. A significant portion of these metastases will be clinically relevant and require treatment (*see Chapter 111*, Table 8).[2] Once a patient develops skeletal metastases, cure is very unlikely and it must be understood by both the patient and the treating physicians that the goal of treatment is palliation and not cure.[2] The five most common cancer types that metastasize to bone are breast, prostate, lung, renal, and thyroid. Almost any cancer subtype can metastasize to bone; however, multiple myeloma is the most common malignancy originating in bone and is responsible for significant skeletal-associated morbidity. As in cases of metastatic carcinoma, cure is unlikely, though systemic control is possible and survival times are improving with evolving therapies. The treatment of problems arising from malignant disease affecting bone requires a multidisciplinary approach involving medical, orthopedic, and radiation oncologists.

Evaluation of a patient with bone lesions

Evaluation of a patient starts with a careful history and physical examination. Location of pain, inciting and alleviating factors, prior history cancer, and of prior treatments are all required to formulate an appropriate treatment plan. In addition to metastases being the potential source of disability, coexisting arthritis and other orthopedic conditions may be the cause of the patient's pain while the presence of the metastasis may be purely incidental. Imaging of the bone affected by metastatic disease is first done with orthogonal plain radiographs visualizing the entire length bone as the process may be multifocal (Figure 1). Bone lesions may be purely lytic (where only bone destruction is seen, as is

typical of lymphoma, multiple myeloma, lung, renal, and thyroid cancer metastases), blastic (where abnormal bone deposition is seen, as is common in metastatic prostate cancer), or mixed (usual for breast cancer metastases). While radioactive technetium bone scans and MRI are very sensitive modalities for detecting metastases, a noncontrast computed tomography (CT) is superior for the evaluation of bone integrity and is often needed to make decisions regarding potential need for surgical intervention. Again, the entire length of the involved bone should be imaged in order to accurately assess fracture risk and help guide potential surgical intervention.

Solitary lesions of bone

Special attention needs to be drawn to the patient with a solitary bone lesion but no biopsy-proven metastatic disease. While prior cancer history makes it likely that the newly seen lesion is a metastasis of that cancer, there is no guarantee of that, so a thorough evaluation is required before any intervention. One of the worst errors one could make is to presume that a patient has metastatic disease and failing to recognize a primary bone sarcoma that might be curable. While sarcomas usually affect teenagers and young adults, they can occur in all age groups. The treatment of sarcoma is radically different from treatment of metastatic carcinoma, multiple myeloma, and lymphoma. Bone sarcoma surgery usually entails wide resection of the tumor with curative intent, while most metastatic lesions are treated with intralesional procedures where palliation is the goal. One of the most common orthopedic procedures done for metastatic disease is intramedullary nailing. An intramedullary nail inadvertently placed through a bone sarcoma leads to contamination of the entire length of the bone as well as of the surrounding soft tissues. A patient in whom limb salvage maybe have been possible before intramedullary nailing will require a much more disabling resection at best and a high-level amputation such as a hemipelvectomy at worst. In addition, reaming of the medullary canal pushes sarcoma cells into the systemic circulation and the lungs, making metastatic disease and death more likely.[3] Even in the presence of a pathologic fracture through a sarcoma, limb salvage with modern chemotherapy and surgical modalities is possible in most cases if fracture healing can be achieved with cast immobilization or minimally invasive fixation methods that do not lead to tissue contamination.[4] Knowledge of the exact tumor diagnosis is required to guide appropriate treatment.

Thus, when presented a patient with an uncertain cancer diagnosis, in addition to evaluation of the affected bone, further staging studies should be undertaken. A CT of the chest, abdomen, and pelvis with oral and IV contrast should be performed to look for visceral metastases and a potential primary tumor. Other skeletal metastases can be detected with a technetium-99 whole body bone scan while detection of a monoclonal spike in serum and/or urine

Holland-Frei Cancer Medicine, Ninth Edition. Edited by Robert C. Bast Jr., Carlo M. Croce, William N. Hait, Waun Ki Hong, Donald W. Kufe, Martine Piccart-Gebhart, Raphael E. Pollock, Ralph R. Weichselbaum, Hongyang Wang, and James F. Holland.
© 2017 John Wiley & Sons, Inc. ISBN: 978-1-118-93469-2

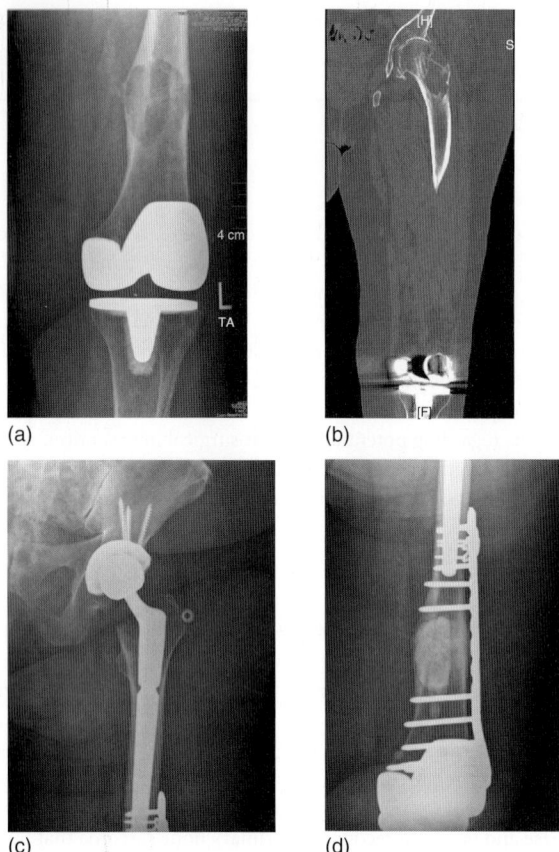

(a)   (b)

(c)   (d)

Figure 1 (a) An 81-year-old woman with metastatic breast cancer with a chief complaint of knee pain. Note the destructive lesion in the distal femoral metaphysics above a well-fixed total knee arthroplasty (b) A noncontrast CT of the entire femur was obtained, demonstrating an additional destructive lesion in the femoral neck. While the lesion was asymptomatic, it was at high risk of sustaining a displaced pathologic fracture. Significant degenerative changes are also seen in the hip joint. (c) and (d) The distal femoral lesion was treated with intralesional curettage, internal fixation with a locking plate, and packing with PMMA bone cement. A press-fit long stem total hip arthroplasty was performed to treat the femoral neck lesion and the arthritis. Note the overlap of the two implants that minimize the risk of periprosthetic fracture and protects the entire length of the bone.

by immunofixation or protein electrophoresis can help establish the diagnosis of multiple myeloma.[5] Bone scintigraphy detects new bone deposition in response to tumor activity, trauma, or degenerative joint disease. While it is a sensitive modality for detecting skeletal metastases in most cases, multiple myeloma, metastatic renal cell, and thyroid carcinomas are usually purely lytic in nature where there is little bone deposition. Lesions from these tumors can be missed by bone scintigraphy. When one of these diagnoses is suspected, a skeletal survey (which consists of AP radiographs of the long bones, chest, and pelvis and lateral radiographs of the spine and skull) should be obtained. Positron emission tomography (PET) CT is another sensitive modality for staging, though its exact indications are still being determined. All discovered sites of skeletal involvement should be further evaluated for risk of fracture that may require treatment. Prostate-specific antigen (PSA) levels, usually elevated in patients with metastatic prostate cancer, should be checked in men where this diagnosis is suspected.

This systematic approach will distinguish patients with multiple bone and visceral lesions in whom metastatic disease or multiple myeloma or lymphoma is suspected from the rare patients with solitary bone lesions in whom suspicion of primary bone sarcoma is higher. There are additional benefits to this evaluation algorithm. The most accessible site for biopsy can be found, which can be different from the site of the patient's original complaint. Metastatic renal cell and thyroid carcinomas are well known to be hypervascular and can hemorrhage significantly during biopsy. Prior knowledge of these diagnoses is useful, as preoperative tumor embolization can be performed and preparations made accordingly.

The final diagnosis, though often suspected based on the radiographic evaluation, is confirmed with a tissue biopsy. If the treating physician is confident of the diagnosis before surgical intervention based on radiographic findings or a known history of metastatic carcinoma or multiple myeloma with confirmatory laboratory findings, an intraoperative frozen section can be used to confirm the diagnosis. Care must be exercised, though, as frozen section is not 100% accurate and provides the correct diagnosis only in 86–94% of biopsies of skeletal lesions.[6] If a sarcoma is suspected, then definitive treatment should be delayed until final histologic diagnosis is made. In addition, the reliability of frozen section is dependent on the experience of the pathologist. Most pathologists have limited experience with primary bone tumors. It is important to note that the biopsy tract, especially in cases of an open biopsy, is contaminated by tumor cells and needs to be resected. While that is of little consequence in metastatic disease or multiple myeloma, in cases of sarcoma, inappropriate placement of the biopsy has been shown to adversely affect outcomes, even leading to unnecessary amputations in 4.5% of cases.[7] Therefore, biopsy should be performed at a tertiary referral center by, or at least in coordination with, a surgeon with training and expertise in the treatment of bone sarcomas.

Options for treatment of skeletal lesions

A range of treatment options exists for skeletal lesions: it spans the spectrum from observation for asymptomatic lesions that do not present a fracture risk to operative intervention for displaced and impending pathologic fractures. In addition to systemic therapy for the cancer, treatment with bisphophonates or denosumab has been shown to reduce the number of skeletal events, such as compression fractures of the vertebrae and need for surgery or radiotherapy in patients with metastatic bone disease and multiple myeloma.[8] Radiation therapy provides pain relief in about 70% of treated lesions. Various therapeutic regimens exist: 8 Gy single-dose treatments have shown similar efficacy to the more traditional and longer 30 Gy 10-day course. Occasionally, the cancer pain recurs, requiring repeat treatment, which is easier to perform with the single-dose treatments.[8] Tumors of different histology have different sensitivity to radiation. Multiple myeloma, lymphoma, prostate, and breast cancers are known for their radiosensitivity while renal cell carcinoma is relatively radioresistant.[9] Sensitivity to systemic and radiation therapies is one of many factors when choosing most appropriate treatment for a patient with a skeletal lesion. Radiation is most appropriate for lesions that do not present a significant fracture risk. The pelvis, spine, ribs, and scapulae are appropriate sites for radiation treatment in the majority of cases, while lesions of the long bones, especially in the lower extremity, present a higher fracture risk and should be evaluated for potential surgical intervention.

In patients with small lesions that are not structurally significant, where radiation has not provided pain relief, radiofrequency ablation (RFA) and cryoablation are useful minimally invasive treatment options. Under CT guidance, a probe is placed into the lesion to allow local treatment. In RFA, the needle probe delivers a high-frequency alternating current into the surrounding tissues, resulting in heat necrosis. Polymethyl methacrylate (PMMA bone cement) may be injected into the void left by the tumor to provide structural support and additional pain relief.[10] Cryoablation is a thermal technique that is conceptually similar to RFA, in which the tumor cells are destroyed not by heating but by cycles of rapid freezing with pressurized argon gas passing through the probe placed in the lesion, followed by slow thawing. Unlike RFA, the zone of thermal necrosis can be visualized on CT. Both modalities can be combined with percutaneous PMMA injection.[11] Such image guided thermal ablation techniques are most appropriate for lesions that present minimal risk of fracture, such as vertebral body, sacral and iliac wing lesions, and many acetabular lesions. Once fracture is present or the bone is at significant risk of fracture due to loss of structural integrity, surgery is usually required. Where clinical considerations weight against surgical intervention, particularly in vertebral metastases, PMMA stabilization can relieve pain and restore patient mobility.

Principles of pathologic fracture treatment

The goals of pathologic fracture treatment are to improve function and provide pain relief. The patient and his or her family must be informed and have to understand that the goal of treatment is palliative in nature and will not result in cure. Risk of complications has to be carefully balanced against the potential benefit. Though survival time of cancer patients is difficult to predict, it should exceed the expected surgical recovery time. Pathologic fractures often fail to heal and when they do heal, they are slow to do so. In a series of 123 patients with 129 pathologic fractures, the overall fracture healing rate was only 35%. In patients who survived for more than 6 months, that rate went up to 74%.[12] This, and the fact that patients with pathologic fractures have multiple systemic comorbidities, must be kept in mind when selecting the optimal treatment approach. Unlike conventional fractures without an underlying malignancy, where union is likely after a relatively short period of restricted weight bearing, in pathologic fractures, such expectation cannot be made. Fixation must be sufficiently durable to allow nearly immediate almost unrestricted weight bearing and last for the entire lifetime of the patient. Multiple surgeries are not a desirable option. Chemotherapeutic regimens are cytotoxic and are often interrupted to allow wound healing from surgery. As systemic disease can progress during such interruptions of systemic treatment, all efforts should be made to minimize the duration and number of interruptions by minimizing the need for multiple surgeries.

The bone affected by tumor is of poor structural integrity, which is what led it to fracture in the first place. Intralesional resection of the tumor and augmentation of the fixation with PMMA bone cement are often required to both provide sufficient stability to the fixation construct and to obtain better local control of the tumor. Addition of bone cement to internal fixation has been shown to provide pain relief that is superior to internal fixation alone[13] and provides a more biomechanically stable construct.[14] Bone grafting is not used in the treatment of metastatic disease or multiple myeloma as the bone graft cannot be expected to incorporate in a patient being treated with chemotherapy and radiation. PMMA bone cement provides immediate stability, is cheap and easy to use, making it preferable to bone grafting. Fracture healing can occur in the presence of bone cement (Figure 3). In addition to tumor

debulking with curettage and high-speed burring to lower risk of recurrence, cryosurgery can be used as a treatment modality in cases of relatively radioresistant tumors where prolonged patient survival is likely, such as in cases of oligometastatic renal cell carcinoma.[15]

Treatment options for pathologic fractures consist of intramedullary nailing, fixation with plates and screws, endoprosthetic replacement, and resection of bone without reconstruction. Choice of treatment depends on tumor biology, location, and surrounding bone integrity. For example, a pathologic fracture of the clavicle due to multiple myeloma, which is both chemo- and radiosensitive, will usually respond well to nonoperative treatment, whereas the same clavicle fracture due to metastatic renal cell carcinoma is best treated with resection of the clavicle. Radiation treatment is an important adjunct to surgical treatment of bone lesions as it reduces the likelihood of tumor progression that might require reoperation and improves function. In one series, it has been shown to reduce the need for reoperation from 15% seen in the group that received surgery alone to only 3% in the group that had radiation treatment after surgery.[16]

Intramedullary nailing

Intramedullary nailing is the most commonly used surgical method of treatment of metastatic disease affecting appendicular bones because of its many advantages. The entire length of the bone is protected by the length of the nail, so if other lesions develop within the same bone, further surgery may not be necessary. The surgery can be done in a minimally invasive manner, allowing for a quicker recovery and a lower surgical risk. In some cases though, depending on fracture characteristics and the sensitivity of the tumor to chemotherapy and radiation, an open approach and placement of PMMA bone cement is required. Relatively radiation-resistant tumors such as metastatic renal cell carcinoma are more likely to require an open approach to lower the risk of complications associated with local tumor progression. The nail can be embedded into the bone cement that has been injected along the entire length the intramedullary canal to enhance construct stability (Figure 2) or, alternatively, cement can be packed around the nail into the defect left by the tumor (Figure 3).

The femur is the most common bone to be treated with intramedullary nailing. A cephalomedullary nail is preferable as the lag screw provides fixation of the femoral neck, a site that is commonly affected by metastatic disease or multiple myeloma. Metaphyseal and diaphyseal humeral lesions are also amenable to intramedullary nailing. The tibia is rarely affected by metastatic disease or multiple myeloma, but intramedullary nailing can be performed in those rare cases. Even more rare are lesions of the long bones of the forearm; however, in selected cases, intramedullary nailing of pathologic forearm fractures can be used safely and effectively instead of the more traditional fixation with plates and screws used in that location.

There must be sufficient bone in both the proximal and distal aspects of the long bone to allow the nail to have sufficient fixation and biomechanical stability. While it is best suited for diaphyseal lesions, intramedullary nailing can be safely used in metaphyseal locations where there is sufficient distance from the joint to allow good fixation. Lesions of the femoral neck are best suited for treatment with arthroplasty and lesions of the humeral head are treated with arthroplasty or plate and screw fixation with cement augmentation.

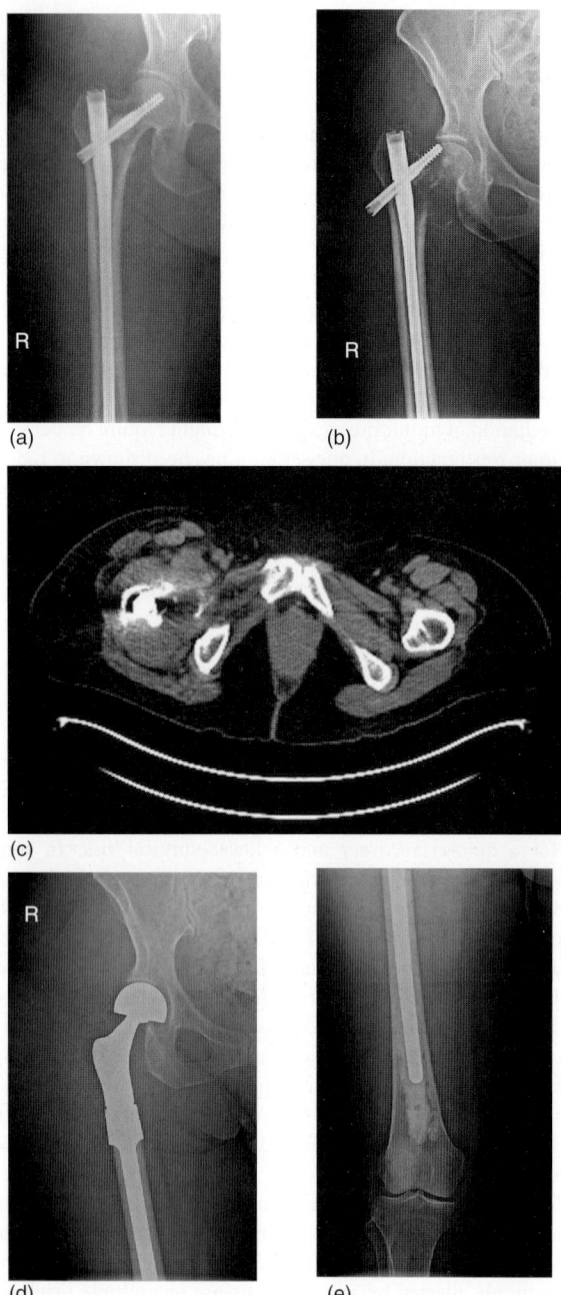

(a)　　　　　　　(b)

(c)

(d)　　　　　　　(e)

Figure 2 (a) A 67-year-old lady who underwent an intramedullary nailing at an outside institution for a painful lesion in the right femoral neck. No preoperative staging was performed. Femoral canal reamings that were sent to pathology showed metastatic renal cell carcinoma. Note the minimal amount of bone destruction present. A small amount of bone cement was injected along the lag screw at the time of surgery. (b) X-rays obtained 6 weeks after surgery show rapid progression of the tumor and destruction of much of the femoral neck and greater trochanter with failure of hardware. (c) CT of the pelvis demonstrates a large tumor mass engulfing the proximal femur. (d) and (e) The patient underwent resection of the tumor, removal of hardware, and a modular proximal femoral replacement. This case underscores the importance of a preoperative staging evaluation of a patient with bone lesions. Had it been performed and the diagnosis of renal cell carcinoma been known at the time of the initial procedure, extensive tumor curettage with an adjuvant and a hemiarthroplasty could have been done, saving the patient from the morbidity of a second more extensive surgical procedure.

Plate and screw fixation

The locking plate technology has revolutionized fracture fixation in general and has also become an invaluable tool in the treatment of pathologic fractures. In contrast to traditional plating techniques that rely on friction of the plate against bone, locking plate technology creates a fixed-angle device where the head of each screw is secured into the plate. Thus, for the construct to fail, all the screws need to fail together, requiring far greater force. In conventional plating, screws can fail sequentially, requiring less force for failure of the entire construct. Locking plates have been shown to be an excellent choice for treatment of fractures close to joints where traditional fixation methods have not provided optimal results.[17] Locking plates in conjunction with liberal use of PMMA bone cement should be used in preference to conventional plates whenever possible. They are best suited for locations near a joint, such as the distal femur, proximal tibia, and proximal and distal humeri where there is insufficient fixation for an intramedullary nail. They are preferable to a joint arthroplasty as they potentially provide better functional results.[18] In addition, this fixation method can be used when another implant, such as a total joint arthroplasty or previous fracture fixation would interfere with placement of an intramedullary device (Figure 1).

Arthroplasty

Joint arthroplasty is reserved for lesions that are so close to the joint that neither intramedullary nailing nor plate and screw fixation will provide reliable stable fixation. It is most commonly used for lesions of the femoral head and neck, especially because even conventional displaced fractures in the geriatric patients have a low union rate. Arthroplasty has even been shown to have superior results to internal fixation for intertrochanteric and subtrochanteric lesions, though the subgroup of patients in whom tumor was removed and internal fixation was augmented with PMMA bone cement fared much better than those in whom internal fixation alone was performed.[19] In cases of diaphyseal fractures where the tumor involves the point of interlocking screw fixation, the use of arthroplasty is preferred over the use of an intramedullary nail as the interlocking screws will not have sufficient support within bone weakened by tumor and are likely to cut out of the bone (Figure 4). Pain from acetabular wear is not a significant concern in oncology patients with a limited life expectancy, so the higher dislocation risk and the longer surgical time associated with a total hip arthroplasty are not justified. A hemiarthroplasty is preferable except in cases of severe pre-existing arthritis or an acetabular lesion requiring surgical intervention (Figure 1). Hemiarthroplasty can also be used for lesions of the proximal humerus where there is not sufficient bone stock to allow fixation with joint sparing implants.

For isolated lesions of the head and neck of the femur, a conventional arthroplasty is used by some surgeons while others use a cemented long stem hemiarthroplasty to protect much of the length of the femur from progression of metastatic disease. In lesions affecting much of the proximal femur, a long stem hemiarthroplasty is needed (Figure 4). This procedure is affected by an approximately 2% risk of intraoperative cardiac arrest and 1% risk of intraoperative or early postoperative mortality associated with the use of pressurized bone cement. As the risk of such an adverse event can be lowered, communication with the anesthesia team is mandatory before and during cementation of the prosthesis. Placement of venting holes in the distal femur before cementation has been shown to lower the

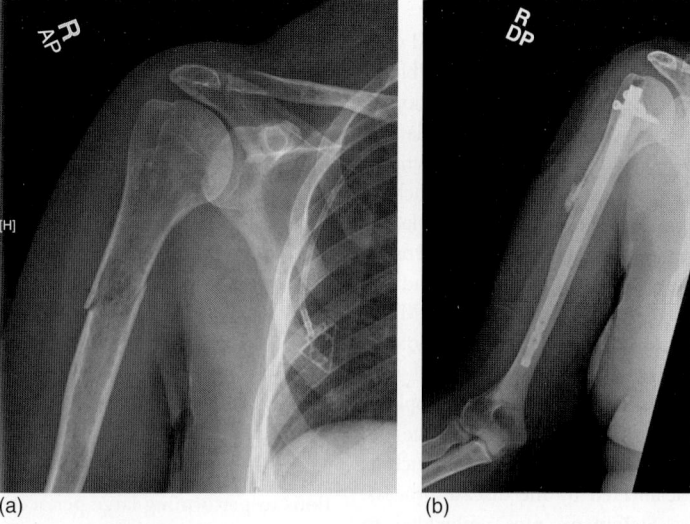

(a)   (b)

Figure 3 (a) A 49-year-old woman with multiple myeloma who sustained a pathologic right proximal humerus fracture. (b) The fracture was sufficiently distal to allow the use of a cemented intramedullary nail. Note the cement mantle going up to the proximal diaphysis. Distal interlocking screws were not used as the entire nail is supported by bone cement.

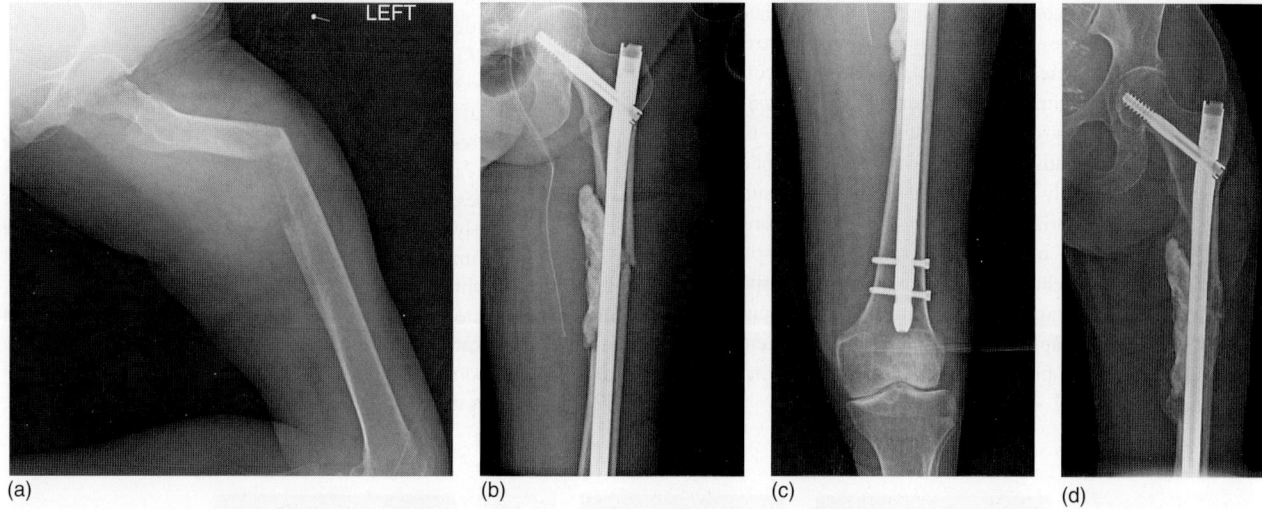

(a)   (b)   (c)   (d)

Figure 4 (a) A 57-year-old woman with metastatic cancer who sustained a left femoral midshaft diaphyseal fracture. (b) and (c) The patient underwent resection curettage of the tumor, intramedullary nailing, and packing of PMMA bone cement around the nail into the defect left by the tumor. (d) 4 months later, the fracture line over the lateral cortex is no longer visible and bone callus is seen, indicating healing of the fracture. Note the fracture callus forming on the medial side around the cement.

intramedullary pressure, but unfortunately no data exist that would demonstrate that this translates into a lower clinical risk of intraoperative cardiac arrest.[20] The venting hole can theoretically act as a stress riser, leading to a fracture distal to the prosthesis.

Megaprostheses

While large oncologic endoprosthetic devices are usually used to reconstruct the large defects left by resection of bone sarcomas, occasionally their use is required in the treatment of metastatic disease and multiple myeloma. The main indications for their use are threefold. One is when the tumor is so extensive and bone stock is so poor, that neither an osteosynthetic device nor conventional arthroplasty is feasible. The second indication is for prior failed fixation due to tumor progression or hardware failure due to a nonunion. The third indication is for the rare patient with a solitary metastatic lesion where resection of the lesion may improve long-term survival. While megaprostheses are an appropriate choice in selected cases, they are associated with a longer operative time, higher complication rate, such as infection and dislocation, and prolonged recovery. Location of the lesion also plays a role as excellent function can be expected in the distal and proximal femoral replacements, while the function of proximal tibial and proximal and distal humeral replacements is inferior. In cases where there is a large diaphyseal defect, an intercalary prosthesis can be used instead of an intramedullary nail. This device has been shown to be more biomechanically stable than an intramedullary nail even with cement augmentation.[21] At least 5 cm of intramedullary canal length is required on each side of the prosthesis to allow the cementation of the stems.

Treatment of periacetabular lesions

Surgical treatment of periacetabular lesions can be associated with significant morbidity, complications, and intraoperative blood loss. Fortunately, many of these lesions respond well to nonoperative measures such as weight bearing restrictions and radiation. Small lesions resistant to radiation may be treated with cementoplasty that can be combined with ablative techniques such as cryosurgery or RFA. However, surgery is required in selected patients with sufficient life expectancy who fail nonoperative treatment. In cases where there is sufficient bone stock and the subchondral plate is preserved, intralesional curettage and PMMA cement packing can be effective. In cases of displaced pathologic acetabular fractures or large lesions affecting the medial wall and/or the subchondral plate, a complex total hip arthroplasty is required. The goal of the reconstruction is to distribute the forces from the acetabulum to the portions of the pelvis, such as ilium and ischium, that are not affected by the disease process. Antiprotrusio acetabular cages, Steinmann pins embedded in the ilium, and bone cement to fill the defect left by the tumor are commonly used. In rare cases where bone destruction is so significant that even reconstruction with a cage will not provide sufficient mechanical support, the use of a partial pelvic prosthetic replacement can be considered, though it is associated with a high complication rate. The last surgical option for treatment of acetabular lesions is resection arthroplasty without reconstruction. It is associated with limb length inequality of about 5 cm and a decline in ambulatory capacity, though ambulation is not precluded, but holds the advantages of having a low complication rate and being a technically quick and relatively simple surgery. This option is most appropriate for patients in whom a more extensive reconstruction would be medically contraindicated or who are nonambulatory at baseline.[22] Periacetabular tumors, especially due to multiple myeloma and renal cell and thyroid carcinoma may be quite vascular, so appropriate preparation for potential transfusion is required and preoperative tumor embolization should be considered.

Resection without reconstruction

While metastatic disease most frequently affects the axial skeleton and proximal femora and humeri, there are instances of metastatic disease to smaller bones such as the clavicle, proximal radius, distal ulna, and proximal fibula. These bones are very slender and implanted hardware has a high risk of failure, even if fixation is augmented with bone cement. Fortunately, excellent function can be obtained with resection of bone from these locations without reconstruction. Once the fractured bone segment or the entire bone is resected, there is no fracture to heal, and excellent pain relief is obtained. This approach allows reduction of surgical time and lower risk of complications while providing results that are equivalent, if not superior, to fracture fixation. As discussed earlier, resection of the femoral head and hip joint without reconstruction is also a good surgical option for patients with large painful periacetabular lesions whose baseline performance status is poor or if there are medical contraindications to performing large periacetabular resections with extensive reconstruction.

Spine lesions

While the spine is the most common site of metastatic disease, fortunately most spine metastases do not require surgery. They are usually incidentally detected on staging studies such as bone scintigraphy or CT of the chest, abdomen, and pelvis. Mechanical integrity of the spine is usually not compromised, so radiation therapy for axial back pain is usually effective. In cases of compression fractures without neurologic compromise, kyphoplasty combined with radiation has been shown to provide pain relief in over 90% of cases.[23] Kyphoplasty is a technique in which a balloon is percutaneously inserted into the vertebral body through the pedicle under image guidance and inflated to restore vertebral body height, which is then maintained by injection of PMMA bone cement into the resultant void. Surgical decompression and fusion are indicated in cases of severe and progressive deformity or neurologic compromise from compression of neural structures (Figure 5). In cases of spinal cord or caudal equina compression,

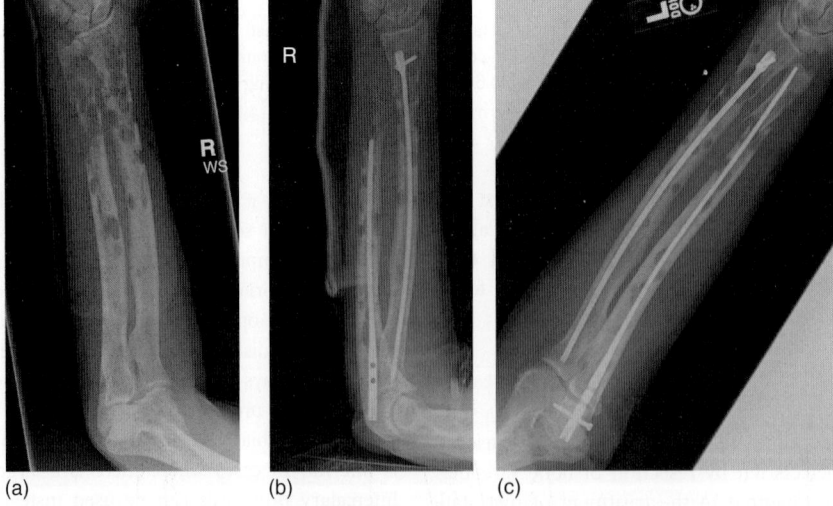

(a)　　　(b)　　　(c)

Figure 5 (a) A 69-year-old man with multiple myeloma who sustained bilateral pathologic forearm fractures through one of multiple radiolucent lesions involving much of the length of bilateral radii and ulnae. (b) and (c) Intramedullary nailing of bilateral radii and ulnae was performed. There was insufficient bone stock to allow fixation of the right distal ulna, so it was resected with minimal functional compromise. Intramedullary nailing was done in a minimally invasive manner and was preferable to fixation with plates and screws that would have required exposure of the entire length of the radius and ulna bilaterally in this already debilitated patient.

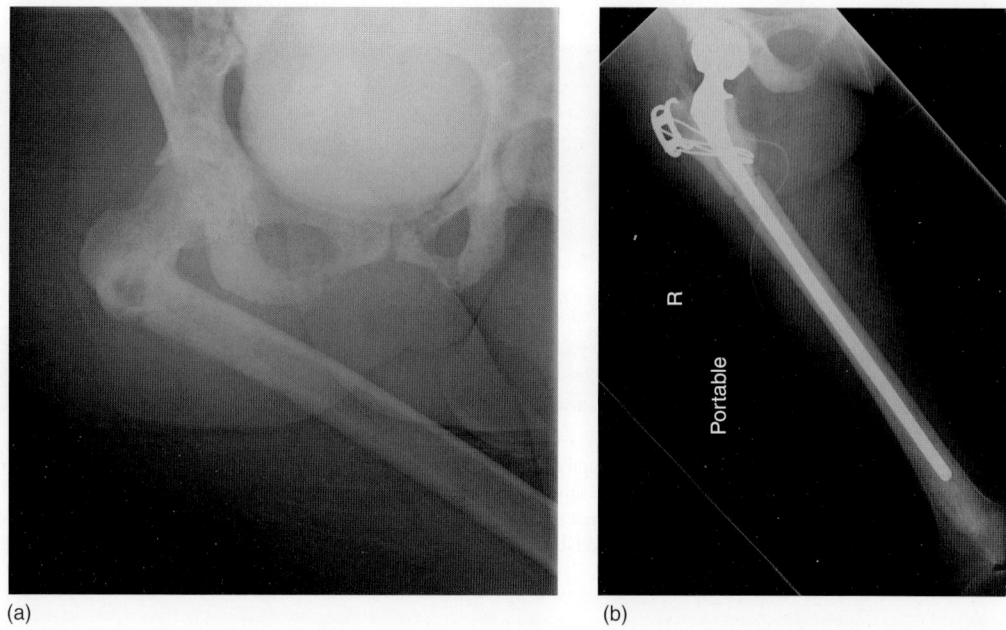

(a)   (b)

Figure 6 (a) A 40-year-old woman with metastatic breast cancer who sustained a subtrochanteric right femur fracture. Note the mixed lytic and blastic changes seen in the femoral head as well as in much of the pelvis. (b) A long-stem cemented hip hemiarthroplasty was performed. A femoral nail would not have been an appropriate choice for this patient as the bone in the femoral head is compromised by metastatic tumor. With an intramedullary nail, risk of lag screw cut-out would have been unacceptably high. The arthroplasty stem serves the same function as a nail in fixing the fracture while the compromised bone in the head of the femur is replaced with the prosthetic head.

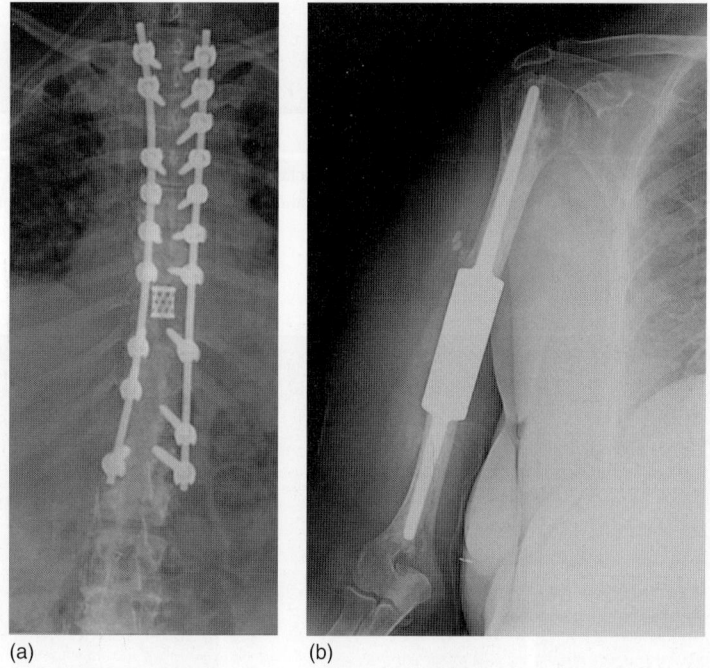

(a)   (b)

Figure 7 (a) A 71-year-old woman with metastatic renal cell carcinoma and a pathologic fracture through a large area of bone destruction in the diaphysis of the humerus. (b) There was not enough bone support for the use of an intramedullary nail or plate and screws, so an intercalary prosthetic replacement was used to reconstruct the defect. Stems cemented into the distal and proximal diaphyseal segments make the construct similar to a fully cemented nail.

surgical intervention provides superior pain relief and is more likely to allow the patient to maintain or even restore ambulatory capacity compared to radiation therapy alone.[24] Timely surgical decompression before irreversible neural damage is critical. In cases of neurologic compromise from radiosensitive lesions such as multiple myeloma and lymphoma, emergency radiotherapy is the preferred treatment modality. Corticosteroids should be administered to relieve edema around the spinal cord and attempt to preserve neurologic function while treatment is being instituted (*see* Ref. 24).

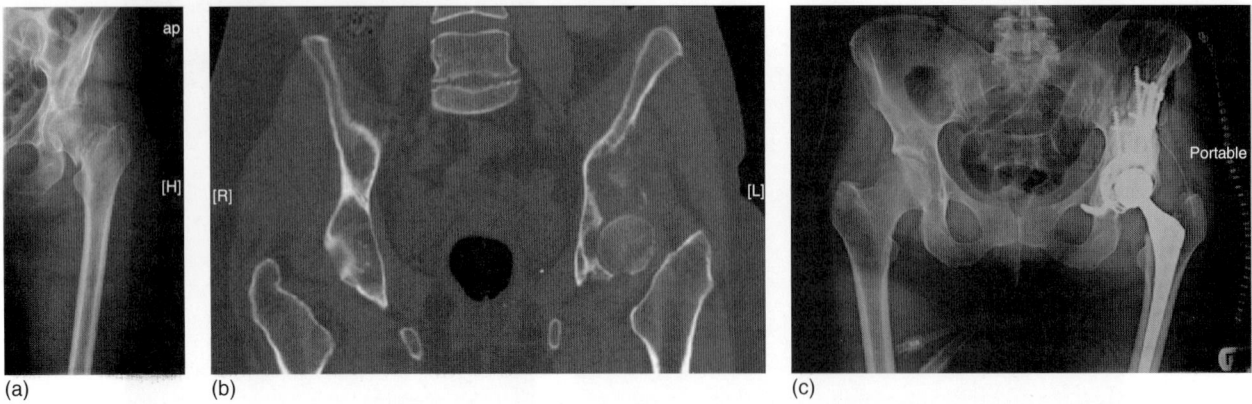

(a) (b) (c)

Figure 8 (a) A 60-year-old woman who sustained a displaced femoral neck fracture in a fall. Note the subtle cortical irregularity at the lateral border of the acetabulum. (b) Coronal CT shows a large destructive lesion in the supra-acetabular area with destruction of the subchondral plate. Biopsy revealed this to be due to metastatic breast cancer. The femoral neck fracture was not related to the patient's cancer. (c) The patient underwent curettage of the tumor and reconstruction of the defect with a total hip arthroplasty with an acetabular cage. The void left by the tumor was filled with PMMA bone cement.

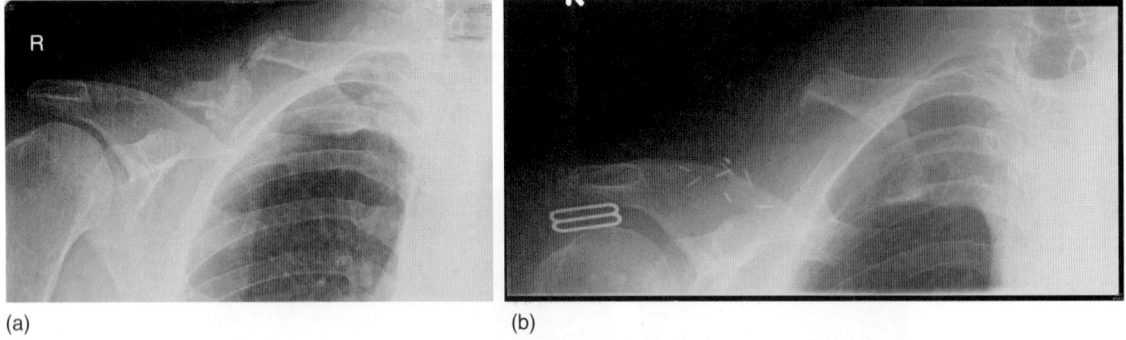

(a) (b)

Figure 9 (a) A 60-year-old woman who sustained a pathologic fracture of her right clavicle through a radiolucent lesion. As a teenager she had a traumatic clavicle fracture that went on to asymptomatic nonunion. (b) Resection of the lateral clavicle, which included the pathologic fracture site, was performed, allowing the patient to return to her baseline status within 2 weeks of surgery.

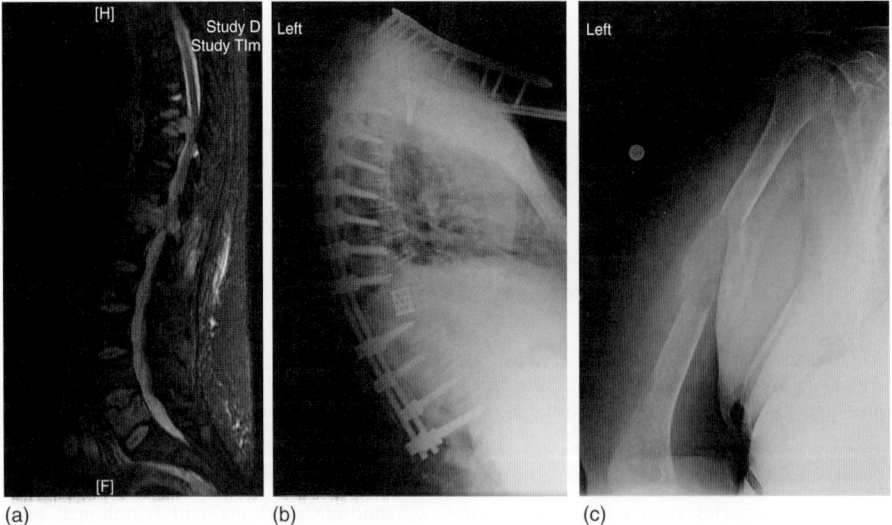

(a) (b) (c)

Figure 10 (a) A 56-year-old woman with metastatic endometrial carcinoma who developed significant lower extremity weakness due to spinal cord compression from a pathologic fracture of the T9 vertebral body. Metastatic deposits in other vertebral bodies are seen. (b) and (c) The patient underwent resection of the T9 vertebral body and fusion with a cage, posterior T8–T10 hemilaminectomy, and instrumentation and fusion from T1 to L1.

Treatment of painful metastases and impending fractures

Besides a displaced pathologic fracture, the indications for surgery are impending pathologic fractures and painful lesions that are not responsive to radiation or other nonoperative treatments. Prophylactic surgical intervention has been shown to be associated with a quicker recovery and superior functional results compared to treatment of a fracture that has already occurred.[25,26] Several systems have been devised to identify the patients at risk of fracture. The one used most commonly was described by Mirels in 1989. The lesion is assigned a score based on four categories (*see Chapter 111*, Table 4A).[27] A score of 1 to 3 is given in each category and the sum of the scores is obtained (Figures 6–10). The parameters are:

1. Location of the lesion. The peritrochanteric femur experiences the highest forces and is assigned a score of 3, whereas the upper extremity is nonweight bearing and is thus assigned a score of 1.
2. Pain quality. Pain exacerbated by activity is the most ominous sign as it implies a mechanical instability at the site of the lesion. All patients with activity-related pain went on to fracture in Mirels' study, whereas only 10% of patients without functional pain sustained fractures.
3. Lesion type. Lytic lesions are the most susceptible to fracture as native bone is destroyed by tumor and not replaced, so a score of 3 is assigned. Blastic lesions are composed of abnormal tumor bone that does not undergo normal remodeling. It is therefore weaker than native bone, but stronger than bone affected by purely lytic lesions, so a score of 1 is given.
4. Size of the lesion as seen on plain radiographs. Larger lesions present a higher fracture risk and therefore get a higher score.

The scores from the four categories are added up to obtain a total score from 4 to 12. Score of 9 is associated with a 33% fracture risk, so surgery is recommended for scores of 9 and above, whereas radiation is recommended for scores of 7 or less. Score of 8 is associated with a 15% fracture risk, so patient factors, such as activity level, body weight, life expectancy, and sensitivity of the tumor to chemotherapy and radiation must be considered (*see Chapter 111*, Table 4B). While Mirels system is 91% sensitive, its specificity is only 35%,[28] so more specific CT-based systems are being sought.[29]

References

1 American Cancer Society. *Cancer Facts & Figures 2015*. Atlanta: American Cancer Society; 2015.
2 Coleman RE. Clinical features of metastatic bone disease and risk of skeletal morbidity. *Clin Cancer Res*. 2006;**12**(20):6243s–6249s.
3 Gaston CL, Nakamura T, Reddy K, et al. Is limb salvage surgery safe for bone sarcomas identified after a previous surgical procedure? *Bone Joint J*. 2014;**96**(5):665–672.
4 Abudu A, Sferopoulos NK, Tillman RM, et al. The surgical treatment and outcome of pathological fractures in localised osteosarcoma. *J Bone Joint Surg Br*. 1996;**78**(5):694–698.
5 Rougraff BT, Kneisl JS, Simon MA. Skeletal metastases of unknown origin. A prospective study of. *J Bone Joint Surg Am*. 1993;**75**:1276–1281.
6 Bui MM, Smith P, Agresta SV, et al. Practical issues of intraoperative frozen section diagnosis of bone and soft tissue lesions. *Cancer Control*. 2008;**15**(1):7–12.
7 Mankin HJ, Lange TA, Spanier SS. The hazards of biopsy in patients with malignant primary bone and soft tissue tumors. *J Bone Joint Surg*. 1982;**64A**:1121–7.
8 Henry DH, Costa L, Goldwasser F, Hirsh V, et al. Randomized, double-blind study of denosumab versus zoledronic acid in the treatment of bone metastases in patients with advanced cancer (excluding breast and prostate cancer) or multiple myeloma. *J Clin Oncol*. 2011;**29**(9):1125–1132.
9 Schocker JD, Brady LW. Radiation therapy for bone metastases. *Clin Orthop*. 1982;**169**:38–43.
10 Toyota N, Naito A, Kakizawa H, et al. Radiofrequency ablation therapy combined with cementoplasty for painful bone metastases: initial experience. *Cardiovasc Intervent Radiol*. 2005;**28**(5):578–583.
11 Callstrom MR, Charboneau JW, Goetz MP, et al. Image-guided ablation of painful metastatic bone tumors: a new and effective approach to a difficult problem. *Skeletal Radiol*. 2006;**35**(1):1–15.
12 Gainor BJ, Buchert P. Fracture healing in metastatic bone disease. *Clin Orthop Relat Res*. 1983;**178**:297–302.
13 Laitinen M, Nieminen J, Pakarinen TK. Treatment of pathological humerus shaft fractures with intramedullary nails with or without cement fixation. *Arch Orthop Trauma Surg*. 2011;**131**(4):503–508.
14 Pugh J, Sherry HS, Futterman B, Frankel VH. Biomechanics of pathologic fractures. *Clin Orthop Relat Res*. 1982;**169**:109–114.
15 Kollender Y, Bickels J, Price WM, et al. Metastatic renal cell carcinoma of bone: indications and technique of surgical intervention. *J Urol*. 2000;**164**(5):1505–1508.
16 Townsend PW, Rosenthal HG, Smalley SR, et al. Impact of postoperative radiation therapy and other perioperative factors on outcome after orthopedic stabilization of impending or pathologic fractures due to metastatic disease. *J Clin Oncol*. 1994;**12**(11):2345–2350.
17 Friess DM, Attia A. Locking plate fixation for proximal humerus fractures: a comparison with other fixation techniques. *Orthopedics*. 2008;**31**:1183.
18 Siegel HJ, Lopez-Ben R, Mann JP, Ponce BA. Pathological fractures of the proximal humerus treated with a proximal humeral locking plate and bone cement. *J Bone Joint Surg Br*. 2010;**92**(5):707–712.
19 Wedin R, Bauer HC. Surgical treatment of skeletal metastatic lesions of the proximal femur: endoprosthesis or reconstruction nail? *J Bone Joint Surg Br*. 2005;**87**(12):1653–1657.
20 Patterson BM, Healey JH, Cornell CN, Sharrock NE. Cardiac arrest during hip arthroplasty with a cemented long-stem component. A report of seven cases. *J Bone Joint Surg Am*. 1991;**73**(2):271–277.
21 Henry JC, Damron TA, Weiner MM, et al. Biomechanical analysis of humeral diaphyseal segmental defect fixation. *Clin Orthop Relat Res*. 2002;**396**:231–239.
22 Issack PS, Kotwal SY, Lane JM. Management of metastatic bone disease of the acetabulum. *J Am Acad Orthop Surg*. 2013;**21**(11):685–695.
23 Gerszten PC, Germanwala A, Burton SA, et al. Combination kyphoplasty and spinal radiosurgery: a new treatment paradigm for pathological fractures. *J Neurosurg Spine*. 2005;**3**(4):296–301.
24 Patchell RA, Tibbs PA, Regine WF, et al. Direct decompressive surgical resection in the treatment of spinal cord compression caused by metastatic cancer: a randomised trial. *Lancet*. 2005;**366**(9486):643–648.
25 Katzer A, Meenen NM, Grabbe F, Rueger JM. Surgery of skeletal metastases. *Arch Orthop Trauma Surg*. 2002;**122**:251–258.
26 Ward WG, Holsenbeck S, Dorey FJ, Spang J, Howe D. Metastatic disease of the femur: surgical treatment. *Clin Orthop*. 2003;**415**:230–244.
27 Mirels H. Metastatic disease in long bones. *Clin Orthop*. 1989;**249**:256–64.
28 Damron TA, Morgan H, Prakash D, Grant W, Aronowitz J, Heiner J. Critical evaluation of Mirel's rating system for impending pathologic fractures. *Clin Orthop Relat Res*. 2003;**415S**:S201–S207.
29 Snyder BD, Hauser-Kara DA, Hipp JA, Zurakowski D, Hecht AC, Gebhardt MC. Predicting fracture through benign skeletal lesions with quantitative computed tomography. *J Bone Joint Surg Am*. 2006;**88**:55–70.

129 Hematologic complications and blood bank support

Richard M. Kaufman, MD ▪ *Kenneth C. Anderson, MD*

Overview

Many of the fundamental therapies used to treat cancer (chemotherapy and stem cell transplantation) disrupt normal hematopoiesis in the bone marrow. As a result, blood transfusion for patients with cancer is an essential supportive modality. The primary focus of this chapter is on "classical" blood component support: how red cells, plasma, platelets, and granulocytes are collected, tested, stored, and administered to address specific deficiencies in patients with cancer. Particular attention is paid to studies of prophylactic platelet transfusion, which over the past several decades has been critical in allowing myelosuppressive treatments to be applied to a variety of malignant disease states. Current infectious risks of blood products are reviewed.

Hematologic complications occur commonly in patients with cancer, related either to the underlying disease or to its treatment.[1,2] Abnormalities in the red blood cell (RBC), leukocyte (WBC), and platelet number and function require transfusion medicine expertise for the provision of appropriate blood component support.[3,4] Indeed, the therapeutic advances made using high-dose combination chemotherapeutic approaches to date would not have been possible without the parallel development of technology to support patients through the hematologic complications of therapy.

Causes of pancytopenia

Cancer and its treatment may alter normal hematopoiesis either by direct effects on hematopoietic stem cells or by inhibiting production of and responsiveness to hematopoietic growth factors (Table 1).

Disease related

Bone marrow hematopoietic cells can be replaced either by primary tumor derived from marrow cells, or by metastatic spread of tumor to the marrow from neoplasms of other organs. Hodgkin and non-Hodgkin lymphoma (NHL), malignant melanoma, neuroblastoma, as well as carcinoma of the breast, prostate, lung, adrenal, thyroid, and kidney commonly manifest marrow involvement. Ultimately, diffuse involvement of marrow with tumor can lead to either marrow fibrosis or necrosis, which may be associated with splenomegaly, thrombocytopenia, and immature cells of all lineages in the peripheral blood.[5]

Chemotherapy related

The role of treatment in marrow injury and recovery varies both with the drugs employed and with the normal turnover rate of cells of different hematologic lineages. The characteristic effects of several drugs on marrow are shown in Table 2. The bone marrow

has a storage compartment that can supply mature cells to the peripheral blood for 8–10 days after the stem-cell pool has ceased to function. Events in the peripheral blood are therefore a week behind the events in the bone marrow. In previously untreated patients, leukopenia and thrombocytopenia are described on the ninth or tenth day after treatment, with the nadir of counts on days 14–18. Recovery of counts is evident by day 21 and complete by day 28. The cytotoxic dose–response effect is usually related to the nadir WBC and platelet count, not the duration of cytopenia. This is due to the resting state of the stem cells of normal bone marrow, which protects them from damage.

Gamma radiation related

Cells damaged by irradiation may divide one time or more before all progeny are rendered reproductively sterile; thus, an irradiated cell will not appear damaged until it divides.[6] At the time of the first postirradiation subdivision, the cell may die, divide aberrantly and produce unusual forms, be unable to divide and remain physiologically functional, or give rise to one or more generation of progeny until cells become sterile. As bone marrow stem cells have a very low capacity for repair of sublethal irradiation damage, multiple smaller radiation fractions may preserve other normal tissues (e.g., lung and intestine), but will not spare bone marrow.

Associated processes

It is essential to remain cognizant of derangements in normal physiology that may occur in the setting of cancer and/or treatment and that contribute to pancytopenia. These include nutritional factors, such as folate, iron, or vitamin deficiencies. There may be abnormal feedback loops in hematopoiesis, such as cell-mediated suppression of hematopoiesis in aplastic anemia or stimulation of thrombopoiesis in the setting of antibody-mediated platelet destruction.[7] Fibrosis can occur either as part of a disease process or as a reaction to therapy, thereby compromising bone marrow reserve. Immunologically mediated destruction of cells and other factors, such as splenomegaly, can result in cytopenias. Moreover, occult bleeding must always be considered as a cause of persistent anemia and refractory thrombocytopenia. These clinical examples emphasize the importance of carefully assessing patients with cancer for treatable medical etiologies of their hematologic complications before attributing these effects to their underlying neoplasms.

Abnormalities of red cells and red cell support

Anemia

Anemia in patients with cancer can be mild to severe and may be attributable to many causes. Hematopoiesis in patients with early stages of cancer may be normal. On the other hand, replacement of marrow cells by tumor is not essential for the development of anemia, even in patients with metastatic cancer. Most commonly, the incidence and magnitude of anemia in patients with cancer increase

Holland-Frei Cancer Medicine, Ninth Edition. Edited by Robert C. Bast Jr., Carlo M. Croce, William N. Hait, Waun Ki Hong, Donald W. Kufe, Martine Piccart-Gebhart, Raphael E. Pollock, Ralph R. Weichselbaum, Hongyang Wang, and James F. Holland.
© 2017 John Wiley & Sons, Inc. ISBN: 978-1-118-93469-2

Table 1 Causes of anemia, thrombocytopenia, and leukopenia in cancer.

Bone marrow replacement by primary tumor (e.g., leukemia)
Bone marrow involvement by metastatic tumor (e.g., breast and
  prostate)
Derangement of normal physiology
• Nutritional (e.g., folate, iron, and negative nitrogen
  balance)
• Abnormal feedback (e.g., stimulation/inhibition of
  hematopoiesis)
• Bone-marrow reaction (e.g., fibrosis)
• Peripheral destruction (e.g., immune hemolysis, diffuse
  intravascular coagulation, and splenomegaly)
• Blood loss

Myelosuppression by chemotherapy or radiotherapy

Table 2 Characteristic effects of drugs and treatments on bone marrow.

Treatment	Hematologic complication
Most chemotherapeutic agents	Leukopenia and thrombocytopenia at 9–10 days; nadir counts at 14–18 days; recovery of counts at 21–28 days
Nitrosourea	Myelosuppression at 4–6 weeks
Vincristine, 1-asparaginase, bleomycin, myelosuppression methotrexate with leucovorin	No myelosuppression
Gamma irradiation	Chronic lymphopenia
Whole-body irradiation	Profound suppression of humoral and cellular immune response

as the disease progresses. This anemia is designated as anemia of chronic disease only if the cellular pattern in the marrow is nearly normal, the serum iron and iron-binding capacity are low, the iron content of the marrow is normal or increased, and the serum ferritin is elevated.[8] The coexistence of low plasma iron levels with adequate amounts of storage iron helps distinguish anemia of chronic disease from iron-deficiency anemia. Moreover, other causes of anemia, for example, overt hemolysis, bleeding, nutritional deficiency, or marrow replacement, must be ruled out. In some patients, such as those with Hodgkin disease (HD), erythrophagocytosis or hypersplenism may account for this decrease in red-cell survival, but in others its etiology is unclear.

Red-cell transfusion

Red-cell transfusions are indicated to increase oxygen-carrying capacity in patients with anemia that is not adequately compensated by normal physiologic mechanisms. Sufficient oxygen-carrying capacity to maintain cardiopulmonary function can be met by a hemoglobin of 7 g/dL (a hematocrit of approximately 21%) when the intravascular volume is adequate for perfusion.[9] In a multicenter randomized trial of critical care patients, a restrictive transfusion strategy (maintaining hemoglobin levels between 7 and 9 g/dL) was demonstrated to be at least as safe as a more liberal transfusion strategy, with the possible exception of patients with acute myocardial infarction or unstable angina.[10] Subsequent randomized trials have compared restrictive versus liberal RBC transfusion strategies in patients with cardiovascular disease having hip surgery[11] or cardiac surgery,[12–14] in patients with sepsis,[15] and in patients with upper gastrointestinal bleeding.[16] A restrictive transfusion strategy (hemoglobin transfusion threshold of 7–8 g/dL) appears to be safe and appropriate for the vast majority of hospitalized inpatients. Currently, however, high-quality clinical trial data to guide RBC transfusion in patients with malignancy are still awaited. Overall,

there is no single hemoglobin level that can be universally applied as a "transfusion trigger." In deciding whether to transfuse a specific patient, the physician should consider the patient's age, degree of anemia, the intravascular volume, and the presence of coexisting cardiac, pulmonary, or vascular conditions.[17] To meet oxygen needs, some patients may require RBC transfusions at higher hemoglobin levels. In particular, hemoglobin levels are commonly maintained at levels of 8 g/dL in the setting of cancer and its therapy. Transfusing one unit of RBC will usually increase the hemoglobin by 1 g/dL and the hematocrit by 2–3% in the average adult weighing 70 kg.

Packed red blood cells (PRBC) are prepared either from whole blood (WB) by the removal of plasma or by erythrocytapheresis. Red cells can be depleted of leukocytes by filtration to produce leukoreduced red cells (LRBC). Leukoreduction can prevent a significant percentage of febrile nonhemolytic transfusion reactions and cytomegalovirus (CMV) infection in transfusion recipients.[18] In the United States and internationally, there is a trend to universally transfuse leukoreduced cellular components to avoid the multiple adverse sequelae of leukocytes. Washed RBCs are prepared by further removal of plasma from PRBCs. These products are sometimes indicated to prevent allergic reactions to plasma proteins.[19] PRBCs are currently stored for up to 42 days at 4°C. Retrospective studies have suggested that transfusing older stored PRBC units may be associated with adverse consequences for the recipient.[20] However, older RBC units have not been demonstrated to increase morbidity or mortality when compared with fresher RBC units in multiple randomized controlled trials.[21–23]

Leukopenia and white cell support

Leukopenia

Leukopenia may occur related to cancer and its treatment. In 1965, Hersh and colleagues summarized the causes of death in patients with acute leukemia treated at the National Cancer Institute and noted a marked decline in fatal hemorrhage, owing to the availability of platelet transfusions, with a concomitant increase in the occurrence of infection alone as a cause of death.[24] A quantitative relationship between circulating leukocytes and infection was established in patients with leukemia; in particular, the probability of being infected is proportional to both the severity and duration of leukopenia.[25]

Granulocyte transfusion

Therapeutic granulocytes were first utilized nearly 30 years ago in leukemic patients with leukopenia and serious infection. The earliest trials, which demonstrated the potential value of granulocyte transfusions, utilized granulocytes harvested from patients with chronic myelogenous leukemia and achieved cell dosages never approached when normal donors were utilized.[26] The importance of dose was defined: less than 10^{10} granulocytes were ineffective whereas greater than 10^{11} cells were effective. Indeed, in an afebrile, uninfected man, the half-life of granulocytes in the circulation is 6.7(4–10) h and the daily turnover rate is 230%. Parallel work in canine models had also demonstrated that dogs deliberately made leukopenic by irradiation and given Gram-negative bacteremia and pneumonia could be successfully treated with granulocyte transfusions.[27]

There have been six randomized prospective trials of prophylactic leukocyte transfusions, given to prevent infections in leukopenic recipients.[28,29] However, none of the studies demonstrated improved survival because alloimmunization, transfusion reactions, CMV infection, and pulmonary infiltrates occurred more frequently in the transfused group. These studies have been criticized owing to inadequate donor-recipient matching and inadequate doses of granulocytes transfused. A large randomized trial of high-dose granulocytes collected from donors mobilized with a combination of G-CSF and dexamethasone has been completed.[29] Currently, the role for granulocyte transfusions remains controversial. When granulocytes transfusions are used, the products must irradiated to prevent graft-versus-host disease (GVHD) when transfused to an immunocompromised host.

Thrombocytopenia and platelet support

Thrombocytopenia
Thrombocytopenia in cancer patients is usually attributable to treatment with chemotherapy and radiotherapy. Impaired production of platelets due to a decrease or absence of megakaryocytes is therefore the most common cause of thrombocytopenia in patients with cancer (Table 3). However, thrombocytopenia may also be due to splenic sequestration in patients who have splenomegaly as part of their primary neoplastic process. In this setting, increased numbers of megakaryocytes are evident unless extensive marrow infiltration is present. Immune-mediated thrombocytopenia may also occur related to antihuman leukocyte antigen (anti-HLA) or antiplatelet-specific alloantibodies. Finally, thrombocytopenia may be related to diffuse intravascular coagulation (DIC), especially in patients with acute myelocytic leukemias, lymphomas, and carcinoma of lung, breast, gastrointestinal, or urologic origin. DIC commonly complicates acute promyelocytic leukemia owing to the presence of both thromboplastic material and fibrinolytic proteases in the promyelocytic subcellular components.[30]

Table 3 Causes of thrombocytopenia.

Acute thrombocytopenia due to increased
- Platelet depletion (utilization, sequestration, or destruction)
- Massive blood replacement
- Cardiac surgery
- Splenomegaly

Immune destruction of platelets
- Self-limited acute idiopathic thrombocytopenia purpura (ITP)
- Post-transfusion purpura
- Drug purpura
- Chronic idiopathic thrombocytopenia purpura
- Consumptive thrombocytopenia

Hereditary defects
Thrombocytopenia with decreased platelet production
- Aplastic anemia
- Acute leukemia

Idiopathic megakaryocytic aplasia
Marrow infiltration
- Malignant
- Nonmalignant—Gaucher disease and granulomatous diseases

Following radiation or myelosuppressive drugs
Drugs producing specific suppression of platelet production (e.g., thiazides, ethanol, and estrogens)
Nutritional deficiency—megaloblastic anemia and severe iron deficiency (rare)
Viral infections
Paroxysmal nocturnal hemoglobinuria

Abnormalities in platelet function
Platelet function can be abnormal in several chronic myeloproliferative disorders. Although most bleeding in patients with acute myeloid leukemia (AML) is related to thrombocytopenia, intrinsic abnormalities in platelet function have been described including decreased platelet procoagulant activity and decreased aggregation and serotonin release responses to ADP, epinephrine, or collagen.[31] Platelet dysfunction is evident in a fraction of patients with IgA myeloma or Waldenstrom macroglobulinemia, multiple myeloma, and monoclonal gammopathy of undetermined significance.[32]

Platelet transfusion support
In 1910, fresh WB was first transfused to thrombocytopenic patients, resulting in a significant rise in the platelet count, hemostasis, and improvement of the bleeding time.[33] In the 1950s, platelets were first used for the treatment of thrombocytopenia related to combination chemotherapeutic treatments of leukemias.[34] Data from the National Cancer Institute in the early 1960s clearly demonstrated that leukemia patients died of hemorrhage during induction of remission with chemotherapy and established the quantitative relationship between platelet count and hemorrhage.[35] It was shown that platelet therapy could modify the course of hemorrhage in both pediatric and adult settings, the only difference being the doses required. Two recent randomized trials compared a prophylactic platelet-transfusion strategy with a therapeutic platelet-transfusion strategy in patients with hypoproliferative thrombocytopenia. Both studies demonstrated a benefit, albeit limited, of platelet prophylaxis, and both showed that prophylaxis has a greater effect on bleeding risk in patients treated with chemotherapy for leukemia compared with autologous stem cell transplant recipients.[36]

Single- and multiple-donor platelets
In the United States, one unit of platelet concentrate is obtained from one unit of WB by centrifugation, and contains approximately 5.5×10^{10} platelets/unit. (This method of preparing platelets is known as the "platelet-rich plasma" (PRP) method. In other countries, platelet concentrates are prepared from WB using the alternate "buffy coat" method.) Concentrates from multiple (4–6) donors are pooled to produce a single component for transfusion. Apheresis technology has permitted harvesting the equivalent of several platelet concentrates from a single donor during a single donation. A single-donor platelet unit typically contains at least 3×10^{11} platelets/unit. The use of single-donor platelets is increasing; they are generally considered to be the platelet product of choice for patients being treated for malignancy.[37] Single-donor platelet collections are utilized to provide HLA-matched donors for alloimmunized recipients who have not responded to platelets from random donors. In the United States, platelet units may be stored at room temperature for up to 5 days.

Indications for therapeutic and prophylactic platelet transfusion
Platelets are commonly transfused to patients with cancer. The majority of platelet transfusions are given prophylactically to prevent bleeding, as opposed to therapeutically, to treat active bleeding.[38] The appropriate indications for transfusion of platelets have been the subject of a recent clinical practice guideline from the AABB.[39] At present, one dose of one apheresis platelets (or equivalent pool of random donor-platelet concentrates) is routinely transfused to cancer patients with platelet counts less

than 10,000/mm³ to reduce the risk of hemorrhage. Data from Gmur and colleagues suggested that the threshold for prophylactic platelet transfusion can safely be set at 5×10^9/L in patients with acute leukemia without fever or bleeding manifestations and at 10×10^9/L in patients without such signs.[40] Prospective clinical trials have shown that the risk of major bleeding was similar whether 10×10^9/L or 20×10^9/L was used as the platelet-transfusion threshold in patients with acute leukemia, and that the lower threshold reduced platelet use.[41-43]

The risk of bleeding at a given platelet count may vary in distinct clinical settings. For example, patients with thrombocytopenia due to AML were reported to have increased bleeding at less than 10,000/mm³ platelets, in contrast to patients with acute lymphocytic leukemia (ALL), who had similar risk of hemorrhage at less than 20,000/mm³ platelets.[44] Patients with chronic thrombocytopenia due to decreased platelet production (i.e., myelodysplastic disorders) may require transfusions, in contrast to patients with accelerated destruction but active production of platelets (i.e., idiopathic thrombocytopenic purpura), who may not require routine platelet transfusions. Moreover, patients with chronic thrombocytopenia may tolerate lower absolute platelet counts without transfusion. In patients with abnormalities of platelet function, it is not the absolute platelet count but rather the number of functional platelets that is important for the prevention of bleeding. Thus, it is difficult to define an absolute platelet threshold for transfusion for all patients, and both the timing and the dose of prophylactic platelet transfusion must therefore be determined on a clinical basis.[39,45-47]

The multicenter randomized PLADO (PLAtelet DOsing) study demonstrated that prophylactic transfusion with low-dose platelets does not increase the risk of Grade 2 or higher bleeding as compared with standard-dose prophylaxis among inpatients with hypoproliferative thrombocytopenia. Patients receiving low-dose prophylaxis do require more frequent platelet transfusions, although fewer total platelets are required overall.[48]

Clinical and laboratory assessment of the effectiveness of platelet transfusion

The effectiveness of platelet transfusion can be assessed by laboratory parameters (the platelet count increment 1 h or 10–15 min after transfusion) and by the observed clinical outcome after transfusion.[49-52] The corrected count increment is defined as the increment in platelet counts from pre- to post-transfusion corrected for the number of units transfused and for the body surface area of the recipient. A CCI of 15,000–20,000/mm³ is usual at 18–24 h, provided fresh, properly stored platelets have been transfused.[52]

Post-transfusion increments in platelet count may be lesser than expected due to splenic sequestration, especially in the setting of splenomegaly.[50] Drug-induced platelet antibodies, which mediate immune destruction of platelets, have been demonstrated. The survival of transfused platelets can also be compromised if the recipient possesses antibodies against donor antigens of HLA-A and HLA-B loci, the ABO system, or platelet alloantigens. Response to platelet transfusion in recipients of hematopoietic stem-cell transplantation has been specifically studied.

Alloimmunization

Platelets bear HLA-A and -B but lack HLA-C and -DR Antigens, and there is a high correlation between the development of lymphocytotoxic anti-HLA antibodies in the recipient and refractoriness to random-donor platelets.[53] Currently, anti-HLA antibodies are most easily detectable using the patient's serum in a flow cytometry assay using HLA antigen-coated beads.

Yankee and colleagues first demonstrated that platelets obtained from HLA-identical siblings or from unrelated donors matched at the HLA-A and -B loci (grade A or B matches) could result in satisfactory post-transfusion increments in alloimmunized recipients who were refractory to random-donor platelet transfusions.[54] Subsequently, Duquesnoy and colleagues found that donors whose HLA antigens were the same (B match) or cross-reactive with the patient's antigens (BX match) were equivalent.[55]

The recognition of the refractoriness associated with the development of anti-HLA antibodies led to attempts to either avoid or delay alloimmunization by modifying the platelets to be transfused. As HLA antigens are expressed on leukocytes, and platelets themselves are poor immunogens, investigators have attempted to (1) remove WBCs from platelets or treat platelets with ultraviolet (UV) irradiation to abrogate the leukocyte antigen-presenting function; (2) use single rather than multiple-donor platelets to minimize exposure to HLA; and (3) transfuse only HLA-matched or leukocyte-depleted HLA-matched platelets. The multicenter prospective Trial to Reduce Alloimmunization to Platelets (TRAP) study confirmed that the incidence of anti-HLA and platelet-specific antibodies alone, as well as the incidence of antibodies associated with platelet refractoriness, was reduced in leukemic recipients who received either filtered or UV-treated pooled random-donor concentrates or filtered single-donor platelets compared to similar patients who received nonfiltered pooled random-donor concentrates.[56] Only 13% of patients developed platelet refractoriness associated with lymphocytotoxic antibodies, suggesting that the majority of unresponsiveness to platelet transfusion is related to other factors. When sensitized recipients remain refractory to HLA-matched platelets, cross-matched platelets are sometimes provided. A third method of dealing with HLA immune refractoriness is to provide antigen-negative platelets, analogous to providing antigen-negative RBCs for patients with RBC alloantibodies.

ABO blood group determinants are intrinsic to platelet membranes.[57] Unlike the case with RBC transfusion, ABO mismatch between donor and recipient is not an absolute contraindication to platelet transfusion. That said, ABO-identical platelet transfusions are preferred. Transfused ABO major-incompatible platelets (e.g., A donor and O recipient) demonstrate recoveries that are about one-third lower than those seen with ABO-identical transfusions.[58,59]

In addition, passively transfused high-titer isohemagglutinins present within the plasma in the transfused platelet concentrates (e.g., donor O and recipient A) have occasionally caused severe hemolysis. The United Kingdom, notably, has instituted routine screening of platelet units for anti-A/B to prevent this problem. Other countries, including the United States, have not adopted a uniform strategy of prevention.[59]

Other therapeutic modalities

Transfusion of fresh frozen plasma

Fresh frozen plasma is the fluid portion of 1 unit (450 mL) of WB that is centrifuged, separated, and frozen at −18°C or lower. It contains physiologic levels of coagulation factors. Fresh frozen plasma is utilized to correct coagulation factor deficiencies; to reverse warfarin effect; and to treat thrombotic thrombocytopenic purpura, disseminated intravascular coagulation, coagulopathy of liver disease, thrombolytic agent overdose, and protein C or S deficiency.[60,61] In addition to the plasma obtained from donated

WB, it can be collected using plasmapheresis procedures for the production of derivatives: coagulation factors (factors VIII and IX), immunoglobulin, and albumin preparations.

Effects of transfusion on the immune system

Alloimmunization

The most firmly established effect of transfusion is the stimulation of antibodies in the recipient against antigens in the transfused products. Both cellular and plasma antigens in transfused blood expose the recipients to hundreds of known alloantigens.

Over 400 RBC antigens have been identified, yet we routinely ensure compatibility for only three of them: A, B, and D. More than 100 HLA antigens, as well as granulocyte- and platelet-specific antigens, have also been identified. Genetic alleles can result in structural and therefore antigenic differences among all plasma proteins, leading to recipient alloantibodies to the donated immunoglobulins. Most alloantigens are ignored in transfusion therapy, as they are poor immunogens. However, studies clearly demonstrate that the development of recipient antibodies to antigens in transfused products relates not only to the number of transfusions but also to their timing. Specifically, individuals who receive equal numbers of transfusions are more likely to develop antibodies if the transfusions are given repeatedly over a longer period than if given within a shorter interval. Some cancer patients, by virtue of receiving repeated transfusions over a longer period, may therefore be more likely to become alloimmunized. Alloantibodies to RBCs can lead to recipient morbidity and shortened RBC survival; antibodies to leukocytes are associated with febrile transfusion reactions and can impair effectiveness and survival of transfused granulocytes.[62] Anti-HLA-A and -B antibodies as well as platelet-specific alloantibodies impair survival of transfused platelets. Finally, anti-IgA sometimes causes anaphylactic reactions in IgA-deficient recipients, but anti-IgG or -IgM or antilipoproteins are not clinically significant.[63]

Transfusion-associated GVHD

Historic perspective

GVHD is commonly observed after allogeneic bone marrow transplantation (BMT), but is rarely recognized after transfusion or transplantation of other organs. Transfusion associated (TA)-GVHD usually occurs in the immunosuppressed recipient (e.g., BMT recipients), but it can also occur in immunocompetent recipients in the setting of a one-way HLA mismatch.[64] The clinical manifestations include fever and skin rash, anorexia, nausea, vomiting, and watery or bloody diarrhea with or without elevated liver enzymes and hyperbilirubinemia. As there are no pathognomonic features of GVHD, this syndrome is sometimes difficult to distinguish from viral infections or drug eruptions. TA-GVHD is usually severe, and, unlike the situation after allogeneic BMT, it frequently results in pancytopenia secondary to marrow aplasia. The majority of reported cases of TA-GVHD have not responded to immunosuppressive therapies and have been fatal.

Definition of those at risk

In 1986, the National Institutes of Health Consensus Development Conference defined patients who have undergone BMT or those with other forms of immunodeficiency as candidates for irradiated platelet concentrates to avoid GVHD. Patients with leukemias and other cancers who may be immunosuppressed secondary to chemotherapy and/or radiation therapy, or due to intrinsic immune dysfunction (e.g., HD), may be at risk for TA-GVHD. Among patients with HD, it had previously been assumed that combined radiation and chemotherapy were necessary as predisposing factors for the development of TA-GVHD, but several cases of TA-GVHD have recently been documented in patients with HD who were treated with chemotherapy alone. Patients receiving high-dose chemotherapy followed by autologous bone-marrow support are also at risk for TA-GVHD.[65] Finally, immunocompetent patients who share an HLA haplotype with HLA-homozygous blood donors also appear to be at risk for TA-GVHD.[66,67] Homozygosity for HLA types is more likely to occur among first-degree family members (e.g., parents, children, and siblings). It has, therefore, recently been recommended that cellular blood components from such donors be irradiated with at least 25 Gy before transfusion. Indeed, products from all family member-directed donors should be irradiated, given that TA-GVHD has now been reported after transfusion of blood from a second-degree relative.[68] Reports of TA-GVHD after transfusion of cellular blood components from homozygous blood donors to heterozygous nonblood relatives suggest that indications for gamma irradiation may need to be broadened.[69,70] The risk of transfusion of blood from HLA homozygous donors to unrelated HLA heterozygous patients is 1 in 874 in Japan and may be as high as 1 in 7174 in the United States.[71] Finally, reports confirm that all HLA-matched cellular components should be irradiated.[69-72]

Strategies for prevention

The only currently effective method to prevent TA-GVHD is gamma irradiation of blood products before transfusion. Studies suggest that irradiation at 15–20 Gy can reduce mitogen-responsive lymphocytes by 5–6 logs compared to unirradiated controls.[71] The standards of the AABB (formerly, the American Association of Blood Banks), as well as those of the FDA, now require that blood and cellular components be irradiated with a midplane dose of a minimum of 25 Gy.[72] Studies to date suggest no adverse effects of irradiation on storage of platelets, but the clinical significance of potassium release on storage of irradiated red cells is not yet defined, and post-transfusion red-cell recovery of irradiated units may be decreased.[73,74]

Transfusion-related infectious diseases

Hepatitis B

Although hepatitis B (HB) was formerly a common transfusion-related infection, the use of several generations of HB surface antigen assays to screen potential donors and the use of volunteer versus commercial donors has markedly reduced the incidence of HB transmitted by transfusion.[75] Nucleic acid testing (NAT) is now often performed to test for HB as well. The current estimated per-unit risk of HB is approximately 1 in 200,000 (Table 4).[76]

Hepatitis C

Following the identification of hepatitis A and HB viruses, it was quickly appreciated that neither agent was responsible for most cases of post-transfusion hepatitis. Thus, the term non-A non-B Hepatitis (NANBH) was introduced. In the mid-1980s, donors were screened for alanine aminotransferase (ALT) as well as anti-HBc; these served as "surrogate" markers for individuals having a 20% chance of transmitting NANBH.[77,78]

Table 4 Risks of transfusion.

Complication	Frequency (episodes:unit)
Reactions	
Febrile nonhemolytic	1–4:100
Allergic	1–4:100
Transfusion-related acute lung injury	1:10,000
Acute hemolytic	1:250,000
Delayed hemolytic	1:1,000
Anaphylactic	1:150,000
Infections	
Hepatitis C	1:2,000,000
Hepatitis B	1:200,000
HIV-1	1:2,000,000
HIV-2	None reported
HTLV-I and II	1:250,000–1:2,000,000
Malaria	1:4,000,000
Bacteria red cells	1:500,000
Bacteria platelets	1:75,000
Other complications	
RBC allosensitization	1:100
HLA sensitization	1:10
Graft-versus-host disease	Rare

Abbreviations: HIV, human immunodeficiency virus; HLA, human leukocyte antigen; HTLV, human T-cell leukemia/lymphoma virus; RBC, red blood cell.

The causative agent of NANBH was finally discovered by cloning a fragment of viral cDNA from a chimpanzee infected with NANBH.[79] Subsequently, the entire genome of what is now called hepatitis C virus (HCV) was cloned. A specific assay was developed for bloodborne NANBH, in which a recombinant HCV polypeptide is used to capture viral antibodies.[80] Subsequent testing using multiple-antigen HCV enzyme assays confirmed that nearly all cases of post-transfusion NANBH are caused by HCV. Uniform screening of blood donors for anti-HCV antibodies was implemented in 1990. NAT is now being employed to enhance sensitivity in detecting infection.[81] Along with HIV (discussed below), all blood donations in the United States are now screened for HCV. By narrowing the preseroconversion window period from about 75 days to less than 30, the use of NAT has reduced the per-unit risk of HCV to approximately 1 in 2,000,000.[76]

Cytomegalovirus

Cellular blood components transfused from CMV-seropositive donors to CMV-seronegative transplant recipients and neonates can cause CMV seroconversion and infection. Although equivalent numbers of autologous and allogeneic BMT recipients either seroconvert to or excrete CMV, recipients of autologous BMT rarely develop clinical sequelae. The traditional CMV-seronegative blood products are red cells and platelets harvested from CMV-seronegative donors. LRBC and platelets have been shown to decrease transfusion-acquired CMV infection in infants, in patients undergoing treatment for acute leukemia, and in autologous and allogeneic BMT recipients.[82–85] A multicenter-randomized trial compared seronegative with filtered cellular blood components in CMV-sero-negative patients undergoing autologous BMT and seronegative patients receiving allografts from CMV seronegative donors.[82] Rates of CMV seroconversion and infection were equivalent in recipients of seronegative and filtered components, but significant clinical sequelae were noted only in those patients receiving filtered, unscreened components. These results suggest that filtering can markedly reduce CMV transmission, and filtered components are now considered "CMV safe"; however, it may be premature to conclude that filtered and seronegative components are exactly equivalent.

West Nile virus

West Nile virus (WNV) is a mosquito-borne flavivirus that can be transfusion transmitted. The vast majority of WNV infections result from mosquito bites. About 80% of individuals infected with WNV are asymptomatic. Of the 20% who manifest symptoms, most will have a mild illness (WNV fever). Less than 1% of infected individuals develop a severe meningo-encephalitis, with advanced age being the strongest risk factor.[86] WNV first appeared in the United States in 1999. In 2002, over 4000 clinically significant cases of WNV were reported, including 23 cases determined to have been transfusion associated. In 2003, NAT of blood products was begun nationwide under an FDA investigational new drug (IND) protocol. This testing has eliminated most of the risk of transfusion-transmitted WNV.

Bacterial sepsis

Bacteria very rarely survive in WB stored at 4°C. In contrast, platelets are stored at room temperature on an agitator and are a potential source of bacterial contamination, which can result in transfusion-related sepsis.[87] Blood collection facilities in the United States are now required by AABB to both detect and limit bacterial contamination of platelets.[76] A variety of screening techniques to address bacterial contamination within platelets, such as automated culture systems, are now in use.[88,89]

Human immunodeficiency virus (HIV)

Since 1985, all American blood donors have been screened for anti-HIV antibody using ELISA. Transfusion-transmitted HIV is now exceedingly rare; the few cases that do occur result almost exclusively from seronegative window period donations. Following the initial implementation of HIV antibody screening, improvements in the sensitivity of the HIV-1 and HIV-2 ELISA limited the seronegative window period to approximately 22 days[90] All units donated in the United States are now tested by minipool NAT. NAT (transfusion-mediated amplification, TMA, or polymerase chain reaction, PCR) is performed on pools of 16–24 samples; this technology shortens the window period to approximately 10 or 11 days from the time of exposure. It is estimated that the current residual per-unit risk of HIV transmission is less than 1 in 2,000,000.[76]

Human T-cell lymphotrophic virus type 1

Human T-cell lymphotrophic virus type 1 (HTLV-1) is associated with adult T-cell leukemia/lymphoma (ATL) and tropical spastic paresis (TSP)/HTLV-1-associated myelopathy (HAM), and clusters geographically in endemic areas such as parts of Japan and the Caribbean. In the United States, ATL incidence is similar to that in the Caribbean, as the cases in the United States are all among African-Americans or in patients born outside the United States.[91]

In 1988, blood-collection agencies initiated testing of all blood donors for anti-HTLV-1 antibodies at the time of all donations, with permanent deferral of individuals with confirmed seropositivity. Studies in the United States document that HTLV-1 has been transmitted via transfusion and demonstrate the efficacy of screening. The risk per unit transfused is between 1 in 250,000 and 1 in 2,000,000.[76]

Parasitic diseases

As there is no practical laboratory screening test for malaria, exclusion of donors who have either traveled to or emigrated from endemic areas is the only effective measure to prevent transfusion-related infection. Other parasitic diseases, such as babesiosis or Lyme disease, can be transmitted by an asymptomatic donor who has been bitten by a tick and may be of particular importance in immunocompromised or asplenic patients. Transfusion-transmitted babesiosis is a regional disease. At this time, there are seven endemic US states: Massachusetts, Connecticut, Rhode Island, New York, New Jersey, Wisconsin, and Minnesota.[92] Although transmission of syphilis by transfusion is possible, it requires that blood be drawn during the rather short period of spirochetemia and that the organisms remain viable at the time of transfusion. Although performing a serologic test for syphilis does not prevent transmission of syphilis because this test does not become positive until well after the brief period of infectivity, US federal regulations do require its use as a screening test of potential donors.

Another recognized transfusion-related infection is Chagas disease.[93] In the majority of cases, spontaneous resolution occurs, and patients enter the indeterminate phase with lifelong, low-grade parasitemia, antibodies to parasite antigens, and absence of symptoms. Between 10% and 30% of persons in the indeterminate phase eventually develop symptoms. However, in immunocompromised patients, this illness may take a more fulminant course. The diagnosis of acute infection is made by detection of parasites on blood smear and the diagnosis of chronic infection by the detection of serum antibodies.

Creutzfeldt–Jakob disease

Prospective donors of blood products who have a familial history of dementia and have undergone corneal or brain surgery are deferred.[94-97] Owing to the identification in 1996 of a variant Creutzfeldt–Jakob disease (vCJD), which may be associated with bovine spongiform encephalopathy (BSE), or "mad cow disease," potential donors who resided in the United Kingdom for 3 months from 1980 to 1996 are deferred from donating. Donors residing in Europe for 5 years cumulatively from 1980 onward are also deferred. These travel restrictions are expected to eliminate 90% of person-days of exposure to the causative agent of vCJD at a cost of eliminating 5% of US blood donors. In the United Kingdom, a small number of human cases of transfusion-transmitted vCJD have been reported. Universal use of leukoreduced components for transfusion is recommended in many countries, based on the fact that the vector for transmission of vCJD appears to be the B lymphocyte.

Blood Component Support Post-transplantation. After BMT, there is a period of pancytopenia, when patients require multiple RBC and platelet transfusions. In cases of donor-recipient ABO incompatibility (about one-third of allogeneic transplants), particular care must be paid to blood provision. In these situations, blood products are selected to be ABO-compatible with both the donor and recipient.

ABO incompatibility between marrow donor and recipient may be either major, with isohemagglutinin in the recipient directed against donor RBC antigens, or minor, with isohemagglutinin in the donor directed against recipient RBC antigens. Major ABO incompatibility has the potential risk of severe hemolytic reactions, graft rejection, or delayed engraftment.[98-100] Attempts to overcome major ABO incompatibility have included depletion of RBCs from the bone-marrow graft before BMT and/or removal of isohemagglutinin from the recipient by large-volume plasma exchanges or immunoadsorption, but these maneuvers are not done routinely.[101,102] Although studies suggest that major ABO incompatible HLA-matched transplants have resulted in no increase in patient mortality, incidence of rejection, delayed reconstitution, or GVHD compared to ABO compatible controls, some reports suggest that RBC reconstitution can be delayed in this setting.[98,103] Red-cell engraftment may be especially delayed in the setting of major ABO-incompatible nonmyeloablative stem-cell transplantation, where host antidonor isohemagglutinin levels tend to decrease more slowly than in myeloablative BMT.[104]

Potential adverse outcomes of minor ABO incompatibility between marrow donor and recipient include rapid immune hemolysis at the time of infusion of donor marrow resulting from passive transfer of isohemagglutinin in the marrow plasma, or delayed immune hemolysis caused by anti-RBC antibodies produced by donor lymphocytes.[105] There is no effect of minor ABO incompatibility on graft rejection, the incidence and severity of GVHD, or patient survival. Although exchange transfusion of the recipient before BMT using red cells of the donor's blood group has been utilized to prevent hemolysis caused by passive transfer of isohemagglutinin in the marrow product, this is rarely a clinically significant problem and can more easily be avoided by removing plasma from the marrow before infusion. Minor ABO incompatibility can result in adverse reactions owing to the production of anti-A and/or anti-B antibodies by donor-marrow lymphocytes early (1–3 weeks) following transplantation, particularly in patients on cyclosporine therapy or those receiving T cell-depleted allografts.[106,107] In this setting, transfusions of either group O or donor group RBCs are utilized to dilute the recipient red cells; in some cases, exchange transfusion has been required owing to very rapid engraftment of donor lymphocytes and production of anti-RBC antibodies.

Conclusion

The development and implementation of new and aggressive therapies for patients with cancer to date would not have been possible without parallel developments for the provision of blood-component support. In the future, the blood-component laboratory will provide specialized cellular components to facilitate the use of new and promising transplantation and cellular therapies for patients with hitherto incurable diseases.

Key references

The complete reference list can be found on the Wiley Companion Digital Edition of this title (see inside front cover for login instructions).

10 Hebert PC, Wells G, Blajchman MA, et al. A multicenter randomized, controlled clinical trial of transfusion requirements in critical care. Transfusion Requirements in Critical Care Investigators, Canadian Critical Care Trials Group. *N Engl J Med.* 1999;**340**:409–417.

11 Carson JL, Terrin ML, Noveck H, et al. Liberal or restrictive transfusion in high-risk patients after hip surgery. *N Engl J Med.* 2011;**365**:2453–2462.

14 Murphy GJ, Pike K, Rogers CA, et al. Liberal or restrictive transfusion after cardiac surgery. *N Engl J Med.* 2015;**372**:997–1008.

15 Holst LB, Haase N, Wetterslev J, et al. Lower versus higher hemoglobin threshold for transfusion in septic shock. *N Engl J Med.* 2014;**371**:1381–1391.

16 Villanueva C, Colomo A, Bosch A, et al. Transfusion strategies for acute upper gastrointestinal bleeding. *N Engl J Med.* 2013;**368**:11–21.

21 Fergusson DA, Hebert P, Hogan DL, et al. Effect of fresh red blood cell transfusions on clinical outcomes in premature, very-low-birth-weight infants: the ARIPI randomized trial. *JAMA.* 2012;**308**:1443–1451.

22 Steiner ME, Ness PM, Assmann SF, et al. Effects of red-cell storage duration on patients undergoing cardiac surgery. *N Engl J Med.* 2015;**372**:1419–1429.

23 Lacroix J, Hebert PC, Fergusson DA, et al. Age of transfused blood in critically ill adults. *N Engl J Med.* 2015;**372**:1410–1418.

35 Gaydos LA, Freireich EJ, Mantel N, et al. The quantitative relation between platelet count and hemorrhage in patients with acute leukemia. *N Engl J Med.* 1962;**266**:905–909.

36 Wandt H, Schaefer-Eckart K, Wendelin K, et al. Therapeutic platelet transfusion versus routine prophylactic transfusion in patients with haematological malignancies: an open-label, multicentre, randomised study. *Lancet.* 2012;**380**(**9850**):1309–1316. doi:10.1016/S0140-6736(12)60689-8. Epub 2012 Aug 8. PMID: 22877506.

39 Kaufman RM, Djulbegovic B, Gernsheimer T, et al. Platelet transfusion: a clinical practice guideline from the AABB. *Ann Intern Med.* 2015;**162**:205–213.

40 Gmur J, Burger J, Schanz U, et al. A safety of stringent prophylactic platelet transfusion policy for patients with acute leukemia. *Lancet.* 1991;**338**:1223–1226.

41 Rebulla P, Finazzi G, Marangoni F, et al. The threshold for prophylactic platelet transfusions in adults with acute myeloid leukemia. *N Engl J Med.* 1997;**337**:1870–1875.

42 Wandt H, Frank M, Ehninger G, et al. Safety and cost effectiveness of a 10×10^9/L trigger for prophylactic platelet transfusions compared with the traditional 20×10^9/L trigger. A prospective comparative trial in 105 patients with acute myeloid leukemia. *Blood.* 1998;**91**:3601–3606.

48 Slichter SJ, Kaufman RM, Assmann SF, et al. Dose of prophylactic platelet transfusions and prevention of hemorrhage. *N Engl J Med.* 2010;**362**(7):600–613.

51 O'Connell B, Lee EJ, Schiffer CA. The value of 10-minute posttransfusion platelet count. *Transfusion.* 1988;**28**:66–67.

54 Yankee RA, Graff KS, Dowling R, Henderson ES. Selection of unrelated compatible platelet donors by lymphocyte HLA matching. *N Engl J Med.* 1973;**288**:760–764.

56 Slichter SJ. Leukocyte reduction and ultraviolet B irradiation of platelets to prevent alloimmunization and refractoriness to platelet transfusions. *N Engl J Med.* 1997;**337**:1861–1869.

58 Julmy F, Ammann RA, Mansouri T, et al. Transfusion efficacy of ABO major-mismatched platelets (PLTs) in children is inferior to that of ABO-identical PLTs. *Transfusion.* 2009;**49**:21–33.

76 Stramer SL. Current risks of transfusion-transmitted agents: a review. *Arch Pathol Lab Med.* 2007;**131**:702–707.

81 Stramer SL, Caglioti S, Strong DM. NAT of the United States and Canadian blood supply. *Transfusion.* 2000;**40**:1165–1168.

82 Bowden RA, Slichter SJ, Sayers M, et al. A comparison of filtered leukocyte-reduced and cytomegalovirus (CMV) seronegative blood products for the prevention of transfusion-associated CMV infection after marrow transplant. *Blood.* 1995;**86**:3598–3603.

89 Kaufman RM. Platelets: testing, dosing and the storage lesion. *Hematology Am Soc Hematol Educ Program.* 2006:492–496.

130 Coagulopathic complications of cancer patients

Maria T. De Sancho, MD, MSc ▪ Jacob H. Rand, MD

Overview

Bleeding and thrombotic complications are common in cancer patients. The bleeding complications usually result from abnormalities in platelets or deficiency of coagulation factors and require specific blood or coagulation factor replacement. Thromboembolic events including deep venous thrombosis and pulmonary embolism are common and associated with serious complications. New biomarkers, diagnostic imaging approached and anticoagulant therapies have significantly improved the care of these patients. Ongoing research in the understanding of the various disturbances in hemostasis, application of innovative treatment modalities, and use of appropriate thromboprophylaxis in cancer patients should lead to further decreased morbidity and improved survival.

Bleeding and thrombotic complications are major causes of morbidity and mortality in cancer patients. As a result of advances in cancer treatment, the prevalence of these complications has been progressively rising in recent years. Bleeding is common in patients with leukemias, particularly those with acute promyelocytic leukemia (APL); however, due to improved targeted therapies, early hemorrhagic deaths have decreased to 5–10% within the context of clinical trials, but not replicated in clinical practice as evidenced from recent-population-based registries.[1] In general, bleeding complications occur relatively infrequently in patients with solid tumors, except those with melanoma, germ cell tumors, carcinoma of the cecum and prostate cancer,[2] although carcinomas of the kidney, bladder, endometrium, and cervix may first time be recognized by bleeding. In particular, gemcitabine and bevacizumab-based therapies are associated with an increased risk of high-grade hemorrhage in patients with solid tumors.[3,4] Cancer-mediated hypercoagulability occurs as a consequence of direct activation of procoagulant pathways by cancer cells. Cancer patients account for about 20% of newly diagnosed venous thrombosis events (VTEs) and in up to 50% in postmortem studies.[5] This chapter reviews the physiology of normal hemostasis, and then discusses the relationship of the coagulation system and cancer, and the pathophysiology of bleeding and thrombosis in the cancer patient. Next, the diagnostic and treatment approaches to the disorders most frequently encountered in cancer patients are described. Finally, the new generation of direct oral anticoagulants (DOACs) such as anti-Factor Xa and anti-Factor IIa inhibitors are addressed.

Physiology of normal hemostasis

Hemostasis dependent on both cellular components and soluble plasma proteins is the physiologic mechanism that halts bleeding after injury to the vasculature. Circulating platelets adhere and aggregate at sites of blood vessel injury. Platelet adhesion is dependent on the presence of the von Willebrand factor (vWF) and is followed by an aggregation response. Activation of platelets results in a flipping of the polarity of inner and outer leaflets of the cytoplasmic membrane and consequent exposure of anionic phospholipids that serve as platforms for the assembly of blood coagulation enzyme complexes. The extrinsic pathway of blood coagulation is initiated when blood is exposed to tissue factor (TF), a transmembrane protein expressed in the deeper portions of the blood vessel wall that may also be present in stimulated endothelial cells. Thrombus propagation occurs via incorporation of active, blood-borne TF into the growing clot.[6] TF binds activated factor VII (factor VIIa) and the resulting complex activates factors X and IX. Activated factor IX (factor IXa) combines with factor VIIIa to provide a second pathway to activate factor X. Factor Xa complexes with factor Va and prothrombin to form prothrombinase, which cleaves prothrombin to generate thrombin, the key enzyme in hemostasis. In the final step of the coagulation cascade, thrombin cleaves fibrinogen to generate fibrin monomers, which then polymerize. This polymer is covalently cross-linked by factor XIIIa (itself generated from factor XIII by thrombin) to form a chemically stable clot. Thrombin also feeds back to activate cofactors V, VIII, and XI further amplifying the coagulation system.[7]

Fibrin deposition is limited by an endogenous anticoagulant system. Antithrombin (AT) is a plasma protein member of the serpin (serine protease inhibitor) family that inhibits the activities of all of the activated coagulation enzymes particularly factors IIa and Xa. Protein C is a vitamin K-dependent protein that proteolyzes factors Va and VIIIa to inactive fragments. Protein C binds to an endothelial cell protein C receptor (EPCR)[8] and is activated by thrombin bound to thrombomodulin, another endothelial cell membrane-based protein, in a reaction that is modulated by a cofactor, protein S. TF pathway inhibitor is a plasma protein that forms a quaternary complex with TF, factor VIIa, and factor Xa, thereby inhibiting the extrinsic coagulation pathway.

There has been increasing intriguing evidence that, in addition to its role in hemostasis, factor XI plays a role in venous thrombosis. This has been supported by a recent clinical trial of a factor XI antisense oligonucleotide in patients who were at increased risk for DVT because of knee replacement surgery in which this strategy significantly reduced venous thrombosis. This type of anticoagulant strategy has the possibility of yielding important clinical benefits for cancer patients as it appears that factor XI level did not need to be reduced below a homeostatic level of 20% in order to gain a prophylactic effect. It is therefore possible that this strategy may be able to reduce the rate of thrombosis without significantly increasing the risk of bleeding.[9] However, this possibility will require testing in well-designed clinical trials.

The fibrinolytic system refers to a cascade of serine proteases that result in fibrin degradation and clot dissolution. The final step in this process is the conversion of the circulating zymogen

Holland-Frei Cancer Medicine, Ninth Edition. Edited by Robert C. Bast Jr., Carlo M. Croce, William N. Hait, Waun Ki Hong, Donald W. Kufe, Martine Piccart-Gebhart, Raphael E. Pollock, Ralph R. Weichselbaum, Hongyang Wang, and James F. Holland.
© 2017 John Wiley & Sons, Inc. ISBN: 978-1-118-93469-2

plasminogen into its active form plasmin. In the circulation, this is mainly achieved by tissue-type plasminogen activator (t-PA). This catalysis is highly dependent on the presence of fibrin, as binding of both plasminogen and t-PA to fibrin increases plasmin generation by more than two orders of magnitude. Mechanistically, plasminogen binds to exposed lysine residues formed in fibrin and these binding sites increase in number during fibrin cleavage allowing more plasminogen binding to occur, thereby amplifying the process allowing more plasmin to be generated. Naturally occurring plasma inhibitors [α2 antiplasmin, plasminogen activator inhibitor (PAI)-1, and PAI-2] also exist to limit plasmin activity or its generation in the circulation. The most potent of these is α2 antiplasmin. Plasmin is largely protected from α2 antiplasmin while bound to fibrin, allowing fibrin cleavage to occur. Other key regulatory steps occur at the level of the plasminogen activators, as the activity of t-PA and also urokinase-type plasminogen activator (u-PA), the second important endogenous plasminogen activator, are both regulated by PAI-1 and PAI-2.

The most recently described mechanism that limits the fibrinolytic system is via "thrombin activatable fibrinolysis inhibitor." The protein, thrombin activatable fibrinolysis inhibitor (TAFI), is a carboxypeptidase that specifically removes exposed lysine residues from fibrin, thereby removing the ability of plasminogen and t-PA to dock onto lysine binding sites in fibrin. As it requires activation by thrombin, TAFI becomes engaged as a direct consequence of coagulation to stabilize and protect clots from premature removal by the fibrinolytic system.[10]

Relationship of coagulation system, inflammation, and cancer

The relationship between blood coagulation and cancer was first described in the medical literature during the latter half of the nineteenth century with Trousseau's classic report of the association of migratory thrombophlebitis and gastric carcinoma.[11] In 1878, Billroth demonstrated cancer cells within a thrombus and theorized that tumor cells were spread by thromboembolism.[12] The interaction between blood coagulation and tumor angiogenesis and growth is supported by the involvement of several coagulation factors, specifically TF and thrombin in cancer neoangiogenesis, growth, and dissemination. Cancer cells or host cells in response to the neoplastic process cause local and systemic inflammatory stimuli that can switch the endothelium to a prothrombotic surface.[13] Endothelial damage leads to exposure of subendothelial VWF and TF. VWF in turn induces platelet and tumor cell adhesion, with subsequent platelet activation and aggregation. TF plays a key role in the initiation of the coagulation cascade. TF is aberrantly expressed on the surface of activated endothelial cells, monocytes, and tumor cells.[14] TF is upregulated in endothelium in pathologic states such as cancer as evidenced by the expression of TF and cross-linked fibrin on the endothelium of newly formed blood vessels within human tumors.[15]

Microparticles

Cell-derived vesicles, in particular extracellular vesicles (EVs) such as microparticles (MPs) and microvesicles, besides exosomes, are raising more and more attention as a novel and unique approach to detecting diseases.[16] MPs are generally defined as 0.1 to 1 μm membrane particles that expose the anionic phospholipid phosphatidylserine and membrane antigens representative of their cellular origin. Platelet-derived microparticles (PMPs) represent the most abundant MP subtype. Their presence reflects platelet activity, physiopathology, and the thrombotic state of cancer patients. Because platelets play a key role in cancer progression, as well as formation of metastasis, PMPs also may be important in the proliferation of cancer cells, cancer cell interactions, metastatic progression, angiogenesis, and inflammation.[17]

While this is of great research interest and has diagnostic potential, the methodology(ies) for MP analysis has not yet been sufficiently standardized for routine clinical use. The authors of a recent consensus workshop concluded that there was significant variability among laboratories even when a common protocol was utilized.[18]

Bleeding disorders

Cancer can cause both quantitative and qualitative changes in platelets.[19] Reactive thrombocytosis occurs in approximately 60% of cancer patients, while thrombocytopenia occurs in up to 11% of patients with untreated malignancy (Table 1).

The major bleeding problems are commonly caused by tumor invasion of blood vessels and adjacent organs, complications of treatment, and vitamin K deficiency. Bleeding in the cancer patient may present as either localized bleeding usually as a result of tumor invasion or as generalized bleeding diathesis caused by thrombocytopenia, thrombocytopathies, specific coagulation factor deficiencies, disseminated intravascular coagulation (DIC), or hyperfibrinolysis.[19] Appropriate treatment of bleeding in cancer patients needs to address the underlying disorder responsible for the bleeding.

Thrombocytopenia

Thrombocytopenia is the most frequent hemostatic disorder in cancer patients, occurring in approximately 10% of cases, even before starting chemotherapy. In the acute setting, thrombocytopenia is usually caused by decreased production either secondary to chemotherapy and/or radiation therapy or bone marrow infiltration, platelet sequestration in the spleen, or increased peripheral destruction, as in sepsis, disseminated DIC, and thrombotic microangiopathies (TMA)[20] (Table 2). Bortezomib, a proteasome inhibitor used in newly diagnosed and relapsed multiple myeloma, causes a transient, cyclical, and reversible thrombocytopenia.[20] Thrombocytopenia as a result of bone marrow infiltration commonly occurs in patients with small-cell lung cancer, breast cancer, and prostate cancer, as well as in patients with acute leukemia. On the other hand, thrombocytopenia secondary to splenic sequestration is usually observed with myeloproliferative disorders and less commonly with lymphomas and chronic lymphocytic leukemia. Clinically evident bleeding episodes are more likely to occur when thrombocytopenia is caused by diminished production of megakaryocytes rather than by immune destruction.

The most common clinical manifestation of thrombocytopenia is mucocutaneous bleeding. This can occur in the form of petechiae, or ecchymoses, and epistaxis, oral, gastrointestinal, or genitourinary bleeding. Spontaneous bleeding usually does not occur unless the platelet count is less than 5000–10,000/mm^3. However, in the presence of sepsis, uremia, trauma, or surgery, bleeding complications, including into the central nervous system, may occur with a higher platelet count.

The clinical history, physical examination, review of medications, and timing of prior chemotherapy, immunotherapy, or radiation therapy must be reviewed. In addition, examination of the peripheral blood smear is vital in the diagnostic work-up of thrombocytopenia. Spurious thrombocytopenia manifested by platelet clumping on the peripheral smear or platelet satellitism

Table 1 Hemostatic abnormalities in cancer patients.

Abnormality	Mechanism
Platelets	
Thrombocytopenia	Marrow infiltration by tumor
	Chemotherapy effects
	Biological response modifiers
	Monoclonal antibodies and immunotoxins
	Proteasome inhibitor (bortezomib)
	Disseminated intravascular coagulation (DIC)
	Hypersplenism
	Immune mediated (autoimmune, alloimmune)
	Thrombotic microangiopathies (TMA)
Thrombocytosis	Increased production:
	• reactive
	• primary
	° myeloproliferative disorders
Platelet function abnormalities	Uremia
	Acquired von Willebrand syndrome
	Myeloproliferative disorders
Abnormalities in coagulation factors and clinically available coagulation activation markers	
Hypofibrinogenemia	Asparaginase, DIC
Dysfibrinogenemia	Hepatocellular carcinoma
Factor X (decreased)	Amyloidosis
Decreased coagulation factors	Impairment in hepatic synthesis, DIC, vitamin K deficiency
Elevated D-dimer and fibrin degradation products	Inflammation, thrombosis, fibrinolysis, DIC, renal insufficiency, hepatic failure
Elevated prothrombin fragment 1 + 2	Disseminated malignancies, DIC
Fibrinolysis	
Increased secretion of plasminogen activators	Acute promyelocytic leukemia (APL)
Overexpression of annexin II	APL
Decreased levels of plasminogen activator inhibitors	Increased fibrin(ogen) degradation products and D-dimer
Acquired thrombophilias	
Antithrombin deficiency	Impaired hepatic synthesis of anticoagulant proteins, DIC, L-asparaginase, unfractionated heparin (UFH), and low-molecular-weight heparin (LMWH)
Protein C deficiency	Impaired hepatic synthesis, DIC, vitamin K antagonists (VKA)
Protein S deficiency	Impaired hepatic synthesis, DIC, VKA
Tissue factor pathway inhibitor deficiency (TFPI)	Impaired hepatic synthesis, DIC
Cytokines and hemostasis	
Proinflammatory cytokines (IL-1, IL-6, TNF)	Key role in tissue factor expression in monocytes and endothelial cells

Elevated microparticles have increasingly been associated with thrombosis in cancer; however, these tests have not yet been sufficiently standardized to be useful.
DIC, disseminated intravascular coagulation; TMA, thrombotic microangiopathy; IL, interleukin; TNF, tumor necrosis factor.

(platelets surrounding the polymorphonuclear leukocytes) must be excluded.

The treatment of bleeding associated with thrombocytopenia in the cancer patient is often managed empirically even when a specifically defined cause cannot be identified. Table 3 lists the critical platelet counts in various situations and general guidelines for platelet transfusion. Prophylactic transfusion of platelets is not indicated in patients who are asymptomatic for bleeding unless the platelet count is below 5000/mm^3. However, in cancer patients undergoing chemotherapy and those with leukemia, prophylactic platelet transfusions are generally beneficial in decreasing the risk of bleeding when the platelet count is below 10,000/mm^3.[21,22] For cancer patients undergoing major surgery or invasive procedures such as central venous catheterization, bronchial or endoscopic biopsy, lumbar puncture, thoracentesis, thoracostomy tube placement, and abdominal paracentesis, it is generally recommended that platelet transfusions should be administered in thrombocytopenic patients to a target level of greater than 50,000.[23] For minor invasive procedures such as arterial puncture or cannulation, prophylactic transfusion is not necessary if the platelet count is at least 20,000/mm^3 and local pressure is applied at the puncture site until hemostasis is achieved.[23] Platelet transfusions are usually indicated in thrombocytopenic patients to keep the platelet count above 50,000/mm^3 when evidence of microscopic or gross bleeding

is detected, as manifested by either occult blood stool tests and mucocutaneous bleeding. The risk of central nervous system bleeding is generally low and bleeding depends on several factors such as concurrent anticoagulant therapy, etiology of thrombocytopenia, coagulation abnormalities, impaired renal or hepatic function, severe sepsis, trauma, and the use of mechanical ventilation. Subdural and intracerebral hematomas occur in approximately 2.5–5%[24] and 2%, respectively, of leukemic patients following hematopoietic stem cell transplantation.[25,26] Comparative studies show that platelets derived from single or random donors produce similar posttransfusion increments, hemostatic benefits, and side effects.[23]

Thrombocytopathies

In addition to quantitative platelet changes, cancer can also cause qualitative platelet abnormalities. The main disorders are described in the following sections.

Acquired von Willebrand Syndrome

Several types of cancer have been reported in association with acquired von Willebrand syndrome (aVWS). Among the lymphoproliferative disorders, monoclonal gammopathy of undetermined significance (MGUS) is the condition most frequently associated

Table 2 Differential diagnosis of thrombocytopenia in cancer patients.

Decreased platelet production
- Metastases to bone marrow
- Acute and chronic leukemias
- Lymphomas
- Plasma cell dyscrasias
- Medications including cytotoxic chemotherapy and targeted therapies
- Radiation therapy

Platelet destruction
- Medications
- Immune mediated
- Bacterial sepsis
- Viral, fungal, and protozoal infections
- DIC
- Heparin-induced thrombocytopenia
- Thrombotic microangiopathies

Splenic sequestration
- Myeloproliferative disorders
- Myeloproliferative disorders
- Lymphomas
- Chronic lymphocytic leukemias

Combination of the above mechanisms

DIC, disseminated intravascular coagulation; HUS, hemolytic uremic syndrome; TTP, thrombotic thrombocytopenic purpura.
May consider adding liver insufficiency as etiology of thrombocytopenia due to decrease in thrombopoietin synthesis.

Table 3 Critical platelet counts and recommendations for transfusion in cancer patients[a].

Platelet count threshold	
Mucocutaneous or gastrointestinal bleeding	>50,000
Leukemias	
Preinduction chemotherapy	>20,000
Acute promyelocytic leukemia	>5000 to 10,000
Prophylaxis	
Asymptomatic	>5000
Major surgery	>50,000
Invasive procedures	
Major	>50,000
Minor	>20,000

[a]These are intended to serve as general guidelines. Actual treatment will vary depending on specific circumstances.

with aVWS. It can also be associated with multiple myeloma, Waldenstrom macroglobulinemia, chronic lymphocytic leukemia, hairy cell leukemia, and non-Hodgkin lymphoma. Among the myeloproliferative disorders, essential thrombocythemia (ET) is the most common while polycythemia vera (PV) and chronic myeloid leukemia are less frequent. Solid tumors including Wilms tumors and carcinomas have also been associated with aVWS.[27]

The clinical manifestations of aVWS are similar to those seen in patients with the hereditary form of the disease except for the notable absence of a family history or lifelong personal history for bleeding. Spontaneous mucocutaneous and gastrointestinal bleeding may be present. Postsurgical bleeding may also occur. Laboratory screening tests generally reveal a prolonged activated partial thromboplastin time (aPTT) and a normal or borderline prolonged bleeding time, or by prolonged closure times of the PFA-100. Treatment is directed to the underlying malignancy and supportive measures such as corticosteroids, deamino-8-D-arginine

vasopressin (desmopressin acetate or DDAVP), factor VIII/vWF concentrate, and intravenous immunoglobulin.[27,28]

Acquired hemophilia (factor VIII autoantibodies)

Patients with solid tumors, plasma cell dyscrasias, and lymphoproliferative disorders may develop an acquired hemophilia as a consequence of autoantibodies against factor VIII, often referred to as "acquired inhibitors." The inhibitors are almost always immunoglobulin G (IgG) molecules. The most common presenting complaint is bleeding into the skin or muscles in patients with no previous history of bleeding diathesis. The hallmark finding is a prolongation of the aPTT in the presence of a normal prothrombin time (PT) along with plasma mixing studies that demonstrate an aPTT that remains prolonged after incubation at 37 °C for 1–2 h. In contrast, in patients with coagulation factor deficiencies, plasma mixing studies normalize the aPTT. Contamination of the blood sample with heparin, which frequently is the inadvertent result of instillation for maintaining vascular access line patency, may artifactually prolong the aPTT and affect the mixing tests. Heparin that has entered the sample may be removed in the testing laboratory with the enzyme heparinase or resin absorption, after which the plasma may be retested. The acute bleeding can be managed with desmopressin acetate if there is a low inhibitor titer [<5 Bethesda units (BU)] or with human or porcine factor VIII. Factor VIII bypassing agents such as recombinant human factor VIIa or activated prothrombin complex concentrate are used in case of moderate- to high-titer inhibitor (>5 BU). Immunosuppressive therapy such as corticosteroids, cyclophosphamide, vincristine, cyclosporine, and intravenous immunoglobulin (IVIg) may be used in addition to the treatment of the underlying neoplasm. Rituximab should be considered in patients who are resistant to first-line therapy or cannot tolerate standard immunosuppressive therapy.[29]

Uremia

Platelet dysfunction is common in cancer patients with chronic renal failure and causes significant bleeding. The pathophysiology of uremic bleeding is multifactorial and includes dysfunctional vWF, increased levels of cyclic adenosine monophosphate and nitric oxide generated by platelets, uremic toxins, and anemia that causes the platelets to be displaced from the vascular endothelium, thereby decreasing their ability to adhere and aggregate in response to endothelial damage.[25] Treatment is recommended for patients with active bleeding or for those undergoing an invasive procedure, such as placement of hemodialysis catheters. Patients usually respond to hemodialysis and administration of DDAVP at a dose of 0.3 µg/kg intravenously; cryoprecipitate (10 bags given intravenously over 30 min) and conjugated estrogens (0.6 mg/kg over 30–40 min once daily for 5 consecutive days) may occasionally be required. Erythropoietin-stimulating agents such as recombinant human erythropoietin and darbepoetin have been shown to reduce and prevent bleeding in uremic patients and have a more sustained effect than either DDAVP or conjugated estrogens.[30]

Myeloproliferative disorders

Among the myeloproliferative conditions, PV and ET are the most likely to be associated with hemorrhagic and thrombotic complications. Thrombosis represents the initial manifestation for 12–39% of patients with ET and PV[28] Increasing age (>65) and a previous history of thrombosis were identified as major risk factors for thrombosis.[31] An acquired point mutation in the pseudokinase domain of Janus kinase 2 (JAK2(V617F)) is found in approximately 97% and 50% of patients with PV and ET, respectively.

Other potential determinants of thrombotic risk include cardiovascular risk factors. Leukocytosis was reported to be an independent risk factor for thrombosis and survival both in PV and ET.[32,33] All patients with PV are managed with phlebotomy and low-dose aspirin. The recommended HCT target is below 45%[34] ET patients at low risk for major vascular complications should be observed without treatment. Low-dose aspirin is given in the presence of microvascular symptoms. A careful correction of concomitant cardiovascular risk factors should be pursued. In high-risk patients, hydroxyurea (HU) remains the first choice drug for most PV and ET patients requiring a cytoreductive therapy because it is the only treatment proven to be effective in reducing life-threatening thrombotic complications.[34,35] IFN-α and anagrelide may be considered in younger patients, pregnancy (for IFN-α), and in cases resistant or intolerant of HU. JAK2 inhibitors with limited side effects can be considered for patients with PV and/or ET if therapy is required.[36]

Coagulation factor deficiencies

Cancer patients may develop various coagulation factor abnormalities resulting from vitamin K deficiency as a consequence of malnutrition, diarrhea, liver disease, biliary obstruction, use of oral anticoagulants, and antibiotic therapy. Patients with primary or metastatic hepatocellular carcinoma have deficiency of vitamin K-dependent factors (factors II, VII, IX, and X and proteins C and S), similar to that seen with liver cirrhosis. These patients almost always have increased levels of fibrinogen, unlike patients with cirrhosis or acute liver failure who have decreased fibrinogen levels. Acquired inhibitors of coagulation factors are frequently seen in multiple myeloma and other plasma cell dyscrasias.

The treatment of cancer patients with coagulation factor deficiencies, aside from the treatment of the underlying neoplasm, is generally supportive, and consists of vitamin K, fresh-frozen plasma, and cryoprecipitate. Oral vitamin K is the treatment of choice. Cryoprecipitate is administered IV, generally at a dose of 1 unit of cryoprecipitate for every 5 kg of body weight.[37]

Amyloidosis

Haemostatic disorders are common in amyloidosis. Laboratory abnormalities include a prolongation of the PT and the aPTT. Moreover, prolongations of the thrombin time (TT) that have been associated with hepatic amyloid infiltration and reptilase time (RT) have also been found. The PT, but not the TT, appears to be a clinically useful predictor of bleeding tendency.[38]

Drug effects (L-asparaginase)

L-Asparaginase is used in combination with other agents, for induction of remissions in acute lymphocytic leukemia. L-Asparaginase can cause depletion of many of the coagulation factors with an associated risk for thrombosis and hemorrhage. Levels of t-PA and PAI were increased during treatment while cross-linked fibrin degradation products remained within normal limits, excluding the presence of DIC.[39]

Acute promyelocytic leukemia

APL-associated hemostasis disorders result from at least two distinct mechanisms, the release of procoagulant activities and plasminogen activators from the leukemic cells. The T15–17 translocation induces hyperexpression of TF and renders the patient hypercoagulable. It appears that plasmin-dependent primary fibrinogenolysis is the major etiologic factor for low fibrinogen levels in APL patients. *In vivo* differentiation therapy with all-trans-retinoic acid induces a rapid decrease in plasmin activation and a normalization of fibrinogen level, and was associated with a significant decrease in TF gene expression in bone marrow cells.[40] Administration of heparin in APL has been discontinued in current treatment regimens that include ATRA. Heparin has been thought to control the coagulopathy associated with APL by inhibiting intravascular fibrin formation and reducing the consumption of clotting factors and platelets, thereby decreasing the bleeding tendency.[1]

Thrombotic complications

The pathogenesis of thrombotic complications in cancer patients is multifactorial. In addition to the common predisposing factors for thrombosis such as immobility, venous stasis, advanced age, history of previous thrombosis, sepsis, and the use of central venous access devices, tumor cells have unique prothrombotic characteristics. Transformed malignant cells can induce platelet abnormalities, abnormal activation of the coagulation cascade, decreased hepatic synthesis of anticoagulant and coagulant proteins, fibrinolytic abnormalities, acquired thrombophilias, and expression of inflammatory and angiogenic cytokines (Table 1). Multiple biomarkers have been linked to cancer-associated thrombosis. The highest level of evidence currently exists for pre-chemotherapy-elevated platelets and leukocyte counts and low hemoglobin levels. D-Dimer is also predictive of cancer-associated VTE. Many cancer patients have elevated D-dimer levels without obvious thrombosis and there is no consensus on the cutoff levels that would be predictive of cancer-associated thrombosis. TF, the physiologic initiator of hemostasis, is widely expressed across many types of cancer. TF is released into the circulation in the form of MPs, and levels can be detected in cancer patients. There is no consensus "standard" TF assay however. Initial reports suggested a significant association of elevated TF with subsequent VTE. The majority of these data were derived from patients with specific cancers, particularly pancreatic cancer.

Several factors contribute to the increased risk for bleeding and thrombotic complications in the cancer patient (Table 4). Thrombotic manifestations in cancer patients may present as one of the following: migratory thrombophlebitis or Trousseau syndrome, venous thromboembolism (VTE), thrombotic microangiopathy (TMA), arterial thrombosis, and DIC.

Migratory thrombophlebitis (Trousseau syndrome)

Trousseau syndrome is a classically described variant form of venous thrombosis characterized by a recurrent and migratory pattern preferentially involving superficial veins of the arms and chest.[11] This syndrome should precipitate the search for an occult malignancy, especially in patients with recurrent and migratory venous thrombosis affecting unusual sites such as subclavian veins, or veins of upper extremities, axilla, or neck. Trousseau syndrome is highly associated with mucin producing adenocarcinomas.[41] Its clinical manifestations also include chronic DIC associated with microangiopathy, non-bacterial endocarditis, and arterial emboli in patients with cancer. Migratory thrombophlebitis has also been associated with the use of somatostatin or octreotide therapy for malignant carcinoid syndrome.

Table 4 Risk factors for bleeding and thrombotic complications in cancer patients.

Use of indwelling catheters—*Thrombosis*
Systemic inflammatory response syndrome (SIRS)—*Thrombosis*
Sepsis—*Thrombosis and bleeding*
Prior chemotherapy and radiation treatment—*Mainly bleeding but also thrombosis*
Selective estrogen receptor modulators (SERMs): tamoxifen, raloxifene
Concomitant use of hormone replacement therapy or oral contraceptives—*Thrombosis*
Antiangiogenic agents (thalidomide, lenalidomide, bevacizumab[a] , sunitinib, sorafenib) — *Thrombosis*
Erythropoiesis-stimulating agents—*Thrombosis*
Metastatic disease to the liver and/or bone marrow—*Mainly bleeding*
Vitamin K deficiency—*Mainly bleeding*
Acute peptic ulcer—*Bleeding*
Slipped ligatures from recent surgery—*Bleeding*

[a]Also bleeding.

Table 5 Wells criteria for pulmonary embolism.

Variables	Points
Previous DVT or PE	1.5
Heart rate ≥ 100 per minute	1.5
Surgery or immobilization within the past 4 weeks	1.5
Hemoptysis	1
Active cancer	1
Clinical signs of DVT	3
Alternative diagnosis less likely than PE	3

0–1 point: low clinical probability; 2–6 points: intermediate clinical probability; ≥7 points: high clinical probability for PE.
Source: Wells et al. 1997.[47] Reproduced with permission from Elsevier.

Venous thromboembolism

VTE, involving DVT and pulmonary embolism (PE), may occur in 4–20% of cancer patients and is one of the leading causes of death. The overall incidence of cancer-related VTE in postmortem studies has been reported as high as 50%. In patients presenting with *de novo* idiopathic VTE, there is a high risk for a concurrent cancer, especially within the first year after the diagnosis of thromboembolism. Cancer patients at greatest risk for VTE include those with mucin-secreting tumors (e.g., pancreatic and gastrointestinal cancer), cancers of the lung, brain, prostate, breast, and ovary, and patients with APL and myeloproliferative disorders, specifically PV and ET. VTE often complicates the care of cancer patients after major surgery and of patients receiving chemotherapy and/or hormonal therapy.[5]

The risk of developing thrombosis in cancer patients is influenced by the age and hormonal status of the patient. Postmenopausal women with advanced breast cancer receiving tamoxifen or aromatase inhibitors in addition to adjuvant chemotherapy have a higher risk for thrombotic events than do premenopausal women with breast cancer.[42] Thromboembolic events have also been reported with angiogenesis inhibitors (thalidomide, lenalidomide, and bevacizumab).[15,43] The pathogenic mechanisms of thromboembolic events associated with thalidomide are thought to be related to the development of acquired activated protein C resistance and a reduction in thrombomodulin level.[15,44] Endothelial injury produced by the combination of thalidomide with chemotherapy and subsequent restoration of endothelial cell PAR-1 expression are probably factors that promote thrombosis.[45] Cancer patients receiving erythropoiesis-stimulating agents for anemia have also been reported to have increased risks of thrombotic complications.[46]

Major advances in the diagnosis of VTE generally—that is, not cancer-specific—include the development and validation of a standardized clinical model (Table 5)[47] to determine the pretest probability of VTE and the measurement of plasma D-dimer. The integration of these two advances has resulted in the formulation of safe, diagnostic algorithms that decrease the need for serial and/or invasive testing.[48] A study in oncologic patients has shown that D-dimer results have high negative predictive value and sensitivity for PE and, if negative, can be used to exclude PE in this population.[49]

As with other patients, the majority of DVT in cancer patients originate in the iliofemoral venous system. Diagnostic imaging modalities for DVT include ascending contrast venography, compression ultrasonography, and magnetic resonance venography. Ascending contrast venography remains the gold standard for diagnosing DVT, but this procedure is invasive and requires contrast material, which is frequently irritating and may result in

complications. The finding of an intraluminal filling defect caused by thrombus surrounded by contrast is diagnostic for DVT. Non-compressibility of a proximal lower limb vein on compression ultrasonography has a diagnostic sensitivity rate of 97% and a specificity rate of 94%.[50] Although compression ultrasonography is highly sensitive for detecting proximal DVT, it is not as accurate for diagnosing isolated distal DVT. Magnetic resonance venography has sensitivity and specificity rates of 92% and 95%, respectively, for proximal DVT.[51] It is useful in diagnosing pelvic vein DVT, especially isolated iliac vein thrombosis, which is difficult to diagnose with compression ultrasonography.

Several studies conducted in cancer patients with suspected DVT have demonstrated that two of the following studies can reliably exclude DVT and decrease the need for invasive testing: a low pretest probability, a normal D-dimer level, and a normal compression ultrasonogram.[47]

The standard treatment of VTE outside the setting of malignancy is to initiate anticoagulation with either intravenous or subcutaneous unfractionated heparin (UFH) or subcutaneous low-molecular-weight heparin (LMWH) or fondaparinux (an indirect Xa inhibitor) at therapeutic doses followed by oral warfarin therapy for a minimum of 3 months to achieve an international normalized ratio (INR) between 2.0 and 3.0.[52] However, in patients with active cancer, continued anticoagulation is recommended following the first episode of VTE.[52] Intravenous UFH can be started with an initial bolus of 80 U/kg followed by a continuous IV infusion of 18 U/kg/h, adjusted to maintain the aPTT at 1.5–2.5 times the control value. Alternatively, LMWH can be administered in weight-adjusted, once- or twice-daily subcutaneous doses without the need for laboratory monitoring. Warfarin therapy can be commenced within 24 h after heparin treatment is started. Heparin therapy is continued for at least 5 days until the INR is within the therapeutic range for 2 consecutive days. However, in patients with large iliofemoral vein thrombosis or major PE, some investigators have recommended extending heparin treatment to 7–10 days.

Retrospective and prospective clinical trials have demonstrated a survival advantage in cancer patients treated with LMWH for established thrombosis.[53,54] LMWHs have several advantages when compared to UFH: laboratory monitoring is rarely required, only subcutaneous injection is necessary, and there are lower incidences of bleeding, heparin-induced thrombocytopenia (HIT),[55] and osteoporosis.[56] The use of long-term LMWH as an alternative to warfarin therapy in cancer patients with acute VTE has been analyzed in two clinical trials. The CANTHANOX trial compared 3 months of warfarin versus enoxaparin anticoagulation in cancer patients with DVT and/or PE. Although the risk of recurrent VTE was lower in the enoxaparin group, the difference was not statistically significant. Warfarin was associated with a high bleeding rate.[57] In the CLOT trial, which continued treatment for 6 months, the cumulative risk of recurrent VTE was reduced from 17% in the oral anticoagulant group to 9% in the LMWH group resulting in a statistically significant risk reduction for VTE.[58] Overall, there were no differences in bleeding between the groups. Current guidelines recommend the use of LMWH for the first 3–6 months as long-term treatment of VTE in cancer patients.[52] Cancer patients with recurrent VTE tend to have a short survival. Escalating the dose of LMWH has not been shown to be effective for treating cases that are resistant to standard, weight-adjusted doses of LMWH or a vitamin K antagonist (VKA).[59]

The use of systemic thrombolytic agents such as t-PA should be restricted to patients with massive iliofemoral DVT or massive PE and hemodynamic instability because of the significant risks of bleeding associated with thrombolysis.[52] Furthermore, despite the proven efficacy of thrombolytic agents in achieving more rapid resolution of radiologic and hemodynamic abnormalities in patients with PE, studies to date have not shown any survival benefit with thrombolysis. At the present time, catheter-directed thrombolysis for initial treatment of VTE should be confined to selected patients requiring limb salvage. In general, thrombolytic therapy is contraindicated in cancer patients with brain metastases who develop VTE because of their significant risk for intracranial bleeding.[60] Surgical thromboembolectomy is restricted to patients with massive PE in extremis, or who have contraindications to or who do not respond to thrombolysis.[52] For cancer patients with VTE who have contraindications to anticoagulant therapy or those with recurrent VTE despite anticoagulation, placement of a retrievable or permanent inferior vena cava (IVC) filter is generally recommended. However, IVC filters are associated with undesirable side effects, such as debilitating leg symptoms caused by filter-related thrombosis.[61] A recent study reported that IVC filters were safe and highly effective in preventing PE-related deaths in patients with cancer with VTE disease.[62] However, patients with a history of DVT and bleeding or a metastatic/disseminated stage of disease had the lowest survival after IVC filter placement.

The major concern about treatment of VTE in cancer patients is the higher risk of bleeding and VTE recurrence compared to non-cancer patients. A prospective cohort study demonstrated that the 12-month cumulative incidence of recurrent VTE in cancer patients was 20.7% versus 6.8% in patients without cancer, and the parallel estimate for major bleeding was 12.4% versus 4.9%, respectively.[63] Recurrence and bleeding were both related to cancer severity and occurred predominantly during the first month of anticoagulant therapy and, remarkably, could not be explained by sub- or overanticoagulation. The risk of recurrent VTE has been reported to be two- to threefold higher and the risk of major bleeding is three- to sixfold higher in cancer patients than in patients without cancer.[58]

Routine anticoagulant prophylaxis for central venous catheters is not recommended.[64] Recombinant t-PA is effective in restoring flow to indwelling catheters occluded by thrombus.[65] Perioperative cancer patients, particularly those with breast cancer undergoing chemotherapy or on selective estrogen receptor modulators and patients with advanced cancers that are associated with high risk of VTE such as brain tumors, and colorectal, pancreatic, lung, renal cell, and ovarian adenocarcinomas, should receive antithrombotic prophylaxis with intermittent pneumatic compression devices or compression elastic stockings and LMWH. The recommended doses are dalteparin 5000 U SC daily, enoxaparin 40 mg SC daily, or fondaparinux 2.5 mg SC starting 8–12 h postoperatively.[64,65] Two trials in cancer patients undergoing surgery reported that continuation of LMWH prophylaxis for 3 weeks after hospital discharge reduced the risk of late venographic DVT by 60%. Finally, cancer patients who are immobile or bedridden with an acute medical illness also should receive antithrombotic prophylaxis with low-dose UFH or LMWH. However, ambulatory cancer patients do not require VTE prophylaxis. Cancer patients receiving chemotherapy or hormonal therapy also do not require routine primary thromboprophylaxis.[66] Of note, thromboprophylaxis with aspirin, warfarin, or LMWH is widely used by clinicians for patients with multiple myeloma receiving thalidomide or lenalidomide in combination with chemotherapy or high-dose steroids.[67,68]

General prophylaxis and treatment

A recent consensus clinical practice guideline from ASCO described recommendations for VTE prophylaxis and treatment in patients with cancer, and based on a systematic review of the literature recommended that most *hospitalized* patients with cancer require thromboprophylaxis throughout hospitalization. Thromboprophylaxis was not routinely recommended for outpatients with cancer. It may be considered for selected high-risk patients. Patients with multiple myeloma receiving antiangiogenesis agents with chemotherapy and/or dexamethasone should receive prophylaxis with either LMWH or low-dose aspirin. Patients undergoing major cancer surgery should receive prophylaxis, starting before surgery and continuing for at least 7–10 days. Extending prophylaxis up to 4 weeks should be considered in those with high-risk features. LMWH is recommended for the initial 5–10 days of treatment for deep vein thrombosis and PE as well as for long-term (6 months) secondary prophylaxis. Use of novel oral anticoagulants is not currently recommended for patients with malignancy and VTE.[66]

Anticancer effects of anticoagulation treatment

Experimental and indirect clinical evidence suggests that anticoagulants, particularly LMWH, may have antineoplastic effects. It has been suggested that anticoagulants can interfere with tumor angiogenesis, proliferation potential of cancer cells, and the immune system by augmenting the antitumor activity of tumor necrosis factor and interferon mediated by NK cells.[69] Anticoagulants may also interfere with the various stages of the metastatic cascade.

Heparin-induced thrombocytopenia (HIT)

HIT is an immune-mediated thrombocytopenia that occurs in approximately 1–5% of patients receiving heparin.[70] The decrease in platelet count typically occurs 5–10 days after starting heparin but may develop within 24 h if there has been exposure to heparin during the preceding 3 months. Occasionally, the platelet count starts to fall only after heparin has been stopped (delayed-onset HIT). The frequency of HIT varies according to the type of heparin preparation (bovine UFH > porcine UFH > LMWH), the exposed patient population (postoperative > medical > pregnancy), and gender (female > male).[70] HIT is caused by heparin-dependent, platelet-activating antibodies that recognize platelet factor 4 (PF4) bound to heparin. The resulting platelet activation is associated with increased thrombin generation. Venous or arterial thromboses including deep venous thrombosis, PE, limb artery thrombosis, thrombotic stroke, and myocardial infarction can occur. A clinical pretest probability score known as the 4T's (degree of thrombocytopenia, timing of thrombocytopenia, other etiologies of thrombocytopenia, and thrombosis) is useful in clinical practice. HIT should be suspected and treatment rapidly instituted in a patient with an intermediate of high test probability.[71] In clinical practice, the laboratory diagnosis of HIT is made with a positive PF4-dependent immunoassay. Management consists of discontinuing all forms of heparin and using direct thrombin inhibitors such as lepirudin or argatroban, which do not have any cross-reactivity to HIT antibodies. For patients receiving warfarin at the time of diagnosis of HIT, reversal of warfarin anticoagulation with vitamin K is recommended.

Thrombotic microangiopathies

TMAs involve hemolytic anemia, thrombocytopenia, neurologic symptoms, renal dysfunction, and fever. The majority of these cases are reported in patients with adenocarcinoma, particularly gastric cancer; however, TMA also occurs in patients with breast cancer and lung cancer, and in Hodgkin and non-Hodgkin lymphomas.[72] Thrombotic thrombocytopenic purpura/hemolytic uremic syndrome also occurs in association with cancer chemotherapy, especially with mitomycin C, bleomycin, cisplatin, and tamoxifen,[73] use of cyclosporine,[74] and interferon,[75] after hematopoietic stem cell transplantation,[76] and with Sunitinib maleate, an oral multitargeting tyrosine kinase inhibitor approved for the treatment of metastatic renal cell carcinoma.[77]

The pathophysiology of cancer-associated TMA is postulated to be similar to that of usual primary TMA. It involves injury to vascular endothelium with release of ultralarge vWF multimers due to a deficiency of a vWF-cleaving protease (ADAMTS-13) causing platelet aggregation.[78,79]

Typically, the microangiopathic hemolytic anemia and thrombocytopenia are severe and reticulocytosis is usually present, with increased levels of lactic acid dehydrogenase, reflecting intravascular hemolysis. The peripheral blood smear demonstrates numerous schistocytes. Renal failure and neurologic and pulmonary dysfunction are common. Standard treatment of TTP is plasmapheresis. Other treatment modalities that may be used in refractory cases include vincristine, intravenous gamma globulin, rituximab, and splenectomy.[80–82] Platelet transfusions are usually contraindicated because infused platelets may amplify the extent and severity of the formation of microvascular thrombi. Regardless of treatment, the prognosis of cancer patients with TMA is generally poor.

Arterial thrombosis and nonbacterial thrombotic endocarditis

The association between arterial thrombosis and cancer is less well described. Isolated cases have been reported and chemotherapy has been implicated as a cause.[83] The selective estrogen receptor modulators tamoxifen and raloxifene increase the risk of stroke,[84] especially in postmenopausal women at increased risk for coronary events and in current smokers.[85] Importantly, patients with acute ischemic stroke in the setting of active cancer (especially adenocarcinoma) have a significant short-term risk of recurrent ischemic stroke and other types of thromboembolism.[86]

Nonbacterial thrombotic endocarditis (NBTE) represents a form of consumptive coagulopathy most commonly seen with adenocarcinomas of the lung and pancreas. The diagnosis should be suspected in any cancer patient who presents with ischemic embolic events. Echocardiography is diagnostic with the finding of sterile thrombotic vegetations on cardiac valves. In addition to valvular vegetations, ventricular segmental wall motion abnormalities resulting from silent embolization to the coronary arteries

have been reported in 18% of cancer patients with NBTE. Management is essentially supportive and consists of treatment of the underlying cancer and anticoagulant therapy with unfractionated or low-molecular-weight heparin.

Disseminated intravascular coagulation (DIC)

DIC is a clinicopathological syndrome that complicates patients with malignancy. Patients with solid tumors (prostate, pancreas, lung, stomach, colon, and breast) and those with leukemia, especially APL, may be complicated by DIC that is manifested primarily by bleeding. Patients with hematologic malignancies often present with a state of chronic DIC in the absence of active thrombosis and/or bleeding. The bleeding disorder in APL is thought to be due to the abnormally high levels of expression of annexin A2 on APL cells, which leads to increased production of plasmin and ensuing bleeding from unopposed fibrinolysis. Annexin A2 is a phospholipid-binding protein on the surface of endothelial cells that serves to bind plasminogen and its activator, tPA. In APL cells, the t_{15-17} translocation induces hyperexpression of TF in the leukemic cell, linking the primary oncogenic event with induction of hypercoagulability.[87]

Plasma MP-associated TF procoagulant activity may play an important pathogenic role in the evolution of overt DIC in various types of malignancy.[88]

The thrombotic disorders associated with DIC include recurrent venous thrombosis, peripheral arterial thrombosis, cerebrovascular thrombosis, disseminated arterial disease with organ failure, peripheral limb ischemia, and gangrene. Chronic forms of DIC are characterized by less florid clinical findings and more subtle, but persistent, laboratory abnormalities. Metastatic cancer is a common cause of chronic DIC. Over time, approximately 25% of patients with metastatic cancer develop a thrombotic event. In cancer patients, the diagnosis of DIC is made clinically and corroborated by a constellation of laboratory abnormalities (Table 6).[89] There is no single laboratory test that can establish or exclude the diagnosis of DIC. In most cases, a combination of tests in a patient with a clinical condition that is associated with DIC can be used to diagnose the disorder with reasonable certainty. In the presence of an underlying disease associated with DIC, an initial platelet count of less than 100,000/mm^3 or a rapid decline in the platelet count and prolongation of the PT and aPTT is seen in about 50–60% of cases of DIC, and the presence of fibrin(ogen) degradation products and D-dimers in plasma. Fibrinogen levels may remain in the normal range in the face of its consumption because of increased synthesis of this acute-phase reactant. A finding of hypofibrinogenemia is only useful diagnostically in very severe cases of DIC. The peripheral blood smear may also demonstrate the presence of red cell fragmentation or schistocytes, but rarely >10% of the red cells. Soluble fibrin (SF) monomer, which is only generated intravascularly, is a sensitive but not specific test for the diagnosis of DIC.[90] There appears to be no added value measuring the natural anticoagulant protein C and/or AT.[91] The International Society of Thrombosis and Hemostasis (ISTH) sub-committee of the Scientific and Standardization Committee (SCC) on DIC has recommended the use of scoring system for overt DIC.[91] The sensitivity and specificity of the ISTH overt DIC score are 91% and 97%, respectively.[92] It is important to repeat the tests to monitor the dynamically changing scenario based on the laboratory results and clinical manifestations.

In general, the treatment of DIC is directed against the underlying cancer but supportive management to the bleeding or thrombotic manifestations is required. Cancer patients with DIC who are

Table 6 Abnormalities in cancer patients with disseminated intravascular coagulation.

Thrombocytopenia
Prolongation of PT and aPTT
Hypofibrinogenemia[a]
Decreased levels of factors V and VIII[b]
Presence of fibrin(ogen) degradation products and D-dimer[c] with secondary interference with fibrin polymerization and platelet aggregation
Presence of schistocytes or fragmented red blood cells in the peripheral blood smear indicating microangiopathic hemolysis

[a]Fibrinogen levels may remain in the normal range despite consumption because of increased production: a finding of hypofibrinogenemia is only useful diagnostically in very severe cases of DIC.
[b]Factor VIII levels may be increased in some patients with early DIC because of thrombin activation of factor VIII.
[c]Plasma D-dimers are specific cross-linked fibrin derivative generated when the endogenous fibrinolytic system degrades fibrin.

bleeding or at high risk for bleeding (patients undergoing surgery or invasive procedures) should receive platelet transfusions to maintain the platelet count greater than 50,000/μL and FFP (initial doses of 15 mL/kg, although a dose of 30 mL/kg produces a more complete correction of coagulation factor levels) if the PT or aPTT is prolonged. The administration of purified coagulation factor concentrates in DIC is not generally recommended unless patients are fluid overloaded and cannot receive FFP. Coagulation factor concentrates contain only specific factors, whereas in DIC, there is a global deficiency in coagulation factors. Severe hypofibrinogenemia (<1 g/L) needs to be treated with cryoprecipitate or fibrinogen concentrates if available. A dose of 3 g would raise plasma fibrinogen by 1 g/L, this can be given as two cryoprecipitate pools (10 donor units) or as 3 g of a fibrinogen concentrate. The response to the supportive transfusion therapy should be monitored clinically and with laboratory tests.[89] The bleeding associated with DIC in APL oftentimes responds dramatically to treatment with all-trans-retinoic acid.[86]

Although there are no clinical randomized controlled trials demonstrating that the use of heparin in patients with DIC results in improved clinical outcome, intravenous heparin may be used in cancer patients with DIC-associated thrombosis for stabilization while the cancer is being treated unless moderate to severe thrombocytopenia or bleeding is present. The recommended dose of heparin is 10 U/kg/h by continuous IV infusion without a loading dose. Monitoring aPTT may be complicated but monitoring for signs of bleeding is important. In critically ill, nonbleeding patients with DIC, pharmacological thromboprophylaxis with either unfractionated or low-molecular-weight heparin is recommended.[89] In general, patients with DIC should not be treated with antifibrinolytic agents. However, in patients with DIC and bleeding secondary to primary fibrinolysis (e.g., prostate cancer), the fibrinolytic inhibitor, epsilon aminocaproic acid, can be administered with an initial IV loading dose of 4–6 g over 1 h followed by an IV infusion of 1 g/h while monitoring the clinical response. The recommended oral dose of aminocaproic acid is 50–60 mg/kg every 4–6 h.[93] However, in those patients with a primary thrombotic presentation and secondary fibrinolysis, fibrinolytic inhibitors should be avoided until the thrombotic process is controlled.[89]

Drugs for treatment of bleeding and thrombotic disorders

Recombinant factor VIIa
Recombinant factor VIIa (rFVIIa) is FDA approved for patients with bleeding secondary to hemophilia A or B who have inhibitors

against factors VIII and IX and in patients with hereditary factor VII deficiency.[94] It has also been shown to be effective in controlling bleeding due to thrombocytopenia, thrombocytopathies, acquired coagulation factor deficiencies, and in patients undergoing cancer surgery. There is increasing evidence on the use of rFVIIa in patients with hematological malignancies and in patients who develop critical bleeding associated with hematopoietic stem cell transplantation.[95]

Thrombopoietin receptor agonists
Thrombopoietin receptor agonists (TPO-RAs), romiplostim and eltrombopag, are FDA approved to increase platelet counts in patients with chronic immune thrombocytopenic purpura (ITP). They have shown benefit in splenectomized and nonsplenectomized patients. TPO-RAs are approved to treat thrombocytopenia in the setting of hepatitis C and cirrhosis and recently in aplastic anemia. Both agents, although not licensed yet, have efficacy in the treatment of MDS and in nonmyeloablative chemotherapy. Short-term efficacy and safety are well documented and long-term efficacy and safety are emerging. Potential risks include thrombosis, myelofibrosis, development of hematologic malignancies, and liver toxicity with eltrombopag.[96]

Direct oral anticoagulants (DOACs)
Oral direct factor Xa inhibitors such as rivaroxaban, apixaban, and edoxaban and oral direct thrombin inhibitors such as dabigatran are being used in clinical practice for prevention of stroke and systemic embolism in the setting of nonvalvular atrial fibrillation and for the prevention and treatment of VTE. In the context of cancer patients, current clinical practice guidelines all recommend the use of therapeutic doses of LMWHs for the initial and long-term treatment of cancer-related thrombosis. The use of vitamin K antagonists (VKA) is acceptable if LMWH is not available. For the long-term treatment of VTE in patients with cancer, LMWH compared with VKA reduces venous thromboembolic events but not mortality. The decision for a patient with cancer and VTE to start long-term LMWH versus oral anticoagulation should balance the benefits and harms and integrate the patient's values and preferences for the important outcomes and alternative management strategies.

DOACs have been shown to be comparable to conventional therapy for the acute treatment of VTE but their efficacy and safety in cancer patients remain uncertain. Their use cannot be supported until trials comparing them with LMWH are available.[97,98]

Summary

Bleeding and thrombotic complications are common in cancer patients. Significant advances in the understanding of the interrelationship between cancer, blood coagulation, and tumor angiogenesis have occurred in recent years. Bleeding complications usually result from abnormalities in platelets or deficiency of coagulation factors and require specific blood or coagulation factor replacement. Thromboembolic events including deep venous thrombosis and PE are not only common but also serious complications seen in cancer patients. Advances in novel biomarkers, diagnostic imaging, and availability of newer anticoagulant agents have greatly facilitated the care of these patients. Ongoing research in the understanding of the various disturbances in hemostasis, application of innovative treatment modalities, and use of appropriate thromboprophylaxis in cancer patients should ultimately lead to decreased morbidity and improved survival.

Key references

The complete reference list can be found on the Wiley Companion Digital Edition of this title (see inside front cover for login instructions).

1 Choudhry A, DeLoughery TG. Bleeding and thrombosis in acute promyelocytic leukemia. *Am J Hematol.* 2012;**87**(6):596–603.

5 Donnellan E, Kevane B, Healey Bird BR, Ni Ainle F. Cancer and venous thromboembolic disease: from molecular mechanisms to clinical management. *Curr Oncol.* 2014;**21**(3):134–143.

21 Estcourt L, Stanworth S, Doree C, et al. Prophylactic platelet transfusion for prevention of bleeding in patients with haematological disorders after chemotherapy and stem cell transplantation. *Cochrane Database Syst Rev.* 2012;**16**:5.

23 Slichter SJ. Evidence-based platelet transfusion guidelines. *Hematology Am Soc Hematol Educ Program.* 2007;**2007**:172–178.

27 Sucker C, Michiels JJ, Zotz RB. Causes, etiology and diagnosis of acquired von Willebrand disease: a prospective diagnostic workup to establish the most effective therapeutic strategies. *Acta Haematol.* 2009;**121**(2-3):177–182.

34 Marchioli R, Finazzi G, Specchia G, et al. Cardiovascular events and intensity of treatment in polycythemia vera. *N Engl J Med.* 2013;**368**(1):22–33.

35 Kiladjian JJ. The spectrum of JAK2-positive myeloproliferative neoplasms. *Hematology Am Soc Hematol Educ Program.* 2012;**2012**:561–566.

37 O'Shaughnessy DF, Atterbury C, Bolton Maggs P, et al. Guidelines for the use of fresh-frozen plasma, cryoprecipitate and cryosupernatant. *Br J Haematol.* 2004;**126**(1):11–28.

38 Mumford AD, O'Donnell J, Gillmore JD, Manning RA, Hawkins PN, Laffan M. Bleeding symptoms and coagulation abnormalities in 337 patients with AL-amyloidosis. *Br J Haematol.* 2000;**110**(2):454–460.

41 Varki A. Trousseau's syndrome: multiple definitions and multiple mechanisms. *Blood.* 2007;**110**(6):1723–1729.

46 Bennett CL, Silver SM, Djulbegovic B, et al. Venous thromboembolism and mortality associated with recombinant erythropoietin and darbepoetin administration for the treatment of cancer-associated anemia. *JAMA.* 2008;**299**(8):914–924.

47 Wells PS, Anderson DR, Bormanis J, et al. Value of assessment of pretest probability of deep-vein thrombosis in clinical management [see comments]. *Lancet.* 1997;**350**(9094):1795–1798.

49 King V, Vaze AA, Moskowitz CS, Smith LJ, Ginsberg MS. D-dimer assay to exclude pulmonary embolism in high-risk oncologic population: correlation with CT pulmonary angiography in an urgent care setting. *Radiology.* 2008;**247**(3):854–861.

51 Huisman MV, Klok FA. Diagnostic management of acute deep vein thrombosis and pulmonary embolism. *J Thromb Haemost.* 2013;**11**(3):412–422.

52 Kearon C, Akl EA, Comerota AJ, et al. Antithrombotic therapy for VTE disease: antithrombotic therapy and prevention of thrombosis, 9th ed: American College of Chest Physicians Evidence-Based Clinical Practice Guidelines. *Chest.* 2012;**141**(2 **Suppl**):e419S–e494S.

53 Siragusa S. Low molecular weight heparins as antineoplastic agents. *Recent Pat Anticancer Drug Discov.* 2008;**3**(3):159–161.

58 Lee AY, Levine MN, Baker RI, et al. Low-molecular-weight heparin versus a coumarin for the prevention of recurrent venous thromboembolism in patients with cancer. *N Engl J Med.* 2003;**349**(2):146–153.

60 Goldhaber SZ. Thrombolysis for pulmonary embolism. *N Engl J Med.* 2002;**347**(15):1131–1132.

62 Wallace MJ, Jean JL, Gupta S, et al. Use of inferior vena caval filters and survival in patients with malignancy. *Cancer.* 2004;**101**(8):1902–1907.

64 Holbrook A, Schulman S, Witt DM, et al. Evidence-based management of anticoagulant therapy: antithrombotic therapy and prevention of thrombosis, 9th ed: American College of Chest Physicians Evidence-Based Clinical Practice Guidelines. *Chest.* 2012;**141**(2 **Suppl**):e152S–e184S.

66 Lyman GH, Bohlke K, Khorana AA, et al. Venous thromboembolism prophylaxis and treatment in patients with cancer: American Society of Clinical Oncology clinical practice guideline update. *J Clin Oncol.* 2015;**33**(6):654–656.

70 Linkins LA, Dans AL, Moores LK, et al. Treatment and prevention of heparin-induced thrombocytopenia: antithrombotic therapy and prevention of thrombosis, 9th ed: American College of Chest Physicians Evidence-Based Clinical Practice Guidelines. *Chest.* 2012;**141**(2 **Suppl**):e495S–530S.

71 Lo GK, Juhl D, Warkentin TE, Sigouin CS, Eichler P, Greinacher A. Evaluation of pretest clinical score (4 T's) for the diagnosis of heparin-induced thrombocytopenia in two clinical settings. *J Thromb Haemost.* 2006;**4**(4):759–765.

76 Tsakiris DA, Tichelli A. Thrombotic complications after haematopoietic stem cell transplantation: early and late effects. *Best Pract Res Clin Haematol.* 2009;**22**(1):137–145.

82 Riedl M, Orth-Höller D, Würzner R. An update on the thrombotic microangiopathies hemolytic uremic syndrome (HUS) and thrombotic thrombocytopenic purpura (TTP). *Semin Thromb Hemost.* 2014;**40**(4):413–415.

83 Javid M, Magee TR, Galland RB. Arterial thrombosis associated with malignant disease. *Eur J Vasc Endovasc Surg.* 2008;**35**(1):84–87.

85 Mosca L, Grady D, Barrett-Connor E, et al. Effect of raloxifene on stroke and venous thromboembolism according to subgroups in postmenopausal women at increased risk of coronary heart disease. *Stroke.* 2009;**40**(1):147–155.

89 Levi M, Toh CH, Thachil J, Watson HG. Guidelines for the diagnosis and management of disseminated intravascular coagulation. *Br J Haematol.* 2009;**145**(1):24–33.

91 Toh CH, Hoots WK, SSC. on Disseminated Intravascular Coagulation of the ISTH. The scoring system of the scientific and standardisation committee on disseminated intravascular coagulation of the international society on thrombosis and haemostasis: a 5-year overview. *J Thromb Haemost.* 2007;**5**(3):604–606.

93 Mannucci PM, Levi M. Prevention and treatment of major blood loss. *N Engl J Med.* 2007;**356**(22):2301–2311.

96 Mitchell WB, Bussel JB. Thrombopoietin receptor agonists: a critical review. *Semin Hematol.* 2015;**52**(1):46–52.

97 Carrier M, Cameron C, Delluc A, Castellucci L, Khorana AA, Lee AY. Efficacy and safety of anticoagulant therapy for the treatment of acute cancer-associated thrombosis: a systematic review and meta-analysis. *Thromb Res.* 2014;**134**(6):1214–1219.

98 Akl EA, Kahale L, Barba M, et al. Anticoagulation for the long-term treatment of venous thromboembolism in patients with cancer. *Cochrane Database Syst Rev.* 2014;**7**:CD006650.

131 Urologic complications

Rachel A. Sanford, MD ▪ *Ala Abudayyeh, MD* ▪ *Christopher J. Logothetis, MD* ▪ *Nizar M. Tannir, MD, FACP*

Overview

The management of patients with cancer requires anticipation and timely intervention for urologic complications including urinary tract obstruction, cystitis, nephritis, and nephrotoxicity from chemotherapeutic agents. In patients with limited-stage disease receiving therapy with curative intent, skilled management of urologic complications is crucial for delivering adequate doses of chemotherapy and avoiding dose reductions that may compromise the likelihood of cure. In the metastatic setting, skillful management of urologic complications including urinary obstruction can provide significant palliation of symptoms. This chapter reviews the diagnosis and management of urinary tract obstruction occurring at the level of the ureters, the bladder, and the urethra. Mechanisms of chemotherapy- and radiation-induced cystitis and nephritis and their management are reviewed. Finally, an overview of the most commonly used potentially nephrotoxic therapeutic agents is provided, with an emphasis on diagnosis, treatment, and prevention. In addition to cytotoxic chemotherapy, the nephrotoxicity caused by targeted therapies is discussed, and emerging insights into immune-related adverse events (irAE) that may affect the kidney are reviewed.

Introduction

Anticipation and timely intervention for urologic complications of cancer and its therapy may facilitate treatment of patients with localized disease and expand opportunities for the treatment of patients with metastatic disease. Management of obstructive uropathy, prompt detection of drug-induced renal toxicity, and the management of such toxicity without excessive dose reduction are critical to the successful treatment of cancer patients. Renally based dose adjustment and the monitoring of multiple agents with nephrotoxic potential are nuanced yet essential components of oncologic practice, and management of urologic complications often requires coordinated multidisciplinary care. This chapter reviews the most frequent urologic complications of cancer and its therapy.

Urinary tract obstruction

Obstruction of the urinary tract may occur at multiple levels (ureter, bladder, or urethra) due to direct extension, encasement, or invasion of these structures by cancer. The natural history and management of obstructive uropathy are determined by the obstruction's location, time course (acute versus chronic), and the anticipated responsiveness to therapy of the malignancy implicated in the obstruction. For curable cancers whose therapies contain essential components that are nephrotoxic [cisplatin, ifosfamide, and methotrexate (MTX)], prompt reversal of obstructive uropathy is important to permit adequate chemotherapy dosing. In patients with advanced cancers of the GU tract resulting in obstruction and debilitating urinary symptoms that compromise quality of life, urinary diversion is an important palliative procedure aimed at relieving suffering and prolonging survival. In both scenarios, a range of less invasive interventions including stenting and external drainage of the urinary tract, which are performed by an urologist or an interventional radiologist, may allow early intervention and reduce the need for extensive surgical procedures.

The first suggestion of the presence of an obstructive uropathy may be a rising serum creatinine level, particularly in ureteral obstructions, which are often painless. Bladder outlet or urethral obstruction resulting in a distended bladder may be palpable on physical exam. Acute unilateral hydronephrosis may cause hypertension, due to activation of the renin-angiotensin system;[1] this hypertension is reversible with relief of the obstruction. Urinalysis may be bland, or may reveal significant hematuria.[2] The cornerstones of diagnostic imaging are ultrasound and CT with contrast, with the former often pursued first to avoid the potential nephrotoxicity of IV contrast and exposure to radiation. Detailed anatomic imaging may be obtained by MRI, but the use of this modality is limited in patients with GFR < 30 due to concerns about nephrogenic systemic fibrosis (NSF).

Regardless of the location of the urinary obstruction, with time, the inability to pass urine leads to increased pressure on the renal pelvis, hydronephrosis, and renal tubule atrophy. If allowed to continue, irreversible injury may occur.[3] Urinary obstruction may also provide a nidus for infection. The radiographic appearance of the kidney under conditions of acute and chronic obstruction is distinct, with the former appearing as an enlarged kidney with a normal-to-thickened renal cortex, and the latter appearing smaller than average with a thinned cortex. Relief of the obstruction is unlikely to result in significant improvement in renal function with chronic obstruction, and the visualization of a small kidney with thinned cortex on ultrasound should usually halt a planned intervention.

Following relief of an acute obstruction, return of renal function is anticipated in 7–10 days, although longer periods of recovery may be observed.[4] In the period immediately following relief of the obstruction, the renal tubule's concentrating capacity is abnormal, which may cause a period of postobstructive diuresis. This is most commonly observed with acute high-grade obstructions.

Ureteral obstruction

The ureters are located in the retroperitoneum, making them particularly vulnerable to mechanical obstruction by pathologic retroperitoneal lymphadenopathy or retroperitoneal fibrosis. Such obstructive uropathy is most frequently the result of either primary nodal diseases (lymphomas) or periaortic lymph node metastases of urologic neoplasms, particularly prostate cancer and germ cell tumors. In the case of retroperitoneal adenopathy due to highly

Holland-Frei Cancer Medicine, Ninth Edition. Edited by Robert C. Bast Jr., Carlo M. Croce, William N. Hait, Waun Ki Hong, Donald W. Kufe, Martine Piccart-Gebhart, Raphael E. Pollock, Ralph R. Weichselbaum, Hongyang Wang, and James F. Holland.
© 2017 John Wiley & Sons, Inc. ISBN: 978-1-118-93469-2

chemotherapy-responsive malignancies, particularly some germ cell tumors or aggressive lymphomas, the expected prompt response to therapy may allow the clinician to avoid acute intervention to relieve the obstruction, particularly in the case of unilateral or partial obstruction. The need to administer nephrotoxic curative-intent chemotherapy (for example, cisplatin) may require intervention to bypass the obstruction even in chemoresponsive disease. The rate and degree of anticipated response to therapy and the degree of compromise in renal function together indicate whether placement of a percutaneous nephrostomy is necessary or whether a reasonable expectation exists that relief of obstruction can be achieved with cytotoxic chemotherapy alone.

When mechanical bypass of a ureteral obstruction is required, a ureteral stent or percutaneous nephrostomy may be employed. Multiple sites of ureteric obstruction, long occlusions, or a tortuous ureter may be indications to proceed directly with percutaneous nephrostomy.[5] While a unilateral percutaneous nephrostomy may preserve adequate renal function for palliative therapy, patients whose long-term disease-free survival is dependent on nephrotoxic therapy require maximal preservation of renal function and bilateral percutaneous nephrostomy is often required in this setting. Although they may be key to the delivery of therapy, percutaneous nephrostomies are not without risk and are a potential source of infection that may complicate, delay, or even require modification of treatment plans.[6,7] Attention to detail in the placement and care of nephrostomies is required. This includes the optimal placement of catheters to reduce pain, frequent changes of the catheter, and care of the insertion site.

During nephrostomy tube placement, the intrarenal collecting system is imaged with ultrasound and/or fluoroscopy to select a site of renal entry. In experienced hands, an appropriate nephrostomy tract can be established in 98% of cases, with major complications occurring in approximately 4%.[5] Major complications may include hematoma formation, hemorrhage, vascular injury, sepsis, bowel or lung injury, or death. Following relief of the obstruction and the resultant intrarenal pressure by nephrostomy tube placement, an internal double-J stent may be placed. This is performed in an antegrade manner using the nephrostomy as an entry point. While intervention with percutaneous nephrostomy or stenting may allow for delivery of curative-intent treatment in a patient who might not otherwise be able to receive therapy, the risk-benefit analysis may be markedly different in a patient with advanced incurable disease. Recent studies show that intervention for urinary obstruction results in patients with metastatic cancer spending a significant percentage of their remaining life hospitalized,[7,8] and it has long been recognized that progressive uremia due to renal failure may provide a peaceful death for highly symptomatic patients suffering from terminal disease. A patient with severe pain (unrelated to obstruction) and very short life expectancy may be best served by no intervention, but rather implementation of comfort measures. This difficult decision requires careful communication between physician, patient, and the patient's family members.

Bladder outlet and urethral obstruction

Malignant bladder outlet and urethral obstructions are most commonly caused by prostate or bladder cancers, and may also be seen with ovarian, cervical, and uterine cancers. While ureteral obstruction is frequently asymptomatic, patients with bladder outlet and urethral obstruction often present with troublesome symptoms resulting from bladder irritation and distension. These may have a significant impact on a patient's perceived quality of life.[9,10] Prostate cancers that arise from the portion of the prostate immediately adjacent to the intraprostatic urethra need not be

large to cause marked symptoms. Urine output may fluctuate, with periods of both relative oliguria and increased urinary output because of overflow incontinence.

The management of obstructions due to prostate cancer is guided by the stage of the prostate cancer. Newly diagnosed prostate cancer is likely to be exquisitely sensitive to hormonal manipulation, and prompt androgen deprivation therapy (ADT) with temporary foley catheter placement may result in relief of the obstruction with fairly prompt removal of the indwelling foley. In contrast, castrate-resistant prostate cancer, which nearly invariably develops after a period of response to ADT, will not exhibit this prompt response to therapy and will likely require more permanent relief of obstruction, either by nephrostomy or suprapubic catheter. In addition, very large prostate or bladder tumors, regardless of their anticipated response to therapy, may be indications to proceed directly with placement of percutaneous nephrostomy tubes.[3] Bladder outlet or urethral obstruction may be managed by the placement of a suprapubic urinary catheter. Generally, this technique provides palliation of symptoms and should not be pursued in patients being treated with curative intent as it violates normal anatomic barriers of the GU tract.

For patients with urethral obstruction, symptoms are often difficult to relieve. Although percutaneous nephrostomies and suprapubic catheters can divert urinary flow, they do not fully relieve symptoms related to urgency, hematuria, dysuria, and frequency. Transurethral resection of the prostate may be considered for palliation of symptoms in advanced disease, and definitive prostate surgery may provide significant relief in prostate cancers treated with curative intent. The management of these symptoms remains a therapeutic challenge for clinicians.

Cystitis and nephritis

Hematuria can be a frightening event for the cancer patient. Hematuria may result from bleeding anywhere along the urinary tract, and gross hematuria may require palliation to prevent excessive blood loss. The location of bleeding may be suggested by the appearance of the hematuria: long, vermiform clots typically indicate upper tract bleeding, while bright red blood without clots that partially clears with urination usually indicates a lower tract bleed. Recurrence of hematuria after treatment of malignancy may herald relapse within the GU tract.

Management of hematuria focuses on controlling blood loss and preventing retention of blood clots which may cause urinary obstruction and renal damage. The most common initial management of lower urinary tract bleeding is continuous bladder irrigation with normal saline. Cystoscopic evacuation of clots may be required for palliation. In selected patients, a bleeding tumor may be brought under control with radiation.[11] The management of cyclophosphamide-, ifosfamide-, or radiation-induced cystitis and bleeding is a challenging clinical problem. Embolization of bladder vessels or instillation of steroids has occasionally palliated such patients, but treatment is frequently unsatisfactory. Diluted formaldehyde may denature and fix superficial tissue layers. Emergency cystectomy has been undertaken to avoid exsanguination. Other treatments include hyperhydration,[12] bladder irrigation, oral or intravesical aminocaproic acid (for lower urinary tract bleeding only),[13] intravesical alum,[14] and intravesical prostaglandins.[15,16] Experimental approaches include argon laser coagulation,[17] amifostine,[18] hyperbaric oxygenation,[19] and conjugated estrogens.[20]

Chemotherapy-induced cystitis

Cyclophosphamide and ifosfamide are the most commonly used oxazaphosphorines. Other therapeutic agents that can produce gross hematuria include intravesical treatment with doxorubicin, mitomycin, and bacillus Calmette-Guérin.[21] Both cyclophosphamide and ifosfamide are metabolized to acrolein, an urothelium-toxic metabolite.[22] Chemotherapy-induced thrombocytopenia may exacerbate bleeding. Sterile hemorrhagic cystitis has been reported in up to 20% of patients receiving high doses of cyclophosphamide and in approximately 8% of patients receiving ifosfamide.[23] With conventional doses of cyclophosphamide, cystitis can be prevented by encouraging abundant oral hydration at the time of chemotherapy. With ifosfamide, this complication can be reduced with intravenous hyperhydration and the use of uroprotective mesna. Mesna is given as an intravenous bolus equal to 20% of the ifosfamide dose 15 min before ifosfamide administration, as well as 4 and 8 h later (the total dose of mesna should be equivalent to 60% of the ifosfamide dose). Mesna may also be given as a continuous infusion at a dose equivalent to the ifosfamide dose. Continuous infusion of mesna should be maintained for 4–8 h after completion of ifosfamide infusion. When given with cyclophosphamide, mesna is predominantly used with high-dose chemotherapy in bone marrow transplantation. The dose of mesna used is approximately 60–160% of the cyclophosphamide dose and is given intravenously in 3–5 divided doses or by continuous infusion.[21,24]

Hemorrhagic cystitis may occur with chemotherapy regimens that do not contain cyclophosphamide due to chemotherapy-associated thrombocytopenia, and the presence of a GU malignancy may serve as a nidus for bleeding. Hemorrhagic cystitis in bone marrow transplantation due to chemotherapeutic regimens must be differentiated from infectious hematuria as a result of adenovirus[25] or BK human polyomavirus[26] infection.

Radiation-induced cystitis

Although relatively uncommon, hemorrhagic cystitis may develop following the treatment of pelvic neoplasms with either external beam radiation or brachytherapy. The pathophysiology of radiation-induced cystitis involves damage to vascular endothelium and endarteritis leading to progressive ischemia, inflammation, fibrosis, and ultimately tissue necrosis.[27] It may appear from 6 months to several decades following completion of radiation, and in one study, affected 6.5% of patients receiving pelvic radiation.[28] Total-body irradiation for bone marrow transplantation is associated with hemorrhagic cystitis in 10–17% of patients.[14,29] Patients at highest risk are those receiving concurrent cyclophosphamide or who have undergone urologic interventions. Radiation cystitis may develop decades after the completion of radiation therapy, but as this scenario may also represent disease recurrence, thorough investigation must be undertaken before ascribing new hematuria to radiation cystitis.

Radiation nephritis

Radiation is often delivered near the kidneys to control nodal metastasis from radiation-sensitive tumors (e.g., lymphomas and seminomas). Radiation-induced nephritis may develop as a result of irradiation of the kidneys, and is related to both the total dose of radiation and the volume treated.[30] However, modern shielding techniques have dramatically decreased the incidence of this complication. Renal dose tolerance (TD5/5) is estimated to be 20 Gy in adults, with glomerular function declining at 15 Gy and function nearly completely lost at 25–30 Gy. Radiosensitizers such as cisplatin, carmustine (BCNU), and actinomycin D tend to lower normal tissue radiation tolerance. Symptoms are rarely seen acutely (within 6 months of treatment). Six to twelve months after radiation, signs and symptoms including hypertension, edema, albuminuria, active urinary sediment, and rise in BUN and serum creatinine may be noted. In the chronic phase (>12 months), hypertension is the most common finding. Eventually, patients may develop hyperreninemic hypertension related to renal scarring, atrophy of cortical tubules, and glomerulosclerosis. Rarely, patients may develop progressive deterioration of renal function requiring hemodialysis or renal transplantation.[31] Avoiding these debilitating complications is an essential aspect of sophisticated modern radiation techniques.

Total-body irradiation in bone marrow transplantation has been associated with dose-dependent long-term renal toxicities including hypertension, anemia, decreased glomerular filtration rate (GFR), hematuria, and proteinuria. Pathologic findings include necrosis of vascular structures and disruption of both endothelial and epithelial cells of the basement membrane.[32] In a review of bone marrow transplant patients receiving total-body irradiation with 14 Gy, the incidence of nephropathy decreased with increased renal shielding: 30% of patients treated without shielding developed nephropathy, 15% of patients treated with partial shielding developed nephropathy, and no patients developed nephropathy with 30% shielding.[33]

Diagnosis, treatment, and prevention of nephrotoxicity of cancer therapeutic agents

Many widely used chemotherapy agents have the potential for renal toxicity (Table 1). Adverse effects include tumor lysis syndrome, paraneoplastic glomerulonephritis, obstructive uropathy, and direct nephrotoxicity resulting in renal failure and electrolyte disturbances. These are more common in the geriatric population secondary to polypharmacy and comorbid conditions. The nephrotoxic effects of these agents are more commonly observed in bone marrow transplantation due to high-dose chemotherapy, polypharmacy, and total-body irradiation. In the following sections, we describe commonly used agents that cause serious renal toxicity. Table 2 lists additional agents that may cause nephrotoxicity. Table 3 lists the mechanism of renal injury for several drugs. Drug–drug interaction is another crucial consideration in the administration of potentially nephrotoxic agents; Table 4 highlights some of these drug interactions. These tables are not comprehensive, and careful review of all prescription and over-the-counter medications is essential to the prevention of renal toxicity in the cancer patient. Dose adjustment for several essential chemotherapy agents is summarized in Table 5.

Cisplatin

The introduction of cisplatin to the clinic highlighted the potential hazards of nephrotoxic chemotherapies.[34] Effective prevention and management of cisplatin's renal toxicity is critical to appropriate delivery of this drug, and development of platinum analogues has in part been motivated by cisplatin's renal toxicity. The study of cisplatin, the modification of its delivery, and the anticipation of and screening for nephrotoxicity provide a paradigm for the study of nephrotoxic agents in general.

Cisplatin is principally excreted by the kidneys; however, only a small portion of the total cisplatin dose can be identified in the urine in the first few days of therapy.[35] Much of the drug is irreversibly bound to protein, but active metabolites including the aquated diamino derivative and the parent are found in the ultrafiltrable plasma fraction. Clearance of this plasma component

Table 1 Therapeutic agents associated with nephrotoxicity.

Alkylating agent
  AZQ (diaziquone)
  Carboplatin
  Cisplatin
  Cyclophosphamide
  Ifosfamide
  Nitrosoureas (streptozocin, carmustine, lomustine)
  Oxaliplatin
Antitumor antibiotic
  Mitomycin C
  Plicamycin
Antimetabolite
  5-Azacytidine
  Clofarabine
  Gemcitabine
  High-dose methotrexate
Folate antagonist
  Pemetrexed
Targeted therapies
  VEGF inhibitors (bevacizumab, sunitinib, sorafenib, pazopanib, axitinib, cabozantinib)
  mTOR inhibitors (everolimus, temsirolimus)
  Cetuximab
Biologic agent
  Aldesleukin (IL-2)
  Interferon
Immunotherapies
  Ipilimumab
Other
  Asparaginase
  Cyclosporine
  Gallium nitrate
  Gefitinib
  Imatinib
  Pentostatin
  Tacrolimus

is triphasic, with nearly all drug eliminated in 4 h, but with a terminal half-life exceeding 24 h. Cisplatin nephrotoxicity is a result of necrosis of the proximal convoluted tubules, and its severity can be abrogated with aggressive hydration. As cisplatin is a highly emetogenic medication, brisk intravenous fluid administration and aggressive anti-emetics are central to avoiding dehydration, which may potentiate nephrotoxicity.[36,37]

Clinically, cisplatin-induced nephrotoxicity may be identified by a rise in serum creatinine and a decline in GFR. Other signs may include hypomagnesemia and moderate proteinuria, which is attributed to a tubular defect.[38] Hemolytic-uremic syndrome (HUS) has also been described, particularly when cisplatin is combined with bleomycin.[39] Routine monitoring of GFR as well as electrolytes including calcium, magnesium, and phosphorus is recommended. A minimum interval of 7 days between cisplatin doses is also recommended, as maximal nephrotoxicity frequently does not manifest in less than 7 days. A significant decline in the creatinine clearance should result in a delay of therapy.

Prevention of toxicity with hydration is crucial. Administration of normal saline supplies abundant chloride ions, which diminish the formation of the aquated species by mass action, thereby lessening nephrotoxicity. Conflicting reports exist about the role of mannitol[40] and furosemide (Lasix)[41] in cisplatin hydration. Coadministration with other nephrotoxic medications including ifosfamide and MTX can potentiate renal damage, and adequate hydration is crucial in this setting. Concurrent cisplatin and aminoglycoside antibiotic use have been reported to result in a significantly greater reduction in

renal function.[42] Meticulous attention to laboratory findings, adequate hydration, and avoidance of drug–drug interactions, when possible, are critical.

Methotrexate

Methotrexate (MTX) is principally excreted by renal glomerular filtration. Renal toxicity due to MTX may be particularly devastating, as prolonged exposure to the drug substantially increases bone marrow toxicity and mucositis. The renal toxicity of MTX is a dose-dependent phenomenon, and renal failure has been implicated in deaths associated with the use of this agent.[43] As it is highly protein bound, it is not readily cleared by dialysis in case of overdose.[39] The nephrotoxicity of MTX manifests primarily in the renal tubule, where extensive necrosis of the convoluted tubules occurs. The lesion has been termed crystalline hydronephrosis and has been attributed to deposition of the agent. The precipitation of MTX and its less soluble principal metabolite, 7-hydroxy-MTX, in the renal tubule results in changes in preglomerular vascular pressure and a direct decrease in glomerular filtration.

Avoidance of MTX nephrotoxicity can be accomplished by selecting patients with adequate renal function, ensuring appropriate hydration, and alkalinizing the urine to pH 7 or higher. MTX may accumulate in fluid collections; therefore, drainage of pleural effusions or ascites before administration is indicated. Before administration of MTX, adequate renal function should be ensured (normal serum creatinine and minimum urinary flow of 100 mL/h). Additional protective measures include administration of leucovorin starting 24–36 h after the start of therapy and continuing until plasma MTX levels fall to <0.1 micromolar. Monitoring for potential drug–drug interactions is crucial; weak organic acids such as salicylates increase MTX levels by displacing the drug from binding sites on plasma proteins. In addition, renal tubular transport is diminished by probenecid and salicylates. These agents should be avoided during MTX infusion.

Nitrosoureas

Each of the nitrosoureas (lomustine [CCNU], methyl-CCNU, and BCNU) was predicted to have significant nephrotoxicity[44,45] and this has been confirmed in large phase 3 trials.[46,47] Unlike MTX and cisplatin, nitrosoureas cause interstitial nephritis. Hydration does not appear to prevent nitrosourea-induced nephrotoxicity, and limiting the cumulative dose administered is the primary method of preventing renal damage.

Mitomycin C

Mitomycin C is an antibiotic isolated from *Streptomyces caespitosus*. Although it has demonstrated significant activity in a variety of tumors, its current use is limited due to adverse effects including prolonged thrombocytopenia. Mitomycin C has also been associated with HUS with a widely varying interval between drug exposure and onset of HUS.[48] Patients receiving mitomycin C should be carefully monitored for any early signs or symptoms suggestive of HUS (rising creatinine or LDH, anemia). Total cumulative doses of less than 30 mg/m^2 of body surface area are rarely associated with HUS and most cases occur with doses >60 mg.[49] While steroids can reduce the pulmonary toxicity of this agent, they have demonstrated no clear nephroprotective effect.

Targeted therapies

Mammalian target of rapamycin (mTOR) inhibitors, everolimus and temsirolimus, may produce proteinuria and acute kidney injury (AKI)[50] via a mechanism of biopsy-proven focal segmental glomerulosclerosis[51] as well as acute tubular necrosis.[52] Cases of

Table 2 Clinical and pathologic features of chemotherapy-associated nephrotoxicity.

Drug	Type of injury	Clinical features	Urine analysis	Time of toxicity	Treatment/outcome	Prevention
5-Azacytidine	Acute tubular	Renal tubular acidosis	Bland, hypoosmolar on therapy	Polyuria and rising creatinine 7–10 days post dose	Replace HCO_3, PO_4, Mg; recovery is complete	Daily creatinine, BUN, and electrolytes
Bevacizumab	Glomerulopathy	Proteinuria	Proteinuria	Increasing with cumulative dose	Discontinue if nephrotic syndrome; hold therapy if urinary protein	Monitor regularly
Carboplatin	Tubular	Mg wasting	Bland	Rising creatinine 5–10 days after therapy	Cessation of drug; dialysis as necessary; recovery usually incomplete	Avoid other nephrotoxic drugs; Mg may increase in patients previously treated with cisplatin
Cisplatin	Acute tubular	Mg wasting	Bland	Rising creatinine with cumulative dose	Cessation of drug; dialysis as necessary; recovery usually incomplete	Vigorous hydration; Cl diuresis, mannitol diuresis, Na thiosulfate; avoid aminoglycosides
Cyclosporine	Tubular and afferent arteriole vasoconstriction	Increased K and decreased Mg; renal tubular acidosis; edema; hypertension	Proteinuria	Rising creatinine from days to months after initiation of therapy	Cessation of drug; dialysis as necessary; recovery usually complete	Periodic drug level; monitor creatinine, BUN, and electrolytes
AZQ (diaziquone)	Tubular and glomerular	Anuria, proteinuria, and renal tubular acidosis	Proteinuria	Rising creatinine 5–10 days after therapy	Cessation of drug; dialysis as necessary; recovery usually complete	Avoid doses >245 mg/m²
Gallium nitrate	Glomerulopathy	Proteinuria and occasional azotemia	Proteinuria	Proteinuria followed by rising creatinine during and shortly after therapy days	Cessation of drug; recovery usually complete	Daily urine flow >2 L; avoid doses >300 mg/m²/day for 7 consecutive days
Ifosfamide	Acute tubular	Oliguria	Bland	Rising creatinine within 1–2 days after therapy	Supportive dialysis; recovery usually complete	Oliguria may be increased in patients with prior cisplatin therapy; mesna
Interleukin-2	Prerenal azotemia	Oliguria and hypotension	Proteinuria and hematuria	Rising creatinine during therapy	Stop drug when creatinine ≥4.5 mg/dL or >4 mg/dL with acidosis, fluid overload or increased K; creatinine >1.5 mg/dL with oliguria; recovery usually within 1–2 weeks	Dopamine at renal doses and fluids
Ipilimumab	Interstitial nephritis	Rising creatinine	Proteinuria, few WBC, few RBC	Weeks	Drug withdrawal, steroids may be necessary	Careful monitoring or serum creatinine
Methotrexate	Acute tubular	Oliguria	Bland	Rising creatinine within 1–2 days of dose	High-dose leucovorin based on methotrexate level; high-volume urine output and alkalinization; recovery is complete	Vigorous hydration and urine alkalinization; dose reduction on renal dysfunction; avoid aminoglycosides and nonsteroidal anti-inflammatory; leucovorin
Plicamycin	Acute tubular	Abrupt renal failure	Mild proteinuria	Rising creatinine during dosing	Cessation of drug; re-treat, if recovery complete	Alternate-day dosing; check creatinine and BUN daily
Mitomycin C	Renal vascular lesions	Hypertension, anemia	Hematuria, proteinuria	Rising creatinine after two or more doses (12–40 weeks from start)	Permanent cessation of drug; SPA immunoperfusion and dialysis; poor recovery	Stop drug at cumulative dose of 60 mg
mTOR inhibitors	Acute tubular, FSGS	Rising creatinine	Proteinuria	Weeks to months	Cessation of drug; recovery may not be complete in patients with comorbidities	Regular monitoring
Nitrosoureas	Interstitial fibrosis, glomerular sclerosis	Late complications	Bland	Rising creatinine months to years after therapy	Supportive dialysis; recovery is complete	Stop BCNU at cumulative dose of 1200 mg/m²
Streptozocin	Tubular	Proteinuria, occasionally severe	Proteinuria, aminoaciduria	Proteinuria followed by rising creatinine during dosing	Cessation of drug; recovery usually complete	Stop drug at first evidence of proteinuria; hydration will not prevent injury
VEGF inhibitors	Tubular, capillaries	Proteinuria, hypertension	Proteinuria, may be nephrotic range	Weeks to months	Hypertension: aggressive medical management Proteinuria: hold for moderate proteinuria until resolution. Nephrotic-range proteinuria should prompt permanent discontinuation	Regular monitoring

Abbreviations: BCNU, carmustine; BUN, blood urea nitrogen; SPA, staphylococcal protein A; FSGS, focal segmental glomerulosclerosis.

Table 3 Types of renal injury caused by cancer chemotherapeutic agents.

Pathologic finding	Causative agent
Acute glomerulonephritis	None reported
Acute tubular necrosis	Plicamycin mTOR inhibitors Cisplatin
Interstitial nephritis	Nitrosoureas, ipilimumab
Membranous glomerulonephritis (protein losing)	AZQ (diaziquone), bevacizumab
Obstructive uropathy	Methotrexate
Renal tubular acidosis	5-Azacytidine
Renal vasculitis	Mitomycin C

Table 4 Drug interactions that can increase serum levels of antineoplastic agents or add renal toxicity.

Axitinib	CYP3A4/5 inhibitors
Cabozantinib	CYP3A4 inhibitors
Capecitabine	Leucovorin
Carboplatin	Cyclophosphamide, aminoglycosides, topotecan
Cisplatin	Any nephrotoxic agent,[a] melphalan, paclitaxel,[b] rituximab, topotecan[b]
Cladribine	Cyclophosphamide (high dose)
Cyclophosphamide	Allopurinol
Cyclosporine	Any nephrotoxic agent,[a] vancomycin, melphalan, cimetidine, potassium-sparing diuretics, naproxen, sulindac, diclofenac, allopurinol, cytochrome P-450 inhibitors,[c] methotrexate
Etoposide	Aprepitant, cyclosporine, valspodar
Everolimus	Selected strong CYP3A4 inhibitors, many antivirals, ketoconazole
Gefitinib	Cytochrome P-450 3A4 inhibitors
Gemcitabine	5-Fluorouracil
Ifosfamide	Cytochrome P-450 inhibitors,[c] aprepitant
Interleukin-2	Any nephrotoxic agent[a]
Melphalan	Buthionine
Methotrexate	Organic acids, penicillins, cisplatin, NSAIDs, amiodarone, aspirin, ciprofloxacin, cotrimoxazole, cyclosporine, doxycycline, mercaptopurine, probenecid, procarbazine
Mercaptopurine	Allopurinol, methotrexate, TPMT inhibitors
Mitomycin	5-Fluorouracil-related hemolytic-uremic syndrome
Pazopanib	CYP3A4 inhibitors and inducers
Streptozocin	Any nephrotoxic agent[a]
Sunitinib	CYP3A4 inhibitors and inducers
Temsirolimus	CYP3A4 inhibitors and inducers, many antivirals, dexamethasone
Tacrolimus	Any nephrotoxic agent,[a] cyclosporine, cisplatin, drugs metabolized through cytochrome P-450 3A
Thioguanine	TPMT inhibitors
Topotecan	Cisplatin,[b] carboplatin[b]
Trimetrexate	Cimetidine, cytochrome P-450 inhibitors[c]

Abbreviations: NSAIDs, nonsteroidal anti-inflammatory drugs; TPMT, thiopurine methyltransferase.

[a]For example, aminoglycosides, amphotericin B, intravenous contrast, NSAIDs.
[b]Related to sequence of administration.
[c]Azoles antifungals, macrolides, calcium channel blockers, corticosteroids, grapefruit juice.

irreversible renal injury requiring dialysis have been reported. AKI due to mTOR inhibitors should prompt drug withdrawal, and guidelines for medication rechallenge are lacking. As the likelihood of irreversible kidney injury is higher in patients over 65 with hypoalbuminemia, hypertension, or preexisting chronic kidney disease (CKD), these patients should not be rechallenged with mTOR inhibitors.[51]

Targeted therapies that inhibit angiogenesis via the VEGF pathway (bevacizumab, sunitinib, sorafenib, pazopanib, axitinib, and cabozantinib) may produce proteinuria and hypertension due to renal effects. VEGF is expressed by podocyte cells of the glomerulus as well as capillary cells, and VEGF inhibitors are thought to decrease podocyte tight junction expression, leading to proteinuria. The effects are dose dependent and reversible with drug withdrawal. Patients on VEGF inhibitors should have frequent monitoring of blood pressure, and antihypertensive medications should be initiated promptly if hypertension is noted. It is not uncommon to prescribe 2–3 medications for control of blood pressure; however, with aggressive medical management of blood pressure, VEGF therapy can be continued. The presence of both hypertension and proteinuria should prompt the use of an ACE inhibitor as first-line antihypertensive therapy. The management of proteinuria is by grade outlined in the package insert of each individual VEGF inhibitor; in general, therapy is temporarily suspended for moderate proteinuria, and permanently discontinued if the proteinuria reaches nephrotic range.[53]

Immunologic agents

Interleukin-2 may cause renal insufficiency via a prerenal azotemia from capillary leak syndrome. This renal toxicity is reversible with discontinuation of the drug, intravenous hydration, and if needed, pressors and renal dose dopamine.[43] Cyclosporine produces renal vasoconstriction primarily at the afferent arteriole, causing arterial hypertension and renin-mediated renal dysfunction.[54] Acute nephrotoxicity is reversible with dose modification. In contrast, chronic administration may cause irreversible renal failure secondary to renal tubular fibrosis.[55]

In the past few years, immune checkpoint blockade has become a very attractive strategy in cancer therapy. Ipilimumab, a fully human, IgG1 monoclonal antibody blocking cytotoxic T-lymphocyte-associated antigen 4 (CTLA-4), nivolumab, a fully human IgG4 antibody blocking the programmed death-1 (PD-1) receptor, and pembrolizumab, a humanized monoclonal IgG4-kappa isotype antibody against PD-1, have all become the new arsenals against cancer. Significant tumor regression is achieved by inhibition of T-cell activation (CTLA-4), T-cell exhaustion (PD-1), and blocking the negative immune regulatory signaling of the PD-1 receptor expressed by T-cells.[56] Ipilimumab has been associated with a number of autoimmune phenomena including colitis, pneumonitis, and rarely nephritis.[57] The injury is associated with infiltration of highly activated CD4 and CD8 T cells and elevated levels of inflammatory cytokines.[58] The mechanism of renal injury is usually interstitial nephritis, with rare reports of nephrotic syndrome.[59,60] Renal function returns to normal with drug withdrawal; steroids may be necessary.[61] Nivolumab and pembrolizumab toxicity have been immune mediated; their toxicity has been less severe when compared with ipilimumab. A possible explanation is that PD1/PD-L1 checkpoint interaction takes place at the tumor site, whereas the CTLA4/B7 interaction occurs mostly in the lymphoid organs with more systemic effects,[62] which may then spare the kidneys. Building on the efficacy of these drugs as monotherapy, and the potential synergy of PD-1 and CTLA-4 blockade, a natural next step was to combine agents that target these two immune pathways. A phase I study in patients with advanced melanoma used a combination of ipilimumab and nivolumab, yielding 53% of patients having an objective response, all with tumor reduction of 80% or more.[56] The incidence of grade 3/4 adverse events (AEs) was the highest reported in the concurrent-regimen patients (53%), which was higher than reported with monotherapies. Serious AEs related to the treatment were hepatic events (in 15% of patients), gastrointestinal events (in 9% of patients), and renal events (in 6% of patients).[56]

Table 5 Adjustment of antineoplastic agents based on renal insufficiency.

Azacytidine	Unexplained increase in creatinine or blood urea nitrogen; delay treatment until back to baseline, then reduce dose by 50%
Blemomycin	Creatinine clearance 10–50 mL/min: reduce dose by 25%
	Creatinine clearance <10 mL/min: reduce dose by 50%
Capecitabine	Creatinine clearance 30–50 mL/min: reduce dose by 25%
	Creatinine clearance <30 mL/min: not recommended
Carboplatin	Adjust according to Calvert formula:
	$\quad$ Total dose (mg) = (target AUC) × (GFR + 25)
Carmustine	Creatinine clearance <60 mL/min: omit dose
Cisplatin	Creatinine clearance 10–50 mL/min: decrease dose by 25%
	Creatinine clearance <10 mL/min: decrease dose by 50%
Clofarabine	Use with extreme caution
Cyclophosphamide	Creatinine clearance 10–50 mL/min: reduce dose by 25%
	Creatinine clearance <10 mL/min: reduce dose by 50%
Cytarabine	Creatinine clearance <60 mL/min, use caution; may decrease dose or change schedule
Daunorubicin	Creatinine >3 mg/dL: decrease dose by 50%
Etoposide	Creatinine clearance 15–50 mL/min: decrease dose by 25%
	Creatinine clearance <15 mL/min: consider 50% dose reduction
Fludarabine	Creatinine clearance 30–70 mL/min: decrease dose by 20–50%
	Creatinine clearance <30 mL/min: not recommended
Gefitinib	Use caution with severe renal impairment
Gemcitabine	Use caution with severe renal impairment
Hydroxyurea	Creatinine clearance <10 mL/min: reduce dose by 80%
Ifosfamide	Creatinine clearance 46–60 mL/min: reduce dose by 20%
	Creatinine clearance 31–45 mL/min: reduce dose by 25%
	Creatinine clearance ≤30 mL/min: reduce dose by 30%
Lomustine	Creatinine clearance <60 mL/min: omit dose
Melphalan	Dose reduction may be necessary; IV: BUN >30 mg/dL or creatinine >1.5 mg/dL: consider 50% dose reduction
Mercaptopurine	Decrease dose or increase interval
Methotrexate	Creatinine clearance 10–50 mL/min: reduce dose by 50%
	Creatinine clearance <10–30 mL/min: avoid use
Mitomycin C	Creatinine clearance <10–60 mL/min: reduce dose by 25%
	Creatinine clearance <10 mL/min: reduce dose by 50%
Oxaliplatin	Use with caution in mild to severe renal impairment
Pemetrexed	Hold therapy if creatinine clearance <45 mL/min: patient with grade 3/4;
	$\quad$ nonhematologic toxicity should decrease dose by 25%
Pentostatin	Creatinine clearance <30–60 mL/min: dose reduction may be necessary
Plicamycin	Creatinine clearance 10–50 mL/min: reduce by 25%
	Creatinine clearance <10 mL/min: reduce dose by 50–70%
Procarbazine	Creatinine clearance <30 mL/min: omit dose
Ralitrexed	Creatinine clearance <25–30 mL/min: reduce dose by 50%
	Creatinine clearance <25 mL/min: omit dose
Streptozocin	Use with caution
Teniposide	Dose reduction may be necessary
Thiotepa	Dose reduction may be necessary
Topotecan	Creatinine clearance 20–39 mL/min: decrease dose to 0.75 mg/m^2
	Creatinine clearance <20 mL/min: insufficient evidence
Tretinoin	Maximum dose of 25 mg/m^2
Trimetrexate	Hold therapy if creatinine >2.5 mg dL; dose adjustment may be necessary

Abbreviations: AUC, area under the curve; BUN, blood urea nitrogen; GFR, glomerular filtration rate; IV, intravenous.

Other agents

Other agents with potential for nephrotoxicity are listed in Table 2.

Monitoring for drug-induced nephrotoxicity

The anticipated mechanism of renal injury should guide what monitoring tests are employed. For example, tubular defects resulting from cisplatin nephrotoxicity may not be immediately reflected in GFR, whereas hypermagnesiuria and hypomagnesemia are characteristic of cisplatin nephrotoxicity. Monitoring patients for nephrotoxicity with agents that can cause interstitial nephritis (nitrosoureas) requires routine and frequent urinalyses, whereas agents that may cause HUS (mitomycin C and gemcitabine) should prompt attention to the relevant laboratory parameters. The appearance of microhematuria should lead physicians to further investigate drug-induced renal injury.

Table 6 Cockcroft formula.

(14 – Age) Weight (kg)
72 × Serum creatinine

The most common renal functional abnormality as a result of cytotoxic therapy is a decline in GFR, and this may prompt a dose adjustment or a change of therapy. Particular attention should be paid to the correct calculation of renal function by adjusting for weight. The creatinine clearance calculated by the Cockcroft-Gault formula (Table 6) is accurate in patients of average body habitus, but may result in erroneous predictions in patients who are significantly under- or overweight. The wide fluctuations in weight that may occur in patients undergoing cancer therapy require frequent monitoring of weight and recalculation of GFR with each chemotherapy dose.

Key references

The complete reference list can be found on the Wiley Companion Digital Edition of this title (see inside front cover for login instructions).

2 Gutmann FD, Boxer RJ. Pathophysiology and management of urinary tract obstruction. In: Rieselbach RE, Garnick MB, eds. *Cancer and the Kidney.* Philadelphia: Lea & Febiger; 1982:594–624.

6 Bahu R, Chaftari AM, Hachem RY, et al. Nephrostomy tube related pyelonephritis in patients with cancer: epidemiology, infection rate and risk factors. *J Urol.* 2013;**189**(**1**):130–135.

7 Misra S, Coker C, Richenberg J. Percutaneous nephrostomy for ureteric obstruction due to advanced pelvic malignancy: have we got the balance right? *Int Urol Nephrol.* 2013;**45**(**3**):627–632.

8 Little B, Ho KJ, Gawley S, Young M. Use of nephrostomy tubes in ureteric obstruction from incurable malignancy. *Int J Clin Pract.* 2003;**57**(**3**):180–181.

12 Trotman J, Nivison-Smith I, Dodds A. Haemorrhagic cystitis: incidence and risk factors in a transplant population using hyperhydration. *Bone Marrow Transplant.* 1999;**23**(**8**):797–801.

14 Kohno A, Takeyama K, Narabajashi M, et al. Hemorrhagic cystitis associated with allogeneic and autologous bone marrow transplantation for malignant neoplasm in adults. *Jpn J Clin Oncol.* 1993;**23**:46–52.

16 Abt D, Bywater M, Engeler DS, Schmid HP. Therapeutic options for intractable hematuria in advanced bladder cancer. *Int J Urol.* 2013;**20**(**7**):651–660.

18 Srivastava A, Nair SC, Srivastava VM, et al. Evaluation of uroprotective efficacy of amifostine against cyclophosphamide induced hemorrhagic cystitis. *Bone Marrow Transplant.* 1999;**23**:463–467.

21 Drake MJ, Nixon PM, Crew J. Drug-induced bladder and urinary disorders. Incidence, prevention and management. *Drug Saf.* 1998;**19**:45–55.

22 Brade WP, Herdrich K, Varani M. Ifosfamide—pharmacology, safety and therapeutic potential. *Cancer Treat Rep.* 1985;**12**:1–47.

24 Abudayyeh A, Abdelrahim M. Current strategies for prevention and management of stem cell transplant-related urinary tract and voiding dysfunction. *Curr Bladder Dysfunct Rep.* 2015;**10**(**2**):109–117.

27 West NJ. Prevention and treatment of hemorrhagic cystitis. *Curr Opin Support Palliat Care.* 2014;**8**(**3**):235–240.

28 Levenback C, Eifel PJ, Burke TW, Morris M, Gershenson DM. Hemorrhagic cystitis following radiotherapy for stage Ib cancer of the cervix. *Gynecol Oncol.* 1994;**55**(**2**):206–210.

30 Krochak RJ, Baker DG. Radiation nephritis. Clinical manifestations and pathophysiologic mechanisms. *Urology.* 1986;**27**(**5**):389–393.

31 Perez C, Brady L. *Principles and Practice of Radiation Oncology,* 3rd ed. Philadelphia: Lippincott-Raven; 1998.

32 Kapur S, Chandra R, Antonovych T. Acute radiation nephritis. Light and electron microscopic observations. *Arch Pathol Lab Med.* 1977;**101**(**9**):469–473.

33 Lawton CA, Cohen EP, Murray KJ, et al. Long-term results of selective renal shielding in patients undergoing total-body irradiation in preparation for bone marrow transplantation. *Bone Marrow Transplant.* 1997;**20**:1069–1074.

34 Walker EM, Gale GR. Methods of reduction of cisplatin nephrotoxicity. *Ann Clin Lab Sci.* 1981;**11**:397–410.

35 Speer RJ, Ridgway H, Hall LM. Coordination complexes of platinum as antitumor agents. *Cancer Chemother Rep.* 1979;**59**:629–641.

36 Ozols RF, Cordon BJ, Jacobs J, et al. High-dose cisplatin in hypertonic saline. *Ann Intern Med.* 1984;**100**:19–24.

37 Gonzales-Vitale JC, Hayes DM, Cvitkovic E, Sternberg SS. The renal pathology in clinical trial of cisplatinum (II) diamminodichloride. *Cancer.* 1977;**39**:1362–1371.

38 Buamah PK, Howell A, Whitby H, et al. Assessment of renal function during high-dose cisplatin therapy in patients with ovarian carcinoma. *Cancer Chemother Pharmacol.* 1982;**8**:281–284.

39 Berns J, Ford P. Renal toxicities of antineoplastic drugs and bone marrow transplantation. *Semin Nephrol.* 1997;**17**:54–66.

41 Santoso JT, Lucci JA 3rd, Coleman RL, Schafer I, Hannigan EV. Saline, mannitol, and furosemide hydration in acute cisplatin nephrotoxicity: a randomized trial. *Cancer Chemother Pharmacol.* 2003;**52**(**1**):13–18.

42 Gonzales-Vitale JC, Hayes DM, Cvitkovic E, Sternberg SS. Acute renal failure after cis-dichlorodiammineplatinum (II) and gentamicin-cephalothin therapies. *Cancer Treat Rep.* 1978;**62**:693–698.

43 Jariwala P, Kumar V, Kothari K, Thakkar S, Umrigar DD. Acute methotrexate toxicity: a fatal condition in two cases of psoriasis. *Case Rep Dermatol Med.* 2014;**2014**:946716.

44 Denine EP, Harrison SD, Pechkam JC. Qualitative and quantitative toxicity of sublethal doses of methyl-CCNU in BDF1 mice. *Cancer Treat Rep.* 1977;**61**:409–417.

45 Carter SK, Broder L, Friedman M. Streptozotocin and metastatic insulinoma. *Ann Intern Med.* 1971;**74**:445–446.

46 Harmon WE, Cohen HJ, Schneeberger EE, Grupe WE. Chronic renal failure in children treated with methyl CCNU. *N Engl J Med.* 1979;**300**:1200–1203.

47 Ellis ME, Weiss RB, Kuperminc M. Nephrotoxicity of lomustine. *Cancer Chemother Pharmacol.* 1985;**15**:174–175.

48 Medina PJ, Sipols JM, George JN. Drug-associated thrombotic thrombocytopenic purpura-hemolytic uremic syndrome. *Curr Opin Hematol.* 2001;**8**(**5**):286–293.

49 El-Ghazal R, Podoltsev N, Marks P, Chu E, Saif MW. Mitomycin-C-induced thrombotic thrombocytopenic purpura/hemolytic uremic syndrome: cumulative toxicity of an old drug in a new era. *Clin Colorectal Cancer.* 2011;**10**(**2**):142–145.

50 Hudes G, Carducci M, Tomczak P, et al. Temsirolimus, interferon alfa, or both for advanced renal-cell carcinoma. *N Engl J Med.* 2007;**356**(**22**):2271–2281.

51 Izzedine H, Boostandoot E, Spano JP, Bardier A, Khayat D. Temsirolimus-induced glomerulopathy. *Oncology.* 2009;**76**(**3**):170–172.

52 Izzedine H, Escudier B, Rouvier P, et al. Acute tubular necrosis associated with mTOR inhibitor therapy: a real entity biopsy-proven. *Ann Oncol.* 2013;**24**(**9**):2421–2425.

53 Izzedine H, Rixe O, Billemont B, Baumelou A, Deray G. Angiogenesis inhibitor therapies: focus on kidney toxicity and hypertension. *Am J Kidney Dis.* 2007;**50**(**2**):203–218.

56 Wolchok JD, Kluger H, Callahan MK, et al. Nivolumab plus ipilimumab in advanced melanoma. *N Engl J Med.* 2013;**369**:122.

57 Voskens CJ, Goldinger SM, Loquai C, et al. The price of tumor control: an analysis of rare side effects of anti-CTLA-4 therapy in metastatic melanoma from the ipilimumab network. *PLoS One.* 2013;**8**(**1**):e53745.

58 Kaehler KC, Piel S, Livingstone E, Schilling B, Hauschild A, Schadendorf D. Update on immunologic therapy with anti-CTLA-4 antibodies in melanoma: Identification of clinical and biological response patterns, immune-related adverse events, and their management. *Semin Oncol.* 2010;**37**:485–498.

59 Fadel F, El Karoui K, Knebelmann B. Anti-CTLA4 antibody-induced lupus nephritis. *N Engl J Med.* 2009;**361**(**2**):211–212.

60 Forde PM, Rock K, Wilson G, O'Byrne KJ. Ipilimumab-induced immune-related renal failure—a case report. *Anticancer Res.* 2012;**32**(**10**):4607–4608.

61 Izzedine H, Gueutin V, Gharbi C, Mateus C, Robert C, et al. Kidney injuries related to ipilimumab. *Invest New Drugs.* 2014;**32**(**4**):769–773.

62 Robert C, Soria JC, Eggermont AM. Drug of the year: Programmed death-1 receptor/programmed death-1 ligand-1 receptor monoclonal antibodies. *Eur J Cancer.* 2013;**49**:2968–2971.

132 Cardiac complications

Michael S. Ewer, MD, MPH, JD, LLM, MBA ▪ Steven M. Ewer, MD ▪ Thomas Suter, MD

Overview

Patients with malignant diseases often have coexisting cardiovascular disorders or may face serious cardiovascular complications in the course of their disease. The disorders may result from underlying conditions such as atherosclerosis, hypertension, or valvular abnormalities, or they may result directly from cancer or its treatment (Table 1). In addition, cardiovascular disorders that are unusual in patients not afflicted with cancer may be more common in the cancer patient and sometimes are unsuspected. Furthermore, cardiovascular diseases common in the general population must not be overlooked in patients with cancer; the presentation of such entities may be unusual, and the diagnosis often is more complex. Increased clinical scrutiny is therefore necessary in this vulnerable population. Multiple clinical problems may also coexist and defy a simple illumination because of the complex interactions between the malignancy, its treatment, and the cardiovascular system; what affects one often alters the presentation and course of the others. This chapter will look at some of the more common cardiovascular complications of cancer and its treatment, and will also address some of the dilemmas encountered in cancer patients with concomitant cardiac conditions.

Evaluation of the cardiovascular system in the cancer patient

The evaluation of the cardiovascular system in patients with cancer begins with a detailed history and a complete physical examination. Signs or symptoms suggestive of heart failure, dysrhythmia, ischemia, or pericardial disease—all of which are common in the cancer patient—trigger a more rigorous cardiovascular assessment.[1] The individual approach should be targeted to include the specific clinical entities that are enumerated in Table 1. If clinical assessment of the patient indicates possible cardiac disease, further evaluation may include an electrocardiogram, chest X-ray, and echocardiogram. Additional imaging techniques or invasive modalities such as coronary angiography and electrophysiologic evaluation may be required for specific instances. The cardiac ultrasound or echocardiogram has enjoyed the widest usage in evaluating cancer patients. It plays an important role in evaluating cardiac contractile dysfunction and assessing the integrity of cardiac structures.[2] A complete echocardiographic evaluation involves several complementary techniques, each of which provides information about cardiac abnormalities from a different vantage point. Transthoracic two-dimensional echocardiography images large regions of the heart, and in some views, all four cardiac chambers can be seen and wall motion abnormalities reflecting regional or global dysfunction can be assessed. Localized or loculated pericardial effusions as well as primary and metastatic tumors can be appreciated using two-dimensional echocardiography although

other imaging modalities may also supplement and reinforce information initially obtained from the cardiac ultrasound.[3] In situations where ultrasound imaging is suboptimal, echo contrast agents may be employed to augment the echocardiographic interface. Such agents are increasingly used and are generally regarded as safe.[4]

Spectral and color flow Doppler studies, which are performed routinely as part of a cardiac ultrasound evaluation, show the direction and velocity of blood flow in the cardiac chambers and across the valves. This information is graphically depicted and is often superimposed on the two-dimensional echocardiogram. Valvular hemodynamics, intracardiac shunts, turbulent blood movement, and abnormal direction of blood flow are best evaluated using Doppler studies. Doppler studies provide important information regarding diastolic function, an aspect of cardiac physiology that has become increasingly important. Strain (deformation) echocardiography provides information regarding active and passive repositioning of myocardial segments. While these newer techniques improve the predictive value of the ultrasound examination, their role in the routine management of cancer patients is evolving.[5] Transesophageal echocardiography provides a higher resolution view of certain cardiac structures than does the transthoracic study. Although the technique is semi-invasive, the increased diagnostic sensitivity of the transesophageal studies often offsets this disadvantage. Transesophageal studies are especially useful in identifying vegetations and other valvular lesions or myocardial involvement of cancer, which may be extremely difficult to assess on transthoracic studies (Figure 1). The transesophageal study, in part because of the position of the probe, is an important adjunct for the evaluation of posterior accumulations of pericardial fluid, as may be seen post-operatively; they are also of considerable value in defining and monitoring intracardiac masses and thrombi (Figure 2).[6] Intraoperative transesophageal echocardiography is helpful in documenting the extent of an inferior vena caval tumor as well as the result of resection of such tumors (Figure 2).[5] Three-dimensional cardiac ultrasound now is available in many centers and provides enhanced information regarding spatial relationships of intracardiac structures including the cardiac valves. The technique allows the two-dimensional image to be rotated around a selected axis, providing images of improved special orientation.[6]

Nuclear imaging techniques provide important information concerning both cardiac function and evaluation of ischemic heart disease. The multigated (MUGA) cardiac blood pool scan remains a common assessment tool for following left ventricular ejection fraction in patients being treated with agents known or suspected of being cardiotoxic. Nuclear imaging techniques may have a lower intra- and interobserver variability than do echocardiographic assessments. The technique requires electrocardiographic gating that can be problematic in patients with dysrhythmia; in addition, MUGA scans acquire data over a period of several minutes, and therefore depend on patients being able to remain immobile during

Holland-Frei Cancer Medicine, Ninth Edition. Edited by Robert C. Bast Jr., Carlo M. Croce, William N. Hait, Waun Ki Hong, Donald W. Kufe, Martine Piccart-Gebhart, Raphael E. Pollock, Ralph R. Weichselbaum, Hongyang Wang, and James F. Holland.
© 2017 John Wiley & Sons, Inc. ISBN: 978-1-118-93469-2

Table 1 Important cardiovascular complications of cancer.

– Primary cardiac neoplasia
  ○ Malignancy
    ■ Cardiac tumors
    ■ Pericardial tumors
– Metastatic cancer
  ○ Pericardial metastasis
    ■ Pericardial effusion
    ■ Pericardial tamponade
  ○ Myocardial metastasis
    ■ Cardiomyopathy
    ■ Arrhythmias
      • Tachyarrhythmias
      • Conduction system disease
– Complication of cancer treatment
  ○ Coronary vasospasm
    ■ Myocardial infarction
  ○ Arrhythmias
    ■ Supraventricular
    ■ Ventricular
      • QT prolongation
  ○ Cardiomyopathy
    ■ Type I dysfunction (irreversible)
      • Chronic heart failure
      • Sudden cardiac death
    ■ Type II dysfunction (reversible)
    ■ Disorders of diastolic filling
  ○ Hypertension
  ○ Effects of radiation
– Miscellaneous entities
  ○ Cardiac amyloidosis
  ○ Carcinoid heart disease
  ○ Thromboembolic phenomena
  ○ Pulmonary hypertension

acquisition. Once the imaging data is acquired, it provides an estimation of ejection fraction, information regarding wall-motion abnormalities, and parameters of cardiac relaxation (diastolic function). While MUGA scans have previously been used to assess cardiac function in large oncologic clinical trials, the improvement in cardiac ultrasound imaging and the concerns regarding radiation exposure are providing an impetus toward the wider use of ultrasound in following patients both in and out of clinical trials.

Regardless of the method used, it must be emphasized that the results of any estimation of cardiac function are affected by many noncardiac factors, and that alterations in cardiac function for a specific patient must be interpreted with some caution.[7] Furthermore, it should be noted that small changes in the left ventricular function (LVEF changes of 10% points or less) frequently reflect conditions not associated with the cancer or its treatment but rather by physiological variations of cardiac function or by unrelated conditions such as metabolic state, anemia, or other conditions.

Magnetic resonance imaging (MRI) can delineate intracardiac pericardial, and great vessel anatomy, and can delineate intracardiac and pericardial masses.[8] Rapid-acquisition MRI, MR angiography, and contrast-enhanced MRI techniques, while not having usurped cardiac ultrasound, are assuming a broader role in the routine evaluation of cancer patients.[9,10] To some extent, it now can be considered the new gold standard for quantification of ventricular volumes, function, and mass.[11] The cost of MRI remains considerable, and acquisition times are problematic for some patients; the technique is increasingly utilized to estimate ejection fractions for patients who cannot be otherwise evaluated. Cardiac computerized tomography is increasingly being used as an imaging modality and, like MRI, allows for excellent visualization of the pericardium and nearby extracardiac structures. Positron emission tomography (PET) has theoretical advantages over more traditional imaging techniques and is increasingly used to evaluate myocardial viability in cancer patients.[12]

Metastatic involvement of cardiac structures

Metastatic involvement of cardiac structures is common and is seen in approximately 8–10% of patients with cancer; the incidence is somewhat less in elderly patients.[13] Involvement may constitute an incidental finding at autopsy or may be the initial catastrophic presentation of cancer. There are wide variations among primary disease sites and tumor types. Newer imaging techniques have made it possible to recognize cardiac involvement much earlier than was previously possible, often at a time when intervention can be efficacious. Tumor spread to cardiac structures may be by direct invasion (i.e., lung or esophagus), by retrograde lymphatic spread (i.e., lung and breast), or by hematogenous seeding (i.e., melanoma, leukemia, or lymphoma). In view of the relatively high incidence of lung and breast cancers, these neoplasms are the most common primary sites of metastatic lesions to cardiac structures.

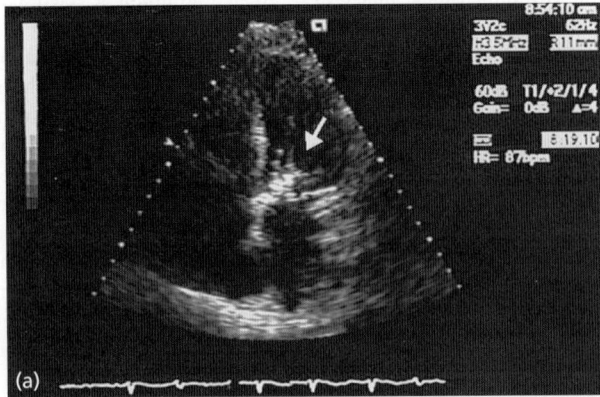
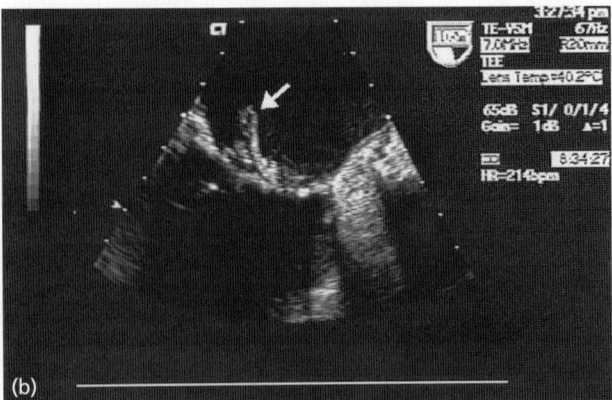

Figure 1 Echocardiogram frames of a patient with infective endocarditis involving the mitral valve. (a) Transthoracic 5-chamber image from a patient with suspected infective endocarditis involving the aortic valve. Note significant thickening of the aortic cusps. (b) Transesophageal image from the same patient recorded the same day, more clearly showing the bulky aortic valve vegetation.

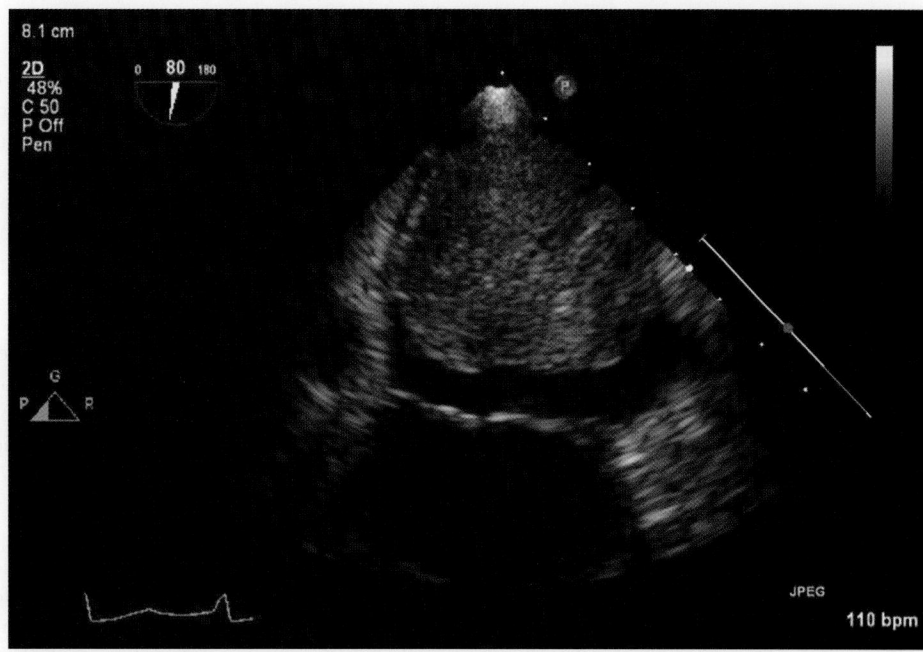

Figure 2 Transesophageal echocardiogram demonstrating a large left atrial mass in a patient who presented with angina. Echocardiographic features were consistent with tumor, and pathology was consistent with a pleomorphic myxoid sarcoma.

Malignant melanoma, once metastatic, is particularly likely to involve cardiac structures.[14] While spread to the pericardium is much more common than is spread to other cardiac structures, metastatic involvement has the potential to involve myocardial and endocardial sites. The heart, therefore, should be included in routine examinations that seek metastatic involvement in patients with Hodgkin and non-Hodgkin lymphomas, leukemias, gastrointestinal, gynecologic cancers (especially ovarian), multiple myeloma, and sarcoma (Figure 2).[15] In addition, renal cell cancer may spread to the inferior vena cava and extend into the right atrium and right ventricle; these lesions often are amenable to surgical resection.

Pericardial involvement

Pericardial effusion

Pericardial effusion in cancer patients may be malignant or nonmalignant in nature and may be related to the tumor, its treatment, or to underlying cardiac or systemic disease. Malignant pericardial effusion is defined as an effusion associated with pathologic evidence for tumor invasion of the pericardium. A malignant pericardial effusion, however, may still be present even when malignant cells are not demonstrable by routine cytologic examination of the fluid. Pericardial effusion is also seen following radiation, anticancer treatment, lymphatic obstruction, altered oncotic balance, or infection. Fluid may demonstrate considerable variability with regard to both the quantity of fluid that accumulates and the pressure exerted on the pericardium and the cardiac chambers. The rate of accumulation and the distensibility of the pericardial sac determine the hemodynamic effect and the symptoms of these effusions.[16] As little as 100 mL of fluid may cause symptoms in a patient with a scarred or infiltrated nondistensible parietal pericardium, whereas large effusions containing as much as 1 L may remain relatively indolent when the pericardial sac is elastic and the effusion accumulates gradually. The finding of malignant pericardial effusion generally implies a poorer prognosis.[17]

Generally, pericardial fluid is not static but is in equilibrium with other body fluids. Abnormal fluid build-up occurs when fluid enters the pericardial sac more rapidly than can be reabsorbed. This disequilibrium may occur when the efferent lymphatic vessels are obstructed, or when subcarinal lymph node metastases mechanically prevent effective drainage. Malignant effusions are usually serosanguinous or frankly bloody and often (but not always) contain cytologically identifiable cancer cells. When chylous effusions are malignant, the most likely cause is lymphoma; chylous effusions also have been reported following radiation for gynecologic malignancy.[18]

The onset of symptoms in patients with malignant pericardial effusion may be insidious. Indeed, many patients with large effusions are totally asymptomatic, the effusion only suspected when cardiac silhouette enlargement is noted on the chest radiograph. Decreased mean electrocardiographic QRS voltage also suggests a pericardial effusion, but other causes of decreased voltage are common in cancer patients, making this finding less useful; a recent drop in voltage should raise suspicion of the presence of pericardial effusion. Pericardial effusions are often first discovered as incidental findings on ultrasound, radionuclide, or other cardiac imaging studies, with the fluid appearing as a relatively inactive area separating the cardiac from the hepatic and pulmonary blood pools. Occasionally, a rocking motion of the heart suggesting hemodynamic compromise (cardiac tamponade) is noted. Computed tomographic (CT) images of the chest also may demonstrate pericardial effusions but are not especially helpful for estimating the fluid volume. CT of the chest is frequently used to evaluate pulmonary or mediastinal tumor involvement, and therefore may provide the first indication of an unsuspected pericardial effusion. Once suspected, the diagnosis is usually confirmed by echocardiography, and its progression or resolution may be followed with serial studies.[19-21]

Cardiac tamponade

The accumulation of pericardial fluid may lead to an increase in global or localized intrapericardial pressure and compromise cardiac output (tamponade).[22] The symptoms include dyspnea and exertional intolerance; signs include hypotension, tachycardia, neck-vein distention, hepatomegaly, and cardiogenic shock. Heart sounds are often, but not always, distant and difficult to auscultate, and pericardial friction rubs may or may not be present. Vague chest discomfort or fullness is frequently noted. Most patients with significantly increased intrapericardial pressure also demonstrate an exaggeration of the decrease in pulse pressure during inspiration; when the systolic blood pressure decreases more than 10 mm Hg with normal inspiration, *pulsus paradoxus* is deemed to be present. A highly characteristic finding of cardiac tamponade is electrical alternans, whereby the electrocardiographic QRS voltage becomes larger and smaller on alternate complexes. This phenomenon is caused by physical movement of the heart toward and away from the electrode as the heart rocks back and forth within the fluid-containing pericardial sac. While electrical alternans is not always seen in cases of cardiac tamponade, when present it is a very helpful finding. Cardiac tamponade can almost always be diagnosed on the basis of physical findings and noninvasive studies. Echocardiography confirms the diagnosis and characterizes the extent and location of accumulated fluid, which may vary considerably. Systolic inward motion (collapse) of the right atrium is a sensitive but not specific finding; collapse becomes more specific when it extends for more than one-third of the cardiac cycle. Diastolic collapse of the right ventricular wall becomes more pronounced as hemodynamic compromise progresses and is a much more specific finding. A dilated, incompressible inferior vena cava is uniformly present in the setting of tamponade. Doppler flow studies show exaggerated respiratory variation in aortic outflow and mitral inflow velocities. Cardiac catheterization is usually not required to confirm the diagnosis but may show a graphic representation of pulsus paradoxus, and elevation and equalization of the diastolic pressures in the cardiac chambers ensues as tamponade progresses. With tamponade, the pulse becomes weak or totally absent during inspiration, and patients develop symptoms of low-output cardiogenic shock. Death, sometimes preceded by profound bradycardia, may ensue if tamponade is not resolved promptly.

Management of malignant pericardial effusion and pericardial tamponade

The management of malignant pericardial effusion depends on a number of factors, including the likelihood of the tumor responding to local (surgical, radiotherapeutic, or intracavitary) or systemic anticancer therapy; the extent of and the symptoms attributable to the effusion; and the overall anticipated survival of the patient.[23,24] Patients with tumors highly likely to respond to the systemic therapy may proceed with their treatment; sometimes, the malignant effusion resolves in responses to the systemic anticancer therapy alone. Pericardial effusion diagnosed in patients with tumors unresponsive to treatment may require local intervention. In patients who have a more favorable oncologic prognosis and who are sufficiently strong to undergo general anesthesia and surgery, creation of a pleuropericardial window is both effective and generally considered the procedure of choice. Although the transthoracic and the subxyphoid approaches are equally efficacious, in-hospital mortality was significantly greater for patients treated with the subxyphoid approach.[25,26] Using either approach, the communication formed usually remains patent, and the larger surface area available in the pleural space permits more effective reabsorption of the excess fluid. Pericardial needle drainage may be required before surgery as a stabilizing measure in patients who have very large effusions or evolving tamponade. Symptoms often resolve dramatically after removal of fluid,

allowing patients to again engage in activities that had become impossible.

Needle drainage is now almost always undertaken with either echocardiographic or fluoroscopic confirmation of the position of the draining catheter, whereby newer instrumentation using smaller penetrating devices and improved imaging techniques have lowered the pericardiocentesis risk.[27] Some patients experience transient left ventricular dysfunction after resolution of cardiac tamponade, and thus, a period of careful monitoring is important.[28] The advantages of the pericardial window over percutaneous pericardiocentesis have not been fully evaluated, but some studies suggest little advantage to the more invasive pericardial window procedure. The advisability of routine drainage of large pericardial effusions in patients without tamponade has also been questioned; Merce et al. point out the low diagnostic yield and the lack of therapeutic benefit.[29] The clinical management of such patients should be determined by their overall performance status, oncologic prognosis, and the expertise at the treatment center.

Sclerosis may be considered following needle drainage but is now employed much less frequently than heretofore, in part due to the significant patient discomfort associated with this procedure. A number of sclerosing agents have been studied, including hyperosmolar glucose, radioactive gold, bleomycin, sterile talc, doxycycline, and triethylenethiophosphoramide (thio-TEPA®).[30,31] Doxycycline, used at a dose of 250–500 mg, has received considerable attention as an effective sclerosing agent.[32] In many instances, daily draining the fluid until the residual effusion is <50 mL without instilling a sclerosing agent is highly effective in preventing recurrent accumulations.[33] Balloon pericardiotomy has been largely replaced by surgical pericardiotomy, an intervention that can often be accomplished with minimal invasion.[34]

Metastatic involvement of the myocardium

The spread of malignant tumors to the myocardium is being increasingly recognized *in vivo* through the broader use of imaging studies. While previously myocardial involvement was most commonly found at autopsy, this is no longer the case. Many patients in whom metastatic disease to the myocardium is identified before death also have evidence of concomitant pericardial involvement.

The most dramatic manifestation of myocardial metastatic disease is sudden dysrhythmia.[35,36] Sudden cardiac death can occur in this setting but is unusual. Cardiac perforation and erosion of the coronary vessels with hemorrhage or infarction may also occur but are exceedingly rare. More commonly, patients with myocardial involvement demonstrate signs of loss of functioning muscle mass and present with progressive shortness of breath or exercise intolerance; a decreased ejection fraction may be seen. The electrocardiographic representation of loss of electrical potential can be seen and may be indistinguishable from changes typically encountered with myocardial infarction due to coronary occlusion (Figure 3). ST segment elevations, T-wave inversions, or Q waves may be seen in such cases, even when the coronary arteries are normal angiographically.[37]

The diagnosis of metastatic involvement of the myocardium may be difficult to establish. A high suspicion may prompt special imaging, and MRI studies may be helpful in determining the presence and extent of metastatic myocardial disease. Although treatment of metastatic disease to the myocardium often is supportive, large lesions or those with impending valvular obstruction should be considered for surgical removal.[38,39]

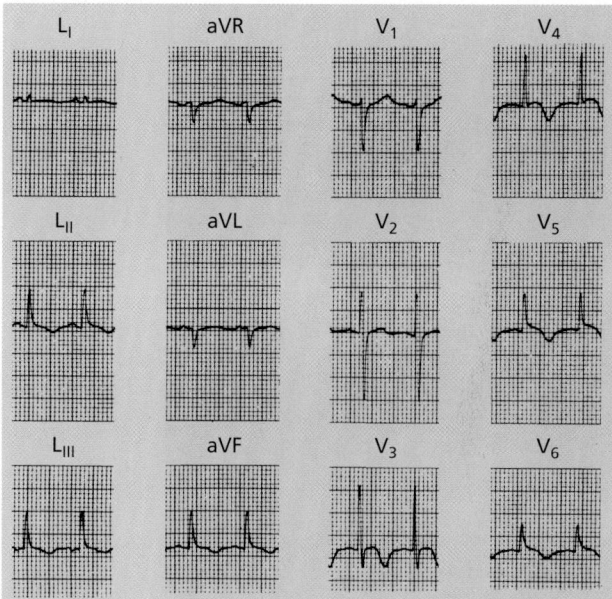

Figure 3 Electrocardiogram suggesting ischemia in a 26-year-old man with documented (by magnetic resonance imaging) myocardial metastatic disease and no history to suggest other causes of the electrocardiographic abnormality. Note T-wave inversions in the inferior leads (2, 3, and AVF) as well as in the precordial leads (V_4–V_6).

Cardiac effects of mediator release, high output states, and infiltrative disorders in cancer patients

Metabolically active mediators commonly are associated with some forms of neoplastic diseases and frequently are the immediate cause of a patient's presenting signs and symptoms.[40] Such mediator-associated diseases, or paraneoplastic syndromes, may have a direct or indirect effect on the cardiovascular system.

Carcinoid heart disease

Carcinoid tumors arise from enterochromaffin cell-derived neuroendocrine tissue, most commonly in the gut or lungs; oncologic considerations regarding these tumors are considered elsewhere in this text. Carcinoid heart disease results from prolonged release of biologically active mediators from the tumor that stimulate the formation of a distinctive fibromuscular plaque that destroys the integrity of the cardiac valves.[41-46] Carcinoid heart disease is seen most commonly in patients who have ileocecal carcinoid tumors that have metastasized to the liver. Rarely, it occurs in patients with bronchial or ovarian carcinoid tumors, and, if outside the confines of the portal venous system, carcinoid heart disease may develop in the absence of hepatic metastases. The exact mechanism of plaque formation and cardiac injury remains elusive, but a number of possible mediators, including kinins, serotonin, 5-hydroxytryptophan, histamine, and prostaglandins, have been suggested; another as yet unidentified compound or combination of compounds may also contribute.[47]

Mediator release into the hepatic vein from metastatic liver disease predisposes patients to right-sided cardiac lesions. Because these mediators are eliminated by the lungs, the left heart is spared unless a right-to-left shunt is present. The lesions generally appear along the intima of the great veins, the right atrium, and the coronary sinus. The margins and distal (ventricular or downstream) aspect of the tricuspid leaflets are often thickened, and the *chordae tendineae* may also be involved. The pulmonic valve may be thickened and retracted. The damage appears to be aggravated by turbulent blood flow, which explains the characteristic location of the lesions. When the primary tumor or metastasis is in the lung, the mediators are released directly into the pulmonary venous bed and bypass the inactivating properties of lung tissue; left-sided valvular lesions are seen in such cases.[48] Left-sided lesions are less frequent than right-sided ones but are more likely to result in hemodynamic compromise. A review of surgically excised valves noted considerable variation in the histological appearance of the material.[49-51]

The most important consequence of carcinoid plaques is thickening and fibrosis of the valves with resultant distortion of the valvular apparatus and ring. Tricuspid regurgitation and pulmonic stenosis are typically seen, but in the case of progressive destruction, a rigid tricuspid valve with hemodynamic abnormalities reflecting both stenotic and regurgitant characteristics may be encountered. Significant pulmonic regurgitation is rare. Stiffening of the right atrium may be noted and contributes to the neck-vein distention commonly seen in patients with the carcinoid syndrome. A high-output state, probably due to mediator release, has also been described.[52]

The clinical manifestations of carcinoid heart disease vary considerably. Some patients are able to tolerate the hemodynamic consequences of their valvular lesions well, whereas others develop symptoms early; this is especially so in the elderly or those with predisposing cardiac abnormalities.[53] Early symptoms include fatigue, dyspnea on exertion, and palpitations owing to a high-output state, dysrhythmias, or to both. Later, symptoms of right-sided congestive heart failure, including edema, hepatomegaly, and ascites, predominate. Cardiac murmurs often predate symptoms, and the murmur of tricuspid regurgitation may be an early finding. Most frequently, the murmur is appreciated as a loud, holosystolic, blowing sound heard along the left lower sternal border. The murmur may be augmented during inspiration. The murmur of pulmonic stenosis cannot always be distinguished from that of the often coexisting tricuspid regurgitation; when heard, the pulmonic murmur is usually harsher and is appreciated most prominently in the second left intercostal space.

The chest radiograph may reveal prominence of the right ventricle. Unlike congenital pulmonic stenosis, which often includes poststenotic dilatation of the pulmonary trunk, this finding is usually not seen with carcinoid heart disease. Electrocardiographic findings include changes suggestive of right ventricular volume or pressure overload with or without right atrial abnormalities, right ventricular hypertrophy, right bundle-branch block, and/or right axis deviation; low voltage in the standard (limb) leads may also be seen.

Echocardiography is the most useful noninvasive tool for diagnosing carcinoid heart disease (Figure 4). It not only identifies the valvular abnormality, but, when coupled with Doppler ultrasonography studies, also provides hemodynamic data for estimating the degree of valvular involvement.[54] Along with the thickening and loss of mobility of the tricuspid leaflets, increased flow velocity across the tricuspid valve during diastole is often evident. A regurgitant jet can be seen in the right atrium during systole. Furthermore, echocardiography can quantify the right atrial and ventricular enlargement that is characteristic of this condition. When of sufficient size, echocardiography is helpful in recognizing metastatic carcinoid tumors that involve the heart.[55]

The management of patients with carcinoid heart disease must be individualized and is often challenging. Although the carcinoid plaque is largely irreversible, controlling or eliminating the offending mediators can delay plaque progression. In this respect, treatment of the primary tumor or metastatic disease is crucial. Once

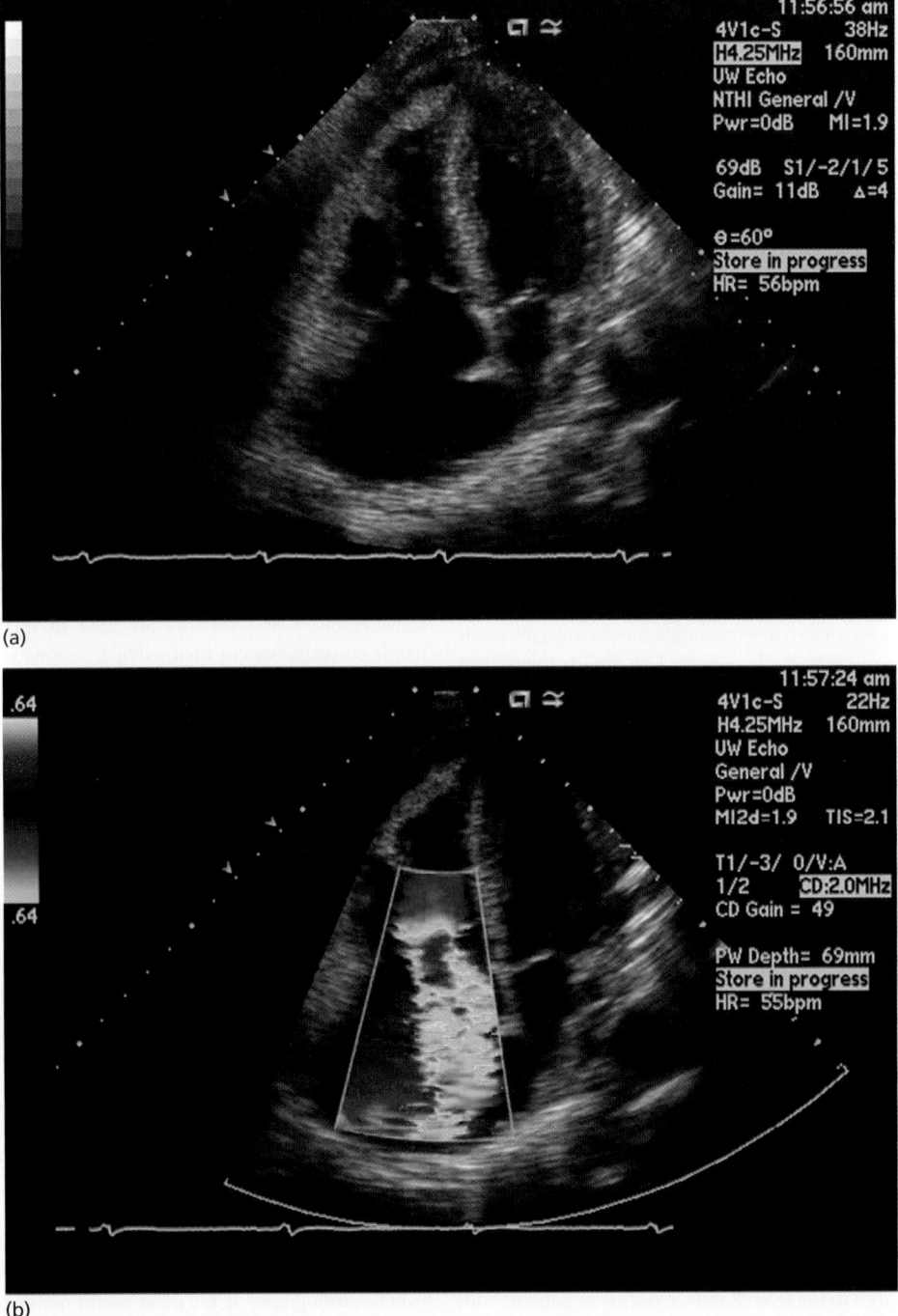

Figure 4 Carcinoid heart disease: (a) two-dimensional four-chamber study showing the thickened retracted and mal-coapting tricuspid valve leaflets. (b) Image from the same study with color-flow Doppler views showing severe tricuspid regurgitation. Also evident is right atrial and right ventricular chamber enlargement and a small pericardial effusion.

the diagnosis is established, carcinoid heart disease is initially managed pharmacologically with diuretics, afterload reduction, and salt restriction; the benefit of β-adrenergic blockade is unproven. Surgical intervention in the form of valvuloplasty or replacement is being considered more frequently than heretofore and with improved outcome, and some suggest early intervention.[44]

High-output states and high-output cardiac failure

Increased cardiac output occurs in many cancer patients and is most commonly due to anemia, hyperthyroidism, the syndrome of inappropriate antidiuretic hormone secretion, or the shunting of blood through tumors. High-output states are relatively common in patients with multiple myeloma.[56] In addition, liver disease (nutritional cirrhosis or infectious hepatitis), fever, emotional excitement, and hypoxemia are also common causes of increased cardiac output and hyperdynamic states. High-output states are seen as well following treatment with a number of biologic response modifiers, including the interferons (possibly related to fever and the influenza-like reaction) and interleukins, in which case the phenomenon usually is of short duration.

High-output states are associated with a moderately increased heart rate (usually 85–110 beats per minute, but sometimes higher) and with increased stroke volume. Physical examination typically reveals neck veins of normal appearance as right-sided pressures are generally not increased. Peripheral pulses, however, are often bounding and have a rapid upstroke and fall; systolic blood pressure is elevated, and diastolic blood pressure often is reduced. Auscultation may reveal a systolic murmur and demonstrate a presystolic (S4) gallop. Pulmonary congestion is not uncommon in severe hyperdynamic states.

Echocardiography or radionuclide imaging is helpful in establishing the diagnosis. Two-dimensional ultrasound studies show increased wall motion in all views. In extreme cases, the images appear to suggest an almost total obliteration of the left ventricular cavity during systole; the ejection fraction is increased. Doppler examination reveals uniformly increased flow across all four valves. MUGA scans may also offer important data concerning the left ventricular ejection fraction and cardiac output. Right heart catheterization with the measurement of cardiac output confirms the diagnosis, but the procedure is rarely justified. It is important not to confuse this clinical picture with that of the more commonly encountered low-output congestive heart failure, with which it shares a number of characteristics. The treatment of high-output states should be directed toward the underlying cause; in the cancer patient, metastatic disease with or without shunting, hyperthyroidism, hypoxia, anemia, and infection are the most common considerations. High-output states often respond to blood transfusion, diuretics, oxygen administration, or antipyretics. In selected cases, β-adrenergic blockers may be useful. Unless patients are symptomatic, the high-output state does not require specific therapy, and efforts should be directed at managing the underlying cause.

Cardiac amyloidosis

Amyloidosis, or the deposition of amyloid proteins, may occur in a variety of organs including the heart, and may be caused by a number of pathologic processes.[57] Amyloid proteins are made up of fibrils consisting of anti-parallel beta-pleated sheets that deposit in the interstitial spaces and are resistant to proteolysis. They are formed from a wide variety of precursor proteins.[57,58] Clinically, significant cancer-related amyloidosis is encountered in patients with multiple myeloma and, rarely, in patients with Hodgkin lymphoma. The amyloid protein associated with these diseases is known as AL amyloid and is derived from light-chain immunoglobulin (both Igλ and Igκ). AL amyloid accumulates in the atrial and ventricular myocardium and leads to either a restrictive or less commonly a dilated cardiomyopathy. Endocardial deposition resulting in valvular abnormalities has also been described.

Clinically, patients with cardiac amyloidosis experience fatigue and show signs of decreased cardiac output. Dyspnea and edema are common symptoms, and anorexia, weight loss, and presyncope are also encountered. In addition to heart failure, atrial or ventricular dysrhythmias or cardioembolic events are reported. Physical signs include elevated jugular venous pressure, edema, hepatic congestion, ascites, hypotension, macroglossia, and periorbital purpura. Conduction abnormalities are seen and, when associated with low effective heart rates or low-output states, may be symptomatic; stress-precipitated syncope may be a precursor of sudden cardiac death.[59,60] Both systolic and diastolic function may be impaired. Restrictive cardiomyopathy can be difficult to distinguish from constrictive pericarditis clinically; even findings at cardiac catheterization are not always conclusive in establishing the correct diagnosis. The chest radiograph shows a normal-sized or slightly enlarged cardiac silhouette. When cardiac

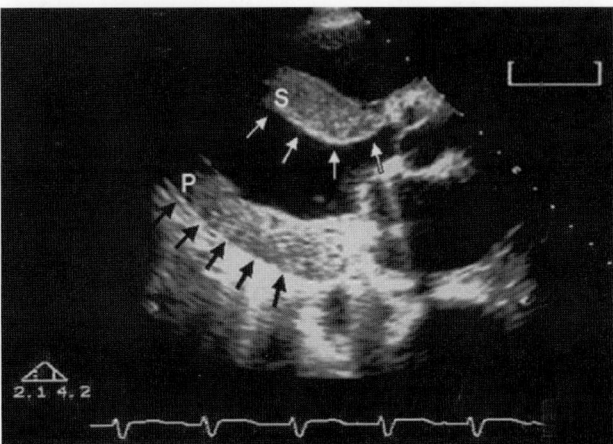

Figure 5 Long-axis echocardiographic view from a patient with cardiac amyloid infiltration. Note thickened septum (S) and posterior wall (P) with stippled appearance (arrows).

failure appears, pulmonary congestion or pleural effusion may be seen. Electrocardiographic findings can include decreased voltage, a pseudo-infarction pattern, conduction system abnormalities, and atrial arrhythmias.[61] The echocardiogram is often helpful in suggesting the diagnosis of amyloidosis (Figure 5). Ultrasonic images may demonstrate a thickened septum and posterior wall with normal internal dimensions of the left ventricle; diastolic relaxation is often impaired. In addition, a spotted or stippled echogenic appearance is often seen, and pericardial effusion is not uncommon. Atria are enlarged and may show markedly reduced mechanical function, even in the absence of atrial dysrhythmias. The paradox of left ventricular hypertrophy on cardiac ultrasound with decreased electrocardiographic voltage should suggest cardiac amyloidosis.[62] Antimyosin scintigraphy, showing left ventricular thickening and diffuse myocardial antimyosin uptake, has been reported to be highly suggestive of amyloid heart disease. Cardiac MRI may be a useful adjunct in diagnosing amyloid infiltration, as a characteristic pattern of late gadolinium enhancement helps distinguish amyloid heart disease from other cardiomyopathies.[63]

Cardiac catheterization demonstrates elevated intracardiac pressures in all chambers, with the minimum left ventricular pressure often increased to at least 10 mm Hg. The "dip and plateau" pattern seen on intraventricular pressure tracings in patients with constrictive pericarditis may be absent. Prominent papillary muscles are demonstrated with angiography. Endomyocardial biopsy with specimens stained with Congo red are helpful in confirming the diagnosis.[64]

The therapeutic interventions for cardiac amyloidosis are limited. Loop diuretics serve as the mainstay of medical treatment. Cardiac glycosides are dangerous in that they contribute to dysrhythmia; sudden death has been reported following their use.[65] Beta blockers and non-dihydropyridine calcium channel blockers can exacerbate a low cardiac output state and angiotensin-converting enzyme inhibitors can precipitate profound hypotension. In instances where malignant dysrhythmia is triggered, implantable defibrillators have been offered, but current evidence does not support their use in amyloid cardiomyopathy.[66] Clinical improvement may parallel control of the underlying process in patients with reactive forms of amyloidosis, and systemic treatment of myeloma may delay or alleviate the symptoms of myeloma-related cardiac amyloidosis.[67] Intracardiac thrombosis is a significant risk in patients with amyloid infiltration. In one autopsy series, thrombosis was encountered in 33% of patients coming to autopsy. Anticoagulation in the presence of significant cardiac amyloidosis has been suggested. Therapy with a number of antineoplastic agents, including melphalan, cyclophosphamide, carmustine, and vincristine, have been attempted, as has hematopoietic stem cell transplantation.[58] Restrictive cardiomyopathy due to light-chain deposition disease may, in rare cases, be reversible. Cardiac transplantation followed by autologous hematopoietic stem cell transplant has been successfully performed in selected patients.[68]

Cardiac dysrhythmia in the cancer patient

Cardiac rhythm disturbances are common in cancer patients. Dysrhythmias may be caused by the tumor, but more often, they are a consequence of anticancer treatment, the result of metabolic abnormalities, or from a reduced dysrhythmic threshold associated with underlying heart disease. The rhythm disturbances seen in cancer patients are morphologically and functionally identical to those seen in patients without malignancy. In some settings, it is essential to suppress a cardiac dysrhythmia vigorously, whereas in others, rhythm disturbances may be a transient manifestation of a temporary disturbance in homeostasis requiring little or no intervention. Many antineoplastic agents are associated with transient dysrhythmia, and because such rhythm disturbances are often asymptomatic, the phenomenon is not fully appreciated. Such chemotherapy-related rhythm disturbances generally are of short duration and little immediate clinical importance, yet they may be an indication of actual myocardial involvement that may become overtly manifest only at a later time. When associated with cancer treatment, most instances of dysrhythmia do not constitute an absolute indication to alter the chemotherapeutic regimen.

When faced with clinical decisions regarding which patients to treat, at what point in their management to initiate therapy, how long to continue treatment, and what form of therapy (pharmacologic or electrical) to use have been the focus of considerable debate. The wide assortment of antidysrhythmic drugs has not simplified these decisions. One useful approach is to distinguish dysrhythmias resulting from toxic substances or other metabolic abnormalities from those associated with structural abnormalities directly related to cardiac structures.[36]

Categories of dysrhythmia: primary (structural) versus secondary (metabolic)

The structural abnormalities within the heart that can result in cardiac abnormalities encompass a broad group of cardiac disorders. Ischemic heart disease, muscle hypertrophy, valvular disease, and infiltrative processes all fall within this group of disturbances. In cancer patients, tumor infiltration, cell loss following chemotherapy, pharmacologically induced ischemia, and fibrosis following radiation should also be included. Severe dysrhythmias, both supraventricular and ventricular, may appear with little warning and progress to hemodynamic instability and sudden cardiac death. Sudden death is more common in the presence of infiltrative processes such as amyloidosis.

Dysrhythmias in cancer patients also may be the result of nonstructural abnormalities. Most commonly, these include alterations in volume status, electrolyte disturbances, drug effects, and hormonal alterations, but other metabolic abnormalities that effect cardiac pacemaker and conduction tissue should also be considered.

Treatment of cardiac rhythm disturbances

Acute rhythm disturbances that result from metabolic abnormalities and that are not life threatening may be managed conservatively; in

such cases, careful observation during treatment of the underlying abnormality may suffice. Active intervention is required when the dysrhythmia results in significant hemodynamic embarrassment, when the rhythm disturbance is likely to progress and become life threatening, or when a protracted rhythm disturbance is of the type that results in an increased likelihood of a thromboembolic event. Ventricular ectopy is seen commonly and ranges from isolated ventricular extrasystoles and benign accelerated idioventricular rhythm to malignant forms such as ventricular tachycardia or fibrillation. Coexisting conditions, such as fever or debilitation, which may augment tissue hypoxia, especially in anemic patients, predispose patients to ventricular ectopy. Unexpected death in cancer patients is usually attributed to dysrhythmia. Hemodynamic instability, regardless of the underlying cause, constitutes a medical emergency requiring the use of advanced cardiac life-support protocols.

Once the decision has been made to treat a patient experiencing dysrhythmia, the choice between pharmacologic intervention and the use of internal nonpharmacologic therapy such as implantable pacemakers or defibrillator or the use of ablation therapy generally follows the usual guidelines for these therapies. In difficult cases, electrophysiologic studies or pharmacologic threshold analysis may be useful. Implantable devices increasingly are being used in cancer patients; malignant disease *per se* should not be considered a barrier to their use, but should be balanced with the patient's prognosis.

An ever-increasing number of drugs are being implicated in causing a well-recognized variant form of ventricular tachycardia known as *torsades de pointes*. This polymorphic ventricular tachycardia (Figure 6) is frequently preceded by a prolonged QT interval on the standard electrocardiogram. The QT interval is measured from the onset of the QRS complex to the end of the T wave and is then corrected for heart rate. This form of ventricular dysrhythmia is also associated with some antibiotics (erythromycin, clarithromycin, and pentamidine) psychotropic drugs (haloperidol), anti-emetics, some forms of high-dose chemotherapy, and bone marrow transplantation.[69-71] Arsenic trioxide, which is most commonly used in the treatment of acute promyelocytic leukemia, also prolongs the QT interval, and patients should be observed carefully for QT prolongation during treatment with this agent.[72,73] Prompt recognition of this potentially malignant dysrhythmia and withdrawal of the offending agent may be the most appropriate therapy. Anecdotally, *torsades de pointes* may be more likely in African-Americans. QT prolongation has been reported to be more frequent in male patients as well as in those with hypokalemia. Serial monitoring of the QT interval is advised in high risk individuals.[74] Table 2 lists the most important agents associated with QT prolongation.

Acute treatment of unstable patients with *torsades de pointes* is nonsynchronized electrical defibrillation. First-line medical management is intravenous magnesium sulfate, regardless of the serum magnesium level. Isoproterenol infusion or overdrive pacing can suppress *torsades de pointes* by increasing the heart rate and thus shortening the QT interval. Lidocaine and phenytoin are additional treatment options.[75,76] Maintenance of potassium and magnesium homeostasis is crucial in preventing recurrences of this dysrhythmia. The offending QT-prolong agent should identified and discontinued, and other potential QT-prolong drugs avoided.

Cardiac complications of cancer treatment

Nonsurgical therapies used to treat patients with cancer can impact the heart in a variety of ways. These therapies consist of chemical and biologic agents as well as physical agents such as ionizing radiation

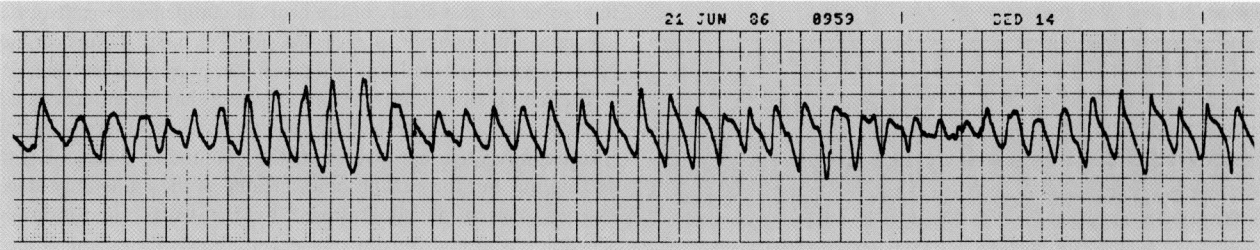

Figure 6 Rhythm strip of a patient with episodes of *torsades de pointes*. A previous rhythm strip (not shown) demonstrated prolongation of the QT interval.

Table 2 Drugs associated with QT prolongation and known risk of *torsades de pointes*.

Amiodarone	Halofantrine
Anagrelide	Haloperidol
Arsenic trioxide	Ibutilide
Astemizole	Levofloxacin
Azithromycin	Levomethadyl
Bepridil	Mesoridazine
Chloroquine	Methadone
Chlorpromazine	Moxifloxacin
Ciprofloxacin	Ondansetron
Cisapride	Pentamidine
Citalopram	Pimozide
Clarithromycin	Probucol
Cocaine	Procainamide
Disopyramide	Propofol
Dofetilide	Quinidine
Domperidone	Sevoflurane
Dronedarone	Sotalol
Droperidol	Sparfloxacin
Erythromycin	Sulpiride
Escitalopram	Terfenadine
Flecainide	Thioridazine
Fluconazole	Vandetanib
Grepafloxacin	

Adapted from the Arizona Center for Education and Research on Therapeutics. Reference: https://crediblemeds.org/ (accessed March 1, 2015).

Table 3 Anticancer treatments associated with cardiotoxicity.

I. Drugs associated with Type I myocardial depression
   Anthracyclines
      Doxorubicin
      Pirarubicin
      Idarubicin
      Epirubicin
      Daunorubicin
   Anthraquinones
      Mitoxantrone
   Potential toxicity intensifiers
      Cyclophosphamide
      Ifosfamide
      Mitomycin C
      Etoposide
      Melphalan
      Vincristine
      Bleomycin
      Paclitaxel
   Toxicity inhibitors
      Dexrazoxane
II. Drugs associated with Type II myocardial depression
   Trastuzumab
   Lapatinib
   Sunitinib
   Gleevec
   Other monoclonal antibodies/tyrosine kinase inhibitors
III. Other cardiodepressant agents
   Cyclophosphamide (high dose)
   α-Interferon
IV. Antineoplastic agents associated with ischemia
   5-Fluorouracil (5-FU)
   Capecitabine
   Vinblastine
   Vincristine
   Bleomycin
   Cisplatin
   Biological response modifiers
V. Antineoplastic agents associated with hypotension
   Interleukin-2
   Omacetaxinemepesuccinate-2
VI. Antineoplastic agents associated with hypertension
   Bevacizuamab
   Sunitinib
VII. Antineoplastic agents associated with pulmonary hypertension
   Desatinib
VIII. Miscellaneous agents with known or suspected cardiac toxicity
   Paclitaxel (bradycardia)
   Arsenic trioxide (prolonged QT interval/*torsades de pointes*)
   Bleomycin
   Actinomycin D
   Mitomycin C
   Alkylating agents
      Cyclophosphamide
      Ifosfamide
IX. Radiation (dose dependent; may affect any cardiac structure)

(Table 3). Individual modalities and combinations may act independently, additively or synergistically; for example, the combination of cardiac irradiation and anthracyclines produces additive or synergistic toxicity. Damage resulting from cancer treatment may affect the pericardium, the myocardium, the vasculature, the conduction system, and the heart valves. With some modalities, the heart may incur subclinical damage, and later insults or sequential stress may then trigger clinically relevant cardiac dysfunction.[77]

Cardiotoxic anticancer agents

Cardiotoxic anticancer agents may cause permanent or temporary contractile dysfunction, ischemia, rhythm disturbances, and fluctuation in blood pressure. The discussion will review the subject of specific cardiotoxic anticancer agents according to this classification.

Agents associated with left ventricular dysfunction

Anthracyclines and their related anthraquinones are the most widely studied agents associated with contractile dysfunction, but other agents may affect cardiac function through different mechanisms. From a functional standpoint, anticancer agents can be divided into two types, type I and type II, according to a number of characteristics.[78] Type I agents are associated with primary, or direct myocyte cellular injury that may progress to cell death with

Table 4 Type I and type II treatment-related cardiac dysfunction.

Type I (e.g., doxorubicin)	Type II (e.g., trastuzumab)
Cellular death	Cellular dysfunction
Damage starts with the first administration	
Biopsy changes (typical of anthracyclines)	No typical anthracycline-like biopsy changes
Cumulative dose related	Not cumulative dose related
Permanent damage (myocyte death; bad prognosis)	Predominantly reversible (myocyte dysfunction; good prognosis)
Risk factors:	Risk factors:
– Combination CT	– Prior/concomitant anthracyclines or paclitaxel
– Prior/concomitant RT	– Age
– Age	– Previous cardiac disease
– Previous cardiac disease	– Obesity (BMI > 25 kg/m²)
– Hypertension	

CT, computed tomographic; RT, radiation therapy; BMI, body mass index.

ongoing exposure or stress. Cardiac damage, once it has progressed beyond the threshold of cell death, is permanent. Type I drugs cause damage that is cumulative and dose related and is associated with typical endomyocardial biopsy changes. Agents associated with type II treatment-related cardiac dysfunction may cause myocyte dysfunction that resembles hibernation or stunning and are more likely to be reversible; in addition, they may contribute to injurious increases in wall stress through other mechanisms such as increased afterload or fluid retention that may compromise vulnerable myocytes. Type II agents do not demonstrate toxicity that is cumulative or dose related and they are not associated with the typical endomyocardial biopsy changes that are seen with anthracyclines.[77] These differences are summarized in Table 4.

Type I anticancer treatment-related agents: anthracyclines and related agents

The effects of anthracyclines on the heart have been the most extensively studied of all of the cardiotoxic agents; doxorubicin cardiotoxicity serves as a model for understanding anthracycline-associated and related type I cardiomyopathies.

Doxorubicin cardiotoxicity may be recognized early or late during a course of treatment, or it may present months or even years after the completion of treatment. Early manifestations of toxicity include electrocardiographic abnormalities and myopericarditis. Significant early cardiac dysfunction is rare with current dosing regimens, but cases of heart failure occurring within weeks of the first administration of the drug have been reported.[79,80] Early toxicity is more likely to occur in elderly patients or in patients who have received large single doses and has been reported more commonly in patients treated with daunorubicin than with doxorubicin. Sudden death following doxorubicin administration also has been reported but is rare. Both ventricular and supraventricular cardiac dysrhythmias may be seen during the administration of doxorubicin but are seldom life threatening. It is now believed that these phenomena are manifestations of cell injury and death associated with anthracyclines, and this is supported by the finding that markers of acute cardiac damage such as troponin T are increased following exposure.[81,82] Early manifestations, therefore, may be more important than had heretofore been appreciated and troponin release following administration is an important marker and quantifier of early cell death. This initial damage marks the beginning of an ongoing process that may go largely unrecognized

in view of the vast ability of the heart to compensate for myocyte loss, and our inability to measure small changes in myocardial reserves with the usually utilized parameter of ejection fraction.[83]

The cumulative dose of anthracycline has been correlated with risk of clinically significant heart failure. Overt clinical manifestations are unusual when the cumulative dose is below 400 mg/m², but the risk becomes greater as the cumulative dose exceeds 450 mg/m² administered by the usual rapid-infusion schedule.[84] Cardiomyopathy may occur at lower doses when other cardiotoxic drugs are administered concomitantly (see later discussion). Considerable interpatient variability exists that often cannot be explained by the known risk modifiers of prior cardiac injury or conditions known to increase susceptibility to injury, and genetic differences may play a role—a subject of on-going interest and research. It follows that if cardiac decompensation occurs early, that is, <4 weeks from the last doxorubicin administration, it is much more likely to be serious or have a fatal outcome; patients who experience early toxicity probably have had more severe initial damage and or less baseline cardiac reserves. Doxorubicin cardiomyopathy may become manifest months, and even years, after an uncomplicated course of chemotherapy at or near the usual maximum recommended dose. Such late cardiomyopathy may involve additional insults or stresses.[77] Sequential stress or injury may explain some of the cases heretofore thought of as late cardiotoxicity. As the anthracyclines have been in use for more than 40 years, some of the patients cured of leukemias, lymphomas, sarcomas, and breast cancer may harbor subclinical cardiac damage that now makes them particularly prone to symptomatic heart failure in the event of additional cardiac insults. The effect of doxorubicin exposure on the genesis of coronary artery disease, myocardial infarction, and other cardiac injuries that occur with aging is unknown. In one older review, 12 of 43 patients with doxorubicin-induced cardiomyopathy died owing to progressive cardiac dysfunction.[85]

Mechanism of anthracycline-associated cardiotoxicity

The mechanism of the cardiac damage caused by anthracycline exposure has not been fully elucidated; however, free radical formation is believed to be an important factor. Free radicals can injure lipid structures in the myocardial cell, and the resultant peroxidation of these lipid structures impairs the function of the sarcoplasmic reticulum and mitochondria. Cardiac myocytes are more prone to these degenerative changes as they lack catalase and superoxide dismutase and thus are less able to metabolize free radicals than are other cells.[86] Cell necrosis is the end result of this damage. It is evident that the mechanisms for cardiotoxicity are sufficiently different from those of oncologic efficacy that cardioprotection is possible. While the generation of the oxygen free radicals is associated with cardiotoxicity, there is increasing evidence that topoisomerase IIß plays a major role, and that inhibition of topoisomerase, as may be associated with dexrazoxane, is cardioprotective.[87,88] It has been suggested that the level of atrial natriuretic peptide is increased in at least some patients with doxorubicin-associated cardiotoxicity, and this appears to correlate more with changes in diastolic than with changes in systolic function.[89]

Clinical manifestations of anthracycline-associated cardiotoxicity

The clinical manifestations of doxorubicin-related cardiomyopathy are indistinguishable from other forms of congestive heart failure. Patients may be asymptomatic in the early stages or may exhibit only minimal signs of cardiac dysfunction. In many patients, the first sign of a cardiac abnormality may be a failure to return to baseline cardiac rate promptly following exertion. Resting tachycardia and loss of respiratory variation in heart rate may also be seen. As cardiac failure progresses, patients experience increasing dyspnea, with dyspnea at rest a poor prognostic sign.

The cardiac examination of a patient with fully developed cardiomyopathy often reveals an S3 gallop, an enlarged area of cardiac dullness, an exaggerated increase in cardiac rate with minimal activity, and, when pulmonary congestion ensues, diffuse rales. The chest radiograph shows nonspecific findings of an enlarged cardiac silhouette and engorged vasculature. Pleural effusion may be noted. The electrocardiogram may show nonspecific repolarization changes. B-type natriuretic peptide (BNP), a marker of volume expansion and high ventricular filling pressures is usually elevated, the elevation proportional to the degree of cardiac failure.[90,91] The left ventricular ejection fraction remains the most widely used parameter with which to monitor the cardiac status in patients receiving doxorubicin or related agents.

The structural changes in myocardial tissue seen on examination of cardiac biopsy specimens can provide vital information concerning the toxicity of doxorubicin and related compounds.[92–94] In highly selected patients, biopsy may provide the essential information and is generally regarded as safe.[95] The cardiac biopsy specimens are graded according to ultrastructural changes seen by electron microscopy with both the degree and the extent of the abnormalities considered in determining the final grade. With the presently used anthracycline regimens, cardiac biopsy is no longer undertaken.

Several groups of patients are known to be at greater risk of developing cardiac dysfunction at relatively lower cumulative doses of anthracyclines. Among these are elderly patients, pediatric patients, those with pre-existing cardiovascular disease and those with low baseline ejection fraction.[96] It is now postulated that any patient with diminished cardiac reserve or where increased oxidative stress is present is at increased risk for anthracycline-associated cardiotoxicity.[81] Despite some reports to the contrary, anthracyclines are generally not considered to be associated with coronary spasm or primary myocardial ischemia.[97] For all patients in whom an increased risk is present, heightened surveillance and implementation of cardiac-sparing regimens should be considered, as should, when feasible, nonanthracycline regimens. Irradiation through portals that include the heart is a well-documented risk factor for cardiomyopathy, and patients who are expected to undergo concomitant or sequential cardiac irradiation should be considered for cardioprotection and additional monitoring.[98,99]

A number of antineoplastic drugs have also been associated with increased anthracycline toxicity. Cyclophosphamide (discussed further below) may augment the cardiotoxic effect of doxorubicin toxicity, a matter of particular clinical importance because the drugs are often used together.[100] Dactinomycin, plicamycin, dacarbazine, and mitomycin C, all reportedly augment doxorubicin, but the evidence for the first three has not been persuasive.[100] Mitomycin C, however, appears to add substantially to the toxicity of doxorubicin, even when given after the completion of doxorubicin therapy.[101] Paclitaxel has also been reported to increase the cardiotoxic effect of doxorubicin. In one study, however, patients receiving the combination at cumulative doses of doxorubicin of below 340–380 mg/m^2 did not demonstrate the additive effect.[102] The higher incidence of cardiac toxicity observed when the two drugs are administered within a short time may be due to the fact that paclitaxel interferes with the pharmacokinetics of doxorubicin, leading to higher systemic levels

of both doxorubicin and doxorubicinol, a metabolite.[103] Alternatively, the apparent increase in toxicity may simply be the result of increased surveillance using imperfect tests in patients undergoing frequent monitoring of cardiac function. Other anthracyclines and related agents, such as mitoxantrone (an anthraquinone), demonstrate intrinsic cardiac toxicity that is additive; as is noted below, changing from one anthracycline to another does not provide cardioprotection.[104,105]

Various strategies can lower the extent of doxorubicin cardiotoxicity. Limiting the cumulative dose is a strategy that grew out of the observation that clinically apparent cardiotoxicity is unusual at cumulative doses of <300 mg/m^2 and that the incidence is about 5% at a cumulative dose of 400 mg/m^2.[84] Limiting the cumulative dosage to these levels in patients without risk factors helps to keep the cardiotoxicity within an acceptable range. Dose limitation also decreases the need for cardiac monitoring, as the likelihood of cardiotoxicity is lower; the risk of stopping effective therapy early because of false-positive testing results may exceed the benefits of such testing. Dose limitation, however, does not take into consideration patients who are still responding after receiving the limiting dose. Most patients, including many who are identified as having "risk factors" tolerate 300 mg/m^2 of doxorubicin or the cardiotoxic equivalent of other anthracyclines.[96]

Encapsulating the parent anthracycline compound in liposomes reduces the incidence and severity of cardiotoxicity.[106–108] Both pegylated and nonpegylated preparations have been studied, and the pegylated preparation is approved for the treatment of Kaposi's sarcoma, ovarian carcinoma, and multiple myeloma in the United States. Pegylated liposomal doxorubicin is also effective in the treatment of breast and ovarian cancer; comparisons of liposome encapsulated and conventional doxorubicin in the treatment of that disease confirmed cardioprotection with comparable antitumor activity.[109,110] Pegylated liposomal doxorubicin appears to have a clinical efficacy similar to its parent compound in a subset of anthracycline-sensitive tumors.[111] Both pegylated and nonpegylated liposomal doxorubicin are clearly cardioprotective.[112,113] With the pegylated form, cardioprotection has been demonstrated both by cardiac biopsy as well as by noninvasive studies.[110] The degree of cardioprotection is difficult to quantify, but studies suggest that at least twice the number of cycles of pegylated liposomal doxorubicin can be given with the same degree of cardiotoxicity as is seen with the unprotected parent compound (Table 5). The spectrum of oncologic efficacy may be slightly different for the liposomal-encapsulated preparation; the degree of stomatitis and hand-foot syndrome is higher.[114]

Modification of the dose schedule has been clearly shown to decrease anthracycline cardiotoxicity. A series of trials of continuous-infusion doxorubicin using infusion times of 24–96 hours, gauging the cardiotoxicity on the basis of endomyocardial biopsy findings have been undertaken.[115,116] Patients treated with continuous infusions showed a significantly lower incidence of high-grade endomyocardial pathology in their biopsy specimens despite receiving a significantly higher cumulative dose. Efficacy is not compromised, but infusions longer than 96 h are limited by increasingly troublesome mucositis and hand-foot syndrome.[117] Continuous infusion has also been evaluated in the pediatric population with conflicting reports as to cardioprotection.[118,119] The relative cardioprotection of various doxorubicin administration schedules is depicted in Table 5. Despite clear evidence of cardioprotection, the inconvenience of portable infusion pumps and indwelling catheters that are required for continuous infusion as well as the trend to use lower cumulative dosages

Table 5 Relative toxicities of anthracycline: a comparison of relative toxicities of different cardiotoxic drugs and dosage schedules.

Drug	Schedule	Relative myelosuppressive potency compared with doxorubicin administered by standard schedule	Approximate relative cardiotoxicity[a]	Cardiotoxicity index compared with doxorubicin administered by standard schedule[b]	Recommended maximum dose (mg/m^2)[c]
Doxorubicin	Rapid infusion (20 min)	1	1	1	400
Doxorubicin	Weekly	1	0.73	0.73	550
Doxorubicin	24-h infusion	1	0.73	0.73	550
Doxorubicin	48-h infusion	1	0.62	0.62	650[d]
Doxorubicin	96-h infusion	1	0.5	0.5	800–1000[d]
	Rapid infusion	1	(substantial)		
Pegulated liposomal doxorubicin	Rapid infusion	1	Uncertain Probably <0.7	Uncertain Probably <0.7	Uncertain
Epirubicin	Rapid infusion	0.67	0.66	0.44	900
Mitoxantrone	Rapid infusion	5	0.5	2.5	160
Daunorubicin	Rapid infusion	0.67	0.75[e]	0.5[e]	800[e]
Idarubicin	Rapid infusion	5	0.53	2.67	150
Pirarubicin	Rapid infusion	1	0.62	0.62	650[e]
Doxorubicin + dexrazoxane	Rapid infusion	1[e]	0.5	0.5[e]	800–1000[e]
Doxorubicin, 300 mg/m^2 + dexrazoxane	Rapid infusion	1[e]	0.73[e]	0.73[e]	550[e]

[a]Factor by which the cardiotoxic effects of the cumulative dose of rapid infusion doxorubicin can be compared with the cumulative dose of the agent, combination, and schedule listed, when given at an equivalent myelosuppressive dose.

[b]Derived by dividing 400 mg/m^2, the recommended maximum dose of rapid-infusion doxorubicin, by the recommended maximum dose for the agent in question. The cardiotoxicity index represents a factor by which to multiply the cumulative dose of a drug administered to obtain an approximation of toxicity that might be expected had the resultant amount of doxorubicin been given by rapid infusion. For example, if a cumulative dose of 120 mg/m^2 mitoxantrone had been administered, the patient would be expected to demonstrate cardiac damage approximately equal to 300 mg/m^2 of doxorubicin given by rapid infusion ($120 \times 2.5 = 300$). This value is useful when changing from one cardiotoxic regimen to another. When the sum of the products of the indexes and the cumulative doses administered exceeds 400, the risk of clinically significant cardiotoxicity exceeds 5%.

[c]Dose-producing clinically significant congestive heart failure in 5% of patients.

[d]Less toxic by endomyocardial biopsy.

[e]Inadequate data.

of doxorubicin has made many clinicians reluctant to use such schedules.

A number of compounds with possible cardioprotective properties have been investigated. The single approved cardiac protector to date is the iron chelator dexrazoxane. In a study of 92 patients randomly assigned to receive a doxorubicin-containing regimen (50 mg/m^2 doxorubicin with 500 mg/m^2 cyclophosphamide and 500 mg/m^2 fluorouracil given every 21 days) or the same regimen together with dexrazoxane, the investigators found a significant decrease in cardiotoxic effects demonstrated by ejection fraction measurements, biopsy grades, and clinical signs or symptoms of cardiac dysfunction.[120] Other toxicities and antitumor effects were unaffected. However, one subsequent study that confirmed the cardioprotective activity of dexrazoxane showed a decrease in antitumor effect as well.[121] There was no suggestion of diminished antineoplastic activity, however, in patients given dexrazoxane after they had received 300 mg/m^2 of doxorubicin.[122] Other studies have not found the efficacy of anthracyclines to be decreased by dexrazoxane. Dexrazoxane also has been studied in conjunction with epirubicin and mitoxantrone.[123,124] These studies suggest that dexrazoxane also reduces the cardiotoxicity of agents other than doxorubicin. Dexrazoxane also is used in children where there are special concerns regarding late toxicity.[125] Recent investigations suggest that dexrazoxane interferes with or inhibits topoisomerase II complexes, providing a possible explanation as to why dexrazoxane is cardioprotective while other antioxidants have not been shown to do so.[126]

Cardiac monitoring of patients receiving doxorubicin

Most patients undergoing treatment for cancer, even elderly patients and those with known cardiac disease, can tolerate at least some doxorubicin.[96] Patients with significant dilated cardiomyopathy and patients who have experienced cardiotoxicity from the prior use of an anthracycline or related drug are the major exceptions. Most patients with reduced ejection fractions as the result of prior myocardial infarctions tolerate doxorubicin when it is given with some form of cardioprotection and when the cumulative dose remains below 300–400 mg/m^2; increased monitoring in those settings is prudent. Patients being considered for doxorubicin therapy generally undergo a cardiac evaluation including a determination of ejection fraction and a standard (12-lead) electrocardiogram to provide a basis for later comparison.[127–130]

Patients without risk factors and who are without signs or symptoms suggesting cardiac compromise need not be reassessed before receiving a cumulative dose of 300–350 mg/m^2 by standard infusion or its equivalent when using alternate agents or administration schedules (Table 5). Thereafter, reassessment after each two additional cycles of treatment is appropriate. When cumulative doses exceed those noted in Table 5, additional scrutiny is essential. At any dose level, patients with increased risk factors for early toxicity should be monitored more closely. At dosages suggested in Table 5, the risk of heart failure approaches 5% in the absence of other cardiac risk factors.

Patients whose ejection fractions fall below 50% are at increased cardiac risk. If the ejection fraction has not changed, they may be treated up to 300 mg/m^2 with careful monitoring. For those whose ejection has either fallen by more than 15% points or has fallen to a value below 45%, strong consideration should be made to stop doxorubicin and substitute alternative therapy using noncardiotoxic agents.

Other anthracyclines and related (type I) agents

Clinically, the cardiotoxic effects of daunorubicin, idarubicin, epirubicin, pirarubicin, and mitoxantrone are identical to those of doxorubicin. As is the case with oncologic efficacy of these agents, the cumulative dosages, expressed in milligrams per square meter, that cause cardiotoxicity differ between the various agents. The cardiotoxicity of these agents has not been studied as extensively as has that of doxorubicin. Nevertheless, on the basis of ejection fractions and findings from cardiac biopsy specimen evaluation at equivalent oncologic doses, some data has emerged. Epirubicin is associated with a decrease in the incidence of cardiac toxicity compared with that seen for doxorubicin given by rapid infusion (Table 5).[131,132] The cardioprotection afforded by epirubicin, which is being used increasingly for the treatment of breast cancer, allows an additional margin of safety that may be especially important in populations at increased cardiac risk; a Cochrane review noted cardioprotection, however, suggested that the degree of protection may not be as high as was previously thought.[133] Some investigations have suggested that the combination of paclitaxel and epirubicin causes less cardiotoxicity than the combination of doxorubicin and paclitaxel, and they attribute this to the fact that paclitaxel interferes less with the metabolism of epirubicin than with the parent compound.[134,135] Available data regarding idarubicin suggest that 150 mg/m^2 is a safe cumulative dose for patients who have not yet been exposed to anthracyclines.[136] Data for pirarubicin (THP doxorubicin), a doxorubicin analog used extensively in Japan and France, but not approved for use in the United States, suggest that the agent is significantly less cardiotoxic than doxorubicin given by standard-infusion schedules.[137] Mitoxantrone, an anthraquinone, is considered less cardiotoxic than doxorubicin in equi-myelosupressive dosages.[104,138] Switching from one agent to another does not offer cardioprotection, and considerable care must be exercised when considering a new cardiotoxic treatment in a patient who has previously been treated with other type I cardiotoxic agents, even remotely.

Type II anti-cancer treatment-related agents

Type II agents by definition do not demonstrate cumulative dose-related toxicity, and therefore, the cardiotoxic expression is much less predictable. The best studied of these agents is trastuzumab, but other agents should also be considered in this grouping. Trastuzumab, a humanized monoclonal antibody directed against HER2, is effective for the treatment of breast cancers and other cancer types that overexpress this antigen (approximately 20–25% of breast cancers). Cardiomyopathy, with clinical signs and/or symptoms initially thought to be similar to those seen with anthracyclines, was observed in early clinical studies with trastuzumab. Concerns regarding cardiotoxicity led to a number of large multicenter trials that included more than 10,000 patients who received trastuzumab. A summary of the trials and their respective treatment arms is given in Table 6.[139–141] Several important conclusions have emerged, the most important from the perspective of cardiotoxicity are as follows: (1) cardiac dysfunction in treatment arms that include an anthracycline followed by trastuzumab are higher than similar arms without trastuzumab; the difference, however, is <4% but has, nevertheless, been of concern; (2) cardiac toxicity is largely but not invariably reversible; (3) cardiac deaths are extremely rare; (4) regimens that include trastuzumab without pretreatment with an anthracycline have a smaller incidence of cardiac dysfunction; and (5) the cardiotoxicity associated with trastuzumab, while different from that of doxorubicin, is clinically indistinguishable using MUGA or echocardiographic parameters of decreased systolic function. An additional factor that emerged from these trials is that the interval between the anthracycline and trastuzumab may be a crucial factor.[129,142]

Although the precise mechanism of trastuzumab-induced cardiomyopathy is not well understood, its specific binding to HER2 and disruption of the ErbB-2 signaling pathway in the heart is thought to be the primary event. ErbB-2 (HER2/neu) belongs to the epidermal growth factor receptor (EGFR) family of receptor tyrosine kinases, of which there are four members: EGFR, HER2/neu, HER3, and HER4. These receptors are activated by the EGF family of ligands, including EGF itself, heregulin and neurogulins, which are expressed in the heart. Binding of these EGF ligands to EGFR, HER3, or HER4 induces heterodimer formation with HER2, triggers receptor autophosphorylation, and initiates downstream signaling. Among those pathways activated are Ras/Raf, PI3K/Akt, JNK, and MAPK, all important regulators of transcription in cardiac myocytes. An extensive body of work

Table 6 Summary of cardiotoxicity in adjuvant trials involving trastuzumab.

Trial	Number of patients	Entry criteria	Arms	Reported cardiac events (%)	Reported reversibility	Follow-up (year)
NSABP B-31	2043	Node+	A) AC-T B) AC-TH	A) 0.8 B) 4.1	Yes	7
BCIRG 006	3222	Node + or high-risk node Age < 70	A) AC-T B) AC-TH C) TPH	A) 0.4 B) 1.9 C) 0.4	N/A	3
NCCTG N9831	1944	Node + or high-risk node	A) AC-T B) AC-T-H C) AC-TH	A) 0.3 B) 2.8 C) 3.3	Yes	3
HERA	3386	Node + or high-risk node	A) Std B) Std-H	A) 3.6 B) 0.6	Yes	8
FinHer	232	Node + or high-risk node Age < 66	A) V/T-FAC B) V/T(H)-FAC	A) 3.4 B) 0	N/A	5

A, anthracycline; C, cyclophosphamide; T, taxane; H, trastuzumab; P, carboplatin; Std, standard (neo)adjuvant regimen (94% contained anthracycline); V/T, vinorelbine or taxane; F, 5-fluorouracil; N/A, not applicable.
Follow-up time reflects most recently reported data.

has implicated these pathways in cardiac development, maintenance of normal cardiac function, response to stress, hypertrophy, and regulation of apoptosis. Indeed, targeted deletion of HER2 in murine models has demonstrated a specific role for this receptor in mediating the growth, repair, and survival of cardiomyocytes after stress.[143] Temporary disruption of the HER2 signaling pathway by trastuzumab thus results in an inadequate or even maladaptive response to cardiac stress that can lead to systolic dysfunction and congestive heart failure.[144] Interference by trastuzumab in cardiomyocyte repair may also explain why patients previously exposed to anthracyclines are more susceptible to trastuzumab toxicity.

Cardiac dysfunction related to trastuzumab appears to be largely reversible.[7,139–142,145] As it is an insult that involves an organ often previously damaged by exposure to an anthracycline, the question as to how great a portion of the observed dysfunction is likely to return arises. The dilemmas of whether and when to temporarily hold or permanently stop trastuzumab, how to assess the risk of restarting after functional recovery, and how to monitor such patients is under consideration. Several groups have suggested guidelines, all of which are based on expert opinion rather than on concrete data derived from prospective clinical trial.[129,146]

Other type II agents

In addition to trastuzumab, lapatinib, sunitinib, imatinib, and other agents have raised concerns of possible cardiotoxicity. Specifically myocardial dysfunction, QT interval prolongation, and ischemia have been considered as potential adverse events in these agents. To date, none have shown biopsy changes as are characteristic for anthracyclines, although some alterations in mitochondrial structure have been reported. Interestingly, these agents do not exhibit cumulative dose-related toxicity and can be given for extended periods of time in many patients. With regard to myocardial depression, a secondary effect may be implicated; in the case of sunitinib, significant hypertension is noted, and in the case of imatinib fluid, retention may be the crucial factor.[142,147–149]

Varying degrees of QT prolongation have been noted with a number of these agents, but severe lengthening as well as the need to hold or stop the medication due to QT prolongation is rare, as are ischemic events.[70] Lapatinib cardiac dysfunction was reported in 2.2% of patients previously treated with anthracyclines and 1.5% of patients without prior exposure to cardiotoxic regimens; most patients (88%) experienced some degree of reversibility with regard to cardiac dysfunction.[147]

Other drugs that demonstrate a decrease in cardiac function

Significant decreases in myocardial function are occasionally noted for other agents that do not clearly fit within either the type I or type II classification. Rarely, α-interferon has been associated with a dramatic decrease in ejection fraction.[149] The mechanism is unknown; however, inflammation and increased metabolic requirements have both been implicated; patients who survive the initial episode usually go on to recover cardiac function.[150] An unusual form of cardiac damage is associated with high-dose cyclophosphamide administration. When severe, the damage takes the form of a hemorrhagic myocarditis.[151] The process is often acute, is related to high individual doses (usually $4.5\,g/m^2$ or more) rather than to the cumulative dose, and is associated with decreased ejection fractions and mean QRS voltage. Although severe hemorrhagic myocarditis may be fatal, milder presentations may be asymptomatic and reversible.

Treatment considerations of patients with treatment-related cardiac failure or dysfunction

The most important treatment consideration in patients who develop anthracycline-associated cardiac dysfunction is the avoidance of additional anthracyclines. Once established, anthracycline-associated cardiac dysfunction differs little from other forms of cardiomyopathy and it is treated in a similar way. The American College of Cardiology and the American Heart Association have issued guidelines for the diagnosis and management of chronic heart failure in adults.[152] Patients who have been treated with anthracyclines but show no symptoms of cardiac dysfunction should have other conditions that exacerbate cardiac dysfunction aggressively treated. Hypertension should be controlled and lifestyle changes encouraged. Pharmacological intervention should also be considered for those who have ejection fractions below 45–50%. Some evidence suggests that medical therapy is most effective when given early, and therefore should be initiated as soon as LV dysfunction is appreciated.[153] Angiotensin-converting enzyme (ACE) inhibitors and β-adrenergic blockers are indicated for patients with LV dysfunction. For patients with symptomatic heart failure, salt restriction and diuretics may be added. Digitalis preparations may offer symptomatic relief and are useful in controlling the ventricular response in patients who experience atrial fibrillation; they probably do not prolong life. Anticoagulation may be appropriate if atrial arrhythmias are present. There is no specific therapy for anthracycline-related cardiomyopathy. An underlying malignancy should not, however, be considered a contraindication to aggressive heart failure therapy and, in selected patients, mechanical assist devices and cardiac transplantation may be considered for those who have achieved oncologic stability or cure.[154] Cardiac failure associated with type II agents different, in that there is higher likelihood of recovery, and rechallenge after recovery can be considered.

Agents associated with myocardial ischemia or thromboembolic events

A number of agents have the potential to cause myocardial ischemia, with or without frank myocardial infarction. The most extensively studied such agent is 5-fluorouracil (5-FU), especially when the agent is administered in combination with cisplatin.[155] Capecitabine, a fluoropyrimidine carbamate, is currently used in the treatment of gastrointestinal and breast malignancy, and is an orally administered prodrug, which is enzymatically converted to 5-FU. Myocardial infarction and dysrhythmia have been reported with both drugs.[156,157] Ischemia is triggered through coronary artery vasoactivity or spasm. Isolated cases of myocardial ischemia have also occurred after the administration of vinblastine, vincristine, bleomycin, cisplatin, and biologic response modifiers. The wide spectrum of ischemic responses suggests that ischemia accompanying anticancer treatment is more common than is generally appreciated. Nonspecific electrocardiographic changes may be seen in nearly half the patients treated with 5-FU and as many as 16% show electrocardiographic evidence of ischemia including ST-segment depression or elevation and changes suggesting myocardial infarction (Figure 7). Many of the affected patients have underlying coronary artery disease, which suggests that pre-existing coronary artery abnormalities augment the ischemic potential of 5-FU and related agents. The use of a calcium channel blocker has been reported to prevent the ischemia.[158] Selected patients may also be treated with intravenous nitroglycerin while receiving 5-FU to prevent myocardial

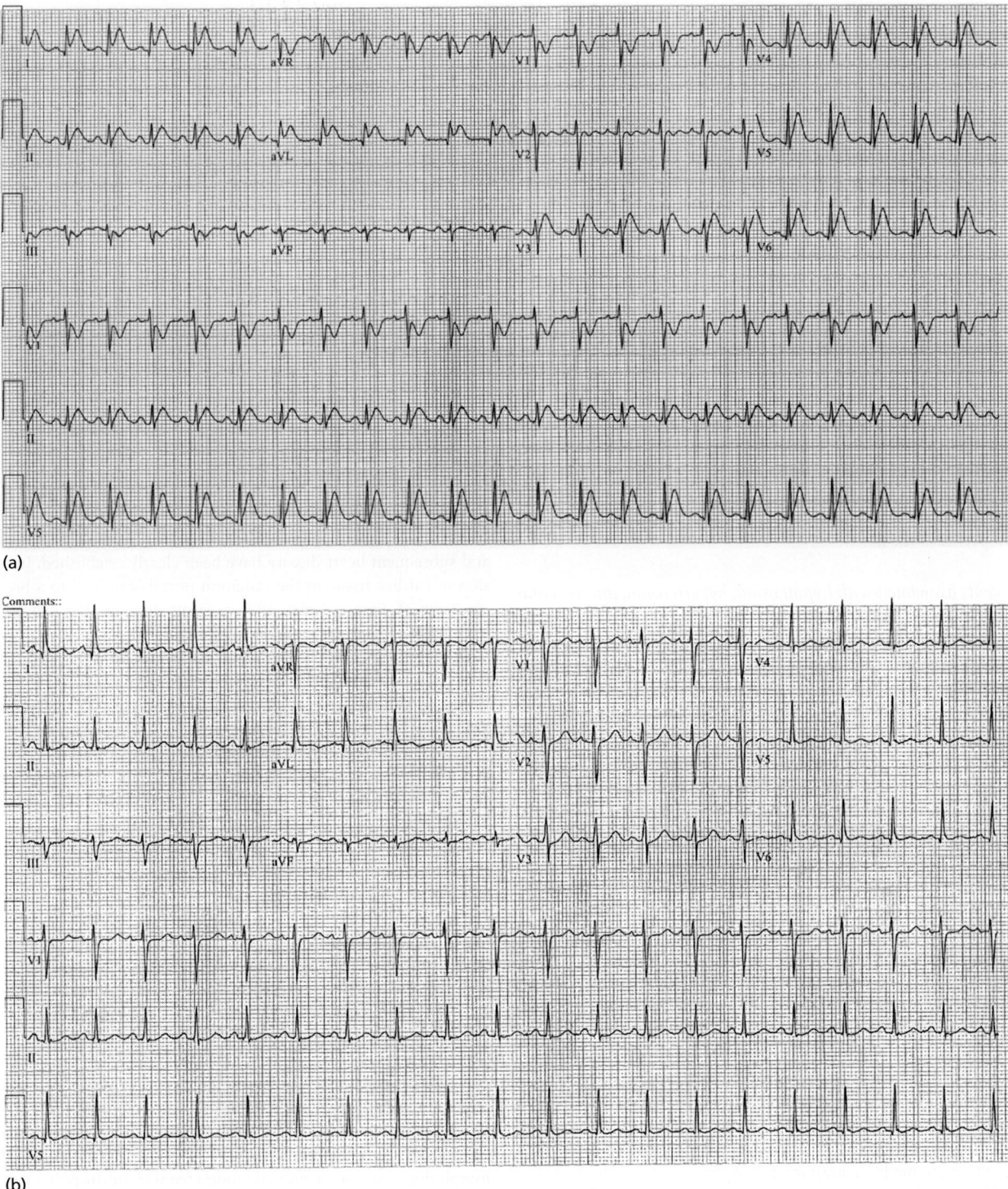

Figure 7 An electrocardiogram in a 44-year-old woman during an episode of chest pain while receiving 5-fluorouracil. Acute anterolateral ST elevation was due to coronary vasospasm (a). Electrocardiographic changes normalized shortly after nitroglycerin administration, with resolution of symptoms (b).

ischemia or infarction. When ischemia can be controlled treatment may be continued, albeit with increased monitoring and caution.

Treatment-related high-output states may also result in myocardial ischemia in patients with fixed atherosclerotic lesions that preclude increasing the blood supply because the vessels cannot dilate, a phenomenon known as "coronary steal." The interferons are especially likely to initiate ischemia in this manner. Ischemia may also result from fever, often produced by biologic modifying agents, and from hyperthyroidism. Tumor necrosis factor has been associated with a hypercoagulable state, which suggests vascular occlusion as a possible alternative explanation for the ischemia that occurs in patients being treated with cytokines and other biologic response modifiers. Anemia is an important coexisting factor, as any cause of ischemia can be exacerbated by a diminished oxygen-carrying capacity.

Patients with evidence of myocardial ischemia, regardless of the mechanism, should be observed closely for rhythm disturbances, although the level of observation and intervention depends on the overall prognosis. Individuals with known preexisting coronary artery disease can be treated with β-adrenergic blockers and/or a long-acting nitrate to help reduce the likelihood of an ischemic event. Controlled underlying ischemia or evidence of ischemia associated with a particular therapy should not be considered an absolute contraindication to further treatment with the implicated agent or agents. Cancer patients with underlying coronary artery disease are often candidates for revascularization, which can significantly improve the patient's ability to tolerate therapy and their overall quality of life.

The cardiac events associated with hormonal therapy have been studied in large groups of postmenopausal breast cancer patients. Tamoxifen is associated with decreased cholesterol, and this may offer some cardioprotection; the agent, however, is associated with an increased risk of thromboembolic events. The aromatase inhibitors anastrozole, letrozole, and exemestane have been associated with hypercholesterolemia and have been shown to carry a small increased risk of cardiovascular disease when compared with tamoxifen; this observation may in part be related to the protective properties of the latter.[159]

Agents associated with hypotension, hypertension, and vascular toxicity

Some degree of hypotension develops in many patients as a consequence of their chemotherapy. The most frequent cause is volume depletion, often as a result of nausea and/or vomiting. Other causes of hypotension related to chemotherapy are decreased cardiac output, loss of vascular tone, and increased permeability of the small vessels and capillaries (capillary leak). Most instances of hypotension in patients receiving chemotherapy are transient and can be managed with careful monitoring and the administration of fluids or vasopressor agents. Rare instances of life threatening and profound hypotension have been reported.

Interleukin-2 use is associated with significant, but usually transient, hypotension, frequently requiring pressor agents.[160,161] Capillary leak has been implicated. Interleukin-2–related myocardial ischemia is possibly related to the hypotension, although a direct toxic effect has not been excluded. Interleukin-2 is also associated with an increased incidence of supraventricular dysrhythmias and myocarditis.[162] The vasodilation that occurs in response to interleukin-2 appears to be mediated by the release of nitric oxide. Evidence has suggested that NG-monomethyl-L-arginine, an inhibitor of nitric oxide synthase, reverses the hypotension caused by interleukin-2, lending support to the role of nitric oxide in the production of hypotension and indicating the therapeutic potential of NG-monomethyl-L-arginine as well.[163]

Omacetaxine mepesuccinate, previously called homoharringtonine, was approved for the treatment of refractory chronic myeloid leukemia. The drug is associated with dose-related, sometimes severe, hypotension arising immediately after its intravenous administration.[164] Intravenous epinephrine has been helpful in stabilizing patients in this setting.

Considerable interest has surrounded the possible cardiac effects of paclitaxel. In one study, asymptomatic bradycardia occurred in 29% of patients treated with maximally tolerated doses of paclitaxel. More severe rhythm abnormalities have also been reported, but they usually are seen in patients with underlying cardiac abnormalities or in the presence of electrolyte imbalance.[165] Serious cardiac problems are rare with paclitaxel, and most patients can be treated without

special monitoring.[166] Hypersensitivity reactions are also known to occur.[167]

Cisplatin, an agent widely used to treat genitourinary malignancy, head and neck tumors, and non-small cell lung cancer is known to induce hypertension. Thalidomide and paclitaxel may induce hypotension. Bevacizumab, a monoclonal antibody against vascular endothelial growth factor, has been associated with significant increases in blood pressure in more than 25% of treated patients. Serious and sometimes permanent hypertension has been reported in up to 14% of treated patients; rarely patients develop hypertensive crises. Patients with baseline hypertension are at increased risk and should be monitored during therapy.[168] Antihypertensive therapy and consideration of alternate treatment is appropriate for patients in whom the blood pressure is difficult to control. All antiangiogenic agents, including sunitinib, alemtuzumab, gemtuzumab, infliximab, muromanoab-CD3, rituximab, and sorafenib, are associated with increased incidence of hypertension, usually reversible upon holding or stopping the medication. Once hypertension is controlled rechallenge may be initiated, and many patients are able to continue treatment with acceptable cardiac risk.

Cardiac complications of radiation therapy

Links between radiation to the chest in the treatment for malignancy and subsequent heart disease have been clearly established. Inclusion of cardiac tissue in the radiation portals can lead to a broad spectrum of disease, which often presents decades after exposure. Recognition of these risks has led to dramatic improvements in radiation techniques over the years, but the degree to which the heart can be spared has not been fully determined, as long-term follow-up studies in patients treated with modern techniques are still underway.

The pathophysiology of ionizing radiation's cardiotoxic effects involves both DNA damage and generation of reactive oxygen species. Cells with higher turnover are more susceptible, particularly the vascular endothelium. Small vessel damage then leads to inflammation and ultimately fibrosis of cardiac tissue. All layers of the heart are involved, leading to acute and chronic pericardial disease, accelerated coronary artery disease, cardiomyopathy, valvular disease, and conduction system abnormalities. Secondary cardiac malignancies attributed to radiation therapy (RT) have even been reported.[169] The heart responds to the radiation insult over time with late-presentation and chronic progressive functional decline showing a direct correlation with the radiation fraction to the heart. Animal models have demonstrated a radiation dose-dependent chronic congestive myocardial failure with damage to the myocardial microvasculature; histological examination shows a marked reduction in capillary density, myocardial degeneration, and necrosis with interstitial fibrosis.[170,171] Cell kinetic studies show increased endothelial cell proliferation about 30–100 days postradiation. The morphologic changes in animal models parallel the drops in cardiac output and left ventricular ejection fraction.

Human data on cardiac effects of RT have come mostly from patients with Hodgkin's lymphoma and breast cancer, who historically received significant doses of cardiac radiation and who also are available for long-term follow-up studies. In contrast, survival in lung cancer is generally too poor to allow significant development of cardiac complications. Risk factors include total radiation dose, volume of the heart exposed, and specific techniques used, but other factors play a role, including age at the time of exposure (younger patients are at higher risk), concurrent treatment with anthracycline-containing chemotherapy regimen, and traditional cardiac risk factors. Although exposure of the heart to >35 Gy is commonly considered to increase risk, recent studies have shown

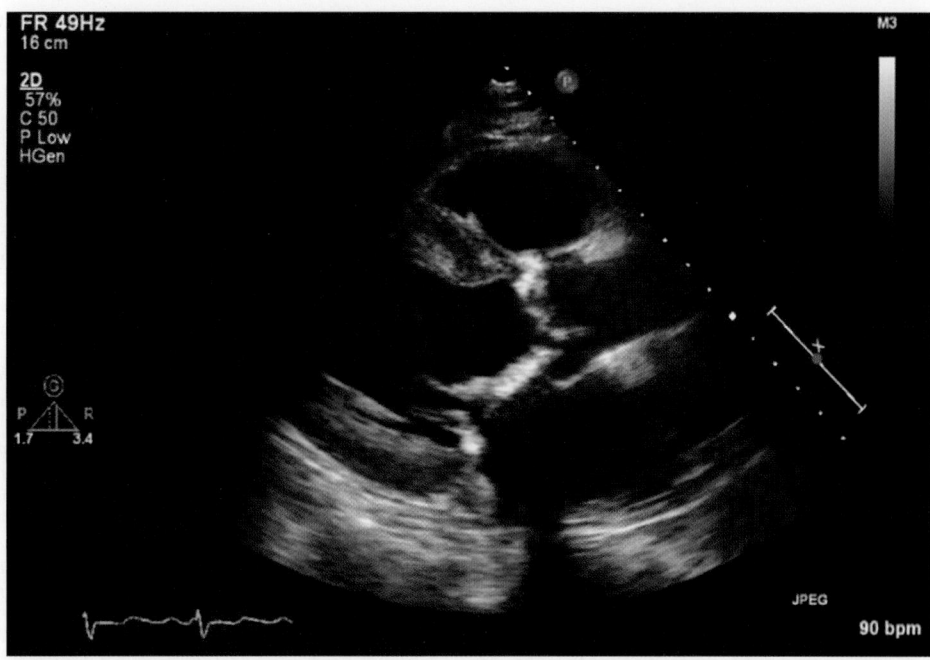

Figure 8 Parasternal long-axis echocardiographic view from a 40-year-old patient who received mantle radiation for lymphoma two decades prior. Note the severe thickening and calcification of the aortic and mitral valves. This patient also had severe coronary artery disease, cardiomyopathy, and abnormal pericardial thickening, all likely sequelae of his prior cancer treatment.

risk with lower doses as well. The Childhood Cancer Survivor Study found a greater than twofold increase in risk of heart failure, myocardial infarction, pericardial disease, and valve disease at radiation doses of 15–35 Gy.[172] Another smaller study found a relative risk of 12.5 for cardiac death for those exposed to cardiac doses of 5–15 Gy and relative risk of 25 at >15 Gy.[173]

Radiation treatment for Hodgkin's lymphoma carries the highest risk of cardiac complications owing to proximity of mediastinal nodes to the heart, younger age at diagnosis, and good potential for long-term survival. The relative risk of fatal cardiac events has been reported as 7.2 after radiation-containing treatment.[174] Because it may take years or even decades for radiation-related heart disease to become clinically manifest, the discovery of major complication may not appear until late follow-up assessments are undertaken; in some instances, this may be years or decades after the initial exposure. The most common complications are valvular lesions (predominantly regurgitant) and myocardial infarction and also seen are restrictive cardiomyopathy, dysrhythmia, and autonomic dysfunction (Figure 8). Pericardial disease has become less prevalent with better cardiac shielding and other technical improvements.[175]

Breast cancer cohorts provide us with the richest body of evidence regarding radiation effects on the heart, owing to both the overall disease prevalence and the opportunity to compare right-sided versus left-sided disease. Several studies have utilized this natural control group to distinguish between systemic effects of chemotherapeutics and those of localized cardiac radiation. A strong correlation between RT and increased cardiovascular mortality was established by many early randomized trials.[176] Improved techniques, including better cardiac shielding, tangential fields, and respiratory gating, have certainly reduced or delayed cardiac morbidity and mortality, yet significant risk probably remains, especially for left-sided cancers. Inclusion of the right or left internal mammary lymph node chain in the radiation field increases cardiac exposure and has been shown to increase subsequent cardiovascular complications. Similar to the data for Hodgkin's lymphoma, risk of cardiac events after RT

increases with duration of follow up, treatment with anthracyclines, and traditional cardiovascular risk factors.

Clinical manifestations of radiation cardiotoxicity are broad. Acute pericarditis can occur at the time of radiation treatment, and pericardial effusion is commonly seen in the acute and subacute setting, but can also be chronic. Distinction from malignant pericardial effusion can be difficult and occasionally necessitates fluid analysis by cytology. Cardiac tamponade is rare. Chronic inflammation can manifest as constrictive pericarditis, which can be challenging to diagnose and carries a grave prognosis unless the patient is well enough to undergo surgical pericardiectomy.

Coronary artery disease after radiation can present as angina, myocardial infarction or sudden death; the risk increases with time. At least two mechanisms appear to be involved in macrovascular disease. First, radiation induces thickening of the arterial wall secondary to intimal and adventitial proliferation; the luminal area is thereby reduced. Second, radiation greatly accelerates atherosclerosis and acts synergistically with that process to enhance cholesterol deposition and luminal ulceration.[177] Thus, as noted earlier, traditional cardiac risk factors such as smoking and dyslipidemia play a key cooperative role in the pathogenesis. Because of its location, the left anterior descending artery is the most frequently affected.

The treatment of radiation-associated vascular injury is similar to the conventional treatment of ischemic cardiac disease; nitrates, β-adrenergic blockers, platelet inhibitors, and calcium channel blockers are the mainstays of pharmacological therapy. Invasive approaches for the management of ischemic heart disease are also often helpful; balloon angioplasty, however, often requires inflation pressures that are higher than those ordinarily used, and longer periods of balloon inflation may be required. Bypass surgery may prove more difficult than usual from a technical standpoint because of the smaller vascular lumens and because the surgeon must work in a previously irradiated field. Nevertheless, bypass surgery remains an important option for these patients.

The spectrum of radiation-induced cardiomyopathy includes diastolic dysfunction, restrictive cardiomyopathy, and systolic dysfunction. Small vessel ischemic disease and fibrosis are the predominant underlying pathology, with subsequent ventricular remodeling possible. Restrictive cardiomyopathy can be very difficult to distinguish from pericardial constriction—especially as both may be present in the same patient. Endomyocardial biopsy is sometimes employed before pericardiectomy to rule out coexisting myocardial disease, which carries a prohibitive operative mortality.

Valvular involvement, while common, is usually not severe. Nevertheless, valve injury is progressive and can contribute to significant morbidity that accompanies the irradiated heart. The most common lesions found are tricuspid regurgitation, mitral regurgitation, and aortic regurgitation, but aortic stenosis is occasionally encountered.[178,179] Histologically, the valves show endocardial thickening resembling fibroelastosis.[180]

Radiation injury to the cardiac conduction system has also been noted and is usually suggested by abnormalities on the electrocardiogram. Prolongation of the PR interval is often seen, as are supranodal and infranodal atrioventricular blocks. Complete heart block is occasionally encountered, and pacemaker implantation may prove lifesaving for such patients. Autonomic dysfunction can manifest with inappropriate sinus tachycardia, bradycardia, or inadequate heart rate response to exercise.

References

1 Ewer MS, Benjamin RS, Yeh ET. Cardiac complications. In: Holland J, Frei E, eds. *Cancer Medicine*, 6th ed. Hamilton, Ontario: BC Decker; 2003.

5 Plana JC, Galderisi M, Barac A, et al. Expert consensus for multimodality imaging evaluation of adult patients during and after cancer therapy: a report from the American Society of Echocardiography and the European Association of Cardiovascular Imaging. *J Am Soc Echocardiogr*. 2014;**27**(9):911–939.

7 Ewer M, Gibbs H, Swafford J, Benjamin R. Cardiotoxicity in patients receiving trastuzumab (Herceptin): primary toxicity, synergistic or sequential stress, or surveillance artifact? *Semin Oncol*. 1999;**26**(suppl 12):96–101.

21 Klein AL, Abbara S, Agler DA, et al. American Society of Echocardiography clinical recommendations for multimodality cardiovascular imaging of patients with pericardial disease: endorsed by the Society for Cardiovascular Magnetic Resonance and Society of Cardiovascular Computed Tomography. *J Am Soc Echocardiogr*. 2013;**26**:965–1012.

22 Spodick D. Current concepts: acute cardiac tamponade. *N Engl J Med*. 2003;**349**:684–690.

36 Ewer SM, Yusuf SW. Arrhythmia in the cancer patient. In: Ewer MS, Yeh ETH, eds. *Cancer and the Heart*, 2nd ed. Shelton, CT: Medical Publishing House-USA; 2013:190–209.

51 Strickman N, Rossi P, Massumi A, Hall R. Carcinoid heart disease: a clinical, pathologic and therapeutic update. *Curr Prob Cardiol*. 1982;**6**(11):1–41.

66 Kristen AV, Dengler TJ, Hegenbart U, et al. Prophylactic implantation of cardioverter-defibrillator in patients with severe cardiac amyloidosis and high risk for sudden cardiac death. *Heart Rhythm*. 2008;**5**:235.

70 Kim PY, Ewer MS. Chemotherapy and QT prolongation: overview with clinical perspective. *Curr Treat Options Cardiovasc Med*. 2014;**16**:303–308.

78 Ewer MS, Lippman S. Type II chemotherapy-related cardiac dysfunction: time to recognize a new entity. *J Clin Oncol*. 2005;**23**(13):2900–2902.

82 Cardinale D, Sandri MT, Colombo A, et al. Prognostic value of troponin I in cardiac risk stratification of cancer patients undergoing high-dose chemotherapy. *Circulation*. 2004;**109**(22):2749–2754.

84 Swain S, Whaley F, Ewer M. Congestive heart failure in patients treated with doxorubicin: A retrospective analysis of three trials. *Cancer*. 2003;**97**:2869–2879.

87 Zhang S, Liu X, Bawa-Khalfe T, et al. Identification of the molecular basis of doxorubicin-induced cardiotoxicity. *Nat Med*. 2012;**18**:1639–1642.

92 Ewer MS, Ali MK, Mackay B, et al. A comparison of resting and exercise ejection fractions with cardiac biopsy grades in patients receiving adriamycin. *J Clin Oncol*. 1984;**2**:112–117.

99 Von Hoff D, Layard M, Basa P, et al. Risk factors for doxorubicin-induced congestive heart failure. *Ann Intern Med*. 1979;**91**:710–717.

114 O'Brian M, Wigler N, Inbar M, et al. Reduced cardiotoxicity and comparable efficacy in a phase III trial of pegylated liposomal doxorubicin HCL (CAELYX/Doxil) versus conventional doxorubicin for first-line treatment of metastatic breast cancer. *Ann Oncol*. 2004;**15**:440–449.

116 Hortobagyi G, Frye D, Buzdar A, et al. Decreased cardiac toxicity of doxorubicin administered by continuous intravenous infusion in combination chemotherapy for metastatic breast carcinoma. *Cancer*. 1989;**63**:37–45.

119 Lipshultz SE, Miller TL, Lipsitz SR, et al. Continuous versus bolus infusion of doxorubicin in children with ALL: long-term cardiac outcomes. *Pediatrics*. 2012;**130**:1003–1011.

121 Swain S, Whaley F, Gerber M, et al. Cardioprotection with dexrazoxane for doxorubicin-containing chemotherapy in advanced breast cancer. *J Clin Oncol*. 1997;**15**(4):1318–1332.

125 Lipshultz SE, Scully RE, Lipsitz SR, et al. Assessment of dexrazoxane as a cardioprotectant in doxorubicin-treated children with high-risk acute lymphoblastic leukaemia: long-term follow-up of a prospective, randomised, multicentre trial. *Lancet Oncol*. 2010;**2010**:950–961.

133 van Dalen EC, Michiels EMC, Caron HN, Kremer LCM. Different anthracycline derivates for reducing cardiotoxicity in cancer patients. *Cochrane Database of Systematic Reviews*. 2010;(**5**. Art. No.: D005006). doi: 10.1002/14651858.CD005006.pub4.

134 Gennari A, Salvadori B, Donati S, et al. Cardiotoxicity of epirubicin/paclitaxel-containing regimens: role of cardiac risk factors. *J Clin Oncol*. 1999;**17**:3596–3602.

139 Tan-Chiu E, Yothers G, Romond E, et al. Assessment of cardiac dysfunction in a randomized trial comparing doxorubicin and cyclophosphamide followed by paclitaxel, with or without trastuzumab as adjuvant therapy in node-positive, human epidermal growth factor receptor 2-overexpressing breast cancer: NSABP B31. *J Clin Oncol*. 2005;**23**:7811–7819.

140 Suter T, Procter M, Van Veldhuisen D, et al. Trastuzumab-associated cardiac adverse effects in the Herceptin Adjuvant Trial. *J Clin Oncol*. 2007;**25**:3859–3865.

141 Joensuu H, Bono P, Kataja V, et al. Fluorouracil, epirubicin and cyclophosphamide with either docetaxel or vioorelbine, with or without trastuzumab as adjuvant treatment of breast cancer. Final results of the FinHer Trial. *J Clin Oncol*. 2009;**27**:5685–5692.

142 Ewer MS, Ewer SM. Cardiotoxicity of anticancer treatment. *Nat Rev Cardiol*. 2015;**12**(9):547–558.

144 Crone S, Zhao Y, Fan L, et al. ErbB2 is essential in the prevention of dilated cardiomyopathy. *Nature Med*. 2002;**8**:459–465.

145 Ewer MS, Vooletich M, Durand J, et al. Reversibility of trastuzumab-related cardiotoxicity: new insights based on clinical course and response to medical treatment. *J Clin Oncol*. 2005;**23**:7820–7827.

147 Perez EA, Koeler M, Byrne J, Preston AJ, Rappold E, Ewer MS. Cardiac safety of lapatinib: pooled analysis of 3689 patients enrolled in clinical trials. *Mayo Clin Proc*. 2008;**83**:679–686.

148 Ewer MS, Suter TM, Lenihan DJ, et al. Cardiovaxcular events among 1090 cancer patients treated with sunitinib, interferon or placebo: a comprehensive adjudicated database analysis demonstrating clinically meaningful reversibility of cardiac events. *Eur J Cancer*. 2014;**50**:2162–2170.

159 Forbes JF, Cuzick J, Buzdar AU, Howell A, Tobias JS, Baum M. Effect of anastrozole and tamoxifen as adjuvant treatment for early-stage breast cancer: 100-month analysis of the ATAC trial. *Lancet Oncol*. 2008;**9**:45–53.

168 Zhong J, Ali AN, Voloschin AD, et al. Bevacizumab-induced hypertension is a predictive marker for improved outcomes in patients with recurrent glioblastoma treated with bevacizumab. *Cancer*. 2015;**121**(9):1456–1462. doi: 10.1002/cncr.29234.

172 Mulrooney DA, Yeazel MW, Kawashima T, et al. Cardiac outcomes in a cohort of adult survivors of childhood and adolescent cancer: retrospective analysis of the Childhood Cancer Survivor Study cohort. *BMJ*. 2009;**339**:b4606.

173 Tukenova M, Guibout C, Oberlin O, et al. Role of cancer treatment in long-term overall and cardiovascular mortality after childhood cancer. *J Clin Oncol*. 2010;**28**:1308–1315.

133 Respiratory complications

Vickie R. Shannon, MD ▪ George A. Eapen, MD ▪ Carlos A. Jimenez, MD ▪ Horiana B. Grosu, MD ▪ Rodolfo C. Morice, MD ▪ Lara Bashoura, MD ▪ Scott E. Evans, MD ▪ Roberto Adachi, MD ▪ Michael Kroll, MD ▪ Saadia A. Faiz, MD ▪ Diwakar D. Balachandran, MD ▪ Selvaraj E. Pravinkumar, MD, FRCP ▪ Burton F. Dickey, MD

Overview

The respiratory system is particularly susceptible to complications of cancer and cancer therapy. This vulnerability arises from the stringent architectural requirements for gas exchange, the continuous exposure of the respiratory tract to the external environment, and the severe symptoms that can accompany respiratory compromise. Gas exchange requires patent airways, an effective musculoskeletal ventilatory pump, a thin alveolocapillary membrane, and adequate blood flow through the pulmonary circulation. In cancer patients, primary and metastatic tumors of the chest compromise major airways; pleural effusions externally compress the lungs and impair diaphragmatic function; direct, hematogenous, or lymphangitic spread of tumor replaces functioning lung parenchyma; resectional surgery reduces parenchymal volume; nonresectional surgery can transiently impair lung function; radiotherapy, chemotherapy, stem cell therapy, and infection injure the vulnerable alveolocapillary membrane; tumors directly or indirectly compromise the musculoskeletal pump; and venous thromboembolism (VTE) and pulmonary vasculopathy obstruct pulmonary blood flow.

The normal respiratory system contains considerable physiologic reserve, such that surgical loss of one lung is generally well tolerated. However, in cancer patients, insults to multiple components of the respiratory system may result in progressive loss of physiologic reserve and increasing dyspnea. Dyspnea, cough, wheezing, stridor, chest pain, and hemoptysis are common symptoms in the cancer setting that lead to pulmonary consultation.

In this chapter, we will discuss the pathophysiology, diagnosis, and management of the major respiratory complications of cancer and its therapy. We begin with the direct effects of cancer and cancer therapies on the lungs, review major indirect effects of cancer on the lungs, and end with respiratory failure in the cancer patient.

Malignant airway obstruction

Malignant airspace disease may be central or peripheral, focal or diffuse, or endoluminal or extraluminal or both. The dominant symptom complex associated with this process depends upon the location and extent of disease, which also dictates therapy.

Common cancer types and clinical presentation

The most common cause of malignant airway obstruction is direct extension from an adjacent tumor, particularly bronchogenic carcinoma. Esophageal and thyroid malignancies also frequently extend directly into the airways. Primary tumors of the major airways are relatively rare, with squamous cell carcinoma, adenoid cystic carcinoma, and carcinoid tumors most often implicated.[1,2] Airway compromise can also occur from metastatic renal and breast carcinomas or intrathoracic lymphomas. Both endoluminal disease and extrinsic compression by tumor may severely compromise airway luminal diameter. Reduction in airway caliber and architectural distortion synergistically impair airflow obstruction and mucus clearance, leading to increased work of breathing and dyspnea.[3] Luminal narrowing of the trachea and mainstem bronchi typically manifests as dyspnea, cough, wheeze, stridor, and atelectasis. Airway obstruction beyond the mainstem bronchi usually results in atelectasis, postobstructive pneumonitis, cough, and dyspnea. Individual patient presentations range from asymptomatic discovery on staging work-up to frank respiratory failure due to critical airway obstruction.[4] Exertional dyspnea typically occurs when tracheal diameter is reduced below 8 mm. Further reduction in tracheal diameter to <5 mm is usually associated with dyspnea at rest.[5] Chronic obstructive pulmonary disease (COPD) exacerbations or mucosal edema and increased secretions that accompany superimposed pneumonias may precipitate respiratory failure, even in patients with only moderate tumor-related airflow limitation. Symptoms may thus improve with measures directed at treating the infection or COPD exacerbation.

Differential diagnosis

While critical airway obstruction is not usually a diagnostic challenge, the clinical presentation of subcritical obstruction can be. Stridor indicates pathognomonic significant tracheal obstruction. Other findings, including dyspnea and wheezing, are prominent but nonspecific clinical symptoms that denote airflow limitation. Concurrent conditions such as congestive heart failure, pleural effusions, and pulmonary emboli may produce similar symptoms, obscuring the diagnosis.

Diagnostic evaluation

The diagnostic work-up is aimed at establishing a definitive diagnosis, quantifying airflow limitation, and delineating anatomic extent in an effort to optimize therapeutic strategies. The characteristic blunting noted in the flow-volume loop upon pulmonary function testing (PFT) often provides an indication of tracheal obstruction. However, this is a relatively insensitive test, with positive findings noted only with tracheal diameters below 10 mm.[6] Spirometry may also precipitate frank respiratory failure in patients with severe airway obstruction and should be used with caution in this subgroup of patients. Rarely, deviation or compression of the trachea may be seen on plain chest radiographs. Plain chest films are otherwise not helpful in defining the anatomic extent of tumor or therapeutic options. Standard chest computed tomography (CT) as well as the latest iterations of low-dose multidetector scanners and advanced airway imaging techniques that allow multiplanar and three-dimensional (3D) reconstruction provides

Holland-Frei Cancer Medicine, Ninth Edition. Edited by Robert C. Bast Jr., Carlo M. Croce, William N. Hait, Waun Ki Hong, Donald W. Kufe, Martine Piccart-Gebhart, Raphael E. Pollock, Ralph R. Weichselbaum, Hongyang Wang, and James F. Holland.
© 2017 John Wiley & Sons, Inc. ISBN: 978-1-118-93469-2

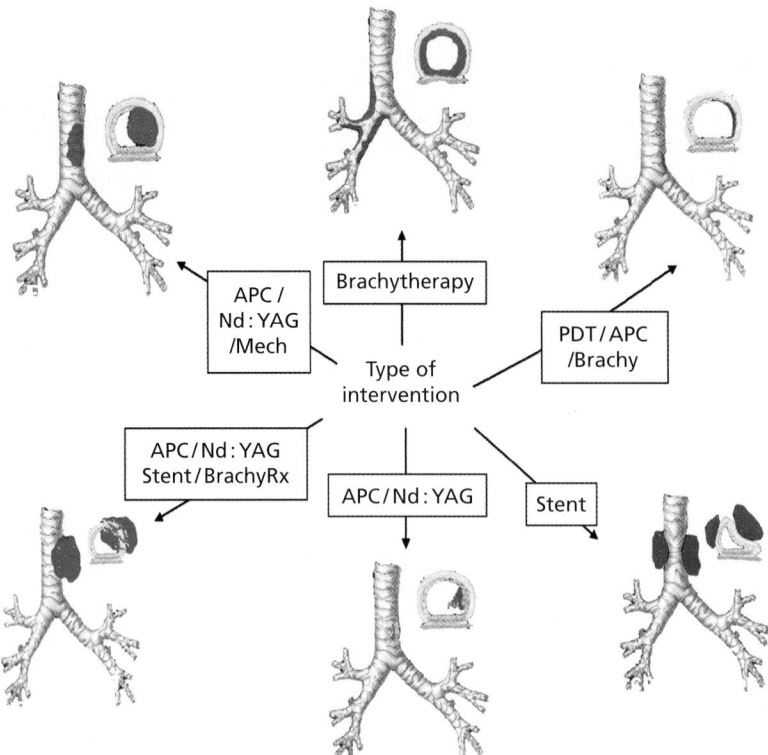

Figure 1 Approach to airway obstruction using interventional bronchoscopic therapy.

valuable additional information regarding the extent of the lesion and guidance in optimizing therapeutic strategies.[7] Bronchoscopy, either flexible or rigid, remains the gold standard in the work-up of airway obstruction. Histologic confirmation of malignancy can be obtained at the time of the examination. Furthermore, bronchoscopy offers direct visualization of the lesion, which permits precise characterization of tumor vascularity and the extent of obstruction, as well as the degree of obstruction attributable to endoluminal versus extraluminal disease. Recent reports have also supported the use of endobronchial ultrasonography as an adjunctive tool in treatment planning.[8]

Management of malignant airway obstruction

Tumor characteristics, including histologic type, stage, and location, and patient attributes, such as urgency of presentation and performance status, dictate management. Therapeutic strategies vary based on the location and type of obstruction, as well as the local expertise and available institution-specific resources. Surgical resection provides the best prospect for long-term disease control and should be considered in all patients during the initial evaluation. Localized involvement of the small airways and lung parenchyma is best treated by surgical resection, if feasible. In many cases, however, external beam radiotherapy or systemic chemotherapy may be the only treatment options. Patients with central airway obstruction often present with either medically or surgically unresectable disease. While a comprehensive review of the various modalities is beyond the scope of this chapter, some basic principles are outlined (Figure 1). In emergent cases, the barrel of the rigid bronchoscope may be used to mechanically core out the tumor and dilate the airways, providing palliation. Flexible bronchoscopy and balloon bronchoplasty may be used to dilate the airways in less urgent cases.[9] Electrocautery, argon plasma coagulation, laser therapy, cryotherapy, brachytherapy, and photodynamic therapy are reasonable approaches for predominantly endoluminal

disease (Figure 2). Extraluminal-predominant disease may be best treated with external beam radiotherapy and endobronchial stent placement (Figure 3). Since most lesions are mixed with endo- and extraluminal components, multimodality therapy, using endobronchial laser therapy with mechanical debulking followed by stent placement and subsequent consolidation with external beam radiotherapy, for example, is quite common. Symptom palliation, resulting in reduction in levels of care, may be accomplished in most instances with the judicious application of endoscopic techniques.[10] Patients should be evaluated carefully with an early referral to an experienced bronchoscopist who can match the various therapeutic modalities available to the individual patient.

Malignant pleural effusions

Malignant pleural effusion is a common clinical problem in the cancer setting that signifies distant spread of tumor and, hence, advanced disease. Malignant pleural effusions have significant therapeutic and prognostic implications. Estimates of the incidence of malignant pleural effusions in the United States approach 150,000 cases annually.[11] Malignant pleural involvement without effusion occurs in up to 45% of patients with metastatic disease to the pleura.[12] In primary pleural malignancies, such as malignant mesothelioma, pleural effusions may be absent. Nearly any type of neoplasm can affect the pleura. Lung cancer accounts for up to half of all malignant effusions, followed in frequency by breast carcinoma and lymphoma. Pleural effusions may occur with acute and chronic leukemias and myelodysplastic syndrome (MDS). Pleural effusions in patients with leukemia are most often due to infection and to a lesser extent leukemic infiltration of the pleura.[13] Unfortunately, in 5–10% of patients, a primary tumor cannot be identified.[14,15] Most pleural malignancies arise from tumor emboli to the visceral pleura. The parietal pleura may be involved secondarily, presumably by seeding from the visceral

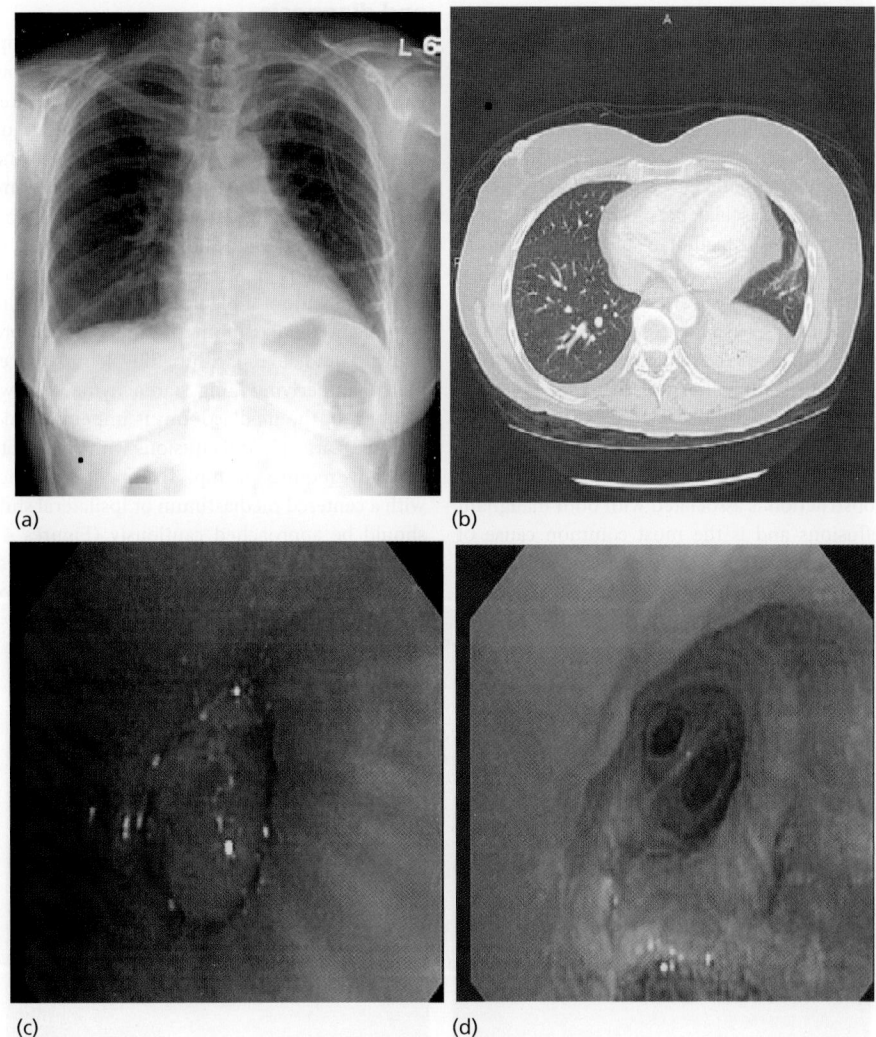

Figure 2 Left lower lobe collapse secondary to metastatic sarcoma (a and b). Complete obstruction of the LLL basilar segments due to a large obstructing tumor was noted at bronchoscopy (c) which was removed using snare forceps and argon plasma coagulation, revealing a patent distal airway (d).

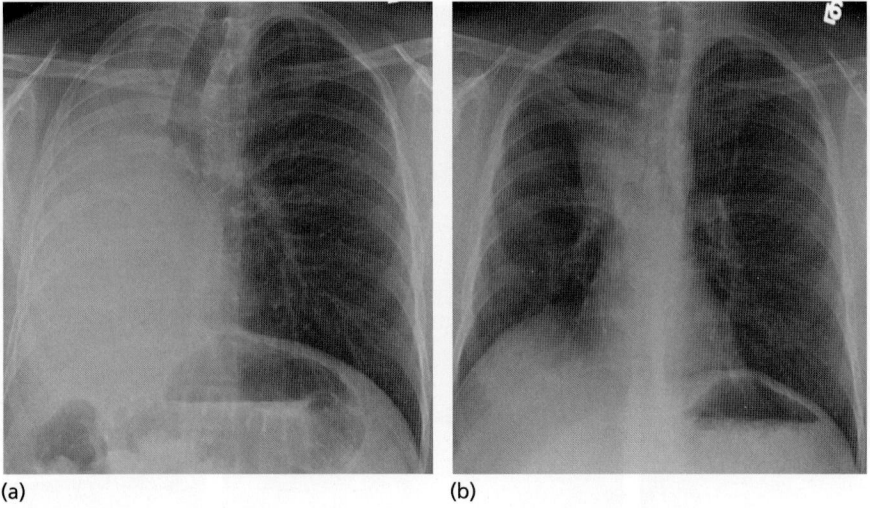

Figure 3 Complete opacification of the right thorax secondary to obstruction of the right mainstem bronchus by a large, predominantly extraluminal mass (a). A wire stent was placed into the bronchus intermedius (b), resulting in partial reexpansion of the right lung.

pleura. Direct extensions of tumor from the lung, chest wall, mediastinal structures, or diaphragm and hematogenous metastasis to the parietal pleura are other mechanisms that contribute to the genesis of malignant pleural fluid formation.[16] In addition to direct tumor involvement of the pleura, malignant pleural effusions can result from lymphatic blockage anywhere between the parietal pleura and the mediastinal lymph nodes.[17] Elevations in the local production of vascular endothelial growth factor (VEGF), a potent mediator of increased vascular permeability, also play a significant role in the formation of malignant pleural effusions.[18] Among VEGF homologs, VEGF-D showed a 92.6% rate of positive expression in a study of malignant pleural effusion and may be a useful marker in the diagnosis.[19] Seventeen percent of all pleural effusions in patients with cancer are "paramalignant," a term used for effusions that occur in the setting of cancer that are not caused by direct malignant involvement of the pleural space.[16] These effusions develop as a result of local or systemic effects of the tumor, complications of cancer therapy, or concurrent nonmalignant disease.[20] Lymphatic obstruction is associated with both malignant and paramalignant effusions and is the most common cause of paramalignant effusions. Other common causes include bronchial obstruction, trapped lung, and pulmonary embolism (PE).

Clinical manifestations, imaging studies, and diagnosis

Most commonly, patients present with symptoms of progressive exertional dyspnea. Cough may also be a troubling symptom with large effusions. Constitutional symptoms are common signals of advanced disease, and thus malaise, weight loss, and poor appetite may become more frequent as the performance status worsens. Hemoptysis and chest wall pain are less common symptoms and may indicate malignant endobronchial disease and tumoral invasion of the chest wall. Standard chest roentgenograms and bilateral decubitus films of the chest provide critical information in the initial evaluation of pleural effusions, including effusion size, position of the mediastinum and diaphragms, presence of loculations and air fluid levels within the pleural space, and characteristics of the underlying lung parenchyma. Knowledge regarding the position of the mediastinum is imperative in therapeutic decision making. Large pleural effusions with contralateral mediastinal shift typically require prompt therapeutic thoracentesis, while those with a centered mediastinum or ipsilateral shift of the mediastinum should be approached cautiously (Figures 4 and 5). In addition to pleural effusions, other disease processes that may cause an ipsilateral shift of the mediastinum or a centered mediastinum with

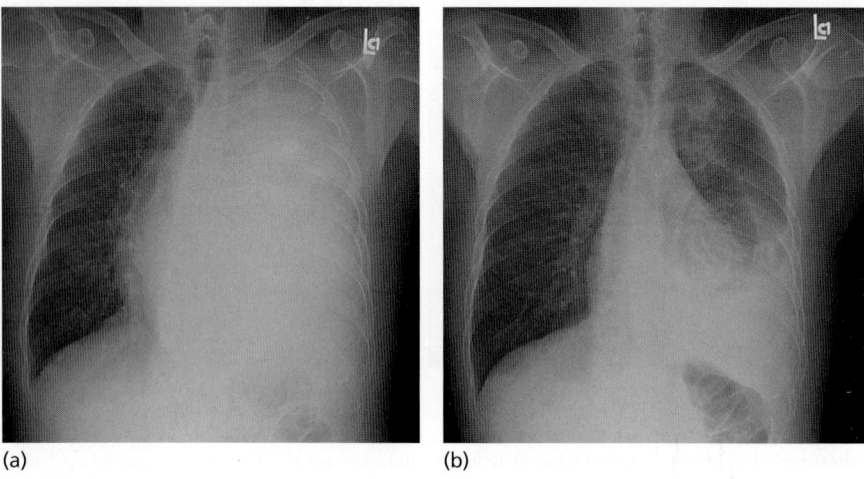

(a)   (b)

Figure 4 Large left-sided pleural effusion causing opacification of the left hemithorax and contralateral shift of the mediastinum (a). Following thoracentesis (b) the mediastinum shifted back the midline.

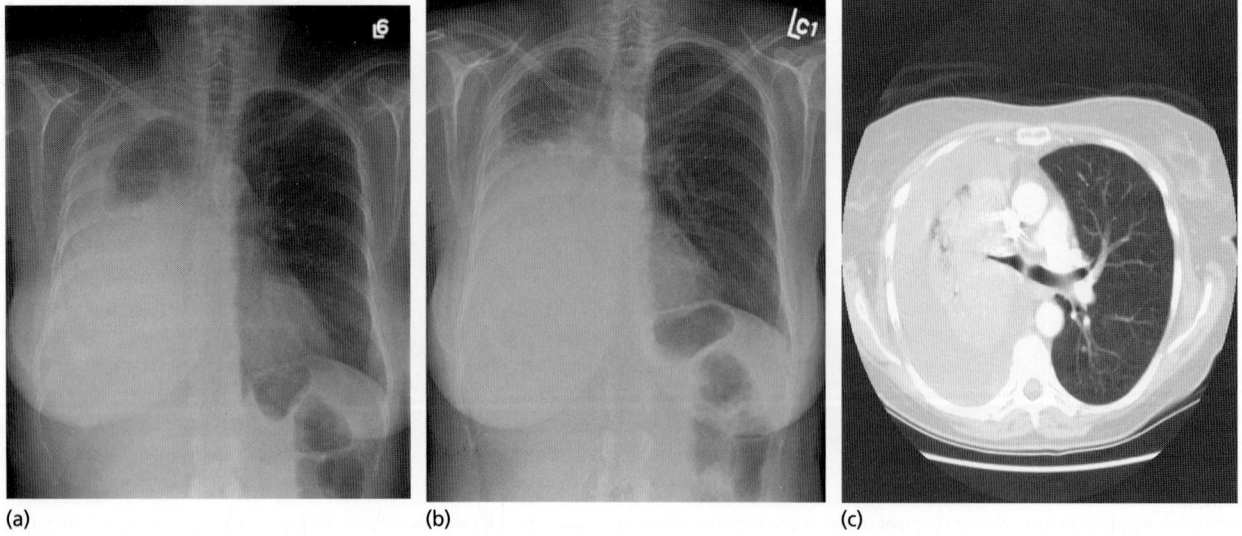

(a)   (b)   (c)

Figure 5 Large right-sided pleural effusion (a) with ipsilateral shift of the mediastinum following thoracentesis (b), indicating volume loss secondary to atelectasis or mass. A CT scan of the chest (C) demonstrates a large mass compressing the right mainstem bronchus.

hemithorax opacification include a frozen mediastinum associated with malignant mesothelioma or lymphoma, atelectasis related to occlusion of the ipsilateral central airway, or extensive tumoral infiltration of the ipsilateral lung simulating a large effusion.[20] CT is helpful in identifying loculated effusions; offers better anatomical information of the chest wall, parietal and visceral pleura, mediastinal structures, and lung parenchyma; and is especially valuable in delineating alternate diagnoses.[21] Ultrasonography provides guidance in locating the optimal site for thoracentesis and is particularly helpful in the setting of loculated pleural effusions. The identification of entrapped lung by ultrasonography using tissue movement may permit deformation (strain) analysis prior to thoracentesis.[22,23] Positron emission tomography (PET) with ^{18}F-fluorodeoxyglucose (FDG) and magnetic resonance imaging (MRI) are both helpful in highlighting extrapleural extension of disease.[21] PET imaging provides valuable information associated with malignant mesothelioma; however, its utility in the evaluation of other malignant pleural diseases has not been established. Chemical analysis reveals an exudative effusion in most cases, with only 5% of malignant pleural effusions being transudates.[20] Positive pleural fluid cytology, noted in 62% of cases, represents the diagnostic cornerstone of malignant pleural effusions.[24] Tumor marker measurements improve the diagnostic yield of cytologically negative effusions by 33% and are particularly valuable when lymphoma, leukemia, or multiple myeloma is suspected.[25,26] The role of flow cytometry in the study of mesotheliomas remains controversial.[27] Pleuroscopic pleural biopsies have a 95% sensitivity in the diagnosis of pleural malignancies, and diagnostic yield increases only incrementally (1%) when combined with pleural fluid cytology. By contrast, closed pleural biopsy has a diagnostic yield of only 44% but improves to 77% when combined with an analysis of pleural fluid cytology.[24]

Management of malignant pleural effusions

Because malignant pleural effusions often signal advanced disease and incurability, treatment efforts are frequently directed toward palliation. Hence, awareness of available therapeutic options tailored to individual patient needs is important. The patient's performance status and information regarding prior thoracenteses, including the volume of fluid evacuated, whether lung reexpansion and symptom palliation were obtained, and the time interval between repeated taps, are important components of the evaluation that help to guide further therapy. Performance status is the best predictor of survival in patients with recurrent malignant pleural effusions.[28] The presence of local chest wall abnormalities, future cancer treatment plans, the patient's preferences, and the availability of family support influence the approach to these patients. Palliation with simple therapeutic thoracentesis represents a reasonable approach to patients with newly diagnosed chemo- or radiosensitive tumors, such as lymphoma and breast, small-cell lung, germ cell, ovarian, prostate, and thyroid neoplasms, while awaiting response to definitive therapy. After the initial clinical and roentgenographic evaluation, a symptom-limited therapeutic thoracentesis is recommended. A recent consensus statement by the American Thoracic Society and the European Respiratory Society recommends that not more than 1.0–1.5 L of fluid be slowly evacuated from the pleural space in one sitting and that drainage should be discontinued if the patient develops symptoms of dyspnea, cough, or chest discomfort.[11] In our experience, patients with radiographic evidence of contralateral mediastinal shift from large pleural effusions may safely tolerate the removal of 2–2.5 L of fluid in one sitting as long as there are no procedure-related symptoms of chest pain, cough, or dyspnea. However, large-volume pleural fluid

drainage during a single procedure should be carried out cautiously, especially when radiological studies reveal a centered or ipsilaterally shifted mediastinum. Measurement of pleural pressures during the evacuation of large amounts of fluid may reduce procedure-related complications.[29] However, in light of the safety of symptom-limited evacuation, pleural pressure measurement may not be necessary, and its role requires further study. Lung reexpansion following thoracentesis may be assessed with posterior–anterior (PA) and lateral chest radiographs. Repeat thoracenteses spaced 1–2 days apart may be necessary to properly assess lung reexpansion associated with large effusions.[30] In 97% of patients, malignant pleural effusions will recur within 1 month, with most of these effusions reappearing within 1–3 days following fluid evacuation.[31] Patients with limited life expectancies (<30 days) and poor performance status or those in which pleural fluid reaccumulation is slow are best treated with repeated therapeutic thoracentesis. Repeated thoracentesis is a reasonable approach for patients with malignancies that are expected to respond to chemotherapy and/or radiation therapy (RT). However, frequent thoracentesis may trigger the production of local cytokines and fibrin, resulting in pleural fluid loculation, which not only complicates further thoracenteses but also limits future modes of palliation.[32] The use of indwelling pleural catheters has been accepted over the past few years as an alternative palliative option for patients with recurrent malignant effusions. Ideal candidates for this palliative modality include patients with life expectancies in excess of 30 days and in whom prior thoracenteses effected symptomatic relief. Considerations for pleural catheter implantation are valid in this group of patients regardless of lung reexpansion following thoracentesis. Indwelling pleural catheters may be placed in an outpatient setting. Following documentation of proper catheter position, the patient, trained family members, or caregivers may drain the fluid intermittently at home. Daily pleural fluid drainage is recommended initially. During each session, which typically lasts less than 15 min, drainage should be continued until the patient develops cough or chest discomfort, or the fluid stops flowing spontaneously, presumably because the pleural space has been emptied. At our institution, 92% of patients treated with indwelling catheters reported significant relief of dyspnea, and 52% achieved effective pleurodesis. The mean time from catheter insertion to catheter removal was 32 days. Catheter-related complications were observed in only 4% of the patients, including one patient with empyema and two patients with persistent pain at the insertion site. In another study, only 6% of patients required additional drainage of fluid following removal of the catheter.[33] Patients who have chemotherapy or radiation after catheter placement and those who are more short of breath at baseline have greatest improvements in utility.[34] In a subgroup analysis, patients meeting criteria for a pleurodesis procedure achieved 70% effective pleurodesis after insertion of indwelling pleural catheter.[35]

Traditionally, chemical pleurodesis has been the most widely used method to control recurrent malignant pleural effusions. Unfortunately, the lack of prospective studies precludes comparative analyses of efficacy, safety, and cost of the existing chemical agents and pleurodesis techniques. The results from available literature suggest that nonchemotherapeutic agents are more efficacious and the most cost-effective sclerosants.[11] Sterilized, asbestos-free talc is the preferred pleurodesing agent. Complications vary with the surface characteristics of the talc particles. The use of talc particles that are less than 5 mm in size has been associated with pulmonary injury, including acute pneumonitis and respiratory failure associated with adult respiratory distress syndrome, and should be avoided.[36] The safety of large-particle talc for pleurodesis was recently confirmed in a European multicenter trial in which no association with adult respiratory distress syndrome was identified.[37] The superiority of thoracoscopic talc insufflation over talc slurry as a method of administration of the sclerosant is a matter of debate. Success rates of >90% have been reported for both techniques, without significant differences in the rate of overall complications or disease recurrence.[11] The largest published prospective randomized trial comparing thoracoscopic talc insufflation and talc slurry included 501 patients with a performance status of 1 or 2. Results showed no difference in 30-day survival rates and pleurodesis success rates between chest tube talc slurry and thoracoscopic talc poudrage. Unexpected high morbidity and mortality rates were reported in both groups. A subset analysis suggested that thoracoscopic talc insufflation may be advantageous for patients with lung or breast cancer.[38] Based on the available information, our group considers all patients with a good performance status (ECOG 0, 1, or 2), and in whom symptomatic relief and lung reexpansion was achieved after initial drainage of the pleural fluid, for either indwelling pleural catheter placement or pleurodesis with pleuroscopic talc poudrage as the preferred palliative modalities. Rarely, alternative modalities such as pleuroperitoneal shunts and parietal pleurectomy are used in the management of recurrent symptomatic effusions following pleurodesis failures or effusions associated with trapped lung. Chylous effusions associated with malignancy are controlled by treating the primary tumor. Prolonged loss of chyle, a protein-rich, fat-laden, and lymphocyte-predominant fluid, may result in lymphopenia, severe nutritional depletion, and water and electrolyte loss. Mortality due to chylothorax can be as high as 50%. Among those patients with recurrent symptomatic chylothorax and cancer relapse or progressive disease despite adequate treatment, parenteral alimentation and talc pleurodesis[39] and indwelling pleural catheter placement represent reasonable treatment alternatives.[40]

Pleuroperitoneal shunt placement is an attractive option, since chyle is not lost but mobilized from the thorax to the peritoneum where it is reabsorbed, thus mitigating the risk of malnourishment and immune suppression. Unfortunately, the pleuroperitoneal shunt pump mechanism displaces only 1.5–2.5 mL at a time, making its use cumbersome. In addition, the incidence of obstruction of the pump is high. Peritoneal tumor seeding through the shunt is a theoretical concern, although this has not been clearly documented. Embolization of the thoracic duct represents an alternative strategy in the management of recurrent chylous effusions. This procedure appears to be well tolerated, but definitive evidence of its efficacy in the cancer population is not available. Parietal pleurectomy, decortication, and pleuropneumonectomy are associated with high mortality rates and do not provide better symptom control than other palliative options.[11] The utilization of compounds to block VEGF either alone or in combination with other palliative modalities is promising. Theoretically, decreasing production of pleural fluid with VEGF blockade followed by drainage of the pleural effusion and instillation of a chemical agent to obtain pleural symphysis could accelerate pleurodesis and reduce hospital stay.[41] Regrettably, the final results of a single-arm phase II clinical trial of the VEGF receptor inhibitor, vandetanib, combined with intrapleural catheter placement in patients with non-small-cell lung cancer (NSCLC) and recurrent malignant pleural effusion did not significantly reduce time to pleurodesis.[42]

In summary, in patients with limited life expectancies, modalities that offer the best chance for palliation of symptoms, the lowest procedure-related morbidity and mortality, and the shortest hospital stay represent a reasonable approach to the management of recurrent malignant effusions. A multidisciplinary approach (Figure 6), involving oncology, pulmonary medicine, interventional radiology, and thoracic surgery, offers the best opportunities to achieve these goals.

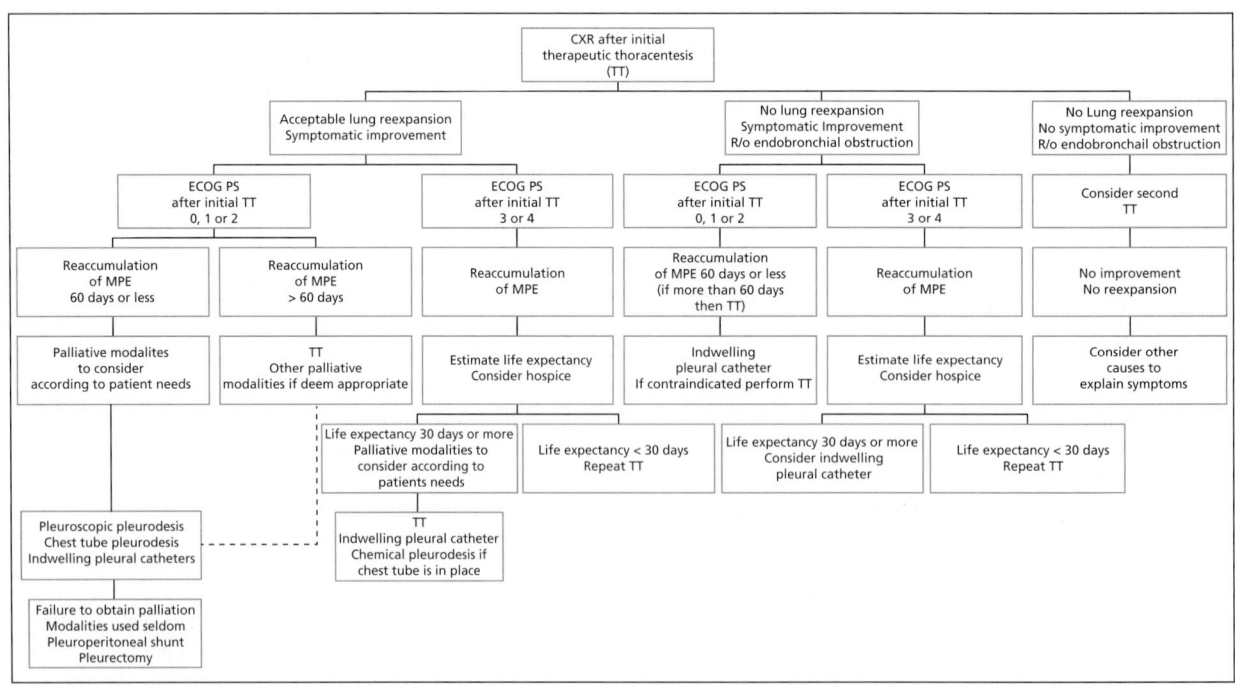

Figure 6 Management of malignant pleural effusions (MPE). Patients with chemo- or radiosensitive tumors on initial treatment (lymphoma, breast cancer, small-cell lung cancer, germ cell cancer, ovarian cancer, prostate cancer, and thyroid neoplams) may be candidates for therapeutic thoracentesis while awaiting systemic treatment results.

Postsurgical respiratory insufficiency

Diagnostic evaluation

The initial approach to the patient with an anatomically resectable tumor includes strategies to determine the patient's functional operability and the predicted long-term pulmonary disability following the loss of the resected lung. This may be accomplished through pulmonary-specific testing as well as a general assessment aimed at identifying and optimizing control of any coexisting systemic diseases. The pulmonary evaluation consists of three sequential steps: (1) measurement of baseline pulmonary function, (2) quantitative radionuclide regional ventilation/perfusion (V/Q) pulmonary studies to calculate postoperative lung function, and (3) exercise testing for patients that do not meet acceptable results on the two previous steps.[43] Among the PFTs that have been used as predictors of postoperative outcome, reduced values of forced expiratory volume in 1 second (FEV_1) and diffusing capacity for carbon monoxide (DLCO) are the most reproducible and most frequently used for predicting complications of lung resection.[44] For decision making, values of FEV_1 reported as percent of predicted that take into account variations in patients' height, gender, and race are preferred over values reported in absolute units (L). In our laboratory, more than half of patients with an FEV_1 between 60% and 80% of predicted have an estimated postpneumonectomy FEV_1 by radionuclide studies that is below acceptable values for safe resection (<40% of predicted). Therefore, we recommend that only those patients with baseline FEV_1 and DLCO ≥ 80% of predicted and no clinical evidence of contralateral pulmonary disease be considered for resection without further testing. All other patients should undergo a "split function" evaluation, which is a quantitative radionuclide assessment of regional lung ventilation and/or perfusion. In this study, the uptake of radioactive ions by various regions in each lung is measured by inhalation of ^{133}Xe or by intravenous administration of ^{133}Xe dissolved in saline or ^{99}Tc macroaggregates. In practice, estimates of lung perfusion alone are easiest and most commonly measured. The percentage of radioactivity contributed by each lung correlates with the contribution to the overall function by that lung. The predicted postoperative FEV_1 (FEV_1ppo) and predicted postoperative DLCO (DLCOppo) are calculated by subtracting the percent functional uptake of the region to be resected from the total uptake. Several

investigators have documented the usefulness of split function studies for predicting both the risk of complications and the loss of pulmonary function after pulmonary resection.[45,46] In these studies, preoperative predicted values are close to measured postoperative values for pneumonectomy and for resections involving more than three segments.[47] Pulmonary function remains relatively stable after pneumonectomy. Predictions for a smaller resection, such as a lobectomy, however, are less reliable, owing to a disproportionate early loss, followed by significant functional improvement with time.[48] Kearney et al.[49] also described a low FEV_1ppo as the only significant independent predictor of complications. Other variables, including age ≥ 60, male sex, history of smoking, pneumonectomy, hypercarbia, (pCO_2 ≥ 45 mm Hg), desaturations on exercise oximetry (SaO_2 ≤ 90%), and a preoperative FEV_1 ≤ 1 L were not predictive of complications. Markos et al.[50] reported that a DLCOppo <40% of predicted was associated with higher morbidity and mortality and was the best predictor of postoperative respiratory failure. In summary, an FEV_1ppo and DLCOppo of ≥ 40% of predicted on split function studies represent safe preoperative criteria for lung resection, including pneumonectomy. Patients that do not meet these criteria but are candidates for lesser surgeries, such as a lobectomy or segmentectomy, should undergo further evaluation with exercise testing.

The rationale for using exercise testing in these high-risk patients is based on two concepts: (1) lung function is not the only determinant of performance, and (2) losses for lobectomies or lesser resections improve over time and tend to be overestimated by radiospirometric studies.[43] Exercise testing also offers the advantage of examining cardiopulmonary and musculoskeletal interactions during stress in a single study. The most validated form of exercise testing is cycle ergometry with incremental workloads to the symptom-limited maximum ($\dot{V}O_{2peak}$). Using this method, Smith et al.[51] found that only 1 of 10 patients with a $\dot{V}O_{2peak}$ > 20 mL/kg/min developed complications postoperatively, whereas all patients with a $\dot{V}O_{2peak}$ < 15 mL/kg/min had complications. We conducted two studies on patients that had been considered inoperable because of FEV_1 ≤ 40% of predicted, FEV_1ppo ≤ 33% of predicted, and/or arterial PCO_2 ≥ 45 mm Hg. Patients that reached a $\dot{V}O_{2peak}$ ≥ 15 ml/kg/min underwent surgical treatment; others were referred to radiation and/or chemotherapy. All surgically treated patients were extubated within 24 h, and the

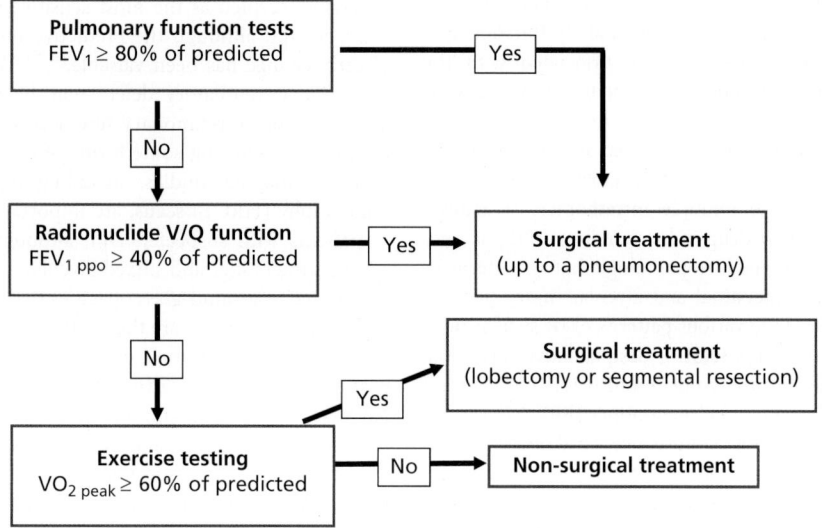

Figure 7 Approach to preoperative evaluation for lung resection.

median time to discharge following surgery was 8 days. There were no inhospital deaths, although reversible postoperative complications occurred in 40% of the patients. Moreover, a survival benefit among these high-risk patients treated surgically was noted.[52,53] More recently, we determined that values of $\dot{V}O_{2peak}$ expressed as percent of predicted more accurately estimated surgical risk and helped to maximize the number of patients that can safely undergo lung resection. We concluded that high-risk patients that achieve a $\dot{V}O_{2peak} \geq 60\%$ of predicted during exercise have an acceptable outcome after lung resection, even if $\dot{V}O_{2peak} < 15\,mL/kg/min$.[33] Our approach to preoperative assessment for lung resection is summarized in Figure 7. In addition to an estimation of surgical risk and postoperative function, the goals of preoperative assessment include the development of strategies to reduce the risk and maximize the number of patients that can benefit from surgical therapy. Finally, one must keep in mind that there is no test that will predict all complications and that the patient and the surgeon should make the final decision regarding the risk/benefit of surgical treatment.

Chemotherapy-induced lung injury

Conventional chemotherapy, as well as a growing list of molecularly targeted antineoplastic agents, is frequently implicated in lung injury. Lung toxicity in this setting may be idiosyncratic, unpredictable, and highly variable from one therapeutic class of drugs to the next. In addition, individual agents within a certain therapeutic class may induce similar patterns of lung injury with widely varying frequencies. For example, among the class of small-molecule tyrosine kinase inhibitors (TKIs) that target the epidermal growth factor receptor (EGFR), gefitinib and erlotinib have been associated with sometimes fatal interstitial pneumonitis (IP), while lung toxicity following use of the dual EGFR-HER2 TKI lapatinib is very rare.[54] Similarly, fatal lung injury following administration of the cytotoxic alkylating agents busulfan and cyclophosphamide is well recognized, whereas lung injury from the alkylating agent chlorambucil is very unusual and has been confined to isolated case reports.[55-57]

Lung injury associated with conventional chemotherapy

The pathogenesis of chemotherapy-related lung injury is poorly understood. Proposed mechanisms include direct cytotoxicity to type II pneumocytes and/or the alveolocapillary endothelium, cytokine release resulting in endothelial dysfunction and capillary leak syndrome, oxidative injury associated with the release of free oxygen radicals, and/or cell-mediated lung mechanisms.[58-60]

Individual drug toxicities may be confined to the pulmonary interstitium, alveoli, pleura, pulmonary circulation, or airways, or, alternatively, may involve multiple intrathoracic structures. The response of the lung to drug-induced injury (DLI) is very limited, resulting in stereotyped histopathologic injury patterns or syndromes. Predominant interstitial and alveolar injury patterns are most common and include various patterns of IP, such as nonspecific interstitial pneumonitis (NSIP), desquamative interstitial pneumonia (DIP), hypersensitivity pneumonitis (HP), organizing pneumonia (OP), and eosinophilic pneumonia (EP). Noncardiogenic pulmonary edema (NCPE), diffuse alveolar damage (DAD), acute respiratory distress syndrome (ARDS), and diffuse alveolar hemorrhage (DAH) are other forms of DLI-related injury patterns. In addition to direct lung injury, chemotherapy-induced immune suppression may predispose patients to life-threatening infections, of which pneumonia is most common. Drug-induced granulomatous disease and lymphadenopathy have also been described. These lung injury patterns have been reported following conventional chemotherapeutic regimens as well as molecular targeted and immune modulator therapies. Patterns of lung injury associated with conventional and molecularly targeted cancer therapies are shown in Tables 1 and 2, respectively.

Estimates of the incidence of DLI caused by individual agents are hampered by the frequent use of complex multidrug and multimodality regimens given either concomitantly or sequentially. Predisposing factors such as older age, cumulative dose, concomitant or sequential radiotherapy, oxygen administration, prior lung injury, and the use of multidrug regimens significantly influence both the occurrence and latency periods between drug exposure and the development of clinical symptoms.

Overlapping clinical, radiographic, and pathologic manifestations of lung injury caused by cardiogenic and NCPE, infections, cancer relapse, or RT confound clinical distinctions between these entities and also render precise estimates of DLI difficult. Other conditions that may mimic DLI include aspiration pneumonitis, cardiogenic pulmonary edema, acute lung injury (ALI), and ARDS.[61,62] Clinical symptoms range from low-grade fever with dry cough and dyspnea to fulminant disease which may rapidly progress to respiratory failure and ARDS. Skin rash, flushing, and bronchospasm, when present, may suggest either an allergic hypersensitivity reaction or a non-IgE-mediated pseudoallergic reaction. These symptoms may occur within minutes to hours of therapy. In a recent study, direct activation of mast cells by cationic drugs was found to be the cause of pseudoallergic reactions.[63] Allergic reactions typically require a sensitization period, with symptom onset during the second or subsequent cycles of therapy. Pseudoallergic reactions, by contrast, may occur within minutes after administration of the first cycle of chemotherapy. Clinical manifestations of other forms of DLI, including IP, typically occur early, within weeks to a few months after initiation of therapy.[59,60] Delayed pulmonary fibrosis, occurring months to years after exposure to bleomycin, busulfan, cyclophosphamide, gemcitabine, and the nitrosoureas as a late manifestation of DLI, has also been described.[64-67]

Systemic markers of inflammation, such as leukocytosis, elevated erythrocyte sedimentation rate, and C-reactive protein, are common but nonspecific findings. Derangements on PET are nonspecific but nonetheless important in assessing the degree of DLI-related pulmonary impairment. Reductions in the DLCO are generally accepted as the most sensitive parameter in the assessment of DLI, although the predictive potential for the detection of early change has been variable.[68-73] With disease progression, a restrictive ventilatory defect may be seen.[65,74] Near-complete normalization of pulmonary function within 2 years of exposure is common following some forms of chemotherapy-induced lung injury.[73] Imaging studies, including high-resolution computed tomography (HRCT) scans, are important tools in the evaluation of patients with suspected DLI, although the findings are nonspecific. Interstitial and mixed alveolar–interstitial abnormalities, manifested as ground-glass opacities that localize to the peripheral and lower lung zones, are the most frequent radiographic findings on CT. Upper lung zone predominant infiltrates are also seen, particularly following drug-induced hypersensitivity reactions. Nodular lesions may mimic underlying malignancy. Reticular lines, septal thickening, and mosaic attenuation are also observed. Pulmonary fibrosis associated with traction bronchiectasis and honeycomb patterns may be seen as the disease progresses. Diffuse uptake of 18F-FDG on PET–CT imaging has been observed in patients with radiographic changes suggestive of pneumonitis

Table 1 Major clinical syndromes and histologic patterns of chemotherapy-induced lung injury.

Agent class	Specific agent	DAD, ARDS, DAH	Hemoptysis (unrelated to DAH)	NCPE	IP	EP	Granuloma formation	Bronchospasm/IR	BOOP	PHTN (PVOD, PAH)	VTE/PE	Pleural disease	Opportunistic infections	MetHgb	Radiation recall pneumonitis
Alkylating agents	Busulfan	✓			✓	✓			✓						
	Cyclophosphamide	✓			✓	✓			✓			✓		✓	
	Ifosfamide	✓												✓	
	Temozolomide	✓		✓					✓						
	Oxaliplatin	✓		✓	✓	✓	✓	✓	✓				✓		✓
	Carboplatin							✓							
	Cisplatin							✓							
	Melphalan	✓			✓	✓	✓		✓			✓			
Antimetabolites	Methotrexate	✓		✓	✓	✓		✓					✓		
	Azathioprine	✓		✓	✓	✓									
	Cytarabine	✓		✓	✓	✓									
	Fludarabine	✓		✓	✓	✓							✓		
	Azacitabine			✓											
	Gemcitabine	✓		✓	✓	✓	✓	✓				✓			✓
	Pentostatin				✓	✓									
	Pemetrexed	✓		✓	✓	✓		✓							
Cytotoxic antibiotics	Zinostatin	✓			✓	✓		✓	✓	✓					
	Bleomycin	✓			✓	✓		✓		✓					
	Mitomycin C	✓		✓	✓			✓		✓					
	Amrubicin									✓					
	Liposomal doxorubicin							✓							
Topoisomerase inhibitors	Irinotecan				✓	✓		✓							
	Topotecan	✓			✓	✓		✓	✓						
Podophyllotoxins	Etoposide	✓			✓	✓		✓							
	Teniposide	✓			✓	✓									
Nitrosoureas	BCNU														
	CCNU														
Taxanes, microtubule inhibitors	Paclitaxel	✓			✓	✓		✓	✓	✓					✓
	Docetaxel	✓			✓	✓		✓				✓			✓
	Vincristine	✓						✓							
	Vinblastine	✓						✓							
	Vindesine	✓						✓							
	Vinorelbine	✓						✓							
	Ixabepilone							✓							
Other	All-trans-retinoic acid	✓			✓	✓					✓	✓			
	Arsenic trioxide	✓			✓	✓						✓			
	Procarbazine				✓	✓	✓		✓			✓			
	L-asparaginase														

DAD, diffuse alveolar damage; ARDS, acute respiratory distress syndrome; DAH, diffuse alveolar hemorrhage; NCPE, noncardiogenic pulmonary edema; IP, interstitial pneumonitis; EP, eosinophilic pneumonia; IR, infusion reaction; BOOP, bronchiolitis obliterans with organizing pneumonia; PHTN, pulmonary hypertension; PVOD, pulmonary venoocclusive disease; PAH, pulmonary arterial hypertension; VTE/PE, venous pulmonary embolism/pulmonary embolism; MetHgb, methemoglobinemia.

Table 2 Major clinical syndromes and histologic patterns of lung injury associated with molecularly targeted agents.

Agent class	Specific agent	DAD, ARDS, DAH	Hemoptysis (unrelated to DAH)	NCPE	IP	EP	Granuloma formation	Bronchospasm (IR/CR)	BOOP	PHTN (PVOD, PAH)	VTE/PE	Pleural disease	Opportunistic infections	MetHgb	Radiation recall pneumonitis
Monoclonal antibodies	Cetuximab	✓			✓			✓							
	Panitumumab	✓			✓				✓			✓			✓
	Bevacizumab		✓					✓	✓		✓				
	Alemtuzumab	✓	✓	✓	✓			✓					✓		
	Rituximab	✓	✓		✓			✓					✓		
	Obinutuzumab							✓							
	Ofatumumab	✓						✓							
	Ibritumomab	✓						✓							
	Trastuzumab	✓						✓							
	Pertuzumab							✓							
	Gemtuzumab			✓				✓							
	Ipilimumab						✓								
Tyrosine kinase inhibitors	Gefitinib	✓			✓				✓						
	Erlotinib	✓			✓				✓						✓
	Imatinib	✓		✓	✓						✓	✓			
	Dasatinib											✓			
	Bosutinib											✓			
	Ponatinib										✓				
	Sorafenib	✓	✓	✓	✓										
	Sunitinib		✓		✓						✓				
	Pazopanib		✓		✓										
	Vandetanib				✓										
	Idelalisib				✓								✓		
	Trametinib						✓				✓				✓
	Crizotinib	✓			✓										
	Vemurafenib				✓								✓		
	Ruxolitinib												✓		
Rapamycin inhibitors	Everolimus	✓		✓	✓	✓									
	Temsirolimus	✓			✓										
Proteasome inhibitors	Bortezomib	✓			✓				✓	✓					
	Carfilzomib				✓					✓					
Immune modulators	Thalidomide										✓				
	Lenalidomide		✓	✓	✓	✓	✓		✓	✓		✓			
	Pomalidmine		✓												
	IL-2		✓	✓											
	TNF		✓												
	IFN-g		✓												

DAD, diffuse alveolar damage; ARDS, acute respiratory distress syndrome; DAH, diffuse alveolar hemorrhage; NCPE, noncardiogenic pulmonary edema; IP, interstitial pneumonitis; EP, eosinophilic pneumonia; IR, infusion reaction; BOOP, bronchiolitis obliterans with organizing pneumonia; PHTN, pulmonary hypertension; PVOD, pulmonary veno-occlusive disease; PAH, pulmonary arterial hypertension; VTE/PE, venous pulmonary embolism/pulmonary embolism; MetHgb, methemoglobinemia.

following bleomycin-, etoposide-, and rituximab-based therapies. Similar findings may also be seen with lymphangitic spread of tumor.[75,76]

Bronchoscopy with performance of bronchoalveolar lavage (BAL) may be helpful in excluding competing diagnoses of infection or background disease. Studies have shown diagnostic yields as high as 70–90% for pulmonary infections and 35–70% for lymphoma and lymphangitic spread of lung cancers.[77,78] BAL fluid in DLI is typically hypercellular with increased numbers of neutrophils or lymphocytes. Decreased CD4/CD8 ratios on BAL fluid are supportive findings; however, ratios vary widely and cannot distinguish sufficiently between drug-induced versus other causes of interstitial lung diseases (ILDs).[79] Drug-induced HP is suggested by BAL lymphocytosis of greater than 50%, with a low CD4 to CD8 ratio. BAL eosinophilia of greater than 25% is supportive of drug-induced EP. The presence of DAH is supported by progressively bloody BAL samples on sequential saline aliquots and/or cytologic evidence of increased numbers of hemosiderin-laden macrophages on BAL fluid. Transbronchial and surgical lung biopsies may be helpful in documenting IP, DAD, EP, and OP and excluding competing diagnoses such as vasculitis, infection, and underlying malignancy. Although pathologic findings attributable to DLI may be seen in 20% of tissue biopsies, histopathologic criteria for DLI have not been established, and no findings are considered pathognomonic. Nonetheless, lung biopsies are useful in excluding competing diagnoses and characterizing the histopathologic pattern of lung injury. This information is not only useful in diagnosing DLI but also in guiding therapeutic options. The diagnosis of DLI is usually based on the temporal association between drug exposure and the development of pulmonary injury; the integration of compatible clinical, radiographic, and laboratory findings; and the exclusion of competing diagnoses.

Treatment of chemotherapy-related DLI remains anecdotal and empiric, rather than evidence based. Withdrawal of the suspected offending agent is the mainstay of treatment in the majority of cases. Spontaneous improvement may be seen in most patients following drug withdrawal, although disease progression may occur even after withdrawal of the offending agent. General recommendations suggest discontinuation of the culprit drug once sufficient clinical suspicion to support its association with pneumotoxicity has been established. One clear exception to this recommendation has been in the setting of the differentiation syndrome following all-trans-retinoic acid (ATRA) or arsenic trioxide therapies for treatment of acute promyelocytic leukemia.[80] Systemic steroid therapy along with de-escalation of drug dose rather than drug withdrawal has been associated with successful resolution of toxicity in patients with mild to moderate forms of this syndrome.

Systemic glucocorticoids and supportive care (including inhaled bronchodilators, supplemental oxygen, and mechanical ventilation) should be initiated if clinically indicated. Corticosteroids have been shown to abrogate symptoms of DLI in certain steroid-responsive lung injury patterns, such as HP, EP, and bronchiolitis obliterans with organizing pneumonia (BOOP). In other entities, including pulmonary fibrosis, pulmonary vascular disease, and bronchiolitis obliterans (BO), corticosteroids have no beneficial role. Current expert opinion advocates close surveillance with high-resolution CT scans and continued therapy without dose interruption for asymptomatic ILD. For symptomatic patients, the grade of pneumotoxicity should be used to guide management decisions, which may include dose modification or interruption, with or without the institution of corticosteroid therapy.[81] For patients with moderate (grade 2 or greater) IP, drug interruption and initiation of

corticosteroid therapy, dosed at 0.75–1 mg/kg/day of prednisone or its equivalent, are recommended. Steroids are typically maintained at the higher dose until symptom improvement is established and then tapered over a 1–3-month time period, pending the response to therapy. Bronchoscopy with alveolar lavage is recommended to rule out competing diagnoses of infection and/or alveolar hemorrhage.[82] Drug rechallenge is generally not recommended, except in specific settings, such as ATRA and arsenic-related differentiation syndrome.[80,83] The decision to reintroduce the offending targeted agent following the development of IP must be must on a case-by-case basis and should be based upon the individual agent, the severity of the reaction, and the availability of alternative therapies.

Lung injury associated with molecular targeted and immunotherapies

The identification of aberrant proteins which are either overexpressed or dysregulated in cancer cells has resulted in a rapidly growing class of molecularly targeted antineoplastic agents. Because of their narrow spectrum of inhibition, these agents were thought initially to cause minimal end-organ toxicity, unlike conventional chemotherapeutic agents. Although the spectrum of toxicities due to targeted therapies (dermatologic, vascular, coagulation, ocular, pulmonary) may be dissimilar to that seen with conventional cytotoxic agents (alopecia, mucositis, severe myelosuppression, nausea, vomiting, pulmonary), the frequency and intensity of toxicities are similar between the two major classes of antineoplastic therapies. ILD, infusion reactions (IRs), vasculopathies, and pleural effusions are common sequelae of targeted therapies. Lung injury associated with targeted therapies may arise from on-target (inhibition of the intended targets) or off-target (inhibition of unintended targets) mechanisms. Overlapping toxicities may also occur, due to cross-interaction of multiple signaling pathways.

Radiographic detection of ILD may be seen as early as 2 months following therapy, with clinical pneumonitis typically occurring within the first 6 months of targeted therapy. Symptoms of dry cough, dyspnea, and fever are most common. Fulminant respiratory failure is rare but has been described following rituximab therapy and also as a complication of mammalian target of rapamycin (mTOR) and EGFR inhibitors (Figure 8).

Drug-induced lung syndromes

Interstitial lung disease (ILD)
NSIP represents the most frequent morphologic pattern of ILD caused by DLI. Injury is signaled by the insidious development of a nonproductive cough and dyspnea, which typically occurs within weeks to months following drug exposure. Symptom development may precede radiographic findings by days to weeks. Common radiographic changes include interstitial and mixed alveolar–interstitial abnormalities that localize to the peripheral and lower lung zones. Nodular lesions, reticular lines, septal thickening, mosaic patterns, and ground-glass attenuations are also observed. Risk factors for drug-induced ILD varies with the individual agents but in general include advanced age, concurrent radiation or multiagent therapy, preexisting lung disease, and the need for high-inspired supplemental oxygen. Early on, damage to epithelial and endothelial cells leads to alveolar edema and DAD, which may progress in some cases to end-stage fibrotic lung disease and respiratory failure despite drug withdrawal and corticosteroid therapy.

Bleomycin-induced pneumonitis (BIP) is seen in up to 20% of bleomycin-treated patients, with higher rates associated with total

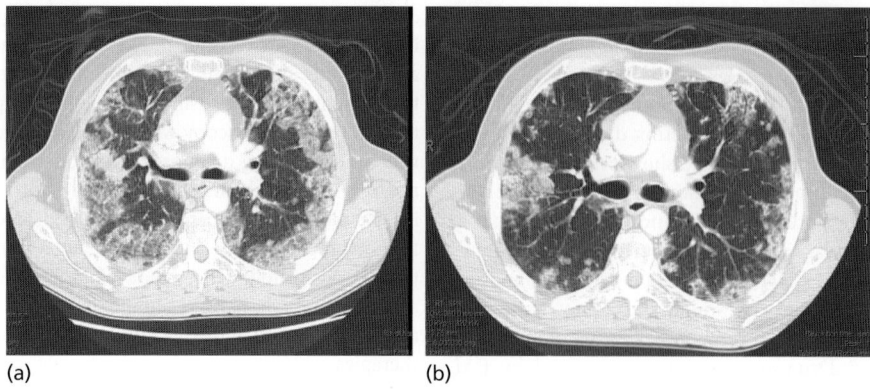

Figure 8 60-year old man presents with a maculopapular rash and progressive dry cough with shortness of breath that developed 12 weeks after starting erlotinib for advanced pancreatic cancer. The extensive, ground glass, and nodular pleural-based infiltrates (a) significantly improved within 2 weeks of discontinuation erlotinib and initiation of systemic steroid therapy (b).

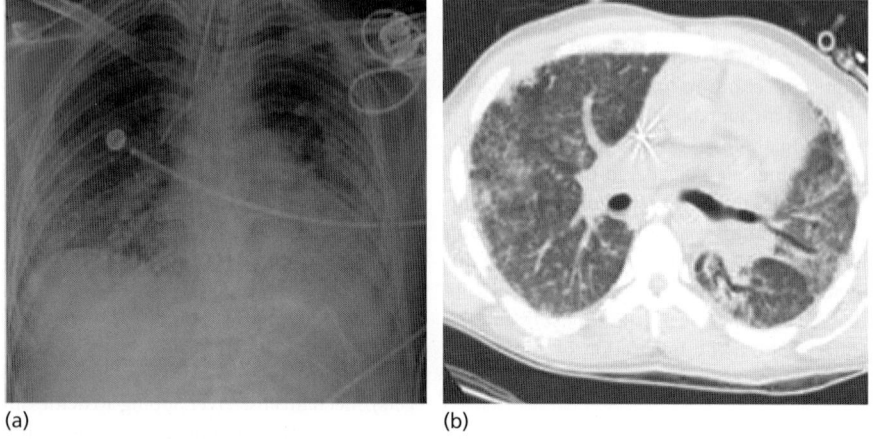

Figure 9 24-year old woman who developed respiratory distress following abdominal surgery for an unrelated illness 3 months after completing bleomycin-based treatment for Hodgkin's lymphoma. CXR (a) and CT scan (b) showed bilateral patchy reticulonodular and airspace disease. Work-up was consistent with ARDS associated with bleomycin toxicity, presumably triggered by hyperoxia during surgery.

cumulative doses above 400 U. In addition, age greater than 70 years, uremia, bolus administration, multiagent therapy, multimodality therapy with concomitant or sequential radiation, and high-inspired oxygen administration have been associated with an increased incidence and severity of BIP.[58,84,85] Evidence to suggest that high-inspired fractions of oxygen may provoke or exacerbate pulmonary toxicity in bleomycin-exposed patients is largely anecdotal. A threshold fraction of inspired oxygen or duration of oxygen therapy that increases the risk of lung injury has not been definitively established. In addition, the time interval following bleomycin treatment after which the risk of hyperoxia-associated bleomycin toxicity is mitigated is unknown. Nonetheless, careful titration of supplemental oxygen to achieve an oxygen saturation at or above 89–92% is recommended. Symptoms of dry cough and exertional dyspnea typically evolve over 1–6 months after bleomycin exposure but have been described during therapy as well as a late manifestation (>6 months) of bleomycin toxicity (Figure 9). Bleomycin causes a predictable decline in DLCO, which was thought initially to be an early marker of lung injury and an indication for drug withdrawal. However, threshold cutoffs for drug withdrawal based on a declining DLCO have not been established. Furthermore, only a small percentage of bleomycin-exposed patients with changes in DLCO will develop clinical toxicity.[86] In our practice, monitoring DLCO with serial PFTs is reserved for patients with known lung disease and/or compromised lung function at baseline. Serial monitoring of DLCO is performed as cumulative doses of bleomycin approach 400 U or if clinical symptoms suggestive of bleomycin toxicity develop. The optimal dosing of corticosteroid therapy is not well defined. Starting doses of prednisone or its equivalent at 0.75–1 mg/kg (based on ideal body weight) per day to a maximum of 100 mg/day for the first 4–6 weeks is reasonable. Tapering of prednisone is usually accomplished over a few months, in accordance with the patient's condition and clinical response. Resolution of BIP typically occurs over time, with most patients showing improvements in pulmonary function and radiology at 15 months or greater. Delays in diagnosis, continuation of bleomycin, or the development of fibrosis portends a worse prognosis. Mortality rates are low (1–3%) but increase to 10% among patients with cumulative doses above 550 U.

The nitrosoureas bis-chloroethylnitrosourea (BCNU) also cause a dose-dependent IP, with rates as high as 50% among patients whose cumulative dose exceeds 1500 mg/m². Unlike other forms of drug-induced IP, BCNU-induced lung injury exhibits a predilection for the middle and upper lobes. Upper lobe-predominant fibrosis and pneumothorax may occur years after completion of BCNU therapy. Late-onset pneumonitis has been reported also following cyclophosphamide and busulfan administration. Acute and subacute IP developing within hours or weeks following the taxane drugs, paclitaxel and docetaxel, has been well documented.[87] Although the pneumonitis is typically mild, severe reactions, progressing to pulmonary fibrosis and death, have been reported with both drugs. The incidence and severity of taxane-related IP is influenced by dose and dosing schedule. The presence of prior fibrosing lung disease and the concomitant use of other agents that potentiate lung toxicity (such as gemcitabine) and concurrent RT increase the incidence of this disease.

IP has been reported following treatment with many classes of targeted agents, including mTOR inhibitors (everolimus, temsirolimus), EGFR inhibitors (gefitinib, erlotinib, cetuximab, panitumumab), multikinase angiogenesis inhibitors (sorafenib, sunitinib), the HER2 inhibitor (trastuzumab), multikinase Bcr-Abl inhibitors (imatinib, dasatinib, nilotinib, bosutinib), proteasome inhibitors (bortezomib, carfilzomib), the ALK inhibitor (crizotinib), c-Met inhibitor (tivantinib), and immunomodulatory agents (thalidomide, lenalidomide, pomalidomide). ILD is most common following mTOR therapy, occurring in up to 39% of mTOR-treated patients with solid tumors.[81,88–90] Most patients are asymptomatic: however, fulminant respiratory failure has been described. Recent studies suggest that the appearance of mTOR-induced ILD in patients with renal cancer may correlate with antitumor activity.[81] This observation, if confirmed, should help to guide treatment strategies for asymptomatic patients with radiographic evidence of mTOR-related IP. Successful rechallenge following dasatinib, everolimus, and temsirolimus-related IP has been reported.[81,91]

Hypersensitivity pneumonitis (HP)

HP-like reactions are typically characterized by fever, dyspnea, dry cough, headache, fatigue, rash, and BAL lymphocytosis following repeated exposure to the offending agent. IP may evolve over the first 3–4 weeks after drug exposure and wax and wane without adjustments in therapy. Poorly formed granulomas with mononuclear cell infiltration are common histologic findings in subacute and chronic HP. Hilar adenopathy and pleural effusions occur in up to 10% of patients. Histologic evidence of ill-defined granulomas, together with a skin rash and radiographic findings of hilar adenopathy or pleural effusions, may help to distinguish methotrexate-induced lung injury. Radiographic changes include homogeneous opacities with upper lobe predominance, particularly in chronic forms of the disease. Among the drugs that have been implicated in the development of HP, methotrexate has been the most studied. Lung injury has been reported following oral, intravenous, intrathecal, and intramuscular routes of methotrexate administration. Overall, the prognosis for patients with chemotherapy-induced HP is very favorable. Complete resolution of clinical symptoms and radiographic findings is typical following steroid therapy in early-stage disease.

Alveolar processes

Noncardiogenic pulmonary edema (NCPE), diffuse alveolar damage (DAD), and adult respiratory distress syndrome (ARDS)

NCPE occurs as a result of injury to the alveolocapillary membrane, resulting in capillary leak and a noncardiogenic (permeability) pulmonary edema. With disease progression, severe physiological impairment consistent with ARDS and its histologic hallmark, DAD, may ensue. Drug-induced NCPE often occurs as an idiosyncratic reaction, unrelated to drug dosage or duration of therapy. Patients typically present with acute dyspnea, hypoxia, and alveolar infiltrates in the absence of heart failure. Reactions are typically mild and self-limited, although progression to ARDS with fatal outcomes occasionally occurs. Drug withdrawal, supplemental oxygen, and the judicious use of diuretics usually effect a rapid recovery. With the exception of ATRA- and arsenic-induced NCPE (see section titled "Lung Injury Associated with Conventional Chemotherapy"), drug rechallenge with the offending drug often results in recrudescence of symptoms and is not recommended. Aggravating factors that potentiate disease progression to ARDS include multiagent protocols and the concomitant or sequential use of radiation or oxygen therapy, particularly following therapy with bleomycin or busulfan.[92,93] Once established, the response of ARDS to drug withdrawal and corticosteroid therapy is variable. Progressive respiratory impairment, leading to respiratory failure and death, has been reported with some agents (busulfan, cyclophosphamide, bleomycin) despite drug withdrawal. Among molecular targeted therapies, ARDS has been best described following agents that inhibit the EGFR (gefitinib, erlotinib, cetuximab), the antilymphocyte monoclonal antibodies (mAbs) (rituximab, alemtuzumab, ofatumumab), and the rapamycin inhibitors (everolimus, temsirolimus). Acute withdrawal of the JAK2 inhibitor, ruxolitinib, has been associated with the development of ARDS as a result of a cytokine rebound reaction. Preemptive use of corticosteroids, along with supportive therapy and a slow taper off this agent, is recommended to mitigate this potential problem.[94,95]

Diffuse alveolar hemorrhage (DAH) and other bleeding disorders

Drug-induced DAH most often occurs as a result of injury to the alveolocapillary membrane but may occasionally be seen as a consequence of bland alveolar hemorrhage without distortion of the lung architecture. DAH in the absence of DAD is a rare complication of rituximab[96] and alemtuzumab.[97] Tumor cavitation with sometimes fatal bleeding complications has been described during treatment of central airway tumors with bevacizumab therapy.[96]

Eosinophilic pneumonia (EP)

EP is characterized by fever, dyspnea, hypoxia, and homogeneous ground-glass opacities that have a predilection for the periphery and upper lobes. Alveolar and peripheral blood eosinophils are common features. A leukocyte composition of >20% eosinophils of the total leukocytes recovered by BAL is consistent with EP. The "reverse pulmonary edema pattern" is a classic radiographic feature but is seen in only 33% of patients. A growing list of agents has been implicated in the development of EP, including bleomycin, busulfan, methotrexate, procarbazine, fludarabine, and, more recently, oxaliplatin- and taxane-based therapies. Drug withdrawal and initiation of high-dose steroids are associated with favorable outcomes.[61,98–101]

Pleural disease

Pleural effusions and fibrosis

Drug-induced pleural disease is typically a manifestation of a generalized pleuroparenchymal abnormality but may occur as an isolated event.[102] Isolated pleural effusions are seen occasionally following administration of methotrexate, dasatinib, bosutinib, docetaxel, ATRA, and granulocyte-colony stimulating factor (GCSF).[103,104] An exudative, lymphocyte-predominant effusion is typical, which may be unilateral or bilateral and small to moderate in size. Optimal therapy for drug-induced pleural effusions is not well defined, but thoracentesis, diuresis, and steroid therapies have been employed with varying rates of success. Spontaneous resolution of the pleural effusion may occur following drug withdrawal in some cases. Pleural thickening may accompany pulmonary fibrosis as a late manifestation of cyclophosphamide, BCNU, or bleomycin toxicity.

Pulmonary vascular disorders (PVD)

Thromboembolic disease, pulmonary hypertension, and pulmonary veno-occlusive disease

The adverse effects of chemotherapeutic agents on the pulmonary vasculature may result in thrombosis, pulmonary hypertension (PH), or pulmonary veno-occlusive disease (PVOD). The diagnosis of pulmonary vascular disease is suggested by an isolated reduction in DLCO or a DLCO that is disproportionately decreased relative to other lung function parameters on PFT. The prothrombotic effects of tamoxifen appear to be related to drug-related decrements in protein C and antithrombin III levels.[105] Combined therapy with tamoxifen and other chemotherapeutic agents, such as cyclophosphamide, methotrexate, and 5-fluorouracil, confers a threefold increased risk of thromboembolic phenomenon.[106,107] Thromboembolic events, with rates ranging from 14% to 43%, have been reported among recipients of thalidomide-based chemotherapy, given in combination with steroids, doxorubicin, or BCNU.[108–111] The VEGF inhibitors, bevacizumab, sunitinib, and sorafenib, are also associated with thromboembolic events (Figure 10).[2,96,112,113] Pulmonary arterial hypertension (PAH) is a rare complication of antineoplastic agents, suggesting possible individual susceptibility. Severe PAH has been reported following treatment with the Bcr-Abl TKI dasatinib, which, in most cases, is only partially reversible after drug withdrawal.[114–117] An off-target mechanism of drug-induced PAH following use of this multikinase inhibitor has been postulated. There have been no reports of PAH following exposure to the more selective Bcr-Abl TKIs. In fact, the safe use of selective Bcr-Abl TKIs, such as nilotinib and imatinib following dasatinib-associated

PAH, is well described.[115,118] Once dasatinib-associated PAH is suspected, the drug should be withdrawn, and rechallenge is not recommended.[119] PH following interferon therapy has been attributed to potential interferon-induced endothelial dysfunction.[120,121] Zinostatin, an antitumor antibiotic, causes hypertrophy of the pulmonary vascular wall leading to PH, possibly as a result of direct toxicity to the pulmonary endothelium.[122] Chemotherapy-related PH may also present as PVOD, a process characterized by fibrous obliteration of pulmonary venules and small pulmonary veins (see section titled "Pulmonary Hypertension in the Cancer Patient"). Although several drugs have been implicated in the development of PVOD, bleomycin and BCNU have been associated with the most incriminating data.[123,124]

Drug-induced airway disease

Bronchospasm

Bronchospasm with associated dyspnea, wheezing, and hypoxia is a common and sometimes life-threatening manifestation of chemotherapy-related acute IRs. Virtually all chemotherapeutic agents may trigger an IR, defined as an adverse reaction that is temporally related to drug infusion with signs and symptoms inconsistent with the known toxicity profile of the drug. Until recently, all adverse events associated with drug infusions were referred to as "hypersensitivity reactions." However, an allergic component is absent in many of these reactions, and, thus, "IR" is the preferred term. Acute IRs typically occur within the first few minutes to hours of drug exposure, although late reactions, occurring 10–12 h following drug administration, have also been reported. Events typically occur as an IgE-mediated hypersensitivity response to foreign proteins (type 1 hypersensitivity reaction) or as a non-IgE-mediated pseudoallergic response. The latter is caused by certain cationic drugs which may trigger the activation of mast cells and subsequent cytokine release (anaphylactoid reaction).[63] Following exposure to some agents, such as carboplatin, oxaliplatin, and L-asparaginase, IgE antibodies are produced and bind mast cells and basophils. Subsequent reexposure to the drug may reduce an explosive release of vasoactive mediators (histamines, leukotrienes, and prostaglandins) from basophil and mast cells, triggering a type 1 hypersensitivity reaction and anaphylaxis. Type 1 reactions typically occur within minutes of infusion. Associated respiratory symptoms include cough, dyspnea, wheezing, and chest tightness. Stridor due to oropharyngeal and laryngeal edema may also occur. As the disease progresses, bilateral pulmonary infiltrates associated with permeability pulmonary edema may develop, which may progress to ARDS. Occasionally, these reactions may be sufficiently severe to lead to respiratory failure, shock, and death.[125]

IRs associated with taxane administration (paclitaxel, docetaxel) are clinically similar to IgE-mediated type 1 reactions; however, the proposed mechanisms underlying taxane IRs may be different. Paclitaxel is formulated in a highly allergenic polyoxyethylated castor oil solvent, Cremophor EL, which may trigger mast cell/basophil activation and subsequent hypersensitivity reaction. Polysorbate 80, which is the vehicle used in formulating docetaxel, may induce IRs via similar mechanisms.[126] IRs due to taxane administration have been attributed to the taxane component as well as the vehicle used to solubilize these agents. Nonetheless, other antineoplastic agents that are formulated in Cremophor EL (cyclosporine, teniposide, ixabepilone) or polysorbate 80 (etoposide) should be avoided in patients with a history of IRs following taxane administration.[127] Typically, taxane-associated IRs occur early during the first or second infusion. Standard prophylaxis with histamine receptor antagonists and steroids has reduced the incidence of

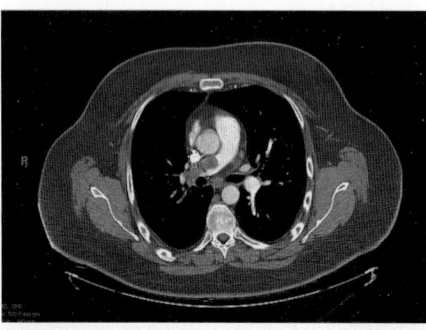

(a)

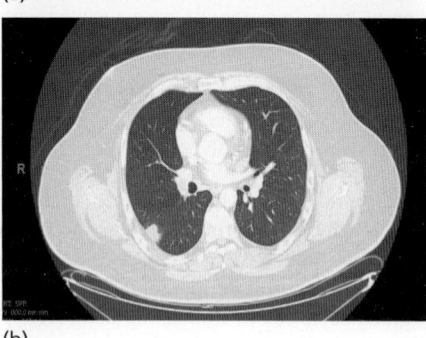

(b)

Figure 10 CT angiogram showing large central embolus in a patient treated with bevacizumab-based chemotherapy for cholangiocarcinoma (a). Associated pulmonary infarct is suggested by the wedge-shaped subpleural density overlying the lateral segment of the right middle lobe (b).

paclitaxel-induced bronchospasm from 30% to 2%.[128] Recent studies have shown the presence of BRCA1/2 mutations to be an independent risk factor for the development of IRs among women treated with carboplatin-based chemotherapies for breast or ovarian cancer. IRs in this setting tend to occur at lower cumulative dose exposure.[129]

The infusion of most mAbs may provoke a cytokine release syndrome, an immune response characterized by dyspnea, wheezing, and "flu-like symptoms" which typically occurs within the first few hours of administration.[130] Symptoms are typically mild, with fatal reactions occurring in a minority of patients. The percentage of mouse protein is thought to correlate with the immunogenic response, including IRs. Thus, the earliest mAbs were murine derived and highly immunogenic in humans. One strategy to decrease the immunogenicity of mABs has been the development of chimeric mouse–human (cetuximab, rituximab, brentuximab), partially humanized (bevacizumab, trastuzumab, alemtuzumab, gemtuzumab, obinutuzumab), and fully humanized (ipilimumab, ofatumumab, panitumumab, ramucirumab) antibodies. Reduced immunogenicity based on murine content of the mAB was suggested in a recent study in which the severity of IRs following panitumumab therapy (0.5%) was fourfold less than that following cetuximab therapy (2%).[131] Risk factors for mAB-induced IRs include a prior history of allergic reaction to the drug, the route and rate of administration, drug form, and multiagent therapy. Test dosing prior to infusion does not reliably predict subsequent IRs. Mild IR events following mAb therapy may be managed with supportive care (supplemental oxygen, antihistamines, steroids, and nebulized β-agonists) either with or without cessation of therapy. Premedication with antihistamines, corticosteroids, and antipyretics is generally recommended for the chimeric mouse–human mAbs, such as rituximab and cetuximab. Among several of the humanized mAbs (alemtuzumab, trastuzumab) and fully human mAbs (ramucirumab, ofatumumab), the risk of IRs is also sufficiently high to warrant premedication therapy. Typically, decisions regarding the need for prophylaxis and safety of drug rechallenge are based on the severity of the hypersensitivity reaction and are made on a case-by-case basis.[132] Breakthrough IRs may occur despite prophylaxis. Thus, close monitoring during and immediately following drug infusion is recommended.

One other class of agents that has been associated with bronchospasm includes the vinca alkaloids. Although vinorelbine and other vinca alkaloids are rarely associated with lung toxicity, acute reactions characterized by cough, bronchospasm, flushing, dyspnea, abdominal pain, and hypotension have been described when these agents are given either concurrently or sequentially with mitomycin chemotherapy.[133,134]

Other clinicopathologic syndromes

Granulomatous disease
The development of noncaseating granulomas is a rare manifestation of drug-induced lung injury that has been described most often following methotrexate and interferon therapy.[135,136] Methotrexate- and interferon-induced granulomatous lymphadenopathy is indistinguishable from sarcoidosis. In addition to methotrexate and interferon, procarbazine, ipilimumab, and sirolimus may also incite a granulomatous pneumonitis. Drug withdrawal may result in disease regression.

Pulmonary complications of thoracic radiation: Radiation pneumonitis and fibrosis

One of the many challenges of RT is the precise delivery of the radiation dose to target organs while sparing critical surrounding normal tissues. In thoracic neoplasms, where anatomical changes during treatment and tumor motion associated with respiratory variation are common, clinically significant lung injury following conventional thoracic radiation occurs in 5–20% of patients. Radiation-induced lung injury (RILI) is, in fact, the most common dose-limiting complication following thoracic radiation and chemoradiation regimens. Recent advances in radiation techniques, imaging, and delivery systems, such as proton therapy, 3D conformal radiation therapy (CRT), intensity-modulated radiation therapy (IMRT), and stereotactic body radiation therapy (SBRT), have the potential to achieve higher target doses of radiation while mitigating radiation exposure to adjacent normal tissues. Radiation damage does occur with the newer radiation strategies, however, and the associated radiographic patterns and severity of RILD may differ from lung injury caused by conventional radiotherapy. Factors such as total radiation dose, dose per fraction, the volume of irradiated lung, and beam characteristics and arrangements all influence the development of radiation pneumonitis (RP). Preexisting lung disease, underlying poor pulmonary reserve, prior radiotherapy, and rapid steroid withdrawal also influence the clinical appearance and severity of lung injury.[137] Multimodality regimens that combine radiation with chemotherapeutic agents such as mitomycin, cyclophosphamide, vincristine, adriamycin, bleomycin, gemcitabine, the taxanes, and actinomycin D may not only potentiate radiation pneumotoxicity but also shorten the latency period following radiation exposure.[138] Although data regarding optimal dose–fractionation and dose–volume relationships that mitigate lung injury are still evolving, it is generally agreed that a hyperfractionated course of radiation delivered to the smallest lung volume offers the lowest possibility of lung toxicity. Radiographically apparent lung damage is common with total doses of radiation that exceed 40 Gy. At doses >70 Gy, unusual pulmonary complications, including bronchial stenosis, bronchomalacia, mediastinal fibrosis, and injury to the recurrent laryngeal nerve, have been reported. Lung injury at radiation doses below 20 Gy is rare.[139]

RP and radiation fibrosis (RF) represent acute and late phases of RILI, respectively, and are the most frequent forms of radiation toxicity. Acute pneumonitis is heralded by fever, dyspnea, and nonproductive cough which may develop insidiously 1–3 months after completion of RT and may precede the radiographic changes of RP. Radiographic changes may be seen as early as 3–4 weeks following RT, characterized by discrete ground-glass opacities, ill-defined patchy nodules, or consolidation with air bronchograms and volume loss within the irradiated field. In mild cases of acute RP, these changes may resolve within 6 months, leaving a linear scar. Regional scarring is seen in nearly all patients, including those without clinical symptoms. Measurable changes in PETs, including a reduction in lung volumes and diffusing capacity, may be seen as early as 2–3 months after irradiation. Histopathologic features of early RP include interstitial edema, hemorrhage, and fibrinous exudates with reactive type II pneumocytes. With more severe injury, RF develops. RF is signaled by the appearance of a well-demarcated area of volume loss, linear densities, bronchiectasis, retraction of the lung parenchyma, tenting and elevation of the hemidiaphragm, and ipsilateral pleural thickening. Like RP following conventional RT, these changes usually occur within the irradiated field. RF usually evolves over 6–12 month posttreatment and stabilizes within 1–2 years following completion of RT. RP detection methods using 18[F]-2-fluoro-2-deoxyglucose positron emission tomography (FDG-PET) imaging permits quantitative assessment of RP, which manifests as enhanced FDG uptake. Higher standard uptake values (SUV) derived from PET–CT imaging have been associated with increased risks of symptomatic RP.[140,141] The utility of this imaging modality in identifying individuals at high risk for developing symptomatic RP is currently being investigated.

A less predictable or sporadic form of RP has also been recognized.[116] Sporadic pneumonitis occurs in a minority (5%) of patients and is thought to represent a type of HP characterized by a bilateral CD4+ T-lymphocytic alveolitis that diffusely involves both lungs. Hence, radiation changes on imaging studies may extend well beyond the irradiated field. Patients present at 1–3 months following thoracic irradiation with symptoms of dyspnea and dry cough that are disproportionate to the volume of lung irradiated. This form of pneumonitis and its associated symptoms typically abate in 6–8 weeks without significant long-term sequelae.[116,142,143]

Radiation recall pneumonitis describes a rare but well-recognized inflammatory reaction that occurs within a previously irradiated area of pulmonary tissue after application of certain chemotherapeutic agents. Recall pneumonitis has been observed most often following taxane- and anthracycline-based therapies. Gemcitabine, etoposide, vinorelbine, trastuzumab, and erlotinib have also been implicated as triggers for this disease (Tables 1 and 2).[144,145] Patients typically present with dry cough, low-grade fever, and dyspnea during the initiation of the precipitating agent or following several courses of therapy. Lung injury in recall pneumonitis typically occurs shortly after administration of the inciting antineoplastic agent, which may be weeks to years following completion of radiotherapy. Radiographically, ground-glass opacities and areas of consolidation that conform to the radiation treatment portal are seen. Drug withdrawal and initiation of corticosteroids and supportive care usually result in a favorable outcome. Rechallenge with the offending agent has been successful in some cases.[146]

Radiation-related pleural effusions may occur as an early complication (within 6 months) of radiation pleuritis or as late sequelae (1–5 years) of mediastinal irradiation with associated mediastinal fibrosis, systemic PH, or lymphatic obstruction. These effusions are typically small, ipsilateral, and asymptomatic. Occasionally, patients may complain of shortness of breath or pleuritic chest pain. Pleural fluid cytology is negative. Reactive mesothelial cells within the pleural fluid are common. PVOD has also been reported as a rare complication of radiation-induced lung toxicity. Radiation-induced OP and EP involving nonirradiated areas in patients with breast cancer have also been documented.[147,148] Radiation-induced OP is thought to represent an immunologically mediated, lymphocyte-predominant hypersensitivity-like reaction. Both EP and OP may produce migratory pulmonary opacities on chest radiographs, which typically develop 1–3 months following radiotherapy. The presence of blood or tissue eosinophils, coupled with a prior history of asthma or atopy, favors the diagnosis of EP. Corticosteroid therapy is associated with prompt recovery of radiation-induced OP and EP, although relapsed disease may rarely occur after steroid withdrawal. Another intrathoracic complication of RT includes pulmonary congestion, which may occur as a sequela of radiation-induced myocardial and/or valvular dysfunction.

Factors such as the location, type, and extension of the primary tumor as well as the corresponding beam configuration and portals directly influence the shape and distribution of radiation-induced lung damage. RILD associated with the newer modes of RT delivery and imaging, such as 3D-CRT and IMRT, may not result in the stereotyped straight-edged infiltrate but rather, assume a mass-like or whorled appearance or, alternatively, appear as poorly marginated and irregular nodules. Thus, lung injury following newer radiation techniques may be remarkably difficult to distinguish from competing disease entities such as infection or recurrence of the underlying malignancy.[149] Postradiation volume loss, bronchiectasis, and consolidation may occur with these modes of RT delivery but typically are less extensive than injury patterns following conventional radiation.[150] Proton radiotherapy improves delivery of radiation dose to the tumor with less dispersion before reaching the tumor target. This observation may permit safe escalation of radiation dose to tumoricidal levels while sparing critical normal lung tissues.[151,152] In one small study, patients that received proton therapy for medically inoperable NSCLC tolerated higher doses of radiation with reduced rates of pneumonitis versus those who underwent conventional radiotherapy.[151] Further studies are needed to investigate these radiation modalities and their true impact reducing the risk of RP.

Infection, drug toxicity, and recurrent tumor are major mimickers of RILI. Correlation with radiation treatment plans, knowledge of expected patterns of RILI, and temporal correlation with RT are important in the diagnosis of radiation damage. Lung opacities that develop prior to the completion of radiation should suggest an alternative diagnosis. Cavitation within the fibrotic area of irradiated lung may be due to a superimposed infectious process such as tuberculosis or Aspergillus species, recurrent tumor, or postradiation necrosis. The loss of bronchiectasis due to filling of the airways with tumor or infection is also an important radiographic indication of superimposed disease.

RILI represents a continuum of changes initiated by an inflammatory pneumonitis, which progresses to fibrosis, although whether pneumonitis and fibrosis represent a continuum or separate entities has not definitively resolved. Unfortunately, definitive pharmaceutical strategies in the successful prevention and treatment of RILI remain elusive. RP may respond to steroid therapy. Although evidence-based recommendations regarding dosing schedules and strategies are not available, in general, 40–60 mg of daily prednisone over several weeks, followed by a several-week taper provides relief of symptoms in most patients. There is no conclusive evidence that successful treatment of acute pneumonitis mitigates the later development of RF. Once established, steroids have not been shown to be of benefit in the treatment of this late sequela of RT.

Pulmonary complications of hematopoietic stem cell transplantation

Hematopoietic stem cell transplantation (HSCT) is the only curative option for many patients with relapsed and high-risk hematologic malignancies. Despite advances in treatment regimens and supportive care, pulmonary complications occur in up to 60% of HSCT recipients, accounting for significant morbidity and mortality.[153–155] Pulmonary complications of HSCT are divided into "early" (those that occur during the first 100 days posttransplant) and "late" (those that occur > than 100 days posttransplant) (Table 3). These complications are due primarily to direct toxicities from conditioning regimens, delayed bone marrow recovery, prolonged immunosuppressive therapy, and graft versus host disease (GVHD). Infectious complications occur most commonly after allogeneic HSCT due to the high incidence of GVHD and prolonged use of immunosuppressive therapy. As successful prophylactic treatment strategies have effectively reduced the rates of infectious pulmonary complications, noninfectious pulmonary complications have emerged as a major cause of post-HSCT morbidity and mortality.

Table 3 Noninfectious pulmonary complications following hematopoietic stem cell transplantation.

Early (<100 days)	Late (>100 days)
• Pulmonary edema • Idiopathic pneumonia syndrome • Diffuse alveolar hemorrhage • Periengraftment respiratory distress syndrome • Secondary pulmonary alveolar proteinosis (rare) • Pulmonary venoocclusive disease (rare)	• Bronchiolitis obliterans • Cryptogenic organizing pneumonia • Posttransplant lymphoproliferative disorders • Lymphocytic interstitial pneumonitis (rare)

Early-onset noninfectious complications of HSCT

Pulmonary edema and pleural effusions
Diffuse pulmonary edema is one of the most common early complications after transplantation. Etiologies include increased hydrostatic capillary pressure associated with the administration of large volumes of fluid and cardiac dysfunction. Increased pulmonary capillary permeability and NCPE owing to the preconditioning regimen also occur.[155,156] Hydrostatic and permeability etiologies of posttransplant pulmonary edema may be present simultaneously and overlap with other early-onset pulmonary complications. The abrupt onset of dyspnea, hypoxia, and bilateral pulmonary infiltrates coupled with the absence of infection on diagnostic evaluation are supportive findings. Pleural effusions may accompany pulmonary edema. Bilateral pleural effusions associated with weight gain may be approached conservatively without the need for diagnostic thoracentesis.

Periengraftment respiratory distress syndrome (PERDS)
Periengraftment respiratory distress syndrome (PERDS) is characterized by fever, NCPE, erythematous skin rash, and hypoxemia and occurs during the neutrophil recovery phase of HSCT. The NIH-sponsored Blood and Marrow Transplant Clinical Trials Network includes PERDS within the definition of idiopathic pneumonia syndrome (IPS); however, there may be value to considering it separately because of its favorable prognosis and lower mortality.[156] The reported incidence varies widely with disease definition and the population studied but generally occurs in 5–10% of autologous HSCT recipients when stringent diagnostic criteria are used.[157,158] While the pathophysiology is not well understood, proposed mechanisms include the release of proinflammatory cytokines during the engraftment period and endothelial damage from the conditioning regimen. Risk factors include the use of growth factors, the number of infused mononuclear or CD34 positive cells, the speed of neutrophil recovery, type of conditioning regimen, underlying disease, and peripheral blood as the source of stem cells. Some studies have shown improvement with corticosteroid therapy.[158,159]

Idiopathic pneumonia syndrome (IPS)
In 1993, a panel convened by the NIH proposed a broad working definition of IPS as widespread nonlobar radiographic infiltrates in the absence of congestive heart failure or evidence of lower respiratory tract infection.[160] IPS occurs in 10% of HSCT recipients, usually 14–90 days following transplantation. Mortality rates range from 50% to 70%.[161–163] Risk factors include transplantation for malignancy other than leukemia, older age, total body irradiation, type of pretransplant chemotherapy, high-grade GVHD, CMV

(cytomegalovirus)-seropositive donor, HLA (human leukocyte antigen) disparity, and lower performance status.[162] Possible etiologies of IPS include direct toxic effects of the chemoradiation conditioning regimen, occult infection, and release of inflammatory cytokines. However, the association of IPS with the presence of acute GVHD after allogeneic transplantation suggests that alloreactive T-cell injury may also be an important contributor.[162,163] The clinical presentation is nonspecific, with symptoms of acute dyspnea, cough, and fever associated with diffuse infiltrates on chest radiograph. The diagnosis of IPS relies largely on the exclusion of infection and absence of cardiac, renal, or iatrogenic fluid overload. Treatment includes high-dose intravenous corticosteroids and supportive care with supplemental oxygen and broad-spectrum antibiotics. Earlier preclinical and clinical data suggested a potential role for tumor necrosis factor-α (TNF-α) in the pathogenesis of IPS. However, a recent randomized trial found high early response rates to systemic corticosteroid therapy but no further increase in response to treatment with the addition of etanercept, a TNF receptor fusion protein.[164]

Diffuse alveolar hemorrhage (DAH)
Posttransplant DAH is characterized by widespread lung injury and diffuse radiographic infiltrates in the absence of identifiable infection following allogeneic and autologous stem cell transplants.[165–169] The Blood and Marrow Transplant Clinical Trials Network includes DAH within the definition of IPS. DAH has also been described in one-third of patients during the periengraftment period.[157,170] Bronchoscopically, DAH appears as progressively bloody returns on lavage fluid taken from three or more subsegmental bronchi. The bronchoscopic criteria for DAH diagnosis have expanded to include cytologic evidence of >20% hemosiderin-laden macrophages in the BAL fluid. Increased hemosiderin-laden macrophages and bloody lavage fluid may be seen in association with diffuse lung injury from a wide variety of causes in the posttransplant setting. Bloody BAL fluid is, thus, neither sensitive nor specific for DAH and may simply represent an index of severity of alveolar injury and concomitant hemostatic defects rather than a separate syndrome. More important, prognosis and therapy are determined by the underlying pathophysiologic process (engraftment syndrome, IPS, sepsis, etc.).[171] There are no associations between the development of DAH and coagulopathy or thrombocytopenia. Furthermore, platelet transfusion does not improve respiratory status. Treatment of DAH includes high-dose intravenous corticosteroids and supportive care, such as supplemental oxygen, mechanical ventilation, and platelet transfusion. Recombinant human factor VIIa (rFVIIa) has been used to enhance hemostasis, but a recent retrospective analysis showed no survival advantage with the addition of rFVIIa to high-dose corticosteroid therapy.[172]

Pulmonary venoocclusive disease (PVOD)
PVOD is a rare complication of HSCT in which progressive occlusion of pulmonary veins and venules caused by intimal proliferation and fibrosis leads to PH.[173] High-dose chemotherapy and infections are implicated as causes of PVOD. The onset is typically insidious, with progressive dyspnea and fatigue occurring several weeks to months after transplant.[124,174,175] Current treatment options are limited, and mortality rates can reach up to 100% within 2 years.

Late-onset noninfectious complications of HSCT

Posttransplantation bronchiolitis obliterans syndrome (BOS)
Bronchiolitis obliterans syndrome (BOS) is the most common pulmonary complication among long-term survivors of allogeneic HSCT. It is a late manifestation of GVHD that leads to progressive respiratory insufficiency and sometimes death. BOS almost never occurs in the absence of GVHD and, thus, affects only allogeneic transplant recipients.[154,176,177] The incidence of 5–26% varies with the diagnostic criteria used.[178] BOS affects small airways, causing chronic inflammation, epithelial mucous metaplasia, submucosal scarring, smooth muscle hypertrophy, and concentric bronchiolar fibrosis. The most commonly identified risk factors are chronic GVHD, older age, viral infections during the first 100 days after transplant, the presence of airflow limitation before transplant, low serum IgG, and the use of methotrexate or busulfan in the conditioning regimen.[157,179] Patients may be asymptomatic in early stages of BOS, which delays the diagnosis. Late presentations, including dyspnea, cough, and wheezing, are more common, as airflow obstruction progresses.[180,181] Chest radiographs are usually normal, but high-resolution CT scans may show evidence of air trapping, thickened or dilated small airways, and mosaic attenuation. Bronchoscopy with BAL and transbronchial lung biopsy is generally not helpful in establishing the diagnosis. PFTs are the primary tools used for diagnosis and follow-up. Evidence of airflow obstruction with reduction in FEV_1 and FEV_1/forced vital capacity (FVC) are supportive PFT findings. The NIH consensus guidelines for diagnosing PTCB include (1) FEV_1/FVC < 0.7 and FEV_1 < 75% of predicted, residual volume on PFTs > 120% predicted; (2) evidence of air trapping, small airway thickening, bronchiectasis on HRCT, or pathological confirmation of constrictive bronchiolitis; and the (3) absence of any infectious process on radiographic, laboratory, or clinical testing.[179] Typically, these diagnostic criteria are associated with delayed diagnosis, severe airflow obstruction, and development of airway fibrosis which contribute to poor prognosis and limitation of therapeutic interventions. Recent publications have proposed revising these criteria to facilitate the diagnosis of BOS at earlier stages.[178]

Treatment options for BOS have not been evaluated in any prospective trials. Traditionally, augmentation of systemic immunosuppression with corticosteroids and calcineurin inhibitors has been the mainstay of therapy.[163] However, two retrospective analyses indicate that inhaled high-dose corticosteroid therapy is effective in stabilizing FEV_1 and reducing symptoms significantly.[182,183] A beneficial effect of azithromycin, possibly due to its anti-inflammatory effects, has also been reported in an observational study.[184] A recent retrospective analysis suggested the use of a less toxic combination (fluticasone, azithromycin, and montelukast) which helped in reducing systemic immunosuppressive therapy within a shorter period of time.[185] Lung transplantation is an option in selected patients. Chronic GVHD continues to be a major cause of mortality and morbidity in long-term survivors of HSCT. BOS is an important contributor to this process. The clinical course and disease progression are variable, but persistent airflow obstruction is associated with a significantly increased risk of death.[176] Early detection and properly conducted prospective trials for the management of BOS are crucial to improve survival.

Cryptogenic organizing pneumonitis (COP)
Also known as *idiopathic bronchiolitis obliterans organizing pneumonia (BOOP)*, Cryptogenic organizing pneumonitis (COP) occurs mostly in allogeneic HSCT recipients with GVHD. COP is a distinct entity that should not be confused with BOS.[177,186–188] It is less common than BOS, with an incidence of 1–2% in long-term survivors. Dry cough, dyspnea, and fever accompanied by patchy infiltrates on chest radiograph and CT scan are the predominant presenting signs and symptoms. The diagnosis is made with surgical lung biopsy. COP is usually responsive to corticosteroids with more favorable prognosis; however, no standard treatment guidelines are currently available.[156]

Posttransplant lymphoproliferative disorder (PTLD)
Posttransplant lymphoproliferative disorder (PTLD) is an uncontrolled expansion of donor-derived Epstein–Barr virus (EBV)-infected B lymphocytes that develops in response to inadequate cytotoxic T cell function.[154,189] It occurs in approximately 1% of HSCT patients, usually within the first 4–12 months after transplant. The lung is involved only 20% of the time, most commonly with ill-defined nodular infiltrates. Treatment includes reduction of immunosuppressive therapy anti-CD20 monoclonal antibody (rituximab), antiviral drugs, and infusion of EBV-specific cytotoxic T lymphocytes.

Pneumonia
Pulmonary infections frequently complicate cancer and its therapy.[190,191] Classic clinical indicators to suggest the presence of lower respiratory infections include the development of pulmonary parenchymal infiltrates, leukocytosis, fever, and expectoration of purulent secretions. However, as a consequence of impaired immune responses, these typical clinical observations may be absent in cancer patients with pneumonia. Therefore, a high index of suspicion is required to avoid overlooking the diagnosis. Further, early radiographic imaging, often including CT scanning, is indicated in cancer patients with unexplained clinical deterioration or new infiltrates on conventional imaging.

The diagnosis of pneumonia is confirmed by recovery of the likely pathogen from an otherwise sterile source (e.g., blood, urine, pleural fluid) or isolation of a noncommensal organism in respiratory secretions. Although the utility of expectorated sputum in the diagnosis of pneumonia is debated, cytologically confirmed lower respiratory samples appear to be diagnostically useful. Fiberoptic bronchoscopy with BAL is considered the diagnostic tool of choice for obtaining lower respiratory samples. While this procedure is safe for most cancer patients,[192] traditional culture methods yield the responsible pathogen in only 25–51% of cases.[193–196] The benefit of BAL may be enhanced by early bronchoscopic evaluation, particularly if obtained before the initiation of antimicrobial therapy. Microscopic examination of transbronchial biopsy specimens can identify angioinvasion of commensal microbes (e.g., *Aspergillus* spp.). Culture of biopsy material, however, has not been proved diagnostically superior to BAL and is often precluded in cancer patients due to coagulopathy and/or thrombocytopenia. Culture results from BAL, or biopsy can be difficult to interpret due to frequent microbial colonization of the upper airway. Conversely, sterile respiratory tract cultures do not exclude an infectious etiology, particularly in the setting of recent administration of broad-spectrum antibiotics. Molecular techniques, including polymerase chain reaction (PCR) testing for pathogen genomic material or antigen detection methods (e.g., serum galactomannan, urinary *Histoplasma* antigen), can also supplement the diagnostic evaluation.

Early and accurate diagnoses are critical to a successful outcome, although treatment should not be withheld while diagnostic interventions are undertaken. Antimicrobial selections are based on knowledge of the infecting pathogen, if available, pneumonia severity, underlying immune status, and the presence of comorbid conditions[197,198] (see section entitled "Infection in the cancer patient"). Delays in appropriate antimicrobial therapy increase the risk of secondary complications and infection-associated deaths, especially in severely immunosuppressed individuals. Therefore, it is common practice to initiate empiric and/or preemptive antimicrobial therapy in patients in which the suspicion of infection is high. However, the clinician is cautioned to recall that cancer patients are prone to numerous causes of fever and pulmonary infiltrates other than infectious pneumonias, including toxicities of therapy, systemic inflammation associated with extrapulmonary infections, heart failure, parenchymal cancer involvement, or intrapulmonary hemorrhage.

Venous thromboembolism

PE and deep venous thrombosis (DVT) are manifestations of VTE. Approximately 20% of all VTEs are associated with cancer, and cancer increases the risk for VTE 4–6 fold. Surgery, chemotherapy, hormonal therapy, growth factors, angiogenesis inhibitors, erythropoietic agents, and central venous catheters (CVC) contribute to cancer-associated VTE.[199] The diagnosis and therapy of VTE may delay, discontinue, or preclude many forms of cancer therapy.[200,201] Cancer-related VTE is associated with significant overall mortality but is an infrequent cause of death.[202] One study found that 3.5% of cancer patients die from VTE.[203]

The clinical presentation of VTE is nonspecific. Scoring systems developed to estimate the pretest probability of DVT and PE (such as Well's scores) in combination with D-dimer testing can be used to rule out VTE in cancer patients; however, the likelihood of finding normal D-dimer levels among cancer patients is less than 30%. Furthermore, an elevated D-dimer has no significant positive predictive value in the cancer setting.[204] Doppler/compression ultrasound is the preferred method to diagnose DVT, although MRI and CT may be required in special circumstances, such as internal iliac vein or vena cava thrombosis. HRCT or CT angiography is the best method for diagnosing PE and offers the advantage of providing additional information regarding thoracic pathology that may confound the diagnosis.[205] Urgent bedside echocardiography should be considered for diagnosis and risk stratification of unstable patients with suspected massive PE.[206]

Pharmacological VTE prophylaxis should be considered in every hospitalized patient with cancer.[207] Cancer patients undergoing abdominal or pelvic surgery should receive low molecular weight heparin (LMWH) prophylaxis extended for 4 weeks.[208] Routine prophylaxis in ambulatory cancer patients undergoing active chemotherapy is recommended only for patients with myeloma receiving thalidomide or lenalidomide as part of combination chemotherapy.[208] There is no evidence that anticoagulation prevents catheter-associated thrombosis and guidelines recommend against it.[207]

Routine VTE induction therapy is used in cancer patients. LMWH is the preferred drug for initial treatment of VTE in this setting. Unfractionated heparin should be used in patients with impaired renal function. Thrombolytics have not been studied systematically in patients with cancer, but their use may be considered in cases of massive PE. An IVC filter should be placed when anticoagulation is contraindicated.[207,209] Based on limited evidence, VTEs found incidentally should be managed as symptomatic VTE.[210] For maintenance therapy, LMWH rather than vitamin K antagonists (VKA) is preferred because LMWH is better at preventing recurrences.[199] When tolerated, maintenance therapy can be continued

indefinitely for patients with active cancer.[202–204] The use of the new oral anticoagulants in cancer patients is generally discouraged, as few patients with cancer were included in the major trials, and there are no established procedures for monitoring these agents.[205]

Pulmonary hypertension in the cancer patient

PH, defined as a mean pulmonary artery pressure (mPAP) ≥25 mmHg at rest, may be an underrecognized problem in the cancer setting. Transthoracic doppler echocardiography (TTE) provides an estimation of pulmonary artery systolic pressure (PASP) and serves as a noninvasive screening tool for PH. PAH denotes a subpopulation of PH characterized by the presence of precapillary PH based on an end-expiratory pulmonary artery wedge pressure (PAWP) ≤ 15 mm Hg and a pulmonary vascular resistance > 3 Woods unit.[207] Right heart catheterization (RHC) is required for diagnosis of PH or PAH.[208] RHC allows assessment of hemodynamic impairments and evaluation of vasoreactivity of the pulmonary circulation, which may guide subsequent classification and management. In acute presentations of PH, secondary causes, such as acute thromboembolic disease, hypoxemic respiratory insufficiency, airway bronchoconstriction, or cardiac dysfunction, must be excluded.

PH may precede the cancer diagnosis or occur at any point along the continuum of cancer care. PH occurring after completion of cancer therapy has also been described. Estimates of cancer-related PH vary broadly with specific cancers, associated cancer therapies, and detection methods. Nonspecific signs and symptoms of exertional dyspnea and fatigue early in the disease process render diagnostic evaluations notoriously difficult and result in substantial delays in treatment. Therefore, a high degree of suspicion is needed to detect PH early, when treatments are more efficacious. Syncope, angina, peripheral edema, abdominal distention, and hemodynamic instability are signs of advanced disease which is often refractory to therapy. In acute presentations of PH, secondary causes, such as acute thromboembolic disease, hypoxemic respiratory insufficiency, airway bronchoconstriction, or cardiac dysfunction, must be excluded.

In the revised 2013 World Health Organization clinical classification scheme, PH is categorized into five groups which share similar etiologies, hemodynamic characteristics, and therapeutic approaches. These include PAH (Group 1), PH due to left heart disease (Group 2), PH due to lung diseases and/or hypoxia (Group 3), chronic thromboembolic pulmonary hypertension (CTEPH, Group 4), and PH with unclear multifactorial mechanisms (Group 5).[209] Cancer-related PH is represented in several of these categories. For example, the TKI, dasatinib, is now considered a risk factor for PAH and is included in Group 1.[209] This drug causes moderate to severe precapillary PH, which may improve or fully resolve following drug cessation.[115] PVOD, a rare cause of PH that is characterized by occlusion or narrowing of the pulmonary veins, represents a subgroup of Group I PH. Infection, chemotaxins, thoracic radiation, and stem cell transplantation are postulated risk factors for PVOD, although no clear causal relationship has been established.[101,174,211] The prognosis for PVOD is poor. Although some patients may tolerate arterial vasodilators, fatal pulmonary edema precipitated by pulmonary vasodilator therapy has been observed.

Chronic myeloproliferative disorders (MPDs) constitute a rare cause of PAH. Several potential mechanisms of MPD-associated PH include high cardiac output, splenectomy, direct obstruction of pulmonary arteries, chronic thromboembolism, portal hypertension, and congestive heart failure.[209,212] Other cancer- and cancer treatment-related entities that involve the pulmonary vasculature may also cause PH. These include external compression and/or entrapment of large pulmonary veins by adenopathy, neoplasms, or mediastinal fibrosis. Hodgkin's lymphoma and germ cell tumors underlie most causes of PH due to mediastinal compression. Fibrosing mediastinitis related to radiation and infection (*Aspergillus*, *Mycobacterium tuberculosis*, blastomycosis, mucormycosis, and cryptococcosis) has also been reported to cause PH.[213–215] The principal primary malignances involving the pulmonary vasculature are sarcomas. Typically, these rare and frequently fatal tumors arise from the main pulmonary arteries, although pulmonary venous sarcomas have also been described.[216] Patients with pulmonary arterial sarcomas often present with signs and symptoms that mimic CTEPH (dyspnea, chest pain, cough, hemoptysis). However, associated findings of unexplained fever, weight loss, clubbing, anemia, and elevated ESR should raise suspicion of malignancy. Secondary tumoral involvement of the pulmonary vascular bed may present as macrovascular central tumor emboli or tumor cell aggregates that occlude small vessels. The latter may occur with or without lymphangitic spread of disease. Choriocarcinomas and mucinous tumors originating in the breast, lung, gastrointestinal tract, and kidneys are associated with the highest rates of tumor embolization.[217] Clinical symptoms of tumor emboli range from the abrupt onset of dyspnea, chest pain, and cardiovascular collapse to subacute symptoms of cough, exertional dyspnea, and exercise intolerance associated with unexplained PH. Pulmonary tumor thrombotic microangiopathy (PTTM) is an unusual cause of malignancy-related PH that is most often seen in patients with adenocarcinomas, particularly of the stomach.[218] Patients present with severe, refractory PH that rapidly progresses to sudden cardiovascular collapse and death. Findings on pulmonary microvascular cytology are diagnostically useful; however, the diagnosis of PTTM is most often made at necropsy. No definitive treatment has been identified thus far. Although in most major medical centers, CT angiography has replaced V/Q scans in the evaluation of thromboembolic events; in the setting of suspected tumor emboli, V/Q scans may be of greater diagnostic utility than the chest CT. Multiple subsegmental mismatched defects on V/Q scintigraphy are supportive findings. Pulmonary microvascular cytology of samples obtained from a wedged pulmonary artery catheter during RHC may offer additional support for tumor embolization.[217]

Leukemic sequestration and leukocyte thrombus formation within the pulmonary microvasculature are rare complications of hyperleukocytosis (WBC > 50,000/dL) and blast crisis associated with myeloid and lymphocytic leukemias. Patients typically present with dyspnea, nonproductive cough and hypoxemia associated with interstitial infiltrates, and signs of PH and cor pulmonale. The clinical manifestations of macrovascular tumor emboli resemble acute pulmonary thromboembolic disease. Microvascular tumor embolization, however, typically presents with insidious symptoms of dyspnea, nonproductive cough, hypoxemia, and severe pulmonary artery pressure elevations. Cor pulmonale and diffuse interstitial infiltrates, suggestive of lymphangitic spread of disease, are common findings that worsen the already poor prognosis. Acute hypoxemic respiratory failure has also been reported following the initiation of chemotherapy for treatment of acute nonlymphocytic leukemia. This syndrome, known as leukemic cell lysis pneumopathy, typically occurs during the initial 48 h of treatment and is thought to be caused by chemotherapy-induced pulmonary leukostasis and perivascular hemorrhage. Measured PaO_2 may be artificially low in patients with hyperleukocytic leukemias in the absence of lung involvement, owing to leukocyte metabolism of oxygen within the arterial blood gas syringe. In this setting, oxygen saturations obtained by pulse oximetry are normal. Rapid analysis of an iced arterial blood gas specimen or the addition of cyanide to the blood gas syringe eliminates this problem.

The evolution of therapy guidelines for PAH over the past two decades has resulted in evidence-based treatment strategies that favorably impact survival and significantly improve the quality of life of these patients.[219] Treatment of PH should address the underlying cause. The need for supportive therapies, including supplemental oxygen, diuretics, anticoagulant therapy, and exercise should be assessed in all patients. More advanced therapies are directed at PAH itself and should be initiated based on the results of further testing and national guidelines. Current and emerging therapies for PAH target the endothelin, nitric oxide, and prostaglandin pathways. Specific treatment strategies may include monotherapy or, more frequently, combination therapy.[220] Unfortunately, no cure exists for this devastating condition. Caution in extrapolating PAH treatment guidelines to other forms of PH is warranted. No studies have addressed the utility of pulmonary vasodilator therapy in the management of cancer-related PH. Dobutamine, milrinone, intravenous prostacyclin, inhaled vasodilators, and extracorporeal life support are accepted therapies for PH with hemodynamic decompensation in the general population.[221] Specific guidelines regarding the optimal use of vasopressor therapy in the critically ill cancer patient with PH and associated hemodynamic deterioration have yet to be delineated.

Sleep disorders in cancer patients

Sleep disturbance and chronobiology have important implications throughout the continuum of care of the cancer patient, impacting cancer prevention, treatment, and survivorship.

Cancer prevention

Prolonged sleep duration and disturbed circadian rhythms of sleep are associated with an increased risk of cancer. In a large Japanese cohort study, sleep durations of less than 5 h or greater than 9 h per night conferred higher cancer prevalence.[222] Chronic sleep disturbance caused by rotating and nocturnal shift work may also increase the risk of cancer. Nurses who worked rotating shifts for more than 30 years had an increased relative risk of breast cancer in one study. Suppression of melatonin, a naturally occurring hormone with oncostatic potential, occurs with nocturnal light exposure and may contribute to the increased cancer risk among patients with chronic sleep disturbance.[223–225] Sleep disruption and abnormal circadian rhythms have been associated with impaired immune system-mediated tumor surveillance which may also increase cancer risk.[226,227] Obstructive sleep apnea (OSA) appears to confer an increased cancer risk, with higher rates associated with more severe nocturnal hypoxia.[228–230] These findings implicate a link between sleep disturbance and cancer and highlight good sleep hygiene and treatment of sleep disorders as potential targets for cancer prevention.

Cancer treatment

Excessive daytime sleepiness and fatigue are associated with increased plasma cytokines, such as IL-6. A good night's sleep can decrease the levels of this cytokine. Inflammatory mediators produced by specific cancer interventions or the cancer itself may exacerbate sleep disruption. For example, chemotherapy regimens used to treat breast cancer may induce elevations in VEGF which is

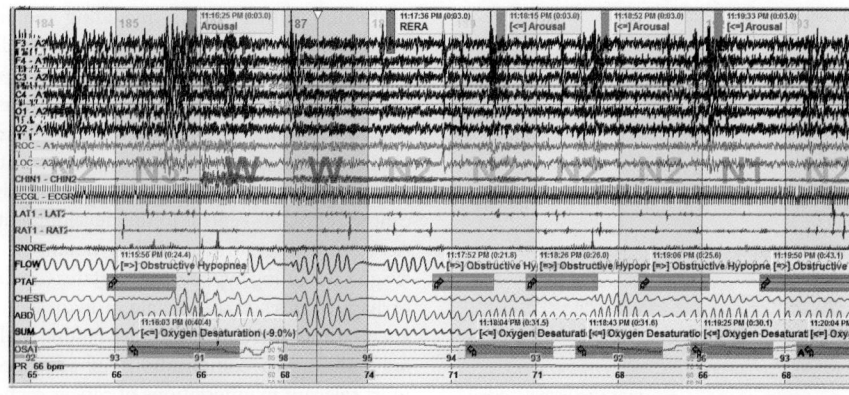

W = awake; N1, N2, N3 = sleep stages

Figure 11 76-year old man who presented with loud snoring, witnessed apneas, and daytime hypersomnolence 9 years following completion of chemoradiation therapy for tonsilar squamous cell carcinoma. BMI at presentation was $22\,kg/m^2$. Severe obstructive sleep apnea–hypopnea syndrome with an apnea–hypopnea index of 32 events/hour of sleep and an oxygen saturation nadir of 72% was observed on polysomnography (5 min view).

associated with disturbed sleep.[231] Sleep loss and, in particular, loss of rapid eye movement (REM) sleep are known to be hyperalgesic. Thus, reduced sleep conditions, including REM sleep deprivation, which is common in many cancer patients, confer increased sensitivity to pain.[232]

Primary sleep disorders, including restless leg syndrome and periodic leg movement disorders, are often associated with insomnia and daytime hypersomnolence. These disorders are more common among certain cancer subgroups, perhaps due to chemotherapy-related anemia and peripheral neuropathy.[233] The OSA syndromes may also be more prevalent in certain cancers. In a study of 56 patients with tumor of the head and neck region, 84 percent met clinical criteria for OSA (Figure 11).[234] Opioids are known to worsen symptoms of central sleep apnea. This form of sleep-disordered breathing may be problematic in cancer patients, as many are on opioid medications for cancer-related pain.[235]

Chronobiology and chronotherapy attempt to optimize the effects of cancer chemotherapy while minimizing toxicity by taking advantage of the differences in the circadian rhythm of the cell cycle of tumor cells versus host tissues. Clinical and animal studies have shown that dose intensity can be increased while simultaneously reducing toxicities and improving treatment outcomes.[236,237]

Cancer survivorship

Disturbed sleep, fatigue, and insomnia may occur in up to 51% of some cancer survivors.[238] Cognitive and behavioral therapy (CBT) is the treatment of choice for insomnia and have been shown to improve symptoms of insomnia, decrease sedative-hypnotic medication use, and quality of life. CBT can also impact immune function in cancer patients by increasing levels of IL-1β and γ-interferon, which are thought to promote sleep.[239]

Pulmonary rehabilitation

Pulmonary rehabilitation (PR) represents a multidisciplinary strategy that incorporates exercise training, patient and family education, psychosocial and behavioral interventions, and outcome assessment in the management of patients with chronic respiratory diseases. Evidence-based support for PR in the care of patients with COPD has led to the implementation of this treatment strategy as standard of care in the management of this group of patients. The systemic effects and comorbidities associated with cancer, in

particular, fatigue, dyspnea, anemia, skeletal muscle impairment, muscle wasting, poor exercise intolerance, depression, deconditioning, and anxiety, add substantially to the burden of the disease. PR targets many of these symptoms, resulting in reductions in symptoms of dyspnea and fatigue, and improvements in exercise tolerance and quality of life. Poor exercise tolerance confers worse surgical outcomes following lung resection and limits the ability to withstand the potential toxicities of chemotherapy.[240,241] Thus, the rationale for providing PR to patients with cancer is quite strong, particularly in the setting of lung cancer, where COPD and lung cancer often coexist. Recent small studies suggest that PR may impact lung cancer management favorably by improving a variety of clinically meaningful outcomes, such as performance status, chemotherapy-related fatigue, oxygen consumption, exercise tolerance, and health-related quality of life.[242] In a study by Bobbio and colleagues, an increase in work rate and oxygen consumption (VO_{2max}) following a 4-week course of preoperative PR permitted patients who were considered nonoperative based on presurgical VO_{2max} to undergo successful lung resection surgery.[243] In other investigations, improvements in exercise endurance, muscle strength, and dyspnea scores following 6–8 weeks of postsurgical PR have led to reduced hospital stay and increased quality of life among patients that underwent thoracotomy and resection for lung cancer.[243–248] In the nonsurgical setting, several small reports have suggested a beneficial role for PR in countering chemotherapy- and radiotherapy-related fatigue, ameliorating performance status, and reducing the length/frequency of hospitalizations among patients with cancer.[249–252]

Acute respiratory failure

Acute respiratory failure (ARF) is the most common reason for ICU admission among adult patients with cancer. Predisposing conditions for both acute and chronic respiratory insufficiency in cancer patients can be divided into those that cause "lung" failure or "pump" failure. Lung failure is typically associated with ventilation/perfusion abnormalities, shunts, or alterations of alveolocapillary diffusion and leads primarily to hypoxia, at least in its early stages. A classic example of lung failure is ARDS. Lung failure may also develop in the absence of ARDS as a consequence of ventilation/perfusion mismatch associated with pneumonia, atelectasis, or PE or as a result of shunt associated with pulmonary edema. Other common causes of lung failure are listed in Table 4.

Table 4 Lung versus pump failure in acute respiratory failure: characteristics and underlying causes.

	Lung failure	Pump failure
Characteristic features	Hypoxemia	Severe hypercapnia and acidosis Mild hypoxemia
Pathogenesis	Ventilation/perfusion mismatch Shunts Alterations in alveolocapillary membrane	Exhaustion of ventilatory pump (CNS, PNS, or respiratory muscles)
Underlying conditions	Acute lung injury/ARDS Pneumonia Atelectasis Pulmonary embolism/tumor emboli Lymphangitic spread of tumor Chemotherapy Radiation therapy Pulmonary leukostasis Transfusion-related lung injury Postoperative respiratory insufficiency	Coexisting COPD Intrinsic or extrinsic airway compression Obstructive sleep apnea associated with head and neck malignancy

CNS, central nervous system; PNS, peripheral nervous system.

Pump failure, by contrast, results from primary failure of alveolar ventilation and leads to severe hypercapnia and acidosis with only mild hypoxemia. Multifactorial causes of ARF, such as severe COPD exacerbation with superimposed pneumonia, may lead to both lung and pump failure. This mixed picture is a common occurrence in the cancer patient and requires a systematic approach to each component of respiratory failure to devise appropriate treatment strategies.

Causes of pump failure

Central nervous system disorders: impaired drive

Isolated central depression of ventilatory drive is a rare cause of pump failure that may result from insults to the central nervous system, such as medullary tumors or infarction and sedating or narcotic medications. Acquired central hypoventilation may occur following neurosurgical procedures for brainstem tumors, particularly those that are close to the fourth ventricle. Radiation to the base of the skull may have similar adverse effects. Occult hypothyroidism may also contribute to central hypoventilation and ventilatory failure, particularly in elderly women and following treatment for head and neck carcinoma. More often, respiratory failure owing to depressed central drive occurs as an additional insult, superimposed on chronic respiratory insufficiency. In this setting, small doses of narcotic or sedating medications may have a profound effect on alveolar ventilation. Respiratory muscle fatigue may also contribute to central hypoventilation by sending inhibitory signals to the respiratory center in the CNS to reduce drive, thereby protecting the muscles from injury and mitigating further muscle fatigue.

Peripheral nervous system disorders: inadequate neuromuscular competence

Transmission of signals from the CNS to the respiratory muscles occurs via the spinal cord and peripheral nerves. Hence, conditions causing neuromuscular dysfunction, such as primary neurologic diseases, spinal cord lesions, neuromuscular blocking drugs, and muscle weakness, may precipitate ventilatory failure. Systemic anesthetics cause potent neuromuscular blockade and ventilatory

depression. Other agents, including sedatives, anxiolytics, hypnotics, and aminoglycosides, typically produce severe respiratory depression only in the setting of preexisting neuromuscular diseases such as myasthenia gravis and myasthenic paraneoplastic syndrome or after massive overdose. One exception to this principle is methadone, which may cause ventilatory insufficiency with chronic administration. Muscle fatigue, a pervasive problem in the cancer setting, is central to the development of respiratory failure. An extensive list of factors may potentiate cancer-related muscle fatigue, including hypoperfusion states (cardiogenic, septic, or hemorrhagic shock), excess lactate or hydrogen ion production, severe anemia, and, thereby, respiratory failure. Malnutrition and cachexia are well-known complications of advanced cancer. One of the most relevant manifestations of cancer cachexia is muscle wasting, which contributes to markedly depressed strength and endurance of the skeletal muscles, including the diaphragm.[253] Overinflation of the thorax and flattened diaphragms associated with COPD, a common comorbidity of lung cancer, further contribute to compromised respiratory muscle performance and ventilatory failure. Electrolyte disturbances such as hypophosphatemia, hypokalemia, and hypomagnesemia frequently complicate chemotherapy and may cause profound muscle weakness in the cancer patient. In addition, many of the drugs used in the treatment of ventilatory failure, including beta-agonists, diuretics, and corticosteroids may exacerbate hypophosphatemia and aggravate muscle weakness. Chemotherapeutic agents and other drugs used in cancer treatment may also have deleterious effects on the neuromuscular system. Although corticosteroid-induced myopathy has been well described, the role of these drugs in potentiating respiratory muscle dysfunction has been recognized only recently.[254,255] Among the chemotherapeutic agents, vinca alkaloids, cisplatin, and the taxanes are most frequently associated with peripheral neurotoxicity. The clinical manifestations of these drugs on lung function may be subtle in the absence of predisposing factors, such as preexisting neuromuscular abnormalities. In addition to their CNS effects, the use of anesthetic agents, in particular halothane, propofol, and nitrous oxide, may induce respiratory depression by decreasing diaphragmatic contractility.[256,257] Injury to the phrenic nerve following surgery for head and neck cancer or surgery to the anterior mediastinum, esophagus, or lungs may cause persistent diaphragmatic dysfunction and ventilatory failure. Loss of diaphragmatic function from direct phrenic nerve invasion by tumor may also be seen, particularly among patients with lymphoma or cancers of the lung or head and neck. Diffuse neural dysfunction resulting from paraneoplastic syndromes is another cause of respiratory failure in the cancer setting. Lambert–Eaton myasthenic syndrome, which affects about 3% of patients with small-cell lung cancer, myasthenia gravis, which occurs in 10–15% of patients with thymoma, and demyelinating peripheral neuropathy, seen in 50% of patients with the osteosclerotic form of plasmacytoma, are the most common types of paraneoplastic disorders of the peripheral nervous system. These disorders typically have a subacute and debilitating course that may lead to ventilatory failure.

Increased work of breathing: increased respiratory system load and chest wall abnormalities

A variety of cancer-related factors may result in acute or chronic escalations in the respiratory system load. Elevations in airway resistive workloads, characterized physiologically by abnormal airway resistance and increased elastance, are cardinal features of COPD, airway inflammation, airway edema, or physical obstruction by mucous, blood, or tumor. Upper airway obstruction caused by tracheal stenosis associated with prior intubation or radiation to the head and neck and intubation with a small (<7.5 mm internal diameter) endotracheal tube contributes significantly to increased airflow resistance and respiratory failure. Abnormalities involving the chest wall and thoracic spine caused by tumor, radiation, or surgery may cause increased chest wall elastic loads, increased work of breathing, and respiratory failure.

Lung failure (pulmonary edema, ARDS, ALI)

Pulmonary edema/acute respiratory distress syndrome/acute lung injury

The predilection for pulmonary edema in the setting of cancer arises from a broad array of insults to the lungs that may be sorted according to the underlying permeability characteristics of the microcirculation and the presence or absence of DAD histopathologically. In normal permeability pulmonary edema, increased hydrostatic pressure caused by an imbalance in Starling forces leads to fluid filtration into the lungs. Pulmonary edema of cardiogenic and neurogenic etiologies, as well as lung edema caused by lung reexpansion, lymphatic obstruction, and relief of upper airway obstruction, are typically associated with normal microvascular permeability.

The histopathologic hallmark of increased microvascular permeability is the accumulation of proteinaceous fluid within the interstitium and alveoli resulting from a breach in the integrity of the alveolar and microvascular surfaces. Increased permeability pulmonary edema, occurring in the absence of DAD, is referred to as capillary leak syndrome. In the cancer setting, this type of pulmonary edema may occur following the administration of cytokines such as interferon, IL_2, and TNF, which disrupt capillary endothelial integrity. These drugs may also cause direct toxicity to the myocardium, resulting in mixed or overlap edema associated with normal and increased permeability etiologies. Neurogenic and reexpansion pulmonary edema represent two other causes of mixed edema, which are observed frequently in the cancer setting. The frequent need for transfused blood products (packed red blood cells, platelets, and granulocytes) in the cancer setting predisposes the cancer patient to the syndrome of transfusion-related lung injury (TRALI), another form of NCPE. PH with normal left ventricular end-diastolic pressures is also a cardinal feature of this syndrome. The treatment is supportive. Resolution of clinical symptoms and radiographic changes typically occurs within 2–3 days of symptom onset without permanent pulmonary sequelae, although in 20% of patients, symptoms and radiographic changes may persist for a week and may be associated with lung injury (ALI/ARDS—see following text).[258,259]

ALI and ARDS are terms used for varying severity of pulmonary edema accompanying the histopathologic finding of DAD. ARDS is reserved for severe lung injury in which bilateral pulmonary infiltrates and severe hypoxemia (as defined by a ratio of the partial pressure of arterial oxygen to the fraction of inspired oxygen < 200) occur in the absence of clinical evidence of left atrial hypertension.[260] ALI is reflective of a lesser injury, as indicated by a PaO_2/FiO_2 ratio between 200 and 300. The list of cancer-related precipitating conditions associated with ARDS is extensive. An etiological dichotomy that sorts the causes of ARDS into conditions that provoke direct lung injury (pneumonia, gastric aspiration) and those that are associated with systemic diseases that promote indirect lung injury (sepsis, TRALI) provides a simplistic approach to ARDS but is confounded by inciting events that are often multifactorial or unknown. Clinically, patients may present with ARF and associated hypoxemia within 24–48 h of the predisposing event. Fever and leukocytosis, owing to the inflammatory response associated with lung injury, may be prominent findings, even in the absence of infection. Although the radiographic changes in ARDS are not distinctive, the chest X-ray is important, nonetheless, in ruling out competing diagnoses such as pneumothorax, infections, and congestive heart failure. Patchy areas of lung involvement may be seen as ground glass opacifications early on which may progress to diffuse areas of consolidation. Radiographic findings suggestive of cardiogenic pulmonary edema such as Kerley B lines, cardiomegaly, and apical vascular redistribution are typically absent. Progression to the fibroproliferative phase is common, resulting in persistent hypoxemia associated with poor lung compliance, increased dead space, V/Q imbalance, and PH.

Management of respiratory failure

Medical therapy

The management of the critically ill cancer patient with respiratory failure involves aggressive supportive care as well as strategies that target the precipitating cause. Standard supportive measures include the provision of supplemental oxygen, inhaled bronchodilators, nutritional support, chest physiotherapy, and pulmonary toilet and the prudent use of diuretics, vasopressors and antibiotics, where indicated. Although fluid loading augments oxygen consumption and tissue oxygen delivery, careful attention to fluid homeostasis is imperative, as a persistent positive fluid balance has been associated with a poor outcome.[261,262] More specific interventions, such as administration of helium–oxygen (heliox) mixtures, may provide temporary relief of acute respiratory distress associated with proximal airway obstruction and serve as a bridge to more definitive therapy. Patients with DAH may benefit from the early use of high-dose steroids, DDAVP, and aggressive blood and blood product support.[263] Recombinant factor VII (rFVIIa) and antifibrinolytics such as aminocaproic acid have been used to treat transplant-related DAH, although convincing evidence supporting this practice is not available.[264-266] The effect of activated protein C administration in reducing sepsis-related ARDS mortality has been exciting; however, conflicting results in subgroup analysis and concerns regarding serious bleeding have led to removal of this from the market.[267-269]

Advances in supportive care coupled with early identification and management of precipitating condition(s) and strategies that attenuate ventilator-associated lung injury have contributed to significant increases in ARDS-related survival rates over the past decade.[270] Several trials of high-dose corticosteroids for early-phase ARDS failed to demonstrate a survival benefit. A salutary effect of high-dose glucocorticoids given during the fibroproliferative phase of ARDS was suggested in several small studies, though not borne out in a large, multicenter, NIH-sponsored (ARDS-Net) trial.[271-274]

Mechanical ventilation

Noninvasive ventilation (NIV)

Assisted ventilation is often required to manage ARF that is nonresponsive to conservative medical therapy. Newer modes of mechanical ventilation as well as the use of noninvasive ventilation (NIV) have shown promising results and gained broad acceptance in the management of cancer patients with respiratory failure. The efficacy of NIV has been clearly demonstrated in several randomized, controlled studies in the management of pump failure[275,276] as well as selected cases of lung failure.[275] In a recent retrospective study of the outcome of cancer patients following ICU transfer for ARF, the use of NIV was associated with marked improvements in patient survival.[277] In addition, significant reductions in the need for conventional mechanical ventilation and declines in both ICU and post-ICU hospital mortality have been linked to the use of intermittent NIV during the early stages of hypoxemic ARF (PaO_2/FiO_2 ratio <250).[278–280] Evidence favoring the early use of NPPV for ARF among immunocompromised patients is derived from several small studies which purport reduced rates of endotracheal intubation, length of ICU stay, and ICU mortality.[278,281,282] Immunocompromised patients with respiratory failure who require mechanical ventilation have notoriously poor prognoses, with an estimated 1% increase of risk for pneumonia per day of mechanical ventilation.[283] Thus, NIV in this setting has quickly gained broad acceptance in the management of cancer patients with respiratory failure.

Invasive mechanical ventilation (IMV)

Intermittent mandatory ventilation remains the standard of care for severe ARF and for NIV treatment failures. Overdistension of the lungs at end-inspiration and repetitive collapse of the lungs at end exhalation that occurs with conventional mechanical ventilation at high tidal volumes may trigger further lung injury. This observation prompted the development of lung-protective ventilator strategies that mitigate alveolar overdistension and enhance recruitment of atelectatic alveoli, thereby reducing the incidence of ventilator-induced lung injury. Lung-protective ventilator strategies may be accomplished with conventional modes of ventilation such as assist-controlled and pressure-controlled ventilation with or without inverse ratio ventilation or alternative methods, such as biphasic positive airway pressure ventilation (BIPAP), airway pressure release ventilation (APRV), jet and high frequency oscillatory ventilation, and differential lung ventilation. None of these modes of ventilation have proven to be superior to conventional ventilatory strategies. Convincing evidence favoring the use of protective ventilator strategies is derived from the National Institutes of Health ARDS Network trial where lower tidal volumes (6 mL/kg of predicted body weight) and limited static inspiratory pressures (<30 cm H_2O) resulted in a 22% improved survival compared to patients mechanically ventilated using higher tidal volumes and inflation pressures.[284,285] Other adjuncts to ventilator management of patients with ARF, including extracorporeal membrane oxygenation (ECMO) and partial liquid ventilation (PLV), prone positioning, and surfactant instillation, have been proposed; however, the merits of these therapies over conventional treatment strategies have not been proven definitively. Early tracheostomy may be associated with improved outcomes in critically ill patients. Practice guidelines regarding the appropriate timing of tracheostomy in patients that require prolonged mechanical ventilation are based on a consensus statement, nearly two decades old, that suggested that tracheostomy be considered after 21 days of mechanical ventilation. Although these recommendations were based only on expert opinion, modern practice broadly continues to follow them. In a recent meta-analysis, an 8.5 day decrease in total mechanical ventilation days and significant reduction in ICU length of stay was seen among patients that underwent early tracheostomy (within 7 days of initiation of invasive mechanical ventilation) compared to those in which tracheostomy was performed late, although mortality was not altered significantly.[286]

Respiratory failure outcomes

The mortality rate of critically ill cancer patients with respiratory failure is at least threefold higher than that of concurrently admitted cancer patients without respiratory failure.[287–289] Conditions common to the critically ill cancer patient, such as cardiac, renal, or hepatic dysfunction, disseminated intravascular coagulation, hemodynamic instability, and the need for mechanical ventilation, are independent predictive variables that portend a poor outcome.[287,288,290] Early reports documented mortality rates in excess of 90% among mechanically ventilated cancer patients with ARF, especially among patients with hematologic malignancies and recipients of hematopoietic transplants.[291–294] More recent investigations have offered a more favorable perspective, with mortality rates of 69–84%.[288,289,295,296] Survival gains may be attributable to better infection prophylaxis measures, improved transplantation techniques, standard use of preventive measures that mitigate aspiration, more aggressive use of hematopoietic growth factor support following transplantation, and trends toward the use of peripheral stem cells rather than bone marrow as a source of donor stem cells. In addition, the newer ventilation strategies including NIV and lung-protective ventilator strategies may play a role in improved survival.[289] Finally, the implementation of programs for early identification and management of deteriorating patients on general hospital wards and improvements in ICU admission and triage criteria may not only contribute to overall improved ICU survival but also to the appropriate use of hospital resources.[297,298]

Key references

The complete reference list can be found on the Wiley Companion Digital Edition of this title (see inside front cover for login instructions).

2 Keefea D, Bowena J, Gibsonb R, Tanc T, Okerac M, Stringer A. Noncardiac vascular toxicities of vascular endothelial growth factor inhibitors in advanced cancer: a review. *Oncologist*. 2011;**16**:432–444.

13 Faiz SA, Sahay S, Jimenez CA. Pleural effusions in acute and chronic leukemia and myelodysplastic syndrome. *Curr Opin Pulm Med*. 2014;**20**(4):340–346.

34 Ost D, Jimenez CA, Lei X, et al. Quality-adjusted survival following treatment of malignant pleural effusions with indwelling pleural catheters. *Chest*. 2014;**145**:1347–1356.

37 Janssen JP, Collier G, Astoul P, et al. Safety of pleurodesis with talc poudrage in malignant pleural effusion: a prospective cohort study. *Lancet*. 2007;**369**(9572):1535–1539.

40 Jimenez C, Mhatre A, Martinez C, et al. Use of an indwelling pleural catheter for the management of recurrent chylothorax in patients with cancer. *Chest*. 2007;**132**:1584–1590.

44 Datta D, Lahiri B. Preoperative evaluation of patients undergoing lung resection surgery. *Chest*. 2003;**123**(6):2096–2103.

52 Morice RC, Peters EJ, Ryan MB, Putnam JB, Ali MK, Roth JA. Exercise testing in the evaluation of patients at high risk for complications from lung resection. *Chest*. 1992;**101**(2):356–361.

53 Walsh GL, Morice RC, Putnam JB Jr, et al. Resection of lung cancer is justified in high-risk patients selected by exercise oxygen consumption. *Ann Thorac Surg*. 1994;**58**(3):704–710; discussion 711.

58 Sleijfer S. Bleomycin-induced pneumonitis. *Chest*. 2001;**120**(2):617–624.

78 Shannon V, Andersson B, Lei X, Champlin R, Kontoyiannis DP. Utility of early versus late fiberoptic bronchoscopy in the evaluation of new pulmonary infiltrates following hematopoietic stem cell transplantation. *Bone Marrow Transplant*. 2010;**45**(4):647–655.

80 Rogers J, Yang D. Differentiation syndrome in patients with acute promyelocytic leukemia. *J Oncol Pharm Pract*. 2012;**18**(1):109–114.

82 Dy G, Adjei A. Understanding, recognizing, and managing toxicities of targeted anticancer therapies. *CA Cancer J Clin*. 2013;**63**(4):249–279.

87 Nagata S, Ueda N, Yoshida Y, Matsuda H, Maehara Y. Severe interstitial pneumonitis associated with the administration of taxanes. *J Infect Chemother*. 2010;**16**(5):340–344.

88 Duran I, Goebell PJ, Papazisis K, et al. Drug-induced pneumonitis in cancer patients treated with mTOR inhibitors: management and insights into possible mechanisms. *Expert Opin Drug Saf*. 2014;**13**(3):361–372.

93 Shannon V, Price K. Pulmonary complications of cancer therapy. *Anesthesiol Clin North Am*. 1998;**16**(3):563–585.

95 Beauverd Y, Samii K. Acute respiratory distress syndrome in a patient with primary myelofibrosis after ruxolitinib treatment discontinuation. *Int J Hematol.* 2014;**100**(5):498–501.

114 Godinas L, Guignabert C, Seferian A, et al. Tyrosine kinase inhibitors in pulmonary arterial hypertension: a double-edge sword? *Semin Respir Crit Care Med.* 2013;**34**(5):714–724.

115 Montani D, Bergot E, Gunther S, et al. Pulmonary arterial hypertension in patients treated by dasatinib. *Circulation.* 2012;**125**:2128–2137.

129 Moon D, Lee JM, Noonan AM, et al. Deleterious BRCA1/2 mutation is an independent risk factor for carboplatin hypersensitivity reactions. *Br J Cancer.* 2013;**109**(4):1072–1078.

140 Castillo R, Pham N, Ansari S, et al. Pre-radiotherapy FDG PET predicts radiation pneumonitis in lung cancer. *Radiat Oncol.* 2014;**9**(74):1–10.

146 Ding K, Ji W, Li J, Zhang X, Wang L. Radiation recall pneumonitis induced by chemotherapy after thoracic radiotherapy for lung cancer. *Radiat Oncol.* 2011;**6**(24):1–6.

153 Diab KJ, Yu Z, Wood KL, et al. Comparison of pulmonary complications after nonmyeloablative and conventional allogeneic hematopoietic cell transplant. *Biol Blood Marrow Transplant.* 2012;**18**(12):1827–1834.

164 Yanik GA, Horowitz MM, Weisdorf DJ, et al. Randomized, double-blind, placebo-controlled trial of soluble tumor necrosis factor receptor: enbrel (etanercept) for the treatment of idiopathic pneumonia syndrome after allogeneic stem cell transplantation: blood and marrow transplant clinical trials network protocol. *Biol Blood Marrow Transplant.* 2014;**20**(6):858–864.

172 Elinoff JM, Bagci U, Moriyama B, et al. Recombinant human factor VIIa for alveolar hemorrhage following allogeneic stem cell transplantation. *Biol Blood Marrow Transplant.* 2014;**20**(7):969–978.

178 Chien J, Duncan S, Williams KM, Pavletic SZ. Bronchiolitis obliterans syndrome after allogeneic hematopoietic stem cell transplantation-an increasingly recognized manifestation of chronic graft-versus-host disease. *Biol Blood Marrow Transplant.* 2010;**16**(1 **Suppl**):S106–S114.

185 Norman BC, Jacobsohn DA, Williams KM, et al. Fluticasone, azithromycin and montelukast therapy in reducing corticosteroid exposure in bronchiolitis obliterans syndrome after allogeneic hematopoietic SCT: a case series of eight patients. *Bone Marrow Transplant.* 2011;**46**(10):1369–1373.

187 Nakasone H, Onizuka M, Suzuki N, et al. Pre-transplant risk factors for cryptogenic organizing pneumonia/bronchiolitis obliterans organizing pneumonia after hematopoietic cell transplantation. *Bone Marrow Transplant.* 2013;**48**(10):1317–1323.

189 Rasche L, Kapp M, Einsele H, Mielke S. EBV-induced post transplant lymphoproliferative disorders: a persisting challenge in allogeneic hematopoetic SCT. *Bone Marrow Transplant.* 2014;**49**(2):163–167.

199 Lee AY, Peterson EA. Treatment of cancer-associated thrombosis. *Blood.* 2013;**122**(14):2310–2317.

203 Lyman GH, Khorana AA, Kuderer NM, et al. Venous thromboembolism prophylaxis and treatment in patients with cancer: American Society of Clinical Oncology clinical practice guideline update. *J Clin Oncol.* 2013;**31**(17):2189–2204.

204 Carrier M, Khorana AA, Zwicker JI, Noble S, Lee AY, Subcommittee on Haemostasis and Malignancy for the SSC of the ISTH. Management of challenging cases of patients with cancer-associated thrombosis including recurrent thrombosis and bleeding: guidance from the SSC of the ISTH: a reply to a rebuttal. *J Thromb Haemost.* 2014;**12**(1):116–117.

205 Yeh CH, Gross PL, Weitz JI. Evolving use of new oral anticoagulants for treatment of venous thromboembolism. *Blood.* 2014;**124**(7):1020–1028.

209 Simonneau G, Gatzoulis MA, Adatia I, et al. Updated clinical classification of pulmonary hypertension. *J Am Coll Cardiol.* 2013;**62**:D34–D41.

230 Nieto FJ, Peppard PE, Young T, Finn L, Hla KM, Farre R. Sleep-disordered breathing and cancer mortality: results from the wisconsin sleep cohort study. *Am J Resp Crit Care Med.* 2012;**186**:190–194.

234 Faiz SA, Balachandran D, Hessel AC, et al. Sleep-related breathing disorders in patients with tumors in the head and neck region. *Oncologist.* 2014;**19**:1200–1206.

242 Mujovic NMN, Subotic D, Marinkovic M, et al. Preoperative pulmonary rehabilitation in patients with non-small cell lung cancer and chronic obstructive pulmonary disease. *Arch Med Sci.* 2014;**10**(1):68–75.

245 Granger CLCC, McDonald CF, Berney S, Denehy L. Safety and feasibility of an exercise intervention for patients following lung resection: a pilot randomized controlled trial. *Integr Cancer Ther.* 2013;**12**(3):213–224.

274 Steinberg K, Hudson LD, Goodman RB, et al. Efficacy and safety of corticosteroids for persistent acute respiratory distress syndrome. *N Engl J Med.* 2006;**354**(16):1671–1684.

282 Caples S, Gay PC. Noninvasive positive pressure ventilation in the intensive care unit: a concise review. *Crit Care Med.* 2005;**33**(11):2651–2658.

296 Kew A, Couban S, Patrick W, Thompson K, White D. Outcome of hematopoietic stem cell transplant recipients admitted to the intensive care unit. *Biol Blood Marrow Transplant.* 2006;**12**(3):301–305.

Robert S. Bresalier, MD ▪ H. Franklin Herlong, MD ▪ Boris Blechacz, MD, PhD

Overview

Gastrointestinal and hepatic complications represent some of the most common and potentially life-threatening disorders associated with treatment of the cancer patient. The expansion of therapeutic options for these patients has been accompanied by a growing number of direct and indirect consequences that effect the rapidly dividing cells of the GI tract. Cytotoxic, immunologic, and infectious insults often combine to increase toxicity. Recognition of these complications, together with proper evaluation and management, is key to the well being of these patients.

A growing spectrum of treatments is available to combat cancer. Chemotherapy, radiotherapy, and molecular targeted therapies including immunotherapies lead to adverse effects in several organs systems, including those of the gastrointestinal (GI) tract. GI complications are very common in patients undergoing cancer treatment. Some of these complications can be life threatening and require prompt and appropriate diagnosis and treatment. This chapter addresses common GI complications that result from cancer treatment and focuses on the evaluation and management of these problems.

Esophageal disorders

Esophagitis

Esophagitis in patients with cancer may be due to the direct cytotoxic effects of chemotherapy or radiation, or by infections due to immunosuppressive effects of cancer therapy (Table 1). Cell death leads to mucosal atrophy, ulceration, and initiation of the inflammatory response. Reactive oxygen species, proinflammatory cytokines, and metabolic byproducts of colonizing organisms may also play a role in amplifying tissue injury.[1,2] Synergy between chemotherapy and radiotherapy may increase the severity and extent of esophagitis observed with combined modality therapy. Esophagitis may also be due to pill-induced injury, acid reflux disease, and graft-versus-host disease (GVHD) in hematopoietic stem-cell transplant recipients. When esophagitis is suspected, particularly in an immunocompromised patient, prompt evaluation with endoscopy with biopsies and/or brushings is indicated to allow for early diagnosis and therapy.

Radiation-induced esophagitis

Radiation-induced esophagitis can occur during external beam radiation treatment of lung, head and neck, and esophageal cancers. Acute radiation esophagitis is primarily due to injury to the rapidly dividing cells of basal epithelial layer, which subsequently leads to thinning and denudation of esophageal mucosa. The severity of esophagitis depends on radiation dose and is exacerbated by the concurrent use of chemotherapeutic agents such as cisplatin.[3-5] Patients generally complain of odynophagia, dysphagia, and chest pain. Endoscopy findings include erythema, edema friable mucosa, ulcerations, or stricture formation. Treatment of acute esophagitis includes the use of local anesthetics such as oral viscous lidocaine hydrochloride, systemic narcotic analgesics, and acid suppression with proton pump inhibitors. Symptoms in some patients are so severe as to require temporary percutaneous gastrostomy (PEG) placement. Some patients undergoing extensive head and neck surgery and chemoradiation may benefit from PEG placement before treatment in anticipation of severe symptoms. A recent consensus statement of the Multinational Association of Supportive Care in Cancer (MASCC) and the International Society of Oral Oncology (ISOO) suggested the use of intravenous amifostine to prevent esophagitis induced by concomitant chemotherapy and radiation in patients with nonsmall cell lung cancer.[1] Esophageal strictures are treated by endoscopic dilation. In patients with tracheo-esophageal fistula due to esophageal cancer, covered stents (self-expanding metal or plastic stents) are the treatment of choice, and can achieve fistula closure in 70–100% of patients.[6]

Fungal infections

Esophageal candidiasis is very common in immunocompromised patients, with *C. albicans* being the most common causative organism for esophageal and oropharyngeal candidiasis (OPC). Patients complain of odynophagia and/or dysphagia. On endoscopy, esophageal candidiasis is identified by white plaque-like lesions with surrounding erythema on the esophageal wall. Esophageal biopsies or brushings may confirm the presence of invasive yeast or hyphal forms of *C. albicans*. An empiric course of antifungal therapy is recommended in immunocompromised patient with odynophagia or dysphagia. Endoscopy should be performed if symptoms do not improve within 72 h. The general duration of antifungal treatment is 14–21 days. Candida esophagitis in immunocompromised patients requires systemic antifungal therapy; it cannot be treated with topical agents.[7-10] Patients unable to tolerate oral agents require intravenous therapy. The treatment of esophageal candidiasis includes azoles, echinocandins, or amphotericin B.[7-15] Azoles inhibit cell membrane formation by inhibiting the synthesis of ergosterol, a principal component of fungal cell membrane. Fluconazole, an azole, is the recommended first-line agent due to its efficacy, ease of administration, and low cost. For patients with fluconazole-refractory esophageal candidiasis who can tolerate oral therapy, newer azoles (voriconazole and posaconazole) are available. Itraconazole has been found to be as effective as fluconazole for the treatment of esophageal candidiasis, however its

Holland-Frei Cancer Medicine, Ninth Edition. Edited by Robert C. Bast Jr., Carlo M. Croce, William N. Hait, Waun Ki Hong, Donald W. Kufe, Martine Piccart-Gebhart, Raphael E. Pollock, Ralph R. Weichselbaum, Hongyang Wang, and James F. Holland.
© 2017 John Wiley & Sons, Inc. ISBN: 978-1-118-93469-2

Table 1 Common causes of esophagitis in patients receiving cancer therapy.

Infectious agent/injury	Endoscopic appearance	Treatment
Candida albicans	White plaque-like lesions with surrounding erythema on the esophageal mucosa	Systemic antifungal treatment with fluconazole, itraconazole, voriconazole, or echinocandins
Herpes simples virus	Small vesicles, coalescing to form ulcers	Acyclovir and foscarnet sodium
Cytomegalovirus	Linear or serpiginous ulcers	Ganciclovir, foscarnet sodium and valganciclovir
Varicella–Zoster virus	Small vesicles, similar to HSV ulcers	Intravenous acyclovir
Polymicrobial oral flora	Bacteria mixed with necrotic epithelial cells in biopsy samples	Broad-spectrum antibiotics
Injury due to chemotherapy and radiation	Friable mucosa with erythema and edema	Lidocaine hydrochloride, narcotic analgesics, proton pump inhibitors, and endoscopic dilation/stents (for strictures), PEG[a]

[a]Percutaneous gastrostomy.

use is limited by significant nausea and by its potential for drug interactions owing to inhibition of the cytochrome p 450 enzymes.

Patients requiring intravenous therapy should be treated with fluconazole or one of the echinocandins (caspofungin, micafungin, or anidulafungin), rather than amphotericin B, because of their better toxicity profiles. Echinocandins inhibit synthesis of β(1,3)-D-glucan, an essential component of the fungal cell wall. Mammalian cells do not require β(1,3)-D-glucan, thereby limiting potential toxicity. Relapse rates are higher with echinocandins compared to azoles, and these are used as second-line therapy if treatment with azoles has failed. Amphotericin B is reserved for esophageal candidiasis during pregnancy and in individuals with drug-resistant candidiasis. OPC is a local infection. Risk factors include radiation, chemotherapy, antibiotics, and steroids. Treatment is with local agents such as nystatin or clotrimazole troches. Patients at risk of developing OPC may be given antifungal prophylaxis. Topical antifungals, such as clotrimazole or miconazole, are effective for prophylaxis.[16]

Viral infections

Viral infections of the esophagus are caused by herpes simplex virus (HSV), cytomegalovirus (CMV), and, rarely, varicella-zoster virus (VZV).[8,17] Patients usually present with odynophagia and dysphagia. Less-frequent symptoms include nausea, vomiting, heartburn, epigastric pain, and fever. In the case of HSV esophagitis, some patients may have coexistent herpes labialis or oropharyngeal ulcers. Diagnosis is made by endoscopy and biopsy (Figure 1). In the early stage, HSV lesions may appear as small vesicles, although they are rarely seen. The vesicles eventually coalesce to form large ulcers, which are usually less than 2 cm in size. The ulcers are well circumscribed with normal-appearing intervening mucosa. CMV will cause ulcers that are linear or serpiginous and deeper than HSV-related ulcers. Exudates may also be present. Biopsies taken from the edge of an HSV-related ulcer will show intranuclear inclusions and multinucleated giant cells. Inclusions can also be detected by immunohistochemistry using monoclonal antibodies to HSV. Viral cultures are helpful in identifying resistant strains in patients who do not respond to acyclovir. VZV can produce esophagitis in adults with herpes zoster, usually in the setting of disseminated infection. Endoscopically, VZV ulcers are similar to those seen with HSV. On biopsy specimens, distinction from HSV will require immunohistochemistry or culture.

CMV infects endothelial cells and fibroblasts, but not epithelial cells as with HSV and VZV. Routine biopsies in a CMV-infected patient show intranuclear inclusions in fibroblasts and endothelial cells. Immunohistochemistry with anti-CMV antibodies is also helpful for diagnosis.

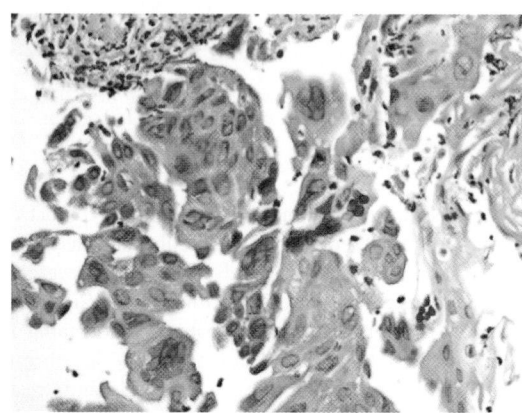

Figure 1 Herpes simplex virus (HSV) esophagitis. High-power view of esophageal mucosa shows squamous cells with ground glass nuclear viral inclusions and multinucleated giant cells in a background of neutrophilic exudates.

For patients with HSV esophagitis, acyclovir (400 mg orally five times daily for 14–21 days or 5 mg/kg intravenously every 8 h for 7–14 days) is the therapy of choice.[8,9,18,19] Acyclovir-resistant HSV result from mutations in the thymidine kinase (TK) gene of HSV. Viruses with TK mutations are generally cross-resistant to valacyclovir, but remain susceptible to agents that act directly on DNA polymerase such as foscarnet (80–120 mg/kg/day IV in 2–3 divided doses until clinical response). Cases of severe persistent infection with acyclovir-resistant HSV occur almost exclusively in immunocompromised hosts. Famciclovir or valacyclovir can be considered in patients able to tolerate oral therapy, although there is limited clinical experience with these drugs for the treatment of HSV-associated esophagitis. VZV esophagitis is initially treated with intravenous acyclovir as these patients usually have disseminated infection. After clinical improvement, treatment may be changed to oral agents used for HSV esophagitis. CMV esophagitis is treated with intravenous ganciclovir (5 mg/kg twice daily) or foscarnet sodium (68 mg/kg IV every 8 h or 90 mg/kg every 12 h) for 3–6 weeks.[8,20–22] The patient may be switched to valganciclovir 900 mg every 12 h once the patient can absorb and tolerate oral therapy. Valganciclovir is an oral precursor of ganciclovir. Valganciclovir is an oral precursor of ganciclovir. At a dose of 900 mg daily, valganciclovir produces systemic drug exposure equivalent to 5 mg/kg of intravenous ganciclovir. The role maintenance treatment after the clearance of infection is not well defined.

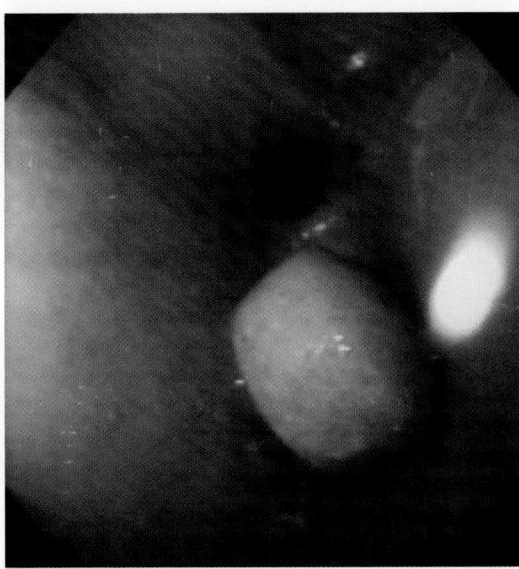

Figure 2 Pill-induced esophageal damage. A pill is seen at endoscopy lodged above an esophageal stricture.

Bacterial infections

Bacterial esophagitis can occur in the immunocompromised patient and is usually polymicrobial and derived from oral flora. The diagnosis is made by endoscopic biopsies and treatment is broad-spectrum antibiotics.

Pill-induced esophagitis

Pill-induced esophagitis can occur in patients taking medication at bedtime with insufficient liquid or in the recumbent position. The most common medications associated with this disorder include potassium chloride, tetracyclines, aspirin, nonsteroidal anti-inflammatory drugs, quinidine, iron, and alendronate. Injury is caused by prolonged contact of the caustic contents of the medication with the esophageal mucosa. Patients will often present with sudden onset of odynophagia, which may be severe enough to make even the swallowing of saliva difficult and painful. Endoscopy is helpful in making a diagnosis; but more importantly, it serves to rule out other diagnoses such as infectious esophagitis and malignancy. On endoscopy, there is usually a discrete, single ulcer located in the proximal esophagus. On occasion, the injury appears as a nodular, polypoid lesion, suggestive of a neoplasm, or as a stricture (Figure 2). Esophageal biopsies are nonspecific and may show acute inflammatory changes only. There is no specific therapy for this disorder, as pill-induced ulcerations can heal spontaneously within a few days without any intervention. Strictures will require endoscopic dilation

Malignant dysphagia

Patients with esophageal cancer often present at an advanced, incurable stage. For those who are not candidates for chemoradiation or surgery and for those who develop recurrent dysphagia after treatment, a variety of endoscopic techniques have been developed to improve esophageal luminal patency.

Esophageal dilation can be performed with through-the-scope balloons, mercury-filled rubber bougies, or wire-guided polyvinyl bougies (Savary-Gilliard dilators), but dilation, to be successful, must be repeated every few weeks and the procedure carries a risk of perforation. Self-expanding metal stents (SEMS) are used increasingly as an effective nonsurgical option for the palliation of obstructive, advanced esophageal tumors.[23–27] SEMS are made of a variety of metal alloys in different shapes and sizes to adjust to the length and position of the malignant stricture. Furthermore, approved devices are available in the uncovered, partially covered, and fully covered design. Additionally, they vary as to construction (nitinol vs surgical steel vs plastic) and function (fully patent vs "antireflux"). SEMS are placed under endoscopic guidance with or without fluoroscopy (Figure 3). Newly designed double-layered nitinol (Niti-S) stents are associated with longer survival time and fewer complications than previous designs. Once a metal stent is deployed, it cannot be removed. There have been several randomized trials comparing different stents in patients with malignant esophageal strictures.[24] Advantages of SEMS include relative ease of insertion, larger stent diameters, and low risk of perforation with elimination of the need for excessive dilation. Disadvantages include high cost, tumor ingrowth and overgrowth, stent migration, maldeployment, inadequate expansion, airway obstruction, and hemorrhage. The rate of tumor ingrowth has now been reduced with the introduction of stents covered by a polyurethane coating. Covered stents are the device of choice in the management of patients with tracheo-esophageal fistulas.[6] A recent additional option for palliation of esophageal cancer has resulted from the development of self-expanding plastic stents (SEPS). SEPS have been reported in some cases to have a higher failure rate of stent placement and higher migration rate, and to conform less easily to strictures. Stents are also effective at providing symptom relief in patients with esophageal malignancies after chemoradiation. The risk of complications, such as esophagorespiratory fistula, increases with radiation dose. Biodegradable stents, which gradually dissolve over time, are being developed. Stents have also been proposed as a bridge to surgery in those receiving neoadjuvant therapy.

Ablative techniques such as lasers, photodynamic therapy (PDT), and high-dose brachytherapy have been successfully applied for palliation of malignant esophageal obstruction, but for the most part have been supplanted by SEMS. Laser energy produced by the neodymium:yttrium-aluminum garnet crystal, or Nd:YAG, delivered endoscopically through a quartz fiber has been extensively used for the palliation of esophageal cancer in the past. This approach may require prior esophageal dilation to allow passage of the endoscope. Major complications include esophageal perforation, development of tracheo-esophageal fistula, hemorrhage, and bacteremia. Disadvantages of Nd:YAG laser therapy include difficulties in treating long, tortuous lesions or lesions located in the proximal esophagus, number of treatment sessions required, and high cost. PDT uses a photosensitizing agent and low-power laser to achieve tumor necrosis and luminal patency. Porfimer sodium (Photofrin®) is the only photosensitizer approved by the Food and Drug Administration for the treatment of esophageal cancer. Photofrin® is administered as an intravenous bolus and is selectively retained at a high concentration by neoplastic tissue. Approximately 48 h after injection, patients are exposed to monochrome laser light at 630 nm via cylindrical diffuser attached to the tip of a quartz optical fiber placed through the accessory channel of an endoscope, initiating a photochemical reaction in the tissue leading to the formation of oxygen radicals, ischemia, and tumor necrosis.

A recent Cochrane Collaboration analysis extensively reviewed 53 studies on interventions for dysphagia in esophageal cancer.[28] This analysis concluded that SEMS are safe, effective, and quicker in palliating dysphagia compared to other modalities, but that high-dose intraluminal brachytherapy is a suitable alternative and may provide additional survival benefit with a better quality of life. Combinations of brachytherapy and SEMS may reduce the need

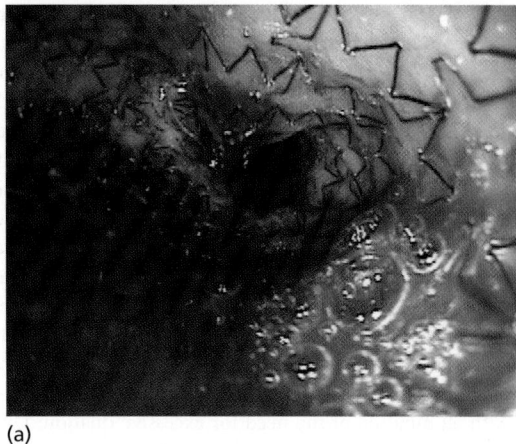 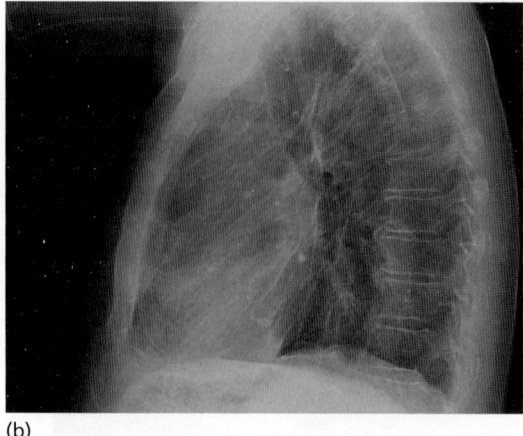

(a)   (b)

Figure 3 Self-expanding esophageal stent. (a) Endoscopic view of a self-expanding stent deployed in the esophagus for treatment of an esophageal stricture. (b) Chest radiograph showing stent deployed in the esophagus.

for reinterventions. Rigid plastic stent insertion, dilation alone or in combination with other modalities, and chemotherapy alone were not recommended for palliation of dysphagia owing to a high incidence of complications and recurrent dysphagia.

Diarrhea

Chemotherapy and radiation

Diarrhea is a common complication of cytotoxic therapy, and has been described with fluoropyrimidines (5-fluorouracil and capecitabine), irinotecan, methotrexate (MTX), and cisplatin (Table 2).[29-31] Diarrhea also commonly occurs in patients receiving small-molecule epidermal growth factor receptor-tyrosine kinase inhibitors (erlotinib and sorafenib). Diarrhea can be very debilitating and in severe cases it can lead to treatment delays, reduced quality of life, and diminished compliance. It is the dose-limiting factor and the major toxicity of regimens containing a fluoropyrimidine and/or irinotecan. The severity of chemotherapy-induced diarrhea is often described, particularly for study purposes, using the National Cancer Institute Common Toxicity Criteria (NCI CTC). Grading is based on number of stools per day, presence of nocturnal stools, and the need for parenteral support or intensive care.

The severity of diarrhea with 5-FU is increased by the addition of leucovorin. Moreover, diarrhea can be worse when 5-FU is administered by bolus injection as opposed to intravenous infusion. Irinotecan can cause an early-onset diarrhea accompanied by abdominal cramping, lacrimation, salivation, and other symptoms that appear cholinergic-mediated. The late diarrhea associated with irinotecan is unpredictable and can occur at all dose levels. It is seen less often when given in the every 3-week schedule compared to every week. Significant diarrhea has been reported with a combination of irinotecan, 5-FU, and leucovorin compared to 5-FU and leucovorin alone. Grade 1 to 2 diarrhea has been reported in up to 56% of patients receiving erlotinib, and 34% of patients taking sorafenib.[32,33]

Radiation therapy can produce injury to the GI mucosa. Symptoms typically occur during the third week of fractionated radiotherapy. Pelvic or abdominal radiation can lead to acute enteritis, characterized by abdominal cramping and diarrhea in approximately 50% of patients. These symptoms are made worse by concomitant chemotherapy.[1]

Table 2 Differential diagnosis of diarrhea in the cancer and hematopoietic cell transplant patient.

Chemotherapy-related (fluoropyrimidines, irinotecan, methotrexate, cisplatin, small-molecule epidermal growth factor receptor-tyrosine kinase inhibitors: erlotinib and sorafenib), and others
Colitis secondary to immune-modulatory agents (ipilimumab, nivolumab, lambrizumab), and others
Radiation therapy
Conditioning regimen
Graft-versus-host disease
Infection
Bacterial (including *C. difficile*)
Viral (including CMV)

Opioid agonists are the cornerstone of therapy for chemotherapy-induced diarrhea.[34] Loperamide and diphenoxylate are both widely used and are approved by the US Food and Drug Administration (FDA) for this indication. Loperamide is more effective. For mild-to-moderate diarrhea, an initial dose of 4 mg loperamide hydrochloride may be given, followed by a further 2 mg every 4 h or after every stool. Severe diarrhea often requires a more aggressive regimen, with an initial dose of 4 mg loperamide hydrochloride followed by a further 2 mg every 2 h or 4 mg every 4 h until the patient is diarrhea-free for 12 h. This high-dose loperamide has been used effectively for the control of irinotecan-induced diarrhea. Octreotide, a synthetic long-acting somatostatin analog, has been used as second-line therapy in opioid-resistant patients.[1] It decreases the secretion of vasoactive intestinal peptide, prolongs intestinal transit time, and reduces secretion of intestinal fluid and electrolytes. The recommended initial dose of octreotide is 100–150 g given subcutaneously three times per day, or 25–50 g every hour if given as an intravenous infusion. Octreotide can be titrated to higher doses (500–2500 g three times daily) for the treatment of those individuals who do not respond to lower doses.

Other drugs used as adjunctive therapy in chemotherapy or radiation-induced diarrhea include absorbents such as kaolin and charcoal, deodorized tincture of opium, paregoric, and codeine phosphate.

Because of the well-recognized risk of diarrhea associated with irinotecan, several recent studies have investigated prophylactic regimens to prevent chemotherapy-induced diarrhea. Long-acting, slow-release formulation of octreotide (octreotide LAR) can be administered by intramuscular injection once a month. Once steady-state levels have been achieved, a 20-mg intramuscular dose of octreotide LAR every 4 weeks produces the same pharmacologic effects as 150 μg octreotide tid by SC injection and dramatically reduces fluctuations in peak and trough octreotide concentrations. Additionally, octreotide LAR (at a starting dose of 20 mg) effectively controls diarrhea associated with carcinoid syndrome,[31] and monthly doses of 20–30 mg are currently being investigated for the treatment and prevention of chemotherapy-induced diarrhea.

For patients undergoing hematopoietic stem-cell transplantation (HCT), diarrhea may be due to the conditioning regimen (total body irradiation and/or high-dose chemotherapy). Pretransplant conditioning regimens can injure the GI mucosa, causing secretory diarrhea that resolves after mucosal restitution. After day 20, acute GVHD is the most common cause of diarrhea in these patients. GVHD will be discussed separately.

Clostridium difficile-associated diarrhea

If diarrhea is not directly the result of chemotherapy or radiation and particularly if it occurs in a hospital setting, *Clostridium difficile* infection should be considered as this is the most common cause of infectious diarrhea in hospitalized patients. Although commonly associated with use of antibiotic therapy, risk factors for *C. difficile* diarrhea or colitis also include bowel surgery, immunocompromised state, and any process that suppresses the normal flora including antifungal and chemotherapeutic agents. Cancer patients receiving chemotherapy appear predisposed to *C. difficile*-induced diarrhea even in the absence of antibiotics. In a study of such patients, MTX, doxorubicin, and cyclophosphamide were the drugs most frequently associated with *C. difficile* infection. Clinical presentation may vary from mild diarrhea without colitis, colitis with systemic manifestations, pseudomembranous colitis with or without protein-losing enteropathy, and fulminant colitis with development of toxic megacolon. Diagnostic testing for *C. difficile* has rapidly evolved.[35] Previously rapid EIA tests for toxin A or B were the most widely used diagnostic tests. These tests have a sensitivity of 75–95% and specificity of 83–98%. Two major advances in the laboratory diagnosis of *C. difficile* are the use of glutamate dehydrogenase (GDH; an enzyme produced by *C. difficile*), detection in stool (75% to >90% sensitivity with a negative predictive value of close to 100%), and nucleic acid amplification

tests (PCR) for toxin genes. Endoscopically, pseudomembranes can be seen as adherent yellow plaques that vary in diameter from 2 to 10 mm (Figure 4). The rectum and sigmoid colon are typically involved, but in approximately 10% of cases, colitis is only present in the more proximal colon and can be missed during sigmoidoscopy.

Therapy for *C. difficile diarrhea* depends on disease severity.[35] Standard therapy for *C. difficile*-associated diarrhea is oral metronidazole or oral vancomycin. Metronidazole at a dose of 500 mg three times daily either orally or intravenously for 10–14 days is as effective as oral vancomycin given at a dose of 125 mg four times daily. The lower dose of vancomycin 125 mg four times a day is as effective as the higher dose of 250 mg four times a day in mild-to-moderate case and is much less expensive. Metronidazole has some advantages over vancomycin including its lower cost and the observation that it can reduce selection of vancomycin-resistant enterococci (VRE). Metronidazole is therefore the initial therapy of choice in nonsevere cases of *C. difficile*-induced diarrhea. If there is no improvement in 3 days, treatment with vancomycin should be initiated. In patients with severe *C. difficile* infection and signs of systemic toxicity, the recommended treatment regimen is initial therapy with vancomycin 125 mg orally four times daily, with dose escalation at 48 h intervals up to 500 mg four times daily if patients fail to improve. If patients do not respond to oral vancomycin, the addition of intravenous metronidazole 500 mg every 8 h, or vancomycin retention enemas (0.5–1 g of vancomycin dissolved in 1–2 L of normal saline every 4–12 h), should be considered. The use of antiperistaltic agents is not recommended as they may obscure symptoms and there is evidence that decreased transit time can lead to complications and lengthen the duration of illness. Relapse of CDI is common, occurring in up to 10–25% of all patients with CDI. Relapses usually occur within 1–3 weeks after termination of initial therapy, and are probably caused by failure to eradicate the organism rather than development of antibiotic resistance. These patients are likely to relapse repeatedly. First relapses should be treated with a second 10–14-day course of oral metronidazole or vancomycin. If a patient relapses after taking a second course of antibiotics, different approaches have been suggested, including tapered or pulsed antibiotic therapy, longer duration of treatment (several weeks), and the use of toxin-binding resins such as colestyramine or colestipol hydrochloride alone or in combination with vancomycin. Fidaxomicin is an alternative agent

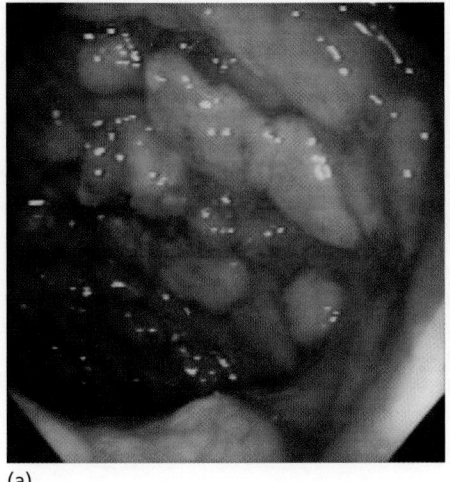
(a)

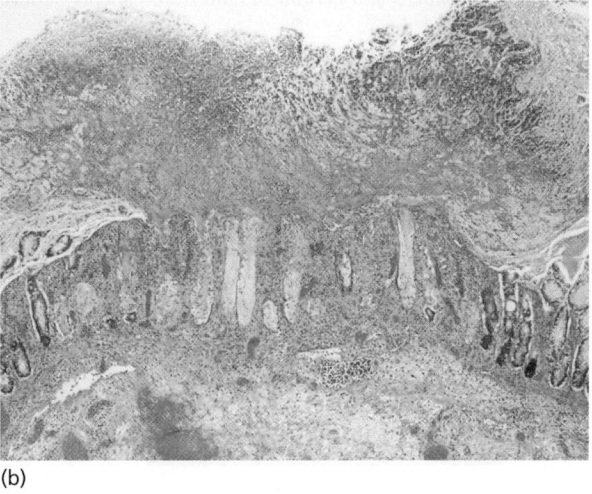
(b)

Figure 4 Pseudomembranous colitis. (a) Pseudomembranes adherent to the colonic mucosa seen at colonoscopy. (b) Low-power view of colonic mucosa shows a typical volcano (mushroom)-like appearance with luminal inflammatory exudates.

for treatment of an initial recurrence of CDI. For treatment of initial recurrence of CDI, the initial response to therapy with fidaxomicin and vancomycin is comparable, but the likelihood of subsequent recurrence is lower with fidaxomicin than vancomycin (20% vs 36%). If there is a third recurrence, fecal microbiota transplant should be considered. In small series, 2 weeks of vancomycin followed by 2 weeks of rifaximin has proven successful in controlling recurrent disease. A recent study used two neutralizing, human monoclonal antibodies against *C. difficile* toxins A (CDA1) and B (CDB1) in 101 symptomatic patients who were receiving either metronidazole or vancomycin, and the rate of recurrence of *C. difficile* infection was significantly lower among patients treated with the monoclonal antibodies.[36]

Other infectious diarrhea

In the posthematopoietic cell transplant patient, infectious diarrhea is relatively uncommon. Viruses are the most common organisms found (astrovirus, adenovirus, CMV, and rotavirus), followed by nosocomially acquired bacteria (*C. difficile* and Aeromonas). CMV deserves a special mention as it can cause diarrhea and bleeding because of mucosal ulceration. The diagnosis of CMV is made by endoscopic biopsy (Figure 5); specimens should be sent for immunohistochemistry and viral culture. Infectious diarrhea related to *Salmonella*, *Shigella*, and *Campylobacter* species are very rare in hospitalized transplant patients. Diarrhea related to parasites (*Cryptosporidium*, *Giardia lamblia*, and *Entamoeba histolytica*) is also a rare cause of diarrhea; most of these patients are infected pretransplantation.

Colitis

Neutropenic enterocolitis

Neutropenic enterocolitis is characterized by fever and right lower quadrant pain in neutropenic patients. It is seen in children and adults with hematologic malignancies, aplastic anemia, and after myelosuppressive therapy for solid malignancies.[37–42] Histologic examination of biopsy samples from patients with neutropenic enterocolitis is characterized by a thickened bowel wall, edema, mucosal ulcerations, focal hemorrhage, and mucosal or transmural necrosis. Numerous bacterial and/or fungal organisms have been identified in surgical specimens and peritoneal fluid from patients

with neutropenic enterocolitis, A diagnosis of neutropenic enterocolitis is usually established by computerized tomography (CT). Abnormal findings on CT and ultrasound include a fluid-filled, dilated cecum, a right lower quadrant inflammatory mass and pericecal fluid, or inflammatory changes in the pericecal soft tissues Treatment consists of bowel rest, intravenous fluids, and broad-spectrum antibiotics. Cytopenias and coagulopathy associated with oncologic treatment should be corrected as neutropenia contributes to the pathogenesis of the disease, and coagulopathy can be associated with blood loss from mucosal hemorrhage. Recombinant granulocyte colony-stimulating factor (G-CSF) may be used to hasten leukocyte recovery, which contributes to the resolution of neutropenic enterocolitis. Surgery has been recommended for patients with persistent GI bleeding despite correction of cytopenias and coagulopathy, and for patients with perforation or clinical deterioration despite pharmacologic therapy.

Colitis secondary to immune-modulatory, antineoplastic agents

Immune-modulatory agents enhance tumor-directed immune responses through modification of immune checkpoint pathways, T-cell stimulatory pathways, or with adoptive cell therapy.[43] However, this approach has also been associated with intestinal adverse effects, in particular with therapeutic agents targeting immune checkpoint pathways (i.e., cytotoxic T-lymphocyte antigen-4 (CTLA-4) and PD-1). CTLA-4 is a key negative regulator of T-cell activation in the adaptive immune response. Transient, antibody-mediated CTLA-4 inhibition has been shown to enhance T-cell response. Ipilimumab and tremelimumab are fully humanized, monoclonal IgG1 antibodies targeted against CTLA-4. While the GI adverse effect profile of tremelimumab was similar to ipilimumab, tremelimumab had no survival benefit over chemotherapy for melanoma in a recent randomized controlled phase III trial.[44] CTLA-4 inhibitors have predominantly been used for melanoma although they have also been evaluated in other solid malignancies such as pancreatic carcinoma, prostate carcinoma, renal cell, ovarian, and small-cell lung cancer.[45,46] Given the regulatory role of inhibitors such as CTLA-4 and PD-1 in adaptive immune response, they have a broad spectrum of immune-mediated Adverse Events (imAE) including enterocolitis, hepatitis, dermatitis, hypophysitis, uveitis, and nephritis; enterocolitis is the most common adverse event.[47] The majority of immune-related adverse events have been observed during the induction and reinduction periods.[46] The development of ipilimumab-associated enterocolitis is independent

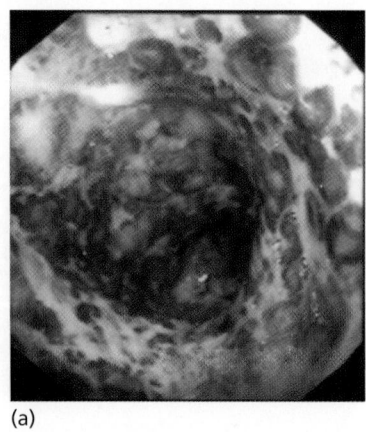
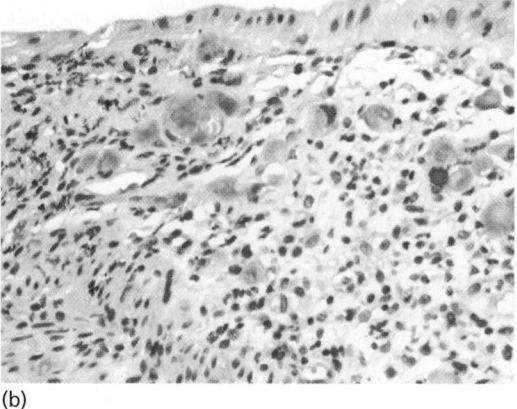

(a)   (b)

Figure 5 Cytomegalovirus (CMV) colitis. (a) CMV colitis as seen at endoscopy. (b) High-power view of inflamed colonic mucosa demonstrates multiple viral inclusions in stroma cells.

of the number of cycles, but appears to be dose dependent.[47,48] There is some evidence that the development of enterocolitis might be a positive predictor for tumor response in patients with melanoma and renal cell cancer treated with ipilimumab.[47] Enterocolitis most commonly presents with diarrhea but abdominal pain, nausea/vomiting, fever, anal pain, and constipation have been reported as well.[5] The majority of patients who develop enterocolitis do so within 21 days following their last dose.[47] Overall, up to 33–51% of ipilimumab-treated patients experience diarrhea, including 16% with grade 3 and <1% with grade 4.[44–46,48] Intraluminally, the colon is particularly involved with up to 8% of patients developing colitis, including 4–5% and 0–1% with grade 3 and 4 colitis.[45,46] Diarrhea is usually watery with few leukocytes and only rarely positive for blood.[49] Radiologically, ipilimumab-associated colitis is characterized by mesenteric vessel engorgement, colonic wall thickening, mucosal enhancement, and fluid-filled colonic distension. Colitis can either develop diffusely or as segmental colitis associated with diverticulosis (SCAD). While panenteritis has been described, the colon is the most commonly involved area.[49,50] Endoscopic presentation of ipilimumab-associated colitis is unspecific and severity dependent showing macroscopic findings such as mucosal erythema, friability, edema, and ulcerations.[47] In the majority of patients, histologic findings include neutrophilic inflammation with cryptitis and occasional crypt abscesses, or a mixed neutrophilic–lymphocytic inflammatory picture. In few patients, lymphocytic predominant inflammation is seen with increased numbers of CD8+ T-cells in crypts and CD4+ cells in the lamina propria.[47,49] 0.7–6.6% of ipilimumab-treated patients develop colonic perforation or require colectomy.[5] Mortality of patients developing enterocolitis secondary to ipilimumab treatment has been reported as high as 5%.[47] Treatment of ipilimumab-associated adverse events is guided by severity (Table 3), but other etiologies need to be ruled out.[51] Mild GI symptoms can be treated symptomatically without discontinuation of ipilimumab; however, frequent reassessment is imperative to identify the development of more severe symptoms or life-threatening complications. In cases of moderate enterocolitis, ipilimumab should be withheld and can be restarted 7 days after significant symptom-improvement or -resolution. If moderate symptoms persist after 7 days, initiation of treatment with systemic corticosteroids is recommended (e.g., 0.5 mg/kg/d prednisone or equivalent) until improvement to

mild symptoms or symptom-resolution is observed. Once symptoms are mild and corticosteroid dose has been tapered to ≤7.5 mg daily, ipilimumab can be resumed. Severe enterocolitis and life-threatening complications require permanent discontinuation of ipilimumab. In these cases, systemic corticosteroids should be administered (e.g., 1–2 mg/kg/d prednisone or equivalent) once intestinal perforation is ruled out.[51] In corticosteroid-refractory cases, the successful use of infliximab has been reported in a limited number of patients.[47,52,53] Prophylactic initiation of budesonide concurrent with ipilimumab did not significantly decrease rates of diarrhea or colitis.[54,55] Programmed cell death protein-1 (PD-1) is a receptor expressed on T-cells, which attenuates T-cell activation upon binding of its ligands PD-L1 (B7-H1) and PD-L2 (B7-DC). While PD-L2 is frequently expressed by APC, PD-L1 overexpression has been observed in tumors.[43,56] Nivolumab and lambrizumab are PD-1-targeted, humanized monoclonal IgG4 antibodies currently evaluated in ongoing or planned randomized controlled phase II and III trials.[43] In a recent nonrandomized controlled trial, the most common GI adverse event in patients treated with Nivolumab was diarrhea with an incidence of 18%, with grade 3–4 diarrhea in 2%. Other GI adverse events included nausea, vomiting, abdominal pain, and dry mouth observed in 5–8% of patients.[15] Rates of GI adverse events were not considerably higher with nivolumab/ipilimumab combination therapy compared to monotherapy.[57] In two clinical trials including 173 and 135 patients, lambrizumab-associated diarrhea was observed in only 1–20%.[56,58] Given the novelty of these agents, there is currently insufficient experience in regard to optimal management, but a severity-guided, conservative approach similar to ipilimumab-induced enterocolitis has been proposed.[43]

Radiation-induced proctitis and colitis
Patients receiving radiation therapy to the abdomen and pelvis for the treatment of gynecologic, genitourinary, GI, and other malignancies are at risk of developing acute or chronic intestinal injury. Acute radiation injury in the rectum and distal colon usually occurs within 6 weeks of therapy and is characterized by diarrhea (see above), rectal urgency, tenesmus, and, occasionally, rectal bleeding. These symptoms usually resolve within 6 months without the need for therapy. Chronic radiation proctitis or coloproctitis has a delayed onset, occurring approximately 1 year or later after

Table 3 Management of ipilimumab-induced enterocolitis.

Severity	Definition	Management	Advanced management
Mild		• Continue ipilimumab • Symptomatic management	*If progression in symptom severity:* See below
Moderate	• 4–6 stools/day over baseline • Abdominal pain • Blood or mucus in stool	• Hold ipilimumab • Symptomatic management • Consider endoscopic evaluation	*If no resolution after 7 days:* • systemic corticosteroids (0.5 mg/kg/d or equivalent) • Resume ipilimumab once symptoms have improved to mild PLUS corticosteroids ≤7.5 mg/d. *If progression to severe symptoms:* See below
Severe or life threatening	• ≥7 stools/d over baseline • Peritoneal signs • Ileus • Fever	• Discontinue ipilimumab • permanently • Consider endoscopic evaluation • Systemic corticosteroids (1–2 mg/kg/d or equivalent)	*Ongoing symptoms:* • Continuous evaluation for perforation or peritonitis • Consider repeat endoscopy • Consider alternative immunosuppressive therapy (e.g., infliximab)

Source: Adapted from Gangadhar TC, Vonderheide 2014[43] with data from Squibb 2011.[51] Reproduced by permission of Macmillan Publishers Ltd.

exposure to radiation. It is caused by obliterative endarteritis and chronic mucosal ischemia, resulting in epithelial atrophy and fibrosis. It may end in stricture formation and bleeding within the colon and rectum. Patients with radiation proctitis often present with diarrhea, bleeding, tenesmus, urgency, difficulties with defecation, and less commonly fecal incontinence.

The diagnosis of radiation proctitis is made by colonoscopy or sigmoidoscopy. Endoscopic findings include mucosal edema, erythema, friability, and the presence of telangiectasias. In severe cases, mucosal ulcerations and strictures can be observed.

Treatment for radiation proctitis depends on symptoms.[1] In some studies sucralfate enemas have been used to treat chronic radiation-induced proctitis but may increase the risk of rectal bleeding, other treatments that have shown some benefit in small clinical trials include hyperbaric oxygen and short-chain fatty acid enemas. Various thermal endoscopic therapies have also been used successfully to treat bleeding associated with radiation proctitis and include argon plasma coagulation (APC). Surgery should be considered for patients with intractable symptoms such as strictures, pain, or bleeding. A detailed discussion of the endoscopic and surgical treatment of radiation proctitis is beyond the scope of this review. The selection of treatment for radiation proctitis should be based on the type and severity of symptoms as well as local expertise. Intravenous amifostine has been recommended at a dose of >340 mg/m^2 to prevent radiation proctitis in patients receiving radiation therapy.[1]

Intestinal manifestations of graft-versus-host disease

The use and indications of allogenic hematopoietic cell transplantation (HCT) have significantly increased throughout the past decades with approximately 25,000 procedures per year.[59] The main complication of HCT is GVHD with GI involvement in 54% of those undergoing transplantation.[60,61] GVHD occurs as a response of donor T cells to genetically defined recipient cell surface proteins. Human leukocyte antigens (HLAs) are class I HLA (A, B, and C) and class II (DR, DQ, and DP) proteins. The former are expressed by all nucleated cells, while the latter are predominantly expressed by hematopoietic cells; however, HLA class II protein can also be expressed by other cell types in the setting of inflammation and injury. HLA class I and II mismatch is positively correlated with the frequency of acute GVHD.[62,63] However, HLA-matched patients can still develop GVHD owing to individual differences in ubiquitously expressed minor histocompatibility antigens (i.e., HY and HA-1).[64–66] Interestingly, incidence rates of acute GVHD following mismatched umbilical cord-derived HCT are similar to rates of matched bone marrow-derived HCT, but incidence rates of chronic GVHD are higher after peripheral stem cell versus bone marrow stem-cell transplant with 53% versus 41% incident reported.[67,68] Autologous GVHD is a distinct entity describing an autoimmune GVHD-like syndrome that develops after autologous stem-cell transplant, and has been associated with drugs such as cyclosporine and alemtuzumab.[69,70]

On the basis of its chronologic correlation to the time of cell transplantation, GVHD has been classified as acute (≤100 days post-transplant) or chronic (>100 days post-transplant). The latter form can be an extension of acute GVHD, reoccurrence of a successfully treated acute form, or can occur *de novo*. However, this classification has been found inaccurate owing to changes in condition regimens, resulting in later onset of acute GVHD and overlap syndromes.[59,71] Therefore, an expert panel has suggested a new classification for GVHD (Table 4).[73]

Table 4 Modified classification of acute and chronic graft-versus-host disease (GVHD).

Categories	Time of symptom onset post-HCT	Presence of acute GVHD features	Presence of chronic GVHD features
Acute GVHD:			
Classic acute GVHD	≤100 days	Yes	No
Persistent, recurrent, or late-onset acute GVHD	>100 days	Yes	No
Chronic GVHD:			
Classic chronic GVHD	No time limit	No	Yes
Overlap syndrome	No time limit	Yes	Yes

Source: Filipovich AH, Weisdorf D, Pavletic S, Socie G, Wingard JR, et al. 2005.[72] Reproduced with permission from Elsevier.

Acute GVHD

The most common presentation of acute GVHD is high-volume, secretory diarrhea. GI hemorrhage has been associated with a poor prognosis; it can be indicative of mucosal ulceration in the setting of GVHD but other causes have to be considered.[74,75] GVHD-associated diarrhea has been described as an exudative, protein-losing enteropathy; however, sensitivity and specificity of fecal α1-antitrypsin in the diagnosis of stage 2–3 GI-GVHD are only 79% and 62%, respectively.[76] Occasionally GI-GVHD can also result in pancreatic insufficiency, thereby potentially contributing to diarrhea. Other common GVHD-associated symptoms include anorexia, nausea, vomiting, abdominal pain, and ileus. The absence of such symptoms does not exclude the presence of GVHD, and the differential diagnoses for these symptoms are broad in HCT patients, given the aggressive conditioning regimens, their multidrug use, and their susceptibility to infections owing to severe neutropenia following HCT. Hence, a high level of suspicion is required. On physical examination, sequelae of GVHD manifestations and complications should be assessed such as cutaneous GVHD, dehydration and weight loss, and failure to thrive. Occasionally, patients can develop ascites. Oropharyngeal manifestations of GVHD can include gingivitis, mucositis, and erythema.[72] Radiologic features of intestinal GVHD include bowel wall thickening, intestinal dilatation, mucosal enhancement, and gastric wall thickening. Diffuse small bowel wall thickening has been associated with worse prognosis, and any colon involvement on CT correlates with GVHD severity.[77,78] Radiologic findings do not significantly differ between acute and late-onset GVHD.[79] Endoscopic findings in GVHD include a spectrum from mild erythema to mucosal edema and diffuse mucosal loss. In particular, mucosal sloughing has been reported to be highly specific.[80] While endoscopy has been shown to be highly predictive for the diagnosis of GVHD, approximately one-fifth of patients with histologically confirmed GVHD have no significant macroscopic findings on endoscopic evaluation.[81] Therefore, a tissue diagnosis is usually required in the diagnosis of acute GVHD. Typical histologic findings include crypt epithelial cell apoptosis, crypt destruction ("exploding crypt cells"), and variable lymphocytic infiltration of the epithelium and lamina propria (Figure 6). Importantly, similar findings can also be observed in the absence of GVHD within the immediate post-transplant period secondary to pretransplant regimens. However, non-GVHD-related histologic changes have usually resolved 20 days after transplant.[24] Other differential diagnoses that need to be excluded in the evaluation of GVHD-like symptoms and histologic findings include infectious etiologies (i.e., CMV and cryptosporidium) and iatrogenic adverse effects (i.e., mycophenolate mofetil and proton pump inhibitors). Histologically, GI-GVHD has historically been classified as grades 1–4

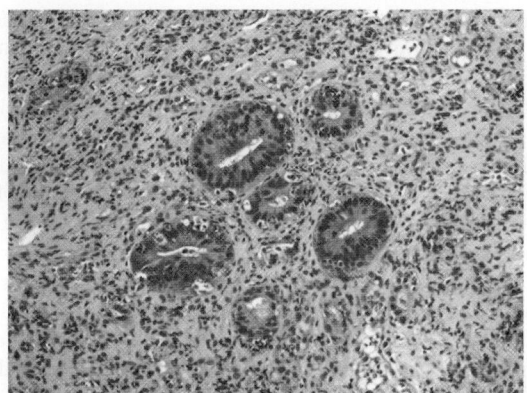

Figure 6 Graft-versus-host disease involving the colon. The colonic mucosa shows prominent crypt apoptosis and focal crypt dropouts in a background of granulation tissue.

based on severity.[71] Controversies around endoscopic evaluation include the extent of endoscopic evaluation. Discordance between upper intestinal biopsies and rectal biopsies has been reported in up to 45% of patients with GI-GVHD. Symptoms are not predictive of site of involvement. While some studies suggested that rectal biopsies are sufficient, other studies reported gastric biopsies as providing higher yields in diagnosing GI-GVHD. Distal colonic evaluation is frequently sufficient and associated with lower complication rates than colonoscopy.[82] Reduced-intensity conditioning regimens were effective in reducing tissue injury and were shown to delay onset of acute GVHD to >100 days but have been associated with higher rates of relapse in some patients.[83,84] The mainstay of GVHD prevention is pharmacologic calcineurin inhibition (i.e., cyclosporine, tacrolimus, or sirolimus) in combination with other immunosuppressants (i.e., MTX or mycophenolate mofetil) in the early post-transplant phase[85,86]; however, a recent Cochrane database analysis concluded that high-quality RCTs are needed to define the optimal GVHD prevention strategy.[87] Frequently, patients who develop acute GVHD on calcineurin-inhibitor prophylaxis do so in the second month after transplant. Any form of visceral GVHD requires high-dose corticosteroid treatment, which results in resolution of acute GVHD in up to 60%.[1,2,31] For cases with corticosteroid-refractory cases of GVHD, therapeutic strategies such as extracorporeal photopheresis and anti-TNFα agents (e.g., etanercept) have been evaluated, but further studies are required.[59] In addition to immunosuppressive therapy, supportive management such as infection prophylaxis, rehydration, and nutritional supplementation is required.

Chronic GVHD

The prevalence of chronic GVHD in long-term survivors of HCT is >50%.[73] It is the major cause of late nonrelapse mortality in HCT patients.[59] Risk factors associated with its development include age, prior acute GVHD, time from transplantation to chronic GVHD, donor type, disease status at transplantation, GVHD prophylaxis, and gender mismatch.[88] Unfortunately, the pathomechanisms, diagnostic criteria, and optimal management are poorly understood. Recently, the National Institute of Health (NIH) developed several consensus documents on criteria for clinical trials in chronic GVHD.[72] In this chapter, the diagnosis is based on diagnostic signs of chronic GVHD, or distinctive signs (defined as manifestations not typical for acute GVHD but not sufficient to establish the diagnosis of chronic GVHD without further testing) with confirmation by biopsy, laboratory test, or radiology. Similar to acute GVHD, chronic GVHD can manifest as anorexia,

nausea, vomiting, diarrhea, weight loss, and failure to thrive.[72] Oropharyngeal manifestations of chronic GVHD include lichen planus-like changes, hyperkeratotic plaques, xerostomia, mucosal atrophy, mucoceles, pseudomembranes, and ulcers. Esophageal findings can include esophageal webs, strictures, and concentric rings. Other findings include mucosal erythema, edema, and erosions. Histologic evaluation can also show epithelial apoptosis and crypt cell loss, but these changes are not specific, and, therefore, not considered diagnostic for chronic GVHD. Supportive care is one of the key elements in the management of chronic GVHD. Patients need to be monitored for infectious complications. Oropharyngeal lesions in HCT patients developing 3 years after transplant should be evaluated for squamous cell carcinoma and other secondary malignancies. Similarly, patients with dysphagia and odynophagia need to be evaluated for other etiologies such as pill or radiation esophagitis and viral esophagitis. Dysphagia due to strictures can be managed by careful endoscopic dilatation; unfortunately, studies regarding perforation rates are lacking. Patients with diarrhea need to be evaluated for infectious etiologies, malabsorption, pancreatic insufficiency, and nutritional deficiencies. Forty-three percent of patients with chronic GVHD are malnourished and 14% severely malnourished; therefore, nutritional assessment and support should be provided.[89,90] A key element in the treatment of chronic GVHD is immunosuppression. Topical corticosteroids can be attempted (i.e., budesonide and beclomethasone) in mild cases of chronic GVHD.[91,92] However, moderate or severe chronic GVHD and GVHD of nonaccessible areas require systemic corticosteroids usually at a dose of 1 mg/kg/day for 2 weeks followed by a 6–8 weeks taper; patients should be thoroughly reassessed at 3 months to decide on further tapering versus maintenance or second-line therapy.[93]

Hepatic complications of cancer treatment

Chemotherapy-associated liver injury is an unfortunate consequence of the treatment of many cancers. Consequently it is important to assess liver function carefully before and during therapy (Tables 5, 6).

Effect of pre-existing liver disease on cancer therapy

Pre-existing liver disease can not only affect the choice of therapeutic options, but for drugs that are metabolized by the liver, necessitate dosage modification. Measurement of hepatic enzymes, commonly referred to as "liver function tests," does not assess functional capacity of the liver. They are sensitive indicators of acute liver injury but do not measure the liver's ability to metabolize drugs or synthesize important proteins. The albumin and bilirubin concentrations are surrogate markers of the liver's synthetic and biotransformation potential, but are influenced by external factors limiting their sensitivity and specificity. Consequently, a reliable assessment of liver function should not be based on a simple profile of a few laboratory tests, but a composite picture based on clinical, laboratory, and radiographic data. In addition, none of the frequently used hepatic laboratory tests can accurately assess hepatic fibrosis. Common hepatic disorders, such as nonalcoholic fatty liver disease, can progress silently to cirrhosis with normal or minimally elevated transaminases and bilirubin. The only evidence for chronic liver disease might be evidence of portal hypertension on the physical exam or nodularity of the liver on imaging studies.

For some drugs, published guidelines describe usage restrictions and dosing on the basis of readily available hepatic serologic tests.

Table 5 Causes of hepatic abnormalities in cancer patients.

Pre-existing liver disease
Viral hepatitis
Nonalcoholic fatty liver disease
Alcoholic liver disease
Hemochromatosis
Autoimmune hepatitis
Wilson disease
Celiac disease
Alpha-1-antitrypsin deficiency
Direct effects of the tumor
Hepatic metastases
Portal vein thrombosis
Biliary obstruction
Indirect effects of the tumor
Paraneoplastic syndromes
Causes of liver disease during cancer treatment
Drug-induced liver disease
Graft-versus-host disease (acute and chronic)
Sinusoidal obstruction syndrome
Viral hepatitis
Sepsis-induced cholestasis
Ischemic liver injury
TPN
Liver disease affected by cancer treatment
Hepatitis B
Nonalcoholic fatty liver disease
Autoimmune hepatitis

Table 6 Differential diagnosis of hepatic biochemical tests abnormalities associated with cancer therapy.

	AST/ALT	Alkaline phosphatase	Bilirubin
Drug-induced liver disease	2–10× ULN	2–10× ULN	2–20× ULN
Viral hepatitis	2–10× ULN	2–3× ULN	2–10× ULN
Sinusoidal obstruction syndrome	2–5× ULN	2–3× ULN	2–10× ULN
Graft-versus-host disease	2–5× ULN	2–10× ULN	2–20× ULN

Abbreviations: AST, aspartate aminotransferase; ALT, alanine aminotransferase; and ULN, upper limit of normal.

However, for many therapeutic agents, the clinician must use subjective data on which to design a treatment regimen. Many treatment protocols require dosage modification based on the bilirubin concentration, but relying on the bilirubin concentration alone can be misleading. Gilbert's syndrome, a benign disorder of bilirubin metabolism, can spuriously raise the total bilirubin concentration leading to an inappropriate modification of a treatment regimen.

Up to 30% of patients undergoing cancer therapy have evidence of pre-existing liver disease, with nonalcoholic fatty liver the most common. Many drugs can exacerbate fat deposition in the liver. The most common are hormonal therapies used to treat breast cancer and prostate cancer. Hepatic steatosis develops in up to one-third of women treated with tamoxifen but it is usually asymptomatic and not associated with progressive liver disease.[94] Antiantigen therapy for prostate cancer can exacerbate components of the metabolic syndrome, resulting in accelerated hepatic steatosis.[95]

Chemotherapy or chemoradiation can lead to reactivation of underlying hepatitis B caused by intensification of the immune response to the hepatitis B virus (HBV) when immunosuppressive therapy is withdrawn. While HBV reactivation can occur with any chemotherapy regimen, the risk is highest with anti-CD20 monoclonal antibodies (rituximab and ofatumumab).[96] Reactivation can occur in patients with inapparent hepatitis B infection manifested only by a positive core antibody (anti-HBc) in the absence of detectable surface antigen (HBsAg). In one report, 5 of 21 HBsAg negative/anti-HBc positive patients receiving rituximab developed reactivation.[97] Several major societies have published guidelines for the evaluation and treatment of HBV infection in patients undergoing cancer treatment.[98–100] Most recommend prophylactic antiviral therapy at the onset of cancer treatment and for at least 6 months after completion of therapy. Lamivudine can be used in patients with no detectable HBV DNA and with a short duration of immunosuppression (<12 months).[101] Because of potential viral resistance, tenofovir or entecavir should be used when there is detectable HBV DNA or when anticipated therapy is greater than 1 year.[102]

Patients with underlying hepatitis C appear to respond differently to chemotherapy compared to those with hepatitis B.[103] Modest increases in transaminase and HCV RNA levels develop in approximately half of HCV infected patients, but a severe hepatitis flare is rare. Consequently, dose modification is usually not indicated. Effective oral antiviral regimens for the treatment of HCV that do not require interferon suggest that many more patients with HCV infection who are undergoing cancer therapy will become candidates for antiviral treatment.

Hepatotoxicity caused by cancer therapy

Adverse drug reactions occur commonly in patients undergoing cancer treatment. Recognizing hepatotoxicity can be challenging as this population of patients is frequently on multiple medications and there can be many potential causes of abnormal liver including tumor progression, systemic infection, or parenteral nutrition.

Most hepatotoxic reactions are idiosyncratic and caused by either metabolic disruption or an immunologic reaction to the drug or one of its metabolites.[104] Typically these reactions occur in patients without underlying liver disease and resolve when the drug is discontinued without significant fibrosis or impaired synthetic function. With more severe drug toxicity, often manifested by elevations in the serum bilirubin, the offending agent has to be discontinued even when therapeutic alternatives may be limited.

The antimetabolites commonly used in cancer therapy include cytosine arabinoside (Ara-C), 5-FU, 6-mercaptopurine (6-MP), azathioprine, 6-thioguanine, and MTX. Hepatic metabolism plays an important role in the processing of these drugs, and dose reductions are usually necessary in patients with liver dysfunction. Ara-C, used in the treatment of acute myelogenous leukemia (AML), has on rare occasions been associated with cholestasis, which appears reversible.[105] Intra-arterial administration of the 5-FU metabolite floxuridine (fluorodeoxyuridine [FudR]) has been associated with two types of toxicity: one suggestive of hepatocellular injury and the second one consistent with sclerosing cholangitis, with stricturing of the intra and extrahepatic bile ducts, and elevations of alkaline phosphatase and bilirubin.[106–108]

Combinations of 5-FU and oxaliplatin or irinotecan are used for neoadjuvant therapy in patients with colorectal cancer before the resection of liver metastases. These neoadjuvant regimens, particularly those with oxaliplatin, have been associated with steatosis and injury to the hepatic vasculature causing a disorder with features of chronic sinusoidal obstruction syndrome (SOS).[109–112]

6-MP is often used for maintenance therapy in acute lymphoblastic leukemia (ALL). Two patterns of toxicity have been reported: hepatocellular injury and cholestasis.[113] Toxicity occurs more commonly when the daily dose of 2 mg/kg is exceeded. Azathioprine is a nitroimidazole derivative of 6-MP. Its toxicity is less frequent and less dose dependent compared with 6-MP. Three different patterns of toxicity are described: a hypersensitivity reaction, a cholestatic reaction, and endothelial cell injury with development of elevated portal pressures, SOS, and peliosis hepatis.[114]

High-dose MTX therapy has been associated with reversible elevations in aminotransferases.[115] Patients taking chronic low-dose MTX therapy for psoriasis or rheumatoid arthritis are at risk for developing hepatic fibrosis and cirrhosis. The risk is low in patients who receive less than 1.5 g of MTX as cumulative dose.[116]

Alkylating agents uncommonly cause hepatotoxicity. With the exception of cyclophosphamide and ifosfamide, patients receiving alkylating agents do not require dose reduction. Temozolomide, an alkylating agent used to treat brain tumors, has caused severe hepatotoxicity, prompting an FDA recommendation for monitoring hepatic enzymes throughout the course of therapy.[117]

Other alkylating agents (including melphalan, chlorambucil, nitrogen mustard, and busulfan) are not dependent on the liver for their metabolism and are not frequently associated with hepatotoxicity.

The antitumor antibiotics include doxorubicin and daunorubicin. Doxorubicin can cause hepatocellular injury and steatosis. Dose reduction has been recommended in patients with cholestasis to avoid greater toxicity.[118] Similar guidelines are followed for daunorubicin.

Asparaginase, used to treat acute lymphocytic leukemia, causes a form of mitochondrial injury in the liver, particularly in those with underlying fatty liver disease. Some patients with asparaginase liver injury respond to carnitine.[119] The breakdown of asparagine can also cause hyperammonemia.[120]

Many of the molecularly targeted kinase inhibitors are metabolized in the liver and require dose adjustment in patients with underlying liver disease. Lapatinib, a dual inhibitor of both human epidermal growth factor receptor 2 and EGFR, causes hepatotoxicity in approximately half of the patients receiving the drug with several reports of potentially fatal reactions.[121] The presence of certain HLA alleles is associated with an increased risk for hepatotoxicity.[122] Pazopanib targets multiple tyrosine kinases and causes a severe hepatitis in approximately 20% of patients.[123] It is also associated with a more benign form of hyperbilirubinemia in individuals with underlying Gilbert's syndrome.[124]

Checkpoint inhibitors are immunomodulatory antibodies that target cytotoxic T-lymphocyte-associated antigen 4 (ipilimumab and tremelimumab) and the programmed cell death-1 receptor (nivolumab and pembrolizumab). By enhancing the immune response to tumor antigens, these agents have improved survival in patients with advanced melanoma. Elevations in the transaminases, developing around 8 weeks after initiation of therapy, are seen in less than 10% of patients receiving either class of checkpoint inhibitors.[56,125,126] Because the hepatotoxic reaction shares clinical and histologic features of autoimmune liver disease, immunosuppression with corticosteroids is started promptly once other potential sources of liver injury have been excluded.[126]

Sinusoidal obstruction syndrome

SOS, formerly called veno-occlusive disease (VOD), occurs most commonly after HCT, but can also result from exposure to toxins (Senecio alkaloids), nontransplant chemotherapeutic agents, high-dose radiation therapy to the liver, or after liver transplantation.[127,128] It is characterized clinically by tender hepatomegaly, jaundice, and weight gain with ascites. The prevalence of SOS varies widely in published studies, but has been estimated at around 20%. The clinical presentation of SOS mimics the Budd Chiari syndrome where occlusion of the hepatic veins results in postsinusoidal portal hypertension. However, in SOS it is the sinusoidal

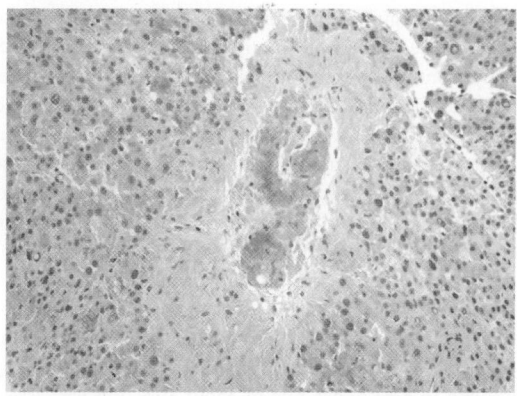

Figure 7 Sinusoidal obstruction syndrome (veno-occlusive disease) of the liver. The small hepatic vein demonstrates fibrous obliteration with fibrin deposits. The perivenular hepatocytes show prominent sinusoidal congestion.

and terminal hepatic venule endothelial cells, not the hepatic veins, that are targeted.[129,130] Following injury to the endothelial cells, there is activation of the coagulation cascade with clot formation. Fibrin plugs, intracellular fluid entrapment, and cellular debris progressively occlude the sinusoids, causing intrahepatic sinusoidal hypertension (Figure 7).

Pretransplant risks factors for the development of SOS include older transplant recipient age, female gender, poor performance status, donor-recipient HLA disparity, advanced malignancy, prior abdominal radiation, second myeloablative transplant, reduced pulmonary diffusion capacity (DLCO), and prior liver disease.[131–134]

The type and intensity of the transplant conditioning regimen are the greatest risk factors for developing severe SOS. Risk increases with total body irradiation dose and the use of certain drugs such as 6 mercaptopurine (6-MP), 6-thioguanine, actinomycin D, azathioprine, busulfan, cytosine arabinoside, cyclophosphamide, dacarbazine, gemtuzumab-ozogamicin, melphalan, oxaliplatin, and urethane.[130,131]

SOS typically presents initially with unexplained weight gain and tender hepatomegaly within the first week post-transplant. Ascites develops in about 25% of patients. Moderate elevations in the transaminases, with direct hyperbilirubinemia, follow with peak bilirubin levels less than 20 mg/dL.[135]

The diagnosis can be made frequently on the basis of typical signs and symptoms after ruling out other conditions such as viral infection, GVHD, systemic infection, and tumor infiltration. Two systems for the diagnosis of SOS, the Baltimore and Seattle criteria, have been published but the accuracy of these criteria has not been established.[135,136] Liver biopsy, rarely required for the diagnosis of SOS, typically shows sinusoidal dilatation with zone 3 hemorrhagic necrosis. Fibrin deposition with congestion is seen in the sinusoids and centrilobular venules. With time, collagen is deposited in the sinusoidal and venular lumens with occlusion of the terminal hepatic veins. If a biopsy is necessary for diagnosis, transjugular access is the safest route and can be accompanied by measurement of the hepatic venous gradient (HVPG).[137] Assessing the HVPG can discriminate between GVHD and SOS as the HPVG is greater in the latter.

Prevention of SOS should be a goal in all HCTs. Minimizing the use of potentially hepatotoxic agents and reduced-intensity conditioning regimens can potentially limit the severity of SOS. Pharmacologic prophylaxis is used routinely in many transplant centers. With allogeneic HCT, ursodeoxycholic acid, started before the preparative regimen and continued for 3 months, resulted in a reduced incidence of SOS when compared with placebo. Some centers use continuous infusion of low-dose heparin in autologous HCT. Mild-to-moderate SOS can be treated with supportive therapy including analgesics for right upper quadrant pain relief and diuretics to control extravascular fluid accumulation. Patients with severe SOS rarely respond to supportive therapy alone. On the basis of the histological presence of microthrombosis and fibrin deposition in the hepatic venules of patients with severe SOS, therapies that promote fibrinolysis with or without anticoagulation have been used. These treatment strategies include the use of alteplase (recombinant tissue-type plasminogen activator or tPA) alone or in combination with heparin and defibrotide. Treatment with alteplase and heparin resulted in a response rate of about 30%, but was associated with a significant risk of life-threatening hemorrhage, particularly in patients with multiorgan failure.[138–140] Defibrotide is a polydeoxyribonucleotide with antithrombotic, anti-ischemic, and thrombolytic properties without causing significant anticoagulation. Defibrotide given intravenously in doses ranging from 5 to 60 mg/kg per day for a minimum of 14 days results in a response in 42–55% of patients, without significant treatment-related toxicity.[141] Predictors of survival with defibrotide therapy included younger age, autologous stem-cell transplantation, and abnormal portal vein flow, while regimens based on busulfan and the presence of encephalopathy predicted worse outcomes.[142] Insertion of a transjugular intrahepatic portosystemic stent-shunt (TIPS) has been reported in small number of patients with severe SOS. TIPS was effective in improving portal pressure gradient; and in some patients, it was associated with clinical improvement of hepatic and renal symptoms. Nonetheless, these effects may be transient and may not improve overall survival.[143–145] Orthotopic liver transplantation (OLT) has been reported anecdotally as a rescue therapy in patients with SOS after stem-cell transplant, when there has been no response to medical therapy. However, the majority of patients with severe SOS are not candidates for OLT, because of the presence of malignancies and/or multiorgan failure.[146,147]

Graft-versus-host disease of the liver

The liver is the second most commonly involved organ in acute GVHD affecting approximately 50% of patients. Severe hepatic GVHD without other organ involvement is rare. The earliest biochemical findings are elevations in the conjugated bilirubin and alkaline phosphatase concentrations, reflecting the underlying pathologic injury.[72] Typically, there is extensive bile duct damage with degeneration and atypia of the bile duct epithelium, cell dropout, and a mixed cellular infiltration of small bile ducts leading to cholestasis.[148] While clinical and laboratory data can be highly suggestive of hepatic GVHD, a liver biopsy may be required for a definitive diagnosis and to rule out confounding diagnoses such SOS, infection, or drug toxicity. In some cases a percutaneous liver biopsy may not be feasible because of the risk of bleeding owing to thrombocytopenia soon after hematopoietic cell transplant. In these instances, if a liver biopsy is deemed to be necessary for diagnosis, a transjugular approach may be the preferred option. For acute GVHD, the first and most effective treatment option is the use of corticosteroids alone or in combination with tacrolimus. If this combination is unsuccessful in controlling hepatic GVHD, second-line treatments include antithymocyte globulin and mycophenolate mofetil.[149,150] Chronic hepatic GVHD can develop after previous acute GVHD or de novo without a history of previous acute GVHD. Approximately 50% of patients with chronic GVHD have hepatic involvement most often with asymptomatic elevations of the bilirubin and alkaline phosphatase

concentrations.[151] The histologic appearance of chronic hepatic GVHD mimics that of another immune-mediated liver disease, primary biliary cirrhosis, with injury to septal and interlobular bile ducts by chronic inflammatory cells.[148,152] The initial treatment of chronic hepatic GVHD is the same as acute GVHD with corticosteroids and tacrolimus. Patients with refractory chronic hepatic GVHD may respond to thalidomide.[153]

Other GI complications of cancer therapy

Constipation

Constipation is a common problem in patients undergoing cancer treatment. In this setting, constipation is usually caused by a combination of poor oral intake, decreased physical activity, and antiemetic agents such as ondansetron and opioid analgesics. Opioid-induced constipation is one of the most frequent adverse effects of opioid therapy.[154] These agents slow intestinal transit time. Constipation has also been reported in patients taking vinca alkaloids, in particular vincristine and thalidomide.

Impaction, bowel obstruction, and colonic pseudo-obstruction must be ruled out before initiating pharmacologic therapy for constipation. Constipation should be anticipated in the cancer patient, and steps taken to avoid this complication. Electrolyte abnormalities and other reversible causes of constipation should be corrected. Drugs that cause constipation should be discontinued if possible. Laxatives, with or without stool softeners, can be used in the initial treatment of constipation. Stimulant laxatives such as bisacodyl and senna alter electrolyte transport by the intestinal mucosa and increase intestinal motor activity. If these agents are not effective, osmotic agents such as lactulose or sorbitol can be effective at improving stool frequency and consistency. Polyethylene glycol solutions are available in powder form and have been found to be effective at improving chronic constipation. The use of drugs to improve colonic transit has been disappointing. Metoclopramide seems to be ineffective, and tegaserod (a 5-hydroxytryptamine receptor agonist) has significant cardiovascular adverse effects, and is not available in the Unites States outside of an emergency investigational new drug (IND) process from the FDA. Lubiprostone, a chloride channel activator, is FDA approved for the treatment of chronic idiopathic constipation. It is a bicyclic acid that works locally on the apical part of the intestine and helps to increase intracellular fluid and intestinal motility. It may be useful in the patient with constipation whose symptoms are increased with opioid use, and with constipation induced by chemotherapy. It is FDA approved for treatment of opioid-induced constipation related to noncancer pain. Methylnaltrexone, a micro-opioid-receptor antagonist for the treatment of opioid-induced constipation in advanced-illness patients, is approved for use in the United States. The agent, a derivative of naltrexone, selectively antagonizes the peripheral microreceptors in the GI tract without effects on the CNS. In clinical trials, subcutaneous methylnaltrexone reversed opioid-induced constipation after the first dose in approximately 50–60% of the patients.[155] In most of the cases, effective laxation occurred within 1 h. It does not affect opioid analgesic effects or induce opioid-withdrawal symptoms. Recent advances in neurogastroenterology are leading to the development of new classes of medications, which may aid in the treatment of severe constipation.[156] Peripherally active μ-opioid receptor antagonists (PAMORAs) allow preservation of the central analgesic effects of these drugs, while antagonizing peripheral effects on the GI tract. Naloxegol and TD-1211 are prototypes in this class. Naloxegol is an oral PEGylated conjugate of naloxone. Naloxegol has recently been approved to treat opioid-induced diarrhea in adults with noncancer pain.[157]

Nausea and vomiting

Nausea and vomiting frequently occur after administration of chemotherapeutic agents. The likelihood of developing nausea and vomiting following chemotherapy depends on several factors including the chemotherapy dose and the intrinsic emetogenicity of a given agent.[158] The emetogenic potential of intravenously administered antineoplastic agents can be assigned to five levels, ranging from minimal or less than 10% risk (e.g., bevacizumab) to a high or greater than 90% risk (e.g., cisplatin). Emesis can be acute (i.e., occurring within the first 24 h of receiving chemotherapy) or delayed.

Various antiemetic agents are now available for the prevention and treatment of chemotherapy-induced nausea and vomiting. These include agents with a high therapeutic index such as 5-hydroxytryptamine-3 (5-HT$_3$) receptor antagonists (e.g., ondansetron, granisetron, dolasetron, tropisetron, and palonosetron), neurokinin-1-receptor antagonists (e.g., aprepitant), and corticosteroids (usually used in combination with other agents). Agents with a low therapeutic index are also used, such as metoclopramide hydrochloride, butyrophenones, phenothiazines, cannabinoids, and olanzapine. The preferred agent and regimen depend on the emetogenic level of a given chemotherapeutic drug. For drugs with a low emetogenic risk, antiemetics are given only before chemotherapy, while antiemetics are provided before and after chemotherapy for those chemotherapy drugs with a high emetogenic risk (levels 3 or higher).

Gastrointestinal perforation, fistula formation, arterial thrombosis, and bleeding

GI perforation, fistula formation, arterial thrombosis, and bleeding have been reported with bevacizumab, a monoclonal antibody against VEGF. Intestinal perforation has been reported in 1–2% of patients treated with bevacizumab for metastatic colorectal cancer.[159,160] Risk factors associated with perforation include an intact primary tumor, prior irradiation, acute diverticulitis, intra-abdominal abscess, and GI obstruction.

Acute pancreatitis

Acute pancreatitis in patients with cancer or in those who have undergone hematopoietic stem-cell transplantation can be caused by conditions present in the general population, including gallstones and alcohol. However, other etiologies should be taken into consideration when managing cancer patients who have acute pancreatitis, including medications and chemotherapeutic agents.

Drug-induced pancreatitis has no distinguishing clinical features, and therefore taking a careful drug history and excluding other etiologies are essential to make a diagnosis. Some of the most common drugs known to cause acute pancreatitis include metronidazole, sulfonamides, tetracycline, furosemide, thiazides, estrogen, and tamoxifen. During the course of chemotherapy, pancreatitis has been reported with the use of azathioprine, prednisone cytosine arabinoside, and various regimens of combination chemotherapy including vinca alkaloids, MTX, mitomycin, 5-FU, cyclophosphamide, cisplatin, and bleomycin. Associated illnesses and multidrug regimens often make it difficult to determine a cause and effect relationship.[161]

Oral mucositis or ulceration of the oropharynx

Oral mucositis or painful ulceration of the mucosal lining of the oropharynx occurs frequently in individuals undergoing radiation and chemotherapy for solid malignancies. It occurs in 20–40% of patients receiving conventional chemotherapy, 80% of patients receiving high-dose chemotherapy, and has been reported in up to 98% of individuals undergoing hematopoietic stem-cell transplantation. Evidence-based recommendations for prevention and treatment of oral mucositis have been recently published.[1] Palifermin, a recombinant human keratinocyte growth factor-1, decreases the incidence and duration of mucositis in patients with hematologic malignancies who are receiving chemotherapy and requiring stem-cell transplantation support, and has been approved by the FDA for this indication. New guidelines recommend that this agent be used to prevent oral mucositis in patients receiving high-dose chemotherapy and total body irradiation followed by autologous stem-cell transplantation for hematologic malignancies.[1] Oral cryotherapy is also recommended to be used to prevent oral mucositis in patients receiving bolus 5-fluorouracil chemotherapy. Low-level laser therapy has been recommended to prevent oral mucositis in patients receiving human stem-cell transplantation conditioned with high-dose chemotherapy. Benzydamine mouthwash (but not other antimicrobial mouthwash or lozenges) should be used to prevent oral mucositis in patients with head and neck cancer receiving moderate dose radiotherapy without concomitant chemotherapy. Zinc supplements may be beneficial to prevent oral mucositis in oral cancer patients receiving radiation or chemotherapy. Sucralfate mouthwash is not recommended to prevent or treat mucositis in those receiving chemotherapy or radiation for head and neck cancer owing to demonstrated lack of benefit.

Key references

The complete reference list can be found on the Wiley Companion Digital Edition of this title (see inside front cover for login instructions).

1 Lalla RV, Bowen J, Barasch A, et al. MASCC/ISOO clinical practice guidelines for the management of mucositis secondary to cancer therapy. *Cancer.* 2014;**120**:1453–1461.

3 Konig CC, Wouterse SJ, Daams JG, et al. Toxicity of concurrent radiochemotherapy for locally advanced non-small-cell lung cancer: A systematic review of the literature. *Clin Lung Cancer.* 2013;**14**:481–487.

8 Masur H, Brooks JT, Benson CA, et al. Prevention and treatment of opportunistic infections in HIV-infected adults and adolescents: updated guidelines from the Centers for Disease Control and Prevention, national Institutes of Health, and HIV Medicine Association of the Infectious Diseases Society of America. *Clin Infectious Dis.* 2014;**58**:1308–1311. (see also http://aidsinfo.nih.gov/guidelines/html/4/adult-and-adolescent-oi-prevention-and-treatment-guidelines/0).

15 Villanueva A, Gotuzzo E, Arathoon EG, et al. A randomized double-blind study of caspofungin versus fluconazole for the treatment of esophageal candidiasis. *Am J Med.* 2002;**113**(4):294–299.

24 Didden P, Spaander MCW, Kuipers EJ. Esophageal stents in malignant and benign disorders. *Curr Gastroenterol Rep.* 2013;**4**:319–328.

28 Dai Y, Lee C, Xie Y, et al. Interventions for dysphagia in oesophageal cancer (review). *Cochrane Database Syst Rev.* 2014;(**10**.Art. No. CD005048.). doi: 10.1002/14651858.CD005048.pub4.

35 Surawicz CM, Brandt LJ, Binion DG, et al. Guidelines for diagnosis, treatment and prevention of *Clostridium difficile* infections. *Am J Gastroenterol.* 2013;**108**:478–498.

36 Lowy I, Molrine DC, Leav BA, et al. Treatment with monoclonal antibodies against Clostridium difficile toxins. *N Engl J Med.* 2010;**362**(3):197–205.

37 Nesher L, Rolston KV. Neutropenic enterocolitis, a growing concern in the era of widespread use of aggressive chemotherapy. *Clin Infect Dis.* 2013;**56**:711–717.

38 Ebert EC, Hagspiel KD. Gastrointestinal manifestations of leukemia. *J Gastroenterol Hepatol.* 2012;**27**:458–463.

43 Gangadhar TC, Vonderheide RH. Mitigating the toxic effects of anticancer immunotherapy. *Nat Rev Clin Oncol.* 2014;**11**:91–99.

50 Kim KW, Ramaiya NH, Krajewski KM, et al. Ipilimumab-associated colitis: CT findings. *AJR Am J Roentgenol.* 2013;**200**:W468–W474.

51 Squibb B-M. YERVOY™ *(ipilimumab): Immune-mediated Adverse Reaction Management Guide* [online], 2011; www.hcp.yervoy.com/pdf/rems-management-guide.pdf (accessed 12 August 2015).

56 Hamid O, Robert C, Daud A, et al. Safety and tumor responses with lambrolizumab (anti-PD-1) in melanoma. *N Engl J Med.* 2013;**369**:134–144.

58 Robert C, Ribas A, Wolchok JD, et al. Anti-programmed-death-receptor-1 treatment with pembrolizumab in ipilimumab-refractory advanced melanoma: a randomised dose-comparison cohort of a phase 1 trial. *Lancet.* 2014;**384**:1109–1117.

59 Ferrara JL, Levine JE, Reddy P, Holler E. Graft-versus-host disease. *Lancet.* 2009;**373**:1550–1561.

62 Fernandez-Vina MA, Klein JP, Haagenson M, et al. Multiple mismatches at the low expression HLA loci DP, DQ, and DRB3/4/5 associate with adverse outcomes in hematopoietic stem cell transplantation. *Blood.* 2013;**121**:4603–4610.

67 Anasetti C, Logan BR, Lee SJ, et al. Peripheral-blood stem cells versus bone marrow from unrelated donors. *N Engl J Med.* 2012;**367**:1487–1496.

71 Washington K, Jagasia M. Pathology of graft-versus-host disease in the gastrointestinal tract. *Hum Pathol.* 2009;**40**:909–917.

72 Filipovich AH, Weisdorf D, Pavletic S, et al. National Institutes of Health consensus development project on criteria for clinical trials in chronic graft-versus-host disease: I. Diagnosis and staging working group report. *Biol Blood Marrow Transplant.* 2005;**11**:945–956.

76 Rodriguez-Otero P, Porcher R, Peffault de Latour R, et al. Fecal calprotectin and alpha-1 antitrypsin predict severity and response to corticosteroids in gastrointestinal graft-versus-host disease. *Blood.* 2012;**119**:5909–5917.

85 Cutler C, Logan B, Nakamura R, et al. Tacrolimus/sirolimus vs tacrolimus/methotrexate as GVHD prophylaxis after matched, related donor allogeneic HCT. *Blood.* 2014;**124**:1372–1377.

87 Kharfan-Dabaja M, Mhaskar R, Reljic T, et al. Mycophenolate mofetil versus methotrexate for prevention of graft-versus-host disease in people receiving allogeneic hematopoietic stem cell transplantation. *Cochrane Database Syst Rev.* 2014;7:CD010280.

88 Arora M, Klein JP, Weisdorf DJ, et al. Chronic GVHD risk score: a Center for International Blood and Marrow Transplant Research analysis. *Blood.* 2011;**117**:6714–6720.

93 Wolff D, Gerbitz A, Ayuk F, et al. Consensus conference on clinical practice in chronic graft-versus-host disease (GVHD): first-line and topical treatment of chronic GVHD. *Biol Blood Marrow Transplant.* 2010;**16**:1611–1628.

96 Mitka M. Increased HBV reactivation risk with of atumumab or rituximab. *JAMA.* 2013;**310**:1664.

99 Artz AS, Somerfield MR, Feld JJ, et al. American Society of Clinical Oncology provisional clinical opinion: chronic hepatitis B virus infection screening in patients receiving cytotoxic chemotherapy for treatment of malignant diseases. *J Clin Oncol.* 2010;**28**:3199.

101 Loomba R, Rowley A, Wesley R, et al. A systematic review: the effect of preventive lamivudine on hepatitis B reactivation during chemotherapy. *Ann Intern Med.* 2008;**148**:519.

103 Torres HA, Davila M. Reactivation of hepatitis B virus and hepatitis C virus in patients with cancer. *Nat Rev Clin Oncol.* 2012;**9**:156.

121 Azim HA, Agbor-Tarh D, Bradbury I, et al. Pattern of rash, diarrhea, and hepatic toxicities secondary to lapatinib and their association with age and response to neoadjuvant therapy: analysis from NEoALTTO trial. *J Clin Oncol.* 2013;**31**:4504.

123 Shibata SI, Chung V, Synold TW, et al. Phase 1 study of pazopanib in patients with advanced solid tumors and hepatic dysfunction: a National Cancer Institute Organ Dysfunction Working Group study. *Clin Cancer Res.* 2013;**19**:3631.

149 Martin PJ, Rizzo JH, Wingard JR, et al. First- and second-line systemic treatment of acute graft-versus-host disease: recommendations of the American Society of Blood and Marrow Transplantation. *Biol Blood Marrow Transplant.* 2012;**18**:1150.

150 Wolff D, Ayuk F, Elmaagacli A, et al. Current practice in diagnosis and treatment of acute graft-versus-host disease: results from a survey among German-Austrian-Swiss hematopoietic stem cell transplant centers. *Biol Blood Marrow Transplant.* 2013;**19**:767.

154 Siemens W, Gaertner J, Becker G. Advances in pharmacotherapy for opioid-induced constipation-a systematic review. *Expert Opin Pharmacother.* 2014;**16**:515–532. Dec 24, epub ahead of print.

156 Camilleri M. Novel therapeutic agents in neurogastroenterology: advances in the past year. *Neurogastrowenterol Motil.* 2014;**26**:1070–1078.

157 Corsetti M, Tack J. Naloxegol, a new drug for the treatment of opioid-induced constipation. *Expert Opin Pharmacother.* 2015;**16**:399–406.

158 Hesketh PJ. Chemotherpay-induced nausea and vomiting. *N Engl J Med.* 2008;**358**:2482–2494.

160 Scott LJ, Chakravarthy U, reeves BC, Rogers CA. Systemic affect of anti-VEGF drugs: a commentary. *Expert Opin Drug Saf.* 2014;**14**:379–388. Dec 9; epub ahead of print.

161 Morgan C, Tillet T, Braybrooke J, et al. Management of uncommon chemotherapy-induced emergencies. *Lancet Oncol.* 2011;**12**:806–814.

135 Oral complications of cancer and their treatment

Stephen T. Sonis, DMD, DMSc ▪ Anna Yuan, DMD

Overview

The mouth is a frequent site of direct and indirect adverse side effects of cancer therapy. In myelosuppressed patients, its diverse microbiota makes the oral cavity both a site of local infection and a potential source of bacteremias and sepsis. While about half of all patients being treated with chemotherapy or radiation therapy will develop some form of oral toxicity or infection, almost every patient receiving an aggressive myeloablative regimen or local radiotherapy to the head and neck manifests acute and chronic toxicities. The diversity of the tissues found in and around the mouth—keratinized and nonkeratinized mucosa, bone, salivary glands, and teeth—contributes to the range of susceptibility, acuity, and clinical implications of regimen-related oral complications. In almost all instances, precancer treatment elimination or control of existing oral diseases and aggressive management of oral health during cancer therapy favorably impacts outcomes.

The mouth is a frequent site of acute and chronic adverse side effects of cancer therapy. These range broadly in their nature, incidence, severity, and course, but all adversely affect patients' quality of life, ability to tolerate therapy, overall cost of treatment, risk of local and systemic infection, and rehabilitation. Oral complications of cancer therapy are perceived as common in some cohorts such as patients with head and neck cancer (HNC), but relatively rare in others. This perception has been largely fueled by under-reported patients who worry that mentioning toxicity symptoms during treatment might, as a consequence of dose de-escalation, result in a compromise of their optimum anticancer therapy. While this phenomenon is not unique to oral complications, data surrounding the underestimates of oral toxicities are substantial. Additionally, oral side effects have been reported with many forms of developing therapies including cetuximab, antiresorptive medications, and mTOR inhibitors. It has also become clear that oral complications rarely occur in isolation. Rather, probably because of common biologic underpinnings, they predictably occur with other regimen-related toxicities.[1]

Overall, about 40% of patients being treated for cancers, not of the head and neck, develop some form of mouth-related problems, which range from xerostomia to mucositis.[2] The frequency escalates to more than 75% for patients being treated for HNC, those who develop graft-versus-host disease (GVHD), and patients receiving aggressive myeloablative chemotherapy regimens. The symptomatic and functional consequences of oral complications include increases in analgesic and antibiotic use, length of hospital stays, hospitalizations for pain and fluid management, nursing resource use, diagnostic treating, and need for parenteral feeding. The impact on charges and costs is dramatic. In a study population of patients receiving treatment for HNC and nonsmall cell lung cancer, the incremental cost of oral mucositis alone was found to be $17,244.[3] In the past, oral complications were largely considered to be inevitable, often were not recognized early, and were treated retrospectively rather than in a prospective or preventive manner. Significant progress has been made in the past decade to better define the biology and epidemiology of oral complications of treatment. As a result, interventions that target mechanisms have evolved, as has a better understanding of at-risk populations.

Pretreatment assessment

The risk of many of the side effects that impact the mouth can be successfully reduced by the elimination of existing sites of dental disease before anticancer treatment is initiated.[4-6] A pretreatment dental visit is strongly recommended as it serves a range of purposes. First, it provides an opportunity for the identification and elimination of sources of active and chronic dental or periodontal infections or chronic irritation when the patient is best able to tolerate treatment with the least risk of undesirable post-treatment sequelae, such as infection or osteonecrosis. Second, oral manifestations of the primary cancer may be detected. Third, it provides an opportunity for patient education and discussion regarding the impact of the cancer and its treatment on short- and long-term oral health. Fourth, for the patient about to undergo surgical intervention for tumors about the mouth, pretreatment evaluation is critical to optimize the fabrication of prostheses. The construction of protective appliances before the start of radiation therapy may reduce the impact of treatment on scatter-induced injury.

Not surprisingly the frequency of dental disease or faulty prostheses or restoration reported on screening of patients with cancer reflects the incidence of these conditions in the general population. While positive findings of less-than-optimal oral health were reported in two-thirds of patients evaluated before stem cell transplantation (HSCT),[7] pathology of such severity as to require intervention is only required in about a third of screened patients.[7] Similarly, of patients with cancers of the head and neck who were screened before radiation therapy, between half and two-thirds required dental extractions, primarily because of diagnoses associated with periodontal disease.[8,9] Although elimination of possible oral and dental sites of infection before chemotherapy had a significant, favorable impact on morbidity relative to local infection and sepsis,[4] definitive data demonstrating that preirradiation elimination of oral foci of infection favorably impacts outcomes is needed.[10] Effective dental screening with appropriate treatment before the onset of cancer therapy results in significant cost savings, by reducing the incidence of infection during periods of granulocytopenia.[11]

Holland-Frei Cancer Medicine, Ninth Edition. Edited by Robert C. Bast Jr., Carlo M. Croce, William N. Hait, Waun Ki Hong, Donald W. Kufe, Martine Piccart-Gebhart, Raphael E. Pollock, Ralph R. Weichselbaum, Hongyang Wang, and James F. Holland.
© 2017 John Wiley & Sons, Inc. ISBN: 978-1-118-93469-2

Timing of assessment and dental treatment

If oral screening is performed so close to the initiation of cancer therapy as to preclude dental intervention, the value of the process is nullified. The ideal interval between the completion of dental treatment, particularly extraction, and the initiation of radiation therapy has been the subject of much debate. Nonetheless, given the rate by which wounds of the mouth heal, particularly extraction sites, it appears that a minimum of 2 weeks is acceptable and 3 weeks desirable.[12] For patients about to undergo chemotherapy, sufficient time between the completion of dental treatment and the patient's anticipated granulocyte nadir (<500 cells/mL) is required. In general, nonemergent dental treatment should not be performed in a typical ambulatory setting if the patient is significantly thrombocytopenic (<100,000 platelets/mL).[13]

Because of the acute onset of some hematologic malignancies and the need for immediate chemotherapy, pretreatment dental and oral screening in this high-risk population may not be possible. In these cases, oral assessment should be performed as close to the initiation of therapy as possible for two reasons: first, such an examination provides an important baseline for oral health and second, the finding and elimination of active oral infection in this markedly myeloablated group is often critical to their overall clinical course. Eradication of identified sources of odontogenic infection should not be delayed, as there is significant data to support the conclusion that dental extractions may be performed safely in this group if they are managed well, preferably in a hospital setting.[10] The complication rate for extractions in patients with hematologic malignancies is reported to be 13%, with no effect on length of hospital stay or mortality. The most common complications include pain and bleeding. It is important to note that there is no evidence to suggest that an aggressive strategy of extraction of *asymptomatic* teeth has any benefit in the prevention of systemic infection.

Components of the pretreatment assessment include baseline data such as medical and dental histories; laboratory data—such as antibody status relative to herpes simplex type 1 virus—and a clinical assessment that should include an extraoral examination of the head and neck, intraoral soft-tissue examination, periodontal disease screening, and dental evaluation. Radiographic evaluation should include those films that are necessary to definitively diagnose periodontal disease and caries, periapical pathology, and impacted teeth. It is also important to assess the patient's knowledge of, and motivation for dental maintenance. Teeth that demonstrate evidence of untreated periapical pathology, or advanced caries, or periodontal disease should be eliminated.

Patients with removable prostheses should be encouraged to minimize their use or leave them out during their cancer therapy as even subtle mucosal trauma accelerates the risk and onset of mucositis. Similarly, the removal of orthodontic bands before the start of chemotherapy is an essential component in preventing trauma to atrophied mucosa.[14]

Oral complications of radiotherapy

Oral complications of radiation therapy are primarily the result of acute and chronic local tissue injury. In addition, radiation-induced xerostomia may result in secondary effects on the teeth and periodontium. The dose rate, total dose of radiation, use of concomitant chemotherapy, the size of, and structures within, the radiation field are the major determinants of oral toxicity. As a result, patients being treated for tumors of the mouth, oropharynx, tongue, nasopharynx, and salivary glands are at highest risk. Patients with hypopharyngeal or laryngeal tumors are also often affected, although at a slightly

lower rate. Brachytherapy tends to be more stomatotoxic than external beam irradiation. Although intensity-modulated radiation therapy (IMRT) (*see **Chapter 83***) may spare some structures, its impact on oral mucosa is significant. Oral tissues that are directly affected by radiation include mucosa (epithelium and tissues in the lamina propria), salivary glands, bone, and muscle. In children, radiation that includes the jaws negatively affects craniofacial and dental development.[15]

Mucositis

Both radiation and chemotherapy can produce significant damage to the oral mucosa as a side effect of treatment. The term mucositis (ICD9 code 528.1) is preferred over stomatitis when describing mucosal injury caused by antineoplastic therapy as the latter is a generic term and can be associated with a range of infectious or traumatic etiologies unrelated to chemo- or radiotherapy. The severity and kinetics of radiation-induced oral mucositis are related to dose rate and total dose that target the oral mucosa. Local mucosal irritation, secondary infection, and xerostomia are factors that amplify the damaging effects of radiation to the tissue.

Three themes have characterized the mucositis discussion in the past 5 years: first, the pathobiology has been more fully defined; second, the commonality in mechanisms by which mucosal injury occurs has been applied to all parts of the alimentary canal; and third, mucositis rarely occurs as an isolated toxicity.[16] In addition, the impact of genomics on toxicity risk, including mucositis, has become clear and is being more fully defined.

Historically, mucositis was viewed as the result of direct radiation or chemotherapy-mediated injury to stem cells in the basal layer of the oral mucosa. It was proposed that these rapidly dividing cells were indiscriminately damaged, resulting in atrophy and subsequent ulceration. Simultaneously, connective tissue injury was thought to lead to an increase in vascular permeability and tissue edema. However, studies defining the mechanisms by which mucositis occurs reveal a process that is biologically more complex. Although epithelial stem cells are the ultimate mediators of mucosal injury, it is now clear that their demise occurs by indirect, as well as direct, mechanisms.[17,18] In fact, direct clonogenic cell death of these cells is insufficient to produce the extent of clinical injury that is typically observed. Rather, a sequence of events[18] triggered by the generation of reactive species in cells of the lamina propria produce a cascade of events in the endothelium, connective tissue, extracellular matrix, and the inflammatory infiltrate. This sequence begins almost immediately, following the initial exposure of the mucosa to radiation, and results in a range of molecular mediators and signals that permeate to the epithelium and cause injury, apoptosis, and necrosis.

Radiation-induced oral mucositis typically begins within the first 2 weeks of therapy, at cumulative doses of 10–20 Gy. Although clinical changes are observed at these doses, the cellular and tissue events producing these changes begin almost immediately following initial dosing (see below). Mucosal erythema, mild epithelial sloughing, and the formation of islands of hyperkeratosis characterize early changes of mucositis. These changes are accompanied by relatively mild symptoms characterized by a painful burning sensation that is analogous to a food burn such as that caused by hot cheese. Patients often have difficulty tolerating spicy foods. With the exception of the dorsal surface of the tongue, hard palate, and the gingiva, any mucosal surface of the mouth is susceptible. Most commonly affected areas are the buccal mucosa (cheeks), ventral and lateral surfaces of the tongue, and the floor of the mouth (Figure 1). The soft palate and oropharynx are also frequently involved and are consistent drivers of symptoms associated with

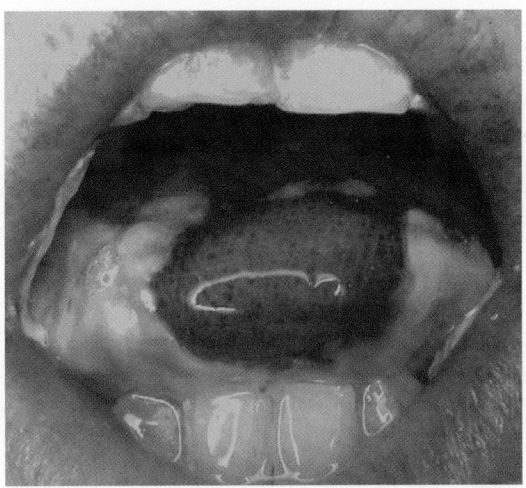

Figure 1 Severe oral mucositis with ulceration and pseudomembrane formation of the lateral and ventral surfaces of the tongue and buccal mucosa induced by myeloablative chemotherapy for conditioning before HSCT.

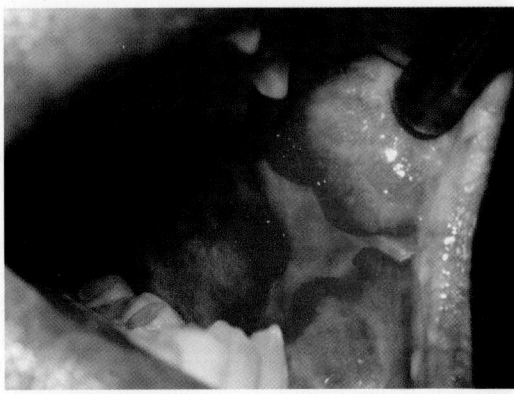

Figure 2 Severe oral mucositis with ulceration, erythema, and pseudomembrane formation of the left buccal mucosa induced by radiation therapy for treatment of an oral carcinoma.

pain on swallowing. Consequently, patients may complain of a sore throat early in their treatment.

At cumulative doses of about 30 Gy, the integrity of the mucosa breaks down and ulceration occurs. Ulcers typically begin as isolated lesions, but then coalesce forming large, contiguous breaks in the mucosa, often covered by a collection of dead cells and bacteria in a pseudomembrane. In severe cases, the lesions may bleed (Figure 2). Ulcerative mucositis is extremely painful. Not only do ulcers cover large mucosal surface areas, but they are also deep. Patients who have undergone radiation therapy and have developed mucositis describe this complication as the most significant of their treatment.[19] In many cases, mucositis results in breaks in radiation treatment, hospitalization for fluid support or pain management, and the need for parenteral feeding.[20] The incremental economic cost of oral mucositis in this population is significant.[3] It is important that patients about to begin treatment have some concept of the severity of mucosal injury that they are likely to develop. The typical pretreatment characterization of mucositis as "mouth sores" seems to trivialize their significance to patients. It seems likely that a more realistic description and management plan would be advantageous. In most patients, ulcerative mucositis is self-limiting and resolves spontaneously 4–6 weeks following the completion of radiation.

Evaluation of mucositis

Comparisons of the stomatotoxicity of treatment regimens and efficacy assessments of mucositis interventions have been hindered by the lack of a universally acceptable scoring system for the condition. Currently, the grading systems most commonly used to describe oral mucosal toxicity are the World Health Organization (WHO) and National Cancer Institute's common terminology criteria for adverse events (NCI-CTCAE) scales. The WHO scale combines objective findings of erythema and ulceration with the patients' ability to eat solids, liquids, or nothing by mouth (Table 1). In its latest iteration (v.4) the CTCAE scale eliminates objective assessment of mucosal health and relies completely on symptomatic and functional (oral intake) endpoints. While this approach minimizes the clinician's effort to assess mucositis, the dependence on patient-reported symptoms and function is complicated by analgesic use, individual pain perception, and nonmucositis-related function modifiers such as edentulism, nausea, and so on.

Prevention and treatment

There is currently no approved, active preventive or treatment intervention for radiation-induced mucositis in the United States. There is consensus that improved oral status may reduce the risk or severity of mucositis. Maintaining a high level of oral hygiene during treatment is thought to be beneficial.

As mucosal injury is related to the extent of mucosa exposed to radiation, the use of midline radiation blocks[22] and three-dimensional radiation treatment[23] may reduce the extent of stomatotoxicity.

Benzydamine hydrochloride is a nonsteroidal rinse with anti-inflammatory, analgesic, and anesthetic properties that is approved for use in the prevention and treatment of radiation-induced mucositis in Canada, Australia, and Europe. Results of a number of studies suggest its efficacy in this application.[24,25] The MASCC panel recommended the use of benzydamine among patients receiving moderate dose radiotherapy.[26] There are no data to support its use in patients receiving concomitant chemotherapy.

A number of palliative barrier agents have been suggested to alleviate symptoms associated with oral mucositis. Gelclair, which has FDA approval as a device, purportedly forms a barrier on injured mucosa.[27] Sucralfate, an agent that has wide use in the treatment of gastric ulcers, forms a protein-drug complex on the site of ulcerated mucosa. Its use as a rinse in the treatment of mucositis has been reported in a number of studies, although its efficacy seems inconsistent.[28,29] It is specifically not recommended in the MASCC guidelines. MuGard, a hydrogel, demonstrated significant palliation in a multi-institutional, randomized, placebo-controlled trial.[30]

A variety of topical agents exist for mucositis pain management. These include viscous lidocaine, benzocaine in Orabase, and suspensions of Benadryl in Kaopectate or milk of magnesia. Caphosol, a rinse originally developed as a tooth-remineralizing solution for patients with xerostomia, is an electrolyte solution of sodium phosphate, calcium chloride, sodium chloride, and purified water, which purportedly lubricates the mucosa and thereby attenuates mucositis. The solution is approved as a device, but the results of clinical trials are inconsistent.[31–33] Oral aloe vera has been available for some time as a palliative agent. However, it failed to demonstrate efficacy in a phase 2, double-blind, randomized, placebo-controlled study.[34] Topical palliative rinses are typically effective only for mild forms of the condition. Systemic pain management following the WHO pain ladder is often necessary. Additionally, cold foods, such as ice cream or Popsicles, may be soothing. Patients should be instructed to remove dental prostheses.

Table 1 Staging and management of medication-related osteonecrosis of the jaw.

Stage	Clinical presentation	Management
At risk	No exposed bone	Patient education
0	No clinical evidence of necrotic bone, but nonspecific clinical findings, radiographic changes, and symptoms	Systemic management, including the use of pain medication and antibiotics
1	Asymptomatic exposed and necrotic bone, or fistulae that probes to bone with no evidence of infection	Patient education; antibacterial rinses; careful follow-up
2	Exposed and necrotic bone, or fistulae that probes to bone, associated with infection as evidenced by pain and erythema in the region of the exposed bone with or without purulent drainage	Patient education; antibacterial rinses; antibiotics; pain control; superficial debridement of bone to dislodge loose fragments and smooth rough contours; careful follow-up
3	Exposed bone with pain and usually with associated soft-tissue inflammation or infection; may see osteolysis extending to the inferior border of mandible or pathologic fracture; may see extraoral fistula	Patient education; antibacterial rinses; antibiotics; pain control; palliative surgery; careful follow-up

Source: Ruggiero et al. 2014.[21] Reproduced with permission from Elsevier.

The role of microbes on the severity and course of radiation-induced mucositis is unclear.[35] The strategy of mucosal decontamination as a mucositis intervention has produced conflicting results. Chlorhexidine gluconate rinses do not appear to have a role in mucositis prevention or treatment in radiation mucositis and, in fact, might exacerbate the condition.[36] Lozenges containing polymyxin E, tobramycin, and amphotericin have been studied and seem to of marginal value and are not recommended.[37]

Given its importance as an unmet need, the development pipeline for mucositis is rich with agents that target key elements in its pathogenesis. Clinical trials are currently in progress in which drugs targeting oxidative stress, the innate immune response, and proinflammatory elements are being studied.[38] Low-level laser therapy is also being investigated for its potential utility as an intervention of oral mucositis. While results of clinical trials are encouraging, the lack of substantive studies defining its biological effects as related to tumor response is troubling. More investigation is clearly needed to assure that its impact on premalignant and malignant tissue is benign.[39]

Xerostomia

Xerostomia is one of the most consistent and bothersome side effects of radiation therapy in which the salivary glands are included in the field of treatment,[40] and may be exacerbated by concomitant chemotherapy. The effects of radiation on salivary flow are variable, and symptoms of dry mouth may not correspond to observed salivary flow. Xerostomia is caused by the effects of radiation on acinar cells, especially of the serous glands (parotid). Consequently, inflammation, degeneration, and fibrosis of the glandular parenchyma occur. The extent, duration, and degree of recovery are functions of the dose rate, total dose, and radiation port. Onset of xerostomia may be noted as early as 1 week following the start of radiation (cumulative dose of 10 Gy).[41] The saliva turns thick and ropey as serous function is diminished, but mucous production remains. Patients whose radiation to the ear and neck is in cumulative doses of 60 Gy more often develop irreversible xerostomia, with an 80% loss in salivary gland function.[42] Spontaneous recovery is unlikely for patients with xerostomia persisting for 12 months or longer.[43] With lesser doses of radiation, however, inflammation and edema of glandular tissue often spontaneously disappear within a year of the completion of treatment.[44]

In addition to functional changes caused by xerostomia, such as dysphasia and alteration in taste, loss of saliva is also associated with a reduction in oral clearance, diminished salivary immunoglobulin A (IgA) levels, and salivary antibacterial enzymes. Consequently, patients with xerostomia are susceptible to increases in local oral infections including caries, periodontal disease, and candidiasis.

Aggressive oral hygiene to reduce the tooth-borne bacterial load is critical to reducing the risk of dental disease.

Radiation-induced caries can be a common problem in patients with xerostomia.[42] Changes in salivary composition, decreases in buffering capacity, and loss of the cleansing action of saliva result in the accumulation of bacteria, increases in local cariogenic flora, and tooth decalcification with consequent caries development.[45,46] Typically, radiation caries present with lesions at the cervical margins of teeth, which then rapidly progress. Decalcification (white, chalky enamel) of the incisal edges of the teeth may also be noted. In addition to tooth loss, a major consequence of uncontrolled caries may be abscess formation in patients who are at risk for osteoradionecrosis (ORN).

Four goals should be considered for the prevention and treatment of xerostomia. Preservation of salivary function is critical. Whenever possible, tissue-sparing techniques aimed at minimizing the amount of salivary tissues exposed to direct radiation should be used. While bilateral field radiation may result in an 80% reduction of salivary flow, mantle irradiation typically causes only a 30–40% decrease. Parotid sparing using three-dimensional treatment or intensity-modulated radiotherapy techniques offers the greatest chance of glandular repair.[47] Stimulation of salivary flow should start simultaneously with radiation therapy (XRT), as should an anticaries regimen to protect the dentition. Replacement of reduced secretions may be introduced as soon as needed.

Stimulation of salivary flow may be accomplished through local or systemic means. Sucrose-free lemon drops or sugarless chewing gum may be used. Cinnamon- or mint-flavored mints or gum should be avoided as they may irritate the mucosa.

Drug therapy may also help to stimulate parotid flow.[48] Of the cholinergic agents, pilocarpine has been best studied and found to stimulate parotid function, but not submandibular or sublingual gland function in patients with Sjögren syndrome and radiation-induced xerostomia.[49,50] Other agents such as bromhexine, anetholtrithion, bethanechol HCl, potassium iodide, neostigmine, and reserpine have been used for salivary stimulation, but data substantiating their efficacy are scant. In contrast, substantial data exist to support the use of pilocarpine HCl tablets to stimulate salivary flow in patients with radiation-induced xerostomia.[51] In cases in which pilocarpine is used after patients have completed radiation treatment and are symptomatic, at least some residual salivary function must be present, and patients should be cautioned that clinically significant improvements in salivary flow may not be realized for up to 3 months following the initiation of treatment. Alternatively, pilocarpine may be prescribed to start simultaneously with radiation therapy. In either case, the typical dose of 5 mg given three times daily may be titrated depending on the patient's response and manifestation of side effects.

Amifostine, a nonprotein, free-radical scavenger has been approved as a cytoprotective agent for salivary glands to prevent radiation-induced xerostomia.[52] The recommended dose for amifostine is 200 mg/m^2, administered once daily as a 3-min infusion, starting 15–30 min before standard fraction radiation therapy. The need for intravenous infusion, frequency of dosing, cost, and potential side effects have limited amifostine's adoption. Furthermore, the results of a recent meta-analysis suggest that amifostine's efficacy is tempered among patients receiving radiation regimens in which concomitant chemotherapy is also administered.[53]

Salivary replacement can be accomplished with the use of saliva substitutes or artificial saliva.[54] Most of these materials contain carboxymethylcellulose and may provide transient symptomatic relief of mucosal dryness. Saliva substitutes are available as over-the-counter rinses or sprays and are most effective if used before meals and at bedtime. A number of toothpastes and chewing gums have been developed specifically for use in patients with xerostomia.

Exciting new regenerative approaches to restore salivary gland function have recently been reported, but are still limited to preclinical studies.[55]

The most effective protective strategy for radiation-induced caries is the aggressive use of topical fluorides.[56] Topical fluoride supplements should be initiated at the start of radiation treatment. Continuation of fluoride following the completion of radiotherapy is critical, especially in patients who develop xerostomia. Fluorides for dental use come in three forms: rinses, gels applied by tooth brushing or in customized trays, and drops also used in trays molded to fit over patients' teeth. Patients in whom xerostomia is anticipated should have fluoride trays fabricated before the initiation of radiotherapy. Fluoride gel or drops are placed in the trays and applied by the patient each day. Use of tray-borne application can be supplemented with acidulated fluoride rinses; generally, the use of rinses in the morning and trays before sleep is most effective and easiest for patients. Acidulated fluorides tend to work best, although neutral fluoride rinses are available for patients with mucositis in whom acidulated material might be irritating, or for patients with porcelain prostheses in whom pitting of the restorations might occur. The supplemental use of a remineralizing toothpaste should also be considered.[57] Aggressive oral hygiene is to be encouraged, and patients should be seen by a dentist frequently. Regular dental visits are critical to insure early detection and intervention of caries and periodontal disease.

For patients who cannot tolerate trays because of gagging or mucositis, fluoride gels may be applied with a toothbrush, either as 1.1% sodium fluoride or as 0.4% stannous fluoride. The latter appears to be more efficacious. Patients should be instructed to avoid sucrose.

Loss of taste is a transient, but bothersome, sequelae of head and neck radiation.[58] The severity of taste loss increases rapidly up to doses of 30 Gy, but then usually plateaus. Patients who receive doses of 30 Gy or more may lose their ability to distinguish salt or sweet tastes. Fortunately, hypogeusia is typically transient and taste begins to return within 1–2 months after the completion of treatment. Total recovery may take up to a year. If there does not seem to be progression to improvement following radiotherapy, candidiasis should be ruled out.

Osteoradionecrosis

Of all of the oral complications of head and neck radiation, one of the most significant is ORN.[59] First described in 1927, ORN

results in the denudation of soft tissue and exposure and necrosis of bone.[60,61] Although not limited to the jaws, it frequently occurs at this site. ORN causes a painful, chronic, open, and foul-smelling wound that is typically of great distress to the patient. Most cases ultimately heal with conservative treatment, but the course is usually prolonged. ORN was attributed to a triad of trauma (often tooth extractions), radiation, and infection.[62] Subsequent studies suggest, however, that ORN represents a defect in wound healing rather than a true osteomyelitis.[63] The etiology appears to relate to diminished vascularization as a consequence of XRT.[64] Histologic changes of thickened arterial and arteriolar walls substantiate this hypothesis. The finding of cultivable and noncultivable bacteria may suggest an infectious component.[65]

No consensus exists concerning the overall frequency of ORN, although reported ranges vary between 4% and 44%. While approximately 15% appears to be the preponderant experience,[59,63] a recent meta-analysis reported that only 2% of HNC patients are at risk.[66] The mandible is involved more often than the maxilla, which probably reflects the difference in blood supply and vascularity of the two bones. Time until onset of ORN following XRT is variable. Some authors have described ORN as early as 2 weeks after XRT, others report it as a late condition. Most cases occur within the first 3 years after XRT (74%). Equally controversial is the rate at which ORN risk diminishes with time after the completion of XRT, although it seems clear that the risk never reaches zero.[67]

A number of risk factors for ORN have been positively identified.[68] Men have been reported to have a risk for ORN that is threefold higher than women.[61] Patients who are edentulous are twice as likely as patients with teeth to develop ORN. Furthermore, the frequency of ORN increases dramatically in individuals with active dental disease (e.g., periodontal disease, caries, periapical disease, and poorly fitting prostheses).[59] Fifty percent of cases appear to be associated with tooth extraction following radiation. These findings strongly support pre-XRT dental evaluation and aggressive repair and removal of diseased teeth. The field size, dose rate, and total dose of XRT have a marked effect on the frequency of ORN. Patients who receive cumulative doses of 65 Gy or more to the mandible or maxilla are more likely to develop ORN than are patients receiving lesser doses. Use of three-dimensional radiation techniques has resulted in a slight reduction in ORN risk.[69] Patients with tumors that are adjacent or contiguous with bone are also at higher ORN risk. It is likely that this finding is due to the inclusion of bone in the radiated field as the volume of bone exposed to XRT has a direct impact on ORN risk. Poor nutrition and immune status also appear to predispose to the condition. Diagnosis of ORN is usually based on clinical findings. In cases in which the diagnosis is questionable, magnetic resonance imaging may be of value.[70]

Treatment of ORN is based on the severity and chronicity of the condition.[71] Fortunately, most lesions (up to 60%) eventually heal in approximately 6 months with conservative therapy consisting of local debridement, saliva irrigation, and oral antibiotics.[72] Results of studies in which pentoxifylline, used for its anti-TNF activity, was assessed are inconsistent.[73,74]

Lesions showing no improvement or demonstrate progression require more aggressive therapy. For these cases, surgical debridement and hyperbaric oxygen (HBO) may be indicated.[75,76] In extensive cases, radical resection of involved bone with immediate microvascular reconstruction has been used successfully in patients who have failed more conservative treatment, including HBO.[77] The use of autologous bone marrow aspirate concentrate coupled with allogeneic dental pulp stem cells with platelet rich plasma was recently reported to be successful in patient's refractory to conventional approaches.[78]

Because most cases of intra-oral ORN are associated with dental disease and post-XRT extractions, eliminating potential sites of odontogenic pathology before the start of radiation is the basis for prevention. Teeth with periodontal disease, advanced caries with a risk of impingement on the dental pulp, fracture, or periapical disease should be removed before the initiation of XRT. Teeth adjacent to or involved in potential surgical sites (for tumor resection) also should be extracted. Because of the consequences of ORN, even suspiciously diseased teeth, especially in the XRT area, should be eliminated. The timing of dental extractions in patients being treated with XRT has been the subject of much analysis, discussion, and controversy; however, the consensus is that teeth should be extracted before XRT.[13] Ideally, a minimum 21-day healing period is desirable, although a shorter time may be dictated by circumstances. In either instance, extraction before XRT is much more desirable than extraction after the start of therapy, because a number of studies suggest that post-XRT extractions carry significant risk of ORN, no matter how long after XRT they are performed. In all cases, extraction should be performed as atraumatically as possible, with special care given to the soft tissue, primary closure if possible, and good local postoperative wound management. Perioperative use of antibiotics is also recommended.

Aggressive oral hygiene, use of fluorides, and dental care are important components in preventing the development of dental disease once XRT has started. If dental disease develops after XRT and a tooth is restorable, endodontic therapy is more desirable than extraction. Inevitably, extractions are sometimes required of teeth in radiated fields.[79] The risk of ORN in these cases has been reported to be reasonable (5.6%), even without the use of HBO. The efficacy of HBO in these cases is unresolved. One study found that, among patients having teeth removed within the first year following radiation, 98.5% of extraction sites treated pre- and postoperatively with HBO healed without complications. However, the efficacy of HBO reportedly decreased the farther out from where radiation extractions were performed.[80] The utility of HBO, with its incurred cost and multiple visits, warrants additional study.[81]

Oral complications of chemotherapy

Oral complications of cancer chemotherapy result from the effects of the drug acting on the oral mucosa (direct or primary stomatotoxicity), the patients' inability to contain local, minor oral disease during myelosuppression (indirect or secondary stomatotoxicity), or some combination of the two.

Risk factors

Not all patients who undergo cancer chemotherapy are at equal risk to develop oral complications. This is especially true of oral mucositis. Although a number of variables have been identified that bear on the frequency and severity of oral problems, their predictive value, in general, has yet to be definitely defined. Risk factors can be divided into those that are associated with the patient and those that are related to the treatment regimen.[82]

Patient-related risk factors include tumor diagnosis, patient age, gender, body mass, genetics, the patient's oral condition before cancer therapy, the level of oral care during therapy, baseline xerostomia, and baseline neutrophil numbers. Patients with hematologic malignancies (i.e., leukemia and lymphoma) are at greater risk of oral complications than are patients with nonhead and neck solid tumors. For example, more than 66% of patients with leukemia and 33% of patients with non-Hodgkin lymphoma develop oral problems. It seems likely that tumor-related myelosuppression is at least partly the basis for this observation.[83] Almost all patients with

tumors of the head and neck who receive local therapy develop problems after treatment.

The role of age as a risk factor for mucositis is unclear as there are few studies that compare the rate of mucositis among patients of varying ages with similar diagnoses. Among children, nadir of the neutrophil count, lower body weight, and higher peak creatinine levels have been observed to be associated with higher rates of mucositis.[84] Among adult patients with solid tumors being treated with 5-fluorouracil (5-FU), mucositis appears to be more severe and persistent among older persons.

Sex may affect risk. There are reports to suggest that women are more likely to have toxicities associated with 5-FU than are men.[85] This trend was also reported in patients receiving high-dose chemotherapy (BEAM) or high-dose melphalan followed by autologous HSCT.[86] A mechanism to explain this phenomenon has yet to be determined. Genetics may affect mucositis risk in at least two ways.[87] Patients with genetic defects, which affect drug metabolism, are at increased risk for mucositis.[88,89] For example, among a population of patients being treated with methotrexate for chronic myelogenous leukemia, increased toxicity (including mucositis) was observed in those individuals with lower methylenetetrahydrofolate reductase activity (TT genotype). Similarly, deficiencies in dihydropyrimidine dehydrogenase (DPD) predispose to toxicities mediated by 5-FU. Alternatively, genetics may affect and regulate the mechanisms, which provide the biological basis for chemotherapy-induced mucosal injury. For example, proinflammatory cytokine production varies among the population and is genetically controlled. These cytokines play a role and track closely with nonhematologic toxicities. Consequently, patients who are predisposed to be high producers of these proteins may also be at increased risk for mucositis and other toxicities. For example, among a cohort of allogeneic HSCT recipients, specific tumor necrosis factor polymorphisms conferred a relative risk (RR) of severe toxicities in excess of 17-fold.[90] The results of a recently reported study in a pediatric cohort being treated for a variety of malignancies suggest an association among ABO blood types. The RR of oropharyngeal mucositis was 2.86 among patients with type O compared to 0.47 for type A and 0.59 for type B.[91] Further study is needed to fully elucidate the impact of functional genes on mucosal injury, but it promises to be important in determining both risk and predicting responsiveness to mechanism-based interventions.[92] It is generally agreed that patients whose pretreatment oral condition is poor are at greater risk for some, but not all, oral complications.[93] Chronic irritation for poorly fitting prostheses or faulty restorations predisposes patients to the development of ulcerative mucositis. Patients with advanced periodontal disease, pulpal disease, or low-grade soft-tissue infections such as those associated with partially erupted third molars (i.e., wisdom teeth) are at increased risk for developing sepsis of oral origin once they become myelosuppressed. However, elevated risks of infection are not associated with asymptomatic radiographically demonstrable periapical lesions in endodontically treated teeth.[94]

The level of oral care during therapy has a marked influence on outcome relative to oral complications and infection.[95] The ability of the patients and their healthcare providers to reduce the load of oral bacterial flora favorably affects the risk of both local and systemic infection.[96] Aggressive techniques of oral hygiene, including mechanical debridement of the teeth and soft tissue, and antimicrobial rinses are effective.

Xerostomia before and during chemotherapy may be associated with an increased risk of mucositis.[97] It has been suggested that alterations in the health of desiccated oral mucosa and an overall increase in the resident oral microflora may contribute to increasing the probability of mucositis. Studies evaluating treatment strategies aimed at replenishing saliva or mouth moisture have had very mixed results. The favorable effect of pilocarpine on chemotherapy-induced mucositis reported in one study was not replicated in a similar trial[98] or among recipients of autologous HSCT.[99]

The extent of mucositis correlates negatively with neutropenia. Baseline neutrophil counts of less than 4000 are associated with higher rates of mucositis.[97] This finding may explain, in part, the observation of increased rates of mucositis among patients with hematologic malignancies.

Risk of complications also relates to the form, schedule, and dose of chemotherapy used.[16] Concomitant radiation, including TBI, also enhance the risk of oral problems. For example, the incidence of mucositis has been reported to be markedly lower in reduced intensity stem cell transplant recipients (30.9%) compared to patients who received conventional conditioning regimens (90.2%).[97] Significant differences exist in the degree of stomatotoxicity of drugs used for chemotherapy.[16] Drugs or regimens containing anthracyclines, taxanes, platinum, and 5-FU are consistently stomatotoxic. Conditioning regimens in which TBI is used also cause mucositis at high rates. There are 17 specific drugs or combinations in which oral mucositis rates (grade 3–4) affect a significant percentage of patients (>25%):

- Docetaxel/5-FU
- Docetaxel + XRT
- Paclitaxel + XRT
- Docetaxel + 5-FU
- Paclitaxel/5-FU + XRT
- Docetaxel/platinum + XRT
- Paclitaxel/platinum + XRT
- Docetaxel/platinum/5-FU
- Paclitaxel/platinum/5-FU
- Oxaliplatin + XRT
- Platinum/taxane + XRT
- Platinum/methotrexate/leucovorin
- 5-FU/platinum
- 5-FU/leucovorin/taxane
- Irinotecan/5-FU CI + XRT
- Ara-C/idarubicin/fludarabine
- Methotrexate
- Isofamide/etoposide
- Melphalan

In viewing the above list, it is important to remember that the incidence of oral complications, particularly mucositis, tends to be vastly under-reported in terms of occurrence and severity. Virtually every chemotherapeutic agent in the current armamentarium has the potential to produce a stomatotoxic response in at least some portion of the treated population.

Repetitive, low-dose regimens tend to be less toxic than do bolus doses of the same agent. Toxicity that is secondary to radiation is dependent on cumulative dose; pulsed application of therapy does not significantly reduce stomatic changes.

Ulcerative mucositis usually occurs 5–8 days following the administration of chemotherapy and it lasts approximately 7–14 days. Lesions heal spontaneously and without scar formation. Chemotherapy-induced mucositis is confined to the movable oral mucosa: the mucosa of the cheeks, lateral and ventral tongue, inner aspects of the lips, floor of the mouth, and soft palate. Unlike radiation-induced mucositis, that produced by chemotherapy does not affect the hard palate or gingival. The dorsal surface of the tongue is also not affected. This observation is likely to be attributable to the differences in the character of the epithelium on each mucosal surface. Of the sites in the mouth, the buccal mucosa (cheeks), lateral and ventral surfaces of the tongue, and the floor of the mouth are the most commonly involved. In patients who receive multiple cycles of chemotherapy, lesions tend to reappear in the same sites. Numerous studies have confirmed that mucositis is not of infectious (particularly viral) origin.

The biologic mechanisms, which underlie chemotherapy-induced mucositis, are currently the topic of intense investigation.[18,100] As noted above, mucositis was viewed as the result of nonspecific toxicity of chemotherapy directed against the rapidly dividing cells of the oral basal epithelium. Although data exist to support the hypothesis, the observation that agents could alter the course of mucositis with little or no epithelial activity suggests a more broadly based pathogenesis. It appears that mucositis represents a clinical outcome due to a complex interaction of local tissue toxicity (endothelium, connective tissue, and epithelium), the level of myelosuppression, and the local environment. Disruption of connective tissue and endothelial cells initiated by free radical formation likely leads to the activation of a range of transcription factors and increased expression of a number of genes that result in stimulation of proinflammatory cytokine production and tissue damage. Simultaneous activation of other signaling pathways and enzyme activation results in increases in ceramide, proteolytic enzymes, and other mediators of direct and indirect epithelial injury. Thus, in addition to clonogenic death of basal cells caused by direct DNA injury, secondary pathways produce a barrage of mechanisms that lead to apoptosis or necrosis. Therefore, the epithelium first becomes atrophic, as its renewal ceases, and then eventually completely breaks down to form an ulcer. It is noteworthy that in some patients, the extent of cumulative injury to the basal epithelium does not reach the threshold needed for ulceration to occur. In these patients, the thinned mucosa is mildly to moderately symptomatic (grade 1 mucositis). In cases when ulceration does occur, secondary colonization by oral bacteria (both gram positives and gram negatives) occurs. Cell wall products from these bacteria make their way into the underlying connective tissue where they effectively stimulate additional proinflammatory cytokine production by infiltrating macrophages.

The better understanding of the pathobiology of mucositis has served as the basis for the development of mechanistically based interventions.[38] The first of these agents to gain approval was palifermin (keratinocyte growth factor-1, Kepivance, Amgen) for the prevention and treatment of oral mucositis in patients receiving conditioning regimens in preparation for HSCT to treat hematologic malignancies. In a phase 3 trial in 212 HSCT recipients receiving a stomatotoxic conditioning regimen, palifermin, administered in multiple doses before and after transplantation was successful in significantly reducing the duration, incidence, and severity of oral mucositis, favorably affecting patient-reported quality of life outcomes, and in reducing days of opioid use and fever.[101] It seems likely that palifermin's effect was the consequence, not only of its ability to stimulate epithelial proliferation, but also because of its cytoprotective activates mediated through increased expression of mediating transcription factors. Of the 450,000 patients who develop mucositis each year in the United States, the HSCT population comprises only 5%. Consequently, extension of these and other agents to other tumor populations is a major objective.

Low-level (helium-neon) laser therapy (LLLT) has demonstrated efficacy in reducing the severity and symptoms associated with oral mucositis.[102] While additional studies are needed to confirm its value, the cost and logistics of LLLT may limit its overall utility. As more is learned about the ability of LLLT to impact a wide range of cellular and molecular pathways known to be associated with tumor progression and growth mandates studies demonstrating its lack of activity relative to impacting tumor response.

A number of cytoprotective strategies and agents have been suggested as mucositis interventions. Oral cryotherapy is inexpensive and without risk, its use for 30 min starting 5 min before the infusion of bolus 5-FU, edatrexate, or melphalan may be helpful in reducing the severity of mucositis.[26] Pentoxifylline has been evaluated in a number of studies with mixed results. The topical application of trefoil factor was reportedly beneficial in mitigating mucositis in patients with colorectal and HNCs.[38,103] The development of biologics, gene transfers, and other therapies targeting specific biological pathways is also under investigation.[38]

Because the presence of oral micro-organisms is thought to adversely affect the course of mucositis, antimicrobial therapy has been studied extensively as an approach to intervention.[36] In general, the weight of data suggests that reduction of the oral bacterial load through medication does not bear significantly on the incidence or severity of mucositis. The use of topical antimicrobials such as chlorhexidine gluconate has consistently failed to improve the frequency or course of mucositis in randomized, blinded trials.[104,105]

Palliation has been the most widely used approach for the management of mucositis. Saline 0.9% has been used for years and is more effective than hydrogen peroxide, and at least as good as "magic mouthwashes."[106] Barrier-type palliatives such as sucralfate suspension and Gelclair are available, although their benefit has not been convincingly shown. Topical lidocaine or Benadryl in Kaopectate or milk of magnesia may offer some topical relief, but often do not eliminate the need for parenteral analgesia.

Effects of targeted therapies

Ulceration associated with mTOR-inhibitor use

Inhibitors of the mammalian target of rapamycin (mTOR) have demonstrated encouraging results in clinical trials as an intervention for advanced malignancies. Oral ulceration is among the most significant dose-limiting toxicities associated with these agents[107] and has been reported as mucositis. However, the clinical course, behavior, appearance, and likely pathogenesis mTOR inhibitor-induced oral ulcers strongly suggest that they are profoundly different from mucositis induced by radiation or cytotoxic agents.[108]

Unlike typical chemotherapy-induced mucositis, aphthous lesions present as discrete, ovoid, relatively shallow ulcers, and surrounded by a characteristic erythematous margin (Figure 3). Lesions develop more quickly after drug administration and typically resolve spontaneously after an extremely painful course. Although randomized trials have not yet been performed, treatment approaches similar to those used for major aphthous stomatitis may be effective.

Dysesthesia associated with mTKIs

Multitargeted tyrosine kinase inhibitors (mTKIs) offer a specifically directed approach to cancer therapy for an increasing number of malignancies. These small molecular inhibitors have been associated with oral discomfort without evidence of physical findings. The term dysesthesia is more precise and descriptive; it is preferred to stomatitis, which is nonspecific but was used in previous studies. These dysesthesias can present as mucosal sensitivity, burning, dysgeusia or hypogeusia, xerostomia (with

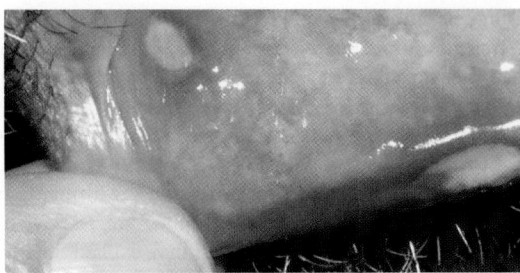

Figure 3 Oral mucosal ulcers associated with the administration of an mTOR inhibitor. Note that the lesions are well defined and oval with a central area of necrosis and an erythematous periphery reminiscent of aphthous stomatitis.

adequate salivary flow), and other altered sensations such as paresthesia and anesthesia. These symptoms can occur in up to 60% of patients on mTKI therapy and can be associated with other side effects of therapy including the development of palmar-plantar erythrodysesthesia.[109]

Calcineurin-induced inflammatory fibrovascular hyperplasia

Calcineurin inhibitors used for immunosuppression can induce inflammatory fibrovascular hyperplasias in the oral cavity. While cyclosporine is associated with a more diffuse, generalized overgrowth of densely fibrous gingival tissue, tacrolimus-induced pyogenic granulomas present as localized fibrous polyps more often seen on the tongue and buccal mucosa.[110]

Osteonecrosis

Bisphosphonates and the RANK-L inhibitor denosumab have been administered concomitant with chemotherapy as a strategy to reduce metastases to bone. Among patients being treated in this way, osteonecrosis of the jaws, particularly of the mandible (twice as common compared to maxilla), has been reported with increasing frequency.[111] The frequency of the condition has been reported to be between 3% and 8.5%.[112] Newer cases have been reported with angiogenesis inhibitors such as sunitinib and bevacizumab, prompting the nomenclature designation as medication-related osteonecrosis of the jaw (MRONJ).[21] The presentation of osteonecrosis in this population varies in symptomatology. Although some patients experience pain, others do not. The majority of cases appear to be associated with dental manipulation, such as extraction, or soft-tissue trauma. The mechanism underlying this pathology is yet to be defined, as is a full appreciation of the natural history of the condition. Conservative treatment seems to be most appropriate (Table 1). Presently, the most judicious strategy is to assure aggressive dental screening and treatment before the initiation of treatment so that the possible need for dental intervention is minimized.

Infections

Simultaneous with the breakdown of the oral epithelium, the patients' ability to deal with the abundant oral microbial flora is compromised by their myelosuppression. Thus, the mouth becomes an important source of bacteremia and sepsis in the granulocytopenic cancer patient, as well as locoregional secondary infection. These manifestations of indirect stomatotoxicity parallel the bone marrow status; hence, they are maximal at, or just proceeding toward the patient's granulocyte nadir. Systemic invasion of oral viridans streptococci is particularly common. Of these, *Streptococcus mitis* is associated with the most serious sequelae.

Fungal infections

Local oral infections in myelosuppressed patients are attributable to fungal, viral, and bacterial organisms, in order of descending frequency. Candidiasis is the most frequent oral infection and may appear in its characteristic white, curdy form or as erythematous, macular lesions.[113] It most frequently occurs on the palate, tongue, and corners of the mouth. Poorly controlled oral candidiasis increases the risk of aspiration and the development of candidal esophagitis or fungemia. In addition, aspergillosis and mucormycosis are not uncommon in myelosuppressed patients; these lesions can appear as invasive oral ulcerations that are painful and may involve bone.

As systemic candidiasis is associated with high rates of morbidity and mortality,[114] antifungal prophylaxis may be a reasonable consideration among patients in whom prolonged neutropenia is anticipated, that is, HSCT or stomatotoxic, myeloablative chemotherapy recipients. In general, topical agents are ineffective in this group. Treatment options include fluconazole, caspofungin, and micafungin.[115]

Topical antifungal prophylaxis directed against *Candida* may be beneficial for patients receiving head and neck radiation and promotes xerostomia, and in patients who are immunosuppressed with steroids. The polyene antifungal agents (e.g., nystatin) or the imidazole agents, clotrimazole (Mycelex) are equally efficacious. Nystatin is formulated as a thick, cherry-flavored suspension that is not a favorite of chemotherapy-nauseated individuals. Mycelex is dispensed as a troche. For pediatric patients, nystatin popsicles made by putting the drug plus water into an ice cube tray seem to work well. Two other imidazoles also are available: ketoconazole (Nizoral) and fluconazole (Diflucan); both have demonstrated efficacy for the prophylaxis and treatment of existing disease. The requirement of an acidic environment for ketoconazole, however, may limit its usefulness in patients who have difficulty eating. Azole resistance may be of relevance in the treatment of fungal infections. Some of the candida species such as *Candida glabrata* and *Candida krusei* are inherently less sensitive to azole antifungal medications.[116]

The efficacy of chlorhexidine gluconate rinses as a topical antifungal agent is unclear.[117] In vivo data suggest that chlorhexidine reduces the activity of nystatin.[118] Hence, its simultaneous use with nystatin is not recommended.

While the use of surveillance cultures for predicting the presence or course of fungal infection has long been shown to be of little value, PCR may have a role in the rapid diagnosis and speciation of oral candidal infections.[119]

Viral infections

Herpes simplex virus type (HSV-1) is the most common oral viral infection in patients receiving chemotherapy or head and neck radiation, and determination of antibody status is an important part of risk assessment. Oral HSV-1 infection can result from a primary infection with the virus or the reactivation of latent virus in a previously exposed host.[120] It is the latter that is most frequent in patients receiving cancer therapy. Individuals with prior HSV-1 exposure who are seropositive for the virus are at much greater risk than are patients who are negative. The most common manifestation of infection with HSV-1 is oral ulceration. While this may appear to be clinically similar to other forms of mucositis, it usually differs in its course and distribution.

The timing of HSV-1 infection in patients receiving chemotherapy or HSCT is typically quite consistent.[121] Lesions generally are seen approximately 18 days following the start of therapy. This temporal relationship is important in differentiating lesions that

likely result from HSV-1 from those that result from direct stomatotoxicity, which are noted 5–7 days after the start of treatment, and from secondary surface infection (usually bacterial) that are seen at the patient's maximum myelosuppression (i.e., granulocyte nadir), which occurs around 12–14 days. Lesions can appear on any mucosal surface including the most heavily keratinized tissues of the hard palate and gingiva. Viral culture is the most definitive way to diagnose HSV-1 infection, and aggressive culturing is recommended, especially in patients who are seropositive. Systemic acyclovir remains the treatment of choice for prophylaxis and treatment of HSV infection.[121]

Herpes zoster also may present with oral lesions in patients who receive therapy for cancer.[115] These lesions tend to be crop-like. Although they begin as vesicular lesions, they quickly rupture and form painful, small, ulcerative lesions. Unlike those from HSV-1, these lesions usually are unilateral and linear, often following one of the branches of the fifth cranial nerve.

Bacterial infections

The oral cavity may be a frequent source of local and systemic bacterial infection in the myelosuppressed patient with cancer, as evidenced by the increasing frequency of streptococcal infections among patients with granulocytopenic cancer.[115] Bacterial infections may be of soft tissue or gingival or odontogenic origin. Patients receiving cancer therapy often have increased numbers of oral organisms as a consequence of reduced hygiene and xerostomia. Additionally, the composition of the oral flora shifts from one in which gram-positive organisms predominate to one with an abundance of gram-negative pathogens.

Most often, odontogenic infections result from degeneration and infection of the dental pulp subsequent to bacterial invasion secondary to caries. Because of a patient's inability to mount an inflammatory response, conventional signs of dental infection (e.g., abscess formation, swelling) are absent, and patients complain of localized tooth pain. Percussion or thermal sensitivity with clinical and/or radiographic evidence of caries progressing into the pulp is diagnostic. Neurotoxicity may cause dental pain that mimics odontogenic infection in patients receiving plant alkaloids. Odontogenic infections predominantly result from anaerobic species that are similar to those found in dental plaque. Treatment should consist of eliminating the source of infection, and in most cases, this involves tooth extraction. The safety of tooth extraction in the face of myelosuppression has been reported by a number of investigators.[122] These studies indicate that extraction may be performed with antibiotic coverage, platelet transfusion if needed, attention to tissue management, and good closure. Use of hemostatic agents such as Gelfoam in extraction sockets is discouraged, because they may act as foci of infection. Generally, platelet transfusion is not necessary for counts greater than 50,000 cells/mL. Systemic antibiotic coverage is indicated until the wound is epithelialized.

Gingival infections are relatively common in patients receiving myelosuppressive therapy. Some are localized, such as those that are associated with partially erupted third molars (i.e., wisdom teeth), whereas others tend to be more diffuse. Acute gingival and periodontal infections are worse in patients with pre-existing chronic gingival inflammation or periodontal disease.

The clinical appearance of acute gingival infections, which occur during periods of granulocytopenia, resembles that seen in acute necrotizing ulcerative gingivitis. Pain and loss of the gingival architecture, particularly necrosis of the interdental papillae, are characteristic. These lesions tend to be of a mixed bacterial nature, and include a variety of pathogens, such as *Staphylococcus epidermidis*, *Pseudomonas aeruginosa*, and bacteria typically associated with periodontal disease such as bacteroides and veillonella.

Treatment should include local debridement in addition to systemic antibiotics. Local culture of lesions may be more useful than blood culture, because invasion of intact organisms may not occur. Empirical treatment is recommended regardless of culture results.

Mucosal infections in the myelosuppressed patient often are superimposed on ulcerated areas that have broken down as the result of direct stomatotoxicity. Ulcers may appear to be penetrating, with rounded borders and yellowish-white necrotic centers. Because of the lack of an inflammatory response, erythematous borders are usually absent. If the ulcerations are precipitated by trauma, secondary hematoma formation may occur in the patient with thrombocytopenia. Soft-tissue infections tend to be of gram-negative etiology, although HSV-1 must be ruled out. Treatment should include debridement, palliation, and antimicrobial therapy. Bacterial and viral cultures should be performed as well.

Strategies for the prevention of oral infection include eliminating sources of mucosal irritation and reducing the quantity of the local oral flora.[6] In addition, treatment of low-grade, asymptomatic infection before the start of therapy minimizes the risk of acute episodes once myelosuppression occurs. Reduction in the oral flora may be accomplished by mechanical and/or chemical means. Local debridement of the teeth can be accomplished with conventional tooth brushing; soft brushes should be used. Thrombocytopenia is not a contraindication to mechanical debridement if common sense is used. Brushing should be discontinued in the face of significant bleeding. Alternatively, cotton swabs or a towel-wrapped finger may be used to clean the teeth. Dental floss is an excellent adjuvant for cleaning but may be difficult for patients to use if they are unfamiliar with it. It also may be used until patients become profoundly thrombocytopenic. Essentially, anything that the patient or provider can use to physically wipe debris and micro-organisms from the teeth will be beneficial. Cotton swabs, sponges, and rubber tips all may be of use.

Rinses are of varying degrees of help in maintaining oral hygiene. Any fluid that flushes the mouth, including water, will be of some help. Saline and diluted peroxide are frequently used. Generally, mouth rinses containing alcohol as their active agent cause burning of the atrophic mucosa and are not recommended. Mixed results have been reported with chlorhexidine gluconate rinses. If chlorhexidine is used, its administration should be timed to avoid contact with nystatin, because the effects of the latter may be inactivated by chlorhexidine. Similarly, povidone iodine rinses have demonstrated efficacy in reducing the resident oral flora. Other drugs have been tried as preventatives, and fluoride rinses reduce the ability of oral bacteria to adhere to teeth. Consequently, they also may be helpful.

Patients with removable prostheses should be instructed to remove them during periods of myelosuppression. Oral bleeding during such periods most often is of gingival origin. Spontaneous gingival bleeding is a rare occurrence when platelet counts exceed 20,000 cells/mL. Slow oozing may be noted at lower platelet levels, especially in areas with preexisting periodontal disease. Local treatment of gingival bleeding includes initial debridement, nondisturbance of formed clots, and topical application of thrombin under pressure. Gingival bleeding usually is interpreted as evidence that the platelet count is low enough to allow other, more threatening hemorrhage.

Hematoma formation often occurs in areas of trauma, especially the buccal mucosa, alveolar mucosa, or edentulous areas. Areas of submucosal hemorrhage form bluish, blister-like areas, which then form a yellowish-white, tumor-like mass of fibrin. Epithelialization occurs beneath the mass. If bleeding occurs before healing is complete, topical therapy may include thrombin, microfibrillar collagen, or other hemostatic gel. Before healing is complete, the clot may serve as a focus for microbial growth. It should be checked daily and removed as soon as epithelialization is complete. Unchecked sublingual bleeding may cause respiratory embarrassment by elevating the tongue.

Oral complications associated with HSCT

Mucositis

The risk of mucositis in the HSCT population is largely dependent on the intensity of HSCT conditioning regimen and varies widely to a high incidence of 76%.[123] The inclusion of total-body irradiation also impacts the risk of developing mucositis.[16] As with other forms of chemotherapy-induced mucositis, lesions are localized to the movable oral mucosa and are most frequent in the floor of the mouth, lingual frenum, and labial and buccal mucosae (Figure 1). There appears to be no significant difference in either the onset of mucositis following transplantation or the duration of mucositis among recipients of autologous or allogeneic HSCT. Woo and colleagues[124] reported a mean time of mucositis onset as 5 days following HSCT for autologous recipients, as compared to 6 days for allogeneic recipients. The mean duration of mucositis for both groups was approximately 6 days, with resolution in 10–12 days. In another study in which autologous HSCTs were performed in patients who received cyclophosphamide and TBI, the duration of WHO grade 3/4 mucositis was longer. Mucositis almost always resolves by 3 weeks after transplant, an important diagnostic observation when patients go on to develop GVHD. There is an association between absolute neutrophil count (ANC) and mucositis resolution. Unless patients have extremely severe lesions, mucositis usually spontaneously resolves with an ANC of greater than 500 cells/mL. However, it does not appear that the administration of either GCSF or GM-CSF prevents or minimizes the mucositis development.

The mechanism of mucositis induction is discussed elsewhere in this chapter. It is important to note that the condition occurs independently of oral mucosal infections with either viral or fungal etiology. As noted above, palifermin has recently been approved for the prevention and treatment of oral mucositis in autologous HSCT recipients (see above).

Infection

Oral infection is a major cause of morbidity among HSCT recipients. Of special importance in this patient population is the oral cavity as a source of systemic or distant infection.[125] The incidence of streptococcal infections in HSCT recipients has increased dramatically. Consequently, pretreatment screening to identify and eliminate asymptomatic, dormant, or potential sources of dental infection or irritation should be mandated for HSCT recipients.

In addition to bacterial infections, HSCT recipients are at risk for oral viral and fungal infections during the period of their granulocytopenia. As with other myelosuppressed patients, the clinical presentation of these infections in the BMT population often varies from the classic descriptions typically associated with these lesions. Consequently, early and aggressive culturing is mandated. Members of the herpes group account for most viral infections; herpes simplex, varicella, and herpes zoster are associated with oral infections in HSCT patients. The routine practice of acyclovir prophylaxis,

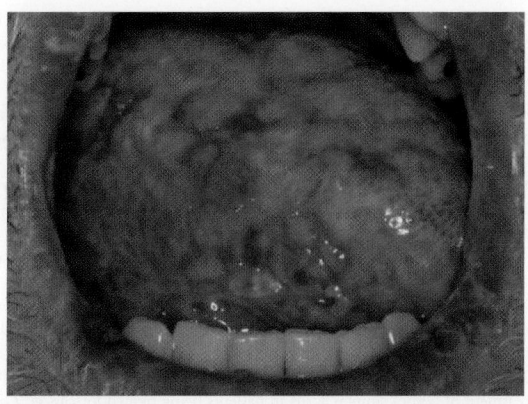

Figure 4 Oral manifestations of graft-versus-host disease characterized by mucosal blistering and lichenoid changes. Source: Courtesy of Dr. Nathaniel Treister.

however, generally has been discontinued. In addition, acyclovir resistant mucocutaneous herpes simplex infections have been reported in HSCT populations. Candidiasis is the most common fungal infection, although both mucormycosis and aspergillosis have been reported. Lesions of the deep fungal infections generally present as nonhealing gingival ulcerations. Biopsy is the diagnostic method of choice.

Graft-versus-host disease

The mouth is a common site for manifestations of both acute and chronic GVHD.[126,127] Although there are relatively few reports on the oral manifestations of acute GVHD, three clinical patterns of oral lesions have been described and are noted as early as 3 weeks following transplantation and almost 1 week after the onset of skin lesions (Figure 4). Initially, multiple, small, white, and papillated lesions are present on the movable mucosa. These progress to the development of keratotic, white, and lacey lesions that clinically resemble lichen planus and, in fact, have been described as lichenoid in appearance. Desquamative lesions may then develop. These also are similar to the lesions of erosive or bullous lichen planus, and unlike the other two forms, these tend to be symptomatic and require intervention.

The mouth is only second to the skin as a site for manifestations of chronic GVHD. The oral lesions of chronic GVHD appear approximately 3 months or later following transplantation. Approximately 70% of patients with GVHD develop oral lesions, which most typically are lichenoid in appearance. Symptomatic lesions usually present as erosive, vesiculobullous lesions of the oral mucosa, with peripheral areas of keratotic striations. Additionally, xerostomia is a frequent finding among patients with chronic GVHD. Both mucosal and salivary gland changes result from lymphocytic infiltration; the resulting tissue changes are analogous to those seen in other autoimmune changes in the mouth.

Biopsy of the minor salivary glands of the lip appears to be an accurate and sensitive way to confirm the diagnosis of chronic GVHD, and it is more predictive than either biopsy of the buccal mucosa or the parotid gland. Technically, minor salivary gland biopsy is easily performed in an office setting with local anesthesia and a minimum of tissue manipulation. Histologically, one notes acinar atrophy and/or destruction accompanied by a lymphocytic infiltrate that is rich in CD3+ T cells.

Lichenoid lesions generally respond to topical or systemic steroid therapy. Ultraviolet A light therapy reportedly has benefit in the treatment of severe, nonresponsive lesions. Therapy for xerostomia was discussed earlier in this chapter. As with other patients having

xerostomia, patients with GVHD are at increased risk for caries and should be managed accordingly.

Additional late effects of HSCT and GVHD also affect the mouth. Of sites for secondary malignancies in this population, the mouth is among the most common. Consequently, patients should receive routine and thorough oral examinations to screen for the development of squamous cell carcinoma. Pediatric HSCT has also been reported to be associated with significant long-term oral and craniofacial complications. Early referral and aggressive follow-up care by pediatric dental specialists are recommended.

Key references

The complete reference list can be found on the Wiley Companion Digital Edition of this title (see inside front cover for login instructions).

2 Epstein JB, Guneri P, Barasch A. Appropriate and necessary oral care for people with cancer: guidance to obtain the right oral and dental care at the right time. *Support Care Cancer.* 2014;**22**:1981–1988.

6 Elad S, Raber-Durlacher JE, Brennan MT, et al. Basic oral care for hematology-oncology patients and hematopoietic stem cell transplantation recipients: a position paper from the joint task force for the Multinational Association of Supportive Care in Cancer/International Society of Oral Oncology (MASCC/ISOO) and the European Society for Blood and Marrow Transplantation (EBMT). *Support Care Cancer.* 2015;**23**:223–236.

8 Jham BC, Reis PM, Miranda EL, et al. Oral health status of 207 head and neck cancer patients before, during and after radiotherapy. *Clin Oral Investig.* 2008;**12(1)**:19–24.

15 Jawad H, Hodson NA, Nixon PJ. A review of dental treatment of head and neck cancer patients, before, during, and after radiotherapy: part 1. *Brit Dent J.* 2015;**218**:65–68.

16 Sonis ST, Elting LS, Keefe D, et al. Perspectives on cancer therapy-induced mucosal injury: pathogenesis, measurement, epidemiology and consequences for patients. *Cancer.* 2004;**100(9 Supp)**:1995.

17 Russi EG, Raber-Durlacher JE, Sonis ST. Local and systemic pathogenesis and consequences of regimen-induced inflammatory responses in patients with head and neck cancer receiving chemoradiation. *Mediators Inflamm.* 2014:1–14, Article ID 518261.

18 Sonis ST. The pathobiology of mucositis. *Nat Rev Cancer.* 2004;**4**:277.

21 Ruggiero SL, Dodson TB, Fantasia J, et al. American Association of Oral and Maxillofacial Surgeons position paper on medication-related osteonecrosis of the jaw — 2014 update. *J Oral Maxillofac Surg.* 2014;**72**:1938–1956.

26 Lalla RV, Bowen J, Barasch A, et al. MASCC/ISOO clinical practice guidelines for the management of mucositis secondary to cancer therapy. *Cancer.* 2014;**120**:1453–1461.

38 Yuan A, Sonis S. Emerging therapies for the prevention and treatment of oral mucositis. *Expert Opin Emerg Drugs.* 2014;**19**:343–351.

42 Agular GP, Jham BC, Magalhaes CS, et al. A review of the biological and clinical aspects of radiation caries. *J Contemp Dent Pract.* 2009;**10**:83–89.

51 Saleh J, Figueiredo MA, Cherubini K, et al. Salivary hypofunction: an update on aetiology, diagnosis and therapeutics. *Arch Oral Biol.* 2015;**60**:242–255.

53 Gu J, Zhu S, Li X, et al. Effect of amifostine in head and neck cancer patients treated with radiotherapy: a systematic review and meta-analysis based on randomized controlled trials. *PLoS.* 2014;**9**:e95968.

54 Villa A, Connell CL, Abati S. Diagnosis and management of xerostomia and hyposalivation. *Ther Clin Risk Manag.* 2015;**11**:45–51.

56 Hong CH, Napenas JJ, Hodgson BD, et al. A systematic review of dental disease in patients undergoing cancer therapy. *Support Care Cancer.* 2009;**2010(18)**:1007–1021.

58 Hong JH, Omur-Ozbek P, Stanek BT, et al. Taste and odor abnormalities in cancer patients. *J Support Oncol.* 2009;**7**:58–65.

59 Reuther T, Schuster T, Mende U, Kubler A. Osteoradionecrosis of the jaws as a side effect of radiotherapy of head and neck tumour patients—a report of a thirty year retrospective review. *Int J Oral Maxillofac Surg.* 2003;**32**:289–295.

62 Lee IJ, Koom WS, Lee CG, et al. Risk factors and dose-effect relationship for mandibular osteoradionecrosis in oral and oropharyngeal cancer. *Int J Radiat Oncol Biol Phys.* 2009;**75**:1084–1091.

63 Jacobson AS, Buchbinder D, Hu K, et al. Paradigm shifts in the management of osteoradionecrosis of the mandible. *Oral Oncol.* 2010;**46**:795–801.

66 Nabil S, Samman N. Risk factors for osteoradionecrosis after head and neck radiation: a systematic review. *Oral Surg Oral Pathol Oral Med Oral Radiol.* 2012;**113**:54–69.

71 Rice N, Polyzois I, Ekanayake K, et al. The management of osteoradionecrosis of the jaws — A review. *Surgeon.* 2015;**13**:101–109.

72 McCaul JA. Pharmacologic modalities in the treatment of osteoradionecrosis of the jaw. *Oral Maxillofac Surg Clin North Am.* 2014;**26**:247–252.

75 Fritz GW, Gunsolley JC, Aubaker O, et al. Efficacy of pre- and postirradiation hyperbaric oxygen therapy in the prevention of postextraction osteoradionecrosis: a systematic review. *J Oral Maxillofac Surg.* 2010;**68**:2653–2660.

79 Koga DH, Salvajol JV, Alves FA, et al. Dental extractions and radiotherapy in head and neck oncology: review of the literature. *Oral Dis.* 2008;**14**:40–44.

81 Chuang SK. Limited evidence to demonstrate that the use of hyperbaric oxygen (HBO) therapy reduces the incidence of osteoradionecrosis in irradiated patients requiring tooth extraction. *J Evid Based Dent Pract.* 2012;**12**(3 Suppl):248–250.

82 Peterson DE, Keefe DM, Sonis ST. New frontiers in mucositis. *Am Soc Clin Oncol Educ Book.* 2012;**2012**:545–551.

89 Schwab M, Zanger UM, Marx C, et al. Role of genetic and nongenetic factors for fluorouracil treatment-related severe toxicity: a prospective clinical trial by the German 5-FU Toxicity Study Group. *J Clin Oncol.* 2008;**26**:2131–2138.

92 Sonis S, Antin J, Tedaldi M, et al. SNP-based Bayesian networks can predict oral mucositis risk in autologous stem cell transplant recipients. *Oral Dis.* 2013;**19**:721–727.

102 Oberol S, Zamperlini-Netto G, Beyene J, et al. Effect of low level laser therapy on oral mucositis: a systematic review and meta-analysis. *PLoS One.* 2014;**9**(9):e107418.

105 McGuire DB, Fulton JS, Park J, et al. Systematic review of basic oral care for the management of oral mucositis in cancer patients. *Support Care Cancer.* 2013;**21**:3165–3177.

108 Sonis S, Treister N, Chawla S, et al. Preliminary characterization of oral lesions associated with inhibitors of mammalian target of rapamycin in cancer patients. *Cancer.* 2010;**116**:210–215.

109 Boers-Doets CB, Epstein JB, Raber-Durlacher JE, et al. Oral adverse events associated with tyrosine kinase and mammalian target of rapamycin inhibitors in renal cell carcinoma: a structured literature review. *Oncologist.* 2012;**17**:135–144.

113 Worthington HV, Clarkson JE, Eden OB. Interventions for treatment of oral candidiasis for patients with cancer receiving treatment. *Cochrane Database Syst Rev.* 2007;**18**:CDOO1972.

115 Lerman MA, Laudenbach J, Marty FM, et al. Management of oral infections in cancer patients. *Dent Clin N Am.* 2008;**52**:129–153.

120 Djuric M, Jankovic L, Jankovic T, et al. Prevalence of oral herpes simplex virus reactivation in cancer patients: a comparison of different techniques of viral detection. *J Oral Pathol Med.* 2009;**38**:167–173.

121 Glenny AM, Fernandez MLM, Pavitt S, et al. Interventions for the prevention and treatment of herpes simplex virus in patients being treated for cancer. *Cochrane Database Syst Rev.* 2009;**21**:CD006706.

122 Filmore WJ, Leavitt BD, Arce K. Dental extraction in the thrombocytopenic patient is safe and complications are easily managed. *J Oral Maxillofac Surg.* 2013;**71**:1647–1652.

125 Herbers AHE, de Haan AFJ, van der Velden WJFM, et al. Mucositis not neutropenia determines bacteremia among hematopoietic stem cell transplant recipients. *Tansplant Infect Dis.* 2014;**16**:279–285.

126 Imanguli MM, Alevizos I, Brown R, et al. Oral graft-versus-host disease. *Oral Dis.* 2008;**14**:396–412.

136 Gonadal complications

Vignesh Narayanan, MD ■ Catherine E. Klein, MD

Overview

Improvements in cancer therapy over the past 50 years have allowed survivors of pediatric sarcomas and leukemias, and young adults with high-grade lymphomas, Hodgkin disease, and testicular tumors to reach adulthood but suffer the long-term consequences of those therapies. Alterations in gonadal function are frequent and distressing side effects of modern cancer therapy. Women face symptoms of premature ovarian failure, including menopause, sterility, and presumably accelerated osteoporosis and possible early heart disease. Men experience oligo-azoospermia and subclinical Leydig cell dysfunction, leading to infertility and long-term effects of "andropause" including decreased bone density, lean muscle mass, decreased libido, and increased risk of coronary artery disease.

With recognition has come better documentation of the frequency and severity of these complications, more effective patient counseling, and innovative approaches to attenuate gonadal toxicity. Options include hormonal manipulation, selection of alternative treatments, and pretreatment cryopreservation of embryos or germ cells, but these choices must be offered pretherapy, and patients remain uninformed of potential loss of fertility or options to preserve it. As cancer therapies improve and the number of cancer survivors increases, the practicing oncologist must address these issues in a timely and sensitive manner.

Improvements in cancer therapy over the past 50 years have allowed survivors of pediatric sarcomas and leukemias, and young adults with high-grade lymphomas, Hodgkin disease (HD), and testicular tumors to reach adulthood but some suffer the long-term consequences of those therapies. Alterations in gonadal function are frequent and distressing side effects of modern cancer therapy. Women face symptoms of premature ovarian failure (POF), including menopause, sterility, and presumably accelerated osteoporosis and possible early heart disease. Men experience oligo-azoospermia and subclinical Leydig cell dysfunction, leading to infertility and long-term effects of "andropause" including decreased bone density, lean muscle mass, decreased libido, and increased risk of coronary artery disease.

With recognition has come better documentation of the frequency and severity of these complications, more effective patient counseling, and innovative approaches to attenuate gonadal toxicity. Options include hormonal manipulation, selection of alternative treatments, and pretreatment cryopreservation of embryos or germ cells, but these choices must be offered pretherapy, and patients remain uninformed of potential loss of fertility or options to preserve it. As cancer therapies improve and the number of cancer survivors increases, the practicing oncologist must address these issues in a timely and sensitive manner.

Historical background

Radiation impact on gonadal function was recognized a century ago. Atomic Energy Commission studies of normal men in the 1960s confirmed exquisite sensitivity of spermatogonia to as little as 10 cGy of irradiation.[1] Oocytes were more resistant but also displayed a dose-dependent sensitivity, which resulted in sterility and POF with an age-related frequency. Research published in 1939 demonstrated that 500 cGy to human ovaries was associated with amenorrhea that persisted up to 18 months. All women over the age of 40 became permanently infertile.[2]

Initial reports suggesting detrimental effects of chemotherapy on reproductive function were confirmed by a pathologic study of testicular tissue of 30 men who received nitrogen mustard in the 1940s. Twenty-seven of these men had testicular atrophy and absent spermatogenesis.[3]

The first convincing report of menstrual irregularities in women undergoing chemotherapy appeared in 1956.[4] Four women starting busulfan for chronic leukemia developed menopausal symptoms within 3 months. Ovarian and endometrial tissue showed findings consistent with POF. Gonadal toxicity from other drugs was soon recognized, and the list continues to grow (Table 1).

Assessment of gonadal function after gonadotoxic therapy

Assessment in males

Semen analysis has been the cornerstone of assessment of gonadal function in men, and measurement of gonadotropins (FSH, LH), anti-Müllerian hormone (AMH), and inhibin-B levels are used in children and prepubertal boys.

AMH is produced by Sertoli cells and impacts male sexual differentiation by causing regression of Müllerian ducts.[5] After age 9, AMH levels decline indicating androgen effect on Sertoli cells and early spermatogenesis.[6] In prepubertal boys older than 9 years, Inhibin-B and basal testosterone levels assume more relevance. Leydig cells are more resistant to the effects of chemotherapy than germ cells, thus childhood survivors of cancer may have normal testosterone despite being azoospermic.[6]

Semen volume, sperm concentration, mobility, and morphology are markers of testicular function in adult men. Markers of spermatogenesis such as FSH and inhibin-B levels fluctuate widely and are not predictive of reproductive outcomes. Low or normal testosterone levels along with elevated LH levels are seen commonly in adult survivors of cancer,[7] but are also subject to interindividual variability and lack sensitivity to detect small but meaningful changes in testicular function. Novel biomarkers including sperm messenger RNA, micro-RNAs, histone modifications, and DNA methylation patterns are under development.[7] Genetic testing of sperm using fluorescent *in situ* hybridization (FISH) and DNA

Holland-Frei Cancer Medicine, Ninth Edition. Edited by Robert C. Bast Jr., Carlo M. Croce, William N. Hait, Waun Ki Hong, Donald W. Kufe, Martine Piccart-Gebhart, Raphael E. Pollock, Ralph R. Weichselbaum, Hongyang Wang, and James F. Holland.
© 2017 John Wiley & Sons, Inc. ISBN: 978-1-118-93469-2

Table 1 Probability of decreased gonadal function associated with commonly used antineoplastic agents.

Frequency	Men	Women
Common	Cyclophosphamide	Cyclophosphamide
	Nitrogen mustard	Nitrogen mustard
	Procarbazine	Procarbazine
	Nitrosoureas	Nitrosoureas
		Busulfan
		Melphalan
		Thalidomide
Possible	Vinblastine	Vinblastine
	Etoposide	Etoposide
	Cisplatin	Cisplatin
	Carboplatin	Carboplatin
	Corticosteroids	Chlorambucil
	Ifosfamide	Hydroxyurea
	Interferon	Actinomycin D
	Cytosine arabinoside	Tamoxifen
	Imatinib	Imatinib
		Taxane
	Thioguanine	Thioguanine
		Interferon
		Cytosine arabinoside
Rare	Vincristine	Methotrexate
	Doxorubicin	Doxorubicin
	Bleomycin	Bleomycin
	Methotrexate	Vincristine
	5-Fluorouracil	5-Fluorouracil
	Azathioprine	Dacarbazine
Inadequate information	Navelbine	Navelbine
	Taxanes	Etoposide
	Gemcitabine	Gemcitabine
	Interleukin	Pemetrexed
	Gefitinib	Ifosfamide
	Alemtuzumab	Bevacizumab
	Pemetrexed	Gefitinib
		Alemtuzumab

fragmentation identify chromosomal aneuploidy in the sex chromosomes and assess the extent of DNA damage after gonadotoxic therapy. A higher incidence of sperm aneuploidy was noted in men treated with BEP chemotherapy for testicular cancer as well as the ABVD regimen for HD.[8,9] Aneuploidy returned to baseline values within a few months, but some patients had persistent abnormalities for up to 2 years after therapy. Future impact of these measurements is potentially intriguing.

Assessment in females

Oocyte numbers are fixed at birth and are not replenished.[10] Advancing age and anti-neoplastic therapy quantitatively and qualitatively decrease this pool and adversely affect fertility. Assessing ovarian reserve before fertility preservation is important, especially in women aged over 35.

Measurement of FSH, inhibin B, clomiphene citrate challenge test, antral follicular count (AFC), and AMH assess ovarian reserve and predict the oocyte yield with assisted reproduction. Elevated FSH (>20 mIU/mL) in the early follicular phase of the menstrual cycle indicates impaired ovarian reserve and predicts failure of assisted conception.[11] However, FSH level varies during the menstrual cycle, and neither FSH nor inhibin-B levels are reliable in prepubertal girls. The AFC can be quantified by transvaginal ultrasound to assess ovarian reserve but is not useful in determining oocyte quality or predicting pregnancy outcomes with IVF.[12]

The granulosa cells of ovarian antral follicles produce AMH, and serum levels are a surrogate for the number of developing ovarian follicles. AMH levels decline toward menopause. Unlike FSH and inhibin-B, serum AMH levels do not fluctuate through the menstrual cycle and are valid in children.[10]

Low serum AMH levels were first described in women with prior childhood cancer who still had regular menses indicating low ovarian reserve.[13] Well-conducted studies have found low AMH levels in breast cancer and childhood HD survivors with a clear dose–response relationship between the number of chemotherapy cycles and serum AMH levels.[14,15] Therapy with alkylating agents and pelvic/total-body irradiation often results in low or undetectable AMH levels.[16] Women with low pretreatment AMH levels are more likely to develop amenorrhea after chemotherapy for breast cancer.[17] Nomograms incorporating age and AMH levels have been developed to predict postchemotherapy ovarian recovery in newly diagnosed breast cancer patients and accurately gauge the need for fertility preservation techniques. AMH levels do not predict spontaneous conception of pregnancy or pregnancy outcomes.

Effects of cytotoxic chemotherapy on gonadal function

Effects in boys

Early reports of therapy in prepubertal and pubertal boys suggested relative resistance of the less mature testicle to chemotherapy-induced effects. The frequency of testicular dysfunction, however, varies widely among studies. Three major factors determine the extent of testicular damage among prepubertal boys receiving cytotoxic chemotherapy: the specific drug, the cumulative dose of the drug, and the pubertal stage. The majority of boys progress normally through puberty without supplemental androgen.[18,19] Testicular volume may be reduced, however, and elevated LH levels indicate some degree of Leydig cell dysfunction.[6]

Years after treatment with single-agent cyclophosphamide, the prevalence of normal adult sperm counts has been reported in small, heterogeneous case series to range between 0% and 100%.[20,21] Oral cyclophosphamide cumulative doses of 0.7–52 g caused gonadal damage in 16% of prepubertal boys, but 67% of pubertal boys had evidence of gonadal dysfunction.[22] Chlorambucil and azathioprine for renal disease in patients aged 6–15 years produced azoospermia in 17 of 21 patients for up to 11 years after cessation of treatment.[23]

Most available data relate to multiagent chemotherapy. MOPP chemotherapy in boys with HD impairs subsequent spermatogenesis, a defect reported to last for years.[19,24]

A meta-analysis of 30 studies comprising 456 patients who received cyclophosphamide for renal disease, HD, or leukemia found that fewer than 10% of prepubertal boys receiving less than 400 mg/kg (total dose) of cyclophosphamide had gonadal dysfunction, whereas 30% of those over 400 mg/kg did.[25] Gonadal dysfunction ranged from 0% to 24% in prepubertal boys, but was 68–95% in sexually mature men. A recent analysis of 214 adult male survivors of childhood cancer treated with alkylating agents found the incidence of oligospermia and azoospermia to be 28% and 25% respectively.[26] Impaired spermatogenesis was unlikely when the cumulative cyclophosphamide equivalent dose (CED) was less than 4000 mg/SqM. CED was associated with a statistically significant increase in the risk per 1000 mg/SqM for azoospermia and oligospermia.[26] Unfortunately, poorly understood exceptions to these general trends and lack of reliable predictions for any given patient are problematic. Even small doses of alkylating drugs in prepubertal children can cause permanent sterility.

Whether Leydig cell function is affected in pubertal males is less clear. Gynecomastia with elevated FSH and LH has been reported in pubertal boys receiving MOPP treatment.[19] Other studies find normal basal and stimulated gonadotropin tests,[18] and abnormal testosterone responses to human chorionic gonadotropin (hCG) challenge are uncommon. Gonadotropin secretion was normal in 29 of the 32 patients studied in a cohort of 40 men treated in childhood for HD; 26 of 28 had elevated gonadotropin levels but normal serum testosterone and secondary sexual characteristics. Eleven of thirteen were azoospermic and remained so for up to 17 years.[27] Seventeen adult survivors of childhood sarcoma demonstrated azoospermia in 58%, oligospermia in another 30%, but normal testosterone in 94%. LH was elevated in 92% (40% of those with normal testosterone levels), suggesting Leydig cell insufficiency.[6] Although levels of LH, FSH, and serum testosterone following chemotherapy in prepubertal boys may be normal, testicular biopsies after combination chemotherapy for acute lymphoblastic leukemia or HD commonly show seminiferous tubular damage and interstitial fibrosis.

Effects in men

Single-agent alkylating drugs induce permanent damage to adult seminiferous epithelium. Cyclophosphamide cumulative doses over 9 g result in universal azoospermia; with doses over 18 g that change is irreversible.[28] Multiple studies of HD patients receiving combination chemotherapy with or without procarbazine indicate that this drug is uniquely gonadotoxic. In one study of 19 patients treated with cyclophosphamide, vincristine, procarbazine, and prednisone (COPP) regimen, all remained oligospermic 11 years after therapy; 7 of 10 treated with COPP without procarbazine had return of spermatogenesis within 3 years.[29,30]

Methotrexate causes minimal long-term reproductive toxicity. That vincristine may be less toxic than vinblastine is inferred from the slightly lower incidence of infertility following MOPP therapy than MVPP (mechlorethamine, vinblastine, procarbazine, and prednisone). Although studies of single-agent daunorubicin are not available, it appears to have minimal long-term effect when used in combination therapy not containing cyclophosphamide. When used with cyclophosphamide, however, daunorubicin appears to potentiate gonadal toxicity. Long-term administration of azathioprine does not seem to affect semen quality.

Most data has been derived from studies of combination chemotherapy and indicate permanent infertility among HD and some nonseminomatous testicular cancer survivors. Complicating the interpretation of these studies is the observation that before therapy as many as 30% of men with HD and 50% with germ cell tumors are oligospermic; disorders of sperm motility and morphology are more common.[31-33] Multivariate analysis found that elevated erythrocyte sedimentation rate and advanced stage are predictors of pretherapy infertility among HD.[34] Pretreatment FSH levels may provide a prognostic marker for subsequent spermatogenesis in young men with germ cell cancer.[35] MOPP or MOPP-like regimens to treat HD render all men infertile during therapy, and recovery is unlikely (Table 2). In a prospective study of 37 men receiving MVPP, 12 had low sperm counts before treatment, but all were azoospermic after two cycles and remained so for the first 12 posttreatment months.[38] Longer term follow-up finds only 5–15% ever regain spermatogenesis. Studies comparing MOPP chemotherapy to ABVD (doxorubicin, bleomycin, vinblastine, and dacarbazine) conclude that the latter combination produces less gonadal toxicity.[22,36] For patients with advanced HD, BEACOPP (bleomycin, etoposide, doxorubicin, cyclophosphamide, vincristine, procarbazine, and prednisone) is increasingly employed. The German Hodgkin study group (GHSG) found that the incidence of azoospermia was significantly

Table 2 Gonadal effects of combination chemotherapy.

Disease	Regimen	n	Azoospermia/ amenorrhea (%)	References
Males				
Hodgkin disease	MOPP (adults)	150	73–95	[25,30,36]
	MOPP (pubertal)	18	78	[25]
	MOPP (boys)	27	14–80	[25,37]
	ABVD	13	0	[25]
	ChlVPP	13	87	[27]
	MVPP	210	84–100	[32,33,38–40]
	PACEBOM	12	0	[41]
	NOVP	21	5	[42]
	Stanford V	79	<85	[43,44]
Non-Hodgkin lymphoma	BEACOPP	15	93%	[45]
	COPP	7	66–100	[46]
	VAPEC-B	14	14	[30]
	MACOP-B	15	0	[47]
Testis cancer	PVB	112	15–28	[48,49]
	PVB + Dox	36	17–39	[50,51]
	PEB	42	12	[42]
Acute leukemia	Standard dose	48	3–75	[52]
	High dose	104	14–32	[52,53]
Sarcomas	Dox/MTX (rt)	222	6–90	[54,55]
Females				
Ovarian cancer	P + others	66	0–8	[56–58]
Breast cancer	L-pam + FU	98	21–72	[59,60]
	CMF	549	54–96	[61,62]
	Mitomycin	15	26	[63]
Hodgkin disease	MOPP (adults)	95	55–71	[38,64]
	MOPP (pubertal)	15	7	[25]
	MVPP	72	36	[19]
	ABVD	24	0	[27,36]
	PACE BOM	15	0	[65]
	Stanford V	63	<60	[43,44]
Acute leukemia	Various	47	15	[66]
Non-Hodgkin lymphoma	Various	36	44	[67,68]
	High-dose	Case reports of pregnancies		[40,49,69,70]

Abbreviations: ABVD, Adriamycin (doxorubicin), bleomycin, vinblastine, dacarbazine; ChlVPP, chlorambucil, vinblastine, prednisone, procarbazine; CMF, cyclophosphamide, methotrexate, 5-fluorouracil; COPP, cyclophosphamide, vincristine, prednisone, procarbazine; 5-FU, 5-fluorouracil; MACOP-B, methotrexate, doxorubicin (Adriamycin), cyclophosphamide, vincristine (Oncovin), prednisone, bleomycin; MOPP, mechlorethamine, Oncovin (vincristine), prednisone, procarbazine; MVPP, mechlorethamine, vinblastine, prednisone, procarbazine; NOVP, mitoxantrone, vinblastine, vincristine, prednisone; PACE BOM, doxorubicin, cyclophosphamide, etoposide, bleomycin, vincristine, methotrexate, prednisolone; PEB, cisplatin (Platinol), etoposide, bleomycin; L-PAM, L-phenylalanine mustard; PVB, Platinol (cisplatin), vinblastine, bleomycin; PVB + dox, cisplatin, vinblastine, bleomycin, doxorubicin; VAPEC-B, vincristine, doxorubicin, prednisone, etoposide, cyclophosphamide, bleomycin.

higher among those treated with eight cycles of BEACOPP or four cycles of COPP/ABVD compared to two cycles of COPP/ABVD (93%, 91%, and 56%, respectively).[45] An update of the Stanford V regimen (vinblastine, doxorubicin, vincristine, bleomycin, mustard, etoposide, and prednisone) reported 19 conceptions in 13 male survivors.[43]

Data on outcomes after treatment for non-Hodgkin lymphoma (NHL) are less robust, but evidence suggests that the cyclophosphamide, vinblastine, and prednisone regimen is less toxic than MOPP.[30] A report of 14 men treated with vincristine, doxorubicin, prednisone, etoposide, cyclophosphamide, and bleomycin suggests that this may be an effective, relatively nontoxic regimen for NHL.[47] Leukemia therapy appears less toxic,[71] although both allogeneic and autologous stem cell transplant (SCT) increase the likelihood of long-term infertility. Kreuser found 100% recovery during maintenance therapy among 10 patients aged 14–38 years treated with combination chemotherapy.[39,52]

The majority of men presenting with testicular tumors are oligospermic. In 41 patients studied prospectively, Drasga reported that 77% were oligo-azoospermic and 17% were azoospermic; only 6% had adequate sperm counts for cryopreservation.[48] Abnormalities of sperm motility are at least as prevalent. Following 2 months of therapy with cisplatin, vinblastine, and bleomycin, with or without doxorubicin, 94% of men in Drasga's study were azoospermic.

Recovery of spermatogenesis following chemotherapy for testis cancer is common. Most studies show a time-dependent recovery of spermatogenesis, with nearly 50% of patients recovering some sperm production after 2 years (Table 2).[50,51] Longer follow-up has shown no adverse effects on fertility or sexual function.[51] Recovery seems to be partly related to the cumulative dose of cisplatin. In those who receive over 400 mg/m^2, permanent infertility should be anticipated. Limited data suggest that ifosfamide may cause less irreversible infertility than its similarity to cyclophosphamide might predict.[70,72]

As in boys, Leydig cell function is more resistant and is usually well compensated; despite frequently elevated gonadotropin levels, few men require androgen replacement.[24,30] Subclinical Leydig dysfunction may have underrecognized sequelae, including excess cardiovascular morbidity increased hypercholesterolemia and obesity, in conjunction with lower testosterone and elevated LH/FSH.[73]

Effect in prepubertal girls

The ovarian effects of chemotherapy in prepubertal girls are variable and depend on the drug, dose, and duration of therapy. Single-agent cyclophosphamide for nonmalignant disorders rarely causes either a delay in puberty or permanent sterility.[74] Most girls treated with procarbazine or nitrosoureas for brain tumors show biochemical evidence of primary ovarian dysfunction, but progress normally through puberty. Ovarian function returns to normal over a period of years, and elevated gonadotropin levels decrease to baseline in most women. Eighty percent of girls treated for ALL also proceed normally through puberty.[75] In a large study of survivors of childhood cancer, the likelihood of premature menopause was 13-fold higher when compared with siblings: 8% by age 40.[76] This increase was associated with higher doses of alkylating agents, ovarian radiation, and a diagnosis of HD. In Ewing sarcoma survivors, 67% developed POF at a median follow-up of 5.7 years. All who underwent pelvic irradiation had POF.[77]

Histologically, however, prepubertal ovaries are significantly damaged by cancer chemotherapy. Follicular maturation arrest, stromal fibrosis, and a partially depleted ova population have all been reported following single-agent cyclophosphamide as well as cytosine arabinoside (ara-C)-based antileukemic therapy.

Effects in women

The effects of antineoplastic agents on the female gonadal function have been inferred from the incidence of amenorrhea, gonadotropin levels, and long-term fertility rates and outcomes. One autopsy series of acute leukemia patients showed no difference in the number of primary follicles, but secondary follicles were markedly depleted.[51] Clinically, women receiving these agents develop POF: vaginal dryness with dyspareunia, endometrial hypoplasia, decreased libido, hot flashes, oligomenorrhea evolving into amenorrhea, and low serum estrogen levels with compensatory elevations of serum FSH and LH levels.[33,78]

The frequency of amenorrhea and infertility depends on the drug, its total dose, concomitant radiation, and the patient age when treated. Single-agent alkylating drugs are those most consistently associated with POF. Small series report that 50–75% of women treated with cyclophosphamide develop amenorrhea within a month of starting therapy, although there is a strong age-related susceptibility. In one study, the total dose of cyclophosphamide received before the onset of amenorrhea was 5.2 g for patients over 40, 9.3 g for those 30–39, and 20.4 g for those 20–29. Menses returned in 50% of women under 40.[63] Return of menstrual function was correlated with the dose administered after the cessation of menses.

Old studies of adjuvant chemotherapy with L-phenylalanine mustard for breast cancer showed significant, age-related POF: 73% of the women aged 40–49, but only 22% of the women under 39, developed amenorrhea during therapy.[59] Single-agent treatment with busulfan or chlorambucil is associated with well-documented age and dose-related ovarian toxicity.[79,80]

Sarcoma patients treated with high-dose methotrexate rarely report amenorrhea and serum gonadotropin levels remain normal during and after therapy.[54] Lower dose methotrexate for gestational trophoblastic tumors appears to exert no significant toxicity, although one survey from England found that menopause occurred on average 3 years earlier in chemotherapy-treated women.[81] Fluorouracil, daunorubicin, and bleomycin as single agents are also well tolerated.

Few data are available for etoposide, but ovarian dysfunction has been reported among women receiving the drug for gestational tumors.[82]

Tamoxifen appears to exert a mild estrogenic effect associated with decreased gonadotropin levels in both premenopausal and postmenopausal women treated for breast cancer. Menstrual irregularities are common, but the incidence of persistent amenorrhea is unclear. Successful pregnancies have been reported among women on chronic interferon therapy for a variety of malignant and nonmalignant diseases.[65]

Most reported outcomes come from studies of multiagent therapy. The incidence of amenorrhea in women treated with MOPP, MVPP, or COPP ranges from 15% to 80% (Table 2).[29,35,44,83–85] Two-thirds develop amenorrhea during therapy. A dose–response relationship is unclear. In one study, there appeared to be no difference between three and six cycles of MOPP.[86] Age at the time of treatment, however, is an important variable affecting the incidence and onset of permanent amenorrhea. Sixty to hundred percent of patients over age 25 develop permanent amenorrhea during therapy. POF occurs with initiation of therapy in 5–30% of women under 25 and in an additional percentage over the next months. Younger women experience at least a 50% likelihood of POF 5–10 years of therapy.[87] Preliminary reports suggest that HD regimens such as ABVD or doxorubicin, cyclophosphamide, etoposide, bleomycin, vincristine, methotrexate, and prednisolone may have lower rates of prolonged amenorrhea.[38,56] Horning has reported 24 conceptions among 19 women treated with the Stanford V regimen V.[43] Women receiving methotrexate, doxorubicin cyclophosphamide, vincristine, prednisone, and bleomycin for aggressive lymphomas appear, in small series, to maintain fertility.[41] Women treated with four cycles of Mega-CHOP for NHL had recovery of ovarian function.[88] Eight of these patients conceived spontaneously. In a second study of women younger than age 40 receiving CHOP therapy for NHL, only 2 of 36 women developed POF.[89] Fifty percent of these women conceived in first remission of their disease.

Women receiving cisplatin-containing therapy for germ cell tumors typically become amenorrheic during treatment, but over 90% resume menstruation within a few months of completing treatment.[57,90–92] Among women with breast cancer, who may already have age-related decreased reproductive potential, 80% receiving adjuvant therapy with cyclophosphamide, methotrexate, and 5-fluorouracil (CMF) become menopausal within 10 months of beginning therapy.[61,62] The reported ranges, however, vary between 20% and 100%.[93] Those given doxorubicin and cyclophosphamide usually become anovulatory within 3 months; sooner if they are perimenopausal. Few women under age 30 treated with doxorubicin-containing regimens experienced amenorrhea; about one-third of women aged 30–40 years, and nearly all those over 40 years of age do so. Epirubicin-containing regimens are similar. Adjuvant docetaxel with doxorubicin and cyclophosphamide resulted in a 61% rate of amenorrhea in a patient population whose average age was 49.[94]

Fertility following high-dose chemotherapy

Case reports and small series have documented the recovery of fertility in very few patients treated with high-dose regimens. A retrospective survey of over 37,000 SCT patients found that only 0.6% subsequently conceived.[95] Follow-up of 187 young women previously treated with SCT for either aplastic anemia or leukemia found the anticipated age-dependent effect of cyclophosphamide on ovarian function.[53] Fifty-seven percent of female patients had fertility impairment at 2.3 years following SCT. Only 7% of 144 patients recovered fertility, and recovery took longer in women than in men. A longitudinal study of 217 childhood allogeneic SCT patients found that 56% of men had fertility impairment with elevated FSH/LH and low testosterone after a median of 2.6 years. Azoospermia was documented in 14 of 15. Only 3% recovered fertility 3.4 years after SCT.[96] Patients transplanted for aplastic anemia overall do somewhat better, particularly those under age 25.

Effects of radiation therapy on gonadal function

Effects in men

Therapeutic irradiation in boys with acute leukemia was a standard practice to prevent testicular relapse. Doses below 1200 cGy were insufficient to control disease, and early protocols were replaced by those delivering 2400 cGy to both testes. This dose induced permanent Leydig cell damage, puberty was delayed, testosterone levels were diminished, and gonadotropin levels were increased in most patients.[97]

In adults, single 400–600 cGy doses of testicular radiation may produce azoospermia for 5 years or longer.[1] Berthelsen evaluated men undergoing prophylactic radiotherapy for seminoma and found that two-thirds became azoospermic from scatter dose of 201–130 cGy.[98] Shapiro has documented oligospermia/azoospermia lasting up to 24 months after as little as 27 cGy.[99] Adult Leydig cell dysfunction, with elevated LH values, occurs at radiation doses greater than 2000–3000 cGy, and can require hormone replacement. Fractionated radiation appears to produce tubular damage equivalent to that seen with single doses. Recovery occurs in the majority of those who are treated for germ cell tumors; series report 37–66% success rates in men wishing to conceive a pregnancy.[100]

TBI for SCT conditioning is routinely associated with permanent azoospermia. Secondary infertility has been reported in association with radiation administered to the hypothalamus or pituitary in conjunction with chemotherapy for intracranial neoplasms.[101]

Whether there are permanent effects on the surviving germ cells of men receiving radiation remains uncertain. Most studies have been unable to document an increase in malignancies in offspring.[102]

Effects in women

The radiation sensitivity of the human ovary has not been well defined. Small primordial oocytes are considerably more sensitive than large follicles, and ovarian sensitivity to radiation is dose and age dependent. In adult women, single doses of 500 cGy produce menstrual irregularities in women of all ages. For women over 40, 600 cGy reliably induces menopause. Women aged 20–30 can tolerate up to 3000 cGy if fractionated over 6 weeks.[103] Uterine radiation in childhood increases risk for nulliparity, spontaneous abortions, and intrauterine growth retardation, so fertility is not assured even if ovarian function is preserved. In a retrospective study of 162 patients with stage II/III colorectal cancer, the incidence of amenorrhea in patients was higher among women with rectal cancer compared to colon cancer (94% vs 4.2% respectively), possibly related to pelvic irradiation in rectal cancer patients.[104]

Effects of targeted therapies on gonadal function

In the era of molecularly targeted therapy, several new drug classes have entered clinical use, but there is a paucity of data regarding their effects on fertility. Furthermore, cytotoxic agents are often used concurrently, and the effect of combination therapy on gonadal function has not been studied.

Effect of TKIs

Imatinib inhibits c-KIT, crucial for Leydig cell function, and platelet-derived growth factor receptor (PDGFR) essential for gonocyte migration. c-KIT and PDGFR are also expressed in oocytes and have important roles in fulliculogenesis and female fertility. Oligozoospermia, gynecomastia, and testicular failure have been described in prepubertal boys.[105] Case reports document oligospermia in men, but most men father normal offspring.[106] Women treated with imatinib appear to conceive normally but may have an increased risk of congenital malformations, hence discontinuation of therapy before pregnancy is recommended.[107]

Rapid onset of hypogonadism and low testosterone has been described in men treated with crizotinib.[108] A follow-up study documented low testosterone levels with reductions in sex-hormone binding globulin, LH, FSH, and free testosterone, suggesting central hypogonadism.[109] Dasatinib and sunitinib have been associated with gynecomastia, but their effects on fertility are unknown.

Effects of M-TOR inhibitors

Sirolimus and everolimus also inhibit c-KIT. The reproductive side effects of m-TOR inhibitors are inferred from organ-transplant patients. Men treated with sirolimus and everolimus have low testosterone and oligospermia, with elevated FSH and LH; effects are reversible after discontinuation of therapy.[110] In human ovarian cortical strips treated in vitro with rapamycin, oocyte destruction by granulosa cells was discovered, although previous reports had implicated m-TOR inhibitor-mediated apoptosis as the mechanism for oocyte loss.[111]

Effects of monoclonal antibodies and immunotherapy

Alemtuzumab, a monoclonal antibody against CD52, causes immobilization and agglutination of sperm because CD52 is also expressed on the surface of the sperm.[112] Cytotoxic T-lymphocyte-associated antigen 4 (CTLA-4) blockade with ipilimumab and programmed cell death-1 (PD-1) receptor agents for the treatment of melanoma can cause hypophysitis and hypopituitarism. In the sentinel trial of ipilimumab in melanoma, the incidence of serious hypopituitarism was low at 1.8%.[113] The incidence of reproductive side effects with CTLA-4 and PD-1 blockade is not known.

Protective measures

Protection for men

It has long been speculated that halting spermatogenesis through hormonal manipulation might ameliorate testicular damage, as most chemotherapy agents are selectively toxic to dividing cells. In clinical trials of men receiving chemotherapy for HD, two attempts using GnRH analogs have been unsuccessful.[114,115] For men who desire fertility following combination chemotherapy for advanced HD, ABVD is clearly preferable to MOPP.[38] Use of GnRH analogs does not shorten the recovery time to spermatogenesis. Masala et al. documented some protection with the use of testosterone in patients treated with cyclophosphamide. ASCO Guidelines indicate this procedure to be experimental.

Men anticipating cancer therapy should consider semen cryopreservation. The process of sperm cryopreservation is no more detrimental to sperm quality in cancer patients than in noncancer controls.[116] Because of the high prevalence of abnormal pretherapy semen analyses, many patients have been considered poor candidates, but successful impregnation has been achieved following artificial insemination using semen with quite low sperm counts and poor sperm motility.[117] With meticulous reproductive assistance, fertilization may be effective in up to 45% of cases. In addition, *in vitro* fertilization and subsequent implantation has been successful in cases of even lower sperm counts and motility.[118] With the advent of intracytoplasmic sperm injection (ICSI), where only a single live spermatozoon is selected and injected into an oocyte, the chance of conception can be greatly enhanced despite exceedingly low sperm counts. Garcia compared ICSI in patients with malignancies with noncancer patients who underwent the same assisted reproductive procedure. The cumulative pregnancy and cumulative live birth rates in cancer patients were 69% and 62%, respectively, comparable to noncancer patients.[119] Fertilization has been reported using spermatozoa retrieved by testicular biopsy and with sperm extracted from the vas deferens at the time of orchiectomy in several azoospermic testis cancer survivors.[120] Many centers nonetheless report that the overall success rate among men who elect to preserve semen may be somewhat limited, and perhaps is influenced by factors other than semen quality. One series from Memorial Sloan-Kettering Cancer Center reported locating 48 of 69 men who had banked sperm, but at a median of 27 months posttreatment only 11 had attempted to use their sperm for artificial insemination. Of these, only three achieved successful pregnancies.[117,121]

Penile vibratory stimulation and electro-ejaculation may provide an option for pubertal boys.[122] Very preliminary studies of testicular circulatory isolation suggest that this mechanical procedure is protective in a rat model and might be feasible in human clinical trials.[123]

Testis sperm extraction is reported to recover spermatozoa in 55–85% of men with nonobstructive azoospermia of various etiologies. Damani reported a series of men azoospermic after chemotherapy. Spermatozoa were found in 65%. A total of 26 ICSI cycles were performed in 12 couples. Fertilization rate was 65%. All babies born to date have had normal neonatal examinations.[124]

Testicular tissue biopsy and cryopreservation is experimental, as is isolation of germ cells from testicular tissue for storage. Gonadal shielding remains the mainstay of protection from therapeutic radiation. No convincing studies to suggest benefit from scrotal cooling are currently available.

Protection for women

Reversible suppression of ovarian function by oral contraceptives or GnRH analog might offer gonadal protection to cycling women about to undergo potentially sterilizing radiation or chemotherapy. Some animal models have validated the hypothesis, both in protection from radiation and in chemotherapy-induced ovarian damage.[125] Results of such trials in humans have been conflicting, however, and the number of patients studied remains small. Most promising of these reports is that of Chapman and Sutcliffe, who administered oral contraceptives to women anticipating receiving MVPP therapy for HD. Five of six women had resumption of normal menses at a mean follow-up of 26 months.[126]

Pacheco administered leuprolide acetate to 12 patients aged 15–20 anticipating treatment for lymphoma.[127] Suppression was continued monthly with depot administration until 1 month after cessation of chemotherapy. All 12 treated patients resumed normal menstrual cycling within 6 months, compared to none of the four women in this study who did not receive leuprolide suppression. Three pregnancies were reported. In a meta-analysis of six randomized controlled trials (RCTs) that examined reproductive outcomes among women with HD and ovarian and breast cancer, administration of GnRH analogs with chemotherapy was associated with a statistically significant increase in resumption of spontaneous menstruation and ovulation (OR 3.46 and 5.70, respectively).[128] Subsequent meta-analyses of RCTs exclusively among patients with breast cancer have yielded conflicting results regarding prevention of POF and spontaneous resumption of menses with GnRH agonists.[129–131] In a large trial evaluating the effect of adjuvant chemotherapy in premenopausal women with node positive breast cancer (NSABP-B-30 trial), those with prolonged amenorrhea had better disease-free survival and overall survival.[132] Thus, ovarian suppression in breast cancer patients for fertility preservation is controversial.

The highest live birth rates are reported following ovarian stimulation and embryo cryopreservation, and are therefore the best current option for women in stable relationships. Superovulation is required before fertilization, and neither the time required nor the hormone manipulation necessary may be acceptable. The implantation rates range from 8% to 30%. The cumulative pregnancy rate can be more than 60%.[133]

Cryopreservation of ovarian tissue remains experimental but could be considered in women who require urgent cancer treatment. Ovarian cortical tissue also has the advantage of containing large numbers of follicles and thereby increasing the potential for successful future pregnancies. The ovarian tissue can ultimately be transplanted back in to the patient, thus restoring ongoing fertility. Transplanted tissue has been reported to restore normal menstrual cycling[134] and live births have been reported following orthotopic transplantation of cortical strips to the remaining ovary. In 114 Belgian women treated for various malignancies who underwent cryopreservation, a total of 49 spontaneous pregnancies in 33 patients and two induced pregnancies were reported after a mean follow-up of 50 months.[135] This technique may ultimately offer an option for young girls as well as sexually mature young women.

Recently, the Edinburgh selection criteria for identifying patients at risk for POF after gonadotoxic therapy was validated and may be useful in selecting patents for intervention.[136] Unresolved medical and ethical issues have fueled debate regarding these techniques.[137]

For patients undergoing pelvic radiotherapy, oophoropexy can be considered. At the time of exploratory or staging laparotomy, the ovaries are moved either medially behind the uterine fundus or laterally out of the radiation port. Radiation exposure is decreased 90%, and hormonal function is preserved in 55–95% of patients; however, fertility is still compromised, possibly owing to the abnormal tubo-ovarian anatomy or radiation scatter. A small trial of laparoscopic propriosacral ovariopexy offers the possibility of a less invasive approach to fertility preservation.[138] One option in this setting is the transposition of only one ovary and removal of the second for cryopreservation.[139] Specific ovarian shielding may be useful in some cases.

Protection for children

No proven methods for protection of future fertility in children are available at this time. Some centers offer ovarian tissue or testicular tissue cryopreservation as an experimental approach, but research in this area is fraught with ethical problems. Many excellent reviews of the technical and ethical issues of fertility preservation are available (Table 3).[127,135]

Outcomes of pregnancy

Chemotherapy

Case reports document successful conception and delivery of normal infants to patients who have received even the most aggressive of chemotherapy regimens; neither male nor female permanent infertility can be presumed following chemotherapy for cancer. Several retrospective series have evaluated the outcome of pregnancy in women treated with chemotherapeutic agents as children or young adults who completed therapy and then became pregnant.

One large study evaluating offspring of children treated for a variety of cancers found that in a total of 286 subsequent pregnancies there was no increase in congenital anomalies, and chromosomal analysis was normal in 23 of 24 children tested.[140] Pregnancies in women previously treated for trophoblastic tumors also appear to

have no associated increased risk of congenital anomalies, spontaneous abortions, or neonatal mortality.[141]

Holmes evaluated women treated for HD and compared the 93 pregnancies in their chemotherapy-treated patients to 288 sibling-control pregnancies. Overall, there was no difference between the groups, although when the subgroup that received both radiation therapy and chemotherapy was analyzed separately, it appeared that combined treatment produced more spontaneous abortions in wives of male patients, and those female patients were slightly more likely to produce abnormal offspring than control women.[142]

Offspring of fathers treated with prior chemotherapy likewise appear to be normal. When large series are combined, nearly 1400 live-born children have been reported to have a congenital defect incidence of about 4%, not significantly different from the general population. Most of these anomalies represent common, nongenetic abnormalities.[142]

Further follow-up suggests that offspring growth, development, and school performance are probably normal. A National Cancer Institute study to address the question of cancer in offspring of treated patients found a slight and statistically insignificant excess of cancers in these children when compared to offspring of sibling-matched controls (0.3% vs 0.23%), numbers not different from those expected in the general population. When analyzed by age and sex, however, it appeared that there was an excess of cancers diagnosed in male offspring under age 5.[143]

Risk to the fetus exposed *in utero* to chemotherapy agents depends on gestational age and the drug and dose administered. Folate antagonists should not be administered during the first trimester. Other antimetabolites have rarely been associated with congenital abnormalities. First trimester exposure to 5-fluorouracil, cyclophosphamide, busulfan, and chlorambucil has been associated with low birth weight in infants and other abnormalities on rare occasion.[144] Fetal myocardial necrosis has been reported following maternal administration of anthracyclines.[145] Imatinib has demonstrated teratogenicity in animal models, but case reports have documented successful pregnancies in women who conceive during treatment.[146] Rituximab given unintentionally to a pregnant woman resulted in an uncomplicated pregnancy delivering an apparently healthy infant. Interferon-a has been given safely during pregnancy in a small number of women.[147]

Whether the risk to the fetus is further increased with drug combinations is uncertain. Case reports and small series indicate that exposure in the second and third trimesters is associated with minimal risk to the fetus and that long-term development of these offspring is normal.[148,149] Nonteratogenic effects including low birth weight, intrauterine growth retardation, and more subtle developmental abnormalities remain to be defined. *In utero* exposure to diethylstilbestrol has been linked to the development of genital clear cell carcinomas in the female offspring of these women, but other clear documentation of carcinogenesis from *in utero* exposure to

Table 3 Options for preservation of fertility in patients with cancer.

	Males	Status	Females	Status
Children	Testicular tissue cryopreservation	Unproven	Ovarian tissue cryopreservation	Unproven
Adults	GnRH analog	Unproven	GnRH analog suppression	? Effective
			OCP suppression	Unproven
	Sperm cryopreservation	Accepted	Oocyte cryopreservation	Experimental
	Testicular sperm extraction	Experimental	Ovarian tissue cryopreservation	Available
			Embryo cryopreservation	Available
			Ovarian tissue transposition	Experimental

Abbreviations: GnRH analog, gonadotropin-releasing hormone analog; OCP, oral contraceptives.

chemotherapy is lacking. No information is available on the reproductive potential of these children.

Radiation therapy

Most of what is known about the genetic effects of radiation therapy is inferred from data on survivors of atomic bomb exposure. The increase in untoward outcomes of pregnancies (major congenital defects, stillbirth, and death during the first week of life) is small, estimated at 0.00182/gonadal rem (roentgen-equivalent–man)—the quantity of any ionizing radiation equivalent to the biologic effect of 1 rad (cGy).

Among women treated with radiation therapy below the diaphragm, preterm delivery in up to 20% of pregnancies and an excess of low birth-weight infants have been reported. That these adverse outcomes are often clustered in the first posttreatment year suggests they may result from local uterine or hormonal factors and may not be because of genetic defects.[46,150]

In utero exposure to irradiation produces the greatest risk of teratogenesis during the period of organogenesis from the second to the eighth week, with growth retardation, eye problems, and microcephaly appearing as the predominant abnormalities. A safe dose has not yet been defined, but generally, a therapeutic abortion is recommended for any uterine dose of 10 cGy during the first trimester. Supradiaphragmatic irradiation is associated with considerable scatter to the fetus, much of which can probably be prevented with abdominal shielding. Local irradiation of the neck and axilla may be safe during the first trimester.[144]

Psychosocial issues

The psychosocial issues of disfigurement, loss of fertility, anxiety about birth defects, sexual performance, and recurrence of tumor all have important impacts on the unmarried patient facing dating and mate-selection issues, as well as on married patients in a stable relationship, for whom the separation rate may be fourfold of that of the general population.[46,149,150] Detailed discussion of these important issues is beyond the scope of this publication, but excellent reviews are available for the interested reader seeking further information.[42,149,151–155]

For physician assessment of sexual functioning, Andersen has proposed a model that helps the provider address many issues before they arise.[42]

Summary

- Gonadal dysfunction is related to drug-dose and is age-related
- Younger patients are more likely to preserve fertility
- Alkylating drug therapy causes damage in all age groups
- Children of both genders enter puberty normally after chemotherapy
- Traditional endocrine measures of gonadal toxicity are insensitive
- Alkylating drugs appear to be the most toxic; procarbazine particularly
- Many cytotoxic drugs are not well-studied
- ABVD for HD should replace MOPP if possible for young patients with HD
- Perimenopausal women with breast cancer are likely to become menopausal with chemotherapy
- New agents have theoretical risks but are not well-studied
- Risks to fertility should be part of chemotherapy consent discussion
- Proven options to preserve fertility in men are limited to semen cryopreservation

---

(Summary box, top right)

- Many men with HD or testicular tumors are oligospermic at presentation
- Oligospermia should not prevent cryopreservation
- New and effective options to preserve fertility in women are under development
- Fetal exposure to most chemotherapy agents is safe after the first trimester
- Outcomes of pregnancy during chemotherapy are good
- Outcomes of pregnancy after childhood chemotherapy are normal
- Early fetal exposure to folate antagonists must be avoided

Key references

The complete reference list can be found on the Wiley Companion Digital Edition of this title (see inside front cover for login instructions).

3 Gilman A. The initial clinical trial of nitrogen mustard. *Am J Surg.* 1963;**105**:574.

5 Josso N, Cate RL, Picard JY, et al. Anti-Müllerian hormone: the Jost factor. *Recent Prog Horm Res.* 1993;**48**:1–59.

7 Dere E, Anderson LM, Hwang K, Boekelheide K, et al. Biomarkers of chemotherapy-induced testicular damage. *Fertil Steril.* 2013;**100**:1192–1202.

10 Dewailly D, Andersen CY, Balen A, et al. The physiology and clinical utility of anti-Müllerian hormone in women. *Hum Reprod Update.* 2014;**20**(**3**):370–385.

16 Gracia CR, Sammel MD, Freeman E, et al. Impact of cancer therapies on ovarian reserve. *Fertil Steril.* 2012;**97**:134–140 e131.

17 Anderson RA, Cameron DA. Pre-treatment serum anti-Müllerian hormone predicts long term ovarian function and bone mass after chemotherapy for early breast cancer. *J Clin Endocrinol Metab.* 2011;**96**:1336–1339.

18 Shalet SM, Hann IM, Lendon M, et al. Testicular function after combination chemotherapy in childhood for acute lymphoblastic leukaemia. *Arch Dis Child.* 1981;**56**:275–278.

19 Whitehead E, Shalet SM, Jones PH, et al. Gonadal function after combination chemotherapy for Hodgkin's disease in childhood. *Arch Dis Child.* 1982;**47**:287–291.

24 Aubier F, Flamant F, Caillaud JM, et al. Male gonadal function after chemotherapy for solid tumors in childhood. *J Clin Oncol.* 1989;**7**:304–309.

26 Green DM, Liu W, Kutteh RW, et al. Cumulative alkylating agent exposure and semen parameters in adult survivors of childhood cancer: a report from the St Jude lifetime cohort study. *Lancet Oncol.* 2014;**15**:1215–1223.

34 Rueffer U, Breuer K, Josting A, et al. Male gonadal dysfunction in patients with Hodgkin's disease prior to treatment. *Ann Oncol.* 2001;**12**:1307–1311.

36 Viviani S, Santoro A, Ragni G, et al. Gonadal toxicity after combination chemotherapy for Hodgkin's disease: comparative results of MOPP vs ABVD. *Eur J Cancer Clin Oncol.* 1985;**21**:601–605.

43 Horning SJ, Hoppe RT, Breslin S, et al. Stanford V and radiotherapy for locally extensive and advanced Hodgkin's disease: mature results of a prospective clinical trial. *J Clin Oncol.* 2002;**20**:630–637.

44 Horning SJ, Hoppe RT, Kaplan HS, Rosenberg SA. Female reproductive potential after treatment for Hodgkin's disease. *N Engl J Med.* 1981;**304**:1377–1382.

45 Sieniawski M, Reineke T, Josting A, et al. Assessment of male fertility in patients with Hodgkin's lymphoma treated in the German Hodgkin study group (GHSG) clinical trials. *Ann Oncol.* 2008;**19**:1795–1801.

48 Drasga RE, Einhorn LH, Williams SD, et al. Fertility after chemotherapy for testicular cancer. *J Clin Oncol.* 1983;**1**:179–183.

51 Hansen PV, Trykker H, Helkjaer PE, Andersen J. Testicular function in patients with testicular cancer treated with orchiectomy alone or orchiectomy plus cisplatin-based chemotherapy. *J Natl Cancer Inst.* 1989;**81**:1246–1250.

54 Shamberger RC, Rosenberg SA, Siepp CA, Sherins RJ. Effects of high-dose methotrexate and vincristine on ovarian and testicular functions in patients undergoing post-operative adjuvant treatment of osteosarcoma. *Cancer Treat Rep.* 1981;**65**:739–746.

64 Santoro A, Bonadonna G, Valagussa P, et al. Long-term results of combined chemotherapy-radiotherapy approach in Hodgkin's disease: superiority of ABVD plus radiotherapy versus MOPP plus radiotherapy. *J Clin Oncol.* 1987;**5**:27–37.

66 Meirow D. Reproduction post-chemotherapy in young cancer patients. *Mol Cell Endocrinol.* 2000;**169**:123–131.

70 Dominik B, Burkhard FC, Mills R, et al. Fertility and sexual function following orchiectomy and 2 cycles of chemotherapy for stage I high risk nonseminomatous germ cell cancer. *J Urol.* 2001;**165**:441–444.

73 Meinardi MT, Gietema JA, van der Graaf WTA, et al. Cardiovascular morbidity in long-term survivors of metastatic testicular cancer. *J Clin Oncol.* 2000;**18**:1725–1732.

75 Quigley C, Cowell C, Jimenez M, et al. Normal or early development of puberty despite gonadal damage in children treated for acute lymphocytic leukemia. *N Engl J Med*. 1989;**321**:143–151.

89 Elis A, Tevet A, Yerushalmi R, et al. Fertility status among women treated for aggressive non-Hodgkin's lymphoma. *Leuk Lymphoma*. 2006;**47**:623–627.

90 Marchetti M, Romagnolo C. Fertility after ovarian cancer treatment. *Eur J Gynaecol Oncol*. 1992;**13**:498–501.

93 Bines J, Oleske DM, Cobleigh MA. Ovarian function in premenopausal women treated with adjuvant chemotherapy for breast cancer. *J Clin Oncol*. 1996;**14**:1718–1729.

94 Martin M, Pienkowski T, Mackey J, et al. Adjuvant docetaxel for node-positive breast cancer. *N Engl J Med*. 2005;**352**:2302–2313.

96 Pfitzer C, Orawa H, Balcerek M, et al. Dynamics of fertility impairment and recovery after allogeneic hematopoietic stem cell transplantation in childhood and adolescence: results from a longitudinal study. *J Cancer Res Clin Oncol*. 2015;**141(1)**:135–142.

109 Weickhardt AJ, Doebele RC, Purcell WT, et al. Symptomatic reduction in free testosterone levels secondary to crizotinib use in male cancer patients. *Cancer*. 2013;**119**:2383–2390.

111 McLaughlin M, Patrizio P, Kayisli U, et al. mTOR kinase inhibition results in oocyte loss characterized by empty follicles in human ovarian cortical strips cultured in vitro. *Fertil Steril*. 2011;**96(5)**:1154–1159.

116 Hallak J, Kolettis PN, Sekhon VS, Thomas AJ, Agarwal A. Sperm cryopreservation in patients with testicular cancer. *Urology*. 1999;**54**:894–899.

124 Damani MN, Masters V, Meng MV, et al. Postchemotherapy ejaculatory azoospermia: fatherhood with sperm from testis tissue with intracytoplasmic sperm injection. *J Clin Oncol*. 2002;**20**:930–936.

127 Pacheco BP, Ribas JMM, Milone G, et al. Use of GnRH analogs for functional protection of the ovary and preservation of fertility during cancer treatment in adolescents: a preliminary report. *Gynecol Oncol*. 2001;**81**:391–397.

139 Martin JR, Kodaman P, Oktay K, Taylor HS. Ovarian cryopreservation with transposition of a contralateral ovary: a combined approach for fertility preservation in women receiving pelvic radiation. *Fertil Steril*. 2007;**87**:189.e5–189.e7.

150 Doll DC, Ringenberg S, Yarbro JW. Management of cancer during pregnancy. *Arch Intern Med*. 1988;**148**:2058–2064.

137 Sexual dysfunction

Leslie R. Schover, PhD

Overview

Sexual problems related to cancer are usually caused by physiological damage from treatment, but are exacerbated by psychosocial issues such as poor communication, relationship conflict, or preexisting sexual dysfunction. Sexual dysfunction affects almost two-thirds of the estimated 14 million cancer survivors in the United States, including over 50% of those treated for pelvic or breast cancers and at least 25% for other sites. Optimal treatment is multidisciplinary, addressing both physical damage and coping skills. If a committed relationship exists, it is best to include the partner in education and intervention.

Historical perspective

Sexual dysfunction has been recognized as a morbidity of cancer treatment since the 1950s. Early publications focused on mutilating surgery for breast cancer, impaired body image, and loss of feminine identity.[1] Research later revealed that systemic therapy plays a much greater role in sexual morbidity than local treatment of the breast.[2]

By the 1980s, radical pelvic surgery was redesigned to spare autonomic nerves responsible for penile blood flow.[3] However, nerve-sparing radical prostatectomy resulted in a return to baseline erectile function in less than 25% of men.[4] More recently, robotic-assisted laparoscopic prostatectomy (RALP) has claimed to increase the accuracy of nerve-sparing and enhance recovery of normal erections. Although RALP shortens hospital stays and decreases acute complications, two large studies using Medicare and Surveillance, Epidemiology, and End-Results (SEER) databases found no advantage over open surgery in preserving sexual function and a disadvantage in urinary incontinence.[5,6]

Attempts to minimize sexual consequences of pelvic radiotherapy began with the introducing brachytherapy[7] or computerized three-dimensional conformal fields for external beam treatment.[8] Long-term preservation of sexual function again proved disappointing, as did later efforts using intensity-modulated radiation therapy or proton beams.[8,9]

In the 1980s, sexual function began to be considered in women with gynecological malignancies.[10] As in men, attempts were made to spare nerves and tissues contributing to sexual pleasure and function during surgery or adjuvant radiation therapy.[9] However, premature ovarian failure and exacerbation of vulvovaginal atrophy by pelvic radiotherapy were increasingly recognized as risk factors for sexual dysfunction.[11] Techniques from cognitive behavioral sex therapy, a short-term, action-oriented type of psychological treatment[12] were used with male and female cancer patients, including efforts to enhance relationship satisfaction and sexual communication.[13]

Nevertheless, fewer than 20% of cancer patients/survivors currently seek help when they have a sexual problem.[14,15] Few cancer centers offer treatment for sexual problems and sexual dysfunction remains a long-term unmet need for cancer survivors.[16,17]

> Although recognition of cancer-related sexual problems began in the 1950s, most men and women still do not seek professional help for their dysfunctions and attempts to modify cancer treatment to spare sexual function have been disappointing.

Incidence and epidemiology—local and worldwide

About 59% of an estimated 14 million male cancer survivors in the United States, and 66% of women were treated for pelvic or breast tumors[18] with at least a 50% prevalence of long-term, severe sexual dysfunction.[19] Sexual problems affect at least 25% of survivors of treatment for nonreproductive cancers, including hematologic malignancies[20] and cancers of childhood.[21,22]

Given comparable prevalence and types of cancer in Europe and other industrialized nations, the risk for sexual dysfunction is similar.[23] Little information is available on sexual consequences of cancer in countries with low medical resources, but cancers potentiated by the human immunodeficiency virus (HIV) and the human papillomavirus (HPV) such as cervical, vulvar, anal, and penile cancer are more common, with a high likelihood of sexual morbidities.[24] The diagnosis can lead to divorce and ostracism in rural areas where cancer is stigmatized.[25]

Sexual problems related to cancer are severe and generalized, including loss of desire for sex or ability to get aroused and reach orgasm, and interference from fatigue, pain, or incontinence.[19] Without professional treatment, most problems do not resolve with time. Most dysfunctions are caused by cancer treatment,[19] including damage to autonomic nerves in the pelvis, reducing genital blood flow during sexual arousal,[3,4] especially for men,[26] and direct damage to genital blood vessels and tissue from pelvic radiation therapy.[9] Male erectile dysfunction also results from decreased genital blood flow after surgical interruption of blood vessels[27] or radiation damage.[9] Without regular inflow of oxygenated blood, erectile tissue in the penis atrophies. As a result, too much blood drains into the venous system, limiting erectile rigidity.[27]

Although the vagina expands and the clitoris swells with sexual arousal in women,[28] damage to hemodynamics is poorly understood. It is clear that estrogen deprivation plays a major role in female sexual problems,[19,29,30] decreasing the lubrication produced during sexual arousal by the vaginal mucosa. With vulvovaginal atrophy, sexual caressing and penetration become painful, often leading to loss of desire to engage in sex and difficulty reaching orgasm.[31]

Holland-Frei Cancer Medicine, Ninth Edition. Edited by Robert C. Bast Jr., Carlo M. Croce, William N. Hait, Waun Ki Hong, Donald W. Kufe, Martine Piccart-Gebhart, Raphael E. Pollock, Ralph R. Weichselbaum, Hongyang Wang, and James F. Holland.
© 2017 John Wiley & Sons, Inc. ISBN: 978-1-118-93469-2

In both men and women, loss of desire frequently ends with avoiding sexual encounters.[19] Low androgen levels are sometimes a factor in loss of desire for men, for example, during anti-androgen therapy for prostate cancer,[32] after intensive chemotherapy,[33] or after radiation that damages the testes.[34]

> Toxicity from cancer treatment leads to severe and long-term sexual dysfunction affecting desire, arousal, orgasm, and pain.

Risk factors—premorbid sexual function, cancer treatments, and behavioral characteristics

Many people have sexual problems before their cancer diagnosis, especially men. Erectile dysfunction is strongly associated with age-related cardiovascular disease, hypertension, diabetes, smoking, sedentary lifestyle, and obesity.[35,36] Erectile dysfunction is the most common reason that aging couples stop having sex.[37] At least half of women over age 50 are no longer sexually active because of lack of a functional sexual partner.[38] Being sexually active and functional at cancer diagnosis increases distress about new sexual problems in men and women.[39,40]

Cancer treatments with a high risk of sexual dysfunction include intensive chemotherapy, total body irradiation, graft versus host disease after allogeneic transplant,[41] treatments leading to abrupt ovarian failure in premenopausal women,[30] pelvic radiation therapy,[9] radical pelvic cancer surgery in men,[4–6,42] chemoradiation for pelvic tumors,[43] anti-androgenic therapy for prostate cancer,[32] and aromatase inhibitors for breast cancer.[40] Although penile and vulvar cancers are rare in Western nations, radical surgery removing major areas of genital tissue obviously also causes problems.[44,45] Vaginal reconstruction for advanced cervical or rectal cancer often fails to restore women's sexual pleasure.[46]

Psychosocial or behavioral factors also contribute to cancer-related sexual problems. Patients with a history of sexual abuse or trauma may have difficulty coping with cancer treatment, especially if the malignancy is in the reproductive system.[47] Relationship conflict and poor communication is also associated with poor sexual outcomes.[4] Traditional beliefs on masculinity and suppression of emotion may contribute to deterioration of sexual function after treatment for prostate cancer.[48] Both men and women scoring high on neuroticism, a personality trait involving depression and anxiety, have higher rates of sexual problems after cancer.[49,50]

Prevention—surgical, medical, behavioral

Modifications of cancer surgery to prevent sexual dysfunction have included sparing autonomic nerves near the prostate,[3–6] not only during radical prostatectomy but also in radical cystectomy or surgery for colorectal cancer.[42,51] Enhancement has had limited results, as has avoiding damage to accessory arteries to the penis during pelvic surgery.[52] Animal research and theoretical models support penile rehabilitation after surgery, using treatments for erectile dysfunction to promote penile blood flow, but benefits on recovery of erections in humans are unclear.[27] Nerve-sparing in radical hysterectomy has little impact on female sexual function.[26] Tissue-sparing surgery has been used instead of partial penectomy to treat localized penile cancer[44] or substituted for radical surgery in women for vulvar cancer,[45,53] but a majority of patients still have

major sexual problems. Breast conservation or reconstruction also has few advantages over mastectomy in preserving women's sexual pleasure and desire.[2]

Cancer treatments that preserve ovarian function in younger women, such as conservative surgery for low-grade ovarian cancer[54] or local therapy alone for ductal carcinoma *in situ*,[55] leave most women with normal sex lives. Intensive chemotherapy increases sexual dysfunction in both men[33] and women,[56] but less toxic regimens rarely achieve equivalent survival benefits. One exception is treating early-stage Hodgkin lymphoma with nonalkylating chemotherapy.[57] The trend toward personalized medicine and use of biological response modifiers may eventually lessen sexual morbidity, but little information is yet available on their sexual side effects.

Behavioral strategies may help prevent cancer-related sexual problems. Staying sexually active or stretching genital tissues with vacuum erection devices or vaginal dilators may prevent atrophy.[27,58,59] Counseling that promotes more open sexual communication, and continued, noncoital sexual intimacy, certainly may prevent a loss of satisfaction within a couple's relationship or a reduction in sexual self-esteem.[60,61]

> Risk factors for sexual dysfunction after cancer include:
> - Intensive chemotherapy
> - Radiation damage to the gonads or genitals
> - Hypogonadism due to cancer treatment
> - Removal of areas of genital tissue
> - History of sexual trauma
> - Relationship conflict
> - Personality factors such as neuroticism or traditional gender beliefs
>
> Prevention may include:
> - More conservative cancer surgery
> - Less toxic chemotherapy
> - Using behavioral strategies to preserve genital tissue or promote intimacy

Screening

Patients should be screened for sexual concerns and problems across the continuum of cancer care. During treatment planning, potential damage to sexual function from cancer treatment should be explained, including a mention of any conservative treatments. Although most patients rank survival over sexuality, a few would risk poorer cancer control for a treatment that would preserve sexual function. During treatment and at follow-up visits, sexual function should be monitored, at least with a periodic question, for example: "Sexuality is one important part of quality of life. Do you have any questions or concerns today about changes in your sex life since your cancer treatment?" In a study of patients in palliative care, about half wanted to continue sexual activity, despite a very high prevalence of sexual problems.[62] In 2013, a new National Comprehensive Cancer Network survivorship guideline recommended systematic screening for sexual dysfunction by interview or questionnaire, followed by further evaluation and referrals for treatment. Although the guideline was categorized under survivorship, it includes patients at any point of care.[63]

A brief questionnaire can be used to screen for sexual dysfunction. The National Cancer Institute sponsored creation of the Patient-Reported Outcomes Measurement Information System

(PROMIS) Brief Sexual Function profiles for men and women. These multiple choice questionnaires with 8 and 10 items, respectively, can be administered as an entire scale or using computer adaptive software, only by asking relevant items.[64]

Diagnosis

Because sexual dysfunction is most typically measured by self-report, diagnostic nomenclature has been varied and controversial.[65] Many labels do not help clinicians in choosing evidence-based treatments for problems. It is helpful to categorize sexual problems as affecting the following:

- ability to desire sex and experience subjective arousal
- ability for the genitals to engorge with blood during sexual arousal (i.e., erection in men and vaginal lubrication and expansion in women)
- ability to experience a satisfying orgasm
- problems with pain interfering with sexual pleasure
- urinary or fecal incontinence during sex

Most people treated for cancer have more than one specific sexual problem. For example, a woman who had chemoradiation for localized cervical cancer may have vulvovaginal atrophy and vaginal stenosis, causing dryness and acute pain with sexual caressing or penetration. As a result, her desire for sex and ability to reach orgasm are also impaired. A man may be unable to get or keep firm erections after radical prostatectomy. Urine may also drip from his penis with arousal and at orgasm. If he uses a medical treatment for erections, he may realize that his penis has shrunk in size or developed a curvature.[66] These problems lead him to avoid sex.

Taking the time to elicit a full description of the patient's sexual problems remains the most important aspect of diagnosis. For women, a pelvic examination with attention to pain and atrophy on the vulva and inside the vagina is crucial.[67] For men with erectile dysfunction, urologists may conduct a color duplex ultrasound imaging studies of the penis, before and after injecting drugs to create an erection.[68] Such testing may identify venous insufficiency due to atrophy of the erectile tissue, which can limit the efficacy of oral medication or penile injection therapy. However, many urologists prescribe treatments empirically for erectile dysfunction, starting with oral medication and proceeding if necessary to penile injection therapy, a vacuum device, or a urethral suppository, with a penile prosthesis as the final step.[69] In many aging men, cardiovascular disease complicates the treatment of cancer-related sexual problems.[70]

> Screening and diagnosis should be multidisciplinary, using brief questionnaires, a careful interview, and relevant focused examinations to get a full picture of the type of problem and its medical and psychosocial causes.

Prognostic factors

Only a few prognostic factors for sexual rehabilitation have been identified. Men or women who were not sexually active before cancer diagnosis are unlikely to seek help after cancer, unless they had previously sought treatment for their problems.[37,40] Younger men who start out with normal erections are more distressed and likely to seek help after surgery for prostate cancer.[71] Having a partner who still enjoys sex is also crucial.[72] For women, being in a sexual relationship is key to help-seeking.[40]

Poor general and sexual communication are barriers to success with cognitive-behavioral treatment of sexual problems.[13] In fact, couples with troubled relationships are less likely to enter clinical trials of sexual counseling.[73,74] Research on treatment outcomes is not available for people who are single or in a same-sex relationship.[75,76]

> Since research focuses on medical or counseling treatments that are short term, it is not surprising that barriers to success include a history of sexual problems, lack of a motivated partner, and poor sexual communication.

Multidisciplinary care

Research suggests that a multidisciplinary approach, combining medical and psychosocial care, is the most effective for cancer-related sexual problems.[72,74] Table 1 lists common sexual problems and suggested treatment components. Resuming a satisfying sex life requires good communication,[104,105] acceptance that intimacy may include noncoital sexual stimulation,[72,74,104] and ability to cope with some "performance" limitations. On the other hand, intervention programs using brief counseling without any medical treatments may reduce distress about sexual problems or improve sexual satisfaction somewhat, but do not resolve sexual dysfunction.[72,105,106]

Unfortunately, specialty clinics that include a psychologist and physician providing integrative treatment are rare even at comprehensive cancer centers. Mental health professionals trained in psychooncology typically lack expertise in treating sexual dysfunction. Most sex therapists have little knowledge about cancer and its treatments.

Psychosocial factors and management

In addition to the sychosocial factors already mentioned, a clinician should also assess the influence of culture,[25] sexual orientation,[75,76] ethnicity,[107–109] and religion on sexual issues. Good treatment outcomes are unlikely if interventions are incompatible with patients' sexual attitudes.

Survivorship and follow-up

Continued assessment of sexual problems and referral for treatment is important during survivorship, particularly given the long-term nature of cancer-related sexual dysfunction.

Unmet needs, future directions, and conclusions

Although sexual problems have often been dismissed as an unfortunate, but minor side effect of cancer treatment, they affect 25–50% of cancer survivors and have negative impacts on quality of life. Improvements are needed in the availability of cost-effective solutions for assessment, patient education, and multidisciplinary care. For patients with reasonable levels of literacy, education and self-help tools can be provided in high-quality, online interventions.[72,74] Patients from underserved communities may need additional guidance from peer counselors[108] or patient navigators. When first-line interventions do not resolve sexual problems, a stepped care approach can be used to refer patients for more intensive treatment.

Table 1 Components of multidisciplinary care for common, cancer-related sexual problems in men and women.

Sexual problem	Patient education	Brief sexual counseling	Physiological treatments
Male low desire	Problem often multifactorial, not simply hormonal (shame about erections, fatigue, medications, poor body image)	Help with loss of masculine self-esteem, poor body image, relationship conflict	Androgen replacement only if hypogonadal,[33,34] controversial after prostate cancer;[77] change medications that may contribute
Erectile dysfunction	Aging, premorbid risk factors, and cancer treatment all can damage erections	Help with decision-making on medical treatments; inclusion of partner; help with sexual communication to increase adherence[14,78]	PDE5 inhibitors, vacuum erection devices, penile injection therapy, urethral suppositories;[78] penile prosthesis surgery[79]
Changes in orgasmic pleasure	Cancer treatment may lead to orgasms without erection or ejaculation, weakened orgasmic sensation, inability to reach orgasm (central nervous system damage)[66]	Relearn how to reach orgasm, or intensify sensations, use of vibrators or erotica[80]	Treatment of hypogonadism or hyperprolactinemia, change medications that can interfere with orgasm[80,81]
Premature ejaculation	Erectile dysfunction can be misperceived as premature ejaculation if need prolonged stimulation to get an erection and then ejaculate quickly	Sex therapy techniques such as stop-start or squeeze[80]	Oral medication, though not very effective;[80] treatment for erectile dysfunction may correct problem[80]
Penile curvature	Cancer treatment can create penile curvature, understand timeline of pain with erection and changes in curvature[82]	Counseling about depression and body image issues	Use medical treatments to reduce curvature; surgical correction of curvature with or without penile prosthesis[82]
Pain during sex	Causes of genital pain during sex and interference with sex from chronic nongenital pain	Sensate focus exercises or mindfulness to focus on sexual pleasure and away from pain[83]	Treat chronic nongenital pain with medication or other modalities; medical treatments for pain at orgasm or testicular pain[84,85]
Incontinence during sex	If has stoma, consult with specialty nurse on minimizing interference with sex; urinary incontinence common after radical prostatectomy	Counsel on coping with incontinence during sex, use of mattress pads and other aids	Oral medications or penile tension loop to prevent urinary leakage during sex;[86] collagen injections;[87] surgery to insert artificial sphincter;[88] control of fecal incontinence using diet and medication[89]
Female low desire	Understanding that problem often multifactorial, not simply hormonal[90]	Help with poor body image, relationship conflict, coping with history of traumatic sexual experience,[47] coping with chronic fatigue and life stress	Treatment for pain that may lead to avoidance of sex;[67,74] changing medications that may contribute;[90] androgen replacement rarely helpful and may increase breast cancer risk[91]
Vulvovaginal dryness and pain with sex	Vulvovaginal atrophy is common after normal menopause and more severe after some cancer treatments[67,74]	Counseling on medical treatment options and on better sexual stimulation and communication to maximize sexual arousal, positions for penetration that may help avoid pain[67,80,92]	Regular use of vaginal moisturizers and water- or silicone-based lubricants during sexual activity;[67,74] use of graduated vaginal dilators;[59,93] low-dose vaginal estrogen if cancer is not hormone sensitive;[94] ospemifene[95]
Difficulty reaching orgasm	Women normally reach orgasm more easily with clitoral stimulation, genetic contribution to ease of reaching orgasm[96]	Training on reaching orgasm with self-stimulation or vibrator; transition to partner sex[97]	Change in medications that can interfere with orgasm[81,97]
Incontinence during sex	If has stoma, consult with specialty nurse on minimizing interference with sex; urinary incontinence commonly interferes with sex;[98] fecal incontinence frequent after pelvic radiation[99]	Behavioral bladder training and pelvic floor therapy[100]	Use of oral medications[101] or bulking agents[102] to prevent urinary leakage; sacral neuromodulation for neurogenic or overactive bladders;[103] control of fecal incontinence using diet and medication[89,99]

Key references

The complete reference list can be found on the Wiley Companion Digital Edition of this title (see inside front cover for login instructions).

4 Salonia A, Burnett AL, Graefen M, et al. Prevention and management of post-prostatectomy sexual dysfunctions. Part 1: choosing the right patient at the right time for the right surgery. *Eur Urol.* 2012;**62**:261–272.

5 Hu JC, Gu X, Lipsitz SR, et al. Comparative effectiveness of minimally invasive vs open radical prostatectomy. *JAMA.* 2009;**302**:1557–1564.

9 Incrocci L, Jensen PT. Pelvic radiotherapy and sexual function in men and women. *J Sex Med.* 2013;**10(Suppl 1)**:53–64.

12 Schover LR, Evans RB, von Eschenbach AC. Sexual rehabilitation in a cancer center: diagnosis and outcome in 384 consultations. *Arch Sex Behav.* 1987;**16**:445–461.

14 Prasad MM, Prasad SM, Hevelone ND, et al. Utilization of pharmacotherapy for erectile dysfunction following treatment for prostate cancer. *J Sex Med.* 2010;**7**:1062–1073.

15 Hill EK, Sandbo S, Abramsohn E, et al. Assessing gynecologic and breast cancer survivors' sexual health care needs. *Cancer.* 2011;**117**:2643–2651.

17 Holm LV, Hansen DG, Johansen C, et al. Participation in cancer rehabilitation and unmet needs: a population-based cohort study. *Support Care Cancer.* 2012;**20(29)**:13–24.

19 Schover LR, van der Kaaij M, van Dorst E, Creutzberg C, Huyghe E, Kiserud CE. Sexual dysfunction and infertility as late effects of cancer treatment. *EJC Suppl.* 2014;**12**:41–53.

21 Bober SL, Zhou ES, Chen B, Manley PE, Kenney LB, Recklitis CJ. Sexual function in childhood cancer survivors: a report from Project REACH. *J Sex Med.* 2013;**10**:2084–2093.

26 Pieterse QD, Kenter GG, Maas CP, et al. Self-reported sexual, bowel and bladder function in cervical cancer patients following different treatment modalities: longitudinal prospective cohort study. *Int J Gynecol Cancer.* 2013;**23**:1717–1725.

27 Fode M, Ohl DA, Ralph D, Sønksen J. Penile rehabilitation after radical prostatectomy: what the evidence really says. *BJU Int.* 2013;**112**:998–1008.

31 Kingsberg SA, Wysocki S, Magnus L, Krychman ML. Vulvar and vaginal atrophy in postmenopausal women: findings from the REVIVE (REal Women's VIews of Treatment Options for Menopausal Vaginal ChangEs) survey. *J Sex Med.* 2013;**10**:1790–1799.

33 Kiserud CE, Schover LR, Dahl AA, et al. Do male lymphoma survivors have impaired sexual function? *J Clin Oncol.* 2009;**27**:6019–6026.

38 Lutfey KE, Link CL, Rosen RC, Wiegel M, McKinlay JB. Prevalence and correlates of sexual activity and function in women: results from the Boston Area Community health (BACH) survey. *Arch Sex Beh.* 2009;**38**:514–527.

39 Steinsvik EA, Axcrona K, Dahl AA, Eri LM, Stensvold A, Fosså SD. Can sexual bother after radical prostatectomy be predicted preoperatively? Findings from a prospective national study of the relation between sexual function, activity and bother. *BJU Int.* 2012;**109**:1366–1374.

40 Schover LR, Baum GP, Fuson LA, Brewster A, Melhem-Bertrandt A. Sexual problems during the first 2 years of adjuvant treatment with aromatase inhibitors. *J Sex Med.* in press.

41 Wong FL, Francisco L, Togawa K, et al. Longitudinal trajectory of sexual functioning after hematopoietic cell transplantation: impact of chronic graft-versus-host disease and total body irradiation. *Blood.* 2013;**122**:3973–3981.

44 Kieffer JM, Djajadiningrat RS, van Muilekom EA, Graafland NM, Horenblas S, Aaronson NK. Quality of life in patients treated for penile cancer. *J Urol.* 2014;**192**:1105–1110.

46 Scott JR, Liu D, Mathes DW. Patient-reported outcomes and sexual function in vaginal reconstruction: a 17-year review, survey, and review of the literature. *Ann Plast Surg.* 2010;**64**:311–314.

55 Bober SL, Giobbie-Hurder A, Emmons KM, Winer E, Partridge A. Psychosexual functioning and body image following a diagnosis of ductal carcinoma in situ. *J Sex Med.* 2013;**10**:370–377.

56 Rosenberg SM, Tamimi RM, Gelber S, et al. Treatment-related amenorrhea and sexual functioning in young breast cancer survivors. *Cancer.* 2014;**120**:2264–2271.

57 Behringer K, Mueller H, Goergen H, et al. Sexual quality of life in Hodgkin lymphoma: a longitudinal analysis by the German Hodgkin Study Group. *Brit J Cancer.* 2013;**108**:49–57.

64 Flynn KE, Lin L, Cyranowski JM, et al. Development of the NIH PROMIS® Sexual Function and Satisfaction measures in patients with cancer. *J Sex Med.* 2013;**10**(**Suppl 1**):43–52.

66 Frey A, Sønksen J, Jakobsen H, Fode M. Prevalence and predicting factors for commonly neglected sexual side effects to radical prostatectomies: results from a cross-sectional questionnaire-based study. *J Sex Med.* 2014;**11**(**9**):2318–2326.

67 Carter J, Goldfrank D, Schover LR. Simple strategies for vaginal health promotion in cancer survivors. *J Sex Med.* 2011;**8**:549–559.

69 Montorsi F, Adaikan G, Becher E, et al. Summary of the recommendations on sexual dysfunctions in men. *J Sex Med.* 2010;**7**:3572–3588.

72 Schover LR, Canada AL, Yuan Y, et al. A randomized trial of internet-based versus traditional sexual counseling for couples after localized prostate cancer treatment. *Cancer.* 2012;**118**:500–509.

74 Schover LR, Yuan Y, Fellman BM, Odensky E, Lewis PE, Martinetti P. Efficacy trial of an Internet-based intervention for cancer-related female sexual dysfunction. *J Natl Compr Canc Netw.* 2013;**11**:1389–1397.

79 Tal R, Jacks LM, Elkin E, Mulhall JP. Penile implant utilization following treatment for prostate cancer: analysis of the SEER-Medicare database. *J Sex Med.* 2011;**8**:1797–1804.

80 McMahon CG, Jannini E, Waldinger M, Rowland D. Standard operating procedures in the disorders of orgasm and ejaculation. *J Sex Med.* 2013;**10**:204–229.

81 Gitlin M. Sexual dysfunction with psychotropic drugs. *Expert Opin Pharmacother.* 2003;**4**:2259–2269.

82 Tal R, Heck M, Teloken P, Siegrist T, Nelson CJ, Mulhall JP. Peyronie's disease following radical prostatectomy: incidence and predictors. *J Sex Med.* 2010;**7**:1254–1261.

84 Seyam R. A systematic review of the correlates and management of nonpremature ejaculatory dysfunction in heterosexual men. *Ther Adv Urol.* 2013;**5**:254–297.

86 Mehta A, Deveci S, Mulhall JP. Efficacy of a penile variable tension loop for improving climacturia after radical prostatectomy. *BJU Int.* 2013;**111**:500–504.

92 Kao A, Binik YM, Amsel R, Funaro D, Leroux N, Khalifé S. Biopsychosocial predictors of postmenopausal dyspareunia: the role of steroid hormones, vulvovaginal atrophy, cognitive-emotional factors, and dyadic adjustment. *J Sex Med.* 2012;**9**:2066–2076.

95 McLendon AN, Clinard VB, Woodis CB. Ospemifene for the treatment of vulvovaginal atrophy and dyspareunia in postmenopausal women. *Pharmacotherapy.* 2015;**34**(**10**):1050–1060.

97 Meston CM, Hull E, Levin RJ, Sipski M. Disorders of orgasm in women. *J Sex Med.* 2004;**1**:66–68.

100 Rutledge TL, Rogers R, Lee SJ, Muller CY. A pilot randomized control trial to evaluate pelvic floor muscle training for urinary incontinence among gynecologic cancer survivors. *Gynecol Oncol.* 2014;**132**:154–158.

108 Schover LR, Rhodes MM, Baum G, et al. Sisters Peer Counseling in Reproductive Issues After Treatment (SPIRIT): a peer counseling program to improve reproductive health among African American breast cancer survivors. *Cancer.* 2011;**117**:4983–4992.

138 Endocrine complications and paraneoplastic syndromes

Sai-Ching Jim Yeung, MD, PhD, FACP ▪ *Robert F. Gagel, MD*

Overview

Transformation of normal cells results in activation and/or suppression of a number of hormonally active genes. This chapter outlines the several clinical endocrine paraneoplastic syndromes and their appropriate management. Treatment of cancer results in a number of endocrine or metabolic manifestations, most of which are related to hormone deficiency or drug-related toxicity. The introduction of targeted therapy that disrupts signaling pathways and immunotherapy, contrary to expectations, has actually increased the number of endocrine manifestations. This chapter will chronicle the major new endocrine toxicities in addition to those observed with older cytotoxic chemotherapies and radiation.

Introduction

This chapter is divided into two major sections. The first focuses on endocrine complications in cancer patients and the second on endocrine paraneoplastic syndromes. Cancer and its treatment can lead to endocrine dysfunction or clinical and laboratory abnormalities that obscure or mimic endocrine diseases. Paraneoplastic syndromes are a group of diverse clinical syndromes seen in cancer patients caused by circulating biologic/humoral factors that include hormones, immunoglobulins, cytokines, and other agents.

Endocrine complications

Hypothalamic–pituitary dysfunction

Radiotherapy is a common cause of hypothalamic–pituitary dysfunction in cancer patients. There is no strong direct evidence to implicate chemotherapy as a cause of permanent dysfunction of the anterior pituitary, although some of the newer targeted therapies may affect pituitary function. Metastasis to the hypothalamic region or the pituitary gland is uncommon,[1] and clinical manifestations of endocrine dysfunction because of metastatic disease in this region are rare. However, benign tumors such as pituitary tumors and craniopharyngiomas frequently affect this anatomic region and cause endocrine dysfunction. The introduction of immunotherapy by immune checkpoint blockade [anti-CTLA4 antibodies (ipilimumab and tremelimumab) and anti-PD-1 antibody (nivolumab)] has been associated with development of autoimmune hypophysitis that requires hormonal replacement (corticosteroids or thyroid hormone) in 2–3% of treated patients.

Development of radiation-induced hypothalamic dysfunction is insidious; hormonal deficiency can manifest years after radiation. In general, the rapidity of onset and severity of dysfunction depend on the total dose of radiation and the rate of delivery. The sequence and frequency of dysfunction among the axes of hypothalamic–pituitary functions vary. The somatotropic axis is the most susceptible, while the thyrotropic axis is the least susceptible (Figure 1).[2–5] The diagnosis of hypothalamic–pituitary dysfunction requires vigilance of the physician because most presenting symptoms (e.g., fatigue and weakness) are nonspecific and attributable to other causes common among cancer patients. A diagnostic screen for hypothalamic/pituitary dysfunction may include serum growth hormone (GH) and insulin-like growth factor-1 (IGF-1) measurement and evaluation for gonadal failure. Signs of overt hypopituitarism include hypoglycemia, hypotension, and hypothermia.

In children and adolescents, evaluation of sexual development is a useful diagnostic tool. Staging sexual development according to Tanner's criteria, menstrual history in girls and penile/testicular size in boys should be evaluated. In children who have had cranial irradiation, height and weight should be measured every 6 months. In children treated with spinal and craniospinal irradiation, local rather than general growth abnormalities may be present and, if so, require specific evaluation. Foot size is a reliable indicator of growth that can be easily measured. Deviation from normal growth curves should be evaluated for GH deficiency, hypothyroidism, and adrenal insufficiency. If the initial evaluation of GH, IGF-1, thyrotropin (TSH) and free thyroxine (T_4) levels, and radiographic bone age reveal abnormality, then detailed dynamic testing to evaluate the hypothalamic/pituitary axes should be performed (Table 1).

In adults who have received cranial or head and neck irradiation, detection of hypothalamic–pituitary abnormalities is more challenging. One strategy to detect hypothalamic–pituitary abnormalities in adults consists of routine screening for GH deficiency and gonadal failure. It is recommended that measurements of IGF-1 and testosterone levels in males and documentation of menstrual history in females be obtained annually for 5 years, and then at 5-year intervals for another 10 years. Any abnormalities noted on the screening tests should be pursued with further dynamic testing to evaluate all the axes of hypothalamic–pituitary functions.

Immunotherapy-induced hypophysitis

The development of immunotherapeutic approaches to treat melanoma and a growing list of other malignancies has resulted in a number of bystander effects. Prominent among these side effects is immunotherapy-induced hypophysitis (IH). In the phase III clinical trial of ipilimumab, 2.3% of patients developed symptoms of IH and evidence of hormonal deficiency including glucocorticoid, thyroid, gonadal, and GH deficiency, necessitating long-term replacement therapy. The pituitary-related events were grade 3 or 4 in 1.9% of these patients, necessitating urgent treatment or hospitalization. The onset of pituitary failure ranged from 11 to 19 weeks, following

Holland-Frei Cancer Medicine, Ninth Edition. Edited by Robert C. Bast Jr., Carlo M. Croce, William N. Hait, Waun Ki Hong, Donald W. Kufe, Martine Piccart-Gebhart, Raphael E. Pollock, Ralph R. Weichselbaum, Hongyang Wang, and James F. Holland.
© 2017 John Wiley & Sons, Inc. ISBN: 978-1-118-93469-2

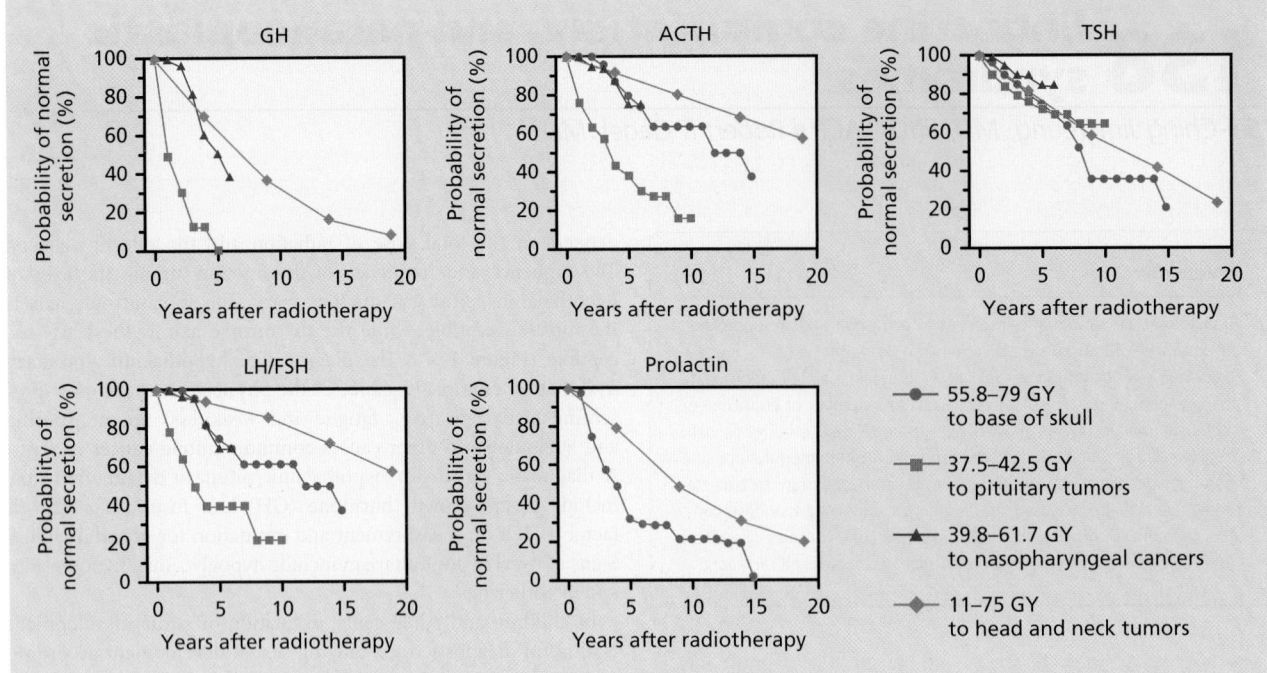

Figure 1 Probability of normal pituitary hormone secretion over time after radiation exposure to the hypothalamic–pituitary areas. Data from four studies were replotted on this single figure. The first set of values (*closed circle*) are from Pai et al.,[3] where the patient received 55.8–79 Gy to the base of the skull. The second set of values (*solid square*) are from Shalet et al.,[83] where patients with pituitary tumors were treated with 37.5–42.5 Gy. The third series (*open triangle*), from Lam et al.,[2] shows the effect of radiation treatment for nasopharyngeal carcinoma with 39.8–61.7 Gy. The final series (*open diamond*) represents data from Samaan et al.,[4] in which 11–75 Gy was administered to treat head and neck tumors.

initiation of ipilimumab therapy. Common presenting complaints include headache, mental status alterations, abdominal pain, modified bowel habits, and hypotension; it is often difficult to distinguish IH from brain metastasis or symptoms associated with widespread metastatic disease. This difficulty suggests that clinicians initiating therapy with immunotherapy agents should obtain baseline thyroid (free T_4 and TSH), adrenal (ACTH, adrenocorticotropic hormone and 8 a.m. serum cortisol), gonadal [luteinizing hormone (LH), follicle-stimulating hormone, and estradiol in females or testosterone in males], and growth-related hormones (GH and IGF-1) as baseline before initiating therapy. These measurements should be repeated if a patient develops symptoms suggestive of endocrine deficiency or acute symptoms of hypophysitis (headache and visual disturbance). In patients with symptoms or physical findings consistent with IH, an MRI (magnetic resonance imaging) of the pituitary gland and repeat hormone testing as described above should be performed together with dynamic testing of the adrenal endocrine axis (e.g., low-dose cosyntropin stimulation test). A recent report highlighting a larger experience in a single center indicates that IH is observed not only with anti-CTLA4 agents (ipilimumab and tremelimumab),[6] but also with an anti-PD1 agent (nivolumab). In a report describing 968 patients treated with these agents for melanoma, prostate cancer, and renal cell carcinoma at a single center, 2.7% (27 subjects) had one or two hormonal deficiencies together with either pituitary enlargement in MRI scans or headache.[6] In these 27 patients, central adrenal deficiency was identified in 77%, central hypothyroidism in 89%, and central hypogonadism in 79%. An abnormality of the pituitary gland was found by MRI in 85%.[6] After a median follow-up period of 17 months (range: 1–76), none of the patients recovered normal adrenocortical function, whereas 12–13% recovered thyroid or gonadal function. Clearly, this is a significant and evolving issue; it is unclear at this time whether combinatorial therapy with two or more immunotherapeutic agents, currently under development, will be associated with higher incidence and/or severity of toxicity.

Thyroid disorders

Thyroid disorders and abnormalities in thyroid function are commonly associated with cancer and its therapy.

Serum thyroid hormone-binding protein abnormalities

The levels of thyroid hormone-binding proteins [thyroxine-binding globulin (TBG), prealbumin, and albumin] can be modified by sex hormone levels and nutritional factors; abnormalities of both are encountered frequently in cancer patients. Several chemotherapy drugs affect thyroid function test results. L-Asparaginase appears to reversibly inhibit synthesis of albumin and TBG, resulting in low total thyroxine (T_4), but normal free T_4 levels.[7] The combination of podophyllin and alkylating agents has also been reported to decrease TBG.[8] Both 5-fluorouracil[9] and mitotane[10] increase the total T_4 and triiodothyronine (T_3) levels without suppressing TSH, suggesting that these drugs increase thyroid hormone-binding capacity in the serum.

Euthyroid sick syndrome

Alterations in thyroid hormone metabolism occur in patients with cancer and other serious systemic illnesses.[11] Low serum T_3 levels, which may be found in up to 70% of moderately to seriously ill cancer patients, are caused by a decrease in the extrathyroidal conversion of T_4 to T_3. Serum concentrations of free T_4 are usually normal or high, while concentrations of free T_3 are below normal or low. The patients are clinically euthyroid, and serum TSH level and TRH stimulation test results are normal.

In most patients with euthyroid sick syndrome, T_3, T_4, and TSH levels are normal. Clinical manifestations of hypothyroidism are

Table 1 Dynamic testing of the hypothalamic/pituitary axes.

Test	Dose/sampling	Contraindications
Growth hormone axis		
Insulin hypoglycemia	0.075–0.1 U regular insulin/kg IV to achieve glucose ≤40 mg/dL. Sample for glucose and GH at 0, 30, 45, 60, and 90 min	Coronary heart disease or seizures
Arginine	0.5 g/kg (up to 30 g) IV over 30 min. Sample for GH at 0, 30, 60, 90, and 120 min	Liver disease or renal disease
L-Dopa	500 mg by mouth. Sample for GH at 0, 30, 60, 90, and 120 min	Systolic blood pressure <100 mm Hg or age > 60 years
Arginine and GHRH	Arginine dose as above. GHRH 1 µg/kg IV push. Sample for GH at 0, 30, 60, 90, and 120 min	Liver disease or renal disease
Clonidine stimulation protocol	Clonidine 0.15 mg/m² by mouth. Collect GH samples at baseline, 30, 60, 90, and 120 min	
Growth hormone-releasing hormone (GHRH) stimulation protocol	GHRH at 1.0 µg/kg body weight IV push. Collect GH samples at baseline, 15, 30, 45, 60, 90, and 120 min	
Growth hormone suppression test	The test should be performed after an overnight fast with the patient maintained at bed rest. The patient should drink a solution of 100 g glucose. Collect GH samples at baseline, 60, and 120 min	
Adrenal axis		
ACTH stimulation test, 1-h	Synthetic ACTH 1–24 1 or 250 µg IM or IV. Draw blood for cortisol at 30 and 60 min after injection	
ACTH stimulation test, 48-h	Beginning at 9 a.m., obtain baseline 24-h urine for 17-hydroxycorticosteroids (17-OHCS) and creatinine. Collect 24-h urine as on day 1. Beginning at 9 a.m., start IV and give 250 µg synthetic ACTH 1–24 in 250 mL normal saline over 8 h every 8 h for 48 h. Alternatively, 40 IU of depot formulation of purified bovine ACTH in gelatin IM every 12 h for 48 h. Repeat 24-h urine as on days 1 and 2. Days 4 and 5: Collect 24-h urine as on previous days	
Corticotropin-releasing hormone (CRH) stimulation test	Fast for at least 4 h before the test. Human CRH at 1.0 µg/kg IV bolus over 30 s. Blood samples should be collected at 15 and 1 min before CRH administration and at 15, 30, 45, 60, 90, and 120 min after for measurements of cortisol and ACTH	
Low-dose dexamethasone test, overnight	Dexamethasone 1.0 mg (adult) or 20 µg/kg (children) PO between 11 p.m. and midnight. Serum cortisol is collected at 8–9 a.m. the next morning. A cortisol level <1.8 µg/dL essentially excludes Cushing syndrome	
Low-dose dexamethasone test, 48-h	Serum cortisol is collected at 8–9 a.m. Dexamethasone 0.5 mg (adult) or 10 µg/kg (children) PO immediately after the cortisol is drawn and again every 6 h for 48 h. A second plasma cortisol is drawn at 9 a.m., 6 h after the last dexamethasone dose. Serum cortisol concentrations <1.8 µg/dL exclude Cushing syndrome	
High-dose dexamethasone test, 48-h	Serum cortisol is collected at 9 a.m. Dexamethasone is administered (2.0 mg; 50 µg/kg in children) every 6 h for 48 h. A second plasma cortisol is drawn at 9 a.m., 6 h after the last dexamethasone dose. Patients with functional adrenal adenomas show no suppression of cortisol levels in the 48-h sample relative to the initial (baseline) sample. Seventy-eight percent of patients with pituitary source of excess ACTH showed >50% suppression of plasma cortisol, while only 11% of patients with an ectopic source of excess ACTH had a >50% suppression	
Comprehensive, 6-day, low-/high-dose dexamethasone test	This protocol incorporates the low- and high-dose dexamethasone tests in succession. 24-h urinary free cortisol and/or 17-hydroxycorticosteroid (17-OHCS) measurement can help verify the results of serum cortisol and ACTH	
Gonadotropin-releasing hormone (GnRH) stimulation test	GnRH 100 µg IV. A sample for serum LH should be collected at baseline and 40 min after GnRH administration	
Metyrapone stimulation (overnight) test	At 11 p.m., metyrapone 30 mg/kg (maximum 3 g) PO with a snack. On the following morning, at 8 a.m., measure serum cortisol and 11-deoxycortisol	

GH = growth hormone; GNRH = growth hormone-releasing hormone; IV = intravenous; IM = intramuscular; PO = by mouth.

usually absent, but assessment may be confounded by obtundation, edema, and hypothermia that may accompany severe illness. Low free T_4 levels in the context of euthyroid sick syndrome usually indicate a grave prognosis, with a mortality rate of more than 50%. Although it is generally accepted that thyroid hormone therapy has no benefit, in practice it is sometimes difficult to differentiate between the euthyroid sick syndrome and secondary hypothyroidism. Judicious replacement of T_4 at physiologic levels in these uncommon patients may be appropriate if there are no contraindications (e.g., active ischemic heart disease).

Hypothyroidism

Thyroidectomy
Thyroidectomy may be performed for a variety of oncologic reasons in the management of thyroid cancer, head and neck cancer, or thyroid metastasis. Thyroid replacement is needed in this group of patients. In thyroid cancer patients, supraphysiologic doses of thyroid hormone are adjusted to suppress TSH without overt hyperthyroid symptoms. In others, the dose of thyroid hormone should be adjusted to keep TSH in the normal range.

Table 2 Incidence of hypothyroidism (including compensated hypothyroidism) after radiotherapy.[a]

Type of malignancy or conditions	Radiation dose	% with hypothyroidism
Hodgkin disease	30–60 Gy	30–50
Head and neck cancer	40–72 Gy	25–50
Lymphoma	20–40 Gy (median 36 Gy)	30–42
Breast carcinoma	?	15–21
Total-body irradiation in BMT	13.75–15 Gy	15–43

BMT = bone marrow transplantation.
[a]Data based on Refs 4 and 12–22.

Radiation

Irradiation is an important cause of hypothyroidism [primary (thyroid), secondary (pituitary), and tertiary (hypothalamic)]. Radiation-induced primary hypothyroidism is caused by thyroid cell destruction, inhibition of cell division, vascular damage, and possibly an immune-mediated phenomenon. Factors that increase the risk of developing primary hypothyroidism include a high radiation dose to the vicinity of the thyroid gland, duration since therapy, lack of shielding of the thyroid during therapy, and combined irradiation and surgical treatments.[12]

The incidences of hypothyroidism after radiation therapy for various cancers and conditions are tabulated in Table 2.[4,12–22] A relationship between radiation dose and the prevalence of hypothyroidism is based on studies of patients with Hodgkin disease.[15,18] Long-term follow-up of patients treated with low-dose radiotherapy suggests that the threshold for causing clinically evident hypothyroidism is approximately 10 Gy. For Hodgkin-disease patients who received >30 Gy, the actuarial risk of hypothyroidism was up to 45%, 20 years after irradiation.[15] Patients with frank or subclinical hypothyroidism should receive thyroid hormone-replacement therapy.

Chemotherapy

The diagnosis of hypothyroidism in 14% of BMT (bone marrow transplantation) patients who received chemotherapy but did not receive total-body irradiation[23] suggests a causal relation between hypothyroidism and high-dose combination cytotoxic chemotherapy. This notion is also supported by studies that showed an increased incidence of primary hypothyroidism in patients treated with multiple combination drug regimens[24,25] with or without radiation.[24] L-Asparaginase, in addition to inhibition of TBG synthesis discussed above, may also inhibit TSH synthesis reversibly and lead to temporary hypothyroidism with decreased free T_4 levels.[26]

Thyroid dysfunction is a recognized side effect of cytokine treatments. Treatment with interleukin-2 produces thyroid dysfunction in approximately 20–35% of patients.[27] These patients have hypothyroidism, hyperthyroidism, or hyperthyroidism followed by hypothyroidism.[28] Approximately 10% of interferon-treated patients develop primary hypothyroidism.[29] Pituitary enlargement secondary to interferon-induced hypothyroidism has also been reported.[30] Patients with antithyroid antibodies before therapy are at higher risk of cytokine-induced thyroid dysfunction.

Retinoid X receptor (RXR) ligands may be used in the treatment of certain malignancies such as cutaneous T-cell lymphoma. Bexarotene (a RXR-selective ligand) caused secondary hypothyroidism dose-dependently.[31] A single dose can rapidly suppress TSH in healthy subjects.[32] In addition to suppressing transcription of TSH by an RXR-mediated thyroid hormone-independent mechanism, bexarotene also increases metabolic clearance of thyroid hormones by a nondeiodinase-mediated pathway.[33]

Tyrosine kinase inhibitors

The rapid introduction of small organic molecules that inhibit kinase activity (tyrosine kinase inhibitors, TKIs) into cancer therapy over the past decade has led to the recognition that many of these agents affect thyroid function in profound ways. The first mechanism is a direct effect of these agents on thyroid function. A number of TKIs target receptor tyrosine kinases with well-defined functions in the thyroid gland including the vascular endothelial growth factor receptor, the epidermal growth factor receptor, RET, KIT, and MET. Other agents target downstream signaling pathways such as RAF, PI3K, and mTOR. These signaling pathways are operative in the thyroid and important for normal thyroid cell growth and function. It is not surprising that disruption of these pathways has effects on thyroid cell growth and death and thyroid hormone synthesis. Indeed hypothyroidism occurs at significant incidence rates with a number of agents: sunitinib, 7–85%; pazopanib, 12%; nilotinib, 22%; axitinib, 20–100%; cabozantinib, 15%; sorafenib, 8–39%; dasatinib, 50%; and imatinib, 0–25%.[34] Routine measurement of thyroid function (free T_4 and TSH) at regular intervals during the first year of therapy with one of these agents seems prudent as it is often difficult to differentiate nonspecific side effects of TKI therapy from primary hypothyroidism or effects of metastatic cancer.

There is a second mechanism for development of hypothyroidism in patients treated with specific TKIs for metastatic thyroid carcinoma who have also undergone total thyroidectomy. Specific agents approved (vandetanib, cabozantinib, sorafenib, and lenvatinib) or studied (pazopanib, motesanib, and sunitinib) for treatment of differentiated or medullary thyroid carcinoma cause an elevation of the serum TSH concentration and low serum T_4 levels with high percent incidences: vandetanib, 49%; cabozantinib, 57%; sorafenib, 41%; and lenvatinib, 57%. As each of these agents causes diarrhea and malabsorption, one presumed mechanism for this effect is reduced absorption of thyroid hormone, although effects on thyroid hormone metabolism have not been excluded. Increasing the thyroid hormone dosages by as much as one-third generally resolves the problem. It is important to note that there may also be malabsorption of calcium, magnesium, and vitamin D, causing worsening hypocalcemia or hypomagnesemia in patients with mild thyroidectomy-associated hypoparathyroidism.[35] Routine measurement of free T_4 and TSH should be incorporated into management as more than 50% of these patient will require a dose modification of thyroid hormone (as well as magnesium, calcium, and vitamin D supplementation). It is important to note that primary hypothyroidism, hypocalcemia, or hypomagnesemia can be readily treated, and their appearance, if addressed promptly, should not limit the use of the TKIs. However, in patients with hypothyroidism, hypocalcemia, or hypomagnesemia, all of which can prolong the QT interval, it may be necessary to withhold TKIs that prolong QT interval, that is, vandetanib,[35] lenvatinib,[36] and sorafenib in patients with QT prolongation until the QT abnormalities are resolved.

^{131}I-containing compounds

The use of ^{131}I for treatment of thyroid cancer requires a high serum TSH level. High TSH level is achieved by either withholding thyroid hormone replacement or increasingly by administration of recombinant human TSH. The use of ^{131}I-containing compounds in the treatment of other tumors may result in hypothyroidism. For instance, using high-dose (100–1000 mCi) [^{131}I]-metaiodobenzylguanidine to treat unresectable pheochromocytoma may result in primary hypothyroidism.[37]

Metastasis to the thyroid

Hypothyroidism secondary to metastatic infiltration and replacement of the thyroid by cancer is extremely rare.

Screening

Children who have received either head and neck or cranial irradiation should have a free T$_4$ and a TSH measurement annually for 5 years, and every 2 years thereafter. Early detection of abnormal T$_4$ and TSH levels will permit medical intervention before hypothyroidism adversely affects physical and intellectual development and growth. In adults, neck irradiation for treatment of lymphoma and various head and neck tumors is associated with a high incidence of primary hypothyroidism. Patients who have received irradiation should have free T$_4$ and TSH levels measured annually for 5 years, and then every other year for 10 years, and thereafter every 5 years for another 10 years. Once hypothyroidism is diagnosed, the patient should receive thyroid hormone-replacement therapy.

Hyperthyroidism

Radiation-induced painless thyroiditis with hyperthyroxinemia is an uncommon side effect of external-beam radiotherapy to the head and neck area. Transient hyperthyroidism may occur as a result of inflammation and destruction of thyroid tissue with release of thyroglobulin (containing T$_4$ and T$_3$), and is usually followed by hypothyroidism. Transient hyperthyroidism has been reported after mantle radiotherapy in Hodgkin disease patients, and occurs usually within 18 months of treatment.[38] A low uptake of radioiodine in most of these cases suggests a diagnosis of silent thyroiditis, but some have Graves' disease. In one series of Hodgkin disease patient treated with radiation, the risk of Graves' disease in these patients was estimated to be at least 7.2 times that in a healthy population.[15]

Ophthalmopathy similar to that in Graves' disease has been reported within 18–84 months of high-dose radiotherapy to the neck for lymphoma, breast cancer, and nasopharyngeal or laryngeal cancer. Ophthalmopathy may occur without hyperthyroidism and in the absence of the human leukocyte antigen-B8.[39] This suggests that radiation-induced thyroid injury may induce an autoimmune process that is similar to Graves' disease.

There have also been examples of TKI-associated hyperthyroidism, including two deaths (sorafenib and sunitinib associated).[40] The presumed mechanism of hyperthyroidism is thyroiditis. Patients with severe hyperthyroidism should be treated aggressively for thyroid storm; consideration should be given to holding TKI therapy until the patient is stabilized in such cases.[34]

Thyroid nodules and cancers

Low-dose radiation increases the risk of thyroid nodules and cancer. The association between thyroid cancer and low-dose irradiation has been extensively examined,[41] and is discussed in the chapter about thyroid cancer (*see **Chapter 80***).

Energy balance and glucose metabolism

Obesity and metabolic syndrome

Cancer treatments may lead to obesity and the metabolic syndrome.[42–44] The metabolic syndrome is a cluster of abnormalities consisting of central obesity, dyslipidemia, hyperglycemia, and hypertension that increases the risk of type 2 diabetes and cardiovascular disease. Obesity is a modifiable risk factor for carcinogenesis as well as cancer progression. The mechanisms by which obesity promotes cancer include: hyperinsulinemia due to insulin resistance, high IGF-1, adipokines, low adiponectin, increased production of estrogens by adipose tissue, and increased inflammation. Obesity in cancer survivors may place them at increased risk for poor disease outcomes.[42,45,46] Obesity increases the risk of colorectal and genitourinary second primary cancers.[47] Although low levels of physical activity in cancer survivors can contribute to obesity, the pathophysiologic basis of the weight gain is unclear. As obesity is an adverse prognostic factor for many cancers and is a modifiable risk factor, secondary obesity after cancer treatment needs to be addressed.

Diabetes mellitus

Diabetes mellitus type 2 (DM2) is associated with an elevated risk of pancreatic, liver, colon, gastric, breast, and endometrial cancer.[48–53] Extensive epidemiologic data suggest important roles of diabetes in carcinogenesis[48–53] and cancer survival.[54] The strongest association is perhaps with pancreatic cancer.[55–59] Apart from the frequently coexisting obesity, the mechanisms by which diabetes promotes cancer include: hyperinsulinemia, high IGF-1, and hyperglycemia. Hyperglycemia per se has a promoting effect on cancer proliferation. In male, cancer survivors with a fasting serum glucose concentration ≥ 126 mg/dL had a higher relative risk for hepatopancreatobiliary second primary cancer.[47] Evidence-based guidelines for the management of DM2 in cancer patients to optimize patient survival are lacking.

The administration of glucocorticoids (e.g., in combination therapy regimens, for edema of brain metastasis, for prevention of transplant rejection, for graft-versus-host disease in BMT, and for nausea/vomiting) is probably the most common cause of diabetes mellitus in cancer patients. Therefore, patients who receive glucocorticoids must be periodically screened for diabetes with evaluation of fasting glucose levels during therapy. Treatment with streptozocin[60] or L-asparaginase[61] may result in insulin-deficient diabetes mellitus. Although there is no evidence of a delayed onset of diabetes mellitus following treatment with streptozocin, follow-up has been limited and short term. For long-term survivors treated with streptozocin, periodic screening for delayed development of diabetes mellitus may be indicated. Diabetes mellitus may also develop as a consequence of serious pancreatitis secondary to treatment with L-asparaginase. Immunotherapy for cancer using cytokines such as interleukin-2 and interferons may cause toxicity to pancreatic β cells and lead to insulin-dependent diabetes.[62] Tacrolimus, an immunosuppressive agent used to prevent graft-versus-host disease in BMT, also increases the incidence of diabetes, perhaps by damaging pancreatic β cells.[63] Patients who received allogenic BMT are likely to be receiving both glucocorticoids, cyclosporine A and tacrolimus, and are particularly at risk for developing diabetes mellitus.[64] Management of the blood glucose levels would depend on the severity of the blood glucose level abnormality and on the underlying pathophysiologic mechanism of the increase in blood sugar. In general, insulin will be needed in patients who are insulin deficient.

Metabolic bone diseases

Osteoporosis

Four groups of adult patients are at particular risk for accelerated bone loss and osteoporosis: (i) patients with lymphoma, myeloma, or leukemia; (ii) women with breast cancer treated with cytotoxic chemotherapy frequently undergo an early menopause[65] and cannot receive estrogen-replacement therapy; (iii) postmenopausal women with estrogen-receptor positive breast cancer; and (iv) men with prostate cancer who are on antiandrogenic therapy and made hypogonadal. Normal bone remodeling involves a delicate balance between bone formation by osteoblasts and bone resorption by osteoclasts. Antineoplastic therapy is toxic to osteoblast function and decreases bone formation. Production by the tumor of hormonally active substances [e.g., parathyroid hormone-related protein (PTHrP), lymphotoxin, interleukin-1, and interleukin-6] may contribute to bone loss. In most cases, it is not clear whether bone loss is caused by antineoplastic therapy or by the underlying disease process and its effects (including cachexia, malnutrition, poor calcium and vitamin D intake, or a combination of these). In patients with breast or prostate cancer, sex steroid hormone deficiency induced by therapy is the most important cause of bone loss. Bone loss is prominent in patients with several disorders (myeloma, leukemia, and lymphoma), affecting the hematopoietic cells, perhaps because of cytokine production and an intimate relationship of hematopoietic cells with bone-forming cells or the use of high-dose or prolonged therapy with glucocorticoids.

A number of drugs can induce osteoporosis.[66] In cancer patients, glucocorticoids, methotrexate, and cytotoxic drugs that cause renal loss of calcium, magnesium, or phosphorus (e.g., platinum compounds, cyclophosphamide, and ifosfamide) have significant impact on bone density. Osteoporosis (generalized or localized) is observed in children receiving methotrexate therapy for acute lymphoblastic leukemia (ALL).[67] The osteoporosis improves significantly after cessation of methotrexate therapy. Longitudinal study of ALL patients showed that the leukemic process, high-dose glucocorticoids, and hypomagnesemia (owing to renal wastage following cyclical glucocorticoid and nephrotoxic chemotherapy or antiinfective agents) contributed to the impairment of calcium and vitamin D metabolism and decrease in bone mass at different stages of the treatment process.[68] Adjuvant chemotherapy for breast cancer (usually involving 5-fluorouracil, cyclophosphamide, and doxorubicin or methotrexate) is associated with low bone mass in premenopausal patients.[69] Bone loss during chemotherapy is substantial and may lead to increased risk of fracture. Posttreatment hypogonadism appears to be a major factor in these adult women with osteoporosis. While tamoxifen has a slight protective effect on bone loss, the opposite is true for aromatase inhibitors. BMT usually involves treatment with high-dose cytotoxic drug, glucocorticoids, and immunosuppressive agents. In 24 patients who underwent BMT with high-dose chemotherapy, profound effects on bone biomarkers were observed.[70]

Prompt investigation of gonadal dysfunction in cancer survivors and prompt replacement of gonadal steroids (in the absence of contraindications) in young hypogonadal men or women are recommended to decrease the risk of future bone fractures. The bone mass of long-term cancer survivors should be assessed when the patient is about 30 years old, the age at which most people have attained peak bone mass.[71] If bone mass is normal, no further evaluation is needed beyond the usual recommendations for prevention of osteoporosis. If it is abnormal (more than 2 standard deviations below normal), the patient should be referred for evaluation of the multiple reversible causes of osteoporosis.

A key point in the management of the osteoporosis syndrome in cancer patients is the use of bone mineral density measurement (e.g., by dual-energy X-ray absorptiometry) to assess fracture risk and to monitor the effects of therapy. This measurement should be performed early in the course of management of the malignancy

so that appropriate preventive measures can be implemented. The oncologist who is prescribing medications that are likely to decrease bone mass should consider active use of bisphosphonates (e.g., alendronate, risedronate, ibandronate, or zoledronate), calcitonin, selective estrogen-receptor modulators (SERMs), or denosumab, in addition to a daily intake of 1200–1500 mg elemental calcium and vitamin D supplementation. Bisphosphonates and denosumab are effective therapies for prevention of bone loss. While osteoporosis in children with leukemia will frequently reverse because the children are in the formative years of bone development, in adults more active measures such as bisphosphonate or teriparatide therapy to prevent bone loss should be considered, rather than waiting for the development of a fracture syndrome.

Another key point is correction of abnormal mineral and vitamin D metabolism by dietary supplements. Nutritional deficiency in teenagers and young adults results in lower bone mass. Treatment of hypocalcemia, hypomagnesemia, and vitamin D deficiency is integral to the successful therapy of osteoporosis in cancer patients. Recent studies document that clinically relevant vitamin D deficiency is present in 50% of the normal population; the percentage is almost certainly higher in patients undergoing cancer therapy.

Osteomalacia

Osteomalacia, a condition characterized by unmineralized bone matrix, is a rare complication of chemotherapy, but should be considered in osteopenic patients and those with osteomalacic clinical syndrome (bone pain and proximal myopathy). The most common cause is a decrease in the serum calcium and/or phosphorus concentrations caused by nutritional deficiency and renal wasting of phosphorus and calcium. Patients who have received chemotherapeutic agents that cause hypophosphatemia, hypomagnesemia, or hypocalcemia are particularly at risk. Investigation of the levels of serum ionized calcium, phosphorus, magnesium, and vitamin D metabolites should be included in the initial evaluation. Appropriate replacement therapy of these vitamins and minerals should be instituted once deficiencies have been identified. Other contributing factors include systemic acidosis and drugs such as anticonvulsants and aluminum.[66] Tumor-induced osteomalacia will be addressed in the section that follows discussing paraneoplastic syndromes.

Ifosfamide causes tubular damage leading to renal phosphate wasting, hypophosphatemia, and rickets/osteomalacia.[72] The toxic effects of ifosfamide on renal tubular function include Fanconi syndrome in adults and children. Tubular damage is seen most commonly when ifosfamide is administered in doses of 50 g/m^2 or more, or when it is used in combination with cisplatin.[73] Rickets is reported most commonly in children. Estramustine, used in the treatment of prostate cancer, has been reported to increase bone resorption and at the same time cause hypocalcemia, hypophosphatemia, and secondary hyperparathyroidism.[74]

Adrenal diseases

Adrenal metastasis

Hematogenous metastasis to the adrenal glands is common, exceeded in frequency only by hematogenous metastasis to the lung, liver, and bone.[75] Autopsies have documented that 9–27% of patients who died from malignant illness had adrenal metastasis, with bilateral involvement in one-half to two-thirds of patients with adrenal metastasis.

The presence of adrenal metastasis may have important implications for diagnostic and therapeutic planning. When patients with cancer have an adrenal mass but no evidence of metastasis elsewhere, it is important to determine whether this mass represents a metastatic tumor or a separate, unrelated adrenal lesion. Recent advances in imaging techniques have allowed the identification of adrenal lesions antemortem as part of the tumor-staging evaluation. The location of the adrenal glands in the perinephric fat allows the detection of almost all normal glands and contour-deforming masses as small as 5–10 mm. Computed tomography (CT) has a sensitivity and specificity in the detection of adrenal masses. Characteristics on CT examination that suggest adrenal metastasis rather than primary adrenal disease include heterogeneity, contrast enhancement, bilaterality, and size >3 cm.[76]

Without other evidence of metastatic disease, whether the adrenal mass is actually a metastatic tumor is critical information in determining the appropriate therapy for the cancer. Evaluation of a patient who has a malignant adrenal mass should include a history and physical examination to elicit evidence of adrenal insufficiency, Cushing syndrome, mineralocorticoid excess, or pheochromocytoma. Biochemical assessment should include a short ACTH stimulation test with measurements of serum cortisol to rule out adrenal insufficiency. A 24-h urine collection should be obtained to measure urinary free cortisol, aldosterone, catecholamines, and metanephrines. Pheochromocytoma must be excluded, especially if there is hypertension, or an operative procedure of any type is contemplated. It has been reported that one-half of the patients who had a clinically unsuspected pheochromocytoma had clinical deterioration or even death immediately following a non-adrenal-related surgical procedure.[77]

If the biochemical assessment for pheochromocytoma is negative, CT-guided fine-needle aspiration should be considered. This procedure has a sensitivity of 85% in detecting cancer.[78] MRI may be helpful in the diagnosis of pheochromocytoma. Functional scintigraphy using ^{131}I-6-iodomethyl-19-*nor*-cholesterol (NP-59) may be used in conjunction with CT and MRI to aid in the diagnosis of a unilateral adrenal mass >2 cm.[79]

Adrenal insufficiency

Despite the relatively high prevalence of adrenal infiltration by many common cancers, clinically evident adrenal hypofunction occurs infrequently, except when both adrenal glands are affected by metastatic disease.[80] It is estimated that more that 80% of adrenal tissue must be destroyed before corticosteroid production, under both basal and stress conditions, is impaired.[81] Because the clinical manifestations of adrenal insufficiency are nonspecific and overlap findings in cancer patients, a high index of suspicion is required to detect this treatable condition. The cachexia and weakness seen in patients with adrenal insufficiency can mimic the general wasting seen in patients with extensive metastatic disease. Electrolyte abnormalities can easily be explained by poor intake, malnutrition, side effects of chemotherapeutic agents, or paraneoplastic syndromes. Adrenal insufficiency may develop gradually and therefore be confused with cancer-associated cachexia.

Approximately 20–30% of the patients with bilateral adrenal metastasis will develop adrenal insufficiency.[80] These patients should all be evaluated by the ACTH stimulation test with serum cortisol measurements and should receive glucocorticoid- and mineralocorticoid-replacement therapy when adrenal insufficiency is suspected and until normal adrenal function is documented. Patients who are stable should receive 20 mg of hydrocortisone in the morning and 10 mg in the early afternoon. In the event of circulatory instability, sepsis, emergency surgery, or other major complications, stress dosages of parenteral glucocorticoid should be given (e.g., hydrocortisone succinate 100 mg intravenously every 8 h).

Other causes of primary adrenal insufficiency in cancer patients include autoimmune adrenalitis, adrenal hemorrhage, and granulomatous diseases. Many cancer patients may be immunocompromised. For example, patients with leukemia or lymphoma or patients who have undergone BMT are immunosuppressed. In these patients, infection of the adrenal glands by cytomegalovirus, mycobacteria, or fungi may lead to adrenal insufficiency.

Adrenal insufficiency may be drug induced. Etomidate,[80] a common intravenous anesthetic, and ketoconazole, an antifungal drug, both inhibit the production of cytochrome P450-dependent enzymes in the glucocorticoid synthetic pathway. Aminoglutethimide and metyrapone are drugs that inhibit enzymes in steroidogenesis, and may cause adrenal insufficiency when used in the treatment of prostate, breast, and adrenocortical cancers. Mitotane, structurally related to the insecticide dichlorodiphenyltrichloroethane (DDT), has selective toxicity for adrenocortical cells. Adrenal insufficiency is commonly observed when mitotane is administered in doses necessary to treat adrenocortical cancer; glucocorticoid replacement therapy is mandatory in such patients.[10] Increased protein binding is observed in mitotane-treated patients, and may lead to an increased daily requirement of glucocorticoids during replacement therapy. Suramin, recently proposed as an anticancer agent based on its activity against the tumor growth factors, may also cause adrenal insufficiency.

Secondary adrenal insufficiency because of metastasis to the pituitary or hypothalamus may also occur. The most common cause of secondary adrenal hypofunction, however, is exogenous glucocorticoid therapy that suppresses hypothalamic–pituitary adrenal function. A prolonged course of therapy may lead to hypothalamic–pituitary suppression lasting for many months. Short periods of steroid therapy (i.e., 1, 2, or 4 weeks) in patients with leukemia and lymphoma suppress adrenal function for 2–4 days in most patients, and for longer in some patients. In patients who have received glucocorticoids for more than 2 weeks, a tapering period of 10–14 days should be considered. This is especially true for chemotherapy regimens that included high-dose glucocorticoids such as those used in the treatment of acute leukemia and lymphoma. In addition, patients who have been treated within the past year with prolonged glucocorticoid courses should receive stress dosages of glucocorticoid if acute medical or surgical complications occur (e.g., neutropenic fever with hypotension and acute typhlitis). Irradiation of the hypothalamic–pituitary region causes ACTH deficiency and secondary adrenal insufficiency in 19–42% of treated patients (Figure 1). Several diagnostic approaches have been used to evaluate secondary adrenal insufficiency, including basal 8 a.m. serum cortisol measurements and dynamic tests with 1 μg of synthetic $ACTH_{(1-24)}$, insulin-induced hypoglycemia, or metyrapone. The effects of immunotherapy on pituitary ACTH production were discussed earlier in this chapter.

Disorders of growth hormone secretion and growth

Childhood cancer or its treatment commonly impairs growth. Medulloblastoma and ALL, common childhood malignancies, are frequently treated with cranial or craniospinal irradiation and/or chemotherapy. Close to 40% of adult survivors of childhood brain cancer are below the tenth population percentile for height, and the risk factors for short stature are young age at diagnosis and radiation treatment affecting the hypothalamic–pituitary axis.[82] GH deficiency and damage to the osseous growth plates are two common mechanisms of growth retardation.

Cranial irradiation may cause hypothalamic or pituitary dysfunction. The hypothalamus appears to be more radiosensitive than does the pituitary gland and may be damaged by lower radiation doses (<40 Gy). Higher doses (>40 Gy) are likely to damage both hypothalamic and pituitary function. Deficiency of one or more pituitary hormones following irradiation of the hypothalamic/pituitary area occurs in almost 100% of patients 5 years after irradiation (Figure 1).

GH deficiency is the most frequently noted and often the first pituitary manifestation to arise after cranial irradiation. Isolated GH deficiency following irradiation is common, and the effects are dose related. At lower doses (20–24 Gy), the only effect may be an altered GH secretory pattern and subnormal response to insulin-induced hypoglycemia. With intermediate and higher doses, the GH response to the stimulatory effect of arginine is impaired, and the frequency and amplitude of pulsatile GH secretion are decreased.[5] At doses up to 30 Gy, abnormal GH secretion and growth retardation are observed in more than 35% of patients, necessitating GH treatment.[83]

In addition to growth retardation caused by GH deficiency, craniospinal or spinal irradiation for hematologic malignancy or central nervous system tumors and total-body irradiation before BMT may cause two other effects. First, irradiation affects the growth plates in vertebral bodies and in the pelvis and decreases vertebral growth. Second, irradiation causes resistance to GH or IGFs.

Children treated with chemotherapy for malignancy frequently have a period of reduced growth velocity, followed by a "catch-up" growth phase. Systemic illness seems to be the most important component of growth retardation in these children, although chemotherapy may play a significant role. Both growth velocity and height are lower in children who are treated with higher doses of chemotherapy and for a longer duration with combination chemotherapy than in those who receive regular therapy or less-intensive chemotherapy. If there is no catch-up growth after 1.5–2 years, it is important to exclude GH deficiency.

In adults, GH deficiency is thought to cause decreased bone and muscle mass, lower exercise capacity, increased adipose tissue, fatigue, a poor sense of well-being, impaired myocardial function, and increased cardiovascular risks. GH replacement may be indicated to improve the patients' quality of life and sense of well being,[84] but the concern over IGF-1-induced reactivation of malignant disease should be factored into the decision.

Disorders of electrolyte/mineral metabolism

Hyponatremia

Risk factors for hyponatremia include treatment-induced nausea and vomiting, certain chemotherapy agents, hydration with hypotonic fluid, pain, opiates, and stress (both physical and psychological). In a prospective study of in-patient cancer patients, the incidence of hyponatremia is 3.7% with sodium depletion and syndrome of inappropriate antidiuretic hormone (SIADH), each accounting for about one-third of all causes.[85] SIADH is characterized by low serum osmolality and inappropriately high urine osmolality in the absence of diuretics, heart failure, cirrhosis, adrenal insufficiency, and hypothyroidism. In cancer patients, SIADH may be caused by vasopressin secreted by tumors [e.g., up to 15% of small-cell lung cancers (SCLCs)], abnormal secretory stimuli (e.g., intrathoracic infection and positive pressure ventilation), or cytotoxicity affecting paraventricular and supraoptic neurons. It is also possible that chemotherapy-induced lysis of vasopressin-containing cancer cells leads to or worsens SIADH. Drug-induced renal salt wasting or tumor-induced salt wasting

(mediated by atrial natriuretic peptide)[86] can also cause hyponatremia, hypoosmolality, elevated urinary sodium, and urinary osmolality. These SIADH-like syndromes are difficult to distinguish from SIADH when signs and symptoms of fluid volume depletion are subtle or absent. Nonetheless, there are convincing reports that provide evidence of chemotherapy-induced hypothalamic or pituitary damage in the context of SIADH. There are at least seven reports associating vincristine with SIADH, and some of these reports document inappropriately high serum levels of vasopressin.[87] Vinblastine has also been reported to cause severe hyponatremia and SIADH.[87] The presumed mechanism of vinca alkaloid-induced SIADH is paraventricular or supraoptic cell microtubular damage.

Cyclophosphamide therapy has been associated with hyponatremia and SIADH. Autopsy findings in a case of fatal hyponatremia induced by cyclophosphamide (1800 mg/m^2) suggest that cyclophosphamide directly affects the hypothalamus.[88] Those findings included infundibular necrosis, decreased intraaxonal secretory granules, and depletion of posterior pituitary vasopressin. Patients treated with lower doses of cyclophosphamide also develop hyponatremia, hypotonicity, urinary hypertonicity, and increased plasma vasopressin levels. Damage to the renal tubules and resulting defects in salt and water transport may be the major cause of hyponatremia associated with low-dose cyclophosphamide therapy.[89]

There are many reports of cisplatin-induced hyponatremia caused by renal salt wasting.[90] Several reports claim that cisplatin induces SIADH. The mechanism of cisplatin-induced hyponatremia is unclear, but it has been suggested that renal toxic effects of cisplatin, that is, decreased papillary solute content and maximal urinary osmolarity are the major factors, rather than a direct effect of cisplatin on vasopressin secretion. In a majority of the patients who have elevated vasopressin levels, the vasopressin levels became suppressed after correction of hypovolemia.[90] Therefore, the stimulus for vasopressin release in these patients was probably hypovolemia caused by renal salt wasting.

Figure 2 outlines the algorithm for evaluation and treatment of hyponatremia. For hypovolemia and sodium loss, fluid and sodium replacement is the primary treatment. The AVP-receptor antagonists directly block the binding of AVP with its receptors. In clinical trials, conivaptan, lixivaptan, tolvaptan, and satavaptan effectively correct hyponatremia associated with SIADH, cirrhosis, or congestive heart failure, and this new class of drugs are likely to be useful for cancer-related hyponatremia.[91]

Hypernatremia

Hypernatremia secondary to central diabetes insipidus occurs frequently as a complication of neurosurgery or destruction by the tumor of the anterior pituitary or the related hypothalamic nuclei. Nephrogenic diabetes insipidus can result from the effects of ifosfamide or streptozocin on tubular reabsorption of water. Ifosfamide has broad nephrotoxic effects, although tubular damage predominates. Distal tubular defects develop in about half of patients treated with ifosfamide. However, frank nephrogenic diabetes insipidus leading to hypernatremia is not common.[92] Streptozocin is another nephrotoxic drug; in addition to causing glomerular defects (proteinuria) and tubular defects (Fanconi syndrome), streptozocin therapy has been reported to cause nephrogenic diabetes insipidus.[93]

Hypocalcemia

Hypocalcemia may be one of the features of tumor lysis syndrome. Hypocalcemia can also be caused by primary hypoparathyroidism

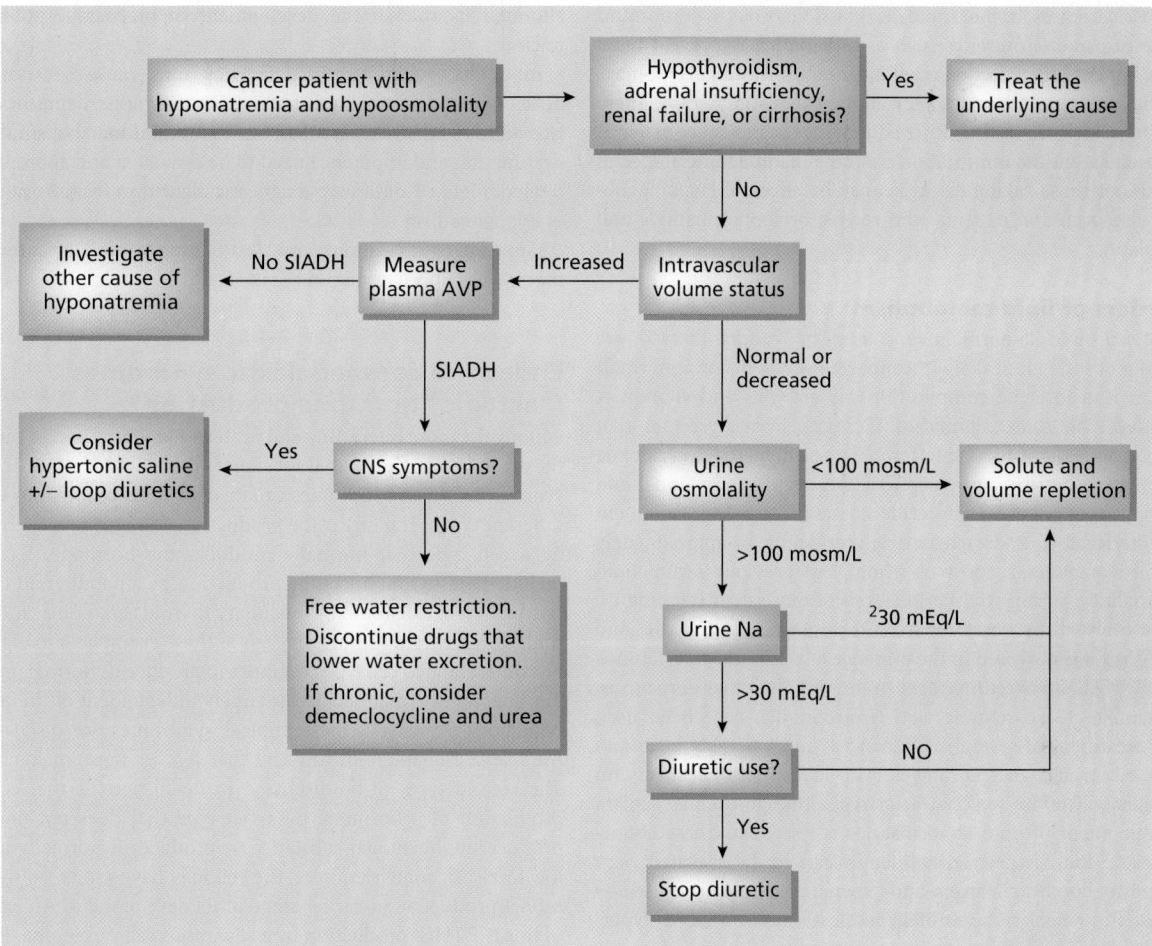

Figure 2 Approach to evaluation of hyponatremia in a cancer patient.

after surgical procedures in the neck that sacrificed or damaged the parathyroid glands (e.g., total laryngectomy and total thyroidectomy). Hypocalcemia is also a common complication of chemotherapy.[87] Hypocalcemia has been reported in 6–20% of cisplatin-treated patients. Effects of cisplatin on renal tubular function, magnesium metabolism, bone resorption, and vitamin D metabolism may explain the hypocalcemia. Profound hypomagnesemia causes a decrease in the secretion of parathyroid hormone and a reduction in the calcium-mobilizing effects of parathyroid hormone. Hypomagnesemia also inhibits formation of 1,25-dihydroxy vitamin D_3 (1,25-dihydroxycholecalciferol). Cisplatin may inhibit the mitochondrial function in the kidneys and thereby inhibits conversion of 25-hydroxycholecalciferol to 1,25-dihydroxy cholecalciferol by the enzyme 1-alpha-hydroxylase. In addition, cisplatin may have a direct inhibitory effect on bone resorption. Carboplatin therapy, similar to cisplatin therapy, is associated with a 16–31% incidence of hypocalcemia. Dactinomycin is another antitumor antibiotic that blocks DNA-directed RNA synthesis, causing hypocalcemia in animals. Dactinomycin also abolishes the calcium-mobilizing effect of thyroid hormone, presumably by interfering with osteoclast-mediated bone resorption. Asymptomatic hypomagnesemia, hypocalcemia, and hypoparathyroidism have also been reported in patients treated with a combination of doxorubicin and cytarabine.

Hypercalcemia

The incidence of hypercalcemia in cancer patients is approximately 1%.[94] Hypercalcemia in cancer patients is a poor prognostic sign associated with a shortened survival. The paraneoplastic syndrome of hypercalcemia of malignancy is discussed under the section titled "Endocrine Paraneoplastic Syndromes ('Ectopic' Hormone Production)." No chemotherapy has been identified as a cause of hypercalcemia. However, there is a clear association between low-dose (usually 2–7.5 Gy) external-beam irradiation of the head and neck area and subsequent development of primary hyperparathyroidism. There is a 2.5- to 3-fold increase in the incidence of primary hyperparathyroidism after low-dose irradiation of the neck.[95] Among patients who developed primary hyperparathyroidism, 14–30% had prior exposure to radiation. The interval from irradiation to development of hyperparathyroidism ranges from 29 to 47 years. Primary hyperparathyroidism also develop in the context of multiple endocrine neoplasia, types 1 and 2. Surgery is the principal treatment for primary hyperparathyroidism. Removal of adenoma is usually curative, but in the context of MEN1, the surgical procedure of choice is 3.5-gland parathyroidectomy.[96]

Hypomagnesemia

Cisplatin causes morphologic changes and necrosis in the proximal tubule, an important site of magnesium reabsorption. Hypomagnesemia occurs in approximately 90% of patients treated with cisplatin,[97] and 10% of the hypomagnesemic patients have symptoms of muscle weakness, tremors, and dizziness. Vigorous hydration and the use of osmotic diuretics such as mannitol may prevent renal failure, but has little effect on renal magnesium wasting. Hypomagnesemia may persist long after cessation of cisplatin therapy. There are no large series in the literature addressing the incidence of hypomagnesemia, but the information from the manufacturer indicates that 60% of those taking cisplatin may be affected. Hypomagnesemia also occurs in patients who receive cyclophosphamide and carboplatin.

Disorders of lipid metabolism

Short-term lipid abnormalities caused by cancer therapy are generally of little clinical significance. However, major abnormalities can lead to acute complications. Interferons and vitamin A derivatives can cause significant increases in triglycerides that can lead to pancreatitis. Interferons cause hypertriglyceridemia by increasing hepatic and peripheral fatty acid production[98] and by suppressing hepatic triglyceride lipase.[99] Long-term treatment with interferon-α_2 causes hypertriglyceridemia in approximately one-third of patients, most of whom had previous serum lipid abnormalities. Serum triglyceride levels of more than 1000 mg/dL are not unusual. In a case report, a therapeutic effect of diet and gemfibrozil was observed in the presence of continued interferon-α therapy.[100] All-*trans*-retinoic acid (tretinoin) and other derivatives, for example, 13-*cis*-retinoic acid (isotretinoin), have been used in the treatment of several malignancies, most notably head and neck cancers and acute promyelocytic leukemia. The effects on lipid metabolism are well characterized, although the mechanism of development of lipid abnormalities is less clear. These abnormalities include hypertriglyceridemia caused by elevated very low-density lipoprotein levels, and hypercholesterolemia caused by increased low-density lipoprotein level. Retinoid-induced hypertriglyceridemia can cause stroke and pancreatitis. Hyperlipidemia associated with retinoid therapy has been treated with gemfibrozil or fish oil.

Sexual dysfunction

Radiation treatment to the head may cause a broad spectrum of hypothalamic–pituitary abnormalities (Figure 1). The resultant thyroid, GH, or adrenal deficiency may indirectly affect reproductive function. Sexual function is directly affected by hyperprolactinemia or gonadotropin deficiency, commonly observed in patients treated with <40 Gy of cranial irradiation.

Hyperprolactinemia occurs commonly (up to 50% incidence within 2 years) following head and neck irradiation with a median hypothalamic–pituitary radiation exposure of 50–57 Gy.[4] Radiation damage to the hypothalamus leading to a loss of the normal inhibition of prolactin secretion is the proposed mechanism of hyperprolactinemia. Hyperprolactinemia inhibits the secretion of gonadotropin by the pituitary and decreases the responsiveness of the pituitary to gonadotropin-releasing hormone (GnRH), thereby causing secondary hypogonadism. Treatment with dopamine agonists (bromocriptine and cabergoline) inhibits prolactin secretion, and it may be reasonable to proceed with a therapeutic trial if other anterior pituitary functions are normal.

Gonadotropin deficiency occurs commonly (up to 61%) in patients treated with irradiation for brain tumors.[101] In children, delayed puberty, absent menarche, and inadequate sexual development are significant problems related to gonadotropin deficiency. Early or even precocious puberty has been reported in patients treated with combined chemotherapy and cranial irradiation for ALL[102] or brain tumor.[103] This phenomenon occurs more frequently in female patients. Concomitant GH deficiency is frequently noted, although its role in the development of precocious puberty is unclear.

In adults, gonadotropin deficiency may cause sex hormone deficiency and sexual dysfunction. Sex hormone deficiency may alter libido and adversely affect bone and lipid metabolism. Sexual dysfunction and impotence need to be evaluated and appropriately treated. Figure 3 outlines a diagnostic algorithm for the evaluation of hypogonadism.

Gonadal complications and dysfunction caused by anticancer therapy have been reviewed.[87]

Endocrine paraneoplastic syndromes ("ectopic" hormone production)

Among the more interesting and protean manifestations of cancer is the production of hormonal substances that produce unique clinical syndromes. These syndromes can be classified broadly into several different types. The first is the production of a hormonal substance by a cell type that normally produces the hormone. Examples include parathyroid hormone production by a parathyroid cancer, production of calcitonin by medullary thyroid carcinoma, and serotonin by carcinoid tumors. In each of these examples a malignancy of a differentiated cell type continues to produce its normal product, but does so in a manner that is largely independent of the normal regulatory processes. These clinical syndromes are discussed in the relevant chapters in this text that discuss these malignancies. The second type, to be discussed in detail here, is the "ectopic" production of a hormone by a cell type that does not normally produce the hormonal substance or produces it normally at very low levels. In some examples, the cell may have produced the hormonal product at an earlier stage in its development. An example of this is PTHrP production by a squamous cell carcinoma. PTHrP is normally expressed in differentiating squamous cells, but is not expressed or is expressed at low levels in differentiated squamous epithelium.[104] Another example of "ectopic" hormone production occurs in a hormone-producing cell whose machinery has been co-opted to produce another hormone. An example of this is the production of ACTH by a wide spectrum of neuroendocrine tumor types, small-cell carcinoma of the lung being one example.

Production of peptides by neuroendocrine tumors comprises the most common of the "ectopic" hormone syndromes. Neuroendocrine cells are dispersed throughout nearly all organs. Prominent are lung, gastrointestinal tract, pancreas, thyroid gland, adrenal medulla, breast, prostate, and skin. The list of hormones produced by tumors derived from members of this group of neuroendocrine cells includes ACTH, calcitonin, vasoactive intestinal peptide (VIP), bombesin, growth hormone-releasing hormone (GHRH), pancreatic polypeptide, corticotropin-releasing hormone (CRH), neurotensin, somatostatin (SRIH), and other small peptides.

Defined clinical syndromes

There are clearly defined clinical ectopic hormone syndromes that occur with some frequency. Their recognition may help in the definition of the cancer type and lead to appropriate management approaches. In addition, these syndromes are a major cause of morbidity and mortality; treatment approaches are available for many of these syndromes and can improve both quality and duration of survival.

Ectopic ACTH production

Inappropriate secretion of ACTH, although uncommon, is an important cause of morbidity and mortality in certain types of

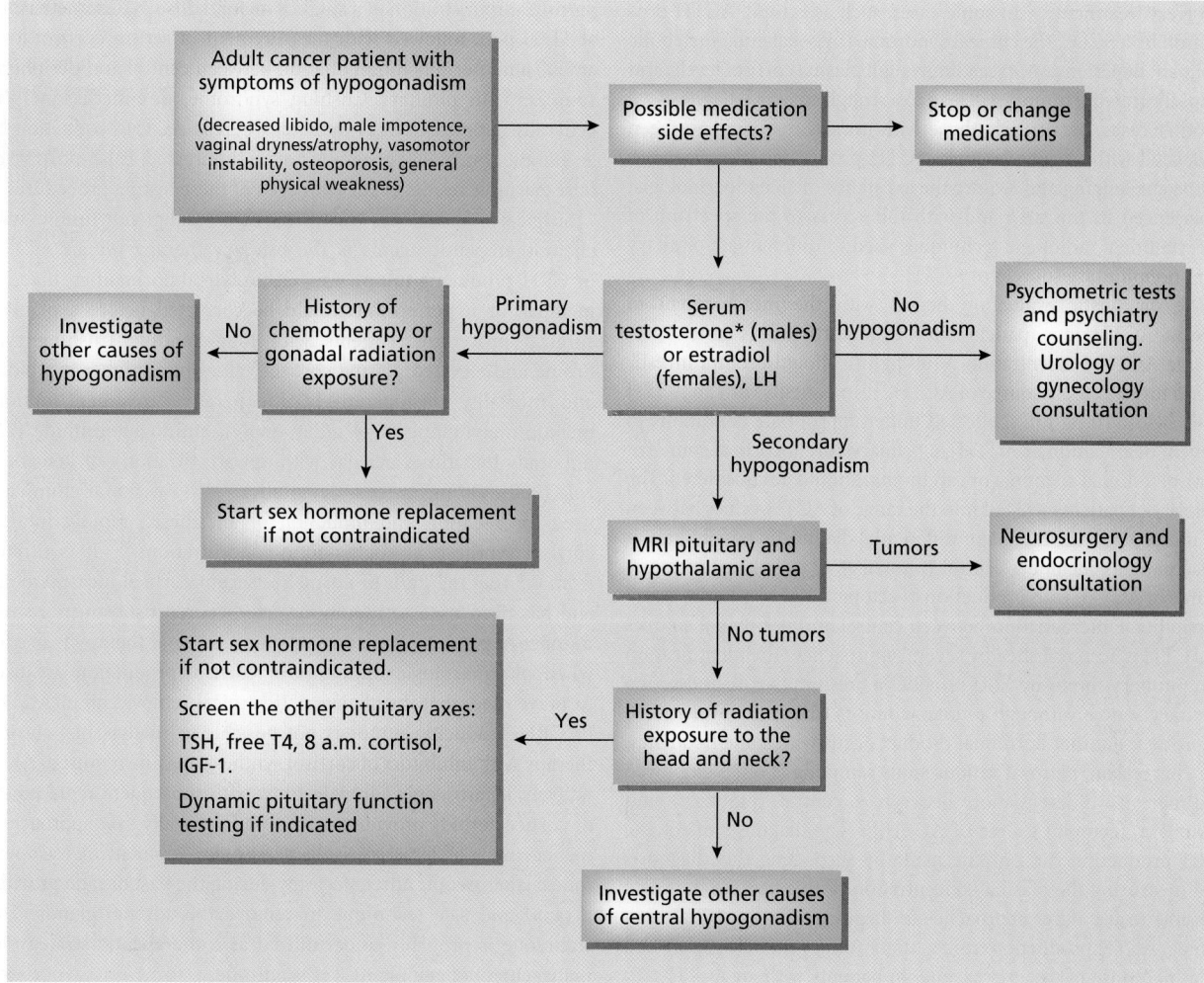

Figure 3 Approach to evaluation of hypogonadism in a cancer patient.

malignancies. There are at least two different mechanisms: ectopic ACTH production or ectopic production of CRH, the hypothalamic peptide that normally stimulates ACTH synthesis and release.

The most common cause of ectopic ACTH production is the expression of proopiomelanocortin (POMC) by a tumor. Post-translational processing of POMC normally proceeds down one of two mutually exclusive pathways.[105] The POMC precursor can be cleaved in two different ways to produce peptides with very different biologic activities. The pathway that leads to ACTH production and Cushing syndrome is one in which POMC is cleaved to produce big melanocyte-stimulating hormone and ACTH. Fortunately for cancer patients, the enzymes that cleave POMC to produce ACTH are expressed uncommonly outside of the normal pituitary gland. Most malignant tumors expressing the POMC gene produce peptides that cause no identifiable clinical syndrome. The most common tumor type that overexpresses POMC and the proteolytic enzymes that cleave it to produce ACTH is SCLC, although a broader spectrum of tumors including pulmonary carcinoid, medullary thyroid carcinoma, islet cell malignancy, pheochromocytoma, and occasional ganglioneuromas will produce this hormone. Cushing syndrome produced by "ectopic" production of ACTH is characterized by adrenal cortical hyperplasia and hypercortisolism.[106]

The second cause of excessive ACTH production is tumor production of CRH.[107] Ectopic production of this peptide causes a

clinical syndrome characterized by pituitary corticotrope hyperplasia leading to adrenal cortical hyperplasia and Cushing syndrome. Identification of excessive CRH production requires that the clinician consider this possibility and measure CRH in blood. Neoplasms that can produce CRH include medullary thyroid carcinoma, paragangliomas, prostate cancer, and islet cell neoplasms. There are examples of cancers that produce both ACTH and CRH.

Patients with ectopic ACTH syndrome may present with clinical features of Cushing syndrome—easy bruising, centripetal obesity, muscle wasting, hypertension, diabetes, and metabolic alkalosis predominate. Alternatively, patients with rapidly growing SCLC may present with a clinical syndrome characterized by cachexia, muscle atrophy, profound hypokalemic metabolic alkalosis, and hypertension without the other clinical findings of Cushing syndrome.

The hallmark of ectopic ACTH syndrome is the finding of an elevated plasma ACTH concentration. However, in the differential diagnosis of hypercortisolism in a cancer patient with an elevated plasma ACTH concentration, one should also consider an ACTH producing pituitary tumor.[108] Differentiation between pituitary ACTH production (a primary pituitary tumor) and ectopic tumor production of ACTH or ectopic CRH production, mimicking a pituitary tumor, is among the most difficult diagnostic workups in the discipline of endocrinology. There are numerous examples where failure to correctly differentiate between ectopic ACTH production and a pituitary tumor producing ACTH has led to incorrect treatment.[109] In some cases, such as ectopic ACTH production by a SCLC, the clinical syndrome (hypokalemia, metabolic alkalosis, hypertension, exceedingly high plasma cortisol levels, and a rapidly growing tumor) will lead to a straightforward diagnosis.[110] In other cases, particularly those with tumors that have not been associated with frequent ectopic ACTH production, the diagnosis can be challenging and require the assistance of an endocrinologist experienced in this area and with full access to the spectrum of interventional radiologic techniques used to differentiate pituitary from nonpituitary sources of ACTH.

The diagnostic evaluation begins with the measurement of plasma ACTH in a patient with hypercorticism (Figure 4). A plasma ACTH concentration >100 pg/mL should prompt investigation for an ectopic source of ACTH.[111] In patients with an ACTH value below 10 pg/mL (collected under appropriate conditions to prevent degradation of ACTH), a primary adrenocortical source of cortisol (adrenal adenoma or carcinoma) should be considered. The majority of patients will fall into the range of ACTH values between 10 and 100 pg/mL. The major differential diagnostic possibilities in these patients include a central (pituitary) or peripheral (ectopic) source of ACTH, with production of ectopic CRH by a tumor a rare possibility. Differentiation between central and peripheral sources of ACTH is accomplished by several approaches. The identification of a pituitary tumor by MRI provides a presumptive diagnosis of a pituitary source, although pituitary tumors that are nonfunctional or produce another hormonal product occur with some frequency. For this reason, petrosal venous sinus sampling is often employed and permits differentiation between a central (pituitary) and peripheral (ectopic) source of ACTH.[112] The diagnosis of ectopic CRH production can only be made by suspecting this diagnosis and measuring the plasma concentration of this peptide. It is also possible to use other approaches to diagnose ectopic ACTH syndrome. ACTH production from a tumor is not generally suppressed by a high dose of dexamethasone. In patients with an ACTH >10

pg/mL, administration of a single 8 mg oral dose of dexamethasone at 11:00 p.m. followed with measurement of serum cortisol level at 8:00 a.m. permits differentiation between central and peripheral sources.[106] In pituitary Cushing syndrome, dexamethasone will generally suppress ACTH by 50%, whereas ACTH production by an ectopic source will generally not be suppressed. False-positive or false-negative results occur with each of these testing procedures.

Surgical removal or treatment of a malignant tumor with chemotherapeutic agents is the primary therapy for an ACTH- or CRH-producing tumor. Any electrolyte abnormalities, diabetes mellitus, or hypertension should be corrected before a planned surgical procedure. Patients with long-standing Cushing syndrome and elevated plasma cortisol values have higher morbidity and mortality postoperatively. Preoperative treatment options include metyrapone (1–4 g/day orally), aminoglutethimide (250 mg orally four times per day with upward titration), or ketoconazole (200–400 mg twice a day orally).[113,114] Parenteral etomidate, used for sedation and induction of anesthesia, rapidly inhibits cortisol synthesis at subhypnotic concentrations.[115] It is titrated from 0.3 to 4 mg/kg/h to normalize serum cortisol measurements and has been used to rapidly reverse hypercortisolism in a small number of patients. Replacement glucocorticoid therapy is needed when pharmacologic inhibitors of cortisol production are used to prevent adrenal insufficiency. If surgical removal of an ACTH- or CRH-producing tumor is not possible or inadvisable, chronic therapy with inhibitors of cortisol synthesis may be required. Alternatively, laparoscopic adrenalectomy with subsequent replacement of corticosteroids provides a rapid and generally safe approach to management of hypercortisolism. The development of retroperitoneal laparoscopic adrenalectomy during the past decade provides a rapid and safe technique to remove the adrenal glands. This technique is probably underutilized as a therapeutic strategy for management of ectopic ACTH syndrome.

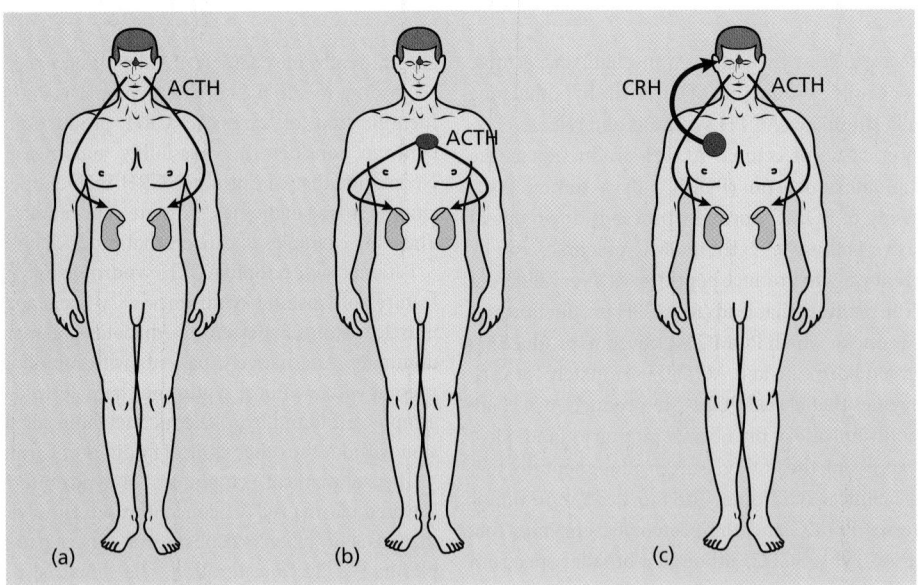

Figure 4 Differential diagnosis of adrenocorticotropin (ACTH)-dependent Cushing syndrome. It is difficult to differentiate between a pituitary (a) and ectopic (b) source of ACTH, the most common causes of ACTH-dependent Cushing syndrome. To differentiate with certainty, placement of catheters in veins draining the pituitary gland (inferior petrosal sinuses) combined with stimulation by exogenous corticotropin-releasing hormone permits differentiation with certainty (discussed in text). Ectopic corticotropin-releasing hormone (CRH) production by a tumor results in increased ACTH production by the pituitary gland (c). It is difficult to differentiate between ectopic CRH production and pituitary-dependent Cushing syndrome, necessitating the measurement of CRH in peripheral blood to make the diagnosis with certainty. Malignant tumors occasionally produce both CRH and ACTH, further complicating the diagnostic evaluation (not shown).

Patients with rapidly progressive SCLC and ectopic ACTH syndrome form a unique subset of patients because of the need to initiate chemotherapy on a timely basis. Unfortunately, these patients are also highly susceptible to opportunistic infections, and initiation of therapy will often lead to death or serious morbidity related to infection.[116] The central dilemma in these patients is that a period of 1–2 weeks may be required for pharmacologic inhibitors of cortisol synthesis to normalize the serum cortisol (and a longer period may be required for normalization of immunity), a delay in the initiation of chemotherapy that is generally deemed unacceptable from an oncologic perspective. Retroperitoneal laparoscopic adrenalectomy, a straightforward and well-tolerated technique following normalization of electrolyte abnormalities and hypertension, may provide a strategy for rapid normalization of excessive cortisol secretion. Prophylactic therapy for opportunistic infections caused by pneumocystis carinii or fungi should be considered if chemotherapy is initiated shortly after normalization of the serum cortisol.

Hypercalcemia caused by malignancy

Hypercalcemia is a common and serious cause of morbidity and mortality in cancer patients.

The most common causes of hypercalcemia in patients with cancer are PTHrP-mediated hypercalcemia, increased production of the active metabolite of vitamin D, calcitriol or 1,25 dihydroxy vitamin D3, and localized osteolytic hypercalcemia.[117,118] Ectopic production of PTH is a rare cause of cancer-associated hypercalcemia. Other common causes of hypercalcemia, most notably primary hyperparathyroidism, should be considered in the cancer patient with hypercalcemia. Measurement of serum intact parathyroid hormone (iPTH) permits differentiation between hyperparathyroidism and a number of other causes of hypercalcemia. The combination of hypercalcemia and an elevated parathyroid hormone level combined with increased urinary calcium excretion provides reasonable evidence for primary hyperparathyroidism. Suppression of the iPTH below the normal range is found in PTHrp or calcitriol-mediated hypercalcemia. Other less-common causes of hypercalcemia in cancer will be discussed below.

Parathyroid hormone-related protein

PTHrP is a small peptide in which 8 of the first 16 amino acids are identical to PTH. This small peptide causes hypercalcemia by binding to the PTH receptor and activating the expression of an osteoblast-specific cell surface protein, RANK ligand (RANKL). Interaction between RANKL and the RANK receptor on the osteoclast precursor causes increased osteoclast differentiation, bone resorption, and hypercalcemia. Other PTH-like actions of PTHrp include hypophosphatemia and increased urinary calcium excretion. PTHrp-mediated hypercalcemia is characterized by a suppressed iPTH level and a low or normal calcitriol level. This contrasts with the finding of elevated iPTH and calcitriol levels in primary hyperparathyroidism. PTHrP production is found commonly in squamous cell carcinomas; other tumors that produce it include: breast, neuroendocrine, renal, melanoma, and prostate tumors.

Calcitriol production by malignant tumors

Lymphoma commonly produces calcitriol, leading to increased gastrointestinal absorption of calcium. Lymphomatous tissue, such as granulomatous tissue seen in sarcoid, berylliosis, silicone-induced granulomatous, tuberculosis, and fungal infection, expresses 1α-hydroxylase, the enzyme that converts 25-hydroxy vitamin D3 to calcitriol. Clinical studies show that a high percentage of lymphoma patients have hypercalciuria at the time of diagnosis; a smaller percentage have frank hypercalcemia.[119] The characteristic clinical features of hypercalcemia in the context of lymphoma include a suppressed serum iPTH, a normal or slightly increased phosphorus level (caused by the suppression of PTH), hypercalciuria, absence of bone metastasis, and an elevated serum calcitriol level in approximately one-half of hypercalcemic patients.[119]

Localized osteolytic bone resorption causing hypercalcemia

Certain malignancies metastasize to bone frequently, and some cause hypercalcemia. Hypercalcemia associated with breast cancer and myeloma is common. In contrast, prostate cancer, despite its more frequent presence in bone, rarely produces hypercalcemia. Malignancies that cause hypercalcemia produce cytokines, PTHrP, or other factors that stimulate increased bone resorption.[117,118] Perhaps, the best characterized is the production of PTHrP by breast carcinoma cells. There is compelling evidence in animal models that PTHrP production by breast cancer cells stimulates osteoclastic resorption and release of transforming growth factor (TGF)-β from normal bone. In this animal model, TGF-β release from bone stimulates proliferation of breast carcinoma growth, setting up a loop in which PTHrP production not only stimulates increased osteoclastic resorption, but also accelerates growth of adjacent breast cancer.[120,121] Indeed, this thought process led to an examination of and subsequent approval of bisphosphonates and denosumab, classes of drugs that inhibit osteoclast bone resorption, for prevention of cancer metastasis.[122,123]

In multiple myeloma, several factors contribute to localized osteolysis. Increased expression of RANKL causing localized osteoclast proliferation appears to be the most important cause. Other factors that may contribute to osteoclast proliferation in myeloma are interleukin-6 and macrophage inflammatory protein 1α.[118]

Impact of malignancy-related hypercalcemia

Severe hypercalcemia in the context of hypercalcemia is associated with a shortened life span. The average survival for patients with severe and unresponsive hypercalcemia can be measured in weeks to months. The causes of death include complications of hypercalcemia (coma and renal failure) and progression of tumor. The development of hypercalcemia is often, although not always, an indicator of tumor progression in the face of adequate therapy. As it is not always possible to predict which patients will respond to oncologic therapy, it is important to treat hypercalcemia in all newly diagnosed patients with cancer. Whether to continue to treat recurrent and/or refractory hypercalcemia is a decision that should be based on response of the causative tumor to oncologic therapy and the overall prognosis of the patient. Severe hypercalcemia frequently causes depression of cerebral function or coma, a clinical situation that may reduce suffering in a dying patient.

Therapy of hypercalcemia

Dehydration is a common finding in hypercalcemic patients. Increased urine excretion of calcium causes a concentrating defect, leading to increased fluid loss. Initial management should focus on the reversal of dehydration by infusion of a solution of normal saline at rates between 100 and 300 mL/h. Hydration will commonly lower the serum calcium by 10–40% over a period of 6–12 h. Patients with severe hypercalcemia, defined as a serum calcium concentration >13 mg/dL (3.25 mmol/L), an alteration of mental status, or evidence of renal dysfunction attributable to hypercalcemia should be treated with either intravenous pamidronate (60–90 mg over 4 h) or zoledronate (4 mg over 30 min),[124] glucocorticoids (40–60 mg/day prednisone equivalent), or gallium nitrate (200 mg/m²/day, infused daily for 7 days).[125,126] Salmon calcitonin may lower the serum calcium concentration by 1–2 mg/dL early in the treatment course, but is rarely effective long term. These drugs are sometimes used in combination or sequentially in a patient who is poorly responsive. Glucocorticoids, which inhibit calcium absorption, are most commonly used as primary therapy for lymphoma, whereas bisphosphonate therapy is more likely to be effective in hypercalcemia associated with solid tumors. Zoledronate is generally more effective than pamidronate because of its increased potency.[127] Use of bisphosphonates for long-term treatment of bone metastasis has been associated with development of osteonecrosis of the jaw in 1–2.5% of treated patients. This has not been an issue in patients treated short term for hypercalcemia associated with malignancy.

A monoclonal antibody directed against RANKL (denosumab) prevents its interaction with the RANK receptor on osteoclast precursors, thereby reducing osteoclast-mediated bone resorption.[128] Denosumab is an effective inhibitor of bone resorption, and recent clinical studies have established its efficacy in patients with hypercalcemia and bone metastasis, particularly those patients who have become unresponsive to bisphosphonate therapy.[128]

Human chorionic gonadotropin

Human chorionic gonadotropin (HCG) is formed from two different protein subunits encoded by separate genes. The first is the α subunit that is shared by all members of the pituitary class of glycoprotein hormones including HCG, LH, follicle-stimulating hormone (FSH), and thyroid-stimulating hormone (TSH). The second, the β subunit, is unique for each of these hormones. Production of HCG is found in trophoblastic tumors (choriocarcinomas, testicular embryonal carcinomas, and seminomas) and, uncommonly, in tumors of the lung and pancreas. In younger children, precocious puberty, caused by HCG stimulation of ovarian function, is seen. In adult males, gynecomastia is a common occurrence. Hyperthyroidism may develop from an interaction of HCG with the thyroid-stimulating hormone receptor (TSHR), particularly when β-HCG is expressed at high levels.

Removal or effective therapy for the underlying tumor is the most effective therapy for clinical syndromes caused by excessive β-HCG production. Hyperthyroidism can be treated short term with thionamide therapy if there is belief that chemotherapy or other strategies to treat the underlying malignancy are likely to be effective. In patients with less-responsive tumors, thyroidectomy or radioactive iodine may be required.

Hypoglycemia

Tumor-induced hypoglycemia is an uncommon but challenging cause of morbidity for cancer patients. Three different clinical syndromes have been identified. First, insulin can be produced by islet cell malignancy. Islet cell tumors commonly produce low levels of insulin that are clinically insignificant until large tumor burdens, most commonly in the form of hepatic metastasis, develop. A second cause is insufficient gluconeogenesis, seen in patients with near complete replacement of hepatic parenchyma by tumor, interfering with or eliminating glucose production. The third form is caused by increased concentrations of insulin-like growth factor II (IGF-II), a peptide that activates the insulin receptor. This syndrome is most commonly seen in patients with fibrosarcomas, hemangiopericytomas, or hepatomas. In these patients IGF-II levels are most commonly elevated, the result of a failure of insulin-like growth factor binding protein 3 (IGFBP3) and acid labile subunit to form a complex capable of binding IGF-II efficiently. The elevated circulating IGF-II activates the insulin receptor and causes hypoglycemia.[129–131]

The most common presentation for each of these clinical syndromes is fasting hypoglycemia, and patients are most likely to develop symptoms during normal periods of fasting, particularly during nocturnal hours. Measurement of a plasma insulin, proinsulin, and C-peptide during a period of hypoglycemia is the most important diagnostic tool for separating the first clinical type (insulin production) from the second (replacement of liver by tumor) and third (IGF-II) types. The findings of elevated insulin, proinsulin, and C-peptide in the face of hypoglycemia (and the absence of any drugs that might stimulate insulin release from normal pancreas) make a compelling case for unregulated insulin production as a cause of the hypoglycemia. In contrast, insulin, proinsulin, and C-peptide levels will be low in tumor replacement of the liver or IGF-II-mediated hypoglycemia. Laboratory findings in IGF-II-mediated hypoglycemia include an elevated serum IGF-II, low or normal insulin, proinsulin, and C-peptide measurements, low IGF-I levels, and generally normal IGFBP3 or acid labile subunit measurements in the context of a large sarcoma or retroperitoneal tumor.

Surgical excision or antineoplastic therapy to reduce tumor mass is effective in insulin or IGF-II-mediated hypoglycemia; there is little effective therapy for hepatic replacement by tumor other than providing glucose. Hypoglycemia is treated with frequent meals. Patients may remain symptom-free by being awakened for caloric intake during nocturnal hours. A continuous infusion of 20% dextrose through a central venous line may be required to maintain normal blood glucose in patients, particularly those with hepatic replacement by tumors. Glucagon infusion (0.5–2 mg/h) to stimulate hepatic gluconeogenesis is also an effective therapy for patients with insulin-producing tumors or those with IGF-II-mediated hypoglycemia. It is important to document a response to glucagon (1 mg subcutaneously with measurement of plasma glucose at 30 and 60 min following injection) before trying this therapeutic approach. Glucagon can be administered in small volumes (1–5 mL over 24 h), making it possible to use small infusion pumps.[132] Patients treated with glucagon may develop the characteristic rash associated with glucagonoma, necessitating discontinuance of this treatment modality. Other therapies that have been applied with periodic success include recombinant GH (3–6 μg/kg subcutaneously daily) or glucocorticoids (20–40 mg prednisone equivalents per day). Octreotide or lanreotide have been used in patients with insulin-producing islet cell tumors, generally without success. The lack of success may relate to the fact that SRIH analogs currently available are more effective for inhibiting glucagon than insulin secretion. Diazoxide (3–8 mg/kg/day in 2–3 divided doses) has been used successfully to inhibit insulin secretion, but causes fluid retention, thereby limiting its usefulness at effective doses.

Hypoglycemia may also occur in patients with lactic acidosis in the context of end-stage leukemia or lymphoma. This clinical syndrome occurs in patients with end-stage or extensive disease and leukemic/lymphomatous involvement of the liver. It is hypothesized that lactic acid production by tumor cells exceeds the ability of the liver to clear it. The etiology of the hypoglycemia is unclear, but may result from impaired hepatic gluconeogenesis.[133]

Syndrome of inappropriate antidiuretic hormone

SIADH was discussed earlier (see the section titled "Disorders of Electrolyte/Mineral Metabolism: Hyponatremia") as a side effect of cancer therapy. In addition, approximately 15% of SCLC, 1% of other lung cancers, and 3% of squamous cell head and neck cancers produce vasopressin in an unregulated manner, leading to hyponatremia, hypoosmolality, increased urine sodium excretion, and an inappropriately high urine osmolality relative to the plasma tonicity.[134] In addition, other benign or malignant neoplasms that include primary brain tumors, hematologic neoplasms, skin tumors, and gastrointestinal, gynecologic, breast, and prostate cancers, and sarcomas can produce this clinical syndrome.

Most patients who develop this syndrome are asymptomatic. In cases where the serum sodium concentration falls <120 mEq/L, altered mental status and seizures may develop. In particular, women of reproductive age who develop hyponatremia may develop profound cerebral degeneration. Fluid restriction can be used effectively for short-term management, but treatment with demeclocycline (150–300 mg/day), an agent that inhibits the effects of vasopressin on the kidney, is preferable for long-term treatment. Vasopressin receptor antagonists, conivaptan, lixivaptan, tolvaptan, and satavaptan, have shown efficacy in clinical trials and at least one, conivaptan, is currently FDA-approved in the United States in an intravenous form (20 mg intravenously over 30 min, followed by 20 mg over 24 h). Tolvaptan (15–60 mg/day) is approved for oral use. Both of these agents are highly effective and it is important to monitor the serum sodium concentration carefully after initiation of therapy.

A consideration in the long-term use of demeclocycline and the V2 receptor antagonists is the cost of therapy. In a patient with a serum sodium concentration <120 mEq/L, use of intravenous conivaptan results in improvement or normalization of the serum sodium over a 24–48 h period and may be most appropriate in this emergent situation; demeclocycline effects are seen over several days. For longer-term therapy, particularly when it is not possible to reduce tumor mass, consideration should be given to the less-expensive demeclocycline, which is generally well tolerated and effective.

Other ectopic hormone syndromes

Tumor-induced osteomalacia

Severe hypophosphatemia caused by renal phosphate wasting is the hallmark of tumor-induced osteomalacia. This clinical syndrome is characterized by osteomalacia, caused by inadequate mineralization of osteoid, and moderate to severe proximal myopathy.[135] Tumors that produce this clinical syndrome include mesenchymal tumors (osteoblastomas, giant cell osteosarcomas, hemangiopericytomas, hemangiomas, and nonossifying fibromas)[136] and, rarely, malignant tumors such as prostate or lung cancer. There is compelling evidence that fibroblast growth factor-23, a member of the fibroblast growth factor family that is mutated in autosomal dominant osteomalacia,[137] is overexpressed by some neoplasms causing tumor-induced osteomalacia.[138] Oral or intravenous supplementation of phosphate combined with vitamin D therapy is generally effective for eradicating or improving clinical symptoms. Complete surgical removal of the tumor is generally curative.

Erythropoietin, thrombopoietin, leukopoietin, or colony-stimulating factor production

Polycythemia caused by ectopic erythropoietin production is a rare clinical syndrome. It is found in cerebellar hemangioblastoma, uterine fibroids, pheochromocytomas, and renal cell, ovarian, and hepatic cancers.[139,140] Treatment can include surgical or chemotherapy reduction of tumor mass or phlebotomy. Other less well-defined syndromes include production of thrombopoietin, leukopoietin, or colony-stimulating factor by some tumors. These conditions are treated by appropriate chemotherapy to reduce its size or by surgical removal.

Renin production

Production of renin by renal (Wilms tumor, renal cell carcinoma, or hemangiopericytoma), lung (SCLC and adenocarcinoma), hepatic, pancreatic, or ovarian carcinomas can produce a clinical syndrome characterized by hypertension, hypokalemia, and evidence of increased aldosterone production.[141] Therapy with spironolactone, angiotensin-converting enzyme inhibitors, or angiotensin receptor antagonists may lower the blood pressure and normalize electrolyte abnormalities in patients in whom the tumor cannot be resected.

Growth hormone and prolactin

Acromegaly is a condition characterized by elevated GH and IGF-1 values, most commonly caused by a pituitary tumor. There are uncommon examples of GH production by lung and gastric adenocarcinomas. Ectopic production of GHRH, the hypothalamic peptide that normally regulates GH production by the pituitary,[142] has been demonstrated for islet cell tumors, bronchogenic carcinoids, and SCLC. It is unlikely that treatment with SRIH analogs, one of the mainstay therapies for pituitary tumors producing GH, will be effective. However, the GH antagonist, pegvisomant, is likely to be effective for treatment of GH excess. Ectopic prolactin production is found rarely in gonadoblastoma,[143] lymphoma,[141] leukemia,[144] and colorectal cancer.[145] The clinical syndrome includes galactorrhea and amenorrhea in women and hypogonadism and gynecomastia in men. Dopamine agonists (bromocriptine, quinagolide, or cabergoline), effective for treatment of pituitary prolactinomas, are generally ineffective for treatment of ectopic prolactin production.

Key references

The complete reference list can be found on the Wiley Companion Digital Edition of this title (see inside front cover for login instructions).

1 Fassett DR, Couldwell WT. Metastases to the pituitary gland. *Neurosurg Focus.* 2004;**16**:E8.

2 Lam KS, Tse VK, Wang C, Yeung RT, Ho JH. Effects of cranial irradiation on hypothalamic-pituitary function—a 5-year longitudinal study in patients with nasopharyngeal carcinoma. *Q J Med.* 1991;**78**:165–176.

3 Pai HH, Thornton A, Katznelson L, et al. Hypothalamic/pituitary function following high-dose conformal radiotherapy to the base of skull: demonstration of a dose-effect relationship using dose-volume histogram analysis. *Int J Radiat Oncol Biol Phys.* 2001;**49**:1079–1092.

4 Samaan NA, Schultz PN, Yang KP, et al. Endocrine complications after radiotherapy for tumors of the head and neck. *J Lab Clin Med.* 1987;**109**:364–372.

5 Shalet SM. Disorders of the endocrine system due to radiation and cytotoxic chemotherapy. *Clin Endocrinol (Oxf).* 1983;**19**:637–659.

11 Chopra IJ. Clinical review 86: euthyroid sick syndrome: is it a misnomer? *J Clin Endocrinol Metabol.* 1997;**82**:329–334.

13 Grande C. Hypothyroidism following radiotherapy for head and neck cancer: multivariate analysis of risk factors. *Radiother Oncol.* 1992;**25**:31–36.

16 Constine LS, Donaldson SS, McDougall IR, et al. Thyroid dysfunction after radiotherapy in children with Hodgkin's disease. *Cancer.* 1984;**53**:878–883.

30 Vecil GG, Papadopoulos NV, Vassilopoulou-Sellin R, McCutcheon IE. Interferon-induced hypothyroidism causing reversible pituitary enlargement. *Endocr Pract.* 2008;**14**:219–223.

31 Sherman SI. Etiology, diagnosis, and treatment recommendations for central hypothyroidism associated with bexarotene therapy for cutaneous T-cell lymphoma. *Clin Lymphoma.* 2003;**3**:249–252.

32 Golden WM, Weber KB, Hernandez TL, et al. Single-dose rexinoid rapidly and specifically suppresses serum thyrotropin in normal subjects. *J Clin Endocrinol Metab.* 2007;**92**:124–130.

34 Illouz F, Braun D, Briet C, Schweizer U, Rodien P. Endocrine side-effects of anti-cancer drugs: thyroid effects of tyrosine kinase inhibitors. *Eur J Endocrinol.* 2014;**171**:R91–R99.

35 Wells SA Jr, Gosnell JE, Gagel RF, et al. Vandetanib for the treatment of patients with locally advanced or metastatic hereditary medullary thyroid cancer. *J Clin Oncol.* 2010;**28**:767–772.

36 Schlumberger M, Tahara M, Wirth LJ, et al. Lenvatinib versus placebo in radioiodine-refractory thyroid cancer. *N Engl J Med.* 2015;**372**:621–630.

37 Quach A, Ji L, Mishra V, et al. Thyroid and hepatic function after high-dose 131 I-metaiodobenzylguanidine (131 I-MIBG) therapy for neuroblastoma. *Pediatr Blood Cancer.* 2011;**56**:191–201.

40 Haraldsdottir S, Li Q, Villalona-Calero MA, et al. Case of sorafenib-induced thyroid storm. *J Clin Oncol.* 2013;**31**:e262–e264.

43 Makari-Judson G, Judson CH, Mertens WC. Longitudinal patterns of weight gain after breast cancer diagnosis: observations beyond the first year. *Breast J.* 2007;**13**:258–265.

46 Kroenke CH, Chen WY, Rosner B, Holmes MD. Weight, weight gain, and survival after breast cancer diagnosis. *J Clin Oncol.* 2005;**23**:1370–1378.

48 Nilsen TI, Vatten LJ. Prospective study of colorectal cancer risk and physical activity, diabetes, blood glucose and BMI: exploring the hyperinsulinaemia hypothesis. *Br J Cancer.* 2001;**84**:417–422.

59 Everhart J, Wright D. Diabetes mellitus as a risk factor for pancreatic cancer. A meta-analysis. *JAMA.* 1995;**273**:1605–1609.

75 Abrams H, Spiro R, Goldstein N. Metastasis in carcinoma—one thousand autopsied cases. *Cancer.* 1950;**3**:74.

82 Gurney JG, Ness KK, Stovall M, et al. Final height and body mass index among adult survivors of childhood brain cancer: childhood cancer survivor study. *J Clin Endocrinol Metab.* 2003;**88**:4731–4739.

87 Yeung SC, Chiu AC, Vassilopoulou-Sellin R, Gagel RF. The endocrine effects of nonhormonal antineoplastic therapy. *Endocr Rev.* 1998;**19**:144–172.

95 Cohen J, Gierlowski TC, Schneider AB. A prospective study of hyperparathyroidism in individuals exposed to radiation in childhood. *JAMA.* 1990;**264**:581–584.

97 Stewart AF, Keating T, Schwartz PE. Magnesium homeostasis following chemotherapy with cisplatin: a prospective study. *Am J Obstet Gynecol.* 1985;**153**:660–665.

101 Constine LS, Woolf PD, Cann D, et al. Hypothalamic-pituitary dysfunction after radiation for brain tumors. *N Engl J Med.* 1993;**328**:87–94.

104 Maioli E, Fortino V. The complexity of parathyroid hormone-related protein signalling. *Cell Mol Life Sci.* 2004;**61**:257–262.

108 Newell-Price J. Cushing's syndrome. *Clin Med.* 2008;**8**:204–208.

114 Nieman LK, Ilias I. Evaluation and treatment of Cushing's syndrome. *Am J Med.* 2005;**118**:1340–1346.

116 Dimopoulos MA, Fernandez JF, Samaan NA, Holoye PY, Vassilopoulou-Sellin R. Paraneoplastic Cushing's syndrome as an adverse prognostic factor in patients who die early with small cell lung cancer. *Cancer.* 1992;**69**:66–71.

117 Stewart AF. Clinical practice. Hypercalcemia associated with cancer. *N Engl J Med.* 2005;**352**:373–379.

118 Roodman GD. Mechanisms of bone metastasis. *N Engl J Med.* 2004;**350**:1655–1664.

119 Seymour JF, Gagel RF, Hagemeister FB, Dimopoulos MA, Cabanillas F. Calcitriol production in hypercalcemic and normocalcemic patients with non-Hodgkin lymphoma. *Ann Intern Med.* 1994;**121**:633–640.

120 Guise TA, Yin JJ, Thomas RJ, et al. Parathyroid hormone-related protein (PTHrP)-(1-139) isoform is efficiently secreted in vitro and enhances breast cancer metastasis to bone in vivo. *Bone.* 2002;**30**:670–676.

122 Wang Z, Qiao D, Lu Y, et al. Systematic literature review and network meta-analysis comparing bone-targeted agents for the prevention of skeletal-related events in cancer patients with bone metastasis. *Oncologist.* 2015;**20**:440–449.

128 Hu MI, Glezerman IG, Leboulleux S, et al. Denosumab for treatment of hypercalcemia of malignancy. *J Clin Endocrinol Metab.* 2014;**99**:3144–3152.

129 Baxter RC, Holman SR, Corbould A, et al. Regulation of the insulin-like growth factors and their binding proteins by glucocorticoid and growth hormone in non-islet cell tumor hypoglycemia. *J Clin Endocrinol Metab.* 1995;**80**:2700–2708.

134 Flombaum CD. Metabolic emergencies in the cancer patient. *Semin Oncol.* 2000;**27**:322–334.

138 Jonsson KB, Zahradnik R, Larsson T, et al. Fibroblast growth factor 23 in oncogenic osteomalacia and X-linked hypophosphatemia. *N Engl J Med.* 2003;**348**:1656–1663.

139 Infections in patients with cancer

Lior Nesher, MD ■ *Kenneth V. I. Rolston, MD, FACP*

Overview

Patients with cancer have an increased risk of developing infections, owing both to their underlying disease and its treatment. This risk appears to be greatest in patients with hematologic malignancies and in hematopoietic cell transplant recipients. This is due primarily to the development of various immunologic defects such as neutropenia and impaired cellular and/or humoral immunity, each associated with a unique spectrum of infection. Newer therapeutic modalities for the treatment of some cancers are changing the spectrum of infections as are the increasing use of catheters and other medical devices. While bacterial infections are documented most often, opportunistic fungal and viral infections are being encountered with increasing frequency. The morbidity and mortality of infections in cancer patients is generally greater than in the general population. Thus, early diagnosis and the prompt administration of appropriate therapy are of paramount importance. Antimicrobial resistance among these pathogens has become a worldwide problem, which can only be partially tackled by the development of novel agents. Consequently, the importance of conducting frequent epidemiologic surveillance in order to detect local epidemiologic shifts and of infection prevention, infection control, and antimicrobial stewardship cannot be emphasized enough. The number of cancer survivors is steadily increasing. Many of these patients remain immunosuppressed for substantial periods of time. Keeping these survivors healthy and infection free will continue to be a challenge for years to come.

Infection remains a common problem in patients with cancer. The frequency and nature of infection depend on the type of underlying neoplastic disease.[1] Multiple episodes of infection are not uncommon. Neutropenia, impaired cellular or humoral immunity, the use of catheters and other medical devices, splenectomy, surgery, radiation, nutritional status, and local factors such as obstruction increase the susceptibility of these patients to infection. Each risk factor is associated with a unique set of infections, although there is some overlap. Multiple factors often exist in the same patient. Table 1 lists defects in host defense mechanisms and the infections associated with those defects.

Infections primarily associated with neutropenia

Types of febrile episodes

A specific causative pathogen is identified in about 20–25% of febrile episodes in neutropenic patients (microbiologically documented infections). An additional 20–25% of episodes have identifiable sites of infection (e.g., pneumonia, cellulitis, and enterocolitis) but have negative cultures (clinically documented infections). Approximately 40–45% have neither an obvious clinical focus of infection nor positive cultures, and are referred to as episodes of unexplained fever (Figure 1). The majority of these are presumed to be due to an occult infection and respond to antibiotic therapy. Fewer than 5% of febrile episodes are due to non-infectious causes such as transfusion reactions, tumor fever, or drug fever.[2,3]

Sites of infection

The most common sites of infection encountered in neutropenic patients are the respiratory tract followed by the bloodstream (including central line-associated bloodstream infection-CLABSI), the urinary tract, skin and skin structure infections (SSSIs), and infections originating from the oro-pharynx and the gastrointestinal tract (Figure 2). Less frequent but clinically important sites include the central nervous system, bones, joints, and end organs such as the liver and spleen. Most microbiologically documented infections are caused by the patient's own microflora with a minority being acquired from exogenous sources/environmental exposure.

Infections primarily associated with impaired cellular and humoral immunity

Defects in cell-mediated immunity are common in patients with hematologic malignancies including malignant lymplomas, in allogeneic hematopoietic cell transplant (HCT) recipients, in recipients of high-dose corticosteroid therapy, and in patients treated with newer modalities (nucleoside analogs, monoclonal antibodies, and temozolomide) and result in an increase in infections caused by bacterial pathogens such as *Legionella* spp., *Salmonella* spp., *Nocardia* spp., *Listeria monocytogenes*, and *Rhodococcus equi*.[4-6] Mycobacterial infections (*Mycobacterium tuberculosis* and non-tuberculous mycobacteria) are also relatively common in such patients. *Aspergillus* spp., *Pneumocystis jiroveci*, and the endemic fungi (*Cryptococcus neoformans*, *Histoplasma capsulatum*, and *Coccidioides immitis*) cause most of the fungal infections in this setting.[7,8] Viral infections are predominantly caused by the herpes group of viruses with cytomegalovirus (CMV) being the most frequent. The community respiratory viruses are important causes of morbidity and mortality in allogeneic HCT recipients. Parasitic infections such as toxoplasmosis, strongyloidosis, and babesosis are also seen more frequently in patients with impaired cellular or humoral immunity.[9-11] In patients with impaired humoral immunity, infections caused by encapsulated organisms such as *Streptococcus pneumoniae* and *Haemophilus influenzae* are common.

Infections in patients with solid tumors

Patients with solid tumors who are not significantly immunosuppressed also develop infections frequently. Risk factors include

Holland-Frei Cancer Medicine, Ninth Edition. Edited by Robert C. Bast Jr., Carlo M. Croce, William N. Hait, Waun Ki Hong, Donald W. Kufe, Martine Piccart-Gebhart, Raphael E. Pollock, Ralph R. Weichselbaum, Hongyang Wang, and James F. Holland.
© 2017 John Wiley & Sons, Inc. ISBN: 978-1-118-93469-2

Table 1 Defects in host defense mechanisms and common infections associated with malignant diseases.

Disease	Prominent defect	Predominant infections
Acute leukemia, aplastic anemia	Prolonged neutropenia	Gram-positive cocci, Gram-negative bacilli, fungi (*Candida, Aspergillus, Zygomycetes, Fusarium, Trichosporon*)
Hairy cell leukemia	Neutropenia, impaired lymphocyte function	Gram-negative bacilli, Gram-positive cocci, mycobacteria (including nontuberculous)
Chronic lymphocytic leukemia, multiple myeloma	hypogammaglobulinemia (impaired humoral immunity)	Encapsulated organisms, *Streptococcus pneumoniae, Haemophilus influenzae, Neisseria meningitides*
Hodgkin disease	Impaired T-lymphocyte response	*Pneumocystis jiroveci, Cryptococcus* spp., mycobacteria, *Toxoplasma, Listeria monocytogenes, Cryptosporidium, Candida,* CMV
Hematopoietic stem cell transplant recipients	Neutropenia, impaired cellular and humoral immunity	Gram-positive cocci, Gram-negative bacilli, cytomegalovirus, *Candida, Aspergillus,* herpes viruses (HSV, VZV, CMV)
Breast cancer	Tissue necrosis, radiation damage, foreign bodies	Gram-positive cocci, Gram-negative bacilli, anaerobes (polymicrobial infections common)
Lung cancer	Local obstruction, tissue necrosis	Gram-positive cocci, Gram-negative bacilli, anaerobes (polymicrobial infections common)
Gynecologic malignancy	Local obstruction, tissue necrosis	Mixed aerobic and anaerobic enteric flora including *Enterococcus* spp. (polymicrobial infections common)

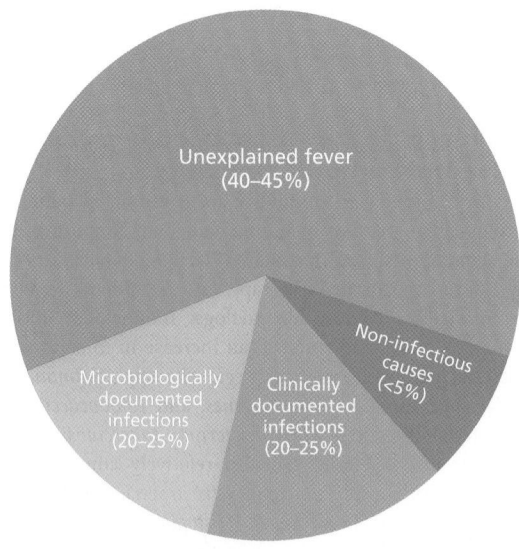

Figure 1 Types of febrile episodes in patients with neutropenia.

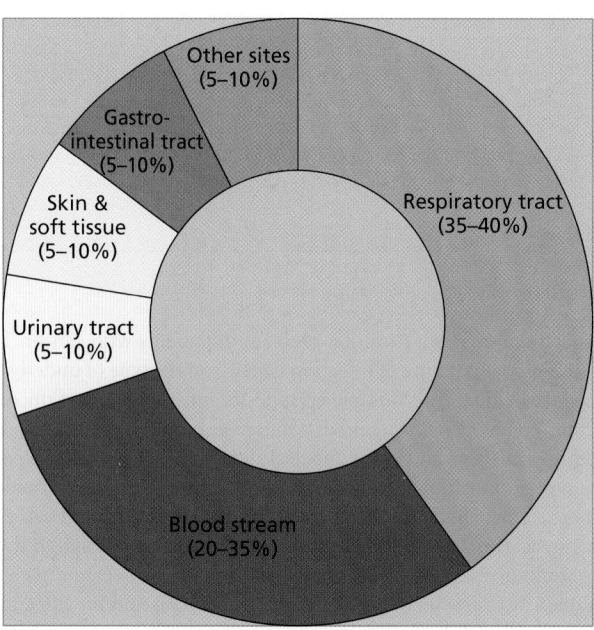

Figure 2 Common sites of infection in patients with neutropenia.

neutropenia that is generally short lived, disruption of normal anatomic barriers (skin and mucosal surfaces), obstruction caused by bulky or rapidly expanding tumors, radiation damage, surgical procedures, and the presence of various medical devices. The common sites of infection seen in patients with various solid tumors are summarized in Table 2. The site of infection depends on the location and size of the tumor or the site and nature of the medical device, radiation, or surgical procedure. Surgical site infections and catheter-related infections are caused most often by organisms colonizing the skin, although opportunistic pathogens such as *Pseudomonas aeruginosa* and other Gram-negative bacilli are beginning to emerge in this setting.[12] Removal of the offending device and complete or partial relief of obstruction are important aspects of the management of infections in patients with solid tumors. If this is not feasible, prolonged suppressive therapy might be necessary.

Spectrum of infection

Bacterial infections

Currently, Gram-positive organisms cause ~50% of bacterial infections in neutropenic patients (Table 3). Gram-negative bacilli account for ~18%, and a substantial proportion, especially deep tissue infections, is polymicrobial.[13–16] Bacteria commonly isolated from neutropenic patients are depicted in Table 4. Geographic and institutional variations do exist.[17] Consequently, clinicians should consider local epidemiology and resistance patterns when initiating empiric antibiotic therapy.

Table 2 Common infections in patients with solid tumors.

Tumor location	Infection site or type
Breast	Wound infection; cellulitis or lymphangitis related to axillary node dissection; mastitis; breast abscess; bacteremia
Central nervous system (brain, meninges)	Wound infection; epidural/subdural infection; brain abscess; meningitis/ventriculitis; proximal and distal end-shunt-related infections; aspiration pneumonia; urinary tract infection; bacteremia
Genitourinary and prostate	Cystitis; urethritis; acute/chronic pyelonephritis ± bacteremia; catheter-related complicated urinary tract infection (nephrostomy/stents); wound infection; acute/chronic prostatitis; epididymitis; orchitis; pelvic abscess
Hepatobiliary-pancreatic	Wound infection; peritonitis; ascending cholangitis ± bacteremia; hepatic, pancreatic, or subdiaphragmatic abscess
Head and neck	Cellulitis; wound infection; deep facial space infection; mastoiditis/osteomyelitis; sinusitis; aspiration pneumonia; bacteremia; suppurative intracranial phlebitis; meningitis; brain abscess; retropharyngeal and paravertebral abscesses
Musculoskeletal (muscles, bones, joints)	Wound infections; pyomyositis; lymphangitis; bursitis; synovitis; septic arthritis; osteomyelitis; wound infection; prosthesis-related infections; bacteremia
Upper gastrointestinal	Esophagitis; tracheoesophageal fistula with pneumonitis/lung abscess; gastric perforation and abscess; feeding tube-related infections; mediastinitis/osteomyelitis
Lower gastrointestinal	Wound infection; intra-abdominal or pelvic abscess; peritonitis (perforation); enterocolitis; urinary tract infection; perianal/perirectal infection; sacral/coccygeal osteomyelitis

Table 3 Bacterial infection in 2223 febrile episodes in neutropenic patients.

Infection type[a]	2002–2003		2012–2013	
	No.	%	No.	%
Microbiologically documented	262	26	321	26
Gram-positive	134	51	163	51
Gram-negative	51	20	55	17
Polymicrobial	71	27	92	29
Anaerobic	6	2	11	3
Clinically documented	210	21	298	24
Unexplained fever	521	53	611	50

[a]These data are derived from surveys conducted at the University of Texas MD Anderson Cancer Center, Houston, Texas, USA.

Table 4 Common infectious agents in patients with cancer.

Neutropenia
  Bacteria
    Gram-positive organisms
      Coagulase-negative staphylococci
      Staphylococcus aureus (including MRSA)
      Enterococcus spp. (including VRE)
      Viridans group streptococci
    Gram-negative organisms
      Escherichia coli
      Klebsiella pneumoniae
      Pseudomonas aeruginosa
      Other *Enterobacteriaceae*
      Stenotrophomonas maltophilia
  Fungi
    Candida spp.
    Aspergillus spp.
    Zygomycetes
    Fusarium spp.
Cellular immune dysfunction
  Bacteria
    Listeria monocytogenes
    Rhodococcus equi
    Salmonella spp.
    Mycobacteria
    Nocardia spp.
    Legionella spp.
  Fungi
    Aspergillus spp.
    Cryptococcus spp.
    Histoplasma capsulatum
    Coccidioides immitis
    Pneumocystis jiroveci
  Protozoa
    Toxoplasma gondii
  Helminth
    Strongyloides stercoralis
  Viruses
    Cytomegalovirus
    Herpes simplex virus I and II
    Varicella-zoster virus
    Epstein–Barr virus
Humoral immune dysfunction
  Streptococcus pneumoniae
  Haemophilus influenzae

Gram-positive bacteria

Coagulase-negative staphylococci (CoNS) are isolated most often and predominantly cause CLABSI.[18] *Staphylococcus lugdunensis* is a more virulent species and needs more aggressive management.[19,20] *Staphylococcus aureus* is often associated with deep-seated infections (deep abscesses and endocarditis), and all patients with *S. aureus* bacteremia should be evaluated for such foci.[21] Other sites of infection include SSSIs, pneumonia, bone and joint infections, and septic thrombophlebitis. Of concern is the increasing rate of methicillin resistance among *S. aureus* isolates, which is now >50% at many centers.[22] Many of these isolates have developed tolerance or reduced susceptibility to vancomycin (referred to as the MIC creep), thereby reducing the efficacy of this agent.[23–27] Alternative therapeutic agents include daptomycin, telavancin, dalbavancin, oritavancin, linezolid, tedizolid, and ceftaroline.[28–30]

Viridans group streptococci (VGS) are encountered often in patients with acute leukemia undergoing intensive chemotherapy and in allogeneic HCT recipients.[31,32] Risk factors include chemotherapy with agents that induce severe oral mucositis, prophylaxis with fluoroquinolones that can promote the selection of these organisms, and treatment of chemotherapy-induced gastritis with antacids or histamine type 2 (H2) antagonists.[33,34] *Streptococcus mitis* is the predominant species. Bacteremia is the most common manifestation. Some patients develop a rapidly progressive disseminated infection involving the bloodstream, lungs, central nervous system, and skin (Figure 3). This is associated with 25–35% mortality despite aggressive therapy.[35] Of concern are reports that 20–60% of VGS are penicillin resistant at some institutions.[31,36] Beta-hemolytic streptococci also cause infections in neutropenic patients, but less often than VGS.[37]

The enterococci colonize the lower intestinal tract.[38,39] Common sites of infection are the bloodstream, urinary tract, and intra-abdominal infections. *Enterococcus faecalis* is the predominant species accounting for 60–70% of isolates. Most *E. faecalis* strains are susceptible to penicillin, ampicillin, and vancomycin although these agents may lack bactericidal activity. Consequently, combinations of these agents with aminoglycosides are recommended for

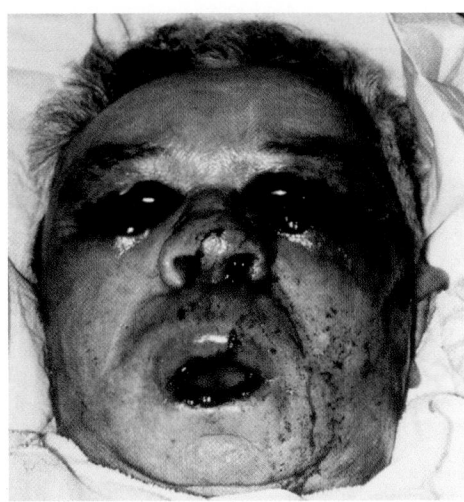

Figure 3 Invasive infection caused by α-hemolytic (viridans) streptococci. Note the hemorrhagic nature of the lesions in this patient with thrombocytopenia.

serious enterococcal infections. *Enterococcus faecium* isolates often express high-level resistance to the aminoglycosides, ampicillin, and vancomycin-resistant enterococcus (VRE). Risk factors for infection with VRE include intestinal colonization and the use of antimicrobial agents with significant activity against anaerobes (metronidazole, clindamycin, and imipenem).[40] The administration of vancomycin (both oral and parenteral) is also a risk factor. Established therapeutic options for VRE include linezolid, daptomycin, oritavancin, and quinupristin/dalforpristin.[41–43] Combination therapy may be necessary. Less common but important Gram-positive pathogens include *Bacillus* spp., *Corynebacterium* spp., *Micrococcus* spp., and *Stomatococcus mucilaginosus*.[44,45] Nocardiosis is caused by several *Nocardia* spp. (*Nocardia asteroides* complex, *Nocardia brasiliensis*, and *Nocardia otitidiscaviarum*). The most common sites of infection are the lungs (70%) and soft tissue sites (16%).[46] Establishing a specific microbiologic diagnosis is of paramount importance as the differential diagnosis is wide. Trimethoprim/sulfamethoxazole remains the backbone of therapy although it is often combined with the carbapenems, tetracyclines, or aminoglycosides. *L. monocytogenes* is primarily acquired by the consumption of raw milk or products (cheese) made from raw milk. Bacteremia (75%) and meningoencephalitis (20%) are the most common manifestations.[47]

Immunoglobulins play an important role in the immune systems response to various infections by either opsonization or complement activation. Impaired humoral immunity leads to increased susceptibility to infections caused by *S. pneumoniae* and other encapsulated organisms.[37] The widespread use of the conjugate pneumococcal vaccine has led to a reduction in the frequency of pneumococcal disease especially in pediatric populations.

Gram-negative bacteria

The intestinal tract serves as an important source of infection in neutropenic patients with the predominant pathogens being enteric Gram-negative bacilli. *Escherichia coli*, *Klebsiella* spp., and *P. aeruginosa* remain the three primary pathogens.[13,48] Other Enterobacteriaceae (*Citrobacter* spp., *Enterobacter* spp., *Proteus* spp., and *Serratia* spp.) are less common. Despite a decline in the frequency of Gram-negative infections due to antibacterial prophylaxis, the proportion caused by non-fermentative Gram-negative

bacilli (NFGNB) such as *P. aeruginosa*, *Stenotrophomonas maltophilia*, and *Acinetobacter* spp. has increased.[49] *P. aeruginosa* is the most frequently isolated and the most virulent NFGNB and causes between 15% and 20% of Gram-negative infections. It is also the most common Gram-negative organism isolated from polymicrobial infections.[16] Infections caused by *S. maltophilia* are being documented more often in patients with hematologic malignancies and in HCT recipients.[50,51] The switch from trimethoprim/sulfamethoxazole (TMP/SMX), which is active against *S. maltophilia*, to the fluoroquinolones, which generally are not, as preferred agents for prophylaxis, may account for this increase. Other infrequent but important NFGNB include *Achromobacter* spp., *Alcaligenes* spp., and non-aeruginosa pseudomonads such as *Pseudomonas putida* and *Pseudomonas fluorescens*. Bacteremia is the most common site of infection followed by pneumonia and urinary tract infection. Fever is often the only manifestation of infection. Other manifestations such as ecthyma gangrenosum are uncommon (Figure 4). Polymicrobial infections and infections that are complicated by deep tissue involvement (pneumonia, neutropenic enterocolitis (NEC), and perirectal infections) are associated with greater morbidity and mortality.[16,52] The emergence of resistance to β-lactam agents and carbapenems is of great concern.[53–55] Some organisms, especially *P. aeruginosa* and *Acinetobacter* spp., have become multi-drug resistant.[56,57] Very few options to treat such organisms (colistin, tigecycline, and combination regimens) currently exist, and very few novel agents are in the developmental pipeline.[58,59] Many institutions now conduct surveillance studies in high-risk patients looking for fecal colonization with VRE, *P. aeruginosa*, extended spectrum beta-lactamase (ESBL) producers, and carbapenem-resistant *Enterobacteriaceae* (CRE), because positive surveillance cultures often predict subsequent infection.[60–63]

Impaired cellular immunity is a risk factor for legionellosis. The most common *Legionella* species causing infection is *Legionella pneumophila*. Hospital water systems often harbor *Legionella* spp. and many cases of hospital-acquired legionellosis can be traced to such sources.[64] Pneumonia is the most common manifestation. The detection of urinary antigens or recovery of the organisms on special media is required to make a specific diagnosis. The fluoroquinolones and macrolides are used most often for treatment and there appears to be no advantage to using them in combination. Non-typhoidal *Salmonella* and *Campylobacter* spp. infections are also seen with increased frequency in patients with impaired cellular immunity.[65]

Cell-mediated immunity plays an essential role in the control of mycobacterial infections. The association of tuberculosis and Hodgkin's disease or hairy cell leukemia has been well established.[66]

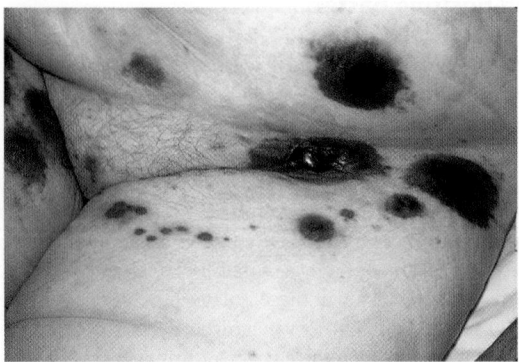

Figure 4 Multiple skin lesions (ecthyma gangrenosum) in a patient with *Pseudomonas aeruginosa* bacteremia.

Tuberculosis can precede the diagnosis of these malignancies, occur concomitantly, or develop during or after their treatment. Pulmonary infection that produces fever, cough, and weight loss is common. Diffuse pulmonary infiltrates with or without mediastinal enlargement are the most common radiographic findings. Nontuberculous mycobacterial infections are less common.[67,68] They produce pulmonary infections, lymphadenitis, SSSIs, catheter-related infections, and disseminated disease. The species isolated most often are *Mycobacterium avium-intracellulare, Mycobacterium abscessus, Mycobacterium chelonae, Mycobacterium fortuitum, Mycobacterium kansasii,* and *Mycobacterium marinum.* Prolonged, multiple drug therapy is usually administered for progressive infection.[69]

Anaerobes

Anaerobes are frequently involved in deep-seated, polymicrobial infections such as abdominal/pelvic abscesses, NEC, peri-rectal infections, complicated SSSIs, and pneumonia.[52,70] The organisms isolated most often include *Peptococcus* spp., *Fusobacterium nucleatum, Bacteroides* spp., and *Prevotella* spp.[71] *Clostridium difficile* infection (CDI) is the leading infectious cause of diarrhea in cancer patients in whom there is increased severity of illness, higher mortality, and an increased risk of relapse and complications. Newer diagnostic tests are available including polymerase chain reaction (PCR)-based assays.[72] Metronidazole is now considered inferior to vancomycin for the treatment of CDI.[73] Agents such as rifaximin and nitazoxamide have been used with limited success.[74-76] Fidaxomycin is an oral macrocyclic antibiotic that has been recently approved by the FDA for the treatment of CDI in adults, especially those individuals at greatest risk for relapse.[77,78] Fecal transplants have also been used successfully in this setting and appear to be promising.[79] Preventive measures include strict enforcements of infection control practices, appropriate antimicrobial usage, and improved environment cleaning methods.

Fungal infections

Prolonged neutropenia (>7 to 10 days) is a key risk factor for the development of invasive fungal infections (IFIs). The most common causes of IFIs in neutropenic patients are *Candida* spp. and *Aspergillus* spp.[80] The epidemiology of IFIs has changed substantially over the past 10–15 years.[81,82] Before the availability of agents such as fluconazole, invasive candidiasis was quite common with *Candida albicans* being the predominant species. The routine use of azole prophylaxis has led to a decrease in the frequency of candidiasis with manifestations such as oro-pharyngeal candidiasis (thrush), esophagitis, and chronic systemic (hepatosplenic) candidiasis becoming almost of historical interest. Candidemia, often catheter-related, is now the most common manifestation, with the alimentary tract being the predominant portal of entry. Recent studies have demonstrated a major shift from *C. albicans* to non-albicans *Candida* spp. (*Candida glabrata, Candida tropicalis, Candida krusei,* and *Candida parapsilosis*).[82-84]

There are no characteristic physical signs and symptoms of disseminated candidiasis. Often, the only indication is persistent fever and a gradual worsening of the patient's clinical condition. Some patients have ocular infection causing blurred vision, pain, scotomata, or loss of visual acuity. Nearly 10% of patients develop characteristic erythematous macronodular skin lesions (Figure 5). A chronic form of *Candida* infection known as chronic disseminated candidiasis has been described, usually after neutrophil recovery. Patients remain febrile and debilitated with substantial weight loss. Symptoms including right upper quadrant or

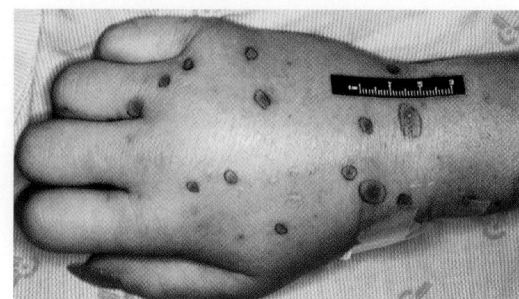

Figure 5 Characteristic macronodular cutaneous lesions in a patient with acute leukemia and disseminated *Candida krusei* infection.

shoulder pain may appear. Alkaline phosphatase levels are usually elevated. Hepatosplenomegaly may be detected. Imaging of the liver and spleen reveals multiple lesions. Approximately 90% of the patients respond to appropriate antifungal therapy.[62] This type of infection has virtually disappeared from institutions where azoles or echinocandins are used for antifungal prophylaxis. Treatment should be guided by *in vitro* antifungal susceptibility data.[85] Breakthrough *C. parapsilosis* fungemia may develop during echinocandin therapy, as may *C. glabrata* infection during azole therapy. Echinocandin resistance among *C. glabrata* isolates appears to be increasing.[86] *C. krusei* isolates are resistant to fluconazole. The mortality associated with systemic candida infections is ~40%. Guidelines for the management of candidiasis have been published by various societies.[87-90]

Aspergillosis is also frequent in patients with persistent neutropenia. Other risk factors include prolonged high-dose corticosteroid therapy, graft-versus-host disease (GVHD), repeated cycles of neutropenia, respiratory viral infections, and advanced age.[91] The most common pathogen is *Aspergillus fumigatus.*[92] Infection is usually acquired by inhalation of spores. Outbreaks of aspergillosis associated with construction within or adjacent to the hospital have occurred. More than 70% of infections involve the lungs (IPA, invasive pulmonary aspergillosis), and approximately 35% of patients have hematogenous dissemination to other organs.[93] Often, the only evidence of infection is prolonged fever with pulmonary infiltrates that fail to respond to antibacterial therapy. High-resolution CT scanning of the lung is helpful in the early diagnosis of aspergillosis.[94,95] Characteristic findings in early stage disease are multiple nodules with a halo of surrounding ground-glass attenuation that represents hemorrhage surrounding a region of pulmonary infarction (Figure 6).[94-96] As healing occurs, the infarcted tissue becomes necrotic and retracts from the viable tissue leaving an air crescent. *Aspergillus* sino-orbital infection is being diagnosed with increasing frequency in patients with acute leukemia and in HCT recipients, accounting for at least 15% of cases of aspergillosis (Figure 7). Infections may erode through the base of the skull and invade the brain or cause destruction of the paranasal and facial structures and the eye. A localized form of aspergillosis has been described in association with intravascular catheters.[97] *Aspergillus* spores may be deposited at the time of insertion or may be impregnated in materials used for catheter dressings. These infections are potentially serious because they can disseminate.[97,98] Skin lesions, manifested as sharply defined black eschars, occur in about 5% of patients with disseminated infection. Voriconazole is the preferred agent for the treatment of invasive or disseminated aspergillosis. Posaconazole and lipid preparations of amphotericin B are used more often for salvage therapy or when voriconazole intolerance occurs. Combination therapy with a triazole and an echinocandin may be useful for salvage

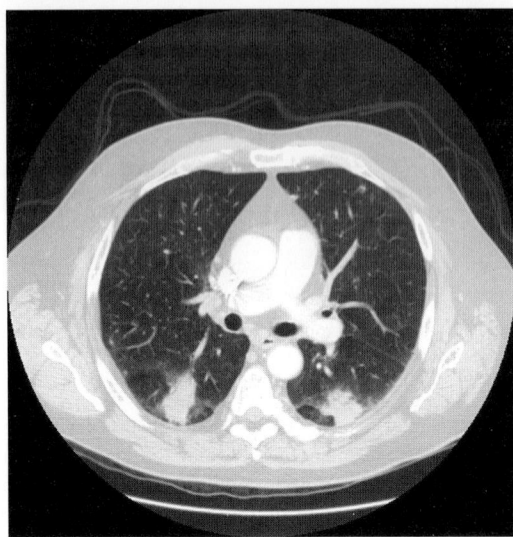

Figure 6 Rounded pulmonary lesions with surrounding halo, compatible with invasive pulmonary aspergillosis.

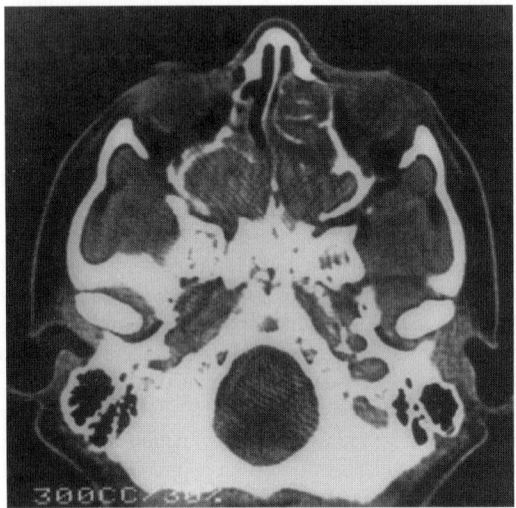

Figure 7 Pansinusitis caused by *Aspergillus* spp. in an allogeneic bone marrow transplant recipient with persistent fever.

therapy of invasive aspergillosis.[85,90,99,100] A recent randomized trial has shown higher survival in patients with invasive aspergillosis treated with voriconazole and anidulafungin than those treated with voriconazole monotherapy.[101]

Cryptococcosis is caused by two sibling species, *C. neoformans* and *Cryptococcus gatti*. The primary site of infection is the lung, which follows the inhalation of spores. Dissemination usually involves the central nervous system (meningoencephalitis and cryptococcoma). Fever and meningeal symptoms are common. Cerebrospinal fluid (CSF) abnormalities include raised opening pressure, lymphocytosis, elevated proteins, and low glucose levels. Cryptococcal antigen is also detected in the CSF and serum in most cases. Induction therapy with amphotericin B or its lipid formulations plus 5-fluorocytosine followed by maintenance therapy with fluconazole is the current standard of care.[102] Histoplasmosis and infections caused by other endemic fungi are less common.[8] They usually cause pulmonary, CNS, or disseminated infection and should be considered in the differential diagnosis in endemic areas. Pneumonia caused by *P. jiroveci* has traditionally been associated

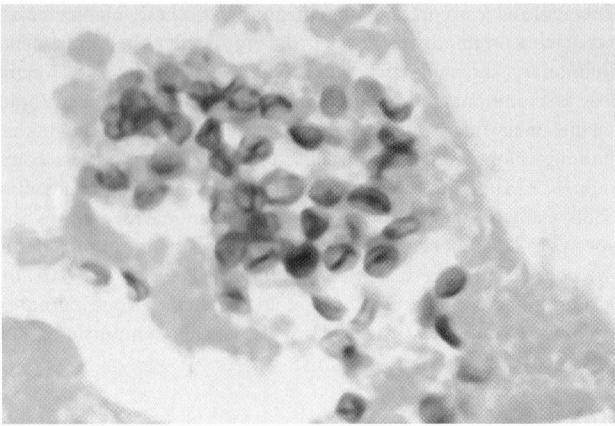

Figure 8 Gomori methenamine silver (GMS) stain from a bronchoalveolar lavage specimen demonstrating multiple organisms in a patient with *Pneumocystis carinii* pneumonia.

with impaired cellular immunity, which results in the reactivation of dormant infection.[103,104] The clinical presentation is usually subacute. Clinical features include fever, a non-productive cough, and progressive dyspnea. The most common CT findings are diffuse bilateral ground glass pulmonary infiltrates with apical predominance and peripheral sparing.[105] The diagnosis is often made by demonstrating the organisms on respiratory specimens including biopsy tissue using stains such as methenamine silver or toluidine blue (Figure 8). Staining methods have been supplanted by sensitive molecular techniques including semi-quantitative or quantitative PCR.[106,107] High-dose TMP/SMX remains the agent of choice for prophylaxis and treatment. Alternative agents include pentamidine, atovaquone, clindamycin plus primaquine, and dapsone plus trimethoprim.[108]

Other opportunistic fungi

Mucormycosis (zygomycosis) is still relatively uncommon with the most common pathogens being *Rhizopus* spp., *Mucor* spp., *Lichtheimia* (formerly *Absidia*) *corymbifera*, *Rhizomucor* spp., and *Cunninghamella bertholettiae*. Invasive pulmonary infection is the most common form of infection. Some patients develop sinopulmonary, rhinocerebral, gastrointestinal, cutaneous, or disseminated infection.[109,110] The clinical presentation of mucormycosis is often indistinguishable from aspergillosis. Mucormycosis should be considered in patients who are immunosuppressed and who develop sinusitis or IFI after prolonged exposure to voriconazole, which is not active against these organisms.[111–113] Early diagnosis and administration of antifungal therapy is critical along with surgical debridement of infected tissue. Control of underlying diseases and reversal of risk factors when feasible is also of paramount importance.[85,114] Amphotericin B products and posaconazole are the only antifungal agents with reliable activity against Mucorales.[115] Isavuconazole has also just been approved for the treatment of mucormycosis. Lipid preparations of amphotericin B are preferred for initial therapy, and there is some evidence to suggest that combining these preparations with an echinocandin might be beneficial.[116] Therapy is often switched to posaconazole when feasible. *Trichosporon beigelii* can cause disseminated infection particularly in patients with severe neutropenia. A variety of skin lesions have been described and occur in approximately 30% of patients. Portals of entry include the gastrointestinal tract, respiratory tract, and intravenous catheter sites. *Fusarium* spp. have emerged as significant pathogens in patients with neutropenia.[117]

Localized infections of the lung, sinuses, and skin occur, but most patients have disseminated infection. Cutaneous and subcutaneous skin lesions are frequent.[118] Similarly to *Aspergillus* spp., these organisms invade blood vessels, causing thrombosis and infarction. Usually *Fusarium* spp. can be isolated readily from blood culture or tissue specimens. It may be difficult to distinguish *Fusarium* from some other fungi on histopathologic examination. Recovery from this infection depends on resolution of neutropenia, and currently available antifungal agents are at best only marginally effective.[119,120]

Various other fungi cause significant infection in neutropenic patients. These organisms include *Blastoschizomyces capitatus*, *Scedosporium* spp., *Geotrichum candidum*, and *Malassezia furfur*.[121] The majority of patients who are infected have hematologic neoplasms, especially acute leukemia.[122]

Viral infections

Viral infections are uncommon in patients with neutropenia unless they are HCT recipients. Herpes viruses are identified most frequently, especially herpes simplex viruses (HSV), varicella-zoster virus (VZV), and CMV. Most adults are HSV seropositive, and reactivation can occur in ~60–80% of patients undergoing HCT or intensive chemotherapy for hematologic malignancies. Reactivation generally occurs while patients are still severely neutropenic with oral mucositis/ulceration being the most common manifestation. Esophagitis indistinguishable from *Candida* esophagitis occurs occasionally. Encephalitis and dissemination are uncommon. HSV prophylaxis is recommended in patients undergoing HCT or remission induction therapy for leukemia.[123] Reactivation of latent VZV also occurs and prophylaxis to prevent recurrence of VZV infection in seropositive patients is recommended for the first year following allogeneic HCT.[124,125] Community respiratory viruses, including RSV, influenza A and B viruses, parainfluenza viruses, human metapneumovirus, human coronaviruses, and human rhinoviruses, are common among HCT recipients and patients with acute leukemia in whom upper respiratory tract infection can progress to pneumonitis, which is associated with substantial morbidity and mortality.[126] Testing for respiratory viruses is recommended in high-risk patients. Specimens include nasopharyngeal swabs, washes, or aspirates, tracheal aspirates, and bronchoalveolar lavage specimens. Optimum treatment for most of these viral infections, except for influenza viruses, remains to be determined. Ribavirin therapy for upper respiratory infection with RSV deters progression to pneumonia and may improve overall outcome in HCT recipients.[127]

Reactivation of EBV may occur after HCT or following chemotherapy with purine analogs such as fludarabine. EBV infection may be responsible for Richter transformation or development of Hodgkin disease in patients with chronic lymphocytic leukemia. In recipients of HCT or solid-organ transplants, uncontrolled proliferation of EBV infected B cells may occur, producing post-transplant lymphoproliferative disorders (PTLDs). In younger patients, a mononucleosis-like syndrome is a common presentation. Fever, sore throat, and lymphadenopathy are typical findings. Dissemination can occur from localized nodular lesions and can be fulminant and rapidly fatal. It is important to monitor high-risk patients (umbilical cord blood transplants, haploidentical transplants, and T-cell-depleted transplants) for EBV DNA viral load using PCR assays. Rituximab is recommended for preemptive therapy or the treatment of PTLD.[128,129]

HHV-6 is being recognized as an important pathogen in HCT recipients.[130,131] Serologic reactivation accompanied by specific

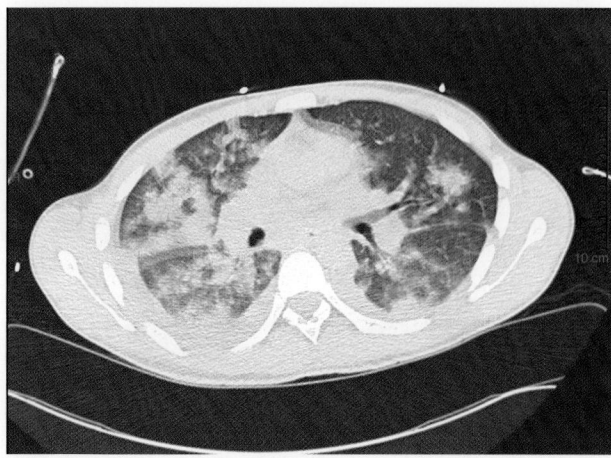

Figure 9 Computerized tomography scan of an allogeneic HCT recipient with CMV pneumonitis, showing diffuse bilateral pulmonary infiltrates.

manifestations, including fever, rash, pneumonitis, hepatitis, myelosuppression, and neurologic dysfunction, have been described in recipients of bone marrow, kidney, and liver transplants. HHV-6 viremia is not necessarily associated with increased mortality, and routine screening is not necessary.[132,133] Ganciclovir and foscarnet inhibit viral replication, and therapy with these agents may be useful in patients with severe infections. Immunotherapeutic prevention and treatment strategies are being developed.[134,135]

CMV infection occurs frequently in immunocompromised patients, especially those with impaired cellular immunity. It is a common complication in patients undergoing allogeneic HCT and has a negative impact on overall survival after transplantation.[136] CMV seropositivity in HCT recipients is a major risk factor. Without prophylaxis, 50–80% of seropositive patients undergoing HCT reactivate latent infection. CMV seropositivity, in both the HCT recipient and the donor, has an impact on the subsequent development of CMV end organ disease.[137] Other risk factors for CMV infection include total body irradiation, umbilical cord blood transplantation, the use of T-cell-depleted stem cells, treatment with purine analogs (fludarabine and cladribine), and monoclonal antibodies against CD20 (rituximab), CD52 (alemtuzumab), GVHD, and advanced age.[138] CMV pneumonia is the most common manifestation (Figure 9). Other manifestations include retinitis, esophagitis, enteritis, hepatitis, myocarditis, and encephalitis. In addition to end organ disease, CMV infection has been associated with GVHD and secondary bacterial and fungal infections. Early detection of CMV infection is of paramount importance, in order to deploy preventive measures. These measures consist of CMV prophylaxis that has now fallen out of favor when compared to preemptive therapy. The preemptive strategy consists of the administration of antiviral therapy (ganciclovir and foscarnet), which is initiated upon detection of CMV, using either the phosphoprotein 65 (pp 65) antigenemia assay or the PCR assay. Viral load-based, risk-adapted, preemptive treatment strategies have successfully prevented CMV disease, with a very low incidence of breakthrough disease.[139] Unfortunately, the treatment of established end organ disease, especially pneumonia is not very satisfactory. Currently available systemic antiviral agents include ganciclovir, foscarnet, cidofovir, and leflunomide in addition to some novel agents such as letermovir and brincidofovir that are in the developmental pipeline.[140,141]

Varicella has been recognized as a serious infection in children undergoing cancer chemotherapy. Nearly 30% of children receiving cancer chemotherapy develop serious complications during varicella infection, with around 7% fatality rate. Characteristic

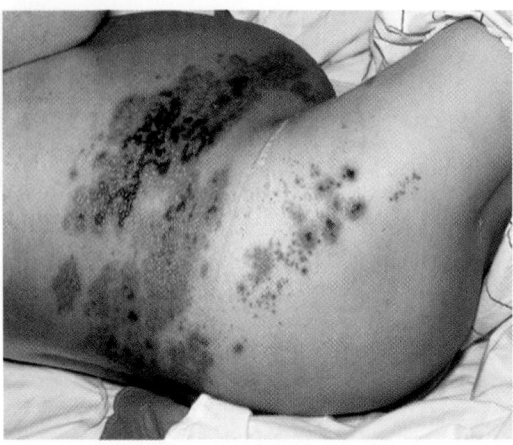

Figure 10 Typical vesicular rash caused by varicellazoster virus. Note the dermatomal distribution and the hemorrhagic nature of lesions in this patient with thrombocytopenia.

manifestations of varicella include a generalized vesicular rash and fever. Lesions appear initially on the face and scalp and subsequently spread to the trunk and extremities. New lesions continue to appear as older lesions crust. Infection may be unduly prolonged in patients with cancer. The vesicles become hemorrhagic and necrotic in patients with thrombocytopenia. Around 10% of children develop a bacterial superinfection. Disseminated visceral infection may result in widespread pneumonia and focal necrosis of the liver, pancreas, or adrenal glands.

Herpes zoster occurs most often in patients with lymphoproliferative disorders. The infection is characterized by a unilateral vesicular rash in the distribution of one or two adjacent sensory dermatomes (Figure 10). Occasionally, patients develop a generalized varicelliform eruption. The rash is accompanied by pain (zoster-associated pain) that can last for several weeks or months. Cutaneous dissemination of herpes zoster occurs in approximately 35% of patients with cancer, as compared with only 4% of those without cancer. Therapy with adrenal corticosteroids, radiation, or antitumor agents facilitates dissemination.

Laboratory confirmation of the diagnosis is generally not required. VZV can be recovered from the vesicular fluid for a few days after the onset of the eruption. Cultures are positive 30–60% of the time. Detection of VZV antigens in skin scrapings using fluorescence microscopy and detection of VZV DNA, in the CSF or other tissues, using PCR, are more rapid and sensitive diagnostic techniques.

Therapy of VZV infection shortens viral shedding, accelerates healing of lesions, and reduces the frequency of visceral disease. Oral valacyclovir and famciclovir are better absorbed and more effective than acyclovir. Severe infections such as meningoencephalitis and pneumonitis require intravenous acyclovir therapy. Therapy with foscarnet or combination therapy with foscarnet and acyclovir should be considered for patients who fail to respond to acyclovir alone. Varicella-zoster immune globulin must be given within 96 h of exposure to be effective. Varicella vaccine is available for universal immunization and postexposure prophylaxis.[142,143] The vaccine is safe, immunogenic, and effective in leukemic children at risk for serious disease, if chemotherapy is interrupted for 1 week before and after administration; approximately 50% developed a mild rash. A 1-week course of antiviral therapy following exposure may be useful for patients who are at risk.[144] A heat-treated vaccine has been shown to be safe and immunogenic in immunocompromised adults.[145]

Hepatitis viruses

Hepatitis B virus (HBV) reactivation occurs primarily in patients receiving anti-CD20 agents (rituximab and ofatumumab) and in HCT recipients with clinical manifestations ranging from asymptomatic elevation of hepatic enzymes to fulminant hepatic failure and death. The risk of reactivation is higher with chronic HBV infection (positive HBsAg) than in individuals with resolved infection (positive HBsAb and negative HBsAg). Diagnostic tools such as quantitative HBV DNA measurements and newer antiviral agents (entecavir, lamivudine, and tenofovir) have improved the detection of HBV reactivation and the treatment of reactivated infection. Universal screening of cancer patients for HBV versus risk-based screening remains a matter of debate. Many societies including ASCO and NCCN currently recommend risk-based screening for patients who will be receiving immunosuppressive therapy including anti-CD20 therapy.[146,147] Hepatitis C virus (HCV) causes chronic infection in more than three million individuals in the United States and is a major risk factor for the development of liver cancer. HCV reactivation has been described primarily among patients with hematologic malignancies and recipients of rituximab therapy.[148] However, reactivation occurs less frequently than with HBV, and the role of screening cancer patients for HCV has not yet been established.[149,150]

Other infections

Toxoplasmosis is one of the most common parasitic infestations in man. Disseminated disease generally occurs in immunocompromised individuals with the CNS, heart, and lungs being involved most often.[151] Computerized tomography (CT) or magnetic resonance imaging (MRI) of the brain reveals multiple hypodense lesions, often with moderate contrast ring enhancement. The diagnosis can be confirmed by serologic testing or biopsy, if feasible. Specific therapy consists of pyrimethamine plus sulfadiazine or spiramycin. Alternative agents such as clindamycin, atovaquone, and TMP/SMX have also been used for treatment and/or prophylaxis.[152] *Strongyloides stercoralis* is a soil transmitted helminth and lymphoma is the most common malignancy associated with strongyloidiasis. Many infestations are asymptomatic and some produce only eosinophilia.[153] Common clinical features include fever and gastrointestinal symptoms such as diarrhea and abdominal pain/cramping. Immunosuppression often induced by corticosteroids can trigger the development of hyperinfection of dissemination.[10,154] Pulmonary infiltrates and pleural effusions that are often hemorrhagic can develop, followed by respiratory insufficiency/failure. Polymicrobial bacteremia cause by enteric Gram-negative bacilli and anaerobes is not uncommon. Diagnostic tests include demonstration of the organisms in stool and respiratory specimens, and serological enzyme-linked immunosorbent assay (ELISA) methods. Ivermectin is the therapeutic agent of choice. Screening of high-risk patients (allogeneic HCT recipients and corticosteroid usage) is recommended especially in endemic areas.[155]

Special situations

Abdominal infections

An acute abdomen is one of the most difficult problems that physicians caring for patients with cancer encounter.[156] Causes of acute abdomen include appendicitis, cholecystitis, diverticulitis, peritonitis, abdominal abscesses, splenic infarcts, NEC, and tumor lysis/perforation. Patients usually have abdominal pain, distention, guarding, rebound, and diminished or absent bowel sounds. These signs/symptoms may be blunted in neutropenic patients and those receiving immunosuppressive agents. Supportive measures, antibiotics, and occasional surgical intervention are needed for management.

NEC is seen primarily in patients with hematologic malignancies but is now being seen with increasing frequently in patients with solid tumors due to the use of agents such as the taxanes, which produce severe intestinal mucositis.[52] Common presenting features include fever, abdominal pain or cramping, distention, and diarrhea. Complications include bacteremia that is often polymicrobial, hemorrhage, bowel wall perforation, and abscess formation. The disease may be limited to the cecum (typhlitis), but usually involves the entire lower intestinal tract. Radiographic examination (preferably CT) usually reveals evidence of a paralytic ileus with lack of bowel gas in the right lower quadrant, minimal distention of the terminal ileum, and >4 mm thickening of the bowel wall, which is considered a hallmark of NEC. Initial management is supportive and includes bowel rest, intravenous fluids, correction of cytopathies and coagulopathies, and broad-spectrum antibiotics that include coverage for *P. aeruginosa* and anaerobes. Surgical intervention may be necessary to manage complications such as hemorrhage or bowel perforation.

Perianal infections

Perianal infections are estimated to occur in 6% of patients with hematologic neoplasms. More than 90% of patients are neutropenic.[157] The major presenting symptom is pain that is aggravated by defecation. Erythematous, indurated, or ulcerated lesions with extensive tissue necrosis and sloughing extending into the rectum are common. The infection often occurs at a site of a fissure or hemorrhoid. Most of these infections are caused by aerobic Gram-negative bacilli, especially *P. aeruginosa* and *E. coli*. Therapy includes general measures such as sitz baths, warm compresses, stool softeners, analgesics, along with broad-spectrum antibiotics. Empiric antifungal therapy is not recommended. Abscesses, if present, should be drained.[158] Resolution of infection often depends on recovery of the neutrophil count. Patients with hematologic diseases who recover from perianal infections caused by hemorrhoids or anal fissures should undergo surgical correction when feasible, to avoid recurrent infections.

Catheter-related infections

Central line-related bloodstream infections have become relatively common.[159] The majority of these infections are caused by *Staphylococcus* spp. and other Gram-positive organisms that colonize the skin, *P. aeruginosa*, *Enterobacteriaceae*, *S. maltophilia*, and *Candida* spp. Quantitative blood cultures and time to positivity help establish the diagnosis of CLABSI, although neither method is foolproof.[160–164] Sequential time to positivity can also be a predictor of outcome and prognosis.[165] Some episodes, especially those caused by CoNS can be successfully treated without the removal of the catheter.[166] However, catheter removal is usually necessary for CLABSI caused by *S. aureus*, *Acinetobacter*, *Pseudomonas* spp. *S. maltophilia*, *Candida* spp., and non-tuberculous mycobacteria. In addition, if there are signs of localized infection at the catheter insertion site, or if fever or bacteremia persists despite adequate therapy, catheters must always be removed.[160] Antimicrobial lock therapy may be useful particularly if catheter removal is not feasible.

The most serious complications of CLABSI are septic thrombophlebitis and endocarditis. Antimicrobial impregnated catheters have been shown to reduce the frequency of catheter-associated infections.[159,167]

Therapy of infections in patients with neutropenia

Initial patient evaluation

Febrile neutropenic patients should receive prompt, empiric, broad-spectrum antimicrobial therapy generally via the intravenous route and at maximal therapeutic doses.[168] Pretreatment evaluation should be performed as expeditiously as possible, as a delay in instituting empiric therapy can result in diminished response rates.[169] Pertinent historical information should be obtained, and a thorough physical examination should be performed. Particular attention should be paid to sites that are frequently infected or serve as foci for the dissemination of infection. These include the oro-pharynx, lower esophagus, perineum, paranasal sinuses, fingernails, and skin including the armpits, groin, and vascular catheter insertion sites. Cultures from all appropriate sites (blood, urine, and throat) should be obtained. In patients with central venous catheters cultures from a peripheral site and from all lumens of the catheter should be obtained.[170,171] Neutropenic patients with pneumonia may have normal appearing radiographs. CT scans of the chest and paranasal sinuses should be performed if these sites are potential sources of infection. Complete blood counts and determinations of baseline values for renal and hepatic function should be obtained. Finally, risk assessment should be performed in order to determine whether the patient requires hospitalization or not.[172] Low-risk febrile neutropenic patients can be treated with out-patient parenteral or oral antibiotic regimens if the infrastructure for out-patient management of such patients is in place.[173–175] All other patients should receive hospital-based therapy. Outpatient therapy can be administered after a short period of hospitalization or for the entire febrile episode.[176–179] It has been shown to be safe and effective in both adults and children.[180–182] Outpatient therapy is associated with substantial cost savings, a lower incidence of superinfections with resistant nosocomial pathogens, and improved quality of life for patients and convenience for their families and caregivers.[173,183] Various societies including the Infectious Diseases Society of America, the National Comprehensive Cancer Network, and the American Society of Clinical Oncology have published recent guidelines for the management of infections in patients with cancer, which include algorithms for outpatient therapy in low-risk patients.[168,184,185]

Initial antibiotic therapy

The empiric regimen should be based on local epidemiologic and resistance patterns and should provide potent coverage against Gram-negative organisms including *P. aeruginosa* and Gram-positive pathogens. This is usually achieved by administering either a single broad-spectrum agent (monotherapy) or antibiotic combinations.[168,185] Tables 5 and 6 list the common antibiotic agents and regimens used in this setting. No single regimen is optimal and various factors dictate the choice of one regimen over another. Monotherapy with agents such as the Group 2 carbapenems, cefepime, and piperacillin/tazobactam is considered appropriate for up to 60% of febrile neutropenic episode especially if no obvious focus of infection can be identified.[168] If resistant Gram-positive infections are likely (e.g., in patients colonized with

Table 5 Common empiric antibiotic regimens for febrile neutropenic patients.

Regimens for low-risk patients
   → Oral
      Quinolone + amoxicillin/clavulanate
      Quinolone + clindamycin or azithromycin
      Moxifloxacin or levofloxacin (monotherapy)
   → Parenteral
      Ceftriaxone or ertapenem ± amikacin
      Aztreonam + clindamycin
      Quinolone ± clindamycin
      Ceftazidime or cefepime
Regimens for moderate to high-risk patients
   Combination regimens
      Aminoglycoside + antipseudomonal penicillin/beta-lactamase inhibitor or cephalosporin or carbapenem, or quinolone (if patient not on quinolone prophylaxis)
      Vancomycin(or linezolid or daptomycin) + antipseudomonal penicillin, or cephalosporin, or carbapenem, or quinolone (if patient not on quinolone prophylaxis)
   Single-agent regimens (monotherapy)
      Extended-spectrum cephalosporin (cefepime)
      Carbapenems (imipenem, meropenem, or doripenem, but not ertapenem)
      Antipseudomonal penicillin/beta-lactamase inhibitor (piperacillin/tazobactam)

Table 6 Antimicrobial agents commonly used in patients with neutropenia.

Aminoglycosides	
Amikacin	5 mg/kg q8 h or 15–20 g/kg/day (single daily dose)
Antipseudomonal penicillins + β-lactamase inhibitor	
Piperacillin + tazobactam	3.375 g q6 h, IV
Extended-spectrum cephalosporins	
Cefepime	1–2 g q8 h, IV
Carbapenem	
Imipenem/cilastatin	500 mg q6 h, IV
Meropenem	1 g q8 h, IV
Monobactam	
Aztreonam	1.5–2.0 g q6–8 h, IV
Quinolones	
Ciprofloxacin	200–400 mg q8h[a]
Levofloxacin	500 or 750 mg q24 h[a]
Moxifloxacin	400 mg q24 h[a]
Others	
Vancomycin	1 g q12 h, IV (monitor levels) target trough 15–20
Trimethoprim-sulfamethoxazole	2.0–20.0 mg/kg/day (trimethoprim) IV q6 h[a]
Metronidazole	500 mg IV q6–8 h[a]
Linezolid	600 mg IV q12 h[a]
Daptomycin	6–8 mg/kg/day
Tigecycline	Initial loading dose 100 mg, then 50 mg IV q12 h
Antifungal agents	
Azoles:	
Fluconazole	200–800 mg q24 h[a]
Itraconazole	200 mg q12 h[a]
Voriconazole	6 mg/kg loading dose q12 × 2 doses, then 4 mg/kg q12 h[a]
Posaconazole	Suspension 200 mg q 8 h with food, tablets/IV 300 mg q 12 h × 2, then 300 mg q24 h[a]
Isavuconazole	iv/po loading dose of 200 mg q 8 h x 6 doses, then 200 mg q24 h
Echinocandins:	
Caspofungin	70 mg day 1, then 50 mg q24 h
Micafungin	100 mg q24 h
Anidaulafungin	200 mg day 1, then 100 mg q24 h
Polyenes:	
Amphotericin B deoxycholate	0.3–1 mg/kg/day once daily
Amphotericin B liposomal (ambisome)	1–10 mg/kg/day once daily
Amphotericin B lipid complex (abelcet)	5 mg/kg/day once daily
Anti viral agents	
Acyclovir	5–12 mg/kg q8 h[a]
Valacyclovir	1 g q8 h
Ganciclovir	5 mg/kg q 12 h
Valganciclovir	Oral 900 mg q12 h
Foscarnet	90 mg/kg q12 h
Cidofovir	5 mg/kg IV once a week, must be given with probenecid 3 g before infusion and 1 g 2&8 h post infusion
Ribavirin	Oral 10–20 mg/kg q 8 h, available in inhalation, note drug is cytotoxic and teratogenic

Abbreviations: IV, intravenously; PO, orally.
[a]Preparations are available for both intravenous and oral administrations, check dosing for each specific preparation.

MRSA (methicillin-resistant *Staphylococcus aureus*) or VRE), a combination of these agents with vancomycin, linezolid, or daptomycin is considered appropriate. However, studies have shown that the addition of these agents after a resistant Gram-positive infection has been identified just as effective as empiric usage. Vancomycin may no longer be adequate at some institutions owing to changing susceptibilities, and alternative agents such as daptomycin, dalbavancin, and telavancin may be considered, although clinical experience with these agents in neutropenic patients is limited.[23,27–29] Combinations of antipseudomonal beta-lactams and aminoglycosides are generally used to try and provide synergistic bactericidal activity against Gram-negative pathogens such as *P. aeruginosa*. Agents with potent anaerobic activity should be administered when anaerobic infections (e.g., perirectal infections and NEC) are likely or have been documented. The initial regimen may need to be altered during the course of the febrile episode, depending on the susceptibility of microorganisms isolated from clinical specimens, the development of bacterial, fungal, or viral superinfections, or lack of apparent efficacy after administration of the regimen for 3 days. Consequently, all patients need to be carefully monitored for response, toxicity, and the development of other complications, and appropriate changes should be made if the clinical situation or microbiologic data indicate the need.[186] Initial empiric therapy is usually associated with response rates of 65–85% (higher in low-risk patients).[180] A substantial proportion of patients will respond after modification of the initial regimen including the addition of antifungal therapy after 5–7 days.[168]

Duration of therapy

Some authorities recommend continuation of antibiotic therapy in patients with documented infections until recovery of the neutrophil count (i.e., an absolute neutrophil count >500 cells for two consecutive days). This approach is expensive and may not be needed in many patients. It actually represents broad-spectrum prophylaxis after resolution of infection in many patients. This may result in an increased number of resistant superinfections requiring further modifications of antibacterial therapy and/or the addition of antifungal therapy, and adds to the overall cost of therapy. Another approach is to continue antibiotics until all sites of infection have resolved, the causative pathogen, if isolated, has been eradicated, and the patient has been treated for a minimum of 7 days and has remained free of significant symptoms or signs of infection for at least 4 days. This is indeed the case in most patients with unexplained fever. Antibiotic therapy may be discontinued safely at this point despite the persistence of neutropenia. This approach is less expensive and may be associated with fewer superinfections.

Persistent fever

Patients who remain febrile despite antibacterial and antifungal therapies pose a difficult challenge. These patients may have bacterial infections that are resistant to therapy or infections by other pathogens (viruses and parasites). Drug-related fever or tumor fever may also be present. Aggressive, often invasive, diagnostic maneuvers are sometimes necessary in order to make a specific diagnosis and provide specific therapy to such patients. In patients unable to tolerate invasive diagnostic procedures, continuation of the empiric antibacterial and antifungal regimens and the addition of empiric antiviral or antiparasitic therapy might be necessary.

Other therapeutic modalities

Nearly 15–25% of infections occurring in patients with neutropenia fail to respond to appropriate antimicrobial therapy. In most cases, profound neutropenia persists. The availability of the hematopoietic growth factors has rekindled interest because the administration of granulocyte colony-stimulating factor (G-CSF) to donors increases the number of neutrophils that can be collected.[187–189] Preliminary clinical studies suggest that this approach to white blood cell collection has produced therapeutic benefit in selected recipients.[190,191]

The administration of hematopoietic growth factors to patients receiving cancer chemotherapy reduces the severity and duration of neutropenia and, hence, the frequency of infectious complications. Guidelines for this use of these agents have been prepared by the American Society of Clinical Oncology.[192] The efficacy of these factors as adjuncts to antibiotic therapy for patients who are neutropenic after they have become infected has not been clearly established. It is reasonable to administer these agents to patients with neutrophil counts <500/mm^3 who develop pneumonia, septic shock, sepsis syndrome, or fungal infection, because these patients have a poor prognosis without recovery of their neutrophils. These agents should also be considered for patients with documented infections who are failing to respond to appropriate therapy after 24–48 h. The role of granulocyte colony-stimulating factors appears to be expanding.[193] IFN-γ may be beneficial for some bacterial or fungal infections that are not responding to appropriate therapy.[194]

Infection prevention

Suppression of the endogenous microflora, from which most infections arise, is usually achieved using antimicrobial prophylaxis (bacterial, fungal, viral, or protozoal) during the periods of risk. The acquisition of new organisms is accomplished by various techniques, including strict infection control, the use of well-cooked foods, which reduces contamination with Gram-negative bacteria, and various isolation techniques or protected environments.

Antibacterial prophylaxis

Prophylactic antimicrobial regimens achieve a major reduction in the patients' microbial burden. The quinolones (ciprofloxacin and levofloxacin) are the most commonly used agents for antibacterial prophylaxis resulting in significant reduction in the frequency of Gram-negative infections, but with little impact on the frequency of Gram-positive infections.[195,196] Although quinolone prophylaxis is associated with reduced mortality related to Gram-negative infections, and in reduced all cause mortality in some studies, it has also resulted in the emergence of quinolone resistance among enteric Gram-negative bacilli including *E. coli*.[197–199] Its use remains controversial and it is therefore not recommended for routinely in neutropenic patients, but must be considered only in patients at high risk for bacterial infection, such as those with prolonged periods of neutropenia.[168,184,185] Discontinuation of prophylaxis when indicated is critical. Surveillance for the emergence of resistant organisms is also of utmost importance.[200,201]

Antifungal and antiviral prophylaxis

Increasing frequency of IFIs in high-risk patients has led to the use of antifungal prophylaxis.[202] Fluconazole (and itraconazole) prophylaxis has been shown to decrease both superficial colonization and systemic *Candida* infections. The selection of resistant species (*C. krusei* and *C. glabratta*) is a potential problem, although these organisms are also seen in "azole naïve" patients. Prophylaxis against molds including *Aspergillus* spp. is less successful although newer agents such as micafungin, voriconazole, and posaconazole with more potent activity against molds than older agents have been evaluated.[203–205] Increased voriconazole administration has already been associated with the emergence of breakthrough zygomycotic infections, cautioning against the widespread adoption of this strategy. TMP/SMX remains the agent of choice for *P. jiroveci* prophylaxis.[108] Alternative (but less effective agents include pentamidine, dapsone, and atovoquone.

Prophylactic acyclovir has been shown to prevent reactivation of HSV infection in patients undergoing intensive chemotherapy (with or without radiation therapy) before HCT or induction therapy for leukemia or lymphoma. Preemptive therapy (rather than prophylaxis) with ganciclovir or foscarnet is the current recommendation for high-risk patients with positive CMV antigenemia.[139]

Isolation

Reduction of the acquisition of new organisms has been attempted by putting patients at risk into reverse isolation. Patients are also given well-cooked foods and are asked to avoid fresh fruits and vegetables (e.g., tomatoes and salads) that are naturally contaminated with Gram-negative bacilli such as *P. aeruginosa*, *Klebsiella pneumoniae*, and *E. coli*. More elaborate regimens are expensive and time consuming and have not been shown to be more effective than strict adherence to hand-washing techniques.

Protected environments provide a combination of the two approaches, that is, the use of isolation units to protect the patient against nosocomial contamination plus antibiotic regimens to reduce the patient's endogenous flora. The protected environment generally consists of isolation units, which provide a barrier between the patient and the hospital environment, using aggressive decontamination techniques and filtered air. The patient's food is specially prepared or sterilized to minimize contamination. Disinfection of the patient is achieved using intensive regimens, which include oral nonabsorbable antibiotics. Patients bathe with germicidal soaps and apply topical antibiotic ointments or sprays to areas of heavy microbial contamination.

Because attempts at suppressing the endogenous microflora and those at preventing the acquisition of organisms have not been overwhelmingly successful, other means for infection prevention need to be developed. The hematopoietic growth factors [granulocyte-macrophage (GM)-CSF and G-CSF] have been demonstrated to shorten the duration of neutropenia and to reduce the number of febrile days and of documented infections in selected subpopulations of patients with neutropenia. Current guidelines suggest that the primary use of these agents is not indicated in patients who were previously untreated and receiving most chemotherapy regimens. The secondary administration of growth factors can decrease the probability of febrile neutropenia after a documented occurrence in an earlier cycle. It can also

Table 7 Antimicrobial stewardship strategies.

Continuing education for all healthcare providers
Guidelines/pathways for appropriate antimicrobial usage based on local microbiology and susceptibility/resistance
Formulary interventions restricting specific agents
Audits of antimicrobial usage with feedback to prescribers
Introduction of surveillance and decision support programs
Monitoring outcomes (morbidity, mortality, and length of stay) and resistance patterns
Comprehensive infection control program

reduce the period of neutropenia and the frequency of infectious complications in patients undergoing high-dose cytotoxic therapy with autologous marrow transplantation.

Antimicrobial stewardship

Antimicrobial resistance results in increased morbidity, mortality, and cost of healthcare. Antimicrobial stewardship has become an essential part of the management of patients with cancer, particularly in an age where the development of novel antimicrobial agents is at a standstill. The major goal of antimicrobial stewardship is to optimize antimicrobial usage while reducing unwanted consequences such as toxicity and the selection of resistant organisms.[206,207] Strategies for effective antimicrobial stewardship are listed in Table 7. These strategies are best implemented by an independent, multidisciplinary, antimicrobial stewardship team (MAST).[208-210]

Perspectives

Infection remains a serious complication for many cancer patients. The spectrum of infection continues to change, and the emergence of multidrug-resistant pathogens has posed serious challenges, especially as new drug development is rather limited. Disseminated fungal infections have become the leading cause of death in patients with hematologic malignancies, and in HCT recipients. Despite some improvements, the early diagnosis and adequate treatment of many IFIs remain unsatisfactory. Viral infections represent a growing threat particularly in patients with hematologic malignancies and HCT recipients. Newly emerging global threats (such as MERS and Ebola) can have a devastating impact on patients with cancer who are immunosuppressed. Reliable methods for the rapid diagnosis of these and other viral infections, and effective means for their prevention and treatment still need to be developed. Parasitic infections remain uncommon except in endemic areas. Although effective therapies are available, toxicity and the need for prolonged maintenance or suppressive therapy can be problematic. The development of risk-assessment strategies has led to the recognition of a "low-risk" subset among patients with neutropenia. Newer treatment strategies such as outpatient oral therapy have resulted in substantial cost savings, reduction in healthcare-associated infections, and improved quality of life. Protected environments, prophylactic programs, infection control strategies, and the CSFs have reduced the risk of infection in patients with cancer. Antimicrobial stewardship may delay the development of resistant organisms. Newer technologic advances should lead to further progress. Nonetheless, the recognition, prevention, diagnosis, and treatment of infections in patients with cancer will continue to challenge us in the foreseeable future, as we work toward the larger goal of eliminating cancer.

Key references

The complete reference list can be found on the Wiley Companion Digital Edition of this title (see inside front cover for login instructions).

2 Bow EJ. Neutropenic fever syndromes in patients undergoing cytotoxic therapy for acute leukemia and myelodysplastic syndromes. *Semin Hematol.* 2009;**46**:259–268.

3 Zell JA, Chang JC. Neoplastic fever: a neglected paraneoplastic syndrome. *Support Care Cancer.* 2005;**13**:870–877.

7 Roblot F, Imbert S, Godet C, et al. Risk factors analysis for Pneumocystis jiroveci pneumonia (PCP) in patients with haematological malignancies and pneumonia. *Scand J Infect Dis.* 2004;**36**:848–854.

12 Rolston KV, Nesher L, Tarrand JT. Current microbiology of surgical site infections in patients with cancer: a retrospective review. *Infect Dis Ther.* 2014;**3**(**2**):245–256.

13 Wisplinghoff H, Seifert H, Wenzel RP, et al. Current trends in the epidemiology of nosocomial bloodstream infections in patients with hematological malignancies and solid neoplasms in hospitals in the United States. *Clin Infect Dis.* 2003;**36**:1103–1110.

14 Nesher L, Rolston KV. The current spectrum of infection in cancer patients with chemotherapy related neutropenia. *Infection.* 2014;**42**:5–13.

16 Rolston KV, Bodey GP, Safdar A. Polymicrobial infection in patients with cancer: an underappreciated and underreported entity. *Clin Infect Dis.* 2007;**45**:228–233.

22 Liu C, Bayer A, Cosgrove SE, et al. Clinical practice guidelines by the infectious diseases society of america for the treatment of methicillin-resistant *Staphylococcus aureus* infections in adults and children. *Clin Infect Dis.* 2011;**52**:e18–e55.

34 Bochud PY, Eggiman P, Calandra T, et al. Bacteremia due to viridans streptococcus in neutropenic patients with cancer: clinical spectrum and risk factors. *Clin Infect Dis.* 1994;**18**:25–31.

37 Shelburne SA, Tarrand J, Rolston KV. Review of streptococcal bloodstream infections at a comprehensive cancer care center, 2000–2011. *J Infect.* 2013;**66**:136–146.

41 Dubberke ER, Hollands JM, Georgantopoulos P, et al. Vancomycin-resistant enterococcal bloodstream infections on a hematopoietic stem cell transplant unit: are the sick getting sicker? *Bone Marrow Transplant.* 2006;**38**:813–819.

50 Safdar A, Rolston KV. Stenotrophomonas maltophilia: changing spectrum of a serious bacterial pathogen in patients with cancer. *Clin Infect Dis.* 2007;**45**:1602–1609.

52 Nesher L, Rolston KVI. Neutropenic enterocolitis, a growing concern in the era of widespread use of aggressive chemotherapy. *Clin Infect Dis.* 2013;**56**:711–717.

53 Boucher HW, Talbot GH, Bradley JS, et al. Bad bugs, no drugs: no ESKAPE! An update from the Infectious Diseases Society of America. *Clin Infect Dis.* 2009;**48**:1–12.

54 Bushnell G, Mitrani-Gold F, Mundy LM. Emergence of New Delhi metallo-β-lactamase type 1-producing enterobacteriaceae and non-enterobacteriaceae: global case detection and bacterial surveillance. *Int J Infect Dis.* 2013;**17**:e325–e333.

58 Boucher HW, Talbot GH, Benjamin DK, et al. 10 x '20 progress—development of new drugs active against gram-negative bacilli: an update from the Infectious Diseases Society of America. *Clin Infect Dis.* 2013;**56**:1685–1694.

67 Chen CY, Sheng WH, Lai CC, et al. Mycobacterial infections in adult patients with hematological malignancy. *Eur J Clin Microbiol Infect Dis.* 2012;**31**:1059–1066.

72 Cohen SH, Gerding DN, Johnson S, et al. Clinical practice guidelines for Clostridium difficile infection in adults: 2010 update by the society for healthcare epidemiology of America (SHEA) and the infectious diseases society of America (IDSA). *Infect Control Hosp Epidemiol.* 2010;**31**:431–455.

80 Lewis RE, Cahyame-Zuniga L, Leventakos K, et al. Epidemiology and sites of involvement of invasive fungal infections in patients with haematological malignancies: a 20-year autopsy study. *Mycoses.* 2013;**56**:638–645.

87 Pappas PG, Kauffman CA, Andes D, et al. Clinical practice guidelines for the management of candidiasis: 2009 update by the Infectious Diseases Society of America. *Clin Infect Dis.* 2009;**48**:503–535.

89 Groll AH, Castagnola E, Cesaro S, et al. Fourth European Conference on Infections in Leukaemia (ECIL-4): guidelines for diagnosis, prevention, and treatment of invasive fungal diseases in paediatric patients with cancer or allogeneic haemopoietic stem-cell transplantation. *Lancet Oncol.* 2014;**15**:e327–e340.

90 Mousset S, Buchheidt D, Heinz W, et al. Treatment of invasive fungal infections in cancer patients-updated recommendations of the Infectious Diseases Working Party (AGIHO) of the German Society of Hematology and Oncology (DGHO). *Ann Hematol.* 2014;**93**:13–32.

94 Caillot D, Latrabe V, Thiébaut A, et al. Computer tomography in pulmonary invasive aspergillosis in hematological patients with neutropenia: an useful tool for diagnosis and assessment of outcome in clinical trials. *Eur J Radiol.* 2010;**74**:e172–e175.

101 Marr KA, Schlamm HT, Herbrecht R, et al. Combination antifungal therapy for invasive aspergillosis: a randomized trial. *Ann Intern Med.* 2015;**162**:81–89.

103 Kamel S, O'Connor S, Lee N, et al. High incidence of Pneumocystis jirovecii pneumonia in patients receiving biweekly rituximab and cyclophosphamide, adriamycin, vincristine, and prednisone. *Leuk Lymphoma.* 2010;**51**:797–801.

108 Cooley L, Dendle C, Wolf J, et al. Consensus guidelines for diagnosis, prophylaxis and management of Pneumocystis jirovecii pneumonia in patients with haematological and solid malignancies, 2014. *Intern Med J*. 2014;**44**:1350–1363.

123 Zaia J, Baden L, Boeckh MJ, et al. Viral disease prevention after hematopoietic cell transplantation. *Bone Marrow Transplant*. 2009;**44**:471–482.

126 Hirsch HH, Martino R, Ward KN, et al. Fourth European Conference on Infections in Leukaemia (ECIL-4): guidelines for diagnosis and treatment of human respiratory syncytial virus, parainfluenza virus, metapneumovirus, rhinovirus, and coronavirus. *Clin Infect Dis*. 2013;**56**:258–266.

134 Zerr DM, Boeckh M, Delaney C, et al. HHV-6 reactivation and associated sequelae after hematopoietic cell transplantation. *Biol Blood Marrow Transplant*. 2012;**18**:1700–1708.

136 Ljungman P, Griffiths P, Paya C. Definitions of cytomegalovirus infection and disease in transplant recipients. *Clin Infect Dis*. 2002;**34**:1094–1097.

139 Green ML, Leisenring W, Stachel D, et al. Efficacy of a viral load-based, risk-adapted, preemptive treatment strategy for prevention of cytomegalovirus disease after hematopoietic cell transplantation. *Biol Blood Marrow Transplant*. 2012;**18**:1687–1699.

145 Mullane KM, Winston DJ, Wertheim MS, et al. Safety and immunogenicity of heat-treated zoster vaccine (ZVHT) in immunocompromised adults. *J Infect Dis*. 2013;**208**:1375–1385.

160 Mermel LA, Allon M, Bouza E, et al. Clinical practice guidelines for the diagnosis and management of intravascular catheter-related infection: 2009 update by the Infectious Diseases Society of America. *Clin Infect Dis*. 2009;**49**:1–45.

168 Freifeld AG, Bow EJ, Sepkowitz KA, et al. Clinical practice guideline for the use of antimicrobial agents in neutropenic patients with cancer: 2010 update by the infectious diseases society of america. *Clin Infect Dis*. 2011;**52**:e56–e93.

172 Klastersky J, Paesmans M, Rubenstein EB, et al. The multinational association for supportive care in cancer risk index: a multinational scoring system for identifying low-risk febrile neutropenic cancer patients. *J Clin Oncol*. 2000;**18**:3038–3051.

184 Flowers CR, Seidenfeld J, Bow EJ, et al. Antimicrobial prophylaxis and outpatient management of fever and neutropenia in adults treated for malignancy: American Society of Clinical Oncology clinical practice guideline. *J Clin Oncol*. 2013;**31**:794–810.

185 Baden LR, Bensinger W, Angarone M, et al. Prevention and treatment of cancer-related infections. *J Natl Compr Canc Netw*. 2012;**10**:1412–1445.

192 Smith TJ, Khatcheressian J, Lyman GH, et al. 2006 update of recommendations for the use of white blood cell growth factors: an evidence-based clinical practice guideline. *J Clin Oncol*. 2006;**24**:3187–3205.

195 Bucaneve G, Micozzi A, Menichetti F, et al. Levofloxacin to prevent bacterial infection in patients with cancer and neutropenia. *N Engl J Med*. 2005;**353**:977–987.

196 Cullen M, Steven N, Billingham L, et al. Antibacterial prophylaxis after chemotherapy for solid tumors and lymphomas. *N Engl J Med*. 2005;**353**:988–998.

197 Gafter-Gvili A, Fraser A, Paul M, et al. Antibiotic prophylaxis for bacterial infections in afebrile neutropenic patients following chemotherapy. *Cochrane Database Syst Rev*. 2012;**1**:CD004386.

203 van Burik JA, Ratanatharathorn V, Stepan DE, et al. Micafungin versus fluconazole for prophylaxis against invasive fungal infections during neutropenia in patients undergoing hematopoietic stem cell transplantation. *Clin Infect Dis*. 2004;**39**:1407–1416.

205 Cornely OA, Maertens J, Winston DJ, et al. Posaconazole vs. fluconazole or itraconazole prophylaxis in patients with neutropenia. *N Engl J Med*. 2007;**356**:348–359.

206 Dellit TH, Owens RC, McGowan JE, et al. Infectious diseases society of America and the Society for Healthcare Epidemiology of America guidelines for developing an institutional program to enhance antimicrobial stewardship. *Clin Infect Dis*. 2007;**44**:159–177.

209 Tverdek FP, Rolston KV, Chemaly RF. Antimicrobial stewardship in patients with cancer. *Pharmacotherapy*. 2012;**32**:722–734.

Sai-Ching Jim Yeung, MD, PhD, FACP ■ *Carmen P. Escalante, MD*

Overview

Cancer and its treatment can lead to oncologic emergencies. This chapter discusses the approach to acute emergency problems in cancer patients. A list of emergent problems has been selected for focused discussion. Sudden cardiopulmonary arrest is discussed along with special consideration in resuscitation of cancer patients. Arrhythmia, superior vena caval syndrome, pericardial tamponade, and acute hemorrhage are important cardiovascular emergencies. Tumor lysis syndrome can be rapidly fatal, and early recognition and treatment are very important in preventing disastrous outcomes. Pulmonary problems include airway obstruction, pleural effusion, hemoptysis, pneumothorax, and pulmonary embolism. Neurological emergencies include spinal cord compression, brain herniation, and status epilepticus. Neutropenic fever is perhaps the most frequently discussed important topic in oncologic emergency. Other important issues such as perforated viscus, anaphylaxis, and cytokine release syndrome are also discussed. Oncologists and emergency physicians must be aware of these potentially serious acute complications of cancer patients in order to initiate appropriate treatments in a timely manner.

Introduction

An oncologic emergency is an acute condition that is caused by cancer or its treatment and that requires intervention as soon as possible to avoid mortality or severe morbidity. Cancer patients are more likely to require emergency care than noncancer patients. Physical debilitation, altered hemostasis, and impaired immunity due to malignancy or its treatment also make cancer patients vulnerable to accidents and mishaps in everyday life. Because cancer patients have unique concerns and changes in physiological status, emergency care providers need to adapt to their special needs.

The emergency care of cancer patients is evolving into a hybrid discipline—a cross between oncology and emergency medicine. There are many types of problems for which cancer patients present to an emergency care facility, and in-depth discussions would fill volumes.[1-3] Because of page constraints and coverage of some relevant topics in other chapters of this book, this chapter will cover only selected topics.

Approach to acutely Ill cancer patients

Cancer patients often have comorbidities such as coronary heart disease, diabetes mellitus, and chronic obstructive pulmonary disease. Some of these may be attributable to the same risk factors for carcinogenesis (i.e., old age, diet, cigarette smoking, or sedentary lifestyle). Emergency care providers caring must assess the extent of the malignancy, the response to treatment, the overall prognosis, and the patient's and family's wishes in order to formulate an appropriate treatment plan (Figure 1). The majority of cancer patients who are approaching their ends of life do not want "heroic" measures, and addressing advance directives and do-not-resuscitate (DNR) orders in a timely manner may improve the quality of life in the weeks before death.[4]

First, the patient should be rapidly assessed. This assessment should include the chief complaint, a focused history, vital signs, and a quick overall physical assessment. If the patient is unable to relay the history of present illness, a family member, companion, or caregiver may provide pertinent information. Intervention for unstable vital signs should be initiated immediately. In case of cardiopulmonary arrest, appropriate guidelines are followed (http://www.acls.net/aclsalg.htm).[5] Once the patient is stabilized, thorough history and physical examination should be completed. For the majority of cancer patients with emergencies, a comprehensive evaluation is necessary. The emergency may be due to the cancer, cancer treatments, or comorbid conditions, all of which should be considered in the differential diagnosis.

Circulatory oncologic emergencies

Sudden cardiopulmonary arrest

Most deaths are preceded by cardiopulmonary arrest. Resuscitation is more likely to succeed when cardiopulmonary arrest was caused by an acute reversible insult rather than by a steady irreversible decline in bodily functions. The success rate of resuscitation and the hospital discharge rate of resuscitated patients are similar for cancer patients and noncancer patients.[6] A meta-analysis of inpatient resuscitation (including cancer patients) estimated that the probabilities of successful resuscitation and being discharged alive are about 30% and 12%, respectively.[7] Similarly, for cancer patients with out-of-hospital arrest who received resuscitation at the Emergency Department of a cancer center, the probabilities of successful resuscitation and being discharged alive are 43% and 17%, respectively.[8] The mortality rate of cancer patients in intensive care is about 50%, which is similar to that of severely ill non-cancer patients.[9] If a cancer patient has good performance status and is not expected to die soon, reluctance to resuscitate the patient or admit the patient to intensive care is unjustified. A non-end stage cancer patient in cardiopulmonary arrest should be resuscitated with the same level of intense effort as any noncancer patient. However, when cardiopulmonary arrest occurs as the expected final event, resuscitation is generally futile.

Oncologists should ensure that advance directives (medical power of attorney, living will, and out-of-hospital DNR orders) are discussed with cancer patients and their families. Many informed patients readily sign living wills or appoint health care proxies. Timely recommendation of DNR status may avoid unnecessary trauma to patients, futile efforts, wasted resources, and anguish

Holland-Frei Cancer Medicine, Ninth Edition. Edited by Robert C. Bast Jr., Carlo M. Croce, William N. Hait, Waun Ki Hong, Donald W. Kufe, Martine Piccart-Gebhart, Raphael E. Pollock, Ralph R. Weichselbaum, Hongyang Wang, and James F. Holland.
© 2017 John Wiley & Sons, Inc. ISBN: 978-1-118-93469-2

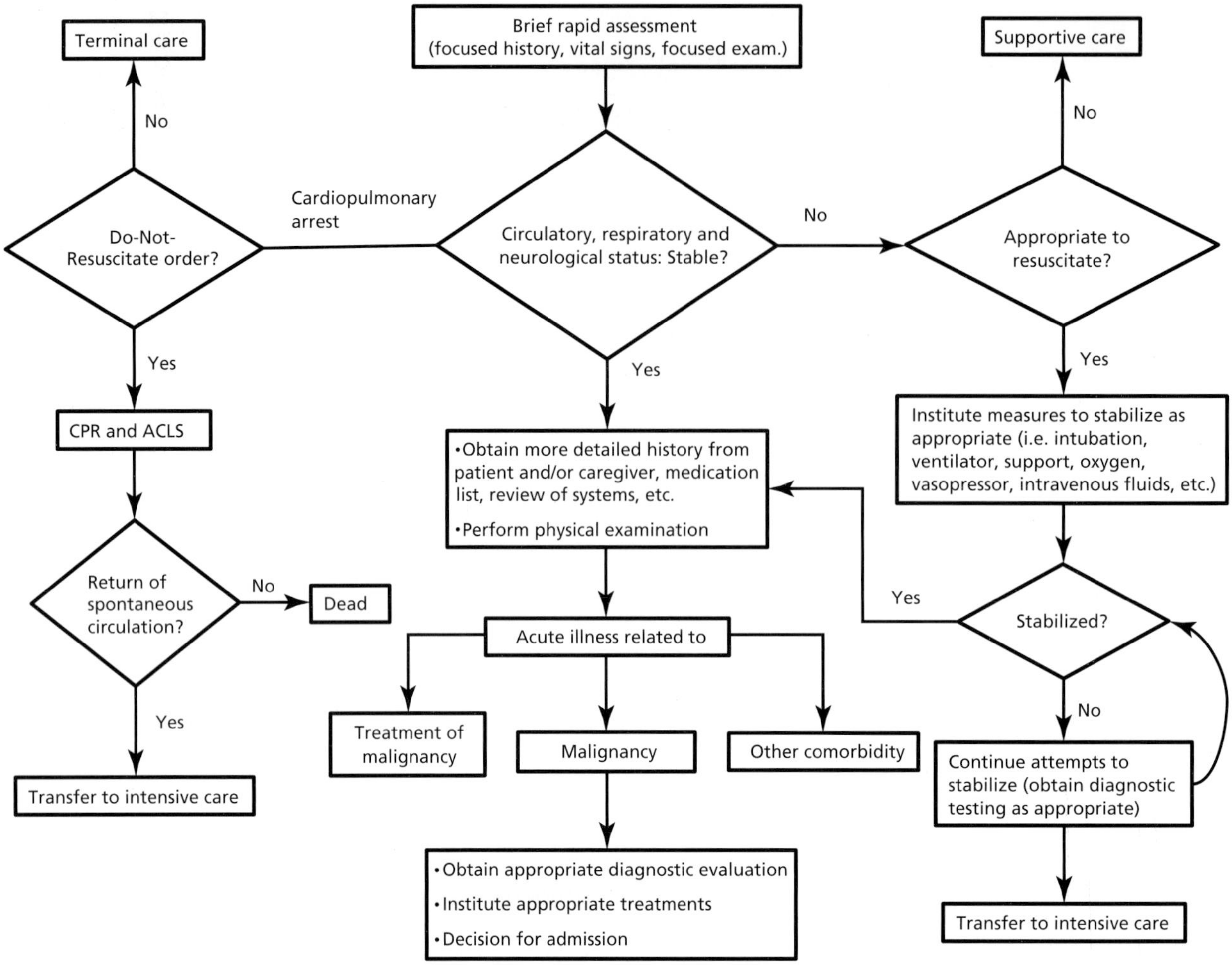

Figure 1 Approach to acutely ill cancer patients.

for family members; this also provides time for open discussion to settle disagreements among the patient and family members.

When a cancer patient presents to a health care facility in impending or full cardiopulmonary arrest, the emergency physician may have never seen the patient before, and assessment of prognosis is difficult and often impossible. The decision to initiate or continue resuscitation should be based on a rapid assessment of the patient's physical condition, a brief history of the events preceding the arrest, and the following factors: (1) duration of arrest, (2) initial cardiac rhythm, (3) rigor mortis or algor mortis, (4) type, stage, and prognosis of cancer, (5) history of cancer treatment and prospects for its success, (6) expressed directives of the patient or family, (7) comorbid conditions, (8) performance status and nutritional status, (9) potential quality of life if the patient survives, and (10) advanced age.

The fact that the patient was transported to an emergency center may indicate that death is unexpected, that the family has not yet accepted the patient's grave prognosis, or that the patient or family is seeking relief of symptoms or suffering at the last moments of life. Demands for resuscitation may be motivated by denial of the terminal condition. A questionnaire-based study has found that most cancer patients want to be resuscitated despite poor survival rates, and that they want themselves and their next of kin to be involved in the decision-making process.[10] In the absence of clear advance directive, resuscitation may be needed to give the family "closure" by knowing that "everything possible has been done."

However, resuscitation of patients with advanced refractory malignancies may be inappropriate when it will only prolong pain and suffering.

Special consideration in resuscitation of cancer patients

Most physicians and health care providers follow the resuscitation algorithms outlined in the advanced cardiac life support (ACLS) protocols (http://www.acls.net/aclsalg.htm).[5] However, identification of specific causes of cardiopulmonary arrest may enable physicians to target efforts to reverse or control the specific causes. Carcinoid crisis is a good example of an uncommon but preventable and treatable cause of cardiopulmonary arrest in cancer patients. The crisis may be precipitated by anesthesia, biopsy, surgery, chemotherapy, or adrenergic drugs (e.g., dopamine and epinephrine). Affected patients may develop refractory hypotension, arrhythmias, and bronchospasm due to massive release of serotonin and other vasoactive peptides from the tumor. Carcinoid crisis can be aborted or treated with octreotide acetate, a somatostatin analog, 150–500 μg intravenously (IV).[11] Cardiac tamponade is another example. If a patient has pulseless electrical activity due to tamponade by a malignant pericardial effusion, resuscitation will not succeed until the pressure on the cardiac chambers is relieved by pericardiocentesis.

Causes of cardiac arrest in cancer patients

In the general population, undiagnosed neoplasm is a rare cause of sudden death. In cancer patients, a review of causes of death found that 4% of patients died of cardiac problems and that 90% of these died from atherosclerosis-related ischemic heart disease.[12] Most causes of cardiopulmonary arrests in cancer patients are related to cancer or antineoplastic therapy, rather than primary cardiac disease.

Tumor-related causes

Tumor-related cardiac problems are usually the result of pericardial involvement (e.g., neoplastic pericarditis and cardiac tamponade). Tumors can induce arrhythmias by secretion of hormone mediators (e.g., catecholamines by pheochromocytomas and serotonin by carcinoid tumors) or by direct mechanical irritation of the heart or pericardium. Arrhythmias associated with myocardial tumors, coronary obstruction by tumor, and massive tumor embolization have been reported to cause sudden cardiopulmonary arrest. Cardiac amyloidosis can also lead to intractable congestive heart failure, arrhythmias, conduction disturbances, and sudden death.[13] Other tumor-related causes of arrest include hemorrhage, loss of ventilatory function, and organ failure.

Systemic therapy-related causes

Antineoplastic agents can cause complications (angina, myocardial infarction, congestive heart failure, hypotension, arrhythmia) leading to cardiopulmonary arrest.[14] Doxorubicin may cause electrocardiographic and rhythm changes (mostly benign) in about 30% of patients[15] and sudden cardiopulmonary arrest in almost 1% of patients.[16] Some drugs (e.g., imatinib, trastuzumab) may interfere with myocardial remodeling after cytotoxic myocardial damage, causing cardiomyopathy and heart failure.[15] High-dose cyclophosphamide may cause ventricular arrhythmia, cardiomyopathy, pericardial effusion, and cardiac arrest.[17] Fluorouracil and capecitabine are associated with acute coronary vasospasm leading to angina and myocardial infarction; they have also been reported to cause acute cardiogenic shock. Hypotension, arrhythmia, and sudden death have been reported with cytokines (interleukin-2 [IL-2], interferons) and monoclonal antibodies.

Radiotherapy-related causes

Radiation can damage the pericardium and heart.[18] Pericarditis may occur shortly or months to years after exposure of the chest to radiation. Radiotherapy can lead to valvular diseases, pericardial effusion, tamponade, pericardial fibrosis, or restrictive cardiomyopathy. The direct toxic effect of radiation can cause electrocardiographic changes, including T-wave abnormalities and atrial arrhythmias. Exposure of the heart to radiation is also associated with coronary artery problems (accelerated atherosclerosis, endarteritis, medial fibrosis, intimal proliferation), leading to myocardial infarction and sudden death.[19]

Arrhythmia

Arrhythmia is a common problem in cancer patients that needs emergency care. Sustained arrhythmia can lead to cardiopulmonary arrest and death; otherwise, the symptoms of intermittent arrhythmia can be subtle. The symptoms are primarily due to the hemodynamic effects. Significant signs and symptoms include isolated or recurrent loss of consciousness (syncope), light-headedness (dizziness), palpitation, chest pain, dyspnea, and acute neurologic deficits.

Sustained arrhythmia can be diagnosed electrographically readily. However, arrhythmia is often transient or intermittent, causing difficulty in diagnosis. An electrocardiographic rhythm strip or a brief period of continuous monitoring does not exclude latent and potentially serious rhythm disorders. When symptoms suggest arrhythmia, Holter monitoring for 24–48 h or event recorders (continuous loop, postevent, or real-time continuous) are indicated to capture the arrhythmia. Analysis of cardiac rhythm may be complicated in cancer patients because they often have exaggerated respiratory variations of the electrical axis and changes in mean QRS voltage that can be confused with heart rhythm irregularity. Such changes may be due to pleural or pericardial effusions, pulmonary surgery (pneumonectomy or lobectomy), or radiation-induced lung damage.

Primary arrhythmia

Primary arrhythmia arises from cardiac and pericardial structures. Common causes of primary arrhythmia in all patients include ischemic disease; increased intracardiac pressure and wall stress; congestive, hypertrophic, and infiltrative cardiomyopathy; and fibrosis. In cancer patients, the causes of primary arrhythmia are primary or metastatic intracardiac tumors, amyloid infiltration, myocarditis, pericarditis, pericardial constriction, and cardiomyopathy related to antineoplastic agents (especially anthracyclines and anti-HER2 therapy).[14]

Secondary arrhythmia

Secondary arrhythmia arises from toxic reactions to drugs; increased sympathetic states (severe anxiety, hyperthyroidism, pheochromocytomas, carcinoid tumors, etc.); abnormal electrolytes; and radiation-induced heart damage. Some cancer drugs are arrhythmogenic (Table 1).[20-24] In addition to chemotherapy, antifungal agents, antiprotozoans, and antibiotics, which are commonly used to treat infectious complications in cancer patients, may prolong the QT interval [listed at http://www.qtdrugs.org (Arizona Center for Education and Research on Therapeutics)], potentially leading to arrhythmia.

Treatment of arrhythmia

Treatment of arrhythmia should be based on both urgency and etiology. For hemodynamically stable arrhythmias of secondary origins, the primary treatment should focus on correcting metabolic derangements (particularly potassium, calcium, and magnesium) and discontinuing culprit drugs. Specific treatment to reverse the causative factor should be administered. When treatment aimed at controlling the cardiac rhythm is necessary, standard guidelines for management of arrhythmia may be followed.[5] Commonly used IV antiarrhythmic drugs are listed in Table 2.

Paroxysmal supraventricular tachycardia (SVT) may be converted back into sinus rhythm in a considerable proportion of cases by vagal maneuvers. Adenosine administered as one or two doses of rapidly injected boluses under electrocardiographic monitoring is frequently effective in restoring sinus heart rhythm. Adenosine is also used to determine the mechanism of the arrhythmia when the diagnosis is unclear on electrocardiograms.

Stable secondary arrhythmia is unlikely to deteriorate into a life-threatening catastrophe. Frequently, secondary arrhythmia presents as ventricular ectopy (sometimes in bigeminy, trigeminy, or other coupled patterns), or supraventricular ectopy (often as intermittent or sustained SVT). Isolated premature ventricular complexes do not require any treatment. Complex forms of ventricular ectopy are often controlled by β-adrenergic blockers.

Table 1 Antineoplastic drugs associated with cardiovascular side effects.

	Pulmonary HTN	Systemic HTN	Ischemia	Reduction in LVEF	QT prolongation	VT/Sudden death	Bradycardia	AF/SVT
Tyrosine kinase inhibitors								
Imatinib	Reported			0.5–1.7%				
Dasatinib	Reported			2–4%	<1–3%			
Cabozantinib		33%			Mean increase of QTcF by10–15 ms; No QTcF >500 ms			
Lapatinib				1.5–4%	16%			
Erlotinib			2.3%					
Nilotinib	Reported	10–11%			1–10%; QTcF > 500 ms in 1%	Reported		
Pazopanib		40–42%		8–11%	QTcF > 500 ms in 0.2–2%	Torsades de pointes in <1%		
Sorafenib		9–43%	2.7–3%	12%	No large changes (i.e., <20 ms)			
Sunitinib		5–47%		2.7–27%	Dose-dependent	Torsades de pointes in 0.1%		
Vandetanib		33%			QTcF > 500 ms in 1%	Reported		
Antibodies								
Bevacizumab		4–35%	0.6–1.5%	1.7–3%				
Trastuzumab		4%		2–28%				
Alkylating agents								
Cisplatin	Reported	Reported	Reported	Reported		Reported		Reported
Ifosfamide				17%				Reported
Cyclophosphamide			Reported	7–28%				Reported
Busulfan				Reported				
Mitomycin				Reported				
Anthracyclines/anthraquinones								
Daunorubicin				Reported				
Doxorubicin				3–26% 5% at the cumulative dose of 400–450 mg/m²		6%	Reported	2.2–10.3%
Idarubicin				5–18%				
Epirubicin				0.9–3.3%				
Mitoxantrone				Reported				
Antimetabolites								
Capecitabine			3–9%	Cardiogenic shock reported		2.1%		
5-Fluorouracil			1–68%	Cardiogenic shock reported				4.2–6.5%
Gemcitabine								8.2%
Cytarabine				Reported				
Clofarabine				27%				
Topoisomerase I inhibitors								
Irinotecan							Reported	
Taxanes								
Paclitaxel			<1–5%			0.26%	<0.1–31%	0.18%
Docetaxel			1.7%	2.3–8%				
Vinca alkaloids								
Vincristine			Reported					
Vinblastine			Reported					
Miscellaneous								
IL-2				Reported		0.2%		17.4%
Arsenic trioxide					26%			
Vorinostat					3.5–6%			
Interferon-α			1%	Reported				1%
Tretinoin (retinoic acid)				Reported				
Bortezomib				2–5%				
Thalidomide							0.12–55%	
Pentostatin				Reported				

Abbreviations: AF, atrial fibrillation; HTN, hypertension; LVEF, left ventricular ejection fraction; QTcF, QT interval corrected by Fridericia's formula; SVT, supraventricular tachycardia; VT, ventricular tachycardia.

Source: Data from Yeh et al. 20, Lenihan and Kowey 21, Guglin et al. 22, Yeh and Bickford 23, and Ewer and Ewer 24.

Table 2 Commonly used IV antiarrhythmic drugs.

Name	Class	Dose[a]	Indication[a]
Adenosine	Nucleoside	6 mg IV over <3 s followed by NS 20 mL bolus; second dose and third dose of 12 mg 2 min apart as needed	Narrow complex PSVT; PSVT due to AV node or sinus node reentry
Amiodarone	Class III antiarrhythmic	Cardiac arrest: 300 mg IVP; 150 mg IVP q 3–5 min up to 2.2 g/day	
		Stable wide-complex tachycardia: 150 mg IV over 10 min; repeat q 10 min as needed; maintenance infusion 0.5 mg/min; up to 2.2 g/day	Supraventricular or ventricular tachyarrhythmias; control of rapid atrial tachyarrhythmia in patients with low LVEF when digoxin is ineffective
Atropine	Anticholinergic	0.5–1 mg IVP q 3–5 min as needed, up to 0.04 mg/kg	Symptomatic sinus bradycardia; Mobitz type 1 AV block; asystole
Digoxin	Digitalis glycoside	Loading dose: 10–15 μg/kg lean body weight in divided doses	To slow ventricular response in A. fib. or A. flutter; PSVT
Diltiazem	Calcium channel blocker	0.25 mg/kg IV over 2 min; second dose 0.35 mg/kg IV over 2 min in 15 min prn; maintenance: 5–15 mg/h by titration	To slow ventricular response in A. fib. or A. flutter; PSVT; to terminate AV nodal re-entrant tachycardia
Esmolol	β-Blocker	0.5 mg/kg over 1 min; then infuse at 0.05 mg/kg/min; titrate up to maximum of 0.3 mg/kg/min	PSVT, A. fib. or A. flutter; Reduce incidence of VF in MI or USA
Ibutilide	Class III antiarrhythmic	1 mg IV over 10 min; repeat in 10 min prn	SVT including A. fib. A. flutter; effective for conversion of A. fib. flutter of relatively brief duration
Isoproterenol	β-Agonist	Infuse 2–10 μg/min; titrate	Symptomatic bradycardia; torsades de pointes refractory to Mg; β-blocker overdose
Lidocaine	Local anesthetic	1–1.5 mg/kg IVP; repeat 0.5–0.75 mg/kg IVP q 5–10 min up to total of 3 mg/kg prn; maintenance: 30–50 μg/kg/min IV	VT or VF; wide-complex tachycardia; significant ventricular ectopy; torsades de pointes
Metoprolol	β-Blocker	5 mg slow IVP q 5 min up to a total dose of 15 mg	PSVT, A. fib., or A. flutter; Reduce incidence of VF in MI or USA
Procainamide hydrochloride	Class IA antiarrhythmic	20–50 mg/min up to a total dose of 17 mg/kg	Recurrent VF or VT
Propranolol	β-Blocker	0.1 mg/kg slow IVP in three divided doses 2–3 min apart	PSVT, A. fib., or A. flutter; Reduce incidence of VF in MI or USA
Quinidine gluconate	Class IA antiarrhythmic	Intermittent bolus doses of 80 mg every 5–10 min or 10 mg/min IV infusion up to 400 mg	Supraventricular and ventricular arrhythmias
Verapamil	Calcium channel blocker	2.5–5 mg IV over 2 min; repeat q 15–30 min prn up to a total dose of 20 mg	PSVT, A. fib., or A. flutter

Abbreviations: A. fib., atrial fibrillation; A. flutter, atrial flutter; AV, atrioventricular; IV, intravenous; IVP, intravenous push; LVEF, left ventricular ejection fraction; MI, myocardial infarction; NS, normal saline; prn, as needed; PSVT, paroxysmal supraventricular tachycardia; USA, unstable angina; VF, ventricular fibrillation; VT, ventricular tachycardia.
[a]Source: From ACLS Provider Manual.[5]

Amiodarone should be considered for patients with a low left ventricular ejection fraction, but with caution for patients with hepatic insufficiency or underlying thyroid diseases. Rarely, amiodarone can cause hypotension, bradycardia, and QT prolongation that may precipitate torsades de pointes. Except for β-adrenergic blockers, many antiarrhythmic drugs, especially types 1A, 1C, and 3, are potentially proarrhythmic.[25] Cardiac monitoring during the initiation of antiarrhythmic therapy should be considered because cancer patients may have an increased susceptibility to proarrhythmic effects due to metabolic derangements and concomitant use of other QT-prolonging drugs.

SVT is the most common arrhythmia in cancer patients. Although pharmacological agents are used for sustained SVT with stable hemodynamics, elective synchronized cardioversion under conscious sedation should be considered early and planned appropriately. The initial energy level for synchronized cardioversion recommended by the American Heart Association is 100 J, but an initial shock with an energy level of 200 J has been recommended by others for the conversion of atrial fibrillation.[26] Higher energy levels for cardioversion are appropriate when cancer patients have concomitant effusions or are significantly overweight. If sinus rhythm can be restored within 48 h of the onset of SVT, anticoagulation therapy may be avoided. However, the time of onset of arrhythmia is not always clear. Intracardiac thrombosis may be excluded by transesophageal echocardiography. In lack of clear evidence for the time of onset, the patient should be anticoagulated prior to cardioversion.

Arrhythmias of structural origin in cancer patients are more difficult to control than arrhythmias of metabolic etiology. In the emergency setting, the therapeutic goals are stabilization of hemodynamics and respiratory status, discovery of correctable pathologic conditions, and control of symptoms. Depending on the etiology of the arrhythmia, emergent consultation with cardiologists and emergent diagnostic or interventional procedures may be required.

Patients with unstable arrhythmia should be treated with aggressive pharmacological or electrical interventions. The interventions should follow established algorithms such as those by the American Heart Association.[27] These interventions include administration of a vasopressor, such as vasopressin or epinephrine (if required); administration of antiarrhythmic drugs such as amiodarone, lidocaine, and procainamide; electrical cardioversion or defibrillation; airway management; ventilation with oxygen; administration of IV fluid; and chest compression (if required). Emergency treatment of torsades de pointes varies from the standard algorithms for ventricular tachycardia; it entails expedient use of IV magnesium sulfate, electrical overdrive pacing, pharmacological overdrive with isoproterenol, or administration of phenytoin or lidocaine.

Tumor lysis syndrome

Tumor lysis syndrome (TLS) consists of severe hyperphosphatemia, hyperkalemia, hyperuricemia, azotemia, hypocalcemia, and metabolic acidosis (out of proportion to renal insufficiency) due to the massive release of cell contents and degradation products of dead tumor cells into the bloodstream.[28] TLS can occur spontaneously, but it usually occurs within 72 h after chemotherapy in patients with leukemia and lymphoma, but new therapeutic regimens may alter the timing of onset. TLS can also occur in patients with nonhematologic malignancies, including small cell carcinomas, nonsmall cell lung cancer, breast cancer, and ovarian cancer.

The symptoms of TLS are nonspecific. Common symptoms include nausea, vomiting, cloudy urine, weakness, fatigue, and arthralgia. Other signs and symptoms related to metabolic and electrolyte abnormalities include neuromuscular irritability, seizures, muscle weakness, and arrhythmia. Arrhythmia may cause sudden death in patients with TLS.[29] Precipitation of uric acid in the renal tubules may lead to nephropathy and acute renal failure.[30] The acute cause of death in TLS is arrhythmia secondary to severe electrolyte abnormalities (especially hyperkalemia) and renal failure. Early recognition of metabolic abnormalities and prompt treatment can avoid fatal outcomes.

Factors associated with increased risk of TLS include the type of malignancy (e.g., acute lymphocytic leukemia, acute myeloid leukemia with white blood cell count > 75,000/μL, Burkitt's lymphoma), responsiveness to therapy, rapid malignant cell turnover, and large tumor burden.[31] Other risk factors are preexisting renal insufficiency, acute renal failure developing shortly after the treatment, and poor response to hydration. Pretreatment serum lactate dehydrogenase levels, which tend to correlate with tumor bulk in lymphoma or lymphocytic leukemia, can predict the development of posttreatment azotemia, but pretreatment hyperuricemia is not predictive. A predictive scoring system for TLS has been proposed based on data from acute myelocytic leukemia patients undergoing induction therapy.[32,33] The score may potentially be used in a risk-based prophylaxis for TLS. Preventive measures should be started early in patients at risk. Aggressive hydration with IV crystalloid fluid up to 3 L/m^2/day may maintain a urine output >100 mL/h with or without diuretics. The xanthine oxidase inhibitor allopurinol (100–300 mg/day orally) may prevent severe hyperuricemia. The role of febuxostat, a new xanthine oxidase inhibitor, remains to be studied.

The diagnosis of TLS requires a high level of suspicion because there are few signs or symptoms in the early stage. Routine uric acid and electrolyte screening (including measurement of calcium and phosphorus levels) is indicated in patients with high tumor bulk or hematologic malignancies. The diagnosis of TLS may be based on the Cairo–Bishop definition.[31,34] Once diagnosed, patients with severe TLS should have continuous monitoring of hemodynamic and electrocardiographic parameters in intensive care. The allopurinol dose may be increased up to 900 mg/day. Rasburicase, a recombinant urate oxidase that converts uric acid to allantoin, is highly efficacious in reducing uric acid level. Rasburicase (150–200 μg/kg IV daily or one-time dosing with a rescue dose as needed) may be used to prevent or treat urate nephropathy.[35] Increased IV fluid hydration may be coupled with diuresis using loop diuretics (e.g., furosemide, 20–200 mg IV every 4–6 h) and acetazolamide (250–500 mg IV daily). Urinary alkalinization by sodium bicarbonate or acetate IV infusion to increase the solubility of urate in urine should only be considered in cases of severe hyperuricemia when rasburicase is not available. Frequent electrolyte measurements (every 4–6 h) may be required. Hyperkalemia should be treated with insulin plus dextrose, calcium, and bicarbonate IV along with oral potassium ion-exchange resins (sodium polystyrene sulfonate). In hyperphosphatemic patients with hypocalcemia, the addition of an oral calcium-based compound (e.g., calcium acetate or calcium carbonate) will reduce phosphate absorption and enhance calcium absorption. IV calcium infusion can potentially cause calcium phosphate precipitation in the presence of severe hyperphosphatemia and should be used cautiously. Dialysis may be required for patients with symptomatic hypocalcemia and a serum phosphorus level >3.3 mmol/L (>10.2 mg/dL). Other indications for dialysis include persistent or refractory azotemia, hyperkalemia, hyperuricemia, oliguria, anuria despite diuretic use, acidemia, and volume overload. Prompt dialysis should be instituted with continued monitoring until biochemical abnormalities resolve. Hemodialysis is the most common mode of dialysis; prolonged hemodialysis sessions, continuous arteriovenous hemodialysis, continuous veno-venous hemofiltration, and continuous renal replacement therapy at a high dialysate or replacement fluid flow rate (>3 L/h) are alternative methods.

Pericardial tamponade

Pericardial tamponade occurs when a pericardial effusion impairs hemodynamics. Accumulation of excess fluid in the pericardial space in cancer patients is due to obstruction of lymphatic drainage and/or excess fluid secretion from tumor nodules on pericardial surfaces. Mesothelioma is the most common malignancy that arises from the pericardium. Carcinoma of the lung and malignant thymoma may involve the pericardium by direct extension. More frequently, malignancies arrive at the pericardium by retrograde lymphangitic spread or hematogenous dissemination. Melanoma is the malignancy most likely to metastasize to the heart. Lymphomas, leukemias, and gastrointestinal neoplasms may also cause pericardial effusions.[36] Cytologic examination of pericardial fluid reveals metastatic disease in 70–80% of cancer patients with pericardial effusion. Nonmalignant causes of pericardial tamponade include pericardial abscess, Candida pericarditis, and complications of central venous catheterization.

Malignant pericardial effusion usually occurs in advanced malignancy and is associated with poor prognosis (median survival time: about 6 months; 1-year survival rate: 28%).[37] More than two-thirds of patients with malignant pericardial effusion are asymptomatic. In symptomatic patients, common complaints are shortness of breath, dyspnea on exertion, chest pain, orthopnea, and general weakness. Findings on physical examination may vary from normal to hemodynamic collapse. Tachycardia, hypotension, jugular venous distention, organomegaly, and edema may indicate compromised cardiac output. The classic findings of cardiac tamponade are determined by both the quantity of pericardial fluid and the rapidity of fluid accumulation. Pulsus paradoxus, an exaggeration of the physiological decrease in systolic blood pressure with inspiration, is a classic but nonspecific finding of cardiac tamponade because it is seen also in patients with lung cancer, significant lung disease, or cor pulmonale.

Diagnosis of pericardial tamponade usually requires additional testing. Low QRS voltage and electrical alternans in electrocardiographs are suggestive findings. Chest radiographs may reveal widening of the mediastinum and cardiac silhouette (Figure 2a, b). Computed tomography (CT) or magnetic resonance (MR) imaging studies frequently detect pericardial effusions as an incidental finding. These studies provide information on the location (loculated or not) and size of pericardial effusions but do not adequately assess the hemodynamic significance. Two-dimensional echocardiography is the most useful test for diagnosing pericardial effusion and

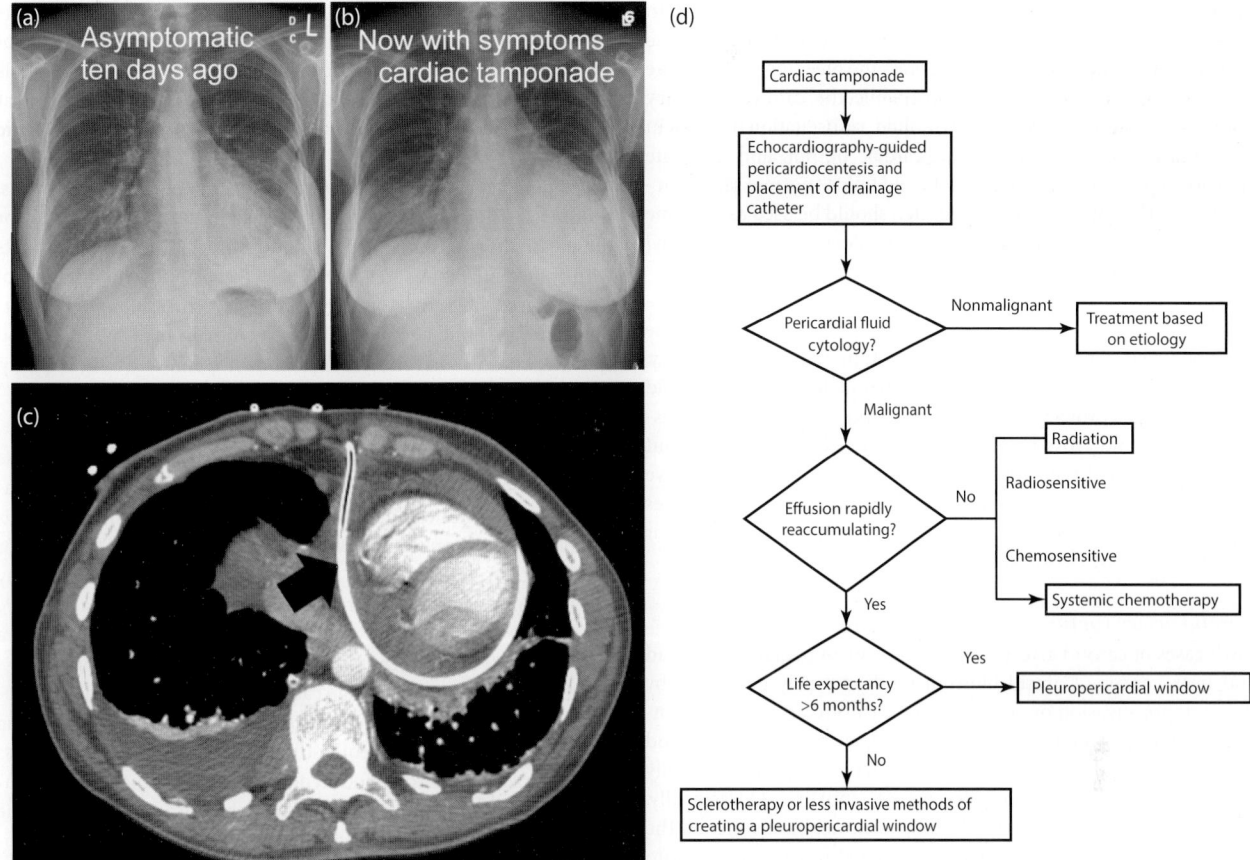

Figure 2 Chest imaging of patients with pericardial tamponade and management algorithm. Widening of mediastinum and cardiac silhouette is evident (b) when compared with a prior chest radiograph (a). Chest CT of a different patient with pericardial tamponade shows the presence of an indwelling drainage catheter (c). An algorithm for management of pericardial effusion is shown (d).

evaluating its hemodynamic significance, that is, the presence of cardiac tamponade. Collapse or compression of the right atrium, diastolic collapse of the right ventricle, and cardiac "rocking" (side-to-side or front-to-back movement) are often observed in cardiac tamponade. Alterations in the respiratory variation of flow across the mitral valve as measured by Doppler shift are also helpful in evaluating the hemodynamics.

Initial management of malignant pericardial effusion depends on the hemodynamic stability. A scoring system may guide the decision for urgent pericardiocentesis.[38] In patients with hemodynamic compromise, ultrasound-guided pericardiocentesis, with placement of a drainage catheter into the pericardial space (Figure 2c), may be performed emergently in the emergency center or intensive care unit (Figure 2d). Complications are rare and may include massive pericardial bleeding and pneumothorax. Pericardial fluid can be drained from the catheter, and the catheter can stay until <50 mL/day of fluid is drained. Fibrinolytic agents may be used to unclog the catheter to facilitate drainage and avoid repeat pericardiocentesis or replacement of the catheter.[39] However, pericardial fluid will usually reaccumulate after removal of the catheter.

Long-term management of malignant pericardial effusion focuses on preventing reaccumulation of fluid, which occurs in >50% of patients. Because the long-term survival for most patients with malignant pericardial effusion is limited, an effective therapy with limited discomfort and risk to the patient should be employed. Creation of a pleuropericardial window using a variety of approaches can avoid repeated pericardiocentesis. This surgical procedure is usually done in an operating room, but it can be performed in a

hospital room or intensive care unit using local anesthesia. The use of a percutaneous intrapericardial balloon catheter to create a pleuropericardial window has had some success.[40] A laparoscopic transdiaphragmatic approach to create a pericardioperitoneal shunt has also been described.[41] In stable patients, systemic chemotherapy, pericardial radioactive colloid, or thoracic external-beam irradiation may be used for tumors that are sensitive to these treatment modalities. Additional radiotherapy should be avoided in patients with significant prior exposure of the heart to radiation. Local application of cytotoxic agents or sclerosing agents to the pericardium can prevent fluid reaccumulation in many patients,[42] but sclerotherapy can be very painful.

Acute hemorrhage

Acute gastrointestinal bleeding and genitourinary bleeding are discussed in other chapters. Hemoptysis, which can rapidly compromise respiratory function, will be discussed later in this chapter. This section will cover some less frequent but serious bleeding events: carotid arterial rupture, splenic rupture, and retroperitoneal hemorrhage.

The manifestations of acute hemorrhage depend on the rate and the site of bleeding. In most cases, the site of bleeding is obvious, but sometimes bleeding can be internal and difficult to diagnose. Signs and symptoms of hypovolemia and hypoperfusion include tachycardia, hypotension, oliguria, and depressed mental status. Very often, diagnostic imaging studies or procedures, such as CT scans, ultrasonography, arteriography, or endoscopy, are necessary to diagnose internal bleeding.

The primary management objectives for acute hemorrhage are to rapidly identify the bleeding source and achieve hemostasis. In the acute setting, direct pressure to compress the bleeding vessel or site should be applied whenever feasible while the cardiopulmonary status is assessed expeditiously. IV fluid resuscitation is vital in maintaining intravascular volume, cardiac output, and adequate vital organ perfusion. Isotonic crystalloid fluids (normal saline, lactated Ringer's solution, PlasmaLyte, etc.) should be used as first-line agents because colloids (e.g., gelatins, dextrans, hydroxyethyl starches, albumin) have not been proven to improve survival.[43] Coagulopathy or thrombocytopenia should be corrected immediately by transfusion of blood products. The decision to transfuse red blood cells depends on the hematocrit, hemodynamic stability, persistence of hemorrhage, estimated blood loss, and comorbid diseases (e.g., coronary artery disease and cerebrovascular disease). Typed and cross-matched red blood cells are preferred, but noncross-matched type-specific blood or type-O blood may have to be used in life-threatening cases. Specific therapeutic procedures to control bleeding, such as embolization, balloon tamponade, or surgery, should be performed in a timely manner.

Carotid artery rupture

Most cases of carotid artery "blowout" occur in patients with head and neck cancers. Carotid blowout syndrome may be caused by direct tumor invasion or erosion into the carotid artery or by complications of cancer treatment, for example, postsurgical wound infection, postradiation necrosis, or orocutaneous fistula. It usually occurs as a sudden and massive arterial spurting. Occasionally, ominous minor and transient bleeding (sentinel bleeds) herald the massive blowout. In some cases, bleeding through a fistula into the esophagus or trachea may manifest as massive hematemesis or hemoptysis. Without prompt management, the patient's condition will rapidly deteriorate to hypotension, hypovolemic shock, loss of consciousness, and death.

Hemostasis is of utmost importance. As neck vessels are accessible to direct manual compression, continuous firm compression should be applied at the site of the carotid artery rupture until the patient arrives at the operating room for surgical treatment. Crystalloid IV fluid resuscitation, prompt transfusion of blood products, and administration of vasopressors should be performed to maintain perfusion of vital organs. Carotid artery rupture has limited surgical options, and surgical ligation of the bleeding carotid artery is associated with high morbidity (25% of patients have neurologic sequelae) and high mortality (40%).[44] Endovascular treatment with vessel sacrifice (embolization or balloon occlusion) or stent placement (covered stent) has become major treatment options.[45,46]

Splenic rupture

The spleen is fragile and vulnerable to rupture from trauma. In cancer patients, spontaneous splenic rupture is relatively rare and is associated with acute leukemia, non-Hodgkin's lymphoma, chronic myelogenous leukemia, hairy cell leukemia, and Hodgkin's lymphoma. Metastases to the spleen in patients with solid tumors such as gastric, prostate, and lung cancer can also cause rupture. The mechanism of spontaneous splenic rupture is not clear. Minor trauma to the spleen may contribute in some cases. Other contributing factors include splenomegaly, infiltration of the splenic capsule by malignant cells, splenic infarction, thrombocytopenia, coagulopathy, anticoagulation therapy, and disseminated intravascular coagulation.

The typical clinical presentation of splenic rupture involves pain in the left shoulder or abdomen (left upper quadrant), tachycardia, and hypotension. The severity of the signs and symptoms may depend on the extent of bleeding. Diagnostic peritoneal lavage is rarely used in nontraumatic cases; thus, the definitive diagnosis of splenic rupture relies on imaging studies. Contrast-enhanced CT is the diagnostic study of choice; ultrasonography can be performed at bedside for hemodynamically unstable patients to diagnose splenic rupture.[47]

For patients with splenic rupture and hematologic malignancies, prompt splenectomy is necessary because the mortality rate for these patients is extremely high without surgery. In selected patients with contraindications to surgery, selective arterial embolization of the ruptured site may stop the bleeding.[48] Other supportive treatments are IV fluid, supplemental oxygen, pain medications, blood transfusion, and correction of thrombocytopenia and coagulopathy.

Retroperitoneal hemorrhage

Damage to retroperitoneal organs or structures may cause retroperitoneal hemorrhage. Malignancies rarely cause spontaneous retroperitoneal hemorrhage; in such cases, the culprit is usually renal cell carcinoma or adrenal gland neoplasm (primary or metastatic). Anticoagulation, thrombocytopenia, and coagulopathy are predisposing factors. Retroperitoneal or intraperitoneal invasive procedures and placement of a central venous catheter through a femoral vessel can also cause severe retroperitoneal hemorrhage.

Retroperitoneal hemorrhage causes nonspecific signs and symptoms that vary according to the rate of bleeding and the underlying disease. Patients may present with abdominal pain, a tender mass in the flank, tachycardia, and hypotension. Some may have hematuria or hematochezia if the blood somehow finds its way into the ureter or gastrointestinal tract. It is difficult to establish a diagnosis of retroperitoneal hemorrhage on the basis of clinical findings. Maintaining a high level of clinical suspicion and performing early imaging studies are keys to the successful management of retroperitoneal hemorrhage. CT of the abdomen and pelvis is the noninvasive study most commonly used to diagnose retroperitoneal bleeding (Figure 3). Bedside ultrasonography may also rapidly diagnose retroperitoneal bleeding.

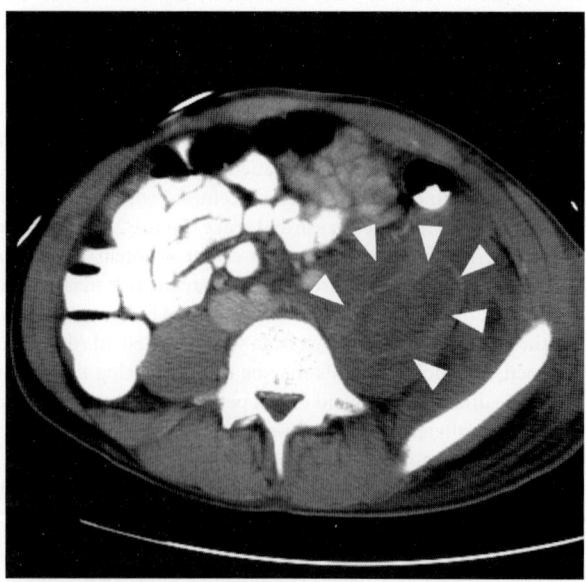

Figure 3 Retroperitoneal bleeding. The CT scan of the abdomen and pelvis of a thrombocytopenic leukemia patient showed a large inhomogeneous retroperitoneal collection (white arrowheads) consistent with a hematoma in the left psoas muscle displacing bowel loops to the right.

The management of retroperitoneal hemorrhage depends on the severity of bleeding and the underlying cause. After the initial stabilizing treatments for acute hemorrhage, the patient should be monitored closely for hemodynamic stability and continuation of blood loss. In life-threatening situations, most patients require emergent laparotomy to remove the bleeding tumor or organ.[49] Renal cell carcinomas are often hypervascular, and selective arterial embolization may control the bleeding of a renal lesion. External-beam radiation treatment of a bleeding tumor is another option in hemodynamically stable patients with a relatively stable hematocrit.[50]

Superior vena cava syndrome

Superior vena cava (SVC) syndrome refers to a constellation of signs and symptoms resulting from partial or complete obstruction of blood flow through the SVC to the right atrium. The obstruction may be caused by compression, invasion, thrombosis, or fibrosis of this vessel. Lung cancer is the leading cause of SVC syndrome; non-Hodgkin lymphoma is the second most common cause.[51,52] Although Hodgkin lymphoma commonly involves the mediastinum, it rarely causes SVC syndrome. Primary mediastinal malignancies such as thymoma and germ cell tumors account for <2% of SVC syndrome. Breast cancer is the most common metastatic disease that causes SVC syndrome;[53] other metastatic cancers include gastrointestinal adenocarcinoma, prostate adenocarcinoma, sarcomas, and melanoma. Nonmalignant causes of SVC syndrome include retrosternal goiter, pyogenic infections, sarcoidosis, teratoma, pleural calcification, silicosis, postradiation fibrosis, chemotherapy-induced fibrosis, constrictive pericarditis, and idiopathic mediastinal fibrosis.[52] An increasing cause of SVC syndrome in cancer patients is central venous catheter-induced thrombosis.

Obstruction of the SVC causes a rise in venous pressure in the SVC. Collateral venous circulation often flows through the azygos venous system. Obstruction below or at the entrance of the azygos veins forces blood to travel in the opposite direction down the azygos and chest wall veins to reach the inferior vena cava. SVC obstruction caused by tumors often develops insidiously over weeks. However, thrombosis may cause a rapid onset of obstruction. Sudden SVC obstruction is a true emergency because the rapid elevation of pressure in the SVC causes increased intracranial pressure, resulting in cerebral edema, intracranial thrombosis or bleeding, and death.

Common symptoms of SVC syndrome are a sensation of fullness and pressure in the head, cough, dyspnea, chest pain, and dysphagia. More significant symptoms include visual disturbances, hoarseness, stupor, seizure, and syncope. Typical signs include venous distention of the neck and chest wall, nonpitting edema of the neck, facial edema, facial plethora, tongue edema, proptosis, retinal vessel dilatation, stridor, and upper extremity edema. The signs and symptoms are exacerbated by lowering the upper body relative to the heart (i.e., bending forward, stooping, or lying down).

CT, especially contrast-enhanced spiral CT, is the most useful diagnostic study. It not only reveals the site of obstruction and collateral flow but also differentiates extrinsic compression of SVC by tumor from thrombosis. CT also provides anatomical details about the tumor and its surrounding structures, helping to guide biopsy procedures if a histologic diagnosis of the tumor has not been established previously. CT can also detect other emergent complications—such as proximal airway obstruction and pericardial effusion—that frequently coexist with SVC obstruction. If IV iodine contrast is contraindicated, radionuclide venography and MR imaging are alternatives. 3-D contrast-enhanced MR venography may be superior to CT, digital subtraction angiography,

and Doppler ultrasonography in detecting and determining the extent of thrombo-occlusive disease in chest vessels.[54] Contrast angiography for diagnosis of SVC syndrome is rarely indicated.

An algorithm for SVC syndrome is available (http://www.factsoncancertreatment.org.uk/index.php?option=com_alresource&keyword=S&catid=1&Itemid=107). The method for establishing the histologic cancer diagnosis may depend on the working diagnosis, location of the tumor, physical status of the patient, comorbid conditions, and available expertise of the health care facility. CT-guided needle biopsy is an alternative to surgical biopsy by thoracotomy or mediastinoscopy.[55] Bronchoscopy may provide the cancer diagnosis in up to 50% of patients with SVC syndrome. If lymph nodes are accessible, excisional biopsy can establish the diagnosis with minimal morbidity. Excisional biopsy is preferred if lymphoma is suspected because the histologic classification of lymphoma is firmly based on lymph node architecture.

In rare emergent situations of impending airway obstruction or increased intracranial pressure, endovascular interventions,[56] including angioplasty, SVC stenting, and pharmacomechanical thrombolysis, should be employed immediately. Stenting provides rapid symptomatic relief in the majority of patients and improves the quality of life. These stents usually remain patent for the rest of the patient's life.[57] Some authors recommend stenting as first-line treatment of SVC syndrome.[57,58] Stenting may relieve severe symptoms while the histologic diagnosis of the malignancy is being pursued, or when radiation or chemotherapy has failed or not yet taken effect.

Supplemental oxygen, bed rest with upper body elevation, and sedation may help to lessen the symptoms by lowering venous pressure and cardiac output. The use of diuretics may transiently decrease edema, but the efficacy of diuretics has not been proven, and overdiuresis causes dehydration, which should be avoided to minimize the risk of thrombosis. Corticosteroids (e.g., dexamethasone) may be useful in the presence of airway compromise or increased intracranial pressure. Anticoagulation is controversial despite the presence of superimposed thrombosis in up to 50% of SVC syndrome. Anticoagulation and thrombolysis may be beneficial in situations such as indwelling catheter-induced thrombosis or propagation of the thrombus into the brachiocephalic or subclavian system. However, anticoagulation increases the risk of intracranial bleeding, especially when intracranial pressure is elevated, and may complicate or delay biopsy procedures; therefore, it should be avoided unless a clear indication is identified.

Radiotherapy remains the principal treatment for many patients with malignant SVC syndrome, especially in recurrent disease after chemotherapy or chemo-insensitive tumors such as nonsmall cell lung cancer.[59] In general, radiotherapy is well tolerated, and SVC syndrome symptoms begin to improve in about 1 week. Radiotherapy is also justified if a histologic diagnosis cannot be established in a timely manner. Chemotherapy is the preferred initial treatment of SVC syndrome caused by chemosensitive tumors such as small cell lung cancer and lymphoma. Most small cell lung cancer patients experience partial or complete resolution of the signs and symptoms within a couple of weeks. Although SVC obstruction recurs in approximately 25% of cases, salvage chemotherapy and/or radiotherapy can achieve prompt resolution of symptoms in most patients. After chemotherapy for lymphoma, local consolidation with radiotherapy may be beneficial in patients with large cell lymphoma and large mediastinal masses. Cancer invasion of SVC is no longer considered unresectable.[60] Surgical treatment with reconstruction may be indicated for certain tumor types or selected patients.[61]

Respiratory oncologic emergencies

Massive hemoptysis

Approximately 5% of hemoptysis episodes are considered massive. The definition of massive hemoptysis ranges from the expectoration of >100 mL of blood in a single episode to >600 mL in 24 h.[62] Airway bleeding leading to life-threatening airway obstruction, hypotension, aspiration, or anemia is also considered massive hemoptysis. The mortality rate of massive hemoptysis is about 30%, ranging from 5% to 71% depending on the volume of blood expectorated and the rate of bleeding.[63–67] Other factors associated with mortality include low pulmonary reserve and large amount of blood retained in the lungs.[64] Death attributable to endobronchial and alveolar hemorrhage is usually due to asphyxiation rather than exsanguination.

The primary causes of massive hemoptysis in cancer patients are malignancy, infection, and hemostatic abnormalities. Bronchogenic carcinoma is the most common cause of massive hemoptysis in cancer patients over 40 years old. About 3% of lung cancer patients have fatal hemoptysis,[68] which occurs more commonly in necrotic squamous cell carcinoma than other types of lung cancer. Hemoptysis secondary to lung metastases is most commonly associated with melanoma, breast, kidney, laryngeal, and colon cancers. Other tumors, such as esophageal tumors, may cause massive hemoptysis by direct extension to the tracheobronchial tree. In immunocompromised patients (e.g., patients with hematologic malignancies, bone marrow transplantation, or prolonged neutropenia), necrotizing, angioinvasive fungal infections (aspergillosis and mucormycosis) may cause massive pulmonary hemorrhage.[64] Hemostatic abnormalities such as severe thrombocytopenia and coagulopathy may result from malignancy or its treatments and contribute to hemorrhage. Another factor that can contribute to massive hemoptysis in cancer patients is lung injury by radiation or chemotherapy.

In addition to hemoptysis, symptoms may include dyspnea, hypotension, tachycardia, central cyanosis, clammy skin, or chest pain. Hemodynamic instability may require volume resuscitation. The respiratory status should be initially supported by supplemental oxygen. The American College of Chest Physicians Guidelines recommend securing the airway by endotracheal intubation with a single-lumen tube, and emergent bronchoscopy to identify the bleeding site for endobronchial interventions such as laser or plasma coagulation and electrocautery.[69] Endobronchial interventions may also include administration of topical agents (thrombin), iced saline lavage, injection of epinephrine 1:20,000, and tamponade with a balloon catheter. Although rigid bronchoscopes offer improved airway control, ability to suction, and the ability to remove large clots, fiber optic scopes offer improved access and visualization of the distal airways. Other airway management options include unilateral intubation via the bronchoscope or a double-lumen endotracheal tube to isolate the unaffected lung. For massive right-sided pulmonary bleeding, the left main stem bronchus is intubated over the bronchoscope, but unilateral intubation of the right lung in patients with massive left-sided bleeding is not recommended due to the risk of right upper lobe occlusion. For patients bleeding from one lung, lateral decubitus positioning with the affected lung in the dependent position may help to minimize aspiration to the unaffected side. Underlying coagulopathies must be corrected, and cough suppressants may be helpful.

Noe et al. have proposed an algorithm for management of massive hemoptysis, in which CT angiography plays an important role.[70] Bronchial artery embolization is becoming first-line treatment for massive or recurrent hemoptysis. Together with bronchoscopy and chest X-ray, CT angiography provides information about the tumor, bleeding site, and anatomy of the bronchial and extrabronchial arteries for planning the endovascular intervention. Bronchial artery embolization is safe and effective. Embolization of the bleeding vessel may be performed with Gianturco steel coils, absorbable gelatin pledgets, polyvinyl alcohol foam, or isobutyl-2-cyanoacrylate. Patients in whom embolization fails may benefit from radiotherapy. Emergency lung resection is feasible in selected patients and is generally performed in patients with refractory hemoptysis in whom other treatments have failed or bleeding from the pulmonary vessels.[71]

Massive pleural effusion

Approximately 10% of pleural effusions are massive when there is near-complete opacification of the hemithorax on chest X-ray. About two-thirds of massive pleural effusions (Figure 4) have underlying cancer.[72] The malignant causes are lung carcinoma (36%), breast carcinoma (25%), lymphoma (10%), and ovarian carcinoma (5%).[73] Adenocarcinoma accounts for 79% of lung carcinoma cases that metastasize to the pleura.[74] In young adults, lymphoma is the most common cause of malignant pleural effusions.[74] After pneumonia, malignancy is the second leading cause of exudative pleural effusions, and malignancy is the cause of 8–20% of transudative pleural effusions.[75] Other factors causing pleural effusions include local tumor effects (hilar and mediastinal lymphadenopathy causing impaired lymphatic drainage from the pleural space), systemic tumor effects, hypoalbuminemia, complications of cancer treatment [radiotherapy and chemotherapy (e.g., methotrexate, procarbazine, cyclophosphamide, mitomycin, bleomycin, and IL-1)], and congestive heart failure.

For some patients, the pleural effusion may be the presenting sign of the malignancy. Common symptoms are cough, dyspnea, and orthopnea, but about one-fourth of malignant pleural effusions are asymptomatic. The presence and severity of these symptoms depend on the volume and the rapidity of fluid accumulation. Fever is occasionally present and may be due to atelectasis or pneumonia. Pleuritic chest pain and pleural friction rubs are not common; when

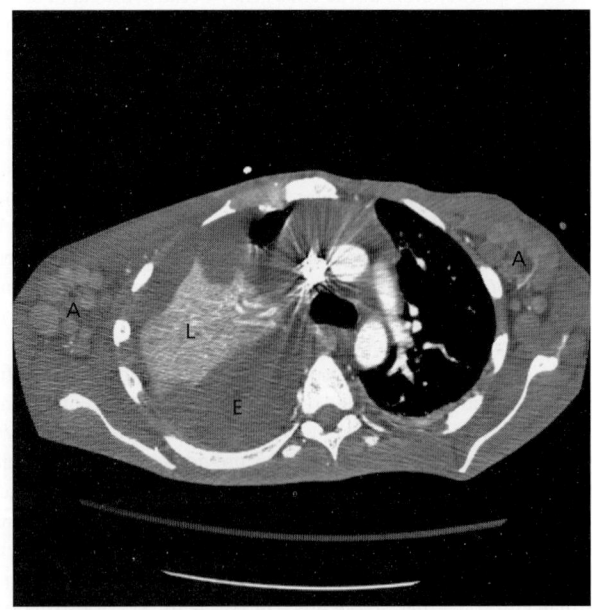

Figure 4 Massive pleural effusion. The CT scan of the chest of a patient with a massive pleural effusion is shown. L, collapsed lung; E, pleural effusion; A, extensive axillary lymphadenopathy.

present, they indicate extensive neoplastic involvement of the pleura and chest wall.

A pleural effusion is diagnosed by clinical examination and confirmed with radiography. On examination, patients with pleural effusion exhibit dullness to percussion, decreased breath sounds in the area of the effusion, and decreased diaphragmatic excursion and tactile and vocal fremitus on the affected side. Sometimes crackles may be auscultated immediately above the percussed dullness. Patients with large-volume effusions (>1500 mL) may have an inspiratory lag, contralateral tracheal deviation, and intercostal fullness. The pleural effusion caused by lung carcinoma is generally on the same side as the primary lesion.[72] The cause of a pleural effusion is generally diagnosed by thoracentesis. Malignant effusions may appear serous, serosanguinous, or bloody. Fluid analysis discriminates between exudative and transudative effusions.[76] Cytology is more sensitive than percutaneous pleural biopsy to diagnose the cause of the effusion.[74,77] Other more invasive diagnostic options include bronchoscopy, pleuroscopy, video-assisted thoracoscopy, and open pleural biopsy.

Treatments are chosen based on severity of symptoms, rate of fluid accumulation, overall prognosis, performance status, and responsiveness of the malignancy to treatment. Massive pleural effusion causing hemodynamic instability, significant dyspnea, hypoxemia, or mediastinal shift should be treated emergently by thoracentesis. However, the benefits of a therapeutic thoracentesis without pleurodesis are usually temporary; in approximately 70% of cases, fluid reaccumulates within 30 days unless effective systemic chemotherapy is administered. If there is no symptomatic improvement after thoracentesis in cancer patients with a lung trapped by visceral pleura encasement, placement of an indwelling pleural catheter is not indicated.[78] Otherwise, an indwelling pleural catheter will allow outpatient periodic drainage of pleural fluid to improve symptoms,[79,80] particularly dyspnea, and improve quality-adjusted survival.[81] Some patients may also achieve pleurodesis over time. Chemical pleurodesis should be considered in patients with life expectancy of more than a few months and symptomatic relief after thoracentesis. The effective sclerosing agents, with success rates of 72–90%, are doxycycline, minocycline, bleomycin, and talc.[82,83] Tube thoracostomy may be indicated depending on clinical and radiographic findings and the biochemical characteristics of the effusion:[84] empyema, infected pleural fluid as confirmed by culture or microscopy (e.g., Gram stain), or complicated parapneumonic effusions. Patients in whom thoracoscopic treatment fails and patients with chronic complicated parapneumonic effusions should be considered for open thoracotomy and decortication.

Acute airway obstruction
Acute airway obstruction usually involves the upper airway. Tumors that obstruct by direct extension are primary tumors of the head and neck (base of tongue, larynx, hypopharynx, thyroid, or trachea) and mediastinum (lung cancer, thymoma). Metastatic tumors that may cause upper airway obstruction are cancers of the breast, esophagus, kidney, colon, melanoma, sarcoma, and mediastinal lymphoma. The mechanisms causing the obstruction include extrinsic compression, tumor encroachment, tumor-associated airway edema, and hemorrhage. Nonmalignant causes include food or foreign body aspiration, severe tracheomalacia, tracheal stenosis or stricture, and airway edema (due to hypersensitivity and infections). Severe drug-induced angioedema may occur with angiotensin-converting enzyme inhibitors and paclitaxel. The most common cause of lower airway obstruction is primary bronchogenic carcinoma. Other rare causes of lower airway obstruction are metastases from cancers of the colon, breast, thyroid and kidney, melanoma, lymphoma, and

sarcoma. Patients with carcinoid tumors may experience severe bronchospasm due to release of hormone mediators.

Dyspnea may be the only early symptom of airway obstruction. When dyspnea occurs with exertion, the upper airway diameter is usually decreased to 8 mm, whereas when dyspnea occurs at rest, the airway diameter is usually decreased to 5 mm, often coinciding with the development of stridor. As obstruction progresses, orthopnea, tachycardia, diaphoresis, wheezing, stridor, and intercostal muscle retraction may be noted. Stridor is an ominous finding that may be rapidly followed by cyanosis, obtundation, bradycardia, and death.

The oral cavity should be quickly visualized to exclude foreign body aspiration. In most cases of upper airway obstruction, the clinical examination provides the diagnosis. The clinical examination is often corroborated by direct visualization via either laryngoscopy or bronchoscopy depending on the location of the lesion. For lower airway obstruction, chest radiographs identify the obstruction in 75% of cases. CT of the neck and/or chest is very helpful in diagnosing obstruction by tumors. Edema caused by acute infection in a previously narrowed airway should also be considered in the differential diagnosis.

The management of airway obstruction is to reverse or bypass the obstruction. In addition to supplemental oxygen, supportive therapies may include administration of corticosteroids, inhaled racemic epinephrine, bronchodilators, helium–oxygen mixtures, and antibiotics (if infection is suspected). Laryngoscopy or bronchoscopy may be necessary to guide endotracheal intubation in upper airway obstruction.[85] Patients with obstructions involving the upper third of the trachea may require a low tracheotomy. Decisions for surgical interventions depend on extent of the malignancy, responsiveness to antineoplastic treatment, performance status, and comorbid conditions. For central airway obstruction, interventional pulmonary treatments may use rigid or flexible bronchoscopes[86] and may include placement of tracheobronchial stents, balloon bronchoplasty, laser bronchoscopy, endobronchial argon plasma coagulation, photodynamic therapy, cryosurgery, and brachytherapy. Other treatment options include CT-guided radiofrequency ablation, external-beam radiotherapy, and surgical debulking or resection.

Pneumothorax
Pneumothoraces in cancer patients are iatrogenic or spontaneous. The majority of pneumothoraces treated in hospitals are iatrogenic.[87] Procedures that may cause a pneumothorax include percutaneous lung biopsy, transbronchial biopsy, insertion of central venous catheters, and insertion of pulmonary artery catheters. Spontaneous pneumothorax is most commonly due to chronic obstructive pulmonary disease. Both primary and metastatic pulmonary neoplasms may also cause pneumothorax. Chemotherapeutic agents associated with pneumothorax include bleomycin, carmustine, and lomustine. Infectious agents associated with pneumothorax include *Staphylococcus*, *Klebsiella*, and *Pseudomonas* species, *Pneumocystis carinii*, and *Mycobacterium* species. Rupture of mycetoma into the pleural space may result in pneumothorax and is associated with *Aspergillus fumigatus* infection, coccidioidomycosis, cryptococcosis, and mucormycosis.

The severity of symptoms at presentation is related to the patient's underlying pulmonary status. Patients may present with respiratory distress, tachypnea, tachycardia, cyanosis, diaphoresis, and agitation. Patients with underlying lung disease often cannot tolerate decreases in vital capacity and have an increased risk for respiratory failure secondary to pneumothorax. Dyspnea is often unrelated to the volume of pneumothorax; however, dyspnea and chest pain are present in almost all cases of significant pneumothorax. The chest pain is frequently acute and pleuritic on the affected side. Cough, hemoptysis, and orthopnea are less frequent.

Small pneumothoraces are usually undetectable on physical examination. Examination usually demonstrates tachycardia, absent tactile fremitus, hyperresonance, and absent or decreased breath sounds on the affected side. Patients with large or tension pneumothoraces may have contralateral deviation of the trachea, asymmetrical hyperexpansion, and decreased movement of the affected hemithorax. Patients with a tension pneumothorax may have elevated central venous, pulmonary artery, and right atrial pressures. Hypotension, severe hypoxemia, and respiratory acidosis occur when increased intrapleural pressure impedes venous return.

The diagnosis of pneumothorax is confirmed when an upright chest radiograph reveals a visceral pleural line with the absence of lung markings beyond the line. For patients with a small pneumothorax, the pleural line may be difficult to discern. Previous work has shown that one-third of pneumothoraces are undetected on semi-erect and supine chest radiographs.[88] Pleural ultrasonography may be more accurate than chest radiography to diagnose pneumothorax.[89]

Patients with small pneumothoraces may be closely observed with supplemental oxygen and serial chest radiographs 3–6 h after the initial radiograph. If there is no expansion of the pneumothorax, the patient may be discharged from observation with appropriate follow-up instructions and repeat radiograph in 12–48 h.[90] For symptomatic, rapidly expanding, and moderate to large (>15% of the ipsilateral pleural space) pneumothoraces, catheter aspiration should be done. Outpatient management with small caliber intercostal catheters and Heimlich valves has a success rate of 78%.[91] Failure to re-expand or recurrence following catheter aspiration requires tube thoracostomy. Tube thoracostomy is indicated as initial treatment for traumatic pneumothorax, hemothorax, pneumothorax occupying >15% of the ipsilateral pleural space with retained secretions, pneumothorax with lung infections on the affected side, and pneumothorax related to mechanical ventilation/barotrauma. Patients with a persistent air leak due to bronchopleural fistula and patients with only partial lung expansion 5–7 days after a tube thoracostomy should be considered for surgical repair. Chemical pleurodesis may be indicated for recurrent pneumothorax.[92]

Pulmonary embolism

Pulmonary embolism can be difficult to diagnose in cancer patients because the signs and symptoms may be masked by the neoplastic process or complications of cancer treatments. Cancer is an independent risk factor for thromboembolism in addition to other factors such as major trauma/surgery, advanced age, recent myocardial infarction, cerebral vascular accident, immobility, obesity, and history of thrombosis. Compared with patients without malignancies, cancer patients have higher rates of initial thrombosis, thrombosis recurrence, and fatal pulmonary embolism.[93] The risk of thromboembolism in cancer patients without other comorbid conditions is 15–20%. Compared with noncancer patients undergoing similar procedures, cancer patients undergoing surgery have two to three times the risk of developing postoperative deep venous thrombosis.[94]

In most cases, symptoms of pulmonary embolism are vague. Dyspnea, pleuritic chest pain, and tachypnea were present in 97% of patients with confirmed pulmonary embolism.[95,96] The most common presenting symptom is dyspnea. Frequently, patients also have tachycardia. Massive pulmonary embolism may cause syncope. Angina may occur due to right ventricular ischemia. Hemoptysis may rarely occur due to pulmonary infarction 12–36 h after the

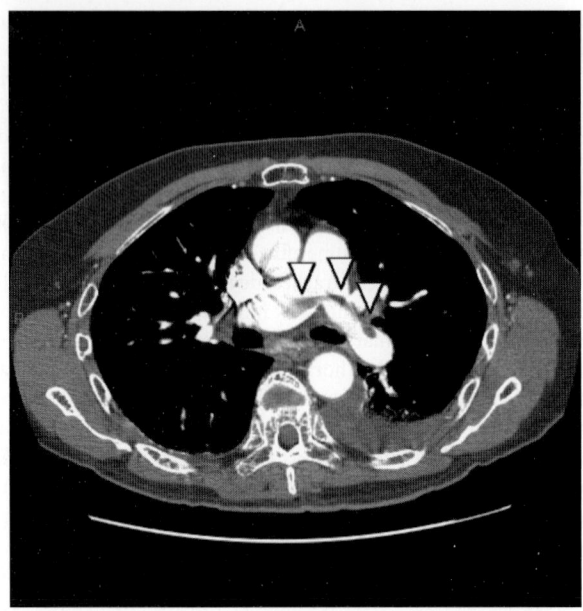

Figure 5 Saddle embolus. This CT scan shows a saddle embolus (below the three arrowheads) at the bifurcation into the pulmonary arteries.

embolic event. Deep venous thrombosis in the lower extremities is found in <50% of patients with pulmonary embolism. Sometimes, fever and a pleural rub may also be detected.

Pulse oximetry or arterial blood gases may demonstrate hypoxemia for which supplemental oxygen should be provided. Chest radiography is helpful in excluding other causes of the symptoms, and occasionally may suggest pulmonary embolism by the presence of a Hampton's hump (dome-shaped and pleura-based lung opacity) or Westermark sign (peripheral radiolucency due to decreased blood flow with or without central pulmonary vessel dilatation).

An electrocardiogram commonly shows sinus tachycardia, inverted T waves, or nonspecific ST-T wave abnormalities. Right axis deviation, atrial arrhythmia, right bundle branch block, and P-pulmonale may occur, but the classical S1-Q3-T3 pattern is unusual. In cancer patients, D-dimer has a high negative predictive value and sensitivity for pulmonary embolism, and a normal D-dimer result can exclude pulmonary embolism.[97] In another study that included cancer patients, a D-dimer concentration >3000 ng/mL is associated with centrally located pulmonary emboli and death within 15 days.[98]

High-resolution CT pulmonary angiography or spiral CT is the first-line diagnostic test (Figure 5); in case of IV iodine contrast allergy, MR angiography is an alternative. For diagnosis of pulmonary embolism, CT and MR angiographies have a sensitivity and specificity of about 80% and 90%, respectively.[99,100] The negative predictive value of CT angiography is 98%.[101] The radionuclide ventilation-perfusion (V/Q) scan is second line when CT or MR angiography is contraindicated because of renal dysfunction or hypersensitivity. As emboli in the distal pulmonary vasculature are not reliably detected with CT or MR angiography, patients with strong suspicion of pulmonary embolism but negative findings on either imaging modalities should be considered for contrast pulmonary angiography, the diagnostic gold standard.

Hemodynamically unstable patients should be stabilized by administration of IV fluid and/or inotropic agents as guided by central venous pressure monitoring in intensive care. Oxygen at high concentration via mask or endotracheal tube may be necessary for massive pulmonary embolism. Treatment options for patients with massive pulmonary embolus and hemodynamic instability (i.e., occlusion of >40% of the pulmonary vasculature, right ventricular dysfunction according to echocardiography, and severe hypoxemia) include systemic thrombolysis, catheter-directed thrombolysis, and embolectomy. In pulmonary embolism causing acute right ventricular dysfunction, thrombolytic therapy is associated with decreased all-cause mortality despite increased major bleeding and intracranial hemorrhage.[102] Thrombolysis demands special attention to contraindications related to bleeding risk (especially in the presence of brain metastasis). Due to increased risk for massive bleeding and intracranial hemorrhage but no reduction in mortality, thrombolysis should not be used for most normotensive patients with pulmonary embolism.[103] Although systemic thrombolysis may be beneficial in massive pulmonary embolism, catheter-directed thrombolysis may cause less major bleeding complications than systemic thrombolysis; the role for catheter-directed thrombolysis remains to be clearly defined.[104] Surgical or catheter embolectomy is reserved for patients in whom other approaches of clot removal have failed.

There are published guidelines for the management of venous thromboembolism in cancer patients.[105,106] Low-molecular-weight heparin (LMWH) is recommended for the initial 5–10 days of anticoagulation for cancer patients with newly diagnosed pulmonary embolism and creatinine clearance >30 mL/min. Unfractionated heparin (IV bolus of 80 units/kg followed by continuous infusion at 18 units/kg/h) can be an alternative to LMWH. LMWH has the advantages of not requiring partial thromboplastin time monitoring and IV access. IV unfractionated heparin may be preferred in patients who very probably will need invasive interventions because of its short half-life. IV unfractionated heparin is administered in a bolus injection of 5000–10,000 units, followed by a continuous infusion of 1000–1500 units/h with adjustments to maintain the activated partial thromboplastin time at 1.5–2.0 times the control value.[107] For long-term (≥6 months) anticoagulation, LMWH is preferred over vitamin K antagonists (e.g., warfarin) because it is less likely to interact with other drugs and chemotherapy, needs no monitoring, is associated with fewer recurrence of venous thromboembolism, and may prolong survival of cancer patients.[108] Treatment with vitamin K antagonists to an international normalized ratio between 2 and 3 is an acceptable alternative for long-term therapy when LMWH is not possible. Extending anticoagulation beyond 6 months may be considered for patients with active malignancy until cancer treatment has completed and the malignancy has become inactive.[109] A number of new antithrombotic agents are currently under investigation for applications in cancer patients.[110] Their use for either prevention or treatment of pulmonary embolism in cancer patients is not recommended at this time.

Anticoagulation is contraindicated in the presence of active intracranial bleeding, recent surgery, thrombocytopenia (platelet <50,000/µL), or coagulopathy. Inferior vena cava filters may be considered when anticoagulation is contraindicated or when pulmonary embolism recurs or existing thrombus worsens under optimal therapy with LMWH, but end-stage cancer patients may gain little benefit.[111] Contraindications for anticoagulation should be periodically reassessed so that anticoagulation can resume when it is safe. Filters are not recommended for primary prophylaxis in cancer patients.[105]

For patients with primary brain malignancies, anticoagulation is recommended in the same manner as for patients with other cancers. Many cancer patients with pulmonary embolism may be safely treated as outpatients, especially cases of incidental pulmonary embolism, which are clinically unsuspected and are discovered in CT scans ordered for treatment response evaluation or staging.[112] As the rates of recurrence, morbidity, and mortality in incidental cases are comparable to symptomatic cases, incidental pulmonary embolism should be treated in the same way with initial and long-term anticoagulant therapy as for symptomatic pulmonary embolism except for peripheral subsegmental emboli that are judged to be highly probable imaging artifacts.[106,110,113]

Neurologic oncologic emergencies

Spinal cord compression

Spinal cord compression occurs in 3–5% of cancer patients and should be considered an emergency because treatment delay may result in irreversible morbidity, including paralysis.[114] In 95% of cases, spinal cord compression is caused by metastases involving the vertebral column (70% in the thoracic spine, 20% in the lumbosacral spine, and 10% in the cervical spine). Metastasis to the thoracic vertebrae is likely to cause problems because of the vulnerable local blood supply and the fact that the spinal canal is narrowest here. Spinal cord compression occurs more frequently in patients with lung, breast, unknown primary, prostate, and renal cell cancer than other malignancies.

Back pain is the most common symptom in spinal cord compression, and patients may present with pain localized to the spine or radicular pain due to neural compression. The pain may worsen with movement, recumbence, coughing, sneezing, or straining. Muscle weakness follows pain and may be accompanied by sensory loss. Once symptoms of autonomic dysfunction, urinary retention, and constipation develop, irreversible paralysis rapidly follows. Paralysis and urinary retention before treatment are predictive of poor outcome. Clinical findings include tenderness elicited by palpation over the involved vertebral segments, muscle weakness, abnormal reflexes, and sensory loss in the distribution of the involved spinal segment and below. Leg ataxia may be present prior to muscle weakness. Patients with autonomic dysfunction may have a palpable bladder, an increased postvoid residual urinary volume, or decreased rectal tone.

Clinical guidelines for diagnosis and management of spinal cord compression are available.[115,116] Patients with spinal cord compression often have abnormalities (e.g., bony erosion and pedicle loss, partial or complete vertebral collapse) on plain radiographs of the spine. However, normal spine radiographs do not exclude epidural metastasis. MR tomography of the spine is the best method for evaluating epidural spinal cord compression (Figure 6). Gadolinium enhancement should be used when there is suspicion of cord compression due to epidural abscess or neurological symptoms due to leptomeningeal metastasis. Gadolinium enhances inflamed tissues and defines anatomic margins. Myelography accompanied by CT may be performed with minimum discomfort. However, when metastatic disease completely blocks the flow of cerebrospinal fluid, myelography does not allow definition of the upper margin of tumor involvement.

Treatment of spinal cord compression aims to improve or prevent loss of neurologic function, provide local tumor control, stabilize the spine, and pain control. Analgesics, especially opioids, should be administered promptly and judiciously because inadequate pain control often delays appropriate physical examination and diagnostic imaging study. When spinal cord compression is suspected, corticosteroid therapy should be administered. Dexamethasone is often used as it has good gastrointestinal absorption and a 36-h half-life. It is controversial whether a high-dose (100 mg) IV bolus

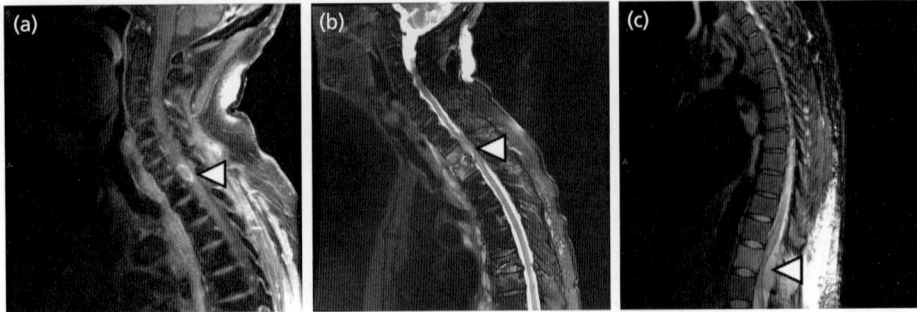

Figure 6 Spinal cord compression. Sagittal MRI images of the spine from three different patients demonstrate an intramedullary lesion (*arrowhead*) in low cervical spine (a), compression of the lower portion of the thoracic spinal cord by metastatic disease in the vertebral body (*arrowhead*) (b), and compression of the upper portion of the lumbar spinal cord by an epidural tumor (*arrowhead*) (c).

followed by maintenance doses (usually 16 mg every 6 h) is necessary.[117] Low doses (4–10 mg every 6 h) may be just as effective with fewer side effects.[116,118] For most patients with spinal cord compression by a radiosensitive malignancy, radiotherapy alone is the standard initial treatment. The outcome of radiotherapy depends on the pretreatment neurologic status and radiosensitivity of the malignancy. Surgical decompression may be appropriate for patients requiring spine stabilization, patients who have had prior radiotherapy in the area of the compression, patients who need tissue for diagnosis, and patients with progression despite appropriate treatment with steroids and radiation, but may not be appropriate for patients with advanced malignancy and a limited life expectancy. A meta-analysis has shown that surgical resection followed by radiotherapy may improve ambulation ability and survival better than radiotherapy alone.[119] Chemotherapy may be effective for compression by a chemosensitive malignancy and may also be used in combination with other treatments or sometimes as an alternative when other choices are not appropriate (e.g., high operative risks, or near-maximum radiation doses already delivered to the affected area).

Brain herniation

Patients with possible brain herniation should be rapidly assessed, and those with hemodynamic instability should be stabilized with appropriate therapies.[120] Symptoms and physical findings suggestive of brain herniation include changes in the level of consciousness, papilledema, pupillary and eye movement irregularities, nausea, vomiting, meningismus, decorticate or decerebrate posturing, and Cushing reflex (hypertension and bradycardia). If there are findings suggestive of herniation or increased intracranial pressure, an imaging study such as a noncontrast CT of the brain should be performed emergently. MR imaging can provide additional diagnostic information after the patient has been stabilized.

On recognition of clinical signs of brain herniation, treatment to decrease intracranial pressure should be instituted immediately, even before brain herniation is documented by imaging studies. Emergency treatments include hyperventilation and administration of mannitol and steroids. Hyperventilation is the most rapid way to decrease intracranial pressure. Sedate, intubate, and ventilate to achieve a PCO_2 of 25–30 mm Hg, which causes cerebral vasoconstriction, decreases cerebral blood volume, and subsequently decreases intracranial pressure. The benefit of hyperventilation is generally short-lived, and equilibration may occur within a few hours. Mannitol 20–25%, a hyperosmotic agent, is effective within minutes of administration and remains effective for several hours by forming an osmotic gradient between the blood and brain to drive water from the brain to the blood. Mannitol 20–25% is administered IV at 0.5–2.0 g/kg over 20–30 min. Additional doses may be necessary if the patient continues to deteriorate. Corticosteroids should be administered and may be helpful especially when herniation is due to vasogenic edema surrounding intracranial metastases.[121] Dexamethasone is commonly administered at an initial bolus dose of 40–100 mg IV, then 40–100 mg/day in divided doses.

Further treatment in intensive care may include IV infusion of hypertonic saline, propofol, and hypothermia.[120] Neurosurgical intervention such as placement of a ventricular drain or decompressive craniectomy may be necessary if the patient has neurologic deterioration despite appropriate medical management. Treatment should be directed at the underlying cause once intracranial pressure is controlled.

Status epilepticus

Status epilepticus is defined as >5 min of continuous seizure activity or >2 sequential seizures without full recovery between seizures.[122] It can lead to devastating neurologic and systemic consequences, such as neuronal injury and cell death, neurogenic pulmonary edema, and rhabdomyolysis with renal failure. Tumors in the brain causes about 7% of cases of status epilepticus, and these cases have higher short-term mortality than status epilepticus unrelated to tumors.[123]

The etiology of seizures in cancer patients may include structural, metabolic, infectious, and treatment-related causes. In a review of 50 cancer patients presenting to an emergency center with seizures, 16% had seizures due to a new structural lesion and 52% had previously documented central nervous system lesions.[124] Seizures commonly occur in patients with intracranial tumors. The cancers that commonly metastasize to the brain are lung cancer, breast cancer, melanoma, genitourinary malignancies, and gastrointestinal malignancies.

Neurologic function is often suppressed (confused or unresponsive) postictally. Clinical findings after seizure activity may include bruising or tongue bites, signs of urinary or fecal incontinence, and increases in lactic acid and muscle enzyme levels. It is important to determine whether the patient has previously had seizures and, if so, the type of seizure and medications used for control. The status, extent, and treatment of the malignancy should also be reviewed. If the event precipitating seizure activity cannot easily be determined, a diagnostic workup should be initiated. Evaluation may include measurement of electrolytes, serum glucose, calcium, and magnesium, and hepatic and renal function testing. A complete blood cell count, blood cultures, measurement of electrolytes, urea nitrogen, creatinine, glucose, calcium, magnesium, blood gases, anticonvulsant drug levels (if prescribed), drug screens, and electroencephalography are appropriate. CT brain imaging without IV contrast is necessary.[125] Lumbar puncture may also be indicated depending on the suspected seizure precipitant, the patient's condition, findings on imaging, and whether convulsions have stopped to allow the procedure to be performed.

When patients present with status epilepticus, airway, breathing, and circulation should be assessed immediately (Figure 7).[122,125] Cardiopulmonary status should be supported and stabilized according to ACLS algorithms. Hypoglycemia as the cause of seizure must be first excluded or diagnosed and treated. Anticonvulsant therapy with an IV benzodiazepine (e.g., lorazepam or midazolam) should be administered to halt seizure activity. Generally, lorazepam (typically 4–8 mg IV) is used because of its rapid onset of action and longer duration of efficacy. After seizure has stopped, an unconscious patient should be placed on his or her side in the recovery position to prevent aspiration. Airway suctioning and supplemental oxygen may be required. Reversible medical causes of seizures should be corrected. These patients will likely not require long-term anticonvulsant therapy. Patients with status epilepticus due to other causes will require prolonged treatment with an anticonvulsant. Some clinicians prefer levetiracetam in cancer patients because it is not metabolized by the liver and has minimal drug interactions with antineoplastic therapy. For patients with continuing seizure activity despite initial anticonvulsant treatment, therapy can be escalated in steps to high-dose anticonvulsant therapy (e.g., pentobarbital,

thiopental, propofol, and midazolam) with complete sedation, intubation/ventilator support, and electroencephalography monitoring in intensive care.

Other oncologic emergencies

Perforated bowel

Perforation along the gastrointestinal tract is a serious emergency. In cancer patients, common causes are spontaneous perforation secondary to tumor (primary or metastatic) and iatrogenic perforation secondary to endoscopy or cancer treatment. If the wall of the gastrointestinal tract is significantly infiltrated or replaced by tumor, radiotherapy- or chemotherapy-induced tumor necrosis may lead to bowel perforation. Antiangiogenic therapies such as bevacizumab and small molecule inhibitors such as imatinib and sorafenib have been associated with bowel perforation.[126] Bowel perforation can be caused by severe infections such as typhlitis and neutropenic enterocolitis.[127] Severe gastroenteritis due to radiotherapy or chemotherapy may lead to severe bowel dilatation/distention and subsequent perforation. Common causes of bowel perforation unrelated to cancer include appendicitis, diverticulitis, and peptic ulcer disease.

Typically, perforation causes acute pain that prompts emergent evaluation. In cases of cervical esophageal perforation, symptoms at presentation may include neck pain, dysphagia, hoarseness, and subcutaneous emphysema. In thoracic esophageal perforation, upper abdominal rigidity, severe retrosternal chest pain, odynophagia, and hematemesis are common. In gastric perforation, acute onset of severe abdominal pain is usually the first symptom. The pain may be associated with nausea and vomiting, and in about 15% of patients, significant bleeding is present. Referred pain to the shoulders may occur because of irritation of the diaphragm. In cases of free perforation into the peritoneal cavity, abdominal distension and signs of peritonitis (severe rebound abdominal tenderness, guarding/rigidity, and absent bowel sounds) may be present.

Fever and leukocytosis with left shift may be present in patients with peritonitis, mediastinitis, or abscess. However, the white blood cell count should be interpreted in the context of recent chemotherapy or use of neutrophil-stimulating cytokines. Amylase levels may be high in intestinal, esophageal, or gastric perforation, and lipase levels may be high in gastric perforation. In cervical esophageal perforation, a plain radiograph of the neck in the lateral view may show air in the deep cervical tissues. Plain radiographs of the chest are also valuable in esophageal perforation as pneumomediastinum may be evident. Free air detected by plain radiographs (upright chest X-ray or abdominal series with upright or decubitus views) (Figure 8) can provide evidence of bowel perforation. As for duodenal perforation, plain abdominal radiographs may show air in the retroperitoneal space. Other radiographic signs of perforation include outlining of both sides of the bowel wall by air and visualization of the hepatic ligament. If bowel perforation is highly suspected clinically and the initial studies do not show evidence of perforation, CT scan with oral water-soluble contrast agent (e.g., diatrizoate) is very accurate in diagnosing bowel perforation and can provide detailed information about the location and surrounding anatomy of the perforated structure.

Management of a perforated viscus may be expectant management, expectant management followed by surgery, or immediate surgery. Factors influencing the management are the etiology, size, location and containment of the perforation, the clinical course (development of sepsis), the patient's performance status and quality of life prior to the perforation, the prognosis based on the status

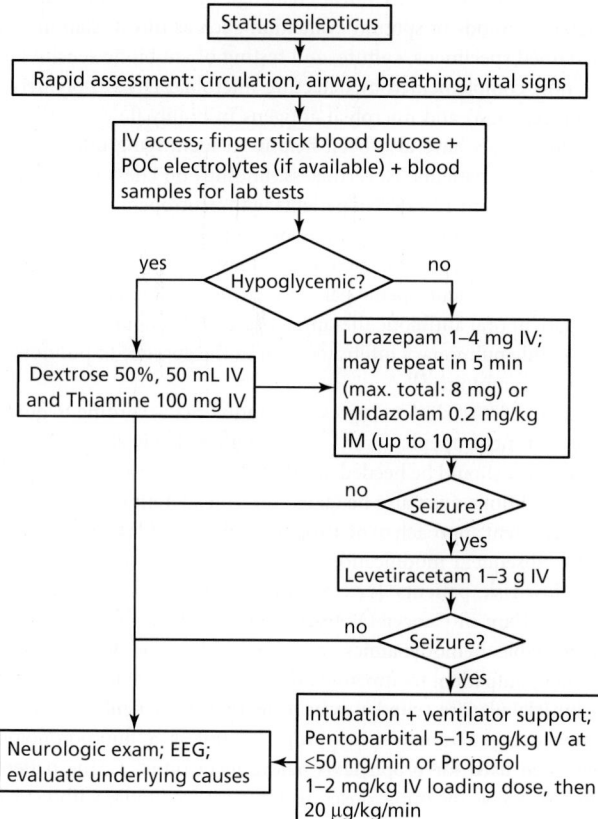

Figure 7 Algorithm for management of status epilepticus adapted for cancer patients. *Abbreviations*: EEG, electroencephalogram; POC, point-of-care bedside testing; IV, intravenous; IM, intramuscular. (Source: Modified from Brophy et al. 2012[122] and Claassen et al. 2012.[125])

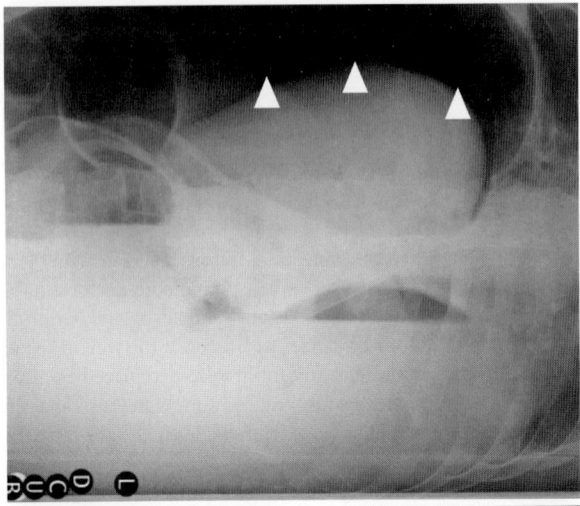

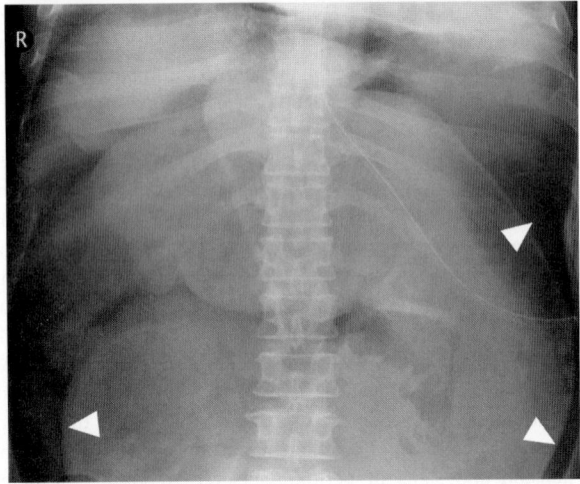

Figure 8 Pneumoperitoneum. A 53-year-old man with multiple myeloma and amyloidosis involving the gastrointestinal tract, undergoing treatment with thalidomide and dexamethasone, presented with acute abdominal pain and abdominal distention. Abdominal radiographs showed intraperitoneal free air (*arrowheads*). Laparotomy revealed bowel perforation secondary to massive colonic distention.

of the malignant disease, and comorbid conditions that increase the risk of perioperative mortality. Nonsurgical treatment measures include nasogastric tube suction, administration of broad-spectrum IV antibiotics, IV hydration, parenteral nutrition, and close monitoring.[128] If the patient's condition deteriorates during expectant treatment, then a decision to operate can be made.

Neutropenic fever

Neutrophils are phagocytic white blood cells that defend the human body against infections. Neutropenia is defined as a neutrophil count of ≤1000 cells/μL, absolute neutropenia as neutrophil ≤500 cells/μL, and profound neutropenia as neutrophil ≤100 cells/μL.[129] Neutropenia often occurs in cancer patients as a consequence of intensive chemotherapy or the malignancy. Infection is the leading cause of morbidity and mortality in neutropenic patients. Fever [defined as a single oral temperature >38.3°C (101°F) or >38.0°C (100.4°F) for >1 h] in a neutropenic cancer patient often resolves after empirical systemic broad-spectrum antibiotics (up to about 60% of cases).[130] Neutropenic fever is a true medical emergency, and timely administration of antibiotics may prevent sepsis and death.

Neutropenic patients are immunocompromised and lack the ability to mount a full inflammatory response to infections. Therefore, any symptom or sign of infection should be investigated fully.[131] Physical examination should include careful inspection of commonly infected sites such as mouth, pharynx, perineum, eyes, vascular access sites, percutaneous catheter sites, and skin. Initial laboratory evaluation should include: complete blood cell count, serum creatinine, blood urea nitrogen, transaminases, blood cultures from a peripheral vein and vascular access ports or catheters, urinalysis, urine culture. Chest radiography is indicated for patients with respiratory signs or symptoms.

Further evaluation should be guided by physical findings, signs, and symptoms. Lesions on the mucous membranes and the skin can be viral (e.g., herpes simplex and varicella zoster), bacterial (e.g., ecthyma gangrenosum), or fungal (e.g., disseminated candidiasis, aspergillosis, or *Fusarium*) infection. Any site of a localized infection should be pursued with aspiration or biopsy for pathogen identification to guide treatment. Sinus symptoms may be due to bacterial or fungal infections, some of which may be invasive and fatal. Abdominal pain, distention, bloody diarrhea, nausea, and vomiting are typical findings in neutropenic enterocolitis.[132] In the presence of diarrhea, stool specimens should be evaluated with for *Clostridium difficile* infection by a toxin assay or polymerase chain reaction. Perianal symptoms may suggest the presence of a perianal abscess. The differential diagnosis of pulmonary disease in febrile neutropenic patients is broad: infection (viral, bacterial, fungal, and protozoan), radiation-induced pathologic conditions, chemotherapy-induced side effects, hemorrhage, and infarction. Correlation of pulmonary symptoms and findings on chest radiographs is a clinical challenge in neutropenic patients. Classic methods of sputum evaluation such as direct examination of stained specimens, culture, and testing of antibiotic sensitivities are now complemented by detecting microbial DNA (polymerase chain reaction) and microbial antigens in bodily fluids or tissues. Serologic tests have also been helpful in identifying infections in neutropenic patients. Nevertheless, findings on chest radiography are abnormal in 17–25% of patients with neutropenic fever despite the absence of pulmonary signs or symptoms,[133] and lung infiltrate on chest X-ray can predict a complicated clinical course.[134] Therefore, if a neutropenic patient is being considered for possible outpatient oral antibiotic therapy, a chest X-ray should be obtained to exclude pulmonary infiltrates even in the absence of pulmonary signs or symptoms.[131]

About 80% of clinicians prescribe antibiotics according to guidelines for neutropenic fever.[135] Although guidelines and general statements should be heeded, local epidemiology and clinical practice conditions must also be taken into consideration.[136] The initial management approach of neutropenic fever should be based on risk with subsequent modification based on clinical response.[130,137–139] For low-risk patients [i.e., Multinational Association for Supportive Care in Cancer (MASCC) score ≥21 or Talcott group 4] with stable hemodynamics, no comorbidity and low symptom burden, outpatient treatment with oral fluoroquinolone plus amoxicillin/clavulanate (clindamycin if allergic to penicillin) as initial empiric regimen may be appropriate unless a fluoroquinolone has been used for prophylaxis before fever onset.[140] The patients should receive the initial doses of empirical antibiotics within 1 h of triage. Eligibility for outpatient management should be determined by monitoring the patient's condition for at least 4 h. However, successful outpatient management relies on coordination among primary care, oncology and emergency departments to ensure a rapid response and close follow up during the outpatient treatment period as well as effective communication between clinicians and patients and their care takers.[141]

The standard approach for neutropenic fever is inpatient treatment with IV antibiotics. Factors associated with prolonged hospital stay in adults with neutropenic fever include hematologic malignancies, high-intensity chemotherapy, long duration of neutropenia, and cultures growing Gram-negative multidrug-resistant bacteria.[142] Monotherapy with broad-spectrum β-lactam antibiotics, such as piperacillin-tazobactam, carbapenems or the fourth-generation cephalosporin cefepime, is recommended. Adding other antimicrobials (e.g., aminoglycosides, fluoroquinolones, vancomycin, colistin, daptomycin) to the initial regimen in cases with suspected or known antibiotic resistance or serious infections is also indicated. Empirical coverage for Gram-positive organisms with vancomycin is acceptable if a Gram-positive bacterial infection is suspected or known, for example, cellulitis, central venous catheter-related infection, mucositis, or the use of prophylactic antibiotics against Gram-negative bacteria.[130] Vancomycin use in neutropenic fever has more than tripled to 55% in 2010 over 10 years.[135]

If a febrile neutropenic patient does not respond to the initial broad-spectrum antibiotic therapy, additional antibiotics or antifungal therapy is recommended. Fluconazole may be used as initial empirical therapy in patients who have not received prior antifungal prophylaxis. Amphotericin B is beneficial for patients with persistent fever during broad-spectrum antibiotic treatment without antifungal prophylaxis, persistent neutropenia for more than 15 days, or a documented fungal infection. *Candida albicans* and nonalbicans Candida species are important pathogens in leukemia patients and bone marrow transplant recipients, and *Aspergillus* infection causes significant problems in patients with prolonged and profound neutropenia. Other fungi, such as *Fusarium* and *Trichosporon*, are emerging as important pathogens, perhaps owing to increased prevalence of antifungal prophylaxis.

In high-risk patients, especially leukemic patients, a de-escalation approach may be employed instead of the escalation approach discussed above.[138] Patients at risk for infection with resistant pathogens (e.g., methicillin-resistant *Staphylococcus aureus*, vancomycin-resistant *Enterococcus*, extended spectrum β-lactamase-producing Gram-negative bacteria, and carbapenemase-producing organisms) and patient with unstable hemodynamics should be treated initially with broad-spectrum antibiotic combinations. Major risk factors for infection with resistant pathogens include prior colonization or infection by resistant organisms and a high local prevalence of resistant pathogens in cultures obtained when fever started in neutropenic patients. De-escalation of antibiotic therapy is based on the culture results and clinical response 72–96 h after initiation of antibiotic therapy.

The adjunct therapy of a myeloid colony-stimulating factor to increase leukocytes in chemotherapy-induced neutropenic fever does not improve overall mortality, although such therapy is associated with shorter durations of fever, neutropenia, and antibiotics use.[143] Although prophylactic colony-stimulating factors should be considered if the risk of chemotherapy-induced neutropenic fever is >20%, starting these factors after fever onset in a neutropenic patient is generally not recommended.[130]

Anaphylactic reactions to chemotherapy drugs

Anaphylactic reactions to chemotherapy drugs are another important type of emergency in cancer patients. Urticaria and angioedema occur in 90% of anaphylactic reactions. Other manifestations are chest tightness, upper airway obstruction, abdominal pain, bronchospasm, and hypotension. The National Institute of Allergy and Infectious Diseases and the Food Allergy and Anaphylaxis Network have established diagnostic criteria for anaphylaxis; depending on the probability of allergen exposure, a different number of criteria based on acute onset and involvement of the tegumentary, respiratory, cardiovascular, or gastrointestinal systems are used.[144] Important elements in anaphylaxis treatment are early recognition, airway maintenance, and hemodynamic support (Table 3).[145-149] Common chemotherapy drugs that may cause anaphylaxis include: L-asparaginase, taxanes (paclitaxel and docetaxel), etoposide, teniposide, procarbazine, platinum compounds (cisplatin and carboplatin), ifosfamide, cyclophosphamide, anthracyclines (daunorubicin, doxorubicin, and idarubicin).

Systemic reactions to cytokines and monoclonal antibodies

Biological drugs are protein drugs produced using biotechnology, which include monoclonal antibodies, fusion proteins, and cytokines. Several cytokines (interferons and ILs) and monoclonal antibodies have been approved for the treatment of specific malignancies. A new classification of adverse reactions to biological agents differentiates five types: (α)—reactions due to massive release of cytokines, (β)—hypersensitivity because of an immune reaction against the biological agent, (γ)—immune or cytokine imbalance syndromes manifesting as immunosuppression, autoimmune, or inflammatory diseases, (δ)—symptoms due to cross-reactivity, and (ε)—symptoms not directly involving the immune system.[150] The toxic effects associated with cytokines may be serious. Monoclonal antibodies may induce massive release of cytokines, which may lead to fever, rigor, dyspnea, hypoxia, hypotension, or even death. Reactions vary widely from skin reactions to anaphylaxis, and reactions to some of these biological agents have been reviewed.[151]

Interferon-α

Acute adverse effects of interferon-α (IFN-α) occur during the first 2–8 h, but they rarely limit treatment, and severity lessens with subsequent doses in most patients. Flu-like symptoms, hypotension or hypertension, tachycardia, nausea, and vomiting are common side effects. With chronic administration, fatigue, anorexia, and weight loss can become severe.[148] Mild granulocytopenia develops gradually after the first week. Immune hemolytic anemia and thrombocytopenia are rare. Ischemic colitis, ischemic optic neuropathy, and congestive heart failure have also been reported. Neurologic, behavioral, and cognitive changes may limit treatment. Flu-like side effects may be managed with acetaminophen or nonsteroidal anti-inflammatory drugs. Other supportive care measures may be provided depending on the symptoms.

Interleukin-2

High-dose IL-2 (aldesleukin) is associated with cardiovascular and hemodynamic adverse effects that resemble septic shock.[152] High-dose IV IL-2, which should be given in an inpatient setting, can lead to hypotension, vascular leak syndrome, and respiratory insufficiency. Support of peripheral vascular resistance with vasopressors, endotracheal intubation, and fluid resuscitation may be necessary during therapy. Acute neurologic side effects (psychosis, disorientation, and behavioral changes) may occur and require discontinuation of therapy. Guidelines for administration of high-dose IL-2 have been suggested.[153] Low-dose IV and subcutaneous IL-2 regimens can be administered in an ambulatory care setting with observation for several hours after administration. Common symptoms include fever, chills, nausea, vomiting, anorexia, malaise, fatigue, myalgia, arthralgia, and pruritus. Prophylaxis includes

Table 3 Recommendations for acute management of anaphylaxis in adults.

1. Remove the antigen or delay the absorption of the antigen
2. Assess airway; intubate if there is evidence of laryngeal edema or impending severe airway obstruction; in extreme circumstances, when orotracheal intubation or bag/valve/mask ventilation is not effective, cricothyrotomy or catheter jet ventilation may be needed
3. Assess hemodynamics; position the patient supine (or semi-reclining in a position of comfort if dyspneic or vomiting) and elevate the legs
4. Administer epinephrine as first-line treatment
   ○ In case of a less severe episode: 0.3 mg SQ, 1 mg/mL, repeated at 10- to 20-min intervals
   ○ In case of a more severe episode: 0.3–0.5 mg IM, 1 mg/mL, repeated at 5- to 10-min intervals
   ○ In case of shock or airway obstruction: 1 mg/100 mL IV, 0.01–0.02 mg/min, up to a total dose of 0.1 mg
   ○ In case of persistent shock: may repeat dose or start an IV drip infusing at 2–10 μg/min
   ○ If patient is over 50 years old or has a history or cardiac problems and life-threatening symptoms exist: test dose of 0.1–0.15 mg SQ or IM
5. Administer IV crystalloid fluid (normal saline or lactated Ringer's solution)
   ○ In case of hypotension, administer 1 L over 15 min, then reassess; repeat as needed up to 3 L
6. Administer glucocorticoid
   ○ Methylprednisolone 125 mg IV push; may repeat every 4 h if symptoms persist (alternative: hydrocortisone 500 mg, dexamethasone 20 mg, or other potent corticosteroids)
7. Administer antihistamines (both H1 and H2 blockers)
   ○ Diphenhydramine 25–50 mg IV or IM; repeat every 2–4 h as needed
   ○ Cimetidine 300 mg IV or famotidine 20 mg IV
8. Inhaled racemic epinephrine via a nebulizer can reduce laryngeal swelling; β-agonists for bronchospasm and wheezing
9. In case of resistant hypotension,
   ○ Military antishock trousers, or Trendelenburg's position may be helpful
   ○ Infuse dopamine 5–20 μg/kg/min IV by titration
   ○ Administer naloxone 0.4–2.0 mg IV every 2 min (maximum 10 mg)
10. In case of β-blocker-accentuated epinephrine-resistant anaphylaxis
   ○ Administer glucagon 1–5 mg IV over 2–5 min
   ○ Administer terbutaline 0.25 mg SQ
   ○ Administer isoproterenol 2–10 μg/min IV by titration

Abbreviations: IM, intramuscularly; IV, intravenous; SQ, subcutaneously.
Source: Data from Simons et al.,[145] Lieberman et al.,[146] Boyce et al.,[147] and Muraro et al.[149]

Table 4 Antibody therapies approved by the US Food and Drug Administration.

Pharmaceutical agent	Target antigen	Monoclonal antibody type	Conjugated moiety	Indication	Acute side effect[a]
Alemtuzumab (Campath-1H)	CD52	Humanized	—	B-cell chronic lymphocytic leukemia	Cytopenias, infections, cardiomyopathy
Bevacizumab (Avastin)	VEGF	Humanized	—	Colorectal cancer	Epistaxis, headache, hypertension, rhinitis, back pain, exfoliative dermatitis, taste alteration, rectal bleeding
Brentuximab vedotin (Adcetris)	CD30	Chimeric	Monomethyl auristatin E	Hodgkin lymphoma, anaplastic large cell lymphoma	Cytopenias, peripheral sensory neuropathy, fatigue, upper respiratory tract infection, diarrhea, rash, cough, nausea, and vomiting
Cetuximab (Erbitux)	EGFR	Chimeric	—	Colorectal cancer, head and neck cancer	Skin toxicity (acneform rash), interstitial lung disease, infection, diarrhea, nausea, conjunctivitis, pulmonary embolus
Denosumab (Prolia, Xgeva)	RANK ligand	Human	—	Bone metastasis	Hypocalcemia, hypophosphatemia
Gemtuzumab ozogamicin (Mylotarg)	CD33	Humanized	Calicheamicin	CD33-positive acute myeloid leukemia	Cytopenias, infection, bleeding, mucositis, hepatotoxicity
Ibritumomab tiuxetan (Zevalin)	CD20	Murine	Radiolabeled (yttrium-90 or indium-111)	Non-Hodgkin lymphoma	Cytopenias, fatigue, nasopharyngitis, nausea, abdominal pain, cough, diarrhea
Ipilimumab (Yervoy)	CTLA-4	Human	—	Melanoma	Fatigue, diarrhea, pruritus, rash, colitis
Ofatumumab (Arzerra)	CD20	Human	—	Chronic lymphocytic leukemia	Neutropenia
Panitumumab (Vectibix)	EGFR	Human	—	Colorectal cancer	Skin toxicity, paronychia, fatigue, nausea, diarrhea, bowel obstruction
Pertuzumab (Perjeta)	HER2	Humanized	—	HER2-positive breast cancer	Diarrhea, alopecia, neutropenia, nausea, fatigue, rash, peripheral neuropathy
Rituximab (Rituxan)	CD20	Monoclonal antibody	—	B-cell non-Hodgkin lymphoma	Infection, cytopenias, hypogammaglobulinemia
Tositumomab (Bexxar)	CD20	Murine	Radiolabeled (I-131)	Non-Hodgkin lymphoma	Cytopenias, infection, hypothyroidism
Trastuzumab (Herceptin)	HER2	Humanized	—	HER2-positive breast cancer	Cytopenias, diarrhea, fatigue, stomatitis, upper respiratory tract infections, mucosal inflammation, nasopharyngitis, dysgeusia

[a]In addition to cytokine release syndrome.

acetaminophen 650–1000 mg 1 h before therapy and 4 and 8 h later and histamine type 1 and 2 receptor antagonists (e.g., diphenhydramine 50 mg orally 1 h before therapy and 25 mg 4, 8, and 12 h later plus cimetidine 800 mg orally before therapy). Meperidine (25–50 mg IV) may be given as needed for rigor and chills.

Monoclonal antibodies

The list of antibody pharmaceuticals has grown (Table 4). Immediate reactions appear during the first hour after administration and are heterogeneous in etiology and presentation (nausea, vomiting, skin reactions, respiratory symptoms, and hypotension).[151] Some involve release of cytokines (type α); others involve an IgE-mediated hypersensitivity (type β). Anaphylaxis, urticaria, and angioedema can occur. Patient-related risk factors for having a reaction include the malignancy, concomitant treatments, and current immune status; drug-related factors include the degree of humanization, method of production, glycosylation pattern, and the allergenic potential of the excipients. Delayed hypersensitivity can appear between 2 h and up to 14 days after infusion [151] and is often serum sickness-like (e.g., rash, vasculitis, and erythema multiforme).

Although the incidence rates of reactions vary (e.g., 40% for trastuzumab and 77% for rituximab), the general precaution and treatment of the antibody infusion syndrome are the same. Transient symptoms may be treated and supported similar to anaphylaxis (Table 3). Prophylactic treatment with acetaminophen and diphenhydramine may attenuate this antibody infusion syndrome. Reactions generally resolve by slowing or interrupting the infusion. After symptoms resolve, infusion may be restarted at 50% of the previous rate.

Key references

The complete reference list can be found on the Wiley Companion Digital Edition of this title (see inside front cover for login instructions).

1 Perkins JC, Davis JE (eds). *Hematology/Oncology Emergencies, An Issue of Emergency Medicine Clinics of North America*. Philadelphia, PA: Elsevier Health Sciences; 2014.

5 American Heart Association. *Advance Cardiovascular Life Support (ACLS) Provider Manual*. Dallas, TX: American Heart Association, Inc.; 2011.

8 Hwang JP, Patlan J, de Achaval S, Escalante CP. Survival in cancer patients after out-of-hospital cardiac arrest. *Support Care Cancer*. 2010;18:51–55.

9 Staudinger T, Stoiser B, Müllner M, et al. Outcome and prognostic factors in critically ill cancer patients admitted to the intensive care unit. *Crit Care Med*. 2000;28:1322–1328.

10 Ackroyd R, Russon L, Newell R. Views of oncology patients, their relatives and oncologists on cardiopulmonary resuscitation (CPR): questionnaire-based study. *Palliat Med*. 2007;21:139–144.

21 Lenihan DJ, Kowey PR. Overview and management of cardiac adverse events associated with tyrosine kinase inhibitors. *Oncologist*. 2013;18:900–908.

23 Yeh ET, Bickford CL. Cardiovascular complications of cancer therapy: incidence, pathogenesis, diagnosis, and management. *J Am Coll Cardiol*. 2009;53:2231–2247.

24 Ewer MS, Ewer SM. Cardiotoxicity of anticancer treatments: what the cardiologist needs to know. *Nat Rev Cardiol*. 2010;7:564–575.

27 Kern KB, Halperin HR, Field J. New guidelines for cardiopulmonary resuscitation and emergency cardiac care: changes in the management of cardiac arrest. *JAMA*. 2001;285:1267–1269.

28 Howard SC, Jones DP, Pui CH. The tumor lysis syndrome. *N Engl J Med*. 2011;364:1844–1854.

31 Wilson FP, Berns JS. Tumor lysis syndrome: new challenges and recent advances. *Adv Chronic Kidney Dis*. 2014;21:18–26.

38 Ristic AD, Imazio M, Adler Y, et al. Triage strategy for urgent management of cardiac tamponade: a position statement of the European Society of Cardiology Working Group on Myocardial and Pericardial Diseases. *Eur Heart J*. 2014;35:2279–2284.

43 Annane D, Siami S, Jaber S, et al. Effects of fluid resuscitation with colloids vs crystalloids on mortality in critically ill patients presenting with hypovolemic shock: the CRISTAL randomized trial. *JAMA*. 2013;310:1809–1817.

45 Haas RA, Ahn SH. Interventional management of head and neck emergencies: carotid blowout. *Semin Interv Radiol*. 2013;30:245–248.

58 Fagedet D, Thony F, Timsit JF, et al. Endovascular treatment of malignant superior vena cava syndrome: results and predictive factors of clinical efficacy. *Cardiovasc Intervent Radiol*. 2013;36:140–149.

69 Simoff MJ, Lally B, Slade MG, et al. Symptom management in patients with lung cancer: Diagnosis and management of lung cancer, 3rd ed: American College of Chest Physicians evidence-based clinical practice guidelines. *Chest*. 2013;143:e455S–e497S.

78 Sweatt AJ, Sung A. Interventional pulmonologist perspective: treatment of malignant pleural effusion. *Curr Treat Options in Oncol*. 2014;15:625–643.

81 Ost DE, Jimenez CA, Lei X, et al. Quality-adjusted survival following treatment of malignant pleural effusions with indwelling pleural catheters. *Chest*. 2014;145:1347–1356.

89 Alrajab S, Youssef AM, Akkus NI, Caldito G. Pleural ultrasonography versus chest radiography for the diagnosis of pneumothorax: review of the literature and meta-analysis. *Crit Care*. 2013;17:R208.

90 Baumann MH, Strange C, Heffner JE, et al. Management of spontaneous pneumothorax: an American College of Chest Physicians Delphi consensus statement. *Chest*. 2001;119:590–602.

97 King V, Vaze AA, Moskowitz CS, Smith LJ, Ginsberg MS. D-dimer assay to exclude pulmonary embolism in high-risk oncologic population: correlation with CT pulmonary angiography in an urgent care setting. *Radiology*. 2008;247:854–861.

98 Klok FA, Djurabi RK, Nijkeuter M, et al. High D-dimer level is associated with increased 15-d and 3 months mortality through a more central localization of pulmonary emboli and serious comorbidity. *Br J Haematol*. 2008;140:218–222.

102 Chatterjee S, Chakraborty A, Weinberg I, et al. Thrombolysis for pulmonary embolism and risk of all-cause mortality, major bleeding, and intracranial hemorrhage: a meta-analysis. *JAMA*. 2014;311:2414–2421.

103 Riera-Mestre A, Becattini C, Giustozzi M, Agnelli G. Thrombolysis in hemodynamically stable patients with acute pulmonary embolism: A meta-analysis. *Thromb Res*. 2014;134:1265–1271.

105 Farge D, Debourdeau P, Beckers M, et al. International clinical practice guidelines for the treatment and prophylaxis of venous thromboembolism in patients with cancer. *JTH*. 2013;11:56–70.

106 Lyman GH, Khorana AA, Kuderer NM, et al. Venous thromboembolism prophylaxis and treatment in patients with cancer: American Society of Clinical Oncology clinical practice guideline update. *J Clin Oncol*. 2013;31:2189–2204.

113 van Es N, Bleker SM, Di Nisio M. Cancer-associated unsuspected pulmonary embolism. *Thromb Res*. 2014;133(Suppl 2):S172–S178.

114 Robson P. Metastatic spinal cord compression: a rare but important complication of cancer. *Clin Med*. 2014;14:542–545.

116 O'Phelan KH, Bunney EB, Weingart SD, Smith WS. Emergency neurological life support: spinal cord compression (SCC). *Neurocrit Care*. 2012;17(Suppl 1):S96–S101.

119 Lee CH, Kwon JW, Lee J, et al. Direct decompressive surgery followed by radiotherapy versus radiotherapy alone for metastatic epidural spinal cord compression: a meta-analysis. *Spine*. 2014;39:E587–E592.

120 Stevens RD, Huff JS, Duckworth J, et al. Emergency neurological life support: intracranial hypertension and herniation. *Neurocrit Care*. 2012;17(Suppl 1):S60–S65.

122 Brophy GM, Bell R, Claassen J, et al. Guidelines for the evaluation and management of status epilepticus. *Neurocrit Care*. 2012;17:3–23.

123 Arik Y, Leijten FS, Seute T, Robe PA, Snijders TJ. Prognosis and therapy of tumor-related versus non-tumor-related status epilepticus: a systematic review and meta-analysis. *BMC Neurol*. 2014;14:152.

125 Claassen J, Silbergleit R, Weingart SD, Smith WS. Emergency neurological life support: status epilepticus. *Neurocrit Care*. 2012;17(Suppl 1):S73–S78.

130 Freifeld AG, Bow EJ, Sepkowitz KA, et al. Clinical practice guideline for the use of antimicrobial agents in neutropenic patients with cancer: 2010 update by the infectious diseases society of america. *Clin Infect Dis*. 2011;52:e56–e93.

137 Alp S, Akova M. Management of febrile neutropenia in the era of bacterial resistance. *Ther Adv Infect Dis*. 2013;1:37–43.

138 Averbuch D, Orasch C, Cordonnier C, et al. European guidelines for empirical antibacterial therapy for febrile neutropenic patients in the era of growing resistance: summary of the 2011 4th European Conference on Infections in Leukemia. *Haematologica*. 2013;98:1826–1835.

145 Simons FE, Ardusso LR, Bilò MB, et al. World Allergy Organization anaphylaxis guidelines: summary. *J Allergy Clin Immunol*. 2011;127:587–593.e1-22.

148 Campbell RL, Li JT, Nicklas RA, Sadosty AT. Emergency department diagnosis and treatment of anaphylaxis: a practice parameter. *Ann Allergy, Asthma Immunol*. 2014;113:599–608.

151 Corominas M, Gastaminza G, Lobera T. Hypersensitivity reactions to biological drugs. *J Investig Allergol Clin Immunol*. 2014;24:212–225; quiz 211p following 225.

PART 13

The Future of Oncology

141 A vision for twenty-first century healthcare

Leroy Hood, MD, PhD ▪ Kristin Brogaard, PhD ▪ Nathan D. Price, PhD

Overview

The convergence of system medicine, big data, and patient-activated social networks is leading to a medicine that is predictive, preventive, personalized, and participatory (P4). P4 medicine has two central thrusts—optimizing wellness and demystifying disease. To bring P4 medicine into the healthcare system, we initiated a longitudinal pilot study generating individual data clouds for 108 well people. The integration of the individual data clouds identified "actionable possibilities" that allow individuals to optimize wellness or avoid disease. We believe that this approach will transform healthcare by decreasing costs, increasing quality, and promoting innovation in a new healthcare sector—scientific wellness.

A vision for healthcare

Healthcare is one of the most significant challenges of our time. Costs are rapidly growing worldwide and are not delivering commensurate improvements in health.[1] For example, even though the United States is the biggest healthcare spender in the world, it ranks near the bottom of the top 17 developed nations in survival among those 50 years of age and older.[1,2] Moreover, studies on the drivers of health and disease show that approximately 30% is attributable to genetic causes, 60% to environmental and behavior causes, and only about 10% to healthcare itself, with interactions among these factors.[3] Thus, the focus of today's healthcare—which is almost entirely on disease—ignores major aspects of the actual drivers of health. This focus is problematic because once biological systems are altered in disease, they often cannot be restored to their fully functional pre-disease state. Clearly, major systemic changes are needed to provide the healthcare we need for the twenty-first century.

Quantifying wellness and demystifying disease

To transform the current healthcare system, we suggest the adoption of two major thrusts—*quantifying wellness* and *demystifying disease* by studying its origins. Wellness is critical to both optimizing human potential (or capital) and providing fundamental insights into disease and disease prevention through its ability to examine the earliest wellness to disease transitions so as to study disease at the point of detectable inception. On the contrary, contemporary healthcare generally analyzes and treats patients only after they become sick.

The key to this transformation is to take a systems biology approach to disease, which leads naturally to systems medicine and its conviction that healthcare of the future must be predictive, preventive, personalized and participatory—P4 medicine. The

fundamental question is how to apply P4 medicine to patients and introduce it into the contemporary healthcare landscape.

In this chapter, we outline a powerful new approach to quantifying wellness and minimizing disease that will serve as a model for transforming healthcare. It will be introduced through an extended, data intense, longitudinal study of 100,000 "well" people. This model will provide the basis for establishing quantitative metrics of wellness and for identifying the transition states from wellness to most common diseases.

The emergence of P4 medicine

As background, we provide a personal view of how this P4 vision of medicine has emerged over the past 40 years, and how its implementation will impact the healthcare system of the twenty-first century.

The early stages

Let us review the state of biomedical research five decades ago. When one of us (Lee Hood) began as an assistant professor at Caltech in 1970, it was obvious that biology and disease were far more complex than most researchers assumed at that time—and that studying biological systems one gene or one protein at a time was not likely to decipher this complexity.[4] The well-known parable of the elephant and six blind men is apt: each man felt a different part of the elephant (trunk, leg, tusk, etc.) and characterized the elephant by that observation. So, to one person the elephant was like a snake (trunk) while to another it was like a fan (ear) and so forth. Understanding the elephant requires a holistic approach that integrates the data. The study of biology and medicine suffers from analogous complexities, where we measure one or a few genes or proteins and fail to see the whole picture. We need to integrate different global or comprehensive types of biological information to decipher disease complexity. The emergence of this new integrative discipline—now called systems science—has led to the transformation of biology and medicine.

What became obvious in the 1970s was that scientists lacked the approach (systems science), the technologies, and the systems-driven strategies to address biological complexity. During this period, I read Thomas Kuhn's *The Structure of Scientific Revolutions*,[5] which highlighted the difficulties in catalyzing paradigm changes in physics due to scientists' conservatism and reluctance to move beyond conventional wisdom to think outside the box. It became clear to me that there needed to be paradigm shifts in the field of biology, to move beyond reductionist thinking to a broader systems approach. At that point I made a decision to dedicate my career to deciphering in various ways biological complexity. Most of these efforts were initially viewed with considerable skepticism—as predicted by Kuhn.

Facing these challenges, I participated in five paradigm changes over the next four decades that addressed biological complexity and

Holland-Frei Cancer Medicine, Ninth Edition. Edited by Robert C. Bast Jr., Carlo M. Croce, William N. Hait, Waun Ki Hong, Donald W. Kufe, Martine Piccart-Gebhart, Raphael E. Pollock, Ralph R. Weichselbaum, Hongyang Wang, and James F. Holland.
© 2017 John Wiley & Sons, Inc. ISBN: 978-1-118-93469-2

led to the emergence of systems biology, systems medicine, and the concept of a medicine that was predictive, preventive, personalized, and participatory—P4 medicine.[6,7] These paradigm changes were as follows:

1. Bringing *engineering to biology* through the development of six instruments that allowed the reading and writing of DNA and proteins. These instruments introduced the concept of high-throughput biological data generation and its associated big data and analytics.[8-10]
2. One of these instruments, the automated DNA sequencer, enabled the *Human Genome Project*, which produced a complete list of genes, and by inference proteins—parts lists that made systems science possible.[9,11,12]
3. The emergence of *cross-disciplinary biology*—bringing together biologists, chemists, computer scientists, engineers, mathematicians, physicists, and physicians under one roof—learning one another's languages and working together in effective teams to enable "big biology" efforts to solve very complex biological problems. This collaborative effort fueled the cycle of biological discovery driving technology that, in turn, drives analytics to understand the mechanisms of biology. Bill Gates played a critical role in catalyzing the shift to cross-disciplinary biology in 1992 by recruiting me to establish the Department of Molecular Biotechnology at the University of Washington Medical School, which pioneered key technologies and analytics in genomics, proteomics, cell sorting, and large-scale DNA synthesis.[13] This department also produced two of the 16 centers involved in sequencing the human genome.
4. In 2000, I co-founded the Institute of Systems Biology to pioneer *systems science* and its necessary technologies and analytics.[14,15] This global systems approach was the key to addressing biological complexity. Its application to disease led to the fifth paradigm change.
5. *Systems medicine and P4 medicine* emerged from the application of systems science to disease.[16-18] Thus, the first four paradigm changes led to a revolutionary new approach to study disease, wellness, and medicine.

In retrospect, these experiences generated the following useful insights about how to catalyze paradigm changes in modern society:

- New ideas need new organizational structures—each of these five changes required the creation of new organizational entities to serve as their champions. Longstanding bureaucratic cultures can only rarely adopt new ideas as they were honed by outdated needs and experiences of the past, and thus often have trouble adapting to the present, let alone the future.
- If you want to persuade organizations to adopt new ideas, you must engage the organization's leadership. Middle-level managers often fail to understand the paradigm changes as they are mired in day-to-day operations.
- Each of these ideas was initially met with considerable skepticism. Determined optimism is essential for moving ideas forward in the face of widespread resistance.
- Each of these changes fundamentally altered how we viewed and practiced biology and medicine.
- It is essential to bring new ideas to the broader community of biological scientists, and ultimately to the public. At the Institute for Systems Biology (ISB), the Logan Center for Education is committed to bringing modern science to these audiences—and to promoting K-12 science education in this new context.

The book of life—four levels of biological information

These paradigm changes provided the conceptual framework and the tools to understand information in biology in a far more holistic manner than ever before—as four discrete levels of information—DNA, RNA, proteins, and biological networks or systems (Figure 1). They also demonstrated the need to be able to integrate and model biological information to address its complexity.

The genome can be described as a book containing the digital instructions for life.[11] The genome is a four-letter language of DNA (G, C, A, T) and is packaged in 23 pairs of human chromosomes that are present in each of an individual's 10^{13} cells. The human genome (diploid) contains about 6 billion letters or about 6 m of DNA. Since your body contains 10^{13} cells, it has sufficient DNA to reach from the earth to the sun 600 times. The genome is divided into about 20,000 units of information termed genes.

The genes can be read as digital four-letter copies (or transcripts) of the DNA language—these copies are termed RNA. The genes can be modified chemically or through their interactions with proteins,

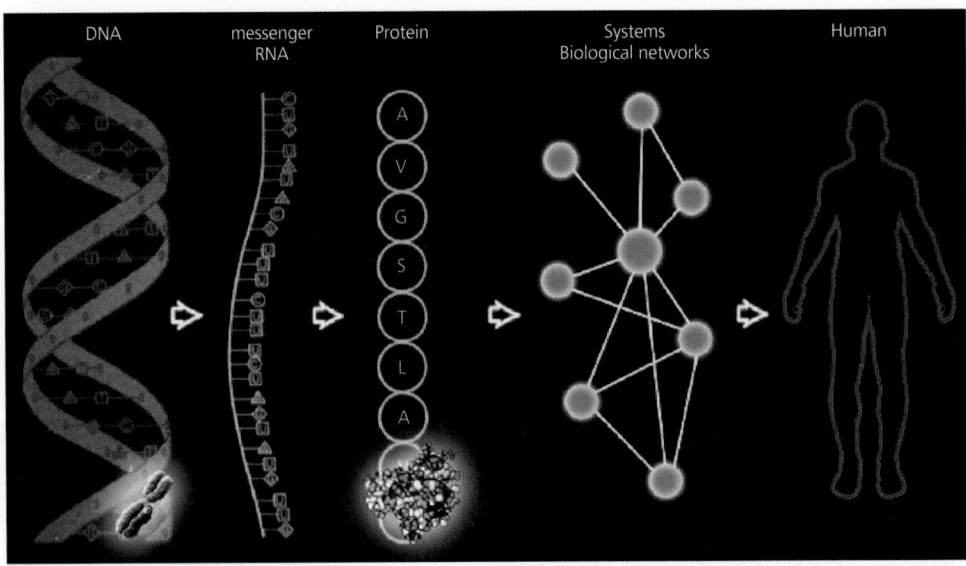

Figure 1 A schematic representation of the many different data types that are present in individual data clouds.

thus modifying their ability to be expressed. These are termed epigenetic modifications. The generation of RNA transcripts for individual genes allows for their differential amplification according to their use needs (up to millions of RNA copies per cell) and it allows the transcripts to be altered chemically to modify their information content. For example, we studied one human gene, neurexin, that had at least 2000 different RNA transcripts—and the fascinating question was how many of these unique transcripts represented different units of information (the others are presumably noise).[19]

Most RNA transcripts can be translated by a complex biological machine into proteins, which represent the third level of information. A 20-letter language corresponding to the 20 amino acids encodes proteins. This language directs the folding of each protein into a unique and complex three-dimensional structure that executes the specific functions of life. Proteins may function alone or through interactions with other proteins and/or informational molecules to create complex molecular machines or biological networks.

Networks, the fourth level of information beyond DNA, RNA, and proteins, arise from interactions between proteins and DNA, RNA, other proteins, and small molecules of life (metabolites) in the context of the various biological networks of life (e.g., gene regulatory networks, protein interaction networks, and metabolic networks). These networks are dynamical, changing over time, and are formed both by the information from their genes and the information from their environment. Thus networks encode the dynamics of life that occur *via* the integration of both genetic and environmental information. Biological networks mediate critical life processes including development, physiology, and aging. Perturbations in biological networks cause human disease.

Classical molecular biology involves the study of life, analyzing one or a few genes or proteins at a time. Systems biology involves analysis of the dynamics of networks in developmental processes, physiological responses, and aging. To facilitate systems analysis of these dynamical networks, it has been critical to begin developing tools that enable the sequence analysis of all genes in the genome;

all gene modifications (epigenome); all RNAs (transcriptome); all the proteins in a given cell, organ, or creature (the proteome); and the metabolites present in a given cell, organ, or creature (the metabolome). These collectively are termed "omic" analyses. It is also important to measure at least some higher level physiological and psychological phenotypes.

Today, there are several approaches to understanding biology and medicine. For example, the term genomic medicine is very popular and it addresses the role that the genome plays in disease. In contrast, systems medicine (a systems approach to disease) takes a holistic and integrative approach to the dynamics of life and disease, which includes the genome but also the transcriptomes, epigenomes, proteomes, metabolomes and more complex phenotypes. Systems medicine focuses on understanding the roles that both the genome and the environmental changes play in wellness and disease, in part through a study of its dynamical biological networks.

Systems medicine: a tipping point

Systems medicine has two central features.

First, each individual will have a virtual, personalized, dynamical cloud of billions of data points (Figure 2). The data are heterogeneous in type and multiscale in dimension. They range from molecular, cellular, and organ data to social networks that link individuals together—and these data are dynamical in that they change with time and environmental perturbations. The ISB is developing the analytical tools to integrate and model these data to identify "actionable possibilities" that will enable each individual to respond to these opportunities in order to optimize their wellness and/or minimize the severity or chances of disease.

These big-data clouds present an enormous signal to noise challenge stemming from the inherent variability (noise) in biological information that is irrelevant to the health questions at hand. Thus, systems approaches are critical to mining these large datasets for

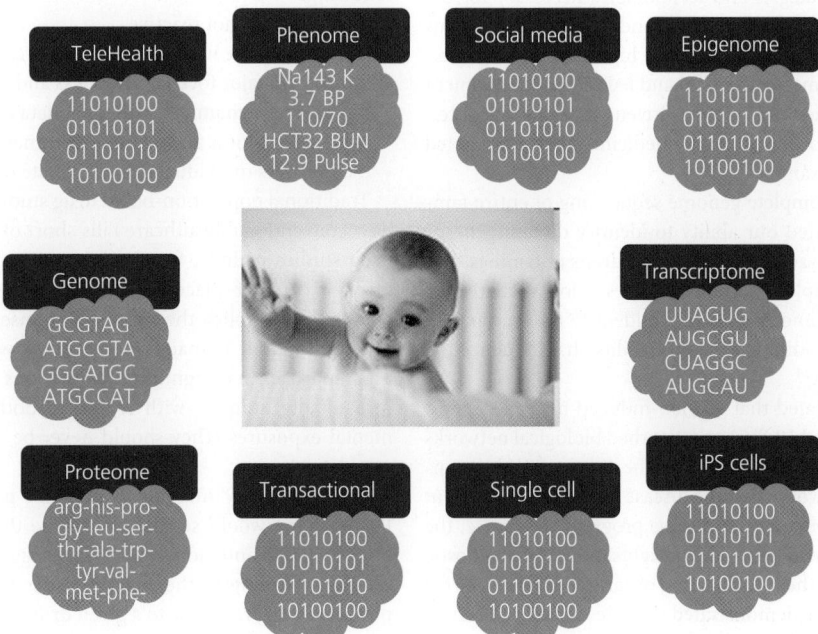

Figure 2 A schematic diagram of the "network of networks." Biological networks can operate at the level of genes, of proteins and other molecules, of cells, of organs, and even of social networks of individuals. In disease, some of these networks are altered to become disease perturbed. The difference between normal and disease-perturbed networks provides insights into disease mechanisms, early diagnosis, and improved identification of drug target candidates.

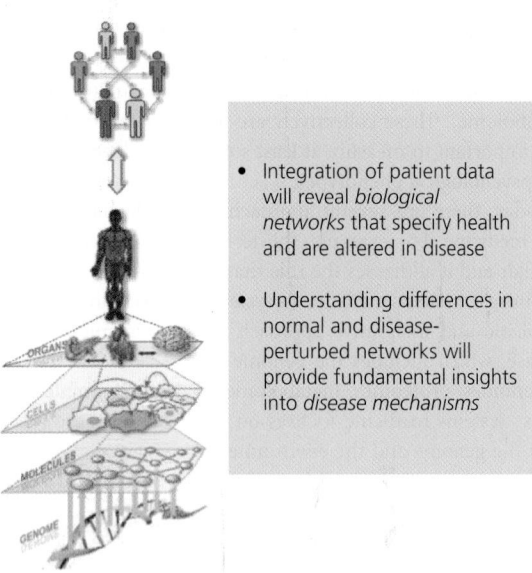

- Integration of patient data will reveal *biological networks* that specify health and are altered in disease

- Understanding differences in normal and disease-perturbed networks will provide fundamental insights into *disease mechanisms*

Figure 3 A schematic diagram of the four hierarchical levels of biological information—DNA to RNA to proteins to interactions, networks, and biological systems.

actionable information, identifying potentially small signals from amidst large amounts of noise.[20]

Second, dynamical biological networks manage, integrate, and transport biomolecules and associated information in living organisms, and these in turn mediate normal development and physiological responses. These networks become perturbed in disease,[21,22] and thus alter the information they process (Figure 3). Assessing the differences between normal and disease-perturbed networks provides deep insights into disease mechanisms, novel diagnostics approaches, and new therapeutic target candidates.

In 2008, ISB initiated a $100 million partnership with the state of Luxembourg. It provided $20 million annually to ISB for 5 years to develop the strategies and technologies necessary for the advancement of systems medicine. This funding was flexible, thus allowing the institute to pursue high-risk high-reward strategies. These efforts were extremely successful and led to the development of nine novel technologies and systems-driven strategies that accelerated the enablement of translational medicine, as demonstrated by the following three examples.

- First, we pioneered complete genome sequencing of entire families and this accelerated our ability to identify disease genes.[23] To date, we have analyzed 23 diseases, hundreds of families, and more than 9000 complete human genomes. Most recently, we employed family genome sequencing to identify rare variants in a cluster of genes encoding neural excitability that influence the risk of bipolar disease.[24]

- Second, we demonstrated that a prion-induced neurodegenerative disease in mice had 10 disease-perturbed biological networks that emerged over the 22-week course of the disease.[25] We demonstrated that these networks became disease perturbed at different points during the course of the disease progression. Hence, the earliest changing networks provided insights into early diagnostic possibilities as well as the identification of early therapeutic target candidates. We further demonstrated that the dynamics of these 10 different networks collectively explained virtually every aspect of the pathophysiology of this disease. These results provide fundamental insights into early disease mechanisms, as well as into the later stages of disease progression.

- Third, we used a systems approach to blood protein diagnostics to develop a panel of 13 blood proteins that enabled us to distinguish benign lung nodules from cancerous lung nodules[26] via a test that is now clinically available through the ISB spinout company, Integrated Diagnostics. Over-diagnosis of lung cancer from identified nodules is a huge problem, leading to as many as 40% of surgeries being performed on benign nodules. Thus, broad implementation of this test could save the healthcare system billions of dollars in unnecessary surgeries, in addition to significantly reducing the morbidity and unnecessary risk to the health of the patients. Twelve of these 13 proteins map into three disease-perturbed networks of lung cancer—opening up the possibility for new approaches to identify drug target candidates and blood protein diagnostics that can follow the progression of the disease as a nodule turns from benign to malignant. In this regard, we have also demonstrated (as discussed above) that one could follow brain-specific blood proteins to reveal from the *blood* the progressive disease perturbations of four major networks in prion-induced neurodegeneration, including the first disease-perturbed network.[25] Together, these results support the idea that diagnostic biomarkers can be identified for the very earliest stage of the disease and that these biomarkers can follow disease progression.

P4 medicine: a revolution in healthcare

The novel strategies and technologies that resulted from ISB's successful Luxembourg partnership led to the insight that the "new medicine" must be predictive, preventive, personalized, and participatory—P4 medicine. Indeed, P4 medicine emerged from a convergence of three powerful forces in science and technology: (1) systems medicine; (2) big data and analytics; and (3) patient/consumer activated social networks. The four Ps each accurately describe the general features of this "new medicine" and how it differs strikingly from conventional medicine. Distinguishing features of P4 Medicine from contemporary medicine include the following:

- It is proactive, not reactive.
- It focuses on the individual and not averaged patient populations.
- It places a major focus on wellness and not just disease.
- It generates dynamical individual data clouds that can be used to optimize wellness and avoid or eliminate disease.
- It empowers individuals to participate in their own health.

Traditional population-based drug studies are classic examples of how conventional healthcare falls short of P4 medicine. Currently, drug studies include, for example, up to 30,000 patients that are given a drug or placebo; their responses are extrapolated into curves that establish the average responses of the population; and a determination is made on this basis whether the drug works. This approach has significant limitations because each patient is individually unique—with regard to both genetics and environmental exposures. They should never be studied only as averaged populations.

We must study individuals and not populations. Accordingly, P4 medicine would separately analyze the individual data clouds of the 30,000 individuals and then aggregate them into related groups according to the characteristics that are of interest to the physician (e.g., response to a given drug, adverse reaction to a given drug). This view also argues that experiments with single patients ($N = 1$) can be incredibly useful, especially if there are longitudinal measures in place that enable patients in their "well" state to serve as their own control as disease manifests and progresses.

P4 medicine also harnesses the power of patient (consumer)-activated social networks. Individuals will become empowered through networks that communicate and engage them in the opportunities of P4 medicine. Empowered patients will be the driving force for bringing an understanding of the new medicine to physicians and will be the major instigator of change in contemporary healthcare. These patient-driven social networks also enable patients to participate in crowd sourcing to optimize their own health—by sharing valuable lessons and learning from others' experiences. Ultimately, these networks will be a powerful social force for driving physicians and a conservative healthcare system to accept change.

P4 medicine: quantifying wellness and demystifying disease

P4 medicine has two central thrusts—wellness and disease.[27-29] Today's healthcare focuses almost entirely on disease and is where the vast majority of society's healthcare dollars are currently spent. However, studies about the drivers of health and disease show that approximately 30% is attributable to genetic causes, 60% to environmental and behavioral causes, and only about 10% to healthcare, with considerable interactions among these factors.[3] To catalyze an effective twenty-first century healthcare system we need to more fully address the remaining 90% of the drivers of health. This requires a reorientation toward maintaining and optimizing wellness—and not just reacting to disease once symptoms manifest or become severe. The key to making wellness a credible scientific study is to quantify it. We will outline how this might be done later in this chapter. Our view is that that over the next 10–15 years two separate healthcare industries will emerge—the scientific wellness industry and the disease industry (current healthcare industry). Further, the scientific wellness industry will far exceed the disease industry in market cap during this time. We are now at the earliest stages of the emergence of this transformational science-based wellness industry.

The importance of wellness can be further articulated by the following observation. If the rate of increase in lifespan seen over the past 15 years continues, approximately one half of the children born in 2015 will live to be 100.[30] The question arises as to what physical and intellectual condition they will be in during the last 20–30 years of life. Clearly, a move toward wellness is essential for our future.

A pilot wellness program

Once the systems medicine tipping point was reached and P4 medicine delineated, the question arose as to how it might be brought to the current healthcare system. We realized that we needed a compelling pilot program that included all of the principles of the four Ps and that focused on both wellness and disease. We termed this scientific wellness as it employed the dense, dynamic, personal data clouds.

100,000 Person Wellness Project

In 2013, we proposed a systems-based project that included the four Ps, generated dynamical patient data clouds, and focused on the scientific wellness and disease conditions relevant to each individual—namely, a longitudinal, data-rich study of 100,000 well people over a multi-decade timeframe.[27,31] We proposed to (1) determine the complete genome sequence of each individual; (2) study blood, saliva, and urine every 3 months to delineate clinical

chemistries, 700 metabolites, and about 400 proteins; (3) analyze the gut microbiome every 3 months; and (4) include descriptive assessments of past medical history, current physical and psychological states, and quantified self-measurements (activity, pulse and quality of sleep with a fitbit and blood pressure and weight). The overarching concept is to analyze the individual measurements and to integrate various combinations of these data types into models for each individual that reveal "actionable possibilities" that if acted upon could improve their health or allow them to avoid disease (see below).

As these measurements are assessed over time it could soon become possible to divide the individuals into two groups—first, those who remained well or improved in health and, second, those who transitioned into disease (Figure 4). From those who remained well, or improved, we can identify metric panels that should allow us to quantify wellness. We are convinced that these metrics will allow us to delineate physical and psychological aspects of wellness. One might imagine that each individual has a conceptual "well of wellness" and we believe that many of us are low down in our wells. Acting on personalized actionable possibilities brings us up toward the top of our wells—optimizing both our physiological and psychological health. How effectively individuals optimize their own wellness is a function of how effectively they respond to their personalized actionable opportunities.

For those who transitioned into disease we could analyze the longitudinal data back to identify the wellness to disease transition point, allowing us to study the earliest perturbations to relevant disease-perturbed biological networks (Figure 4). These insights would lead to the possibility of understanding the earliest disease mechanisms, of developing pre-symptomatic diagnostic agents and of possibly identifying drug target candidates that could be deployed in preventive medicine to avoid the downstream cascade of negative events leading ultimately to the manifestation of disease. In time, this would make it possible to change individuals early on in the disease trajectory back to the wellness trajectory—and thus save healthcare systems significant dollars. Accordingly, this wellness study not only studies wellness, but it also studies disease at precisely the time medicine should study disease—at its point of inception. Conventional medicine generally studies only sick patients, long after the wellness to disease transition has occurred—an often-ineffective process. Many systems, even after

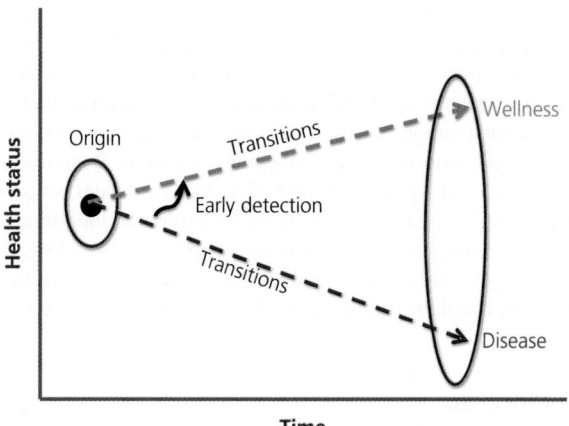

Figure 4 Health status change over time. Individuals can move in a trajectory that leads to maintaining or increasing wellness, or can transition to being less well and into disease. Early detection and actionable possibilities can aid in transitioning individuals from a disease trajectory and into a wellness trajectory as well as optimizing wellness for each individual.

disease is treated, cannot return to their same level of effectiveness from before the disease. The study of wellness will let us both optimize human capital and identify the wellness to disease transitions that will let us terminate disease early and bring individuals back quickly from the disease initiation and back onto their wellness trajectories.

Actionability is a central concept for connecting data to behavior, that is, by identifying items that are actionable; we are not just providing a risk of a negative future event (which has few demonstrated effects on behavior) but rather providing in depth information into what is happening in an individual's body now and providing a roadmap for what can be done immediately (and consistently over time) to have a material impact on his or her body in the present (which does motivate behavior). The actionable possibilities would be brought to the individuals by coaches who could clearly explain the actionable possibilities and how the individual could respond appropriately to them in the context of their own desires for their health. The coaches would be supported by physicians for clinical advice through the established healthcare system. The coaches are an incredibly important part of this process to aid people in improving their own health.

Importance of data accessibility from the longitudinal 100K Wellness Project

Our view of data accessibility is quite simple. It is essential that all of the patient de-identified data be available to qualified investigators who will mine it for the predictive and preventive medicine of the future.

One's children and grandchildren, accordingly, will be the beneficiaries of the analysis of one's data—each of us individually contribute to the medicine of the future that will improve the health of our children—optimizing wellness and avoiding disease. We would argue that it is one's social obligation to allow their data to be used to invent the future medicine. George Church in his Personalized Genome Project (PGP)[32] has made a similar plea. If consumer and patient data are to be made widely available to qualified investigators, two important concerns must be considered.

First, it is essential to have strong security in place to protect the data. Appropriate methods such as encryption are available for protecting the data and must be employed.

Second, there are federal and state laws in place that aim to protect individuals against genetic discrimination, including the Genetic Information Nondiscrimination Act (GINA). GINA prohibits health insurance companies from denying coverage or charging higher premiums solely on the basis of genetic information. GINA also prohibits employers from using genetic information for hiring, firing, promotion, and other employment decisions. There are, however, significant types of discrimination that GINA does not protect against, including discrimination for life insurance, long-term care insurance, and disability insurance. Congress should address these issues by expanding GINA and enacting other relevant legislation to ensure that there is no discrimination on the basis of genetic data.

Scaling up

One of our primary goals was to understand how to scale the wellness program to 100,000 well individuals. Our initial thought was to scale in four tranches—going from 100 to 1000 to 10,000 and finally to 100,000—each over a period of a year or so. However, we had many questions about this strategy:
- What measurements should be made? How often?

- How would we develop all of the analytical tools?
- How much would a project for 100,000 individuals cost?
- How could we scale this project up from 100 to 100,000?

Hundred Person Wellness Project

With these questions in mind, we launched the effort with a 10-month pilot study of 108 individuals (100 Pioneers) in March of 2014 and completed the data gathering at the end of the year. Accordingly, we have gone through three data tranches (every 3 months) and are now in the process of analyzing these data. We discuss here some of the initial striking results that the pilot study generated.

Hundred Pioneer pilot study results

The study required a sophisticated team to manage a host of scientific, logistical, organizational, and participant engagement issues. These included sample collection procedures, decisions about the appropriate assays to include (for discovery as well as clinical utility), sample distribution for analyses (vendors and ISB), the development of analytical tools to integrate and model the Pioneer data to reveal actionable possibilities, the recruitment and training of wellness coaches, and the formation of an MD advisory panel to oversee this process. Of the 108 Pioneers who enrolled in the study, all remained in the study throughout its duration and the majority have expressed interest in continuing the study into its next phase. Seventy percent of our Pioneers were compliant to the coaching recommendations of their actionable possibilities. Our high retention and engagement rates were influenced by three elements: (1) the coach was incredibly effective in explaining each individual's actionable possibilities and in encouraging individuals to act upon them in accordance with their own health objectives; (2) understanding how one's own genes interacted with and impacted other types of data was particularly persuasive in encouraging people to change behavior; and (3) observing the positive (and appropriate) changes in one's data cloud over time in response to specific lifestyle changes was an enormously reinforcing experience.

The first data tranche of clinical chemistries revealed that 91% of the Pioneers had specific nutritional deficiencies and 68% had inflammatory indicators (both correctable). Three Pioneers had extremely high levels of mercury. Two of these ate significant amounts of tuna sushi, while one had mercury arising from old dental fillings. One substituted salmon for tuna sushi and within 2 months his mercury level had dropped by half—and the other two had similar experiences in dealing with their mercury sources.

We had several indications of likely disease transitions. For example, two of the Pioneers were homozygous for the variant that causes hemochromatosis (C282Y). In a small proportion of such individuals, this disorder can lead to high iron and ferritin levels in the blood. High blood iron levels can attack the joints, pancreas, the liver, and/or the heart—potentially leading to arthritis, diabetes, liver cirrhosis/cancer, and/or cardiac decompensation in various combinations. Since this disease often presents with the cardiac complications, individuals may be already chronically ill with diabetes or liver disease before they are diagnosed.

The treatment is simple. Send the individuals with the C282Y mutations to their physician for a work-up for the diagnosis; if indicated, the individual can have regular blood draws until normal iron levels are reached. We identified the two individuals with homozygous C282Y genotypes only with the earliest changes, before any serious tissue damage had been done, thus over time saving the healthcare system significant dollars—by avoiding what could have been chronic hemochromatosis. Further, the children of these individuals are being genetically tested—stopping the progression of an undiagnosed and treatable disease to the next generations.

Using standard cutoff values for fasting serum glucose, we identified 53 of the 108 participants who had fasting glucose in the prediabetic range at baseline (e.g., were prediabetic). After only 5–6 months of health coaching, seven of these individuals had reverted to normoglycemia and the overall trend in glucose levels in the population was decreasing.

The integration of two or more different data types (e.g., blood, microbiome, genetics, activity) was also informative. For example, using Genome-wide Association Studies (GWAS), we could place the 108 Pioneers into five, low to high risk categories according to their genetic (GWAS) propensity for Crohn's disease. When the bacterial populations in the gut microbiome were compared against these genetic propensities—two strains of more "pathogenic" bacteria increased as the genetic risk for each group of individuals increased. Thus, there is an association between the genetics of Crohn's disease susceptibility and changing microbial populations in the gut microbiome. It is not yet clear what the causal association might be or whether there is a strong actionable possibility here.

What is clear is that every one of the 107 Pioneers had multiple actionable possibilities. There was a remarkable compliance, with more than 70% of the Pioneers acting upon their actionable possibilities. Thus, this program can optimize wellness and/or reduce disease for each individual.

Many participants came to three conclusions as a result of these studies:

- Your genes determine your potential, not your destiny. For many conditions, a change in behavior can address genetic limitations.
- Personalized, comprehensive and real-time data are empowering. With this knowledge, it is easier and more motivating for one to take responsibility for one's health. This is the key to beginning to control healthcare costs.
- Many of the Pioneers are interested in continuing with the next phase of the longitudinal study (which we will outline shortly). This is a measure of how convinced most were that this study had profoundly "changed their lives."

Benefits of the 100,000 (100K) person and 107 Pioneer wellness studies for healthcare

1. We will create a catalog of actionable possibilities for optimizing wellness and minimizing disease, and for aiding others in launching similar studies. This catalog of exponentially increasing actionable possibilities (analyzing new data identifies new actionable possibilities) will be a central focus of optimizing individual wellness in the future.
2. We will generate the dynamical, personalized data clouds that permit the extraction of individual actionable possibilities, which, if acted upon, allow individuals to optimize wellness and minimize disease.
3. We will generate a multiparameter, biomarker panel for wellness that in time, we believe, will allow us to disentangle the physiological and the psychological components of wellness quantitatively from the blood. It will facilitate individuals moving up their well of wellness to maximize their own human potential.
4. We will delineate the wellness to disease transitions for the common diseases and open the possibilities for early diagnosis followed by early treatment—thus moving individuals quickly from

their early disease trajectories back to their wellness trajectories. Analysis of this dataset will thus catalyze opportunities focused on the predictive and preventive aspects of P4 medicine.

5. We will push the development of miniaturized, highly parallelized, microfluidic-based, fully automated and less costly assays that will eventually be migrated to a smart phone, so that the assays may be done at home and transmitted to analytical centers for evaluation. This will lead to a digitalization of medicine that will catalyze the large cost reductions and democratization of use benefits previously seen in the digitization of communications and IT.
6. We will create a database that will have an enormous amount of information for wellness and for disease transitions. These data will provide the raw material for innovation and the creation of companies in the wellness and the disease transition fields.
7. The 100K Person Wellness Project will help catalyze three major benefits of P4 medicine to the healthcare system: facilitating lower costs, introducing more effective healthcare, and accelerating innovation and company creation.

How do we plan to proceed?

We have two major strategies for moving the 100K Wellness Program forward:

1. ISB plans to push the 100K Wellness Project forward by bringing in partners, both national and international, that will manage smaller groups of Pioneer-like projects on wellness and employ patients that are predisposed to certain diseases to enable us to follow disease transitions more quickly. We have several potential partners in the European Union and are exploring additional possibilities with countries in Asia and the Middle East. These would be academic efforts that could also drive the development of new assays (see above) and analytical tools.
2. We have launched a company, Arivale, which will provide a scientific path to wellness for consumers. Our goal is that this company will, in time, significantly help reduce the cost and improve the efficacy of maintaining or enhancing wellness. We already see this digitization of medicine taking place, through the process of determining how to effectively optimize the types of data that need to be aggregated, and by building out the data analytics capabilities for extracting the actionable knowledge from these data. In the first 6 months of its existence, Arivale without advertising attracted more than 1000 consumers in the Seattle area.

Systems medicine and cancer: a postscript

A reader of this book might ask just what systems medicine (and P4 medicine) might offer cancer. It is clear that the systems approach to cancer has much to offer and we will briefly outline a few examples.

1. Cancers shed rare cells into the blood that can be isolated and characterized, especially with the new techniques of single-cell analysis. These cells may provide new opportunities for early diagnosis, following the progression of the cancer, identifying the recurrence of cancer, and possibly even localizing the distant sites of metastases.
2. One can assess the network dynamics of cancer progression in mouse model systems (as we did for prion-induced neurodegeneration) and gain insights into early disease-perturbed networks, which in turn provide opportunities for developing early diagnostics and potential therapeutic targets to attack cancer at its early inception. We have studies underway in mouse models for glioblastoma with striking results that demonstrate

that disease-perturbed networks explain many of the most fundamental properties of cancer.

3. One can develop blood diagnostics for cancer, follow its progression, follow the response to therapy, identify recurrences, and even identify disease-perturbed networks that provide insights into possible therapeutic drug candidates (see our earlier description of an approach to lung cancer diagnostics).

4. One form of RNA, micro (mi)RNA, plays a very important role in cellular regulation. These miRNAs interact with important regulatory networks and provide yet another systems-driven approach to identifying molecules that could be drug target candidates.

5. A key aspect of future cancer treatment will be triple drug therapies that are initiated at the outset of the treatment of the disease. Cancer and HIV/AIDS (human immunodeficiency virus/acquired immunodeficiency syndrome) are diseases exhibiting excessive mutation rates. Just as triple drug therapy converted HIV/AIDS from a fatal to a chronic disease, triple drug therapy for cancer will have the opportunity to do the same. An understanding and analysis of the disease-perturbed networks of cancer is the key to identifying multiple potential drug target candidates that can act synergistically with one another. Moreover, systems strategies can be deployed to identify appropriate combinations of three or more drugs through combinatorial analyses.

6. The longitudinal study of well people as described above will ultimately allow us to identify the wellness to disease transitions in cancers and begin to investigate early disease-perturbed networks. An understanding of these early transitions will open new possibilities for early diagnostics and therapies.

7. We can apply longitudinal wellness studies to individuals undergoing cancer treatment to optimize their wellness during this difficult process. Wellness is never seriously considered as part of cancer treatment today. Moreover, we can do the same for patients that have already undergone successful (cytotoxic, chemotherapeutic) cancer treatments to once again optimize their wellness.

These are just a few examples of how P4 medicine can address cancer—and we are just at the beginning of imagining all of the P4 opportunities that lie ahead of us for cancer research. The key is to bring P4 medicine into the healthcare systems rapidly so that medicine can begin to exploit these opportunities. A major challenge, quite obviously, is how to bring an understanding of these opportunities to physicians—who often can be quite conservative in their willingness to accept new ideas.

The democratization of wellness and healthcare

Our vision for the future of healthcare is that patients will participate by taking responsibility for their own health, the digitization of medicine, and our more effective understanding of how to use personalized data clouds to optimize wellness and avoid disease that we can substantially reduce the cost of healthcare while enhancing its effectiveness.

We are convinced that this will happen through a focus on wellness and the early identification of disease transitions that can be identified and treated rapidly and effectively. As costs come down and concrete discoveries are made, P4 medicine will be brought not only to the developed world but to the developing world as well. Who would have thought in 1990 that a woman in a rural village in India could make a living for her family using a cell phone? Yet, this is precisely what has happened through the digitization of communications. In a similar manner, the digitization of medicine, together with the other changes noted above, will strikingly reduce the costs of healthcare and that, in turn, will democratize P4 healthcare for the poor as well as the rich. It is difficult to comprehend, within the next decade, how many individuals, rich and poor alike, might be in a position to transform their human potential through optimizing wellness and minimizing disease. These are indeed exciting times for advancing medicine. As we move into the twenty-first century, medicine will increasingly become predictive, preventive, personalized, and participatory. It will focus on each of us as individuals and optimize our health according to each of our individual and unique characteristics.

Acknowledgments

We thank the individuals in the Pioneer 100 project for their participation in this adventure and the many wonderful team members (too numerous to mention) who have made this project possible. We thank Gretchen Sorensen and Jennifer Lovejoy for many valuable comments on the manuscript. We also thank the Institute for Systems Biology for providing philanthropic support to this project, the Robert Wood Johnson Foundation, and the M.J. Murdock Charitable Trust for grants that helped to partially fund the study.

References

1 de la Maisonneuve C, Martins JO. Public spending on health and long-term care: a new set of projections. OECD Economic Policy Papers; 2013.

2 Woolf S, Aron L (eds). *US Health in International Perspective: Shorter Lives, Poorer Health*. National Research Council and Institute of Medicine. Washington, DC: National Academies Press; 2013.

3 Schroeder SA. Shattuck Lecture. We can do better—improving the health of the American people. *N Engl J Med*. 2007;**357**(**12**):1221–1228.

4 Hood L. Biological Complexity under Attack. 2011: Genetic Engineering and Biotechnology News.

5 Kuhn T. *The Structure of Scientific Revolution*. **264**. 1962: University of Chicago Press, Chicago.

6 Hood L, Heath JR, Phelps ME, Lin B. Systems biology and new technologies enable predictive and preventative medicine. *Science*. 2004;**306**(**5696**):640–643.

7 Flores M, Glusman G, Brogaard K, Price ND, Hood L. P4 medicine: how systems medicine will transform the healthcare sector and society. *Per Med*. 2013;**10**(**6**):565–576.

8 Hood L. Systems biology: integrating technology, biology, and computation. *Mech Ageing Dev*. 2003;**124**(**1**):9–16.

9 Hood L. A personal view of molecular technology and how it has changed biology. *J Proteome Res*. 2002;**1**(**5**):399–409.

10 Hood L. Biotechnology and medicine of the future. *JAMA*. 1988;**259**(**12**):1837–1844.

11 Hood L, Galas D. The digital code of DNA. *Nature*. 2003;**421**(**6921**):444–448.

12 Smith LM, Sanders JZ, Kaiser RJ, et al. Fluorescence detection in automated DNA sequence analysis. *Nature*. 1986;**321**(**6071**):674–679.

13 Hood L. A personal journey of discovery: developing technology and changing biology. *Annu Rev Anal Chem (Palo Alto Calif)*. 2008;**1**:1–43.

14 Hood L, Rowen L, Galas DJ, Aitchison JD. Systems biology at the Institute for Systems Biology. *Brief Funct Genomic Proteomic*. 2008;**7**(**4**):239–248.

15 Kitano H. Systems biology: a brief overview. *Science*. 2002;**295**(**5560**):1662–1664.

16 Hood L. Systems biology and p4 medicine: past, present, and future. *Rambam Maimonides Med J*. 2013;**4**(**2**):e0012.

17 Hood L, Friend SH. Predictive, personalized, preventive, participatory (P4) cancer medicine. *Nat Rev Clin Oncol*. 2011;**8**(**3**):184–187.

18 Tian Q, Price ND, Hood L. Systems cancer medicine: towards realization of predictive, preventive, personalized and participatory (P4) medicine. *J Intern Med*. 2012;**271**(**2**):111–121.

19 Rowen L, Young J, Birditt B, et al. Analysis of the human neurexin genes: alternative splicing and the generation of protein diversity. *Genomics*. 2002;**79**(**4**):587–597.

20 Sung J, Wang Y, Chandrasekaran S, Witten DM, Price ND. Molecular signatures from omics data: from chaos to consensus. *Biotechnol J*. 2012;**7**(**8**):946–957.

21 Ideker T, Galitski T, Hood L. A new approach to decoding life: systems biology. *Annu Rev Genomics Hum Genet*. 2001;**2**:343–372.

22 Ideker T Thorsson V, Ranish JA, et al. Integrated genomic and proteomic analyses of a systematically perturbed metabolic network. *Science*. 2001;**292**(**5518**):929–934.

23 Roach JC, Glusman G, Smit AFA, et al. Analysis of genetic inheritance in a family quartet by whole-genome sequencing. *Science*. 2010;**328**(**5978**):636–639.

24 Ament SA, Szelinger S, Glusman G, et al. Rare variants in neuronal excitability genes influence risk for bipolar disorder. *Proc Natl Acad Sci U S A*. 2015;**112**(**11**):3576–3581.

25 Hwang D, Lee IY, Yoo H, et al. A systems approach to prion disease. *Mol Syst Biol*. 2009;**5**:252.

26 Li X-J, Hayward C, Fong PY, et al. A blood-based proteomic classifier for the molecular characterization of pulmonary nodules. *Sci Transl Med*. 2013;**5**(**207**): 207ra142.

27 Hood L, Price ND. Demystifying disease, democratizing health care. *Sci Transl Med*. 2014;**6**(**225**):225ed5.

28 Hood L., Price ND. Promoting Wellness and Demystifying Disease: The 100K Project. Clinical Omics; 2014.

29 Hood L, Lovejoy JC, Price ND. Integrating big data and actionable health coaching to optimize wellness. *BMC Med*. 2015;**13**(**1**):4.

30 Office for National Statistics. *Historic and Projected Data from the Period and Cohort Life Tables, 2012-Based Revised*. UK: Office for National Statistics; 2014.

31 Gibbs WW. Medicine gets up close and personal. *Nature*. 2014;**506**(**7487**):144–145.

32 Church GM. The personal genome project. *Mol Syst Biol*. 2005;**1**:2005.0030.

Index

A

ABC (ATP binding cassette) family proteins, multidrug resistance, 603, 608, 609, 733, 734–735, 737
abdominal infections, cancer patients, 1872–1873
abdominoperineal resection (APR), 1167, 1179, 1182, 1184, 1185
Abelson murine leukemia virus (A-MuLV), 344
abemaciclib/ribociclib (CDK 4/6 inhibitors), metastatic breast cancer, 1425
ABL gene *see* BCR-ABL fusion gene
absorption, pharmacokinetics, 618
ablation therapies
access to health care, US health disparities, 884, 886
acetyl-coenzyme A (acetyl-CoA), cancer cell metabolism, 191, 192, 193, 194
acinar cell carcinoma, exocrine pancreas, 1133
acral erythema (AE), dermatological complications of chemotherapy, 1719, 1724–1725
acral melanoma, 1443
acromegaly, growth hormone-secreting pituitary adenomas, 949, 953–954
ACTH *see* adrenocorticotropic hormone
acupuncture, integrative oncology, 545–546
acute generalized exanthematous pustulosis (AGEP), 1717, 1718
acute lymphoblastic leukemia (ALL), 1581–1593
  adolescents and young adults, 1589
  chemotherapy, 1586–1587
  chromosomal aberrations, 122–124
  clinical presentation, 1581–1582
  CNS prophylaxis, 1586, 1588–1589
  cytogenetic/molecular abnormalities, 1583–1585
  diagnosis, 1582–1585
  disease subtypes, 1589–1590
  epidemiology, 1581
  etiology, 1581
  eye infiltration, 940–941
  hematopoietic cell transplantation therapy, 831, 832, 837–838
  immunophenotyping, 1582–1583
  induction therapy, 1586–1587
  karyotype analysis, 1584–1585
  lymphoblastic lymphoma relationship, 1620
  methotrexate therapy, 625, 629
  minimal residual disease, 1589
  morphology/cytochemistry, 1582
  newly diagnosed patients, 1585–1587
  novel therapies, 1590–1592
  pediatric, 845–848
    Down syndrome, 846–847
    genetic/chromosomal factors, 846–847
    genomic/epigenetic factors, 848
    infiltration of the eyes, 940–941
    relapsed/refractory, 848

signs and symptoms, 847–848
  therapies, 848
postremission therapy, 1587–1588
prognostic factors, 1585
radiotherapy, 1588–1589
relapse, 1589
salvage therapy, 1589
stem cell transplantation, 1587, 1588, 1589
therapy 1585–1592
acute monocytic leukemia (M5), 1550, 1554
acute myeloid leukemia (AML) 1545–1569
  see also acute promyelocytic leukemia
  3 + 7 therapy regimen, 1556–1558
  anthracycline + cytarabine 3 + 7 regimen, acute myeloid leukemia, 1556–1557
  chemotherapy related, 1547
  classification
    cytogenetic, 1548
    FAB, 1548–1551, 1552–1555
    morphologic, 1548–1550
  clinical presentation, 1555–1556
  CNS involvement, 1566–1567
  complications, 1566–1567
  cytogenetics/chromosomal abnormalities, 1532
  de novo, chromosomal aberrations, 121–122
  extramedullary acute myeloid leukemia (myeloid sarcoma), 1552
  FLT3 ITD mutations, 1545, 1548, 1550, 1553, 1558, 1565
  genetic mutations, 1547
  hematopoietic cell transplantation therapy, 831, 832, 837
  induction therapy, 1556–1559
  M0-minimally differentiated, 1549, 1552
  M1-AML without maturation, 1549, 1550, 1552
  M2-AML with maturation, 1549, 1552
  M3-acute promyelocytic leukemia, 1549, 1552–1553
  M4-myelomonocytic leukemia, 1549, 1553
  M5-monocytic leukemia, 1550, 1554
  M6-erythroleukemia, 1550, 1554
  M7-megakaryocytic leukemia, 1550, 1554–1555
  with MDS-related changes, 1550, 1552
  metabolic complications, 1567
  methotrexate therapy, 629
  mixed phenotypic leukemia, 1555
  myelodysplastic syndrome, 1529, 1532, 1537–1538
  older patients and poor prognostic subgroups, 1558–1559
  ophthalmic complications, 1567
  pathogenesis/etiology, 1545–1547
  pediatric, 848–849
  postrelapse therapy, 1556, 1561–1562
  postremission therapy, 1556, 1559–1561
  pregnancy, 1567
  prognosis, 1547–1548

relapsed/refractory disease therapy, 1556, 1561–1562
risk factors, 1547
signs and symptoms, 1555–1556
therapy, 1556–1566
transformation, from myelodysplastic syndrome, 1537–1538
tyrosine kinase mutations, 1545–1546, 1565
acute pancreatitis, cancer patients, 1819
acute promyelocytic leukemia (APL/M3), 1549, 1552–1553
  differentiation therapy, 153–156
  hemostasis disorders, 1745, 1749
  leukemogenesis, 155–156
  PML-RAR fusion proteins, signaling pathway aberrations, 142
  in pregnancy, 871
  therapy, 153–155, 1562–1564
acute respiratory distress syndrome (ARDS), 1788, 1792, 1793, 1801, 1804
adamantinoma, bone tumors, 1487–1488
Adcetris® *see* brentuximab vedotin
Addisonian crisis (hypocortisolism), 955
adeno-associated virus (AAV), gene therapy vectors, 818
adenoid cystic carcinoma of the lacrimal gland, 946
adenomatosis polyposis coli gene (*APC*), 61, 75–77, 93, 94, 1160, 1161
  see also familial adenomatous polyposis
adenomatous hyperplasia, endometrium, 1306
adenomatous (malignant) polyps, colorectal cancer, 1164–1165
adenosarcoma, gynecological, 1361, 1363, 1366
adenosine antimetabolites, 645–648
adenosquamous carcinoma
  cervix, 1285
  endometrium, 1307
  lung, 1014
S-adenosylmethionine (SAM), cancer cell metabolism, 191, 194
adenovirus vectors, gene therapy, 183, 818–819
ADH *see* antidiuretic hormone
adolescents and young adults (AYAs)
  acute lymphoblastic leukemia, 1589
  gonadal complications of cancer therapy, 1833, 1834, 1836, 1837
adoptive cellular therapy (ACT), 793–800, 805–807, 820–822
  see also tumor-infiltrating lymphocytes
ado-trastuzumab-emtansine (TDM-1; Kadcyla®), 769, 1432
adrenal insufficiency, cancer patients, 1855
adrenal medulla, pheochromocytoma, 979
adrenal metastases, from other cancers, 1854–1855
adrenocortical cancer (ACC), 967–969

Holland-Frei Cancer Medicine, Ninth Edition. Edited by Robert C. Bast Jr., Carlo M. Croce, William N. Hait, Waun Ki Hong, Donald W. Kufe, Martine Piccart-Gebhart, Raphael E. Pollock, Ralph R. Weichselbaum, Hongyang Wang, and James F. Holland.
© 2017 John Wiley & Sons, Inc. ISBN: 978-1-118-93469-2

experimental models *see* animal models; models
exponential growth
exposome/exposomics, chemical carcinogenesis, 302, 304, 305
exposure..., *see also* environmental exposure to carcinogens; occupational exposure to carcinogens; radiation exposure
exposure-response relationships
  drug efficacy, 615
  drug safety, 604, 615–617
  pharmacological studies, 615–617
extracellular matrix (ECM), tumor microenvironment, 251
extracellular microenvironment *see* tumor microenvironment
extracellular signaling, normal cell proliferation control, 187
extracellular signal-related kinase (ERK), 141
  MEK inhibitors, melanoma therapy, 474, 1452–1453
extracellular vesicles (EVs), microRNAs, 133–134
extracorporeal photopheresis (ECP), mycosis fungoides, 1632
extragonadal germ cell tumors (EGCTs)
  cancer of unknown primary site, 1679
  male, 1248, 1265–1266
extramedullary hematopoiesis (EMH), 1662–1663
extravasation reaction
  chemotherapy complications, 1721–1722
  vinca alkaloids, 688
extrinsic systems biology, 247, 248, 251–253
eyelid tumors, 944, 946
  nonmelanoma skin cancer, 1463, 1465, 1466, 1470
eyes
  see also ocular diseases
  cancer-associated retinopathy, 945
  lacrimal gland tumors, 946
  melanoma, 1450–1451
  ophthalmic complications of acute myeloid leukemia, 1567
  ophthalmic neoplasms, 935–946
  retinoblastoma, 935–940
    pediatric, 858
    soft tissue sarcoma risk, 1500
    tumor suppressor genes, 69–71
  uveal melanoma, 1450–1451

F
FAB *see* French/American/British study group classification
factorial experiments, statistical design, 263–264
factor VIII
  autoantibodies, 1748
  hemostasis, 1745
  recombinant, bleeding disorder treatment, 1753
factor XI, hemostasis, 1745
fadrozole, 722, 723
fallopian tubes
  epithelial cancer, 1317–1338
  fimbriae, 1318
  ovarian cancer origins, 1318
  sarcomas, 1367
false discovery rate (FDR), bioinformatics analysis, 239, 240
familial..., *see also* congenital syndromes; genetic predisposition; germline mutations; hereditary cancer syndromes
familial acute myeloid leukemia, 1547
familial adenomatous polyposis (FAP), 75–77
  see also adenomatosis polyposis coli gene
  bone tumors, 1496
  brain tumors, 921
  colon adenocarcinoma risk, 1152, 1160
  Gardner syndrome, 75, 921, 1160, 1496, 1500

gastric polyps, 1092
  pancreatic cancer risk, 1130
  screening, 471
familial atypical multiple-mole melanoma (FAMMM), pancreatic cancer risk, 1130
familial medullary thyroid carcinoma (FMTC), 55–56, 67, 959, 960, 978
familial melanoma, 1442
familial pancreatic cancer, 1129–1130
familial patterns
  chronic lymphocytic leukemia, 1595
  gastric cancer, 1091
familial tumor syndromes of the CNS, 920–921
families, cancer survivor care, 914
family history
  breast cancer risk, 1370–1371, 1374
  breast/ovarian cancer, 1318–1319
  colorectal cancer risk, 1159
  hormone-related cancer risk, 316
  screening and prevention, 471–472
FAMMM *see* familial atypical multiple-mole melanoma syndrome
Fanconi anemia (FA), hormone-related cancer risk, 316
FAP *see* familial adenomatous polyposis
Fareston *see* toremifene
Faslodex *see* fulvestrant
Fast Healthcare Interoperability Resources (FHIR), 279
fat consumption
  breast cancer risk, 309–310, 422–424
  colorectal cancer risk, 421, 422
fatigue, cancer/treatment effects, 911
favorable/good risk neoplasms
  cancer of unknown primary site, 1678–1680
  early stage Hodgkin lymphoma, 1610–1611
  male disseminated germ cell tumors, 1255–1256
FCR *see* fludarabine–cyclophosphamide–rituximab regimen
FDA *see* Food and Drug Administration
FDG-PET scans *see* ^{18}fluorodeoxyglucose–positron emission tomography
FdUrd *see* 5-fluorodeoxyuridine
febrile episodes, neutropenia in cancer patients, 1865, 1866, 1873–1875
fecal immunochemical tests (FITs), 445
fecal occult blood tests (FOBTs), 445
Federation of Gynecology and Obstetrics (FIGO)
  cervical cancer staging, 1290
  gynecological sarcoma staging, 1363
  ovarian cancer staging, 1326–1327
females
  cancers of unknown primary site, 1678–1679
  gonadal complications of therapy, 1835–1839
  gonadal function assessment, 1834
  Hodgkin lymphoma gonadal complications, 1836
  peritoneal carcinomatosis of unknown primary site, 1678–1679
  protection from therapy effects, 1835–1838
  urethral carcinoma, 1240–1241
Females United to Unilaterally Reduce Endo/Ectocervical Disease (FUTURE), HPV vaccination, 436
fertility
  breast cancer, 1438–1439
  cancer therapy effects, 1833–1841
  germ cell malignancies, 1346–1347
  gonad function assessment after therapy, 1833–1834
  ovarian cancer, 1318, 1346–1347
  preservation measures prior to therapy, 1838–1839
  testicular cancer, 1263–1264
fetal effects
  chemotherapy, 632, 867, 1839–1840

radiotherapy, 1840
fever
  see also febrile episodes
  AIDS-related non-Hodgkin lymphoma, 901
  cancer presentation, 5
  infections in cancer patients, 1875, 1894–1895
FGF-1 *see* acidic fibroblast growth factor
FGF-2 *see* basic fibroblast growth factor
FGFR, drug targets, 65
FGFs *see* fibroblast growth factors
fiber consumption *see* dietary fiber intake
fiber exposure, mineral fiber carcinogenesis, 1037–1038
fiberoptic bronchoscopy (FOB), lung cancer, 1019
fibrin deposition, normal hemostasis, 1745
fibrinolytic system, normal hemostasis, 1746
fibroblast growth factors (FGFs)
  angiogenesis regulation, 208, 210–211
  receptor dimerization, 138–139
  receptor gene *FGFR* drug targets, 65
fibroelastomas, cardiac tumors, 1064, 1065
fibroepithelial polyps, benign vaginal lesions, 1280
fibrohistiocytic tumors *see* nonossifying fibroma
fibromas
  chondromyxoid fibroma, 1482
  granulosa-stromal cell tumors, 1347
  nonossifying fibroma, 1483
  ossifying fibroma (osteofibrous dysplasia), 1484
fibromellar hepatocellular carcinoma, 1106–1107
fibrosarcomas, breast, 1379
fibrosis
  see also primary myelofibrosis
  bone marrow, 1663
  pulmonary therapy complications, 1793–1796
fibrotic transformation
  essential thrombocythemia, 1661
  polycythemia vera, 1667
fibrous bone tumors, 1482–1484
fibrous cortical defect, bone tumors, 1483–1484
fibrous dysplasia, 1482–1483
  congenital syndromes, 1495–1496
  osteofibrous dysplasia, 1484
fibrous morphology (sarcomatoid) type malignant pleural mesothelioma, 1039
field carcinogenesis, chemoprevention, 433
FIGO *see* Federation of Gynecology and Obstetrics
fimbriae of fallopian tubes, ovarian cancer origins, 1318
financial costs
  bioinformatics, 234–236
  breast screening, 1384
  health services, 549, 557–558
finasteride, prostate cancer chemoprevention trials, 315, 435–436, 1220–1221
fine-needle aspiration (FNA), 496
  breast cancer, 1382, 1385–1386
  lung cancer, 1019
  pancreatic cancer, 1136
finger/toe-nail reactions, chemotherapy complications, 1721, 1722
first-generation aromatase inhibitors, 722, 723
FISH *see* fluorescence *in situ* hybridization
fish oils, cancer prevention, 428
fistulas
  anal, 1178
  esophagorespiratory, 1089
  gastrointestinal, 1819
FLAIR *see* fluid-attenuated inversion recovery imaging
flat noninvasive urothelial carcinoma *in situ*, 1195, 1196, 1198
flexible sigmoidoscopy (FSIG), colorectal cancer, 445, 1162
floor of mouth (FOM), 984, 990

skeletal metastases of unknown primary site, 1679
  urethral carcinoma, 1240–1241
malignancy theories, incompatible with observations,
  589–590
malignant adnexal neoplasms *see* sebaceous
  carcinoma
malignant airway obstruction, 1781–1782, 1783
malignant conversion, 287, 289–290
  see also neoplastic transformation
malignant dysphagia, 1809–1810
malignant esophagorespiratory (tracheoesphageal)
  fistulas, 1089
malignant fibrous histiocytoma (MFH) *see*
  undifferentiated pleomorphic sarcomas
malignant hepatoma *see* hepatocellular carcinoma
malignant mastocytosis, 1568
malignant melanoma *see* melanoma
malignant myeloid diseases, chromosomal
  aberrations, 117, 119–122
malignant pericardial effusion (pericardial
  tamponade), 1880, 1881, 1884–1886
malignant peripheral nerve sheath tumors (MPNST),
  neurofibromatosis link, 1499–1500
malignant pleural effusion, 1782, 1784–1786
malignant pleural mesothelioma (MPM), 1037–1050
  biologic/novel therapy agents, 1047–1048
  biomarkers, 1040
  diagnosis, 1039
  extrapleural pneumonectomy, 1042–1043, 1044
  histologic subtypes, 1039
  imaging, 1040–1041
  intrapleural chemotherapy, 1047
  laboratory evaluation, 1039
  low grade types, 1039
  molecular biology, 1037–1038
  radiation therapy, 1044–1046
  supportive care, 1041–1042
  surgical diagnosis and staging, 1041
  surgical treatment, 1042–1044
  symptoms and signs, 1039
  systemic chemotherapy, 1046–1048
  treatments, 1041–1048
  trimodality therapy, 1043, 1046
  unresectable, 1047
malignant rhabdoid tumors, pediatric, 851, 852
malignant tracheoesophageal (esophagorespiratory)
  fistulas, 1089
malignant transformation *see* neoplastic
  transformation
malnutrition *see* cachexia
MALTs *see* mucosal-associated lymphoid tissues
mammalian target of rapamycin (mTOR), pathway,
  renal cell carcinoma, 1191
mammalian target of rapamycin (mTOR) inhibitors
  dermatological complications, 1719
  gonadal complications, 1837–1838
  oral ulceration, 1828
  overcoming breast cancer endocrine therapy
    resistance, 730
  renal cell carcinoma treatment, 1192
  renal toxicity/nephrotoxicity, 1760
Mammary Prevention 3 trial, 435
mammography
  breast cancer screening, 311–312, 441–445,
    1382–1384
  pregnancy, 868
mantle cell lymphoma (MCL), 1615, 1619, 1623,
  1626–1627
MAP *see* MYH-associated polyposis
MAPK *see* mitogen-activated protein kinase
MAPs *see* microtubule-associated proteins
marginal zone lymphoma (MZL), 1615, 1618–1619
marijuana
  appetite stimulation, 1690

head and neck cancers risk from smoking, 982–983
marine sponges (*Halichondria okadai*), 707
  see also eribulin mesylate
massage, integrative oncology, 545
mass balance studies, pharmacokinetics, 618–619
massive hemoptysis, emergencies, 1888
massively parallel sequencing, 98, 99, 108, 112
  see also next generation sequencing
massive pleural effusion, emergencies, 1888–1889
mass spectrometry
  novel cancer biomarkers, 476
  protein analysis, 40, 41
mast cell hyperplasia, 1567
mast cell leukemia, 1567, 1568
mastectomy
  breast cancer
    conservation therapy comparison, 1396
    early stage, 1390, 1393–1394
    locally advanced disease, 1397
  contralateral prophylactic mastectomy, 1436
  ductal carcinoma *in situ*, 1383
matching, minimizing confounders and bias, 552–553
maternal age
  at first birth, breast cancer risk, 309
  molar pregnancy and gestational trophoblastic
    neoplasia risk, 1353
matrigel, matrix components for three-dimensional
  tumor models, 252
mature B-cell acute lymphoblastic leukemia (Burkitt
  leukemia), 1590
maximal cytoreductive procedures, malignant pleural
  mesothelioma, 1042
maximally tolerated dose (MTD), phase I trials, 575,
  580, 581–582, 583
maytansine/analogs, antibody-drug conjugate
  payloads, 710
Mazabraud's syndrome, 1496
M-CSF *see* macrophage colony-stimulating factor
MD Anderson Cancer Center, hepatocellular
  carcinoma, 1109
MDR1 (multidrug-resistance protein 1) *see*
  p-glycoprotein
MDS *see* myelodysplastic syndrome
meat
  public health guidelines, 419
  stomach cancer risks of cooked preserved meats,
    426
mechanical ventilation, acute respiratory failure,
  1803–1804
mechanism of action (MOA)
  anticancer therapies, 613, 614
  biomarkers for personalized medicine, 562, 563
  kinase inhibitors, 613, 614
mechanistically based therapies *see* targeted therapies
mechanistic principles of cancer, biological hallmarks,
  7–16
mechlorethamine (mustine), 649, 650
mediastinal germ cell tumors, 1069–1073
  benign, 1069
  chemotherapy, 1070, 1071, 1072
  clinical characteristics, 1069–1070
  epidemiology, 1069
  evaluation/staging, 1070
  histopathology, 1069
  male, 1243, 1247, 1248, 1255
  malignant, 1069–1072
  nonseminomatous, 1069, 1070, 1071–1072
  radiation therapy, 1070–1071
  seminoma, 1069, 1070–1071
  surgery, 1071, 1072
  treatment, 1070–1072
mediastinoscopy, lung cancer, 1020
mediator release, cardiac disease in cancer patients,
  1767–1768

medical devices, Internet of Things, 281
medical oncologists, cancer patient management,
  512–513
medical oncology
  adjuvant therapy, 516
  cancer prevention, 513–514
  cancer surveillance, 517
  cancer suspicion and diagnostics, 511–512
  clinical trials, 516–517
  drug resistance, 514, 516
  early stage versus late stage, 516
  evolving therapeutics, 514–516
  palliative and end-of-life care, 517–518
  patient management understanding, 512–513
  principles, 511–519
  therapeutics, 514–518
medical orders for life-sustaining treatment (MOLST),
  522–523
medical power of attorney, 517, 1879–1880
medication review, polypharmacy evaluation in older
  patients, 879
meditation, integrative oncology, 544, 545
medroxyprogesterone acetate (MPA)
  cachexia in cancer patients, 1690
  endometrial cancer, 1313–1314
medullary breast carcinoma, 1378
medullary thyroid carcinoma (MTC), 959, 971
  familial/hereditary, 55–56, 67, 959, 960, 978
  multiple endocrine neoplasia syndrome MEN-2,
    978
medulloblastomas, pediatric, 856–857
megakaryocytic leukemia (M7), 1550, 1554–1555
megaprosthesis, metastatic bone disease, 1731
megestrol acetate (MA)
  cachexia in cancer patients, 1690
  endometrial cancer, 1313–1314
MEK (MAP/ERK pathway) inhibitors, melanoma
  therapy, 474, 1452–1453
melanoma, 1441–1459
  adjuvant therapies, 1448–1449
  advanced disease, 1451–1458
  amelanotic lesions, melanoma, 1442, 1443
  anorectal, 1185
  choroidal, 942–944
  clinical implications of genomics, 110–111
  clinical presentation, 1442–1443
  CNS metastases, 1457
  congenital melanocytic nevi (CMN), melanoma
    risk, 1442
  drug resistance evolution, 111–112
  dysplastic nevi/dysplastic nevus syndrome, 1243,
    1442
  epidemiology/etiology, 1441
  eyes, 1450–1451
  genetic basis, 108
  genetic predisposition, 1442
  genomic landscape, 108–110
  genomics and evolution case study, 108–112
  immunotherapy, 1448–1449
  interferon therapy, 752
  interleukins, 746, 747, 748, 750–751
  in-transit/locoregional recurrent disease,
    1447–1448
  iris, 942
  molecular biology, 108–112, 1444–1445
  nevi relationship, 1441–1442
  nodular melanoma, 1442, 1443
  ocular, 942–944
  ovarian metastases, 1351
  pathological features, 1443
  pediatric oncology, 860
  in pregnancy, 871–872
  prognostic factors, 1442
  risk assessment, 1442

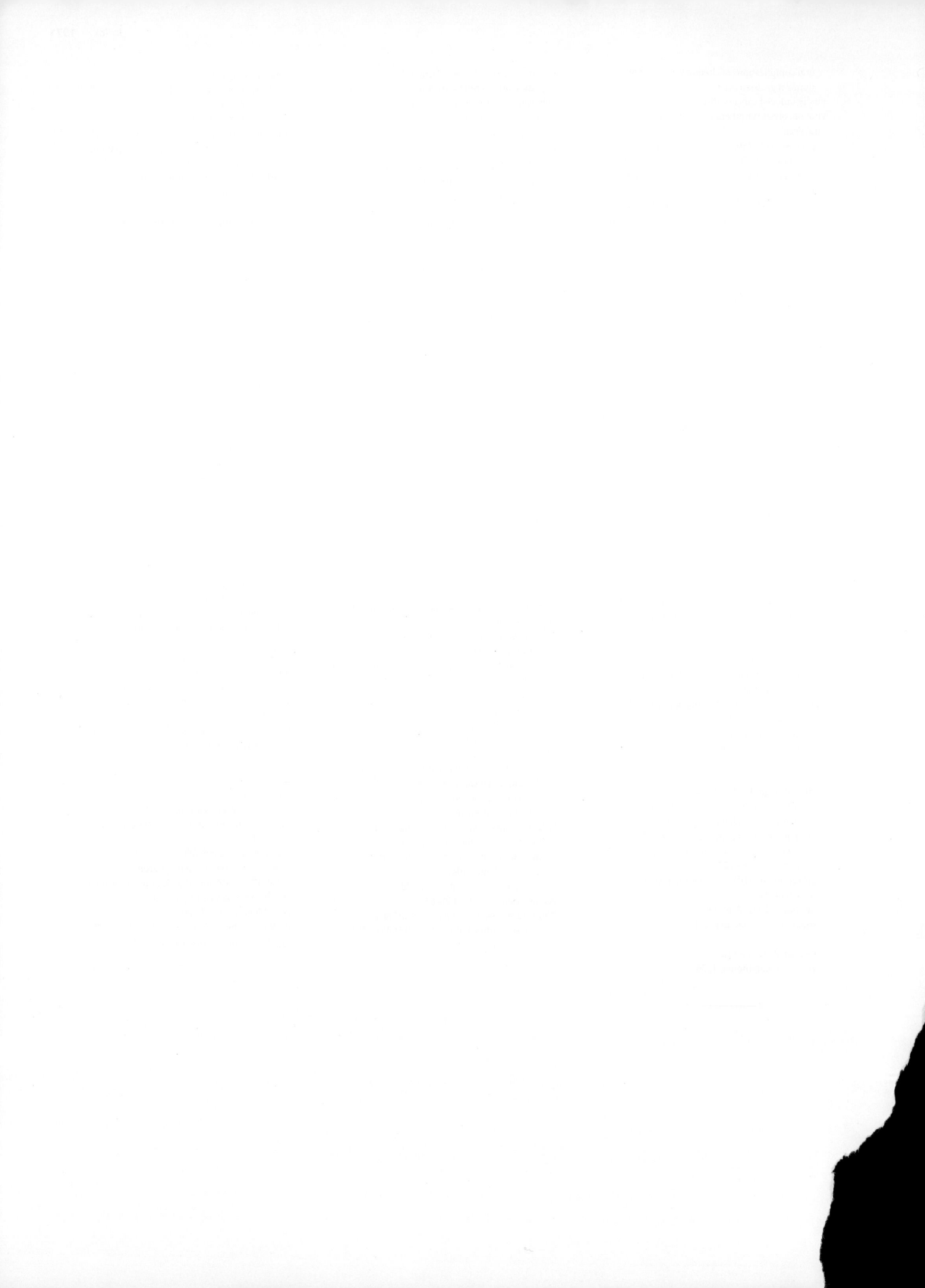